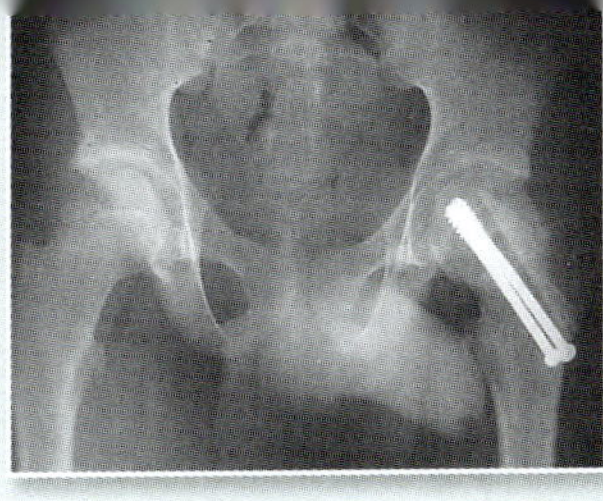 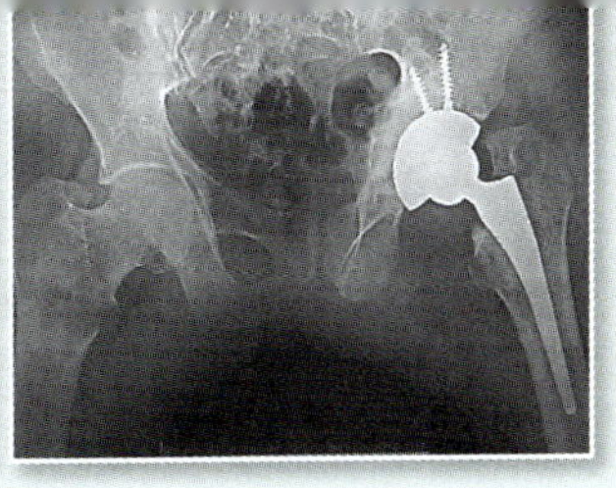 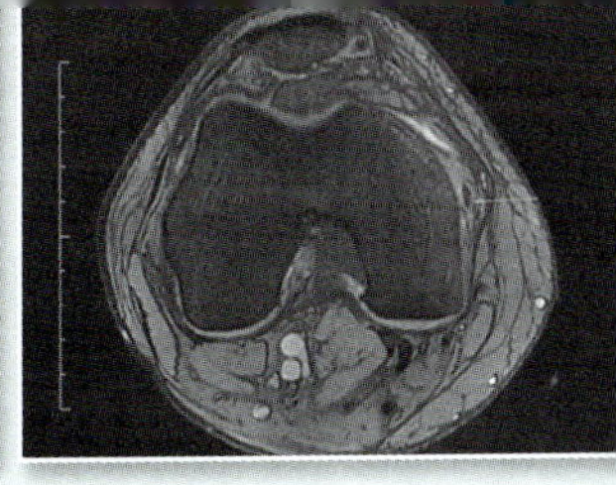

Essential
ORTHOPEDICS
Principles and Practice

VOLUME 1

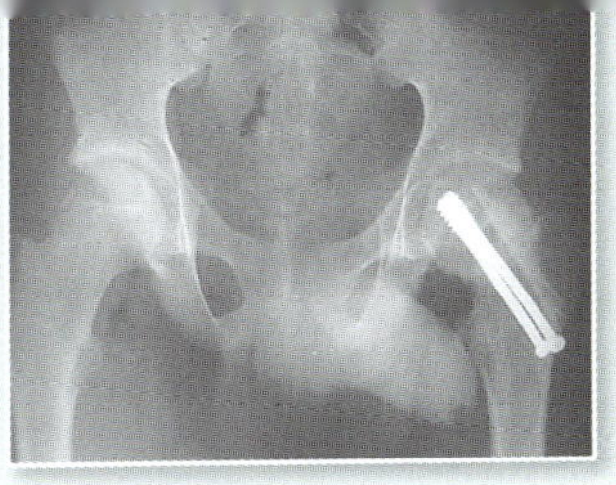

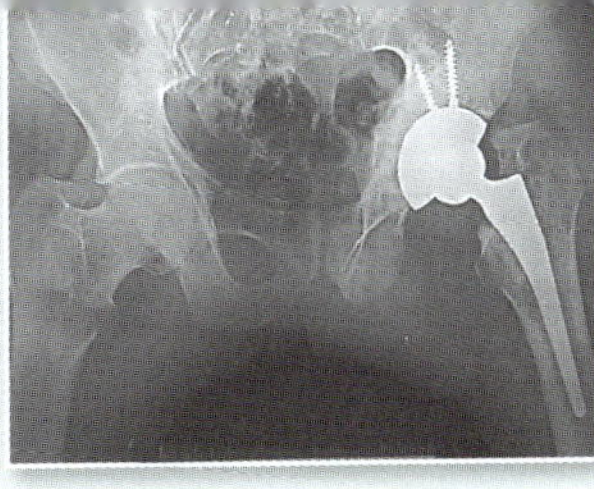

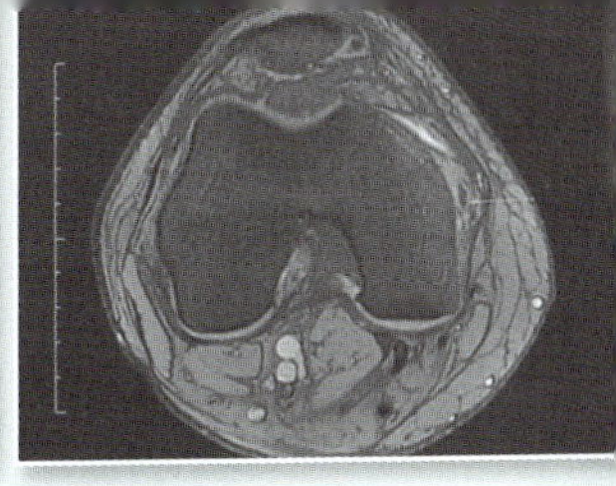

Essential ORTHOPEDICS Principles and Practice

THIRD EDITION

Manish Kumar Varshney
MS (Orth) DNB (Orth) MNAMS MRCS (Glasgow)
Senior Consultant Orthopedic Surgeon
SMVD Narayana Superspeciality Hospital
Reasi, Jammu and Kashmir, India

JAYPEE

JAYPEE BROTHERS MEDICAL PUBLISHERS
The Health Sciences Publisher
New Delhi | London

Jaypee Brothers Medical Publishers (P) Ltd.

Headquarters
EMCA House
23/23-B, Ansari Road, Daryaganj
New Delhi 110 002, India
Landline: +91-11-23272143, +91-11-23272703
+91-11-23282021, +91-11-23245672
Email: jaypee@jaypeebrothers.com

Corporate Office
4838/24, Ansari Road, Daryaganj
New Delhi 110 002, India
Phone: +91-11-43574357
Fax: +91-11-43574314
Email: jaypee@jaypeebrothers.com

Overseas Office
J.P. Medical Ltd
83 Victoria Street, London
SW1H 0HW (UK)
Phone: +44 20 3170 8910
Email: info@jpmedpub.com

EU GPSR Authorised Representative
Logos Europe, 9 rue Nicolas Poussin
17000, La Rochelle, France
Phone: +33 (0) 6 67 93 73 78
E-mail: Contact@logoseurope.eu

Website: www.jaypeebrothers.com
Website: www.jaypeedigital.com

Essential Orthopedics: Principles and Practice (Volumes 1 and 2)

First Edition: 2016

Second Edition: 2018

Third Edition: 2022, ***Reprint:*** **2025**

ISBN: 978-93-5465-105-2

Printed at: Samrat Offset Pvt. Ltd.

Dedicated to

All my students, my teachers from
whom I learned Orthopedics,
both my sons—Siddhant and Mrigank
who taught me how to teach,
and my loving wife—Neeta
who spared me from my homely duties
while being engaged in preparing this book.

Contributors

Avinash Razdan
DMRD DMB (Radio Diagnosis)
Associate Consultant
SMVD Narayana Superspeciality Hospital
Reasi, Jammu and Kashmir, India
avinash.razdan@gmail.com

Jaydip Patel
DNB FIAS FISS
Director
Trinay Hospital
Ahmedabad, Gujarat, India
jaydipshyani.js@gmail.com

Manish Kumar Varshney
MS (Orth) DNB (Orth) MNAMS MRCS (Glasgow)
Senior Consultant Orthopedic Surgeon
SMVD Narayana Superspeciality Hospital
Reasi, Jammu and Kashmir, India
drmkvarshney@gmail.com

Mohinder Singh Chib
MBBS MS FIAS FIAP
Consultant Orthopedics and Trauma
Gupta Hospital
Kathua, Jammu and Kashmir, India
drmohindersinghchib@gmail.com

S Pavan MS
Chief Consultant and Head
Department of Orthopedics
Tata Motors Hospital
Jamshedpur, Jharkhand, India
pavan.sudarshan@tatamotors.com

Shafiq Hackla
MS (Orth) DNB FNB (Sports Medicine)
Attending Consultant
Artemis Hospital
Gurugram, Haryana, India
hacklashafiq17@gmail.com

Shalinder Kumar Sharma MS (Orth)
Associate Professor
Government Medical College
Rajouri, Jammu and Kashmir, India
drshalinder@gmail.com

Preface to the Third Edition

In a nutshell, the third edition of *Essential Orthopedics: Principles and Practice* is a thoroughly revised edition. I am glad that readers pointed to some critical mistakes in the previous editions, and the same have also been included. The revision and upgradation do not involve only the clinical text but even the grammatical and spelling mistakes are thoroughly corrected. The book has been revised literally word by word. Upgradation of clinical knowledge involves incorporation of the latest developments that have made a significant impact on orthopedics (leaving behind the investigational approaches/methods to minimize cluttering and confusion). The clinical and core text changes significantly involve:

- General orthopedics as lots of changes have been made in the diagnosis for diseases, tools used (e.g., for slipped upper femoral epiphysis, etc.), and therapies based on molecular targets (rheumatoid arthritis, osteoporosis, etc.).
- Various new diseases (scurvy, chronic renal disease, etc.) and techniques (electrospinning, etc.) have been added that were omitted in previous editions. Annexure 1 for Upper Limb Trauma is revised for newer treatment methods and expanded to include small bone injuries of wrist and hand.
- Regional orthopedics have also undergone changes with respect to better understanding of diseases and their management (viz. Shoulder Instability, Imaging of Shoulder Joint, Total Hip Replacement, etc.). Certain previously omitted conditions (patellar tendon rupture, etc.) have been added or expanded.
- Totally new additions include chapters on Musculoskeletal Imaging, Preoperative Planning, Nanotechnology, Orthopedics in Digital Renaissance, Neglected Trauma to Bones and Joints (Annexure 4), expansion on Malunions, etc.
- Addition of lots of relevant figures and photographs along with tabulation and compression of details in text considered too descriptive to be of any use.

Most importantly the *chapter organization of the book has massively changed* as there was discontinuity in previous presentation and mis-positioning of related topics. Various chapters have been merged to maintain comprehensiveness and provide space for adding newer chapters without increasing overall numbers of chapters! The total number of chapters have been in fact reduced compared to previous edition (to partly reduce scare amongst the readers). I hope the current text will meet the comprehensive need of readers to learn and repair orthopedic knowledge.

Happy reading!

Manish Kumar Varshney

Preface to the First Edition

Orthopedics like other medical faculties is a growing branch. The growth is, however, much faster than other fields. Till the beginning of the last century, the orthopedics as a discrete was nonexistent to this world but the efforts of pioneers in the field gave birth to the baby that boomed possibly the fastest to become one of the most favored surgical branches to new entrants in the postgraduation. Orthopedics is the most glamorous and preferred surgical faculty for all youngsters aspiring to quickly gain sort of "superspecialization" as not much is available or required after one does his postgraduation in orthopedics, the regionwise faculty development into knee, shoulder, hip, pediatric orthopedics, orthopedic oncology and spine surgery are mostly fellowship dependent.

The scenario in orthopedics was not similar when the faculty started and in the beginning most of the evidences were mere "possibilities" as propounded in the replete literature of the older times written by the eminent persons in the field. Soon it came to be realized that opinions do not count and are often deleterious to general practice that may be true only for certain circumstances, so the era of "evidence-based practice" gradually evolved. With a few hitches then dawned the time where evidence was sought for most of the prevailing practices that were repeatedly questioned by surgeons around the world. This was pioneered by efforts of Association for Osteosynthesis (AO) Foundation and others and did help to some extent. In the beginning, however, the evidence was more of confusion rather than leading and the laid down facts had to be constantly changed and adjusted more due to poverty in exactness of the previously laid principles and less also to the emerging evidence as is evident from changing AO philosophy and the glaring failure of metal-on-metal hips. As a postgraduate, it became difficult for me to comprehend the historical errors and practice, changing philosophy and emerging new evidence and importantly remember them all. It was even more difficult to be accurate in orthopedic examinations to rationalize my understanding and teachings to that of the senior examiners who had started the practice even in a more bleak and confused environment prevailing at their time. However, I did realize during the course that some fundamentals were constantly getting lost in these times of evolution that could not be passed on to the youngsters and clinical examination has by now become a mere formality due to higher dependence/pervasiveness on advanced imaging and some illicit activities. The beginning of this century was marked by two major developments I feel—the development of improved implants and instrumentation (particularly the locked plate-screw constructs) and higher importance laid down for minimally invasive surgery. It became quickly evident to me that we need a text that encompasses all these facts so that the student gets a "One Stop" text where he can refer to most of his queries. This encouraged me to write down the current text and incorporate the most significant of previous practices and the current developments, some attempts have been made to incorporate the futuristic techniques but it is limited by unavailability of "evidence-based practice", so I have personally restricted that.

I feel that the future of orthopedics lies in correct and prudent diagnosis (aided solidly by sound knowledge and clinical examination) and ethical practice (not just money making as is considered an important practice nowadays); the basis of which should be correct and true literature and not polluted one. I found that some youngsters in the race of just publishing even resort to unethical practice and publish skewed and incorrect findings that pollute the sacred literature which has access to all and even amateur people who may not be able to rationalize and fall prey to wrong practice. This, I feel, also is the reason that newer meta-analysis and even systematic reviews are unable to yield evidence in favor of one or the other method rather often end in saying "no statistically significant different in practice".

The current text will help a practicing surgeon to acquaint himself with the alternatives available for a particular condition. I have tried to integrate most of the methods that are in practice or known currently for different orthopedic conditions and also organize the text in the form of answers to common theory questions for use to a postgraduate student. I tried to make a sincere effort in producing a text that can give an orthopedic surgeon insight into the orthopedic practice importantly the basic sciences and how diseases are based on faults in them. The textbook has been organized in the form of regional disposition to capture the region-specific conditions. There is vast emerging evidence and will keep emerging even at the time of this writing in the form of modern and new molecular markers that aim to diagnose disorders correctly and fast. The future for treatment of some of these disorders might also lie in the molecular level by using microinstruments such as nanotechnology and gene therapy, so I tried to cover that topic also comprehensively.

I would like to thank from my heart to all those who have contributed to the text. Particularly, Professor Alok Sud from Lady Hardinge Medical College and Associated Hospitals, New Delhi, India, who stood by the commitment once made and put constant efforts in providing me the text in pediatric orthopedics and helped till end in organizing some photographs despite ourselves being only formally introduced and worked for a short duration together. The other person who has helped in preparing the text is Dr S Pavan, who stood always by my side whenever required and also relieved me of my duties often at even hectic times to prepare the text. My juniors Dr Jaydip Patel, Dr Amit Singh and Dr Swapnil Sharma have provided help at difficult times when I needed them for text correction and improvement despite some of them being engaged in their own academic work. Especially, I would thank Dr Jaydip, who even woke-up untiringly at nights despite his duties to correct the text and add to the base work done by others and Dr Swapnil, who provided support regardless of his examinations going on. The contribution of others is not nevertheless small and Dr Ashok Jadon, Dr Sanjay L Srivastav, Dr Ankit Data and Dr Sachin Bharti have contributed thoroughly to the nonorthopedic topics and Dr Aditya Soral, Dr Ram Kinkar Jha and Dr S Dutta, without their help the text could never be completed. My family had been very supportive in displaying immense courage to face social restrictions and my untimely absence from home due to writing work, sometimes when my kids needed me most to play, read, learn and enjoy and my wife missing me sometimes altogether in important festivals and ceremonies. There are, however, some sour memories also and it is also important to mention that the writing had not been easy at all, with minimal help coming from persons I thought would contribute the most. The most respected and dear ones from my earlier relations in the field got too busy or otherwise to provide any help but this was to my best use and possibly advantage that it made me write all the topics by myself, which gave me further knowledge and confidence in areas where I was lacking in my training.

Lastly, I am highly thankful to Shri Jitendar P Vij (Group Chairman), Mr Ankit Vij (Group President), Ms Sunita Katla (PA to Group Chairman and Publishing Manager), Ms Samina Khan (Executive Assistant to Director–Publishing), the artists and all the team members who untiringly worked to bring out this wonderful text despite various delays and hitches from my end. It is only with the help of the publishing team at M/s Jaypee Brothers Medical Publishers (P) Ltd, New Delhi, India, that I could produce the text with confidence. Especially Shri Jitendar P Vij has grown in respect and stature in my thoughts who gave me the opportunity and initiated me for writing giving timely broad outlines, similarly production team has constantly assisted me in sorting out nitty-gritty problems that an author would usually encounter.

Providing an updated and correct text is always a challenge and some concepts would keep changing over time—is a fact. To this end, I reiterate all the readers of this text to kindly keep posting me in case, they find fundamental errors in the text or some critical updates that should be incorporated so that we can help all others in their future reading. I am open to all the criticism as they are bound to arise by difference of opinion that should be freely communicated to me at my e-mail—drmkvarshney@gmail.com. One may also reach me at the so-called in fashion social sites such as Facebook® or WhatsApp. In the name of Almighty, I present the text as an endeavor to promote the proficiency of both the neophyte and experienced orthopedic surgeon, bearing in mind to the truest of an attempt to present contradictory accumulation of discernment into logical concepts and the fact that condensing the mountain of knowledge may not be possible in the lifetime with ever-evolving concepts.

Manish Kumar Varshney

Acknowledgments

I am extremely thankful to Shri Jitendar P Vij (Group Chairman), Mr Ankit Vij (Managing Director), Mr MS Mani (Group President), Ms Chetna Malhotra Vohra (Associate Director—Content Strategy), Ms Pooja Bhandari (Production Head), and Ms Nikita Chauhan (Senior Development Editor) of M/s Jaypee Brothers Medical Publishers (P) Ltd, New Delhi, India, for giving the go-ahead at the very beginning and helping us in every way possible to bring out this book.

Contents

VOLUME 1

VOLUME 2

SECTION 6 Sports Medicine

SECTION 7 Regional Orthopedics: Shoulder

SECTION 8 Regional Orthopedics: Hip

SECTION 10 Regional Orthopedics: Spine

SECTION 1

Bone Anatomy, Physiology, Pathology, and Related Diseases

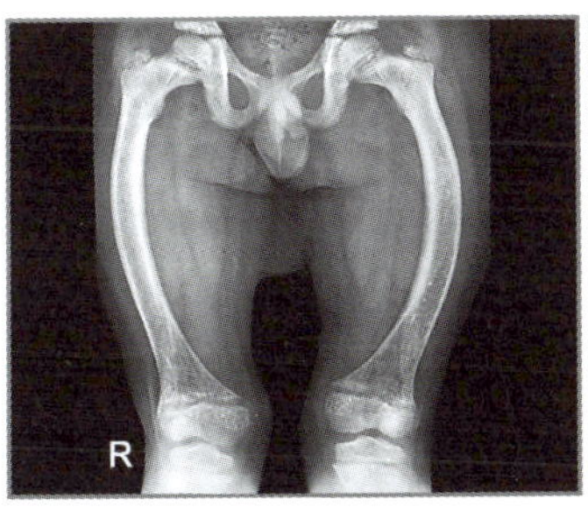

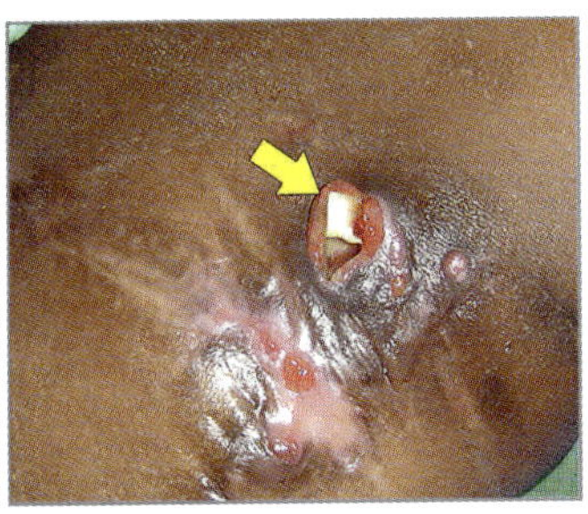

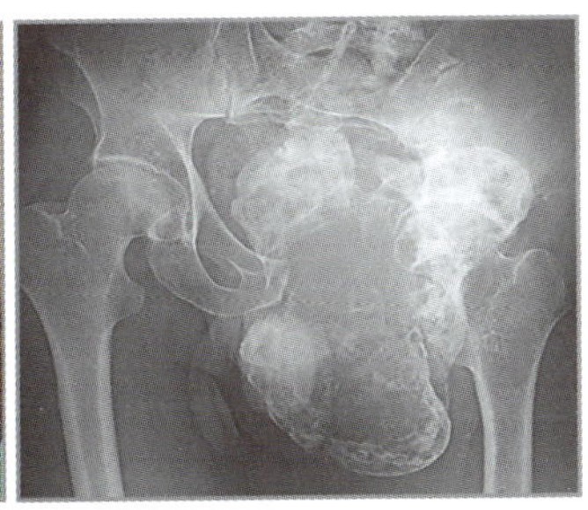

CHAPTER 1

Bone Structure, Physiology, Metabolism, and Associated Disorders

Manish Kumar Varshney

INTRODUCTION

Orthopedics is a science that deals with bones and its disorders primarily; but it has its extension into surgical management of disorders of joints, nerves, and muscles due to their close association. The literal meaning of orthopedics [Orthos (L.) = "straight", "pedios" (L.) = "children"—straightening a (crooked) child] does not qualify to the scope of current practice of the faculty dealing with prevention and treatment of bone and joint disorders, deformities, and deficiencies. Bone is a connective mesenchymal tissue that is distinctively recognized as "hard tissue" of the body. Contrary to the common notion in a layman that hard "objects" are abiotic, bones are lively, and have active metabolism, so they also get involved in various metabolic disorders similar to other body tissues. Additionally bones are susceptible to fracture due to characteristic hardness. In this chapter, we will study the macro- and microscopic structure of bones and their cellular elements, bone biology, growth, and its metabolic regulation. Briefly, we will also discuss some disorders that involve bones due to altered metabolism and control.

BONE STRUCTURE

Bone is a composite tissue (in strict engineering sense) consisting of organic matrix, inorganic minerals, cells, and water. Biologically, it is a dynamic mesenchymal (specialized connective) hard tissue that undergoes continuous formation, deformation, and remodeling throughout life. The size of bone increases by growth (skeletal modeling) during initial life till physeal closure but the shape of bone changes throughout life by virtue of the dynamic process of remodeling. While modeling gives initial shape and structure to bones during the growth phase the process of remodeling occurs in adulthood and is essentially a mechanism that differentiates living tissue from nonliving tissue. Remodeling gives capacity to bone to "repair" itself and renew the lost internal structure that continuously happen from wear and tear process. It also enables bone to adapt itself to changing environment resulting from altered activity levels and aging (Wolff's law, see bone remodeling detailed later). Both modeling and remodeling occur via "coupling" of bone resorption and bone formation that occurs simultaneously. Structurally, the bone per se consists of **(Fig. 1)** predominant inorganic (60%) and organic components (40%).

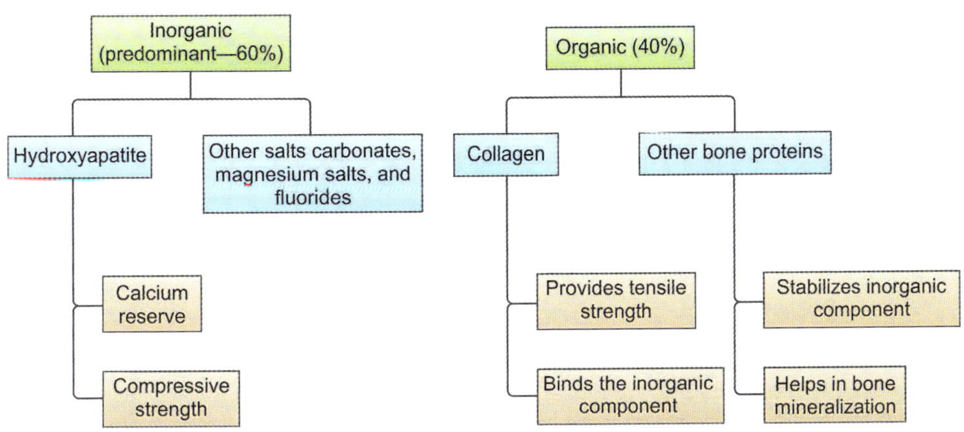

Fig. 1: Broad constituents of bone.

- The inorganic portion comprises of crystalline calcium phosphate salts, present in the form of hydroxyapatite [$Ca_{10}(PO_4)_6(OH)_2$] with minor contribution from carbonates, fluorides, and other magnesium salts.
- The organic component is dominated by type I collagen that forms the basic architecture of bone on which inorganic portion is deposited. Support to collagen is provided by derived protein components such as proteoglycans, glycoproteins, phospholipids, and phosphoproteins that serve specific functions (discussed below).

Both the components give bone its unique mechanical, biological, and electrical properties. Loss or inadequacy of either the mineral component (osteomalacia or rickets) or the organic component (like osteogenesis imperfecta) produces structurally weak bones that fail easily. The human and primate bones comprise **(Figs. 2A to E)** of typical distribution of hard (compact) bone outside, supported internally by softer (cancellous) bone that has nine times the metabolic activity. This distribution of hard (cortical/compact bone) and spongy (cancellous bone) components in tandem gives bone mechanical advantage of discrete rigidity and flexibility together. Such a structure is called a "composite" (in engineering terms) mentioned initially.

- And is in turn covered by the periosteum (green envelope here). Illustrated are the dispositions of cortical and cancellous components.
- Of human bone in a typical long bone (tibia here), the cancellous bone typically occupies the epiphysis and metaphysis of a long bone while cortical bone predominates in the diaphysis. The microstructure of mature cortical (compact) bone comprises of [concentric rings around Haversian (longitudinal) and Volkmann (transverse) canal system] within the osteoid (C), also shown are the osteocytes arranged in the lamellations (D) that form the largest network of cells connecting skeletal system to the outside environment through their processes (E), and also maintains homeostasis within bone.

FUNCTIONS OF BONE

The bone functions to:

- Provide a rigid framework of all vertebrates to support the body.
- Act as levers for muscles.
- Give shape to soft tissues and protect vital organs of body by forming rigid or flexible cavities.
- Provide minerals in time of need as it has mineral reserve for calcium and phosphate.
- It helps in the hematopoiesis (formation of blood cells) by virtue of its marrow content.

With the overview of basic composition of bone in mind, now we can delve into the more intricate aspects of orthopedic osteology (scientific study of bones).

CLASSIFICATION OF BONE BY APPEARANCE

The human body has 206 bones at skeletal maturity that evolve from nearly 270 bones at birth by a process of fusion, but all these can be grouped broadly into five different types of bones **(Figs. 3A to E)**.

Long Bones

The long bones are formed by endochondral ossification. The bones of arm, forearm, thigh and legs, viz., femur, ulna, tibia, radius, humerus, and fibula, are typical examples. These have two ends (*epiphysis*), a cylindrical tube in the middle (*diaphysis*), and a transitional zone between them (*metaphysis*). The long bones develop from cartilage enlarge through a process of endochondral ossification. The ossification centers for epiphysis and the diaphysis are different and are separated by growth plate also known as physis which is basically a layer of hyaline cartilage organized into different layers.

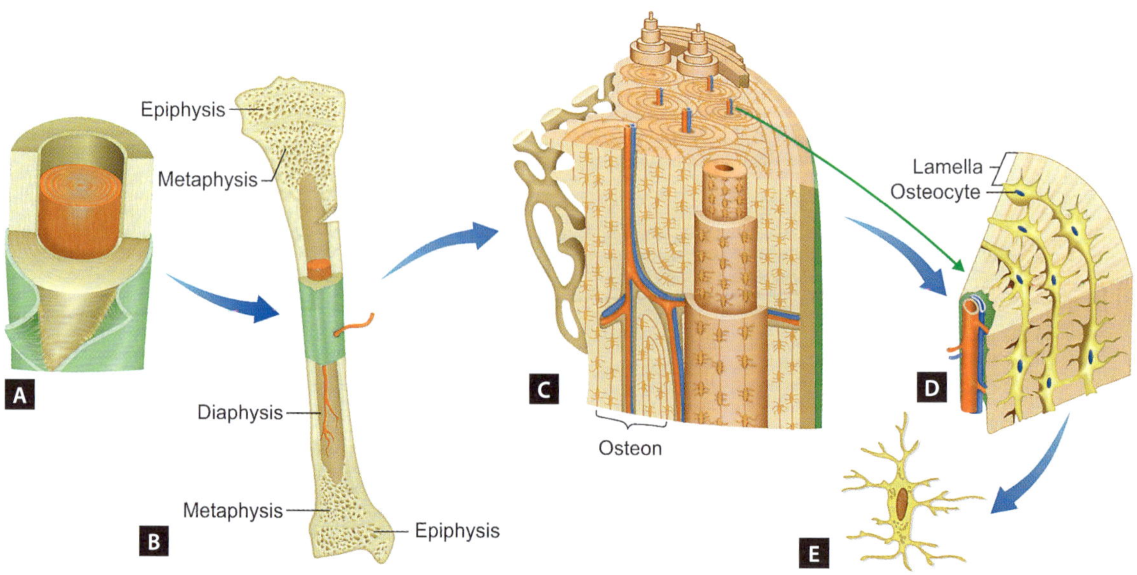

Figs. 2A to E: The gross appearance (A to C) to microstructure (D and E) of bone. The cortex forms a cylinder encircling the medullary cavity.

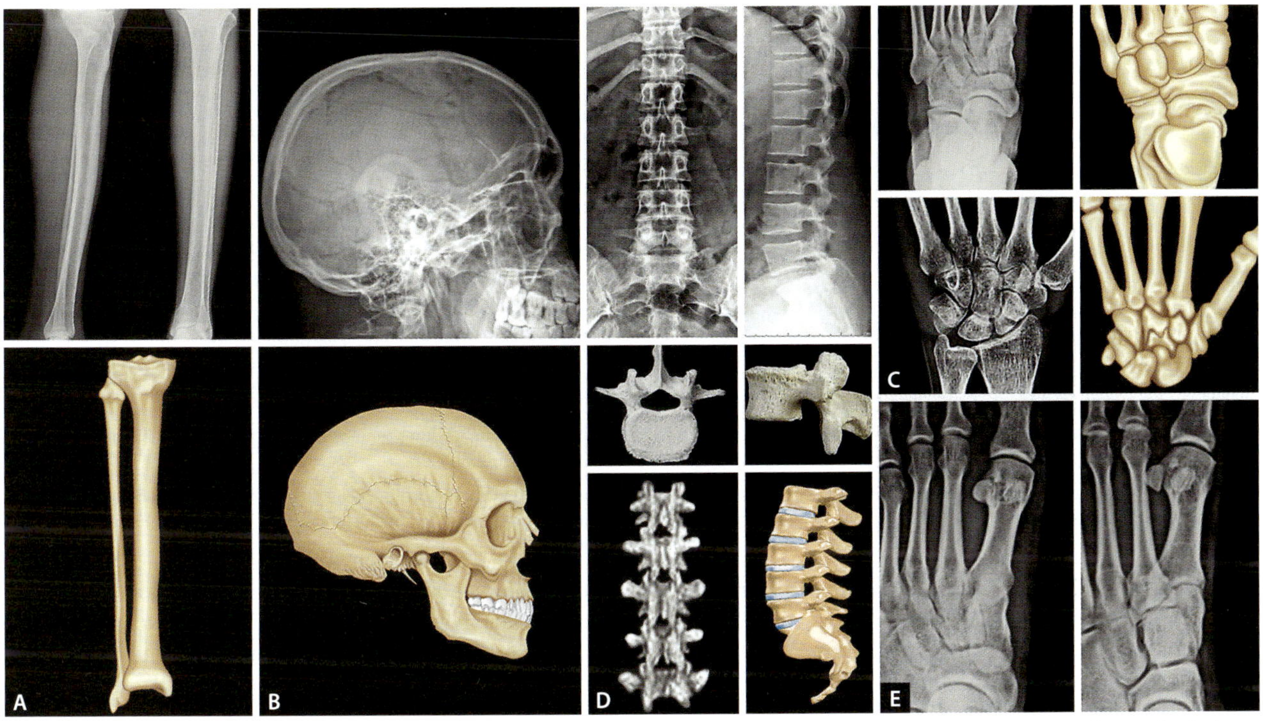

Figs. 3A to E: The five types of bones in human body. Long bones here exemplified by tibia and fibula (A) have expanded metaphysis at both the ends capped by epiphysis that is separated by physis from metaphysis in an immature bone and a cylindrical shaft in middle. Flat bones are typified by skull (B) bones that have an outer and an inner table. The carpal and metatarsal bones (C) represent the short bones. Vertebrae (D) are best examples of irregular bones with multiple irregular processes and parts. Sesamoid bones develop later in life commonly at the wear and tear sites of tendons or where the tendons need some mechanical advantage for their action, here are shown the sesamoid bones in the tendon of flexor hallucis brevis beneath the first metatarsal of foot (E).

Flat Bones

The flat bones as against long bones develop from a discrete process called intramembranous ossification. Scapula and sternum are the representative examples. The flat bones have an inner and an outer table of cortical bone intervened by trabecular bone as are exemplified by skull bones.

Short Bones

Carpal and tarsal bones are representative examples. They are predominantly composed of trabecular bone that is shelled by a thin layer of cortical bone.

Irregular Bones

They are like short bones in cut sections, but unlike them they have no smooth structure resembling any geometrical shape (hence, irregular). Vertebrae are classic examples.

Sesamoid Bones

These bones also resemble short bones, but form without ossification center (except patella) due to undue stress in the region. They are found embedded in tendons or ligaments and serve specific functions.

GROSS FEATURES OF BONE

As evident from the above classification the bones are either shaped as a hollow tube (long bones) or bilaminar plate of bone (flat bones) containing variable cortical or trabecular structures. Cortical (compact) bone is dense and calcified bone forming hard outer structure of bone providing most of the mechanical strength. It is also referred to as "cortex" commonly by surgeons and consists of aggregations of concentric lamellar bone in the form of osteons. Osteons at their center contain Haversian and Volkmann vascular canal systems, individual nerves, and one or two lymphatic channels (discussed in detail later). One can say that well-developed osteons define cortical or compact bone and its presence is the hallmark. The marrow cavity is the space inside the cortical walls that contains hematopoietic marrow tissue, fat, and bony spicules. Trabecular bone consists of these slender spicules and trabeculae (not >0.2–0.4 mm) that are separated by marrow spaces. Trabeculae of bone support the marrow elements by increasing surface area and providing scaffold for attachment of the cells and they also lighten the bone. It fills the metaphyseal and epiphyseal region of bones by virtue of gaps in between. Trabeculae are also composed of lamellar bone with longitudinal arrangement, but the osteons are not formed **(Table 1)**. These spongier regions develop according to the lines of stress giving bone ability to deform (elastic nature) before failing (tensile strength). In addition to the ability to withstand the tensile forces, bone robustly resists compression forces also avidly which is primarily a function of the cortical/compact bone present in outer cortex (composite design).

The bone can be divided into following anatomical parts (these are also functionally and physiologically distinct units, **Figures 2A to E**):

TABLE 1: Differences between cortical and cancellous bone.

Cortical bone	*Cancellous bone*
Forms the outer part or "shell" of bone	Contained within shell
Predominantly found in diaphyseal region	Predominantly seen in metaphyseal and epiphyseal regions
Concentric lamellar structure around Haversian system—osteonal formation	Contains lamellae, but osteons are missing
Provides compressive strength to bone	Provides tensile strength to bone and resilience
Provides attachment to tendons, ligaments, and periosteum	Provides scaffolding to marrow cavity and space for osteoprogenitor cells
Metabolically less active	Nine times more metabolically active than cortical bone
Slow remodeling. Thickening occurs on the concave side (compression), while convex side (tensile side) undergoes thinning and resorption	• Complete trabecular structure changes with continuous remodeling • Trabecular hypertrophy under compressive forces and even with tensile forces. They atrophy and disappear with reduction of these forces
Usually minimal change in osteoporosis	Undergoes great amount of resorption in osteoporosis
When used as a graft mainly provides strut support and compressive strength—less osteogenic potential	Preferred in bone grafting for higher osteogenic potential and remodels by creeping substitution
Cortical bone undergoes remodeling through "cutting cones" led by osteoclasts followed by osteoblasts	Remodeling in cancellous bone occurs directly on the surface of trabeculae by "creeping substitution"

Epiphysis—part of bone that lies between physis or physeal scar and articular cartilage. The part is usually intra-articular and takes part in joint formation and function. The periosteum in intra-articular region lacks the cambium layer that contains totipotential cell rests responsible for periosteal callus formation. This explains the reason why joints containing significant region of epiphyseal bones (like hip joint containing neck of femur) are more prone to nonunion, because callus formation is minimal.

Physis—this is the growing structure consisting of flat portion adding length to bone and the circumferential portion of the growth plate adding to width of bone and physis itself as it grows (discussed later for detailed structure).

Metaphysis—this is the funnel-like part at ends of diaphysis that predominantly comprises of trabecular bone. The metaphysis lies between physis and diaphysis and is quite susceptible to osteoporotic fractures due to high metabolic (catabolic) bone loss and lack of cortical bone which is less prone to such catabolic bone wasting. Being metabolically active metaphysic is also susceptible to remodeling defects like multiple osteochondromatosis. Radiologically, the extent of metaphysis is defined by a square drawn from epiphysis and the length of line being derived from the greatest horizontal dimension at metaphysis.

Diaphysis—this is the predominant central tubular portion of long bones giving them the characteristic form. Most cortical bone is found on this region giving tensile (partly) and compressive strength (predominantly) to the region. It is the strongest part of bone and is susceptible to fractures by virtue of extreme levered forces being transmitted through it. Also, it is subject to direct trauma in the center of limb.

Bone marrow—it fills the medullary cavity and is responsible for most of the hematopoietic activity from the contained progenitors. The marrow gradually changes from red (hematopoietic) in adolescents to yellow or white (fatty) in adults. The red marrow persists in the vertebrae, some metaphyseal regions, and flat bones in adults.

Periosteum—it is a thick fibrous membrane that covers the bone all-over like a laminating membrane (except at articular cartilage and dense tendon attachments). The membrane is divided histologically into outer fibrous (collagen) and inner cellular layer. The latter is important structure responsible for bone repair and is referred to as the "cambium" layer. It contains totipotent (in young children) or multipotent (in adolescents and adults) cells that serve as osteoprogenitor cells capable of forming new bone and callus with traumatic disruption. Periosteum also serves to add thickness to bone by appositional bone deposition; this is especially true at the sites of tendon attachment through Sharpey's fibers that give a traction force on bone. Sharpey's fibers are thick collagen bundles that anchor the periosteum to circumferential bony lamellae and dominate in the regions of tendon attachment.

Endosteum—there is no microscopic or macroscopic structure distinctly seen inside the bone that can be referred to as endosteum. The outer resting layer of marrow and its interface with bone is what is referred to as endosteum commonly. Electron microscopically there is a thin arrangement of highly cellular osteoblastic and osteoclastic elements but is devoid of characteristically distinguishable membrane.

MICROSCOPIC ANATOMY

Based on collagen fiber arrangements, bones have two distinct histological appearances—woven bone and the lamellar bone.

Woven Bone

Woven bone is also called immature bone, coarse bundled bone, or sometimes fiber bone. It is made from randomly-oriented collagen fibers in interlacing or "burlap" (coarse canvas) fashion, with numerous osteoblasts and osteoprogenitor cells (so-called immature bone cells). When viewed under polarized light, it shows haphazard structural organization. Woven bone is much more cellular than the organized lamellar bone and has higher number of cells per unit area. Woven bone is the major bone type in the developing fetus that matures to lamellar bone in adult. In adults, immature bone is still found at remodeling sites, in the alveolar socket (mouth), fracture repair (callus), and at tendinous intersection. It occurs pathologically in osteosarcoma, fibrous dysplasia, and several other tumors. The synthesis of woven bone is triggered by platelet-derived growth factor (PDGF-A and PDGF-B) and insulin-like growth factor (IGF-I and IGF-II) and is seen in areas of fast bone growth.

Lamellar Bone

Lamellar (thin plate) bone (mature bone) on polarized light microscopy has characteristic well-organized arrangement of collagen fibers seen as parallel bundles (2–4 μm) of deposited bone. Lamellar bone develops during remodeling of immature bone by replacement of the latter. Continuous secondary organization (remodeling) is pathognomonic of mature lamellar bone. Lamellar bone is deposited in slow growing regions, but the control mechanisms have not been fully understood. In the cortex, the lamellae have concentric tubular arrangement containing 5–15 concentric lamellae. Outer circumferential lamellae **(Figs. 2A to E)** lie next to the periosteum, while inner circumferential lamellae lie near endosteum. The interstitial lamellae **(Figs. 2A to E)** represent archaic remnants of old concentric lamellae. These variable size (thick or thin) tubes of concentric lamellar arrangement are called osteon and a number of them are closely packed with few gaps, if any, to form compact bone. The fibers of each lamella run in a spiral fashion rather than concentric cylinders around the canal. The osteons surround a central Haversian canal (Haversian systems—after Clopton Havers who defined it in 1691) that contains vascular bundle of capillaries and venules and also nerves, lymphatic canals, and a loose connective tissue encompassing osteoprogenitor cells **(Figs. 2A to E)**. It is a branching system of cylinders arranged longitudinally in the bone. Volkmann's canals (transverse perforating canal system) are vascular channels that interconnect Haversian canals and also the Haversian system to periosteal blood vessels and intramedullary vascular supply **(Figs. 2A to E)**. Osteocytes are located in the interlaminar regions with their processes arranged in a radial pattern into the canaliculi. The osteons act like fibers of bamboo that resist deformation.

CELLULAR ELEMENTS OF BONE

Osteoblasts, osteocytes, and osteoclasts are predominant cells in bone **(Table 2)**. Osteoblasts serve the purpose of bone formation (osteogenesis), while osteoclasts are mainly accountable for bone resorption; their combined action contributes to progressive mineralization and remodeling. The osteocytes maintain the milieu of bone and its homeostasis through vast network of canalicular system that communicates with external environment through Haversian–Volkmann system. The three types of cells have different origins; while osteoblasts and osteocytes (along with chondrocytes, adipose cells, fibroblasts, and myocytes) originate from mesenchymal stem cells (MSC), the osteoclasts are related to monocyte or macrophages, and hence, derived from hematopoietic stem cells. Bone mineralization is a chemical process that is facilitated by the cellular elements, so we can call it biochemical process. The bone resorption and bone formation are to be tightly coupled with favorable chemical milieu (controlled by

TABLE 2: Cellular elements of bone.

Cell type	*Transcriptional factors for differentiation and function*	*Physiological function*	*Associated disorders*
Osteoblasts (mesenchymal origin)	• *Runx2/ATF4* • *Osf2/Cbfa1* • Osterix • Wnt/β-catenin pathway • Parathormone (PTH) • Dkk1 and sclerostin from osteocytes negatively influence osteoblastogenesis	• Bone formation (osteoid synthesis, mineralization, skeletal development, and remodeling) • Osteoclast differentiation • Formation of osteocytes	• Osteogenesis imperfecta • Fibrodysplasia ossificans progressive • Cleidocranial dysostosis • Osteoid osteoma • Osteoblastoma • Osteosarcoma
Osteoclasts (monocyte/ macrophage lineage)	• RANK expression (RANK-L from osteoblasts) • C-fos • M-CSF (monocyte colony stimulating factor) • Osteoprotegerin (OPG) • PTH and calcitonin • Tumor necrosis factor-α • Estrogen • Prolactin • IL-17 and IL-6 • Transforming growth factor-β (TGF-β)	Bone resorption (increased by vitamin D, PTH, PTHrP, prolactin, IL-6, and TNF-α; decreased by estrogen, calcitonin, TGF-β, IL-17, and OPG)	• Osteopetrosis • Pycnodysostosis • Paget's disease • Tumor-induced osteolytic bone disease
Osteocytes (mesenchymal origin)	• miR-23a cluster • TGF-β • Dentin matrix protein-1 (DMP-1)	• Mechanosensing (stress and strain on bone) • Cell-signaling and regulation of bone metabolism • Regulate osteoblast and osteoclast activity by producing (sclerostin, cathepsin K, WNTs, DKK1, DMP1, IGF1, and RANKL/OPG)	• Sclerosteosis • van Buchem disease • Hypophosphatemic rickets • WNT1 and plastin 3 mutation-related disorders • Craniodiaphyseal dysplasia (lionitis) • Bone tumor metastasis • Osteoporosis and osteoarthritis

various extraneous and intrinsic processes) to result in proper physiological mineralization.

Osteoblasts

Osteoblasts are derived from pluripotent mesenchymal stem lineage. These mesenchymal progenitors can differentiate into various cell types including fibroblasts, chondrocytes, adipocytes (PPARγ2 stimulant), myoblasts (MyoD stimulant), and bone marrow stromal cells. Under appropriate stimulation [by Cbfa1 (core-binding factor α1) and/or runt-related transcription factor 2 (Runx2)], the stem cells first differentiate into osteoprogenitor cells (pluripotent cells) and then into osteoblasts **(Fig. 4)**. The osteoblast pathway can be induced by bone morphogenetic protein (BMP) 2, 4, and 7 that upregulate the Cbfa1 messenger ribonucleic acid (mRNA). The osteoprogenitor cells are dispersed into various bone elements and this has a purpose. They are found in:

- The inner layer (cambium) of the periosteum (predominant source)—responsible for callus formation
- Bone marrow (regenerative and intramedullary callus formation)
- The endosteum—endosteal callus formation
- Haversian and Volkmann's canals—direct or primary healing of bone and remodeling
- Perivascular tissue adjacent to bone—ill-defined function, but may form ectopic bone, e.g., post-traumatic/postsurgical or pathologic bone formation in myositis ossificans.

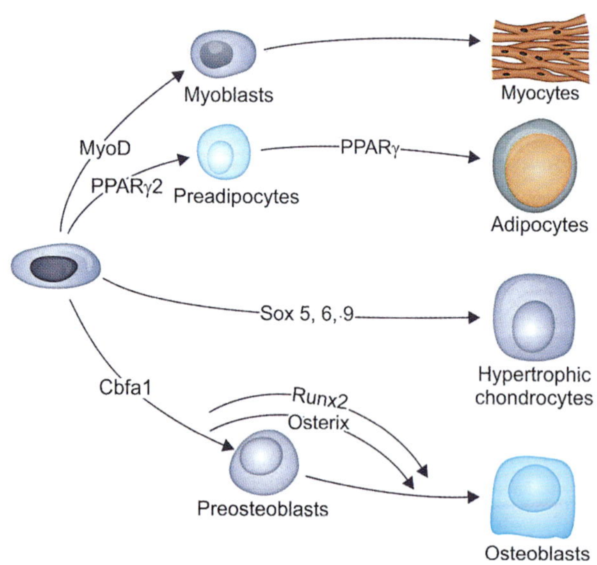

Fig. 4: The differentiation pathway for mesenchymal stem cell and generation of osteoblasts. Note the stem cell can transform into different cells under appropriate influences. For generation of osteoblasts the stem cells first differentiate into osteoprogenitor cells (pluripotent cells) induced by BMP 2, 4, and 7 that upregulate the Cbfa1 mRNA. There is also a possible flux mechanism that operates simultaneously and it has been found that inhibitor of PPARγ that reduces adipocytogenesis increases osteoblastogenesis and, hence, bone formation. This may find therapeutic utility in future management of osteoporosis. (PPARγ: peroxisome proliferator-activated receptor gamma)

Osteoblasts measure 15–20 μm in diameter and contain copious cytoplasm. They are cuboidal to columnar, and form a single layer of cell over bone surface where new matrix is being laid down. The cells deposit new bone or new osteoid (*the osteoid seam*) along the surface adjacent to bone only—a property called polarization, bone is not deposited at the free or superficial surface. The mineralization front lies deeper to the osteoid seam, where organized mineralization of the newly formed osteoid is being carried out. Osteoblasts are connected to each other by adherens type tight junctions, the desmosomes, and tight junctions. The high metabolic activity of osteoblasts is suggested by presence of abundant rough endoplasmic reticulum and bulky golgi apparatus (involved in protein synthesis) and abundant mitochondria required for fulfilling energy requirements and staining basophilic with hematoxylin and eosin stain.

Osteoblasts serve two main functions:

1. They produce the organic component of bone matrix—the osteoid by synthesizing and secreting type I collagen along with proteoglycans or glycosaminoglycans. Each new layer is laid down upon existing layer of osteoid (appositional growth) separated by a distinct cementing or watermark line.
2. Osteoblasts facilitate subsequent mineralization of osteoid by secreting matrix vesicles. They create a conducive milieu for deposition of calcium and phosphate in the organic matrix. Osteocalcin secretion is at its peak during mineralization.

The accessory functions (also important) of osteoblasts include:

- Production of noncollagenous proteins including the osteocalcin, osteopontin, bone sialoprotein, and osteonectin that takes part in bone mineralization and maintenance
- Regulating bone metabolism—this is made possible by responding to alteration in levels of hormones involved in calcium metabolism through receptors for parathyroid hormone (PTH) and 1,25-dihydroxyvitamin D3 present on mature cells
- Paracrine activity by secretion of various cytokines such as IL-6 and IL-11, and granulocyte colony-stimulating factor (G-CSF) and macrophage colony-stimulating factor (M-CSF) (thus play a role in myelopoiesis also). The osteoblasts also secrete a number of growth factors such as transforming growth factor-β (TGF-β), IGF, BMP and PDGF
- Differentiation of osteoclasts—this is now considered a primary function with increasing understanding of osteoporosis. The osteoblasts secrete receptor activator of nuclear factor-kappa B (RANK) ligand to regulate the activation and differentiation of osteoclasts that then effect remodeling. The pathway is also the culprit for increased bone resorption in osteoporosis and drugs targeting the same are increasingly becoming popular for treatment of osteoporosis.

Process of Mineralization as a Function of Osteoblasts (Fig. 5)

Alkaline phosphatase (ALP) produced by the osteoblast acts as a pyrophosphatase and is the primer for initiation of the mineralization process. The matrix vesicles secreted actively by osteoblasts (discussed above) are the centers for synthesis of crystalline hydroxyapatite from amorphous calcium phosphate though this also takes place outside of vesicles after mineralization has been initiated. The crystals within vesicles act as needle to rupture the membrane of vesicles when they come in contact. These free crystals induce further the precipitation of crystalline hydroxyapatite over the entire organic matrix surface which is lying in a supersaturated solution of calcium and phosphate.

The progressive changes can be described in a pathway as follows:

Expression of cell cycle and histone genes (initial proliferative phase) → upregulation of genes linked to formation of bone matrix (viz., for type I collagen and ALP) → expression of genes for osteocalcin and bone sialoprotein that are associated with mineralization (final stage of osteoblast maturation).

Markers of Osteoblastic Activity

- Alkaline phosphatase enzyme levels and activity is increased with osteoblast activity.
- The noncollagenous proteins (discussed above) also mark osteoblast phenotype and are expressed uniquely during osteoblast differentiation.

It is observed that with osteoblast maturation the proliferative capacity keeps constantly decreasing.

Osteoblast Differentiation and Regulation

Osteoblast proliferation or differentiation is under paracrine and endocrine control with the predominant control of the former. There is a fine control of relative strengths of opposing signaling pathways within a complex system. Osteoblasts also respond to chemical and mechanical stimuli (Wolff's law). The chemical regulators include growth factors (usually proliferation and maturation factors) such as TGF-β, BMPs, fibroblast growth factors (FGFs), and transcription factors (differentiation factors) such as *Runx2/Cbfa-1* [core-binding factor alpha (1)] and osterix predominantly.

- *Runx2* transcription pathway target genes include osteocalcin, bone sialoprotein, osteopontin, and collagen alpha-1 (a1) that is responsible for mineralization front mainly and also somewhat for production of cartilage anlage. Mutations causing dysfunction or loss of function of the *Runx2* gene causes cleidocranial dysplasia.
- Osterix basically acts further downstream of *Runx2* pathway and is also responsible for osteoblast differentiation affecting mineralization.

Other regulators of osteoblast differentiation and function include:

- Dickkopf (Dkk1)—this is a negative regulator of bone formation. Reduced *Dkk1* (gene deletion) increases trabecular and cortical bone thickness and volume. It is a lucrative target for osteoporosis treatment.
- Osteocalcin (gamma-carboxyglutamic acid protein), osteopontin (secreted phosphoprotein 1), and osteonectin (secreted acidic cysteine rich protein)—osteopontin and osteocalcin are negative regulators of bone formation, deficiency of former leads to ectopic calcification of tunica media of arteries and resistance to estrogen deficient bone resorption, while deficiency of latter produces higher bone mass of good quality without impairing bone resorption. Osteonectin is a positive regulator and its deficiency produces severe osteopenia, cataracts, and weak lens capsule.
- *Wnt/β-catenin pathway:* Signaling by the Wnt family of secreted glycolipoproteins via the transcription

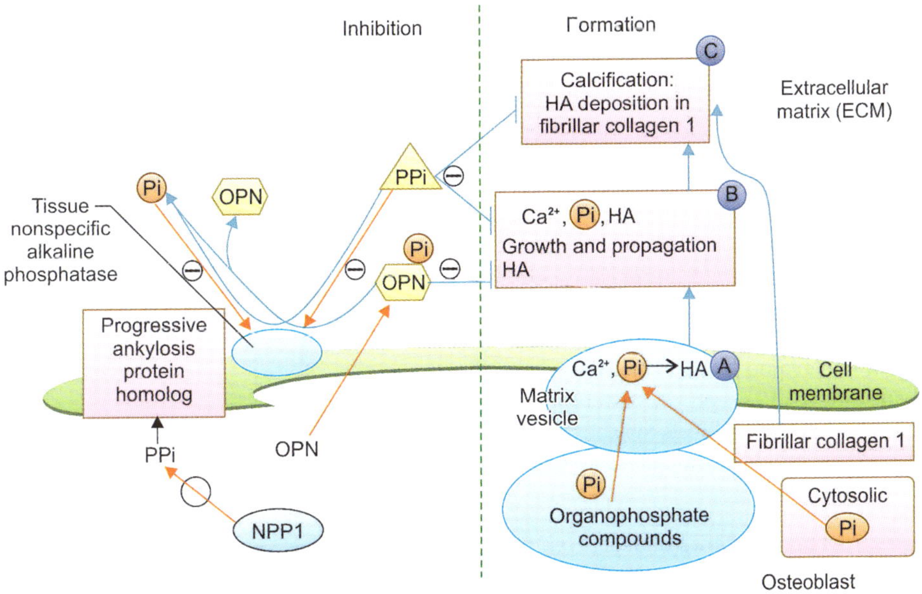

Fig. 5: Role of osteoblasts in bone mineralization; also depicted is the complex interaction of the alkaline phosphatase and pyrophosphate along with the role of vesicles. (OPN: osteopontin; PPi: pyrophosphate; Pi: inorganic phosphate; HA: hydroxyapatite; NPP1: nucleotide pyrophosphatase/phosphodiesterase 1)

coactivator β-catenin controls embryonic development and adult homeostasis (canonical pathway). This pathway promotes osteoblast commitment and proliferation, finally culminating into its differentiation. Wnt binds to a coreceptor low-density lipoprotein receptor-related protein (LRP5 or LRP6) activating the pathway which is comediated by one of the frizzled family member (Fz). The activity and binding of LRP5/6 is antagonized by sclerostin (product of osteocytes) and the Dickkoppf (Dkk) family, thus they are now being targeted for osteoporosis therapy and prevention by inhibiting their action. This is discussed in detail under pharmacotherapy of osteoporosis in Chapter on "Metabolic Diseases of Bone".

- Leptin has long known to be synthesized by adipocytes. Leptin mediates its effects of osteoblast differentiation and mineralization by inhibiting glycogen synthase kinase-3β (GSK-3β). This mechanism seems to be centrally regulated, but overall effect is negative regulation on bone formation. The leptin-hypothalamic axis control pathway is not fully elucidated as to how it controls bone deposition or bone mass. It is a common finding that patients with generalized lipodystrophy (absence of adipocytes and white fat) develop osteosclerosis and accelerated bone growth.
- *Mechanical regulation of osteoblast function:* Osteoblasts also respond to mechanical stress to mediate changes in bone size and shape, a property that has been exploited in some treatment forms like Ilizarov osteosynthesis and possibly also in electrical or sonological stimulation of bone formation. Calcium hydroxyapatite crystals have a piezoelectric effect possibly modulating the osteoblast activity, but complete understanding and science behind this effect is lacking. This process is essential component of bone remodeling.

  In adult and aging bone where many of the bone surfaces are inactive, osteoblasts become flattened resembling squamous cells lining bone surfaces (quiescent osteoblasts). This quiescent reservoir gets reactivated into functional forms during remodeling, fracture repair, and neoplasia when active bone formation occurs.

Role of Osteoblasts in Various Disorders

Osteoarthritis (OA): Subchondral bone metabolic changes have been suggested as a major pathogenic factor for development of OA. There is fivefold increase in leptin expression in OA that modulates the osteoblasts to actively produce reactive bone at the degenerated ends. This effect is observed in the form of elevated levels of bone formation markers (osteocalcin and ALP) seen in osteoblasts of osteoarthritic bone. Type I collagen levels synthesis is also increased in OA producing subchondral sclerosis that is a radiological hallmark of OA.

Osteoporosis and glucocorticoid therapy associated bone loss is related to osteoblast function: Osteoprotegerin (OPG)/RANK/RANK ligand (RANKL) system represents the main regulatory factors of bone remodeling and are involved in the pathogenesis of osteoporosis though all the mechanisms are not fully clear. DKK-1 mRNA is overexpressed in osteoblasts treated with glucocorticoid suppressing the mineralization function.

Effects of smoking and alcohol osteoblast: Moderate amount of nicotine and alcohol both seem to stimulate osteoblast to produce bone. Moderate alcohol consumers have low levels of osteoporotic fractures. Excess of everything though is bad and leads to increased bone resorption.

Osteocytes

They are the most abundant cells of bone (90–95% of all bone cells). Around 10% of the embryonic osteoblastic population is lost by getting trapped and enclosed in their own synthesized matrix. These then become osteocytes **(Fig. 6)**. Their cytoplasm also contains spherical granules stainable with periodate-leukofuchsin like osteoblasts suggesting common origin. The spaces which they occupy are known as lacunae. The lacunae *(L. "pit or depression")* are flat to oval cavities containing fine apertures called canaliculi *(L. "tiny dust")* through which cytoplasmic processes of osteocytes pass **(Figs. 2A to E)**. Baud and Auil classified the lacunae into four types as follows:

1. *Inactive:* Small lacunae with smooth borders largely seen in cortical bone.
2. *Osteolytic:* Large lacunae with irregular borders present in cancellous bone.
3. *Osteoplastic:* Large lacunae with recently formed matrix present at sites of remodeling and fracture repair.
4. *Empty:* Lacunae only containing cellular debris following death of osteocytes.

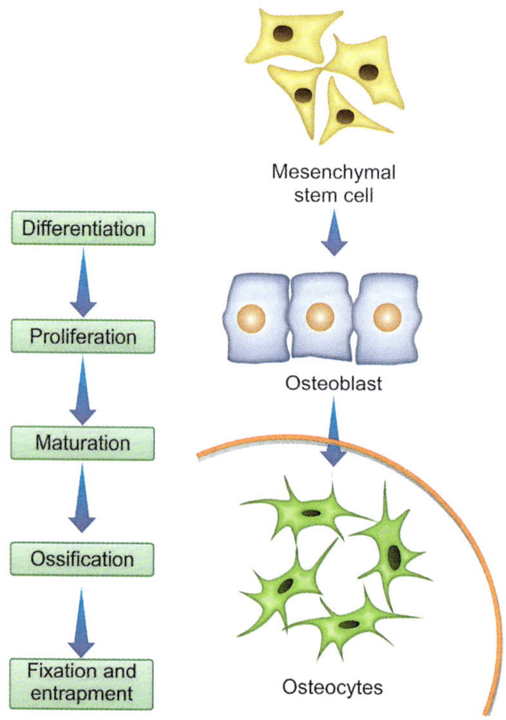

Fig. 6: Formation of osteocytes: These cells are none other than osteoblasts that get entrapped in the bone matrix with deposition of it around the cells. The cells then develop and communicate with other cells through processes.

Osteocytes are not dead or nonfunctional cells and their vitality is essential to the maintenance of bone. When the osteocyte dies, the bone around it also becomes nonfunctional and is eventually removed. The processes of osteocytes intercommunicate and these cells are also connected to surface osteoblasts through the network of canaliculi, hence, in all they form a large network inside the bone. Unlike osteoblasts the processes of osteocytes are joined by gap junctions [connexins (CX43 and CX45); and hemichannels, the tubular membrane protein connections] which help them "talk" to each other and with cells far off and outside of the bone matrix. They serve following functions:

- Cell signaling (because of vast network) and maintaining the viability of bone matrix. Osteocytes also have N-methyl-D-aspartate (NMDA) neural receptors and may be involved in central mechanisms of bone mineral metabolism like bone resorption in reflex sympathetic dystrophy (RSD)
- Regulates the mineral exchange between the extracellular fluid (ECF) and bone by means of the widespread canalicular system
- Osteocytes express osteoblast-specific factor-1 (OSF-1) that serves to stimulate osteoblasts. The secreted OSF-1 accumulates on bone surface and binds to N-syndecan (receptor for OSF-1) located on osteoblast progenitor cells.
- Osteocytes similar to osteoblasts are also known as mechanosensory cells. The thin layer of unmineralized matrix around osteocyte cell body and processes mediate the mechanical influence by loading derived flow of interstitial fluid across the osteocyte membrane (primarily facilitated by connexins). This affect translation of mechanical stress to cellular events culminating in bone formation and remodeling.

Regulation of Bone Metabolism and Mineralization as a Function of Osteocytes

- *The bone-renal axis for bone mineral metabolism:* Patients with autosomal recessive hypophosphatemic rickets display a hypomineralized bone phenotype manifesting as rickets or osteomalacia. There is isolated renal phosphate wasting associated with elevated FGF23 (a phosphatonin) levels and normocalciuria. Similar, phenotype is displayed in animal models having deficient dentin matrix protein 1 (DMP1) which is otherwise highly expressed in osteocytes. In patients with hypophosphatemic rickets there is a mutation affecting the DMP1 start codon, while some patients display a seven base pair deletion damaging the functional C terminus of DMP1. These findings suggest close relation of renal function and osteocyte in bone mineral metabolism.
- Osteocytes possess receptors for PTH, which regulates mineral ion homeostasis.
- Human osteocytes secrete sclerostin that inhibits bone formation. In the absence of sclerostin a disorder called sclerosteosis develops in which the skeleton develops high bone mass characterized by increased osteoblast activity. Uninhibited osteoblastic activity results from loss of the *SOST* gene product, sclerostin.
- Osteocytes possess ability to transform into chondrocytes. Signaling pathway modulation through drugs may prevent depletion of chondrocyte precursors in osteoarthrosis and provide therapy for fracture nonunions.

Osteoclasts

Osteoclasts are multinucleated cells related to the monocyte/macrophage lineage found at bone remodeling site. Their cytoplasm is acidophilic and contains β-glucuronidase. They are derived from hematopoietic progenitor cells unlike the osteocytes or osteoblasts. Despite having discrete origin for osteoclasts their differentiation requires the presence of osteoblasts at various steps. Differentiation and maturation of osteoclasts also need a variety of hematopoietic cytokines such as tumor necrosis factor (TNF), interleukins (ILs) 1, 3, 6, and 11, stem cell factor and CSF. Development of osteoclasts and their maturation (the osteoclastogenesis) needs hormonal support from PTH and 1,25-dihydroxyvitamin D_3 and cytokines like TGF-α and epidermal growth factor (EGF). Osteoclastogenesis is inhibited by calcitonin, estrogen, and TGF-β **(Fig. 7)**. The main function of osteoclasts is bone resorption that is in contrast to osteoblasts at first glance, but in fact both processes are complementary in normal physiology of bone. The characteristic features of osteoclasts are as follows:

- They are found within pits called Howship's lacunae—these are the sites of active bone resorption or may

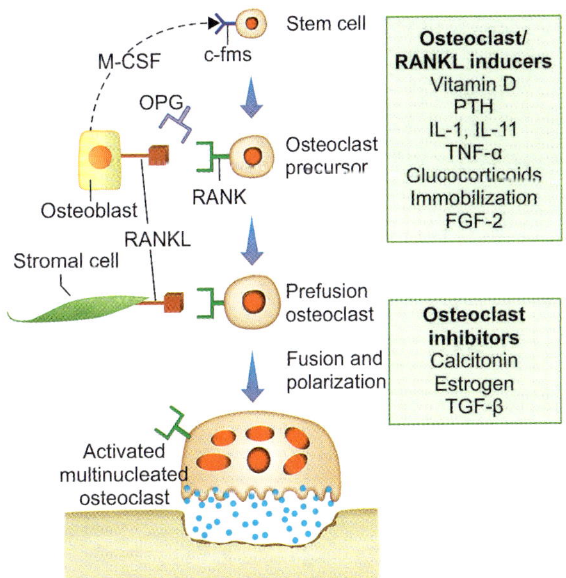

Fig. 7: Role of various cytokines and factors in production of osteoclasts (osteoclastogenesis). Osteoclastogenesis is inhibited by calcitonin, estrogen, and TGF-β. [RANK: receptor activator of nuclear factor κ; RANKL: receptor activator of nuclear factor κ ligand; M-CSF: monocyte-colony stimulating factor; OPG: osteoprotegerin; IL: interleukins; TNF-α: tumor necrosis factor alpha; FGF: fibroblast growth factor; PTH: parathormone; TGF-β: transforming growth factor beta; c-fms: colony-stimulating factor 1 receptor (also known as CSF1R)]

represent quiescent cavities where bone resorption has already occurred.

- Osteoclasts like osteoblasts are highly polarized cells with only one site of activity where bone resorption is occurring. The nuclei gather away from the resorbing bone surface **(Fig. 8)** as the space near to resorptive site will be occupied by vesicles and organelles involved in active resorption.
- "Ruffled border"—it is the cell surface in direct apposition to the bone with numerous infoldings of the plasma membrane **(Fig. 8)**. Ruffled border disappears when the cell is in the resting state. The cytoplasmic region between the conglomerated nuclei and the ruffled border (site of bone resorption) is rich in carbonic anhydrase and in tartrate-resistant acid phosphatase (TRAP), lysosomes, mitochondria, vesicles, and free ribosomes.
- Clear zone—At the site of active bone resorption osteoclast attach to bone matrix in a ring-like fashion sealing the area. This ring-like area of the cell membrane that forms the perimeter of the ruffled border is called "clear zone" or "sealing zone". This attachment to the bone matrix involves participation of actin filaments and the alpha-v beta-3 ($\alpha_V\beta_3$) integrin.

Osteoclast-mediated Bone Resorption

Bone resorption is a systematic process that involves sequential steps as follows:

Mineral resorption: Bone resorption requires the creation of acidic media via secretion of hydrogen ions [aided by adenosine triphosphate (ATP) driven proton pump] around the ruffled border of osteoclasts in the sealed off clear zone. The process requires the enzyme carbonic anhydrase II to generate hydrogen ions. Acid phosphatase is produced by osteoclasts. These dissolve the alkaline mineral phase of bone.

Removal of organic matrix: Lysosomes release acid hydrolases into the acidified extracellular space and collagenase.

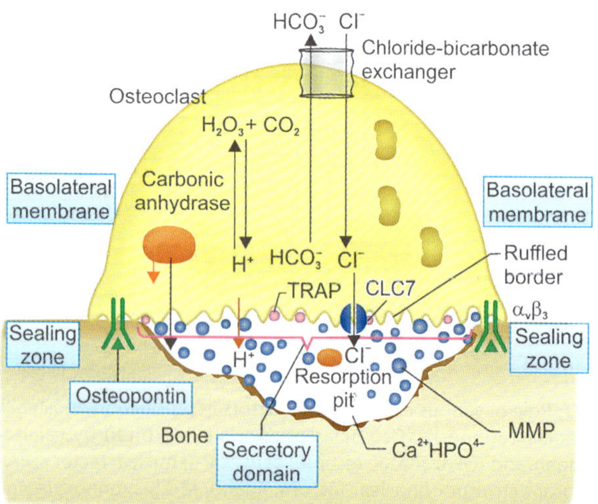

Fig. 8: Illustration depicting the structure and function of osteoclasts. (TRAP: tartrate-resistant acid phosphatase; CLC7: chloride channel 7; MMP: matrix metalloproteinase)

Degradation of collagen may also be helped by oxygen-derived free radicals. There is disruption of mineralized matrix to a depth of 1–2 μm. Osteoclasts migrate over the bone surface (migration front lead by osteoclasts followed by osteoblasts) creating many resorption pits in their path which is followed by mineralization front lead by osteoblasts recreating bone (coupled bone resorption and formation).

Regulation of Osteoclastic Bone Resorption

The process is highly regulated otherwise all the bone of body will dissolve away in an uncontrolled manner. Osteoclasts are stimulated primarily by IL-6 and RANKL (and are the targets for antiresorptive therapy). These cytokines are produced locally by the osteoblast under the influence of PTH, vitamin D3, TGF-β, IL-1, and TNF-α. Osteoclasts have calcitonin receptors that can directly influence the cells, but PTH or vitamin D receptors (VDRs) are missing from osteoclasts so their influence is indirect. Bone resorption is also influenced by interactions of the cell membrane integrins and bone matrix proteins that contain amino acids RGD (arginine, glycine, asparagine) such as the type I collagen, fibronectin, bone sialoprotein II, and osteopontin. These proteins bind to cell membrane integrins and initiate outside-in signaling pathways that finally culminate in bone resorption. In pathological state like in giant cell tumor (osteoclastoma), the osteoclasts are stimulated for bone resorption by IL-6.

Pathological bone resorption: TNF-α and IL-1 secreted by T-cells and macrophages in rheumatoid arthritis (RA) and other pathological conditions also stimulate bone resorption. These cytokines bypass the normal cell-to-cell contact required for osteoclast formation (in physiological state) instead they directly stimulate osteoclast progenitors to differentiate and mature into osteoclasts. This produces uncoupling of the process of bone resorption and formation.

Regulation of Osteoclastogenesis

Interferon-gamma (IFN-γ): It suppresses osteoclastogenesis. The T-cell-mediated osteoclastogenesis is supported by suppressor of cytokine signaling 1 (SOCS1). SOCS1 counteracts inhibitory cytokines such as IFN-γ so it is a positive regulator for osteoclastogenesis, but not always. SOCS1 is induced by RANKL stimulation during osteoclastogenesis. But osteoclast precursor cells develop tolerance or resistance to IFN-γ-mediated inhibition only if they are first stimulated by RANKL that induces SOCS1. This order of stimulation suggests that the ultimate fate of osteoclast precursor cells is determined not only by the balance of cytokines, but also by the cytokine first encountered.

Osteoclastogenesis: It is negatively regulated by IFN-β. RANKL induces IFN-β in osteoclast precursors. IFN-β inhibits the expression of c-Fos which is an essential transcription factor for osteoclastogenesis. c-Fos also negatively modulates the influence of IFN-β setting up a negative feedback loop, thus RANKL-induced IFN-β induces its own inhibitor.

Regulation of Osteoclast Differentiation

The RANK/RANKL/OPG axis: The proliferation and survival of osteoclast precursors, cells of the monocyte-macrophage lineage, is dependent on M-CSF secreted by osteoblasts **(Figs. 7 and 9)** and marrow stromal cells. Osteoblasts under the influence of PTH, vitamin D, prostaglandin E2 (PGE2), or IL-11 express RANKL mRNA. Both osteoblasts and stromal cells produce RANKL that binds to the RANK receptor on osteoclast precursors. M-CSF primes hematopoietic progenitor cells to become osteoclasts that are activated by RANKL to differentiate into mature or functional osteoclasts. The RANK and RANKL interaction on osteoclast precursors and on osteoblasts or stromal cells, respectively, requires cell-to-cell contact for further development of osteoclast precursors and maturation **(Fig. 9)**. In the cytoplasm, RANK undergoes complex interaction with TNF receptor associated factor (TRAF). TRAFs have different effects, while TRAF2 induces osteoclast differentiation TRAF6 is involved in osteoclast activation. Osteoblasts also secrete soluble protein OPG that prevents osteoclast activation by interfering with above RANK/RANKL interaction as it falsely attaches to RANKL (hence, it acts as a decoy receptor). OPG, thus, modulates the process of osteoclastogenesis and it strongly blocks osteoclastic bone resorption.

Clinical Implication

Osteoclasts and RA: Osteoclasts are the major culprit cells for RA and cause three types of bone changes:

1. Focal bone loss—seen at the joint margins producing the characteristic erosive changes and cysts.
2. Periarticular osteopenia—seen more prominently around inflamed small joints of hands and feet.
3. Generalized bone loss—this involves the axial and appendicular skeleton and is cytokine-mediated property of systemic involvement. TNF-α is responsible for reduction in ALP activity, decreased osteocalcin expression and perturbed collagen type I synthesis that prohibits mineralization of tissue, while bone resorption is continued. It also directly inhibits the osteoblast function in RA.

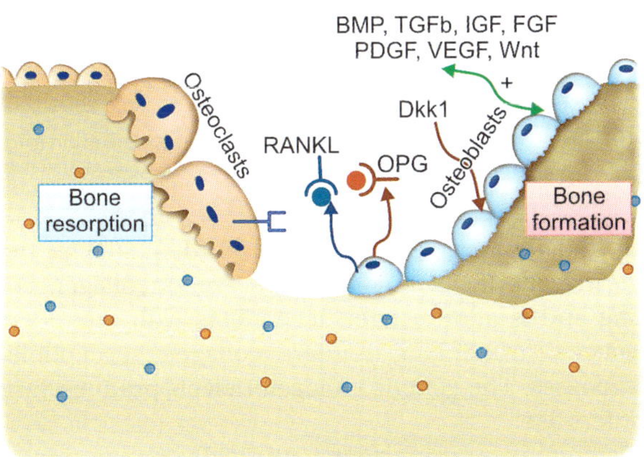

Fig. 9: The bone resorption-synthesis coupling due to interaction between osteoclasts and osteoblasts mediated by RANK-RANKL interaction and osteoprotegerin (OPG) protein that is essential for remodeling. (RANKL: receptor activator of nuclear factor κ ligand; OPG: osteoprotegerin; Dkk: dickkopf-1; BMP: bone morphogenic protein; TGF: transforming growth factor; IGF: insulin-like growth factor; FGF: fibroblast growth factor; VEGF: vascular endothelial growth factor; Wnt: portmanteau of int and Wg and stands for "Wingless-related integration site")

Targeting RANK/RANKL: As the RANKL/RANK interaction is so important to osteoclast activation, differentiation, and maturation, it is a hot target to prevent increased bone resorption in metabolic bone diseases such as RA and osteoporosis and even neoplasia (like GCT). In recent studies, it has been also found to be involved in bone resorption in osteoclastoma. It has been conjured that inhibiting the RANKL/RANK interaction or RANK-mediated signals would prevent pathological bone loss by tipping the balance to mineralization. Patients from familial Paget's disease of bone have been found to have altered first exon of RANK. Denosumab, a novel drug, is found to be effective in preventing attachment of RANKL to RANK receptor, hence, opening the possible role in above-mentioned diseases.

Marrow adipocytes: Marrow adipocytes are not just filler or replacement cells but they are now considered important and active element of bone cell milieu. They are different from other white, brown, or beige fat found elsewhere in the body. They increase with age and are correlated with reduced bone mass induced through modulation of PPARγ and *RUNX2* proteins. They also negatively affect hematopoiesis and are now sought-after targets for bone disease therapies.

COMPOSITION AND STRUCTURE OF BONE MATRIX

Collagen

Bone is a connective tissue. Like all other connective tissues it also contains varying amounts and combination of collagen, elastin (a related fibrous protein), glycosaminoglycans and proteoglycans. Collagen is the most abundant protein component in all these. Collagens have a unique triple helix composed of three component polypeptide alpha chains. There are several subtypes each produced by a different gene and differ in their biochemical structure. Some 28 different types of collagen have been identified, important ones are listed in detail in **Table 3**. Type I collagen is the most abundant type of collagen in bone (easy to remember; b-one).

Type I collagen, also known as alpha-1 type I collagen, is a protein that in humans is encoded by the *COL1A1* gene. It is a fibrillar type collagen that is also present in other tissues such as skin, menisci, tendon and ligaments, intervertebral disk annulus fibrosus and synovial joint capsules. Most (≈90%) of bone organic matrix is made up of type I collagen. Type I collagens have several subtypes. The type I collagen specific to bone has predominantly galactosyl-hydroxylysine amino acid configuration in contrast to glucosyl-galactosyl-hydroxylysine predominant conjugate found in dermal collagen. Also hydroxylation and glycosylation as post-translational modifications of collagen are found only in bone specific collagen that partly explains mineralization property of this tissue and not at other places where type I

TABLE 3: Different types of collagen and characteristics.

Types of collagen	*Remarks*	*Disorders*
I	Most abundant, bone, teeth, tendon, skin, vessels, cornea, and fibrocartilage	Osteogenesis imperfecta, Ehlers–Danlos syndrome, and Caffey's disease
II (fibrillar)	Hyaline cartilage, vitreous humor of eye and nucleus pulposus of intervertebral disk disorder (IVD)	Chondrodysplasias and collagenopathy types II and XI
III (fibrillar)	Granulation tissue, skin, intestines, and large vessels (30%)	Ehlers–Danlos syndrome, Dupuytren's contracture
IV	Lens of eye, renal glomeruli, and basement membranes	Alport syndrome and Goodpasture disease
V (fibrillar)	Interstitial tissue associated with collagen I and large vessels (5%)	Ehlers–Danlos syndrome
VI	Short chain collagen of interstitial tissue	Atopic dermatitis and ulrich myopathy
VII	Anchoring fibrils of dermoepidermal junctions	Epidermolysis bullosa dystrophica
VIII	Endothelial cells	Corneal dystrophy type II
IX	Fibril-associated collagens with interrupted triple helix (FACIT) collagen, cartilage (10–20%)	Multiple epiphyseal dysplasia type 2 and 3
X	Mineralizing cartilage	Schmid metaphyseal dysplasia
XI (fibrillar)	Cartilage	Collagenopathy types II and XI
XII	FACIT collagen	
XIII	Transmembrane collagen	
XIV	Undulin	
XVII	Transmembrane collagen	Bullous pemphigoid and junctional epidermolysis bullosa

collagen is found. The type I collagen is composed of basic structure comprising of repeating tripeptide sequence (Gly-X-Y). The X and Y are commonly proline and hydroxyproline and only to a lesser extent lysine/hydroxylysine. The Gly-X-Y is organized in a left-handed supertwisted helix (the "α" chain) contributing majorly to the strength of collagen. As a comparison of strength collagen fibers are said to have tensile strength greater than steel wire of equivalent cross-section. Collagen synthesis is controlled by over 20 genes. The single collagen fibril is made of three polypeptide chains arranged in a helical fashion making up the fundamental units. Aggregate of three units of these fundamental collagen fibril forms tropocollagen. This tropocollagen then aggregates in a staggered fashion to form a collagen microfibril. A collagen fibril is formed by removal of N- and C-propeptides from collagen microfibrils causing their rearrangement. Between two tropocollagen molecules there is electron microscopically identified "dark area" which is termed a "hole". It measures about 41 nm and is considered to be the site where mineralization is initiated **(Fig. 10)**. The cross-linking of collagen fibrils imparts stability and improves structural integrity. Cross-linking in collagen is a chemical process involving aldol reaction. Initially, aldehyde is generated by an amino oxidase enzyme which condenses with a lysyl or hydroxyl group to produce a Schiff base forming a cross-link. The aldehyde may also condense with a similar aldehyde in an aldol reaction to generate a stronger bond. The amino oxidase enzyme can be blocked by nitriles. These nitriles are alkyl cyanide substances responsible for producing the disorder lathyrism. Poor collagen quality of collagen in lathyrism leads to development of various spinal coronal and sagittal plane deformities, demineralized bones, recurrent joint dislocations, aortic aneurysms, and various nervous system manifestations. On the other hand, extensive "cross-linking" between α-chains as is found in

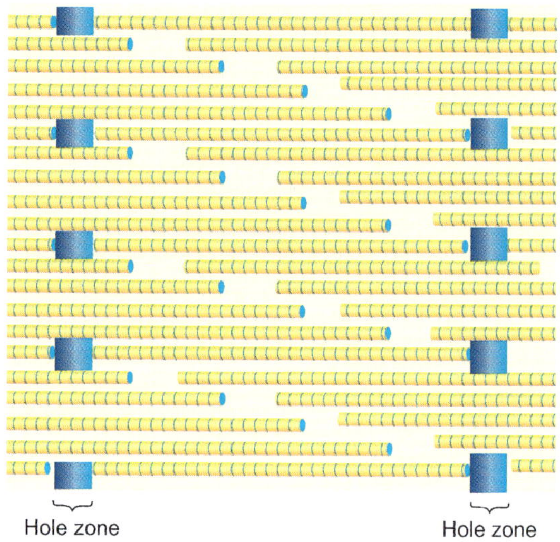

Fig. 10: Illustration of the structure of collagen fibril distribution (organic phase of bone) and concept of hole zone that is the space available for mineralization (inorganic phase).

aging individuals gives a rigid and brittle character to the connective tissue. Penicillamine prevents collagen cross-linking and is administered to patients with scleroderma. Defective cross-linking renders collagen susceptible to collagenases. The genetic collagen defects produce various disorders like:

- Osteogenesis imperfecta [clinically presenting with brittle bones that fracture easily, characterized by a glycine to cystine change though various other varieties are found (discussed later)]
- Ehler–Danlos syndrome (clinically present with loose joints that frequently dislocate and also relocate, characterized by a glycine to serine substitution).

Clinical marker—for estimating bone turnover, urinary excretion of hydroxyproline (found exclusively in collagen) and other products of collagen degradation (such as pyridinoline and deoxypyridinoline) are assessed in osteoporosis. These are markers of collagen breakdown and the level of collagen degradation by these degradation products in urine or serum indirectly reflect amount of bone turnover.

Other Noncollagenous Matrix Proteins

Calcium Binding Proteins

Osteopontin: Osteopontin is a sialylated and highly phosphorylated phosphoprotein, which exists in multiple forms and is important in cell attachment. This protein is regulated by substances such as 1,25-dihydroxyvitamin D, TGF-β, PTH, etc. Osteopontin binds to the integrin receptor on osteoclasts and activates the phospholipase C pathway resulting in increased intracellular calcium through Src tyrosine kinase. Osteopontin is found in high amounts in the extracellular matrix (ECM) of developing intramembranous and endochondral bones, and is present in good amount in osteoblasts, osteocytes, osteoclasts, and chondrocytes.

Bone sialoprotein II (BSP II): BSP II is a bone specific protein having cell attachment properties due to its RGD sequence (but less than osteopontin).

Osteonectin: This is a 32 kilodalton (kD) phosphorylated glycoprotein that regulates the extracellular calcium hydroxyapatite formation and mineralization. Osteonectin is also known by other names like SPARC that stands—"secreted protein acidic rich in cysteine", culture shock protein or basement membrane-40 (BM-40), and is encoded by *SPARC* gene. Osteonectin links mineral to collagen (by binding to both to Ca^{2+}, collagen type I, and hydroxyapatite) and thrombospondin. It also promotes mineralization by initiating hydroxyapatite crystal growth. Recently, osteonectin has been found to have involvement in pleotropic functions such as morphogenesis, tissue remodeling, angiogenesis, and cell migration. The last function may be explained by its function as an antiadhesive protein by virtue of involvement in cell matrix interactions that is possibly linked to prostate carcinoma metastasis. Osteonectin is expressed in various tissues, but its concentration is particularly high in osseous tissue (up to 10,000 times compared to other tissues). The second peculiarity is that it is the most abundant noncollagenous bone protein and quantitatively it increases with bone maturity. The functions of this protein for bone tissue are:

- Mineralization of nascent bone
- Support to osteoblasts in development, maturation, and survival
- Crystallization of inorganic solutes and binding to collagen matrix
- Cell migration, proliferation, and possibly differentiation

Gamma-carboxyglutamic acid proteins ("Gla" proteins): Osteocalcin (bone Gla protein) comprises significant portion of about 20% of the total noncollagenous proteins in bone. It is the second most predominant noncollagenous protein of bone. Osteocalcin is an osteoblast-specific protein with characteristic 3-gamma carboxyglutamic acid residues (Gla) that serves to negatively regulate osteoblasts itself (self-check mechanism). Its synthesis is vitamin K-dependent and is enhanced by 1α,25-dihydroxyvitamin D3. The circulation and excreted protein concentration indirectly reflects metabolic cellular activity. Osteocalcin serves following functions:

- Regulates crystal growth and osteoclast recruitment
- Inhibitor of osteoblast function
- May attract osteoclast progenitors in the area for maturation into osteoclasts, thus acting as chemoattractant.

Osteocalcin is encoded by *BGLAP* gene. It is synthesized by osteoblasts following stimulation from 1α,25-dihydroxyvitamin D3 regulated by TGF-β and secreted into the osteoid during mineralization. Osteocalcin is required to stimulate bone mineral maturation. Hence, it serves as a marker for mineralized tissue (like ALP) and increased bone turnover. Apart from ALP it is a good and specific marker for increased osteoblastic activity. It should, however, be clearly understood that both these markers do not correlate with each other as they are synthesized by osteoblasts during different stages of development. The early differentiation marker is ALP, while osteopontin and osteocalcin are late differentiation markers. Clinical utility lies in following the progress of patients with osteosarcoma, and as a marker for its recurrences or metastases in patients with anabolic therapy for osteoporosis the serum levels correlate well with bone turnover and increases in bone marrow density (BMD). Other than bone osteocalcin acts as a hormone that stimulates pancreatic β cells to secrete insulin and increases synthesis of testosterone that may have a role in male fertility.

Fibronectin (FN) and Thrombospondin

These proteins contain an arginine-glycine-aspartic acid (RGD) amino acid sequence (like osteopontin) and mediate the attachment to integrins, located on cell surfaces. Fibronectin (FN) is prominent and versatile ECM glycoproteins. FN is involved in cell adhesion, development and growth, proliferation, differentiation, and cell migration. It is responsible for wound healing, development of carcinoma lung, embryonic growth, and development of various tissues. FN mutation and deficiency are incompatible with life. Thrombospondin (TSP 1, 2, 3, 4, and 5) is an antiangiogenic protein first isolated from α-granules of platelets. TSP acts as an autocrine growth factor and takes part in prominent role in organization of the ECM by binding substrates at various binding sites. It also mediates platelet aggregation. TSP is deposited into the bone matrix, where it regulates the ECM proteins. It is also expressed by osteoblasts and chondrocytes besides platelets.

Connective Tissue Growth Factor

Connective tissue growth factor (CTGF) also called CCN2 is matricellular protein of the CCN family of ECM associated with heparin binding proteins that regulates various cellular functions such as cell adhesion, migration, proliferation, and differentiation. It also regulates matrix production and cell survival. CTGF is involved in bone cell (especially osteoblast) differentiation and maturation. The angiogenic activity (chemotaxis of endothelial cells and vascular smooth muscle cells) of CTGF is responsible for neovascularization of the mineralized cartilage in the process of endochondral ossification. CTGF stimulates the production of extracellular matrix (ECM) proteins in fibroblasts and osteoblasts such as type I collagen and fibronectin. It is also mitogenic for fibroblasts and chondrocytes and also promotes their differentiation. CTGF blocks apoptosis where cell adhesion is prevented, so supports cell migration and improves cell survival. This feature especially gathers importance in various tumorigenesis (cartilaginous tumors), development of atherosclerosis, and other fibrotic diseases.

Osteoactivin

Osteoactivin (OA) expression increases during matrix maturation and mineralization. OA is expressed in various malignant tumors such as in glioma and hepatocellular carcinoma facilitating tumor invasiveness.

Alkaline Phosphatase

This enzyme is a hydrolase that causes dephosphorylation in alkaline medium. It is produced by osteoblasts in bone and has three-related isozymes. The isozymes are tissue related and are associated with three separate genes. These are:

1. The placental (regan isozymes)
2. Intestinal form (ALP-3) is seen in a variety of tissues such as bone (ALP-2), liver (ALP-1), kidney [proximal convoluted tubules (PCT)], and skin.
3. Tissue nonspecific form—found in bone osteoblasts is associated with a single gene at chromosome 1. ALP is adhered to the cell membrane, via phosphatidylinositol that can be broken by phospholipase C and the enzyme is released free from cell membrane.

All three isozymes require zinc and magnesium ions for their activity. ALP is a glycoprotein that catalyzes the splitting (by hydrolysis) of phosphates (such as pyridoxal-5'-phosphate) at an alkaline pH between 8 and 10. This makes enzyme inactive in blood. Bone specific ALP reflects the biosynthetic activity of osteoblasts. The synthesis of tissue nonspecific ALP is increased by vitamin D and thyroxin, whereas glucocorticoids and PTH inhibit its production. In physiological states, the expression of ALP is cell cycle dependent, where its activity is high in G1 through S phases and reduces in G2 through M phases. The most interesting fact is that despite such a long period of identification of this enzyme the exact role of ALP in bone mineralization is still not fully understood and most explanations are theories. The enzyme has been demonstrated in matrix vesicles, but its role is elusive and may involve degradation of pyrophosphate that is otherwise an endogenous inhibitor of apatite crystal formation by precipitation. Serum ALP activity is raised in various orthopedic and nonorthopedic conditions as follows:

- Orthopedic conditions where serum ALP is raised:
  - Growing children (physiological rise)
  - Primary and secondary hyperparathyroidism
  - Rickets and osteomalacia
  - Healing fractures
  - Neoplasias like osteosarcoma
  - Paget's disease
  - Osteoblastic metastasis from prostate
  - Treatment of osteoporosis by anabolic agents
  - Hyperthyroidism
  - Herpes zoster
- Nonorthopedic causes of raised ALP:
  - Neoplasias—leukemia and Hodgkin's lymphoma
  - Pregnancy
  - Oral contraceptives
  - Hepatitis
  - Hepatic malignancies
  - Amyloidosis
  - Inflammatory bowel disease
  - Septicemia
  - Sarcoidosis
  - Myocardial and pulmonary infarctions (acute injuries)
  - Pancreatitis
- The ALP serum levels are reduced in hypophosphatasia.

BLOOD SUPPLY OF BONE

Bone receives around a fifth (10–20%) of the cardiac output. The two predominant vascular systems for blood supply include **(Fig. 11)**:

1. The periosteal system.
2. The endosteal system (misnomer as there is no endosteum, better called intramedullary system).

Minor contributions come from:

- Epimetaphyseal system.
- Articular ligaments (like obturator ligament in hip).

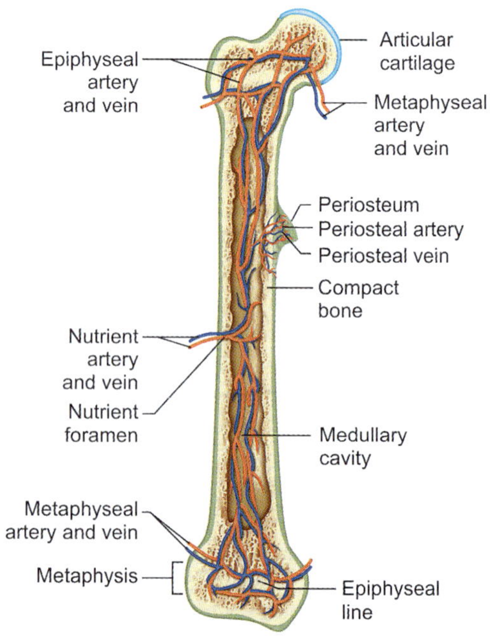

Fig. 11: Illustration depicting the blood supply of bone, nutrient artery—diaphyseal circulation, metaphyseal, and epiphyseal vessels supply the respective zones; periosteum supplies the peripheral one-third of the cortex.

Periosteal System

The periosteal system (also called accessory nutrient arterioles) supplies only the outer third of the cortex. Entire long bone except its cartilage ends is covered by periosteum with deficiencies only in the region of capsular attachments and nutrient vessels. The periosteum has an inner cellular osteogenic layer (cambium) containing osteoprogenitor cells. This layer serves to increase bone girth by appositional bone deposition before skeletal maturity. The outer layer of periosteum consists of fibrous tissue that is predominantly supportive and imparts stiffness to it. The periosteum is thick in children due to the presence of active cambium (cellular layer) with blood supply in the form of longitudinal arterioles incorporated within. However, with aging the cambium gets hypotrophied and becomes thin, also the vascularity reduces with absence of prominent longitudinal arterioles. This has important surgical implications with respect to higher incidence of nonunion and delayed union in fractures fixed after ripping periosteum, especially in adults. Over most of the surface of long bones in an adult the periosteum is loosely attached beneath muscle bellies. The only periosteal blood vessels in those areas are venules and capillaries. Periosteal supply is a low pressure system compared to intramedullary system of blood supply. So, the normal flow in mature bone is centrifugal with excess blood exiting from the periosteal venules. In vascular stress situations like acute embolism of the intramedullary system or reaming of intramedullary canal, the blood flow of the periosteum increases many fold compensating for the loss in blood supply. In such situations, the blood flow becomes centripetal.

Intramedullary System

Diaphyseal nutrient arteries (one or two) enter through the cortical bone often in an oblique direction. The common ports of nutrient artery entry are the fascial regions firmly attached to the diaphysis of long bones or along anatomical bony ridges like linea aspera of the femur. Perivascular fat supports and protects the afferent blood vessels in these regions so that the vessels can approach directly the cortical surface and enter. The principal nutrient artery to bone is formed of these afferent vessels. The afferent vessels after entering the intramedullary system divide into ascending and descending branches that supply inner two-thirds of the cortex (outer thirds being supplied by periosteal supply, discussed above) and whole of the medullary cavity. The above system holds true for most long bones, except large irregular bones, flat bones, and some short bones that receive a major blood supply from the periosteum superficially or otherwise from large nutrient arteries that directly penetrate into the medullary bone. The intramedullary and periosteal systems of blood supply anastomose freely.

Metaphyseal and Epiphyseal Arteries

This system supplies blood to the ends of bones, diaphysis being supplied by the above mentioned systems. They arise as principle branches from adjacent articular supply or periarticular plexus. This system also freely anastomoses with the diaphyseal or intramedullary system terminating in bone marrow, trabecular bone, cortical bone, and articular cartilage. In immature skeleton, growth plate (end plates of cartilage component of physis) separates these arteries from intramedullary system. Near the growth plate (physis) a few vessels make hairpin bend and retreat back upon themselves, while most enter into an open circulation. In the past, this arrangement of hairpin bends was considered to reduce the rate of blood flow to cause localization of blood-borne bacteria and serve as focus of onset of hematogenous osteomyelitis, especially in children. This concept is challenged now (discussed under bone infection section). After closure of growth plate in adult, the entire expanded end of the long bone becomes the metaphysis. This metaphysis receives superficial blood supply from periosteal arteriolar vessels entering all over, except in regions covered by articular cartilage. The longitudinal afferent arterioles seen in periosteum of immature skeleton in metaphysis and diaphysis disappear with age-related atrophy of the cambium layer of the periosteum. Throughout life of individual this layer remains dormant and atrophic until activated by specific stimulus like trauma.

Venous and Lymphatic Drainage

From bone, the blood is drained by collateral venous system that accompanies the afferent arteries. These veins leave through foramina near the articular ends of the bones commonly. Lymphatic vessels are also abundant in the periosteum.

Direction of Blood Flow

The intramedullary system of vessels represents a high pressure system within the long bone. This system is derived from the nutrient artery that is a branch of systemic circulation, so the intravascular pressure is higher in the medulla or marrow of bone than in the periosteal system, where vasculature mainly comprises of venules and capillaries. As is commonly known from laws of physics fluid that current flows from high to low pressure region, consequently, the direction of normal blood flow in physiological state in bone through the diaphyseal cortex of a long bone is centrifugal, i.e., from medulla to periosteum (inside-out). Under some pathologic conditions the intramedullary vascular pressure may get diminished resulting in reversal of blood flow through the vascular channels of the diaphyseal cortex, so that it becomes outside-in or centripetal. This flow reversal can happen with:

- Occlusive vascular disease
- Osteoarthritis
- Displaced fracture
- Reaming of intramedullary canal—as while performing intramedullary nailing.

Under above conditions, the blood flow reversal primarily occurs through existing normal vascular channels though studies demonstrate opening up and development of new vascular channels also.

NERVE SUPPLY OF BONE

Bones have rich nerve supply, especially at the articular ends of the long bones, the vertebrae and larger, flat bones. The nerve fibers supplying bones accompany nutrient blood vessels to reach the interior of bones and Haversian system. Also, accompanying the arteries inside the Haversian system are vasomotor nerves that control blood flow through them as in physiological state in most other body systems by vascular constriction or dilation. The periosteal nerves have nociceptive ends so it is pain sensitive (common experience is needed for anesthetizing periosteum, while placing Steinmann pin). Bones are also innervated by sympathetic fibers originating from the sympathetic ganglion that again enters bone along with nutrient vessels. Blood flow in bones reduces by 80% in stressful conditions and shock. Neurotransmitters released by various nerve endings not only regulate the blood flow, but also they have a role in bone development and remodeling. Dopamine transporter gene (DAT) (-/-) deletion mice demonstrated 30% reduction in bone mass and strength.

The endogenous cannabinoids (anandamide, 2-arachidonoylglycerol) have been found to regulate bone remodeling to some extent. They activate the G protein-coupled; central and peripheral cannabinoid receptor type 1 (CB1) and type 2 (CB2), respectively. CB1 is responsible for the typical cannabinoid-associated psychotropic and analgesic effects, but CB2 is of interest and plays role in liver fibrosis and atherosclerosis. Endocannabinoids inhibit lipogenesis (effect opposite that of corticosteroids and alcohol). So they have trophic effect on bone formation and remodeling **(Fig. 12)**. CB2 receptor null mice show accelerated age-related trabecular bone loss with minimal change in cortical thickness (osteoporosis like changes). This is partly explained by increased osteoclast number in the trabecular bone. CB2-specific agonist increases osteoblast number and activity, while simultaneously restraining osteoclastogenesis in trabecular bone. They inhibit proliferation of osteoclast precursors directly and also restrict the differentiation and maturation of osteoclasts by suppressing expression of receptor activator of NF-κβ ligand in bone marrow-derived osteoblasts or stromal cells. Thus, it appears that endocannabinoid system maintains normal bone mass by CB2 signaling. In addition to other modalities being tried, CB2 receptor system may serve a molecular target for the diagnosis and treatment of osteoporosis in future.

BONE DEVELOPMENT

In human embryo bone appears after seventh week. Typically two forms of bone formation are evident in the system. The bones of the entire axial and appendicular skeleton develop through either intramembranous or endochondral bone formation (ossification). The two processes differ in absence or presence of a cartilaginous intermediary, respectively. A cartilage model is first formed and which ossifies in latter process **(Fig. 13)**, while it is conspicuously absent in former. A third mode of physiological bone formation during development is appositional ossification that is mainly responsible for increasing thickness of long bones and increasing bone size in intramembranous ossification.

Intramembranous Bone Formation

In this process a modeled primordial cartilage anlage forms, but it is not ossified and for new bone to be formed the anlage needs to be completely resorbed. The flat bones of the skull and face are typical examples of intramembranous (membranous) ossification. On the preformed scaffold of cartilage the osteoprogenitor cells aggregate at the sites of new bone formation (preosseous condensation) that are

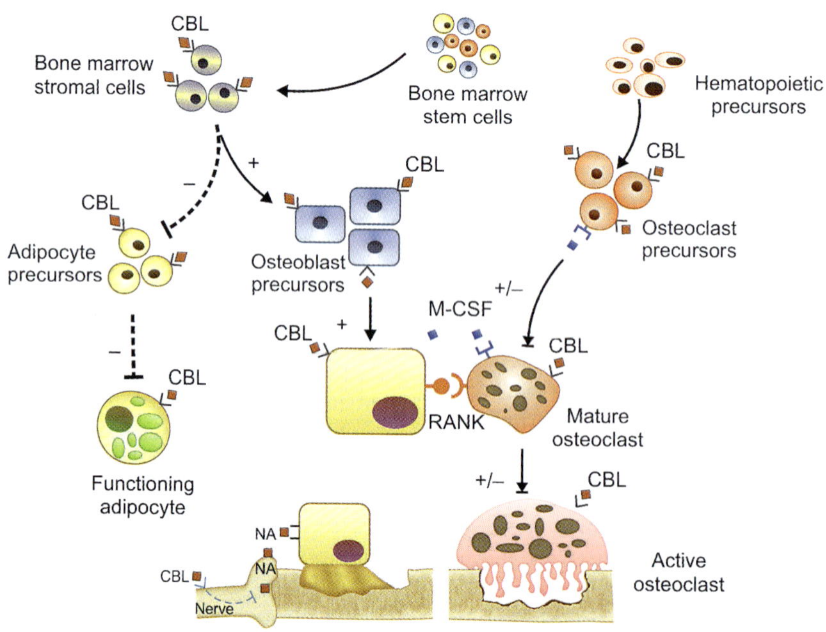

Fig. 12: The endocannabinoid system and its effect on bone formation. (CBL: cannabicyclol; M-CSF: monocyte-colony stimulating factor; RANK: receptor activator of nuclear factor κ; NA: sodium channels)

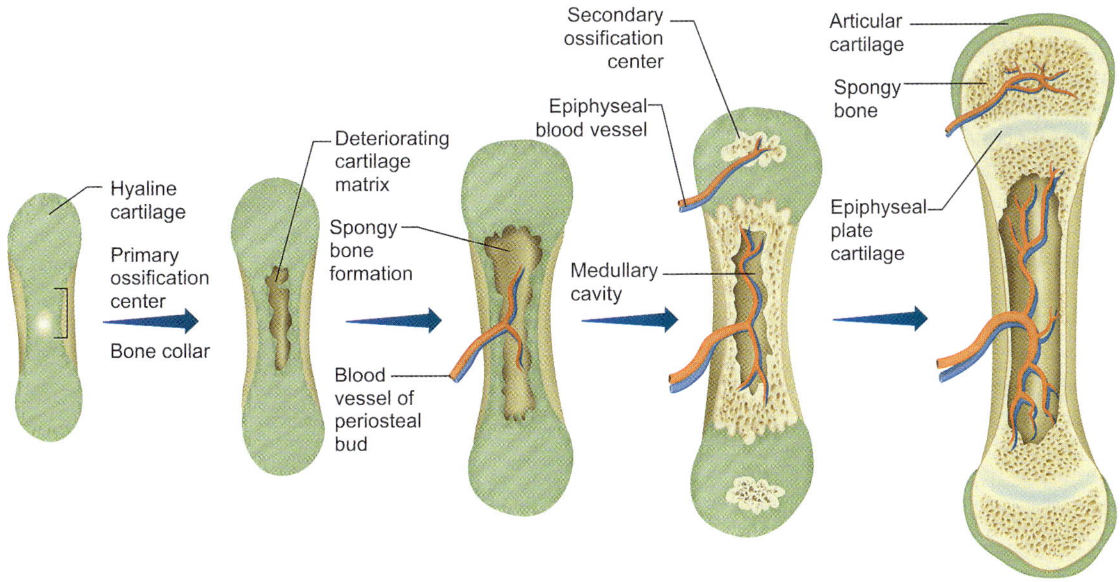

Fig. 13: The illustration depicting process of endochondral bone formation from a cartilage model.

usually centrally located and differentiate into osteoblasts that actively synthesize new bone matrix advancing radially peripherally. Osteoblasts then lay the bone successively on this scaffold in layers, a process called apposition (deposition upon prior bone). Ossification centers develop within the bone and enhance the rates of mineralization. The surrounding mesenchyme condense into periosteum and lays down bone beneath it. The bones take on a lamellar character gradually. In the adult, similar process is called Haversian remodeling. Chondroid bones of the skull (Wormian bones) that are seen in association with suture closure are developmentally intermediate between cartilage and bone. They contain both types I and type II collagen. Here, the scaffold is formed by chondroid bone upon which lamellar bone is deposited. It is not replaced by bone as in the endochondral ossification. Many factors (all not known) play potential roles regulating bone formation. Core-binding factor alpha-1 (cbfa-1) or *Runx2* transcription pathway (discussed above) is responsible for osteoblast differentiation and binding to the osteocalcin promoter. This causes osteocalcin expression essential for processing of mineralization front.

This pathway is also responsible partly for formation of cartilage anlage. Cbfa-1 mutation causes cleidocranial dysplasia in which there is delayed ossification of cranial sutures and absent or hypoplastic clavicles.

Endochondral Bone Formation

Here, a cartilage tissue first forms as a model (cartilage anlage) from aggregated mesenchymal cells and is subsequently ossified. The appendicular skeleton, vertebral column, and pelvis develop via endochondral ossification. This discrete complex process can be divided into five stages.

First Stage

This stage begins with differentiation of MSC to become cartilage progenitors. At molecular level, this involves expression of transcription factors, Pax1, and scleraxis by activation of cartilage-specific genes.

Second Stage

This stage (the precartilaginous state) involves condensation of the committed MSC to form compact nodules and these cells differentiate into chondrocytes by the progression of activity of Pax1 and scleraxis in stage one. The condensation of committed cells is affected by N-cadherin. This precartilaginous state also involves expression of *SOX9* gene (sex reversal Y-related high-mobility group box protein) that encodes a deoxyribonucleic acid (DNA)-binding protein. *SOX9* expression is an essential step that is required for proper organization of further complex interactions. Mutations of the *SOX9* gene are generally incompatible with life and it has been found that infants with specific mutations of the *SOX9* gene die from respiratory failure due to poorly formed tracheal and rib cartilages.

Third Stage

This stage is marked by chondrocytes proliferation forming the cartilage model (precartilage condensation). Chondrocytes secrete a cartilage-specific ECM.

Fourth Stage

In this stage, the chondrocytes hypertrophy produces collagen type X and fibronectin, so that mineralization can be proceeded by calcium carbonate.

Fifth Stage

This stage is marked by vascular invasion of the cartilage model and apoptosis of hypertrophic chondrocytes. The osteoprogenitor cells after proper stimulation differentiate into osteoblasts that begin to lay down osseous matrix on the mineralized cartilage remnants that have been partially degraded. This process occurs in the cartilage model first at the region forming future diaphysis of long bone and is known as the primary center of ossification. From the primary ossification center, the endochondral ossification spreads vertically along the axis of the developing bone in both directions. Secondary centers of ossification form at the ends of each bone (the epiphysis) eventually leaving an area of cartilage between the primary and secondary ossification centers called growth plate or physis. It is here that continued growth in length occurs at both ends of the developing bone.

Nonphysiological Bone Formation

Bone can also form in various other forms and processes, but not involving the skeletal development. Callus formation and regenerate development are physiological forms of bone formation that occur in specific conditions and are not a part of developmental ossification process. Similarly, ectopic ossification and myositis ossificans are pathological forms of bone formation.

STRUCTURE OF PHYSIS

The commonly used term "epiphyseal plate" or "epiphyseal growth plate" should be discarded as they actually confuse with "epiphysis". Rubin introduced the term "physis" or "physeal segment" and is preferable. Two forms of growth plates exist in long bones one horizontal and the other spherical. The horizontal growth plates are responsible for increase in length of bone, while the spherical growth plates take part in growth of epiphysis and the physis itself circumferentially and contributes also to thickness of bone. The fully developed cartilaginous growth plate in the human long bone typically comprises of various anatomically discrete tissues acting together as a composite unit to perform one specialized function, and thus is referred as an organ by many researchers. The physis for physioanatomical description can be divided into three components **(Flowchart 1)**:

1. The cartilaginous component of growth plate contains three predominant regions **(Fig. 14)**:
   a. Reserve zone—contains spherical, single, or paired chondrocytes involved in matrix production. They are full of glycogen and have predominantly anaerobic environment due to low PO_2.
   b. Zone of chondrocyte proliferation—this zone serves three purposes—matrix production, cellular proliferation, and longitudinal growth. Latter is equal to the combination of former two. It has flattened chondrocytes arranged in distinct columns. The endoplasmic reticulum occupies progressively increasing percent of the cytoplasmic area that rises from 14.9% at the top of the zone to 40.1% at the bottom of the zone of chondrocyte proliferation. Biochemical analysis reveal that this zone contains the highest content of hexosamine, inorganic pyrophosphate, and has highest lysosomal activity. The chondrocytes in this zone are the only cells of growth plate that divide (proliferate). Longitudinal growth in the physis is directly proportional to the product of rate of production of new chondrocytes at the top of the proliferating zone to maximum size of the chondrocytes in the lowermost layer of the hypertrophic zone. Due to heavy demand and consumption oxygen tension is maintained higher in the proliferating zone of physis at mean of 57 mm Hg (± 5.8 mm Hg) compared to any other zones.

Flowchart 1: Structure of physis and involvement in various disorders.

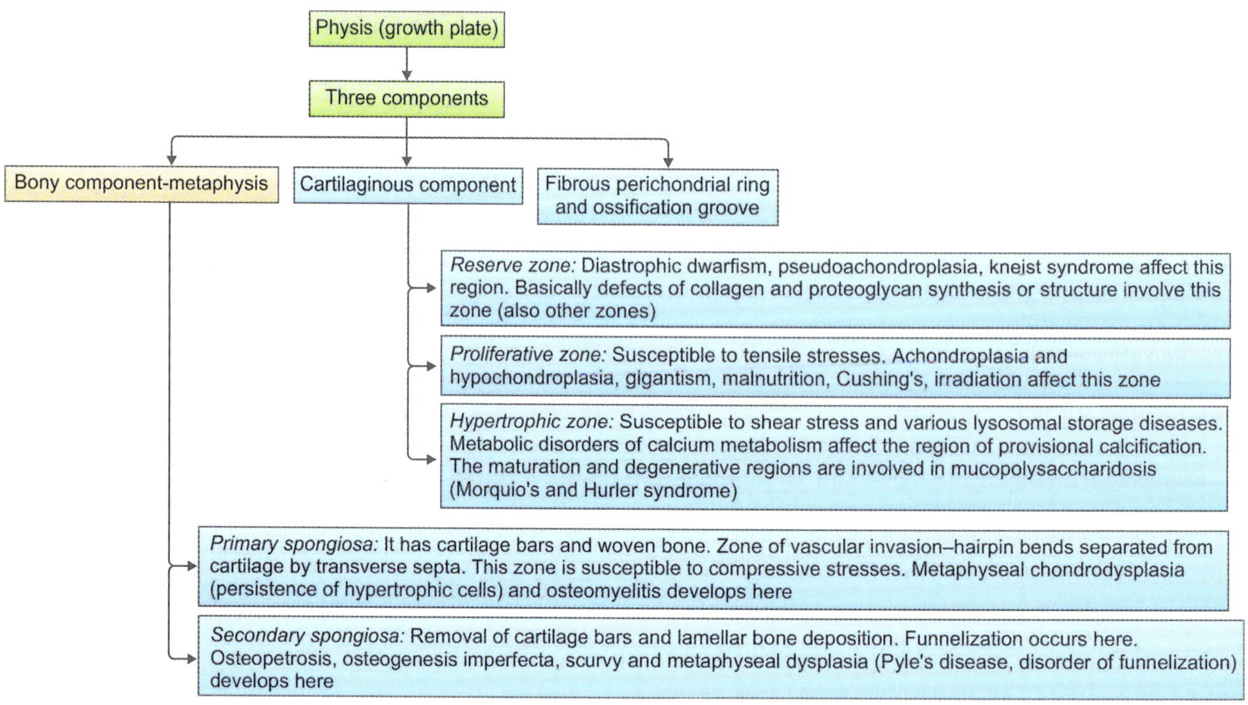

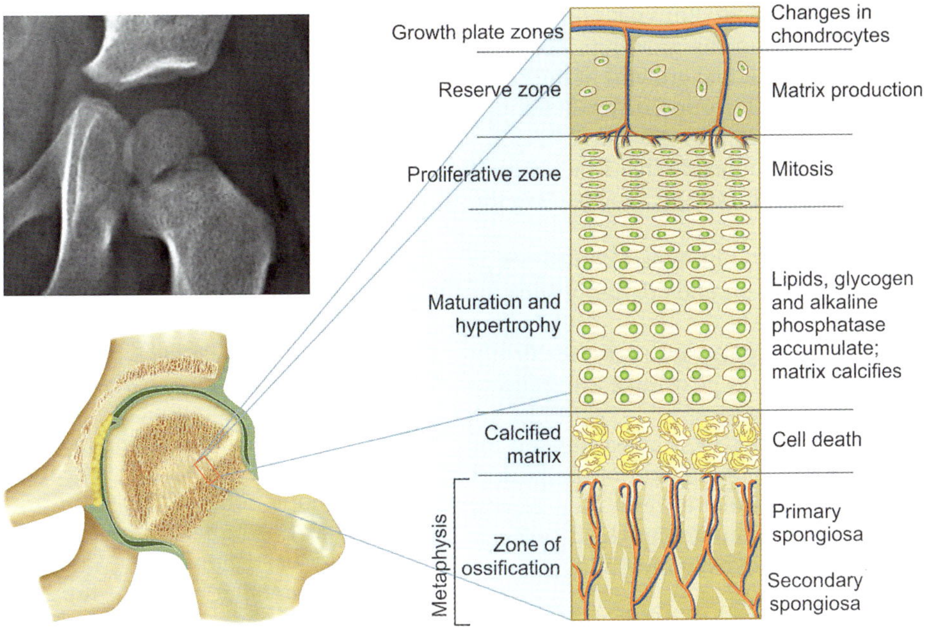

Fig. 14: Structure of growth plate of bone—the physis, the illustration depicts various zones, and associated disposition of vasculature.

c. Zone of chondrocyte hypertrophy—this zone has three discrete functional and histological regions namely the maturation zone, degenerative zone, and zone of provisional calcification. The function of this zone is to prepare the matrix for calcification and to calcify the matrix. The chondrocytes show progressive vacuolation and increase in size with disintegration. The mitochondria instead of forming ATP start to accumulate calcium. The initial calcification (seeding) occurs at the bottom of the hypertrophic zone (zone of provisional calcification) within physis. This is initiated by matrix vesicles around which then mineralization progresses. As noted above, matrix vesicles are rich in ALP that destroys pyrophosphate which is an inhibitor of calcium phosphate precipitation. Destruction of pyrophosphate tips the balance to precipitation of calcium and phosphate, and hence, facilitates mineralization. Matrix vesicles also simultaneously accumulate calcium from the calcium lost through mitochondria at the same level in the middle of the hypertrophic zone. The following sequence of events occurs for final calcification:
   - Mitochondrial calcification
   - Reduction of nutrients and oxygen supply to the hypertrophic chondrocyte with mitochondrial death
   - Anaerobic glycolysis (this occurs due to distance from vascular supply, and hence, oxygen tension this hypertrophic zone is very low to a mean of 24.3 ± 2.4 mm Hg). Entire stored glycogen is consumed.
   - Calcium is released from mitochondria
   - Nucleation of mineralization in matrix vesicles
   - Matrix calcification

The cartilaginous matrix gets calcified as the cells hypertrophy. This calcified cartilage then serves as a scaffold for bone matrix deposition by osteoblasts. The lacunae that remain after apoptosis of hypertrophic chondrocytes are utilized by blood vessels. Abnormalities in chondrocyte development or function can disrupt this organized sequence of physeal growth and maturation producing abnormal bones usually stunted in growth and having crooked shape. Achondroplasia is such a condition causing dwarfism and possibly involves a mutation in FGF.

2. The bony component or metaphysis serves few important functions—it is involved in vascular invasion of transverse septa at the bottom of cartilaginous portion of growth plate providing blood supply, the other functions are new bone formation and bone remodeling. It has two predominant components, the primary spongiosa and the secondary spongiosa. There is internal (histologic) remodeling with removal of calcified cartilage bars (primary spongiosa) and lamellar bone deposition (secondary spongiosa). The external or anatomic remodeling gives funnel shape to metaphysis (funnelization). Near the transverse septa separating metaphyseal from cartilage component there is low oxygen tension (19.8 ± 3.2 mm Hg) and high degree of rouleaux formation of RBCs due to vascular stasis. High levels of phosphoglucoisomerase (enzyme compatible with anaerobic metabolism) are found in this region. The low oxygen tension inhibits WBC activity which is highly oxygen dependent, while it is favorable for pathogens. This may explain the reason for hematogenous osteomyelitis in ends of bone and not vascular stasis per se; the concept is still, however, challenged.
3. A fibrous sheath surrounds the growth plate at periphery that comprises of perichondrial ring of LaCroix and the ossification groove of Ranvier. These two structures are structurally different and serve different functions.

It appears that the groove of Ranvier contributes chondrocytes to the physis for the growth in diameter (appositional growth or latitudinal growth) of the plate. There are three distinct cell groups in the Ranvier's ossification groove:

1. Progenitor cells for osteoblasts—this is a group of densely packed cells that forms the bony band in the perichondrial ring.
2. Undifferentiated cells and fibroblasts contribute to appositional chondrogenesis and are responsible for diametrical growth of physis.
3. Fibroblasts cover the groove and serve to firmly anchor the perichondrium of hyaline cartilage to growth plate.

The perichondrial ring provides mechanical support for the otherwise weak bone-cartilage junction of the growth plate. It is a dense fibrous band that encircles the growth plate at the bone-cartilage junction and in which collagen fibers run vertically, obliquely, and circumferentially.

Blood Supply of the Physis

The three components of growth plate have distinct blood supply. The proliferative zone receives blood supply from branches of epiphyseal vessels that penetrate the top 4–10 columns. These vessels arise perpendicular to the main perichondrial epiphyseal artery and pass through micro spaces in the reserve zone to finally terminate in the proliferative zone at the summit of cell columns. These vessels do not pass across the proliferative zone into hypertrophic zone. The nutrient supply for hypertrophic zone instead comes indirectly from terminal branches of nutrient artery which is also supplied by metaphyseal arteries or plexus of vessels at places. The nutrient artery is the main supply for the central metaphyseal region and as much as four-fifths of the metaphysis receives nutrition and oxygen through it. The metaphyseal blood vessels supply only peripheral portions of the metaphysis, especially through the periosteum. As mentioned earlier also, the nutrient and metaphyseal arteries terminate into vascular loops or capillary tufts. The terminal branches pass vertically toward the bone-cartilage junction of physis and turn back sharply forming hairpin bends just below the last intact transverse septa at the base of the cartilage portion of the plate. The venous branches from hairpin bends descend via several progressively larger veins to finally drain into the large central vein of the diaphysis. Here, again we see that no vessels penetrate the bone (metaphysis) cartilage (hypertrophic zone) junction beyond the last intact transverse septa, hence, hypertrophic zone is not directly penetrated by any vessel and most nutrients reach it via diffusion or open circulation. Hence, in a fully-developed growth plate, hypertrophic zone is entirely avascular. Compared to above the groove of Ranvier and the fibrous perichondrial ring of LaCroix are richly supplied from perichondrial arteries.

Regulation of Growth Plate (Physis)

The chondrocytes elsewhere in body are not responsible for organ growth as in bone. So, the chondrocytes of the growth plate are functionally different from articular cartilage cells. Even the chondrocytes within different parts of the growth plate show different response to similar stimuli. Growth plate is regulated by a host of systemic and local factors.

- Systemic factors regulating the metabolism and development of growth plate include growth hormone (GH), vitamin D and glucocorticoids, IGF-I, thyroid hormone, and estrogens (in females). These factors affect the linear growth of bone and also maturation of physis (maturation is enhanced by estrogen so females grow longer earlier and physis closes also faster terminating the linear growth earlier)
- Parathyroid hormone, IGF, and vitamin C influence the whole cartilage component
- The GH and thyroid hormones are trophic to reserve proliferative zone and the maturation region of hypertrophic zone
- Gonadal hormones stimulate the hypertrophic and metaphyseal regions
- Local factors that influence the growth and function of physis include TGF-β, PTH-related protein (PTHrP), Indian hedgehog (IHH), and FGF receptor type 3 (FGFR3) **(Fig. 15)**:
  - TGF-β inhibits chondrocyte proliferation, hypertrophic differentiation, and matrix mineralization
  - Indian hedgehog induces the expression of PTHrP in the perichondrium. PTHrP inhibits chondrocyte differentiation, thus acting as a negative feedback loop
  - Proliferative zone is controlled by FGF, PDGF, and TGF-β. The maturation of chondrocytes occurs under the influence of PGs and IGF.

Appositional Ossification

The enlargement of bone in diameter occurs by appositional bone growth. The osteoblasts deposit additional bone on the existing bone surface. There is continuous bone resorption from inside until the desired bone thickness is reached.

PROCESS OF BONE MINERALIZATION

Calcification of cartilage and osteoid as a physiologic process is called mineralization. The inorganic matrix is laid down in a specific pattern along the organic matrix. The process is complicated and poorly understood. Calcium hydroxyapatite predominates mineral phase in humans (invertebrates contain calcium carbonate, whereas plants have oxalate) that is deposited along the long axis of the collagen fibrils. The inorganic matrix is deposited in the hole zone of collagen matrix created by the space left between staggered arrangement of fibrillar structure. The individual collagen macromolecules are staggered by one-fourth of their length leaving around 400 Å long and 15 Å wide hole zones. The mineral is initially deposited as randomly and poorly-oriented amorphous calcium phosphate. The amorphous phase undergoes a series of organized solid phase transformations that ultimately lead to production of crystalline hydroxyapatite which is the stable solid phase. Various factors are important in mineralization **(Table 4)**.

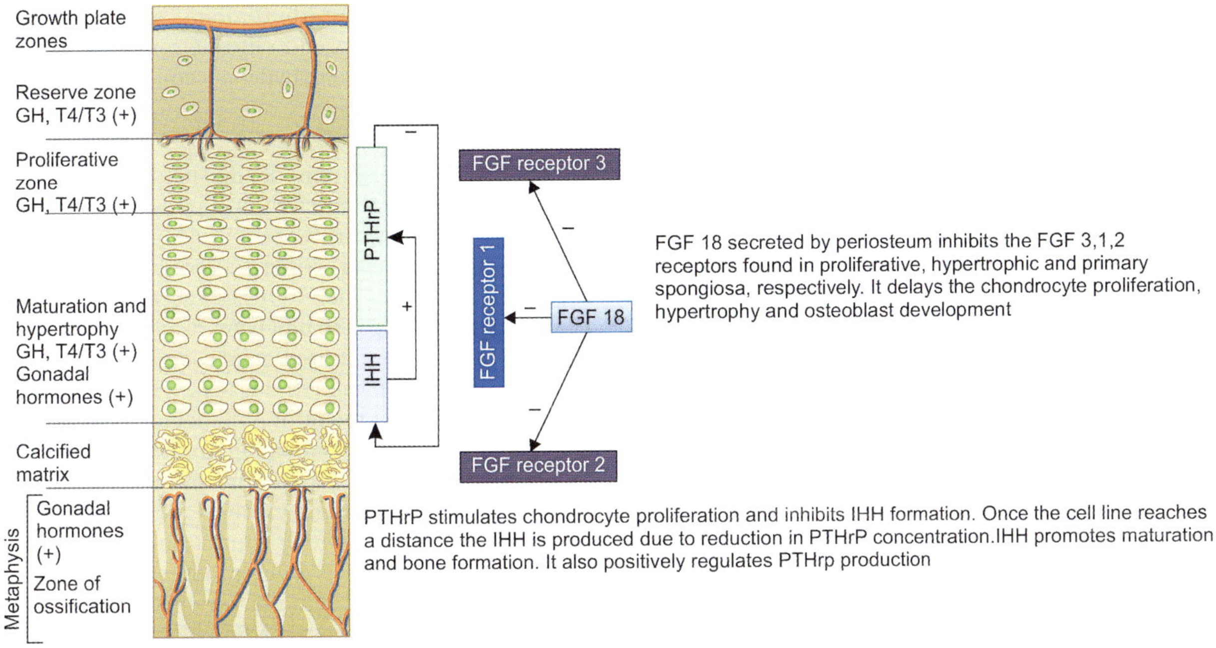

Fig. 15: The effect of various growth factors and cytokines locally on the different zones of physis. (FGF: fibroblast growth factor; GH: growth hormone; T4/T3: tetraiodothyronine and triiodothyronine hormones)

TABLE 4: Role of various constituents in bone mineralization.

Component	*Remark*
Collagen	Provides support to crystal deposition. Collagen can initiate crystal precipitation. Facilitates formation of solid phase crystals from solution. Does not nucleate crystal deposition
Calcium-binding protein	• These phosphoproteins may nucleate crystal deposi tion and promote polymerization • Proteoglycan inhibits calcification by sequestering the calcium ions or shielding collagen
Gla proteins	Osteocalcin and other Gla proteins bind calcium by virtue of Gla residue
Pyrophosphate	Inhibits calcification and increases the solubility of calcium phosphate preventing precipitation
Alkaline phosphatase	Possibly degrades pyrophosphate to aid in crystal precipitation and mineralization

The initiation of mineralization is caused by heterogeneous nucleation. There is active binding of calcium, phosphate, and calcium phosphate complexes at the nucleation site and not just simple precipitation of the mineral. Matrix vesicle provides the requisite environment for this process. The physiologic state of extracellular fluids is supersaturated with respect to octacalcium phosphate. Pyrophosphate and serum proteins act as crystal inhibitors. Phosphatases and proteases are essential to locally remove these inhibitors and facilitate apatite formation. Still crystallization would need local increase in concentration of substrates (calcium and phosphate) far beyond supersaturation levels to overcome the energy of the reaction of crystal formation and real mechanism is elusive and may involve quantum biologics in essence. Many theories have been propounded by eminent researchers for explaining mineralization initiation and propagation, but for that the role of matrix vesicles should be understood first.

Role of Matrix Vesicles in Initiation

Matrix vesicles are the membrane bound cell free structures derived from chondrocytes and osteoblasts serve these requisites and initiate mineralization. The trilamellar membrane bound matrix vesicles secreted by chondrocyte seed the calcium phosphate salt in matrix. Probably derived from mitochondria, they can either store calcium or ATP. In the proliferative zone with high oxygen availability, the mitochondria synthesizes ATP for cellular requirement. While progressing down to hypertrophic zone, the oxygen concentration falls and the mitochondria store calcium instead of ATP. These are extruded out at zone of provisional calcification with degeneration of cells and burst releasing microcrystals of calcium phosphate (possibly hydroxyapatite also). Under supersaturated conditions the mineralization is, hence, initiated.

Mineralization Propagation

After nucleation hydroxyapatite crystal formation undergoes propagation (multiplicative proliferation) leading to progressive ossification of calcification. These are matrix vesicle-mediated and collagen-mediated hydroxyapatite precipitation.

For theories regarding bone mineralization one school of thought gives primacy to matrix vesicles. The other school gives bone matrix the primacy for initiating and propagating mineralization. These two theories have tried to explain the intermediate mechanisms between calcium, phosphate, and hydroxyl ions in blood stream and eventually formation of hydroxyapatite.

The Urist Triphasic Hypothesis

In first phase, a soluble calcium protein substrate is formed. The calcium disrupts hydrogen bonds in collagen and reacts to form calcium complexes. These anionic complexes in phase II react with phosphate to form soluble protein calcium phosphate complex. In phase III, the neutralized calcium-protein-phosphatase complex reacts with Ca^{2+} and HPO_4^{2-} depending on the solubility product which is kept at metastable state (supersaturated) at the mineralization front.

The Glimcher Hypothesis

Proposes the stereochemical disposition of collagen components to be primarily responsible for nucleation. The nucleation occurs with respect to the physical organization of the collagen physical and chemical properties.

Pathological Calcification

Unlike the physiological calcification of bone described above there are lots of pathological conditions where calcium deposition occurs:

- Damaged tissues have pathologic extracellular or intracellular "dystrophic" calcification. The calcium deposition within the soft tissues (both dystrophic and metastatic) in myeloma, metastases, fat necrosis, trauma, sarcoidosis, scleroderma, hyperparathyroidism, etc., is caused by calcium hydroxyapatite.
- "Metastatic" calcification occurs in association with altered serum levels of calcium and phosphate.
- Crystal deposition in joints—this deposition is rarely massive and simulates tophaceous deposits, hence, called tophaceous pseudogout. The linear calcification seen along menisci and articular cartilage or in the intervertebral disk radiographically is mostly due to calcium pyrophosphate deposition (CPPD disease).
- *Tumor calcinosis:* This is a "tumor-like" calcium deposition that occurs in extracapsular soft tissue around hip, shoulder, elbow, and knee without an obvious associated metabolic mineral disorder. It is not a neoplasia and the use of term "tumor" should be dropped. The deposition is reactive or metabolic simulating a neoplasm seen commonly in African Americans. The disease is asymptomatic producing only symptoms from surrounding soft tissue compression. Radiologically, there is a well demarcated circular to oval and nodular calcific mass formed from coalescence of multiple nodules into single concretion. Serum phosphate and calcitriol levels are usually elevated. Treatment consists of complete excision of masses as incomplete excision causes recurrence.
- Soft tissue calcifications are commonly seen in disorders associated with hypercalcemia such as primary and secondary hyperparathyroidism, scleroderma, and hypervitaminosis D and chronic renal disease (here, mechanisms other than hypercalcemia are involved).

BONE REMODELING

Semantically, the term remodeling stands for the constant recycling of minerals (calcium and phosphate) from bone to maintain homeostasis. Over a prolonged period of time the term has, however, come to recognize correction of angulation and translation to restore acceptable alignment. The term remodeling is so much engraved in understanding of the orthopedic literature that its use has to be continued in the incorrect form even in this text. What we understand as evolved version of the term remodeling is actually "bone modeling". The terms remodeling and modeling are often used interchangeably and without proper understanding. With evolution, remodeling came to mean "restructuring" the fractured bone to its prefracture form, modeling on the other hand is a continuous process that extends even beyond the native structure of bone is regained. Bone modeling adapts osseous structure to loading by changing bone size and shape and removes damage in a way this process is a part and parcel of even normal bone that maintains its strength. Despite being incorrect the term remodeling will continue to be used to avoid any confusion with the current inappropriate usage of the term. Remodeling (actually bone modeling) is a process that involves tight coupling of bone resorption and formation to adjust to constantly changing requirements with activity and aging **(Fig. 16)**. It is essential for the bone to change its form in response to stress and strain else, it will never leave its infantile form or be able to bear the increasing weight with growth. Persons doing active labor need to have stronger bones supporting muscles so on and so forth. Also, remodeling acts like regular maintenance work healing the microtrauma and fractures that keep occurring in this "hard" tissue. Bone undergoes remodeling throughout life which is primarily a function of trabecular bone arrangement, but is actively also seen in healing compact bone of immature bone fractures, while minimally in adult compact bone. To put it in figures nearly 25% of the metabolically active cancellous bone and some 3% of the cortical bone gets renewed each year. It is an essential process as without remodeling (that also entails repair of microfractures) bone would exceed its elastic tolerance limits within a short period of time. The remodeling is not constantly occurring throughout the skeleton at once, but it occurs in discrete packets termed bone remodeling units (BRU) by Frost, scattered throughout the skeleton. Each packet takes 3–4 months to complete. There is, however, some quantitative bone loss with age (senile osteoporosis) as bone formation always lags temporally and quantitatively from bone resorption possibly due to decreased number of osteoblasts. The process of remodeling of bone involves three discrete steps of activation, bone resorption, and bone formation that need discrete cellular and molecular components to complete. Bone remodeling is prominent at endosteal and periosteal surfaces and is also seen within Haversian canal systems that contain osteoprogenitor cells.

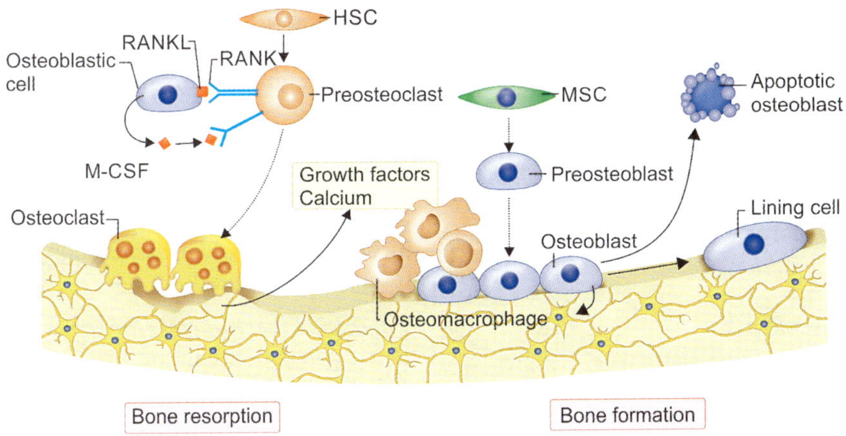

Fig. 16: Concept of bone remodeling as a function tight coupling of two alternating opposing processes, the bone formation, and bone resorption. Also shown is the effect of various growth factors and cytokines. (RANK: receptor activator of nuclear factor κ; RANKL: receptor activator of nuclear factor κ ligand; HSC: hematopoietic stem cell; MSC: mesenchymal stem cell; M-CSF: monocyte-colony stimulating factor)

The width of tubular bones and also the bone mass are controlled by cortical bone remodeling.

Resorption of bone is interestingly activated by stimulatory cytokines IL-1 and IL-6 produced by osteoblasts (that are ironically really meant for bone formation) and also involves modulation of the integrin RGD sequence interaction. Bone resorption takes approximately 10 days carried out by a "cutting cone" of osteoclasts. The defect created after resorption is filled in by fibrovascular tissue containing pericytes (later forming Haversian and Volkmann's canals), monocytes or macrophages, MSC, and undifferentiated osteoprogenitor cells in loose connective tissue. Histopathologically, basophilic line—the "cement" or the "reversal" line marks the outer edge of the osteon (where bone formation is initiated). The resorption front of cutting cone does not follow osteonal arrangement and progresses randomly, so that in a single go it can take down multiple osteons. With mineralization front, the osteons are partially repaired and form new interconnected channels depending on the stress pattern. The lamellae that remain as reminiscent of cutting cone activity persist as interstitial lamellae and keep accumulating over the age of person. The interstitial lamellae are less active metabolically and are, hence, unable to repair promptly. This is partly responsible for senile osteoporosis.

Bone formation is a function of osteoblasts taking approximately 3 months that varies with age and nutritional status of the individual. The osteoblastic activity is mediated by differentiation regulators such as TGF-β, PDGF, IGF, and Gla proteins (discussed above). More important is, however, the linking or "coupling" of bone resorption and bone formation and this is immensely complex. We understand at least three mechanisms that explain this coupling:

1. The current postulated model is that "osteoclastogenic" and "osteoblastogenic" cytokines are stimulated simultaneously by the same signal transduction pathway mediated by glycoprotein 130. Glycoprotein 130 is increased by the influence of PTH and vitamin D, whereas sex steroids inhibit it.
2. During the osteoclastic process some osteoblast stimulating factors such as IGF-I and IGF-II and TGF-β are released that would stimulate formation of osteoblasts from the osteoprogenitor cells by the time bone resorption process is completed.
3. The most fascinating and studied mechanism for coupling bone resorption and formation is the RANK/RANKL interaction, where osteoblasts regulate osteoclastogenesis.

Whatever the mechanism, coupling has been exploited by giving intermittent PTH therapy to treat osteoporosis so successfully.

Why and how osteoclastic activity precedes osteoblastic activity always? The most logical answer to this is that the ground needs to be cleared by osteoclastic activity for new bone to form in an organized robust way by osteoblasts rather than just a namesake patch work to be done—the body systems are more honest, organized, and authentic. The osteoclasts are fast workers, so they finish their work early and bone synthesis should be more meticulously and gradually done so osteoblasts come late, it is apparently perceived that the bone resorption occurs early even though both started the race at same time. Also, the RGD sequence may be directly stimulated in response to stress or strain (discussed below) stimulating the osteoclasts first followed by osteoblasts.

Effect of Stress and Mechanosensory Systems on Remodeling (Wolff's law)

The mechanobiology of bone modeling is discussed in greater detail in the Chapter on "Fracture Repair, Bone Grafting, and Bone Banking", a primer is presented here for completion purpose. Wolff's law described by Julius Wolff in 1882 in strict accordance with mathematical laws states, *"every change in form and function of bones is followed by changes in the internal architecture and external conformation"*. Since long it has been known that mechanical forces influence morphology of skeleton. If the stresses on a limb are taken off say in immobilization the tissues undergo atrophy and the bones undergo "disuse" osteoporosis. On the other hand, it is seen that children with malunited fractures of long bones nearly always remodel into almost normal appearing bones (except for some rotational under correction), while poliomyelitis limbs with poor stress on bones stay malunited. Similarly, weightlessness in space causes rapid decrease in bone mass, equivalent to the reduced amount of stress on them reflecting the need for constant force in maintaining skeletal health.

Pathways Affecting the Wolff's Law

Stress response: Under conditions of load there is an altered bone metabolism and DNA synthesis. These responses are mediated by electrical or chemical messengers (cytokines). Two separate components mediate this stretch sensory pathway. The cell network consisting of osteocytes and their processes communicate with surface cells through connexins that play a dominant role in the mechanosensing of strain by the osteocyte dendritic processes, modulating osteoblast bone formation according to mechanical load. Osteoblasts and fibroblasts exhibit stretch sensitive ion channels. The mineralized matrix is responsible for stream-generated potentials when fluid flowing through the matrix carries along particular ions (in the presence of different ones attached to the matrix). These stretch sensitive and stream-generated potentials may be responsible for the signaling altered cellular metabolism. A "piezoelectric" effect produced due to compression of the hydroxyapatite crystal that has been so commonly highlighted is actually much less important in signaling, but may be responsible for the coupling of mechanical-electrical phenomena in bone.

Strain response: Osteoblast proliferation in response to strain is mediated by the inositol 1,4,5-trisphosphate system. Neomycin-mediated inhibition of phospholipase C blocks inositol trisphosphate production and, hence, subsequent osteoblast proliferation.

Combined mechanism (for stress and strain): Cells maintain a constant milieu or basal equilibrium state for stress. This equilibrium is defined by the number and quality of intercellular focal adhesions, intracellular cytoskeleton polymerization, and the amount of externally applied deformation (stress-strain equilibrium). The mechanism involves activation of G proteins and other kinase cascade by load stimulus detected by mechanoelectrochemical sensory system. This specific sensory system includes stretch sensitive ion channels, integrin cytoskeletal machinery, and load-conformational sensitive receptor tyrosine kinase. Integrins form important components of this mechanical sensory system. The $\alpha v\beta 3$ integrins bind to RGD sequence of osteopontin that triggers osteoclastic resorption. The matrix proteins having RGD sequence undergo conformational change in response to tension strain. The matrix tension is then "communicated" to bone cells via previously detailed osteocyte network. Nitric oxide (NO) might also be a part of this signaling process.

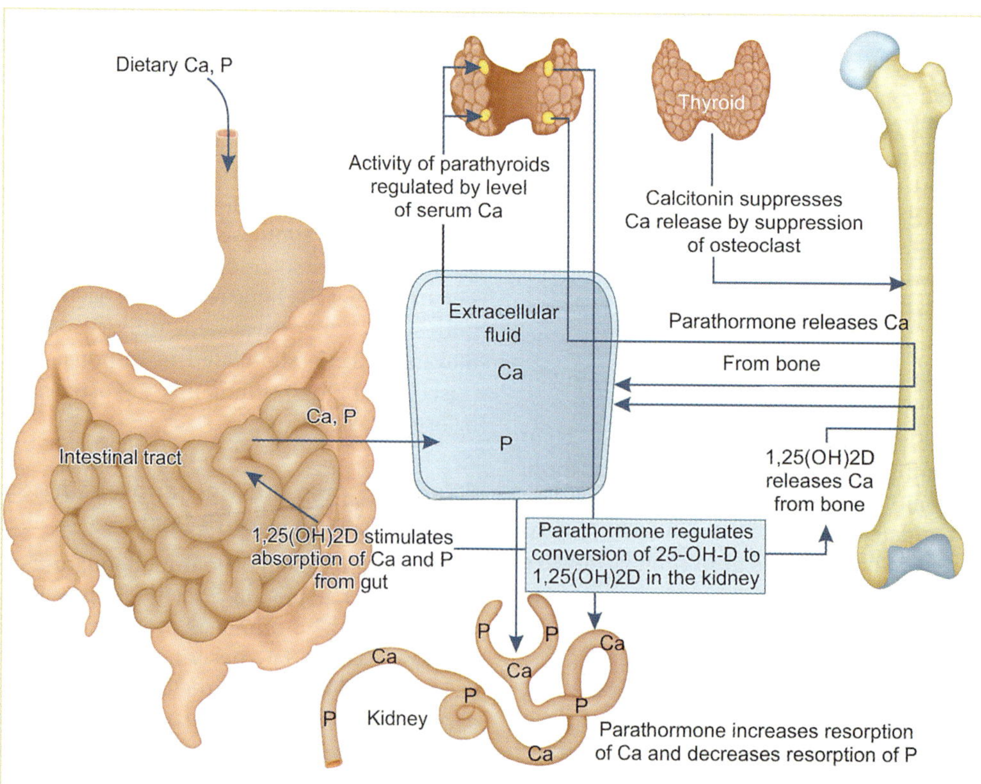

Fig. 17: Illustration depicting the endocrine control of bone calcium and phosphate metabolism. Shown are the effects of PTH and vitamin D on intestine and bones. (Ca: calcium; P: phosphorus)

REGULATION OF BONE METABOLISM

Endocrine Control (Fig. 17)

Systemic and local factors maintain:

- Balance between bone formation and loss
- Homeostasis in calcium levels in the body for various physiological functions, especially muscle contraction
- Maintenance of a reservoir of phosphate required for generating energy.

Parathyroid Hormone

Parathyroid hormone produced from the parathyroid gland is a polypeptide hormone synthesized from pro-PTH. PTH maintains calcium homeostasis by stimulating bone resorption. In fetal and neonatal animals, PTH is required for normal formation and development or remodeling of cancellous bone. PTH also impacts intestine and kidney function. Reduced serum calcium is the strongest stimulator of PTH release from parathyroid glands. The physiologic role of PTH includes:

- Increase in osteoclastic activity which results in calcium and phosphate release from the bony skeleton (mediated through osteoblasts and RANK and RANKL).
- In kidney, PTH reduces calcium excretion, but increases phosphate excretion. It also stimulates 1,25-dihydroxy vitamin D production.

These measures increase serum calcium concentration which suppresses the secretion and synthesis of PTH. PTH controls the serum calcium levels on a minute to minute basis probably because we live in low calcium-high phosphate environment and the calcium levels are important with respect to sustaining life. Interestingly, despite being bone resorptive hormone; receptors for PTH are found on preosteoblasts, osteoblasts, and chondrocytes, but are absent from osteoclast which supports the notion that PTH mediates osteoclastogenesis and bone resorption is osteoblast-dependent and mediated via cytokines (discussed above). The ultimate effect of this action, however, is osteoclast activation, initiation of bone resorption, and maintaining adequate blood calcium levels for optimal functioning of dependent organs like contractile tissues by calcium release from bone. Simultaneous osteoblast stimulation might be a check mechanism preventing too much bone resorption and "policing" the action of osteoclasts against excessive calcium stealth. Clinical use of PTH analog has demonstrated that in certain situations PTH stimulates bone formation. It has been shown that in continuous administration of PTH there is increased osteoclastic resorption with simultaneous suppression of bone formation. The effect reverses to bone formation instead when PTH is administered in low doses, intermittently. This anabolic effect is also probably indirectly mediated via IGF-I and TGF-β. Constant high serum PTH levels initiate osteoclast formation resulting in bone resorption that over-rides the effects of activating genes that direct bone formation indicating that osteoclast function and formation requires persistently high PTH levels due to indirect action. The action on osteoblasts is more direct, but possibly the bone resorption is much more efficient process than the slower bone formation so that persistent elevated levels produce predominantly bone resorption. PTHrP is expressed early in the osteoblast progenitor cells and regulates bone formation in a paracrine manner. This process persists longer so that pulsatile stimulation by even low doses of PTH will stimulate osteoblasts escaping bone resorption that needs high persistent levels.

Calcitonin

Calcitonin is a peptide hormone synthesized by parafollicular cells of thyroid. Its secretion is regulated by extracellular calcium levels and gastrin. The calcitonin acts to tone down calcium from blood maintaining normocalcemia by removing excess calcium. Calcitonin blocks PTH-mediated bone resorption by osteoclasts. This is done through increased adenylate cyclase and cyclic adenosine monophosphate (cAMP) or as mitogen acting on bone cells. It promotes renal calcium excretion. Calcitonin acts as an "emergency hormone" protecting against sudden hypercalcemia. The hypocalcemic effects of calcitonin are temporary and with continuous infusion of calcitonin "escape phenomenon" is seen where the effects of PTH supersedes that of calcitonin. The actions of calcitonin are independent of vitamin D levels. Calcitonin receptors are present on osteoclasts and its precursors, and certain tumor cells. Increased levels result in a temporary fall in plasma calcium.

The physiological role of calcitonin on bone morphology and ultimate function is not fully clear. Decline or overproduction of calcitonin does not have any significant alterations in bone density. The uncertainty may arise from possible recently identified dual action of calcitonin bone formation and resorption. Calcitonin and alpha calcitonin gene-related peptide (alpha-CGRP) deficiency (Calca-/- -) exhibits high bone mass mediated by increased bone formation with normal bone resorption in animals. However, with only alpha-CGRP (alpha CGRP-/-) deletion osteopenia was seen. These may explain why alterations of calcitonin serum levels in humans do not result in major changes in bone mineral density. Calcitonin does, however, has some therapeutic role, it is used in management of hypercalcemia of malignancy, pain control in osteoporosis (the effect on bone mineral alteration is meagre if any) and in Paget's disease (osteoclasts from Paget's patients are hyper-responsive to calcitonin).

Vitamin D

Vitamin D_2 = ergocalciferol and vitamin D_3 = cholecalciferol. The common layman term for vitamin D refers to and includes cholecalciferol (diet and even the drug supplements); 1,25-dihydroxyvitamin D = calcitriol. Vitamin D can be synthesized in skin epithelial cells, and therefore by definition it is not a vitamin. The predominant source of vitamin D normally is synthesis within skin and depends on the conversion of 7-dehydrocholesterol to vitamin D_3 (cholecalciferol) from UV-B radiation (wavelength 290–320 nm). Ergosterol (naturally derived) and 7-dehydrocholesterol (derived from cholesterol and stored in skin) are the precursors for vitamin D. In the skin, they are activated by ultraviolet light to previtamin D that is thermally converted to ergocalciferol (D_2) and cholecalciferol (D_3). The reaction involves rapid formation of previtamin D_3 (photochemical reaction), which is then slowly converted to vitamin D_2 or D_3. These compounds are transported in the body via an alpha-globulin binding protein also known as vitamin D-binding protein (DBP or Gc protein). DBP is vital in maintaining stable serum levels for vitamin D and its metabolites. It also modulates the rate of bioavailability, activation, and end organ responsiveness of vitamin D. If the exposure to UV light is prolonged then previtamin D_3 gets converted to lumisterol and tachysterol that are photoisomers and do not bind to DBP. They get wasted with skin slough. Vitamin D_2 and D_3 undergo hydroxylation in liver to yield 25-hydroxyvitamin D in the presence of magnesium. This is the most abundant circulatory form of vitamin D. The hydroxylation in liver is not stringently regulated so measurement of 25-hydroxyvitamin D_3 is the standard method for determining a patient's vitamin D status. Further hydroxylation is done in PCT of kidney forming 1,25-dihydroxyvitamin D (calcitriol) and 24,25-dihydroxyvitamin D (less active and produced under the influence of calcitonin). The most active form of vitamin D is 1,25-dihydroxyvitamin D. The normal plasma level of 25-hydroxycholecalciferol is about 30 ng/mL, and that of 1,25-dihydrocholecalciferol is 0.03 ng/mL. This hormone (calcitriol) has various functions including:

- Calcium and phosphorus metabolism:
    - Stimulates synthesis of calcium binding protein (cholecalcin—transports calcium from luminal to basal layer in intestine)
    - Affects osteocalcin production
    - Osteoid mineralization
    - Osteoclastic bone resorption and maintenance of blood calcium levels
    - Increased active transcellular absorption of calcium from proximal part of intestine
    - Increased phosphorus absorption from distal part of small intestine
    - Reduced calcium and phosphorus excretion from kidney
- Skin growth
- Insulin secretion
- Reproduction
- Combating tuberculosis, viral infections, and influenza by stimulation monocyte maturation

Deficiency of calcitriol is related to:

- Precipitation of autoimmune diseases and death due to heart disease
- Stroke secondary to hypertension
- Inflammatory bowel disease
- Muscle weakness and falls
- Fractures
- Cancers of colon, breast, and prostate

Calcitriol is primarily responsible for controlling calcium metabolism in the intestine, proximal tubule of kidney, and bone. 1,25-dihydroxyvitamin D [1,25-$(OH)_2$ D_3] production is in turn regulated by other metabolic regulators such as PTH and calcium concentration itself. Formation of calcitriol is facilitated by PTH when the plasma Ca2+ level is low. Low calcium levels actually increase the PTH levels responsible for majority effect. When the plasma Ca2+ level is high, renal 1-α-hydroxylation is inhibited producing only little 1,25-dihydroxycholecalciferol and instead majority is directed at producing the relatively inactive metabolite 24,25-dihydroxycholecalciferol instead **(Fig. 18)**. The production of 1,25-dihydroxyvitamin D_3 [1,25-$(OH)_2$ D_3] is also increased by low levels of plasma PO^{3-} while high levels inhibit the same which is mediated by a direct inhibitory effect of PO^{3-} on 1α-hydroxylase. The third route for control of 1,25-dihydroxycholecalciferol formation is the direct negative feedback effect of the metabolite [1,25-$(OH)_2$ D_3] on 1α-hydroxylase, a positive feedback effect on 24-hydroxylase producing 24,25-dihydroxycholecalciferol and a direct effect on the parathyroid gland to inhibits the production of mRNA for PTH.

Lack of vitamin D results in rickets in children and osteomalacia in adults due to impaired mineralization of newly formed bone. There is accumulation of excessive

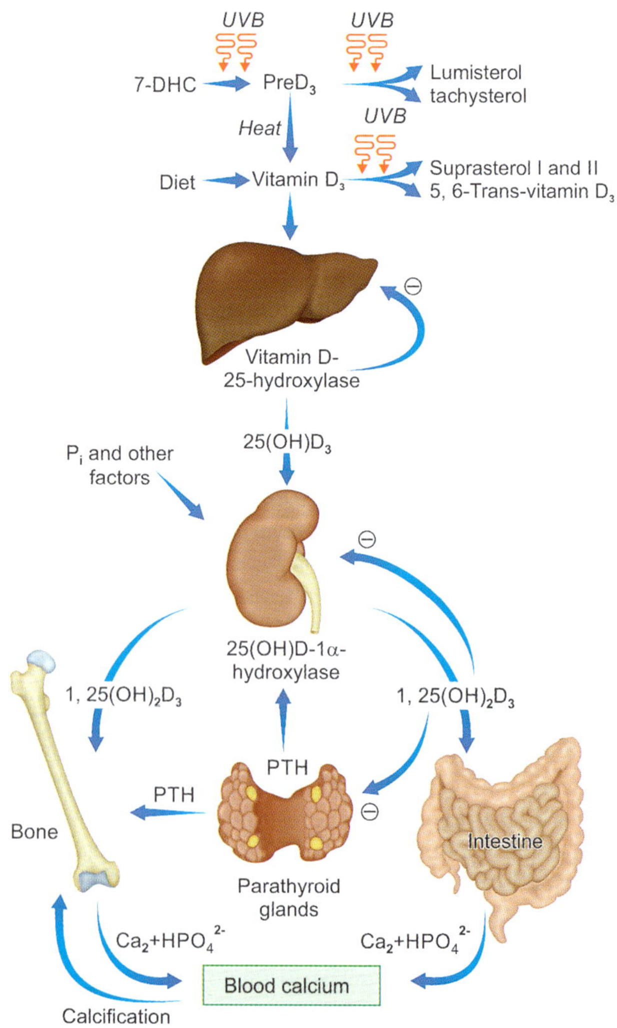

Fig. 18: Formation and metabolism of vitamin D in body. (7-DHC: 7-dehydrocholesterol; Pi: inorganic phosphorus)

proteinaceous bone matrix which fails to mineralize. Excessive vitamin D would instead increase bone resorption and cause hypercalcemia. Vitamin D activity is mediated by VDR present on several cell types. The VDR is complex arrangement that forms homodimers or heterodimers with members of the steroid hormone receptor superfamily of which the retinoic acid receptor (RXR) is most notable. VDR ultimately forms a transcription factor. Rickets has been reported to result from errors or mutations in genes that code for this steroid hormone receptor superfamily of nuclear receptors. Polymorphism of *VDR* gene has been recently portended to be responsible for postmenopausal osteoporosis making it genetically predetermined. VDR manifests most of the functions—calcium transportation, prodifferentiation, antiproliferative, and immunomodulatory activities. The VDR II especially has a role for vitamin D in bone metabolism. The VDR II deficiency or mutation may also be responsible for progressive alopecia. The marrow mononuclear cells fuse to form osteoclasts on exposure to vitamin D only in the presence of osteoblasts as only the latter contain VDRs and not the osteoclast precursors. PTH has synergistic action to that of vitamin D mediating this activity.

Role of vitamin D in osteogenesis: As noted above, calcitriol acts to resorb bone by stimulating the formation of osteoclasts. That involves close association of osteoblasts containing the VDR. Vitamin D_3 is responsible for stimulation of osteoblast differentiation through induction of osteocalcin and expression of ALP. Osteocalcin and ALP serve as markers of mature osteoblasts. Osteoblast differentiation through release of ALP is mediated via intermediary MAPK (mitogen-activated protein kinases)/ERK (extracellular signal-regulated kinase) signaling (also known as Ras-Raf-MEK-ERK pathway) pathway. Osteoclast formation is stimulated via cell-cell contact between osteoblasts and osteoclast precursor cells involving the RANK/RANKL pathway upregulation that represents osteoclast differentiation factor. It also involves downregulation of OPG expression which is an inhibitor for osteoclastogenesis via "decoy" RANK receptor mechanism (discussed above). 1,25-$(OH)_2$ D_3 mediates bone resorption and remodeling by secondary stimulation of osteoclasts. In addition, 1,25-$(OH)_2$ D_3 also inhibits osteoblast proliferation and may instead stimulate its apoptosis through induction of TNF-α. 1α-hydroxylase system (mainly renal) responsible for synthesis of calcitriol is also seen in macrophages, monocytes, keratinocytes, and lymphocytes which are not regulated by negative feedback mechanisms and amount to hypercalcemia seen in various conditions. Mutations in the human 1α-hydroxylase gene cause pseudovitamin D deficiency rickets.

Vitamin A

Vitamin A decreases the formation of bone and cartilage matrix. These effects are mediated by retinoic acid (RA—the most active metabolite of vitamin A). RA is a potent regulator of osteoblast growth and differentiation. RA acts on nuclear receptors that belong to the steroid hormone receptor superfamily (wide above in description and functioning of VDR). Alterations in RA levels during embryonic skeletal development result in prominent abnormalities of the appendicular and craniofacial skeleton. RA increases levels of osteopontin and osteocalcin mRNA in osteoblasts, hence, acting trophic to its formation. The retinoid signaling pathway also prominently affects the expression of the skeletogenic regulatory factors such as Sox9 and Cbfa1 that act like band masters for bone formation and development in the embryological ossification process.

Gonadal Hormones and Growth Hormone

Estrogen promotes longitudinal growth and excess of it leads to premature fusion of the physis. So therapeutic doses will produce a growth spurt, but it will be soon arrested due to premature fusion of physis. Reduced estrogen leads to bone loss by directly affecting osteoblasts and possibly osteoclasts, and may be mediated via PTH and calcitonin. In hypogonadism, the physes remain open and produce a long, slender, and poorly muscled person (eunuchs are typical example). Androgens maintain bone mass via receptors on osteoblasts and possibly by strain from strong and developed muscles, so common in androgen abusers.

Excess GH causes rapid growth without having any effect of maturation of physis. The actions are likely mediated on bone primarily by IGF. Gonadal hormones though may exert direct effect through GH receptors found on osteoblasts and chondrocytes.

Growth Factors in Regulation of Bone Metabolism

Transforming Growth Factor-beta

Transforming growth factor exists in two forms, TGF-α and β. TGF-α is now called EGF and is not present in bone. TGF-β increase synthesis of DNA, plays important osseous metabolic effects like it enhances the synthesis of bone matrix proteins like type I collagen and fibronectin, proteoglycans and it also reduces the activity of ALP. TGF-β plays an important role in intramembranous and endochondral ossification and also enhances fracture and wound healing. The effects are mediated by inhibiting production of hydrogen peroxide, deactivating proteolytic enzymes, and upregulating integrin receptors for ECM proteins. TGF-β1 enhances the proliferation and early differentiation of osteoblasts and a high rate of collagen synthesis, but inhibits terminal differentiation and mineralization of culture matrix. TGF-β binds to TGF-β specific type I and type II receptors initiates a sequence of events → phosphorylation of SMADs 2 and 3 → complex formation of SMADs 2/3 with SMAD 4 → translocation of SMAD 2/3/4 complex into the nucleus → finally transcriptional activation of specific target genes. TGF-β1 specifically increases intracellular calcium ion transport which enhances expression of a5 integrin that is necessary for osteoblast adhesion. Following osteoblast adhesion, its proliferation is also enhanced by TGF-β1 by inhibiting p57 cyclin-dependent kinase inhibitory protein (CKI) that is negative regulator of the cell cycle. TGF-β1 also increases production of collagen, while suppressing its maturation in effect increasing the collagen content quantitatively.

Bone Morphogenetic Proteins (See Chapter on Fracture Repair, Bone Grafting, and Bone Banking) and Osteogenesis

Bone morphogenetic proteins are osteotropic factors that belong to TGF-β superfamily. BMP-2 is responsible for gene expression and synthesis of osteoblast differentiation markers, viz., ALP and osteocalcin, in preosteoblast cells in the developing fetus. BMP-2 exposure for a very short duration itself is sufficient to induce cellular effects most of which are signaled through specific type I and type II serine/threonine kinase receptors. BMP receptor type IB (BMPR-IB) plays an essential role in osteoblast commitment and differentiation. BMP signals to inhibit myogenic differentiation and facilitate osteoblast differentiation in MSC that is mediated through BMPR-I acting through SMAD 1, 5, and 8. Additionally, BMP-2 induces osteoblast differentiation through *Runx2* that, as previously detailed, is a global mediator for osteogenesis. *Runx2* and BMP-2-induced SMAD proteins together lead to osteoblast differentiation.

Insulin-like Growth Factors I and II

Insulin-like growth factors are final pathways for many cell lines to promote proliferation, differentiation, and matrix production of bone and cartilage. Osteoblasts and chondrocytes produce them and the activity of GH has been closely linked to them. GH binds to specific receptors in target tissues that then produce IGF-I. IGF-I in turn has endocrine, paracrine, and autocrine effects on the stimulated cells and MSC. For its endocrine actions, IGF-I has to be transported by IGF-binding proteins (IGFBPs carrier proteins). IGFBP III appears to be the most important of them and it is postulated that deficiency of IGF or IGFBP III may be responsible for Laron-type dwarfism.

Other Growth Factors

Platelet-derived growth factors have been competed to be one of potent osteogenic growth factors and have been diversely utilized in orthopedic disorders from osteonecrosis to nonunion (effects though have never been fully substantiated). PDGF is important mitogens for osteoblasts and also have a chemotaxis effect. PDGFs are typically thought to play important role in bone remodeling. The role of FGFs in osseous development and metabolism are not fully elucidated, but mutations of FGF are thought to induce certain skeletal deformities such as Pfeiffer syndrome, Apert syndrome, achondroplasia, Jackson-Weiss syndrome, and Crouzon syndrome.

ENDOCRINOPATHIES AND BONE INVOLVEMENT

Primary Hyperparathyroidism

Primary hyperparathyroidism is not an uncommon endocrine disorder, incidence of which keeps rising with advancing age peaking at sixth decade. It is characterized by increased production of PTH following failure of negative feedback loop resulting in increased renal absorption of calcium, increased vitamin-D synthesis, phosphaturia, and bone resorption. Affected pediatric patients suffer from the disease more severely than the adult counterparts and also have higher incidence of end organ damage. Pediatric patients can be classified into those with neonatal onset of the disease and others with onset in childhood.

Causes

Neonatal disease may arise from autosomal recessive inheritance or may be secondary to maternal hypothyroidism. Childhood and adult forms commonly arise from parathyroid adenoma, less commonly from parathyroid hyperplasia, or rarely parathyroid carcinoma, and as part of multiple endocrine neoplasia (MEN) syndrome.

Associated Mutations

Mutations in *MPRT2* gene and retinoblastoma gene.

Epidemiology

Asymptomatic cases represent around 1% of population; patients >60 years represent 0.2% of the incident disease. Asymptomatic cases are increasingly detected due to multiple point screening commonly done while visiting physician (serum calcium levels, PTH levels for osteoporosis management, etc.)

Signs and Symptoms

Classical patients with "stones (renal), abdominal groans, psychiatric moans, and bones" are rare to find and most patients are now asymptomatic at detection. The classical manifestations are mentioned below:

Renal manifestations—deposition of calcium in renal parenchyma (nephrocalcinosis) or recurrent nephrolithiasis, diabetes insipidus, and renal failure.

Abdominal groans—constipation, vomiting, peptic ulcer disease [may be associated with Zollinger-Ellison syndrome (MEN)] and acute pancreatitis.

Psychiatric moans—result from memory loss, fatigue, depression, and delirium.

Bones—the characteristic findings are osteitis fibrosa cystica (brown tumor), which occurs in 10–20% of patients. Histologically, there are increased giant multinucleated osteoclasts in scalloped areas on the surface of the bone (Howship's lacunae) and the normal cellular and marrow elements are replaced by fibrous tissue. Radiological changes usually include areas of subperiosteal cortical resorption which is evident radiologically replacement of the usual sharp cortical outline of the bone in the digits by an irregular outline. Endosteal resorption, also known as cortical tunneling, is seen as a lacy pattern of the inner cortex of the bone. There is also resorption of the phalangeal tufts (acro-osteolysis), osteopenia, and coarsening of trabeculae. Subligamentous bone resorption is also seen typically in distal femur and proximal tibia. Other findings include loss of lamina dura dentes, mineralization of soft tissues (metastatic soft tissue and visceral calcifications, and chondrocalcinosis), development of bone cysts, "salt and pepper" appearance of skull due to trabecular resorption, and development of genu valgum (less common) or slipped capital femoral epiphysis (uncommon).

Some people add to this *"thrones"* referring to polyuria and constipation.

Diagnosis

- Elevated immunoreactive PTH level in asymptomatic hypercalcemia
- Hypercalcemia, hypophosphatemia, increased urinary phosphate, increased ALP, and increased excretion of hydroxyproline in the urine.

Treatment

Usually, the asymptomatic patients are managed conservatively with adequate hydration and reduced calcium intake. The patients should be followed annually for serum calcium levels, BMD test, and serum creatinine. There is a growing concern for cardiovascular deterioration, neuropsychiatric dysfunction, the adverse effects of osteoporosis, and reduced bone quality favoring early surgery. Prophylactic parathyroidectomy is, however, debated and there is no clear consensus. Currently, surgery is indicated in patients with sustained serum calcium >1 mg/dL above normal, creatinine clearance <60 mL/min, age <50, and bone density t-score <–2.5 at any of the three sites.

Pediatric patients are commonly managed with bilateral neck exploration and biopsy of the parathyroid glands. If a single parathyroid adenoma is discovered then exploration and excision of single-affected gland can be performed.

Surgical removal of the functional parathyroid lesion results in a rapid decrease in circulating PTH levels, due to rapid bone formation by uninhibited osteoblasts (hungry bone). It may acutely result in severe hypocalcemic tetany since the half-life of PTH in plasma is approximately 20 minutes. Postoperatively, if hypercalcemia persists for a week or more or recurs after showing initial improvement one should suspect a second adenoma or metastases from carcinoma.

Secondary Hyperparathyroidism

This is a condition of increased (but not autonomous) PTH secretion in response to hypocalcemia. The most common cause of increased PTH secretion by parathyroid glands is secondary to chronic renal failure. The mechanism is not very clear and though on initial thought 1,25-$(OH)_2$ D_3 deficiency appears to be the cause; the real picture is much broader:

- There is resistance to normal levels of PTH in blood resulting in hypocalcemia.
- There is increased phosphatonin (FGF23) secretion by osteocytes that inhibits 1α-hydroxylase that is responsible for reduced 1,25-$(OH)_2$ D_3 levels.

Patients usually have chondrocalcinosis at knee and pubic symphysis, bone pains, joint pains, deformities, and pathological fractures (renal osteodystrophy), ectopic calcification, and pruritus.

Secondary hyperparathyroidism may also arise due to calcium malabsorption (as in malabsorption syndromes, bariatric surgery, chronic pancreatitis, and nutritional deficiency) and osteomalacia, but these cases are rare. Especially important is identification of secondary hyperparathyroidism in patients of osteoporosis (due to associated vitamin D deficiency) who are to be started on teriparatide as the effect will be blunted in these patients due to baseline elevated PTH levels.

Treatment

This disease differs from primary hyperparathyroidism in the fact that the hormonal secretion and hyperplasia of the gland can be suppressed by appropriate therapy. The patients should be given calcitriol (0.25–2 μg/day) and phosphate-restricted diet. Calcimimetics (cinacalcet) have been introduced and approved for use in patients on dialysis. They act by allosteric activation of calcium sensitive parathormone receptors. Long-term management and maintenance of normocalcemia depends on renal transplantation, but even then a few patients may develop tertiary hyperparathyroidism.

Pseudohyperparathyroidism

This results from excessive PTH-like polypeptides secreted in circulation from malignant tumors of nonparathyroid origin. Characteristic findings include persistent hypercalcemia and hypophosphatemia, absence of bone metastasis, atrophy of parathyroid glands, and remission of hypercalcemia on extirpation of tumor which is also the treatment.

Hypoparathyroidism, Pseudohypoparathyroidism, and Pseudopseudohypoparathyroidism

In calcium metabolism, it is expected that low levels of serum calcium would stimulate PTH secretion but in hypoparathyroidism there remain low serum levels of PTH in spite of hypocalcemia and secondary hyperphosphatemia. Idiopathic hypoparathyroidism can occur in familial or sporadic forms and may be associated with syndromes, like DiGeorge syndrome (congenital absence of the parathyroid glands). Other causes are autoimmune disorders and postsurgical resection. Pseudohypoparathyroidism is a hereditary disease is clinically similar to hypoparathyroidism, but here the parathyroid glands are normal with elevated PTH. There is primarily end organ resistance to PTH. Pseudopseudohypoparathyroidism (PPHP) is the normocalcemic form of PHP.

The face and the skull are areas that are frequently involved in affected pediatric patients. Radiographs commonly show generalized or focal osteosclerosis (20% patients), particularly in the skull, pelvis, and proximal femur. There is thickening of the cranial vault and facial bones, sutural diastasis due to associated increased intracranial pressure and abnormal tooth development with delayed eruption or supernumerary teeth. Additional uncommon findings include premature physeal fusion, dense metaphyseal bands, and soft tissue, tendons, and spinal ligament calcifications. Premature physis fusion typically manifests as shortening of one or more of the metacarpals and metatarsals affecting most commonly the fourth and fifth rays. This finding is more characteristic of PPHP and most commonly involves the hands. Other inconsistent and rare findings include diaphyseal exostoses, coxa valga or vara, osseous bowing, cone epiphyses, and accelerated skeletal maturation.

The majority of cases of pediatric pseudohypoparathyroidism are managed with the administration of calcium and vitamin D analogs. Nonresponders may be managed with PTH replacement therapy can be used, however, concerns of developing osteosarcoma with this therapy remain.

Chronic Kidney Disease-Mineral Bone Disorder (Previously Known as *Renal Osteodystrophy*)

Chronic kidney disease (CKD)-mineral bone disorder (MBD) describes a histomorphometric group of metabolic bone disorders and characteristic musculoskeletal manifestations secondary to chronic renal failure. There are four disorders that are classified in this category:

1. *Hyperparathyroid bone disease:* Both glomerular and tubular dysfunctions contribute to the development of hyperparathyroidism and MBD. Tubular dysfunction causes hypocalcemia because of deficient vitamin D synthesis, whereas impaired glomerular function results in phosphorus retention. Both result in hypocalcemia that then triggers secondary hyperparathyroidism in a physiological feedback mechanism to restore calcium levels **(Fig. 19)**. Hyperparathyroid bone disease is the major metabolic abnormality in CKD-associated MBD. The bone effects of rising PTH are nonlinear due to possible interplay of confounding molecular interactions (FGF23, serum phosphorus concentration, degree of chronic metabolic acidosis, levels of 1,25 dihydroxyvitamin D and 25 hydroxyvitamin D). As the disease progresses, rickets and osteomalacia develop.
2. *Osteomalacia:* Histomorphometrically, it is classified as:
   - Presence of abundant osteoid (>80% of osteoid surface)
   - Thick osteoid seams (>14 μ)
   - Prolonged mineralization lag time (>100 days)

   Histological characterization requires simultaneous assessment of mineralization osteoid thickness or osteoid volume and mineralization lag time or osteoid maturation. Cardinal clinical finding for diagnosis is elevated ALP. Osteomalacia always has a diagnosis so other causes should always be borne in mind and evaluated **(Box 1)**. The usual clinical profile in osteomalacia is raised ALP, biopsy proven osteomalacia, a normal 25 hydroxyvitamin D, low 1,25 dihydroxyvitamin D levels, and elevated FGF23 levels. This may, however, be also seen in oncogenic osteomalacia but notably in CKD serum phosphate is high but in oncogenic osteomalacia it is very low.
3. *Adynamic renal bone disease:* As the name suggests the disease is characterized by absence of bone turnover identified histologically as absence of any tetracycline labels through thin microtome slices of cortical and cancellous bone. It may occur due to iatrogenic or idiopathic causes. Iatrogenic adynamic renal bone disease is seen in the context of chronically suppressed PTH concentrations, <100–150 pg/mL due to treating physician medications and can be reversed by reducing the amount of calcium containing phosphate binders, the dialysate calcium bath concentration, or active vitamin D analogs or cinacalcet. Idiopathic form seems to arise more commonly in severe form of disease and has apparently no cause. Diabetes mellitus has been suggested as a cause although. Aluminum accumulation in bone also mimics adynamic bone disease.
4. *Mixed renal bone disease:* This has features of other three forms described above and may represent transitions between these forms during the course of CKD.

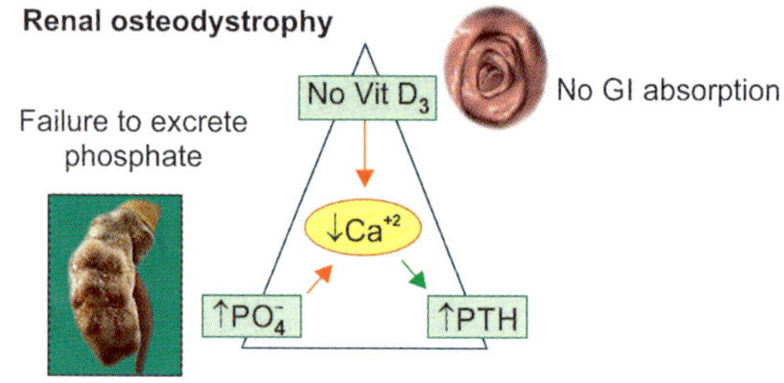

Fig. 19: The reduced serum calcium in chronic kidney disease arises from combined dietary and renal effects resulting in reduced vitamin D levels and increased phosphate (PO_4^{3-}). Hypocalcemia leads to elevated parathormone (PTH) levels and resulting bone changes.

BOX 1: Osteomalacia mostly always has an identifiable cause.

- Severe 25(OH)D deficiency (<8 ng/mL)
- Chronic hypophosphatemia
- Vitamin D-resistant rickets
- Renal tubular acidosis
- Oncogenic osteomalacia (low serum PO_4, elevated FGF 23, low, 1,25D, phosphaturia)

Radiographic features of CKD-associated MBD come from hyperparathyroidism-induced osteoclastic bone resorption and classically include subperiosteal, endosteal, and subligamentous bone resorption as well as osteopenia with coarsening of the trabecular pattern. Subperiosteal resorption is most frequently seen in the middle phalanges of the hand, distal clavicle, and distal femur and proximal tibia. Acro-osteolysis is terminal tuft bone resorption of the digits. Subchondral resorption adjacent to physeal cartilage (osteitis fibrosa) manifests as lucency at the edge of the physis, simulating rickets, and predisposing to epiphyseal slippage. Osteosclerosis also is a common manifestation that causes diffuse chalky bone density, which in the spine affects the vertebral end plates, producing the rugger jersey spine. Bone mineral density can be measured by dual X-ray absorptiometry to assess bone mass in the pediatric population. The specific treatments of the three forms of disease are outlined in description of pathologies above.

Heavy Metal Poisoning

Heavy metals (metals having specific density of >5 g/cm^3) implicated in bone disorders include lead, mercury, aluminum, arsenic, cadmium, and nickel. They are widely distributed in the earth's crust and also normally present at very low concentrations in the body. They have potential of accumulation and produce cumulative deleterious chronic degenerative changes in the nervous system, liver, kidney, and bones.

Most of the heavy metals produce their effects by enzymatic inhibition, impaired antioxidant metabolism, oxidative stress, and free-radical formation. These days the heavy metal poisoning commonly occurs due to industrial activity and consequential water and land pollution and also it is seen as occupational hazard (dyeing, hiding, and allied industries). Lead poisoning is a serious concern in children. Lead has industrial use but no physiologic use; therefore, any evidence of lead in the body should be considered contamination. In children accidental ingestion (lead-based paints in households and toys) most frequently occurs in toddlers and it is absorbed through calcium absorption sites. Although it is poorly absorbed through the gastrointestinal (GI) tract but chronic exposure to very small amounts of lead is enough to cause pathological changes. The most common childhood presentation of lead poisoning (plumbism) is central neurotoxicity. Other symptoms include anemia, anorexia, abdominal pain, vomiting, and growth delay.

The diagnosis of heavy metal toxicity is by measuring the blood levels of the metal in question. The radiological manifestations of lead poisoning are prominent and include:

- Dense transverse metaphyseal lines mostly around the knee (due to the increased deposition of calcium along with lead). These may, however, be normally be present in femur and tibia so the presence of fibular bands is more specific to diagnosis. These bands can be also seen in other sites of the axial and appendicular skeleton. Slowly with growth these dense bands migrate to the diaphysis and disappear in a few years. The differential diagnosis for dense metaphyseal bands include other heavy metal poisoning, scurvy, rickets, and treated leukemia.
- Abnormal tubular bone remodeling—this is characteristically seen in distal femur producing metaphyseal widening and sutural widening in skull (raised intracranial pressure).

Identified heavy metal poisoning in pediatric patients with markedly elevated blood levels of the metal should be handled as emergencies and treated immediately with appropriate therapy and specific chelating agents.

Sickle Cell Disease

Sickle cell disease (SCD) is the first human inherited disease that was understood at the protein and the DNA level. SCD is an autosomal recessive hemoglobinopathy that results in formation of abnormal polymer of hemoglobin in hypoxic environment that can take large shape in severe oxygen-stress. The RBC's assume abnormal sickle shape when viewed end-on and cause occlusion of small blood vessels. This produces the characteristic vaso-occlusive crisis and bone infarcts. Most of the skeletal manifestations are secondary to the infarcts and bone necrosis produced at various sites and can present acutely or in a chronic manifestation. Acute manifestations of SCD include painful vaso-occlusive crisis, osteomyelitis, bone marrow infarcts, stress fractures, and vertebral collapse ("fish-type" or "H-shaped" vertebrae). Chronic manifestations are mainly related to osteonecrosis and secondary bone collapse and deformity.

Vaso-occlusive crisis occur frequently in the bone marrow and affects virtually all pediatric patients with SCD, commonly starting in late infancy. The resulting bone marrow infarction typically occurs in the medullary cavity or epiphyses and produce localized or multifocal intense pain, edema, and erythema with or without fever and leukocytosis. Dactylitis is considered a classic presentation of vaso-occlusive SCD (children between 1 and 2 years of age). Because bones of digits of hands and feet contain hematopoietic marrow in children so they present with a swollen and painful digit. Osteonecrosis results from vaso-occlusion of the epiphyses and may involve the articular surfaces. Joint effusion is seen with epiphyseal involvement and may be associated with adjacent soft-tissue edema.

Radiographs are of no significant value in acute crisis but bone scintigraphy or better an MRI would reveal the correlative changes. Bone scintigraphy is especially helpful in assessing multifocal involvement showing increased uptake in areas of acute bone marrow infarction. Whole-body MRI with diffusion-weighted imaging sequences can evaluate not only the extent of disease but also the acuity of the infarcts. MRI is typically more helpful in the localized involvement because whole body scans are cumbersome and not easily feasible. Acute bone infarcts are hyperintense on fluid-sensitive sequences and hypointense on T1-weighted MR images and display no enhancement after contrast. The more chronic infarcts tend to be predominantly hypointense with a peripheral bright halo on fluid-sensitive sequences and hypointense with fatty elements on T1-weighted MR images.

Plain radiographs demonstrate chronic marrow infarcts as serpiginous lytic lesions with a peripheral sclerotic line and diffuse or patchy osteosclerosis. In the epiphyses, a subchondral crescentic lucency is quite characteristic.

Acromegaly

This is due to excess pituitary GH secretion (primary or due to excess GH release hormone).

Causes

Pituitary adenoma (>98% cases), MEN1, GH cell carcinoma, and metastasis, McCune-Albright syndrome, ectopic sphenoid or parapharyngeal sinus pituitary adenoma, excess GH release hormone secretion—hypothalamic hamartoma, choristoma, etc.

Clinical Findings

The patients are usually diagnosed after 10 years of age. Characteristic features include:

- Increased hand and foot size (increased shoe and glove size)
- Prognathism and increased mandibular size
- Frontal bossing
- Broad chest
- Pituitary gigantism if hypersecretion occurs before physeal closure
- Increased heel pad thickness
- Carpal tunnel syndrome
- Macroglossia
- Increased gap between lower incisors
- Broad joints (due to increased growth of epiphysis and cartilage hypertrophy)

In adults, the bones are thickened due to appositional bone deposition while in children the bone length also increases. Bones that develop late ossification centers such as scapula, sternum, mandible, and ischium are unusually enlarged as they are in the influence of increased hormonal level for longer duration. The joints of these individuals due to unusual biomechanics and shape are prone to OA.

Treatment

The goal is to control the GH and IGF-I hypersecretion, arrest tumor growth, and reduce comorbidities. Surgical resection (trans-sphenoidal and high cure rate) is preferred modality for most patients. Somatostatin analogs (octreotide and lanreotide) are used for patients with invasive macro-adenomas (for tumor shrinkage) and for those requiring immediate control of symptoms or those who cannot undergo surgery for various reasons. Other drugs like bromocriptine or GH antagonist (pegvisomant) are indicated for patients who cannot tolerate somatostatin analogs. Latter is highly effective, but cost is a concern. Radiation therapy is reserved for indicated patients only and has disadvantage of late-onset hypopituitarism and inability to control IGF-I levels.

BONE IN HEALTH AND DISEASE

Bone health is affected by many physiologic, pharmacologic, and demographic factors that affect bone resorption and formation **(Fig. 20)**. Physiological processes (like age) and common pathological states (like diabetes mellitus, smoking, and nonosseous malignancy) that affect the bone tissue quality will be discussed below.

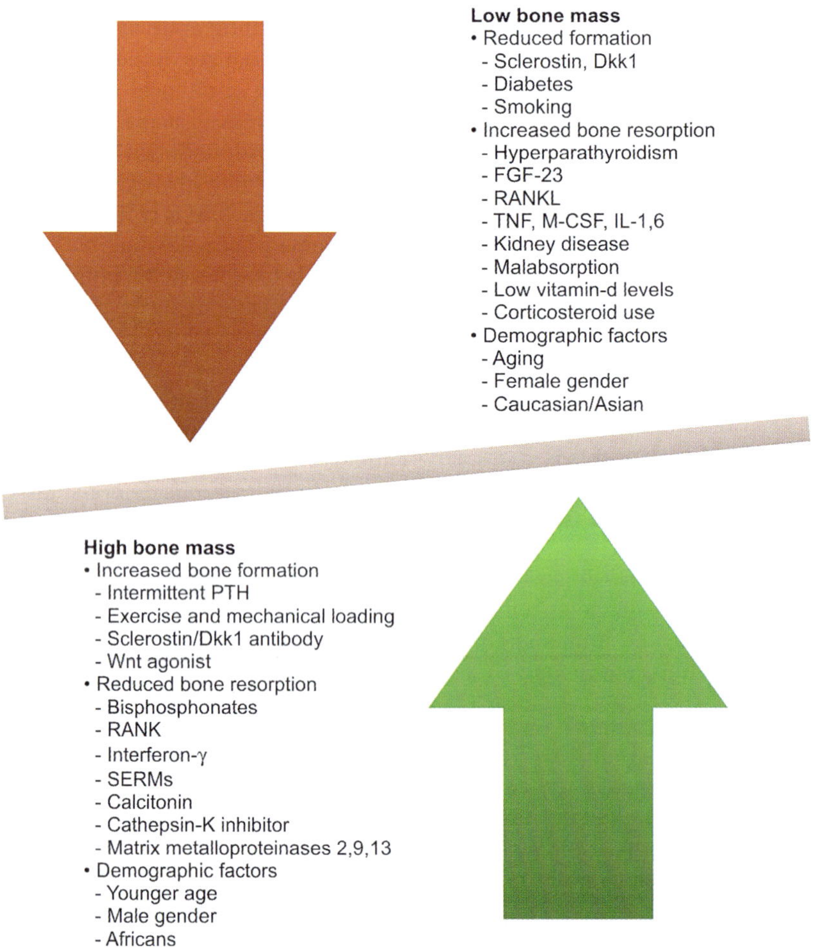

Fig. 20: Various determinants of bone mass and bone health. The factors may act to increase or reduce the bone mass.

Aging

Bone undergoes many remodeling cycles throughout life. With each cycle the amount of new bone formation reduces slightly reducing the accrued bone mass. The predominant factors responsible for this are:

- Increased osteocyte apoptosis
- Reduced number of precursor cells with age
- Reduced mechanical loading of bone due to reduced activity levels
- Accumulation of reactive oxygen species reducing quality of organic tissues and cellular components
- Increased collagen cross-linking reducing elasticity
- Reduced trabecular mass, thinned cortices, and changed center of gravity altering mechanics and predisposing to fractures with loading

Diabetes

Diabetes has been associated with poor healing of bone and increased risk of infection. Apart from end-organ damage in diabetes mellitus there is also widely recognized impairment in bone function in the disease that may be ascribed to:

- Derangements in anabolic factors and inhibition of osteoblast function
- Decreased bone formation and turnover
- Reduced osteoblast proliferation and reduced remodelling
- Reduced IGF-I
- Increased levels of sclerostin (inhibits Wnt and preventing osteocyte differentiation and bone formation)
- Accumulation of advanced glycosylation end products (AGE) including glycosylated type 1 collagen that interferes with osteoblast and osteocyte function contributing to instability of the bone matrix
- AGEs also activate nuclear factor-κβ (NF-κβ) inflammatory pathway increasing bone resorption via osteoclastogenesis
- Diversion of MSC into adipocyte lineage
- Thiazolidinediones also divert (MSC) into adipocytes via PPAR-γ modulation
- Increased incidence of falls due to retinopathy and neuropathy
- High rates of orthopedic infection due to impaired leukocyte function

Malignancy

Nonosseous cancers affect bone in two primary ways—metastasis and treatment related (like radiotherapy):

- Radiation-induced inflammation, vascular fibrosis, and reduced tissue circulation impairs bone metabolism directly
- Radiation bone necrosis results from hypoxia, hypovascularity, tissue breakdown, and disrupted healing predisposing to pathological fractures and chronic infections
- Bone metastasis produces osteolysis through increased expression of RANK-L, matrix metalloproteinases and PTHrP.
- Tumor cells can cause osteoclastic mimicry by fusing with osteoclast precursors and directly causing bone resorption
- Osteolysis in-turn facilitates cancer progression via TGF-β release, increased calcium, and hypoxia
- Prostate cancer metastasis may also produce immature woven bone (blastic metastasis) via tumor cell epithelial-to-mesenchymal transdifferentiation and osteomimicry

Smoking

Smoking has been widely implicated in developing bone nonunion. It is also associated with poor bone quality and osteoporosis.

- Smoking generates reactive oxygen species, impairs mitochondrial activity, impairs fibroblast migration, and reduces blood flow to the site of injury
- It increases osteoclast numbers and reduces bone growth
- Chondrogenesis in fracture healing is directly hampered by smoking reducing chances to good union producing pseudarthrosis
- Smoking also increases chances of infection and osteomyelitis.

CONCLUSION

- The human skeleton is made of a strong and stable framework of bones that are finely engineered composite tissue present in various shapes and forms.
- Bone is a living tissue with active synchronization and evolution of its cellular elements chiefly composed of osteoblasts, osteoclasts, and osteocytes. The osteocytes form the largest network of connecting cells throughout the body. Osteoblasts and osteoclasts act in synchronization to form and reform the bone.
- The basic framework of the bone is formed by the collagen molecules and a lot of them are available serving minutely different purposes but type 1 collagen predominates in bone. Mineralization of collagen is specific and unique to bone giving it the "hard" consistency a property found only for bone.
- Bone is an active metabolic tissue with quite predominant blood supply and like other tissues also has neural supply that has trophic influences. In immature skeleton the bone grows at the ends for increase in length while perimetric growth also occurs by appositional bone formation. Physis or growth plate of the bone is a specialized tissue which is very sensitive to metabolic influences and genetic factors—any error at some or the other stage is responsible for various malformations and osseous defects.
- The process of bone formation, remodeling, and calcium metabolism is highly regulated by local and systemic factors chiefly hormones (endocrinopathies have their discrete manifestations on skeleton), but one of the unique influences comes from mechanical factors like the stress on the skeleton (Wolff's law).

CHAPTER 2

Fracture Repair, Bone Grafting, and Bone Banking

Manish Kumar Varshney

INTRODUCTION

Injury to bone and resulting insufficiency is a common occurrence needing attention of orthopedic surgeon. Bone is a living tissue as we learnt thoroughly in previous chapter, so it has the capacity to repair itself like all other living tissues but the process is quite sensitive and small derangements derail the same. Successful regeneration of bone and ultimate osseous repair involves numerous modifications in the expression of several gene pathways in correct sequence. We should, hence, be proficient in understanding the biological processes behind bone repair so that the outcome can be optimized. Also one should be able to determine the reason for suboptimal outcome if it unfortunately happens. This will help in reviving and balancing future strategies to redirect treatment so that the morbidity is minimized. Bone grafting and use of extra bone to fill defects of improving biology is a common procedure in trauma and elective orthopedics. It is also a very important component of managing complications of bone healing like delayed and nonunion. Biology of bone grafts, their types, and discreet usage should be also understood to provide the best option to the patient in need. Bone banking is a good concept that is foreseen to resolve the issue of filling bone defects as needed in orthopedic oncology, revision arthroplasty, and complicated reconstructions. The facility is, however, quite limited in its evolution in India but is expected to improve substantially in near future due to increasing awareness.

DEFINITION AND CLASSIFICATION

Fracture is a break in the continuity of a bone along with partial or complete disruption of blood supply to the region, visible radiologically as a uni- or bicortical break. Philosophically experts define fractures as a soft tissue injury in which bone is incidentally involved—highlighting the importance of soft tissue handling and preservation for optimal results of fracture management.

To describe fracture complete information need to be deciphered from the information provider to the others. This should also be documented comprehensively. A useful guide is provided to fracture description including following headings:

- Side and bone involved—left/right femur and humerus
- Condition of skin—open fracture (Gustilo-Anderson—**Table 1**)/closed fracture
- Location within bone—proximal third or middle or distal third or otherwise metaphyseal or diaphyseal fracture. In skeletally immature bone epiphyseal and/or physeal involvement should be communicated (Salter- Harris classification—**Table 2, Fig. 1**)
- Extent of involvement—complete/incomplete fracture
- Displacement (distal fragment with respect to proximal, **Figs. 2A to E**)—anterior, posterior, medial, lateral, overlapping (bayonetting), and distraction
- Angulation (defined by the direction of apex, **Figs. 2A to E**)—anterior/posterior and medial/lateral
- Rotation (distal fragment with respect to proximal, **Figs. 2A to E**)—internal or external rotation
- Fracture pattern **(Fig. 3)**—transverse, oblique, spiral, comminuted, greenstick, torus, etc.

TABLE 1: Classification of open fractures.

Gustilo and Anderson (1976) classification [modified by Gustilo, Mendoza, and Williams (1984)]	***Risk of infection***
Grade I: Clean wound <1 cm in diameter or puncture wound that appears clean with a simple fracture pattern, no skin crushing, or internal degloving	0–12%
Grade II: A laceration >1 cm but <10 cm, without significant soft-tissue crushing, including no flaps, degloving, or contusion. Fracture pattern may be more complex. High velocity trauma	2–12%
Grade III: An open segmental fracture or a single fracture with extensive soft-tissue injury (>10 cm). Injuries older than 8 hours, farm injuries, gunshot injuries, segmental fractures, and fractures with diaphyseal bone loss are also included in this type. Type III injuries are subdivided into three subtypes: 1. *Type IIIA*: Adequate soft-tissue especially periosteal coverage of the fracture despite high-energy trauma or extensive laceration or skin flaps. 2. *Type IIIB*: Inadequate soft-tissue coverage with periosteal stripping and bone damage or bone loss. There is often gross contamination. Soft-tissue reconstruction is necessary. 3. *Type IIIC:* Any open fracture (irrespective of wound size or bone loss/type of fracture) that is associated with vascular injury that mandates repair.	9–55%

TABLE 2: Salter and Harris classification (1963) of physeal fractures.	
Type I	A transverse fracture through the growth plate typically through the hypertrophic zone. This manifests as increased width of physis. As the germinal portion remains intact, there is no growth disturbance
Type II	A fracture through the growth plate and the metaphysis sparing the epiphysis
Type III	A fracture through growth plate and epiphysis sparing the metaphysis. The line of fracture passes from hypertrophic zone of physis and exits through epiphysis damaging the germinal layer. Being intra-articular prompt reduction and fixation is mandatory. Tillaux fracture is a typical example
Type IV	A fracture through all three elements of the bone, the growth plate, metaphysis and epiphysis. The straight fracture line passes through the whole width of physis and is prone to growth disturbances at healing by virtue of linear bony bar formation
Type V	A compression fracture of the growth plate due to crushing force. This results in a decreased height of the growth plate radiologically. The growth disturbance is very common and has a poor prognosis
Type VI (Rang, 1968)	Injury to the peripheral portion of the physis (zone of Ranvier) and a resultant bony bridge formation which may produce an angular deformity
Type VII (Ogden, 1982)	Isolated injury of the epiphysis only—no involvement of physis or metaphysis
Type VIII (Ogden, 1982)	Isolated injury of the metaphysis at the primary and secondary spongiosa region with possible impairment of endochondral ossification
Type IX (Ogden, 1982)	Injury of the periosteum (periosteal avulsion—usually iatrogenic) which may impair intramembranous ossification

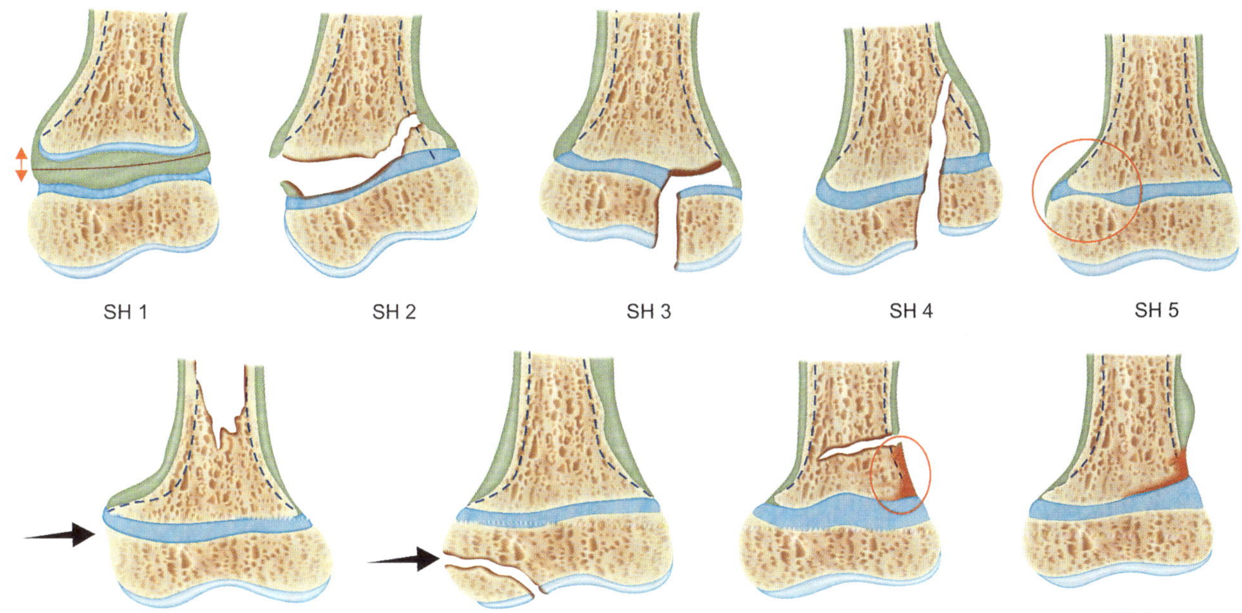

Fig. 1: The Salter–Harris (SH) classification of physeal injuries in skeletally immature patients. (Easy to remember mnemonic with the word "SALTER"—Type-1: **S**lipped epiphysis; Type-2: **A**bove passing fracture line through metaphysis; Type-3: **L**-shaped fracture through epiphysis; Type-4: **T**hrough the physis fracture line across epiphysis-physis-metaphysis; Type-5: **R**ammed physis).

- Condition of joint—intra-articular and extra-articular
- Duration—fresh fracture or old fracture (≥3 weeks)

Fractures can be "incomplete" where the fracture line is not seen to pass through the opposite cortex, viz.

- "Stress fracture" (fatigue fracture) occurring due to excessive compressive stress (usually) or tensile loading
- "Greenstick fracture" of immature skeleton where cortex and periosteum are intact on concave side
- "Cortical rupture" in bone tumors
- Other types of incomplete fractures "may not show break in bone" structure at all, viz. "impaction fractures" due to compression force at cancellous bone and "torus fracture" in immature skeleton.

"Complete fractures" can be closed (with skin intact) or "open" ("compound" is misnomer) with a break in overlying skin that can occur from outside in (trauma force) or inside out (sharp bone spike).

"Pathological fractures" occur in structurally abnormal bone such as neoplastic and metastatic lesions, infection, metabolic bone disease (radiopenic bone) or osteopetrosis and bisphosphonate-associated fractures (radiodense bone).

Fractures occurring near bone can be termed "juxta-articular" (just near the articular surface), "intra-articular" (fracture line communicating with joint space) or "extra-articular" (outside joint altogether).

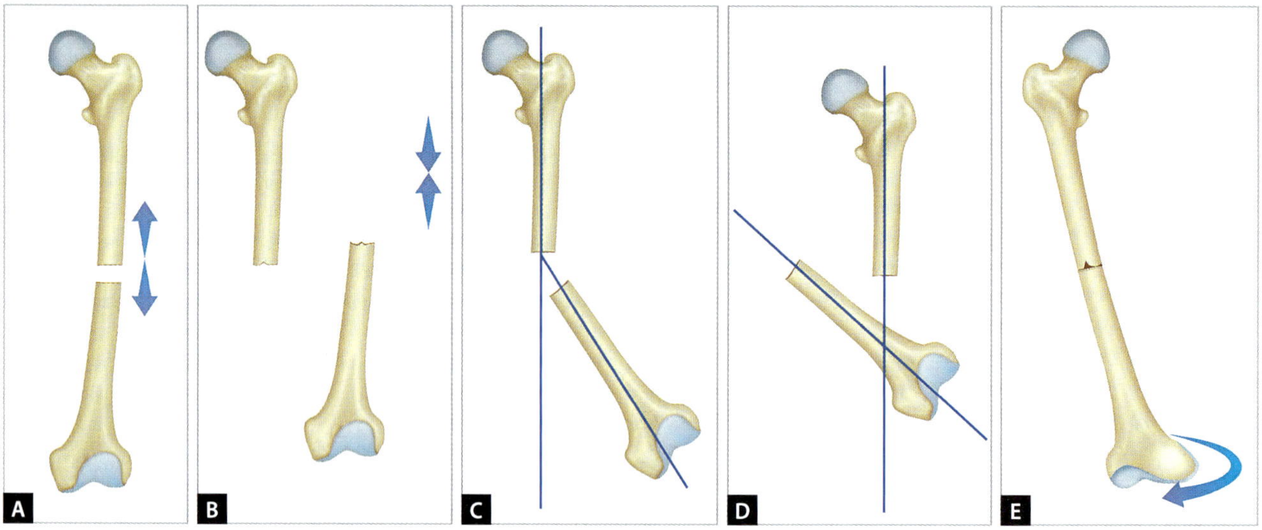

Figs. 2A to E: Common displacements incurred in fractures of long bones.

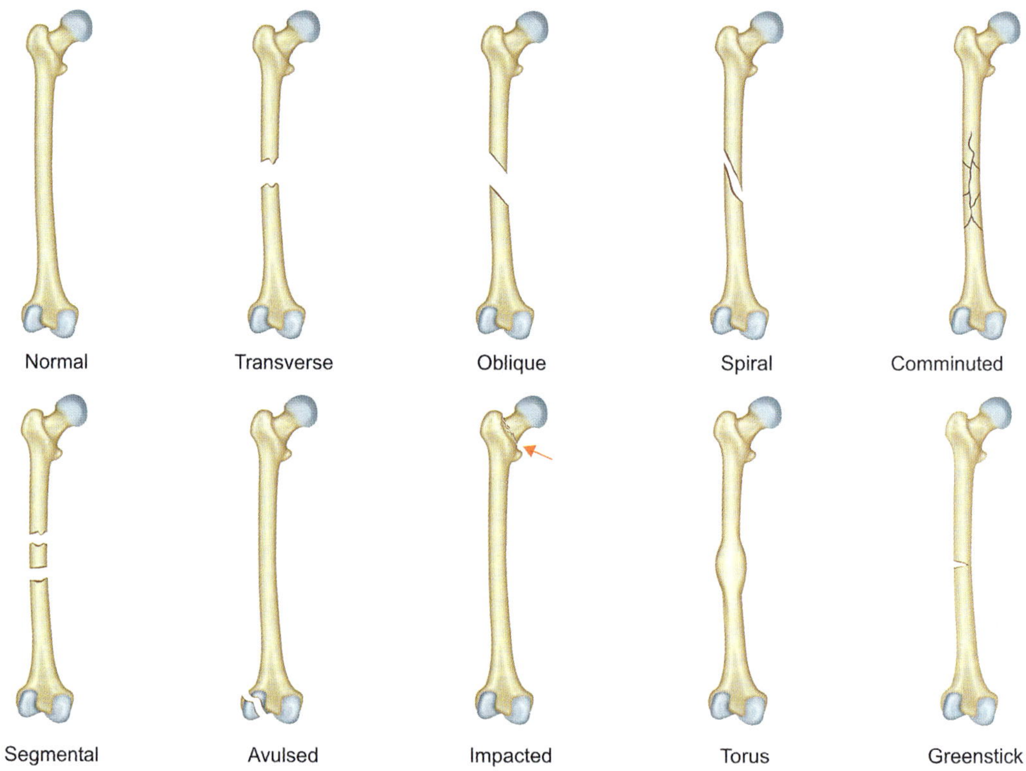

Fig. 3: Various fracture patterns.

Corner or bucket-handle fractures occur in child abuse resulting from violent shaking of the extremity.

"Fracture dislocation" results when the joint surfaces also separate in association with fracture of one or both bones.

Sometimes bone may shatter into pieces at the fracture site into more than two pieces resulting in a "comminuted fracture".

"Avulsion fractures" (traction fractures) occur at the attachment site of ligaments, tendons, or capsule, here, the bone fragment is pulled with the soft tissue.

Fractures impose lot of added physiological demand on body, also there can occur complications if the fractures are not treated properly **(Table 3)**. Conventionally fractures were stabilized by cast treatment or prolonged splinting that led to development of local and systemic complications collectively called "fracture disease" **(Table 4)**. Modern orthopedics deals predominantly with reducing the morbidity of fractures by rationally using operative and various stabilization procedures that are still evolving.

TABLE 3: Complications of fractures and repair process.

Local	*Systemic*
Vascular injury	Shock
Orgonal and muscle injury	Fat embolism
Neural injury	Deep vein thrombosis and thromboembolism
Ligament and capsular injury	SIRS
Compartment syndrome and Volkmann's ischemic contracture	ARDS
Nonunion and malunion	Septicemia
Fracture disease	Gangrene and tetanus (open fractures)
Myositis ossificans (heterotopic ossification)	Pulmonary complications (atelectasis and pneumonitis) for bed-ridden patients
Reflex sympathetic dystrophy (CRPS)	
Osteomyelitis	
Growth disturbances pressure ulcers	

(ARDS: adult respiratory distress syndrome; CRPS: complex regional pain syndrome; SIRS: systemic inflammatory response syndrome)

TABLE 5: Local and systemic factors influencing fracture repair.

Local factors	*Systemic factors*
• Type of bone (reduced with pathologic fractures) • Type of fracture (open and comminuted, and bone loss) • Intra-articular fracture • Surrounding soft tissue injury and devascularization • Single or both bone fracture (maintained fibula can produce tibial nonunion) • Soft tissue interposition and distraction • Local bone pathologies such as cysts, fibrous dysplasia, malignancies (neoplastic cells keep eating away the repair response and cells) • Infection (misdirection of energy and inflammatory cells to counter infection rather than healing of bone) • Venous stasis • Type of treatment and fixation (rigid, soft tissue stripping, etc.)	• Age • Activity level (immobilization in the form of bed rest and "space" flight) • Nutritional status • Hormonal factors • Vitamin and mineral deficiencies • Diseases such as diabetes mellitus, anemia, and neuropathies • Drugs (NSAIDs, cytotoxic chemotherapy, fluoroquinolones, phenytoin, calcium channel blockers, steroids, and tetracyclines) • Smoking • Alcohol abuse • Head injury

(NSAIDs: nonsteroidal anti-inflammatory drugs)

TABLE 4: Fracture disease.

George Perkin coined the term fracture disease for morbidity following prolonged immobilization and nonweight bearing	
Stiffness	Of joints by fibrosis and capsular contracture and synovial adherence
Muscle atrophy	Disuse atrophy
Skin atrophy	Due to immobilization and altered sympathetic stimulus, associated with hyperhidrosis later
Circulatory dysfunction	Predominantly due to sympathetic dysfunction, if excessive sympathetic stimulus results RSD can develop
Osteopenia	Under remodeling due to released stress according to Wolff's law

(RSD: reflex sympathetic dystrophy)

PHYSIOLOGY OF FRACTURE REPAIR

"Fracture repair" [if not augmented {by fixation or bone morphogenic protein (BMP)} or interfered (gross displacement, loss of vascularity, etc.)] is a systematic and organized complex cascade of regenerative tissue formation with influences of local and systemic factors, in which bone heals by primary or secondary mechanisms. For a successful fracture repair appropriate cells need to be recruited with simultaneous activation of appropriate genes at a right time in a correct anatomical location. Fracture repair is essentially a "regenerative" process rather than healing as the defect is actually replaced by new bone and not by scar tissue (so fracture "healing" could be a misnomer). The potential of skeleton to regenerate is astounding. Notwithstanding with the healing of other adult tissues that leave a scar tissue, new bone is formed, replaced, and continuously remodeled/modeled until the original site of injury is barely recognizable. Surrounding soft tissue injury is an important determinant to fracture repair by virtue of maintaining good blood supply to the region. Repair may be disrupted at inception (slow union), or "immediately after inception in initial period" (delayed union) or interrupted (nonunion) anytime during the process depending on healing of surrounding soft tissue and synchronization of bone repair. Colloquially it is said that fracture is a soft tissue injury where the bone is incidentally broken. Various other local and systemic factors are also responsible for proper fracture repair **(Table 5 and Fig. 4)**. Three types of fracture repair are noted:

1. Direct intramembranous repair
2. Creeping bone substitution
3. Indirect fracture repair (intramembranous + endochondral bone formation)

Intramembranous Repair (Direct Bone Healing, Gap Healing, Osteonal Remodeling, Contact Healing, and Haversian Remodeling)

There is no callus formation (no cartilaginous/endochondral bone repair phase) and the bone heals directly without any intervening tissue or callus mainly due to rigid fixation. Bones when apposed together anatomically under physiological compression loads heal without any intervening tissue. This is the ideal situation for fracture repair and is the natural course when the gap is below critical limit of 400 μm (some take it to 500 μm). The cutting cones cross from one side to another across the fracture **(Fig. 4)** and the following ossification front heals the fracture in turn. Healing passes through the following stages (see also below in the determinants of fracture repair):

- *Resorption of bone ends*: Compression at fracture, damage to blood supply at the fracture site causes partial resorption of the bone ends.
- *Fibrous tissue formation*: Fibrous tissue forms from the healing hematoma or lying down of inflammatory tissue

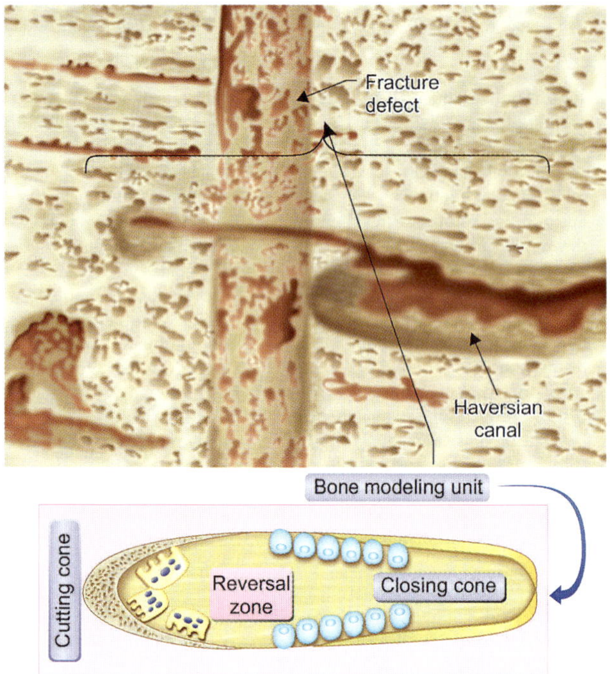

Fig. 4: Repair of fracture defect by a bone modeling unit (primary bone healing) that works across a well-apposed fracture with less than critical fracture defect.

at the gap. It is a very thin layer and predominantly comprises of collagen. The stages of inflammation after granulation tissue are not followed in this type of healing and by virtue of absolute stability, the bone assumes as if it is not broken at all.

- *Maturation to lamellar bone*—because of the close apposition of bone ends the normal process of Haversian remodeling occurs across the fracture site. The advancing osteoclastic migration front in the form of cutting cones cross the fracture site and the fibrous tissue followed by the osteoblastic ossification front and thin capillary vessels that seal the gap.

The above described process of direct bone healing requires anatomic approximation of bone ends and absolute rigidity as in open reduction and internal fixation (ORIF). This minimizes the strain. "Primary cortical healing" occurs at coapted bone ends apposing each other intimately where cortical continuity is established by "cutting cones". Osteoclasts lead the cutting cones leaving void filled by new blood vessels that deposit stem cells at fracture site. Progenitor cells then differentiate into osteoblasts that secrete matrix and bridge fracture gap and also this microcallus is replaced by new osteons. The "cutting cones" thus allow for "direct Haversian remodeling". Common occurrence after ORIF is persistence of small gaps (micrometer sized) at point of contact. Gaps may also arise from resorption of fracture ends fixed under compression. These interstices are repaired by "gap healing". Angiogenesis occurs in these gaps and mesenchymal cells differentiate into osteoblasts repairing the bone as above. This is also the mode of healing in "stress fractures".

Creeping Substitution

Second type is "creeping substitution" (term first used by Phemister) and is primarily seen in cancellous bone. It is typical of intra-articular and periarticular fractures stabilized by rigid fixation anatomically. Creeping substitution is also seen during incorporation of cancellous bone graft. Creeping substitution is the process of resorption of the trabecular network of bone and lying of new bone by appositional ossification on the surface of the scaffold, hence, left (both processes occurring simultaneously). The inside of the newly laid bone microtubes is hollow filled with resorptive material and is gradually replaced with bone. The inflammatory cells and granulation tissue creeps into the tubes and new bone formation occur. They provide the pluripotent cells needed for new bone formation and remodeling. This sandwich architecture of necrotic bone surrounded by viable new bone is remodeled by osteoblastic activity from granulation tissue. Gross architecture of the bone is maintained, hence, the scaffold (dead trabecular bone) is copy-pasted (substituted) by new living bone.

Repair with Bone Callus Formation (Endochondral Repair, Secondary Bone Healing, Indirect Bone Healing)

This is the most common pathway for bone repair and is typical of diaphyseal fractures. This requires some instability and micromotion at the fracture site instigating response in periosteum and neighboring soft tissues. Secondary bone repair involves combination of intramembranous and endochondral ossification. Probably we have been so engrossed by seeing fracture callus in patients treated with cast immobilization and from our classical teaching that we think this to be the standard method of fracture repair. However, this is not so most probably as this requires formation of extraneous tissue (cartilage) and takes longer time to heal. Callus is a preossification cartilage tissue that forms in response to controlled motion rather micromotion at the fracture site and is inhibited by rigid immobilization. Endochondral fracture repair process is also termed secondary bone repair (because there is need for "intermediate tissue" the callus) and can be broadly classified into three main "R" stages **(Fig. 5)** as below (modified from Cruess–Dumont). The modern understanding of the molecular interactions involved is presented in **Table 6** that has bearing on complications of fracture repair and may serve as potential therapeutic targets.

Reactive Stage (Inflammatory Stage)

This stage is akin to inflammatory response seen in response to tissue injury and comprises of two phases:

1. *Hematoma formation and induced inflammation*: Hematoma immediately forms due to blood leak into surroundings from disrupted vessels, periosteum, and endosteum. Blood in a free state (outside vessels) is a reactive tissue and immediately induces local inflammation. This hematoma is vastly responsible for further stages and osteogenesis as demonstrated

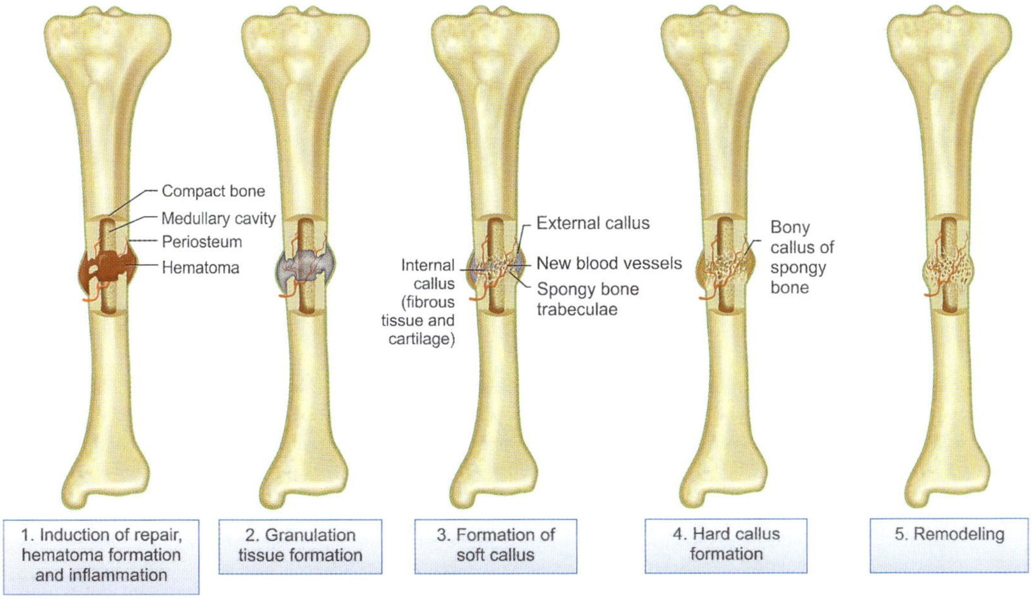

Fig. 5: Fracture repair by callus formation (secondary bone healing).
Note: This is not the primary mode of fracture healing, formation of callus shows a compromised state wherein bone has to take help of complementary tissue (callus) for healing the defect.

TABLE 6: The involvement of molecular mechanisms in various stages of indirect bone repair. Also mentioned is their role in pathogenesis of complications of bone repair and possible therapeutic targets for improving bone repair process.

Cellular elements	*Factors/enzymes/mediators*	*Pathophysiological role*	*Remarks*
Reactive/inflammatory phase:			
Macrophages, polymorphonuclear leukocytes (PMNs), and T-lymphocytes	Interleukin (IL)-1, IL-6, and tumor necrosis factor (TNF)-α	Establishing inflammation and inception of bone repair	
Platelets	• Transforming growth factor (TGF)-β family including bone morphogenic protein (BMP) and growth and differentiation factors (GDFs) • Platelet derived growth factor (PDGF)	• BMP-2 and GDF-8 expressed as early response genes • BMP-2 activates endochondral ossification by inducing chondrogenesis and periosteal osteogenesis	
	Integrins like plasma fibronectin	• Found within 3 days • Bridges for cell-to-cell and cell-to-ECM interaction • Associated with callus establishing provisional fibers and attachments in developing cartilaginous matrices • Integrins also activate signal transduction pathways for cell life cycle, cellular shape, and motility	• Upregulates new cell membrane receptors such as vascular endothelial growth factor (VEGF), PDGF, and epidermal growth factor (EGF) • Forces cellular decision for future biological action such as cellular attachment, movement, death, and differentiation. Cell adhesion through integrin and α-actinin helps differentiation into osteoblastic lineage
	• Arachidonic acid metabolism • Cyclooxygenase (COX)-1 and COX-2 metabolize arachidonic acid into prostaglandin (PG) G2 and H2, respectively • 5-lipoxygenase (5-LO) metabolizes arachidonic acid into leukotrienes	• Platelet aggregation • Vasoconstriction • Leukotrienes have chemotactic effect, increase vascular permeability, and phagocytosis, cause edema	• COX-2 is specific to inflamed tissue, so COX-2 inhibitors are a risk factor for fracture healing • 5-LO inhibitors accelerate fracture bridging time, increase callus size and its mechanical properties. Inhibiting 5-LO increases COX-2 expression accelerating chondrogenesis and reducing healing time
	• Wnt pathway • All 3 pathways activate by binding of wnt protein ligand to frizzled receptors activating protein "disheveled" inside cell	• Effect on TGF-β transcription • Canonical pathway important for conversion of undifferentiated MSCs to osteoblastic lineage	• Inducing wnt increases bone healing while inhibiting, it causes osteopenia. Antisclerostin antibodies (romosozumab) promote bone formation and increase callus. Parathyroid hormone and PGE2 inhibit sclerostin production. Calcitonin increases sclerostin production

Contd...

Contd...

Cellular elements	Factors/enzymes/mediators	Pathophysiological role	Remarks
	• Sclerostin (produced by osteocyte) is Wnt-inhibitor. Antagonism of BMP-induced bone formation by sclerostin is mediated by Wnt signaling and not BMP-signaling pathways		• Lithium can be used to modulate β-catenin stimulating bone healing
Reparative stage:			
Chondroprogenitor MSCs, chondrocytes, revascularization, cartilage-specific matrix proteins, and type-II collagen		Soft callus formation	Protein synthesis is complete by 2 weeks and calcium is released into extracellular matrix by hypertrophic chondrocytes for mineralization
Platelets	• Platelet concentrate (α-granules) containing PDGF-AA, -BB, -AB, TGF-β (β1 and β2 isomers), platelet factor-4, IL-1, platelet derived angiogenesis factor, vascular endothelial growth factor (VEGF), epidermal growth factor (EGF), and epithelial growth factor, platelet-derived endothelial growth factor, insulin like growth factor (IGF), osteocalcin, osteonectin, fibrinogen, vitronectin, thrombospondin, and fibronectin • BMP-2 and GDFs	• PDGF and TGF-β have important role in soft callus formation • TGF-β activates fibroblasts (collagen formation), endothelial cells for angiogenesis, chondroprogenitor cells for cartilage • PDGF induces mitogenesis and improves life of MSCs and osteoprogenitor cells. It also activates macrophages that produce tissue debridement • BMP-2 induces chondrogenesis and periosteal osteogenesis (intramembranous ossification). GDF-8 guide MSCs to chondro-osteogenic lineage. GDF-5 and TGF-β 2 and 3 play role in chondrogenesis	• Platelet concentrate is being used at delayed union and nonunions to stimulate bone repair • Recombinant PDGF has been approved by FDA as an alternative to autograft for ankle and hindfoot fusions • Recombinant BMP is used in spinal fusions and treatment of recalcitrant nonunions
Mature and hypertrophic cartilage, budding membrane structures, matrix vesicles, neovascularization, osteoblast progenitors, and chondroclasts		Mature (hard) callus formation	Calcification of matrix occurs as the chondrocyte proliferation stops
	• Matrix vesicles from chondrocytes are produced a budding membrane structures. They contain enzymes for mineralization such as phosphodiesterase and phosphatases, and proteolytic enzymes • Chondroclasts remove calcified cartilage allowing neovascularization and migration of osteoprogenitor cells	• Proteoglycans inhibit mineralization so they are cleaved by proteolytic enzymes. Phosphatases degrade matrix phosphodiesters to release phosphate ions required for precipitation with calcium • Action of chondroclasts remodel primary spongiosa (early calcified cartilage) into secondary spongiosa (woven bone) which is further converted to lamellar bone	
Remodeling phase:			
Osteoblast and osteoclast	• Receptor activator of nuclear factor-kappa B ligand (RANKL) found on osteoblasts activates RANK in monocytes (osteoclast precursors) modulating their fusion to form multinucleated osteoclasts and also stimulates osteoclasts • Macrophage colony stimulating factor activate RANKL expression in fractured bone	• Osteoblast-osteoclast interaction produces remodeling • Activation of RANK by RANKL promotes maturation of preosteoclasts into osteoclasts	• Native bone has minimal RANKL-RANK activity. It increases manifold in fractures. RANKL overproduction is also seen in rheumatoid arthritis and psoriatic arthritis • Denosumab mimics natural action of OPG reducing differentiation of osteoclast precursors into osteoclasts and regulating bone resorption of osteoclasts • Strontium ranelate increases bone deposition by osteoblasts and regulates

Contd...

Contd...

Cellular elements	Factors/enzymes/mediators	Pathophysiological role	Remarks
	• Osteoprotegerin (OPG) is endogenous RANKL inhibitor serving as decoy receptor for RANKL. It reduces osteoclast activation and bone loss • Estrogen suppresses RANKL signaling • PTH stimulates osteoblasts to increase expression of RANKL and inhibits OPG expression. This increases osteoclastic activity and bone resorption if given continuously. Intermittent administration of PTH activates osteoblasts much more than osteoclasts producing net increase in bone formation • PTHrP is found in all body tissues and regulates cell growth, survival, and differentiation. It stimulates bone formation without increasing bone breakdown (only anabolic effect seen)		bone resorption by osteoclasts (dual action bone agent). It increases OPG secretion by osteoblasts • Effects of estrogen are responsible for accelerated bone healing seen in fetus (second and third trimester). Progesterone helps bone formation and healing in first trimester. Hyperdynamic circulation might also have similar role • PTH is used off-label to speed fracture healing and treat nonunions. It increases fracture callus volume, increases bone mineral content, and total osseous volume • Bisphosphonates inhibit osteoclastic activity. Animal studies have shown increased callus volume, trabecular bone volume, and bone mineral content after bisphosphonate treatment but this is associated with delayed maturation and remodeling of callus so the effects on bone repair are unclear

(ECM: extracellular matrix; MSC: mesenchymal stem cell; PGE2: prostaglandin E2)

by Mizuno et al. They demonstrated that as early as fourth day, the hematoma has "osteogenic power" that progressively increases. Hematoma at fracture site lifts periosteum and underlying cells die, also pressure effect of hematoma produces ischemia. The fibroblasts survive bone necrosis, the extent of which is determined by degree of impact. Cellular toxicity induces chemotactic cytokine response and is responsible for the "regional acceleratory phenomenon" (RAP) as described by Frost. Complicated cellular process of cellular recruitment, migration, multiplication, osteoblast and osteoclast differentiation, mineralization control, and remodeling control ensues as part of RAP. Osteoblast progenitors are recruited by osteogenic induction of undifferentiated cells from bone marrow and mesenchymal cells from "cambium" layer of periosteum. Osteoclasts come from hemopoietic cells of bone marrow. BMPs help in differentiation of cells to osteoblasts, clasts, and cytes. These cells then migrate to fracture focus. Under the influence of platelet-derived growth factor (PDGF) and transforming growth factor-β (TGF-β); the progenitor cells proliferate into colony forming unit fibroblasts (CFU-F), all collectively forming granulation tissue. Other cytokines and paracrine influences on the cells are derived from inhibin, activins, BMPs, nodal related genes, glial derived neurotropic factor, αFGF, βFGF and IGF-1. Most of these are mitogenic (some authors have cited uncontrolled activation from these factors to cause "tumor formation and neoplasia development" later—as a practicing orthopedic surgeon we so commonly find trauma at the site related by the patients to neoplasia. Personally I am unsure of this relationship but true is the fact that many patients do report local trauma months/weeks ago and logical could be the derivation that uncontrolled activation of mitogens could cause neoplasia formation). Mineralization is controlled by systemic factors regulating calcium and phosphorus metabolism. Inflammation usually reaches its peak at 48 hours and then is modulated according to the treatment a fracture is receiving.

2. *Granulation tissue formation*: The hematoma is infiltrated by developing vessels from surrounding healing tissue under effect of vascular endothelial growth factor (VEGF) and fibroblast growth factor (FGF). The proliferating fibroblasts (that survive ischemia) along with ingrowing vessels evolve into fibrovascular granular tissue rich in type II collagen. This stage lasts some 2 weeks. This is biochemically "mesenchymal" step and is predominated by collagen type 1, 2, 3, and 5. Access to substrate molecules (oxygen, glucose, and amino acids) and clearance of metabolic products (CO_2, lactate, and urea) are of critical importance to cell survival. The processes by which molecules are moved in and out of a fracture or graft site are collectively referred to as "mass transport". This process may be mediated by fluid flow (convection, e.g., with muscle contraction) or by diffusion of molecules along concentration gradients or in response to electromagnetic forces. At distances greater than 200 μm, the transport of oxygen and other nutrients rapidly becomes a limiting factor for cell survival. As a general rule, there is an inverse square relationship between cell concentration and the depth of cell survival, such that fourfold reduction in the concentration of implanted cells will double the depth of their survival within an implant.

Reparative Stage

This stage essentially comprises of reparative tissue deposition and can be divided into following phases:

Phase of callus formation: Callus is the bone regenerative tissue that forms in response to micromotion at the bone injury site aimed to naturally unite the two opposed stabilized bone ends. Formation of callus reduces the interfragmentary strain by increasing surface area and thus improving local environment toward healing. The formation of callus is a combined effect of four distinct healing responses as outlined by Einhorn emanating from the bone marrow, the periosteum (most important), bone cortex proper, and external soft tissues (response mounted by surrounding muscles and mesenchymal tissue). There are two histologically varied forms of callus that can be recognized:

1. *Soft callus (primary callus)*: After 2 weeks the periosteal derived cells few millimeter proximal from fracture develop into chondroblasts to form hyaline cartilage, distally somehow the cells from cambium layer develop into osteoblasts and deposit the organic matrix (osteoid substance with disorganized collagen fibers) and woven bone rapidly. New osteoblasts can be derived from many cells such as periosteum (cambium layer), muscle derived cells, blood vessel cells (pericytes), and bone marrow fat mesenchymal stem cells (MSCs). The osteoblasts are modulated by various factors throughout fracture repair **(Fig. 6 and Table 6)**. This is biochemically "chondroid-osteoid" step predominated by collagen type 1, 2, and 10. In contact with periosteum, the bone lamina forms proximally creating bone bridge. At the fracture site the cells deposit hyaline cartilage and as the focus solidity increases the cartilaginous cells hypertrophy and cartilage progressively mineralizes by endochondral ossification. This is biochemically "chondroid" step predominated by type two and nine collagen. There are three types of callus formation at the site of fracture. (1) "Periosteal bridging callus" typically develops in the above described fashion. It should be realized that amount of periosteal callus has no relation to the size of initial hematoma, but reflects the need for ancillary stabilization required if blood supply is adequate and is inversely related. In addition to the periosteal callus a slowly developing (2) "intramedullary callus" is laid down from inside the bone supplied by medullary arterial system. This has double concave shape with periphery adhered to endosteum and is the predominant response during "gap repair". (3) Third type is the "intercortical uniting callus" occupying the space between the opposed cortices of fractured ends. Its size is totally dependent on reduction and apposition of bone ends so that it is absent in compressed plating. Apart from above a fourth type of tissue is also seen called "external soft tissue" response (not a true callus) that develops from vascular mesenchymal tissue like muscles and is important in fracture repair as absence of the same has been cited as one of the reasons for nonunion of distal third tibial fractures. These four types of callus responses have been incorporated in the philosophy of "fracture healing process" propounded by McKibbin (see below). Differentiation of progenitor cells depends on type of strain delivered (see also Parren Theory below) and oxygen tension. High strain and/or low oxygen produce fibrogenic differentiation and fibrous tissue. Rigid fixation with low strain and high oxygen promotes direct woven bone formation (intramembranous ossification); intermediate strain, and low oxygen promotes cartilage formation (endochondral ossification). Mobile regions (relative stability, e.g., with nailing) with hydrostatic loading (compressive stress) at fracture produces cartilaginous differentiation, while tensile loading produces fibrocartilaginous differentiation. The mineralization progresses from immature bone bridge toward focus. The fracture during this stage is "sticky", i.e., it is deformable (can be angulated) but not displaceable (ends cannot be separated) by physiologic loads. Supervised mobilization can begin during this stage. As this step involves prominent migration of osteoprogenitor cells from cambium layer of periosteum, the areas of bone lacking this remain deficient in the

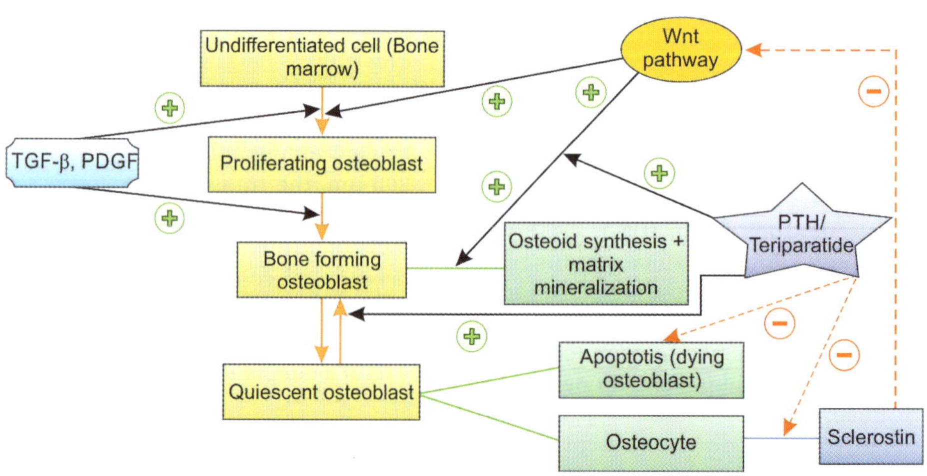

Fig. 6: Illustration depicting the influences from various factors modulating the function of osteoblasts during fracture repair. Also depicted is the potential impact of various therapeutic drugs. (PDGF: platelet-derived growth factor; PTH: parathyroid hormone; TGF: transforming growth factor)

soft callus response like the neck of femur; making them vulnerable to nonunion.

2. *Hard callus*: As the immature bone grows strong the woven bone gradually transforms into primary lamellar bone. This bone, however, grows in many directions. The transformation usually commences in fourth week and finishes around 16th week. The amount of callus formation is dependent primarily on oxygen tension but also on strain pattern (treatment) at the fracture site.

Phase of consolidation (lamellar bone deposition): There is resorption of bone ends with bridging callus formation. The fracture line becomes vague. The initially-deposited collagen is predominantly type 2 that is gradually replaced by type 1 collagen on which mineral phase quickly deposits. This is biochemically "osteoid" step and is predominated by type 1 collagen. The process of formation of lamellar bone in hyaline cartilage is termed endochondral ossification while formation of lamellar bone from woven bone is called bony substitution and both processes occur simultaneously in consolidation. Mineralization of fracture callus is an essential step in bone formation that depends on degradation of proteoglycans affected by endopeptidase and deposition of crystals affected by alkaline phosphatase.

Remodeling

Semantically remodeling is the constant recycling of minerals (calcium and phosphate) from bone to maintain homeostasis. Over a prolonged period of time the term has, however, come to recognize correction of angulation and translation to restore acceptable alignment that is though incorrect but widely accepted and followed. We will continue to use the word "remodeling" for same impression without complicating the issue further. Remodeling is the process of slow restoration of normal bone structure, passing through stages of primary lamellar bone (multidirectional osteons) to secondary lamellar bone (longitudinal osteons). The stage starts during reparative stage and continues even after clinical bone union (up to 7 years). Remodeling is based on the special units called "bone modeling units" described by Frost. This is spearheaded by osteoclasts covering the bonnet shape capillary vessels cutting into the previous bone, resorbing the bone in areas of depression called "Howship lacunae". These "cutting cones" are followed by osteoblasts depositing new mature bone (concentric lamellar). This structural modification continues indefinitely according to the functional load and stress pattern on the bone (Wolff's law). Factors and medications modulating the osteoclastic activity are depicted in **Figure 7**.

The potential for remodeling is influenced by a number of factors as follows:

- *Proximity to appendicular skeleton*: Proximal humerus is more apt for remodeling than distal radius or ulna.
- *Juxtaphyseal deformities*: Usually the physes are aligned perpendicular to long axis of bones. So any deformity that places physis out of place would correct readily. This is affected by increased growth at the concave side while reduced growth at the convex side of deformity, following the Hüeter–Volkmann law. Such type of remodeling would correct 75% of the angular deformity. Diaphyseal correction following Wolff's law would correct the rest of 25% of deformity provided growth potential remains. According to Wolff's law bone would be deposited on the concave side where it is required more mechanically due to stress concentration while resorption would take place at the convex side where tensile strain predominates.

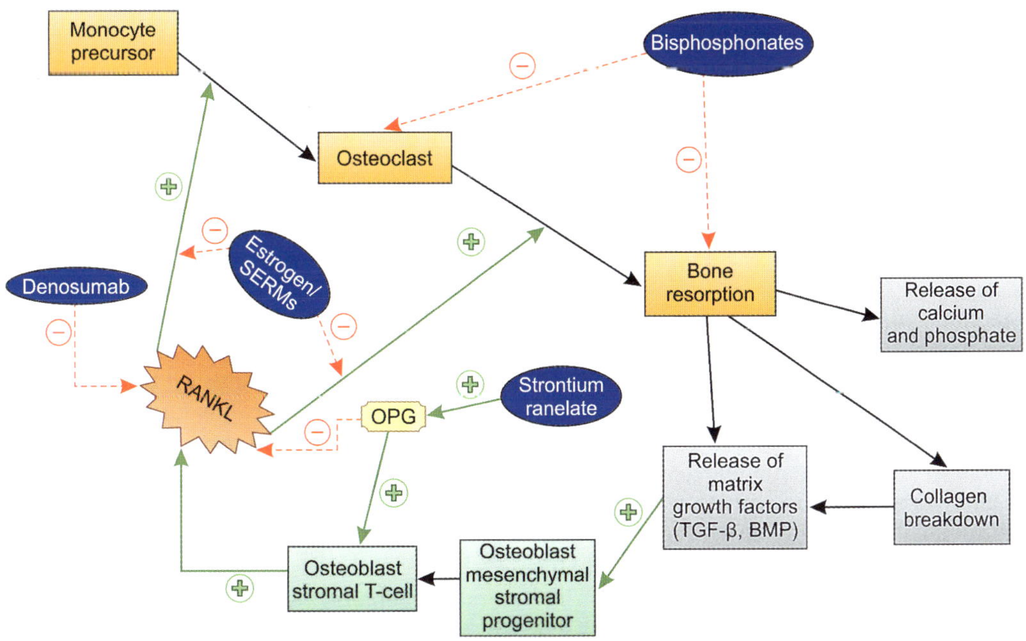

Fig. 7: Modulation of osteoclasts during fracture repair and remodeling. Also depicted are the effects of various therapeutic drugs. (BMP: bone morphogenic protein; OPG: osteoprotegerin; SERM: selective estrogen receptor modulators; TGF: transforming growth factor)

- *Place of the affection of physis*: The physes that grow rapidly and contribute to the overall growth of skeleton most would help to remodel a fracture fast. Considering this fact proximal humerus fractures (proximal humerus physis contributes to 80% of humeral growth), distal radius fractures (75% contribution to radius growth), distal femoral fractures (70% growth contributed for femur). Tibial growth is more evenly distributed with 55% occurring proximally and 45% distally so remodeling potential is more evenly distributed.
- *Fracture location*: Metaphyseal fractures would remodel better and faster due to high bone turnover than diaphyseal deformities.
- *Geometry of deformity*: Deformities that occur in the same plane as the predominant motion at the adjacent joint would remodel fastest and to fullest. This explains why rotational malalignments would remodel the least in limbs.
- *Age of patient*: It is well understood that girls stop growing in height by around 14 years of age while skeletal maturity is reached in boys by 16 years of age after which remodeling potential reduces drastically and is minimal.
- *Pathological bone*: Remodeling potential of bone is compromised heavily under the influence of metabolic bone diseases such as rickets, osteomalacia, osteogenesis imperfecta, skeletal dysplasia, etc. Correction of deformity under such circumstances by interventionist measures (surgical or otherwise) is a must rather than relying on the intrinsic capability of bone to do so.

Strength at the fracture site gradually improves overtime and is further classified into four progressive stages depending on the physical strength gained at the fracture site:

- *Stage 1*: Torsional testing causes failure at the fracture site in a low-resistance pattern
- *Stage 2*: Similar to stage 1 but in a high-resistance pattern
- *Stage 3*: In torsional testing the bone fails partly at the original fracture site and partly in the previous intact bone.
- *Stage 4*: Failure does not occur at the original fracture site.

Alternative Proposed Patterns of Fracture Repair

Apart from above commonly accepted pattern of fracture repair, "Frost" also proposed stages of fracture repair that delineates five stages, viz.

1. Stage of hematoma formation
2. Stage of granulation tissue (inflammation and cellular proliferation)
3. Stage of callus
4. Stage of remodeling

Stage of modeling—the terms remodeling and modeling are often used interchangeably and without proper understanding. While remodeling simply means "restructuring" the fractured bone to its prefracture form, modeling on the other hand is a continuous process that extends even beyond the native structure of bone is regained. Bone modeling adapts osseous structure to loading by changing bone size and shape and removes damage in a way this process is a part and parcel of even normal bone that maintains its strength. So, bone modeling is under the influences of mechanical stress/strain (as explained by Wolff's law, etc.) that adapts the biological form. One should remember, however, that same mechanical stress/strain principles and Wolff's law also apply for process of remodeling. Modeling is, however, a continuous process where bone "models" itself depending on the needs whether mechanical or functional. So, in essence, fracture repair should end at end of remodeling stage but as remodeling and modeling are overlapping processes stage of modeling is mentioned as a continuum of the repair process. The "fracture healing process" as propounded by McKibbin incorporates the basis of four types of callus responses described above to explain the process of fracture repair.

1. *Primary callus response (involves part of periosteal bridging callus and intercortical callus)*: Viable osteoblasts from apposed bone fragments incorporate in the soft callus. Unable to bridge the fracture gap completely and failure will produce horse hoof nonunion. This response is very swift to initiate and progress and quickly resolves the tolerance to movement; it also is predominant response in total rigidity.
2. *External bridging callus (incorporates the periosteal bridging callus and external soft tissue response)*: By far this is the most predominant callus response manifested by extensive callus tissue formation and clinically palpable swelling at the fracture site by 2–3 weeks and later. This is the predominant response of osseous tissue in closed treatment methods and cast immobilization. Periosteal totipotent and pluripotent cells take part in the callus response. It forms fast (less than previous response) but has marvelous ability to bridge the fracture gap. If total rigidity (rigid fixation) prevails, this response will be absent absolutely. The external bridging callus develops in accordance with Wolff's law. Larger the diameter higher is the torsional and bending resistance. Torsional resistance is proportional to four times the radius (4 × R) so increased callus diameter as seen in functional cast bracing of long bones due to cyclic muscular movements will have higher resistance to strain and loading.
3. *Late-medullary callus (involves intramedullary callus)*: This is a combination of appositional and endochondral ossification and is an essential step to formation of hard callus. It is slow to develop but has the best ability to bridge the fracture gap. The response is seen both in closed treatment of fractures and rigid fixation.
4. *Primary cortical response (involves intercortical callus)*: This is slowest to develop and is dependent on rigid fixation and hard callus formation. It is seen by 50–80 days and progresses very slowly at the rate of 1 mm every 3 weeks.

IMPORTANT DETERMINANTS OF FRACTURE REPAIR

Fracture repair is a sensitive process and can be easily altered by various intrinsic, extrinsic, and treatment-related factors **(Flowchart 1)**. Some commonly seen important influences are described below.

Method of Treatment

Stability at the fracture site determines the differentiation of progenitor cells and the amount of callus formation. Different modalities used provide for different types of repair and knowledge can be used for our clinical use **(Table 7)**. With absolute stability, rigid fixation, and low strain environment there is no movement (500–2,000 microstrain) at the fracture site and fracture heals with "primary fracture repair" at diaphyseal site (even where secondary bone repair usually is the rule). Primary fracture repair (intramembranous repair) does not pass through above-mentioned stages. Primary fracture repair is not inferior or superior method of repair but is essential normal process of fracture repair in dense cancellous bone (no or minimal callus forms) and intracapsular fractures where cambium layer of periosteum is deficient as in fracture neck of femur. With plating a fracture and establishing absolute stability we remove the local hematoma and create a periosteal wound this suppresses callus formation. This is desired in intra-articular fractures where callus would disturb intra-articular congruity. There are two fate of this fixation, if a gap is left between the fracture ends a gap repair occurs; else with compressed ends a primary contact repair ensues.

1. *Gap primary fracture repair (gap <400* μm): Intramedullary callus plays a predominant role in this repair. By 6 weeks marrow callus completely occupies the canal and vessels grow from it up to the cortical gap surrounded by granulation tissue. Over this the osteoid and woven bone is laid out filling the gap. This immature bone is continuous with the marrow callus and is oriented transversely to the longitudinal axis of bone and Haversian system. In the second stage that takes months, Haversian longitudinal remodeling occurs and normal bone structure is restored. This second stage consists of "cutterheads" passing from one side of fracture to other (diaphyseal cortex) according to ARF scheme (activation, resorption, and formation), welding the fracture.
2. *Contact primary repair (primary cortical healing and Haversian remodeling)*: With compression at fracture site the osteons at both ends are opposed so close that the first stage of gap repair is omitted and "cutterheads" follow the ARF scheme from start "osteonal remodeling". Tunneling produced by "cutterheads" is followed by

Flowchart 1: Determinants and various inhibitory influences (left-hand side) on fracture healing.

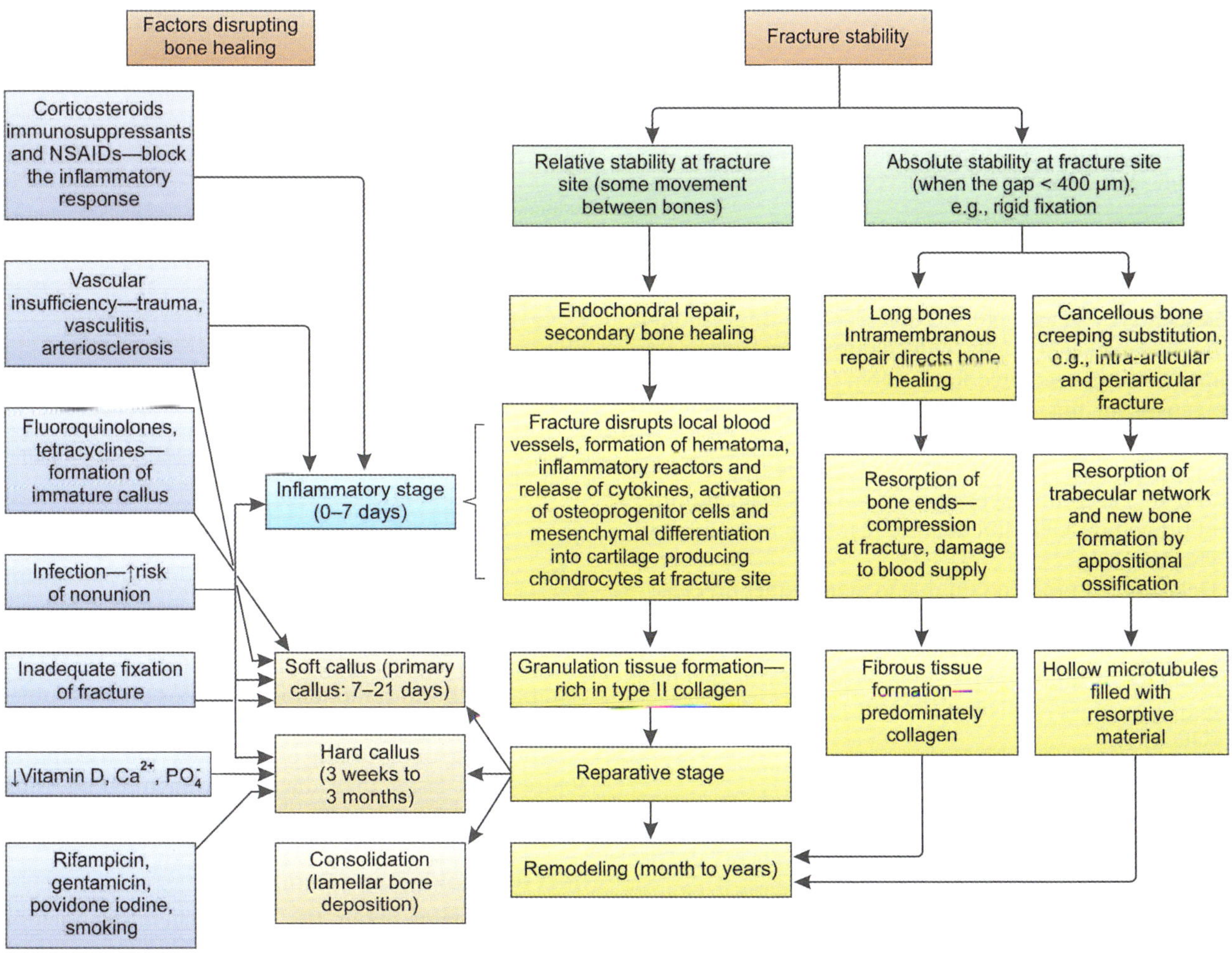

(NSAIDs: nonsteroidal anti-inflammatory drugs)

TABLE 7: Type of stabilization and its impact on fracture repair (it is assumed that no nonunion results).

Type of stabilization	*Predominant type of repair*
Plaster of Paris cast	Endochondral ossification
DCP plating	• Gap repair without compression • Primary cortical repair (Haversian remodeling) with compression • Endochondral repair can occur on opposite side
Locked plating in rigid mode and compression	Primary cortical repair
Open reduction and locked plate in "elastic mode"	Combination of primary cortical repair and endochondral repair (predominates)
MIPPO	Endochondral repair
Intra-articular fractures fixed with plate	Creeping substitution at cancellous surface and primary cortical repair (no callus)
Intramedullary nail	Early periosteal callus and endochondral repair. Late intramembranous repair
External fixator	• *Elastic*: Endochondral repair through periosteal bridging callus • *Rigid*: Primary cortical repair
Wire loops	Creeping substitution at cancellous bone and endochondral repair at diaphysis

(DCP: dynamic compression plate; MIPPO: minimally invasive percutaneous plate osteosynthesis)

capillaries and activated osteoblasts eventually forming the Haversian system. This also explains why we should achieve compression of fracture ends if we are aiming for absolute stability. It should be, however, recognized that the side opposite to plate fixation still can produce secondary bone repair by callus formation commonly seen as it is difficult to achieve "absolute" stability and uniform compression always.

Endocrine Influence and Effect of Local Growth Factors on Fracture Repair

The various influences of local growth factors and hormones are detailed in **Table 8**.

Effect of Age and Site of Fracture

Fracture healing is faster in younger patients (children and adolescents) by a factor of 1.5–2 times, i.e., the time required for fracture to heal in elderly (older than 60 years) will be 1.5–2 times than that required for children for similar fracture. The causes for this difference have been studied and are possibly as follows:

- Delay in onset of periosteal reaction (due to periosteal and its cambium layer atrophy)—decreased number of progenitor cells and delayed response to TGF-β and vitamin D.
- Delay in cell proliferation due to aging effect on cells—decrease in the division capacity of cells.
- Decreased bone formation—lower osteoinductive capacity of bone matrix, increased ratio of receptor activator of NF-κB ligand (RANKL) to osteoprotegerin (OPG).
- Delayed angiogenic invasion of cartilage—decreased blood vessel formation. There is reduced expression of PDGF-BB in endothelial progenitor cells in elderly. Hypoxia-inducible factor-1α and transcripts of "VEGF" are expressed promptly in young patients early in course of fracture repair. This is partly mediated by expression of MMP9 and 13 that are also expressed early (3–7 days) in the young but take 21 days in elderly.

TABLE 8: Endocrine and paracrine influence on fracture repair.

Growth factors/hormones	*Action*
TGF-β (platelets, inflammatory cells, chondrocytes, and osteoblasts)	Progenitor cell stimulation
BMPs (chondrocyte and osteoblasts)	Cartilage formation, recruitment, proliferation, differentiation, and enhancement
FGF (inflammatory cells, chondrocytes, and osteoblasts)	Mesenchymal cell proliferation
PDGF (platelets, inflammatorycells, and endothelial cells)	Stimulation of type-I collagen synthesis
IGF chondrocytes and osteoblasts)	Production of type-I collagen stimulation
Cortisone	Decreased callus proliferation
ACTH	Reduce or stop consolidation
Thyroxine	Stimulates consolidation
Growth hormone	Stimulates callus formation
PTH	Stimulates consolidation and remodeling

(ACTH: adrenocorticosteroid hormone; BMP: bone morphogenetic protein; FGF: fibroblast growth factor; IGF: insulin-like growth factor; PDGF: platelet-derived growth factor; PTH: parathyroid hormone; TGF-β: transforming growth factor beta)

- Protracted period of endochondral ossification—changed local and systemic milieu of signaling molecules. Decreased antioxidant levels and higher oxidative damage to regenerating cells.
- Impaired bone remodeling—apoptosis of osteoblasts with aging and glycation of matrix disturbs bone healing.

Depending on location of fractures, the metaphyseal fractures heal faster than diaphyseal fractures and upper limb fractures unite faster than lower limb fractures.

Effect of Smoking and Radiation

Cigarette contains about 109 known chemicals including nicotine, benzene, tar, etc., which harm bone. Nicotine depresses osteoblast activity, may inhibit revascularization of bone graft, has a negative impact on fracture repair, and inhibits the expression of a wide range of cytokines including those associated with neovascularization and osteoblast differentiation. It increases the risk of bone fractures by inducing osteoporosis, reduces estrogen effectiveness, and can counter the antioxidant properties of vitamins C and E. Nicotine has direct effect on arteriolar blood flow and collagen synthesis. Additional suppression of bone anabolism due to smoking comes from chronic hypoxia, hypercarpnia, and increased arteriolar vasospastic activity. Hypoxia affects osteogenic differentiation of human MSCs. The incidence of nonunion is substantial in active smokers. Radiation produces long-term suppressive effects on Haversian system by reducing the vascularity and cellularity. Postoperative radiation reduces bone graft incorporation and should be delayed for 3 weeks. High dose radiation also reduces the structural integrity of bone. Radiation also affects the bone structure, function, and metabolism. Exposing bone to radiation can result in four major types of complications: (1) osteoradionecrosis, (2) fractures, (3) bone growth changes, and (4) radiation-induced cancers. Radiation itself is called a "complete carcinogen", in that it can cause the four phases of cancer's formation: (1) initiation, (2) promotion, (3) progression, and (4) metastatic activity of transformed cells. The minimum latency period for radium-caused tumors is around 3 years with a peak time of about 8 years. Children who receive radiation for cancers (other than those of bony origin) are at particular risk if their growing bones receive large doses of radiation [*see* Chapter on "Orthopedic Oncology (Bone Tumors and Metastasis) and Heterotopic Ossification"].

Miscellaneous Influences on Fracture Repair

- Nonsteroidal anti-inflammatory drug (NSAID) usage during fracture repair is associated with higher incidence of nonunion due to COX-2 inhibition. They are also associated with longer healing times.
- Glucocorticoids also hamper proper fracture repair due to combined anti-inflammatory effect and alteration of calcium metabolism. It is shown to inhibit fracture healing, reduce callus strength, and prolong healing times if taken during fracture repair process.
- Nutritional deficiencies of calcium and vitamin D are associated with impaired fracture repair and nonunion. Similar effects are seen in untreated or decompensated chronic renal and liver disease.
- Diabetes mellitus (DM) impairs fracture healing but pathomechanisms are not very clear. Peripheral vascular disease producing hypoxia and its negative effect on osteoblast proliferation and function reduces healing capacity. Glycosylated collagen has poor strength and its synthesis is also hampered in DM. Type X collagen synthesis is reduced in fracture callus and deficient scaffolding production prevents soft callus response. DM reduces early cellular proliferation, macrophage function, delays endochondral ossification, and reduces biomechanical strength of fracture callus. Treatment with metformin itself slows bone repair. Insulin combined with parathyroid hormone (PTH) may help improve bone repair in DM.
- Alcohol intake independently influence various elements of initial inflammatory response. It has also immunosuppressive effects predisposing to infection and nonunion.
- Local nonmodifiable factors that compromise fracture healing include excessive injury to bone and surrounding soft tissues, interruption of local blood supply, soft-tissue interposition, inadequate reduction or/and immobilization, bone death due to thermal, chemical, radiation burns, or infection.
- Interfragmentary micromotion and low amount of strain stimulate callus response, ossification, and repair. Large amounts of strain and excessive mobility only deposit connective fibrous tissue due to damaged vascularity and deficient inflammatory response producing frank nonunion. These are discussed in great detail below.

LAWS ASSOCIATED WITH FRACTURE REPAIR AND BONE REMODELING

Mechanobiology is the study of the influence of mechanics on biological processes. While we know that bone structure and form is influenced by mechanical factors, hardly do we understand the mechanism by which the mechanical influences translate into biological form completely. For example, we know that interfragmentary micromotion is needed for callus formation but we do not understand as to why physiological axial compressive forces favor the bone formation while interfragmentary strain is detrimental. We, hence, need to understand the repair path under the mechanical influences well and determine ways of limiting interfragmentary strain to improve fracture repair by the surgical methods we adopt/plan.

Wolff's Law

Meyer demonstrated that the spongiosa of cancellous bone shows a well-motivated structure which is closely connected with the statics and mechanics of bone (his drawings stimulated not only orthopedic surgeons but even engineer's like Culmann). Wolff was influenced by Meyer's ideas and in 1869, he claimed that some physiological properties of bone can be proven by the concept that "bone aligns itself along directions of principle stresses". I will here strictly encourage the reader to go through the description of Wolff's law as detailed under "Effect of Stress and Mechanosensory Systems on Remodeling" at the end of topic of remodeling in Chapter on "Bone Structure, Physiology, Metabolism, and Associated Disorders".

The principal directions of a stress tensor at any given point are orthogonal and the trabeculae in bone seem to intersect at right angles. He proposed four principles based on the mechanism of which the last two have been proven wrong:

1. There is perfect mathematical correspondence between the structure of cancellous bone in the proximal femur and trajectories of Culmann's crane. Carl Culmann

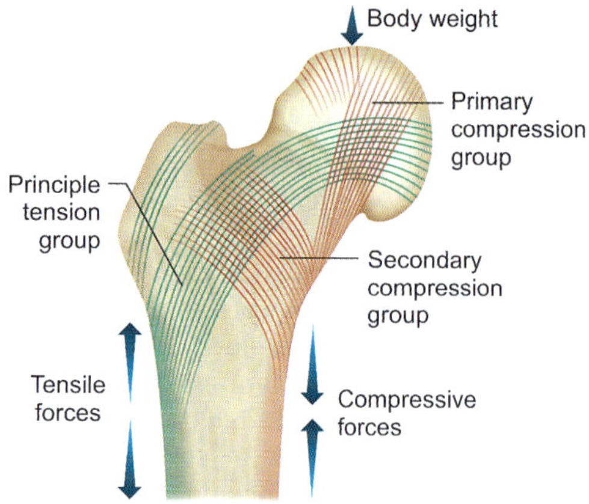

Fig. 8: *Wolff's law*: In accordance with this law the trabeculae in the bones are distributed.

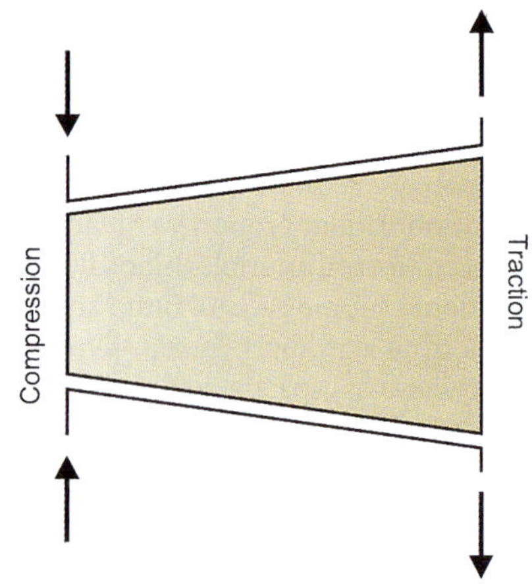

Fig. 9: The Hüeter–Volkmann law for physeal growth (see text for description).

was a German engineer who worked on "graphic mechanics" and pointed out that the lines in Meyer's drawings resembled the principle stress trajectories in cantilever beams. His student made a crane with a curved beam stimulated by Meyer's drawings of internal bone structure of cancellous bone.

2. There is statistical importance and necessity of the trajectory structure of the bone.
3. Bone growth can occur only in the interstitial space (proved wrong).
4. The compact bone is nothing but a compressed cancellous bone (proved wrong).

Wolff concluded from his observations that increased compressive and distraction forces stimulated bone osteoblasts, whereas reduced compressive and distraction forces inhibited them. Moreover, he considered compressive forces to be more important and was impressed by the callus formation at the concave (compression) side of angulated fractures. "Wolff's law of bone transformation" is related to remodeling and states that the bone's trabecular structure adapts to the types of stress it is subjected to, so that structure of bone is dictated by the functional demands. Taking it further a fully developed bone, hence, must serve the function at that part of body as it has developed in response to the functional demands there. So, in short, Wolff's law can also be extended to simply state that "form dictates function" **(Fig. 8)**.

Hüeter–Volkmann Theory (1862)

This is relevant to the physis (growth plate) and physeal growth; it should not be misinterpreted with Wolff's law that applies to bone remodeling. According to this principle excessive compression leads to tissue atrophy and inhibits the physeal growth, whereas decreased compression and moderate distraction enhances osteogenesis promoting bone growth. The effect is such that a physis subjected to angulatory forces will show retarded growth at the compression side **(Fig. 9)** and increased growth at the distraction side (tensile forces). Finely analyzed the bone is adapting itself in the direction of applied force finally and is in congruence with Wolff's law. So essentially both laws tell the same thing that bone develops according to applied forces. Classic relation of Hüeter–Volkmann theory can be seen with the development of congenital scoliosis (and Blount's disease) where the vertebral physis develops according to compression and tensile forces and hence wedge vertebrae with bent spine result.

Mechanical Effects on Fracture Repair

There are various theories that give an understanding into type of tissue response under various forces (stress/strain) acting at the fracture site. This mechanobiological correlation dates back to 1800s when the work of Roux (theory of functional adaptation) attracted the attention of then surgeons engaged in exploring ways to better fracture repair. Pauwels expanded this initial work to suggest some basic principles of tissue histogenesis at fracture site. Before we embark on descriptions we should understand the mechanical terms used as the terminology gets increasingly confusing.

Stress: This defines force acting per unit area (dimensions similar to pressure). If the stress tends to expand an object so that the force acts outward then it is called tensile stress, while stress acting to compress an object with force acting in inward direction is called compressive stress. The term hydrostatic stress is used to describe a state of tensile or compressive stress equal in all directions within or external to a body. Hydrostatic stress causes a change in volume of a material.

Strain: Simply stating strain refers to change in length upon original length. This is a dimensionless factor so has no units. Strain is related to change in dimensions and shape of a material but not necessarily always a change in volume. Due to the fact that the changes in length are quite small so strain in commonly expressed in microstrain ($\times 10^{-6}$). Tensile strain along a linear object would result in increased length while compressive strain would result in shortening changing the dimensions of the object. These types of strains are called *normal strains*. The other type of strain is shear strain where the force is applied parallel to one of the surfaces so that the object gets deformed and, hence, changes in shape this causes changes in the angles but not necessarily change in volume.

The following gives a brief description of the various correlations derived by different researchers in the field of mechanobiologics, most of them though incomplete but do give some insight into the type of tissue expected under different stress/strain conditions or combinations.

Pauwels' Concept

Continuing with the mechanobiologics of bone repair, Pauwels, first, suggested that cellular or extracellular matrix deformation associated with distortional stress (shear strain and pure shear) stimulates mesenchymal cell differentiation into fibroblasts (fibrous tissue) while hydrostatic compression (hydrostatic stress) which causes a volume change favors mesenchymal cell differentiation into chondrocytes (cartilage). Secondly, he suggested that varying combinations of shear and hydrostatic pressure would stimulate differentiation into fibrocartilage (i.e., combination of the two, **Fig. 10**). Lastly, he proposed that primary bone formation requires a stable low strain (not to confuse with shear!) mechanical environment (minimal change in length) so as to successfully complete endochondral bone formation.

Perren Interfragmentary Strain Theory

Perren (1979) and Perren and Cordy (1980) proposed a brilliant hypothesis, the "interfragmentary strain theory", which related the tissue response to the local mechanical environment. With the Pauwels hypothesis we understood that some strain is needed at the fracture site for bone formation but the upper limit of such strain (how maximum) is explained by Perren and Cordy theory of interfragmentary strain. The theory was initially devised to explain the mechanism of "gap healing" or "contact healing" without formation of fracture callus based on longitudinal strain. Perren conceptualized the existence of particular tissue in the fracture gap based on the strain, the region. With progressively increasing strain, the tissue changes from granulation to fibrous to cartilage to osseous. So at very low strains bone would form (in line with Pauwels postulates) while large strain would be only borne by granulation tissue that would never ossify. This theory is better understood if we keep fracture repair by cast immobilization. Understanding the Perren's theory in another way we can consider that as the tissue at the fracture site stiffens (hematoma → granulation tissue → soft callus → hard callus, etc.) the strain at the gap would increasingly reduce thus favoring bone formation ultimately. In other words, a tissue will not be produced in the fracture gap if the strain exceeds permissible limit for that tissue. Though this is a given fact that forces in numerous directions and types apply in a fracture gap, so considering only longitudinal strain is insufficient; which it is indeed but nevertheless good for basic understanding. The interfragmentary strain was defined as the ratio of the relative displacement of fracture ends versus the initial gap width.

- Interfragmentary strain (ε gap) = fracture gap displacement/initial gap width
- $\Delta l/L$

This definition of gap strain corresponds to a small deformation definition of strain. Perren theorized that interfragmentary strains above 100% would lead to nonunion. Strains between 10 and 100% would produce and sustain initial fibrous tissue formation **(Fig. 11)**. Strains between 2 and 10% would lead to cartilage formation and an endochondral ossification formation. Strains under 2% would lead to direct bone formation and primary fracture repair **(Fig. 12)**. Perren believed that once set in progress tissues once formed would stiffen the fracture gap, which in turn, would lead to lower strains, this would allow formation of the next stiffest tissue and the cycle would repeat until all bone was formed. Though easy to understand the interfragmentary strain theory of Perren suffers from significant limitations. Firstly, it is an oversimplified model of tissue formation. Secondly, only axial strain is considered completely neglecting the normal strain or shear that commonly occurs at all fracture sites. Lastly, though the theory explains the incremental change in tissue at the fracture site along with changes in strain it fails to explain the various types of tissue in different regions found in the fracture callus and the basic heterogeneous nature of regenerative tissue always formed.

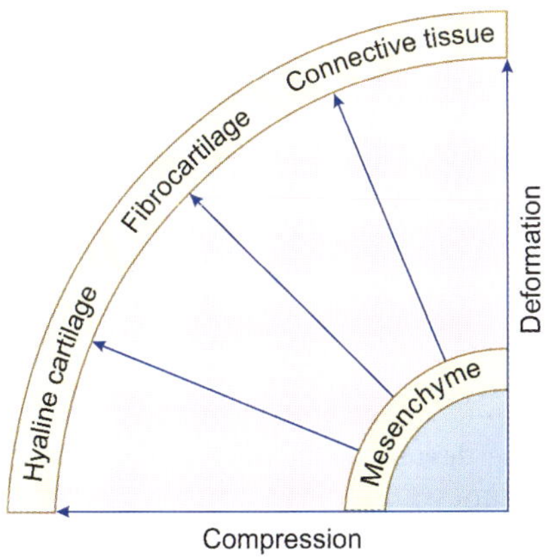

Fig. 10: The Pauwels' concept of tissue differentiation based on different types of stress/strain patterns.

Carter and Blenman Theory

Their theory differs from Perren's theory in that it not only predicts that the magnitude of mechanical stimulus will affect fracture tissue differentiation, but also the type of mechanical stimulus (cyclic, compressive, tensile, or shear). In addition, Carter and Blenman believed that vascular supply to tissues was the primary factor determining tissue differentiation. Based upon the level of vascularity, they believed that both the magnitude and type of mechanical stress, basically hydrostatic pressure versus octahedral shear stress (stress acting along a particular plane), would affect the type of tissue within fracture sites. If a good vascular supply was available to tissues, Carter and Blenman believed that the following sequence would occur **(Fig. 13)**:

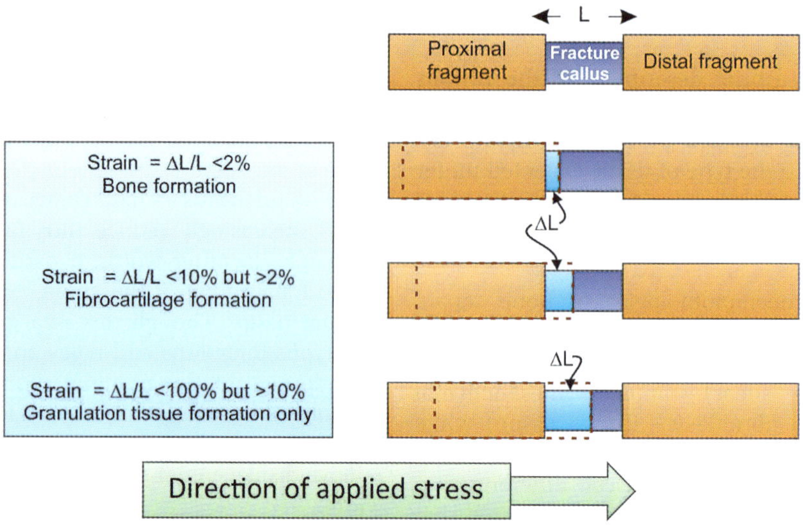

Fig. 11: Perren's interfragmentary theory (see text for description).

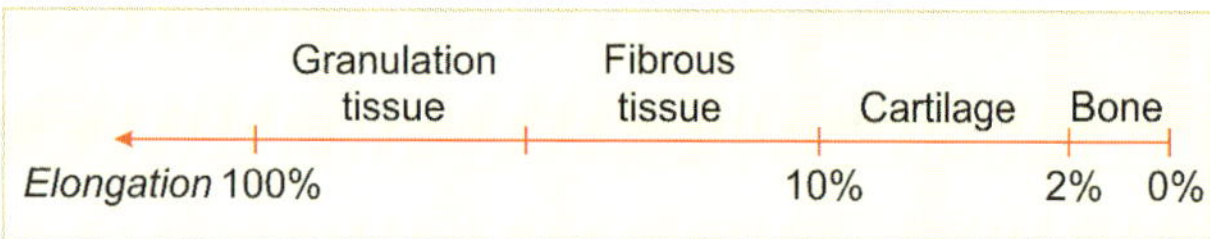

Fig. 12: Schematic diagram of the concept of possible types of tissue formation based on Parren's interfragmentary strain theory.

- Fracture elicits osteogenic stimulus.
- If minimal cyclic stresses are present with good blood supply, bone will form directly.
- If high hydrostatic compressive stresses were present, fibrocartilage would form. One should remember that this is volume changing stress and not axial compressive stress. Volume changing stress that is applied from all surfaces would also reduce vascularity and, hence, cartilage formation due to low oxygen in the region.
- If high tensile or shear stresses were present, fibrous tissue would form.
- If fibrocartilage forms, subsequent shear stresses would lead to bone formation.

Carter and colleagues developed the osteogenic index:

$$I = \sum_{i=1}^{c} ni\,(Si + kDi)$$

where "I" is the scalar value of the index, i is a given load case, c is the total number of different load cases, ni is the number of loading cycles for a given load case, and Si is the cyclic octahedral shear stress (always positive), Di is the cyclic hydrostatic stress (negative if compression, positive if tension), and k is an empirical factor weighing the relative contributions of hydrostatic and shear stress to tissue differentiation. The higher the value of "I", the more likely that the tissue will ossify. The observers realized that the load will never be constant at fracture site as callus is a 3D tissue with heterogeneous development. The osteogenic index will hence be a summation of various mechanical stimuli at different load situations. This equation correlates the osteogenic index to summative and differently applied hydrostatic stress and octahedral shear stress. Vascularity plays an important role with well perfused regions requiring significantly high amounts of hydrostatic stress to produce cartilage while very less amount is needed for poorly perfused regions.

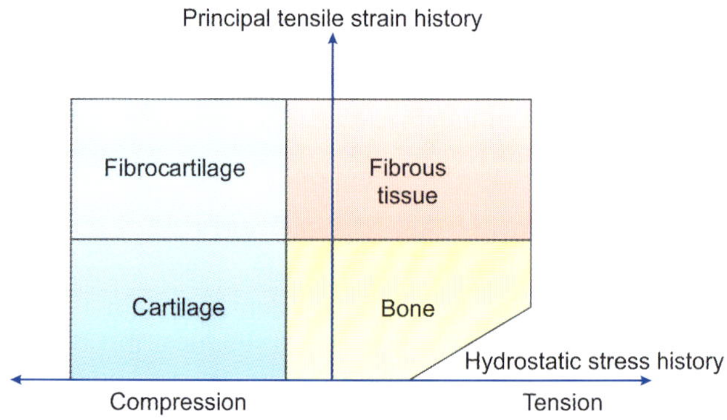

Fig. 13: Carter and Blenman concept of variability in tissue expression with different combination of stress and strain.

Prendergast and Huiskes

Their hypothesis differentiates osteogenic index between the linear-elastic or poroelastic material properties for healing tissues. Biological tissues by virtue of containing fluid are a mixture of fluid and solid phases that is more akin to poroelastic material properties. They arrived at a new theory that the relative velocity between fluid, solid, and shear strain, rather than hydrostatic pressure and shear strain determines tissue differentiation. This can be represented by equation:

$$S = \gamma/a + v/b$$

where, γ is the deviatoric shear strain (strain that changes shape at constant volume), v is the solid/fluid velocity, and a and b are constants varying for different tissue types.

The relationship defines a summation of maximal distortional strain and relative velocity between fluid and

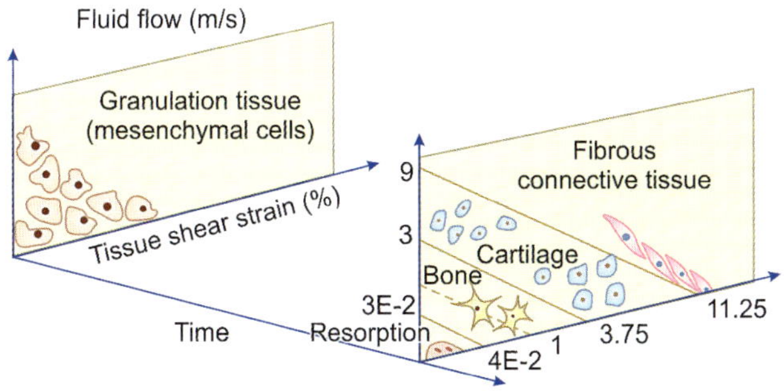

Fig. 14: Prendergast and Huiskes hypothesis of summation of maximal distortional strain and relative velocity between fluid and solid.

solid. In this case the following conditions are satisfied **(Fig. 14)**:

- Bone will be formed if S < S bone
- Cartilage will be formed if S bone < S < S cartilage
- Fibrous connective tissue will be formed if S > S cartilage

Claes et al. Review and Expansion of Pauwels' Concept

They comparatively studied the tissue distribution of healing tibial fractures in an animal with that of an equivalent finite element (FE) study. They created FE models, which represented the healing callus at different stages of development and tried to correlate the stress and strain values from these models with detailing of the histological sections from parallel animal study. They further sorted out some combination in values of hydrostatic pressure and axial strains that produced specific tissue differentiation. According to them hydrostatic pressure of 0.15 MP and strain <5% stimulates intramembranous ossification while compressive hydrostatic pressure >0.15 MP and strain <15% would stimulate endochondral ossification **(Fig. 15)**. Values outside of these regions would result in either fibrous tissue or cartilage. They also proposed from the animal studies that ossification only occurs on an existing bony surface.

COMBINED INTERPRETATION OF CONCEPTS

From above theories, it can be inferred that a combination of "vascularity", "stability" at fracture, and "stress/strain" modulate the biological tissue formation. The combinations of factors influence tissue formation as follows:

- As a rule the fracture repair and consolidation is inversely proportional to the amount of mobility at fracture site. Higher the mobility greater is the cartilage formation. Callus and cartilage as intermediary stage of fracture union are commonly perceived, this is due to the fact that conventional cast immobilization permits fragment mobility and, hence, formation of intermediary cartilage. With growing stability at fracture site overtime and reducing mobility due to callus formation, the cartilage undergoes metaplasia into bone.
- If there is no mobility, then cartilage does not develop and with gap less than critical defect the bone heals directly by remodeling. This healing is nine times faster than healing through callus intermediary.

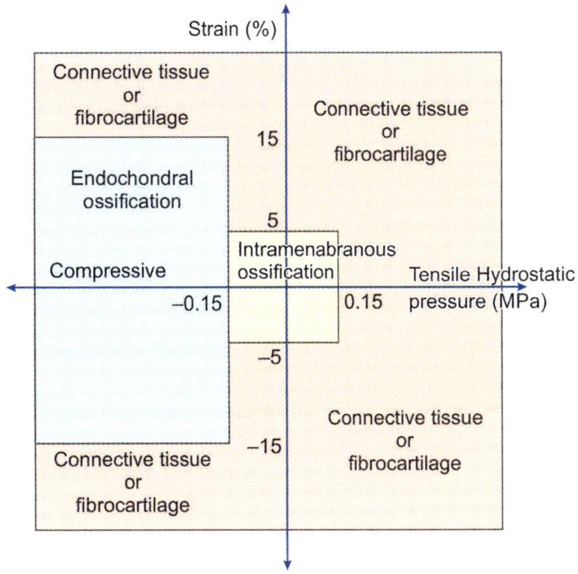

Fig. 15: Claes et al. expansion of Pauwel's concept of differing tissue formation with various stress/strain patterns.

- Compression at fracture has dual effects. Physiological compression stimulates bone formation (like thickening of cortex on the concave side of bone—in accordance with Wolff's law). However, as demonstrated by Hüter-Volkmann excessive compression produces bone atrophy and tensile force stimulates bone growth though this is more suited to growth plate. Also Ilizarov demonstrated that moderate distraction and reduced compression supports bone formation in tissue and osteogenesis. Influence of compression also varies with the type of bone—compression is useful for spongy bone while harmful for diaphyseal bone.
- Compressive stress (not exceeding the elastic limits of bone) produces endochondral ossification—osteogenesis at fracture site. Continuous physiological compressive loading with good vascularity produces bone hypertrophy (as seen with tibialization of fibula)—this process will fail if vascularity is inadequate. Reduced compression with maintained vascularity produces osteopenia (as in space walkers). Reduced load and vascularity both retards bone formation (as in poliomyelitis).
- Intermittent compressive stress or minimal shear stress in a stabilized fracture (controlled micromotion) promotes osteogenesis.
- Intermittent compressive hydrostatic stress (pressure) at fracture site "without" controlled motion/stabilization produces gross chondrogenesis (pseudoarthrosis) that does not ossify.
- Constant excessive loading of the fracture site (compressive stress) forms cartilage at the fracture site and inhibits endochondral ossification due to bone necrosis (this is the rationale for "accordion maneuver" where the compression is released intermittently alternating with distraction). This may be true as reported by Ilizarov but in studies by AO group application of axial compressive stress did not result in necrosis of fractured

sheep bone even if the bone is overloaded. This finding got translated into the concept of dynamic compression plating (DCP) where axial compression stress (and not hydrostatic stress) was given to appose the bone fragments so as to facilitate primary cortical bone repair. Axial compression of the fractured ends would inhibit endochondral ossification so repair would be faster and indeed bone repair after DCP fixation is faster than PC-fix or newer LCP plate fixation.

- Tensile stress (as in distraction histiogenesis) produces intramembranous ossification.
- Strain at fracture site, i.e., shear stress favors fibrogenesis—fibrous nonunion or fibrous ankylosis.
- Low levels of mechanical stimuli (micromotion) at the fracture site:
    - Good vascularity settles into ossification (osteogenesis)
    - Poor vascularity at fracture site produces chondroid tissue

Methods to Enhance Fracture Repair

Before embarking on the methods of enhancing fracture healing the physical and electrical properties of bone should be understood. The compact bone is required to bear stress of muscular contractions and loading stress of the body weight continuously. It also serves to protect the internal soft organs. This entails requirement of good compressive and tensile strength. The compact bone has specific gravity, 1.92–1.99; tensile strength, 13,000–17,000 psi; compressive strength, 18,000–24,000 psi (compressive strength parallel to the long axis, 7,150 psi; and at right angles to the long axis, 10,800 psi). The strength of cancellous bone has linear relationship to its elastic modulus. The strength is proportional to strain rate raised to power 0.06. Range for values is wide for cancellous bone depending on the method of testing, size of bone, origin, etc., shear strength ranges from 1 to 17 MPa. The cancellous bone is less stiff in tension than compression so the tensile strength is less than its compressive strength and tensile strength of compact bone.

The "electrical properties" of bone depend on a number of factors. The bone is "dielectric" (applying voltage produces current across ends determining the "capacitance") and "anisotropic" (charge flowing in all directions in a branching pattern rather than unidirectional flow in a metal wire/rod) with respect to its electrical properties. This means that they are semiconductive (dielectric) themselves but properties differ, "impedance" is lowest in the longitudinal direction and highest in the radial direction. The electrical properties of fully hydrated bone are significantly different from those of dry and partially wet bone and these properties are highly frequency-dependent, they also vary with moisture content, methods of measurement, temperature, and pH of the fluid. In general the cancellous bone has lower resistance than cortical bone. The metaphysis of long bones is negatively charged in relation to diaphysis. The fracture site is more electronegative than surrounding bone. "Conductance" is a property of the bone marrow and a normal value indicates establishment of intramedullary canal. Piezoelectricity is a coupled field effect meaning application of stress/strain are coupled to electrical field generating current and polarization (like thermoelasticity—application of heat produces expansion and vice versa). These gradient effects are now referred to as "flexoelectric", however, the term piezoelectric effect will be used here for common understanding. Bones exhibit "piezoelectric properties" meaning that when stress is applied to the bone, the bone produces a current within itself—the piezoelectric effect, this is due to deformation of hydroxyapatite (HA) crystals. Under the effect of a tensile strain the bone develops electronegativity at the compression site (electrons grouped nearer) while it becomes electropositive at the tension side (electrons deviate farther). Reverse piezoelectric effect (an applied current produces material compression) is a property exhibited by some materials exhibiting piezoelectric effect like bone. This piezoelectric property implies that a voltage could be applied to the bone and the bone itself would compress (develops strain). Compression across fracture improves healing (mechanical property of bone). But the dielectric property (capacitance) would lead to generation of current with the applied voltage and could damage the cells if it exceeds the impedance. So it is imperative that standard protocols must be used. Compact bone in addition exhibits a permanent electric polarization as well as "pyroelectricity" (which is a change of polarization with temperature) determined by polar structure of collagen and orientation in bone. Electric properties and variation with fracture occurrence (development of electronegativity) and restoration (of electrical properties) with healing have been exploited to develop impedance imaging that may possibly indicate development of nonunion or delayed union early. Conductance measures indicate fracture healing at 8 weeks but the values depend tremendously on the cross-sectional area and volume of bone. Inductance though independent of these variables is still not standardized.

Fracture repair may not progress the ideal way always and various methods are utilized to improve or enhance the fracture repair. These are broadly classified into:

- Biophysical stimulation (mechanical and electrical methods)
- Biological methods

Biophysical Stimulation

The various "biophysical methods" rely on the interactions between biophysical stimuli and cellular responses to effect bone repair or enhance the callus maturation. The basis of using various methods is the effect of mechanical stimulation on induction of fracture repair or at least alteration of its pathway. Repetitive loading under small strain and high frequency or overloading through excessive exercise causes bone hypertrophy. This was also influenced by the direction and magnitude of mechanical stimulation. It is envisaged that mechanical stimuli possibly alter cytoplasmic processes or paracrine influences on the cells and if it is so then mechanical stimulation can consistently produce desirable effects. The commonly used methods are discussed as follows:

Ultrasound

This is a noninvasive method transmitting mechanical energy through skin. High-intensity ultrasound (500 mW–3 W/cm^2) induces an intense warming of tissues. This form is effective for reducing pain and controlling muscular spasm. Initially same high-intensity waves were employed for treatment of nonunion in Germany (1960s) but it carries risk of bone necrosis. Low-intensity pulsed ultrasound (LIPUS) has minimal, if any, heating effects and accelerates fracture repair in normal and osteoporotic bone by controlling inflammation and enhancing differentiation of cells. LIPUS increases cell proliferation, protein synthesis, membrane permeability, integrin expression, increased cytosolic calcium levels, and stimulates angiogenesis.

- The mechanical strength of callus improves along with torque and stiffness possibly through piezoelectric effect.
- Osteoprogenitor cells favorably respond to mechanical energy transmitted by ultrasound, possibly by alteration in ionic permeability of cell membrane and changes in the second messenger activity.
- There is increased incorporation of calcium in cultured cartilage and bone cells, improvement in local blood flow (angiogenesis), and stimulation of expression of numerous genes involved in repair process such as aggrecan, insulin like growth factor (IGF), and TGF-β.

The modern LIPUS consists of 1.5 MHz sine wave administered in a burst of 200 μs, with a pause of 800 μs (pulsed 1:4), repeated 1,000 times per second (rate of 1 KHz). The average intensity over space and time is 30 mW/cm^2 and the average intensity over the "on" period is 150 mW/cm^2. It is administered daily through a nonmoving transducer for 20 minutes. LIPUS has been found to be effective for fresh cases, delayed unions, and nonunions with healing rates of 94%, 90%, and 83%, respectively. They have been approved by Food and Drug Administration (FDA) in 1994 for treatment of fresh fractures. Recently, these have been found effective for treatment of infected and noninfected nonunion.

Electrical Stimulation

"Electrical properties of bone and cartilage" can be modulated to enhance fracture repair. "Stress generated potentials" are produced in calcified matrix by virtue of piezoelectric effect of deformed dry collagen molecules and HA crystals. Streaming potentials are generated by interstitial fluids forced through calcified matrix by dilation/compression. Both the dry and hydrated bone has electrical properties, when mechanically stimulated the bone cells produce electrical field that mediates cell proliferation. Friedberg/Brighton introduced the concept of "bioelectric steady state potential" generated in areas of active growth and repair in "nonstressed" bones. Compression site in a stressed bone and area of active bone growth is electrodense (electronegative) while the tension side in a stressed bone or areas of minimal osseous activity are electropositive. There is bone deposition on the compression side as it becomes slightly alkaline while the tensile side shows mineral resorption. This mechanism is altered with fracture and the fracture site itself becomes negatively charged. Yashuda demonstrated that externally applied charge (electricity) can induce or stimulate new bone formation around cathode (negative electrode) that mimics compression-induced bone charges (compression causes electronegativity while tensile forces produce electropositivity). Typically they are indicated for delayed union of a well-positioned diaphyseal fracture in a patient who has undergone many surgeries. This has also been shown to be useful for nonunions especially those with hypertrophic callus formation.

Mechanism **(*Figs. 16A to C*)**: Like most incidental findings in medical science the mechanism of new bone formation through electrical or magnetic field is largely unknown. Cyclic adenosine monophosphate (cAMP) and alteration in intracellular calcium levels have been implicated but never consistently confirmed. Stimulation by "direct current" stimulates neo-osteogenesis by direct effect of current, release of hydroxyl ions locally (chemical reaction), reducing vicinity PO_2 and increased pH. Low PO_2 stimulates new bone growth and higher pH favors calcium deposition. The mechanisms of "inductive coupling" and "capacitive coupling (CC)" are even more unclear but possibly related to direct effect of the current.

- *Direct current* **(*Fig. 16A*)**: Constant application of 20 μA at 1 V to cathode applied directly to the bone surface (Dwyer/Wickham) induces bone by electric, chemical, and mechanical effect. The anode is placed in the adjacent soft tissue or skin surface. Electric current is the primary stimulator but the production of hydroxyl ions (electrochemical) locally increases the pH and lowers PO_2 at cathode. This prevents bone resorption and increases bone formation by stimulating the osteoblastic activity. There is additionally production of H_2O_2 at cathode which enhances osteoclast differentiation. Osteoclast bone resorption additionally stimulates the osteoblasts. The H_2O_2 may also stimulate the macrophage to secrete VEGF that indices angiogenesis and fracture healing. Direct current stimulation may induce formation of BMP 2, 6, and 7 by osteoblasts to stimulate bone formation. Mechanical effects of cathode insertion and electrode movement can possibly help bone formation. Inflammatory reaction (stage I of fracture repair) is produced in the tissue. The method is invasive and vigilant measures and regular monitoring needs to be done to prevent infection. Direct current leads to warming effect in tissues and blistering at anode while pitting at cathode. This may also be responsible to inflammatory effect at fracture site at low strengths. Brighton used similar DC current but applied to percutaneous electrodes reporting bone union in 84% uncomplicated (no infection or synovial pseudoarthrosis) cases.
- *Inductive coupling or pulsed electromagnetic field (PEMF) developed by Bassett et al.*: Here, a time varying electric field is applied to a pair of coils placed on opposite sides of fractured extremity. This produces time-varying magnetic field between coils and in turn secondary time-varying electric field of 10 μA/cm^2 at 20 mV gets generated in the tissues. PEMF acts by both electrical and mechanical influence on the bone **(Fig. 16B)**. Electrical

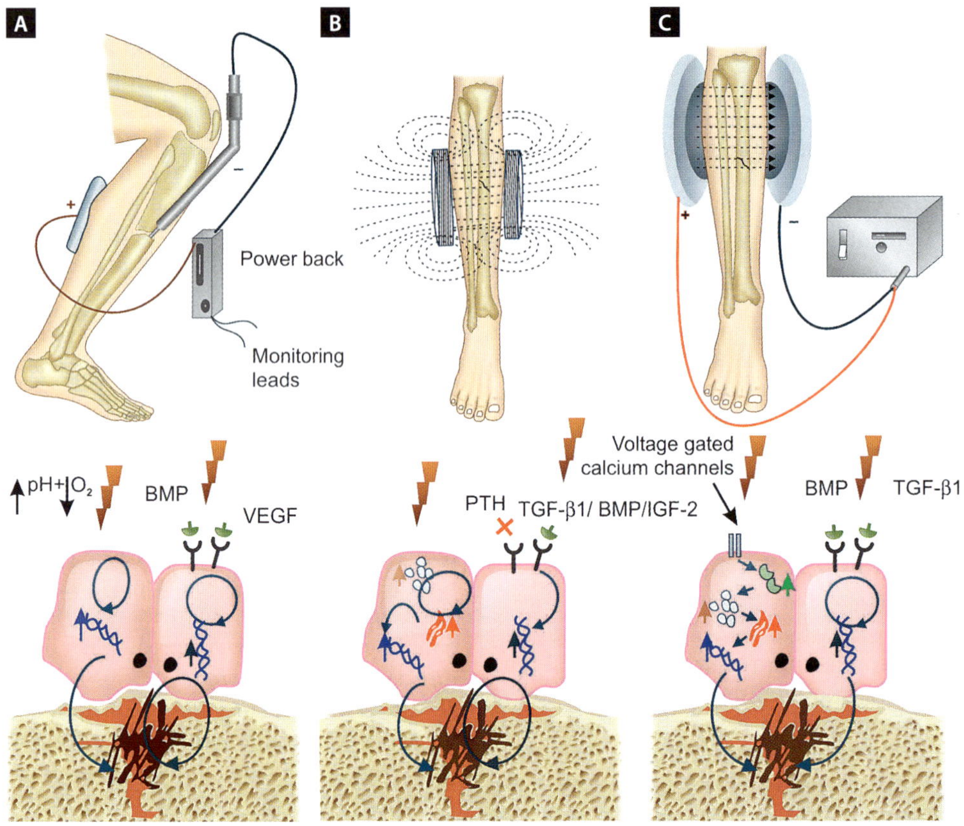

Figs. 16A to C: Mechanism of electrical and magnetic stimulation of bone formation as used in various contemporary methods to stimulate bone formation. (A) Stimulation of bone formation by direct current; (B) Pulsed electromagnetic field-induced bone formation; (C) Capacitive coupling for enhancing bone formation. (BMP: bone morphogenic proteins; IGF: insulin like growth factor; PTH: parathyroid hormone; TGF: Transforming growth factor; VEGF: vascular endothelial growth factor)

current helps as described in the direct current, while pulsed electrical field generates piezoelectric effect compressing and relaxing the fracture site. This generates micromotion and compressive strain at the fracture site. This induces calcification of fibrocartilage and hyaline cartilage (fibrous tissue is not induced at all). PEMF has also been found to upregulate the genes related to bone formation (*hOXA10* and *AKT1*), collagenous, and noncollagenous matrix proteins (*COL1A* and *SPARC*), genes for cytoskeletal component (*FN1* and *VCL*), and genes at transductional level (*CALM1* and *p2RX7*) in in-vitro cell culture of osteoblasts. They are also found to downregulate the genes related to degradation of extracellular matrix (MMP-11 and *DUSP4*). PEMF has direct inhibitory influence on PTH signaling. The PEMF prevents store of cAMP to build up inside cell normally associated with PTH activity. This increases increased calcium uptake by the cell. Also there is direct increase in intracellular levels by a mechanism different from CC. This is a noninvasive method but requires frequent and prolonged sittings and visits to hospital. Double-blinded studies have shown efficacy of PEMF on osteotomy healing and delayed union.

- *Capacitive coupling (CC)*: A time-varying electric field is applied to paired electrodes (not coils), generating time-varying electric field (capacity coupled generators) across tissue in a symmetrical sine wave pattern with peak-to-peak amplitude of 5 V and frequency of 60 kHz. This is due to dielectric property of bone. This produces average electric field of 80 mV/cm (range 20–150) at 5–10 mA in the fracture callus. Here the role of any magnetic field (as in inductive coupling) is negligible. CC causes an increase in cytosolic calcium through voltage-gated calcium channels increasing intracellular calcium **(Fig. 16C)**. This enhances calmodulin stores and induces cell proliferation and callus formation and maturation. CC also enhances bone formation by activation of bone formation through expression of mRNA for BMP 2, 4, 5, 6, and 7. Collagen synthesis and production of cAMP is induced in the tissues enhancing calcification on reparative stage.

Indications of electrical stimulation:
- Hypertrophic nonunion
- Stable fixation with fracture in acceptable alignment
- Patient who does not want surgical procedures or unfit for surgical procedure, having untreatable skin disease at the site of nonunion or poor skin condition (grafted skin), and coexisting infection.

Contraindications for electrical stimulation:
- Pseudoarthrosis
- A vascular nonunion

- Coexisting deformity
- Nonunion of upper limb as need for simultaneous immobilization may compromise function at joints permanently.
- Humerus and femur fractures with large gaps (gaps equal to width of the bone) and also possibility of pseudoarthrosis in these bones is inherently high. Additionally, it is difficult to immobilize the humerus completely.

Complications:
- Infection with implanted electrodes
- Skin irritation at position of electrodes
- Incorporation of the electrode in the new bone requiring surgical removal

Extracorporeal Shock Wave Therapy

This is a relatively newer mode studied for mechanical enhancement of fracture repair, this requires higher frequency and energies for stimulation of repair. Breaking down of stones in kidney that have same structure as HA might have similar effects of microstimulation (creating microfissures, cavitation with liberation of energy, and increased local blood flow) at the osteogenic and nonunion sites. Mechanism though is still not clear and some attribute the benefit to be biased by prolonged immobilization itself. It was first used in Bulgaria (1980s) by Valchanov and Michailov. This is given by means of electrohydraulic or electromagnetic devices under C-arm control. The power of trains of shock waves is adjusted to the size of the skeletal segment—for large bones the power is 2 kV using electrohydraulic devices, 0.6–1 mJ/mm^2 using electromagnetic devices.

Mechanical Stimulation

Distraction histiogenesis (osteogenesis): Developed by GA Ilizarov, this concept entails use of controlled distraction to new tissue genesis/formation. Theoretically indefinite amount of tissue can form with the technique, if applied to bone then osseous tissue will form. One should realize that tissue should be present from beginning that can be stretched rather "distracted" not to confuse with fractures initially fixed in distraction (gap) that are actually the cause of nonunion. Under optimal conditions the "regenerate" that forms is distracted somewhere 1 mm/day till the desired length is achieved. Bone forms in "intramembranous ossification" (so it is not called callus) fashion else with unstable environment pseudoarthrosis results. The tissue is left to consolidate for twice as long as the distraction phase while physiologic stress bearing can be allowed anytime during treatment. For optimal results 5–7 days latency followed by continuously applied distraction (ideally motorized) throughout the day and stable fixation is mandatory. The technique has been successfully utilized for treatment of nonunions, limb lengthening, deformity correction, and segmental bone loss, primary fixation of comminuted fractures and open fractures, varicose ulcers, trophic ulcers, and arthrodesis of joints. Carrying the fixator and cosmesis is the primary concern.

Controlled axial micromotion: Controlled axial (mechanical) stimulation (by using Wagner type frame) had been used by few authors for treatment of tibial fractures and had shown reduced time to union and secondary surgeries.

Intermittent pneumatic soft tissue compression: In animal model (rabbit), the method has been found to increase callus area. Though elusive and not substantiated, reduced venous stasis, and increased interstitial fluid return to circulation may increase NO and local prostacyclin levels improving callus density.

Functional cast bracing of Sarmiento: This is based on the concept of maintaining the limb in near physiological state throughout the fracture repair process. The brace is applicable to nearly cylindrical body parts like the arm and leg where free motion is allowed at the proximal and distal joints. The concept of Wolff's law is mostly applicable to the method as early weight bearing is begun and also cyclic muscular movements have been found to enhance the development of external callus response along with trophic effect on periosteal callus thus enhancing the fracture repair. It should be remembered that the brace should be a "total contact brace" else fracture would displace during weight bearing and may even fail. Total contact brace forms a closed compartment that prevents fracture displacement by maintaining the hydrostatic pressures within compartment exceeding the displacing forces at the fracture site. The other concern is that this bracing is ineffective and may complicate the venous drainage when there is acute swelling at the site and in the limb. For a typical functional knee brace the proximal portion is trimmed to resemble a PTB prosthesis with anterior portion at the level of inferior pole of patella, the posterior wall extends one fingerbreadth below the anterior impression of patellar tendon anteriorly. Lateral wings of the brace remain high for providing rotational stability.

Biological Methods

Osteoinduction (term introduced by Marshall R Urist) is a process that supports the mitogenesis of undifferentiated mesenchymal cells, leading to the formation of osteoprogenitor cells that form new bone **(Box 1)**. Osteoconduction is a property of a matrix that supports the attachment of bone-forming cells for subsequent bone formation **(Box 1)**. Osteogenic property can be defined as the generation of bone from bone-forming cells.

Bone Morphogenic Protein

Bone inducing principal was first postulated in 1952 by Marshall Urist et al. New bone formation was demonstrated by him in rabbit muscle by implanted demineralized lyophilized segments of bone in 1965. He pioneered the concept of presence of a substance naturally present in the bone responsible for regeneration and repair activity in the bone, and called this substance BMP. The "bone-inducing component" or BMP, also as it was later called, was isolated

BOX 1: Biological methods to improve bone regeneration.

- *Osteoconductive*: Bone graft substitutes
- *Osteoinductive*:
  - Bone morphogenic proteins
  - Platelet rich plasma
  - Conditioned plasma
- *Osteogenic*:
  - Bone grafts
  - Bone marrow infiltration
- *Systemic agents*:
  - Prostaglandins
  - Fibronectin

in 1981 from demineralized bone matrix (DBM) by using acid and chaotropic agents. The isolated component was cloned and tested form in vivo activity. This "bone inductive extract" was found to be a family of dimeric molecules having highly conserved seven-cysteine TGF-β domain in their C-termini. They are a group of growth factors also known as cytokines and also as metabologens. The evolution in understanding of BMP is represented in **(Table 9)**. Till now, around 20 types have been recognized, BMP 2–7 belongs to TGF-β superfamily while BMP1 is a metalloproteinase. These proteins are secreted as homodimers or heterodimers of 110–140 amino acid peptides linked by one disulfide bond (molecular weight of approximately 30 kd). They are now found not to be responsible only for bone formation from cartilage but constitute important pathway signaling in morphogenesis since birth, throughout the body (so "BMP" may be a misnomer). BMP signaling plays critical roles in heart, neural, and cartilage development, as expected because TGF-β superfamily is involved in vast cellular processes of fundamental importance. Paradoxically, BMP3 has in fact shown to be an inhibitor of osteoinductive activity in the rat, and ironically this is the most abundant BMP in body. BMP in bone is produced by osteoblasts, chondrocytes, osteoprogenitor cells, chondrocytes, and platelets.

BMPs seem to be involved in the regulation of cell proliferation, survival, differentiation, and apoptosis, but their hallmark is their ability to induce bone, cartilage, ligament, and tendon formation at both heterotopic and orthotopic sites. This is affected by inducing differentiation of multipotent mesenchymal stem cells into osteoblasts and osteochondrogenic lineages. Recombinant human bone morphogenetic protein-2 (rhBMP-2) blocks the differentiation of osteoblast precursor cells into myoblasts or adipocytes. Sampath and collaborators demonstrated that when OP-1 (BMP-7) is added to cultures of bone cells enriched with osteoblasts at different stages of differentiation it stimulates cell proliferation, collagen synthesis, induction of alkaline phosphatase, PTH-mediated production of cAMP, and osteocalcin synthesis. The effects of BMP are mediated by canonical and noncanonical signaling mediated by the mature C-terminal mature peptide binding to receptor **(Fig. 17)**. In the canonical pathway, the BMP binds to cell-surface receptors (six types have been identified) forming mainly two broad groups of dimers namely type-I (BMPR-I) and type-II (BMPR-II) serine/threonine kinase receptors. The six receptors are grouped into type I and type II receptors broadly having three subtypes each. Type-I receptors include activin receptor type IA (ActRIA), BMP receptor type IA (BRIA), and BMP receptor type IB. These form heterotetrameric complexes with type II receptors namely BMP receptor type II (BRII), activin receptors type IIA and IIB (ActRIIA and ActRIIB). The activated type I receptors phosphorylate the intracellular effector proteins

TABLE 9: Historical evolution of development in understanding of BMP (the wonder molecule).

1965	Marshall Urist has discovered that demineralized bone matrix (DBM) can induce bone formation
1971	Urist conceptualizes bone morphogenic proteins (BMPs)
1981	Extraction and reconstitution of BMP activity for bioassay
1991	First use of BMP with DBM
October 2001	FDA grants humanitarian device exemption (HDE) approval for osteogenic protein-1 (OP-1; rhBMP-7)
July 2002	FDA approves rhBMP-2 (INFUSE) for a single level spine fusion (L4-S1)
April 2004	FDA grants HDE approval for OP-1 putty for revision spinal fusion
May 2004	FDA approves rhBMP-2 (INFUSE) for treating acute open tibial shaft fractures
2008	FDA approval to rhBMP-2 for treatment of posterolateral lumbar pseudoarthrosis

(FDA: Food and Drug Administration; rhBMP: recombinant human bone morphogenetic protein-2)

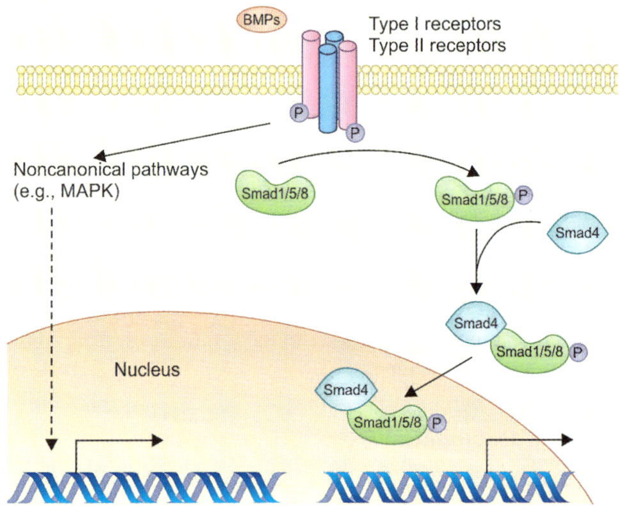

Fig. 17: The action of bone morphogenic protein (BMP) molecules through canonical and noncanonical pathways. The canonical pathway involves binding of BMP to type 1 or 2 receptors forming a complex of four nonconforming subunits (heterotetrameric). This complex then phosphorylates the Smad proteins activating them and enabling their union to co-Smad allowing for translocation into the nucleus. In the nucleus the complex then mediates gene-regulation. In noncanonical pathway the same is mediated through involvement of variety of pathways of which the most studied are mitogen-activated protein kinase (MAPK). The regulation of genetic pathways basically is directed toward bone formation regulation. The mesenchymal cells are stimulated to differentiate down the osteogenic lineage to this end by increased expression (transcription and translation regulated by BMP) of runt-related transcription factors 2 and osterix.

chiefly the receptor regulated Smads (activated Smad 1/5/8). These activated Smads then form complexes with comediator Smad (Smad 4) that translocate into the nucleus functioning as transcription factor and regulating gene expression. In the noncanonical pathway, the osteoinductive signals are mediated by Smad independent pathways namely p38 mitogen-activated protein-kinase pathway and phosphatidylinositol 3-kinase/protein kinase b pathway (details are out of the scope of current text). Whether canonical or noncanonical both seem to converge at the runt-related transcription factor 2 and *Osterix genes* that are fundamental to osteoblast differentiation. At the cellular level the BMPs migrate along concentration gradient inducing differentiation and proliferation along defined spatial arrangement. The cells are stimulated to form chondrocytes within 5–7 days that upon capillary invasion get calcified and replace with bone in 9–12 days. The mineralized bone gains functional bone-marrow elements by 14–21 days. Clinically rhBMP-7 (OP-1) has been approved as alternative to allograft for treatment of nonunion which was extended in 2004 to its use as an alternative to allograft for posterolateral spine fusion. The rhBMP-2 (Infuse) has been approved for use in anterior lumbar interbody fusion with a fusion device (LT cage—lumbar tapered titanium interbody fusion device). In 2008, this has been extended to its use for posterolateral lumbar pseudoarthrosis, open tibia shaft fractures with intramedullary nail fixation. There is, however, extensive off label use of BMP (cervical discectomy and fusion, etc.) which has recently raised concern particularly as to hypertrophic bone formation at the site and induction of colon cancer and Barrett's esophagus. Various delivery systems have been evaluated notable of which are DBM, polylactic and glycolic acid, hyaluronic acid gel, ceramics, calcium phosphate based cements, depot injectable carriers, viral vectors, and gene guns. Carrier for BMP needs to maintain a critical threshold concentration of BMP at implantation site for the required period (temporal distribution), act as scaffold over which bone growth can occur and contain the BMP at the localized site and prevent extraneous bone formation (spatial containment). The current typical dosage of rhBMP-7 is 3.5 mg which is generally administered bound to 1 g of bovine collagen granules acting as scaffold. The complications of BMP like excess bone formation and immunologic response (anticollagen and anti-rhBMP protein formation) are linked to the dose administered. New delivery methods like oxidized alginate hydrogels that allows lower concentration of BMP to be used may ameliorate these problems. Treatments that combine the use of BMPs for fusion or nonunion have been found to be as effective as the use of autogenous bone grafts minus the morbidity and complications associated with harvesting the latter. Apart from bone formation BMP could help in cartilage regeneration in osteochondral defects and reverse diabetic renal disease. For anterior interbody fusion a total dose of 4.2–12 mg of rhBMP-2 at concentration of 1.5 mg/mL is recommended. The recommended total dose of OP-1 as humanitarian device exemption for recalcitrant posterolateral fusion nonunion is 7 mg for both sides. The recommended dose of OP-1 for recalcitrant long bone nonunions is 7 mg. Recent studies have identified specific BMP antagonists (i.e., noggin and chordin) and members of the DAN family (i.e., gremlin and follistatin). These antagonists may be used therapeutically in pathological conditions characterized by excessive bone formation.

Prostacyclins

These are mainly only research molecules and clinical utility is still not substantiated. PGE1-increase cortical thickening (limbs/ribs of neonates) and PGE2-increase bone formation. Normal fracture healing is demonstrably impaired by PG inhibitors. CP533 and 536 are nonprostanoid EP2 receptor selective PGE2 agonist that stimulates local bone formation/ enhance fracture healing.

Platelet Concentrate and Bone Marrow Injections and Stem Cells

After Goujon reported formation of ectopic bone in 1869 with the application of bone marrow, the technique has been used with various modifications and refinements. Bone marrow aspirate (BMA) from "red active marrow (RAM)" (typically posterior iliac crest) contains MSC in the strength of 1:100,000. Volumes ranging from 15 to 150 mL have all been used. Aspiration is done in volumes of <4 mL (ideally 2 mL) from every 2 to 3 mm depths in a fan like fashion to capture as many MSCs without dilution. It is estimated that typical BMA from RAM contains 70 million marrow cells of which 700 would be MSCs. It is postulated that MSCs act synergistically with BMP to produce effective fracture repair response (osteoinductive and osteogenic) and can also be used for delayed and nonunions. Transpedicular harvest from vertebral bodies has also been described. For optimum clinical efficacy it is recommended that a high-degree open pore scaffold with interconnected geometry is used to deliver the BMA. Ceramic HA, β-tricalcium phosphate (TCP) and ultraporous β-TCP have been studied to be effective. The BMA can be ultracentrifuged to yield high concentration of stem cells in a lower volume that can be incorporated with scaffolds to produce similar effects. Composite grafting of BMA with BMP is found to yield better results. Recently the isolated MSCs have been induced by dexamethasone in vitro to enhance the ability of BMP-2 modified MSCs in osteogenic conversion as part of stem cell therapy.

Sclerostin domain-containing protein 1 (Sostdc1) prevents activation and skeletal differentiation of MSCs. So, MSCs need specific activation before usage as protein factories. Injecting MSCs to fracture site provides molecules that enhance fracture repair in a continuous supply. An alternative is to use MSC exosomes. These are extracellular vesicles that contain the protein content of cytoplasm. Skeletal stem cells are now being increasingly identified and used for bone repair.

Platelets are a source of a variety of growth factors many of which are relevant to fracture repair. Some 30 different factors and cytokines have been identified like platelet-derived growth factor (PDGF-bb, -ba, -aa isoforms), TGF-β (β1 and β2 isoforms), platelet factor 4, IL-1, VEGF, EGF, IGF, osteocalcin, osteonectin, thrombospontin-1, etc. Platelet rich plasma (PRP) is used as a liquid from 50 to 100 mL of full blood passed through two-stage centrifuge process yielding 1/10th the original volume with platelet concentrated of 1,000,000 platelets/μL. This is mixed with bovine thrombin and $CaCl_2$ for activation in vivo. Although in vitro stimulation of mitogenic (i.e., transforming) response to PRP in human trabecular bone is found the same has not been translated into clinical efficacy in vivo, though its supportive role to fracture repair cannot be fully denied and is under study. PRP has also been used to treat chronic elbow tendinosis (tennis elbow) and diabetic foot ulcers with some success.

Parathyroid Hormone

Parathyroid hormone and PTH-related peptide (PTHrP) have been documented to be potent in the expansion of progenitor populations and in the regulation of differentiation of these cells. Recent research indicates that both PTH and PTHrP play an important role in regulating the pool of undifferentiated MSCs available for growth plate expansion and fracture callus formation. It appears that PTH or PTHrP is required to prevent the depletion of progenitor cells needed in the formation of the growth plate or fracture callus. Thus, it would be expected that exogenously administered PTH may have an important biologic function at sites of healing bone. Moreover, recent reports have documented that PTH can reverse the effect of aging on depleting osteoblast progenitor cells. Both chondrogenic and osteogenic precursor cells seem to be targets of PTH. Because both cell types contribute to normal fracture repair, it is likely that PTH has a beneficial effect on fracture repair. Cost is a deterring factor and studies have yet to document the low cost to benefit ratio.

Ultra Concentrate of Centrifuged Blood

This is composed of leukocytes and platelets and is often referred to as PRP or autologous conditioned plasma. There is little clinical evidence for its use from centrifuged blood. There is a recent concern about enhancement of bone healing due to high concentration of leukocytes that have been found to inhibit bone formation in animal studies.

Anabolic Supplementation and Minerals

High protein diet promotes fracture healing in animal models; there is some weak evidence of improved fracture repair with essential amino acid supplemented diet rich in arginine. Zinc supplementation also similarly increases bone protein component but is more effective at later stages of fracture repair.

Bone Grafts and Bone Graft Substitutes

Bone grafts provide a latticework for ingrowth by host bone and supply living osteogenic cells to the host and growth factors induce bone formation. History dates back to 1668 and first bone graft was a xenograft (no more used today) where the skull of a soldier was reconstructed using a dog's skull by Job van Meekeren. After Lane and Sandhu introduced internal fixation, Albee, Kushner, Henderson, Campbell, and others added principle of osteogenesis to develop bone grafting for nonunion. Bone grafting is in principle a surgical procedure that replaces missing bone in bone defects due to complex fractures or to augment bone healing/repair/strength when it fails to heal properly (delayed and nonunion). Bone graft incorporation occurs through five stages (Urist) **(Table 10)**. Cancellous and cortical grafts incorporate by different mechanisms and have fundamental differences **(Table 11)**.

Biological mechanism of effect of bone grafting: The bone grafts tend to improve bone healing or fracture repair by one or combination of following mechanisms:

- *Osteoinduction*: It is the property by which the graft causes stimulation of osteoprogenitor cells to differentiate into osteoblasts that then begin new bone formation. BMP is a typical example. Autogenous bone especially cancellous bone carries with it the factors and cellular elements that can act for "osteoinduction" in paracrine manner. These grafts serve as a scaffold for currently existing osteoblasts and also trigger the formation of new osteoblasts promoting faster integration of the graft. Bone reamings are example of pure osteoinductive grafts.
- *Osteoconduction*: It is the property where the bone graft material serves as a scaffold (framework) for new bone growth. Osteoblasts from the host bone use the bone graft material as a framework upon which it generates new bone.
- *Osteogenesis*: It is the process of bone formation by the osteoblasts from bone graft itself in addition to the bone formation by osteoblasts of host bone. For this the bone graft should be sufficiently vital enough and free of immunological response. Though exact interval time for bone graft to remain outside and retain its osteogenic activity is not known but this should be minimized and done immediately, if possible.
- *Osteopromotion*: It is enhancement of osteoinduction without the possession of osteoinductive properties. DBM could fall into this category to some extent.

Theories of Bone Graft Incorporation

Phemister introduced the term "creeping substitution" which is the mechanism for cancellous bone graft incorporation (and even cancellous bone repair). Granulation tissue invades the areas of resorption and pluripotential mesenchymal cells differentiate into osteoblasts laying seams of new osteoid along the dead trabeculae of the bone graft forming an "osteoid tube" on the existing scaffold. The surface cells

TABLE 10: Stages of bone graft incorporation.

Stage	***Description***
Inflammation	Bone resorption and chemotaxis by necrotic tissue and inflammation
Osteoblast differentiation	From cells in graft or marrow precursors
Osteoinduction	Support and growth of bone cells
Osteoconduction	Scaffold to guide cells for bone formation
Remodeling	Graft modification to the innate bone structure

TABLE 11: Difference between cancellous and cortical bone grafts.

Cancellous bone graft	*Cortical bone graft*
Consists predominantly of soft spongy bone	Consists predominantly of hard cortical bone
Contains higher number of living bone cells	Contains more of bone matrix and less cells
Mainly acts as a filler to obliterate cavities	Mainly acts as structural support
Poorly resists compression or bending force	Good compressive strength and provides tensile strength also
Cannot be used to augment strength of bone	Can be used to augment bone strength as in fixation of osteoporotic fractures
Provides biological support to healing as in cases of comminuted fractures primary bone grafting with cancellous bone supports fracture repair	Less of biological support but is used to fill bone gaps in diaphyseal defects
These grafts gather strength overtime	They tend to become weaker with time
Incorporates faster (3–9 months)	Slow incorporation and is often incomplete (union to parent bone takes 3–6 months while complete incorporation of graft may take 2 years to even a decade depending on the length of graft)
Creeping substitution is the primary mode of incorporation	Reverse creeping substitution and a process similar to remodeling is the way this graft incorporates
Can be used in places that have potential for being infected as the graft will be quickly resorbed, if infection prevails	Should not be used at infected sites as there is a high chance of organisms making these metabolically inactive grafts their home gathering shelter and complicating treatment

TABLE 12: Structural properties of bone grafts.

Grafts type	*Osteoconduction*	*Osteoinduction*	*Osteogenesis*	*Structural integrity*
Cancellous autograft	+++	++	+++	± (fair if impaction bone grafting done)
Cortical autograft	+	+	±	+++
Allograft	+	+	–	++
Calcium phosphate	+	–	–	+
Demineralized bone matrix	+	++	–	±
Xenograft	+	–	–	++
Bone marrow	–	–	++	–

of the trabecular bone from graft survive and take part in actively forming the new bone (Abott). The necrotic tissue in marrow spaces and Haversian canals is removed by macrophages. The debris and necrotic bone inside the tube is resorbed by migrated macrophages that differentiate into osteoclasts converting them into "hollow tubes". These tubes are then invaded by granulation tissue and form new bone inside. In cortical bone the process is much slower as the osteoclasts have to resorb the dense bone along Haversian system. This is invaded by the granulation tissue and new bone is laid (reverse creeping substitution). The bone grafts can be classified according to the type of bone or the type of source and vary in their basic structural or compositional properties **(Table 12)**. Following are the common terms used:

- *Cancellous*: Predominantly cancellous bone.
- *Cortical*: Predominantly cortical bone.
- *Corticocancellous*: Combination of both for faster repair and structural integrity.
- *Autograft*: Obtained from same individual.
- *Syngraft (previously isograft)*: Obtained from twin.
- *Allograft (previously homograft)*: Obtained from different person from same species.
- *Xenograft (previously heterograft)*: Obtained from different species usually bovine.
- *Synthetic*: Synthesized completely in laboratory or industrially.

Autogenous Bone Graft

Better called "transplants", these are still the "gold standard" and can be used in various forms according to the need. Advantages and disadvantages of autograft versus allograft bone are provided in **Table 13**. A brief description of various common forms of usage is as follows:

- *Multiple cancellous (or corticocancellous) chips*: Most widely used for stacking, stuffing voids, filling defects, nonunion, delayed union, fusion, etc. in onlay fashion Has highest osteogenic potential. Can be morcellized and used for impaction bone grafting (amount is the limiting factor). Ilium is the most common site for procurement proximal and distal femur, proximal and distal tibia, distal radius, and olecranon can be used as required.
- *Single onlay cortical grafts*: Treatment of nonunions before development of good internal fixation methods. Tibia or split fibula was commonly used. Spinal fusion (rare) is the only modern use, principally because of donor site morbidity and development of fixation.

TABLE 13: Advantages and disadvantages of autograft versus allograft methods.

Autograft	***Allograft***
Advantages: • Readily available • Quick and reliable incorporation • No immunogenicity • No clearance hassles for authority • No risk of "transmitting" infections as with allografts • Different forms—cortical, cancellous, and combined available for various uses	*Advantages*: • Quick and easy to use • Available now in various sizes and shapes for different use • Cortical versus cancellous can be chosen • Large amount for massive reconstruction available • Shortens operative time
Disadvantages: • Increase time of surgical procedure • Limited in amount for large reconstructions and defects • Pain at operative site, morbidity, and increased length of stay • Increased cost of surgery • "Second" surgery and potential risks like infection • Chronic pain may persist • Possibility of hernia and secondary complications	*Disadvantages*: • Requires setup and maintenance • Not readily available in India • Various regulatory clearances needed • Risk of infection especially the clostridial and viral infections has still not been eliminated • Weak osteogenic potential though provides good structural support (osteoconductive) • Procurement, processing, and preservation need expertise and dedication

- *Dual onlay cortical bone graft (of Boyd 1941)*: Classically described for congenital pseudoarthrosis tibia. No indication in modern orthopedics, however, modified allograft can be used for augmenting cortical insufficiency in revision arthroplasty in this fashion.
- *Inlay bone grafting*: Principally described as a sliding and graft reversal inlay technique to treat nonunion tibia by Albee (superseded now by rigid fixation and cancellous bone grafting). Extended indications in current practice are typically utilized for ankle arthrodesis and anterior spinal fusion. Typically local tibia, fibula, ribs, or iliac crest are used.
- *H-grafts*: Typically used for anterior cervical spine in past and uncommonly for scaphoid nonunion.
- *Dowel grafts and peg grafts*: Corticocancellous grafts used in past for treatment of nonunions in regions where onlay grafting is not possible. For neck of femur ilium was used in conjunction with screw fixation (now people use fibula as curvature of ilium limits practical utility). Carpal scaphoid nonunion have also been treated by cancellous pegs prepared from dense bone. Nowadays, vascularized pedicle or free grafts are commonly used.
- *Medullary grafts*: Used to augment screw purchase in osteoporotic bones, commonly humerus. Intramedullary fibula provides two additional cortices for screw purchase. With locked screw plate constructs the utility has reduced.
- *Hemicylindrical grafts*: Massive cortical hemicylindrical grafts supplemented with cancellous bone are placed to bridge the defect. As with most other grafting techniques, this is also hardly ever used (may be used in some cases of bone tumor excision).
- *Fibular head graft*: This is typically used to recreate distal radius articular surface. In cases where distal radius is sacrificed as in giant cell tumor same side fibula is harvested and fixed in a reversed fashion.
- *Vascularized pedicle grafts*: These grafts carry their own vascular supply so that the incorporation and remodeling is faster. Local rotation pedicle grafts are more popular as they are easy to use like periosteal and muscle pedicle-based grafts for hip, scaphoid (pronator quadratus based), intercompartmental supraretinacular artery-based bone pedicle for scaphoid. Free microvascular fibular grafts can be placed at remote site for femoral neck and other diaphyseal defects following tumor excision, infection, or traumatic bone loss are popular but require expertise.
- *Intercalary graft*: Usually allografts are used for large diaphyseal defects; however, vascularized fibula can be used along with bridge plate fixation with better results.

The various sites for obtaining cancellous bone graft are:

- *Iliac crests (anterior and posterior)*: Usually cancellous chips are obtained from the inner table and cancellous portion of anterior ilium, however, sometimes requirement for tricortical graft necessitates removal of a wedge. Bicortical chips are harvested after lifting the iliac crest cap. The graft is taken from the outer table and cancellous bony region underneath the gluteus maximum muscle when harvesting is done from posterior iliac crest.
- Proximal tibia
- Trochanteric region of femur
- Distal condylar region of femur
- Olecranon process of ulna
- Distal radius styloid process

The cortical autografts are obtained from:

- *Fibula*: Entire proximal two-thirds bone may be utilized but care should be taken to avoid injury to the peroneal nerve and peroneal muscles. Distal fourth fibula must be left in place to maintain a stable ankle joint. Middle third fibula is commonly used as a vascularized graft also.
- Tibia proximal half region (Phemister graft).

Allografts and Allogenic Bone Grafts

Better called "implants", these differ from transplants as the bone is nonviable. They are available in various forms. Supply in our country is limited for awareness and lack of banking facilities. A graft may be orthotopic (transplanted to the same site in the recipient that it occupied in the donor, e.g., distal femur to distal femur); heterotopic (transplanted to a different site but one occupied by the same tissue as in the donor, e.g., fibula to spine); or ectopic (transplanted to a site normally occupied by a different type of tissue, e.g., fascia lata as a tendon graft). Ectopic sites are mainly investigational for bone grafting. The various types of allografts are as follows:

- Fresh—no clinical use due to high immunogenic potential.
- Fresh-frozen—less immunogenic but needs secondary procedure for sterilization. Preserves BMP.
- Freeze-dried (lyophilized)—bone should be extracted from donor within 8 to 12 hours of death. The bone loses its inductive factors and BMP due to enzymatic autodigestion by intracellular and extracellular enzymes. Antigen-extracted allogeneic (AAA) bone as advised by Urist may retain inductive factors. Here, chloroform-methanol is used to extract lipids and cell membrane lipoproteins (4 hours); hydrochloric acid extracts acid-soluble proteins and demineralizes the surface in 24 hours; and neural phosphate buffer is used to remove endogenous intracellular and extracellular transplantation antigens. The bone is then frozen and freeze dried and stored at -60°C.
- *Demineralized bone matrix (or bone matrix gelatin, BMG)*: This is a digested source of BMP, used as bone graft extender. DBM is available in two forms, dry or injectable. DBM is mixed with a carrier. Carriers (inert with regards to bone generation) include hyaluronic acid, collagen, glycerol, gelatin, and actual derivatives of DBM itself. Second generation DBM putties (carrier is loaded with BMP) have higher concentrations of BMP and are possibly better.
- *Osteochondral allografts*: Bony chunk with cartilage cover, used for large articular defects in osteochondroses of knee.
- *Shell allografts*: Biologic resurfacing of articular defects using devascularized osteoarticular graft with a small bony component.
- *Large composite allografts*: Usually required for excision of large tumors or reconstruction of defects in revision arthroplasty after freeze thawing.

Indications for use of allograft: Reconstruction of massive bone defects arising from trauma, infection (debridement), osteolysis or revision arthroplasty, and resection of bone tumors requiring amount of bone that cannot be supplied by extended autografting procedures. The following are the typical common procedures for which allografts are used (some are common indications for bone grafting in general):

- Reconstruction of skeletal defects following tumor resection
- Reconstruction of bone defects as a result of primary joint arthroplasty osteolysis
- Reconstruction of extensor mechanism of knee
- Reconstruction of congenital or developmental bone and joint defects (protrusio acetabuli and dysplastic hip) and deformities. Acetabular plastical arthrosis (remodeling) is required to improve coverage of the femoral head
- Obliteration of cystic cavities of bone
- Repair of fresh comminuted fractures with bone loss
- Treatment of nonunion and complicated osteoporotic fractures
- Arthrodesis of large joints
- To provide bone blocks for limiting joint motion (arthrorisis), e.g., flail joint in poliomyelitis
- Treatment of scoliosis and spinal fusion
- Repair of massive segmental bone defects
- Repair of periodontal osseous defects

"Xenografts (heterogeneous bone grafts)" have been used but are now out of favor because of easier access to allografts. Bovine bone xenograft is harvested and washed in water, extracted with peroxide to oxidize proteins, and washed with acetone to remove fats. After gamma sterilization the product (kiel bone) mainly serves to be osteoconductive scaffold.

Bone Graft Substitutes

They are also called 'alloplastic bone grafts' but less commonly. These are materials that can be used in place of bone grafts but are purely osteoconductive unless they act as a carrier for delivery of some inductive materials like BMP (see elsewhere). Typically, they are comprised of silicon, calcium, or aluminum.

- *Calcium-based products are widely used*:
    - *Calcium-phosphate based grafts (tricalcium phosphate)*: Calcium phosphate naturally occurs in bone as HA [$(Ca_5(PO_4)_3OH$ or $Ca_{10}(PO_4)_6OH_2)$]. Synthetic HA is osteoconductive but very slow to absorb taking years to incorporate. Calcium phosphate-based grafts are, hence, synthesized in different forms to improve biological characteristics and are available as ceramics, powders, and cements. "Ceramics" are highly crystalline structures created by a process known as "sintering" (heating nonmetallic mineral salts at temperatures greater than 1,000°C). Sintering increases the strength of mineral substitute but reduces the resorption and remodeling capacity. These phosphate materials have variable rates of osteointegration based on their crystalline size and stoichiometry. They have the advantage of incorporating at a slower rate than calcium sulfate materials but faster than HA. Pore size is important and defines the integration properties. Recommended pore size is 100–150 μm. Higher pore size permits faster ingrowth but reduces strength. This results in a faster degradation of the mineral substitute. Mineral substitutes with a smaller pore size allow the platelets and leukocytes to congregate within the pores and secrete cytokines to induce and implement bone formation. Mineral substitutes are osteoconductive only; however, they may be combined with DBM (osteoinductive) or BMA (osteogenic) to form a composite bone graft substitute. TCP is one such bioceramic that is available in α and β forms. TCP absorbs faster than synthetic HA but is less strong. The α form resorbs faster than beta which is (β-TCP) preferred. β-TCP is available as blocks, granules, and

powders. The resorption rates vary from 6 months to 2 years. β-TCP is available for dental procedures, posterolateral spinal fusion, and as bioresorbable screws. Basic calcium phosphates are defined mixes of bioceramics to balance biomechanical properties and absorption rates, e.g., BoneSave® (Stryker corporation) is a 80–20 parts by weight mix of β-TCP and HA. Ion-substituted ceramics—HA of native bone is not a pure form of HA and contains various impurities. To increase the biological activity there is interest in producing ceramics that resemble native impure as closely as possible. The "phase purity" of bioceramics refers to these substitutions and relative distributions of different phases in the material. A number of materials have been produced by substituting ions such as silicate, carbonate, fluoride, magnesium, and strontium. Silicate-substituted calcium phosphate results from substitution of the phosphate ions by silicate ions. The impurity substitutes only 0.8% by weight of the material and has been shown in animal studies to cause more rapid bone formation and histopathological features of bone formation equivalent to autogenous bone graft. "Synthetic HA" is a crystalline calcium phosphate osteoconductive bone substitute not commonly used for slow bone formation. Calcium phosphate can also be manufactured as "cement", by adding an aqueous solution (containing sodium carbonate) to dissolve the calcium, which is followed by a precipitation reaction in which the calcium phosphate crystals grow (in the presence of calcium carbonate—premixed) and the cement hardens. The primary advantage of cements over blocks, granules, or powders is the ability to custom-fill defects and increased compressive strength (55 MPa), but has the disadvantage of leaking through the fracture and into joint from where the resorption is poor and can lead to functional deficit, difficulty in extraction if infection occurs, poor resistance to torsion, and sheer forces.
- Coralline ceramics are formed by thermochemically treating coral with ammonium phosphate, leaving TCP with a structure and porosity that are similar to those of cancellous bone. Pore size and porosity are important characteristics of bone graft substitutes. No osseous ingrowth occurs with pore sizes of 15–40 μm. Osteoid formation requires minimum pore sizes of 100 μm, with pore sizes of 300–500 μm reported to be ideal for osseous ingrowth. Calcite (magnesium containing calcium carbonate) is obtained from sea urchins having characteristics similar to bone HA.
- Calcium sulfate and calcium carbonate are not very popular for bone grafting. Calcium sulfate is commonly known as "plaster of Paris" as it was used in Paris for coating walls to make them fire resistant. Calcium sulfate ($CaSO_4.2H_2O$) partially dehydrates to produce a hemihydrate ($CaSO_4.½H_2O$). Calcium sulfate rapidly absorbs within few weeks following insertion and has been used clinically as autograft extender in short segment posterolateral spinal fusions.

- *Bioactive composites*:
  - *Silicate-based grafts*: Available as bioactive glasses are usually now available for carrier purpose and have good structural strength.
  - Bioactive composite of polyethylene reinforced with HA has been used for orbital floor repair and as middle-ear implants.
  - Newer materials being studied include biodegradable polymers such as polylactic and glycolic acids that are completely degraded by hydrolysis later into nontoxic metabolites eliminated as CO_2 and water.
  - Aluminum-based grafts like aluminum oxide binds to bone in response to stress and strain between implant bone interfaces.

Engineering principles for synthesis of bone graft substitutes: The bone grafts to be successful must have some architectural and surface properties that provide it strength and biological viability (allow penetration of nutrients, removal of by-products and cell migration and colonization) to use as bone growth. Some technical concerns are as follows:
- Reproduce the highly porous architecture of cancellous bone for homing and colonization by MSCs. This is very important as changing pore size alters response of cells—pore diameters of 15–50 μm stimulate fibrovascular growth, 50–150 μm causes osteoid formation, and 150–500 μm pores are the most optimal size resulting in mineralized bone.
- Surface properties need to be so reproduced that fibrin clot is well-stabilized and osteoprogenitor cells become associated with matrix scaffolds.

Complications of Bone Grafting (Autograft and Allograft)

Bone grafting is an enticing procedure and a life savior for orthopedic surgeons at times of complicated reconstructions but it is not without complications that can be troubling at times. The following is a list of complications associated with the bone grafting procedure and two of them will be discussed in detail.
- Additional surgical and anesthesia time
- Added costs
- Morbidity in the form of pain and delayed mobilization
- Development of incisional hernia
- Vascular injury
- *Neurological injury*: Posterior iliac grafting—cluneal nerves and anterior iliac grafting—lateral femoral cutaneous grafting
- Fracture of donor bone
- Hematoma and seroma formation
- Additional site for potential infection
- Logistic—limited amount of bone available for grafting
- Cosmetic concern and chronic pain
- Ureteral injury
- Transmission of infection (allograft)
- Rejection of allografted bone
- Very rarely tumor cell transplantation.

Infections associated with bone allografts: Use of allografts has increased tremendously over last decade especially with the availability of bone banking facility and standardization. Allografts act as porous, noncellular, and avascular foreign bodies that are prone to bacterial adhesion. Upon attachment bacteria protect themselves by secreting a thick glycocalyx matrix rendering them inaccessible to immune surveillance and local cellular defense mechanisms. The issue of allograft-associated sepsis rose after identification of a 23-year-old man with *Clostridium sordellii* sepsis was attributed to allograft transplantation. By 2002, the Center for Disease Control (United States) had reported 26 cases of clostridial infections associated with musculoskeletal tissue allografts probably a result of decomposition of tissues in donor. Varied infections have been reported form implanted allograft bone including viral [hepatitis B and C, and human immunodeficiency virus (HIV)], bacterial [*Clostridium* species, *S. aureus*, (group-A beta-hemolytic *streptococci* (GABHS), *Pseudomonas*, *Enterococcus* organisms] and fungal. Aseptic processing of allografts has improved but does not completely sterilize the tissue from organisms or spores. Even practice of submerging the bone in antimicrobial solutions does not ameliorate the spores. To destroy the spores, gamma radiation and treatment with ethylene oxide or a low-temperature chemical sterilization should be done at the time of implantation (at the cost of decreased integrity of the graft and possible synovitis). Irradiation has been proposed to reduce bacterial transmission and may also inactivate HIV but the efficacy has not been quantitatively studied. Strict guidelines for processing the bone grafts and establishing standards for testing aerobic and anaerobic organisms and fungi as well as reporting of infections should be laid down.

Over the past years, the use of "antibiotic-impregnated bone grafts (AIBGs)" has become a popular procedure in the treatment of bone and joint infections. A major advantage of AIBGs involves the possibility of impregnation of various antibiotics depending on the sensitivity profile of the causative organism, and also an additional surgery for removal of the antibiotic carrier is not necessary, as in the use of antibiotic-loaded bone cement. Vancomycin is the most common antibiotic used (VAN-BG) but others like tobramycin, gentamycin, clindamycin, cephalothin, and rifampicin have also been used. Antibiotics are incorporate by manual mixing or by placing the bone grafts into antibiotic-containing solutions. Better of the two methods is, however, unknown. There is a higher amount of antibiotic uptake in demineralized bone compared to native one. Furthermore, there exist great discrepancies regarding the exact antibiotic/bone graft ratio. From various studies, vancomycin is found to significantly better elute from cancellous bone in comparison with tobramycin. Rifampicin elutes longest; for up to 21 days while beta-lactamase are the shortest to do so. Although high local concentrations are eligible for a successful eradication of the infection, it should be borne in mind that such high concentrations might be associated with an accompanying toxic effect on cells. High concentrations of vancomycin have been reported to substantially reduce osteoblast replication and even cause cell death. In case of a biantibiotic combination, a synergistic effect has been described between aminoglycosides and glycopeptides when eluted from acrylic bone cement. However, the amount of vancomycin eluted from vancomycin-netilmicin-loaded grafts was significantly reduced compared with those loaded only with vancomycin, whereas the release of netilmicin is not hampered. Moreover, the addition of blood significantly slowed down the antibiotic elution over the first 7 days in vitro. In clinical practice, AIBGs might be used in the prophylaxis as well as in the treatment of bone and joint infections. The prophylactic use of antibiotic-loaded bone grafts for prevention of wound infections after orthopedic surgery has been though only sparsely done.

Rejection of allograft: Allografts can induce immune response and are liable for rejection. The rejection process, however, is not as prominent as that of other soft tissue transplantation. Allografts possess cell surface glycoproteins typically from the contained bone marrow cells, endothelial cells, and retinacular activating cells. These are recognized by innate "cell-mediated immunity" of the host. T-lymphocytes recognize class I and II antigens to mount host immune response. Collagen possibly incites mild cell-mediated and humoral immune response, while noncollagenous portion (proteoglycans, osteopontin, osteocalcin, etc.) produce cell-mediated immunity but to even a lesser extent. Mineral phase (HA) is nonimmunogenic. The implanted graft is surrounded by inflammatory cells restricting the incorporation. Inflammatory cells also get sensitized and may possibly lead to increased reaction on future implantation but the effects have not been specifically studied. The degree of the host response is related to the antigen concentration and total dose which is significant in fresh allografts. Modern allograft processing kills most of the resident cells and washes away the surface proteins to a large extent. This is the cause of frequent seroma formation and persistent serous discharge from the operative site as the incorporation is dependent on cellularity and MHC compatibility between host and donor following massive allograft transplantation.

BONE BANKING

A bone bank provides usable bone grafts (implants) on demand that serve predictable function, and are free from transmissible disease. An increase in the demand of bone grafts due to higher number of complex (spinal fusion and tumor resection reconstruction) and revision surgeries have pressed the need for developing storage and procurement facilities for allograft bone. Autograft alone cannot specifically supply the demand in large tumor excisions, complicated articular, and extra-articular reconstructions in revision arthroplasty, etc. Several centers are storing bone using nonuniform methods in our country as a central regulatory authority does not exist. Also, there is no intercommunication between the centers and they function autonomously. There are lots of advantages for the use of allografts **(Table 12)**, but there needs to be strict regulatory mechanisms for development and induction of bone banking facility like the use of blood products. This is important because the techniques and regulatory keep evolving.

Need for constant updation in screening methods and regulation: With the initial use there was not much focus on screening the donors. This came into focus with transmission of hepatitis B infection in a medical student who received bone from above knee amputee (Shutkin 1954). Then other infections like transmissions of HIV infection in 1984, hepatitis C virus in 1992 and 1995, and new infections like SARS in 2004 have been reported. Thus, the screening methods need to be constantly updated to incorporate unusual and new infections. Also like other organ transplantation unethical activities like "trafficking" can ever become prominent so regulation of all human tissues should be strict and traceable. This also encourages registration of complications.

The Bone Banking Protocol

Ideally a protocol should be developed by the responsible person from department of orthopedics (preferably the HOD), organ donation and retrieval unit or a bone banking administrator, operation theater nurse, hematological laboratory technician, pathologist, and microbiologist in a combined effort depending on the needs and availability of resources for that center and surroundings. They also comprise the team or organizational unit of bone bank. The bone banking administrator need not be a medical personnel but should have adequate training to handle the bone bank.

Donor Selection

Informed consent from the person is a must before retrieving the tissue if says he is undergoing hip arthroplasty (for obtaining femoral head). For cadaveric bone retrieval, it is ideal if the person has expressed his wish for donation premortem but deviation may be legally obtained if closest of the relatives freely and voluntarily give consent to do so (depending on state laws) postmortem. The criteria used to judge if bone can be reasonably obtained from the patient are tabulated in **Box 2**.

Excision of Graft Bone, Processing, and Storage

- The removed femoral head is inspected and capsule and synovial tissue are cultured on aerobic and anaerobic bacteria. In order to exclude malignancies, autoimmune inflammatory processes, or infections, a biopsy of 1 cm^3 of representative bone and capsule is sent for histopathological examination (HPE) (though HPE as a routine standard procedure is debated by agencies and really not mandatory for lacking literature support of utility). The dimensions are noted and it is wrapped using double jar technique (described by Nather). The graft is washed in normal saline or biofiltered water followed by hydrogen peroxide to remove grossly visible fat and debris and dipped in 2% aqueous iodine solution for 15–30 minutes followed by a thorough repeat wash with normal saline. The excess water is then drained and the graft put in a smaller sterile glass jar with a screw-on cap. This is then put in a larger glass bottle with air seal lock, both the jars are sterile. Due labeling of the graft is done with dimensions and it is sent to storage deep-freezer within 30 minutes. The freezer has a temperature of –80°C and that has a continuous temperature registration device charting temperature changes round the clock. The ambient storage temperature range is between –90°C and –70°C to protect against temperature-induced

BOX 2: Criteria used for excluding patient from bone donation (not a comprehensive list and can be modified from center-to-center).

Specific exclusion criteria:
- No consent
- HIV, HBsAg, HCV, and CMV positive patient (serologically and clinically proven)
- Men having homosexual intercourse after 1977
- Immigrants (after 1977) from countries in which heterosexual intercourse is an important factor for HIV transmission
- Persons indulging in or suspected to be involved in prostitution (or their partners) since 1977
- Intravenous medication/narcotics use (documented or suspected)
- Hemophilic patients who received clotting factor concentrates
- Individuals who received blood transfusion before 1980
- Individuals who had a skin tattoo or did piercing <6 months ago
- Individuals who stayed in a severe acute respiratory syndrome (SARS) epidemic area or individuals who had face-to-face contact with a SARS patient

General exclusion criteria:
- Language barrier or patient unable to understand and give consent for any reason (mental retardation and psychiatric patients)
- Age <18 years
- Active or recent systemic infection
- Patients with severe burns or contaminated wounds
- Meningitis/encephalitis
- Tubercular infection of bone or joints
- Leprosy
- Active "slow-virus" infection (suspected or documented) or patients suffering from dementia
- Previous undocumented infection with hepatitis B or C and HIV
- Active or past syphilis infection
- Recent (<4 weeks) vaccination with live vaccine (measles, yellow fever, mumps, polio, oral typhoid, and rubella)
- Patients with rheumatoid arthritis or connective tissue disorders/autoimmune diseases
- Documented or suspected metabolic disorders
- Patients with insulin-dependent diabetes mellitus or those treated with growth hormones in past
- Patients on chronic medication (phenytoin and corticosteroids)
- Recent exposure to toxic substances (lead, aluminium, or other substances known to home bone)
- Patients with malignancies and those treated with anticancer chemotherapy
- Significant radiation exposure to bone as in radiotherapy

BOX 3: Recommended tests that should be performed on donor's blood sample and tissues.

- Blood and rhesus typing
- Hemogram including erythrocyte sedimentation rate (ESR) and C- reactive protein
- *Viral (hepatitis)*:
  - HBsAg, hepatitis B core antigen, and hepatitis B antibody
  - Anti-HCV antibody (repeat after 180 days for living donors)
  - Viral nucleic acid
- *Viral markers for*:
  - HIV1 and HIV2 (repeat for living donors after 180 days)
  - HTLV (repeat for living donors after 180 days)
  - CMV
- Syphilis (VDRL, venereal disease reaction laboratory)
- *Microbiology (of soft tissue specimen and bone)*:
  - Gram stain and Ziehl Neelsen stain
  - Aerobic culture (nutrient agar, blood agar, and chocolate agar)
  - Anaerobic culture (thioglycolate broth)
- Histopathological examination

(VDRL: venereal disease research laboratory)

damage to the tissue. As a backup measure nitrogen tank should be installed in case the freezer fails. In any case, if the cold chain for storage fails at any time then the whole batch of bone graft has to be discarded. In deep frozen condition, the unprocessed allogenic bone tissue can be preserved for a maximum of 5 years. Blood samples are collected simultaneously while harvesting the bone graft to determine blood type and routine hemogram **(Box 3)**. During surgery, bacterial culture swab samples from the soft tissues (hip capsule) are collected. Serological screening for infectious diseases is reperformed 6 months after surgery to exclude infections with window period. This takes care of persons that might be recently infected.

- For harvesting cadaveric bone, the donor's limbs are prepped and draped using standard surgical principles, and the tissue is recovered by trained persons. Bones are commonly retrieved from ilium, femur, humerus, tibia, ribs, and vertebrae. Many other types of tissues can be recovered, including stem cells, soft tissues (tendon and ligament), and skin. Fresh articular cartilage is initially refrigerated and then placed in a culture medium to maintain its viability for up to 28 days. Small bones and soft tissues are collected using the described "double jar" technique while long bones should be triple wrapped in sterile packaging. The three layers consist of inner gamma irradiated polyethylene bag, middle layer of autoclaved linen where the bone is tied at ends with cotton tape and outer again a sterile polyethylene bag. The dimensions of bones should be measured and put on the label (to match in future with recipient). All obtained graft material is swab cultured immediately upon retrieval prior to processing. The periosteum is immediately stripped, cleaned as above, and the grafts from hereon are kept frozen at –80°C for all further processing and storage (fresh frozen graft). The method for lyophilization is different (preferred for cadaver allografts) and is described below. If gross bacterial contamination is identified or suspected, the material is kept under surveillance and newer techniques, such as bacterial extraction, are used to confirm the results. There is high chance of both false-positive and false-negative results with swab culture. All the materials are discarded if bacterial contamination is confirmed or suspicion unsettled. For cadaveric donors, as it is not possible to reobtain blood samples after 6 months, the blood samples are also stored with the grafts and serological tests reperformed at 6 months before release into storage facility.

Sterilization of Graft

The sterilization techniques differ at various setups and keep evolving. Regardless of the technique used, the objective is to remove all infectious elements with minimal impact on the performance of the allograft. Tissue can either be processed aseptically or be secondarily "sterilized". In all the safest method appears to be aseptic harvesting with strict monitoring. To be considered sterile, allografts should have fewer than 10^6 microorganisms; for medical devices, the requirement is fewer than 10^3 microorganisms. For fresh frozen grafts the above described method is followed. For freeze-dried allograft preparation the method is as follows. Commonly the harvested graft bone is cut and washed with biofiltered water (with or without pressurization) followed by pasteurization (shaker bath at 60°C for 3 hours) and centrifugation with alcohol (70% for 3 hours) or detergent solution. Pasteurization (not necessarily required and should be omitted if aseptic precautions are followed) removes most bacteria, fungi, and viruses including HIV (heating >60°C damages the healing properties of bone so should be avoided). Alternatively, aqueous solution of iodine may be used to similar effect but prolonged exposure is cytotoxic. Alcohol therapy is effective against HIV, bacteria, and spores. Antibiotics have not been shown to give an additional benefit in reduction of contamination. Some authors have even demonstrated adverse effects of some antibiotics. The lyophilized graft after terminal sterilization (see later) is stored at room temperature.

Terminal sterilization is usually done by gamma irradiation. Gamma radiation is effective in killing bacteria, fungi, spores, and, to a lesser degree, viruses. Depending on the dose, however, gamma radiation can weaken the graft. Doses below 1.5 Mrad do not adversely affect the tissue strength. A minimum dose of 2 Mrad is required to kill bacteria and 4 Mrad for killing viruses. After such high dose irradiation the bone is discolored and fibrillar network of bone is destroyed. Solubility of collagen and proteoglycans increase reducing structural strength and inductive capacity is greatly reduced. A dose of 2.5 Mrad is chosen for processed bone giving priority to sterilization and is given by Co^{60} gamma generators. After processing the grafts are sent to quarantine for final storage. Grafts are stored at the tissue bank during the quarantine period (6 months) until the second stage serologic and bacteriologic test results and autopsy reports (when required) are received and cleared. The graft is then released for human use after proper labeling and sent to definite storage.

Choice of Freeze Dried versus Fresh Frozen Graft

The shelf life in storage depends on the method of processing and storage; commonly either Freeze drying (lyophilization—infinite) or deep freezing (5 years) is used. Fresh frozen grafts are obtained under strict sterile conditions and may not be processed (though most units process them with above method to minimize chances of infection). Freezing an allograft has little impact on the mechanical properties and reduces its immunogenicity; however, it does reduce viability of articular cartilage unless cryopreserved. Lyophilization removes >95% of the water enabling biological material (arresting the enzymatic lysis) to be stored for long periods of time even at room temperature. This process is achieved by first freezing the graft and then sublimated in vacuum; the drying is achieved by water evaporation from the specimen and condensation in the condenser. Freeze drying further diminishes the immunogenicity of the graft and also eliminates the bacterial contamination but does alter mechanical properties (especially if not rehydrated properly). Freezing at –15 to –30°C is not recommended as ice crystals develop very fast.

All freeze—dried and frozen tissue requires "reconstitution". The length of reconstitution time varies according to the type of tissue. Reconstitution of lyophilized bone grafts is done aseptically at 4° temperature before use. Sterile normal physiological saline or Hartmann Ringer—lactate solution is commonly used. Some surgeons use antibiotic solution (amoxicillin and cloxacillin solution) but the efficacy and need is unknown. Any bone which requires modification before use or is intended for load-bearing purposes should be reconstituted for longer periods of time preferably 24 hours. Freeze-dried tissue is brittle (lack of water) which can be reduced by prolonged reconstitution. All reconstituted grafts must be used within 24 hours. Graft incorporation usually follows the steps as for an autograft. The fresh frozen grafts intended to be used are allowed to thaw in operation theatre in situ for 1 hour before surgery. It is then soaked in 1 liter of normal saline and prepared by removing all soft tissues and remaining periosteum if any. The articular cartilage should be removed before cutting or morcellization of the graft. This is then again washed thoroughly before surgical use. Culture swabs should be obtained at the time of graft usage also.

Quality control of bone banking: As stated above, as lot many procedures are involved in bone banking so a stringent protocol should be followed that needs regular monitoring. A few are discussed below.

- *Histopathological screening*: The HPE establishes good quality bone being stored and used. HPE has not been mandated by all agencies and few centers omit it altogether. The rationale is that it has never been documented to be cost effective and makes hardly any difference in patient management or to recipient. Most of the findings have been over-diagnostic for suspicion of malignancy or inflammatory disorders that got hardly documented in the donors on follow-up. Also it has been found that with 100% sensitivity and 99.9% specificity surgeon can preoperatively and during surgery with gross examination rule-out exclusions. There have been a few instances on the contrary where malignancies in early stages have been found that were missed on routine hematological or clinical examination. Equalizing evidence exists that suggest presence of occult findings (B-cell lymphoma, myeloma, sarcoma, Paget's disease, ochronosis, metabolic disease, osteonecrosis, and Gaucher's disease) to a significant instance and recommend HPE. Thus, a HPE of bone grafts should be carefully institutionalized. We would recommend HPE only when there is critical suspicion that cannot be settled otherwise.
- *Culture swab*: This is a mandatory requirement. The culture specimen obtained at the time of graft implantation and usage serves purpose of quality control check on banking procedure. The policy decision needs to be determined for the use of better culture methods as swab cultures have been often found to show false-negative results. There are two ways one by taking multiple specimens and culturing them after processing or otherwise using routine antibacterial processing of the graft before surgical use.

CONCLUSION

- Fracture is a break in continuity of otherwise normal bone (fracture in abnormal bone will be termed pathological fracture) that induces a host of inflammatory and reparative processes to incite metabolic changes in this hard tissue of body.
- Bone regeneration depends on three essential elements: (1) progenitor cells, (2) growth factors (osteoinduction), and (3) osteoconduction. The process of osseous repair is primarily a direct healing which is possible in exact apposition of the fractured fragments under compression.
- If the fragments are not apposed well then fracture repair occurs by indirect or secondary healing involving the intermediary tissue called callus.
- The repair process in either case is stereotyped and follows a predetermined path governed genetically and discrete cellular processes, however, extrinsic control is exercised in the form of mechanical, cytokine (paracrine), and hormonal (endocrine) influences; any discrepancy of which would produce abnormal process resulting in slow, delayed repair, or nonunion. To provide optimal outcome, the surgeon should have a clear understanding of the stepwise process along with various influences such as Wnt pathway, RANKL, NSAIDs, etc., that can be modulated at appropriate time.
- In modern day practice the treatment variable has specific influence on the fracture repair and it is of utmost importance not to disturb the local biology of fracture healing and maintain vascularity for optimal outcome whatever the method used for fracture fixation.
- In case the fracture repair does not follow the desired path constitutionally or due to treatment variables, various methods are available for improving the possibility of fracture repair that broadly fall into biological and nonbiological methods. Bone grafting is the most widely accepted method of improving fracture repair.
- Due to increased number of surgeries being performed, the need of bone grafts is constantly increasing necessitating the deployment of bone banking facilities.

CHAPTER 3

Metabolic Diseases of Bone

Manish Kumar Varshney

OSTEOPOROSIS

INTRODUCTION

Osteoporosis ranks as number one metabolic bone disease that affects population and its prevalence at any given point of time exceeds the collective prevalence of major medical diseases (diabetes, breast cancer, and hypertension) combined together when considered with respect to total number of persons affected. The terms "osteoporosis" and "osteomalacia" were coined by Pommer in 1885 and he also avidly differentiated between them. "Osteoporosis" was considered as reduction in the amount of bone that is qualitatively normal while "osteomalacia" was deemed to be a normal amount of bone that is in adequately mineralized. This differentiation was, however, wrong because osteoporosis is now proven to be a qualitative defect of bone in addition to quantitative reduction of the bone mass. A restrictive and inappropriate definition commonly followed by clinicians in general practice is "fragility fractures"—fractures in bones occurring with nonviolent trauma (such as falling with standing height). This definition essentially does not indicate or refer to primary prevention and should not be used to clinically define osteoporosis. Some terms should be clarified before using in common practice as they are commonly wrongly referred:

- "Bone strength" relates to bone quantity, quality, and turnover. It also depends on bone shape, distribution of bone mass, and the manner in which load is applied to bone.
- "Bone density/bone mineral density (BMD)" is primarily a derivative of mineral component, and hence reflects bone mass (approximately).
- "Bone size" is probably a constitutional and genetic function with secondary environmental and lifestyle influences.
- "Bone quality" is an accrual term that varies with age. It is determined by bone architecture (microanatomy), mineralization, collagen molecule and fiber formation, damage accumulation (e.g., microfractures) and bone age. Increasing age reduces compositional heterogeneity and toughness of bone while capacity to heal microfractures is also reduced.

DEFINITION

Osteoporosis is both a qualitative and quantitative defect of bone that usually affects all the bones of the body. It can be more precisely defined (Circa, 1991) as a "progressive (often), systemic (commonly), and skeletal disease characterized by overall low bone mass (quantitative) predominated by microarchitectural deterioration (qualitative) of bone tissue that results in increased bone fragility, and hence susceptibility to fracture **(Figs. 1A and B)**". World Health Organization (WHO) definition for osteoporosis based on elevated fracture risk is more objective and is detailed below and stresses solely on the BMD that has ingrained in the minds of physicians. Newer definition of osteoporosis considers it to be a skeletal disorder characterized by low bone strength and increased risk of fracture (National Institutes of Health Consensus Development Panel on Osteoporosis Prevention, Diagnosis, and Therapy) which puts into perspective the changing scenario of a relation much larger and varied than BMD. It must be remembered that there are no symptoms from low bone mass unless fracture occurs.

PROBLEM STATEMENT, PREVALENCE, AND INCIDENCE

Osteoporosis is an ongoing slow pandemic. Nearly one-third of women aged between 60 and 70 years and around 70% older than 80 years have osteoporosis (rest have osteopenia). Primary undesirable consequence of osteoporosis is fragility fracture. Fracture would occur only if a failing force is applied to bone. The magnitude of failing force required is inversely proportional to bone strength. Weaker the bone, hence higher will be chance of fracture. This is at best a rough correlation. Elderly people gradually lose balance during walk and later may fall even during standing. Fall from standing height has been cited the most common cause of osteoporotic fractures. But, there are a variety of factors (bone strength, the fall, and the impact of fall) intrinsic to cause a fracture **(Flowchart 1)**.

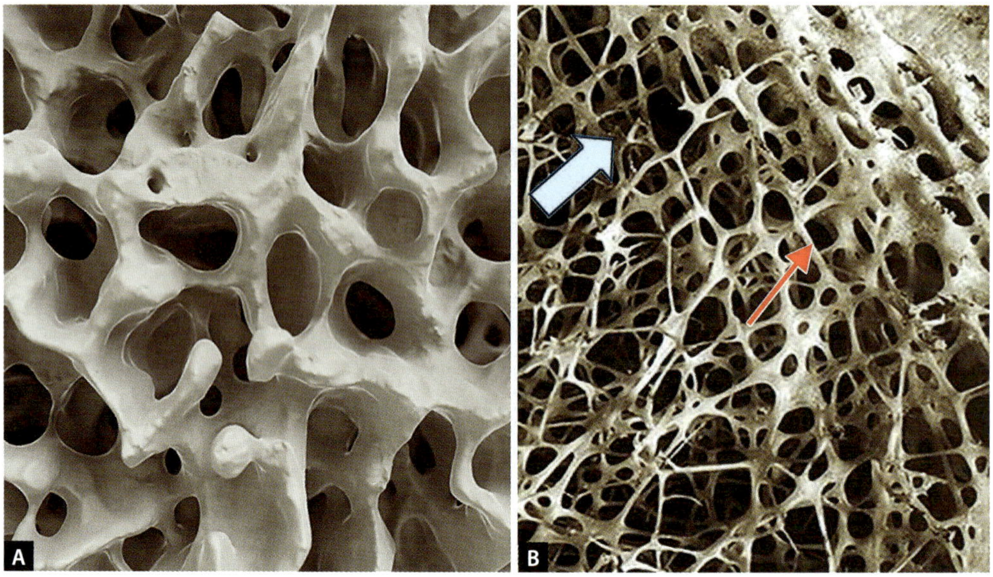

Figs. 1A and B: Microscopic cross-section of cancellous bone. (A) Microstructure of normal healthy human bone with thick trabecular architecture and interconnecting trabeculae; (B) Microscopic appearance of an osteoporotic bone with thinning of trabeculae (arrow). If the trabeculae get broken it is called "perforation" (block arrow). Both - "thinning and perforation" cause weakening of bone making it susceptible to fractures from minimal impact - "fragility fractures".

Flowchart 1: Pathogenesis of osteoporotic fracture.

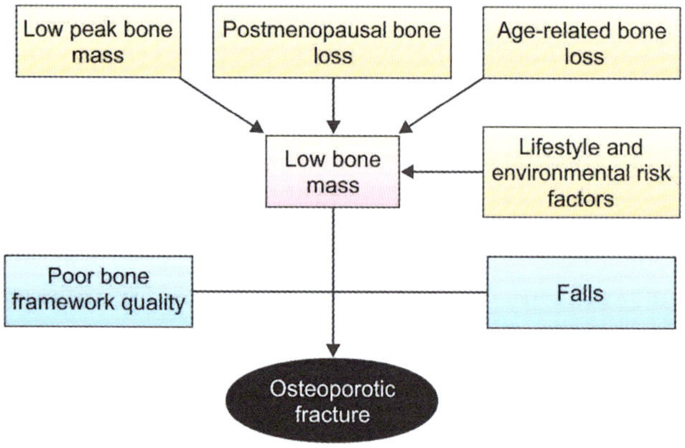

These explain the significantly less prevalence of fractures despite widely prevalent osteoporosis.

Common fractures that occur in osteoporosis are **(Figs. 2A to C)**:

- Fractures of distal radius **(Box 1)**
- Fractures of proximal femur—femoral neck and intertrochanteric **(Box 2)**
- Fracture of vertebral bodies **(Box 3)**
- Other fractures related to low BMD are of metatarsals, proximal humerus, ribs, toes, leg, pelvis, hand, and clavicle.

Ninety percent of all hip and spinal fractures in old age are related to osteoporosis. Thoracolumbar junction (T12 and L1) and mid-thoracic spine are the most frequent areas for vertebral fractures. The lifetime risk of having one or more vertebral fractures in females over age of 50 years is one in three compared to one in five for males of same age. In white women and men aged 50 years or older, the lifetime risk of any osteoporosis-related fracture in the hip, spine, or distal forearm is nearly 40% and 13%, respectively as commonly reported in contemporary literature. With increasing age, the incidence of osteoporotic-related fractures increases. Osteoporotic fractures are less common in nonwhite females and in men. Osteoporosis and consequent fractures are major public health concerns and pose immense economic burden. The costs of burden for fractures are estimated to be USD 21,000 during the first year of a hip fracture and USD 1,200 for a vertebral fracture (Indian data not available). This indicates that cost of osteoporosis-related hip fracture is similar to that incurred for stroke (relative comparison for highlighting severity). Other untoward effects of an osteoporotic fracture include reduced height, poor functional status, residual pain, loss of independence, reduced tidal volume (thoracic spine fractures), reduced metabolism, frailty, increased mortality, poor remaining quality of life **(Fig. 3)**, and fear and depression. Not only the functional disabilities but mortality associated with vertebral fractures is also greater than expected in the general population **(Table 1)**. Vertebral fracture-related mortality exceeds that of hip fracture despite a much higher mortality ratio associated with hip fractures as the former exceeds hip fractures in the mean number of bed days and limited activity days. We will first understand the dynamics of bone loss and development of osteoporosis in next section and preliminary understanding of the objective definition of osteoporosis. Details will then be gradually built upon.

NATURAL HISTORY OF BONE MASS CHANGES IN HUMAN BODY, OPERATIONAL DEFINITION OF OSTEOPOROSIS, AND ITS CLASSIFICATION

Human skeleton is made of cancellous and cortical bone in a ratio of 1:4 by mass (20:80%) while the ratio is reversed (80:20%) when one considers the surface area. This increased surface area also means that the turnover rate will be higher for cancellous bone (25% each year) compared to cortical

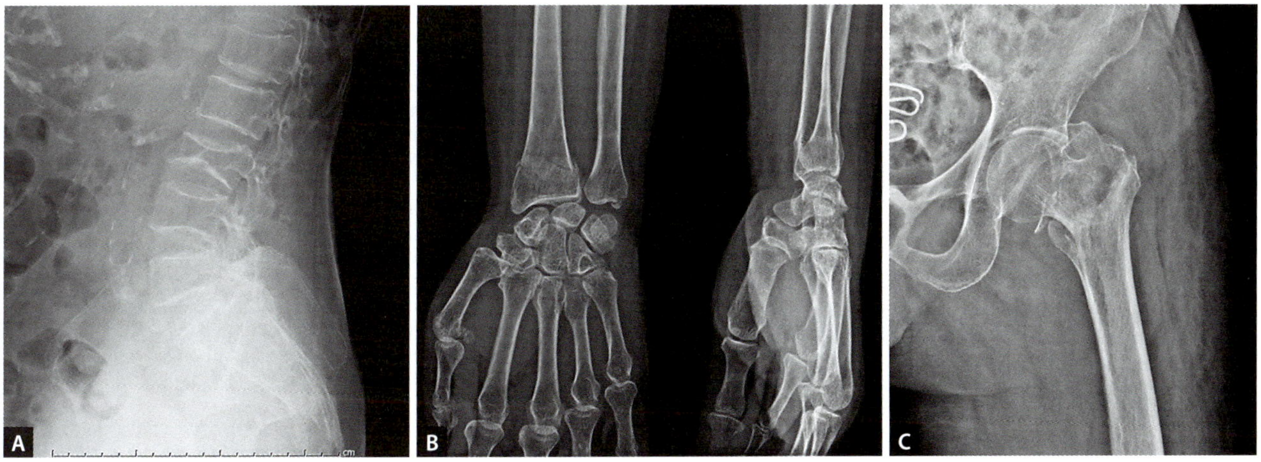

Figs. 2A to C: Osteoporotic fractures: (A) Osteoporotic wedge compression fracture of 3rd lumbar vertebra; (B) Colles fracture of distal radius with fracture of ulnar styloid; (C) Intertrochanteric fracture of left femur.

BOX 1: Distal radius osteoporotic fractures.

- Third most common osteoporotic fracture
- Prior fractures indicate high chances of future fracture
- They tend to occur early (**Box 4**: Bone mass and bone loss) so should alert the treating physician from preventing future more serious fractures
- Caused by fall on outstretched hand as in perimenopausal period the protective mechanisms from fall are still intact
- *Complications:*
  - Pain, temporary disability (dressing, eating, meal preparation, doing hair, toileting, etc.)
  - Long-term degenerative arthritis
  - Complex regional pain syndrome
  - Poor functional recovery in one-fourth patients at 6 months

BOX 2: Hip fractures.

- Second most common osteoporotic fracture
- Marker of future fracture
- Mostly caused by fall from standing height (only 1% falls cause fracture)
  - 5% can also occur spontaneously
- Easily diagnosed clinically and radiologically
- *Complications:*
  - High disability rate in survivors (nearly half of the patients are incapacitated)
  - High mortality rate (similar to breast cancer)

bone (3%). At any given time up to 10% of human skeleton is being remodeled **(Box 4)**. Peak adult bone mass reaches at about the age of 35 years for cortical bone (varying by genetic and environmental factors by a couple of years) and a little earlier for trabecular bone. Bone mass is accumulated from the age of 8 years till the end of 2nd decade. In cortical bones, the bone mass subsequently declines with aging at the rate of 0.3–0.5% per year in both men and women **(Fig. 4)**. This is a universal phenomenon occurring in all races. Over a lifetime a female loses 30% of cortical bone and 50% of trabecular bone; males lose two-thirds of above values. Endosteal diameter of bone increases rapidly than periosteal diameter due to increased trabeculation of cortical bone. Women at peak bone mass have less cortical bone area (6–25% less) than would be expected based on body size explaining

BOX 3: Vertebral fractures.

- Most common osteoporotic fractures
- Strong predictor of future fractures
- Many occur with common daily activities such as lifting weights, pulling, pushing
- Many fractures (25–30%) are only reveled radiologically while remaining clinically silent
- *Complications:*
  - Back pain
  - Loss of height and deformity (kyphosis), costopelvic syndrome
  - Reduced pulmonary function
  - Reduced quality of life (distorted body image, sleep disorder, loss of self-esteem, and depression)
  - Increased mortality

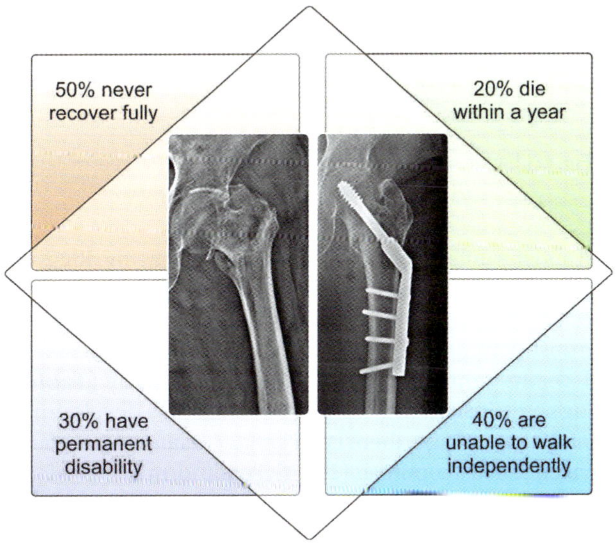

Fig. 3: Long-term morbidity and mortality associated with an osteoporotic hip fracture.

the reduced bone strength in females compared to males. At menopause, the loss of bone mass accelerates in females not taking hormone replacement therapy from an average of 1% initially to 5% over the decade which then again slows. At any given period of time, women have less bone mass than do

TABLE 1: Standardized mortality ratio after a spine fracture.

	Age-standardized mortality ratio	
Fracture	***Women***	***Men***
Proximal femur	2.2	3.2
Vertebral	1.7	2.4
Other major	1.9	2.2
Other minor	0.8	1.5

BOX 4: Bone mass and bone loss.

- Women have lower peak bone mass than men
- Whites have lower peak bone mass than blacks
- *Bone loss occurs:*
  - With advancing age
  - Because resorption is greater than formation
- As bone loss occurs, there is loss of quality as well as quantity
- Rate of cortical bone loss is more or less constant while cancellous bone loss occurs at accelerated rate between 50 and 70 years. Initially, there is higher incidence of wrist fractures (55–65 years of age) which then gives way to spine fractures (65–75 years of age) finally the risk of hip fractures rise (75–85 years of age) when the cancellous bone loss is more or less stabilized to a constant rate

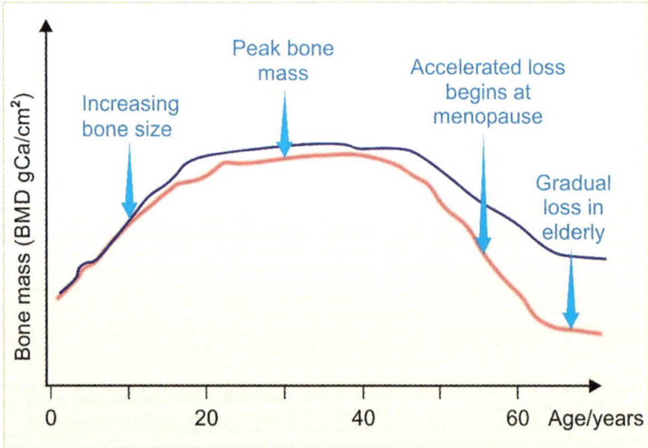

Fig. 4: Change of bone mass with age (red: females; blue: males). (BMD: bone mineral density)

men and the difference gets accentuated with aging. Riggs and Melton classified osteoporosis into primary and secondary types **(Box 5)**. The primary type is further classified into type 1 or postmenopausal and type 2 or senile forms. The senile and postmenopausal forms differ conceptually **(Table 2)** giving some insight into the process of disease development. After 80 years of age, there is no gender-related difference in prevalence of osteoporosis **(Fig. 4)**. Senile form is also referred as involutional osteoporosis. Similar to postmenopausal osteoporosis men have "postclimacteric" osteoporosis as seen in gradual testicular failure. This differs from postmenopausal form only in the sense that clinical evidence of osteoporosis develops some 15 years later and is slow to develop.

The operational definition of osteoporosis (densitometric definition) given by the WHO is in terms of BMD (and hence bone mass). Although BMD is not the only factor that determines fracture risk, but it is the strongest predictor identified for fracture. Hence, osteoporosis is defined for

BOX 5: Classification of osteoporosis.

Primary:
- Type 1 (postmenopausal)
- Type 2 (senile or involutional)
- Type 3 ("postclimacteric", it is not a part of original classification, but is similar to type 1 osteoporosis but occurring in males)

Secondary:
- *Hormonal:* Hypogonadism, thyrotoxicosis, Cushing's syndrome, hyperprolactinemia, and diabetes mellitus
- *Drugs:* Steroids, phenobarbital, anticonvulsants, anticoagulants, cytotoxic agents, etc.
- *Nutritional:* Calcium deficiency, vitamin C and D deficiency, malabsorption, alcohol intake, and malnutrition
- *Metabolic diseases:* Osteogenesis imperfecta, homocystinuria, Marfan's syndrome, etc.
- Chronic liver and renal disease
- *Miscellaneous disorders:* Multiple myeloma, rheumatoid arthritis, mastocytosis, thalassemia, Wilson's disease, hemochromatosis, etc.

Source: Modified from Riggs and Melton.

TABLE 2: Conceptual differences in types of primary osteoporosis.

Type 1 (postmenopausal osteoporosis)	***Type 2 (senile osteoporosis)***
Age >50 years	Age >75 years
Female to male ratio around 5:2	Female to male ratio around 2:1
Involves mainly trabecular bone	Proportionately involves both trabecular and cortical bone
Usually high turnover osteoporosis	Usually low turnover osteoporosis
Predominantly vertebral fractures	Predominantly proximal femoral fractures
PTH normal to low	PTH increased
Estrogen withdrawal main etiology	Age-related reduced bone turnover is the main cause

diagnostic and communication standardization **(Fig. 5 and Table 3)** as a BMD ≥ 2.5 standard deviations below the peak BMD of gender and ethnicity matched 30-year-old healthy Caucasian women (T-score; discussed below). Epidemiologic data that relate "incidence of fracture to BMD" in white women was observed to define the "T-score". It was seen that when BMD > 2.5 standard deviation below peak bone mass was associated with significant increase in fracture incidence so a value of 2.5 was chosen.

There are limitations to using this "BMD-based" definition universally:

- Proper BMD cutoff values have not been estimated for all ethnic and gender groups so cannot be universally applied.
- Bone mineral density values represent (very narrow) densitometric criteria only for diagnosing osteoporosis and do not provide any differential diagnosis of the causes of low bone mass (that can arise from various metabolic abnormalities instead).
- Because BMD is a continuous measure of fracture risk, the chosen cutoffs are a bit arbitrary and in no way a person with value at 2.4 standard deviation is safe against an osteoporotic fracture or a person with value 2.6 will definitely develop a fracture.

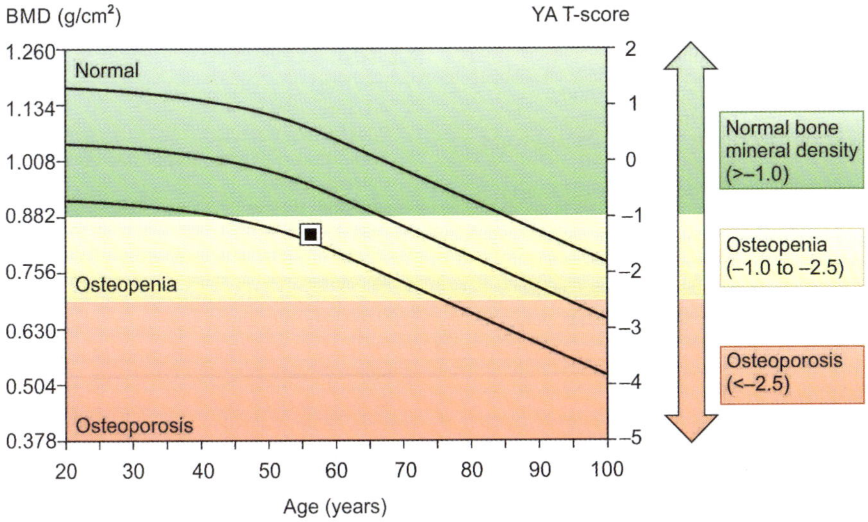

Fig. 5: BMD assessment and defining osteoporosis. (BMD: bone mineral density)

TABLE 3: The densitometric definition of osteoporosis [the World Health Organization (WHO)].

DEXA T-score (note indicated T-scores are negative here so > and < are truly mathematical)	***Bone mineral density (BMD)***	***Interpretation***
T-score > –1	BMD value within 1 standard deviation below mean peak bone mass for a young adult reference population	Normal
Between –1 and –2.5	Between 1 and 2.5 SD below that of the mean level for a young adult reference population	Low bone mass (osteopenia)
T-score ≤ –2.5 (i.e., "numerical values" higher than 2.5 say 3 or 3.2, etc.)	BMD value ≥ 2.5 SD below mean peak bone mass of a young adult reference population	Osteoporosis
T-score ≤ –2.5 and osteoporotic fracture(s)	BMD value ≥ 2.5 SD below mean peak bone mass of a young adult reference population with fractures	Severe or established osteoporosis

(DEXA: dual-energy X-ray absorptiometry; SD: standard deviation)

GENETICS OF OSTEOPOROSIS

Half of the BMD is attributable to inherited factors and some 62 genome-wide loci have been attributed to development of osteoporosis of which 15 genes are identified as causative. Genes for the *TCIRG1* (encodes the APT6i subunit of the osteoclast-specific proton pump), vitamin D receptor (VDR), the Wnt/β-catenin signaling pathway, *CLCN7 (encodes chloride channel),* the estrogen receptor, transforming growth factor alpha (TGF-α), interlukin-6, collagen type I, Cbfa1 [(*core binding factor alpha 1) or* Runt- related transcription factor 2 (Runx2)—regulates osteoblast differentiation] and collagenase are a few. Most of the genes are located in the estrogen pathway, the Wnt/β-catenin signaling pathway and the receptor activator of nuclear factor kappa-B ligand (RANKL)/RANK/osteoprotegerin (OPG) pathway. Mutations in a gene coding for the type 2a sodium-phosphate cotransporter (NpT2a) predisposes to both osteoporosis and kidney stones. A partial form of the fragile X mutation leads to early menopause and increases risk of osteoporosis. Lifestyle risk factors (discussed below), however, modify the genetic influence on BMD significantly.

RISK FACTORS FOR LOW BONE MINERAL DENSITY AND FRACTURE RISK ASSESSMENT

A number of risk factors have been identified and used to predict the risk of developing osteoporosis for development of osteoporosis. The risk factors can be categorized into modifiable and nonmodifiable ones **(Table 4)**. The risk factors for development of osteoporotic fracture are not the same as those for development of osteoporosis **(Box 6)**. It is now understood that these factors predict the risk of fractures much better than solely using BMD as evaluation tool. Using only T-score for assessment of risk of osteoporotic fractures would miss half of the patients who will fracture. Using some combination of these validated risk factors and clinical assessment tools, the risk to fracture in a patient can be estimated as low (<10% chance to fracture in next 10 years), moderate (10–20% in next 10 years), or high (>20% in next 10 years). Three such tools are available developed by different agencies to give an approximate measure of chance to suffer from osteoporosis-related fracture over next 10 years (10-year fracture risk in a given patient).

1. FRAX® tool (accessible at http://www.shef.ac.uk/FRAX/tool.aspx), developed by the WHO.
2. The QFractureScores
3. CAROC produced by the Canadian Association of Radiologists and Osteoporosis Canada.

Fracture risk assessment tool (FRAX®) is a web-based calculator that includes a number of clinically identified risk factors (BMD can be optionally included). FRAX® has been developed to calculate the 10-year probability of a hip fracture taking into account the femoral neck BMD and clinical risk

TABLE 4: Risk factors for possible development of osteoporosis.

Nonmodifiable	***Modifiable***
• Advanced age • Frailty • Parental history of fragility fracture • Early menopause (<45 years) • Primary androgen (males) and estrogen (females) deficiency • *Hypogonadal states:* Androgen insensitivity, anorexia nervosa, athletic amenorrhea, hyperprolactinemia, panhypopituitarism, premature menopause (<40 years), and Turner and Klinefelter syndrome • Ethnicity • Genetic factors (discussed later)—cystic fibrosis, Ehlers–Danlos syndrome, Gaucher's disease, glycogen storage disorders, hemochromatosis, homocystinuria, hypophosphatasia, Marfan syndrome, Menkes steely hair syndrome, osteogenesis imperfecta, parental history of hip fracture, porphyria, and Riley–Day syndrome • Small stature • Rheumatologic and autoimmune diseases—rheumatoid arthritis, ankylosing spondylitis and systemic lupus • Gastrointestinal disorders—peptic ulcer disease, celiac disease, gastric bypass, gastrointestinal surgery, inflammatory bowel disease, malabsorption, pancreatic disease, and primary biliary cirrhosis • Endocrine disorders—diabetes mellitus type 1 and type 2, central obesity, Cushing's syndrome, hyperparathyroidism, thyrotoxicosis and acromegaly • Hematological disorders—hemophilia, leukemia and lymphoma, monoclonal gammopathy, multiple myeloma, sickle-cell disease, systemic mastocytosis, other lympho- and myeloproliferative disorders • Neurological and musculoskeletal risk factors—spinal cord injury, epilepsy, multiples sclerosis, muscular dystrophy, Parkinson's disease, and stroke • Chronic liver and renal disease • Epidermolysis bullosa	• Hyperthyroidism and hyperparathyroidism • BMI < 20 kg/m² in women (<25 in men) • Low body weight [<127 lb (57.6 kg) in women, <154 lb (69.9 kg) in men] • Glucocorticoid intake • Secondary estrogen and androgen deficiency • Smoking • Alcohol consumption >3 units (1 unit = 5 oz. spirits, 12 oz. beer) • Caffeine intake >4 cups/day • Inadequate calcium and vitamin D intake • Prolonged immobility • Lack of sunlight exposure (indoor work) • Sedentary lifestyle • Excessive exercise (impaired hypothalamic-pituitary axis) • Excess protein intake • Anorexia nervosa • Medications [aluminum in antacid preparations, anticoagulants (heparin), antiepileptics, aromatase inhibitors, barbiturates, depot medroxyprogesterone (premenopausal contraception), chemotherapeutic and cytotoxic agents, glucocorticoids (≥5 mg/day prednisolone or equivalent for ≥3 months), gonadotropin-releasing hormone (GnRH), tacrolimus, methotrexate, proton pump inhibitor (PPI) (omeprazole, etc.), lithium, methotrexate, parental nutrition, tamoxifen, thiazolidenediones, and selective serotonin reuptake inhibitor (SSRI), etc.] • Space travel and prolonged low gravity exposure

(BMI: body mass index)

factors shown in **Table 5**. It can also be used to calculate the 10-year probability of other major osteoporotic fractures (defined as clinical vertebral, hip, forearm, or proximal humerus fracture) using the mentioned clinical risk factors. FRAX® tool is most useful in patients with low BMD at femoral neck, when the same is included. It has been found, however,

BOX 6: Risk factors for development of osteoporotic fracture (*not* osteoporosis).

- Low BMD
- Advancing age
- Prior fragility fracture
- Family history of osteoporotic fracture in a first-degree relative
- Current smoker
- Low body weight
- Falls
- Sarcopenia (low muscle mass)
- Dementia

(BMD: bone mineral density)

TABLE 5: Risk factors included in WHO fracture risk assessment model.

Clinical risk factors included in WHO FRAX® tool	
Current age	Gender
Rheumatoid arthritis	Secondary causes of osteoporosis type 1—type 1 DM, osteogenesis imperfecta in adults, untreated long-standing hyperthyroidism, hypogonadism or premature menopause (<40 years), chronic malnutrition, malabsorption, and chronic liver disease
Prior osteoporotic fracture	Parental history of hip fracture
Femoral neck BMD	Current smoking
Low BMI (kg/m²)	Alcohol intake (three or more drinks per day)
Oral glucocorticoids ≥5 mg prednisolone per day for 3 months	

(BMD: bone mineral density; BMI: body mass index; WHO: World Health Organization)

that FRAX® underestimates the fracture risk in patients with multiple osteoporosis-related fractures, recent fractures and those at increased risk for falling. Also, when FRAX® underestimates risk when applied to patients with low BMD at vertebral body but relatively normal BMD at femoral neck. The WHO algorithm is not validated for use of lumbar spine BMD. Benefits and limitations of FRAX® tool are detailed in **Box 7**. The specific applications for FRAX® tool are:

- FRAX® is intended to use in postmenopausal women and men aged 50 years or older.
- FRAX® may be calculated with total hip BMD or femoral neck BMD, but the latter is preferred. Other sites are not recommended.
- FRAX® has not been validated for use in currently or previously treated patients with pharmacotherapy for osteoporosis. Patients of the pharmacotherapy for 1 year or more may be considered untreated.

QFractureScores do not require laboratory measurement. It utilizes simple parameters that are known to the individual and are easily accessible without rigorous testing such as age, sex, height, weight, previous fracture, parental history of hip fracture, current smoking, glucocorticoid treatment, rheumatoid arthritis, and secondary osteoporosis and use of alcohol (>3 units/day). It has the biggest advantage of not requiring any BMD score. Being simple there is likelihood of its use as a systematic population-based program to identify high-risk patients. The inclusion of risk factors such as history of falls, type 2 diabetes, cardiovascular disease, use of tricyclic antidepressants (TCA), hormone replacement therapy, and menopausal symptoms make QFracture a more individualized tool. Unlike FRAX® tool that has been adapted for international use, the current version of QFracture is designed only for use in the United Kingdom.

The CAROC takes into account age, sex, fracture history, and glucocorticoid use to determine a 10-year absolute risk of all osteoporotic fractures. Here, BMD is mandatory to calculate risk. Regardless of the tool used it is important to understand that all these highlight the importance of patient's age (higher the age higher the risk), bone density (lower the density higher the risk), and previous history of osteoporosis-related fracture (higher the risk in such patients) as important determinants of possibly suffering from osteoporosis-related fracture.

Some important risk factors for osteoporotic fractures are further discussed here.

Low Bone Mineral Density

Bone mineral density has been considered the strongest predictor of sustaining a primary osteoporotic fracture (secondary and future fractures are better predicted by having a primary fracture itself). Vertebral fracture risk is inversely correlated to bone mineral content. It is estimated that roughly for a decline of 1 standard deviation in bone mass, there is a 1.3-fold to 2.5-fold increase in risk of osteoporosis-related fracture. One percent increase in BMD decreases fracture risk by about 4%. But, the expectation and relation is nonlinear and nonuniversal. National Osteoporosis Foundation (NOF) study itself revealed that 82% of postmenopausal females that presented with a fracture within 1 year had a T-score above -2.5, and 67% had a T-score above -2.0 as measured with peripheral densitometry. Each standard deviation decrement in femoral neck BMD has been found to increase the risk of fracture 2.6-fold. BMD at the femoral neck is a better predictor of hip fracture than BMD at other places. Patient with previous fracture and current low BMD would have additive influence and is more likely to suffer with a fracture than either factor alone. The risk of fractures in women with two fractures is 75-fold greater, if their BMD currently is less than -2.5 standard deviation compared to those with no fractures and normal BMD.

BOX 7: Benefits and limitations of FRAX® tool.

Benefits:
- Provides quantitative assessment that is better than qualitative predictions
- Fracture probability individualizes patient risk instead of just reporting relative risk
- Can be applied to population beyond Caucasian women (limitation of BMD) so more universal
- Can be combined to cost-utility analysis

Limitations:
- Assessment limited to hip only (vertebral fracture risk not validated)
- "Dose effect" not considered for input of risk factors (like number/site/severity of prior fracture, smoking, glucocorticoids, alcohol, etc.)—only "yes" or "no" input is taken, but individuals vary with "dosage" and "frequency" of these factors that have bearing on fracture risk
- Does not apply to premenopausal women
- Applies only to untreated patients in the age range 40–90 years
- "Secondary osteoporosis" is a dummy risk factor that does nothing if BMD is provided
- Rate of bone loss, bone turnover, falls, and other medications have not been included

Epidemiological Factors

Bone mineral density decreases with age in both sexes. The risk of hip fractures exponentially rises in older age. The lifetime risk of fracture is approximately twice in women than in men. In females, the risk of distal forearm and vertebral fracture increases after menopause. Though often linked to osteoporosis and increasing age the incidence of Colles' fracture actually plateaus with age. Osteoporotic fractures are twice more common in whites than in blacks. White women are more prone (1.5-fold to 4.0-fold) to have a hip fracture than African-Asian women after 40 years of age.

Body Weight and Composition

Higher body mass protects from osteoporosis partially that may be explained by the protective effect of fat on bone tissue mediated, via leptin. Weight gain during adult life would, hence, protect against hip fracture, but voluntary or involuntary weight loss would predispose to fragility fracture at all sites. Voluntary weight loss has not been linked that decisively to hip fracture.

History of Prior Fractures

A previous insufficiency fracture is the most important predictor of future fractures **(Fig. 6)**. Both Multiple Outcomes for Raloxifene Evaluation (MORE) and Vertebral Efficacy with Risedronate Therapy (VERT) trials have shown that a prevalent fracture increases risk of new vertebral fracture by

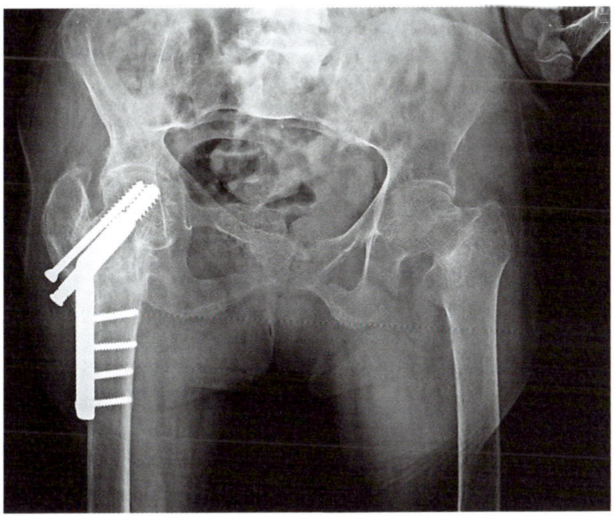

Fig. 6: Previous osteoporotic fracture is the strongest predictor for next fracture. This patient had osteoporotic right intertrochanteric fracture fixed 20 months ago came back with a "fall" and fracture at neck of left femur.

TABLE 6: Probable risk of subsequent fracture in an osteoporotic patient who has sustained a prior osteoporotic fracture.

	Risk of subsequent fracture			
Site of prior fracture	***Hip***	***Spine***	***Forearm***	***Minor fracture***
Hip	2.3	2.5	1.4	1.9
Spine	2.3	4.4	1.4	1.8
Forearm	1.9	1.7	3.3	2.4
Minor fractures	2.0	1.9	1.8	1.9

20% over 3 years and an incident fracture increases risk of new vertebral fracture by 19% over 1 year. Single site vertebral fracture increases the risk of an additional vertebral fracture by fourfold to fivefold, while the risk increases by 12-fold with more than two such fractures as mentioned in **Table 6**. Similar increase in risk of secondary osteoporotic fractures have been reported with any (forearm and hip) prevalent or incident osteoporotic fracture.

Hormonal Influence

Estrogen deficiency increases osteoclast number and bone resorption by secondarily elevated blood cytokine levels such as interleukins-6 and tumor necrosis factor-α (TNF-α). Oral contraceptives used for ≥6 years have been found to increase BMD at the vertebral and femoral neck regions reducing the risk of hip fracture by half. Estradiol hormone body concentrations <5 pg/mL is associated with higher risk of osteoporosis-related vertebral and hip fractures as is the higher sex hormone binding globulin concentrations (≥1.0 μg/dL) as this reduces free hormone levels. This effect is not seen at distal wrist. Tubal ligation interestingly has been associated with estrogen deficiency, but not low BMD or fractures. Amenorrhea, as it is commonly seen in athletes and individuals with anorexia nervosa (psychogenic dietary disorder), is associated significantly with decreased BMD. In contrast to the proposal made by some researchers, there is no evidence to support that breastfeeding or the number of pregnancies is directly associated with alteration in BMD. Pregnancies, however, appear to have a protective factor for BMD, lowering the risk of fracture ultimately. Menopause in females has a significant association with osteoporosis onset and progression. The longer the time to menopause, the higher is the ultimate bone mass. When measured at distal radius each 5-year delay in menopause has been found to be associated with 1.3% higher bone mass.

Medications

A lot of medications are known to reduce BMD. Glucocorticoids, carbamazepine, and phenytoin (barbiturates and valproic acid may induce hyperparathyroidism by accelerating metabolism of vitamin D causing rickets and osteomalacia), heparin, warfarin, thiazide diuretics, aromatase inhibitors, methotrexate, depoprogesterone, proton pump inhibitors (interfere with calcium absorption), and thiazolidinediones (pioglitazone and rosiglitazone) all have been implicated to cause osteoporosis.

Smoking and Alcohol Abuse

Compared to nonsmoking twins, the females who smoke one or more pack per day have a 5–10% reduction in perimenopausal bone mass. Smoking causes increased hydroxylation of estradiol in liver with a decrease in bioactive content. Ethanol in alcohol directly inhibits osteoblast proliferation and function reducing bone formation, maintenance and mineralization, if used over long period (chronic abuse).

Role of Beverages

Caffeine consumption has a mild but definite effect on bone mass. Consumption of 10 cups of coffee per day for 30 years is associated with a 1.1% decrease in distal radial bone mass. In contrast to coffee, high 10-year tea intakes increase BMD possibly due to a benefit from flavonoids, fluoride, or phytoestrogens found in tea. Phosphorated and carbonated drinks leach out calcium from bones and produce calciuria. Chocolates and high sugar-containing meals also have similar effect. Dark chocolates may have some protective effect in contrast.

Calcium and Other Minerals

Aluminum intake in antacid preparations or in dialysis patients, cadmium toxicity, and patients consuming lithium from metered dose inhaler (MDI) are at increased risk of osteoporosis. Higher teenage calcium and milk intake was associated with higher BMD at the spine and hip. Similar effect is noted in adults. Protein is traditionally considered bad for bones due to its calciuric effect, but may be beneficial, if it is consumed with sufficient calcium. Routine fluoridation of drinking may decrease the fracture risk. Boron, magnesium, and selenium have been found to have trophic influence on BMD.

Vitamin D, Vitamin A, and Vitamin B

For obvious reasons vitamin D deficiency impacts BMD negatively and is associated with fractures. Vitamin D deficiency when associated with low calcium intake produces secondary hyperparathyroidism resulting in bone resorption and weakening. Vitamin D excess, however, has a toxic effect and is also associated with low BMD. Excessive vitamin A also is deleterious to bone. Deficiency of vitamin B in elderly has been associated with higher homocysteine levels. Also in patients with homocystinuria due to metabolic defect there is early onset of osteoporosis. Elevated plasma homocysteine levels are associated with higher risk of fracture, but not completely associated to low BMD. Low vitamin B levels and higher homocysteine levels stimulate osteoclasts, while inhibiting osteoblasts simultaneously shifting bone metabolism toward resorption. In addition, homocysteine inhibit the enzyme lysyl oxidase responsible for collagen cross-linking. These may explain the higher than normal risk of fractures in osteoporosis with vitamin B deficiency and raised homocysteine levels despite minor effects on BMD.

Activity Levels

Regular workouts and weight-bearing exercises improve BMD in accordance with Wolff's law. Disuse osteoporosis is common in long-term immobilization, space travelers, and even absolute sedentary inactive population. However, athletes may develop premature osteoporosis due to excessive stress on bone beyond reparative capacity as has been seen in marathon runners. In female athletes, prolonged amenorrhea due to deranged hypothalamic-pituitary axis may contribute.

Falls

Factors predisposing to falls are predictors of osteoporotic fractures not osteoporosis **(Table 7)**. A fall in the last year strongly independently predicts possibility of fall and consequent fracture. The type and pattern of fall varies with age, alertness and intactness of reflexes and affects the site of pathological fracture **(Figs. 7A and B)**.

Bone Morphology

Bone geometry and variations by themselves also predict fracture risk.

Hip-axis length (HAL): It is positively correlated with hip fracture. It is defined as the distance from the greater trochanter to the pelvic brim. With one point increment in standard deviation of HAL, the risk of femoral neck and trochanter fracture nearly doubles. This implicates that tall thin women will be at the highest risk of hip fracture. Other morphological features that have also been identified to independently predict fracture risk (but are not commonly used due to availability of less cumbersome and more standardized measures) include thickness of the femoral shaft and/or neck cortex (reduced thickness predicts fracture), tensile trabecular index (reduced numbers or quantity predicts fracture), and width of trochanteric region (wider trochanter is related to osteoporotic fracture).

Femoral neck width or neck/shaft angle do not have any correlation.

TABLE 7: Causes of falls in elderly.

Personal intrinsic factors	*Extrinsic and environmental factors*
• *Balance and gait:* – Joint disease – Reduced proprioception – Cerebrovascular disease – Neuropathy – Parkinson's disease • *Aging:* – Poor postural control – Kyphosis – Weakness of muscles/ sarcopenia – Slow reaction time – Defective proprioception • *Visual impairment:* – Cataract – Glaucoma – Retinal degeneration • *Cognitive impairment:* – Alzheimer's disease – Stroke – Depression – Deconditioning – Previous falls and fear of falling • Hypoglycemia • Postural hypotension • Arrhythmia • Dehydration • Vitamin D deficiency • Anxiety and agitation • Epilepsy	• *Personal hazards:* – Inappropriate footwear – Clothing • Sedatives and hypotensive drugs • Psychotropic medications • *Hazards at home:* – Bad lighting – Slippery floors – Obstacles in the walking path – Loose rugs – Lack of railing – Uneven pavements

CLINICAL PRESENTATION AND EVALUATION OF OSTEOPOROSIS

Awareness, knowledge, and commitment are required to manage this pandemic. The dismal part of medical care is that only 20% of patients who had a previous fragility fracture would receive treatment for osteoporosis ever. There are no specific clinical signs or symptoms for osteoporosis. Patients generally have nonspecific, nonlocalized, and mild bone pains usually in central skeletal system that slowly progress in intensity and distribution. The back pain is due to microfractures and ligament stretching and in late cases due to iliocostal impingement from kyphotic deformity. The paraspinal muscle constantly remains under strain due to altered sagittal structure of the spine getting spasm and soreness over a period of time. Kyphosis is usually the earliest sign associated with loss of height **(Fig. 8)**. Loss of 2 inches in height sensitively indicates vertebral compression. The number of missing teeth has also been correlated with reduced BMD. All older persons should be evaluated for fall risk. They should be observed as they stand up from chair without using arms and walk few steps and return (get up and go test). Those who have difficulty need assessment for fall circumstances, medications, medical problems, vision, gait and balance, lower extremity evaluation (proprioception and reflexes), mobility tests, basic neurological function (cortical, pyramidal and extrapyramidal, and cerebellar), mental status, and cardiovascular functions. It is very important to assess the risk factors that were responsible to cause osteoporosis and risk factors that may be responsible for development of osteoporotic fracture **(Tables 4 and 5, Box 6)** in the primary evaluation of the patient. Proper mitigation plan can only be developed once this holistic evaluation is performed. Just labeling patient as having senile or postmenopausal osteoporosis is not enough as it has been systematically studied that more than half of the patients initially thought to be primary osteoporosis have in fact secondary causes that need treatment. Previously undiagnosed disorders are quite common.

Differential Diagnosis of Osteoporosis

- *Vertebral deformity:*
    - Osteomalacia
    - Paget's
    - Pott's spine
    - Metastasis

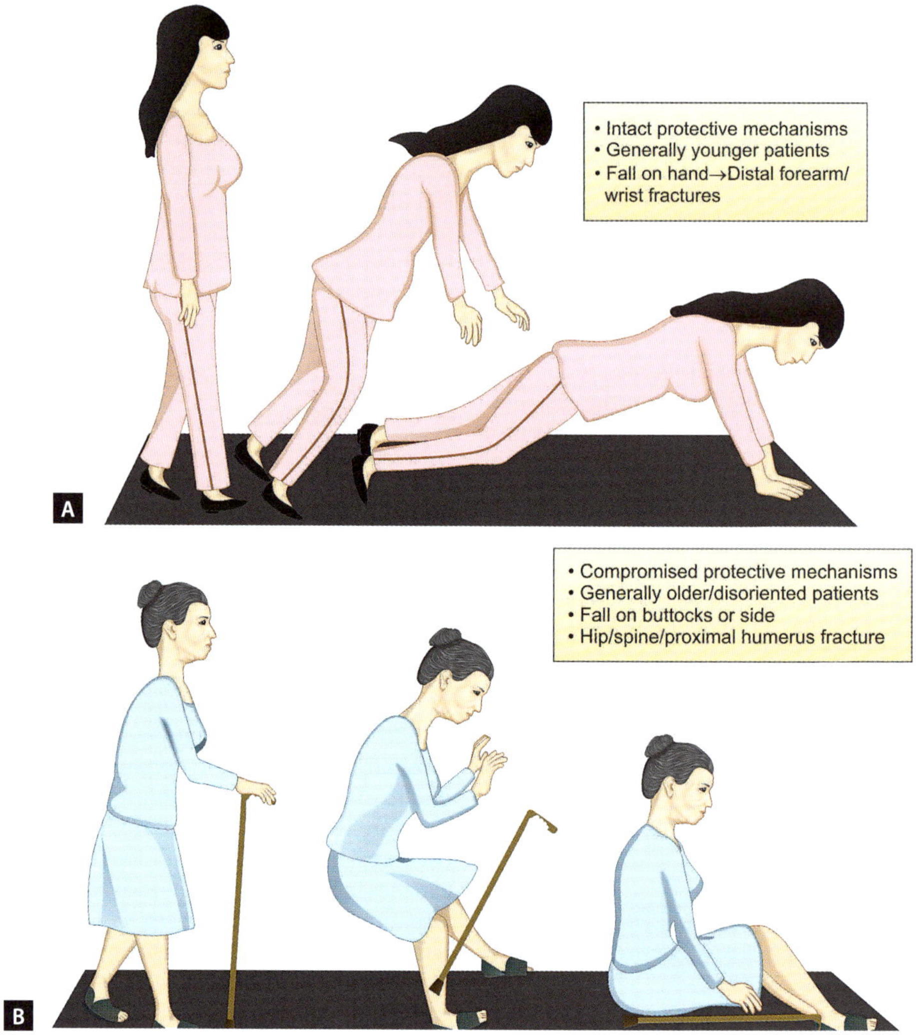

Figs. 7A and B: Types of fall impacting the fracture site.

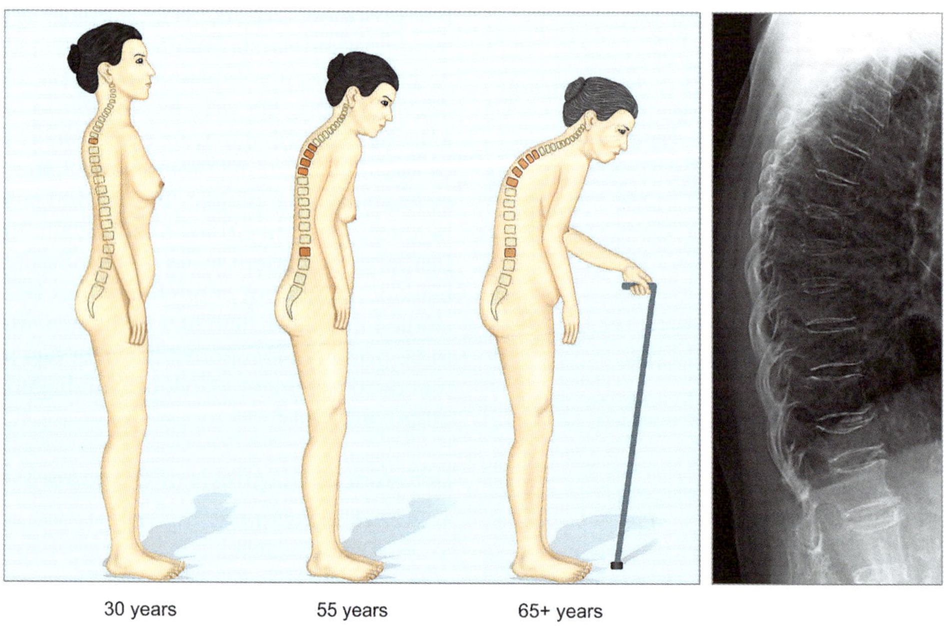

Fig. 8: With osteoporosis there is gradual and progressive loss of height.

- Myeloma
- Traumatic fracture early in life
- Histiocytosis
- *Low-trauma fracture:*
  - Metastasis
  - Myeloma
  - Bone cyst
  - Brown tumor
  - Osteomyelitis

Laboratory Tests

These primarily help in evaluating or excluding secondary causes of osteoporosis and are *never* required for primary evaluation or diagnosis. Protein electrophoresis and urine Bence–Jones proteins help in excluding multiple myeloma. Serum calcium, phosphorus, and parathyroid hormone (PTH) assay are useful to evaluate hyperparathyroidism (high PTH and serum calcium) and are also advised before starting recombinant human parathyroid hormone (rhPTH) treatment. Serum calcium may be obtained before giving zoledronic acid to exclude hypocalcemia that may precipitate tetany. High calcium may be seen in metastasis, but PTH is normal to decreased. Renal panel is used to exclude renal impairment and dose adjustment of injectable bisphosphonates and homocysteine levels may be estimated for suspected homocystinuria. Thyroid- stimulating hormone (TSH), free T4, 24-hour free cortisol, free testosterone may be ordered to evaluate suspected endocrine pathology. Vitamin D deficiency is quite prevalent and levels can be estimated to initiate proper treatment. It has been suggested that low levels of insulin-like growth factor 1 (IGF-1) in women around 40 years of age could identify at-risk patients for future low bone mass and osteoporosis. Serum IGF-1 levels below 1.5 standard deviation may indicate BMD measurement by DEXA.

Bone Turnover Markers

These give an assessment of dynamic aspects of skeletal metabolism and can also be used to monitor the effectiveness of instituted therapy. They also provide insight to evaluate fracture risk but *cannot* diagnose osteoporosis. The *markers of bone formation* include (all are serum markers) the procollagen I carboxyl and amino terminal propeptide (PICP and PINP), bone specific alkaline phosphatase (ALP), and serum osteocalcin (bone Gla protein). The *markers for bone resorption* include plasma tartarate resistant acid phosphatase (TRAP), amino and carboxyl terminal telopeptide of type I collagen (COL1A1) (so-called serum sNTx and sCTx), cross-linked C-telopeptide of type 1 collagen (ICTP) and urinary N-telopeptide (uNTx), bone sialoprotein, urinary collagen [pyridinoline (uPYR) and deoxypyridinoline (uDPD)] cross-links, urinary hydroxylysine glycosides, urinary calcium, and hydroxyproline. Circulating microRNAs (miRNA) are being studied for their utility in identifying the patients with osteoporosis. The miR-133a in circulating monocytes is a potential biomarker under evaluation and quantification for postmenopausal osteoporosis.

Utility of bone markers:
- These predict quite reliably the rapidity of bone loss in untreated patients.
- Bone markers may predict fracture risk in untreated patients (independent of BMD).
- Bone markers can categorize an individual as having fast or slow bone turnover. Fracture risk is higher in the former.
- During treatment follow-up, reduction in markers of bone resorption indicates reduced bone turnover with antiresorptive therapy. This effect is considered parallel to reduced fracture risk independent of changes in BMD. Specifically studies report that decreased urinary pyridinoline and deoxypyridinoline crosslinks after 6 months on alendronate therapy have been associated with increases in BMD at the hip and spine after 2.5 years of treatment.
- Bone markers can be used as a check mechanism on the patients on antiresorptive therapy. The compliance with antiresorptive therapies can be monitored by using these markers as minimal or no reduction in urinary N-telopeptide concentrations suggest poor compliance, though this effect may also arise with impaired drug absorption that should be considered. Urinary N-telopeptide of COL1A1 has shown the most significant association between BMD and response to hormone replacement therapy (HRT).
- Finally, they help to determine duration of "drug holiday" and also as to when the medication should be restarted.

ANALYSIS OF THE BONE MINERAL DENSITY

The BMD is measured predominantly at cancellous sites. The cancellous component of bone being highly metabolic is considered a more sensitive measure of estimating bone loss and regain. The bone transforms early and due to rapid turnover represents the disorders of metabolism early. Cortical bone loss, on the other hand, determines severity of bone loss (total accrued loss). The skeleton can be subdivided into (for DEXA purposes) central (spine and proximal femur, ribs, pelvis, and shoulder) and peripheral (appendicular skeleton minus hips and shoulder). Very importantly, it should be understood that bone mass testing (especially DEXA) is indicated only when the results will influence a treatment decision and should not be used as a business tool as is the common practice. I feel one can justifiably follow the current recommendations as provided by the National Osteoporosis Foundation (2014) that are detailed in **Box 8**. Additional recommendations for analysis of BMD can be:
- Estrogen deficient women (oophorectomized females, prolonged amenorrhea, anorexia nervosa, etc.) at clinical risk of osteoporosis, especially for assessment of early postmenopausal osteoporosis as an indication to start estrogen replacement therapy.
- Primary hyperparathyroidism
- Monitoring response to a Food and Drug Administration (FDA) approved medication for osteoporosis
- Repeat BMD evaluations at >23 months interval, or more frequently, if medically justified.

BOX 8: Indications for BMD testing [National Osteoporosis Foundation (NOF), 2014].

Bone material density (BMD) testing should be considered in following individuals:
- Women aged 65 years and older, men aged 70 years and older, regardless of clinical risk factors
- Younger postmenopausal women, women in menopausal transition, and men aged 50–69 years with clinical risk factors for fracture
- Adults who have fracture at or after the age of 50 years
- Adults with a condition (like rheumatoid arthritis) or taking a medication (like glucocorticoids) associated with low bone mass or bone loss

Bone mineral density analysis had been classically available for central and peripheral skeleton sites as mentioned above. Different devices have been used for assessing BMD at these positions.

- Central skeleton BMD measuring devices (measures hip and spine BMD):
  - Dual energy X-ray absorptiometry
  - Quantitative computed tomography (QCT)
- Peripheral skeleton BMD measuring devices (measures BMD of phalanges, metacarpals, forearm, calcaneus, primarily involves utilizing X-ray and ultrasound)
  - Radiographic absorptiometry
  - Digital X-ray radiogrammetry (DXR)
  - Single X-ray absorptiometry (SXA)
  - Peripheral DEXA (pDEXA)
  - Peripheral QCT (pQCT)

Principle of absorptiometry: Denser tissue will have higher number of electrons in a given volume. Such a tissue will be able to produce higher attenuation (reduction in number and energy of photons in an X-ray beam) of the photons coming from energy source. If the degree of attenuation can be measured then it can be reciprocated to tissue density. Dual-energy scanners release photons in two energy bands:

1. Low energy (30–50 keV)
   - Bone attenuation more than soft tissue attenuation
2. High energy (>70 keV)
   - Bone attenuation similar to soft tissue attenuation
   - Allows to suppress impact of overlying soft tissue

Such dual-energy scanners are, hence, able to better differentiate between bone and soft tissue and also partially correct the presence of varying fat amount. Such dual-energy bands can be produced either by K-edge filtering technique (GE and Norland) or by voltage-switching (Hologic). The various types of scanners also use different DEXA acquisition techniques such as pencil beam (DPX, QDR1000, QDR2000, and XR series), wide fan beam (QDR4500, Delphi, Discovery, and Horizon), or narrow fan beam (Prodigy/iDXA and Stratos). Because different scanners use different techniques, so not all DEXA scanners are same and their values are not intercomparable. Even for follow-up scan in a patient, it is preferable to rely on the same scanner (used to acquire DEXA in past) else the values would be misinterpreted.

Dual-energy X-ray Absorptiometry

Dual-energy X-ray absorptiometry involves very limited radiation exposure. It affords fast, reliable, and fairly accurate measurement of bone mass so is commonly used in screening population and also defining osteoporosis according to the WHO criteria. One must remember that the WHO classification cannot be applied to T-scores from measurements other than DEXA at the lumbar spine, femoral neck, total hip, and distal one-third radius. DEXA has replaced dual-photon and single X-ray absorptiometry and is now the most widely used bone mass measurement tool sort of becoming the currently gold standard for diagnosis, evaluation, and follow-up of osteoporosis patients (discussed above in indications of obtaining BMD). Soft tissue radiation exposure and attenuation is compensated in DEXA by using a combination of high and low X-ray energies. Pencil beam has less scatter, requires less dose (≈1 μSv), and reduces operator or patient radiation compared to cone pencil-beam or fan-beam systems, where the required dose is around 18 μSv. However, the fan-beam systems improve image quality and possibly the accuracy of measurement also. DEXA gives a two-dimensional measure of BMD. It does not, however, measure true volume density as obtained with QCT. Bone mass is reported as an absolute value in grams per square centimeter in DEXA and is then presented as T-score and Z-score as defined below:

- Z-score compares patient's value to an age-matched and sex-matched reference range. The Z-score is of less clinical value and is used in young adults and postmenopausal females less than 50 years of age, Z-scores significantly deviating from normal may indicate an alternative cause of a metabolic bone disease. Z-scores are also useful in diagnosing osteoporosis in children (5–19 years of age). A Z-score of –2.0 or lower is defined as "below the expected range for age" and a Z-score above –2.0 is "within the expected range for age". In children, the conventional sites of BMD measurement (like total hip) are not reliable due to significant variation in skeletal development. These patients should have spine and total body less head (TBLH) BMC (bone mineral content) and areal BMD measured. The diagnosis of osteoporosis in these age groups needs a combination of low BMC or BMD and a clinically significant fracture history (not just low BMD). T-score should *not* be printed in reports of these age groups.
- T-score is a comparison to mean bone mass of young adult normal individuals defined as "healthy Caucasian women population 20–40 years of age". Thus, T-score may be called young adult Z-score. Women are chosen specifically as they represent the lower normal values of healthy population (without any increased risk of fracture, while reference from male population will fallaciously put even some of normal females into osteoporotic category). T-scores are used to both predict fracture risk and classify disease status as in WHO definition. This score was suggested to avoid confusion between different BMD measurement technologies. The score is calculated by the formula:

$$T\text{-}score = \frac{mBMD - YN}{SD}$$

Where, mBMD is the measured bone density, YN is the normal value from young population (reference), and SD is the standard deviation of young adult population.

Quantitatively, a change of 1 standard deviation in either the T-score or Z-score corresponds to a change of approximately 0.06 g/cm^2 (about 10% BMD). T-score of ≤ -2.5 has been used to define osteoporosis as per WHO criteria. Such a cutoff value identifies approximately 30% of postmenopausal women as having osteoporosis using measurements made at hip, spine, or forearm. This is approximately equivalent to the lifetime risk of fracture at these sites. One should remember however that T-score ≤ -2.5 is not always due to osteoporosis only. Nonosteoporotic causes of low BMD include:

- Osteomalacia
- Osteogenesis imperfecta
- Renal bone disease
- Multiple myeloma
- Marrow infiltrative diseases like mastocytosis

Some advice using Z-score in these scenarios but there is no evidence to support use of a specific Z-score cut-point to determine when secondary cause evaluation is needed.

The T-score is applicable for diagnosing osteoporosis "only" in postmenopausal women using "only" central DEXA and forearm DEXA if applicable. For premenopausal women and children (5–19 years of age) T-score is not applicable (and should not appear on DEXA reports) and one has to use Z-scores. For diagnosis in children, spine and total body less head (TBLH) bone mineral content (BMC) and areal BMD are measured but not solely relied to make diagnosis. The diagnosis is made by a combination of low BMC or BMD (Z-score ≤ -2.0) along with clinically significant fracture history defined as:

- Long bone fracture of the lower extremities and/or
- Vertebral compression fracture and/or
- Two or more long bone fractures of the upper extremities

T-scores can, however, be used for perimenopausal women.

Dual-energy X-ray absorptiometry can be used to measure bone mass at central (vertebral and proximal femur) and peripheral sites, the choice of site(s) being primarily guided by the anticipated or expected rates of change in bone mass within these skeletal locations. The choice is also influenced by precision of the testing device at these discrete sites. The central DEXA sites of the hip and spine are commonly preferred because it has:

- Higher precision
- The quantity of trabecular bone at central sites is usually indicative of the osteoporosis burden, and hence fracture risk.
- Bone loss begins early in the trabecular bone as it is highly metabolically active compared to cortical bone and is predominant in central skeleton.
- Ward's triangle has lowest BMD, but is much less predictive or reproducible, so BMD at other locations like the femoral neck (preferred), trochanter or total hip should be measured.

Measurement of forearm BMD should be done only if:

- Lumbar spine and/or hip cannot be measured or interpreted.
- Hyperparathyroidism is suspected.
- Very obese patients (over the weight limit for DEXA table)

Regular follow-up with serial DEXA scan to monitor therapy is controversial. One school of thought recommends yearly scan, while others site benefits of osteoporosis therapy beyond change in BMD and hence rendering repeat DEXA futile. This is substantiated by the fact that minimum 2.77% change in BMD is required between two successive DEXA studies to reach statistical significance for estimating difference with 95% confidence ($p < 0.05$). Not only this, but the measured changed value needs to be multiplied by the "precision error" of the measuring device. If the device has a 2% precision error, a change in BMD of about 5.6% is needed to substantiate BMD change not by chance. Any clinician would know that no currently available modality would achieve this improvement by 1 year of treatment making repeat estimation futile. If the clinician still wishes to get serial measurements done then get DEXA done from same center and know the "least significant change (LSC)" from it before evaluating the report (Ideally DEXA should be repeated only when expected BMD improvement exceeds LSC for the center.). Also, it is better to use grams/cucm values to determine if a significant BMD change has occurred instead of just concentrating on the T-score.

Pitfalls in Dual-energy X-ray Absorptiometry Measurement

Osteoporosis though systemic occurs inhomogeneously across the body with significant discordance between sites, especially in the elderly. Imaging only one site may thus be misleading. Osteophytes due to high prevalence of facet and posterior element spinal osteoarthritis in elderly may yield a falsely elevated bone mass in anteroposterior projection. This is circumvented by measurement of the spine BMD in lateral projection or measuring hip DEXA. Lateral spine scan is still limited in accuracy by soft tissue attenuation due to greater thickness and nonuniformity of soft tissues in this projection.

Relative Contraindications of Central Dual-energy X-ray Absorptiometry

- Pregnancy
- Recent contrast study (generally <72 hours)
    - Measurement of spine BMD will yield false higher values
- Recent nuclear medicine scan
- Extensive orthopedic instrumentation
- Body weight greater than table limit
    - Measure forearm BMD

Peripheral Dual-energy X-ray Absorptiometry

It is commonly used as a cheaper substitute or mass promotion for DEXA. It measures real bone density at either forearm, finger or heel as per machine calibration. Measurement by validated peripheral DEXA (pDEXA) devices can help to predict vertebral and overall fracture risk in postmenopausal women, but the prediction in men is not proven or supported. The radiation risk is trivial. It is not a good method to monitor BMD after therapy.

Trabecular Bone Score

The information provided by trabecular bone score (TBS) is additive and independent to that provided by BMD and clinical risk factors. TBS is a DEXA program that estimates the trabecular (cancellous) bone texture information from a regular posteroanterior (PA) spine DEXA scan. It measures the microarchitectural structure of bone tissue and may improve the ability to predict the risk of fracture **(Fig. 9)**. Because this is derived index it has no units (just a number). Higher TBS correlates with better bone microstructure while lower TBS is associated with worse bone microstructure. TBS is lower in postmenopausal women and in men with prior fragility fracture than their nonfractured counterparts. TBS predicts fracture risk as well as lumbar spine BMD measurements. TBS results are independent of BMD and FRAX® but when combined to BMD and clinical risk factors TBS enhances fracture risk prediction **(Fig. 10)**. TBS data can be used to

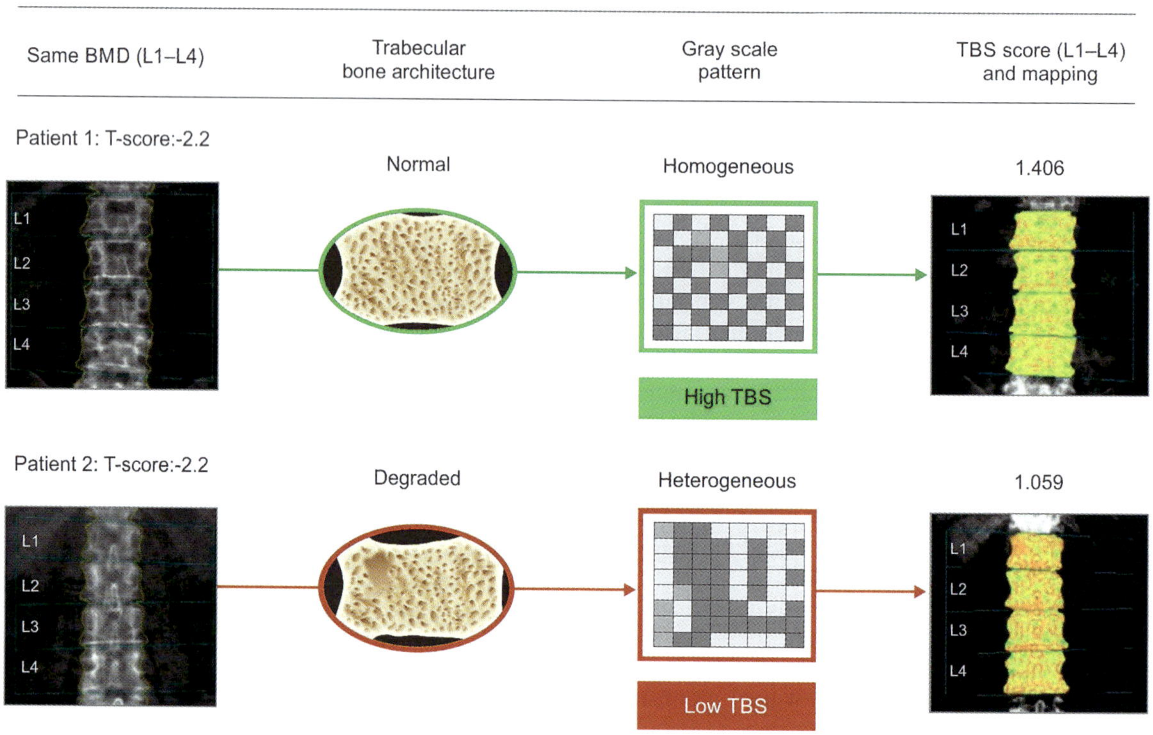

Fig. 9: Principle of assessing trabecular bone score (TBS). The figure explains that with same bone mineral density (BMD) T-score (in patient 1 and 2) the bone microstructure may differ individually affecting the fracture risk. Patient 2 will be at higher risk of osteoporotic fracture. This difference can be captured in TBS assessment and the fracture risk can be hence modified despite same BMD.

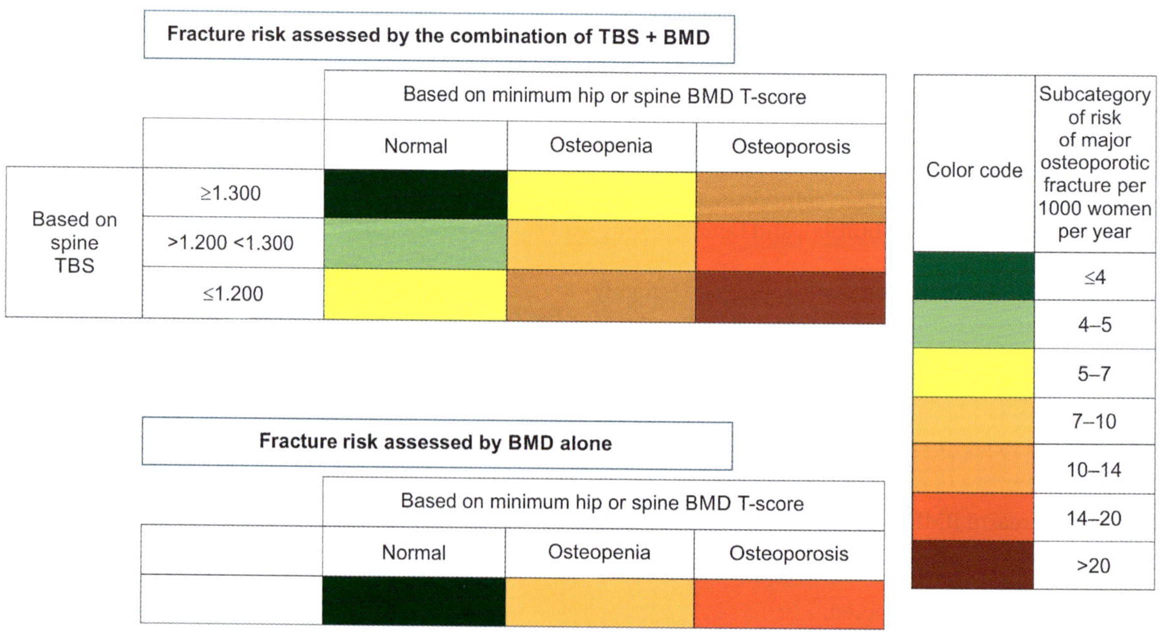

Fig. 10: Possible trabecular bone score (TBS) interpretation table. The interpretation based only on bone mineral density (BMD) (lower table) is very limited and categorizes patients into three broad groups (normal, osteopenia, and osteoporosis). If TBS is added to the BMD assessment (upper table), the interpretation can be fine-tuned and improved to individualize patients with better interpretation of the fracture risk probability.

adjust/improve the FRAX® tool where lower TBS increases the calculated 10-year risk of fracture while higher TBS reduces the 10-year risk of fracture. It is primarily being popularized as a practical, noninvasive, surrogate technique for assessing cancellous bone microarchitecture and trabecular bone properties.

Vertebral Imaging

The current indications for vertebral imaging according to NOF are provided in **Box 9**. Bone loss must exceed 30–40% before it is visible by conventional radiography so plain radiographs are insensitive method and due to wide variability in evaluation and nonstandardization; often inaccurate **(Figs. 11A to C)**. An *incident vertebral fracture* is defined by McCloskey-Kanis method as a minimum height decrease of 4.6 mm and a decrease of 15% in absolute height on a subsequent film (nowadays by common definition, 20% or more reduction in height of any vertebral body at any segment, viz., anterior, middle, or posterior from the nonfractured height is taken significant). Morphologically, the compressed vertebral body appears to be having wedge, biconcave, or crushed appearance.

The diagnosis of acute osteoporotic vertebral fracture is made by one of the following radiological findings:

BOX 9: Indications for vertebral imaging.

Vertebral imaging should be considered for following individuals:
- All women aged 70 years or older and all men aged 80 years or older, if bone mineral density (BMD) T-score at the spine, total hip or femoral neck is < –1.0
- Women aged 65–69 years and men aged 70–79 years, if BMD T-score at the spine, total hip, or femoral neck is <–1.5
- Postmenopausal women and men age ≥50 years with specific risk factors:
  - Low trauma fracture during adulthood (age 50 years and older)
  - Historical height loss of 1.5 inch or more (4 cm)
  - Prospective height loss of 0.8 inch or more (2 cm)
  - Recent or long-term ongoing glucocorticoid therapy

- *Demonstrating a new fracture by imaging:* Conventional radiograph or CT scan that demonstrates a sharp cortical break. CT scan may also demonstrate presence of intravertebral cleft filled with air—intravertebral vacuum cleft phenomenon that may also be seen on lateral radiographic projections in long-standing cases **(Figs. 12A and B)**.
- Finding a change in vertebral configuration by comparing current radiograph and pre-existing films.
- MRI scan can show signal changes suggestive of vertebral fracture. MRI may demonstrate presence of intravertebral cleft/cavity filled with fluid (fluid sign) on T2-weighted images.
- Apart from the above conventional methods, another way is to diagnose vertebral fractures using a DEXA machine—the technique is called "vertebral fracture assessment (VFA)". Though it uses DEXA machine but the methodology if VFA is different from BMD. The three common methods to identify a vertebral fracture in VFA are:
  1. *Quantitative visual assessment:* The interpreter (radiologist/orthopedician) decides if a vertebra is normal or fractured.
  2. *Quantitative morphometry:* This is done by placing six dots to delineate the vertebral body on lateral projection **(Fig. 13)** providing more quantitative assessment and can also be automated using computing devices. The problem is that it may overdiagnose abnormalities that are not fractures and may underdiagnose mild endplate abnormalities.
  3. *Semiquantitative visual:* This utilizes Genant visual grading of fracture type and severity **(Fig. 14)**. The details are provided below in discussion on "spinal deformity index".

Spinal Deformity Index

It incorporates both number and severity of fractures by adding the severity grades of spine from T4 to L4 described

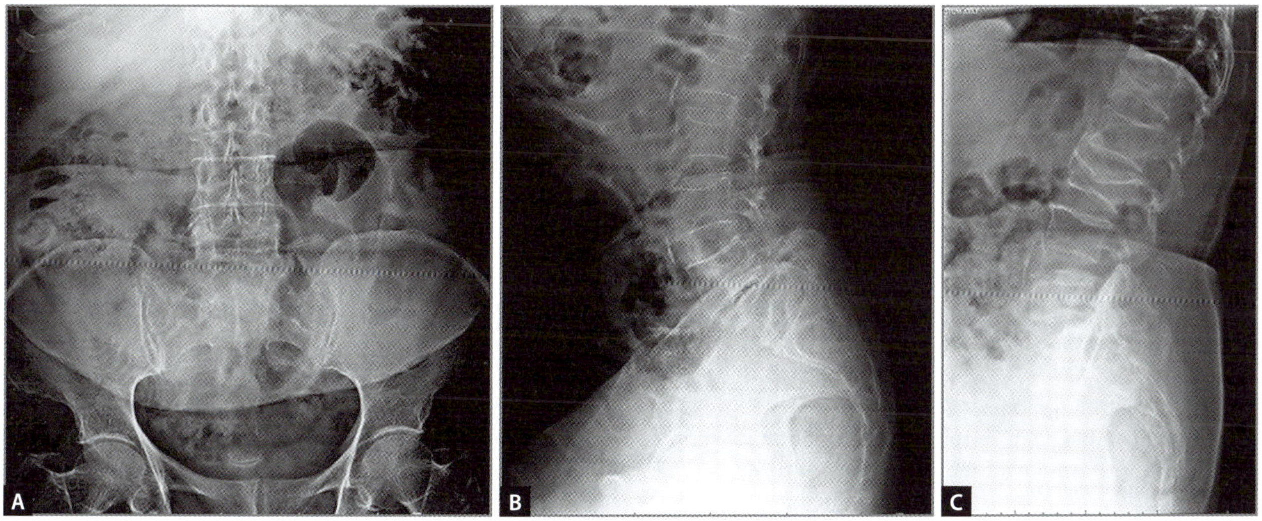

Figs. 11A to C: The (A) anteroposterior (AP) and (B) lateral view of spine and pelvis showing gross osteopenia and washed out appearance of bone with only silhouette appearance. The vertebrae have biconcave appearance but no osteoporotic fracture is seen; (C) The radiograph shows multiple osteoporotic fractures in spine falling into definition of severe osteoporosis [once bone mineral density (BMD) is done].

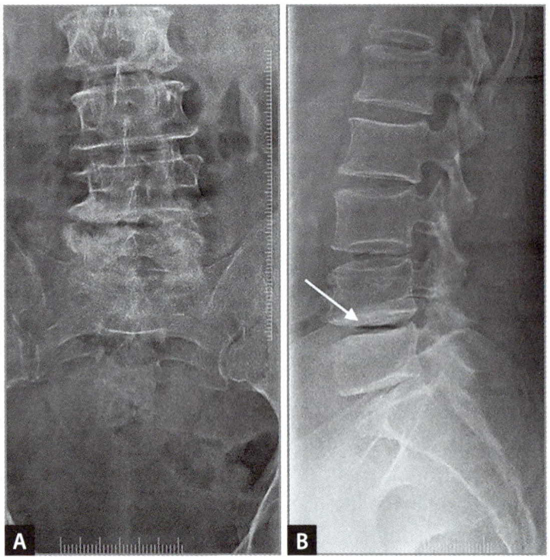

Figs. 12A and B: Vacuum phenomenon appearing as a lucency in disk space at the L4–L5. The space may be filled with gas or fluid as the case may be and appears as a void in standard radiographs especially on lateral projection (arrow).

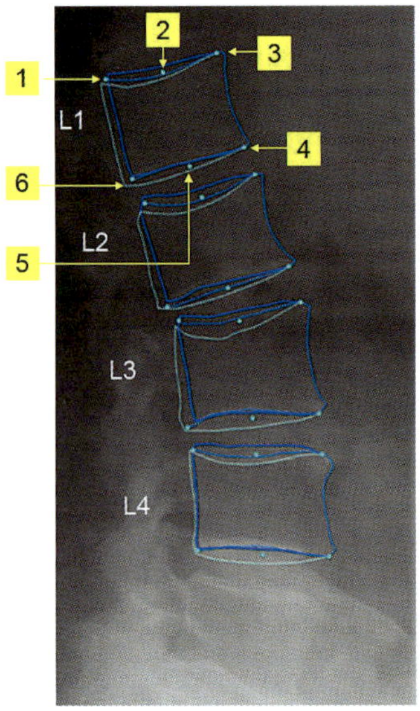

Fig. 13: The quantitative vertebral morphometry is done by identifying six points in the vertebral image [clockwise: (1) Superior posterior rim center; (2) Superior cortical endplate; (3) Superior anterior rim center; (4) Inferior osteophyte handle; (5) Inferior cortical endplate; and (6) Inferior posterior rim center] and comparing with standards.

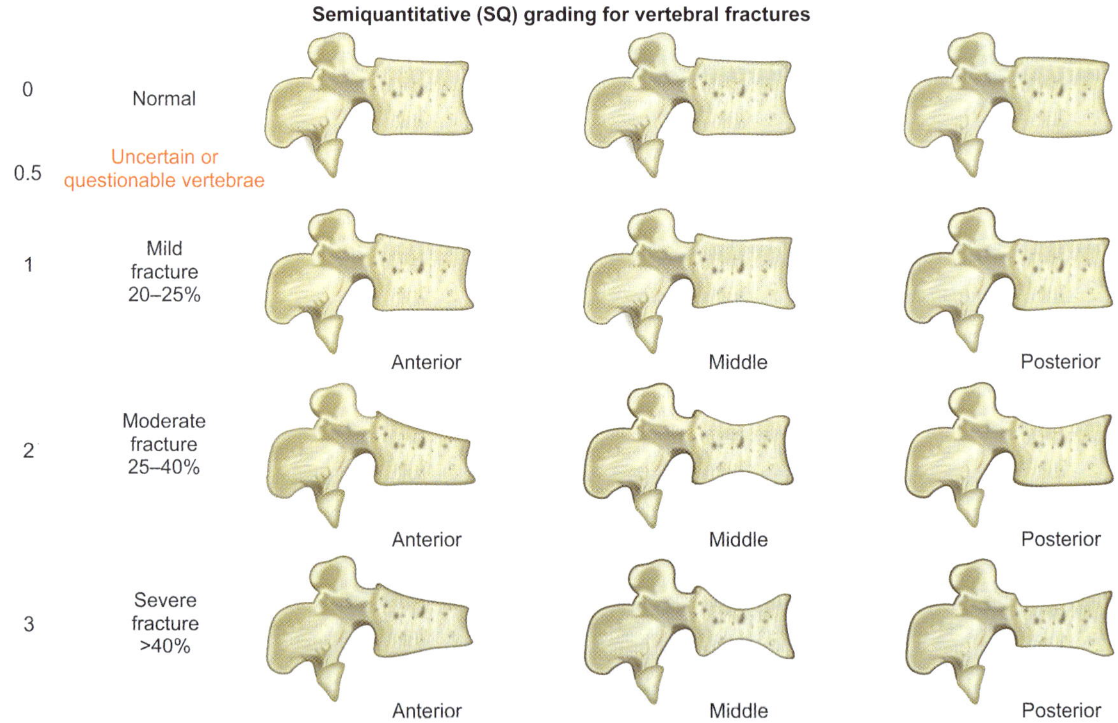

Fig. 14: The Genant chart for identifying the fracture morphology and grading.

on lateral spine radiographs. It was described by Minne et al. and Genant et al. For each vertebra a semiquantitative grade is assigned after visual evaluation. There are three grades: (1) grade 1 is 20–25% decrease in vertebral height, (2) grade 2 (moderate) is 25–40% reduction in height, and (3) grade 3 (severe) is ≥40% reduction in height, while grade 0 is normal vertebra **(Figs. 15A and B)**. The scores are then added up for T4–L4 vertebrae. The spinal deformity index (SDI) value ranges between 0 and 39, higher the SDI greater is chance of incident fracture. Appreciate the osteopenia on a radiograph based on following patterns:

- *Change in radiolucency:* Compare with adjacent soft tissues, amount of trabeculation and overall estimate of osteopenia.

- *Change in trabecular pattern:* Increased vertical striations and thin subchondral plate (superior and inferior endplates).

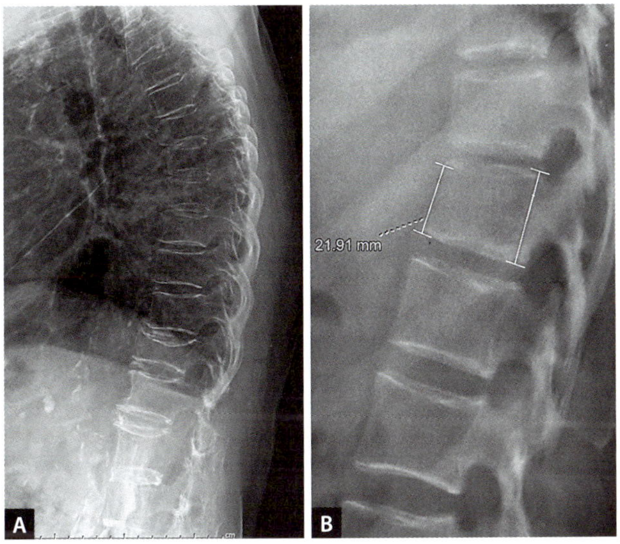

Figs. 15A and B: (A) Spinal deformity index (SDI)—grade the vertebrae from T4 to L4 and add the grades. This X-ray has osteoporotic "central wedge" fracture of L1 with grade 2 deformity. L3 and L4 had been fused previously for unrelated disorder; (B) It is imperative to understand the fact that "anterior wedging" may be seen even in normal spine even up to 25% of the posterior body height as in 12th dorsal vertebra in this asymptomatic patient.

- *Change in shape:* Normal difference in anterior and posterior heights of vertebral body is taken as 1–3 mm, a difference of ≥4 mm is abnormal. The shape changes could be wedge-shaped compression, central compression, or pancake compression. Wedge compression is when the posterior portion of body (central column) is intact compared to burst fracture when both anterior and posterior portions of body get compressed. The biconcave pattern of vertebrae commonly referred to as fish vertebrae resemble the normal biconcave shape of vertebral body of fish (though this is abnormal for humans). Fish vertebrae are seen in osteoporosis, Paget's disease, osteomalacia, and hyperparathyroidism.

Singh Index

Based on the completeness and presence of tensile and compressive trabeculae in proximal femur the index divides femurs radiologically into six grades **(Fig. 16)**:

- *Grade 6:* All normal trabecular groups are visible.
- *Grade 5:* Prominent ward triangle; principal tensile trabeculae attenuated, while principal compressive trabeculae normal. Attenuated secondary compressive. Trochanteric trabeculae vanish.
- *Grade 4:* Marked reduction, but continuous tensile trabeculae. Secondary compressive trabeculae lost.
- *Grade 3 (definite osteoporosis):* Definite break in the continuity of tensile trabeculae

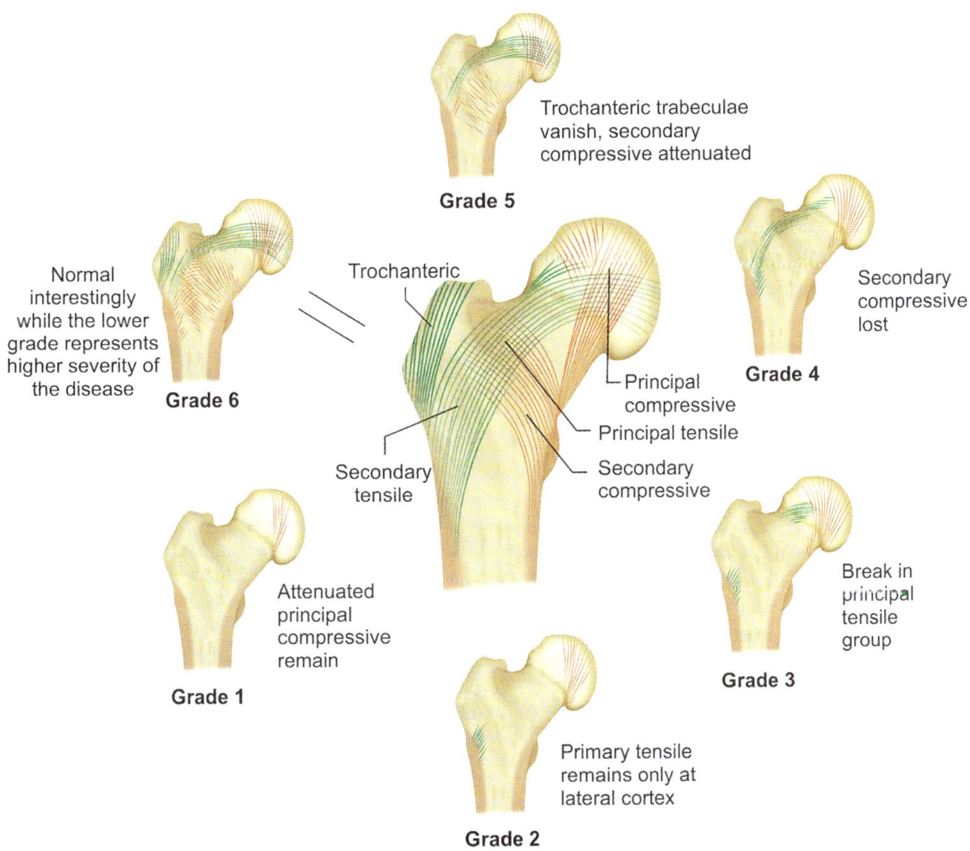

Fig. 16: Singh's index. Note the trabecular disposition in normal femur that gets progressively thinned and disappear sequentially with progression of osteoporosis. Grade 6 is normal interestingly while the lower grade represent higher severity of the disease.

- *Grade 2:* Primary tensile trabeculae remnants visible along lateral cortex, rest vanish. Principal compressive trabeculae present and prominent.
- *Grade 1:* Attenuation of even principal compressive trabeculae, essentially empty proximal femur.

The Singh index correlates with histologic grading of the iliac crest, but has not been found to predict BMD of the proximal femur accurately. It has low sensitivity, but relatively high specificity. Various other methods have also been proposed to predict the fracture risk and include HAL (discussed above), reduced thickness of the femoral shaft cortex, diminished index of tensile trabeculae and wide trochanteric region or a combination of these measurements.

Quantitative Computed Tomography

Quantitative computed tomography gives an accurate assessment of fracture risk and measurement of bone loss, but is seriously limited by radiation dose and running cost. QCT uses any standard computed tomography scan machine to measure volumetric integral, trabecular, and cortical bone density and gives a true three-dimensional (3D) view of BMD. Newer 3D volumetric spine QCT precision measurements are so accurate that they have been used to calibrate other modalities. It utilizes dedicated analytical software that converts Hounsfield's units to volumetric BMD values in mg/cm^3. The precision error is <1% and radiation dose is in range of 150–300 μSv. Volumetric BMD values of >120 mg/cm^3 are considered normal while <80 mg/cm^3 are interpreted as osteoporosis. In-between, values are taken as osteopenia. These values should *not* be interpreted using WHO T-score guidelines for fracture risk categorization. QCT is best done for spine, but marrow fat increases with age and glucocorticoid use giving an overestimation for the extent of bone loss in these two clinical settings. pQCT (peripheral) is done at the forearm bones or tibia and high-resolution pQCT (HR-pQCT) provides accurate and reproducible measures of bone architecture, volumetric density, and microarchitecture. QCT measure of spine trabecular BMD predicts vertebral fractures in postmenopausal women, while pQCT of forearm and ultradistal radius predicts hip, but not vertebral fractures. QCT at proximal femur (neck and total) provides areal BMD (mg/cm^2) that can be used in FRAX® tool optionally to improve fracture risk assessment. There are fundamental differences in QCT and DEXA that must be understood before clinical application of the technologies **(Table 8)**.

Ultrasound

Quantitative ultrasound (QUS) has advantages of portability, lower cost, simple instrumentation, and absence of ionizing radiation. Ultrasound has distinct advantage of providing additional information about bone quality that is not possible with other methods. The typical measurements include speed of sound (SOS) and broadband ultrasound attenuation (BUA). SOS depends on speed and elasticity and is measured in meters/sec while BUA depends on density and scattering architecture (bone structure) and is measured in dB/Mhz/cm. *Stiffness or quantitative ultrasound index* is a combination of SOS and BUA, but it does not reflect a biochemical property of bone so is ineffective. Ultrasound assessment **(Figs. 17A and B)** is most commonly performed

TABLE 8: Fundamental differences between quantitative computed tomography (QCT) and dual-energy X-ray absorptiometry (DEXA).

Central QCT	*Central DEXA*
Three-dimensional volume image	Two-dimensional projection image
True volumetric BMD at spine; areal BMD at hip	Areal BMD at all sites
Spine and hip measurements	Spine, hip, forearm, and total body
Trabecular bone only at spine, integral bone at hip	Integral bone at all sites
Error sources: • Osseous fat	*Error sources:* • Osseous fat • Spine degenerative changes • Soft tissue background
Spine + Hip dose of around 500–800 μSv	Spine + Hip dose of around 1–10 μSv

(BMD: bone mineral density)

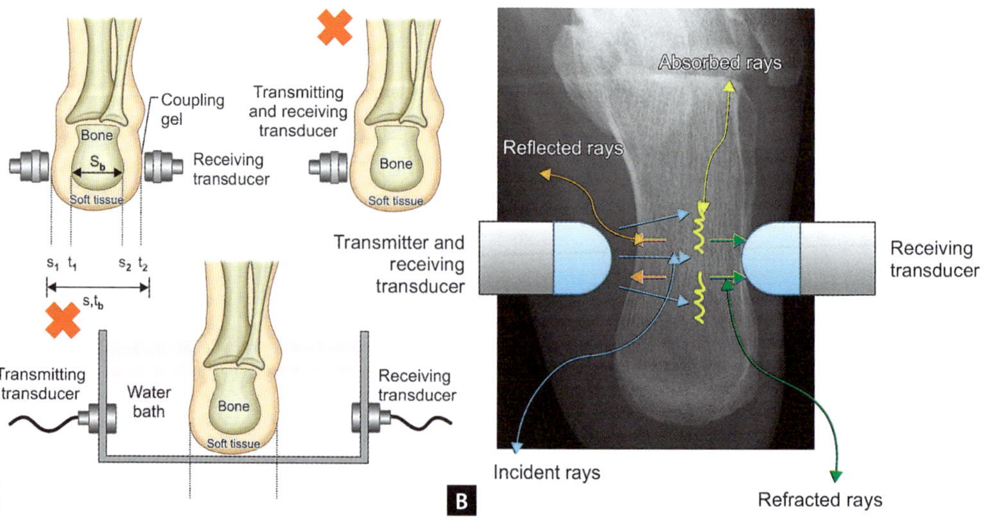

Figs. 17A and B: Quantitative ultrasound. (A) The basic setup consists of transmitter and receiver in a water bath or gel-based coupler. The system (B) captures the transmitted (refracted) and reflected rays thus analyzing the absorbed rays (energy) which depends on bone architecture.

for calcaneus (finger and tibia are other sites) and it has been extrapolated that validated heel ultrasound predicts vertebral, hip, and overall fracture risk in postmenopausal women and hip and nonvertebral fractures in men ≥65 years. The advantages for calcaneus ultrasound are that it has two nearly parallel sides and is surrounded only by a thin layer of soft tissue minimizing errors. The fracture risk doubles for 1-standard deviation reduction in BUA or SOS when measured in standard conditions. QUS does not match central BMD and is highly site specific so correlation of QUS at peripheral sites and BMD at central sites is modest. QUS cannot be used to estimate density at main fracture sites. In general, ultrasonic measurements of the calcaneus are better only for identifying patients with fracture of the hip than of the spine. The limitations of ultrasound include inferior precision of ultrasound measurements, changes in ultrasonic properties of bone with age, and slow rate of bone mass change with treatment needing long intervals for documentation.

Magnetic Resonance Imaging

Magnetic resonance imaging could be a useful investigation for the evaluation of osteoporotic vertebral fractures as it can also differentiate with metastatic spine disease. It can reflect marrow edema quite avidly and define presence of intravertebral cleft/fluid sign. Involvement of pedicle and posterior vertebral elements with soft tissue shadows in the paraspinal and/or epidural region is suspicious of malignancy. Involvement of paradiskal region or vertebral body signals suggestive of abscess would favor infective pathology. Osteoporotic vertebral body involvement is instead suggested by low signal intensity band on T1- and T2-weighted images with spared normal marrow, retropulsed fractured posterior body wall fragment, and multiple vertebral body involvement. Presence of "fluid sign" (high signal on T2-weighted images) is highly suggestive of osteoporosis rather than a metastatic disease.

Quantitative magnetic resonance imaging (QMRI) and structural analysis are research tools only.

Novel early detection techniques for osteoporosis: The following are currently research-based investigations, but may soon be available for early detection of osteoporosis. The details are beyond the scope of current text and reader can refer dedicated text for details.

- Bone fracture detection microsensor—assesses the mechanosensitivity of bone cell and stress in bone. Newer techniques study the brittleness of bone.
- Microfluidic channels (uses biomarkers)—analyze and assess total ALP.
- Biochemical-based BioMEMS (microelectromechanical system) chip—detects osteoprotegerin (OPG) based on gold nanoparticles.
- BioMEMS-based sensors—use electrochemical immunoassay with microfluidic system to study ALP.
- Spectroscopic techniques:
  - Fourier transform infrared spectroscopy (FTIR)
  - Ultraviolet-visible spectroscopy (UV-Vis)

PREVENTION AND TREATMENT OF OSTEOPOROSIS

Reduction of Risk Factors and Nutritional Modifications

Risk Reduction

Patient education is primary mechanism to modify the environmental factors at home and elsewhere. The primary goal in the initiating treatment of osteoporosis is to prevent bone loss beyond the fracture threshold. Measurements of BMD and evaluation using available fracture risk assessment tools (see above for detailed discussion) can be used to assess the risk of a fracture with a high degree of specificity. The perimenopausal transition is a good opportunity to initiate discussion about risk factors for osteoporosis and to consider a BMD test. A careful history and physical examination should be performed to identify risk factors for osteoporosis. A low Z-score increases the suspicion of a secondary disease. Thorough review of the medications and necessary adjustments should be made. Identification of hypogonadal state and thyrotoxicosis by laboratory tests, orthostatic hypotension by clinical methods, and treatment of visual impairment are some of the key measures. Height loss >2.5–3.8 cm (1–1.5 inch) is an indication for radiography to rule out asymptomatic vertebral fractures, as is the presence of significant kyphosis or back pain, particularly if it began after menopause.

The clinical history, physical examination, and radiological evaluation/biological tests are aimed at:

- Excluding a disease that can mimic osteoporosis
- Elucidating causes of osteoporosis and contributory factors
- Assessing the severity of osteoporosis and the risk of subsequent fractures
- Selecting the most appropriate form of treatment

Control of Risk Factors

The following are common measures initiated for most patients:

- *Lifestyle:* Walk briskly for a minimum of 1 hour, three times a week. Enhance practice of muscle-strengthening exercises to improve muscle mass. Aerobics, weight-bearing, and resistance exercises are effective at increasing BMD at spine. Walking improves BMD at hip.
- Smoking cessation
- Alcohol cessation

Supportive Treatment for Fractured Patients

Pain Control and Bracing

Nonsteroidal anti-inflammatory medications, non-narcotic analgesics (paracetamol, tramadol, etc.), low-dose TCA, and other neurotropic agents (such as carbamazepine and gabapentin) should be judiciously used on individual basis. Localized nerve blocks can be used in refractory situations. Transcutaneous electrical nerve stimulation, fomentation of heat and cold, and the use of therapeutic ultrasound have been variably suggested. Calcitonin and some bisphosphonates have been suggested to relieve pain from compression fracture, however, the effect of calcitonin is weak and may not last long. Bracing of the spine for osteoporosis pain control is commonly prescribed despite lack of objective data on effectiveness. Excessive reliance on bracing can adversely lead to muscular weakness and loss of postural support. Weight-bearing exercises are important elements of osteoporosis management. Stress-induced or exercise-induced bone mass improvement is most commonly seen in weight-bearing sites such as the tibia (runners), and in the spine (weight lifters). Spinal extension exercises are preferred over flexion exercises as the latter may predispose to spinal compression fractures and deformities.

Principles of Surgical Management of Osteoporotic Fractures and Effect of Pharmacotherapy

- Manage not just the fracture, but the geriatric patient as a whole, so balance the outcome of inflicting surgical trauma on biology of body system.
- Quick and precise surgeries by expert in the field are preferable. Also one should focus on modalities that afford quickest mobilization, for example, in octogenarians with even minimally fracture of femoral neck doing a quick hemiarthroplasty is beneficial over screw fixation **(Figs. 18A and B)**. For relatively younger patients with osteoporosis total hip replacement would be better.
- The rate of bone union is not affected by osteoporosis per se, but due to old age the prolongation of healing process is possibly due to age-related blunting of reactionary process. However, it is the implant holding strength that influences stabilization of fracture and union. Implants may fail as they have to maintain fracture for prolonged periods due to longer healing time and poor holding strength. Locked screw plate constructs at variable angle are preferable to dynamic compression plates **(Figs. 19A to D)**. Absolute stability and lag screw techniques are not effective in osteoporotic bones. Focus should be strain reduction by utilizing relative stability techniques. Providing wide buttress to juxta-articular fractures is also a good option rather than fixing the fracture fragment.
- Plating is beneficial at juxta-articular and intra-articular fractures, however, for diaphyseal fractures intramedullary nailing should be preferred **(Figs. 20A to C)** for biology preservation, dynamic load sharing, relative stability, and less invasive nature.
- Augmentation with bone cement to improve screw purchase at trabecular bone (delta bolt for hip, cannulated screws with side openings for humerus, femoral condyle, and vertebrae) could be considered to improve strength of fixation. Hydroxyapatite-coated implants with deliverable growth factors, such as bone morphogenetic proteins (BMP), TGF-β could provide improved fixation in future.
- Some people prefer intramedullary fibula graft to improve screw purchase, but the published literature on this method is scanty.
- Comminuted fractures at metaphyseal or periarticular regions could be better managed by arthroplasty, for example, proximal humerus and proximal femur.

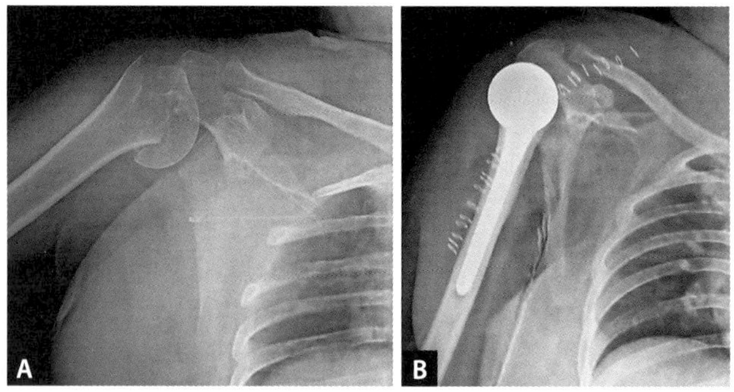

Figs. 18A and B: Shoulder arthroplasty.

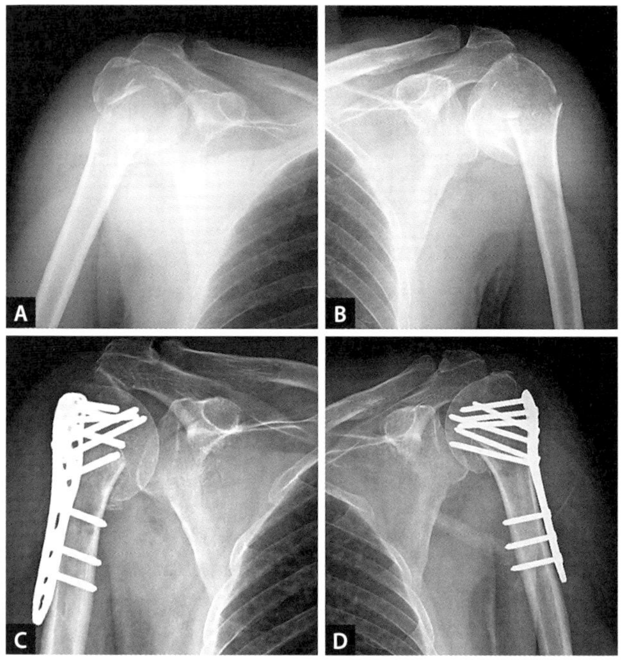

Figs. 19A to D: (A and B) Proximal humeral locking plate; (C and D) Bilateral proximal humerus fractures in a patient treated with proximal humerus locking plate osteosynthesis.

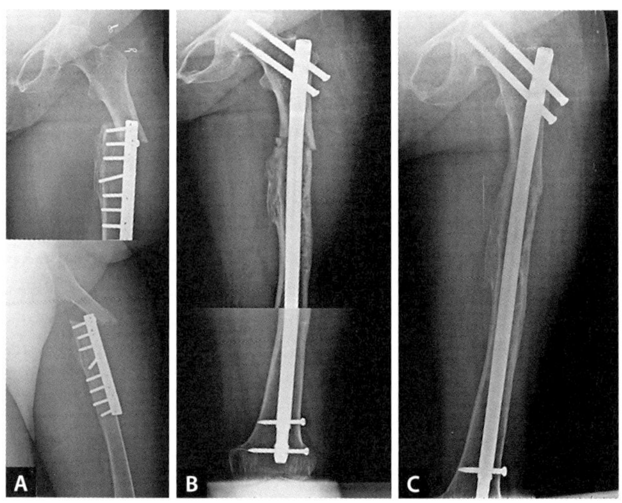

Figs. 20A to C: (A) Patient with osteoporotic proximal femoral fracture. The femur was treated with open reduction internal fixation (ORIF) 20 years ago elsewhere for treatment of fracture of shaft; (B) The implant was removed and intramedullary nailing with (C) reconstruction nail was done that led to complete union.

Pharmacotherapy in Surgery

- Bisphosphonates and anabolic therapy—patients on bisphosphonates can definitely undergo fracture fixation. The question is for those patients who are osteoporotic and identified with a fracture. Though bisphosphonates suppress bone resorption, and hence the coupled process of bone formation, but they have not been primarily found to alter the rate of fracture healing. Increased callus size and mineralization, reduced remodeling, and improved mechanical strength have been observed in animal studies. Improved implant fixation and strength have also been observed. As regard the concern on retarding remodeling, they have not been found to have any adverse effect. Scheduling first dose is the controversy. Oral drugs can be given at any time, however, delaying by 3 weeks is considered better for compliance issues and theoretical concern of formation and organization of fracture callus. Injectable drugs should be preferably delayed for 3–4 weeks or more or withheld (oral drugs are preferable) as drugs like zoledronic acid have localizing effect so they may concentrate at the fracture site immediately after administration and systemic advantages on other bones may be lowered till next dose.
- Teriparatide has not been shown to alter fracture healing and although anabolic has also not been definitely shown to improve fracture healing though the effect is overall positive. Sclerostin and Dickkopf-1 (DKK1) antibodies (discussed below) have also been shown to have beneficial effect on fracture healing.

Osteoporotic Fragility Fractures of Vertebra and their Management with Vertebroplasty and Kyphoplasty (See also Vertebra Plana)

Osteoporotic fragility fractures are associated with significant morbidities such as reduced vital capacity of lungs (thoracic vertebral compression fractures), chronic low back pain (continuous strain on back muscles due to poor posture), shift of sagittal balance, stooping posture and increased tendency to fall, chronic low back pain, and further associated increased risk of vertebral fractures (19.2% increased risk in subsequent year). Overall there is increased mortality that emanates due to variable combination of these but more related to severity of kyphosis. It is not that all of the compression fractures have a bleak outlook and indeed majority heal spontaneously and are clinically silent (silent vertebral fracture). Somewhere one-third of the fractures become painful that gradually reduces over 6–12 weeks. Fractures that fail to heal get filled with fluid typically near the superior endplate in the anterior region. This gradually results in true intravertebral "pseudoarthrosis" formation that is associated with sclerosis of the superior endplate. The fluid is then gradually resorbed to be replaced by "air" and the surrounding bone gets necrosed with replacement of hematopoietic cells with marrow edema and fibrosis. The intravertebral pseudoarthrosis is associated with "dynamic mobility" due to the presence of cleft filled with air or fluid. On performing the supine extension of radiographs, it has been noted that some 87.5% of osteoporotic vertebral fractures are mobile that could restore height by 62.6% if maintained. The intravertebral cleft is responsible for spinal instability but provides an opportunity to restore height by procedures like cement augmentation. After the diagnosis of osteoporotic vertebral fracture is made on radiographs and/or MRI scan, clinician may obtain CT scan to look for posterior vertebral wall fracture or ankylosing spine both of which are contraindications for cement augmentation.

Impregnation of polymethyl methacrylate into the vertebral body (vertebroplasty) provides improved pain relief and rehabilitation **(Fig. 21)**. Vertebroplasty is the direct injection of low-viscosity liquid polymethyl methacrylate (PMMA) cement into the osteoporotic vertebral body fracture. The cement then sets and provides the vertebral body with requisite strength under compressive forces. It was first performed for vertebral hemangioma by Deramond in 1984 (reported by Galibert). The indications of vertebroplasty for osteoporosis include:

- Failed conservative management in symptomatic acute osteoporotic vertebral fracture
- Symptomatic osteoporotic vertebral fracture that is progressively collapsing as seen on imaging
- Symptomatic vertebral fragility fracture with dynamic mobility

The procedure is performed in prone position under local anesthesia usually. Commonly unipedicular approach is used where the vertebral body is accessed through one pedicle or some prefer bipedicular approach where another needle is passed through the other pedicle. Bipedicular approach is helpful where one is suspecting vascular malformation so that before injecting cement one may confirm by injecting contrast in the vertebral body flushed by normal saline before injecting cement. In case of a cavity or cleft there is free flow of contrast or saline from the other needle. Extrapedicular approach may be used for thoracic vertebra where the pedicles are smaller. Commonly two patterns of cement distribution are observed after vertebroplasty—(1) the trabecular or interdigitation pattern [*see* **Figure 4** in Chapter on "Miscellaneous Disorders (Vertebra Plana, Balloon Kyphoplasty, CT-guided Biopsy and Intervertebral Disk Calcification)" in Regional Orthopedics: Spine section], and (2) the cleft or lump pattern **(Fig. 21)**. Trabecular pattern represents cementation into the cancellous trabecular bone rather than void filling. Lump pattern instead

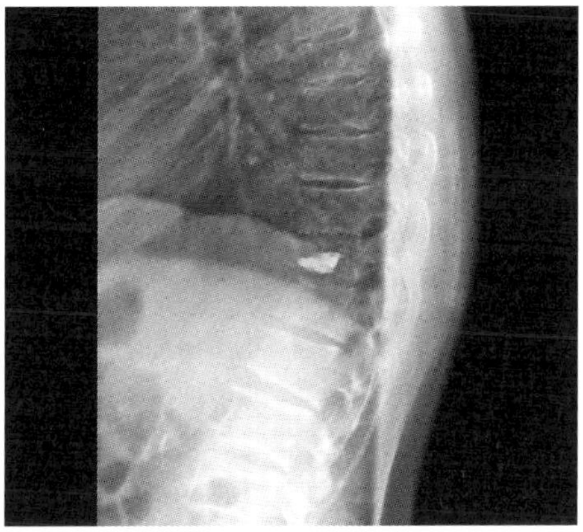

Fig. 21: Vertebroplasty.

represents filling of the intravertebral cleft or fluid cavity of pseudoarthrosis. Lesser amount of cement is injected in the trabecular pattern compared to the void filling pattern and on an average 4 mL of cement is needed considering all cases. One must not try to achieve complete filling of the vertebral body under pressure from endplate to another endplate which is rarely achievable and has high chances of cement leak.

The dreaded complications of vertebroplasty are extradural extravasation of bone cement that would cause neurological compromise and formation of cement emboli that may migrate in the spinal canal. Kyphoplasty (balloon kyphoplasty or balloon-assisted vertebroplasty) is considered to be a more effective procedure as it involves inflating a balloon inside the vertebra restoring vertebral height and then bone cement is injected into the balloon. This potentially ameliorates cement extravasations. Pain relief is prompt and lasting, however, there are concerns of compression fractures of adjacent vertebrae and cost with kyphoplasty.

Balloon kyphoplasty can be performed by orthopedic surgeon or interventional radiologist under general anesthesia or deep sedation **(Figs. 22A to G)**. The majority of vertebral osteoporotic compression fracture occurs at the thoracolumbar junction. The primary indications for balloon kyphoplasty are:

- Painful fractures with a back pain score of 4 points or more on a 0–10 scale not responding to conservative treatment for 6 weeks
- Compression fracture due to osteoporosis (primary or secondary), osteolytic metastatic tumors (D5–L5 levels), multiple myeloma
- *Junctional lesions:* "Adjacent vertebra" of a fractured and treated one at the level of D12 or L1 in severely osteoporotic patient, older than 75 years of age with good Karnofsky performance status score (>70). This is preventive treatment as it has been found that at D12–L1 level if one of the vertebra is treated then the other one shows a fracture within 18 months.

Contraindications for balloon kyphoplasty:

- Age <21 years
- Previous vertebroplasty of the same vertebra
- Pedicular fracture
- Severe disease:
  - Radicular pain
  - Neurological deficit
  - Evident spinal cord compression
- Patients on uninterruptible anticoagulation therapy
- Allergy to any of kyphoplasty instrumentation
- Nonambulatory before fracture
- Fractures due to primary bone tumors, osteoblastic metastasis, and high-energy trauma

Principles of procedure: The procedure is performed as short admission of 24 hours. The success relies on regular expansion of the vertebral body that can be stabilized by intraosseous cement. Injection pressure and the cement viscosity are hence the most important parameters. It has been identified that higher viscosity and lower injection pressures are important for uniform expansion of the bone and optimal filling.

Operative Technique

These are:

- The surgery is done under anesthesia. The patient lies prone and best worked under O-arm or two C-arms to give continuous anteroposterior and lateral views.
- Pedicle is localized under fluoroscopy.
- After making stab incision, 11-gauge biopsy needle is advanced into the fractured vertebral body by transpedicular approach.

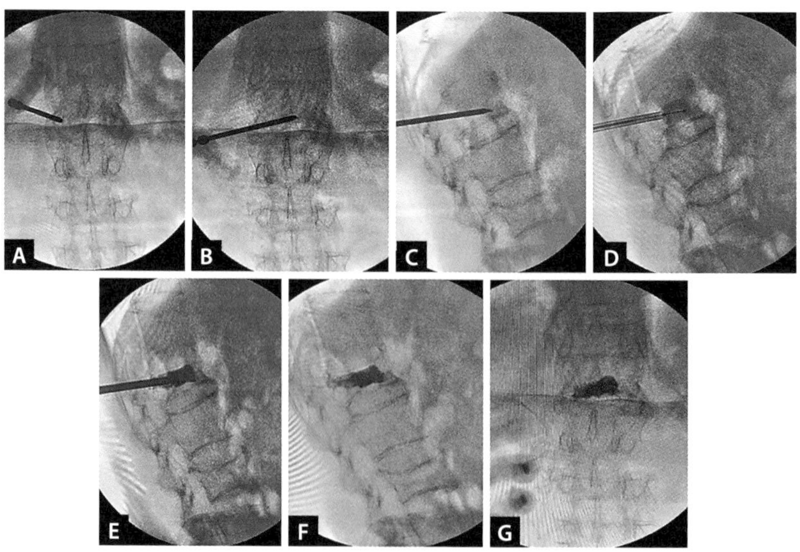

Figs. 22A to G: Technique of performing kyphoplasty in managing osteoporotic vertebral compression fractures. The pedicle of involved vertebra is located in PA fluoroscopy projection (A), the cannula-trochar is advanced till it is located centrally in the vertebral body on PA projection (B); it may cross midline slightly, on lateral projection (C) it is placed not farther than M/3rd anterior third junction of vertebral body for safety. The cannula is removed and sleeve is placed on the trocar that crosses pedicle (D) and balloon is advanced confirming complete deployment in front of cannula (both marker dots beyond cannula), the balloon is inflated with diluted radiopaque dye till recommended pressure to create uniform space (D). Liquid cement is then pushed in the created cavity (E) confirming its placement in the expanded vertebral cavity (F and G) in perpendicular projections.

- Working cannula is introduced and needle is removed.
- Inflatable balloon tamp is introduced under the collapsed end plate.
- Balloon tamps are then inflated under fluoroscopic control measuring the pressure through inbuilt manometer.
- Maximum fracture reduction is achieved and inflation is stopped when the balloon reaches the cortical wall or one obtains the "balloon kissing" position (two balloons introduced through each pedicle touching each other in the vertebral body center).
- Cement is prepared and loaded in syringes.
- At semisolid state (3–5 minutes after mixing, depends on product), the cement is introduced carefully under fluoroscopy control.
- At cement setting, the cannula is removed and wound closed.

Complications of balloon kyphoplasty procedure:

- Minor—transient bradycardia and desaturation are most common.
- Serious—cement pulmonary embolus (0.01–1%), extravasation to epidural space (7–10%). To prevent the latter, one should push cement only when it is semisolid and cannula should be removed in a rotating maneuver slowly.

Vertebroplasty versus Kyphoplasty

Before comparing the two procedures it is best accepted that both the procedures are effective and safe in providing pain relief from osteoporotic fragility fractures. The improvement in quality of life and physical function is quite rapid along with reducing the disability. The comparison between procedures can be based on the following points:

- *Reduction of disability and pain relief:* Most studies and meta-analysis have demonstrated comparable pain relief and functional recovery in the patients with a slight bias toward the former in vertebroplasty and the latter in kyphoplasty. Generally, considering as reported by Han et al., pain relief is better within short-term by vertebroplasty (say 7 days), while kyphoplasty is better in improving the disability in medium term (say 3 months); in long-term there is relatively no discernible difference between the procedures when assessing pain relief and disability reduction.
- *Restoration of vertebral height:* It appears that by the procedure itself if pressurized balloon improves the vertebral body height then kyphoplasty must be able to restore the vertebral height better but in studies there has been quite significant evidence of finding improvement in vertebral height by vertebroplasty also (possibly the prone position by itself improves height during vertebroplasty). Currently, literatures do support improvement in height and sagittal balance by the procedures but exact amount and superiority of one over the other has not been fully determined.
- *Complications and sequelae: Cement leakage* is a significant complication of vertebroplasty with incidence as high as 41% (20–41%) as compared to kyphoplasty (7–9%). Most of the cement leakages are asymptomatic so no further intervention is needed but a leakage into spinal canal (epidural space) causing compression of the neural structures would need emergent decompression. Cement may leak into paravertebral space, diskal, pulmonary space or into segmental veins also. To prevent cement leaks during vertebroplasty, high viscosity cement is recommended and it is suggested that stopping cement injection when it reaches middle and posterior third junction of vertebral body would further prevent leakage into spinal canal. As far as the *adjacent vertebral body fracture* is considered, both procedures have been found to be associated with an increased incidence compared to general population. There is a relative risk of 4.6 for fracture of an adjacent vertebra compared to vertebra located not adjacent to the treated level. It must be mentioned, however, that most of the studies have found a reduction in the incidence of subsequent fractures following treatment by any of the two methods possibly by improvement in the sagittal balance. *Refracture of treated vertebral fractures* and this is the way too common (as high as 78%) in patients demonstrating pericement halo phenomenon. These patients are prone to recollapse of the treated vertebra especially in the kyphoplasty group. The recollapse rate is proportional to the development of osteonecrosis which is conceivably higher in compacted bone from balloon pressure and exothermic cement reaction.

Kyphoplasty is comparatively much expensive than vertebroplasty and for this reason in developing countries like ours we tend to prefer vertebroplasty. Also kyphoplasty needs general anesthesia and longer admission while vertebroplasty could be performed in local anesthesia itself as a day-care procedure.

PHARMACOTHERAPY FOR OSTEOPOROSIS

Nonpharmacological Agents, Calcium, Vitamin D, and Minerals

Calcium alone may somewhat reduce, but not fully prevent bone loss. Despite unclear mechanism of benefit, several controlled clinical trials of treatment with calcium given concomitantly with vitamin D have documented decrease in osteoporosis-related fractures (20–30% risk reduction). Bone loss in men is not modified or controlled by calcium and vitamin D intake significantly, however. Most studies on osteoporosis pharmacotherapy include supplementation with calcium and vitamin D. Thus, it is a standard practice to ensure an adequate calcium and vitamin D intake in patients with osteoporosis irrespective of other antiosteoporosis treatment. There is a heated debate on enhanced vascular disease risk (myocardial infarction and adverse cardiovascular events) with calcium supplementation. The current evidence from various studies and meta-analysis is, however, insufficient and controversial and expert opinion is divided. There has been an often-repeated question of impact of calcium supplementation on stone formation in urinary tract. In patients with a history of nephroureterolithiasis, it has been found that high intake of dietary calcium reduces the risk of stone formation marginally, whereas intake of high doses of supplemental calcium may modestly increase risk (weak relation). Dietary calcium exerts its beneficial effects by binding to oxalate, and hence, preventing the formation or precipitation of calcium oxalate—a primary ingredient in most renal stones. It is recommended that these patients (positive history of renal stones) should be evaluated by 24-hour urinary calcium determination before starting supplementary calcium to avoid hypercalciuria. The recommended daily dosage of elemental calcium is:

- 1,200 mg/day for women aged 51+ years and men aged 71+ years of age (No evidence supporting higher doses > 1,200 mg/day as previously used).

The role of vitamin D is more obscure. Vitamin D supplementation may have a role in prevention of glucocorticoid-induced osteoporosis. Studies failed to show beneficial effects of low-dose vitamin D on osteoporosis-related fractures. Also, the hypercalciuria and hypercalcemia associated with vitamin D preparations limit their routine use (they are still used as essential supplementation without documented indication in most prescriptions). One important note on clinical testing for vitamin D levels. It has been now accepted worldover that 25-OH vitamin D levels of 20–50 ng/mL (≡ 50 - 125 nmol/L) are considered safe and sufficient. There is no need to do repeat testing if adequate supplementation is being done. Even testing of vitamin D levels before initiating supplementation is not strictly recommended and low vitamin D levels are not solely responsible for osteoporosis or allied symptoms. The current recommendation stands at supplementing 800–1,000 IU of vitamin D_3 per day for adults above 50 years of age. It has been, however, my experience that creating iatrogenic vitamin D toxicity is quite uncommon despite irrational use. Individuals with documented vitamin D deficiency should be supplemented with higher doses of vitamin D.

Vitamin K supplementation has been shown to improve BMD possibly due to role in carboxylation of osteocalcin. Vitamin K2 (menaquinone) itself includes many types of vitamin K2. Menaquinone-4 (MK-4) and menaquinone-7 (MK-7) are most studied osteoporosis. Vitamin K1 in the testes, pancreas, and arterial walls is converted to MK-4. MK-4 has been approved for the prevention and treatment of osteoporosis as it has been shown to reduce fracture risk by 87%. MK-4 also prevents bone loss and fractures caused by steroid therapy, anorexia, cirrhosis of liver, and postmenopausal osteoporosis. Patients are rarely, if ever deficient in *magnesium* due to its high availability in diet, but some patients with malabsorption syndrome may need supplementation. *Phytoestrogens* derived primarily from soy products and legumes have recently gained interest available in various ayurvedic preparations and have shown beneficial effects for improving BMD. Of the various plant extracts studied, a natural isoflavone genistein has been found to reduce bone resorption, while simultaneously increase bone formation in postmenopausal women. *Zinc, copper, manganese,* and *boron* have trophic influence on osteoblasts and collagen so could be included in various preparations though strong evidence of clinical effect is lacking.

Osteoporosis-specific Pharmacotherapy and Biological Agents

There are various classes of medicines commonly used for treatment of osteoporosis that act at different stages of intercellular interaction for their effect **(Fig. 23)**. The drugs basically fall into antiresorptive and anabolic groups with few overlapping functions also. The treatment is ideally aimed at increasing bone mass, improve bone architecture and strength and reduce risk of fracture. The usage of the specific drugs should be expertly advocated for different patients. In general, the different drug class, their indications, and their pros and cons are provided below.

Indications: Postmenopausal women and men aged ≥50 years with following clinical features have been indicated to undergo pharmacotherapy as recommended by the NOF:

- Hip or vertebral fracture
- Other prior fractures and low bone mass (T-score between –1.0 and –2.5 at the femoral neck, hip, and spine)
- T-score ≤ –2.5 at the femoral neck, hip, or spine after appropriate evaluation to exclude secondary causes
- Low bone mass (T-score between –1.0 and –2.5 at the femoral neck, hip, or spine) and secondary causes associated with high risk of fracture (such as glucocorticoid use or immobilization)
- 10-year probability of hip fracture ≥3% or a 10-year probability of any major osteoporosis-related fracture ≥20% based on FRAX®.

Some specific risk factors have been included by NOF that should be looked in a patient who is considered a likely candidate for future osteoporotic fracture. These include:

- History of fracture (especially vertebral body) as an adult
- First-degree relative sustaining any fragility fracture
- Low body weight (<127 pounds)
- Current smoker
- Glucocorticoid use for >3 months
- Visual impairment
- Dementia
- Poor health and morbidities
- Estrogen deficiency in late adulthood (before age of 45 years in females)
- History of recent falls suggesting poor balance
- Poor or inadequate calcium intake (lifelong)

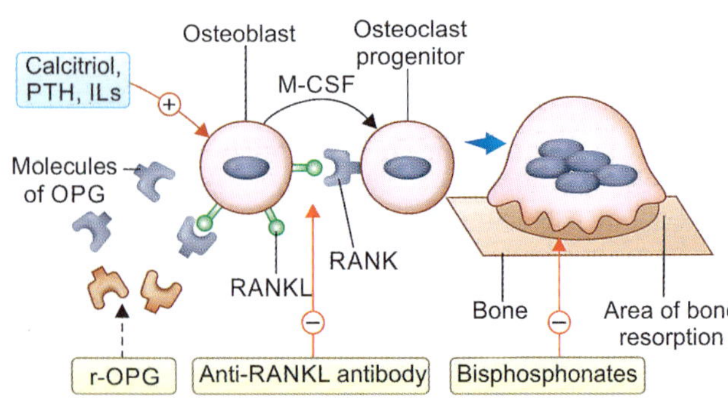

Fig. 23: The interaction of various bone cells and typical sites of action of chief class of drugs commonly used in treatment of osteoporosis. (PTH: parathormone; IL: interleukins; OPG: osteoprotegerin; RANK: receptor activator of nuclear factor κ; RANKL: receptor activator of nuclear factor κ ligand; M-CSF: monocyte-colony stimulating factor)

- Restricted physical activity especially in early years of life that changes to sedentary work later
- Alcohol intake >2 drinks per day

Estrogen

Now largely historical only, the Food and Drug Administration (FDA) has withdrawn the approval of hormone replacement with estrogen for osteoporosis prevention, except in selected cases of postmenopausal osteoporosis. Estrogen replacement therapy (ERT) historically has been used in postmenopausal women to prevent osteoporosis-related fractures before the age of 60 years or within 10 years after menopause based on the premises that there is accelerated bone loss in postmenopausal women. ERT improves bone mass through receptors on osteoclasts lowering bone turnover and resorption. The effect is most prominent when therapy is initiated soon after menopause and used continuously. There is increased lumbar spine BMD of 1–4% at 1 year in women receiving conjugated estrogen at 3.0–0.625 mg/day in combination with calcium. Compared to other available agents, the effect is however modest. ERT raises high-density lipoproteins (HDLs) and lowers low-density lipoproteins (LDLs) to the extent of 10% in postmenopausal women, however, there has been an increase in coronary heart disease (CHD) and thromboembolic events in the first 2 years of therapy. Venous thromboembolic events are 2.7–4.0 times more common among estrogen users than among nonusers. In heart and estrogen or progesterone replacement study (HERS), some of the women were hypercoagulable manifest by prothrombotic gene mutations. There are also important concerns like hyperplasia of endometrium (potentially leading to endometrial cancer) and an increased risk for breast cancer. In addition to a fracture benefit, estrogen lowers the risk of colorectal cancer by 24% and reduces mental stress, estrogen plus progestin, however, increases probable dementia. Addition of progesterone (HRT) diminishes the increased risk of endometrial cancer and cardiovascular events, but increases possibility of developing breast cancer and might also partially blunt the already modest benefit of estrogen on bone. High-dose estrogens are not a preferred initial pharmacotherapy for osteoporosis. HRT may have a role in postmenopausal women in combination therapy with bisphosphonates.

Selective Estrogen Receptor Modulators

Tamoxifene is the first generation selective estrogen receptor modulator (SERM), but not indicated or preferred for treatment or prevention of osteoporosis. Raloxifene (second-generation SERM) is a benzothiopene derivative with estrogenic effects on the skeleton and lipid profile and antiestrogenic effects on the breast and uterus. It has been shown to lower the biochemical markers of bone remodeling and it also increases lumbar spine BMD. It also reduces LDLs, total cholesterol, and triglycerides while raising HDLs. Raloxifene therapy for 4 years appears to reduce cardiovascular events in higher risk women as against estrogen therapy. In the heart (RUTH trial), raloxifene had no significant effect on the risk of coronary events and there was no difference in overall stroke risk, however, it was associated with an increased risk of fatal stroke (HR: 1.49) and venous thromboembolism (HR: 1.44). Important drawbacks to use of raloxifene, however, are its relative inefficiency to reduce fracture risk at nonvertebral sites and that the beneficial effects of raloxifene on BMD dissipate after withdrawal. It reduces the risk of invasive breast cancer, however, there is a roughly threefold increased risk of deep venous thrombosis. Bazedoxifene (third-generation nonsteroidal, indole-based SERM) is approved in Europe for treatment of postmenopausal osteoporosis and may have a beneficial role in dyspareunia and painful sexual intercourse. Lasofoxifene is another potent third-generation SERM (naphthalene derivative) with good oral bioavailability and higher potency. Lasofoxifene specifically binds to human ERα (similar to other SERMs) with high affinity (10 times higher than raloxifene). It has been found to reduce the bone turnover markers significantly as well as the symptoms of dyspareunia and vaginal atrophy.

The combination of raloxifene with alendronate result in greater increase in BMD, but the ultimate effect on fracture prevention is unknown.

Calcitonin

Calcitonin is a naturally occurring peptide hormone produced by the parafollicular C cells of thyroid gland and it directly inhibits osteoclasts. The antiresorptive effects are however mild. A synthetic preparation—the Salmon calcitonin is 40–50 times more potent than human calcitonin and has also the longest half-life among all synthetic preparations. Salmon calcitonin can be administered either subcutaneously or intranasally (preferred) in a dose of 200 IU daily. It is recommended that calcitonin should always be administered with adequate calcium (at least 1 g) and vitamin D (400 IU/day). Large clinical trial has failed to show any benefit of calcitonin on prevention of osteoporosis-related fractures (Henrisken et al., 2016). The clinical effects of intranasal calcitonin on BMD improvement have been reported to be modest only and it is unsure as to whether they represent the effect of drug of supplemental calcium. Long-term administration leads to development of calcitonin-specific antibodies. Neutralizing antibodies may retard the long-term effects of this agent. Interestingly, many studies have reported analgesic effect for acute compression fracture pain and now this drug is more popular for this indication rather than antiosteoporosis effect. European Medicines Agency Committee for Medicinal Products for Human Use have recommended that calcitonin should no longer be used for osteoporosis (July 2012) due to increased overall cancer risk as found in meta-analysis. FDA panel also recommended against use of calcitonin for osteoporosis treatment. Soon this drug will be dropped from the list of therapeutic drugs for osteoporosis.

Bisphosphonates (Diphosphonates)

They are the current first-line drugs for prevention and treatment of osteoporosis. The bisphosphonates are analogs of pyrophosphates (P-O-P) characterized by a phosphorus-carbon-phosphorus bond (so, P-C-P instead of P-O-P). They evolved from industrial use (the textile and oil industries) where it was used as an antiscaling and anticorrosive agent for over a century. They have the basic property of inhibiting precipitation of calcium carbonate. The medical use initiated with the identification of naturally occurring polyphosphate (inorganic pyrophosphate) in urine and plasma by Fleisch et al. that prevent calcification of tissues and stone formation. This pyrophosphate (PPi) is a known by-product of many biosynthetic reactions in the body and its concentration is regulated by hydrolytic enzymes predominantly the ALP. Deficiency of ALP as in hypophosphatasia is associated with increased PPi and mineralization defects. The elementary problem with the use of synthetic pyrophosphates and polyphosphates was that they were effective only when injected and ineffective orally due to hydrolysis in gastrointestinal tract (GIT). It was during this search for stable pyrophosphates that attention got diverted to bisphosphonates (wrongly called diphosphonates) that had good osseous affinity and prevent calcification both in vitro and in vivo. The carbon atom connecting the two phosphate atoms (P-C-P) imparts them stability from chemical and enzymatic hydrolysis. Their clinical use, however, began only with the identification of their unique property of inhibiting dissolution of hydroxyapatite crystals. Bisphosphonates are potent inhibitors of bone resorption.

Pharmacokinetics and Pharmacodynamics

Bisphosphonates are poorly absorbed so that only 1% of the administered dose enters circulation. If taken along with a divalent cation (like calcium supplements) the absorption will be completely blocked. So, they must be taken on an empty stomach to maximize absorption. To reduce gastrointestinal irritation and maximize absorption, the pills should be swallowed with 250 mL of water on an empty stomach, remaining upright for 30 minutes (60 min for ibandronate) after swallowing the tablet, and having nothing to eat or drink for 30 minutes (60 min for monthly ibandronate) after ingesting each pill. Of the absorbed amount, 50% binds to bone and rest is excreted by kidney unchanged. The bisphosphonates are not metabolized in the body due to unfamiliar and strong P-C-P linkage. The phosphonate groups serve two functions. Firstly, they are required both for binding to bone mineral for executing cell-mediated antiresorptive activity. Secondly, varying the R2 substituents result in differences in antiresorptive potency of several orders of magnitude **(Fig. 24)**, while the R1 side chain substituents (hydroxyl or amino) enhance chemisorption to mineral. Although plasma half-life is short, 30–180 minutes, once incorporated into bone they can remain bound to exposed hydroxyapatite crystals and active for up to 10 years (property conferred by R1 side chain). Risedronate can remain in bone for 30 years, whereas zoledronic acid can remain up to 60 years. The variations in efficacy and potency are determined by the structure of the amino side chains **(Table 9)**.

Classification and Mechanism of Action

Bisphosphonates can be classified into two groups regarding their routes of administration—oral (alendronate, risedronate, and tiludronate) or intravenous (pamidronate and zoledronic acid), or both (ibandronate and clodronate). The other classification divides them based on the presence or absence of nitrogen.

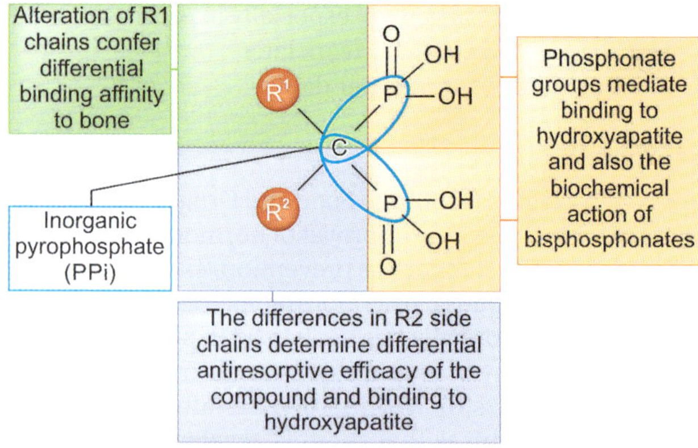

Fig. 24: Bisphosphonate structure.

TABLE 9: Antiresorptive potency of different bisphosphonates.

Drug	*Relative potency*
Etidronate	1
Clodronate	10
Tiludronate	10
Pamidronate	100
Alendronate	1,000
Risedronate	5,000
Ibandronate	10,000
Zoledronate	100,000

There are two basic categories of bisphosphonates:

1. The non-nitrogen-containing bisphosphonates, for example, clodronate, etidronate, and tiludronate—they are metabolized in the cell to compounds that replace the terminal pyrophosphate moiety of adenosine triphosphate (ATP), and thus get incorporated into intracellular analogs of ATP directly. They inhibit osteoclastic activity by producing toxic analogs of ATP (that competes with natural ATP) and cause cell death (thus, apoptosis is the primary effect.).
2. The nitrogen-containing bisphosphonates (alendronate, neridronate, olpadronate, pamidronate, risedronate, ibandronate, and zoledronate)—they inhibit the prenylation and function of (GTP) guanosine triphosphate-binding proteins required for osteoclast formation, function, and survival (osteoclast dysregulation is primary effect.). They alter cholesterol metabolism in osteoclast by inhibiting the enzyme farnesyl diphosphate synthase **(Fig. 25 and Flowchart 2)**, leading to cytoskeletal alterations, disappearance of ruffled border and premature osteoclast cell death, via apoptosis. Inhibition of this enzyme interferes with the prenylation (a process of addition of 15- and 20-carbon side chains that anchor GTP-binding proteins to osteoclast cell membrane). This reduces not only the resorptive capacity of osteoclasts, but also induces apoptosis.

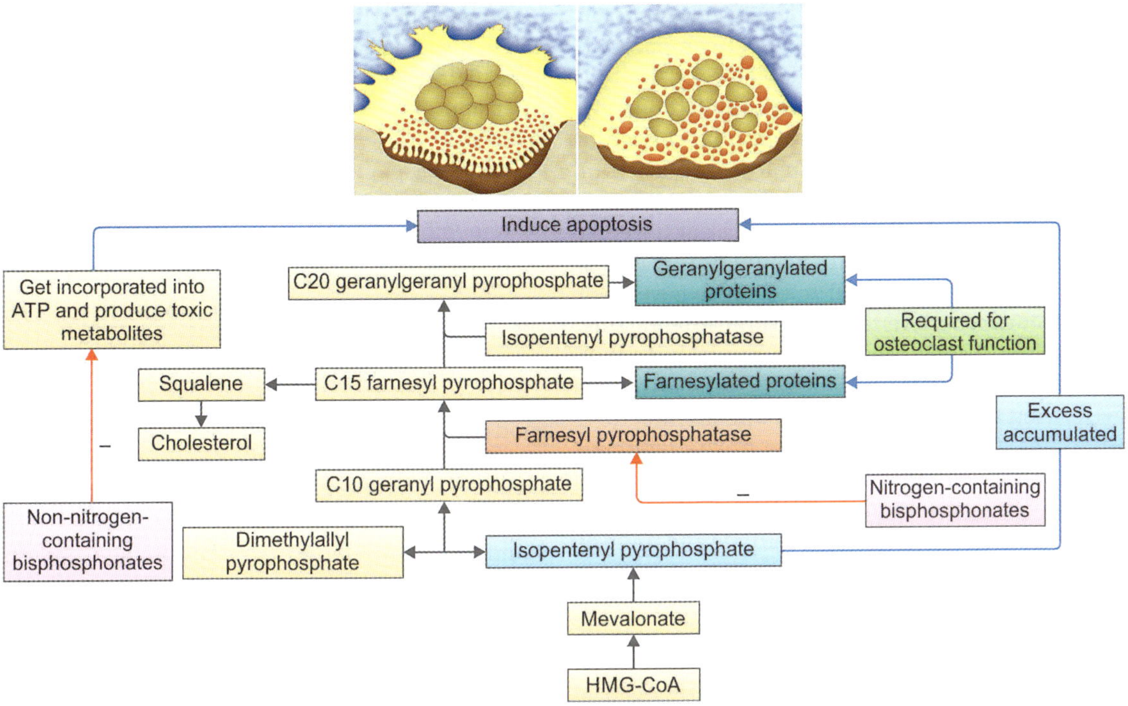

Fig. 25: Mechanism of action of bisphosphonates.
(ATP: adenosine triphosphate; HMG-CoA: 3-hydroxy-3-methylglutaryl-coenzyme A)

The main effect of bisphosphonates, be it of any group, is to reduce bone resorption and bone turnover, required for treatment of osteoporosis. The secondary effects are reduction of angiogenesis by depression of blood flow and a significant reduction in vascular endothelial growth factor (VEGF). Inhibition of epithelial keratinocytes is also observed. The net effect of these actions is reduced healing capacity and the bone sort of becomes metabolically inactive (metabolic freeze). They reduce the recruitment and activity of osteoclasts reducing their lifespan. The rank order of potency for inhibiting farnesyl pyrophosphate synthase is zoledronate > risedronate > ibandronate > alendronate **(Table 9)**, with the more potent heterocyclic bisphosphonates (zoledronate and risedronate), being more potent than the compounds with an alkyl side chain (alendronate and ibandronate) though this does not have equivalent bearing on the antiresorptive capacity. Over prolonged administration, a regional paracrine effect of continuously deposited and recycled bisphosphonates may have persistent effect seen on discontinuation of medication. Bisphosphonates with higher mineral binding affinity, such as alendronate and zoledronate, are associated with greater reduction of bone turnover and have a longer duration of effect after treatment is stopped as conferred by R1 side chain **(Fig. 24)**. Bisphosphonates with lower mineral binding affinity, such as risedronate and etidronate are less effective and their effect is more readily reversible when therapy is stopped. Though unclear and not identified, but they may also have additional unrecognized anabolic effects which would correlate to the findings of persistent increase in BMD realized even beyond stopping the drug after first year of therapy.

Flowchart 2: The overall effect of prolonged administration of bisphosphonates.

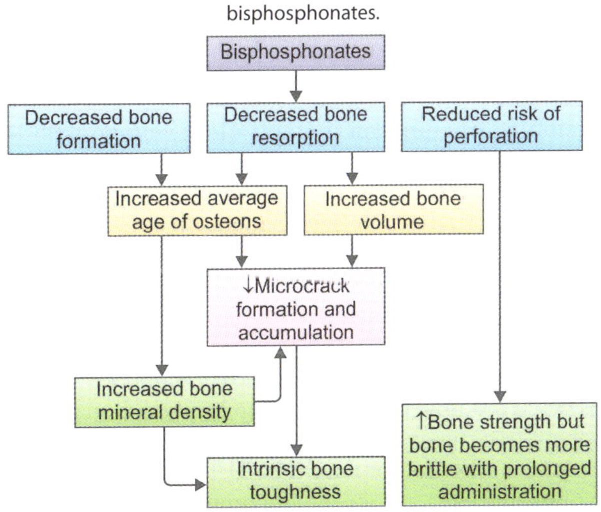

Clinical Uses

Osteogenesis imperfecta: Bone strength is improved by administration of bisphosphonates significantly and it constitutes an important therapy in this disease irrespective of age or clinical presentation.

Osteoporosis: Second-generation bisphosphonate alendronate was the first aminobisphosphonate approved by the US-FDA for the treatment and prevention of osteoporosis. Alendronate inhibits bone resorption without much deleterious effects on mineralization. Spinal BMD shows continuous improvement after alendronate therapy up to 7 years of daily therapy. A once-weekly dosing is most popular, but has been randomly decided.

Risedronate is a third-generation pyridinyl bisphosphonate with somewhat inferior antiresorptive effect compared to alendronate, but similar fracture reduction efficacy.

Tiludronate is ineffective when administered intermittently. Zoledronate (third-generation bisphosphonate) has the highest potency and very good efficacy similar to or better than alendronate. It is given as a yearly injection. Ibandronate is effective in reducing fracture risk at vertebral sites, however, nonvertebral fracture reduction is not as good. Alendronate, risedronate, and zoledronate have been shown to be effective at both vertebral and nonvertebral sites (predominantly hip). Bisphosphonate therapy acts by various mechanisms (discussed earlier) that primarily lower activation frequency slowing the deterioration in bone architecture. Bisphosphonates cause bone metabolic freeze reducing bone turnover, of which there is an earlier decrease in bone resorption than bone formation improving bone strength. The magnitude of response depends on the type and route of administration of the drug. The increase in BMD results from filling in of the remodeling space, and hence relative increase in mineralization of bone tissue. When associated with biological effects and improvement in the bone quality there is also reduction in fracture risk. The effect is more marked in postmenopausal women with osteoporosis. Answer to the long elusive question of duration of bisphosphonate therapy has started to emerge. In 2016, ASBMR has published guidelines for long-term use of bisphosphonate for osteoporosis. In general, oral bisphosphonates can be given for 5 years and injectable ones for 3 years following which reassessment as to further need should be made. If the patients are high risk for developing osteoporosis- related fractures [patients developing fractures on therapy, older woman with low T-score or those with previous major fracture(s)] then therapy may be continued up to 10 years for oral drugs or 6 years of intravenous agents. In such patients, the risk of atypical fractures or osteonecrosis of jaw is outweighed by the benefits from therapy for osteoporotic fracture risk reduction. In patients that are not high risk for developing osteoporotic fractures, a drug holiday for 2–3 years can be given after 3–5 years of therapy. The other questions that cannot be definitely answered are how best to combine bisphosphonates with anabolic treatments and if there are any benefits of treatment in patients who do not have a BMD T-score below –2.5. If bisphosphonates are given concomitantly with anabolic agent like teriparatide then effects of both drugs are mitigated reducing efficacy of any therapy alone. However, it has been found that if teriparatide is given in a pulsed fashion of 3 months alternating on and off in patients already receiving oral weekly bisphosphonates, the BMD increase is higher than bisphosphonate only therapy possibly due to the prudent utilization of the anabolic 3 months window. In general case, however, still bisphosphonates are only recommended sequentially to teriparatide therapy and not simultaneously.

Hypercalcemia of malignancy and antiresorptive effect in cancer patients: Bisphosphonates are the drug of choice for all patients with multiple myeloma and radiologically confirmed bone metastases from breast cancer. Bisphosphonates are to be started in these cases immediately as soon as the diagnosis is made and are continued indefinitely. Other bone metastasis should also be treated with bisphosphonates when appropriate. The effects of bisphosphonates have been twofold:

- Reducing pain
- Prevention of pathological fractures. It should be remembered that they are approved only for cancer with metastasis.

Paget's disease of bone: Interestingly, the antiresorptive effect of bisphosphonates was first demonstrated in Paget's disease. Use of bisphosphonates showed dose-dependent inhibition of bone resorption, and hence remodeling. As good efficacy has been established since 1980s the treatment with bisphosphonate class of drugs for Paget's disease is currently the preferred modality. The primary drug used for the treatment of Paget's has been alendronate, intravenous. Palmidronate (preferred), oral residronate, and tiludronate usually along with calcitonin.

Pediatric uses:

- *Fibrous dysplasia and McCune-Albright syndrome:* Radiological improvement has not been demonstrated, but pain relief has been reported by most patients. Definitive role is not known.
- *Perthes' disease:* Studies have been sparse, but there is a suggestion that possibly they may restrict deformation of the head and collapse similar to osteonecrosis.
- *Osteoporosis in children:* Primary osteoporosis is unknown, but secondary osteoporosis does respond to the effects of bisphosphonates. It reduces occurrence of fractures and increase BMD.

Other uses:

- *Postsurgical:* In enhancing implant fixation
- Prevention of bone collapse in osteonecrosis at various sites, but commonly used at hip joint
- *"Bone scanning":* Bisphosphonates by virtue of their strong affinity for bone mineral get accumulated at sites of increased bone turnover acting as bone scanning agents. Also, their ability to be linked to a gamma-emitting technetium isotope serves an important advantage for detecting bone metastasis and other bone lesions.
- Prevent heterotopic ossification following hip replacement surgery
- Treatment for calcification in renal failure and vascular disease

Pamidronate has been used most commonly for the treatment of lytic bone metastases, Paget's disease, and osteogenesis imperfecta.

Adverse effects: The adverse effects are–

- Approximately 30% of the patients experience influenza-like illness (pyrexia, chills, myalgia, and arthralgia) that tend to resolve within 3–7 days. Treatment with acetaminophen is sufficient for concerned patients and symptomatic relief.
- *Ocular inflammation:* Conjunctivitis, uveitis, iritis, episcleritis, and scleritis occur in <1%. Treat with corticosteroids and avoid use, especially of the intravenous agents.

- *Gastrointestinal adverse effects:* Gastritis, esophageal ulceration, etc.
  - They should be used cautiously in patients with chronic kidney disease. Segmental glomerulosclerosis has been reported with use of palmidronic acid while tubular dysfunction and interstitial nephritis have been reported with use of zoledronic acid. Hypocalcemia is a serious concern that may get acutely precipitated during or immediately after IV infusion of the drug. One must check serum creatinine and calcium levels before treating (especially with IV drugs).
  - They are not recommended in women of childbearing age who are not using adequate contraception.
  - Achalasia and esophageal strictures are absolute contraindications to oral bisphosphonate therapy. Though concern had been raised for development of esophageal cancer in patients taking bisphosphonates but current literature does not support this.
- *Atrial fibrillation (AF):* This serious adverse effect (especially with zoledronic acid) has been reported sporadically but FDA has not found any direct association between AF and bisphosphonate use.
- *Bone joint and muscle pains:* Shift to lower potency bisphosphonate and give supportive care.
- *Bisphosphonate-related osteonecrosis of the jaws (BRONJ):* Osteonecrosis of jaw (ONJ) now better called painful exposure of mandible and maxilla has been mainly reported in cancer patients receiving intravenous preparations and very rarely from patients on oral therapy. Bisphosphonates produce osteopetrosis like picture ("freeze" the skeleton) that leads to osteonecrosis. Injectable bisphosphonates inhibit neoangiogenesis and inhibit VEGF-induced vessel sprouting leading to avascular necrosis. Also, bisphosphonates get concentrated in the jaws as teeth need continuous remodeling at sockets. Inhibition of osteoclast activity inhibits the remodeling and bone is not resorbed. This inhibits new osteoblasts to come and the resident cells die as they have limited life (150 days for osteoblasts and osteoclasts). The osteon, hence, becomes necrotic and the vessels involute causing osteonecrosis. Patients should undergo dental checkup before initiation of the therapy as dental infection has been linked to development of ONJ and all required dental procedures should be completed before bisphosphonate therapy. Treatment by debridement and coverage by flap have been all ineffective including hyperbaric oxygen. These patients have to live with exposed bone sadly as of now. Preventive measures include regular dental care (every 6–12 months) in cancer patients and patients deemed to undergo osteoporosis treatment. At risk patients like diabetics and those on corticosteroid use may consider prophylactic antibiotics and mouth rinses.
- *Atypical insufficiency fractures (AIF):* These have been found to occur at sacrum, femoral shaft, and proximal femur (more likely bilateral). A lot of reports have creeped up mentioning "atypical" fractures associated with the long-term use of bisphosphonates after their first description by Odvina et al. in 2005. A task force was created by American Society for Bone and Mineral Research (ASBMR) to identify and categorize these fractures and address key questions associated with their finding. They defined major and minor features of incomplete and complete atypical femoral fractures and recommended the following major features (at least four of the following five major features should be present in a fracture for classifying as atypical femoral fracture located along the femoral diaphysis from just distal to the lesser trochanter till just proximal to the supracondylar flare, see also Annexure 2: Subtrochanteric fractures):
  - Localized periosteal or endosteal ellipsoid thickening of the lateral cortex present at the fracture site as "beaking" or "flaring"
  - Transverse or short oblique orientation
  - Minimal or no associated trauma
  - A medial spike when the fracture is complete
  - Absence of comminution

The minor features (not needed for diagnosis) include:
- Cortical thickening
- Prodromal dull or aching pain in thigh
- Bilateral incomplete or complete femoral diaphysis fractures
- Delayed fracture healing
- Comorbid conditions
- Concomitant drug use, including bisphosphonates or other antiresorptive agents, glucocorticoids and proton pump inhibitors.

Bisphosphonate-induced subtrochanteric fractures are a serious complication. Due to the bone "freezing" effect of bisphosphonates, the microcracks keep accumulating in the bone and do not get repaired for absence of remodeling due to inhibition of osteoclasts. These are low turnover fractures due to reduction in bone remodeling induced by long-term bisphosphonate therapy. It has been found that the incidence of atypical femoral fractures is around 1–2/100,000/year in patients exposed to bisphosphonate therapy for <2 years while it increases to >100/100,000/year for those kept on bisphosphonates for >8 years. The stress fractures develop over time on the tensile side of femur (lateral cortex). Such fractures typically accumulate in the dense cortical bone. Subtrochanteric region of femur near isthmus contains highest percentage of compact bone so gets weakened enough to fail under repeated stress. It must be, however, mentioned here that the atypical femoral fractures have distinctive characteristics in comparison to exercise-induced femoral fatigue fractures. The latter develop on the medial side and are often more oblique (30–60° pattern) than the bisphosphonate-related atypical femoral fractures. These are transverse fractures without thickening of the cortices (stress fractures usually have thickened cortex). The risk to fracture reduces rapidly as the treatment with drug is discontinued. This suggests that a process other than inhibition only of remodeling is involved as absence of remodeling would only explain the delayed healing or failure to healing of the fracture and not the inception of fracture. Fracture without significant trauma would occur due to poor matrix and mineral properties such as reduced heterogeneity of the organic matrix, increased advanced glycation end products (AGEs like pentosidine) and reduced bone quality (alteration of pyridinoline/deoxypyridinoline ratio and collagen cross-linking reducing postyield deformation of bone and its toughness). This would suggest that the bone at the tensile surface would be unable to bear the physiological stresses and microcracks would develop which in the absence of regular fracture remodeling propagate and coalesce to form larger gaps. These gaps are high strain areas around which the osteocytes die (an effect due to high strain mechanically and reduction of angiogenesis by direct biological effect of bisphosphonates) and ultimately a stress fracture is created that gives way later. Mechanical factors such as the geometry of femur also play a role. Bowing of femur at the upper thirds of femoral shaft is quite common in older females and may be related to the concentration of tensile stress in this region predisposing them to regular microfractures that in oversuppression of bone remodeling would give way ultimately. Other limb alignment features such as smaller femoral neck-shaft angle (higher femoral offset), higher femoral torsion, and short height have also been found in such patients. A causal association between bisphosphonates and atypical fractures has not been completely established though there is a very strong correlation. However, recent observations imply that the risk rises with increasing treatment duration. Bisphosphonates are known to accumulate at the fracture site so continued dosing leads to inhibition of repair of microfractures. However, with drug withdrawal and no new drug available for binding to further new fractures will heal in standard way. The ellipsoid cortical thickening found in patients with AIF represents a suboptimal osteoblastic response to physiologic microfractures which generate a larger callus with greater mineral content but less lamellar bone. The microfractures accumulate resulting in clinical symptoms of pain that precedes complete fracture. The tendency to unite after fixation is also subdued having high chances of delayed or nonunion, if treatment is continued. This effect is possibly related to delayed or incomplete maturation of calcified callus into mature bone by inhibition of osteoclastic remodeling by bisphosphonates. The atypical fractures are treated in a standard way as for shaft femur fracture with strict withholding of the drug. Role of anabolic agents in the treatment of bisphosphonate-associated atypical femoral fractures is emerging and it is considered that such patients may be put on anabolic therapy to improve the outcome (union) as reported in sporadic studies and small case series. For patients who have not developed atypical fractures but are experiencing prodrome (common in more than half of such patients) evaluate the other limb also by radiographs and if possible MRI, while the ipsilateral limb would definitely need prophylactic fixation **(Flowchart 3)**. If a fracture is identified (marrow edema/cortical thickening) then in symptomatic patients prophylactic fixation is recommended with or without anabolic therapy. In patients where there is no pain but radiological evidence of fracture or vice versa in the contralateral limb then observation with protective weight bearing for 2–3 months may be continued (usually with anabolic therapy) until they heal or symptoms

Flowchart 3: Diagnostic and management algorithm for atypical insufficieny femoral fractures (AIF)/impending fractures.

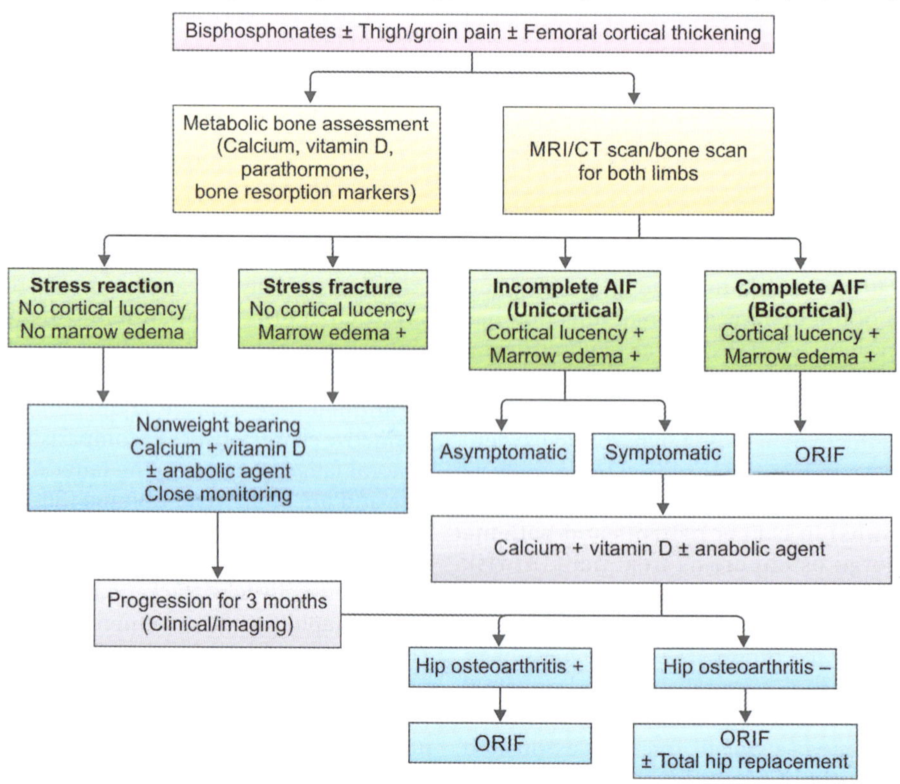

(ORIF: open reduction and interanal fixation)

subside. If this fails then these should also be prophylactically fixed. The pertinent question is regarding seriousness of the problem (AIF) vis-à-vis duration of bisphosphonate therapy. To answer this one can look at risk to benefit ratio of prolonged use of bisphosphonates—for every AIF due to bisphosphonate use (>5 years of continuous use in highly compliant tertiary referral population) nearly 15–100 typical osteoporotic fractures can be prevented. So use of drug for <5 years in nonspecialized center or in less compliant population will have much lesser risk of AIF. I strongly feel the case for use of bisphosphonate longer than 5 years only if there is expected good benefit from it (see below).

Combination Therapy

Combination approaches to osteoporosis therapy (utilizing bisphosphonates) are constantly emerging. Use of two antiresorptive agents is not recommended as no additional benefit has ever been documented while it adds to cost and side effect profile of the agents.

- *Bisphosphonate + estrogen/SERM:* Alendronate is superior to ERT and combination therapy of both is better than either therapy alone. This additive effect is more prominently seen for those on ERT when alendronate is added later. The effect is also seen for patients in whom alendronate is combined with raloxifene. The specific advantage is that alendronate can diminish the loss of BMD seen after stopping HRT.
- *Bisphosphonate + anabolic agent:* Current recommendation is to start antiresorptive drugs, such as bisphosphonates as first-line agents for reducing fracture risk in patients with osteoporosis. In patients with severe osteoporosis (that have enhanced risk of fracture during antiresorptive therapy), starting anabolic agents first is recommended. This is based on the strategy that starting with a bone anabolic substance (like teriparatide) at early stages of osteoporosis and sealing the benefit with antiresorptive agent could first improve the bone mass rapidly, while keeping bone microarchitecture intact may also counter the rapid loss of gains from anabolic therapy as seen on stopping these agents.

Quite often clinicians switch to anabolic agents after they find that the benefit from antiresorptive agents like bisphosphonates is weak or not discernible. This approach causes additional delay in response to PTH though the effect of anabolic agent eventually always comes. There is no recommendation to wait for some time after stopping antiresorptive agent before starting anabolic therapy.

Simultaneous antiresorptive and anabolic agents (like teriparatide): This approach is more tricky and clinician should have a clear understanding. I must admit that no simultaneous combinations have shown convincing results to suggest their use and should be currently avoided.

- *Combining teriparatide with oral bisphosphonates:* This is logically not a good idea as effect of both drugs is reduced causing blunting of effects.
- *Teriparatide + IV bisphosphonate:* This shows primarily early benefit (mostly derived from bisphosphonate only).
- *Teriparatide + SERM:* The combined effect is better than single therapy alone. Same goes with teriparatide + estrogen.
- *Teriparatide + Denosumab:* The effects have been found to be additive exceeding the beneficial effects of single drug alone. This effect has been not only evident at the spine but also at the proximal hip and distal radius (where teriparatide is seemingly less effective). The effect at proximal hip, in fact, appears to be superadditive. It should be noted here that sequential therapy of teriparatide after denosumab is contraindicated and significant transient bone loss is seen with this approach.

Bisphosphonate Holiday

Continuing treatment for 5 years has good clinical support, however, whether the drug should be continued after this duration and for how long is unsettled. Some simple decision making guide can be obtained from following findings:

- Patients with low BMD at femoral neck (T-score < –2.5) after 3–5 years of treatment are at high risk for vertebral fractures and therefore appear to benefit most from continuation of bisphosphonates.
- Patients who have existing vertebral fracture having T-score between –2.0 and –2.5 may also benefit from continued therapy.
- Patients with a femoral neck T-score above –2.0 have a low risk of vertebral fracture and are unlikely to benefit from continued treatment.
- Patients with mild osteoporosis may be considered for "drug holiday" after 5 years of stability.
- Patients at high identified fracture risk may be considered for 1–2 years drug holiday after 10 years of therapy.
- If bone density decreases substantially during drug holiday or a fracture occurs then reinitiate therapy. Patients should be followed for serial BMD measurements (and/or bone turnover markers).

Thiazide Diuretics

Low-dose thiazide diuretics reduce calcium excretion and lead to a significant increase in BMD. They have adverse effects on lipid profile and can cause electrolyte imbalance. Compliance is poor due to intolerable side effects by the normotensive patient and with their relatively weak effects on bone in nonhypercalciuric patients, they are not commonly prescribed.

Receptor Activator of Nuclear Factor Kappa-B Ligand Inhibitors

Denosumab (AMG-162) is a recombinant fully human immunoglobulin G2 (IgG2) monoclonal antibody functionally similar to OPG with affinity and specificity for RANKL **(Fig. 26)**. Denosumab inhibits the RANKL/RANK formation on the osteoblast, and hence preventing the osteoblast–osteoclast interaction decreasing bone resorption. One might recall that RANKL produced by osteocytes and osteoblasts regulate osteoclast number and activity. The inhibitory effect of denosumab on RANK/RANKL interaction results in increased

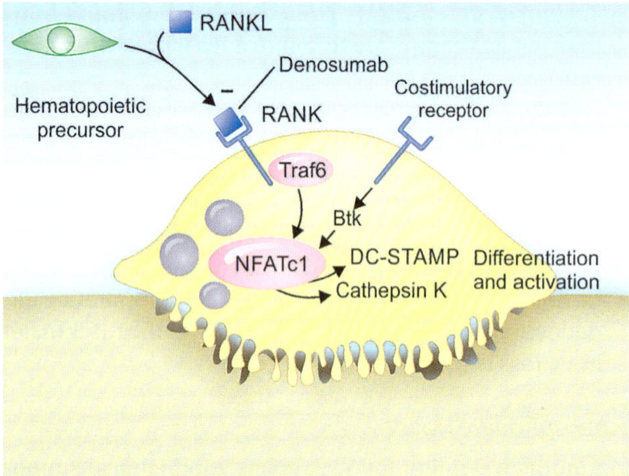

Fig. 26: RANKL inhibitor prevents stimulation and proliferation of osteoclasts, inhibiting bone resorption.
(DC-STAMP: dendritic-cell-specific transmembrane protein; NFATc1: nuclear factor of activated T-cells, cytoplasmic 1; RANKL: receptor activator of nuclear factor kappa-B ligand)

bone mass and strength in both cortical and trabecular bone primarily by antiresorptive action and minimal, if any anabolic effect (it is hence not an anabolic agent). Suppression of bone resorption is seen within first 24 hours. In freedom trial, development of new morphometric vertebral fractures was chosen as the primary endpoint whereby denosumab showed significant reduction in the new vertebral fractures at 3 years (7.2 vs. 2.3%, –68%, $p < 0.0001$). The incidence of hip and nonvertebral fractures was chosen as secondary endpoints. It was demonstrated in the freedom trial that denosumab additionally reduced the nonvertebral fractures also at 3 years (1.2 vs. 0.7%, –40%, $p = 0.04$, and 8.0% vs. 6.5%, –20%, $p = 0.01$, respectively), so in essence there was an overall reduction in the fracture risk. The efficacy of denosumab to reduce fracture risk has been shown to be consistent across patients with varying degrees and types of osteoporosis and fracture risk. It is currently indicated to treat osteoporosis in men and postmenopausal women at high risk of fracture, have multiple risk factors for fracture, are intolerant to other therapies, or in whom previous osteoporosis therapies have failed. Denosumab in a dose of 60 mg administered subcutaneously every 6 months also increases bone mass in men at high risk for fracture who are receiving androgen deprivation therapy for nonmetastatic prostate cancer or in females receiving adjuvant aromatase inhibitor therapy for breast cancer. Patients suffering from autoimmune and inflammatory arthropathy develop osteoporosis due to overactivity of RANKL where denosumab may act as first-line therapy. As denosumab is not significantly metabolized or excreted by kidneys it may be a very good alternative in patients with renal failure where other therapies are either contraindicated or need titration/monitoring. Denosumab is generally well tolerated, but some notable adverse events are:

- Osteonecrosis of the jaw
- Risk of hypocalcemia
- Potentially increased risk of severe infections
- Atypical fractures and delayed fracture healing
- Pancreatitis
- Neoplasia of the breast, reproductive system, and gastrointestinal system are seen more frequently with denosumab treatment although the causal relationship has not been established.

ALX-0141 is another RANKL inhibitor, currently under clinical development.

ANABOLIC AGENTS

This is a new approach altogether as none of the antiresorptive agents activate new bone formation. This is due to the tight coupling of osteoblastic and osteoclastic activity, and hence bone formation will be inhibited, if osteoclast is inhibited. The anabolic agents try to improve the bone formation primarily rather than inhibiting bone resorption.

Parathyroid Hormone

When first introduced (November 2002, FDA approval) the therapy with PTH was hyped as a "cure for osteoporosis" that is only partially true. Currently, the recombinant human full length PTH, rhPTH (1–84), its N-terminal segment rhPTH (1–34), and PTH-related protein (PTHrp) analogs are all available (in different parts of world) that exert their anabolic effect (*osteoanabolic therapy*) on bone by binding to the PTH receptor on osteoblasts. Only "teriparatide"—the N-terminal segment rhPTH (1–34) is, however, approved for treatment of osteoporosis by FDA in men and postmenopausal women at high risk of fracture or those intolerant to other osteoporotic treatments or who fail to improve upon bone mass on previous therapy. The other indication is treatment of steroid-induced osteoporosis (approved in 2009). The "high risk" has been defined by the Hodsman et al. proposed criteria as follows:

- Pre-existing osteoporotic fractures
- Very low bone density (T-score < –3.5)
- Above and/or an unsatisfactory response to antiresorptive therapy

Continuous infusions of PTH and analogs cause persistent elevation of the serum PTH concentration and result in bone resorption, the usual effect of PTH. However, interestingly and contrary to the conventional thinking, exogenously administered intermittent PTH is a potent anabolic agent that stimulates skeletal remodeling and improves BMD. RhPTH (1–34) has significant effect on reducing the risk of vertebral fractures and nonvertebral fractures in postmenopausal women. The increase in BMD is, however, noted most prominently at vertebral sites with little benefit for hip region when given in a dose of 20 µg/day (weekly doses of 56.5 µg have also shown similar benefits). Teriparatide has been shown to reduce the spine fusion failure and pedicle pull-out rates by 50%. There is an initial reduction in cortical bone density possibly due to initial increase in intracortical porosity. The appositional new bone formation is also stimulated that increases the cross-sectional area of bone and cortical bone strength. Due to its unique efficacy profile, some people even recommend the use of teriparatide as first-line treatment for postmenopausal women and for men with severe osteoporosis.

The effect of teriparatide is mediated in a multifactorial manner possibly involving Wnt pathway (stimulating Wnt10b and inhibiting sclerostin), IGF-1 mediated anabolic effect, etc.

The therapeutic effect is also site-specific. While good gains in BMD and trabecular bone volume are seen at vertebral bones (spine) and ilium with initiation of therapy, the effect is subdued at hip region in the first year showing benefits only after 18–24 months. At distal radius and tibia there is, in fact, a reduction in DXA-derived areal BMD. At the distal radius and tibia, teriparatide increases trabecular volumetric BMD but progressively decreases cortical volumetric BMD and increases cortical porosity for up to 24-month, however, the estimated bone strength is improved. Currently, the treatment with teriparatide is recommended for a maximum of 2 years whereby the gains in bone mass are quite secure and significant and also there are concerns of possible development of osteosarcoma with prolonged therapy. The biggest concern is "osteoblast fatigue" seen with the use of rhPTH. The teriparatide-induced stimulation of bone formation peaks after 6–12 months of therapy, after which serum markers of both osteoblast and osteoclast activity slowly revert toward baseline levels. The reduced effect is seen even after introducing drug holiday of 1 year in patients. So, the building consensus is giving treatment with teriparatide for "therapeutic window" of 1 year (no longer duration like 2 years) and after stopping treatment the gains in bone mass may be additionally secured by bisphosphonate therapy.

Availability of only injectable preparation is a potential limitation to the acceptability and compliance with teriparatide. Nasal spray and teriparatide-coated microneedle patch system of rhPTH (1–34), have been found to be effective in improving bone mass. Ostabolin-C is a cyclicized parathyroid hormone analog that only stimulates the adenylyl cyclase avoiding the phospholipase C pathway thus reducing the adverse effects (available in some countries like Canada). Combination therapy of rhPTH with other agents for osteoporosis management has been discussed in detail above under bisphosphonates. There is a suggestion for the use of this drug in fracture repair and also promotion of union in atypical femoral fractures for which it may get clinical use approval in future.

Full length 1–84 PTH is available in Europe and there is currently no reason to prefer over its shorter analog. In an Austrian study, the use of rhPTH (1–84) showed increased rate of union and the speed of fracture repair when used in osteoporosis. In USA, the 1–84 PTH is approved only for use in hypoparathyroidsm.

Parathyroid hormone-related protein (PTHrP) is an equipotent protein analog to 1–84 PTH which has physiological functions, such as stimulation of bone resorption, control of calcium metabolism in lactating women, and allowing tooth eruption. Abaloparatide is a synthetic peptide analog of PTH-related protein (rhPTHrP 1–34) that binds to the PTH/PTHrP receptor with a greater selectivity. It uses similar receptors and intracellular signaling pathways as that of PTH. Interestingly, however, while the continuous administration of PTH (or even rhPTH) leads to bone resorption (a net loss of bone mass, discussed above), the continuous administration of PTHrP (abaloparatide) preferentially stimulates bone formation suggesting that PTHrP could most likely be the endogenous skeletal ligand for the PTH or PTHrP receptor acting as bone anabolic agent. This apparently contradictory finding could be possibly explained by existence of two different activated states of PTH receptor one of which involves continuous cyclic adenosine monophosphate (cAMP) secretion following PTH binding and the other has burst cAMP secretion after PTHrP binding. This latter receptor type mimics the effects of intermittently administered PTH possibly explaining anabolic action. The interest in use of PTHrP for use in osteoporosis has risen due to this pure anabolic effect (only osteoblastic activity) that is different from the mixed anabolic and catabolic effect (combined osteoblastic and osteoclastic activity) of PTH. This anabolic effect is maintained even at very high dose (750 μg/day), and surprisingly at such doses it also stimulates 1,25-dihydroxyvitamin D production. Abaloparatide is available as subcutaneous injectable preparation (80 μg/day) that has shown significant reduction of new vertebral and even nonvertebral fractures (hip and distal radius unlike teriparatide) in postmenopausal women in ACTIVE (the Atrial fibrillation Clopidogrel Trial with Irbesartan for prevention of Vascular Events) trial. The improvement in BMD at vertebral sites has been shown to be better compared to teriparatide and this effect is also observed at nonvertebral sites such as hip and distal radius.

Adverse effects of teriparatide:

- Tiredness and depression
- Palpitation, nausea, vomiting and constipation or diarrhea
- Leg cramps
- Joint pains
- Osteosarcoma [therapy >2 years in rats only, (dose-dependent osteosclerosis, extramedullary hematopoiesis, and increased risk of osteosarcoma when administered at doses greater than the human equivalent starting at a young age) not demonstrated in monkeys or humans (three cases reported, but not linked definitively)]. The "black-box" warning is extended to ostabolin-C and abaloparatide.
- Hypercalcemia

Contraindications to use of rhPTH include:

- Children with open epiphysis
- Patients with history of prior radiation exposure
- Unexplained elevations of serum ALP
- Paget's disease of bone
- Pre-existing hypercalcemia or raised endogenous PTH
- Severe renal impairment
- Pregnancy and breastfeeding mothers
- Presence of bone metastasis or bone tumors

Tibolone

Tibolone is a synthetic steroid with estrogenic, androgenic, and progestin properties. There are reported increases in lumbar BMD in early postmenopausal women. The use is not very common due to other available effective drugs.

Strontium Ranelate

Strontium is a divalent alkaline element that is combined with (combination to malonate is under study) ranelic acid to make it more palatable. The compound contains two atoms of nonradioactive strontium. Strontium usually acts as calcium agonist in most of physiologic process. It is absorbed from the

GIT by either passive diffusion or carrier- mediated absorption. The carrier system is common to calcium and strontium, but has greater affinity for former. After absorption, it is distributed into plasma extracellular fluid, soft tissue and superficial zone of bone tissue, and bone itself. Within bone and calcified tissues it is adsorbed on surface of hydroxyapatite crystals and may participate in bone mineralization. Higher amounts of strontium are found in cancellous bone than in cortical bone. The actions of strontium are mainly mediated via bone selective calcium-sensing receptors (CaSR) on the osteoblasts to stimulate their activity through the phospholipase C-dependent phosphatidylinositol (4,5)-bisphosphate-diacylglycerol-inositol triphosphate pathway. The final effect is downregulation of the OPG/RANK/RANKL signaling; while at the same time upregulation of the Wnt/β-catenin canonical signaling (see below—antagonists of Wnt-inhibitors). It has both anabolic and modest antiresorptive affects, so it is actually a dual action compound rather than being only anabolic one. Strontium ranelate decreases osteoclast differentiation and activity **(Fig. 27)**. Strontium appears to result in uncoupling of bone remodeling (by competing with calcium at the calcium binding site) and increases bone formation by separate mechanism **(Fig. 27)**. It stimulates preosteoblast replication and increases matrix synthesis. In spinal osteoporosis therapeutic intervention (SOTI) study, the risk of new vertebral fractures was found to be halved in strontium group while some fracture risk reduction at hip is also identified. There is also a suggestion that strontium reduces the bone loss associated with estrogen deficiency. Salt-like taste and high doses are concerns for compliance, as are the most common side effects—nausea and diarrhea. Nausea and diarrhea disappear after third month of treatment. There is a rising concern for significantly higher and unacceptable thromboembolic events with the use of this drug. It should be avoided in individuals who have high tendency to develop venous thromboembolism, current or past history of ischemic/coronary heart disease, peripheral arterial disease and/or cerebrovascular disease, those with poorly controlled hypertension, and temporary or permanent immobilization. Some also doubt that higher weight of the cation might spuriously raise the BMD. The use of this drug is not very popular compared to other well-established drugs, it is currently not approved by the FDA, but available in India and European union.

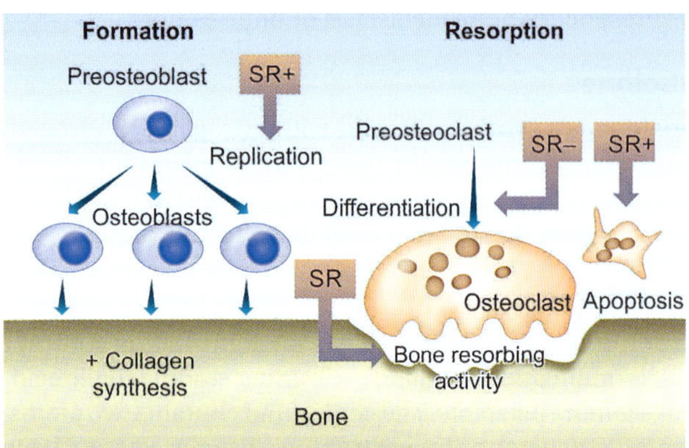

Fig. 27: Mechanism of action of strontium ranelate (SR) in osteoporosis.

Prostaglandins

They have a local paracrine action. They show the effect and are metabolized in the tissue, where they are synthesized (from arachidonic acid by cyclooxygenase pathway). Prostaglandin production is regulated by mechanical stress, cytokines, growth factor, and systemic hormones. They have both inhibitory and stimulatory effect on bone structure. Prostaglandin E2 (PGE2) stimulates bone resorption and formation through the cell surface E4 receptor. Systemic PGE2 administration stimulates proliferation of osteoblast precursors or differentiation of osteoprogenitor cells in bone marrow **(Fig. 28)**. Misoprostol, a methylene analog of prostaglandin E1 (PGE1) (used for treatment of gastric ulcer for its inhibitory effect on acid and pepsin secretion and cytoprotective effect) when administered to oophorectomized rats, significantly reduced oophorectomy- related bone loss at site of lumber spine. This is, hence, quite significantly useful in treatment of postmenopausal osteoporosis where HRT is not feasible or contraindicated. Misoprostol is administered in dose of 800 μg/day.

Statins

These 3-hydroxy-3-methylglutaryl-coenzyme A (HMG-CoA) reductase inhibitors are primarily used as effective cholesterol lowering agents for cardiovascular diseases. As a side effect, these drugs have bone anabolic effects as shown in several observational studies. Osseous effects are possibly mediated by suppressing the formation of the mevalonate.

This compound is an important precursor for osteoclastic activity, and hence reduced substrate controls the bone resorption as seen with bisphosphonates. Additionally, the important anabolic effects are mediated by stimulation of

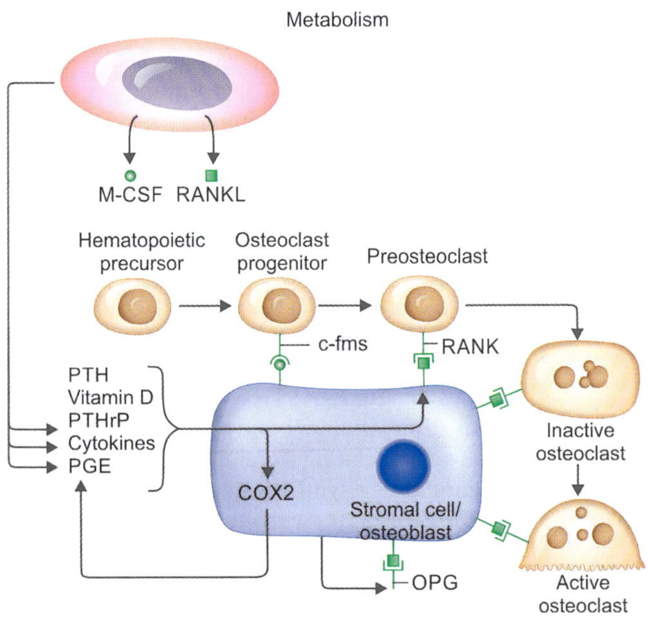

Fig. 28: Mechanism of action of prostaglandins in bone metabolism. [M-CSF: monocyte-colony stimulating factor; PTH: parathormone; OPG: osteoprotegerin; RANK: receptor activator of nuclear factor κ; RANKL: receptor activator of nuclear factor κ ligand; c-fms: colony-stimulating factor 1 receptor (also known as CSF1R); COX: cycloxygenase; PGE: prostaglandin-E]

VEGF expression from osteoblasts by hydrophobic statins such as simvastatin, atorvastatin, and cerivastatin. This effect is affected through reduced protein prenylation and the phosphatidylinositide-3 kinase pathway which also promotes osteoblastic differentiation. The effect of statins is an added advantage to patients' primarily on lipid lowering therapy, but mass usage for osteoporosis may not be cost effective.

Sesamin

Obtained from sesame seeds this is a lignin compound having direct effects on osteoblasts. It stimulates expression of essential genes and key enzymes of the bone mineralization. Also osteoblast differentiation is stimulated by activation of the p38 and ERK/MAPK (mitogen-activated protein kinase) pathway. The alternative pathway (indirect) could also be through osteoclast development, via the expression of OPG and RANKL in osteoblasts. Studies are needed to prove clinical efficacy, however.

Sodium Fluoride

Fluoride is an anabolic agent that stimulates new bone formation via a mitogenic effect on the osteoblast. It typically leads to a rapid increase in vertebral BMD. However, there is usually a BMD loss in peripheral bones. The increased BMD does not translate into reduced fracture risk and in fact a heightened risk of both vertebral and nonvertebral fractures is observed. There is increased incidence of stress fractures of weight-bearing bones, lower extremity pain syndrome, osteomalacia, arthralgia and arthritis, and an increased risk of femoral neck fractures. The routine use of fluoride is not recommended. A different formulation of fluoride, the monofluorophosphate, has been suggested which when administered in lower doses produce lesser GI side effects.

Androgens

Synthetic androgens, such as nandrolone and stanozol, have been tried; however, virilizing side effects in females, lowering of HDL, hepatotoxicity, and the need for parenteral administration limit their utility.

Growth Factors

Growth hormone modulates longitudinal bone growth and when studied in vitro and in vivo it has been found to regulate both bone formation and bone resorption. Administration of biosynthetic growth hormone cyclically with or without calcitonin has been found to significantly increase central BMD, especially in insulin-like growth factor-1 (IGF-1) deficient patients **(Fig. 29)**. Combination therapy of biosynthetic growth hormone with estrogen, calcium, and vitamin D also improves BMD in postmenopausal women. Growth hormone increases bone formation by:

- Direct interaction with GHRs on osteoblasts [IGF-BP5 (binding protein-5) potentiates the effect of IGF on osteoblasts]
- Induction of endocrine and autocrine or paracrine IGF-1.

Recombinant human growth hormone (rhGH) has effects on bone mineral metabolism in postmenopausal females.

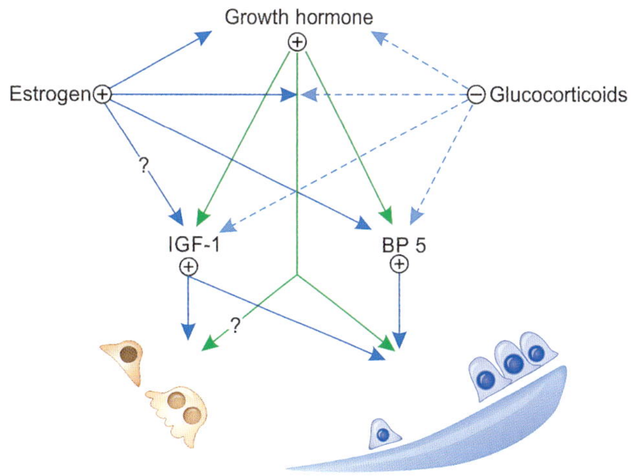

Fig. 29: Effect of growth hormone on bone metabolism and IGF-1 as intermediary. The left part of figure shows osteoclast bone resorption while the right part shows bone formation by osteoblasts.
(BP: binding protein; IGF: insulin-like growth factor)

Growth hormone, however, also results in increased bone resorption, but over a period of time bone mineralization is predominant. It is speculated that the predominant effects of growth hormone are mediated through modulation of IGF-1.

Bone is the second richest source of IGF-1 in the body. IGF-1 may have more rigorous effect in men with idiopathic osteoporosis, however, there is relatively high incidence of unacceptable experiences, like gynecomastia and edema. There is also a theoretical concern of potentiation of prostate and breast cancer with its use. Despite these concerns, it has been found that low levels of IGF-1 may result in greater risk of hip and spine fractures. The beneficial effects on bone metabolism may outweigh the side effects (especially, when given in low doses) and is better than growth hormone in the following ways:

- More direct stimulation of bone formation
- Bypass of skeletal growth hormone resistance that can be present
- A reduction in growth hormone induced side effects, such as carpal tunnel and diabetes mellitus

Low doses of rhIGF-1 may directly increase osteoblastic function with only a minimal increase in bone resorption. Low levels of IGF-1 may identify at risk patients for osteoporosis (discussed above).

Bortezomib

This targets osteoblast proteasome. Proteasome inhibitor bortezomib (Bzb) is anabolic to skeleton in patients with multiple myeloma. The mechanism is, however, unclear. Bzb with lenalidomide or thalidomide has been proposed to increase bone formation by stimulating osteoblast activity and inhibiting osteoclastic bone destruction **(Fig. 30)**.

Oxytocin

It increases osteoblastic bone formation. The effect is prominent during pregnancy and lactation where they not only enhance bone resorption by increasing the number of

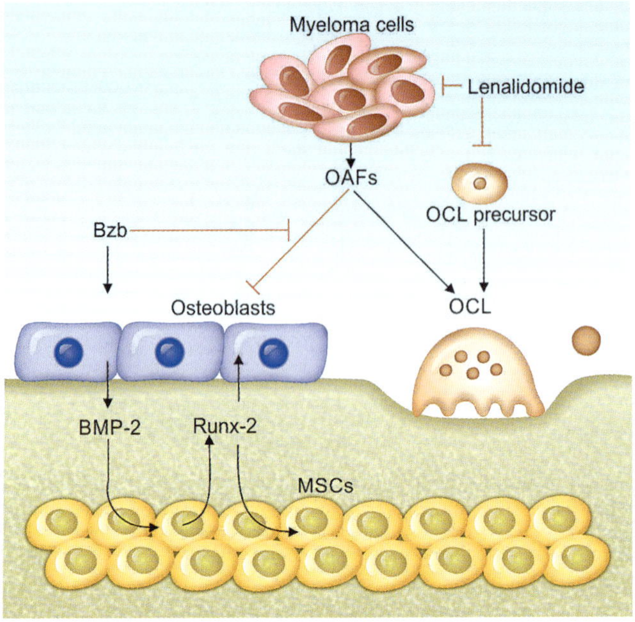

Fig. 30: Effect of bortezomib in patients with multiple myeloma. (BMP: bone morphogenetic protein; MSCs: mesenchymal stem cells; OAF: osteoclast activating factor; OCL: osteoclast)

osteoclasts to make maternal calcium (shunted to the fetus or infant), but also prevent unrestricted bone removal by inhibiting the activity of mature osteoclasts. Their anabolic action may have potential role in human osteoporosis.

Lithium

Therapy with lithium carbonate may improve BMD and bone mass. It has been found that in patients treated with lithium the serum total ALP, serum osteocalcin, and serum CTX were lower representing a reduced bone turnover. There is higher bone density reported at spine, femoral neck, and trochanter in these patients.

Calcilytics

Calcilytics (CaR antagonists) are unique agents that modulate PTH secretion by antagonizing the calcium receptor (CaR, a seven-pass transmembrane G-protein coupled molecule) found on parathyroid cells and shifting the set point down (thus enhancing endogenous PTH secretion at even normal or supernormal calcium concentrations). They work by allosteric modulation of the CaR where a conformational change is induced in the target by related (but not original) molecule that attaches mostly to another site than the original modulator. There are two classes of molecules— one that may mimic the function of calcium on CaR thus serving as calcimimetics like cinacalcet. This mechanism and associated drug will not be useful in osteoporosis. The other molecules that are negative allosteric modulators of CaR—the *calcilytics* (parathyroid selective short-acting calcium-sensing receptor antagonists) will cause release of endogenous PTH and possibly work like teriparatide or rhPTHrP (abaloparatide). These act like osteoanabolic agents. Though available for over 10 years these are still under development. The most focused compounds are oral calcilytics, such as JTT-305/MK-5442 and SB-423557 (amino-alcohol calcilytic Ronacaleret) that have been shown to stimulate endogenous transient PTH secretion, and hence bone formation. The effect of reducing bone loss was also seen in ovariectomized rats indicating that this is estrogen independent. These may represent future therapeutics for osteoporosis. As calcilytics increase secretion and release of PTH, their effect should be temporary and pulsed (like injectable teriparatide) else osteoclastic activation would predominate. They also should have a short half-life so that the parathyroid gland is not exhausted or hyperplasia is induced causing catabolic state. However, the development of MK-5442 was halted in 2011 for unreported reasons in phase III trials. Ronacaleret (SB-423557) has shown promising results in animal trials (rats) by increasing cortical and trabecular bone formation. It has a mean half-life of 4–5 hours with postdose peak increase in PTH by 300–900% in a dose-dependent manner. The phase-II trials of this drug were also discontinued due to lack of any efficacy in postmenopausal females. The concept is logical and is likely to pave way for future research and drug development.

Antagonists of Wnt-inhibitors (Inhibitors of Endogenous Inhibitors–Antisclerostin and Antidickkopf-1 Antibodies)

The Wnt proteins comprise a large family of extracellular cysteine-rich glycoproteins involved in a myriad of unrelated cellular differentiation and proliferation processes. The Wnt signaling pathway has three components, the Wnt/β-catenin or canonical pathway, the Wnt/Ca^{2}+ pathway, and the planar polarity cell pathway of which the first one is specific to bone. The canonical pathway **(Fig. 31)** is strongly osteoblastogenic and reduces the osteoclast activation and activity and regulation of embryogenic remodeling. The binding of Wnt proteins to the LRP5/6-frizzled coreceptor on osteoblast cell membrane causes stabilization of intracellular β-catenin. This, in a way, regulates gene transcription and promotes bone formation by osteoblasts. It is also responsible for reduced adipocytogenesis and redirecting the mesenchymal cells to osteocyte lineage rather than becoming adipocytes. Beta-catenin thus appears to be a desirable intracellular protein for stimulation of bone formation but is very tightly regulated. It is constantly inactivated by glycogen synthase kinase 3 (GSK-3) by phosphorylation if found in a free state (this is actually needed else unregulated activation of transcription by β-catenin would cause excess bone formation as occurs in sclerosteosis or van Buchem disease). The phosphorylated β-catenin is further degraded by ubiquitin/proteosome pathway. This canonical pathway mediated by Wnt liganding to its frizzled receptor involves recruitment of axins to the membrane away from cytoplasm causing inactivation of GSK-3 (axins are essential for its activation) and hence degradation of β-catenin is inhibited that then translocates to nucleus producing desirable anabolic effects.

Sclerostin (encoded by *SOST* gene) and Dkk1 are endogenous inhibitors of the above-mentioned canonical (β-catenin-dependent) Wnt/β-catenin pathway which is found only in bone. These inhibitors prevent exposure of

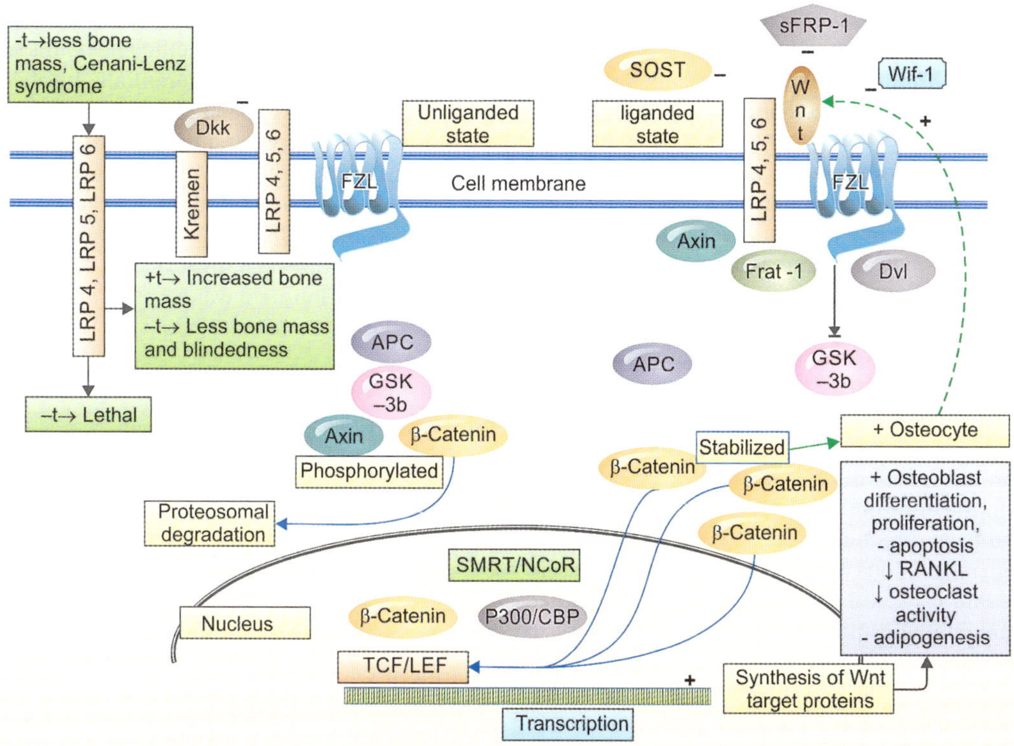

Fig. 31: The Wnt canonical signaling pathway—(right hand side, liganded state) when Wnt (name derives from wingless drosophila and int-1 mouse) bind to Frizzled protein (FZL) and LRP5/6 (LDL receptor-related protein) in a ternary complex at the cell surface, GSK-3b (glycogen synthase kinase 3b) is inhibited and β-catenin is stabilized. This inhibition is affected by Frat (mammalian homolog of GSK3b) and GBP (GSK binding protein) when Dvl (Disheveled) receive signal from Fzl/LRP complex. β-catenin then accumulates in the nucleus and activates lymphoid enhancer factor (LEF)/T-cell factor (TCF)-mediated gene transcription of Runx-2 and cbfa-1 responsible for further effects on osteoblasts (+) and (-) RANKL. In the absence of Wnts (left hand side), β-catenin is phosphorylated by mainly glycogen synthase kinase 3b (GSK-3b), leading to proteosomal degradation. This phosphorylation and degradation is affected through Axin which serves as a scaffolding protein to assemble APC (adenomatous polyposis coli) and Casein kinase (not shown) required to phosphorylate β-catenin. When Wnt binds to LRP the axins are recruited to membrane disturbing the complex formation and preventing the phosphorylation. Inhibitors of Wnt signaling are responsible for reduced bone formation. The inhibitors include Sclerostin/wise (encoded by SOST, sclerosteosis gene responsible for sclerosteosis and van Buchem disease). Sclerostin is synthesized by osteocytes. It inhibits BMP-stimulated bone formation in a pathway different from BMP antagonists. Mechanical stimulation and PTH treatment reduces sclerostin secretion. Mutation in sclerostin or inhibition of this protein leads to release of inhibition of Wnt pathway and increased osteogenesis. The Dkk (Dickpofs)/Kremen are secreted glycoprotein developmental regulators. The Dkk forms a complex with Kremen (a transmembrane protein) that binds to and internalizes LRP, removing it from cell surface. Both Dkk1 and -2 have high affinity for Kremen but complete absence of Dkk2 (or its inhibition) results in osteopenia and increased unmineralized osteoid surprisingly suggesting that it is required for final mineralization and may not be a true inhibitor of the pathway only. Secreted frizzled-related proteins (sFRPs) are expressed by osteoblasts. They are capable of binding Wnt and preventing it from binding to the LRP5/6-frizzled receptor. They also have effect similar to OPG that prevent the binding of RANKL and regulate osteoclasts. Wnt inhibitory factor-1 (WIF-1) is a secreted protein that binds to Wnt proteins and inhibits their activities.

the osteoblast precursors to a Wnt signal. In the absence of this signal or stimulation, osteoblast differentiation and recruitment are stopped. Inhibiting these endogenous inhibitors by antibodies against sclerostin or Dkk1 would, hence, prevent this inhibition to bone formation pathway and should be trophic to osteoblasts and anabolic to bone. Blosozumab and romosozumab are two such fully human antisclerostin antibodies are under study. The subcutaneous administration of a single dose of romosozumab (high-affinity IgG2 human recombinant sclerostin monoclonal antibody) has shown dose-related improvement in bone formation markers and decrease in serum C-telopeptide, CTx a bone resorption marker. This suggests an anabolic effect on bone and potential therapeutic agent. These biochemical changes were supplemented by BMD increases at the lumbar spine and hip within 3 months after the single dose. A dose-finding randomized placebo-, teriparatide- and alendronate-controlled 12-month phase II study in postmenopausal women with low BMD has recently completed, and "Romosozumab" has been found to be as effective as teriparatide and alendronate. Nonspecific hepatitis and neutralizing antibodies to the agent have been reported, but in general it is well tolerated. The most notable effect is that this bone formation is not related to amount of bone resorption or its influence. The development of sclerostin antibodies, hence, unfolds the perspective of uncoupling bone formation and resorption and of restoring bone microarchitecture. This would prove to be a unique method in the future management of osteoporosis where influence of related factors is minimal. The concern is, however, that of neoplasia, the Wnt signaling pathway has been associated with many forms of cancer, such as gastric, kidney, liver, lung, ovarian, and bone cancer itself. Sclerostin inhibition may increase susceptibility to osteosarcoma as also Wnt inhibiting factor-1 has been identified as tumor suppressor gene in human osteosarcoma. This theoretical concern needs to be fully analyzed before mass usage of the sclerostin antibody.

Serum Dkk1 concentrations are significantly higher in patients with low BMD and in women with postmenopausal osteoporosis and also it has broad expression in multiple myeloma and other osteolytic malignant tumors. Considering with its functional roles as an osteoblast formation inhibitor and a potential myeloma growth enhancer, DKK-1 might become an ideal and universal target for immunotherapy. The concept is also interesting in light of the recent finding that waning effect of teriparatide treatment on bone turnover has been shown to be associated with an increase in serum Dkk1. The fully human anti-DKK-1 mAb (BHQ880) has demonstrated improvement in the bone parameters of murine models and also appears to have direct effects on the MM cell growth, possibly through interactions with the bone marrow stem cells and the interleukin-6-related pathways. Both romosozumab and BHQ880 are anabolic and antiresorptive in mechanism for controlling osteoporosis.

"Another interesting though unrelated finding is that romosozumab could enhance the fracture repair process. In monkeys, more bone and less cartilage have been observed in osteotomy models on treatment with romosozumab. Wnt/β-catenin pathway is well known for fracture healing process where it enhances endochondral ossification.

Romosozumab seems to enhance the same through improvement in fracture callus. In animal studies, it also improves intramembranous bone formation. Thus, romosozumab may have future role in treatment of nonunions or delayed unions."

Cathepsin K Inhibitors

Odanacatib is a highly selective orally bioactive cathepsin K inhibitor reversibly binding to cathepsin K. Cathepsin K is the primary osteoclast produced protease that is involved in the degradation of *COL1A1* during bone resorption (congenital absence of this enzyme produces pycnodysostosis—an autosomal recessive disorder with increased bone mass). Odanacatib is a powerful, reversible, and neutral (unlike basic inhibitors) nonpeptidic biaryl inhibitor of cathepsin K that inactivates the proteolytic activity. This neutral inhibition prevents its accumulation in acidic lysosomes, and hence avoiding nontargeted inhibition of cathepsin K. The efficacy of odanacatib has been proven in clinical trials that reported 50% lower urine N-terminal telopeptide (NTx) resorption marker compared with placebo at doses of 50 mg once weekly, whereas the formation markers were increased by 18% at 3 years. The effect is, however, reversible with return on increased bone turnover at 1–2 years after stopping therapy. The increases in spine and hip BMD with odanacatib have been comparable to those observed with zoledronate or denosumab. There is a decoupling between bone formation and resorption possibly due to suppression of osteoclast function and viability resulting from suppression of cathepsin K without altering bone formation. Unlike the generalized suppression of bone resorption seen with bisphosphonates, odanacatib displays site-specific effects on trabecular and cortical bone formation preferentially improving the more deranged form. ONO-5334 is a new cathepsin K inhibitor with little or no suppression on bone formation markers while reduction in the bone resorption markers. There are no clinically relevant safety concerns. With a significant increase in BMD ONO-5334 is a new potential agent for treating osteoporosis. Balicatib (less selective cathepsin K inhibitors) development was stopped due to the appearance of scleroderma-like skin lesions.

Src–Kinase Inhibitors

Src-kinase is a nonreceptor tyrosine kinase enzyme of the Src family of protein kinases. It is essential for osteoclastic bone resorption activity, activation, motility, and survival. Saracatinib (AZD0530) is a novel orally available competitive inhibitor of the enzyme Src-kinase and Abl-kinase family, implied in cell proliferation, differentiation, and response to oxidative stress. Drug-specific randomized, double-blind, placebo-controlled, multiple ascending—dose phase I trial treatment with saracatinib have shown that it inhibited osteoclast-mediated bone resorption, thus, saracatinib could be a good antiresorptive agent.

FUTURE APPROACHES

Soluble activin receptors are being studied on the premises that mutations in *ACVR1* gene (encoding activin receptor type A (*ACVR1*) or activin receptor-like kinase 2 causes fibrodysplasia ossificans progressiva where ectopic bone formation occurs in muscles. *ACVR1* is a key receptor for BMP and mutations in it produce an active receptor that activates intracellular BMP signaling. It would appear that activin promotes bone formation as was previously reported also but investigations deciphered controversial role and more prominently a negative role for activin in osteogenesis especially that of activin A. The mechanism by which activin acts is complex and involves formation of heterotetrameric complexes by sequentially binding of type II and then type I receptors followed by downstream activation of smads and cellular effects of transcription by binding of these to promoter region. Activin A promotes RANKL-mediated osteoclastogenesis while inhibin, follistatin, BAMBI, Cripto, etc., antagonize the effects of activin. Strategically, using soluble activin receptors to bind activin could inactivate activin while balance would then shift to endogenous antagonists of activin. Chimeric antibodies against activin have been produced by fusing extracellular domain of the human activin receptor type IIA and of the Fc fragment of human IgG, injection of single dose of which has been found to improve bone strength and architecture and diminish bone resorption. This could have a dual antiresorptive and anabolic action.

Glucagon-like peptide-2 (GLP-2) has been shown to alter the bone resorption circadian rhythm. Bone resorption occurs with overnight fasting which is seen to be inhibited by GLP-2 in postmenopausal women by reduction in nocturnal CTx concentrations (marker of bone resorption). Though one might ask that this reduced bone resorption would affect bone formation due to resorption-formation coupling in bone remodeling, such an effect was not observed with therapy as the osteocalcin levels (marker of bone formation) remained steady. The effects translated into higher hip bone density. Larger trials are awaited.

MicroRNAs (miRNA)—regulate a number of bone formative pathways by double inhibition. These regulate the BMP, TGF-β, and Wnt/β-catenin signaling pathways of osteoblast formation and differentiation by suppressing the inhibitory signaling mechanisms. The miR-218 is upregulated during osteoblastogenesis, while miR-148a is upregulated during osteoclastogenesis. A lot of osteogenic mi-RNAs are found to be downregulated during pathological conditions and abnormal osteoblast differentiation while others get upregulated. Defining and identifying the specific miRNA may help to synthesize the strategies for future diagnostic and treatment methods. Free circulating miRNA, such as miR-21, miR-23a, miR-24, miR-25, miR-100, and miR-125b have been found to be significantly elevated in the serum of osteoporotic patients and can serve as biomarkers for development of osteoporosis. Circulating monocytes develop into osteoclasts; higher levels of miR-133a and miR-382 have been found in these cells from postmenopausal osteoporosis, especially the former and have been implicated for use as diagnostic assay [real-time reverse transcription polymerase chain reaction (qRT-PCR)]. Inhibition of these and stimulation of "osteosynthetic" miRNAs may help to treat the disease in future also.

SUMMARY OF CURRENT RECOMMENDATIONS TO PREVENT AND TREAT OSTEOPOROSIS (BASED ON NATIONAL OSTEOPOROSIS FOUNDATION)

Universal Recommendations

- Counsel on the risk of osteoporosis and related fractures
- Advise on diet that includes adequate amounts of total calcium intake (1,000 mg/day for men aged 50–70 years, 1,200 mg/day for women aged 51 years and older and men 71 years and older), incorporating dietary supplements, if diet is insufficient.
- Advise on vitamin D intake (800–1,000 IU/day), including supplements, if necessary for individuals aged 50 years and older
- Recommend regular weight-bearing and muscle-strengthening exercises to improve agility, strength, posture and balance, maintain or improve bone strength, and reduce risk of falls and fractures
- Assess risk factor for falls and offer appropriate modifications
- Advise on cessation of tobacco smoking and avoidance of excessive alcohol intake

Diagnostic Assessment

- Measure height annually, preferably with wall mounted stadiometer
- Bone mineral density testing as mentioned in **Box 8**.
- Vertebral imaging as mentioned in **Box 9**.

Monitoring Patients

- Perform BMD testing 1–2 years after initiating medical therapy for osteoporosis and every 2 years thereafter:
  - More frequent BMD testing may be warranted in certain clinical situations.
  - The interval between repeat BMD screenings may be longer for patients without major risk factors and who have an initial T-score in the normal or upper low bone mass range.
- Biochemical markers can be repeated to determine, if treatment is producing expected effect.

Pharmacological Treatment

- Initiate treatment in:
  - Those with hip or vertebral fractures
  - Those with T-scores ≤ –2.5 at the femoral neck, total hip, or lumbar spine by DEXA
  - Postmenopausal women and men aged 50 years and older with low bone mass (T-score between –1.0 and –2.5) at the femoral neck, total hip or lumbar vertebra by DEXA score and a 10-year hip fracture probability ≥3% or a 10-year major osteoporosis-related fracture probability ≥20% based on FRAX® tool.
- No pharmacological therapy should be considered indefinite in duration. After initiation of treatment a comprehensive risk assessment should be done. The decisions are individualized. I feel justifiably one should begin with and antiresorptive agent (bisphosphonate/denosumab) in cases with high bone-loss osteoporosis (type 1 osteoporosis) as occurs in postmenopausal osteoporosis in females and in postclimacteric osteoporosis in males (type 3), this is especially true when disease is detected early or when providing primary prevention. SERMs may be combined or preceded with this therapy as they have additive effect and in females would partially control the perimenopausal symptoms also. Patients who have severe osteoporosis or low bone turnover should be treated with anabolic agents of which teriparatide is the most studied. I feel alternating therapy with an anabolic agent and antiresorptive drug as 3 or 4 monthly cycles could provide better benefit than continuing one agent alone. Abaloparatide might get available in the recent future but its superiority needs to be established. Other agents are still under investigation and need to prove superior again to teriparatide before acceptance. When available and proven safe romosozumab would be indicated both for types 1 and 2 osteoporosis. In any case, the bone mass gained from anabolic agent therapy could be maintained through use of antiresorptives as follow-up therapy. There is still a subset of patients in whom treatment may ultimately fail (**Box 10**); no clear guidelines are available for these unfortunate patients but development in pharmacotherapy is expanding horizons of treating difficult cases also.

BOX 10: Osteoporosis treatment failure.

- Treatment of osteoporosis may be considered failing or failed under any of the following circumstances (and entails change of instituted therapy):
  - Two or more incident fragility fractures:
    - "Incident" implies "during the course of ongoing treatment"
    - Fractures of hand, skull, digits, feet and ankle are not fragility fractures
    - Falls are an important cause of fragility fractures and should be considered while analyzing response to treatment
  - One incident fracture and elevated CTX or P1NP at baseline with no significant reduction during treatment a significant decrease in BMD or both
  - No significant decrease in serum CTX or PiNP or significant decrease in BMD
    - A significant bone turnover marker is a response of 25% decline from baseline for antiresorptive treatments and increase for anabolic agents after 6 months of treatment
    - Decline in BMD should exceed the least significant count of the measuring device
- No evidence is available on the effectiveness of changing treatment when one has been deemed to have failed
- Almost no studies are available to address the issue
- The following general rules are proposed:
  - Weaker antiresorptive is replaced by a more effective/potent drug of the same class
  - Oral drug is changed to injectable drug
  - Strong antiresorptive drug is replaced by anabolic agent
  - Consider evidence for newer drugs and if conventional drugs are ineffective then drugs with different mechanism of action (newer drugs) may help

- In adults, age of 50 years and older after a fracture, institute appropriate risk assessment and treatment measures for osteoporosis as indicated.

ATYPICAL FORMS OF OSTEOPOROSIS

These are not grouped with classical osteoporosis discussed above which is a systemic disease. Most of these atypical forms are localized osteopenic conditions containing the term "osteoporosis" that is actually a misnomer. The following are some of them:

- *Immobilization and disuse related (atrophic osteoporosis):* The primary trophic component to bone remodeling and maintenance is stress. Prolonged immobilization takes away the muscular and pulling stress from the bone. This leads to bone resorption and attenuated bone formation so that there is a net loss of bone mass. This is commonly seen in polio limb, stroke, plaster disease, etc.
- *Sudeck's osteodystrophy (RSD/CRPS; discussed elsewhere)*
- *Regional migratory osteoporosis (RMO):* First described by Duncan et al. in 1969, it is a sequential polyarticular arthralgia of the weight-bearing joints associated with severe focal osteoporosis. RMO primarily affects the lower limbs in middle-aged men, but combined axial skeleton involvement has also been described. Regional osteoporosis is a distinctive feature of the disease. Its presentation and clinical course are identical to those of transient osteoporosis (TO). This clinical entity involves the lower extremities, especially the knee, ankle and foot, with lesser involvement of the hip joint, differentiating it from transient osteoporosis. Migration may occur in the same or a different joint and in an inconsistent time interval after the onset of the first symptoms. Usually, the joint nearest to the diseased one is the next to be affected. There is generalized tenderness with decreased range of motion due to severe pain. The overlying skin is characterized by inflammatory changes and muscle atrophy is frequently found which differentiates it from transient osteoporosis. "Transient regional osteoporosis" is a term used by some authors that combines both RMO and transient osteoporosis.
- *Malignancy-related osteoporosis:* This is mediated by endocrine and paracrine effects in the form of paraneoplastic syndrome. Dkk has been recognized as a common mediator to development of malignancy-related osteoporosis so antibodies against it would be the primary therapy once available. Currently, antiresorptives (like Zoledronic acid) are the agent of choice to prevent bone loss in malignancy.

Transient Osteoporosis (Transient Osteoporosis of Hip, Abortive Osteonecrosis of Hip and Bone Marrow Edema Syndrome)

Transient osteoporosis is an idiopathic condition mostly affecting young and middle-aged males and rarely females in third trimester or immediate postpartum period. Transient osteoporosis involves only the lower extremities, especially the hip joint and, less frequently, the knee, ankle, and foot. Transient osteoporosis of hip and other local osteoporosis syndromes are subtypes of transient osteoporosis. There is sudden onset, spontaneous pain of the affected joint which increases on weight-bearing and is associated with limping and disability. These symptoms gradually subside within 4–9 months. Recurrence may involve the same or adjacent joints. Physical examination is quite unremarkable and there is minimal restriction of range of movement and pain only at the extremes of range. The disjunction between physical examination and disability may help in diagnosing this self-limiting condition, avoiding unnecessary diagnostic and therapeutic measures.

Pathogenesis

The cause and pathogenesis remain obscure till date. Various inclusive theories are presented in literature, like Curtiss and Kincaid neurogenic compression theory and the venous obstruction and secondary localized hyperemia proposed by Rosen. Based on electromyographic findings, indicative of denervation during pain attacks of transient osteoporosis pathology of the proximal nerve roots has been proposed as a possible pathogenic mechanism of transient osteoporosis. This is possibly due to some undefined ischemia in the small vessels proximal to nerve roots and later restoration of blood flow may be responsible for the limited clinical course of transient osteoporosis, which usually lasts ≤9 months. Repetitive occurrence of such ischemic events elsewhere may explain the migratory character of RMO. Regional accelerated phenomenon (RAP) activation has been shown to be a recent possibility. RAP is a process by which the rate of bone modeling and remodeling in local areas may be accelerated up to 10 times the normal rate in response to noxious stimuli. The pathogenesis is unclear, however, it is thought that bone tissue microdamage and consequent microfracture may trigger RAP. Prolonged activation of bone foci where normal bone repair mechanisms are most active may result in transient osteoporosis. Supported by other investigators, these findings may support Frost's theories of prolonged active bone foci as a cause of transient osteoporosis explaining the influence of local and systemic factors in both causing and reversing osteoporosis. Bone marrow edema (BME), as shown on MRI and focal osteopenia, as shown on plain radiographs, are typical findings in the patient with transient osteoporosis.

Laboratory Tests

As such no utility for contextual diagnosis, blood tests are done to distinguish transient osteoporosis from aggressive clinical entities, such as metastatic or metabolic bone disease. Histologic examination of the lesion is necessary only when these other pathologies are suspected.

Conventional radiography: Radiographs may be normal in the early stages of transient osteoporosis. Usually at 3–6 weeks from the onset of symptoms there is periarticular osseous demineralization manifest as osteopenia. These findings may persist even weeks after the symptoms have resolved (sometimes up to 2 years). The joint space remains intact with preserved bony margins and there are no subchondral erosions. In advanced stages of transient osteoporosis, the femoral head may seem to completely disappear in osseous architecture—the "phantom appearance" of the femoral head. The trochanter, acetabulum, and iliac wings are rarely affected.

Bone scintigraphy: Though nonspecific, the findings of technetium Tc-99m methylene diphosphonate scintigraphy are useful in the early diagnosis of transient osteoporosis. Increased uptake (seen in all three phases) in the affected joint usually precedes radiologic features and can appear within a few days after the onset of symptoms. Bone scanning is sensitive, but not specific for detection of transient osteoporosis and can be used in symptomatic period when radiographs are normal. Scintigraphy, however, appears to be very useful both for monitoring the progression of the disease and therapeutic response. It is also helpful in differentiating transient osteoporosis from other conditions that are characterized by regional osteopenia. With subsidence of symptoms reduced activity on the perfusion and blood pool phases are noted that indicate resolution of disease. Increased activity in the delayed bone phase may still persist for many months due to repair activity. Differential diagnosis includes osteonecrosis of the femoral head, trauma or stress fracture of the femoral neck and infection (tubercular infection or osteomyelitis).

Computed tomography: Not a useful investigation for transient osteoporosis, however, findings such as spotty defects without any cortex involvement may be useful for distinguishing transient osteoporosis from other clinical entities.

Magnetic resonance imaging: It is the modality of choice. On MRI, BME is characterized by increased signal intensity on fat-suppressed T2-weighted and short tau inversion recovery images. These are complemented by low signal intensity on T1-weighted images. BME is, however, a nonspecific finding and enhancement of the BME area after intravenous administration of contrast agents is indicative of hypervascularity and increased permeability of the capillary bed. Vasodilation and increased permeability may constitute a result rather than a cause of the BME disclosed on MRI. Differentiation from osteonecrosis is important as early stages may mimic transient osteoporosis lesion. The lack of subchondral changes other than BME on both T2-weighted and contrast-enhanced T1-weighted highly suggests transient lesions. Subchondral area of low signal intensity at least 4 mm thickness on either T2-weighted or contrast-enhanced T1-weighted images suggests osteonecrosis. Presence of contour deformity and areas of subchondral low signal intensity further support osteonecrosis.

Treatment

Transient osteoporosis is a self-limiting disease and treatment is mainly supportive primarily aimed to reduce pain and protect the bone due to reduced mechanical strength. Protected weight-bearing, mild analgesics, and administration of nonsteroidal anti-inflammatory drugs are main therapeutic approaches. Glucocorticoids are not found to be effective for remineralization though they improve pain symptoms. Sympathetic blockade provided no improvement of results in the treatment of transient osteoporosis. Bisphosphonates (especially intravenous) may help in reducing pain and improving bone strength. Calcium and corrective doses of vitamin D should be started. Iloprost, a prostacyclin analog, has shown pain relief in patients with transient osteoporosis of hip and bone marrow edema syndrome by possibly dilating the vessels and reducing permeability.

DISEASES OF OSTEOCLASTIC DYSFUNCTION

PAGET'S DISEASE OF BONE

Paget's disease of bone (PDB) is one of the osteoclast cell disorders, the other common one being osteopetrosis. This section covers both these disorders. After osteoporosis, PDB is the second most common metabolic bone disorder. PDB is a chronic disorder characterized by focal or multifocal disorganized remodeling and bone structure due to osteoclast dysfunction. It was initially described as "osteitis deformans" by Sir James Paget in 1876, however, the term "osteodystrophica deformans" is now preferred. The disease has been reported world over but is common in Caucasians and those of British descent with a peak incidence in 5th decade of life. Males are slightly more commonly affected than females. The prevalence and severity of the disease appears to be reducing and it is encountered less frequently possibly due to environmental changes, such as different migratory patterns, improved diet, sedentary lifestyle, and decrease in the exposure to viral infections and zoonoses. PDB is most commonly discovered in the pelvis (58–80%), spine and skull (40%), femur (32%), and tibia (16–20%). Some cases may have single bone (monostotic disease) involvement but mostly in patients of several noncontiguous bones (polyostotic disease) have the disease. Being a disorder of osteoclasts, the hallmark feature of PDB is focal or multifocal increased bone density (radiographically) and core pathology is characterized by focal areas of increased and disorganized bone turnover (remodeling process), coupled with increased bone formation.

Etiology

The etiology of PDB is still unknown and currently it is considered as a complex, multifactorial disease combining genetic predisposition with environmental factors acting synergistically. Genetically, it is an autosomal dominant condition with variable penetration which appears more commonly in first-degree relatives of affected patients. As PDB is a focal disease with asymmetric distribution, it is suggested that somatic mutations at the early stage of the zygote could be responsible for the mosaicism detected in the patients. Osteoclast precursors could be sensitized by an unknown environmental factor (variably considered a paramyxovirus but it has never been isolated). The genetic conditioning later determines individual susceptibility to ultimately develop the disease. *SQSTM1* mutations are associated with susceptibility to develop PDB. Nearly 40% of the relatives of affected individuals with this mutation appear to be suffering from disease. A number of mutations in the gene *SQSTM1* at locus 5q35 have been related to PDB. Most of these variants affect the ubiquitin-associated (UBA) domain of the protein, which is involved in autophagy processes. SQSTM1 protein (also called p62) directs ubiquitinated molecules to degradation in autophagolysosomes. It interacts with autophagy protein LC3, located in the ruffle border of the osteoclasts. Mutations identified out of the UBA domain of *SQSTM1* also increase NF-κB signaling activating osteoclasts. Seven other mutations have been identified in PDB patients. Genome-wide association studies combined with functional analysis further identified Valosin-containing protein (VCP), *OPTN*, and *RIN3* as causal genes for Paget's disease. Similar to p62, VCP (also known as p97) also indirectly binds to cytoplasmic portion of RANK that regulates osteoclastic differentiation. *OPTN* gene acts as a negative regulator of osteoclast differentiation. The inhibitory effect is mediated by a CYLD-dependent pathway, which is important for the inhibition of NF-κB activation. *OPTN* also inhibits osteoclast differentiation by modulating INF-β signaling pathway. Thus, inactivation of *OPTN* or its mutation results in enhanced osteoclast differentiation and is associated with juvenile PDB. Mutations associated with *RIN3* are linked to GTPases, like Ras and Rab, important for osteoclast function.

Genetics of Paget's Disease of Bone Severity

A combination of risk alleles identified by genome-wide association studies led to the development of a score to predict disease severity, which could improve the management of the disease. In patients without *SQSTM1* mutations, a combination of risk GWAS alleles in the highest tertile was associated with a 27% increase in disease extent, defined by the number of affected bones, and 25% increase in disease severity score, which includes complications secondary to the disease. *SQSTM1* positive patients showed a highly significant increase in disease extent, severity, and number of previous treatments received.

Pagetic Sarcoma

Missense mutation in the *ZNF687* gene (p.P937R) is linked to appearance of giant cell tumor (GCT) in PDB. This mutation is a gain-of-function change, producing an accumulation of the protein in the nucleus and subsequent transcription of the pathway downstream.

Environmental Triggers

Measles virus is the strongest contender as inclusion bodies similar to measles virus nucleocapsid (MVN) protein have been found in cell nucleus. Some people suggest these MVN bodies could just be protein aggregates in the dysfunctional cells, however, recently MVN protein is associated with the upregulation of IL-6 and IGF-1 in osteoclasts from mouse models and PDB patients so still viral factor cannot be completely denied. PDB has also been linked weakly (and possibly not very scientifically) to other factors such as poor calcium and vitamin D intake, consumption of uncontrolled beef meat during childhood, consumption of not purified water, contact with dogs during early years, an excessive mechanical loading on the skeleton and exposure to some environmental toxics.

Pathology

The overall bone volume is markedly increased in PDB manifests due to increase in bone turnover. Osteoclasts are the primarily affected cells demonstrating an increase in number and size and containing more nuclei than normal osteoclasts. These metabolically active cells produce greater osteolysis in turn coupled with increased bone formation by osteoblasts, but in the haphazard process deviating from normal osseus anatomy and mechanobiological laws for bone formation thus, altering bone structure. The disease progresses in waves initiated by intense pathological osteoclastic activity that is quickly followed by activated osteoblasts to lay down new bone visualized as cement lines and the process gets repeated. Due to accelerated bone turnover, new collagen fibers are placed in a chaotic fashion, unlike the laminar distribution of the adult mature bone resulting in characteristic mosaic pattern of the pagetic bone, combining an abnormal woven bone, with some areas of lamellar bone, and numerous disorganized cement lines from previous osteolytic phases. There is increased number of trabeculae and osteoid volume thickness but without mineralization alterations. Increased plasticity of bone facilitates tendency to deform and propensity to fracture.

Clinical Features

Not uncommonly, the disease is incidentally discovered and has a long asymptomatic phase in up to 70% of patients throughout disease evolution. Those who have clinical symptoms present with bone pains, deformity, and complications such as pathological fractures, arthropathy, deafness, vision problems, cardiac, electrolyte and renal problems, etc. Pain is the most common symptom and can be primary or secondary. Primary pain due to PDB per se is dull and deep and mostly nocturnal. Secondary pain is more frequent and is predominantly related to complications such as fracture, neurological entrapment or joint involvement, and sarcomatous change in PDB. Long bones like femur bend as a result of the increased bone volume and malleability while skull shows enlargement and demonstrates facial deformities altering the physical appearance of patients at late age. Kyphosis of spine may be increased. The most common complications of PDB is arthropathy due to pathological alteration of the subchondral bone, microfracture accumulation, neurologic compression and dysfunction secondary to bone growth, vascular steal syndrome, and bone hypervascularization. The latter also manifests as increased focal heat in the superficial bones such as the tibia and high output congestive heart failure. Hypercalcemia and hypercalciuria occur in immobilized patients with formation of renal stones. Sensorineural hearing loss occurs due to compression of vestibulocochlear nerve in internal auditory canal and loss of bone mineral density of cochlear capsule. Conductive hearing loss is due to fixation of middle ear ossicles. Cranial nerve paresis may occur due to foraminal narrowing and basilar invagination may occur in advanced cases with hydrocephalus or brainstem compression.

Pagetic sarcoma is a dreaded and known complication where malignant bone neoplasm develops in the involved bone. Less than 1% of the patient will develop this complication but is devastating as it has poor prognosis. Osteosarcoma is the most common secondary malignancy followed by fibrosarcoma, giant cell tumor, and rarely chondrosarcoma. Pelvis, femur, and humerus are involved in descending order for sarcoma development. A 5-year survival for metastatic Paget's sarcoma is <10% despite prompt and radical measures such as wide surgical resection and chemotherapy. Eighty percent of patients diagnosed with GCT die in 10-year time.

Radiology

General radiological features seen in PDB include coarsened trabeculae with blastic appearance of bone, loss of corticomedullary differentiation, bowing of long bones, and complications of the disease such as fractures, arthritic changes, etc. Radiologically, three phases can be identified:

1. *Lytic phase:* This is marked by intense osteoclastic activity. The pagetic bone lesion could be identified in radiographs as a lytic lesion (osteolytic pagetic phase).
2. *Mixed phase:* Phase of excessively disorganized bone. There is resorption of the bone which is nearing its end along with compensatory bone formation which is gaining momentum. Radiographically, the lesions evolve into a mixture of osteosclerosis (woven bone) and hyperostosis (lamellar bone) due to new bone formation by osteoblasts and osteolysis (mixed phase). Histologically, this stage is identified by presence of cement lines.
3. *Sclerotic phase:* In the final stages, the osteoblastic bone formation predominates forming radiologically sclerotic bone. There is also a reduction in bone turnover and cells.

All three phases may also coexist in same bone instead of appearing sequentially. Different radiographic patterns at various bones that could be observed in each stage are presented in **Table 10**.

Diagnosis

As mentioned above the diagnosis of PDB is incidental in most cases. An elevated level of alkaline phosphatase is detected in the absence of liver disease suggesting elevated bone turnover. It can alternatively be also monitored by procollagen type 1 amino-terminal propeptide (P1NP) levels, considering ALP, bone-specific alkaline phosphatase (bone ALP), and C-terminal telopeptide (CTX) as good alternative markers for disease activity in untreated patients. Serum calcium levels are normal.

Plain radiography features are easily recognizable. The border between healthy and disease areas appears as a lytic image (blade of grass, or candle flame sign in the shaft of long bones). CT, MRI, and PET imaging may be useful to detect suspected sarcomatous degeneration. Tc-99 bone scan demonstrates increased uptake and is nonspecific but has high sensitivity to detect lesions, even at the very early

TABLE 10: The radiographic features of Paget's disease as specific to different phases of disease in various bones.

Phase	*Radiographic findings*
Osteolytic	• Osteoporosis circumscripta in skull (well-defined radiolucent regions of the skull on plain radiographs) • Track sign of femur (two parallel lines running along the long axis of bone—The "linea aspera-pilaster complex" running posteriorly along the bone is seen as radiodense lines) • Blade of grass or candle flame signs in long bones (lucent leading edge in long bone)
Mixed	• Mosaic bone pattern (jigsaw pattern of bone)—coarsened trabeculae and bony enlargement mixed with osteolytic zones • Cotton wool appearance of the skull (coarse fluffy sclerotic patches in lucent area of bone) • Tam O' Shanter sign—Diploic space widening (inner and outer calvaria tables) + platybasia + basilar invagination and appearance of skull falling over facial bones (also called falling hat sign) • Vertebral frame sign (picture frame vertebral body)—results from thickening of vertebral body cortex • Squaring of vertebrae • Coarse vertebral trabecular thickening • Ivory vertebrae (diffuse and homogeneous increase in opacity of a vertebral body) • Enlargement of the pubic rami and ischium
Sclerotic	• Frontal bone enlargement • Cortical thickening and sclerosis of the iliopectineal and ischiopubic lines • Acetabular protrusio • Lateral curvature of the femur • Anterior curvature of the tibia • Looser zones • Banana fracture in long bones (horizontal fracture in deformed bone commonly "femur")

stages of PDB. Lincoln sign (uptake of the radiotracer from one mandibular condyle to another mimicking a man with a black beard on the anterior view) and Mickey-mouse signs (increased radiotracer uptake on the bone scan in the spinous process and pedicles) have been characteristically described for bone scan features of PDB.

Bone biopsy is not typically required for diagnosis, but it may be useful for differentiating other suspected pathologies. Features suggesting Paget's are the presence of abnormal trabeculae, irregular cementation lines with a typical "mosaic" image, increase in vascularity, and increased number and size of osteoclasts.

Differential Diagnosis

- Enchondroma
- Bone island
- Bone infarct
- Metastatic bone disease
- Myeloma
- Lymphoma
- Nonossifying fibroma and fibrous dysplasia
- Eosinophilic granuloma
- Sessile osteochondroma

Treatment

The only absolute indication for treatment of uncomplicated PDB is pain in the affected bone. Bisphosphonates are effective in managing pain in PDB patients. Zoledronic acid is currently the first choice medication. Single 5 mg infusion of zoledronate has been shown to be better than 2 months of oral alendronate. Calcitonin is effective in reducing pain and expression of bone formation and resorption markers but is less effective than bisphosphonates so sparingly preferred. Denosumab also has mechanism similar to bisphosphonates and appears to be effective in treatment but not widely explored for this purpose. Teriparatide should not be used due to concerns of osteosarcoma. Disease progression is best monitored by procollagen type 1 N-terminal propeptide levels but if not available then alkaline phosphatase, bone specific alkaline phosphatase, or N-telopeptide can be used as alternatives. If disease is active, then treatment is continued.

Complications are managed on standard protocols and specific indications. Deformity correction for cosmetic reasons is not commonly performed. Osteosynthesis is, however, needed for Pagetic fractures of bone or prophylactic fixation is done for impending fractures. In latter cases, deformity correction through metaphyseal osteotomy or at CORA (center of rotation of angulation) may be simultaneously performed. Higher chances of nonunion are reported at osteotomy site and fracture healing often goes into delayed union so one must be careful in not disturbing the soft tissue envelop to minimize this complication. Spinal stenosis limiting function/neurology needs decompression. Arthroplasty is done for pagetic osteoarthritis. The degenerative joints in PDB are a challenge to reconstruct due primarily to excessive bleeding during surgery especially during total hip replacement. Total knee arthroplasty patients often have been reported to have suboptimal alignment. It is recommended to defer the surgical reconstruction till medical remission is obtained with bisphosphonates to reduce complications of joint reconstruction.

Treatment of asymptomatic PDB patients showing only biochemical activity is debatable. Current scientific evidence does not support preventive treatment of complications in such patients [Program of Resources, Information and Support for Mothers (PRISM) trial]. ZiPP (Zoledronate in the prevention of Paget's) study is underway for the same.

OSTEOPETROSIS

Synonyms: Marble bone disease, Albers-Schönberg disease (refers to an adult autosomal dominant type 2 milder form of disease), and stone bone.

Definition

Osteopetrosis is a group of heterogeneous inherited sclerosing bone disease characterized by generalized increase in the bone mass (osteosclerosis) primarily resulting from osteoclast dysfunction.

Classification and Types of Osteopetrosis

At least eight different types have been recognized based on various genetic mutations **(Table 11)** and clinical presentations. Important ones are mentioned below—

- Classical types:
  - Autosomal recessive (infantile and malignant)
  - Autosomal dominant (adult and benign) types I and II
  - Autosomal recessive intermediate form
- Variants:
  - Osteopetrosis associated with renal tubular acidosis and cerebral calcification (carbonic anhydrase II deficiency)

TABLE 11: The genetic defects identified in osteopetrosis.

Pattern of inheritance	*Gene target*	*Comments*
Autosomal dominant	*CLCN7*	Varies from asymptomatic to lethal
	LRP5	Mild disease
	PLEHKM1 missense mutation	Mild disease
Autosomal recessive	Carbonic anhydrase II	Loss of function mutation, disease with intermediate severity, brain calcifications seen
	TCIRG1	Various mutations seen, severe disease and replacement of marrow
	RANKL	Loss of function mutation, severe disease
	OSTM1	Loss of function mutation, severe disease with neural and ophthalmologic involvement
	PLEHKM1	Loss of function mutation, intermediate severity disease
	CLCN7	Missense mutation, severe disease with retinal and optic nerve involvement
X-linked	*NEMO*	Severe disease, immunodeficiency, lymphedema

- Osteopetrosis associated with neuronal storage disease
- Drug-induced osteopetrosis
- *Syndromic form:* Variable combination of osteopetrosis, lymphedema, anhidrotic ectodermal dysplasia and immunodeficiency syndrome.

Etiology and Pathophysiology

The disease basically results from modeling and remodeling defects arising out of osteoclast dysfunction. The osteoclasts fail to resorb bone due to defects at various levels resulting from genetic mutations affecting discrete gene products in different forms. For a single form different mutations may result in the phenotype so the disease is heterogeneous. The following are some important identified mutations:

- Adult type I osteopetrosis results from activating mutations of *LRP5* gene. This indicates that the form may not be true osteopetrosis as this mutation does not result in osteoclast dysfunction. The set point (threshold) for bone resorption and remodeling in response to mechanical loading is increased so that the process does not get initiated at physiological loading.
- Half of the cases of adult type II osteopetrosis (the form originally described by Albers-Schönberg in 1904) are attributed to mutations of *CLCN7,* the type 7 chloride channel. The chloride channel is responsible for acidification of extracellular resorption lacuna necessary for bone resorption.
- Some patients with malignant infantile osteopetrosis (autosomal recessive) have a mutation in the *TCIRG1* gene encoding the osteoclast-specific α3 subunit to which H^+ATPase of the vacuolar proton pump is anchored. Others have *CLCN7* and *OSTM1* mutations that together form a chloride channel or chloride/proton-exchanger. These are responsible for acidification of the milieu and bone resorption. In contrast, above few patients have been found to have mutations in *TNFSF11* gene encoding for the osteoclast differentiation factor RANKL, this results in decreased number of osteoclasts itself. Mutations in the RANK receptor also cause osteoclast poor osteopetrosis with additional immunological abnormalities.
- Intermediate form of autosomal recessive osteopetrosis may result from mutations in the *PLEKHM1* gene. A variant of autosomal recessive intermediate form result from mutation of carbonic anhydrase II gene (*Car2*). Carbonic anhydrase catalyzes the formation of carbonic acid that acidifies the lacunae.

The modeling defects are most pronounced in autosomal recessive form and the phenotype develops by second trimester itself. Modeling of bone is responsible for expansion of medullary canal, foramina, etc., during bone development, and hence, hematopoiesis and giving the typical shape to bone metaphysis. The bone marrow develops inside the intramedullary cavity. Defect in bone modeling produces loss in hematopoietic function and resultant anemia and immunodeficiency, skull foramina fail to expand resulting in various cranial nerve palsies and blindness. Remodeling is the process of continued turnover of bone (resorption and reformation) in adult live that is influenced by various mechanical and endocrine factors (discussed in Chapter on "Bone Structure, Physiology, Metabolism, and Associated Disorders"). Defective remodeling results in accrual of microfractures in the bone and qualitative weakness of bone to withstand stress. Such structurally weakened bone though appearing radiodense fails under mild stress and impacts.

Epidemiology and Clinical Features

Benign Adult Form

The adult type 2 autosomal dominant form is the most common form that was recognized by Albers-Schönberg with a prevalence of 5.5/100,000. This is also the most common form in India. It is diagnosed in late adolescence or early adulthood. Clinically, it presents with bone pains, nontraumatic fractures of long bones **(Figs. 32A and B)**, cranial nerve palsies (deafness and facial palsy), carpal tunnel syndrome, and osteoarthritis of the hip and mandibular osteomyelitis. The serum acid phosphatase levels are raised. Bone marrow function is normal. There may be visual impairment due to retinal degeneration and psychomotor retardation affecting school performance. The type I autosomal dominant form is (reported in only three families) characterized by generalized osteopetrosis, especially of the cranial vault with normal acid phosphatase levels, the disease is less severe than type 2 form.

Infantile Malignant Form

This has varied presentations and is uniformly fatal with some patients succumbing in infantile period, while others fortunate just enough to touch end of first decade. Incidence varies from 1 in 200,000 to 1 in 500,000 live births. The patients show failure to thrive and suffer from growth retardation. Cranial nerve neuropathies (multiple) are very common and progressive due to compression of nerves in narrow foramina resulting in deafness, blindness, proptosis, etc. Children have sleep apnea, stuffy nose, and recurrent sinusitis (due to paranasal sinus malformation) that may be associated with maxillomandibular osteomyelitis bringing them to physician earliest and multiply. Bone marrow failure results in pancytopenia, reduced incident immunity, and easy bruising due to thrombocytopenia. Children have growth retardation due to skeletal defect, anemia, recurrent infections, and psychomotor retardation due to hydrocephalus and general growth retardation. Dentition is delayed and bones fracture with minimal impact. Extramedullary compensatory hematopoiesis produces hepatosplenomegaly and hypersplenism.

Investigations

Laboratory Findings

In infantile form, the serum tartrate-resistant acid phosphatase and creatine kinase-BB (CK-BB) (brain isoform) are elevated due to release from defective osteoclasts into systemic circulation. Nutritional calcium deficiency produces hypocalcemia, rickets, and secondary hyperparathyroidism. In adult benign form, the acid phosphatase and CK-BB levels are often increased in type II but normal in type I form.

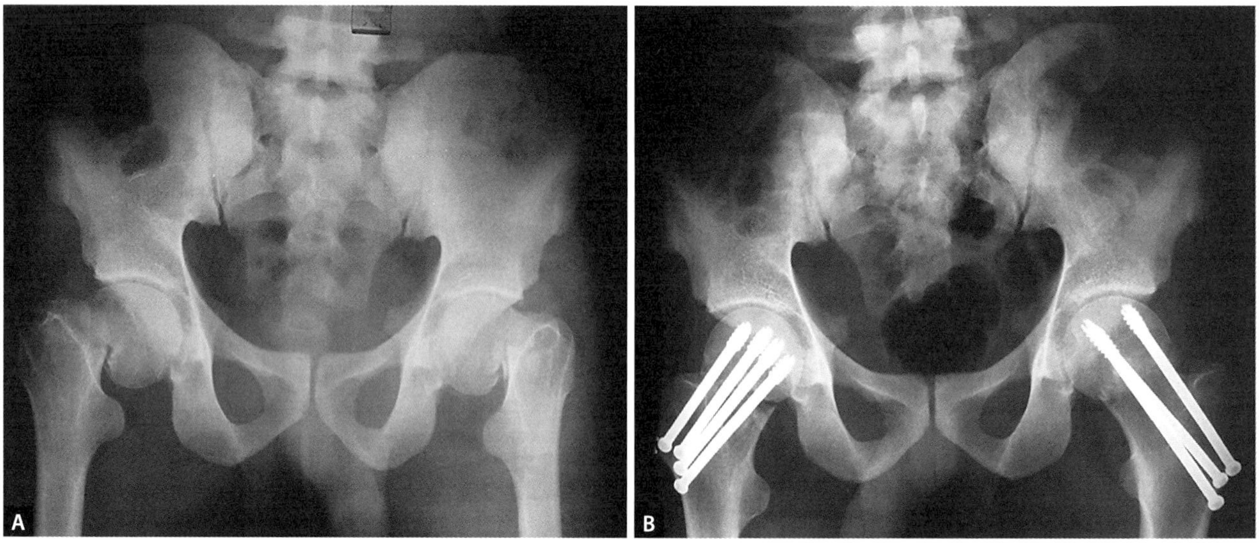

Figs. 32A and B: A 19-year old patient suffering from osteopetrosis fractured both his femoral neck (A) following fall from height of 3 feet. The patient was managed with closed reduction and multiple cannulated screw fixation (B) osteosynthesis (the screw placement is not very optimal!).

Radiology

This has typical findings but differ in individuals due to heterogeneous nature of disease. Generalized osteosclerosis with thickening of both cortical and cancellous bones is common to all, but may vary in extent of involvement, like predominant cranial vault involvement in type 1 adult osteopetrosis without spine involvement.

- Infantile form:
  - Small and under pneumatized sinuses
  - Absent medullary canal
  - Cube-like bones (carpals and tarsals)
  - Erlenmeyer flask deformity of metaphysis with broadening
- Adult form (type 2):
  - Alternating sclerotic and lucent bands:
    - "Rugger–Jersey" spine
    - Endobone formation (bone within bone appearance) in iliac wings and subcristal sclerosis
    - Transverse banding of ends of long bones (metaphysis) this is pathognomonic of type 2 adult form differentiating from type 1 radiologically.

Differential Diagnosis

All possible causes of diffuse osteosclerosis including pyknodysostosis, hypoparathyroidism, pseudohypoparathyroidism, Paget's disease, and myeloproliferative disorders, such as leukemia, sickle-cell disease, osteoblastic metastasis, and poisoning (fluoride, lead, and beryllium).

Treatment

Infantile osteopetrosis is uniformly fatal and the only chance to survival and cure is bone marrow transplantation. The treatment cannot be offered to all due to cost and logistic restraints and nonuniform success rates. The allogeneic human leukocyte antigen (HLA)-matched bone marrow transplant provides normal osteoprogenitor cells that form normal osteoclasts capable of resorbing bone. The transplant should be done before the age of 4 years. Studies have documented good benefit from treatment with interferon γ-1β and high dose calcitriol. Calcitriol stimulates osteoclasts with low calcium intake. Low calcium diet may stimulate osteoclasts, but restriction should be avoided if rickets develops. Interferon therapy improves white blood cell function, increasing bone marrow volume, and increases hemoglobin and platelet counts. Erythropoietin and corticosteroids have been used to treat anemia.

Surgical treatment is required only to correct the complications of disease, such as fracture fixation, decompression of cranial nerves, deformity correction, and arthroplasty for degenerative joint disease. There is high complication rate of iatrogenic fractures, infection, implant loosening, and nonunions in these patients. Osteomyelitis is treated on the principles laid in Chapter on "Infections of Bone (Typical and Atypical) and Surgical Site Infection". Very rarely surgical intervention may be asked for correcting facial deformity and improving cosmesis.

BONE MINERAL AND VITAMIN D DISORDERS

RICKETS

Definition

It is a defect in mineralization of osteoid matrix caused by inadequate calcium and phosphate deposition prior to closure of physis. Rickets is a disease of growing bone that occurs in children (before fusion of epiphysis) and clinical features arise from unmineralized matrix at the growth plate. Cartilage and osteoid continue to expand the growth plate that fails to mineralize. The growth plate thickens, widens, and increases in circumference of metaphysis. There are various causes of rickets **(Box 11)**. A few of them have their own set of clinical, laboratory, diagnostic features, and prognosis that can be grouped into "varieties" or "type" of rickets, detailed below.

BOX 11: Etiological classification of rickets.

Vitamin D disorders:
- Nutritional deficiency of vitamin D
- Vitamin D-dependent rickets type 1
- Vitamin D-dependent rickets type 2
- Congenital vitamin D deficiency
- Secondary vitamin D deficiency:
  - Malabsorption
  - Decrease liver 25-hydroxylase
  - Increase degradation
- Chronic kidney disease

Renal losses:
- Autosomal dominant hypophosphatemic rickets
- Autosomal recessive hypophosphatemic rickets
- X-linked hypophosphatemic rickets
- Hereditary hypophosphatemic rickets with hypercalciuria (HHRH)
- Excess production of phosphatonin:
  - Neurofibromatosis
  - Tumor-induced rickets
  - McCune–Albright syndrome
  - Epidermal nevus
- Dent disease
- Fanconi syndrome
- Distal renal tubular acidosis

Calcium deficiency:
- Decrease intake
- Malabsorption

Phosphorous deficiency:
- Premature infants (rickets of prematurity)
- Aluminum—containing antacids

Pathophysiology

Vitamin D undergoes successive hydroxylation in the liver and kidney to 1, 25-dihydroxycholecalciferol. Its main action is to increase the absorption of calcium from intestine (see regulation of bone metabolism in structure and function of bone). PTH secreted by parathyroid glands mobilizes calcium from bone and increases urinary excretion of phosphate. The third hormone calcitonin secreted by parafollicular cells (C cells), inhibits bone resorption. Although the role of calcitonin seems to be relatively minor. All three hormones operate in concert to regulate the calcium levels in body fluids. A fourth local hormone, PTHrP, acts on one of the PTH receptors and is important in the skeletal development in utero.

A brief review of vitamin D and hydroxycholecalciferol (also see endocrine and paracrine regulation of bone metabolism in Chapter on "Bone Structure, Physiology, Metabolism, and Associated Disorders").

Vitamin D_3 is produced in mammals from 7-dehydrocholesterol by ultraviolet B radiation from the sun. Vitamin D_3 and its hydroxylated derivatives are transported in the plasma bound to a globulin vitamin D binding protein or globulin (DBP), which is also known as Gc protein and binds G-actin. The affinity of DBP for previtamin D_3 is low, but for vitamin D_3 is high. In the liver, 25-hydroxylase converts vitamin D (cholecalciferol) to 25-hydroxycholecalciferol. The final step occurs in kidney where 1α-hydroxylase adds the second hydroxyl group and 25-hydroxycholecalciferol is converted to 1,25-dihydroxyvitamin D (calcitriol). There is upregulation of 1α-hydroxylase that occurs by PTH and hypophosphatemia; hyperphosphatemia, and calcitriol inhibit this enzyme. Most calcitriol circulates bound to DBP. Calcitriol (1, 25-dihydroxycholecalciferol) is also synthesized in placenta, the keratinocytes in the skin, and in macrophages. Person with sarcoidosis and pulmonary alveolar macrophages also produce 1, 25-dihydroxycholecalciferol, on stimulation by interferon-γ. The less active metabolite 24, 25-dihydroxycholecalciferol is also synthesized in the kidneys.

Clinical Features

Below is a comprehensive regionwise list of the clinical signs and symptoms seen in a patient with full blown rickets neglected for long duration (commonly poor socioeconomic conditions). Most patients in clinical practice present with only few of the features.

Head

- Craniotabes—softening of cranial bones a sensation similar to pressing a ping pong ball on applying pressure on occiput or the parietal bones. Craniotabes can also be seen in osteogenesis imperfect, hydrocephalus, and syphilis.
- Frontal bossing
- Delayed dentition and tooth caries
- Delayed closure of fontanel
- Craniosynostosis

Chest

- Rachitic rosary—widening of osteochondral junction, feels like beads of rosary on moving finger along the osteochondral junction from rib to rib.
- Harrison's groove—occurs due to pulling of softened ribs in inspiration by diaphragm. Softened ribs also predispose to atelectasis and pneumonia because of decreased air entry.
- Pectus carinatum (pigeon breast)—sternum projects forward.

Spine

- Scoliosis (uncommon)
- Kyphosis (rachitic cat back)
- Accentuation of lumbar lordosis

Limbs and Joints

- Bone pain and tenderness
- Coxa vara
- Genu valgum or varum
- Windswept deformity
- Bowing of tibia, femur, radius, and ulna
- Widening of wrist, elbow, knee, and ankle because of enlargement of ends of long bones
- Rachitic saber shins
- Sausage-like enlargement of ends of phalanges and metacarpals, with regular constrictions corresponding of the joints string of pearls deformity
- Double malleoli sign

General

- Failure to thrive
- Protuberant abdomen
- Apathy, listlessness and irritability
- Proximal muscle weakness
- Ligament laxity
- Symptoms of hypocalcemia—tetany, seizures, and stridor due to laryngeal spasm
- Bilateral lamellar cataract (Vitamin D deficiency in early infancy)

The clinical features also vary depending on type of deficiency:

- Lower extremity changes predominate in X-linked hypophosphatemic rickets.
- Rickets that is associated with decreased serum calcium levels is associated with symptoms of hypocalcemia, e.g., dietary vitamin D deficiency, vitamin D-dependent rickets (VDDR) types I and II, chronic kidney disease, and dietary calcium deficiency.

Radiological Signs

On radiographic examination, rickets is characterized by:

- Generalized osteopenia
- Bowing deformities of the long bones **(Fig. 33)**, particularly the femur and tibia
- Widening of the growth plate (secondary to deficient mineralization in the provisional zone of calcification) and cupping or flaring of the metaphysis **(Figs. 34A to D)**, particularly in the proximal humerus, distal radius and ulna, and distal femur as explained. Widened growth plate is due to continued hypertrophy of cartilage cells. Normally, capillaries grow from metaphysis to epiphysis via tunnels in the zone of provisional calcification. This growth of capillaries destroys the cartilaginous cells in zone of hypertrophy, thereby limiting the growth of epiphyseal plate. In rickets, tunnels are not formed in the zone of provisional calcification because of defective mineralization, the cartilaginous cells continue to proliferate, but do not die, thus leading to thickened growth plates. The metaphysis is soft due to absent mineralization, hence, the epiphysis is pushed into metaphysis with axial pressure causing cupping. The metaphysis widens under axial pressure and defective modeling of bone causing flaring. Irregular calcification leads to fraying of metaphysis that instead of appearing smooth takes the form of "trees on plateau top" viewed from a distance.
- The radiographic findings in vitamin D resistant rickets are similar to those in infantile rickets. Bowing deformities and shortening of the long bones are, however, more pronounced in early rickets. They are best seen in the rapidly growing distal ends of radius and ulna (more so in ulna). Changes in the shaft appear a few weeks later than metaphysis. The epiphysis is cloudy and indistinct and periosteum is thick. The shaft shows diffuse rarefaction, thin cortices with coarse texture of spongiosa. Sometimes

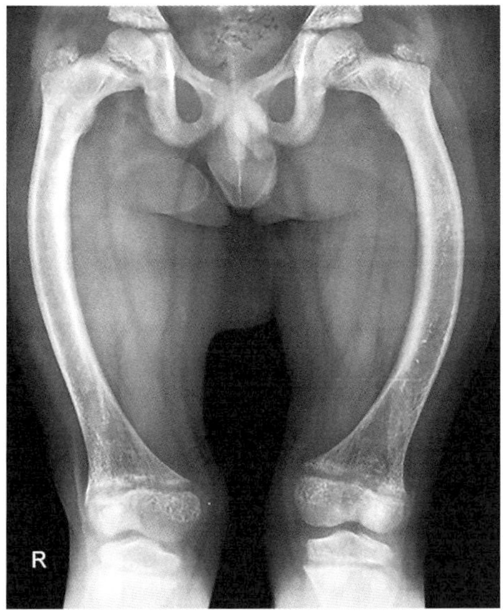

Fig. 33: The bowing of long bones in rickets.

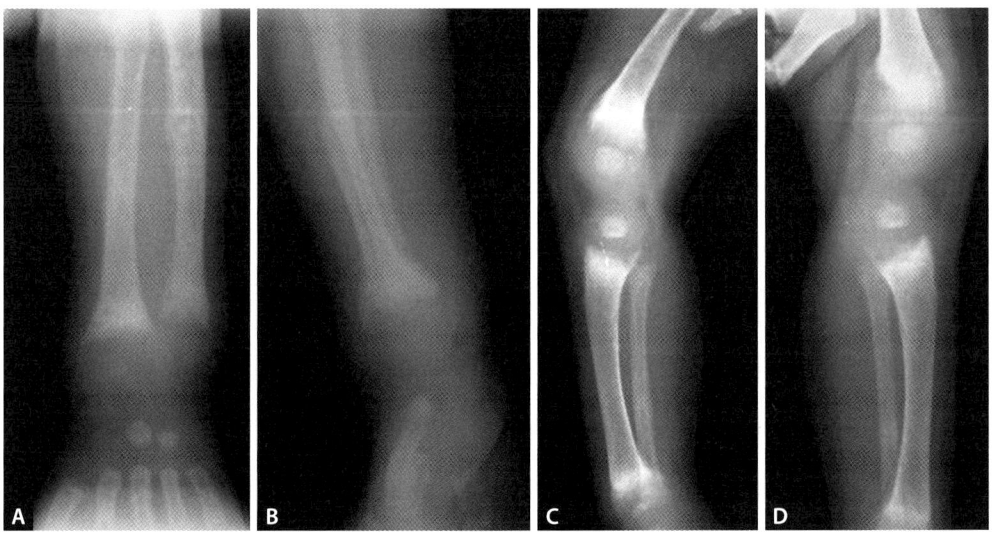

Figs. 34A to D: Radiographs of rickets.

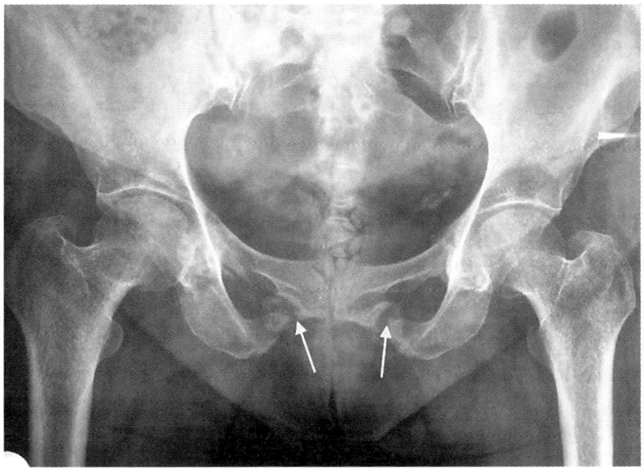

Fig. 35: The radiograph depicts classic appearance of Looser's zones. This is a case of osteomalacia in an adult and not of rickets but the Umbau/Looser's zones are characteristic in their location (here in inferior pubic/ischial rami) and appearance (arrows).

Umbau zones (Looser's zones) are seen as sharply defined radiolucent transverse zones **(Fig. 35)**. The circumflex artery pulsating against soft bone may produce Looser's zone in proximal humerus.

In severe rickets, the margins of tarsal and carpal ossification centers may disappear.

- *Findings of healing rickets:*
  - Earliest finding the reappearance of the provisional zone of calcification, which gradually thickens into a transverse band
  - This is followed by recalcification of the spongiosa in the metaphysis.
  - A dense line appears at the end of metaphysis.
  - Epiphyseal shadow is clearly defined.
  - The end of shaft and epiphysis become clearly differentiated.
  - Finally, the bone appears to be normal.

Nutritional Deficiency of Vitamin D

Globally, vitamin D deficiency remains the most common cause of rickets. Most patients have a combination of risk factors that lead to vitamin D deficiency as it can be obtained from dietary sources or from cutaneous synthesis.

Etiology

Deficiency of vitamin D most commonly occurs in infancy because of a combination of poor intake and inadequate cutaneous synthesis. Infants who receive formula receive adequate vitamin D, even without cutaneous synthesis. Transplacental transport of vitamin D, mostly 25-D, provides enough vitamin D for the first 2 months of life unless there is severe maternal vitamin D deficiency. Breastfed infants, because of the low vitamin D content of breast milk (almost 90% females in India are vitamin D deficient); rely on cutaneous synthesis or vitamin supplements. Cutaneous synthesis can be limited due to the ineffectiveness of the winter sun and cultural practices.

Most infants present in late winters and spring, due to the impact of winter sun. Vitamin D deficiency rickets may also occur secondary to unconventional dietary habits, such as use unfortified soy milk or rice milk.

Clinical Features

These children have an increased risk of pneumonia and muscle weakness, leading to a delay in motor development. The clinical manifestations are typical of rickets with a few presenting even with symptoms of hypocalcemia and prolonged laryngospasm is life-threatening.

Laboratory Findings

Hypocalcemia is variable as blood calcium levels are kept normal by secondary hyperparathyroidism. Hypophosphatemia is secondary to PTH-induced renal loss of phosphate and also decrease in intestinal absorption of phosphate.

The calcitriol levels may be low, normal or high, secondary to the upregulation of renal 1α-hydroxylase due to associated hypophosphatemia and hyperparathyroidism. The serum levels of calcitriol are normally much less than the levels of 25-D so even in moderate vitamin D deficiency states there is enough 25-D present to act as a precursor for calcitriol synthesis in the presence of an upregulated 1α-hydroxylase. In severe vitamin D deficiency, the level of calcitriol will be low. There may be metabolic acidosis and generalized aminoaciduria.

Diagnosis and Differential Diagnosis

The diagnosis of nutritional vitamin D deficiency is based on the combination of a history of poor vitamin D intake and risk factors for decreased cutaneous synthesis, radiographic changes consistent with rickets and typical laboratory findings **(Box 11)**. A normal PTH level is almost never seen with vitamin D deficiency and if present then suggests a primary phosphate disorder. Calcium deficiency may occur with or without vitamin D deficiency. A normal level of 25-D and a dietary history of poor calcium intake support a diagnosis of isolated calcium deficiency.

Treatment

Adequate intake of vitamin D, calcium, and phosphorous is the mainstay of treatment in nutritional vitamin D deficiency rickets, which can be administered by the following methods:

- *Stoss therapy:* 300,000–600,000 IU of vitamin D is administered orally or intramuscularly as 2–4 doses over 1 day. Because the doses are observed, Stoss therapy is ideal in situations where adherence to therapy is questionable.
- *Alternate therapy:* High-dose vitamin D, with doses ranging from 2,000 to 5,000 IU/day over 4–6 weeks.

Either strategy should be followed by daily vitamin D intake of 400 IU/day (for child <1 year of age, else 600 IU/day for age >1 year), typically given as a multivitamin combination. It is important to administer adequate dietary calcium and phosphorus; common sources for which are milk, formula diets, and other dairy products.

For the symptoms of hypocalcemia, patient may need intravenous calcium acutely (IV calcium gluconate 100 mg/kg), followed by oral calcium supplements, which typically can be tapered over 2–6 weeks in children receiving adequate dietary calcium. Alternatively, a continuous intravenous calcium drip may be tried in some patients, which is titrated to maintain the desired serum calcium level followed by conversion to oral calcium of approximately 1,000 mg/day. Transient use of intravenous or oral calcitriol (0.05 μg/kg/day) is often helpful in reversing hypocalcemia in the acute phase by providing active vitamin D during the delay as supplemental vitamin D is converted to active vitamin D.

Prognosis

The prognosis of nutritional rickets is excellent provided the cases are diagnosed early and are followed up thoroughly. The radiological signs of improvement start appearing within a few months and the laboratory parameters also normalize within few weeks. Children with severe deformities are the ones that are diagnosed late or are neglected; they sustain permanent deformities. An orthopedic intervention may only be required to correct these residual deformities, but is undertaken only after the bone disease is healed.

Prevention

In breastfed children, daily administration of multivitamin containing 200–400 IU of vitamin D can prevent nutritional rickets, and for others the diet should ensure adequate vitamin D.

Secondary Vitamin D Deficiency

Etiology

The deficiency of vitamin D occurring from causes apart from inadequate intake (nutritional deficiency) is termed as "secondary vitamin D deficiency", which may be due to:

- Inadequate absorption
- Decreased hydroxylation in the liver
- Increased degradation

Because vitamin D is fat-soluble and its absorption from GIT is dependent on bile acids, a variety of diseases of GIT may decrease its absorption, such as defects in metabolism of bile acids, liver diseases, malabsorption syndromes, cholestatic liver disease, cystic fibrosis, and celiac and Crohn's disease. Malabsorption of vitamin D can also occur with intestinal lymphangiectasia and after intestinal resection. Apart from decreased vitamin D absorption, a decreased vitamin D synthesis occurs in severe liver disease, (also associated with malabsorption), a decrease in 25D formation due to insufficient enzyme activity. The reserve of 25-hydroxlase activity is large and requires a loss of >90% of liver function for any significant impairment.

Treatment

Treatment of vitamin D deficiency due to malabsorption requires high doses of vitamin D. 25-D (25–50 μg/day or 5–7 μg/kg/day) is superior to vitamin D_3 as it is better absorbed. Alternatively, calcitriol may be used which is better absorbed in the presence of fat malabsorption, or with parenteral vitamin D. The dose is adjusted based on monitoring of serum levels of 25-D. The treatment is the same for children with secondary vitamin D deficiency due to activation of P450 in the acute stage, and is followed by prolonged administration of high dose of vitamin D (>800 IU/day), titrated based in serum vitamin D levels. Doses of even up to 4,000 IU/day may be needed in some resistant patients.

Congenital Vitamin D Deficiency

Congenital rickets is seen with severe maternal vitamin D deficiency during pregnancy. The maternal risk factors are similar to nutritional vitamin D deficiency and include poor dietary intake of vitamin D, closely spaced pregnancies and lack of adequate sun exposure. These newborns along with classic rachitic changes have:

- Decreased bone ossification
- Symptomatic hypocalcemia
- Intrauterine growth retardation

There may be a defect in the dental enamel, neonatal bone density, and birthweight. These infants are predisposed to hypocalcemic tetany. Treatment of congenital rickets includes vitamin D supplementation and adequate intake of phosphorous and calcium.

Vitamin D-Dependent Rickets Type I

Vitamin D-dependent rickets type I or pseudovitamin D deficiency is a genetic disorder with an autosomal recessive mode of inheritance. The disorder is the result of mutation in 1α-hydroxylase gene causing reduction in the available enzyme for ultimate hydroxylation step. This prevents conversion of 25-D into calcitriol. Those patients who present within first 2 years of life can have any of the classic features of rickets, including symptomatic hypocalcemia. Typical laboratory findings include elevated PTH levels, decreased serum calcium, low or undetectable serum concentrations of calcitriol 1, 25-$(OH)_2$ D despite normal or increased concentrations of calcifediol (25OHD) **(Table 12)**.

Treatment

Long-term treatment with calcitriol is the treatment for VDDR type I. Initial doses are 0.25–2 μg/day, with lower doses used once the rickets has healed, with adequate intake of calcium. The dose of calcitriol is adjusted to maintain a low normal serum calcium level, a normal serum phosphorus level, and a high normal serum PTH level to prevent possible complications of hypercalciuria and nephrocalcinosis. Patient is monitored during the therapy with urinary calcium excretion with a target of <4 mg/kg/day.

Vitamin D-Dependent Rickets Type Ii

This occurs due to mutations in the gene encoding the VDR an autosomal recessive disorder, preventing a normal physiologic response to calcitriol because of end-organ resistance. More severely affected patients present in infancy whereas less severely affected patients may not be diagnosed until adulthood. A less severe disease is associated with a partially functional VDR. In a percentage of patients, it may

TABLE 12: Laboratory findings in various "varieties" of rickets.

Disorder	Ca	Pi	25-OHD	1,25-(OH)$_2$D	PTH	AlkPhos	Urinary Ca	Urine Pi
Vitamin D deficiency	N, ↓	↓	↓	↓, N, ↑	↑	↑	↓	↑
VDDR, type 1	N, ↓	↓	N	↓	↑	↑	↓	↑
VDDR, type 2	N, ↓	↓	N	↑↑	↑	↑	↓	↑
Dietary calcium deficiency	N, ↓	↓	N	↑	↑	↑	↓	↑
X-linked hypophosphatemic	N	↓	N	RD	N	↑	↓	↑
Dietary Pi deficiency	N	↓	N	↑	N, ↓	↑	↑	↓
Chronic renal failure	N, ↓	↑	N	N	↑	↑	N, ↓	↓
ADHR	N	↓	N	RD	N	↑	↓	↑
HHRH	N	↓	N	RD	N, ↓	↑	↑	↑
Tumor-induced rickets	N	↓	N	RD	N	↑	↓	↑

(ADHR: autosomal dominant hypophosphatemic ricket; HHRH: hereditary hypophosphatemic ricket with hypercalciuria; N: normal; RD: relative decrease; VDDR: vitamin D-dependent rickets)

be associated with alopecia (ranging from alopecia areata to alopecia totalis), which tends to be associated with a more severe form of the disease. Epidermal cysts may be associated, but is a less common manifestation. Levels of calcitriol are extremely elevated and serve to differentiate type II from type I VDDR.

Treatment

A 3–6 months trial of high dose of vitamin D_2, 25-D or calcitriol and oral calcium is given for less severe form of disease, especially those without alopecia. This response is due to a partially functional VDR. The initial dose of calcitriol should be 2 µg/day. Oral calcium doses range from 1,000 to 3,000 mg/day. Unresponsive patients may be treated with long-term intravenous calcium with possible transition to very high dose oral calcium supplements. Patient not responding to vitamin D is difficult to treat.

Rickets in Chronic Renal Failure and Renal Osteodystrophy

Renal osteodystrophy applies to combination of secondary hyperparathyroidism and osteomalacia due to complicated of specific metabolic abnormality associated with chronic renal insufficiency. Nearly 90–100% of patients with advanced renal failure (mostly on maintenance dialysis) develop renal osteodystrophy. Recalling from Chapter on "Bone Structure, Physiology, Metabolism, and Associated Disorders", we know that adequate renal function is imperative in calcium-phosphorus metabolism and in regulating levels of magnesium, aluminum, and other metal ions. Being a pivot point in regulating metal ion metabolism and target organ for PTH even small changes in renal function drastically alter mineral homeostasis.

Etiopathogenesis

Due to alteration of calcium-phosphate mineral metabolism, the homeostasis may shift toward rickets predominant or hyperparathyroidism dominant or osteoporosis dominant pathology. The causes and pathogenesis of each of these are summarized below:

- *Rickets/osteomalacia predominant:* In chronic renal failure, the activity of 1α-hydroxylase in the kidney is decreased, leading to diminished production of calcitriol [producing rickets (pediatric patients) or osteomalacia (adults)]. Along with inadequate calcium absorption and secondary hyperparathyroidism, the rickets may be worsened by the metabolic acidosis of chronic renal failure. In addition, failure to thrive and growth retardation may be accentuated because of the direct effect of chronic renal failure on the growth hormone axis.
- *Hyperparathyroidism predominant:* In chronic renal failure, unlike the other causes of vitamin D deficiency, patients have hyperphosphatemia as a result of decreased renal excretion. The dominant picture may be that of secondary hyperparathyroidism [due to phosphate retention, hypocalcemia, and diminished production of 1,25(OH)2D], osteoporosis, osteomalacia or—in advanced cases—a combination of these. Additionally, the calcium deficiency negatively impacts bone mineralization producing a dynamic bone disease. In long term, the bony consequences may tilt to either of two ways—either high turnover secondary hyperparathyroidism or low-turnover secondary hyperparathyroidism **(Flowchart 4)**. In the former (high turnover) variety, one finds high phosphate, high PTH, high creatinine and BUN, increased urinary phosphate, and low vitamin D levels. In the low-turnover variety, one finds excess aluminum deposition and demineralized matrix in bone with normal or reduced PTH levels.
- *Osteoporosis predominant:* In older patients, the effects of postmenopausal osteoporosis may be superimposed; in some, there are concomitant changes due to glucocorticoid medication; and in patients with end-stage renal failure, bone changes can be aggravated by aluminum retention or contamination of dialyzing fluids.

Histopathology

Apart from the classical features of rickets, the high-turnover hyperparathyroidism shows osteitis fibrosa lesions with numerous enlarged osteoclasts and increased numbers of Howship lacunae. The low-turnover variety shows typical

Flowchart 4: Pathogenesis of renal osteodystrophy.

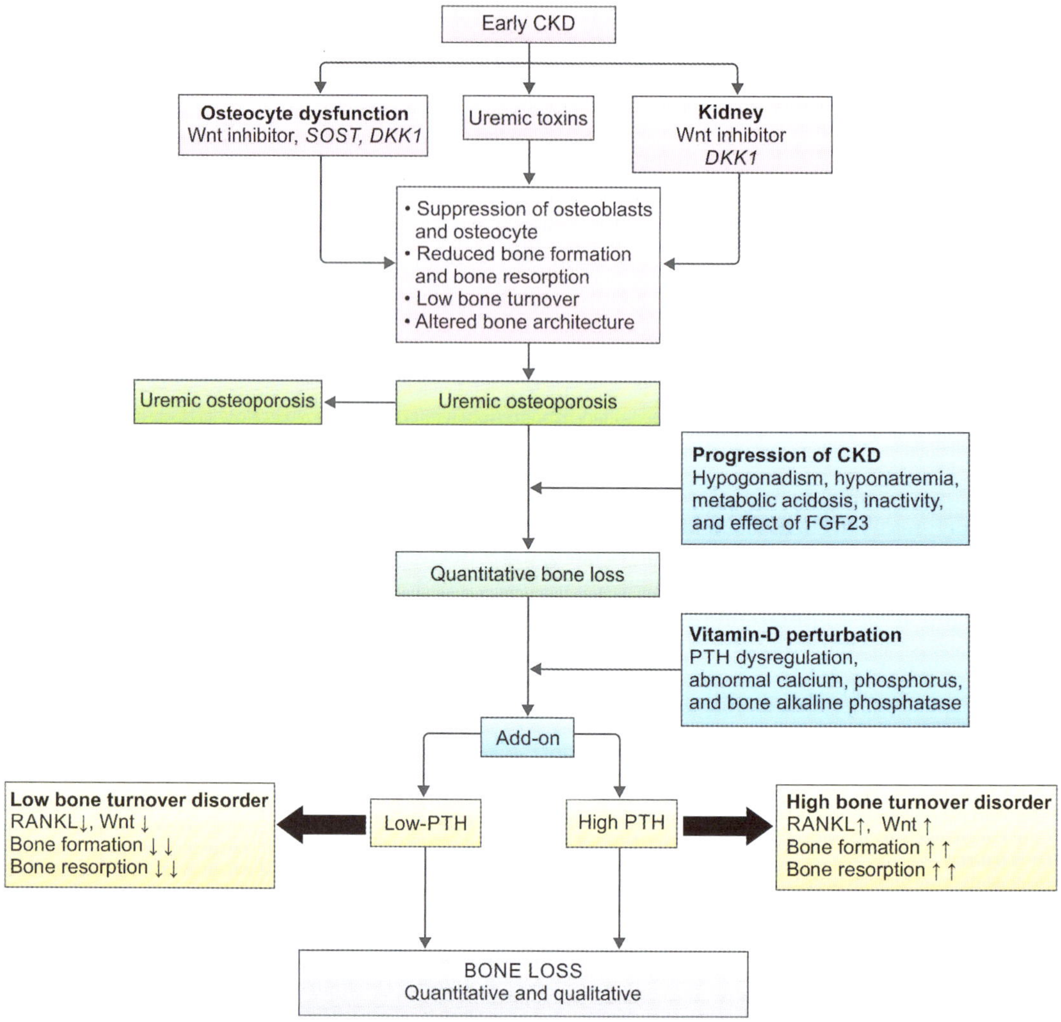

(SOST: gene for sclerostin; DKK1: gene for dkkopf, Wnt: Wnt pathway; FGF23: fibroblast growth factor 23; PTH: parathormone; RANK: receptor activator for nκ; CKD: chronic kidney disease)

osteomalacia along with redundant osteoid accumulation and reduced osteoblastic activity.

Clinical Features and Radiology

Renal abnormalities usually precede the bone changes by several years. Adults usually have nonspecific bone pains, muscle weakness (truncal and girdle region) compromising balance, movement disorder, fragility fractures in ribs, and vertebrae.

- Children have growth retardation, short height; they are pasty-faced and have marked rachitic deformities (frontal bossing, rachitic rosary, bowing of long bones, ulnar deviation of wrist, metaphyseal enlargement, etc.) along with myopathy. X-rays show widened and irregular epiphyseal plates (changes of rickets). In adolescents with long-standing disease, there may be displacement of the epiphyses (epiphyseolysis) presenting with slipped upper femoral epiphysis (SUFE).
- Osteosclerosis is seen mainly in the axial skeleton and is more common in young patients; it may produce a "rugger jersey" appearance in lateral X-rays of the spine due to alternating bands of increased and decreased bone density.
- Adults present with skeletal deformity and heterotopic calcification (periarticular and vascular calcification mostly).
- In all patients, signs of secondary hyperparathyroidism may be widespread and severe.
- In severe renal osteodystrophy, patient may have calciphylaxis—a rare disease presenting with ischemic necrosis of skin, subcutaneous tissues and skeletal muscles.

Biochemical features are low serum calcium, high-serum phosphate, and elevated alkaline phosphatase levels. Urinary excretion of calcium and phosphate is diminished. Plasma PTH levels may be raised (except in low-turnover variety).

Treatment

The aim is maintaining calcium-phosphate homeostasis, avoiding aluminum toxicity and preventing heterotopic calcification. Calcitriol is the treatment of choice. This permits adequate absorption of calcium and directly suppresses the parathyroid gland. Sevelamer hydrochloride, a phosphate binder used orally, and dietary restriction of phosphate to regulate serum phosphate levels can be used individually or in combination as hyperphosphatemia is a stimulus for PTH secretion. In addition, metabolic acidosis may be corrected with alkalis. More recently a calcimimetic drug, cinacalcet, has been introduced which acts directly on the parathyroid glands increasing the sensitivity of calcium receptors and inducing a reduction in serum PTH levels. Aluminum toxicity is managed with deferoxamine during dialysis. Surgical measures may be needed for different indications as follows:

- Renal transplantation should be considered in patients with irreversible long-standing disease.
- Epiphyseolysis may need internal fixation and residual deformities can be corrected once the disease is under control.
- Corrective surgery for deformity and growth disturbance in pediatric patients
- Osteosynthesis in adults for pathological fracture
- Adult patients with steroid-induced osteonecrosis may need joint arthroplasty.

Patients with limited ambulation, marked deformity requiring extensive surgery and decreased BMD compromising implant stability should be preferred toward nonsurgical treatment.

Calcium Deficiency and Rickets

Pathophysiology

- *Poor weaning:* One of the common causes of calcium deficiency rickets especially occurs in children who are weaned from breast milk early. The diet of these children is low in calcium content (juice, soda or calcium-poor soy drink, without an alternative source of dietary calcium), typically <200 mg/day. There is little intake of dairy products or other sources of calcium. Also, the diet may be rich in phytates, oxalates, and phosphates, e.g., green leafy which decreases absorption of dietary calcium from GIT.
- Calcium deficiency rickets may also develop in children who receive intravenous nutrition without adequate calcium.
- Malabsorption syndromes, such as celiac disease, intestinal a β-lipoproteinemia, and after small bowel resection predisposes to calcium malabsorption. Along with other micro- and macronutrients there may be concurrent malabsorption of vitamin D.

Clinical Manifestations

Children have the classic signs and symptoms of rickets. Classically, the diet is deficient in dairy products. Presentation may occur during infancy or early childhood. Because, calcium deficiency occurs after the cessation of breastfeeding, it tends to occur later than the nutritional vitamin D deficiency that is associated with breastfeeding.

Diagnosis

Laboratory findings include increased levels of PTH, calcitriol, and ALP **(Table 12)**. Serum calcium levels may be normal or low, although symptomatic hypocalcemia is uncommon. The urinary excretion of calcium is decreased and due to secondary hyperparathyroidism serum phosphorus levels may be low due to renal wasting of phosphate, which may also cause aminoaciduria. In some children, there is coexisting nutritional vitamin D deficiency; 25-D levels would then be low.

Treatment

Children with dietary calcium deficiency respond dramatically to oral calcium supplementation. Typically the dietary supplement doses of 350–1,000 mg/day of elemental calcium are effective. Vitamin D supplementation is necessary, if there is concurrent vitamin D deficiency. In cases of malabsorption syndrome, calcium supplementation is done parenterally followed by high oral calcium supplements. Prevention strategies include discouraging early cessation of breastfeeding and increasing dietary sources of calcium.

Hypophosphatemic Rickets

Phosphorous Deficiency

Pathophysiology

Inadequate intake: As phosphorous is present in most of the foods, dietary deficiency of phosphorous is extremely rare, except in conditions of prolonged starvation or severe anorexia.

Malabsorption: In malabsorption syndromes, there is decreased absorption of phosphates along with the decreased absorption of other minerals also. Rickets develop in these cases due to simultaneous malabsorption of vitamin D and/ or calcium.

Isolated phosphorous malabsorption: Rare cases of isolated malabsorption of phosphorus occur in patients with long-term ingestion of aluminum-containing antacids. Chronic aluminum exposure results in hypophosphatemia with rickets in children and secondary osteomalacia in adults. This entity responds to discontinuation of the antacid and short-term phosphorus supplementation.

Role of phosphatonin in hypophosphatemic rickets: Phosphate plays a vital role in a number of other biological processes, such as signal transduction, nucleotide metabolism and enzyme regulation, and also phosphate ions are critical for normal bone mineralization. Our understanding on role of phosphate in calcium homeostasis comes from the study of rare disorders associated with renal phosphate wasting. A number of proteins (collectively called phosphaturic peptides or phosphatonins) have been discovered like fibroblast growth factor (FGF)-23, FGF-7, the secreted frizzled-related protein-4 (SFRP-4) and matrix extracellular phosphoglycoprotein that have shown to reduce renal sodium-dependent phosphate transport. Also, among the mentioned phosphatonins, FGF-23 and SFRP-4 inhibit 1, 25-dihydroxyvitamin D synthesis, which leads to a decline in absorption of phosphates from the intestine and also reduce reabsorption of phosphate from kidneys.

X-linked Hypophosphatemic Rickets

X-linked hypophosphatemic rickets (XLH) also known as familial vitamin-D resistant rickets (VDRR) is the most common genetic disorder among the genetic disorders causing rickets due to hypophosphatemia, with a prevalence of 1/20,000. It is an X-linked dominant disorder, the defective gene lies on the X chromosome and so the female carriers are also affected.

Pathophysiology

The defective gene is called *PHEX* because it is a phosphate regulating gene with homology to endopeptidases on the X chromosome location Xp22.2-p22.1. The *PHEX* gene produces a protein that regulates FGF-23 produced from *FGF-23* gene, the latter appears to have either a direct or an indirect role in inactivating a phosphatonin or phosphatonins. If the *PHEX* gene is absent, the degradation of the phosphatonin is inhibited, thus leading to increase in phosphate excretion and decreased production of calcitriol. Also, in the absence of *PHEX* enzymatic activity, osteopontin (mineralization inhibiting protein) may accumulate in the bone to contribute to the osteomalacia. Laboratory investigations in XLH reveal hypophosphatemia and inappropriately low level of 1,25-$(OH)_2$ vitamin D_3. A person affected by this disease usually cannot touch both knees and ankles together by adducting the lower limbs. It also affects their equilibrium in standing position that can be maintained only when the lower limbs are farther apart.

Clinical Features

The clinical features are that of rickets with abnormalities of lower extremity more pronounced as compared to upper limb and is associated with poor growth. Delayed dentition and tooth abscesses are also common. Some patients have hypophosphatemia and short stature without clinically evident bone disease.

Laboratory Findings

Patients have high renal excretion of phosphate, hypophosphatemia, and increased ALP while the PTH and serum calcium levels are normal. Hypophosphatemia upregulates renal 1α-hydroxylase, so it is logically expected that there should be increased calcitriol, but these patients have low or inappropriately normal levels possibly due to normal PTH and calcium levels that are potent regulators.

Treatment

A combination of oral phosphorus and calcitriol is given to get an appropriate response. The daily need for phosphorus supplementation is 1–3 g of elemental phosphorus divided into 4–5 doses. Frequent dosing helps to prevent prolonged decrements in serum phosphorus because there is a rapid decline after each dose also the side effects of high dose phosphorous, such as diarrhea is avoided. Calcitriol is administered 30–70 ng/kg/day divided into two doses.

There may be complications associated with treatment, if an adequate balance between phosphorus supplementation and calcitriol is not maintained. Excess phosphorus, by decreasing enteral calcium absorption, leads to secondary hyperparathyroidism, with worsening of the bone lesions. In contrast, excess calcitriol causes hypercalciuria and nephrocalcinosis; it may even cause hypercalcemia. Hence, laboratory monitoring of treatment should include serum calcium, phosphorus, ALP, PTH, and urinary calcium, as well as periodic renal ultrasounds to evaluate patients for nephrocalcinosis. Normalization of ALP levels is a useful method of assessing the therapeutic response than serum phosphorous. Growth hormone is an effective option for children with significant short stature. Children with severe deformities may need osteotomies, but this should be done only when treatment has led to resolution of the bone disease.

Prognosis

Girls, generally, have less severe disease than boys, probably due to the X-linked inheritance. The response to therapy is usually good, although frequent dosing may lead to problems with compliance. Short stature may persist despite healing of the rickets. Adults generally do well with less aggressive treatment, by receiving some calcitriol alone. Adults with bone pain or other symptoms improve with oral phosphorus supplementation and calcitriol.

Autosomal Dominant Hypophosphatemic Rickets

This disorder is much less common than XLH. There is incomplete penetrance and variable age of onset. In autosomal dominant hypophosphatemic rickets (ADHR), the gene encoding for *FGF-23* is mutated. The mutated *FGF-23* escapes degradation by the proteases, thus elevating its concentration. The actions of *FGF-23*, i.e., decreased reabsorption of phosphates in the PCT and inhibition of 1α-hydroxylase are overwhelmed, thus leading to hypophosphatemia and decreased levels of calcitriol.

In ADHR, as in XLH, abnormal laboratory findings are hypophosphatemia, an elevated ALP level and a low or inappropriately normal calcitriol level. Molecular genetic testing confirms the diagnosis. Treatment is similar to the approach used in XLH.

Hereditary Hypophosphatemic Rickets with Hypercalciuria

It is a rare disorder that is mainly described in the Middle East. It is an isolated real phosphate wasting disorder leading to low serum phosphate levels. Inherited in an autosomal recessive form this is the second type of vitamin-D resistant rickets. The distinguishing feature of HHRH from other forms of hypophosphatemia is that, in HHRH the serum levels of 1,25-dihydroxyvitamin D are elevated which result in hypercalciuria.

Pathophysiology

On chromosome-9, the candidate region contained a sodium-phosphate cotransporter gene, *SLC34A3,* which has been shown to be expressed in proximal tubules cells. Sequencing of this gene revealed disease-associated mutations in five families, including two frame shift and one splice site mutation. Loss of function of the *SLC34A3* protein presumably results in a primary renal tubular defect and is compatible with the HHRH phenotype. The phosphaturic factor FGF-23, which is increased in X-linked hypophosphatemic rickets and carries activating mutations in ADHR, is at normal or low-normal serum levels in the patients with HHRH, further supporting a primary renal defect.

Clinical Manifestations

The dominant symptoms are rachitic leg abnormalities, muscle weakness, and bone pain. Patients may have short stature with a disproportionate decrease in the length of the lower extremities. The severity of the disease varies and some family members have no evidence of rickets, but have kidney stones secondary to hypercalciuria.

Laboratory Findings

Like other phosphate wasting disorders, HHRH is characterized by reduced tubular reabsorption of phosphate (TRP) and hypophosphatemia. However, in contrast to the characteristics of XLH and ADHR, serum levels of calcitriol in HHRH are appropriately elevated for low serum phosphorus levels despite suppressed parathyroid, there is elevated calcium excretion in urine.

Treatment

Therapy relies on oral phosphorus replacement (1–2.5 g/day of elemental phosphorus in five divided oral doses). Treatment of the hypophosphatemia decreases serum levels of calcitriol and corrects the hypercalciuria. The accurate diagnosis of HHRH has important therapeutic implications. Unlike for XLH and ADHR, phosphate supplementation alone can cause a complete remission of HHRH and an addition of vitamin D may lead to complications, such as hypercalcemia, nephrocalcinosis, and renal damage. The response to therapy is usually excellent with resolution of pain, weakness, and radiographic evidence of rickets. There is also an increase in growth.

Overproduction of Phosphatonin

Overproduction of phosphatonins is one of the pathogeneses in tumor-induced osteomalacia (TIO). It is more common in adults than in children. It is a type of paraneoplastic syndrome. If at all it develops in children, the manifestations are characteristic of hypophosphatemic rickets. Tumors associated with TIO are usually mesenchymal in origin, usually benign, small, and located in bone. These tumors secrete a number of different putative phosphatonins (FGF-23, frizzled-related protein 4, and matrix extracellular phosphoglycoprotein), with different tumors secreting different phosphatonins or combinations of phosphatonins. These phosphatonins produce a biochemical phenotype that is similar to XLH and ADHR, including urinary phosphate wasting, hypophosphatemia, low or inappropriately normal calcitriol levels, and elevated ALP levels. Cure can be achieved by excision of the tumor. If the tumor is not resectable, the line of treatment is similar to that of XLH.

Renal phosphate wasting leading to hypophosphatemia and rickets (or osteomalacia in adults) is a potential complication in McCune-Albright syndrome. Triad of McCune-Albright syndrome includes fibrous dysplasia, hyperpigmented macules, and polyendocrinopathy. There are inappropriately low levels of calcitriol and elevated levels of ALP. Patients have elevated levels of the phosphatonin FGF-23, presumably produced by the dysplastic bone. The renal phosphate wasting and inhibition of calcitriol synthesis are related to the polyostotic fibrous dysplasia. Hypophosphatemic rickets can also occur in children with isolated polyostotic fibrous dysplasia. Although a rare possibility, removal of the abnormal bone can cure this disorder in children with McCune-Albright syndrome. The treatment is same as that for XLH. Additionally, bisphosphonate treatment decreases the fracture risk and pain associated with the bone lesions. It also decreases the elevated ALP level.

HYPOPHOSPHATASIA

Hypophosphatasia (also known as phosphoethanolaminuria) is an inborn error of metabolism arising due to loss-of-function mutation in the *ALPL* gene encoding tissue nonspecific alkaline phosphatase (TNSALP). TNSALP is needed for mineralization of bones and teeth so these are the primary targets of abnormality. In addition, the accumulation of inorganic pyrophosphate produces rickets or osteomalacia like clinical presentation. Manifestations include bowing of limbs (can occur in utero), postnatal bowing and shortening of limb, Bowdler bone spurs and generalized poor ossification.

The disease can be inherited either as autosomal dominant (AD) or autosomal recessive (AR) patterns. Five categories of disease are recognized depending primarily on age at diagnosis. The younger the age at diagnosis the severe is the disease. Perinatal disease (AR) is fatal shortly after birth while infantile form (AR) is diagnosed by 6 months of age also having substantial mortality. Childhood disease (usually AR) manifests after 6 months of age with delayed milestones and static myopathy. The children have premature loss of deciduous teeth before 5 years. Adult form (AD or AR) presents with recurrent or slow-to-heal metatarsal fractures or subtrochanteric femoral pseudofractures. Odontohypophosphatasia (usually AD) is the mildest for of disease presenting only with dental abnormalities.

The hallmark finding in these patients is low blood level of alkaline phosphatase (can also be seen in antiresorptive therapy, however). Additionally, hypercalcemia, hyperphosphatemia, hypercalciuria, and elevated phpsphoethanolamine and pyridoxal 5'-phosphate (substrate for TNSALP) is seen.

Treatment is enzyme replacement therapy with recombinant tissue nonspecific alkaline phosphatase (Asfotase alfa) modified to target and anchor to bone. Bone marrow transplant and stem cell therapy have not provided long-term improvement. Supportive therapy may be instituted, viz., vitamin B_6 for responsive seizures, hydration, restriction of dietary calcium, and vitamin D. Thiazide diuretics may be given for hypercalcemia. One must remember that adults with hypophosphatasia should not be given antiresorptive therapy for osteoporosis.

FLUOROSIS

Introduction

Skeletal fluorosis is an endemic metabolic disease of bones, widely prevalent in India and many other countries around the world. Fifty-six million people living in 200 districts are at risk of developing fluorosis. Skeletal fluorosis occurs due to excessive intake of fluoride both from drinking water and food. The optimum upper safe limit is not >6 mg/day. Epidemiological and experimental studies on fluorosis have greatly helped in understanding the disease and provided a rational approach of management of the menace of fluoride toxicity. States known to be endemic in various parts of India include Assam, Andhra Pradesh, Bihar, Delhi, Gujarat, Haryana, Jammu & Kashmir, Karnataka, Kerala, Maharashtra, Orissa, Punjab, Rajasthan, Tamil Nadu, Uttar Pradesh, and West Bengal. The first case report of endemic skeletal fluorosis was from Prakasam district, Andhra Pradesh in 1937, a province in south India. There was also a report of neurologic manifestations of fluorosis, which usually occurs in the later stages of the disease. The fluoride levels in these areas were surprisingly low, i.e., in a range of 1–3 ppm, which is unusual as skeletal fluorosis rarely occurs at levels <6 ppm. The possible mechanisms through which fluorosis occurred in these areas are as follows:

- High atmospheric temperatures (115–116°F) during summer months so people drink a lot of water.
- Hard physical labor activity again leads to increased water intake.
- Poor nutrition, deficient in calories and also vitamin C
- Impaired renal function
- Abnormal concentrations of certain trace elements, such as strontium, silica, uranium, calcium, magnesium, etc. in high concentration in water and food could influence fluoride toxicity.

Clinical Features

Clinical manifestations of fluoride toxicity have uniformity in the clinical presentation. Fluorosis in humans is predominantly dental and skeletal. Dental fluorosis occurs early in the disease process followed by a prolonged symptom free period of nearly 10–30 years which is ultimately followed by a crippling skeletal fluorosis and neurologic abnormalities. During the apparent symptom free stage, the body keeps on accumulating excess fluoride and the patient suffers from vague gastrointestinal symptoms. The neurological manifestations in skeletal fluorosis are dominated by radiculomyelopathy that arise primarily due to mechanical compression of the nerve roots and also the spinal cord from osteophytes, sclerosed vertebral column, and ossified ligaments. The cervical cord is involved earlier than the dorsal cord. The lumbar spine is the first to show skeletal changes, but the involvement of cauda equina is rare. Minor trauma may precipitate neurologic deficits.

In skeletal fluorosis, higher mental function defects and cranial nerve palsies are extremely rare. The motion of the spine is restricted. Sodium fluoride has antimuscarinic and curare like effect on myoneural tissue, although it has no effect on normal muscle membrane potentials even in the endplate region. There is yet no evidence of direct neurotoxicity of fluoride.

Pathogenesis

Inorganic fluoride replaces the hydroxyl groups of calcium hydroxyapatite forming calcium fluorapatite and gets deposited in bone. Osteons become irregular in shape, size, and distribution in compact bone and there is gross reduction in spongiosa. The Haversian canals get enlarged with concomitant irregular distribution of osteocytes and increased irregular interstitial lamellae. Excess fluoride makes invasion by capillaries difficult in the bone forming uneven paths and resulting in isolated cartilage islands. Bone marrow becomes fibrous and poor in cells, while there is secondary hyperparathyroidism due to reduced systemic calcium, producing a high bone turnover state. This may also be aided by osteoblast activation from enhanced expression of transcription factors such as activator protein-1 (AP-1) and Cbfa1, as well as upregulation of cytokines or growth factors such as bFGF, BMP-2, IGF, transforming growth factor β (TGFβ), platelet-derived growth factor (PDGF) and osteoprotegerin ligand (OPGL).

Although fluoride is known to stimulate bone formation, the underlying mechanisms are not fully understood. Recent studies have implicated the Wnt/β-catenin pathway as a major signaling cascade in bone biology. The current study determined the involvement of Wnt/β-catenin signaling in fluoride-induced osteoblastic differentiation, fluoride significantly promoted osteoblasts proliferation and ALP expression as well as the mRNA expression levels of bone differentiation markers, including COL1A1, ALP, and osteonectin. The positive effect of fluoride on ALP activity and mRNA expressions of COL1A1, ALP, osteonectin, and Runx2 was abolished by DKK-1, a blocker of the Wnt/β-catenin receptor. Taken together, these findings suggest that fluoride promotes osteoblastic differentiation through Akt- and GSK-3B-dependent activation of Wnt/β-catenin signaling pathway (see also osteoporosis).

Diagnosis

Urinary and Bone Fluoride

Urinary fluoride levels are the best indicators of fluoride intake. Since, fluoride excretion is not constant throughout the day, 24-hour samples of urine are more reliable than random or morning samples. In normal individuals, urinary fluorides fluctuate widely between 0.1 and 2.0 ppm (average 0.4 ppm) when the fluoride content of drinking water is 0.3 ppm. There is a linear relation between urinary fluoride levels and fluoride intake.

Normal blood fluoride levels in nonendemic regions vary between 0.002 and 0.008 mg/100 mL and in endemic regions the levels range between 0.02 and 0.15 mg/100 mL, whereas in patients with skeletal fluorosis the levels vary between 0.02 and 0.19 mg/100 mL. It is much less a useful reference for detecting fluoride toxicity as major portion is mineral bound. Also, flash blood samples fail to capture the varying fluoride levels with bone metabolic activity that is better studied from 24-hour urinary levels.

Retention of fluoride is measured by the bone fluoride levels and it can be used to monitor the fluoride treatment of osteoporosis. The value varies from 6,000 to 8,400 ppm in bone ash in fluorosis, normal between 500 and 1,000 ppm or mg/kg.

Radiology

The radiographic findings are parallel to pathological changes. The bone tissue continues to be formed, but the trabeculae thus formed have uncalcified borders and are resistant to reabsorption by osteoclasts.

Radiological stages of skeletal fluorosis:

- Stage I—axial skeleton involvement and ground-glass appearance of cancellous bone.
- Stage II—thick primary trabeculae merge with sclerotic secondary trabeculae to make bone homogeneously dense, bone contours become uneven and calcification of paraspinous, sacrospinous, and sacrotuberous ligaments is seen.
- Stage III—axial skeletal bones demonstrate the typical radiological features, marked calcification at the insertion of muscles and tendons. There may be overlap of radiological features.

Osteosclerosis (dense bone) is the typical feature of involved axial skeleton [spine, pelvis **(Fig. 36)**, and ribs], whereas as osteoporosis mainly involves the appendicular skeleton. Skeletal fluorosis produces a spectrum of bone changes, including osteoporosis, exostoses, osteomalacia, changes resulting from secondary hyperparathyroidism and their combination. Interosseous membrane calcification is also a prominent features of the disorder **(Fig. 37)** although this may also be seen in X-linked hypophosphatemic rickets, osteogenesis imperfecta type V, bone metastasis, Paget's disease, and osteopetrosis.

Imaging: The best imaging modality to appreciate bony pathology is computed tomography. Computed tomography provides more details than plain radiographs. Calcified ligaments, spinal canal stenosis, and root canal stenosis are also better appreciated with computed tomography.

A fluorotic vertebrae appears hypointense in both T1- and T2-weighted images.

Prevention of Fluorosis

Prevention of fluorosis is better than cure, as no cure is possible once the disease sets in.

Endemic Fluorosis

Defluoridation of drinking water supplies are based on Nalgonda method (named after the village in India where the method was pioneered) of lime and alum, employs the flocculation principle and uses domestic units. The method is based on filtration of fluoride rich water with activated alumina (PAC granules). There is criticism to this technique for possibility of aluminum toxicity also aluminum has been incriminated in the causation of amyotrophic lateral sclerosis (ALS) and Parkinson's disease. Other methods of defluoridation include electrochemical methods, cation exchange resins, florex, etc. Nutrition has a crucial role in the severity of fluorosis, and hence a balanced diet having adequate calcium and vitamins could reduce the toxicity to fluoride.

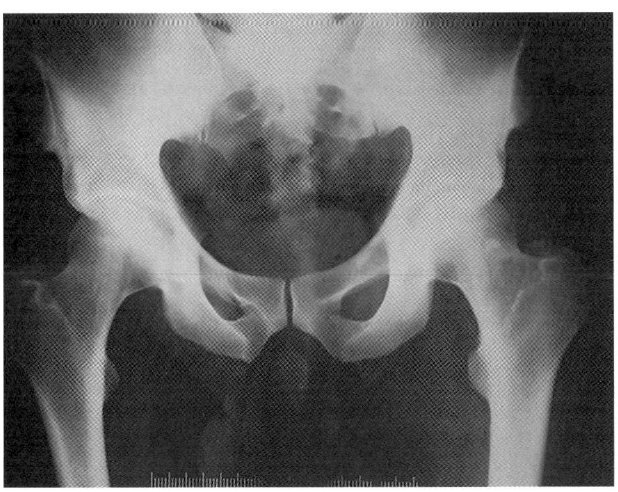

Fig. 36: The plain anteroposterior radiograph of pelvis appears to be an 'underexposed' film but in reality the patient is suffering from fluorosis demonstrating osteosclerosis of pelvic bones and proximal femora.

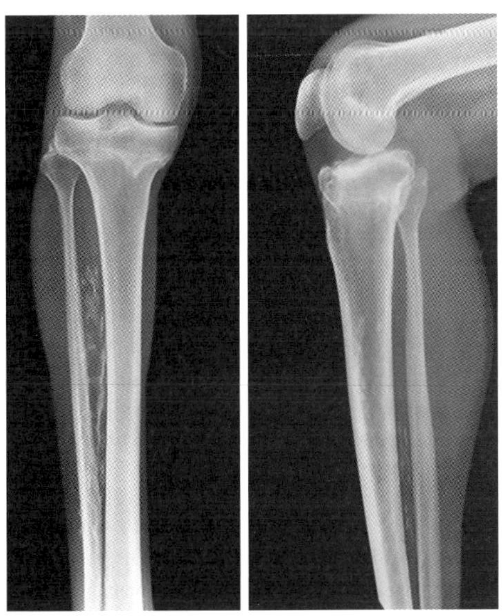

Fig. 37: The tibiofubular interosseous membrane (of the same patient having osteosclerosis of pelvic bones above) demonstrates ectopic calcification which is a prominent feature of fluorosis.

Industrial Fluorosis

A monitoring of urinary fluoride levels should be done in workers in industries and mining exposed to fluorides to keep the levels below 5 ppm. It is observed that skeletal fluorosis does not occur in well-nourished individuals unless the levels exceed >5,000 ppm.

Spine Surgery in Skeletal Fluorosis

Surgery in spine fluorosis is beneficial in the early stage of the disease when only a few spinal segments are involved. The neurological deficits in fluorosis are mainly mechanical. The challenges encountered in operating a fluorotic spine include:

- Difficulty in positioning of the spine during surgery
- Difficulty in intubation during anesthesia because of the rigid cervical spine
- High risk for postoperative respiratory complications because of restricted chest movements and reduced vital capacity.

Operative outcomes with cervical spine operation are better as compared to dorsal spine. Compression at lumbar vertebrae rarely requires decompression.

Causes of cord compression at the level of cervical spine:

- Canal stenosis
- Calcification of ligamentum flavum
- Osteophytes compressing the cord anteriorly
- Ossification of posterior longitudinal ligament (OPLL)
- A combination of these lesions. OPLL is very common in skeletal fluorosis.

Cord compression at the level of dorsal spine is of three types:

1. Localized posterior osteophytes spread over many vertebral levels, though technically feasible for excision, the results are not so rewarding.
2. Localized posterior osteophitic or ossified ligamentous compression, where results are likely to be excellent.
3. Diffuse, extensive where surgery is not beneficial.

INBORN ERRORS OF METABOLISM AFFECTING BONES

GAUCHER'S DISEASE

This autosomal recessive genetic disorder, first described by Gaucher over 100 years ago, is now known to be caused by lack of a specific enzyme glucosylceramide β-glucosidase, which is responsible for the breakdown and the excretion of the cell membrane products from defunct cells. Persistent work on the understanding of pathogenesis of disease has led to development of an effective treatment.

Pathogenesis

On the death of a cell in the body, a glucocerebroside is released from the cell membrane. Before the excretion of the glucocerebroside, the glucoside bond is split by the enzyme glucosylceramide β-glucosidase, which releases the glucose molecules. If there is deficiency of this enzyme, the glucocerebroside are not excreted out of the lysosomal bodies of macrophage of reticuloendothelial system and keeps on accumulating, mainly in the marrow, spleen, and liver. These abnormally accumulated macrophages in the marrow, spleen, and liver are mostly responsible for their enlargement and also secondary changes in the marrow and bone.

Depending on the presence and absence of neurologic involvement, Gaucher's disease is divided into three subtypes:

1. *Type 1:* Non-neuronopathic form
2. *Type 2:* Acute neuronopathic form
3. *Type 3:* Chronic neuronopathic form

Most patients suffer from a chronic form of disorder, with changes predominantly in the marrow, bone, spleen, and varying degree of pancytopenia. A rare form of the disease affecting central nervous system, appear in infancy and usually causes death within a year.

Like other storage disorders, Gaucher's disease is transmitted as an autosomal recessive trait. Males and females are affected equally with relative high incidence in Jewish people of Ashkenazi descent. The phenotype is associated with a large number of different gene defects, five of which appear in the majority of cases.

Clinical Features

In the most common form of disease (type I), patients present in the childhood or adult life with anemia, thrombocytopenia, hepatosplenomegaly or bone pain, about two-thirds of affected people develop skeletal abnormalities. Back pain due to vertebral osteopenia and compression fractures may be the predominant complaint in older patients. Femur neck fractures also are not uncommon; however, diaphyseal fractures are rare. The hemoglobin concentration and platelet counts are usually diminished, there may be elevation of serum acid phosphatase level which is present and is suggestive of diagnosis. The diagnosis can be confirmed by demonstrating low glucocerebrosidase activity in the blood or by identifying abnormal gene mutation in DNA tests.

The orthopedic manifestations of Gaucher's range from osteomyelitis to osteonecrosis. An orthopedic surgeon should recognize them early. Patients with Gaucher's disease are at increased risk of pathological fractures and abnormal bone remodeling, there is increased incidence of delayed and nonunion and there may be increased intraoperative bleeding. Two most common complications of Gaucher's disease are osteomyelitis and osteonecrosis of femoral head, femoral condyle, and proximal humerus. The presentation of osteonecrosis and osteomyelitis may overlap, warranting an accurate diagnosis and appropriate treatment at the earliest. The patients (usually a child or adolescent) may present with an acute bone crisis, with unrelenting pain, local tenderness and restriction of movement, accompanied by pyrexia, leukocytosis, and elevated erythrocyte sedimentation rate (ESR).

Imaging

X-ray shows a variable pattern of radiolucency or patchy density, more marked in cancellous bone. The distal end of femur may be expanded, producing Erlenmeyer flask appearance. A skeletal survey may lead to reversal of osteonecrosis of femoral head, femoral condyles, talus or humeral head.

A radioisotope bone scan may help to distinguish a crises episode from infection, the former is usually "cold" and the latter is "hot". MRI is the most reliable way of defining marrow involvement.

Treatment

Osteonecrosis of femoral head usually results in progressive deformity of the hip. However, most patients manage quiet with symptomatic treatment, and surgery should be deferred for as long as possible. Bone pain may need symptomatic treatment. Specific therapy is in the form of alglucerase enzyme replacement. It has been shown to reverse the blood changes and reduce the size of liver and the spleen. For acute episodes, analgesics and bed rest may relieve the symptoms.

MUCOPOLYSACCHARIDOSES

Introduction

Mucopolysaccharidoses (MPS) are a part of lysosomal storage disease family which occurs due to deficiency or malfunctioning of lysosomal enzymes required for breakdown of glycosaminoglycans (GAGs, formerly called mucopolysaccharides). These GAGs help to build bone, cartilage, tendons, corneas, skin, joint fluid, and other connective tissues. People with MPS, either do not produce enough of one of the eleven enzymes required to breakdown these sugar chains into simpler molecules or they produce defective enzymes resulting in accumulation of partially degraded GAGs in lysosomes and causing symptoms.

Epidemiology

It affects 1 in 25,000 babies and is autosomal recessive disorder, except MPS II which is inherited in X-linked recessive manner. Over time GAGs collect in various organs and connective tissues affecting their function.

Clinical Features

The clinical features are often not apparent at birth, but appear later with progressive storage of GAGs damaging the target organs (bone, connective tissue, and other organs). Damage to neurons from compression of nerves or nerve roots in the spinal cord or in the peripheral nervous system causes pain and impaired motor function. CNS deterioration depends on MPS subtype and affected individuals may have normal intellect or variable retardation of mental functions. Individuals also have variable hearing loss (conductive or sensorineural or both). Recurring respiratory infection are common and many affected individuals have cardiac disease. Vision is affected by cloudy cornea along with degeneration of retina.

Physical symptoms generally include:

- Coarse facial features **(Fig. 38)** (flat nasal bridge, thick lips and enlarged mouth, and tongue)
- Thickened skin

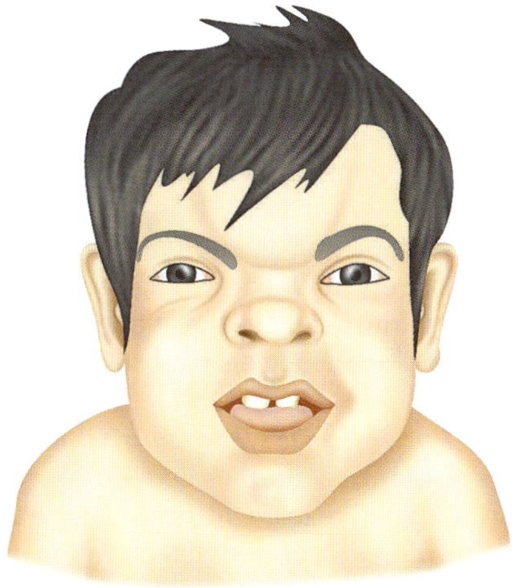

Fig. 38: Rough facial features of mucopolysaccharidosis, also note the frontal bossing, gaped teeth, and gingival hypertrophy with a thickened protruding tongue. The patients are mentally retarded. There is hypertelorism and depressed nasal bridge.

- Excessive body hair growth
- Claw-like hands
- Joint stiffness
- Carpal tunnel syndrome
- Short stature with disproportionately short trunk (dwarfism), dysplasia (abnormal bone size and/or shape), and other skeletal irregularities
- Hepatosplenomegaly
- Hernia

Various types of MPS have been described (MPS V and MPS VIII are no longer recognized): In general, the clinical features of MPS can be grouped as under that present with varying severity.

- *Ophthalmologic disease:* Corneal clouding, glaucoma, chronic papilledema, and retinal degeneration
- *Vestibulocochlear system:* Deafness
- *Central nervous system involvement:* Hydrocephalus and myelopathy, especially in cervical spine due to stenosis
- *Cardiovascular disease:* Hypertension, cardiomegaly, valvular dysfunction, and congestive cardiac failure
- *Abdominal:* Hepatomegaly, umbilical hernia, and inguinal hernia
- *Pulmonary disease:* Airway obstruction, sleep apnea, respiratory compromise, recurrent infections, and cor pulmonale
- *Musculoskeletal disease:* Short stature, joint stiffness, and skeletal abnormalities
- *Peripheral nervous system:* Nerve root compression and peripheral nerve compression neuropathies

MPS I: MPS I is further subdivided into three types (all three types result from an absence of or insufficient levels of enzymes, alpha-L-iduronidase) based on severity of the symptoms:

- *MPS IH (Hurler's syndrome):* It is the most severe of the MPS I subtypes and though normal at birth they usually stop developing between ages of 2 and 4 years. There is progressive mental retardation, limited language development (hearing loss and macroglossia), and loss of physical skills. Vision loss occurs early due to corneal clouding. Children with Hurler's syndrome often die before 10 years from obstructive airway disease, respiratory infections, and cardiac complications.

- *MPS IS (Scheie syndrome):* It is the mildest form of MPS I. The disease is not diagnosed until adulthood as the symptoms are very mild. The average age of presentation is 10–20 years. Intellectually, the children may be normal or may have mild learning disability or severe psychiatric problems.
- *MPS I H-S (Hurler–Scheie syndrome):* It is less severe than Hurler's syndrome. Symptoms generally start appearing between 3 and 8 years. Children may have normal intelligence or moderate mental retardation and learning difficulties. The life expectancy is generally limited till teens or late twenties.

MPS II [Hunter syndrome, iduronate sulfatase deficiency, iduronate-2-sulfatase (IDS) deficiency, sulfoiduronate sulfatase deficiency, SIDS deficiency]. Incidence is 1 in 100,000–150,000 male births.

- Patients with Hunter syndrome are normal at birth, but develop either of the two clinical subtypes by age 2–4 years. Since, it shows X-linked recessive inheritance, the mother alone can pass the defective gene to a son.
- *MPS IIA:* Onset of the disease is at 2–4 years of age. It is a more severe form of Hunter syndrome. The clinical features are similar to that of Hurler's syndrome (MPS I H), but with milder symptoms and no corneal clouding is seen. Whitish skin lesions (Pebbly ivory skin lesions) may appear on upper arms back and upper legs. Cardiomegaly, carpal tunnel syndrome, and cardiac valve abnormalities are common in this disorder. Death from upper airway disease or cardiovascular failure usually occurs by age of 15 years.
- *MPS IIB:* Physical characteristics of MPS IIB are less obvious and progresses at a much slower rate with no hydrocephalus. Persons with MPS IIB may live into their 50s or beyond.

MPS III (Sanfilippo syndrome): The incidence of Sanfilippo syndrome is about 1 in 70,000 births. It is the most common MPS disorder characterized by severe neurological symptoms including progressive dementia, hyperactivity, seizures, aggressive behavior, and inability to sleep for more than a few hours at a time and only minimal somatic involvement. Brain and spinal cord are the main targets. During early disease, the affected children show a marked decline in learning between 2 and 6 years, followed by eventual loss of language skills and loss of some or all hearing. With growth the children acquire an aggressive behavior, hyperactivity, profound dementia and irregular sleep, making them difficult to manage particularly those who retain physical strength. Later children become increasingly unsteady on their feet and most are unable to walk by the age of 10 years. Thickened skin and mild changes in facial features, bone and skeleton structures become noticeable with age, but are much less pronounced. By the age of 10 years, the growth usually stops. Mutations in the *GNS, HGSNAT, NAGLU,* and *SGSH* genes occur in MPS III. There are four distinct types of Sanfilippo syndromes.

1. *Sanfilippo A (mutation of SGSH gene):* Most severe of the MPS III and is caused by missing or altered enzyme heparan N-sulfatase. Children with Sanfilippo A have the shortest survival rate among with those with MPS III disorders.
2. *Sanfilippo B (mutation of NAGLU gene):* Caused by deficient alpha-N-acetylglucosaminidase.
3. *Sanfilippo C (mutation of HGSNAT gene):* Results from mutations in the encoding gene for acetyl-CoA-alpha-glucosaminide acetyltransferase.
4. *Sanfilippo D (mutation of GNS gene):* Due to deficiency of N-acetylglucosamine-6-sulfatase.

Little clinical difference occurs between the four types, but symptoms appear most severe with type A and they live for 8–10 years, following onset of symptoms. For other subtypes, the patients live into their teenage years and some even longer.

MPS IV: Morquio syndrome is a progressive disease that occurs in 1 in 700,000 births and mainly affects skeleton. Its two subtypes result from the missing or deficient enzymes, N-acetylgalactosamine-6-sulfatase (type A, mutation of *GALNS* gene) or beta-galactosidase (type B, mutation of *GLB1* gene) which are required for the breakdown of the keratin sulfate sugar chain. Clinical features though similar in both types are milder in Morquio type B. Symptoms start appearing between age of 1 and 3 years. Skeletal abnormalities include a bell-shaped chest, a flattened curvature of spine, dysplasia of hips, shortened long bones, knock knees and ankles, and wrists. In patients with odontoid hypoplasia and spinal cervical spine, fusion is mandatory. Neurological complications include spinal nerve root compression, conductive and neurosensory loss of hearing, and clouded corneas. Intelligence is normal, but physical growth slows and often stops between 4 and 8 years.

MPS VI: Maroteaux-Lamy syndrome shares physical features as in Hurler's syndrome and usually has normal intellectual development. The disease is progressive with organomegaly that becomes inflamed and scarred later. Complications include deafness, clouded corneas, thickening of the dura and pia compressing nerve roots. Growth is normal at first, but stops suddenly around 8 years. These patients also have dysostosis multiplex (multiple radiologically seen skeletal abnormalities). Nearly all children have some form of heart disease, usually involving valve dysfunction.

MPS VII: MPS VII, Sly syndrome, one of the least common forms of MPS, interestingly was the first autosomal MPS for which chromosomal assignment was achieved. It is caused by deficiency of enzyme β-glucuronidase. In rarest of its forms, there occurs hydrops fetalis, in which large amount of fluid is retained by the body.

MPS IX: Natowicz syndrome or online Mendelian inheritance in man (OMIM) results from hyaluronidase deficiency arising out of heterozygous mutation in the *HYAL1* gene on chromosome 3p21. It is an autosomal recessive disorder.

TABLE 13: The enzyme serum assays and urinary excretion of degradation products in various MPS.

MPS type	*Enzyme deficiency*	*Urinary excretion product*
MPS IH (Hurler's syndrome)	α-L-Iduronidase	Dermatan sulfate, heparan sulfate
MPS IS (Scheie syndrome)	α-L-Iduronidase	Dermatan sulfate, heparan sulfate
MPS I-H/S (Hurler–Scheie syndrome)	α-L-Iduronidase	Dermatan sulfate, heparan sulfate
MPS IIA (Hunter syndrome, severe and mild)	Iduronate sulfatase	Dermatan sulfate, heparan sulfate
MPS IIIA (Sanfilippo syndrome A)	Heparan *N*–sulfatase	Heparan sulfate
MPS IIIB (Sanfilippo syndrome B)	*N*–acetylglucosaminidase	Heparan sulfate
MPS IIIC (Sanfilippo syndrome C)	Acetyl-coenzyme A: Alpha-glucosamine-*N*-acetyl transferase	Heparan sulfate
MPS IIID (Sanfilippo syndrome D)	*N*-acetyl alpha-glucosamine-6-sulfatase	Heparan sulfate
MPS IVA (Morquio syndrome A)	*N*-acetylgalactosamine-6-sulfatase	Keratan sulfate
MPS IVB (Morquio syndrome B)	β-galactosidase	Keratan sulfate
MPS VI (Maroteaux-Lamy)	*N*-acetylgalactosamine-4-sulfatase	Dermatan sulfate
MPS VII (Sly syndrome)	β-glucuronidase	Dermatan sulfate, heparan sulfate

Symptoms include nodular soft tissue masses located around joints with episodes of painful swelling of the masses and pain, the pain that ends spontaneously within 3 days. These arise from the accumulation of nodular aggregates of histiocytes around and within joints.

Diagnosis

Diagnosis is usually established by clinical examination. Urine test [excess mucopolysaccharides are excreted in the urine, **(Table 13)**] and enzyme assays **(Table 13)** are helpful in confirming the diagnosis. Prenatal diagnosis, using amniocentesis (15th–16th week) and chorionic villus sampling (9th week), can verify the fetus either carries a copy of defective gene or is affected with this disorder.

Treatment

At present there is no cure for these disorders. Physical therapy and daily exercises may delay joint problems and improve the ability to move. Changes to the diet will not prevent the disease progression, but limiting milk, sugar, and dairy products has helped some individuals experiencing excessive mucus. Medical treatment is directed at treating systemic conditions and improving the person's life quality. Enzyme replacement therapy has proved useful in reducing non-neurological symptoms and pain. Limited number of enzyme therapies has been introduced with partial benefits demonstrated in various disorders:

- Laronidase is a recombinant human alpha-L-iduronidase polymorphic variant that has been used for treatment of MPS IH and MPS H-S forms. Improved walking capacity and pulmonary function have been reported in these patients.
- Idursulfase is a purified form of human lysosomal IDS and has been used in MPS II with limited success.
- Elosulfase alfa is recently approved for treatment of Moriquio A syndrome (MPS IVA). The treatment has been shown to improve the walking distance in these patients.

Surgery can be done to repair hernia and ventriculoperitoneal shunting to drain excessive cerebrospinal fluid from the brain and decompress nerves (carpal tunnel release). Corrective osteotomy for deformity correction at knee and hip containment surgeries can be done in specific patients. Spinal fusion can prevent progression of kyphosis and scoliosis. Corneal transplantation may improve vision among patients with significant corneal clouding. Bone marrow transplantation (BMT) and umbilical cord blood transplantation (UCBT) have met with limited success in treating MPS. Abnormal physical characteristics other than for those affecting the skeleton and eyes may be improved, but neurological outcome may have varied improvement.

SCURVY

The first concise account of scurvy was written in the 13th century that appeared in Jacques de Vitry's history of the Crusades. Popular accounts of the disease are detailed in descriptions of "Great potato famine" of Europe (1845–48), Portuguese expedition to India in 1497 led by Vasco da Gama and in the "new disease of affluence" (1877–1917) affecting infants in well-to-do families. Scurvy is disease that results from dietary or metabolic vitamin C (ascorbic acid) deficiency. There is failure of collagen synthesis and osteoid formation that ultimately culminates into osteopenia, osteoporosis, and sequelae of spontaneous bleeding.

EPIDEMIOLOGY

The disease is not very common due to improved nutrition and awareness but it is seen in localized areas with high number of migrant population and refugee camps. Classical scurvy has an incidence of nearly 5–8% mostly having bimodal age distribution with male to female ration of 4:3. The first peak is seen during the weaning period of infancy (6 months to 1 year of age) also called infantile scurvy. This is mostly due to orthodox dietary practices prevailing in communities where the weaning diet is deficient in vitamin C. The second peak is seen in patients aged above 60 years where it is often a part of multiple deficiency diseases emanating from malnutrition (Whipple's disease, inflammatory bowel disease, cancer chemotherapy, etc.). Sporadic occurrence of the disease is seen in nomads (dependent on animal milk and donated food), refugee population fed on blended meals and diets primarily comprising of rice, maize, and porridge. Refugees typically depend on external food aids, they have no purchasing power of fresh fruits and vegetables and overcrowding of camps cause rapid disease spread increasing vitamin C requirements.

The daily recommended dose of vitamin C is 30 mg but scurvy can be prevented by 8–10 mg daily intake. Overcooking of food (prevalent in some African population) and deep frying destroys the vitamin C in food causing relative deficiency. Chronic alcoholics are also susceptible due to poor dietary habits. Other at risk population for vitamin C deficiency are people on fad diet, prisoners, widowers living alone unaccustomed to cooking and surprisingly hospital patients! Because vitamin C has a role in iron absorption so scurvy is commonly associated with iron-deficiency anemia.

PATHOPHYSIOLOGY

Invoking collagen metabolism from Chapter on "Bone Structure, Physiology, Metabolism, and Associated Disorders", we know that collagen synthesis and crosslinking depends primarily upon the hydroxylation of proline and lysine. Vitamin C (L-ascorbic acid) is an important cofactor for this process. Humans cannot synthesize L-ascorbic acid because the enzyme L-gluconolactone oxidase is nonfunctional so we solely depend on dietary sources.

When the whole blood vitamin C content falls to a level below 0.3 mg/100 mL (total body pool <300 mg), the metabolic abnormalities arise and clinical signs of scurvy appear. Vitamin C deficiency prevents hydroxyproline and hydroxylysine formation and there is deficiency of chondroitin sulfate. These "nonhydroxylated" proline and lysine residues prevent hydrogen bond formation and crosslinking so the mechanical stability of structure is quite low. Also the mineralization holes within collagen matrix are missing so osteoid mineralization does not occur. Cartilage cells of the epiphyseal plate multiply and orientate themselves normally. Intervening matrix becomes partly calcified, but osteoblasts fail to properly lay down osteoid so demineralized bone deposition occurs. The calcified cartilaginous matrix is also not completely resorbed due to metabolic abnormality. In a nutshell, hence, there is failure to lay down bony matrix, associated with persistence of an unabsorbed calcified cartilage lattice. Radiologically, this appears as osteopenia and epiphyseal plate widening and irregularity (see below for details). Also, the irregular matrix calcification appears as spicules of calcified cartilage that fracture and a very irregular radiologically dense zone arises at the junction of epiphysis and shaft. Failure of cartilage matrix resorption also makes ring sign.

NATURAL HISTORY AND CLINICAL PRESENTATION

Adults have stores for 160–200 days of vitamin C even if dietary deficiency occurs. Mild vitamin C deficiency (total body vitamin C pool of <600 mg and plasma levels of <0.75 mg/dL) is common in general population with intermittent occurrence due to dietary inconsistencies but this never leads to full-blown disease. The signs are lassitude, fatigue, anorexia, muscular weakness (due to reduced carnitine production), and increased susceptibility to infection. There is some suggestion of increased risk of ischemic heart disease or hypertension. This is the period of latent scurvy occurring before manifest disease.

Mild deficiency can progress to marginal deficiency where there is a combination of low dietary intake with factors such as smoking, stress, chronic disease, and diabetes mellitus. There may additionally be shortness of breath and dry and rough skin along with symptoms of latent disease.

Clinical presentation of full blown scurvy (total blood pool levels <300 mg and plasma levels of <0.3 mg/100 mL) can be summarized as follows:

- Infants are irritable
- The skin is dry and rough
- Peripheral edema
- Hemorrhagic manifestation:
  - Gums may bleed spontaneously.
  - Subperiosteal hemorrhage in bones may cause excruciating pain and tenderness.
  - Joints are painful and swollen with intra-articular hemorrhages and reactive synovitis producing limb deformities. The child refrains from moving the limbs—pseudoparalysis.
  - Hemorrhage around erupting teeth and loosening of tooth.
- Fractures or epiphyseal separation may occur.
- Variable degree of anemia (iron absorption abnormalities and folic acid metabolism alteration) + hemorrhages
- Moeller-Barlow disease in infants (5–6 months of age)—(some texts mention Barlow disease as combination of Scurvy and Rickets)
  - Irritability, tenderness of the legs, and pseudoparalysis, usually involving the lower limbs
  - "Pithed-frog" position—legs flexed at the knees and hips partially flexed
  - Costochondral beading (Scorbutic rosary)—there is angular step-off at the costochondral junction that is different from the rounded and nodular thickening of rickety rosary.
  - Petechial hemorrhages in the skin
- Adults develop follicular hyperkeratosis in skin along with petechial hemorrhages
- Poor wound healing
- Hematuria, hematemesis, and bloody diarrhea may occur.
- Severe joint pains and difficulty in breathing
- Myocardial disease due to scorbutic hemorrhages

RADIOLOGICAL FEATURES OF MANIFEST SCURVY

The radiological changes are most marked at wrists, knees, sternal ends of ribs, and in areas of rapid bone growth in children **(Fig. 39)**.

- *Generalized bone rarefaction:* Most prominent in long bone metaphyses (may be associated with pathological fracture or deformity). It appears as ground-glass osteopenia due to reduced trabeculations.

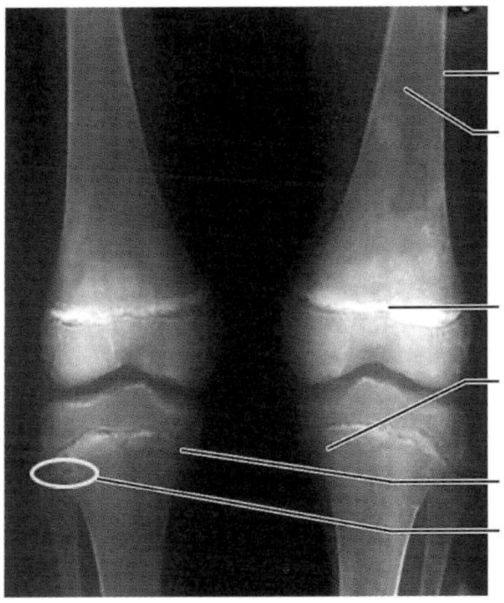

Fig. 39: Common radiological features of scurvy.

- The cortices of bones thin out (pencil thin cortices) merging subtly into the intramedullary region.
- *Metaphyseal lucency (Trummerfeld zone, scorbutic zone):* This is present adjacent to calcified physeal zone of Frankel as a lucent line (because of metaphyseal rarefaction it is even more distinctive due to contrasting calcification). It is so common to find that it has got distinctive identity of "scurvy line".
- Metaphyseal spongiosa is weak and corner fractures occur through the weakened lucent parts results in cupping of the metaphysis.
- The osteopenic metaphyseal clefts at the edges appear due to infarction of meta-epiphyseal junction ("corner sign" of Park).
- Zone of provisional calcification may extend beyond the outer margins of metaphysis causing periosteal elevation and appears as marginal spur formation (Pelkan spurs). These extend at right angles away from the shaft axis and may also fracture from the zone appearing separate from it.
- Normal calcification in growing cartilage produces dense transverse bands:
  - *At juxtaepiphysial zones (Frankel white line):* This is the widened zone of provisional calcification distinctively separating metaphysis from epiphysis.
  - Around ossific centers of the epiphyses (Wimberger's ring sign)
- Subperiosteal hematomas appear as soft tissue swellings or periosseous calcification due to lifting of periosteum and associated periosteal reaction.

DIAGNOSIS

- Classical history of dietary deficiency
- Clinical features as above
- Low levels of vitamin C in plasma/serum (maximum levels are 1.4 mg/100 mL and levels below 0.1 mg/100 mL (= 0.3 mg/100 mL of whole blood) are mostly associated with scurvy)
- Low urinary excretion rate

PREVENTION AND TREATMENT

Since a long time antiscorbutic foods have been identified and recommended by all kith-and-kins. These include apple, peas, pomegranates, cucumbers, citrons, lemons, muscats, onions, berries, and pickled vegetables. Awareness of these classically originated from sailors accounts that prevented development of bleeding gums and foul smell of mouth by use of these dietary addendums.

Vitamin C was initially identified as "hexuronic acid" and later named Ascorbic acid the "L"-form of which is equated with vitamin C. L-ascorbic acid is reversibly converted to dehydroascorbic acid, which together constitutes the active form of vitamin C. The recommended daily allowance of vitamin C has not been defined, but generally, it is considered to be around 30 mg. Indian goose berry (amla) and green chillies are rich sources of vitamin. It is a heat labile vitamin so overcooking destroys it. The fresh fruits should be consumed raw for optimal absorption. Fortification of food items with vitamin C is common and has reduced the incidence of latent and manifest disease to a large extent. Medical supplementation of vitamin C should be done in patients with chronic malnutrition and population at risk as previously discussed. Even still if a manifest disease occurs then the treatment is symptomatic including rest to body parts and splinting to reduce limb pains supplemented with large doses (250 mg oral three to four times daily) of vitamin C bring prompt relief. Megadoses of 1 g/day intravenous are indicated in malabsorption where oral doses will not get absorbed.

CONCLUSION

- Though bone is a hard tissue it is a metabolically active tissue taking part actively in calcium and phosphate metabolism among others.
- The bone is subjected to various metabolic disorders by virtue of active participation in mineral metabolism. Osteoporosis is probably the most rampant of the disorder in the world and is the most common metabolic disorder of bone. Every orthopedic surgeon, whether trauma specialist or reconstruction or sports physician will encounter the disorder in his practice and should be well versed in identifying and treating the disorder meticulously to prevent associated morbidity and mortality.
- One must also try to keep abreast with the drug interactions and use of newer drugs for the management of osteoporosis as they are emerging.
- Rickets is a common disorder in India, especially in the underprivileged population and must be handled in association with pediatrician for associated abnormalities and complete management.
- Metabolic disorders due to enzyme deficiencies are quite challenging to manage, however, supportive care should be provided to the patients as best as we can. Emerging therapies will possibly provide the unfortunate patients with cure someday.

CHAPTER 4

Infections of Bone (Typical and Atypical) and Surgical Site Infection

Manish Kumar Varshney

INTRODUCTION

Orthopedic infections include septic arthritis, prosthetic joint infections, spinal infections [diskitis, vertebral osteomyelitis (OM), and epidural abscess], osteitis/OM, atypical foot infections, diabetic foot OM, and part of surgical site infections (SSI). These infections are becoming more common because of an aging population, an increase in prosthetic joints and increased prevalence of operative orthopedics, and medical comorbidities like diabetes. This chapter deals with the infections of bone (typical and atypical) along with atypical feet infections and SSI. Osteitis/OM is common and remains challenging to treat. Presence of prosthetic devices, hardware from trauma and corrective surgeries, and instrumentation is the major cause of more than doubling of incidence of bone infections and the accrued costs. It is imperative to make a small differentiation between osteitis and OM as it becomes confusing to read different texts that refer these terms discretely. Osteitis is a pyogenic infection mostly that propagates centripetally beginning from the bone surface (cortex) progressing inward. It mostly results from exposed bone that subsequently gets infected like in open trauma or from poor surgery. The surrounding soft tissue is also additionally involved with the primary infection. Some authors define purulent and nonpurulent osteitis that is further subdivided into acute purulent, subacute purulent, and chronic purulent osteitis based on clinical findings. Hofmann proposed two clinical presentations of osteitis.

1. *Acute postoperative osteitis:* Here, the bacterial infection occurs within 8 weeks of trauma or an operation.
2. *Chronic osteitis:* Here, the infection in bone and surrounding soft tissues occurs >8 weeks after treatment or injury.

Osteomyelitis is a more common presentation of bone infection seen in children and immunocompromised adults where the primary infection is in the metaphyseal region of bone very close to marrow or stay within it; that then propagates peripherally to involve the bone and surrounding structures. If arrested in early stages by proper treatment then bone cortex may not be involved per se. Anyway both osteitis and OM are similar in presentation in later stages and "osteitis" is not a preferred term in literature. So, the discussion of osteitis will be rested here and throughout the text the term "osteomyelitis" will be used and described.

HISTORY AND EPIDEMIOLOGY

The oldest known evidence of OM is found in the fractured spine of a *Dimetrodon* Permian reptile, which existed 291–250 million years ago. Bromfield, in 1773, used the term "abscessus in medulla" and advised early decompression. Smith used the term "necrosis" indicating the death of bone. Nelaton introduced the term "osteomyelitis" in 1844. Pasteur used the term "a boil of bone" to describe bone infection. Winnett Orr is credited with the use of both conservative and radical measures to treat OM in preantibiotic era. Recently, the incidence of acute hematogenous OM is decreasing in incidence, whereas the incidence of OM due to direct inoculation or contiguous focus of infection is increasing. Possibly this is related to improvement in general health and increased vehicular trauma and orthopedic surgery. OM secondary to open fractures occurs in 3–25% of cases, usually in young men. 15% of patients with diabetic foot develop OM. Osteomyelitic affection of spine occurs in 2–4% of all cases of OM and is usually hematogenous. Elderly men are more commonly affected than women.

OSTEOMYELITIS

"Osteomyelitis" refers to a primary infection of the bone marrow (myelitis) with subsequent affection of the bone (cortex) and periosteum. The term was coined by Nelaton in 1844. OM is generally categorized into acute or chronic forms based on histopathological findings. Using these pathological and anatomical criteria, the differentiation between acute and chronic hematogenous OM and acute and chronic exogenous (post-traumatic or postoperative) osteitis has been elucidated by many authors. I will refer to infection of bone as OM throughout the chapter and the book as distinction between these two terms is very difficult in clinical practice and it hardly ever makes any difference in management. The acute and chronic forms of OM strictly represent a spectrum (developing temporally) of bone infection that should be understood in continuity.

Only rarely chronic OM will develop without acute form (like in subclinical implant related OM). The distinction between acute and chronic forms is "strictly *not* based on duration". The presence of necrotic bone, as determined by absence of living osteocytes, defines chronic OM. However, as the chronic form takes some time (few weeks to 6 weeks) to develop (recognized by necrotic bone and reactive bone formation) so quite often surgeons refer to chronic form as developing after 6 weeks. The diagnosis of these forms is based on specific findings **(Boxes 1 and 2)**. Because bone necrosis sets in 10 days (histopathologically) following persistence of pus/acute OM, it should be considered that chronic form has begun and practically also treatment alteration is required in patients with persistent symptoms after 10–14 days of treatment for acute OM. Chronic OM is defined with the identification of sequestrum that requires 4–6 weeks for identification on radiographs so this is the often quoted time duration for chronic OM to develop in various texts. The differentiation of acute from chronic can be summarized under following clinical features:

Acute Osteomyelitis

- Infection present for <6 weeks
- *Inflammatory symptoms and signs:* Fever with or without chills, malaise. Presence of pain, limited range of motion (ROM), and redness, and warmth or swelling at infection site.

BOX 1: Diagnostic criteria for acute osteomyelitis.

Peltola and Vahvanen's criteria (Two of the listed findings must be present for establishing the diagnosis):
- Pus on aspiration from affected bone
- Positive bacterial culture from bone tissue or blood (50% cases)
- *Clinical features (signs and symptoms) of acute osteomyelitis (OM) (often absent in adults):* Lethargy, irritability, fever, local bone tenderness, local limb swelling, local erythema, local rise of temperature, pseudoparalysis, and effusion in nearby joint or reduced movements
- Typical radiographic changes of OM

Morrey and Peterson's criteria (Determines the likelihood of having OM):
- *Definite:* Pathogen isolated from bone or adjacent soft tissue or there is histologic evidence of OM
- *Probable:* A blood culture is positive in the setting of clinical and radiographic features of OM
- *Likely:* Typical clinical settings and definite radiographic evidence of OM are present and there is a response to antibiotic therapy

BOX 2: Diagnostic criteria for chronic osteomyelitis (OM) (the list represents diagnostic ability of the characteristics in decreasing order).

- Imaging studies demonstrating sequestrum and contiguous soft tissue infection
- Clinical signs
  - Discharge of bone pieces from sinus tract
  - Exposed bone
  - Persistent sinus tract with or without frank pus discharge
  - Necrotic tissue overlying bone
  - Nonhealing wound exposing surgical hardware
  - Nonhealing wound overlying fracture
- Laboratory evaluation
  - Positive blood cultures
  - Increased C-reactive protein level
  - Increased erythrocyte sedimentation rate

- Decompression, evacuation of pus, and antibiotic treatment targeted to the specific infectious organism are the primary treatment.

Chronic Osteomyelitis

- Infection presents usually for >6 weeks
- Demonstrable sequestrum formation
- Symptoms are nonspecific but few characteristic ones should be looked for **(Box 2)**
- Patients with associated morbidity such as diabetes mellitus (DM), immunosuppression, rheumatoid arthritis, etc. are at higher risk for chronic OM
- Treatment is surgical debridement of the infected bone along with antibiotics and reconstruction of structural bone damage.

Subacute Osteomyelitis

Apart from the above two, a third "primary subacute pyogenic OM" (sometimes called "primary chronic OM") has also been recognized (described by Harris and Kirkaldy-Willis in 1965) that develops within one to several months. They described two types, one with abscess formation (metaphyseal) and the other without (diaphyseal, **Fig. 1**). The latter may have "onion skin" type periosteal reaction confusing with Ewing's sarcoma. The classification by Robert et al. (modified Denhill classification) classifies subacute OM into six types depending on morphology, location, and bone reaction to infection **(Box 3)**.

The above classification of OM into acute, subacute, and chronic forms is an oversimplification but is quite practical (for management perspective). The Lew and Waldvogel system **(Box 4)** divides OM into the categories of hematogenous, contiguous, and chronic. The other best known and popular staging system is the University of Texas Medical Branch (UTMB) clinical staging system for adult OM introduced by Cierny et al. **(Box 5 and Fig. 2)**. The Lew-Waldvogel system classifies the affection of bone arising out of hematogenous seeding (endogenous) or contiguous spread

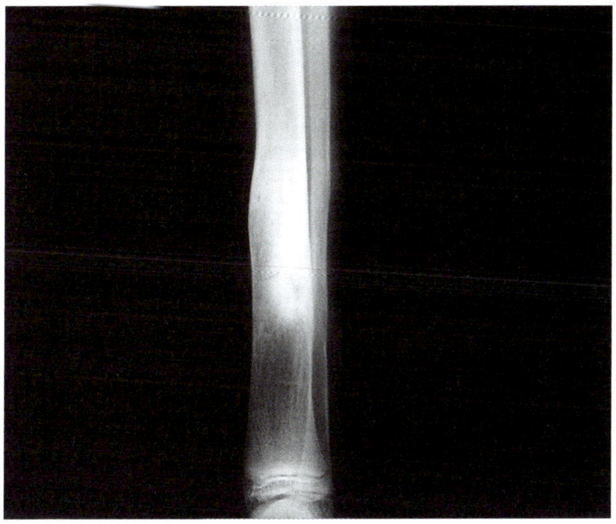

Fig. 1: Subacute osteomyelitis.

BOX 3: Classification for subacute osteomyelitis (Roberts et al.).

- *Stage 1a:* Solitary punched out radiolucency (margins normal)
- *Stage 1b:* Localized radiolucent zone with sclerotic margins (Brodie's abscess)
- *Stage 2:* Large radiolucent lesion usually metaphyseal with cortical erosion
- *Stage 3:* Localized cortical and periosteal reaction
- *Stage 4:* Linear single or multiple (onion skin) periosteal reaction
- *Stage 5:* Central lucency in epiphysis with fine sclerotic margins
- *Stage 6:* Destructive process involving vertebral body

BOX 4: Lew and Waldvogel classification system for osteomyelitis.

- *Hematogenous osteomyelitis (OM):* Bacterial seeding of bone occurs from blood (bacteremia). More than 95% cases in children (discussed in detail in pathophysiology) and 20% in adults. Metaphysis of long bones in children and vertebrae in elderly (>50 years) are common sites on affection. Vertebral OM could be pyogenic (10–15%, including diskitis) or chronic granulomatous (80–85% cases, often tubercular) and rarely fungal or actinomycotic. In intravenous (IV) drug abusers (young adults) the common sites of affection are vertebra, pubic symphysis, sternoclavicular joints, and sacroiliac joints.
- Osteomyelitis secondary to contiguous focus of infection (surgical procedure, trauma, open fractures, chronic soft tissue infection, decubitus ulcer, diabetic foot, and cellulitis)
  - No generalized vascular disease
  - Generalized vascular disease—usually diabetics and generalized atherosclerosis and neuropathic joints
- Chronic OM (necrotic bone)

BOX 5: Cierney–Mader system for classifying osteomyelitis (OM).

*Anatomic type **(Fig. 2)**:*
- *Type 1:* Medullary OM—limited to medullary cavity, usually single organism, hematogenous or intramedullary implants
- *Type 2:* Superficial OM—involves cortex but not marrow or endosteum (akin to osteitis), contiguous soft tissue infection is the cause, often mixed microbiology and local vascular compromise common.
- *Type 3:* Localized OM—involves a part of bone but in entire thickness (from cortex to medulla)
- *Type 4:* Diffuse OM—involves whole diameter of bone and involvement could be extensive

Physiologic class:
- *A host:* Healthy with normal physiologic, metabolic, and immune functions. Good prognosis
- *B host:*
  - *Bs:* Systemic compromise
  - *Bl:* Local compromise
  - *Bls:* Local and systemic compromise
- *C host:* Treatment worse than the disease, health does not allow full treatment

Factors affecting immune surveillance, metabolism, and local vascularity:
- *Systemic factors (Bs):* Anemia and hypoxemia, malnutrition, renal or hepatic failure, DM, chronic hypoxia, immune disease, extremes of age, immunosuppression or immune deficiency, and steroid abuse
- *Local factors (Bl):* Chronic lymphedema, venous stasis, peripheral vascular disease, major vessel compromise, arteritis, extensive scarring, radiation fibrosis, small-vessel disease, neuropathy, and tobacco abuse

(exogenous) and the vascular insufficiency (ischemic form arising from traumatic, pathological, or iatrogenic event). In common practice, the diabetic foot may represent "ischemic form" of OM. The system recognizes chronic OM as a distinct form. The Cierny and Madar system is a comprehensive system that is based primarily on the part of affected bone, physiological status of the patient, and the risk factors that affect immunity, metabolism, and vascularity. Although it does not recognize chronic form of bone infection but in our view, it is best suited for classifying chronic OM itself. The few other authors have also classified the OM for their study purpose but are not as popular **(Table 1)**. The distinction

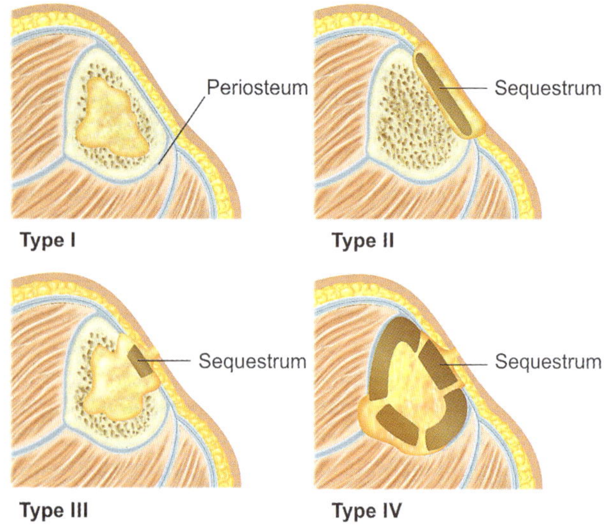

Fig. 2: Anatomic types of osteomyelitis (*see* **Box 5** for details).

TABLE 1: Other less popular classification systems for osteomyelitis (OM).

Author	*Classification and its basis*
Ger R (1977)	Soft-tissue condition: • *Type 1:* Simple sinus • *Type 2:* Chronic superficial ulcer • *Type 3:* Multiple sinuses • *Type 4:* Multiple skin lined sinuses
Kelly et al. (1984)	Etiopathogenesis: • Hematogenous OM • Post-traumatic (united fracture) • Post-traumatic (nonunited fracture) • Postsurgical anatomopathological • *Type 1:* Open, without bone infection • *Type 2:* Circumferential, cortical, and endosteal infection • *Type 3:* Cortical and endosteal infection associated with segmental bone loss
Weilan (1984)	Weilan defined chronic OM as a wound with exposed bone, positive culture, findings, and drainage for >6 months • *Type I:* Open exposed bone without evidence of bone infection but positive soft tissue infection • *Type II:* Circumferential, cortical, and endosteal infection with sequestration and involucrum formation • *Type III:* Cortical and endosteal infection with segmental bone defect
Gordon et al. (1988)	Bone defect: • *Type A:* Tibial defect and nonunion without segmental loss • *Type B:* Tibial defect <3 cm, intact fibula • *Type C:* Tibial defect >3 cm, no intact fibula
Romano et al. (2006)	Bone defect: • *Type 1:* Cavitary defect • *Type 2:* Epiphyseal defect • *Type 3:* Segmental defect
Romano et al. (2011)	"Seven item classification system" of bone and joint infection

of OM into "primary" and "secondary" forms representing endogenous and exogenous infection is practically succinct but nondescriptive and confusing; so it should be dropped.

PATHOGENESIS

The older theories for development of OM have been traditionally engrained in the minds of orthopedic surgeons that it is imperative for a comprehensive text to mention them.

Hobo's observations and hypothesis: Japanese researcher Teruo Hobo published a paper in German which suggested that acute OM developed in the metaphysis of long bones because of "poor phagocytic activity" in metaphysis **(Fig. 3)**. He injected Chinese ink in the nutrient artery system that was evenly distributed throughout for first 6 hours but after that the ink disappeared from diaphysis persisting in metaphysis however. He concluded that phagocytosis is much active in diaphysis compared to metaphysis leading to persistent bacteria developing OM. Other investigators (Trueta), however, related these findings due to sluggish circulation through the "hair-pin bends" of arterioles at metaphysis (see criticism to this view further in modern concept). The infection then develops in the "blood lakes" of slow metaphyseal circulation.

"Starr from Toronto" explained the progression and course of abscess **(Fig. 4)**. He stated that the inflammatory reaction and abscess formation at metaphysis under pressure travels through Haversian and Volkmann's canals to erupt under the periosteum. The adjacent joints are protected by the tight attachment of periosteum to the growth ring. The periosteal vessels get thrombosed and intramedullary vessels are already disrupted thus the blood supply to the cortex is lost and the part of bone becomes avascular. The pus then re-enters the cortex at some other place infecting the medullary cavity setting up another focus. He also supported the concept that individual's general resistance to bacterial aggression somehow determines susceptibility to develop OM.

Wilenski concept: He proposed that the site of bone involvement purely depends on the occlusion of blood vessel at particular site by the septic embolus. If main artery is involved then whole bone is affected **(Fig. 5)**, however, if upper or lower branch is involved then corresponding part will be affected. Embolism of terminal arterioles produces lesion at bone ends and subperiosteal abscess results if periosteal vessels are predominantly involved.

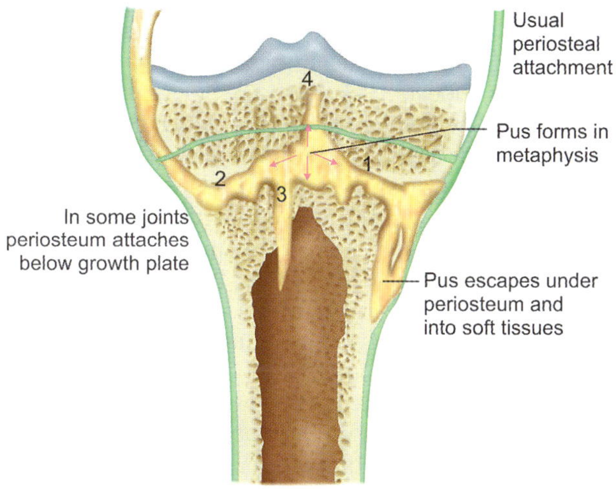

Fig. 4: Pathways of progression of pus: (1) The usual route is, for the pus, to break under periosteum reaching the space through the Haversian system or perivascular space around nutrient vessels. If the periosteum is thick and hard and does not give way; it gets lifted shutting the blood supply to underlying bone forming a cylindrical sequestrum as in infants and young children as seen in **Figure 5**; (2) In some joints (see text), the metaphysis is intra-articular and pus may enter the joint space; also in younger children, the joint capsule is not very strongly adherent to the bone so that the pus under tension can track to joint causing septic arthritis; (3) If the pus does not find its way underneath periosteum and forms proximally in metaphysis, it may directly track into medullary canal causing extensive myelitis as depicted in **Figure 3** also; (4) In infants and adolescents around puberty, the transphyseal vessels are open paving a path for pus to travel to epiphysis and joint causing septic arthritis.

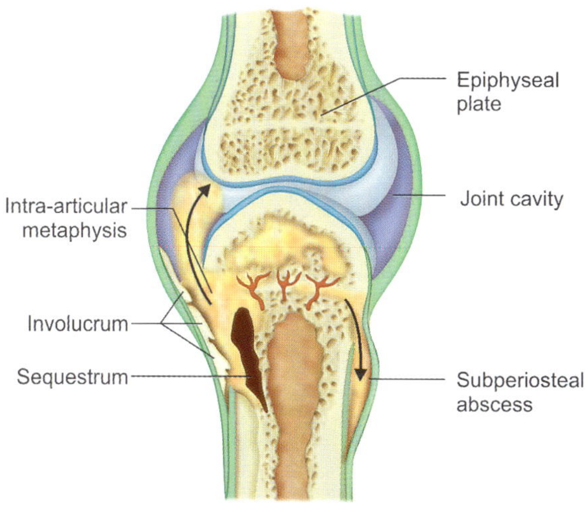

Fig. 3: The common method of development and progression of unchecked acute osteomyelitis.

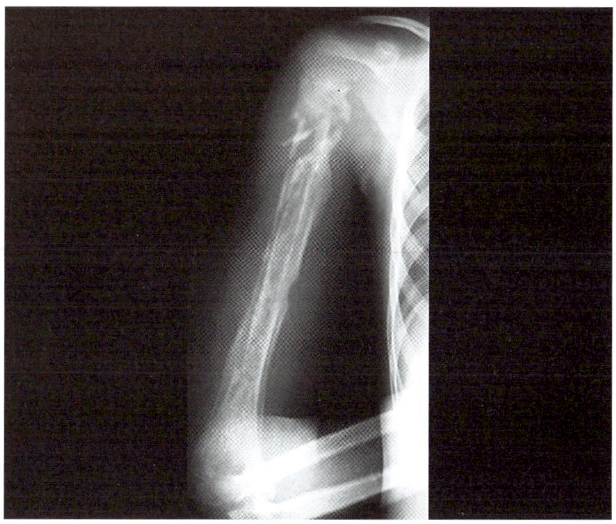

Fig. 5: Whole humerus shaft becoming a sequestrum.

Trueta's hypothesis: Trueta (1968) in his attempt to correlate the clinical features with his hypothesis of underlying pathology described three clinical stages.

1. *Stage I:* He described this as a "boil" in the bone. There is severe constant pain described as "deep" or "in the bone" and is often "not" localized (a bit diffuse) at the focus of infection. Exquisite tenderness is but accurately localized. The inflammatory signs are absent. The exudate passes through the cortex but not to the diaphysis.
2. *Stage II:* There is pus in the medulla and the subperiosteal space. The symptoms and signs are more marked, and systemic symptoms such as malaise, fever, other aches, and pains appear.
3. *Stage III:* The inflammation spreads to soft tissues with characteristic signs of acute inflammation.

The above proposed staged progression may seem logical but this prolonged development and subperiosteal appearance of pus from the formation of exudate and slow transgress through the cortex has been challenged by consistent findings of pus within 48 hours beneath the periosteum. Also, his view of no or late involvement only of diaphysis is also not supported.

Trueta is also credited with the recognition of three types of OM (1959) based on the blood supply, the infantile, childhood, and the adult form of disease. There is a difference in OM in children and adults (summarized in **Table 2**). The site of involvement varies in children according to the blood supply, described in detail by Trueta is presented briefly here:

- In infants, the metaphyseal blood vessels cross the growth plate thus the infection can traverse the physis involving the epiphysis in the process (*see* also Chapter on Septic Arthritis). This can quickly involve the joint also. There is commonly a growth disturbance later as a sequel **(Fig. 6)** to involvement and destruction of the physis if treatment is not prompt (otherwise also the morbidity is high). The bone is thin, weak, and immature giving way easily to the pus under pressure so extensive devascularization and large sequestrum formation do not occur. Pus is, however, copious. Cortical damage is transient while a large involucrum forms due to high regenerating potency of periosteum.
- In childhood, the growth plate and the epiphysis are usually spared and the infection remains limited to metaphysis and proximally. The subperiosteal extension of pus and endosteal thrombosis produce extensive devascularization of the bone and large sequestrum (sometimes whole diaphysis—cylindrical sequestrum) are seen in late presentations **(Fig. 5)**. The cortical damage is hence extensive with prompt involucrum formation. Growth disturbance is rarely seen only with extensive aggressive disease reaching the germinal layer of growth plate, else in common presentations some growth stimulation is common due to increased vascularity. Joint involvement is rare but can occur if:
  - Metaphysis is intracapsular—hip, **(Fig. 7)** proximal humerus, proximal radius, and distal fibula.
  - Iatrogenic seeding occurs while drainage of pus/aspiration.
  - Vessels cross to epiphysis from metaphysis (as in infants).
  - Some envisage weak adherence of periosteum to growth ring as a reason for "leak" of pus beneath periosteum from metaphyseal to epiphyseal and intra-articular region.
- *The adult form:* Osteomyelitis is often due to contiguous spread. Long bone involvement in hematogenous spread is rare. Infected bone is resorbed leaving behind a cavity **(Figs. 8A to D)**. Whole bone involvement and later development of chronic OM are common.

"Morrisey and Haynes" proposed the concept of trauma (as focalizing influence) to delicate metaphyseal circulation

TABLE 2: Differences in the osteomyelitis (OM) in children and adults.

Osteomyelitis in children	*Osteomyelitis in adults*
Usually hematogenous	Usually due to direct inoculation
Metaphyseal location	• Hematogenous (20%)—vertebral commonly other bony sites are commonly seen in IV drug abusers • Traumatic or direct inoculation—any site
Periosteal reaction—frequent and copious	Periosteal reaction—infrequent/subdued
Sequestrum formation is frequent	Bone is often resorbed forming a lytic cavity
Systemic features are common	Less pronounced
Blood cultures often positive	Blood culture often negative
Conversion to chronic form—less common	Commonly converts to chronic form
• *Organisms—Infants:* Group B streptococci • *Children: Staphylococcus aureus, Streptococcus pyogenes, H. influenzae*	• Polymicrobial in 30–50% cases, coagulase positive and negative staphylococci, Gram-negative bacilli (vertebral OM) • *IV drug abusers: P. aeruginosa, Candida* • *Prosthetic infection: Staphylococcus epidermidis*

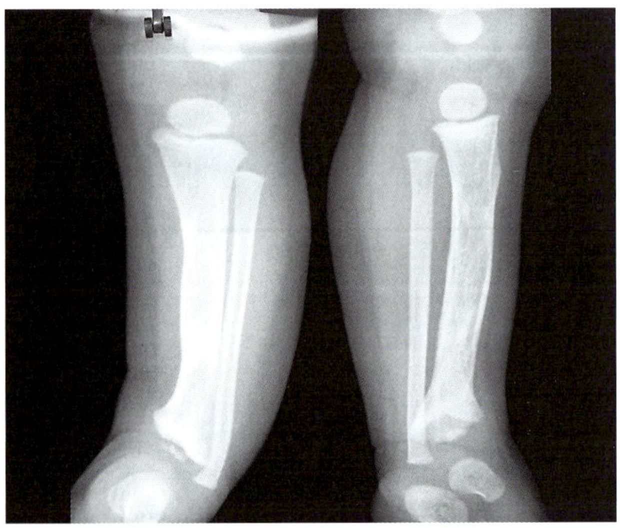

Fig. 6: Postosteomyelitic deformity.

that possibly leads to hematoma formation. This along with local immune deficit supports a lodged bacterium to preferentially localize and thrive; thus, developing infection.

MODERN CONCEPT AND UNDERSTANDING OF OSTEOMYELITIS

Compared to the classical concepts, in the present era there is a very discrete understanding of the development of bone infections. The condition may arise from trauma, bacteremia (distant focus of infection), contiguous focus of infection (nearby abscess or cellulitis) such as those associated with diabetic foot ulcerations and surgery, or orthopedic implants that disrupt the integrity of the bone. But, mere presence of bacteria does not lead to development of bone infection. Once the homeostasis (the equilibrium/stability in the normal body states) of the body has been altered even an innocuous bacteria can enter the body and proliferate.

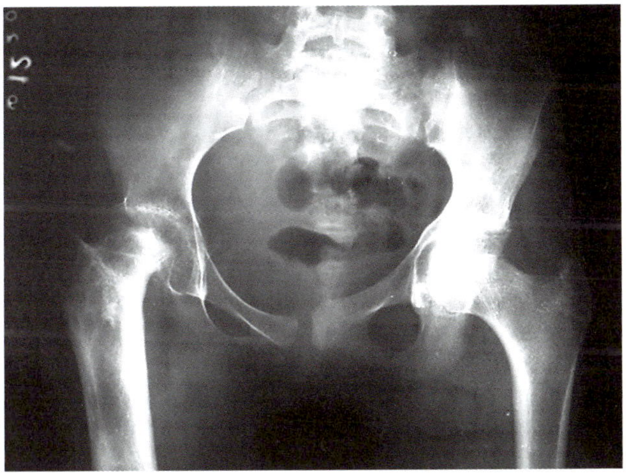

Fig. 7: Patient with osteomyelitis of right proximal femur with secondary hip involvement causing chondro-osteolysis of the femoral head. The hip joint is part of intracapsular so the infection from proximal femur can easily percolate into the joint.

Pathogenesis of acute OM: The bacteria lodge adjacent to the physis, probably in relation to terminal metaphyseal vessels. These vessels are "open-ended" (and *not* looped or "hair-pin bends" as visualized by Trueta and Hobo), as they tunnel between the columns of dividing and decaying physeal cartilage cells. The fact that the vessels enter into "open-circulation" is important for chondrotropic pathogenic bacteria to adhere to cartilage cells at the junction between the physis and metaphysis (see "homing of bacteria" below to understand localization of bacteria to these places). The sluggish flow may not be important at all. With bone growth the branches develop from the extended vessels and may anastomose (that Hobo and Trueta visualized). The bacteria here divide thriving on dead chondrocytes; produce acute inflammation and tissue death secondary to ischemia from either venous or arterial obstruction. There is liquefactive necrosis of medullary tissue. The trabeculae of cancellous bone lose their vascularity and die remaining in the pus as small sequestra **(Figs. 9A to D)**. Second concept is with

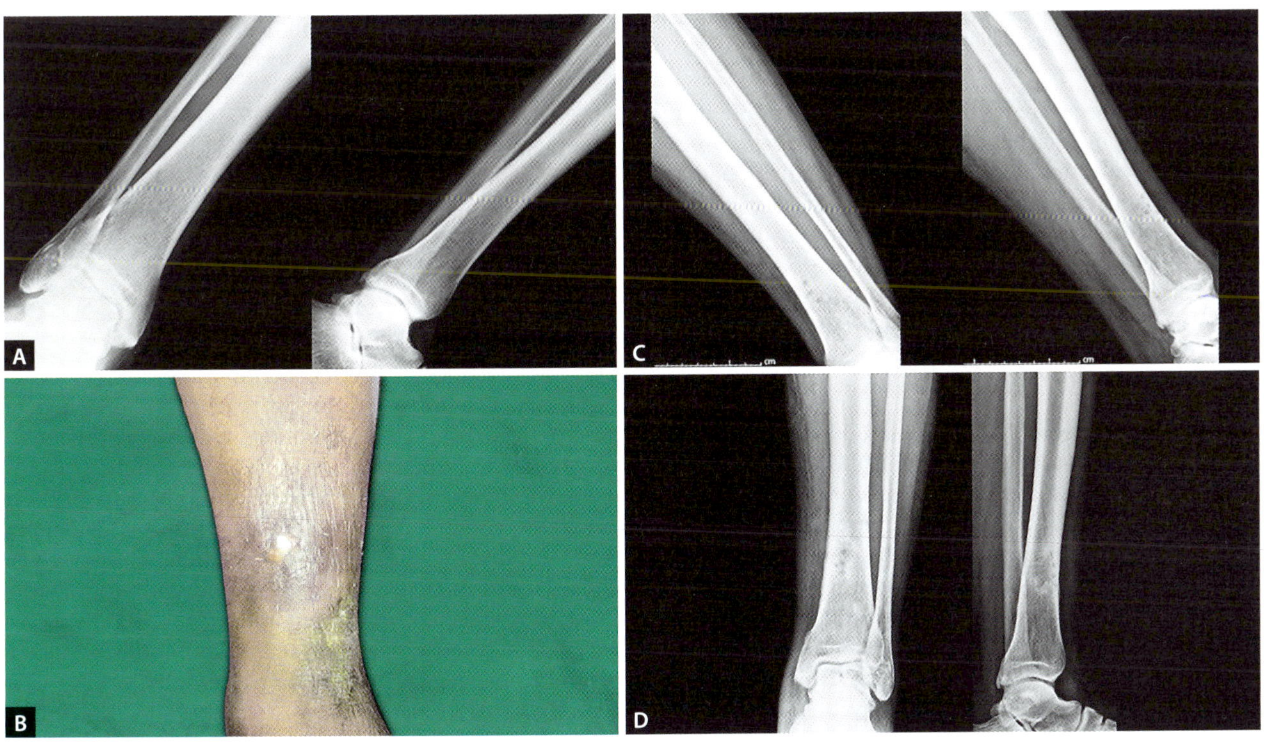

Figs. 8A to D: The patient is an elderly male having pain on anteromedial aspect of tibia. X-rays (A) appear unremarkable but on closer examination one can see osteopenia with mild cortical scalloping on the fibular cortex of tibia in anteroposterior view and anteriorly on lateral X-ray. Decompression had been attempted in the form of multiple drill holes (B) trying to drain pus but patient returned a year later with chronic osteomyelitis, frank pus discharge (C) and intramedullary endosteal reaction (D) to myelitis that resulted in view of unchecked infection. Patient also has nearby eczematous lesion on ankle.

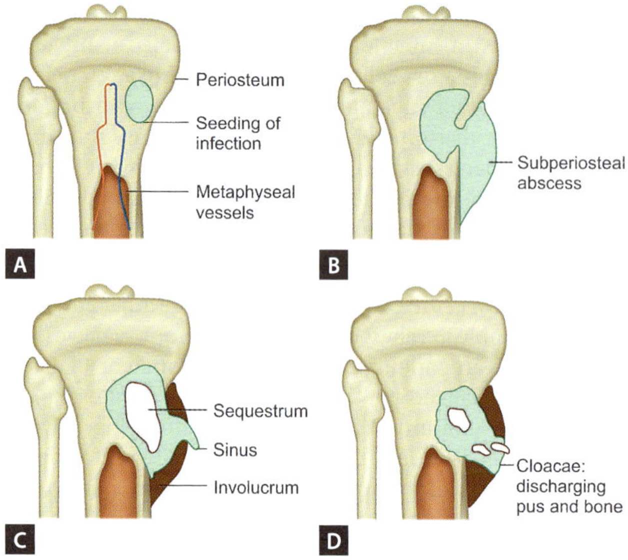

Figs. 9A to D: The microbe lodges into metaphysis commonly through hematogenous seeding (hair pin "bends" may or may not be involved), forming pus (A) causing acute inflammation, systemic illness, and bacteremia. The pus breaks through cortex causing wither joint infection or progression of osteomyelitis or both. In progressive osteomyelitis, the pus accumulates beneath periosteum elevating the same stripping and devitalizing the bone (B). Till here, prompt intervention may prevent development of chronic osteomyelitis. Dead bone starts separating from the parent bone in the abscess cavity and granulation tissue forming sequestrum that usually has a discharging sinus associated with it (C). Reactive bone (involucrum) formation is a reparative process to cover the infection and improve bone stability but is always insufficient punctuated by small holes (cloacae) through which the pus, granulation tissue, and dead bone keep discharging (D) until radical intervention to arrest this smoldering process is undertaken.

respect to finding of predominant periosteal supply in the animal bone model that hypothesizes the *centripetal concept* of developing infection. Initially, there is lodging of bacteria in periosteal circulation with subsequent development of subperiosteal abscess. This then ruptures through or progresses and involves the cortical circulation, producing thrombosis of the nutrient artery and leads to development of characteristic acute OM. The concept is supported by finding of early subperiosteal pus and predominant involvement of cortex than the medulla in most cases of acute OM.

Pathogenesis of chronic OM: Chronic OM is usually (now direct inoculation at surgery with subacute smoldering type infection is increasing) the persistence of acute OM (except points 4, 5, 6, and 7 below, where it may develop de novo) and is a recurring condition difficult to treat completely. It develops in one of the following ways (sometimes a combination of few):

1. Incomplete treatment of acute OM (most common)
2. Trauma and open fractures (now increasing)
3. Implant related infection (probably the second most common now)
4. A hematogenous type of OM
5. Vascular and neurogenic insufficiency (Charcot's) related
6. Infection with chronic persisting type of microbes *Mycobacterium tuberculosis*, *Treponema* species, fungal

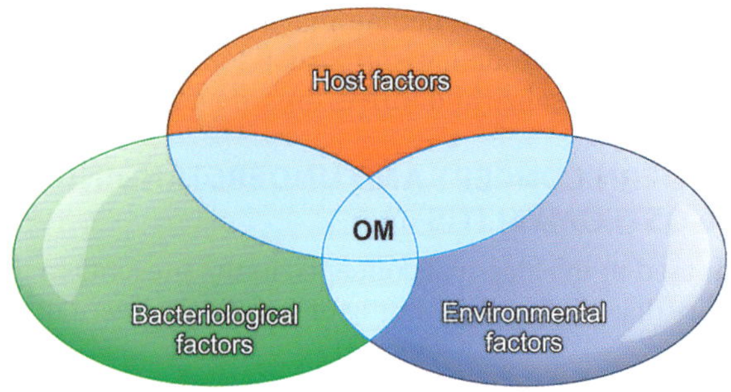

Fig. 10: The interaction of host, bacterial, and environmental factors determines the development of osteomyelitis (OM) not just the presence of bacteria.

7. Osteomyelitis associated with diabetic foot, vascular disease, etc.

Once the bone is infected, the ensuing inflammatory process causes relative ischemia by obliteration (vasculitis) and compression of the vascular channels. This causes necrosis of bone if not treated in time which is walled off by granulation tissue and pus as a sequestrum. Cytokines [interleukin-1β (IL-1β) and macrophage inflammatory protein-2 (MIP-2)] take predominant part in initial inflammatory response and bone necrosis while tartrate-resistant acid phosphatase (TRAP)-positive cells are prominent later (sequestration and involucrum formation). The abiotic components—implants and sequestrum provide a base for formation of the biofilm and result in a smoldering infection that is not amenable to treatment by antimicrobial agents only. Healing produces reactive bone to improve stability in the form of involucrum that has communicating channels with pus and granulation tissue in the form of cloacae.

Modern system recognizes the "close interaction of host factors, bacteriological factors and environment" in a particular fashion that finally settles into infection **(Fig. 10)**. Robson envisaged infection as an "imbalance between germ and host" and was partially correct in suggesting that OM is due to certain predisposing factors.

Host Factors

The host defense comprises innate and adaptive immune response. The innate immune system (neutrophils and macrophages) and complement remove pathogens in various ways. Besides phagocytosis, neutrophils use oxidative burst, protease release, proinflammatory cytokines, and chemokines to kill planktonic forms. Ingeniously they produce neutrophil extracellular traps (NETs) consisting of nuclear contents expelled with antimicrobial proteins deposited on chromatin released outside cell. NETs inactivate virulence factors, immobilize bacteria, promote phagocytosis, and enhance complement activation. Activated (M1) macrophages directly remove bacteria by recognition of surface targets and indirectly by recognizing immunoglobulin or complement on bacterial surface. They also activate innate immune system. Adaptive immunity is conferred by T and B cells. Th1, Th2, and Th17 cells have specific roles. Th17 cells express IL-17A,

IL-17F, and IL-22 and are important in epithelial function and mucosal surface immunity to bacterial and fungal pathogens along with clonotypic TNF/IFN-γ producing $\gamma\delta$ T-cells. B-cell immunity has been exploited in vaccination strategies against *Haemophilus influenzae*. But, for *S. aureus* vaccination strategies have not worked primarily because it is a commensal in 30% population so antibodies are present in majority but the pathogenic variant utilizes alternative strategies to evade defense. There are various defects in above detailed host defense that comprise factors for development of OM.

The "host factors" were grouped by Schmidt (modified here) into the two broad categories:

1. *Endogenous factors [for a comprehensive list see also the Bs physiological group of Cierny-Madar classification* ***(Box 5)****]:*
    - Age >65 years and infancy and childhood
    - Sex—male:female = 4:1 (? due to higher incident trauma)
    - Obesity
    - Nicotine and alcohol abuse
    - Diabetes
    - Vascular diseases
    - Certain fevers like smallpox, scarlet fever, measles, diphtheria, influenza, and typhoid
    - *Immunosuppressive states:* Neutrophil count < 55/mm^3 predisposes to staphylococci, *Candida, Aspergillus,* and gram-negative bacilli. Hypogammaglobulinemia and complement deficiency predispose to infection with streptococci, *Haemophilus,* and *Neisseria,* mycoplasma, and *Ureaplasma urealyticum*. Deficient cell-mediated immunity predisposes to mycobacterial and fungal infections, herpes infection, and *P. carinii*. Hyper-IgE syndrome with IL-17 deficiency predisposes to *S. aureus* infection.
    - Congenital immunosuppressive states such as chronic granulomatous disease, sickle-cell hemoglobinopathy (*Salmonella* infection), and leukocyte adhesion deficiency are associated with acute OM.
    - Cancers and hematological malignancies such as lymphoma and leukemia: possibly also related to cachexia.
    - Steroid and immunosuppressive therapy
    - *Poor hygiene and nutrition (leads to a suppression of the cellular and humoral response):* Albumin level < 3.4 mg/dL, absolute lymphocyte count < 1,500, serum transferrin < 150 mg/dL, arm muscle circumference < 80% of standard, and anergy to a skin test battery indicate poor nutrition. For elective surgery, nutritional support is required in these patients. Various clinical, laboratory, and anthropometric measures should be used to assess patient nourishment. Nutritional index can be calculated by the Rainey-McDonald formula = [(1.2*serum albumin) + (0.013*serum transferrin)]—6.43. A value of 0 or negative indicates malnourishment and high risk for sepsis. Survival into adulthood living under poor hygiene may confer increased immunological tolerance to infection due to repetitive subcritical exposure to infectious agents and conditioning of immunity.
    - *Role of exercise:* Exercise helps the immune system by increasing natural killer cells, macrophage count, cytokines, neutrophil count, and lymphocyte count. There is a small time frame (open window) when athletes are immunosuppressed after an intense physical activity, when ciliary action, immunoglobulin A levels, natural killer cells, T lymphocyte count, and CD4/CD8 ratio are decreased. This susceptibility to infections in athletes in the past was called the "J-curve", but has been recently updated and termed the "S-curve".
2. *Exogenous factors (see also* ***Box 5*** *for Bl physiological factors):*
    - Damage to soft tissue barriers (skin and fascia)
    - Bacterial invasion by a virulent strain or hospital acquired infection
    - Super bugs (multidrug resistant forms)
    - Dead necrotic tissue (due to loss of vascularity from trauma or surgery).

Bacteriological Factors

The quantity and virulence of bacteria (ability to attach, reproduce, and damage the host tissue) are important determinants for infection. Most of the pathogenic bacteria have special features that help them circumvent the immunity, invade the tissues, attach to host tissues, proliferate, and grow even in hostile environment.

- *Evasion of prophylactic antibiotic therapy:* Half of the pathogenic *Staphylococcus* strains exhibit plasmid mediated resistance to antimicrobial agents. Resistant genes in bacteria can be transferred through conjugation (direct transfer from one cell to another), transduction (gene transfer through bacteriophage virus), and transformation [uptake of naked free deoxyribonucleic acid (DNA)]. Staphylococcal chromosomal cassettes (SCCs) are mobile genetic elements that insert into *rlmH* gene. Methicillin-resistance gene *mecA* is common in SCC conferring β-lactam resistance. Plasmids provide resistance to erythromycin, chloramphenicol, tetracycline, β-lactams, aminoglucosides, and macrolides in staphylococcal species. Development of superbugs due to prolonged use of antibiotics and misuse of antibiotics renders prophylactic antibiotic therapy ineffective.
- *Homing of bacteria immunoevasion and persistence:* Most *Staphylococcus* species, *Pseudomonas* species, and gram-negative bacteria have specific factors that mediate adherence to biomaterials and host immunoevasion **(Table 3)**.
    - Trauma to bone (iatrogenic or otherwise) or the "growing ends of bone" exposes the collagen matrix and acellular crystal faces, making it easier for bacteria to adhere to these surfaces using adhesins

TABLE 3: Some cell membrane associated and secreted proteins involved in *S. aureus* pathogenesis.

Protein/protein family	*Function*
MSCRAMM-Clfs-Sdr	
• Clumping factor A (ClfA)	Adhesion to fibrinogen; degradation of C3b Immune evasion
• Clumping factor B (ClfB)	Fibrinogen, keratin, and loricrin binding. Nasal colonization by adhesion to desquamated epithelial cells
• SdrC	β-neurexin binding. Adhesion to desquamated nasal epithelial cells
• SdrD	Adhesion to desquamated nasal epithelial cells
Fibronectin-binding protein A and B (FnBp)	
• FnBpA	Fibrinogen, fibronectin, and elastin binding. Adhesion to extracellular matrix; cell host invasion
• FnBpB	Fibronectin-binding. Adhesion to extracellular matrix; cell host invasion
Collagen adhesion (Cna)	
• Cna	Collagen binding. Adhesion to extracellular matrix
Near iron transporter motif (NEAT)	
• IsdA	Heme, fibrinogen, fibronectin, cytokeratin, and loricrin binding. Heme capture and iron uptake; nasal colonization
• IsdB	Heme, hemoglobin, and 3-β integrins binding. Heme capture and iron uptake; invasion of nonphagocytic cells
• IsdH	Heme, hemoglobin binding. Heme capture and iron acquisition; immune evasion by C3b degradation
Three helical bundle	
• Protein A	IgG, IgM, and TNFR-1 binding. Evasion of immunity; increased inflammation during pneumonia and skin infection
G5-E	
• SasG	Adhesion to desquamated epithelial cells; formation of biofilm
α-, β-, hemolysin (pore-forming toxin) and γ-hemolysin (sphingomyelinase)	Lyse RBC, leukocytes, alter immune signaling
Leukocidins	Pore-forming toxins. Lyse neutrophils, monocytes, and macrophages
Autolysin (Atl), aureolysin, staphylokinase, nuclease	Cell separation, generates extracellular DNA in biofilm matrix. Inactivate neutrophil extracellular traps (NETs)
Phenol-soluble modulins	Lyse neutrophils, breakdown biofilm matrix, important for biofilm disassembly
Superantigenic exotoxins	Stimulate T-cells, nonspecifically, can cause toxic shock syndrome, activate bone resorption, inhibit host immunity in OM
Chemotaxis inhibitory protein of *S. aureus* (CHIPS)	Inhibits neutrophil migration and activation, prevents complement activation

(DNA: deoxyribonucleic acid; IgG: immunoglobulin G; IgM: immunoglobulin M; MSCRAMM-Clf: microbial surface component recognizing adhesive matrix molecules-clumping factor; OM: osteomyelitis; RBC: red blood cells; TNFR-1: tumor-necrosis factor receptor 1)

and other proteins **(Table 3)** in a receptor-ligand fashion.

- Bacterial adhesion to necrotic bone and implants is also mediated by charged properties and van der Waals forces between the bacteria tissue and implants.
- Adult OM has a high rate of treatment failure due to immunoevasion and possibly persistent bacterial reservoirs. The bacteria especially *S. aureus* may persist in submicron cracks and canaliculi through active process of bacterial deformation and replication (challenging the age old concept of *S. aureus* being nonmotile microbe). The bacterium can also persist in cells such as neutrophils and macrophages apart from osteoblasts, -clasts, and -cytes to serve as additional reservoirs for a long time (justifying the use of local antibiotics and prolonged use for sterilizing the area).

- *Evasion of local host defense (the biofilm model to explain the persistence of OM):* The body's own defense is rendered ineffective especially at the implant surfaces and within sequestrum. Biofilm protects bacterial cells from immune cell invasion and antibiotic penetration, facilitates nutrient transport, cell-to-cell communication, and provides mechanical stability. Most bacteria and few fungi have ingenious capacity to synthesize inert glycocalyx capsule (described in 1984) that forms a "biofilm" (concept introduced in 1980) inert to host defense (see also prosthetic joint infection). "Biofilm formation is a process whereby microorganisms of the same species attach to and grow on a surface and produce extracellular polymers that facilitate attachment and matrix formation, resulting in an alteration in the phenotype of the organisms with respect to growth rate and gene transcription" **(Flowchart 1 and Fig. 11)**. The polysaccharide intercellular adhesin (PIA) is mainly responsible for formation of extracellular polysaccharide matrix that makes biofilm. Biofilm is typically quickly and copiously produced by *Pseudomonas aeruginosa*, *Staphylococcus aureus*, and *S. epidermidis*. The glycocalyx is an extracellular polysaccharide molecule that shields from "*host*" molecules in an immunological sense. This glycocalyx (exopolysaccharide) together with

Flowchart 1: Biofilm formation and various influences on the same.

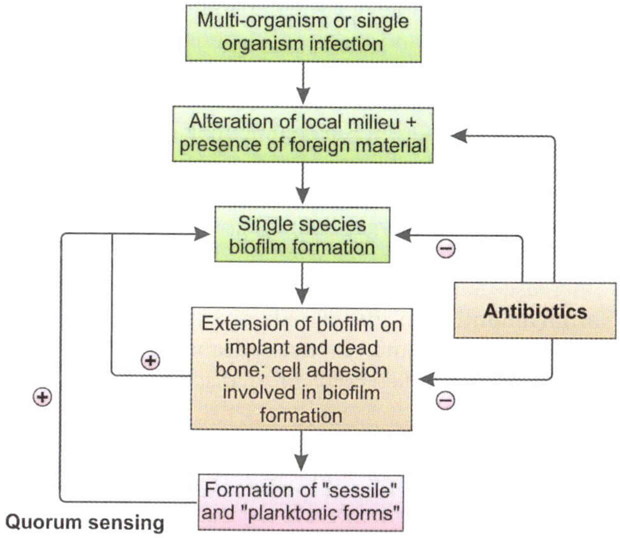

eDNA, proteins, and lipids form the extracellular matrix commonly termed "*slime*" and serves as protective physical barrier for microbes. The biofilm has a base layer that is near the implant and fosters adherence to target surface. The pH and local environment encourage formation of sessile variants of bacteria that collectively develop a colony. The outer layers form discrete structures such as "columns" and "mushrooms". "Streamers" can form in the outer layers that may break off to infect contiguous areas **(Fig. 11)**. Intercellular signaling through the extracellular matrix occurs via "quantum packets" that are transported via nanotubes formed within matrix and these nanotubes are also involved in conducting cell-to-cell electric signals. In chronic bone infections, the lifecycle of the infecting microbe (whether bacteria or fungi) passes through a common sequence as detailed below:

Single cell adhesion → incipient biofilm (immature, formed within 15 minutes of surface adhesion, "crowd behavior" causes aggregation of microbes and slime production) → mature sessile biofilm (within 48 hours there is altered molecular and cellular behavior, reduced cell replication, pillar and mushroom formation increases vertical and horizontal thickness of the biofilm) → mature biofilm with genetic diversity (every other opportunistic microbe from any strain, species or kingdom utilizes the produced biofilm and colonizes it with discrete close

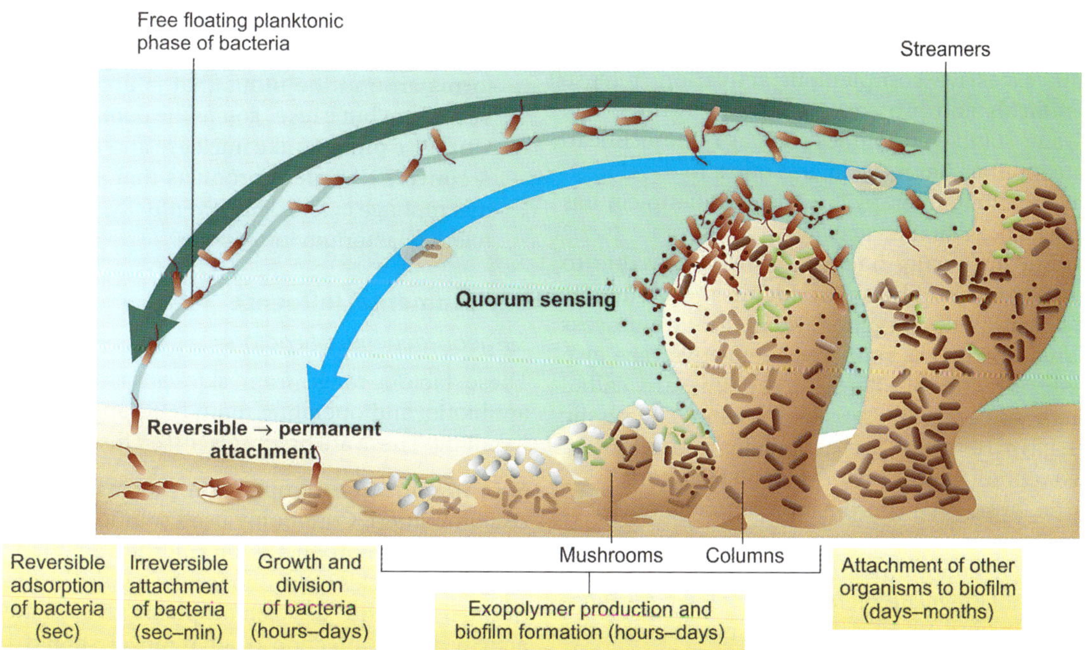

Fig. 11: The structure and formation of biofilm. The biofilm producing bacteria attach quickly to the implant surface or dead bone facilitated by various factors. The attachment to extracellular matrix is mediated via Fbe/SdrG (fibrinogen binding), GehD (collagen binding), and Embp (fibronectin binding) while inhibited by higher concentration of β-lactams (partially justifies use of cocktail in implant arthroplasty). Attachment to polymer surface is facilitated by SSP-1 and 2 (staphylococcal surface proteins-1 and 2) while inhibited by δ-toxin. Once this attachment becomes permanent, the next step is cell-to-cell adhesion having the common motive of thriving on surface; this is mediated by polysaccharide intercellular adhesin (PIA) and accumulation of associative protein. The cells then mature and have keen review of mechanisms for increased proliferations. The colonies grow into mushrooms and columns into which planktonic and sessile variants thrive. The former are facilitated by reduced immunity and absence of antibiotics while the latter suppressed forms develop in inhibitory milieu. To shorten the formation of colonies, the columns constantly release streamers that bypass the stage of temporary adhesion and intercellular interaction. The planktonic bacteria keep getting released from the settled colonies and may lead to intermittent septicemia and or abscess formation.

spatially structured regions, there is fast horizontal genetic transfer that occurs at a rate 10,000 times faster between these groups than in planktonic form. This unique combined genetic characteristic (pangenome) prevents host from developing adaptive immune response) → development of extended phenotype (the biofilm has uniquely altered host and environmental factors that cause variety of changes such as altered pH, O_2 tension and ion concentration that are favorable only to biofilm and host cells will not survive here) → surface dispersion (microbes near the surface regularly detach and are free to colonize other areas of host in remote places, also flow of biofilm due to viscoelastic nature of the slime causes streaming and spread of the biofilm to adjacent surface). Biofilm disassembly in *S. aureus* is mediated by accessory gene regulator (*agr*) system which is a well-characterized two-component peptide quorum sensing system. Initially, there is secretion of autoinducing peptide into the extracellular environment. This triggers increased production of proteases, toxin, and phenol-soluble modulin (PSM) which breakdown the biofilm matrix. PSM are surfactant like peptides that are critical in biofilm dispersal especially *S. aureus*. Following are some of the mechanisms responsible for persistence of infection:

This mix-up of host and bacterial antigens hides the specific bacterial antigens and is not recognized by host immunity.

- The biofilm is impermeable to antimicrobial agents typically the beta-lactams.
- There is a reduced local immunity by inhibition of phagocytes that cannot penetrate the biofilm and in the process they lose their ability to phagocytose. Also with excessive complement activation, release of free radicals and proteases apoptosis results. The highly water-soluble antibiotics such as rifampicin can penetrate biofilms but resistance is quick to develop so combination chemotherapy is advised. Rifampicin has antistaphylococcal biofilm activity.
- The biofilm producing bacteria grow slowly due to highly anaerobic conditions reducing the metabolic activity so antibiotics targeting the replication process (fluoroquinolones) are rendered ineffective (see also prosthetic infections). These organisms are called "persisters" or better the "sessile" variants. The sessile variants have 10^3 times less sensitivity to antibiotics, restricted reproduction, and are difficult to culture.
- The sessile forms keep coordination among themselves by "quorum sensing" (lactone containing molecules that establish communication between intra- and interspecies that regulate metabolic activity in response to population density via signaling molecules) and slowly develop increasing resistance to administered drugs. Quorum-sensing is also involved in production of toxins from the microbes that cause direct lysis of host lead inflammatory response cells like the neutrophils, thus causing nearby tissue damage also. Once the local immunity falls low the return to "planktonic form" (free-floating, virulent, reproductive form, and triggering host systems) can occur accounting for clinical recurrences and acute on chronic episodes (***see* Flowchart 1**). When planktonic forms encounter a devitalized surface coated with protein they quickly home in it. The host immunity already "confused" about the method of dealing with them mounts a common inflammatory reaction that is either ineffective (viz., T_h2 cell humoral response against *P. aeruginosa*) or self-damaging and misdirected (viz., T_h1 and T_h17 inflammatory reaction against *S. aureus*) that causes further tissue damage and increases adhesion surface for microbes. These biofilms are thus a permanent source of virulent pathogens insensitive to immune system and progressively resistant to antibiotics.
- *Development of "pangenome"*: As mentioned earlier the development of microbe diversity in biofilm causes immense changes in the genetic make-up, so much so that different organisms due to horizontal transfer of genetic material develop a similar overt genome or a de facto genome larger than that of any one strain. This genome is termed as "pangenome". The pangenome gives increased survival ability to the biofilm and prevents host from mounting an effective adaptive immune response.
- Small colony variants play a significant role in persistence of infection (detailed mechanism discussed in prosthetic joint infection).
- *S. aureus* is also able to form staphylococcal abscess communities (SACs) which help in forming soft-tissue abscesses, a hallmark of musculoskeletal infection. In SAC, a central replicative group of bacterium is formed that is protectively surrounded by a pseudocapsule of fibrin created by *S. aureus* coagulase cleavage of fibrinogen. A peripheral ring of necrotic neutrophils forms around the nidus that is unable to remove the bacterium but causes soft tissue damage. Staphylococcal virulence proteins like nuclease and adenosine synthase A convert NETs into products that additionally induce macrophage cytotoxicity. Eventually, the SACs rupture to release bacterium into tissues.

Environmental Influence

Surgeon-dependent Factors

These factors range from skin preparation, prophylactic antibiotic, and operating room (OR) environment to tissue handling. These are briefly discussed here.

Skin preparation: Proper skin preparation decreases the contamination. Commonly used solutions such as alcohol, iodine, hexachlorophene, or chlorhexidine fail to sterilize the hair follicles and sebaceous glands where bacteria normally reside. Hexachlorophene has better residual activity for disinfection. Hair removal should be done in the OR. Handwashing is the most important procedure for prevention of nosocomial infections. Hand scrubbing for 2 minutes is now recommended instead of 5 minutes. Double gloving decreased skin contamination and the surgical gloves should be changed every 2 hours.

Operating room environment: Vertical laminar-airflow systems and personnel-isolator systems are recommended for orthopedic surgery. The efficacy can be improved with ultraviolet (UV) light for reducing the number of airborne bacteria. A large number of microscopic particles are dispersed within the OR that commonly originate from the personnel, linen, footwear, etc. serving as favorable attachment site for pathogens. The bacteria are continuously shed from external surface of the persons working there. The sum total of bacterial load in OR can be represented by the following equation:

$$TBL = P\,(SR_p) + [n^*X(SR_x)]$$

Where, TBL is total bacterial load, P = patient, SR = shedding rate, n = number of persons, X = any person. A significant fraction of this is exposed to surgical wound. So, higher the mobility in the OR higher is the basal bacterial load. In-between opening of doors and movements disturb the laminar flow and can be detrimental by creating eddy currents lifting the floor bacteria into air. This bacterial cloud concentration should be kept minimum by strict discipline (**Table 4**). Continuous removal of bacteria by high efficiency particulate air (HEPA) filters is a preferable method. Use of personal OT suites with individualized airflow systems is getting more popular but clinical advantage is yet to be demonstrated.

Prophylactic antibiotic therapy: Following surgery in the first 2 hours, the host defense mechanism works to decrease the bacterial counts. During the next 4 hours, numbers of bacteria increasing by multiplication remain same as those being removed by host defenses. These first 6 hours are called the "golden period", after which the bacteria increase rapidly. Antibiotics increase this window by decreasing bacterial growth and reproduction. Prophylactic antibiotics are directed against the common skin pathogens. Ideally, antibiotic prophylaxis therapy should be administered immediately before surgery (within 30 minutes of skin incision). The dose can be repeated every 4 hours intraoperatively or whenever the blood loss exceeds 1,000–1,500 mL. After surgery, antibiotics have a role only for first 48–72 hours. Continuing antibiotics beyond 72 hours, it leads to fallacious suppression of infection and contributes to development of hospital-acquired infections and superinfections.

Tissue handling: Minimum of the localized necrotic/avascular tissue should remain in the operative site and as clean a wound as possible should result from surgery, which comes from experience and observing meticulous senior surgeons. All dead spaces should be closed and bleeding secured to prevent hematoma formation. Unwanted and prolonged retraction should be avoided.

To these, one should add the "local environment" responsible for persistence of infection. These inappropriate environmental conditions include:

- Presence of orthopedic metallic implants
- Dead space (see the management)
- Presence of bone grafts
- Scar tissue and sinuses

TABLE 4: Operating room (OR) discipline and postoperative wound management practice to reduce chances of infection

Measures	*Comments*
Operating room discipline	
Follow "OT time out": Place all necessary implant and instruments in OR before surgery, no staff rotation, no door opening till end or surgical procedure	Limits the personnel movement, bacterial load, eddy currents, turbulent air flow and reduces surgical time
Follow and propagate proper sterile technique	All subordinates should follow the standard sterile technique reducing risk of wound contamination
Change the OR clothes whenever leaving the confines of OR suite	Avoid fomite contamination
Fresh OT clothes daily (no reuse without wash)	Reduce fomite contamination
Clean the unsterile equipment to be used for patients regularly (like tourniquets)	Reduce cross contamination
The unscrubbed personnel should wash hands before entering OR	Reduce outside contamination
Thorough cleaning of OR including backside of lights	Reduce basal contamination and remove the resistant bacteria from previous patient, cross-contamination
Regular culture surveillance of OR	"Quality control"
All OR personnel should take bath in morning	Reduce bacterial shedding
Wound care	
Layered wound closure	Prevent deep contamination from skin sutures by bacteria tracking along sutures
Isolated room for prosthetic patients	Prevent cross contamination and reduce HAI with resistant bacteria from other patients
Minimize use of drain by meticulous intraoperative bleeding control	All open conduits are direct bacterial entry routes
Keep wounds dry with frequent dressings	Bacteria thrive and multiply in moist regions
Clean wound edges and apply bacteriostatic solution	Reduce contamination from surrounding skin
Screen high-risk patients for MRSA	Ideally, hospital policy should include screening healthcare personnel for MRSA

(HAI: healthcare-associated infection; MRSA: methicillin-resistant *Staphylococcus aureus*)

Role of orthopedic implants in development of osteomyelitis: Orthopedic surgeons should consider the specific implant related features with respect to development of implant related infection:

- The implant site infection rates are different between porous and dense materials with porous materials having a much higher rate.
- Bacteria adhere more to grooved and braided materials compared with flat ones, probably partially due to increased surface area.
- Depending on the "hydrophobicity of bacteria" and "material surfaces" (determined by water contact angles), bacteria adhere differently to materials with different hydrophobicities. The higher the water contact angle greater is hydrophobicity of material. Generally, bacteria with hydrophobic properties (most implant adhering bacteria are hydrophobic) prefer hydrophobic material surfaces (and usually win this "race to surface") before being caught by innate defense cells; the ones with hydrophilic characteristics prefer hydrophilic surfaces and hydrophobic bacteria adhere to a greater extent than hydrophilic bacteria. Hydrophobic materials are more susceptible to bacterial colonization and biofilm formation than hydrophilic ones. In staphylococcal species, these hydrophobic areas are provided by proteins that are covalently bound to the cell wall. The hydrophobicity reduces with cellular ageing in *E. coli* and *P. aeruginosa*. Hydrophobicity of bacteria also reduces with antibiotic therapy (prophylactic or antibiotic containing implants) by virtue of increasing exopolysaccharide synthesis (hydrophilic compound). The hydrophobicity of surface can be reduced along with reduced bacterial adhesion by coating implant with bovine serum albumin, diamond-like carbon coating of PVC, etc.
- There is adsorption of native proteins as soon as implantation occurs and bacteria adhere to these proteins avidly. This process can be reduced by local infiltration of antibiotics.
- The metallic foreign body interacts with the tissue (foreign body reaction). These involve the redox reaction (an electron exchange) at the interface, the hydrolysis (a proton exchange) of oxide hydrate. In water and tissue fluid, corrosion occurs as an electrochemical process in which oxidation (electron loss of the metal) is coupled with reduction (electron gain of electrolyte components). Reduction of oxygen produces hydroxides, and oxides on the metal surface. There is formation of metal organic complexes in the electrolyte as a result of this corrosive process. This reaction can also result in changes of pH and local tissue toxicity, both of which interfere with differentiation of osteoblasts and osteoclasts and reduce the phagocytic activity of neutrophils and the oxidative burst needed to kill microbes (typically caused by metal ion oxides of cobalt-chrome steel). Thus, there is higher possibility of delayed healing and OM. Titanium and tantalum have a reduced foreign body effect and this reduces susceptibility to infection of tissues by 900% (nine times approximately).

DIAGNOSIS

Clinical

Acute hematological OM in children is a clinical diagnosis with typical symptoms **(*see* Box 1)**. In adult's history of open fracture, presence of nonhealing ulcers, contiguous sites of infection, predisposing factors for infection should be sought and physician should have high index of suspicion. Tenderness to deep palpation, thrust tenderness (vertebral OM) at the site, and painful ROM are only the usual clinical features.

Chronic OM is often already diagnosed due to protracted nature of disease and symptoms **(*see* Box 2)** and patient comes usually only for treatment being fed up of previous ones. Pain is the ubiquitous symptom (very long-standing partially healed cases will not complain of pain). Some patients give classical history of "Walenkamp phenomenon" where the pain gradually increases over variable period of time to become unbearable and suddenly relaxes with opening up of sinus and pus discharge. Presence of nonhealing ulcer with exposed bone at base (better detected with sterile steel probe), adherent sinus tract with discharging pus or discharge of bone pieces **(Fig. 12)** strongly suggest chronic OM. On examination, the surrounding ulcer margins are dusky, thin shiny skin (undermining suggests tubercular OM), the base is covered with unhealthy slough. Sinus tract may be indurated and often invaginated **(Fig. 13)**. The bone is tender to deep palpation and irregularly thickened (if involucrum formation is prominent). There is muscle atrophy.

Hematological Investigations

Blood culture is positive in half of acute OM cases in children. In adults, it is commonly negative. Total leukocyte counts, erythrocyte sedimentation rate (ESR), and C-reactive protein (CRP) are elevated and sensitive but nonspecific. CRP could be a better measure and a value of >100 mg/L should prompt physician to aspirate the pathological site.

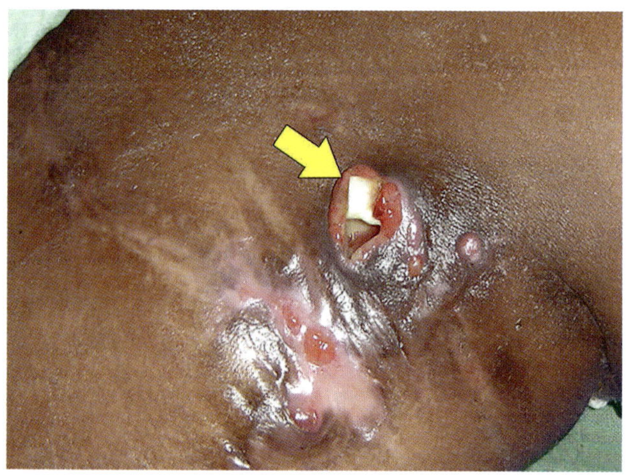

Fig. 12: The photograph shows multiple sinus openings with bone sequestrum at the largest opening (block arrow). The patient has osteomyelitis of the ilium.

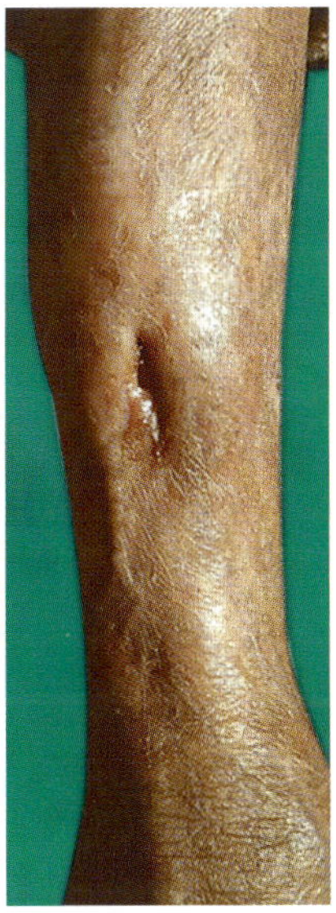

Fig. 13: The clinical photograph depicts a discharging sinus with invaginated margins that connect to the chronic osteomyelitis of underlying tibial diaphysis.

Bacteriological Evaluation

The most definitive evidence for infection is isolation and culture of the pathogenic organism (rest all investigations tell probability). Gram-staining may provide results after 45 minutes but definitive microbiological examination (culture) takes about 48 hours. It is recommended that aspiration and bacteriological investigations should be done before starting antibiotic therapy. In chronic OM, the patients are usually already on antibiotic therapy that should be stopped for 7 days before taking pus samples. Needle aspiration from the lesion under aseptic precautions is the most recommended method or a swab culture should be taken from exposed pathological bone. It should be collected in syringes that are air free. Wrong identification mostly occurs with superficial or wound margin sampling. False negative reports are common with patients on antibiotic therapy. The common bacterial isolates from different age groups and clinical scenario are presented in **Table 5**. Tissue biopsy (see also bone biopsy and difficulty with biofilms further) may be taken from edge of the lesion and kept in CO_2 filled container to reduce exposure to air. Rapid diagnostic methods include Gram stain, acridine orange stain, 10% KOH mount in fungal infection, and monoclonal antibodies to specific bacterial antigens such as *H. influenzae, N. meningococci, Streptococcus pneumoniae,* etc.

After organism has been isolated, the antimicrobial effectiveness is tested by:

- In vitro susceptibility testing of a bacterial isolate
- Measurement of patient's inhibiting or bactericidal serum level against his own infecting bacteria
- Measurement of actual serum concentration of antibiotic.

Lowest concentration of antibiotic that inhibits the growth of isolate is minimum inhibitory concentration (MIC). If MIC levels can be achieved in patients' serum, it is called sensitive. Minimum bactericidal concentration (MBC) is the lowest concentration of antimicrobial agent that allows survival of <0.1% of original cultured inoculum.

TABLE 5: The microbiology of osteomyelitis (OM).

Age-related microbial flora from osteomyelitis	***Common microorganisms isolated from osteomyelitis***
Infants: • Group B streptococci • *Staphylococcus aureus* • *Escherichia coli* *Children (1–16 years):* • *Staphylococcus aureus* • *Streptococcus pyogenes* • *Haemophilus influenzae* *Adults (>16 years):* • *Staphylococcus epidermidis* • *Staphylococcus aureus* • *Pseudomonas aeruginosa* • *Serratia marcescens* • *Escherichia coli*	*Common (>50% of cases):* • *Staphylococcus aureus* • Coagulase-negative staphylococci *Occasionally encountered (>25% of cases):* • Streptococci • Enterococci • *Pseudomonas* spp. • *Enterobacter* spp. • *Proteus* spp. • *Escherichia coli* • *Mycobacterium tuberculosis* • Atypical *mycobacteria* • Anaerobes (*Clostridium* spp. and *Bacteroides* group) *Rarely encountered (<5% of cases):* • *Brucella* spp. • *Salmonella* spp. • Dimorphic fungi • *Candida* spp. • *Aspergillus* spp. • *Mycoplasma* spp. • *Tropheryma whipplei* • *Actinomyces* • *Treponema spp.*
Clinical scenario related common organisms	
Most common organism isolated primary or secondary infection, including adult OM	*Staphylococcus aureus*
Foreign body and implant related infections, contiguous focus of infection	Coagulase negative staphylococci, Gram-negative bacilli, *Propionibacterium* spp.
Nosocomial infections	*Enterobacteriaceae spp., Pseudomonas aeruginosa*
Bite or fist injuries. Diabetic foot lesions, decubitus ulcers	*Streptococci*, anaerobic bacteria
Sickle cell disease	*Salmonella* spp., *Streptococcus pneumoniae*
HIV infection	*Bartonella henselae*
Human/animal bites	*Pasteurella multocida, Eikenella corrodens*
Immunocompromised patients	*Aspergillus* spp., *Mycobacterium avium-intracellulare* or *Candida* spp.
Rare endemic lesions	*Brucella* spp., *Coxiella burnetti*
Intravenous drug abusers	*Pseudomonas aeruginosa, Candida*

(HIV: human immunodeficiency virus)

Serum bactericidal concentration (SBC) is the activity of patient's serum against the infecting organism. Lowest dilution of patient's serum that kills 99.9% of the inoculum is called the SBC. Oral dose is adjusted to give SBC of 1:8 or 1:16.

Molecular Markers

Typically two types of molecular methods are used: (1) amplified and (2) nonamplified. Amplification methods include:

polymerase chain reaction (PCR), reverse transcriptase polymerase chain reaction (RT-PCR), ligase chain reaction, and branched chain reaction. Monoclonal antibodies, direct detection of ribosomal ribonucleic acid (rRNA), and hybridization of rRNA are nonamplified techniques. The molecular methods target specific macromolecules unique to infecting pathogens (like *M. tuberculosis*) and can provide rapid results with high accuracy.

Radiological Imaging

These are easy, sensitive, noninvasive, specific, and patient friendly screening test for infection. The following are used in variable sequence often beginning with the simplest first. Morphological imaging using X-rays, CT-scan, MRI, and USG provide anatomical localization. Functional imaging enables visualization of pathological process. These mainly involve the use of radiopharmaceuticals that trace the physiological changes. Plain scintigraphy, single, photon emission computed tomography (SPECT), and positron emission tomography (PET) are the modalities used. No investigation is absolutely perfect or specific for diagnosis of infection and their use vary depending on evolution of disease and planning. The general specificities and sensitivity of each is mentioned in **Table 6**.

X-rays

The sensitivity and specificity increases temporally with evolution of disease. In general, OM must involve 1 cm of bone and compromise 30–50% of mineral content to produce noticeable changes in plain radiographs. Once prominent it is usually assumed that the changes are present for past 2–3 weeks. It has limited roles in acute OM, but good for radiological evaluation of chronic OM. The various terms used radiologically for chronic OM are detailed in **Box 6**.

- Within a few days (some authors say 48–72 hours), soft tissue changes such as muscle swelling and blurring of the soft tissue planes can be appreciated.
- Periosteal thickening, lytic lesions, endosteal scalloping, osteopenia, loss of trabecular architecture, and new bone apposition take 5–7 days in children and 10–14 days in adults to develop.
- Periostitis, involucrum formation **(Fig. 14)**, sinus tracts, soft tissue fistulas, and most importantly sequestrum formation (for definitions see **Box 6**) are indicative

BOX 6: Some terms and definitions related to chronic osteomyelitis.

Sequestrum: It is a separated, microscopic, or macroscopic necrotic fragment of usually cortical bone (which appears radiodense on X-ray) and is surrounded by infected granulation tissue and pus (radiolucent) from parent viable bone.

Types of sequestrum:

- *Shape:*
  - Pencil like—infants
  - Cylindrical/tubular—infants
  - Ring—external fixator pins, Schanz screws and Ilizarov wires
  - Conical—amputation stump
  - Annular—amputation stump
  - Trapezoid and irregular—adolescents
  - Coralliform—Perthes
  - Flake like—tuberculosis
  - Button sequestrum—calvarium
- *Consistency*
  - Coke like—tuberculosis
  - Feathery—syphilis
  - Sand like (coarse)—tubercular OM in metaphysis
  - Sand like (fine)—viral OM
- *Colored*
  - Black—amputation stump and long exposure of necrotic bone to air while also attached to parent bone (formation of ferrous sulfide), fungal infection, actinomycosis
  - Green—pseudomonal OM

Differential diagnosis of sequestrum: Radiation necrosis, eosinophilic granuloma, metastatic carcinoma, primary lymphoma of bone, fibrous tumors of bone. Mineralization in primary tumor of bone such as osteoblastoma, osteoid osteoma, chondroblastoma, fibromyxoma, and desmoplastic fibroma.

Involucrum (involucre—wrapping, cover): It is a subperiosteal, reactive, viable, immature (woven) new bone formation around a dead bone. It has a rough inner and smooth outer surface.

Differential diagnosis of involucrum: Physiologically seen in infants, neuroblastoma, metastatic leukemia, hypervitaminosis A.

Cloacae: These are single or multiple openings in involucrum that serve as pus discharging sites from the reactive bone. Small sequestrate are also extruded through these holes. They are *not* sites of entrance of vessels.

TABLE 6: Imaging methods used for osteomyelitis (OM).

Imaging modality	*Sensitivity*	*Specificity*	*Comments*
Plain X-rays	10–50%	~60–70%	High rate of false negative (early disease) and false positive (numerous mimicking conditions). The first investigation to guide further evaluation
Ultrasonography	20–50%	40–70%	Highly user dependent and undefined criteria
CT scan	67%	50%	Recommended for identification of sequestrum and where MRI is contraindicated
^{99m}Tc scintigraphy	80%	20–30%	Good investigation if used in combination otherwise low specificity. Multifocal lesions are better identified due to whole body scan. Does not have implant artifact as seen with CT or MRI
111In and 67Ga leukocyte scanning	60–80%	60–70%	The gallium scans are slow to acquire. Indium scans are faster and more efficacious. Quite useful in combined scans where differentiation from aseptic lesions is required. It should be combined with three-phase bone scintigraphy
MRI	80–90%	60–90%	Investigation of choice for identification and planning of OM treatment
PET scan (68Ga, 18F)	95%	90%	Possibly the investigation of choice in future due to fast processing and wonderful spatial resolution combined with PET. Expensive, limited access
Radiolabeled immunoglobulins	91%	70%	Under study and available for research purpose

(111In: indium-111; 67Ga: gallium-67; PET: positron emission tomography)

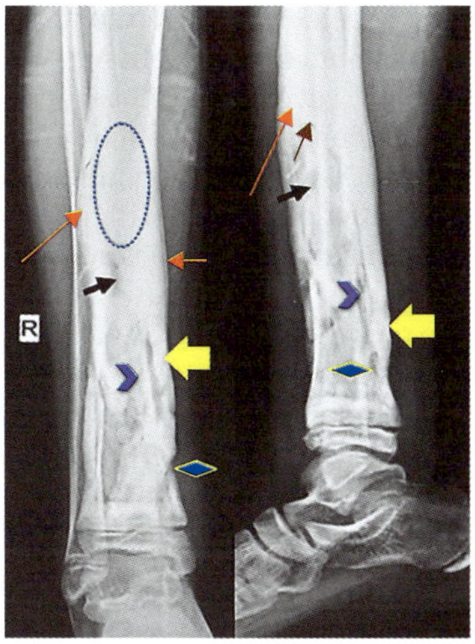

Fig. 14: The radiograph of leg demonstrates primary pathology involving the lower two-thirds of right tibia. There is irregular thickening of cortices *(brown arrow)* with loss of corticomedullary differentiation *(round dotted ellipse)*. Distinctive mixed lytic-sclerotic regions can be observed *(bold arrows)* with areas of sequestrum formation *(chevron pointers)*. There is remarkable involucrum *(block arrows)* with cloacae formation *(diamond pointers)*, periosteal reaction *(red arrows)*, and osteopenia of the nearby bones. The distal physis appears preserved and fibula is comparatively spared from the disease. The features are suggestive of chronic osteomyelitis of tibia.

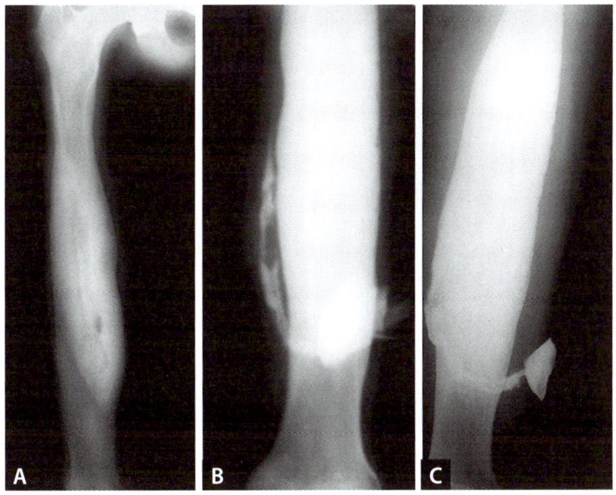

Figs. 15A to C: Sinogram. Look at the fine detached pencil like sequestrum seen well engulfed by dense sclerotic bone all around. In these cases, sinogram helps to delineate the path from sinus to sequestrum that should be excised and also localized the epicenter of involucrum to aid approach. Not surprisingly the path was found well on the other side of sinus (this is usually the case with OM—the path is often indirect).

of chronic OM. Formation of sequestrum is the hallmark of chronic OM, its formation takes 10 days histopathologically, but is evident radiologically only after 3 weeks. It takes further 2–3 months for sequestrum to separate from parent bone and involucrum to engulf and strengthen. They are radiodense due to surrounding hyperemic osteopenia, presence of surrounding lucent granulation tissue for contrast, and sclerotic nature due to absence of bone resorption.

Sinogram

Injecting radiopaque dye through a flexible catheter radiologically reproduces the track of discharging sinuses which may influence the surgical approach and plan **(Figs. 15A to C)**. They demonstrate the branching patterns (not always) that should be removed during debridement, and the culprit sequestrum (in case there are many), that is the focus of pus formation and discharge. The investigation is only used in chronic OM.

Ultrasonography and Doppler Sonography

Ultrasonography (USG) and Doppler sonography are a rapid, easily available, noninvasive, radiation-free, cheap and reasonably accurate diagnostic modality for screening and early diagnosis of OM. It can also detect concurrent septic arthritis. Deep soft tissue swelling adjacent to bone is the earliest to appear (within 48 hours), followed by a thin layer of subperiosteal fluid, subperiosteal abscess (hypoechoic or anechoic shadow), and periosteal reaction.

Ultrasonography is helpful for differentiating conditions such as soft tissue abscess, pyomyositis, and cellulitis. It can be used for guided aspiration of pus. USG can detect features much earlier than radiographs. The technique is but inherently limited by observer and expertise. Doppler sonography can detect hyperemia around periosteum and surrounding soft tissue abscess. The technique is useful in acute OM only and there is no role in chronic OM.

CT Scan

This is a useful three-dimensional (3D) modality that demonstrates abnormal thickening of the affected cortical bone, with sclerotic changes, encroachment of the medullary cavity, and chronic draining sinus. CT scan is favored less than MRI due to poor soft tissue contrast and also radiation effect. Sequestrum is conspicuously seen on CT scan. In this respect, CT scan is even superior to MRI in demonstrating sequestrum, cloacae, involucrum, or intraosseous gas. It should be used in vertebral OM for diagnostic aspiration or tissue diagnosis. There is beam hardening effect in the presence of implants losing the resolution. It is useful only for chronic OM, and has no role in acute OM.

Magnetic Resonance Imaging

This is a highly sensitive investigation to detect OM and assesses the extent of involvement and activity of the disease in cases of chronic bone infection with reliable specificity. Marrow fat is replaced by edema and cellular infiltrates which are lower in signal than fat in T1-weighted images and higher in signal than in T2-weighted images **(Figs. 16A and B)**. The classic findings of MRI in OM are:

- Reduction in normally high marrow signal on T1-weighted images
- Normal or increased signal on T2-weighted images.

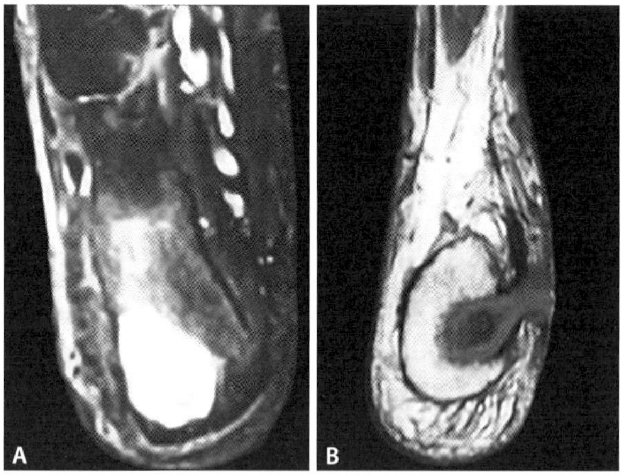

Figs. 16A and B: MRI show conspicuous abscess cavity in calcaneum with surrounding osseous edema (A) and it can also demonstrate connecting sinus tracts (B) obviating the need for sinograms.

The changes in marrow are evident within 3–5 days of onset of symptoms. Combination of short tau-inversion sequences and T1 spin echo images have the highest sensitivity and specificity to detect the disease. Marrow inflammation can be detected within 1–2 days using this combination. The sequestrum and ossified periosteal shell has low intensity on all pulsed sequences, however, the surrounding granulation tissue and the pus have high signal on T2 and STIR images. The distinction is further enhanced by using gadolinium contrast. Periosteal reaction and cortical bone are separated by linear intermediate to high signal intensity on T2-weighted or STIR images. A cloaca is appreciated as a linear low signal intensity periosteum that is elevated from the cortical bone or the thickened cortex that is interrupted by a high signal intensity gap on T2-weighted images. This may be connected to soft tissue forming a sinus. The other advantages beyond detection of OM include:

- Plan the optimal surgical management
- Assess the extent of devitalized tissue and hence the extent of debridement
- Defining the involvement of critical adjacent structures involved that need reconstruction and possible options can be rehearsed beforehand.

Disadvantages of MRI include difficult evaluation in presence of metallic implants due to interference and occasional inability to distinguish infections from reactive inflammation. This has limited role in acute OM, more useful for chronic OM.

Functional Imaging

Nuclear Imaging

They may show pathological changes as soon as 48 hours after the onset of the infection and are being developed for improving the specificity. The gamma emitters include 111In, ^{99m}TC, and 67Ga while the clinically useful positron emitters include 68Ga and 18f. These techniques are useful for chronic OM only.

Three Phase Bone Scintigraphy

The concept is developed on the accumulating property of phosphates (and pyrophosphates in particular) by adsorption and binding to collagen. Methylene diphosphonate (^{99m}Tc-MDP) is the most popular diphosphonate used in clinical practice. ^{99m}Tc-MDP accumulates sequentially in the perivascular space, then in the bone fluid space, and finally in the bone marrow. Depending on requirement and clinical setting one, three, or four phase scan is done.

- The first phase (injection phase) is similar to angiogram (reflecting the local vascular flow) where the dynamic images of the region of study are captured in 2–5 seconds frames for 60 seconds.
- Second phase is the blood pool phase (taken within 5 minutes of injection) where the static images are taken from the region of interest. It shows the relative vascular flow and distribution of isotopes in extracellular space. The intravascular and extravascular activity is clearly distinguished allowing better spatial resolution of bone, joint, and soft tissue. Blood pool better images reflect the level of soft tissue involvement.
- The third phase is performed after a gap of 2–4 hours, which highlights the bone (excess isotope in blood is cleared by kidney) and involved pathology, this reflects the osteoblastic response. During the first two phases, diffuse increase uptake occurs in cellulitis and local increased uptake in all three phases in OM **(Fig. 17)**. Other conditions in which third phase is positive are osteoarthritis and degenerative joint disease, bone neoplasms, post-traumatic bone, and postsurgical state in which bone was operated.
- Delayed scans (so-called fourth phase) taken 24 hours later demonstrate the persistent increased activity in affected regions only due to poor washout of the radiopharmaceutical (decreased vascularity) and continued uptake of radiopharmaceutical by immature woven bone.

Typically for OM, a three-phase bone scan is obtained. In infants a "cold" area may be seen due to reduced delivery of the isotope because of edematous occlusion of flow in intramedullary vessels. In patients with prosthesis, the modality is superior for demonstrating activity over MRI without interference from the artifact. If a bone scan is negative it essentially rules out infection and there is no need to proceed with leukocyte scans. False-positive bone scans are common with neuropathic joint, gout, postsurgical changes, degenerative joint disease, aseptic inflammatory process, and stress fracture or a healing fracture.

Gallium Scintigraphy Scan

Gallium-67 citrate (rarely performed now) shows intense uptake in infection, aseptic inflammatory conditions, and malignancy by their direct leukocyte and bacterial uptake, lactoferrin and transferring binding, accumulation at areas of increased vascularity, and increased bone turnover. The transferrin leaks into the active inflammation regions upon injection and the scans are performed 18–72 hours later. They may reveal abnormal accumulation in regions that were "cold" on ^{99m}Tc scans (due to poor osteoblastic response). They are however limited by poor bone resolution. Gallium scans are considered positive if they show increased uptake than ^{99}Tc-MDP scans or they show incongruent uptake.

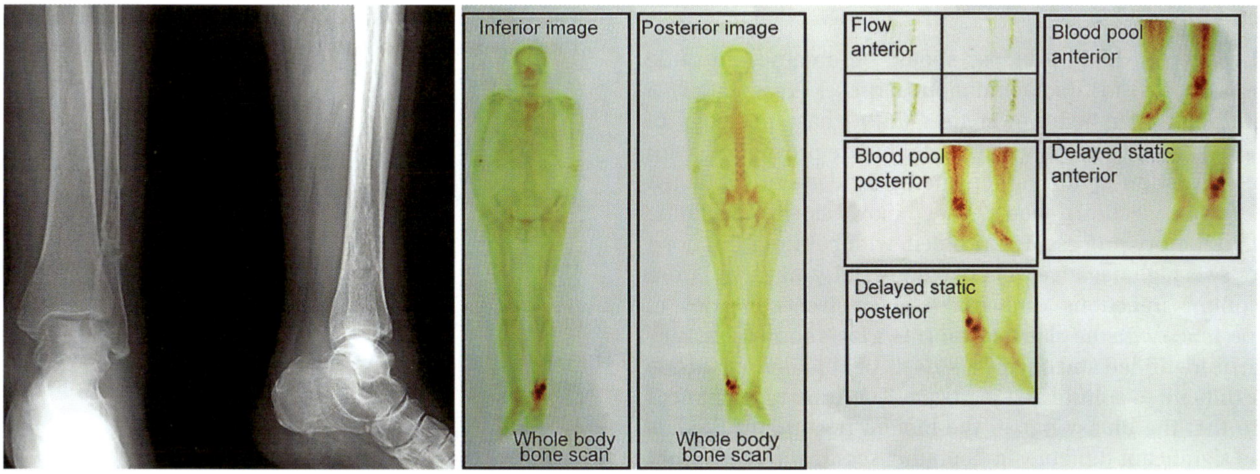

Fig. 17: Three-phase bone scan in a patient with distal fibula lesion. The radiographs demonstrate fracture with attempt at healing and moth-eaten appearance around the fracture site. Three-phase bone scan demonstrated increased uptake in the region along with distal tibia. It is not possible to differentiate osteomyelitis from stress fracture or old trauma really by a bone scan. The patient clinically had local rise of temperature in a swollen ankle and fever. Patient was managed for acute on chronic osteomyelitis successfully.

Labeled Leukocyte Imaging

This is performed either using Indium-111 or with ^{99m}Tc-hexamethyl-propyleneamine oxime (HMPAO)-labeled white cells. There is marked improvement in specificity compared with that of bone scans, particularly when complicating conditions (aseptic inflammation) are superimposed. Labeled leukocyte imaging is the radionuclide procedure of choice for diagnosing so-called "complicating" OM. The technique is limited by requirement of extensive set-up and trained personnel. There is also a risk of contracting human immunodeficiency virus (HIV)/hepatitis-B infection. Newer in vivo methods of labeling leukocytes by peptides and antigranulocyte antibodies are being developed and are called "infection probes". BW 250/183 is a monoclonal antibody against nonspecific cross-reacting antigen-95 (NCA-95) antigen present on leukocytes that has good detection rate for lower limb OM. "Sulesomab" is a monoclonal antibody against NCA-90 antigen of leukocytes. They have also shown to be having good specificity. Similarly "besilesomab (Scintimun)" imaging has been found comparable to ^{99m}Tc-HMPAO scan. ^{99m}Tc-fanolesumab has been withdrawn due to deaths during the trial.

Combined Techniques

Due to inherent limitations of specificity and spatial resolution of various techniques the combined ^{99m}Tc-MDP/111 In-WBCs and combined ^{99m}Tc sulfur colloid bone marrow/111 In WBCs are considered the "method of choice" for OM diagnosis. The sulfur colloid is rapidly taken up by physiological or metabolically active marrow (say traumatic injury to bone or aseptic inflammation) and is nonspecific for increased vascularity (infected marrow is hypervascular but metabolically subnormal due to infection and edema). Infection-related necrosis is cold in these scans but are highlighted by labeled WBC scans. There is noncongruent (mismatching) colloid and WBC uptake in case of sepsis compared to congruent (matching) uptake in an aseptic inflammation or trauma. Similarly, the gallium-67 and ^{99}Tc-MDP scans are combined. If the gallium scan is more intense than Tc-MDP scan then there is likelihood of OM. Reverse suggests reactive lesion (traumatic/aseptic). Incongruous uptake of two scans suggests OM.

Radiolabeled Antibiotics

^{99m}Tc-ciprofloxacin is the most common studied probe and method is gaining popularity for specific binding to the bacterial component. They thoroughly differentiate infective from aseptic process and are taken up by the microbes preferentially. The use and efficacy is debated in literature. They may be associated with radiopharmaceutical misbehavior due to poor recognition by bacterial efflux pumps.

"Radiolabeled immunoglobulins" are under study. One such molecule is ^{99m}Tc-labeled murine immunoglobulin M monoclonal antigranulocyte antibody that binds to human polymorphonuclear leukocyte CD15 antigen. They have 91% sensitivity and 70% specificity but need further standardization.

Positron Emission Tomography Scans

They are highly specific and can be very useful in the detection of osteomyelitic foci and the presence of chronic OM. Fluorine-18 fluorodeoxyglucose (FDG) is the most commonly used compound and has demonstrated that FDG-PET has the highest diagnostic accuracy for confirming or excluding the diagnosis of chronic OM in comparison with other techniques. Inflammatory cells demonstrate increased expression of glucose transporters. This is a fast technique with results available within 30–60 minutes and is unaffected by metallic implants. Vertebral lesions are also better evaluated by FDG-PET. It can also be a good modality to monitor the treatment response or disease activity (periprosthetic infections).

Bone Biopsy

Whenever in doubt a biopsy should be obtained to settle the issue and for documentation purpose. Presence of >5 neutrophils per high-power field (HPF) has specificity of 93–97%. These are especially useful before proceeding with reconstruction or during repeated debridement (obtained as frozen section) where they show slowly declining inflammatory process. The problem with culture from bone biopsy is high negative yield of culture (false-negative) from "biofilm" infections discussed above. Over centuries of experience with the planktonic forms, a lot is known and they can be identified and treated also well, but biofilm organisms are difficult to culture and segregate. There are high chances also that the biopsy misses the biofilm region and there is also significant difficulty in liberating sessile microbes from biofilm even with sonication or subcultures, lastly we have developed only methods to identify the planktonic variants and not the sessile forms in laboratory so we will eventually miss them with current methods. Methods such as phase contrast microscopy, fluorescence staining, PCR, DNA array, RNA, and in situ hybridization probes are needed that are not a regular armamentarium of any standard setup.

PRINCIPLES OF THERAPY

Acute Hematogenous Osteomyelitis

Until the beginning of the 1920s, surgical treatment was the only treatment for OM (ubi pus ibi evacua). The principle is still applicable but antibiotic therapy is the basis for treatment of acute hematogenous OM. Nade outlined following principles (especially pertaining to antibiotic use) for management of acute OM:

- Antibiotic therapy is effective before pus formation (<48 hours).
- Antibiotics cannot sterilize avascular tissue.
- Antibiotics prevent formation of pus once evacuated.
- Evacuation of pus restores periosteum and blood flow.
- Antibiotic should be given following surgery.

Immediately after bacteriological diagnosis, the empirical broad-spectrum antibiotic coverage should be started and then with availability of specific reports the treatment should be narrowed down. If there is no response in 48 hours then surgical evacuation of pus or decompression should be strongly considered to prevent bone necrosis and sequel of acute OM. Surgical indications in acute hematogenous OM are as follows:

- Abscess formation (strongest indication, as soon as pus is aspirated or demonstrated by any diagnostic modality the pus should be evacuated as the antibiotics will not be effective and continuing damage will ensue)
- Concomitant septic arthritis
- Persistence of symptoms without any improvement after 48 hours of antibiotic therapy
- Slow progression as clinically deemed after 72 hours of adequate, directed antibiotic therapy
- Multifocal OM with pus formation especially in an ill and moribund child
- Delayed presentation >7–10 days. Here, the bone is more or less dead and immediate pus evacuation and decompression should be done to preserve as much bone.
- The antibiotic therapy duration is usually for 3 weeks in children. In adults, surgical debridement is usually required for adequate control of infection and treatment courses are typically longer say 4–6 weeks if intravenous therapy.

Drainage of Abscess (Principles Only)

The operation consists of multiple drillings away from epiphyseal line, until pus free marrow is obtained. Periosteum should not be elevated because it not only adds to cortical ischemia but also opens up further tissue planes for pus to traverse. After drainage, the wound is closed primarily to prevent sinus formation and secondary infection. In addition, supportive treatment is given in the form of immobilization, hydration and electrolyte replacement, protein-rich diet, and adequate analgesia. Protein replacement is given to compensate for negative nitrogen balance created by tissue destruction. Hemolysis may need blood transfusion. Immobilization reduces muscle action and blood flow thereby decreased the spread of infection. Splinting is continued even after acute stage has passed to prevent deformity and to keep joints in a good functioning position if there is any likelihood of ankylosis.

Intravenous antibiotics are preferred over oral and should be given for initial 5–7 days (irrespective of surgical drainage) followed by 3–4 weeks of oral therapy. The time is arbitrary but there is some sense in continuing the therapy for 4 weeks as revascularization of bone takes 4 weeks so it should be protected for that period plus 1 week. There is no recommendation for intravenous drug therapy for 6 weeks [except possibly for methicillin-resistant *Staphylococcus aureus* (MRSA) infection]. Clinical improvement is the best way to monitor patient. Children <4 years usually have mixed infections, hence second generation cephalosporins like cefuroxime or cephamandole should be started. Patients with sickle-cell disorder with *Salmonella* usually respond to cotrimoxazole, 4-hydroxy-quinolones, or amoxicillin with β-lactamase inhibitor. Heroin addicts and immunocompromised patients usually have unusual infections such as *Pseudomonas*, *Proteus* or *Bacteroides* where desirable antibiotics include third-generation cephalosporins with gentamicin/flucloxacillin. The improvement occurs within 24–48 hours. Fever should settle within 2–3 days. Erythema and swelling (which should be recorded with a tape measure) should settle and the range and rhythm of movement recover. White cell count should decline within 1 week; ESR should reduce by minimum 20% and CRP to 50% within 1 week. "Tunis protocol" was developed by Essadam and Hammou that defined treatment according to evolution of disease as identified on USG. Based on the sonography done on day 1, surgery is indicated for development of stage 2.

For patients presenting late adequate initial drainage should be supplemented with some procedure that facilitates further drainage of the debris and continuous formation of pus. This is achieved by wide drainage and removal of major discernable sequestrae and dead bone. Medullary cavity should be freely drained in order to relieve medullary tensions and minimize sequestrum formation. The affected segment of bone is exposed by an incision in the periosteum. After drainage of subperiosteal abscess, the medullary cavity is exposed. The cortical bone overlying the metaphysis is excised with an osteotome/gouge/nibbler. The opening is then enlarged for adequate drainage. The X-ray changes in the course of a successful treatment include extensive decalcification which progresses for 70–140 days. Subperiosteal bone formation is limited, small sequestrae are absorbed, and ultimately recalcification is complete. Subperiosteal resection is performed at a late stage of OM when whole/considerable part of bone is necrosed and forms a sequestrum or is riddled with infection. Diaphysectomy is reserved for one of the bones of leg or forearm where the other bone still remains to maintain configuration of the limb. The limb is protected in a cast or brace after bone resection.

Chronic Osteomyelitis

Since its recognition various means of the management have evolved and been reported in the medical literature for treatment of chronic OM. Like malignant tumors the disease is difficult to eradicate fully, likely to recur, destroys the parent bone, and damages surrounding structures. As with the treatment of malignant tumors, one has to distinguish between specific local and systemic therapies. OM treatment also requires multimodality approach with primary disease removal (effective) and supplementary therapy (less effective) combined together **(Figs. 18A to F)**. The treatment of OM is based on three principles (oncologic approach), analogous to the treatment of aggressive tumors:

- Radical surgical eradication of the affected bone and soft tissue (and reconstruction for a stable functional limb)
- Systemic and local chemotherapy (with antibiotics) and adjuvant therapy to eradicate infection
- Retain limb function.

Winnette Orr (World War I) is credited with laying the foundation for developing the principle of wide drainage by good wound debridement and rest (immobilization) to limb. He popularized the cast method. He advocated thorough debridement and cleaning the wounds with Carrel-Dakin solution. The wound is then packed with petroleum soaked gauge to prevent sticking of dressing and setting the bone in a plaster of Paris (POP) cast. The cast was then removed after 3 weeks or if there was complication like foul smell or systemic signs of infection.

At best most of the times even with the best of aggressive management it is considered a satisfactory outcome if the disease can be reduced to a nonsymptomatic state (under remission), always bearing in mind that acute episodes may recur anytime later. It should be realized that any therapeutic approach should not compromise the physiology and limb function to worsen the current situation and should be planned accordingly.

Timing the Intervention

Chronic OM should be treated as soon the patient is ready mentally and physically for sustaining multiple and extensive operations. Careful evaluation should be done before prescribing the whole surgical plan and taking the patient to operation theater. Prerequisites for performing surgery in a symptomatic patient with chronic OM:

- Acute phase should subside and there should be no fever.
- Discontinue antibiotics 1 week before surgery.
- The dead bone (sequestrum) should have separated from parent bone (takes 2–3 months to separate on radiographs though bone dies within 10 days of loss of vascularity).
- The involucrum should be strong enough (radiologically seen in three of the cortices on two perpendicular views)

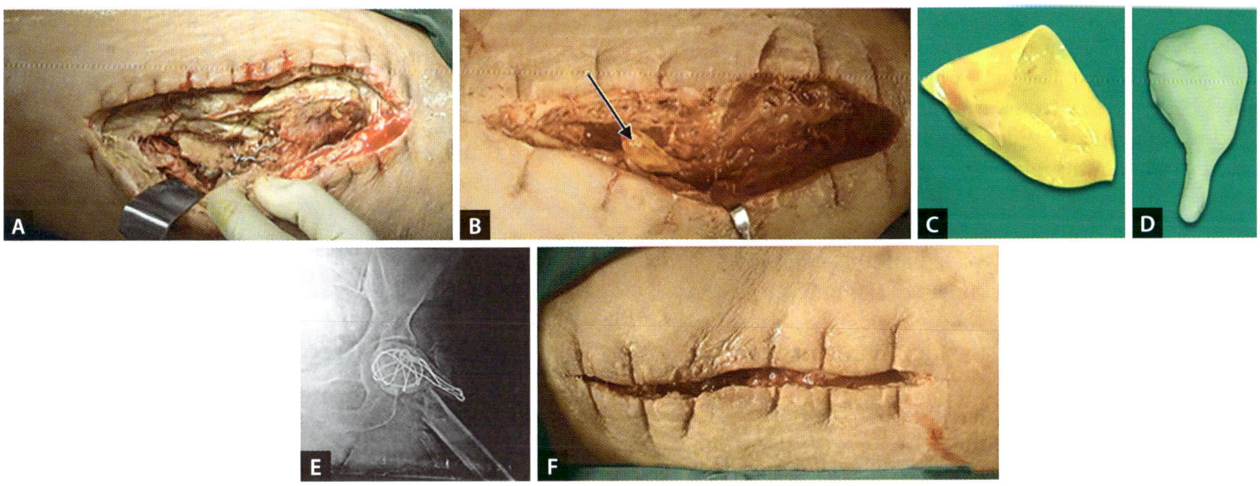

Figs. 18A to F: Sometimes infections have to be dealt on war-footing. This patient was operated somewhere for open nailing of the proximal femur fracture but developed copious discharge from the wound. She was managed with thorough debridement (A) whence two retained hand glove pieces (B and C) were retrieved from the intramedullary canal. Whole proximal femur was debrided (more effective approach) and replaced with antibiotic laden cement spacer (D and E). The wound was closed over suction dressing (supplementary lesser effective approaches). The wound looked better (F) on repeat debridement but the patient succumbed due to septicemia with comorbidities.

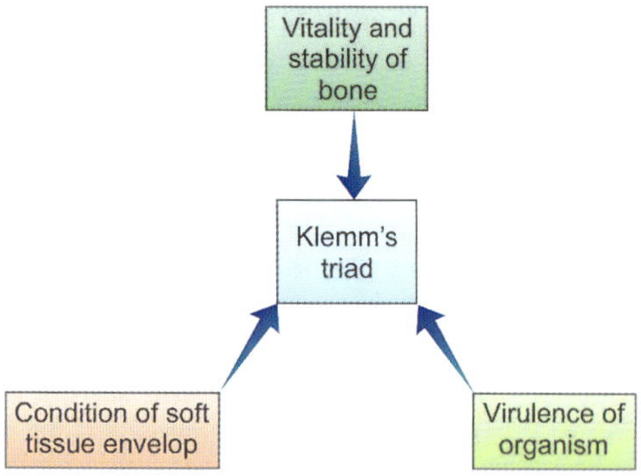

Fig. 19: Klemm's triad.

to support remaining bone after excision. Minimum 70% circumferential strong involucrum (assessed with CT) is required for supporting the bone without need of supportive fixation. As the assessment is difficult so often assistive fixation is done.

- *Salvageable limb:* Klemm's triad **(Fig. 19)** may help in roughly identifying a salvageable limb. Surgeon needs to evaluate the vitality and stability of bone, virulence of organism and sensitivity to antibiotics, and condition of soft tissue envelop. If two or more components are compromised, the chances of providing a functional limb are low.
- Patient should be willing for multiple operations—on an average the number of operations required for treatment of a patient with chronic OM is around 4.

For postoperative wounds even slightest suspicion of infection is enough to consider surgical exploration and re-explorations. The earlier revision surgery is performed, the greater the likelihood of eradication of the infection. This is even more imperative for osteosynthesis or arthroplasty where a foreign implant or material is in place that cannot be reached by systemic antibiotics. The "prophylactic" use of antibiotics in these cases is only suppressive at most and prolongs the time period until surgical revision is ultimately performed. Only in very rare cases, does the innate immunity clear infection while it is kept from flaring up by antibiotics. The use of antibiotics in such situations should be for definitive treatment and clearly goal directed else development of resistance and complications of the treatment will continuously accrue.

Newer antibiotics like daptomycin (a cyclic lipopeptide) have broad-spectrum activity against resistant gram-positive bacteria. Next generation of oxazolidinone such as tedizolid (increased bioavailability) and antibiotics with prolonged half-life such as oritavancin and dalbavancin improves dosing strategies compared to older antibiotics.

SURGICAL MANAGEMENT OF CHRONIC OSTEOMYELITIS

The surgical management of chronic OM needs to be highly tailored depending on patient's needs but a general outline based on classification of OM is presented in **Table 7**. Local surgical treatment for chronic OM is primarily based on five principles:

TABLE 7: Different treatment strategies with respect to the type of osteomyelitis.

Anatomic type	*Usual treatment strategy*
Type I: Medullary	Cortical unroofing, intramedullary curettage and/or medullary reaming
Type II: Superficial	Superficial decortication + Soft tissue coverage (Pedicle or free flap)
Type III: Localized	Excision of focus—Sequestrectomy + medullary decompression + scar excision + bone decortication + stabilization (often necessary)
Type IV: Diffuse	Tumor like approach—Excision of focus + repeat procedure + stabilization of bone + soft tissue coverage
These may be individually combined with either or a combination of: • *Antibiotic beads/cement spacers* • *Antibiotic intramedullary nail (Masala nail)* • *Bone-grafts ± Local antibiotic powders*	

1. Bone and soft tissue debridement removal of infected and necrotic tissue and drainage (wound toileting)
2. Removal of metal implants, hardware, and foreign body
3. Stabilization of the bone throughout
4. Local antibiotic therapy
5. Dead space management
   i. Reconstruction of the soft tissues
   ii. Reconstruction of the osseous defect.

Tissue Debridement

It is better termed "excision of focus" as all the necrotic tissue (bone, periosteum, and surrounding soft tissue) responsible for persistence of infection should be excised thoroughly. To obtain a healthy vascular bleeding bed, rarely the area may need to be excised fully and step 3 (stabilization of bone) will be imperative especially for osseous tissue.

"Sequestrectomy" and removal of infected nonviable bone is another essential component **(Figs. 20A to J)**. The sequestrum is a preferable homing nidus for bacteria as systemic antibiotics cannot reach the necrotic bone, avascular tissue, and puss filled cavity. Also new bone formation is inhibited by the sequestrum that first needs to be absorbed taking a long time. So, sequestrectomy will remove not only the infective focus but also aid in quick healing and bone formation. This involves removal of the visible sequestrum(s). They are identified by their ivory white color and brittle nature.

- To aid identification of nonviable tissue and sequestrum methylene blue can be injected through one of the communicating sinuses (identified on sinogram). The dye stains viable tissue gray but nonviable tissue appears blue. Alternatively dead tissue may be identified by preoperative injection of sulfurous blue which will color all the tissues green, except the devitalized, which will remain uncolored.
- Under tourniquet control, the infected area is exposed and sinus tract incised. The incision for debridement and saucerization extends into normal healthy tissue beyond the diseased area, to allow complete visualization of diseased tissue and preservation of neurovascular structures.

If sequestrum extends beyond its original gutter, then involucrum should be incised longitudinally at either end by knife or osteotome.

- Granulation should be curetted out.
- Progressive nibbling of involucrum and bone is performed till a punctate bleeding bone is reached ("pepper" appearance of bone, "paprika sign"). It is imperative that the tourniquet is deflated at the time of bone debridement. Some people have indicated the use of intraoperative laser Doppler for identifying the viable bone but use is cumbersome and not very accurate.
- *Saucerization:* The resulting defect is burred to have smooth borders that are not undermined (i.e., it is shaped into an open cavity). The covering involucrum if pliable may be invaginated or collapsed to fill the cavity else measures to fill the bone defect/cavity (as described below) are undertaken. This later process is termed "saucerization" and is akin to "wide resection" in tumor excision. A marginal bone excision of around 5 mm is recommended.
- The resulting cavity should be thoroughly inspected for remaining or persisting bone pieces.
- The sequestrae should be inspected for completeness and should not be fractured or broken while removal **(Figs. 20A to J)**. They have a roughened surface facing the granulation tissue. The surface facing the pus is smooth.
- If a bone window needs to be created for removal of covert sequestrum then one should create a surface marking on the parent bone in an "oval" fashion using multiple drill holes that covers 10–15% more length than the measured length of sequestrum **(Figs. 21A to D)**. The bone window is then completed using an osteotome. The above procedure is then completed.
- At the end of sequestrectomy and saucerization, the medullary canal should be completely opened using awls or burrs if there is a sclerotic bony block and thoroughly lavaged with ample saline. This brings in the healing factors for subsequent bone formation.
- The soft tissue debridement is also important. All grossly visible necrotic tissue and slough should be excised.

Limb is splinted till wound has healed. It is protected further to prevent a pathological fracture. Nonweight-bearing ROM exercises are begun soon after wound healing. Antibiotics are generally continued for at least 6 weeks.

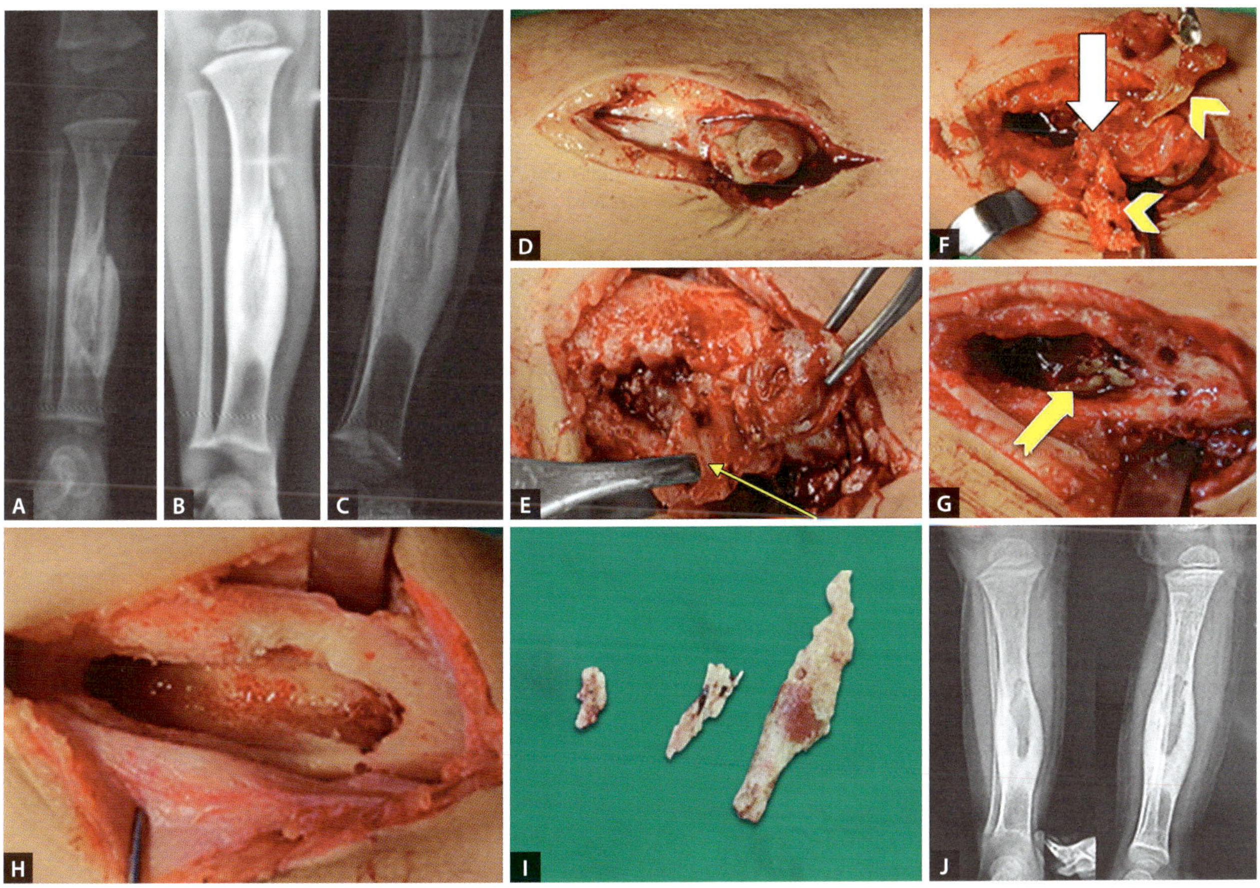

Figs. 20A to J: Chronic osteomyelitis developing in a 4-year-old patient of chronic renal disease on dialysis following episode of acute osteomyeitis (OM) managed with antibiotics initially. The evolution of chronic OM showing separation of sequestrum (A), formation of cloaca (B), partial resorption of sequestrum (C), but development of severe pain due to closure of cloaca and built-up of pus in closed cavity of tibia. Sequestrectomy was planned with removal of sinus tract (D), elevation of bone window (E; arrow), curettage of granulation tissue (block arrow) with careful removal of sequestrae (F; chevrons), identification of remaining sequestrae in the cavity (G; notched arrow), completion of the procedure and smoothening of the edges of cavity (saucerization, H), inspection of the removed sequestrae for completion of procedure (I), postoperative radiographs demonstrating completion of sequestrectomy and smooth bordered cavity (J).

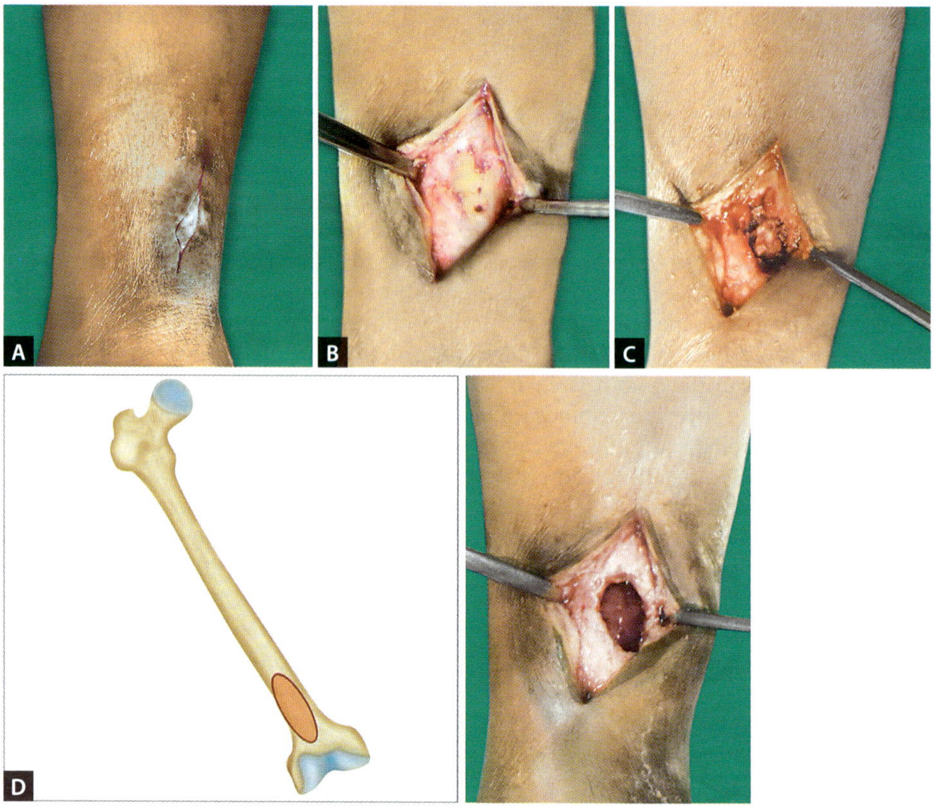

Figs. 21A to D: Sinus tract excision and sequestrectomy. (A) The sinus tract is taken out in the bone deep skin incision to remove the epithelialized tract; (B) The bone is exposed subperiosteally only as much required to prevent devascularization, sequestrated bone is visible as creamish white bone with previous decompression holes surrounded by reactive white bone partially engulfing and partially eating into it; (C) The sequestrated bone is excised and deep infected bone removed. Being predominantly intramedullary form no frank sequestra were visible inside the bone; (D) Note the final oval shape of sequestrectomy.

Removal of Metal Implants, Hardware, and Foreign Body

Metallic implants are almost always involved and need to be removed, only in exceptional cases when the debridement is done very early, infection is not very profuse or from a virulent organism, titanium implants have been used and the implants are well fixed they may be retained. Typically for chronic OM, the intramedullary nailing performed to stabilize the fracture must be removed, the medullary canal reamed and the reaming material examined microbiologically and histologically. Plates must also be removed and the area debrided. After surgical debridement of the osteomyelitic focus, thorough irrigation preferably with a pulsatile delivery system is done. Alternatively for closed cavities the Weber and Lautenbach method **(Fig. 22)** may be used. The Lautenbach method involves:

- Radical debridement of avascular infected tissue
- Debridement of infected endosteum (reaming)
- Insertion of double lumen local antibiotic delivery system
- Delivering high concentration of appropriate antibiotics usually mixed with enzymatic solution to prevent blockage of tubes
- Monitoring effluent for changes in flora and modifying the therapy with subcultures done at 7 days. Less virulent, fastidious organisms should be especially looked for and anaerobic cultures should also be done.

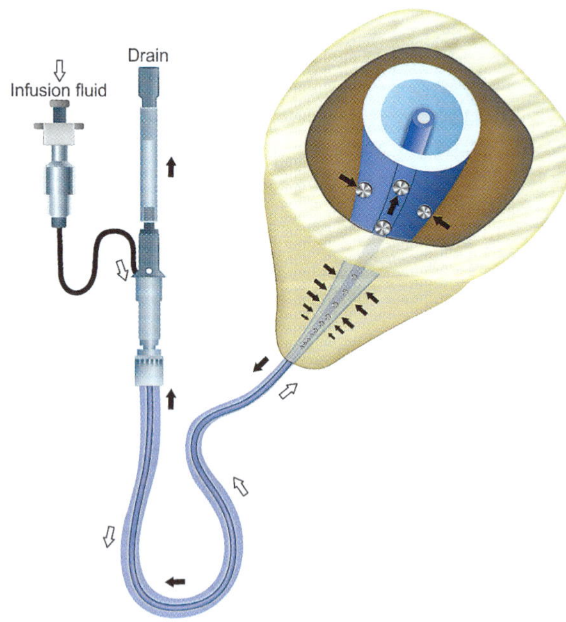

Fig. 22: Lautenbach method.

- Endpoint is when the three consecutive irrigates are sterile, there is improvement in blood parameters and obliteration of the cavity.

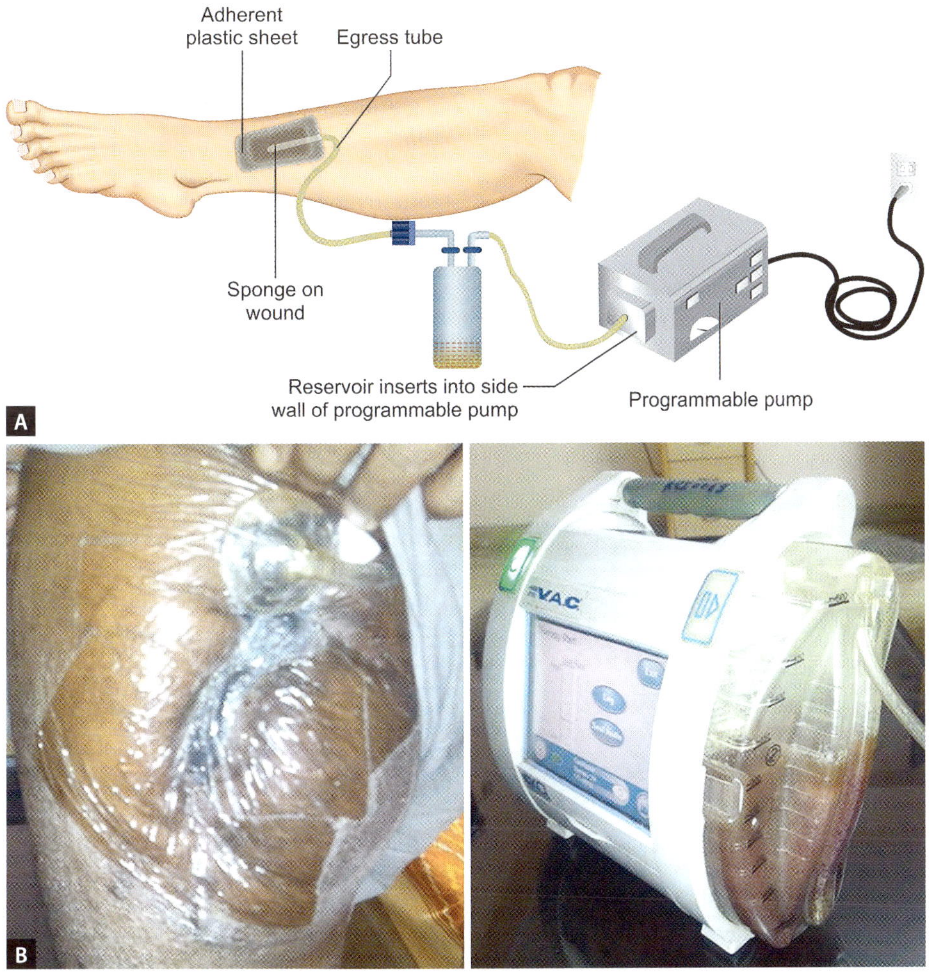

Figs. 23A and B: The principles involved in the management of wound by negative pressure wound therapy (NPWT) as illustrated in (A); the commercially available (B) vacuum-assisted closure system (VAC®).

Primary wound closure is not essential but arrangements should be made or planned for future closure of wound. "Vacuum-assisted closure" **(Figs. 23A and B)** is helpful in:

- Reducing the contamination providing good wound toilet (drainage)
- Avoiding dead space
- Contracting the wound
- Enhancing the granulation tissue
- Improving local vascularity

If soft tissue is difficult to obtain or extensively damaged that needs resection then primary shortening of bone can also be considered as an option especially in upper limb to protect soft tissue and reduce tension on wound/vascularity. Generally, the debridement is repeated every 48 hours until the samples taken from the wound return sterile and local condition of wound looks healthy. Laboratory parameters are usually not relied upon. Local tissue intraoperative biopsies (frozen biopsy) is a useful guide and debridement may not be required if the biopsies do not indicate acute inflammation.

Bone Stabilization

This is an important step as this prevents further tissue damage, stabilizes the wound for supportive healing and better nursing of patient. Commonly the external fixators are used but it may be preferable to use Ilizarov frames for complex reconstructions and thinner wires reducing the chance of infection. External fixators are easy to apply but cumbersome to patient for prolonged duration and possibility of pin site infection. Applying a slab or cast is often inadequate and has to be changed frequently.

Local Antibiotic Therapy

The delivery of local antibiotics for the treatment of musculoskeletal infection has become increasingly popular for following reasons:

- High local levels of antibiotics facilitate delivery of antibiotics by diffusion to avascular areas of wounds.
- Microbes resistant to drug concentrations achieved by systemic antibiotic are susceptible to the extremely high local drug concentrations provided by local antibiotic delivery.
- The MIC for planktonic variant of bacteria is hundreds of order of magnitude lower than the mean-biofilm-eliminating-concentrations (MBEC) needed for managing most chronic orthopedic infections. These high MBEC cannot be achieved by systemic therapy with antibiotics.

TABLE 8: The various available local antibiotic delivery systems.

Delivery system	***Antibiotics generally used***
Nonbiodegradable	
Bone cement (PMMA)	Gentamicin, vancomycin, ciprofloxacin, and β-lactams
PMMA beads	Gentamicin, tobramycin, vancomycin, and β-lactams
Biodegradable	
POP pellets	Gentamicin, teicoplanin
Calcium sulfate cement	Tobramycin
Calcium phosphate cement	Teicoplanin
Hydroxyapatite	Vancomycin
Collagen sponge	Gentamicin
Fibrin	Ciprofloxacin
Polymers: Polylactide/ polyglycolide, dilactide	Gentamicin, fluroquinolones (pefloxacin, ciprofloxacin), vancomycin
Cancellous bone graft	Vancomycin, ciprofloxacin
Fibers	Tetracycline
Chitosan	Vancomycin
Polyurethanes	Gentamicin, ciprofloxacin
"Smart" systems like gelatin	Gentamicin with growth factors

(PMMA: polymethylmethacrylate; POP: plaster of Paris)

- Newer bioabsorbable agents might serve well for dead space management.
- Additional osteoconductive and osteoconductive agents can be used as delivery system helping bone healing.

They provide an efficient delivery of higher levels of antibiotics to the site of infection and yet minimize the risks of systemic toxicity. The current concerns for various delivery systems include:

- Delivery technique
- Antibiotic compatibility
- *Pharmacokinetics:* The current concern is rapid elution of drug early that needs to be converted to sustained release. Strategies principally described to overcome the problem of rapid drug release include the entrapment of the hydrophilic drug within a hydrophobic substance to delay water penetration and drug diffusion and enhancement of drug bonding to the carrying matrix. Drug bonding is achieved either by selecting or modifying a matrix material that forms covalent bonds, Van der Waals, dispersion forces, hydrogen bonds, or ionic interactions between the drug and the matrix.
- Ability to combine with other simultaneous osteo-inductive and osteoconductive measures deployed (like bone grafts)
- Adverse effects

The currently available systems can be divided into biodegradable and nonbiodegradable systems **(Table 8)**, although none is still perfect.

Nonbiodegradable Drug Delivery Systems

"Nonbiodegradable bone cements—antibiotic bone cement [polymethylmethacrylate (PMMA)]" is the current gold standard for local antibiotic delivery in orthopedic surgery. They also have high compression strength so can provide good structural strength that can be used for advantage in membrane-induced technique. It is imperative here to mention and differentiate the two "modes" of using antibiotic loaded bone cements (ALBC). One is the very popular method among arthroplasty surgeons of using ALBC in each and every arthroplasty case as a "preventive" measure. This prophylactic mode is unscientific and ill-founded and gives false sense of security among surgeons for protection against SSI that may easily develop later. These preparations are low-dose ALBC preparations that do not compromise the cement strength (70 MPa: ISO 5388) but do provide local antibiotic concentrations higher than MIC for nearly 40 hours. Logically, a well-performed clean surgery should not need this type of protection as that is simultaneously provided by systemic antibiotic administration. Concurring to this there are no reports suggesting protection over and above systemic antibiotic therapy offered by the use of these low-dose ALBC. The second "mode" of using the bone cements with high dose antibiotic as a "therapeutic modality" in chronic infections and dead-space management does have rationale. The antimicrobial powder acts as a poragen in these preparations (high-dose) creating microvoids in the cement allowing fluid to penetrate but drastically reducing cement strength. In contrast, the low-dose ALBC traps most of the antibiotic and does not allow fluid penetration or elution to provide local antibiotic concentrations. The antibiotic elution from the high-dose ALBC containing >10% v/v antibiotic approaches 75% at 30 days maintaining concentrations >100 times MIC and approaching or exceeding the MBEC concentrations. There are two ways for using an antibiotic with bone cement (nonbiodegradable).

1. One is mixing the antibiotic with bone cement to be used for implantation with prosthesis. This will be permanent implantation, till obviously need for revision arises.
2. The other is temporary where the cement is usually formed into beads that are then implanted for variable duration in the wound **(Figs. 24A to D)**. The implantation can be for short term (see bead pouch technique), or intermediate to long term. In the latter, beads are usually implanted for dead space management and infection control for 2–3 weeks (intermediate term) and removed altogether thereafter or kept for 3 weeks and pulled daily at the rate of 1 bead/day that extends to 2–3 weeks (long term). There is a concern of biofilm producing bacteria thriving on the "foreign material", should they be kept for prolonged period (>4 weeks). There is no role of permanent implantation of beads or use for >6 weeks in the wound in any case. Bead removal is more difficult (especially in long-term cases) because of local tissue scaring and adhesions and may predispose to infection again due to both local and systemic factors. The major drawback is requirement of additional surgery for subsequent removal **(Figs. 25A and B)**. The second procedure puts patient to additional pain and anesthetic complications, and billing costs for second procedure.

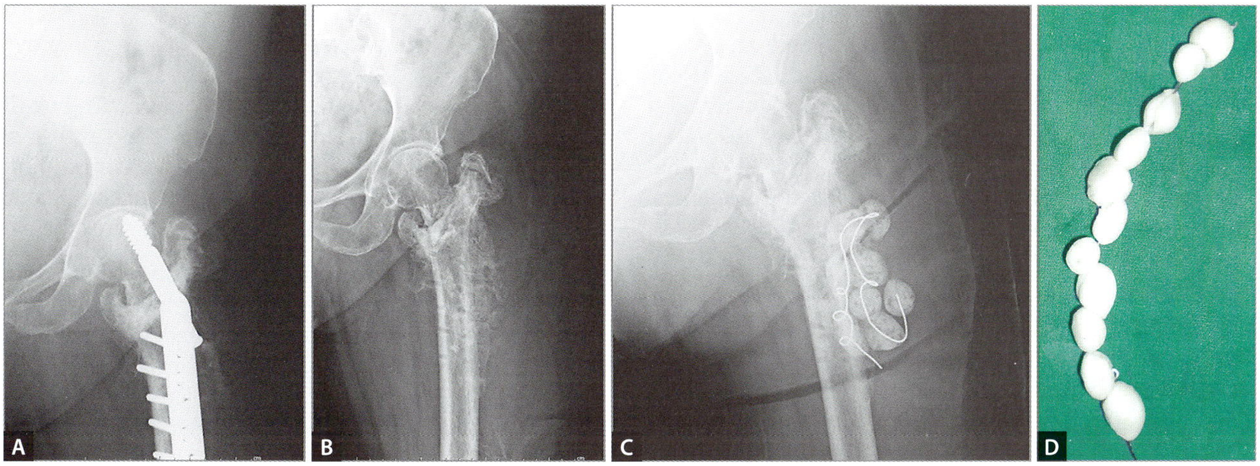

Figs. 24A to D: Antibiotic bead implantation—a patient with dynamic hip screw (DHS) fixation done elsewhere 2 years ago for treating left hip intertrochanteric fracture got infected. The radiographs depict failing implant to construct with superior cut-out and profuse reactive bone formation in proximal femur (A). The screw has collapsed fully. The DHS implant was removed (B) and the infection controlled with temporary implantation of antibiotic beads (C). The antibiotic beads can be prepared in the operation theater (D).

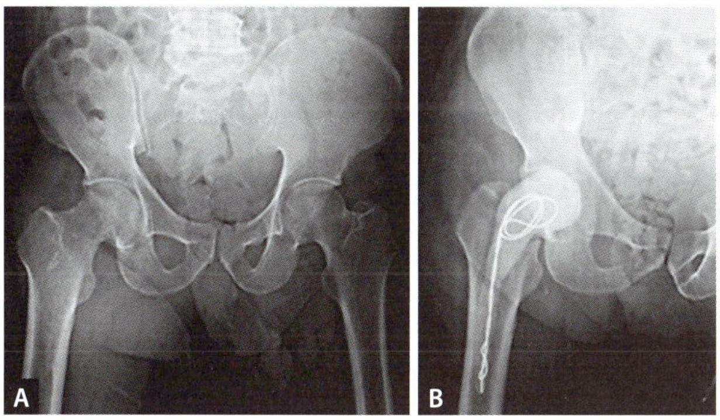

Figs. 25A and B: This right hemi-paretic patient was planned for cemented hemiarthroplasty for pathological fracture neck of right femur but was found to have osteomyelitis with pus formation of the proximal femur. Intraoperative gram-staining demonstrated gram-positive organism. Through intramedullary lavage and antibiotic (4 g vancomycin) cement spacer implantation was done.

The PMMA beads are available premanufactured in fixed dose strength and are liable to wastage. They can be synthesized in operation theater **(Fig. 24D)** using commercial PMMA bone cement mixed with desired antibiotic and rolled into beads fixed over an 18-G or 20-G wire. High viscosity cement should be used rather than liquid low-viscosity cements. Combination of antibiotics has been also attempted. Adding vancomycin powder (4 g) and 480 mg of liquid gentamicin (powder is 20 times more costly) enhances elution of vancomycin by 146% while elution of gentamicin is enhanced by 45%. This is advantageous and cost effective when used for antibiotic beads but the strength of cement is reduced drastically so that this mixture would not be effective for arthroplasty uses. Some considerations for use of antimicrobial agents:

- The antibiotic should be stable at body temperature.
- As good clinical outcomes have been reported with use of ALBC containing <10 vol% poragen, it is recommended that antibiotic weight should not exceed 10% of the weight of cement (2 g for 20 g cement and 4 g for 40 g high viscosity cement) to preserve the integrity and limit systemic toxicity of the drug.
- The antibiotic should be water soluble (for easy diffusion).
- Broad antibacterial spectra, including gram-positive and gram-negative organisms.
- Should be active against the most common bacterial flora.
- Should be able to achieve 10 times or more MIC for the concerned pathogens (i.e., should have good bactericidal effect in low concentrations).
- Should be localized and not enter systemic circulation.
- Should have low rate of primary resistance.
- Should have low rate of development of resistances.
- Should have low affinity to protein.
- Should be readily available in powder form.
- Should have low allergic potential (Sensitivity testing should be done beforehand.)
- Little or no effect on the carrier mechanical or biological properties.

The antibiotics that have been found useful for impregnation with PMMA include (in order of preference)—aminoglycosides (gentamicin and tobramycin), vancomycin, cephalosporins, quinolones, rifampicin, linezolid, doxycycline, β-lactams, macrolides, and antifungal agents such as AmBisome, amphotericin deoxycholate, voriconazole, or fluconazole.

There are some disadvantages of using bone cement:

- High local yield is sustained only for 2–4 weeks and after that the organism may become resistant if not eradicated.
- Second surgery is needed for removal.
- Bacterial colonization may occur as the PMMA surface is quickly coated with fibrin.
- Hypersensitivity reaction may preclude their use or need quick removal.
- Leachable methyl-meth-acrylate monomer has been implicated in local tissue toxicity and systemic effects such as blood pressure lability, hypoxia, and mental confusion.

A BisGMA-TEGDMA-based bone cement, Cortoss™, has been cleared by the United States Food and Drug Administration for vertebral augmentation and has advantages of reduced temperatures while setting and reduced shrinkage. New silorane cements have displayed low exothermicity and good biocompatibility in animal studies along with ability to be incorporated with antibiotics. Recommendations and indications for use of ALBC:

- *Low-dose ALBC:*
  - Implant fixation for aseptic revision arthroplasty (use tobramycin 1.2 g + vancomycin 1 g, or, tobramycin 2.4 g, or commercially premixed ALBC with gentamicin)
  - Implant fixation for second stage reconstruction postinfection
  - Dead-space management only in first-stage PJI—use only commercially available fabricated spacer implant or better use high-dose alternatives as below.
- *High-dose ALBC:*
  - Management of retained biofilm fragments following debridement (use tobramycin 3.6 g + vancomycin 4 g, or, tobramycin 4.8 g/9.6 g, use tobramycin 3.6 g + vancomycin 1 g + 3 g cefoxitin or equivalent for suspected gram-negative infection (i.e., replace 3 g vancomycin with gram-negative active antibiotic), or, for polymicrobial infection with fungi use tobramycin 3.6 g + vancomycin 3 g + ambisome 800 mg/voriconazole 300 mg).
  - Dead space management following debridement in prosthetic joint infections, OM, and open fractures.

Biodegradable Systems

The primary advantage of a biodegradable system is the avoidance of this second surgical procedure. A second advantage is that they can be used initially for management of dead space and eventually may also facilitate repair if combined with newer osteoconductive and osteoinductive carriers. The biodegradable systems can also be modified to vary the magnitude and duration of antibiotic delivery. The biodegradable systems are classified into four broad categories:

1. The bone graft and bone substitutes
2. The protein-based materials (natural polymers)
3. The synthetic polymers
4. Miscellaneous materials

The most acceptable agents include aminoglycosides, β-lactam agents, quinolones, and vancomycin. The elution for water-soluble agents like β-lactams depends on the surface area of the carrier and on the initial concentration of the drug while for relatively insoluble agents like the quinolones porosity of the matrix decides the rate of release.

Bone grafts and bone substitutes: Antibiotics can be added as a powder to morselized cancellous bone (preferable) **(Figs. 26A to G)** or the graft may be soaked in antibiotic-loaded solution (less preferred). Tobramycin, netilmicin, vancomycin, clindamycin, and rifampicin are commonly used. Drug elution and high local antibiotic concentration persist for around 7 days.

Osteoconductive biomaterials [calcium sulfate, calcium phosphate, hydroxyapatite, or tricalcium phosphate (ceramics)] have also been impregnated with antimicrobial agents that also serve to aid dead space management. These materials loaded with antibiotics have the following advantages:

- High steady and extended release
- Thermolabile antibiotics can also be used allowing wider selection of antibiotics.
- Reduced morbidity as second surgery is not needed to remove the ceramic.
- Increases osteoconduction and facilitation of bone regeneration.
- These additionally avoid the risk of transmitting disease pathogens associated with the use of allograft bone.

Calcium sulfate has been typically mixed with 3.64% vancomycin or 4.25% tobramycin per weight (=1 g of vancomycin or 1.2 g for tobramycin per 25 g of calcium sulfate). Other antibiotic-loaded biomaterials include the calcium hydroxyapatites, bioactive glasses, and antibiotic-loaded blood-coated demineralized bone.

Natural polymers: These protein-based substances include antibiotic-loaded collagen sponge, fibrin, thrombin, etc. They work by providing a physical scaffold around the antibiotic mechanically limiting fluid flow, or the protein binds to the antibiotic. Elution of antibiotic ranges vastly from

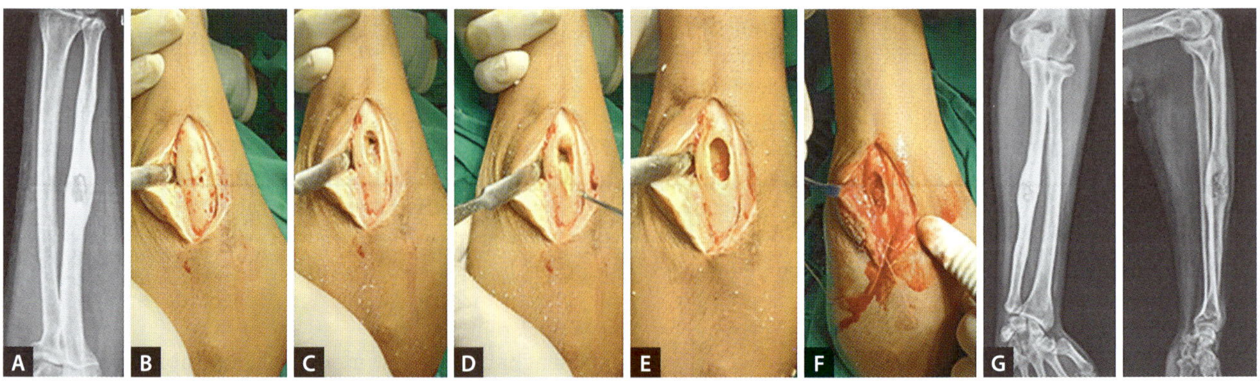

Figs. 26A to G: The patient was suffering from chronic osteomyelitis of ulna (A) with sudden exacerbation of pain and sinus formation. There is distinctive sequestrum formation within ulna (A). The cavity was opened (B and C), sequestrum removed (D), thoroughly curetted with power burr (E) and packed with autogenous bone grafts (F) mixed with antibiotic powder. It went on to complete healing (G).

few hours to days. Collagen sponge produced from animal skin or tendo-Achilles is biocompatible and nontoxic. The porosity of the matrix can be controlled by treating it with chemicals. It can stimulate the proliferation of osteoblasts, thereby promoting callus formation and mineralization. The liposome encapsulated antibiotics have up to three times increased duration of drug release. Polymyxin-B and amikacin are commonly used against *Pseudomonas aeruginosa*. Gentamicin impregnated collagen sponge shows up to 600 times MIC as compared to PMMA beads at 300 times MIC.

Fibrin sealants are being used increasingly as delivery system for antibiotics with low water solubility (tetracycline base) presumably because the precipitated drug dissolves and diffuses slowly from the fibrin clot. They are prepared by the combination of fibrinogen and thrombin solutions that forms a cross-linked clot quickly. The system is better than PMMA in following respects:

- No foreign body response
- Crosslinks to the tissue
- Resorbed by the host

The antibiotic delivery is by way of either diffusion of the antibiotic or by dissolution of the fibrin clot. There is 85% elution of the antibiotic in first 72 hours that is the major disadvantage as remaining drug might be insufficient for persisters.

Synthetic polymers: Biodegradable polymers from glycolide and lactide typically the polylactide/polyglycolide (copolymer in 90:10 ratio) releases the drugs in a controlled manner and dissolves at physiological pH. Tobramycin, clindamycin, vancomycin, ampicillin, gentamicin, polymyxin B, and quinolones have been commonly used with this system. A second advantage is that the kinetics of the release of the antibiotic can be modified by the selection of copolymers of varying monometric composition and molecular weight as well as by alteration of the geometry of the implant. Polymers are available in different patterns such as polylactides, copolymers of lactide and glycolide, polyanhydride, and polycaprolactone. Copolymers are preferred and produce their peak release after 15 days.

Miscellaneous: These materials are developed for different rates and timing of antibiotic release, provision of osteoconduction, osseous integration, and sufficient structural properties. Antibiotic-loaded POP pellets containing gentamicin, fusidic acid, and teicoplanin are well-tolerated and spontaneously absorbed over a period of weeks to months, being replaced by bone ultimately. Chitosan has excellent biodegradable and immunologic activity. Hyaluronic acid and fibrin gel with bone marrow derived mesenchymal stem cells and monoolein-water gels have been used as an alternative treatment for bone and soft tissue infections. Under study are a combination of unconventional marine biomaterials (sponge skeleton, coral, and snail slime) and conventional systems with stem cells to develop smart biomaterials that provide sufficient concentration of antibiotic at the target site, act as a bone strut, and fill dead space and be osteoconductive, osteoinductive, and osteogenic all together. Biodegradable gelatin delivery system has been used that combines the use of gentamicin with growth hormone. A lot more are bound to come but the search for the ultimate is yet on.

Dead Space (Cavity) Management

This often requires the help of expert plastic reconstruction for covering the extensive defects, microbiologist for directed chemotherapy along with the orthopedic surgeon.

Reconstruction of the osseous defect: There are various options **(Flowchart 2)** that can be considered alone or in combination to fill the resulting osseous defect resulting from a successful debridement. These include:

1. Allowing healing with secondary intention from bone bed (not preferred)
2. Local muscle flaps (myoplasty), microvascular muscle free flap
3. Myocutaneous flaps (rotational or free vascularized)
4. Osteocutaneous flaps
5. Osteomyocutaneous flaps
6. Autogenous cancellous bone graft
7. Antibiotic bead pouch technique
8. *Biodegradable antibiotic delivery systems (see above):* Wound can be directly closed over these systems or flaps can be closed over it.

A few are described below:

- *Autogenous cancellous bone grafts:* This is the oldest known technique for reconstructing a bone defect. The prerequisites for successful use of this technique are:

Flowchart 2: Dead space management "toolbox".

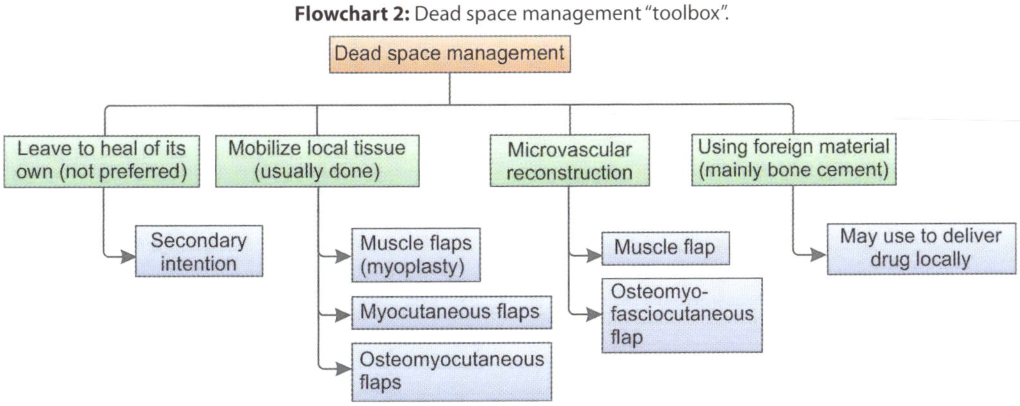

- Critical defect size of 4–5 cm can be reconstructed with cancellous bone graft. Larger defects require other options.
- Optimal vascular situation in soft tissue and bone
- Optimal contact between cancellous graft and living cancellous bone
- Infection-free bone bed in the defect.

▪ *Rhinelander-Papineau technique:* This is a method of open bone grafting of vascularized bone bed defect **(Fig. 27)** that is based on the following principles:
  - Autogenous cancellous bone grafts are rapidly incorporated and resist infection, even if they get infected they are quickly resorbed compared to the cortical bone that persists as sequestrum and prolongs chronic OM.
  - Granulation tissue is resistant to infection.
  - There is no remaining avascular bone and soft tissue.
  - Infected tissue is completely debrided.
  - There is adequate wound drainage.
  - Bone is adequately supported and immobilized.
  - Prolonged use of antibiotics prevents infection.

  The technique has been described in three stages classically:

  1. In the first stage, the wound is excised using above principles and repeated till deemed healthy. In-between, the wound is packed with antibiotic-soaked dressings or bead-pouch technique. The wound is irrigated with normal saline frequently (except the bead-pouch technique) to encourage healthy granulation tissue. Although nailing was originally recommended by Papineau but external fixator is commonly employed. Rhinelander used POP cast. Debridement may be repeated every 5–7 days if there is unhealthy tissue or slough formation. Second stage is delayed till healthy granulation is obtained.
  2. Second stage consists of grafting the healthy granulating bone bed with cancellous iliac bone graft strips of 3–4 mm thickness and 4–6 cm length (some call it pencil grafts) packing them tightly concentrically to recreate the diaphysis shape. The ends of bones are petalled to increase the surface area of contact. Pack the wound with antibiotic-soaked dressings, changing them after 4–5 days when grafts stabilize and incorporate in the granulation tissue. Vacuum-assisted closure (VAC) may be considered to hasten healing and remove serous discharge. Frequent dressings are done till granulation tissue engulfs the grafts and the surrounding skin covers them, in-between the edges may need to be freshened if the epithelium tends to dig into the grafts.
  3. Large wound defects >3–4 cm could take a very long time for spontaneous coverage in these cases, a third stage of providing wound coverage with skin grafts, muscle pedicle flaps, or free microvascular flaps may be done.

  In mini-Papineau technique, after bone grafting instead of waiting for granulation tissue to form, attempt is made to improve vascularity by local muscle pedicle flap so that incorporation is faster and skin coverage can be provided early.

▪ *Bead-pouch technique:* The wound is debrided as above and the defect is filled with commercially available or OT prepared beads on a circlage wire **(Figs. 28A and B)**. It is imperative to count and record the number of

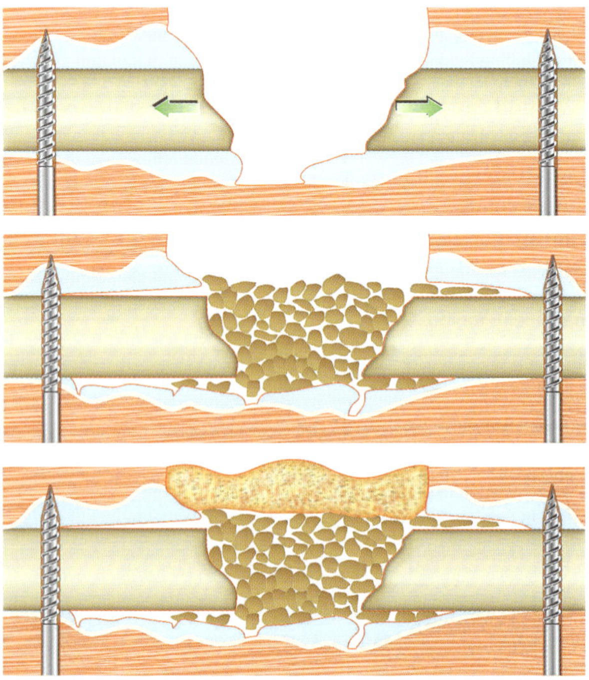

Fig. 27: Papineau technique.

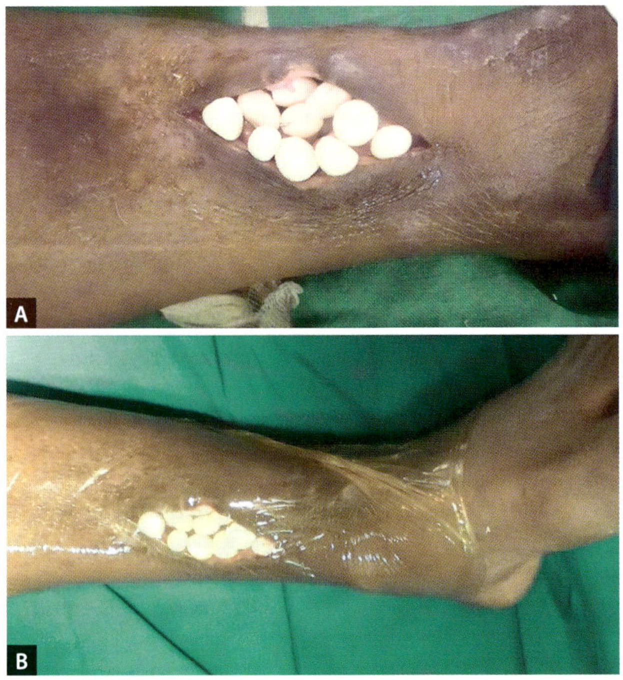

Figs. 28A and B: Bead pouch technique.

beads so that all are removed at next surgery. The wound extensions are closed and edges freshened. Tincture benzoin is applied to the surrounding skin and the prepared defect with beads covered with adhesive sheet. A larger sheet is then wrapped around the limb. This provides a closed bead-hematoma-antibiotic environment for the lesion and controls infection. The dressing is repeated every 48–72 hours depending on the fluid accumulation. Suction drainage is ineffective and in fact counterproductive. Every repeat dressing is followed with the same course as above including debridement till a healthy granulating bed is obtained. When satisfactory wound is obtained a soft tissue coverage is planned.

Reconstruction of Specific Segmental bone Defects

Segmental bone defects arise under following circumstances:

- *Primary diaphysectomy:* Spontaneous discharge of a large segment of the shaft of bone as a result of extensive infection. The periosteum is completely destroyed, therefore, there is no involucrum and the child loses capacity of new bone formation.
- *Late sequestrectomy:* When the entire shaft has been sequestrated with almost no involucrum formation. After removal of sequestrum, a bone defect will appear which is not reformed due to destruction of periosteum.
- *Neonatal disease:* This happens rarely when an extensive defect may develop in spite of the normal capacity of an infant to achieve spontaneous reconstruction.
- Bone loss during open fracture where segment is lost during primary trauma while the preserved limb develops infection and is treated as osteomyelitic limb.

Open bone grafting: This is an acceptable method of reconstructing small to moderate bone defects (up to 3 cm) in children. In upper limbs, defects in humerus can be adequately addressed with fibular (nonvascularized/vascularized) grafting. The results will be good if the growth plate is viable at the more severely affected end. In the forearm, small defects are usually bridged by open bone grafting. However, in large defects, conversion to single bone forearm is an accepted modality. In lower limbs, a bone defect in femur in a small child may be treated with single or double fibular grafting. In tibia, open bone grafting, fibular grafting, and tibiofibular synostosis (single bone leg) are performed depending upon the length of the defect.

The concept of critical bone defects and its management: Key et al., in 1953, described significant bone defect that would not heal by just bone grafting. This defect is described in absolute terms to be a gap that is 1.5 times the diameter of the bone at the place of the defect in the host bone. One can also call it to be "critical defect" as this would need intervention over and above simple bone grafting for successful consolidation. Commonly in an adult, the value for this critical defect is 4–5 cm as for defects larger than this the bone graft tends to get resorbed and the defect would persist. One of the following techniques may be utilized in such circumstances.

1. *Induced membrane technique (Masquelet technique):* Masquelet (2000) reported on a series of 35 cases of large diaphyseal bone defects reconstructed by autologous bone grafting. The technique is aimed at helping to solve the problems of bone graft containment around the bone defect and the commonly desired need for growth supplementation using proteins. They successfully repaired wide diaphyseal defects (≤25 cm) with concurrent severe soft tissue loss using fresh autologous cancellous bone grafts in two-step (first step is more or less mechanical while second step is biological) surgical procedure. In the first step (membrane induction), a PMMA cement spacer is inserted into the defect (after repeated debridement and obtaining clean bed) inducing formation of an encapsulation membrane. The bone is stabilized using external fixator or intramedullary nail. We have used internal fixators (locked plates) for smaller bones of forearm, hand **(Figs. 29A to L)**. After 4–6 weeks, the spacer is removed and the cavity filled with autologous cancellous graft from iliac crest. Morselized cancellous autograft harvested from the iliac crests is preferred but if this amount is not sufficient then demineralized allograft can be added to the autograft in a ratio that does not exceed one part of allograft: three parts of autograft. Bone formation and union occurs in approximately 8–9 months. The advantages of this technique are:

- Prevention of encroachment by adjacent soft tissues into the bone defect
- Stable placement of the graft in place
- Prevention of resorption of graft material by or local production of osteoinductive substances maintains graft volume and helps in augmenting the bone formation (Masquelet).

Biology of induced membrane technique: Nearly 4–5 weeks are needed for development and maturation of a biologically active membrane around the cement-filled nidus that slowly becomes strong enough for bone grafting later. The cement spacer also maintains the defect and inhibits fibrous ingrowth. Masquelet and Begue proposed that this membrane prevents bone graft resorption (but this has not been found always true for filling large bone defects) and improves vascularity and corticalization. Biomembrane formed around PMMA is actually a pseudosynovial membrane that can be 0.5–1 mm thick and has microscopic characteristics of being both hypervascular and impermeable. Histologically, it comprises stratified tissue where the cells are orientated relative to the interface with PMMA. Deeper into the membrane, the fibroblastic cells derived from mesenchymal tissue are arranged in a random fashion. They play an important role in the laying down of extracellular matrix forming the organized pseudosynovial membrane that has been found to express bone morphogenic protein 2 (BMP2), transforming growth factor-beta (TGF-β), vascular endothelial growth factor (VEGF), von Willebrand factor (vWF), interleukin-6 (IL-6), and IL-8. While VEGF is crucial for angiogenesis the vWF has been implicated in the regulation and normal formation of blood vessels and in the membrane it assists in new tissue growth.

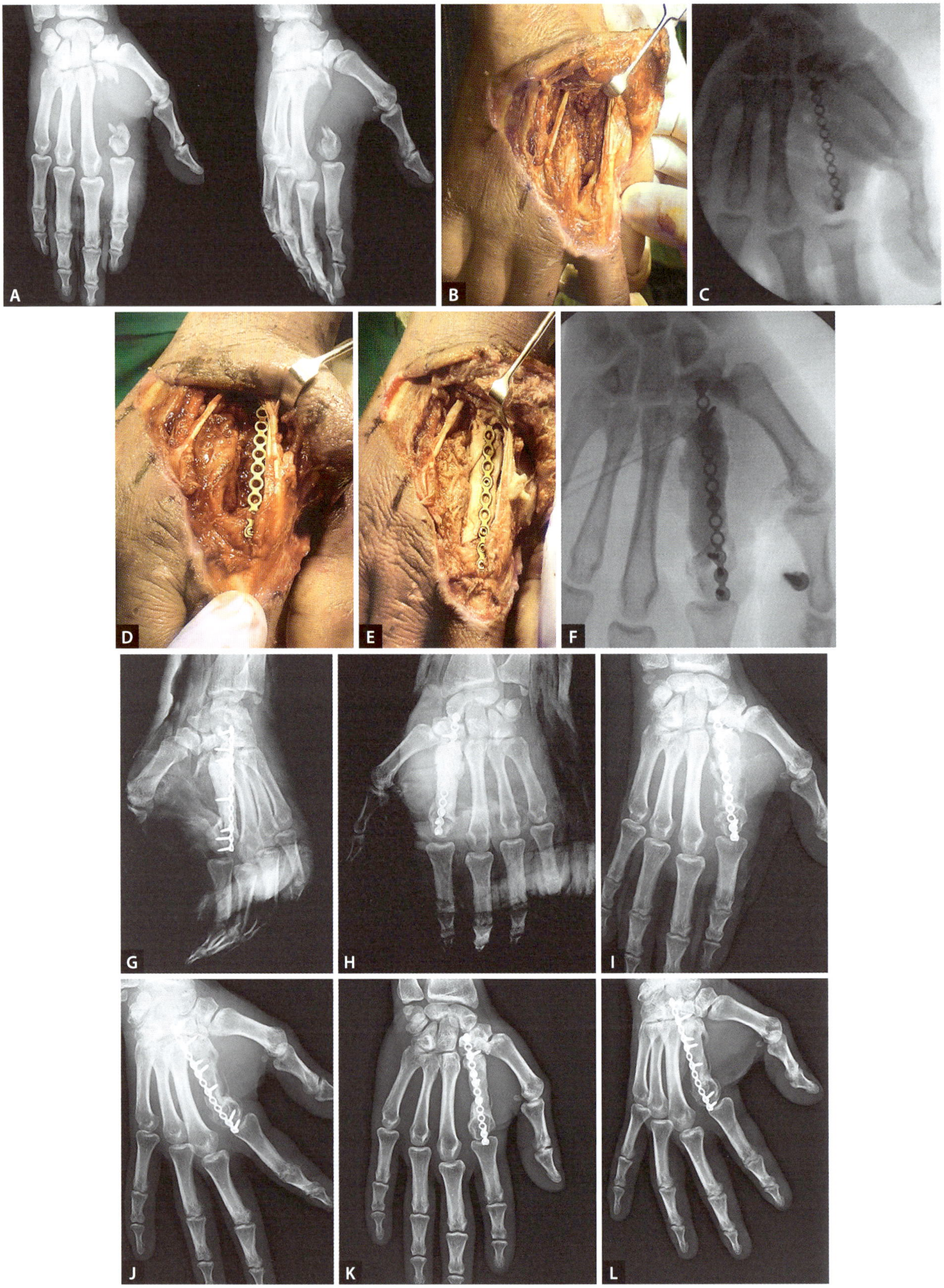

Figs 29A to L: Induced membrane technique (Masquelet technique). Young male with lost middle 3/4th of second metacarpal bone (A) in a road accident was debrided (B). Length obtained under fluoroscope using a plate fixation (C and D) and the gap filled with antibiotic bone cement (E and F). The cement spacer was well maintained and at 8 weeks (G and H). The spacer was removed and cavity filled with cancellous bone graft that showed good consolidation and bone formation after 6 weeks (I and J) and complete union at 3 months (K and L). The plate was removed and patient joined again as car mechanic.

The TBF-β has a stimulatory role instead of a usual catabolic one within the induced tissue type. IL-6 may also stimulate bone formation rather than its regular role in inflammation. Presence of IL-8 may suggest weaning foreign body inflammatory reaction. Fibroblast growth factor-β, platelet-derived growth factor, and insulin-like growth factor-1 found in autogenous bone graft may also help in osteogenesis. The overall construct produces a combination of intramembranous and endochondral ossification histologically producing a progressive healing response. It must be remembered that the membrane alone has been found inadequate to heal a defect greater than critical bone defect. But when autologous bone graft was placed within the membrane nearly all the defects would heal (few defects >15 cm would show premature bone graft resorption). Reconstruction of the femur seems to be specifically associated with a risk of graft resorption. It has also been demonstrated that the 1-month-old membrane has higher osteogenesis-improving capabilities compared to 2-month-old membrane so some have recommended that optimal time for performing second-stage surgery may be within a month after PMMA implantation. I prefer to do the second-stage surgery between 4 and 6 weeks after the first stage of PMMA implantation.

Large amount of graft and sometimes repeated surgery is needed in some patients.

2. *Callus-distraction and distraction histiogenesis (Ilizarov method):* The callus-distraction technique is considered today the gold standard for the reconstructing osseous defects **(*Figs. 30A to F*)**, especially if the defect is >4 cm but <15 cm. The technique is based on the techniques and principles described by Ilizarov.

   Many different techniques for callus distraction have been described and practiced. Each technique has its own specific advantages and disadvantages in terms of stability, secondary soft tissue reconstruction, and ROM of the affected limb. These methods include:
   - Monorail (Wagner type)
   - Lengthening over intramedullary nail (rail-road lengthening)
   - Unilateral external fixators and hybrid fixators
   - Three-dimensional fixators for multi-plane deformity correction
   - Ring fixators (classical Ilizarov technique).

   The advantages of callus distraction are as follows:
   - Bone formation in the distraction zone is autogenic and healthier.
   - A single low risk surgical procedure is performed.
   - Deformity correction can be simultaneously done.
   - Resulting increase in vascularity improves surrounding soft tissue and controls infection.
   - Early weight bearing can be allowed.

   The local soft tissue situation influences type of procedure employed. General guidelines are as follows:
   - Closed and adequate soft tissue envelope + good vascularity with remission of infection + shortening and uniplanar deformity—callus distraction by closed bone transport.
   - Closed and adequate soft tissue envelope + good vascularity with remission of infection + shortening and multiplanar deformity—3D multiplane (single site or multisite osteotomy) or ilizarov method.
   - Difficult soft tissue coverage, open wound or invaginating soft tissues—open bone transport followed by or combined with simultaneous soft tissue coverage.
3. *Microvascular graft osteosynthesis:* Defects larger than 6 cm require vascularized grafts. Advantages of vascularized bone grafts include:
   - Good bone healing due to vascularity with simultaneous cortical bone support
   - Can be used for larger defects >6 cm
   - Can be used for previously failed cases tried with cancellous grafts

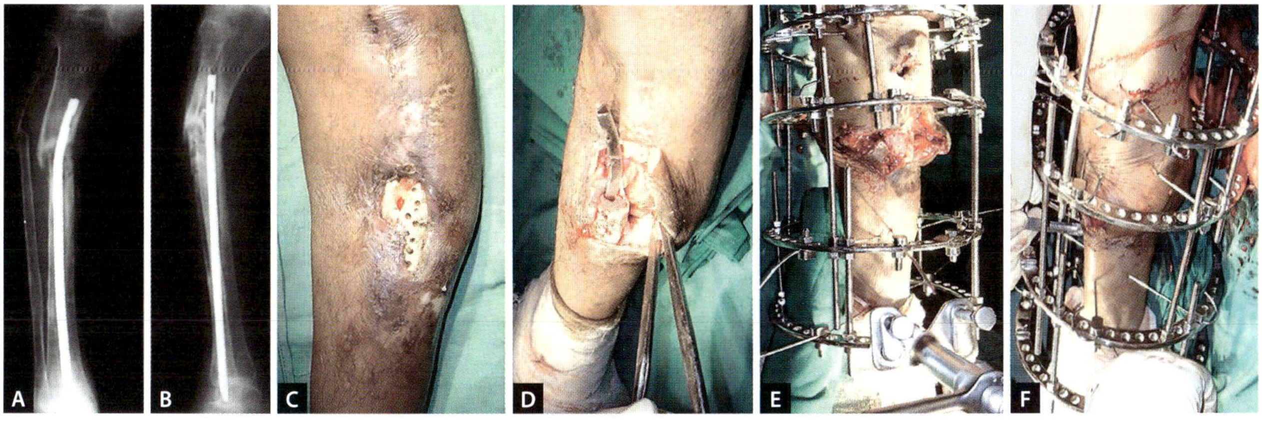

Figs. 30A to F: Ilizarov technique. Messed up case of a poorly fixed open tibial fracture with lots of things to learn from. There is infected nonunion, chronic osteomyelitis with sequestration in upper one-third of tibia. The nail (V-nail) is short, thin and malpositioned fixing the ankle joint instead of fracture. The nonunion is accompanied by deformity and malunited fibula. There is defect in soft tissue coverage and osteopenia of bone. The multiple holes are drill holes attempted to drain pus and allow formation of granulation tissue that also actually failed. For obvious reasons, the ankle was stiff but knee was also stiff due to prolonged immobilization. She was treated with nail removal and excision of nonunion resulting in a gap of 5 cm. Ilizarov fixation with acute docking and intramedullary fibula was used along with Hemisoleus flap to cover the bone and a proximal metaphyseal corticotomy to lengthen bone.

- Can be used in patients with poor soft tissue envelop
- They maintain their mass, architecture, and strength.
- With endurance of load get hypertrophied (undergo remodeling).

Vascularized fibula graft is commonly used; however, vascularized rib and scapular and ilium grafts have been described. The method requires skill and experience in microvascular surgery reconstruction else the success rate is low.

Fibula is straight bone with adequate cortical support and is a composite tissue that makes the use in humerus, tibia, and forearm quite feasible. Double barrel reconstruction is required for femur. Reconstruction up to 26 cm has been reported in literature. The nutrient artery arises from peroneal artery and enters the bone in center. Distal fibula contributes to stability of the ankle mortice so proximal two-thirds is better for reconstruction. The bone can also be used as osseo-myo-fascio-cutaneous flap as it has more of periosteal blood supply. Arteriogram should be obtained before the procedure as peroneal arteria magna is seen in around 5% of cases where the peroneal artery is the dominant artery of foot and harvesting the graft could produce severe ischemia of foot.

4. *Huntington's procedure (ipsilateral fibula transfer, tibialization of fibula):* Unlike transplanting a free fibula, the ipsilateral fibula can be transposed to the tibial defects (fibula pro tibia). The concept was first used by Kahn in 1884 for pseudoarthrosis of tibia. Huntington described the procedure for treating the tibial defect using the ipsilateral fibula transposition in 1903. This method has been used to treat post-traumatic tibial defects; OM produced defects, pseudoarthrosis, and congenital deformities. The original procedure was described as having two steps (now often performed in one step). In the first stage, the distal part of fibula is osteotomized and inserted into medullary canal of tibia or into a trough created on surface for fibula **(Figs. 31A and B)**. The construct may be stabilized with cortical screws of K-wires. The second stage is done at 2–4 months where the proximal portion of the fibula is cut and approximated to tibial surface in a slot created for the same. This can also be stabilized with screws. The bone union occurs at around 6 months. Till then some protection is legible in the form of plaster cast or fixator. Nowadays it is often performed as a single stage procedure. It is imperative to preserve the blood supply to bone. Advantages of the procedure include:
   - Requires less expertise than free microvascular fibula transfer
   - Bone remodels with weight-bearing and hypertrophies
   - Union and bone uptake is more certain that avascular fibula transplant as the graft is vascular here
   - Union bypasses the stage of creeping substitution.

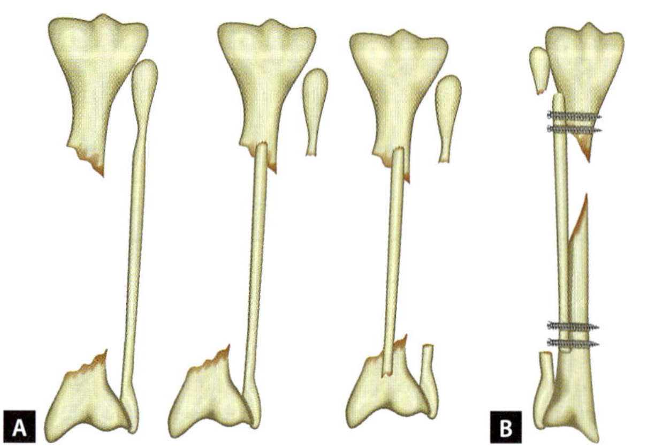

Figs. 31A and B: Huntington's procedure. Either the fibula can be placed centrally into tibia (A) if medullary canal allows or else it can be screwed to it in cases of blocked sclerotic canals (B).

Reconstruction of the Soft Tissue

The planning of covering soft defect is done in the initial surgical planning itself and is carried out when the infection has undergone remission (the term "healing" is not used and complete extirpation of infection is possibly never achieved), usually after 6–8 days of definitive tissue debridement. The soft tissue coverage options depend on the following criteria (Heppert et al.):

- The type of osteosynthesis
- The site and size of the soft tissue defect
- The local vascular status
- Patient compliance

The spectrum of treatment options for soft tissue coverage range from split skin grafts to free vascularized myocutaneous flaps depending on above factors.

Amputation

This is reserved for unrelenting and multiply failed cases or in whom there is no possibility of reconstruction or in whom the reconstructed limb will fare worse that prosthetic fitted amputated limb. Thorough discussion with the family and explaining the patient is a must before undertaking this. It should be fully logically supported and only prescribed when all options have exhausted even in the best of available expertise else patient should be referred to a better equipped and dedicated center. Mere patient in despair and depression demanding amputation is not an indication at all.

ADJUVANTS AND INNOVATIVE STRATEGIES FOR MANAGING OSTEOMYELITIS

Hyperbaric Oxygenation

This is achieved when a patient breathes 100% oxygen in an environment with elevated atmospheric pressure (>1 atm absolute, usually 2–4 atm). The therapy is typically given for 90–120 minutes. Based on Boyle, Dalton's, and Henry's principles, there is an increase in the plasma volume fraction of transported oxygen which is available for cellular metabolism. Increased oxygenation has beneficial physiological effects in the treatment of chronic wounds. Chronic and therapy resistant OM is a good indication for the use of hyperbaric oxygenation. In oxygen deficient environment, the osteoblasts and osteoclasts are inhibited that can be partially reversed by hyperbaric oxygen.

BOX 7: Newer strategies in management and prevention of osteomyelitis.

Implant treatment:
1. Polycationic hydrophobic-coating treated implants to reduce microbial adhesion
2. *Silver-coated orthopedic implants:* They preliminary appear useful in two-stage revisions for infection. Silver-hydroxyapatite (Ag-HA)-coated implants may additionally enhance the osteoconductive property of the implant. Local and systemic toxicity of silver can be reduced by nanoparticle-based delivery strategies to reduce the off-target effects
3. *Implant coating with antibiotic nanoparticles and bone growth factors:* Covalent bonding of antibiotic to surface of titanium implant reduces biofilm formation
4. *Development of vancomycin incorporated chitosan/gelatin coatings coupled with the TiO_2–Sr-HAP surface modified Cp-titanium:* These implants have dual layer—inner one of TiO_2 metal oxide and Sr-HAP ceramic oxide (for integration) over which is laid the antibiotic-gelatin/chitosan layer
5. Coating implants with monocyte chemoattractant protein-1 (MCP-1) has been found to reduce *S. aureus* infection by directly recruiting macrophages to the infection site

Improved antibiotic drug-delivery system:
1. Bioactive glass has dual ability to elute antibiotics and provide scaffolding for bone ingrowth thus eliminating need for bone grafting. It can be especially formulated to produce a bactericidal effect by itself or combined with silver Ag (known antibacterial)
2. *Three-dimensional (3D) composite biodegradable drug delivery scaffolds as antibiotic delivery system and a regenerative device for bone:* They are available as preformulated, injectable, or moldable systems. Preformulated 3D-printed scaffolds with rifampicin and vancomycin have been used to treat *S. aureus* infections and disrupt biofilms. Moldable 3D scaffold can be cut into desirable length, hydrated, and deployed for fitting and curing the bone defect. Injectable composite scaffolds obtained from lyophilization are highly porous and allow hydration in blood or other body fluids. It is easy to administer them through cannula and even fill irregular cavities

Specific strategies against S. aureus:
1. Chlorhexidine gluconate scrub (antiseptic detergent) is better in eradicating methicillin-resistant *Staphylococcus aureus* (MRSA) from implants compared to iodine, saline, and saline with bacitracin
2. Cholesterol biosynthesis inhibitor blocks *S. aureus* virulence, its gene expression, and biofilm formation in animal studies
3. Anti-*S. aureus* antibody-antibiotic conjugates have been used to kill intracellular *S. aureus*

Immunotherapy strategies:
1. Active immunization has been achieved for *H. influenza* and *Streptococcus pneumoniae*. This strategy has failed for other organisms or components of bacterial cell wall/membrane like poly-N-acetyl glucosamine, LTA capsular polysaccharides, and IsdB. Vaccine against IsdB (*S. aureus*) contrarily increased mortality in patients
2. Passive immunization strategies **(*see* Box 8)**

Biofilm dispersal:
1. Enzymatic treatments such as trypsin, dispersin B, lysostaphin, and DNAses lead to dispersal of staphylococci from biofilm
2. Streptokinase or nattokinase decrease the minimum biofilm eradication concentration (MBEC) of available systemic antibiotics by breaking down biofilm-associated fibrin matrix
3. *Targeting quorum sensing system:* Deploying autoinducing peptide type-1 triggers dispersal of MRSA

(DNAses: deoxyribonucleases; isdB: iron-regulated surface determinant; LTA: lipoteichoic acid)

BOX 8: Passive immunization studies under preclinical stages of development.

1. *Targeting biofilm:* Disrupting the shelter of bacteria has strongest influence on winning strategies against infection
   a. Monoclonal antibody (mAb) against DNA-binding proteins from the DNABII family (component of biofilm) is active against many bacterial species. This along with antibiotics like daptomycin reduces the planktonic and adherent bacterial population
   b. Monoclonal antibodies against α-toxin and ClfA prevent biofilm formation reducing the colony forming units from bone/joint tissue, reduced propensity to infection, and less biofilm aggregates
   c. Targeting the glucosaminidase (Gmd) subunit of autolysin (Atl)
2. *Targeting intracellular reservoirs of S. aureus:* This approach aims at reducing the reservoir in tissues to eradicate the infection
   a. *Using antibody-antibiotic conjugate (AAC) composed of monoclonal antibody recognizing specific sugars on wall teichoic acids + rifamycin class derived antibiotic:* The AAC binds to *S. aureus* and upon opsonization the active form of antibiotic gets released within the bacteria due to proteolysis inside the phagolysosome

Also, there is synergistic effect of hyperbaric oxygen and antibiotic therapy on infection control. Other effects include stimulating angiogenesis and suppressing the anaerobic organisms. Recently, it is believed that the use of hyperbaric oxygen is not evidence-based and there is no distinct benefit of the therapy. It is not used as a routine measure in most of the centers.

Role of Growth Factors

Role of BMP in OM is not fully settled and not well appreciated by all. Reports have been encouraging for the use of BMP to improve bone healing. Recently, attempts have been made to deliver the *BMP-2* gene at the defect site using adenoviral vector that improved formation of callus in animal model. Other intriguing research models include use of VEGF, placental growth factor, sonic hedgehog, etc. for improving bone healing.

Inhibiting Biofilm Formation

"Quorum sensing" (see in bacteriological factors above) inhibition by use of ribonucleic acid III inhibiting peptide (RIP) has shown inhibition of biofilm formation by staphylococci.

Other adjuvants include the use of low-intensity pulsed ultrasound (LIPUS), pulsed electromagnetic field (PEMF), platelet rich plasma, etc. for improving bone healing **(Box 7)**.

COMPLICATIONS OF OSTEOMYELITIS

Untreated or poorly treated OM evolves into complicated disease.

Acute Osteomyelitis

- Chronic OM
- Septic arthritis

- Limb length disturbances
- Septicemia
- Endocarditis
- Deep vein thrombosis
- Pyonephritis
- Pulmonary embolism

Chronic Osteomyelitis

- Recurrences and relapses
- Limb length discrepancy
- Pathological fractures
- Infected nonunion
- Implant failure
- Septic arthritis
- Septicemia
- Joint stiffness
- Soft tissue abscess formation and cellulitis
- Soft tissue contractures
- Amyloidosis
- Squamous cell carcinoma of the sinus tract **(Fig. 32)**
- Hansen's 7 Ds (despair, divorce, destitute, depression, delinquency, default, and death)

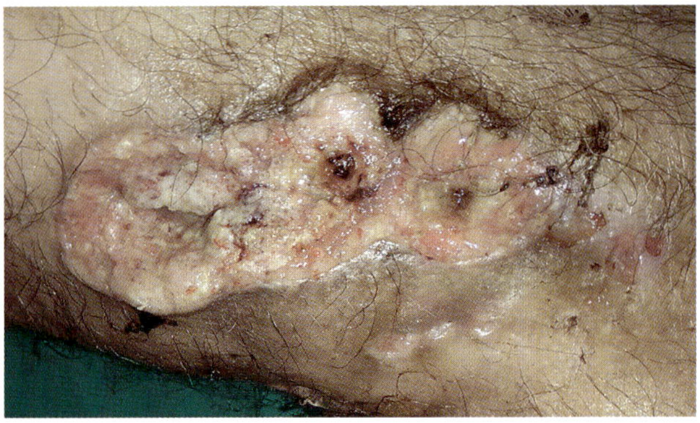

Fig. 32: The formation of squamous cell sarcoma in the sinus tract of chronic osteomyelitis.

PREVENTION OF EXOGENOUS BONE INFECTION

We feel that prevention of OM is cost effective, reduces morbidity, and avoids the long-drawn agony of multiple treatments and possible complications especially if one keeps in mind that amputation is also a possibility patient may land up with. The cycle of infection can be broken at various steps **(Fig. 33)** and then healing phase could be meticulously superimposed. For every set-up, the first step will be to define the patient population at risk for OM so that specific strategies could be defined. The following could serve as a general guide:

Diabetic foot: Prevent diabetic foot itself with excellent foot hygiene and nutrition, meticulous and supervised glycemic control, and use of protective footwear. Patients should be instructed to examine their feet daily. Injuries and any suspected infection should not be neglected **(Fig. 34)** and prompt medical care should be sought. Complete examination of the lower extremities is recommended annually and inspection of feet at interim routine follow-up visits. Measures to prevent diabetic foot ulcers should be re-emphasized at each visit.

Patients with Charcot's joints: They require special shoes preferably custom made as the feet and other joints are deformed. In patients undergoing foot surgery or amputation, the use of protective footwear postoperatively is essential in preventing subsequent ulceration and infection and proper uneventful healing.

Patients with open fractures: Thorough copious lavage with 10–14 L of saline is the first and most effective basis to prevent infection by reducing the bacterial load. Administration of antibiotics within 6 hours of injury and prompt surgical treatment are associated with a reduced risk of developing OM. The intravenous antibiotics could be prolonged in such cases possibly though there is no concrete evidence.

"Patients undergoing orthopedic surgery" especially with the use of implants: Assess the immune status and loco-regional

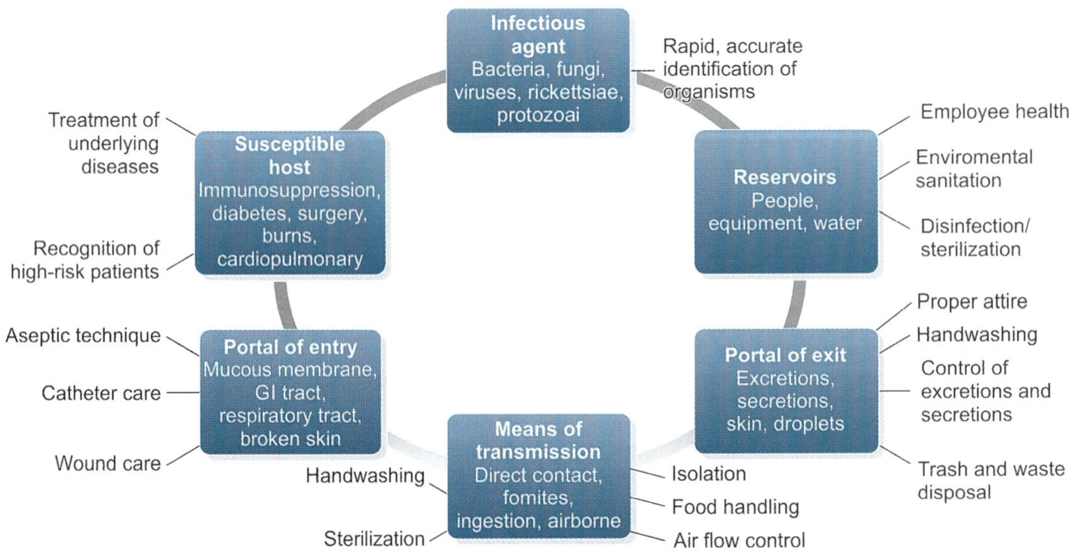

Fig. 33: The chain of infection and possible avenues to break it.

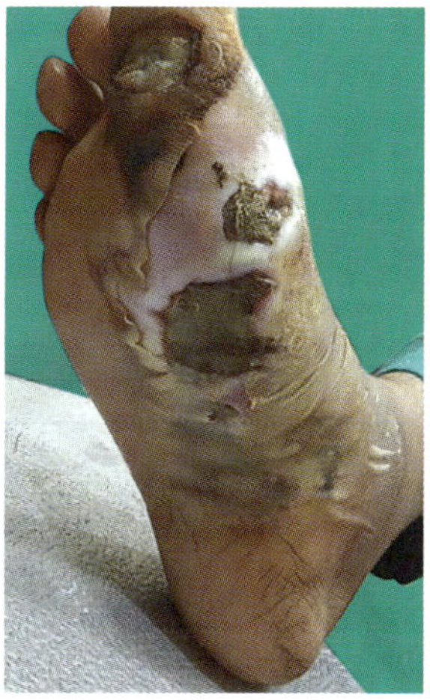

Fig. 34: A patient with diabetic foot developing necrosis and complications following neglected trauma.

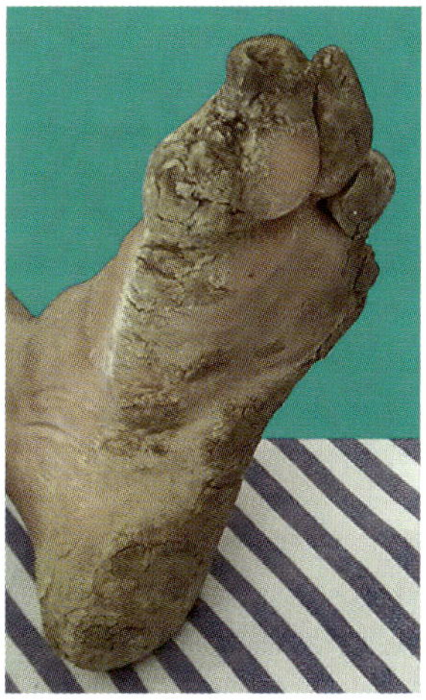

Fig. 35: Poor foot hygiene. One should avoid doing implant-related surgeries in these patients.

TABLE 9: Commonly recommended antibiotics as prophylaxis for orthopedic surgery.

Procedure	*Drug and dose*	*Comments*
ORIF	Ceftriaxone 2 g IV	Add gram negative (amikacin or netilmycin) and anaerobic coverage for open fractures
Spine surgeries and hip arthroplasty	Ceftriaxone (1–2 g IV), or Vancomycin 1 g IV	• Initial dose within 30 minutes of incision • Single preoperative dose recommended, however, for institutes with increased SSI or HAI coverage can be extended up to 48 hours. • Repeat dose if surgical time exceeds 3 hours • Vancomycin or teicoplanin should be reserved for MRSA endemic institutes. Consider intranasal mupirocin ointment for decontamination preoperatively (doctor and patient both)
Joint arthroplasty other than hip	Ceftriaxone or cefazolin or vancomycin as above	Continue antibiotics for 24 hours but not more

(HAI: healthcare-associated infection; MRSA: methicillin-resistant *Staphylococcus aureus;* ORIF: open reduction internal fixation; SSI; surgical site infections)

hygiene **(Fig. 35)** of patient for elective cases. Administration of prophylactic antibiotics preferably within 30 minutes of incision or tourniquet inflation whichever is earlier **(Table 9)**. Standard preoperative procedures, such as the use of antimicrobial shower, shaving, and topical disinfectants, should be followed.

Care by surgeon: It should be emphasized that a lot of infections can be prevented if proper care is taken by the surgeon by proper handwash **(Fig. 36)**, wearing gloves in sterile manner, using antiseptics between patients' examination, etc. following universal precautions is recommended in all high-risk cases.

SOME SPECIAL FORMS OF OSTEOMYELITIS

Subacute Osteomyelitis

Brodie's abscess and Garre's OM (see later) are classic examples.

Vertebral OM (some forms) in adults is an example in modern world. This disease is common in Africa and some 60% patients with bone infection have this type of presentation. Increased host resistance and decreased virulence of bacteria have been proposed to result into this form of disease. Initial homing and proliferation of bacteria is quickly arrested by the local immunity and host reaction walls off the lesion at variable stage of evolution. Alternatively, "trauma hypothesis" states that local injury produces hypoxia and hematoma formation. This serves as a site for lodged bacteria to grow and proliferate. The surrounding bone being relatively healthy resists the infection and walls it off. The inciting cause, however, is itself difficult to support let apart the evolution. In this type of disease there has been no acute attack and the patient has not received specific treatment before presentation. The onset is insidious and as a rule the infection does not produce the systemic features of infection. Pain, the most common presenting symptom, usually presents for months that remits spontaneously in-between for variable durations. Night pains and relief from acetylsalicylic acid is also frequently reported. Localized tenderness and swelling are the only physical signs, though even they "may" be absent. The symptoms and signs often are more prominent after activity and subside thereafter. Sequestrum formation and sinus are conspicuously absent. The distribution of subacute OM is much wider than the acute type, and the disease occurs at various sites. The lower limb is affected much more often than the upper limb. The most commonly affected site is the metaphysis and diaphysis is only occasionally affected in children but the distribution

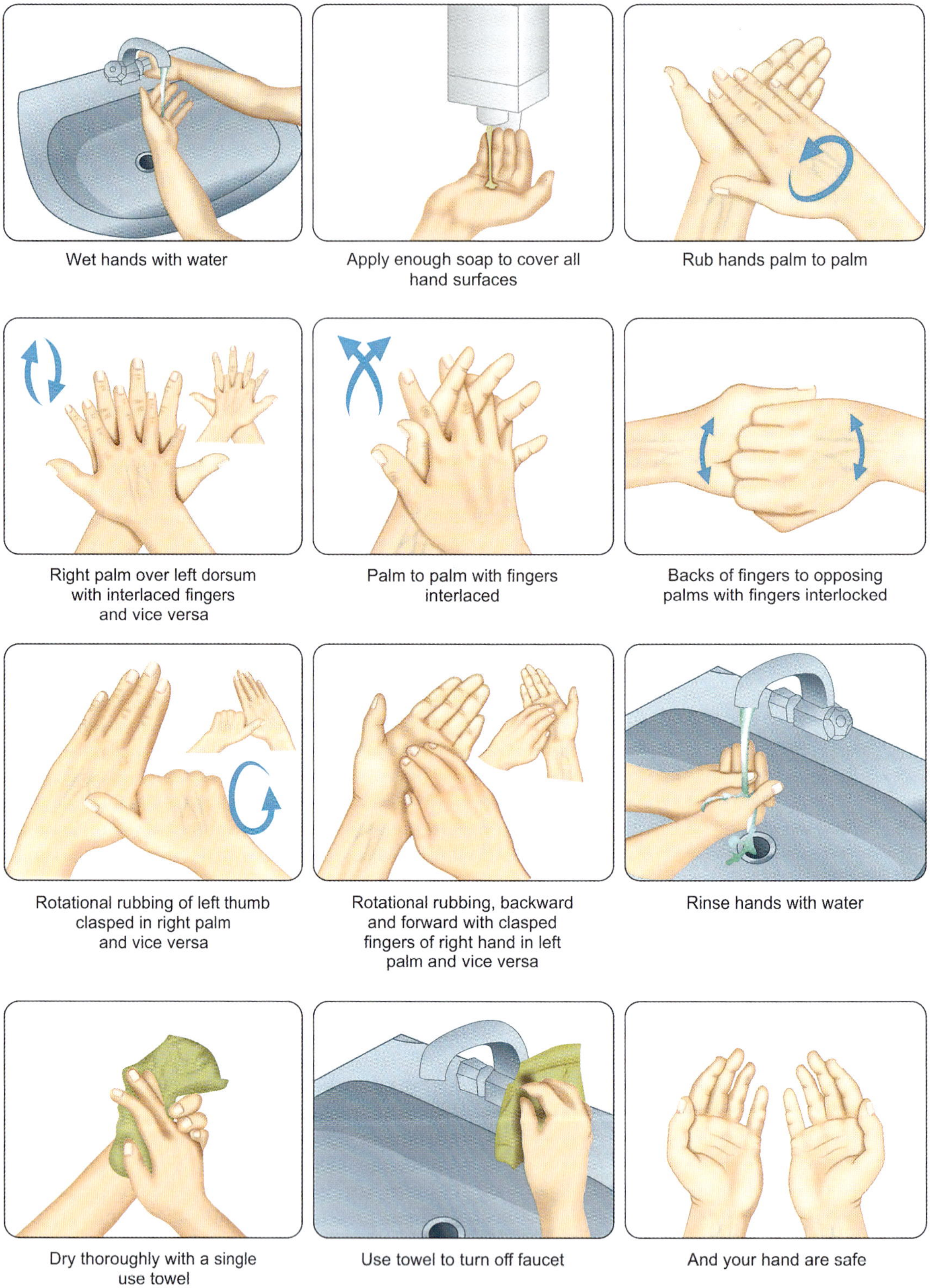

Fig. 36: Handwash technique that should be mandatorily followed.

is equal in adults. Vertebral lesions are more common in adults. Metaphyseal-equivalent locations are also commonly affected and include pelvis, the vertebrae, the calcaneum, the clavicle, and the talus. In small bone such as metacarpals, metatarsals, and tarsals, the lesion is usually subchondral. Multifocal subacute OM is reported but occurrence is rare. Bacterial identification from the lesion is quite difficult and is absent in 30–50% cases. Identified organisms are similar to acute forms and include coagulase-positive *Staphylococcus* (most common >50%), *Streptococcus, Pseudomonas,* and coagulase-negative *Staphylococcus*.

Differential diagnosis (subacute OM): The lesions should be differentiated from Ewing sarcoma, Langerhans cell histiocytosis and osteosarcoma (diaphyseal lesion with onion-skin periosteal reaction); chondroblastoma, aneurysmal bone cyst, giant cell tumor, fungal OM, tuberculous OM, pigmented villonodular synovitis (PVNS) erosions, gout (epiphyseal lesions); nonossifying fibroma, chondromyxoid fibroma (metaphyseal eccentric lesions); osteoid osteoma and intracortical hemangioma.

Investigations: "Laboratory investigations" are often not helpful. On "radiographs", the characteristic lesion is a lytic cavity surrounded by sclerosis **(*see* Fig. 1)** and they can be classified according to Robert et al. **(*see* Box 3)**. Occasionally the communicating metaphyseo-diaphyseal lesions grow as elongated "serpentine" lesions to epiphysis (serpentine sign of Letts). The spinal lesions common in adults require magnetic resonance imaging (MRI) for better characterization and differentiation. Radiographs are nonsensitive and nonspecific, often healing is seen by the time they are appreciated on X-ray films. They are differentiated from tuberculosis by sclerosis of vertebral body. "Contrast-enhanced MRI" is especially helpful. "Penumbra sign" has been described characteristically for Brodie's abscess. In an otherwise doubtful case, radionuclide imaging may help in localizing and differentiating the lesion in combination with other modalities. "Fine-needle aspiration cytology (FNAC) or trephine biopsy" of the lesion is a must for documentation and diagnosis.

Treatment: Treatment is controversial and most people opine for a prolonged course of antibiotic therapy in children before proceeding to surgery. In adults, however, most agree that surgical treatment is preferable. We consider that formation of pus by itself is a hindrance to effective antibiotic therapy and hence simple incision and drainage type treatment producing low morbidity should be initiated early to reduce, also the duration of antibiotics and associated complications. This approach would also ascertain the lesion diagnosis and patient returns to function faster. Surgical indications for subacute OM typically include:

- Poor response to antibiotic therapy
- Doubtful lesions that appear as potential threats
- Impending joint involvement
- Presence of subperiosteal pus or synovitis.

Intralesional curettage of the lesion is adequate for small lesions (<3 cm). For larger lesions or those with weak bony wall support, additional bone graft packing is recommended. It is imperative that the drainage is done as far from the joint capsule as possible for epiphyseal and metaphyseal lesions and where possible indirect approach is better.

Sclerosing Osteomyelitis of Garre

This is a sclerosing form of OM that causes thickening of bone cortex often in irregular fashion without ever identified suppuration in tissue or bones, sequestration of bone, sinus formation or fistulation. The thickening and marked sclerosis is due to closely packed lamellar periosteal reaction in response to chronic low-grade infective pathology (though organisms have not been isolated so far). The term "proliferative periostitis" better represents the pathology that was first described by C. Garre in 1893 although he described this without radiographs (not available at that time). Other terms used to describe the condition include periostitis ossificans, chronic OM with proliferative periostitis, and OM sclerosans Garre's. The disease commonly affects children and young adults. Mandibular affection from periapical inflammation from first molar has also been described exclusively in children. Patients usually present with pain that aggravates with activity and in night. The bone is deformed and thickened. Systemic signs of inflammation are usually absent and uncommonly patients present with recurrent bouts of extreme pain with mild fever.

Radiographs typically demonstrate increased bone density sometimes complete obliteration of the cavity of long tubular bones. There is marked cortical thickening and lamellated periosteal reaction. Typical onion-skin periosteal reaction has been described in mandible.

Differential diagnosis: The relationship to SAPHO (Synovitis, Acne, Pustulosis, Hyperostosis, and Osteitis) syndrome is not clear but some consider this to be a part of the same. The disease should be differentiated from osteoid osteoma, osteoblastic osteosarcoma, Ewing's sarcoma, and eosinophilic granuloma.

Treatment usually involves a course of antibiotics that gives temporary relief (similar to SAPHO syndrome and hence the correlation). In few cases, decompression of the medullary canal is required to relieve symptoms. In extreme unusual cases, surgical removal of a segment of bone or complete removal is required. Bone grafting of the excised area and reconstruction with bone transport or free bone transfer is subsequently needed.

Brodie's Abscess

Brodie's abscess is the most common type of subacute OM **(Figs. 37A and B)**. Nonorthopedic literature (radiology and pathology) often refers this as to a chronic form of OM; however, most orthopedic surgeons believe this to be

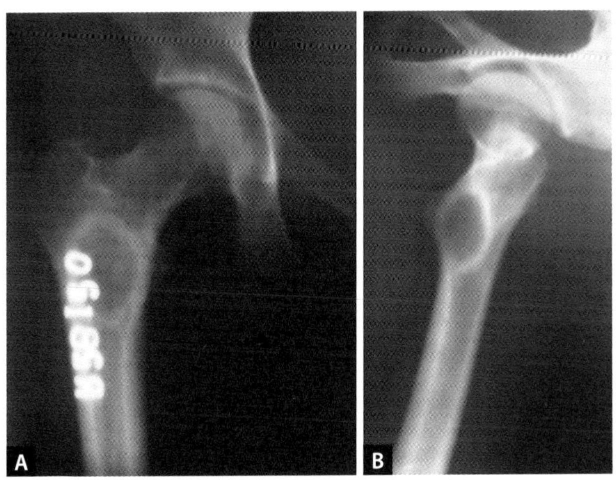

Figs. 37A and B: Well-circumscribed abscess cavity with marginal sclerosis localized in proximal femur (A and B). The differential included calcified cyst (cysticercosis/hydatid) but on excision of the lesion there was pus with granulation tissue.

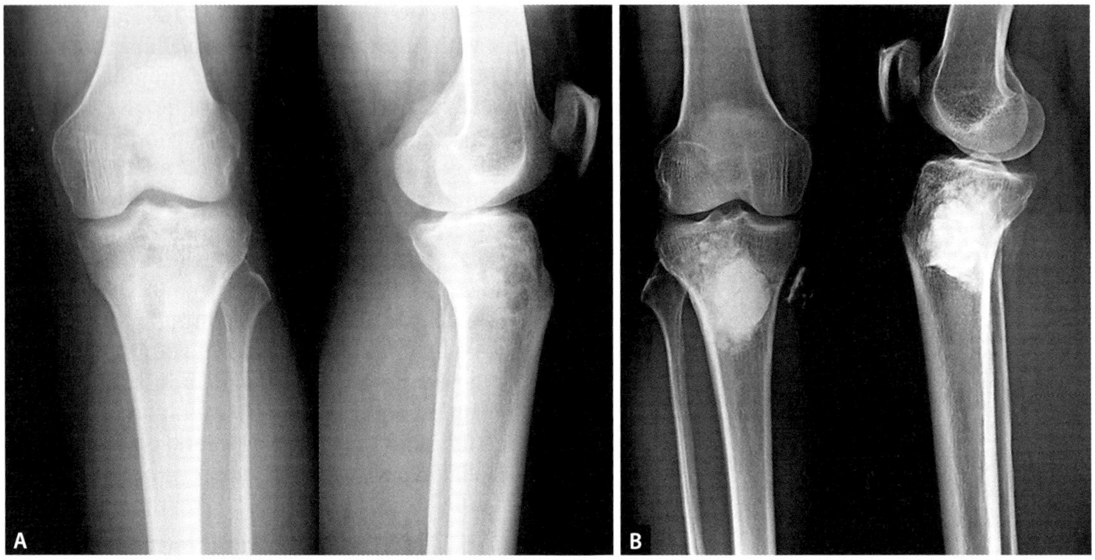

Figs. 38A and B: Brodie's abscess—the abscess cavity (A) was curetted and filled with bone grafts and polymethyl methacrylate cement (B).

a form of subacute OM. Sir Benjamin Brodie (surgeon in St George's Hospital, London, United Kingdom), first described subacute OM in 1,832 (unfortunately from an amputated leg in a man with intractable pain) from dissected specimen. Brodie found a cavity as the size of a walnut filled with dark-colored pus surrounded by whiter and harder dense bone. The inner surface of the cavity appeared to be highly vascular). Typically, it occurs in children more common than in boys. It has a predilection for ends of tubular bones of lower limb. The abscess rarely ever crosses the growth plate or physeal scar. Pain is the common presenting symptom often appearing after playful activities or exertion. Night pains are often noted when the child is at rest. Pain responds to common analgesics. On a radiograph, there is a lytic lesion often in an oval configuration that is oriented along the long axis of the bone surrounded by thick dense rim of reactive sclerosis **(Figs. 38A and B)** that fades imperceptibly into surrounding bone but sclerotic rim may be absent. Pathognomonic feature includes finding of a lucent tortuous channel (serpentine sign) extending toward growth plate. There may be associated periosteal new bone formation with or without adjacent soft tissue swelling. The lesion needs differentiation from giant cell tumor, aneurysmal bone cyst, nonossifying fibroma, chondromyxoid fibroma, etc. (see subacute OM for differential diagnosis). MRI is a good investigation to characterize the pathology. The "target sign" as described by Marti-Bonmati et al. consists of central two rings and a peripheral halo. The "penumbra sign" is comprised of four sections; namely, a central core (the abscess cavity) that appears as low signal intensity on T1-weighted and high on T2-weighted and STIR images surrounded by the first layer of granulation tissue which is isointense to the muscle. The second layer of reactive new bone formation is hypointense on all sequences and the outermost layer appears as a peripheral halo of low signal intensity ring due to edema on T1-weighted images. The penumbra sign may be seen in eosinophilic granuloma, chondrosarcoma, benign cystic lesions of the bone and intraosseous ganglion and has a sensitivity of 75% and specificity, positive and negative predictive values of >90%. Treatment is as detailed in subacute OM above.

Tubercular Osteomyelitis

This is an uncommon affection compared to the frequent articular and vertebral column affection. Primary epiphyseal OM is a rare disease caused by mycobacteria occurring in pediatric population and infants. The disease is commonly suspected when there is no response to conventional antibiotics. BCG OM is again a rare disease that occurs following BCG vaccination in a normal patient with normal immune response and it also occurs in healthy children. We will restrict the details to emphasize the distinguishing features from pyogenic OM. The infection is commonly indolent and present as nonspecific bone pain. Over a period of time, the overlying tissue reveals formation of abscess that forms a persisting sinus. Pus discharge from the sinus is often infrequent, watery, and little unless secondary infection usually pyogenic sets in. The sinus is tethered to the underlying bone with suppressed signs of inflammation in surrounding tissue. The mouth of sinus is often bluish with pouting granulation tissue that frequently blocks the pus discharge. Radiologically, the lesion is lytic with reactive dense bone in periphery due to slow indolent process. If secondary pyogenic infection sets in then osteopenia appears due to inflammation. Flake or coke like and feathery sequestrum **(Figs. 39A to C)** can be identified in the cavity which is commonly empty. Treatment had been classically curettage of the lesion and bone grafting, however, small lesions can heal well with antitubercular chemotherapy.

Neonatal Osteomyelitis

It may present in two forms. In one form, the patient is severely ill with septicemia. The causative organisms are

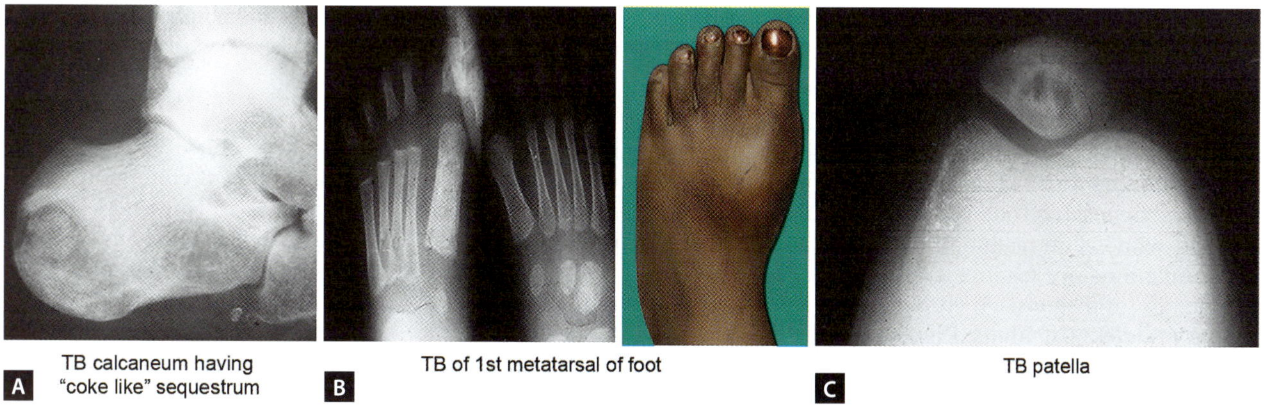

Figs. 39A to C: Tubercular (TB) osteomyelitis.

beta hemolytic streptococci and *Staphylococcus aureus*, common source of infection being the umbilical cord. The other form of presentation is a mildly affected child who is not even febrile. Clinical signs include pseudoparalysis and local signs of inflammation. Radiological signs are similar to those of acute OM. Treatment is usually conservative. These children should be followed up for angular deformities occurring in the adolescence.

Acute Multifocal Osteomyelitis

It is a rare but characteristic condition occurring in infancy where there is lack of constitutional symptoms even in the presence of multiple foci in the long bones. It runs a relatively benign course. The investigations reveal hypogammaglobulinemia and requires correction of this feature along with the regular treatment of OM. Some infants develop recurrent foci of infection as soon as antibiotics are stopped. Such cases should be looked for a primary source of infection elsewhere in the body.

Salmonella Osteomyelitis

Chronic OM may follow salmonella infection in immunocompromised subjects and in children with hemoglobinopathies like sickle-cell anemia. The bacteria enter the bloodstream through the gut. In sickle cell anemia, multiple thromboses occur in the bones and may predispose to infection. Frequently affected bones include vertebrae, ribs, sternum, and calcaneum. The clinical features resemble those of subacute OM with protracted course and may be confused with tubercular infection. Surgical intervention is usually not required until an abscess has to be evacuated or sequestrum has to be removed.

Chronic Recurrent Multifocal Osteomyelitis

It is a well-known entity with multifocal and recurrent osteomyelitic lesions characterized by subacute and chronic features. The etiology is unknown and cultures for bacteria are negative. Radiographs show osteolytic and sclerotic bone lesions with minimal or no subperiosteal bone formation. Often involved bones include spine, tibia, femur, and clavicle. Antibiotics are of no use and an episode generally subsides by 6 weeks with little or no sequelae.

Viral Infection of Bones (and Joints)

Role of viruses as infective agents of bones and joints has never been seriously emphasized and continues to remain out of focus even today. The bone had been a reservoir of viral genome since ages and it has been aptly said that "bones hold the key to DNA virus history and epidemiology". The interaction, pathogenesis, and sequelae of viral infection of bones and joints have not been clearly described but the following is a detail of current understanding (very superficial indeed) of osseous effects of viral infection.

- Smallpox virus (variola virus, now extinct) infection of bones resulted in viral OM, short stubby metacarpals and phalanges, joint ankylosis, joint multidirectional instability, and hypoplastic femoral condyles described as "osteomyelitis variolosa". Acute skull OM after Varicella-Zoster virus (VZV) reactivation and *Propionibacterium acnes* coinfection has been described.
- HIV virus has been implicated in osteonecrosis, increased bone resorption by modifying the structure and function of sealing zone of osteoclasts, and increased incidence of peri-prosthetic joint infections.
- Arthralgias are hallmark of viral infections such as dengue, chikungunya, and Zika virus. Similar arthritides with bone lesions are seen in infections with other members of alpha-virus family (not seen in India) such as Sindbis virus, o'nyong-nyong virus, Mayaro virus, and Barmah Forest virus. Epstein-Barr virus is usually associated with polyarthralgia, or monoarthritis of the knee. Some even associate this with congenital/developmental diseases of bones such as Perthes' disease and developmental dysplasia of the hip (DDH) but the evidence has never been gathered. VZV can be involved in children pauciarticular arthritis. Mumps virus can be associated with small or large joint synovitis. Adenovirus or coxsackieviruses have been associated with recurrent episodes of polyarthritis. Most of the arthritis in viral infections have been attributed to autoimmune inflammatory process however.

SAPHO Syndrome (Pustulotic Arthroosteitis and Sternocostoclavicular Hyperostosis)

This is an acronym for combined occurrence of synovitis, acne, pustulosis, hyperostosis, and OM. It was initially described by Chamot et al. in 1987. Hidradenitis suppurativa may be associated with SAPHO. All components need not be present for diagnosis and often the osteoarticular component is present without dermatological manifestations. Aseptic skeletal inflammatory features are, however, the common denominator for diagnosis. It classically tends to present in young to middle-aged adults. Presentation in the pediatric population is not uncommon.

Pathogenesis

No infective or immune pathology has been identified till date, however, bacterial and viral antigens and autoimmune disease have been commonly implicated as causative agents. Also, the relation to dermatologic features is not clearly established. The pustulosis could represent a spectrum of psoriasis and the skeletal features could be the classical psoriatic arthritis. But, there is less destruction of the peripheral joints and presence of multifocal osteomyelitic changes go against the psoriatic association. Some authors group chronic recurring multiple OM in SAPHO.

Clinical Findings

The disease occurs with equal frequency in both males and females. Pustulosis occurs in around 50% of patients with SAPHO syndrome. It is characterized by chronic eruption of yellowish, intradermal, and sterile pustules on palm and soles. Acne is seen in 15% patients and when present it is severe. The bone and joint lesions present as pain, soft-tissue swelling, and limitation of motion. There is multifocal osteitis/OM notably in chest wall, pelvis, and spine. The mean number of affected bony lesions is five. SAPHO and related conditions have been described to have three stages of progression as follows:

1. Costoclavicular ligament ossification.
2. Arthropathy of the sternoclavicular joint, medial end clavicle osteitis which may also be seen in the first rib and sternum. There may well be a noticeable hypertrophy of the costal cartilages.
3. The osteitis transforms into hyperostosis and ultimately ankylosis.

Plain Film

Sternocostoclavicular region is the most frequently affected region. Hyperostosis and osteosclerosis (sometimes lysis) are seen. Soft tissue involvement may be seen around the lesion. Spine is the second most common region affected. Osteosclerosis of vertebral body with syndesmophyte formation and bridging osteophytes are commonly seen. Long bone involvement is seen in 30% cases. Metaphyseal osteosclerosis and osteolysis with enlargement of bone can be appreciated. Synovitis and arthritis can also be found. The knee, hips, and ankle are commonly affected joints that demonstrate juxta-articular osteoporosis in early stages followed by joint narrowing, erosions, and hyperostosis in advanced stage.

Diagnosis

Diagnosis requires meticulous history and clinical examination. Obtaining radiographs of commonly affected joints may suggest the diagnosis. However, it should be realized that the development of osseous lesions is disjunctive from skin lesions and may be separated by years.

Prognosis and Course of Disease

The disease runs a benign course though patients may have recurrent bouts of attacks. Generally, good response is shown to nonsteroidal anti-inflammatory drugs (NSAIDs) for pain relief. Immunosuppressive therapy and steroid have been shown to be effective in selected reports. Bisphosphonates have been found effective in various studies especially in pediatric patients. Anecdotal improvement with antibiotic therapy has been reported.

ACTINOMYCOSIS

It is a rare, subacute to chronic, suppurative granulomatous bacterial infection, characterized by the development of indurated swellings, contiguous spread, and formation of multiple sinuses and discharge of sulfur granules. Israel described the first human case in 1878; however, the occurrence of yellow granules was previously reported by Bollinger in jaw masses of cattle in 1877. Actinomycosis in human beings is an endogenous infection (and no risk of person-to-person transmission) arising from the pathogen normally presents in the mouth, intestine, and vagina. There are four main clinical forms and various minor presentations have also been reported.

1. *Cervicofacial (lumpy jaw):* This accounts for 50–70% of the reported cases. Initially, there is swelling in the perimandibular area followed by direct spread to adjacent tissues and development of fistula or sinuses.
2. *Thoracic:* This is seen in 15–20% cases usually occurring by aspiration of oropharyngeal secretions. Occasional cases occur following perforation of the esophagus or by direct spread from abdomen or neck lesions. The pulmonary involvement may spread to pleura, pericardium, and chest wall forming multiple sinuses in the end.
3. *Abdominal and pelvic form:* They represent 10–20% cases with often a recent or remote bowel surgery for perforated viscus (appendix, diverticulum, or trauma). It may also be associated with the ingestion of chicken or fish bones. The ileocecal region is most frequently involved. The infection then spreads to nearby structures and abdominal wall with pus discharge. Pelvic form (some include this as a distinct form) is observed in females associated with intrauterine contraceptive devices (IUCD) use.
4. *Vertebral actinomycosis:* Disease almost always has a contiguous focus of infection usually abdominal cavity or from thoracic cavity. Differentiation from tuberculosis

is important. In actinomycosis, the intervertebral disk is usually spared. Also the disease often involves the adjacent pedicles, transverse processes, and heads of neighboring ribs. Kyphus and collapse are unusual. The pus tracks do not respect tissue plane (unlike tubercular abscess that follow regular planes).

Other minor forms include the meningitis, tendinitis, epidural abscesses, endocarditis, pericarditis, pneumonia, bronchiectasis, gingivitis, sublingual plaques, and periodontitis in isolation.

Epidemiology

The disease is seen worldwide with higher occurrence in low socioeconomic status areas and agriculture-based economies and with the exception of pelvic form it occurs frequently in males in the ratio 3:1.

Organism and Pathogenesis

Trauma, presence of foreign bodies like IUCD, and poor oral hygiene may favor tissue invasion following break in the mucous membrane. The causative organisms are nonmotile, nonspore forming, nonacid fast, and gram-positive pleomorphic, anaerobic-to-microaerophilic filamentous bacterial rods that lie latent in body (crevices of tonsil, gingivae, carious tooth, vagina, abdominal organs, etc.) and are typically nonvirulent. The most common organisms identified are:

- *Actinomyces israeli*
- *Actinomyces odontolyticus*
- *Actinomyces viscosus*
- *Actinomyces gerencseriae*
- *Actinomyces naeslundii*
- *Actinomyces turicensis*
- *Actinomyces meyeri*
- *Propionibacterium propionicus*

There are some companion bacteria that are almost always associated with the infection. These include *Actinobacillus actinomycetemcomitans, Peptostreptococcus, Bacteroides, Fusobacterium,* staphylococci, streptococci and *Enterobacteriaceae.* The prevalence and type of companion bacteria depend on the location of disease and they magnify the pathogenicity of actinomycetes. The nonvirulent actinomycetes gain access to the deeper tissue following break in mucous membrane and colonize on devitalized tissue, the companion bacteria may help to demolish host immunity by secreting the enzymes and toxins. The host tissue then mounts inflammatory response with suppuration and subsequent fibrosis. The infection often spreads contiguously ignoring tissue planes. Uncommonly hematogenous spread to distant tissues is also seen.

Clinical Features

Patients usually have history of recent or past dental manipulation, abdominal surgery for perforated viscus, aspiration, trauma to mouth, and dental caries or radiation treatment. There is history of local swellings that enlarge and frequently painlessly form discharging sinuses with characteristic yellow granule (sulfur granule) discharge. The symptomatic history ranges from discharging facial sinuses with indurated swelling, vaginal bleeding, change in bowel habits, abdominal discomfort, or of nausea, or of vomiting, dry or productive cough, shortness of breath, chest pain, fever, weight loss, fatigue and anorexia. On examination, depending on the location of disease one may find—hard multiple nodular lesions, multiple abscesses, and multiple sinuses, sulfur granules typical absence of lymphadenopathy, abnormal breath sounds, cough, scar(s) from antecedent abdominal surgery, low-grade fever, and cachexia. Abdominal mass located often in right lower quadrant, firm to hard in consistency, nontender and fixed to underlying structures. Vertebral actinomycosis presents with localized symptoms and is painful (unlike other forms). There are features of associated contiguous lesion. Gibbus and kyphus are rare. Neurological symptoms are often absent but may be affected with advanced disease. Cerebrospinal meningitis has also been reported.

Radiology

The bone around the infection is osteopenic (due to virulent companion organisms) with variable surrounding sclerosis. There is a variable combination of lysis and sclerosis that gives rise to different clinical types. Vertebral OM presents with a myriad of radiological features that in early stage may show mere absorption of superficial part of vertebral body. In advanced stages, the vertebra has a "honeycombed" appearance with a dense network of suppurating channels surrounded by radiodense bone.

Laboratory Diagnosis

There is anemia with mild leukocytosis. ESR and CRP are usually elevated. Definite diagnosis rests only on demonstration or isolation of the infecting organism from clinical specimen or from sulfur granules. The material can be obtained from the active discharge, needle aspirate, or biopsy material. In pulmonary disease, sputum may be collected but is often considered inappropriate. Sulfur granules may be demonstrated in pus, by shaking it up in a test tube with some saline. The granules sediment on prolonged standing and can be withdrawn with a capillary pipette. The granules are white or yellowish and range in size from minute specks to about 5 mm. They represent the bacterial colonies and consist of dense network of thin gram-positive filaments, surrounded by peripheral zone of swollen radiating club-shaped structures, presenting a sun-ray appearance. Clubs possibly represent the antigen-antibody complexes. Gram-stain smear of the specimen between slides demonstrates the beaded, branched, gram-positive filamentous rods, suggesting the diagnosis. Else, the granules can be crushed between slides and stained with 1% methylene blue. Cultures are done in anaerobic conditions and may need 2–3 weeks for the identification of actinomycetes. Serological diagnosis is irrelevant. Papanicolaou test had been used in the past for identification of actinomycetes like organism.

Histopathology

The sulfur granules are cauliflower-like particles seen on microscopy. These are pathognomonic of actinomycetes but may be seen in nocardiosis, botryomycosis (*Staphylococcus*), and infection with *Streptomyces madurae*.

Treatment

Penicillin (12–20 million U/day) given intravenously for 1–2 weeks followed by oral medicine for up to 6 months is the most effective and commonly used drug unless the person is sensitive to it. Other drugs effective for treatment include the ceftriaxone, imipenem, amoxicillin/clavulanic acid, fluoroquinolones, clindamycin, doxycycline, chloramphenicol and tetracyclines. Surgery is indicated to obtain specimen or drain abscess or excision of fibrotic sinus tract. A recurrent or nonhealing fistula may need excision and reconstruction. Sometimes for late cases removal of intraspinal or intracranial space occupying lesions may require surgery.

MYCETOMA (MADURAMYCOSIS)

Introduction

Mycetoma or maduramycosis is a chronic infection of exogenous origin often localized to foot. "Madura foot" (term used by Colebrook in 1946) possibly originates from the modern reporting of disease from Madurai, Tamil Nadu predominantly committing to feet. Carter used the term "Mycetoma" relating it to fungal etiology. Other names for the disease include morbus *Tuberculosis pedis,* fungus foot disease of India, Godfrey and Eyre's disease, endemic degeneration of the bones of the foot, fungus foot, and morbus pedis entophyticus-affection singulière. The disease has been described in "Atharva veda" referring to "pada valmikam" (literally meaning "anthill foot"). The infection evolves from multiple nodules beneath the skin followed by formation of cavities within the mass and sinuses (6–12 months) with oozing and colored granules. "Tumefaction" refers to the formation of tumor-like masses following long asymptomatic incubation period (5–6 years).

Etiopathogenesis

Literature reports some 30 and more species of bacteria and fungi causing mycetoma. The infecting agents belong to actinomycetes, eumycetes, eubacteria, and dermatophytes. The pathogenic organisms vary from region to region but most commonly *M. mycetomatis* is the infecting organism followed by *M. grisea* and *Aspergillus nidulans*. The risk factors for developing mycetoma include:

- A minor trauma or thorn prick
- Walking without protective footwear (barefoot)
- Agricultural work and farming, thorny sharp vegetable material
- Arid hot regions with prolonged hot sunshine and tropical climate predispose to maduromycosis
- *Immunocompromised patients:* HIV infection, postrenal transplant patients, and diabetic patients.

Following initial injury and inoculation (thorn prick or abrasion), the causative organisms develop grains that are derived from host material predominantly. The host reaction in the form of granulomatous inflammation attempts to engulf the pathogens. Greater frequency in males is related to deficiency of progesterone that inhibits the growth of *M. mycetomatis*, *P. romeroi*, and *N. brasiliensis.* The higher vascularity of eumycetoma is related to upregulation of hypoxia-inducible factor-1α that regulates VEGF and adrenollodullin-2. The actinomycotic infections are fast to grow and quickly involve the surrounding tissue compared to the eumycotic infections.

The mycetoma is classified into two groups depending on primary fungal infection (true mycetoma or eumycetoma) or actinomycotic infection.

Eumycetoma is commonly caused by:

- *Madurella mycetomati, Madurella grisea, Leptosphaeria senegalensis, Curvularia lunata—they have* "dark hard" grains. *Scedosporium apiospermum, Neotestudina rosatii,* and *Fusarium* spp. have pale soft grains.
- Actinomycotic mycetoma (bacterial infection) commonly implicated in the disease include: *Actinomadura madurae* (White grains), *Actinomadura pelletieri* (Red grains), *Streptomyces somaliensis* (Yellow grains) and *Nocardia brasiliensis* (small soft yellow-orange or off-white grains).

The organisms spread following the fascial planes, the conventional routes of spread viz., hematogeneous and lymphatic spread are uncommon but may be seen in immunocompromised patients.

Clinical Features

The disease is an exogenous infection. The disease begins as a single, small, and painless nodule. Slowly the nodule increases in size and becomes fixed to the underlying tissue. The granules grow toward skin and attach to it. The ensuing inflammatory reaction produces cavities and sinuses that discharge typical grains and pus. This process may take months to years and is faster in actinomycotic form. Although it is rarely fatal, mycetoma causes deformities and potential disability at its advanced stage. The earliest sign of mycetoma is a painless subcutaneous swelling that slowly transforms into a nodule. Pain may be seen in late stages of disease with bony involvement or infection with virulent organisms. The nodule breaks-up into sinus with scant but regular pus discharge. Pus is usually a viscous translucent yellowish fluid resembling oil. Constitutional signs and symptoms are rare if at all. With further progression, the regional lymphatic obstruction and fibrosis cause lymphedema and erythema. Primary osseous mycetoma may develop from direct inoculation of organisms into bones (usually following trauma) especially in tibia and calcaneous bones. The condition is painful unlike typical form.

Diagnosis

The clinical feature of subcutaneous swelling $\rightarrow$ sub-cutaneous nodule $\rightarrow$ sinus formation and pus discharge is characteristic. Attention should be given to the prolonged duration of disease, sinuses discharging grains, absence of pain and involvement of regional nodes. Culture (MacConkey agar, malt extract agar, mannitol salt agar plates aerobically incubated at 37°C for 48 hours—actinomycetes take 48–72 hours to grow so respective instruction is legible with sample) are the gold standard for any infectious disease for diagnosis but may be absent and in this instance the triad of "tumefaction", "fistulation with abscess formation", and "extrusion of colored granules" will help. Also histopathology will help in diagnosis. FNAC demonstrates foreign body giant cells and grains with polymorphous inflammation. The grains are surrounded from inside out by neutrophils, monocytes and macrophages, giant cells, and granulation tissue. Histopathological examination of the subcutaneous tissue reveals granulomas surrounded by neutrophil zone and palisading histiocytes with missed inflammatory infiltrate in eumycetoma. The actinomycetoma demonstrates chronic abscess with polymorphs surrounding the granulation tissue and fibrosis. The matted colonies (grains) of organisms are Gram positive and periphery terminates in club. Splendore-Hoeppli reaction (homogeneous eosinophilic material coating the grains) is found around the grain. This represents the antigen-antibody precipitates with immunoglobulin, complement component, cellular debris (plasma cells, macrophages, lymphocytes, and eosinophils). Dark grains are found only with eumycetoma. The Gram-staining is useful for actinomycetoma while Gömöri methenamine silver and Periodic acid Schiff (PAS) stain are better in eumycetoma. Serodiagnosis can be done with immunodiffusion enzyme-linked immunosorbent assay (ELISA) (highly sensitive) or counterimmunoelectrophoresis.

Radiology

In early stages, the soft tissue granuloma appears as a soft tissue shadow with calcification and obliteration of fascial planes. Bone scalloping from external pressure may be seen. Periosteal reaction may appear with increase in inflammation and Codman triangle may be seen. In late stages, the punched out cavities often multiple may appear that have well-defined margins. The actinomycotic cavities are small and more numerous with no definite margins (moth-eaten appearance). In later stages, the bones have "melting snow" appearance. The following stages of Madura foot are described in literature:

- *Stage 0:* Soft tissue swelling (no bony involvement)
- *Stage 1:* Pressure effects of swelling on bone
- *Stage 2:* Periosteal reaction present
- *Stage 3:* Cortical erosion and medullary invasion
- *Stage 4:* Infection spreads along single ray
- *Stage 5:* Horizontal spread across other rays
- *Stage 6:* Multidirectional and random uncontrolled spread.

CT scan assesses the bone involvement quite precisely. The "dot in circle" sign is quite specific for this.

Treatment

Treatment should be initiated after differentiating fungal from bacterial infection. Combination drugs are the standard modality of treatment. The therapeutic endpoint is clinical and radiological cure. For actinomycetoma trimethoprim-sulfamethoxazole (TMP-SMX), dapsone (diaminodiphenyl sulfone), amoxicillin/clavulanic acid, gentamicin and cefotaxime, streptomycin, amikacin, kanamycin, etc. are used in variable combinations. Recurrences are treated with different drugs. Before initiating dapsone G-6PD, deficiency should be evaluated. Welsh regimen comprises using amikacin with TMP-SMX that had been effective for treating the actinomycotic infection. Recently, a two-step regimen (Palit et al.) with high efficacy to treat this infection has been proposed. The intensive phase comprises TMP-SMX with amikacin for 4 weeks followed by oral TMP-SMX and doxycyline. Usually, this is given for 6–8 months. Addition of rifampicin to Welsh regime produces prolonged remission. For resistant infection, streptomycin can be used that is also the drug of choice for advanced disease. *Nocardia* spp. are particularly sensitive to amoxicillin/clavulanic acid combination. Reduction in duration of treatment has been achieved by Ramam two-step regime. This consists of giving penicillin, gentamicin, and TMP-SMX in intensive phase for 5–7 weeks followed by amoxicillin and TMP-SMX in the maintenance phase (2–5 months). Eumycetoma is a typical fungal infection that responds to standard antifungal therapy. This consists of ketoconazole 400–800 mg daily and/or itraconazole 400 mg (*P. boydii*) given for years. *Madurella mycetomatis* responds to itraconazole 400 mg daily for 3 months followed by 200 mg daily for 9 months. Other drugs effective are ketoconazole and amphotericin B. Surgery is required for complete removal or reducing the size of lesion to ease the medical treatment and deformity. It usually requires excising the surrounding healthy tissue for extended margins in view of the fact that actinomycetomas extend their filaments beyond the lesion and are ill-defined. Extensive fibrosis and deformed limb may have to be amputated.

Prognosis

The bacterial infections usually cure successfully with treatment but the fungal infections frequently recur. Frequent surgical debridements are needed for eumycetomas along with antifungal therapy. It is imperative to prevent secondary bacterial infections on fibrotic poorly vascular tissue that may prove to be fatal if septicemia ensues.

Prevention

Health education and improvement in hygiene should be taught to the resident endemic population.

SURGICAL SITE INFECTION

According to the Centers for Disease Control and Prevention (CDC, United States), SSI is an infection that occurs after surgery in that part of the body where surgery took place within 30 days of a procedure or within 90 days (up to 1 year if the implant is left in place) if an open reduction, spinal fusion or implantation of hip/knee prosthesis is done and the infection appears to be related to the procedure. The diagnostic criteria for SSI include:

- Purulent discharge
- Positive culture from aseptically obtained fluid or tissue in organ space
- An abscess or other evidence of infection such as pain, tenderness, local swelling, redness or heat requiring surgical reopening
- Diagnosis of infection by the surgeon.

The SSIs have been classified by CDC into superficial (subcutaneous), deep (deep soft tissue, muscle, and fascia) or organ/space (bone and joints are considered organ/space). All orthopedic SSIs come under the category of organ space SSI. Organ space or implant infections are essentially all biofilm-based requiring removal of all surfaces and implant involved with an established infection for eradication. Few wound categories have been defined to guide the extent of preventive measures like debridement needs to be undertaken with primary injury/procedure. Closed fractures are clean wounds, open fractures are contaminated wounds, established infections (OM, infected nonunion ± hardware) are dirty wounds, and minor break in the sterile surgical field is a clean contaminated wound. A stab wound that gets infected is not a SSI and it may be classified as soft tissue or superficial infection depending on the extent. The various described risk factors for SSI with their optimization are as follows:

Perioperative Patient Optimization and Assessment of Risk Factors for Surgical Site Infections

It is understood that 40–60% of the SSIs can be prevented using several interventions such as carrier eradication, antimicrobial prophylaxis, and skin antisepsis. Operative environment modifications and factors have been dealt separately in joint infections. *S. aureus* is the most common cause of orthopedic SSI and commonly originates from the native skin. In fact, skin antisepsis is considered to be the second most important factor after optimization of operating environment. However, the routine practice of bathing with antisceptic like chlorhexidine before arthroplasty has been shown to be of no clear benefit in reducing infections despite reducing the bacterial counts.

Staphylococcal Colonization

For *S. aureus* infections, nasal carriage is a strong marker for skin colonization and it is deemed that such patients have 2–9 times higher chances of contracting SSI. Now indeed, nasal carriage is considered an independent risk factor for SSI in orthopedic implant surgery. Whether methicillin sensitive *S. aureus* (MSSA) or MRSA decolonization protocols have been found to reduce the SSI by half or even less making universal decolonization an acceptable practice. The most acceptable protocol to this regard is the use of topical intranasal mupirocin ointment for 5 days applied twice daily and giving chlorhexidine bath (for 5 days) immediately before surgery.

Operating Room Personnel Associated Risk Factors

Mostly importantly two factors have been found to reduce SSI—good handwashing and surgical site skin preparation. It is here important to emphasize that postoperative dressings have not been substantiated to reduce SSI. For hand-antisepsis, some unscientific thoughts and practices prevail that must be clarified. Alcohol rubs are NO superior to aqueous-based scrubs in preventing SSI and to this effect chlorhexidine as aqueous rub is more effective in removing pathogens than povidone-iodine. Surgical site skin preparation—as a time honored recent practice performing hair clipping in the surgical preparation area just before surgery is preferred to performing shaving with razors. There is no scientifically proven benefit for plastic adhesive surgical films with or without iodophor impregnation for preventing SSI.

Modifiable Patient Risk Factors

Diabetes Mellitus

It has a strong association with SSI. DM as a risk factor is not strictly modifiable but blood glucose levels should be controlled for sure. Blood glucose levels of >140 mg/dL in postoperative period (*Note:* This is not preoperative levels as usually the anesthetists require for fitness!) are associated with up to three times increased risk of SSI. To be more specific for blood glucose levels it is found more than or equal to two readings of 200 mg/dL (diabetic or nondiabetic patient) or a hyperglycemic index of >1.76 predicts SSI. This is due to impaired humoral and cell-mediated immune functions (chemotaxis, cell adherence, and phagocytosis) and impaired tissue oxygen delivery associated with micro- and macrovascular disease. To optimize patients in preoperative period, exact and universally accepted guidelines are not available but American Diabetes Association recommends fasting blood glucose levels between 90–130 mg/dL and postprandial levels of <180 mg/dL and HbA1C level < 7%.

Obesity

The association of obesity to SSI is multifactorial. Need of larger incisions, increased dissection, increased blood loss, fat necrosis, and longer surgeries are partly associated with SSI. Most of these patients also have associated comorbidities like DM and cardiac problems.

Malnutrition

Albumin level < 3.5 g/dL, total lymphocyte count < 1,500/mm^3, and serum transferrin < 200 mg/dL predict SSI.

Rheumatoid Arthritis

Rheumatoid arthritis (RA) association with SSI can be direct due to disease-specific impairment of wound healing and immune response to pathogens or indirect due to use of various immunosuppressant medications. The association is stronger for late infections rather than acute SSI. Some general recommendations appear in literature for optimization of patient with respect to the medications:

- Corticosteroids have been traditionally associated with increased risk of SSI. But, no definite association has been proven in small studies so there is no recommendation to their use but one should delay restarting them as late as possible.

- Conventional disease-modifying antirheumatic drugs (DMARDs) (nonbiological agents)—despite traditional thought based on the fact that methotrexate causes immunosuppression, there is no scientific evidence that their use causes immunosuppression and its role in SSI is minimal, if any. There is consensus that they should not be discontinued in the perioperative period. Sulfasalazine is normally discontinued 2 days before surgery and restarted 1–3 days postoperatively (check renal and hepatic function), same holds true for leflunomide.
- For biological agents, preliminary evidence suggests increased risk of SSI associated with them and is in particular true for anti-TNF agents. Use of surgical drains is not recommended. The anti-TNF agents should be discontinued at least 4 weeks before the index procedure and restarted around 1–3 weeks postoperatively or as needed, other agents are commonly discontinued 2 weeks before surgery [for a list of agents used, *see* Chapter on "Joint Disorders Including Inflammatory and Noninflammatory Arthritis and Infective Arthritides (Including Mycobacterial infection and Prosthetic Joint Infection)"].

Cigarette Smoking

Smoking doubles the risk of trading SSI compared to nonsmokers in implantation orthopedic surgeries. The effects are mediated by left shift of oxygen-dissociation curve, nicotine-mediated hypoperfusion, reduced collagen synthesis, and decreased immunoglobulin and phagocytosis levels. It is recommended to quit smoking altogether and encourage patients for same possibly also by counseling them.

Human Immunodeficiency Virus infection

It is recommended that CD4 counts > 400/mm^3 and an undetectable viral load are the appropriate measures to ward off increased SSI risk in arthroplasty surgery on such patients.

Dental Procedures

There is no good clinical evidence that dental procedures would cause SSI. The bacterial load with them is 10^4 CFU/mL which is very less compared to that needed for seeding of implanted sites in studies (>3–5 × 10^5 CFU/mL). Such transient bacteremia is even associated with routine procedures like brushing teeth and chewing. "Poor dental hygiene" is but associated with increased risk for SSI after arthroplasty.

Urinary Tract Infection

There is no clear understanding of the relationship between deep SSI and UTI though most researchers do consider it important. One must realize that "bacteriuria" is different from UTI and mere obtaining urine culture does no good as is commonly practiced. Patients with symptomatic UTI (frequency, urgency, and burning micturition) should be properly evaluated and if in these patients CFUs > 10^3/mL are found then surgery needs to be postponed. For asymptomatic bacteriuria, postoperative oral antibiotics would suffice.

Anemia

This is the second most common modifiable risk factor after obesity. By itself it may not be important in increasing the risk of SSI but most patients with preoperative anemia have increased requirement of postoperative blood transfusion and this allogenic transfusion has been shown to increase the risk of SSI.

CONCLUSION

- Infections in orthopedic practice (as is also true for other faculties) are a fearful complication and commonly it is said that bone once infected never gets cured. This notion has made surgeons quite concerned about preventing the infections that appear to be the best method to deal with this fearsome complication.
- There are situations, however, when the infection is unavoidable and happens "spontaneously" (hematogenous spread) or "inevitably" (viz., bad contaminated wound from road traffic accident). In such circumstances, the surgeon has to use his experience and knowledge to get rid of the infection and reconstruct the limb as functionally as possible.
- Infection in orthopedic practice takes a long time to heal provided proper management and healing environment is created/available. More often than not patient or the surgeon loses patience if the infection is not getting controlled, which should be restrained by proper communication.
- It is important to realize that microorganisms in situ do not respond as we have been classically trained during graduation. The organisms develop their own comfortable environment (like biofilms) to suit their survival changing their form and function which is drastically different from the planktonic forms we have been acquainted with. This portends that the treatment modality will also be very different and not just relying on antimicrobial chemotherapy.
- The intent should be, therefore, to disrupt the environment created by the microorganisms which will make their survival difficult and then control the infection. Debridement of the dead tissue and creating a vascular healing environment are the most useful tools that form the basis of dealing infection in orthopedic practice. Advances in strategies that counter these host-hostile and microbe-cozy environment should be readily deployed at first opportunity.
- Later all infections need to be managed on a case-to-case basis as per the persisting conditions, requirements, and individual demands.

CHAPTER 5

Orthopedic Oncology (Bone Tumors and Metastasis) and Heterotopic Ossification

Manish Kumar Varshney

INTRODUCTION

The bone tumors represent specialized region of orthopedics that involves meticulous evaluation, extensive treatment, and comprehensive communication with different specialties. Bone tumors are sarcomas that is an unfortunate occurrence in a patient, getting rid from which requires immense patience and lots of hospital visits all associated with the uncertainty of ever achieving a cure. Conventionally due to dismal prognosis, immature understanding, inadequate surgical methods, lack of adjuvants, and poor evolving methods, the neoplastic disease of bone yielded ultimately into limb or life loss. The recent diagnostic and staging improvements along with advances in medical and surgical management (still evolving in modern science and rapidly too as we will learn below) have enhanced chances of limb-salvage surgery and better patient outcomes in terms of life expectancy and function. Putting this in numbers for survival, some 70% of patients with bone and soft tissue sarcomas 40 years ago would have succumbed to the ultimate truth but now >70% successfully fight and not only this but most of the patients who had amputations are now managed with limb-sparing surgery (LSS). The LSS though challenging is the current preferred method for treating primary bone and soft tissue malignancies. To make this feasible, early recognition, proper evaluation, and timely management are essential. A comprehensive overview of dealing the neoplastic diseases of bone is presented before a discussion on individual conditions.

STAGING

This is the first and most important step to learn as much about the pathology clinically and its possible differential diagnosis *before* performing biopsy. This avoids wrong decisions that may be otherwise made and could likely worsen the eventual outcome of management. A comprehensive routine for staging conventionally needed skeletal survey, a total body scan (to look for other bony lesions or metastasis), a high-resolution computed tomography (CT) scan of the chest and a magnetic resonance imaging (MRI) of the primary lesion and most importantly thorough clinical examination. Nowadays most of the ancillary investigations are (for metastasis) replaced by positron emission tomography (PET) scan.

Staging systems resolve a neoplasia in terms of size, site, grade, and metastasis. The staging systems of the "Musculoskeletal Tumor Society" (also called the "Enneking system") and the American Joint Commission on Cancer (AJCC) are quite popular. Both are useful for tumor evaluation planning strategies and predicting prognosis.

Enneking System

Enneking system is based on knowing the histologic grade of the lesion (G, see below), tumor site (T, intracompartmental or extracompartmental) and metastases (M). Enneking system is simple and the three broad categories based on low grade (I), high-grade lesion (II), and metastatic lesion (III) are further divided into subgroups based on intracompartmental (IIIA) or extracompartmental (IIIB) location **(Table 1)**.

TABLE 1: Staging system of the musculoskeletal tumor society (Enneking system).

Stage	*Grade [G, low (1), high (2)], tumor location [intracompartmental (1), extracompartmental (2)], and metastasis [absent (0), present (1)]*	*Description*
IA	G1 T0, T1 M0	• Low grade • Intracompartmental • No metastasis
IB	G1 T2 M0	• Low grade • Extracompartmental • No metastasis
IIA	G2 T0, T1 M0	• High grade • Intracompartmental • No metastasis
IIB	G2 T2 M0	• High grade • Extracompartmental • No metastasis
IIIA	Any GT1 M1	• Any grade • Intracompartmental • Metastasis
IIIB	Any GT2 M1	• Any grade • Extracompartmental • Metastasis

Note: For description of G, T, and M, see text.

Defining "T"

Tumor located within the bone compartment, more specifically a tumor that remains bounded by "natural barriers" to extension such as bone, fascia, cartilage, muscle aponeurosis, and synovium is called intracompartmental (T1) while those extending beyond the confines of the bone or "natural barriers" are extracompartmental (T2) **(Figs. 1A and B)**. The location of the tumor is established using a combination of specialized procedures, including radiography, tomography, nuclear studies, CT, and MRI. Compartments are specified to describe the tumor site. Compartments are defined on the basis of fascial borders in the extremities. It should be noted that the skin and subcutaneous tissues are classified as a compartment. The potential periosseous space between cortical bone and muscle (containing periosteum, subperiosteal space, and vessels and nerves) is also considered a compartment. For any intra-articular tumor (T1), any soft tissue extension is extracompartmental (T2), any tumor located superficial to deep fascia (T1) will become extracompartmental as soon as it extends into deep fascia (T2). Similarly, a paraosseous (T1) tumor will become extracompartmental (T2) if it extends into bone or extends through fascia. T0 lesions are confined within the tumor capsule and within its compartment of origin. T1 tumors have extracapsular extension into the reactive zone around it, but both the tumor and the reactive zone are confined within the compartment of origin. T2 lesions extend beyond the anatomic compartment of origin by direct extension or some other means (e.g., trauma and surgical seeding). Tumors that involve major neurovascular bundles are classified as T2 lesions. Most bone sarcomas are bicompartmental at presentation (have violated the bone cortex migrating into the soft tissues). Sometimes the tumor may remain within the compartment but break through the pseudocapsule to form *"skip" metastasis* (within same anatomical compartment). These skip nodules (skip foci) are *not* in continuity with the main tumor mass **(Fig. 2)**. These are locoregional metastasis that did not enter circulation. Traditionally, metastasis across a joint has been referred to as a skip lesion. Metastasis across a joint is now deemed to arise from hematogenous spread and considered systemic metastasis. *"Satellite" nodules* form "within" the pseudocapsule separated from the main mass by intervening normal tissue of pseudocapsule **(Fig. 2)**. Benign tumors are covered by true capsule comprising compressed normal cells compared to "pseudocapsule" of sarcomas that is formed from reactive tissue composed of compressed neoplastic cells and fibrovascular zone of reactive cells that contain a variable amount of inflammatory tissue and interacts with the surrounding normal tissue. High-grade and fast-growing tumors have thin reactive zone. For growth of a sarcoma, epiphyseal or growth plate does not pose any resistance or anatomical barrier as there are numerous vascular channels that pass through the epiphyseal plate to the epiphysis. The hyaline articular cartilage does provide an anatomical barrier to local tumor extension, which is very rarely violated by the growing tumor often allowing intra-articular resection (i.e., single compartment resection) of sarcomas. Nearby

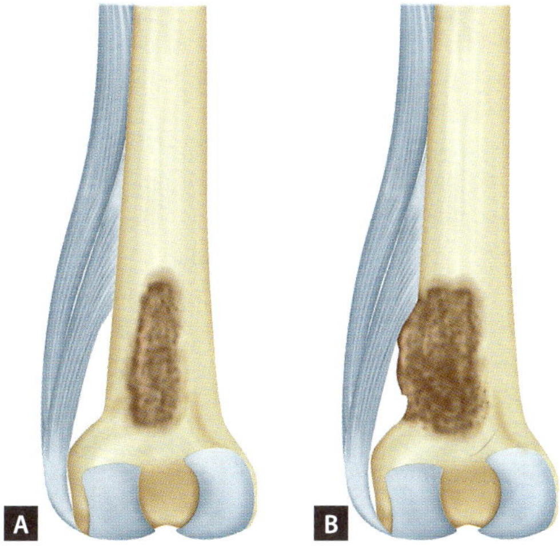

Figs. 1A and B: Bone acts as a compartment itself and any neoplasia inside the bone will be intracompartmental (T1); with breach of periosteum, it becomes extracompartmental (T2).

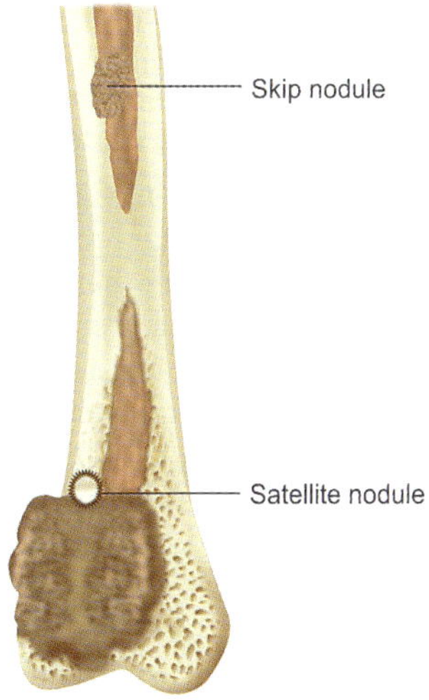

Fig. 2: The tumor growth at the distal metaphyseal region has breached the capsule and reactive zone at multiple places resulting in development of "skip lesion" within the same compartment. Also one can note a "satellite lesion" in the peripheral capsular and reactive zone of the primary tumor mass separated by its own capsule.

joint can still get involved by one of the following routes **(Figs. 3A and B)**:

- Pericapsular spread and secondary capsule breach
- Fracture hematoma extending into joint
- Intra-articular structures like knee ligaments (cruciate)
- Skip metastasis (from direct seeding)
- Direct articular extension of tumor mass

Defining "G" (also see "Grading of Bone Tumors" below) and "M"

Intermediate-grade, high-grade, and undifferentiated lesions are all included in G2. Low-grade and well-differentiated tumors are kept in G1 lesions. Both locoregional and distal metastases are grouped under M1 as any metastasis (whether to nearby tissues or nodes or to far away organs) has poor prognosis and changes management.

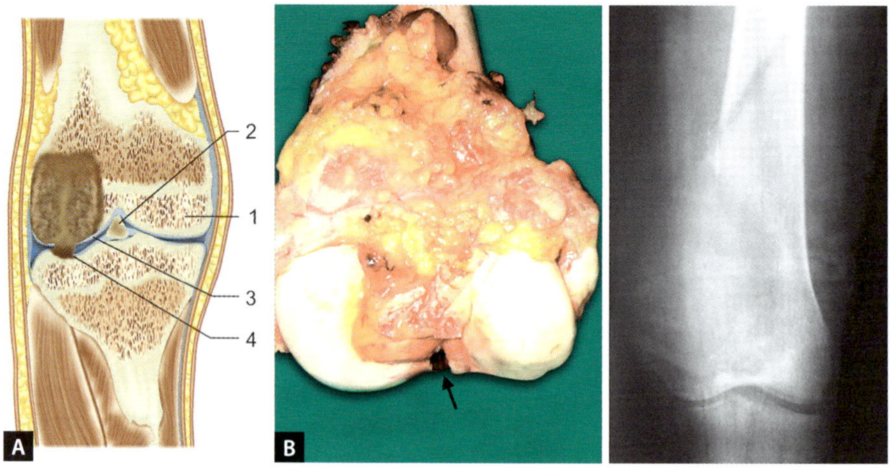

Figs. 3A and B: (A) Tumor spread to joint. A tumor-like giant cell tumor can spread to joint space through various routes—commonly the capsular attachments are the sites for tumor spread (1). Intra-articular ligaments are the other sites for metastasis (2), if the strong subchondral bone is breached then intra-articular seeding can produce skip metastasis (3) while a fast growing malignant tumor (4) can grow into the joint space itself. Traumatic injury can fracture the weakened bone leading to intra-articular hematoma formation and seeding of the joint with tumor cells; (B) The giant cell tumor of distal femur breaches the subchondral bone barrier in the notch region (arrow) to spread into joint. It was not very well-appreciated on radiographs.

American Joint Committee on Cancer System

The American Joint Committee on Cancer (AJCC) system **(Table 2)** has become more popular recently for its similarity to various TNM classifications (for other neoplasms) popular among medical oncologists and many orthopedic oncologists. To use this system, the clinician must know the grade (see below), the size, the presence or absence of discontinuous tumor (skip metastases), and the absence or presence of systemic metastases. Unlike the TNM classification of other tumors, the prominent characteristic of bone and soft tissue sarcoma is the necessity of knowing histological grade and its incorporation into TNM classification. Also unlike the Enneking system, involvement of regional nodes is a separate category for staging. The biological behavior of bone neoplasms varies highly on the histological grade so prognosticating just on the basis of T, N, and M is not legible. The variables in the AJCC staging system have differing importance: stage of tumor is most important followed by metastases, discontinuous tumor, grade, and size in that order.

Based on the poor performance of seventh edition of AJCC system (2011) of classification of bone and soft tissue sarcomas; a revised system **(Table 2)** has been proposed in eighth edition of AJCC classification of tumors (2017). The major changes in the eighth edition for bone and soft tissue sarcomas are:

1. Tumors are described separately according to the primary sites.
   i. For bone sarcoma, three tumor locations are described:
      a. Appendicular skeleton, trunk, skull, and facial bones
      b. Spine
      c. Pelvis
   ii. Four tumor locations are described for soft tissue sarcoma:
      a. Trunk and extremity
      b. Retroperitoneum
      c. Head and neck
      d. Visceral sites
2. Histologic grading system in bone sarcoma is changed to three-grade classifications (see previous edition for 4 grade system).
3. For soft tissue sarcoma, any TN1M0 tumor in the trunk and extremity is now classified as stage IV, whereas for the retroperitoneal tumor, any TN1M0 remains as stage IIIB.
4. For soft tissue sarcomas in the trunk, extremity and retroperitoneum, tumor size is classified into four categories:
   a. ≤5 cm
   b. >5 cm and ≤10 cm
   c. >10 cm and ≤15 cm
   d. >15 cm
5. The notation about the depth of the tumor (superficial or deep from the superficial fascia) has been eliminated.

In the TNM classification for bone sarcomas arising in the appendicular skeleton, trunk, skull, and facial bones, a tumor is first divided into stage I (grade 1) and stage II or more (grade 2 or 3) according to the histologic grade. Then the T factor, i.e., tumor size (T1, ≤8 cm; T2, >8 cm; T3, discontinuous tumors in the primary bone site), determines the stage. Regional lymph node metastasis (N1) and distant organ metastasis (M1a, lung; M1b, bone or other distant sites) are assessed as stage IV regardless of histologic grade or tumor size. However, because lymph node metastasis or extrapulmonary metastasis including bone (M1b) has a poorer prognosis than lung metastasis, lung metastasis (M1a) is classified as stage IVA and regional lymph node metastasis or extrapulmonary metastasis as stage IVB **(Table 2)**.

CLINICAL EVALUATION

Benign tumors in children are usually noticed incidentally by parents. Otherwise, most patients with bone tumors present

TABLE 2: American Joint Committee on Cancer (AJCC) classification of bone and soft tissue sarcoma of extremities (retroperitoneum head and neck and visceral organs have not been described in this text for lack of relevance).

AJCC staging of bone tumors

Stage	*Primary tumor (T)*	*Regional lymph node (N)*	*Distant metastasis (M)*	*Histologic grade (G)*
IA	T1	N0	M0	G1 or GX
IB	T2 or T3	N0	M0	G1 or GX
IIA	T1	N0	M0	G2 or G3
IIB	T2	N0	M0	G2 or G3
III	T3	N0	M0	G2 or G3
IVA	Any T	N0	M1a	Any G
IVB	Any T	N1	Any M	Any G
	Any T	Any N	M1b	Any G

(A) Appendicular skeleton, trunk, skull, and facial bones

Defining tumor size (T)		***Defining regional lymph nodes (N)***	
T category	*Criteria*	*N category*	*Criteria*
Tx	Primary tumor cannot be assessed	Nx	Regional lymph node cannot be assessed
T0	No evidence of primary tumor	N0	No regional lymph node metastasis
T1	Tumor ≤ 8 cm in greatest dimension	N1	Regional lymph nodes metastasis
T2	Tumor > 8 cm in greatest dimension		
T3	Discontinuous tumors in the primary bone site		

Defining M (distant metastasis)		***Histologic grading of tumor***	
M category	*Criteria*	*G criteria*	*Definition*
M0	No distant metastasis	Gx	Grade cannot be assessed.
M1	Distant metastasis present	G1	Well differentiated, low grade
M1a	Lung	G2	Moderately differentiated, high grade
M1b	Bone or other distant sites	G3	Poorly differentiated, high grade

(B) Spine

Defining tumor size (T)

T category	*T criteria*
Tx	Primary tumor cannot be assessed.
T0	No evidence of primary tumor
T1	Tumor confined to one vertebral segment or two adjacent vertebral segments
T2	Tumor confined to three adjacent vertebral segments
T3	Tumor confined to four or more adjacent vertebral segments, or any nonadjacent vertebral segments
T4	Extension into the spinal canal or great vessels
T4a	Extension into the spinal canal
T4b	Extension of gross vascular invasion or tumor thrombus in the great vessels

AJCC staging for soft tissue sarcoma in the trunk and extremity

Stage	*Primary tumor (T)*	*Regional lymph node (N)*	*Distant metastasis (M)*	*Histologic grade (G)*
IA	T1	N0	M0	G1, GX
IB	T2, T3, and T4	N0	M0	G1, GX
II	T1	N0	M0	G2, G3
IIIA	T2	N0	M0	G2, G3
IIIB	T3, T4	N0	M0	G2, G3
IV	Any T	N1	M0	Any G
	Any T	Any N	M1	Any G

Trunk and extremity

Defining primary tumor (T)

T category	*T criteria*
Tx	Primary tumor cannot be assessed
T0	No evidence of primary tumor
T1	Tumor 5 cm or less in greatest dimension
T2	Tumor > 5 cm and ≤10 cm in greatest dimension
T3	Tumor > 10 cm and ≤15 cm in greatest dimension
T4	Tumor > 15 cm in greatest dimension

Defining regional lymph nodes (N)

N category	*N criteria*
N0	No regional lymph node metastasis or unknown lymph node status
N1	Regional lymph node metastasis

Defining M (distant metastasis)

M category	*M criteria*
M0	No distant metastasis
M1	Distant metastasis present

Histologic grading of tumor

G criteria	*G definition*
Gx	Grade cannot be assessed.
G1	Total differentiation, mitotic count, and necrosis score of 2 or 3
G2	Total differentiation, mitotic count, and necrosis score of 4 or 5
G3	Total differentiation, mitotic count, and necrosis score of 6, 7 or 8

Contd...

Contd...

(C) Pelvis	
Defining primary tumor size (T)	
T category	*T criteria*
Tx	Primary tumor cannot be assessed.
T0	No evidence of primary tumor
T1	Tumor confined to one pelvic segment with no extraosseous extension
T1a	Tumor ≤ 8 cm in greatest dimension
T1b	Tumor > 8 cm in greatest dimension
T2	Tumor confined to one pelvic segment with extraosseous extension or two segments without extraosseous extension
T2a	Tumor ≤ 8 cm in greatest dimension
T2b	Tumor > 8 cm in greatest dimension
T3	Tumor spanning two pelvic segments with extraosseous extension
T3a	Tumor spanning two pelvic segments with extraosseous extension
T3b	Tumor spanning two pelvic segments with extraosseous extension
T4	Tumor spanning three pelvic segments or crossing the sacroiliac joint
T4a	Tumor involves sacroiliac joint and extends medial to the sacral neuroforamen.
T4b	Tumor encasement of external iliac vessels or presence of gross tumor thrombus in major pelvic vessels

with musculoskeletal *pain,* which is variably followed by or is associated with *swelling.* Patients often recall a *history of trauma* but that is possibly an incidental correlation but the history is quite prompt in many and needs research.

Pain is the most common symptom of malignant tumors while for benign lesions its absence is the most notable negative feature. When present, it is typically deep-seated, dull, aching increasing in night (sometimes on full moon!), and often resembles toothache. Pain may initially be intermittent and related to activity that quickly progresses in intensity and becomes constant. Initially, the pain is quite responsive to nonsteroidal anti-inflammatory drugs (NSAIDs) and mild narcotics but flare-up require strong analgesics. Sudden increase in pain may represent malignant transformation of benign tumors or hemorrhage in an existing lesion or a pathological fracture. Sometimes, the malignant lesions compress nearby neurovascular bundle often infiltrating and impinging the nerves that produce radicular symptoms. Physician should clearly distinguish between activity-related (due to surrounding inflammation, altered body mechanics, arthritis/bursitis, etc.) and nonactivity-related pain which raises red-flag if present at rest and aggravates at night. Typically, patients with high-grade sarcoma present with a 1–6 months history of pain while with low-grade tumors, such as chondrosarcoma, the history of mild-to-moderate pain is often prolonged for 6–24 months.

Swelling is better examined than explained but some notable points in history include duration of presence of mass, rapidity of increase in size, and presence of pain and tenderness. Progression of swelling should be noted and its relation to pain. Constant increase in size with increasing pain, sudden increase in swelling, and association with fungation indicate aggressive lesion. Pain usually precedes swelling by months, but pain appearing with swelling may indicate pathological fracture in an often benign lesion with ensuing hematoma. Firm to hard, deep mass usually indicates bone pathology whereas a lump that moves with movement of adjacent joint indicates soft-tissue tumor deep to investing fascia while superficial tumors are poorly defined and move freely.

Functiolesia (loss of function) is not commonly seen but may be a presentation of benign lesions. Pathological fracture from lytic lesions like bone cysts is a common presentation. Compression from tibifibular joint ganglion cyst may cause foot drop. Osteochondroma may protrude into soft tissue causing snapping, painful bursitis, or restriction of joint motion.

Syndromic association of few typical tumors should be carefully evaluated based on the associated features. A useful list is provided in **Table 3**. Oncogenic osteomalacia is a very rare presentation of bone tumors seen only with uncommon malignant mesenchymal chondrosarcoma or hemangiopericytoma sometimes. The characteristics of oncogenic osteomalacia are presented in **Box 1**.

PHYSICAL EXAMINATION

A careful examination is imperative to understand the site, size, extent or tumor and possibly determining the benign and malignant process. Site is inspected for soft tissue masses, overlying skin changes, adenopathy, and general musculoskeletal condition. Skin should also be examined for lesions such as hyperpigmented patches of fibrous dysplasia

TABLE 3: Syndromes associated with bone tumors.

Syndrome	*Characteristic features*
Bloom syndrome (autosomal recessive)	Growth deficiency, immunodeficiency, early development of cancer including osteosarcoma
Familial expansile osteolysis (autosomal dominant)	Osteosarcoma
Li Fraumeni syndrome (autosomal dominant)	Osteosarcoma and other soft tissue sarcomas (early onset in affected patients)
Mazabraud syndrome (sporadic)	Polyostotic fibrous dysplasia, osteosarcoma, and intramuscular myxoma
McCune–Albright syndrome (sporadic)	Polyostotic fibrous dysplasia, osteosarcoma, endocrine disorders, and skin pigmentation
Familial Paget's disease (autosomal dominant)	Osteosarcoma, early onset of Paget's disease
Retinoblastoma (autosomal dominant)	Osteosarcoma, retinoblastoma, and other soft tissue tumors
Rothmund–Thomson syndrome (autosomal recessive)	Increased cancer risk—osteosarcoma, poikiloderma, sparse hair, small stature, skeletal abnormalities
Langer–Giedion syndrome (sporadic)	Multiple osteochondromas, chondrosarcomas, + tricho-rhino-phalangeal syndrome II
Multiple osteochondromas (autosomal dominant)	Multiple osteochondromas, secondary chondrosarcoma, secondary osteosarcoma
Maffucci syndrome (sporadic)	Multiple enchondromas, chondrosarcoma, hemangioma, spindle-cell hemangioma, and angiosarcoma
Ollier's disease (sporadic)	Multiple enchondromas
Werner's syndrome (autosomal recessive)	Premature aging, increased risk of various soft tissue and osseous sarcomas

(FD) and fibromatosis. A shiny adherent skin that is tethered to the underlying mass (uncommon) with dilated superficial veins indicates aggressive pathology. Features that indicate malignant pathology include a short clinical history, rapidly progressive lesion, pain not reduced by analgesics, general debility, large size of tumor, shiny skin with dilated veins or fungation and presence of pathological fracture. When metastatic disease is suspected, examine the thyroid gland, prostate, abdomen, and breasts for possible primary tumor.

RADIOLOGICAL EVALUATION

Despite advances in techniques, radiographs are first investigation to be performed and can reveal significant information. They are primarily used to detect and characterize bone pathology. Stepwise assessment **(Box 2)** of the radiographs yields provides uniformity and reduces ambiguity among observers. The radiographs are evaluated for:

- Detection of pathology
- Diagnosis including metastatic disease
- Staging
- Treatment evaluation

They are also the primary modality to follow a patient after treatment until some complications (like recurrence) need further evaluation.

A number of bone lesions are first noticed. Usually, these are focal osseous lesions. Multiple primary bone lesions are uncommon and are often defining by themselves (FD, metastatic, multiple osteochondromatosis, multiple exostoses, Paget's disease, etc.). Some neoplasms such as adamantinoma, osteofibrous dysplasia (OFD), and intramedullary osteosarcoma involve whole of the bone. Few neoplasms characteristically involve only a part of bone such as involvement of posterior cortex distal femur by parosteal osteosarcoma and periosteal desmoid (also known as cortical desmoid, avulsive cortical irregularity).

BOX 1: Oncogenic osteomalacia, tumor-induced osteomalacia (TIO), oncogenic hypophosphatemic osteomalacia.

Oncogenic osteomalacia is a paraneoplastic syndrome characterized by bone pain, fractures, and muscle weakness. There is increased renal phosphate excretion, hypophosphatemia, and low levels of circulating 1,25-dihydroxy vitamin D. The condition is primarily caused by increased levels of phosphate and vitamin D-regulating hormone, fibroblast growth factor-23 *(FGF-23)*. In majority of the patients, a fibronectin-1 *(FN-1)* and fibroblast growth factor receptor-1 *(FGFR-1)* fusion gene has been identified that may be responsible for high FGF-3 levels.

The patients present with bone pain, fractures, gait abnormalities, and muscle weakness. Because of nonspecific symptoms, misdiagnosis into various rheumatologic, orthopedic, or neuropsychiatric cases is common. Often in investigations, no significant abnormality is revealed as also most panels do not include phosphate levels so patient is long treated symptomatically without benefit. The condition can be seen with benign, malignant, or metastatic neoplasms. In any case, histopathologically, a primitive mesenchymal cell has been identified that has the ability to secrete the hormone.

Management

The treatment is primarily based on two lines—one is the normalization of hematological parameters such as correction of serum inorganic phosphate and correction of serum vitamin D levels [and, in turn, the serum parathyroid hormone (PTH) levels]. The other is identification of the neoplastic lesion. As soon as clinical suspicion is made, diagnosis is made by hematological investigations and demonstration of renal tubular wasting of phosphate and exclusion of familial forms must be done [Fanconi syndrome, Fanconi–Bickle syndrome, X-linked hypophosphatemic (XLH) rickets and autosomal dominant/recessive hypophosphatemic rickets autosomal dominant hypophosphatemic rickets/autosomal recessive hypophosphatemic rickets (ADHR/ARHR) by *PHEX*, *FGF-23*, and *DMP-1* gene identification]. While *FGF-23* is elevated in XLH, ADHR, and ARHR, it is found normal or low in Fanconi syndrome, Dent's disease, and XLHR. Tumor localization is done by functional imaging [PET scan or 111-Indium octreotide scintigraphy + single-photon emission computed tomography (SPECT)] followed by anatomical imaging with MRI/CT scan. Ga-DOTANOC PET/CT may be more sensitive to identify TIO. Radiographs usually demonstrate generalized osteopenia and "reactivation" of growth plate as transverse lucent lines in the region of physeal scar. Venous sampling (for *FGF-23*) from the draining site may be added for more assurance if needed. The identified lesion should be excised on standard procedure for type of neoplasm.

If no neoplasm is identified, then corrective treatment is continued in the form of phosphate [15–60 mg/kg/day (1–3 g/day for adults); divided into 4–5 times/day to improve tolerance] and vitamin D supplementation to achieve target serum phosphate and vitamin D/PTH levels. The monitoring is done every 3 months in the form of serum calcium, phosphorus, PTH, urinary calcium, and creatinine. Relocalization of tumor is attempted after 1 year.

BOX 2: Four-step guide to evaluate radiographs for diagnosis.

1. Identify whether monostotic/polyostotic, solitary/multiple lesion, and whether appendicular or axial skeleton or both involved (metastasis/lymphoma).
2. Identify bone segment involved (epiphysis, metaphysis or diaphysis).
3. Identify the predominant area of bone involvement: medulla, cortex, or both.
4. Characterize the matrix of lesion (mineralization within tumor substance) and its margin and cortical destruction. Identify the reaction of the native bone to the lesion (and periosteal reactions).

Next step for focal osseous lesions is to define the bone involved, the lesion's appearance within the bone (matrix type, depending on the characteristics of the neoplasm and what it does to bone), the lesion's margin, reaction of bone to the neoplasms, and upon adjacent soft tissues (including periosteal reaction). To improve making diagnosis and justify differential diagnosis, one must read radiological findings in concert with the clinical parameters (age, sex, symptoms, and pre-existing conditions).

Lesion Location and Size

The typical locations (according to predominance) are given in **Table 4**. The location of lesion within the skeleton (appendicular/axial), within the bone (epiphysis, metaphysis, or diaphysis) and part of the bone (medullary cavity, cortex, juxtacortical bone, or periosteum) is most significant and should be carefully evaluated for differential diagnosis **(Figs. 4 and 5)**. Although most primary bone neoplasms arise in the metaphyseal region; a few are typically defined for the diaphysis (Ewing's sarcoma, neuroblastoma, and other primitive neuroectodermal tumors). Nonossifying fibroma and fibrous critical defect usually span whole metadiaphysis. Metastasis, lymphoma, osteoid osteoma, and histiocytosis X have no specific anatomical predilection. The size of a lesion is usually considered a prognostic feature as it is linked to the disease burden. It has been shown that disease-free survival is much better for neoplastic lesions < 100 cm^3 in volume. The axial lesions affecting the vertebral column have characteristic distribution of lesion **(Table 5)** that can come in handy for differential diagnosis and histopathological correlation.

TABLE 4: Most common/representative location of focal bone lesion (anatomic bone region).

Epiphyseal lesions	*Metaphyseal lesions*	*Diaphyseal lesions*
Chondroblastoma Giant cell tumor (the tumor begins in metaphyseal region and progress to epiphysis settling below the articular cartilage)	Chondrosarcoma giant cell tumor aneurysmal bone cyst	Campanacci's disease or osteofibrous dysplasia
Clear cell chondrosarcoma	Fibrosarcoma	Ewing's tumor
Aneurysmal bone cyst	Osteochondroma	Osteoid osteoma
Langerhans cell histiocytosis*	Osteosarcoma	Osteoblastoma
	Malignant fibrous histiocytoma	(Metastatic disease, lymphoma/myeloma, eosinophilic granuloma, Paget's disease, unicameral bone cyst, hemangioma, fibrous dysplasia, and enchondroma)*
	Nonossifying fibroma or metaphyseal cortical defect	
	(Metastatic disease, enchondroma, fibrous dysplasia, lymphoma/ myeloma, Langerhans cell histiocytosis, hemangioma, Paget's disease, and unicameral bone cyst)*	

*Represents entities that are not specific to the region but are more likely to be present there.

Lesion Margin

Evaluating margins help us to understand what tumor does to the bone. This usually reveals the "nature" of lesion in terms of aggressiveness. Lytic (blastic) processes *do not affect the bone directly*, but act via the native osteoblasts and osteoclasts within the bone through various signaling pathways. Ultimate outcome depends on the balance struck between bone tumor vagaries and attempt at maintaining homeostasis by bone (ability of bone to repair or limit the destruction). A slow-growing lesion will hence show relatively sharp, sclerotic, and well-defined edges while an aggressive lesion due to infiltration and destruction will show ill-defined margins. Lodwick classified radiographic lytic lesions into five grades **(Fig. 6)**. There are three predominant grades (I, II, and III). Grades II and III are difficult to differentiate but both represent aggressive lesion so differentiation and characterization is hardly required.

- *Grade I:* A lesion with geographic destruction has a sharp and well-defined margin. These are slowly growing lesions that progressively eat away all the bone in the space they occupy slowly; producing radiologically a "geographic" pattern of bone destruction. The lesion is well-circumscribed with a narrow zone of transition from normal bone and the actual edge of tumor is closely related to the radiologic margin seen. Of the radiographic features that characterize a lesion, its margin provides perhaps the most information. The next step is to evaluate the margin of these lesions:
  - *Grade IA:* These are lesions with discrete sclerotic margins on radiographs separating them from normal bone. Lesions having a nonsclerotic margin are classified into grade IB, e.g., chondroblastoma, nonossifying fibroma, simple (unicameral) bone cyst, chondromyxoid fibroma, and enchondroma.
  - *Grade IB:* These are lesions with either nonsclerotic margins or those having an expanded cortical shell that exceeds 1 cm, e.g., giant cell tumors (GCTs), aggressive

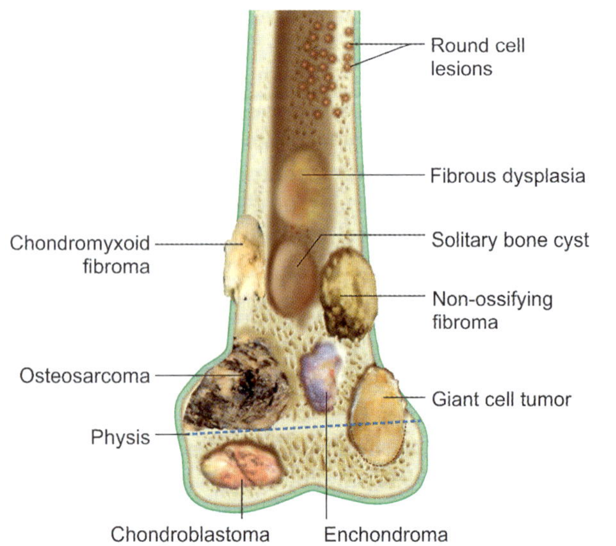

Fig. 4: Osseous location of various bone tumors.

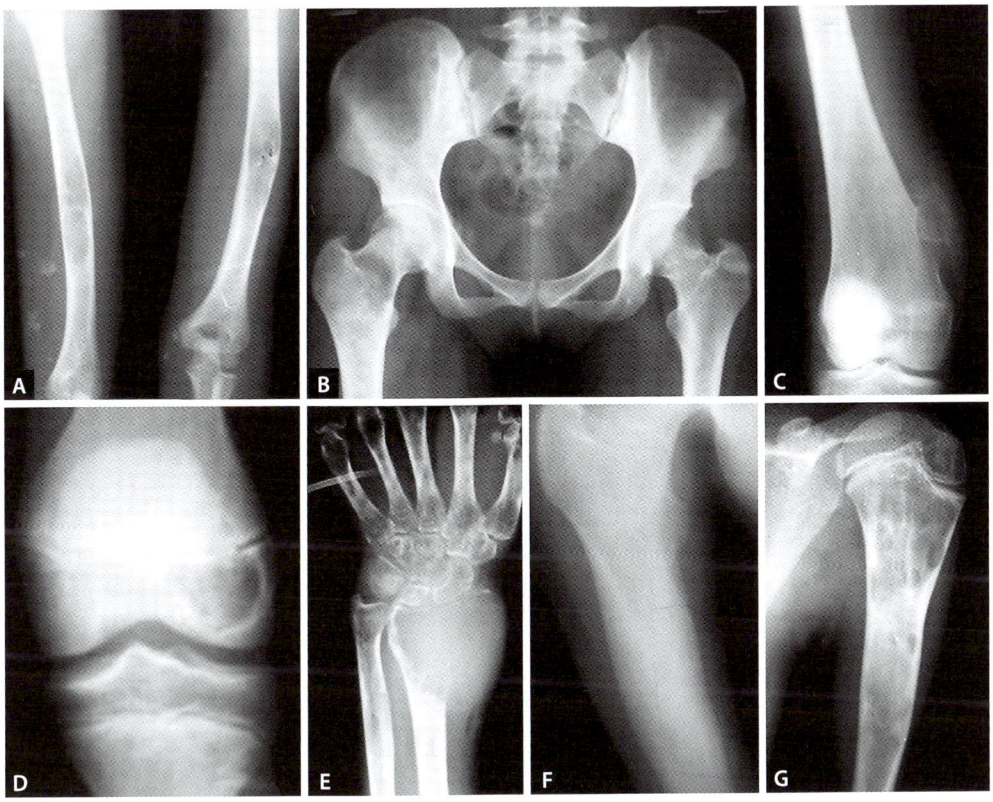

Figs. 5A to G: Some classic radiographs showing typical location of bone tumors in various osseous locations. (A) Diaphyseal simple bone cyst; (B) Metaphyseal chondromyxoid fibroma; (C) Metaphyseal exophytic growing away from the physis—osteochondroma; (D) Epiphyseal chondroblastoma; (E) Epiphyseo-metaphyseal—giant cell tumor; (F) Intracortical lytic lesion surrounded by excess sclerosis of osteoid osteoma; (G) Metaphyseal abutting the growth plate expanding bone—aneurysmal bone cyst.

TABLE 5: Tumors affecting the vertebral column.

Vertebral body	*Posterior elements*
Giant cell tumor	Aneurysmal bone cyst
Hemangioma	Osteoid osteoma
Eosinophilic granuloma	Osteoblastoma
Metastases	
Chordoma	
Multiple myeloma	

aneurysmal bone cyst (ABC), and telangiectatic osteosarcoma.

- *Grade IC:* These lesions have indistinct margins but should not be confused for grade II or grade III lesions. They are focally destructive and locally infiltrative, e.g., aggressive osteoblastoma and malignant fibrous histiocytoma (MFH).

- *Grade II:* Moth-eaten destruction is similar to moth-eaten clothes (multiple small lytic scattered "holes" of destruction in the involved bone). This is a more aggressive pattern than geographic destruction. The scattered areas of bone holes represent the active destructive process separated by areas of normal bone. Later the scattered holes coalesce to form larger areas of bone destruction. In cortical bone, the holes represent the areas of complete cortical destruction. This is seen commonly with aggressive/malignant neoplasms such as Ewing's sarcoma, chondrosarcoma, primary lymphoma and fibrosarcoma, etc.
- *Grade III:* Permeative destruction is an ill-defined, diffuse, somewhat subtle destructive process of bone. It represents an aggressive pattern with bone destruction by a rapidly enlarging/growing tumor. The margins are indistinguishable and merge with normal bone in an infiltrating pattern. The growth is usually parallel to bone axis while transverse growth may represent blow out and imminently result in fracture. The destroyed regions are completely filled with tumor tissue and are possibly created by accelerated osteoclastic activity, e.g., high-grade chondrosarcoma, aggressive primitive neuroectodemal tumor (PNET). Apart from aggressive neoplasms, this pattern is also produced by inflammatory, infectious, and metabolic pathologies.

A special problem is that extremely rapid growth in a cancellous bone may be represented by an "invisible margin". In osteoporotic bones, margins of neoplastic lesion are difficult to appreciate that is also a problem in metabolic bone diseases, and post-traumatic osteoporosis where margins of even benign lesions may appear aggressive, mimicking rapidly growing tumors. Combinations of patterns around a single lesion are frequent and often indicate acquired aggressive behavior. In these cases, the clinical implications of lesion must be considered to be a representation of its most aggressive appearing margins. Changed patterns are often

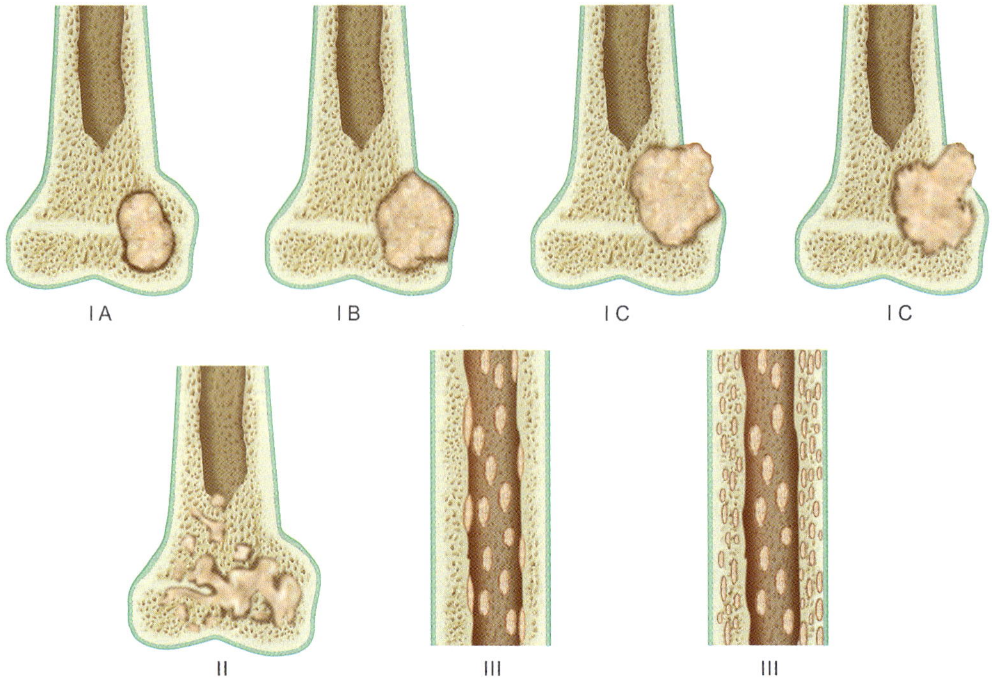

Fig. 6: Lodwick classification for tumor margins.

found with malignant transformation of benign bone tumors or dedifferentiation of malignant lesions.

Cortical Destruction

The high-grade aggressive lesions penetrate through the cortex and periosteum (and its reaction), leaving nothing behind. Intermediate grade lesions often develop into focal cortical defects with eccentrically located soft tissue mass resulting from "spillage" of tumor from the site. Lower grade lesions "expand" the cortex from within with new bone forming on the surface in an attempt to remodeling. Lesions can have varying patterns of cortical destruction; in such cases, the highest grade of cortical destruction represents the true nature of lesion.

Matrix

Matrix represents the proliferative characteristics of bone tumors. Usually, the tumors are nonproductive.

- *Matrix mineralization usually involves the inbuilt physiologic pathways (i.e., ossification on cartilage or osseous backgrounds):* Typically a chondroid matrix radiographically appears as a dot-like or popcorn-like, full rings or partial arcs of calcifications (these represent mineralized lobules of the mulberry-shaped cartilage matrix) seen in enchondroma, chondrosarcoma, and chondroblastoma. Osteoid matrix has a cloud-like, wispy appearance, and is seen in osteoid osteoma and osteosarcoma. The more the mineral in general the more mature and differentiated is the lesion.
- *Dystrophic (degenerating fibrous, myxoid tissue, or fat):* Intraosseous lipoma. Bone infarcts or ossifying lipoma represent osseous matrix production in ischemic bone.
- Metastatic (upon connective tissues altered by a metabolic disease)

  Metaplastic osseous matrix formation is seen in FD.

Bone Reaction

Bone reaction explains what bone does to tumor. This proliferation may be medullary or periosteal **(Fig. 7)**. Very aggressive processes will have no medullary reaction as they "eat-up" everything. Reactive shell (thin or thick) around the lesion in medullary cavity indicates slow-growing lesion. Aggressive processes may show areas of scattered mottled sclerosis in the adjacent bone. Periosteal reactions occur as the lesion approaches a bone's cortex stimulating the periosteum to thicken and become cellular. The configuration of a periosteal reaction depends on the nature of the inciting process, its intensity, aggressiveness, and duration. The pathogenesis of various forms of periosteal reactions in benign and malignant tumors is explained in **Flowcharts 1 and 2**. Simply stating the periosteal reactions can be classified as solid or interrupted.

Slow-growing lesions produce an amorphous (thick) or closely laminated solid periosteal response in comparison to aggressive processes that generate a widely laminated (onion skinned) or sunburst response. A focal process that breaks through cortical shell and the containing periosteal reaction leaves a characteristic Codman angle or triangle at its margins. Expansile lesions with relatively slow growth (simple bone cyst or ABC) may have a thin layer of periosteal bone replacing the destroyed, old cortex. Intra-articular bone-end lesions do not show periosteal reaction as periosteum here is replaced with joint capsule. Below is representation of Ragsdale expanded classification.

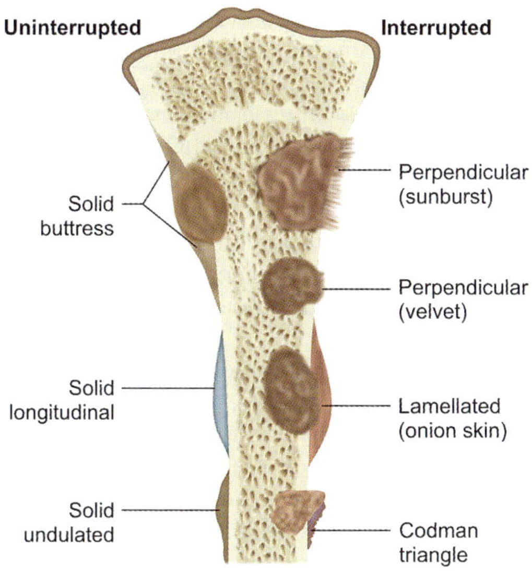

Fig. 7: Types of periosteal reactions.

Solid Periosteal Reactions

Shell formation occurs when slow expanding lesions remove endosteal bone that is replaced by subperiosteal bone deposition, thickening the original bone contour. The thickness of the shell depends on the speed of destructive process relative to the rate of periosteal new bone formation.

Smooth shell: They have smooth outer contour and result from lesions (usually benign) applying uniform pressure on the cortex, e.g., osteoid osteoma.

Ridged shell: Represents trabeculated, septated, or soap-bubble reaction that develops from uneven growth of benign aggressive process, such as nonossifying fibroma, ABC, GCT, and enchondroma, and slow-growing malignant process such as condrosarcoma, plasmacytoma and metastases from renal, thyroid, and melanoma. The ridges represent intermediary remaining/persisting/compressed bone and not trabeculae.

Lobulated shells: In contrast to ridged shell, they result from uneven growth of a relatively slow process (ABC) within the

Flowchart 1: Pathogenesis of periosteal reactions in benign bone lesions.

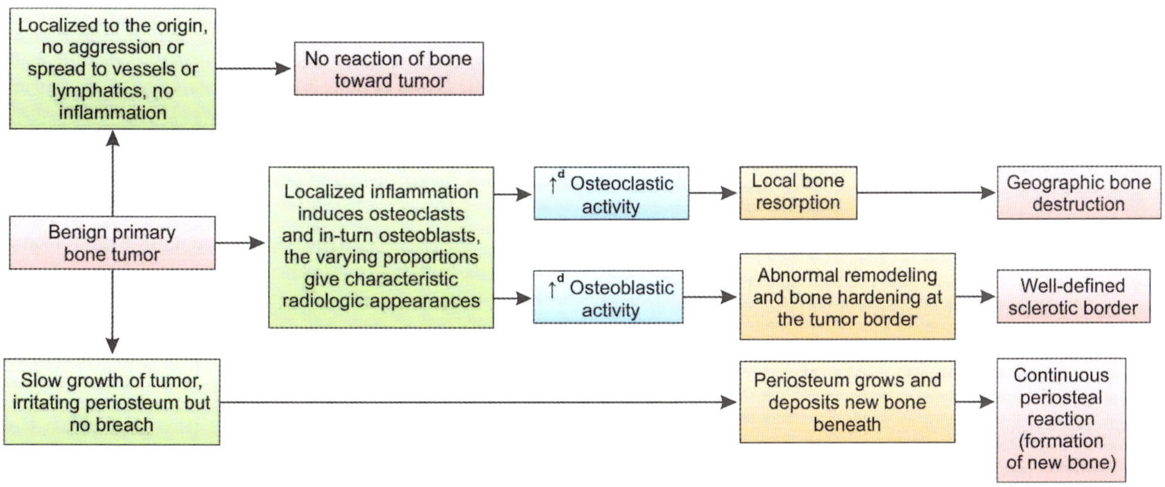

Flowchart 2: Pathogenesis of periosteal reactions in malignant bone lesions.

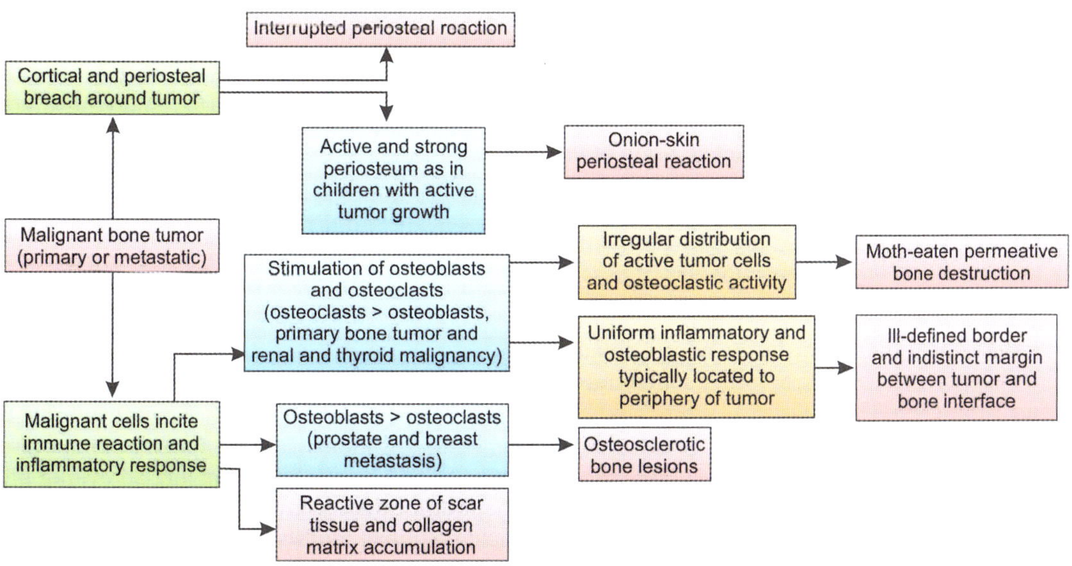

lesion. The faster growing areas are radiopenic and represent cortical bulges while slower growing regions destroy less bone visible as crescents and arcs (they are less destroyed bone and new bone not deposited there).

Continuous Periosteal Reaction

In these reactions, the cortex usually is radiologically intact although varying degree of subperiosteal tumor penetration occurs in the laminated and parallel-speculated forms.

Solid periosteal reaction (cortical thickening or hyperostosis): Multiple layers of new bone are deposited as a single-solid mass due to chronic periosteal stimulation by a relatively innocuous lesion, e.g., intracortical osteoid osteoma, and chronic low-grade infection (Garre's osteomyelitis).

Single lamellar reaction: This is a single uniform radiodense line separated from the underlying cortex and may or may not join the cortex at its proximal and distal extremes. This is pathognomonic of benign process and is seen with osteomyelitis, histiocytosis X, and fractures. Dense undulating periosteal reactions (variant of unilamellar reaction) are seen with chronic osteitis, low-grade osteomyelitis and hypertrophic osteoarthropathy.

Lamellated reactions: This continuous reaction consists of multiple concentric planes of ossification with radiologically appreciable spaces in-between forming the typical "onion-skin". Active bone destroying lesions such as acute osteomyelitis, Ewing's sarcoma, and osteosarcoma form these.

Parallel spiculated reaction (hair-on-end): This is usually seen with malignant processes resulting from new bone formation along the radially oriented periosteal vessels that extend from the periosteum to the cortex, e.g., osteosarcoma, thalassemia (hyperactive marrow lesion).

Interrupted Periosteal Reactions

Codman angle: The Codman angle is seen in the aggressive bone destroying lesions. Codman angle results from any process (whether malignant or benign aggressive) that aggressively lifts the periosteum causing subperiosteal bleeding. Reactive bone forms beneath the periosteum at margin while the aggressive lesion destroys and perpetuates through the adjacent cortical bone leaving a radiopenic area. This process leaves an angle of dense reactive bone at the corners. The density of Codman's angle is less than buttress (see later) and is free of tumor itself. It was originally described by Ribbert in 1914 and later elaborated upon by Codman in 1926 and can be seen with acute osteomyelitis, few aggressive ABCs, chondrosarcomas and osteosarcomas and osteomas.

Buttress: For lesions that expand slowly, the bone formed at the corners becomes dense over time to form a solid buttress (called Codman "triangle"). The buttress is more solid and dense than Codman angle and indicates a benign pathology.

Complex Periosteal Pattern

Divergent spiculated pattern (the sunburst pattern): Results from combined simultaneous reactive bone formation and malignant osteoid production forming "rays of sun" that seem to emanate from the central tumor mass. The space in-between is filled with tumor mass. It is seen commonly with aggressive bone-forming lesions such as osteosarcoma, osteoblastic metastases, and hemangioma and sometimes even with Ewing's sarcoma.

For a working diagnosis, clinician needs to correlate the detailed radiological findings with the age of patient, type of matrix production, site of lesion in skeleton and within bone and so on. Some pathognomonic and most common findings are as follows:

- Metastatic neuroblastoma and Wilm's tumor in diaphysis in the infant and young child.
- Multiple lytic and oval lesions in the same extremity are probably vascular tumors (hemangioendothelioma).
- Metastasis, multiple myeloma (MM), non-Hodgkin's lymphoma (NHL) or Hodgkin's lymphoma in the middle-aged (40–60 years of age), and elderly (60–80 years of age).
- *Diaphyseal lesions:* Ewing's sarcoma are the most typical lesions here especially in the long bones of children and early adolescents. Simple bone cyst may arise in metaphysis that migrate to diaphysis with growth often being asymptomatic earlier in nascent stage.
- *Metaphyseal-epiphyseal lytic lesion:* GCT in a young to middle-aged adult (20–50 years of age) is the most typical lesion.
- Corduroy appearance of vertebral body—hemangioma
- Fallen fragment (leaf) sign—seen with simple bone cyst, ABC
- Presence of gas intralesionally in a juxta-articular lesion is representative of subchondral cyst such as a degenerative cyst or intraosseous ganglion cyst.
- An expanded/enlarged bone with irregular, coarse trabeculae, and cortical thickening—Paget's disease
- Chondroid matrix (typical gross lesional appearance of "lobulated mulberry-like pattern" with fleck-like calcifications is characteristic) in a geographic lytic matrix in small bones of hand—enchondroma.
- Vertebra plana in a child—eosinophilic granuloma (EOG)
- Cockade sign in the calcaneus—intraosseous lipoma
- Cauliflower-like extraosseous growth at metaphyseodiaphyseal junction pointing away from growth plate—exostosis.

Radiographs are also used to restage the tumors following radiotherapy or chemotherapy. The Union for International Cancer Control (UICC) and the World Health Organization (WHO) systems are based on radiographs and scintigraphy respectively **(Table 6)**.

Magnetic Resonance Imaging

MRI is highly effective in evaluating the medullary and soft tissue components of tumor and defining the limits accurately but is also the most misused investigation for diagnosis of benign bone pathologies. Advising MRI should be based on general indications **(Box 3)**. It can evaluate tumor in axial, coronal, and sagittal plane giving an overall picture of the shape and extent of involvement and anatomic features. It is most definitive method to plan surgical margins. Usually, a margin of 1–2 cm for soft tissue and 1.5–2 cm for bone beyond

TABLE 6: Evaluation of treatment response for bone tumors (radiography-based systems).

Response type	WHO (radiographs and scintigraphy)	UICC (radiographs)
Complete	Disappearance of all lesions and negative scans for at least 4 weeks	Disappearance of all lesions and lytic lesions reossify
Partial	Partial reduction in size of lytic lesions, reossification of lytic lesions or decreased density of blastic lesions for at least 4 weeks	*Objective improvement* in evaluable or nonmeasurable lesions. At least *50% reduction* in size of measurable lesions. No new lesions or progression of lesions.
No change (stable disease)	"No change" for at least 8 weeks	Unchanged or <25% increase or <50% decrease in size of measurable lesions
Progressive	Increased size of existing lesions or appearance of new lesions	Mixed—some lesions persist while others progress or new lesions appear. Failure—some or all lesions progress and/or new lesions appear, none regress

BOX 3: Indications for performing MRI in musculoskeletal oncology.

Bone pathology:
- Permeative margins
- Cortical disruption
- Soft-tissue extension
- Unclear etiology/matrix on radiograph

Soft-tissue tumor:
- Pain
- Size > 5 cm
- Deep to muscle fascia
- History of growth

the MRI demonstrated limit is taken as safe for tumor resection. MRI preferably should include the involved portion of the extremity and the joint above and below. The signal intensity of a tumor is compared to adjacent soft tissues (specifically skeletal muscle and subcutaneous fat). A T1-weighted coronal MRI is helpful to determine the intramedullary extent of the tumor and also to detect skip lesions. Contrast-enhanced imaging better evaluates the relationship of tumor to adjacent blood vessels and characterizing cystic lesions. MRI is disease defining for lipomas, liposarcomas, pigmented villonodular synovitis (PVNS), hemangiomas, fibromatosis, and synovial cysts where additional biopsy may not be required for characterization.

MRI is an excellent modality for screening the spine for occult metastases, myeloma, or lymphoma. Tumor viability and response to chemotherapy can be judged by MRI to some extent. Viable tumor is generally bright on T2-weighted images. Signal intensity reduces on T2-weighted images after effective treatment. Uniformly dark signal on T2-weighted images predict good to complete response but is rare and often the treated tissue appears bright. For soft-tissue tumors, MRI is most helpful as radiology is ineffective, in particular, it helps in distinguishing a lipoma from other etiologies.

Computed Tomography Scan

Computed tomography (CT) scan not always required but when a doubt exists for cortical continuity, this is the investigation of choice for demonstration of cortical breach. Some tumors are better diagnosed on CT scan than MRI such as osteoid osteoma.

Bone Scintigraphy (Technetium-99m-MDP)

Bone scintigraphy (Technetium-99m-MDP) was classically used for detecting bony metastasis and later to determine the metabolically active intramedullary extent of the tumor. A surgical margin of 6 cm was chosen for resection from the depicted extent. It is still an excellent modality to determine polyostotic nature of disease and metastatic disease and secondary involvement of bone by primary soft tissue pathology like infection or neoplasia. Margins, however, are better evaluated by MRI. Bone scintigraphy can also be used to assess response to chemotherapy.

Angiography

Angiography is a comprehensive evaluation method for large tumors that likely displace the neurovascular bundles, have a predominant vascular supply by prominent vessel or branch or for evaluation of alternative vascularity for distal extremity in case ligation is required for main vessels. Angiography can also help in planning preoperative embolization for axial tumors or metastatic vascular tumors found to have main single source of vascularity **(Figs. 8A to D)**.

Fluoro-(F-18)-Deoxyglucose Positron Emission Tomography

It is being increasingly used to stage the tumors and assess response to chemoradiotherapy. There is high correlation between uptake and tumor grade. Sodium fluoride labeled PET scan is also being increasingly used (see later in "Metastatic Bone Disease").

The utility of MRI and CT scans is not limited to diagnostic work-up only. Now they have been thoroughly incorporated into a system for evaluation of treatment response also **(Table 7)**.

GRADING OF BONE TUMORS

Grading is based on nuclear anaplasia (degree of loss of structural differentiation), pleomorphism (variations in size and shape), and nuclear hyperchromasia (increased nuclear staining).

Most grading systems are based on three grades:
1. Grade I (low grade): Well-differentiated.
2. Grade II (intermediate grade): Moderately differentiated.
3. Grade III (high grade): Poorly differentiated.

Tumor grade is most strongly correlated with the potential for metastasis. Grade I lesions have <10% potential for metastasis while grade II and grade III lesions have 10–30% and >50% potential, respectively. Most malignant lesions are high grade (Enneking grade G2); low-grade malignant (Enneking grade G1) lesions are less common. Common tumors according to their grades and age distribution are presented in **Table 8**. Grading a tumor follows the staging investigations are completed to minimize the imaging artifacts from biopsy methods.

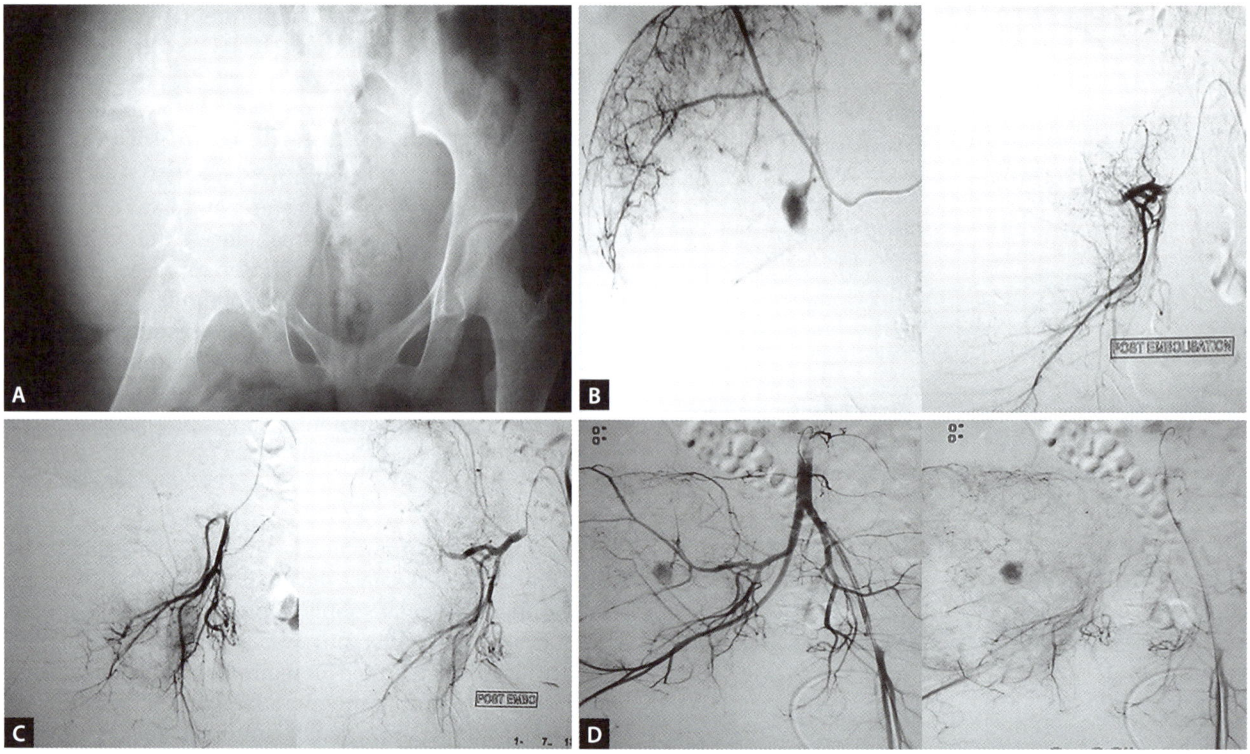

Figs. 8A to D: Angiography and embolization for large neoplastic lesion involving right hemipelvis (A). The patient was planned for surgical resection and reconstruction. Angiography-assisted embolization of the lesion was done by multiple selective branch embolization (B and C) and then main branch embolization also attempted (D). This helps in surgical resection by controlling the bleeding intraoperatively.

TABLE 7: MDA criteria for assessment of treatment response (this incorporates CT scans and MRI that are commonly used for evaluation of neoplastic lesions).

Response type	*Description*
Complete	• Complete fill or sclerosis of lytic lesion on radiograph or CT scan • Disappearance of hot spots (tumor signal) on scintigraphy, CT, or MRI • Normalization of osteoblastic lesion on radiograph and CT scan
Partial	• Sclerotic rim around initially lytic lesion or sclerosis of previously undetectable lesion on radiograph or CT scan • Partial fill-in or sclerosis of lytic lesion on radiographs or CT scan • Regression of measurable lesion on radiographs, CT scan, or MRI • Regression of lesion on scintigraphy (excluding rapid regression—this would later come in complete response) • Decrease in blastic lesion of radiographs or CT scan
Stable lesion	• No change in measurable lesion on radiograph, CT scan, or MRI • No change in blastic lesion on radiographs, CT scan, or MRI • No new lesion on radiographs, scintigraphy, CT scan, or MRI
Progressive disease	• Increase in size of any existing measurable lesions on radiographs, CT scan, or MRI • New lesion on radiographs, scintigraphy, CT scan, or MRI (excluding flares) • Increase in activity on scintigraphy (excluding flares) or blastic/lytic lesion on radiographs or CT scan

TABLE 8: Age at occurrence of various bone lesions.

	Type of lesion	
Age	*Malignant*	*Benign*
Birth to 5 years	• Leukemia • Metastatic neuroblastoma • Metastatic rhabdomyosarcoma	• Osteomyelitis • Osteofibrous dysplasia
10–25 years	• Osteosarcoma • Ewing's tumor • Leukemia	• Eosinophilic granuloma • Osteomyelitis • Enchondroma • Fibrous dysplasia
40–80 years	• Metastatic bone disease • Myeloma • Lymphoma • Chondrosarcoma • Malignant fibrous histiocytoma • Paget's sarcoma • Postradiation sarcoma	• Hyperparathyroidism • Paget's disease • Mastocytosis • Enchondroma • Bone infarct

Bone Biopsy

Tumors can be graded only on the histological sample obtained from the representative tissue. There are different methods to obtain tissue sample from the representative lesion. The biopsy techniques include percutaneous fine-needle aspiration cytology (FNAC), trephine bone biopsy (also called "Tru-Cut® biopsy", the latter is more automated, however) and open (incisional and excisional) tissue biopsy **(Figs. 9A to C)**. The ideal biopsy technique is one that provides

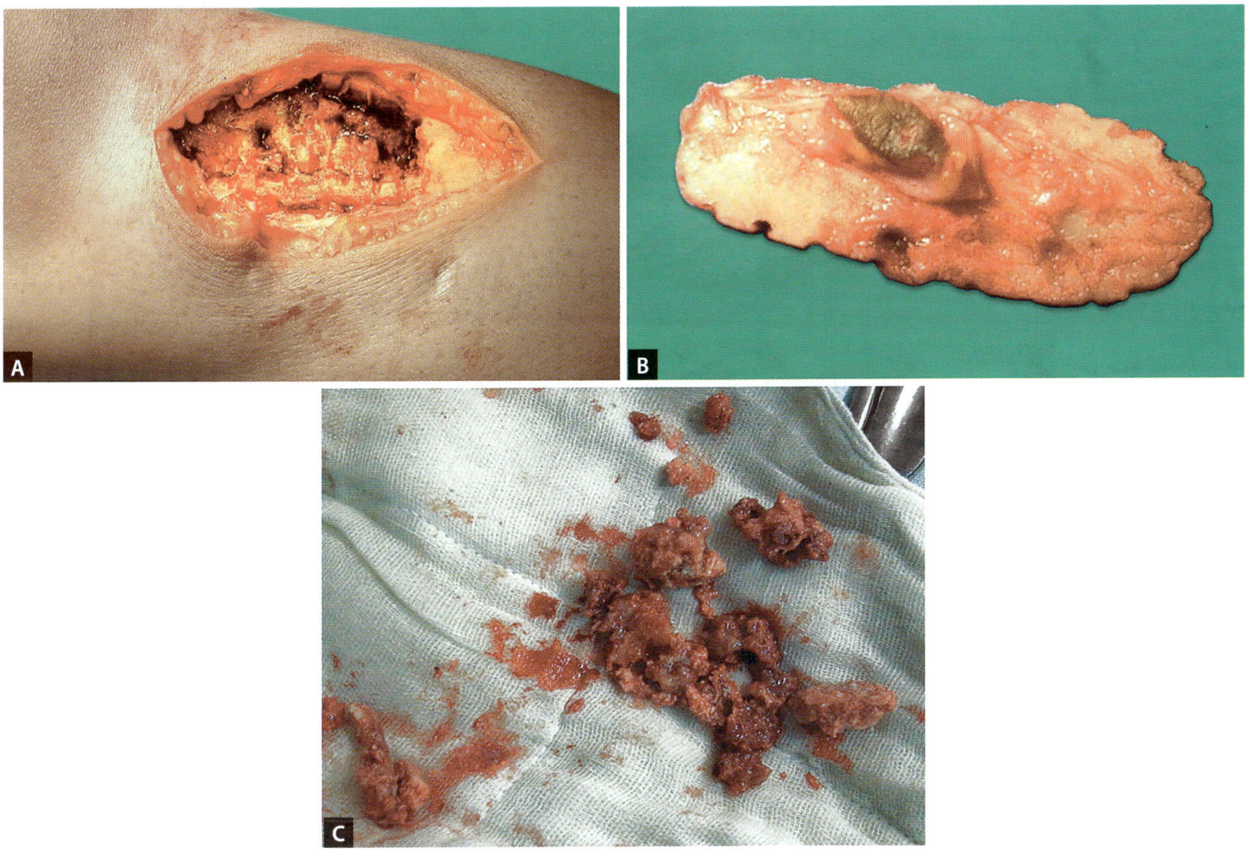

Figs. 9A to C: Open biopsy from a tibial shaft lesion following failed two attempts at obtaining diagnosis by core biopsy. This procedure is equivalent to intralesional excision if a thorough curettage of the lesion is done. The only difference from comprehensive management will be absence of bone grafting the lesion (defect management) in case only biopsy is planned. Note the creation of oblong window (A) and removal of skin tag with the window (B).

sufficient tissue required for proper histologic diagnosis and does not affect subsequent management. FNACs are done for "soft" lesions or expansile lesions that have marched into soft tissues that can be radiologically or palpably localized. They have limited utility and low yield (diagnostic yield is best for a homogeneous tumor). Trephine needle biopsies **(Figs. 10A and B)** are optimal for initial sampling of lesions especially when the nature of the lesion is obvious on the basis of the radiographic features and when adequate tissue can be obtained with a needle also the needle biopsy technique is safe to use in anatomically inaccessible areas such as the spine or pelvis. The advantages of percutaneous needle biopsies are:

- Minimal soft tissue damage or contamination
- Can be done in little or no anesthesia.
- Can be performed under CT or ultrasound guidance for proper localization under radiologic control.
- Careful correlation of the small tissue sample with the radiographs often yields the correct diagnosis.

The main disadvantages of this technique are:

- The amount of tissue yield is small for histopathological purpose and it can frequently be nondiagnostic. The pathologist must be experienced and comfortable with the small sample of tissue.
- The primary bone neoplasms are notoriously heterogeneous—making some areas nonrepresentative of the tumor or may reveal a secondary change masking the original pathology (like secondary ABC). This introduces a great potential for sampling error.
- The relation of bone tumor to soft tissue cannot be commented (soft tissue penetration, etc.).
- Hard tumors are difficult to negotiate and optimal sample may not be obtained.

When the diagnosis of needle biopsy and imaging studies do not correlate or radiographs are difficult to interpret, an open biopsy should be performed to establish the diagnosis. Open biopsy is also necessary with low-grade tumors and when the needle biopsy cannot provide a definitive diagnosis as in ABC due to inherent limitation of not revealing relationship to surroundings. Open biopsy should be performed keeping some basic rules/principles in mind:

- Biopsy should be performed at near conclusion of staging (i.e., all imaging studies have been done to determine extent and characteristics of tumor).
- Biopsy should be done at a center and by the surgeon who is versed with the definitive procedure to be performed **(Fig. 11)**.
- Use smallest possible incision placed over the representative lesion.
- Plan the shortest and most direct path to reach tumor so that soft tissue dissection is limited for possible contamination.

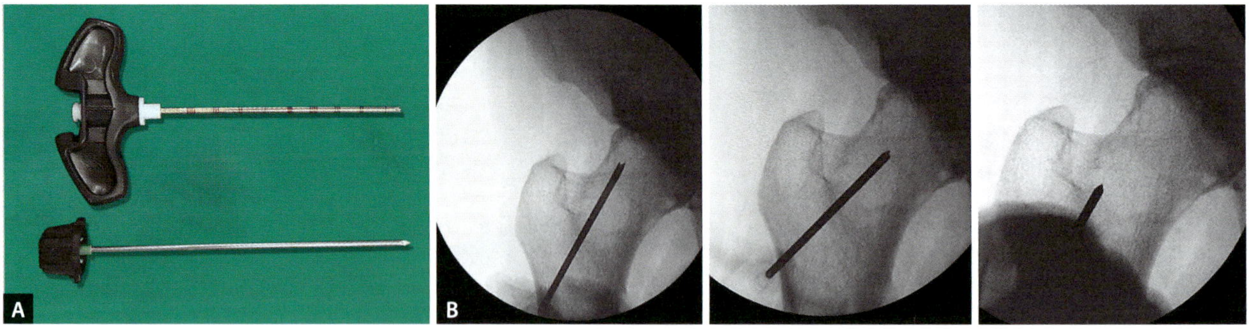

Figs. 10A and B: (A) Bone biopsy needle (for trephine biopsy); (B) The biopsy tissue sample is taken from multiple places of the lesion to improve the yield.

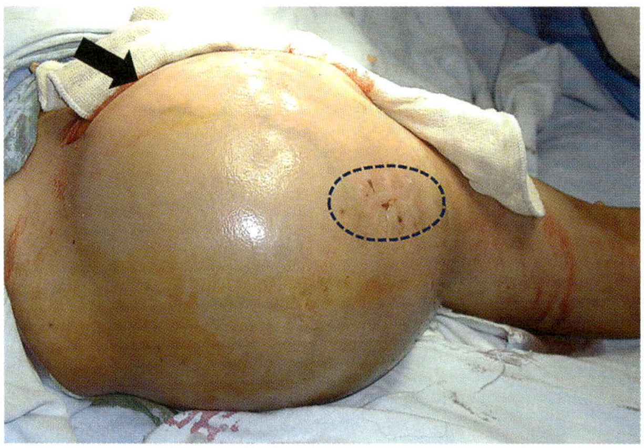

Fig. 11: Biopsy should be aptly planned and done by experienced surgeon. This patient diagnosed as giant cell tumor of proximal humerus from biopsy taken through lateral approach (*dotted ellipsoid*) was in no way planned as to the future need of surgery and surgical approach (*block arrow*). The intended exposure for tumor resection would be deltopectoral approach so the biopsy should also be in line with the incision. Now the distant biopsy site would mean additional excision of skin tag (possibility of tract seeding). Hence, it is suggested that biopsy should be always dealt like interim part of surgical management of neoplasia and be done by experienced surgeon or at the place deemed to be the ultimate destination for management.

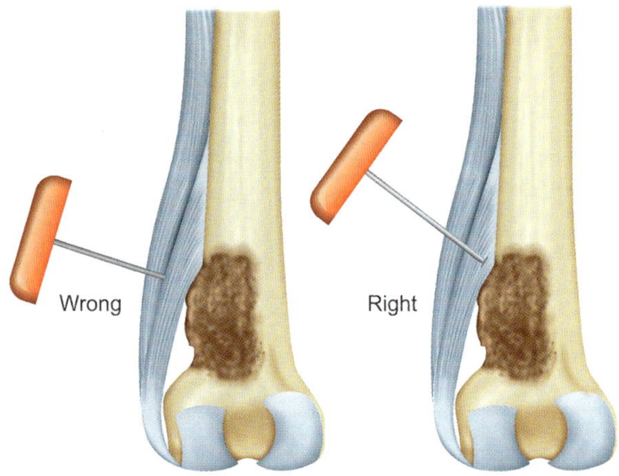

Fig. 12: Do not violate multiple planes or intermuscular planes (left side) during biopsy, restrict to minimum planes or better single least important muscle that can be excised during index procedure (right side).

- The incision should be longitudinal on the extremities and planned to be part of later surgical incision so should be done in guidance of surgeon going to undertake the final reconstruction.
- Use a tourniquet for extremity tumor to improve vision and minimize bleeding and contamination.
- Esmarch bandage should be avoided as it may rupture the tumor into the surrounding tissues.
- The tumor capsule should be closed after the procedure.
- Avoid a plane close to or through a neurovascular bundle when possible.
- Do not violate major flap structures (e.g., gluteus maximus, groin flap, soleus muscle, etc.) that can be helpful for later reconstruction.
- It is better to go through a single muscle belly (violate only one compartment) if unavoidable (better to choose subcutaneous site) and it should be large enough than to go between muscle planes that contaminates both **(Fig. 12)**.
- Do not go through functionally important structures (e.g., rectus femoris, biceps brachii) that may be sacrificed later just because of biopsy tract and compromise function at definitive reconstruction.
- Utilize minimal retraction to limit soft tissue contamination.
- Use a knife or curette to take sample to avoid distorting the sample texture and morphology.
- Obtain multiple samples ideally minimum of four as sarcomas tend to be heterogeneous and have regional morphologic variations (as opposed to carcinomas), especially the bone-forming lesions are quite variegated.
- Regarding biopsy hole shape, an oblong hole with rounded edges affords best residual strength than a rectangular hole with corners **(Fig. 13)**. Increasing width reduces bone strength while increasing length does not so much.
- It is essential to obtain good hemostasis by a meticulous multilayered watertight closure. Remove tourniquet before wound closure. Large tumors may put the closure under pressure and oozing blood predisposes to subsequent drainage contaminating the whole area. Wound dehiscence increases the risk of secondary infection that may delay subsequent chemotherapy or radiotherapy.

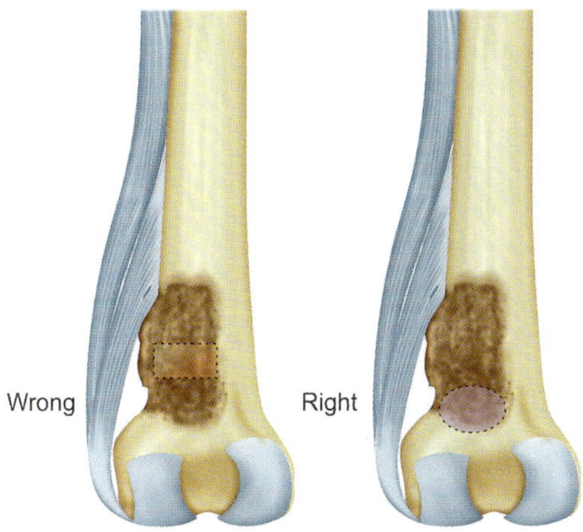

Fig. 13: Correct and wrong method of tumor biopsy. The tumor biopsy should be taken from the edge to evaluate the relationship with surroundings and avoid taking biopsy sample from nonrepresentative central necrotic tissue of rapidly growing tumors. This also identifies zonation seen with osteosarcoma. The window should be oval and not rectangular to avoid stress concentration and reduce fracture risk.

- Drains should be avoided as far as possible. If absolutely necessary, they should be chosen to be the thinnest possible and brought out in line and 1–2 cm beyond one end of the incision so that the drain track can be easily resected with the biopsy track.
- Although optional but a better way is to obtain a frozen section during the procedure from the lesion and not normal tissue to ensure that diagnostic material has been obtained. With large tumors, often the most representative radiologic region is already necrotic producing a negative or nondiagnostic biopsy. Further samples can be obtained when the patient is still draped.
- The operating surgeon should ideally accompany the specimen to the pathology department with radiological studies done so that a clinicopathoradiological correlation can be immediately obtained for the best possible diagnosis
- All biopsy samples should be submitted for bacteriologic analysis if the frozen section does not reveal a neoplasm. Antibiotics should not be delivered until the cultures are obtained.

LABORATORY EVALUATION AND MOLECULAR DIAGNOSTICS

There are no specific guidelines, however; for older patients' complete hemogram with differential counts and erythrocyte sedimentation rate should be obtained. Routine blood chemistry should be obtained along with serum calcium, phosphate, and liver function test. In addition, serum electrophoresis and urinalysis with estimation of Bence Jones proteins should be ordered.

Evaluation of biopsy specimen is the most important aspect in evaluation of neoplastic pathology. Standard microscopy reporting a lesion as benign or malignant bone or cartilage forming neoplasia does not suffice however. Advances in molecular diagnostics provide detailed assistance in understanding, diagnosis, and classification of bone and soft tissue sarcoma. It has further revolutionized into prognostication of the pathology and providing precise therapeutic targets for managing primary neoplasia, its relapse or metastasis. The journey **(Fig. 14)** began with detailing the pathology through electron microscopy describing tissue ultrastructure and aiding in classification. This was, however, quickly superseded by immunohistochemistry that enabled characterization of expressed proteins to define tumor subtype **(Table 9)**. It formed the basis of numerous evolving classifications but could not provide information beyond this (like prognostication and treatment). Cytogenetics then evolved that identified large chromosomal defects but was limited by requirements of viable cells (fresh samples) that can be grown in a cell culture. This limited the utility to few centers and also often the results were uninterpretable until development of FISH (fluorescence in situ hybridization). FISH could detect chromosomal alterations in interphase not requiring culture of tumor cells. It enabled identifying gene copy number changes (amplifications) and detecting gene rearrangements and fusions through specific detection probes. Immediately following FISH more sensitive methods of identifying genomic alterations in DNA extracted from tumor tissue were developed and marked the dawn of era of *molecular cytogenetics*. Polymerase chain reaction (PCR) among them gained popularity and wide application in clinical pathology. Originally, it needed fresh samples but now it is deployed as a standard on clinical grade formalin-fixed paraffin embedded samples. PCR has been further improved to detect mutations (single nucleotide base substitutions), short gene insertions and deletions, and gene fusion and rearrangements. The other popular modality in clinical use is the reverse transcriptase PCR (RT-PCR) that enables RNA-based profiling but it has only limited clinical utility for orthopedic oncology. The most modern modality in use currently is genomic sequencing and comprehensive gene profiling for sarcomas. This was initially based on Sanger technique that quickly evolved into PCR-based methods for identification of hot-spots in cancer-related genes. Then next-generation sequencing was introduced that utilized similar technique but was much faster. It was found necessary to obtain sequence of entire coding region rather than just the hot spots so hybrid capture technique was introduced and it allowed information on all four classes of genomic alterations, viz., base substitutions, short indels, copy number alterations, and gene fusion rearrangements. To further improve sensitivity and range of detection of gene fusion, RNA sequencing has been added to DNA sequencing of sarcomas.

These techniques and their results/interpretations have summarily altered our perspective toward neoplasia and congenital diseases in three major ways:

1. *Classification and diagnosis of tumors:* Utilizing modern methods, the focus has shifted to classification of sarcomas toward therapy-related targets from the earlier mere biological identification. This has identified various molecular alterations **(Table 10)** in oncogenes and tumor-suppressor genes important of which are:
   a. Cell-cycle regulating genes
   b. Tyrosine kinase growth factors

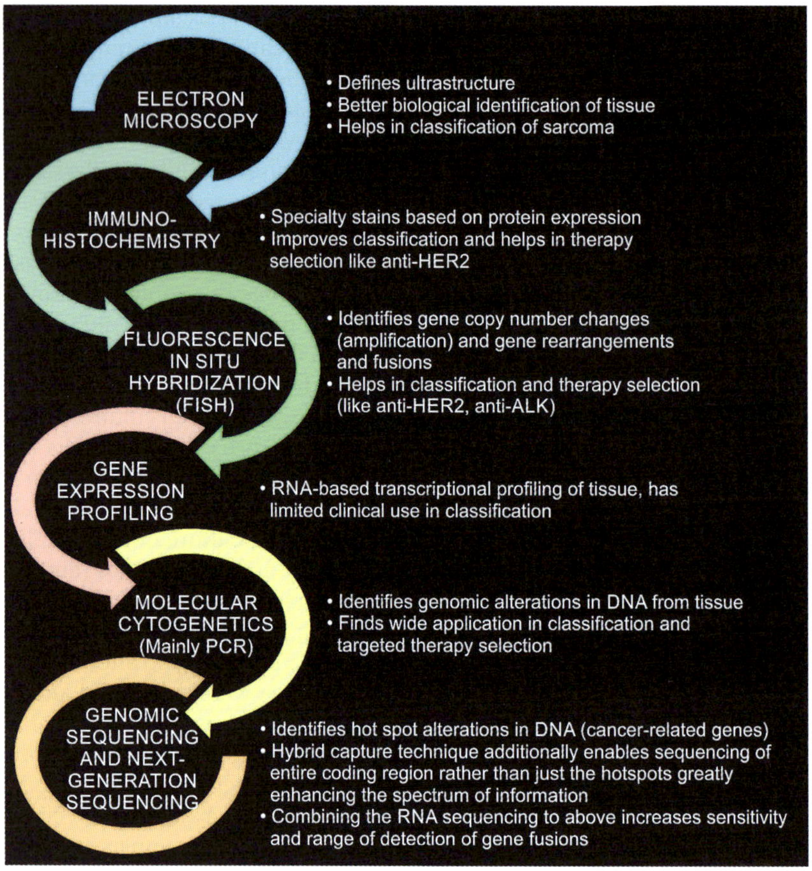

Fig. 14: The evolution of techniques used in diagnostics of bone and soft tissue sarcomas. (ALK: anaplastic lymphoma kinase; HER2: human epidermal growth factor receptor 2; PCR: polymerase chain reaction)

TABLE 9: Immunostains helpful in establishing diagnosis for bone tumors.

	Importance
Immunohistochemical marker	
Mesenchymal marker vimentin	Limited value in differential diagnosis but often used to assess antigen loss during processing as it survives most decalcification procedures. Osteosarcoma and most cartilage tumors.
Epithelial markers	
• Cytokeratins • Epithelial membrane antigen	Epithelioid and synovial sarcomas. Chordomas express both cytokeratin and S-100. Cytokeratin is expressed in adamantinoma.
Neuronal, nerve sheath, and melanocytic markers	
S-100	Neurofibromas, neurilemmomas, liposarcomas, ossifying fibromyxoid tumor, chondroblastoma, chondrosarcomas, clear cell sarcomas, chondromyxoid fibroma
Neurofilament protein	Neuroblastoma, medulloblastoma, retinoblastoma, focally in rhabdomyosarcoma, and malignant fibrous histiocytoma
Leu-7 (CD57)	Chondrosarcoma, neuroblastoma, and rhabdomyosarcoma
Synaptophysin	Neuroblastoma and ganglioneuroblastoma
Endothelial and vascular markers	
CD31	Angiosarcomas and hemangiomas
CD34	Epithelioid hemangioendotheliomas, angiosarcomas
CD20	Lymphomas
Factor VIII antigen	Useful as a confirmatory marker
Fibrohistiocytic marker	
CD68	Malignant fibrous histiocytoma (leiomyosarcoma is CD68)
Miscellaneous markers	
MIC2 gene product (CD99)	Ewing's sarcoma, peripheral neuroepitheliomas, and ependymomas
Osteonectin, osteocalcin, and collagen	Osteosarcoma, cartilage tumors express type II collagen, type X collagen is expressed in zonal fashion in osteochondromas.

TABLE 10: Molecular classification of bone and soft tissue sarcoma.

Tumor	*Translocation/Mutation*	*Gene(s)*	*Additional comments*
Ewing sarcoma; Primitive neuroectodermal tumor (PNET)	t(11;12)(q24;q12) t(21;22)(q22;q12) t(7;22)(p22;q12) t(2;22)(q33;q12) t(17;22)(q12;q12) inv(22)(q21;12) t(16;21)(p11;q22)	*EWSR1-FLI1* *EWSR1-ERG* *EWSR1-ETV1* *EWSR1-FEV* *EWSR1-E1AF* *EWSR1-ZSG* *FUS-ERG*	Activation of oncogene (e.g., *MYC, ID2, CCND1*, and IGF-1). Diagnostic *EWSR1* associated with good prognosis
Angiomatoid fibrous histiocytoma	t(12;22)(q13;q12) t(2;22)(q33;q12) t(12;16)(q13;p11)	*EWSR1-ATF1* *EWSR1-CREB1* *FUS-ATF1*	Activation of oncogenes, diagnostic
Clear-cell sarcoma	t(12;22)(q13;q12) t(2;22)(q33;q12)	*EWSR1-ATF1* *EWSR1-CREB1*	Activation of oncogenes *ARNT2, ATM, GPP34, MITF*, diagnostic
Low-grade fibromyxoid sarcoma/ HSCT	t(7;16)(q33;p11) t(11;16)(p11;p11)	*FUS-CREB3L2* *FUS-CREB3L1*	Oncogene activation, diagnostic
Desmoplastic small round cell tumor	t(11;22)(p13;q12)	*EWSR1-WT1*	Activation of oncogenes (*PDGF, IL2Rβ, BAIALP3, TALLA1, MLF1*), diagnostic and therapeutic (PDGF inhibitors)
Extraskeletal myxoid chondrosarcoma	t(9;22)(q22;q12) t(9;17)(q22;q11) t(9;15)(q22;q21) t(3;9)(q11;q22) Rearrangements of 9q22	*EWSR1-NR4A3* *TAF2N-NR4A3* *TCF12-NR4A3* *TFG-NR4A3* *NR4A3*	Oncogene activation, diagnostic
Myoepithelial tumor of soft tissue and bone	t(6;22)(p21;q12) t(19;22)(q13;q12) t(1;22)(q23;q12	*EWSR1-POU5F1* *EWSR1-ZNF444* *EWSR1-PBX1*	Activation of oncogenes, diagnostic
Epithelioid hemangioendothelioma	t(1;3)(p36;q25)	*WWTR1-CAMTA1*	Diagnostic, oncogene activation
Mesenchymal chondrosarcoma	t(8;8)(q13;q21)	*HEY1-NCOA2*	Diagnosis, oncogene activation
Synovial sarcoma	t(X;18)(p11;q11)	*SS18-SSX1, SSX2, SSX4*	Diagnosis, better prognosis for SS18-SSX2
Undifferentiated small round blue cell tumor	t(4;19)(q35;q13) t(10;19)(q26;q13)	*CIC-DUX4*	Diagnosis, oncogene activation
Osteosarcoma, low grade (parosteal and intramedullary)	12q14-15 (ring chromosomes, giant marker chromosomes)	Amplification of *CDK4, MDM2, HMGA2, GLI, SAS*	Diagnosis
Aneurysmal bone cyst	t(16;17)(q22;p13) t(1;17)(p34.3;p13) t(3;17)(q21;p13) t(9;17)(q22;p13) t(17;17)(q21;p13)	*CDH11-USP6* *THRAP3-USP6* *CNBP-USP6* *OMD-USP6* *COL1A1-USP6*	Diagnosis, cell cycle dysregulation and cell adhesion dysfunction
Tenosynovial giant cell tumor/ pigmented villonodular synovitis	t(1;2)(p13;q35-37)	*COL6A3-CSF1*	Diagnosis, cell cycle dysregulation
Well-differentiated liposarcoma/ atypical lipomatous tumor/ dedifferentiated liposarcoma	12q14-15 (ring chromosomes, giant marker chromosomes)	Amplification of *MDM2, CDK4, HMGA2, GLI, SAS*	Diagnosis
Dermatofibrosarcoma protuberans	t(17;22)(q21;q13)	*COLIA1-PDGFB*	Activation of oncogene *PDGFR*, diagnosis, therapeutic (imatinib and newer drugs)
Giant cell fibroblastoma	t(17;22)(q21;q13)	*COLIA1-PDGFB*	Oncogene activation
Inflammatory myofibroblastic tumor	t(1;2)(q22;p23) t(2;19)(p23;p13) t(2;17)(p23;q23) t(2;2)(p23;q13) t(2;11)(p23;p15) inv(2)(p23;q35)	*TPM3-ALK* *TPM4-ALK* *CLTC-ALK* *RANBP2-ALK* *CARS-ALK* *ATIC-ALK*	Oncogene activation
Alveolar rhabdomyosarcoma	t(2;13)(q35;q14) t(1;13)(p36;q14) t(X;2)(q13;q35)	*PAX3-FKHR* *PAX7-FKHR* *PAX3-AFX*	Oncogene activation
Fibrous dysplasia	Gene mutation at 20q13.2-q13.3	*GNAS*	Diagnosis by PCR, activating point mutation
Desmoid-type fibromatosis	Activating point mutation	*CTNNB1*	β-catenin serves as surrogate marker.

(IGF: insulin-like growth factor; PCR: polymerase chain reaction; PDGFR: platelet-derived growth factor receptor)

   c. Molecular targets of rapamycin (mTOR) pathway genes
   d. Genes in the RAS/RAF pathway
   e. Gene fusions that activate kinases such as ALK, *ROS1*, and *NTRK1*.
2. *New therapeutic targets:* Next generation sequencing has helped us in identifying newer therapeutic targets identified from genomic alterations; replacing the classical nontargeted chemotherapy. Tumor heterogeneity has not come across as a limitation in this targeted approach because it has been seen that the correct driver alteration identified from small biopsy sample quite aptly represents whole tumor tissue and even its metastasis. Some of the currently processed targeted chemotherapy include:
   a. Trastuzumab for *ERBB2* targeted therapies for *ERBB2 (HER2)* amplified osteogenic sarcomas.
   b. Antiepidermal growth factor receptor (EGFR) small molecule drugs/antibodies for *EGFR* overexpressing tumors (primarily of importance in pulmonary carcinoma)
   c. Denosumab targeted against receptor activator for nuclear factor kappa-beta ligand (RANKL) for treatment of GCT
   d. Figitumumab targeted against insulin-like growth factor (IGF)-1R for management of Ewing sarcoma and osteosarcoma. Phase 3 trials have been stopped, however, due to lack of afficacy in non-small cell lung cancer.
   e. Sorafenib targeted against c-kit, FGFR, PDGFR, Ret, VEGFR is being tried for osteosarcoma with modest results.
   f. Crizotinib (kinase inhibitor) for sarcomas expressing activating gene fusions of kinases such as *ALK* and *ROS1*.
   g. Palbocilib against liposarcoma expressing amplified *CDF4* and *CDK6* genes
   h. mTOR inhibitors like ridaforolimus against sarcomas exhibiting mTOR pathway genes such as *P13KCA*.
   i. Imatinib and dasatinib have been successfully used against gastrointestinal stromal tumors (GIST) focusing on *KIT* activation. Based on the same now nilotinib, sunitinib, and regorafinib have been approved for treatment of GIST.
3. *Detection of germline variants in congenital orthopedic diseases:* Utilizing next-generation sequencing various inherited, congenital, and premalignant orthopedic disorders can be identified **(Table 11)** that helps in genetic counseling and planning treatment of these conditions.

TREATMENT

A well-planned approach is required before execution. One should be clear of the future requirements and understand possible complications and their management.

Intent for Surgery

Surgery is done for any of the four requirements of treatment:
1. Diagnostic
2. Definitive
3. Palliative
4. Adjunctive

TABLE 11: Gene defects resulting in congenital and inherited orthopedic conditions.

Disease	*Gene defect (transmission)*	*Cancer risk*
Neurofibromatosis	*NF1* (Autosomal dominant) *NF2* (Autosomal dominant)	High
Enchondromatosis	Unknown (Sporadic)	High
Osteochondromatosis	*EXT1* (Autosomal dominant) *EXT2* (Autosomal dominant)	High
Gardner syndrome	*APC* (Autosomal dominant)	High
Epidermolysis bullosa	*DSP* (Autosomal recessive)	Low
Fibrodysplasia ossificans progressiva	*ACVR1* (Autosomal dominant)	Low
Osteogenesis imperfect	*COL1A* (Autosomal dominant)	Low
Albright syndrome	*GNAS1* (Uncertain)	Low
Ehlers–Danlos syndrome	*COL3A* (Autosomal dominant) *COL5A* (Autosomal dominant)	Low
Marfan syndrome	*FBN1* (Autosomal dominant)	Low

A diagnostic procedure could be an open biopsy or excisional biopsy (marginal excision). Palliative procedure provides temporary pain relief or debulk disease for general well-being and improving function. Palliative procedure may be combined with chemotherapy or radiotherapy for additional relief and are undertaken when no therapeutic procedure is possible. Adjunctive procedure (rarely done in orthopedics) provides local control but is followed by definitive procedure. Definitive procedure is done for complete control and/or reconstruction of the limb intended to completely cure the patient. For malignant neoplasms, chemotherapy and/or radiotherapy are commonly used as adjuvants. The therapeutic surgical intervention culminates into either limb salvage or limb sacrifice surgery ultimately. The following discussion details the principles and practice of "limb salvage surgery (LSS)" in orthopedic neoplasms. An LSS is performed if:
1. Adequate margin for resection of tumor can be obtained with low risk (<10%) of local recurrence.
2. Functional outcome of the reconstructed limb is better than or comparable to that achieved by amputation and prosthetic fitting.

The *primary goal of LSS* is acceptable degree of function in reconstructed limb. Secondary objectives being durability, sustained remission of disease, painless limb, and cosmetic appearance. Decision to reconstruct is individualized based on the tumor location and extent, experience, support available, and the psychosocial characteristics of the patient. In developing nation, the LSS is often precluded due to delayed presentation. Patients and local physicians are unaware of the diagnosis and then do not know correct lace to send the patient, poverty, and illiteracy are superseding factors most of the times. "Fear" of almighty's wrath, availability and access to quack medicines and claims, and poor family support for extensive surgery are prohibiting factors in some ethnic groups. Misguidance by mediocre doctors and local practitioners is another factor for late presentation. Finally, if patient reaches the specialized center, limited number of expertise to handle so many cases becomes the terminal factor for timely management.

Limb-sparing surgery is, however, contraindicated in specific situations **(Box 4)**. "Three-strike rule" is quite efficient in quickly screening is a patient is suitable for limb salvage **(Fig. 15)**. Access the status of bone, nerves, vessels, and soft tissue envelop. If any three of the structures are involved at the planned site for LSS, then probably it is not worth considering. Even with advancements in surgical technique and reconstruction procedures, the morbidity is unacceptably high, limiting the possibility of functional reconstruction. For skeletal reconstruction, bone grafts [avascular **(Figs. 16A to C)** and vascularized bone grafts (fibula, rib, and iliac crest)] are the primary modality used, and it is preferable to have bone banking facilities (allografts) for adequate coverage of patient population.

BOX 4: Contraindications for limb-salvage surgery.

Inability to achieve wide surgical margins due to any or combination of:

- Invasion of major neurovascular structures whose resection will compromise either the viability or functionality of limb terminally.
- Involvement or contamination of multiple compartments with extensive muscle involvement.
- Patients with extensive skin involvement.
- Pathologic fractures where the risk of recurrence increases several folds.
- Sepsis jeopardizing the effectiveness of adjuvant chemotherapy.
- Inappropriate or improper biopsy contaminating normal tissue planes and compartments.

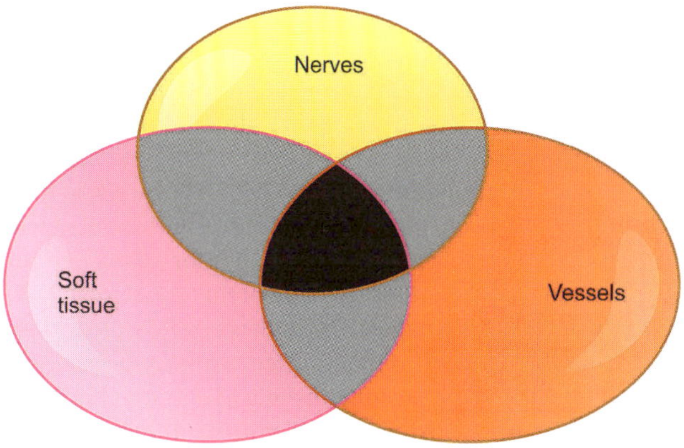

Fig. 15: Three-strike rule. Out of the four critical structures namely bone reconstruction, soft tissue reconstruction, nerves, soft tissue envelop (coverage) if "all" three of the structures are limited (central dark area) simultaneously then limb salvage is possibly not worth considering.

After assessing the resectability of osseous neoplasm, the primary and most important aim is to achieve R0 (R-zero) resection of tumor for optimal local control and prevent recurrence. The R classification (1987, UICC) denotes absence or presence of residual tumor (R) after treatment. Residual tumor may be localized in the area of the primary tumor and/or as distant metastases. R0 corresponds to resection for cure or complete remission. R1 indicates microscopic residual tumor remaining, while R2 refers to macroscopic residual tumor in the surgical field.

Surgical margins often mentioned in different LSS procedures are primarily based on the relationship of the dissection plane to the tumor and its pseudocapsule. They are classified into four types **(Fig. 17)**:

1. *Intralesional margins* (excision) have plane of dissection within the tumor mass removing only a portion of the lesion. Gross tumor and its pseudocapsule (containing satellites), and skip lesions in the surrounding normal tissues are all left behind. This is usually suited for benign bone lesions such as simple bone cyst, ABC, and enchondroma. According to R-classification this is a R2 resection. Depending on intent for surgery, most metastatic lesions operated for palliative surgery are treated with intralesional excision (but for curative excision, such as removing solitary metastasis, a wide margin is preferred).
2. *Marginal excision* margins have dissection plane through the pseudocapsule aiming to remove the lesion en bloc, but leaves behind the skip lesions and possibly microscopic satellite lesions making this an R1 resection. This is also suited for less aggressive lesions such as ABC and GCT.
3. *Wide margins* are the en bloc excision of the lesion where the plane of dissection passes outside the reactive zone of the lesion through the normal tissue removing the tumor

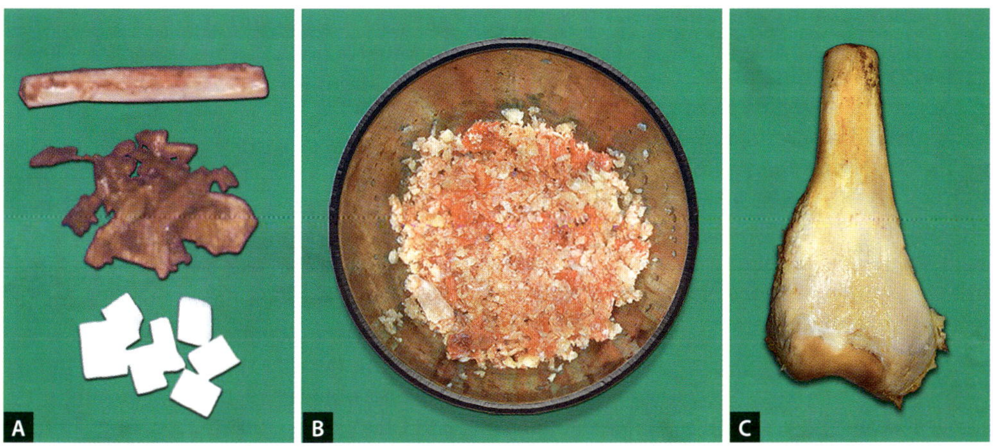

Figs. 16A to C: Various bone grafts in common use for reconstruction after tumor excision. (A) Autologous fibula, cancellous bone chips, and synthetic calcium phosphate cubes; (B) Morselized allograft; (C) Autoclaved graft from excised tumor.

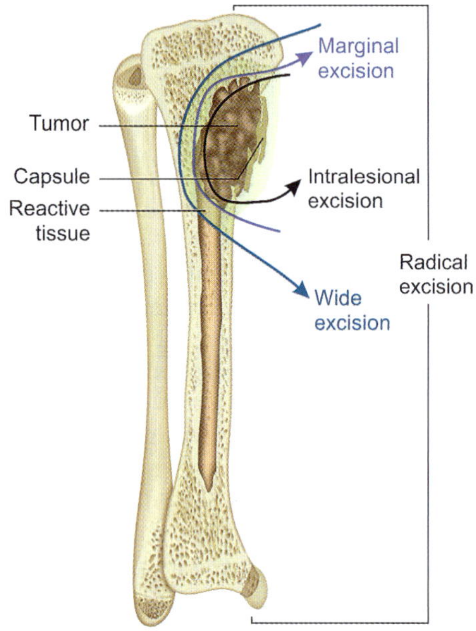

Fig. 17: The surgical resection margins.

with its pseudocapsule and cuff of normal tissue. This is the desired margin for most primary bone sarcomas, but it leaves behind the skip foci so by definition this would also be an R1 resection although most oncologists tend to consider it R0 (incorrect). The distance away from the tumor required to achieve this margin is usually 1-2 cm and depends on type of tissue involved.

Lesser of normal tissue is removed with "resistant" tissue to tumor spread such as cartilage, bone, and thick fascia but some liberal margin is needed for "soft tissue" like the loose areolar tissue or fat. Also a high grade or aggressive tumor that poorly responds to chemotherapy requires wide margin of normal tissue. With advances in imaging, the margins can be shrunk in future preserving the normal tissue as much.

4. *Radical margins* involve removing the entire compartment(s) in which the tumor has extended and in turn also obliterates the possibility of leaving any skip lesions causing recurrence making it R0 resection following the R-classification. This excision type, however, does not define the true margins of excision and can be "marginal" or a "wide excision" depending on the location of the tumor within compartment and its proximity to borders. If the tumor extends till the border of compartment, then by definition, this so-called radical excision (through compartment borders) will just be a "marginal excision". Similarly, "amputation" is not necessarily a radical surgery—it is just a means of obtaining specific margin depending on how close or how far the plane of amputation passes from the primary tumor.

Role of Prophylactic Fixation

Some bone tumors (especially lytic lesions) are large enough to weaken the bone if left untreated. Lytic lesions in bones subjected to high tensile stress like proximal femur often need to be stabilized. Patients often report increased pain on mechanical loading of the extremity that indicates impending fracture and should be promptly treated. The classical radiographic features beyond which prophylactic fixation is prominently suggested include lesions longer than 3.3 cm or wider than 2.5 cm or a lesion involving >50% of the bone cortex. Comparative analysis with quantitative CT scan suggests that these radiological features often overestimate the fracture risk but alternative guidelines have not been developed classical ones continue to be used.

Reconstruction of the Limb

After completing the surgical resection, the next complex step is limb reconstruction. Ideally, resection-reconstruction is already planned before initiating surgery (some changes are incorporated intraoperatively often depending on frozen-section and revised resection margins). The various modalities for limb reconstruction used are as follows:

- Nonmobile reconstruction—Joint arthrodesis
  - *Turn-o-plasty:* This is one of the various methods of joint arthrodesis after tumor resection. This is commonly practiced for tumors around the knee joint for benign-aggressive bone neoplasms that involve the articular surface but not the whole width of metaphysis where reconstruction with mobile bearing procedures would entail too large a bony resection while intralesional procedures are not indicated. The most common indication is GCT of bone while it can also be utilized in management of epiphyseal tumors like chondroblastoma. Technically, for a distal femoral lesion after adequate excision of the lesion, distal tibia is split into two halves. One half is turned upside down and fixed with the remaining femoral stump proximally while it crosses the joint distally and is attached to the other half of proximal tibia. For a proximal tibial lesion, distal femoral bone is split into two halves and similar procedure followed. To build-up bone stock, additional fibular autograft can be taken. Sometimes both fibulae are needed to build-up bone.
- *Mobile joint reconstruction:* This method often entails reconstruction of the bone stock and/or prosthetic reconstruction. Various modalities are often combined to achieve this:
  - Treated bone as graft:
    - Autoclaved tumor bone—osteoarticular or intercalary
    - Pasteurized bone
    - Irradiated tumor bone—osteoarticular or intercalary
    - Liquid nitrogen treated bone
  - Allograft bone including osteoarticular allograft (*See* bone grafting and bone banking in Chapter on "Fracture Repair, Bone Grafting, and Bone Banking")
  - Bone transfer (ulna and fibula to reconstruct radius and tibia respectively), Huntington's procedure [*see* Chapter on "Infections of Bone (Typical and Atypical) and Surgical Site Infection"]

- Endoprosthetic reconstruction
    - Modular endoprosthesis (previously called megaprosthesis)
    - Custom-made prosthesis
    - Expandable prosthesis
- Allograft endoprosthetic (composite) reconstruction
- Rotationplasty

We will discuss the various mobile joint reconstruction methods in detail here.

Treated Bone as Graft

In this method, the resected bone tumor is treated with some method or procedure that is intended to kill the tumor cells so that recurrence from it does not occur. The residual bone is used as a spacer to fill the defect created by tumor resection. Prerequisite for using this methodology is primarily the presence of mineralized voluminous lesion (osteogenic/osteoblastic lesions). It cannot be used with lytic lesions as then there will be nothing left to reimplant. The procedure has following indications and advantages:

- Economical choice compared to prosthesis
- Mostly devoid of disease transmission and graft rejection complications in allograft bone used
- Acceptable within socioregional beliefs
- The bone maintains anatomical disposition so easy to fit in the topographical space (orthotopic).

Autoclave bone treatment: The excised specimen of bone is cleaned of all soft tissues including intramedullary clearance (to reduce the volume). Cartilage is also commonly denuded as after heat treatment it is obviously totally denatured **(Fig. 18)**. The specimen is then subjected to standard autoclaving procedure. Autoclaving involves heating at 1.1 kg/cm^2 (≡15 pounds/in^2) steam pressure, which yields a temperature of 121°C. At 121°C, the time of autoclaving to achieve sterilization is generally considered to be 15–20 minutes, depending on the volume of the load. Sometimes temperature of 123°C at 0.2 MPa for 10 minutes is used depending on individual protocols. Higher times are needed for large voluminous specimens or if water content is expected to be higher. The autoclaved specimen is then cooled and washed with antiseptic solutions (not necessary) and fixed to the remaining stump using proper osteosynthesis. The autoclaved bone is considered inferior to autogenic or allogenic bone graft due to several reasons:

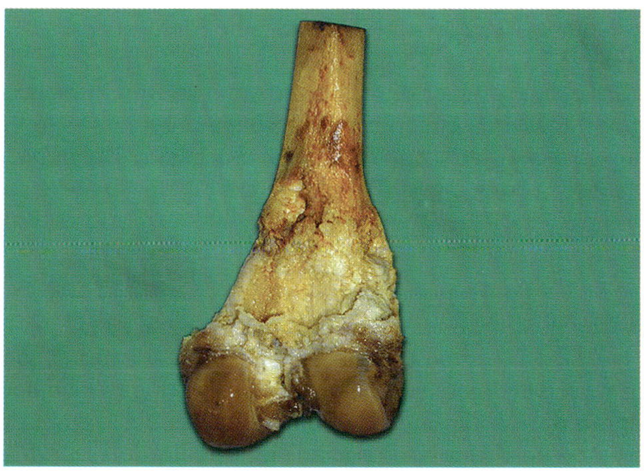

Fig. 18: The autoclave treatment of bone completely denatures the cartilage visualized as charred covering on the femoral condyles here.

- Denaturation of collagen into gelatin
- Mineral degeneration
- Inactivation of bone morphogenetic protein 2 (BMP-2)
- Vascular ischemia
- Damage of bone structure in autoclave temperature, which leads to bone resorption and minimal bone formation after implantation
- Failure of bone healing—high temperatures lead to destruction of bone marrow and totipotent mesenchymal cells precluding bone healing (callus → chondrogenesis → osteogenesis process) from the autoclaved bone

These lead to finding other methods of bone sterilization.

Irradiated tumor bone reimplantation: The excised tumor tissue is swab-cultured immediately upon retrieval prior to processing. The soft tissues and periosteum are immediately stripped and cleaned. The bone is washed thoroughly with saline (betadine and peroxide solution are optional). Terminal sterilization is usually done by gamma irradiation. Gamma radiation is effective in killing bacteria, fungi, spores, and, to a lesser degree, viruses. Depending on the dose, however, gamma radiation can weaken the graft. Doses below 1.5 mrad do not adversely affect the tissue strength. A minimum dose of 2 mrad is required to kill bacteria and 4 mrad for killing viruses but malignant bone cells may not be killed even at 5 mrad. Irradiation at 6 mrad may still contain living cells but devoid of mitotic capability. After such high-dose irradiation, the bone is discolored and fibrillar network of bone is destroyed. Solubility of collagen and proteoglycans increase reducing structural strength and inductive capacity is greatly reduced. Bone neoplasms are a special case as most of the tumors are radioresistant so high doses of irradiation are needed for killing the disease. High-energy X-rays are deployed and commonly 100 Gy irradiation is used for such sterilization (irradiation time is calculated depending on the output of source and bone volume). The irradiated bone is then reimplanted at the site for reconstruction of osseous defect. The main drawback is that the facility is not available everywhere, intraoperative transportation and reserving the facility may not be always feasible and the quality of bone is definitely deteriorated.

Freeze treated bone (cryosurgery): Here, the bone specimen is treated with liquid nitrogen that kills malignant cells primarily by forming ice crystals within cell and ultimate lysis of the cell on thawing. The resected specimen in dipped in liquid nitrogen (15–20 L for 20 min) and may be a free specimen (completely resected) or pedicled at one end (still attached to body at one end) **(Figs. 19A and B)**. It is then thawed at room temperature in warm distilled water at 30° for 15 minutes and reimplanted orthotopically. The advantage of this method is its simplicity, no need for special equipment, can be done in theater itself, and maintains the bone proteins and matrix and also the ligament, and tendon attachments are maintained. Only availability of liquid nitrogen (15–20 L)

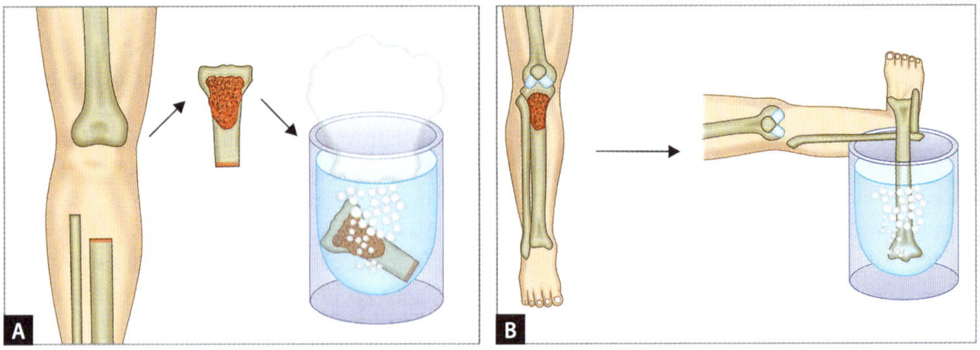

Figs. 19A and B: Cryotreated bone graft. The resected bone may be treated with liquid nitrogen separately [free-preparation (A)] and then reimplanted at the site or it may remain attached to the limb [pedicled graft preparation (B)] while being cryotreated to be replaced later.

is to be assured that is poured in a thermos and specimen can be freeze-treated in it. Specific concerns are protection of the operating and associated staff from cold burns (use a separate workbench) and occurrence of fracture during liquid nitrogen treatment. Fracture occurs due to difference in expansion coefficient of bone and fluids within (matrix, tumor bed, and blood) at freezing temperatures. Hemicortical reconstructions are also possible. Sometimes if the processed bone has large defect, then polymethyl methacrylate (PMMA) bone cement can be used as augment during osteosynthesis.

Pasteurized bone: Due to changes in bone and matrix at high temperatures, alternative method is to use much lower temperature compared to autoclaving. The malignant cells are eradicated using heat treatment at 44°C for 30 minutes, or diathermy heating using a radiofrequency of 13.56 MHz caused tumor destruction. Pasteurization at 60–65°C for 40 minutes in a water bath has also been demonstrated to eradicate malignant cells. The cells after such treatment fail to grow in culture and lack clonogenicity. The main advantage of pasteurization is relatively less effect of the procedure on bone healing and maintenance of bone matrix and strength compared to autoclaving. There is proposal that pasteurization may spare osteoinductive factors in the treated bone.

Endoprosthetic Reconstruction

Megaprostheses are special osteoarticular prostheses that bridge large defects of bones and joints. The term was specifically used in first international workshop on design and application of prosthesis; held at Mayo clinic in 1981. Commercial manufacturers have made prosthesis for all major regions of body including proximal humerus, distal humerus to total humerus, total femur (proximal femur; distal femur, intercalary), proximal and distal tibial, pelvis, and wrist. These commercial prostheses have segmental fixed length extenders that can be used to adjust the length of bony reconstruction needed depending on patient needs **(Figs. 20A to D)**. The osteoarticular prosthesis has a "joint" or articular-metaphyseal fixed component to which length can be added by using extenders. The main advantage is that the prosthesis can be intraoperatively structured (modularity) depending on the osseous defect that patient develops after excision of bone tumor. However, this is also a disadvantage because the fixed length may need either cutting extra bone to "fit" the length or keep limb longer or shorter. This entails using a prosthesis that fits specific patent needs. Custom-made prostheses that fit the patient's needs hence were then used increasingly, where based on patient's parameters the manufacturer would make a prosthesis that is then implanted at index surgery **(Figs. 21A and B)**. The preoperative planning necessitates use of radiological recreation of anatomy (usually a CT scan) and planning the osseous resection site of tumor (using MRI) then passing on the details to manufacturer. The synthesis of prosthesis may take anywhere from 4 to 14 days and then surgery can be done (so this time delay should also be borne in mind while planning). This way a more accurate fit can be given to patient. The difference from modular endoprosthesis is that instead of fitting the "patient to prosthesis"; custom-made prosthesis fits "prosthesis to patient". The custom-made prosthesis can be made as a single block design thus ameliorating the risk of junctional erosions. Material for prosthesis now commonly deploys titanium alloy with hydroxyl-apatite or tantalum coating for bone ingrowth. Alternatively, cemented fixation with smooth surface treated implant can be used. Stainless steel is not recommended as the high nickel content may pose toxicity due to increased exposed surface area. Bearing surfaces are made of highly-crosslinked polyethylene to reduce wear. Ceramic bearing is still not very useful for this purpose. Once implanted the prosthesis is expected to last for 10–15 years and its life is expectedly less than standard joint arthroplasty done for treatment of degenerative joints. One reason is excessive stress at the implant bone interface and at fixation site, the other being younger age of patients in the tumor prosthesis group. Revision surgery would also entail bone loss in the subsequent surgery and further complications. The implant design can be changed to bear some stress at the hinge region by converting it to rotating hinge. One method to address both of the problems is by using a composite implant-bone system.

Composite Allograft-endoprosthetic Reconstruction

It had been commonly observed that there is significant bone formation at the implant bone interface and at the shoulder region of the implant. This encouraged development of "extracortical bone bridging and ingrowth fixation system"—now commonly called composite fixation. The allograft bone has been seen to fuse with the native bone over a period of time

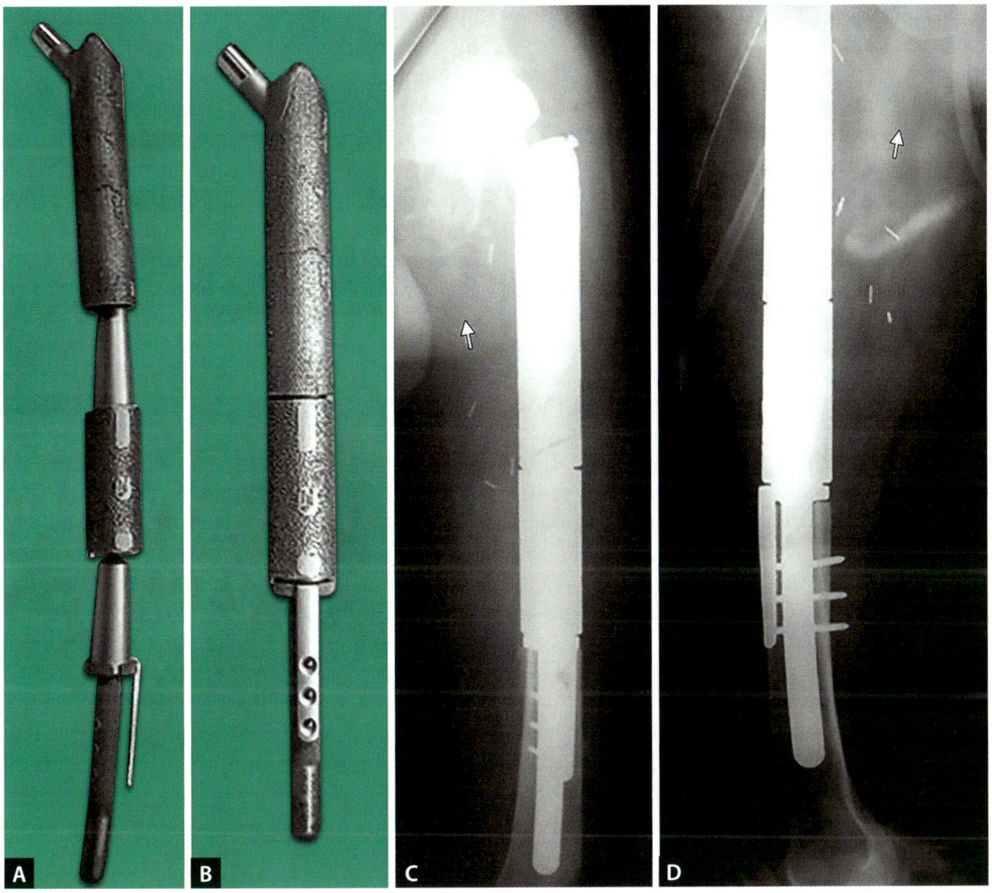

Figs. 20A to D: The commercial megaprosthesis (tumor endoprosthesis) are commonly available as a modular design (A) that can be assembled on table (B) depending on the need of patient for reconstruction. In this case, nearly upper two-thirds of the patient's femur has been replaced with endoprosthesis (C and D).

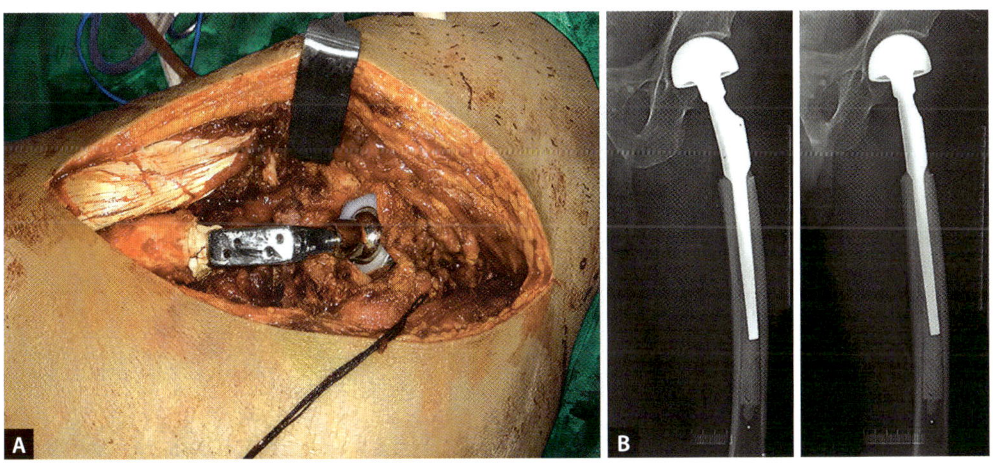

Figs. 21A and B: The custom prostheses are prepared based on patient's specific parameters and are hence available as a monoblock design.

so it was believed that if implant is placed inside bone then this bone will fuse to native bone at one end and will incorporate with the porous-coated implant at the other giving the needed stability. Schematically, the prosthetic implant containing a porous-coated region in the shoulder region is juxtaposed with the allograft or (autologous irradiated/autoclaved) bone. The interface is further sealed with autogenous cancellous bone graft. This bone fuses with the native cortex on one end while biologically fixes to porous-coated implant at the other end. The solid stem is commonly fixed inside bone using cement to achieve initial mechanical fixation. Once bone forms and bridges across the shoulder region of prosthesis it transmits stress from prosthetic segment to the native bone through intermediary allograft (or autologous autoclaved/irradiated) bone and hence partially protects the cement bone interface. The advantages of this composite fixation system are:

1. It allows more effective transfer of stresses from prosthetic segment to bone directly; preventing stress-shielding and bone resorption seen in custom-prosthesis fixation.
2. Reduced stress decreases chances of stem loosening and stem fracture
3. Initial fixation stability achieved with cemented fixation helps in improved bone growth and graft incorporation.
4. Cemented fixation reduces inventory needed to make available the various stem sizes.
5. "*Purse-string effect*": It has been seen that formation of pseudocapsule around the shoulder region of the prosthesis and bone graft incorporation at implant-allograft bone interface prevents wear particles form migrating into the stem-cement-bone interface thus safeguarding against osteolysis. This is called purse-string effect (sealing the region like a constricted area created by purse string).
6. Solid stem-cement fixation would facilitate the removal of implant if revision is indicated compared to bone-ingrown prosthesis.

Expandable Megaprosthesis

A significant number of bone neoplasms are pediatric patients who have growing skeletons. Unfortunately, physis does not pose a significant barrier for most malignant neoplasms and surgical extirpation damages the growing ends of bone that need to be compensated for optimal functional outcome in future. For such patients especially with lower limb malignant tumors who are being considered for limb salvage, future limb-length inequality must be considered. For patients who are near skeletal maturity, the reconstructed limb can be lengthened 1 cm at the initial procedure. Also, epiphysiodesis of the contralateral limb can be done at the appropriate age to preserve limb-length equality (or to minimize inequality). For younger patients that have significant growth remaining, other options should be considered. Historically, amputation (followed by repeated larger prosthetic fitting) and rotationplasty were considered the only reasonable treatments for very young patients with bone sarcomas, advent, and use of expandable prostheses/megaprosthesis gained wide support and popularity. Presently, at all centers this is the preferred modality of limb reconstruction following LSS.

Types of expandable prosthesis: Most endoprostheses are modular, allowing for incremental limb lengthening as an immature patient grows. The conventional technology used in expandable prosthesis is invasive lengthening of the prosthesis based on "screw" mechanism (conversion of rotatory motion into linear motion). The inner threaded rod slides inside of a counter-threaded tube **(Fig. 22A)**. Under short spinal anesthesia, the screw mechanism is manually rotated in the given direction to gain prosthetic length. Usually, these expandable prostheses can gain up to 4–6 cm length in all.

The method that had become popular due to its noninvasive technique for limb lengthening is the use of Repiphysis® Expandable Prosthesis (Wright Medical Technology, Arlington, Tennessee). Cost is the only deterring factor to its common usage. After surgical implantation of this device, the patient is kept under close monitoring for maintaining limb length when leg-length discrepancy (LLD) develops. The device contains a spring-based locking mechanism where energy stored in precompressed spring is used for future lengthening of the prosthesis **(Fig. 22B)**. The procedure is done under fluoroscopy and light sedation. Fluoroscopy is used to identify locking mechanism **(Fig. 22B)** on the prosthesis to position electromagnetic coil **(Figs. 22C and D)**. The coil is then activated for 20 seconds generating a pulsed electromagnetic field (PEMF). Through interference PEMF heats an element in the

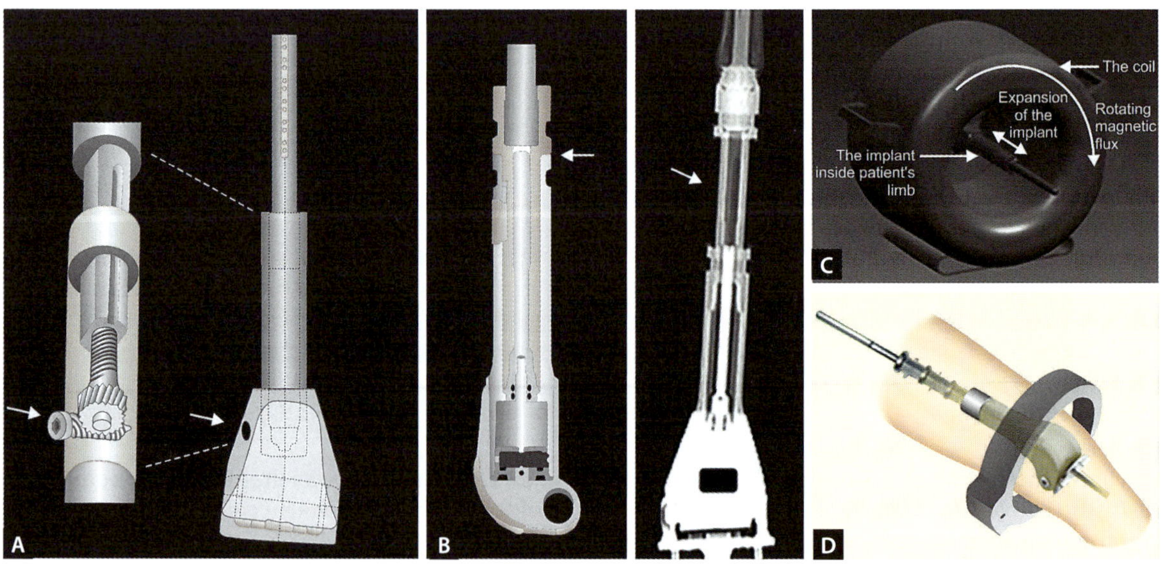

Figs. 22A to D: The Two common types of expandable endoprosthesis. The modular expandable endoprosthesis may be based on a screw-sliding mechanism (A) where the rotatory mechanism of the screw is used to elongate the prosthesis or a more sophisticated pulsed electromagnetic controlled lengthening mechanism is used (B) to manipulate the prosthesis length. The mechanism is located using fluoroscopy and the prosthesis is placed in electromagnetic coil (C and D) that expands the prosthesis through interference.

prosthesis that melts a small segment of polyethylene allowing controlled expansion of the compressed spring, slowly lengthening the prosthesis. LLD is reassessed under fluoroscopy, and the procedure may be repeated one or two times if necessary. Normally, lengths of 0.5–1.5 cm can be gained in each such session. Number of sessions and its frequency can be planned based on LLD. Patients continue to ambulate immediately without an assistive device.

The long-term complications of these prostheses include:

- *Polyethylene wear:* This is still the most limiting factor for articulating surfaces. Even if the prosthesis gains length the overall prosthesis survival is limited by the implanted device that has limited duration articulating surfaces and need to be replaced at appropriate interval.
- Fatigue fracture can occur at the rotating hinge.
- Fatigue fracture at the base of the intramedullary stem where it attaches to the body of the prosthesis.

Rotationplasty (Van Nes Rotationplasty, Van Nes-Borggreve Rotationplasty)

This procedure involves excision of the diseased portion and reattachment of the distal leg with ankle and foot in derotated position to proximal stump to establish ankle as the new knee joint. First described by Borggreve in 1930 for tubercular osteomyelitis of femur, the procedure was popularized by Van Nes in English literature for management of congenital lower limb deficiency (especially proximal femoral deficiency) in 1950. It was adopted for resection-reconstruction in tumor surgery for treatment of osteosarcoma of the distal one-third of the femur by Saltzer and Kotz in Vienna in late 1970s. Modifications to the technique for congenital disorder reconstruction have been described by Brown (attachment of femur to pelvis) and Paley (femoral attachment to acetabulum and Chiari osteotomy) but are not commonly used in orthopedic oncology. The procedure is indicated in the following situations:

1. Malignant tumors around knee joint where resection reconstruction procedures are indicated. As such all lesions of the distal femur and proximal tibia can be surgically managed but situations specifically favoring use of rotationplasty over other reconstruction methods are:
   a. Situation where the expected remaining growth in the opposite healthy leg is >10 cm.
   b. Patients in whom the size of the tumor necessitates removal of so much of the bone or soft-tissue stock as to make any other form of limb salvage impractical.
   c. Involvement of major vasculature near knee (say popliteal vessels) by the neoplasm which can be safely re-established only by segmental resection and reanastomosis.
   d. Patients demanding function and physical or athletic performance over cosmesis.
   e. Revision surgeries due to previous failed reconstruction (infection or local recurrence) in endoprosthesis replacement, provided that the nerve supply can be safely preserved.
   f. Unacceptable sequelae of previous reconstructions like late unmanageable leg length discrepancy or long-term failure of endoprosthetic components with corresponding loss of bone stock.
2. Non-neoplastic reconstruction indications:
   a. Congenital limb deficiencies like proximal focal femoral deficiency
   b. Infected conventional knee arthroplasty implants that cannot be managed by one or two stage revisions.

Technical considerations of rotationplasty: Growth considerations are very important in skeletally immature children. The goal of the surgical procedure is to end up with a thigh segment that will be of the same length as the opposite thigh at the end of skeletal growth. So surgical planning with good understanding of Anderson's growth charts is essential for the surgeon. The other prerequisites of performing rotationplasty are as follows:

- Achieving adequate surgical margins
- Adequate nerve and blood supply to foot and ankle distal must be preservable.
- Ankle and foot must be disease-free.
- Muscle power to ankle must be restorable.
- Adequate preparation and counseling of patient by complete demonstration of the outcome and cosmetic implications.
- Retaining some "over-length" of ankle of the operated leg (as growth compensation is usually subnormal)

Five-patients groups depending on different tumor locations have been described by Winkelmann in 1986—Type AI, being tumors of the distal femur and type AII, are tumors in the proximal tibia. Type BI tumors are situated in the proximal femur, while type BII tumors additionally invade into the acetabulum. Type BIII tumors have total femur involvement. Type A tumors can be reconstructed with "classical" technique but in Type B tumors the hip joint can sometimes be preserved using either a dynamic screw for tibiofemoral fixation or a hemiarthroplasty prosthesis fixed into the proximal tibia. In other cases, involvement of the acetabulum requires an osteotomy of the distal femur. The distal femur is rotated 180° and fixed to the iliac wing resulting in a rotated knee joint replacing hip function (only flexion-extension) and the ankle joint replacing knee function **(Fig. 23)**. Hip flexion is powered by connecting iliopsoas muscle to biceps femoris while hip extension is provided by joining quadriceps tendon to the gluteal muscles. The surgical technique is a topic for dedicated text but let us understand some basic concepts for commonly performed reconstructions:

- *Distal femoral malignancy (Type AI)* ***(Figs. 24A to D):*** Two incisions are placed—one circular circumferential and oval distal incision to match the circumference. Longitudinal medial and lateral incisions are used to dissect the neurovascular structures, isolating the sciatic nerve throughout length. The vessels are either isolated *in toto* or freed proximally and distally to be resected and anastomosed later. Proximally, the quadriceps, adductor group, and hamstring muscles are cut at the planned femoral osteotomy while distally the gastrocnemius heads are cut 1 inch distal to their origins and pes-anserinus tendons are divided near their insertion on proximal tibia. The whole diseased and planned segment is resected as a single mass together with skin and soft tissue cover and osteosynthesis proceeds with plate or intramedullary fixation of femur to 180° rotated tibia. The foot points directly posterior and the vessel reconstruction done if resected. Power to ankle is restored by joining proximal quadriceps to gastrocnemius, hamstring to anterior leg fascia, and adductor group to the lateral leg compartment. Skin flaps are then sutured.

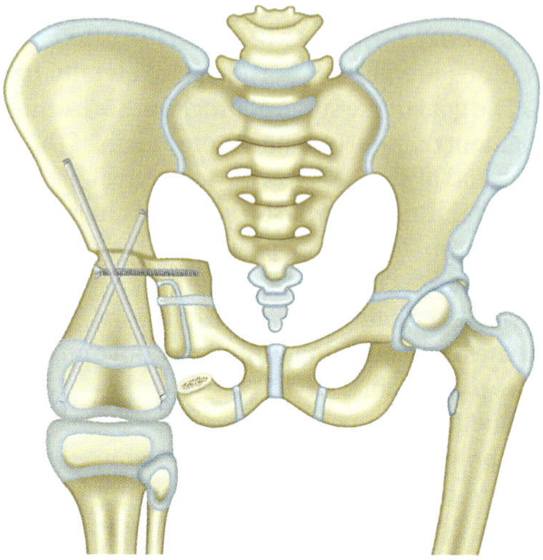

Fig. 23: Rotationplasty can be also performed for proximal femoral malignancies but is uncommonly preferred for this indication. The proximal tumor is resected and the remaining distal stump is attached to the pelvis/acetabular roof commonly with an osteotomy.

- *Proximal tibial malignancy (Type AII):* The skin incisions are usually planned over distal femur and distal tibia. Sartorius, gracilis, and hamstring muscles are divided approximately 5 cm proximal to their insertions. Gastrocnemius heads are released at their origins exposing neurovascular bundle. The anterior tibial artery and deep peroneal nerves are mostly sacrificed and cut distally too. After removing the specimen osteosynthesis is done and muscle to tendon anastomosis done as follows:
  - Biceps femoris and semimembranosus → Tibialis anterior tendon
  - Semitendinosus → Extensor hallucis longus + Extensor digitorum longus tendons
  - Gracilis + Sartorius → Peronei
  - Quadriceps tendon → Achilles tendon
  - Vastus lateralis → Tibialis posterior tendon

Postoperatively the patient is usually managed in intensive care unit for a couple of days. Blood thinners and other precautions for management of blood supply to distal part are especially emphasized. The limb is supported in external brace even better in a cast for 6–10 weeks. Prosthetic fitting is then done. Physiotherapy is essential in training the muscles for maintaining the strength and desired function maintain joint range of motion (ROM), prosthetic rehabilitation,

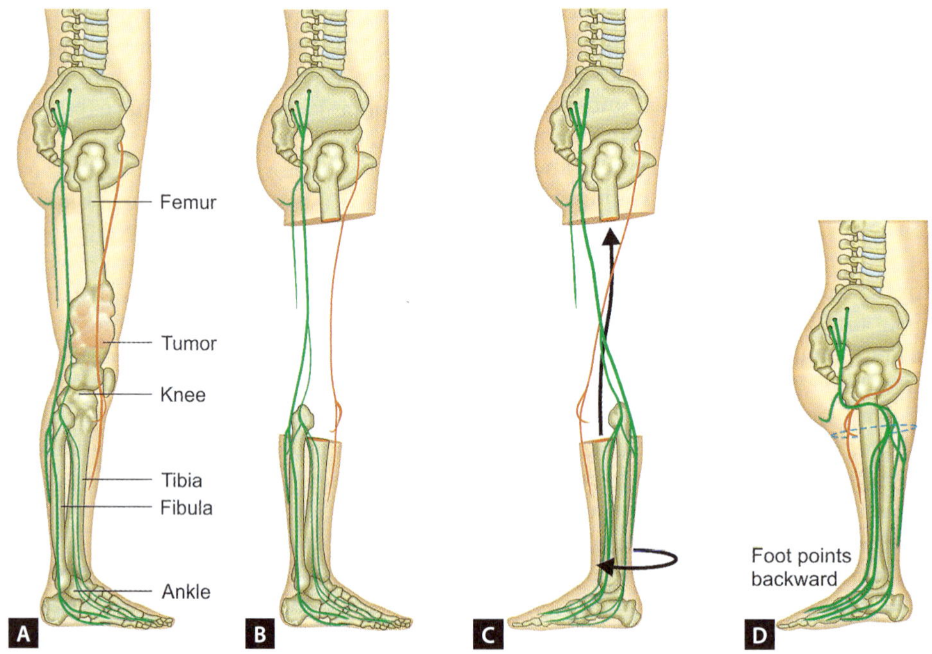

Figs. 24A to D: Schematic drawing showing the common major steps of performing rotationplasty of lower limb for limb salvage from malignant tumor(s) of distal femoral region. (A) Demonstrates the development of tumor in distal femoral region along with disposition of major nerves and vessels. (B) The tumor is meticulously resected according to planning for limb length to keep both knee region (previous ankle) at same height. The specimen is submitted for histopathological evaluation. The nerves are mostly preserved while blood vessels may be divided in the region of tumor infiltration is necessary. (C) The distal part of leg (calf and foot) is rotated by 180° usually clockwise (external rotation), desired shortening done and the vessels are anastomosed if previously resected. (D) The tibia is attached to remaining femur stump creating strudy osteosynthesis. The foot can be fitted in a prosthesis later for mobilization and rehabilitation. Transposition and reattachment of muscles is also done (as described in text) in step (C) and (D) to power the ankle joint now working as knee.

and promote ambulation. This is done by stretching and strengthening exercises, balance training, and prosthetic training.

Complications of rotationplasty:
- Vascular injury and ischemia to distal part
- Nerve injury and insensate limb
- Infection
- Delayed healing/delayed union

Advantages and disadvantages of rotationplasty:
- Limb nonsalvageable limbs can be salvaged by this method.
- Allows functional limb with prosthetic fitting.
- Requires a smaller prosthesis than needed after amputation.
- Sports and ADL are possibly better after rotationplasty.
- Much better ergonomics than an above knee amputation.
- Cosmetic appearance of a posteriorly turned foot is the major repulsion for acceptance of this technique.

ADJUVANT THERAPY

Chemotherapy

Multiagent chemotherapy has been found to increase the survival following LSS for high-grade neoplasms and also it maximizes (in the limits of current resources), the chances for performing LSS. Nearly 10% have metastatic disease at presentation and up to 40–50% will have micrometastasis that is unrecognizable at presentation. Chemotherapy is supposed to help both groups especially the latter. The chemotherapy drugs primarily act by inducing apoptosis (programmed cell death) in the susceptible tumor cells. Adriamycin (cardiotoxic) and its analogs (epirubicin, myelosuppressive but less cardiotoxic) along with ifosfamide (replacing cyclophosphamide used previously) have been essential components for most regimens. Ifosfamide has been effective even in previously treated (but failed) cases of cyclophosphamide with little if any cross-resistance but has to be given with mesna to protect urothelium. With recent addition of high dose of methotrexate, the survival rates and success of LSS have improved to 60–70% in well-managed cases. The chemotherapy can be administered in different forms and regimens and has been found successful for osteosarcoma and Ewing's sarcoma and sometimes for dedifferentiated or mesenchymal chondrosarcomas (other tumors and soft tissue sarcoma poorly respond to chemoagents). Most commonly the chemotherapy is administered after local control of the tumor (as adjuvant) to kill the remaining micrometastasis. The neoadjuvant chemotherapy has become quite popular these days (see below) to downstage the tumor primarily making it better resectable. For patients with unresectable tumors, palliative chemotherapy may be given.

Neoadjuvant Chemotherapy (Induction Chemotherapy)

This approach to chemotherapy involves administering the chemotherapy drugs before local control of the tumor and has evolved from innovative management of osteogenic sarcoma. The local tumor control and rates of limb salvage have been good with this approach. The chemotherapy should be administered through intravenous (IV) route (conventional) or intra-arterial (usually adriamycin/cyclophosphamide) and can be combined with radiation therapy. University of California and Los Angeles regime involves use of IV(continuous infusion for 48 hours) or intra-arterial adriamycin and cisplatin (two cycles), along with ifosfamide (two cycles) and three doses of radiotherapy (2,800 cGy). Other centers, however, use the standard chemotherapy regimens in neoadjuvant period that are to be given as adjuvant period.

Advantages of neoadjuvant chemotherapy are:
- *Attempt arrest of tumor growth:* Interim relief during the prosthesis manufacture period.
- *Controlling micrometastasis and metastasis:* Reducing chances of local recurrence (improving local control of tumor).
- Early defense against possible pulmonary metastases.
- Reduce the emergence of drug resistant tumor cells.
- *Downstage tumor:* Converting nonresectable tumors to resectable category and marginally resectable tumors to adequately resected tumors and preservation of limb function.
- *"Sensitivity testing" of chemotherapy against tumor:* It acts like sensitivity testing of the tumor where failure of neoadjuvant regimen would encourage change or shift to alternative regimen for even the postoperative management.
- Reduce vascularity of tumor.

Disadvantages of this approach however include:
- Systemic toxicity of the drugs and poor preoperative health of patient.
- Possibility of increased infection and poor wound healing resulting from cytotoxic effects of the drugs.
- The waiting period of the primary surgical resection is also increased in case of complication (usually patients have to wait for 3 weeks following neoadjuvant therapy).
- There has been argument based on study by pediatric oncology group that neoadjuvant chemotherapy is equivalent to adjuvant chemotherapy for prolonging patient survival, raising doubts on efficacy of induction chemotherapy. But, there is a significant recognized effect on LSS rate and extremity function following neoadjuvant chemotherapy.

The regimens for induction chemotherapy are still evolving and the best regimen is possibly unknown. Now high-dose methotrexate has also been included in regimens. Radiation therapy needs to be included in the regimen is also unknown. Usually for osteosarcoma, ifosfamide and adriamycin in first cycle followed by two cycles of cisplatin and adriamycin are given in neoadjuvant regimen (aimed to downstage tumor and enhance chances of LSS) followed by surgery and adjuvant therapy of remaining 4, 5, and 6 cycles given after 21 days comprising ifosfamide and adriamycin. Intra-arterial chemotherapy (IAC) has been proposed to improve the results of induction chemotherapy and augment rates of successful LSS. IAC delivers drug predominantly to primary tumor increasing regional drug concentration and possibly better drug penetration in the cells. The systemic concentrations following IAC are similar to intravenous routes to effectively control micrometastasis. Adriamycin is poorly tolerated intra-arterial with local skin necrosis and extensive damage to normal tissue without achieving complete tumor control. Cisplatin is most commonly used medicine for IAC with encouraging results.

Assessment of tumor necrosis following neoadjuvant chemotherapy: The assessment can be done clinically, radiologically, laboratory parameters, and histologic examination for necrosis of the tumor.

Clinically: The reduction in the size, extent, "aggressiveness" of the tumor accompanied with decreased pain, swelling, and temperature is assessed.

Radiological and scintigraphic assessment: Conventional MRI helps in identifying well-established plains between tumor and surrounding tissue, reduction or paraneoplastic edema, and volume of tumor itself. Tumor signal getting isointense (reduced signal intensity on T2-weighted images) to the adjoining normal tissue and identification of necrosis areas in the tumor also help in assessing the chemotherapy response. The scan is very subjective with respect to observer and often inaccurate and inconsistent readings occur. Residual tumor (defined as tumor volume < 10% of original size) cannot be well-appreciated on conventional MRI.

Dynamic contrast-enhanced MRI (calculates inclination of the resultant time–intensity curve from the tumor signal intensity gathered from serial images obtained at 15–20 seconds intervals). This technique is useful for detecting the most viable parts of the tumor and is a good follow-up tool. Brisk slopes (>30%) result from high perfusion in viable tumor. Dynamic MRI can detect small 3–5 mm^3 foci also. Slowly enhancing or nonenhancing regions represent necrotic areas. Responsive tumors in general have gradually or nonenhancing areas. Dynamic MRI is less invasive and has good accuracy for identifying the responsive tumors but cost and logistics are prohibitive factors for routine use. Magnetic resonance spectroscopy as metabolic identifier of viable tumor regions has also been recommended but not recommended for common use.

99Tc-MDP bone scintigraphy (dynamic imaging) done serially can evaluate response (scans are compared to contralateral normal bone). The assessment is very crude and can differentiate between good from poor response only.

Gallium-67 (67Ga)-citrate scans are better than 99mTc-MDP scans for closely defining the actual tumor. A normal gallium scan suggests no residual tumor present.

Thallium-201 scans are further superior due to no residual activity in normal bone, but they have not been routinely studied or evaluated for assessment of tumor response.

PET scans determine the metabolically active regions of tumor cells based on their uptake of radiolabeled glucose [2-(fluorine-18) fluoro-2-deoxy-d-glucose (FDG)]. It can fairly accurately determine the residual disease, but cannot localize the same due to limited spatial resolution, so PET-CT or now PET-MRI appears to be more effective.

On a plain radiograph re-establishment of fat planes, reduction of soft tissue tumor component, healing of pathological fractures and periosteal calcification indicate good response to chemotherapy. The radiographic features are, however, not very conspicuous and underestimate the therapeutic response.

Histological examination: This is the *gold standard* to determine chemotherapy therapeutic response. The resected specimens can be graded for efficacy of treatment based on various systems. The most popular Huvos system (Memorial Sloan-Kettering Cancer Center) is a semiquantitative method performed by grading the extent of necrosis relative to the percentage of residual viable tumor **(Table 12)**. The estimate of tumor necrosis is, however, difficult to calculate based only on the viable cell count per unit area of residual tumor. Picci et al. (Istituto Ortopedico Rizzoli, Italy) developed system that measures the absolute amount of viable tumor cells after chemotherapy which does not change with volume changes of tumor. Salzer-Kuntschik et al. (Cooperative German-Austrian-Swiss Osteosarcoma Study Group) also developed histological grading of tumor response to chemotherapy **(Table 12)**. Akermån stressed that the regional mapping protocol was more important than the type of grading system used **(Fig. 25)**. It is generally considered that if response to chemotherapy is less than the most optimal grade (any system) then the adjuvant chemotherapy needs to be re-tailored and neoadjuvant regimen is not effective. So for Huvos system, any grade less than grade 4 is suboptimal response as it has been found that the prognosis for all other grades is significantly worse than grade 4.

Tumor vascularity response: It is logical to think that a "dying" tumor (say following chemotherapy) will lose its vascularity and has been also seen in research reports that rapid disappearance of tumor vessels is equated well to a favorable response from chemotherapy. Persistence of pathologic vascularity suggests poor response to chemotherapy. Magnetic resonance angiography demonstrates reduction

TABLE 12: Histological grading for response of tumor to neoadjuvant chemotherapy.

Huvos	*Picci et al.*	*Salzer-Kuntschik*
Grade 4: No tumor cells seen	*Total tumor response:* No evidence of viable tumor	*Grade 1:* No viable tumor cells seen
Grade 3: Scattered foci of tumor cells seen	*Good tumor response:* Isolated microscopic foci of viable tumor smaller than the size of a 10x magnification field	*Grade 2:* Single tumor cells or clusters <0.5 cm
Grade 2: Areas of necrosis and tumor cells seen	*Fair tumor response:* Tumor with at least one macroscopic residual nodule of viable tumor	*Grade 3:* Viable tumor cells <10% seen
Grade 1: Little or no tumor response seen	*Poor tumor response:* Easily identifiable or grossly remaining viable tumor areas	*Grade 4:* Viable tumor cells 10–50% seen *Grade 5:* Viable tumor cells 10–50% seen *Grade 6:* No tumor response seen

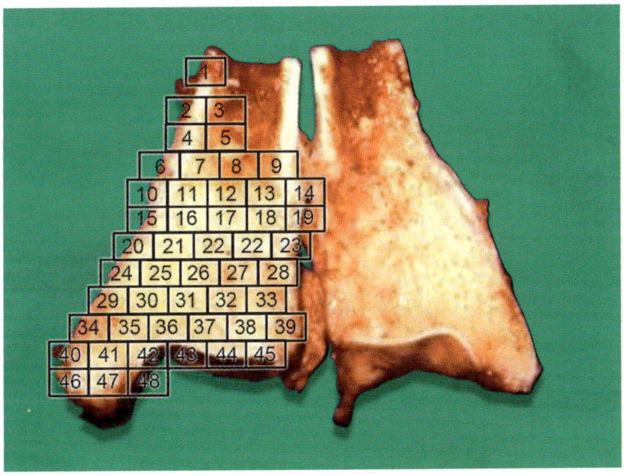

Fig. 25: Assessment of tumor necrosis by regional mapping.

in vascularity in patients showing favorable response. Color Doppler flow imaging (CDFI) estimates the modification of blood flow resistance, no change (reduction) suggests poor response. CDFI estimates qualitative as well as quantitative parameters using spectral analysis. It detects anomalous flow patterns within tumors that determine the qualitative analysis of vascularity, and also provides quantitative estimate of tumor blood supply and intralesional blood flow. The claimed advantages of CDFI over dynamic contrast-enhanced (DCE) MRI and three-phase bone scintigraphy are its apparent superior accuracy, quick examination, low cost, non-invasive nature, and easy accessibility.

Adjuvant therapy is based on the premises that local recurrence and metastasis (up to 80% in amputated limbs) is high following local surgical clearance of the tumor, so chemotherapy may be used as "adjunct" to sterilize the local site and kill metastatic disease. Following success in treating and obliterating the metastasis, chemotherapy has now also been used to remove the micrometastasis and the combination of local tumor control, and adjuvant chemotherapy has consistently improved the survival of well-performed LSS. Usually, a "sandwich" approach to tumor treatment is used where the patient receives 6–18 months of neoadjuvant chemotherapy followed by surgery and reconstruction and 6–8 months of adjuvant chemotherapy. The adjuvant chemotherapy drugs are same as neoadjuvant drugs for patients responding favorable; however for suboptimal responders, the drugs (addition of ifosfamide if not used previously, using a higher dose, adding high-dose methotrexate, etoposide or vincristine, switching to carboplatin from cisplatin, etc.) or rarely, route of administration (intra-arterial instead of intravenous for local control, etc.) are altered.

Adverse effects of chemotherapy: Being general cytotoxic agents, the chemotherapeutic agents have inhibitory and metabolic alteration effects on highly dividing cells. Common temporary side-effects include:

- Nausea, vomiting, and loss of appetite
- Hair loss
- Mucositis and aphthous ulcers

Bone marrow is the site most commonly affected by chemotherapy drugs. Regular monitoring of blood cell counts and prophylactically keeping patients on granulocyte-macrophage colony-stimulating factor (GM-CSF) is recommended. There are higher chances of infection due to low white blood cell (WBC) counts and reduced functionality (immunosuppression), increased chances of bleeding (reduced platelets), and anemia that should be explained to the patient for proper precautions. Ifosfamide had dose-limiting myelosuppression, renal, and CNS toxicity. The CNS toxicity is possibly a part of metabolic encephalopathy related to accumulation of chloroacetaldehyde (metabolite of ifosfamide). This may cause mutism, confusion, blurred vision, auditory and visual hallucinations, seizures, and coma. Vigorous hydration with bicarbonate should be given as prophylaxis and methylene blue can be used to treat neurotoxicity. Ifosfamide and cyclophosphamide can cause hemorrhagic cystitis that can be prevented by giving mesna along with the chemotherapy. Cisplatin may cause ototoxicity (problem hearing high-pitched sounds), neuropathy presenting as numbness, tingling, and even pain in the hands and feet. Nephropathy can also occur after treatment with cisplatin that can be reduced by hydration. Adriamycin is associated with dose-limiting cardiotoxicity that can be reduced without altering efficacy by giving continuous intravenous infusion rather than bolus.

Newer developments and advances in chemotherapy are in accord with other medical faculties and primarily focus on cell biology, immunology, and molecular genetics. There are attempts to improve efficacy and reduce resistance to drugs. There is increasing trend to utilize the specific growth factors countering the adverse effects of most cytotoxic drugs (viz., for high-dose ifosfamide causing thrombocytopenia use thrombopoietin). Peroxisome proliferator activated receptor-gamma (PPAR-γ) and troglitazone have been found to induce differentiation in liposarcoma. IGF-1 is proinductive for osteosarcoma, suppression of the same by reduction of growth hormone release could help to control the tumor growth. Her-2-neu overexpression has been identified in osteosarcoma; there are attempts to treat refractory osteosarcoma with herceptin (rh-mab HER2). Tumor vascularity is a potential site of control of growth and even tumor regression. Matrix metalloproteinase (MMP) inhibitors, vitaxin (monoclonal antibody to endothelial growth factor), anti-VEGF, and thalidomide are all under research for possible utility. Inductively modifying pulmonary macrophages to a tumoricidal state by L-MTP-PE (liposome-encapsulated muramyl tripeptide phosphatidylethanolamine) a mycobacterial component can prevent or reduce lung metastasis. Tumor suppressor genes and disease defining unique mutations are other targets for future therapy.

RADIOTHERAPY

Ionizing radiation (electrons, X-rays, and proton beams) primarily kills tumor cells by DNA damage. This damage results from either of two mechanisms **(Figs. 26A and B)**:

1. Direct double-stranded breaks of DNA accounting for one-third of cellular damage, or

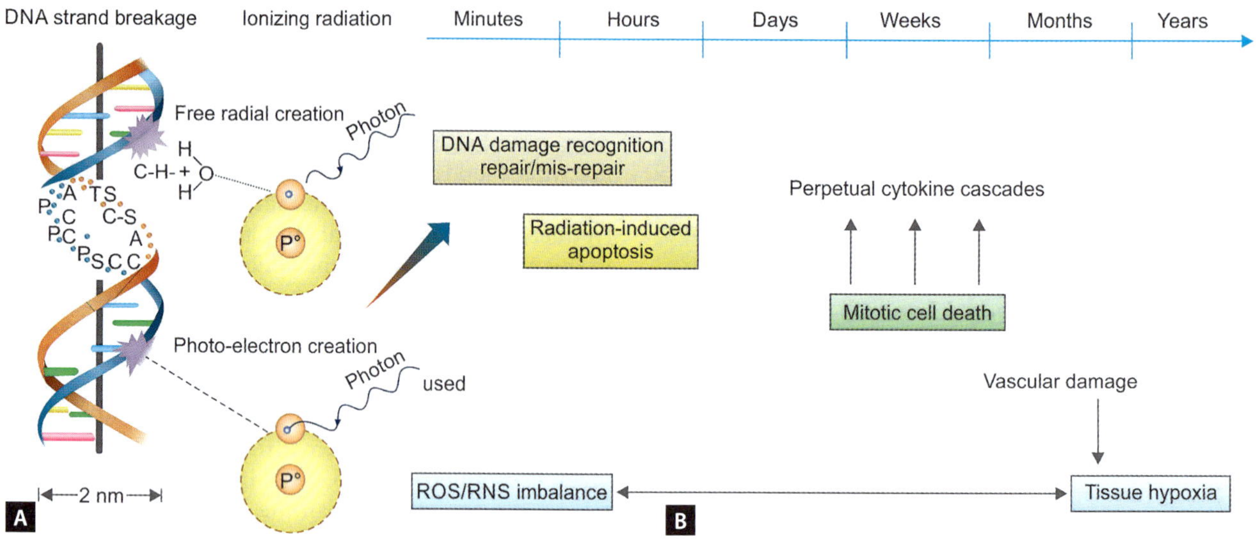

Figs. 26A and B: Effect of radiation on tissues. At cellular level, the radiation causes DNA damage (single- or double-strand damage), which (A) causing cellular necrosis in fast dividing cells or else apoptosis in moderately active cells; (B) Further with mis-repair, there occurs mitotic cell death in dormant cells when they enter cell-proliferation phase. (ROS: reactive oxygen species)

2. Generation of the hydroxyl ions—through interaction with water molecules generating free radicals (remainder damage).

Double-strand break of DNA causes lethal damage to cell, though it can be partially repaired accrual beyond certain limit (dose-dependent and type of tumor cell) causes cell damage. Overwhelming damage (exceeding reparative capacity) results in cell death by apoptosis or during mitosis.

The *dose of radiation* required to achieve desired tumor kill is estimated typically by a clonogenic survival assay as follows. Known number of cells are cultured on plates and exposed to radiation. The number of colonies that then grow is counted and is divided by number of cells seeded giving a survival fraction (SF). The SF at 2 Gy [SF2 General Electric (GE)] has been accepted as a clinically relevant measure of radiation sensitivity for comparison and reference. A plot is obtained for different doses. The tumor cells usually display a shoulder in the low-dose region; the width of which is smaller compared to normal-cell-dose plots. This is due to reduced capability to repair DNA damage of tumor cells.

Repair forms the important step in cell cycle. Radiation damage to mammalian cell can operationally be divided into three subheadings:

1. Lethal damage
2. Potentially lethal damage
3. Sublethal damage

Lethal damage is irreversible and irreparable damage that leads to cell death. *Potential lethal damage* is a component of radiation induced damage that can be modified by postirradiation environment changes. *Sublethal damage* can be repaired in hours unless we add another insult by giving second dose of radiation. Tumor cells have poor mechanism of repair but normal cells recover after radiotherapy, so this forms the basis of fractionated radiotherapy in which gap between two radiotherapy sessions should be at least 6 hours. Reoxygenation also plays an important part in cell kill as oxygenated environment leads to more cell kill and hence oxygen acts as radiosensitizer because oxygenated environment when interacts with radiotherapy leads to production of free radicals which kills tumor cells. Reassortment is required to make cells radiosensitive because as cell divides it moves from S0 phase (most resistant) to G2 M phase (most sensitive). All tumor cells are in different phases of cell cycle and when one fractionation of radiotherapy is delivered it kills all the cells in sensitive phase but cells in the quiescent phase are not killed because they are in most resistant phase. But, when we wait for 6 hours, cell in radioresistant phase of cell cycle moves to radiosensitive phase of cell cycle that can be killed by other delivered fraction. Tumor cell generally under the effect of radiotherapy starts dividing only after 28 days. If unchecked by additional radiotherapy, this would ultimately lead to accelerated repopulation of tumor cells causing radioresistance. Stereotactic radiotherapy that uses very high dose per fraction than conventional fractionation has shown additional direct vascular effects and also activates apoptosis. The latest "R" that is added to 4Rs (repair, reoxygenation, reassortment, and accelerated repopulation) is intrinsic radiosensitivity of tumor toward radiation such as small cell lung cancer, squamous cell, and adenocarcinoma are radiosensitive to radiotherapy in increasing order but bone tumors are least radiosensitive rather intrinsically radioresistant in nature.

Fractionated radiotherapy utilizes this difference in shoulder width for increasing the therapeutic index (adding these low doses will lead to accrual of irreparable damage in tumor tissue while normal cells will repair in meantime). Oxygenation of tumor cells influences the tumor kill by free radical mechanism. Approximately three times more radiation is required to achieve tumor kill in anoxic tissue, although this may also in part be related to aggressive nature of hypoxic tumor tissue. Acridine orange has been found to improve reactive oxygen species in "hypoxic tumors" and enhance tumor kill. The conventional held belief of sarcomas being radioresistant are not recently supported, and in studies these cells have been found to be equally sensitive to radiation. With the availability of *megavoltage beams,* the penetration of radiation has improved compared to older *orthovoltage beams.*

Brachytherapy and teletherapy (external-beam radiation) are primary methods of administering the radiation therapy. Brachytherapy is delivered by implantation of radioactive source in tumor tissue say by catheters filled with substance or by implanted beads or needles. The advantage is direct delivery to the involved region, minimal wastage of radiation as the radiation is primarily absorbed in the affected region, relative sparing of comparatively distant normal tissue (the radiation intensity falls according to inverse square law for distance). The technique though interesting and quite logical is less often used, as it is invasive and required association between surgeon and radiation oncologist. External-beam radiation is administered using linacs (linear accelerators) mounted on gantry that rotates around patient delivering radiation from various angles. X-rays penetrate far into tissue and are used for deep tumors, while electrons deposit most of their energy in a short distance so useful for superficial tumors. Newer agents like *proton beams* (hadrons, charged particles such as carbon, helium, or neon) have useful property of penetrating deep but quickly imparting the energy to the target tissue ("Bragg peak"—improved radiobiological effect by sparing normal tissue) compared to X-rays that keep penetrating and damage the far normal tissue also. Further advancement to this technology has been imparted in the form of "spot-scanning" allowing the use of more intense radiation without increasing the toxicity to patient. Proton beam radiation is, however, expensive.

Radiation dose is measured as "gray" which is equivalent to 1 joule of energy absorbed per kilogram of tissue exposed. This is equal to 100 rad. Usually, patients receiving radiation therapy receive 1.8–2.0 Gy per day that continues for many weeks. Total cumulative dose typically ranges from 60 to 70 Gy for adults. Hyperfractionation has been theoretically poised to further improve the therapeutic index and comprises giving 1.0–1.2 Gy radiation dose twice daily, but practical utility and findings do not depict any advantage on conventional fractionation. Its use has been typically established in head and neck, and lung cancers only but its role is not defined in bone and soft tissue tumors. Delivering radiation to the target tissue requires intense planning to reduce the acute and late toxicity and protecting the normal structures as much. First a simulation is run for specific patient whereby optimal position of the limb is decided and often custom-made splints/cradles (Vac-lock/orfit/Bluebag) are used to positioning. A CT scan is then done in the position (treatment planning CT) where tumor "volume" is outlined, for better assessment it can be merged with previous MRI scans using dedicated software. Classically, three-dimensional conformal radiation therapy (3D-CRT) is used to target tumor and simultaneously sparing the normal tissue. Coplanar beams were used that hit the target tissue through the most direct path, but now with advancement noncoplanar beams (directed at oblique angles) sparing important structures are being used. To target the radiation beams previously, custom-made blocks of metal were mounted on the machine while now multi-leaf computer controlled collimators are used that produce desired pattern for directing the beams. *Intensity-modulated radiation therapy (IMRT)* has developed as refinement of original technique (3D-CRT) where in addition to the target dose, volume, dose to normal tissue, and beam arrangements one also specifies the dose-volume constraints for critical structures and the target volume.

General principles of planning and target delineation depend upon location, size, depth (with respect to fascia), and grade of tumors and these points should be considered before planning the radiotherapy. Bone and soft tissue tumors as seen on imaging along with suspicious surrounding edema should be treated as edema harbors microscopic disease. In preoperative scenario, both CT for delineating primary bone tumor and MRI (to see edema and any soft tissue extension, intramedullary involvement, and skip metastasis) should be done and fused with help of special planning software [such as Monaco **(Fig. 27)**, Pinnacle, etc.]. Certain target volume considerations are looked into planning the disease treatment. Gross tumor volume (GTV) includes gross disease on clinical examination, CT scans, and T1-weighted contrast-enhanced MRI. Using all information, the contours are drawn. Clinical target volume (CTV) includes the subclinical spread and edema. It includes GTV + 3 cm margin in longitudinal dimension and 1.5 cm margin in radial dimension. It also should incorporate any residual disease along with disturbed lesion and violated fascia. In postoperative case give 1 cm margin to scar and include any disease into close by. Planning target volume (PTV) is the margin given to CTV and depends on institutional protocol, it is usually CTV + 0.5–1 cm. In order to prevent lymphedema in patients, small strip of normal tissue should be spared for lymphatic corridor.

There are organs at risk near to PTV and these OARS (organs at risk) should be within the tolerance limit of radiation so that the toxicities should be reduced. The following dose limits to normal tissue are to be respected wherever possible. Dose constraints for some important organs at risk during radiotherapy are as follows:

- Spinal cord: D_{max} 45 Gy
- Heart [V25 (volume of heart to receive <25 Gy) < 10%]: Mean 4–6 Gy
- Liver: Mean dose 18 Gy
- Small bowel (195 cc) < 45 Gy
- Head of femur V50 < 50% (i.e., 50% volume should receive < 50 Gy)
- Achilles tendon V50 < 50%
- Bladder V50 < 60% (i.e., 60% volume should receive <50 Gy)

External-beam radiation is used:

For local control of Ewing's tumor, lymphoma, myeloma, and metastatic bone disease [MBD (palliation)]: High doses (of X-ray therapy, XRT) were used in past for Ewing's sarcoma (60–75 Gy) due to conventional imaging and developing protocols. With standardization and evaluation of previous

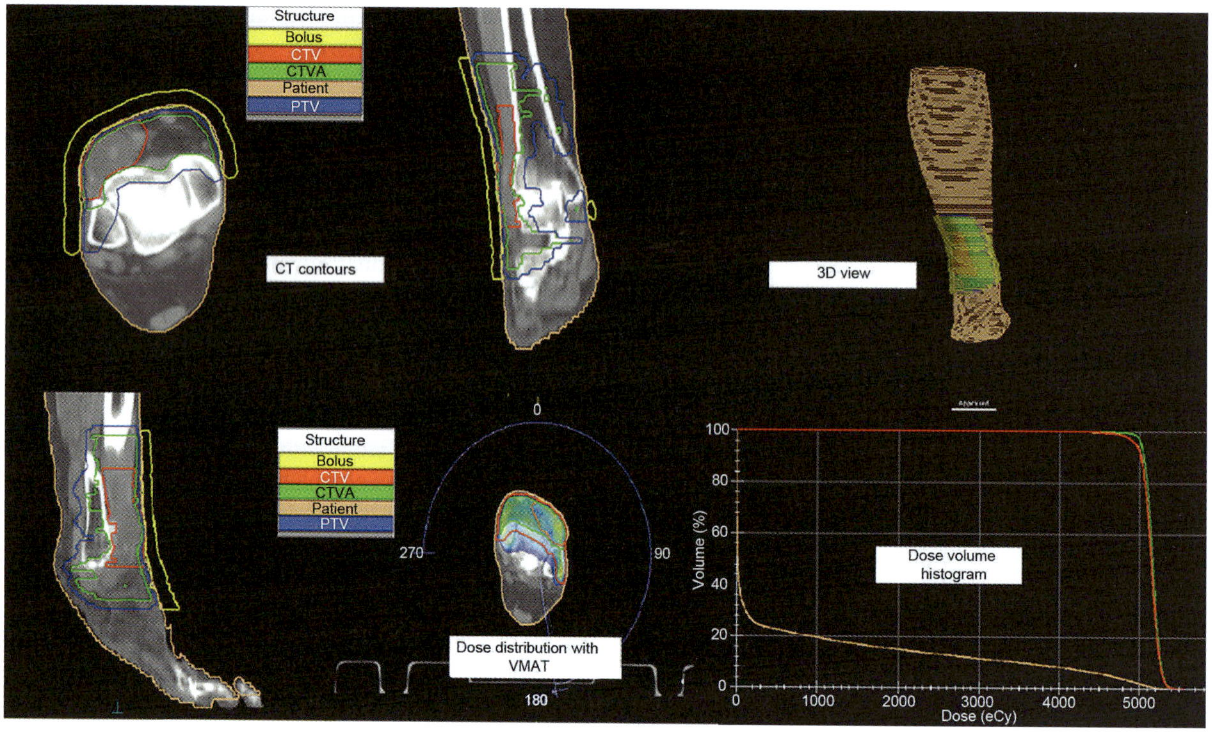

Fig. 27: Steps in radiotherapy planning. (CTV: clinical target volume; GTV: gross tumor volume; PTV: planning target volume; VMAT: volumetric modulated arc therapy)

treatment, the practice of irradiating whole bone was restricted to 40 Gy and giving 16-Gy boost to tumor region, which was found still equivalent to giving approximately 56 Gy to the tumor tissue only. Mostly XRT is begun after 8–12 weeks of chemotherapy when the tumor volume has shrunk drastically taking care to avoid subcutaneous tissue (sparing lymphatics) and not crossing the adjacent joint to preserve function. The most serious complication is development of secondary malignancy (spindle cell sarcoma—commonly osteosarcoma and rarely fibrosarcoma or MFH) that has deterred the use of radiation as primary modality of treatment for Ewing's sarcoma. The incidence of secondary osteosarcoma has been reported from 3 to 22% (higher values for previous high-dose treatment exceeding 60 Gy usually unfractionated and receiving intensive chemotherapy with alkylating agents). All secondary tumors occur near the original tumor. This along with doubts on efficacy on radiation treatment, advancements in orthopedic surgical techniques led to resurgence of surgical modality as the preferred modality of local control. Late stress fractures also can develop in weight-bearing bones exposed to radiation (subtrochanteric and diaphyseal femoral fractures are common sites). Still for difficult surgical sites (pelvis and spine) and secondary clearance of histologically positive margins of surgical resection, radiotherapy is deployed for its higher reward to risk ratio in these situations. Some also use radiotherapy for postoperative adjuvant in tumors showing poor response to chemotherapy. For treating primary osteosarcoma, radiosensitization with adriamycin (daily for 3 days) is followed by 3,500 cGy (10 fractions of 350 cGy) is given followed by LSS (after 2 weeks). Radiotherapy is more frequently, however, used for palliation of metastatic disease or at sites where wide margins were not achieved.

- As an *adjunct* in the treatment of soft tissue sarcomas, in which it is used in combination with surgery: Rhabdomyosarcomas are often treated with radiation therapy for local control. In general, approximately 50 Gy is given for Group III disease (grossly remaining tumor at surgical margin), and 41 Gy for those with Group II disease (microscopic tumor at surgical margins). Radiotherapy is now given at 3 weeks in low-risk patients or at week 12 in intermediate-risk patients. This regimen allows for chemotherapy to be delivered to take care of micrometastatic disease.

Emergency radiotherapy (XRT) at the time of diagnosis is reserved for patients with intracranial extension of their disease. The nonrhabdomyosarcomatous tumors are not as responsive to chemotherapy or radiotherapy and mostly occur in adults. They include MFHs, synovial sarcomas, fibrosarcomas, angiosarcomas, and leiomyosarcomas. For intermediate- and high-grade tumors, adjuvant XRT is given following limb salvage surgery (LSS). Brachytherapy and intraoperative radiotherapy are viable options in these cases. For brachytherapy to be effective, the skin closure should be tension-free, else rotational flap cover should be done. The skin flaps should be thick and vascular. The radioactivity is loaded after at least 6–7 days of surgery with high activity iodine seeds (having less energetic photon) and is regularly monitored limiting dose to skin of <2,000 cGy.

Preoperative radiation has been proposed for improving resectability, better local control of target tumors, reducing the extent of resection, and decreased risk of tumor implantation. There are, however, chances of increased postoperative complications, delay of primary surgical resection, and difficulty in assessing the tumor extent. Postoperative radiation is associated with fewer wound complications, no hindrance to surgery and precise assessment of tumor extent. The diagnosis for postoperative radiation is based on complete histological specimen obtained from surgery while for preoperative radiation, the planning is done from limited biopsy sample and the diagnosis could be incorrect (especially the grade of tumor due to heterogeneous nature of sarcomas).

BENIGN AND MALIGNANT BONE FORMING NEOPLASMS

The different bone pathologies can be grouped as according to WHO classification, however, it is extensive and on a day-to-day basis not followed even by most proficient centers doing tumor surgery. There are a lot of skeletal pathologies that we encounter on a day-to-day basis that mimic neoplasia but are pathologically distinct; a brief mention is done **(Table 13)** for general awareness of orthopedic residents. We will present a simpler differentiation based on predominant tissue seen on histopathology and dividing them into benign, aggressive, and malignant types **(Table 14)** that can be useful to oncologists and orthopedic residents together.

Simple Bone Cyst

Simple bone cyst [unicameral bone cysts (UBC)] also called unicameral, juvenile, or essential bone cyst is not considered a neoplasm and also it is not a true cyst because it lacks endothelial lining. The cyst is primarily a metaphyseal intramedullary lesion that enlarges slowly and is commonly seen in first 2 decades of life. With growth of the child, the cyst may "artifactually" come to lie in diaphysis of bone. The lesion is usually unilocular cavity generally filled with clear or straw-colored fluid though septations may develop in irregular growing cysts or in cancellous bone or with healing of cortical breaches. The lining is composed of thin fibrovascular tissue membrane. Simple cysts are considered either a developmental abnormality (hamartoma) or recently

TABLE 13: Tumor simulators (non-neoplastic conditions that simulate bone tumors).

Patients <20 years of age	*20–50 years of age*	*>50 years of age*
• Chronic osteomyelitis (especially tubercular) • Acute osteomyelitis (sometimes) • Avulsion fractures • Exuberant callus • Myositis ossificans	• Synovial chondromatosis • Ganglionic cyst • Heterotopic ossification • Stress fracture • Pigmented villonodular synovitis • Gout	• Hyperparathyroidism • Paget's disease • Mastocytosis • Bone infarcts • Bone islands • Degenerative cysts of bone • Epidermoid cyst

TABLE 14: Classification and differentiation of bone neoplasia.

Broad tumor group	*Benign lesions*	*Aggressive lesions*	*Malignant lesions*
Tumor-like lesions/ indefinite for neoplasia	• Unicameral (simple) bone cyst • Intraosseous ganglion and subchondral bone cyst	Aneurysmal bone cyst	
Bone-forming lesions	• Osteoma • Osteoid osteoma • Bone island (enostosis)	Osteoblastoma	Osteosarcoma and related variants
Cartilage lesions	• Osteochondroma • Nora's lesion • Enchondroma • Benign chondroma • Subungual exostosis	• Chondroblastoma • Chondromyxoid fibroma • Multiple enchondromatosis	Chondrosarcoma and related variants
Fibrous lesions		Desmoplastic fibroma	Fibrosarcoma
Giant cell lesions	• Giant cell tumor • Giant cell reparative granuloma	Giant cell tumor	
Fibrohistiocytic lesions	Benign fibrous histiocytoma (nonossifying fibroma)		Malignant fibrous histiocytoma
Hematopoietic tumors			• Plasma cell myeloma • Malignant lymphoma
Vascular lesions	• Lymphangioma and hemangioma • Skeletal angiomatosis • Hemophilic pseudotumor • Vascular tumors in the immunocompromised • Glomus tumor	Gorham's disease	• Hemangioendothelioma and epithelioid hemangioendothelioma • Angiosarcoma • Hemangiopericytoma
Miscellaneous mesenchymal lesions	• Fibrous dysplasia • Campanacci's disease (osteofibrous dysplasia) • Fibrocartilaginous mesenchymoma • Intraosseous lipoma • Intraosseous schwannoma	? Adamantinoma	• Adamantinoma • Chordoma • Ewing's sarcoma • Intraosseous liposarcoma • Leiomyosarcoma • Malignant mesenchymoma

the hemodynamic pressure measurements suggest some form of venous obstruction though the chain of events leading to cyst formation is not clear. The normal bone intraosseous pressure is usually around 5–15 mm Hg while intracystic pressure ranges from 15 to 40 mm Hg. The normal bone pressure curves are smooth without any notches while transduced pressure traces from UBC depict systolic, diastolic, and dicrotic notches. ABCs have much higher mean pressures (80–200 mm Hg) and transduced pressure traces can be used for differentiation of these cystic pathologies. Chromosomal anomalies in the form of complex clonal structural rearrangement has been found in chromosomes 4, 6, 8, 12, 16, and 21; however, the significance is unclear.

Clinical Features

The proximal humerus and femur are the most common sites (80%) affected followed by proximal tibia, ilium, and calcaneus. Quite a few are recognized incidentally on radiographs done for other purpose otherwise pain at the site is the most common presentation. Pathologic fractures occur often in young teenagers due to trivial injury while playing, stiffness as a presenting feature is uncommon. Being close to physis an active UBC may be associated with growth arrest, epiphyseal slippage, and limb length inequality.

Radiology

The cysts are visualized as oval or ovoid lytic lesions with thinned cortices in metaphyseal or metadiaphyseal region of the long tubular bones with their long axis aligned parallel to the long axis of bone. The margins are clear and distinct, cortical breach may occur in fast growing cysts or with trauma **(Figs. 28A and B)**. Fallen fragments of bone may be seen within the cyst and is considered pathognomonic.

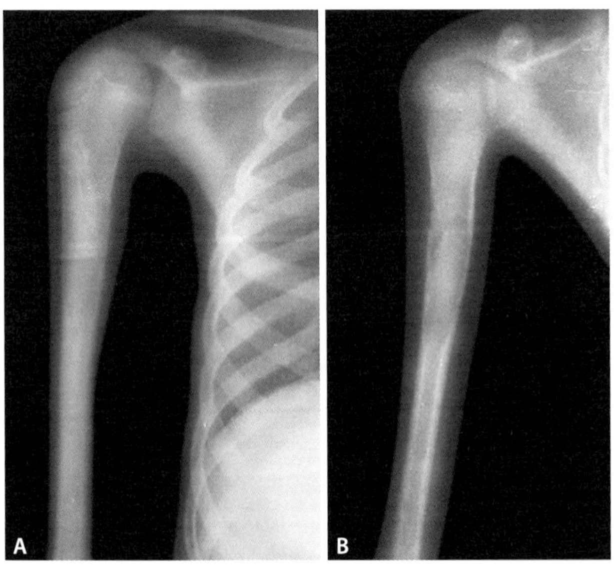

Figs. 28A and B: Unicameral bone cyst (UBC). The patient had an accidental fall with sudden onset of alarming pain in the arm. The radiograph shows a pathological fracture through incidental UBC. Note minimal cortical expansion by the lesion but significant cortical thinning and weakening possibly due to osteoclastic activation by prostaglandins.

Gross and Histopathology

Grossly the cyst is a dilated region of bone containing straw-colored fluid. The walls are generally smooth. The lining of cyst consists of irregular fragments of membranous fibrovascular tissue. Hemosiderin (due to injury), granulation tissue, uncommon giant cells, or scattered chronic inflammatory cells may be additionally present.

Management and Prognosis

Many unicameral cysts heal either spontaneously or following trauma. Pathologic fractures through cyst often heal with healing of cyst unintervened. Impending fracture may be treated with immobilization and aspiration of the cyst along with hydrocortisone injections. For some uncommon cases such as patients with multiple recurrent fractures, lower extremity lesions at-risk of fracture or upper extremity lesions that fail to heal after multiple injections; curettage, with or without bone grafting or cementing may be done. Excision is reserved for recurrent cysts (10% of cases).

Aneurysmal Bone Cyst

Aneurysmal bone cyst also called multilocular or hematinic cyst is a rare (0.14 per 105 individuals) benign neoplastic lesion of bone first recognized by Jaffe and Lichtenstein (1942) that may turn aggressive. It is not a cyst and is called an aneurysm (quite wrongly) only due to characteristic of expanding the bone into "aneurysm" shape and that it is filled with blood. Characteristically, it is seen as multiple fibrous lined communicating spaces that contain hemorrhagic fluid and tissue.

Primary versus Secondary ABC Controversy

Several controversies abound the pathogenesis of ABC but primarily there are two schools of thoughts. One suggests (Tillman and others) that the cysts are *primary* and develop de novo as a result of arteriovenous malformation within the bone. Others (Biesecker and others) do not believe in primary ABC and assert that the cyst is always accompanied by some other tumor into which due to degeneration *secondary ABC* develop. The usual suggestion is that diagnosis of ABC should be made after exclusion of lesions that have tendency toward formation of blood-filled spaces (telangiectasia); that include (these also hence account for most secondary ABCs):

- Giant cell tumor of bone
- Fibrous dysplasia
- Chondroblastoma
- Osteoblastoma
- Nonossifying fibroma (NOF, fibroxanthoma)
- Fibrous histiocytoma
- Electro-oculography (EOG)
- Chondromyxoid fibroma
- Unicameral/simple bone cyst
- Giant cell reparative granuloma
- Telangiectatic osteosarcoma

Support to the de novo pathogenesis has come from cytogenetic studies suggesting that ABCs are true neoplasms.

Abnormalities with coding sequence of the *ubiquitin specific protease 6 (USP6)* gene located at short arm of chromosome 17p13 have been reported. The most common translocation is t(16;17) (q22;p13) that places the *USP6 (TRE2 or TRE17)* oncogene under influence of highly active promoter *CDH11*, but there are many variants **(*see* Table 10)**. These rearrangements are absent in secondary ABCs. Also from the recent studies of successful sclerotherapy for ABC using injectable sclerosants (like polidocanol) instilled directly into cyst support is provided to notion that ABC is a distinct pathological entity. Familial cases of ABC have been distinctly reported and ABCs have been seen as a part of Goltz syndrome and Van Buchem syndrome making possibility of a primary lesion real. ABCs have been, however, frequently found (30–50% of cases) accompanying the mentioned primary pathologies. Possibly both primary (50–70%) and secondary (30–50%) forms exist, we feel, due to common pathogenesis of telangiectasia that can arise either de novo or in pre-existing lesions.

A third variant called *"solid" ABC* has been described (coined by Sanerkin et al.) in 1983 that describes a lesion containing the characteristic reticulated, lacy, chondroid-like material seen in conventional ABC, but without the typical vascular and cyst like cavities. They are closely related to giant cell reparative granuloma (*USP6* gene mutation is seen in them too!) and represent some 5–10% of the ABCs. There are loosely arranged areas of spindle-cell proliferation, scattered giant cells arranged around hemorrhages and abundant reactive new bone formation that may be confused histologically with low-grade osteosarcoma. Although ABCs are commonly found in bone, a fourth variant called the *"soft tissue ABCs"* has also been reported.

Clinical Features

Although, the cyst can be seen in any age (especially secondary ABC), the primary ABC is typically seen to affect the individuals in first 2 decades. The metaphyseal regions in long bones (femur, tibia, and humerus) are commonly affected by the de novo lesion; however, secondary ABC has site predilection according to the primary lesion. In axial spine, the sacrum, pelvis (represent 50% of flat bone lesions), and vertebrae have been reportedly involved. The ABC in vertebrae characteristically involves the posterior elements. The lesion is usually solitary, however, multiple site involvement in same patients has also been reported and can be seen in 5% of patients. Patients commonly have pain and swelling at the site, however, neurological symptoms may be seen as primary complaint in ABCs affecting the vertebrae. Unusually, patients may present with a pathological fracture **(Figs. 29A and B)** at the site of ABC (not uncommon in spine).

Radiology

The radiological features vary with the developmental four stages of ABC also called evolution of ABC. In the incipient phase (usually identified incidentally), there is a small nonexpansile intramedullary (often eccentric) lytic lesion that may have permeative margins **(Fig. 30B)**. There is distinctive

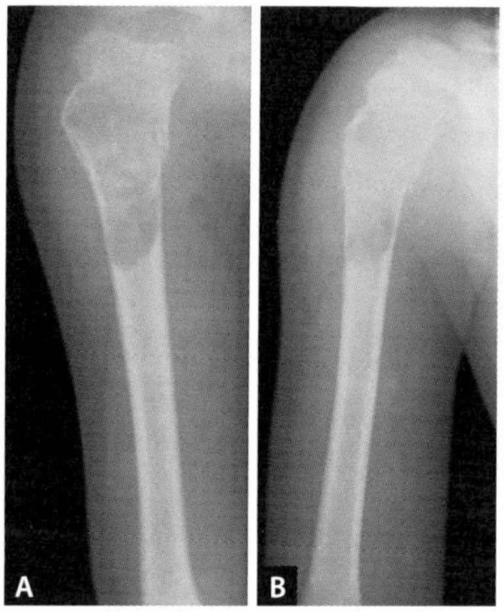

Figs. 29A and B: Pathological fracture of proximal humerus occurring across the aneurysmal bone cyst. The cyst caused thinning of cortices weakening of bone that fractures following a simple fall.

elevation of periosteum. During growth phase, there is rapid growth and lysis of bone that may present as cortical blowout in "accelerated" phenomenon of ABC. The Codman triangles may be prominent at the ends. In the stable phase, there is expanded bone with a "shell" around the lesion along with trabeculations coursing within it (coarse soap-bubble appearance, **Fig. 30A**). The healing cyst (self-resolution or following treatment) shows progressive ossification, resulting in a coarsely trabeculated bony mass often with mineralized matrix. Fluid/blood levels (requires minimum 10 minutes of patient in still position) with multiple internal septae on MRI are a characteristic finding **(Fig. 30C)**. There is increased T1-signal in dependent fluid (due to methemoglobin) while septations are more prominent on T2-weighted images. The cyst may invaginate into normal bone and to epiphysis through growth plate or extend into soft tissue. Capanna et al. described five "morphologic types" (separate from grades mentioned in treatment) based on the radiographic findings:

- *Type I:* Central metaphyseal lesion well-contained within bone with intact bone cortices.
- *Type II:* Lesion gives an inflated appearance to bone with cortical thinning.
- *Type III:* Eccentric metaphyseal location with unaffected cortex.
- *Type IV:* Subperiosteal extension but cortex intact rarely seen in the diaphysis.
- *Type V:* Metadiaphyseal location blowout appearance, cortical breach present, and cyst may invaginate into nearby bone.

Gross and Microscopic Pathology

Intact cut specimens reveal a thin osseous shell surrounding a honeycombed sponge-like mass filled with blood. In secondary ABCs, the solid areas represent the primary bone lesion. On microscopy, the anastomosing cavernous areas filled with blood represent the gross honeycombed structure. These spaces are, however, walled by thin fibrous tissue containing fibroblasts, myofibroblasts, osteoid and

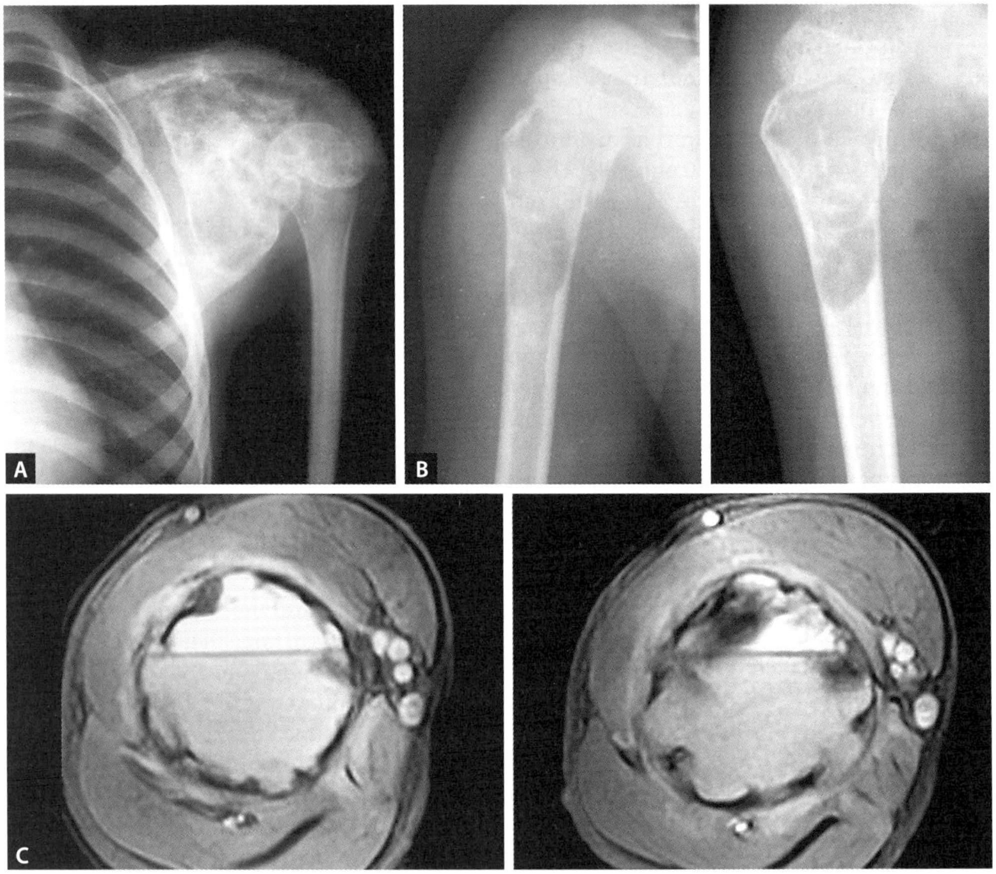

Figs. 30A to C: Aneurysmal bone cyst (ABC). (A) ABC of scapula involving virtually the whole bone in an atypical presentation with the "coarse soap bubble" appearance; (B) Typically located ABC in the proximal metaphyseal region of humerus with pathological fracture; (C) Demonstrates the typical blood fluid levels seen on an MRI of ABC.

chondroid tissue, and osteoclast-like giant cells in varying proportions (instead of smooth muscle wall or endothelial cells of blood vessels of true cavernous vascular spaces). In one-third cases, characteristic reticulated lacy chondroid-like material (described as calcified matrix with a chondroid aura) is seen that actually histologically represents reparative tissue (Campanacci et al.). This has led to the acceptance of ABC as a secondary reparative lesion in primary pathologies (see earlier).

Differential Diagnosis

Telangiectatic osteosarcoma, ossifying hematoma, and hemophilic pseudotumor, large UBC, and Brown tumor.

Treatment

After histopathological diagnosis, the treatment options are multiple and best one for a patient needs to be individualized. Some guide can be taken from Capanna classification of ABC radiologically into three "grades". The inactive cysts have complete periosteal shell and sclerotic bone margins. In contrast, active cysts have incomplete shell and aggressive lesions have indefinite margins. Inactive lesions may be observed as spontaneous regression has been observed. Active and aggressive ABCs are treated by one of the following treatments depending on surgeon's preference.

- Percutaneous methods for inducing sclerosis in the cyst and secondary mineralization (healing) have become recently popular for treatment of extremity and pelvic regions. They have advantage particularly in the juxtaphyseal location and difficult surgical sites **(Figs. 31A to D)**. Alcoholic solution of zein has been investigated by various authors and has good efficacy, but the side effects of percutaneous fistulation, local abscess formation, and sometimes embolization have raised concerns. Polidocanol is an effective, cheap, and reasonably safe alternative that has shown good success in some large studies focused on ABC treatment. Sclerotherapy possibly acts by mechanism same as its role in varicose veins treatment wherein the walls of the cyst containing the active spindle cells are inactivated and the lytic effects subside. Healing of bone then takes precedence, healing the cyst in due course of 6–18 months depending on the size of initial lesion.
- Use of demineralized bone particle instilled into the lesion as a paste of allogenic bone powder and autogenous bone marrow has been reported to induce healing. No curettage or extensive surgery is done, particulated bone allograft is easy to handle and introduce into an irregular cavity. It is expected that the bone grafting material promoting ossification at a pace faster that the native rate

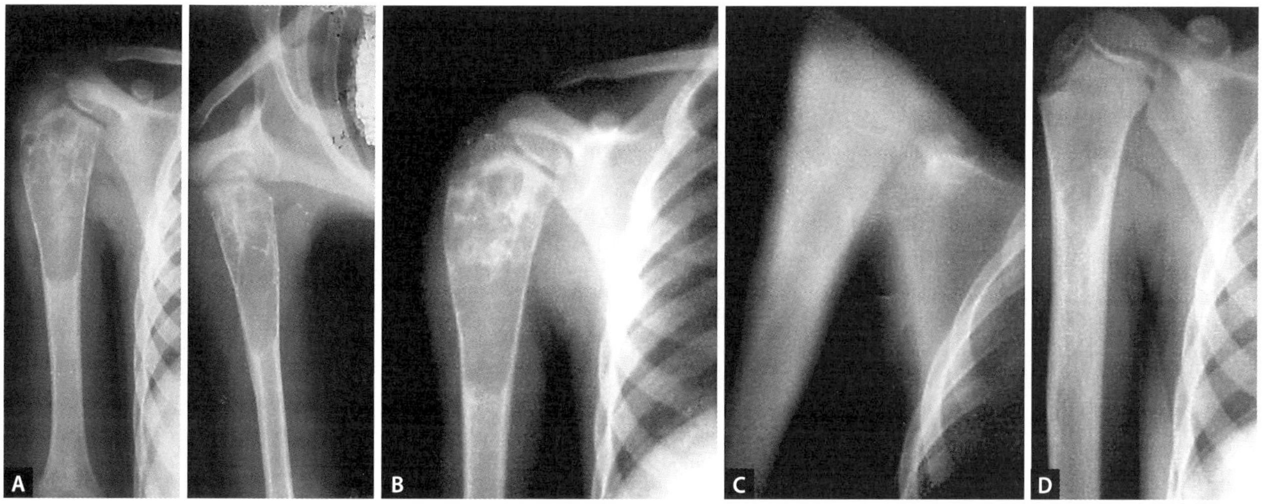

Figs. 31A to D: Sclerotherapy as used to treat aneurysmal bone cyst (ABC)—the resolution is steadily progressive and technique is quite beneficial for juxtaphyseal cysts.

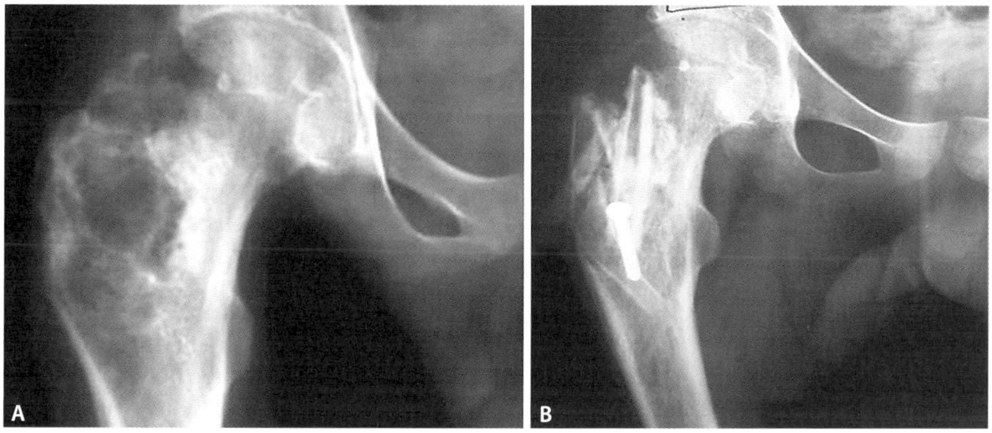

Figs. 32A and B: The long-standing gold standard for treatment of aneurysmal bone cyst is curettage and bone grafting.

of ABC expansion. It also utilizes the repair potential of conventional ABC, in-effect reversing the lesion.
The percutaneous methods are not to be used in patients with rapid expansion of the cyst causing local and distal neurological or vascular symptoms as the time to healing is quite long. It should also be not used in impending fractures and patients allergic to drug.

- Curettage and bone grafting had been the gold standard of treatment that is still used to compare efficacy of other methods **(Figs. 32A and B)**. The curettage can be supplemented with the use of high-speed burr, or extended curettage has been proposed using various adjuvants (peroxide, phenol, cryotherapy, zinc chloride, hypochlorite, and PMMA bone cement) to reduce recurrence rate. The rates of recurrence are quite unacceptable (7–50%) in various series with the use of conventional curettage alone with or without bone grafting, so extended curettage is recommended. Selective arterial embolization has been used for reducing the blood loss in large cysts that are at difficult surgical location but should not be used to rely upon for inducing healing. Growth plate can get damaged while treating the juxtaphyseal lesions **(Figs. 33A and B)**.
- Marginal *en bloc* resection can be done in expendable bones (fibula, clavicle, rib, and pubic ramus) and has got the lowest recurrence rates **(Figs. 34A to C)**. Subperiosteal resection is possible in children which can be simultaneously reconstructed with fibula.
- Radiation therapy though has been found effective in inducing healing and ossification should be abandoned for high likelihood of inducing radiation sarcoma.

Subchondral Cysts and Intraosseous Ganglion

The subchondral cysts ("geodes" radiologically) are well-defined lytic lesion in periarticular region located just below cartilage and associated with degenerative joint disease. They are filled with mucinous fluid and when curetted a thin fibrous lining can be peeled from the periphery. Similar structure when found in epiphyseal or intramedullary location not associated with degenerative joint disease are called intraosseous ganglion (IOG). IOG can present in younger patients and teenagers too **(Figs. 35A and B)**, while subchondral cysts are seen in elderly with degenerated joints or in younger patients with rheumatoid arthritis, CPPD deposition disease or avascular necrosis. Subchondral cysts

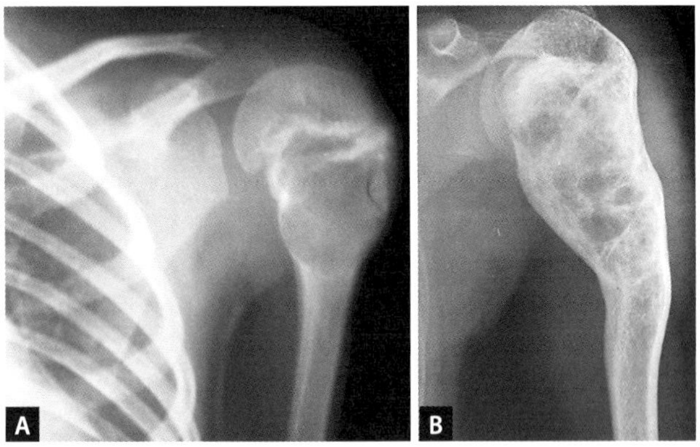

Figs. 33A and B: Complication of curettage and bone grafting for aneurysmal bone cyst (ABC)—the growth plate got damaged during the index surgery leading to premature fusion and growth abnormalities of the bone.

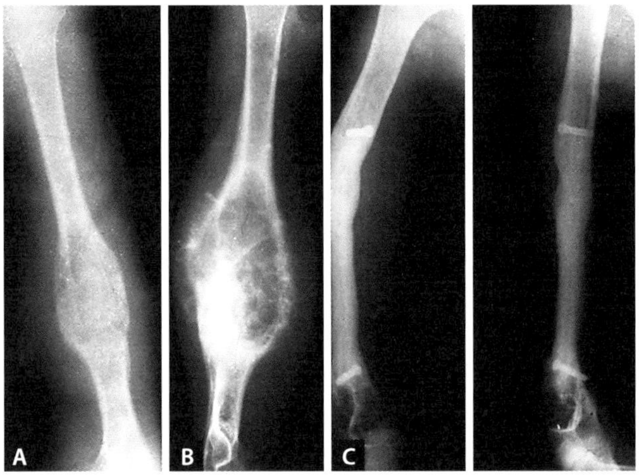

Figs. 34A to C: Excision and bone grafting for treatment of aneurysmal bone cyst (ABC).

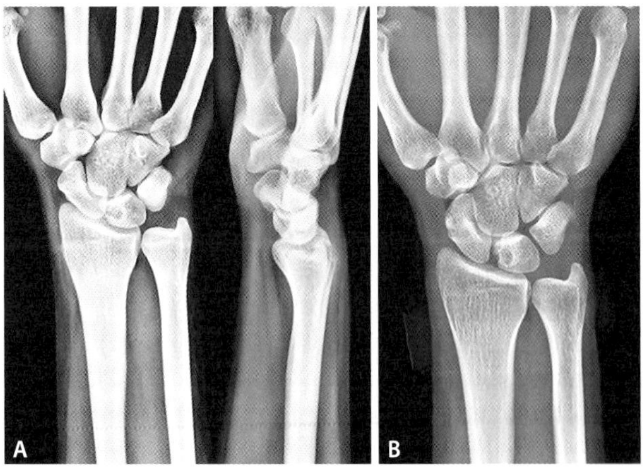

Figs. 35A and B: Intraosseous ganglion. (A) A 19-year-old female presented with severe pain and mild swelling on dorsum of wrist and the lesion was curetted (B) from the lunate bone.

may be confused with chondroblastoma or GCT while IOG should be differentiated from chondromyxoid fibroma. Both entities do not require specific therapy; however, for some symptomatic IOG intralesional excision may be done.

Osteoma

Osteoma consists of abnormally dense lamellar bone deposition typically in craniofacial bones. It may not represent true tumor pathologically, however, the occurrence of multiple osteomas in "gardeners" syndrome suggests some genetic linkage or possible chromosomal abnormality that may qualify for neoplasm. Osteomas in facial sinuses occur in males commonly while that of jaws occurs in females. Spongy variant of osteoma containing fibrofatty component has been described. Osteomas should be differentiated from osteosclerosis, enostosis, osteochondromas, and parosteal osteosarcomas. Some people use term fibro-osteoma and chondro-osteoma for occasional finding of ancillary fibrous or chondroid tissue but these possibly represent degenerated osteochondromas.

Osteoid Osteoma (ICD-O code 9191/0)

Osteoid osteoma is defined by the WHO as a benign bone-forming tumor characterized by small size, limited growth potential and disproportionate pain. It is a painful small osteoblastic lesion first described by Bergstrand. The lesion has a characteristic nidus usually <1.5 cm (lesions > 2 cm are osteoblastomas by definition, in-between size is a gray area until it evolves or regresses into one of the two to match definitions!). Central nidus is the predominant pain producing component. It is surrounded by normal sclerotic bone due to reactive sympathetic bone deposition. The pain is typically nocturnal and responds to aspirin and NSAIDs. Osteoid osteoma has been reported from every bone of body and in all age (1–70 years) groups but has a predilection for large bones of appendicular skeleton usually in first 3 decades of life. Femur and tibia account for most of the cases followed by humerus and axial skeleton. The lesions are classically *cortical* in long bones located in the diaphysis while *periosteal* and *intramedullary* forms can be seen in small tubular bone. Few cases have been reported with the involvement of chromosome 22q13 and loss of part of chromosome 17q.

Clinical Features

Males in first 3 decades are affected more often than females, equalizing later in life. *Pain* is intermittent initially that becomes intensified later to disturb sleep. The localized pain is typically nocturnal and is relieved promptly by acetylsalicylic acid, characteristic of osteoid osteoma. Pain is due to high concentration (100–1,000 times normal) of *PGE2* in the nidus that excites the abundant nerve endings in the nidus. There is often an area of exquisite, localized *tenderness* associated with the lesion, and there may be redness and localized swelling. Radiological identification may be difficult in atypical forms like those in spine where patient may present with painful scoliosis or in periarticular bones where joint contractures, stiffness may be the first presenting features. Osteoid osteomas of hand have been treated with multiple surgeries and even ray amputations for atypical nature of presentation (finger swelling and inflammatory features). Around 5–15% are intra-articular and infrequently respond to salicylates for pain relief. They may cause reactive inflammatory arthritis, secondary osteoarthritis, and ectopic ossification. They are difficult to diagnose radiologically and in the absence of typical symptoms, it may get delayed for months. Bone scan followed by MRI or CT would help diagnose the lesion.

Radiology

Classical presentation is a small lucent round to ovoid lesion in a radiodense area of bone corresponding to the site of clinical pain. The central lucent lesion is commonly 0.5–1 cm in diameter but never >1.5 cm by definition. Larger lesions usually harbinger osteoblastoma so should always raise suspicion. Uncommon lesions with central ossification may have "target" appearance. Radiological localization could be difficult in periarticular regions and in axial skeleton (so rely on other modalities). 99Tc-MDP bone scans consistently reveal hot spot at the osteoid osteoma and can be used to narrow down the site of involvement (especially in above-mentioned radiologically difficult locations). Noncontrast computed tomography (NCCT) is a very good investigation to localize the lesion in all planes especially for surgical or radioablation purpose. On the NCCT, the typical features are small nidus that may have variably extending high density area within **(Figs. 36A to C)**. Reactive peripheral sclerosis surrounds the nidus as usual. Spinal lesions are common in neural arch and may be localized to apophyseal joint or even articular process. On MRI, the lesion appears isoechoic to muscle on T1-weighted images. The T2-weighted image has increased intensity but is still lower than the short tau-inverted images (STIR) sequence where it is hyperintense. Bone marrow edema is seen in around 60% of patients. Intra-articular osteoid osteoma may additionally have synovitis and effusion that is detected on MRI. MRI is better for diagnosis of cancellous bone osteoid osteoma but is inferior to cortical bone osteoid osteoma compared to NCCT. Hypervascularity of the nidus may be misinterpreted for aggressive lesions.

Gross and Microscopic Pathology

With unaided eyes, the nidus appears red, spherical gritty tissue that can be shelled out from the surrounding bone neatly. The nidus appears highly vascular, sharply defined osteoblastic proliferation with poor ossification. The osteoblasts are metabolically active, however, no atypia is seen. Thin fibrovascular tissue surrounds the nidus around which is the normal lamellar dense bone. The previous connotation of "giant osteoid osteoma" possibly represents osteoblastoma.

Differential Diagnosis

Osteoblastoma, salmonella osteomyelitis, sclerosing osteomyelitis of Garre, bone island, and stress fracture.

Treatment

Osteoid osteomas have been known to undergo spontaneous resolution and symptoms may subside over 3–4 years. Most diaphyseal osteoid osteomas, however, require intervention for pain relief. En bloc resection (burr-down technique) followed by intralesional curettage had been the standard approach **(Figs. 37A to C and 38A to F)**; however, various recent modalities to minimize associated surgical trauma have been used. These include radiofrequency ablation (heating to 80°C) under CT or ultrasound guidance, laser-guided interstitial thermal therapy, laser photocoagulation, ethanol injection, and cryotherapy. During surgical excision, identification of the lesion is most important. Several different approaches have been tried. Overpenetrated films give fine detail. Tetracycline labeling the lesion (giving preoperative tetracycline) and localization intraoperatively by ultraviolet light can be done but has low sensitivity. Intraoperative bone scan and using a portable gamma camera has been reported but is too cumbersome. Intraoperative CT scan (modern C-arm has the facility to do intraoperative CT also) identification is the best way to identify osteoid osteoma. This or at some centers ultrasonography is used for radiofrequency ablation (RFA). RFA is now considered the most favorable method for accessible lesions. It has the striking advantages of being minimally invasive and can be performed on a day-care basis. Only issue is inability to obtain histopathological diagnosis with this treatment. Microwave ablation and scanned marking are other strategies. It is anyway imperative

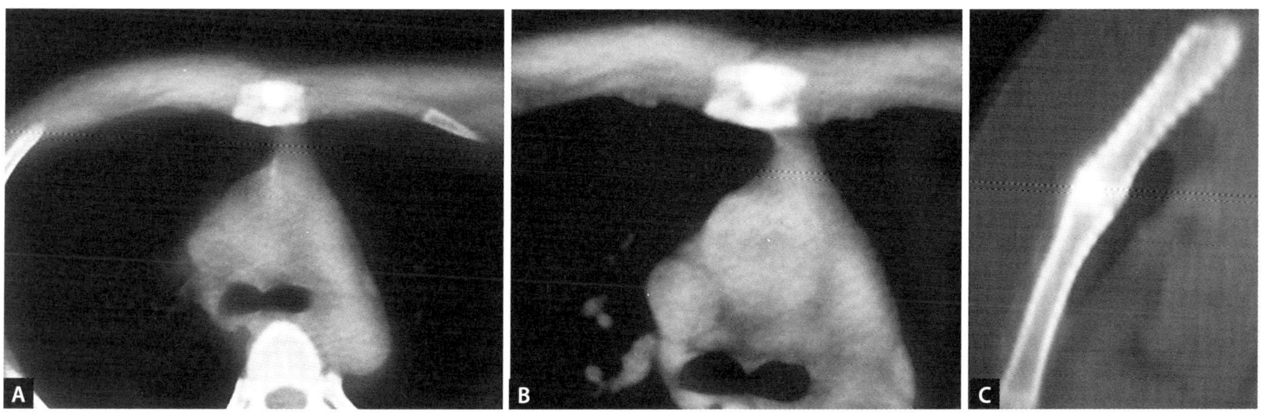

Figs. 36A to C: Osteoid osteoma. Contrast-enhanced CT showing nodular sclerotic thickening at the manubriosternal junction with no contrast enhancement and no soft tissue components.

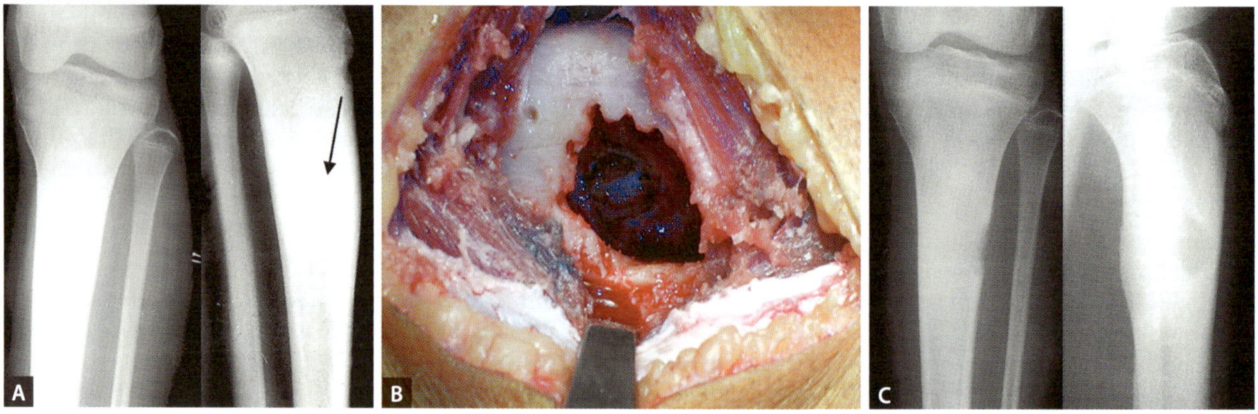

Figs. 37A to C: Osteoid osteoma. (A) There is a predominantly sclerotic lesion of proximal tibia with barely discernable central lucency at the center more appreciable on lateral radiograph (arrow); (B) Intraoperative photograph shows the cauterized oval lesion on posteromedial cortex visible as a target lesion from the lateral cortical window; (C) Postoperative radiograph demonstrating the curetted lesion.

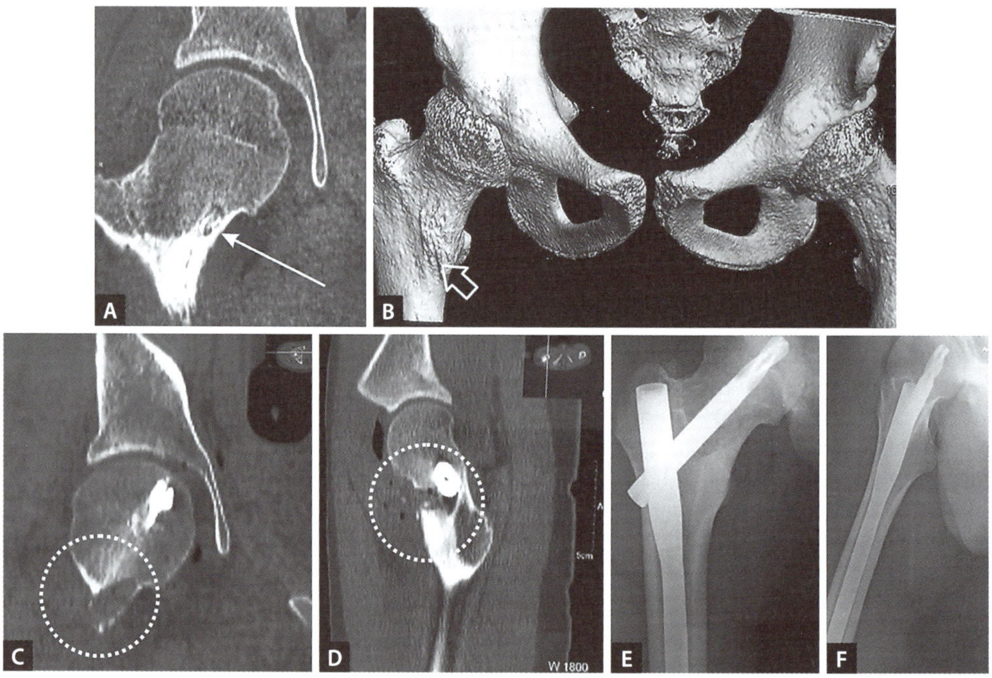

Figs. 38A to F: Osteoid osteoma of proximal femur in the neck region (A) showing well-defined nidus (arrow) and distal hyperostosis near the intertrochanteric line (B, block arrow). The lesion was burred down using intraoperative CT-scan using 8-mm drill over a guidewire with complete destruction of the lesion (dotted oval, C and D) and was prophylactically fixed with intramedullary implant to prevent iatrogenic fracture through the weakened cortex (E and F).

to send the tissue for frozen section confirmation after excision. We additionally cauterize the surrounding bone using standard diathermy to ablate any remaining tissue.

Osteoblastoma

(ICD-O code 9200/0, aka Giant Osteoid Osteoma, Cementoblastoma of Jaw, Ossifying GCT)

The World Health Organization defined osteoblastoma as a rare benign bone-forming neoplasm which produces woven bone spicules, which are bordered by prominent osteoblasts. These are clinically [benign, painful site, male preponderance (2.5:1), majority seen below 30 years] and microscopically (central nidus surrounded by dense lamellar bone) similar to osteoid osteomas with some differences **(Table 15)**. The pain in osteoblastoma is less intense, aspirin is mostly ineffective if pain occurs, they have predilection for axial skeleton (especially posterior elements of spine), may have lobulated margins, higher degree of trabecular haphazardness (instead of orderly zonal pattern of central ossification in osteoid osteoma), and the lesion size is always >2 cm. The osteoblastomas could also become aggressive (malignant osteoblastomas or possibly low-grade osteosarcomas) and are seen in patients above 30 years of age. They are larger than conventional osteoblastomas and have tendency to recur after surgical treatment. The osteoblasts here are large having epithelioid appearance with histiocyte-like vesicular nuclei. Conventional osteoblastomas may be epiphyseal or metaphyseal or diaphyseal and majority are cortical (60%) or intramedullary (35%), while periosteal forms have also been described. The epiphyseal form is most rare occurring in short tubular bones of hands and feet. Microscopically aggressive, malignant, and pseudomalignant forms have been described but their impact on clinical management is undefined.

Radiology

These are uniform, geographic, lytic lesions 3–10 cm in size (range 2–15 cm), having rounded to oval appearance lined by a defined periosteal shell. Lesions of posterior elements of spine have presentation like ABC. Larger tumors in appendicular skeleton usually have secondary ABC (10% of cases). Focal areas of calcification may be seen in 30% of patients that indicate bone tumor mineralization **(Figs. 39A to C)**. At unusual locations, the diagnosis may require obtaining CT scans **(Figs. 40A and B)**. NCCT much better determines the containment of lesion and exact extent.

Rare and inconsistent genetic alterations have been reported some hinting at cell cycle dysregulation related to aggressive potential. Overexpression of hepatocyte growth factor (MET/HGF receptor), MDM2 amplification, and TP53 deletion at splice region has been sporadically reported in aggressive forms.

TABLE 15: Differentiating features of osteoid osteoma and osteoblastoma.

Osteoid osteoma	***Osteoblastoma***
Patient is usually between 5 and 15 years of age	Presents at an older age (range 10–30 years)
Common lesion (10% of benign bone lesions)	Uncommon (1/5th as common as osteoid osteoma)
Reported in every bone of skeleton (the most common proximal femur)	Predilection for spine
Pain is intense and constant, typically nocturnal	Less intense pain and is sporadic
Pain is predictably relieved by NSAIDs (classically aspirin)	Pain unresponsive to NSAIDs
Radiologically central nidus is usually <1 cm and never >2 cm	The nidus by definition is 2 cm or more
There is well-defined and prominent perifocal dense osseous reaction visible as sclerosis	Radiologically, a lytic well-circumscribed lesion confined by a periosteal shell of reactive bone
Cortex is thickened	Cortex is thinned out
Histopathology: • Osteoid trabeculae with zonal pattern of central ossification • Scanty fibrous stromal reaction • Rare multinucleated giant cells	*Histopathology:* • Discontinuous and irregular bone formation • Abundant fibrous stromal reaction • Abundant multinucleated giant cells
Clinically, a benign course	Much aggressive clinical course if untreated

Clinical Features

Axial osteoblastomas present with back pain, scoliosis, and nerve root compression. Cementoblastoma of jaw presents with tooth pain. The characteristic clinical feature that distinguishes them from osteoid osteoma is that aspirin typically does not relieve symptoms. Localized tenderness is present in appendicular lesions (distal femur, proximal tibia, and proximal femur).

Gross and Microscopic Pathology

Grossly, the tumor appears as a red-brownish lesion with gritty consistency due to ossification areas. The tumor has a defined cortical shell or periosteal reactive shell if cortical breach is present that separates the tumor from surrounding soft tissue. The tumor has a "pushing" border unless it grows into aggressive form and may then permeate the periphery but not into nearby tissue which is characteristic of osteosarcoma. Microscopically, the tumor has anastomozing bony trabeculae in a fibrovascular stroma similar to osteoid osteoma. The bony trabeculae have typical osteoblastic rimming that separates this from low-grade osteosarcoma **(Table 16)**. Low-grade osteosarcoma has sheets of osteoblasts. Early osteoblastoma lesions are usually rich in giant cells with occasional chondroid differentiation (if there is a fracture).

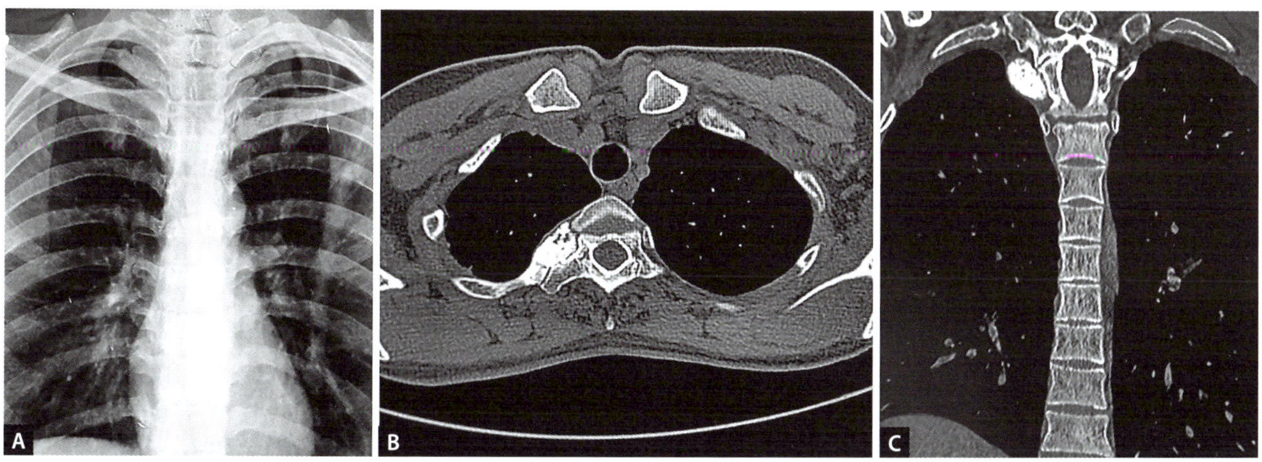

Figs. 39A to C: Unusual osteoblastoma of third rib. The patient presented with pain in the dorsum of back and along right T3 dermatome with some periscapular radiation. On evaluation, she was found to have osteoid producing radiodense mass along head and neck of the third rib (A). The findings were confirmed on NCCT chest (B and C), diagnosed by CT-guided biopsy and treatment was done by resection of the lesion.

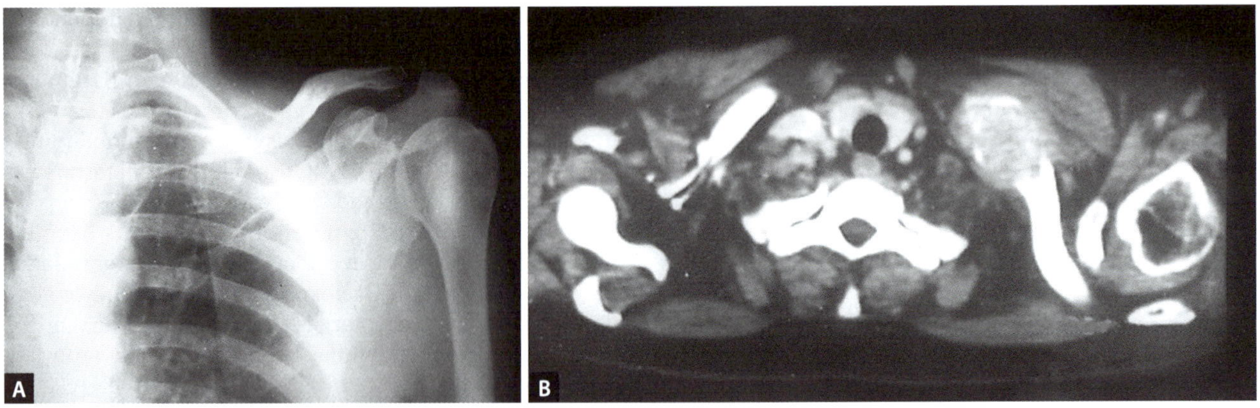

Figs. 40A and B: Osteoblastoma of clavicle better identified on contrast-enhanced computed tomography (CECT) scan.

TABLE 16: Differentiating between osteoblastoma and low-grade osteosarcoma.

Osteoblastoma	*Low-grade osteosarcoma*
Involves short and flat bones and spine	Seen commonly in long bones of skeleton
Long history of intermittent pain with multiple symptomatic treatments	Short history of presentation starting from pain to swelling
Low mitotic rate	High mitotic rate
Atypical mitosis is absent as a rule	Atypical mitosis seen
Microscopically, there is anastomosing bony trabeculae in fibrovascular stroma	Microscopically, lace-like osteoid is seen
Invasion of surrounding structures is not seen	Permeation of surroundings is a common

Secondary ABC may develop in larger tumors with cystic changes (possibly represent degenerative changes).

Differential Diagnosis

Osteoid osteoma (only based on size), low-grade osteosarcoma, GCT, and ABC in spine.

Treatment

Surgical excision is the preferred treatment **(Figs. 41A to C)**. Wide local resection is the usual method but some small lesions may be treated with intralesional curettage or marginal excision. For larger tumors and features of aggressiveness, adjunctive treatment with PMMA cement or cryotherapy should be combined with extended curettage to reduce recurrence rate.

Osteosarcoma (Osteogenic Sarcoma)

These are group of second most common malignant bone neoplasm 2nd only to MM when bone neoplasias are studied overall. They, but, account for the most common primary bone sarcomas. They are also the most common bone-forming malignant neoplasms **(Table 17)** that are characterized by proliferating "neoplastic cells that directly lay down osteoid" (immature bone matrix which is demonstrable at least focally by definition, see later). Not only is this the most common bone sarcoma, it is this tumor that has brought up the "clinico-pathological impression of heterogeneity" in bone tumors as osteosarcoma can have several subtypes, the most typical of which is called conventional osteosarcoma (commonly taught during graduation). WHO defines conventional osteosarcoma as a primary intramedullary high-grade malignant tumor in which the neoplastic cells produce osteoid, even if only in small amounts. Conventional form is divided into several histological patterns depending on the finding of predominant tissue, though they do not have any prognostic significance. Other variants of osteosarcoma apart from conventional form have also been described as follows:

- Conventional osteosarcoma:
  - Osteosarcoma not otherwise specified, conventional central osteosarcoma, medullary osteosarcoma (ICD-O 9180/3)
  - Chondroblastic (ICD-O 9181/3)
  - Osteoblastic
  - Fibroblastic (osteofibrosarcoma ICD-O 9182/3)
  - Fibrohistiocytic (MFH like)
  - Giant cell rich osteosarcoma
  - Osteoblastoma-like osteosarcoma
  - Intracortical osteosarcoma (ICD-O 9195/3)
- Ewing's like osteosarcoma (small cell osteosarcoma)
- Low-grade intramedullary osteosarcoma
- High-grade surface osteosarcoma
- Telangiectatic osteosarcoma (malignant bone aneurysm, hemorrhagic osteosarcoma, ABC-like osteosarcoma)
- Parosteal osteosarcoma
- Periosteal osteosarcoma
- Intracortical osteosarcoma
- Multicentric osteosarcoma
- Secondary osteosarcoma
- Osteosarcoma of the jaw

Some orthopedic oncology groups classify osteosarcoma into surface (parosteal, periosteal, and high-grade surface) and intramedullary forms but this misses other histopathological forms mentioned above. The above comprehensive classification attempts to include as many forms described in literature. Usually, the surface osteosarcomas are low-grade (so high-grade surface is an atypical variant) and intramedullary forms are high-grade (so low-grade intramedullary is atypical).

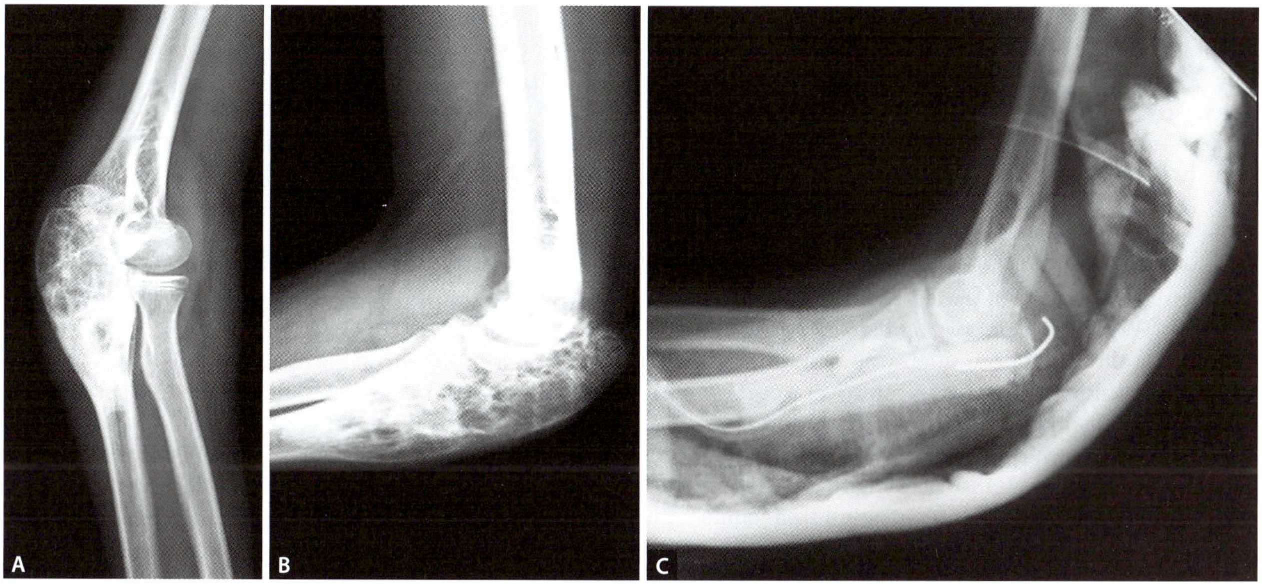

Figs. 41A to C: Osteoblastoma of olecranon—treated with excision and curettage.

TABLE 17: List of most common bone lesions.

Description	***Tumor name***
Most common primary malignant bone tumor	Myeloma
Second most common primary malignant bone tumor	Osteosarcoma
Third most common primary malignant bone tumor	Chondrosarcoma
Most common soft tissue tumor (children)	Hemangioma
Most common bone sarcoma	Osteosarcoma
Soft tissue tumor (adults)	Lipoma
Most common malignant bone tumor in children	Osteosarcoma
Second most common bone tumor in children	Ewing's sarcoma
Malignant soft tissue tumor (children)	Rhabdomyosarcoma
Malignant soft tissue tumor (adults)	Malignant fibrous histiocytoma
Most common primary benign bone tumor	Osteochondroma
Most common secondary lesion in a pre-existing tumor	Aneurysmal bone cyst
Most common secondary malignancies	• Malignant fibrous histiocytoma • Osteosarcoma • Fibrosarcoma
Most common tumor of phalanx	Enchondroma
Most common sarcoma of the hand	Epithelioid sarcoma
Most common sarcoma of the foot and ankle	Synovial sarcoma

Conventional osteosarcoma is distributed throughout the world without any racial or ethnical differences. It is a disease of adolescents and young adults affecting 60% patients under 25 years of age, and 25% cases occur in patients "over 40 years of age—so has a *bimodal distribution*". The second hump of bimodal distribution is lower (less cases) and predisposing conditions should be explored in these cases. There is a conspicuous male preference in younger patients (3:2) that diminishes with increasing age. Three-fourths of all tumors are located in the actively growing (rapid bone turnover) regions of long tubular bones (distal femur, proximal tibia, proximal femur, proximal humerus, distal tibia, and distal humerus). Metaphyseal region is the site for over 85% of these tumors, the diaphysis accounts for some 10% and epiphysis is very rare. Familial and syndromic cases "have been reported, prominent of which are detailed here."

- There is a strong association of *retinoblastoma* and osteosarcoma. Children with bilateral retinoblastomas have very high risk of developing osteosarcoma compared to normal population. There is loss of heterozygosity (LOH) at 13q (long arm of chromosome 13) and corresponding alterations in the Rb1 (retinoblastoma) tumor suppressor gene with poorer prognosis.
- In the *Li-Fraumeni syndrome*, there is an LOH in 17p13.1 (TP53 germline mutations are seen in about 35% of these patients) and is also associated with poorer prognosis.
- Patients with *Rothmund-Thomson syndrome* (also known as poikiloderma congenitale) due to mutations of the *RECQL4* helicase gene on 8q24 have tendency to develop osteosarcoma at a younger age. The patients have characteristic skin findings (e.g., atrophy, telangiectasias, and pigmentation) and other features such as sparse hair, cataracts, small stature, skeletal anomalies, and lastly the significantly higher risk for osteosarcoma.
- *Bloom syndrome* due to *DNA helicase* gene mutation at 15q26.1 [BLM (RECQL3)] is also associated with increased osteosarcoma risk.
- Other syndromes that have been identified to have increased risk for osteosarcoma include *Diamond-Blackfan anemia* (ribosomal protein gene mutation) and Werner syndrome [mutation of *DNA helicase* gene WRN (*RecQL2*)] at 8p12-p11.2.

Secondary osteosarcoma is predisposed on other lesions such as Paget's disease (*LOH18CR1* at 18q21-qa22), autologous stem cell transplantation, osteogenesis imperfecta, bone infarct, chronic osteomyelitis, fibrous dysplasia (especially Albright's syndrome), osteochondroma, GCT or osteoblastoma. Irradiation for various tumors used previously (Ewing's, GCT, ABC, etc.) is a significant risk factor for development of secondary osteosarcoma.

- Postirradiation sarcoma comprises some 3.5–5% of cases. The risk estimated for sarcoma to develop in irradiated bone is 0.03–0.08% with children treated with irradiation at the greatest risk. The prevalence is rising also due to increased survival of patients with primary disease. There should be a latent period between exposure and development of tumor to qualify as radiation induced sarcoma. Median latency is around 11 years though as little as 2 years has also been observed and most sarcomas occur with cumulative dose of 55 Gy or more. Radiologically, these tumors are highly radiodense and sclerotic, radiation osteitis (coarsened trabeculae with lytic cortical areas) can be seen in half of the cases. Though multiple complex genetic alterations are seen but loss of 3p is frequent in postirradiation sarcoma. In general, they have poorer prognosis mostly due to surgically difficult site of occurrence (pelvis and vertebra).
- Sarcomatous change in Paget's disease is seen in 0.7–1% of cases and most of them are osteosarcoma (50–60%). Sarcomatous change occurs in patients with extensive disease but has higher frequency in humerus and much lower in vertebrae. Multifocal disease is also common superimposed on multifocal Paget's. Lytic tumors are more common than blastic or sclerotic patterns on radiology. Histopathologically, the tumors are high grade and mostly osteoblastic or fibroblastic. Genetic alteration in the form of LOH at 18q is common. The prognosis is poor with limited survival and patients with multifocal disease are quick to succumb. Metastasis is present in 25% patients at presentation.
- Bone infarct associated sarcomas are commonly MFH, however, a minority can also be osteosarcomas. This malignant transformation in large and multiple bone infarcts is commonly thought to result from an overly enthusiastic reparative process of osteonecrosis.
- Secondary osteosarcoma also has been reported in literature in pediatric patients from autologous hematopoietic stem cell transplantation. These patients are hence kept under surveillance with skeletal survey.
- Some association possibly exists with orthopedic metallic implants and trauma **(Figs. 42A to E)** which is frequently reported but has not been documented well in the studies, and pathogenesis here is difficult to explain scientifically. The association with cementless total hip replacements have been proposed as quoted in case reports. The majority of such cases have resulted in MFH but few cases of osteosarcoma have also been reported.

Characteristically in secondary osteosarcomas, the incidence of tumor formation, flat bone, and diaphyseal involvement is quite high. One must note that in newer system, osteosarcomas that arise upon an underlying low-grade chondrosarcoma are classified as dedifferentiated chondrosarcoma and no more are they included as examples of secondary osteosarcomas.

Extraosseous osteosarcoma (mentioned here for sake of clarification only) is an uncommon malignant mesenchymal neoplasm that does not have any direct bony origin or attachment to the skeletal system. This rare form of osteosarcoma arises in soft tissue or visceral organs.

Genetics of Osteosarcoma

A lot of genetic alterations are described for the osteosarcoma, however, none is specific for diagnosis. The 17p amplification is quite characteristic of this tumor. The gain of 8q23 seen in around half of the tumors possibly indicates poor prognosis. Similarly, *MYC, FOS,* and *Cathepsin L* are overexpressed in many relapsed and metastatic tumors. Bone morphogenetic proteins-6 (BMP-6) expression and BMP receptor-2 are seen in around half of osteosarcomas.

Radiology

Based on the radiological presentation, osteosarcomas can be broadly classified into three categories: (1) sclerotic osteosarcomas (30%), (2) osteolytic osteosarcomas (25%), and (3) mixed pattern (45%). The classical radiologic appearance is an intramedullary combined lytic and sclerotic lesion with a commonly demonstrable cortical breach and is associated with bone-matrix formation. There is commonly a pattern of permeative invasion of the surrounding bone and soft tissue with calcification **(Fig. 43)**. The borders are poorly defined but are not as aggressive as that of rapidly growing Ewing's sarcoma. Lifting of periosteum by rapidly growing mass breaching the cortices produces the characteristic reactive bone formation—Codman angle (also called Codman triangle). MRI is the modality of choice for defining the intramedullary extent and surrounding infiltration by the tumor **(Figs. 44A to C)**. The investigation guides level of excision of the tumor and the muscle groups that can be spared to retain postoperative function. PET scan has a role in identification of metastasis and prognostication of chemotherapy treatment.

Gross and Microscopic Pathology

Section through bone reveals wide extension within the marrow cavity with variegated appearance. In the same lesion bluish areas of lobular cartilaginous growth and gritty bone with foci of hemorrhage and necrosis, and telangiectatic component may be seen. Rarely, skip areas (skip metastasis) can be found. Microscopically, they are high-grade anaplastic spindle cell tumors with mixed osteoblastic, chondroblastic and fibroblastic differentiation associated closely with presence of epithelioid, plasmacytoid, round and clear cells (pleomorphic) but by definition have definite osteoid production **(Figs. 45A and B)**. Very rarely osteoid may be absent from primary tumor (telangiectatic osteosarcoma), but their metastasis has abundant osteoid production justifying the term osteosarcoma. Both malignant and benign osteoblast-like giant cells can be found in the stroma, abundance of latter is referred to as giant cell rich

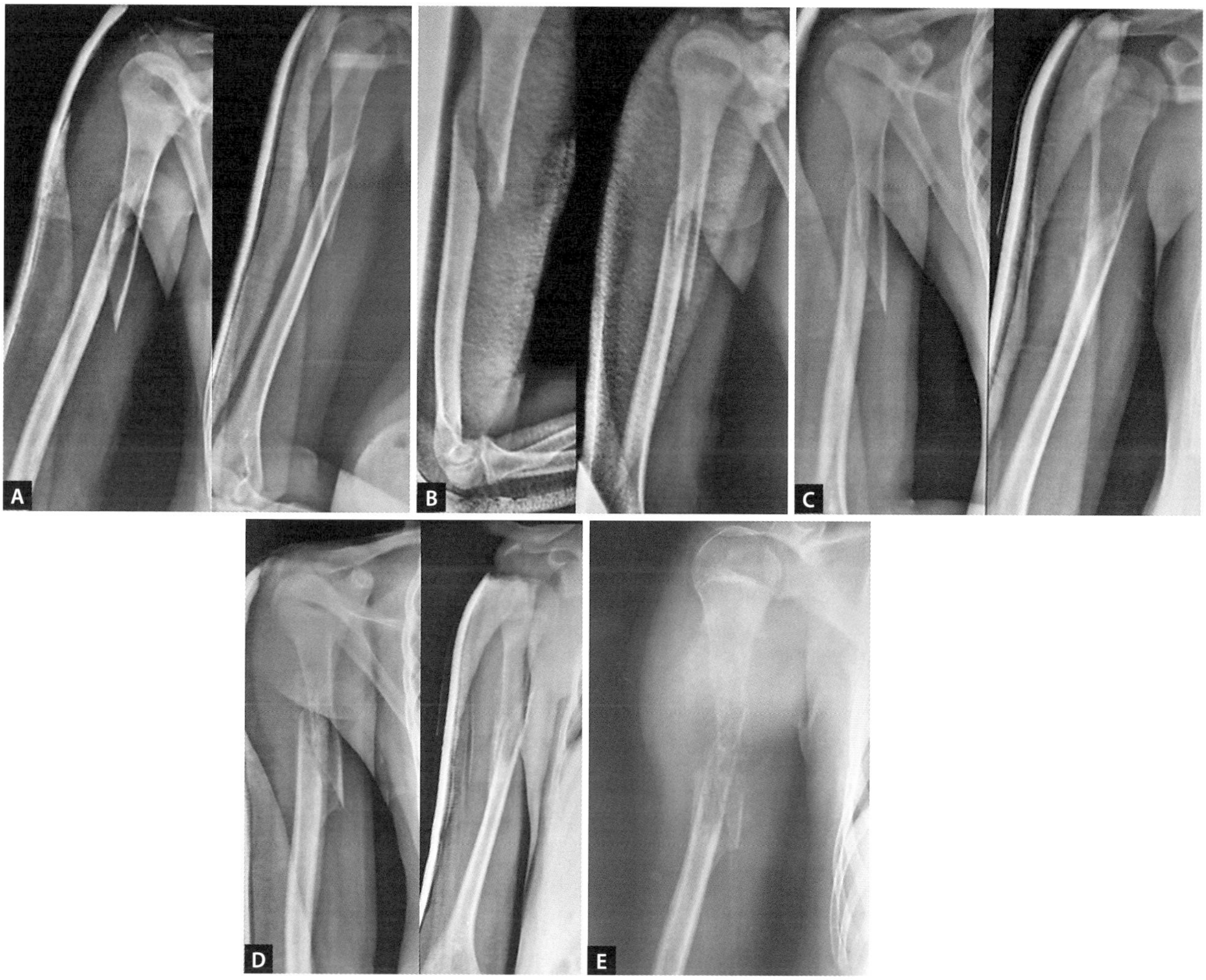

Figs. 42A to E: A 13-year-old male suffered fall from tree injuring right arm and fracturing the humerus on 2nd of January 2013 (A). The treating physician applied POP slab for management and was accepted in the radiographs taken on 25th January 2013. (B) There is evidence of callus formation in radiographs taken on 8th February 2013 (C), that increased in density for radiographs taken on 25th February 2013 (D) but both these radiographs show starting of geographic destruction of the bone around fracture. Radiographs taken on 16th of March show picture of full-blown malignant neoplasia (E) when he presented to us. On biopsy the lesion was found to be a high-grade osteosarcoma. The pathophysiology obviously appears to be trauma in this case as the initial radiograph is innocuous but the precise mechanism for such a progression is unknown and not vehemently defended in literature despite such glaring examples we encounter in our practice.

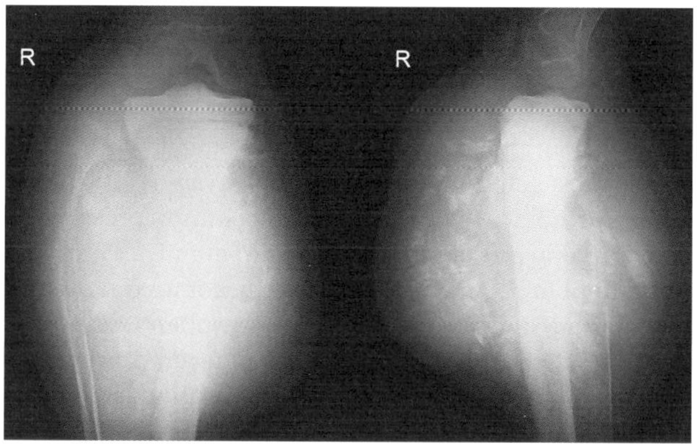

Fig. 43: Osteosarcoma—sclerotic metaphyseal lesion with a sunburst type of periosteal reaction.

osteosarcoma and should be differentiated from GCT. In osteoblastic osteosarcoma, there is predominant production of malignant osteoid. Predominance of malignant cartilage production will be identified as chondroblastic osteosarcoma. Fibroblastic osteosarcoma is characterized by large areas of proliferating fibroblasts arranged in intersecting fascicles representing fibrosarcomas, but foci of osteoid tissue will characterize it as osteosarcoma. Telangiectatic osteosarcoma contains multiple blood-filled cystic and sinusoidal spaces of variable size separated by thin septa. The findings resemble ABC and is the closest differential in terms of treatment and prognosis, so cytologic atypia in the septae and more solid areas should be looked for in histopathology to correctly diagnose telangiectatic osteosarcoma. Phenomenon of "normalization" can be seen in osteosarcoma; this refers

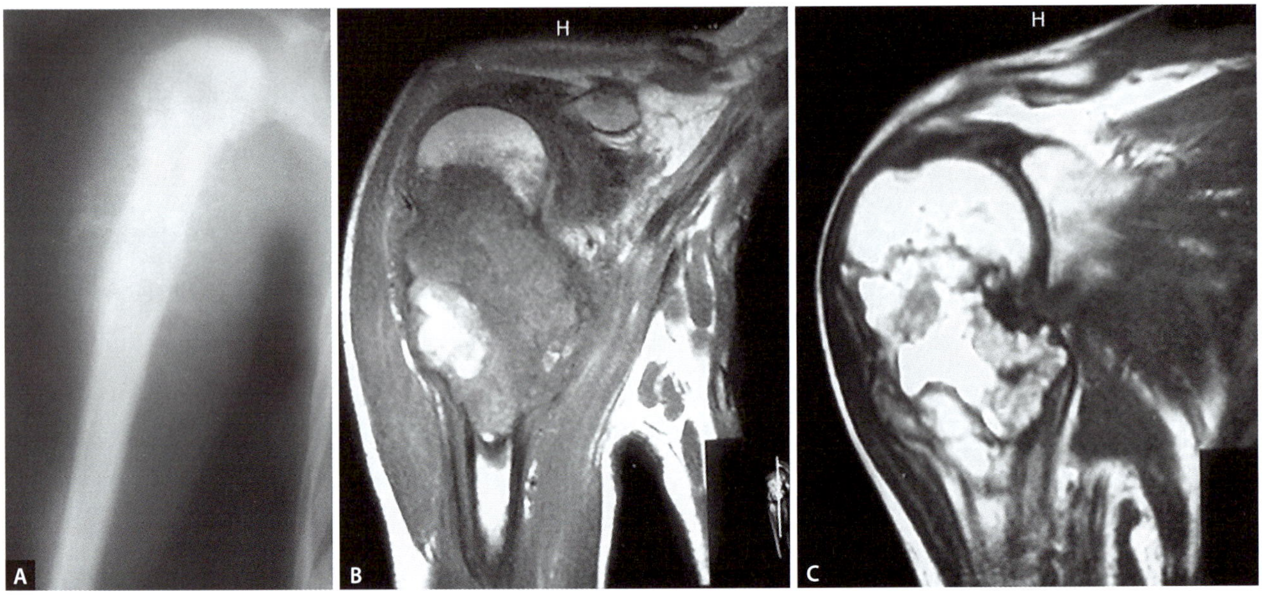

Figs. 44A to C: Magnetic resonance imaging.

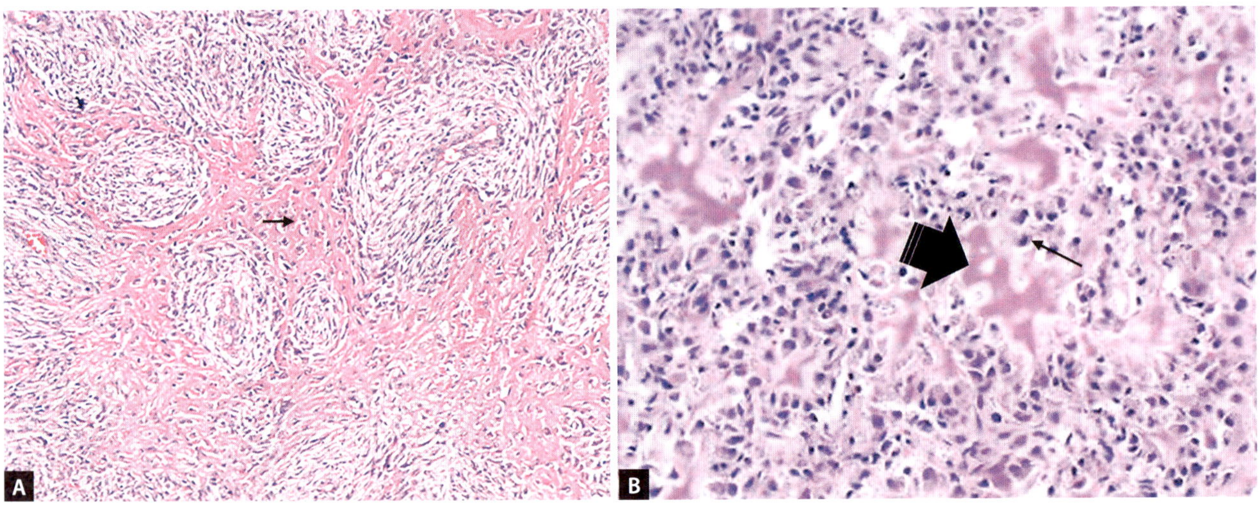

Figs. 45A and B: Histopathology of osteosarcoma. (A) Low-power and (B) high-power microscopic view/photograph of osteosarcoma. (A) There is osteoid formation by tumor cells and it is surrounded by rim of osteoblasts (block arrow); (B) High power view showing characteristic glassy eosinophilic appearance of osteoid (striped arrow) surrounded by plump osteoblasts (thin arrow) without interposition of cartilage.

to osteoblasts becoming smaller and less pleomorphic (regression to normal) as they get incorporated into osteoid. Osteoblastic rimming is however, characteristically absent helping differentiation of neoplastic (absent) from reactive osteoid or osteoblastoma (present). A thin, highly mineralized pattern (the filigreed pattern) is highly suggestive of neoplastic osteoid. There is a tendency of the osteosarcoma to grow in around vessels (angiocentric) giving an overall "basketweave" pattern to tumor. Osteosarcomas of the jaw bones (gnathic osteosarcomas) are usually chondroblastic and have better prognosis. Immunohistochemistry or electron microscopy does not reveal any characteristic features.

Differential Diagnosis

Osteoblastoma, fracture callus, myositis ossificans, GCT, ABC, fibrosarcoma, and MFH of bone.

Clinical Features

Osteosarcoma typically affects the metaphysis of long bones, most common being in frequency of involvement distal femur, proximal tibia, and proximal humerus. Coincidently these are also the most active physes during growth spurt.

Pain without swelling is the most common presentation that is variably present for few weeks to months. The pain is intermittent to begin with but quickly becomes unremitting, deep, boring, and severe. Pain with a swollen tender mass is next most common often seen in delayed presentation or referred cases. Decreased range-of-motion (ROM) and functional limitation are features of delayed neglected cases. Local warmth, telangiectasia, dilated veins, and a bruit on auscultation may be observed particularly in aggressive tumors. There is often a delay of 6–9 months from disease onset to diagnosis. Sudden increase in pain indicates hemorrhage in tumor, secondary changes such as dedifferentiation and rapid growth, pathological fracture, or invasion into nearby neurological structures. Serum alkaline phosphatase (ALP) and lactate dehydrogenase (LDH) are not typically useful for diagnosis but a rise in ALP after tumor excision suggests recurrence.

Treatment

The most apt description is that without appropriate treatment the tumor "is uniformly fatal", and till 1970s the 5-year survival for osteosarcoma was <20%.Conventional tumor has an aggressive local growth pattern and rapid hematogenous spread. Lung is the most common site of metastasis followed by bone although latter occurs only terminally. By the time primary tumor is diagnosed, micrometastasis to lungs is present so osteosarcoma is considered *a systemic disease* at diagnosis now. This is the utmost reason to start contemporary multidisciplinary therapy (chemotherapy, radiotherapy, if required, surgery) focusing on both local and systemic manifestations of osteosarcoma. The drastic improvement in survival rates to 50% appeared after introduction of adjuvant chemotherapy. The initially used drugs such as vincristine, bleomycin, or dactinomycin were quickly replaced by cisplatin, ifosfamide added to doxorubicin and methotrexate that further improved the survival to over 70% in nonmetastatic osteosarcoma.

Patients on chemotherapy are put on protective weight bearing to prevent pathological fractures that could preclude limb-preserving surgery. "With advancements in chemotherapy, the trend shifted to control the micrometastasis with the use of preoperative chemotherapy. This intensive preoperative chemotherapy regimen so-called neoadjuvant chemotherapy combined with assessment of the histological response allowed for better assessment of the surgical margins and early treatment of microscopic disease that would otherwise limit the surgical efficacy. This significant advancement in the current scenario of optimal management of the disease allowed limb-salvage procedures in >80–90% of the cases drastically reducing the need for amputation and producing tumor-free survival of 50–75% even for high-grade osteosarcoma. Analyzing the available data it is found, however, that survival rates improved only between 1973 and 1983 and between 1984 and 1993, but not significantly between 1993 and 2004. This has led some to believe that statistical improvements in "5-year survival" may simply delay the time to recurrence and metastasis that would eventually happen (after the measured 5- or 10-years) in most and also possibly the improvement in results could be mounted by increased intensity of chemotherapy that might still have higher propensity for later side-effects. Overall survival for patients with metastatic disease at presentation ranges from 10 to 40% only, recurrent disease still occurs in 30–40% of patients and >70% of them die of tumor. Even in the survivors of osteosarcoma, there is a significantly increased risk of chronic medical conditions that arise as a result of osteosarcoma-related treatment.

The most important prerequisite for planning a limb-sparing procedures is that LSS should be done only when the preoperative staging indicates that it would be possible to achieve wide surgical margins. To this effect contrary to what is commonly preached a pathologic fracture noted at diagnosis or during preoperative chemotherapy does *not* preclude LSS provided for sure that if wide surgical margins can be achieved **(Figs. 46A and B)**. Although radical margins have been the preferred modality to achieve local control, the advances in chemotherapy have enabled *wide excision* **(Figs. 47 and 48)** to be the desired modality of surgical treatment and limb salvage. Now "navigation" is being increasingly used to achieve clean margins and for intraoperative guidance according to surgical planning. Reconstruction after surgery can be accomplished with many options including:

- Resection and arthrodesis ± bone lengthening **(Figs. 46A and B)**
- Metallic endoprosthesis (and allograft-prosthetic composite) **(Figs. 47 to 51)**
- Allograft (and osteoarticular allograft) ± bone lengthening

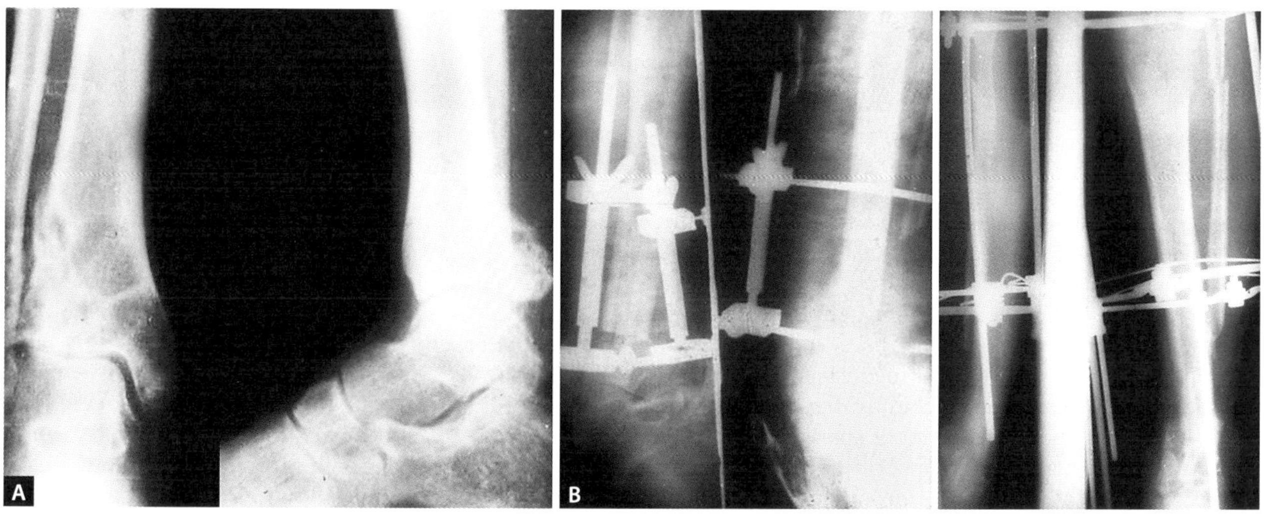

Figs. 46A and B: Giant cell type osteosarcoma of distal tibia with cortical breach—treated with excision and reconstruction by ankle arthrodesis.
Source: S Rastogi, Professor and Head, Department of Orthopedics, Hamdard Institute of Medical Sciences and Research, New Delhi, India.

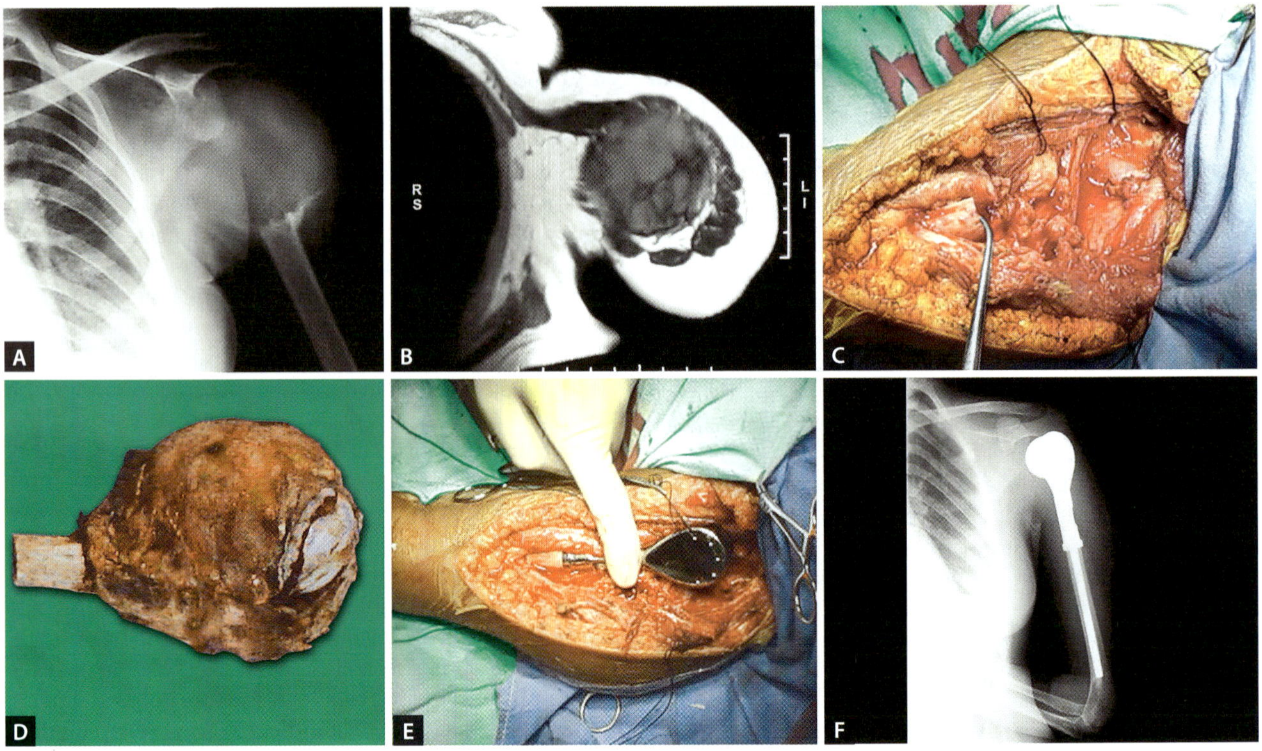

Figs. 47A to F: (A and B) Osteosarcoma of proximal humerus—(C and D) treated with wide excision; and (E and F) Reconstruction by custom prosthesis.
Source: S Rastogi, Professor and Head, Department of Orthopedics, Hamdard Institute of Medical Sciences and Research, New Delhi, India.

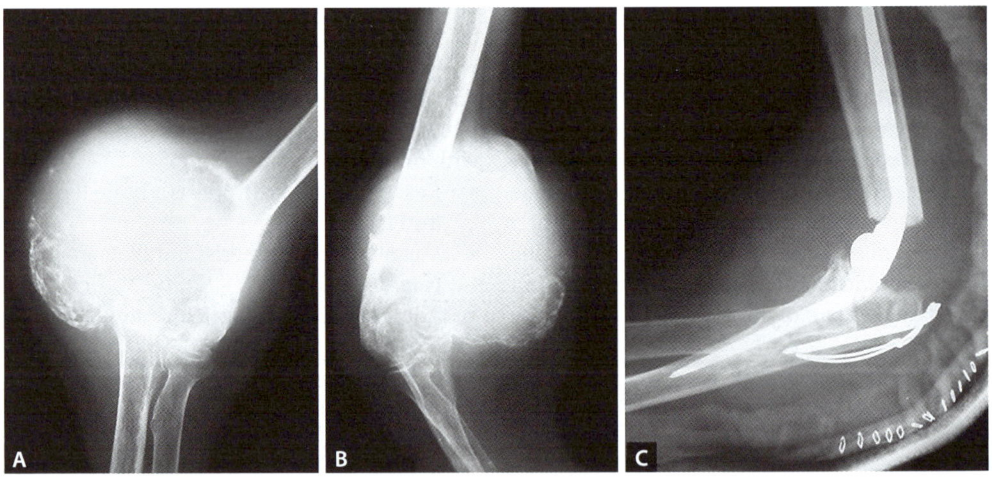

Figs. 48A to C: Osteosarcoma of distal humerus treated with excision prosthetic reconstruction

- Vascularized autologous bone graft ± bone lengthening
- Rotationplasty—cosmetic deformity may not be acceptable to family.
- Wide excision and autoclaved bone graft reconstruction **(Figs. 52A to C)**

The choice of optimal surgical reconstruction is based on various identifiable factors, including the site and size of the primary tumor, the involvement or sparing (or possible reconstruction) of neurovascular supply of the distal extremity, the patient's age and hence potential for additional growth after surgery. One must also try to address the needs and desires of the patient and family as may be involving specific function like participation in sports or future profession, etc. It is now a known fact, however, that delay or prohibition in resumption of systemic chemotherapy after LSS may endanger the chance for cure (increased recurrence), which is quite common when complicated reconstructions are planned for this tumor. This entails making a balanced plan that does not jeopardize chances of tumor-free life over function. Systematic review of retrospective analyses has shown that delay in resuming chemotherapy following definitive surgery is deleterious and is associated with increased tumor recurrence and death. Though considered mutilating and often the last option to resort to, "amputation" remains the optimal choice for saving

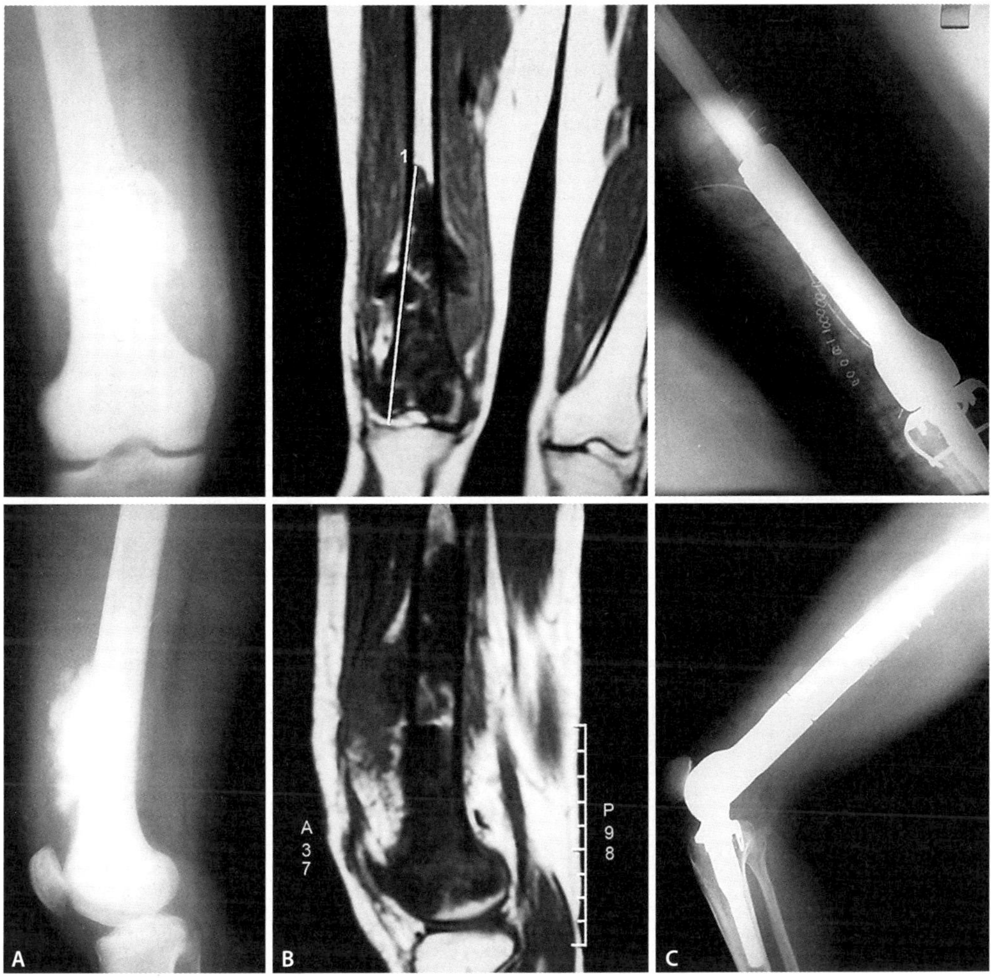

Figs. 49A to C: (A) Osteosarcoma of distal femur (after chemotherapy)—(B) treated with excision (guided by MRI) and (C) endoprosthetic reconstruction.
Source: S Rastogi, Professor and Head, Department of Orthopedics, Hamdard Institute of Medical Sciences and Research, New Delhi, India.

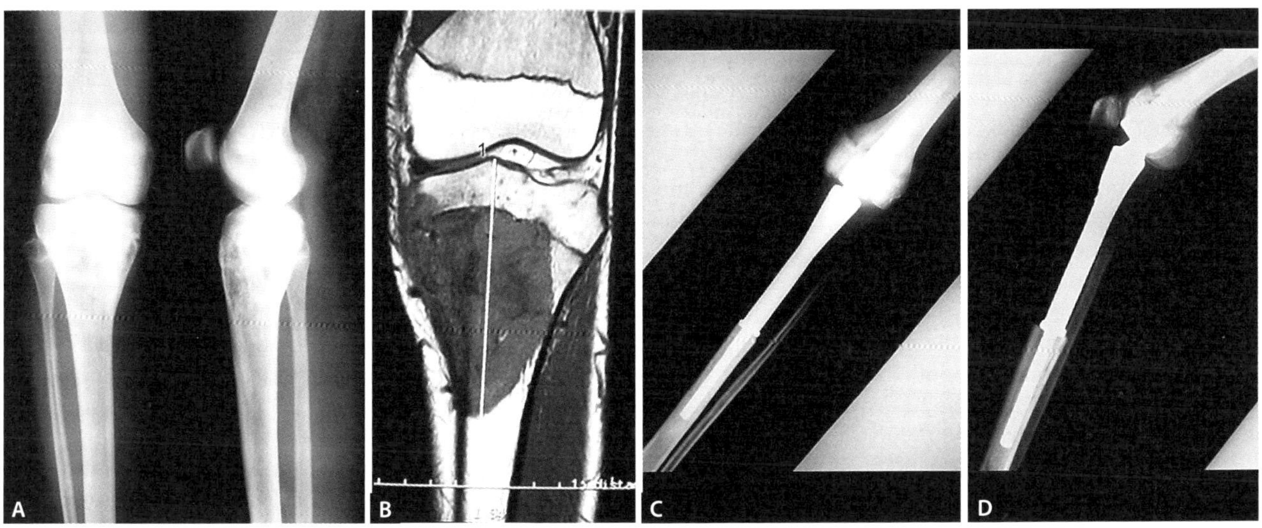

Figs. 50A to D: (A) Osteosarcoma of proximal tibia; (B) Postchemotherapy, treated after MRI planning with (C and D) excision and endoprosthetic reconstruction.
Source: S Rastogi, Professor and Head, Department of Orthopedics, Hamdard Institute of Medical Sciences and Research, New Delhi, India.

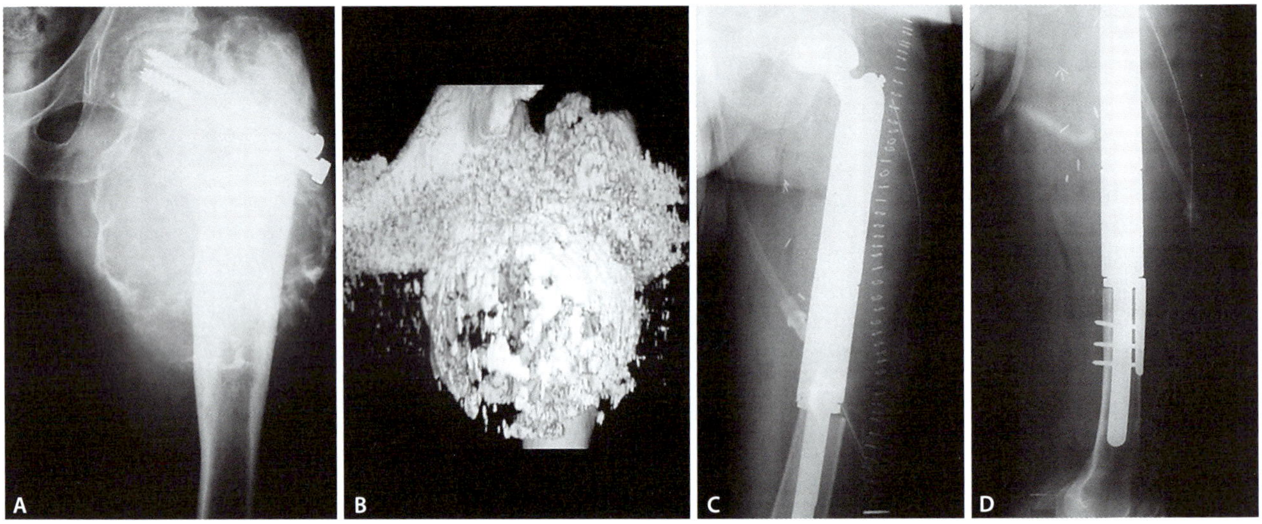

Figs. 51A to D: (A) Osteosarcoma of proximal femur initially treated by screw fixation of neck femur fracture; (B) The shaded surface display (SSD) CT image (shown only for interest); (C and D) Tumor excised and joint reconstructed by custom femoral prosthesis and bipolar prosthesis.
Source: S Rastogi, Professor and Head, Department of Orthopedics, Hamdard Institute of Medical Sciences and Research, New Delhi, India.

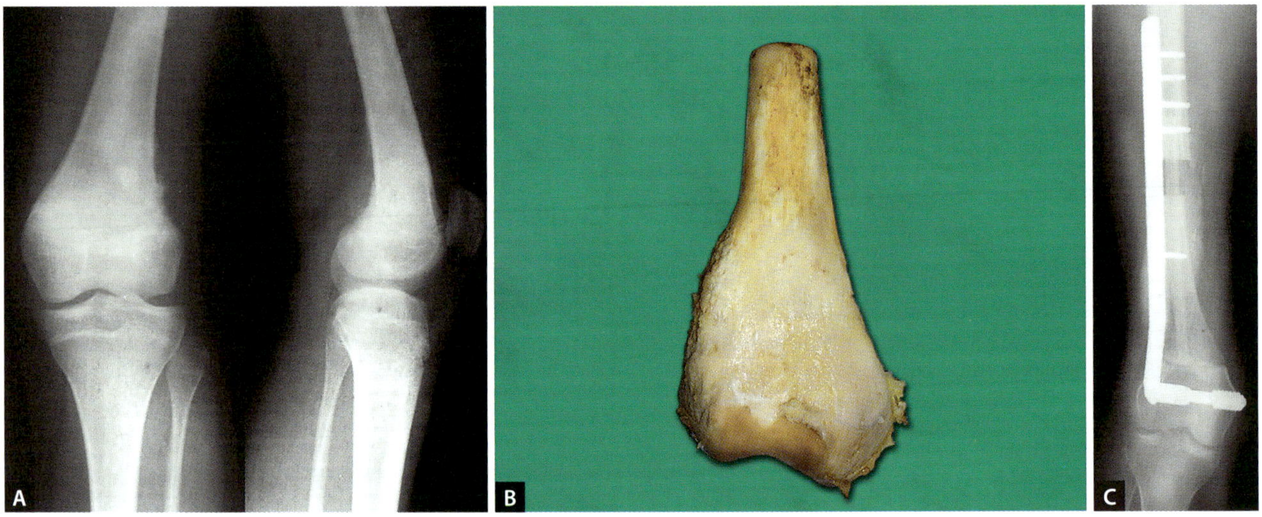

Figs. 52A to C: Osteosarcoma of distal femur, treated by wide excision and reconstruction by using autoclaved bone graft from the excised tumor after cleaning it.
Source: S Rastogi, Professor and Head, Department of Orthopedics, Hamdard Institute of Medical Sciences and Research, New Delhi, India.

life of patient and curing him of the primary tumor in some. This is strongly considered if histopathological examination of surgical specimen shows inadequate margins—plan an immediate amputation. The case is further strengthened if the histologic necrosis following preoperative chemotherapy was poor. The most sensitive indicator till now is response to preoperative (neoadjuvant) chemotherapy. Survival is directly related to chemotherapy response, those with a good response (>90% tumor necrosis) have 80–90% long-term survival while nonresponders (<90% tumor necrosis) survival is usually <15%. One exception to improved survival of responders in osteosarcoma is possibly telangiectatic form where despite extreme sensitivity of the tumor to chemotherapy the survival may not be improved. Current chemotherapy protocols include combinations of the following agents: high-dose methotrexate, doxorubicin, cyclophosphamide, cisplatin, ifosfamide, etoposide, and carboplatin. As for tubercular chemotherapy regimens containing three active chemotherapy agents against osteosarcoma have been found superior to regimens containing two active agents, and also regimens that include high-dose methotrexate are superior. PET imaging during chemotherapy can effectively assess biological response to treatment which directly correlates to prognosis. It would also help clinicians in patient stratification and changing chemotherapy. Pulmonary metastasis and secondary complications are the most common cause of death. Local recurrence in particular is associated with a high risk for death from osteosarcoma. The factors that are associated with increased incidence of local recurrence are:

- Pelvic primary site of tumor
- Doing biopsy at an institution different from the institution performing definitive surgery

- Limb-salvage surgery
- Soft tissue infiltration of the tumor beyond periosteum
- Poor histological response (necrosis) to initial chemotherapy
- Failure/delay in completing planned chemotherapy

It is a known fact that patients who undergo an amputation have lower local recurrence rates than patients undergoing LSS (although not by any means this suggests amputation for all patients). The functional outcome has been similar between amputation and LSS group of patients; this is, however, a strong point favoring amputation at sites where LSS would be difficult or too complex to jeopardize chemotherapy. Radiation therapy is recommended in most patients with osteosarcoma of the head and neck that have been left with positive or uncertain resection margins.

Advances in management of osteosarcoma:

- Radiotherapy
  - *Intensity-modulated radiation therapy:* The radiation beams are modulated to give maximum dose to the tumor area and sparing the surrounding tissues. The sensitive tissues can also be differentially spared.
  - *Proton beam therapy:* Protons do tissue damage after they pass certain distance in soft tissues so that the normal tissue can be spared by adjusting the beam strength. The protons then deliver energy quickly to the tissue.
  - *Carbon ions:* These are heavier protons causing more damage to cancer cells but the treatment is available at select centers (mostly Japan).
- Chemotherapy
  - *Targeted therapy:* Genetic analysis has revealed complex karyotype in osteosarcoma so various possible targets are being explored including Wnt signaling and WWOX as a possible tumor suppressor gene. Chimeric antigen receptor therapies are being developed that facilitate targeting a protein on the surface of cancer cells by engineering the T cells of the patient to target only that protein. Targeting of GD2 glycosphingolipid is interesting as it is expressed in 90% of osteosarcomas. It is being tried in relapsed cases showing good response and can be alternatively or additionally combined with pantyrosine kinase inhibitors, specific IGF-1 inhibitor and mammalian target of rapamycin (mTOR) inhibitor. Saracatinib affecting bone metabolism, bevacizumab, and sorafenib affecting angiogenesis in tumors and drugs such as temsirolimus and everolimus against mTOR protein are being studied. Sorafinib is a multikinase inhbitor that has shown significant response in recurrent/refractory osteosarcoma including metastatic disease and is well-tolerated in young patients at doses of 200 mg twice daily. It can be combined with everolimus for improved effect.
  - Zoledronic acid has been found to act synergistically to paclitaxel in chemotherapeutic regimens against osteosarcomas.

Prognosis

The *pretreatment* factors that influence the prognosis of osteosarcoma include site and size of tumor and presence of metastasis. The degree of tumor necrosis (also see above in "chemotherapy") after chemotherapy is the single most important determinant of outcome *post-treatment*. Site-wise, the distal appendicular lesions fare better than proximal ones. Axial lesions are associated with poor prognosis due primarily to incomplete excision. The craniofacial lesions have better prognosis than appendicular lesion overall for surgical management despite inferior necrosis results. Concerning the size of tumors, larger tumors have a worse prognosis than "smaller ones (<10 cm)". Serum LDH levels that are also related directly to the size of tumor higher levels have poor prognosis.

High LDH is commonly seen at the time of relapse and relapse of osteosarcoma with high serum LDH is correlated with unfavorable prognosis. For metastatic lesions, the prognosis is better for fewer pulmonary nodules and those with unilateral lesions compared to bilateral ones. Metastasis across joint (traditionally incorrectly called "skip lesions") have worse outcome than true skip lesions. Multifocal osteosarcoma has bad prognosis. Of the post-treatment factors, tumor resectability is a key prognostic factor as local adjuvant like radiation therapy is relatively ineffective to control residual disease. Incomplete removal of disease has associated poor survival overall. Patients with limited/less necrosis (<90%) following initial chemotherapy (see earlier) have shown higher rate of recurrence within the first 2 years compared to patients with good response (necrosis ≥ 90%). There is no concluding data to substantiate the prognostic significance of specific chromosomal gains or losses, expression of HER2/c-erbB-2, tumor cell ploidy; LOH of the retinoblastoma gene and *p53* locus, and increased expression of p-glycoprotein.

Some characteristic variants of osteosarcoma are discussed below:

Parosteal osteosarcoma: The tumor arises from the cortical bone on bone surface as a protuberant multinodular mass in older age group (slight female predilection) and is the most common of the surface osteosarcoma. The tumor characteristically is seen on the posterior aspect of femur; other sites being tibia and proximal humerus. They are slow to grow and often present as a mass usually *not* associated with pain. Stiffness in the nearby joint might be the initial presentation. The tumor appears to encircle the bone circumferentially (partially or completely) and may even have a cartilaginous cap-like structure for very slow-growing reasons. Periosteal reaction is rare if at all. Some aggressive ones infiltrate the surrounding tissues **(Figs. 53A and B)**. Metastasis is late to occur as is intramedullary extension. The tumor shows centrifugal differentiation (immature periphery compared to base). Radiologically, the tumor appears as a large and dense irregular exophytic mass attached to parent bone by a wide base. Lucencies within the dense calcification are rare and indicate dedifferentiation (to fibrosarcoma, MFH or osteosarcoma). Deep-seated lucencies indicate aggressiveness. CT is required to determine the intramedullary involvement and "wrapping around" tendency of the bone tumor. The lesion should be differentiated from osteochondroma, myositis ossificans, florid reactive

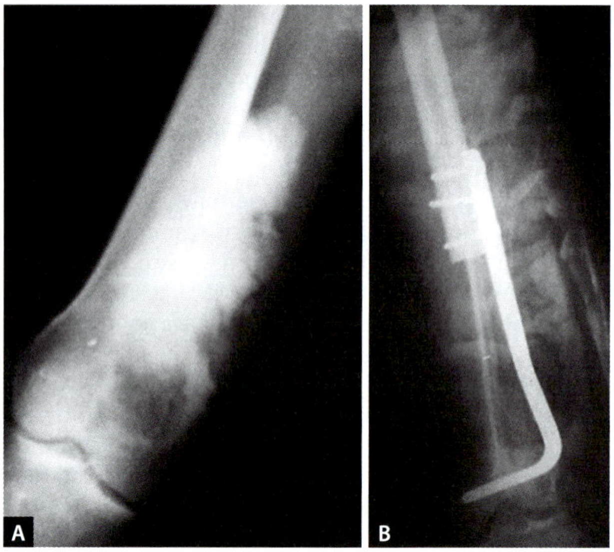

Figs. 53A and B: Parosteal osteosarcoma. The tumor from distal femur appears like a large osteochondroma (an exophytic bone mass) with spiculated radiating calcification. Reconstruction was done after wide excision of tumor.
Source: S Rastogi, Professor and Head, Department of Orthopedics, Hamdard Institute of Medical Sciences and Research, New Delhi, India.

periostitis, periosteal osteochondromatous proliferation (Nora's lesion) radiologically and conventional osteosarcoma and high-grade surface osteosarcoma histopathologically. The parosteal osteosarcoma does not have a contiguous medullary canal as is seen with osteochondroma and also the columnar arrangement of cartilage seen in osteochondroma is missing in parosteal osteosarcoma. Radiologically, the osteochondromas appear lucent in the center. Myositis ossificans shows a centripetal differentiation (periphery more mature, "zonation"). Periostitis is quite painful clinically and has relevant history. The classical histopathological appearance (of parosteal osteosarcoma) is that of irregular osteoid seams surrounded by spindle cells and scattered innocuous fibroblasts, i.e., an overall well-differentiated tumor. Most tumors are grade 1 at diagnosis. Atypia and high-grade lesions correlate with intramedullary spread and metastasis. Parosteal variety differs from conventional variety in that there is one or supernumerary ring chromosome. Unless high-grade, the treatment suffices with well-performed wide excision else neoadjuvant chemotherapy should be given. The prognosis is distinctly favorable with 75–85% survival at 5 years. Recurrences due to inadequate excision are common and are of concern as they are of higher grade that require combined chemotherapy and aggressive surgery for management.

Periosteal osteosarcoma (juxtacortical chondrosarcoma): They are also surface osteosarcomas (originating from cortex), but involve diaphysis of long bones and involve patients of age group similar to conventional osteosarcoma. They are typically described as intermediate-grade chondroblastic osteosarcoma arising on surface of bone. The tibial shaft is the commonly affected region. Clinically, they also initially present as a swelling usually painless to begin with but

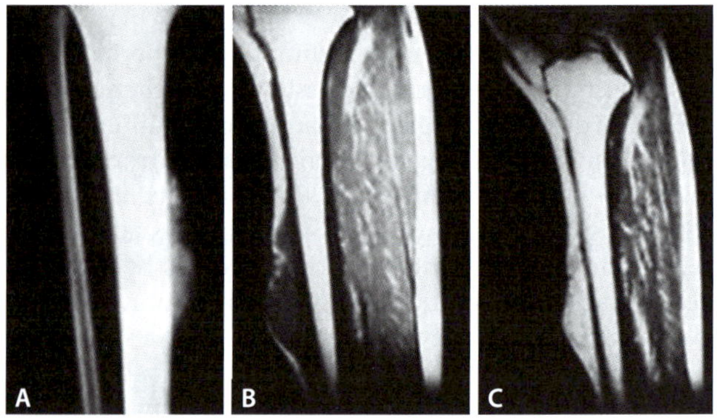

Figs. 54A to C: Periosteal osteosarcoma. This diaphyseal tumor of tibia appears to arise and involve cortex but on MR scanning is seen as a distinct mass.

TABLE 18: Differentiating features of parosteal and periosteal osteosarcoma

Parosteal osteosarcoma	*Periosteal osteosarcoma*
More common surface osteosarcoma	Relatively rare form
Swelling without pain	Swelling quickly accompanied by pain
Metaphyseal femur	Diaphyseal location common
Wraps around the bone	Protrudes into soft tissue
Periosteal reaction uncommon	Periosteal reaction is often seen.
Osteoid formation prominent	Chondroid features common
Zonation seen	Not evident

later develop pain. Rather than wrapping around the bone, they project into the soft tissue as well-circumscribed mass. The cortex is not destroyed but may be scooped and periosteal reaction in the form of Codman triangle is often seen. Radiographically, the lesions are lucent without any intramedullary extension, and mineralization is more or less limited to the tumor base **(Figs. 54A to C)**. The calcification occurs in radiating spiculated pattern. Gross examination of a specimen reveals cartilaginous grayish-blue lobulated mass that contains chondrosarcomatous areas microscopically (resembling intermediate-grade chondrosarcomas); but as per definition of osteosarcoma, there are at least some foci of osteoid formation (often thin and lacy) usually located in the center. High-grade surface osteosarcomas are differentiated on the basis of presence of high-grade anaplastic osteoblasts. Peripheral chondrosarcomas are metaphyseal and lack radiating spicules. Parosteal osteosarcomas are distinguished as per **Table 18** from periosteal osteosarcomas. The periosteal osteosarcoma should be managed like conventional osteosarcoma (wide local resection) with neo- and adjuvant chemotherapy.

Small cell osteosarcoma: Here, the neoplastic cells comprise nest and sheets of small-rounded cells resembling Ewing's sarcoma (however, the characteristic 11:22 translocation is missing). Osteoid surrounds the cells or their groups in a lace-like pattern. This represents a variant of intramedullary conventional osteosarcoma with most cases in first 2 decades.

Radiologically, it is predominantly lytic with permeative margins. It should be differentiated from Ewing's (presence of osteoid), lymphoma (absence of panel of lymphoid and pan-leukocyte markers). Few cases are reported, and radiation, chemotherapy, and surgery are all used depending on surgeon's choice and institutions protocol (osteosarcoma-like treatment or Ewing's sarcoma-like treatment) for no definitive recommendations. The prognosis is worse than conventional osteosarcoma.

Telangiectatic osteosarcoma (Malignant bone aneurysm, hemorrhagic osteosarcoma, ABC-like osteosarcoma): The WHO recognizes telangiectatic osteosarcoma as a malignant bone-forming tumor characterized by large spaces filled with blood with or without septa. The tumor is seen in 4% of cases with the age and site predilection matching to conventional osteosarcoma; however, these patients are more likely to present with pathological fractures (one-fourth patients). Association with Paget's disease and retinoblastoma is strong but not established. Radiologically, it is a purely lytic process without matrix mineralization, only pure destruction of the involved area is seen. Any sclerosis seen on the radiographs should preclude the diagnosis of telangiectatic osteosarcoma **(Figs. 55A and B)**. To differentiate it from ABC features of rapid growth, such as cortical destruction, permeative margins, and soft tissue extension can be often appreciated. Periosteal reaction in the form of Codman triangle and onion-skin are common. ABC-like appearance is seen in some cases. MRI shows frequent fluid levels with extraskeletal extension. Grossly, the tumor has a cystic appearance with the spaces filled incompletely with blood. There is usually no tumor mass available for histopathology. The cystic spaces are lined by benign looking giant cells without endothelial lining that confuses the pathologist to make diagnosis of ABC. Attention to detail lies in septa that are, however, cellular and contain malignant pleomorphic mononuclear tumor cells with atypia that should be carefully looked for diagnosis. Lace-like osteoid is seen but infrequent. Although not so favorable in the past the prognosis is now comparable to conventional osteosarcoma due to effective chemotherapy. The tumor is responsive to current chemotherapy.

Bone Islands (Enostosis)

These represent foci of mature cortical bone within an area of cancellous bone. They possibly reflect failed areas of resorption developmentally during endochondral ossification. Some have likened them to tumor-like condition and others think them to be hamartomas. Typically, they are asymptomatic lesions appearing radiodense round to oval sclerotic 2 mm to 2 cm areas with subtle brush border **(Fig. 56)**. The lesions can appear in any bone but have a preference for pelvis and femur also they may disappear or enlarge with time. They are cold on bone scan. Multiple enostoses are seen in osteopoikilosis.

Giant Bone Islands

The term describes enostosis lesions measuring >2 cm in any dimension. Unlike the small enostosis these are more likely to be symptomatic but are rare and only a few cases have been described in literature. Most are described in adults but sporadically in children. The lesions are associated with increased radionuclide uptake and radiologic appearance could be well alarming. Usually, it appears as an intramedullary oblong, homogeneously dense isolated or multiple foci of sclerosis, oriented along the long axis of bone. The lesion has "paintbrush" or "thorny" appearance due to the radiating spicules seen as pseudopodia exuding from the main lesion. There is no periosteal reaction or invasion of the cortex (bone destruction) suggesting a benign entity radiologically. MRI findings reflect low-signal intensity on all pulse sequences suggesting cortical bone. 99mTc bone scan demonstrates increased radiotracer uptake due to higher bone turnover in the area. Histopathologically, they are composed of compact lamellar bone that subtly blend into the surrounding spongiosa. Symptomatic patient with hot lesion on scintigraphy mandates further evaluation as the differential diagnosis includes various benign and malignant conditions. Benign conditions that may resemble

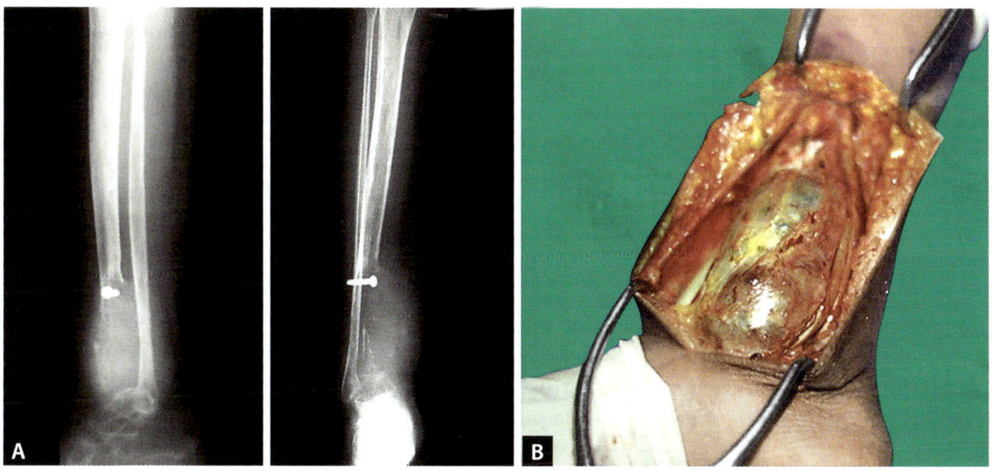

Figs. 55A and B: Telangiectatic osteosarcoma. This is a purely lytic mass of distal tibia initially mistaken and treated as ABC. The patient had to be managed by amputation for gross involvement of surrounding critical structures.
Source: S Rastogi, Professor and Head, Department of Orthopedics, Hamdard Institute of Medical Sciences and Research, New Delhi, India.

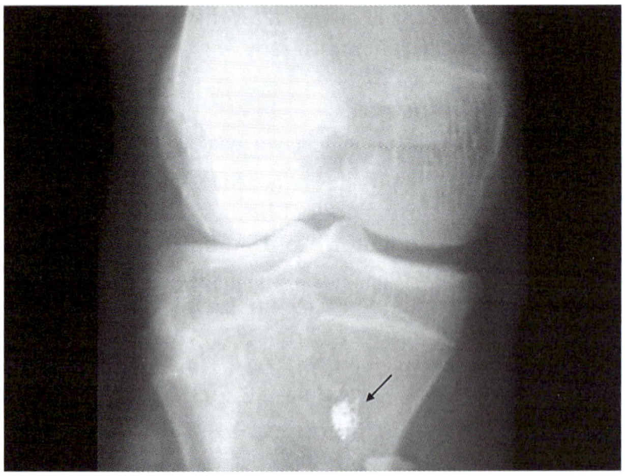

Fig. 56: Bone island (arrow).

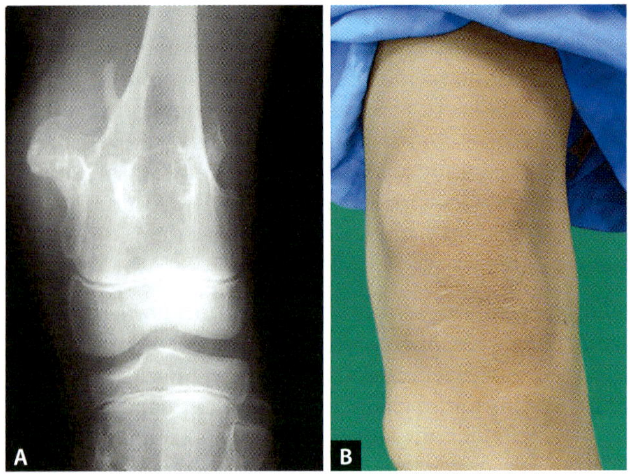

Figs. 57A and B: Osteochondroma around the knee joint. The tumors grow away from the growth plate.

such presentation include atypical sclerotic presentation of nonossifying fibroma, unifocal osteofibrous dysplasia (has bowing deformity but contains fibrous stroma not seen with bone island), giant long bone osteoma (does not include medullary space), osteoid osteoma, osteoblastoma, and osteomyelitis (Garre's). Atypical sclerotic intramedullary osteosarcoma is the closest malignant lesion that may resemble the giant bone islands.

CARTILAGE FORMING LESIONS

Osteochondroma

Osteochondroma (osteochondromatous exostosis, solitary osteochondroma, exostosis, and ICD-O 9210/0) and hereditary form—multiple osteochondromas (hereditary osteochondromatosis, hereditary deforming osteochondromatosis, hereditary chondrodysplasia, diaphyseal aclasis, metaphyseal aclasis, hereditary multiple exostoses, and ICD-O 9210/1).

This is a cartilage-capped metaphyseal exophytic lesion that grows on external surface of the bone pointing away from the joint containing a marrow cavity continuous with that of parent bone. The term *exostosis* is a general term and is used to refer to any outgrowth of a bone from the cortical surface. Osteochondroma is the most common bone tumor even though reported numbers are less due to asymptomatic and clinically unalarming nature of most lesions. Osteochondromas generally arise in bones developed from endochondral ossification. The tumor is thought to arise from:

- Aberrant "pared away" or "displaced" growth plate that possibly rotates and then grows outward from the parent bone. Some suggest herniation of the growth plate (traumatic or otherwise) through lacroix ring and periosteum and continued growth. Support to this comes from the finding that the medullary canal of tumor is continuous with the parent bone and the lesion is covered with periosteum.
- Abnormal epiphyseal rests (Jaffe) separated from the physeal plate during development may grow to produce the tumor.
- Periosteal metaplasia and a defective periosteal ring (Jaffe).
- Recently finding of consistent clonal genetic alterations in these lesions suggests true neoplastic potential. The closest link to the development of benign multiple osteochondromas is made to genes belonging to the EXT family (*EXT1, EXT2*, and *EXT3* located on chromosome 8, 11, and 19, respectively). These genes are considered to be tumor suppressor genes loss of which is possibly responsible for the neoplasia (this lends support to periosteal metaplasia or defective periosteal ring hypothesis).

The tumor grows in a direction away from the growing end of bone (possibly due to attached tendons or muscles pulling it away) with the cartilage cap pointing away from physeal plate **(Figs. 57A and B)**. Tumor growth parallels with growth of skeleton but the size of cartilage cap keeps reducing with age (in the end, cap may be completely eburnated leaving behind only bone). Osteochondroma stops growing at the physeal maturation age (unless malignant change has occurred). Osteochondromas have also been shown to regress.

Secondary osteochondromas have been reported after autologous stem cell transplantation in pediatric patients and also in previously irradiated bones.

Multiple osteochondromas can be sporadic or familial and have autosomal dominant inheritance. These are termed "multiple hereditary exostoses or diaphyseal (or metaphyseal) aclasia". There is often a generalized osseous remodeling defect distributed throughout the body and hence causing limb growth disturbances. Some uncommon syndromes are also associated with development of multiple osteochondromas and include Langer–Giedion (associated with facial dysmorphism and mental retardation) and Potocki–Shaffer (Defect-11) syndrome.

Osteochondroma usually occurs in the first 3 decades with no known sex predilection. Nearly, 15% of all patients with osteochondroma have multiple lesions. The most commonly involved bones are metaphyseal regions of distal femur, upper humerus, upper tibia and fibula and among flat bones, the ilium and scapula account for most of the cases **(Figs. 58A to C)**. Clinically, most of the lesions are detected or noticed incidentally by parents and are asymptomatic, presenting just for worrisome swelling and found while bathing the child. If symptomatic, the most common presentation is that of a hard mass of longstanding duration symptoms (often related to the size and location of the lesion). Multiple osteochondromas usually present as limb growth disturbances. Secondary complications (these are also often painful) are the common reason for surgical intervention and include:

- Mechanical obstruction
- Fracture of the stalk of the lesion
- Nerve impingement
- Pseudoaneurysm of an overlying vessel
- Bursa forming over the osteochondroma and bursitis
- Infarction of the osteochondroma
- Reactive myositis
- Increasing pain and/or rapidly growing mass (possible malignant transformation)

Malignant transformation of osteochondromas (also see secondary chondrosarcoma) has been reported in <1% in patients with solitary and approximately 1–3% in patients with multiple osteochondromas. The features that suggest this include:

- Mass becoming suddenly painful and tender or sudden increase in pain without above changes
- Increase in cartilage cap thickness > 2 cm (seen on MRI or CT, also see histopathology below, and secondary chondrosarcoma for detailed description)
- Excessive cartilage type flocculent calcification seen on radiograph or CT scan
- Lucencies in the bony component or fuzzy border between cartilage and bone on radiograph
- Multiple recurrences in a well-excised lesion

The secondary malignancy is almost always (>95%) low-grade chondrosarcoma though few patients with multiple osteochondromas may develop high-grade chondrosarcoma. Secondary osteosarcoma is seen very infrequently but has been reported.

Radiology

Solitary osteochondromas may be pedunculated or sessile lesions often found in metaphyseal region despite their origin from physeal plate (shift due to continued growth). The characteristic feature is a projection of the cortex in continuity with the underlying bone. The continuity of marrow space into the lesion is evident on CT scan or MRI images. These modalities are also good imaging modalities to estimate the thickness of the cartilage cap that used to have treatment implications previously.

Histopathology

Grossly, the specimens have a well-defined bony narrow or broad stalk (unless sessile) covered by a cartilage cap at the broader end. The cartilage cap is usually thicker in younger patients (adolescents) while a cap larger than 2 cm in an adult should raise suspicion of malignancy. Thickness as an absolute criterion is not very well accepted by experts and is more arbitrary (see also secondary chondrosarcoma). Conventionally, cartilage cap measuring <1 cm is designated for osteochondroma without any validating data. In fact, the mean thickness for cartilage cap has been reported to be 9 mm with a range of few mm to 2.5 cm. On the contrary, chondrosarcomas have been shown to be present even in thinner caps 5–10 mm, so cap thickness is not a good criteria and what some call a “qualitative assessment” of the cartilage cap could better help in differentiation. Microscopically, the chondrocytes show a zonification and superficial ones

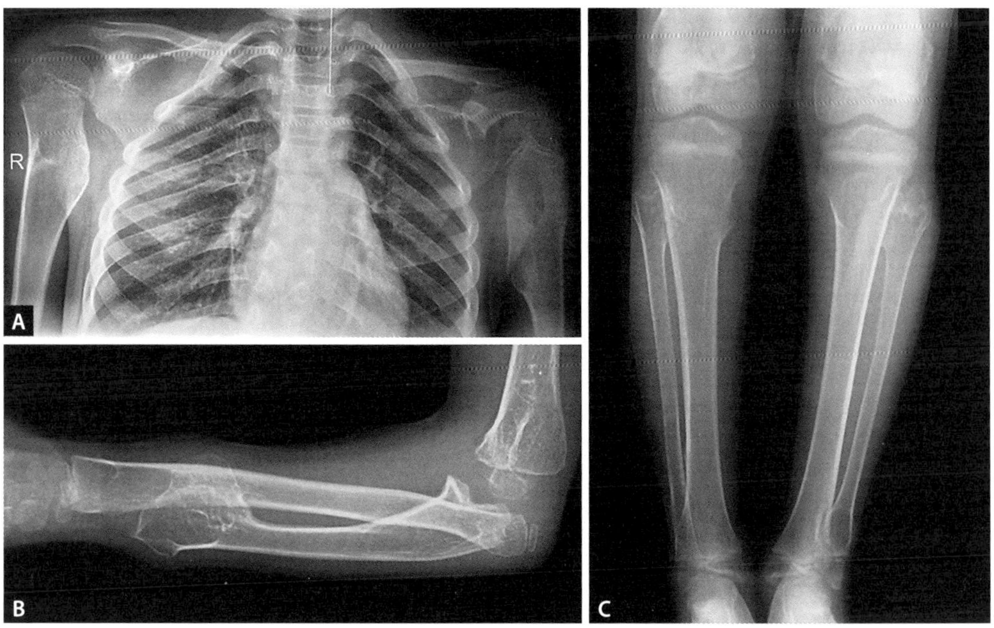

Figs. 58A to C: Hereditary osteochondromatosis showing lesions at multiple sites.

are more clustered and seen in lacunae. The lower ones near the base line-up like in growth plate. Some amount of large disorganized masses of cartilage in the stalk and amorphous calcification with focal necrosis of cartilage is common and should not be mistaken for chondrosarcoma. Chondrosarcomatous cartilage has prominent myxoid change and accentuated cellular and lobular appearance. Permeation of bone and entrapment is pathognomonic of chondrosarcoma.

Differential Diagnosis

Parosteal osteosarcoma and other surface osteosarcoma, supracondylar spur (humerus), malunited fracture, and Nora's lesion.

Management

Excision including the covering periosteum (extraperiosteal resection—the plane of dissection passes outside "extra" the periosteum, or to better remember—not only the tumor but its periosteum is also removed as "extra" precaution) is done for a symptomatic or cosmetically disabling lesion **(Figs. 59A and B)**. The secondary malignancy requires wide excision for cure. Recurrence is common for:

- Incomplete excision (often the cartilage cap is left behind or pathological periosteum inadequately excised) is the most common cause of recurrence.
- The mature bony stalk should be excised completely with periosteum and flange of parent bone at the base, some palisaded cells (at base of stalk) in periosteum might reflect metaplasia and possible recurrence of tumor if not ablated or excised.
- Multiple recurrences in a well-excised lesion indicate malignancy.

Enchondroma (Solitary Enchondroma and Central Chondroma) and Enchondromatosis

Solitary enchondroma are benign hyaline cartilage neoplasms that can occur centrally within the bone (enchondroma) or on the surface (periosteal chondroma). The latter are rare (<2%) benign hyaline cartilage neoplasm formed at bone surface that arises from the periosteum. In the simplest form, solitary enchondroma represents a disruption of endochondral ossification at physeal cartilage that latter proliferates within the metaphyseal bone. Most tumors are solitary, however, variations such as polyosseous involvement (Ollier's disease, see later) or multisite involvement in same bone may be seen. Enchondromas are not uncommon and are responsible for somewhat >10–25% of all benign bone tumors.

Clinical Features

They are found in all ages (5–80 years) but majority of patients present in 2nd to 4th decades. Majority of lesions occur in small bones of hands and feet and enchondroma is indeed the most common bone neoplasm of hand. They are quite uncommon in flat bones such as scapula, pelvis, ribs, sternum or vertebrae, and are undescribed in the craniofacial bones. Typically, patients present with palpable swellings that may or may not be painful. Typically, the lesions do not progress beyond puberty. Pathological fractures are common due to weakened bones. A superficial variant "periosteal chondroma" occurs typically in proximal humerus as a palpable painful mass. Long bone tumors are detected incidentally in radiographs **(Fig. 60)** or bone scans (as hot spot) taken for other reasons.

Radiology

On radiographs, the enchondromas appear as well-marginated tumors that vary from lytic **(Figs. 61A and B)** to tumors with characteristic chondroid mineralization/calcification pattern consisting of punctate, flocculent, or ring and arc calcification patterns. Long bone tumors are commonly centrally located in metaphysis and do not expand the cortex in contrast to small tubular bones where the cortex is expanded and thinned out. At the most mild endosteal scalloping is seen. If any lesion shows extensive endosteal erosion then immediately suspicion for low-grade chondrosarcoma is raised. Soft

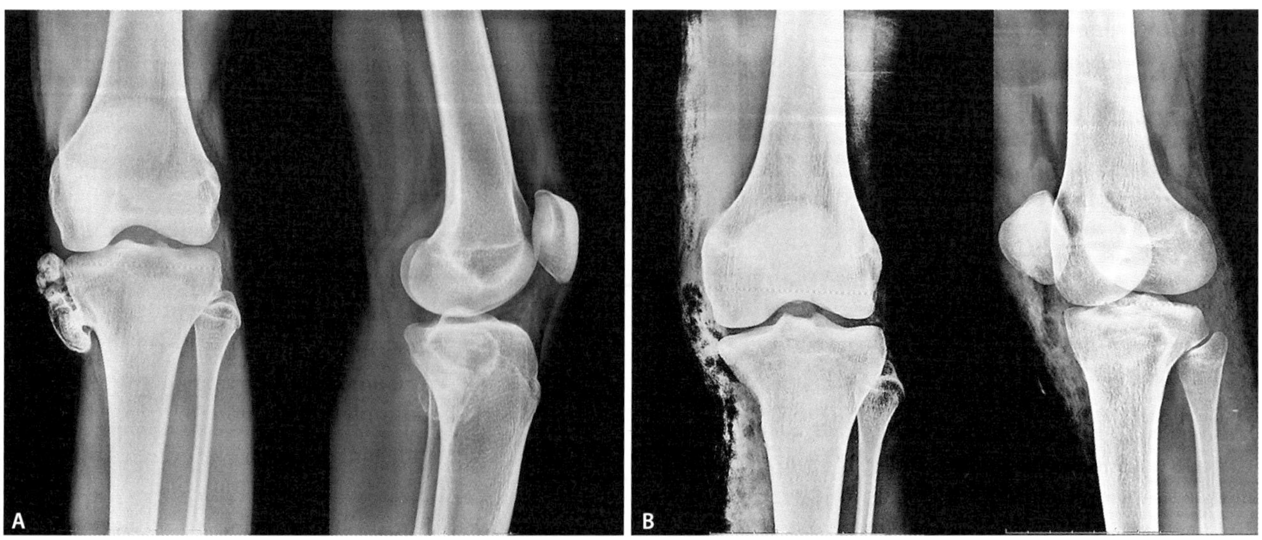

Figs. 59A and B: Exostosis excision. The tumor has been excised with the bone at the base and covering periosteum and cartilage cap.

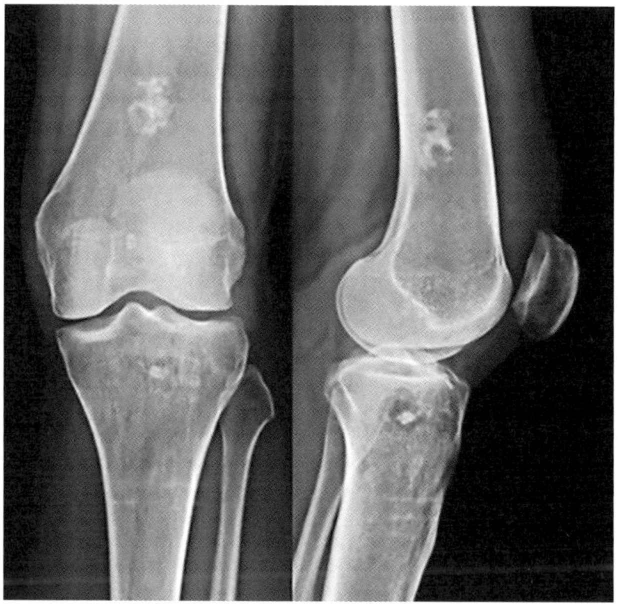

Fig. 60: The incidental finding of enchondromas in femur and tibia seen on (AP and lateral) knee radiograph done otherwise for knee pain. The femoral lesion demonstrates characteristic rings and arc calcifications. The location of the lesions characteristically describes the notion that the solitary enchondromas are basically disorders of growth plate that subsequently proliferate in the metaphyseal bone.

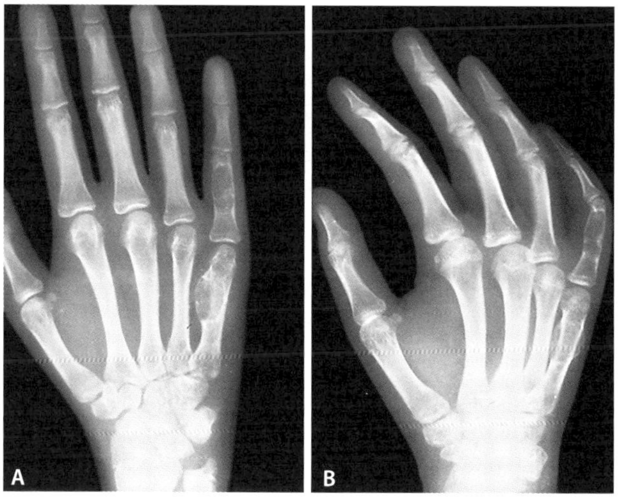

Figs. 61A and B: Enchondroma of small bones seen as lucent lesion within the bone.

tissue invasion as a rule is not seen in enchondromas. The periosteal variant (periosteal chondroma) may demonstrate saucerization of the bone cortex due to pressure effect.

Histopathology

On gross examination, the tumors are usually few mm to 3 cm, larger tumors (>5 cm) are infrequent. The tumor is whitish gray opalescent with gritty yellowish areas of calcification. Long bone tumors have multinodular pattern separated by bone marrow. Microscopically, there is abundant hyaline cartilage with few cells. Myxoid degeneration is frequent. The cells are mononuclear with infrequent binucleate forms and are evenly distributed only occasional clusters are seen. The Haversian system of bone is intact and is not invaded by the tumor cells. Enchondromas of small bones may be more cellular confusing them with low-grade chondrosarcomas.

Management

Most need only radiological surveillance, however, in uncertainties like pain attributed to the lesion or doubtful radiology surgical excision is commonly advised for lesions of long bones. Intralesional thorough curettage suffices in most and resulting void may be but not necessarily filled with cancellous bone graft. Recurrences are rare but may be seen after a long time even low-grade chondrosarcomas have been found to occur in recurrences.

Multiple Enchondromas (Enchondromatosis, Multiple Chondromatosis, Multiple Enchondromatosis, and Chondrodysplasia)

It is characterized by many enchondromas present throughout the skeleton with some syndromic characteristics. Multiple enchondromatosis is a nonhereditary disorder that is characterized by formation of multiple enchondromas in various osseous sites **(Figs. 62A and B)** and has substantial risk of degenerating into chondrosarcoma. The extent of the disease is often highly variable.

Ollier's Disease

The enchondromatosis here has a tendency toward unilaterality. Even in bilateral cases one side of body is predominantly involved. Ollier's disease is a developmental disorder where there is a failure of normal ossification. The large tumors form extensively in the metaphyseal region of multiple bones with varying deformity **(Figs. 63A and B)**. Some studies implicate parathormone receptor and PTH-related peptide gene to Ollier's disease.

Maffucci Syndrome

Maffucci syndrome is a rare and nonhereditary congenital disorder. Here, the multiple enchondromas are associated with hemangiomas (usually cavernous type) of the soft tissues and uncommonly of viscera. Phlebolith formation is common and can be even seen radiologically.

These patients with enchondromatosis are usually younger (severity of disease inversely proportional to age of presentation) and mostly within first 2 decades of life. At presentation, the affected limb is often shortened and deformed. Pathological fractures and bowing deformities are frequent. Any site (diaphysis, metaphysis, or epiphysis) may be involved. Like solitary chondromas, the hands are the most common site followed by feet, femur, humerus, and forearm. The lesions can be intramedullary or periosteal and bony expansion is common in enchondromatosis. Typically, the lesions demonstrate radiolucent columns extending from growth plate into metaphysis radiologically. Though metaphysis is commonly involved, any part of bone including epiphysis or cartilage can be involved. Extension

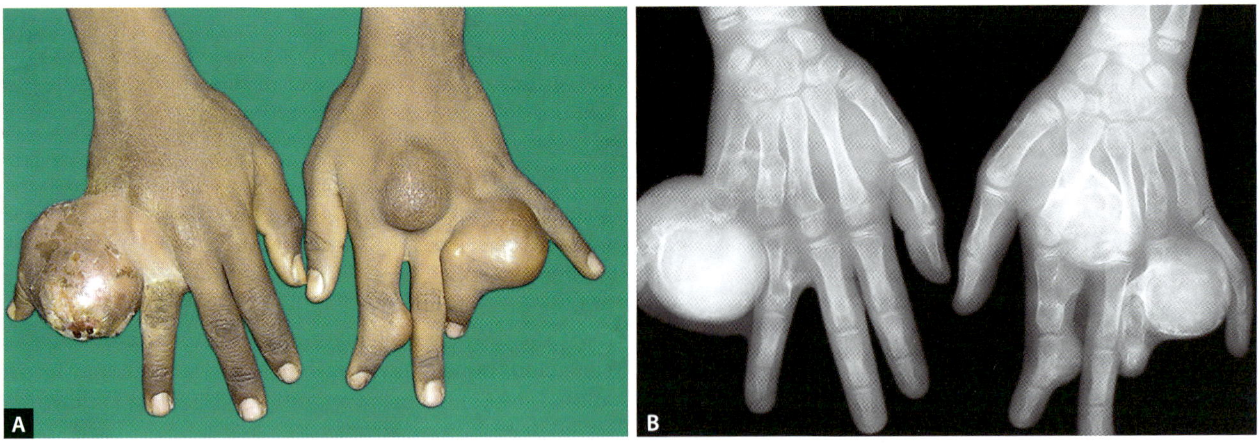

Figs. 62A and B: Enchondromatosis. This is an atypical case of multiple hereditary enchondromatosis. A typical solitary enchondroma looks like the one present on 4th metacarpal of left hand.

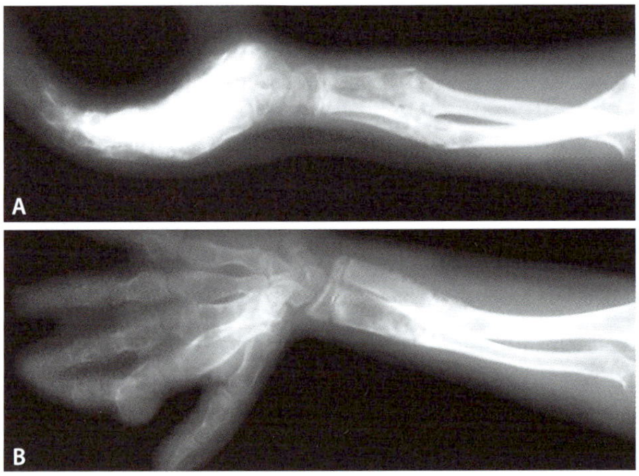

Figs. 63A and B: Ollier's disease. Involvement of left forearm bones with multiple lytic lesions with deformities and pathological fracture.

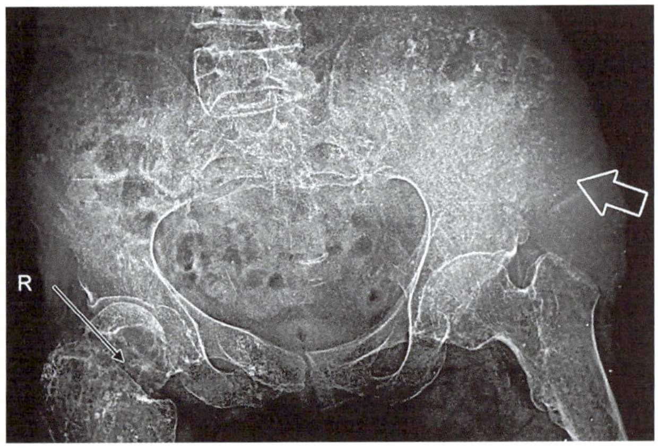

Fig. 64: Development of chondrosarcoma in a patient with Maffucci syndrome. The patient had multiple enchondromatosis and developed blindness at the age of 35 years followed by chondrosarcoma foot after 10 years and of left iliac bone (block arrow) within 1 year. She also developed pathological fracture neck (arrow) and shaft of right femur at this presentation.

beyond cortex into soft tissues heralds development of chondrosarcoma. Necrosis in the tumor tissue and myxoid change suggests chondrosarcoma. By itself, the enchondromas in Ollier's disease are cellular and may also show atypia making differentiation from low-grade chondrosarcoma difficult. Patients should be carefully followed up for possible development of chondrosarcoma. Some 25% patients with Ollier's disease develop chondrosarcoma by age of 40 years **(Fig. 64)**. Patients with Maffucci syndrome are at even higher risk of developing malignancy (possibility of osteosarcoma and dedifferentiated chondrosarcoma) including those of bone and joints.

Chondroblastoma

(ICD-O 9230/0, calcifying giant cell tumor, epiphyseal chondromatous giant cell tumor, and Codman tumor)

This benign cartilage producing neoplasm accounts for <1% of the bone tumors. Codman confused this to chondromatous variant of GCT that was later corrected by Jaffe and Lichtenstein to chondroblastoma as a distinct entity. The tumor usually is seen in skeletally immature patients (10–25 years of age) and classically is located in the epiphysis or apophysis of bones. Metaphyseal or diaphyseal occurrence is unusual. Growth plate is not a barrier for tumor growth and the tumor is often seen crossing across to adjacent metaphysis, but joint penetration is rare if at all. Patients with flat bone (skull, etc.) chondroblastoma present late (3rd to 5th decade). The femur (distal and proximal), tibia, and humerus are the preferred sites but ilium, acetabulum, temporal bones in skull, and tarsal bones are also involved. Lower limb accounts for 70% cases and the proximal femur lesions characteristically involve the greater trochanter rather than the epiphysis. There is confusion as to the origin of tumor and though the most common view of chondrogenic origin is accepted, few researchers have proposed different pathogenesis. Absence of true cartilage matrix and presence of type 1 collagen portend it to be originally a bone-forming lesion (Aigner et al.). Some researchers have suggested that the tumor to be akin to PVNS or GCT of tendon sheath where the tumor originates from intramedullary/endosteal cells similar to tendon sheath cells with preferential differentiation into chondroid tissue.

Clinical Presentation and Radiology

The lesions are solitary and mostly only one bone is involved (multifocal involvement is extremely unusual). Localized pain of long duration is the common presentation while soft tissue swelling and joint effusion can be occasionally seen. Patients with temporal bone lesions might develop tinnitus, vertigo, or hearing loss. The average duration of symptoms (delay in diagnosis) in patients with chondroblastoma is around 20 months. Radiologically, the lesions are small (usually 3–5 cm), eccentrically located in the epiphysis and mostly lytic (70% lesions, calcification is seen in less than third of patients) in a geographic pattern that occupy less than half of the epiphyseal width **(Figs. 65A and B)**. The lesions are sharply demarcated with a thin sclerotic rim that differentiates them from GCT (sclerotic rim absent). The bone is usually not expanded, and there is no periosteal reaction. Secondary ABCs are common. Uncommon large lesions may deform especially in weight-bearing bones due to collapse of the wall. Rare chondroblastomas may metastasize to lungs, however, the excision of the metastasis suffices. These are called aggressive chondroblastomas. The metastasis, however, is nonprogressive.

Histopathology

Gross examination of tissue reveals blue-gray chondroid areas of chondroid tissue with yellow gritty areas of calcification or immature bone. Secondary ABCs may be seen. The chondroblasts are seen with numerous variations. Typically the oval or polygonal cell with a round nucleus that contains prominent longitudinal groove is seen. Chondroblasts are commonly packed in pseudolobulated sheets arranged in a pavement-like pattern. S-100 protein is frequently demonstrable in the chondroblast. Some cells with abundant pink cytoplasm represent epithelioid variant. Syncytial variety lacks most of the typical features. Interspersed are spindle, giant cells, and macrophages that may be hemosiderin positive. Fine network of calcification present around the chondroblasts focally, especially in the necrotic areas results in characteristic "chicken wire" pattern of calcium deposition.

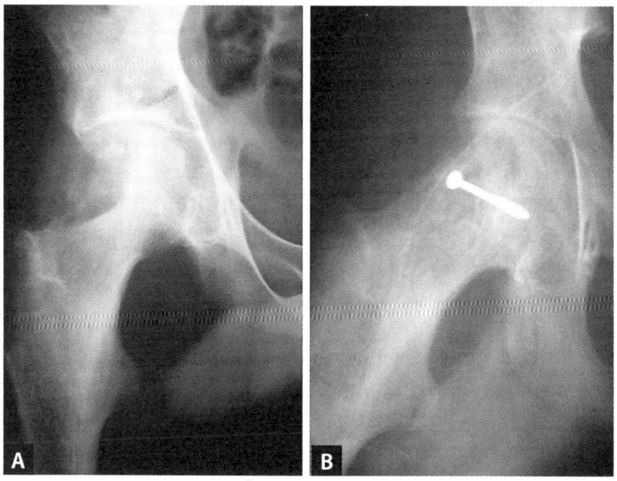

Figs. 65A and B: Chondroblastoma of head of femur treated with intralesional excision and bone grafting.
Source: S Rastogi, Professor and Head, Department of Orthopedics, Hamdard Institute of Medical Sciences and Research, New Delhi, India.

Differential Diagnosis

Radiologically—GCT, chondrosarcoma (clear cell type and low grade), osteomyelitis (Brodie's abscess), EOG, IOG, and histopathologically—osteosarcoma, clear cell chondrosarcoma.

Management

Marginal excision with bone grafting or PMMA cement packing is the usual surgical management. Recurrence is seen in 14–18% cases and is seen within 2 years. Huvos et al. found increased recurrence in lesions associated with ABC though it is not substantiated. For reasons of incomplete curettage to avoid injury to growth plate, the recurrence is more common in pediatric epiphyseal lesions. The curettage can be extended with high-speed burr or cryoablation **(Figs. 65A and B)**. Tissue contamination should be particularly avoided as this is the most common mode of recurrence. Incomplete excision is the most common cause of recurrence (up to 50% within first 2 years) in flat bones, however. For aggressive chondroblastomas, wide excision with excision of metastasis usually suffices **(Figs. 66A to D)**. Recently radiofrequency ablation (Rybak et al.) with a probe has been reported to provide prolonged pain relief in smaller lesions.

Chondromyxoid Fibroma (ICD-O Code 9241/0)

Chondromyxoid fibroma is a rare (<1%) benign locally aggressive tumor first described by Jaffe and Lichtenstein in 1948. Histopathologically, it is characterized by lobules of spindle-shaped or stellate cells in a background of myxoid or chondroid intercellular material. It occurs in males more commonly than females and is seen in 2nd to 3rd decades. Although seen in almost every bone, the common site of occurrence is around knee. A fourth of tumors occur in flat bones especially ilium. Pain usually mild and present for long time is the most common symptom. Flat bone lesions are most often discovered incidentally.

Radiologically, the lesions are geographical, lytic, and grow along the longitudinal axis of bone originating in metaphysis near physis. In a long bone, the location is typically metaphyseal, eccentric, sharply marginated oval lytic zone. In small bones, the lesion appears like a "flame-shaped" lytic lesion. Lesions may extend to epiphysis or diaphysis. Matrix mineralization is not seen (but, if present then it should be suspected for chondrosarcoma).

Histopathology

Gross pathological examination characteristically reveals a solid expansile bluish-gray or white tumor, without necrosis, or cystic changes. The tumor is quite discrete from the surrounding bone. Histopathologically, the classic features are a lobular pattern with stellate or spindle-shaped cells in a myxoid background that have alternating hypercellular and hypocellular patterns. The stellate cells have irregular cell

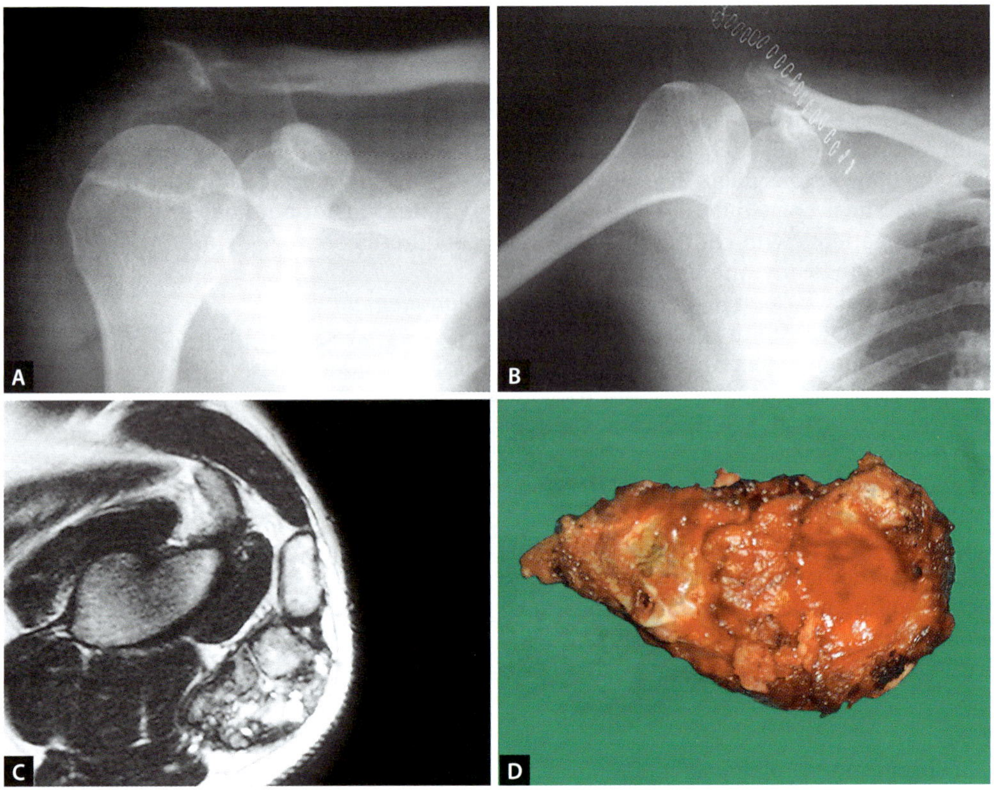

Figs. 66A to D: Chondroblastoma. (A and B) Radiographs demonstrate multicystic, expansile mass localized to acromion and spine of scapula; (C) MRI demonstrates heterogeneously enhancing soft tissue mass with intermediate cystic areas involving the spinous process and acromion of scapula; (D) The lesion was excised and patient kept in aeroplane splint in postoperative period.

processes and scalloped cell membranes, the cytoplasm stains positive for glycogen and prominent cytoplasmic fibrils are seen (combined features of fibroblastic and chondroblastic differentiation). Similarly, hydrated proteoglycans (constituent of the myxoid matrix) and collagen type II (a marker of chondrocytic cell differentiation) are expressed together in the matrix. This combination is quite unique to this tumor. Calcification is seen in tumors from elderly patients and in flat bone tumors. ABC areas are noted in approximately 10% cases. Clonal abnormalities of chromosome 6 particularly the rearrangements of the long arm of chromosome 6 at bands q13 and q25 have been observed in a few patients.

Differential Diagnosis

Chondrosarcoma (permeative growth pattern, involvement of adjacent bone seen), chondroblastoma, and GCT. Fibromyxoma comprises fibrous tissue in a myxoid stroma, but chondroid, osteoid, and bone formation can occur variably. Tumors are predominantly metaphyseal and lack lobulation of chondromyxoid fibroma.

Treatment

Marginal excision with curettage and bone grafting (or PMMA packing) is the standard management of the tumor as the prognosis is excellent. Even recurrences which occur in approximately 15% of cases usually within first 2 years are treated similarly. In some lesions at periarticular sites, the lesion has to be managed with excision and joint reconstruction **(Figs. 67A and B)**.

Chondrosarcoma

Chondrosarcoma is a malignant bone tumor with differentiation of the neoplastic cells to form pure hyaline cartilage. Degenerative changes in the form of myxoid changes, calcification, or ossification may be present. The term chondrosarcoma includes several forms (ranging from milder to aggressive) with diverse morphological features. The different forms are as under:

- Conventional chondrosarcoma
  - Primary
  - Secondary
- Periosteal (juxtacortical)
- Dedifferentiated
- Mesenchymal
- Clear cell

Depending on the tumor location within bone, they are classified as intramedullary (central) or peripheral. Peripheral chondrosarcomas closely resemble periosteal osteosarcomas. Chondrosarcomas tend to occur in older age groups (5th to 7th decades) than the de novo osteosarcomas and do not form the characteristic osteoid. Radiologists classify peripheral chondrosarcoma for differentiating secondary chondrosarcomas that arise on an osteochondroma. Benign cartilage lesions and low-grade chondrosarcomas appear pathologically similar. Also, secondary chondrosarcoma can occur in a previously benign cartilaginous lesion. Dynamic contrast-enhanced MRI has the greatest diagnostic accuracy (93.4% for chondrosarcoma) to differentiating cartilaginous tumors.

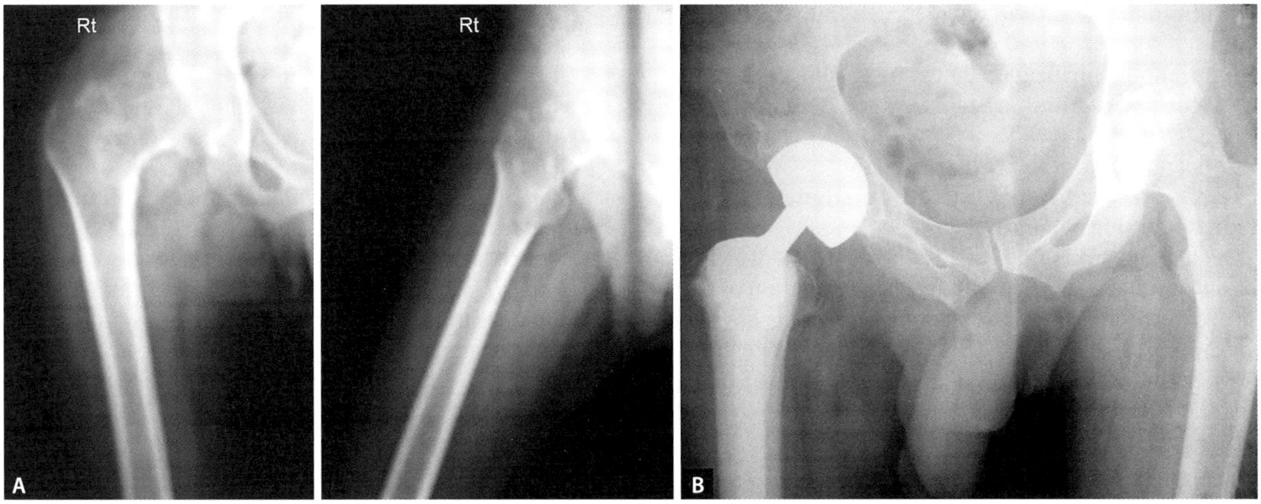

Figs. 67A and B: Chondromyxoid fibroma of proximal femur treated with excision and joint reconstruction.
Source: S Rastogi, Professor and Head, Department of Orthopedics, Hamdard Institute of Medical Sciences and Research, New Delhi, India.

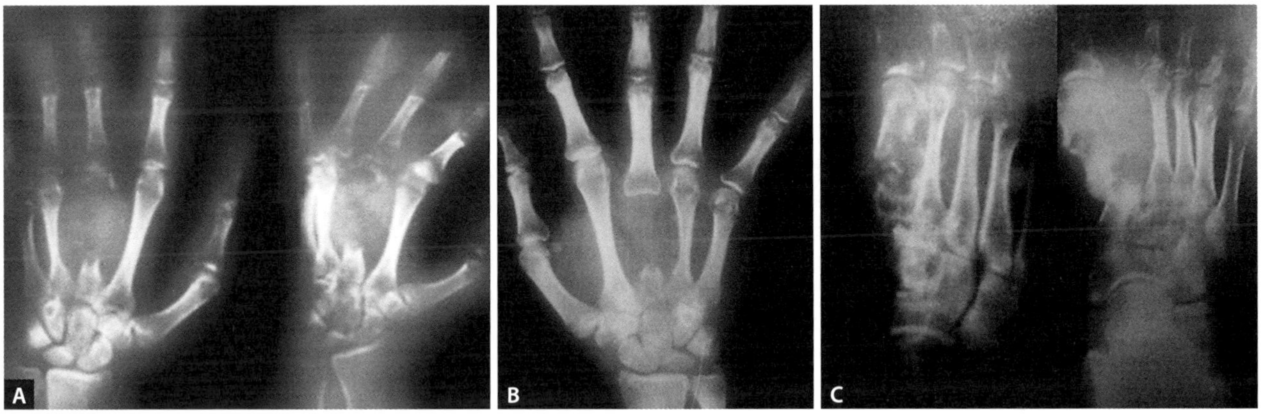

Figs. 68A to C: Chondrosarcoma of small bones. (A and B) Here, the lesions in metacarpal and metatarsals are typified; (C) The metatarsal lesions represent the low-grade chondrosarcoma radiologically.

Primary Chondrosarcoma (ICD-O 9220/3)

This is typically a centrally located tumor arising in a previously normal bone. It is the *third most common* primary bone tumor placed only after myeloma and osteosarcoma in frequency of occurrence. Majority of patients diagnosed with chondrosarcoma are over 50 years of age with a slight male preference. Pelvic bones (typically ilium) followed by the proximal femur and proximal humerus are preferred sites. Girdle regions are hence predisposed for this tumor (around two-thirds of cases). The tumor is extremely rare in spine and craniofacial bones. *Pain* (with or without swelling) is the most common presentation in intramedullary chondrosarcoma, however, painless of painful *swelling* is the most common presentation in peripheral chondrosarcomas. Nerve dysfunction (sciatic or femoral nerves) is seen with pelvic lesions near a neurovascular bundle. Limitation of joint ROM is seen with chondrosarcomas close to a joint. The tumors grow and evolve slowly with metastasis occurring late, recurrent tumors are, however, more aggressive and often dedifferentiated. The mean delay in diagnosis (time from pain to diagnosis) is 19.4 months for grade I and grade II chondrosarcomas and 15.5 months for grade III chondrosarcomas.

Radiologically, conventional chondrosarcomas are often large lesions (>5 cm) that arise in either the diaphysis or the metaphysis. The intramedullary spread is extensive and may involve whole diaphyseo-metaphyseal region or even whole bone **(Figs. 68A and B)** with multiple bone surface erosions (endosteal scalloping). Epiphyseal origin is rare but typical for the clear cell variant of chondrosarcoma as is joint involvement.

Chondrosarcoma is confusing radiologically as it demonstrates both *adaptive* (features suggesting benign lesions) and *aggressive* (malignancy suggestive) radiologic signs. Cortical expansion and thickening are the adaptive changes whereas cortical disruption and development of soft tissue masses represent aggressive radiological changes associated with chondrosarcoma. Cortex is usually thickened and periosteal reaction often absent. The radiological features **(Fig. 68C)** of low-grade lesion on a radiograph include:

- Dense matrix calcifications shaped-like "C (arcs) or O (rings) or spicules" (typical for tumors of cartilage origin), resembling popcorn or commas
- Widespread uniform calcification
- Eccentric lobular growth of the tumor

The radiological features suggesting a high-grade lesion include:

- Amorphous calcification that appears faint on X-ray.
- Larger uncalcified areas or lysis within a previous calcification
- Concentric growth of soft tissue mass
- Endosteal scalloping indicates malignancy (except enchondroma of hand)

Dedifferentiation should be suspected in areas of increased lucency or inhomogeneity. MRI is the investigation of choice to access the extent of tumor for surgical planning. Low-grade chondrosarcomas pose a challenge to diagnosis especially its differentiation from benign chondroid tumors **(Table 19)**. Dynamic contrast-enhanced MR perfusion (DCE-MRI) has been found helpful in them.

Histopathology: Pathologist needs to have good experience in differentiating and diagnosing low-grade chondrosarcomas. Gross examination reveals the typical translucent, blue-gray, or white color corresponding to the presence of hyaline cartilage. The tumors are lobulated with focal hemorrhage and liquefactive (myxoid) changes. Myxoid changes especially if extensive are harbinger of malignant change. Cortical destruction could be evident in flat bones with extension into soft tissues. High-grade lesions are easy to recognize with cellular cartilage matrix showing soft-tissue extension and/or permeation of bone with entrapped pre-existing trabeculae. Aggressive features in chondrosarcoma are suggested by extensive mitotic activity, chondrocyte multinucleation, and necrosis. Myxoid degenerative change is frequent and histopathologically appears like "bubbly transformation" of the cartilage giving the appearance of cyst formation. For low-grade chondrosarcomas some general rules have been developed over large studies done in the past. Whatever the histological picture, the cartilage tumors of sternum are almost always malignant. The chondromas of hands and feet, periosteal chondromas, Ollier's and Maffucci disease associated lesions, and soft-tissue chondromas are dealt as benign despite prominent cellularity. The chondrosarcomas in small bones of hands and feet (rare) present with cortical destruction and permeation into surrounding soft tissues and cancellous bones.

Grading and prognosis: Grading, though not very useful, for other tumors is important with prognostic relevance and

TABLE 19: Radiological features to keep in mind while evaluating chondroid lesions radiologically.

Characteristic	*Enchondroma*	*Chondrosarcoma*
Lesion mineralization	Present	Yes
Bone scan "hot spot"	Less common (one-fifth of lesions)	Common (more than 3/4th of lesions)
Cortical break	Uncommon (<10%)	Present
Soft-tissue extension	Absent	Present
Periosteal reaction	Absent	Present

Note: Important to understand is the fact that lesions in small bones of hands and feet appear more aggressive radiologically and histologically but are less likely to be chondrosarcoma as compared to similar lesions in the axial skeleton (spine and pelvis) that are more likely to be malignant variant.

surgical planning in chondrosarcomas. The tumor is graded as follows *(Mayo clinic and WHO):*

- *Grade I (low grade):* Cytologically, quite similar to enchondroma but with higher cellularity and plump nuclei with open chromatin structure. Occasional binucleate cells are seen.
- *Grade II (intermediate grade):* Prominent cellularity and greater nuclear atypia. Distinct nucleoli are present in most cells, myxoid change may be seen.
- *Grade III (high grade):* High cellularity, prominent nuclear atypia, and pleomorphism. Mitoses are significant and easily located.

Most of the lesions (two-thirds) are grade I while grade II comprise just less than one-third. Grade III is rare. Myxoid change indicates intermediate or higher grade.

Grading (MD Anderson):

- *Grade 1:* The lesion has innocuous hyaline cartilage with scant cellularity. The neoplastic cells have dark, pyknotic nuclei (not larger than lymphocyte).
- *Grade 2A:* More cellular, >20% of cells have nuclei larger than that of lymphocytes. Binucleation and nucleoli may be seen (not prominent), but mitoses are not identified.
- *Grade 2B:* Cellular matrix with abundant binucleate cells, occasional bizarre nuclei, or spindling. The cellular areas are located more toward the periphery of lobules. Mitoses, if found, are <1 every 10 high-power fields.
- *Grade 3:* Lesions have easily identifiable mitosis with a rate of two or more mitoses per 10 high-power fields.

Grade 2B (10–15% chance) and grade 3 (50% chance) have the capability of distant metastasis. Loss of 13q has been associated with metastasis (usually to lungs). Genetically, the periploidy affecting 9p12-22 region found between NOR1 (Orphan nuclear receptor) and EWS (Ewing sarcoma breakpoint region-1) genes is the most common aberration. Grading has a special role in prognostication of chondrosarcoma as high-grade lesion is associated with poor survival other poor prognostic factor is age >50 years.

Chondrosarcoma in situ is used by some authors to describe a symptomatic, intramedullary cartilaginous tumor of a long bone that radiologically appears to be a low-grade chondrosarcoma with lytic areas or high-grade endosteal scalloping but devoid of adaptive or aggressive changes. They have the histologic features of an enchondroma or a low-grade chondrosarcoma. Chondrosarcoma in situ does not metastasize or recur but is considered as a premalignant lesion that should be closely followed clinically and radiologically. These patients can be treated with *intralesional excision* and adjuvant therapy.

Differential diagnosis: Chondroblastomas, enchondromas, chondromyxoid fibromas, fibrosarcoma, fibrous histiocytoma, metastatic disease, Paget's disease, osteochondromas, and Nora's lesion. The differentiating features of chondrosarcoma include an infiltrative margin, entrapment of bone, and infiltration of the Haversian system. Periosteal chondromas are smaller lesions (<3 cm) compared to chondrosarcomas that are usually >5 cm. Chondroblastic osteosarcoma will have malignant osteoid formation. Tophaceous pseudogout may be mistaken as chondrosarcoma and should be differentiated by carefully sampling and processing the specimen. Finding crystals by polarized microscopy and presence of granulomatous response suggests gout.

Management: Wide resection is the surgical margin for treatment of chondrosarcoma. Low-grade chondrosarcomas may be treated by marginal procedures in selected cases if the expected morbidity with wide margins is too high. Use of adjuvant should be considered. Chemotherapy use is controversial, and though for low-grade lesions, it is ineffective, for high-grade lesions in young patient, one may consider chemotherapy to improve outcome. Radiation should be done if wide excision is not satisfactorily performed. Prognosis is primarily dependent on histological grade with 90% survival at 5 years for grade 1 lesions, around 81% for grade 2, and 30% for grade 3 lesions (Evans et al.). Lesions with isolated metastasis (usually lungs) should also be treated with wide resection along with metastasectomy. Lesions that recur (commonly 5 years or later) may show incremental grade and are more aggressive. Newer agent, like BIBR1532, that specifically inhibits the telomerase has been studied to resensitize chondrosarcoma to chemotherapy. Tumor angiogenesis has a role in prognostication and also targeted therapy. Hypoxia inducible factor-1α (HIF-1α) is expressed in chondrosarcoma cells; especially, the increased expression of nuclear HIF-1α is associated with decreased disease-free survival. Inhibition of the angiogenic tyrosine kinase receptors for VEGF, fibroblast growth factor (FGF), and platelet-derived growth factor with oratinib has been shown to reduce tumor size and neovascularity in vivo. Trabectedin induces tumor necrosis and in extraskeletal chondrosarcoma. The role of transcription factor ETV5, micro-RNA, and SOX-9 is actively searched. SOX-9 expression increases in response to low levels of micro-RNA-145 which, in turn, increases expression of ETV5 and subsequently matrix metalloproteinase-2 linked to pathophysiology of chondrosarcoma. Bisphosphonate zoledronic acid has been found to reduce bone pain and improve quality of life in chondrosarcoma patients. Though not in clinical use, third generation bisphosphonate—minodronate has been shown to reduce chondrosarcoma cell growth in a dose-dependent manner in vitro. Similarly, inhibiting estrogen signaling with the aromatase inhibitor exemestane has been shown to inhibit chondrosarcoma cell growth in vitro. Anti-apoptotic proteins Bcl-2, Bcl-xL, and XIAP have been found to mediate radioresistance of chondrosarcoma. Radiosensitivity can be induced in chondrosarcoma by using siRNA to silence the expression of these proteins (*see* Chapter on "Gene Therapy"). Silencing the proteins individually causes up to 9.2-fold increases in radiation sensitivity while silencing two of these genes could enhance the sensitivity even further incrementally. Antisense oligonucleotides against bcl-2 have been found effective for treatment in melanoma and may be possibly helpful for chondrosarcoma too. Acridine orange has been used in radiotherapy to improve generation of reactive oxygen species and enhance tumor kill.

Periosteal chondrosarcoma (Juxtacortical chondrosarcoma, ICD-O 9220/3): This is a rare malignant hyaline cartilage tumor occurring on the surface of bone. The tumor occurs in adults. The tumor occurs in metaphysis or diaphysis usually of distal femur and presents with pain with or without swelling. The tumor erodes the underlying cortex and is covered by the periosteum. Histologically, it is similar to conventional chondrosarcoma and mostly grade 1 or 2 (Mayo). Periosteal chondromas and osteosarcoma are close differential, the former is <5 cm and while latter has malignant osteoid formation.

Secondary Chondrosarcoma

The chondrosarcoma arises in benign precursors [solitary osteochondroma (<2%)/osteochondromatosis (5–30%)], Ollier's and Maffucci syndrome (25–30%). Some say malignancy is a certainty in Maffucci syndrome. The risk factors for development of secondary chondrosarcoma are summarized in **Box 5**. These patients are younger than primary lesions. Girdle bones are more frequently affected **(Figs. 69A to D)**. Features that suggest malignant change include sudden growth of the lesion (increased pain or size of lesion), vanishing calcification and increased lytic permeation, cortical destruction, endosteal erosion, and increase in osteochondroma cartilage cap thickness. Chondrosarcoma arising in enchondromatosis has usually very mucoid/myxoid appearance. The tissue is washed away during fixation due to liquefaction leaving behind cystic cavities. Secondary chondrosarcoma must be distinguished from dedifferentiated chondrosarcoma, which also arises from a pre-existing cartilaginous tumor but characteristically has a high-grade sarcoma adjacent to a low-grade cartilage tumor (see below). The high-grade and dedifferentiated tumor is typically of histology different from chondrosarcoma. Secondary chondrosarcoma, in contrast, is composed entirely of cartilaginous tissue, and it is usually a low-grade malignancy. Furthermore though very rare but dedifferentiated chondrosarcoma can arise in secondary chondrosarcomas. The prognosis of secondary chondrosarcoma is good and comparable to low-grade conventional chondrosarcoma with overall survival of 90% at 5 years. Local recurrence is the only

BOX 5: Risk factors and identifying features for development of secondary chondrosarcoma.

Clinical features:
- *Hereditary conditions:* Ollier's disease, Maffucci syndrome, hereditary multiple exostosis (EXT1, EXT2, and EXT3 mutations)
- Sudden onset of pain or sudden increase in pain
- Male (2:1) in mid-30s
- Sudden increase in size of a dormant lesion
- Pelvic and hip lesions
- Irregular surface to palpation

Radiological:
- Size of osteochondroma >5 cm
- Cartilage cap >2 cm in adults (in adolescents the cap is already quite thick averaging 3 cm in most studies)
- Blurring of osseous border at osteocartilaginous junction suggests invasiveness and is more important than cap thickness
- Inhomogeneous mineralization of cartilage cap

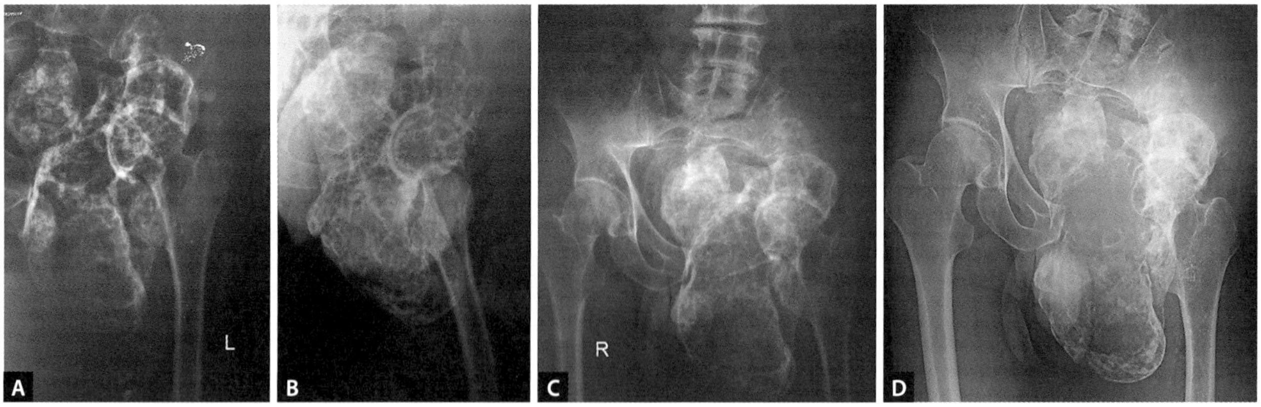

Figs. 69A to D: Evolution and development of chondrosarcoma in unresected large pelvic neoplasia (?osteochondroma). Patient only had radiographs [(year = 2014; A and B), (year = 2018; C)] and no formal attempt at tissue diagnosis was ever attempted. He presented with sudden increase in pain in the pelvic region and was found to develop definite degeneration and increased lucency in the central and inferior portion of the previous neoplastic mass [(year = 2019; D)] compared to previous radiographs (*cf.: A, B,* and *C*). CT-guided biopsy from the lesion was done and demonstrated chondrosarcoma in the current lesion.

concern affecting 10–20% cases so wide excision should be meticulous.

Dedifferentiated chondrosarcoma (chondrosarcoma with additional mesenchymal component): This is characteristically a biphasic lesion containing two clearly defined components, a well-differentiated cartilage tumor which is represented by either an enchondroma or a low-grade chondrosarcoma that is juxtaposed to a high-grade nonchondromatous sarcoma (usually MFH but other lesions such as osteosarcoma, fibrosarcoma, angiosarcoma, and rhabdomyosarcoma have also been reported). Both forms possibly arise from single intramedullary stem cell that evolves to form low-grade chondrosarcoma and with some chromatic aberrations also an anaplastic component (less evolved form). There is histologically abrupt transition between the two components. The patients usually belong to 50–60 years but range from 30 to 85 years. Pain is the most common presenting symptom, however, swelling, paresthesia, and pathological fractures may occur depending on location.

Radiologically these are large, poorly-defined, lytic, intraosseous lesion that often perforate cortex and develop extraosseous extension. The appearance is bimorphic with a lytic mass extending to soft tissues seen in continuation with low-grade chondrosarcoma component with abrupt transition. The cartilaginous portion shows the ring-like opacities that are sharply discrete from the lytic component.

Histopathology: Grossly both cartilaginous and noncartilaginous tumor components can be identified separately in varying proportions, but due to pressure effect or rapid growth, the cartilaginous component may be extremely small. The blue-gray lobulated cartilaginous component is usually central abruptly demarcated from the anaplastic expanded fleshy high-grade component is predominantly extraosseous.

Differential diagnosis: Mesenchymal chondrosarcoma and chondroblastic osteosarcoma.

Management: Dedifferentiated chondrosarcomas are aggressive neoplasms and have a poor prognosis. Metastasis is common and frequently disseminated. Chemotherapy should be used along with aggressive wide resection. Despite this aggressive approach, >90% of patients succumb to disease within 2 years.

Clear Cell Chondrosarcoma (Earlier called Atypical Chondroblastoma)

This is a low-grade malignant, but slow-growing neoplasm, composed of neoplastic chondrocytes having clear cytoplasm in addition to hyaline cartilage. It has a predilection for long bone epiphysis. The tumor is commonly mistaken clinically and histologically for chondroblastomas and osteoblastomas. They represent roughly 2% of all chondrosarcomas. Most patients are in the 3rd or 4th decades (younger than conventional chondrosarcoma), with male predominance (M:F = 3:1). Majority of the lesions are located in humeral and femoral heads (two-thirds of cases), however, any bone of the skeleton may be affected. Pain is the most common presentation, however, due to epiphyseal location joint symptoms also dominate (stiffness, limited ROM, swelling, and effusion). Symptoms may be sometimes prolonged for as long as 5 years.

Radiologically, they are well-circumscribed geographic, lytic, expansile, and focally calcified lesions with epicenter in epiphysis. The resemblance is quite strikingly similar to chondroblastoma. The margins are well-defined.

Histopathology: Grossly, the pathological specimens appear tan, soft, and granular lacking typical chondroid features. Significant amounts of the clear cell arranged in lobular groups are found with focal hyaline cartilage. The "clear cell" chondrocyte has a sharp border and a distinctive large, round, central nucleus containing prominent nucleolus. These prominent clear cells typically stain for S-100 protein (a feature of chondroid cells) and are positive for type 2 collagen. Some cells have a powdery eosinophilic cytoplasm resembling chondroblasts of chondroblastoma. Ultrastructurally, the features of chondrocytes are well-demonstrated that include presence of large, dilated rough endoplasmic reticulum and ample glycogen. The tumor shows rich distribution of multinucleated giant cells. Interestingly, foci of osteoid may also be present but that does not make diagnosis of osteosarcoma as this osteoid is distinctly lined by chondroblasts dissimilar from osteosarcoma.

Differential diagnosis: Radiologically, chondroblastoma, GCT; pathologically, metastatic clear cell carcinoma (renal cell carcinoma).

Treatment: Treatment is by wide surgical resection with overall good prognosis. Late metastasis even after 15 years of initial surgery has been reported.

Mesenchymal Chondrosarcoma (Polyhistioma, Primitive Multipotential Primary Sarcoma of Bone)

Rare bimorphic malignant tumor composed of highly undifferentiated small round cells and islands of well-differentiated hyaline cartilage. The neoplasm occurs in younger age group frequently in the 2nd and the 3rd decades without any sex predilection. Flat bones and axial skeleton is the usual site of involvement typically the craniofacial bones (especially the jawbones), the ribs, the ilium, and the vertebrae. One-fourth of the cases occur in extraskeletal sites and meninges are one of the most common extraskeletal sites of involvement. Longstanding pain and swelling are the common features; oncologic osteomalacia has also been reported. Radiologically, the lesions are lytic and expansile with poor margins and cortical destruction. The small round cells simulate the Ewing's sarcoma arranged in hemangiopericytoma-like pattern. The small cell component is positive for Leu7 and CD99 (similar to Ewing's) and the chondroid component is positive for S-100 protein (like chondrosarcoma). The chromosomal translocations of the Ewing family of tumors are absent from mesenchymal chondrosarcoma. Polymerase chain reaction (PCR) suggests reduced expression of TP53 in one-fifth of the cases. The tumor should be differentiated from Ewing's sarcoma, small cell osteosarcoma, lymphoma, and undifferentiated carcinoma. Mesenchymal chondrosarcoma has an intermediate prognosis with a strong tendency to locally recur after resection. Treatment usually relies on wide resection followed by chemotherapy. Radiotherapy is successful and should be considered for surgically inaccessible tumors. Distant metastasis may occur even after 10 years so a prolonged follow-up is necessary.

FIBROUS LESIONS

Desmoplastic Fibroma (Desmoid Tumor of Bone, ICD-O 8823/0)

This is the osseous counterpart of aggressive soft tissue fibromatosis. It is a nonmetastasizing but locally aggressive neoplasm that comprises typical fibroblasts dispersed in collagenized stroma. Patients usually range in age from 1 to 70 years so it can be said that they have been reported from all age groups but most cases are identified in adolescents and young adults. Lesions commonly occur in metaphysis of long bones. Mandible is the most common site of occurrence but pelvis, ribs, vertebrae, the small tubular bones of the hands and feet have also been reported to be involved. Radiologically, the lesions are lytic and expand bone with coarse trabeculations traveling across **(Figs. 70A to C)**. Periosteal reaction is absent and margins are usually sharp. MRI is preferred diagnostic modality to identify the soft tissue spread and characterization of the lesion. It has low-signal intensity in both T1- and T2-weighted MR images. Grossly the tumor is gray to creamy-white arranged in whorled pattern. The tissue has low cellularity and spindle cells (fibroblasts/myofibroblasts) are separated by abundant collagen. Mitotic figures and atypia are absent or inconspicuous. Similar to soft tissue desmoid trisomy of chromosome 8 and 20 (FISH analysis) is frequently found. The tumor should be differentiated from fibrosarcoma. The tumor is locally progressive and aggressive. Curettage has unacceptably high-local recurrence rates of up to 80% while even after resection 20% cases may recur. Recurrence may occur even years after local excision.

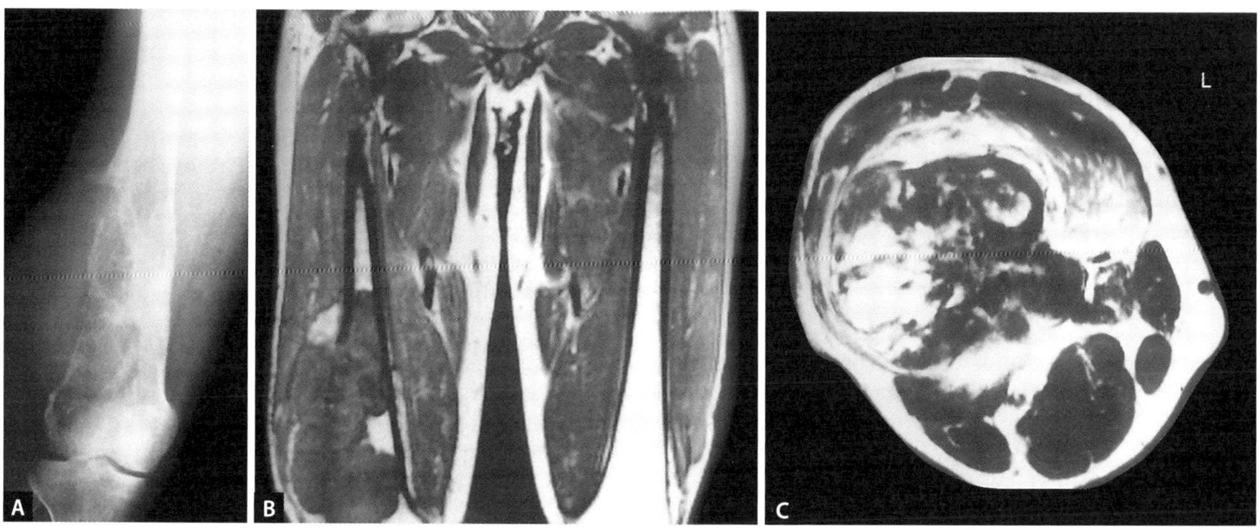

Figs. 70A to C: Desmoplastic fibroma of femur with infiltration into surrounding tissues.

Fibrosarcoma
(ICD-O 8810/3)

This is a malignant spindle cell neoplasm of bone in which the tumor cells are typically organized in a fascicular or "herringbone" pattern. The tumor exclusive has fibrous differentiation without any osteoid or chondroid component. With greater awareness and increasing diagnosis of leiomyosarcoma and rhabdomyosarcomas (previously clubbed with fibrosarcoma), the exact incidence of fibrosarcoma is difficult to determine but they approximately constitute up to 5% of all primary malignant bone tumors. Etiology is unknown but some one-fourth of these tumors have previous associated conditions like prior radiation therapy, Paget's disease, ameloblastic fibroma, GCT, enchondroma, osteochondroma, fibrous dysplasia (FD), bone infarcts, chronic osteomyelitis, and hereditary bone dysplasia.

Clinical Presentation

The tumor is uniformly distributed from 2nd to 6th decades (cases have been even reported from infancy) without any gender preference and cases occurring. The metaphyses of long bones are the most common site typically the distal and proximal femur and proximal humerus. Though pain and swelling are the usual symptoms, significant population (one-thirds) of patients have pathological fracture at presentation.

Radiologically, fibrosarcoma usually appears has a destructive geographic permeative pattern. Some cases may have an ill-defined permeative, "moth-eaten" appearance with cortical destruction, and soft-tissue extension. Periosteal reaction is common.

Histopathology

On gross examination, well-differentiated tumors are white, hard, and gritty due to copious collagen synthesis. The margins are clearly defined. Poorly differentiated tumors are soft with a fleshy consistency and higher cellularity. The spindle-shaped cells are arranged in a fascicular or "herringbone" pattern with a variable amount of collagen production. The undifferentiated forms have more myxoid component justifying the term "myxofibrosarcomas". The higher the grade of tumor, the more cellular it is with less collagen and greater nuclear atypia and mitotic count.

Differential Diagnosis

Malignant fibrous histiocytoma (storiform pattern and epithelioid type cells with "ground-glass" cytoplasm), desmoplastic fibroma (few or absent mitosis).

Treatment and Prognosis

Wide excision is the preferred treatment modality with chemotherapy used in addition for high-grade lesions. Histological grade is the predominant prognostic factor. The high-grade lesions have 5-year survival of the order of only 35% while low-grade tumors are better with 85% survival at 5-years. Presence of metastasis (to lungs), age >40 years, and axial location of the tumor are other poor prognostic factors. Primary fibrosarcoma arising from cortical surface has better prognosis.

GIANT CELL TUMOR
(Osteoclastoma, ICD-O 9250/1)

Giant cell tumor of bone has been known since 1800s, but characterization and differentiation was not done until 1912; Joseph Bloodgood identified it and separated this as GCT, further elaborated later by Lichtenstein in 1940. It is a locally aggressive benign neoplasm characterized by large numbers of osteoclast-like giant cells, distributed uniformly in sheets of *neoplastic* ovoid mononuclear cells (plump epithelioid or spindle cells). The neoplastic cell is the monocyte of preosteoblast lineage that expresses several osteoblastic proteins including RANKL. GCT has propensity to locally recur after treatment (currently 10–20%) but has a low metastatic potential. It occurs slightly more often in females than in males. Young adults are commonly affected and peak incidence is seen around 20–45 years of age. Unlike chondroblastoma and ABC, it is rarely seen in skeletally immature patients (<5% have open physis at diagnosis). The tumor is not uncommon representing around 4–5% of all primary bone neoplasms, and >20% of benign primary bone tumors. The primary areas of involvement are ends of long bones commonly the distal femoral condyles, proximal tibial plateau, proximal humerus, and styloid process of distal radius. The tumor commonly originates from the epiphyseal scar near metaphyseo-epiphyseal junction. Large tumors by their sheer size may grow into the metaphysis and rarely up to even the diaphysis. Multifocal GCTs (synchronous or metachronous) are known to occur (1–2% of all cases) and are more aggressive than conventional form. It should be differentiated from metastasizing GCT **(Figs. 71A to C)**. In axial skeleton (vertebrae and sacrum), anterior column is predominantly involved. The term "benign" represented differentiation of this tumor from other aggressive lesions in older times that required amputation for treatment. This term should be dropped, however, as 3% of GCTs are either primarily malignant or would undergo malignant transformation commonly seen after radiation therapy. Tumors that recur multiple times are also prone to malignant transformation. Rarely, the GCT has also been found to metastasize (benign metastasizing tumor) similar to "benign" chondroblastoma. Some authors consider it to be a low-grade primary bone sarcoma. Few aggressive forms of GCT have been found to be associated with Paget's disease. Genotypically, the reduction in telomere length (500 base pairs) has been demonstrated in GCT. This has been demonstrated at 11p, 13p, 14p, 15p, 19q, 20q, and 21p.

Giant Cell lesions

Several tumors have giant cells as a component and are called giant cell lesions. They are not GCT per se:

- Nonossifying fibromas, metaphyseal fibrous defect **(Figs. 72A and B)**
- Chondroblastoma
- Chondromyxoid fibroma

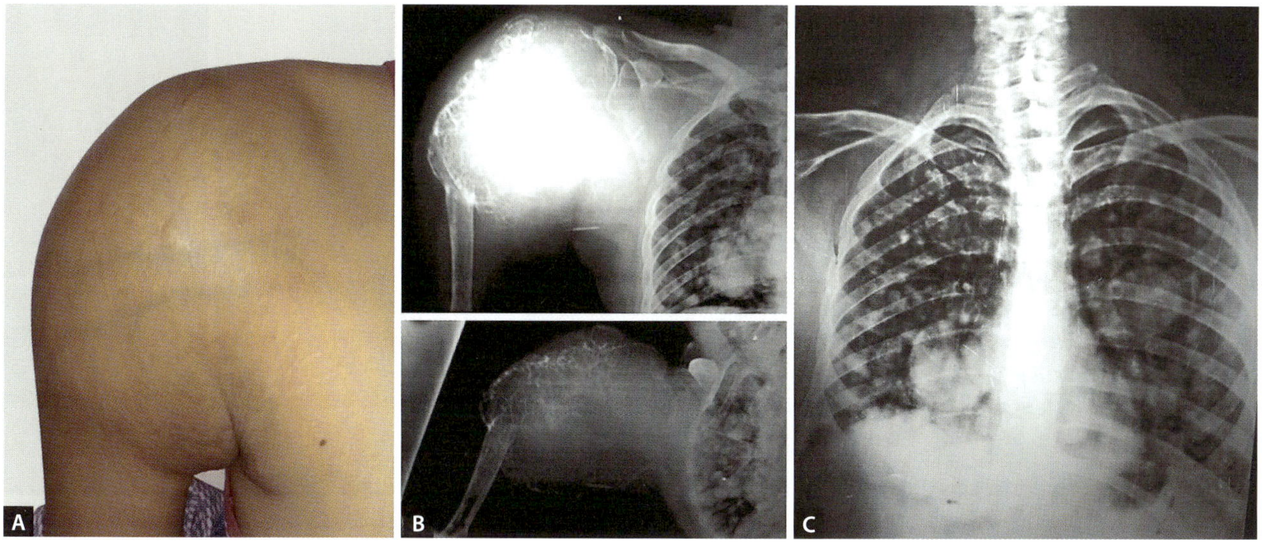

Figs. 71A to C: Metastatic giant cell tumor. This young male presented with large swelling of the left shoulder (A) neglected for various reasons as is common in this subcontinent. The radiograph shows large expansile lytic lesion involving proximal third of humerus with characteristic soap bubble appearance (B). There is loss of shape of the bone and cortical breach. Areas of soft tissue calcifications can also be seen. In the same radiograph one can appreciate pulmonary metastasis but separate chest radiograph (C) is provided for reference showing diffuse metastasis in both pulmonary fields.
Source: Dr Mohinder Chib, Senior Resident, Department of Orthopedics, Government Medical College and Hospital, Jammu, Jammu & Kashmir, India.

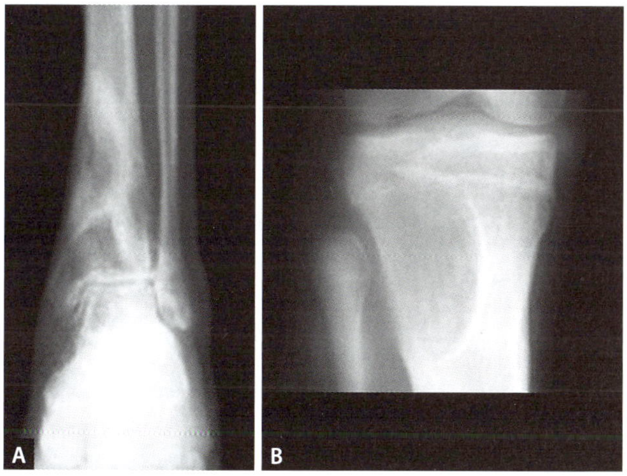

Figs. 72A and B: Nonossifying fibroma. Asymptomatic well-marginated lesions of the bone often an incidental finding.

- Unicameral and ABC
- Hyperparathyroidism
- Paget's disease
- Reparative giant cell granulomas/solid ABC

Radiologically, the characteristic appearance of GCTs is an eccentric geographical lytic lesion without matrix formation typically involving epiphysis and extending to metaphysis **(Figs. 73 to 76)**. The tumors show a well-defined sclerotic transition between the lesion and host bone. Bone response to the pathology in the form of periosteal elevation or reactive bone formation is rare unless a pathological fracture is present. The cortex is expanded and thinned with frequent breach and soft tissue extension. Soft-tissue extensions have thin "egg-shell" of bone remaining. Benign and less aggressive forms have multiple thin trabeculae running as septae across the lytic lesion giving a "soap-bubble" appearance (seen in around 20% cases). The margins of the lesion also vary and hence the tumor has been classified by Campanacci into three radiological subtypes (there is no histopathological correlation though of these radiological subtypes):

- *Type 1 (Quiescent lesions):* Well-defined margin with surrounding sclerosis and little, if any, cortical involvement.
- *Type 2 (Active tumors):* Well-defined margins, but lack surrounding sclerosis. Thin and expanded cortex but no breach **(Figs. 73A to E)**.
- *Type 3 (Aggressive tumors):* Ill-defined margins often with cortical breakthrough and soft tissue extension **(Figs. 74A to D)**.

CT scan provides a good evaluation of cortical continuity. MRI is the investigation of choice for surgical planning especially in axial lesions and aggressive forms or longstanding tumors where soft tissue extension needs accurate assessment. GCT typically shows low to intermediate signal intensity on T1-weighted images and intermediate to high intensity on T2-weighted images. Hemosiderin is associated with attenuation of signals on both T1- and T2-weighted images.

Patients usually present with painful swelling. Juxta-articular tumors may additionally have restriction of joint motion and/or joint effusion. Pathological fractures are seen in around 10% of patients.

Histopathology

Grossly, the GCTs are tan or fleshy rarely crossing the articular cartilage. Joint extension can occur through cruciates or laterally (pericapsular). Histologically, two basic cell types are observed in GCT. The diagnosis rests on stromal cells (neoplastic component) consisting of polygonal to somewhat spindle cells containing central round nuclei. These deemed neoplastic cells originate from mesenchymal stromal cells and express RANKL simulating formation and maturation

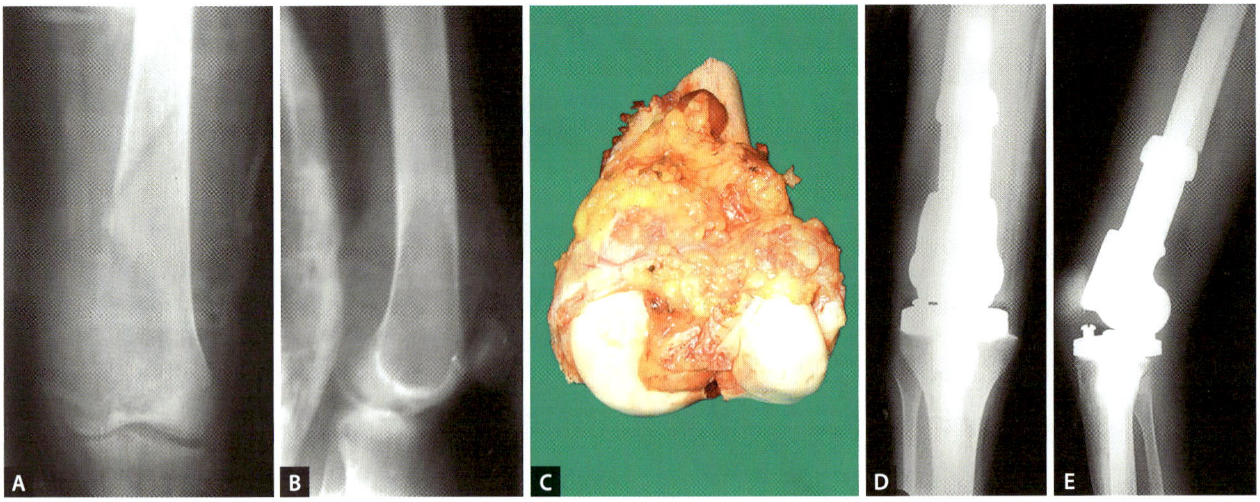

Figs. 73A to E: (A and B) Giant cell tumor of distal femur with minimal subchondral support. Though some may consider an extended curettage and bone grafting but the morbidity and chances of recurrence compromise the functional benefit; (C) So excision, and (D and E) reconstruction with custom prosthesis was done.

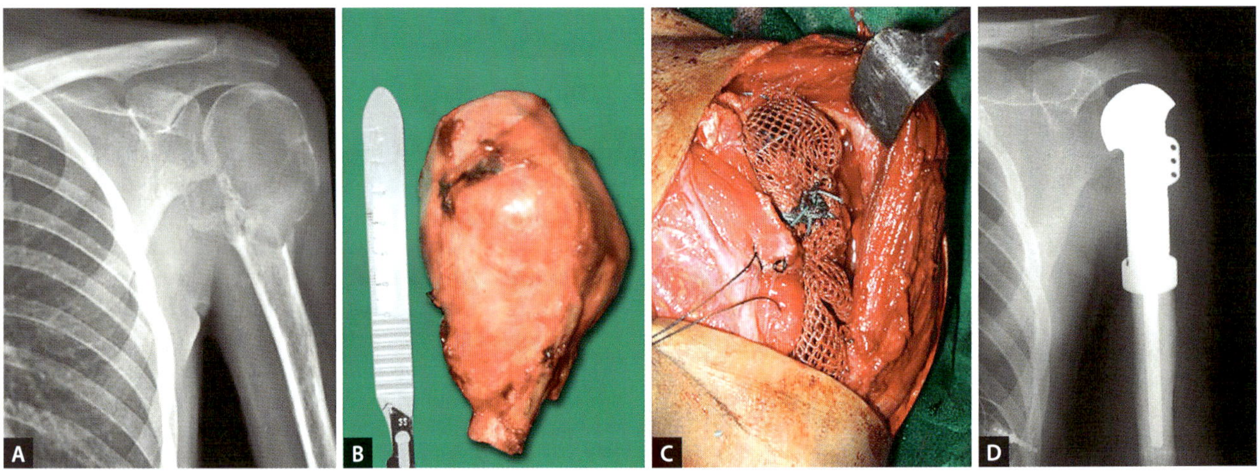

Figs. 74A to D: (A) Type 2 giant cell tumor of proximal humerus; (B) Treated with wide excision; (C) Mesh support for rotator cuff, and (D) Prosthetic reconstruction.

of osteoclasts. Mitotic figures (2–20 per 10 HPF) are often noted but do not correlate with the biological behavior. Dispersed ramblingly throughout the stroma are defining benign multinucleated osteoclast-like giant cells containing 50–100 nuclei. Foci of osteoid matrix may be observed but a chondroid matrix is virtually never seen (pathological fracture is the only exception where chondroid matrix may be seen in the healing callus). The histopathological picture is altered and gets complicated by extensive hemorrhage into the tumor, development of pathologic fracture, or previous surgery where it may resemble a primary bone sarcoma. Areas of ABC may be observed. These cystic areas have surrounding hemosiderin pigment and xanthoma cells. Some 40% of GCT have areas of vascular invasion. A "malignant GCT" is a variegated term. It has been used to describe primary bone sarcomas rich in giant cells (MFH, osteosarcoma). The term also describes "dedifferentiated" GCT that is juxtaposed (*Collision tumor*) with high-grade sarcoma (fibrosarcoma or osteosarcoma). This is better called malignant transformation of GCT. The transformation is usually "secondary" (radiation, etc.), and in this case, the GCT component is "eaten up" by the evolving malignancy. The sarcomatous component is devoid of ordinary GCT features; thus, foci of residual GCT should be looked for which can be found in cases of "primary" malignant transformation. Reviewing old records of patient may help confirming pre-existing GCT to establish diagnosis of malignant GCT rather malignant transformation of GCT. Some people also use "malignant GCT" for lesions that metastasize. The term should be dropped and descriptions should be used rather to describe individual forms.

Differential Diagnosis

Giant cell tumor-like lesions (see above). Giant cell osteosarcoma, carcinomas that have osteoclast-like giant cells—breast, thyroid, and pancreatic should also be kept under differential.

Management

Treatment of GCT is surgical removal using the following different modalities:

- Curettage and bone grafting (no adjuvants)
- Curettage and chemical cytotoxic agents such as phenol, zinc chloride, alcohol, hydrogen peroxide, carbolic acid (5–80% concentration), and trichloroacetic acid.
- Curettage and physical agents (polymethylmethacrylate and cryosurgery)
- Heat cauterization of the walls of the lesion (using electrocautery)
- Extended curettage with high-speed burr and adjuvants
- Primary resection for expendable bones
- Wide excision and reconstruction using grafts or custom prosthesis **(Figs. 73 and 74)**
- Distal radius of GCTs can be variable managed with extended curettage and bone grafting, excision and reconstruction by proximal fibula **(Figs. 75A to F and 76A)**, excision and reconstruction with wrist arthrodesis **(Figs. 76A to G)**
- Radiation therapy for incomplete resection at surgically difficult sites or primarily (used in past) now abandoned for development of sarcomatous transformation (5%)
- Embolization, for unresectable tumors (pelvic and sacral large tumors—usually require multiple sitting as vascularity gets restored eventually). This can also be used prior to surgical excision of large tumors.

Simple curettage, with or without bone grafting, has a significantly high rate of local recurrence of up to 60%. These intralesional and marginal procedures without adjuvants are associated with higher recurrences (the recurrence is actually "persistence" of original disease) due to inability to completely remove the microscopic disease, and recurrence is not correlated with grade or site of lesion. Modern treatment of GCT with extended curettage (making a wide window, using head lamps or dental mirror, angled curettes and high-speed burrs, and pulsatile lavage) and cryosurgery (using liquid nitrogen) to the tumor cavity has achieved a recurrence rate of <3%. Routine use of adjuvants is recommended. Cryotherapy with liquid nitrogen popularized by Marcove has various side effects and has been effectively abandoned due to frostbite of soft tissues and bone necrosis. Bone cement has a tumor kill effect by exothermic reaction and possible chemical reaction (solvent aerosol is cytotoxic) that produces necrosis of tissue for 1–2 mm from contact area. Some people have used methotrexate and adriamycin in the bone cement to augment

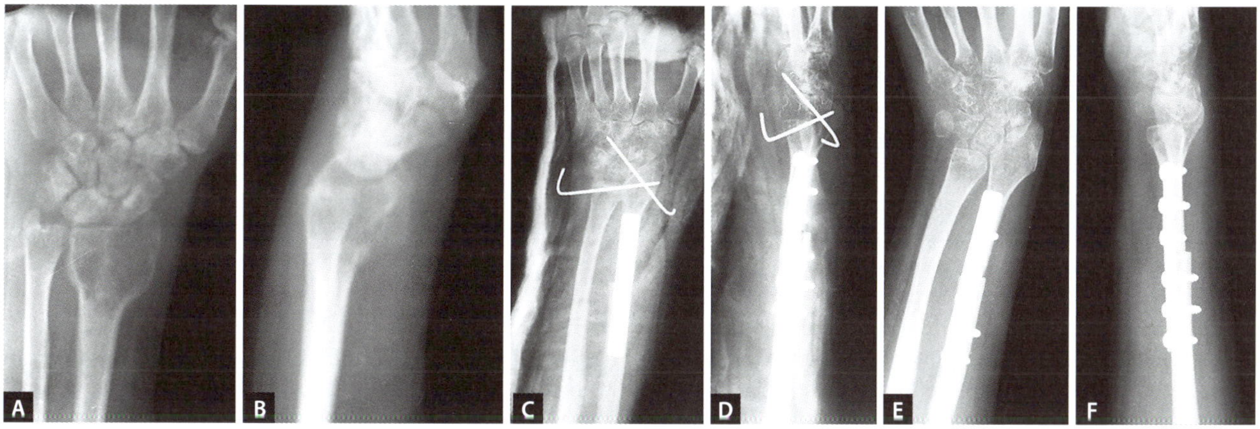

Figs. 75A to F: (A and B) Giant cell tumor of distal radius (C to F) managed with ipsilateral fibular head harvested from the patient and distal radioulnar joint stabilization.

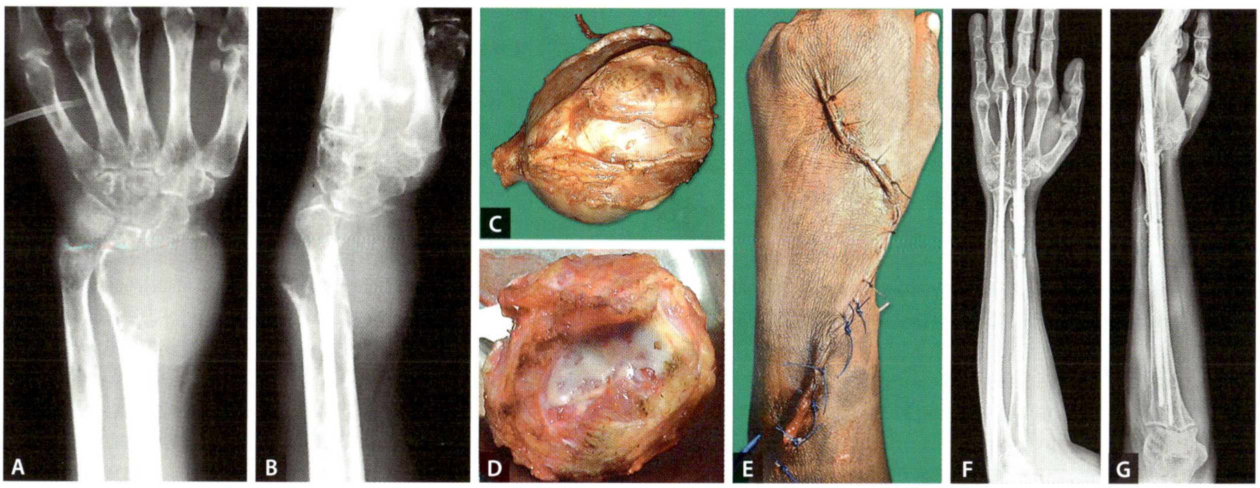

Figs. 76A to G: (A and B) Giant cell tumor of distal radius (C to E) managed with excision and (E to G) fibular grafting and wrist arthrodesis. The bluish discoloration on skin are the "tattoos" common in tribal population.

cytotoxic effect. Bone cement has the advantage of filling the defect and having tumoricidal effect.

Advantages of Cementing

- Cytotoxic (exothermic and monomer aerosol)
- Radiographic detection of recurrence is easier—as a clear lucent line around the cement
- Good structural support and early weight-bearing

Disadvantages of Cementing

- Nonbiological and does not get incorporated in body ever. Cement resists compression but is weak against tensile and torsional forces. It will not provide bone strength in areas such as neck of the femur may result in an increased chance of fractures due to "absolute" deficiency of bone mass.
- Degeneration and crushing of articular cartilage in subchondral lesions—it is recommended to leave 5 mm of subchondral bone, and possibly, using bone grafting to increase bone thickness.

There has been a concern for poor functional outcome in lesions involving large articular surfaces; the larger the articular surface involved the poorer the function. Wide local excision for such larger tumors can be done followed by reconstruction using megaprosthesis (provide mobility but prone to loosening and late failure), arthrodesis (stability but immobility). Arthrodesis reconstruction of limb can be done using standard procedures (internal/external fixation), ilizarov method, osteoarticular allografts, microvascular bone grafts. The role of adjuvants has been questioned in some studies, and it is proposed that adequate tumor removal is more important than just using adjuvants.

Recurrences of GCT occur within 2 years and are less in Campanacci grade 1 and 2 (7%) compared to grade 3 (29%). Total serum acid phosphatase can be used as a tumor marker for monitoring response to the treatment of GCT. TCAP correlates with initial tumor size and normalizes after resection; reappearing with recurrence of tumor. Late recurrence (>5 years) should be suspected for sarcomatous transformation. The recurrences are treated in similar fashion as for primary tumor. Radiation therapy (megavoltage 35–70 Gy) has been used for additional clearance of surgical margins in cases that are difficult to adequately manage surgically (lesions of spine and sacrum) or for aggressive recurrent tumors. Multiple recurrences and use of radiation have been linked to development of malignancy in GCT (secondary malignant transformation apart from primary cases). Pulmonary metastasis seen in 1–5% patients (3–4 years after diagnosis) may regress, grow very slowly (benign pulmonary implants), or progress fast causing death of patient. Metastasis has been associated with surgical manipulation, local recurrence, and location in distal radius and is again not related to the histological grade. Metastasis can be safely resected with good prognosis. Steroids have been used for controlling unresectable metastases. GCT with malignant transformation should be treated like high-grade spindle cell sarcoma (surgical wide excision and chemotherapy) to which it shares the prognosis which is fair. The chemotherapy is similar to that of osteosarcoma and is given for 3–4 months prior to surgical excision.

Newer Treatments

Bisphosphonates especially the newer forms (zoledronic acid and palmidronate) have been proposed to reduce the osteopenia due to osteoclastic effect of giant cells and can be used as adjuvants to extended curettage. Also they have been shown to have in vitro tumoricidal action. With the recognition of osteoclast differentiation factor RANKL on tumor cells, targeted therapy against the receptor has been shown to be promising. Denosumab is the first agent licensed to be used for this purpose by the Food and Drug Administration (FDA) in 2013. It inhibits osteoclast function and prevents bone destruction associated with GCT. Denosumab is strongly considered in treatment of lesions inoperable due to concerns of morbidity and is preferred over radiotherapy.

Giant Cell Reparative Granuloma

Possibly akin to solid ABC, these lesions comprise intraosseous proliferation characterized by granuloma-like aggregates of giant cells in a fibrovascular stroma. The lesions are common in gnathic skeleton and translocations involving *USP6* gene has been demonstrated. In children, phalanges and metatarsals or metacarpals of hands and feet are typically involved. Radiologically, they are expansile lytic lesions. Histopathologically, there are foci of giant cells in a prominent fibroblastic stroma. There may be metaplastic bone but cartilage is absent. Brown tumors should be excluded in differential diagnosis. Intralesional curettage or marginal excision is adequate treatment.

BENIGN FIBROUS HISTIOCYTOMA

(Atypical Fibrous Histiocytoma, Nonossifying Fibroma, Metaphyseal Fibrous Defect, Cortical Fibrous Defect)

This is a group of lesions that have some histopathological features in common such as a storiform pattern of cell organization, presence of histiocyte-like giant cells, foam cells, and a nonspecific polymorphic infiltrate. Metaphyseal fibrous defect represents an eccentric, intracortical proliferation of fibrous tissue, and histiocytes. When they grow large enough, they may involve the medullary cavity of involved bone. With growth, the lesions can migrate to diaphysis. Multiple lesions that grow in association with café au lait spots (neurofibromatosis) and associated with developmental delay comprise Jaffe–Campanacci syndrome. Possibly the lesions represent developmental abnormalities are so prevalent in children (2–14 years of age), and heal within 2 years by sclerosis (the so-called ossifying fibroma). Few cases that fail to heal present with pain or pathological fracture are located most often in lower limb long bones (distal femur and tibia and proximal tibia) **(Fig. 72A)**. Radiologically, they appear as an eccentric, geographically lytic lesion with sclerotic margins **(Fig. 72B)** while in healing phase the lesions are sclerotic by itself. Microscopically, the lesions contain fibrous stroma with cells arranged in storiform fashion.

Foamy histiocytes (xanthoma cells), hemosiderinladen macrophages, and multinucleated giant cells are present in varying proportions. GCT and FD should be kept under differential diagnosis. Treatment is needed only for symptomatic lesions and intralesional procedures suffice.

MALIGNANT FIBROUS HISTIOCYTOMA

(Malignant Histiocytoma, Xanthosarcoma, Malignant Fibrous Xanthoma, and Fibroxanthosarcoma)

A malignant neoplasm composed of cells resembling fibroblasts and pleomorphic cells (resembling myofibroblasts and histiocytes) arranged in a prominent storiform pattern. MFH of bone was initially described by Feldman and Norman in 1972. The tumor accounts for <2% of all primary malignant neoplasms of bone affecting males are more commonly than females. The age of presentation is wide and is distributed through 2nd to 8th decades. Most of the reported cases are seen in adults aged 40 years or older. MFH usually arises as a *primary* bone neoplasm but nearly one-fourth of the cases develop *secondarily over* pre-existing bone conditions (secondary MFH, 28% of cases). These pre-existing lesions reported in literature include Paget's disease, bone infarct or irradiated bone. The most common osseous locations for primary MFH include the long bones of the lower extremities especially femur (30–45%) and tibia; these are followed by humerus. Knee is a common location in appendicular skeleton while the pelvis is most frequently involved in axial skeleton. Secondary MFH is distributed according to the underlying cause, e.g., specific irradiated bone. An uncommon entity associated with MFH is diaphyseal medullary stenosis with malignant fibrous histiocytoma (DMS-MFH). It is an autosomal dominant bone dysplasia/cancer syndrome of unknown etiology. There are significant cortical growth abnormalities manifesting as irregular patterns with diffuse diaphyseal medullary stenosis, metaphyseal striations, and scattered sclerotic bone infarct regions. Malignant transformation has occurred in significant number of cases of the reported DMS-MFH families, and it has been consistently MFH. Genotypically in MFH, LOH was found for markers within the 9p21-22 region.

Clinical Presentation and Imaging

Most patients present with pain and, less frequently, swelling. The average time to diagnosis from onset of symptoms is 7–9 months (1 week to 3 years). Most lesions are metaphyseal lytic lesion that extend up to the epiphysis but never to the subchondral bone. MFH can also be considered a strong differential in an eccentrically located lytic, diaphyseal lesion with cortical destruction and soft tissue extension. Diaphyseal location is infrequent. Though mainly osteolytic, sclerotic areas may be present. Lesion margins are usually ill-defined and a moth-eaten or permeative pattern of bone destruction is observed more prominent in pelvic bones. The osseous cortex is commonly destroyed by the tumor resulting in stress-free soft tissue extension. Bone or periosteal reaction is infrequent if at all. In elderly, the radiological differentials include lymphoma, myeloma or osteolytic metastases, while in younger patients' osteosarcoma and Ewing's sarcoma are possibilities to be considered. MFH should be clinically and histopathologically differentiated from angiomatoid fibrous histiocytoma that is a low-grade tumor and is usually noninvasive, small, often associated with excellent surgical outcome.

Histopathology

Gross appearance is not characteristic and tumor appears as a grayish-white, soft to firm lesion with cortical destruction. Necrosis and hemorrhage are frequent. Microscopically, there is a mixed population of spindle cells, histiocytoid and pleomorphic cells with interspread varying amounts of multinucleated giant cells. Various histological subtypes have been described in MFH including storiform-pleomorphic (most common), histiocytic, myxoid (rare), giant cell, and inflammatory (better prognosis). Most MFH are high-grade tumors.

Management and Prognosis

Due to aggressive and highly malignant nature of the lesion, vascular invasion and metastasis is early. The metastasis is usually to lungs (45–50%). Local control is obtained by wide surgical excision; radiation is commonly employed for incomplete surgical margins or at surgically challenging sites. High-grade resectable lesions are additionally treated with preoperative chemotherapy similar to osteosarcoma. For such patients, tumor necrosis following chemotherapy is an important determinant of prognosis. With localized disease, the 5-year disease-free survival is over 50%. Other favorable prognostic factors are: younger age at presentation (<40 years), histologically a prominent chronic inflammatory infiltrate and low grade.

PLASMA CELL MYELOMA

(ICD-O 9732/3, Myeloma, Multiple Myeloma, Kahler's Disease and Variants, Nonsecretory Myeloma, Indolent Myeloma, Smoldering Myeloma, Plasma Cell Leukemia in addition to Extramedullary Plasmacytoma, and Solitary Plasmacytoma of Bone)

Plasma cell myeloma (PCM) is a monoclonal neoplastic proliferation of plasma cells (B-cells) derived from bone marrow. It is usually multicenter, and infiltrates various organs but rarely produces plasma cell leukemia. PCM is the most frequent primary tumor of bone and the most common lymphoid neoplasm in Blacks and the second most common in Whites after non-Hodgkin lymphoma. It is a disease of elderly presenting usually in the 6th and 7th decades of life and rarely if ever before 40 years of age. Both sexes are equally affected with median age at diagnosis of 68 years in males and 70 years in females. Etiologically, various unproven factors have been proposed that include chronic infections (like chronic osteomyelitis), persistent systemic inflammatory processes as in rheumatoid arthritis, and low-level radiation exposure as in radiologists, nuclear plant workers, etc. Other nonspecific suggested factors are and exposure to asbestos, pesticides, petroleum products, rubber, plastic, and wood products. Kaposi sarcoma (human herpes virus-8 infection) has been associated with POEMS syndrome (polyneuropathy, organomegaly, endocrinopathy, monoclonal gammopathy, and skin changes). A variety of chromosomal alterations with prognostic significance has been found in patients with myeloma that include 13q14 deletions, 17p13 deletions, and translocations t(11;14)(q13;q32) and t(4;14)(p16;q32). Cytokines have been implicated in development of the tumor like interleukin (IL)-6 that drives myeloma cell proliferation.

Clinical Features

Myeloid marrow containing bones in adults are the most frequently involved: vertebrae, ribs, skull, pelvis, femur, clavicle, and scapula. The skeletal lesions are typically well-demarcated osteolytic (osteosclerotic form is also recognized), extensive, and cause *bone pain (70% patients), pathological fractures, hypercalcemia,* and anemia. *Thoracolumbar pain or a compression fracture* is usually the first symptom. *Neurologic symptoms* due to compression of roots or cord often occur and may result from extraosseous extension of the tumor or from a pathological fracture. The osteosclerotic variant of MM commonly presents with *peripheral neuropathy* but this is rare with classic PCM. Loss of bone marrow causes anemia that is exaggerated by amyloid deposition in kidneys causing *renal damage* (and failure) depleting erythropoietin. An M-component (electrophoresis) in γ-globulin region is present in 99% of the patients (serum or urine). Immunoelectrophoresis (qualitative analysis) determines the monoclonal nature. The monoclonal proteins are mainly IgG (50% of the cases) or IgA class (25–20%) and, rarely, of the IgM, IgD, or IgE classes. Antibody concentration of 5 g/L (corresponding to 10^9 cells producing the antibody) is required for accurate determination and quantification by electrophoresis. A monoclonal light chain (Bence Jones protein) is found in the serum in 75% of the patients that results in *renal failure* from light chain proteinuria. *Recurrent bacterial infections* are common due to lack of effective globulin component and ineffective utilization of cells to produce redundant globulins only.

Radiology

Lesions erode the cortex and periosteal new bone formation is not seen. Expansile lesion is usually seen in bones with a small diameter, such as the ribs. Skull radiographs demonstrate the earliest and more severe changes as also evident later in vertebrae, ribs, and pelvis. Generalized osteoporosis may be present in few at presentation. Solitary plasmacytoma lesions are also typically lytic **(Figs. 77A to D)** and may also expand the bone. Presence of sclerotic lesions points typically to the very rare POEMS syndrome that stands for an uncommon cluster of clinical findings—polyneuropathy, organomegaly, endocrinopathy, monoclonal gammopathy, and skin changes. Bone scan is usually negative hence skeletal-survey or full-body staging MRI is more commonly used to examine whole skeleton.

Differential Diagnosis

The differential diagnosis includes:
- Metastasis
- Malignant lymphoma
- Hyperparathyroidism (Brown tumor)
- Langerhans cell histiocytosis

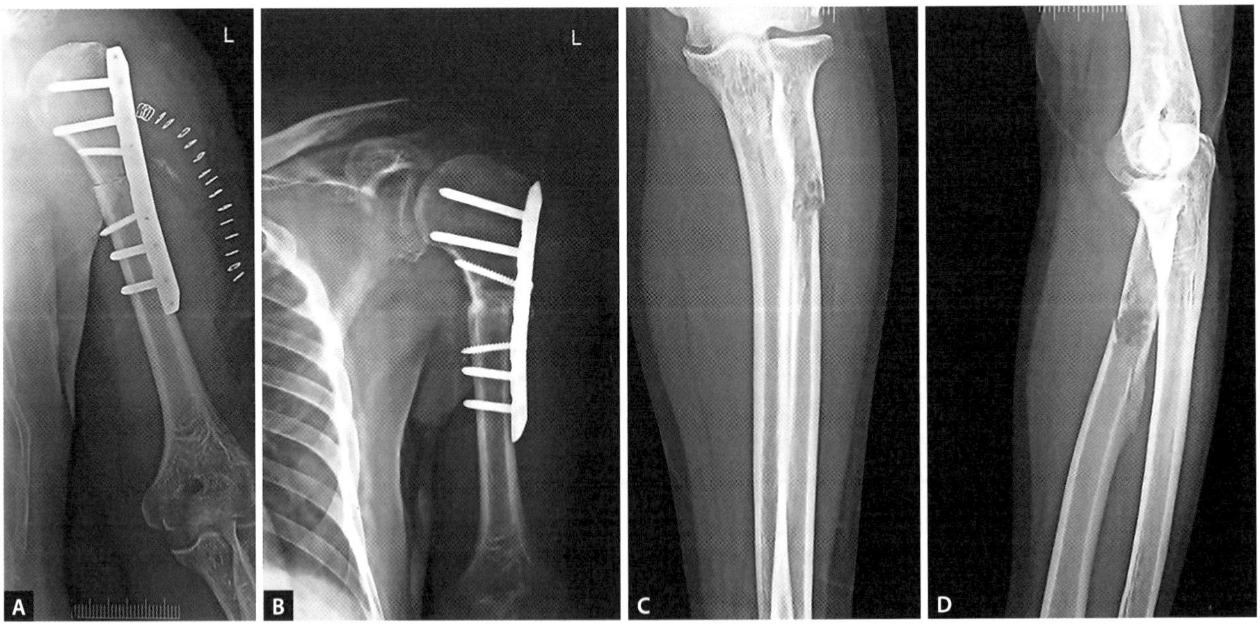

Figs. 77A to D: The 48-year-old male presented with pain in left arm of acute nontraumatic presentation that increases with activity. The area was locally tender and radiology demonstrated pathological fracture through lytic lesion in upper third humerus devoid of any periosteal reaction. Evaluation revealed plasmacytoma of humerus and was treated with resection of the lesion, bone shortening, and osteosynthesis (A). The patient also received local radiotherapy and systemic chemotherapy. PET scan for surveillance was unremarkable and patient was on maintenance therapy. The lesion healed completely in 2 years (B) but unfortunately similar complaints appeared in left forearm and patient was found to have relapse of the disease and new lesion in proximal radius (C and D). Relapse has a poor prognosis.

Histopathology

Histopathologically, the round cells of PCM show variable features of cellular maturity that is closely linked to prognosis. Well-differentiated tumors demonstrate sheets of closely packed cells (resembling normal plasma cells) with little intercellular matrix. These cells have abundant, dense eosinophilic cytoplasm with eccentric nucleus that has characteristic peripherally clustered chromatin in a "cartwheel pattern" **(Figs. 78A and B)**. Intracytoplasmic aggregation of immunoglobulins gives a morular appearance termed "Mott cells". "Russell bodies" is the term used for similar extracellular globules of polymerized immunoglobulins.

Immunophenotype

Myeloma cells express distinct plasma cell associated antigen (PCA, CD38). Malignant lesions express monotypic kappa or lambda immunoglobulin. PCM characteristically expresses monotypic cytoplasmic immunoglobulin and lacks surface immunoglobulin. PCM usually lacks the pan-B cell antigens (characteristically the CD19 and CD20), while CD38 and the immunoglobulin-associated antigen CD79a are expressed mostly.

Investigations

Hematological investigations usually reveal anemia on complete hemogram. Erythrocyte sedimentation rate is prominently elevated and is often around or >100 mm in first hour. Other parameters such as the serum calcium (bone absorption), blood urea nitrogen (catabolism), serum creatinine, and uric acid levels (purine and pyrimidine metabolism) are also often elevated. The most common method to diagnose PCM is by serum protein electrophoresis and measurement of serum immunoglobulins and free light chains. These reveal the characteristic M-spikes which is a sensitive marker though its absence does not rule out myeloma. Bence Jones protein can be detected in urine but 24-hour urine should be collected. *ALP (marker of bone formation) is usually normal* even with extensive bone involvement because of the absence of osteoblastic activity. The diagnosis and differentiation from related disorders is presented in **Box 6**. Plasma cell dyscrasias can be comfortably divided into premalignant and malignant conditions. Monoclonal gammopathy of unknown significance (MGUS) represents a premalignant condition that may (or may not) progress to MM as opposed to asymptomatic MM and active MM that are frankly malignant counterparts. Of these malignant components, asymptomatic MM is distinguished from active myeloma by absence of end-organ compromise identified by the acronym "CRAB" **(Box 6)**. MGUS is approximately 80–100 times more common than MM and is found in 3–5% of general population aged 70 years or older. The MGUS has been found to progress to MM at a rate of around 1% per year. Although similar cytogenetic abnormalities (translocations and deletions) have been observed in patients with MGUS and MM; however, no obvious clinical or conclusions could be drawn based on these chromosome abnormalities. MGUS patients can be stratified to high- or low-risk based on their immunoglobulin isotype; the level of their paraprotein secretion, and the ratio of serum-free light chains. A patient with monoclonal immunoglobulin concentration 1.5 g/dL other than IgG and an abnormally high serum-free light chain ratio would be classified as high risk with 58% risk of progression of MGUS to MM than in one if none of these factors are present. Low-risk MGUS patients can be followed yearly while high-risk MGUS patients should be followed every 3–6 months.

Serum β2-microglobulin has specific role in staging and should be quantitated in all diagnosed cases. The International *Staging System* for myeloma published by the International Myeloma Working Group in 2005 is based on β2-microglobulin concentration:

- *Stage I*: β2-microglobulin (β2M) < 3.5 mg/L, albumin ≥ 3.5 g/dL

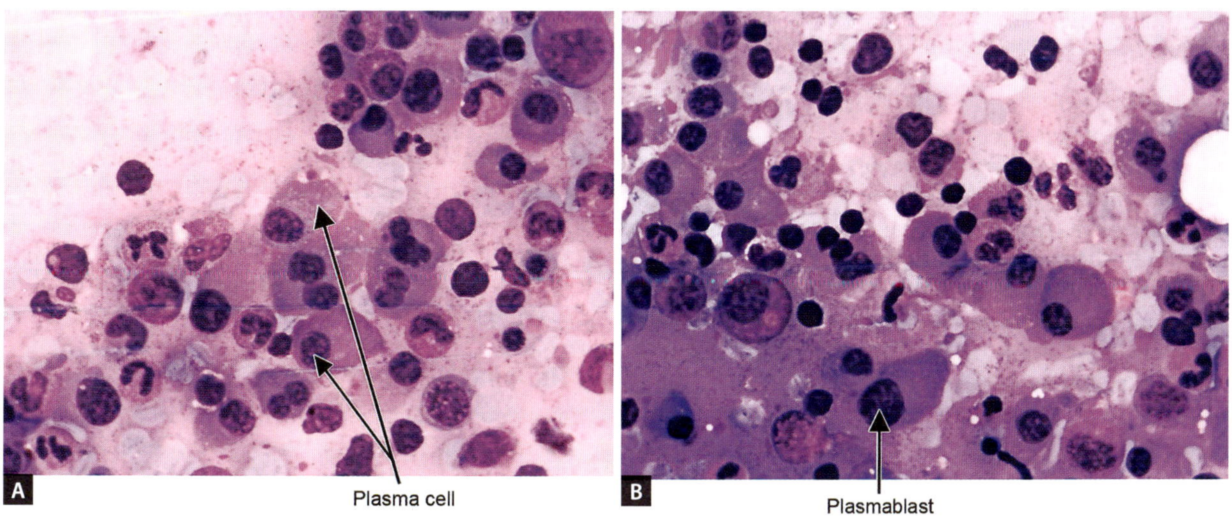

Figs. 78A and B: Multiple myeloma histopathology showing (A) plasma cells with cartwheel pattern in nucleus; (B) An initial plasmablast with higher cytoplasm content and dense nucleus.

BOX 6: Diagnostic criteria for symptomatic multiple myeloma and associated disorders.

Symptomatic multiple myeloma:
- Clonal plasma cells > 10% on bone marrow biopsy or (in any quantity) in a biopsy from other tissues (plasmacytoma)
- A monoclonal protein (paraprotein, M-protein) in either serum or urine (except in cases of true nonsecretory myeloma)
- Evidence of end-organ damage felt related to the plasma cell disorder (*related organ or tissue impairment*, ROTI, commonly referred by the acronym "CRAB"):
  - HyperCalcemia (corrected calcium > 2.75 mmol/L)
  - Renal insufficiency attributable to myeloma
  - Anemia (hemoglobin < 10 g/dL)
  - Bone lesions (lytic lesions or osteoporosis with compression fractures)

Asymptomatic (smoldering) multiple myeloma:
- M-protein (serum) > 30 g/L, and/or
- Clonal plasma cells > 10% on bone marrow biopsy, and
- No myeloma-related organ or tissue impairment

Monoclonal gammopathy of undetermined significance (MGUS):
- M-protein < 30 g/L, and
- Clonal plasma cells < 10% on bone marrow biopsy, and
- NO myeloma-related organ or tissue impairment (ROTI)

Solitary plasmacytoma of bone:
- No M-protein in serum and/or urine
- Single area of bone destruction due to clonal plasma cells
- Bone marrow not consistent with multiple myeloma
- Normal skeletal survey (and MRI of spine and pelvis if done)
- No related organ or tissue impairment (no endorgan damage other than solitary bone lesion)

- *Stage II:* β2M < 3.5 mg/L, and albumin < 3.5 g/dL; or β2M 3.5–5.5 mg/L irrespective of the serum albumin
- *Stage III:* β2M ≥ 5.5 mg/L

Treatment

Multiple myeloma is generally an incurable disease (median survival 3 years; 10% survival at 10 years). β2-microglobulin is the single most strong predictor of prognosis with higher levels associated with shorter survival. Other factors that predict poor or shorter survival include a higher stage at diagnosis, renal involvement causing insufficiency, hypoploidy, chromosome 13q and 17p deletion, translocations t(4;14) and t(14;16), replacement of marrow by neoplastic cells, histopathologically demonstrable cellular immaturity and atypia on bone marrow examination, and high Ki-67 proliferation antigen levels. 10% patients have smoldering disease and require treatment only when symptomatic. Chemotherapy and autologous stem cell transplantation is the mainstay of treatment. Dexamethasone, bortezomib (proteasome inhibitor that targets 26S proteasome), thalidomide, and its immunomodulatory derivative lenalidomide are current employed in varying combinations in patients planned for future stem cell transplantation. Melphalan, prednisolone, and lenalidomide are used in patients not planned for transplantation. Radiation therapy (4,500–5,000 cGy) is effective for solitary plasmacytoma. Autologous hematopoietic stem cell transplantation provides the best chance of event-free survival (EFS) in most patients. High-dose chemotherapy followed by transplantation can be beneficial even in refractory patients. Sequential planned tandem hematopoietic stem cell transplantation with high-dose therapy is an innovative approach that has been quite successful and nearly doubled the sustained remission rates. Newer agents targeting therapy in myeloma patients have been developed. Peferisone is a synthetic alkylphospholipid that interacts and induces cytotoxicity in MM triggered by c-Jun NH2-terminal kinase by inhibiting the Akt/protein kinase B activity (important for MM cell survival and anti-apoptosis). Geldanamycin and tanespimycin are HSP-90 (heat shock protein) inhibitors that show promising results with bortezomib. NPI-0052 is another proteasome inhibitor like bortezomib but with earlier onset of action and different kinetics. Dasatinib (dual Src/Abl inhibitor) showed synergism with antimyeloma drugs in reducing tumor growth in murine models. Everolimus combined with lenalidomide has showed improved efficacy. Inhibitors of activin-A like sotatercept have shown improved BMD and reduced bone pains in patients with MM. Tocilizumab is an IL-6 inhibitor that has been shown effective in murine MM model; other therapies targeting surface receptors includes the anti-CD40, anti-CD56, anti-CD138, antiCS-1, anti-CD70, TGF-β inhibitor, etc. Supportive care is required in patients with respect to the osteolytic lesions, hypercalcemia, and associated pain. Bisphosphonates especially the injectable form has been found effective in this regard. For anemia, erythropoietin has been found effective. Similarly, prophylaxis, evaluation, and treatment are required for patients at risk of developing deep vein thrombosis and infections.

LANGERHANS CELL HISTIOCYTOSIS/ EOSINOPHILIC GRANULOMA

Lichtenstein in 1953 introduced the term histiocytosis X referring to the proliferation of histiocytes (Langerhans cells) due to an unknown etiology which was later renamed as Langerhans cell histiocytosis (LCH). LCH represents a group of disorders that present in various forms, typical of which are:

- *Hand-Schüller-Christian disease:* Syndromic form with disseminated bony and visceral involvement (skin, pituitary gland, lung, brain, liver, spleen, and the gastrointestinal tract). Classically there is a triad of exophthalmos, diabetes insipidus, and osteolytic skull lesions.
- *Letterer–Siwe disease:* Disseminated form of disease usually fatal at a young age. It is characterized by lymphadenopathy, skin rash, hepatosplenomegaly, and pancytopenia.
- *Eosinophilic granuloma:* It is the mildest variant of LCH presenting as isolated bone lesion (90%) or uncommonly as a polyostotic variety (10%).

Eosinophilic Granuloma

The *eosinophilic granuloma (EOG)* is more relevant to an orthopedic surgeon so will be discussed here. EOG presents later than the systemic forms of LCH usually after 20 years of age but spinal EOG may present in a skeletally immature patient as vertebra plana. The disease mostly affects the axial skeleton, namely skull, jaw bone, spine, pelvis, ribs, and long bones. In children, the skull (frontal bone) is the most common site of involvement and if spinal lesion is seen then it is commonly the thoracic spine. In adults, on the other hand, jaw is the most frequently involved site while spinal involvement is mostly localized to cervical spine. The clinical features of EOG depending on the site of involvement include:

- Pain and swelling of the involved bone. The area is tender to palpation and patient has antalgic gait in case of lower extremity or pelvic involvement.
- Pathological fracture of weight-bearing bone
- Back pain, stiffness, kyphosis in cases of spinal involvement. Extensive disease can cause neurological deficits.
- Temporal bone involvement may present with ear canal mass, postauricular swelling, ear discharge, and hearing loss.
- Jaw lesions present with swelling, pain, and loose teeth.

Radiology and Differential Diagnosis

Eosinophilic granuloma mimics several neoplastic and infectious conditions so forms a differential diagnosis to many lytic disorders of bone. It is commonly seen to involve the diaphysis of long bones but metaphyseal (uncommon) and epiphyseal (rare) forms do occur and hence EOG covers a large range of disorders. Also the radiological picture varies with the phase of disease. While the early lesions are mostly uniformly lytic, more active lesions persisting for a longer time develop larger transition zones that may demonstrate permeative or moth-eaten form mimicking a primary sarcoma. Skull lesions are typically punched out lytic lesions. Spinal lesions radiographically look like "coin on edge appearance" due to vertebral collapse (vertebra plana) involving pedicles and posterior vertebral elements. For polyostotic lesions, additional evaluation by PET scan may be done to identify the sites and visceral involvement. Monostotic vertebral involvement should be evaluated by MRI scanning of the lesion and canal. The differential diagnoses of spinal lesions include:

- Multiple myeloma
- Plasmacytoma
- Osteomyelitis
- Tuberculosis
- Leukemia
- Lymphoma

Extremity lesions should be differentiated from:

- Ewing's sarcoma
- Osteoblastoma
- Osteosarcoma
- Malignant fibrous histocytoma
- Paget's disease

Diagnosis and Histopathology

Fine-needle aspiration or CT-guided biopsy of the suspected bone lesion and staining for CD1a and CD207 is done to confirm the diagnosis of EG. Microscopically, the Langerhans cells are distributed in clusters nested within a background of inflammatory cells comprising eosinophils, lymphocytes, and plasma cells. Electron microscopy demonstrates Birbeck granules. In CNS lesions, additional BRAF V600E mutation testing can be done that also helps in targeted therapy.

Treatment

Eosinophilic granuloma is usually self-limiting and usually the polyostotic form without visceral involvement (if encountered) also may be managed with observation or confirmatory biopsy. Patients with a spinal lesion producing pain with no or minimal neurological deficits should be immobilized with brace preferably or by operative fixation. Intralesional methylprednisolone injection (40–160 mg) may be given for symptomatic lesions of the spine and extremities not responding to conservative measures. High-risk patients having poorer prognosis include those with multisystem involvement, skeletally mature patients, more than one bone involvement, and skull-base bone involvement (sphenoid, ethmoid, orbital, and temporal bones). They have a high risk for recurrence and complications so need prompt surgical intervention. Surgical fixation is done for patients with severe pain, restricted ROM, progressive neurological deficits, and spinal instability. Patients with visceral involvement need systemic chemotherapy in the form of vinblastine and high-dose corticosteroids. Low-dose radiation is reserved for refractory cases. The complications of improperly managed orthopedic disease include:

- Musculoskeletal disability or restricted activity
- Growth disturbance
- Pathological fractures
- Methylprednisolone injection associated osteomyelitis

Nonorthopedic related manifestations should be appropriately referred for hearing and vision impairment, neuropsychiatric abnormalities, pneumothorax, pulmonary arterial hypertension, and Increased risk of Hodgkin and non-Hodgkin lymphoma, myeloproliferative disorders, and bronchogenic carcinoma to otorhinolaryngologist, ophthalmologist, neurologist, pulmonologist, cardiologist, and medical oncologist, respectively.

MALIGNANT LYMPHOMA OF BONE (ICD-O 9590/3)

This is an unusual tumor of bone accounting for <7% of bone malignancies. The disease can be present in any age and is more common in males. Portions of bone with active red marrow are involved. Femur is the most common bone while it is also seen in spine and pelvic region. Bone pains are the usual presentation and some patients have palpable mass. The different presentations could be isolated skeletal involvement (with or without regional lymph node involvement), multiple bone involvement without visceral or lymph node involvement, patient presents with bone tumor but is found to have tumor at other sites also, a patient of known lymphoma investigated with bone biopsy.

Radiologically, the features are nonspecific with preferential involvement of diaphysis. There are areas of mixed lysis and sclerosis **(Fig. 79)**. The cortex is usually destroyed and periosteal bone formation is rare. *Histopathologically,* the majority have a diffuse growth

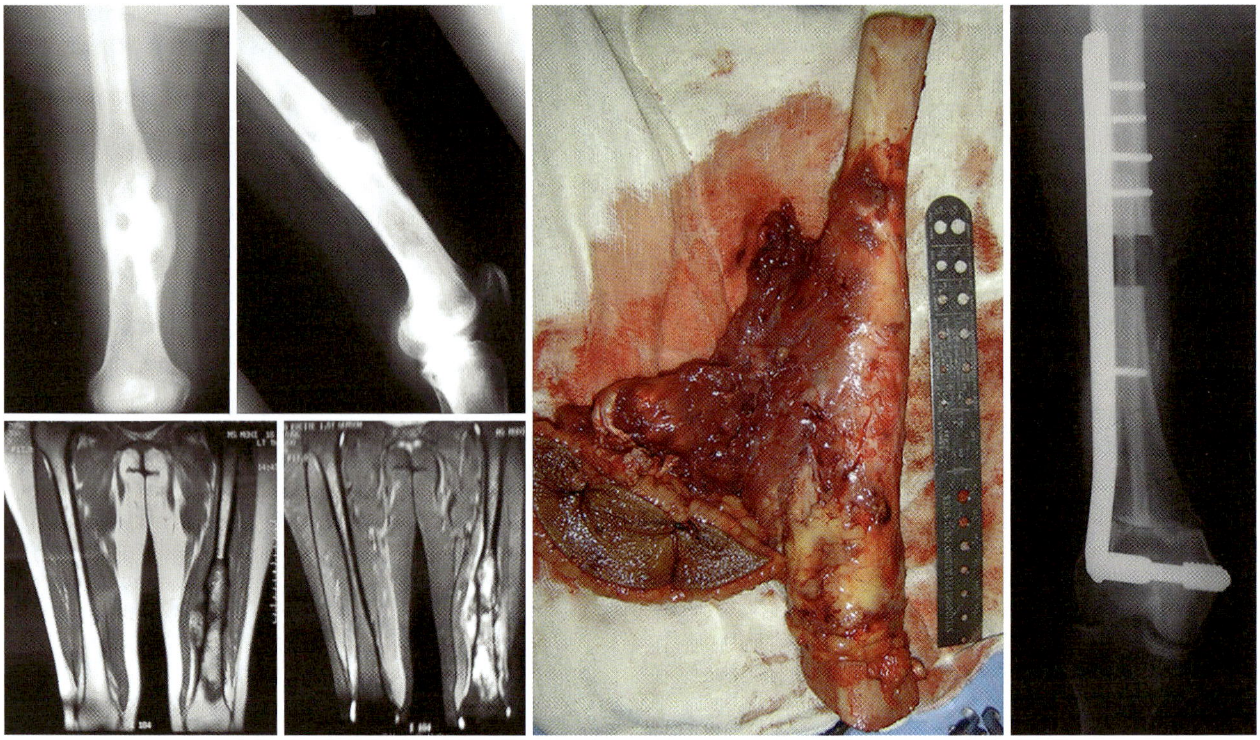

Fig. 79: Malignant lymphoma of bone. The lesion is predominantly diaphyseal with lytic sclerotic lesions. The lesion extends till metaphysis and has soft tissue extension as demonstrated in T1- and T2-weighted MRI. The lesion was excised R0 and striped of soft tissues it was then autoclaved and used again as intercalary graft to reconstruct the bone defect along with autologous fibula.

pattern. The bony trabeculae are normal or thickened. Classical Reed–Sternberg cells with bilobed nuclei are present but difficult to locate. Immunoperoxidase staining is done to classify and characterize the malignant lymphoma. All primary lymphomas stain with CD20.

Treatment

Multiagent chemotherapy and radiation are primary modalities of treatment. Surgical excision of irreversibly destroyed bone or to improve strength of bone is sometimes indicated. Stage of disease is the most important prognostic indicator.

EWING'S SARCOMA

[Ewing's Sarcoma Family of Tumors (EFT) includes: Primitive Neuroectodermal Tumor, Askin Tumor (Ewing's Sarcoma of Chest Wall), Extraosseous Ewing's Sarcoma, Peripheral Neuroepithelioma, Atypical Ewing's and Ewing's Tumor of Bone]

Ewing's sarcoma (named after *James Stephen Ewing*—American pathologist who described it in 1921 in radius of 14-year-old girl) is a primary round and blue cell bone tumor from a family of tumors currently placed under term primitive neuroectodermal tumors (PNET). It is one of the less differentiated tumors from this group of neoplasms (others being neuroepithelioma, neuroblastoma, and Askin tumor), however under tissue culture in the presence of differentiation agents like cAMP, the tumor develops neural features. Ewing's sarcoma per se is restricted for neoplasias that lack any evidence of neuroectodermal differentiation when assessed by light microscopy, immunohistochemistry, and electron microscopy. The term "PNET" is used instead for tumors that demonstrate features of neuroectodermal differentiation by above modalities. Ewing's sarcoma is considered to originate from primordial bone marrow-derived mesenchymal stem cell as identified by various modalities such as cytogenetics, immunohistochemical markers, molecular genetics, and tissue culture. It is interesting to note that in epidemiological studies the incidence of Ewing's sarcoma has remained constant over last 3 decades and is approximately three cases per 1 million per year (United States). In India, the exact incidence is not known but could be higher as it is more common in Caucasians. The median age of patients affected with Ewing's sarcoma is around 15 years most of which (>50%) are adolescents. The tumor is much more common in males. Ewing's sarcoma is commonly distributed (descending order of frequency) in lower extremity (41%), pelvis (26%), chest wall (16%), upper extremity (9%), and spine (6%). The small bones of hands and feet and skull are uncommonly involved (<2%). The extraosseous primary tumors most commonly involves the trunk (32%) and extremity (26%), while head and neck (18%) and retroperitoneum (16%) are also commonly involved. Patients with extraosseous Ewing's sarcoma are more likely to be older, female, nonwhite, occurring more commonly at axial primary sites (less likely to have pelvic primary sites) when compared to patients with skeletal Ewing's sarcoma. Approximately 25% of patients with skeletal Ewing's sarcoma have metastatic disease at diagnosis.

Cytogenetics

The *MIC2* gene product, CD99, is a surface membrane protein that is expressed in most cases of Ewing's sarcoma.

This is though not unique to Ewing's and is also found in synovial sarcoma, non-Hodgkin lymphoma, and gastrointestinal stromal tumors. The detection of a consistent translocation involving the *EWSR1* locus [a member of the TET family (TLS/EWS/TAF15) of RNA binding proteins] on chromosome 22 band q12 and any one of a number of partner chromosomes (number 11 band q24 (*FLI1*), number 21 band q22 (*ERG*), number 7 (*ETV1*), or number 17 (*E1AF*)) is the key feature in the diagnosis of Ewing's sarcoma. The characteristic consistent translocations that result thus include recurrent t(11;22) (q24;q12) chromosomal translocation, t(21;22),[4] t(7;22), and t(17;22). Virtually, all EFTs appear to express some form of *EWS/ETS* gene fusion. The t(11;22) recurrent translocation is an in-frame fusion between the 5′ amino terminus of the *EWS* gene from chromosome band 22q12 with the 3′ carboxy terminus of the 11q24 *FLI1* gene (or other partner chromosome as above), a member of the *ETS* family of transcription factors. *EWS/FLI1* has potent oncogenic activity and the fusion product function as aberrant transcription factors binding to *ETS* target genes. One target is downregulation of expression of TGF-β type II receptor which is a potent tumor suppressor. TGF-β signaling induces apoptosis in many cell types. Inactivation of the INK4a locus encoding the *CDKN2A* cell cycle inhibitor is the second most common genetic alteration in EFTs; important to this finding is the understanding that *CDKN2A* stabilizes the *EWS/FLI1* oncoprotein. Apart from the above-mentioned aberrations that are quite consistent, other abnormalities are also found that involve the *EWSR1* gene at 22q12. Inconsistent but frequent numerical and structural aberrations of chromosomes have been demonstrated in Ewing's sarcoma by various researchers, including gains of chromosomes 2, 5, 8, 9, 12, and 15; nonreciprocal translocation t(1;16)(q12;q11.2); and deletions on 6p. There is a growing consensus that trisomy 20 and *CDKN2A* mutations may indicate a more aggressive subset of Ewing's sarcoma tumors. As molecular diagnosis of Ewing's sarcoma is quite consistent and reproducible, a molecular test based on reverse transcriptase PCR and restriction analysis of PCR products that can be performed on a small tissue sample offers the opportunity to markedly simplify the detection and definition of Ewing's sarcoma.

Clinical Features

There is a delay in diagnosis of ≈6 months from the onset of symptoms in 50% patients, the delay is quite common in pelvic tumors. Pain and a local tender swelling in the involved area are the most common clinical symptoms. The pain precedes swelling by several months. Overlying skin may be red, inflamed, and edematous. Fever (remittent and moderate grade), anemia, leukocytosis, and increase in sedimentation rate are often seen. This may confuse the surgeon to osteomyelitis and has been responsible for few surgeries mistakenly performed to decompress the bone (for acute osteomyelitis). To utter surprise even pus (liquefied tumor) may be found at the time of surgery further reconciling the surgeon for bone infection. Systemic signs often reflect malignant disease that has metastasized, though. Retroperitoneal and spinal tumors may present with back pain and neurological examination should be carefully done in them. Pathological fracture is an uncommon complication but may be seen in neglected cases or those with delayed presentation. Metastatic disease to bone if extensive may lead to petechiae or purpura due to thrombocytopenia. Pulmonary metastasis may be clinically identified with asymmetric breath sounds, pleural rub, etc.

Radiology

An ill-defined osteolytic lesion involving the diaphysis or metaphysis (or both) of a long tubular bone or flat bone is the most common feature. Epiphyseal involvement is extremely rare. Poorly marginated permeative or moth-eaten bone destruction (76%) often associated with "onion-skin" like multilayered laminated periosteal reaction (57%) is characteristic. Occasionally Codman's triangle or sunburst appearance may be seen. The cortex overlying the tumor is irregularly thinned or thickened (40%) and even cystic spaces may be seen in some. A large, ill-defined soft tissue mass is a frequent association in Ewing's tumor. CT scan and MRI are useful investigations and ideally both should be done for staging. Whole body MRI may be done in select cases to guide treatment plan. On T1-weighted images, the tumor appears low to intermediate signal, and on T2-weighted images, there is heterogeneously high signal often with hair-on-end low-signal striations. Gadolinium contrast shows heterogeneous but prominent signal enhancement.

Histopathology

Grossly the tumor is firm, glistening, or more liquefied like pus. Hemorrhage and cystic changes are usual. Microscopically, the classic form comprises cellular sheets and nests of uniform, small, and typical round to polygonal cells with scanty cytoplasm. Areas of necrosis show perivascular cuffing. Rosettes pattern is seen in few patients and have no diagnostic value as they are not at all characteristic. Paying too much attention on them may cause a misdiagnosis of metastatic neuroblastoma. When stained by periodic acid Schiff cytoplasmic glycogen is demonstrated in many (but not all) cases. The glycogen is more prominent if the tumor is fixed in 80% alcohol. Mic-2 (CD99) shows membranous positivity in the large majority of Ewing's sarcoma and PNETs in contrast to cytoplasmic positivity in rhabdomyosarcomas and cells from acute lymphoblastic leukemia. Immunomarkers in Ewing's sarcoma are absent for markers of muscle, leukocyte common antigen (CD45), and blood vessel differentiation. Few histopathological variants of the above classic pattern have been noted including a large cell type variant and a filigree pattern. Large cell variant demonstrated larger cells, and may also have prominent nucleoli. In the filigree pattern, however, the architecture is bicellular (made of two types of cells) that are separated by stroma. "Atypical" Ewing's sarcoma has been described by some authors as lack of glycogen, lobular architecture, or alveolar pattern, frequent (over 2 per high-power field) mitoses, spindling at the periphery of the tumor, and formation of extracellular matrix.

Differential Diagnosis

Differential diagnosis includes neuroblastoma (Homer-Wright pseudo-rosettes and ganglion cell differentiation), non-Hodgkin lymphoma, osteomyelitis, small cell osteosarcoma, rhabdomyosarcoma, non-rhabdomyosarcoma soft tissue sarcomas, and rickets.

Treatment

Like osteosarcoma for reasons of occult metastasis present at diagnosis, Ewing's sarcoma is also considered a systemic disease at presentation to control local disease and kill metastatic disease simultaneously. With current regimens for therapy for localized Ewing's sarcoma, the prognosis is good and patients achieve EFS and an overall survival rate of nearly 70% at 5 years. Current *chemotherapy* regimen includes VAdriaC [*V*incristine, Adriamycin (doxorubicin), and Cyclophosphamide] for 2 days alternating with IE (ifosfamide and etoposide) for 5 days given every 2 weeks (interval compression) or 3 weeks (traditional method). High initial dose of adriamycin (dose intense regimen) has better outcome. Addition of topotecan to above chemotherapy is being studied.

Local control has been deemed to be better with surgery than radiation due to associated growth retardation in young children with radiotherapy. Also surgically resected specimen can be subjected to assess the tumor necrosis that can be then utilized to prognosticate or change chemotherapy (high-dose chemotherapy with stem cell rescue). Positive surgical margins have a poor prognosis. For tumors above the proximal tibia, it is commonly preferable to attempt limb salvage with one of the above techniques or a combination thereof rather than resorting to amputation as the functional and psychological results are much better. These patients if treated with above-knee amputation do poorly over long-term as there is increased energy expenditure compared to limb reconstruction with endoprosthesis. The specific reconstruction technique deployed is determined by the location of tumor, patient's age, and the requirement of additional modalities for comprehensive management (i.e., chemotherapy and/or radiation). Allografts and autogenous vascularized bone grafts in conjunction with endoprosthesis or alone may be used **(Figs. 80A to D)**. Autogenous grafts are associated with donor site morbidity. Allografts are a biological solution without donor site morbidity and will last for lifetime if incorporated. The major drawback is incorporation and union of allografts. Metallic endoprosthetic provides immediately stable reconstruction for mobilization. Expandable prostheses that elongate with time are preferred in children. Newer prosthesis can be lengthened without need of additional surgery. For large defects of lower thigh, rotation plasty is a viable option where the lower leg is rotated and fixed to the thigh, practically converting an above-knee amputation into below-knee amputation. Considering knee fusion/arthrodesis is an acceptable compromise between limb salvage and amputation as far as energy consumption is concerned. This is acceptable especially in patients who are economically compromised as quite prevalent in our nation. For tibial diaphyseal lesions as a case, limb salvage should be considered as a forefront method of reconstruction, unless the benefits of cure by amputation outweigh the possible functional outcomes of limb salvage. For practical purpose and complexity of reconstruction, lesions about the foot and ankle are possibly best managed with below-knee amputation. Before amputation, possibility of treatment for nonreconstructable limb tumor with radiotherapy should be discussed with the family.

Radiation therapy though has been effective especially for unresectable tumors, but there remains always a risk of secondary neoplasms developing in future. Despite these drawbacks that are not certain in all patients who have residual microscopic disease or in whom margins were inadequate, or those who demonstrate viable tumor on histopathological examination of resected tumor specimen should receive adjuvant radiation therapy.

For *metastatic disease* to lungs, standard radiotherapy should be given. For metastatic sites of disease in bone and soft tissues, fractionated radiation therapy doses totaling 45–56 Gy should be given. Pulmonary metastases are managed with whole-lung irradiation (12–15 Gy) even if chemotherapy

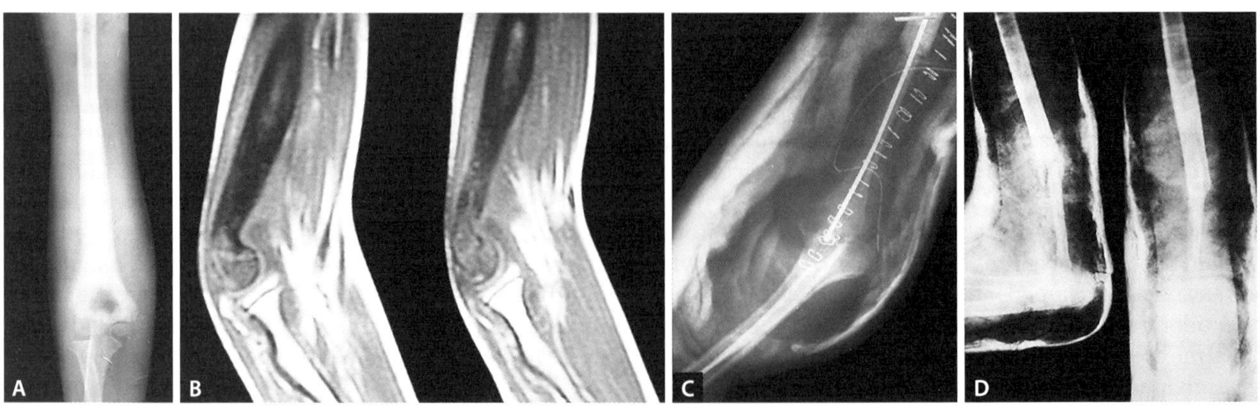

Figs. 80A to D: (A and B) Ewing's sarcoma of humeral shaft in an 8-year-old child postchemotherapy treated with (C and D) excision and reconstruction.
Source: S Rastogi, Professor and Head, Department of Orthopedics, Hamdard Institute of Medical Sciences and Research, New Delhi, India.

has given complete resolution of overt pulmonary metastasis. Currently for patients with metastatic disease, use of high-dose chemotherapy with stem cell rescue for metastatic disease is being studied. Recurrence of tumor usually occurs within 2 years (80%) and prognosis is poor in these cases. Prognosis is further worsened if recurrence is associated with metastasis. There is no standard second-line treatment available at present but a variable combination of cyclophosphamide and topotecan or irinotecan and temozolomide has been found effective in 50% cases. Alternative combination of gemcitabine and docetaxel has also demonstrated activity as is high-dose ifosfamide but they are not primarily used. Modern strategies include figitumumab (monoclonal antibodies against the IGF receptor 1) that has been reported to give favorable response objectively in metastatic recurrent Ewing's sarcoma in nearly 10% of cases. Similarly, a trial of IGF1R antibodies combined with the mTOR (mammalian target of rapamycin) inhibitor temsirolimus demonstrated complete response in two patients and three patients showed minor responses among 17 patients treated for metastatic recurrent Ewing's sarcoma.

Another viable strategy is based on EWS-FLI (a key target now for research). In a nutshell, EWS-FLI binds to RNA helicase A that regulates genetic transcription. YK-4-279 interferes this interaction between EWS-FLI and RNA helicase A proving lethal to Ewing's sarcoma cells in culture and has been demonstrated to reduce tumor growth in an animal model. Antisense oligonucleotide against the EWS-FLI translocation and siRNA (short double-stranded inhibitory RNA of approximately 19–21 base pairs in length that block translation) have been shown to inhibit tumor formation in vitro. CD99 is also a target foe Ewing's sarcoma therapy. Suicide in tumor cells can be induced via programmed cell death (apoptosis) using tumor necrosis factor-related apoptosis inducing ligand (TRAIL) that kills the Ewing's sarcoma cells. TRAIL has a cytokine function that acts by binding to two discrete cell surface receptors namely death receptor 4 (DR4) and death receptor 5 (DR5) activating them and ultimately leading to programmed cell death.

Patients who are treated for Ewing's sarcoma remain at high risk for developing secondary malignancies throughout their life. Of concern are treatment-related acute myeloid leukemia and myelodysplastic syndrome (MDS) that commonly develop 2–5 years after diagnosis in treated patients that occur in 1–2% of survivors of Ewing's sarcoma. Sarcomas develop in previously irradiated field.

Prognostic Factors for Ewing's Sarcoma

Pretreatment Factors

- *Site of tumor:* Distal extremities have the best prognosis followed by proximal part of extremities (intermediate prognosis), the central or pelvic sites (sacrum in particular) have worst prognosis. Pathologic fractures do not appear to be a prognostic factor.
- *Tumor size or volume:* Large volume (100 mL or 200 mL) and/or single dimension > 8 cm tend to occur in unfavorable sites and have poor prognosis.
- *Age:* The younger the patient better is the prognosis. So, infants and younger patients (aged <15 years) fare much better compared to those >15 years of age or adults.
- *Gender:* Females tend to have favorable prognosis.
- *Serum lactate dehydrogenase:* A raised serum LDH levels (particularly >200 IU/L) pretreatment is correlated to unfavorable prognosis. This may be partly also related to large sized primary tumors and metastatic disease that secrete more of this enzyme volumetrically so bad prognosis may be circumstantial.
- *Secondary Ewing's sarcoma:* If Ewing's sarcoma develops as a second malignant neoplasm in patients who have been treated previously for another neoplasm the prognosis is worse. There patients with secondary Ewing's sarcoma are usually older (mean age 47.8 years) compared to those with primary Ewing's sarcoma (mean age 22.5 years) and are likely to have neoplastic lesions in axial skeleton or extraskeletal site.
- *Tumor metastases (detected in about 25% of patients):* It is the *most powerful* predictor of outcome individually. Even considering the distribution of metastasis, if it is solely pulmonary, it fares better than in patients with metastasis outside the lungs. Patients that have single lung involvement again fare better than those with involvement of both lungs. Metastasis to osseous sites only seems to do better than those with metastases combined to both bone and lung. Regional lymph node involvement results in inferior outcome.
- *Cytogenetics:* The *EWS-FLI1* translocation breakpoint is not associated with adverse outcome as had been considered previously. The abnormalities associated with poor outcome identified instead are a complex karyotype (presence of 5 or more independent chromosome abnormalities) and modal chromosome number < 50.
- *Molecular markers:*
    - Detectable fusion transcripts by RT-PCR in morphologically normal marrow is associated with higher recurrence.
    - Poor prognosis has been associated with overexpression of the p53 protein, expression of Ki67, and loss of long-arm chromosome (16q deletion).
    - Increased microsomal glutathione S-transferase expression is associated with resistance to doxorubicin and hence inferior response to chemotherapy.

Treatment Response to Preoperative Therapy

A good response to preoperative chemotherapy is evident in the form of minimal (<5%) or no residual viable tumor left after presurgical chemotherapy that obviously is correlated to significantly improved EFS when compared to patients having residual larger volume of viable tumor left. Better histologic response to preoperative chemotherapy is seen in females and younger patients. PET scans can help to evaluate the response to chemotherapy being a metabolic indicator; decreased PET uptake seen in patients who underwent preinduction and postinduction chemotherapy and were evaluated by PET at both times, correlates well with good histologic response and better outcome.

Histology: Tumors that demonstrate histological variants like filigree pattern have an unfavorable prognosis. However, the degree of neural differentiation has no prognosticating value in Ewing's sarcoma.

FIBROUS DYSPLASIA

(Jaffe–Lichtenstein Syndrome, Fibrocartilagenous Dysplasia, and Generalized Fibrocystic Disease of Bone)

Fibrous dysplasia is a nonheritable, benign, and fibro-osseous lesion that is commonly medullary monostotic (80%), or sometimes polyostotic (20%). Monostotic FD may be present at any age though it is most common in those aged below 30 years while polyostotic FD is seen much early and most commonly presents before puberty. There is equal sex distribution. This was first described by Lichtenstein in 1938 and later further elucidated by Lichtenstein and Jaffe in 1942. It is considered that a developmental failure occurs during remodeling of woven so that mature lamellar bone fails to form. The bone also fails to remodel in response to mechanical stress (i.e., does not follow Wolff's law). Due to loss of maturation, an unorganized mass of immature trabeculae is left enmeshed in dysplastic fibrous tissue. There is not complete failure or absence of remodeling but the turnover is so slow that completion of the remodeling process does not occur. The bone fails to follow Wolff's law and hence trabeculae do not align along the stress line, this is combined with insufficient mineralization causing significant loss in mechanical strength. This causes stress concentration and hence development of pain, progressive deformity, and even pathologic fractures.

Any bone of the skeleton may be involved but generally four forms are considered:

1. Monostotic form affecting single bone (70–80% of cases). The disease is usually asymptomatic until 2nd to 3rd decades, but can be seen even during adulthood. The disease becomes inactive after puberty, and monostotic form has not been found to progress to polyostotic form. Ribs, craniofacial bones, and femur are commonly affected.
2. Polyostotic form affecting multiple bones (20–30% of cases). Usually one side is predominantly involved rather than a uniform distribution **(Fig. 81)**. Lower extremity bones are the most common to be involved (femur, tibia, and pelvis).
3. Craniofacial affecting only the skull and facial bones.
4. Cherubism—distinct from FD in that it is inherited (autosomal dominant), occurs early in life (3–4 years of age), has predominant cosmetic changes in face (symmetric jaw fullness and upward turning of eyes due to bilateral expansile multiloculated cystic masses in mandible and maxilla), and histologically, the tumor resembles giant cell granuloma. They often regress with age.

Associations of Fibrous Dysplasia

- About 2–3% of polyostotic FD are associated with café au lait skin lesions, precocious puberty in girls, with or without fibromyxomatous soft tissue tumors comprising McCune–Albright syndrome (Albright syndrome). Café au lait (French, "coffee with milk") areas of skin pigmentation are observed around the trunk or the proximal parts of the extremities. These areas have characteristic appearance that can be used to differentiate the lesion from other diagnosis. The variegated rough irregular border in FD resembles the "coast of Maine" in contrast to the smooth-bordered (coast of California) areas seen characteristically in diffuse neurofibromatosis (von Recklinghausen disease).
- *Mazabraud syndrome:* There is development of soft tissue or intramuscular myxoma (typically multiple) near most severely affected bone.
- Some cases of polyostotic FD have isolated endocrinopathy (hyperthyroidism, hyperparathyroidism, diabetes mellitus, Cushing's syndrome, and acromegaly) without the full McCune–Albright syndrome precocious puberty in girls.
- Very rarely, secondary sarcomas may develop on FD.

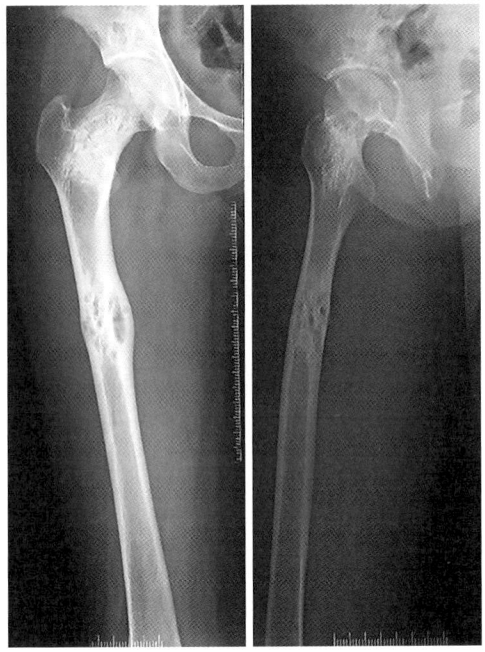

Fig. 81: Polyostotic fibrous dysplasia of bone. The lesions predominantly involve right side of body involving the femur and acetabulum.

Etiopathogenesis

The abnormal replacement of bone with fibro-osseous tissue has been linked to mutation in the gene that encodes the α-subunit of a stimulatory G-protein (Gsα) located on chromosome 20 (*GNAS1* gene). This mutation is present in the lesional tissue only. Even the skin lesions in some cases have been found to have somatic mutations in the signal-transducing guanine nucleotide binding proteins. The mutated protein activates the trimeric stimulatory the G-protein (guanine nucleotide protein) which has three subunits (a, b, and g). In normal functioning, the G-protein is coupled to intracellular effector on stimulation that in-turn causes dissociation of the α-chain of the Gs trimer. The α-chain of the Gs trimer substitutes GTP for GDP following dissociation and activates adenylyl cyclase increasing cAMP intracellularly. The α-chain by virtue of inherent GTPase activity splits phosphate converting GTP to GDP, causing reassociation of the chain to rest of the Gs. This then inactivates the adenylyl cyclase reducing cAMP intracellularly. The point mutation of the *GNAS1* gene on chromosome 20q13.2-13.3 in McCune–Albright syndrome causes an amino-acid substitution where cysteine or histidine amino acids in genomic DNA of osteoblasts are replaced by arginine thus interfering with the GTPase function of α-chain. The Gs, hence, remain constantly activated causing increased adenylyl cyclase activity and increased intracellular cAMP. There is inappropriate hormone secretion and alteration of the local milieu. Mutations were first identified from soft tissue lesions and then later from bony pathology. Interestingly the mutations are only found in the pathological tissue indicating that it is not a germline disorder, and is not heritable. It could be a form of mosaic mutation present in McCune–Albright syndrome originating during fetal development in a variety of cells. In monostotic disease, the genomic mutation probably arises due to unknown factors later in life and producing single tumor. Depending on the cell type where it originates activated Gs produce differential effects like in the skin it causes hyperpigmentation while in the endocrine tissues, there is increased hormonal secretion. Altered local hormonal milieu in bone leads to local bone resorption, and the formation of dysplastic fibro-osseous tissue. The cytokines expressed in FD include mitogens like PDGFs, bone inducing proteins such as BMPs, nuclear transcription regulator like c-fos and IL-6 (increased osteoclast and bone resorption).

It has been found that there is a specific chromosomal abnormality present in all pathological cells from a patient but is not common to all patients suggesting proliferative advantage to a cell line (mutated) producing the lesion, and hence by definition it qualifies for neoplasm. So, FD possibly represents a proliferation of somatically mutated spindle cells occurring either in a mosaic pattern (polyostotic), or at a localized site in bone (monostotic).

Clinical Presentation

It is an incidental finding in majority of monostotic cases as the disease is more often than not asymptomatic. Otherwise pain, deformity, and pathological fracture are the most common presenting features. *Bone pain* has been reported in up to 81% of adults and 49% of children present in dysplastic areas with high stress. A reduction in pain and disease activity with age is seen in many lesions with a possible reactivation at the time of pregnancy in female patients. Bones plastically *deform* under the mechanical pressure from body weight and the type of deformity depends on place and extent of lesion. *Shepherd's crook deformity* (resembling the kyphotic spine deformity of shepherd) is a lateral bow of proximal femur due to passage medially of body weight and developing characteristic deformity in polyostotic disease. Scoliosis develops similarly in spinal lesions. It results in limb shortening, limping and, occasionally, chronic fatigue fracture (seen as a Parrot's beak on medial cortex) accompanied by disabling pain. Other deformities include tibial bow (even saber tibia), protrusio acetabuli, and Harrison's groove (a horizontal depression along the peripheral border diagram in lower thorax, corresponding to its costal insertion). Deformity in monostotic forms halts after skeletal maturity but in polyostotic forms usually continues to progress even after stopping of bone growth. *Swelling* is palpable in subcutaneous bones. Jaw bones are the most common site of involvement, appendicular skeleton is preferentially affected in females while males have predominant skull and ribs lesions.

Investigations

Radiology

The lesions are intramedullary, geographic with well-defined, sclerotic margins and a "ground-glass" matrix. Ground-glass matrix is an area with no or minimally discernable trabecular region having density similar to cancellous bone (lighter compared to cortical region). With continued growth, the sharp cortical border is also lost giving a uniform look to area of lesion. The lesions are often expansile and may contain lucent areas of secondary ABC. Ribs are the most common site of monostotic FD and FD is the most common cause of benign expansile rib lesion. Endosteal scalloping is seen in large lesions and periosteal reaction is absent. Shepherd's crook deformity **(Figs. 82A and B)** develops in proximal femur when the weight of the body acts through the mechanically weakened bone and causes severe varus in the proximal femur. Variegated appearance of skeletal lesions cause some lesions to appear more sclerotic or demonstrate calcified cartilage. Other lesions often show marked bony expansion especially lesions involving the ribs.

Bone scintigraphy and tomography: These are intensely hot on bone scans and may be used to locate the extent and distribution of disease. CT is useful in demonstrating the cortical involvement and continuity.

Magnetic resonance imaging: The lesion has intermediate-intensity on T1-weighted images and is a bit enhanced heterogeneously on T2-weighted images (but less than fluid or malignant tissue).

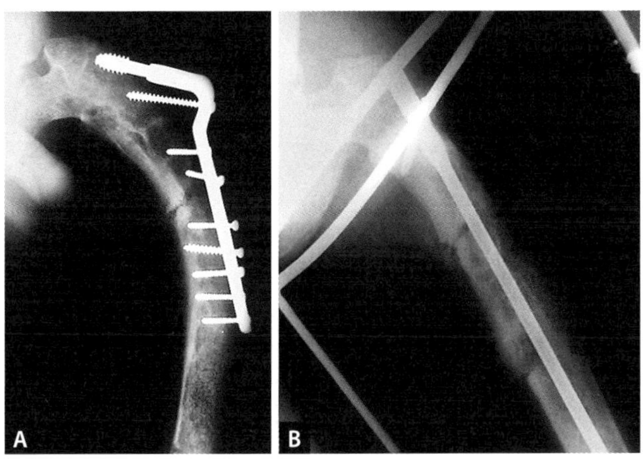

Figs. 82A and B: Fibrous dysplasia. (A) The typical shepherd crook deformity of proximal femur, and (B) its correction done by seekh-kabab osteotomy.

Secondary cysts have high signal intensity. Due to high variability of lesions on MRI, it is not a useful investigation for differentiation of the disease from other lesions.

Histopathology

On gross examination, FD lesion appears firm with variable amount of "grittiness." Cyst formation, if present, is occasional and often secondary (*see* ABC). Some lesions demonstrate cartilage areas grossly. Lesion is easily separable from the encircling shell of bone mostly. On microscopic examination, discrete delicate trabeculae of immature woven bone are dispersed in a background of moderately cellular fibrous tissue. These trabeculae organize into variegated shapes of (Cs, Os) arranged haphazardly and are referred to as forming "Chinese-letters" or "alphabet soup" pattern. Osteoblasts are found interspersed in woven bone but do not rim the trabeculae (differentiating from OFD, fracture callus or myositis ossificans). Occasionally, small foci of lamellar bone may also be seen in a few cases of FD. The background of fibrous stroma is variegated in appearance and is variably cellular, myxomatous, or show prominent collagenization. The fibroblasts in the lesion usually have plump ovoid nuclei. Nonspecific osteoclast-type giant cells may be also found. Cartilage in the form of long islands or rounded nodules with peripheral endochondral ossification is sometimes present (differentiating it from chondrosarcoma). Collections of foam cells are common (should not be confused for metastatic clear cell carcinoma).

Differential Diagnosis

Radiological differential diagnosis includes Paget's disease (different demographics, histologically mosaic pattern on histology), neurofibromatosis type 1 (rare osseous lesions, often axial, and ribbon ribs), OFD (exclusively tibial with anterior bow and cortical lesions), adamantinoma (mostly tibial), nonossifying fibroma, simple bone cyst (more radiolucent, expansile, and thinner lamellar bone surrounding) and enchondromatosis. Pathological differentials include OFD (cortical location, well-organized zonation, and osteoblast rimming), reactive woven bone, well-differentiated intraosseous osteosarcoma (cytologic atypia and permeative growth pattern), and desmoplastic fibroma (extensively heavily collagenized).

Management

For incidental lesions, observation is practiced after confirming that the lesion is FD only especially in monostotic forms as there is minimal risk of pathological fracture or deformity. For polyostotic disease, endocrinology evaluation should be done for endocrine abnormalities and appropriate management. Medical management include mainly use of injectable zoledronic acid (4–5 mg IV every 6 months) or oral (risedronate/alendronate) bisphosphonate. The osteopenic lesions are thought to be mainly due to bone absorption by excess osteoclastic activity that can be effectively inhibited by bisphosphonates. Levels of ALP, fasting urinary hydroxyproline, and urinary type I collagen C-telopeptide) are lower in treated patients and lesions heal in 1–3 years. Clinically, this reduces pain and improves bone strength. Surgical management is directed toward the treatment or prevention of its complications such as deformities and pathological fracture along with surgical extirpation of the disease. Simple curettage and bone grafting **(Figs. 83A to D)** has high failure with local recurrence and reappearance of the lesion in polyostotic disease. Usually, wide procedures are hence adopted as the new bone formed is still dysplastic. For proximal femoral deformity, corrective osteotomy (valgus) and fixation with extramedullary or intramedullary implants is usually done (*see* **Figs. 82A and B**). Cancellous grafts are quickly replaced by dysplastic bones so contrary to the views cortical bone grafts and allografts have a special place in these patients. Reports of secondary neoplasia superimposed on FD are emerging. Malignant transformation into osteosarcoma, fibrosarcoma, MFH, and chondrosarcoma is seen in 0.4–4% cases. Radiation exposure for treatment or patients with Mazabraud's syndrome is at higher risk for malignant transformation.

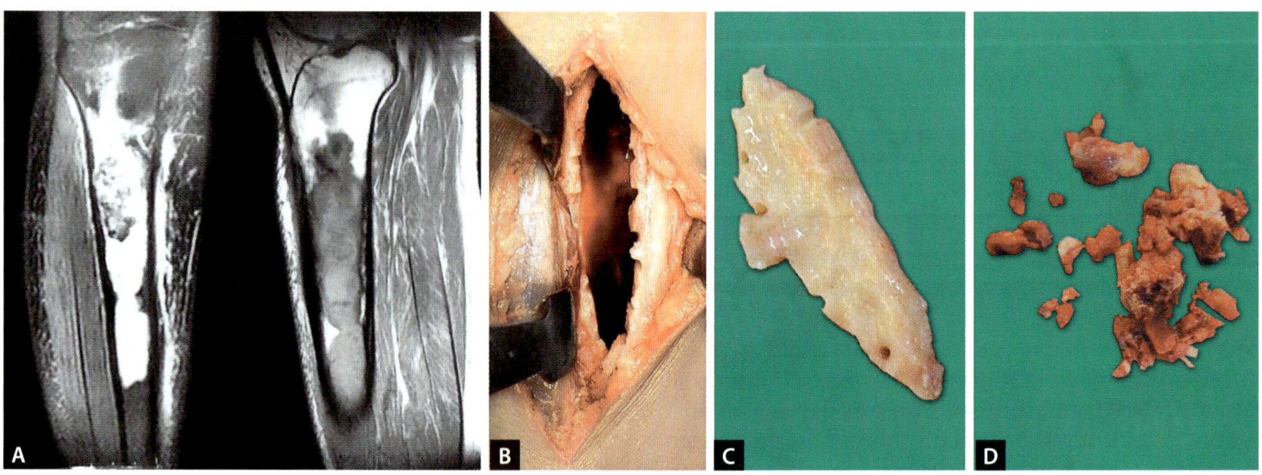

Figs. 83A to D: (A) Fibrous dysplasia of proximal tibial shaft (B and C) treated with extended curettage, and (D) bone grafting.

OSTEOFIBROUS DYSPLASIA (CAMPANACCI'S DISEASE)

Osteofibrous dysplasia is a rare, non-neoplastic fibro-osseous proliferation affecting the cortex of the tibial (commonly) or fibular diaphysis in children and infants. Frangenheim first described the lesion in 1921 as a congenital osteitis fibrosa. Subsequently, Kempson, in 1966, named the lesion ossifying fibroma and described it as an aggressive lesion. In 1981, Campanacci and Laus studied 35 cases recognizing it as a benign disease and coined the term osteofibrous dysplasia of the tibia and fibula. "Dysplasia" is preferred over the use of historical "ossifying fibroma" because it is now considered to be of congenital origin and due to its resemblance to FD; histopathologically, the term expands to osteofibrous dysplasia. The disease is apparently exclusive to tibia and fibula. Few researchers use the term intracortical FD to emphasize its cortical location instead of using Campanacci's disease. Only rarely is OFD and is also referred to as Campanacci syndrome possibly nonpragmatically. Occasional cases involving radius, humerus, and ulna have been reported. The disease is diagnosed in children <10 years of age, with a peak incidence reported among those between 1 and 5 years. Several reports also exist noting there occurrence in new born (hence thought to be congenital). Adults (oldest on record being 39 years of age) with de novo OFD have also been reported. Sex predilection is unclear, some studies do favor male predilection. The etiology of OFD as well as the cell of origin is unknown. Familial occurrence is not popular and only one description of such familial OFD is present in literature.

Etiopathogenesis

The most pertinent hypothesis of occurrence points to origin from a fibrovascular abnormality. Possibly OFD to adamantinoma reflect a spectrum of abnormalities, the two forming extreme ends. A relationship between OFD and adamantinoma has been proposed by Johnson on the basis of common origin of the two—namely, the fibrovascular defect. As proposed by this theory, OFD results from an abnormality in the Haversian canals, whereas adamantinoma is a product of defect of intramedullary vasculature. According to Komiya and Inoue, a deficiency in blood flow within the periosteum results in OFD. Relationship between adamantinoma and OFD is supported by the cytogenetic analysis and finding that both have some extent of chromosomal trisomy. Trisomy of chromosome 7, 8, 12, and 22 has been described in OFD while adamantinoma also has trisomy of chromosome 7 and 12. Strength to this association is provided by report by Sherman et al. coexistent adamantinoma and OFD in the same patient.

Clinical Presentation

The most common presentation is a painless, localized, and firm swelling of the tibia. The tibia frequently is bowed anteriorly or anterolaterally. Pathological fracture may also be present but is uncommon. The symptoms are present for average of 14 months before diagnosis. Pain is present in around one-third of the patients. Some cases are noticed incidentally on radiographs taken for some other reason.

Investigations

Radiology

The lesion is a cortically based, diaphyseal eccentric geographic lucency with well-defined sclerotic margins. There could be multiple lucencies in the cortex separated by areas of sclerosis (multilocular). The anterior cortical surface is usually involved **(Figs. 84A and B)**. There could be anterior bowing of tibia. The cortex is often thickened and the lesion appears expansile. Periosteal reaction is rare and if present it is thick and solid type.

Histopathology

Grossly, the tissue is fibrous gritty contained by the periosteum. Microscopically, the characteristic feature is storiform (cartwheel pattern) fibrous background containing spicules of woven bony trabeculae that are lined by a layer of osteoblasts (osteoblast rimming). Rimming is absent in FD. OFD has additionally zonal architecture (zonification described by Campanacci and Laus) where the immature woven bone is more centrally located while the number and maturity of trabeculae increase toward periphery of lesion so that the center is more fibrous while periphery is more osseous. Focal cytokeratin positivity may be seen raising the possibility that OFD could represent a variant of extragnathic adamantinoma with poorly developed epithelial islands.

Differential Diagnosis

Adamantinoma (soft tissue extension and intramedullary presence), FD (intramedullary, no osteoblastic rimming) (*see* other differences in **Table 20**), and nonossifying fibroma. Other radiological differentials include chondromyxoid

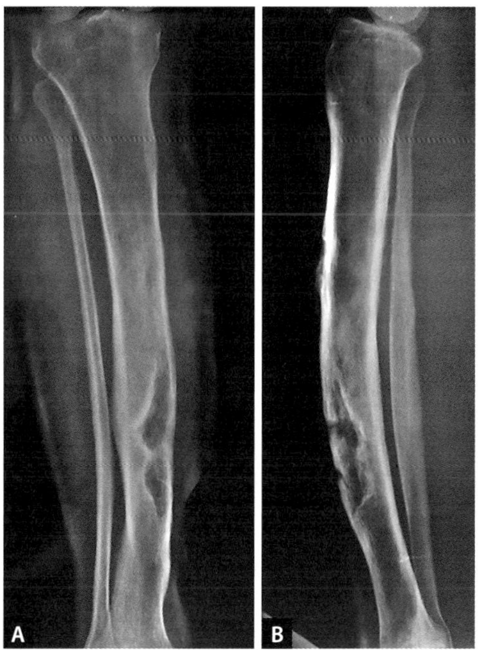

Figs. 84A and B: The anteroposterior (AP) and lateral radiographs of left leg demonstrate cortically based, diaphyseal eccentric geographic lucency with well-defined sclerotic margins typical of osteofibrous dysplasia of tibia with anteromedial bowing of the shaft.

TABLE 20: Differentiating features of fibrous dysplasia from osteofibrous dysplasia.

Fibrous dysplasia	*Osteofibrous dysplasia*
Most commonly presents before puberty (polyostotic form) to up to 30 years (monostotic form)	Presents within 10 years
Can be found anywhere in skeleton—ribs most common	Exclusive to tibia and fibula very rare other sites reported
Intramedullary lesion	Intracortical lesion
Many bones can be involved simultaneously	Limited to one bone
Usually, incidental in monostotic forms, else pain and deformity are the common presentations	Presents as a swelling of tibia with anterior or anterolateral bowing
May be associated with endocrine abnormalities	Not so
Geographical destruction with very fine or lost sclerotic cortical border with growth. Overall a ground glass appearance	Sharp well-defined cortical border around the lesion. Multilocular lesion may also be seen
Alphabet soup appearance on microscopy	Characteristic osteoblastic rimming and zonification seen

fibroma (CMF), ABC, UBC, eosinophilic granuloma (EOG), osteomyelitis, rarely chondrosarcoma, osteosarcoma, and hemangioendothelioma.

Treatment

For OFD, the current recommendation had been to avoid surgical intervention due to high recurrence rates and benign disposition of the lesion. Also the lesion stops growing after skeletal maturity. So apart from biopsy, there is possibly no need for extirpation of lesion. Once the maturity is reached excision with bone grafting may be done. Some advice bracing for prevention of deformity. Surgical management may be done for extensive or deforming lesions or for those having pathological fracture. This view has been recently challenged by Lee et al. and they recommend initial aggressive extraperiosteal resection in all cases. This is typically based on the fact that there is quite a high chance of sampling error in biopsy and finding of high percentage of adamantinoma or adamantinoma-like OFD in resected specimens. Possibly a thorough representative biopsy and vigilant histopathological examination should save patient from such aggressive treatment methods. The prognosis of "true" OFD is excellent and no progression to adamantinoma is seen.

ADAMANTINOMA

Adamantinoma of the long bones (to differentiate it from the jaw lesion) is a clinically low-grade, slow-growing, and primary malignant neoplasm of bone that is histopathologically characterized by epithelial cells dispersed in fibrous or osteofibrous stroma and is radiologically typically located in the diaphyseal region of tibia. The occurrence of this neoplasm is uncommon and it accounts for only 0.1–0.5% of all primary bone tumors and has metastatic potential. Adamantinoma was first reported by Maier in 1900. In 1913, Fischer named the lesion "primary adamantinoma of the tibia". In 1951, Schulenberg clarified the concept and segregated adamantinoma as a separate entity.

Etiopathogenesis

Though still under study the adamantinoma is now considered a tumor of epithelial origin, based on ultrastructural (presence of basal lamina, desmosomes, gap junctions, and epithelial specific keratin) and immunohistochemical studies (strong positive staining with pan-cytokeratin antibody). There are a number of suggestions as to how this "epithelial" abnormality would arise in a mesenchymal tissue [Congenital implantation (Fischer), traumatic (Dockery and Meyerding), and synovial origin (Lederer–Sinclair and Naji)].

Now the most accepted theory is that of displacement of basal epithelium of skin during embryological development to underlying developing bone and later development of the lesion. This is supported by the predominant involvement of anterior tibia which is closest to the skin surface. Adamantinoma to OFD represents possibly a spectrum of disorder a concept that has come in vogue with finding of OFD-like adamantinoma (also called "differentiated adamantinoma"). This lesion differs from classic adamantinoma in its earlier age at presentation (<20 years), intracortical location and predominance of an OFD-like stroma, with only scant small nests of epithelial cells, and indolent, and nonmetastasizing nature. Immunohistochemical staining for keratin, an epithelial marker has been used to demonstrate the epithelial cells. WHO clearly states that an OFD lesion is devoid of epithelial differentiation and one should label a tumor to be OFD-like adamantinoma only if keratin-positive epithelial cells are demonstrated. Most authors now agree that the diagnosis of OFD-like adamantinoma should be based on finding nests of epithelial cells seen on routine tissue staining, whereas OFD lesions would have single, scattered epithelial cells seen only with immunohistochemical staining. To decipher a relationship of OFD to adamantinoma, an expression of several protooncogenes (e.g., c-fos and c-jun) and bone-matrix proteins (e.g., collagen IV, laminin, and galectin 3) in these lesions have been studied. Some of these proteins represent the process of mesenchymal-to-epithelial differentiation, which could explain the origin of the "epithelial" component of the tumor in adamantinoma (possibly from OFD). In adamantinoma, both fibrous and epithelial components express FGF-2 and FGF receptor-1, whereas only the epithelial component expresses high levels of epidermal growth factor (EGF) and EGFR. The expression of epithelial cell markers is higher in adamantinoma than in OFD-like adamantinoma. High levels of Ki-67 (a proliferation marker) are also seen in the epithelial component only. These suggest two things, first that the epithelial portion is likely responsible for tumor growth and malignant behavior. The second is that possibly the epithelial cells acquire higher expression of FGF-2, EGF, and EGFR, as well as higher proliferative activity, as the lesion progresses from benign (OFD) to malignant (adamantinoma) lending support to precursor theory (OFD to adamantinoma spectrum).

Clinical Presentation

Pain and swelling at the site are the most common complaint; there may be discomfort at the swelling lasting months before dull pain appears. The tumor occurs usually in the 2nd to 5th decades with most patients presenting in 25–35 years. It is slightly more common in men than women (5:4). The tumor is typically located in long bones (97% of cases) and tibia specifically (80–85% of cases) represents the most characteristic site. Ipsilateral fibula is involved in 10–15% cases. Other bones have also been reported and include humerus, ulna, femur, fibula, radius, pelvic bones, ribs, spine and small bones of the hand and foot. A history of significant trauma has been noted in about two-thirds of patients. The patient may have bowing deformity of the tibia and pathological fracture is seen in one-fifth of the patients.

Radiology

The lesions are eccentric, diaphyseal, and mostly cortical with soap-bubble appearance with anterior bowing of tibia. Central "intramedullary" lesions are seen in <10% patients though extension to intramedullary region from primary tumor is common. The margins are geographical and may be sharply or poorly delineated with peripheral sclerosis. The multilocular character with septations and ring-like densities produce "soap-bubble" appearance. Cortical breach and soft-tissue extension is seen in 15% patients. Periosteal reaction may be seen in occasional cases.

Technetium pyrophosphate bone scan shows intense uptake that typically corresponds to the extent of lesion. CT scanning details an osteolytic lesion with cortical involvement and intramedullary extension. On MRI, there is homogeneous, intermediate signal on T1-weighted images. The T2-weighted images show a homogeneous or heterogeneous enhancement of the lesion. With gadolinium contrast, there is intense homogeneous signal enhancement. MRI gives critical information regarding distant cortical foci as well as intramedullary and/or soft tissue extension which is useful in determining tumor-free margins and surgical planning and reconstruction.

Histopathology

The tumor is yellow gray to grayish-white well-demarcated fleshy lesion with a lobular growth pattern. Microscopically, the classic tumor shows epithelial islands in a fibrous stroma. The epithelial component may show variety of growth pattern including spindled, basaloid (solid nests of basaloid cells with distinctive peripheral palisading), squamoid and tubular (narrow cords of epithelial cells in a vascular or glandular appearance). The spindled form is differentiated from fibrosarcoma on the basis of atypia. In all, immunohistochemical stains are the best method for diagnosing adamantinoma. OFD-like adamantinoma (differentiated adamantinoma) shows predominantly osteofibrous tissue with few epithelial rests.

Differential Diagnosis

Osteofibrous dysplasia, metastatic carcinoma, epithelioid hemangioendothelioma [von Willebrand antigen, vascular tissue markers (CD34 and CD31), and *Ulex europaeus* would confirm its vascular nature], synovial sarcoma (epithelial component similar to adamantinoma but mesenchymal component is cytologically atypical). Radiological differentials include FD, NOF, ABC, UBC, EOG, and osteomyelitis.

Management

Metastasis (seen in one-fifth of cases) in classic adamantinoma commonly occurs to lungs, lymph nodes, or to other bones and is possibly not a feature of OFD-like adamantinoma. Chemotherapy or radiotherapy is ineffective so surgical extirpation of tumor and metastasis is essential and recommended. En bloc resection with wide margins to clear the tumor is the acceptable method. Appropriate reconstruction with vascularized or nonvascularized autograft or allograft (intercalary and osteoarticular), metallic segmental implants, and distraction osteogenesis can be then done. Local recurrence rates are around 10–30% at average 5 years after treatment. Risk factors for recurrence appear to be shorter duration of pain, pain at presentation, intralesional or marginal excision, patients <20 years of age. With appropriate management, the survival at 10 years has improved to around 90%. Amputation previously considered being treatment of choice has no logical bearing in modern orthopedic practice as it has neither shown an improved survival nor the functional or psychological outcome is acceptable.

CHORDOMA

Chordomas are very rare (0.1/100,000 per year) low-grade malignant tumors of bone having predilection for axial skeleton and in the region of embryonic notochord. They commonly arise from (in descending order of occurrence) the sacrum, skull base (clivus), and the spine. Just about more than half the lesions occur in the sacral region in most series and the other half is localized to the clivus. The most accepted origin is from embryonic rests of notochord that show a dual epithelial-mesenchymal differentiation. Symptoms depend on the anatomic location of the tumor. Tumors of skull base result in headache, development of progressive cranial nerve palsies, visual disturbances, and endocrinopathies. Neoplasms in cervical region cause cord compression and quadriparesis. Sacrococcygeal tumors initially produce lower back pain then progressively bladder or bowel dysfunction, paresthesias finally culminating in a pelvic or sacral mass that would fungate, necrose, and get infected if untreated. Such neglected cases are, however, uncommon and in general the clinical course of disease is slow with typically local symptoms. The chordomas, however, have the potential for metastases and the malignancy would extend to the lungs, bone, and liver in such cases. Radiologically, chordomas are lytic lesions that remain in midline and expand and destroy bone; matrix calcifications may be sometimes seen in the clivus region.

Pathology

The appearance is of chondrosarcoma grossly showing lobulated soft myxoid masses. On microscopic examination, the lesions appear lobulated with a myxoid background.

Fibrous septa separate these lobules that contain cells arranged in cords, sheets or occasionally, haphazardly. At least some of these cells would demonstrate vacuolated cytoplasm (physaliphorous cells). Some of these cells may show eosinophilic cytoplasm or may mimic signet ring cells. Overall nuclear atypia or pleomorphism if present is mild and mitotic activity commonly low or absent. Immunohistochemically, markers for epithelial cells are positive. A newly recognized marker "brachyury" (it is a transcription factor that is involved in notochord development) may be helpful diagnostically.

Variants

- Aggressive, sarcomatous or "dedifferentiated", high-grade variety
- Chordoma of the chondroid variety (contains foci of cartilaginous differentiation) may have a more favorable prognosis than other chordomas. It has predilection for spheno-occipital region.

Differential Diagnosis

Metastatic adenocarcinoma (higher cytologic atypia and lack lobulated growth pattern), liposarcoma (lack lobulated growth pattern, positive fat and mucin stains), myxoid chondrosarcoma (rare axial location and immunostains for cytokeratin negative).

Management

Surgical removal of the tumor has inherent limitations. The main prognostic factor for local failure and survival is quality of surgical margins. There is 70% local failure rate following marginal resection. Due to limited access, an adequate margin can be obtained in roughly only half of sacrococcygeal cases and even more poorly for spine and skull base lesions. Surgical resection at and above S2 for sacrococcygeal lesions result in significant morbidity. Resection of both S2 roots result in incompetent bladder and bowel. The disease-specific survival at 10 years for sacral presentations is around 50% while for tumors arising from the base of the skull; it is only around 30%. Radiation therapy is equally challenging due to unusual sites of the tumor. The tolerance dose of the spinal cord and brainstem, optic pathways, and the rectum is lower than the curative dose of 70 Gy. At suboptimal doses of 40–60 Gy for standard photon beam radiotherapy local control at 5 years is in the 10–40% range. Proton beam therapy fares better with local control at 5 years of 50–60%. Carbon ion radiation therapy may provide the same advantages as protons, possibly with improved biological effectiveness. Stereotactic procedures (radiosurgery), IMRT and use of dynamic arcs (for prosthesis) may improve the result of photon beam therapy especially with radiosensitizing agents. Chemotherapy has long been known to be inactive in chordoma. Recently, interest has regained in the disease with the finding of sensitivity of chordomas to molecular-targeted agents identified in new research. The most effective agent identified and studied is imatinib that has prominent antitumor activity in chordoma. Also EGFR and c-Met are strongly expressed in few chordomas patients and can be potential targets in future. Combinations of cetuximab and gefitinib are being studied as for their antiangiogenic effect.

VASCULAR LESIONS OF BONE

Skeletal Angiomatosis (Cystic Angiomatosis)

This represents multifocal or diffuse intraosseous proliferation of benign vascular or lymphatic channels with concomitant destruction of skeletal architecture. Two variants depending on extent of skeletal involvement are recognized. The regional nonaggressive form involves only a region or part of skeleton while the disseminated form is commonly called "skeletal angiomatosis". The disease is apparently congenital manifesting within first 2 decades of life. There may be associated extraskeletal angiomas (soft tissues, lungs, liver, and spleen) in 60–70% patients. Few authors consider cystic angiomatosis to be less aggressive variant of Gorham's disease in the spectrum of vascular lesions of bone; however, there are characteristic differences (see below in massive osteolysis).

Clinical Features

Patients present with bone pains and swelling but the symptoms are usually not severe. Less commonly the lesions may be painless until bone is replaced by fibrous connective tissue and becomes weak to cause fracture in weight-bearing bone. Vertebral lesions may present with scoliosis and radicular symptoms. Skull, spine, pelvis, ribs, and long bones are all involved in that order. Extraskeletal chylous or hemorrhagic effusions with thrombocytopenia may be present.

Radiologically, lytic lesions appear to contain residual lamellar bone and foci of reactive woven bone. Radiolucent lesions with a soap-bubble or honeycomb appearance are present **(Figs. 85A and B)**. CT scan reveals well-defined lytic lesions with sclerotic margins. Magnetic resonance features are typical of hemangiomas with high intensity on T2-weighted images while on T1-weighted image the lesion

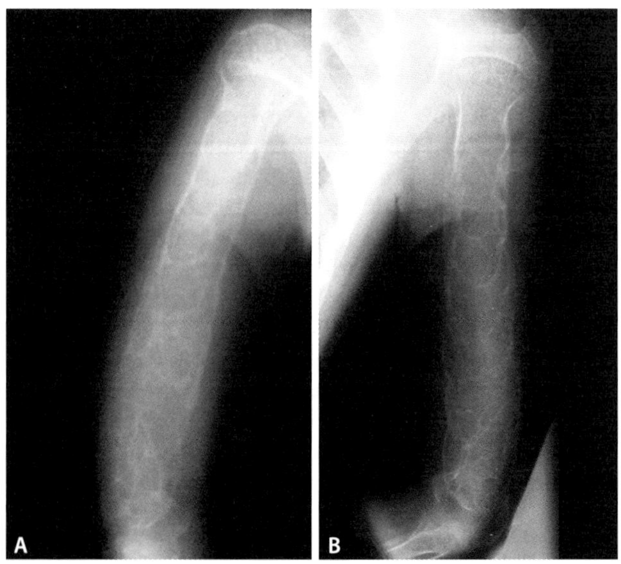

Figs. 85A and B: Cystic angiomatosis replacing the whole bone with multiple blood-filled cysts.

is hypointense. Proton-density weighted images show high intensity but the contrast is reduced due to increased marrow intensity.

Histopathologically, the capillary and cavernous hemangiomas have thin-walled blood-filled vessels (small diameter in capillary and dilated spaces in cavernous) that are lined by a single layer of flat endothelial. Lymphangioma contains dilated, sinusoidal, vessels that are filled with lymph and are also lined by a single layer of flat endothelial cells. The endothelial cell contains Weibel–Palade bodies.

The endothelial cells express vimentin and many cells stain with antibodies to factor VIII, CD31, and CD34.

Management

The disease though aggressive does not show malignant transformation. The morbidity from disease can be controlled with combination therapy of α-interferon, thalidomide (and its derivative lenalidomide), and zoledronic acid. The pain relief is rapid, however, regression of lesion is seen in <70% patients. Moreover, the lesions recur following treatment interruption. Still in many, the lesion is reduced to such an extent that patients successfully get away with small surgical resection. Radiotherapy 50–60 Gy may be applied in resistant cases or for additional local control of disease.

Massive Osteolysis (Disappearing Bone Disease, Essential Osteolysis, Idiopathic Massive Osteolysis, Progressive Massive Osteolysis, Vanishing Bone Disease, Phantom Bone Disease, Gorham's Disease, Gorham's Syndrome, Gorham–Stout Syndrome, Morbus-Gorham-Stout Disease)

It is a rare disorder that can be considered aggressive form of skeletal osteolysis. The disorder is poorly understood and manifests as progressive osteolysis along with proliferation of thin-walled complex, combined lymphatic venous malformation. The bone is replaced by fibrous tissue and may stop also rarely spontaneously. The disease long ago was reported by Jackson in 1838 followed by disease description by Gorham and colleagues (1954) and then again detailed by Gorham and Stout in 1955.

Pathogenesis and Pathophysiology

No evidence of a malignant, neuropathic, or infectious causation has been identified till date as a pathogenic factor producing this disorder, and there is also no documented familial or hereditary predisposition. The mechanism of such rapid and relentless bone resorption is also vague. Gorham's disease is commonly an angiomatosis of blood vessels and quite uncommonly lymphangiomatosis that aggressively expands causing massive bone loss. Some of the suggested theories are as follows:

- *Heyden et al. (1977) local hypoxia and low pH theory:* The unusually wide angiomatosis vessels reduce the blood flow. This slow circulation produces local tissue hypoxia and hence lowers the pH locally. This milieu favors activity of various hydrolytic enzymes and also bone absorption. The theory is supported by high activity of enzymes acid phosphatase and leucine aminopeptidase that have been identified in the mononuclear perivascular cells near the lesions. The calcium ions may get chelated in such acidic environment unable to participate in osteogenesis.
- Cannon and Jacob reported a history of minor trauma in patients of osteolysis. Lereche (1937) had proposed post-traumatic arteriole hyperemia as the mechanism responsible for bone resorption; this was also supported by Gorham and Stout.
- Mundy et al. (1978), however, suggested that local derangement of osteoclastic activity is primarily responsible for the massive osteolysis. He also proposed that the increase in osteoclast formation in Gorham–Stout syndrome is due to increase in the sensitivity of osteoblast precursors to some humoral factors due to unidentified mechanism that promote osteoclast formation and not because of increased circulating numbers of osteoclast precursors. This causes increased bone resorption. Increased local levels of IL-6 have been found by Devlin that also supports osteoclastic bone resorption.
- *Role of thyroid C cells and calcitonin:* There is high likelihood of agenesis of thyroid C cells causing secrete calcitonin deficiency particularly in adolescents and young adults which could induce osteolysis.
- Not well-accepted by others is the proposal by Thomson and Schurman that unrestricted growth of granulation tissue exerts pressure on normal bone resulting in the resorption of bone. This process is similar to that seen in enlarged aneurysms.

Clinical Features

Gorham's disease has been reported to involve persons from any gender or any age group, although most cases manifest in 2nd to 3rd decades. It presents often as dull, aching weakness in involved segments, with increasing deformity, or with pathologic fracture. Following a pathological fracture, there is no callus formation or an osteoblastic response and instead the bone tapers and deforms. Most common sites of involvement are shoulder girdle, thorax, pelvic girdle and skull; while other bones have also been reported to be involved including spine. Contiguous bony involvement is common and joints or intervertebral disks do not serve as barriers at all. Patients with lesions extending outside of bone have a high mortality rate, approaching 50% from chylothorax (results from direct extension and rupture of lymphangiectasia into the pleural cavity or via invasion of the thoracic duct), chylopericardium, chyloperitoneum, and cachexia. It is not uncommon to see few patients presenting with an abrupt onset of pain and swelling, although most present with insidious onset of pain and limitation of motion in the involved limb. If axial skeleton is affected, there can be progressive weakness accompanied with muscle atrophy. In some cases, the disease is as such silent clinically and an innocuous trauma makes the limb painful attracting the attention of patients to seek medical attention that are incidentally detected then with Gorham's disease. Heffez et al. suggested eight criteria for diagnosing massive osteolysis:

1. Positive tissue biopsy demonstrating an angiomatous tissue

2. No or minimal cellular atypia
3. Usually no osteoblastic response (even if seen is mostly inconspicuous) and absent dystrophic calcification
4. Evidence of progressive local bone resorption
5. Nonexpansile and nonulcerative lesion
6. No visceral involvement
7. Regional osteolysis on radiographs
8. Absence of identifiable genetic, metabolic, neoplastic, immunological, and infectious etiology

Radiological

In initial stages of the lesion, intramedullary or subcortical radiolucent foci resemble findings of patchy osteoporosis. With progression, there is osseous atrophy, bone dissolution, appearance of fracture, fragmentation, and even complete disappearance of a portion or whole (advanced cases) of the bone. In cases where part of bone disappears, the remaining bone displays tapering or "pointing" of the ends (sucked candy appearance). The disease can have contiguous spread to nearby bones and even the intervening joints provide no protection to this disease extension. Hence, osteolysis of ilium would be associated with proximal femoral resorption or disease in scapula may be accompanied with destruction of the proximal humerus, clavicle and ribs. This regional osseous destruction pattern is pathognomonic of the disease helping in making diagnosis. The degree of osseous destruction is generally progressive but may also stabilize spontaneously. Computed tomography is the best method to evaluate the extent of bone destruction. Arteriography, venography, and lymphangiography do not demonstrate the intraosseous lesion. MRI features are same as that of skeletal angiomatosis, but the signal characteristics vary, depending on the stage of the disease process. The neovascular tissue is bright on T1 and T2 imaging early, but the predominant fibrous tissue present late in the process is dark on T1 and T2 imaging.

Histopathology

The resorbed bone is replaced by pathological fibrous hypervascular fibrous connective tissue and angiomatous tissue lined by endothelial cells in the early stage of the lesion. There is nonmalignant proliferation of thin-walled vessels in capillary in the involved bones that may also show a sinusoidal or cavernous pattern. The vessels may be empty or contain proteinaceous fluid and/or blood cellular elements. In late stages, the bone is progressively dissolved completely producing massive osteolysis, and ultimately the osseous tissue is fully replaced by fibrous tissue. The histologic changes are similar to benign hemangioma or venous malformation of bone, but there is much more extensive bone destruction with massive osteoclastic activity.

Differential Diagnosis

Infection, inflammatory bone disease, primary malignancy, MBD, angiosarcoma, Langerhans cell histiocytosis, and mastocytosis. Skeletal osteolytic syndromes such as Acro-osteolysis of Hajdu and Cheney, Acro-osteolysis of Joseph, Acro-osteolysis of Shinz, Idiopathic multicentric osteolysis (carpal-tarsal osteolysis), multicentric osteolysis with nephropathy, Farber's disease, osteolysis with detritic synovitis, Winchester's syndrome, hereditary multicentric osteolysis, and neurogenic osteolysis.

Treatment

Some cases, especially those without significant involvement of chest or abdominal cavities, stabilize spontaneously, although return of the "vanished" bone does not occur. The medical treatment for Gorham's disease includes often a combination of radiation therapy, antiosteoclastic medication (bisphosphonates), and alpha-2b interferon. Combination with thalidomide or lenalidomide may help in regression of the lesions. Surgical options include resection of the lesion, and reconstruction using bone grafts and/or prostheses. Local resection and bone grafting, with or without internal fixation, have not been consistently successful, however. Wide resection and limb salvage, with or without prosthetic reconstruction is more appropriate for a good outcome. Amputation may be needed in some cases for a satisfactory wide margin. Definitive radiation therapy in moderate doses (40–45 Gy in 2 Gy fractions) gives good clinical outcome with few long-term complications only. Chylothorax needs to be managed aggressively in these patients of Gorham's disease on priority to save life and minimize future mortality or morbidity. These methods include surgical measures such as pleurectomy and thoracic duct ligation; pleurodesis can be achieved by bleomycin. Ancillary measures include using radiation therapy and oral clodronate.

Epithelioid (Histiocytoid) Hemangioendothelioma and Angiosarcoma

(ICD-O code 9120/3, Hemangiosarcoma, and Epithelioid Angiosarcoma)

These are neoplastic disease of bone that shows *endothelial* differentiation. The tumors show a variable extent of vasoformative features ranging from vacuolization of cells to development of well-formed vascular channels. Hemangioendothelioma and angiosarcoma represent the low-grade and high-grade lesions of the same pathology, respectively.

- Grade 1 hemangioendotheliomas demonstrate well-formed vascular channels. The cells show little or no atypia.
- Grade 2 lesions are more aggressive histopathologically and comprise cuboidal cells with obvious atypia. The vascular channel formation, however, is still evident.
- Grade 3 lesions demonstrate much higher atypical cells than seen in grade 3 lesions but the vascular spaces are much less conspicuous.
- Grade 4 lesions have features similar to poorly differentiated angiosarcomas.

There can be associated soft tissue neoplasms, prominently the pulmonary lesions otherwise now known as the intravascular bronchoalveolar cell tumor. These lesions were previously considered to be pulmonary "metastases" but are now thought to represent the multifocal nature of disease primarily. The tumors are equally divided from 2nd to 8th decade but epithelioid hemangioendothelioma occurs during 2nd and 3rd decades with equal sex predilection. Angiosarcomas are known to occur at previously irradiated sites otherwise etiology is largely unknown.

Clinical Features

These are painful lesions often associated with swelling. Sometimes patients present with a pathologic fracture. The sites commonly affected are the skull and the axial skeleton; in the appendicular skeleton, lower extremity is the most frequently affected.

Radiological Features

The lesions are radiographically purely lytic in appearance and poorly marginated that may have sclerotic borders (low-grade lesions). A soap-bubble appearance and deforming expansile bone appearance is common. The lesions may extend into the soft tissues producing local swellings.

Histopathology

The tumors are bloody and firm (low-grade lesions) to soft (high-grade lesions) in consistency appearing red in cut sections. Both tumors are aggressive and breach the cortex extending into the nearby soft tissue. The neoplastic cells have a vascular space forming prominent histological feature but depending on grade of differentiation some tumors may be difficult to identify as vascular lesions as in poorly-differentiated angiosarcoma. The neoplastic cells have ample cytoplasm that is either amphophilic or faintly eosinophilic. Intracytoplasmic vacuoles are seen in some cells that may occasionally have entrapped erythrocytes. Mitotic figures are not very significant but up to 1–2 mitotic figures per 10 high-power fields may be seen. Eosinophilic inflammatory infiltrate is usually present. Angiosarcomas typically have areas of well-formed anastomosing vascular channels. These channels are lined by atypical endothelial cells containing large hyperchromatic nuclei. The tumor shows reactive osteoid formation in the periphery commonly. Along with the presence of plump osteoblasts, this feature may confuse an otherwise amateur observer with osteoblastoma. The best differentiating feature is, however, the presence of obvious vasoformative cells that should help to establish correct diagnosis. The other differentiating features are positive immunohistochemical staining for vascular markers such as von Willebrand factor (VIII-related antigen), Ulex europaeus lectins, CD31, and CD34 in the tumor cells.

Differential Diagnosis

Metastatic renal cell carcinoma, skeletal adamantinoma, and angiosarcoma.

Management

Surgical resection and reconstruction is the preferred surgical method. The histological degree of differentiation is the most significant factor in the prognosis. Multifocal tumors ironically show a survival advantage possibly related to better differentiation in multifocal tumors.

Hemangiopericytoma

Hemangiopericytoma is a rare low-grade malignant tumor consisting of pericyte-like cells and a prominent vascular pattern. The age distribution is wide and cases have been reported in nearly all age groups. Patients usually present with pain and rarely an association with paraneoplastic syndrome of hypophosphatemic osteomalacia could be found. Commonly pelvis, femur, vertebrae, and mandible are involved but less often tumor has also been reported from clavicle, humerus, scapula, and fibula.

Radiographically, most lesions are predominantly lytic but a trabecular honeycomb pattern similar to hemangioma is also common. The margins of these lesions are usually indistinct.

Histopathology

Grossly, the lesions are generally solid gray or tan. Microscopically, several thin-walled vessels with pericyte-like round or spindle cells are observed. A characteristic "deer-antler"-like branching pattern of vessels is seen typically highlighted by reticulin or von Willebrand antigen stains. Poorly differentiated forms may have areas of cells arranged in ill-defined bundles with mild-to-moderate atypia.

Differential Diagnosis

Mesenchymal chondrosarcomas, MFHs, and small cell osteosarcomas.

Management

Wide resection of tumor and skeletal/prosthetic reconstruction is the treatment of choice **(Figs. 86A to F)**. The role of chemo-radiotherapy is not established.

Glomus Tumor

Glomus tumor of bone is a rare benign but painful highly vascular lesion comprising small uniform specialized smooth muscle cells that resemble the glomus body. They are common in the distal phalanx of digits but may occasionally be seen in the ulna, coccyx, and few other bones. There is slight female predominance and patients have extreme pain.

Histopathologically, the vascular component may either comprise indistinct capillary network or otherwise large blood vessels which in this case are referred to as glomangiomas.

Management

Though marginal excision is commonly done but even intralesional excision is also adequate.

METASTATIC DISEASE OF BONE

The skeleton is third most common site of metastatic disease following lungs (caval circulation) and liver (portal circulation). Overall >50% of patients with any cancer are likely to develop bone metastasis. Breast lung and prostate cancers account for nearly 80% of bone metastasis.

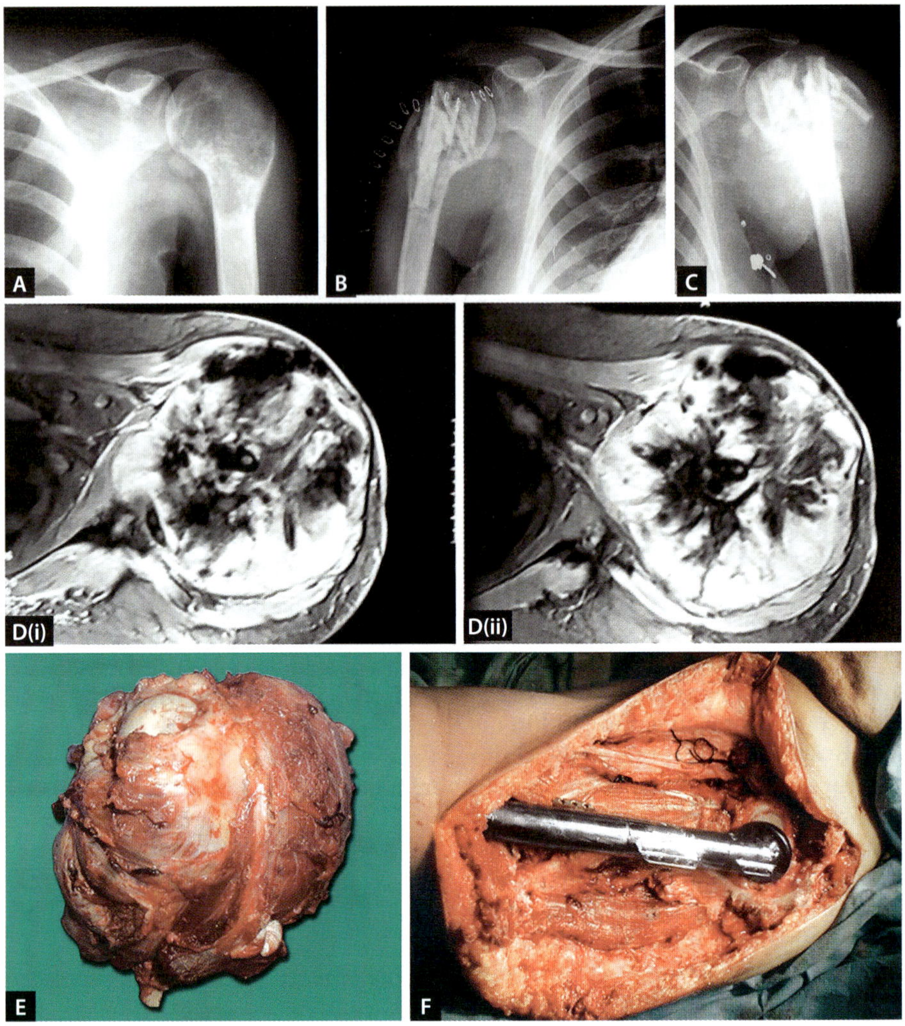

Figs. 86A to F: (A and B) Hemangiopericytoma of proximal humerus treated initially as an ABC that (C) quickly progressed and presented as an angry swelling; [D(i) and (ii)] MRI revealed an aggressive pathology with extensive soft tissue infiltration that was treated with (E) wide excision, and (F) custom prosthesis reconstruction.

Incidence and Site Distribution

Tumors that metastasize commonly to bone are the prostate, breast, and kidney, followed by lung and thyroid other diseases being MM and lymphoma. Bone metastases are seen in over two-thirds of patients with breast (70–75%) and prostate (65–68%) carcinomas (due to protracted nature of these malignancies and higher incidence) and over one-third (28–34%) of patients with renal cell, thyroid, and lung carcinomas. The most common location for bone metastasis is the spine (thoracic spine in particular), followed by the ribs, pelvis, and proximal long bones. Metastasis to spine usually spares the intervertebral disk (as opposed to infection). Most common site for appendicular metastasis is femur bone followed by humerus and then tibia. Metastatic bone lesions noted distal to the elbow or knees are called "acral metastases".

Biology of Bone Metastasis and Routes of Spread

Most of the metastasis are multiple to begin with. The term "solitary metastasis" may be removed in near future as a single metastatic region is extremely rare and possibly does not exist. Primary tumors (lung, breast, prostate, etc.) drive the metastatic process at an early stage itself by stimulating the bone marrow stromal cells to prepare premetastatic niche. This creates favorable microenvironment ("soil") for metastatic cells to settle and grow.

Hematogenous route is the most common mode of spread and is usually arterial seeding but Batson's venous plexus is likely responsible for spread of prostate cancer cells to pelvis and spine. The hematogenous spread is explained by the propensity of malignant tumors toward angiogenesis. This not only helps survival of the primary but also the tumor cells "leak" to distant places and home in the secondary organs. The leak is mediated by cathepsin-K and matrix metalloproteinase enzymes. Meanwhile the epithelial tumor cells often undergo "epithelial-to-mesenchymal phase-transition" that involves morphological and functional remodeling. The tumor cells lose epithelial markers (E-cadherin and cytokeratins) while acquiring mesenchymal-shape and markers like N-cadherin, fibronectin, and vimentin. Such transformed cells serve as potent germinating "seeds" of primary malignancies that can be dispersed as above. These tumor cells then "home" the target organs (like bone) if microenvironment is favorable. Similar "seed and soil theory" was suggested by Paget in 1889 but molecular explanation was obviously missing that time. The bone-homing cells overexpress chemokine receptors like C-X-C motif chemokine-receptor-4 (CXCR-4) whose ligand C-X-C motif chemokine-ligand-12 (CXCL-12) is secreted by stromal. Over a period of time, the tumor cells may acquire osteoblast/osteoclast markers (osteomimicry) evading immune response. The metaphyseal bone (trabecular bone) is the preferred site for bone metastases for the following reasons:

- Increase bone turnover and metabolic activity (hence ample local growth factors)
- Sluggish sinusoidal vascular supply gives the tumor cells ample time and opportunity to move in and home the marrow.
- Focal imbalance at remodeling site
- Uncoupling of bone resorption and bone formation with age (age-related bone cell and metabolic change)

The endothelial cells that line the sinusoidal spaces in metaphyseal region of bone express multiple adhesion molecules which enhance adhesion and extravasation of neoplastic cells into marrow allowing homing. Some of these adhesion molecules of the many identified include intercellular adhesion molecule 1 (ICAM-1), P-selectin, E-selectin, and vascular cell adhesion molecule 1 (VCAM-1). After proper homing supportive bone environment comprising bone-stored IGF-1, transforming growth factor beta (TGF-β), calcium, phosphate, stromal cells, and transient cells (apart from the plethora of growth factors and substrates present in bone—see section on bone biology) provide a supportive milieu for growth of the neoplastic cells. The stromal cells are an important party to this and arise from marrow mesenchymal cells forming adipocytes, fibroblasts, and osteoblasts. They express VCAM-1, syndecan-1, N-cadherin (in contrast to E-cadherin N-cadherin actually stimulate tumor growth) and matrix metalloproteinase-2 (MMP-2) to support the differentiation and proliferation of cancer cells. Transient cells are marrow erythrocytes, T cells and platelets which aid tumor growth and metastases through various pathways.

Metastases produce either osteoblastic or osteolytic or mixed lesions in bone. Osteolytic lesions of breast metastasis are mediated via parathyroid hormone-related protein (PTHrP) that reduces osteoprotegerin (OPG) and increased production of RANKL from osteoblasts. This activates the osteoclast precursors and osteoclasts along with release of bone-stored IGF-1 and TGF-β. IGF-1 promotes breast cancer cell growth and TGF-β promotes the production of PTHrP turning the vicious cycle on. The subsequent osteoblastic activity is blunted, absent, or distorted. The breast cancer cells produce IL-6, IL-11, and prostaglandin E2 and TNF-β that suppress osteoblast while activating the osteoclasts simultaneously producing the lytic lesions. The osteoblastic prostate metastatic lesions are primarily mediated by the tumor-derived peptide ET-1. This stimulates osteoblast cell proliferation via the endothelin-A receptor (ETAR), leading to pathological bone formation. Osteoblastic activity here results in excessive new but disorganized bone formation. ET-1 also suppresses the negative regulator of the Wnt signaling pathway, dickkopfs (DKK1) (*see* Chapter on "Metabolic Diseases of Bone"); hence, supporting the osteoblastic activity. It is notable that like osteolytic breast metastasis high concentrations of PTHrP are also found in prostatic metastasis. Here, their role shifts to osteoblastic activity given the fact that NH2-terminal fragments of PTHrP when activated via the ETAR pathway support osteoblastic potential.

Clinical Presentation and Problem Statement

Prognosis of skeletal metastatic disease substantially depends on the site of primary tumor **(Table 21)**. The reported median survival from diagnosis of bone metastasis varies from 6 months (lung cancer and malignant melanoma) to 12–53 months (prostate cancer). For metastatic breast cancer it is 19–48 months. Survival times following a diagnosis of bone metastases have increased substantially (in 1970s the average survival following recognition of bone metastases was 7 months increasing to 2 years in 1990) placing these patients at higher risk of developing metastatic bone disease (MBD). MBD encompasses symptomatic-skeletal-events (events inducing an exacerbation of cancer related pain) and complications of MBD [termed "skeletal-related events" (SREs)]. The SREs include severe uncontrolled pain, hypercalcemia, limited mobility, pathological fractures, spinal cord compression, and bone marrow infiltration (seen commonly with myeloma and small cell carcinoma of lung) and often are a result of bone resorption **(Flowchart 3)**. Current management is aimed at reducing these SREs (utilizing both locoregional and systematic approaches) but due to inadequate awareness among the medical fraternity less than half of deserving patient only get appropriate treatment. Sharp pain often intermittent that becomes worse at night is experienced by 80% of patients.

TABLE 21: Characteristics of various primary malignancies metastasizing to bones.

Primary tumor	*Radiological characteristic*	*5-year survival*	*Sensitivity to irradiation*
Breast	Lytic/sclerotic	24%	Highly sensitive
Prostate	Blastic/lytic	15%	Highly sensitive
Lung	Lytic	4%	Intermediate
Thyroid	Lytic	54%	Intermediate
Renal	Lytic	12%	Low

Flowchart 3: Pathogenesis of skeletal-related events.

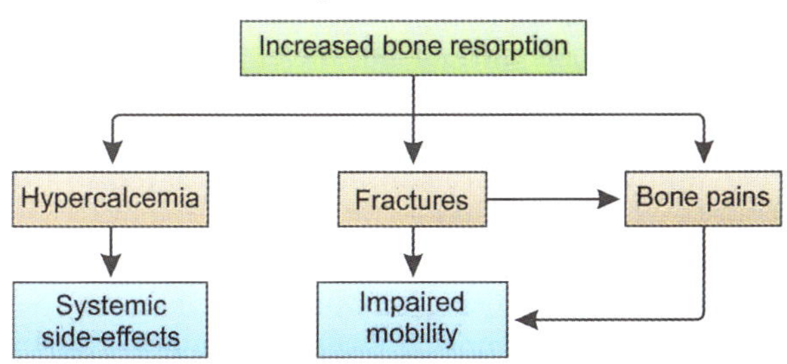

It is expected that around 45% of these patients will experience at least one SRE and in patients who do experience a SRE the survival is low (approximately 4 months). The SREs are often clustered so that a patient undergoing one SRE is more likely than others to undergo another shortly. It has been observed that the outcome for these patients is poor due to:

- Failure to intervene prophylactically and timely in needy patients mainly caused by late referral
- Unavailability of dedicated units/centers for management of patients with skeletal metastasis so that patients usually keep swinging between oncologist and orthopedic surgeon.
- Ignorance about the advanced options available where the patient is deprived of options.
- Poor understanding of the biomechanical basis of orthopedic implants, leading to inappropriate surgery and high-failure rates.

Clinical Evaluation

The patient with a metastatic disease usually presents in one of the following ways:

- Pathological fracture or neurological compromise (spine lesions may even have cauda equina syndrome)
- Referral from oncologist/surgeon/radiologist
- Referral for unexplained generalized musculoskeletal pain.

Pain is the most frequent but most variegated clinical symptom that may range from an intermittent dull ache to deep intense pain. Pain usually gets exacerbated by weight-bearing and is often worse at night or at rest. Pain is usually partially improved with activity unless associated with pathological fracture. The pain is progressive and unrelenting usually nonresponsive to symptomatic treatment. Progressive unrelenting pain usually indicates invasion of adjacent tissues or pathological fracture. There is associated loss of appetite, weight loss, and fatigue with loss of interest in usual activities. The pain is probably due to release of chemical mediators like substance-P, prostaglandins, growth factors, bradykinin, and histamine and stimulation of free nerve endings of bone at mechanically weakened sites.

Hypercalcemia is seen in some 10% of patients with metastatic disease commonly with breast cancer, MM, and squamous lung cancer. Hypercalcemia is mediated by PTHrp from tumor cells.

Bone loss is multifactorial and not just related to the primary metastatic lesions. Treatment of primary cancer also is associated with bone loss. Aromatase inhibitors (used for breast and ovarian cancers), oophorectomy (for ovarian cancers and breast cancer) and orchiectomy (for prostate cancer) and use of GnRH analogs produce hypogonadism leading to bone loss. Use of corticosteroids and radiation therapy has direct effect on bone strength. These contribute to development of pathological fractures in metastatic bone disease.

The following history should be elucidated in these patients as part of evaluation:

- Use of or change in assistive devices for ambulation—loss of ambulatory ability is a poor prognostic factor
- Personal history—smoking, alcohol, and other drug abuse
- Professional history—exposure to asbestos/aerosols
- Details of noticing any shortness of breath, chest pain, pleuritic pain, hemoptysis (pulmonary), hematemesis (esophageal/gastric), gastritis, alteration in urinary (increased frequency or pain) or bowel habits (alternating constipation/diarrhea), rectal bleeding, blood in urine or at end of micturition, and heat or cold intolerance (thyroid neoplasm). Changes or appearance of soft tissue swelling(s) and changes in appearance of skin spots (melanoma) should also be inquired.
- Enquire about the documentation of screening tests—Pap smear, mammogram, prostate examination, colonoscopy, etc.
- Past history of cancer or related treatment (radiotherapy/chemotherapy)
- Family history of cancer

Physical Examination

Accurate note of tender spots, bones, joints, and swellings should be made. Spine tenderness, ROM of involved joints and spine, and deformity should be noted. Presence of limp, sensory—motor deficit should be recorded. Additionally per abdomen, per rectal examination, and examination of breast and thyroid should be thoroughly done for evaluation of any clinically identifiable primary. One should evaluate costovertebral angle (renal lesion) and examine the lymph node chains for localization or lymphoma.

Investigations

A general panel of investigations for patients with metastatic disease is initially prescribed as detailed in **Box 7**. This battery of tests identifies primary in 85% of cases. Specific investigations are additionally done based on the suspicion of pathology.

Laboratory Investigations

For suspected myeloma, urine (Bence-Jones protein), and serum electrophoresis with immunofixation should be done. Beta-2-microglobulin levels should be measured for staging. Based on clinical suspicion, specific blood tests or markers can be done that include CA-19.9 (pancreatic cancer), calcitonin (medullary thyroid carcinoma), CA-15.3/CA-27.29 (breast

BOX 7: The battery of investigations used to identify primary and initially stage the disease.

Blood investigations:
- Complete blood count (CBC)
- Erythrocyte sedimentation rate (ESR)
- C-reactive protein (CRP quantitative may be better)
- Metabolic panel including liver and renal functional tests, electrolytes, and serum calcium with alkaline phosphatase (ALP)
- Urinalysis
- Prostate specific antigen (PSA)
- Carcinoembryonic antigen (CEA)
- Serum protein electrophoresis

Radiographic studies:
- Plain radiograph of the whole bone involved by the lesion
- CT scan of the chest, abdomen, and pelvis with contrast
- Whole body bone scan

cancer), and cancer antigen-125 (ovarian tumor). Urinary N-telopeptide of type I collagen (urinary NTX) correlates with occurrence of SREs and are being increasingly under focus.

Imaging and Radiological Workup

The diagnostic utility of various modalities is summarized in **Table 22**. Completion of staging is done with identification of the primary. Biopsy of the lesion is done at the end of staging. This is important to say if a sarcoma is found then an inappropriate biopsy may preclude limb salvage, likewise if a renal cell carcinoma is found then preoperative embolization is preferred. Biopsy may additionally find 10% of the primary pathology but has poor diagnostic performance if done in isolation. There is a great deal of confusion on evaluation of treatment response—while most physicians utilize sophisticated investigations for evaluation of bone metastasis; the criteria have not till recently included these in treatment evaluation **(*see* Tables 6 and 7)**. The diagnostic algorithm commonly practiced for evaluation is presented in **Flowchart 4**. Detailed radiological workup is discussed below.

Plain X-rays reveal a solitary or multiple, localized or diffuse, small or large usually lytic lesion(s). Skeletal survey had been ordered as a preliminary investigation that includes radiographs of pelvis, long bones, chest, skull, and spine (dorsolumbar region). The lytic lesions are common with metastasis from lung, kidney, thyroid and colonic malignancies and MM, and lymphomas are also osteolytic. Lytic lesions are identified on X-ray with 25–50% loss of bone mineral at the site, hence radiographs are quite insensitive

TABLE 22: Utility of various diagnostic modalities for evaluation of bone metastasis.

Investigation modality	***Pros***	***Cons***	***Utility***
Scintigraphy	• Evaluates whole body • Good sensitivity (62–100%), specificity (80%)	• No anatomic detail • Low specificity • May be negative in purely lytic lesions	Good screening modality
Radiographs	• Bone and lesion anatomic detail • Low cost	• Low sensitivity • Locoregional use	Diagnostic
CT	• Good sensitivity (71–100%), specificity (95%) • Bone and tumor anatomic detail	Locoregional imaging	Diagnostic
MRI	High sensitivity (82–100%), specificity (95%)	• Locoregional imaging • High cost	Diagnostic
PET-CT/MRI	High sensitivity (85–95%), specificity (97%), and evaluation/identification of possible primary	• High cost • Limited availability	Diagnostic

Flowchart 4: Algorithm for diagnostic evaluation of bone metastasis. The box of scintigraphy scanning is painted red because this investigation can be replaced by FDG-PET-CT/MRI if facilities are available and feasible. The PET scans have several advantages over scintigraphy (see text).

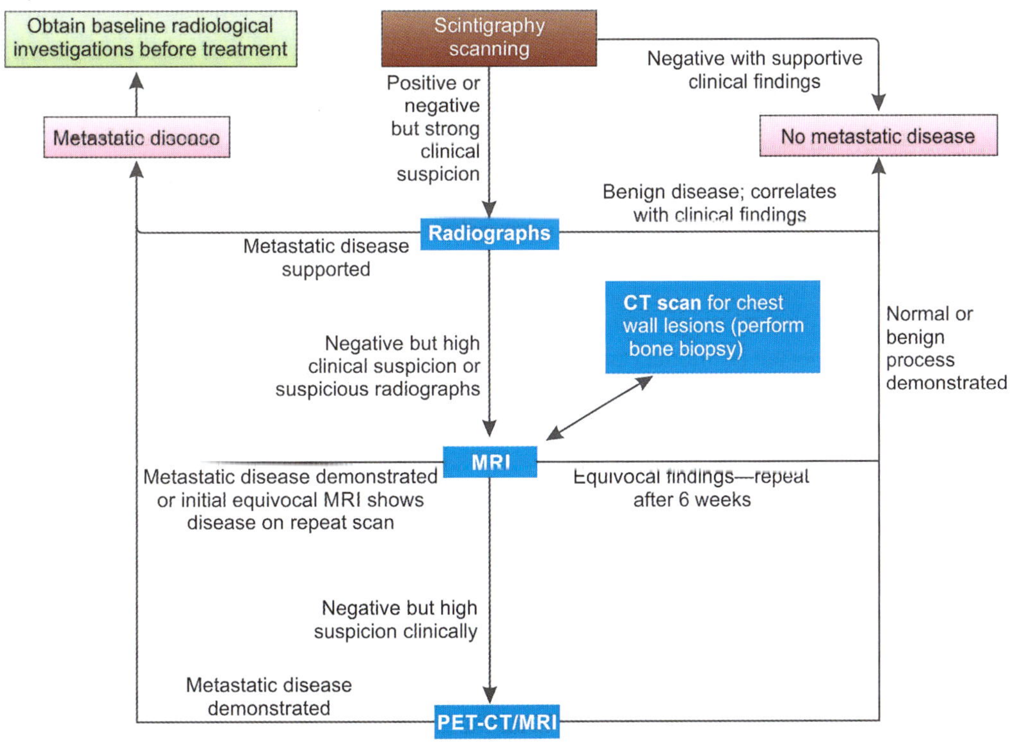

(FDG-PET-CT/MRI: ^{18}F-fluorodeoxyglucose/positron emission tomography/computed tomography/magnetic resonance imaging)

and probably the stage for pathological fracture is already set by then. Pulmonary metastasis may be located to cortical regions of bone. Osteoblastic lesions are seen with prostate and breast malignancy metastasis, but lytic lesions are seen with advanced prostate lesions and mixed appearance is common with breast malignancies.

Technetium Tc-99 bone scan identifies the bone lesion(s) avidly and is quite sensitive. Additionally, it has the advantage of scanning all the skeletal sites at reasonable cost. It can also be used as a guide to identify "easier" site for bone biopsy. It is recommended as the initial modality for investigating bone metastasis. The lesions appear hot on scan unless the metastasis is from pure osteolytic aggressive lesion that has minimal or no osteoblastic activity (few renal cell carcinoma and multiple myeloma). FDG-PET may be used to identify such bone scan negative lesions. Positive scan is defined by:

- Multiple focal typically distributed lesions (random distribution)—obtain radiographs definitely for future assessment of treatment response and SREs.
- Multiple atypical lesions (differential diagnoses—trauma, arthritis, and inflammatory arthropathy)
- Solitary typical lesion (differential diagnoses—osteomyelitis) or small number of typically distributed lesions [differential diagnoses—SAPHO (synovitis, acne, pustulosis, hyperostosis, and osteitis)]
- Diffuse involvement (differential diagnoses—osteoporosis, Cushing's disease, and osteomalacia)
- Photon-deficient lesions

SPECT (single-photon emission computed tomography) has improved sensitivity over conventional bone scan for small metastasis but widespread use of MRI has superseded its use.

CT scan is recommended to evaluate the structural integrity of skeleton.

MRI is highly sensitive to detect small skeletal metastases not detected on bone scans as it reveals abnormal bone marrow. Typical diagnostic feature of a metastatic lesion on MRI is a focal low-signal intensity on a T1-weighted image and a mix-to-high intensity on a fat-suppressed T1-weighted image and high intensity on a T2-weighted image due to marrow edema (high water content). A preliminary ultrasound of abdomen and pelvis followed by contrast-enhanced CT abdomen and pelvis is ordered for unidentified primary. High-resolution CT of chest can be obtained for suspected pulmonary primary.

^{18}Fluorodeoxyglucose-positron emission tomography (FDG-PET): Now FDG-PET is commonly recommended as an initial investigation for identification of primary; and has the additional advantage of mapping the extent of disease and monitoring treatment response. In contrast to bone scintigraphy that detects activity of bone (increased bone formation), FDG-PET detects metabolically active "lesions" in bone so it can detect metastasis that still has not produced structural bony destruction or reactive bone formation. Its use is increasing for initial staging and follow-up of patients typically for lung, breast, and head and neck cancers. The FDG-PET can additionally demonstrate nonskeletal site of tumor metastasis that improves understanding the disease and guide to management. The sensitivity of FDG-PET varies according to the type of metastasis, and for this reason, the sensitivity is higher for osteolytic lesions (multiple myeloma) but less for osteoblastic lesions (prostate) when compared to bone scan. PET using sodium fluoride (NaF-18) is more sensitive than bone scan for osteolytic lesions, but there is higher radiation risk and associated cost. FDG-PET-MRI is still more sensitive as it has been found to additionally detect lesions in 15–20% of cases missed by PET-CT.

The above strategy holds good for evaluation of both solitary or multiple metastasis.

In patients with known history of cancer and a solitary destructive lesion biopsy of the lesion should be done to confirm the metastasis from previous cancer. If there is discrepancy then standard radiological workup is required as above. If there is correlation then the investigations necessary for staging of the tumor are required.

In a patient with multiple visceral and skeletal metastases along with history of cancer one can go ahead with surgery without biopsy confirmation unless the appearance of tumor strongly points to primary bone sarcoma needing confirmation.

Bone Biopsy

As explained previously (see imaging and radiological workup) biopsy from lesion is the last step of metastasis evaluation and may additionally help in identifying 10% of the primary pathologies. Biopsy is performed to confirm the suspicion of primary or to know about the primary lesion itself. FNAC (usually image guided) is the preferred modality in dedicated centers else core biopsy (preferred) or even open biopsy can be done. Principles of bone tumor biopsy should be followed (see above in general principles of bone tumors) but most importantly, it should be done at a center (or at least guided by it) that is going to manage the patient finally. Site errors of biopsy have caused patients to lose their limb in past. Most of the spinal lesions require image guidance in the form of ultrasound or better a CT scan. For a blastic lesion, multiple samples should be obtained to increase yield of biopsy for representative tissue. The tissue should be processed by experienced pathologist and immunohistochemical stains play a predominant role in identification of the tissue.

Differential Diagnosis

Multiple Bony Lesions

- Myeloma
- Osteomyelitis
- Paget's disease and associated sarcoma
- Postirradiation sarcoma
- Chondrosarcoma
- Malignant lymphoma
- Malignant fibrous histiocytoma

Solitary Bone Lesion

- Metastatic carcinoma
- Myeloma
- Infection
- Primary sarcoma/plasmacytoma
- Lymphoma

Management of Bone Metastasis (Flowchart 5)

Bone metastasis is a systemic disease. Currently, the standard of care for skeletal metastasis is a combined multimodality approach that includes pain management, systemic therapy (bone modifying agents, chemotherapy, and hormone therapy), radiation therapy and radiopharmaceuticals, and surgery depending on patient factors (fragility and prognosis of tumor), tumor factors (aggressive lesion vs. moderate, extensive vs. limited disease, sensitivity to chemotherapeutic agents, etc.), site factors (single vs. multiple lesion, location of lesion in skeleton—periarticular, diaphyseal, metaphyseal, etc.). If the patient's life expectancy is longer than the recovery phase for a procedure, intervention will likely improve the remaining quality of life. Recently image-guided percutaneous cryoablation, radiofrequency ablation, focused ultrasound (MRI-guided high-intensity focused ultrasound), and cementoplasty have been variably used and recommended for isolated or limited metastasis. Some of these claim immediate and lasting pain relief but large trials are required for definite indications and recommendations. In all, early and aggressive management yields better quality of life and functional independence.

The Need of the Orthopedic Surgery

The common needs of surgical intervention include:
- Maximize pain control and tumor control locally
- Prophylactic fixation of bones with a risk of pathological fracture due to metastasis
- Stabilization of pathological fracture
- Reconstruction of periarticular metastasis
- Management of spinal instability and neurological symptoms due to cord/nerve compression

The primary *aim of surgical intervention* is to relieve pain and restore function of the limb. The *orthopedic principles* followed for management of pathological fractures occurring in MBD include:
- Providing immediate stability, allowing weight bearing and regaining function. The current standard is to stabilize the entire bone to avoid the need for further surgical intervention.
- Treatment is done assuming that the fracture may not unite.
- The fixation should aim to last the lifetime of the patient.
- To stabilize all the affected parts of bone and all "necessary" bones (as required to achieve above aim).

Fracture Risk Assessment

Plain radiographs are neither sensitive nor reliable to measure cortical destruction and loss of bone strength due to lack of three-dimensional evaluation. Fidler (1973) suggested that a long bone lesion with >50% cortical destruction should be prophylactically stabilized. Harrington (1982) recommended prophylactic surgery to femur if there is:
- Destruction of 50% of a single cortex of any long bone (in any radiological view)
- Avulsion of the lesser trochanter

Flowchart 5: Management algorithm for metastatic disease to appendicular skeleton.

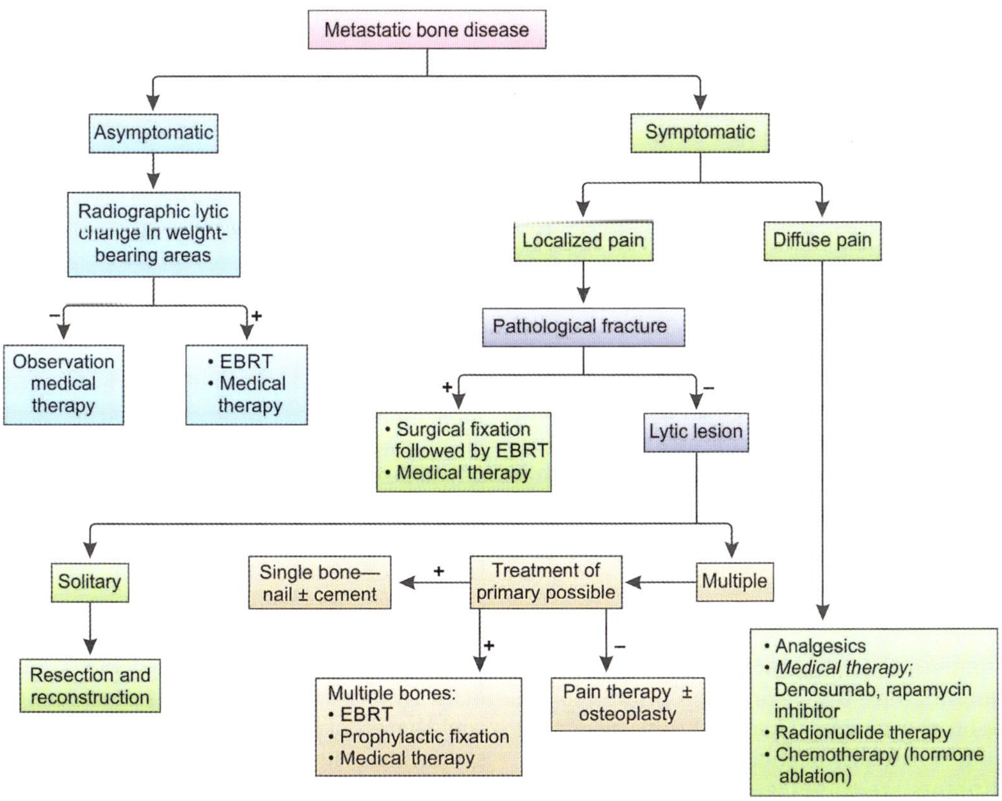

(EBRT: external beam radiation therapy)

TABLE 23: Mirels' scoring system for metastatic bone disease.

Variable	Score 1	Score 2	Score 3
Site	Upper limb	Lower limb	Peritrochanter
Pain	Mild	Moderate	Functional
Lesion	Blastic	Mixed	Lytic
Size*	<1/3 diameter	1/3 to 2/3 diameter	>2/3 diameter

*As seen on plain X-ray, maximum destruction of cortex in any view.
Note: Maximum possible score is 12. If lesion scores 8 or above, then prophylactic fixation is recommended *prior* to radiotherapy.

- Lesion in proximal femur that is ≥2.5 cm in any dimension
- Pain with weight bearing that persists, increases, or recurs following radiotherapy.

Weakened bone produces an "open section" defect where stress gets concentrated and fracture occurs with minor trauma/twisting movement. These fractures are low-energy and soft tissue injury is minor compared conventional traumatic fractures of normal bones. Mirels (1989) devised a scoring system **(Table 23)** that provides a more reliable and reproducible measure of the risk of pathological fracture. Mirel's score of 8 or above indicates high risk for fracture and prophylactic fixation is indicated prior to radiotherapy. Mirel's system has been found to overestimate the need for surgery. CT-based structural rigidity analysis is proposed by musculoskeletal tumor society (MSTS) and appears to substantially improve the accuracy of predicting pathological femoral fracture, it is imperative but to understand that patients with short life expectancy (<6 weeks) rarely gain useful benefit from surgical procedures; however, it is difficult to predict the remaining life so experience and thorough discussion with family should preside. Precision in estimating survival (using externally validated models) is critical in deciding as to which patients would benefit from surgery. Estimating survival and then choosing appropriate implant prevents too extensive surgery in patients with short survival and high percentage of implant failure in those who live longer. In a nutshell, there are three broad categories of surgical management for metastatic bone disease:

1. Prosthetic reconstruction
2. Local excision with or without reconstruction
3. Osteosynthesis

Capanna and Campanacci suggested an easy algorithm in 2001 for guiding adequate treatment of long bone metastases. The patients are divided into four classes **(Table 24)** and treatment decided on the basis of type and stage of tumor, visceral spread, and risk of pathological fracture **(Flowchart 6)**.

Fractures around the Hip

It is the most common pathological fractures that need surgical attention in patients with MBD. For lesion limited to the femoral neck or head, a cemented hemiarthroplasty or total joint replacement is modality of choice for reconstruction. Short-stem implants are the biggest mistake surgeons do and long-stem femoral implants are recommended.

TABLE 24: Different classes of patients as suggested by Capanna and Campanacci for management of metastatic long bone and pelvic disease.

Class	Long bones	Pelvis
1	• Solitary metastatic lesion • Primary with good prognosis (well-differentiated thyroid, prostate, breast sensitive to adjuvants, rectum, clear-cell renal, lymphoma, and myeloma) • Interval over 3 years since detection of the primary	
2	Pathological fracture at any site	Pathological fracture in periacetabular region
3	Impending fracture in a major weight-bearing bone	Supra-acetabular osteolytic lesion
4	• Multiple osteoblastic lesions at all sites • Osteolytic or mixed lesions in nonstructural bone • Osteolytic lesion with no impending fracture in major weight-bearing bone	• Multiple osteoblastic lesions at all sites • Osteolytic or mixed lesions in iliac wing and anterior pelvis • Small periacetabular osteolytic lesions

Flowchart 6: The suggested indications for surgery and conservative treatment by Capanna and Campanacci based on patient classes.

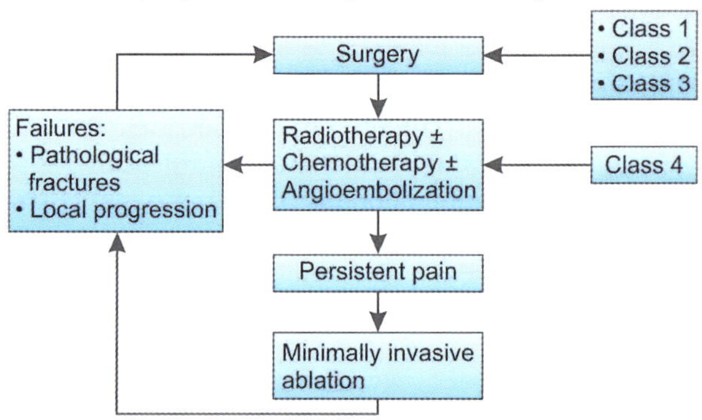

Subtrochanteric fractures or lesions with limited bone loss are best stabilized by "reconstruction" nails or proximal femoral nails that have locking screws up the femoral neck. This also protects neck from the risk of subsequent femoral neck fracture.

Pelvi-acetabular Disease

This region is difficult to approach surgically and prophylactic palliative radiotherapy is commonly used to control symptoms. Angioembolization can provide good devascularization of the lesions and can also be combined with antimitotic agents (adriamycin and platins) to provide prolonged remission and pain relief. Enneking zones 1 and 3 **(Fig. 87)** are nonweight bearing expendable regions that can be excised in toto. Zone 2 lesions may be treated by cementoplasty for constrained, relatively small, lytic usually supra-acetabular lesions that are sites of impending fracture (class 3 patients). Periacetabular lesions have tendency for central migration of the femoral head due to soft acetabular floor. Such lesions could be reconstructed with massive (composite) allograft and special implants with antiprotrusio reconstruction cage, multi hole cups, threaded rods, pins, elastic nails (cut and shaped into the defect), reinforcement rings or saddle prosthesis

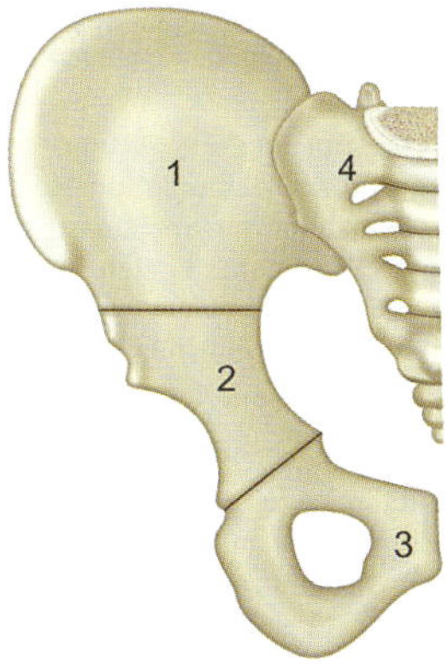

Fig. 87: The Enneking classification of different zones of pelvis as applied to guide treatment.

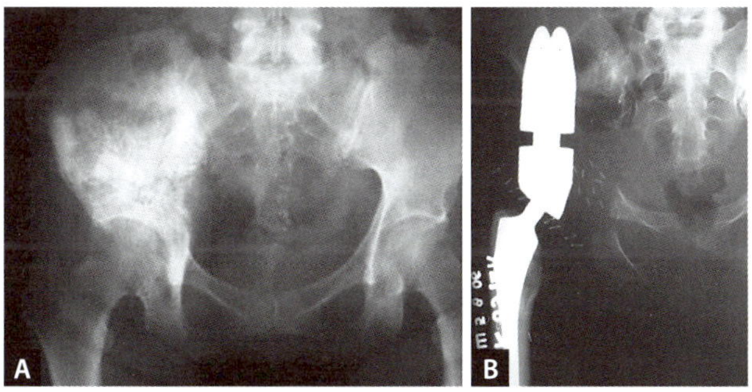

Figs. 88A and B: Metastasis to pelvis. The patient was treated with resection of the metastasis and reconstruction with Saddle prosthesis.

(Figs. 88A and B). Bone cement is often used to augment the construction strength (Harrington technique). For lesions requiring resection of both zones 2 and 3, an inverted ice-cream cone prosthesis or pedestal cup is docked to the remaining intact pelvic bone. In extreme cases, the implant may be inserted in the sacrum. Extensive radiotherapy to this region has high chances of radiation osteonecrosis of the femoral head and subsequent pain.

Shoulder Girdle and Upper Limb

Metastatic lesions of shoulder girdle usually managed with radiotherapy alone. Humeral head lesions are best treated by hemiarthroplasty. Limited glenoid involvement can be managed with total shoulder or reverse shoulder replacement. For forearm bones (acral metastasis), the lesions are limited in size and stresses are low; it is effectively managed with plate fixation and cement augmentation. Elastic nailing with cement augmentation is another option.

Shafts of Major Long Bones (Humerus, Femur, and Tibia)

Reamed interlocked intramedullary nailing (preferably unreamed for renal metastasis) is the modality of choice for treatment of cortical breach or pathological fractures through metastatic lesions of long bones. This prevents telescoping and locked nail gives torsional stability. It is imperative that following reaming the tumor cells that spread through the medullary canal are "controlled" or "killed" by postoperative radiotherapy. The entire bone and operative site should be included in the postoperative radiotherapy field. The benefits of reaming outwit the intramedullary contamination for a palliative therapy, unlike for a primary bone tumor where reaming could be disaster and nailing may spread the tumor throughout the canal ("rodding" a sarcoma) precluding a potentially limb-salvaging surgery (thus biopsy confirmation is a must). Ideally, load-bearing implants are suited for palliation (for immediate mobilization); but plating provides limited length coverage and bones may get weaker in proximal or distal unprotected region with spread of the disease. Large diameter nails (preferably solid, need customization) are a better option that circumvent these problems and give good stability. Some large bone defects can be packed/reconstructed with stainless steel mesh and bone cement in addition to stabilization with an intramedullary nail. It should be remembered that the chosen implant should take care of all the lesions of the bone and none is left through which a fracture can occur. Isolated lesions in diaphysis that are amenable to resection can be excised and filled with "segmental spacers". For lesions of distal humerus and distal tibia, the surgical treatment has to be customized and often is not easy. Functional cast brace as external support with radiation therapy is the recommendation for such nonreconstructable lesions. For "limited lesions" (isolated lesions at these sites, viz., the elbow, ankle, and possibly the knee) a viable option is curettage, cementation, and internal fixation. Distal and proximal tibial isolated lesions are also managed this way. A further method for managing the distal tibial and distal humeral lesions that encroach articular cartilage is endoprosthetic reconstruction especially if the primary can be controlled (better cured) and patient has good prognosis.

Endoprosthetic Surgery

Developed for primary bone tumors, the use of endoprosthesis is increasingly getting popular for metastatic bone lesions. For metaphyseal lesions that are difficult to reconstruct using conventional methods because of extensive bone destruction, it is possible to provide a functional limb with custom-made or modular endoprosthetic systems (sometimes called "megaprostheses"). This is successfully used for the proximal femur and distal femur, proximal tibia, and proximal or distal humerus. Though uncommon but lesions around ankle are also amenable to this (currently, many think that below-knee amputations and prosthetic fitting provides a good functional outcome and is the standard practice).

They are highly effective in maintaining function having a low failure rate (primarily due to limited patient survival) but cost is a prohibiting factor in the developing nations where health insurance penetration is low. Also, dedicated centers regularly treating such patients are missing. The high success rate for any arthroplasty primarily depends on the volume of treated cases, and hence the expertise developed through experience.

Apart from the above, *adjuvant therapy* is an important aspect of patient management; this is detailed below.

Metastatic Disease to Spine

Spine is the most common site for metastasis to skeleton, especially the thoracic spine. The mode of spread is mixed and depends on the primary; while breast thyroid and renal metastasis usually reach by arterial route prostatic and bladder tumor frequently use Batson's venous plexus. Still tumors spreading from pelvis or retroperitoneum may reach directly to spine. Pain, neurological involvement (motor weakness and sensory blunting), and paresis are the usual presenting symptoms. The pain from spinal metastases is disabling and may need good pain physician management for control. Developing motor weakness or paresis leads to high morbidity and associated dependency with high financial impact.

Evaluation of spinal metastasis usually requires MRI scanning in addition to standard radiographs for its limitations. Other evaluation should proceed as detailed above and described for metastatic disease to bone.

Management

Spinal metastasis is usually extensive and that is the common reason for frequent "conservative" management of the disease. Also extensive surgical decompression or stabilization was logically not supported for a compromised patient. Extensive decompression destabilizes spine and fixation methods were cumbersome and quite conventional. However with changing perspective and advances in cancer therapy, this approach is fast changing. Also the availability of newer pedicle screws and rod systems and cages has improved surgical stabilization. For isolated compression, fractures of vertebra kyphoplasty and vertebroplasty achieve good pain relief. A patient with persistent severe pain or having partial neurological deficit is deemed to have unstable spine amenable for surgical treatment unless extensive imaging suggests structural integrity. Such patients should be kept on spinal beds/ripple mattress (to prevent bed sores); a Philadelphia collar should be given for cervical spine lesions.

Few oncological, neurological, systemic, and mechanical factors should be considered before ultimate management plan is fabricated **(Box 8)**. The most common tumors that involve the spine are breast, lung, renal, prostate, thyroid, melanoma, myeloma, lymphoma, and colorectal cancer. The advancements in chemotherapy, radiotherapy, and hormonal therapy have improved patient survival. Classical surgical decompression without stabilization had put surgical intervention into disfavor and radiotherapy used to be classically relied upon intervention. With greater realization of improved mechanical stability and opportunity to surgically decompress spine using anterior and posterolateral combined approaches, the role of surgery has again been emphasized. Surgery is now the preferred treatment for spinal metastasis although role and indications of various techniques need to be better defined. The most important consideration is maintaining the quality of remaining life of the patient which is already compromised by choosing appropriate "aggressiveness" in surgical intervention. So, it is imperative to avoid complications (especially with complex en bloc resections) and gather the maximum benefits of intervention to improve remaining life. We will try to simplify the surgical planning based on the various evaluation systems available **(Flowchart 7)**. The classification and prognosticating systems vary a lot and are based on institutional experiences. The validation is immature and reliability at best debatable but nevertheless they are a useful guide. Staging is the first step to guide future treatment, however, for planning a surgical intervention functional status, expected life remaining, tumor load, and anatomical extent of tumor need to be primarily defined. The scoring systems (Tomita, Tokuhashi, North, and Harrington) avidly define the mentioned criteria barring the anatomical extent. The revised Tokuhashi system is based on six individual scores for the primary site of cancer, presence or absence of paralysis, Karnofsky's performance status, number of extraspinal bone metastases, vertebral body metastases, and visceral metastases, producing a total score in the range 0–15 **(Table 25)**. For a score of 12–15, excisional surgery is recommended with good prognosis, while palliative surgery is suitable for patients with intermediate score (9–11) and patients with score ≤ 8 should undergo only conservative treatment. We find the Weinstein-Boriani-Biagini staging system initially devised for primary vertebral tumors (an improvement over the McLain and Weinstein and Enneking system) useful guide to anatomically define the extent of spinal metastasis. This system divides the axial plane of the vertebral body into 5 concentric and 12 radiating segments **(Fig. 89)** and defines the axial tumor involvement of spine comprehensively. The Spine Oncology Study Group uses a 6-point scale to describe metastatic spinal tumors as follows:

- *Grade 0* defines tumors confined to bone only without epidural extension.
- *Grade 1* is tumor extension up to epidural space but there is no spinal cord abutment (further divided into three categories depending on deformation of epidural fat or thecal sac).

BOX 8: Factors that are assessed for management of spinal metastasis.

Oncologic factors:
- Histological type and responsiveness of tumor to radiation, chemotherapy, and hormonal manipulation. Hematological, small cell lung cancer, choriocarcinoma, and breast carcinoma are radiosensitive, colon and nonsmall cell lung cancer are moderately resistant, and renal cell and melanoma are radioresistant
- Tumor type—high-grade malignant lesion with rapid and progressive destruction (require early surgery)

Neurological considerations:
- Extent of involvement (limited/extensive)
- Duration of compression
- Exact level and direction of compression (for limited involvement)
- Compression with fracture or isolated compression of cord only
- *Staging of epidural extension:* Weinstein-Boriani-Biagini system and Spine Oncology Study Group

Mechanical factors:
- *Spine is unstable if (Fisher et al.):*
  - Movement related pain
  - Symptomatic or progressive deformity
  - Neurological compromise under physiological loads
- Radiological involvement of bilateral facet joints and pedicles

Systemic considerations and patient factors:
- Biological age
- Systemic tumor burden
- Life expectancy (generally should be >3 months)
- General medical condition
- Motivation and understanding of the patient

Flowchart 7: Management algorithm for metastatic disease to spine.

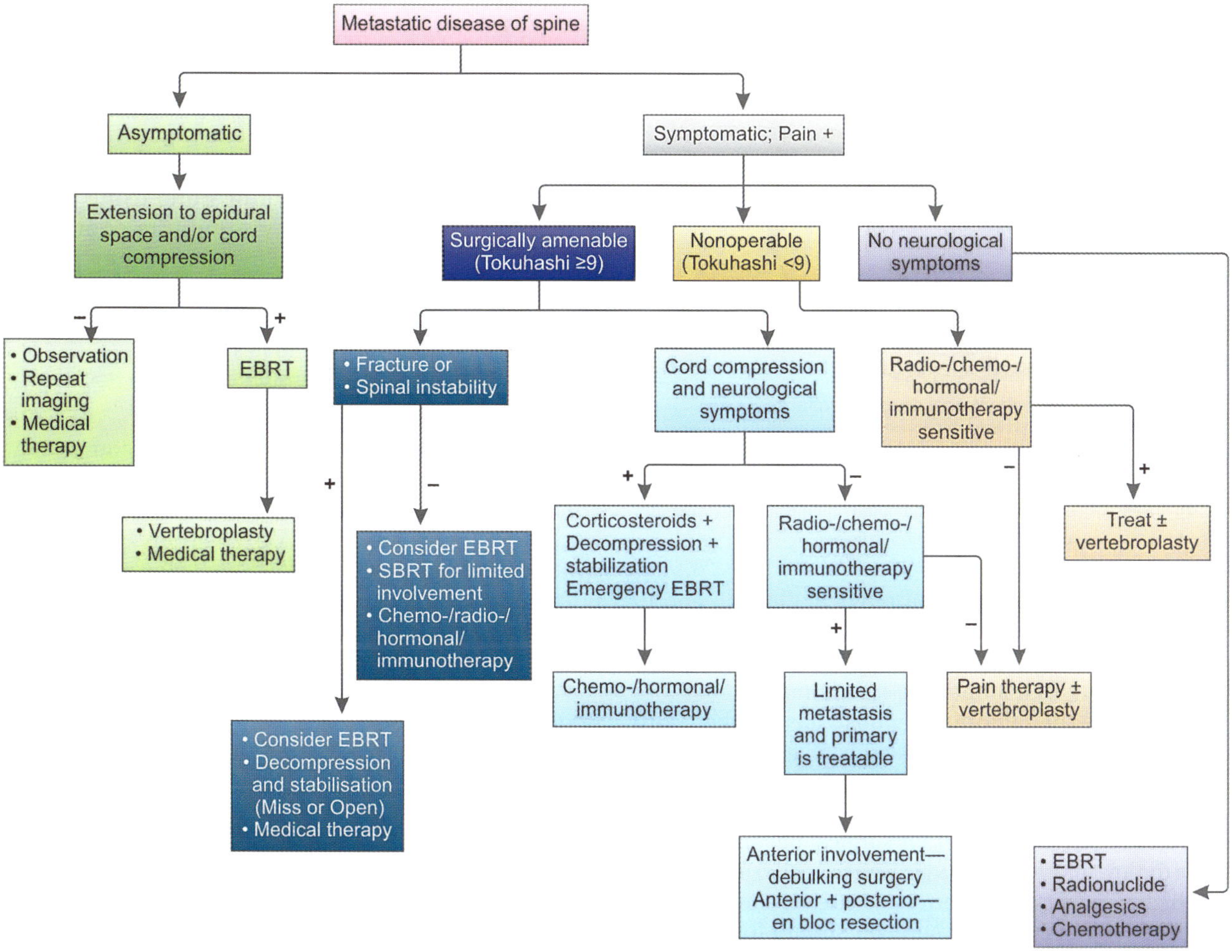

(EBRT: external beam radiation therapy; SBRT: stereotactic body radiation therapy)

TABLE 25: Revised Tokuhashi prognostic score.

Criteria	*Score = 0*	*Score = 1*	*Score = 2*	*Score = 3*	*Score = 4*	*Score = 5*
Karnofsky's performance	10–40	50–70	80–100	–	–	–
Extraspinal bone metastasis	≥3	1–2	0			
Vertebral metastasis	≥3	2	1			
Visceral metastasis	Unremovable	Removable	None			
Primary site	Lung	Liver	Other	Kidney	Rectum	Breast
Palsy	Frankel A, B	Frankel C, D	Frankel D			

- *Grade 2* is spinal cord abutment or even deformation due to pressure but the cerebrospinal fluid remains around the cord.
- *Grade 3* is spinal cord compression with obliteration of any fluid around it.

Grade 2 and 3 tumors are likely to result in neurologic deficits and most likely require surgical decompression (unless radiosensitive). After these evaluations, the primary interventions can be chosen as follows.

Primary radiotherapy is indicated for a multiple level disease in a stable spine with a radiosensitive tumor. The neurological condition should be stable or slowly progressive. Radiotherapy is also done primarily in a patient with poor prognosis and low general condition precluding surgery or as adjuvant to surgical treatment.

Surgical intervention is done with the following goals in mind and planning should be directed to achieve these objectives:

- Decompress the spinal cord or root causing symptoms and restore function
- Stabilize spine
- Preserve the normal motion segments.

Primary surgical intervention is required in patients with grade 2 or 3 tumors, Tokuhashi score of ≥9, progressive or severe neurological deficit, fast advancing deficit, progressive

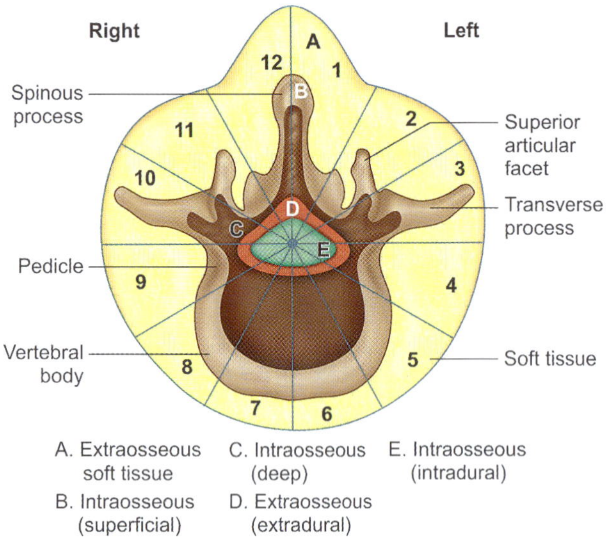

Fig. 89: The Weinstein-Boriani-Biagini staging system for anatomical classification of spinal tumors.

deformity (with or without neurological deficit), and in patients with neural compression predominantly by bone. Patients having metastatic tumor insensitive to radiotherapy or chemotherapy with intractable symptoms, and in those patients, where the radiotherapy dose has reached cord tolerance limits, surgical intervention is relatively indicated due to absence of other effective methods. Intractable pain in patients unresponsive to nonoperative methods may also be another relative indication for surgical decompression. Despite the low threshold for surgical intervention now-a-days due to higher acceptability of error and already compromised and limited life of patient, a surgeon should follow some underlying principles:

- Foremost to bear in mind is that the magnitude of surgical procedure should not exceed (or compromise) patient's ability to survive it or the surgeon's level of competence.
- The surgeon should be familiar with various approaches to spine. Thoracolumbar or cervicodorsal regions require specialized approaches.
- If life expectancy of patient is deemed to exceed the probable stress bearing capability of implant (usually assumed to be 6 months), fusion should be additionally considered.
- It is better to choose titanium implants for possible future need of MRI.
- The planned construct should provide immediate stability for quick functional gain.

In patients with malignant extradural spinal cord compression, the following guidelines apply:

- Give steroids (8–10 mg bolus dexamethasone followed by 16 mg daily) if neurological deficit is suspected or confirmed.
- Patients with compression caused by bone alone and those whose neurological symptoms have developed slowly and not resulted in complete deficits for more than 12–24 hours are the most likely to benefit from surgery. This should be supplemented with radiotherapy.
- Patients treated with radiotherapy alone may be treated with single 8 Gy dose if there is poor life expectancy or with multiple fractionated dose for patients expected to live longer.

Postoperative Management

Focus on wound healing, physical therapy, and thromboembolism prophylaxis should be done using standard guidelines. Adjuvant therapy should be continued in discussion with oncologist. Physical therapy primarily focuses on promoting mobilization and ambulation as early as possible. External-beam radiation therapy after surgery is recommended once the wound has healed.

Adjuvant Therapy

The adjuvant therapy is a very important component of managing MBD whether to spine or long bones. With the growth in understanding of the mechanisms underlying lytic and sclerotic lesions of MBD, various bone targeting agents have been developed and are being studied. These primarily aim at reducing the intractable pain, improve bone strength and quality and few are also being studied to prevent development of metastasis altogether **(Fig. 90)**.

Analgesia

Generally as per the pain profile, the analgesics are chosen with NSAIDs for mild-to-moderate pain and may be added with nonopioid analgesics for top-up or step-up therapy. Calcitonin is a mild antiresorptive agent that has mild analgesic activity but is limited by short half-life and rapid development of tachyphylaxis. Bisphosphonates and denosumab may also help reducing pain by controlling bone destruction. For severe pain, the opioid analgesics are used. Persistent or constant pain for full day will need fixed-dose schedule of analgesics that can be supplemented with short-acting transmucosal lipophilic opioids (like fentanyl citrate) for breakthrough pain. For radicular pain, antiepileptics and tricyclic antidepressants may be given. Ketamine (100 mg daily) has been used successfully in patients that were still uncontrolled with high-dose opioids. Implantable drug-delivery system (IDDS) delivering the drug intrathecally is very effective. IDDS is recommended when the life expectancy is >3 months. Usually, a combination of drugs is given intrathecal opioids are effective by 300 times compared to the oral route. Ziconotide is a synthetic peptide (derived from sea snail *Conus magus*) that selectively blocks N-type voltage calcium channels at presynaptic terminals of the dorsal horn has been validated for cancer pain but is associated with many side effects. Other drugs that have been used include morphine, hydromorphone, fentanyl, meperidine, clonidine, dexmedetomidine, ropivacaine, bupivacaine, tetracaine, baclofen, ketamine, gabapentin, midazolam, etc. in various combinations in IDDS. Finally, unrelenting pain may have to be controlled with nerve block. Supportive therapy in the form of message, TENS, and relaxation techniques also help these patients a lot. In patients with breast cancer, some relief from neuropathic pain has been obtained with dasatinib (an

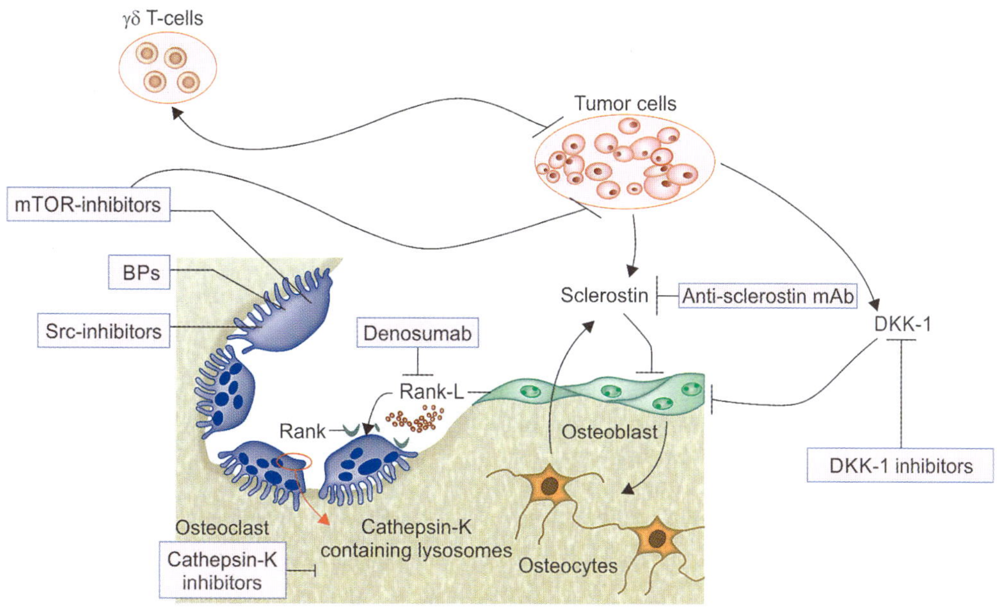

Fig. 90: Mechanisms of action of common and potential therapeutic bone targeting agents for bone metastasis management. (BPs: bisphosphonates; mTOR: mammalian target of rapamycin; DKK-1: Dickkopf-1; mAb: monoclonal antibody)

oral c-Src inhibitor that targets Src-tyrosine kinase) as c-Src is expressed by neurons. Abiratenone acetate and enzalutamide have been shown to improve bone pain and delay the onset of SREs in patients with prostate cancer.

Systemic Therapy

Serious advancements have been made in systemic therapy to reduce SREs, improve bone strength, and treatment/prevention of MBD. Bisphosphonates have a tendency to bind specially at place where active bone resorption is going on and hence controls to some extent bone resorption by inhibiting osteoclast recruitment and activation. Zoledronic acid is most effective compound and controls not only the hypercalcemia but also has shown to lower the incidence of SREs and delay their onset. Injectable bisphosphonates particularly the zoledronic acid (4 mg given every 3 weeks) has been found effective in breast, renal, and pulmonary metastasis. The frequency may be reduced to once every 3 months reducing the adverse effects without reducing efficacy. Denosumab (fully humanized monoclonal IgG-2 antibody that binds to RANK-ligand, inhibiting the interaction between RANK and RANKL interaction) has been found more effective in delaying the time to first SRE. For myeloma and lymphoma, the chemotherapy provides good symptomatic relief and also control of the disease. The concurrent application of radiation therapy and bisphosphonates has shown to bring about a significant pain response, enhanced re-ossification and improved quality of life in patients with bone metastases from a variety of solid tumors. Urinary N-telopeptide of type I collagen (urinary NTX) correlate with an increased risk for SREs and disease progression. They have also been used to assess the response to systemic therapy. The levels normalize in majority of patients treated with zoledronic acid and this in-turn correlates with improved survival. Odanacatib is a cathepsin-K inhibitor that has shown improvement of bone turnover markers in metastatic breast cancer but has been withdrawn due to development of serious atrial fibrillation in patients. Inhibitors of mammalian target of rapamycin (mTOR) like everolimus exert both antiapoptotic and prodifferentiative activities in osteoclasts. Exmestane + everolimus combination has been approved for hormone receptor positive and HER-2 negative advanced carcinoma of breast for reducing SREs. Everolimus in association with bisphosphonates has shown beneficial effect in metastatic lung, prostate, and renal cell carcinoma. Proteasome inhibitor like bortezomib reduces RANK-L-mediated osteoclastogenesis and also promotes osteoblast differentiation. CTCE-9908 is a competitive antagonist of CXCR4, decreased the tumor burden of breast cancer in bone and is being evaluated for possibility of *preventing* bone metastasis. Similarly, inhibitor of TGF-β and inhibitor of integrin receptors (inhibition of integrin αVβ3) are being evaluated as principal inhibitors of bone metastasis. On similar lines, osteoblast modulators like anti-sclerostin antibody (romosozumab, bolosozumab, and BPS804) may prevent onset of multiple-myeloma bone disease especially in combination with bisphosphonates. DKK-1 is another Wnt inhibitor produced by prostate and breast cancer and multiple myeloma. Bi-specific antibody against sclerostin and DKK-1 would be effective in osteoblastogenesis and preventing MBD. ET-1 antagonists like atrasentan significantly delayed the increase in PSA and bone metastasis of prostate cancer. Cabozantinib, a more selective tyrosine-kinase inhibitor, preferentially targets VEGFR2 and hepatocyte growth factor receptor inhibits metastasis in prostate cancer patients and reducing SREs in renal cell carcinoma.

Radiotherapy

Palliative radiotherapy plays an important role in skeletal metastasis to control pain, preventing future fracture, maintaining acceptable quality of life and independence in functions, and preventing tumor progression. After steroids and analgesics, EBRT is the effective and most common method for pain control for localized symptomatic skeletal metastasis. It is often given in multifraction dosage (20 Gy in five fractions, 24 Gy in 6 fractions, or 30 Gy in 10 fractions) and achieves pain relief by destroying tumor cells that reduces inflammatory edema. Single fraction dose of 8 Gy (possibly the standard of care in future) have been found to be equally effective to multifraction doses (for pain relief) and is possibly less toxic. It can produce effective bone healing and sclerosis and may also prevent a pathological fracture from happening by improving bone strength. Stereotactic body radiation therapy (SBRT) is preferred for spinal metastasis for reducing acute side effects but incurs bit higher cost. Single fraction of SBRT has been studied with a dose of 12–20 Gy that provides pain control within 24 hours and pain relief in 2 weeks in >70% cases. Long-term pain relief is obtained in >80% patients. It is being compared to EBRT for up to 3 site disease for pain relief. Multifraction of SBRT is less frequently used but radiation doses of 30 Gy in 10 fractions and 20 Gy in 5 fractions are used by some with good pain relief, and improvement in weakness and paresthesia and minimal toxicity. Fractionated SBRT may be the treatment of choice for select patients with recurrence in the area that was previously treated with radiotherapy. Postoperatively also SBRT is being preferred to EBRT for local tumor control and has a dose response relationship. It should be remembered that radiotherapy will not help control pain of a "mechanical" nature, and only 30–40% of pathological fractures will unite even after radiotherapy. Hemibody external beam irradiation (EBRT) provides rapid pain relief but the use is reducing with the availability of radionuclides.

Radiotherapy is also strongly recommended following nailing or other surgical procedures in patients with metastatic disease for local control of disease.

Radionuclide therapy is particularly useful for osteoblastic metastasis that avidly take-up the bone-seeking radiopharmaceuticals, concentrating, and incorporating them into calcifying areas. These agents are commonly delivered intravenously and quickly home at sites of active bone reaction and remodeling specifically. Excess or unused radionuclides are fast eliminated either through the renal or gastrointestinal system. The indications can be summarized in **Box 9**. Most radionuclides that belong to family IIA of the periodic table are incorporated directly in the bone in lieu of calcium (carrying the same divalent charge). Other radionuclides have to be chelated to organic phosphates to facilitate incorporation into bone matrix. Strontium-89, Rhenium-188, Phosphorus-32 Samarium-153 and Rhenium-186 are the commonly used radiopharmaceuticals. The beta radiation inhibits lymphocyte-associated cytokines or alterations in osteoclast or osteoblast activity giving pain relief. Myelosuppression is a limiting side effect. Phosphorus-32 decays to sulfur-32 isotope likely responsible for its activity but significant myelosuppression has caused loss in interest in this radionuclide. Strontium-89 is rapidly incorporated by body (does not distinguish strontium from calcium). Pain relief is seen at around 3 weeks from injection. It has been combined with chemotherapy for metastatic prostate disease with good results. Samarium-153 belong to lanthanide series and has no inherent bone-seeking property so is provided chelated to organic phosphate (ethylene diamine tetramethylene phosphonate) which targets bone matrix and gets incorporated as polyphosphonate. It is also a gamma-emitter (29%, 103 KeV) so allows for scintigraphy similar to technetium bone scan after injection. Rhenium-186 and -188 are transition metals and are provided attached to hydroxyethylidene diphosphonate. They have shown good pain relief in metastatic breast disease and have been found to control pain better than samarium with quickly reversible myelosuppression. Alpha-emitting radioisotopes are a new category that have lesser myelosuppression. Radium-223 emits helium nucleus that has high energy dissipating capacity over a smaller distance causing extensive damage to the tumor cells but avoiding the surrounding normal tissue for limited penetration. Newer radionuclides are being studied. Lutetium-177 is currently used for radioimmunotherapy and peptide receptor radionuclide therapy for its longer half-life and beta and gamma emission. Thulium-170 has been studied in India as 170-Tm-EDTMP and is found to accumulate in bone (rats). It has high beta- emission and long half-life of 128 days. Tin-117m has affinity to bone in quatravalent (4+) form. It emits low-energy conversion electrons that has high therapeutic window for its short range of emitted conversion electron. EBRT can be combined with radionuclides safely. Radionuclides can be combined with chemotherapy that have improved efficacy possibly by virtue of chemosensitization of tumor cells.

BOX 9: Indications and contraindications of bone-seeking radionuclides.

Indications:
- Diffuse skeletal metastases visualized on nuclear medicine bone scan
- Painful skeletal metastases inadequately treated by analgesics
- Intolerance to prescribed analgesics
- Hormone-insensitive disease (for metastatic prostate cancer)

Contraindications:
- Absolute
  - Presence of epidural spinal cord compression
  - Pending or active pathological fracture of weight-bearing bone
  - Renal failure
  - Pregnancy
  - Breastfeeding
- Relative
  - Uncontrolled extraskeletal disease burden
  - Asymptomatic skeletal metastases
  - Skeletal lesions limited to fewer than three sites
  - Purely osteolytic lesions (no uptake on bone scan)
  - Poor bone marrow reserve
  - Life expectancy < 60 days

MUSCULOSKELETAL SOFT TISSUE TUMORS

Soft tissue tumors are highly heterogeneous group of tumors that arise from the mesoderm with some contribution from the neuroectoderm. Soft tissues considered here are the nonepithelial extraskeletal tissue that includes the skeletal muscles, adipose tissue, fibrous tissue, vascular and lymphatic tissue, and the peripheral nervous system. They are classified on the basis of adult tissue they resemble. Soft-tissue sarcomas are commonly deep seated masses but one-third can be found superficial to fascia. Soft tissue tumors are divided into benign and malignant forms and an additional intermediate category of borderline or low malignant potential within the different histologic categories considered.

Benign tumors have a limited capacity for both autonomous growth and little tendency to local invasion or recur following excision.

Malignant tumors, or *sarcomas*, in contrast, are locally aggressive and are capable of invasive or destructive growth, recurrence, and distant metastasis. It is important to qualify the term "sarcoma" with the histologic grade, for example, "well-differentiated" and "poorly-differentiated" to denote the degree of differentiation or the relative maturity of the tumor with respect to normal adult tissue. Usually, well-differentiated sarcomas are low-grade lesions, whereas poorly differentiated sarcomas are high-grade neoplasms which indicate the likelihood of metastases. Any mass larger than 4 cm and deep and heterogeneous on MRI should be managed as a sarcoma unless proven otherwise. Wide surgical excision remains primary surgical treatment of sarcoma with targeted radiotherapy like IMRT showing good results to reduce rate of recurrence. Surveillance for detecting metastasis using simple chest radiographs is shown to be similar to CT scans. Chemotherapy has no defined role but newer targeted therapies and hypoxia activated alkylating agents combined with doxorubicin may have improved role.

A definite relationship exists between soft tissue tumor type and the age of presentation. For instance, embryonal rhabdomyosarcoma is typically a tumor of infants and children, synovial sarcoma mainly affects adolescents and young adults, and liposarcomas and so-called malignant fibrous histiocytomas (pleomorphic undifferentiated sarcoma) are usually seen in middle-aged and elderly patients. Soft-tissue sarcomas are relatively rare and constituting <1% of all neoplasms when compared with carcinomas and other malignancies.

Pathogenesis

Trauma is frequently implicated in the development of sarcomas. In the majority of cases, trauma merely calls attention to the said part in which the neoplasm was pre-existent. Soft tissue sarcomas have also developed around foreign bodies, such as bullets, shrapnel, and surgically implanted material. The latency period has varied from 2 years to over 50 years, and the most common microscopic types have been so-called malignant fibrous histiocytoma and angiosarcoma.

Environmental carcinogens play a role in the development of soft tissue sarcoma. Asbestos is known to have a causal relationship with the development of mesotheliomas. Other chemicals such as dioxin, phenoxyacetic acid herbicides, and chlorophenols have been linked to tumorigenesis. However, several case control studies have failed to show any significant association among the United States soldiers stationed in Vietnam and exposed to Agent Orange, a defoliant that contained dioxin as a contaminant.

Radiation exposure has been related to the development of sarcomas. However, postradiation sarcomas are extremely uncommon. They can occur sometimes as a result of radiotherapy in the treatment of breast and gynecologic malignancies. MFHs are the most common postradiation sarcoma followed by development of osteosarcoma, fibrosarcoma, malignant peripheral nerve sheath tumor, chondrosarcoma, and angiosarcoma.

Viruses play a significant role in the development of certain soft tissue neoplasms, such as human herpes virus-8 in Kaposi sarcoma, and Epstein–Barr virus in smooth muscle tumors and myopericytomas arising in patients with immunodeficiency.

Some hereditary diseases predispose to the development of soft tissue tumors. Examples include: neurofibromatosis (benign and malignant peripheral nerve sheath tumors); Gardner syndrome (fibromatosis and Gardner fibroma); Li–Fraumeni syndrome caused by germline mutation of the *TP53* gene (various sarcomas), Carney complex (psammomatous melanotic schwannoma and cutaneous myxoma) and tuberous sclerosis (PEComas).

TUMOR AND TUMOR-LIKE CONDITIONS OF FIBROBLASTS/MYOFIBROBLASTS

Nodular Fasciitis

Nodular fasciitis is the preferred term for self-limiting reactive proliferation fibroblasts/myofibroblasts, which was previously known as pseudosarcomatous fasciitis. It is a distinctive lesion because of its ability to simulate a malignant process. Morphologic variants of nodular fasciitis include intravascular and cranial fasciitis.

Epidemiology

It comprises one of the most common soft tissue neoplasms that exceeds in frequency than any other tumor or tumor-like lesion of fibrous tissue. All age groups seem to be affected but the lesion is more often encountered in young adults between 20 and 40 years of age. Both sexes are commonly equally affected. The two variants have distinctive age distribution, whereas intravascular fasciitis commonly affects young adults <30 years of age, the cranial fasciitis develops predominantly in infants under 2 years and is also more frequent in boys.

Sites of Involvement

Nodular fasciitis is commonly encountered in the subcutaneous region, although occasional cases are intramuscular or centered in the dermis. The upper extremity (particularly the flexor aspect of forearms), trunk, and head and neck, are most frequently affected but any part of body can be involved. Intravascular fasciitis is also mostly subcutaneous. Here, most commonly small- to medium-sized veins are affected but occasionally arteries are also involved (rarely both). Cranial fasciitis is generally seen to involve the outer table of the skull and the contiguous soft tissue of the scalp. In some cases, it may spread down through the inner table into the meninges.

Clinical Features

Two important clinical features of nodular fasciitis are a history of rapid growth and its small size. Most of the lesions grow rapidly and have a preoperative duration of 1 month or less. Pain and localized tenderness may be present. The nodules are usually <2 cm and almost always <5 cm. Lesions of intravascular fasciitis, on the other hand, enlarge more slowly but these also normally do not progress >2 cm in size. Cranial fasciitis grows faster akin to nodular fasciitis and may become somewhat larger than them. When the skull is involved in cranial fasciitis, the radiographs demonstrate a lytic defect along with a sclerotic rim.

Etiology

The precise cause is not known. Some patients with nodular fasciitis report local trauma at the site of lesion. Birth trauma has been considered a factor in the production of cranial fasciitis.

Gross and Microscopic Appearance

Nodular fasciitis is not encapsulated and margins are typically infiltrative but may be circumscribed. The cut surface varies from myxoid to fibrous, and occasionally there is central cystic change. Microscopically, this lesion is characterized by cellular proliferation of plump fibroblasts/myofibroblasts set in a myxoid matrix. The lesion may be mitotically active but lacks nuclear hyperchromasia, pleomorphism and atypical mitotic figures. Wide bands of collagen, extravasated red blood cells, lymphocytes, osteoclastic multinucleated giant cells are seen. Foci of metaplastic bone formation may be present. Some highly vascular lesions may resemble granulation tissue.

Treatment

It is cured by lesional excision. Recurrence is very rare. If a recurrence does occur, it may be due to incomplete excision or one should reconsider the original. Intravascular fasciitis and cranial fasciitis also behave in the same benign manner as that of nodular fasciitis despite the sometimes proficient intravascular growth of former.

Ischemic Fasciitis

Other pseudosarcomatous proliferations include ischemic fasciitis and organ-associated pseudosarcomatous myofibroblastic proliferation. Ischemic fasciitis also known as "atypical decubitus fibroplasia" typically occurs over bony prominences, usually in immobilized patients whereas the later can occur anywhere in the genitourinary tract, commonly so in urinary bladder after trauma or surgical instrumentation.

Epidemiology

It most often occurs in chronically immobilized patients and is seen mostly between the 7th and 9th decades of life. Females are affected slightly more frequently than males.

Sites of Involvement

The soft tissues around shoulder are most commonly affected, followed by, those overlying the ribs, sacrococcygeal region, or the greater trochanter.

Clinical Features

Most patients present with a short duration of poorly circumscribed painless mass. The mass usually <10 cm in diameter and is located in the subcutaneous tissue itself. The mass sometimes extends into deeper lying tissues and muscles.

Gross and Microscopic Appearance

Grossly, the lesion is poorly circumscribed and vaguely multinodular, often with a myxoid quality. Histologically, there is central zone of coagulative necrosis surrounded by a ring of newly formed vessels and proliferating fibroblasts/myofibroblasts.

Treatment

Local excision is mostly curative unless local underlying ischemia and injury continues that may pose recurrence.

Fibromas

The common fibromas encountered in orthopedic practice are detailed below.

Fibroma of Tendon Sheath

Fibroma of the tendon sheath represents a slow-growing small, fibrous nodule firmly attached to the tendon sheath. The regions containing most numerous tendons like the hands and feet are commonly affected. The upper extremity is more commonly affected than the lower extremity. Most common sites of involvement in the upper extremity are the fingers (especially the thumb, index, and middle fingers), hand and wrist, i.e., tendon predominant regions with only rare involvement of the forearm, elbow, or upper arm. It is found most commonly in adults aged 20–50 years and is more frequently seen in men. Sites of involvement in the lower extremity are the knee, foot, ankle, and rarely the toe or leg. As many as one-third of patients have slight tenderness, pain, or limited ROM of the affected digit. A history of antecedent trauma has been reported in approximately 9% of cases. It is not clear whether this is a distinct entity or a heterogeneous process representing the end stage of a variety of lesions, particularly tenosynovial GCT or nodular fasciitis.

Elastofibroma

It occurs as a slowly growing, ill-defined deep-seated mass arising between the inferomedial portion of the scapula and the chest wall that only rarely causes pain, tenderness, limitation of motion or scapular snapping. Elderly women are affected more commonly with a peak between the 7th and 8th decades of life. Most arise from the connective tissue between the inferior half of the scapula and the chest wall, and deep to the rhomboids and latissimus dorsi muscles. The lesion is attached to the periosteum and ligaments encompassing the region of the sixth to eighth ribs. Although, usually unilateral, up to 10% of patients have bilateral lesions. Microscopically, it is characterized by a large number of coarse, enlarged elastic fibers. CT and MRI help in diagnosis and simple excision is curative.

Desmoplastic Fibroblastoma (Collagenous Fibroma)

Desmoplastic fibroblastoma is a discrete fibrous neoplasm that characteristically develops in the subcutaneous tissue or voluntary muscle of adults. Most patients are in their 5th or 6th decade of life that present with a slowly growing, painless mass. Men are frequently affected up to three to four times as common than women. The most common sites are the upper extremities, including the shoulder, upper arm, and forearm, followed by the lower extremity; rare lesions arise in the head and neck region. Most are predominantly subcutaneous, but some involve skeletal muscle exclusively. The vast majority of tumors are 4 cm or smaller at the time of excision.

COMMON FIBROUS TUMORS OF INFANCY AND CHILDHOOD

Fibrous lesions that are peculiar to infancy and childhood have no clinical or morphologic counterpart in adult life. They pose a special problem in diagnosis as cellularity and rapid growth may be mistaken for evidence of malignancy.

Infantile Digital Fibromatosis

Infantile digital fibromatosis also known as inclusion body fibromatosis; it typically occurs on the dorsal aspect of digits hands and toes of young children. It presents before 1 year of life and size rarely exceeds 2 cm in diameter. Thumb and big toe are usually not involved. In a minority, more than one digit may be affected. Microscopically, it has characteristic eosinophilic inclusion in the cytoplasm of some of the fibroblasts. Adequate excision is curative.

Fibromatosis

This term applies to a group of related conditions having common features such as fibroblastic proliferation with infiltrative pattern of growth and aggressive clinical behavior with a high tendency for local recurrence, but they never metastasize. They are broadly divided into superficial and deep types. Superficial fibromatoses arise from the fascia or aponeuroses of the palmar and plantar soft tissues are small slow growing whereas deep fibromatoses are large, rapidly growing tumors that involve deep structures, particularly the musculature of the trunk and the extremities.

Superficial Fibromatosis

Palmar fibromatosis also referred to as Dupuytren's contracture (*see* also Chapter on "Common Miscellaneous Conditions of Hand") is the most common fibromatosis that affects adults. The incidence increases with age and rarely affects patients younger than 30 years of age. Superficial fibromatosis affects males three or four times as commonly and is found exclusively in Caucasians. Nearly half of they are bilateral. Around 5–20% of these lesions are associated with plantar lesions, and up to 4% of patients have associated penile fibromatosis (Peyronie's disease). It manifests insidiously as a slow-growing solitary nodule on the palmar surface of hand which develops into cord-like indurations or bands between multiple nodules and adjacent fingers. This often produces to puckering of the overlying skin and develops flexion contractures of the 4th and 5th digits.

Plantar fibromatosis also known as "Ledderhose's disease" has a much greater incidence in children and adolescents as compared to palmar lesions but the incidence increases with age. Although men are generally more affected the incidence in pediatric age is greater in females. Plantar lesions appear as a firm subcutaneous nodule adherent to the skin and is reported by the patient to cause mild pain after longstanding or walking. It is typically located in the medial plantar arch from the region of the navicular bone to the base of the first metatarsal. Plantar lesions only exceptionally result in contraction of the toes. Plantar lesions on microscopy are more cellular and have more chances of recurrence in case of multiple or bilateral lesions or when there is a positive family history.

Aggressive Fibromatosis/Extra-abdominal Desmoid

Extra-abdominal desmoid is a benign but locally aggressive neoplasm of the soft tissue. The patient is commonly a young adult with a variably painful mass in the extremity. MRI demonstrates low/internediate T1 and intermediate T2-weighted heterogeneous mass that extends across fascial compartments.

Microscopically, it comprises a collagenous mass with sparse interspersed spindle cells. Histologically, it is related to familial adenomatous polyposis syndrome, familial dupuytren's contracture, plantar fibromatosis, and Peyronie disease. Characteristically, the lesion easily invades fascial boundaries and compartments proliferating into nearby tissues and even bone.

The treatment of extra-abdominal desmoid is controversial due to poor understanding of natural history. Tamoxifen, chemotherapy, and radiation therapy with or without surgical excision have been variably tried. Surgical resection should achieve wide margins else recurrence is common. Surgical resection is often associated with morbidity due to requirement of extensive dissection **(Figs. 91A to E)** so most surgeons prefer an initial period of aggressive pain management followed by more aggressive measures. Sorafenib and other kinase inhibitors have shown good response to treatment.

Fibrosarcomas

Fibrosarcoma is a malignant tumor of fibroblasts with variable collagen production. They are classified into the adult and infantile types; the latter also known as "congenital fibrosarcomas". The adult type has some distinctive variants namely the myxofibrosarcoma, fibromyxoid sarcoma, and sclerosing epithelioid type.

Clinical Features

The incidence has been declining over time, and this can be attributed to the advances in immunohistochemistry, molecular genetics which makes a distinction from the monophasic fibrous synovial sarcomas, fibromatosis, and other malignant spindle cell neoplasms possible as

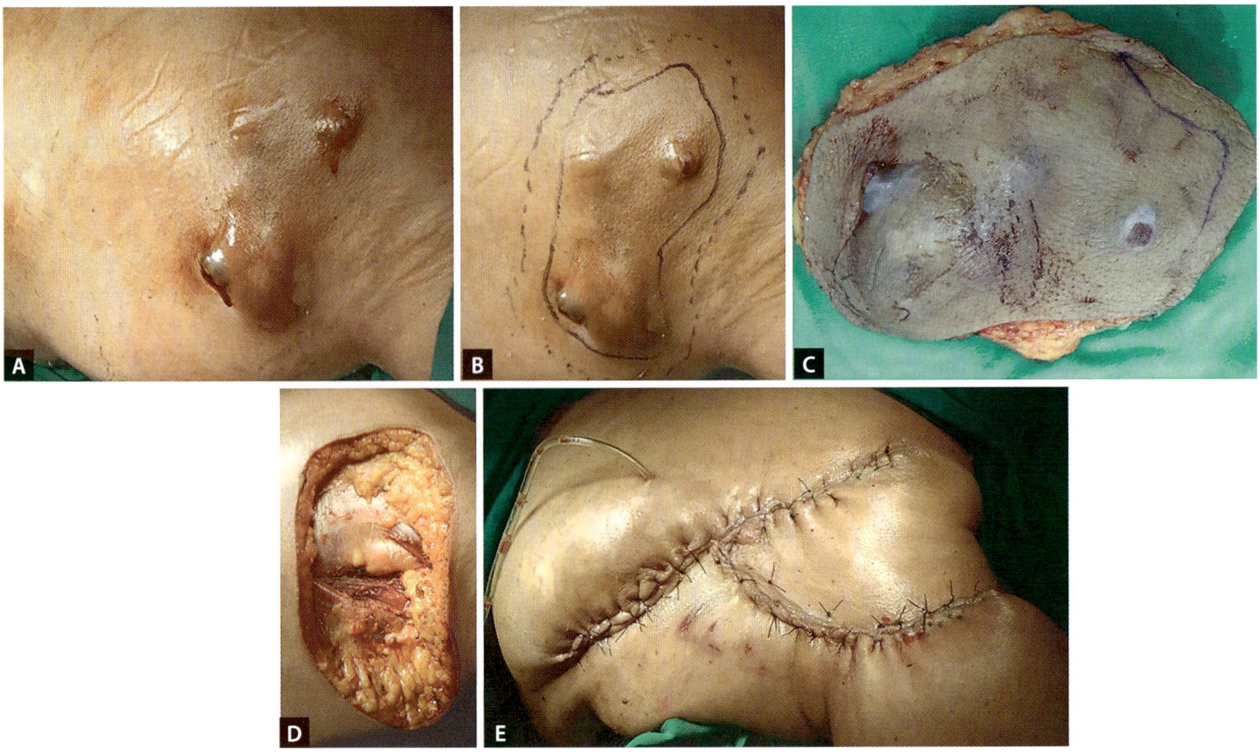

Figs. 91A to E: Aggressive fibromatosis extending from deep fascia lateral to scapular region overlying the latissimus dorsi muscle. The lesion fortunately did not extend deep but involved the skin and showed fungation (A). Wide excision was planned (B and C) along with superficial resection of the latissimus dorsi muscle (D) as a measure of clearance. The defect following R0 resection was then reconstructed with rotation flaps (E) producing uneventful healing.

the diagnosis of fibrosarcomas is mainly by exclusion. Fibrosarcoma may occur at any age but is most common in the 3rd to 5th decades of life with no specific sex predilection. The sites most commonly affected are the deep soft tissues of lower extremities **(Fig. 92)** followed by upper extremities, trunk, head, and neck. The etiology is uncertain though it is known to arise in scar and previously irradiated tissues. It presents as a slow-growing painless mass and hence is diagnosed very late; sometimes after a gap of several years. Weight loss may be present in case of very large tumors with widespread metastases. Hypoglycemia has been reported in some cases.

Gross and Microscopy

The tumor is soft to firm, fleshy, white to tan, and contains areas of hemorrhage of necrosis. They are generally circumscribed except for the very large ones which have irregular infiltrative margins. The cells are arranged in fascicles that intersect each other at acute angles, resulting in a herring-bone appearance and demonstrate variable amount of collagen. The individual cells resemble normal fibroblasts, but some have features characteristic of myofibroblastic differentiation. They are more cellular and fibroblasts have a hyperchromatic nuclei as compared to fibromatosis. The sarcomas with marked pleomorphism and multinucleated giant cells are classified as so-called malignant fibrous histiocytoma (pleomorphic sarcoma) hence low-grade fibrosarcoma is generally a diagnosis of exclusion.

Immunohistochemically, fibrosarcoma should show reactivity for vimentin and type I collagen, positivity for smooth muscle actin, should be taken to indicate incipient differentiation along myofibroblastic lines.

Prognosis and Treatment

The treatment of choice is radical excision. The recurrence rates in literature is highly variable since it is possible that tumors included in the older series also included other entities as immunohistochemical and ultrastructural techniques were not commonly employed. The probability of recurrence depends on the adequacy of surgical margins, local recurrence was 79% in tumors with inadequate surgical margins and 18% in tumors treated by wide or radical excision. The lung followed by the axial skeleton (vertebrae and skull) are the principal metastatic sites.

Metastasis occurs in 9–63% of patients and is dependent on the grade of lesion. Metastasis from fibrosarcomas occurs commonly to lungs and bone (especially axial skeleton), and rarely to lymph nodes. Five-year survival is between 39 and 54%. Poor prognostic factors include a high-grade lesion, high cellularity on microscopy with little collagen production, mitotic rates > 20/10 high-power field and presence of necrosis. The local recurrence rates correlates to completeness of excision so these are reported in a wide range in literature from 12 to 79%. Fibrosarcomas metastasize to lungs and bone, especially the axial skeleton, and rarely to lymph nodes. Adjuvant chemotherapy has been recommended in high-grade lesions.

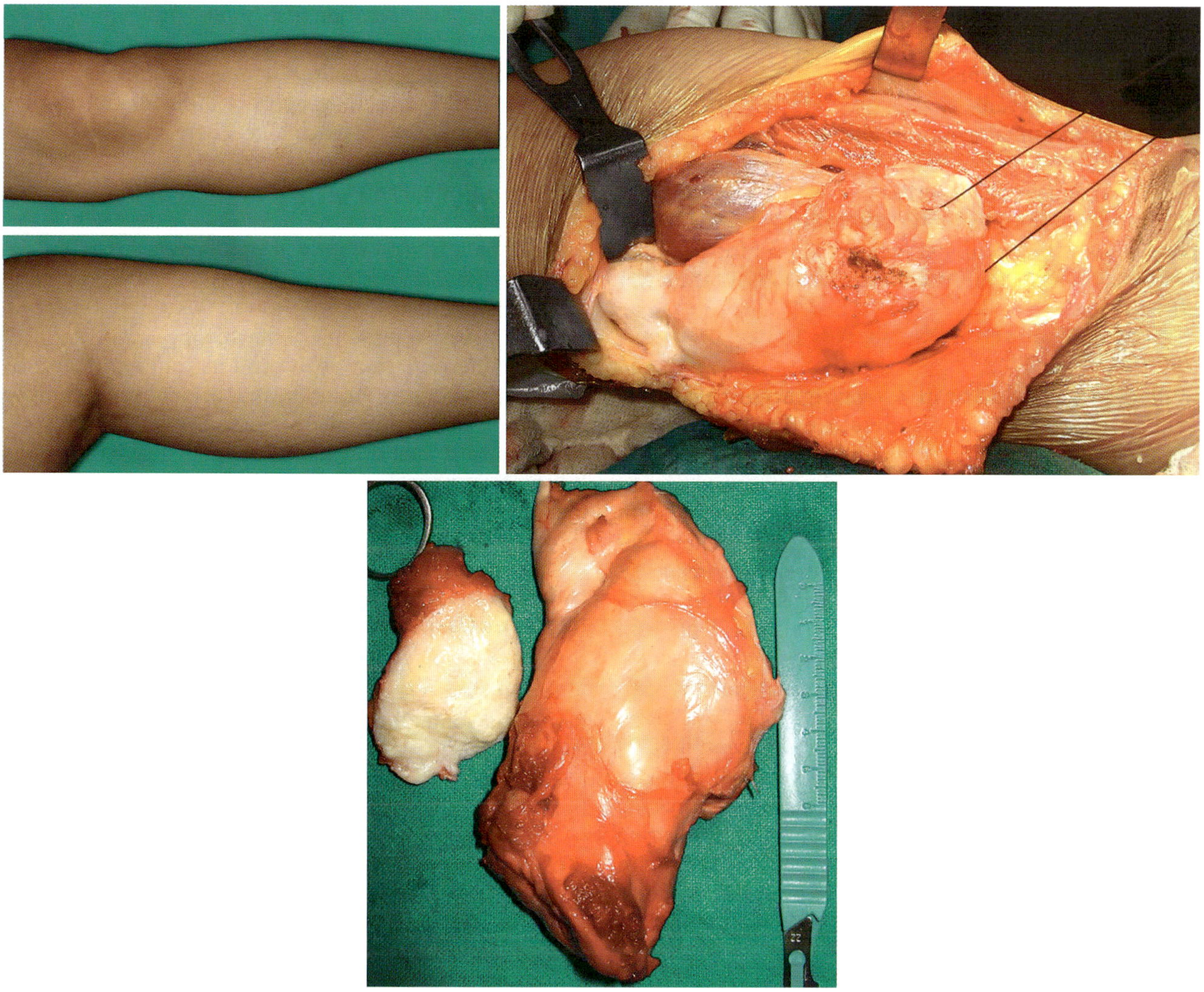

Fig. 92: Fibrosarcoma of calf region. The patient had a painless progressively growing mass of the left calf. The mass was growing over 16 months before the patient developed difficulty in walking and some pain and presented in OPD. The mass was excised in toto.

Nerve Sheath Tumor (Schwannoma)

Schwannoma is a commonly benign nerve sheath tumor arising from Schwann cells of the peripheral nerves. They are also known as "neurilemmoma". They can arise from both cranial as well as spinal nerves. The most common location of occurrence of the tumor is in the inner ear where they present as vestibular schwannoma also known as "acoustic neuromas". They are commonly seen in orthopedic practice with neurofibromatosis type 1 (von Recklinghausen's disease). In NF-1 the gene-encoding neurofibromin is responsible in most of the cases. Neurofibromin is expressed at higher levels in the neural crest during development. Cells from the neural crest migrate to become pigmented cells of the skin, parts of the brain, spinal cord, peripheral nerves, and adrenals, thus explaining the common sites of abnormalities in the disorder. Most commonly arise in 8th cranial nerve and the second most common is 5th cranial nerve. At both sites, the tumor is intradural.

When these tumors are malignant, they are called malignant schwannomas or malignant peripheral nerve sheath tumors or neurofibrosarcomas. These arise commonly in sciatic nerve, brachial plexus, and sacral plexus. There are few variants of schwannoma as follows:

1. Ancient schwannoma
2. Cellular schwannoma
3. Melanotic schwannoma
4. Plexiform schwannoma

Clinical Features

These occur in adults except in von Recklinghausen's disease where they are diagnosed in first decade itself. When they occur in patients with neurofibromatosis type 2 (NF2), schwannomas usually present by the 3rd decade. They occur as a solitary nodule on any sheathed sensory, motor or autonomic nerve (commonly in vagus nerve). Multiple schwannomas are uncommon and occur in von Recklinghausen's disease. The following are the common locations of origin of schwannoma:

- Intracranial schwannomas
  - Cranial nerves
  - Intracerebral (very rare)
- Spinal schwannoma

- Trunk
  - Intercostal nerves
  - Posterior mediastinum
  - Retroperitoneum
  - Gastrointestinal schwannoma
- Limbs
  - Ulnar and peroneal nerves

Common symptoms include hearing loss (vestibular schwannoma), back pain that increases in supine position, paresthesias in lower limb, numbness, weakness of the lower limb, and sciatica.

Diagnosis

The diagnosis is made by investigating according to the presentation. MRI of head and neck will be needed for evaluation of hearing loss in a child. MRI of lumbar and lumbosacral spine is needed in lower back pain with associated symptoms. The schwannoma appears iso- or hypointense on T1-weighted images while it shows intense enhancement on contrast T1-weighted images. On T2-weighted images, it is heterogeneously hyperintense and larger schwannomas show cystic degeneration. Large tumors also have areas of hemosiderin due to intramural hemorrhages (5% cases). "Split-fat sign" is seen in non-fat-suppressed images where a thin rim of fat embraces along the long axis of lesion. Target sign comprising peripheral high signal with low central signal and "fascicular sign" comprising multiple small ring-like structures are seen in peripheral large schwannomas. Imaging in the plane of affected nerve will often demonstrate a "string sign" which is imaging visualization of the mass arising from nerve itself. Histology classically identifies hypercellular areas (Antoni A), hypocellular areas (Antoni B), and Verocay bodies.

Treatment

The vestibular schwannoma is primarily a domain of ENT surgeon and neurosurgeon. Spinal schwannomas are usually managed by surgery for weakness, numbness, or pain. Microsurgery is preferred with intraoperative electrophysiological monitoring. The nerve is opened, and the tumor is carefully excised. Large tumors are managed in addition by radiotherapy (stereotactic spine radiosurgery) that utilizes highly focused radiation beams to target spinal tumor. This is beneficial in the sense that the surrounding tissue is spared of ill-effects of radiation with nearly instant recovery.

HETEROTOPIC OSSIFICATION

The term specifically refers to presence of bone formation (ossification) at a place where it should not be present (heterotopic) that is usually the soft tissue.

The entity is included with bone tumors only for the reason that there is often a clinical, radiological, and histopathological confusion with aggressive bone tumors. Heterotopic ossification (HO) was first described in 1883 by Riedel. HO may be nontraumatic or traumatic arising from still unknown factors that may be local or genetic. There is a lot of confusion between usage of term myositis ossificans and heterotopic ossificans. I feel the term "myositis ossificans" should be dropped as the muscle (use of myo-) may not be involved and inflammation (use of "itis"-) is virtually absent. The term still is virtually so deeply engraved in minds and literature that it is difficult to remove completely, even the readers would have searched the index of this book for "myositis ossificans" to reach here. There are three following types of HO:

1. Heterotopic ossification per se (previously "myositis ossificans circumscripta")
2. Traumatic HO (previously "myositis ossificans traumatica")
3. Fibrodysplasia ossificans progressiva (FOP) (previously "myositis ossificans progressiva")
4. Neurogenic heterotopic ossification

The differentiation of HO and its traumatic form may diminish, however, in future and may become same entity with realization of possible microtrauma events in predisposed patients, with further research insights into pathogenesis. It is more important to differentiate metastatic calcification that occurs in conditions such as hyperparathyroidism from HO of any type.

Heterotopic Ossification (Myositis Ossificans Circumscripta)

It is a localized, non-neoplastic, HO predominantly seen in extremities. It seems to have predilection for mature soft tissue and some degenerated tissue that has less reparative capacity so it is rare in children. Majority of the cases have been described in quadriceps and brachialis muscles. Due to nonclarity on the pathogenesis, it has been variably thought to occur idiopathically associated with certain systemic disorders [tetanus, hemophilia, disseminated idiopathic skeletal hyperostosis (DISH)] or due to trauma (minor injuries as in sports person). Huge amount of controversy exists over trauma as inciting event. There is a possibility that injured muscle (e.g., sports injury) heals with fibrous tissue that degenerates to undergo ossification as for endochondral ossification possibly related to alteration in local growth factors. HO, however, develops in 7–8 weeks but bone formation takes a bit longer so this could be an argument against this hypothesis. Once the lesion is matured (usually 2 months) spontaneous regression is seen in significant number of patients (30%).

Evolution of Disease

Clinicians should be aware of the evolution of disease and as such with all early, intermediate, and late presentations because patients may present anytime during disease evolution. The fever, swelling, erythema, and joint stiffness typically seen in early HO may closely mimic the presentation of cellulitis, osteomyelitis, or thrombophlebitis. Based on the description detailed below a lot of clinicians think that pathogenically HO possibly best represents a localized tissue disruption that stimulates a repair response which in the presence of hematoma gets organized (and follows the stages) in a manner similar to a fracture healing, the pathogenesis is detailed in the description for traumatic HO (see below).

- *Early disease (inflammatory phase):* Early there is swelling and pain similar to an infection or soft tissue aggressive tumor. Radiographs are normal or show a soft tissue density. On ultrasonography, a hypoechoic mass with a central reflective core is seen that may have a lamellar hyperreflectivity at the periphery of the mass. The CT scan reveals enlarged muscle group with normal attenuation. MRI is quite helpful showing isointense to hyperintense on T1-weighted images and intermediate to high signal on T2-weighted images. These features though suggestive of HO may be confused with focal myositis so confirmation comes only when the lesion matures with time.

- *Intermediate stage (consolidation phase):* The lesion becomes clinically firm with constant pain. There may be limitation of movements at adjacent joints if the lesion is large. The radiographs show "dotted veil" calcification confusing with rhabdomyosarcoma or synovial sarcoma. There may be continuous or discontinuous peripheral calcification. CT scan is a better modality and reveals zonal phenomenon with a rim of calcification of varying thickness at the periphery while central area similar to muscle. MRI is more nonspecific with variable signal at the center and decreased signal intensity at periphery on all pulses. Calcific tendinitis is an important differential at this stage if the mass is small as in tendinitis the mass is small with associated calcification.
- *Late stage (maturation phase):* The mass becomes bony hard and easily discernable from its surrounding tissue. The pain reduces dramatically but the swelling and deformity is a concern for most patients. The mass may merge with the adjacent bone resembling osteochondroma. The movements at the associated joints may be limited in a large mass. It is imperative to recognize the pattern of mineralization at the periphery which is more mature than the central region that is still evolving (Zonation phenomenon). This helps in differentiating it from extraskeletal osteosarcoma. The osteosarcomas have an immature periphery while the center is more mature showing dense calcification centrally. The MRI shows overall reduced due to calcification; however, an important differentiating feature could be the presence of central signal intensity similar to marrow favoring the diagnosis of heterotopic ossification.

Differential Diagnosis

Osteomyelitis, osteochondroma, osteosarcoma, myositis, pentazocine-induced myopathy, hematoma formation, intramuscular parasitic cysts, rhabdomyosarcoma, and synovial sarcoma.

Treatment

Absolute prevention is not possible as often they are idiopathic to develop strictly following definition. When identified in early stage bisphosphonates and/or NSAIDs can be started to limit the extent of lesion. The prognosis is good and the lesion usually does not recur after surgical excision if performed adequately.

Traumatic Heterotopic Ossification

This is by far the most common form clinically encountered. It can occur after virtually any type of musculoskeletal trauma. The lesion of HO is extra-articular and develops outside the joint capsule. It is notable that bone formation occurs outside the muscle fibers or spindles (not within them) in the connective tissue between muscle planes. This is against the common belief that ossification occurs within the muscles. HO has been commonly noted to occur after arthroplasty of hip, knee, shoulder, or elbow; fractures; and joint dislocations and periarticular soft tissue trauma. As opposed to circumscripta form, loss of joint motion and resulting functiolesia are the principal complaints after traumatic HO **(Figs. 93A to E)**. The difference is elucidated in the hip HO. There are two main forms of hip HO seen, one the lateral form and other central type. The lateral type is associated with the anterolateral and lateral surgical approach and develops around greater trochanter and gross restriction of mobility. The central type instead has genetic predisposition and is unrelated to surgery-related factors, prior operations, preoperative hip motion, or surgical approach. The incidence of HO after total hip arthroplasty (THA) is around 50% (0.6–90%) though 90% of these are asymptomatic. Common predisposing factors for development of HO after THA include ankylosing spondylitis, Paget's disease, hypertrophic osteoarthritis, and cerebral palsy as also the use of uncemented components are associated with increased incidence of heterotopic ossification.

Pathogenesis

At its essence HO represents transformation of primordial cells of mesenchymal origin, within muscle connective tissue septa into osteogenic cells, though the complete pathway is not recognized. It is generally accepted that three conditions are needed to be fulfilled for development of HO, viz., presence of osteogenic precursor cells, metaplasia inducing agents, and a permissive environment (Chalmers et al.). The role of prostaglandin E2 (PGE2) has been emphasized to mediate the differentiation of the progenitor cells into osteogenic tissue. It has been shown that muscle injury alone will not produce HO and some bone injury is required for its development. The heterotopic bone may begin some distance from normal bone, later moving toward it. Possibly, there is role of BMP in the development of heterotopic ossification.

Gross and Microscopy

They present as a well-defined mass with a soft to firm center and hard gritty periphery ranging in size from 2 to 12 cm. Microscopically, the most important diagnostic feature is provided by the maturation pattern (zonal phenomenon), characterized by a central cellular area, an intermediate zone of osteoid formation, and a peripheral shell of highly organized bone. It must be understood that the zonal pattern develops in lesions that are at least 3 weeks old. In the early phase, lesions are extremely cellular with numerous mitoses and atypical mitotic figures and bear a resemblance to nodular fasciitis microscopically. If biopsied too early, the cellular fibrous proliferation, osteoid, and primitive bone may be mistaken for that of osteosarcoma, as the process evolves, osteoid appears in an orderly pattern initially as ill-defined trabeculae and woven bone which subsequently matures into well-developed lamellar bone. Eventually, the central cellular areas

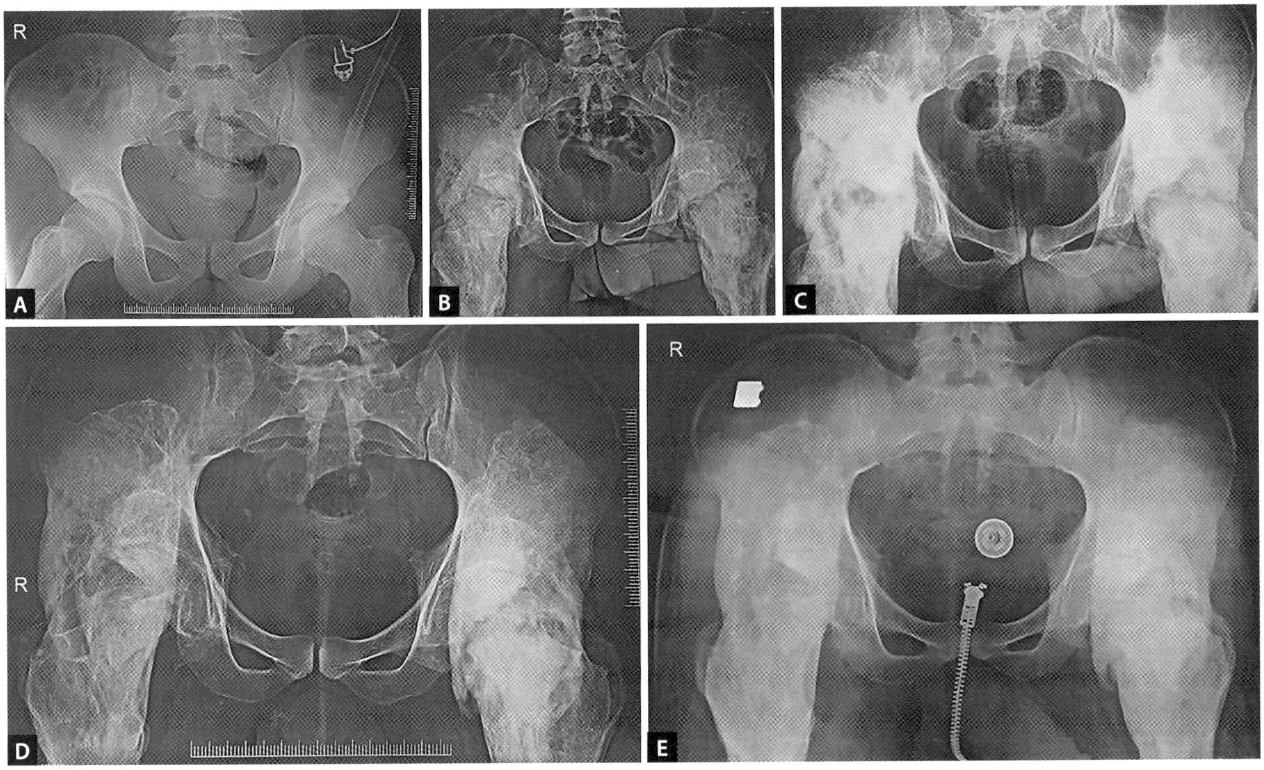

Figs. 93A to E: Post-traumatic heterotopic ossification. The patient suffered from dislocation of both hip joints managed by closed reduction (A). The patient developed florid heterotopic ossification (B) seen at 65 months post-reduction. The mass matured over a period of 1 year (B to E) and patient did not agree for surgical excision of the mass despite both hips being extra-articularly ankylosed.

become progressively collagenized and ultimately undergo ossification. The periphery of HO shows mature lamellated bone surrounded by a pseudocapsule of compressed muscle fibers and connective fibrous tissue. The mature HO resembles true bone with cancellous area and mature lamellar bone with Haversian system, vessels, and even bone marrow that contains minor hematopoietic elements. The spindle cells have the characteristic ultrastructural features of fibroblasts and myofibroblasts and express vimentin and other smooth muscle markers such as actin whereas the osteocytes and osteoblasts express vimentin and osteocalcin. A reactive lesion histologically and pathogenetically probably related to myositis ossificans has been described in the small bones of the hand fingers and less frequently the toes, as fibro-osseous tumor of the digits. In fibro-osseous pseudotumor, the lesional calcification has a more random distribution.

Clinically, traumatic HO also undergoes the previously mentioned three stages for circumscripta with albeit a greater tendency to limitation of joint movements. Joint stiffness and resulting loss of limb function are the principal complications of traumatic HO. Entrapment of peripheral nerve in the organizing mass and development of pressure ulcers due to undue pressure from swelling in an ectopic site are other complications of HO. Overall clinically significant complications of HO develop in 15–20% patients.

Investigations

The extent of lesion is evident on radiographs in late stages, or CT scan in earlier stages or MRI in earliest stages as described above. Hip being the most common site for development of HO has received most attention and few classification systems exist. Metabolic activity of the lesion is evident by scintigraphic scanning that supplements the radiographs if the combination is resorted to instead of complicated investigations. In the early stages, the scintigraphic scan reveals intense uptake at the site of lesion that reduces in intermediate stages and finally becomes cold in late stages. Approximately 2.5 weeks after injury, flow studies and blood-pool images can detect development of incipient HO. The typical findings on delayed scintigrams, however, become positive nearly 1 week later. The bone scans are sensitive enough that they can performed serially to identify metabolically silent lesions that can then be excised.

Laboratory investigations: The levels of alkaline phosphatase are elevated early and are abnormal approximately 2 weeks after injury. The alkaline phosphatase levels have been shown to increase to approximately 3.5 times the normal value after 10 weeks of the inciting trauma and they return to normal by nearly 18 weeks in a typical case due to maturation of mass. These, however, do not reflect the true metabolic activity of the lesion and cannot guide the timing of surgical removal. Also in many cases with limited disease or small lesions, the levels may remain normal. Serum creatine kinase levels correlate with the muscle involvement; with a higher level correlating to severe form of HO. Similar to any inflammatory event rise in CRP early has been reported but is nonspecific. The only value of this marker could be to evaluate the treatment response of NSAIDs, in which case the levels fall with favorable response.

Measurement of the 24-hour urinary excretion of PGE2 has been recommended to identify HO early in predisposed cases. A rise in levels indicates qualifying the lesion metabolism with bone scan.

Treatment

Because the treatment of a well-developed lesion is not very effective (recurrence common) or easy (undefined planes of involvement and possible secondary deficits after excision), it is considered that preventing the development of HO by appropriate prophylaxis or its early treatment early would be the best strategy. The first step to management once the diagnosis of early HO is confirmed is to initiate passive joint ROM exercises to maintain mobility. Early active mobilization versus aggressive delayed mobilization is debated, however, we feel that movements should begin early that may be intensified later as the lesion matures. The following agents have been recommended for prophylaxis of HO:

- Bisphosphonates (etidronate) and specific nonsteroidal anti-inflammatory drugs (such as indomethacin > ibuprofen > diclofenac) have been used for prophylaxis against development of HO or its treatment. Drug dosing, type of drug, timing of dosing, and length of treatment are undefined and surgeons often devise their own protocol. It is logical and recommended to start bisphosphonates as soon as serum ALP or urinary PGE2 levels are noted or imaging studies demonstrate the presence of incipient HO.
- Heterotopic ossification can be successfully prevented and treated by radiation therapy. A single irradiation of 7 Gy has been used successfully in patients who developed HO previously after a surgery. The modality is especially useful in patients having contraindications to receiving indomethacin. Considering the complications of radiation therapy including secondary sarcoma development, the treatment should be reserved only to these high-risk patients.
- *Thalidomide:* Thalidomide has been found to reduce the progression of ossification of soft tissues and may serve to improve functional status. The action may be related to reduction of TNF-α during flare-ups.

Surgical resection of HO should be delayed until when it has matured. This is done with the aim of reducing both the intraoperative complications like identification problem and hemorrhage, and minimizing postoperative HO recurrence. The ideal candidate for surgical resection of HO will hence be one who has clinically silent lesion (no joint pain or swelling), a normal alkaline phosphatase level, and a three-phase bone scan not showing any uptake in flow or blood-pool images suggesting maturation of HO. Variously recommended measures such as serial bone scans, evaluating alkaline phosphatase (ALP), and creatine kinase, or recently urinary PGE2 levels can be followed or developed on institutional basis and should be strictly followed if found adequate. A common guide is presented in **Table 26**. Garland proposed an approach independent of bone scintigraphy, serving as only a rough guide to management. In this approach, surgery is delayed as long as possible depending on the etiology underlying the development of HO. In general, a period of 6 months is recommended after direct trauma to musculoskeletal system, a period of 1 year after spinal cord injury, and 1.5 years after head injury has been proposed. It is imperative here to note that such prolonged delay in managing the patient leaves them at risk of the development of complete joint ankylosis and resulting intra-articular secondary damage or other complications of HO. This approach is hence not very popular due to lack of objective measures for initiation of treatment in this modern world of evidence-based medicine and protocol followed management. This has encouraged attempts to stage and identify the maturity of HO using various imaging studies **(Box 10)**. Quite unfortunately, however, still accurate indicators of maturity have remained elusive. Radiographic findings, ALP levels, and bone scans are at best, an approximation to balance appropriately delayed intervention without the mentioned complications.

TABLE 26: Classification of heterotopic ossification (HO) by Schmidt and Hackenbroch.

Region or grade	*Description*
Region 1	HO strictly below tip of greater trochanter
Region 2	HO below and above tip of greater trochanter
Region 3	HO strictly above tip of greater trochanter
Grade A	Single or multiple HOs <10 mm in maximum diameter without bony contact with pelvis or femur
Grade B	HOs >10 mm without contact with pelvis but with possible contact with femur; no bridging from femur to pelvis, with no evidence of ankylosis
Grade C	Ankylosis by means of firm bridging from femur to pelvis

BOX 10: Guidance criteria for surgical removal of heterotopic ossification.

- Definite presence of severely restricted movements at the joints or progressive loss of movements at the joint
- Absent fever, swelling, erythema or other signs of active heterotopic ossification lesion
- Normal serum alkaline phosphatase
- Reduced or absent uptake in blood flow and blood-pool images in scintigraphy

Neurogenic Heterotopic Ossification

This form was first described by Dejerine and Ceilier (1918) in patients with spinal cord injury (SCI) in times of the First World War. HO is now recognized as a commonly occurring sequelae to SCI, especially the one sustained after trauma. Other conditions associated with neurogenic HO albeit with lesser frequency are head injury (trauma) and injury to brain or spinal cord following many diseases such as stroke, hypoxic encephalopathy, encephalitis, tetanus, polio, tabes dorsalis, syringomyelia, and burns. This form appears 3–12 weeks from the injury and cases as late as 1 year have been described. Associated bony injury is not considered as a prerequisite for development of this type of HO. There are a few characteristic findings with respect to the development of HO location in these patients. Patients with complete injury to cord are more likely to develop HO. HO always develops below the level of injury. Similar to other forms hips are the most common site of involvement. The stages of development evaluation, treatment, and prognosis are similar to traumatic form and circumscripta form described above except that the disease is often more extensive involving various sites together.

Fibrodysplasia Proliferans Progressiva (Fibrodysplasia Ossificans Progressiva, Munchmeyer's Disease, and Previously Myositis Ossificans Progressiva)

This disorder is among the rarest genetic conditions of connective tissue, with an incidence of 1 case per 2 million persons. Transmission is autosomal dominant with variable expression. The condition is characterized by (1) progressive heterotopic endochondral ossification and (2) congenital malformation of the great toe [hallux valgus, malformed first metatarsal (monophalangism)], affected individuals may also have short thumbs. Most mutations are sporadic (that means new mutations rather than inherited ones—as patients hardly reach the age or activity for reproducing). Apart from the two defining conditions for FOP patients might also express some other atypical features (FOP plus) or may present with variation in one or both of them (FOP variants). The disease progresses temporally and has a well-defined unfortunate course. Impending HO is signaled by large painful swellings of highly vascular fibroproliferative tissue developing in various connective tissue sites. These lesions appear often spontaneously but may be triggered by minor trauma and even immunization injections. The lesions mature through endochondral ossification and lead to ankylosis of all major joints of axial and appendicular skeleton.

Pathogenesis

As demonstrated by Urist, formation of bone at ectopic sites is associated with the presence of BMP, so much attention and focus for pathogenesis has shifted to this molecule. The BMP signaling pathway and its dysregulation is considered primary to pathogenesis. FOP cells exhibit dysregulated expression of BMP4 along with reduced expression of BMP antagonists. There are also defects in internalization of BMP receptors causing prolonged/sustained stimulation signals. There appears also an associated increased activation of BMP downstream signaling to further add to the process of metaplasia of mesenchymal cells to osteogenic cells and excessive response to even physiological amounts of BMP present locally. The mutant *FOP* gene has been mapped to chromosome 2 in all sporadic and familial cases of classic *FOP* where point mutation from single nucleotide substitution (c.617G > A; R206H) occurs in the activin receptor A type I/activin-like kinase-2 (*ACVR1; ALK2*) gene. The *ACVR1* gene is involved with production of BMP type I receptors. The gene is found in muscles and cartilage also controlling their growth and development (including the normal ossification of cartilage during skeletal development). Due to structural changes, the receptor somehow is kept continuously on and also fails to internalize when the actual work is finished or not required. The disease development is influenced by both the genetic and environmental influences. Disease phenotype during prenatal development is strongly influenced by genetic factors while environmental factors determine the postnatal development of heterotopic ossification.

Clinical Features

The mesenchymal tissue such as the muscle and connective tissues like tendons and ligaments gets gradually ossified. Bone formation occurs outside the anatomical skeleton (i.e., heterotopic location). When forming around joints, it slowly constrains movement and produces joint stiffness. In terms of distribution of the disease, it has been seen that dorsal, axial, cranial, and proximal anatomic locations are involved before the development of disease in ventral, appendicular, caudal, and distal regions **(Figs. 94A and B)**. The disease starts from the neck and shoulders and flowing down the trunk and into the limbs. The loss of mobility resulting from joint stiffness is the primary disability. With the involvement of head and neck, the inability to fully open mouth from involvement of temporomandibular joints causes difficulty in speech and eating leading to malnutrition. Though the progression rate may vary among patients, most are bedridden

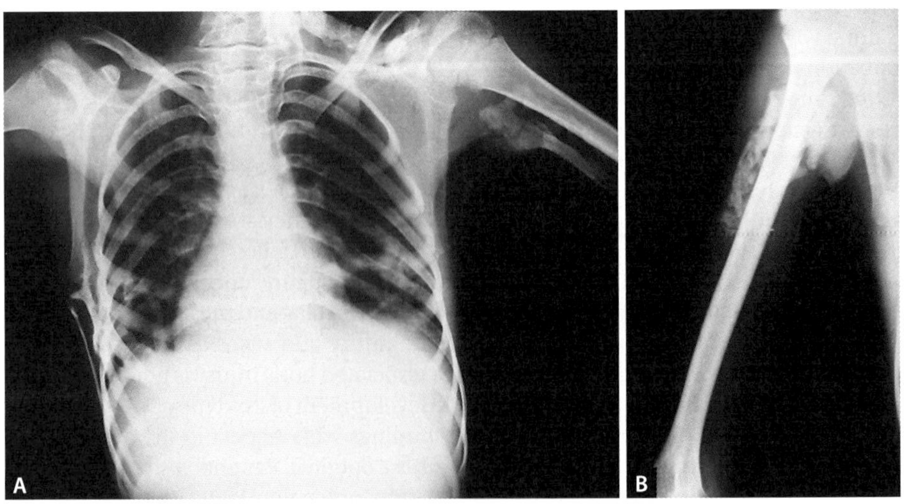

Figs. 94A and B: Fibrodysplasia proliferans progressiva (myositis ossificans). There is extensive bone formation around the (A) chest and (B) arm.

by early twenties and require life-long assistance in household activities and carrying out activities of daily living. During the early childhood, patients develop sporadic episodes of painful soft tissue swellings commonly mistaken for tumors that may spontaneously regress but often lead to bone formation in the connective tissue and muscles. The bone formation does not involve native bone, however, the HO spans the joints and mobile structures limiting their mobility. It is fortunate that the diaphragm, tongue, and intraocular muscles are spared in FOP; however, the mechanisms are elusive. Some phenotypic skeletal abnormalities that exist in patients with FOP include proximal medial tibial osteochondromas, clinodactyly, short broad femoral necks, orthotopic ankylosis of the costovertebral joints, and intercostal muscles/muscle ossification. The latter two features contribute to thoracic insufficiency syndrome. Sensorineural hearing loss due to involvement of cochlea or vestibulocochlear nerve may be seen but is often conductive due to middle ear ossification. Several other features have been described in variants and are grouped under atypical FOP plus. Such features include:

- Head and neck—sparse and atrophic scalp hair (prominent in 2nd decade), cognitive impairment and diffuse cerebral dysfunction causing seizures, craniopharyngioma, cerebellar abnormalities, and cerebral cavernous malformations.
- Ocular features—cataracts, retinal detachment, and childhood glaucoma.
- Skeletal features—synovial osteochondromatosis of hips and/or osteoarthritis, and polyostotic FD.
- Miscellaneous—growth retardation often severe, persistence of primary teeth in adulthood, primary amenorrhea, aplastic anemia, and hypospadias.

Differential Diagnosis

Differential diagnosis includes progressive osseous heteroplasia, Albright hereditary osteodystrophy, aggressive juvenile fibromatosis (histopathologically during intermediate stage), desmoid tumors, brachydactyly, and soft-tissue sarcoma.

Treatment and Prognosis

Most patients die early from restricted lung disease, pneumonia, malnutrition, and right-sided heart failure (thoracic insufficiency syndrome); however, some patients also live productive lives. Median lifespan is around 40 years. There is no treatment for this form of HO. Attempted removal of bone is followed by even more extensive bone formation. Limited benefits have been reported using corticosteroids (short 4-day course given early during acute flare-ups) and etidronate. These can be followed with NSAIDs to control further symptoms. Female patients that get pregnant suffer increased risk during pregnancy and should be appropriately counseled. They can get acute flare-ups, breathing difficulty in third trimester, necessary cesarean section, and risk of general anesthesia. The fetal risks include obviously FOP, prematurity, fetal distress, and cerebral palsy. Preventive strategies are the ones that should be stressed for most patients and include lifestyle modification, restriction of outdoor activity and impact sports in children to prevent trauma though it has risk of compromising independence. Use of household safety measures to prevent falls, protection from respiratory decline (incentive spirometry), etc., should be advised and practiced.

CONCLUSION

- Bone neoplasms represent a vast field of orthopedic subspecialty that requires extensive coordination with various other faculties for comprehensive management.
- Characterization of neoplasms into benign and malignant is essential but not easy as intermediate aggressive benign forms and subtle malignant forms are also seen.
- Patients should be managed only in specialized centers where all facilities for comprehensive management are available and to this end one should refer these patients to dedicated centers rather than doing half-hearted work and then referring with complications.
- Asymptomatic benign bone neoplasms with characteristic features only need observation and radiological surveillance but bone lesions with radiographs concerning malignancy and soft tissue lesions > 4 cm in diameter lying deep to fascia are indications for advanced imaging and referral to dedicated center.
- Biopsy of lesion is a critical step in patient workup and should be performed by the surgeon familiar with the procedure and will be majorly involved in the management of patient especially surgical resection.
- Osteosarcoma and Ewing sarcoma need multidisciplinary approach such as chemotherapy and appropriately timed surgical resection with or without radiation therapy. Chondrosarcoma is primarily a surgical disease and should be aptly planned for surgical resection because other modalities are not effective.
- Newer modalities like biological chemotherapy and molecular markers are being evaluated for better management and prognostication of these patients.
- Soft-tissue sarcomas are best treated by a combination of surgical resection and radiotherapy. Chemotherapy is not as effective.
- Metastatic disease is the most common malignancy affecting skeleton and remains a challenge till now. Surgeons need to appropriately understand the workup, surgical opportunities, and limitations to provide best suited care to the patient individually. Adjuvant therapy is advancing fast and should be properly updated.
- Future lies in providing complete cure to the patients even with metastatic disease with guided therapy.

CHAPTER 6

Osteonecrosis and Osteochondrosis

Manish Kumar Varshney

INTRODUCTION

Until now in the previous chapters we have learnt the various metabolic and neoplastic pathologies affecting the bones. These mainly pertain to the altered physiological and growth-related processes of the bone. We have also understood in Chapter on "Bone Structure, Physiology, Metabolism, and Associated Disorders" that bone being a living and metabolically tissue has its own independent blood supply. Disruption of this blood supply will produce effect similar to myocardial infarction (MI); so, it has been likened to "bone attack". There are characteristic similarities between MI and bone attack viz. variable area of involvement, slow revascularization (if at all), permanent damage in the form of aseptic necrosis [osteonecrosis (ON)] expected in part at least, protracted course of immediate and developing illness, etc. But unlike MI where immediate revascularization helps, this approach is not feasible for ON, instead we attempt to facilitate the regeneration process and support the collapsing bone. Replacing the dead bone is much easier that a heart transplant also so I think the utility of immediate diagnosis and "angioplasty-like treatment" has not been developed in orthopedics. This chapter describes pathophysiology of ON in detail along with common bone regions affected and their treatment options in detail. Some treatment options like arthrodesis that are also part of treating other diseases are covered wholly to avoid repetition elsewhere.

OSTEONECROSIS

Synonym: Avascular necrosis (AVN) of bone, bone infarction (used for metaphyseal or diaphyseal bone), aseptic necrosis of bone, ischemic bone necrosis (used for epiphyseal or subarticular bone), Chandler's disease (hip), and osteochondritis dissecans. The term bone infarction should not be used as ON is reserved for epiphyseal location of bone while bone infarction indicates the process at any location of bone.

Definition: Osteonecrosis is death of living elements of involved bone (cells including marrow) with progressive destruction and alteration of bone architecture as a result of compromised vascularity. The process is purely aseptic but may be incited by loss of vascularity from infection. ON was first described by Hippocrates circa 400 BC. Most of the earlier descriptions were pertaining to ON due to infection—osteomyelitis. First case of aseptic ON was described by Paget in 1970.

Etiology and Classification

First classification system is division of ON into primary (idiopathic) and secondary types (known factors for ON). Though intuitively based on etiological cause it lends little room for stratification of treatment and prognosis for treatment perspective.

Second system is used by pathologists that divide ON into medullary and corticomedullary infarction, the latter one is painful and represents classic ON. Medullary infarction may occur with reaming canal or by nutrient artery embolism. The system is hardly useful as the forms are difficult to identify clinically or radiologically.

Third one is commonly used by surgeons as it has treatment implications. This divides ON into traumatic and atraumatic causes and will be followed in the chapter. Traumatic injury to the vascularity of bone is the most common cause of ON. However, nontraumatic causes are also numerous and can be classified into various categories **(Box 1)**. There are fundamental differences between traumatic and nontraumatic ON that are central to decide current and future treatment options of a patient.

- While the traumatic ON is limited to the extent of initial trauma and disruption of vascularity, nontraumatic causes are progressive and keep progressing till the inciting agent is removed.
- Compromised vascularity due to trauma is often limited to single joint but is complete and it is final occurrence unless later another trauma occurs, it is unilateral or confined to region of injury.
- Nontraumatic causes are diffuse and can involve many bones and the area of ON may keep expanding with involvement of progressively nearby portions of bone in the process and even distant unrelated areas of bone may get involved later.

BOX 1: Etiological factors for development of osteonecrosis. Few factors are definitively (D) linked to development of osteonecrosis while others are still probable (P).

- *Trauma (D):*
  - Fracture neck of femur, fracture dislocation, dislocation of hip (anterior > posterior, but in absolute numbers posterior dislocation outnumber), acetabular fractures
  - Fracture proximal pole of scaphoid or through waist
  - Fracture through neck of talus
  - Fracture of femoral condyle in coronal plane (Hoffa's fracture)
  - Fracture capitellum and fracture lateral condyle of humerus (children)
- *Nontraumatic:*
  - Idiopathic
  - Genetic disorders (P) (with increasing recognition of them the term idiopathic will be ultimately dropped)
  - Drug induced
    - High-dose prolonged glucocorticoids (P)
    - Chemotherapy (D)
    - Alcohol (P)
    - Smoking (P) (>20 pack years)
    - Bisphosphonate use (P)
    - Organ transplantation (D-chemotherapy)
  - Dysbarism and gas emboli (D) (Caisson's disease)
  - Metabolic
    - Gaucher's disease (D)
    - Hyperuricemia (P)
    - Chronic renal failure (P)
    - Hepatic disorders (P)
    - Chronic pancreatitis (P)
    - Hypercholesterolemia and hyperlipidemia (P)
  - Endocrine and related disorders
    - Cushing's disease (P)
    - Pregnancy (P)
    - Hyperparathyroidism (P)
  - Hematological
    - Sickle cell anemia (D)
    - Thalassemia (P)
    - Myeloproliferative disorders (P)
    - Polycythemia (P)
  - Infection and autoimmune disease
    - Systemic lupus erythematosus and other connective tissue disorders (P)
    - Rheumatoid arthritis (P)
    - Human immunodeficiency virus (HIV) infection (P)*
    - Septic arthritis (P)
  - Irradiation (D)

*Osteonecrosis (ON) related to HIV infection is now considered secondary to use of antiretroviral drugs.

- Nontraumatic ON affects the fatty marrow that has reduced blood supply while it leaves the red marrow that contains good blood supply and ample osteoprogenitor cells. Traumatic ON, however, affects both equally.
- Nontraumatic ON is often bilateral and asymptomatic disease may indicate early-stage disease at some other place. In early stage, a specific region of the bone is usually involved like the anterosuperior region of femoral head.

A substantial number of cases have no identifiable etiologic factors for development of ON and have been referred as idiopathic. Few causes of nontraumatic ON have been studied in detail (detailed below) due to higher incidence and interest of researchers to understand the pathogenesis of disorder.

Steroid abuse: At the outset it should be mentioned that there has been *NO documented dose-dependent relation to ON with steroid use* and variously mentioned daily, yearly, or lifetime accrued values are mere speculations. It is interesting to note, however, that oral medication has been likened more frequently to development of ON than parenteral route. On the contrary though, cases of ON developing even after intra-articular administration have also been reported, however, higher doses of the drug consumed (>20 mg/day) early in few months have been related to higher chances of developing ON. Glucocorticoids are *the most common cause of nontraumatic ON*. The interest developed with identification of ON in a case report on a patient with rheumatoid arthritis in 1957. The increased incidence of ON world over appears to parallel the rise in glucocorticoid therapy for treatment of systemic conditions as well as organ transplantation. This lends strongest support to possible direct cause to affect relationship, also observation that the ON may regress if the medication is withdrawn early gives further support to pathogenesis. Patients receiving steroid therapy have an approximately 20-fold increase in their likelihood of developing ON. Clinically, the development of ON takes 6 months to 3 years from the onset of steroid therapy but MRI-based study has revealed development of lesion by around 3 months itself. The pathophysiology of development of ON pathway is still elusive.

Steroid-induced ON is caused by multiple factors that also influence each other during the process of ON development **(Flowchart 1)**. Mutations that affect intracellular steroid transport and metabolism have 9-fold increased risk of ON. These genes include multidrug resistance (MDR1/p-glycoprotein, ABCB1) and cytochrome p4503A (CYP3A4). Proposed hypothesis emphasizes small vessel occlusion by fatty emboli and increased impedance of sinusoidal blood flow secondary to a rise in intraosseous pressure (venous obstruction). This is proposed secondary to fatty infiltration following steroid therapy. Fatty infiltration may arise due to abnormality in bone marrow stem cell function, hyperlipidemia, etc. Abnormalities of lipid metabolism, vascular endothelial dysfunction, apoptosis of bone tissue, and importantly biomechanics of bipedal posture (as ON is not at all common in quadrupeds) are also responsible for development of ON. The following are some of the identified effects of steroids on bone tissue that has also been implicated in the development of ON:

- Glucocorticoid-induced *apoptosis of osteocytes* disrupting the osteocyte lacunar-canalicular system and dependent processes. The effect is considered to stem from increased oxidative stress in cells under the influence of corticosteroids. The same deleterious effect is seen in bone marrow stem cells due to generation of oxygen free radicals that prevent osteogenic differentiation by stimulating extracellular signal-regulated kinases (ERKs) and nuclear factor-κβ.
- *Adipocyte hypertrophy* has been observed in histologic specimens of human femoral heads following short treatment with dexamethasone along with hyperlipidemia, fatty liver, and systemic fat emboli for prolonged period. Fat embolism may be partially responsible for initial localized ON. High-dose

Flowchart 1: Proposed mechanism of development of osteonecrosis as a result of steroid intake/therapy (these are also the in-general effects of steroids on bones).

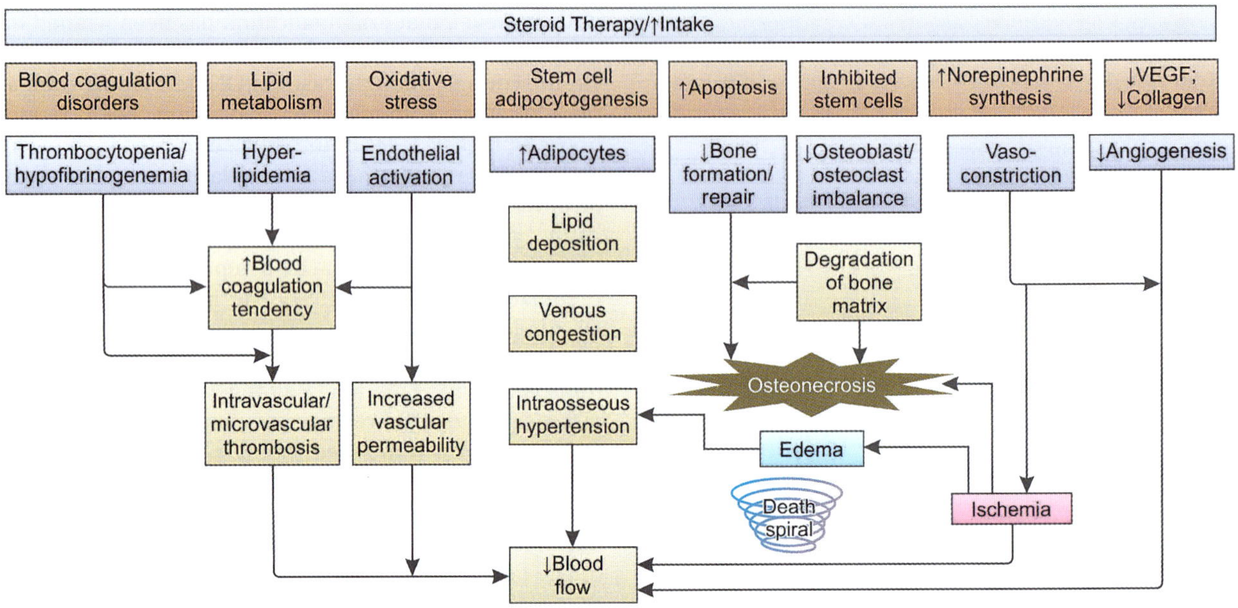

(VEGF: vascular endothelial growth factor)

corticosteroid is also associated with thrombocytopenia, hypofibrinogenemia and hyperlipidemia (increased circulating triglyceride and cholesterol). This results in a bit of blood glutiousness increasing likelihood of thrombosis to vascular walls where already damage due to lipid deposition has happened. *Intravascular coagulation* is one of the most preferred theories of development of ON.

- Dexamethasone induces the differentiation of bone marrow-derived stem cells into adipocytes, while *inhibiting differentiation of bone marrow-derived stem cells into osteoblasts* and osteogenesis. This is affected through activation of PPAR-gamma (peroxisome proliferator-activated receptor gamma adipose-specific 422 and adipsin) path and inhibition of Cbfa1/Runx2-dependent differentiation into osteogenic cells (*see* also Chapter on "Bone Structure, Physiology, Metabolism, and Associated Disorders"). Mesenchymal stem cells from patients with corticosteroid-induced ON of the femoral head have lower proliferative ability and bone regeneration capacity.
- Dexamethasone *inhibits expression of type-I collagen* and *osteocalcin* deteriorating the matrix quality. There is a suppression of osteoblast proliferation and bone resorption by suppression of the recruitment of osteoclasts precursors. This imbalance in osteoblast and osteoclast function causes degradation of bone matrix and ultimately osteoporosis.
- Prednisolone therapy has been found to *decrease bone density* and cancellous bone area while causing trabecular narrowing.
- *Damage to subchondral bone and articular cartilage damage:* In steroid treated animal models the thickness of subchondral bone has been found to be reduced predisposing to subchondral collapse. Articular cartilage also reduced in thickness and there is reduced proteoglycan concentration in the damaged region.
- Progressive ON results from *intraosseous hypertension* due to excessive marrow fat accumulation and adipogenesis in marrow. Increased recruitment of adipocytes results in reduction in the pool of stem cells available for osteoblast production. Dexamethasone has been shown to increase messenger ribonucleic acid (mRNA) expression of PPAR-γ enhancing adipogenesis while simultaneously it decreases mRNA expression of Cbfa1 inhibiting osteogenesis.
- Dexamethasone *impairs angiogenesis* by suppressing the production of vascular endothelial growth factor (VEGF) from osteoblasts. This impairs the reparative capacity of bone leading to progressive ON. This effect is both dose- and time-dependent for steroid therapy. Not only an impairment in neovascularization, corticosteroids have been also implicated in excessive Ca_2^+ uptake in vascular smooth muscles causing vasoconstriction. Increased intracellular calcium further downregulates the expression of nitric oxide synthase making vasoconstriction long lasting and ischemia independent.
- The vessels of bone also have *atypical response to local factors* under the influence of steroids causing local disturbance in blood flow. The vessels show an increased response to endothelin-1 (vasoconstrictor) and a decreased response to bradykinin (vasodilator).
- Lipid-lowering agents counteract the inhibitory effect of steroids on osteoblastic gene expression, and inhibit adipogenesis. Adrenocorticotropic hormone (ACTH) receptors are present on osteoblasts that enhance their proliferation when activated may protect against methylprednisolone induced ON.

Alcohol abuse: There is increased risk of femoral head ON in individuals consuming >400 mL of alcohol per week, but the dose effect is not documented and can vary as detailed below:

- Alcohol increases serum triglyceride and cholesterol levels along with liver and bone marrow fatty infiltration. Also, there is adipocyte hypertrophy and hyperplasia in the bone similar to that seen with steroids but the mechanism is different.
- Triglyceride deposition causes osteocyte pyknosis and ultimately death producing an increased percentage of empty osteocyte lacunae. Bone cells show diminished alkaline phosphatase activity and expression of osteocalcin under influence of ethanol.
- Chinese herb puerarin (antioxidative and antithrombotic) prevents alcohol-induced ON.

Hypercoagulability: Hypercoagulability (especially intravascular) as a cause of ON was first suggested by Paul Jones in 1992. Sickle cell disease, hereditary thrombophilia, and antiphospholipid antibodies syndrome are the classic examples. Formation and propagation of intravascular thrombi may be seen in these disorders. Additionally, the risk is increased by impaired fibrinolysis, hypersensitivity reactions, thromboplastin release during pregnancy, malignant tumors, and inflammatory bowel disease. Ethanol and corticosteroids promote intravascular coagulation producing fat emboli.

- It has been widely accepted that mutations in the factor V Leiden or the *prothrombin 20210A* gene are related to significant increased risk of ON (they are more prevalent and significantly related to ON than steroid or alcohol use).
- Similarly, protein C and protein S deficiencies have been associated with ON of the femoral head.
- Other identified factors for hypercoagulability and ON are gene polymorphisms resulting in increased activity of the *plasminogen activator inhibitor-1 (PAI-1)* gene, alterations in the methylenetetrahydrofolate reductase (MTHFR). They produce hypofibrinolysis and higher homocysteine and lipoprotein levels.

Genetic factors: With the recently identified correlation of hypercoagulability and ON, search for various genetic factors to join the intermediate chains of ultimate pathway to ON began. The mechanisms are many but unified concept linking is still elusive and will develop ultimately. Anomalies such as single nucleotide polymorphism (SNP) play a major role in the etiology and progression of ON due to genetic alterations in key components in the coagulation cascade including protein C, protein S, and PAI-1 as mentioned above. Other possible candidates with increased risk of ON are mentioned below:

- T-786C Drosophila nitric-oxide synthase (dNOS) SNP—this results in decreased activity of nitric oxide, which is responsible for promoting angiogenesis, bone formation, and inhibiting platelet aggregation.
- SNP of the transferrin (TF), vascular endothelial growth factor C (VEGFC), and sterol regulatory element-binding transcription protein (SREBP)-3 (IGFBP3). Angiotensin-I-converting enzyme (ACE) gene SNP is associated with increased chance of progression of steroid induced ON.
- SNP of SREBP-2 gene, interleukin receptor 23 gene, annexin gene family, catalase gene, and promoter polymorphisms in the VEGF gene.
- Polymorphisms in genes that inhibit the tissue factor pathway, vitamin D receptor (VDR) gene, the thymidylate synthase gene (TYMS), and the type II collagen A1 (COL2A1).
- Enhanced P-glycoprotein (P-gp) activity (C3435TT genotype) is associated with resistance to ON probably, this hastens steroid metabolism and clearance before development of ill-effects. SNP in G2677T/A and ABCB1 (c3435t) gene are related to increased sensitivity to steroid-induced ON.
- Genetic polymorphisms are also associated with alcohol-induced ON. Differences in the alcohol metabolizing enzyme genes may be responsible for development of ON due to different allele frequencies of ADH2*1 (alcohol dehydrogenase) and ALDH2*2 (aldehyde dehydrogenase).

Radiation necrosis: Osteoradionecrosis is the death of bone due to radiation. It commonly presents as a local area of bone necrosis in the form of "radiation osteitis".

- The necrosis is primarily induced by vasculitis caused by radiation that leads to thrombosis and occlusion.
- The capillaries are also damaged directly by radiation and endothelial damage makes them leaky. This leads to development of bone edema and further compromises vascular perfusion.
- The osteocytes and the delicate canalicular system get damaged by the high dose irradiation causing direct cell death.

Commonly, the complication is seen in mandible due to precarious blood supply and other risk factors; however, the development of this complication is by itself very rare. The risk of development of osteoradionecrosis is increased in:

- Persons with poor oral hygiene
- Radiotherapy >70 Gy
- Radiotherapy combined with chemotherapy
- Dental trauma or dental repair after completion of radiotherapy

The common symptoms of osteoradionecrosis include:

- Pain
- Joint stiffness and joint pains
- Swelling
- Sloughed skin or nonhealing ulcer
- Exposed necrotic bone
- Fracture at site of radiation not explained by trauma

The osteoradionecrosis is usually managed by debridement and sequestrectomy combined with microvascular reconstructive surgery with or without hyperbaric oxygen therapy (HBOT).

Pathophysiology of Osteonecrosis

Ultimately, ON occurs through one united reason, which is decreased blood flow to bone that leads to ischemia and death The pathogenesis of ON is characterized into four mechanisms: direct cellular toxicity (steroids/radiation), extraosseous (viz. trauma), intraosseous (hemorrhage/edema/marrow replacement), or intravsacular (viz. nitrogen bubbles and lipid emboli). The pathogenesis has not been fully documented and description is lacking due to noncongruence of the described mechanisms and variety of causes that can all not be linked to a common unified pathway. A lot of theories have been presented and accepted in literature in the past only to be superseded later by newer ones. These have nevertheless always supported and acted as ladder step in progress toward better understanding of the pathogenesis.

Older Concepts

- Phemister proposed "aseptic necrosis" as the main cause that results from fractures, radiation and vascular obstruction from thrombosis, or embolization. The concept of primary vascular involvement came later.
- Ficat proposed that ON is due to "compartment syndrome effect" of venous stasis producing ischemia.
- Chandler implicated vascular cause and compared ON to MI introducing the term "coronary disease of the hip" resulting from embolic phenomenon. He was incorrect though, as there is no defined relation of ON with increased age. With increased age the marrow spaces open up due to atrophy of resident adipocytes so in fact there is decreased resistance to blood flow, irrespective of arteriosclerosis.
- Atsumi suggested extraosseous interruption of the superior retinacular arteries and blocked revascularization in areas of subchondral collapse in the weight-bearing region. He was correct for traumatic ON.
- Glimcher and Kenzora, however, found no evidence of primary gross vascular injury and proposed primary metabolic cause to ON. He was partially correct for nontraumatic ON.

Currently, intraosseous hypertension, adipogenesis or embolism, and extravascular compression have all been accepted as mechanisms for development of idiopathic ON. In view of lack of unified single mechanism, support is lending to "multiple hit" theory, with accumulated insults from various causes reaching a critical threshold and initiating the disease process. A possible mechanism for common causes of ON has been presented **(Flowchart 2)**. Whatever may be the hypothesis there is hardly any explanation to

Flowchart 2: The etiopathogenesis of osteonecrosis—an integrated explanation of various proposed etiological causes. Also shown in green boxes are potential "points" of intervention and predominant mechanisms by which the medical interventions act to retard or break the process of ongoing osteonecrosis.

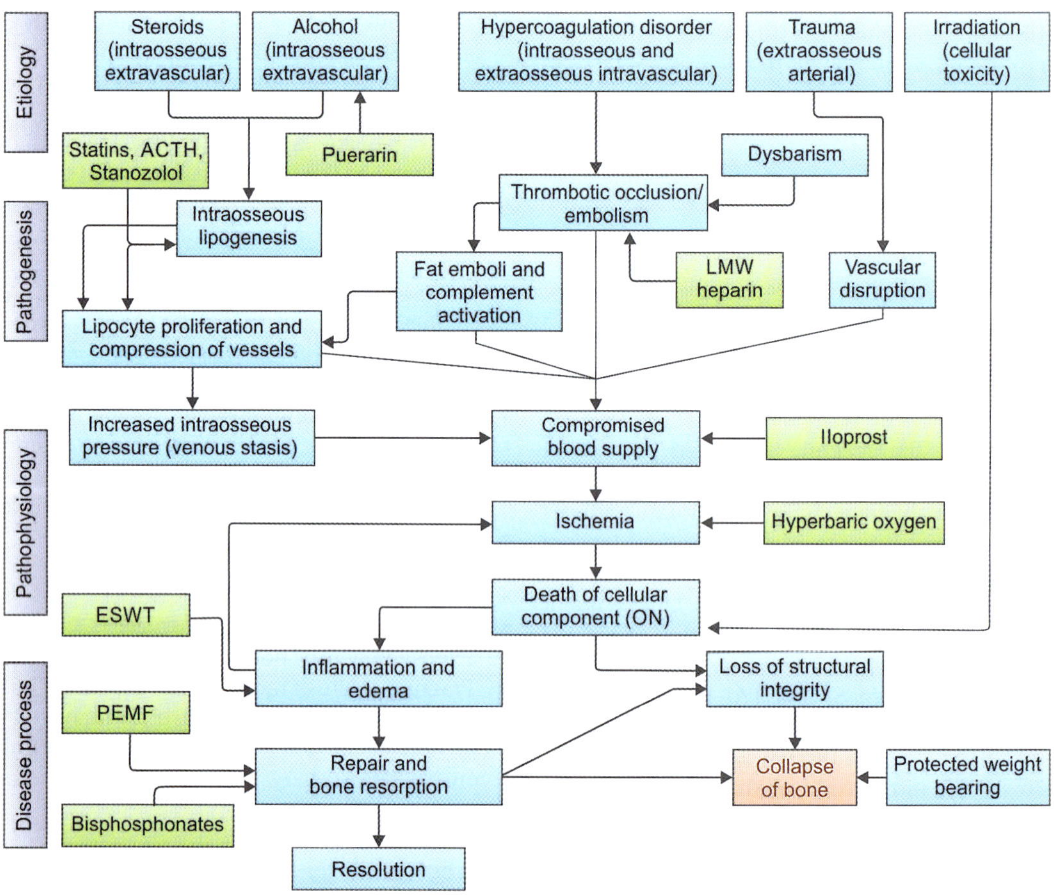

(ACTH: adrenocorticotropic hormone; ESWT: extracorporeal shock-wave lithotripsy; LMW: low-molecular weight; ON: osteonecrosis; PEMF: pulsed electromagnetic field)

occurrence of ON at specific sites of predilection that have been recognized for so long. By above mechanisms it is difficult to explain the occurrence of ON at femoral head or scaphoid or talus. So, the characteristics of these bones and occurrence of ON are discussed separately. There is one thing in common, however, that the blood supply is relatively poorly supplemented by the collateral circulation at these sites so even minimal injury or compromise to vasculature has higher chance of ON here.

OSTEONECROSIS OF FEMORAL HEAD

History and Epidemiology

The condition is a common cause of hip pain and frequently responsible for morbidity, if not recognized early. It represents somewhere around 3% of the hip pathologies with the prevalence peaking around 3rd to 5th decade for nontraumatic ON. The age group of peak incidence is gradually shifting up (older population) due to more justified usage of corticosteroids and steroid sparing drugs. Advancements in management of autoimmune disorders (vasculitis, neurological, and renal disorders), human immunodeficiency virus (HIV) infection, and transplant medicine have resulted in improved life-expectancy and hence larger number of patients with advanced ON. It is responsible for 6–29% of all total hip arthroplasties presently with the numbers bound to increase. The male to female ratio is around 3:1 for nontraumatic ON but it should be higher for traumatic ON and males seem to suffer high velocity injuries more. It is one of the few disorders that when recognized early can be effectively managed to prevent disability and protracted treatment later. Konig noted the condition in 1888 but somehow named it as osteochondritis dissecans. Vascular occlusion as a cause of bone necrosis was thought to be the primary cause of ON and term "AVN" became popular. Later numerous causes of traumatic ON were described but attention to idiopathic ON was drawn by Haenish in 1925. Bone necrosis may still occur in presence of adequate vascularity due to microcirculation changes or direct cell death, so the term "AVN" is inappropriate to describe the whole gamut of the disorder. "ON" is a better term to be used in the descriptive sense that also relates to the ultimate pathology.

Blood Supply of Femoral Head and the "Starling Resistor" Concept

The blood supply of femoral head is peculiar and vulnerable to injuries so it needs a detailed discussion for understanding the cause and effect of post-traumatic ON.

The blood supply to *femoral head* **(Fig. 1)** is derived from three primary sources (as described by Crock), the metaphyseal system, retinacular system, and the foveolar system as follows:

- *Extracapsular arterial ring (ECA):* This is the chief system giving rise to both intramedullary and extramedullary arterial systems. The ECA gives less prominent metaphyseal branches to intertrochanteric region which also supply the head through neck (intramedullary metaphyseal system). It is located at the base of femoral neck and is formed:
    - Posteriorly by branch of medial circumflex femoral artery

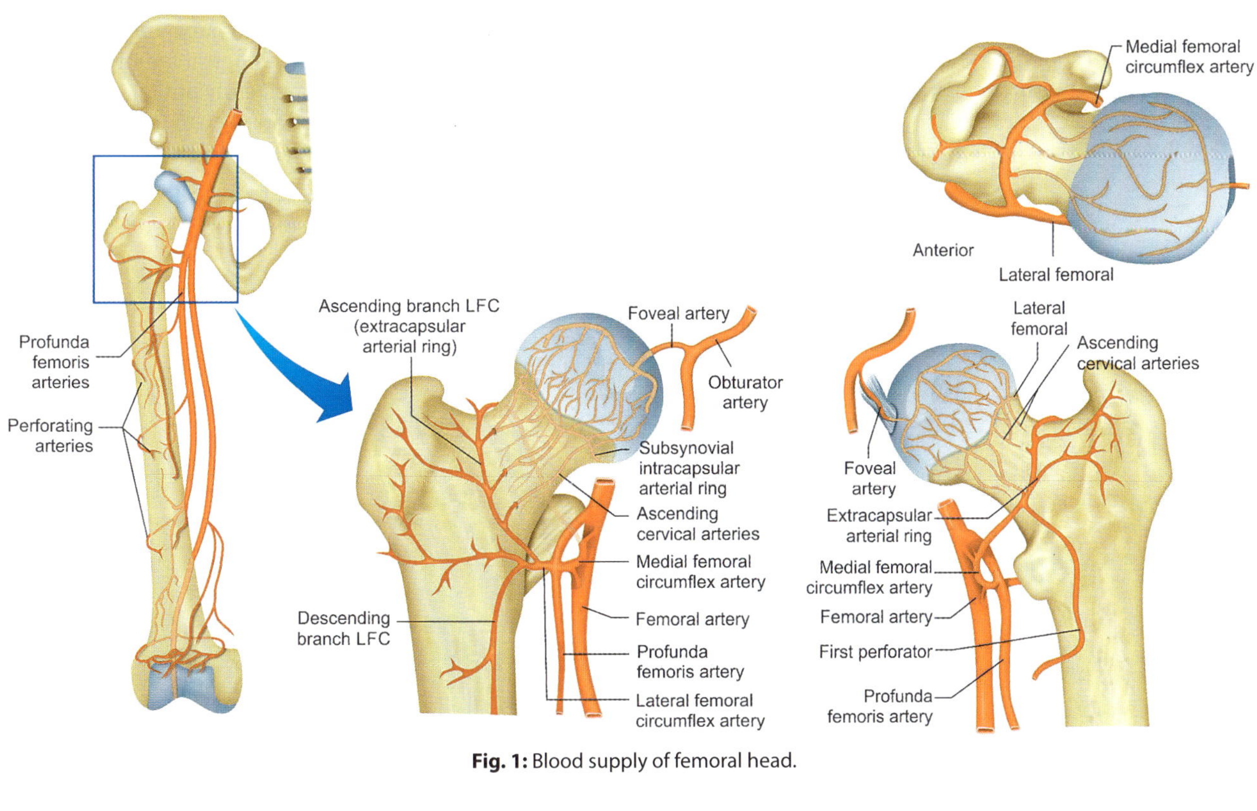

Fig. 1: Blood supply of femoral head.

- Anteriorly by branch of lateral circumflex femoral artery more often a branch of profunda femoris artery (main branch of femoral artery)
- Ascending cervical branches of ECA (also known as epiphyseal arteries of Trueta or retinacular arteries) that arise from ECA (more prominent system) and ascend up the neck partly also supplying the neck in due course:
  - Divided into anterior, posterior, medial, and lateral groups.
  - Anteriorly, these vessels penetrate the capsule at intertrochanteric line while, posteriorly they pass underneath the orbicularis fibers of the capsule.
  - Lateral group (*lateral ascending cervical vessels)* is the most important group carrying major portion of blood supply to head and neck of femur.

- *Subsynovial intra-articular arterial ring of Chung* (*Circulus articuli vasculosus of Hunter)* is formed from lateral ascending cervical vessels:
  - Located at the margins of articular cartilage on surface of neck of femur
  - It is either a complete or incomplete ring
  - Provides epiphyseal vessels (that penetrate the head just outside the articular cartilage to supply major portion of head)
- Artery of ligamentum teres
  - Branch of obturator artery (more often) or medial circumflex femoral artery
  - Variable supply in adults
  - Supply head around the region of fovea

The metaphyseal *femoral neck* is well vascularized in comparison and is supplied by a cruciate-shaped anastomosis between:

- Branches from ascending cervical arteries
- Branches from subsynovial intra-articular arterial ring
- Intramedullary branches of superior nutrient artery system
- Metaphyseal vessels from intertrochanteric region

"Starling Resistor" Concept of Femoral Head

The femoral head (in fact metaphyseal regions of most long bones) functions as a starling resistor. This is a concept to explain the regulation of flow through flexible tubes or pipes by fixing them in a limited volume shell with rigid shell or walls. When the fixed volume shell is filled with fluid, increased, pressure leads to collapse of the passing flexible tubes and the flow through them stops or is reduced. Thus, by controlling the volume of contained liquid in fixed volume space, and hence the pressure inside the shell the flow from tubes is controlled. The femoral head in similar way is bound by rigid shell of cortical bone. The blood vessels inside make a closed loop system which is influenced by the changes in bone marrow pressure **(Fig. 2)**. It is found that in the pathological femoral heads the bone marrow pressure is increased or at higher normal range at resting position and also rise suddenly on minimal increase in fluid volume. This increase in the volume occurs physiologically during activity where the fluid leaks from vessels into marrow space. If the marrow is occupied by pathological tissue like adipocytes as is seen in steroid therapy or alcoholic patients there will be less space available for this physiological fluid and the pressure will suddenly rise inside the closed shell. This increase in pressure will mitigate the flow from vascular system of the femoral head producing ischemia. This intraosseous hypertension has been proposed to develop from various inciting causes and is considered the principal cause of ischemia in nontraumatic ON.

The tests for hemodynamic function can diagnose subtle ischemia before any radiological investigations are positive. Intramedullary pressure in the femoral head normally measures 10–20 mm Hg at rest. In response to saline challenge the pressure rises by 15–20 mm Hg normalizing quickly. The patient is also asymptomatic and does not feel pain on saline challenge. In pathological femoral heads, the resting pressures are not elevated early but later in course of still asymptomatic disease they are seen to be higher by three to four times normal. The saline challenge is also significant

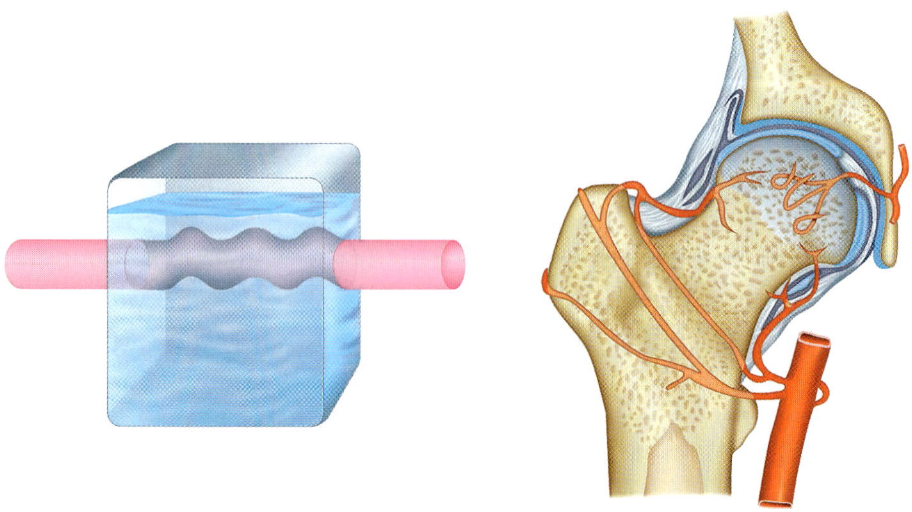

Fig. 2: Starling resistor.

in that the rise in intraosseous pressure is sudden, sharp, and sustained (till 100 mm Hg) and the patient feels pain in the involved hip. If venography is performed, the dye will not mark the small vessels and the distribution is limited to central proximal regions only. The prominence is also slow to develop.

Clinical Presentation

The process of bone infarction is usually asymptomatic and patient hardly ever notices it in early stages, especially the traumatic cases as the trauma overshadows other disease processes. Pain in the affected joint is typically the presenting symptom of ON and is true for most nontraumatic causes of ON. Some patients are totally asymptomatic and have no pain (identified only due to presence of ON in other hip). The reason may be related to size and site of ON lesion. Small lesions <25% of the femoral head located in medial one-third region are less likely to be symptomatic. Larger more lateral lesions are commonly symptomatic and likely to collapse. The pain appears with mobilization and is usually more on standing and walking commonly localized to groin or the buttock region. Continuous pain is uncommon. Some patients may have night pains also. Frequently the ON is recognized on radiographs done for other purposes. The patient notices gradual increase in pain and slowly developing limp that initially subsides with analgesics to only worsen and become nonresponsive later. With collapse of femoral head, the movements of the hip diminish, especially the flexion, abduction, and internal rotation. The clinician should specifically enquire about the prior medications and radiation treatment, metabolic diseases, ischemic pathologies, antitubercular therapy received in past, HIV infection, smoking, and alcohol abuse. ON associated with HIV infection was previously thought to be due primarily to HIV infection *per se* but is now considered secondary to antiretroviral treatment and its incidence is thought to rise significantly in near future. In any case the attending physician should have high index of suspicion for ON as there are no pathognomonic signs for early disease. It is imperative to realize that in nontraumatic causes the *other hip* should be given due attention. Only a few cases may spontaneously regress with resolution of the symptoms, but in them the diagnosis could hardly ever be established. With progression to deformity the pain is present at rest and ultimately the symptoms and signs of osteoarthritis develop in the joint.

Differential Diagnosis

The clinical differential diagnosis is quite broad but the important differentials to keep in mind are:

- Femoroacetabular impingement
- Tuberculosis (TB) of the hip joint
- Labral tear
- Stress fracture of femoral head or neck
- Cartilage disorders and formation of loose bodies and osteochondromatosis
- Transient osteoporosis of the hip joint
- Monoarticular rheumatoid arthritis
- Dysplasia

Evaluation

Radiographs (Fig. 3A)

The bones are radiologically silent in early stages. After a lag of 3–4 months from the onset of symptoms they progressively demonstrate:

- Osteopenia is seen early in the course of disease due to hypervascularity.
- Sclerosis (diffuse) and density changes of the involved region which is invariably the proximal region of the involved bone. This represents gross loss of vascularity, and hence suspended remodeling process. The sclerosis results from initially increased osteoblastic activity suspended remodeling and bone resorption and relative osteopenia of the surrounding bone due to hyperemia.
- Cystic changes and development of irregular dense areas. This represents the attempt at repair by the body

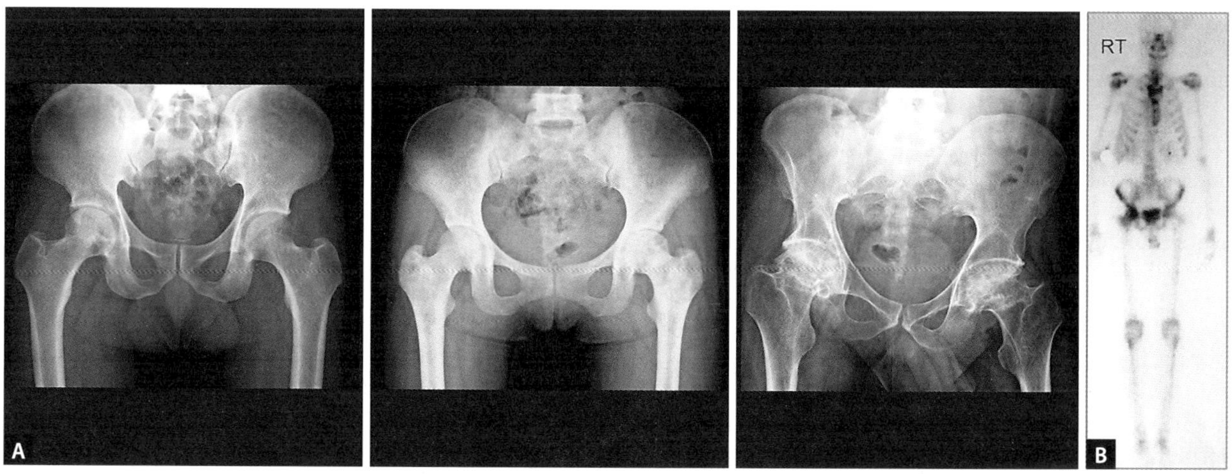

Figs. 3A and B: (A) Osteonecrosis of femoral head showing progressive radiographic features; (B) Scintigraphy scanning picture of a patient with osteonecrosis of femoral head right hip. The scan shows increased uptake in right femoral head without corresponding increase in vascularity. Apart from osteonecrosis, chronic inflammation is a close differential in such finding.

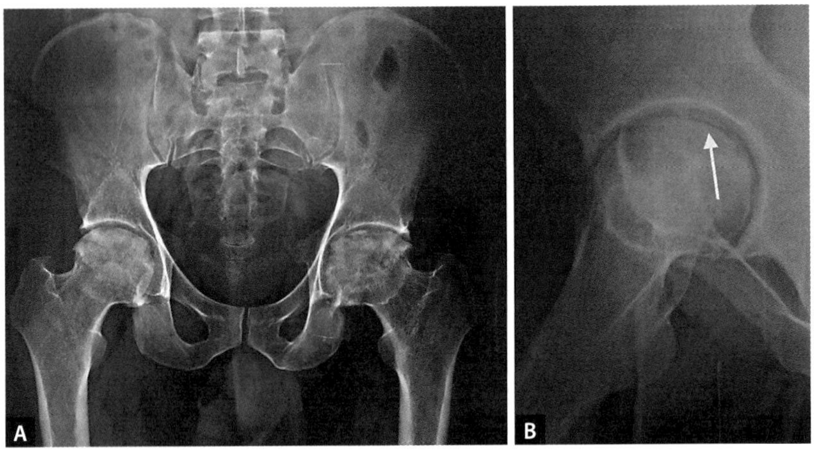

Figs. 4A and B: Osteonecrosis of both hips (A) in a patient with typical crescent sign seen on lateral (B) projection (arrow).

resorbing the bone irregularly with unresorbed areas in between

- Development of subchondral lucencies (crescent sign) and impending collapse **(Figs. 4A and B)**.
- "Half-moon sign" on radiographs represent subchondral fracture and collapse. It should be understood that *collapse is NOT due to reduced vascularity or bone necrosis but mainly due to reparative activity of the regenerative tissue that absorbs the bone and causes weakness and collapse*. Thus, collapse comes late otherwise it should have been present from start if it was due to bone necrosis itself. There are two types of reparative mechanisms that get activated in the femoral head of ON patients. First is the appositional bone formation initiated by osteoblast like cells around necrotic trabeculae that produces reparative osteogenesis, the other one is the destructive repair that is creeping of granulation tissue along the necrotic trabeculae to cause increased bone resorption. The latter form predominates in most patients causing collapse.
- Loss of shape, form, and flattening of the bone then follows
- Secondary arthritis of the joint develops as an end result
- In talus, the appearance of radiolucency in dome indicates "good prognosis"— appearance of vascularity and resulting resorption.

Scintigraphic Scanning (Fig. 3B)

In the initial radiographically silent but clinically painful stage, there is increased vascularity of the affected bone. This is also supplemented with increased osteoblastic activity. Thus, the disease process can be picked up by scintigraphic scan that depend on the metabolic activity of bone.

- Central cold spot is surrounded by peripheral hot region—the resolution of the image should be high "doughnut sign (cold in hot)". It indicates reactive bone formation or granulation tissue developing in the periphery of necrotic or metabolically silent bone. The study should be done using pinhole collimation and *single-photon emission computed tomography* (SPECT) with scatter correction and iterative reconstruction algorithms.
- Later, the area becomes grossly hyperemic with development of reparative tissue and development of osteoarthritic changes.

Magnetic Resonance Imaging

This is the most sensitive (nearly 100%) and specific (90%) investigation to evaluate occurrence of ON or differentiating the disease process from other related disorders.

- There is decreased signal intensity in the subchondral region on both T1- and T2-weighted images **(Figs. 5A to D)** in early stage localized to medial aspect of femoral head causing appearance of cortical thickening (false). Though nonspecific this is the most common finding.
- In next stage of reparative process, the reactive zone shows ring or band of low-signal intensity on T1-weighted scans in subchondral bone appearing high-signal intensity on T2-weighted scans due to edema of reparative or granulation tissue (double-line sign). This finding is diagnostic for ON.
- There can be straightening or depression of the subchondral bone, fluid-filled subchondral fractures (equivalent to the half-moon sign), and geodesic formation.
- *Prognostically* a benign course is indicated by absence of a focal depression of the subchondral bone and absence of deep low-intensity lines. The region is likely to collapse if the involved area exceeds 5 cm^2.

Necrotic lesions are classified into four types, based on their location on T1-weighted images or X-ray images.

1. Type A lesions occupy the medial one-third or less of the weight-bearing portion.
2. Type B lesions occupy the medial two-thirds or less of the weight-bearing portion.
3. Type C1 lesions occupy more than the medial two-thirds of the weight-bearing portion but do not extend laterally to the acetabular edge.
4. Type C2 lesions occupy more than the medial two-thirds of the weight-bearing portion and extend laterally to the acetabular edge.

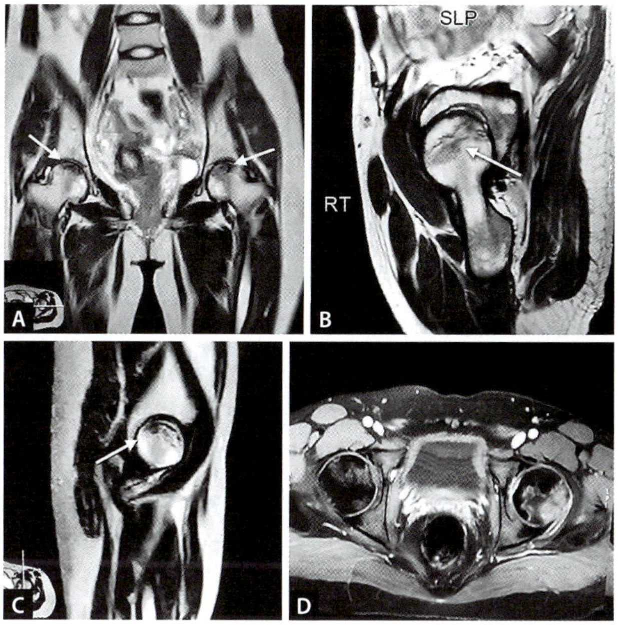

Figs. 5A to D: MRI of osteonecrosis (ON) femoral head. The images show geographical area of destruction in the anterosuperior portion of both femoral heads (stage "C" on right and stage "D" on left on Mitchell grading), surrounded by a low signal intensity lesion in T1-weighted images (arrows, A). Double line sign is evident as an outer low-intensity rim and inner high-intensity band (arrow, B). Crescentic sign is visible as a subchondral fracture (arrow, C). Post-gadolinium images show irregular peripheral enhancement all along the inflammatory changes (D).

Computed Tomography Scan

This is of limited utility now and was used when MRI was not easily available:

- The central dense sclerotic bone appears as "asterisk sign".
- This is a good modality to assess the extent of collapse or the severity of secondary degenerative joint disease and calcification but is superseded by MRI now.

Bone Biopsy

This is the best confirmatory method but mainly intended for research purpose. The histology is diagnostic and can be used exceptionally to settle any debate.

- Presence of marrow infarction and anucleate bony trabeculae are characteristic
- Granulation tissue surrounding areas of bone necrosis
- Areas of creeping substitution and sequestrum formation similar to the ones seen in osteomyelitis
- Fatigue fractures and collapse of subchondral bone cartilage disruption and joint deformity

Guidelines for prescribing radiological investigations:

- A patient at risk for ON develops hip pain. The initial examination should consist of an anteroposterior (AP) pelvis and frog-leg lateral radiograph of the symptomatic hip.
- If the radiograph findings are definite for ON, an MRI is indicated only in clinically suspected and nontraumatic ON cases to judge status of other hip. 80% of asymptomatic hips with an ON lesion on MRI eventually become symptomatic. 90% of asymptomatic hips without an ON lesion on MRI will remain asymptomatic.
- If the radiographic findings are equivocal for ON or are normal on the symptomatic side, then MRI is indicated to confirm the diagnosis of ON and to exclude other differentials.
- If MRI cannot be performed, a bone scan with SPECT imaging is a reasonable alternative.
- Screening of a patient who is at high-risk for ON may be of value *only* if prophylactic treatment of asymptomatic ON is proven useful.

TABLE 1: Modified Ficat and Arlet staging of osteonecrosis of femoral head (can also be used to stage talus and femoral condyle osteonecrosis). The original staging system was a 3-part staging to which 4th stage was added by Ficat himself. Later the modification in the form was stage 0 and subclassification of stage 2 into "A" and "B" came up.

Stage	*Symptoms and signs*	*X-ray*	*Bone scan*
0 (Preclinical)	None	–	↓ uptake
I (Preradiographic)	None or mild	–	↓ uptake
II	Mild	Altered density A. (Precollapse) Sclerosis or cysts or normal joint line, normal head contour B. (Early collapse) crescent sign (subchondral fracture), flattening	↑ uptake
III (Collapse)	Mild to moderate	Loss of sphericity, collapse	↑ uptake
IV (Osteoarthritis)	Moderate to severe	↓ Joint space, acetabular changes	↑ uptake

Staging

Different staging systems have been proposed for ON of femoral head. The systems differ on the use of diagnostic modalities for disease progression. Oldest system was based on the Ficat and Arlet observation from France in 1960s of the progressive radiological changes. This was then modified later in 1970s **(Table 1)**. A comprehensive system was developed from university of Pennsylvania that included MRI in the staging and classification and subclassified according to the region of involvement and extent of the disease **(Table 2)**. The presence of crescent and collapse has not been very well correlated and it has been often found difficult by the orthopedic surgeons as to where to place an X-ray showing crescent. Crescent heralds collapse and is found to quickly develop presenting with collapse rather than before collapse. The "international classification" has combined the two stages (3 and 4) of the Steinberg classification to resolve the issue and also presence of advanced or early

TABLE 2: Steinberg (University of Pennsylvania) classification system for osteonecrosis (ON) of femoral head.

Stage	Clinical and laboratory findings
Stage 0	• Asymptomatic • Radiography or magnetic resonance imaging or scintigraphy normal • Histology or intraosseous pressure measurement only demonstrate osteonecrosis • Used for staging the other normal hip in a diagnosed case of ON hip
Stage I	• Symptoms ± • Radiography and CT scan commonly unremarkable Histology findings are abnormal • Avascular necrosis diagnosed on MRI (or bone scan) and subclassified as percentage of area involved (MRI only): – IA: <15% (minimal) – IB: 15–30% (moderate) – IC: >30% (severe)
Stage II	• Patient is symptomatic (see text) • Radiographs may show osteopenia, osteosclerosis, or cysts subchondral radiolucency is absent • Magnetic resonance imaging findings are diagnostic and subclassified as for stage I
Stage III (critical stage)	• Patient is symptomatic • Radiographic findings include subchondral lucency (crescent sign) and subchondral collapse. The shape and form of the head is maintained • The stage is critical as treatment for restoration surgeries are helpful • Subclassification depends on the extent of crescent on MRI or radiographs: – Stage IIIa: <15% of the articular surface – Stage IIIb: 15–30% of the articular surface – Stage IIIc: >30% of the articular surface
Stage IV	• Flattening or collapse of femoral head is present Joint space may be irregular • CT scanning is more sensitive than radiography Subclassification depends on the extent of collapsed surface (radiographs only): – Stage IVa: <15% of surface is collapsed – Stage IVb: Approximately 15–30% of surface is collapsed – Stage IVc: >30% of surface is collapsed
Stage V	• Radiography findings show changes of secondary osteoarthritis (narrowing of joint space, sclerosis of acetabulum, and marginal osteophytes) • Subclassification is done on X-ray for region of narrowing joint space: Medial, central, and lateral
Stage VI	Findings include extensive osteoarthritic changes and destruction of the femoral head and joint

osteoarthritis does not necessarily change the management so the stages 5 and 6 have also been combined. This system developed by Association of Research Circulation Osseous (ARCO) **(Table 3)** is the current standard to classify and stage the ON of femoral head that should be followed. It is interesting to note that the system looks very similar to Ficat system but crescent and collapse are in stage 3 and not in stage 2B. The stage 4 may need to be split again as the newer cartilage reconstruction strategies have necessitated the early osteoarthritis changes that can be possibly controlled by these methods.

With the development of osteotomy as treatment method it was recognized that the type of osteotomy, its prognosis, and planning depend on the location and extent of necrotic lesion. This subclassification is not properly addressed by any of the classification systems. So, Kerboul et al. developed a system of measuring the arc of articular surface **(Fig. 6)**

TABLE 3: Association of Research Circulation Osseous (ARCO), staging of osteonecrosis of femoral head. This was partial adaptation of the University of Pennsylvania classification but the stages 3 and 4 were combined as the stages 5 and 6. This is based on rationale that crescent sign is almost always associated with some collapse (stages 3 and 4) and osteoarthritis (stages 5 and 6) need not be stratified.

Stage	Radiological features
Stage 0	• All present diagnostic techniques are normal or nondiagnostic. • Only pressure measurements would reveal increased intraosseous pressure, at this stage patient is asymptomatic. • This could be the stage of normal contralateral hip • (Future diagnostic techniques like measurement of resistance to flow may help diagnosing this stage).
Stage 1	• Plain X-ray and CT scan are normal • At least one of the scintigraphy or MRI is positive • An open biopsy will confirm the diagnosis • This stage is subdivided in three categories according to the LOCATION (MRI only) of the lesion and the extension of the lesion under weight-bearing dome of the acetabulum – Medial – Central – Lateral • For further study and follow-up on the results of different forms of treatment and the development of the disease, QUANTITATION (MRI only) can be added. This quantitation is a calculation of the area of femoral head involvement: – Minimal: <15% – Moderate: 15–30% – Extensive: >30%
Stage 2	• Radiographs show areas of abnormalities: Porosis, sclerosis, osteolysis, and focal lysis. • The femoral head remains spherical on anteroposterior (AP) and lateral views on X-ray and CT-scan. Again, scintigraphy and MRI are positive. There is NO subchondral fracture or CRESCENT SIGN or flattening. Subclassification is important, as described in stage 1.
Stage 3	• CRESCENT SIGN visible on the X-ray. The femoral head fails mechanically. • The X-ray (usually more prominent on lateral film) shows a fine radiolucent subchondral fracture line, usually referred to as the "crescent sign". Progressive flattening of the femoral dome will occur. Late radiographs show the articular surface of the femoral head to be flattened, but there is no evidence of joint line narrowing or acetabular involvement. • Subclassification and quantitation (X-ray or CT-scan) is added, but quantitation can also be done by the calculation of the amount of flattening of the femoral dome. • First, it is determined whether the crescent sign appears more prominent in the AP or lateral view. After selection of the most prominent view the length of the crescent is expressed as a percentage of the entire articular surface. • Minimal = <15% involvement or a depression of <2 mm • Moderate = 15–30% involvement or a depression of 2–4 mm • Extensive = >30% involvement or a depression of more than 4 mm
Stage 4	• Appearance of osteoarthritis • The joint-space starts narrowing • This is progressively associated with changes on the acetabular side of the joint and with signs of a beginning osteoarthritis with areas of sclerosis, cysts, and marginal osteophytes. Later on, the radiographic examinations show advanced degenerative changes, and finally, a complete joint destruction is seen.

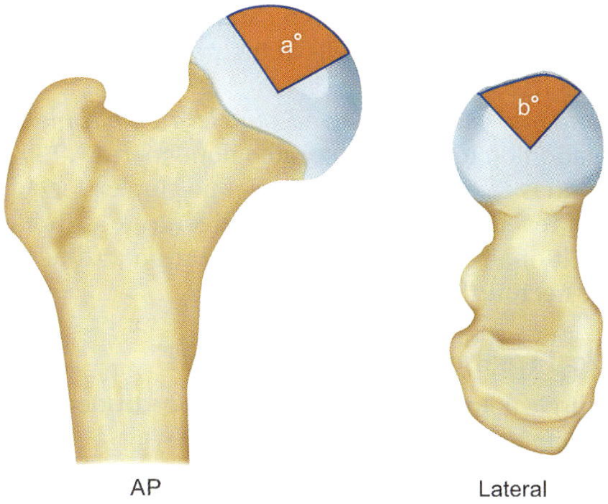

Fig. 6: Kerboul angle = area in angle on AP (a°) + area in angle (b°) in lateral image (MRI or X-ray). (AP: anteroposterior; MRI: magnetic resonance imaging)

involved in AP and lateral radiographs of the femoral head. This is called the combined necrotic angle (CNA) as the arcs on two views are added up and is now better assessed by MRI (though originally demonstrated on radiograph). Original classification was proposed on radiographs where he divided the necrotic region into small, medium, and large regions:

- Small ≤160°
- Medium 161–199°
- Large 200 or more degrees.

The modified classification based on MRI (as measured on midsagittal and midcoronal images) has much higher values as the MRI overestimates the necrotic region:

- Grade 1 is <200°
- Grade 2 is 200–249°
- Grade 3 is 250–299° and grade 4 is >400°

The system has also been used to predict the possibility of collapse of articular surface:

- Combined necrotic angle <190° = low risk for collapse
- Combined necrotic angle 190–240° = moderate risk
- Combined necrotic angle >240° = high risk for collapse

Diagnostic criteria for ON head of femur (2001 revised Japanese criteria, the older criteria were too many and correlation was poor): Two of the following five criteria make disease condition eligible for diagnosis of ON head of femur.

1. Collapse of the femoral head (including crescent sign) without joint-space narrowing or acetabular abnormality on X-ray images.
2. Demarcating sclerosis in the femoral head without joint-space narrowing or acetabular abnormality.
3. "Cold in hot" on bone scans.
4. Low-intensity band on T1-weighted MRI (band-like pattern).
5. Trabecular and marrow necrosis on histology.

Management

The current management is surgical only and is accepted universally. Only a few patients may be managed conservatively bearing specific indications as follows:

- Comorbidities precluding surgery
- Primary lesion is so advanced that joint preservation (stage 3 and above, ARCO) is of no use but patients symptoms do not warrant arthroplasty
- Surgery refused

The *conservative management* includes protecting the hip from transmitted forces and adjuvant therapy:

Protected weight-bearing: This is used to reduce the forces normally transmitted across the hip joint and provide symptomatic relief. Also, this may delay the appearance of osteoarthritis though the natural course of disease is not altered. Protected weight-bearing is an integral part of surgical management of ON with the hip preserving methods to definitively protect the hip during healing or revascularization phase. The indications for protected weight-bearing can be summarized as follows:

- *Definitive:*
  - Following hip joint preserving surgery for ON of femoral head.
  - As a part of conservative management where patient is waiting for definitive management like arthroplasty. This will reduce pain and possibly delay progression of osteoarthritis.
  - Refused surgery, medically unfit to undergo surgery.
- *Alternative:*
  - Deciding to undergo surgery
  - Small lesions

Adjuvant therapy: This entails primarily the use of pharmacotherapy and certain unconventional methods to support or improve the healing process and sometimes supplement the definitive management. The role of definitive measures to improve the disease process is unsure:

- *Analgesics:* They should be judiciously used while reinforcing the need of definitive management.
- *Bisphosphonates:* They have been found to give symptomatic relief from pain and improved quality of life. The rate of collapse has been found lower with the therapy but the effect does not seem to provide critical level of cure enough to replace surgical management. It is interesting to note that bisphosphonates themselves cause ON (BRONJ) of jaw. They probably protect the bone from resorption during healing phase but how sound a bone will form in healing then is unclear without resorption. The effect is akin to homeopathic treatment where the poison of a disease is itself the cure for it!
- *Patients with hyperlipidemias:* Lipid-lowering agents and stanozolol have been found to provide symptomatic benefit and curative effect.
- *Patients with coagulopathies:* Warfarin, low-molecular-weight heparin, and stanozolol have been found to be effective to some extent.
- Transplant patients have been found to get relief from calcium channel blockers but the mechanism is not clear. Nifedipine has by itself also been reported to give symptomatic relief in patients of ON.
- Injectable prostacyclin (PGI_2) analog iloprost has reported relief in isolated study on ON femoral head due to its vasoactive effects.

- *Use of pulsed electromagnetic fields (PEMF):* There have been anecdotal reports of use of PEMF either with core decompression or alone (stage 1 and 2, ARCO). Improvements have been reported in the disease process though confirmation and concrete evidence is lacking. The beneficial effects may be due to following reasons:
  - In short-term implicated to chondroprotective effect from reduced inflammation and reduction of bone edema protecting the perfusion.
  - In long-term the PEMF may promote the osteogenic activity at necrotic area (*see* also methods to enhance fracture repair) and prevent trabecular fracture. This may also prevent collapse of the necrotic fragment.
  - The induction of cell differentiation and production of matrix protein synthesis has been proposed as a mechanism of prevention of progression or development of steroid induced ON as the effects are opposite to that of steroid on osteoblasts.
- *Use of extracorporeal shockwaves in management of ON:* Shock waves may cause neovascularization and cause expression of angiogenic growth factors but the exact mechanism is unclear. It has been compared to core decompression and found to improve function of hip to a greater extent. Longer term follow-up of patients demonstrated threefold reduction in conversion to arthroplasty as compared to core decompression + nonvascularized fibular grafting.
- *Hyperbaric oxygen therapy (HBOT):* Acts by targeting the underlying pathophysiology of femoral head necrosis (FHN). In early stages, HBOT facilitates oxygenation of hypoxic tissue and reduces edema through creating a high concentration of dissolved oxygen and inducing vasoconstriction. This gives early pain relief. HBOT promotes better oxygenation of ischemic bone cells, irrespective of the circulating hemoglobin and without the need for the energy required for dissociation of oxygen from hemoglobin promoting bone resorption, revascularization and osteogenesis. The patients are generally exposed to compressed oxygen at 2.5 atmospheres absolute (ATA) for 45–100 treatment sessions each one lasting around 80 minutes.
- *Bone marrow injections (Hernigou):* This technique of bone marrow grafting is used as a method to augment and better the poor results of core decompression. The bone marrow is aspirated from anterior iliac crest and placed in bags. The pooled aspirate 150 mL is filtered to remove fat and clotted blood from cellular elements. Concentration is done at 400 g for 5 minutes. The leukocytes are removed and marrow gets reduced to 30 mL. This concentrate is injected through the core decompression hole (3 mm) under pressure. The reason for failure of core decompression alone seems to be insufficient creeping substitution from the small number of progenitor cells in the necrotic and surrounding bone. Red marrow contains not only a hematopoietic component but also contains a stromal component in which osteogenic bone cell precursors are found. The osteogenic potential of bone marrow is utilized here to synthesize bone. In vivo osteogenesis is seen when density of implanted cells at the treated site is high and exceeds 3×10^6 per mL.
- *Bone marrow aspirate and platelet-rich plasma (PRP):* In addition to the concentrated bone marrow, 120 mL of blood is centrifuged and platelet portion extracted from it to reveal PRP. The platelet concentrate is thought to additionally enhance revascularization and healing of the necrotic lesion.

Surgical Treatment of Osteonecrosis

The surgical treatment options can be divided into hip preserving and hip sacrificing methods:

- *Hip preserving methods:* They are aimed to relieve patient's pain and to prevent progression of the disease. The indications and contraindications are detailed in **Box 2**. Following are some standard methods:
  - Core decompression (alone or supplemented with allograft, autograft, stem cells, biologics, or tantalum rods)
  - Vascularized and nonvascularized bone grafting and revascularization procedures
  - Osteotomies of proximal femur
  - Application of various osteogenic strategies like growth factors with and without delivery systems
  - Osteochondral reconstruction
- *Hip sacrificing:*
  - Hip arthroplasty
  - Hip arthrodesis
  - Excisional (Girdlestone) arthroplasty.

Before embarking on the surgical procedures there are certain prognostic indicators that can be of help in counseling the patient and decision making which should be properly understood and borne in mind.

BOX 2: The indications and contraindications of hip preserving procedures commonly performed.

Indications of hip preserving procedures:
- Core decompression (with or without adjuvants)
  - Symptomatic Ficat stage I/II lesions, ideally in young, nonobese patients with a Kerboul combined necrotic angle (CNA) >2,000 on MRI
  - Asymptomatic Ficat stage I/II femoral head lesions with a CNA <2,000 on MRI
  - Asymptomatic femoral head lesions in patients with bilateral hip involvement with one symptomatic hip
- Free vascularized fibular grafting
  - Symptomatic Ficat stage II-IV in patients >50 years of age with a CNA >2,000 on MRI
  - Ficat stage IV disease in patients >20 years of age, because of limited treatment options
- Proximal femoral osteotomy
  - Symptomatic Ficat stage II/III in patients >50 years of age with CNA >2,000 on MRI
  - Absence of acetabular involvement

Contraindications:
- Ficat stage III or higher
- Combined Kerboul angle <2,000 on MRI
- Rapidly progressive osteonecrosis (ON)
- Infection

Poor prognostic factors for joint preserving surgery include:

- Crescent involving >30% of the joint surface
- Combined necrotic angle of >240°
- Articular collapse >2 mm
- Large cartilage defect noted on MRI scan
- Unstable patient who is likely to not follow the instructions, especially the nonweight-bearing program postoperatively.

Core Decompression ("Forage" in French Meaning Drilling or Boring)

This process was *discovered by Paul Ficat and Jacques Arlet in the 1960s while they were trying to decipher the cause of pain in ON of hip* and is currently the gold standard for management of stage 1 and 2 ON. They did "functional exploration" of the hips and measured intraosseous pressure and perfusion with venogram. In the process, they discovered that the stress test of injecting saline increased pain while after decompression (drilling) pain in most of the patients disappeared. Core decompression is considered essential component for most of the hip preserving procedures and is basic step to them, with a minority of changes in technique. The classical procedure involves drilling 8–10 mm core into the necrotic region that decompresses the region and provides a vascular channel but nowadays multiple 3.2 mm channels drilled in different directions have become more popular. It is based on the deep-seated notion that there is raised intraosseous pressure in bone caused by venous stasis and needs to be decompressed for proper perfusion.

Indications:

- Stage 1 or 2 ON (ARCO system, i.e., precollapse)
- Initial procedure for deemed intralesional bone marrow, stem cell injection
- Initial procedure for vascularized or nonvascular fibula grafting

Contraindications:

- Advanced disease (stage 3 or 4 ARCO)
- Patients medically unfit for surgery
- Relative contraindication is a patient >50 years of age as the advancements in arthroplasty have improved the quality of life and management perspective beyond this age.

Specific procedure details are as follows:

- On a fracture table or in the supine position hip is draped free. Image intensifier is positioned for AP and lateral views.
- Keep the leg internally rotated about 15° so that operative plane is more or less horizontal and we get a profile AP view.
- Place a 1–2 cm incision on lateral thigh beginning 5–6 cm distal to tip of trochanter.
- Entry point is just proximal to the insertion of the gluteus maximus into the proximal femur on the lateral metaphyseal flare **(Fig. 7)**.

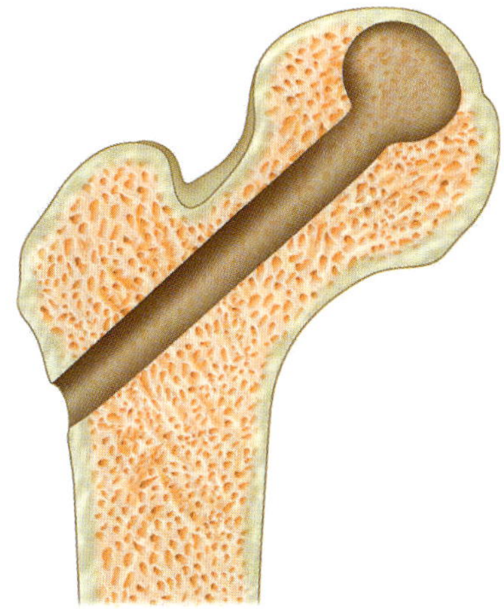

Fig. 7: Core decompression. A path is drilled to the necrotic region and dead bone is curetted out from there.

- Later cortical window is made a bit larger than the drill size (Ficat and Arlet used 8–10 mm diameter Michele Trephine, Hungerford used 12 mm Jewett starter) so that the follow-on drill can be maneuvered to necrotic lesion. A coring device will help obtain core for additional histopathological evaluation.

Postoperative management: Give protected weight-bearing for 6 weeks (crutches) following surgery to prevent incidental fracture from lateral stress riser. In case smaller drill holes are made, this can be shortened to 3 weeks. There is reactive stimulation of bone and hyperemia following drilling, this also weakens bone. Reduced weight-bearing on walking will prevent collapse of the fragment.

It is imperative to take care to:

- *Avoid too distal a window:* If placed below lesser trochanter level then chances of iatrogenic fracture are high.
- Avoid anterior half of the femur shaft for entry point. As the necrotic lesion is centered in anterolateral region so anterior entry point will not enable proper targeting of the necrotic region.
- *Avoid too less drilling or too far drilling:* In the former, the decompression core will not reach the necrotic lesion and in latter, the femoral head will get perforated.

Modifications of Core Decompression

- Making multiple or a single core (s) of 3.2 mm diameter—decompression is effective and has additional following advantages:
  - The small diameter drill can more easily reach the anterior portion of femoral head that is commonly involved with ON
  - Small incision and minimal morbidity
  - Less risk of fracture from stress riser
  - The risk of weakening the bone and accidently penetrating the articular surface is considerably reduced.
- Making branching smaller cores from central larger core (Steinberg)—this tries to cover and decompress a larger area while reducing the risk of fracture **(Figs. 8A and B)**.

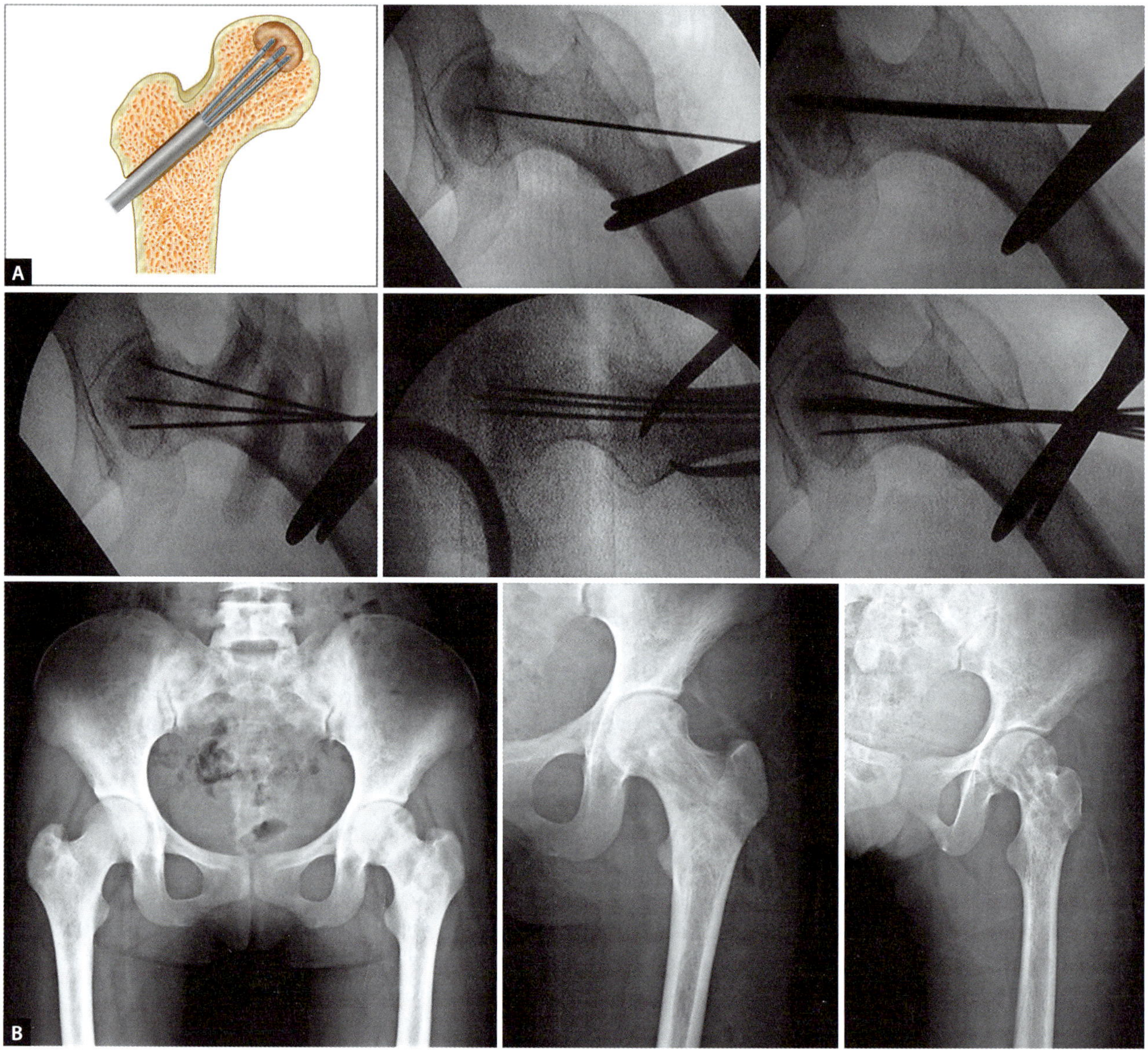

Figs. 8A and B: (A) Multiple channels for core decompression; (B) Multiple channel core decompression—the patient has grade 2b (Ficat) or stage 2 lateral minimal (ARCO) ONFH treated with multiple channel (5 channels) core decompression. There is a large lateral window created with 8 mm reamer through which the smaller channels have been developed as illustrated in Figure 8A. (ARCO: Association of Research Circulation Osseous; ONFH: osteonecrosis of the femoral head).

- *Bone grafting the core:*
  - *Cancellous bone:* This provides osteoinductive process to the drilled channel and enhances the reparative process. Some prefer to push the cancellous blocks in the partially removed necrotic bone to support the subchondral region and produce repair till that region.
  - *Fibula:* The modified Phemister technique is most commonly utilized where a structural graft (such as fibula, intertrochanteric bone, iliac crest, or allograft fibula) is packed into the tract created by trephine. Autologous fibula is commonly used in India after forage **(Figs. 9A to D)**. Though it has no specific recommendation but filling the defect created may be a better idea and may have mechanical and biological role (not substantiated though only hypothesized—described later). Vascularized fibula insertion is uncommonly used but seems to have better prognosis.
  - Bone marrow grafting as detailed above is also now commonly practiced by surgeons but improvements like including PRP or human mesenchymal stem cells may have a better scientific usage.
  - Delivery of erythropoietin in core decompression may enhance the regeneration by virtue of angiogenic properties.
  - Use of stem cells and growth factors—as above.
- *Arthroscopic core decompression:* Multiple drill holes are made in the necrotic region from the head neck junction under fluoroscopic guidance arthroscopically (no lateral

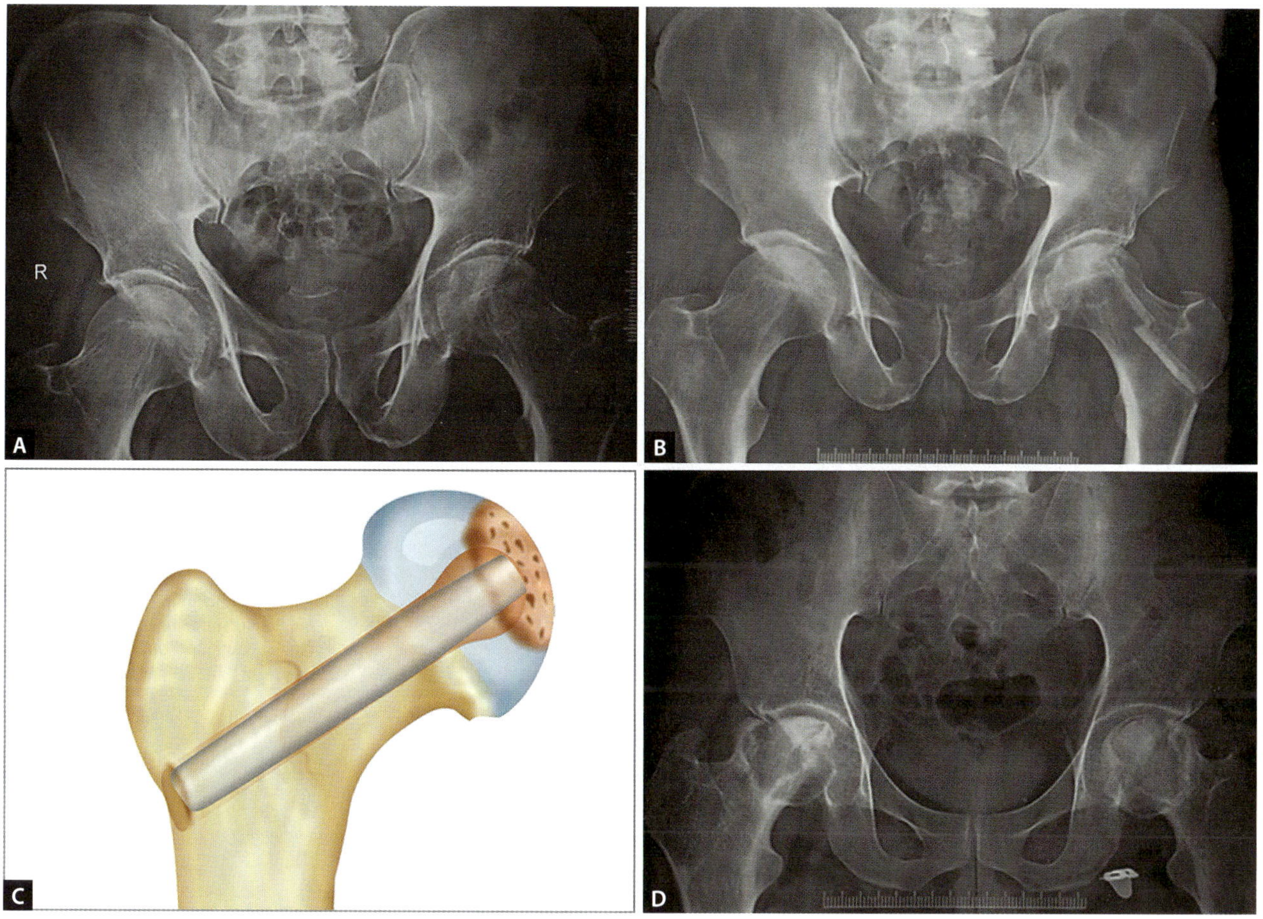

Figs. 9A to D: Forage and fibular grafting. In a patient with osteonecrosis of both hips right hip had stage 1 ARCO while left hip has stage 3 ARCO lesion (A). Right hip was managed with multiple core decompression and left side with addition of fibular cortical graft to support the collapsing lesion. The postoperative radiograph (B) is at 15 months follow-up, showing healing of the collapse and consolidation. Illustration of the simplified technique where fibular cortical graft is inserted into the drilled core (C), however it is not always possible to insert the fibula monoblock and it has to be split instead for insertion. Radiograph (D) is inserted to show the usual progression of the disease if osteonecrosis is left untreated. (ARCO: Association of Research Circulation Osseous).

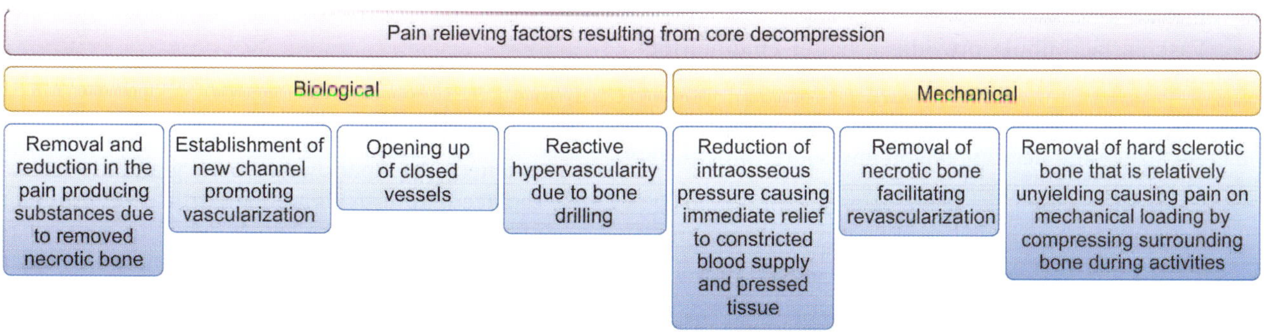

Fig. 10: Pain relief from core decompression.

opening of the proximal femur). The region is then saturated with PRP. For larger lesions the decompression and bone removal are done through a cortical window made at the head-neck junction and a composite of bone graft and PRP is impacted into the region. Fibrin membranes are applied to the window to seal it in the end.

Mechanism of relief from symptoms (Fig. 10): Both biological and mechanical factors interplay to provide relief from symptoms and biological factors help improve vascularity of the head.

- Decompression of the starling resistor so that the compartment syndrome effect is resolved and intraosseous pressure reduced to or within normal (immediate).

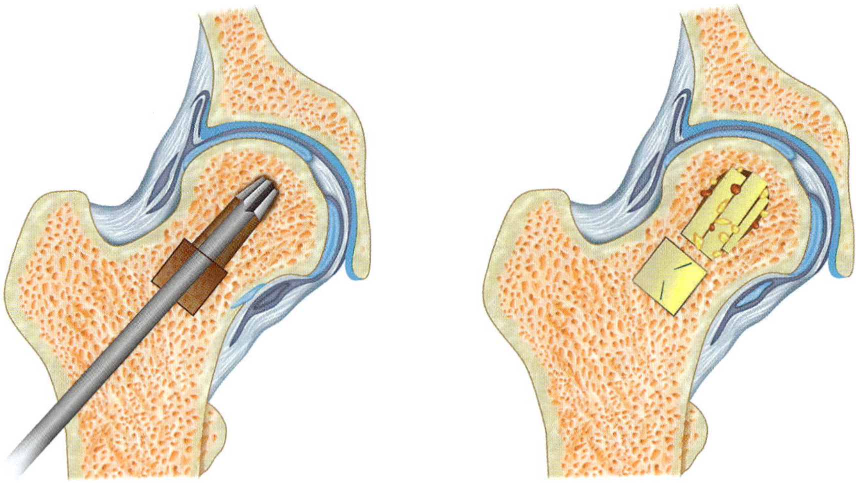

Fig. 11: Light bulb procedure.

- Partial removal of necrotic bone may reduce the local inflammatory mediators of pain reducing the pain (medium term).
- The normal bone and necrotic bone junction is a sclerotic region that secludes the necrotic region from revascularizing and regenerative tissue. Breaking this barrier provides channel for granulation tissue and regenerative tissue to reach and penetrate the necrotic bone (long term).
- Fibula is commonly inserted in Indian subcontinent after core decompression, this has following proposed effects:
  - Mechanical support to the necrotic region to prevent collapse. Being predominantly cortical it is resorbed slowly so long-term support remains.
  - The defect is filled up so lesser regenerative tissue will be required for filling the defect.
  - The medullary canal of fibula will assist in making the granulation tissue reach the defect faster and provide faster revascularization.
  - Vascularized fibula provides a better channel for revascularization into the necrotic region.

Prognostic factors for success of core decompression:

- Larger size of the necrotic region has poorer prognosis (>15% of area of the articular surface or CNA >240°)
- Age—younger patients fare better.

Bone Grafting Procedures

The bone grafting procedures can be grouped under vascularized and nonvascular grafts.

- *Debridement of the necrotic lesion and bone grafting the lesion:* Here the lesion is debrided and the necrotic bone is cleared first. Cancellous bone obtained from iliac crest is grafted into the site and packed. Two approaches are available to perform this technique:
  - *The light bulb procedure (Rosenwasser et al.):* Here the window is made into anterior aspect of the neck of femur. The neck is approached through Watson-Jones or Smith-Peterson's approach and window is created at the level of the junction of the femoral head and neck. After packing the bone graft the window is replaced. To provide strong cortical support small cut fibular cylinders can be used to support the subchondral region **(Fig. 11)** and rotated inside and impacted so that they do not come-out through the window.
  - *The trapdoor procedure **(Fig. 12)**:* Here the window is made through articular surface of femoral head after surgical dislocation of the hip to preserve the blood supply of hip. A "trapdoor" window is made in the femoral head cartilage to access the diseased subchondral bone. After removing the necrotic bone and repacking, the cartilage flap is then replaced and secured back. This directly addresses the necrotic region, however, requires expertise and carries risk of damage to vascularity.

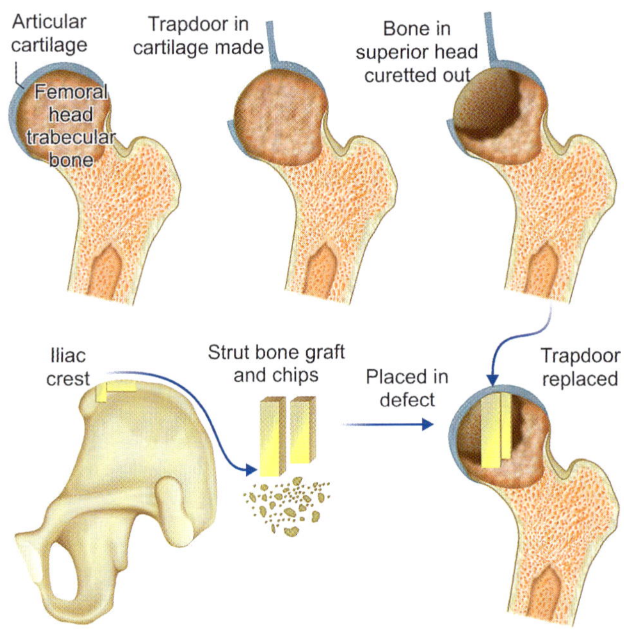

Fig. 12: Trapdoor procedure.

- *Nonvascular bone grafts:* Bone grafts can be harvested from patient's iliac crest or from core track to fill into the lesion. These provide scaffold for new bone formation and are osteoinductive. Harvesting fibula and packing into the core decompression site (Boettcher and Bonfiglio) are discussed before. Similarly, tibial cortical strut grafts (Phemister) can be inserted.
- *Local pedicled vascular bone graft:* They carry with themselves a native source of vascular supply improving and augmenting the reparative process. The bone and the necrotic region are exposed as done for light bulb procedure. The local pedicled graft is then inserted into the cleared defect. The advantage of vascularized bone graft (VBG) is that they revascularize the defective bone without creeping substitution, and thus accelerate fracture healing. The osteocytes are preserved and graft consolidation is accelerated. Vascularized grafts offer superior biological and mechanical properties compared to nonvascular bone grafts by minimizing post-implantation remodeling and resultant bone resorption. These methods are suitable for stage 1 to 3 ARCO classification. A variety of methods and grafts have been utilized in the literature.
    - *Muscle pedicled bone grafts* **(Figs. 13A to C)**: The corticocancellous grafts are harvested from the region along with the muscle pedicle and then inserted into the defect. No dissection of the specific vascular pedicle is required. The graft survives on the periosteal blood supply received from attached muscle. The periosteal blood supply has been demonstrated to reach medullary canal (Crock, 1967) though from the original work of Jonson it was thought that the periosteum supplies not more than outer half of the bone cortex. Berggren, et al. demonstrated that graft surviving on periosteal blood supply fare similar to the grafts receiving medullary supply.
        - *Meyer's Quadratus femoris pedicled bone graft (modified from Judet):* This technique utilizes posterior approach and the graft is obtained from the femoral attachment of quadratus femoris at the posterior intertrochanteric area. This is then inserted into the femoral head-neck defect created by removal of necrotic bone. The graft is based on lateral epiphyseal vessels and medial circumflex femoral artery. The technique may endanger the blood supply of the femoral head that is derived itself from the medial circumflex femoral artery and retinacular vessels. The graft should be pushed into the defect and can be secured with screws. The graft has also been used to treat silent hips (Stage 1) by Lee and Rehmatullah reporting good results. Modification has been done in the form of using titanium mesh to protect the subchondral region and inserting the pedicled bone graft into another cylinder created from the mesh. The approach has the advantage of clearly visualizing the anterolateral necrotic region from posterior aspect (which may be difficult to see from the anterior approach).
        - *Tensor fascia lata muscle based iliac crest bone graft:* Proponents of this technique find it better to localize the necrotic region from anterior approach and using adjacent graft for reconstruction. Also, the damage to native supply of the femoral head is preserved using this method that approaches the hip anteriorly. The flap is based on the ascending branch of lateral circumflex femoral artery. Dr DP Bakshi used a variety of grafts [quadratus, tensor fasciae latae (TFL), sartorius, and gluteus medius] reporting very good results. He even used them for advanced collapse and early osteoarthritis. In advanced collapse, he used to trim the superolateral femoral osteophytes (cheilectomy) and also perform adductor tenotomy variably. He reported that patients with early arthritis also improved significantly with the treatment but steroid-induced ON has poor results.

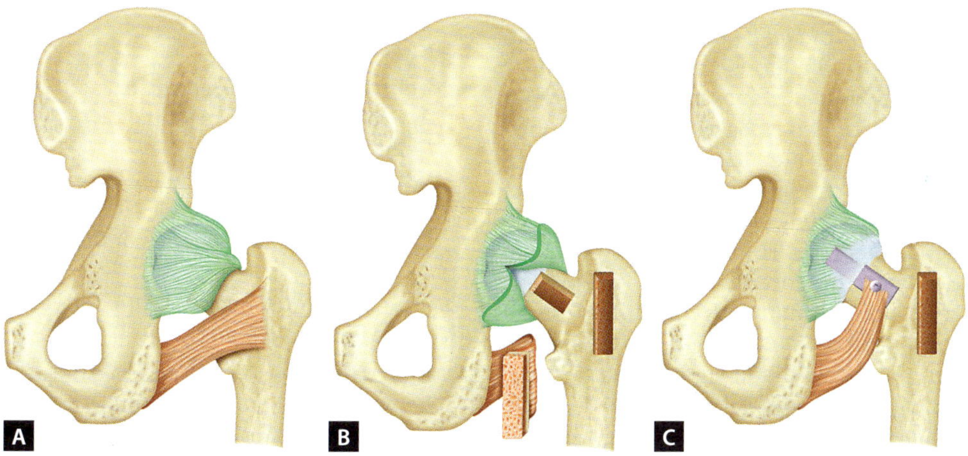

Figs. 13A to C: Illustration depicting quadratus femoris-based vascular bone grafting [muscle pedicle bone grafting (MPBG)] placed in a trough created in neck region for decompression of the osteonecrotic femoral head. The graft is commonly fixed with a screw and the cavity can also be filled with cancellous bone graft (BG).

- *Gluteus medius muscle pedicle based trochanteric bone graft:* The bone is raised from anterior aspect of trochanter and inserted into the defect anteriorly. The graft receives its blood supply from the superior gluteal vessels and lateral circumflex femoral artery.
- *Gluteus medius muscle pedicle based iliac bone graft:* The bone is elevated from the iliac crest rather than trochanter.
- *Sartorius muscle pedicle based anterior bone graft:* They carry stronger cortical component and are preferred in adolescents using the anterior approach. In adults, the TFL-based VBGs are preferred.
- Iliopsoas based muscle pedicle graft have been tried in animals.

- *Muscle pedicle vascularized periosteal grafting:* Based on quadratus femoris muscle has been described for treating nonunion of femoral neck but may be useful for treating ON also. This does not utilize the bone component.
- *Vascular periosteal grafting (Zhu et al. 1992):* Vascularized iliac periosteal grafting has been used in the past for treatment of ON femoral head. This is based on the work by Finley et al. (1978) that vascularized periosteum is capable of producing new bone.
- *Muscle pedicle graft only (no bone attached):* This innovative concept was studied by Forgon and Montsko who utilized the gluteus muscle pedicle from anterior trochanter without bone and compared to similar pedicle with bone. They found that the revascularization of the experimental devitalized head of femur in rabbits was faster and more complete with the muscle pedicle grafts only than when it was attached to bone piece. This contrary finding to our common logic was explained by the concept of muscular metaplasia. Though there are no clinical trials reported on the use of muscle alone but it seems to be an interesting concept.
- *Vascular pedicle-based bone graft (VBGs, microvascular bone grafts, and vital bone grafts):* These are local pedicle-based graft that can be rotated and does not require microvascular anastomosis as for free vascular bone grafts. Two types have been described and used successfully in literature. The *iliac crest bone graft* based on deep circumflex iliac vessels (Iwato et al.) provides a good supply of corticocancellous bone and osteoprogenitor cells. The bone is harvested with its pedicle, rotated, and inserted into the defect. The graft receives predominant intramedullary blood supply as opposed to muscle pedicle bone grafts surviving on periosteal blood supply. Fixation can be achieved with screws for stabilization of the graft; however, this whole surgical procedure requires good knowledge of microvascular surgery. The *trochanteric VBG* has been recently reported by Zhao in 2010 where a 3 cm long and 2 cm wide bone from anterolateral aspect of trochanter based on lateral circumflex femoral artery is used to fill the debrided necrotic tissue. The procedures have been successful in stage 1, 2, and 3 ARCO system for ON femoral head.

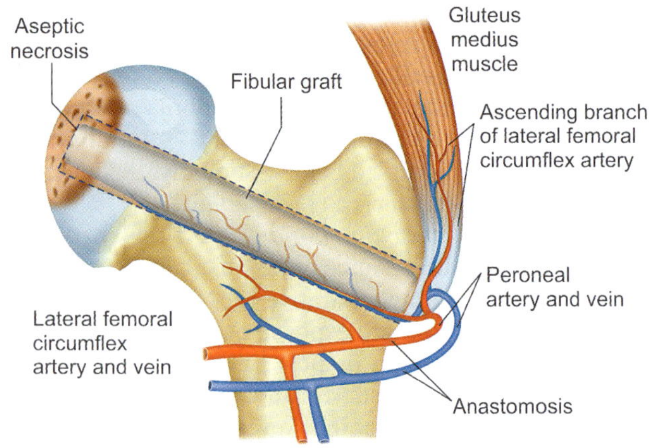

Fig. 14: Free vascularized fibular bone graft (BG).

- *Free vascularized fibula graft* (Judet and Gilbert, Brunelli and Brunelli) is a remotely transplanted microvascular bone graft that has been the most commonly studied graft in this category. The procedure **(Fig. 14)** is aimed to excavating away the necrotic bone, replacing this with viable and structurally sound bone, preserving the femoral head and sparing the hip joint from degeneration and yielding reproducible results with high effectiveness. Typically, the procedure is indicated in adults <50 years of age having ARCO stage 1 or 2 ON femoral head with available expertise and infrastructure for microvascular surgery. The prerequisites for the surgery include:
  - Absence of collapse (though it is commonly also offered to stage 3 ARCO patients) and particularly cystic change in hip
  - No degeneration of joint or reduction of joint space
  - Full range of motion (ROM) of hip
  - Involvement of <15–20% of the femoral head
  - Palpable dorsalis pedis and posterior tibial pulses

Contraindications

- Neuromuscular compromise
- Active infection of hip joint
- Cellulitis around hip
- Venolymphatic insufficiency
- Extensive arterial disease
- Contractures of distal joints or foot

Surgical Technique: Exposure and Preparation of Proximal Femoral Region

- It is better to use epidural anesthesia that additionally helps by vasodilation in addition to pain control.
- Use a curvilinear incision and expose interval between tensor fascia lata and the gluteus medius.
- Reflect vastus lateralis distally for 6–8 cm exposing posterolateral aspect of the proximal femur.

- Interval between the rectus femoris and vastus intermedius is utilized to identify ascending branch of the lateral femoral circumflex artery and its two accompanying veins.
- The vessels are dissected free from vastus intermedius and separated till their origin from profunda femoris artery.
- On a femoral guide pin placed through center of the neck core is drilled and the necrotic region excavated till 4 mm from articular surface (can be narrowed to 2 mm in patients with collapse of the femoral head).

Exposure of the Fibula

- The fibula is harvested using a straight incision from middle third of leg.
- After reflecting the peronei anteriorly, the fibula is dissected free extraperiosteally and anterior intermuscular septum divided. The periosteum is preserved fully reflecting the anterior musculature and exposing interosseous membrane.
- Posterior intermuscular septum is divided and muscles are exposed and dissected free.
- The fibula cuts are made 15 cm apart protecting the peroneal vessels and separating from interosseous membrane close to fibula.
- Quite often the modern surgeons take a "buoy skin flap" as a marker for sustained vascularity of the graft for postoperative and follow-up assessment, this is taken along with the vascularized fibular graft as its extension. The first use of this "buoy flap" was done by Yoshimura et al. for sentinel surveillance of the vascularized fibular graft.
- The vessels are flushed with heparin saline and graft prepared.
- Prepared graft is passed through generously spacious femoral core and anastomosis done.

Postoperative Course

The patients are kept nonweight-bearing for 6 weeks followed by mobilization of the hip joint and static exercises. For patients with preoperative collapse the protected weight-bearing is done for 6 months.

Modification

The above extra-articular technique is most popular and commonly used at dedicated centers. Zhang's technique requires an anterior arthrotomy, with the creation of an anterior cortical trough in the femoral neck. This technique has advantage of requiring shorter fibular pedicle, and hence less dissection at the donor site. The disadvantage is, however, creating a stress riser in the neck of femur and possible hip stiffness due to anterior arthrotomy.

Complications

- Postoperative bleeding (fall of up to 4 g/dL is seen after this surgery not uncommonly)
- Postoperative infection
- Subtrochanteric fracture
- Neurapraxia of peroneal nerve
- Flexor hallucis longus (FHL) induced toe contracture (use a below knee cast with foot platform extension for 2 weeks as preventive measure)
- Ankle pain
- Leg length discrepancies
- Accelerated head collapse
- Transient foot drop

Prognosis

The results have been reported to be good to excellent at the centers performing the surgery. They have variably reported poorer results with steroid induced, alcohol induced, or idiopathic forms. Preoperative collapse has been definitively linked to poor prognosis.

Osteotomy for Management of Osteonecrosis Femoral Head

Osteotomies are done to replace the defective and necrotic collapsible region of head with relatively healthy and sturdy portion.

- They put the damaged painful region out of weight-bearing axis and prevent further collapse
- Also, they give time to the damaged region to heal
- They possibly decompress the starling resistor

Various investigators have developed different techniques reporting varied success and advantages. The *typical indication* to perform an osteotomy is a relatively young patient (<50 years) with stage 2 or 3 disease (ARCO staging) having limited disease in the femoral head that can be substituted by healthier region with fair amount of success. The other indications that should be adhered to while advising the procedure to patient include—(1) patient should not be under treatment with long-term steroids; (2) there should be minimal osteoarthritic changes; (3) small Kerboul necrotic angle; and (4) minimal/no acetabular involvement.

Types of proximal femoral osteotomies: There are two broad categories **(Fig. 15)** classified on the basis of technicalities of the procedure and broad usage for ON of femoral head arc:

1. *Angular osteotomies:* That changes the angle in a given two dimensional plane taking away the head from the weight-bearing acetabular dome. Typically, the varus or valgus osteotomies are done in subtrochanteric region that may be combined with flexion or extension component for "offset" defects. These are relatively easier to perform and commonly used, if osteotomy is the planned method.
2. *Rotational osteotomy:* Done at the transtrochanteric region that moves the head three-dimensionally anteriorly or posteriorly. These are difficult to perform and have not produced consistent results despite logical superiority.

Choice of osteotomy and how does an osteotomy work?

There are some ethnic differences in femoral anatomy that produce preference of one osteotomy over other. The transtrochanteric rotational osteotomy has been classically only performed and studied in Asian countries because the posterior capsule of the hip in Asians may be more lax and may

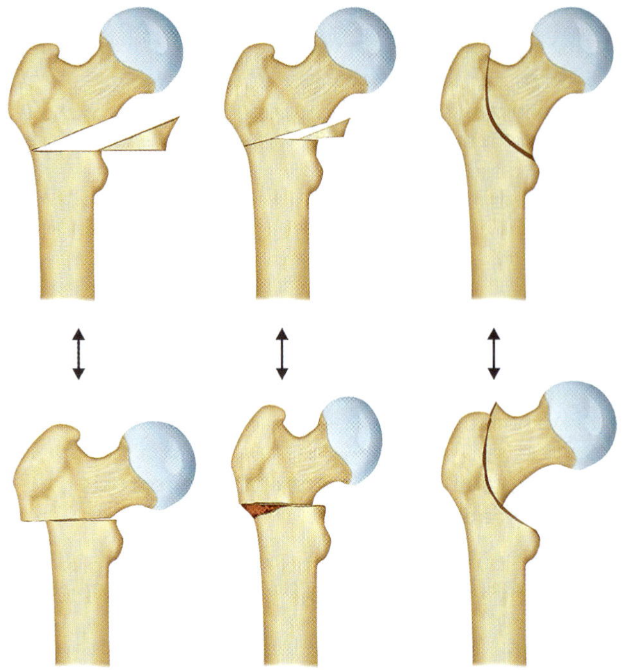

Fig. 15: Femoral osteotomy for osteonecrosis (ON) hip.

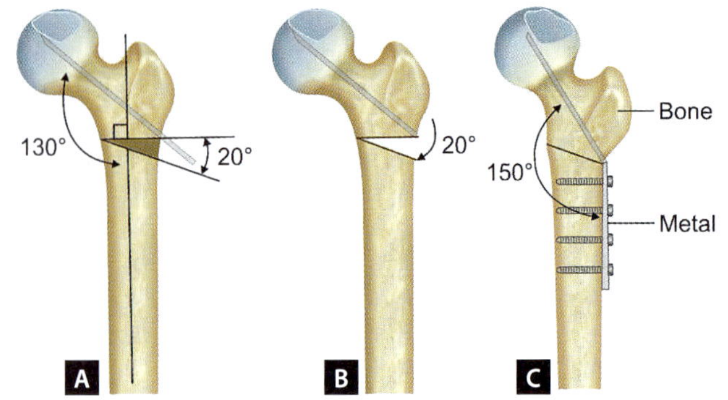

Figs. 16A to C: Illustration depicting valgus osteotomy for moving away the necrotic region of femoral head away from weight-bearing region. The fragments are usually stabilized using fixed-angle implants like blade plate, alternatively dynamic hip screw can be used. Lesions less than 20–25% of the volume of femoral head only should be preferably treated with this method.

allow for better rotation of the anterior portion of the femoral neck. This may also be the reason why results of Sugioka osteotomy were never reproduced in western studies. On the contrary, the intertrochanteric angular osteotomy has been more successful in Caucasians. The osteotomy according to my experience is chosen more prudently based on the location of the osteonecrotic lesion. It should be understood that osteotomy is designed to remove the pathological part from weight-bearing region. This is achieved as follows:

- For any type of angular osteotomy, the distal part of the limb is displaced after the desired cut.
- So, for a varus osteotomy the contextual leg is displaced medially (adducted), i.e., taken toward the midline producing varus at osteotomy and the osteotomy is then fixed. In this case the operated foot will cross over to the other side to produce varus at the osteotomy site.
- When the patient walks the foot tends to take a normal position (i.e., parallel to the other foot placed 4–6 inch away) and the limb hence goes away from midline toward resting position (in a varus osteotomy). This will move the fovea of a normal head (or necrotic lesion) medially bringing the lateral nonweight-bearing healthy part of femoral head under the acetabular dome.

Similarly, for a posterior lesion the limb is positioned behind the midcoronal plane of body producing extension at osteotomy site. When the patient walks and the foot will take normal resting position, the lesion will get displaced more posteriorly and the anterior healthy part will come under the acetabular dome. Thus, for a:

- *Medial lesion:* Varus osteotomy is done
- *Laterally placed lesion:* Valgus osteotomy is done
- *Anterior lesion:* Flexion osteotomy is done
- *Posterior lesion:* Extension osteotomy is done
- *Posterolateral lesion:* Valgus extension osteotomy is done
- *Anterolateral lesion (wrongly called anterosuperior lesion):* Valgus-flexion osteotomy is done
- *Posteromedial lesion:* Varus-extension osteotomy is done
- *Anteromedial lesion:* Varus-flexion osteotomy is done.

It is easier to remember the type of osteotomy by understanding that the distal part of the limb (distal to osteotomy) should be moved in the direction of the lesion (medial lesion → varus osteotomy, anterior lesion → flexion osteotomy).

- For rotational osteotomies the proximal part is rotated to take the lesion away from weight-bearing portion and is simpler to understand. For anterior or anteroinferior lesions the anterior rotational osteotomy is done. For posteriorly located lesions the proximal part is rotated posteriorly.

Pre-requisites to performing osteotomy (methods to improve success):

- The lesions should be small or medium-sized with a CNA of <200° (Kerboul) or with <30% of femoral head involvement.
- There should be 20–30° of normal head region located in the direction of compensatory movement as this will get shifted to occupy the area of lesion.
- More than 30° of flexion or extension or varus-valgus should not be done as this produces discomfort and subluxation of the head.
- There should be no degenerative acetabular changes.
- Patient should be willing for prolonged nonweight-bearing.
- The causative agent (steroid/alcohol) must be discontinued.
- Collapse of femoral head is not a contraindication provided it is limited to a region that can be reasonably moved away from weight-bearing portion.

Valgus osteotomy: It is done in patients with <20–25% lateral lesion and <20% posterior lesion **(Figs. 16A to C)**. Addition of flexion is calculated on the true lateral radiographs. The upper limit of flexion is 30° as more than this will lead to subluxation. The planning and methodology are outlined elsewhere. Briefly after obtaining the cuts the psoas is released with small fragment of lesser trochanter. Bone wedge is placed anterolaterally and osteotomy fixed with angled blade plate. The necrotic region is curetted in "light-bulb" fashion and the collapse is elevated. Bone grafting is done with cancellous bone.

Varus osteotomy: It is done for young patient with stage 2 or 3 ARCO stage, CNA of <200° (Kerboul) and no radiographic evidence of acetabular involvement. After osteotomy, the femoral shaft is brought into adduction and flexion and fixed in position with AO fixed-angle blade plate **(Figs. 17A to C)**. Upon resumption of normal posture, the necrotic area is brought anteriorly, inferiorly, and medially. The flexion or extension component is added from lateral radiographs. The osteotomy is done from base of greater trochanter to just above the lesser trochanter.

Rotational transpositional osteotomies: The main rationale for development of this difficult method of moving the necrotic segment of head out of the weight-bearing region was that the angular osteotomies are limited by the amount of alteration in the femoral neck-shaft angle that can be tolerated without altering the biomechanics of the hip and the mechanical axis. Rotational osteotomies do not alter the neck-shaft angle, hence can be used more liberally for even larger lesions (Kerboul CNA > 200°). Wagner in 1967 described double intertrochanteric osteotomy but abandoned it due to unacceptable results. He concluded that the results were not superior to conventional osteotomy and the procedure was demanding. Sugioka first reported excellent results of transtrochanteric transposition osteotomy with anterior rotation of the head and neck. The results have, however, never been reproduced by subsequent authors. This could be partially due to nonadherence to the strict criteria and precise cuts used by Sugioka in his study. The greatest disadvantage beside is the requirement of prolonged non-weight-bearing that is quite unacceptable to modern young population.

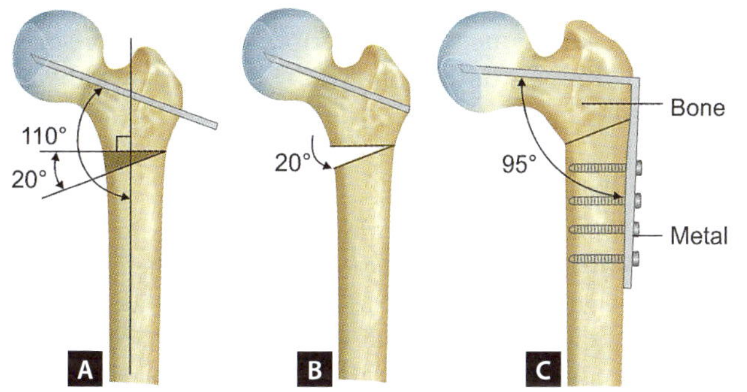

Figs. 17A to C: Illustration depicting varus osteotomy for moving away the necrotic region of femoral head away from weight-bearing region. The fragments are usually stabilized using fixed-angle implants like blade plate, alternatively dynamic condylar screw (DCS) can be used. Lesions <20–25% of the volume of femoral head only should be preferably treated with this method.

As mentioned above that strict adherence to inclusion criteria and surgical procedure is a must to the success of the procedure. Most of the cases have anterolateral necrotic lesion with a relatively healthier posteroinferior bone. If healthier portion of the femoral head occupies >36% of the weight-bearing acetabular dome then anterior rotational osteotomy is used. For larger lesions where the defect is so large that fragment cannot be anteriorly rotated, a posterior rotational osteotomy is done. The steps used by Sugioka **(Figs. 18A to C)** are as follows:

- Expose the hip using modified Ollier's approach (lateral approach).
- Osteotomize greater trochanter and reflect with attached tendons of gluteus medius, minimus, and piriformis **(Fig. 18A)**.
- Expose lesser trochanter.
- Dissect the short external rotators and capsule (anterior and posterior) attached to intertrochanteric ridge widely.

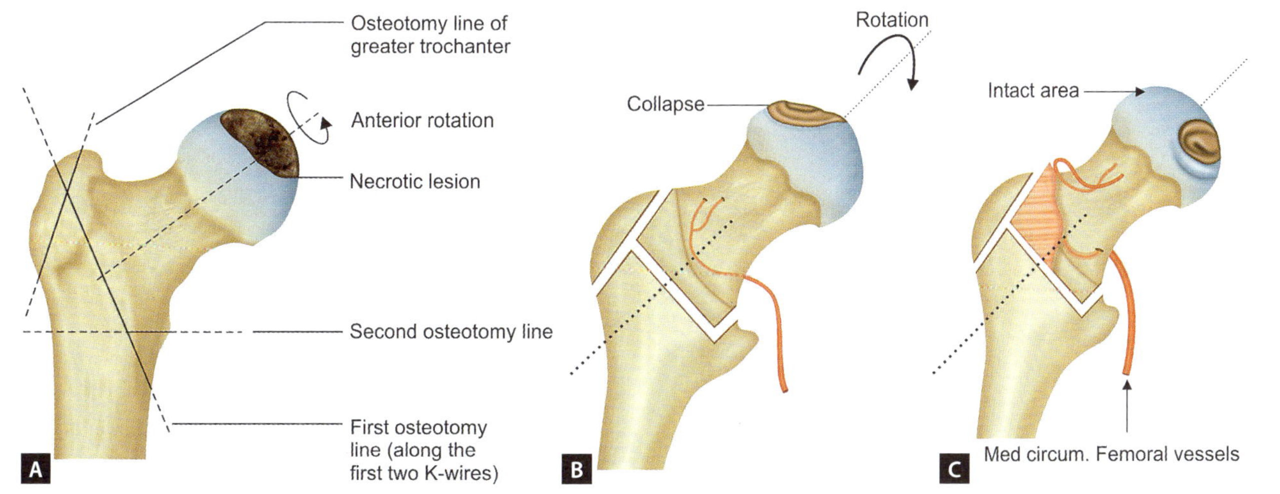

Figs. 18A to C: The illustration demonstrates the various osteotomy lines along which the rotational osteotomy of Sugioka is done (A). The rotation is done along the axis of femoral neck so that the necrotic region goes away from the weight-bearing portion and the vascularity to the region is preserved (B). Final position after the osteotomy completion (C).

- Dissect the quadratus femoris protecting the medial circumflex femoral artery (this can be adequately done by leaving some fibers of the muscle attached to femur).
- Insert a K-wire from 1-cm distal to intertrochanteric crest directed toward inferior aspect of lesser trochanter from the posterior margin of the cut trochanteric surface.
- Insert another K-wire from the anterior margin of the cut surface, parallel to first wire in the AP view. The plane of these wires should be perpendicular to the femoral neck.
- Place a third wire distal and parallel to the second wire.
- Inspect the dome and extent of lesion.
- Perform the transtrochanteric osteotomy along the first two wires **(Fig. 18A)** which is perpendicular to the axis of femoral neck.
- Second osteotomy is performed at the superior edge of lesser trochanter with a wide angle to allow rotation of the proximal fragment **(Fig. 18A)**.
- Place a 3-mm Steinman pin in the superolateral corner of the femoral head from posterior to anterior, to help in rotation of the fragment **(Figs. 18B and C)**.
- Third wire serves as lighthouse to assess the amount of rotation achieved.
- Flex and adduct the distal fragment to appose it with the rotated proximal fragment.
- Fix osteotomy with screws.
- Trim any prominent edges or margins.
- Fix the greater trochanter using tension band.

Posterior rotational osteotomy of Atsumi et al. for larger lesions or inefficient remaining posterior femoral head region:

- Hip is exposed using modified Southern approach.
- Short external rotators and quadratus femoris are incised near the acetabular margin protecting the vessels exposing the joint capsule.
- Osteotomy of greater trochanter is done as above.
- Incise iliopsoas from lesser trochanter to allow hip rotation.
- Incise the vastus lateralis tendon and then release the capsule circumferentially from acetabular margin.
- Insert the K-wires as described above.
- First osteotomy is performed as above, the second osteotomy is done transversely and not in a wide angle.
- Flex and rotate the hip externally. Insert Steinman pin into anterior aspect of the femoral neck to rotate the head posteriorly. Remainder attached capsule and obturator ligament can be cut at this step.
- Fix osteotomy with screws or screw-plate construct (used by Atsumi et al.). Reattach the greater trochanter using tension band.

Postoperative regime: Bed rest is given for 1–2 weeks (Sugioka used traction for 24 hours X 1 week followed by night time traction X 1 week). Begin active ROM exercises after first week that can be extended to active assisted exercises. Target 90° of hip flexion by end of 3 weeks. Atsumi started partial weight-bearing after 5–6 weeks while Sugioka deferred the same till signs of healing were evident in the radiographs (6–8 weeks). Continue the partial weight-bearing till 6–12 months depending on extent of lesion and osteotomy healing.

Advantages of Posterior Rotation Technique

- Rotation does not stretch the posterior branch of medial circumflex femoral artery which gets shifted medially.
- The necrotic lesion is shifted posteromedially and does not encounter the weight-bearing zone even on flexion of the hip. This possibly helps in better remodeling and healing.

Arthroplasty

Some unfortunate patients, however, continue to have the progressive disease and get no relief from the described hip preserving methods. For these symptomatic patients arthroplasty **(Figs. 19A and B)** serves as a reasonable method of achieving good painless function. The resurfacing procedures were as quick to go out as they were introduced and are no more in practice. Till recently the results of total hip arthroplasty were considered inferior in ON patients than those undergoing the same for osteoarthritis hip. But this was primarily due to the younger age of the patients and inability of the older implants to cope with the functional demands of this age group. With the advancements in the bearing design and tribology, various novel lasting options have become available that give very satisfactory results. The results and satisfaction of the patients have reached such a level that the

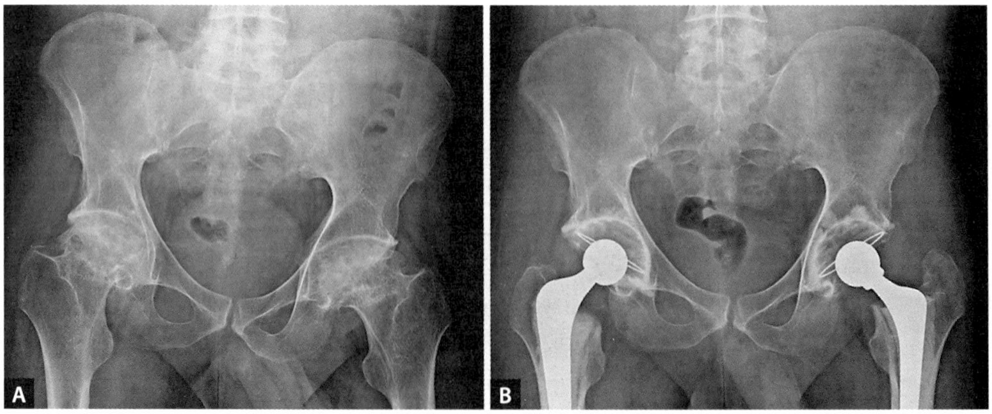

Figs. 19A and B: Arthroplasty for avascular necrosis (AVN) hip.

procedure is offered (sometimes irrationally though) to even early stage (stage ≤3 ARCO) disease in younger patients. The current recommendations for arthroplasty in ON hip are:

- Patients with advanced ON hip—(stage 3 ARCO) any age (patients <30 years of age may still be considered for alternative procedures)
- Older patients (>50 years age) with stage 3 or more disease
- Patients with stage 3 disease who do not want to undergo osteotomy and want to lead an active life
- Combined necrotic angle of >240° where the failure rate of other procedures is significantly high may be now offered arthroplasty
- All cases of failed previous surgery

Contraindications

- It should not be used in all those patients who can be reasonably managed with joint preservation procedures for early-stage disease.
- Very young patients (<30 years) still will have to undergo multiple surgeries with the available implants so should be properly counseled for the procedure and, if possible, the healing potential of other procedures should be utilized unless it is a very advanced disease.
- All patients unfit to undergo the procedure (medical unfitness or unfit from anesthetic point of view).

The principles of arthroplasty, choice of implant, approach, and complications are similar to the ones discussed elsewhere.

Arthrodesis

Arthrodesis as a procedure is not usually indicated for ON hip. It had always been a salvage procedure in contemporary orthopedics. The current indication lies for previously failed reconstructive procedures, especially in infected cases in patients who desire a stable hip. So, a young active male with significant pain and disability who had failed reconstruction or contraindicated for arthroplasty but desires a stable hip will be offered arthrodesis. It should be made clear that the later conversion to arthroplasty is sought with significant failure rates and poorer outcome primarily due to muscle atrophy. The procedure details and contraindications are detailed elsewhere.

Resection Arthroplasty

This is the ultimate treatment of last resort **(Figs. 20A and B)**. The femoral head and neck are removed and intermediary fibrous tissue serves as pseudoarticulation. The procedure is indicated for symptomatic patients with failed arthroplasty procedure or previous failed reconstructions that do not want to undergo further surgery and want to have a mobile hip for daily chores. The patients should be counseled for persistent instability and lurch with shortening and that the hip will not be able to sustain high demands. Despite these obvious and unacceptable disadvantages, the good part of resection arthroplasty is that it can be relatively easily converted into total hip replacement.

Miscellaneous Procedures

Hemiarthroplasty (Femoral Endoprosthesis)

The indications are very vague and results worse than total hip replacement. For inactive elderly patient having limited survival and weak musculature, hemiarthroplasty may be opted.

Acrylic Cement Injection

Like kyphoplasty for vertebral osteoporotic fractures the necrotic femoral head lesion is elevated with a pin or punch and the defect is filled with low viscosity cement to provide strong support to the necrotic fragment. The sphericity of head is maintained and it is believed that remodeling process may ensue healing. The relief in pain is prompt but there is concern of further ON around the injected cement and loss of healing potential due to thermonecrosis of the living bone cells. The procedure had never gained popularity and large trials are unavailable.

Porous Tantalum Rod Insertion

Similar to providing support to the necrotic fragment by cement instillation, there have been attempt to insert a highly porous coated tantalum rod in a fashion similar

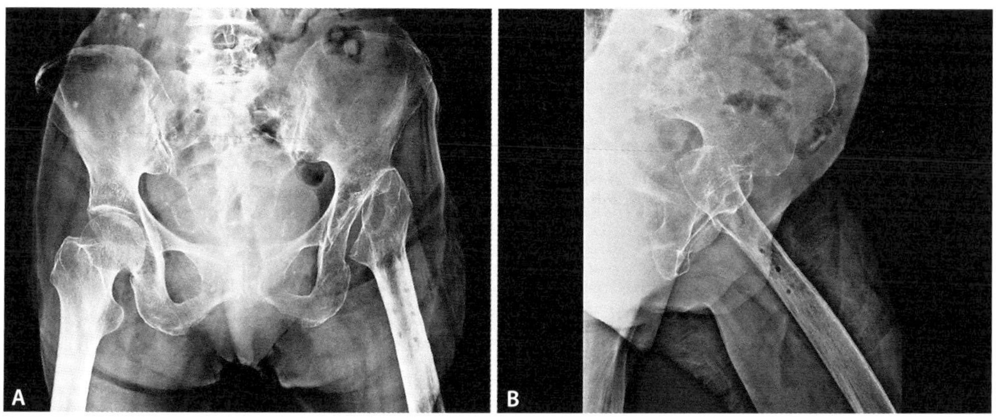

Figs. 20A and B: Resection arthroplasty.

to use of fibula that prevents collapse. The tantalum has been shown to be quickly incorporated with bone and fixes well. The operative time and bleeding are less compared to vascularized fibula and if required the revision to hip arthroplasty is easier. The technique has limited utility for stage 1 or 2 disease (ARCO) in view of available clinical support and may gain popularity later.

Newer Strategies Involving Modulation of Bone Repair Process

With greater insights revealed into the cause of ON femoral head the following deteriorations have been grossly associated with the development of the disorder:

- Aberrant osteoclastic resorption activity (increased initially and reduces later to cause sclerosis)
- Continuous increased vascular permeability
- Slow and inadequate reparative angiogenesis and osteogenesis
- Instead of osseous tissue aberrant connective tissue formation
- Mechanical weakening of the tissue
- Diffusion of necrotic area.

These disorders can be partly controlled by cellular and growth factor strategies that have potential to realign the reparative pathways. A few studied and deployed in research studies are mentioned here.

Cell-based Strategies to Treat Osteonecrosis Femoral Head

Apart from the use of autologous bone marrow, further research is being carried with the use of *in vitro* expanded autologous mesenchymal stem cells seeded directly or on collagen sponge or ceramics. Also, the use of combined expanded mesenchymal stem cells (CD90 positive that can transform into osteoblasts), hematopoietic precursor cells (CD133 positive that can differentiate into marrow elements), and endothelial precursors (CD90 positive that can differentiate into vessels or angiogenic tissue), added to bioengineered β–tricalcium phosphate (β-TCP) granules inserted into the curetted necrotic region has been studied. Novel method of using allogenic mesenchymal stem cells has been done in an attempt to provide the facility off the shelf, but concerns of infection transmission and immunologic rejection are major concerns.

Growth Factor-based Strategies

Various growth factors have been under study to improve the outcome of joint preserving methods. These include the bone morphogenetic proteins (BMP), insulin-like growth factor-1 and -2, transforming growth factor-β1 (TGF-β1), platelet-derived growth factor, and fibroblast growth factor-2 that are involved in bone repair and healing process naturally.

Bone morphogenic proteins: Bone morphogenic proteins (specifically the BMP 2, 4, 7, and 9 are osteoinductive de novo) induces the formation of both bone and cartilage by stimulating mesenchymal progenitor cells. Addition of the demineralized bone matrix and processed allograft chips to BMP-7 has also been studied. Use of combined BMP-2 and 14 has been studied in animal models with encouraging results. It is also possible to genetically synthesize cells that can secrete the desired protein at the lesion location. This is done by either direct delivery of the gene constructs at the location which are taken up by surrounding cells (then synthesizing the osteoinductive proteins) or by previously transducing the cells ex vivo and then transplanting the cells at the target site.

Vascular endothelial growth factor: This strategy helps by angiogenesis induction and secondary bone formation in the improved environment. Similar to above strategy either the plasmids are injected or placed onto carrier (collagen sponge) into the site that transfect the cells locally or the VEGF plasmid transfected carrier (usually some virus) is injected that transfects cells and induces production.

Granulocyte colony-stimulating factor (G-CSF), stem cell factor (SCF) and hepatocyte growth factor (HGF): It has been studied with encouraging results. The latter has been specifically found to act synergistically with VEGF in improving bone formation.

Scaffold-based Treatment Strategy

As there is not just a single mechanism responsible for ON or collapse of femoral head, singular cell-based or growth factor-based therapy would mostly remain suboptimal. Synthetic 3D scaffolds that can deliver cellular mediators, osteogenic, and angioblastic cells or growth factors at the target site would logically be more successful if these modern strategies are progressing in correct path. The scaffold combined with biologics serves as a template to facilitate cellular level interactions and the formation of bone extracellular matrix (ECM) that is expected to be more favorable to reparative angiogenesis and later osteogenesis. For human use, the material used for the scaffold should be nonimmunogenic, nontoxic, controllable, inexpensive, and readily available. Such materials are discussed in detail in Chapter on "Electrospinning, Three-dimensional Printing, and its Application in Orthopedics". As suggested by Dr Scott Hollister the 4Fs determine scaffold properties and these include, form, function, fixation, and formation. Form dictates the closeness of the scaffold to resemble osseous structure and defect while function entails the ability of scaffold to substitute for mechanical properties initially that slowly give way to ingrown bone. Fixation is the attachment of the scaffold to neighboring structures. Formation is the osteoconductive nature of scaffold that would give way to bone grown at the defect site. In late 1990s, porous ceramic with autologous expanded osteogenic cells have been used that showed success and the strategy has been expanded to include growth factors. Use of rhBMP-2 for clinical studies to this purpose has been however, stopped due to the concern of cancer risk identified by some researchers. There are various concerns to the commercial use of scaffolds. Due to huge variability in the patient population and response to synthetic scaffolds it is still unknown as to the trade-off between various components of 4F that need to be incorporated or are acceptable and the critical levels of cellular or tissue factors to be used. Also, the biological release systems have variable response to dose and time scale of carrier delivery into tissue that may have unacceptable side effects or undesirable effects.

Cartilage Reconstruction Strategies for Advanced Stage Disease

In advanced disease (stage 4 ARCO), cartilage damage occurs that is characteristic of degenerative joint disease. For a limited disease or cartilage damage, the localized area can be resurfaced with cartilage as is done for knee chondral lesions. With the increasing use of MRI for diagnosis and staging of the disease small reconstructible defects are being increasingly diagnosed. Once the cartilage reconstruction strategies become successfully established, the ARCO classification of ON will need to be restratified into advanced disease with limited cartilage lesion and extensive joint degeneration stages (as currently exists in university of Pennsylvania classification stages 5 and 6 for ON femoral head). The specific strategies used are:

- Osteochondral transplantation (mosaicplasty)
- Autologous chondrocyte implantation (ACI)
- Matrix-induced autologous chondrocyte implantation (MACI)

These are detailed in section on joint disorders. These strategies require limited and nonprogressive disease. The reports are limited in number and finding such specific patients might be difficult unless hip arthroscopy is routinely performed. The acellular matrix-based technique may be combined with microfracture to additionally gain from the autologous mesenchymal stem cells.

The currently acceptable (though always debatable) treatment algorithm for osteonecrosis of the femoral head (ONFH) is presented in **Flowchart 3**.

OSTEONECROSIS OF THE DISTAL FEMUR (FEMORAL CONDYLES)

Synonyms: Ahlback disease, spontaneous ON of knee, and SPONK

This is the second most common site of ON after ONFH and accounts for 10% of all ON diagnosis. Spontaneous ON of the knee was described by Ahlback in 1968.

Etiology

As is the case with other forms of ON the etiology for ON of distal femur is unsettled and most are proposals as causative agents based on isolated or clustered reports.

- Multiple repetitive trauma and osteoporosis may be a causative factor in spontaneous osteonecrosis of the knee (SPONK)
- Other risk factors (secondary ON)
  - Alcohol abuse
  - Corticosteroid use
  - Sickle cell disease and other hemoglobinopathies
  - Systemic lupus erythematosus (SLE)
  - Gaucher's disease
  - Renal transplantation
  - Microvascular embolism or thrombosis
  - HIV, hepatitis B infection
  - Caisson's decompression disease
  - *Iatrogenic*: Posterior cruciate ligament (PCL) reconstruction, arthroscopy.

Blood Supply of Femoral Condyles (Fig. 21)

As with the precarious blood supply observed at the common sites for occurrence of ON, a peculiar pattern of blood supply to distal femoral condyles is seen. The lateral and medial

Flowchart 3: Treatment algorithm for ONFH based on ARCO (Association of research circulation osseous) staging.

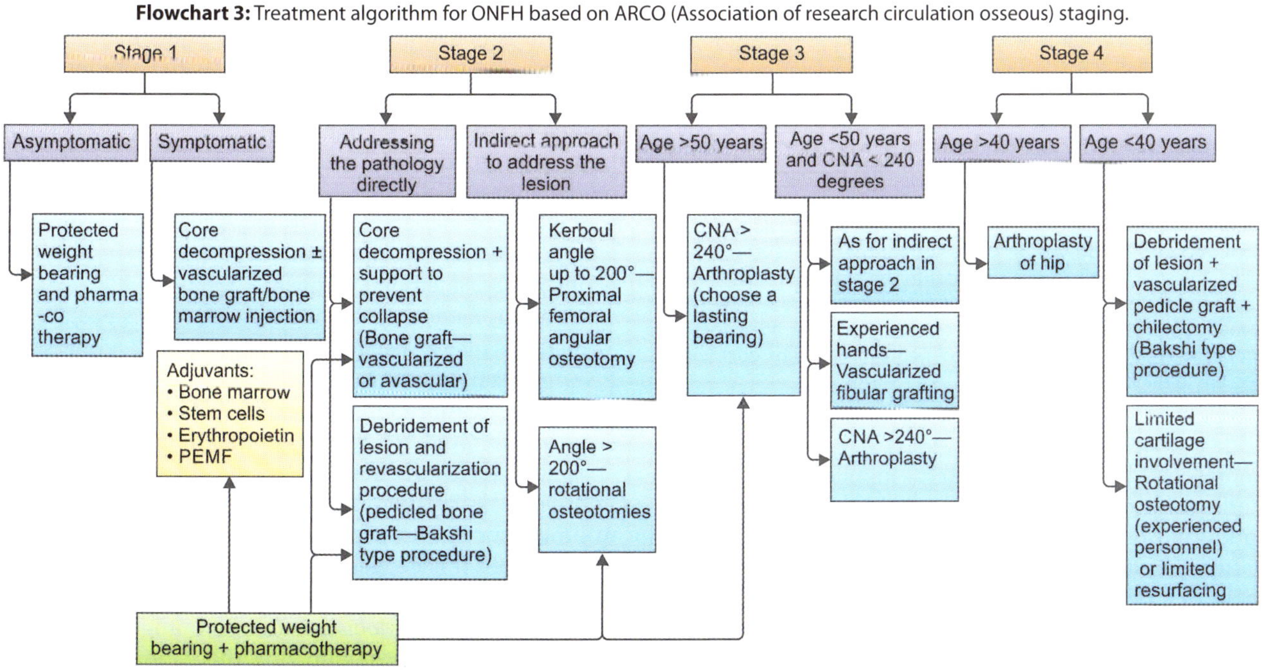

(CNA: combined necrotic angle; ONFH: osteonecrosis of the femoral head; PEMF: pulsed electromagnetic fields)

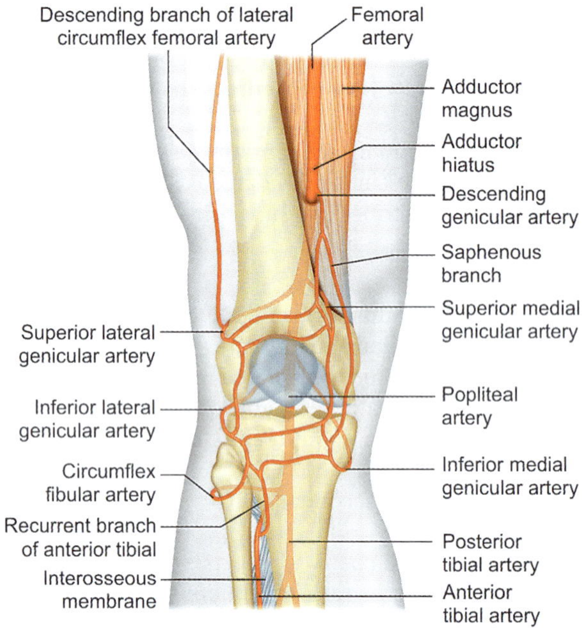

Fig. 21: Blood supply of femoral condyles. The lateral femoral condyle receives supply from superior lateral geniculate artery, the terminal ends of which penetrate the bone from lateral aspect. Branches of the middle geniculate artery reach the bone from the medial wall of the intertubercular notch. The medial femoral condyle is supplied primarily by the superior medial genicular artery and other lesser branches of the popliteal artery. The close proximity of the extraosseous vessels to the medial femoral condyle and the standard femoral tunnel used during posterior cruciate ligament (PCL) reconstruction may explain the occurrence of ON after PCL reconstruction. The subchondral bone of the medial femoral condyle draws its blood supply mainly from the descending geniculate artery. The intraosseous supply to the medial condyle appears to consist of a single nutrient vessel supplying the subchondral bone with an apparent watershed area of limited supply. The blood vessels, which supply the lateral parts of the medial condyle have the longest intraosseous course and reduced vascular density. Branches of the middle geniculate artery penetrate the medial femoral condyle only in the posterior part of the intercondylar fossa. These posterior vessels do not contribute to the supply of the subchondral bone. In the anterior part of the medial wall of the intercondylar fossa, there is the wide femoral insertion of the PCL. The intraosseous supply to the lateral condyle is shown to consist of an arcade of vessels providing multiple branches to the subchondral bone with no obvious "watershed" region of limited vascularity possibly explaining the higher occurrence of ischemic events in medial femoral condyle. The fibrocartilage of the chondral apophyseal insertion of the PCL is avascular and acts as barrier, which impedes blood vessels to penetrate the bony surface in this region. The subchondral bone adjacent to the femoral insertion of the PCL receives its blood supply from vessels that penetrate the bone at the medial wall of the medial femoral condyle. The region adjacent to the femoral insertion of the PCL is the most frequent site for osteochondritis dissecans in the knee joint.

femoral condyles are discretely supplied by genicular arteries with the medial one at poverty of receiving blood (Reddy and Frederick). Lateral femoral condyle is supplied by superior lateral and inferior lateral genicular arteries that form a vascular plexus to give multiple nutrient arteries entering the condyle. The medial femoral condyle on the other hand is supplied primarily by the superior medial genicular artery and other lesser branches of the popliteal artery. Apart from this extraosseous blood supply difference significant differences are also seen in intraosseous circulation. The lateral condyle has a rich arcade of vessels providing multiple branches to the subchondral bone with no obvious "watershed" region of limited vascularity while the medial condyle has a single nutrient vessel supplying the subchondral bone with an apparent watershed area of limited supply. These may explain the higher frequency of ischemic events occurring in the medial femoral condyle. Not only this but there is also the significant finding that the extraosseous vasculature of medial femoral condyle is very near to bone that can get damaged in procedures such as standard femoral tunnel preparation during PCL reconstruction explaining the occurrence of ON with this procedure.

Clinical Features and Classification

Osteonecrosis of knee has been classified (Patel et al.) into two forms based on etiopathogenesis, clinical presentation, and extent of bone involvement:

1. Spontaneous or idiopathic form—localized disease, usually unilateral in elderly age group >55 years.
2. Secondary ON—more extensive disease, known primary cause and is bilateral in 80% patients aged 40–55 years commonly. One should also look for other joint involvement in these patients.

Females are affected three times more than males in both forms. The symptoms relate less to the ON per se but for the development of subchondral collapse of necrotic segment which results in development of incongruity of the articular surfaces and painful secondary arthritis. The collapse of necrotic bone produces sudden localized pain that increases with weight-bearing and stair climbing. The pain is also felt more at night, especially in the secondary ON group where dull aching, diffuse pain may be present for months preceding the collapse of bone. In SPONK, the disease is limited to one knee usually with a predominance of medial femoral condyle involvement. This is more limited to subchondral bone and epiphysis. The secondary form is on the contrary more extensive and often involves metadiaphysis also.

Lotke et al. classified the ON of medial condyle into three groups based on the relative size of lesion with respect to the width of medial femoral condyle.

1. *Group 1:* Radiographs normal, bone scan is positive, and patients may be asymptomatic for up to 15 months.
2. *Group 2:* Lesions measuring <50% of the femoral condyle.
3. *Group 3:* Lesions larger than 50% of femoral condyle and produce rapid collapse. These should be treated early before development of fixed deformity.

This classification based on size gained importance to prognosticate the patients and possibly guide timing of intervention. It is suggested that lesions that are >40% the size of condyle have a poor prognosis. In absolute terms, lesions >5 cm^2 are associated with bad prognosis. This size can be estimated by multiplying the width of lesion (AP projection) to the length obtained from lateral radiographs.

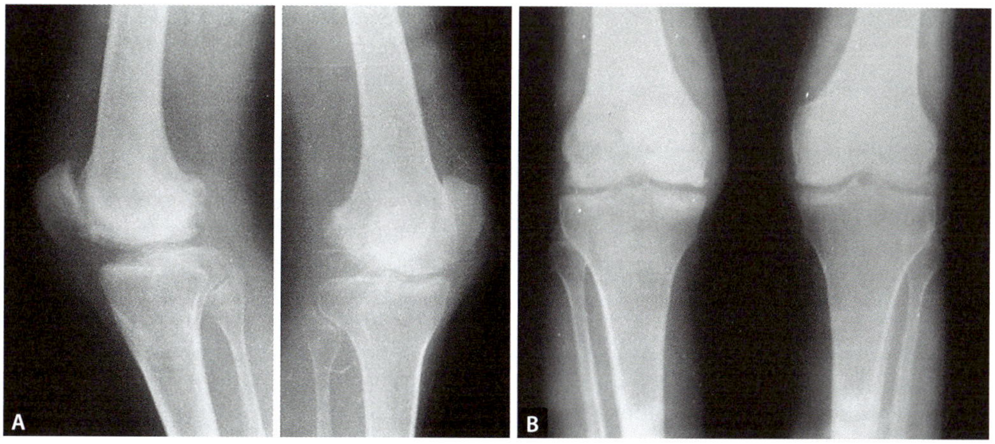

Figs. 22A and B: Radiographs spontaneous osteonecrosis of the knee (SPONK).

Pathophysiology

For secondary ON, the mechanisms of development of the disease are similar to those explained in above sections. Interestingly, the development of SPONK has been partly linked to osteoporosis. These weak bones sustain multiple insufficiency fractures even with normal weight-bearing processes. The injury-healing mechanisms produce intra-osseous edema, hence increased pressure. This may lead to development of ON due to ischemia of subchondral bone whose vascularity may also get cutoff from this process.

Investigations

Laboratory investigations should be done to rule out hemoglobinopathies and various coagulopathies. Screening for viral infection is a routine for surgical procedure. AP, lateral knee radiographs, and tunnel views should be obtained **(Figs. 22A and B)**. Radiolucent area is seen in the subchondral region followed by collapse and development of deformity. The advanced disease is accompanied by arthritic changes in the knee. MRI is a sensitive investigation and lesions are visible on MRI before appearance in the knee. The disease extent and localization are more precise on an MRI and is the investigation of choice **(Figs. 23A to D)**. Bone scans are preferred modality to identify lesions at other locations in cases of secondary ON of distal femur.

Staging and Treatment

Spontaneous ON of femoral condyles staged by Koshino; modified into five stages by Aglietti **(Table 4)** is preferably used by clinicians for categorizing progression of disease. Based on the Ficat and Arlet system of staging of the ONFH radiographic staging of distal femoral ON was proposed by Mont et al. **(Table 5)**. The treatment is commonly based on general guidelines as prescribed for ONFH.

Conservative Management

This is based on the premises that smaller and limited disease may resolve completely over time due to repair and revascularization of the lesion, especially with SPONK. An attempt for supporting the ongoing revascularization should be done along with symptomatic control of the disease.

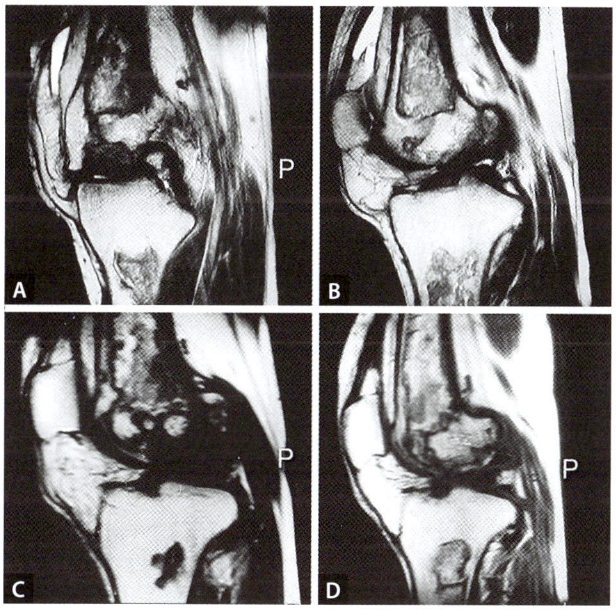

Figs. 23A to D: MRI "spontaneous osteonecrosis of the knee (SPONK)".

TABLE 4: The Koshino and Aglietti staging systems of spontaneous osteonecrosis of the knee.

Stage	***Koshino system***	***Aglietti system***
Stage 1	*Incipient:* Pain (+). Normal radiographs. Positive bone scans	Radiographs normal. If disease does not progress for 6 months then will remain static more likely
Stage 2	*Avascular:* Subchondral radiolucency in weight-bearing area. Distal sclerosis. Minimal articular change at arthroscopy	Area of slight flattening of femoral condyle
Stage 3	*Collapse:* Calcified plate with radiolucency surrounded by sclerotic halo. Collapse of subchondral bone	*Crescent sign:* Radiolucency with distal sclerosis and halo of bony reaction
Stage 4	*Degenerative:* Osteoarthritic changes including joint space-narrowing, osteophyte formation, and sclerosis	Calcified plate, sequestrum with radiolucency and sclerotic halo
Stage 5	NA	Osteoarthritis

TABLE 5: Mont et al. modified Ficat and Arlet-based radiological classification for secondary osteonecrosis distal femur.

Stage 1	Normal joint space, normal joint contour, and areas of mottled osteoporosis
Stage 2	Normal joint space, normal joint contour, and wedge sclerosis
Stage 3	Slightly decreased joint space, subchondral collapse, and sequestrum appearance
Stage 4	Decreased joint space, collapse, and destruction of trabecular pattern

Ahlback et al. found lesions <0.24 cm^2 often resolve taking months. The conservative treatment should be associated with regular follow-up to identify nonresponders so that early intervention could be undertaken. Following are the usual components of a standard conservative protocol varying in duration of submission:

- Protected weight-bearing in a splint or patella tendon bearing (PTB) cast or better rest for 4–6 weeks followed by gradual weight-bearing on splint
- Use of lateral wedge insole in the footwear for affected limb
- Analgesics
- Physical therapy with quadriceps and hamstring strengthening exercises

Operative Treatment

There are a variety of operative treatments reported in literature emanating from the differential needs in patients with different age group, physical demands, and also stage of disease. These factors should guide the management in specialized practice also. Following is a brief on the various methods:

- *Arthroscopy:* This procedure has been used primarily for debridement of the intra-articular pathologies resulting from disease such as cartilage flaps, osteochondral fragments, meniscal tear, and possibly managing the wear on cartilage by creating microfracture simultaneously. It has been postulated that fluid might seep into the bone from joint through subchondral deficiencies and increase intraosseous pressure further causing ischemia and disease progression. Microfracture however, does not alter the natural course of disease.
- *High tibial osteotomy (HTO):* The osteotomy is based to unload the femoral condyle and enhance revascularization. Osteotomy can be done only if one of the condyles is predominantly affected so it is more appropriate option for SPONK variety because the usually progressive other form of secondary ON has larger span of disease within the bone and may pose future complications to HTO (contraindicated). A valgus osteotomy is done for medial femoral condyle while varus osteotomy is done for lateral femoral condyle involvement. Goal of 10° of valgus should be aimed to adequately unload the condyle. The results are poorer for higher Koshino stages so early osteotomy is recommended. The indications for HTO for ON distal femur, hence are:
    - Localized disease or disease limited to one femoral condyle
    - Stage <3 (Koshino system), or stage 3 with <50% of condyle involvement
    - Age <60 years (else prefer replacement)
    - Willing patient
- *Core decompression:* Based on the philosophy for development of disease due to primary increased intraosseous pressure and hence possible improvement by decompression of bone in ONFH by attempting to increase vascularity, the procedure has been used quite commonly for distal femur also. This procedure has, however, not been recommended by Lotke et al. Usually extra-articular core decompression is done by placing a guide pin into the lesion and drilling the track by a 6–8 mm drill. Multiple small drill holes may also be made using thicker K-wires. The core decompression achieves early symptom relief (pain), however, once flattening occurs the procedure is ineffective. Core decompression has been recommended for stage 1 and 2 Ficat, results for stage 3 have been unpredictable. Various additives have been tried to improve the result and prevent progression of the disease. Goitz recommended pushing injectable calcium sulfate-based bone putty into the tract along with bone marrow aspirate to hasten healing. Even stem cell injections have been tried but results seem to be comparable to original technique only.
- *Autologous bone grafting:* Use of osteoperiosteal graft into the femoral defect has been described with reasonable symptomatic relief. This is useful for stage 3 (flattened femoral condyle). The graft is taken from the ilium and press-fit into the defect from articular side. Shape and contour of the graft are matched to the recipient site. The periosteum is retained to utilize the possible chondrogenic potential which is physically aided by continuous passive mobilization after surgery. Prerequisites for performing the surgery are an acceptable alignment and width of defect less than 3 cm. If malalignment is present then corrective osteotomy needs to be done simultaneously. The only positive aspect of this surgery is that it maintains the bone stock even if future surgeries are required.
- *Osteochondral allograft:* Where facilities are available for procurement and storage of osteochondral allograft, this is a promising surgery to restore the articular surface and subchondral bone in younger patients. Elderly patients are possibly better treated with arthroplasty. A good and successful outcome of this surgery depends on the following (as recommended by Meyers et al.):
    - Osteochondral allografts should be fresh and no >0.5–1 cm of subchondral bone should be used. The size is immaterial nowadays with the use of fresh-frozen allografts that reduces the immunogenicity of the graft to a large extent.
    - Donor and recipient sites should be precisely matched.
    - A firm press fit should be obtained.

- Joint should be stable and disease should not be a progressive disorder.
- Synovial membrane should be closed.
- Till complete incorporation the patient should be kept nonweight-bearing.
- Early joint movement should be started to prevent arthrofibrosis.

Arthroplasty: Unicondylar knee arthroplasty (UKA) is preferred for spontaneous disease localized to one compartment in elderly age group. The UKA is unable to make larger changes in resultant axis so there should be no malalignment in the joint prior to performing arthroplasty for successful outcome. With gross malalignments total knee arthroplasty (TKA) should be done. Other prerequisites for success of the procedure include weight <75 kg, low activity level, flexion contracture of <30°, and <10° of angular deformities. The unicondylar ON should be stage 3 or less and with limited disease else implant loosening may happen.

Total knee arthroplasty is the ultimate modality to treat the patients with advanced disease. It remains the most predictable surgical treatment modality, particularly in the elderly patient with ON and those with secondary ON of knee. The results of TKA in ON though are not as good as for osteoarthritis knee treated with TKA.

OSTEONECROSIS OF TALUS

(Latin word *taxillus:* Ankle bones of a horse, these bones were used as playing dice by Roman soldiers)

Talus bone ON is common after high energy injury to ankle joint that results in significant trauma to talus and the ankle mortise (only injury to talus like fracture of neck is a less common cause of ON). It can also occur less commonly from nontraumatic causes but post-traumatic ON is by far the most common due to peculiar anatomy and blood supply of the bone.

Anatomy and Blood Supply

Sixty percent of surface of talus is covered by articular cartilage, and there are no muscular or tendinous attachments. Only a limited area of penetrable bone is available for vascular perforation. Small nutrient vessels, variations in intraosseous anastomosis, and a lack of collateral circulation, predispose the talus to ON when its vascular supply is disturbed. Three extraosseous arterial contributors that branch to supply the bone **(Fig. 24)** are: The posterior tibial artery, the dorsalis pedis artery, and the perforating peroneal artery.

- Posterior tibial artery (dominant supply) supplies majority of the talar body and posterior process.
  - The first branches enter the body from posterior tubercle that along with the perforating peroneal artery supply the medial and lateral tubercles
  - Artery of tarsal canal arises 1 cm beyond the previous branches
    - Anastomoses with the tarsal sinus artery and supplies majority of talar body (central and lateral two-thirds of body) through branches from tarsal sinus.

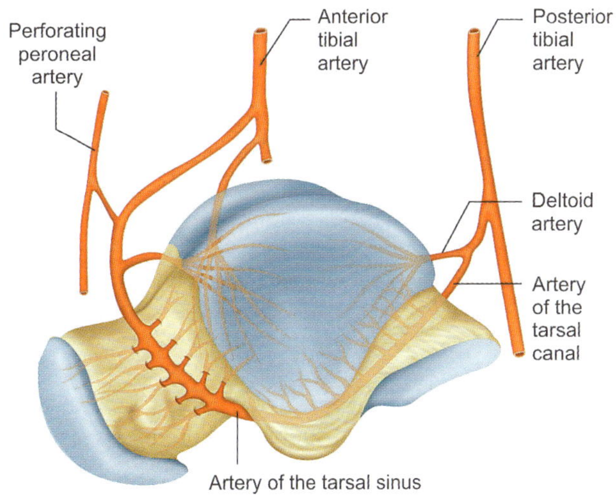

Fig. 24: Blood supply of talus. Talus receives its main blood supply from all three vessels around the bone namely posterior and anterior tibial and the perforating peroneal vessels constituting the extraosseous blood supply. The intraosseous blood supply is derived from the closest extraosseous source. The head and neck regions get rich supply from superior neck vessels through branches of anterior tibial artery and artery of sinus tarsi, so they have rare chances of ON. The body of talus gets rich supply from the six direct vessels that arise from artery of tarsal canal, a branch of the posterior tibial artery. Medial one-fourth to half of body also receives major supply from deltoid artery. The lateral one-eighth to one-fourth talar body receives contribution from artery of sinus tarsi but is highly variable. It is formed from perforating peroneal, dorsalis pedis or an anastomosis of both and anastomoses with artery of tarsal canal. The posterior tubercle receives direct supply from branches of posterior tibial artery. So, from above it appears that only the lateral aspect of talar body has less prominent blood supply than other regions and may undergo ON in an untoward event. Vascular anastomoses are numerous between the three vascular systems around ankle so a vascular insult resulting in ON occurs only in predisposed patients or with talar dislocation stripping all of blood supply.

    - Inferolateral half of head and neck from the tarsal sinus artery or the anastomotic loop.
  - Deltoid branch of posterior tibial artery
    - Supplies medial one-third of talar body
    - May be only remaining blood supply with a displaced fracture
- Anterior tibial artery through its branches
  - Supply superomedial half of head and neck
  - Through dorsalis pedis artery branch (lateral tarsal artery) it supplies the inferolateral part of the head and neck if not supplied as above
- Perforating peroneal artery via artery of tarsal sinus
  - Supplies head and neck
  - Supplies lateral part of body of talus as above

Classification

Osteonecrosis of talus can develop after trauma **(Table 6)** or may be atraumatic (corticosteroids, alcoholism, SLE, renal transplants, sickle cell anemia, hyperlipidemia, irradiation, and inherited thrombophilias), or idiopathic. Trauma is the most common cause of ON talus **(Table 6)**. Talar neck fractures are not the major cause of ON as have been portended for so long, instead complete dislocation from the

TABLE 6: Classification of talus fractures (Hawkins classification).

Type	Description	Risk of osteonecrosis
I	Nondisplaced talar neck fracture	0–15%
II	Displaced fractures with dislocation or subluxation of subtalar joint	20–50%
III	Displaced fractures with dislocation or subluxation of both ankle joint and subtalar joint	20–100%
IV	Displaced fractures with dislocation or subluxation of subtalar, tibiotalar, and talonavicular joints	70–100%

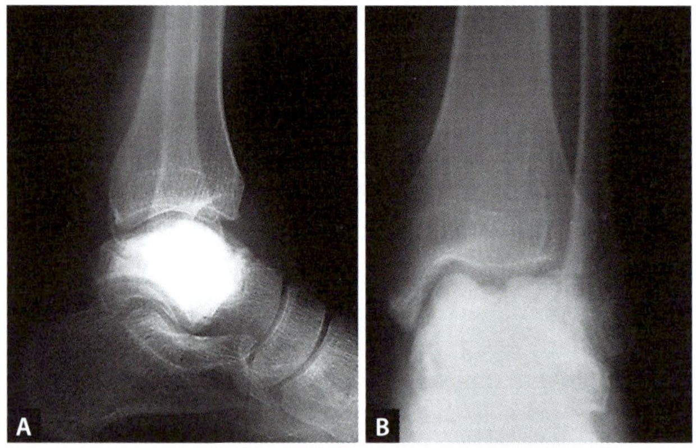

Figs. 25A and B: Osteonecrosis (ON) talus as seen on a plain X-ray.

mortise detaches the blood supply and predisposes to ON. The ON is classified into:

- Small (osteochondral lesion)
- Partial talus involvement
- Total talus involvement

It can also be divided into:

- Early and
- Late stages (after 9–12 months of injury)

Diagnosis and Evaluation of on Talus

Radiologically, the ON develops in the proximal body portion. This is visible as a dense sclerotic bone on AP projection **(Figs. 25A and B)**. MRI is much more sensitive in diagnosing ON but this early diagnosis is hardly ever useful for management of the patient **(Figs. 26A and B)**. It cannot be used to define treatment path for patient or predict the future course. So, radiographs remain the ultimate modality in defining the treatment algorithm for patients. Staging for ON of talus is evaluated similar to Ficat system or ARCO system. The Hawkins sign is still the best predictive method to find if ON is going to settle in the bone. The presence of subchondral lucency (partial or total) under talar dome at 6–8 weeks (viewed best on mortise view) suggest revascularization and a good prognosis and that revascularization process is progressing and patient may not require further surgical intervention(s). Due to revascularization, there is resorption of the bone, and hence osteopenia. Partial Hawkins depicts incomplete ON (usually lateral as medial part is richly supplied). Absence of the same suggests failed revascularization and the attention should be shifted to prevent future collapse of the bone by protection and management alternatives as discussed below. Radiographs are also essential to evaluate the degenerative changes and development of osteoarthritis. With progression of ON there is increased collapse of the dome, fragmentation of body of talus and osteoarthritic changes in the ankle joint. In cases of atraumatic ON of talus, a bone scan should be obtained to assess ON at other sites, the ON of femoral head generally precedes the ON at talus.

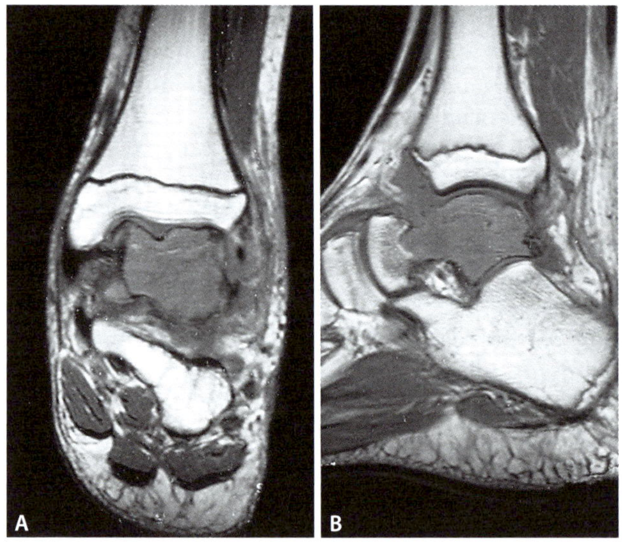

Figs. 26A and B: MRI talus avascular necrosis (AVN).

Management of Osteonecrosis Talus

Based on the premises that there are no established guidelines or staging system for treatment of ON of talus and the fact that clinical progression is highly variable the treatment is mainly symptomatic. If the patient of ON does not have pain then just continue weight-bearing possibly partially protected in patellar tendon-bearing brace so that creeping substitution heals the disease to complete resolution or that collapse develops. If there is collapse or that the patient has pain then decision to surgical intervention is made easier. So, one can argue that the treatment is more or less tailored according to stage of presentation (early vs. late). A simple guide can be as follows.

Early osteonecrosis

- *With fracture:* Protect in cast till fracture union then allow weight-bearing and treat surgically (usually core decompression)
- *Without fracture:* Allow weight-bearing and treat surgically [usually joint preserving methods (see below)].

Late osteonecrosis: This commonly requires joint sacrificing procedures like:

- Arthrodesis of ankle
- Arthroplasty
- Talectomy

Role of weight-bearing on healing of the ON and progression of disease or collapse: The replacement of whole necrotic bone in talus by creeping substitution may take up to 36 months. It is difficult for patients to remain nonweight-bearing for so long, and the fact that it is still not established whether walking full weight-bearing consistently produces collapse makes one reluctant to keep the patient nonweight-bearing. Also, there is no cutoff limit known where the bone gains enough strength to bear weight of the patient. Given all these variables and still the logical thought that bone will collapse only under pressure, surgeons employ partial- or non- or full-weight-bearing at their discretion. It is but shown that poor results of treatment of ON talus are not correlated with either methods of treatment or the time patient is kept nonweight-bearing.

The surgical methods are divided into two types:

1. Joint preserving methods
   - Core decompression
   - Bone grafting
     - Nonvascularized
     - Vascularized
2. Joint sacrificing
   - Arthrodesis
   - Arthroplasty
   - Talectomy

Core Decompression

This is the preferred method for precollapse stage (< stage 3, Ficat or ARCO). The 2.5 mm, 3.2 mm, or 4.0 mm drill is used to make multiple cores in the ON region. Usually, the posterolateral approach between the Achilles and peroneal tendons is used. Uncommonly, lateral or medial one may be used to access unreachable portions. The core decompression may be used with pressure sensors (to localize areas of increased intraosseous pressure) for more focused decompression. The patients are put in a short leg cast for 2 weeks and movements are permitted after wound healing. Full weight-bearing is permitted after 3–4 months till then partial weight-bearing in brace is maintained. Patients usually report prompt pain relief and improved movements. Patients are followed every 3 months for assorting disease progression. Pain relief and absence of collapse indicate resolution. If the pain recurs or is not relieved then usually removal of necrotic bone and a bone grafting procedure is needed.

Bone Grafting for Osteonecrosis of Talus

The following types of bone grafting procedures are commonly performed:

- Nonvascular autografting (or allografting if available)
- Vascularized pedicle grafting
- Vascularized free graft

Nonvascularized bone graft: To closely match the native talar bone, iliac crest graft is commonly used. There is also the need to provide strong enough graft to support weight-bearing. A tricortical iliac crest bone graft, thus will serve the purpose well. The talus is exposed from lateral aspect after fibular osteotomy. The lateral wall is removed and the necrotic bone curetted. Tricortical bone graft is then put inside the talus and window replaced. Patients are kept nonweight-bearing for 6 weeks to 2 months, and then partial weight-bearing is allowed for up to 6 months. The incorporation of graft may take 3 years so patients should be followed till this period. Osteoarticular allograft can be done, if facilities are available.

Vascularized bone grafting procedure: Local vascularized *pedicle graft* is available in the form of:

- Vascularized cuboid bone graft based on transverse pedicle of proximal lateral tarsal artery
- Vascularized cuneiform bone graft based on middle pedicle branch of distal medial tarsal artery—the pedicle is but very short to be used for talus ON
- Vascularized lateral cuneiform bone graft based on distal lateral tarsal artery
- Vascularized lateral malleolus based on anterior lateral malleolar artery

Vascular free graft from iliac crest has been used but is technically demanding. Similarly, free vascularized distal femoral graft consisting of periosteum, cortical bone, and some underlying cancellous bone has been successfully used to prevent collapse of the osteonecrotic talus.

Arthrodeses for Management of Talar Osteonecrosis

The goal of treatment by arthrodeses is achieving a plantigrade painless foot. The poor quality of the talus lends itself unavailable for arthrodesis, and hence unconventional methods have to be employed. The three most common methods employed for arthrodesis in treatment of ON talus are:

1. Tibiotalocalcaneal arthrodesis
2. Tibiocalcaneal arthrodesis
3. Ankle arthrodesis

Tibiotalocalcaneal arthrodesis: This is the preferred method of arthrodesis for treatment of ON talus. The intramedullary device (retrograde intramedullary nail) is the preferred mode of fixation.

Operative technique: The patient is placed in a supine position with bolster under the ipsilateral hip to allow easier access to the lateral and posterolateral ankle. Tourniquet is used to control bleeding. A longitudinal incision is made over the fibula and carried distal to the sinus tarsi that provides access to both the ankle and subtalar joints. The dissection is carried deep in the internervous plane between the lateral branch of the superficial peroneal nerve and the sural nerve. Distal fibulectomy is completed approximately 5 cm above its distal tip and preserved for use as a corticocancellous graft. Debridement of the ankle joint and removal of articular cartilage of talus is done. The subchondral bone is removed from the distal tibia and talar dome. Congruency of the two surfaces is important for large contact area and avoidance of nonunion. Similar process is carried out to denude the subtalar joint. Fish-scaling can be done to aid union. A transverse incision is made on the plantar heel, at a point directly below the midpoint between the anterior and posterior edges of the tibial plafond articular surface. Soft tissue is retracted to avoid injury to the lateral plantar nerve and artery. It should be remembered that the medullary canal of the tibia lies somewhat medial to the insertion site in the calcaneus. The correct position of the hindfoot in both the sagittal and coronal planes should be maintained during nailing. Ankle should be in 5° of valgus, neutral dorsiflexion or plantar flexion, and external rotation equal to that on the opposite side. Prior to placement of the nail, the corticocancellous graft from the fibula should be inserted into both the ankle and subtalar arthrodesis sites. The arthrodesis sites are then covered with Gelfoam.

Complications: Nonunion (tibiotalar or subtalar), fracture of tibia or calcaneum, malunion, and infection.

Tibiocalcaneal arthrodesis: Similar to above the tibial and calcaneal surfaces are prepared after excision of body of talus. Retrograde nail is used to fix the surfaces to each other and anterior surface of tibia to the head and neck of talus **(Figs. 27A and B)**. If there is severe osteopenia or osteoporosis of the calcaneus, or if there is bone loss of the calcaneus, screw fixation should be done. Care should be taken not to disturb the calcaneocuboid joint. Before insertion of the nail or screws the surfaces should be bone grafted. Wounds are closed over drain.

Complications: Malposition and malunion are the most common complications, painful foot due to nerve entrapment, wound dehiscence, and nonunion are also not uncommon.

Ankle arthrodesis: An overall perspective to ankle arthrodesis is presented here to cover the topic comprehensively instead of limiting to ON of talus. Ankle arthrodesis is a procedure to fuse the tibiotalar joint for painful ankle arthritis **(Figs. 28A and B)**. Ankle arthrodesis could be an option for limited collapse in ON of talus. This procedure was compared to ankle arthroplasty for functional outcome recently but due to ill sustained outcome of ankle arthroplasty the ankle arthrodesis retained its position to provide durable pain relief and function.

Many authors have described the procedure with initial descriptions coming from E. Albert and later Lexer in 1906 who described intramedullary fixation for hindfoot and ankle fusion. Sir John Charnley in 1951 described use of two parallel Steinmann pins inserted into distal tibia and talus, respectively and tightened with screw clamps for producing compression apparatus and arthrodesis **(Fig. 29)**. Arthrodesis of ankle has been performed more frequently than arthrodesis of the hip or knee. It can be intra-articular and extra-articular or combined. Extra-articular techniques are useful in children, where joint surfaces are cartilage and in treating patients with active infection like TB.

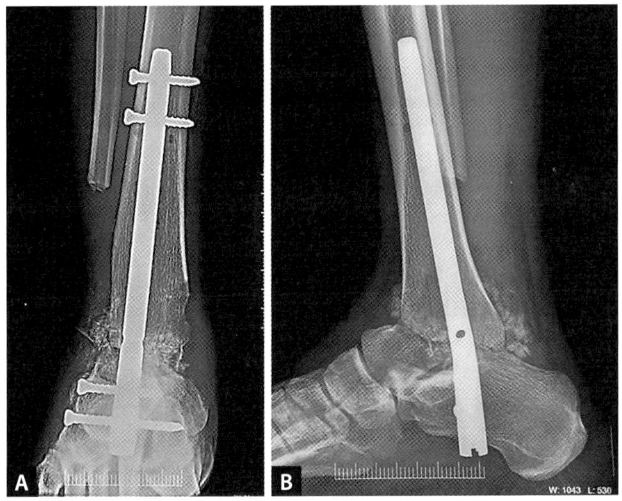

Figs. 27A and B: Tibiocalcaneal arthrodesis. (A and B) Note the extensive use of bone graft derived from talus and also the apposition of anterior surface of tibia to neck/head of talus (B).

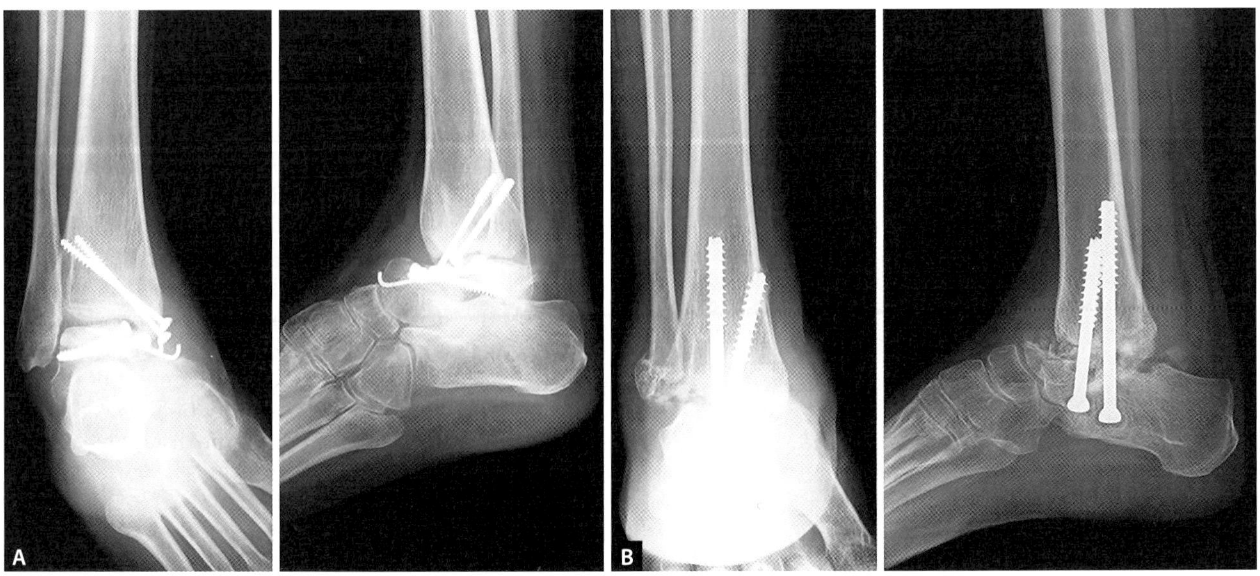

Figs. 28A and B: Ankle arthrodesis.

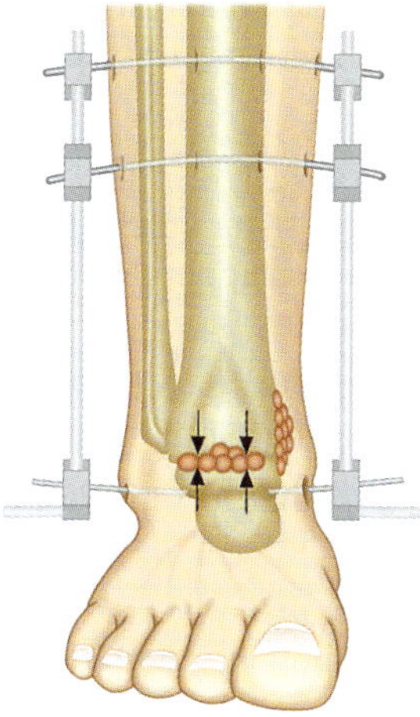

Fig. 29: Charnley's compression arthrodesis of ankle joint using Steinmann pins in tibia and talus attached to external compression apparatus.

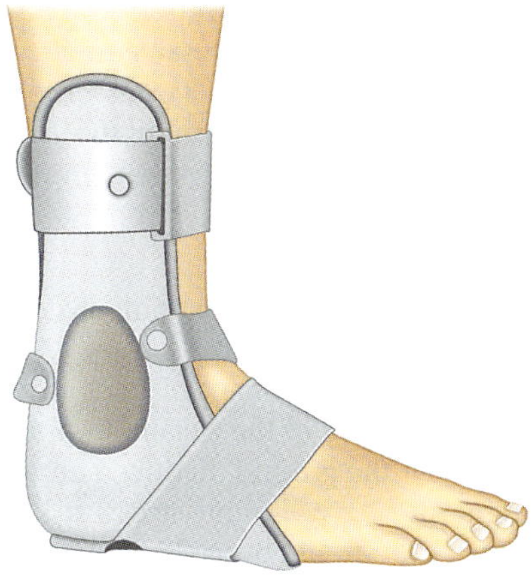

Fig. 30: The patient can be given a trial of orthotics (as shown) or a walker boot to get a feel of arthrodesed ankle and make-up his mind.

Indications: All painful ankle conditions arising from any cause not amenable to reconstruction or conservative measures

- Osteonecrosis of talus
- Post-traumatic osteoarthritis of ankle (most common indication)
- Unstable, painful, or deformed ankles (malunion/congenital)
- Severe rheumatoid arthritis of ankle
- Chronic instability with secondary changes in the joint
- Infection (settled acute or chronic nonresponsive) of ankle joint
- Salvage of failed total ankle arthroplasty
- Severe equinus deformity at ankle
- Hemochromatosis
- Pigmented villonodular synovitis
- Primary osteoarthritis of ankle (rare)

Pathophysiology: The post-traumatic conditions lead to malalignment and malunion with progressive intra-articular cartilage damage. Chronic lateral ankle instability from various causes lead to anterior subluxation of talus and hindfoot varus due to varus tilt of talus in mortise.

Inflammatory arthropathy leads to progressive erosion of the articular cartilage and may be associated with chronic posterior tibial tendinopathy and hindfoot valgus. There is usually a compensatory forefoot varus.

Contraindications:

- Concomitant arthrosis at subtalar or nearby joints—the compensation at these joints will produce pain even after arthrodesis, and the degeneration may increase.
- Active infection at the site
- Severe peripheral vascular disease that cannot be improved
- Relative
  - Neuropathic foot—high chances of failure
  - Poor compliance
  - Presence of nonhealing ulcers of foot

Prerequisites and preoperative planning for performing arthrodesis:

- Assess movements at hip or knee (especially external rotation at hip as patients tend to rotate extremity externally during walking and will need hip external rotation).
- Previous surgical scars should be included into the incision.
- Sensation of the extremity should be evaluated. Diabetic neuropathy is a relative contraindication. Distal peripheral pulses should be palpable, if there is any doubt then perform Doppler examination.
- Heel cord contracture should be noted by maximally inverting and dorsiflexing the foot to lock the subtalar joint.
- *Gait analysis and hindfoot function:* Functional hindfoot is essential for successful ankle arthrodesis as without it patient will have severe morbidity in mobilization. Hindfoot stiffness commonly arises in ankle arthritis due to simultaneous hindfoot arthritis and may be better treated with ankle arthroplasty.
- *Motor function:* Dorsiflexion, plantarflexion, and subtalar movements are important after ankle arthrodesis. Without these the functional outcome of arthrodesis will not be satisfactory. In case of weakness, perform pantalar arthrodesis or Bridle tendon transfer.
- Patient should properly understand the resulting disability—he can be given a trial of orthotics or short leg cast or walker boot to get a feel of arthrodesed ankle and it will also assess the relief in pain that can be obtained with the procedure **(Fig. 30)**. Obtain informed consent with a thorough explanation (after surgery the foot allows dorsiflexion or plantar-flexion of 10–25° only). The following options are available to improve compliance and help patient make-up his decision:
  - A double-upright brace with a patellar tendon bearing support
  - A locked ankle with solid ankle cushion heel (SACH)
  - A rocker bottom sole with ankle foot orthosis (AFO)

- Patient should stop smoking as nonunion rates as high as 16 times have been reported. Patients on anti-inflammatory immunosuppressive medications should also stop the medication for 2–3 weeks prior to procedure
- Perform a radiographic assessment to evaluate the distal tibiofibular joint axis of the lower extremity.

Optimal position of arthrodesis:

- 0–5° of valgus
- Rotation should be matched to uninvolved ankle (usually 5–10° of external rotation)

Slight posterior displacement of talus is recommended to improve the lever arm of the calcaneus and makes easier for the foot to clear the ground. Reduced anterior lever arm reduces fatigue during walk and stress at knee. Excessive posterior translation should be avoided else the contact area reduces for successful fusion.

Approaches of ankle arthrodesis:

Irrespective of method one should aim to create broad cancellous surfaces that are congruent and place the ankle in desired position.

Open:

- *Anterior approach (most commonly used):* Through the anterior tibial tendon sheath. This can be supplemented with anteromedial or anterolateral approach to gain assess to far posterior region.
- *Transmalleolar or transfibular approach:* Gives better access to posterior aspect of ankle.
- *Posterior approach:* For isolated tibiotalar fusion in patients with compromised anterior skin and for tibiotalar calcaneal arthrodesis.

Arthroscopic: Three portals are used to debride the joint and denude cartilage. Anteromedial (just medial to tibialis anterior), anterolateral (just lateral to peroneus tertius), and posterolateral portals (to assess posterior recess and tubercle) are commonly used. Joint distraction is required for smooth passage of the instruments. Denude the articular surfaces of remaining cartilage to expose bleeding subchondral bone maintaining the contour of bony surfaces. Two to three percutaneous, cannulated or noncannulated cancellous screws, are used to fix and achieve compression in situ. The technique is useful only if there is no malalignment and the deformity is correctable.

Miniopen: This is quite similar to arthroscopic technique, except that incisions are given at the site of portals. Debridement, denuding of articular surfaces are done with sharp flat osteotomes and curettes. In situ fixation is done as for arthroscopic technique. Iliac crest bone grafting may be done to achieve safer union. Like the arthroscopic technique this technique limits the morbidity from large incisions, is associated with low blood loss, better and possibly faster healing rates due to minimal disruption of surrounding vascularity. The technique is especially useful in patients with local skin compromise and vascular disease. The technique, however, suffers from the common disadvantage of inability to correct fixed deformities.

Retrograde intramedullary nailing technique: It utilizes a short distal femoral nail (DFN) like nail with helical blade and has shown reasonably good results. This is the preferred approach when simultaneous subtalar arthrodesis is to be achieved.

Other Methods

Blair: This method uses an anterior distal tibial sliding graft, allows nearly normal appearance of the foot with little shortening of the extremity.

Morris: Morris modified Blair's technique by placing a screw in the tibial inlay and using a longitudinal Steinmann pin.

Lionberger: Using a pediatric hip compression screw for fixation.

Principles of performing arthrodesis and technical details

- Approach should allow inspection of joint surface from all around.
- Thorough debridement and denudation of cartilage should be done without exaggerating the deformities.
- Broad and congruent cancellous bone surfaces should be prepared taking care to avoid bone necrosis due to overheating.
- Fixation devices should be strong enough and allow compression of the opposing surfaces so that healing is prompt and bony without intervening fibrous tissue else it will be inadequate and painful.
- If gaps remain fill them with packed cancellous bone grafts.
- Double check the position of ankle joint to provide a plantigrade foot before fixation and align hindfoot to the lower extremity and the forefoot to the hindfoot.
- The malleoli may be preserved for defining the correct position of the ankle, and preserving vascularity but they create a bulbous deformity so shaving to trim the projections is recommended for proper footwear and cosmesis. Preserving malleoli still helps in younger patients, if they require ankle arthroplasty in future by providing appropriate bone stalk and proper landmarks.

Rationale and types of bone grafting: Bone grafting is generally required if the cut surfaces are not congruous or deformity does not permit proper alignment. Bone grafting improves the chances of union, corrects the deformity, and fills any voids left due to bone loss in traumatic deformities. Various types and methods of bone grafting have been described and one is free to choose method or combination depending on the individual case.

- *Full thickness graft from ilium (Chuinard and Peterson):* The block is impacted between tibia and talus and is especially useful in children as it prevents damage to distal tibial physis. This technique can also be used as salvage for failed ankle arthroplasty.
- *Vertical corticocancellous bone graft chips (Campbell):* For large bone defects the corticocancellous grafts are put in place.
- *Dowel technique:* Used only for minimal correctible deformities.
- *Tibial onlay graft (Marcus):* He used dome osteotomy to correct deformities and fixation by staples and screws with tibial onlay bone graft.

- *Anterior sliding graft (Blair):* Corticocancellous graft taken from anterior, medial or lateral tibia 2 cm wide, 1 cm deep and 8–10 cm long is impacted into tunnel created in the talar neck and fixed to tibia proximally.
- *Central bone graft:* Recommended for TB or rheumatoid ankles where the bone is osteoporotic and weak. The core for graft (usually fibula) is drilled into the tibia anterosuperiorly to pass across the joint into talus posteroinferiorly.
- *Use of malleoli (may be avoided if future ankle arthroplasty is envisaged):* Partial fibula onlay (lateral) with the medial one-half of the fibula used as cancellous bone.
- *Free VBG (Bishop):* The cuboid and cuneiform grafts described for ON talus can be used for ankle fusion.
- "Bone slurry" collected during miniarthrotomy approach (Paremain) may be used to fill the spaces before fixation and impaction of the bone surfaces.

Special consideration for ON talus: If the posterior half of the talus is affected by ON, an anterior tibial sliding graft is recommended. If the posterior two-thirds of the talus are affected, the talar body may be removed and a tibiocalcaneal fusion is done. Large slabs of iliac crest graft are required to fill gaps in this type of reconstruction.

Fixation techniques in ankle arthrodesis:

- *External fixator:* Monoplanar, multiplanar frames in various designs can be constructed. Ilizarov frames have also been used and are quite popular for versatility.
  - Advantages:
    - Versatile so can be used for uncommon cases and complicated surgeries where other methods may not be appropriate
    - Can be used in active infection
    - Osteoporotic bones and poor bone quality are not contraindications
    - Can be modulated and compression at raw surfaces reproduced in outdoor, if loosening or resorption of bone ends seen
    - Has the ability to bypass the poor soft tissues
  - Disadvantages:
    - Cumbersome to carry for patient
    - Pin tract care or infection
    - Nonunion may occur, if rigidity not obtained
- *Internal fixation:* This is the most popular and often preferred method if no specific contraindication exists.
  - Parallel or crossed or converging *screws* are the most common methods of fixation often applied in lag fashion. Two to three screws (anterolateral and medial and posterolateral from tibia to talus) are commonly used. Three screws provide better compression strength and stability than two screws. Fibula can be additionally transfixed to talus. Alternative method is use of posterior only screw fixation using cancellous screws inserted obliquely across tibiotalar surfaces with sandwiched iliac crest bone graft.
  - Plate fixation is less commonly preferred due to soft tissue complications
    - Lateral T-plate or pediatric 90° osteotomy plate is a rigid stable construct.
    - Anterior contoured plate (wolf blade plate or tension plate) is preferred for osteoarthritis, joint destruction and for salvage procedures.
    - Posterior plate is uncommonly used due to the need of a posterior approach and limited access. Commonly an osteotomy blade plate fixation is utilized. It has been proposed for segmental bone loss, infected nonunion or collapsed talar body.
    - Intramedullary nails should be reserved for combined ankle and subtalar arthrodesis.
  - Advantages of internal fixation:
    - Ease of insertion
    - Patient convenience
    - Greater independence to manage the joint surfaces and correction of deformity
    - Higher strength
  - Disadvantages and limitation:
    - Skin flap necrosis
    - Infection
    - Prominent hardware
    - Persistence of implant in the body and possible late effects
- *Adjuvant therapy:* Electrical stimulation has been shown to improve the rates of union after arthrodesis.

Postoperative management: Keep the patient in splint or below knee slab for comfort (internal fixation). Wound inspection is done regularly at 3–4 days. At 10–14 days the sutures are removed and patient is given a touch-down short-leg cast. If external fixator is applied compression can be added. At 6 weeks the patient is given a cam boot, if healing has progressed significantly (internal fixation) with evident union else the cast is continued. For patients on external fixation the apparatus is continued with addition of compression. At 12–16 weeks the fixator is removed depending on the union and short-leg cast is added for 2–4 weeks. If internal fixation was used then at 12–14 weeks the patient is shifted to cam boots (if deferred before) or slowly transited to regular footwear.

Complications of operative ankle arthrodesis

- Infection
- Wound dehiscence
- Nonunion (pseudarthrosis)
- Malunion
- Late-onset subtalar arthritis
- Neurovascular injury, neuroma

Ankle Arthroplasty for Management of Talar Osteonecrosis and General Considerations

Total ankle arthroplasty provides a mobile, painless stable alternative to ankle arthrodesis in end-stage diseases of ankle. The development and acceptance of ankle prosthesis has always remained in controversy, especially with the prevailing popularity of ankle arthrodesis. Following success of hip and knee arthroplasty the ankle prosthesis introduced in 1970s met with failure and disappointing results. The first-generation designs were cemented and bulky with large intramedullary stems. These often also required subtalar fusion at the index operation and the results were very disappointing. With design changes the results improved quite substantially and were not that dismal, though some patients did require amputations. These amputations were actually ultimate measures to relieve pain in patients and were not a sole complication of ankle arthroplasty. The failure is attributed to various causes that were not recognized at the time of designing the implant:

- The ankle joint is a relatively small joint bearing the weight of whole body so forces acting per unit area of bone or joint are large. This results in higher moment and higher compressive forces.
- The questionable quality of bone in the distal tibia due to pathology and variable bone strength may preclude stable implant fixation.
- The soft tissues about the ankle are thin and frequently compromised by previous trauma, surgery, systemic disease, and steroid use. The vascularity of these thin soft tissue flaps can be easily impaired with hematoma formation.
- Delayed wound healing has been reported to occur in as many as 40% of patients and most long-term series cite rates of deep infection of 3–5%.
- Subsidence, wear, and loosening occurred within a few years due to poor quality of articular bearings.

Despite all this the high incidence of nonunion, secondary degeneration at adjacent joints, loss of physiological movement of foot and ambulation, development of equinus deformity of feet, and the concern that patients may need other procedures for lower limb that may add to disability in future have regained the interest in ankle arthroplasty. With improved understanding and studies on anatomical design and biomechanics of the native ankle joint the second-generation designs have become popular. The main constrains to use are financial and that the patient often have had multiple prolonged treatment that they are averse to ankle arthroplasty. These second-generation designs are uncemented and provide variable combination of constraint or congruency (see later).

Indications of Ankle Arthroplasty

- Primary degenerative arthritis
- Systemic arthritis (e.g., rheumatoid arthritis, SLE, and mixed connective tissue disorders)
- Patients who would require subtalar fusion or triple arthrodesis in future or has bilateral arthritis requiring treatment—the results of bilateral arthrodesis and pantalar fusion have been dismal
- Secondary osteoarthritis
    - Osteonecrosis talus (less than one-third talus involved)
    - Post-traumatic (if the malalignment and instability are manageable)
- Salvage of malunion and nonunion after ankle arthrodesis
- Salvage of failed ankle arthroplasty
- Low demand patients who are not likely to go for aggressive laborious jobs

Contraindications

Absolute
- Active infection
- Nonreconstructible or advanced peripheral vascular disease
- Unmanageable instability and malalignment
- Charcot arthropathy
- Severe joint hypermobility syndrome
- Suspected or documented metal allergy
- High physical demand activities or sports

Relative
- Severe osteoporosis
- Prior severe trauma with dislocation of the talus (disruption of the mortise and ligaments)
- Osteonecrosis of talus more than one third of bone involvement
- Neuromuscular disorder
- Diabetic patient without polyneuropathy

Design Considerations and Types

The most basic design conformation is based on the method of fixation:
- *Cemented:* It failed fast in younger patients especially, so had been discontinued for poor results **(Fig. 31)**.
- *Uncemented:* Nearly all the current available designs are uncemented.

The other classification is based on the number of components and the bearing type used **(Fig. 32)**:
- Fixed-bearing two component design:
    - *Constrained:* Limit axial rotation
    - *Semiconstrained:* Partially limit axial rotation
    - *Unconstrained:* Permit increased axial rotation but require ligament stability
- A three-component mobile-bearing design.

Ankle arthroplasty has also been classified according to whether there is congruity in the articulating surfaces or not:

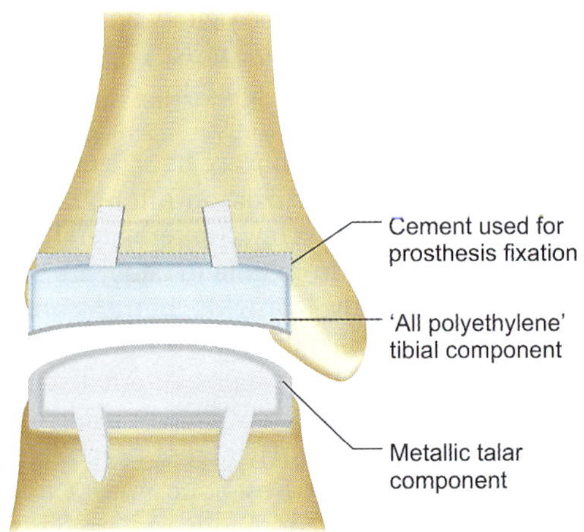

Fig. 31: The older designs were cemented and failed fast.

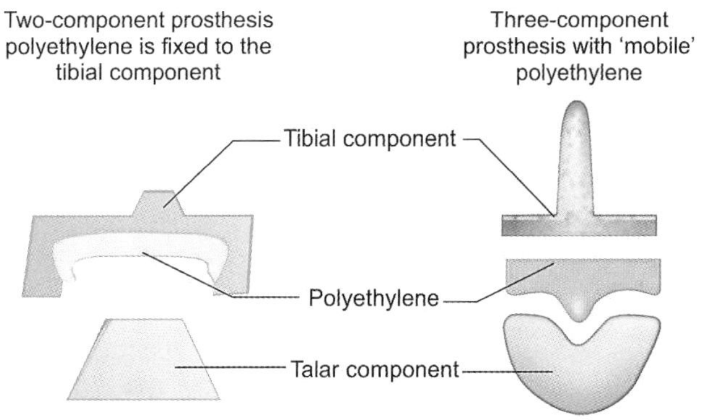

Fig. 32: Illustration of component-based classification of ankle arthroplasty designs.

- *Congruent (preferred):* Spherical, spheroidal, cylindrical, and conical
- *Incongruent designs:* Trochlear, bispherical, concave-convex or convex-convex articulations

Constrained designs limit the axial rotation and AP translation at joint and are more stable, but put higher stress on the implant bone interface due to development and transmittance of the shear forces. Unconstrained designs though give low stress are more susceptible to instability and need precision in placement and patent ligaments. Some designs require synostosis formation at distal tibia and fibula to share the load between bones (agility ankle). Because conformity or congruity is the closeness of fit for articulation surfaces, so fully congruent surfaces will have similar radii of curvature and these will have lowest wear rates as the force per unit area is less and is distributed all throughout the articulation. Ideally hence an implant should have unconstrained design (low implant bone stress) with full congruity (low wear rate). This results in "constraint-conformity or congruency conflict"—for fully congruent surfaces the articulations will naturally have to be constrained so such ideal designs are not possible. An intermediary measure is adopted in the form of putting mobile-bearing implants where the articulation is congruent and constrained but to reduce stress transmission and permit rotations can move independently on its own axis. Such implants though innovative have their share of problems. The mobile bearing has effectively two moving articulations, and hence will have double the wear rate shortening its life. Also, the faster wears will lead to progressive instability and aseptic inflammatory response and loosening. To circumvent this, "quality" of bearing is being improved in the form of highly cross-linked and interlinked poly.

Principles of Surgery and Implant Design

Based on above background the following are some of the considerations for a successful ankle arthroplasty design and surgical procedure:

- Total ankle prosthesis should be anatomically similar (kinetically and kinematically) to the native ankle to replicate the functions.
- Eversion and inversion stability should be provided by the tibiotalar articulating surfaces.
- Anteroposterior stability should be provided by the tibiotalar ligaments.
- Ligament balancing should be done by proper ligament balancing.
- Bony resection should be minimal—to provide subchondral bone support for implant.
- Component should take the support of whole distal tibial flange and transmit the requisite forces across—to prevent subsidence of the implant and future loosening.
- To minimize the contact stress the force should be transmitted across the central thirds of prosthesis articulation.
- Ankle should be well aligned and ligament balancing should be appropriate—this is highly imperative for nonconstrained designs.
- The polyethylene should be congruent to the metal tibial and talar components and should not extend past the metal component, else edge loading and wear occurs fast.

The procedural details of individual joints can be obtained from the designing and marketing company. The following designs are commonly available **(Figs. 33A to K)**:

- The Scandinavian total ankle replacement (STAR) total ankle arthroplasty—three-component, fully conforming mobile bearing
- Buechel-Pappas total ankle arthroplasty—three-component, mobile bearing, Titanium
- The HINTEGRA total ankle arthroplasty
- The Bologna-Oxford (BOX) total ankle arthroplasty
- Ankle evolutive system (AES) ankle total ankle arthroplasty—three-component, Co-Cr HA-coated implant
- The ESKA total ankle arthroplasty
- The Salto and Salto total ankle arthroplasty
- Mobility total ankle arthroplasty
- INBONE total ankle arthroplasty
- Ramses ankle total ankle arthroplasty (France)—spheroidal talar component allowing multiaxial freedom
- TNK total ankle arthroplasty
- The agility total ankle arthroplasty—requires tibiofibular synostosis formation
- Revision agility total ankle arthroplasty

In general, there are three-component designs (except Agility and TNK) and all contain Co-Cr components (except Buechel-Pappas—made of titanium alloy) that are fixed without cement. Most are implanted through anterior approach (ESKA—requires single transfibular approach; agility ankle additional distal fibular incision in addition to anterior approach to do tibiofibular synostosis). Accompanying surgeries in the form of heel-cord lengthening, medial ligament reconstruction, hindfoot fusion, etc., might be required for individual cases.

After Treatment

- Immediately after surgery the ankle is immobilized in a well-padded cast or splint until the incisions have healed adequately to protect from uncontrolled movements.

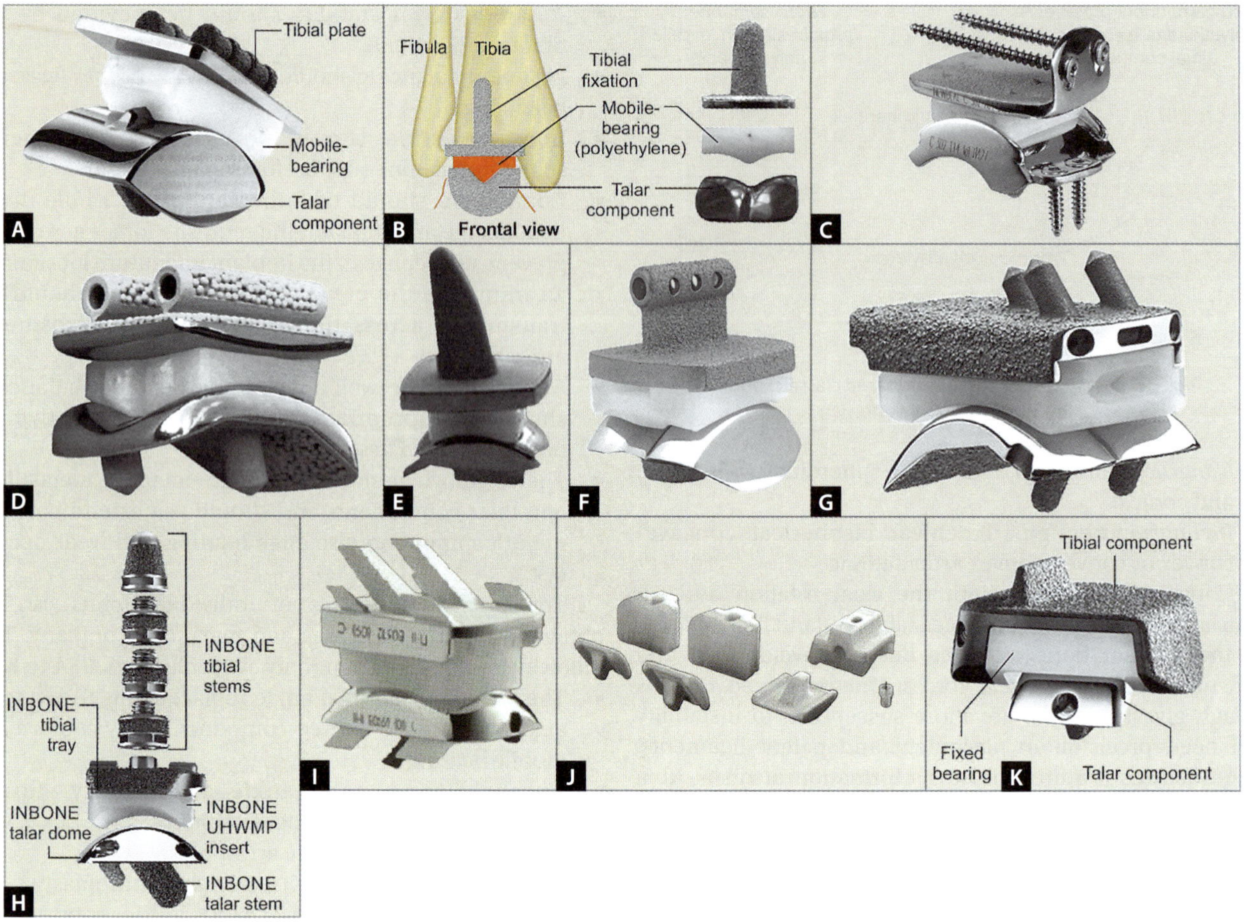

Figs. 33A to K: The various total ankle arthroplasty designs available. (A) Scandinavian total ankle replacement (STAR); (B) Buechel-Pappas; (C) Hintegra; (D) Bologna-Oxford (BOX) ankle; (E) Ankle evolutive system; (F) Salto total ankle; (G) Infinity total ankle; (H) INBONE total ankle; (I) Ramses France total ankle; (J) TNK total ankle; (K) Agility total ankle.

- Weight-bearing to tolerance is begun on the first postoperative day with the splint on.
- The fixed splint is removed on fifth to seventh day with a brace that protects the ankle against the eversion, inversion and rotational stress. A removable controlled ankle motion (CAM) walker boot may be provided to allow initiation of early range-of-motion activities in patients whose surgery has been uncomplicated.
- For patients with additional surgeries or those with poor bone quality a weight-bearing cast is applied for 6 weeks followed by brace application for additional 4–6 weeks.
- No recommendation exists for keeping the patients nonweight-bearing for prolonged period unless some surgical complication or poor fit of the implant was there.
- Stretching program begin immediately for ankle with weight-bearing, to regain mobility.
- The patient is gradually weaned from the CAM boot over 4–6 weeks and allowed regular shoe wearing.

Complications of Ankle Arthroplasty

Intraoperative

Malpositioning: All malpositions reduce longevity of the implant.

- *Varus malalignment:* Medial impingement, stiffness, and edge wear.
- *Valgus malalignment:* Lateral gutter pain due to subfibular impingement, arch pain, and edge wear.
- *Medial translation of the tibial component:* Higher risk of malleolar fracture.
- *Lateral malpositioning:* Fibular impingement and osteolysis, deltoid stretching, and varus tilting of talus.
- *Anterior malposition:* Anterior tilt and subsidence of tibial component, anisometric loading of collateral ligaments.
- *Posterior malposition:* May be in fact useful at these places, the tibial implant under stronger posterior cortex. Concern, however, is always there for posterior tilt and implant subsidence and anisometric loading of collateral ligaments.
- *Proximal displacement:* Higher chance of subsidence due to tibial tray on softer cancellous bone. Shortened gastrocnemius-soleus complex → plantar flexion weakness.
- *Distal displacement:* Lengthened gastrocnemius-soleus complex → loss of dorsiflexion and altered gait.

Improper size of implants: Anisometric stretching of ligaments and impingement.

Malleoli fracture: Produce malposition of the components or poor implant fixation and subsequent loosening. They should be fixed stably with the index surgery.

Tendon injury: Posterior tibial, peroneal, flexor digitorum longus (FDL), flexor hallucis longus (FHL) tendons should be protected and repaired primarily with four-strand repair if cut.

Postoperative

- Wound dehiscence
- Infection
- Deep vein thrombosis (DVT)
- *Syndesmosis nonunion (problem only with Agility ankle):* It is recommended to use two syndesmotic screws for early healing
- *Loss of motion:* Plantar flexion contracture due to existing heel-cord contracture, inadequate posterior capsular release
- Aseptic loosening
- Subsidence
- Polyethylene wear and instability

KIENBOCK'S DISEASE (LUNATOMALACIA)

Definition

An isolated disorder of the carpal lunate arising out of vascular compromise from varied causes manifested radiographically as sclerotic changes followed by progressive fragmentation and collapse.

History

The name of the lunate bone derives from the "crescent-shaped" (Latin: lunatus), from Latin Luna ("moon"), due to bone's resemblance to a crescent moon. Kienbock's disease is a disorder of the wrist named for Dr Robert Kienbock, a radiologist in Vienna, Austria who described "traumatic softening" of the lunate in 1910 (most of the ON and skeletal malformations have been described in detail radiologically around this time as X-ray were discovered and used medically in the first decade of 20th century). He attributed it to traumatic disruption of the blood supply to the lunate and subsequent disturbance of the bony nutrition and called this "lunatomalacia". The condition had, however, been earlier described by Peste in 1843 (French literature). Specifically, Kienbock's disease is another name for ON with fragmentation and collapse of the lunate. This has classically been attributed to arterial disruption, but may also occur after events that produce venous congestion with elevated interosseous pressure.

Anatomical Considerations

Lunate Bone (Latin: os lunatum)

- *Bone structure:* The lunate is found within the proximal row of carpal bones. It is a crescent-shaped carpal bone present within the hand. The proximal surface of the lunate bone is smooth and convex, articulating with the radius. The radial surface is flat and narrow, with a crescent-shaped facet for articulation with the scaphoid. The ulnar surface possesses a smooth and quadrilateral facet for articulation with the triquetral. The palmar surface is rough, as is the dorsal surface. The dorsal surface is broad and rounded. The distal surface of the bone is deep and concave. The distal surface articulates with convex articular surface of capitate (type 1 lunate of Viega, the type 2 lunate additionally articulates with hamate). The convexity of capitate is greater (less radius of curvature) than concavity of lunate. This produces localized stress on the lunate predisposing to the osseous collapse and fragmentation later in the course of disease. It is considered that the transmission of higher stress through bone may lead to coronal split seen at and beyond stage IIIB. The lunate is stabilized by a radial ligament to the scaphoid and an ulnar ligament to the triquetrum. Three types of lunate have been described (Antuña Zapico) on the basis of the angle between the lateral scaphoid side of the lunate and the proximal radial side of the lunate to understand relationship between lunate shape and ulnar length **(Fig. 34)**.
    - Type I lunate had an angle >130° (proximal apex or crest)—this is the weakest with a greater potential for bone fatigue and stress fracture and is seen in ulna negative wrists.
    - Type II lunate had an angle of approximately 100°—seen with ulna zero.
    - Type III lunate has two distinct facets on proximal surface (one for radius and other for TFCC)—seen with ulna plus.

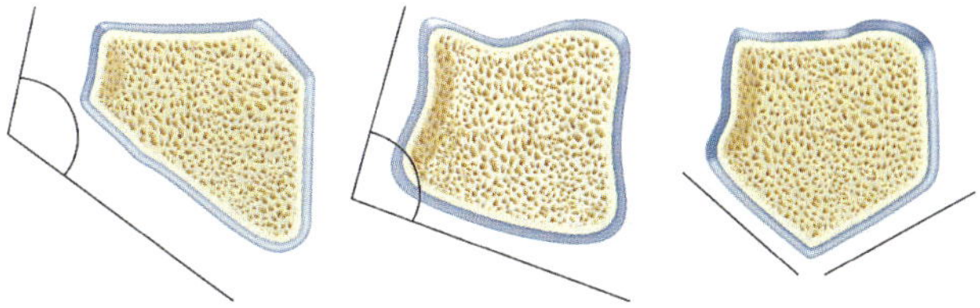

Fig. 34: The three types of lunate as described by Antuña Zapico.

Ligaments between the radius and carpal bone also stabilize the position of the lunate, as does its position in the lunate fossa of the radius. Testut-Kuentz radioscapholunate (RSL) ligament is inserted at the radial proximal side of lunate. This ligament is considered a mesocapsule extending from the palmar radiocarpal joint capsule. One to five nutrient vessels enter through the ligament along with radiolunate-triquetral ligament. Logically, lesions of RSL could lead to ischemia in radial proximal side of bone which is the usual initial site of Kienbock's disease. If there is an anastomosis between the dorsal and volar plexus the chances of ON are minimized.

- Articulations of lunate bone **(Fig. 35)**
    - Radius proximally
    - Capitate and hamate distally
    - Scaphoid on radial side
    - Triquetral on ulnar side

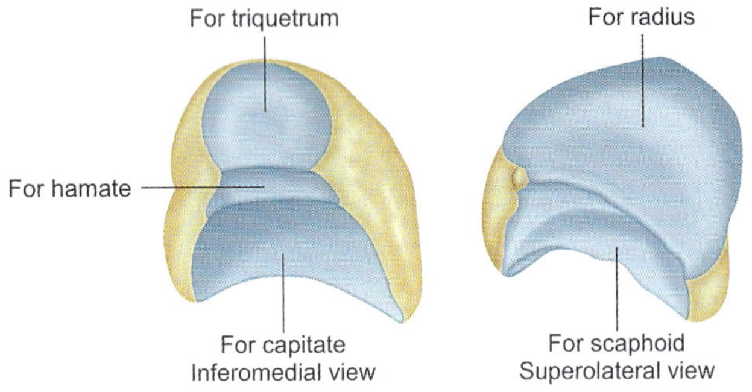

Fig. 35: Articulations of lunate bone.

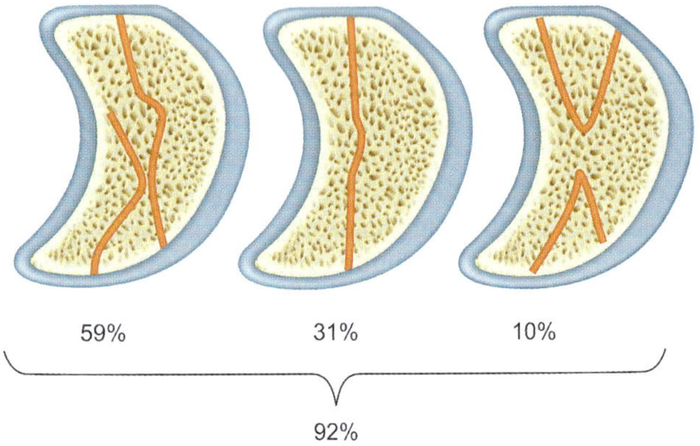

Fig. 36: The different patterns of intraosseous vascular anastomosis of lunate bone supplied by volar + dorsal pedicle. Most patients have an inverted 'Y' pattern (59%) as shown on left, the 'I' pattern in middle is seen in one-third of population. Both these patterns along with patients having single volar pedicle (8% population, not shown) are susceptible for osteonecrosis following fracture of lunate.

- *Blood supply:* The lunate receives its blood supply from dorsal (through dorsal foramen from dorsal intercarpal, radiocarpal, and transverse metacarpal arches forming dorsal plexus) and palmar branches originating from a palmar plexus as well as direct ulnar, radial and anterior interosseous artery. 10–25% lunates receive only either dorsal or volar artery and are at risk of lunatomalacia putting them at higher risk of loss of vascularity from trauma or interruption. The dorsal supply is more inconsistent as also are the dorsal foramina. The volar foramina are higher in number. The blood supply through RSL ligaments has been emphasized before. Apart from the extra-articular anastomosis the intraosseous anastomosis has also been implicated in the development of lunatomalacia. Three patterns of intraosseous anastomosis have been described namely the "X", "Y", and "I" patterns (Gelberman, **Fig. 36**). This anastomosis occurs beyond the midportion of the bone. I and Y pattern are more susceptible for ON following fractures possibly.
- *Function:* The carpal bones function as a unit to provide a bony superstructure for the hand. As a proximal carpal bone, the lunate is also involved in movement of the wrist.

Predisposing Factors

Etiology is still undefined so various factors have been proposed (none proved) as the possible causes of developing AVN of lunate bone (most of them based on case studies), and hence the Kienbock's disease:

- *Aberrant blood supply to lunate:* Problems with arteries [single dominant nutrient arterial supply for lunate (20% patients)]
  - Poorly organized intraosseous circulation—"I" pattern of anastomosis
  - Venous congestion leading to increased intraosseous pressure (Jensen)—this may also be partially responsible to finding Kienbock's in cerebral palsy (5–10% prevalence). The patients maintain a flexed posture of wrist and due to raised muscle tone the blood outflow is impeded producing increased intraosseous pressure.
  - Vasculopathies:
    - Septic emboli
    - Raynaud's disease
    - Scleroderma
    - Systemic lupus erythematosus
    - Dermatomyositis
    - Rheumatoid arthritis
    - Juvenile idiopathic arthritis
- Coagulopathies and metabolic disorders
  - Sickle cell anemia
  - Gout
  - Antiphospholipid antibody syndrome
  - Crohn's enteritis
- Skeletal variations:
  - Small lunate bone (Tsuge and Nakamura)
  - Negative ulnar variance (Huelten) putting extra pressure on the lunate due to large unsupported area of bone in certain wrist motions (extension and ulnar deviation). This extra stress causes microtrauma in the bone and could eventually lead to Kienbock's disease. Huelten advised radial shortening to reduce pressure on lunate while Persson advised ulnar lengthening procedure. The association is supported by finding higher incidence of lunatomalacia in cerebral palsy patients and patients with congenital shortening of the ulna in Langer-Giedion syndrome.
  - Abnormal wrist biomechanics—pointed hammer effect of capitate along with higher force transmission through the bone (35% of forces across the wrist).
- Some diseases may be linked to a greater risk, including lupus, cerebral palsy, sickle cell anemia, and gout. One study found that 9.4% of cerebral palsy patients also had Kienbock's disease.
- Repetitive significant trauma as in power drillers (Jack Hammer), single major trauma as in motor vehicle accident—there are various methods trauma has been proposed to cause AVN.
  - Trauma acting on vascular system directly (avulsion of pedicle)
  - Trauma acting on osseous system (fracture theory)
  - Trauma acting on vascular nervous system

Vasodilatation causes stasis and decalcification while the usual mechanism is vasoconstriction of the vessel and thrombosis and interruption of the vascularity. Repetitive trauma has been proposed to cause trabecular ruptures and multiple osseous lamina form with simultaneous healing and thickening of trabeculae that interfere with vascularity—the "fault-plate hypothesis".

- Endothelial cell dysfunction—steroids and viral disease (HIV and hepatitis B virus infection)
- Chronic scapholunate dissociation has been associated with development of Kienbock's disease.
- There is no compelling evidence, however, suggesting that certain jobs may increase the risk of developing Kienbock's disease.

Pathological Phases of Osteonecrosis Lunate

There are three pathological phases of ON lunate:

1. Early vascular changes commence with *ischemia*, subsequent *necrosis*, and revascularization. Currently, the MRI and bone scan are of value in interpreting the vascular changes.
2. *Intermediate osseous changes:* Lichtman has described this over the last 33 years. The initial radiological changes are of sclerosis followed by *subchondral collapse* appreciated better on CT scan. Subchondral bone plate is critical to progression of collapse and its survival is the key to preservation of form of bone and articular cartilage.
3. *Late chondral stage:* The articular cartilage is soft and can be indented suggesting that it has a false floor. This is followed by lamination and *wear of cartilage* with loss of agility.

Clinical Features

Kienbock's disease is seen most often in young adults (between 20 and 45 years of age), but it is also diagnosed in children as well as in older age groups. It is somewhat more common in dominant wrist of males aged 20–40 years (females tend to have equal involvement of wrists and present later in life—4th decade).

Kienbock's disease is usually unilateral and isolated. A history of trauma is often reported by the patients, often minor or repetitive trauma. The disease is slowly progressive with unspecific signs and symptoms.

- A painful and sometimes swollen wrist
- Passive dorsiflexion of middle finger produces characteristic pain
- Limited ROM in the affected wrist (stiffness)
- Decreased grip strength in the hand
- Tenderness directly over the lunate (on the top of the hand at about the middle of the wrist)
- Pain or difficulty in turning the hand upward.

However, as these things also can occur with many other things, so they are not very specific.

Kienbock's disease in children has two forms:

1. *Infantile form:* Present between 5 and 10 years and have excellent prognosis with conservative therapy and immobilization.
2. *Juvenile Kienbock's disease (Teenbock's disease):* Patient presenting between 10 and 15 years and have prognosis similar to infantile form while those presenting >15 years may need surgical treatment but prognosis is still better than adult types.

Investigations

- X-ray imaging during Stage 1 of the disease will show an apparently normal lunate bone, later sclerosis, fracture, fragmentation, and collapse are seen. The collapse is in the form of scapholunate advanced collapse (SLAC) wrist and is also called Kienbock's disease advanced collapse (K-DAC). The various radiological indices **(Figs. 37A and B)** used by different authors to evaluate the bony involvement include:
  - Stahl's lunate index (normal = 0.50–0.56)

$$= \frac{\textit{Length of lunate on PA}}{\textit{AP diameter of lunate on lateral view}}$$

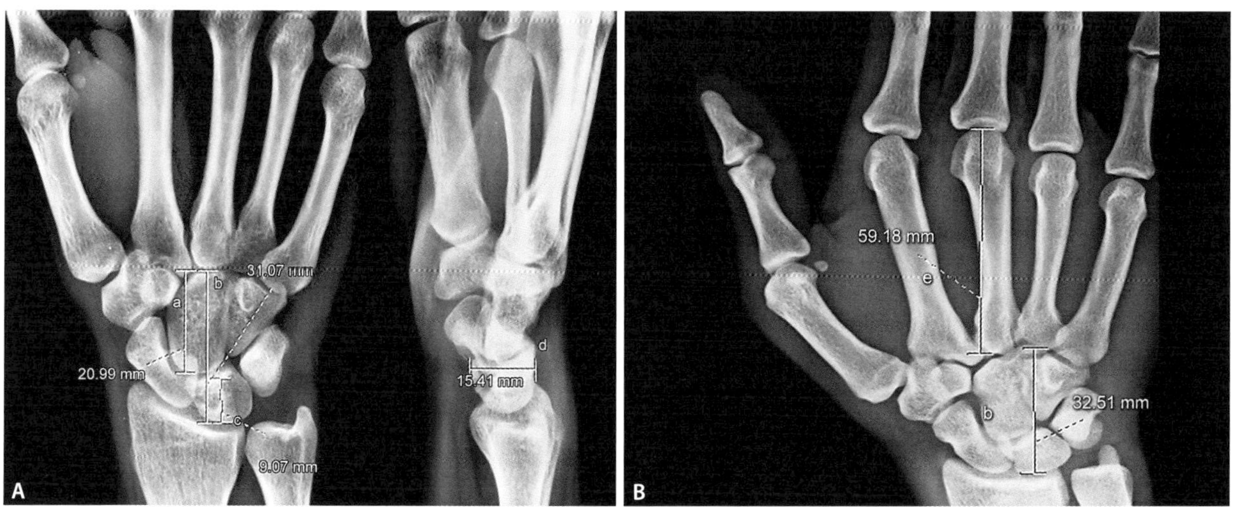

Figs. 37A and B: Radiology of Kienbock's disease and various indices described. (A) Bouman's index and calculation of Stahl's lunate index; (B) Method of calculating Youm's index and wrist showing positive ulna variance.

- Ulnar variance (radioulnar index) = distance between distal point of ulna on radial side and the distal point of radius on ulnar side. Normal is ±2, –2 means ulna is 2 mm shorter than radius.
- Youm's index of carpal height (normal 0.51–0.57)

$$= \frac{\textit{Carpal height}}{\textit{Length of 3rd metacarpal}}$$

- Bouman's index of carpal height (normal 0.62–0.66)

$$= \frac{\textit{Length of capitate}}{\textit{Carpal height}}$$

- Magnetic resonance imaging can help to assess the blood supply to the lunate. The Gadolinium-infused MRI has been used to find the vascular patterns (Schmitt-Lanz) and the following have been found:
    - *Pattern N:* Normal—Normal signal (no enhancement)
    - *Pattern A:* Marrow edema with intact (viable) bone trabeculae. Increased (homogenous) signal (proximal lunate)
    - *Pattern B:* Early marrow necrosis with fibrovascular reparative tissue—mixed (inhomogeneous) signal zones
    - *Pattern C:* Necrotic bone marrow with collapse—decreased (homogenous) signal
- Computed tomography scanning may be used in later stages to determine the number and sizes of the lunate fragments.

Classification

First described by Stahl based on radiographs and modified by Lichtman et al. in 1977 into four stages, the classification now called *Stahl-Lichtman classification* for Kienbock's disease is quite popular. The purpose of this classification system is to guide treatment and to enable comparison of clinical outcomes. The classification system and proposed modification is presented in **Table 7**.

The *American Society for Surgery of the Hand (ASSH) classification* for Kienbock's disease has four stages:

- *Stage 1:* The lunate has lost its blood supply. Radiographs are normal. There is some pain, possibly some swelling as well, and a risk of fracture.
- *Stage 2:* X-rays show that the bone is unusually dense. When bone loses its blood supply it hardens.
- *Stage 3:* The bone starts to shatter (fragments and collapses, **Figs. 38A and B**).
- *Stage 4:* The lunate has completely collapsed. The other bones next to the lunate have also become damaged and arthritic **(Figs. 39A and B)**. Not all patients reach this stage.

Arthroscopic classification of lunatomalacia (Bain and Begg, **Table 8**) has been proposed for the recent consideration

TABLE 7: Modified Stahl-Lichtman classification of lunatomalacia.

Stage "0" (not a part of described classification)	• Intermittent symptoms. Pain with stress. X-ray, MRI normal. Stress test abnormal—can be considered "Angina" of wrist as the patient has pain on stress • *Lunate stress test (similar to coronary stress test):* Repetitive axial loading of the lunate under stress followed by fat suppressed T-1 sequences show Schmittt-Lanz pattern "A" bone edema. Compare this to other side
Stage I	Normal radiograph (possible lunate fracture). Bone scan and magnetic resonance imaging positive
Stage II	Sclerosis of the lunate without collapse. Portions of the lunate begin to deteriorate. This shows as increased density on X-rays
Stage III	Lunate collapse and fragmentation + proximal migration of the capitate • *Stage IIIA:* Proximal carpal row remains aligned • *Stage IIIB:* Proximal carpal row becomes malaligned and destabilizes, fixed flexion deformity of the scaphoid • *Stage IIIC:* (Proposed) presence of coronal fracture in the bone on MRI (the only other bone where such an avascular coronal fracture is seen in navicular bone of foot)—poor prognosis and will need more aggressive treatment like lunate excision or proximal row carpectomy
Stage IV	Lunate disintegrates with radiocarpal and midcarpal arthritic changes

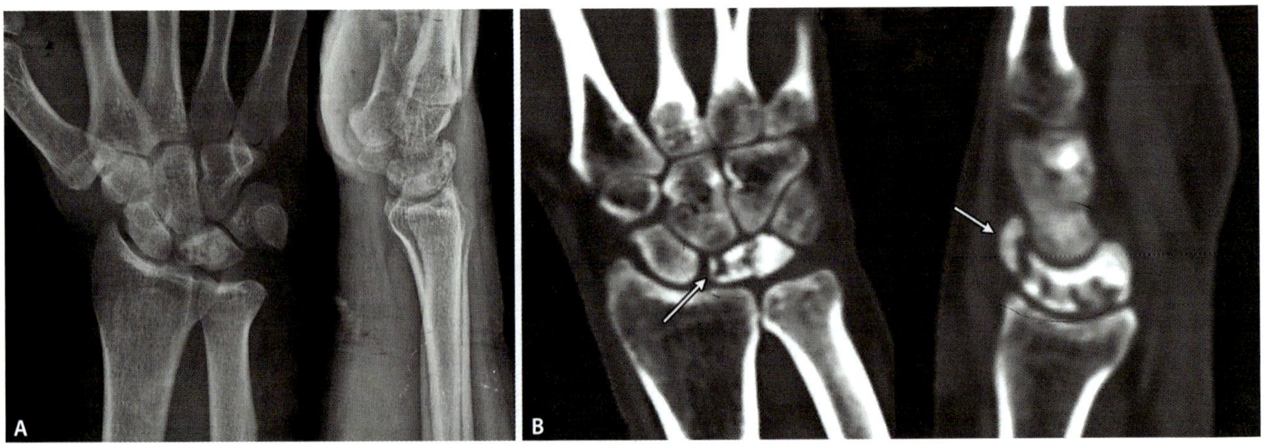

Figs. 38A and B: Stage 3 ASSH Kienbock's disease—radiographic picture (A). The lunate bone has started to shatter as is more clearly evident on NCCT wrist (B, white arrows). It can be classified as stage IIIA Stahl-Lichtman as there is lunate fragmentation along with proximal migration of capitate but minimal disruption of Gilula's arc, sagittal fractures are seen but not coronal fracture. (ASSH: American Society for Surgery of the Hand; NCCT: noncontrast computed tomography)

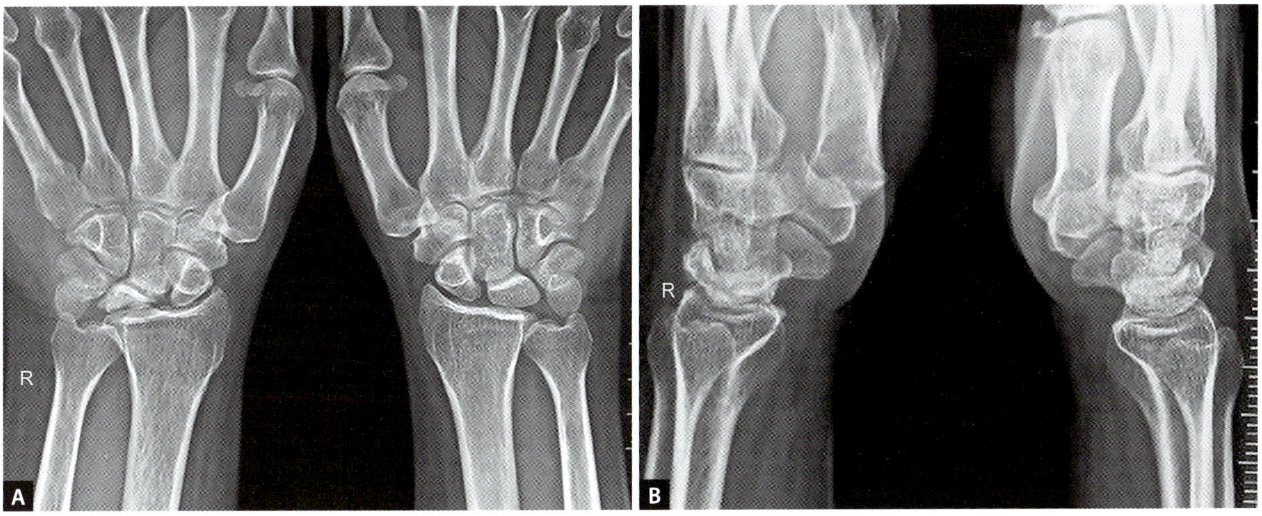

Figs. 39A and B: The AP (A) and lateral (B) radiographs of both wrists demonstrate ASSH stage 4 Kienbock's disease with complete collapse of the lunate bone of right wrist and developing radiocarpal and intercarpal arthrosis (compare from left wrist). (AP: anteroposterior; ASSH: American Society for Surgery of the Hand)

TABLE 8: Arthroscopic classification and proposed treatment based on the system.

Grade	*Arthroscopic finding*	*Treatment recommendation*
Grade 0	Normal articular surface of lunate	None required
Grade 1	Nonfunctional proximal lunate articular surface only	Proximal row carpectomy or radioscapholunate fusion may be indicated
Grade 2	Two nonfunctional articular surfaces	
Grade 2a	The proximal articular surface of the lunate and the lunate fossa are both nonfunctional	A radioscapholunate fusion will remove both nonfunctional articular surfaces and enable the wrist to articulate through the normal midcarpal joint
Grade 2b	The proximal and distal articular surfaces of the lunate are nonfunctional. This typically occurs when there is a coronal fracture in the lunate extending between the radiocarpal and midcarpal joints. The lunate fossa of the radius and the head of the capitate are normal	This is best managed with a proximal row carpectomy. Lunate replacement is another alternative. These patients often do not do well with more complex procedures such as internal fixation or vascularized bone grafting
Grade 3	Three articular surfaces are nonfunctional	Most likely it will be the capitate articular surface which remains functional. This situation could be managed with a hemiarthroplasty. Alternatively, a salvage procedure such as a total wrist fusion or arthroplasty
Grade 4	All four articular surfaces are nonfunctional	A total wrist fusion or arthroplasty is indicated

that cartilage preservation and function are important determinants of outcome rather than radiological features. Also, frequent use of wrist arthroscopy to evaluate the patients has set in the path for use of arthroscopic classification. The various methods used for treatment of Kienbock's disease based on findings at wrist arthroscopy have been presented **(Table 8)**.

The prognostic significance of the main classification systems and the MRI patterns are presented in **Table 9**.

TABLE 9: Prognostic significance of various classification systems and magnetic resonance imaging findings for Kienbock's disease.

Prognosis	*Litchman classification*	*Bain and Begg classification*	*Magnetic resonance imaging findings*
Good	0, 1	0	Normal (N), A
Intermediate	2, 3A	1, 2, 3	B
Poor	3-B, 3-C	4, 2B	C

Treatment

Conservative

Nonoperative treatment has its proponents. The rationale for this approach lies in the observation that spontaneous regression of the signs and symptoms has been observed in early Kienbock. If the stress on the bone is taken away then revascularization can occur spontaneously.

Treatment is primarily directed by the level of symptoms. The primary methods of nonoperative treatment are immobilization (splint or cast) and anti-inflammatory medications. Resting the wrist increases the likelihood of

TABLE 10: Treatment modalities based on various classification systems.

Stahl-Lichtman	*Bain and Begg*	*Magnetic resonance imaging*	*Treatment*
0	0	A	Medical and preventive therapy
1	1	A	Medical and supportive therapy (temporary unloading of lunate), treat underlying disorder (autoimmune disorder and antiviral treatment) Surgical treatment (conservative failure)— *Ulna minus* → radial shortening ± revascularization *Ulna neutral or plus* → capitate shortening + capitohamate fusion ± revascularization
2	0 or 1	A	Joint leveling, revascularization as above
2	2	B	STT fusion ± revascularization procedure
2	4	C	Radiocarpal fusion
3A	1, 2	B	As for stage 2, bias toward doing revascularization
3A	3, 4	C	Wrist arthrodesis
3B	0	A	Salvage lunate—correct the scaphoid subluxation, rotation and perform scaphocapitate fusion to unload lunate ± revascularization procedure
3B	1	B	Proximal row carpectomy
3B	2	C	STT fusion, carbon implant ± wrist denervation
3B	3, 4	C	Wrist arthrodesis
3C (proposed)	2b	C	Proximal row carpectomy ± wrist denervation
4	3,4	C	Wrist arthrodesis

(STT: scaphotrapeziotrapezoid)

restoring blood flow to the lunate bone. However, this is only an option during stage 1 **(Table 10)** when the bone is radiologically silent and cartilage is healthy. Recently, a combination approach utilizing bone marrow injection, ultrasonic therapy while simultaneously unloading the lunate using external fixator has been found to be effective in early stages of disease.

To avoid trauma and collapse is first choice in the earlier stages. Younger patients tend to have a better ability to reestablish blood flow to various areas (see clinical features), so in a very young patient, always start with this approach, especially if the disease is early, in hopes of allowing revascularization of the lunate and prevention of disease progression.

Anti-inflammatory drugs may help manage the symptoms of swelling and pain during the early stages. Wrist injection with steroids may also help. More importantly if the cause is identified then respective medical treatment should be undertaken like treatment of vasculopathies, coagulation, and autoimmune disorders and infection **(Table 10)**. Despite all these measures, there is a definite progression in the collapse seen radiologically. There seems to be dissociation between the symptoms and radiological findings—situation similar to scaphoid nonunion. So, operative treatment should always account for the patient's symptoms.

Operative

The primary indication of surgery is a patient with persistent pain not responsive to conservative treatment. Lots of operative treatments for various stages have been described by different surgeons treating the disease in discrete patients. The methods can be grouped under few distinct categories like:

- Decompression of lunate
  - Joint leveling procedure
- Revascularization procedures
- Prosthetic replacement
- Limited fusion and wrist fusion

The following enumerates reported procedures for treatment of Kienbock's procedure:

- Capitate shortening
- Ulna lengthening and radial shortening
- Metaphyseal osteotomy (core decompression)
- Scaphotrapeziotrapezoid (STT) arthrodesis with or without lunate resection
- Scaphocapitate arthrodesis with or without lunate resection
- Radius-lunate (Chamay) arthrodesis
- Radius-lunate-scaphoid arthrodesis
- Wrist arthrodesis
- Lunate resection with ulnar column arthrodesis
- Lunate resection and capitate lengthening
- Prosthetic replacement of lunate
- Resection of the lunate
- Lunate resection and substitution with the vascularized pisiform
- Direct vessel implantation
- Vascularized bone grafting
- Proximal row resection
- Wrist denervation

Not everything can be done in a patient. Only selected procedures are possible depending on stage of disease. A simplistic approach based on various stages is presented in **Table 10**. One important concept to understand is that lunate is the keystone of the proximal carpal row. Simple resection leads to immediate and severe collapse of the carpus with subsequent osteoarthritis. So, substitution of the space or preservation of bone is necessary. If this cannot be done then arthrodesis should be done to prevent collapse of carpals.

Decompression of the Lunate

Leveling procedures of the distal radioulnar joint (DRUJ): Radial shortening **(Fig. 40)** or ulnar lengthening.

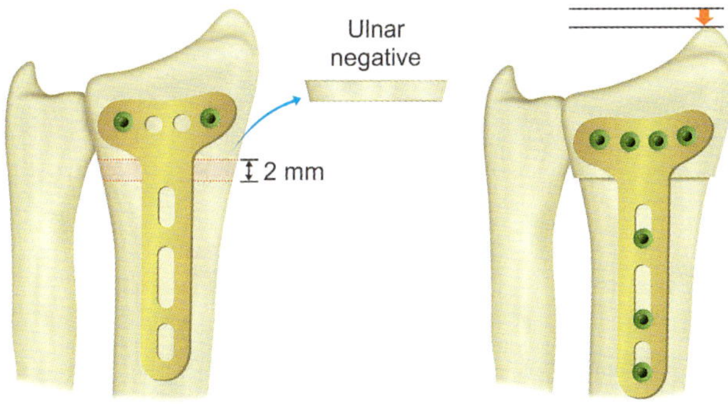

Fig. 40: Radial shortening for ulnar negative patients to equalize joint surfaces.

If the bones of the forearm are uneven in length, a "joint leveling" procedure [shortening the longer bone (Huelten) or lengthening the shorter bone (Persson)] can be done. This procedure applies only for ulna minus wrist (i.e., negative ulnar variance). Ulna can be made longer with bone graft or radius shortened by removing a section of the bone. Radial shortening is preferred due to:

- Lower complication rates
- Ability to change the inclination of radius for improved carpal stability and mobility
- There is a concern of loading the DRUJ with joint leveling procedures induced by DRUJ incongruity. This requires lateral translation of radius, further lending support to this procedure over ulnar lengthening.
- The severe ulna minus patients may have excessive DRUJ incongruity due to joint leveling procedures and in such cases the ulna lengthening is contraindicated.

Mechanism of action of joint leveling procedures:

- This reduces the compressive forces (unloads) on the lunate and seems to halt progression of the disease.
- Partial denervation of the wrist also occurs with the radius shortening and may also account for the pain relief obtained.
- Forces on the lunate, caused by using the hand forcefully, are thought to flatten down the lunate, advancing the stage of the disease. This collapsing force can be reduced by 70% with an appropriate radial shortening or ulnar lengthening.

The procedure is indicated in patients:

- Till stage 3B
- With intact lunate architecture
- Preserved capitolunate joint, of course with ulna minus wrist

In patients with neutral or positive ulnar variance, shortening the radius is a poor idea. In this clinical situation, radial wedge osteotomies designed to decrease the radial inclination have been proposed. The *open wedge* radial osteotomies have been shown to have better effect as the closing wedge osteotomy increases pressure on lunate. The aim is to flatten the slope by 4–6° that essentially produces radial deviation of the carpus. The decreased radial inclination is associated with increased carpalulnar distance and lunate coverage ratio. Patients report good movements and reduced pain with improved grip strength. The joint leveling procedures can be combined with revascularization procedures.

Intracarpal Procedures

Lunate excision: This procedure is mentioned here only, not to be performed. The resulting carpal shift destroys the carpal mechanics producing a painful arthritic joint that ultimately needs salvage by arthrodesis. To prevent the carpal shift, a spacer implant (lunate arthroplasty) had been used extensively before but the results were not satisfactory and silicone synovitis frequently developed further complicating the issue. Replacement with a carbon implant or the head of the capitate (Graner's procedure) while preserving the volar ligaments may be appropriate for stage three patients individually. It is, however, recommended to use other well-studied procedures.

Limited carpal arthrodesis: To ease pressure on the lunate the wrist bones can be fused to form a bigger bone mass, bearing the stresses and preventing their migration due to shear increase in size. A variety of intercarpal fusions for the treatment of Kienbock's disease have been used. The goal of all is to reduce forces on the lunate, crushing it down, and in procedures that involve the scaphoid, to correct and maintain proper scaphoid position.

- *Capitohamate arthrodesis (Chuinard):* Due to progressive collapse of lunate the proximal migration of capitate is inevitable. To prevent this, capitate can be fused to hamate side to side so that the capitate no longer puts axial pressure on the lunate and prevents progressive fragmentation. This also gives time for bone to revascularize. The method has also been recommended to combine with capitate shortening that additionally reduces the pressure from lunate.
- *Scaphocapitate fusion:* Biomechanically, this fusion has been shown to reduce compressive forces at the radiolunate joint by about 10%. Some surgeons prefer this fusion because it requires only one fusion site and is technically easier to perform.
- *Scaphotrapeziotrapezoid arthrodesis/fusion:* This fusion theoretically succeeds in preventing carpal shortening. The STT arthrodesis can also be combined with a VBG or other revascularization procedure (Stage 3A). The authors from Germany and Japan recommend this procedure as a primary treatment commonly. The problem is increased loading of the scaphoid bone and development of radioscaphoid arthrosis. Similar to this radial carpal fusion, the ulnar side carpal limited arthrodesis has been proposed to relieve the proximal migration of the carpus. This triquetro-capito-hamate fusion is combined with lunate resection.
- *Capitate shortening (Almquist):* This procedure can reduce the pressure on lunate when the ulnar variance is either neutral or plus, and hence the radial shortening is not an option. Biomechanically, the load on lunate is reduced by over 60% but with significantly increased load

on scaphoid and trapezoid articulation by some 150%. Combining capitohamate arthrodesis can transfer the load to ulnar aspect and additionally decompress the lunate bone.

If the disease has progressed to severe arthritis of the wrist, fusing the bones will reduce pain and help maintain function, although motion is limited.

Revascularization Procedures

Revascularization techniques, usually involving a bone graft taken elsewhere from the body—often held in place by an external fixator for a period of weeks or months—have been successful at stages as late as 3B, although their use at later stages (like most other treatments for Kienbock's) is controversial. The basic principles involve removing the necrotic bone and replacing it with living bone. Lunate is protected during the revascularization period (usually with temporary stabilization of the carpus) as this makes the bone soft. Healing occurs by either direct revascularization or creeping substitution. The VBGs are indicated for patients with intact cartilage shell and they can also be combined with the conventional methods of management like joint leveling procedure or joint decompression. The various methods for vascularized bone grafting include:

- *Saffar's technique:* The lunate is replaced by pisiform bone pedicled on the ulnar artery
- Second dorsal metacarpal head vascularized graft based on 2nd dorsal metacarpal artery (Hori et al.)
- The pronator quadratus bone flap of Leung
- Kuhlmann vascular bone graft from distal radius based on volar carpal artery (used also for nonunion scaphoid)
- Scaphoid tubercle on abductor pollicis brevis muscle
- Cored decompression and nonvascularized bone grafting
- Free VBGs from the iliac crest (Tamai) and medial femoral condyle have also been used
- Dorsal distal radius pedicle bone grafts [intercompartmental (IC) segmental artery-based bone grafts]—Zaidemberg et al. initially described the use of a pedicled dorsal radius VBG for scaphoid pathology. Anatomical classification of the potential donor grafts was proposed by Sheez et al. The types of grafts from distal radius can be grouped into two categories:
  1. Those within the retinaculum
  2. Those superficial to retinaculum

The vessels form radial and ulnar anterior interosseous and posterior interosseous vessels give rise to three dorsal arches the dorsal intercarpal arch, dorsal radiocarpal arch, and a dorsal supraretinacular (SR) arch **(Fig. 41)**. The extensor retinaculum vessels are subdivided into extensor compartment (EC) vessels versus those between compartments—the so called IC vessels. Vessels on the surface are called SR vessels. Four main vessels have been identified for use as pedicled vascular bone grafts:

1. 1, 2 intercompartmental supraretinacular artery (1, 2 ICSRA—*see* Preiser's disease).
2. 2, 3 ICSRA
3. 4th extensor compartment artery (ECA)
4. 5th ECA

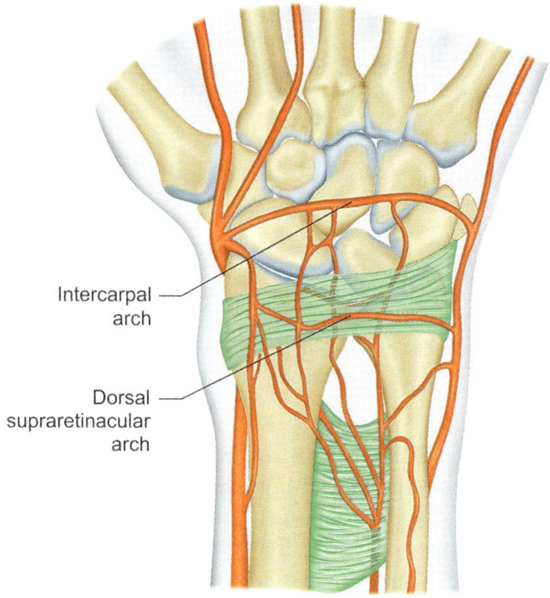

Fig. 41: The disposition of intercompartmental segmental arteries around the wrist joint. Note the intercarpal and dorsal supraretinacular arch and various intercompartmental branches that emerge from the arches.

The 4 + 5 EC vessel is the preferred pedicle where the bone graft from 4th ECA is taken pedicled on 5th ECA. The 4th and 5th ECA are identified and bone graft harvested from the 4th ECA **(Figs. 42A to C)**. The common origin of vessels is identified and ligated proximally to elevate the pedicle. To prevent collapse of the lunate during revascularization the scaphocapitate pinning is performed.

- The 5th ECA has larger diameter to provide as pedicle and the length of combined vessels is long enough to reach any carpus.
- The exposure of 5th ECA is done from ulnar aspect, hence the pedicle is protected from ulnar-sided capsulotomy during rotation.
- In general, dorsal approaches preserve the volar native vascular supply so are preferred.

Metaphyseal Decompression

Just the common understanding of induction of hyperemia due to surgical fiddling of tissues has been utilized by Illarramendi by performing the distal radial and ulnar metaphyseal decompression. The primary pathology in lunate was not addressed. The procedure is based on the premises that hyperemia will lead to secondary increase in vascularity of lunate bone, and hence directly address the primary pathophysiology of decreased or absent blood flow.

Unloading the Lunate

Use of external fixation to unload lunate has been used for early stage Kienbock's disease. This may promote revascularization by reducing the incident pressure but has not been proven in large studies. The effect may be similar to cast treatment for immobilization of the wrist.

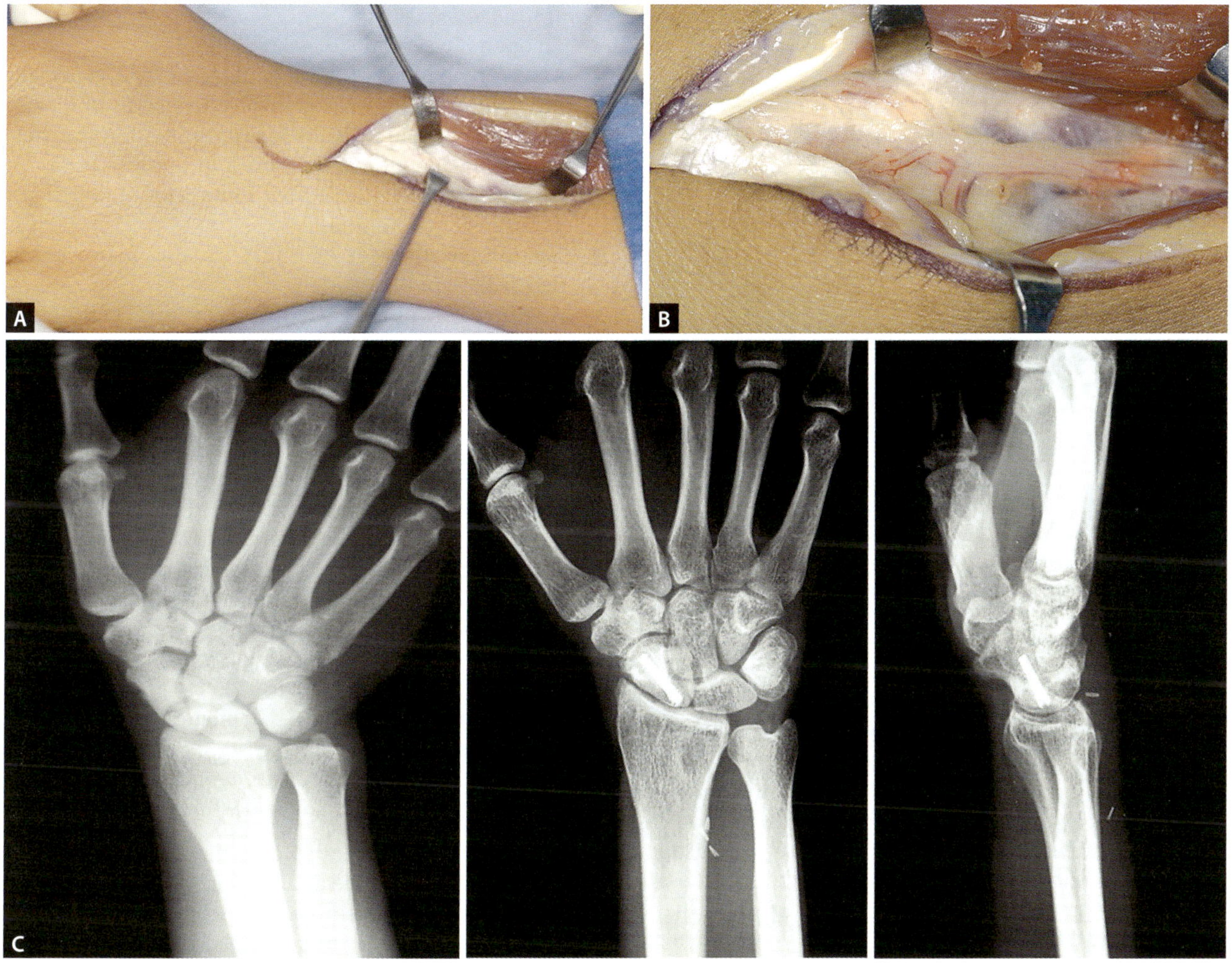

Figs. 42A to C: Exposing and harvesting the 4th extra-compartmental artery (ECA). Incise the skin dorsally in a lazy-S shaped incision (A). Identify and neatly retract extensor digitorum communis (EDC) this directly exposes the 4th ECA lying above the retinaculum (B). This can be used for revascularization procedures (here used for nonunion scaphoid). In this particular example it has been used in a 'reversed' fashion—proximally ligated and distally based pedicle.

Source: Prof. PP Kotwal, Chairman, Institute of Orthopedics and Joint Replacement, Pushpavati Singhania Research Institute, New Delhi, India.

Salvage Procedures for Pain Relief

These include wrist denervation, arthroplasty, arthrodesis, and proximal row carpectomy done in stages 3B and 4. Arthroplasty procedures include partial or complete prosthetic replacement of wrist, or proximal row carpectomy.

Proximal Row Carpectomy (Stamm, 1944)

The procedure is specifically indicated in proposed stage 3C and 3B. This removes lunate along with the other two carpal bones. The preserved capitate head articular surface and cartilage of the lunate fossa favors the outcome after this procedure.

Wrist Denervation

This is usually an adjunctive procedure combined with other procedures. When done alone for advanced procedures the relief is usually not complete.

Wrist Arthrodesis

This is the simplest salvage procedure that is aimed to fuse the radiocarpal, intercarpal and carpometacarpal (CMC) joints and ameliorate pain from arthrosis **(Fig. 43)**. The procedure is also used to treat patients that fail to obtain relief after other surgical procedures. The limitations of wrist movement after arthrodesis are quite well compensated by the movements at hand and elbow. Despite good pain relief in many some patients might continue to have pain. Arthrodesis of the wrist is performed less often nowadays due to trend towards reconstructive surgery.

History of wrist arthrodesis: Arthrodesis of the radiocarpal joint has evolved over the last 50 years. The trend has been toward increasing stability in the method of fixation. Early procedures used cortical or cancellous bone grafting with limited fixation methods, such as pins or screws. Campbell and Keokarn described an inlay bone grafting technique

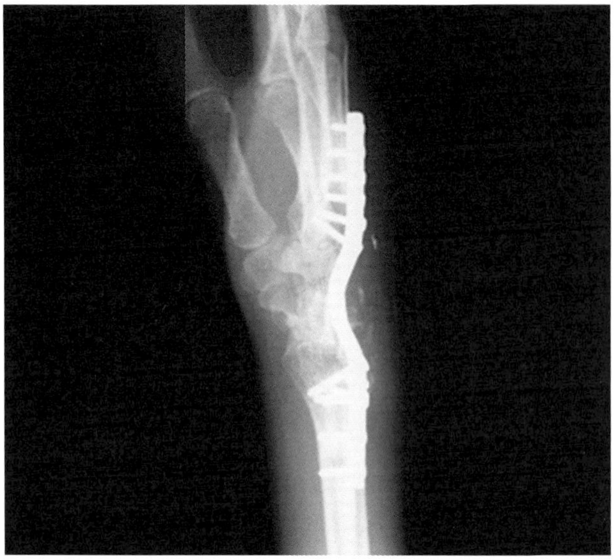

Fig. 43: Wrist arthrodesis done using a hybrid plate containing 3.5 mm screws for radius and 2.5 mm screws for metacarpal.

of wrist fusion in 1964. Haddad and Riordan applied this technique through a lateral (radial) approach.

Various fixation methods have been described, including screws, multiple staples, and multiple Steinmann pins. These methods still are employed frequently, especially in patients with rheumatoid arthritis. Even in these patients, however, the trend has been toward plate fixation for wrist arthrodesis. Rehak et al. compared the results of pin versus plate fixation in 57 patients with rheumatoid arthritis. Successful results were not significantly different in the two groups.

In 1970, the AO group described a rigid fixation method using a dynamic compression plate. In mechanical testing studies, this plate proved to be the most stable fixation, and currently is the most favored and commonly used technique for wrist arthrodesis. The advantages of the dynamic compression plate include excellent fusion rates, decreased incidence of malposition, and increased stability that allows early rehabilitation. The AO plating technique requires less bone grafting than other methods, and often an adequate amount of graft can be harvested from the distal radius. Anderson and Thomas reported the use of dynamic compression plates for wrist arthrodesis without the use of bone graft. All 15 patients in their series achieved wrist fusion by 12 weeks. Iliac crest bone graft is recommended unless an adequate amount of cancellous graft is available from locally resected bone and the distal radius.

Indications

- Severely comminuted intra-articular fractures
- Post-traumatic arthritis with painful destruction of the joint
- Joint destruction caused by infection or tumor resection
- Kienbock's disease
- Rheumatoid arthritis
- Stabilization of a paralytic wrist and hand
- Correction of wrist flexion deformity in patients with spastic hemiplegia
- Failed total wrist arthroplasty

Contraindications

- An open physis of the distal radius
- An elderly patient with a sedentary lifestyle, especially if the nondominant wrist is involved, such as in a patient with rheumatoid arthritis for whom tendon transfer or joint replacement may be more appropriate
- Quadriparetics who use their motors for modified grasp and transfer techniques
- Neurologic diseases or injury causing major sensory deprivation in the hand
- Advanced rheumatoid disease where stabilization techniques are more suitable than formal arthrodesis

Position of arthrodesis: The wrist should be fused in a position that would not be fatiguing and that would allow maximum grasping strength in the hand. This is usually 10–20° of extension (dorsiflexion) with the long axis of the third metacarpal shaft aligned with the long axis of the radial shaft. Clinically, it is determined by the position that the wrist normally assumes with the fist strongly clenched. Several authors recommend the neutral position, which allows full supination and pronation and personal hygiene functions, while providing sufficient grasping strength. Still others favor slight palmar flexion to 25°. In general, neutral to 5° of ulnar deviation is preferred. If bilateral wrist fusions are indicated, the positions of the wrists should be determined by the needs of the patient. The neutral position for both wrists is thought to provide maximal function.

Method: The technique of surgery depends mainly on the quality of bone substance and degree of joint degeneration. Differences between fusion types include the type of bone graft and osteosynthesis being used. The aim is to create a stable joint in an acceptable functional position. The position of arthrodesis depends on the patient's needs as follows:

- A neutral position is generally accepted in patients with rheumatoid arthritis
- Slight wrist extension and ulnar deviation are preferred in patients with degenerative joint disease

Historically, single or multiple screws have been used to hold a cortical bone graft in place in the dorsal aspect of the wrist. The use of a single K-wire to supplement immobilization in a cast has also been described. A technique described for use in patients with rheumatoid arthritis uses a single permanent Steinmann pin advanced retrograde from the third metacarpal into the medullary canal of the radius.

Some methods of internal fixation include the use of multiple staples without an intramedullary pin and the technique of placing a pin from the thenar eminence into the medullary canal of the radius without exposing the wrist. The use of dorsal placement of a 9-hole plate from the second metacarpal to the radius with an additional corticocancellous autogenous iliac crest bone graft was first described in 1972. Later, Larsson described a similar technique that used a 6-hole self-compressing plate. By the early 1980s, a larger 8-hole 3.5 mm dynamic compression plate was advocated to provide more appropriate rigid fixation.

Currently, a specifically designed wrist arthrodesis plate is available, which combines a 3.5 mm dynamic compression plate proximally and 2.7 mm dynamic compression plate distally. This combination AO-ASIF wrist arthrodesis plate allows for improved and stable fixation by using larger screws in the distal radius and provides reduced risk of metacarpal fracture and fragmentation by using smaller 2.7 mm screws into the metacarpal.

Investigations

- *Radiography:* At least three views of the wrist (AP, lateral, and oblique) should be taken to identify the intracarpal and intercarpal joints with arthrosis. Radiographs should be examined for loss of joint intervals, subchondral reactive bone formation, subchondral cysts, and osteophyte formation. Contralateral wrist radiography can be used to assess ulnar variance of the pathologic side. The clenched-fist view stresses the intercarpal ligaments and may reveal an incompetent scapholunate ligament. Failure to address this problem at operation results in the failure of a STT fusion.
- *CT scanning of the wrist:* When plain radiography appears to be inadequate to identify the bony pathology accurately, CT scanning of the wrist can be helpful by exposing malalignment of bony columns and underlying arthropathy.

Complications

- Extensor tenosynovitis most common complication and is related to prominent plate and screws
- Intrinsic contracture
- Carpal tunnel syndrome
- Nonunion of the CMC joint
- Radioulnar joint instability
- Ulnocarpal abutment

OSTEONECROSIS OF SCAPHOID AND PREISER'S DISEASE

The etymology of the scaphoid bone (Latin: os scaphoideum, os naviculare manus) is derived from the Greek *skaphos*, which means "a boat" and *eidos*, which means "kind". The name refers to shape of the bone looking like a reminiscent of a boat. The older literature on human anatomy referred this as "navicular bone" of the hand, representing topological similarity to navicular bone of foot. The bone bears significant structural and functional significant position in wrist joint and is subjected to rigorous stress.

Preiser's disease, or (idiopathic) ON of the scaphoid, is a rare condition where ischemia and necrosis of the scaphoid bone occurs without previous notable event (though the cases originally described by Preiser himself were all traumatic and associated with fractures). The term is sometimes incorrectly used for post-traumatic ON of scaphoid. It is thought to be caused by repetitive microtrauma or side effects of drugs (e.g., steroids or chemotherapy) in conjunction with existing defective vascular supply to the proximal pole of the scaphoid. It was first described by Georg Preiser (1876–1913) in 1910 in five patients, all with previous history of wrist trauma and scaphoid fractures in three of them. Although the term Preiser's disease has now become synonymous with atraumatic ON of the scaphoid, various authors have implemented different unique terms to denote the condition. These terms include idiopathic ON (wrongly termed AVN) of the scaphoid, osteochondritis dissecans of the scaphoid, and avascular nontraumatic necrosis of the scaphoid.

Bony Anatomy

Scaphoid articulates with five bones:

1. Radius proximally
2. Trapezoid bone and trapezium bone distally
3. Capitate and lunate on ulnar aspect

It forms the radial border of the carpal tunnel. The scaphoid bone is the largest of the proximal row of wrist bones, its long axis being from above downward, lateralward, and forward. The palmar surface of the scaphoid is concave, elevated, and forming a tubercle, giving attachment to the transverse carpal ligament. The proximal surface is triangular, smooth and convex, and articulates with the radius and adjacent carpal bones. The lateral surface is narrow and gives attachment to the radial collateral ligament. The medial surface has two facets, a flattened semilunar facet articulating with the lunate bone, and an inferior concave facet, articulating with the head of the capitate bone. The dorsal surface of the bone is narrow, with a groove running the length of the bone and allowing ligaments to attach, and the surface facing the fingers (anatomically inferior) is smooth and convex, also triangular, and divided into two parts by a slight ridge.

Blood Supply

Typically, the scaphoid is supplied by two groups of small vessels **(Fig. 44)**. Majority of its blood supply comes from dorsal vessels at or just distal to waist area perfusing the proximal pole in a retrograde fashion. These are branches of radial artery that enter scaphoid through foramina along its dorsal ridge. It supplies 70–80% of bone, including the

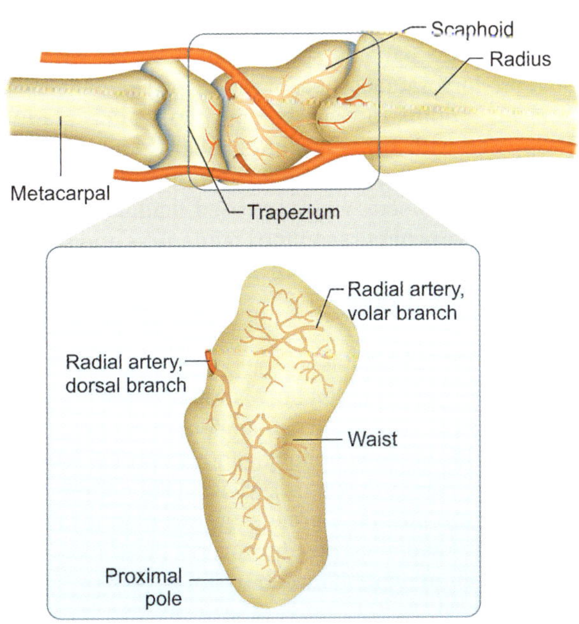

Fig. 44: Blood supply of scaphoid (see text).

entire proximal pole. The second group of vessels arises from palmar and superficial palmar branches of radial artery and enters carpal scaphoid in region of its distal tubercle. This perfuses distal 20–30% of bone, including tuberosity. The vascular supply of clinically distinct proximal and distal scaphoid can be summarized as follows:

- The proximal two-thirds to three-fourths of scaphoid are supplied by vessels entering dorsal surface through dorsal ridge in 79%. Alternatively, the vessels may enter distal to waist in 14% and proximal to waist in 7%.
- *Distal scaphoid:* The tubercle and distal 20–30% of scaphoid are supplied by palmar vessels predominantly. In a few persons, supplying vessels may enter tip of tubercle reaching the waist. There is no anastomosis between the dorsal and palmar vessels.

The simplistic inference from the pattern of blood supply is the fact that fractures through waist of scaphoid or proximally will cutoff blood supply to proximal fragment of scaphoid in majority of the patients. So ON is commonly seen in such cases.

Functions of Scaphoid

The carpal bones provide a bony super structure for the hand. They provide the mobile bearing for the hand to move as an organ over forearm bones

- The scaphoid along with the lunate, articulates with the radius and ulna to form the wrist joint. With all movements and stress bearing, the scaphoid bone takes part in wrist function.
- The scaphoid serves as a link between the two rows of carpal bones. The scaphoid flexes during radial deviation and extends on ulnar deviation of wrist.

Clinical Features

As reported by Kalainov and colleagues, the disease is seen approximately two-thirds of the time in the dominant wrist. Preiser's disease appears to affect adults almost exclusively, with only occasional case report existing in pediatric population. The patients suffer from a vague wrist pain located on dorsoradial aspect of the wrist. The pain is often present for months to years before presentation gradually accompanied with stiffness. Some patients will have mild-to-moderate swelling over the dorsum or radial aspects of the wrist that worsens with increased loading and use of the wrist. There is often a snuffbox tenderness and scaphoid tubercle tenderness. ROM and grip strength are reduced compared with the other wrist.

Diagnostic Imaging

The radiographic examination should start with four plain radiographs of the wrist, including a zero-rotation posteroanterior, lateral, oblique, and scaphoid (clenched fist PA with ulnar deviation) views **(Fig. 45A)**. If the radiographs are normal a bone scan can help localize the problem to the radial carpus; however, a bone scan cannot adequately differentiate between tumors, AVN, or fractures in the scaphoid. Furthermore, after a positive bone scan, patients are often sent for an MRI evaluation, to localize the

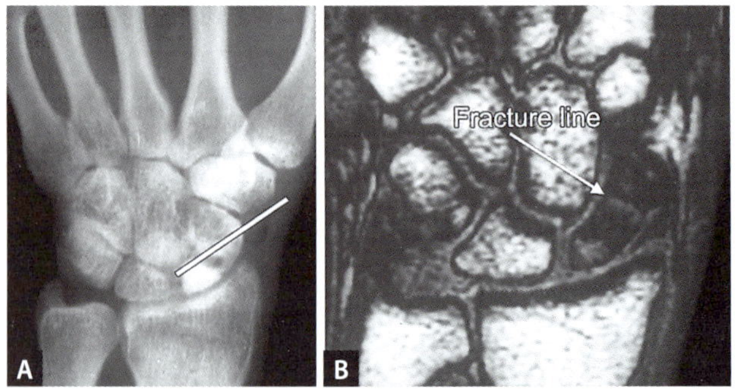

Figs. 45A and B: Radiology of scaphoid osteonecrosis. Note the hyperdense osteonecrotic proximal fractured fragment (A, pointer) which is confirmed on MRI scan (B).

TABLE 11: Classification of Preiser's disease.

Stage	*Findings (based on plain radiographs)—Herbert and Lanzetta*	*Findings (based on plain radiographs)—Kalainov modification*
1.	Normal radiographs but positive bone scan	Normal radiographs
2.	Increased proximal pole density plus generalized osteopenia	Scaphoid sclerosis, lucencies, and fissuring on plain radiographs
3.	Fragmentation of proximal pole ± pathologic fracture	Fragmentation of scaphoid
4.	Carpal collapse with osteoarthritis	Scaphoid collapse and fragmentation with periscaphoid arthritis

pathology and also define its nature **(Fig. 45B)**. Radiographs may reveal changes ranging from sclerosis to fragmentation and collapse (similar to changes discussed with Kienbock's disease). Cystic changes are seen in adjacent bones possibly due to accompanying osteoporosis. MRI remains the gold standard (high sensitivity and specificity for carpus ON) and may be enhanced by the use of intravenous injection of gadolinium to improve resolution. Findings include loss of signal intensity indicating necrosis, which may be localized or diffuse.

Classification

Three classification systems have been devised for grading scaphoids afflicted with Preiser's disease. The first scheme, derived by Herbert and Lanzetta in 1993 **(Table 11)**, is based on the progression of the disease as seen with plain radiographs. Based on four stages, this system starts at stage 1 with normal radiographs but a positive bone scan, and ends at stage 4 with total collapse of the scaphoid and periscaphoid arthritis (similar to Litchman classification of Kienbock's). The classification has been modified by Kalainov and colleagues **(Table 11)**. Kalainov also proposed classification of Preiser's disease based on MRI **(Table 12)**.

Preiser's Disease-associated Injuries or Differential Diagnosis

- Scaphoid fracture
- Scaphoid nonunion

TABLE 12: Preiser's disease classification as proposed by Kalainov and colleagues.

Type	Findings (based on magnetic resonance imaging)
1.	Diffuse ischemia and necrosis of scaphoid
2.	Localized necrosis of scaphoid

- Keinbock's disease
- Ulnocarpal impaction syndrome

Preiser's Disease Complications

- Degenerative changes in adjacent articulations
- Stiffness and motion loss
- Weakness
- Complex regional pain syndrome (CRPS)
- Continued pain
- Instability

Treatment

Based on the similar guidelines as for lunatomalacia the ON of scaphoid can be managed conservatively or surgically. The conservative measures, however, fail more often with Preiser's disease. Unlike Kienbock's disease, however, the operative treatments are limited for Preiser's as there is no relevance of unloading the bone.

- Nonoperative—immobilization is effective in 20% of cases
- Operative treatment of salvageable scaphoid (stage 1 and 2)
  - Microfracture drilling
  - Revascularization procedure (bone grafts)
  - Allograft replacement

Revascularization for Scaphoid (Also Relevant to Nonunion Scaphoid)

- Using the scaphoid tubercle on an abductor pollicis brevis muscle pedicle (Roy-Camille 1965), for scaphoid waist delayed union
- Volar distal radius bone graft based on a pronator quadratus muscle or anterior interosseous artery pedicle (Braun, 1983) for scaphoid nonunions
- Pedicled thumb metacarpal vascular bone graft based on 1st dorsal metacarpal artery
- Kuhlmann's palmar distal radius graft based on a branch of the palmar radiocarpal arch (volar carpal artery)
- *Distal ulna pedicle graft based on a reverse-flow ulnar artery pedicle (Guimberteau):* The technique is demanding and requires an ulnar arterial reconstruction with a vein graft
- *Intercompartmental supraretinacular artery-based bone graft (ICSRA 1, 2):* In 1991, a vascularized pedicle distal radius bone graft was described by Zaidemberg based on the "ascending irrigating branch" of the radial artery and was used successfully in 11 established scaphoid nonunions and is preferred by me for most cases unless specifically contraindicated. The dorsal radial location of this graft allows a single surgical incision for graft harvest, carpal exposure, and placement in the scaphoid for nonunions or AVN.

Technique of harvest of intercompartmental supraretinacular artery graft for scaphoid: Through a curvilinear approach wide exposure of scaphoid vascular bone graft elevation from its bed and ON site are obtained. The ICSRA **(Figs. 46A to K)** is visualized on the surface of the retinaculum (note it is on the surface not in the compartment, **Figs. 46A to K**). When using a pneumatic tourniquet, Esmarch's bandage exsanguination is not recommended as it squeezes the blood out of fine vessels and identification might be difficult, instead just elevate the arm to drain excess blood. The first and second compartments are opened creating a "cuff" of retinaculum and once the ICSRA vessels are dissected and protected, the scaphoid is exposed through a capsulotomy **(Fig. 46D)** all through same incision. A slot is created in the scaphoid for VBG **(Fig. 46E)**. The graft is then elevated based on a retrograde—flow pedicle and tourniquet released to ascertain blood flow **(Fig. 46H)**. The graft is then gently press-fit into the prepared slot trimming as needed.

- Treatment of advanced disease (stage 3 and 4)
  - Proximal row carpectomy (see ON of lunate)
  - Scaphoid excision with four-corner fusion (lunate-capitate-triquetrum-hamate fusion)
  - Wrist denervation (see ON of lunate)
  - Wrist arthrodesis (see ON of lunate)
- Arthroscopic treatment of AVN of the scaphoid

  Arthroscopy in Preiser's disease allows direct visualization and assessment of the exact pathology of the radiocarpal and midcarpal joint and the scaphoid cartilage. Arthroscopic debridement of the necrotic scaphoid can be combined with microdrilling to "decompress" and assist vascularization (similar to core decompression for femur).

OSTEOCHONDROSIS

Synonyms and related keywords: Osteochondritis, epiphysitis, apophysitis, aseptic epiphyseal necrosis, ischemic epiphyseal necrosis, and childhood painful joints.

Introduction

Definition: Osteochondrosis is a self-limiting developmental derangement of normal bone growth due primarily to involvement of centers of ossification in epiphysis; beginning usually in childhood as a degenerative or necrotic condition. Various affected sites have been crudely grouped together under the term osteochondrosis primarily based on their morphological and evolutional similarity on radiographs. Practically, all the epiphyses have been known to be afflicted typically showing many of the features of ischemic necrosis (it is prudent to drop the term "avascular" from AVN as vessels are there but somehow ischemia prevails) not only radiologically but also histologically.

Epidemiology

Frequency of affliction at different sites vary and considering the fact that it is a self-limiting disorder a lot go undiagnosed making exact documentation difficult. Some are so infrequent that a physician may not encounter them in their whole period of practice. There are definite

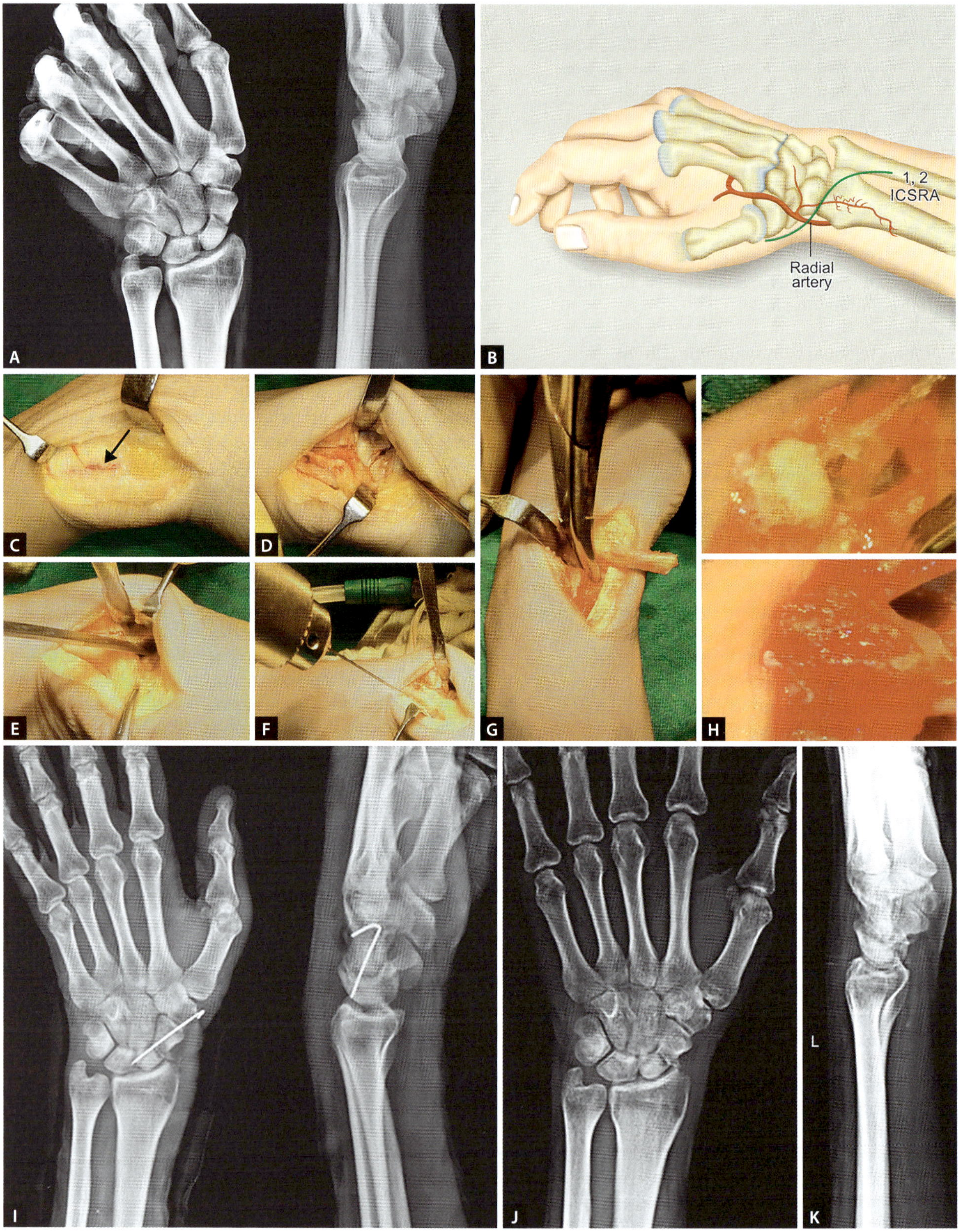

Figs. 46A to K: (A) Nonunion of fracture of scaphoid; (B) Illustration of the 1, 2, intercompartmental supraretinacular artery (1,2 ICSRA); This patient though does not have any overt carpal instability as he was diagnosed early. Long-standing nonunions become unstable and often present with dorsal intercalated segment instability (DISI). The patient was managed by Zaidemberg vascularized graft technique for correction of nonunion and deformity that went into uneventful union; (C) Exposure of the intercompartmental vessels (arrow); (D) Exposure of the nonunion site; (E) Preparation of the nonunion site and measuring the required graft size; (F) Marking the bone graft size by drill holes using K-wire; (G) Elevating the graft and performing partial radial styloidectomy; (H) Ensuring the vascularity of graft by deflating tourniquet; (I) Placement of the graft and fixing with smooth pin; (J and K) Radiograph of patient at 3 months showing well-placed graft and ensuing start of union, also note the partial radial styloidectomy.

ethnic and racial differences when some of the common well studied osteochondrosis are considered. Perthes' disease is uncommon in African and Chinese descendants, whereas Blount's disease is common in African region and uncommon in the West. Most of the osteochondrosis occur shortly after the appearance of bony nucleus around "mid-growth spurt" at the time when epiphysis is mainly cartilaginous and growing rapidly; making it susceptible to injury. The exceptions to this are osteochondritis dissecans, Scheuermann's disease and Osgood-Schlatter disease that predominantly occur during adolescent growth spurt. All osteochondrosis occur more frequently in males barring the exception of Freiberg's disease which is commoner in females, and juvenile osteochondritis dissecans of elbow (capitellum) that is common in female javelin throwers. Delayed appearance and maturation of growth center in males may account for this difference as also the higher activity level, further traumatizing the immature epiphysis.

Problem

Osteochondrosis is not an uncommon disorder; pertinent to this fact is the often-overlooked condition of nonspecific bone and joint pains in a child during growth spurt, many of which may be osteochondrosis.

Osteochondritis dissecans is controversially included in the group osteochondrosis by some. Strictly following the definition, it is not primarily due to ischemic process involving growth center and that it also occurs in adults. Juvenile form, however, may represent a focal ischemic involvement and only those forms should be included. Controversy exists over expanding and including post-traumatic ON and normal variants of ossification into the group, however, it should be realized that with growing knowledge; an etiological basis has been assigned to define the group and one should not congregate etiologically unrelated but morphologically similar conditions.

Etiology

Various factors have been ascribed in an attempt to explain the occurrence of osteochondrosis. Social deprivation, dietary deficiency, and passive smoking ("the unknown industrial factor") have been the oldest and most controversial propositions that are sparsely accepted. The studies were area specific and could be compounded by "etiological fallacy". Genetic predisposition, environmental, thrombotic predisposition, acute or repeated trauma, embolism, copper (trace element) deficiency, and finally infection are by and large in various combinations (multifactorial) or in isolation accepted as most probable causes. Various compounding factors such as hormonal imbalance (hypothyroidism), sickle cell anemia, Gaucher's disease and mucopolysaccharidoses, tetany from magnesium deficiency, cystic fibrosis, etc., have also been identified; however, these are now well-established diseases and should not be linked with osteochondrosis. It is well said that we should think in terms of "syndrome" (e.g., Osgood-Schlatter syndrome rather than disease) for multiple causes some often undeterminable may also be involved; hence, by this corollary it must be patent that cause is largely a matter of hypothesis, what concerns us is the fact that there is a distinct pathological condition which can be "controlled" if not corrected by proper therapy. It is of interest that "infection" which was unanimously discredited as a cause has been shown to either trigger or potentiate the disease process somehow directly or through autoimmune mechanisms. Genetic predisposition producing hypercoagulable state due to deficient tissue factor pathway inhibitor (TFPI), fibrinolysis defects (protein-S, protein-C deficiency, and resistance to activated protein-C) all need to be further substantiated, specified, and strongly correlated. Likewise, there is no consensus on inheritable disorders of thrombophilia due to mutations in G20210A prothrombin gene, factor V (G1691A) Leiden, methylenetetrahydrofolate reductase C677T genes or anticardiolipin antibodies. Second hand smoking may be related by β–fibrinogen gene G-455-A polymorphism to development of Perthes' disease. Some individual mechanical factors may be related to development of specific diseases as long patellae (Grelsamer Type II) and extensor apparatus, external tibial torsion in Osgood-Schlatter, and Sinding-Larsen-Johansson disease. Blount's disease is inherited in autosomal dominant pattern, however inheritance pattern in other potentially inheritable disorders like Scheuermann's needs to be characterized. Further, some trace element deficiencies like copper and zinc have been proposed in animal studies.

Pathophysiology

The initial event(s) remain elusive but clinical and radiological evidence point to ischemic necrosis of ossification center that could be secondary to a definite or multiple additive traumatic event or a primary vascular event. In every circumstance, it would be more definitive to say that osteochondrotic process is essentially a degeneration of osseous nucleus of epiphysis almost certainly the result of an interference of its blood supply leading to necrosis of cartilage canal vessels in subchondral bone and adjacent epiphysis or to a failed enlargement of bony centrum and disordered proliferation of cartilage cells within epiphysis. Secondary changes of fragmentation, collapse, sequestrum formation, etc., follow the strain, pressure, and tension characteristic of respective regions. The disease process can be isolated, involving single epiphysis or in multiple site affections; sequential, or simultaneous. The underlying process in multiple affections seems to be essentially the same; however, presentation may vary depending upon various stresses and strains to which the epiphyses have been subjected. The efficacy of regenerative and reparative process determines the ultimate outcome in terms of long-term clinical presentation. Complete healing leaves little harm done, however partial healing or failure to heal becomes a source of chronic pain and disability later in life, reflecting no credit on the physician who overlooked it in the child.

Ponseti proposed some common denominators in all osteochondrosis:

- Uncertain etiology
- Clinical pattern of progress
- Radiological appearance of ischemic necrosis

Duthie and Houghton proposed a model of development of osteochondrosis:

- Normal epiphysis subjected to extreme trauma, e.g., "pitcher's elbow" with osteochondritis dissecans of capitellum
- Mildly dyschondrotic epiphysis subjected to more than usual stress, e.g., Perthes' disease
- Severely affected dyschondrotic epiphysis subjected to normal stress, e.g., capital femoral epiphysis in Gaucher's disease

Biochemical abnormalities in the form of altered expression of matrix metalloproteinases (MMP-1, 3, 13), altered collagen to proteoglycan ratio, glycosaminoglycans, and aggrecan overexpression consequent upon altered mechanics furthering cartilage damage are all proposed but need further assertion by concrete evidence.

Classification

Previous classifications dividing osteochondrosis into pressure, traction, atavistic (burrows) or compression, tension, and atavistic (Goff) were inadequate. The presently accepted classification divides them into three types as follows:

1. *Articular osteochondrosis:*
   - Primary involvement of articular and epiphyseal, cartilage and subjacent endochondral ossification center—Freiberg's disease and Froelich disease **(Fig. 47B)**
   - Secondary involvement of articular and epiphyseal cartilage as a consequence of ischemic necrosis of subjacent bone—Perthes' disease **(Fig. 48A)**, Kohler's disease, and osteochondritis dissecans.
2. *Nonarticular osteochondrosis:*
   - *At tendon attachment:* Osgood-Schlatter syndrome **(Fig. 48B)**, Monde-Felix **(Fig. 47A)**, and Iselin's disease **(Fig. 47C)**
   - *At ligamentous attachment:* Vertebral ring
   - *At impact sites:* Sever's disease **(Fig. 48C)**
3. *Physeal osteochondrosis:*
   - Long bone—tibia vara (Blount's disease)
   - Scheuermann's disease

Eponyms are so deeply engraved into literature that it is impossible to complete the description without their mention. A comprehensive list of described osteochondrosis is provided in **Table 13**.

Associated Disorders

Various investigators have found major genitourinary disorders associated with Perthes' disease. Also, the risk of inguinal hernia was eight times in these patients.

Slipped capital femoral epiphysis may occur with Scheuermann's disease. Recently, attention has been shifted to the occurrence growth retardation with osteochondrosis substantiated by reduced urinary deoxypyridinoline (DPD) and glycosaminoglycans excretion and low plasma levels of insulin-like growth factor 1 (IGF-1) disturbing collagen metabolism that may later be linked to pathogenesis in syndromic terms.

Clinical Features

Presentation and findings discretely depend not only on the site of involvement but also the stage of progression. Pain that is localized to site viz. pain on kneeling in Osgood-Schlatter disease or referred (to knee in Perthes' disease) is usually present in initial stages; however, it should be remembered that more often than not the affections are asymptomatic and present late during disability. Localized tenderness, limitation of movements of adjacent joints, swelling, gait disturbance (lower limb affections), and sometimes reactive joint effusion in adjacent joint are often found either individually or in combination. Growth disturbance and secondary deformities are late presentations in specific entities such as Blount's disease (shortening and tibia vara), Scheuermann's disease (kyphosis), Perthes' disease (shortening and coxa vara/magna/breva). More important is the realization that presence of systemic symptoms of inflammation such as fever, malaise, weight loss, local redness, and raised temperature should alert physician to search for causes other than osteochondrosis.

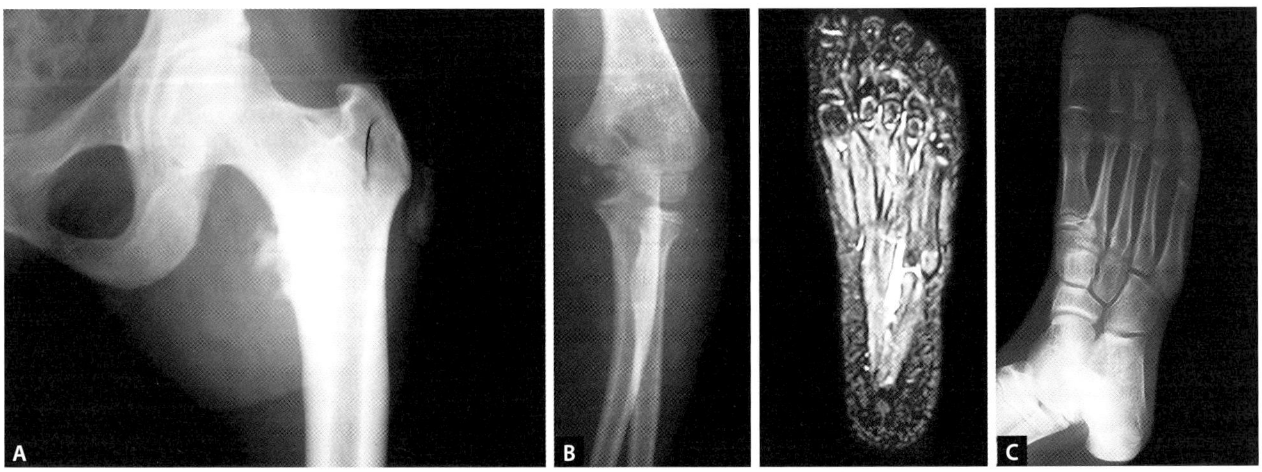

Figs. 47A to C: (A) Osteochondrosis of lesser trochanter (Monde-Felix disease); (B) Osteochondrosis of medial condyle of elbow (Froelich disease); (C) Osteochondrosis of base of fifth metatarsal bone—radiological and MRI picture (Iselin's disease).

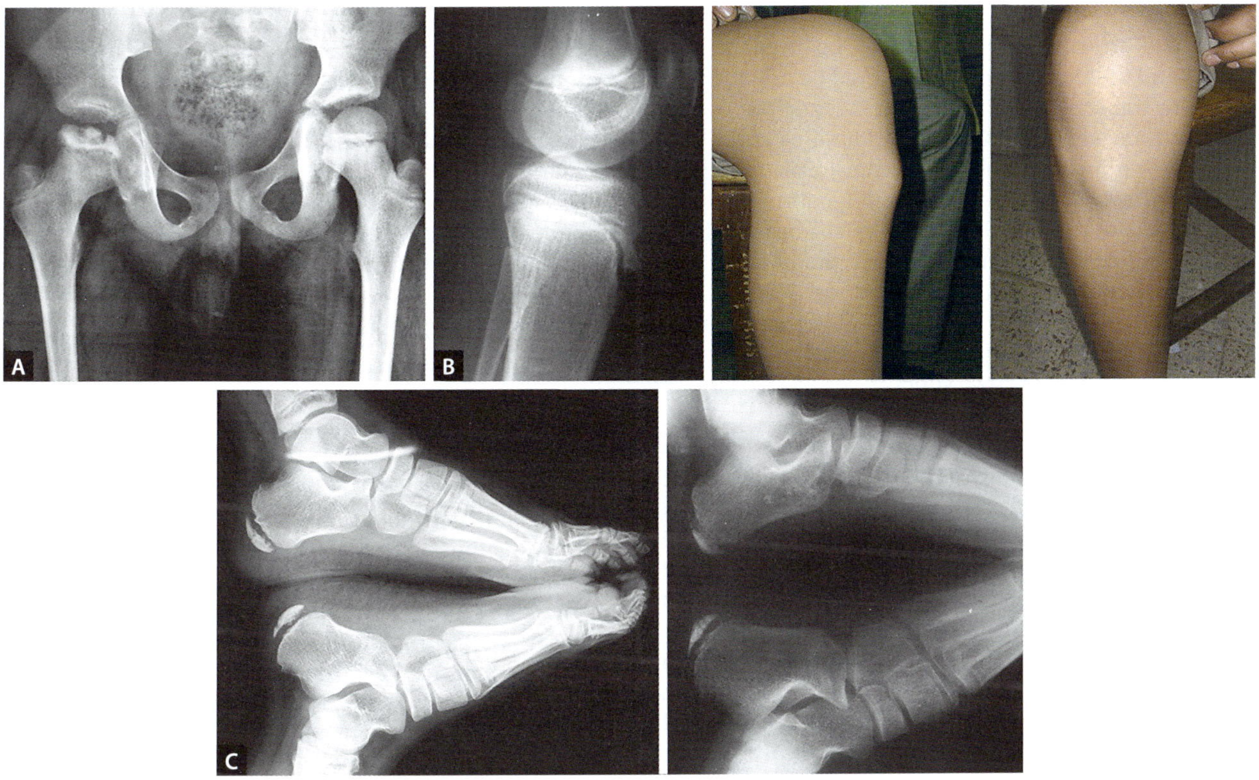

Figs. 48A to C: (A) Osteochondrosis of right femoral head (Perthes' disease); (B) Osteochondrosis of tibial tuberosity (Osgood-Schlatter disease); (C) Sever's disease—initial presentation and later healing phase (note healing can be varied with some showing fusion while some may appear as disease progression with increased fragmentation as in the lower right radiograph.

TABLE 13: Eponyms commonly used for various osteochondrosis.

Primary center of ossification	*Secondary center of ossification*
Carpal scaphoid (Preiser)	Vertebral epiphysis (Scheuermann)
Lunate (Kienböck)	Iliac crest (Buchman)
Medial cuneiform (Buschke)	Symphysis pubis (Pierson)
Patella (Köhler)	Ischiopubic junction (Van neck)
Talus (Mouchet)	Ischial tuberosity (Valtançoli)
Tarsal scaphoid (Köhler)	Calcaneal apophysitis (Sever)
Vertebral body (Calve)	• Accessory tarsal navicular or os tibiale externum (Haglund) • Second metatarsal (Freiberg) • Fifth metatarsal base (Iselin) • Talus (Diaz) • Distal tibial epiphysis (Lewin) • Proximal tibial epiphysis (Blount) • Tuberosity of tibia (Osgood-Schlatter) • Secondary patellar center (Sinding-Larsen) • Lesser trochanter of femur (Monde-Felix) • Greater trochanter of femur (Mandl, Buchman) • Capital epiphysis of femur (Legg-Calve- Perthes) • Phalanges (Thiemann) • Heads of metacarpals (Mauclaire) • Proximal epiphysis of radius (Schaefer) • Distal epiphysis of ulna (Burns) • Medial humeral epicondyle (Froelich) • Lateral humeral condyle (Froelich) • Capitellum of humerus (Panner) • Humeral head (Hass) • Clavicle (Friedrich)

Differential Diagnosis

- Chondroectodermal dysplasia
- Tubercular epiphysitis
- Dysplasia epiphysealis multiplex
- Gaucher's disease
- Mucopolysaccharidosis
- Type V physeal injuries
- Acute transient epiphysitis
- Chondroblastoma
- Rickets
- Osteomyelitis
- Hypothyroidism.

Investigations

Osteochondrosis by themselves does not primarily alter the laboratory parameters. However, it is imperative to rule out other disorders before labeling the patient with osteochondrosis. A complete hemogram with erythrocyte sedimentation rate, blood chemistry, especially focusing on to serum calcium, phosphate and alkaline phosphatase is mandatory; other investigations depend on individual case. Investigations to look for genetic polymorphism, trace element detection (copper, zinc), urinary DPD excretion and plasma IGF-1 are primarily of research interest and should not be used to screen patients.

Plain X-rays

Exact imaging features are descriptive of specific entities; hitherto some features are shared in the group. Early involvement typically presents as reduction in size, increased density, and irregular architecture of involved centrum **(Figs. 47 and 48)**. In addition, there could be asymmetry in size of bony trabeculae and irregular trabeculation.

With advancement, fibrillation and fissures in the cartilage anlage with or without sequestrum formation appear **(Fig. 48A)**. There may be separation of a part of bone with parent nucleus—"crescent" sign. In weight-bearing joints, there may be reduction in the joint space, but is unusual.

Revascularization usually presents as worsening of radiographic picture with development of osteoporosis, absorption of necrotic tissue, and deformation of epiphysis due to loss of underlying support ("step-defect" and "buttressing" phenomenon).

The picture in squeal or "burnt-out phase" depends on the degree of damage by ischemia and its chronologic arrest. Complete and early restoration by reparative process leaves no deformity. Late and incomplete restoration of blood supply compounded by additional assault and poor protection develops into irregular, deformed and deshapened epiphysis with collateral and subsequent changes in metaphysis and joint **(Fig. 47B)**. Resultant specific deformities are mushroom head of Perthes' disease with subluxation, kyphosis (with or without scoliosis) in Scheuermann's disease, tibia vara in Blount's, cubitus valgus in panner's, Madelung deformity in distal radial epiphyseal affection, genu recurvatum and patella alta in Osgood-Schlatter disease, etc. Joint arthrosis is the delayed presentation of usually all articular osteochondrosis that have been poorly restored, due to abnormal distribution of stresses and irregular resulting joint surfaces, e.g., Kienbock's disease and Perthes' disease.

Magnetic Resonance Imaging

Typically, the disease is recognized and staged on the radiographic features as they have long being described thereof. MRI does not help additionally in diagnosing the disorder. However, it is a useful tool in differentiating the disorder from inflammatory conditions such as tubercular involvement and osteomyelitis. Physeal mapping of the growth plate can be undertaken to help surgical correction (Blount's disease). Small fragments can be better revealed along with some comment on their residual attachment to parent bone as well as on vascularity such as juvenile osteochondritis dissecans, Freiberg's disease, Sinding-Larsen-Johansson disease (Jumper's knee), and Osgood-Schlatter syndrome. Associated information like underlying bone defects; their extent, etc., can also be judged on scans.

Early MRI images show focal high signal intensities in epiphysis or neighboring soft tissues due to edema. Variable signal is seen in the avascular fragment due to either edema, seen as hypointensity or sclerosis seen as hyperintensity on T1-weighted images. Marrow edema in parent bone is a regular finding. The signal changes extend to anywhere from peripheral irregularity of ossific nucleus to complete replacement of normal marrow fat. Intra-articular effusion may be seen. Revascularization leads to replacement of necrotic focus with fatty marrow. Loose bodies and residual deformities which are common in osteochondritis dissecans are, however, rare in osteochondrosis. In Scheuermann's kyphosis, Schmorl's nodes are seen as low or high signal alteration in T2 images with neighboring marrow edema. Also, disk herniations and discogenic sclerosis are seen. Similarly, in Kohler's or Freiberg's infarction, deformity, fragmentation, fractures, collapse, and edema are frequently observed. Perthes' may show acetabular labral tears and metaphyseal cysts in addition to above-mentioned features.

Bone Scan Scintigraphy

Bone scan is proven to have high sensitivity and specificity in detecting avascularity, but whether it is not superior to MRI. Scintigraphic changes in Perthes' disease have been extensively studied; however, other osteochondrosis continue to be neglected probably because of lower incidence rates. In Perthes', pinhole images in both AP and lateral views with technetium-99 tracer, should preferably be taken. In the initial stages of ischemia, even before any radiographic changes are seen in a symptomatic patient, striking absence of tracer uptake is noted either focally or in entire epiphysis with a normal uptake in physis and acetabular rim. This represents the growth disturbance in epiphysis when metabolic activity and obviously the blood flow are low, with no reparative response yet from surrounding physis or metaphysis. This helps in early diagnosis months before any radiographic changes become obvious. With reparative response in the form of revascularization from neighboring uninvolved epiphysis and metaphysis, there is increased activity at the margin of hypoactive necrotic focus which gradually decreases in size. There is also increase in activity in neighboring physis and metaphysis, representing an osteoblastic response. Complete healing is heralded by a normal tracer distribution in entire epiphysis compared to opposite side. Increased activity may also rarely be explained by degenerative changes. Scan may be useful in assessing acetabular containment of head, sclerosis, subchondral fractures, intra-articular effusion and fragmentation of chondral surface. Disappearance of previous activity (for example in lateral column in Perthes') indicates collapse or infarct, a poor prognostic marker. Schmorl's nodes show increased tracer uptake in acute phase and a normal or increased activity in later phases.

Histopathology

In general, all stages of process have been described involving necrosis of bone and cartilage, revascularization, granulation tissue formation, osteoclastic resorption of necrotic trabeculae, and formation of mature and lamellar bone. The features are not specific to any particular entity and resemble ischemic necrosis. There is reduced collagen to proteoglycan ratio in electron micrographic studies.

Treatment

Frequently, osteochondrosis respond to symptomatic non-operative treatment with complete or partial resolution. The main aim is to reduce the morbidity and decrease duration of symptoms with supervised treatment, although it may not influence the final outcome that is always to be explained in detail to parents and the patient.

Principles

- Protection and prevention of additional trauma
- Preventing development of secondary deformity
- Reduction of mechanical stress transmission to bone during process of reossification
- Facilitation of reossification process
- Removal of osteochondrotic fragments that have become loose bodies
- Compensating fixed bony deformities by realignment
- Salvage surgery

As to present date there is no mechanism to arrest the process, a close follow-up in the initial phase with specific interventions guided as above is the standard policy. The treatment options can be divided into nonoperative and operative interventions in general; that have to be individualized for specific cases.

Medical Treatment and Supportive Measures

Preventing additional trauma

- Proper counseling of the parents and patient about the disease and natural expected progression
- Providing rest to the affected part(s)
- Avoiding contact sports
- Cold fomentation and analgesics to relieve pain

Preventing secondary deformity and reducing mechanical stress across the joint:

- Traction to relieve pain prevents deformities, counter muscle spasm due to pain, reduce stresses across joint and give rest
- Bracing and plaster of Paris casts to divert the forces to less involved area, containment of involved epiphysis to provide proper scaffold to counterpart in joint during growth and prevent dysplasia
- Assisted weight-bearing

Facilitation of reossification process:

- Supplementing with calcium and multivitamin and trace element preparation

Preventing secondary deformity:

- Counter bracing as for Blount's and Perthes' disease
- Guided physiotherapy program and exercises as for Scheuermann's disease

Operative Intervention

Surgery is usually undertaken when the conservative method fails or is expected to fail during follow-up assessment or is ineffective in management. Also, when it is deemed that surgery may help in restoring the reparative process or at least guide the reparative process to produce a better outcome it can be undertaken, e.g., in unstable osteochondrosis. Sometimes surgery may be undertaken to improve cosmetic appearance.

- Arthroscopic procedures are usually undertaken in large joints:
    - Removal of loose bodies in osteochondritis dissecans either
    - Facilitation of regeneration by "microfracture" technique
    - Pinning or refixation of salvageable fragment
- Open removal of loose fragment (ossicle) in secondary pseudoarthrosis of Osgood-Schlatter disease.
- Refixation using bioabsorbable pegs or pins (e.g., polyglycolide) and screws (preferable) or autologous bone pegs of partially avulsed patellar tendon in Osgood-Schlatter disease and Freiberg's disease.
- Osteotomy to correct the secondary deformity in Blount's disease and Madelung deformity. Valgus-extension corrective osteotomy in Perthes' to correct abduction and flexion deformity, dorsal wedge osteotomy with pin fixation in Freiberg disease to improve congruity of metatarsophalangeal joint.
- Shelf acetabuloplasty (labral support procedures), varus derotation osteotomy of femur and Salter's innominate osteotomy to improve containment and acetabular remodeling in Perthes depend on individual case assessment. Similarly, spinal fusion is done in Scheuermann's disease to control the progression of deformity.
- Salvage surgeries are sometimes required in late cases with poor final outcome to reduce disability. These reconstructive procedures are exampled by Garceau's cheilectomy and shelf augmentation for malformed femoral head in Perthes' disease. Trochanteric advancement in femoral epiphyseal arrest. Tibial lengthening in Blount's disease. Selective carpal or wrist arthrodesis in Kienbock's disease. Interpositional arthroplasty using fascia, membranes, capsule, tendons in Freiberg's disease, and late presenting elbow osteochondrosis with secondary changes have been successfully tried.

The approach to each and every disease has to be individualized based on sound principles. It is imperative that a well-designed regimen is required in the follow-up after surgical intervention consisting of postoperative protection to promote healing and maintain the results achieved. A guided physiotherapy program to reduce disability must be simultaneously undertaken during rehabilitation.

Future Perspectives

RANKL inhibition, immunomodulation of T-helper cells, anti-TNF-α may help limit the progression of disease by individual mechanisms in Perthes' disease. Bisphosphonates (Zoledronic acid) has shown promising results but there are also concerns of alteration in morphology and physeal growth disturbance.

OSTEOCHONDRITIS DISSECANS OF THE TALUS

In 1922, Kappis described osteochondritis dissecans in the ankle joint. Osteochondritis dissecans as detailed above is a localized injury or condition affecting an articular surface that involves separation of a segment of cartilage and subchondral bone. Osteochondritis dissecans of the talus account for 4% of all osteochondral lesions in the body.

Etiology and Natural History of Disease

Although thought originally to be avascular now it is considered mostly traumatic origin. The osteochondral fragment is usually separated from the parent bone. If the fragment is stable new capillaries may cross fracture and revascularize it while if unstable or displaced, ON fragmentation occurs and the fragment becomes separated into a loose body. Lesions are located, either posteromedial or anterolateral on the talus.

- *Posteromedial lesions:* Often asymptomatic, with no history of trauma. There is less risk of osteoarthritis.
- *Anterolateral lesions:* Usually symptomatic, associated with trauma 98% of lateral lesions and 70% of medial lesions are associated with trauma.

Mechanism of Injury

It is mainly caused by inversion injuries of the foot. Mechanisms of injuries for various commonly occurring lesions are as follows:

Anterolateral Lesions

- Result from inversion and dorsiflexion forces, which cause the anterolateral aspect of the talar dome to impact the fibula.
- These lesions are usually shallower and more wafer shaped than medial lesions, possibly because of a more tangential force vector, that results in shearing type forces.

Posteromedial Lesions

Result from a combination of inversion, plantar flexion and external rotation forces, which cause the posteromedial talar dome to impact the tibial articular surface with a relatively more perpendicular force vector.

Clinical Features

- Ankle pain usually localized to the side of the talar lesion
- Intermittent swelling
- Patient may complaint of catching or grinding, instability and frequent giving way
- History of ankle sprain is common
- May have crepitus with movements
- Joint effusion is common
- Tender along tibiotalar joint line either anterolaterally or posteromedially depending on lesion location

Investigations

X-rays

- Lesions appear as a well circumscribed area of sclerotic subchondral bone separated from the remainder of the epiphysis by a radiolucent line
- Nontraumatic lesions should be radiographed for other ankle as disease is bilateral in 10–25% of cases
- Stress radiographs are indicated, if instability detected, on examination

Magnetic Resonance Imaging

Magnetic resonance imaging allows determination of location of lesion as well as integrity of articular cartilage.

CT Scan

Computed tomography provides best definition of bone fragments seen on plain X-ray, but not as helpful at detecting subtle lesions.

Bone Scan

Bone scan can identify lesions, but is not helpful in determining integrity of articular cartilage.

Classification or Staging

Berndt and Harty proposed staging system in 1959 based on progressive involvement of structures with ongoing stress on joint. Newer MRI and arthroscopic systems are more popular however:

Hepple et al. MRI Staging

- *Stage 1:* Only articular cartilage is damaged
- *Stage 2:* Cartilage injury with underlying fracture. This stage can further be divided into following substages as follows:
  - *Stage 2A:* Cartilage injury with underlying fracture and edema
  - *Stage 2B:* Cartilage injury with underlying fracture but no edema
- *Stage 3:* Detached (rim signal) but not displaced fragment
- *Stage 4:* Displaced fragment
- *Stage 5:* Subchondral cyst formation

Cheng et al. Arthroscopic Staging System

- *Stage A:* Smooth, intact but soft or ballotable lesion, stable
- *Stage B:* Rough surface but stable fragment
- *Stage C:* Fibrillation of cartilage seen, but is stable
- *Stage D:* Flap present or bone exposed and is unstable
- *Stage E:* Loose, undisplaced fragment and is unstable
- *Stage F:* Displaced fragment and is unstable

Treatment

Conservative Management

- Conservative management of osteochondral lesions of the talus (OLT) should be attempted first
- Symptomatic patients with negative findings on plain radiographs (but MRI positive) should undergo an initial period of immobilization, followed by physical therapy.

Surgical Management

Surgical treatment depends on a variety of factors, including:

- Patient's profile (activity level, age, and degenerative changes)

- Lesion characteristic (location, size, and chronicity of lesion)

Principles of Surgery (also see Chapter on "Articular Cartilage: Structure, Function, Injury, and Management")

- Loose body removal, with stimulation of fibrocartilage growth (microfracture, curettage, abrasion, or transarticular drilling). Drilling can be accomplished, using existing arthroscopic portals, a curved meniscus repair needle guide and transmalleolar drill holes. Sinus tarsi approaches to posteromedial lesions, also known as retrograde drilling or transtalar drilling, do not disrupt the articular surface.
- Securing lesion to the talar dome, through retrograde drilling, bone grafting, or internal fixation.
- Stimulating the development of hyaline cartilage through osteochondral autografts [osteochondral autograft transfer system (OATS) mosaicplasty], allografts or cell culture (discussed in Chapter on "Articular Cartilage: Structure, Function, Injury, and Management"). The OATS procedure transplants a single plug into lesion and mosaicplasty is used to harvest and transplant multiple circular plugs that closely recreate the lesion architecture. Single plug grafts, result in reduced ingrowth of the fibrocartilage but being large in size are associated with greater donor site morbidity than mosaicplasty. The mosaicplasty procedure is said to provide a better match to the talar dome contour and surface area of the defect, although 20–40% of the defect is filled with fibrocartilage. The donor plugs are classically obtained from femoral notch region or condyles though grafts from ipsilateral medial or lateral articular facet of the talus have been described. ACI and MACI are described elsewhere.

Treatment for Different Stages (Based on MRI)

Stage 1: Posteromedial and anterolateral lesions—conservative (an initial period of nonweight-bearing with cast immobilization, followed by progressive weight-bearing and mobilization to full ambulation by 12–16 weeks). Posterolateral may also be managed with cell culture system if patient demands.

Stage 2A: Conservative as above for both locations. Further treatment depends on restaging.

Stage 2B: Posteromedial lesions prolonged conservative trial as exposure and management of the lesion is associated with morbidity. Large lesions more than 1 cm in diameter with recalcitrant symptoms may be treated with open OATS or mosaicplasty. Anterolateral lesions are managed with arthroscopic debridement and stimulation technique.

Stage 3: Posteromedial lesions treated with immobilization and nonweight-bearing for 3–6 months. Lateral lesions are treated with arthroscopy (stimulation/OATS/refixation of the fragment). Screw fixation typically is used only for anterolateral lesions because of the difficulty in gaining good exposure for posteromedial lesions and inadvertent damage to the articular cartilage.

Stage 4: Displaced fragment is unstable and should be removed. For large lesions (>5 mm anterolateral or >1 cm posteromedial) the defect is covered with OATS or allograft.

Stage 5: Arthroscopically excise the lesion fill the cyst with bone graft and OATS. Retrograde (transtalar) drilling can facilitate bone grafting, which is ideal for large subchondral cystic lesions, with intact articular cartilage.

Coexisting Osteochondral Lesions of the Talus and Ligamentous Instability

The treatment guidelines are less clear. Options include, first repairing the lesion and then repairing the ligamentous injury at another time or repairing the two injuries simultaneously and postponing early ankle motion, until the ligament has healed. Thermal capsular shrinkage may also be a possible treatment solution.

Surgical Exposures

Anterolateral lesions: These lesions are accessed via an anterolateral approach to the ankle joint. Still an anterior plafond bone block may be needed to gain exposure of the tibiotalar joint. Plantarflexion aids in exposing the lesion.

Posteromedial lesions: Need a medial malleolar osteotomy to access the lesion. A separate approach is to use combined anterior and posterior arthrotomy exposure. This approach allows access to 80% of the talar dome, while it avoids the medial malleolar osteotomy in most cases.

Postoperative Care

Rehabilitation can generally begin after healing is demonstrated, which may occur after 6–7 weeks of non-weight-bearing. Ankle active and passive ROM exercises, strength development, and proprioceptive training are main pillars for treatment. Patient should be informed that pain following operative treatment is common for up to a year. After 6 months, a persistent effusion, a catching sensation or severe pain, signifies that healing is not progressing as intended and further investigation and management is indicated. Salvage in the form of ankle arthrodesis or ankle arthroplasty may be proposed.

Complications of Osteochondral Lesions of Talus

- Ankle arthritis
- Chronic pain
- Stiffness
- Resorption of grafts
- Infection
- Transmission of viral diseases in allograft transplants

CAISSON DISEASE

Synonyms: Decompression sickness (DS), bends, chokes and staggers, and nitrogen disease. DS is the preferred term as it indicates the closest pathomechanism of development of disease.

Definition

Decompression sickness is the clinical syndrome produced by formation of bubbles of dissolved supersaturated inert gas during or after decompression. The gas bubbles may, however, form even in nonsupersaturated scenarios as in rapid ascent to high altitudes in unpressurized aircrafts.

History

"Caisson disease" is a term coined by Andrew Smith to describe the illness that he encountered among workers during the construction of the Brooklyn Bridge. The term "Caisson" refers to the engineering term where a high-pressure tube is placed in difficult mining regions (like quicksand). The high pressure pushes away the water and sand from the mining shaft and workers can do mining inside **(Fig. 49)**. For workers to enter into the shaft there is an "air lock" at the surface which is a pressurized box.

The idea of pressurized mining came from Papin (1691) and Coulomb (1779) that was used by Triger (1839)—a French mining engineer who also described the effects of compressed air on human body. Triger noted that persons working in high atmospheric pressures were unable to whistle at 3 atm (1 atm = 33 feet sea water = 14.7 pounds per square inch), there was a nasal tone to voice, deaf miners were able to hear better and could do laborious work better with few developing joint pains. The fact that the disease is problematic only on coming out of the compressed air region was first noted by Pol and Watelle in 1854.

Risk Factors

Personnel working at the following places are at risk of DS:
- Mining
- Tunneling
- Bridge construction
- Deep sea diving
- Aviation

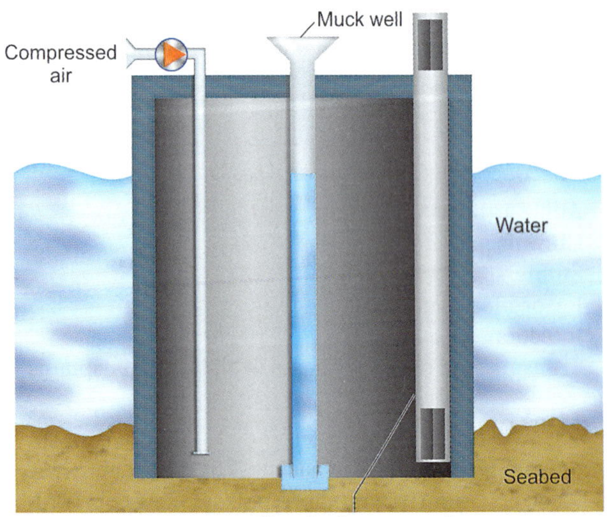

Fig. 49: Caisson disease.

Pathomechanism of Decompression Sickness

Nitrogen gas is the main culprit for development of Caisson's disease. Normally nitrogen gas at a constant pressure is dissolved into the tissues saturating them. The saturation is proportional to atmospheric pressure of the containing environment. If pressure rise more gas dissolves supersaturating the tissues while at lower pressure desaturation occurs. For every 10.13 m depth the ambient pressure increases by 1 standard atmosphere pressure (101.3 kPa) so going to 20 m (65.61ft) the pressure rises to 3 ATA. Pressure changes while rising to surface are usually gradual and during this time the excess gas gets released into vascular system to be disposed by lungs if a patient moves from a high to low pressure region. The rate of creation of equilibrium is constant, and if the pressure changes occur fast, unfortunately, the capacity of body to dispose excess dissolved gas is exceeded. In a critical situation with rapid change in pressure, nitrogen bubbles form that may develop in the tissues or vascular system itself. These bubbles may simply grow from microbubbles already present in the system. Bubble formation also occurs in the potential spaces like joints from which the clearance is typically slow. The myriad of symptoms is due to this bubble formation. The recognition of bubble formation as a cause of caisson was recognized only lately. Boyle (1670) observed bubble in the aqueous humor of a snake. This was reinforced by Hoppe with the finding in animals of intravascular free air with rapid decompression (1857). Mericourt suggested that the severity of disease is related to the depth and duration of stay, the longer the worse and higher are chances. One of the preceding popular hypotheses (now proved wrong) was systemic congestion—central organs, firm and compact structures, and organs within closed cavity are congested under compressed air and malfunction. The other hypothesis was systemic exhaustion (also rejected now)—compressed air super saturated organs with oxygen increasing the work efficiency and exhausting the organs, on decompression the fatigue manifest along with the endothermic effect of decompressing gas.

Types and Clinical Features

The Medical Research Council (MRC) DS panel recognized two types of illness in 1961:
- *Type 1:* This is a "nonserious" illness that commonly manifests as joint and skin symptoms. The joint pains have been called "bends". Interestingly, the "bends" is derived from the Grecian Bend that was a forward stooping posture introduced in 1870s by a popular ladies fashion. With joint pains of DS, the patients assume the same forward stooping posture and term "the bends", hence colloquially came into use.
- *Type 2:* The serious form is characterized by inability to breathe ("chokes") and dizziness (vestibular system "staggers"). These patients also developed various neurological symptoms and, if not promptly addressed the patients died of cardiovascular collapse.
- *Type 3:* It was suggested by Neumann and Bove in 1987 to be added to original system—this represents progressive

and treatment resistant DS. Here the nitrogen gas bubble load is so high that the arterial system collapses and is fatal.

Bubbles may form in tissues and cause various mechanical effects by mechanical distraction of pain fibers. In venous system, small amounts of bubbles are removed by pulmonary capillaries while large quantity may cause endothelial damage and lead to activation of coagulation pathway and symptomatic pulmonary vascular obstruction producing cough, dyspnea, and pulmonary edema that can be fatal, if not treated early. Presence of patent foramen ovale (25% adults) may lead to shunting of the bubbles to arterial circulation producing various cerebral, inner ear, and skin manifestations. In the musculoskeletal system joint pains are the most common manifestation due to formation of bubbles in the joints, bones, and periarticular muscles. Long-term manifestation may include ON at various sites, typically those with precarious blood supply as discussed in the above section. Neurologic manifestations include confusion, visual, and speech disturbances that may arise from cerebral arterial gas embolism. Inner ear disease manifests as hearing loss, vertigo with or without vomiting. Formation of bubbles in spinal cord leads to paralysis, upper motor neuron signs, bladder dysfunction, abdominal, and girdle pain. Involvement of cardiovascular system produces chest pain, arrhythmia, hemoconcentration, coagulopathy, and hypotension. Cutaneous rash, itch, soft tissue edema, and fatigue are other manifestations.

Prevention and Treatment

Use of helium instead of nitrogen drastically reduces the central narcotic symptoms. The divers should follow strict protocol of halting the ascent periodically called the "decompression stops". As soon as the symptoms are identified the patient should be given 100% oxygen that washes out the inert gas from tissues. Definitive treatment in all but very minor cases include recompression and hyperbaric oxygen. Recompression reduces the bubble volume and increases the inert gas partial pressure difference between alveoli and tissue, this increases inert gas diffusion from bubble. Hyperbaric oxygen helps reduce the proinflammatory effects and symptoms of inert gas. The earlier it is introduced the better are the results. Recompression is usually done at 2.8 ATA followed by stepwise decompression over hours (for 5–8 hours usually often repeated on subsequent days) depending on the protocol used. Patients should be adequately hydrated and supported symptomatically.

CONCLUSION

- Osteonecrosis involves death of living elements of bone—both the osseous cellular and marrow elements that ultimately damages the bone architecture (shape, form, and function).
- Osteonecrosis results from ultimate vascular failure to cellular components but the vessels are present so in this sense the commonly used term "AVN" is a misnomer.
- Various causes of ON have been identified but the identification of a particular cause in patient hardly alters the course of treatment which is guided by the stage of progression of the disease. It is better to concentrate on prevention of ON rather, if possible.
- Traumatic ON is common in bones having already precarious blood supply such as the scaphoid, femoral head, and talar body, and humans presently have minimal rather no control over the onset or progression of traumatic ON.
- Early identification of ON is the key to provide the patient with best possible outcome while preserving the native anatomy. In later stages mostly reconstructive procedures or arthrodesis especially in smaller joints are ultimate modalities.

SECTION

2

Joint: Structure, Function, and Related Disorders

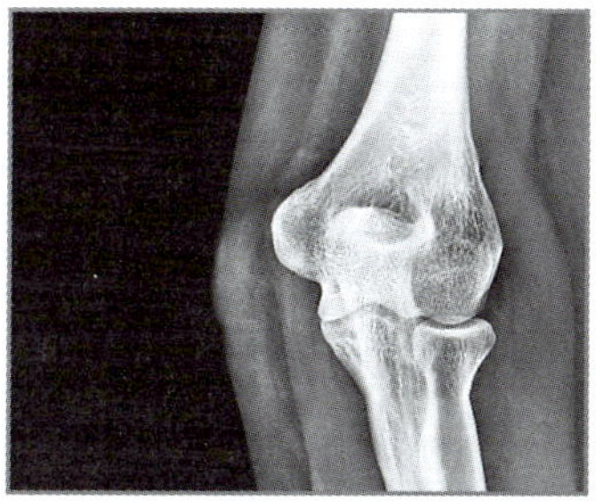

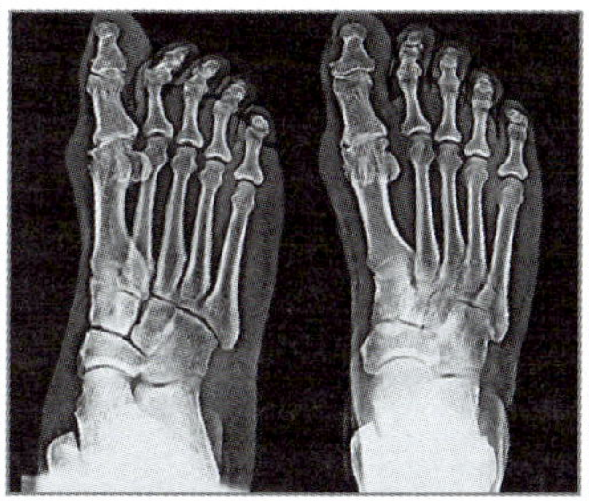

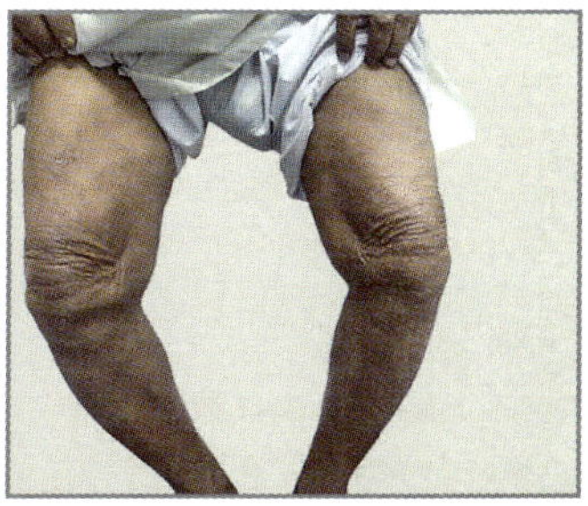

CHAPTER 7

Joints of Skeleton, Synovial Joint Structure and Function

Manish Kumar Varshney

INTRODUCTION

Joints provide assembly units to the bones and provide mobility to otherwise stiff bony skeleton. Due to stress concentration at immobile regions and mobility at specific joints, the age- and activity-related degeneration is evident over time. Some pathologies such as inflammatory and crystal arthropathy characteristically involve synovial joints so their study as a separate unit is imperative.

DEFINITION

A joint is defined as articulation between two or more bones or parts of bones. Joints are essential components of the skeleton.

FUNCTIONS

The functions are:

- They produce segmentation of the skeleton to allow mobility.
- They give segmental growth to the body depending on the needs and roles.
- They provide fulcrum for various muscle action assisting in ergonomics and power utilization.
- They serve as proprioceptive regional centers for balancing and stabilization.
- Indirectly serve as shock absorbers (else one would fall like a log of wood).
- Joints (aka arthroses) are classified according to the intervening material and the way of articulation of the components. The structure of a joint determines its function so the movement of these joint ranges from no movement to freely movable. The term "*diarthrosis*" encompasses all synovial joints and refers to joints designed for movement.

JOINT CLASSIFICATION

The joints in human body can be classified morphologically (rather biomechanically) and functionally **(Flowchart 1)**. The morphological classification takes into account the shape of articulating surfaces and the principal axis of rotation of the junction. Functionally, the joints are classified as synarthrosis (allowing no movement), synchondrosis (allowing some

Flowchart 1: Structural and functional classification of joints. The structural classification is based on the type of intervening tissue. Functional classification represents degree of movement where—synarthrosis allows no movement, amphiarthrosis allows some movement, and diarthroses are mobile joints.

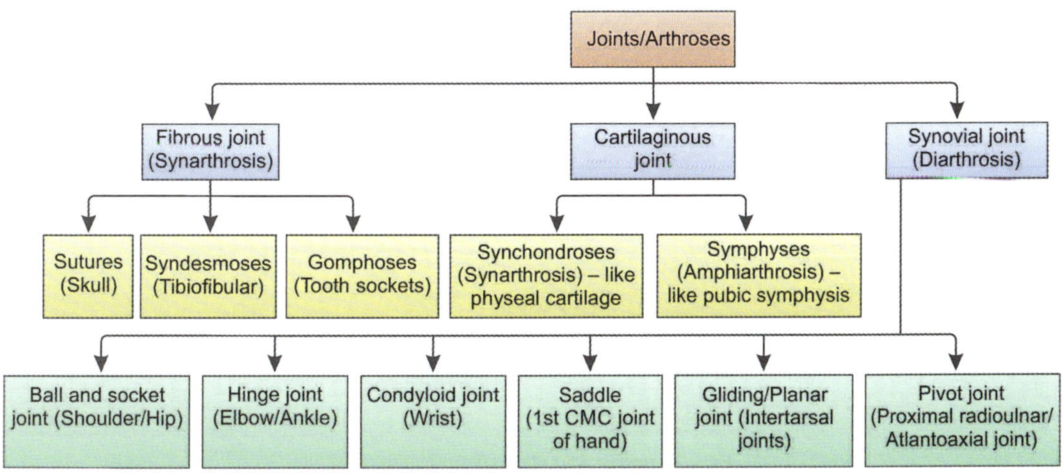

movements), and diarthrosis (that are mobile). Though the synarthroses are immobile, they are the most stable joints of body while diarthroses are weakest in stability but they allow good movements. Specific characteristics of some of the articulations are described here.

Synovial Joints (Diarthrodial Joint; Diarthrosis)

Synovial joints (diarthrodial joint; diarthrosis) are designed for movement **(Fig. 1)**. They are the most common types of joints and typically have a joint cavity. Characteristic of these joints includes hyaline cartilage covering the ends of bones for smooth articulation and joint is enclosed within fibrous capsule. The synovial membrane forming the inner layer of the capsule produces the synovial fluid filling the joint cavity. This articulation is discussed in detail further. Depending on the predominant axis of rotation, the synovial joints have been further divided into six types (*see* kinematic classification and **Flowchart 1**).

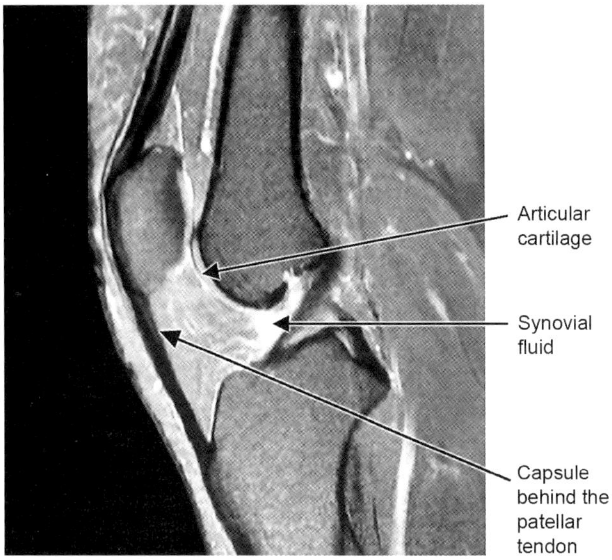

Fig. 1: Synovial joint magnetic resonance imaging (MRI).

Fibrous Joints

Syndesmoses (fibrous joints) have variable thickness of intervening fibrous tissue (a ligament or fibrous membrane) as articulating surface. They allow some movement depending on the length of the fibers connecting the bones. The suture joints of the skull **(Figs. 2A and B)**, the radius and ulna in the forearm, and tibia and fibula in leg joined by the interosseous membrane are examples. The bonds between the teeth and the jawbones known as gomphosis or dentoalveolar syndesmosis also fall in this category.

Synchondroses

Synchondroses are joints united by cartilage with minimal movement. The growth plate is an example of temporary synchondrosis since it ossifies **(Figs. 3A and B)**.

Symphyses

In *symphyses*, hyaline articular cartilage covers the two opposing surfaces and the joints are united by fibrocartilage.

They are also called cartilaginous joints. The strength of the fibrocartilage gives stability, while the hyaline cartilage helps in shock absorption. Pubic symphyses **(Fig. 4)** and intervertebral disks are types of symphyses. These joints may become increasingly mobile during specific conditions such as symphysis pubis laxity during childbirth.

Synostoses

Synostoses are joints that are eventually closed by bony union.

With age, all synchondroses, sutures, and some syndesmoses will ossify with no movement allowed.

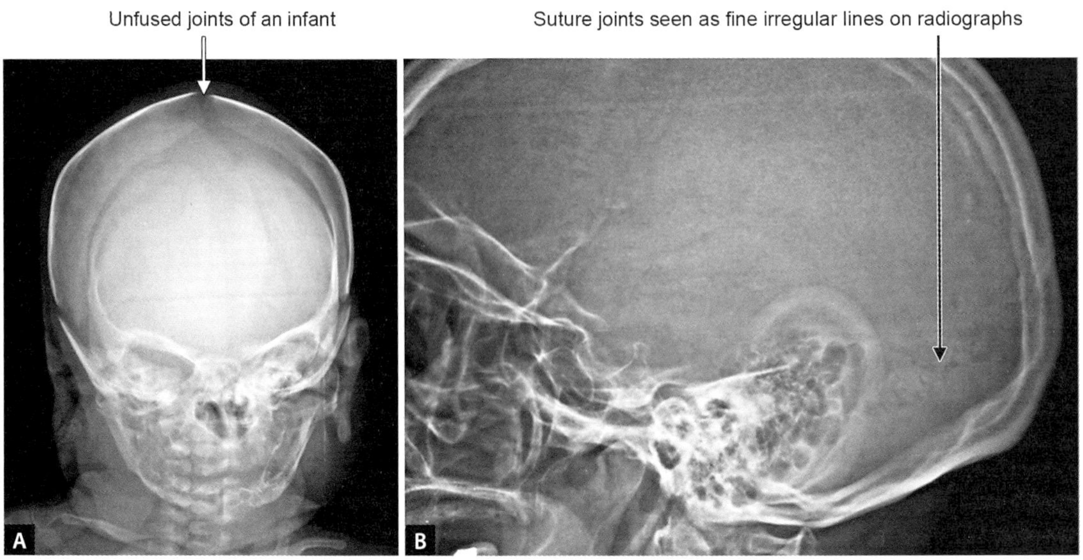

Figs. 2A and B: Gomphosis (suture joints of skull).

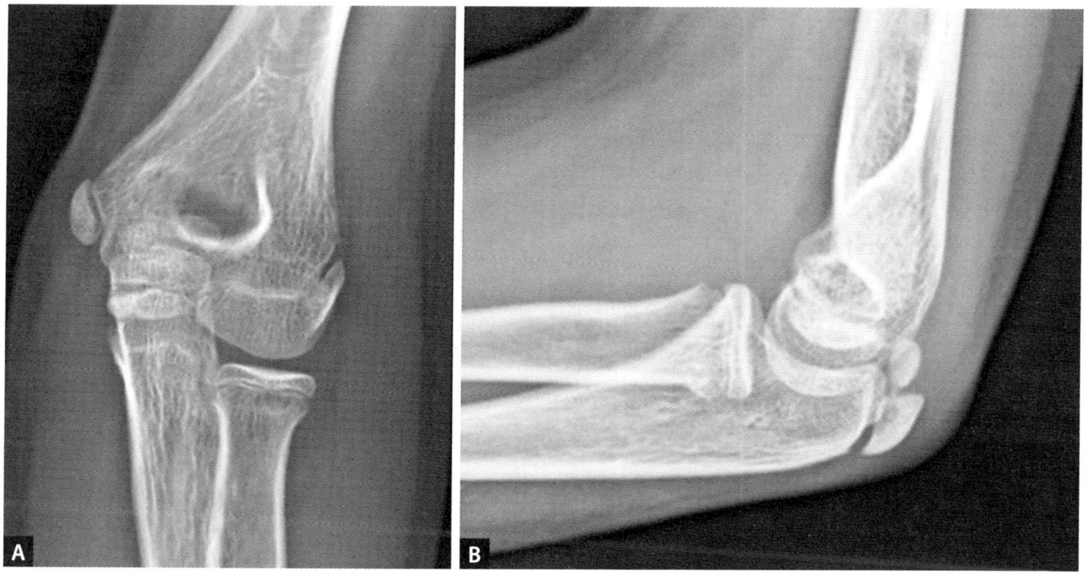

Figs. 3A and B: Synchondrosis (e.g., growth plate).

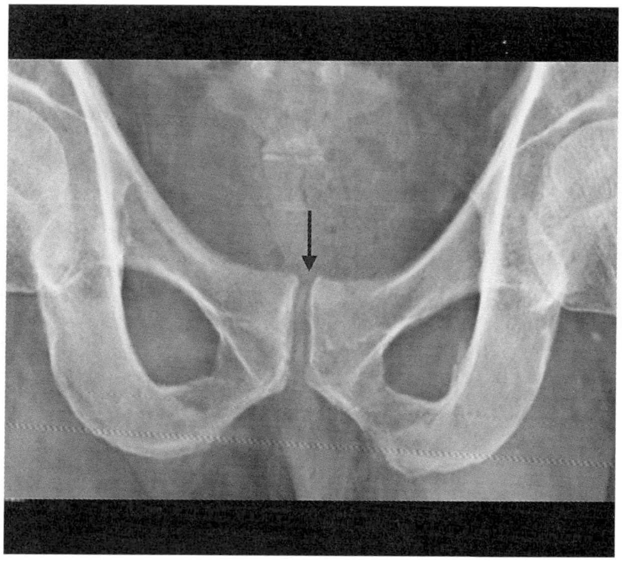

Fig. 4: Symphysis (symphysis pubis).

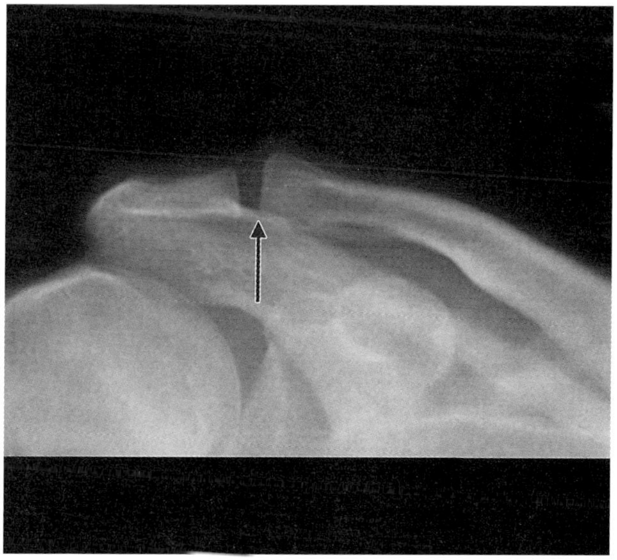

Fig. 5: Plane joint (acromioclavicular).

KINEMATIC CLASSIFICATION AND MOVEMENTS AT DIFFERENT TYPES OF SYNOVIAL JOINTS

Osteokinematics and arthrokinematics are often used interchangeably in the literature and in common parlance but they describe different aspects of joint motion.

- Osteokinematics is the description of the relative movement between two bones on either side of a joint.
- Arthrokinematics describes the movements occurring between the joint surfaces, such as rolling, spinning, and gliding of joint surfaces.

There are six possible degrees of freedom for joint movements (three rotations and three translations) in three-dimensional space but geometrical configuration and soft tissue constraints limit osteokinematics to fewer axes and planes of motion.

Plane joints are characterized by flat articulating surfaces and have gliding (translatory movement) and spinning arthrokinematics. The osteokinematics of plane joint movement ranges from uniaxial to triaxial. The acromioclavicular joint has triaxial **(Fig. 5)**, and the vertebral zygapophyseal (facet) joints are examples of uniaxial joints.

Hinge joints allow movement in one plane (usually sagittal) and about one axis of rotation, usually transverse. The elbow joint **(Figs. 6A and B)** is a hinge joint. They are constrained joints.

Saddle (sellar) joints have opposing concave and convex fitting surfaces. The osteokinematics of saddle joints is predominantly biaxial (motion about two primary axes in two planes) but also have a third axes allowing some rotation (triaxial). The carpometacarpal (CMC) joint of the thumb

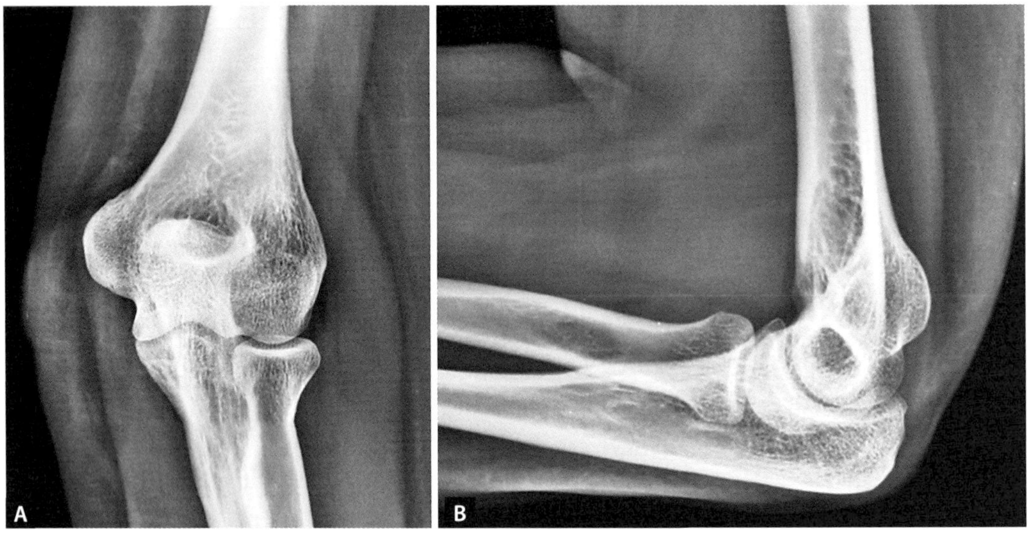

Figs. 6A and B: Hinge (elbow) joint.

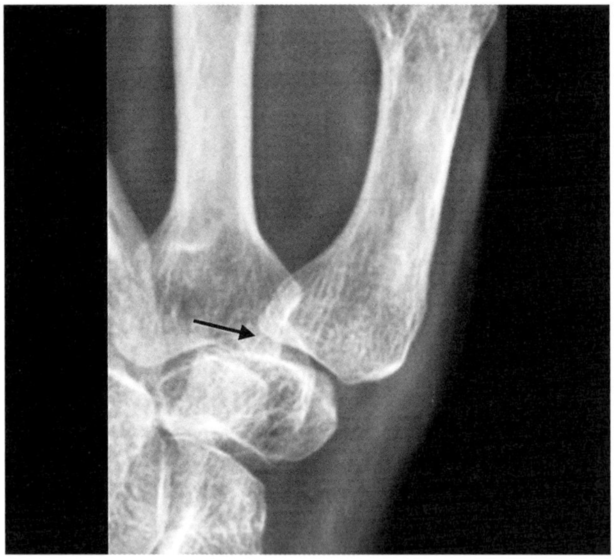

Fig. 7: Saddle (1st CMC) joint. (CMC: carpometacarpal)

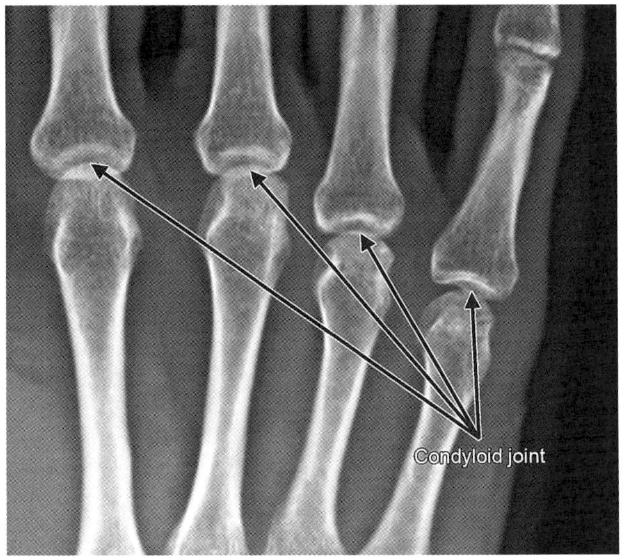

Fig. 8: Condyloid (metacarpophalangeal) joint.

(Fig. 7) allows opposition by adduction-flexion-internal rotation in such a joint.

Condyloid joints have a shallow or flat concave surface opposing a nearly spherical convex surface. These joints have osteokinematics across two axes. The arthrokinematics of condyloid joints is explained by the "concave-convex rule" where rolling and gliding occur simultaneously in opposite direction to prevent bones falling off during movement. The convex condyloid component rolls in the direction of bony movement and glides in the opposite direction with respect to the concave component to maintain congruency of joint surfaces. Metacarpophalangeal joints of the fingers **(Fig. 8)**, the condyles of jaw articulating with base of skull, and the knee joint are some examples. The atlanto-occipital joint is also a condyloid joint.

Ball and socket joints have a convex surface that moves within a relatively deep concave surface. Ball and socket joints have 6° of freedom. The hip **(Fig. 9)** and glenohumeral joints are types of ball and socket joints.

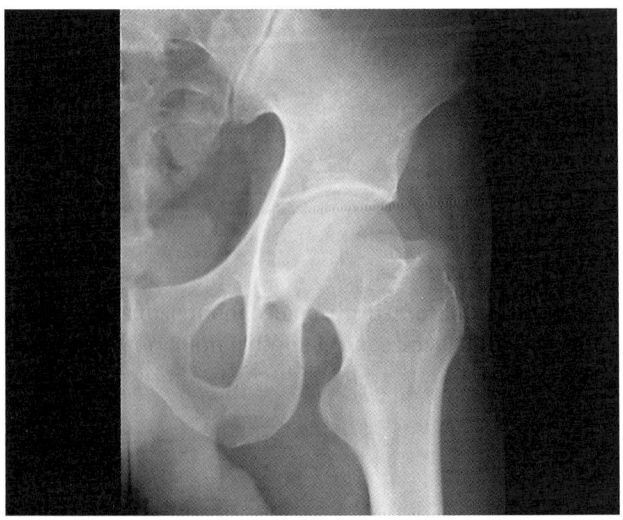

Fig. 9: Ball and socket joint (hip joint).

Pivot joints have a sleeve or ring formed by one bone within which the rounded process of the opposing bone moves. They are uniaxial joints. Atlantoaxial joints and the proximal radioulnar **(Figs. 10A and B)** joints are types of pivot joints.

SYNOVIAL JOINT

Synovial joints consist of fluid-filled cavity containing hyaline cartilage lined bone ends enclosed in a tough fibrous capsule joining and surrounding the adjoining bony surfaces. The joint capsule is lined by a synovial membrane that secretes the synovial fluid.

Detailed Anatomy and Physiology of Synovial Joint (Fig. 11)

The synovial joint is covered all around by *joint capsule* forming the outermost layer. There are two connective tissue layers in the joint capsule. The outer fibrous layer is made up of collagen fibers. The fibrous capsule is thickened at places forming intrinsic ligaments that are different from ligaments outside the capsule (extrinsic ligaments). Both types of ligaments provide vital additional stability to the synovial joint. The fibrous layer surrounds the joint and attaches to the periosteum of the adjacent bones. The joint capsule is supplied by a number of somatic sensory fibers for sensations of proprioception, pressure, pain, and vibration. Sometimes, the joint capsule may be deficient to allow for passage of structures in/out of the joint like the biceps tendon in shoulder joint. The synovial membrane lining the inner layer of joint capsule is poorly innervated but highly vascularized.

Neural Innervation

- *Pain perception:* The joint ligaments, capsule, and the periosteum have pain fibers whereas synovial membrane and the articular cartilage are insensitive to pain. When

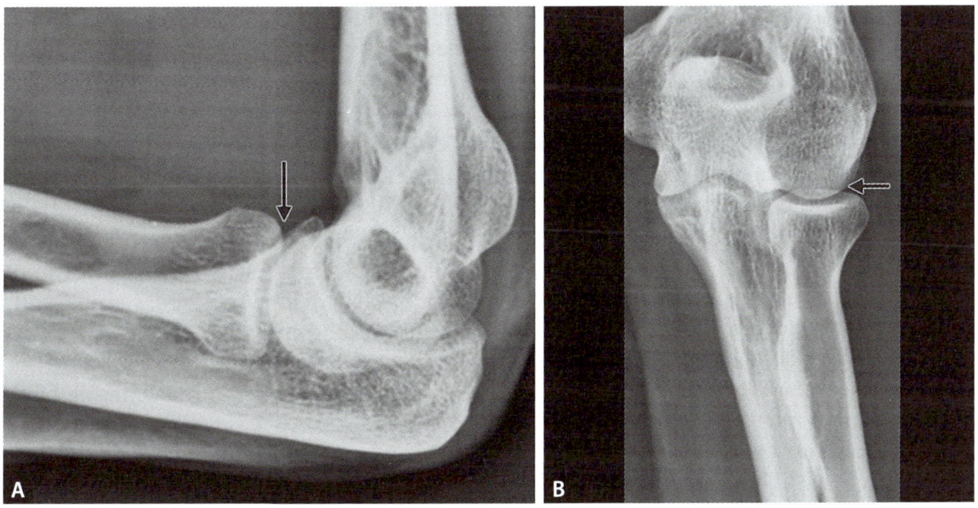

Figs. 10A and B: Pivot joint—proximal radioulnar joint.

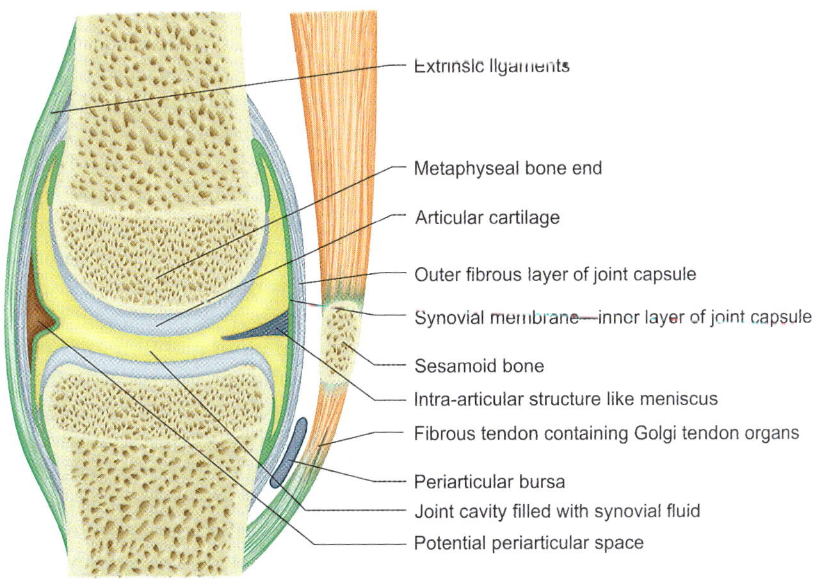

Fig. 11: Synovial joint anatomy.

there is swelling within a joint from disease or trauma, pain endings are stimulated giving rise to the sensation of pain.

- *Proprioception:* The paciniform corpuscles (small, elongated Pacinian corpuscles), Ruffini-type endings, and some of the free nerve endings in the joint capsule respond to the bending of joints (proprioception). They have a protective function against the extremes of hyperextension and hyperflexion. The Ruffini endings [also referred to as Ruffini corpuscles, flower spray organs, and slow adapting type II (SA-II) axons] additionally function as slow adapting mechanoreceptors and detect changes in joint angle and motion.
- *Muscle reflexes:* Muscle and capsule tension are detected by Golgi tendon organs found in the fibrous ends of tendons and adjacent to joint capsule. The terminals of the Golgi tendon organs are compressed when the collagen fibers are stretched by muscle contractions or joint capsule movements, and they discharge to complete local reflex loop.

Synovial Membrane

The synovial membrane is contiguous with cartilage of synovial joints. It forms the inner surface of the fibrous capsule surrounding the joint, and is made up of cuboidal cells or *synoviocytes* arranged one to four cell layers deep. They can absorb and secrete synovial fluid essential for lubrication. There are three types of synovial arrangements: (1) areolar, (2) fibrous, and (3) adipose—

1. The *fibrous type* has a thin cellular layer, which rests on connective tissue fibers and merges with the outer fibrous capsule. It is located over tendons.
2. The *areolar type* has two layers. The outer layer consists of fibroblasts, mast cells, macrophages, along with collagen and elastic fibers. The inner cellular layer consists of fibroblasts and synovial cells. The areolar type is thicker than the other two types and allows movement of the membrane over the fibrous capsule.
3. The *adipose type* is found in area such as the knee joint over the intra-articular fat pads.

The inflammatory cytokines increased in degenerative and inflammatory joint diseases are produced by synovial cells and macrophages of the synovial membranes. The synoviocytes are of three types: (1) type-A cells (macrophage-like), which are phagocytic and act as antigen-presenting cells. (2) Type-B cells (fibroblast-like) are the most predominant and produce synovial fluid including its components such as hyaluronic acid, fibronectin, and collagen. (2) Type C cells have unknown function and may serve as precursor to other cell types. Synovial fluid is produced by serum ultrafiltration that helps to deliver nutrients to chondrocytes and lubricates joint. Collagen and proteoglycan are secreted by the synoviocytes and have a phenotype that includes the strong expression of vascular cell adhesion molecule-1 (VCAM-1). They are immunoreactive for vimentin (an interfilament molecule) and not for epithelial markers. The cells are flexible and permit joint movements, as they line fibrous capsules and cover exposed osseous surfaces and intracapsular ligaments. Rheumatoid arthritis starts in the synovial membrane and becomes a source of matrix metalloproteinases (MMPs) and cytokines in the synovium and synovial fluid. The type-B (fibroblast-like) synoviocytes proliferate aggressively and invade adjacent cartilage and bone forming *pannus*. This hyperactivity of synovial cell eventually destroys both the cartilage and the underlying bone. Other molecular changes associated with synovial inflammation include increased chimerin, increased citrullinated cellular fibronectin, and increased mesenchymal stem cells.

Adaptation of Synoviocytes to Mechanical Stress

The shear forces caused by the motion of synovial fluid during mechanical loading activate the mitogen-activated protein kinase (MAPK) pathways, causing c-jun and c-fos transcription factor activation leading to cell growth and proliferation. These changes let the tissues to adapt to stressful conditions. Mechanical shear forces also induce the production of heat-shock proteins (HSPs) 60 and 70, which protect the stressed and/or injured cells against apoptotic death. The synovial membrane has low rate of cell death from apoptosis and cells adapt to a variety of mechanical stresses successfully, provided additional joint pathologies such as rheumatoid arthritis or osteoarthritis are not present.

Synovial Fluid

Normally, there is little free lubricating fluid in the joints, which varies from <1 to 4 mL in large joints. This synovial fluid is a clear or straw colored, viscous, and fluid-containing hyaluronic acid and lubricin.

- The hyaluronic acid (hyaluronate) is a large, highly polymerized mucopolysaccharide having the following functions:
  - It nourishes chondrocytes in the articular cartilage.
  - It reduces friction between joint surfaces.
  - It provides viscosity.
- Lubricin (lubrican) also known as superficial zone protein is another secreted glycoprotein in the joints encoded by the plasticity-related gene (PRG). It also protects articulating surfaces and controls synovial cell growth thus serving the role of maintaining cartilage structure and extracellular matrix. Camptodactyly-arthropathy-coxa vara-pericarditis syndrome (CACP) is an autosomal recessive disorder in humans in which there is a loss of lubrican function leading to premature joint failure.
- The synovial fluid is similar to plasma in electrolyte composition, but it lacks most proteins, particularly those with high-molecular weight.
- Albumin and globulin are found but in 5–6 times lower concentration than plasma. The A:G ratio in synovial fluid is 20:1. Among globulins, the $\alpha 1$ and β globulins are found in similar concentrations while the $\alpha 2$ and γ globulins are found in much lesser quantity.
- Synovial fluid is paucicellular under normal conditions with a normal cell count of 65–89 cells per mm^3 mostly predominated by lymphocytes and monocytes. In arthritis and other inflammatory conditions, synovial fluid contains

infiltrating immune cells (monocytes/macrophages and T-cells) and inflammatory mediators such as cytokines.

Synovial Fluid Analysis

Synovial fluid analysis can differentiate between noninflammatory, inflammatory, and traumatic conditions. Systematic examination includes macroscopic and microscopic, and biochemical analysis.

- *Microscopic examination:* Differential white blood cell count, total white and red blood cells, evaluation for crystals is done.
- *Physical characteristics:* The fluid volume, color, clarity, and viscosity of the joint fluid are seen.
- *Microbiological studies:* Cultures are done and Gram's and acid-fast bacillus (AFB) stains are performed.
- *Serological studies:* Glucose, proteins, and lactate dehydrogenase.

Collection of Specimen

Arthrocentesis is done avoiding contamination under full aseptic conditions. The syringe is rinsed with sodium heparin (25 U/mL) (EDTA and oxalate are crystalline in the dry state, and are avoided so as to prevent any artifacts while checking for crystals). For cytological evaluation, 2 mg potassium oxalate per mL of synovial fluid is added. Culture for pyogenic bacteria and mycobacteria, Romanowsky stains, and wet preparation for analysis of crystals must be performed. Chemical examination and immunological tests can be ordered on physician consideration or preference.

Gross Examination (Figs. 12A to D)

- *Clarity:* It is normally transparent. Rise in proteins and/or cells makes it cloudy. Depending on appearance, flecks can be rice bodies as in tuberculosis, rheumatoid arthritis. In ochronosis, flecks resemble ground pepper or wear particles from prosthesis.
- *Color:* Normally, it is clear to a light yellow. Xanthochromia is seen in long-standing hemorrhage and pigmented villonodular synovitis. Color may be opaque or cloudy white in inflammations and in chronic arthritis or lymphatic obstruction, it is chylous.
- *Viscosity:* Hyaluronate gives it high viscosity. This is tested by suspending a drop of fluid from a needle tip (syringe drip test) or between two glass slides, a 3–5 cm long "string" is formed. Increased water content leads to a shorter string as in inflammation or sudden edema. The viscosity may also be tested with Hess viscosimeter.
- *Clot formation (rope test):* Glacial acetic acid is used to test for mucin clot formation. A tight clump formation is seen when glacial acetic acid is added to synovial fluid due to aggregation of mucin. The clump is firm, ropy, and does not disintegrate on vigorous shaking. In mild inflammation, the clump is soft and friable. In advanced inflammation, there is cloudy flocculent precipitate formation. Spontaneous clot formation is seen in hemarthrosis.

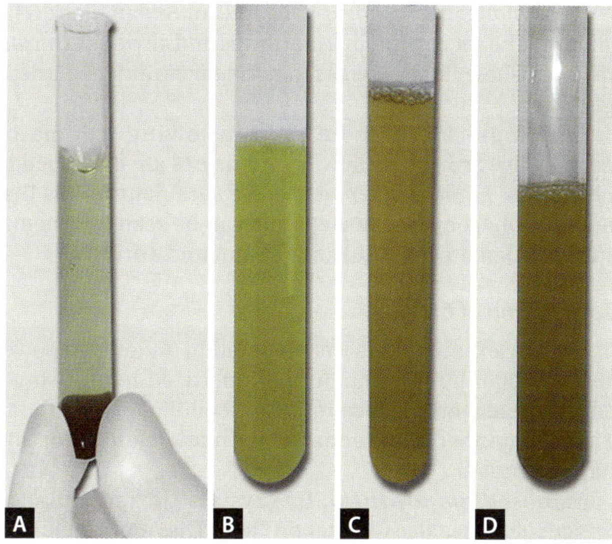

Figs. 12A to D: Synovial fluid gross examination. Color of fluid varies with pathology. (A) Normal straw-colored synovial fluid; (B) Fluid color deepens to yellowish in degenerative arthropathy; (C) Little turbidity is added in crystal arthropathy; (D) Finally, pus-like thicker fluid with greater turbidity is seen in septic arthritis.

Cell Counts and Light Microscopy

Normal synovial fluid does not have many cells. The typical WBC count of normal synovial fluid is <100 mm^3 (normal DLC reads $N_{0\text{-}25}$ $L_{0\text{-}78}$ $M_{0\text{-}71}$ histiocytes$_{0\text{-}26}$ synoviocytes$_{0\text{-}12}$). Red cell counts help to identify hemorrhagic effusion. A standard hemocytometer chamber is used to count cells. In hemorrhagic effusions, RBCs may be lysed using 0.3% saline to aid fluid examination.

Cellular evaluation is done by air-dried smears on a glass slide stained by any of the Romanowsky stains. Normal cellular elements found in synovial fluid include monocytes, lymphocytes, neutrophils, and synoviocytes. Finding *eosinophils* in synovial fluid is abnormal and when seen in excess of 2%, they may represent rheumatic diseases, allergic disease (acute and chronic urticarial), parasitic arthritides, or hypereosinophilic syndromes. Reduced lymphocytes in synovial fluid are seen in patients with rheumatoid arthritis treated with nonsteroidal anti-inflammatory drugs (NSAIDs); injection of contrast media with epinephrine is associated with a leukocytosis.

Erythrophagocytosis, hemosiderin pigment, and hematoidin crystal (intracellular or extracellular golden yellow refractile) are found in intra-articular hemorrhage. Iron-laden chondrocytes suggest hemochromatosis.

Ragocytes or rheumatoid arthritis cells are seen in inflammatory disorders (not specifically rheumatoid arthritis). They are neutrophils containing refractile round cytoplasmic inclusions (phagocytosed immunoglobulins, rheumatoid factor). *Reiter's cells* (not diagnostic of Reiter's disease) are macrophages containing one or more phagocytized neutrophils seen in various inflammatory conditions.

Marrow fragments in synovial fluid indicate fractures involving joints. *Platelets* may be found in rheumatoid arthritis.

Lipid-laden macrophages (Oil red O or Sudan black B fat stain) may be seen in traumatic arthritis and chylous arthritis. Lipid may show "Maltese cross" birefringence under polarized light.

Cartilage cells may be seen following trauma or degenerative arthritis. Yellow chondrocytes are described in ochronosis. *Lupus erythematosus cells* are neutrophils that contain a phagocytized nucleus and can be seen in systemic lupus erythematosus (SLE) and rheumatoid arthritis.

Examination of Crystals

Crystals are examined as a wet preparation under high power (400 or 1,000×) in a compensated polarized light. Using a red compensator, the location (intracellular, extracellular, or both), number (few, moderate, or many), and color and shape are noted.

Monosodium urate (MSU) crystals (intracellular or extracellular) [*see* also Chapter on "Joint Disorders Including Inflammatory and Noninflammatory Arthritis and Infective Arthritides (Including Mycobacterial Infection and Prosthetic Joint Infection)"]:

- Needle shaped
- 5–25 mm long
- *Polarized light* ***(Fig. 13)****:* Strongly negatively birefringent—they appear bright yellow when the long axis of the crystal is oriented parallel to the axis of the red compensator, while color is blue when the crystal is at perpendicular orientation.

If polarized light is not available then MSU crystals can be recognized by their size and color in Romanowsky stain.

Calcium pyrophosphate dihydrate (CPPD) crystals (intracellular or extracellular):

- Rod to rhomboidal shaped
- 1–20 mm in length and up to 4 mm in width
- *Polarized light* ***(Fig. 13)****:* Weakly positive birefringent (appearance opposite that of MSU)—the crystal appears blue with parallel orientation to red compensator, while it appears yellow when perpendicular.

Steroid crystals seen following intra-articular steroid injection usually extracellular (can be intracellular in neutrophils):

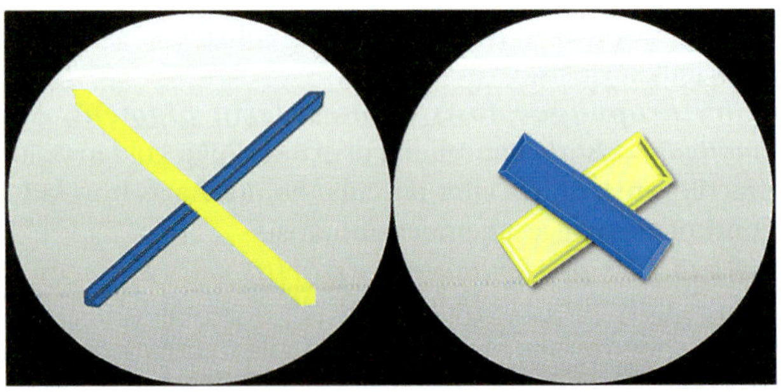

Fig. 13: Crystals of uric acid and calcium pyrophosphate: Birefringence is the property of refractive materials to polarized light. The uric acid crystals are needle-like and negatively birefringent to polarized light (red compensator) appearing blue when aligned perpendicular and yellow when aligned parallel to it. While the calcium pyrophosphate crystals are shorter, rhomboidal and positively birefringent—appearing blue when aligned parallel and yellow when aligned perpendicular to the polarized light (red compensator).

- Mimic MSU crystals. In contrast to MSU, these have ragged edges.
- They are 10–20 mm in length, rectangular to needle shaped.
- *Polarized light:* Negatively birefringent. They dissolve in alcohol fixatives, so examination of a wet preparation is necessary.

Calcium oxalate (CO) crystals are associated with primary oxalosis and chronic renal failure on dialysis:

- Pyramidal, 1–2 mm in size
    - *Polarized light:* Positively birefringent
    - Once identified, oxalate anticoagulation should be stopped in patient.

Cholesterol crystals (extracellular) seen with chylous effusion:

- Large flat rhomboidal plates with notched corners
- *Polarized light:* Strongly positively birefringent
- Do not cause inflammatory arthritis.

Basic calcium phosphate (BCP) crystals and hydroxyapatite—scanning electron microscopy is required to see theses crystals.

Chemical Examination

Glucose

Synovial fluid and plasma specimens are to be collected at the same time. Glucose difference between synovial fluid and plasma is important rather than absolute values. The glucose is estimated using Somogyi-Nelson method that estimates true glucose only. Joint fluid glucose equilibrates with serum levels after 6–8 hours; fasting levels are most reliable. Low synovial fluid glucose can be used to differentiate infection from inflammatory effusion. Normally, there is a glucose difference of <10 mg/dL between serum and joint fluid. With increasing inflammation, glucose levels in joint fluids fall. Infection is to be considered when synovial fluid glucose is <20 mg/dL and difference from serum values exceeds 50%. Significant variations in glucose concentration in inflammations and infections have reduced the usefulness of this investigation.

Lactate

Synovial fluid lactate rises in infections.

Protein

The utility is very limited and does not differentiate between transudate and exudate. An increase in protein concentration >2.5 g/dL is not normal and if >4.5 g/dL, is suggestive of inflammation. The values have very low specificity if at all.

Microbiological and Immunological Examination

Gram's stain is a rapid test to identify and confirm the pathogen in septic arthritis and immediately indicates the antimicrobial treatment to be offered. It may be negative in patients on antimicrobial therapy. Leukocyte esterase reagent (LER) strips may be used for rapid diagnosis of joint infection, especially in periprosthetic infections. If ordered, appropriate transport media to keep vitality of fungal, anaerobic, and tuberculous pathogens should be used. For rapid analysis,

TABLE 1: Typical synovial fluid results in various disorders.

Gross	Normal fluid composition	Noninflammatory (such as traumatic, reactive, and degenerative)	Septic arthritis	Inflammatory arthropathies (such as rheumatoid)	Crystal arthritis
Appearance	Clear, oil-like viscous fluid	Reactive and degenerative effusion—clear Blood stained—post-traumatic	Turbid	Cloudy	Usually cloudy
Viscosity	High	High	Inconsistent	Low	Inconsistent
Color	Straw	Yellow to red depending on hemorrhage	Cloudy to yellow	Cloudy yellow	Cloudy yellow
WBCs per mm^3	<100, usually monocytes	Up to 2,000, usually monocytes	>80,000 usually poly	2,000–50,000 (poly and mono)	2,000–75,000 (poly and mono)
Neutrophil	<25%	<25%	>75%	≥50	≥50
Crystals	No	No	No	No	Yes
Culture	Sterile	Sterile	±	Sterile	Sterile
Gram's stain	–	–	±	–	–
Protein	<2 g/dL	N to (↓ -dilutional) with hemorrhage, the proteins increase but seldom increase above 5 g/dL	↑↑↑ (both albumin and characteristically globulins rise)	N to ↑↑↑ (complement level reduced in rheumatoid arthritis but N in ankylosing spondylitis). A:G ratio may be reversed in rheumatoid arthritis	↑↑↑ (globulins increase in proportion to duration of inflammation but unlike rheumatoid arthritis A:G ratio reduces but does not reverse)
Mucin clot	Firm	Firm	Friable, whole aspirate cloudy	Friable	Friable
Glucose (difference from fasting blood sample)	≈0	≈0	Absolute value of glucose level is less than 20 mg% *and* the difference from serum values exceeds 50%	<50 mg%	>50 mg%

(WBC: white blood count)

stains along with fluorescent detection methods are requested in some cases. Latex agglutination is used for rapid analysis of fungal and bacterial antigens, analysis of metabolites by gas chromatography and Limulus lysate assay for bacterial endotoxin are ordered on physician's discretion. Most immunological tests pertain to rheumatoid arthritis. Estimations such as IgG, IgM, IgA, rheumatoid factor, and complements have been assessed but offer no distinct clinical advantage and are never a routine. The finding of rheumatoid factor in synovial fluid is specific to rheumatoid arthritis.

Differentiation of Inflammatory, Noninflammatory, and Infectious Effusion (Table 1)

With specific questions in mind, the interpretations of fluid analysis can be referenced. Without contributory clinical and other laboratory data, the fluid analysis is nonindicative. Septic versus inflammatory arthritis, crystal-related versus septic arthritis, and gout or pseudogout can be differentiated on fluid analysis; however, two processes may simultaneously exist. Septic arthritis has predominance of white blood cells. The findings resemble pus (antimicrobial treatment modifies the findings) and neutrophils account for 90% of the cells. These findings should be extended for culture of pathogen and Gram's stain. WBC counts in crystal arthritis can resemble septic arthritis with range from 100 mm^3 to >100,000 mm^3 with as much as 80% neutrophils. Therefore, it is important to demonstrate characteristic crystals. WBCs ranging from 2,000 to >100,000 mm^3 with >50% neutrophils in inflammatory noncrystal, nonseptic arthritis. The diagnosis is based on exclusion of organisms and crystals. Low cell counts indicate noninflammatory and nonspecific conditions.

TRAUMATIC ARTHROTOMY

Traumatic arthrotomy refers to opening up of joint externally or internally due to trauma and is more serious than a simple laceration. The articular cartilage undergoes irreversibly damaged by infection, and the joint has limited ability to fight infection. Therefore, all traumatic arthrotomies should be treated urgently. The injury is usually an "outside-in" injury but can be "inside-out" (i.e., periarticular bone pieces piercing the capsule and skin or joint dislocation).

Etiology

Trauma as above, needles, knives, thorns, nails, bullets, and animal or human bites have all been cited. There could be a puncture wound, bite or laceration near a joint, or an open fracture into or adjacent to a joint. One should always look for the possibility of joint contamination and breach of sterility—as a thumb rule, the joint is considered unsterile and contaminated unless proved otherwise, so appropriate treatment should be initiated.

Diagnosis

To determine whether a joint communicates with a laceration or open fracture, saline load test is performed.

Saline (150 cc) with methylene blue is injected aseptically into the joint from an uninjured area. The presence of dye at the laceration site indicates that the sterility of the joint has been compromised. For individuals allergic to methylene blue or patients taking monoamine oxidase (MAO) inhibitors or other serotonergic drugs (methylene blue potentiates serotonin release in brain), either indigo carmine (1:100 dilution) or fluorescein dye should be used. The amount of saline required varies with the size of laceration, site of injection of fluid, etc. It is found that to detect 95% of 1 cm communicating lacerations, around 150 mL of saline needs injected. There is a high incidence of false negatives in small joint lacerations (31–99% reported sensitivity), for this reason, joint sterility should mostly be considered to be compromised unless proven otherwise. The saline load test need not be done in patients whose radiographs show obvious intra-articular air or a foreign body.

Differential Diagnosis

Simple laceration without capsular breach (not extending into the joint).

Treatment

It is imperative to ensure that the joint is sterile so all efforts are directed at removing all possible and known infecting agent. As a secondary measure, any necrotic tissue that may serve as a focus for infection is removed.

- The treatment is formal arthrotomy. Traumatic arthrotomy site can be used for debridement, if it is in a convenient place and allows adequate access to the joint. Otherwise, a convenient standard incision should be made to expose the joint adequately. Debride the original wound to clean edges and then close. If skin cover is doubtful, primary local rotation flap is a better concept rather than keeping the joint open. Irrigation is used to reduce bacterial burden.
- In smaller traumatic arthrotomies, arthroscopy or a standard incision may be used to debride the joint. Antiseptics, surfactants, and saponifying agents used in open fractures are avoided for washing the hyaline cartilage. Local infiltration with broad-spectrum antibiotic solution could, however, serve to control infection.
- If infection is subacute or chronic, include a thorough synovectomy in the surgical debridement.
- It is a very good opportunity to confirm the suspected ligament injuries during the debridement. Ligament injuries, if present simultaneously, should be thoroughly assessed in operating room avoiding additional damage by expert to formulate a plan for later reconstruction. It may not be prudent to reconstruct the ligaments immediately; however, small avulsions or bony avulsions could be repaired in a relatively clean wound.

Support the joint in a plaster of Paris (POP) slab or traction. Continuous passive motion is a good aide to regain early movements and prevent joint stiffness.

CONCLUSION

- Joints provide the mobile units in skeleton.
- Joints are of various types that subserve discrete function at their locations.
- Understanding joints make us understand their kinematics and specialized movements that need to be restored in case of damage.
- Understanding synovial joint anatomy is important, as few of the diseases are quite specific to this joint, viz., rheumatoid arthritis.
- Synovial membrane is a specialized structure that has characteristic physiological functions to maintain the longevity of the joint particularly involving the secretion of nourishing and lubricating synovial fluid.
- As synovial fluid is a product of synovial membrane, its examination provides an avenue to evaluate the joint pathology.

CHAPTER 8

Disorders of Synovium

Manish Kumar Varshney

INTRODUCTION

The synovium is an active component of the joint metabolically. The membrane can be involved in various inflammatory and noninflammatory processes. While the inflammatory processes are discussed later in Chapter on "Joint Disorders Including Inflammatory and Noninflammatory Arthritis and Infective Arthritides (Including Mycobacterial Infection and Prosthetic Joint Infection)", this chapter focuses on the disorders primarily involving the synovium only. So these disorders are mostly mono- or pauci-articular and remain intra-articular pathologies. Tenosynovial giant cells tumors may be localized or diffuse and located in juxta-articular or intra-articular locations. Intra-articular disease is known as pigmented villonodular synovitis (PVNS) which may itself be localized or diffuse. Tenosynovial giant cell tumor (GCT) affecting the tendon sheath is known as GCT of the tendon sheath. These tumors are believed to be benign rather reactive neoplasms. Because synovium is highly vascular so rare disorders causing vascular malformations may arise within synovial lining producing synovial hemangioma. Lipocytes within the synovium may proliferate into villous lipomatous proliferation (lipoma arborescens) in reaction to trauma or metabolic diseases like diabetes or inflammatory arthritides. Bleeding into the joint as a part of coagulopathies secondarily affects the synovium and is basically a chronic synovial reaction that ultimately results in complete articular erosion and destruction of the joint. The hemophilic arthropathy is, hence, discussed with the inflammatory joint disorders and excluded from this chapter. Though completely unrelated but due to shear misnamed nomenclature; "*synovial sarcoma*" is discussed in this chapter for sake of finding no better place!

PIGMENTED VILLONODULAR SYNOVITIS (SYNOVIAL XANTHOMA AND VILLOUS SYNOVITIS)

Pigmented villonodular synovitis is an intra-articular locally destructive fibrohistiocytic proliferation that is considered to be a diffuse counterpart of GCT of tendon sheath. It is an uncommon and benign proliferative disease of the synovial joint, synovial bursa, and tendon sheath seen within 3–8 cases per million per year general population. Of the described two forms—*diffuse* form affecting often the synovium and the *localized* form affecting the tendon sheaths and bursae, the former is far more common in joints and now described as PVNS while the latter is far more common at extra-articular sites and described as GCT tendon sheath or bursa. There are a lot of morphological and genetic similarities between the two as tendon sheaths and bursae (localized form) are also related to synovium (diffuse form) in origin. The term "PVNS" was used by Jaffe to describe idiopathic villous overgrowth of synovial membrane and typical pigmentation usually found in a single joint, but the disease as such was reported as early as 1852 by Chassaignac in flexor tendon sheaths of fingers. The name "PVNS" signifies the color changes due to deposits of cholesterol and hemosiderin on gross examination. It is most commonly seen in the third decade (20–50 years), slightly more often in men. Granowitz and Mankin classified the disease into diffuse and localized forms. The diffuse form tends to occur a bit early (20–40 years) than the circumscribed form (30–50 years). Pediatric age group is very rarely if ever affected but multifocal form is more common and it becomes a lower level differential for juvenile polyarthritis.

Disease Distribution

Two forms are usually easily evident—clinically, radiologically, or on gross examination. Typically, it causes diffuse nodular synovitis throughout the joint but *rarely* may give rise to a circumscribed focal nodular form. It is characterized by the slowly progressive, exuberant, benign proliferative process of synovial tissue and is usually monoarticular. It may affect the synovium of the joints, bursae, and tendon sheaths, and is most commonly observed in the knees (76%), hips, ankles, calcaneocuboid joints, elbows, and small joints of the fingers or toes. The disease may also involve the common flexor sheath of the hands or fingers. Less commonly, temporomandibular joint and the facet joints of the spine and tendon sheaths in the wrist, ankle, or foot may be involved. Extra-articular tumors of the soft tissue and muscle have also been described.

Pathogenesis

Although the cause is unknown but clonal abnormalities (see later) and the capacity for autonomous growth suggest

PVNS to be a true neoplasm. The proliferative nodules have a tendency to bleed, and over time hemosiderin is deposited in the joint giving rise to the characteristic pigmentation of the nodules and the "crank case oil" appearance of the affected joint fluid. Older theories of possible infection (bacterial), lipid metabolic disorder (due to finding of cholesterol), or hemorrhage as inciting inflammatory event are possibly not true because it could not be experimentally produced. Geschickter et al. proposed osteoclast proliferation in associated sesamoid bones to be the cause but this also found no takers or any support from the clinicopathological findings. Jaffe suggested inflammatory response to unknown inciting event leading to xanthoma formation. The macrophages derived from reticuloendothelial system somehow get modified to contain cholesterol. Currently, however, autogenous proliferation is considered to be the primary (i.e., a neoplasm) event rather than ascribing other causes.

A breakpoint in the *colony stimulating factor-1 (CSF-1)* gene at the 1p13 breakpoint and translocation at the *COL6A3* gene at 2q35 are the current contenders found in the development of PVNS. CSF-1 encodes the CSF-1 cytokine that helps in the proliferation and differentiation of monocytes and macrophages, and *COL6A3* encodes a type-IV alpha-3 collagen chain. The t(1;2) translocation, which fuses the *CSF1* gene on chromosome 1p11 to the collagen type VI a3 (*COL6A3*) promoter on chromosome 2q37 results in overexpression of *CSF1*. There is thus increased expression of IL (interleukin)-1b, IL-6, tumor necrosis factor (TNF)-α, and matrix metalloproteinase 9 (MMP-9) possibly resulting from increased CSF-1 cytokine and CSF-1R in studied patients—typically the diffuse form that may be responsible also for the cartilage destruction seen in these patients.

Radiology

The nodules cause appearance of recurrent hemarthroses (hyperdense effusion), smooth cortical saucerized erosions **(Fig. 1)**, and subchondral cysts on X-ray. The joint space is initially preserved but later degenerative changes of osteoarthritis appear **(Fig. 1)**. MRI has proven very useful to make the diagnosis because of the paramagnetic effects of hemosiderin (dark on T1 and T2). Localized PVNS of knee is commonly seen near the Hoffa's fat pad lying behind it. MRI easily demonstrates a globular mass artifact with frond-like appearance of folded synovium **(Fig. 2)**. MRI shows joint effusion with dark signal lining the synovium and internal structures of the joint. This material shows susceptibility effects on gradient echo-imaging resulting in "blooming" of the low signal due to the iron in the hemosiderin deposition. This finding of "blooming artifact" and a low T1- and T2-weighted image signal is diagnostic of PVNS making it one of the few soft tissue pathologies that can be directly diagnosed on MRI without even needing a histopathological confirmation. This said but diagnosis is still established by examination of tissue by microscopy. Calcification is rare in cases of PVNS and if present, alternative diagnoses should be considered, particularly synovial sarcoma.

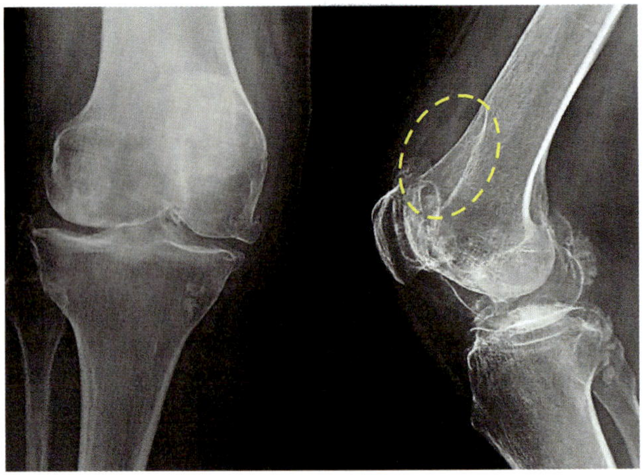

Fig. 1: Localized pigmented villonodular synovitis of right knee. The long-standing lesion eroded the anterolateral cortex of femur with scalloping better visualized on lateral projection (yellow dotted oval). The patient developed osteoarthrosis and underwent total knee arthroplasty.

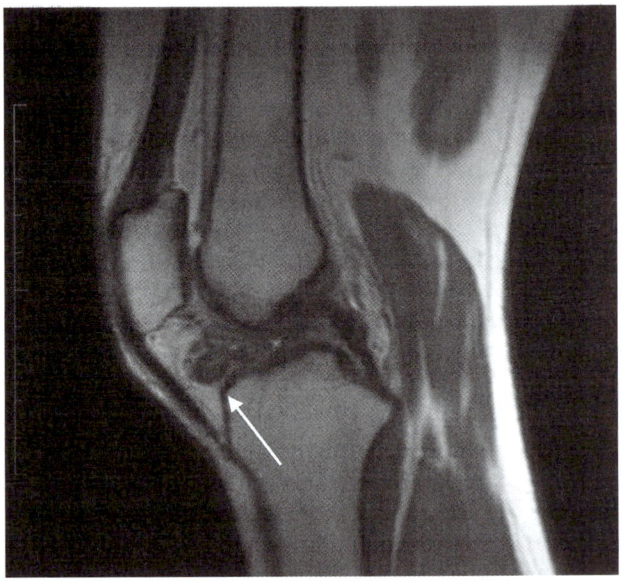

Fig. 2: MRI scan in a patient who presented with knee pain, swelling, and limitation of movements. The scan demonstrates localized globular mass in anterior compartment abutting the Hoffa fat pad, with frond-like folded synovium (arrow).

Differential Diagnosis

Amyloid arthropathy (low signal on MRI but absent blooming artifact), synovial chondromatosis (multiple mineralized intra-articular bodies), synovial hemangioma (intermediate T1-weighted image signal intensity with hyperintensity on T2-weighted imaging), synovial lipomatosis (fatty lobular mass with joint effusion and absent hemosiderin), synovial sarcoma (low intensity on T1-weighted images and high intensity on T2-weighted images), and infection.

Surgical Pathology

Grossly, the mass from localized disease is chocolate-colored with rubbery consistency and is encapsulated lacking any

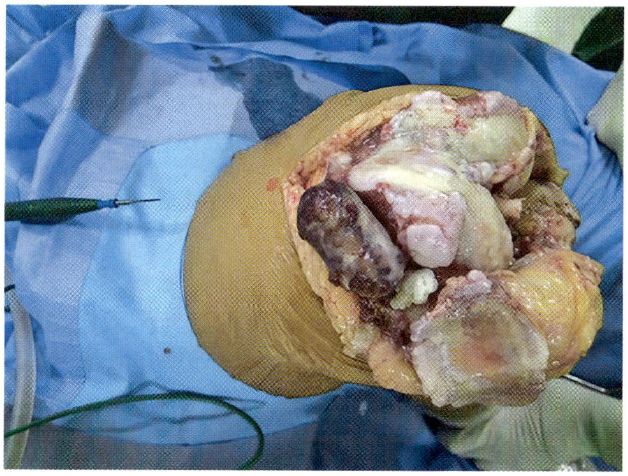

Fig. 3: The mass as visualized grossly during performance of total knee arthroplasty for patient shown in **Figure 1**. The mass was oval-shaped, measured 9 × 3 cm, firm to hard in consistency, and had distinctive chocolate color. One can also note the deeper than usual colored synovial fluid as seen in everted-eroded patellar cup.

villonodular structure **(Fig. 3)**. The masses are nodular and may be large or small, soft or hard. The synovium in diffuse variant is red to brownish in color and has numerous large, finger-like villi that fuse to form pedunculated nodules (often >5 cm). Microscopically:

- *Villi stroma:* Cellular, diffuse, expansile, and somewhat infiltrative sheets of small ovoid, polyhedral or spindle-like synovial cells admixed with larger cells.
- The proliferative synovium invades adjacent cartilage and bone. Cleft-like and blood-filled spaces are relatively prominent. The osteoclastic giant cells are absent or rare in 20% of cases. In the diffuse form, usually two types of mononuclear cells are seen—the small histiocyte-like cells and larger cells. The small histiocyte cells can be round or spindle-shaped, but the predominance of the larger cells may lead this tumor to be mistakenly diagnosed as a sarcoma.
- Hemosiderin granules and lipids are prominent in macrophages. Multinucleated giant cells may be present. The smaller cells are histiocyte-like and often display grooved nuclei. Sheets of foam cells can also be observed. Xanthoma cells are also commonly seen but are more frequent at the periphery of the lesion.
- Mitoses can be quite frequent in rare malignant cases, showing >20 mitoses per 10 high-power fields (HPF) and necrosis. The mitosis, however, is not correlated with metastatic potential. Even histologically benign cases with low mitotic figure have also metastasized.
- Chromosomal studies show that translocations involving chromosome 1p11-13 are common in PVNS and GCT of tendon sheath. Both the mononuclear and multinucleate cells can be positive for CD68. Overexpression of colony-stimulating factor 1 receptor (CSF1R) in both these lesions (the location for CSF1 is chromosome 1) has been recently demonstrated. This possibly represents translocations involving CSF1 and the collagen gene *COL6A3* (which resides on chromosome 2q35).

Clinical Course

Pigmented villonodular synovitis is considered as a benign disease. Localized PVNS occurs most often in the hands, but is also seen in knee and ankle where the diagnosis is usually made while ruling out other causes for swelling. Symptoms may be mild and intermittent and may be present for years before the patient seeks medical attention. Diffuse form is much more aggressive to present with, although patient may still present after 9–12 months of onset of swelling that commonly precedes pain.

- Clinically, PVNS presents with insidious onset of swelling and pain in one joint, most commonly the knee.
  - Limp usually arises later due to advancement of disease.
  - Often the joint as a whole is swollen by the swelling and effusion.
  - On examination, a firm to hard swelling that fills the joint is clinically palpable.
  - Tenderness as a whole is mild-to-moderate with minimal localized inflammatory signs.
  - Radiographs may show joint space narrowing, erosions, and subchondral cysts.
- Mechanical symptoms in the form of locking, snapping or limitation of movement (usually extension) are more often seen with the rare localized variety of disease.
  - Localized disease may present as a small intra-articular tumor.
  - Less common than the diffuse form.
  - Does not show similar destructive joint changes.
  - Aspirate may be normal color due to less frequent hemarthrosis.

The joint fluid contains blood and is dark red or almost black in color "crank case oil" (except sometimes in nodular form). Aspirating such a joint fluid in the absence of trauma quite characteristically represents PVNS. Lipid-containing macrophages may be present in the fluid.

Diagnosis

Ultrasound-guided biopsy is recommended for histopathological diagnosis **(Figs. 4A and B)** else percutaneous biopsy from suprapatellar pouch may be taken.

Treatment

Localized lesion may be observed if they are not causing disturbing symptoms but rarely is this practice followed. Patient's anxiety and satisfaction after complete excision of the localized lesion makes this the most commonly used approach. Extra-articular lesions are rationally treated by open excision of the lesion while for intra-articular lesion open or arthroscopic approach needs to be decided by the access of the lesion by arthroscopy and experience of the surgeon and his comfort. Lesions behind the anterior cruciate ligament (ACL) and far posterior lesions may be treated by open arthrotomy while for posterior approach posterolateral/medial approaches may be still used. The treatment for diffuse form usually consists of complete synovectomy. A treatment algorithm is proposed for management of PVNS

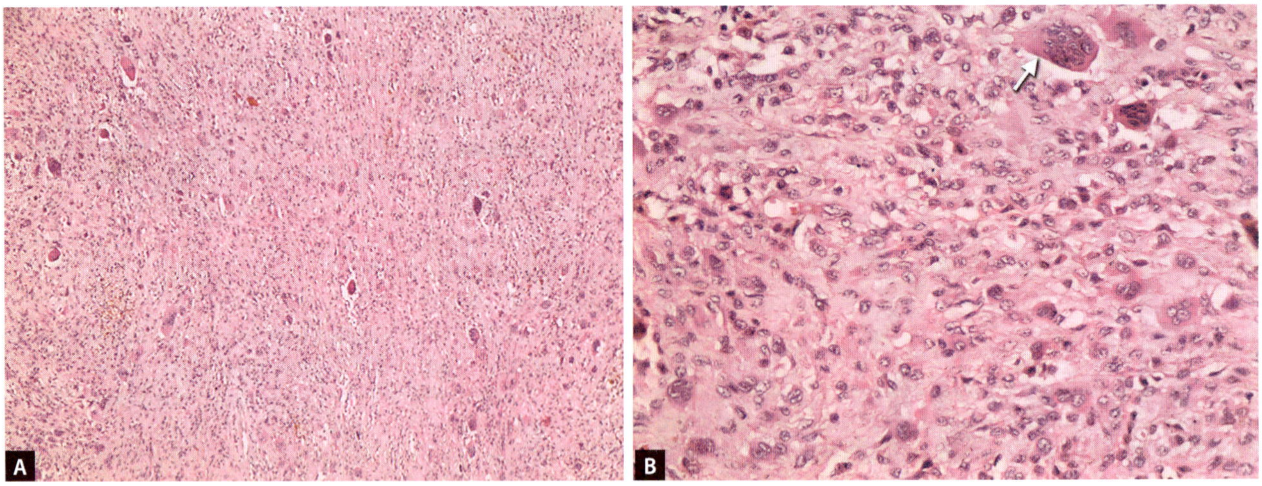

Figs. 4A and B: Histopathology of mass from ankle anterior aspect **(Fig. 1)** that came out to be tenosynovial giant cell tumor (A). Low-power view showing scattered giant cells. The giant cell is marked with arrow on high-power view (B).

Flowchart 1: Management of pigmented villonodular synovitis.

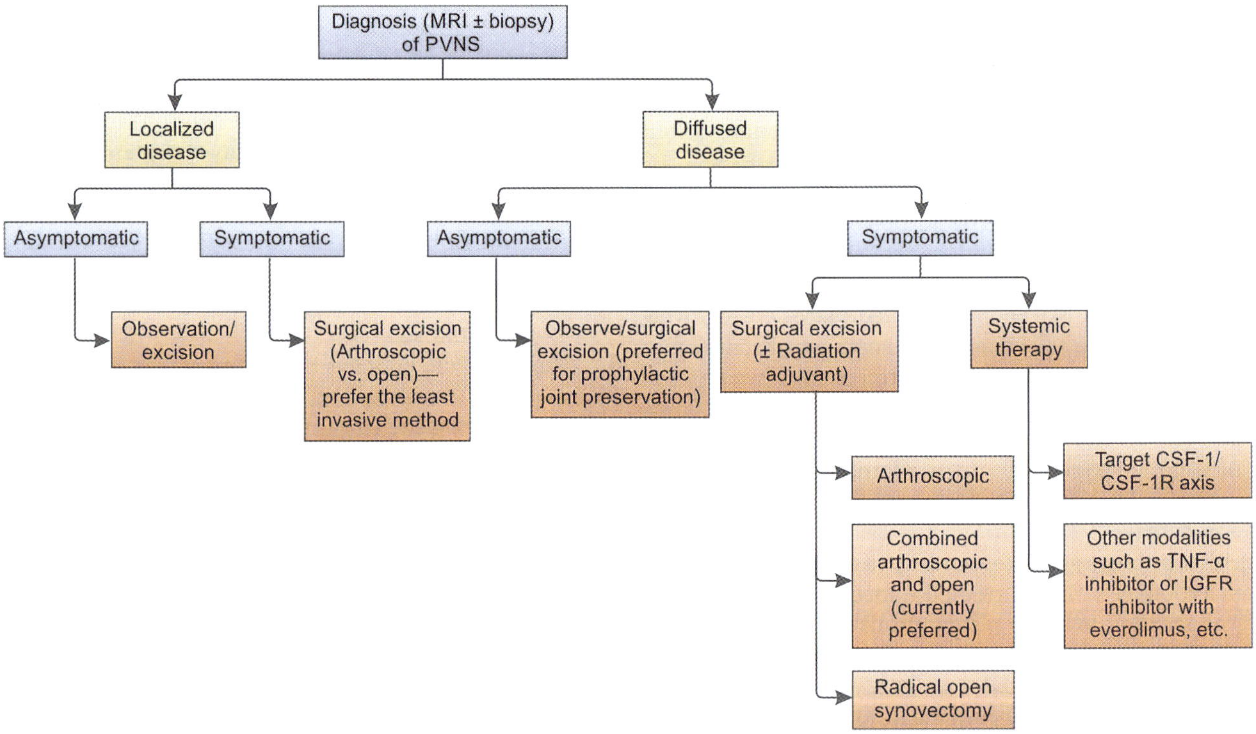

(CSF: colony stimulating factor; IGFR: insulin-like growth factor receptor; PVNS: pigmented villonodular synovitis; TNF: tumor necrosis factor)

in **Flowchart 1**. Partial synovectomy is liable to recur with vengeance. Best current practice seems to be combined arthroscopic anterior extirpation of the disease and posterior lesion excision by open arthrotomy. The disease has a tendency to recur (around 20–30%), sometimes requiring extensive synovectomy and total joint arthroplasty (for aggressive end-stage disease). Median time to recurrence is around 14–18 months. Complete macroscopic resection, female gender, and fresh cases were associated with better local control of the disease while incomplete excision, mitotic activity, bone involvement, and knee location versus hip are associated with increased incidence of disease recurrence. External beam radiation may be used to control recurrent disease but is not a favorable option for primary treatment due to intractable complications such as joint stiffness, skin necrosis, and permanent changes and development of secondary sarcoma. Doses of 30–35 Gy in 15 divided fractions have been used (higher doses of 50 Gy in 25 fractions are possibly overcure) either as primary treatment or adjuvant to surgical management with recurrence rates much below surgical management. Complications, typically the risk of secondary sarcoma that develops at mean 7 years, are the major limitations to its use. Intra-articular yttrium-90 has been also used but is associated with serious complications of skin necrosis and draining sinus. Discovery of newer modalities to treat PVNS based on the discovery of high concentrations of CSF-1 and CSF-1R in the lesion by monoclonal antibodies [imatinib, nilotinib, emactuzumab (RG7155), and pexidartinib] targeting this CSF-1/CSF-1R axis is underway. Imatinib is a tyrosine kinase inhibitor that has been shown to block the Bcr-Abl (breakpoint cluster region-Abelson proto-oncogene) complex, platelet-derived growth factor receptor (PDGFR), c-Kit proto-oncogene, Abl, and Abl-related gene (ARG); nilotinib is a tyrosine kinase inhibitor which targets several members of the type 3 receptor tyrosine kinases, including PDGFR-alpha, c-Kit, and *CSF1R* while emactuzumab (RG7155) is a recombinant, humanized monoclonal antibody of IgG1 subclass directed against *CSF1R* expressed on macrophages. Imatinib was first tried in a few patients with reasonable success but the cost of treatment is too high for this benign disease undue subjecting the patients to complications of chemotherapy. Nilotinib had disappointingly low response rate. Emactuzumab had good response within a few weeks but with significant adverse effects. Pexidartinib (previously PLX3397, Plexxikon) is an orally administered novel small molecule that selectively inhibits *CSF1R*, c-Kit, and mutant FLT3 kinases, by targeting key components of both the tumor and its microenvironment (such as macrophages, osteoclasts, and mast cells) has shown good response and is approved by the Food and Drug Administration (FDA) for use in recalcitrant diffuse forms. One should monitor these patients for cholestatic hepatitis closely. Till date none of the systemic treatments have been approved for treatment of PVNS but if future favorable response is seen they may serve as important adjuvant (to surgery) or even first-line treatment for this disorder either for treatment of primary advanced disease or recurrent/intractable cases. Left untreated, PVNS eventually causes joint destruction needing joint arthroplasty where still the synovial proliferation might develop from inaccessible regions. Amputation is mutilating but is last resort for severe intractable disease. Though metastasis has been reported but malignant transformation or accelerated destruction has not been found.

SYNOVIAL CHONDROMATOSIS

Synovial chondromatosis (synovial chondrometaplasia) is a benign and uncommon disorder characterized by multiple focal metaplastic growths (from subsynovial connective tissue) of normal-appearing cartilage that may develop in the synovial membrane of joints, communicating periarticular bursae or tendon sheath. Calcific degeneration and even ossification may occur in the metaplastic growths that may detach when their pedicles snap forming loose bodies. It is extremely rare for the lesions to degenerate into chondrosarcoma but few cases have been reported. Jaffe restricted the definition to include only those cases that have a chondroid proliferation within the subsynovial connective tissue and not all cases of loose bodies in the knee. The criteria for labeling patients has been, however, extended by Milgram and Schajowicz to include patients with four or more osteocartilaginous loose bodies **(Fig. 5)** even in the absence of synovial metaplasia or in the absence of any other cause. Synovial chondromatosis is an uncommon disorder seen predominantly in men (1.8:1) and most commonly in the knee joint. The disease is seen commonly in third to fifth decade but presentation can occur from the teen years to the seventh decade and is monoarticular. The ectopic foci of cartilage often result in painful joint effusions, cartilage degeneration, and the loose bodies may cause mechanical symptoms.

Milgram (1977) proposed three phases of development of synovial chondromatosis:

1. *Early:* Active intrasynovial disease without loose bodies.
2. *Transitional:* Active disease with loose bodies.
3. *Late:* Multiple loose bodies but no intrasynovial disease.

Clinical Features and Distribution

Symptoms are dull pain, swelling, and stiffness of the joint. Knee is the most common joint affected. Locking and intermittent grating sensation present initially may transform into degenerative arthritis **(Fig. 5)** over time and disease progression. Other large joints such as hip, elbow, and shoulder and very occasionally small joints can be affected. The joint is tender to palpation with nodules palpable as free small marbles along with crepitus. There is usually already an early set-up of degenerative arthritis suggested by joint line tenderness and terminal restriction of 10–15° of movements.

Two forms have been described: (1) Primary, and (2) secondary synovial chondromatosis. The primary form is the typical metaplastic development of cartilage nodules that gradually fuse and enlarge to form larger nodules and may detach to form loose bodies. There are no other identifiable joint abnormalities. There have been reported increased levels of bone morphogenic protein 2 and 4 (BMP-2 and BMP-4) reported from diseased synovium and free bodies. High levels of BMP-2 and BMP-4 mRNA may promote cartilaginous and osteogenic metaplasia. Also Ki-67, a general marker of proliferative activity has been

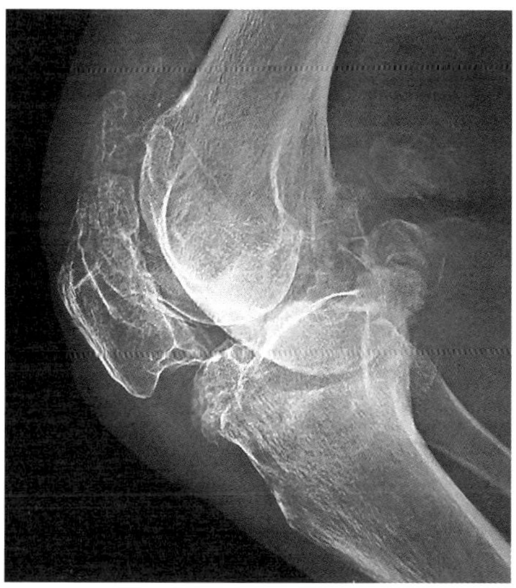

Fig. 5: Synovial chondromatosis. The radiograph demonstrates multiple ossified loose bodies scattered all throughout the knee joint and advanced joint degeneration.

found to be increasingly expressed in the synovial membrane. Elevated levels of chondrocalcin has been reported by Fukuhara et al. in the synovial fluid of patients with synovial chondromatosis that may also assist in the diagnosis of these patients but its widespread use is not popular. Secondary form of the disease is seen where some other joint pathology is already present such as rheumatoid or osteoarthritis, osteonecrosis, osteochondritis dissecans, neuropathic joints, and tuberculosis or osteochondral fractures. The loose bodies develop by inducing metaplastic change following implantation of worn chondral and osteochondral fragments into synovium. The free bodies are far more larger and irregular than the primary form.

Surgical Pathology

At sites of synovial reflection in the stratum synoviale, there is transformation into hyaline cartilage. A number of white and glistening chondroid nodules are seen protruding into the joint. These may be loose in the joint space, but some are pedunculated with tethering to the synovium deriving nutrition from same. The nodules may fuse to form multinodular masses. Segments of cartilage or the spheroidal masses themselves break loose and continue to grow as loose bodies deriving nutrition from fluid **(Fig. 6)**. When calcification and ossification of loose bodies occur, the disorder is referred to as *synovial osteochondromatosis*. Microscopically, the cartilage has a distinct multinodularity and presence of smaller cellular areas that are thought to represent the proliferative foci. The absence of this multifocality should question diagnosis. Eventually, the constant friction and damage to native cartilage leads to development of osteoarthritic changes.

Initially, the chondrogenic process was thought to be metaplasia of primitive mesenchymal cells lying beneath the synovial membrane. More recently, clonal cytogenetic findings with recurring but nonidentical changes in chromosome 6 have been reported, suggesting that this is, in fact, a neoplastic cartilage tumor. Loss of Rab23, an essential negative regulator of the sonic hedgehog signaling pathway, has been demonstrated in synovial chondromatosis. In addition, loss of collagen X and collagen IX genes has been implicated in the pathogenesis. The multifocal nature of chondrocyte growth is explained by the observation that only a subpopulation of cells proliferate and that these cells demonstrate an autocrine growth factor loop consisting of fibroblast growth factor (FGF)-9 and FGF receptor 3.

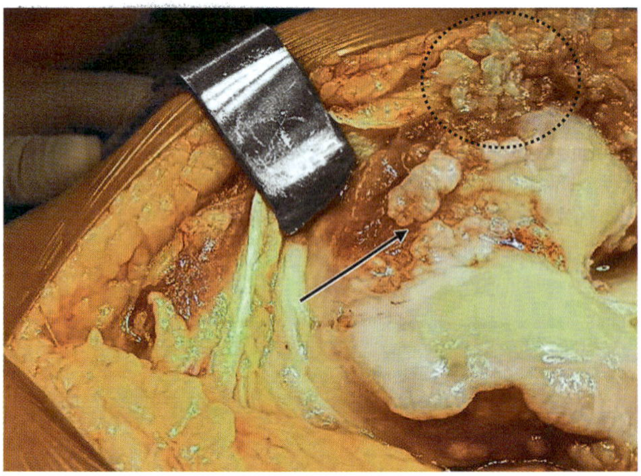

Fig. 6: Synovial chondromatosis of knee gross appearance. The different phases of development of the chondral metaplasia can be seen within the dotted oval, demonstrating small metaplastic regions and coalescing nodules forming larger ones on left half of the oval. Also shown is a loose chondroid body (arrow) lying free in the joint space.

Diagnosis

Plain radiographs are usually normal unless there is calcification in the loose bodies. Uncalcified loose bodies appear as foci with opacity similar to that of water especially in lateral projections of the knee. Finding calcified loose bodies usually entails late disease where degeneration has already set in **Figures 7A to I**. Classically, air contrast arthrogram used to be done to reveal the cartilaginous loose bodies but is obsolete now. MRI has taken precedence now that reveal cartilaginous nodules with intermediate signal intensity on T1-weighted MRI and high-signal intensity on T2-weighted images. Arthrocentesis is commonly done to reduce joint fluid pressure and one must obtain cell count, crystal examination, Gram staining, and cultures for thorough evaluation. Although increased levels of interleukin (IL)-6, vascular endothelial growth factor (VEGF)-A, and chondrocalcin have been reported but their role in establishing diagnosis is limited, if at all.

Differential Diagnosis

The differentials for synovial chondromatosis include lipoma arborescence, PVNS, synovial hemangioma, and rheumatoid arthritis with rice bodies.

Management

Radiographs may show several rounded calcifications within the joint cavity **(Figs. 7A to I)**. Surgical management is indicated in patients having recurrent painful effusions, mechanical symptoms, or both as a consequence of synovial chondromatosis. Treatment is synovectomy; however, the tumor may recur and patient should be warned that osteoarthritis is present at any stage of diagnosis, so knee would ultimately get worn off. The only controversies in management are whether to go for complete or incomplete synovectomy and what approach to use—arthroscopic versus open. In view of the current evidence with the easy availability of arthroscopy it is preferred modality for all joints amenable to this management (commonly knee, hip, shoulder, elbow, and possibly ankle). For all other joints and location of disease not approachable with arthroscope, open approach would be legible. Also arthroscopic approach is somewhat debatable in ankle joint where open approach might be preferred. Surgeons well trained in surgical dislocation of the hip may prefer open to arthroscopic approach, especially if there is need for secondary procedure like labral repair or so for addressing femoroacetabular impingement, which is commonly associated. Complete synovectomy is associated with

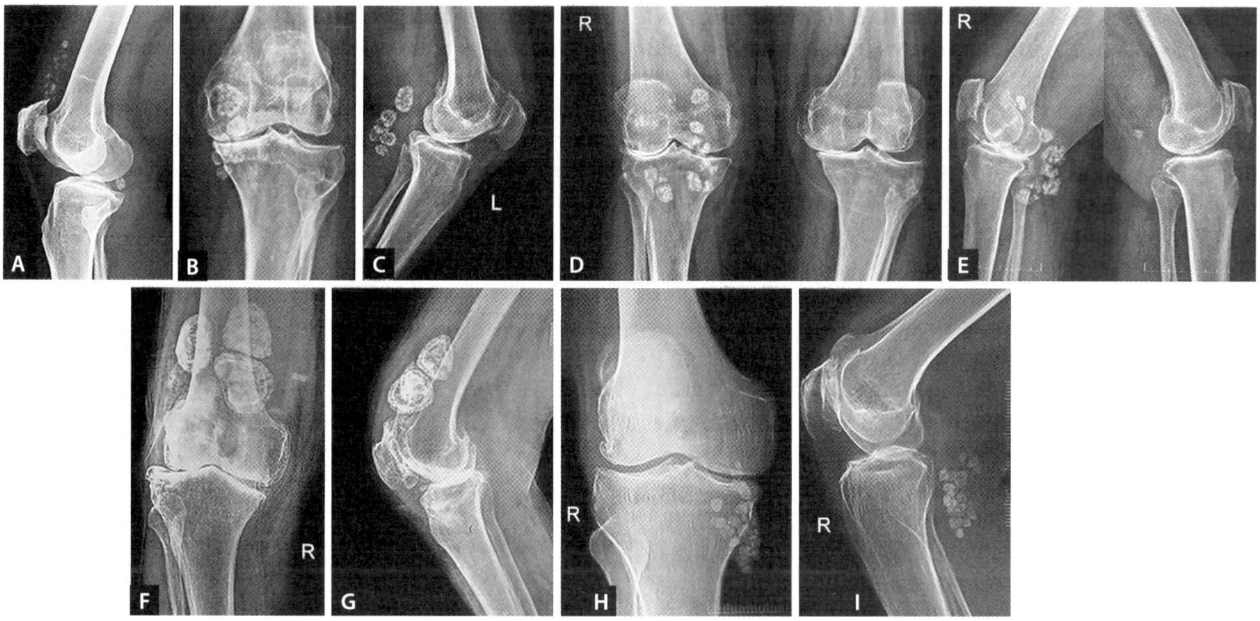

Figs. 7A to I: Radiographs of synovial chondromatosis of the knee. (A) The loose bodies may be localized within a pouch in the joint as seen here they were localized in the suprapatellar recess separated from the joint by a thin membrane that had to be removed for assessing the 18 osteocartilaginous bodies; (B and C) The typical radiographic appearance of synovial chondromatosis appearing as rounded to oval bodies demonstrating chondroid calcification within; (D and E) Anteroposterior and lateral projections of both knees of the same patient demonstrating irregular calcified masses in right knee to stress on the fact that not necessarily the disease is bilateral; (F and G) The loose bodies may grow to grotesque size in neglected cases as is common in this part of the world where seeking treatment and accepting surgery is quite difficult; (H and I) Similar to (A) the loose bodies here are localized in a posterior pouch, however, this was incidentally detected and patient was asymptomatic.

unacceptable joint stiffness later in course of rehabilitation so should be restricted for failed recalcitrant cases. Menisci are usually damaged and removed in the same sitting. With the development of osteoarthritis, joint replacement with synovectomy is the management of choice with good results.

SYNOVIAL SARCOMA

Synovial sarcoma is a malignant mesenchymal neoplasm often found near a large joint of both upper and lower extremities. It is a well-defined clinical entity which despite its name does not arise from or differentiate toward synovium. Synovial sarcomas constitute 5–10% of soft tissue sarcomas. Synovial sarcoma is a highly aggressive malignant slow-growing neoplasm, especially in males that has a peak incidence in the second and third decades of life. It frequently arises from the deep soft tissue adjacent to joints or tendons of extremities. The tumor is believed to arise from primitive mesenchymal tissue that displays variable epithelial differentiation including glandular formation and/or spindle cells. Small foci of calcification may be present in the tumor mass. In older individuals, the lower limb is the most common site of origin. In younger patients, monophasic and poorly differentiated forms predominate over biphasic ones, and like those lesions of younger individuals, size, degree of differentiation, and mitotic indices appear to have prognostic significance. It has also been suggested that proliferation markers such as Ki 67 can be used in prognostication.

Grossly, the lesions are often described as tan-white, firm (depending on the amount of fibrous stroma), and circumscribed multinodular mass of fish-flesh consistency. Rapidly growing tumors have infiltrative margins and a variegated appearance with areas of hemorrhage, necrosis, and cyst formation. It is usually multinodular and also could be multicystic.

Microscopically, two major categories of synovial sarcoma are recognized—(1) monophasic, and (2) biphasic. The ovoid or spindle cells are either distributed in relatively homogeneous pattern (monophasic) or both spindle and glandular epithelial differentiation (biphasic) are seen in tumors. The gland-like spaces are lined by cuboidal (synovial-like) or columnar cells deriving its nomenclature. The sarcomatous component is made up of spindle cells with a fibroblast-like appearance. Specialized subtypes have been identified, including myxoid, hemangiopericytic, and calcifying-ossifying types. The latter form termed as *calcifying synovial sarcoma,* in an intra-articular position, may mimic synovial chondromatosis. *Monophasic* synovial sarcoma is composed of only one of the two components. In the large majority of cases, this applies to the spindle cell sarcomatous component, i.e., monophasic fibrous synovial sarcoma. Purely epithelial *monophasic* synovial sarcoma is extremely rare and can only be confirmed with cytogenetics. A poorly differentiated synovial sarcoma has been recognized, characterized by a greater degree of cellularity, atypia, necrosis, and mitotic activity. Histologically, poorly differentiated synovial sarcoma has three cell types: large cell or epithelioid, small-cell pattern indistinguishable from other round cell sarcomas such as the Ewing's sarcoma/ primitive neuroectodermal tumor (ES/PNET) family, and a high-grade spindle-cell type.

Immunophenotypically, both the monophasic and biphasic forms are immunoreactive with antibodies directed against high-molecular-weight cytokeratin and including CK-7, -8, -14, -18, and -19 (cytokeratins of the Moll classification scheme). There is also immunoreactivity to epithelial membrane antigen (EMA), CD99, epidermal growth factor receptor (EGFR), and BCL2. A small percentage of tumors are known to be positive with anti-E cadherin and S-100 protein. The lesions are CD34 negative, and only small number of cases stain with CD117, h-caldesmon or desmin. Calponin (muscle marker) immunoreactivity [as also identification of metallothionein and melanoma antigen gene (MAGE)] has recently been shown to be of value in separating this lesion from other mimicking conditions.

Cytogenetics: The tumor has a specific translocation t(X;18) (p11:q11). This has been identified as four fusion genes *SS18/SSX* 1 to 4 and is presumably relevant in pathogenesis.

Clinical Features

The tumor presents as a slowly growing mass near a joint, without much pain, and has predilection for lower extremity. It occurs primarily in the para-articular regions of the extremities, usually in close association with tendon sheaths, bursae, and joint capsules, but it is extremely rare for it to invade the joint space and synovial membrane. Intra-articular synovial sarcomas account for <5%. The area of the knee is the most common site, followed by the foot, ankle, elbow, and shoulder. The upper extremities account for around 10–15% of all cases followed by head and neck region. However, synovial sarcomas have been described at every anatomic site. Other primary sites include the buttocks, abdominal wall, retroperitoneum, and mediastinum. Pain may be due to secondary involvement of nerves. The diagnosis is often delayed owing to the slow and insidious growth and preoperative duration varies from 2 years to 4 years, and 20-year histories are known. The tumor spreads along tissue planes. The most common site of visceral metastasis is lung. The diagnosis is made by biopsy.

Radiology

In 15–20% of synovial sarcomas, multiple small, spotty radio-opacities caused by focal calcification are seen on X-ray. Extraskeletal osteosarcoma is the only other sarcoma with focal calcification and bone formation but these tend to occur in an older group of individuals.

Differential Diagnosis

Adenocarcinoma, mesothelioma, carcinosarcoma, fibrosarcoma, malignant peripheral nerve sheath tumor, hemangiopericytoma, malignant solitary fibrous tumor, ES/PNET, round cell liposarcoma, and rhabdomyosarcoma.

Treatment

Treatment is wide resection of the tumor with or without chemotherapy and radiation therapy. Extensive surgery including radical local excision, often with removal of an entire muscle or muscle group, and amputation, depending mainly on the size of the tumor and its location may be required. Because radical local excision is often impossible with tumors situated near a large joint (the favored location of synovial sarcoma), adjunctive radiotherapy in addition to local excision of the tumor is favored. With adequate surgical excision or with adjunctive radiotherapy, the recurrence rate has been reported to be significantly lower (<40%). In most cases, the recurrent growth manifests within the first 2 years after initial therapy. Metastases occur more commonly in the lungs, followed by lymph nodes then bone marrow. Five-year survival is 36–76%, and 10-year survival is 20–63%. Good outcomes are reported by some authors in younger patients (age <15 years), lower extremity, in tumors <5 cm diameter, have <10 mitoses/10 HPF and no necrosis and low stage but this is debatable. Stage (clinical group) and invasiveness at presentation have been shown to be critical prognostic indicators. Prognosis does not differ between monophasic and biphasic tumors as also differences in key demographic features (age and gender) or location (central versus peripheral). However, cases with the *SS18/SSX2* variant gene, which is mostly found in monophasic synovial sarcoma, have a better prognosis. *SYT-SSX1*-containing tumors, however, have a worse prognosis, and this appears to be related to high expression of cyclins leading to increased proliferation. Poorly differentiated synovial sarcoma is aggressive with frequent metastases. The calcifying variant fares better with survival of 83% after 5 years. Currently used chemotherapeutic agents are doxorubicin, ifosfamide, and cisplatin. In particular, regimens that include ifosfamide and doxorubicin or epirubicin are efficacious, resulting in a partial or complete response in about 50% of patients. Amputation of the involved distal extremity may be required in intractable, resistant large tumors, or recurrent cases. Chemotherapy may be beneficial in some patients with metastatic disease. Postoperative radiation has been used in some cases to improve local control. Isolated pulmonary metastasis can be surgically removed. Newer modalities are being tried to improve survival and include gefitinib (EGFR inhibitor) for patients with locally advanced or metastatic synovial sarcomas that overexpress EGFR as overexpression of EGFR has been documented in 55% patients. BCL2 is overexpressed in the vast majority of synovial sarcomas. G3139, an antisense-oligonucleotide that decreases BCL2 expression and induces apoptosis, has been found effective in vivo. Sarcomas overexpressing Her2 may well respond to trastuzumab, having recurrent or metastatic disease.

SYNOVIAL HEMANGIOMA

Synovial hemangioma is a vascular venous malformation within the synovial lining seen in children (most commonly seen between 10 and 12 years of age) and young adults. It is a rare and benign condition most commonly seen in the knee joint. It was first reported by Bouchut in 1856 and few hundred cases have been reported since then. The disease may be intra-articular or extra-articular or rarely combined. True synovial hemangioma may be considered as a subset of soft tissue hemangioma and should be differentiated from hemangiohamartoma that represents an arteriovenous malformation. The lesions can be cavernous, capillary, or mixed. Bennet and Cobey divided intra-articular lesions morphologically into localized (solitary) and diffuse formations that may arise de novo or post-traumatically. They may be associated with Maffucci syndrome or von Hippel-Lindau disease. The localized form is seen commonly at the anteromedial aspect of knee and has minimal cartilage involvement with good prognosis.

The lesions are nearly always symptomatic and patients present with joint effusion, restricted motion at joint, and pain. The intra-articular masses are usually palpable with atrophy of the quadriceps. Joint effusions are mostly due to intra-articular hemorrhages causing hemarthrosis.

Radiological diagnosis is commonly established by MRI that offers superior tissue contrast over CT scan. It demonstrates lobulated mass with low to intermediate signal intensities on T1-weighted sequences. T2-sequence images demonstrate markedly hyperintense background (from pooled blood within vascular spaces) and low signal-intensity linear structures within the lesion from fibrous septae. Sometimes fluid-fluid levels (suggestive of hemorrhage) are evident. Gadolinium contrast shows marked heterogeneous enhancement. Plain radiographs are commonly passed as normal but in later stages may show cortical thickening, scalloping, and variable density soft-tissue shadow. Phleboliths may be seen within the mass as well-circumscribed calcifications that are pathognomonic. Less than 5% of patients have cortical destruction, periosteal reaction, advanced physeal maturation, osteoporosis, leg-length discrepancy or changes similar to hemophilia. So, the clinical differential diagnosis includes PVNS, synovial chondromatosis, meniscus tear, and cruciate ligament injury while radiologically on plain X-ray inflammatory arthropathies such as rheumatoid arthritis, juvenile rheumatoid arthropathy, hemophilic arthropathy and lipoma arborescens, and for MRI additionally cystic synovial hyperplasia are differentials.

Treatment is primarily surgical because the lesions are universally symptomatic. Localized forms are amenable to arthroscopic or open wide excision (preferable) with lesser propensity to recurrence. The diffuse form is difficult to manage due to lack of distinct margins and infiltrative nature of the lesion. Complete synovectomy has to be performed but recurrences are common because it is seldom achieved. Preoperative embolization may be considered in these cases to ease localization and resection. Refractory cases may need adjuvant radiotherapy. Multiple recurrences and joint destruction often need arthroplasty.

LIPOMA ARBORESCENS

(*Other terms:* Diffuse lipoma of the joint, diffuse synovial lipoma, diffuse articular lipomatosis, fatty infiltration of the synovial membrane, or villous lipomatous proliferation of the synovial membrane)

The condition was originally described by Hoffa where he likened the frond-like appearance of lesion to a "tree and leaf" so naming it "arborescens (L. for "tree-forming" or "treelike"). Lipoma arborescens is a rare and chronic nonspecific reactive condition affecting joints and bursae where due to replacement of subsynovial connective tissue by mature fat cells the synovium proliferates into villous lipomatous "frond-like" depositions of fatty tissue. The reaction may often form mechanical, traumatic, or inflammatory insults arising from osteoarthrosis, meniscal tears, synovial cysts, chondromatosis, and medical ailments such as diabetes, rheumatoid arthritis, and psoriatic arthritis. The disease is seen in fifth to seventh decade of life as it is slowly progressive. Most common site is the suprapatellar pouch of the knee **(Fig. 8)** but cases have also been described in hip, shoulder, elbow, ankle, wrist, bursae, and even tendon sheaths. One-fifth of the cases have bilateral involvement and polyarticular disease is very rare. The distinction into idiopathic "primary" form seen in younger patients and reactive "secondary" forms in older population proposed by some authors appears futile for therapeutic or prognostic purposes.

There is no specific gender predilection. The patients usually have joint swelling and painless intermittent joint effusions that may be associated with restriction of joint movements and/or mechanical symptoms. Pain is a variable symptom and is not much bothering in many. Intra-articular hemorrhage is also rare. Differential diagnosis involves synovial hemangioma, synovial lipoma, synovial chondromatosis, and PVNS.

The lesion grossly has appearance of a fatty mass with a branching villous growth pattern **(Fig. 8)** that under a microscope shows synovial hyperplasia with scattered chronic inflammatory cells and abundant mature adipocytes in the subsynovial tissue. Plain radiographs may demonstrate fatty lucencies within soft tissue lesion. Joint commonly demonstrate degenerative changes. CT scan demonstrates low-density intra-articular mass. MRI is diagnostic and demonstrates frond-like villous projections and focal nodules all composed of homogeneous fat signal on all pulse

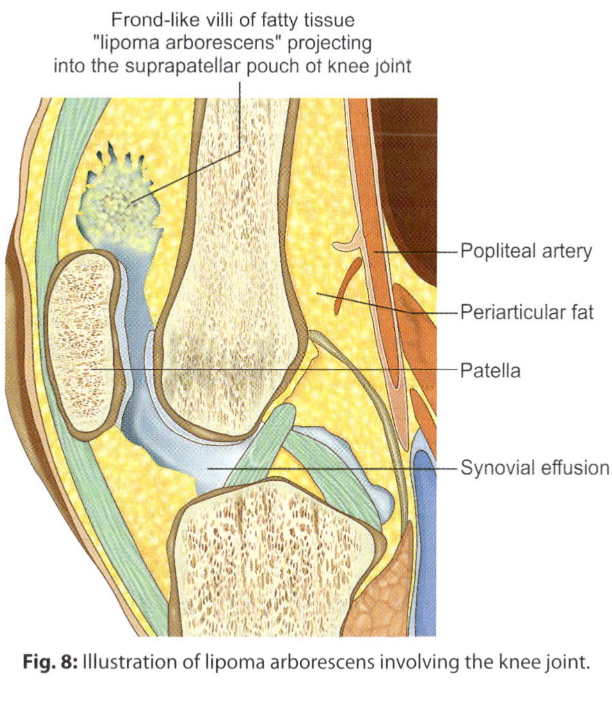

Fig. 8: Illustration of lipoma arborescens involving the knee joint.

sequences (high signal on both T1 and T2 that saturates on fat suppressed sequences). Gradient echo may show chemical artifact at fat-fluid interface.

Treatment is needed only for symptomatic cases. Total or subtotal synovectomy (arthroscopic or open) is therapeutic and recurrences are very uncommon if at all. Nonsurgical management involves local steroid injection and use of intra-articular radioisotopes.

CONCLUSION

- Synovium is an active metabolic component of the synovial joint and is subjected to metabolic and neoplastic disorders.
- Giant cell tumor of the tendon sheath or synovial membrane (pigmented villonodular synovitis) is the most common neoplastic pathology identified that needs surgical management.
- Metaplasia of the synovial membrane is responsible for production of loose intra-articular bodies that are responsible for pain, joint locking, and damage to cartilage and in long run osteoarthritis of the joint like a damaged bearing destroys the wheel bearing or automobile.
- Malignant pathology of synovium occurs commonly in the form of synovial sarcoma and has poor prognosis most often.

CHAPTER

9 Articular Cartilage: Structure, Function, Injury, and Management

Manish Kumar Varshney

INTRODUCTION

Articular cartilage covers the intra-articular ends of long bones and is a highly specialized connective tissue of synovial joints providing a smooth and lubricated surface with an extremely low coefficient of friction. Hyaline articular cartilage is subject to regular wear and tear and is limited in its capacity for self-repair, being avascular, alymphatic, and aneural. Maintaining health of cartilage and optimizing repair following injury is a field of aggressive and active research with limited success achieved till now. We are still far in preventing cartilage degeneration and its medical management, so understanding pathophysiology in detail is imperative.

STRUCTURE AND COMPOSITION

Hyaline cartilage is the chief component of articular cartilage typically (fibrocartilage is seen in repair of damaged articular cartilage, callus and at tendon ligament insertion; fibroelastic cartilage is seen in menisci) and is 1–4 mm thick. It is composed of a dense extracellular matrix (ECM) that comprises the main tissue and only a thin distribution of *chondrocytes*. The cartilage cells or chondrocytes are surrounded immediately by pericellular matrix containing proteoglycan and noncollagenous proteins (no collagen), completely engulfing the chondrocyte **(Fig. 1)**. Surrounding this is the territorial matrix containing collagen fibrils possibly providing mechanical protection to chondrocytes during loading. As a functional unit, the chondrocyte along with its pericellular microenvironment form the "chondron". The chondron has been classically considered to represent primary structural, functional, and metabolic unit of articular and other hyaline cartilages **(Fig. 2)**. The concept of the chondron historically was introduced by Benninghoff (1925) who identified it using polarized light microscopy. Later these structural units were released from tibial cartilage in the mid-1980s by Poole et al. demonstrating the individuality of chondrons. This finding conclusively established that chondron is a microanatomical unit defining the adult articular cartilage. Grossly each chondron is made up of a single chondrocyte that is attached peripherally to transparent pericellular glycocalyx. This is then further enclosed within a fibrillar pericellular capsule serving together as a basic structural unit. Macrostructurally, the chondrocytes are distributed in different zones of articular cartilage together with ultrastructural matrix of collagen fiber and ECM. There are five discrete zones in a hyaline cartilage primarily depending on the collagen fibers alignment, which impart each zone particular function biomechanically **(Fig. 3)**.

1. Superficial zone (gliding zone and tangential collagen fibers)—resistant to shear; has few, if any, metabolic activity. It has the lowest proteoglycan (PG) and highest water content and is covered by fine layer called "lamina splendens".

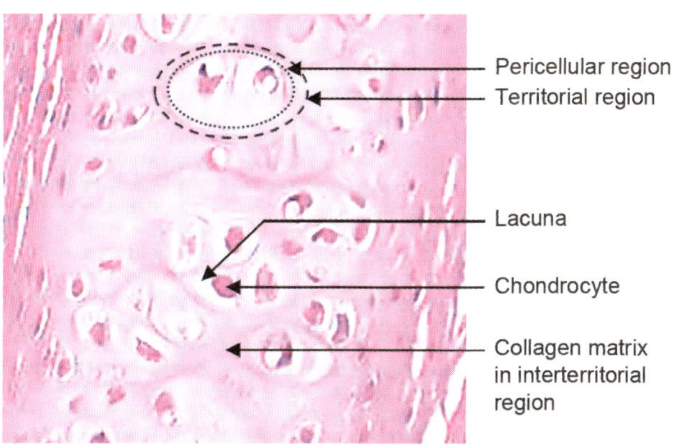

Fig. 1: Cartilage structure.

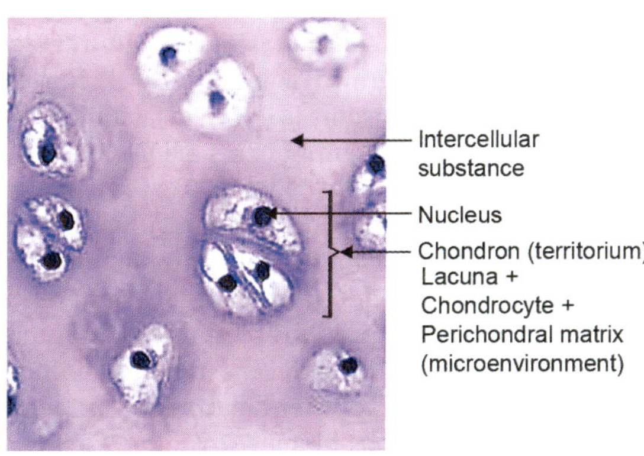

Fig. 2: Chondron.

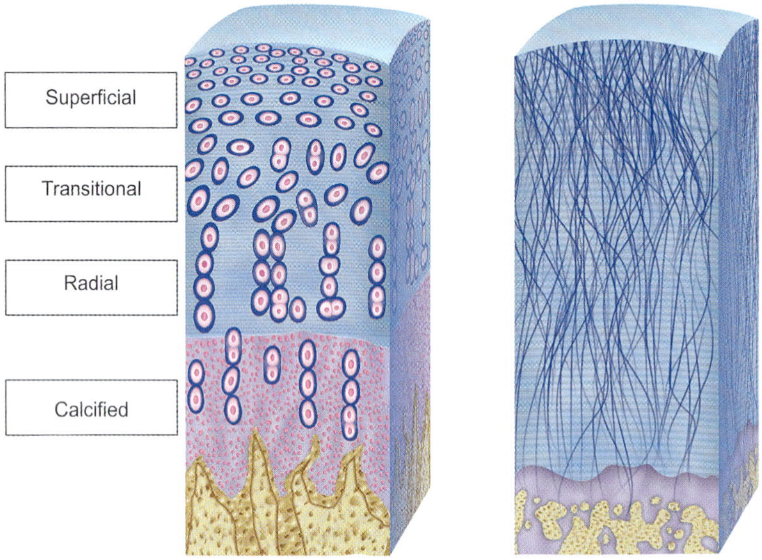

Fig. 3: Articular cartilage structure. Illustration depicting the cellular and fibril disposition within the cartilage.

2. Transitional zone (middle zone and oblique collagen fibers)—resistant to compression, active metabolism of chondrons, and ECM proteins.
3. Radial zone (deep zone and vertical collagen fibers)—resistant to compression, collagen synthesis, and cross-linking zone. It has the highest proteoglycan content and lowest water.
4. Tidemark—resistant to shear.
5. Calcified zone—basically acts to anchor articular cartilage to subchondral bone and prevents transport of nutrients from underlying bone.

When examined under low power microscopy (10x), three theoretical regions can be identified within each zone—the pericellular region, the territorial region, and the interterritorial region (the largest region comprising collagen fibrils with specific spatial distribution in different zones and proteoglycan) which is responsible to most of material properties of cartilage **(*see* Fig. 1)**.

Chondrocytes

Chondrocytes are cells unique to cartilage that represent highly specialized mesenchymal cells dedicated to cartilage formation and function. They contribute 1% to the total volume and 5% to the total weight of the articular cartilage. Derived from mesenchymal stem cells (MSCs) they are regulated primarily by transforming growth factor-β (TGF-β), fibroblast growth factors (FGF), and insulin-like growth factor-1 (IGF-1). They produce the structural components of ECM of articular cartilage primarily composed of collagen and proteoglycans. They are also involved in synthesis of various enzymes. Chondrocytes are found scattered individually throughout articular cartilage enclosed in lacunae. MSCs differentiate into chondrocyte with upregulation of cartilage specific matrix components (collagen II and aggrecan) under the influence of TGF-β1 and 2 primarily. Other factors that induce this differentiation are bone morphogenetic protein (BMP) 2, 4, 6, 7, 9, and 13, FGF-2 and -18, IGF-1, growth differentiation factor-5 (GDF-5) and proteins of Wnt family. Physiological factors are also responsible for this differentiation and include—mechanical loading like deformation, shear stress, etc. (most important trophic factor—so one must keep playing), low oxygen tension, oxidative pressure, and electrical potential of cells. During cartilage growth chondrocytes have a roundish shape. The shape of chondrocyte changes according to the age, pathological state, and the layer in which they are placed.

- Chondrocytes are bit flattish in the superficial zone and lie parallel to the articular surface.
- They are spherical in the intermediate zone and have high metabolic activity.
- In the deep zone, chondrocytes are large with small nuclei and form long perpendicular columns.
- In the zone of calcified cartilage, cells are small and roundish with a large nucleus.

Chondrocytes in arthritic cartilage form clusters of up to 30 cells possibly representing attempt at tissue repair and regeneration that is damaged due to wear and tear. Each chondrocyte forms a specialized microenvironment (*chondron*) that is the responsible functional unit for ECM turnover. There occurs a hostile environment in the vicinity of chondron characterized by deranged synthesis of ECM and increased concentration of matrix metalloproteinases (MMPs). This modified microenvironment traps the chondrocyte and also prevents their migration. The chondrocytes in osteoarthritis (OA) are susceptible to tumor necrosis factor-α (TNF-α) induced cell death and have downregulated nuclear factor kappa beta (NFkβ) that reduces cell survival and also increases production of MMP.

Chondrocytes are anaerobic (oxygen tension in the cartilage is low ranging from 10% at surface to <1% in deep layers) and receive their nutrition primarily via diffusion of substances from synovial fluid. The circulation of synovial fluid is facilitated by joint movements. Glucose is the primary metabolite for chondrocytes and a precursor for glycosaminoglycans (GAGs).

Intercellular Matrix

The intercellular matrix of articular cartilage is composed of structural macromolecules that include—

- Collagens—these form the most abundant component.
- Noncollagenous proteins—predominated by proteoglycans and glycoproteins.
- Small quantities of lipids and phospholipids.

Apart from the macromolecules normal articular cartilage gains its resilience from the tissue fluid that represents between 65 and 80% of the total weight of cartilage. Tissue fluid is distributed nonuniformly within the layers of cartilage (80% at the surface and 65% at the deep zone) to allow deformation of the cartilage under stress by imparting graded viscosity to the cartilage. Collagens and proteoglycans form 20 to 25% of the dry weight of cartilage. Articular cartilage gains its characteristic biomechanical properties by the relative percentage of these main macromolecules. Most of the water is in pore spaces, some 30% is present in the interfibrillar space. The dense interfibrillar matter makes the fluid water behave like a gel. This water shifts across the ECM through micropores by applying a pressure gradient across the tissue. The slowness of this shift imparts viscosity to cartilage. Also, the fluid shift through the matrix pores makes frictional resistance against this flow very high. The frictional resistance increases with applied load so that it acts like a stiff ultimate, but soft initial shock absorber. The permeability of the healthy cartilage to fluid otherwise is also very low. The combination of these two properties namely the frictional resistance to fluid flow and the pressurization of water within the matrix due to low permeability imparts the cartilage its two characteristics that form the basis of synovial joint mechanics:

1. Ability of articular cartilage to withstand loads up to 20 times body weight
2. Ability to deform matching the conformity of surfaces.

Osteoarthritic cartilage has deranged ECM environment causing disruption of these properties, and hence higher fluid volume is seen to compensate for lost space. This results in increased permeability, reduced strength, and cartilage fibrillation ultimately due to poor distribution of biomechanical forces.

Type II collagen represents 90–95% of all types of collagen found in cartilage, others include types VI, IX, X, and XI. Collagens form a superhelix structure. The collagen fibers are highly cross-linked and align in parallel rows with a quasi-staggered pattern. This formation imparts high tensile strength to the structural framework of cartilage. Orientation of collagen fibers varies according to the zones giving extraordinary resilience with strength (***see* Fig. 3**). Type VI collagen stabilizes chondrocytes within the matrix. Normally, the role of this collagen is minimal in young cartilage, but with aging the chondron is rendered unstable and less viable where this collagen synthesis and quantity is greatly increased in OA. Type XI collagen is an adhesive holding the collagen lattice together. Type X collagen is not a normally seen component of healthy tissue and is found in pathological tissues that undergo calcification/ossification like hypertrophic cartilage of physes in rickets, fracture callus, cartilage tumors, and heterotopic ossification, and is associated with cartilage calcification. Schmid metaphyseal chondrodysplasia results from genetic defect of type X collagen.

Proteoglycans (**Fig. 4**) are heavily glycosylated protein monomers providing the compressive strength to the articular cartilage (*proteoglycans and glycoproteins are both composed of proteins conjugated to saccharides, but the fundamental difference is that in proteoglycans the polysaccharides attach to protein with serial repeat units and that the ratio of carbohydrate to protein is very high, while in glycoproteins the ratio is reverse and there are no repeat units*). The compressive strength is primarily provided by aggrecan (large aggregating proteoglycan) that is attached to hyaluronic acid polymers. Aggrecan represents the second largest group of macromolecules in the articular cartilage. They are present in close conjunction in the ECM with collagens and account for 10–15% of the dry macromolecular weight. The typical described structure of proteoglycans comprises a protein core that attaches covalently to one or more linear glycosaminoglycan chains (**Fig. 4**). These chains are large and run a serpentine course occupying most of the free space and may be composed of >100 monosaccharides. The chains extend away from the central protein core. The chains remain segregated from each other because of repulsive electronegative charge forces. A variety of proteoglycans are present in articular cartilage, all having discrete essential function to maintain health of the tissue. These include but not limited to aggrecan (largest proteoglycan in size and also most abundant), decorin, biglycan, and fibromodulin. Aggrecan is particularly important as it interacts with hyaluronan (HA) to form large aggregates determining the water holding capacity of cartilage primarily. Link proteins mediate the interaction between hyaluronan and aggrecan. These aggrecan molecules, like most proteoglycans comprise a central protein core attached to projecting multiple glycosaminoglycans chains. Keratan sulfate, chondroitin 4-sulfate, and chondroitin 6-sulfate form the glycosaminoglycans in aggrecan chiefly (**Fig. 4**). Alteration of the glycosaminoglycans with aging is responsible for altered microstructure and biomechanics of cartilage. For example, the level of chondroitin 4-sulfate decreases with aging, while that of keratan sulfate rises reducing the water holding capacity. Proteoglycan biglycan is found mainly in the immediate surroundings of chondrocytes. Biglycan chiefly interacts with collagen VI, the level of which rises with aging. Other noncollagenous proteins found in cartilage such as anchoring C II, fibronectin, and chondronectin basically stabilize proteoglycan macromolecules and their interaction with other molecules (hyaluronan and collagen) to maintain homeostasis.

METABOLISM AND REGULATION

It is a known fact that the articular cartilage is avascular so in any case the metabolism is anaerobic and that too scanty due to paucity of cellular components. Subchondral bony plate separates articular cartilage from the richly vascular subchondral spaces so there is no direct nutritional supply. Articular cartilage derives its nutrition from diffusion through the synovial fluid. Due to the absence of specialized nutritional

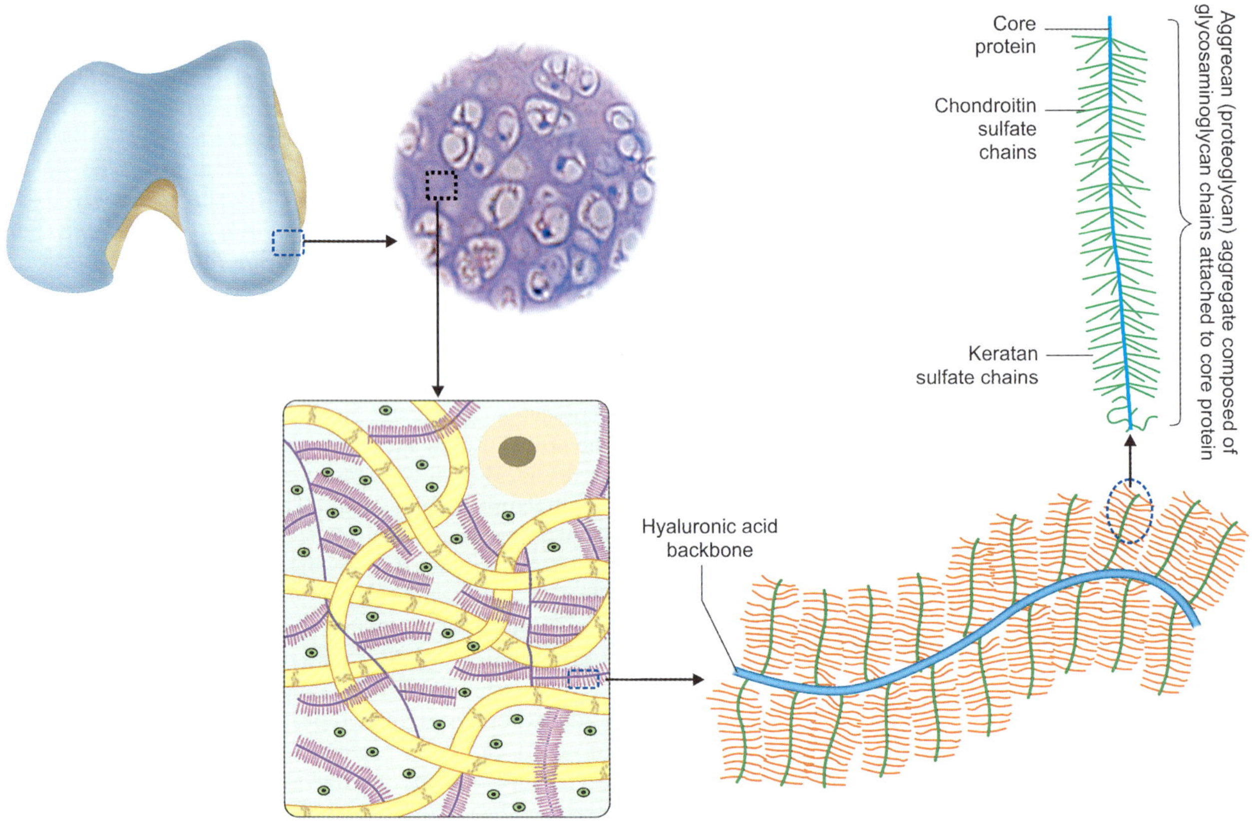

Fig. 4: Cartilage intercellular matrix and structure of proteoglycans.

supply, the cartilage matrix itself takes over the function of selecting nutrition offered. Cartilage matrix restricts diffusion of molecules by their size, charge, and molecular configuration. Though not consistently seen (due to dynamic nature) it is estimated that the mean pore size within the ECM is about 6.0 nm. The anaerobic metabolism of chondrocytes can be altered by a variety of factors. Cytokines and various growth factors mediate the intercellular communications. The factors have autocrine, paracrine, and endocrinal influence. Alteration in the cytokine milieu as is seen in diseases such as rheumatoid arthritis, OA, and osteoporosis due to altered production causes abnormal responses by cartilage cells. They also affect the underlying bone. Some of identified cytokines affecting articular cartilage are:

- *Insulin-like growth factors (IGF):* IGF-1 (somatomedin C) and II. These are trophic to articular cartilage and stimulate deoxyribonucleic acid (DNA) and cartilage matrix synthesis, especially immature cartilage of growth plate.
- *Transforming growth factors (TGF):* TGF-β 1–3 stimulate synthesis of proteoglycans while suppressing the type II collagen synthesis. Stimulates synthesis of plasminogen activator inhibitor-1 and tissue inhibitor of matrix metalloproteinases inhibitor (MMPI), protecting the cartilage from degradation.
- *Fibroblast growth factors acidic and basic (aFGF and bFGF):* They stimulate DNA synthesis in chondrocytes.
- *Interleukins (IL):* IL-1β, IL-6, and IL-8 stimulate chondrocyte as regard the synthesis, secretion, and maintenance of proteoglycans into the ECM by them.
- *Tumor necrosis factors:* TNF-α plays a role in the degradation and synthesis of matrix macromolecules, especially metabolism of proteoglycans.
- *Colony stimulating factor (CSF):* Macrophage-CSF stimulate cartilage repair following injury.
- *Others:* Prostaglandins and parathyroid hormone-related peptide (PTHrP) affect healing of cartilage, especially the degenerative one.

The cartilage macromolecules once formed are rarely recycled. For example, proteoglycan turnover can take up to 25 years and is mostly limited to late adult life. The half-life of collagen ranges from several decades to 400 years. Once damaged, new chains and macromolecules need to be synthesized and integrity restored. MMPs such as the collagenases, gelatinases, and stromelysins, and the cathepsins primarily the cathepsin B and D are mainly involved in cartilage turnover. These enzymes have specific functions such as:

- Degradation of aggrecan by cathepsins
- Degradation of helical collagen fibrils by collagenase that acts at a single site
- Stromelysin degrades the protein core of aggrecan causing disintegration of the molecule
- Gelatinase acts as scavenger and digests denatured types II and IV collagen which is seen in elderly. Gelatinase also digests fibronectin, elastin, and collagen types V, VII, X, and XI to make up space for further protein synthesis and incorporation.

Matrix metalloproteinases are secreted as latent proenzymes that remain inactive until activated extracellularly. This process is inhibited by MMPI. Inactivation of MMP is an emerging trend in prevention of joint degenerative disorders (osteoarthritis) and even RA. Some antibiotics such as doxycycline and minocycline have been found to be useful to this effect.

BIOMECHANICS OF ARTICULAR CARTILAGE

Articular cartilage is capable of storing, transmitting, and dissipating energy during activity. The properties of ECM and its organization give two discrete phases to articular cartilage that helps it adjust to the requirement of maintaining low-friction mobile environment in presence of compressive stress. The functional articular cartilage phases are:

1. Fluid phase—helps to dissipate stress and provides resilience and maintains low friction.
2. Solid phase—maintains structure and bears the compressive forces.

It is the presence of these two phases that the cartilage is said to be biphasic. Water is the principal component of the fluid phase. The solid phase is formed by the macromolecular integrated structure of ECM, which is porous and quasi-permeable. The cross-linking of collagen fibrils is responsible for providing tensile strength to the collagen. The interaction between proteoglycan aggregates and tissue fluid provides the requisite compressive strength to cartilage. The negative electrostatic repulsion forces maintain high pressure within the tissue acting as a shock absorber and tight compartment. When a loading force is rapidly applied as during articular contact there occurs an immediate rise in tissue pressure due to trapped tissue **(Fig. 5)**. Sudden increase in pressure is first resisted by the resilience of tissue then follows slow egress of the fluid out of the ECM through micropores generating a large frictional drag and biomechanically acting as a highly viscous tissue due to low porosity. The low porosity of cartilage retains fluid and prevents it from being quickly squeezed out of the matrix; rather most of the fluid is transplaced instead to a low pressure region within the tissue (much like a bean bag). The cartilage shows differential permeability to different loads and is not constant varying with the speed and direction of applied load also **(Figs. 6A and B)**. As soon as the compressive load is removed, the partly squeezed fluid returns into the place. When subjected to a moving load, the articular cartilage exhibits a viscoelastic property, especially when the applied load is constant or it is a sustained deformation. This viscoelastic property of articular cartilage can be either:

- Flow dependent—which depends upon interstitial fluid volume and interaction with proteoglycan aggregate (micropore intactness) and the frictional drag (biphasic viscoelastic behavior, discussed above) associated with this flow.
- Flow independent—is caused by macromolecular deformation and movement specifically involving the collagen proteoglycan matrix.

This explains the importance of fluid pressure and fluid retention by proteoglycans as a significant component of total

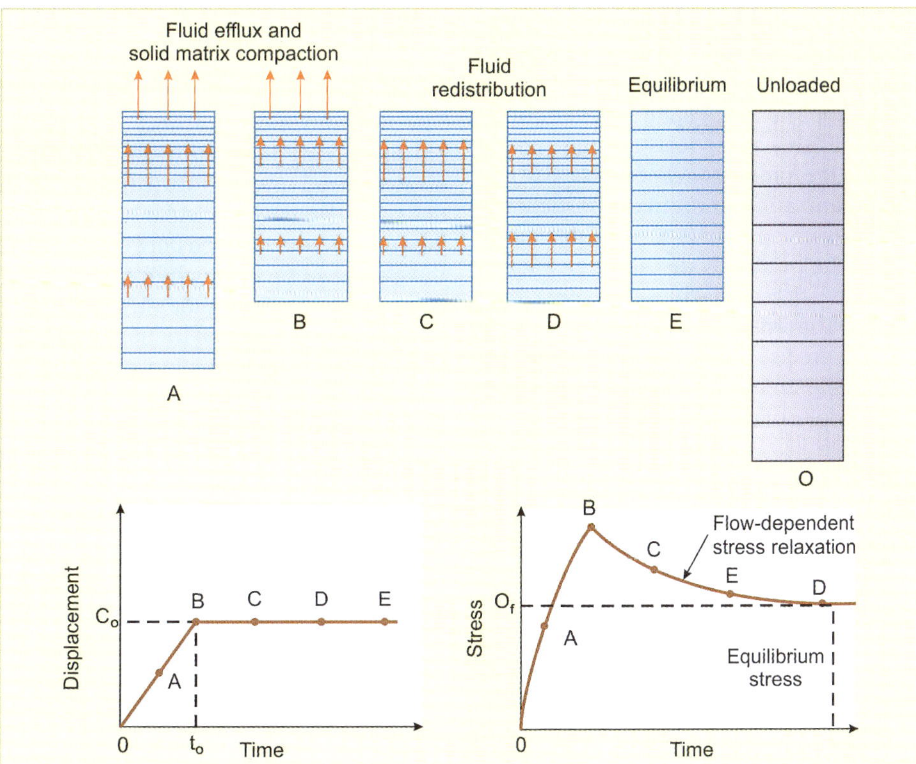

Fig. 5: Effect of applying a load on cartilage. The cartilage tissue passes through stages A to E behaving as a non-Newtonian tissue due to multiphasic tissue and fluid distribution. There occurs displacement proportionate to the load applied with acute rise in stress but the stress quickly readjusts and reduces. This is especially important as chondrocytes are susceptible to high pressures.

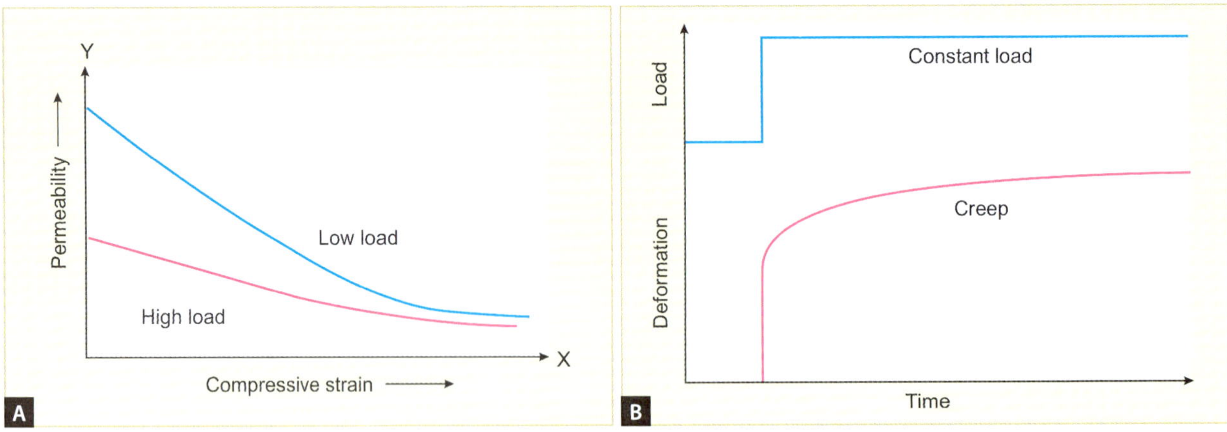

Figs. 6A and B: (A) Differential permeability of cartilage to applied load; (B) Creep in articular cartilage.

load support. Water-imbibed proteoglycans act like numerous micro water balls packed in a place that can displace with applied force in a limited fashion. This reduces the stress acting on a unit area upon the solid matrix by meticulous distribution. Cartilage exhibits an interesting property of *creep,* i.e., increasing deformation with time in response to a constantly applied compressive stress, and this creep occurs until an equilibrium value is reached. When a shear force is applied it produces a constant strain.

The strain is transmitted to cartilage tissue and rises to a zenith in deformed cartilage, if the cartilage structure is not disrupted there follows a slow "stress-relaxation" process to achieve an equilibrium between stress generated for the applied strain. The initial resilient phase of cartilage deformation is important to disperse the shear force and is quickly transformed to viscous phase to maintain integrity. Articular cartilage tends to stiffen with increased strain so that the stress-strain curve is nonlinear and cannot be described by Young's modulus value. This shear-resistant property of cartilage is most evident in the middle zones of cartilage where the composition and organization of matrix is particularly complex. This shear stress response is also imparted by differential stretching of the randomly distributed collagen fibrils that bear the stress at different magnitude of shear force and angle of applied force. The tensile force-resisting property of collagen is a function of precise molecular arrangement of fibrils and the ultimate tensile strength of collagen comes from intramolecular and intermolecular cross-links.

LUBRICATION AND WEAR (SYNOVIAL JOINT LUBRICATION)

Friction occurs whenever two nonlubricated surfaces glide over each other duc to interaction of asperities on the surface. The coefficient of friction depends on the shear strength of the sliding surfaces and area of contact. Typical dynamic dry coefficient of friction for plastic on plastic interface is 0.1–0.3 and for polished metal on metal interface is 0.003–0.04. Articular cartilage is unique in having fluid film interface that reduces friction many times between cartilage interfaces. The fluid interposition produces two broad mechanisms of lubrication **(Figs. 7A to G)**—the fluid film lubrication (hydrodynamic) and the boundary lubrication, depending on whether a continuous fluid film is present that lubricates or the fluid film itself reduces to molecular dimensions (minimum thickness in boundary lubrication) respectively. Often a combination is seen. The efficiency of these lubrication processes (discussed further) means that wear in synovial joints is minimal. Cartilage fibrillation increases the coefficient of friction.

Hydrodynamic Lubrication (Fig. 7A)

When fluid exudes due to gliding of surfaces moving in one direction at high speed, they are separated by hydrostatic pressure of continuous fluid film that lubricates the surfaces in a closed space. This is very transitory as it requires wedge-shaped fluid film to be present between the surfaces, which are impossible in slow-reversing movement of joints.

Elastohydrodynamic Lubrication (Fig. 7B)

The predominant method of articular cartilage lubrication during joint motion (dynamic joint loading) is elastohydrodynamic lubrication. The fluid film pressure deforms/flattens the articular surface by increasing the surface area. The fluid is trapped between the surfaces and lubricates the gliding surfaces much like the formation of thin layer of water when ice-skate glides over solid ice. This is responsible for the low coefficient of friction (0.002–0.04) of human joints **(Fig. 8)**. Fluid film formation, elastic deformation of cartilage, and fluid efflux from cartilage all reduce coefficient of friction. Elastic deformation depresses the surfaces greater than the height of asperities so that few if any asperities rub against each other reducing friction.

Boosted Lubrication (Fig. 7F)

Here the solvent part (water) of the lubricant enters the articular cartilage that is squeezed from joint fluid hyaluronic acid complexes boosting the lubrication of articular cartilage. The synovial fluid is entrapped between articulating surfaces and under hydrostatic pressure within cartilage migration of hyaluronic acid is prevented into articular cartilage while solvent moves in. The solute (hyaluronic acid) remains between the surfaces providing lubrication, the coefficient of friction for this type of lubrication is higher than for elastohydrodynamic lubrication.

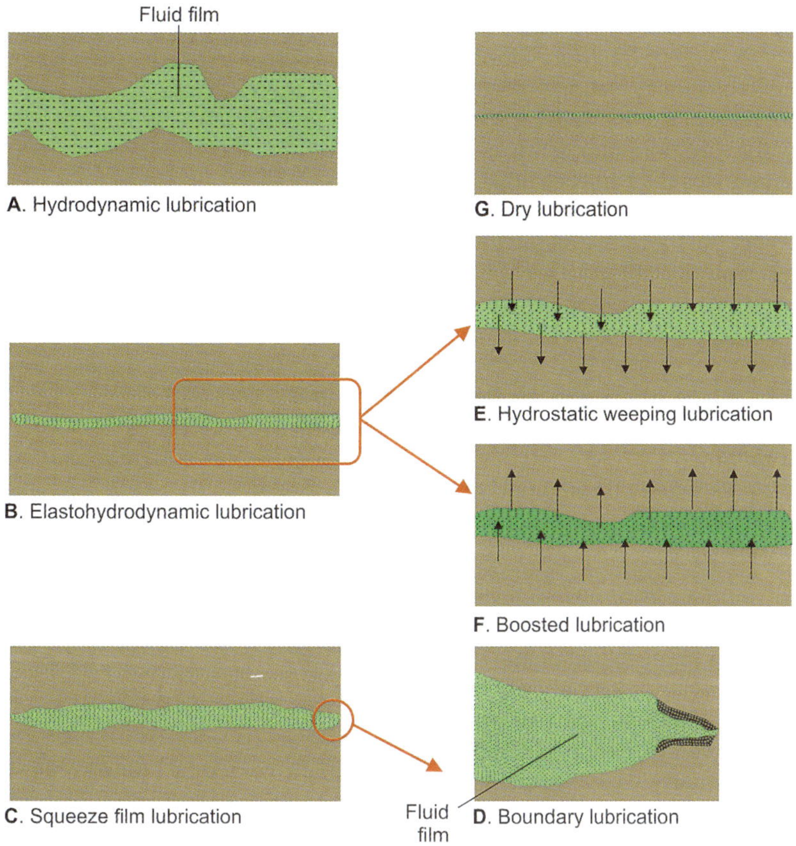

Figs. 7A to G: Lubrication concept and types: The lubrication properties for synovial joint changes in accordance with the synovial fluid film and loading. The lubrication changes from hydrodynamic (A) to dry lubrication (G) with reducing thickness of the fluid film. In-between the elastohydrodynamic (B), squeeze film (C), boundary lubrication (D) are seen with reduced thickness of the film and changes in load properties of the joint. The elastohydrodynamic lubrication is the prime type seen in synovial joints (B) with dynamic loading. The cartilage surface flattens out (along with the fluid film in response to loading) with intervening fluid film providing the rolling lubrication at slow movements between joint surfaces. The cartilage may imbibe the exuded water from synovial fluid increasing the concentration of hyaluronic acid providing a boosted lubrication (F). In other scenario, the fluid quickly moves in and out of cartilage with increased and reduced loading giving "weeping hydrostatic" lubrication (E). The boosted and weeping types are commonly always associated with elastohydrodynamic lubrication. Often with loading the thin fluid film gets squeezed in the form of a convex shape with lesser deformation of cartilage at the edges while greater deformation at the center. This squeezed film (C) provides lubrication at compressive loads that may be associated with shear forces and is combinedly seen with elastohydrodynamic lubrication (see above). Often the cartilage due to its physiological properties will show boosted and weeping lubrication here too. At the edges of the convex fluid film where the cartilage is less deformed, the cartilages from opposing surfaces barely touch each other and have high stress concentration. Boundary lubrication here comes into play (D) with concentrated nonhyaluronic glycoproteins lining the stress concentrated cartilage and providing lubrication. The fluid film is reduced to molecular level thickness. In dry lubrication, the cartilages rub against each other as the fluid film does not practically exist.

Hydrostatic Weeping Lubrication (Fig. 7E)

Describes the ability of articular cartilage to exude or imbibe fluid as the joint surfaces glide over each other providing self-lubrication. Compressed articular surfaces weep (exude water and small ions through pores about 6 nm). The fluid film then produces hydrostatic lubrication where a fluid film is maintained by pressure (in mechanical engineering) of pumps between bearings. In joints, the cartilage maintains this fluid film by virtue of their structural deformation under pressure at places beyond the area of impending contact. When pressure is released the cartilage absorbs the fluid again. This mechanism is called self-pressurized hydrostatic lubrication.

Squeeze-Film Lubrication (Fig. 7C)

Within the elastic cartilage, the fluid film is trapped in a biconvex shape. The cartilage depresses less at periphery than at the center trapping the synovial fluid to provide lubrication.

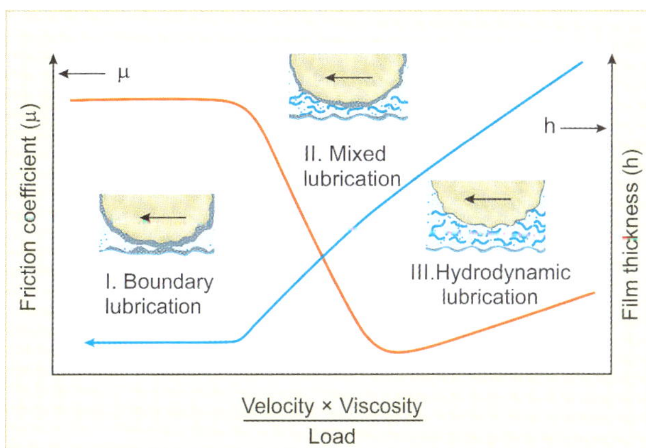

Fig. 8: The coefficient of friction variation with different types of lubrication. The mixed pattern is commonly seen in synovial joints as elastohydrodynamic lubrication.

Boundary Lubrication (Fig. 7D)

Here a hyaluronate free glycoprotein fraction of lubricant prevents direct surface contact of the articulating surfaces. The superficial zones of articular cartilage of opposing surfaces are partially separated by the thin fluid film acting as third slippery surface. The fluid particles slide on each other more readily than they are sheared-off from the underlying surfaces. This mechanism is, however, lost under excessive loads. The coefficient of friction is typically 0.05–0.15 for boundary lubrication.

EFFECTS OF INJURY

Three main patterns of cartilage injury are recognized morphologically and structurally:

1. Superficial matrix disruption
2. Cartilage defects that do not extend throughout the full depth of cartilage (partial thickness cartilage defects)
3. Full thickness cartilage defects.

Natural history of cartilage injuries according to subtypes:

- Varying depth of cartilage damage incur different healing response. Superficial injuries (Type 2) that do not extend below tide mark heal poorly and possibly persist for ever due to avascularity of superficial layers (away from bone) of cartilage although some direct proliferation of chondrocytes may occur. Similarly, type 1 injuries limited to chondrocyte heel poorly.
- Deep lacerations of articular cartilage extending beyond the tidemark (Type 3) heal with fibrocartilage produced by undifferentiated mesenchymal cells derived from subchondral bone.
- Joint instability (ligament injuries) reduces the proteoglycan to collagen ratio initially (4 weeks), however, later (by 12 weeks) proteoglycans are resynthesized. Various changes happen in cartilage in response to aging and degeneration that are summarized in **Table 1**.
- Immobilization of joints leads to atrophy of the articular cartilage and continuous movement has shown trophic influence, so early mobilization after surgery has a critical basis.

There is another way of classifying the cartilage injuries—generalized (degenerative) and focal cartilage defects. The focal cartilage defects may arise secondary to trauma, localized chondromalacia or due to osteochondrosis [*see* Chapter on "Orthopedic Oncology (Bone Tumors and Metastasis) and Heterotopic Ossification"]. Osteochondritis dissecans (OCD) can be taken as a typical example to discuss the focal cartilage defects.

OSTEOCHONDRITIS DISSECANS

Osteochondritis dissecans is defined as a focal, idiopathic alteration of subchondral bone with risk for instability and disruption of adjacent articular cartilage that result in premature OA. The cartilage overlying the fragment survives longer due to nutrition from synovial fluid. Uncommonly, but definitely identified in some cases; is the reincorporation and spontaneous remission of the disease with conservative management. The term "osteochondritis dissecans" was originally coined by Franz Konig (1887) but is apparently a misnomer as there is no inflammatory process associated with pathological fragment or the underlying bone. The underlying bone has normal vascularity and this characteristic distinguishes OCD from osteonecrosis. OCD characteristically affects two distinguished age group of patients—the juvenile form (affecting patients from 5 to 15 years with open physis) and the adult form (affecting patients in adolescent and adult age group). The latter may, however, also represent undiagnosed juvenile lesions.

TABLE 1: Effect of aging and degeneration on cartilage structure (although often the aging process and osteoarthritis are considered similar; however, there are key differences in the molecular pathology that differentiates the two—this should make one realize that osteoarthritis is not really only an age-related disorder).

Component	*Change with aging*	*Change with osteoarthritis*
Hydration and permeability	Reduced	Increased
Collagen (quantitative)	Unchanged	Absolute reduced, relative increased due to loss of proteoglycans
Proteoglycan synthesis	Reduced	Reduced
Proteoglycan degradation	Reduced	Increased
Proteoglycan (quantitative)	Decreased	Decreased
Chondroitin sulfate	Reduced	Increased
Keratin sulfate	Increased	Reduced
Chondrocyte size	Increased	Unchanged
Chondrocytes (number)	Reduced	Reduced
Elasticity	Increased (more friable)	Reduced (stiffened)

Epidemiology

It is an uncommon disorder (15–30 per 100,000 persons), seen more commonly in teenage population (12–19 years of age). Male to female ratio is 3:1. The disease may be bilateral in 40% patients. With increasing involvement in sports, the incidence seems to be increasing in children and females. OCD affects knee (femoral condyles, medial more commonly) most often, but talar dome and capitellum are also significantly involved. Uncommonly reported sites include patella, femoral head, tibial plateau, glenoid, talar head, and even vertebrae. The medial femoral condyle is commonly involved typically at the posterolateral aspect. Lateral femoral condyle accounts for <15% of cases.

Etiology

The proper characterization of the focal separation of the fragment is unknown; however, the possible etiologies include:

- Trauma—as the OCD is increasingly seen with sports person direct injury or microtrauma is the most interesting and cited pathogenic factor. Though direct trauma can cause a subchondral fracture, but this hardly has been the case in any reported patient as the posterolateral aspect of medial condyle is secluded from the direct forces. Microtrauma due to tibial spine impingement has been the proposed classical mechanism of injury. Similarly, inversion in plantar flexion has been proposed to be the development of OCD of talus. The traumatic hypothesis, however, fails to explain the high percentage of bilateral lesions.

- Skeletal maturation (accessory centers of ossification)—some think that the unusual sites of development of OCD might represent accessory/pathological centers of ossification. Abnormal ossification centers are common to occur in children during rapid growth periods.
- Vascular insufficiency/ischemia—interruption of the microvasculature to subchondral bone by repetitive microtrauma and healing could cut-off the lesion from the parent bone vascular supply. The blood supply to subchondral bone is end-arterial and was considered to lack any anastomoses, so sequestration would be fast to occur. However, later extensive osseous circulation studies have refuted this hypothesis by conclusively documenting the intraosseous anastomosis.
- Genetic conditions (e.g., multiple epiphyseal dysplasia)—this is a difficult one to support as no concrete correlation has ever been established.
- Metabolic factors.

Clinical Presentation

Vague and poorly localized pain of insidious onset is the usual complaint. Later with fragment separation clicking, popping or locking may be reported. The symptoms are often associated with activity. Long-standing cases may develop external rotation of tibia as a compensatory mechanism during walking to avoid impingement of tibial spine to OCD lesion. On examination, mild-to-moderate effusion with muscle atrophy is observed. The lesion may be tender to palpation. For knee Wilson's test may be helpful. With legs dangling free from edge of couch in sitting position, ask the patient to extend knee while the leg (tibia) is maintained in internal rotation. Patient reports pain in nearly 30° from extension position that disappears on external rotation of leg (tibia). Subtle restriction of movements (like loss of terminal extension of knee or elbow) is quite characteristic and should caution one to investigate the lesions thoroughly.

Diagnosis

- Characteristic radiographic findings include a well-circumscribed area of subchondral bone separated by a crescent-shaped radiolucent outline of the fragment. In late stages, the lesion may be empty with fragment displaced into joint space **(Figs. 9A to E)**. Radiographs are less sensitive and specific to diagnose early lesions **(Table 2)**. The two-dimensional imaging is liable to miss the lesions with overlapping bony structures of bones in joints. Special views to demonstrate the suspected articular surface should be done like tunnel views for knee and special views for capitellum and talar dome. If radiographs are usually normal, further evaluation is not required, unless very high suspicion remains or if the symptoms are escalating. In general, there are four different radiological classifications for OCD. The Cahill and Berg **(Fig.10)** and the Harding systems **(Fig. 11)** localize the lesion in AP and

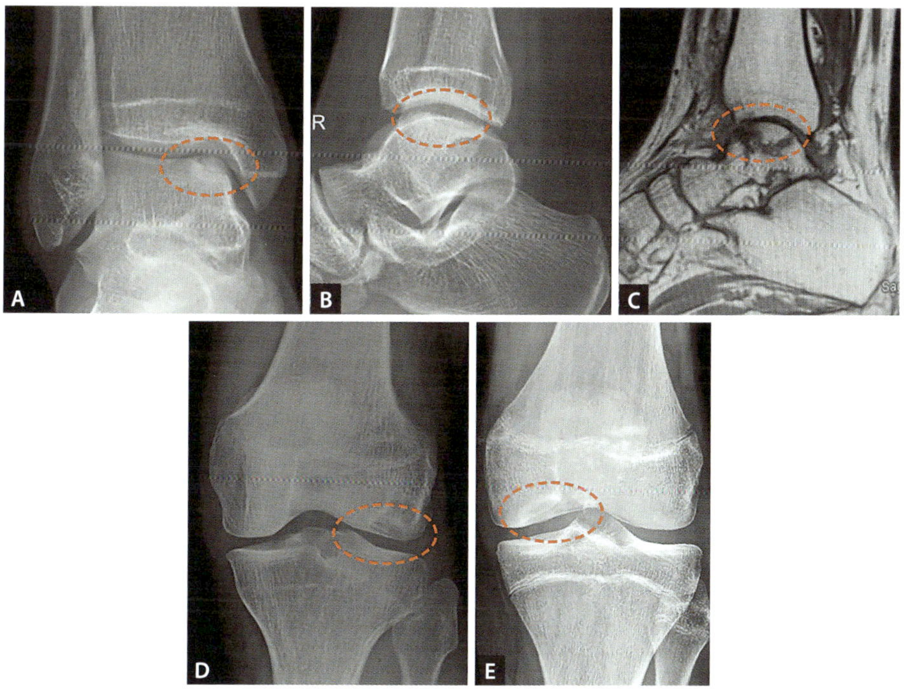

Figs. 9A to E: The various radiological appearances of osteochondritis dissecans (OCD). The anteroposterior (AP) and lateral (Lat) radiographs of ankle (A and B) demonstrating the sharply demarcated fragment with flattening of the region in lateral projection. MRI of the lesion (C) showing the true extent of lesion that appears small on AP larger on lateral projection but still larger on MR scan due to projection limitation in AP view. The lesion may be seen either on lateral femoral condyle (D) or medial femoral condyle (E).

TABLE 2: Staging/grading of osteochondritis dissecans (OCD) lesions.

Radiological staging of OCD (Bedouelle)	*MRI grading of OCD*	*Arthroscopic grading of OCD*	*Surgical staging of OCD*
Stage 1: Incomplete lesion with well-defined image (1a) with more or fewer calcifications within (1b)	*Grade 1:* Thickening of cartilage, no break in cartilage. Low signal changes	*Stage 1:* Irregularity and softening of cartilage. No definite fragment seen	*Stage 1:* Stable lesion in continuity with host bone, intact articular cartilage
Stage 2: Presence of a nodule (2a) with more or less shrinkage of nodule in relation to condyle (2b)	*Grade 2:* Fissure in cartilage. Low signal rim behind fragment indicating fibrous attachment	*Stage 2:* Fissure in cartilage, definite fragment seen, but fragment not displaceable	*Stage 2:* Stable lesion on probing, partly discontinuous from parent bone
Stage 3: Sleigh-bell aspect—the fragment dangling from a thin pedicle and is shaped like a small Christmas bell	*Grade 3:* Cartilage breached, high signal on T2 behind fragment indicating synovial fluid between fragment and underlying bone	*Stage 3:* Discrete fragment, displaceable, but still attached by fibrous attachment or by overlying cartilage	*Stage 3:* Unstable lesion on probing, but fragment in position. Fragment separated from bone completely
Stage 4: Free fragment in the joint with empty bed	*Grade 4:* Loose body	*Stage 4:* Loose fragment and osteochondral defect	*Stage 4:* Dislocated free fragment in the joint

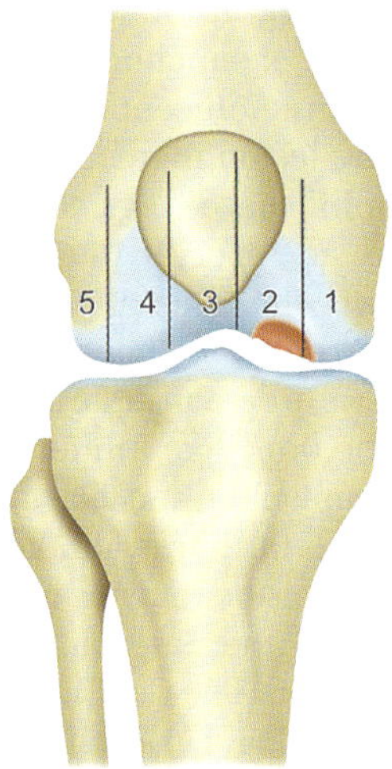

Fig. 10: The Cahill and Berg classification for localization of osteochondritis dissecans lesion on AP projection of knee dividing into five zones. Zone 1: Medial condyle (internal half); Zone 2: Medial condyle (external half); Zone 3: Femoral notch; Zone 4: Lateral condyle (internal half); Zone 5: Lateral condyle (external half).

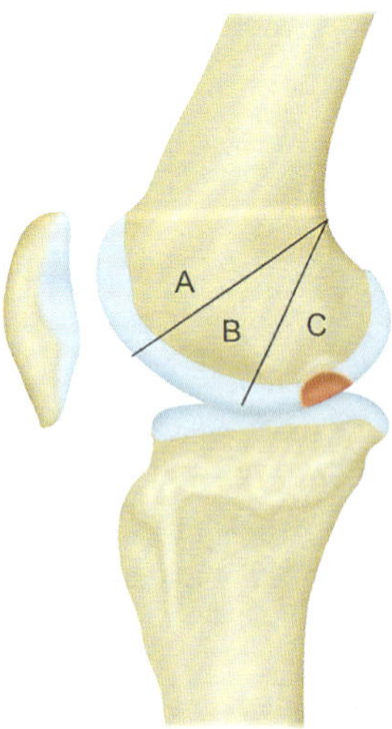

Fig. 11: The Harding classification for localizing the osteochondritis lesion on lateral projection dividing into three zones. Zone A is in front of the Blumensaat line. Zone C is behind the tangential line to the posterior cortex of the femoral diaphysis. Zone B is between zones A and C.

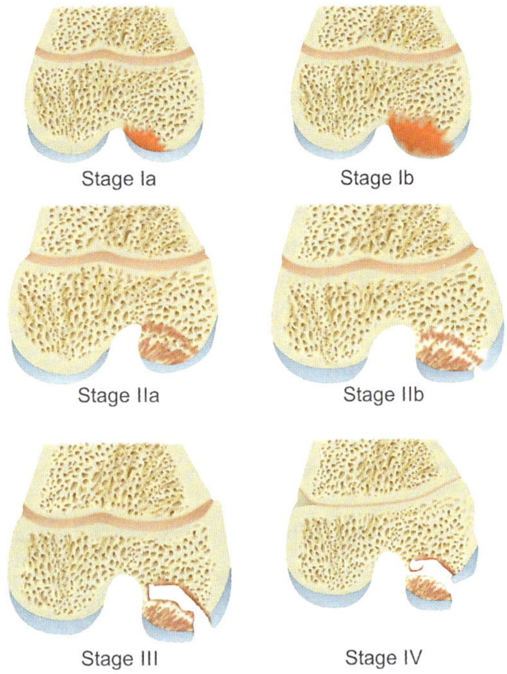

Fig. 12: The Bedouelle's classification for osteochondritis dissecans in children.

lateral projections of the knee, respectively. The Bedouelle **(Fig. 12) (Table 2)** and Hughston et al. systems classify the lesion into pathological stages.

- Magnetic resonance imaging (MRI) seems to be the modality of choice for investigating the lesion, especially staging them **(Table 2)** once demonstrated on radiographs. For a large number of possible bilateral lesions the *contralateral joint* should be examined on identifying pathology in one joint. The MRI staging is also helpful for differentiating the stable lesions from unstable ones (Grade II vs. Grade III) as the latter require definite surgical intervention. Further help can be obtained from arthroscopy.
- Arthroscopy of the joint, quite commonly recommended, is a good therapeutic modality, but may miss initial lesions as the articular cartilage is frequently normal till quite late. The arthroscopic staging closely matches the MRI staging system **(Table 2)**. The ROCK (Research in OsteoChondritis

of Knee) group has developed a classification in common language to communicate the combined MRI-arthroscopic findings. The lesions are primarily divided into immobile and mobile lesions as follows:

- *Immobile lesions:*
  - "Cue ball"—no detectable abnormality arthroscopically
  - "Shadow"—cartilage intact but subtly demarcated
  - "Wrinkle in rug"—cartilage is demarkated with a fissure or wrinkle.
- *Mobile lesions:*
  - "Locked door"—cartilage fissuring at periphery but unable to hinge open
  - "Trap door"—the fissure hinges open
  - "Crater"—exposed subchondral bone defect.
- Technetium bone scans have been proposed to partly determine the possible success of conservative management. If a significantly increased uptake is observed then it suggests marked osteoblastic activity, so that the conservative management would be successful.
- Ultrasonography is highly user dependent and may be useful in evaluating lesions of elbow if done by an experienced person.

Treatment

The treatment depends primarily on the age of patient, stability of lesion, and also on the size of lesion. Stability is the prime determinant of surgical treatment.

- For younger patients (females <11 years and males <13 years)—stable lesion (grade 1 or 2 on MRI)—conservative management usually suffices and should be followed for 4–6 months. Activity modification, cessation of impact activities, and protected weight bearing with crutches or an offloader brace is given to the patient. If symptoms fail to resolve or are progressing at 6 months then resort to simpler operative procedures like debridement and drilling.
- For younger patients with unstable lesions (grade 3 or 4 MRI)—partial takedown of the lesion with debridement of the fibrous tissue and drilling is commonly resorted. Transarticular (to minimize articular cartilage injury) or retroarticular drilling can be done with similar results in either technique. Bioabsorbable pinning can be attempted in selected patients. Metallic screws need removal in future but cannulated headless compression screws offer better fragment compression and sturdy fixation.
- Skeletally mature patients need more aggressive treatment anyway and should be approached as described here for management of focal cartilage loss. A simplistic algorithm is presented for management based on the radiological staging and defect size in **Flowchart 1**.

METHODS TO REPAIR OR RECONSTRUCT FOCAL CARTILAGE DEFECTS

The natural history of chondral injury of the knee is not fully defined including the various influences of physical and chemical factors on it. Articular cartilage integrity may be lost due to trauma, abnormal loading (due to mechanical derangement of joints, e.g., malunion), and aging induced degenerative changes in the cartilage over time. There is loss of cartilage volume (chondropenia) with aging and compromised biomechanical function. This is followed

Flowchart 1: Management of knee osteochondritis dissecans.

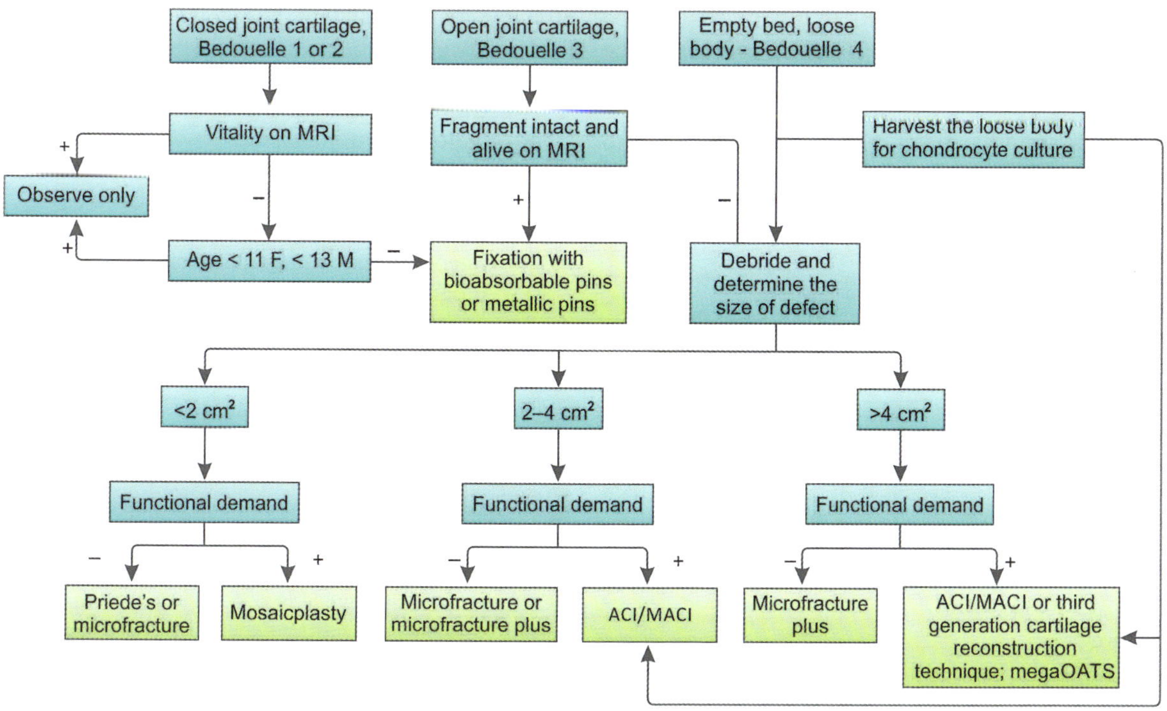

(ACI: autologous chondrocyte implantation; MACI: matrix-assisted chondrocyte implantation; OATS: osteochondral autograft transfer system)

by injury to cartilage and development of partial and full thickness articular cartilage defects. Loss of cartilage function causes increased joint contact pressures between the articulating surfaces quickening the cartilage damage. This further leads to increased friction between joint surfaces following loss of lubrication and accelerated joint degradation as manifested in various stages of osteoarthritis.

The biggest challenge for an interested clinician to recommend chondral repair methods is lack of accurate measurement tools that can objectively define critical cartilage defect or predict future cartilage loss. There are various available cartilage repair techniques that attempt to reduce pain and restore function. The goal of cartilage reconstruction/repair is to provide:

- Durable reconstruction that performs for a long time.
- Reproducing hyaline (ideal) or hyaline like regeneration.

Regeneration of cartilage requires either progenitor cells (to undergo chondrogenesis) or chondrocytes capable of proliferation to ultimately synthesize de novo "hyaline articular cartilage". Not only this but there are other multitude of factors maintaining the fine balance in proper homing of cartilage cells and further proliferation into cartilage **(Fig. 13)**, failure of any one of which may derail success of repair process. Keeping this in mind several repair strategies have been developed varying in complexity and efficacy. The choice of a clinical repair technique in a typical patient depends on:

- Classification of the defects **(Tables 2 and 3)**
- Clinical status of patient (evaluated with SF-36)
- The patient demand—a palliative, reparative or restorative approach.

Size and type of defect is evaluated using radiology. Computed tomography arthrogram, MRI, and arthrogram MRI provide a precise appreciation of the width on AP slices and length on sagittal slices. Arthroscopy can also be used to measure the size. Type of lesion is often graded using the International Cartilage Repair Society (ICRS) grading system **(Table 3)**.

The ICRS system has been developed in an effort to ensure uniform standards of management and introduces a comprehensive method for classifying articular cartilage defects.

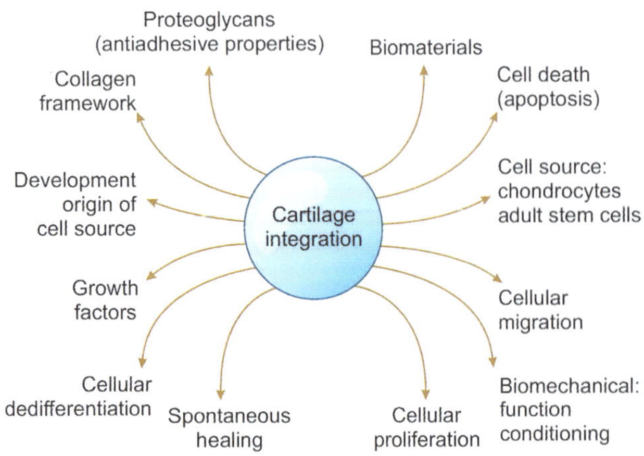

Fig. 13: The multiple fine-tuned factors responsible for successful cartilage integration in repair techniques.

The ICRS system is based on an assessment of nine variables (freely available on internet as "ICRS evaluation package"): etiology (traumatic or chronic), defect thickness **(Table 3)**, lesion size (<2 cm^2 or >2 cm^2), degree of containment, defect location, integrity of knee ligaments, associated meniscal injury, joint alignment, and identification of factors in the patient history. Etiology is classified as either traumatic or chronic. ICRS defines a *contained* defect as one surrounded by articular cartilage on all sides. The defects in the weight bearing surface of the knee are classified by ICRS as either unipolar—isolated or bipolar—combined with a defect on the articulating surface. As highlighted by the ICRS system the articular cartilage should be evaluated as a *functional unit* and for this ligamentous and meniscal integrity are essential. We know from biomechanics of meniscus that loss of as little as 30% of the meniscus increases joint contact pressures by >350%. Included in this "functional unit" assessment is varus/valgus malalignment that should be addressed before cartilage repair to ensure success of specific articular cartilage repair methods. Correct any varus or valgus malalignment. Considering all these factors the indications for surgical reconstruction of cartilage defect (using especially the modern cellular methods) are:

- Age <50 years (biological potential for cartilage to heal) and that arthroplasty may be too early for them
- Stable joint with acceptable alignment
- Nonobese (BMI < 30)
- The International Cartilage Repair Society grade 3 or 4
- Nonkissing lesions
- Lesion must not be too small (<0.5 cm^2) and neither too large (>2–3 cm^2)—although some have attempted repair of up to 4 cm^2 lesions.

There are a lot of modalities that can be used for cartilage reconstruction **(Fig. 14 and Flowchart 2)**. The surgical repair strategies broadly fall into the following groups:

- Palliative:
  - Neglect
  - Arthroscopic lavage
  - Radiofrequency ablation
- Marrow (subchondral) stimulation
- Reconstruction using direct tissue transfer:
  - Mosaicplasty
  - Osteochondral autograft transfer system (OATS)
  - Allograft implantation
- Newer strategies aiming to obtain hyaline cartilage:
  - Cell-based repair
  - Scaffold-based repair
  - Cell + Scaffold-based repair

TABLE 3: The International Cartilage Repair Society (ICRS) grading of cartilage defects.

Grade	Description
Grade 1	*Nearly normal (superficial lesions):* Softening, fibrillations, lacerations, and fissures
Grade 2	Abnormal (<50% of cartilage depth)
Grade 3	Severely abnormal (cartilage defects extending down to >50% of cartilage depth)
Grade 4	Severely abnormal (lesion extending past subchondral plate, bone exposed)

- Cell + Scaffold + Growth factors
- Gene therapy
- Combination strategies.

Following are the commonly practiced methods as discussed in detail.

Masterly Benign Neglect and Medical Management

This strategy could be suitable for an unwilling patient with defects < 1 cm or stable small OCD. Documentation is a must for future medicolegal purpose. The stress on the joint is removed and patient is recommended rest and abstinence from eliciting positions and activities. Graded program of muscle strengthening and lifestyle modification is introduced with supportive medical care. The cartilage that may develop with this approach is at best fibrocartilage that is poor in biomechanical properties and tends to wear off fast. It does not allow high demand activities.

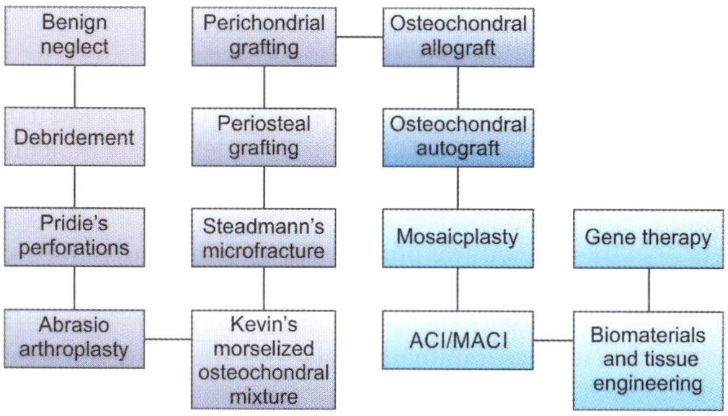

Fig. 14: Reconstruction ladder of modalities available for reconstruction of cartilage/osteocartilaginous defect depending on complexity of technique/technology involved and evolutionary paradigm. (ACI: autologous chondrocyte implantation; MACI: matrix-assisted chondrocyte implantation)

Some medications have been used for enhancing cartilage repair most popular of which are curcumin and procollagen type-II peptide. Curcumin (diferuloylmethane) is obtained as an extract from *C. longa* (turmeric) and is portended to have multiple mechanisms of action to improve cartilage health. Its therapeutic potential covers diseases such as cancer, Alzheimer's disease, osteoporosis, inflammatory bowel disease, depression, arthritis, diabetes, vitiligo, and endometriosis due to anti-inflammatory, antioxidant, antiviral, antibacterial, and antitumor effects. Treatment with curcumin results in reduction of IL-1β, IL-6, IL-8, TNF-α, NF-κB, COX-2, and reactive oxygen species (ROS). It also inhibits the activity of several kinases related to the degradation of the cartilage, including a tyrosine kinase, p21-activated kinase 1 (PAK1), mitogen-activated protein kinase (MAPK), and protein kinase C (PKC) thus protecting cartilage from inflammatory damage. Production of MMP-3, MMP-9, and MMP-13 is suppressed by inhibition of activator

Flowchart 2: Schematic overview of various groups of strategies for repair of cartilage defect with common examples.

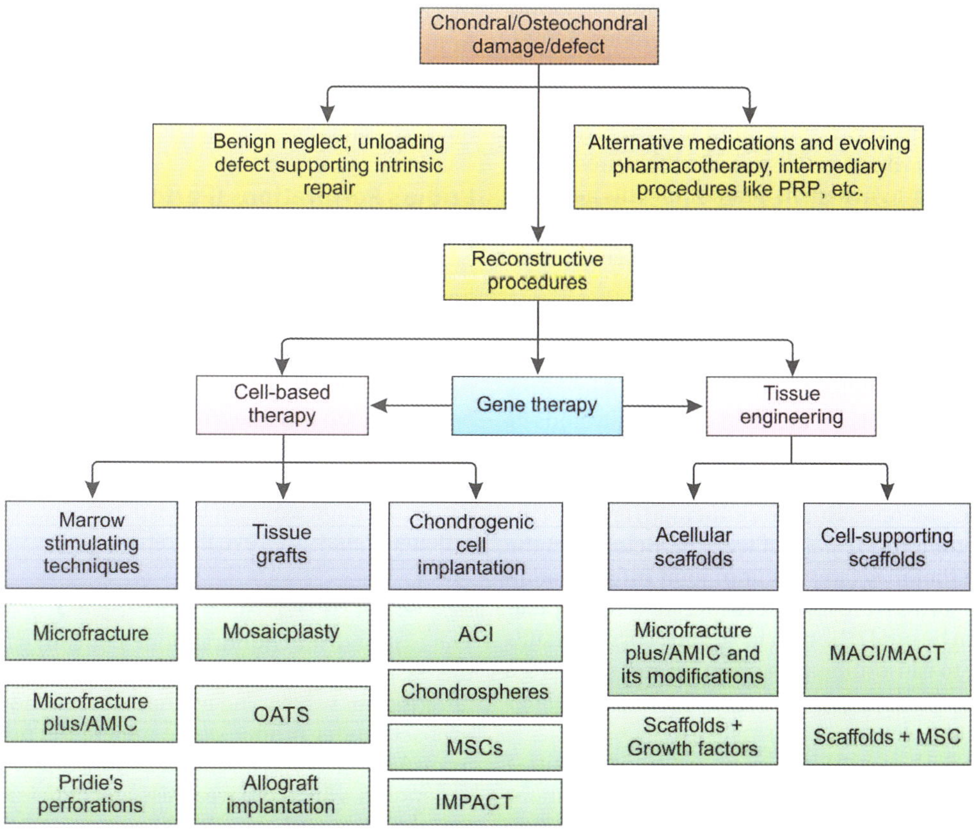

(ACI: autologous chondrocyte implantation; AMIC: autologous matrix-induced chondrogenesis; MACI: matrix-assisted chondrocyte implantation; MACT: matrix-assisted cartilage transplantation; MSC: mesenchymal stem cells; OATS: osteochondral autograft transfer system)

protein 1 (AP-1) pathway and NF-κB protecting cartilage from degradation. Additionally curcumin inhibits the activation of I kappa B kinase (IKK) in chondrocytes, osteoblasts, and synovial cells thus inhibiting the expression of caspase-3 proapoptotic gene in chondrocytes. Procollagen type-II peptide administered orally has shown to experimentally improve cartilage matrix quality and repair in animal models. The synthesis of collagen type II and proteoglycans improve under the therapeutic effect. Currently, the treatment is at best supportive and may be used as interim or supplemental measure with other reconstructive methods.

Joint Lavage and Debridement

Symptomatic patients with chondral lesions of <2 cm^2 diameter have been successfully treated with debridement and lavage. In true sense, they are not to be included in cartilage "repair" technique as they put no attempt at repair of defect. Hypertrophied and inflamed synovial membrane release catabolic enzymes and cytokines (such as IL-1 and IL-2 and TNF-α) into the joint space causing swelling and pain that recur intermittently. Joint lavage and debridement aims at diluting the local factors and washing them away along with removing excess synovium to resolve knee inflammation, pain and the damage incurred. This also includes removal of loose cartilage fragments and osteocartilagenous loose bodies. The technique is generally reserved for elderly lower demand patients that have limited symptoms. Also, patients who are unlikely to follow the postoperative mobility restrictions like lower income group laborers who are sole earners in family may also be managed with lavage and debridement of joint. Although palliative in the sense that no attempt to address the pathology is done, it involves symptomatic treatment only to relief from pain and improvement in function is fast and patient can immediately bear full weight with unrestricted activities though long-term benefit is doubtful. This modality has always been competed to be inferior in providing symptomatic relief that too also wades off fast. There is no significant medium to long-term benefit.

Radiofrequency Energy

Radiofrequency energy (RFE) has been used in many forms and it is interesting to note that this modality usually finds its way for orthopedic conditions where standards of care have yet not been established. RFE melts and removes damaged tissue to produce smooth surface reducing friction. This also prevents continuous release of wear particles from the fibrillated tissue that may later result in joint inflammation later. RFE in two forms—the bipolar (bRFE) or a monopolar (mRFE) wand can be used. The high local ionic current results in tissue heating to cause annealing effect, so essentially RFE is useful only for partial thickness defects. The two modalities mentioned have differing mechanisms.

1. The current path in mRFE goes from the probe tip → through the surface of cartilage → subchondral bone → ground plate or it may "leak" through irrigation solution → the joint capsule → the grounding plate.
2. In bRFE heating electric current passes between the positive and negative electrode tips, thus the conduction remains localized within the irrigation fluid and there is minimal if any possibility of leak. High local current causes vaporization of the irrigating saline producing an "ionic plasma" type milieu. The tissue effects with bRFE are, hence, secondary to combined thermal (resistance to current) and ionic modification.

The biggest advantage of RFE is that it is a simple tool that can be delivered arthroscopically under direct vision; it is inexpensive and safe for operating room personnel. The greatest limitation is that this is a technique only for "partial thickness defects"; one cannot expect cartilage formation at bald surfaces using RFE. Beneficial reports following the use of RFE for treatment of articular cartilage defects are difficult to find and substantiate. Lu et al. advised caution with the use of both mRFE and bRFE during thermal chondroplasty. He also mentioned the potential to damage surrounding cartilage with the device. One should understand, however, that RFE also causes joint lavage and the fact that mechanical debridement does minimal or in fact no attempt to improve pathology, it is unlikely to be of much benefit in intermediate to long-term, as has been shown by various researchers. The recent use of nonablative RFE is portended to be more protective to chondrocytes and cause less death than conventional RFE. Nonablation RFE passes through a bipolar mechanism. It is produced from a monopolar generator and passes via a protected tip to prevent electrode from tissue contact, which is in contrast to ablative RFE (mRFE or bRFE that deliver RFE through a direct electrode to tissue contact). In the best knowledge of current literature, the absence of concrete benefits and understanding of mechanism any recommendation for its use is futile and is willfully avoided till clarity emerges.

Pridie's Perforations (Perforation de Pridie, 1959)

This could be called the first systematic approach to cartilage regeneration. Multiple drill holes are made in the subchondral bone using sharp drill or K-wires to stimulate fibrocartilage formation using a power drill **(Fig. 15A)**. Criticism evolved from the resulting necrosis of surrounding tissues from drilling that could damage the MSCs and also produce greater necrotic bone defect to provide a base for cartilage growth. However, once carefully performed this method is also perceivably similar to microfracture technique in generation of new tissue. Injection of platelet-rich plasma into the holes or intra-articularly may improve the repair.

Johnson's Abrasion Chondroplasty

The exposed subchondral bone beneath cartilage defect at the base is abraded using burr. This exposes mesenchymal intraosseous vessels and multipotent subchondral cells. Once exposed under proper stable milieu, the new cartilage may form. At best, a surgeon can expect an imperfect fibrocartilage generation, which is a weak tissue. There is a strong concern that the strong subchondral bone may get weak and burning may produce thermal necrosis.

Steadman's Microfracture and Continuous Passive Motion

Microfracture technique is considered to be the first-line surgical option at this moment for full-thickness articular cartilage defects. This is also the technique against which most other modalities are compared for assessment of efficacy. The principal difference from Pridie's perforations lies in not using a power drill in microfracture, so that this is a low energy violation of the subchondral bone. Although the heat generation is often cited as the possible cause of osteocyte necrosis, but reverse has been observed in studies. There is a higher amount of osteocyte necrosis with the use of awls due to high pressure induced cellular damage, while in water immersed drilling of subchondral drilling the temperature failed to reach the necrosis threshold of the cells. The reasons for considering this as basic modality used for comparing with different techniques are its advantages considered by many:

- The technique is minimally invasive.
- It is comparatively easy.
- The surgical morbidity is also minimal.
- It is relatively much cheaper.

The cartilage defect is first debrided to stable and smooth edges, so that further flap elevation or damage does not occur. This provides a pool for the clot (superclot) to form. The blood clot provides a scaffold containing growth factors and cytokines. The underlying bone is scraped to remove calcified cartilage layer for better tissue attachment and then penetrated using an awl **(Figs. 15A and B)**. Smaller diameter awls (1-1.2 mm) or "hollow" awls may produce better articular cartilage repair. The holes are placed 3-4 mm apart (to maintain the structural and functional integrity of subchondral bone) and are usually 3 mm deep. Previously used depth of 5 mm is possibly inappropriate. The smaller depth enhances the concentrated growth factors, which are required to initiate and support a chondrogenic repair in full-thickness defects. Higher concentration of FGF-2 is required to produce a hyaline cartilage that is possible in smaller depths only. Also, the MSCs pack better around the smaller portal than a larger portal. Marrow totipotent stem cells that migrate into the clot differentiate under appropriate milieu to form fibrocartilage repair tissue. This tissue is of inferior quality and strength with poorer wear characteristics than hyaline articular cartilage. Steadman himself reported that up to 80% of young patients with isolated post-traumatic, full-thickness chondral defects that were treated with microfracture improved at an average follow-up of 7 years. He noted that *worse outcomes* (I would call them relative contraindications to this technique) were associated with:

- Patients aged >30 years
- Lesions sized >2 cm^2
- Lesions located in the central portion of the medial femoral condyle.

Compared to osteocartilage implant autografts; microfracture alone technique induces less glycosaminoglycan content, lower synthetic activity, and increased glycosaminoglycan expulsion in the defects. We feel that the microfracture technique could be useful in cases with larger lesions in low demand areas or smaller regions in high demand areas and it could be utilized as a first-line technique in the sense, if it fails other usually more aggressive repair techniques can be still deployed.

As it is known that the repair tissue is not that conducive so in an effort to improve the tissue quality and adhesion to underlying bone, a new approach and logical one has been proposed that combines microfracture technique to a membrane/scaffold in order to enhance access of bone marrow stem cells to the defect (called "plus microfracture"). Autologous matrix-induced chondrogenesis (AMIC) uses a collagen (I/III) membrane to cover the microfracture site. The porous side of this matrix membrane remains on the side of microfracture area and membrane is glued to the periphery using fibrin glue. In animal models, a polyglycolic acid (PGA)

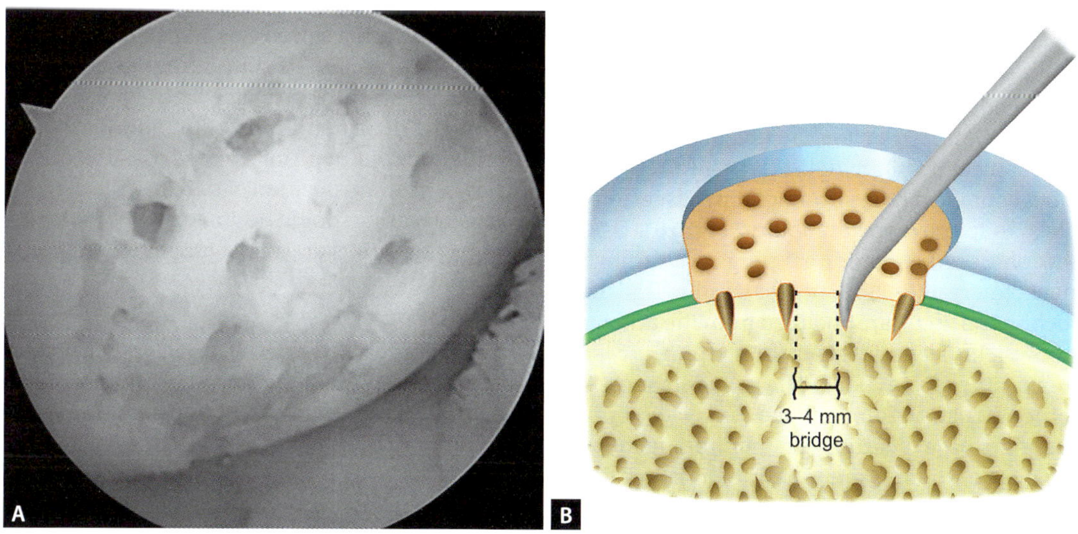

Figs. 15A and B: Microfracture technique. (A) Conventional practice of drilling multiple subchondral holes using low-revolution K-wire (to reduce heat generation and killing the totipotent cells); (B) The holes can be also drilled/impacted by using a dedicated curved awl, conventionally to maintain the integrity of subchondral bone the holes must be drilled 3–4 mm apart. Using awl is also better as this allows proper depth control and also holes can be made as perpendicular to the subchondral bone as possible.

scaffold and the hyaluronic acid have been used to cover microfractured full-thickness articular cartilage defects. The cell-free scaffolds hold the stem cells derived from marrow in the microfracture facilitated environment resulting in development of repair tissue. It has been shown that the repair tissue formed from "microfracture plus" technique contains type II collagen which is much better and closely resembles true cartilage matrix than the tissue formed with microfracture only technique. Alternative "plus technique" adjuvants with similar success include use of BMP-7 or -4 in collagen sponge or by using recombinant Sox-9 [SRY-type high mobility group (HMG) box] bound collagen membrane to cover the defect.

Newer modifications: Attempts are underway to improve the quality of regenerated tissue and make it as close to hyaline cartilage as possible. Following are some of the strategies described in literature:

- Additional use of concentrated bone marrow with scaffold and microfracture may result in hyaline-like cartilage formation.
- Use of platelet-rich plasma or autologous conditioned plasma intra-articularly and various growth factors (like IGF, FGF-18) after microfracture improves quality of tissue formation. Injection of hyaluronic acid produces no improvement over microfracture alone technique. Use of subcutaneous rh-PTH after microfracture inhibits cartilage production so is contraindicated.
- Intra-articular injection of kartogenin that mediates conversion of marrow stem cells into chondrocytes through CBF-β-Runx1 signaling pathway improves quality of fibrocartilage.

Mosaicplasty

Mosaic autografts (mosaicplasty) of Hangody comprise transplanting a collection of small osteochondral cylinders packed side-by-side into the defect. This is now also known as osteoarticular transplant system (OATS) first described by Yamashita et al. OATS helps in maintaining the shape of condyle compared to use of single chunk of osteochondral tissue. Mosaicplasty is normally used to treat full-thickness defects. The procedure is often done in an open fashion with the joint exposed through classical medial parapatellar approach. The central defect is debrided and the defect converted into a contained one surrounded by disease-free healthy cartilage to improve the durability **(Fig. 16)**. Using appropriate trephines, the cylindrical plugs are removed from the defect (to create recipient sites) and cylindrical plugs of osteochondral tissue are obtained from the articular cartilage of nonweight-bearing regions (donor plugs). Mega OATS uses single large plug of bone. The cylinders must be harvested perpendicular to joint surface. This is essential to ensure that grafts have a cartilage cap of homogeneous thickness. The donor cylinders are usually a bit larger than the recipient site for press fit and are inbuilt in the harvesting system, so one must be careful in paying attention to detail of the manufacturer. Some computer-navigated systems are also recently made available to endure proper harvest. It is important to preserve the cartilage cap when the graft is being harvested.

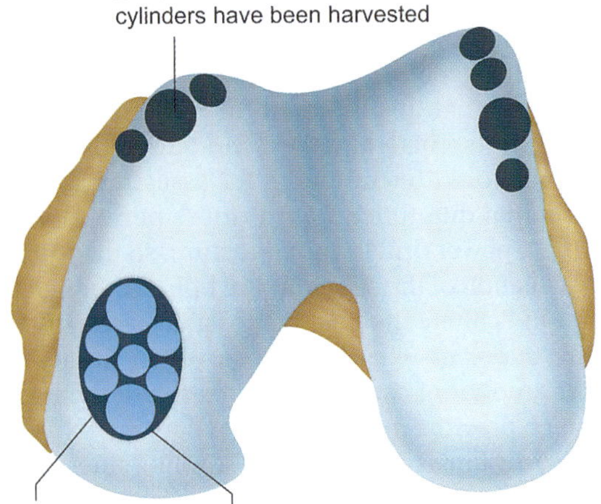

Fig. 16: Mosaicplasty.

While seating into defect the donor central plugs are kept higher than peripheral ones to maintain rounded condylar contour. In case, a graft is too taller than the adjacent articular surface, the spongy bone is shortened until it sits flush with the articular surface. Hangody published a large series of 831 cases of mosaicplasty in humans operated from 1992 to 2002. The results were good to excellent in 92% of patients with femoral condylar implantations, 87% with tibial resurfacing, 79% with patellar and/or trochlear mosaicplasties, and 94% with talar procedures. Mosaicplasty was historically restricted for smaller cartilage defects (<2 cm^2) due to limitation in obtaining the healthy graft tissue that could only be taken from a limited healthy area of the same joint. With proper anatomical knowledge, the procedure is currently now endured also for larger articular cartilage defects (up to 4 cm^2) and the procedure can be performed arthroscopically using calibrated commercial system. It is essential to make the joint rounded contour as anatomical as possible and fill at least 80% of the defect for the procedure to be successful. Some surgeons have used this system for even larger defects (>4 cm^2)—"mega OATS", but infrequently used elsewhere. Postoperatively intra-articular drain is placed for 24 hours. Nonweight-bearing mobilization and joint strengthening exercises are continued for a period of 4–8 weeks, varying with respect to size and position of the cartilage defect. The return to weight-bearing should be gradual. This protocol is essential to protect the grafts and allow proper integration.

Allografts

For a too large cartilage defect an allograft may be considered, especially when the underlying bone is also nonsupportive. Implantation of allografts includes taking osteochondral tissue, chondrocytes or other cells or cartilage from a donor and transplanting it into a different individual of the same species. The allograft has advantages such as:

- Smaller incision is needed
- No donor site morbidity and limitation of graft size/numbers
- Decreased surgical time

- Larger grafts are available
- The grafts can be matched to contour.

The greatest advantage I feel is that allograft can be shaped to fit the contour of the defect irrespective of the size and then press-fitted into place which is not possible with OATS typically. They can be used both as mosaicplasty and as single chunk-shaped like the defect. The concern with their use is that long-term storage significantly decreases cell viability over time. The cells upregulate genes associated with apoptosis including CD30, CD30 Ligand, Fas, Fas ligand, TNF, several caspases, and matrix degradation enzymes leading to chondrocyte apoptosis. The viability can be improved by storing the allograft in culture media rather than conventional lactated ringer solution. Lack of chondrocyte viability, implant rejection, nonunion, graft displacement, disease transmission, availability and processing facility are some of the issues with their use. Z-VAD-FMK [carbobenzoxy-valyl-alanyl-aspartyl-(O-methyl)-fluoromethylketone] (pan-caspase activity inhibitor) has been used to improve the preservation technique and prolong the survival time of chondrocytes. Freeze-drying to –150°C or –190°C is another viable alternative, especially when done in presence of cryoprotectants like glycerol or DMSO (dimethylsulfoxide).

Autologous Chondrocyte Implantation

Autologous chondrocyte implantation (ACI) is a *first-generation* cell-based therapy that involves transplantation of autogenous chondrocytes/chondrospheres into articular cartilage defects. The ACI procedure, first introduced by Brittberg and coworkers, has become the most competent surgical procedure for treatment of cartilage defects. The specific advantage is that it promises to provide complete hyaline repair tissues for articular cartilage repair.

Mechanism of new cartilage formation: The repairing capability not only relies on the cells from chondrocyte progenies, but also from the periosteum derived MSCs. Undifferentiated mesenchymal cells from periosteum, especially the cambium layer are proven to be source of cells in new forming cartilage. Periosteum-derived progenitor cells of the cambium layer can express endogenous TGF-β1 and TBR-I and TBR-II when they are exposed to the exogenous stimulation of TGF-β1. TGF-β1 plays a substantial trigger for an early phase of proliferation and chondrogenesis. Continuous passive motion has been implicated as an important factor for enhanced cartilage repair beside the biological factors. The dynamic fluid pressure studies suggest that low pressures of 13 kPa enhance chondrogenesis, by upregulating the p38 mitogen-activated protein kinases (p38 MAPK) which enhances the expression of chondrogenic markers including Col2α, aggregan, Sox9, and Runt-related transcription factor 2 (Runx2) whereas the cells decreased their expression of chondrogenic markers when exposed to p38 MAPK inhibitor under excessive pressure.

Procedure details: In ACI, cells are taken from nonweight-bearing regions of joint typically the lateral trochlear ridge **(Fig. 17)**. The chondrocytes then are enzymatically isolated from the ECM and cultured in monolayer for 3–4 weeks. This increases the volume of cells available for implantation 30-fold for a yield of approximately 12 million viable chondrocytes. The technique of using chondrosphere consists of generation and implantation of spheroids of autologous or allogenic articular chondrocytes. The expanded chondrocytes are condensed in order to form spheroids, which then are coalesced and can be implanted into the cartilage defect. The defect is prepared into a circular or oval shape by debriding all damaged and unstable tissue down to subchondral bone with a rim of stable healthy cartilage. The walls of the defect are kept as vertical as possible to allow for suture fixation of the graft. Care is taken to avoid penetration of the subchondral bone plate, as this would stimulate a fibrous response. Periosteum harvested from proximal tibia is used to seal the defect. The cambium layer containing multipotent stem cells is sutured facing the defect. The chondrocyte containing solution is injected into the prepared partially sealed cavity and suturing of periosteum completed **(Figs. 18 and 19)**. Further sealing to prevent the leakage of solution can be done by fibrin glue.

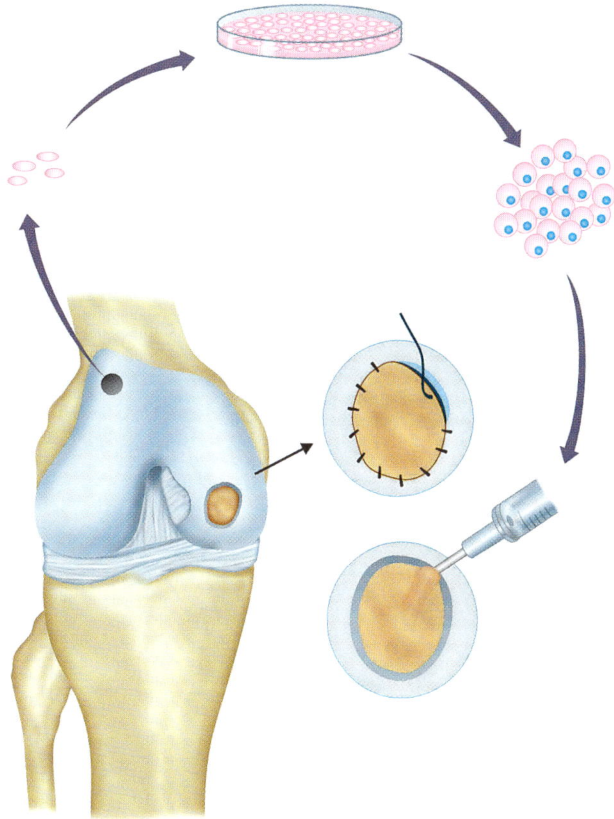

Fig. 17: Autologous cartilage implantation.

The *main drawbacks* of ACI are:

- Need for large open arthrotomy
- The two-stage procedure (one for cell harvesting and the other for implantation)
- The prolonged period of time required to expand sufficient numbers of chondrocytes in vitro
- High cost of cell culture system
- Poor retention and dedifferentiation of cells following implantation

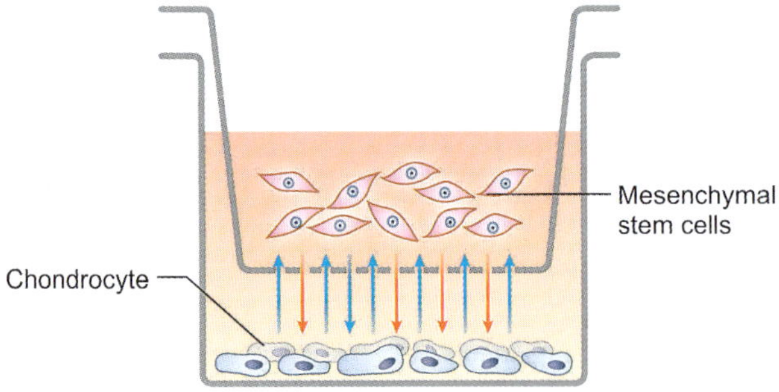

Fig. 18: The chondrocyte mesenchymal stem cell co-culture system.

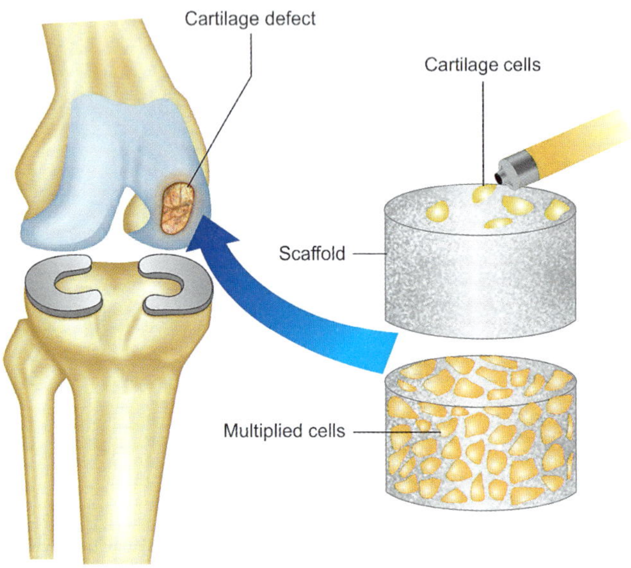

Fig. 19: Illustration depicting the essential scheme of second-generation cell-based cartilage defect repair assisted by matrix—MACI. Here, the obtained chondrocytes are expanded and implanted in suitable matrix that enable uniform distribution of chondrocytes and help in holding and maturing them preventing dedifferentiation.

- Ablation and loss of implanted cells from the defect site
- Prolonged nonweight-bearing
- Periosteal hypertrophy and other problems with the use of periosteal patch (discussed further).

It has been found in comparative study of ACI and mosaicplasty that athletes who are treated with mosaicplasty returned to active sports more quickly, but the durability and clinical improvement is higher with ACI. Most studies for ACI technique in management of cartilage defects report favorable outcomes such as good adherence of the regenerated tissue to underlying bone, seamless integration with adjacent cartilage, and mechanical properties close to adjacent tissue. I personally feel that ACI paves the future for cartilage reconstruction technique and must be given as a viable option when considering articular cartilage defect repair. Efforts are on to simplify the technique and reduce the drawbacks mentioned above that are needed to be addressed. To prevent cartilage hypertrophy at the transplant site, making the procedure single stage and improving cell survival and viability various modifications are underway as described below.

Collagen-covered Autologous Chondrocyte Implantation

There are a lot of undue and not unfrequently seen complications associated with the use of a periosteal flap in ACI procedures which include:

- Graft delamination
- Potential ectopic calcification of the periosteal patch
- Graft hypertrophy—leading to "catching" of the knee joint.

Researchers are focusing to the use of an alternative membrane to seal the cartilage defect. Instead of using periosteum, the collagen membranes are a viable substitute. The collagen membrane has a compact layer to prevent diffusion of the cells out of the pouch and an inner porous layer to encourage cell invasion and attachment. This adaptation avoids the second incision needed in the classic ACI technique (to harvest periosteum) and theoretically reduces the potential for postoperative periosteal hypertrophy. This procedure is termed Collagen Covered Autologous Chondrocyte Implantation (CACI) or ACI-C. The collagen membrane has been found to completely resorb. Although no clinical and functional difference in the patient performance has been found between ACI and ACI-C but incidence of hypertrophy seems to be less with CACI/ACI-C. Though further trials are needed, but collagen appears to be a better substitute to cover the cellular reconstruction defect.

Matrix-assisted Chondrocyte Implantation

This is an advancement over the use of membranes. It is logical to use a scaffold for cells to colonize and develop into tissue rather than just using the membranes. The technique uses adaptation from tissue engineering. MACI is a *second-generation* approach for articular cartilage reconstruction where chondrocytes are combined to a three-dimensional scaffold (matrix) replicating the defect **(Fig. 19)**. The defect shape and size engineered scaffold facilitates chondrocyte migration, adhesion, and replication without losing the phenotypic characteristics. This prevents dedifferentiation which had been a concern observed in previous systems. The matrices can be synthetic [carbone, polylactic (PLA) or polyglycolic acid (PGA), or dacrylen] or natural that are further divided into protein (collagen, fibrin, and gelatin), or polysaccharides (alginate, agarose, and hyaluronic acid). Hyaluronic acid is the favorite among these for various properties. MACI has shown good healing response with better repair than ACI, but some concerns still remain like the inability to treat large cartilage surface defects and the inherent donor site morbidity as well as two stages needed for chondrocyte harvest from native cartilage tissue.

General drawbacks associated with the use of chondrocytes (ACI, CACI, and MACI) in cartilage defect repair:

1. *Limited size of reconstruction achievable:* All the cell-based repair/reconstruction procedures for cartilage defects utilizing chondrocytes (e.g., ACI) are currently limited by the maximum size of defects (2–10 cm^2) they can treat. For successful cartilage synthesis, it is observed that a cell density of 10,000 cells per microliter (μL) is needed in ACI. Need to harvest chondrocytes result in a two-stage procedure and donor site morbidity.

2. The second limitation of chondrocyte-based system of cartilage repair is the absolute requirement for monolayer expansion of the cultured cells to increase cell density in the transplant system. During clonal expansion, the chondrocytes may dedifferentiate into other cell lineages and lose capacity to synthesize cartilage like tissue. It is important to, hence, characterize viable and functional chondrocytes and use only them for the purpose of reimplantation. This method is called characterized chondrocyte implantation or CCI. This is a time-consuming process. To overcome this difficulty, alternative sources of cells (such as mesenchymal cells, co-culture systems, and growth factors biomolecules) for cartilage defect repair are being widely investigated and are discussed later.
3. The chondrocyte culture takes a long time and is a costly process.
4. Some chondrocytes inevitably leak from created pocket at the defect despite best of closure. There is a definite risk then that the number of viable cells may fall below repair density for new cartilage tissue. Also there is theoretical concern of inhomogeneous distribution of cells within the defects.

To address the last issue use of alternative sources of cells (mesenchymal cells, co-culture systems, and growth factors) for cartilage defect repair has been widely investigated and are discussed further.

Third-generation Chondrocyte Grafting

This is still under evaluation and basically involves chondrocyte and matrix culture system **(Fig. 20)**. Principle is culturing chondrocytes in an implantable biological matrix with ideal properties—biocompatible, biodegradable, and bioactive while preserving the phenotypic characteristics, thus favoring the cellular proliferation and synthesis of the ECM, which is permeable, easy to use, and inexpensive. Hyaluronic acid is the principal component for matrix. The cartilage defect is filled in several layers using "mushroom technique".

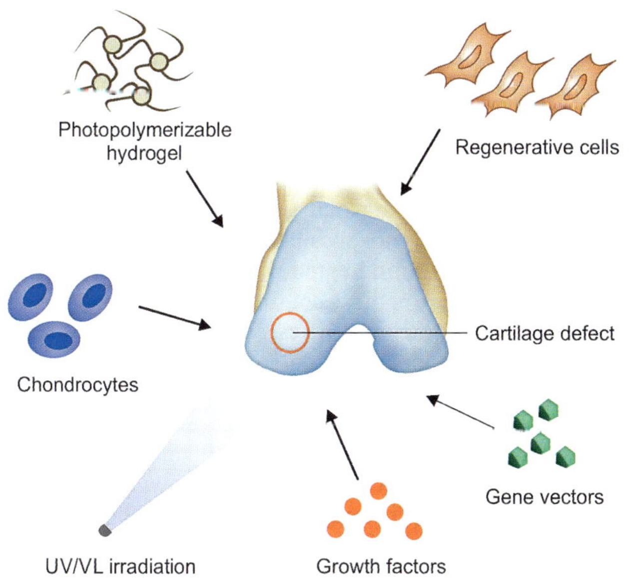

Fig. 20: Illustration depicting the use of various strategies in third-generation chondrocyte grafting where a combination of various strategies is used to improve chondrocyte survival and hasten uptake. To this one can also add three-dimensional (3D) printing where cartilage can be synthesized in several layers reproducing the anatomical layered structure of cartilage. (UV: ultraviolet; VL: visible light)

SCAFFOLDS

Biodegradable scaffold acts as a template to support interaction, proliferation of cells, and deposition of ECM. It is desirable that they maintain the characteristic cellular phenotype and function. They are increasingly being promoted for various newer cartilage reconstruction strategies including the use of MSCs and growth factors (kindly also *see* Chapter on "Electrospinning, Three-dimensional Printing and its Application in Orthopedics"). Scaffolds can be generally grouped into two types:

1. Synthetic
2. Natural

The advantage with synthetic scaffolds is that we can control the structural and mechanical properties and can develop them in many shapes according to requirement. On the other hand, natural scaffolds allow greater cellular interaction by virtue of presence of natural ligands that facilitate cell adhesion.

Synthetic Scaffolds

Polycaprolactone (PCL), poly L-lactic acid (PLLA), and polyglycolic acid (PGA) are the most commonly used *synthetic materials*. In particular, the PCL scaffolds have been used for in vitro chondrogenesis using the MSCs that exhibit or are stimulated to express chondrogenic gene and deposit ECM. In general, the advantages of synthetic scaffolds are:

- They are pathogen free (no risk of disease transmission)
- Very low potential for immunological rejection
- They have controllable and known degradation rate and can be used for labile growth factor delivery
- As mentioned above, they can be synthesized into a range of different forms like particles, meshes, and fibers.

The most important drawback of synthetic scaffolds is possibility of biocompatibility like their degradation products are usually highly concentrated organic acids that can induce localized inflammation or toxify the local milieu and cause cell death.

Scaffolds Derived from Natural Materials

The most widely used natural materials are the polypeptides and polysaccharides due to their biodegradability and nontoxic degradation products (the greatest disadvantage of synthetic scaffolds).

- The most favored substance for researchers despite extensive search has been collagen due to its ubiquitous nature and favorable mechanical properties that excel any of other natural scaffolds tried. The other advantage of collagen is that it can be fabricated to alter its mechanical properties to our use and also degradation rate can be modified using cross-linking treatment. Collagen can interact reliably with various other molecules such as polysaccharides and even protein-based growth factors as in natural existence. Classically, type I/III collagens have been used in natural collagen-based scaffolds, but with advancements and for the purpose of chondrogenesis type II collagen scaffolds and hydrogels are being developed for repair applications. It has been found that the functionality and regenerative capacity of collagen scaffolds can be improved by adding GAGs to these systems.

- Chondroitin sulfate plays an important role in cartilage regeneration by enhancing chondrocyte proliferation and matrix production in vitro, so it has also been used in cartilage defect repair application. Chondroitin sulfate is mostly copolymerized to collagen for this clinical use.
- Hyaluronic acid is the other contender for use as a scaffold. It is a nonsulfated GAG found in native hyaline articular cartilage. The hyaluronic acid interacts positively with CD44 and I-CAM-1. It also negatively influences chondrocyte apoptosis and decelerates oxidative stress and inhibits the catabolic interleukin (IL)-1. Hyaluronic acid has overall chondrogenic effect stimulating chondrocyte differentiation, influencing cellular mobility, differentiation, and development and regulating the matrix structure during chondrogenesis.
- Chitosan has been recently approved for clinical use for use in combination with bone marrow stimulation. It is derived from the crustacean shells.

Scaffold Geometry and Its Effect on Defect Repair

In order for cells to colonize (migration and adhesion) the scaffold and further mature to effect chondrogenesis (matrix synthesis) geometry and microarchitecture of synthetic or natural scaffolds are key determinant factors. The important properties of scaffolds like pore size (porosity) affect cell infiltration and matrix production. The stiffness of scaffold should match that of native matrix so that the cells have a natural "feel". Cells get important feedback through mechanosensitive molecules that are delivered through their substrates by pulling and "feeling" the resistance to deformation as it has been seen that cells in their nascent stage are highly sensitive to the nearby environment and conducive stability. This is established by the findings made by Engler et al. that MSCs express high levels of neurogenic transcriptional factors [nerve growth factor (NGF) and glial cell line-derived neurotrophic factor (GDNF)] on gels with low stiffness (0.1–1 kPa) along with neurogenic specific cytoskeletal factors. Myogenic transcriptional factors (Pax3, MyoD1) are highly expressed by MSCs on gels with intermediate stiffness (11 kPa). Increasing the stiffness of gels to 34 kPa, the seeded MSCs express the highest level of osteogenic factors (BMP1, BMP4, and CBF-α1). So, it is evident that changing the material properties of scaffolds will alter the cell lineage that gets generated. The systems should be optimized to improve the differentiation of implanted MSCs to chondrocyte and improve retention of these implanted cells.

BIOMOLECULES FOR CARTILAGE DEFECT REPAIR

Articular cartilage being avascular relies heavily on the biochemical and biophysical stimuli that affect its homeostasis and regenerative capacity. These soluble growth factors have been utilized for in vitro chondrogenesis and it is suggested that they can improve repair of the cartilage defect in vivo. The following are some of the prominent growth factors that can be used:

- Bone morphogenetic proteins (BMPs)—belonging to TGF-β family, they are the most widely studied and for maintaining chondrogenic phenotype BMP-4, BMP-6, and BMP-7 are identified to be most effective. They also upregulate cartilage matrix synthesis.
- Basic fibroblast growth factor 2 (FGF-2) strongly stimulates the MSCs and chondrocytes by enhancing the chondrogenic capacity (of MSCs) and ECM synthesis (of chondrocytes), especially when deployed in three-dimensional culture systems.
- Transforming growth factor-β and its isoforms (1, 2, and 3) evoke chondrogenic response in progenitor cells and MSCs.

Combinations of above enhance the desired effects. TGF-β, for example, when given with other growth factors, produces a greater chondrogenic response than when given alone. Platelet-derived growth factor (PDGF) also enhances cartilage matrix production by chondrocytes and simultaneously preventing endochondral maturation by inhibiting alkaline phosphatase (ALP) activity (a problem frequently encountered during cell expansion from MSCs during culture—discussed above). This is not without associated limitations, the relatively short half-lives and short-range diffusion of growth factors require a carrier system to enhance their action for tissue regeneration else effect in culture systems is not visible. This endures another use of scaffolds for delivering growth factors—another step advanced from what has been described till now.

Use of Scaffolds for Delivery of Growth Factors

The growth factors are required to continue the growth and proliferation of cartilage and avoid dedifferentiation. These are very labile and have short half-life. Also, there is a problem of quick washout and immediate release, if no slow-release systems are used. The release of desired growth factor from the scaffold on demand is the main goal of using them for growth factor delivery. As it is not possible to store the information in scaffolds, delivery is modulated by ingeniously improvising interactive response of these couture-made delivery systems to isolated or combined physical stimuli such as pH, temperature, and locally available enzymatic activity. The growth factors are incorporated onto scaffolds either through chemical immobilization or by physically encapsulating them or commonly both. Chemical immobilization is achieved through either covalent bonding of the growth factors onto the biomaterial or through noncovalent incorporation where the growth factor is incorporated with direct charge-to-charge interaction with the biomaterial. This is usually followed by secondary incorporation using physical methods. It involves the addition of microparticles encapsulating the desired growth factor into the biomaterial while synthesis. Microparticles developed from chitosan, alginate, and gelatin provide good controlled delivery of growth factors.

Mesenchymal Stem Cells

To address the concern of phenotype alteration in culture systems of chondrocytes, it is proposed to use adult MSCs as an alternative to chondrocytes due to:

- Multipotent cells are capable of differentiating into a variety of connective tissue cells including cartilage-like cells.
- Mesenchymal stem cells are trophic to cells in the sense that they also secrete a range of factors such as cytokines and growth factors. These cytokines facilitate cellular activity that ranges from differentiation to immunological response. The immunological response in vitro is suppressed through inhibition of TNF-α and interferon-γ (IFN-γ) secretion and direct inhibition of T-cell proliferation in vivo as the specific surface markers such as CD80 and CD86 are absent on them. These characteristics offer great advantage to their use in regenerative medicine and future tissue engineering interventions. A novel therapeutic approach involving MSCs is based on combining allogenic MSCs with autologous chondrocytes in their pericellular matrix (chondrons) together known as "Instant MSC Product accompanying Autologous Chondron Transplantation (IMPACT)". The chondrons are obtained from debrided cartilage tissue of the defect itself and recycled. The combination of this recycled chondrons with allogenic human bone marrow MSCs stimulates cartilage regeneration and results in regeneration of tissue qualitatively similar to ACI. IMPACT technique can be done in a single day avoiding multiple admissions and procedures.

Mesenchymal stem cells can be derived from a range of sources such as bone marrow, adipose tissue like Hoffa's fat pad and even synovium. The ideal cell source for cartilage reconstruction procedure is elusive due to conflicting reports in literature. There seems to be some superiority to bone marrow- and synovium-derived MSCs over others. Pleuripotential stem cells obtained from embryonic lineage or can be reprogrammed from somatic cells under influence of various factors such as Oct4, c-MYC, Sox4, Klf4, etc. producing induced pleuripotential stem cells (iPSCs). These programmed cells differentiate to form embryoid bodies that can be implanted to cartilage defect with or without scaffolds.

GENE THERAPY IN CARTILAGE TISSUE ENGINEERING

It appears that all these methods and advancements discussed above should solve the problems of cartilage regeneration and make chondrogenesis viable and easier. A practical look into currently available methods makes us rethink why cartilage repair is not so real still? The conventional methods of growth factor delivery are plagued with:

- Poor maintained concentration in desired levels due to short half-life of growth factors
- Need for repeated application
- Inconsistent delivery of the agent making most systems unreliable
- Diffusion of growth factors away from the desired region of action.

Gene therapy has been developed as a measure to circumvent the problems (specifically local factor availability and supply) associated with growth factor use in various systems.

Gene transfer delivers a therapeutic protein to a target cell or tissue that after incorporation starts acting as a local source of the particular growth factor (*see* also Chapter on "Gene Therapy in Orthopedics"). This provides a constant and regular source for the desired growth factor. Most commonly a plasmid DNA containing a specific reporter gene that can stimulate a desired gene expression (to synthesize a growth factor) is used for incorporation through a virus vector. Scaffolds have been developed that are used as carrier systems for plasmid DNA to develop what are now termed as "gene activated matrices" (GAMs). Specifically, if the plasmid DNA containing reporter genes is designed to elicit a chondrogenic response in the implanted cells, these GAMs can be deployed for cartilage healing. The encoding DNA plasmid can be introduced into the target cell by either viral or nonviral vectors. The viral vectors have proven effective transfection efficiencies and have been used for long, but there have always been concerns regarding the immunogenicity and carcinogenicity. This has warranted more emphasis on nonviral vectors. One such studied possible matrix is the collagen-glycosaminoglycan (CG) scaffold used as a carrier for nonviral vectors containing IGF-1 recombinant protein. When used in vivo it has shown that seeded chondrocytes synthesize significantly higher cartilage-like matrix than control scaffolds. Another logical and useful strategy is to use "dual-axis therapy" that can simultaneously enhance cartilage repair and counter the inhibitory influences. This method has shown greater potential in cartilage defect repair applications. Specifically, they use a combination of anabolic (IGF-1) and anti-catabolic (IL-1 antagonist) proteins to regulate tissue homeostasis using gene therapy. The anabolic proteins stimulate matrix production while simultaneously anticatabolic proteins inhibit expression of genes related to catabolic tissue response. The future therapies are majorly directed to gene therapy, but require capital and clearance of ethical issues. Possibly in future no surgical reconstruction will be required for cartilage defects.

CHONDROCYTE CULTURE AND COCULTURE SYSTEM

Background

Chondrocytes are extremely difficult to culture and proliferate and require strict conditions. The requirements have increased for the current use of these cells in ACI and similar cartilage reconstruction techniques. Chondrocytes give us good insight to investigate intracellular and molecular events associated with chondrocyte differentiation and activation. The main problem during culture is the tedious procedure and that the cultured chondrocytes tend to dedifferentiate into fibroblasts, especially during monoclonal expansion phase. This dedifferentiation during culture can be detected when chondrocytes start synthesizing collagen types I and III instead of collagen type II (articular chondrocytes) or type X (epiphyseal chondrocytes). The dedifferentiated cells also switch synthesis from high molecular weight proteoglycans (aggrecan) to low-molecular weight proteoglycans (biglycan and decorin). Various factors have been identified for this untoward process such as low-density plating, monolayer culturing, extraction from human adult cartilage, extraction from chondrosarcoma or immortalization, etc. To minimize conversion to fibroblasts extensive use of cells from young animals such as rabbits or cattle, which are more stable than human adult chondrocytes, is being promoted. Several immortalized chondrocyte cell lines have been shown to express a chondrocyte specific phenotype with a high proliferation rate. The problem with these is that the phenotypic stability is lost more quickly during expansion in serial monolayer cultures, compared with primary cultures of cells from juvenile animals. Recently, efforts to obtain a better phenotype than that of two-dimensional (2D) cultured chondrocytes have evolved. These include embedding the cells in an artificial matrix commonly made of stabilizers like alginate, agarose, or collagens. The chondrocyte phenotype is improved with their use, but on the flip side cellular growth is slowed making less number of cells available in the same time.

Procedure of Human Chondrocyte Culture

- For human primary articular chondrocytes complete culture medium consists of Dulbecco's modified Eagle's medium (high glucose) supplemented with 4 mM L-glutamine, 100 U/mL penicillin, and 0.1 mg/mL streptomycin and with 10% (v/v) fetal calf serum.
- Place the specimen in collection medium at 4°C. Mince all collected cartilage slices into about 1–3 mm^3 pieces.
- Rinse the cartilage once with sterile Dulbecco's phosphate-buffered Ca^{2+} and Mg^{2+} free saline (PBS).
- Add these to 10 mL of 0.2% trypsin solution. Stir the mixture, rinse, and transfer to 0.2% collagenase solution and centrifuge.
- Wash the cartilage pieces in 10 mL serum-free culture medium.
- Incubate for 90 minutes at 37°C in a CO_2 incubator while shaking.
- Centrifuge for 5 minutes at 200 g and discard the supernatant.
- Resuspend the pellet in 10 mL of complete culture medium and count the cells in a hemocytometer. Seed the suspended chondrocytes onto tissue culture plates or dishes at a density of 1×10^5 cells/cm^2.
- Incubate the culture plates or dishes for 2 days undisturbed at 37°C under humidified conditions and 5% CO_2/95% air to ensure strong attachment.
- Change the medium on the day before harvest.

The most recent advancement in cartilage reconstruction is the development of *co-culture systems.* These systems are emerging as novel methods that are a step ahead to the use of MSCs. They enhance the differentiation and chondrogenesis potential of MSCs. The major drawback of using MSCs only in the reconstruction is possibility of potential mineralization that occur with their use in chondrogenic conditions in vitro. This produces conditions similar to an endochondral ossification pathway. Such misrepresentation of differentiation pattern can be checked by the use of coculture systems by controlling the "crosstalk" between cells. The tendency to hypertrophy of the MSCs is inhibited by chondrocytes that secrete parathyroid hormone-related protein (PTHrP) in coculture (chondrocytes + MSCs) systems. The other interesting advantage of these systems is that MSCs have enhanced the proliferation of chondrocytes and stabilized their phenotype by secreting trophic factors. The chondrocyte-related gene expression and production of cartilage-like matrix in vitro have been seen in these coculture systems by upregulation of the specific pathways. These advantages (that nullify the disadvantages of either cell-culture system individually) make coculture systems current favorites though these are also not without limitations.

CONCLUSION

Articular cartilage is a specialized tissue having unique properties of being able to survive in low oxygen, low nutrition environment with the ability to bear all the stress and wear from continuous mobility. There is no other tissue that could have substituted for this marvellous structure.

- Articular cartilage maintains the low friction essential need for the synovial articulations else the movements would be too energy consuming and noisy!
- The advantage of being able to survive in low oxygen and low nutrition environment, however, makes the repair of the tissue also very difficult if it gets damaged. The reason is that because of low metabolism it is difficult to culture the cells outside the body (though now done at specialized centers) and also that the process is very slow. There are very limited avenues of supplying nutrition or improving vascularity to simulate healing as can be done for osseous or other metabolically active body tissues.
- Most of the therapeutic interventions are surgical only and broadly rely on either transplantation or in modern sense utilizing the totipotential cells for transforming into chondrocytes under proper milieu. AMIC offers single stage possibility to obtain cartilage repair.
- The newer modalities such as ACI, ACI-C, CACI, MACI, CCI, and repair systems using scaffolds ± growth factors or systems combining the use of mesenchymal cells, scaffolds, and growth factors have attracted interest of young and dynamic sports physicians and knee surgeons lately. It is important to realize that though claimed benefits are quite encouraging, proper training, and setup is essential for utilizing the modalities to maximum. There is still no standardization or definite recommendation to the use of one technique over other and not even the so-called "generations" of development of techniques are clear to majority. Some people label ACI, MACI, CACI, and mesenchymal cells with scaffolds as generation 1, 2, 3, and 4 which are incorrect in true sense as one

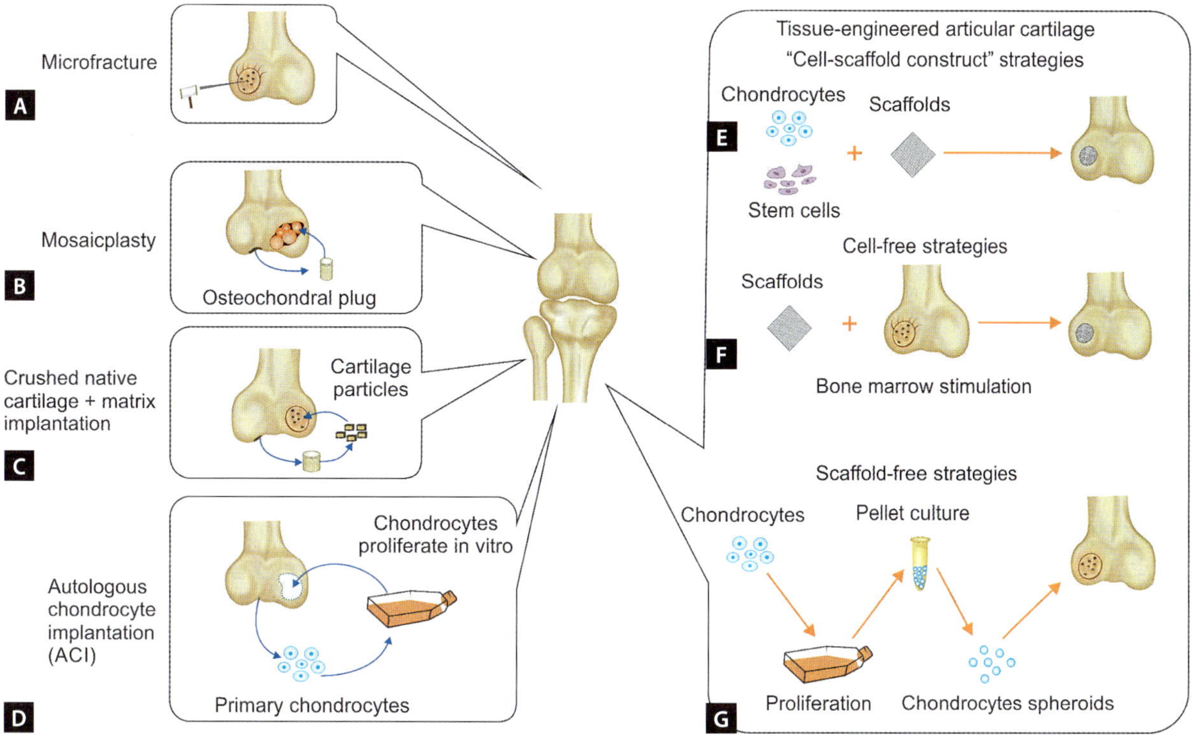

Figs. 21A to G: Illustration depicting various reconstructive methods and strategies used for reconstruction of cartilage defects. Details are available in the text. Specific points are highlighted here. Illustration (C) represents a specific form of matrix-assisted chondrocyte implantation (MACI) where instead of expanding chondrocytes in vitro, the native cartilage from nonweight-bearing region is taken and crushed/minced and reimplanted using suitable matrix into the debrided defect—so it is transplanting the chondrocytes sometimes referred to as MACT (T-transplantation). Illustration (E) demonstrates third generation techniques where chondrocyte health and proliferation is supported by modifying the environment using mesenchymal stromal/stem cells. This may also entail using specific growth factors. Illustration (F) depicts "microfracture plus" technique now quite popular for its simplicity and is also referred to as autologous matrix-induced chondrogenesis (AMIC). Schema (G) demonstrates alternative to ACI where instead of chondrocytes chondrospheres are used.
(ACI: autologous chondrocyte implantation)

technique is evolving from the other using majority of the components from base technique and there is no major shift of technology in ACI and CACI, they are mere variants of a technique. Until more research data and stability on the use of a technique develops it is better to restrict their use for specific patients and those not suitable to other more easier and quicker stable methods like mosaicplasty **(Figs. 21A to G)**.

CHAPTER 10

Joint Disorders Including Inflammatory and Noninflammatory Arthritis and Infective Arthritides (Including Mycobacterial infection and Prosthetic Joint Infection)

Manish Kumar Varshney

ARTHRITIS

Arthritis is a term that encompasses a variety of synovial joint centered inflammatory and noninflammatory disorders. It affects both sides of articulating surfaces (so osteonecrosis is not an arthritis) variably involving cartilage and synovial membrane. The disorders are characterized by painful loss of joint motion, swelling, and joint deformity. When left untreated, these disorders cause severe disability and increased mortality. Because of the noninflammatory nature in many, the use of suffix "itis" is not consistent and instead "osis" is recommended. Still because the term arthr"itis" is so commonly ingrained that it is difficult to altogether modify the terminology. In general, they can be grouped into productive (noninflammatory) and nonproductive (inflammatory) arthritis. In the former, there is significant proliferative bony reaction but inflammation is not the primary inciting factor while in latter joint inflammation is of prime occurrence. There is another way to group the arthritides, based on the presence or absence of rheumatoid factor (i.e., seropositivity) and is commonly followed in the clinics. Those who are positive fall under the group of seropositive arthritis and are commonly rheumatoid arthritis (RA) if clinically supported. The other group (seronegative) can be further classified based on inflammatory or noninflammatory affection of joints. So the classification system can be broadly presented as:

- Arthritis:
  - Seropositive arthritis—RA
  - Seronegative arthritis:
    - Noninflammatory arthritis—Osteoarthritis, hypothyroidism
    - Inflammatory arthritis:
      - Monoarthritis—Gout, septic arthritis, tuberculous arthritis
      - Oligoarthritis—Gout, spondyloarthropathy [(1) ankylosing spondylitis (AS), (2) psoriatic arthritis (PsA), (3) reactive arthritis, (4) arthritis associated with inflammatory bowel disorders (enteropathic arthritis), and (5) undifferentiated SpA], psoriasis
      - Polyarthritis—SLE, psoriasis, RA.

OSTEOARTHRITIS (OSTEOARTHROSIS, ARTHROSIS, AND DEGENERATIVE JOINT DISEASE)

INTRODUCTION

Osteoarthritis is not a suitable term (particularly the use of "itis") but for its contemporary usage the term is retained and slowly we are realizing that the term is not also absolutely wrong. For the classical usage of suffix "itis" depicting inflammatory pathology, a number of authors have suggested using alternative term like osteoarthrosis or degenerative joint disease for this age-related mechanical degeneration of joint. Arthritis implies inflammation of a diarthrodial (synovial membrane-lined) joint, yet in osteoarthritis there is negligible inflammation. As the knowledge advances, however, a lot of inflammatory mediators are being recognized responsible for the development of this disease so osteoarthr "itis" may not be completely wrong.

By definition "osteoarthritis" is a typical productive, progressive arthropathy (better considered syndrome) with heterogeneous clinical presentation that can occur in any synovial joint though it commonly affects the hands, feet, knees, hips, and spine. Osteoarthritis is considered to result from excessive mechanical stress applied to susceptible joints predisposed on chondrocyte dysfunction (that may be genetic or environmental—see below). The susceptibility in turn arises from genetic inheritance, female sex (twice as common than males), family history, ethnicity (Caucasians are prone), higher than normal bone mineral density (BMD), and obesity. Osteoarthritis can arise as:

- A common age-related disorder (primary or idiopathic form), or
- Could be end-result of other arthritis or disorders or trauma (secondary form).

In any case, the primary sites of tissue injury in osteoarthritis are the cartilage of the joint and the subchondral bone. Cartilage damage is primary while the microfractures in subchondral bone lead to proliferation of new bone at the periphery. The microfractures are accompanied by a healing process that increases the density of the bone just under the cartilage surface, resulting in subchondral

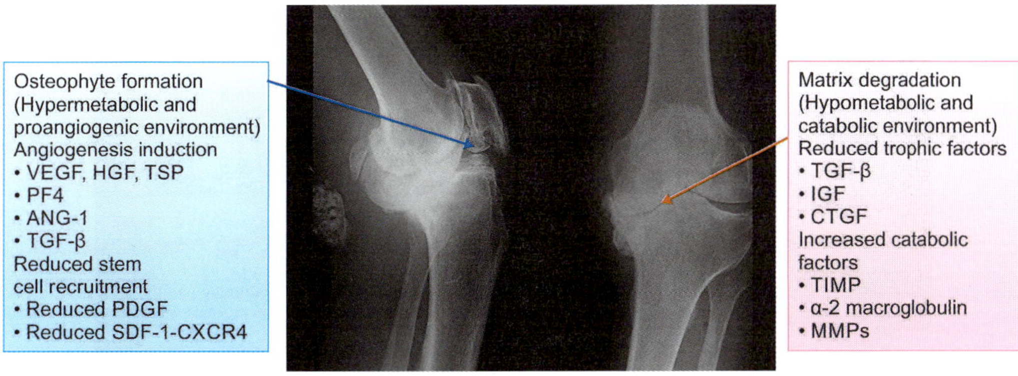

Fig. 1: Osteoarthritis inflammatory pathway (In addition to the mentioned cytokines, interleukin beta-1 produced by chondrocytes, osteoblasts, and synoviocytes play a key role in inflammatory response by magnifying the production of catabolic cytokines and ultimately reducing the production of type-2 collagen and causing aggrecan proteolysis. The inflammatory and catabolic effect gets prolonged in the presence of tumor necrosis factor-alpha). (ANG-1: angiopoietin-1; CTGF: connective tissue growth factor; CXC: chemokine ligand 4; HGF: hepatocyte growth factor; IGF: insulin-like growth factor; MMP: matrix metalloproteinases; PDGF: platelet-derived growth factor; PF4: platelet factor 4; SDF-1: stromal cell derived factor; TGF-β: transforming growth factor; TIMP: tissue inhibitor of metalloproteinases; TSP: thrombospondin-1; VEGF: vascular endothelial growth factor)

sclerosis. The damage to hyaline articular cartilage and associated bony remodeling is visible radiologically as joint space narrowing, osteophytes, and subchondral cysts leading to structural and functional failure of joint ("joint failure" akin to heart failure). Variable degrees of synovitis and thickening of the joint capsule is seen in some patients. Osteoarthritis is classically described as a purely mechanical (disequilibrium between breakdown and repair of the tissues) and noninflammatory arthritis but now it is clearly recognized that inflammatory pathways are upregulated as well with release of inflammatory cytokines by the cartilage **(Fig. 1)**. The chondrocytes release degradative proteolytic enzymes in response to stress, which result in the changes of the cartilage seen in osteoarthritis. The renewed interest in osteoarthritis is due to the realization of the dynamic component of disease, but still the disease is assessed and managed clinically as a structural rather than physiological disorder.

EPIDEMIOLOGY

Osteoarthritis is the most common form of arthritis and a leading cause of disability in the modern world.

- Osteoarthritis of at least one joint occurs in 80% of population above 75 years of age. The fact that the incidence of osteoarthritis increases significantly with age has led to the erroneous conclusion that osteoarthritis is simply an age-related degenerative condition. Osteoarthritis arises due to combined influence of ligamentous laxity, a failure of the periarticular structures such as muscles and proprioceptors to function appropriately, a reduction in matrix production by chondrocytes, or decreased responsiveness of chondrocytes to growth factors.
- There is no gender difference for milder form of disease; however, the severe form favors females. The nodal generalized form of the disease is also commonly seen in females.
- Osteoarthritis of hip is more common in Europeans than Asians (especially Indians).
- Symptomatic osteoarthritis is poorly correlated with radiographic appearance. Half of adults older than 50 years with radiographic osteoarthritis are symptomatic as is also the case with knee osteoarthritis. Radiographic hand osteoarthritis on the contrary is symptomatic in only 3–7% cases.

ETIOLOGY

Osteoarthritis is likely a genetically heterogeneous disease with strong environmental influence. The following are the commonly cited causes (also considered risk factors) for osteoarthritis **(Fig. 2)**.

Age: The single risk factor most strongly correlated with osteoarthritis is increasing age. Osteoarthritis is the most common chronic disease in later life; >80% of persons over age 75 years are affected. The disease progresses with age and the clinical severity and radiological changes get worsened gradually. There are age-related changes in articular cartilage (see Section on cartilage structure and function) that are most probably responsible for this. However, all the age-related cartilage changes do not match the cartilage damage of osteoarthritis so ancillary and genetic factors do play a role. The differences in the cartilage changes between age-related degeneration and osteoarthritis related cartilage changes are tabulated in section on cartilage structure and function.

Genetics: The Framingham Study and the Baltimore Longitudinal Study on Aging clearly support a significant genetic contribution to osteoarthritis, with evidence for a major recessive gene and a multifactorial component, representing either polygenic or environmental factors. There is a significantly higher concordance for osteoarthritis between monozygotic twins than between dizygotic twins. Inherited forms of osteoarthritis may be caused by mutations in several genes that are expressed in cartilage, including those encoding Types IV, V, and VI collagen, as well as cartilage oligomeric matrix protein (COMP). The

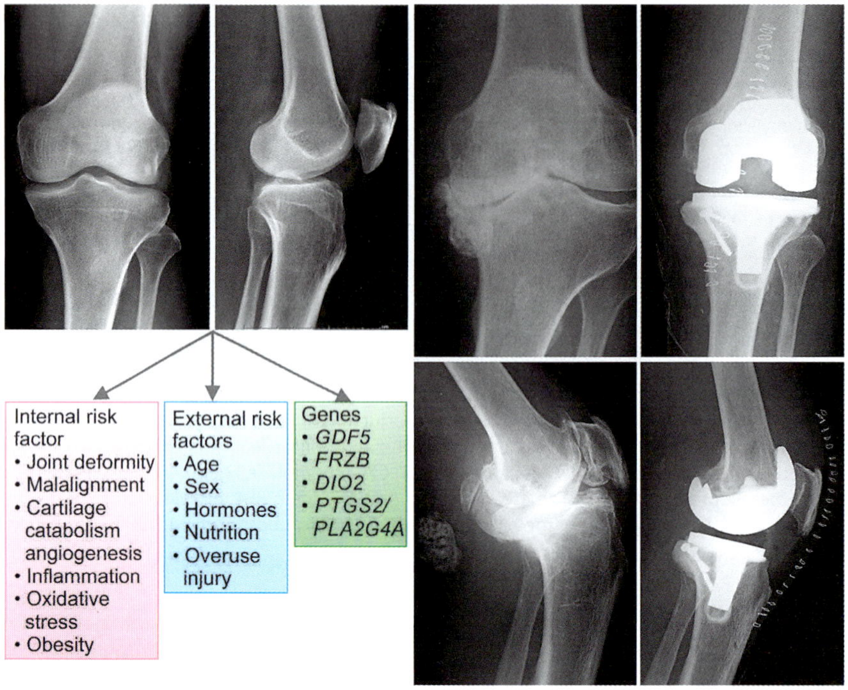

Fig. 2: Various factors responsible for development of osteoarthritis.

haplotype of a vitamin D receptor (VDR) that plays a vital role in controlling BMD appears to be associated with a two-fold risk of knee osteoarthritis (although the VDR locus is very close to the COL2A1 locus on chromosome 12q, so that the association may be due to linkage disequilibrium with the latter).

Familial: Nodal generalized osteoarthritis is seen to run in families.

Joint location: Weight-bearing joints are commonly affected but the effect is differential, e.g., the age-related stress distortions in cartilage increase in femoral head but decrease in talus. This explains occurrence of osteoarthritis in hip and knee with age but not in ankle. Also knee chondrocytes exhibit more interleukin-1 (IL-1) receptors than ankle chondrocytes and that knee chondrocytes express mRNA for matrix metalloproteinase-8 (MMP-8), whereas chondrocytes from the ankle do not.

Trauma (intra-articular fractures): They produce joint incongruence and malalignment. Altered joint geometry may interfere with nutrition of the cartilage, or it may alter load distribution, either of which may result in altered biochemical composition of the cartilage, irrespective of age.

Repetitive joint use: Athletes and contact sports players have higher incidence of osteoarthritis. Repetitive trauma at a subfracture level has been shown to accelerate remodeling in the zone of calcified cartilage, with reduplication of the tidemark and thinning of the noncalcified zone resulting in stiffening of the subchondral bone, increased wear of the overlying cartilage, and ultimately development of osteoarthritis. A lot of factors interplay in the development of post-traumatic osteoarthritis or osteoarthritis due to repetitive use as in athletes **(Fig. 3)**. Occupations that require regular kneeling and squatting are correlated with an increased incidence of knee osteoarthritis.

Obesity: It is the most important modifiable factor for knee osteoarthritis (but not hip) in both the patellofemoral joint and tibiofemoral joint especially in women. There is a close association with new-onset and progression of knee osteoarthritis with obesity. Obesity not only increases the forces at weight-bearing joints, but may also change posture, gait, and physical activity level, any or all of which may further contribute to altered joint biomechanics. Adipokines such as leptin, adiponectin, and visfatin produced by white adipose tissue are proinflammatory cytokines and are also expressed by osteoblasts, synoviocytes, and chondrocytes that are important part of the inflammatory process and matrix degradation. Weight reduction programs have a definite role in management of osteoarthritis. For every 6 kg weight loss [approximately 2 body mass index (BMI)] the risk of developing knee osteoarthritis dropped >50%. It is interesting to note that increased body weight protects against osteoarthritis in birds!

Joint dysplasias, deformations, and malalignment: Perthes disease, genu varum, achondroplasia, developmental dysplasia of hip, and recurrent dislocation of patella all predispose to early development of osteoarthritis. I personally feel that joint instability and/or mechanical derangement is the most important factor for development of osteoarthritis in lower limbs. Even 5° of varus at knee increases 70–90% loading of the medial knee compartment increasing the risk of osteoarthritis fourfold while 5° of valgus increases similar risk in lateral compartment by five times.

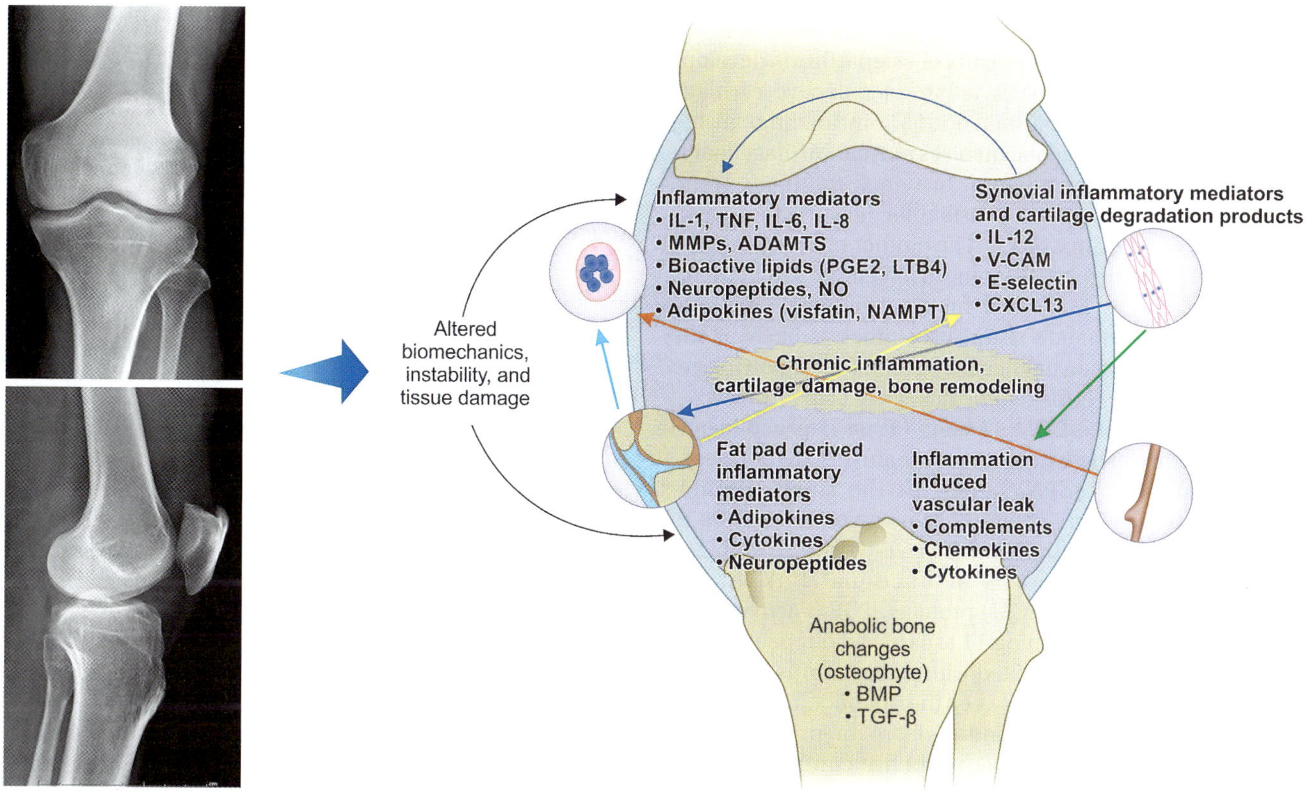

Fig. 3: Trauma and overuse injury to joint. (ADAMTS: alpha-disintegrin and metalloproteinase with thrombospondin motifs; BMP: bone morphogenic protein; CXCL: chemokine ligand-1; IL: interleukin; LTB: lymphotoxin β; MMP: matrix metalloproteinases; PG: prostaglandin; TGF: transforming growth factor; TNF: tumor necrosis factor; V-CAM: vascular cell adhesion molecule)

Preceding crystal deposition and endocrine disorders: They alter the structural integrity of cartilage and predispose for early osteoarthritis.

Smoking: It may have a protective role but rigorous studies required/needed (ethically difficult).

Higher bone density: This has been linked to osteoarthritis of the hip and knee, but not the hand. The stiff subchondral bone deforms less under loading; increasing stress to the cartilage.

Low vitamin C and D: These are associated with progression of knee osteoarthritis.

Gender: Before 50 years of age osteoarthritis is more common in men due primarily to joint injury occurring from sports and accidents. After 50 years women are about twice as likely as men to develop osteoarthritis and this difference is quite startling for severe disease. The gender differences in osteoarthritis incidence after the age of 50 years may be the result of postmenopausal estrogen deficiency. Nuclear estrogen receptors (ERs) have been detected in articular chondrocytes of humans. Chondrocytes express two isoforms of ER-ER-α and ER-β—that may have different organ specific roles; ER-α is expressed more predominantly in cortical bone and ER-β in cartilage and cancellous bone. Estrogen stimulates production of proteoglycan in cartilage. There is a small role of reduced quadriceps strength and increased hand muscle strength to development of knee osteoarthritis in females and hand osteoarthritis in men.

BOX 1: Principal types of osteoarthritis and their putative etiologies.

Primary (Idiopathic) type:
- Genetic
- Chondropathy
- Various intrinsic and extrinsic factors as shown in **Figure 2**

Secondary type:
- Trauma—most important secondary factor especially for osteoarthritis hip in India
  - Joint trauma (intra-articular and otherwise)
  - Ligament injury
- *Metabolic/endocrine:*
  - Hemochromatosis
  - Acromegaly
  - Hyperparathyroidism
  - Ochronosis
- Inflammatory disorders
- *Neuropathic disorders:*
  - Diabetes mellitus
- *Crystal deposition disease:*
  - Calcium pyrophosphate
  - Uric acid
  - Hydroxyapatite
- *Anatomical abnormalities:*
  - Bony dysplasia

Apart from the above etiologies for primary or idiopathic osteoarthritis, there are various identified secondary causes of osteoarthritis provided in **Box 1**.

PATHOPHYSIOLOGY AND PATHOGENESIS

There are two major mechanisms of osteoarthritis development. The first one involves failure of defective cartilage (genetic or otherwise) to sustain normal joint loading causing joint damage. The other one involves normal cartilage that is injured by repeated microtrauma or a single traumatic event.

A *genetic basis* appears possible for polyarticular small joint nodal arthritis in women. The mother of a woman with distal interphalangeal (DIP) joint involvement (Heberden's nodes) is twice as likely to exhibit osteoarthritis in these joints, and the proband's sister three times as likely as the mother and sister of an unaffected woman. The following are some putative targets for genetic linkage of osteoarthritis:

- Mutations in the *COL2A1* gene (Type II procollagen) have been inflicted; however, mechanisms are not clear.
- Asporin gene (*ASPN*) codes for the small leucine-rich proteoglycan subfamily of proteins that binds to transforming growth factor-β (TGF-β) and to collagen and aggrecan. There is a functional link among extracellular matrix (ECM) proteins, TGF-β activity, and disease. *ASPN* containing 14 aspartic acid repeats (D14) was significantly associated with osteoarthritis knee.
- There is an imbalance between the catabolic and anabolic pathways of cartilage metabolism in osteoarthritis **(Fig. 3)**. The catabolic pathways are commonly associated with proinflammatory proteins, including IL-1β, tumor necrosis factor-β (TNF-β), IL-17, macrophage inflammatory protein-1β (MIP), etc. Proteinases (such as cysteine proteinases, metalloproteinases, and serine proteinases) are upregulated in response to stress on cartilage. There is impairment of production of new ECM proteins by chondrocytes under the influence of cytokines while increased degradation of the products already present. Members of MMP include ADAM and ADAMTS (alpha-disintegrin and metalloproteinase with thrombospondin motifs), a haplotype of the *ADAM12* gene polymorphism is associated with osteoarthritis knee (sevenfold increased risk in females).
- Alteration in the canonical Wnt signaling pathway—single nucleotide polymorphism in the *FRZB* (strong association) and possibly *LRP5* (indefinite) is associated with osteoarthritis hip.
- *BMP2* is associated with development of osteoarthritis of knee while *GDF5* (required for formation of bones and joints in the limbs, skull, and axial skeleton) has been associated with hip osteoarthritis in Asian population (Chinese and Japanese).

Traumatic insult and increased IL-1 stimulate chondrocytes to undergo cell division ("cloning") and start repair, producing increased quantities of collagen, metalloproteinases and proteoglycans. This leads to thickening of cartilage in the very early stages of osteoarthritis (because of increased proteoglycan accumulation) but the repaired tissue has qualitatively inferior type 1 collagen and has increased fibronectin. Patchy sclerosis and osteophytes, however, reduce bone elasticity transferring increasing loads to the cartilage causing further damage **(Fig. 3)**. Synovitis occurs in reaction to degraded cartilage and bone and soluble matrix proteins. Lost structural integrity of menisci and anterior cruciate ligament (ACL) (with associated altered joint mechanics), joint incongruence, poor muscle strength, continued physical activity, and excessive biomechanical overload of the joint can lead to development of osteoarthritis after inadequately treated trauma or its residual effects. Cartilage damage can occur through direct impact of trauma in three ways—(1) cartilage only disruption, (2) fracture along tidemark, and (3) fracture through the calcified cartilage into subchondral bone (sort of osteochondral lesion) all of which can progress over time to develop into osteoarthritis. There is a fourfold increased risk of developing osteoarthritis in a previously injured knee. Trauma *is the second most important modifiable risk* factor after obesity for development and progression of osteoarthritis.

Angiogenesis and osteoarthritis: Angiogenesis is related to synovial inflammation and is an intermediary pathway for development of osteoarthritis. Angiogenesis is responsible for immigration of inflammatory cells and release of inflammatory mediators into the joint. The angiogenic factors are released by synovial macrophages, endothelial cells, and synoviocytes with possible interaction of VEGF.

Metabolic changes in the synovial membrane lead to decreased concentration and viscosity of the synovial fluid and poor lubrication characteristics. Endogenous production of growth factors such as TGF-β and BMPs have been implicated in driving osteophyte formation and synovial thickening associated with osteoarthritis.

MICROSTRUCTURAL PROGRESSION OF OSTEOARTHRITIS

The osteoarthritic changes are found to progress in following stages:

Stage 1: Proteolytic breakdown of the cartilage matrix along with altered chondrocyte metabolism. The chondrocytes produce increased amount of catabolic enzymes (metalloproteinases like collagenase and stromelysin) destroying the cartilage matrix. The production of protease inhibitors [tissue inhibitors of metalloproteinases (TIMP) 1 and 2] is reduced.

Stage 2: Fibrillation and erosion of the cartilage, releasing the degenerated and altered proteoglycan and collagen fragments into synovial fluid producing inflammatory reaction.

Stage 3: Chronic inflammatory reaction in the synovium. Production of metalloproteinases, IL-1, and TNF-β by synovial macrophages. Other proinflammatory molecules like free radicals may also be a factor.

Stage 4: Alteration in the joint architecture and compensatory bone overgrowth further irritate the synovium and a vicious cycle gets laid down.

Tissue Biomarkers of Osteoarthritis

It can very well be argued that with the consistent diagnosis of osteoarthritis on radiographs there is no need for biomarkers; however, it is a fact that the patient's symptoms and function (biology) does not always match with the images (radiographs). The term "pre-arthritis" has been used to define cellular and matrix changes that occur before osteoarthritis can be diagnosed by conventional means and may serve in future to identify patients at risk. Tissue markers for break down products of Type II collagen [urinary C-terminal telopeptide II (uCTX-II)] and aggrecan turnover, anabolic peptide of collagen Type-III [serum N-propeptide III (PIIINP)], an index of synovial cell turnover [urinary glucosyl-galactosyl pyridinoline (uGly-Gal-PYD)], metalloproteinases, serum cartilage oligomeric protein (COMP), and tissue cytokines [inflammatory biomarkers—nitric oxide (NO), IL-1β, and TNF-β] may be used to diagnose and assess the burden of disease. Treatment efficacy can be judged by uCTX-II, urinary MMP-1 and 3, and serum hyaluronic acid (sHA) levels. In addition there are some "prognostic biomarkers" that have been related to monitor the progression of osteoarthritis like IL-6, adiponectin, leptin, and previously mentioned uCTX and COMP. MRI is considered the imaging modality of choice to show early changes in cartilage. Nuclei-based MRI techniques using phosphorus, fluorine, or especially sodium allow the capture of high-contrast images of cartilage. Delayed gadolinium enhanced MRI allows measurement of glycosaminoglycan content and can be useful for early detection of OA.

CLINICAL FEATURES AND DIAGNOSIS

Symptomatic knee osteoarthritis is defined as pain on most days with radiographic evidence of joint degeneration. This occurs in 12% of the persons older than 55 years of age. The clinical features of osteoarthritis are varied for different joints. Hip osteoarthritis is uncommon in Indian subcontinent. The shoulders, hips, and knee osteoarthritis were commonly described in miners. Hand involvement had been classically described in craftsmen, construction workers, and miners. The commonly affected knee and hip joints have typical presentations that can be used for diagnostic purposes **(Box 2)**. The diagnostic criteria for knee joint have been elaborated more by ACR **(Table 1)**. The common *symptoms of* osteoarthritis include:

- Pain is undoubtedly the most important symptom of osteoarthritis, especially activity related or mechanical pain. There is another type of pain commonly found in these patients that is inflammatory pain. These two types have specific characteristics that help in distinguishing them **(Table 2)**. The degree of joint pain does not always correlate with the degree of structural changes seen on radiographs (concordance increases with severity of damage however). Young patients often have maximal pain several hours after the physical activities. Pain at night could be present in patients with mild osteoarthritis who have used joints for several hours (sports person), patients with advanced osteoarthritis with severe destructive changes in bone and cartilage breakdown and in acute inflammatory exacerbation of

BOX 2: American College of Rheumatology (ACR) radiological and clinical criteria for knee and hip osteoarthritis.

Knee osteoarthritis (sensitivity = 91% and specificity of 86%):

1. Knee pain "AND" one of the following:
   a. Age >50 years
   b. Morning stiffness <30 minutes
   c. Crepitus
2. "AND" radiologic osteophytes

Hip osteoarthritis (sensitivity of 91% and specificity of 89%):

1. Hip pain "AND" at least two of the following features:
   a. ESR < 20 mm 1st hour
   b. Radiologic osteophytes
   c. Radiologic joint space narrowing

(ESR: erythrocyte sedimentation rate in 1st hour)

TABLE 1: Criteria for classification of osteoarthritis of knee joint.

Clinical and laboratory	*Clinical and radiographic*	*Clinical*
Knee pain + at least 5 of 9 below (92% sensitive and 75% specific)	Knee pain + at least 1 of 3 below (91% sensitive and 86% specific)	Knee pain + at least 3 (ideally 4) of 6 below (95% sensitive and 69% specific)
• Age >50 years • Stiffness <30 minutes • Crepitus • Bony tenderness • Bony enlargement • No palpable warmth • ESR < 40 mm/1st hour • RF <1:40 • Synovial fluid analysis of osteoarthritis	• Age >50 years • Stiffness <30 minutes • Crepitus + Osteophytes on radiographs	• Age >50 years • Stiffness <30 minutes • Crepitus • Bony tenderness • Bony enlargement • No palpable warmth

(ESR: erythrocyte sedimentation rate; RF: rheumatoid factor)

TABLE 2: Joint pain in osteoarthritis.

Mechanical joint pain	*Inflammatory joint pain*
Deep and dull ache, localized to one or a few joints	It is a burning pain that could persist for days. This is infrequent and inconsistent pain and may have relapsing character.
Aggravated by prolonged use or strenuous activity	Could be triggered by weather changes, prolonged walking, minor sprain, or from misplacement of the feet during walking on uneven surfaces.
Pain felt often by end of day or with increased mechanical loading of joint	Pain usually associated with morning stiffness and is felt more at beginning of day but lasts <30 minutes.
Relieved by rest or gentle massage	Relieved by rest and ice but dramatic relief with anti-inflammatory medication.
In advanced disease, the pain is constant and even appears at night. Sudden sharp pain may get superimposed often appearing during movements after a period of rest.	With advanced disease, this is often associated with inflammatory effusion and increased intensity superseding the mechanical pain.

the disease. The pain may be referred from its location sometimes confusing from other disorders. The pain of osteoarthritis hip may be referred to knee, pain of cervical facet joints may be referred to shoulder, arm, forearm, and hand while that of lumbar facet joint pain may radiate to the lower limbs resembling sciatica. The origin of osteoarthritic pain is debatable but one or more of the following factors contribute definitely:

- Subchondral bone microfracture
- Periosteal stretching by osteophytes
- The stretching of ligaments and capsule (cartilage is not innervated so does not cause pain)
- "Bone angina" caused by intraosseous hypertension and intraosseous stasis. This results from reduced functional caliber of blood vessels due to thickened trabeculae. This may be partially responsible for night pains.
- Joint inflammation and irritation of nociceptive receptors in synovium, capsule, and enthesitis.
- Stretching of joint and ligament capsule by altered joint mechanics—varus/valgus laxity and joint opening on the "other" side of joint involvement.
- Bursitis due to constant friction and altered mechanics causing activity related pain.

- Stiffness of short duration ("gelling" of joints) often described as a short-lived stiffness seen after inactivity localized to the joint region (unlike diffuse of RA). It appears after period of prolonged inactivity like watching movie in theater (movie-theater sign, though it was classically described for chondromalacia).
- Reduced movements, crepitus, and swelling (acute on chronic presentation) are features of late and advanced disease—a decrease in joint mobility is the first sign in the course of the disease (decrease internal rotation of the hip, decreased external rotation of the shoulder, decrease in knee flexion). Bony swelling and crepitus stand out as the best signs for clinical differentiation at an advanced stage of the disease. Joint effusion occurs during inflammatory exacerbations and fluid has a high viscosity, a low cell count, and no crystals.
- Joint instability—This is a feeling of instability or buckling (shifting of bone surfaces without actually giving way). This arises due to:
  - Muscle fatigue from increased coefficient of friction in joint and increased work.
  - Muscle inhibition due to pain and so reduced splinting action across joint.
  - Ligament laxity due to abnormal joint opening stresses.

The *physical findings* of osteoarthritis include:

- Joint line tenderness due to myofascial trigger points, adjacent bursitis or tendonitis, and ligament enthesopathy.
- Crepitus on joint movement—palpable cracking or crunching sound.
- Bony enlargement often felt along the joint line (differentiate from enthesopathies that represent calcification of sites of tendon, ligament or joint capsule insertion). In hand Heberden's nodes (DIP) and Bouchard's nodes (PIP) are frequently encountered. They arise form periarticular bony hypertrophy and subchondral gelatinous cyst formation on dorsal surface of involved joints. *Squared hand* appearance may arise from angular deformities of CMC and MCP joints. The notion that Heberden's nodes are characteristic of osteoarthritis and Bouchard's nodes for RA should be dropped. It is true that RA involves PIP but it is an inflammatory and not a productive arthropathy so formation of nodes occurs commonly with osteoarthritis and in secondary joint degeneration with RA. So that there is early appearance of Heberden's nodes in osteoarthritis while Bouchard's nodes appear later or in inflammatory form of osteoarthritis. In RA, on the other hand, the Bouchard's nodes appear with advanced disease but Heberden's nodes will be very rare. Also there is a significant overlap in the pattern of joint involvement in the two diseases so these nodes should not be used as a distinguishing feature.
- Restricted joint ROM—Caused by variable contribution of pain, effusion, capsular contractures, muscle spasm or weakness, loose bodies, joint malalignment, and altered center of rotation. Both active and passive movements should be tested to differentiate them and following points may help:
  - Effusion produces elastic end feeling.
  - Intra-articular loose body often produces sudden stop and then a *springy* bounce back.
  - Hard end feel is commonly due to capsular contracture or involuntary muscle spasm.
  - Bony hard end feel is produced by impinging large osteophytes and joint malalignment.
- Painful ROM especially terminal in early disease that increases in arc with disease progression.
- Joint deformity varus at knee **(Figs. 4A and B)**, angulation at PIP and DIP, flexion, adduction, and external rotation at hip.
- Muscle atrophy

CLINICAL STAGING OF OSTEOARTHRITIS

Early stage: The pain and stiffness are intermittent. Pain is often felt after prolonged activity while stiffness appears following prolonged rest (movie-theater sign). Patients may have acute exacerbations and seasonal changes in symptoms gradually becoming more frequent.

Moderate osteoarthritis: The pain progresses with the passage of day. Symptoms are present daily but relief is prompt with analgesics (use increases progressively) and may have intermittent periods of minimal symptoms needing no medications. Patients, however, usually avoid strenuous and aggressive activity. Joint line tenderness is prominent and joint effusions occur commonly. In dry form of disease, anterior knee pain due to fat pad inoculation of cartilage degradation products with ensuing inflammation is the hallmark.

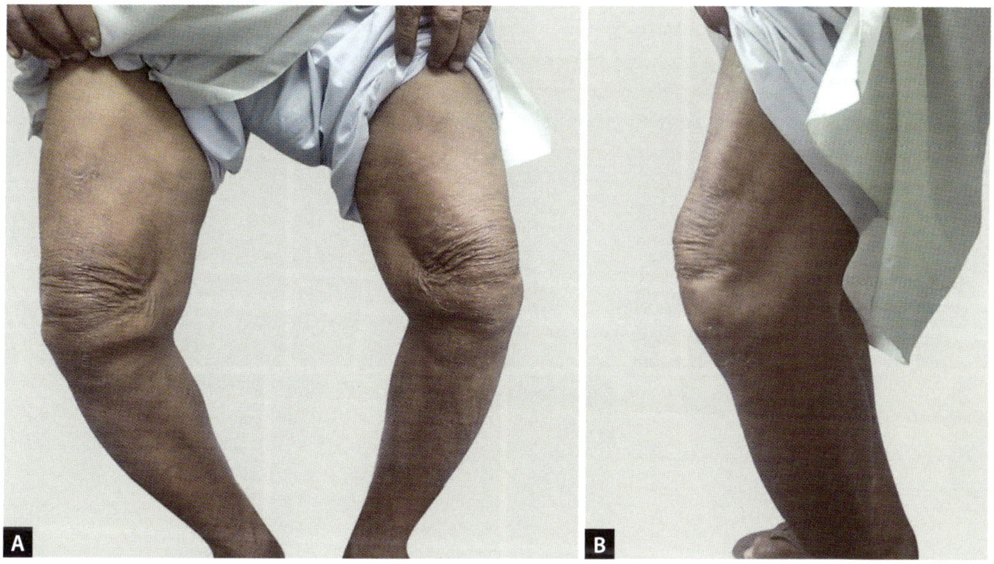

Figs. 4A and B: Osteoarthritis knee. Note the severe varus deformity at (A) knee in the patient with (B) fixed flexion deformity.

Severe or advanced osteoarthritis: There is alteration of the structure of synovial fluid reducing the lubrication. Osteophytes impinge on ligaments producing pain on all movements and restricting them terminally. Joint is felt to have bony excrescences and appears bumpy ("bumpy and wobbly joints"). Pain and stiffness are marked with instability during walk due to joint erosion. Full loss of the cartilaginous joint surface in severe osteoarthritis allows bone to rub on bone. The articular surface becomes polished and sometimes even grooved, a process called "eburnation". There are fixed deformities and gait pattern changes with slow walking and some patients also feel breathlessness. The stress on spine increases causing back pain. Use of analgesics is frequent and later the highest dose of analgesics also fails to relive symptoms fully.

INVESTIGATIONS

Radiographic investigations are the most common investigations performed. There are various staging systems; the commonly used ones for knee and hip are presented in **Tables 3 and 4**. The radiopathologic correlations of osteoarthritis are presented below:

- Cartilage fibrillation and erosion = joint space narrowing (may be localized)
- Subchondral new bone formation = subchondral sclerosis
- Myxoid degeneration = subchondral cysts (geodes formation)
- Trabecular compression = bone collapse/attrition
- Fragmentation of osteochondral surface = loose bodies

In India, primary osteoarthritis of knee is common while that of hip is rare; the various radiographic features for different stages are shown in **Figures 5A to H**. Arthroscopy may be used for confirmation in specific situations (unicompartmental osteoarthritis of knee) or sometimes to stage arthritis, which can show cartilage and synovial membrane abnormalities and also detect osteophytes. CT scan, MRI, and ultrasonography are not recommended for diagnostic purpose.

TABLE 3: Radiographic staging system for osteoarthritis knee.

Kellgren and Lawrence (KL) system	*Ahlbäck classification system*
Grade 0: No discernable radiographic features of osteoarthritis present *Grade 1:* "Doubtful" joint space narrowing and possible osteophytic lipping *Grade 2:* Definite osteophyte(s) and possible joint space narrowing ("minimal") on AP weight-bearing radiograph *Grade 3:* Multiple osteophytes, definite JSN ("moderate"), sclerosis, minimal bony deformity *Grade 4 ("severe"):* Large osteophytes, marked joint space narrowing, severe sclerosis and definite bony deformity disturbing the bony contour or joint alignment	*Grade 1:* Joint space narrowing (<3 mm) [equivalent to grade 3 KL ("moderate") system] *Grade 2:* Joint space obliteration [this and all below are equivalent to grade 4 KL ("severe")] *Grade 3:* Minor bone attrition (0–5 mm) *Grade 4:* Moderate bone attrition (5–10 mm) *Grade 5:* Severe bone attrition (>10 mm)

TABLE 4: Radiological staging of osteoarthritis hip.

Radiographic grading	*MRI grading*
Grade 0: No radiographic evidence *Grade 1:* Possible joint space narrowing and subtle osteophytes *Grade 2:* Definite joint space narrowing, definite osteophytes and some sclerosis, especially in acetabular region *Grade 3:* Significant joint space reduction, small osteophytes, some sclerosis and geodesic formation in femoral head and acetabulum *Grade 4:* Gross loss of joint space with above features plus large osteophytes and increased deformity of the femoral head and acetabulum	*Grade 0:* Normal *Grade 1:* Inhomogeneous high signal intensity in cartilage (T2) *Grade 2:* Inhomogeneity with areas of high signal intensity in articular cartilage (T2); indistinct trabeculae or signal intensity loss in femoral head and neck (T1) *Grade 3:* Above along with indistinct zone between femoral head and acetabulum; subchondral signal loss due to bone sclerosis *Grade 4:* Above plus femoral head deformity

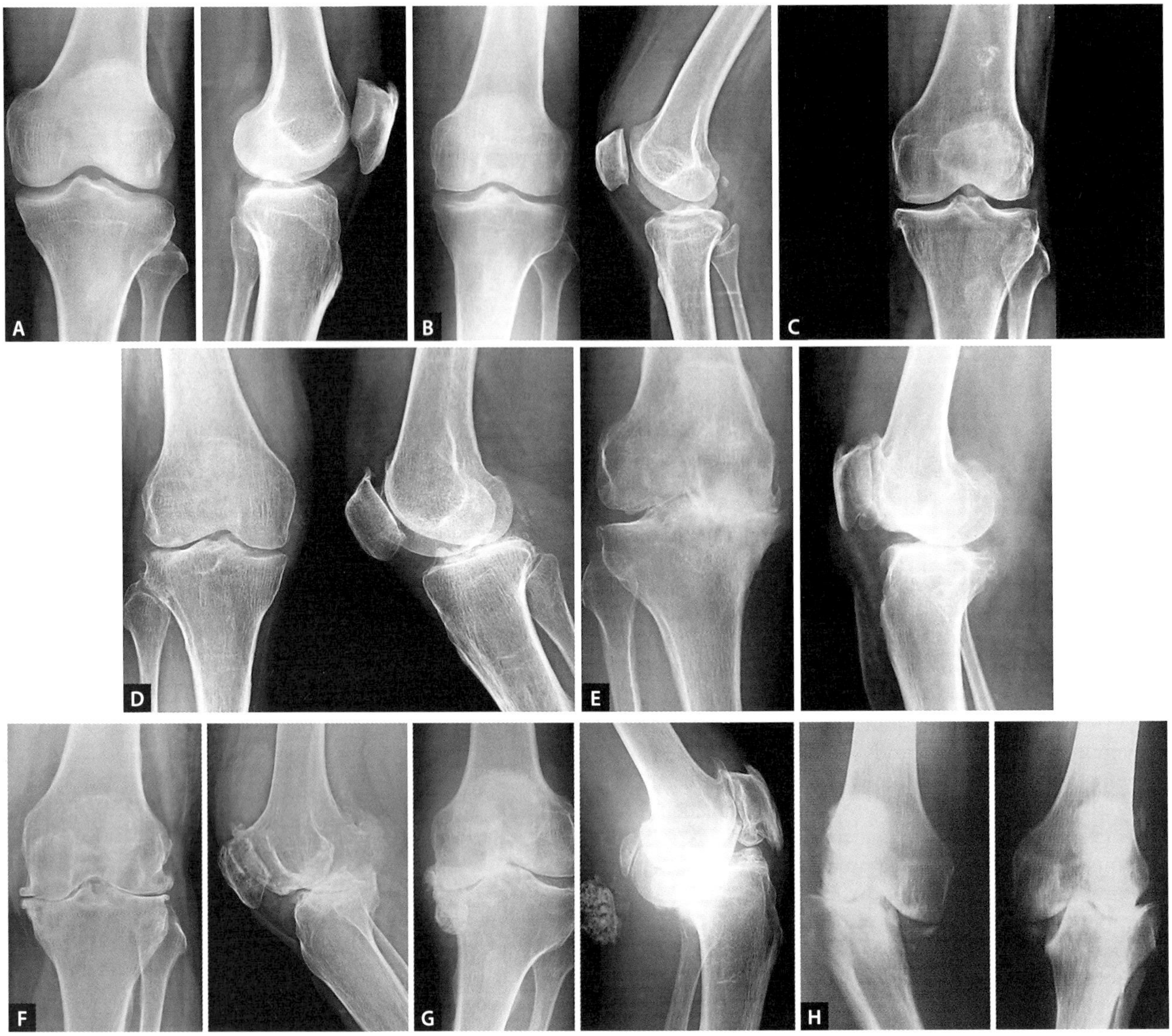

Figs. 5A to H: Osteoarthritis knee stages radiographs. (A) Grade 0—normal knee; (B) Grade 1—medial knee joint and patellar pole lipping; (C) Grade 2—medial tibial and femoral osteophyte, possible joint space narrowing; (D) Grade 3—joint space narrowing including patellofemoral joint space narrowing; (E) Grade (4-KL, 2Ahb)—extensive osteophytes and joint space vanished with subchondral sclerosis; (F) Grade 3 Ahb—minor bone attrition (0–5 mm); (G) Grade 4 Ahb—moderate bone attrition (5–10 mm); (H) Grade 5 Ahb—severe bone attrition (>10 mm). (Ahb: Ahlback; KL: Kellgren & Lawrence)

DIFFERENTIAL DIAGNOSIS

Rheumatoid arthritis, PsA, seronegative spondyloarthropathies, and enthesopathies. For early disease anserine bursitis, iliotibial band friction syndrome (runner's knee), patella tendonitis, patellofemoral pain syndrome, prepatellar bursitis, and semimembranosus bursitis.

ACUTE COMPLICATIONS OF OSTEOARTHRITIS

Commonly the patients keep suffering from symptoms and seek medical help only on aggravation of pain. Various causes of aggravated symptoms in osteoarthritis include:

- Ruptured Baker's cyst
- Microcrystalline arthropathy
- Bursitis
- Meniscal tear
- Labral tear
- Rotator cuff impingement and tear
- Spontaneous osteonecrosis of the knee
- Osteophyte fracture

VARIANTS OF PRIMARY OSTEOARTHRITIS

These clinical patterns arise from involvement of various joints and heterogeneous clinical patterns. The specific pattern may be triggered by diverse constitutional and environmental factors and are discernibly different from each. These subsets have been described according to following clinical characteristics:

- Identifiable causes of osteoarthritis

- Joint sites and number of joints involved
- The pattern of joints involvement
- Associated crystal deposition
- Associated inflammation
- Radiographic changes

Familial primary generalized osteoarthritis (Nodal generalized osteoarthritis): This form has a familial and possibly genetic predisposition to development of osteoarthritis that has female preponderance especially postmenopausal. There is premature development of Heberden's and Bouchard's nodes that is symmetrical, as well as the early degeneration of the articular cartilage at multiple joints. The joints commonly affected are saddle joint, metacarpophalangeal and interphalangeal joints of the thumbs, knee joints, hip joints, acromioclavicular joint, and spine (facet joints). The radiographic change is no different from sporadic form but tends to progress more rapidly and has a severe appearance for age of presentation. There is often an episodic symptomatic phase lasting 1–3 years that subside leaving behind the deformities but little disability.

Inflammatory or erosive osteoarthritis: Here the inflammatory component predisposes with frequent joint effusions, stiffness, and erosion of subchondral bone. This is a rare and more aggressive but limited (in distribution) form of familial primary generalized osteoarthritis. Ankylosis is seen in some cases. Postmenopausal women between 45 and 55 years are frequently affected in this form possibly linked to hormonal predisposition to disease. There is predominant affection of the hand (DIP) joints distributed bilaterally and symmetrically with overt pain, synovial swelling and erythema. The function of hand is quite compromised.

Localized large joint osteoarthritis:

- *Hip joint*: Classically presenting with groin pain and restricted flexion and internal rotation. The presentation is divided into two main subgroups:
  i. *Superior pole osteoarthritis:* The degenerative process affects the superior weight-bearing portion of the joint affecting obese males unilateraly.
  ii. *Central (Medial pole) osteoarthritis:* This is much less common and has a female preponderance usually associated with hand osteoarthritis and primary generalized osteoarthritis. There is central cartilage loss with positive Trendelenburg sign.
- *Knee joint*: This is a commonly involved joint in osteoarthritis that gives rises to significant disability, possibly the most common joint affected with osteoarthritis. Of the three compartments, medial joint compartment is the most commonly involved. The classical presentation is pain on weight bearing especially on climbing stairs and getting up from chair. "Gelling phenomenon" is quite common with the classical signs described above. Baker's cyst is a frequent finding along with pes anserinus bursitis. Involvement of patellofemoral joint is frequently seen in persons habitual of squatting or those who have to frequently climb large flight of stairs. The patellar undersurface cartilage is also more commonly eburnated in middle age females—a condition called chondromalacia. Patellar chondromalacia is described below in detail as it closely resembles degenerative cartilage disorder and osteoarthritis in early stage.

CHONDROMALACIA PATELLAE (CHONDROPATHY)

This is a frequent cause of anterior knee pain associated with crepitus in young adults and is also called "runners knee". There are articular cartilage changes on patella producing the characteristic symptoms and signs. The changes in articular cartilage are similar to early osteoarthritis changes, however, there seems no correlation with the progression to patellofemoral arthritis or tibiofemoral osteoarthritis pattern or coexistence. There is much less data available for prevalence of chondromalacia patellae. The term chondromalacia means "cartilage softness". The term chondromalacia patellae should not ever be used to refer anterior knee pain or patella femoral pain syndrome, it is a specific entity where the cartilage at undersurface of patella gets degenerated. Anterior knee pain provides a description of a symptom rather than a clear diagnosis, and thus encompasses a number of medical conditions (including chondromalacia). Patellofemoral pain syndrome is a diagnosis that should be applied only to individuals who have pain behind the kneecap (retropatellar pain) in the absence of damage to the cartilage or any other distinct pathology.

Pathophysiology of Chondromalacia

The articular cartilage of patella is the thickest in body with around 4–6 mm thickness. The coefficient of friction for cartilage on cartilage is 20% to that of ice on ice. The forces transmitted across the patellofemoral joint are large even in day-to-day activities. During level walking, the forces are 1.8 times the body weight, during climbing upstairs the forces are 3.5 times the body weight, while going downstairs they are five times the body weight. During getting up from squatting position the forces are eight times the body weight and while landing from a jump the forces are as high as 10–12 times the body weight. The exact mechanism of softening and degeneration are unclear; however, microtrauma accumulation in sports injuries or jogging, trauma [to anterior knee, fracture patella, meniscal injury or ligament injury (ies), previous knee surgeries], maltracking due to muscle weakness or malalignment, excessive lateral pressure syndrome due to chronic lateral patellar tilt (doubtful significance as chondromalacia develops on the medial facet first), patella alta, increased Q-angle, overuse (gymnasts, marathon runners), and hormonal alteration have all been implicated. Possibly due to larger thickness the metabolic demands are high and near threshold availability of nutrition and oxygen from synovial fluid may tip the balance toward degeneration making it susceptible to softening, fibrillation, and delamination.

Clinical Features

Patients usually complain of pain, crepitus (popping and cracking), decreased function, and occasionally swelling. The pain is dull and aching discomfort localized in the anterior aspect of the knee around or behind the kneecap. Activities such as running, jumping, stairs, hiking, squats, and lunges will exacerbate the condition. Patients also notice that sitting in one position for a period of time (driving, riding in a plane or a car) brings up pain when they get up (the so-called theater sign). The pain most likely arises from the abnormal force transmission through the softened cartilage to the underlying bone. Other symptoms that may feature are a sensation of catching or giving way, crepitation, and puffiness or swelling of the knee. Examination findings are nonspecific with the frequent presence of effusion, retropatellar tenderness, and patellofemoral joint crepitus. In addition, quadriceps wasting may be discernably present. The correlation of symptoms and signs to cartilage damage is poor and treatment relies heavily on the investigations and direct examination using arthroscope.

Investigations

Radiographs and CT-scans are of little use if any. Radiographs may show tilted patella (as in lateral patellar facet pressure syndrome). MRI is the investigation commonly referred to and may show a variety of morphological changes including diffuse swelling, blister formation, crabmeat appearance, ulceration and U-shaped focal defect, fissuration and linear defects, flap formation, and diffuse thinning of cartilage. The MRI grading for chondromalacia is commonly used and is based on outerbridge criteria **(Table 5)**. The cartilage damage is also graded according to *depth of involvement* on MRI (common for all cartilage lesions not specifically chondromalacia) as follows:

- *Grade I:* Intrachondral changes with intact surface
- *Grade II:* Surface abnormality
- *Grade III:* Loss of <50% of cartilage thickness
- *Grade IV:* Loss of 50–100% of cartilage thickness

Arthroscopy is the investigation of choice for determining both the presence and pattern of degeneration of the cartilage. The pathology can be explored and possibly treated at the same instance. The outer bridge classification is the most commonly used system for staging chondromalacia patellae **(Table 6)** devised specifically for arthroscopic evaluation.

Management of Chondromalacia

Most cases are self-limited and successfully controlled with conservative management. Isometric quadriceps, hamstring stretching, weight loss (1 kg weight loss takes away 4 kg of pressure from patella), activity modification, patellar taping and nonsteroidal anti-inflammatory drugs (NSAIDs) help in long-term control of symptoms. High impact activities (jumping, running, and deep squats), hiking, weight lifting, etc. should be avoided. If these methods fail then surgery to either correct the alignment and mechanics of joint or remove diseased cartilage is commonly resorted to. Various options include:

- Joint lavage and arthroscopic shaving of the cartilage to make it smooth
- Local excision of diseased cartilage and microfracture
- Modern chondroplasty techniques—ACI, MACI
- Realignment procedures for maltracking patella
- Realignment osteotomies of femur or tibia if required
- Patellofemoral arthroplasty
- Rarely patellectomy

TABLE 5: MRI grading (modified outer bridge) of chondromalacia.

Grade I	• Focal areas of hyperintensity with normal contour • *Arthroscopically:* Softening or swelling of cartilage
Grade II	• Blister-like swelling/fraying of articular cartilage extending to surface • *Arthroscopically:* Fragmentation and fissuring within soft areas of articular cartilage
Grade III	• Partial thickness cartilage loss with focal ulceration • *Arthroscopically:* Partial thickness cartilage loss with fibrillation (crab-meat appearance)
Grade IV	• Full thickness cartilage loss with underlying bone reactive changes • *Arthroscopically:* Cartilage destruction with exposed subchondral bone

TABLE 6: Outerbridge grading of chondromalacia.

Grade	*Pathology*
I	Softening and swelling of articular cartilage (closed chondromalacia)
II	Fragmentation and fissuring of articular cartilage affecting an area of <0.5 inches
III	Fragmentation and fissuring of articular cartilage affecting an area >0.5 inches
IV	Cartilage erosion to bone

TREATMENT OF OSTEOARTHRITIS

The *goal* in osteoarthritis or degenerative joint disorder is to maintain a *painless active life* with objectives of control of pain and swelling, minimizing disability. Initially reducing inflammation with NSAIDs and pain control beginning with acetaminophen are appropriate. Exercises to strengthen the muscles and improve flexibility, as well as weight loss, should be stressed immediately. A common algorithm is suggested in **Figure 6**. Before prescribing surgery which is the ultimate modality, education, exercises, weight loss, physical therapy, braces, and orthotics should be given due admission as they all have definite role in improving the quality of life and alleviating symptoms.

Topical Analgesics

Topical NSAIDs and capsaicin may be used as alternative to those having contraindications to their systemic use. Topical diclofenac is effective for long-term pain relief and has lower GI side effects. Topical capsaicin works by depleting the neuropeptide substance P and must be used for >3–4 weeks for optimal benefit.

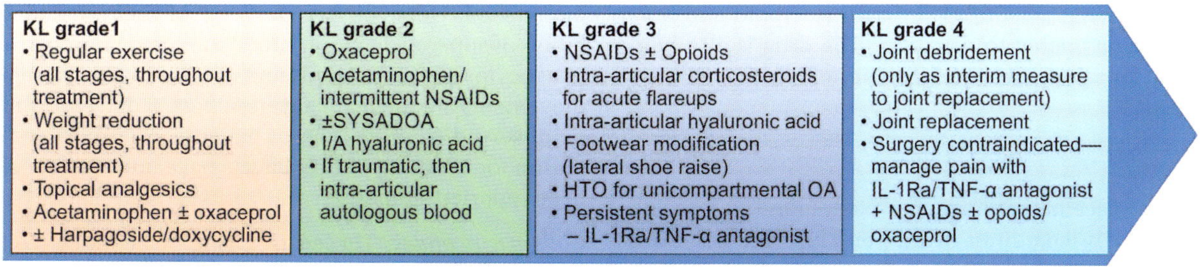

Fig. 6: Algorithm for osteoarthritis management.

Exercise, Weight Loss, and Lifestyle Modifications

Exercise improves flexibility and strengthening muscles supports the affected joints for want of ligament stability, increases aerobic capacity and endurance, and facilitates weight loss. Strengthening the muscles improves joint stability and reduces pain. Low-impact isokinetic and isotonic strengthening exercises (swimming, biking, and walking) are preferable but initially isometric exercises should be introduced gradually escalating to isotonic and resistive exercises. Moderate exercises effectively improve joint symptoms, function, and also there is an improvement in the cartilage glycosaminoglycan content. Weight loss reduces the symptoms of osteoarthritis in weight-bearing joints. Each kilogram of weight loss results in a sixfold to eightfold reduction in the load exerted on the knee per step during daily activities. To improve symptoms of medial joint compartment knee osteoarthritis, lateral wedge orthotics or knee bracing for more muscular, younger patients may provide symptomatic improvement. The use of a cane in opposite hand is beneficial. The use of transcutaneous electrical nerve stimulation (TENS) has been recommended by NICE, this possibly helps by improving muscle strength and coordination and may have negative feedback effect on pain mechanism.

Supportive Devices

Supportive devices partially unload the joint and may improve symptoms. Some of these devices include canes, crutches, walkers, corsets, collars, orthotics for shoes and sometimes cervical traction. Canes, when properly used, can increase the base of support and decrease loading and demands on the affected lower limb and its joints.

- The total length of a properly measured cane should be equal to the distance between the upper border of the greater trochanter of the femur and the bottom of the heel of the shoe.
- This should result in elbow flexion of about 20°.
- The cane should be held in the hand contralateral to and moved together with the affected limb.
- The healthier limb should precede the affected limb when climbing up stairs; when climbing down stairs, the cane and the affected limb should be advanced first.
- The cane can unload the affected hip by 60%.

Analgesics and Anti-inflammatory Drugs

Nonsteroidal anti-inflammatory drugs effectively relieve pain in patients with osteoarthritis. They reduce inflammation associated with osteoarthritis by inhibiting the production of prostaglandins. Acetaminophen provides no significant improvement in pain over placebo. There is potential for gastrointestinal toxicity, including dyspepsia, ulcer, perforation, and hemorrhage and is an important concern for patients taking NSAIDs. Selective COX-2 enzyme inhibitors are as effective as the nonspecific NSAIDs in treating osteoarthritis with decreased incidence of gastric toxicity but increased risk of thrombosis, ischemic cardiovascular disease, heart failure, hypertension, and cardiac arrhythmia. Tramadol and combination of tramadol with acetaminophen can provide improved pain relief in patients that cannot tolerate NSAIDs or are contraindicated.

Prostaglandin sparing anti-inflammatory drugs (PSAIDs) have failed to provide effective pain relief and in patients with renal insufficiency alternatives like tapentadol or nefopam may be used.

Natural inhibitors of neovascularization like *curcumin* and *resveratrol* have been found effective in inhibiting metastatic tumor cell homing and angiogenesis. They are now available and also being used for treatment of osteoarthritis. *Deltonin* and β-chanonine are naturally occurring steroids having good anti-inflammatory and anti-tumor activity and are also being evaluated for use in arthritic joints.

Intra-articular Hyaluronans (Viscosupplementation)

At low load speed, HA acts as a lubricant and during faster movements as a shock absorber. In osteoarthritis, the concentration of HA is reduced by one-half to one-third of normal. HA injections (high or low molecular weight) appear to moderately improve short-term pain but no conclusive benefits have been reported on disease outcome so not recommended. Adverse reactions are rare; however, "pseudoseptic" reactions in 1–1.5% patients have been reported.

Injectable Corticosteroid

Localized osteoarthritis to a joint or acute inflammatory exacerbation can be managed with depot preparations of steroids. Effects last 4–6 weeks then wane-off fast. It should not be used more frequently than once in 4 months as cartilage damage and disease progression occurs.

Harpagoside (Devil's Claw Extract)

This is an iridoid glycoside that has shown anti-inflammatory, anti-rheumatic, and antioxidant effects. The medicine has shown promising relief from osteoarthritic pain and fewer side effects compared to diacerein. The drug is also being evaluated for acute, subacute, chronic, and nonspecific low-back pain.

Estrogens

Estrogen replacement therapy has been found to lower the prevalence of osteoarthritis of knee and hip. The side effects (see "Osteoporosis") possibly limit their use as regular therapy.

Pulsed Electromagnetic Fields and Quantum Magnetic Resonance

There are individual supporters for these modalities but no concrete literature support exists.

Ginger-based Products

These products have been found to control symptoms of osteoarthritis. Isolated reports found reduced pain on standing but long-term effects are doubtful.

Disease-modifying Drugs for Osteoarthritis

Symptomatic Slow-acting Drugs for Osteoarthritis (SYSADOA), Glucosamine, and Chondroitin Sulfate (Chondroprotective)

The term "chondroprotective" is a misnomer as no such concrete effect on preservation or regeneration of cartilage has been demonstrated.

Glucosamine sulfate is the monosaccharide precursor to glycosaminoglycans. Chondroitin sulfate is composed of repeating units of galactosamine sulfate and glucuronic acid. Oral supplementation with glucosamine and/or chondroitin sulfate is thought to stimulate synthesis of glycosaminoglycan and proteoglycans and inhibiting degradative proteolytic enzymes. The results have been mixed and not very encouraging. It is interesting to note that the relief in symptoms has been better in patients with higher grade osteoarthritis (where surgery is better) than those with earlier disease form. Another interesting finding is that in most of the randomized controlled trials (RCTs) done to evaluate the efficacy of drugs where a placebo is used the "placebo effect" is itself very high (around 60%) and therapeutic drugs find it difficult to surpass this high efficacy to produce a significant difference. High placebo effect has suggested most experts to favor a conservative approach for early disease rather than going aggressively at controlling the symptoms.

S-adenosylmethionine (SAM): It is a methyl group donor and oxygen radical scavenger supposed to prevent cartilage damage due to peroxidation and inflammation. The results have been mixed and possibly require prolonged administration.

Diacerein: Diacerein and its active metabolite rhein are anthraquinones related to senna compounds. They inhibit the synthesis of IL-1β in human osteoarthritis synovium in vitro, as well as the expression of IL-1 receptors on chondrocytes. IL-1-dependent stromelysin-1 production is also diminished. Other observed effects of rhein include inhibition of superoxide anion production and chemotaxis and phagocytosis of neutrophils and macrophages. Loose bowel movements are the main adverse effect of diacerein and can be observed in up to 30% of patients—the most common reason for noncompliance. Effects have not been consistent in all reported studies.

Collagen peptides: These are a mix of peptides (collagen hydrolysate) of different length obtained by enzymatic hydrolysis of native collagen obtained from animal connective tissues. They contain abundance of amino acids hydroxyproline, glycine, and proline. They have a high bioavailability and have been found to get incorporated in cartilage on ingestion. They have also been reported to increase synthesis of native collagen and proteoglycans producing modest pain relief but improvement of joint function is conflicting. Often a concoction of collagen hydrolysate with curcumin/ginger or flavinoids is variably promoted.

Doxycycline

Tetracyclines appear to inhibit tissue metalloproteinases (collagenase and gelatinase). This could be due to their ability to chelate calcium and zinc ions. They also prevent proteoglycan loss, cell death, and deposition of Type X collagen matrix. There has also been investigation into the potential role of NO in the mechanism of action of the tetracyclines. Doxycycline may slow the rate of progression of osteoarthritis but there is no pain relief.

Other Inconsistently Administered Therapies

Numerous therapeutics are under development for amelioration of osteoarthritis or control its progression targeting chondrocytes and innate inflammatory pathways **(Table 7)**. Few are discussed below.

- *Use of autologous blood product:* This is aimed to augment tissue healing. These blood products are usually fractionated fragments of blood highly rich in platelet content. The platelets have the capability to release chemokines from β-granules positively influencing the tissues with low healing potential. Intra-articular injection of activated platelet concentrate may enhance cartilage healing and remodeling.
- *Univestin:* This is a combination of plant extracts obtained from *Scutellaria baicalensis*, and *Acacia catechu* that helps in alleviating pain and stiffness. The proposed mechanism is through inhibition of both cyclooxygenase (COX) and lipoxygenase (LOX) though dedicated trials are not available.
- *IL-1 receptor and TNF-β antagonist:* IL-1 receptor antagonist (IL-1Ra) has shown reduced expression of collagenase in cartilage and prevents osteoarthritis progression in animal studies. IL-1Ra (Orthokine, Anakinra) is an example of approaches that inhibit activity of catabolic cytokines. Additional inhibition of TNF-β is associated with cartilage preservation by decreasing release of glycosaminoglycans and increasing

TABLE 7: Emerging pharmacological therapeutic targets to control osteoarthritis and chronic pain and promote regeneration.

Pathophysiological process and mediators	*Effect and its therapeutic strategy*
Cartilage degradation • MMP-13, ADAMTS-5 • DDR2 activation by serine proteinase • Cathepsin-K • ADAM17	*Loss of cartilage and wear* • MMP inhibitor • Serine proteinase inhibitor • Tyrosine kinase inhibitor • Polyphenols (green tea)
Chondrocyte hypertrophy • Hedgehog signaling, IKK-α, ADAM10	*Harbinger of cartilage degeneration* Small molecule inhibitors of Gli, Smo, etc.
Chondrogenesis and inhibition of endochondral calcification • Runx1 • PTH receptor • EGFR signaling	*Improves cartilage regeneration* • Thienoindazole derivative TD-198946 • Kartogenin • Teriparatide, mitogen inducible gene
Cartilage anabolism • IGF-1 • FGFR-2 and -3 • Calcitonin	*Improves cartilage health* • Humanized IGF-1 heparin binding domain fusion protein • rh-FGF18 (Sprifermin) • Oral or intra-articular calcitonin
Autophagy and cell survival • mTOR • AKT/Fox3/PPARγ/CXCR2	*Improve tissue metabolism* • Rapamycin, polyamines, ω-6 polyunsaturated fatty acids • Chemokine antagonists or blocking antibodies
Subchondral bone catabolism • WNT/β-catenin • Adenosine receptors	 • Sclerostin, DKK-1 antibodies • A2AR antagonists
Subchondral bone anabolism • BMP • BMP-7	 • BMP antagonists (Gremlin, follistatin) • Recombinant BMP-7 (Eptotermin)
Mechanical, inflammatory stress • Canonical NF-κβ signaling • JAK/STAT signaling • Reactive oxygen species (ROS) • HIF-2α, MMP, ADAMTS55	*Initiation of cartilage degeneration* • Curcumin, resveratrol, IKK-β inhibitor (SAR113945) • Jakinibs (Tofacitinib) • Antioxidants, iNOS inhibitors, mitochondrial ROS scavengers • Suppressor of cytokine signaling (SOCS)
Calcification and crystals • NPP1, transglutaminase inorganic pyrophosphate • TLRs, NLRP3	*Proinflammatory and tissue degradation* • Phosphocitrates • TLR and NLRP inhibitor
Innate immunity • TLRs • Complement	*Proinflammatory* • 6-Shagoal, Boswellic acid, kaempferol • CR2-factor H (alternative complement pathway)
Angiogenesis and synovitis • VEGF	 Bevacizumab

(ADAM: A disintegrin and metalloproteinase; ADAMTS: a disintegrin-like and metalloproteinase domain (reprolysin type) with thrombospondin type 1 repeats; BMP: bone morphogenic protein; EGFR: epidermal growth factor receptor; FGF: fibroblast growth factor; HIF-2α: hypoxia-inducible factor-2α; iNOS: inducible nitric oxide synthase; JAK/STAT: Janus kinase/signal transducer and activator of transcription; MMP: matrix metalloproteinase; mTOR: mechanistic target of rapamycin; NLRP: nucleotide-binding oligomerization domain, leucine rich repeat and pyrin domain; PTH: parathormone; TLR: toll-like receptor; VEGF: vascular endothelial growth factor; WNT: wingless related integration site)

lubricin production. Tocilizumab and infliximab plus methotrexate (MTX) have shown reduction in synovial VEGF and inflammation.

- *MAP kinase inhibitors (see rheumatoid arthritis):* Mitogen-activated protein kinase regulate production and activity of multiple mediators of joint tissue destruction. Inhibition of this pathway can slow disease progression in osteoarthritis.
- Angiogenic inhibitors like angiostatin and endostatin are being evaluated for inhibition of βVB3-mediated angiogenesis.
- *NF-κβ inhibitors:* NF-κβ transcription factors are triggered by a host of inflammatory cytokines and can be targeted to reduce the disease progression.
- Vitamin E, N-acetyl-L-cysteine (NAC), and superoxide dismutase have the potential to protect the chondrocyte from reactive oxygen species (ROS) released during traumatic insult. These ROS are the primary agents causing chondrocyte death after trauma. The source of these excess ROS seems to be mitochondria. Superoxide and NO are two implicated ROS for induction of apoptosis. NAC is a powerful hydroxyl and hypochlorous radical scavenger and also inhibits activation of c-Jun N-terminal kinase, p38 MAP kinase, redox-sensitive activating protein-1, and NF-κβ transcription factor activities.
- Rotenone inhibits the secretion of superoxide from mitochondria and may have a therapeutic role.
- *Inducible nitric oxide synthase (iNOS) inhibitors:* Substances like N-Nitro-L-arginine methyl ester (L-NAME), N-iminoethyl-L-Lysine (L-NIL) have been found to reduce the progression of post-traumatic osteoarthritis in animals.

- Pan Caspase inhibitors like Z-VAD-FMK [benzyloxy-carbonyl-Val-Ala-Asp (OMe) fluoromethylketone], a cell permeable fluoromethylketone that inhibit caspase enzyme in a broad spectrum prevent apoptosis may benefit when injected intra-articularly but the results have been inconsistent.
- Poloxamer 188 (P188), a nontoxic nonionic surfactant that has a hydrophilic surface and a hydrophobic center, similar to the lipid bilayer composition has been found to protect the cell membranes, repair damaged ones and prevent apoptosis. The compound acts via direct inhibition of IL-6 mediated pathway inhibiting the phosphorylation of Stat1, Stat3, and p38. This prevents their migration to nucleus and hence synthesis of catabolic products is not initiated. Also the glycogen synthase kinase-3 (GSK3) involved in apoptosis is inhibited.

Surgical Management

Various surgical options exist for relieving pain and improving the function of involved joint(s).

Arthroscopic lavage has shown no better lasting results than analgesic therapy. It provides temporary pain relief (similar to injectable steroids and viscosupplementation) by washing away the painful metabolites from synovial fluid full of catabolic mediators and worn fragments of cartilage to relieve inflammation. Mechanical symptoms in early stages of osteoarthritis are the main indications for performing arthroscopy. Although patients with mild disease may obtain 90% improvement of symptoms, with mild disease defined as joint space >3 mm with normal or varus alignment, those with severe disease may only obtain 25% relief of symptoms. In advanced degeneration, results are no better than placebo. Arthroscopic chondral lavage and cartilage regenerative procedures are discussed in section on cartilage repair.

Osteotomy

These correct the resultant or causative misalignment of joint and additionally unload the pathological side of joint involvement. Osteotomies have been previously used for hip osteoarthritis (like the classical McMurray osteotomy) but now hardly anyone uses them for this indication. Knee is still an area for practice of osteotomy for specific indications and patients. The following are the commonly used osteotomies for knee isolated compartment osteoarthritis:

- Varus-producing distal femoral osteotomy is indicated in patients with valgus gonarthrosis and isolated lateral compartment arthritis.
- Valgus-producing high tibial osteotomy (HTO) is indicated in patients with varus gonarthrosis and isolated medial compartment arthritis.

Though popular and commonly used in past, proximal tibial osteotomy [*high tibial osteotomy (HTO)*] is losing popularity as a reconstructive procedure; however, HTO was first described by Lagenback in 1854.

Principle: High tibial osteotomy unloads the affected part of knee joint by correcting malalignment and redistributing stresses hence relieves pain and restores function.

Rationale of doing HTO (realignment procedure):

- *Role of alignment:* Severity of varus directly correlated to radiologic progression. Varus worsens the problem and odds for radiological progression increased fourfold with a varus malalignment.
- *Baseline stage of disease:* Varus affects damaged knees more. In a Kellgren-Lawrence score 3 knee with varus alignment the risk of progression of osteoarthritis is 10-fold.
- *Dynamic loading:* With a varus knee the adductor moment leads to progression of osteoarthritis by dynamically loading the deformed joint.

Indications of high tibial osteotomy:

- Pain and disability from unicompartmental involvement (usually medial) osteoarthritis < grade 4 (Ahlback grading) documented on radiographs (or better arthroscopically) in a high demand young individual. Patellofemoral osteoarthritis should be < grade 3 (Ahlback).
- Age <60 years and varus (or valgus) of <15° at the knee with full extension.
- Motivated patient who can use assistive devices and understands activity limitation for significant period of time.
- In menisectomized knees, HTO is indicated for prevention of long-term overload or as an additional procedure to meniscal transplantation.
- As a protective procedure for chondral resurfacing or various cartilage reconstructive procedures.
- Anterior cruciate ligament, posterior cruciate ligament (PCL), or posterolateral complex insufficiency with varus alignment or thrust.

Patient selection: Ideal patient—40–60 years old active male with varus of <15° having isolated medial activity and no patello femoral symptoms. Should have full extension and >100° of flexion, nonsmoker, BMI < 30 and lateral compartment arthrosis of <grade 3.

Contraindications:

- Absolute:
  - Age >65 years (the risk of failure increases 7.6% per year of age, and in patients over 65 years the relative risk is 1.5 times that of younger patients)
  - Diffuse osteoarthritis
  - Tibiofemoral subluxation—lateral subluxation of tibia > 1 cm.
  - Medial compartment bone loss > 2–3 mm
  - Medial compartment osteoarthritis grade ≥ 4 (Ahlback)
  - Flexion contracture > 15°
  - Inflammatory arthritis
  - Menisectomy in the compartment or other compartment.
  - Rheumatoid arthritis
  - Mediolateral insufficiency
  - Unrealistic patient
- Relative:
  - Obese (BMI > 40)
  - Poor ROM < 90° knee flexion

- Nonspecific knee pain
- More than 20° of correction needed
- Peripheral vascular disease
- Smoker > 15 cigarettes/day
- Osteoporosis

- Extra-articular deformity

Types of high tibial osteotomy: Various techniques have been described for realigning the joint by HTO, oldest one and most popular is the lateral closing wedge, valgus producing osteotomy described by Jackson and Waugh (1961) popularized by Coventry (1965). The different techniques of performing HTO (with or without navigation) are:

- Lateral closing wedge, valgus producing osteotomy
- Medial opening wedge osteotomy with bone graft (Debeyre and Patte in 1951)
- Dual osteotomy
- Dome (barrel vault) osteotomy of Macquet
- Chevron osteotomy (oblique)
- Opening wedge osteotomy using external fixators (hemicallotasis):
    - Ilizarov
    - External fixators

There are technique related advantages for open or a closed wedge osteotomy **(Table 8)**, no head to head comparison for efficacy of one procedure to relieve symptoms is available. The choice is mostly surgeon dependent; lateral closing wedge osteotomy has the longest track record and has been time tested; however, recently with the availability of fixed angle devices and measured blocks of synthetic grafts resurgence in open wedge osteotomy procedure is seen. Hemicallotasis has been also recently preferred by surgeons for being able to gradually correct the varus malalignment under supervision and control on the final correction reached. However, concerns of pin site care and infection and limitation of future total knee arthroplasty (TKA) are the specific concerns.

Site of osteotomy in proximal tibia is also a matter of debate. Classically, the osteotomy was performed above the level of tibial tubercle but now mainly the concern of patella baja and need of future TKA makes most people perform osteotomy below the tibial tubercle. The relative advantages of each site are compared in **(Table 9)**.

Preoperative planning (open or closed wedge): The most essential component for performing HTO is to plan the procedure and rehearse on paper. The aim is to achieve lower limb mechanical alignment of 183–186° range (3–6° valgus at knee from "zero line"—line joining the hip and ankle centers) that gives best results. There is consensus that slight overcorrection achieves better satisfaction among patients. Dugdale recommended 3–5° of valgus, Hernigou (3–6°), Amendola (3–7°), Coventry (10-year survival rates were 63% in knees with 5° valgus angulation, 87% in knees with 6–7° valgus angulation, and 94% in knees with ≥8° valgus angulation). Preoperative knee alignment is assessed for the five criteria—frontal mechanical axis, joint line, sagittal mechanical axis, patellofemoral joint and malrotation. "*Malalignment test*" **(Fig. 7)** is used in patients in whom frontal mechanical axis deviation (MAD) exists. This is done by drawing a z-line (zero line) on full leg AP radiograph taken with patella pointing forward joining the center of femoral head and center of ankle (distal tibia). In a normal

TABLE 8: Advantages of open wedge and closing wedge high tibial osteotomy (HTO).

Closing wedge osteotomy (Coventry)	*Opening wedge osteotomy*
• Time honored • Commonly available jig • Higher union rate • Fixation covered with soft tissue • Decreases tibial slope • No loss of correction due to collapse or graft failure	• Easy exposure • No fibular osteotomy required and tibiofibular joint spared • Options of fixation wide • May increase MCL tension • Restores bone stalk • TKA conversion relatively easier • Relatively easier to control slope • No nerve dissection

(MCL: medial collateral ligament; TKA: total knee arthroplasty)

TABLE 9: Comparative advantages of various sites of high tibial osteotomy.

Above tibial tubercle	*Behind tibial tubercle*	*Below tibial tubercle*
• Large cancellous surface • Close to deformity • Time honored • Minimal learning curve • Smaller incision	• Stable fixation • No step off • Can displace tibial tubercle anteriorly—"Macquet effect" relieving stress on patellofemoral joint • No patellar tendon scarring	• Large proximal fragment • Allows correction in multiple planes • No bone removed • Minimal incision • No retropatellar scarring • Q-angle undisturbed

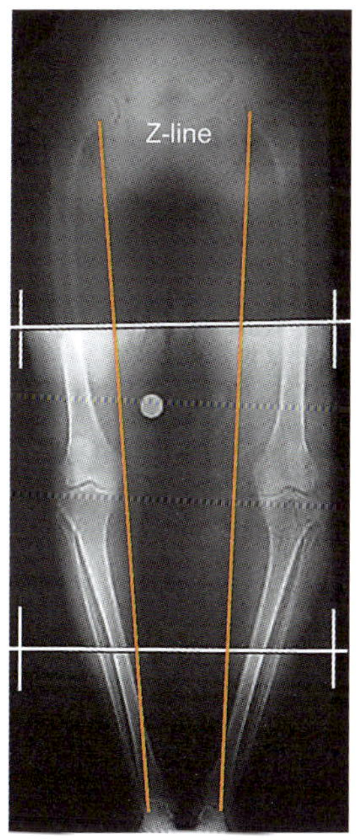

Fig. 7: Malalignment test: The line from center of femoral head to center of ankle passes normally just medial to the knee center depicting but in this case, the line passes medial to knee joint on both sides suggesting significant malalignment. Line can even pass laterally suggesting valgus malalignment. Acceptable deviation range for medial side is 0–15 mm.

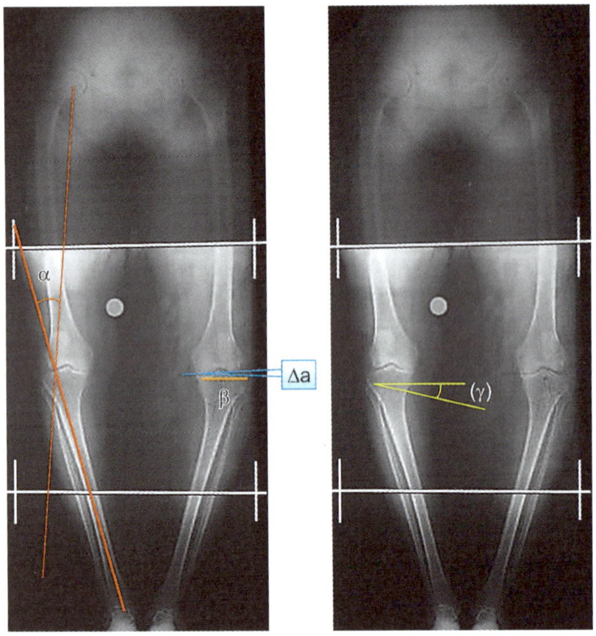

Fig. 8: Measuring the wedge size through radiographic method—α is the angle measured from the intersecting lines at Fujisawa point.
β = Δa × 76.4/b (b = width of tibial plateau)
The angle of wedge (γ) = α − β
The angle is marked and the wedge is calculated on the radiograph, as done here for open wedge osteotomy.

knee, it passes just medial to center of knee joint if not then a MAD is present and measured in millimeter (normal range is 0–15 mm).

Calculation of wedge size:

1. The radiographic method (Dugdale's, **Fig. 8**):
   Step 1: On a long leg film, join the center of head to "Fujisawa point" on tibial plateau and extend distally. Draw another line from Fujisawa point to center of ankle. Measure this correction angle (α) in degrees. *Fujisawa point* lies at the junction of medial two-thirds and lateral one-third on tibial articular surface (it will be 10 mm lateral to midpoint on a 60-mm tibial articular surface). It is also the point at 62.5% of the tibial plateau width on lateral tibial condyle. Some consider static point to be oversimplification and recommend choosing point based on extent of cartilage damage. Jakob and Jakobi suggested that correction of the mechanical axis depends on the thickness of the cartilage in the medial compartment: if one-third of the medial cartilage is lost, the mechanical axis should pass 10–15% lateral from the center of the tibial plateau; if two-thirds of the cartilage is lost, the axis should pass 20–25% lateral; and if all is lost, the axis should pass 30–35% lateral.
   Step 2: Subtract the varus malalignment caused by ligamentous laxity (β). Measure the joint line convergence angle (JLCA) on preoperative full length AP films of both limbs, which is defined as the angle between femoral and tibial joint lines. The difference between the two is "Δa". By using constant "k" of 76.4 the β = k × (Δa)/tibial plateau width. So final correction angle (γ) = α − β.

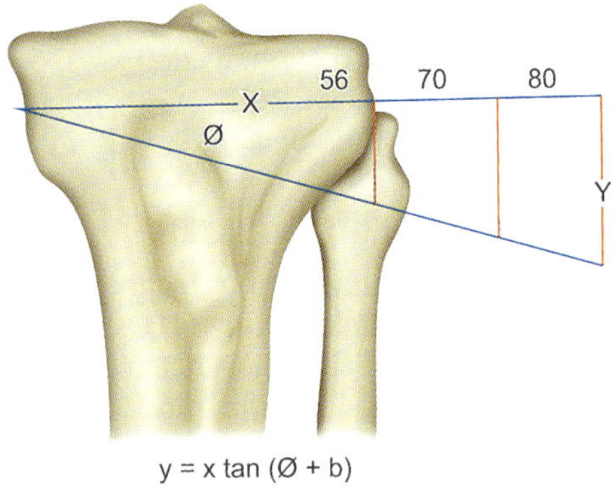

Fig. 9: Trigonometric method for measuring the wedge.

   Step 3: Rotate the angle (γ) to desired position (CORA) for osteotomy on the radiograph. The CORA for medial opening wedge osteotomy lies at fibular head, while for closing wedge osteotomy generally a point 2–2.5 cm distal to medial joint line is chosen.
   Step 4: Measure the required cut length from this superimposed angular wedge. For simplicity step 2 can be avoided.
2. Size of osteotomy wedge could also be measured *trigonometrically* by following formula **(Fig. 9)**:
   $$Y = X \tan(\varphi + b)$$
   Where Y = base-length of wedge, X = width of tibial plateau on AP film, φ = degree of correction. A simpler version of the equation is W (size of wedge) = diameter (tibia at osteotomy site) × 0.002 × angle.
3. *Approximation method:* The classical approximation given by Coventry for calculation of the tibial osteotomy wedge size was equivalence of 1 mm of wedge length for every degree of correction needed, but this holds true only for tibial plateau length of 57 mm and is no longer followed in modern world for need of accuracy.
4. *Computerized methods:* For surgical planning of complex deformities Chao and Sim developed software called osteotomy analysis and simulation software (OASIS). Tool PreOp-plan from Siemens for Tomofix®.

Other factors that should be evaluated for preoperative planning include:

- Gait analysis (valgus thrust predicts failure)
- Rotational deformity of lower limb
- Ligamentous laxity
- Anteroposterior laxity:
  - ACL deficiency—Need simultaneous or sequential correction.
  - PCL deficiency—May consider increasing slope.
- Patient factors (smoking—choose iliac graft instead of synthetic bone grafts)

Surgical procedure: Coventry recommended a lateral closing wedge osteotomy for varus deformity in osteoarthritic knee and medial closing wedge tibial osteotomy for valgus deformity but suggested supracondylar femoral medial closing wedge osteotomy if deformity exceeds 12°. In closing-wedge osteotomy, the proximal osteotomy line is located in parallel with the articular surface and 2–2.5 cm inferior to the joint line. The distal osteotomy line is determined referring to the α angle and the wedge of bone between the osteotomy lines is removed. The proximal tibiofibular joint has to be frequently disrupted for proper wedge (lateral closing wedge for varus deformity) or else inferomedial portion of fibular head can be partially removed. It is helpful to preserve a posteromedial beak of proximal fragment that overrides the distal fragment on closure of osteotomy and provides added support and stability. It is better to use L-plates with compression (preferred) or simply cast immobilization or Steinmann pin fixation (avoid). For opening wedge HTO the proximal osteotomy line is drawn from a point 3.5–4 cm inferior to the medial knee joint line to the tip of the fibular head from which another same length line is drawn obliquely by the α-angle. Various fixation methods are available all in common to avoid collapse of osteotomy gap. Puddu plate with predefined metal blocks, Tomofix® (Synthes, Pennsylvania) with synthetic bone graft wedges, locked plate constructs.

Barrel vault osteotomies (though it is technically difficult and involves creation of inverted "U" osteotomy followed by fragment rotation into desired plane) and hemicallotasis are preferable for larger corrections.

Complications: Various complications can arise from HTO and include:

- Undercorrection
- Thromboembolic disease
- Peroneal palsy
- Nonunion
- Infection
- Vascular injury
- Problems inherent to internal fixation
- Intra-articular fracture
- Patella Baja (this was mainly a risk associated with cast immobilization before the advent of internal fixation and faster immobilization, a closing-wedge osteotomy has been found to increase patellar height while opening-wedge osteotomy reduces it)
- Alteration of tibial slope (see below)
- Increased Q-angle

Impact of HTO on joint kinematics and future procedures (effect on tibial slope): HTO offers pain relief for around 8–10 years. HTO has been shown to have improved results in ACL-deficient knees. This may be related to HTO improving the stability of the knee. All HTOs have been shown to *alter the slope of the tibia*. Lateral closing wedge osteotomies tend to decrease posterior tibial slope, translate the tibia in posterior direction stabilizing knees with anterior instability (ACL deficient) while medial opening-wedge osteotomies increase posterior tibial slope and translate tibia in anterior direction stabilising knees with posterior instability (PCL deficient knees). For patients with chronic ACL insufficiency there is posteromedial tibial wear. Decreased tibial slope reduces tibiofemoral contact area and pressure offloading the tibial plateau. So a closing-wedge osteotomy improves symptoms of anterolateral instability with varus alignment and ACL deficiency. Medial opening-wedge osteotomy heightens the likelihood of increased posterior slope and is recommended in knees with chronic PCL injuries and posterolateral instability that has been inversely correlated with posterior tibial slope. The combination of varus malalignment with posterolateral instability is termed "triple varus" that may be managed with medial opening wedge osteotomy. It should be, however, remembered that slope should not be increased any >10° as this will otherwise produce chronic ACL insufficiency in already PCL deficient knee.

Failed HTO is best addressed with TKA. Main concerns following HTO for performing TKA arises from retropatellar fibrosis, patella baja, deformed proximal tibia and offset tibial shaft (implant placement, probability of varus cut), altered slope, altered joint line, implant related complications, lateral soft tissue scarring and prior incision. The studies initially reported serious concerns and inferior results but most studies now report equivalent functional results for TKA performed after HTO than for otherwise osteoarthritis knee. TKA after lateral closing wedge osteotomy in general requires prolonged operation time and causes some reduction in postoperative knee ROM.

On the other hand, the osteotomy did not have significant influences on clinical outcomes in the mid-term and long-term follow-up. Theoretically, opening-wedge osteotomy is advantageous over closing-wedge osteotomy regarding bone stock preservation and impingement between the tibial component stem and the anterior tibial cortex. It obviates the problem of patella infera, lifts medial condyle, tightens medial collateral ligament (MCL) maintain tibial shaft alignment. In conclusion, HTO is a preferred procedure for management of unicompartmental knee osteoarthritis in young, heavy, and active (particularly male) with good functional range of motion.

Unicompartmental Knee Arthroplasty

The term "unicondylar" refers to a device with two components that resurface the tibiofemoral articulation. "Unicompartmental" refers to the philosophy of resurfacing only one compartment **(Figs. 10A to C)**, with a specific implant; this can be medial, lateral, or patellofemoral. They should not be used interchangeably. Unicompartmental knee arthroplasty (UKA) restores the kinematics without significantly altering the natural alignment or ligament balance.

Principle: Unicompartmental knee arthroplasty removes the diseased painful portion (replacement procedure) of the knee and is a resurfacing arthroplasty (joint preserving) reconstructing the bearing surfaces. It restores natural alignment of the joint and restores ligament tension and joint line.

Rationale: It is prudent to replace the symptomatic compartment rather for limited disease than doing TKA and providing a faster recovery time with minimal invasiveness. Also revising UKA to TKA later is probably easier than after HTO.

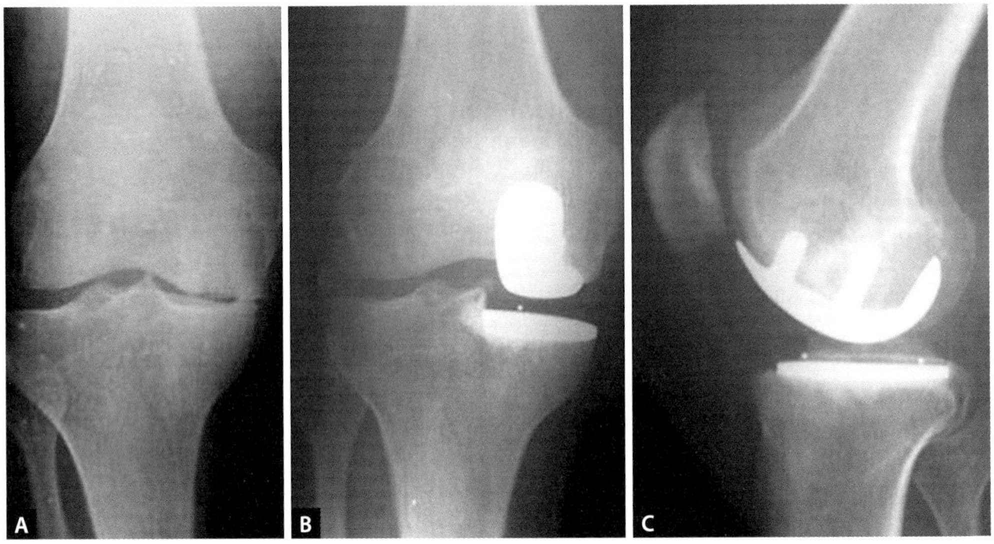

Figs. 10A to C: Unicondylar knee arthroplasty for medial tibiofemoral arthritis.

Indications: Classically UKA is indicated in unicompartmental osteoarthritis of the knee in a low-demand, elderly, thin patient (>55 years) with competent cruciates and collateral ligaments.

Patient selection:
- Patients >55 years
- BMI < 30
- Low level of activity
- Minimal rest pain
- Range of motion (ROM)—minimum arc of 90°
  - Flexion contracture <5°
  - Passively correctible angular deformity ≤ 10° varus or 15° valgus

Contraindications:
- Age <60 years
- Weight >95 kg
- High activity level
- Patellofemoral pain
- Contralateral tibiofemoral joint arthritis
- Menisectomized patient (other compartment)
- Inflammatory arthritis
- Symptomatic ACL insufficiency
- PCL insufficiency
- Collateral ligament insufficiency
- Varus >15°; valgus >15°; flexion contracture >10°

Preoperative planning: Standard AP and lateral radiographs to identify damage to compartments (especially patellofemoral) and possible cruciate damage. Long-leg films to assess alignment. Patellofemoral and stress views to better assess patellofemoral compartment and ligament laxity respectively.

Prosthetic designs and rationale: Two basic designs are available with their advantages and limitations, the clinical results with them seem to be similar:
- A fixed femoral and fixed tibial component with low conformity between the two articular surfaces. This allows relatively unconstrained movement between the femoral and tibial articulations. The ligaments control the movement. Disadvantage is that the limited conformity results in high stresses in the tibial component which produces excessive polyethylene wear and possible early component loosening especially if the polyethylene is thin.
- A free mobile bearing with absolute congruency between the metal femoral and metal tibial articulating surfaces maintained through the full range of movement. Disadvantage of this design is the possibility of a dislocation of the mobile articulating surface.

The components should be placed in such a way that the tibial and femoral components are parallel and in maximum congruency in both flexion and extension. The components should be placed in the center of the compartment as an offset placement will result in weak fixation and early loosening. The posterior slope should be restored as close as possible to avoid strain on ACL. In contrast to HTO undercorrection is recommended in UKA. Minimum 6 mm of poly thickness is recommended.

Performance and results: The cumulative benefits of UKA over TKA and HTO are short hospital stay, full ROM, speedy recovery and unaided walk, able to sit cross-legged on floor, reciprocal stair climbing, brisk walking, jogging allowed, joint preserving, not compromising future surgery and joint preserving. Postoperative morbidity and infection after UKA is less than TKA. The long-term failure rates for UKA are some 1.8 times than TKA. The cumulative revision rates for TKA have reduced, however, remain same for UKA. Component loosening due to malpositioning and various other factors is the most common cause of failure. Disease progression in the other compartments is the second most common cause followed by polyethylene wear. In conclusion, prefer UKA in older, light, and sedentary patient or middle-aged female with unicompartmental osteoarthritis.

TABLE 10: Comparative features of high tibial osteotomy and unicompartmental arthroplasty

Feature	*UKA*	*HTO*
Age	>55 years	<60 years
Activity level	Low demand	Active person
Weight	<30	Obese can undergo
Ideal alignment	<10° and passively correctable	5–15°
ROM	Flexion >90°, <5° flexion contracture	Flexion arc 120°, <5° flexion contracture
Arthrosis severity	Any	Ahlback <3
Joint instability	None tolerated (?ACL deficiency can be tolerated)	Some amount of ACL/PCL deficiency acceptable
Multiplanar deformity	No	Can be corrected
Corrective goal	Undercorrection	Overcorrection
Complications	Less	More
Conversion to TKA	Bone stock loss on both femoral and tibial side. Results UKA → TKA inferior than primary	Tibial component alignment, exposure difficulties. Results HTO → TKA better

(ACL: anterior cruciate ligament; HTO: high tibial osteotomy; PCL: posterior cruciate ligament; ROM: range of motion; TKA: total knee arthroplasty; UKA: unicompartmental knee arthroplasty)

HTO versus UKA: These two techniques are considered alternatives (with strict ingenious patient selection) for management of medial gonarthrosis; however, the principal differences are outlined in **Table 10**.

Cartilage Preserving or Regeneration Procedures

Various modalities are being worked upon for management of localized defect as detailed in **Box 3**.

Total knee arthroplasty is the cornerstone for treatment of advanced arthritis that provides reproducible and sustained pain relief with functional improvement. Arthrodesis is reserved for small joints or where arthroplasty is contraindicated.

BOX 3: Cartilage preserving and regenerative procedures for osteoarthritis (most of these are already discussed in Chapter on "Articular Cartilage: Structure, Function, Injury, and Management" and can be detailed from there). *(It must be remembered that the use and propaganda for stem cell therapy, platelet rich plasma, MSCs and autologous therapies has far outpaced the evidence and is currently experimental only, without any definitive support from research/literature to their indiscriminate usage)*

Chondrocyte transplantation:
- Autologous chondrocyte implantation (ACI and ACI-collagen)
- Matrix-assisted chondrocyte implantation/transplantation (MACI/MACT)

Osteochondral bone grafting: Mosaicplasty and osteochondral autograft transfer system (OATS) can be used for coverage of defects with hyaline cartilage up to 4 cm but for larger defects allografts are commonly needed.

Gene therapy: The gene therapy strategies in focus are: (1) Growth factors like TGF-β, BMP, FGF, IGF-1β, and epidermal growth factor (EGF); (2) SMADs; (3) Inhibition of proinflammatory cytokines like TNFα, IL-1; (4) apoptosis inhibition—Bcl-2, Bcl-XL, inducible nitric oxide synthase (iNOS); (5) Transcription factors like SOX9.

Mesenchymal stem cells (MSCs): They can induce differentiation of resident progenitor cells into chondrocyte regenerating articular cartilage. They can be obtained from bone marrow, adipose tissue, synovium, periosteum, infrapatellar fad pad, umbilical cord, placenta, etc. and express CD105, CD73, and CD90. MSCs are expanded under influence of FGF-2, TGF-β, PDGF, and three-dimensional (3D) culture systems for tissue engineering approaches. The chondrogenic differentiation of MSCs proceeds through 3 main stages, viz., condensation, differentiation, and terminal differentiation (maturation) characterized by expression of N-cadherin, collagen type-II and X, aggrecan and alkaline phosphatase. If growth factors are not used, MSCs can be directed to chondrogenic differentiation by silencing of anti-chondrogenic microRNAs and blockade of proangiogenic factors. 3D microenvironments are also helpful. The induced MSCs can be directly injected into the joint (multiple injections necessary) or they can be implanted on tissue-engineered constructs (better success rate). An additional approach is mixing MSCs with primary chondrocytes or chondrons isolated fresh from articular cartilage.

Platelet-rich plasma (PRP): They have proliferative effect on chondrocytes and MSCs and is a rich source of anti-inflammatory cytokines. PRP reduces the effects of inflammatory cytokines like IL-1β. The outcomes are variable so there is no concrete evidence supporting their use for or against in osteoarthritis. Additional strategies involve use of autologous adipose-derived stromal vascular fraction (SVF) alone or mixed with PRP, etc. There is no concrete evidence to use of these autologous therapies.

TOTAL KNEE ARTHROPLASTY

INTRODUCTION

Total knee arthroplasty is one of the most successful orthopedic procedures in the modern world. As with other joints, total knee replacement (TKR) was initially developed as a salvage option for badly damaged knees mostly due to infections or end-stage arthritis. Over the years, a more demanding lifestyle of patients combined with early successes of TKA has increased the expectations of the patient and in-turn has led to development of newer prostheses simultaneously the threshold for prescribing and accepting the surgery has gone down. This chapter will deal with a brief history of the development of prostheses, contemporary knee prostheses, indications and surgical approaches and techniques for TKA.

History

Earliest attempts at TKA were based on the concepts of interposition. Verneuil and Ferguson were the earliest to rely on various materials interposing between the resected ends of distal femur and proximal tibia. Most of these knees were damaged due to infection and the results of these procedures were uniformly poor. Gluck, a German doctor was the first to use a hinged knee prosthesis made of ivory for patients with end stage arthritis in 1890. Variable early results led to uniformly poor mid- to long-term results due to lack of proper fixation techniques and neglect of basic knee biomechanics.

In the period from 1940 to 1960, encouraged by the success of cup hemiarthroplasty of the hip, many surgeons tried different forms of hemiarthroplasty in the knee. Of importance was the use of acrylic tibial inserts by McIntosh for valgus and varus deformities. The early results of such a prosthesis (later made of metal) were good. However, subsidence and dislocations were frequent on long-term follow-up. Gunston, in the late 1960s, improved on the idea and developed an implant (Polycentric knee) which had metal femoral runners imbedded in the condyles and they articulated with separate medial and lateral polythene tibial troughs. For the first time in the history, acrylic bone cement was used for fixation of the implant. The genesis of modern knee prosthesis began with the work of Freeman et al. The Freeman-Swanson knee was developed in late 1960s. This design laid down three principles which found way in all the future designs based on functional approach: (1) Sacrifice the cruciate ligaments to correct the deformity; (2) Sacrificing the cruciates also simplified the mechanics and the function of stability and mobility was taken over by "roller in trough" design; (3) The implant components were seated on flat cancellous bone surfaces for better and uniform cementing.

Four models in vogue during 1970s as described by Insall with increasing complexity were:

1. Unicondylar
2. Duocondylar
3. Geometric
4. Guepar

Subsequent work on the development of unconstrained surface replacement prostheses was done along two different design philosophies—functional and anatomical.

Functional Approach

Functional approach focused on simplifying the biomechanics and kinematics of the natural knee and aimed at providing an engineering solution for mobility and stability. These designs focused more on reducing the wear and thus the articulations were made more conforming in shape. The mainstay of this philosophy was sacrifice of both cruciate ligaments.

Anatomic Approach

This approach emphasized on the preservation of as much native tissue as possible. The designs based on this approach aimed at recreating the mechanics of the natural knee. Initially, all the designs preserved both the ACL and the PCL, but eventually, all designs aimed at preserving only the PCL. The designs based on this approach focused more on providing less constraints and thus reduce the incidence of loosening.

Contemporary Knee Designs

Though the initial prostheses derived from these approaches carried a clear demarcation between the features, over a period of time desired features were identified and most of the contemporary TKA prostheses have certain common features:

- Asymmetrical femoral components with anatomically oriented trochlear groove
- Multiple sizing options for a better fit across variable anatomy
- Modular components for better soft tissue tension and ease of revision
- Moderately conforming round-on-round tibiofemoral articulation in coronal plane
- Multiple radii of curvature in the sagittal plane of the femoral component

Contemporary Cr Design

- What we have retained:
  - Asymmetrical femur
  - Varied geometry patellar flange
  - Posterior slot for PCL
- What we have changed:
  - Increased conformity of articulating surfaces
  - Compromise between mobility and wear

Contemporary Ps Design

- What we have retained
  - Cam-post mechanism
  - More conforming articulations
  - Metal-backed tray
  - Modularity
- What we have changed
  - Abandoned "spherical on spherical" articulation
  - Added asymmetrical anatomical femoral condyles
  - Varied geometry patellar groove for better patellar articulation. The various comparative features of cruciate retaining versus posterior stabilized knee are presented in **Table 11**.

Special Design Features

Guided Motion Prosthesis

Guided motion prosthesis is defined as a prosthesis which has inherent design features that compel the femoral and tibial components to move in a certain predefined manner. The following are the types:

- *Single-radius femur:* Multiple radii in the sagittal plane help in even distribution of the stress at the femorotibial articulation in early flexion and help to roll-back in deep flexion. However, concerns have been raised about the potential loss of tension in the collateral ligaments while the knee flexes due to sudden change in the radius of the femoral component, changing the length of the collaterals. To offset this disadvantage, the idea of a single sagittal radius was brought into fore. The other proposed advantage was that the posteriorized flexion-extension axis improved the mechanical advantage of the extensor apparatus and thus potentially reduces the incidence of anterior knee pain. Although the concept appears tempting theoretically, current studies do not support an improved result with such prostheses.
- *Medial-pivot knee:* This type of prosthesis aims at recreating the normal knee kinematics. In the natural knee on flexion, the more conforming medial joint acts as the axis for rotation and it is mostly the lateral femoral condyle which rotates and slides posteriorly. Medial-pivot knee aims at recreating the same kinematic phenomenon. Again, although the concept sounds appealing, no long-term study is available to either support or refute the potential advantages of this design feature.

TABLE 11: The comparative features of cruciate retaining versus posterior stabilized knee.

Cruciate retaining bicondylar knee reconstruction designs	*Posterior stabilized bicondylar knee reconstruction designs*
ACL is sacrificed but PCL retained. It should be avoided in inflammatory arthritis or PCL degeneration due to risk of imminent or delayed PCL rupture. Suitable for mild varus/valgus knee.	ACL and PCL both sacrificed. Femoral component box substitutes for PCL. Increased stability in previous patellectomy patients and weak extensor mechanism. It can be used in inflammatory arthritis. Suitable for mild-to-moderate varus/valgus.
Advantages: • Increased quadriceps strength (controversial) • Improved stair climbing • Preserved PCL proprioception (unknown benefit) • Lower shear forces on the tibial component • Smaller box so preserves femoral bone in notch preparation • Near-normal knee kinematics • Theoretically lesser patellar complications • No cam-post jump complication (that exists in PS knee)	*Advantages*: • Theoretically easier to achieve ligament balance in the knee without need to balance PCL • Greater deformity correction (compared to CR) • Better knee ROM (theoretical) • Less polyethylene wear as the articular surfaces are more congruent
Disadvantages: • Future PCL degeneration or rupture can later produce flexion instability • Imbalance/Tight PCL is detrimental for increased wear of polyethylene due to dysfunctional TKA kinematics	*Disadvantages*: • Cam-post jumps over the femoral box—dislocated knee in mid-late flexion instability (increased flexion gap) • Lax knee has increased polyethylene wear on postosteolysis • Patellar clunk (unique complication due to femoral box) • Higher chances of technical error which can involve elevating the joint line

(ACL: anterior cruciate ligament; CR: cruciate-retaining; PCL: posterior cruciate ligament; PS: posterior stabilized; ROM: range of motion; TKA: total knee arthroplasty)

Rotating Platform Knee

Knee prostheses have an inherent conflict between the two potentially devastating complications—wear and component loosening. To reduce wear, it is essential for the femorotibial articulation to be as conforming as possible. Increased conformity undoubtedly reduces wear but at the same time, it also reduces the degree of freedom in the motion of the knee prosthesis. This reduced freedom for motion in an unconstrained prosthesis has the potential to transfer the stresses to the implant-cement-bone interface and cause loosening of the prosthesis. This potential conflict was realized by Buchel and Papas and the came up with a novel idea to tackle the problem. They made the articulation highly conforming to reduce the incidence of wear and to reduce transfer of stresses to the implant-cement-bone interface, they added a component of mobility between the tibial insert and tibial tray. By adding a central pit in the tibial tray and a peg in the insert, they allowed the tibial insert to rotate freely on a highly polished metal tibial base plate. The concept has held itself well against the test of time, however, no long-term study including randomized trials and meta-analyses have shown a distinct advantage of this design feature. Besides, the rotating platform design has its own share of unique complications like bearing "spin-out" if the knee is not properly balanced. There is also a potential for increased back side wear due to the motion between the poly insert and tibial tray. Currently, the rotating platform design is used by surgeons mainly in the relatively younger population which is likely to use the knee for more demanding activities and who require a more natural feel in their replaced knee. Also, the concept has found a good hold in hinged designs where the stresses generated at the implant-cement-bone interface due to increased constraint is offset by the mobility of the tibial poly on the underlying metal tray.

From all above advancements and retentions modern arthroplasty designs available as surgical armamentarium include the following common designs:

- Unicompartmental (uncemented/cemented, rotating/fixed bearing)
- Cruciate retaining bicondylar (fixed/rotating bearing ± patella resurfacing)
- Posterior stabilized bicondylar (fixed/rotating bearing ± patella resurfacing)
- Constrained nonhinged knee for severe deformities and soft-tissue insufficiency
- Constrained hinged prosthetic components for ligament insufficiency, revision knee and severe bony deficiency (rotating hinge vs. fixed hinge)

GOALS OF TOTAL KNEE REPLACEMENT

The goals of total knee replacement are more or less the same as for any other form of arthroplasty, that is:

- To restore the damaged joint surface
- To provide painless free motion at the knee joint

Achieving these goals help in improving the quality of life of patients suffering from end-stage knee arthritis. The surgical objectives set to achieve these goals comprise restoring mechanical axis and joint line, balancing ligaments, and restoring Q-angle.

PRINCIPLES OF TOTAL KNEE REPLACEMENT

Successful total knee replacement requires strict adherence to the following guiding principles:

1. *Alignment:* It has been shown in multiple studies that the femoral and the tibial components have to be implanted in such a manner that the mechanical axis of the lower extremity is restored. The mechanical axis of the limb is defined by a straight line passing through the center of the hip joint, center of the knee joint, and the center of the ankle joint. In a replaced knee, when a straight line is drawn from the center of the hip to the center of the ankle, ideally it should pass through the center of the knee joint. Restoration of this axis equilibrates the load distribution in the medial and the lateral compartment, going by the recommendation of Insall. Hungerford and Kenna have challenged this concept of mechanical alignment

by stating that restoring the prearthritic anatomy of the patient will lead to better patient satisfaction and better joint kinematics. They recommend placing the femoral component in 9–10° of anatomic valgus and the tibial component in 3° of anatomic varus thereby recreating 6–7° of valgus at the knee joint. This concept is known as the concept of anatomical alignment. Although the concept looks appealing, it has not found many takers simply because of the fact that if the surgeon is inexperienced; cutting the tibia in varus intentionally may actually cause an excessive varus, leading to early failure. Slight undercorrection of coronal alignment can decrease ligament imbalance but incurs a risk of varus malalignment. Therefore, aiming for near-normal medial stability with neutral alignment is one of the best solutions in TKA for medial osteoarthritis of the knee.

2. *Soft-tissue balancing:* Coronal plane balancing of soft-tissues is mandatory to maintain equal load transmission across knee in varus and valgus stress. Long-standing disease process produce fixed soft-tissue contractures. Varus knee has tight medial structures while valgus degenerated knee (as in rheumatoid arthritis or lateral condyle hypoplasia) has tight lateral structures that are released appropriately as detailed in **Table 12**.
3. *Gap balance:* The gaps have to be balanced both in coronal (mediolateral) and sagittal plane (flexion-extension gaps). The coronal plane balancing is mostly achieved by ligament releases and proper component rotation. For balancing the knee in sagittal plane, a complex combination of capsular releases, variation of component sizes and extra cuts need to be performed. If the knee is left unbalanced excessive load transfer through one compartment will lead to early loosening and failure. Also, tight compartments will cause the knee to become painful and reduce the range of motion. Loose flexion gap produces flexion instability while loose extension gap leads to recurvatum knee. Tightness of any gap reduces knee movements and is disabling **(Box 4)**.
4. *Joint line preservation:* The amount of bone removed from femur and tibia should be reconstructed by the thickness of implanted components. This optimizes the function of ligaments and muscles around knee.

Preoperative Planning

Preoperative planning requires the standard series of radiographs of the affected knee. A long hip-knee-ankle radiograph is essential to plan tibial and femoral cuts to restore the mechanical alignment. On the femoral side, the angle between the femoral anatomic axis and the line perpendicular to the femoral mechanical axis is called the valgus correction angle. The angle of the distal femoral cut is equal to the valgus correction angle. Usually, it is between 6–7° in a varus knee and 4–5° in valgus knee. The intersection between the femoral anatomic axis and mechanical axis also determines the entry point for the femoral intramedullary jig. On the tibial side, the tibial cut is planned perpendicular to the mechanical axis of the tibia, which often coincides with the anatomic axis with 4–5° of posterior slope in the sagittal plane (more in CR versions).

Surgical Technique

Functional and anatomical approach in the designing of the TKR implant was also instrumental in development of different philosophies in the surgical technique of total knee replacement—gap balancing technique and measured resection technique.

- *Gap balancing technique:* This technique was developed for implanting the PS knees. The main focus of this technique was on the restoration of flexion and extension gap balance, which was achieved by varying the depth of the distal femur cut. Varying femoral distal cut was necessitated by the fact that the restricted sizes of the femoral component often led the surgeon to choose a smaller femoral component in relation to the actual size of the femur. This led to an increase in the flexion gap which required to be balanced by increasing the distal femoral cut. Classic gap balancing technique had the following steps:
  - Initial ligament releases to bring the knee in approximate alignment before bone cuts.

TABLE 12: The typical structures released in a degenerated knee with varus of valgus deformity.

Varus knee	*Valgus knee*
1. Medial osteophyte removal 2. Subperiosteal stripping of the deep medial collateral ligament (MCL) 3. Posteromedial capsular release 4. PCL sacrifice (posterior stabilized knee) 5. Distal tibial anterior or posterior periosteal stripping of the MCL depending on tightness in flexion or extension respectively 6. Pie crusting of MCL for combined flexion and extension tightness of MCL	1. Lateral osteophyte removal 2. Subperiosteal lateral joint capsule release 3. Lateral patellofemoral ligament release 4. "Pie crusting" of the iliotibial band (extension tightness) 5. Popliteus release for knee tight in flexion 6. PCL sacrifice (posterior stabilized knee) 7. Lateral collateral ligament release from its femoral insertion (avoiding complete release and subsequent varus instability)

(ACL: anterior cruciate ligament; PCL: posterior cruciate ligament)

BOX 4: Principles that are currently agreed upon and found to improve outcome in gap balancing.

The following are recommended for ligament balancing in TKA in typical a varus knee:

- The medial extension gap "laxity" should be within 1–3 mm to avoid flexion contracture.
  - Higher permitted laxity than this gives a feeling of instability to patient during ambulation.
  - No permitted laxity usually leaves knee in flexion contracture preventing locking in standing and resulting quadriceps tiredness.
- The medial flexion gap should be equal to the medial extension gap (or 1–2 mm larger) for normal stability
  - Larger medial flexion gap would increase anterior translation and produce mid-flexion/late-flexion instability.
- Lateral extension laxity up to 3° does not cause severe clinical problems.
- The femoral component should never be internally rotated to adjust the flexion gap.

(TKA: total knee arthroplasty)

- Tibia cut perpendicular to the mechanical axis with varying posterior slope. The tibial cut was conservative to prevent creating a large flexion gap.
- Knee flexed and distracted—AP cutting block rotated to make it parallel to the tibial cut and fixed to the femur and flexion gap created.
- Knee extended and distracted. The depth of distal cut determined by the spacer block which filled the flexion space most appropriately.

Varying distal cut in "gap balancing technique" often led to the elevation of joint line which at times could be detrimental.

- *Measured resection technique:* This technique was developed in conjunction with the anatomical approach, which also emphasized retention of PCL. For the PCL to be functional and capable of causing rollback without laxity or tightness, it was imperative to restore the joint line to the prearthritic normal. Therefore, the main focus of this technique was "restoration of the joint line". Going by the philosophy, the bone cuts were planned in such a manner that they remove little bone from femur, just enough for the implantation of the component. The tibial cut in measured resection technique required removal of at least the same thickness of the bone from the healthy side as would be substituted by the implant and therefore the tibial cut was about 9–10 mm deep when measured from the healthy side. The classic measured resection technique had the following steps:
  - No ligament releases before bone cuts.
  - Tibial cut perpendicular to the mechanical axis in coronal plane with a 7° posterior slope (if PS knee is used then slope is kept near neutral = 0 degree to prevent cam jump). The depth ranged from 9–10 mm when measured from the healthy side. Increased tibial slope helps in substituting for PCL deficit but increases flexion gap (can be partially offset by increasing distal cut by 1–2 mm) and also produces tendency to recurvatum deformity if excessive. Higher slope increases tendency toward anterior tibial translation and mid-late flexion instability.
  - Femoral cuts taken independent of the tibial cuts. Fluted intramedullary reference jig rod to reduce pressure is used. Entry hole is overdrilled to 12 mm. Distal cut of depth 9–10 mm depending on the system is made in 5–7° of valgus. Lesser valgus is used for taller patients and in valgus deformed knee. Larger degree of valgus is used for shorter patients and varus deformed knees. Femoral sizing is then done using anterior or posterior referencing **(Table 13)**. Rotation of the component determined by the femoral anatomical points—posterior condylar axis and transepicondylar axis or the Whiteside line **(Table 14)**.
  - Once the trial components are in place—they acted as tensioners and the ligaments are balanced subsequently **(Table 15)**.
  - The classic measured resection technique was more tolerant to slight mismatch in the flexion extension gap balance.

TABLE 13: The comparative features of anterior versus posterior referencing jig for sizing of femoral component.

Anterior referencing system	*Posterior referencing system*
The anterior cortex of femur is kept as a reference standard and paddles can be moved up or down to size the femur **(Fig. 11)**.	Posterior condyles of femur are taken as standard for sizing the femoral component by moving the anterior marker handle up or down **(Fig. 12)**.
It affects the flexion balance as sagittal plane change takes place posteriorly that comes to play during knee flexion. Smaller component will widen flexion gap while larger component chosen will tighten it and reduce flexion range of motion.	It affects the patellofemoral joint more prominently. Larger component chosen will overstuff the patellofemoral articulation and produce anterior knee pain and reduce flexion ROM.
Flexion-extension gap imbalance may happen if not done appropriately.	• Patella femoral overstuffing if larger component chosen • Anterior notching if smaller component chosen

(ROM: range of motion)

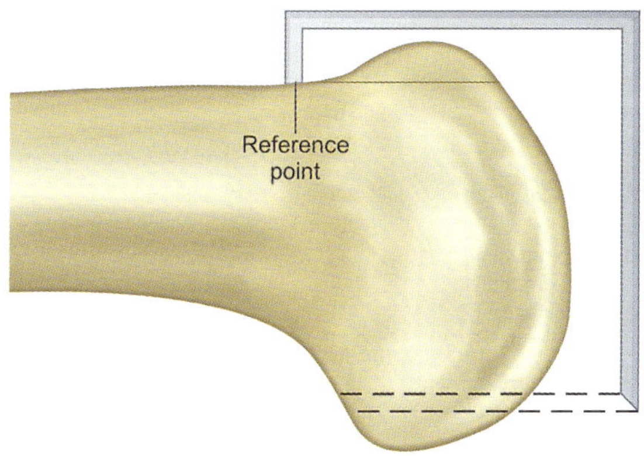

Fig. 11: Anterior referencing system.

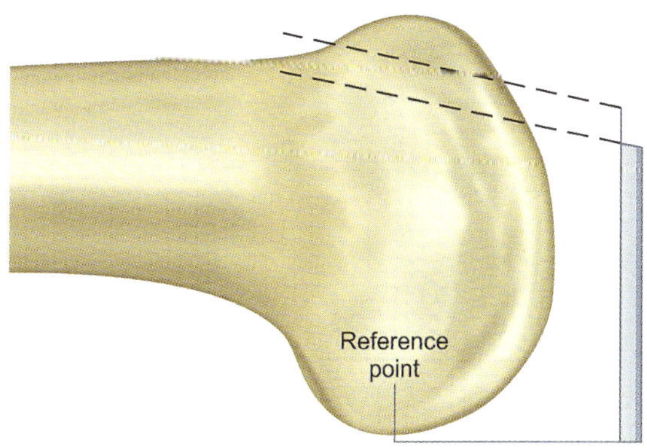

Fig. 12: Posterior referencing system.

Current Surgical Technique

As we can see from above, none of the techniques used were fool-proof. Gap balancing, on one hand, achieved perfect gap balancing in the sagittal plane, compromised on the level of joint line. On the other hand, measured resection technique achieved a perfect joint line but not without tolerating a compromised flexion-extension gap equality. To offset the

TABLE 14: The techniques used to reference neutral femoral implant rotation **(Fig. 13)**.

Transepicondylar axis (TEA, horizontal axis)	*Whiteside line (AP axis)*	*Posterior condylar axis*
Axis—Line connecting lateral epicondyle prominence to medial epicondyle sulcus between superficial and deep MCL. This axis places femoral component in 3° of desired external rotation. Not easily altered with alteration in bone morphology, most accurate if adequately marked. It is perpendicular to mechanical axis so anterior and posterior cuts are placed parallel to this axis. It is also used in revision TKR. *Disadvantages*: 1. Difficult to determine anatomically as instead of points they are small mounts. 2. Difficult to draw line and approximations are used instead.	Axis—Line drawn from the deepest part of the trochlear groove anteriorly to the center of the intercondylar notch (lateral fibers of PCL insertion). This line corresponds with mechanical axis—anterior and posterior cuts must be perpendicular to it. This axis places femoral component in 3° of desired external rotation. *Disadvantages*: 1. Altered by altered femoral anatomy. 2. The central notch point is more approximate than real. 3. Invalid in revision cases.	Axis—Paddles of the femoral size measuring jig placed on the posterior femoral condyles mark this axis. The posterior condylar has to be rotated by 3° externally to obtain desired femoral component placement. *Disadvantages*: 1. Altered in valgus knee, lateral condyle hypoplasia and dysplastic femora. 2. Invalid in revision cases 3. 3° of external rotation addition is not universal.

(MCL: medial collateral ligament; PCL: posterior cruciate ligament; TKR: total knee replacement)

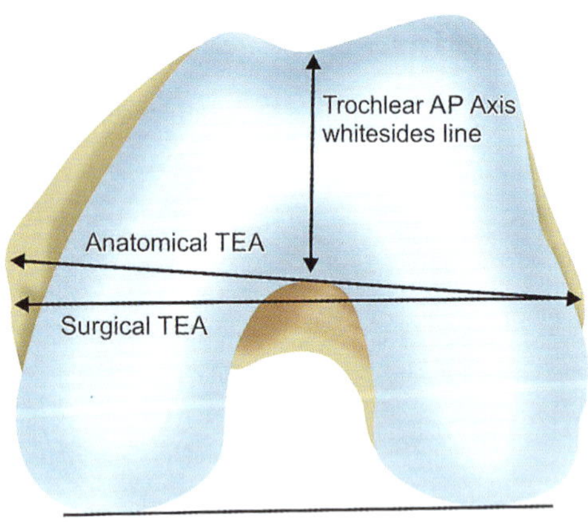

Fig. 13: Techniques used to reference neutral femoral implant rotation: Transepicondylar axis (TEA, horizontal axis), whiteside line (A-P axis), and posterior condylar axis.

disadvantages of each, the current implant systems work on the philosophy of "modified gap balancing technique". This technique incorporates the steps from both the classical approaches making this a hybrid approach. Emphasis is placed on conservative bone cuts and determination of femoral component rotation independent of the tibial cuts. At the same time, efforts are made to achieve a perfect

TABLE 15: The different way-arounds in managing mismatched flexion/extension gaps.

Extension gap	*Flexion gap*	*Possible solution*
Balanced	Loose	• Upsize femur (better with anterior referencing) • Fill cement posteriorly or better use posterior augments
Balanced	Tight	• If tibial slope is neutral or reverse, then increase slope • Downsize femoral component (better option with anterior referencing)
Loose	Balanced	• Add distal femoral augment • Downsize femoral component and use a thicker insert
Tight	Balanced	• Check if posterior femoral osteophytes are removed and perform capsular release from femur • Increase distal femoral cut
Loose	Loose	• Increase tibial poly insert
Loose	Tight	• Downsize femoral component ± add distal femoral augment
Tight	Loose	• Upsize femoral component • Posterior femoral augments • ± Revise (increase) distal femoral cut
Tight	Tight	• Use thinner poly insert • Revise (increase) tibial cut

flexion-extension balance **(Table 16)**. Most of this has been made possible by the increase in the availability of different component sizes which closely match the native femur.

Surgical Approaches

Various surgical procedures have been described for performing a total knee replacement. They can be classified into three types:

1. Routine approaches
2. Minimally invasive approaches
3. Approaches for difficult exposure

Routine Approaches

The traditional approaches for TKR are still the most widely used. Over a period of time these surgical approaches have shown to provide sustained good results although none of the studies support the theoretical benefits of one approach over the other. All the exposures start with an anterior midline or slightly medial longitudinal incision on the knee. The major difference in between the approaches is the site of arthrotomy.

- *Medial parapatellar:* The arthrotomy in this approach extends proximally into the substance of the quadriceps tendon. A cuff of tendon is left on the medial side of the incision for easy and better closure. This approach is the most commonly used surgical approach. It provides the widest exposure and is compatible with primary as well as revision arthroplasty procedures.
- *Midvastus and subvastus:* Medial parapatellar approach has an inherent drawback that it requires violating the sanctity of the quadriceps tendon. Thus, theoretically

TABLE 16: The different structures released for achieving rectangular balanced flexion and extension gaps.

Order of release of soft-tissue contracted structures for achieving rectangular extension and flexion gaps	
Varus deformity (medial structures are contracted and need release while lateral are already lax)	*Valgus deformity* (lateral structures are tight due to contracture and need release while medial structures are already lax)
Routine releases needed in order of increasing severity: • Deep MCL release (it is recommended to release this till mid-coronal plane in mild-to-moderate deformities but in severe deformities usually complete release is needed) • Osteophyte removal • Posteromedial release and removal of posterior oblique ligament • Medial tibial reduction osteotomy	*Routine preparation steps in order of standard sequence:* • Limited but precise bone cuts and reduce femoral valgus cut • Osteophyte clearance • Posterolateral capsule
Still trapezoidal in extension: Release superficial MCL posterior oblique portion from tibial insertion	*Still tight in extension:* • Iliotibial band (ITB) fractional lengthening by pie-crusting • Complete ITB release off Gerdy's tubercle if no improvement
Still trapezoidal in flexion: • Anterior portion of superficial MCL tibial insertion • Consider PCL release/PS implant if started with CR knee • Release semimembranosus	*Tight in flexion:* • Release anterior part of popliteus insertion • Release whole popliteus for severe deformity/contracture
Trapezoidal in both flexion and extension: • Pie crusting with 18-gauge needle • Complete MCL release as a ligamentoperiosteal sleeve from tibia—needs constrained implant	*Tight in flexion and extension both:* • Release both ITB and popliteus (differential vs. complete depending on severity) • Release LCL (some surgeons release it first rather than ITB and popliteus) because this is the only laterally tight structure that effectively tightens both flexion and extension gaps. • If both popliteus and LCL are released, then constrained prosthesis will be needed.

(CR: cruciate-retaining; MCL: medial collateral ligament; PCL: posterior cruciate ligament; PS: posteriorly stabilized)

it can lead to delayed rehabilitation and late return of quadriceps function. The midvastus and subvastus approaches are answers to this problem. In the midvastus approach, the arthrotomy utilizes an incision through the fibers of the vastus medialis muscle and in the subvastus approach; the entire vastus medialis muscle is elevated. Both these approaches are good in maintaining the integrity of the quadriceps tendon and thus theoretically provide better and early rehabilitation. However, with these approaches the exposure can be quite difficult in patients who are obese or those who have a bulky medialis muscle. Studies are yet to show an unequivocal benefit of these approaches over the medial parapatellar approach.

Minimally Invasive Approaches

These approaches aim at reducing the size of the incision and at the same time reducing the amount of damage to the soft tissue and help better and rapid rehabilitation of the patient. These approaches have been made possible due to the advancement in the surgical instrumentation, which have been reduced both in size as well as the profile. The minimally invasive approaches are either the modification of the routine approaches—medial parapatellar, midvastus and subvastus or the novel "quadriceps sparing approach". The quadriceps sparing approach utilizes a small medial or lateral parapatellar arthrotomy and "side cutting" instrumentation for taking the bone cuts.

Although the minimally invasive approaches are attractive, they are associated with higher rate of complications particularly malpositioning of the implant. Also, the spectrum of cases in which these can be use is quite narrow.

Extensile (Difficult) Exposures

In certain primary as well as revision cases, the routine approaches are unable to provide adequate exposure for surgery. This may be either due to the shortening/scarring of the quadriceps mechanism or due to the presence of significant deformities. These approaches invade the quadriceps mechanism in one of the directions—proximally or distally. The approaches are—modified Coonse Adams quadriceps turndown, Insall's quadriceps snip, tibial tubercle osteotomy.

In most of the cases, quadriceps snip is enough for exposing the joint. The approach involves extending the proximal limb of the medial parapatellar arthrotomy incision laterally and proximally. The advantage of this procedure is easy closure.

COMPLICATIONS OF TOTAL KNEE REPLACEMENT

By virtue of being a totally elective procedure where patient optimization is mandatory, TKR is one of the safest orthopedic surgeries. Still, the rate of any major or minor complication varies between 2 and 3%. The complication rate is highest among patients undergoing a simultaneous bilateral TKR. The complications can be divided into:

1. Systemic complications
2. Local complications
3. TKR specific complications

Systemic Complications

- Thromboembolism:
  - Common complication after TKR surgery if no prophylaxis is used
  - Rate of pulmonary embolism—1–28%, no prophylaxis used
  - Rate of fatal embolism—0.1–2%, no prophylaxis used
  - Most of the thrombosis affects the distal veins and therefore the risk of fatal embolism is lesser than THR.
  - However, the rates may be underestimated because the distal clots can grow proximally into popliteal

veins and femoral veins so effect appear late (3–4 weeks after surgery)—delayed deaths at home.
    - No universally accepted prophylaxis regimen
    - AAOS guidelines recommend use of multiple measures—physical and pharmacological
    - Early mobilization is the most effective and cheapest.
    - Pharmacoprophylaxis can be given by using any of these—UFH, LMWH, Xa inhibitors (including oral), and warfarin.
    - Physical measures—calf pumps, anti-DVT stockings.
- Fat embolism:
    - Not a frequent complication
    - Presents with tachypnea, dyspnea, disorientation, hypoxia, anxiety, profuse tracheobronchial secretions
    - May be due to fat embolism during intramedullary instrumentation
    - Treatment is supportive with use of mechanical ventilation and steroids.
    - Prevention is better:
        - Lavage IM cavity before instrumentation and suction of fat
        - Use of fluted rods
        - Navigation—especially in bilateral simultaneous cases

Local Complications

- Wound drainage and delayed wound healing:
    - Prevention of wound complications should be the target.
    - Management starts in the preoperative period by planning the skin incision.
    - Risk factors:
        - Previous scars
        - Postradiotherapy/burns
        - Adherent scar tissue
    - Systemic risk factors:
        - Malnutrition
        - Diabetes mellitus
        - Immunocompromised state
        - Prolonged corticosteroid use
        - Inflammatory arthritis
    - Preoperative measures in case of bad soft tissue:
        - Sham incision—mostly historical interest, not routinely recommended
        - Tissue expanders—a time of 8–10 weeks should be allotted to tissue expansion procedure before TKR is done.
        - Prophylactic flaps—minimum of 12 weeks should be allowed between coverage and subsequent TKR procedure.
    - Tips and tricks in cases with previous skin incisions:
        - Use the most lateral incision as most of the blood supply comes from the medial aspect.
        - Make minimum flaps and that too below the deep fascia.
        - Small transverse incisions can be crossed at 90°.
        - Short oblique incisions can be ignored.
        - If the angle between a long oblique incision and vertical incision is <60° consider—tissue expanders/prophylactic flap coverage or infrequently, sham incisions.
    - Intraoperative measures:
        - Good hemostasis—especially lateral genicular artery
        - Avoid lateral release
        - Timing of tourniquet deflation—still a matter of debate
    - Postoperative care:
        - Identify at risk wounds
            - Ecchymosis
            - Blisters
            - Superficial skin necrosis
            - Prolonged serosanguinous discharge
            - Swollen and painful knee
        - Care
            - Do not prolong antibiotic therapy unnecessarily.
            - Stop pharmacoprophylaxis and use mechanical devices for DVT prevention.
            - Stop physio, compression bandage, and limb elevation.
            - Frequent cold compresses
            - If the discharge still present—second look surgery, thorough wash and watertight closure
            - Consider it as deep infection if there is an opening in the capsular layer and do good thorough lavage.
- Vascular complications:
    - Rare complication
    - Incidence—0.03 to 0.2%
    - Can be either injury to popliteal vessels or perigenicular vessels
    - May present acutely or subacutely as—AV fistula, pseudoaneurysm and aneurysms
    - Treatment includes direct repair in acute cases—most of the limbs can be salvaged.
    - AV fistula, pseudoaneurysms, and aneuryms may require:
        - Thrombin injection
        - Resection and repair
    - Vascular insufficiency can also occur due to acute arterial occlusion. Atherosclerotic plaques can dislodge during surgery and may occlude the circulation downstream. Can be successfully treated by surgical embolectomy.
- Neurological complications:
    - Rare but troublesome complication
    - Incidence—0.3 to 0.5%
    - Risk factors:
        - Significant flexion or valgus deformity
        - Tight postoperative dressing
        - Epidural analgesia
    - Double crush:
        - Happens when TKR is done in continuous analgesia

  - Pressure on nerve due to catheter and second point of pressure due to tourniquet
  - Recommended to restrict tourniquet pressure to less than 320 mm Hg
- Treatment:
  - Complete recovery is rare.
  - Sensory loss more likely to remain
  - Most surgeons recommend conservative treatment.
  - Immediate removal of tight bandages and flexion of knee
  - In valgus knees, postoperatively keep knee in 30 ° flexion
  - Use of AFO and exercises
  - Operative decompression of nerve also shows good result.

Total Knee Replacement Specific Complications

- Instability:
  - One of the most common cause for revision
  - Constitutes 10–22% cases of TKR failure
  - Causes of early instability:
    - Component malalignment
    - Failure to restore mechanical axis
    - Imbalance of flexion-extension space
    - Rupture of MCL, PCL (in CR knees)
  - Late instability is mostly due to poly wear.
  - Other causes of late instability:
    - PCL tear in CR knee and postfracture in PS knee
  - Instability can be in coronal plane, sagittal plane or combined.
  - Symmetrical extension instability—due to over-resection of distal femur:
    - Treatment—revision with distal augments
  - Asymmetrical extension instability:
    - Under-correction of preoperative deformity—more common in severe varus/valgus
    - If excessive release required—in old patients, use constrained implant
    - Other cause—Iatrogenic MCL tear/over-release of tight side
    - Treatment depends upon the underlying cause
  - Flexion instability—early due to gap imbalance and late due to either PCL attenuation (CR knee) or post-wear (PS knee)
  - Commonest problem—over-resection of posterior femoral condyles with reduction in posterior offset or excessive posterior tibial slope
  - Symptoms and signs:
    - Recurrent effusion
    - Instability while climbing stairs/getting up from chair
    - Positive posterior drawer test, posterior sag
  - Treatment—revision with posterior augments, constrained implant
  - Genu recurvatum deformity:
    - Prevention is better than cure.
    - Mostly seen in patients with neuromuscular disease
    - Other patients—patients with RA, preoperative valgus deformity
    - Treatment:
      - Rotating hinge with extension stop
      - Under-resection of distal femur—overstuff the extension space
      - Posterior repositioning of collateral ligament
- Arthrofibrosis:
  - Incidence ranges from 1.2 to 17%
  - Multiple contributory factors—patient and surgical
  - Risk factors:
    - Female sex
    - High BMI
    - Low pain threshold
    - Depressed patient
    - Patient personality
    - Preoperative diagnosis—JRA, post-traumatic
    - Previous knee surgery
    - Previous history of arthrofibrosis
  - Surgical factors—incorrect component position or imbalance
  - Treatment:
    - Begin with adequate pain relief and manipulation
    - If unsuccessful, then attempt manipulation—done at 6 weeks but can be done till 90 days from TKR.
    - If manipulation fails, then do arthroscopic lysis.
    - Open lysis
    - If all fails—revision TKR.
- Component loosening:
  - Aseptic loosening commonly seen on the tibial side
  - One of the most common cause for revision
  - Multifactorial in causation:
    - Malpositioned implant
    - Malalignment of axis
    - High BMI
    - Implant geometry
    - Small tibial component
    - Polythene wear and osteolysis
  - Tibial loosening is design specific. Early tibial designs without a central peg had a high failure rate. Patients with flat-on-flat design have a higher chance of poly wear and subsequent loosening.
  - Incidence of loosening further lessened by use of metal backed tibia probably due to equal stress distribution.
  - Loosening may appear on the X-ray as complete, progressive radiolucent lines below the tibial tray. However, the relation of RLLs with loosening is still not completely established.
  - Femoral component loosening is rare and mostly due to faulty surgical technique or osteoporotic bone.
  - Patellar component loosening—uncommon with all poly cemented components
  - Causes of patellar component loosening:
    - Asymmetric facet resection
    - Malpositioning of button

- Osteoporosis
- Patellar AVN
- Insertion into sclerotic or worn out bone

- Patellar complications:
  - Patellar clunk syndrome:
    - Seen more commonly in PS knees
    - Soft tissue nodule forms at the junction of superior patellar pole and quadriceps tendon. This nodule becomes hyperplastic and rubbery with repeated passage through the femoral trochlea.
    - Sudden passage causes painful clunk on knee extension from a flexed position.
  - *Synovial entrapment/hyperplasia*—less well-defined condition. Patient complains of pain and crepitus on knee extension from 90° flexed position.
  - Treatment of both clunk and hyperplasia:
    - Physical therapy
    - Surgical removal of nodule
    - Arthroscopic debridement
    - Patellar prosthesis revision
    - Open resection through limited lateral approach.
  - Patellar subluxation/dislocation:
    - Multifactorial causation
      - Malpositioned implant
        - Internally rotated femoral/tibial component
        - Malpositioned patellar button
      - Femoral component shape
      - Excessive knee valgus
      - Tight lateral retinaculum
    - Treatment ranges from proximal realignment procedures to revision of malpositioned components.

Contemporary Interventional Techniques to Manage Chronic Knee Pain

Chronic knee pain is very common in middle-aged population due to osteoarthritis or rheumatoid disease. Analgesics like NSAIDs are mainstay in conservative management of pain. However, they became less effective with the progression of disease and often discontinued due to side effects on their prolonged use. Evidence-based knee injections for the management of arthritis have shown that commonly used techniques such as steroid, intra-articular injection of hyaluronate, botulinum toxin Type A, tropisetron, and tanezumab are effective in reducing the arthritic pain. Recently other techniques like radiofrequency ablation of genicular nerves and inter-articular injection of platelets-rich plasma (PRP) are being used. These two techniques are described here.

Radiofrequency Ablation (RFA) of Genicular Nerves

In the knee, nociceptors are located throughout the joint; in the capsule, ligaments, menisci, periosteum, and subchondral bone. Cellular and structural changes within the peripheral joint components promote biochemical sensitization and may activate nociceptors located on the afferent nerve fibers. Inflammatory cytokines may further increase biological function of pain mediators by stimulating their receptors, contributing to clinically symptomatic pain. These painful sensations are carried by nerves innervating the knee joint and skin over it.

TABLE 17: Nerve supply of knee joint.

Major nerve	*Sensory (genicular) branches*
Femoral	a. Nerve to vastus medialis b. Nerve to vastus intermedius c. Nerve to vastus lateralis
Tibial	a. Superior medial genicular b. Inferior medial genicular c. Middle genicular
Common peroneal	a. Superior lateral genicular b. Inferior lateral genicular c. Recurrent genicular
Obturator	Genicular branch from posterior division

The sensory branches from sciatic, femoral, and obturator nerves which carry pain sensation from knee are called genicular nerves. Radiofrequency lesioning of these nerves is effective to control chronic knee pain. There are 10 articular branches **(Table 17)** to knee joint which are responsible for pain sensation from knee joint and skin surrounding it. However, only superior medial genicular and inferior medial genicular (branches from tibial nerve), and superior lateral genicular (branch from common peroneal nerve) are accessible for radiofrequency treatment. These three branches have consistent anatomical presence and have shown effective pain relief after local anesthetic injection or radiofrequency ablation. Other than these genicular nerves, saphenous nerve which carries painful sensation from anterior and medial aspect of knee joint and skin is also accessible to RF treatment in adductor canal.

Technique: The patient is placed in supine position and fluoroscopy is used to visualize the knee joint in anteroposterior view. The landmarks used for the superior medial and superior lateral genicular nerves are the junction of the femoral shaft with the medial and lateral epicondyles. The landmark for the inferior medial genicular nerve is the medial aspect of the tibia at the shaft-epicondyle intersection **(Fig. 14A)**. The skin is anesthetized with 1% lidocaine and a 20–21 gauge 100 mm insulated radiofrequency (cannula) needle with a 5–10 mm active tip is advanced toward each of these locations until the lateral view confirmed that the needle tips at the posterior one-third of the femur and tibia **(Fig. 14B)**. Sensory stimulation at 50 Hz is performed to confirm correct needle position followed by motor stimulation at 2 Hz to confirm the absence of muscle fasciculation. Lidocaine is injected to anesthetize the nerves and RFA is then performed at 80°C for 180 seconds in the lesion mode. The diagnostic genicular nerve block with local anesthetic is usually done before RFA to ensure effectiveness of RFA. The duration of pain relief is expected to last from 6 months to more than a year. RFA can be repeated if pain reoccurs due to regeneration of nerves. This technique is also effective in patients with persistent pain after total knee replacement surgery. To further increase the effectiveness of the RFA, new technologies like "Cooled RF", bipolar RF and RFA under ultrasound guidance have been used recently.

Platelet-rich Plasma Injection Therapy

Platelet-rich plasma is volume of plasma that contains a concentrate of platelets above (usually 4–5 times) that of baseline blood levels (150,000–200,000/μL) In a special container the patient's own blood (20–60 mL) is centrifuged after mixing it with anticoagulants (Hard spin). The RBCs are separated and remaining contents are recentrifuged (soft spin) to get PRP **(Figs. 14C and D)**. Separated PRP (3–7 mL) is injected in the knee joint. Sometime platelets activators (bovine thrombin or 10% calcium chloride) are also mixed to activate the platelets before injection.

Platelet-rich plasma role in osteoarthritis knee: The healing process of osteoarthritis comprises three phases: (1) inflammation, (2) cell proliferation, and (3) remodeling. PRP augments tissue healing through the natural healing cascade. Growth factors are released from the granules of platelets and induce chemotaxis, cell migration, angiogenesis, proliferation, differentiation, and matrix production. PRP also enhances HA secretion and increases release of angiogenic growth factors. This biological therapy uses the patient's own platelets and plasma, which mainly convey fibrin and growth factors as effectors. These growth factors act on the entire joint. They promote restoration of joint homeostasis, have inductive and protective effects on chondrocytes, and stimulate the production of HA by synoviocytes. All these properties help to promote a generative biological environment and to slow down joint and cartilage degeneration, thereby relieving symptoms. The clinical effects are equivocal and there is no definitive guideline for or against its usage. It is still an unproved ancillary technique.

Technique: After application of local anesthesia, a 21-gauge needle is inserted into the joint through the external patellar wing, centered in the central region of the patella in the cranial-caudal plane. After placement of the needle into the joint space, synovial fluid arthrocentesis can be performed if it is necessary. Once arthrocentesis has been carried out and without removal of the needle, 8 mL of PRP is infiltrated. The infiltration is directed into the midpoint area of the femoropatellar region using an external approach (with the help of fluoroscopy or ultrasound) to prevent infiltration

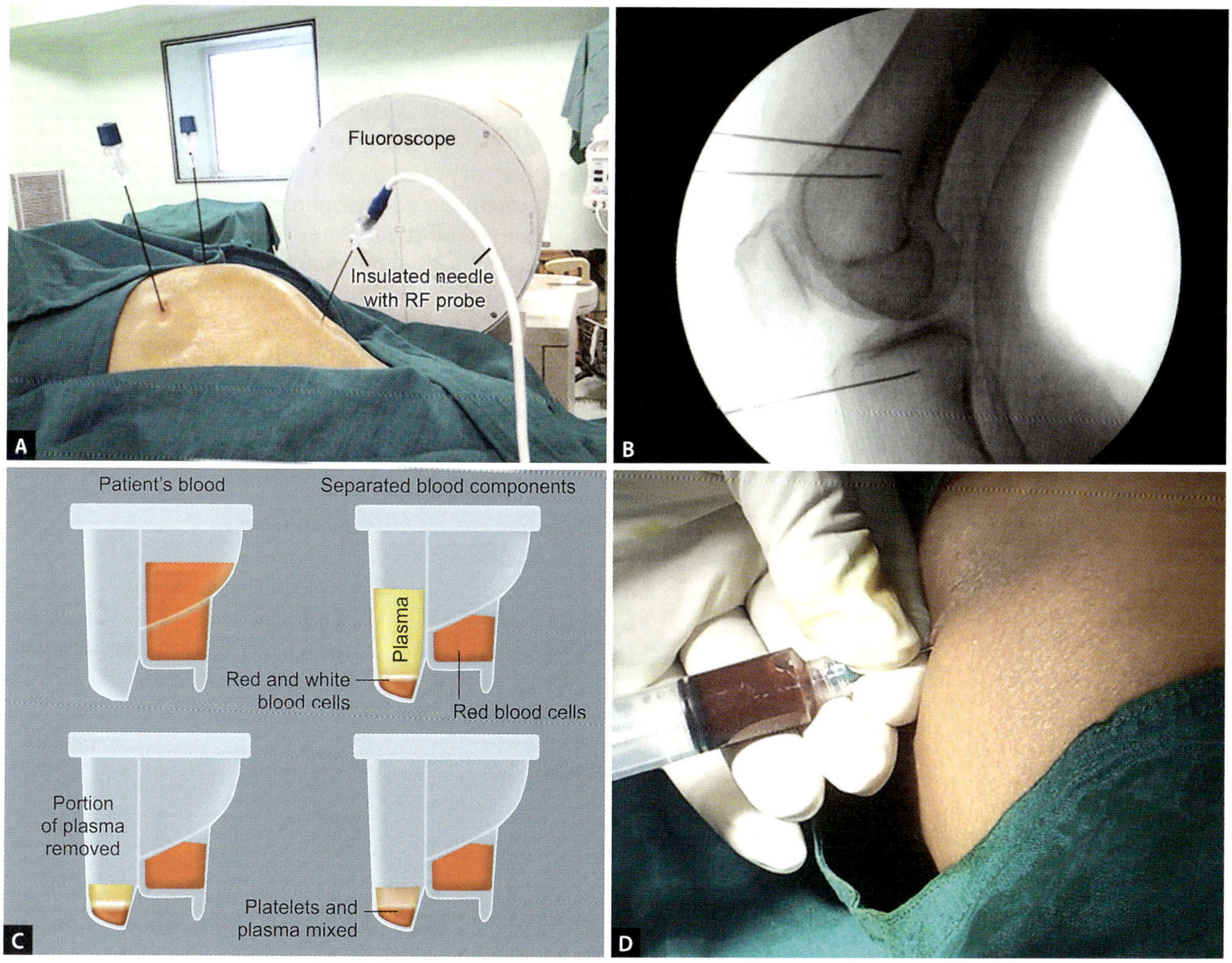

Figs. 14A to D: (A) Radiofrequency ablation (RFA) needle insertion under fluoroscope; (B) Final target of needles in lateral view; (C) Stages of platelet-rich plasma (PRP) preparation; (D) Injection of separated PRP in knee joint.

into the synovial membrane, which would cause pain. Most patients require two treatments, but some patients with severe diseases may require more. Some people respond immediately, but most of the time it takes approximately 6 weeks to respond to the treatment. It is necessary that these patients should avoid anti-inflammatory (NSAIDs and steroid) drugs 2–3 weeks before and after the PRP injection as it may affect the efficacy of PRP treatment. This technique is very safe; however, repeated use should be avoided and a strict asepsis is mandatory during whole procedure to avoid infection.

CALCIUM PYROPHOSPHATE DIHYDRATE CRYSTAL DEPOSITION DISEASE (CPPD DISEASE OR ARTHROPATHY, PSEUDOGOUT, CHONDROCALCINOSIS, AND PYROPHOSPHATE ARTHROPATHY)

INTRODUCTION

This is a nonurate crystal arthropathy caused by deposition of calcium pyrophosphate dihydrate ($Ca_2P_2O_2.2H_2O$, or CPPD) crystals in the loose, avascular connective tissue matrices of articular hyaline cartilage, fibrocartilaginous menisci, and of certain ligaments and tendons that are particularly susceptible to calcification. The $Ca_2P_2O_2.2H_2O$ has calcium to phosphate ratio of 1.0. When associated with acute arthritis the disorder has clinical presentation similar to gout flare so was initially termed pseudogout but has characteristic differences to conclude it as a different entity **(Table 18)**. Although, both urate and CPPD crystals can cause an acute arthritis, the clinical features of articular CPPD deposition, particularly the frequent occurrence of severe cartilage degeneration, suggest that CPPD crystals have far more complex biologic effects in the joint than do gout crystals. CPPD manifests clinically as acute or chronic inflammatory arthritis, and CPPD can promote degenerative joint disease.

- The term chondrocalcinosis (calcification of fibro and hyaline cartilage) refers to the characteristic radiologic features of CPPD crystal deposition in cartilaginous tissue. Other disorders associated with it are:
  - Hypomagnesemia
  - Hypophosphatasia
  - Hemochromatosis
  - Wilson's disease
  - Hyperparathyroidism
  - Possible associations include—gout, ochronosis, hypocalciuric hypercalcemia, diabetes mellitus, and X-linked hypophosphatemic rickets.

The term "pyrophosphate arthropathy" was coined in 1969 by HLF Currey and the term is commonly used in the United Kingdom.

Some related but *distinct crystal deposition disease* include crystals of basic calcium phosphate (BCP), including partially carbonate-substituted hydroxyapatite HA deposited pathologically in articular cartilage, particularly in osteoarthritis. The chemical formula for HA is $Ca_5(PO_4)_3OH{\cdot}2H_2O$, and it has a calcium-to-phosphate ratio of 1.67. Inflammatory conditions also may result from deposition of the closely related BCP crystals octacalcium phosphate [chemical formula $Ca_8H_2(PO_4)_6{\cdot}5H_2O$; calcium:phosphate ratio 1.33], tricalcium phosphate or "whitlockite" [chemical formula $Ca_3(PO_4)_2$; calcium:phosphate ratio, 1.5] in periarticular structures, such as the rotator cuff (calcific tendinitis) and subacromial bursa of the shoulder and calcium oxalate crystals.

PATHOGENESIS

In CPPD deposition arthropathy (CPPDDA), there is excess calcium and pyrophosphate solute with the joint such that crystal precipitates out into the joint spaces and is deposited within the synovium and articular cartilage. Dysregulated proton-pump inhibitors (PPI) metabolism and other factors are at the core of pathogenesis of crystal deposition in idiopathic and other forms of CPPD **(Fig. 15)**. The crystals are 0.5–5 mm in the greatest diameter. They first develop in the articular matrix, menisci, and intervertebral disks. The deposits later enlarge into large chalky white friable masses. They are distinguishable from gout by their

TABLE 18: Differentiation gout and pseudogout.

Pseudogout	*Gout*
The classical features are found in large joints.	Smaller joints of hands and feet are predominantly affected.
The patients have pain similar to osteoarthritis and degenerative joint disease, inflammation is minimal.	Pain characteristically has an intense inflammatory component, felt throughout day but increasing in morning or with change in weather.
The margins of joint are irregular (enlarged joints) with osteophytes and bony swelling.	The joints are inflamed and tender with classical signs.
Radiologically, chondrocalcinosis is seen in advanced cases in the form of fine calcified cartilage line.	Serologically, patients have elevated uric acid levels.
Examination of joint fluid reveals calcium pyrophosphate crystals.	The patients have characteristic uric acid needle like crystals.

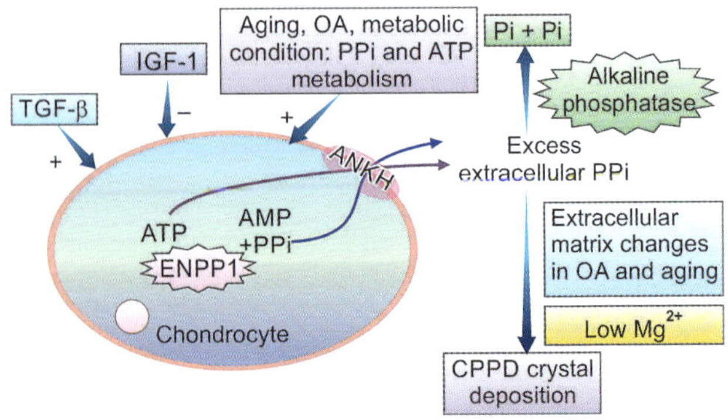

Fig. 15: Calcium pyrophosphate dihydrate (CPPD) pathophysiology. (AMP: adenosine monophosphate; ATP: adenosine triphosphate; IGF-1: Insulin-like growth factor 1; OA: osteoarthritis; PPi: pyrophosphate; TGF-β: transforming growth factor-beta)

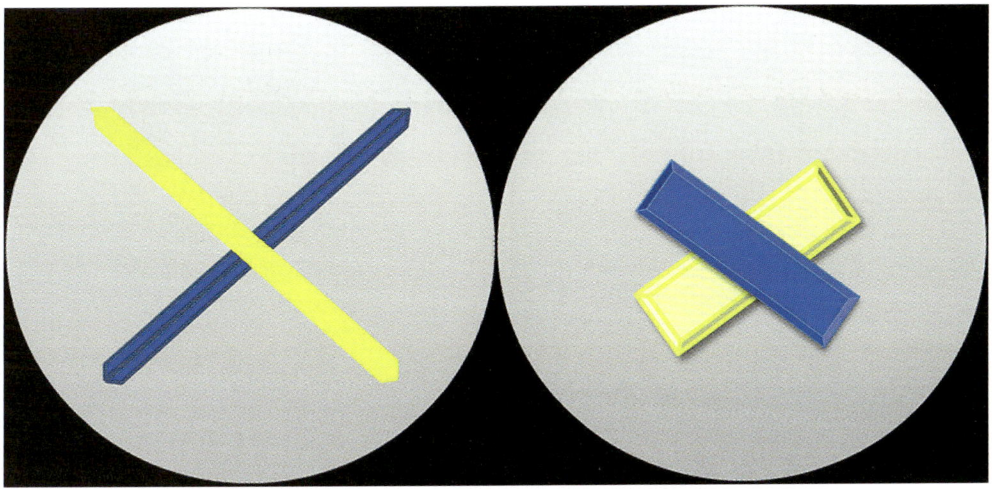

Fig. 16: Crystals of uric acid and calcium pyrophosphate: Birefringence is the property of refractive materials to polarized light. The uric acid crystals are needle like and negatively birefringent to polarized light (red compensator) appearing blue when aligned perpendicular and yellow when aligned parallel to it. While the calcium pyrophosphate crystals are shorter rhomboidal and positively birefringent—appearing blue when aligned parallel and yellow when aligned perpendicular to the polarized light (red compensator).

positive birefringence under polarized light (gout contains uric acid crystals that are negatively birefringent). The difference is explained in **Figure 16**. Articular cartilage matrix calcification can reflect deficiencies of certain physiologic calcification inhibitors or upregulation of mediators that actively drive stereotypical patterns of tissue injury, culminating in calcification within degenerating cartilage. The deposited monoclinic CPPD crystals are more inflammatory than the triclinic crystals producing prolonged joint degeneration similar but more rapid to osteoarthritis. There is a strong linkage of sporadic, aging-associated CPPD crystal deposition disease with excess chondrocyte inorganic pyrophosphate-generating nucleoside triphosphate pyrophosphohydrolase (NTPPPH) activity and augmented inorganic pyrophosphate generation by chondrocytes that promotes cartilage supersaturation with inorganic pyrophosphate. Articular cartilage, unlike growth-plate cartilage, is specially designed and shielded to avoid the process of matrix calcification. Relatively reserved output of PPI by chondrocytes physiologically functions to limit BCP crystal growth. This protective mechanism becomes deleterious by excessive PPI output in CPPD. The NTPPPH plasma cell membrane glycoprotein-1 (PC-1) plays a central role in sustaining and augmenting extracellular inorganic pyrophosphate in chondrocytes along with the multiple-pass, transmembrane protein ankylosis protein homolog human gene (ANKH). PC-1 [also known as ectonucleotide pyrophosphate pyrophosphohydrolase 1 (ENPP1)] is one of three highly homologous NPP family isoenzymes that share NTPPPH catalytic activity. Upregulated PC-1/ENPP1 expression is associated with both calcification and apoptosis in degenerative human cartilages. ENPP1 generates intracellular and extracellular PPI via hydrolysis of ATP and other nucleoside triphosphates. PC-1/NPP1 expression is stimulated by the chondrocyte growth factor TGF-β, which markedly elevates chondrocyte extracellular inorganic pyrophosphate. The capacity of TGF-β to raise chondrocyte inorganic pyrophosphate rises with aging. Intracellular PPI and ATP are transported to the extracellular space by processes involving ANKH. This pyrophosphate could combine with calcium to form CPPD crystals in matrix vesicles or on collagen fibers having decreased levels of glycosaminoglycans that normally inhibit and regulate crystal nucleation (collagens II and I, proteoglycans, and osteopontin). Mg^{2+} helps determine whether more inflammatory monoclinic (predominates in hypomagnesemia) or less inflammatory triclinic CPPD crystals are formed. CPPD crystals in the joint space are phagocytosed by monocyte-macrophages and neutrophils activating the *inflammasome* and propagating inflammation. The inflammatory responses are mediated by NOD-like receptor, pyrin domain containing 3 (NLRP3) inflammasome activation and consequent caspase-1 activation, and interleukin 1-β (IL-1β) maturation, and secretion.

A minority of patients with CPPD crystal deposition disease have metabolic abnormalities like hyper-parathyroidism, hemochromatosis, hypophosphatasia, hypomagnesemia (including the Gitelman's variant of Bartter's syndrome), etc. Presence of CPPD arthropathy in patients <50 years of age should raise suspicion of these metabolic disorders. Patients with familial chondrocalcinosis may have possible linkage to *ANKH* gene mutations at 5p chromosome region. ANKH mediates development and anatomic progression of both early-onset familial CPPD and late-onset disease. Linkage with chromosome 8q of both early onset osteoarthritis and chondrocalcinosis in a New England family was given the designation CCAL1. Chromosome 5p-linked chondrocalcinosis (CCAL2) is broadly distributed and has been studied in greater detail than 8q chondrocalcinosis.

CPPD deposition can develop in different zones of articular cartilage and is typically related to excessive extracellular inorganic pyrophosphate. Abundant cartilage NO production may promote mitochondrial dysfunction, chondrocyte extracellular ATP depletion, and lowering of

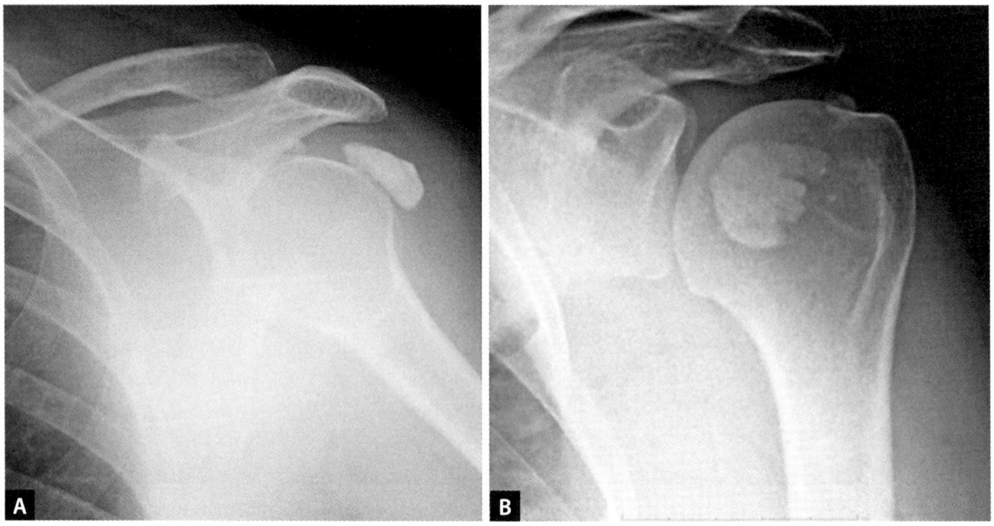

Figs. 17A and B: Calcium pyrophosphate dihydrate (CPPD) deposition at shoulder but no evidence of osteoarthritis (OA). There is a fine white line seen at superior aspect of labrum on anteroposterior (AP) view.

extracellular inorganic pyrophosphate that favors HA over CPPD crystal deposition as seen in *Milwaukee shoulder syndrome*. The shoulder is the most common articular region affected by symptomatic BCP crystal deposition, in part reflecting unique shoulder-structure function. Degenerative changes promoted by biomechanic stress promote calcific tendinitis in the body of the rotator cuff that may eventually either resorb or rupture the tendon. Osteopontin that normally restrains BCP crystal deposition promotes MMP activation, as well as macrophage recruitment and osteoclast activation in calcific tendinitis. Cathepsin K expression and osteoclast-like functions at sites of tendon calcification suggests a mechanism for both resorption of BCP crystal deposits and tendon degeneration leading to rupture.

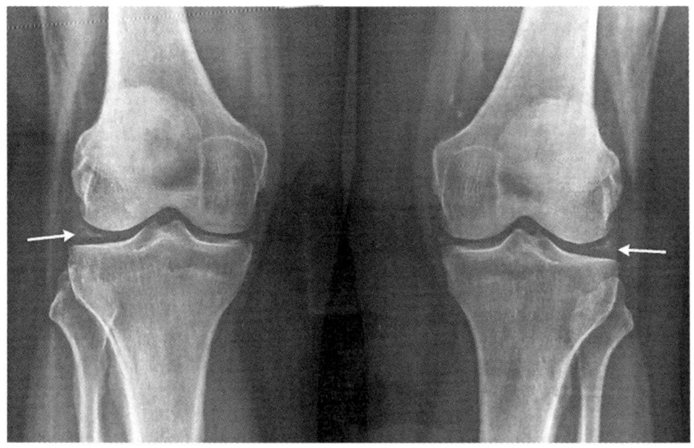

Fig. 18: The radiograph demonstrates characteristic calcification of the lateral menisci of both knees due to calcium pyrophosphate dihydrate (CPPD) crystal deposition in the hyaline cartilage (arrows). There is also initiation of calcification of the medial menisci of both knees.

CLINICAL FEATURES

CPPDDA affects a similar to that of osteoarthritis. It is very often clinically silent, but is a biomarker of aging and connective-tissue degeneration. In most patients, CPPDDA appears to represent a systemic articular and soft tissue pathophysiology disorder in aging. It becomes more prevalent with age and affects about 5% of the population. The disease may be asymptomatic, acute, subacute, or chronic or may cause acute synovitis superimposed on chronically involved joints. The clinical features in many cases are very similar to osteoarthritis: joint pain, crepitus, and stiffness after prolonged rest. However, radiographic evidence of CPPDDA at one joint is frequently associated with the disease at distant joints, whether osteoarthritis is present or not **(Figs. 17A and B)**. CPPDDA has a predilection for joints different from typical osteoarthritis although knee is still the most frequent joint involved. But it is interesting to note that knee osteoarthritis, but not hip osteoarthritis, is associated with radiographic evidence of CPPD at distant joints. Joints susceptible for CPPDDA include the radioscaphoid joint, the scaphotrapeziotrapezoidal joint, the metacarpophalangeal joints (particularly the second and third), the patellofemoral joint, and the talonavicular joint. There is no clear correlation between the extent of calcification and progression of disease. CPPDDA is polyarticular in around 70% patients and radiographic demonstration of punctate and/or linear radiodense deposits in fibrocartilaginous joint menisci or articular hyaline cartilage (called *chondrocalcinosis*, **Fig. 18**) support CPPDDA over osteoarthritis. Other characteristic features include:

- Axial involvement
- Sacroiliac erosions
- Cortical erosions of femur
- Osteonecrosis of medial femoral condyle

It should be borne in mind that chondrocalcinosis is also seen in calcium oxalate deposition. The proposed diagnostic criteria are depicted in **Box 5**. CPPD also has a tendency to present with occasional flares where patients develop acute inflammation in the joint, swelling from a joint effusion and erythema (termed *pseudogout* by McCarty et al.). Other clinical manifestations of CPPD deposition include: (1)

BOX 5: Proposed diagnostic criteria for calcium pyrophosphate dihydrate (CPPD) deposition disease (McCarty et al. 1994)

Criteria:
1. Demonstration of CPPD crystals, obtained by biopsy or aspirated synovial fluid, by definitive means (such as characteristic radiographic diffraction powder pattern)
2. (a) Identification of monoclinic or triclinic crystals showing a weak positive birefringence (or no birefringence) by compensated polarized light microscopy
   (b) Presence of typical calcifications on radiographs (as discussed in text): Heavy punctate and linear calcifications in fibrocartilages, articular (hyaline) cartilages, and joint capsules, especially if bilaterally symmetric
3. (a) Acute arthritis, especially of knees or other large joints
   (b) Chronic arthritis, especially of knee, hip, wrist, carpus, elbow, shoulder and metacarpophalangeal joints, particularly, if accompanied by acute exacerbations.

Diagnostic categories:
A. *Definite:* Criteria 1 or 2a present
B. *Probable:* Criteria 2a or 2b present
C. *Possible:* Criteria 3a or 3b suggests possible underlying CPPD deposition disease

worsening of typical forms of osteoarthritis, (2) neuropathic arthritis like induction of severe destructive disease, e.g., the Milwaukee shoulder, (3) RA like production of symmetric synovitis (sometimes seen in familial forms with early onset), (4) ankylosing spondylitis like intervertebral disk and ligament calcification with restriction of spine mobility (also seen in hereditary forms), (5) spinal stenosis (most commonly seen in the elderly), and (6) rarely periarticular tophus-like nodules.

There are several presentations of CPPD that also afford to classify the disease to some extent:

Type A ("Pseudogout")—Seen in 25% cases presenting as acute pain and swelling of single large joint like knee, wrist, shoulder, etc. It is rare in small joints. The factors that may precipitate acute pseudogout include:

- Intercurrent illness
- Direct trauma
- Surgery (especially parathyroidectomy)
- Blood transfusion and parenteral fluids
- Starting thyroxine replacement therapy
- Joint lavage

Type B ("pseudorheumatoid")—Seen in 5% patients presenting as polyarthritis. The synovitis and joint flares are however out of phase with each other.

C and D ("pseudo-osteoarthritis")—Type C with attacks and Type D without attacks seen in 50% patients. This presents with acute attacks on chronic osteoarthritis like symptoms.

Type E ("asymptomatic")—The chondrocalcinosis is incidentally detected on radiographs.

Type F ("pseudoneuropathic")—This rare presentation is seen as severe joint destruction neuropathy.

Other types include tophaceous CPPD deposits, spinal CPPD: "Crowned dens syndrome" (seen as deposits around the atlantoaxial joint), spinal stenosis, and cervical myelopathy. The BCP deposition disease presents like rheumatic conditions and has been seen associated with erosive arthritis, *Milwaukee shoulder syndrome,* mixed crystal deposition disease, pseudopodagra, calcific tendonitis, and bursitis. Milwaukee shoulder is an uncommon destructive form of disease affecting the shoulder in elderly females. Abundant intra-articular BCP (deposition of hydroxyapatite or octacalcium phosphate or tricalcium phosphate) crystalline material is typically present in the distinctive noninflammatory syndrome of rotator cuff tear and marked cartilage degeneration, an entity termed *Milwaukee shoulder syndrome* (MSS), *cuff tear arthropathy* or *apatite-associated destructive arthritis.* The process may be bilateral but is generally worse on the side of the dominant hand. Substantial glenohumeral joint effusions are typically seen, and synovial fluid is often blood-stained but contains, at most, relatively low numbers of mononuclear leukocytes. Joints other than the shoulder, such as the knee and hip, can be affected by a condition similar to MSS, sometimes in the same individual with shoulder involvement.

Calcium oxalate arthritis is an unusual form of arthritis that is seen associated with various conditions like:

- End-stage renal disease on dialysis
- Short bowel syndrome
- Diet rich in spinach, ascorbic acid
- Thiamine deficiency
- Pyridoxine deficiency

DIFFERENTIAL DIAGNOSIS

CPPD is a great mimic and rheumatologists keep this in differential for most disorders be it osteoarthritis (pseudo), RA (pseudo), hypophosphatemic rickets, hypocalciuric hypercalcemia, ochronosis, gout (pseudo), amyloidosis, septic arthritis (actually it is pseudoseptic arthritis), neuropathic joints (pseudo), Wilson's disease, polymyalgia rheumatic or even meningitis. Deposition of nonpathologic dicalcium phosphate dihydrate (DCPD), which has a chemical formula of $CaHPO_4$ $2H_2O$ (calcium-to-phosphate ratio of 1.0), also known as "brushite" crystals, has been thought to cause some atypical calcifications, but it should be noted that brushite crystals can arise as an artifact of preparation of calcified tissue for pathologic analyses.

RADIOLOGY

The deposition of calcium pyrophosphate within the articular structures, primarily the hyaline cartilage and the meniscal fibrocartilage, can become radiographically visible. The inflammatory component may contribute to some radiographically identifiable erosion at the joint surfaces, particularly in the radioscaphoid joint.

TREATMENT

Aim is to control the acute attacks and lessen chronic and anatomically progressive sequelae of crystal deposition. There is no specific treatment for idiopathic CPPD deposition disease. NSAIDs, steroids through various routes of administration, colchicine, synthetic adrenocorticotrophic hormone (ACTH) are mainstay for controlling acute attacks. Chloroquine has been found to be effective in treating polyarticular crystal deposition disease. Patients with pseudorheumatoid disease may potentially respond to MTX. Arthroscopic irrigation and colchicine help in osteoarthritic CPPD deposition disease. Novel targeting therapies include probenecid that suppresses ANK-induced and TGF-β-induced increases in extracellular inorganic pyrophosphate in vitro. Phosphocitrate is an inorganic pyrophosphate analog that inhibits NO induced calcification of cartilage and suppresses cell-stimulation and recruitment in HA and CPPD crystal deposition. Phosphocitrate also suppresses the ankylosing features of crystal deposition disease but has low bioavailability and needs to be given parenterally. Bisphosphonates (pyrophosphate analogs) can be beneficial in some cases of idiopathic infantile arterial and periarticular calcification, including disease associated with PC-1/NPP1 deficiency.

HEMOPHILIC ARTHROPATHY

INTRODUCTION

Hemophilia is one of the oldest recognized diseases. It is a group of disorders of blood coagulation disorders representing functional deficit in specific plasma clotting factor. Hemophilia A (classic hemophilia) and hemophilia B (Christmas disease) are due to deficiencies of factors VIII and IX respectively. Both are sex-linked recessive diseases, making women asymptomatic carriers of the gene (if heterozygous). Hemophilia A (Factor VIII deficiency) accounts for 85% of the cases while hemophilia B (factor IX deficiency) accounts for 15% cases. The original article describing articular cartilage changes of hemophilic arthropathy is credited to Konig while Albert Key described the "tumor-like" presentation at knee in a 13-year-old boy. Until the development of clotting factor replacement therapy, life expectancy for patients with hemophilia was around 11 years. Since the 1980s, replacement therapy has lengthened patients' lives to 50 or even 60 years.

There are several musculoskeletal manifestations of hemophilia; the most common are hemarthroses and muscle hemorrhage, with some patients developing a chronic arthritis and end-stage arthropathy. Progression of hemophilic arthropathy occurs from hemarthrosis to chronic synovitis to extensive joint surface erosion and ultimately end-stage joint destruction. Joints undergo continual minor daily trauma and so are prone to bleeding. Recurrent hemarthroses may lead to a chronic arthritis in which iron-containing, superficial lining cells of the synovium become hyperplastic. This hyperplastic synovial tissue, usually devoid of inflammatory cells, may form into an invasive pannus tissue, associated with marginal erosions of cortical bone and thinning of hyaline articular cartilage. Hemarthroses occur in 75–90% of patients with hemophilia. The most commonly affected joints are the knees, ankles, elbows, and shoulders. Bleeding into the joints of the fingers, wrists, feet, and axial spine is distinctly unusual. Recurrent hemarthrosis result in chronic proliferative synovitis and is associated with limitation of movements and arthropathy **(Fig. 19)**. Hemophilic arthropathy spares spine. End-stage arthropathy results from chronic arthritis seen radiologically as bony enlargement (squaring of metaphysis) and narrowing of joint space. There are marked flexion contractures, fibrous adhesions in the joint, and marked muscle atrophy. End-stage hemophilic arthropathy is characterized by following features:

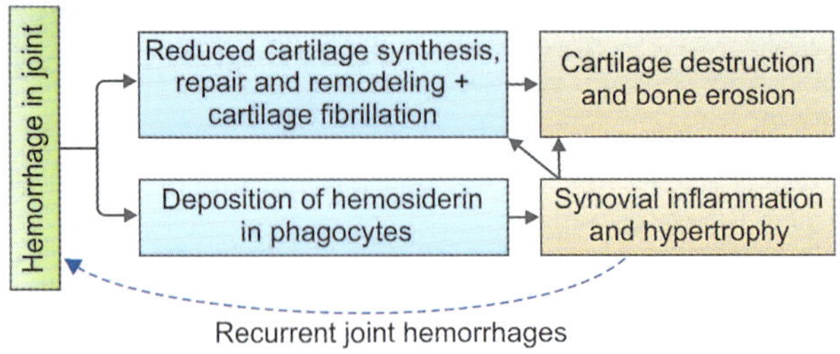

Fig. 19: Pathogenesis of joint changes in hemophilic arthropathy.

BOX 6: Hemophilic arthrofibrosis.

Arthrofibrosis:
- The extent and severity of arthrofibrosis is most severe with hemophilic disease than in any other disease where it develops (like inflammatory, infectious, post-traumatic or postsurgical patients)
- Arthrofibrosis forms within capsule and subsynovial layer of the joint running from capsule to articular surface or between articular surfaces.
- The tissues contain very high population of myofibroblasts.
- Condition aggravates even further following surgery where the healing process is over reactive and persistent beyond the normal period with aggressive fibroplasia and tissue metaplasia.
- It is mediated by cytokines, growth factors, and reactive nitrogen and oxygen species (RONS). RONS stimulates hemorrhage and release of hemosiderin further releasing RONS setting up a vicious cycle. Increased COX-2 levels are also found that are anti-apoptotic supporting synovial hyperplastic hyperplasia.
- Management includes:
  - *Low-dose radiation postoperatively*: This may complicate wound healing and make future surgeries difficult by producing late accelerated fibrosis.
  - *Intra-articular steroids*: Reduces host defenses to infection. Usually, a short course of oral steroids is preferred.
  - *Intra-articular botulinum toxin*: This inactivates IL-1.

- Arthrofibrosis—fibrous adhesions severely restricting movement of joint **(*see* Box 6)**
- Severe flexion contractures
- Angular deformities
- Loss of bone stock due to synovial cysts and mechanical abrasion

Pain is always present but not the most prominent symptom. Patients may also develop hemorrhage into their marrow space, resulting in pseudotumors of bone (also see **Box 7**). These are generally isolated lytic lesions with well-defined margins that may be confused radiographically with other true neoplastic lesions of bone an ignorant surgeon could even amputate for resemblance to osteosarcoma. Hemorrhage into muscles and soft tissues lead to myonecrosis and secondary joint deformities like flexion at knee, talipes at ankle, etc. Compartment syndrome may result from the bleeding diathesis most commonly developing in the volar forearm compartment.

RADIOLOGY

Recurrent hemorrhage into a joint leads to eventual deposition of ferritin within the joint that can be sensitively

BOX 7: Hemophilic pseudotumors.

- Hemophilic pseudotumors are rare complications of hemophilia that develop following intramuscular or intraosseous hemorrhages. Clinically, they resemble tumors but are not neoplastic in pathological sense so called "pseudotumors". They are also called "hemophilic cyst of soft tissue" if occurs within muscle or "hemophilic cyst of bone" if it occurs within a bone to totally segregate them from "tumors". The incidence is low seen in 1–2% of patients with hemophilia typically between 20 and 70 years of age. They develop after recurrent episodes of hematoma formation within muscle or bone whence the previous one fails to resolve completely. Often the bulky muscles with abundant blood supply and juxta-articular regions of bone are involved.
- Intramuscular pseudotumors frequently compress nearby structures that is the common reason for their evaluation and discovery. The most frequent is the development of iliopsoas hematoma producing pelvic pseudotumor. Groin pain that increases with internal rotation of the hip is the main symptom but this may also be seen in bleeding within the hip joint. Pelvic pseudotumors due to iliopsoas hematoma is, however, also sometimes associated with femoral nerve palsy and numbness in saphenous nerve. Hip bleeds are identified with increased femoral head to tear drop distance in anteroposterior view of pelvis. The other important differential is acute appendicitis that can be radiologically (ultrasonography/CT/MRI) differentiated. Hemophilic pseudotumor of bone presents with a slowly growing painless or painful mass that may be associated with pathological fractures in surrounding bones. Radiologically, they appear as well-defined, unilocular or multiloculated, lytic, expansile lesions of variable size that involve metaphysis (more common), diaphysis or epiphysis of long bones. Uncommon findings include endosteal scalloping, perilesional sclerosis, cortical thinning or thickening, trabeculations, and septations.
- Ultrasonography in acute stages shows central anechoic area with increased "fluid" echoes behind the lesion. The thick wall separating the lesion from surrounding structures is better differentiated on CT scan (especially contrast enhanced).
- Management importantly involves distinguishing these pseudotumors from true neoplasms such as chondrosarcoma, liposarcoma, and synovial sarcoma that may develop in these patients. This involves adequate radiological evaluation followed by biopsy from the lesion. Once confirmed to be a pseudotumor various modalities of treatment are described like percutaneous ultrasound-guided aspiration/evacuation (usually unsuccessful), radical surgical removal (preferred), low-dose radiation therapy (only for nonresectable and/or recurrent disease) in fractions of 2 Gy or less until a total dose of 6–23.5 Gy, curettage and bone grafting for intraosseous pseudotumors. Preoperative arterial embolization 2 weeks before surgery is recommended for large pelvic pseudotumors that are likely to cause extensive bleed. Standard surgical precautions for these patients should be taken still there is high chance of infection, fistulation, and pathological fractures in these patients sometimes requiring amputations.

detected on MRI. Hemorrhagic joint effusion also causes increased blood flow to the bone around the joint possibly due to inflammation. This increased flow in turn causes overgrowth of the adjacent epiphyses and early leg length discrepancies. Overgrowth of the femoral condyles leads to widening of the intercondylar notch and overgrowth of the patella causes the appearance of squaring of its inferior pole. There is subnormal gain in height due to premature epiphyseal fusion. Arthritic changes are evident in most by second to third decade depending on disease severity. Radiographic staging of hemophilic arthropathy is done in accordance with orthopedic hemophilia treatment center's modified Arnold and Hilgartner system grades of hemophilic arthropathy as follows:

- *Grade 1:* Soft-tissue fullness indicating joint effusion and synovial thickening. Juxta-articular osteopenia is often present.
- *Grade 2:* Widened epiphysis, surface irregularity and small erosions, normal cartilage interval or "joint space".
- *Grade 3:* Narrowing of cartilage interval with extensive surface erosions. Juxta-articular bony cysts may be present.
- *Grade 4:* Findings of stage 3 but with complete loss of cartilage interval and marked surface irregularity. Reactive sclerosis, squaring of the margins of femoral condyles, and subluxation are often present as well as large synovial cysts.

TREATMENT

The treatment has evolved from plasma transfusion in 1950s, cryoprecipitate in late 1960s for hemophilia A and plasma derived concentrates in 1970s to use of safer recombinant clotting factors in 1990s that persisted for a long time. Replacement of the deficient factor (VIII, costly) or fresh frozen plasma (factor IX) should be started as soon as the prodromal symptoms develop to maintain 50% of activity. This is also required when planning a major surgery. Patients receiving cryoprecipitate are at risk of developing HIV and hepatitis B and C infection so factor VIII concentrate is the preferred modality. The patients undergoing joint replacement should be monitored for deficient factor levels; presence of high titers of factor VIII inhibitor is a contraindication to this surgery. This treatment though effective is cost and time intensive so improvement is sought in the form of extended half-life products like pegylated and fusion proteins that need fewer infusions. Mechanisms other than factor replacement are being developed. Bispecific monoclonal antibody Emicizumab acts by stabilizing interaction of factors IXa and X bypassing need for factor VIII. This is particularly for treatment of hemophilia A patients with an inhibitor to factor VIII. Another approach is siRNA approach that acts by downregulating the anticoagulant antithrombin III to rebalance the coagulation system. Gene therapy is also helping in the therapy of hemophilia where Christmas disease patients have been treated with AAV8 infused gene modified with zinc finger nucleases. Improved gene splicing and joining using CRISPR/Cas9 will further enhance the capability of genetic modification to treat hemophilia A also. Some 15% of patients on replacement therapy develop autoantibodies to the humanized proteins inhibiting their efficacy especially for the factor VIII. These patients have to be managed through immune tolerance program where they are given large doses of clotting factors that overwhelm and suppress the inhibitors but it makes treatment cost intensive. Strategies involving use of factor VIIA and VIII bypassing agent are effective in some of these patients but not all. Newer monoclonal antibodies may be effective in managing these patients.

Muscle hematomas should be evacuated after factor replacement. Ultrasound-guided hematoma evacuation is safe but not infrequently unsuccessful due to excessive viscosity of the content. Untreated they may cause compartment syndrome and nerve compressions.

Radiosynovectomy

Radiosynovectomy or radiosynoviorthesis had been extensively used for treatment of rheumatoid arthritis while a variety of radiocolloids have been also used for chronic hemophilic synovitis. 32P chromic phosphate (or radiocolloid gold or yttrium) is commonly used for radiosynovectomy with dosage of 0.5 millicuries is used for large joints and half dose for small joints in children. In adults, the dosages are doubled respectively. Before injecting the radiocolloid the clotting factor levels are restored to 50–100% of normal. The steps include:

- Prepare the parts using standard aseptic preparation.
- Locally anesthetize the skin and subcutaneous tissues.
- Insert a 23- to 18-gauge needle (prefer smaller gauge for subcutaneous joints) and place it intra-articular. If needed it can be done under ultrasound guidance.
- Inject the selected dose using a separate syringe for precise dose administration. Flush the needle and tract with 5 mL lidocaine and 1 mL dexamethasone solution.
- Immobilize the joint for 2 days avoiding any strenuous activities.
- Biodistribution analysis is then done using Geiger–Müller counter through small window analysis of the target and contralateral joint.
- ^{198}Au had been used in pediatric population without any side effects to growth plate or articular cartilage. Development of late radiation induced neoplasia had been the concern but 32P does not penetrate deep into the tissues (bone mostly remain spared) and also development of intra-articular neoplasia is very rare. Because of low penetrance of 32P chromic phosphate the therapy may be ineffective in hypertrophied synovium whence measures like preprocedure intra-articular steroid to reduce synovial thickness or arthroscopic synovectomy have to be used.

OCHRONOSIS (ALKAPTONURIA)

INTRODUCTION

The term "alkaptonuria" ("alkali" + "kaptein"—to suck up avidly) was coined by Boedeker in 1859, denoting avidity for oxygen in alkaline solution. Ochronosis is a rare hereditary autosomal recessive disease with ineffective homogentisic acid oxidase in the pathway of tyrosine catabolism so that excessive homogentisic acid (*ortho-meta*-dihydroxyphenylacetic acid) is secreted in the urine imparting brownish black color. The kidneys rapidly clear this material and only a small amount remains in the tissues, but eventually it begins to accumulate in the cartilage of the ear, skin, intervertebral disks, and sclera **(Figs. 20A and B)**. Ochronosis denotes this bluish black pigmentation (due to oxidation of pigment) of connective tissue and was coined by Virchow for microscopic appearance of the pigment ("Ochrea"—dark yellow). The relationship between alkaptonuria and ochronosis was first recognized in 1902 by Albrecht. Exogenous ochronosis has been described with the use of topical hydroquinone, phenol, picric acid and exposure to resorcinol, benzene, and antimalarials but are not prominent orthopedically.

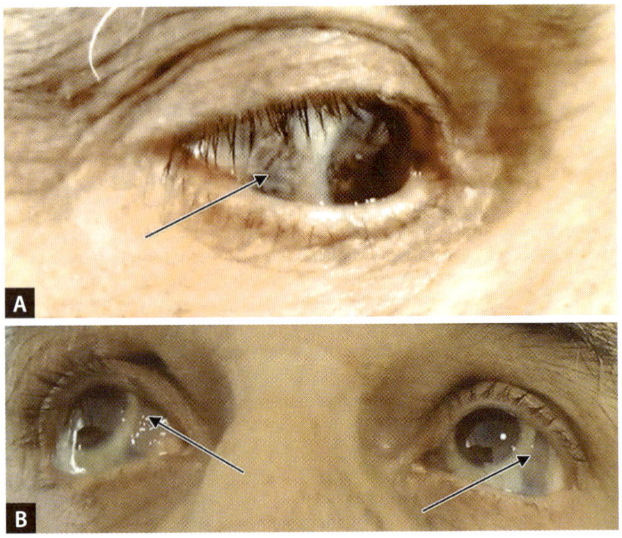

Figs. 20A and B: The deposition (arrows) of bluish black pigment in the sclera of the patient with alkaptonuria.

CLINICAL FEATURES

Alkaptonuria is asymptomatic but clinically identifiable symptoms develop with pigment deposition. By the fourth decade, these deposits begin to calcify causing the synovial joints to show chondrocalcinosis. Eventually, the patients develop secondary osteoarthritis and spondylosis related to disk degeneration caused by the deposition of homogentisic acid in cartilage. In ochronitic spondylitis there is calcification and ossification of intervertebral disks producing rigid spine with stooped posture, loss of lumbar lordosis, knee flexed, and typical stance. There are but little if any osteophytes, the sacroiliac joints are normal and spine is unaffected (no bamboo spine) differentiating this from ankylosing spondylitis. The earliest symptoms are usually localized to lumbar spine and spondylosis, however, with progression the dorsal and cervical spine get involved. Radiographic calcified disks suggest but are not diagnostic of ochronosis as they can be found in pseudogout, hemochromatosis, chronic respiratory paralytic poliomyelitis, and iatrogenic (spinal fusion). Splits in disk material appear to account for radiolucencies in the disks that have been termed vacuum disks. The arthropathy is typical with brittle cartilage fragments and pigmented "shards" in the synovium **(Figs. 21A to C)**. Commonly the knees, shoulders, and hips are affected sparing the small joints of hands and feet. Osteochondral joint bodies are common and occasionally CPPD crystal associated inflammation may be seen. Radiographically, the peripheral arthropathy is indistinguishable from osteoarthritis and demonstrates narrowing of the joint space, small marginal osteophytes, and eburnation. Other features include grayish black discoloration of tympanic membrane, black cerumen, systolic cardiac murmur due to stenosis of aortic and mitral valves. Prostatic calculi are seen in majority of men with ochronosis and can be digitally palpated per rectally.

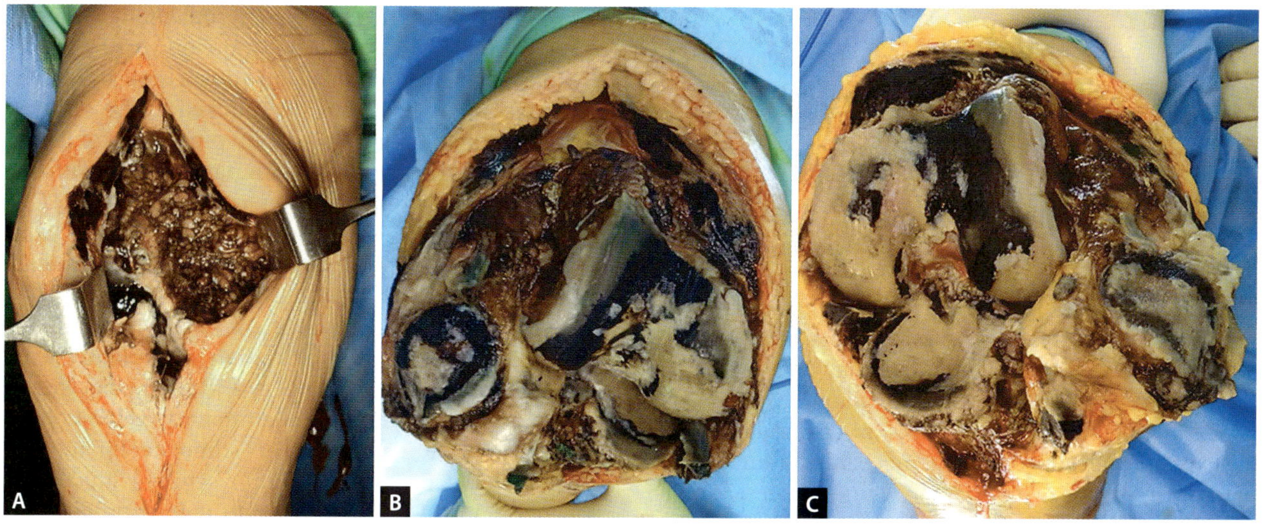

Figs. 21A to C: The clinical appearance of tissues in a patient with alkaptonuria. The photographs were taken when the characteristic black tissues were seen while performing total knee arthroplasty on the patient. The hypertrophic inflamed synovium was tanned (golden brown to black, A). Specifically notable is the fact that the cartilage covering bones was mildly affected while the bone turned pitch black due to deposition of the pigment (B and C). So all the shiny black bony regions represent eburnated bone at subchondral level while the "spared" areas were still covered with cartilage.

TREATMENT

Mainly on the lines of management of osteoarthritis and spondylosis (physiotherapy, braces, analgesics, weight reduction, etc.). Patients often require arthroplasty for large joints. High-dose ascorbic acid is suggested to reduce binding of the pigment to the tissues. Protein or tyrosine restricted diets are unpalatable. Steroids, irradiation, tyrosinase, vitamins, and phenylbutazone have been found ineffective. Nitisinone (reduces production of homogentisic acid by inhibiting 4-hydrophenylpyruvate dioxygenase) may be helpful (need to be studied) and is currently available for treatment of tyrosinemia Type 1.

RHEUMATOID ARTHRITIS

INTRODUCTION

Guillaume de Baillou (1538–1616) was the first to use the word "rheumatism" in the modern sense. Rheumatoid arthritis (RA) is a chronic, inflammatory, autoimmune disease that may involve multiple organ systems but mainly targets the synovial joints. It is more common in women than men (ratio of 2–3:1) and has peak incidence somewhere between 35 and 50 years. There is no "diagnostic criteria" for rheumatoid arthritis. RA is diagnosed in individuals with symmetrical inflammatory polyarthritis affecting the small joints of the hands, feet, and wrists persisting for >6 weeks with characteristic laboratory abnormalities. The American College of Rheumatology has established a set of clinical criteria **(Table 19)** to establish the diagnosis. Patients have swollen joints and early morning stiffness typically lasting longer than 1 hour. They may be positive for rheumatoid factor and/or anticitrullinated peptide/protein antibody (ACPA). The most specific laboratory finding for RA is the presence of anticyclic citrullinated peptide (anti-CCP) antibodies seen in 60–70% patients. Anti-CCP antibody may be present before rheumatoid factor is detected. One must understand that ACPA is an umbrella term that includes anti-CCP, so not all ACPA are anti-CCP. The terms "ACPA" and "anti-CCP" are being used interchangeably and some preference to former is developing. The majority of patients afflicted with RA have ongoing, progressive disease with periods of reduced activity.

TABLE 19: The 2010 revised criteria for the classification (not diagnosis) of RA (for newly presenting patients who have at least 1 joint with definite clinical synovitis that is not better explained by another disease) (Maximum score = 10, score ≥ 6 is definitive RA).

Criteria		*Score*
Joint involvement	1 large joint (shoulder, elbow, hip, knee, and ankle)	0
	2–10 large joints	1
	1–3 small joints (MCP, PIP, thumb IP, MTP, and wrists)	2
	4–10 small joints	3
	>10 joints (at least 1 small joint)	5
Serology	Negative RF and negative anti-CCP antibodies	0
	Low-positive RF or low-positive anti-CCP antibodies (three times upper limit of normal)	2
	High-positive RF or high-positive anti-CCP antibodies (>3 times upper limit of normal)	3
Acute-phase reactants	Normal CRP and normal ESR	0
	Abnormal CRP or abnormal ESR	1
Duration of symptoms	<6 weeks	0
	≥6 weeks	1

(CCP: cyclic citrullinated peptide; CRP: C-reactive protein; ESR: erythrocyte sedimentation rate; IP: interphalangeal; MCP: metacarpophalangeal; MTP: metatarsophalangeal; PIP: proximal interphalangeal; RA: rheumatoid arthritis; RF: rheumatoid factor)

ETIOLOGY

Infections, genetic susceptibility, and environmental factors have been implicated in etiology. The concordance rate in monozygotic twins is high (12–15%) compared to a prevalence of 1% in the general population. Major histocompatibility complex class II loci is the prime culprit that hosts the DR4β chains (*DRB*0401* and *DRB**0404) having greatest association with RA. Other loci that may have a role include the major histocompatibility complex class III genes for TNF-α, heat shock protein 70 (*HSP70*), and complement C4. Although, there is no consistent evidence of any specific microorganism in RA synovium there may be a subclinical infectius trigger outside the synovium. Mycoplasma, Epstein-Barr virus, cytomegalovirus, parvovirus, and rubella virus have all been suggested, but mechanism is undefined. Cigarette smoking is considered the strongest known environmental risk factor for RA and is associated with anti-CCP and RF positive RA. Alcohol consumption may lower the risk of developing RF and anti-CCP positive RA. Data from Finland suggest coffee consumption as a risk factor for seropositive RA. Consumption of olive oil and fish oil may protect against development of the disease similar to statin use in hyperlipidemic patients where the risk is reduced by up to 40%. Nulliparity and early menopause are associated with increased risk of developing RA while breast feeding seems to have protective effect.

PATHOGENESIS

"Immunogenetics of rheumatoid arthritis" has been constantly under study. In a nutshell for an orthopedician to understand initiation or perpetuation of RA, there is an imbalance in the T-helper (Th)17 and T-regulatory (Treg) cells where the former are increased while the latter get reduced in patients with active disease. It is a well-known fact that the Th1, Th2, and Th17 cells specialize in immunity against viral, parasitic and other infections; while Treg cells control the immune response and mediate tolerance against harmless self- and nonself-antigens. Differentiation and function of Treg cells require transcription factor forkhead box p3 (Foxp3) and also inducible Treg can be generated in periphery from CD4+ T-cell. The primary imbalance between ↑Th17/↓Treg cells is primarily responsible for progression of RA and in fact cell-based therapy with Treg cells has been shown to produce durable disease remission in RA patients. Inflammatory cytokines and chemokines are at the heart of development of RA. Classically, it was thought that that RA arises due to imbalance between Th1 and Th2 imbalance, but this is an incomplete story. Within the synovium T-cell expansion and differentiation is dependent on the presence of proinflammatory cytokines. The balance of cytokines produced by Th1/Th2 subsets of Th cells determine what distinct Th subpopulation will develop. So in the presence of IL-1β, IL-6, and IL-23 differentiation into Th-17 is promoted, but presence of TGF-β will inhibit the same and favor differentiation into CD4 + CD25 + Foxp3 + Tregs. Balance to Th17 differentiation will further lead to production of proinflammatory cytokines like IL-2, TNF-α, IFN-γ, IL-17A, macrophage inflammatory protein (MIP)-1, monocyte chemotactic protein (MCP)-1, and IL-1β continuing inflammation and progression of RA. Even the expression of IL-17 has been linked to the severity of RA. Expansion of Treg cells leads to production of IL-4 and IL-10 that are mainly anti-inflammatory and control and downregulate inflammation. Treg cells also secrete TGF-β1 that suppresses T cell, B-cell proliferation and cytokine (IFN-γ) production. It also reduces multiorgan inflammation and excessive lymphocytic infiltration.

Antigen-mediated activation of T-cell (especially the Th17) initiates a cascade activation of endothelial cells **(Fig. 22)**, proliferation of Types A and B synoviocytes, and recruitment of additional inflammatory cells from the bone marrow. TNF-α and IL-1 stimulate inflammatory cells to release oncostatin M into synovial fluid. TNF-α and oncostatin M work together to induce production of collagenases called MMPs by the diseased synoviocytes and chondrocytes resulting in excessive collagen degradation and cartilage matrix collapse. When the immune response is triggered by the antigen, additional antigens may be created and recognized by the T-cell to create an ongoing immune response. The major population of T-cells in the rheumatoid synovium is composed of CD4+ memory T-cells. Although, the T-cells outnumber the B-cells there are active plasma cells in the synovium and the expanded B lymphocyte pool, which suggest a significant humoral component to inflammation that is manifest in the synovial fluid. The antibody, a gamma globulin (rheumatoid factor), is produced in lymph nodes and coats the cell membranes of lymphocytes and plasma cells, which travel to the synovium where they react with the antigen causing acute inflammatory reaction. The synovium is transformed to pannus of synoviocytes, T-cells, and macrophages. This vascular granulation tissue is composed of proliferating fibroblasts, small blood vessels, and a variable number of mononuclear cells and produces a large amount collagenase and stromelysin, producing tissue damage. The cytokines IL-1 and TNF play a key role. The synovitis and vascular proliferation invade adjacent cartilage and bone. These further degrade cartilage and stimulate osteoclasts to promote periarticular bony erosion and osteopenia.

Laboratory Evaluation

Typically, there are no tests that define RA. The utility of common tests is discussed below:

Rheumatoid Factor

These are nearly 59% sensitive and 93% specific for diagnosis of rheumatoid arthritis. These are autoantibodies to the epitopes in the Fc portion of IgG. These autoantibodies may be of the IgM, IgA, IgG, or IgE isotype but commonly the IgM portion of rheumatoid factor is tested which is present in 60–70% of patient population. The association between elevated serum RF and RA was first noted in the late 1930s by Waaler. Substantial evidence favors the view that RF contributes to tissue injury in RA. Both IgM RF and IgG RF can enhance complement activation (both alternate

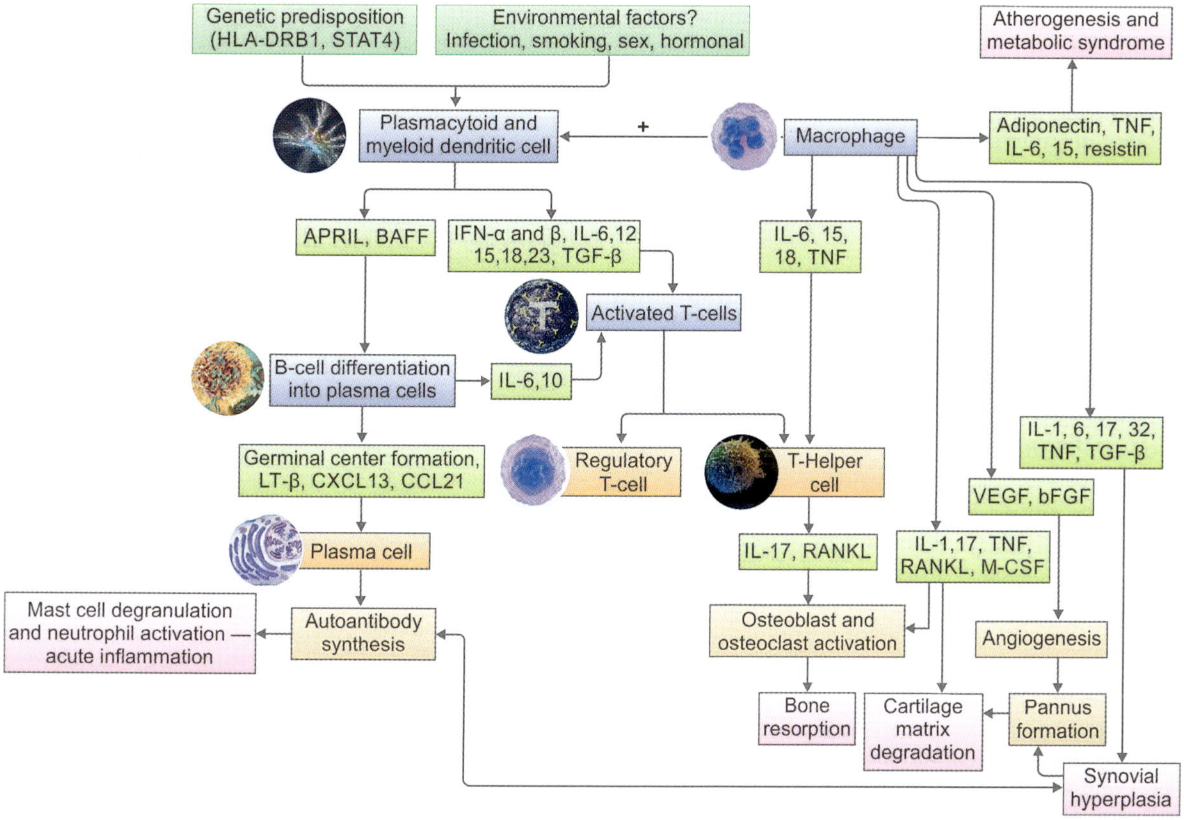

Fig. 22: Pathogenesis of rheumatoid arthritis. [APRIL: a proliferation-inducing ligand; BAFF: B-cell activating factor; CCL21: chemokine (C-C motif) ligand 21; CXCL13: chemokine (C-X-C motif) ligand 13; IL-1: interleukin-1; M-CSF: macrophage-colony stimulating factor; RANKL: receptor activator of nuclear factor kappa-B ligand; STAT4: signal transducer and activator of transcription 4; TNF: tumor necrosis factor; VEGF: vascular endothelial growth factor]

and classic pathways) by IgG complexes. RF may directly activate natural killer (NK) cells stimulating the secretion of TNF and IL-1. It is now clear that at least part of the RF in RA patients originates from B-cells that have undergone T-cell-dependent and antigen-driven germinal center maturation. The most definitive proof of an antigen-driven B-cell response is the finding of clonally-related V sequences (i.e., those that are derived from the same germ line V, D, and J gene segments) that contain shared mutations, and have high affinity for antigen. Approximately, 75% of patients with RA exhibit elevated titers of serum RF when tested by conventional techniques such as the latex fixation test. This is a nonspecific test and false positive test is seen in 5% of normal adult population and 15–20% of patients above 65 years of age. The test may be also positive in unrelated conditions like SLE, Sjögren syndrome, scleroderma, chronic liver disease, sarcoidosis, pulmonary fibrosis, tuberculosis, leprosy, syphilis, influenza, leishmaniasis, malaria, etc. For poor predictive value positive test does not diagnose RA. The RF assay has also been found to have a relatively low positive predictive value for RA (24%) or for any rheumatic disease (34%) in a general hospital-based practice. Because of poor sensitivity and pretest probability of disease RF is not at all a good test to screen asymptomatic patients. If used as a screening test some one-third of the patients will be missed. The negative predictive value (exclusion of disease with a negative test result) is much better (89% for RA and 85% for any rheumatic disease) so that RF assay is more useful in excluding RA than in diagnosing it. Importantly, though the presence of rheumatoid factor indicates poor prognosis as these patients tend to have more severe and progressive disease. Seropositivity is associated with more aggressive articular disease, both radiographically and functionally. Also the higher the titer in suggestive patients greater is the chance of severe systemic disease (including subcutaneous nodules, vasculitis, leg ulcers, and neuropathy). Serum RF decreases with effective pharmacotherapy and improved functional status. Although not performed routinely, IgA RF may be a useful diagnostic and prognostic marker in RA. Elevation of both IgM RF and IgA RF appears to be relatively specific for RA because this combination is rarely found in other rheumatic diseases.

ACPA (Anticitrullinated Peptide Antibodies) and Anti-CCP (Anticyclic Citrullinated Peptide Antibodies)

They are around 98% sensitive and 95% specific for RA. ACPA are antibodies to citrullinated products of various proteins like filaggrin (an intermediate filament-associated protein), vimentin (a cytoskeletal intermediate filament protein found in human spleen or placenta mesenchymal cells), fibrinogen, etc. containing arginine residue. The arginine in these proteins is converted to citrulline by peptidylarginine deiminase (PAD) as a post-translational modification. Several isotypes of PAD have been identified in RA synovium that induce citrullination of synovial proteins, and citrullinated proteins as well as local production of ACPA has been demonstrated in rheumatoid joints. Anti-CCP are specific antibodies against cyclic citrullinated peptides that are commercially tested commonly. The term ACPA is being preferred now-a-days and refer to same thing. Citrullinated peptides have greater affinity for HLA DR4A (DRB1*0401 or *0404) antigen binding grooves relative to corresponding arginine containing peptides. For its high specificity the probability of detecting anti-CCP in patients with early RA approximates 70%, so it may be useful in predicting which patients with early, undifferentiated synovitis are likely to develop RA. Positive test could hence be relied upon to confirm diagnosis in clinically suspected *early cases*. The development of anti-CCP is common in individuals with an RA associated HLA-1β allele and in those who smoke cigarettes, and may occur 1–5 years before the development of clinical manifestations of RA. The presence of anti-CCP appears to be a significant risk factor for predicting erosive disease, equalling or exceeding that of the presence of IgM rheumatoid factor. The presence of anti-CCP in isolation (clinically nonsuspected patients), however, is not useful to predict the future development of RA because it can be found in around 1.5% of normal individuals, most of whom will not develop RA.

Antinuclear antibody with a homogeneous pattern is found in 30–40% of patients with RA. Other laboratory findings that suggest but are not diagnostic of RA include presence of antiperinuclear factor, antikeratin antibodies, elevated erythrocyte sedimentation rate (ESR > 30 mm in first hour), elevated C-reactive protein (CRP) (>0.7 pg/mL), decreased hematocrit level (normocytic normochromic anemia) and/or elevated platelet count.

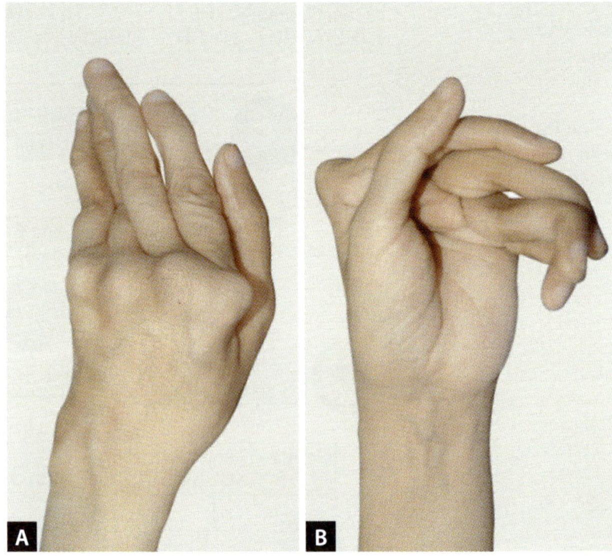

Figs. 23A and B: Rheumatoid deformity of hand—look at the marked ulnar drift of fingers at metacarpophallangeal (MCP) joint with radial deviation of wrist (the "z-deformity"). There is volar subluxation of phalanges at MCP with variable occurrence of swan-neck deformity.
Source: Professor PP Kotwal, Chairman, Institute of Orthopedics and Joint Replacement, Pushpavati Singhania Research Institute, New Delhi, India.

CLINICAL FEATURES AND DIAGNOSIS

Some Definitions

Early RA—RA duration <6 months. *Established RA*—RA disease duration ≥ 6 months or meeting diagnostic criteria **(*see* Table 19)**. *RA remission*—(ACR/EULAR) a tender joint count, swollen joint count, CRP (mg/dL) level, and patient global assessment of ≤1 each or a simplified disease activity score (DAS) of ≤3.3. The DAS is a composite score using the tender and swollen joint count, ESR, and the patient global assessment of disease activity using a 100 mm visual analog scale. The DAS is commonly used in clinical trials to assess the response to treatment (although clinically it is more used in Europe than US). The DAS28 is calculated by surveying the 28 joints [knees + upper extremities (shoulders, elbows, wrists, MCP, and PIP joints)] as follows:

DAS28 = 0.56* (number of tender joints) + 0.28* (number of swollen joints) + 0.70 ln (ESR) + 0.014 * global assessment (in mm).

Classically RA is a symmetric and polyarthritis of small joints. Most patients of RA have weeks to months of insidious onset of fatigue and joint pains that may be transient early but later the joint inflammation becomes more persistent with warmth, effusion, tenderness, and loss of function. The DIP joints are characteristically spared. A tenth of patients experience an acute onset of symptoms. Early morning joint stiffness lasting >60 minutes is seen in most patients that improves over next few hours and physical activity. Duration of morning stiffness usually correlates with the extent of synovial inflammation. Structural damage to the joints begins early, however, manifests usually after a year. With persistent inflammation there is damage to and weakening of ligaments, tendons, and joint capsule. The unopposed physical forces and muscle imbalance lead to development of characteristic deformities in hand namely the z-deformity **(Figs. 23A and B)**, swan-neck deformity, and boutonniere deformity. In the feet, there may be eversion at the subtalar joint, plantar subluxation of metatarsal heads, forefoot widening, and hallux valgus. Extra-articular manifestations of RA are summarized in **Box 8**. Some keypoints that should be understood while making a diagnosis of RA are as follows:

- RA is entirely a clinical diagnosis. Do not hesitate to make a diagnosis of RA even if RF is absent. Nearly 80–85% of the individuals are seropositive (positive for rheumatoid factor) rest are seronegative.
- Mere presence of rheumatoid factor in blood is not at all enough to make a diagnosis of RA, it should be clinically supported.
- Once RF is positive in a given patient, it need not be repeated since it correlates poorly with clinical response to treatment (*see* rheumatoid factor below and also prognostic factors). Titers of RF do not help in monitoring treatment efficacy. A negative RF needs to be repeated 4–6 monthly for the first 2 years of disease, since some patients may take 18–24 months to become seropositive.

BOX 8: Extra-articular manifestations of rheumatoid arthritis (RA).

Skin:
- Rheumatoid nodules—seen in up to 30% patients mainly distributed over extensor aspect of the forearm and other pressure areas of skin. These are not specific for RA but quite useful for diagnosis and prognosis correlating with the seropositivity, disease activity, and progression.
- Leukocytoclastic vasculitis is seen as palpable purpura most often resolving spontaneously. Rheumatoid vasculitis can lead to large ulcerations on the lower extremities although this is uncommon. Other manifestations of vasculitis include splinter hemorrhages, periungual infracts, digital necrosis, mononeuritis multiplex (10%), and symmetric peripheral neuropathy (45%). Vasculitis may be drug induced in a few cases (etanercept).

Amyloidosis

Hematologic:
1. Anemia usually normocytic, normochromic
2. Macrocytic (?MTX)
3. Aplastic (gold, MTX, leflunomide)
4. Leukopenia (triad of leukopenia, splenomegaly and RA = Felty's syndrome seen in 1%)
5. Lymphopenia (usually with lupus overlap or HIV infection)
6. Thrombocytopenia

Cardiovascular:
- Pericarditis
- Myocarditis
- Endocarditis (valvular and valve ring nodules)
- Coronary vasculitis

Respiratory:
- Idiopathic interstitial pneumonitis and fibrosis are rare. This may be associated with the use of MTX.
- Pleuritic and pleural effusion are more a feature seen in older patients
- Bronchiolitis obliterans
- Rheumatoid pulmonary nodules are a feature of seropositive disease but these are asymptomatic findings. Radiologically, they are seen as coin-shaped lesions but need differentiation from malignancy.

Renal—Mesangial glomerulonephritis most common. Renal involvement is the most common organ failure mainly due to amyloidosis:

Neurologic:
- Entrapment neuropathies are common: Carpal tunnel syndrome, tarsal tunnel syndrome, ulnar nerve compression at Guyon's canal
- Mononeuritis multiplex is a peripheral and bilateral neuropathy that can present acutely. Sudden onset of motor neuropathy can signal the presence of aggressive vasculitis and poor prognosis
- Sensorimotor peripheral neuropathy
- Cervical myelopathy (40%, due to atlantoaxial subluxation). Subluxation at lower levels is uncommon but is more likely to cause pain and neurological symptoms. Cervical myelopathy can be fatal. Initial symptoms include paraesthesia, muscle weakness, and later sensory loss, paralysis, incontinence and syncope.

Psychiatric—Depression (40%)

Bone—Secondary osteoporosis due often to inactivity, nutritional deficiency, glucocorticoid use and pre-existing osteoporosis. By itself the cytokines generated due to disease activity are responsible for periarticular osteopenia.

Eye (importantly it should be realized that uveitis and conjunctivitis are not a feature of RA)
- Keratoconjunctivitis sicca (xerophthalmia) is most common.
- Episcleritis is often benign and resolves spontaneously
- Necrotizing keratitis
- Painful scleritis causing scleromalacia

Tendons and ligaments—Spontaneous rupture of tendons is common at wrist, hand, and rotator cuff. Tenosynovitis and weakening of ligaments leads to joint instability and subluxation.

Felty's syndrome—This is the association of splenomegaly and neutropenia with destructive RA. Systemic disease, hepatomegaly, and lymphadenopathy are also common and the occurrence of RA in relatives is quite high. In uncomplicated cases, the treatment is usually conservative, splenectomy remaining controversial and has transient effect only as the cellular destruction is immune mediated.

Contd...

Contd...

LGL syndrome (Large granular lymphocyte syndrome);
This is also associated with neutropenia and splenomegaly. LGL syndrome is differentiated from Felty's syndrome by the presence of large granular lymphocytes and a clonal lymphocytosis. The clonality is demonstrable by PCR of T-cell receptor gamma gene. The arthritis is usually less destructive than seen with Felty's.

(PCR: polymerase chain reaction)

- Do not diagnose RA unless hands are involved. Also DIP joint involvement is exceedingly rare in RA. If DIP joints are involved suspect psoriatic arthropathy, scleroderma or osteoarthritis.
- RA is typically bilaterally symmetrical. Asymmetrical or unilateral involvement should arouse suspicion of other arthritides like psoriatic or seronegative spondyloarthropathy.
- RA is a polyarthritis. Refrain from making a diagnosis of monoarticular RA.
- Lumbar spine is not involved in RA. The presence of inflammatory low backache with monoarticular or oligoarticular involvement especially in lower limbs falls under seronegative spondyloarthropathy.

Palindromic rheumatism: It was described by Hench and Rosenberg in 1942. Pain usually begins in one joint or in periarticular tissues; symptoms worsen for several hours to a few days and are associated with swelling and erythema. Then, in reverse sequence, symptoms resolve, leaving no residua. Up to half of patients with palindromic rheumatism go on to develop RA, particularly those with HLA-DR4.

Around a third of patients have slowly progressive course while other third have waxing and waning cyclical course. The remaining third have prolonged indolent remissions with intermittent exacerbations.

The median life expectancy of persons with RA is shortened by 3–7 years possibly attributed to susceptibility to infections, cardiovascular disorders and drug therapy itself.

Still's disease: Adult onset Still's disease is an autoinflammatory disease. The condition "juvenile-onset Still's disease" is now grouped under juvenile idiopathic arthritis. Typically, this affects patients 16–35 years old and presents with:
- Arthralgia
- "Salmon-pink" rash
- Pyrexia
- Fatigue
- Lymphadenopathy
- Elevated serum ferritin
- Rare pericardial and pleural effusion

Radiographic Findings

In early course of disease, the radiographs are mute or show periarticular/juxta-articular osteopenia **(Figs. 24A and B)**. Cartilage destruction deformities and bony erosions come later and are nonspecific. Only clue to RA could be symmetrical involvement but much before radiologic evaluation clinical evaluation should have established diagnosis. Erosions tend to be marginal (away from the

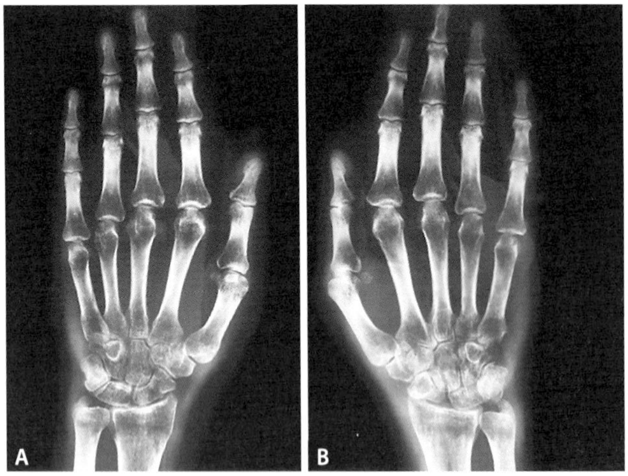

Figs. 24A and B: The anteroposterior (AP) radiographs of hands depicting characteristic periarticular osteopenia across the wrist and interphalangeal joints in a patient with rheumatoid arthritis.

weightbearing portion of the joint). In the hip, the femoral head tends to migrate axially or superomedially, whereas the hip tends to migrate more superolaterally in osteoarthritis. In the shoulder, the humeral head tends to be high-riding. Radiographs are helpful for reconstruction planning and prognostication of patient.

DIFFERENTIAL DIAGNOSIS

- *Diffuse connective tissue disease:* SLE, scleroderma
- Mixed connective tissue disease
- Calcium pyrophosphate dehydrate deposition disease
- Erosive inflammatory osteoarthritis
- Chronic fatigue syndrome
- Polyarticular gout
- Reactive arthritis
- Viral arthritis
- Lyme disease
- Intermittent hydrarthrosis
- HIV infection
- Polymyalgia rheumatica
- Rheumatic fever
- Whipple's disease

TREATMENT

The treatment is aimed to control pain and inflammation, maintain function, prevent occurrence of deformities and joint destruction and control systemic involvement, so in a way the target is either remission or low disease activity if remission cannot be achieved within 6 months. This methodology of therapy is classically called treat-to-target strategy as exemplified for RA.

Counseling and splinting are very important to maintain function and prevent deformities in the patients. With proper awareness and physiotherapy programs, the patients should be made to realize the importance of rehabilitation and need of compliance with pharmacotherapy and assistive devices to avoid joint destruction.

PHARMACOTHERAPY

Pain Relief

NSAIDs are the mainstay for providing acute pain relief and cover for the time until effect of DMARDs develop. Maximum approved doses should be prescribed, and if a satisfactory clinical response is not achieved after 2–3 weeks, another NSAID should be tried. None is superior and usually conventional NSAIDs are started reserving COX-2 specific inhibitors to patients not tolerating the former.

Corticosteroids

They were used as anti-inflammatory agents but have shown good disease modifying activity. Clear decision as to how and when to start them should be the concern instead of their bad reputation. They are rapidly acting drugs and relieve joint inflammation; improve symptoms of stiffness, fatigue, and loss of appetite; reduce ESR and CRP levels; and increase hemoglobin values. They also have protective influence on joint destruction. The improvement in the rate of disease progression appears to be greatest in the first 6 months of treatment with low-dose prednisolone. The glucocorticoid is useful and effective early in the course of disease. Restrict the dose of prednisolone to 10 mg/day in men and 7.5 mg/day in females. Women who take >7.5 mg/day for longer than 3 months risk bone loss. Abrupt withdrawal often induces an acute flare-up of the arthritis, and, rarely, a systemic rheumatoid disease with necrotizing vasculitis and mononeuropathy develops in patients with rheumatoid nodules and strongly positive serum RF tests. Some people use mega doses of methyl prednisolone (3 infusions of 1,000 mg alternate day) but it should be avoided. Single joint effusions can be well managed with intra-articular crystalloid preparation of steroid that gives lasting relief for months. Combining with DMARDs initially for rapid relief and then tapering the glucocorticoids is a useful option.

Doxycycline

Tetracyclines inhibit MMPs and are immunomodulatory. Classically, suspicion on mycoplasma as a causative agent leads to the use of tetracyclines. It is now evident that tetracyclines are useful in RA because of their anti-inflammatory effects and not for antimicrobial effects. Studies reveal mixed results. Recently clinical effects of doxycycline with MTX were found to be superior to MTX monotherapy in RA. Photosensitivity is the main concern.

Statins

These drugs also seem to have anti-inflammatory properties. Statins have been reported to inhibit interactions between leukocytes and endothelial cells, to reduce the production of inflammatory cytokines, and to decrease T-cell activation. Current data on efficacy of statins for treatment of RA are mixed and still preliminary.

Disease-modifying Antirheumatic Drugs (DMARDs) and Biological Agents

They make the central theme in management of rheumatoid arthritis while other therapies mentioned above are temporary and add intermittently to improve the outcome or control the disease exacerbations. The aim of therapy is disease remission or achieving a low disease activity [LDA, Low disease activity state according to any of the validated composite disease activity measures that include joint counts (see above)] if remission cannot be achieved. Based on the Austrian and Dutch rheumatologists' recommendations the DMARDs have been reclassified into synthetic and biological agents as follows:

- *Synthetic DMARDs:* Synthetic DMARDs are traditional, small molecular mass drugs further classified into:
  - *Conventional synthetic DMARDs (csDMARDs):* These include methotrexate (most used first-line drug), leflunomide, sulfasalazine, hydroxychloroquine and uncommonly azathioprine, cyclosporin A, and cyclophosphamide. They were not developed based on a specific mechanism of action to specifically treat a disease/target but were found helpful in treating rheumatoid arthritis later or incidentally.
  - *Targeted synthetic DMARDs (tsDMARDs):* The rational development and design of these newer synthetic medications "targets" specific molecular structure/pathway to control the disease as typified by Janus kinase (JAK) inhibitor. These drugs include baricitinib, tofacitinib, upadacitinib, filgotinib, and peficitinib.
- *Biological DMARDs (bDMARDs):* These are modern drugs developed through genetic engineering. They are also divided into two categories:
  i. *Biological original/originator DMARDs (boDMARDs):* They are the original active agents developed to target specific molecular structures. The agents most effective against rheumatoid arthritis in this category are:
     - *TNF inhibitors (TNFi):* Adalimumab, certolizumab, etanercept, golimumab, infliximab; IL-6Ri: sarilumab, tocilizumab
     - *Costimulation-inhibitors:* Abatacept; anti-B cell (CD20)-rituximab.
  ii. *Biosimilars (bsDMARDs):* They are generic drugs that meet regulatory criteria allowing generic manufacturers to emulate the design of innovator products after patent expiration. Currently, they are available for adalimumab, etanercept, infliximab, and rituximab.

With this new terminology, better understanding of the natural history of disease and increasing experience in treating RA the consensus guidelines (ACR-EULAR-NICE) keep changing nearly every year. It is difficult to keep up with every minor or sometimes even the major alterations in them, but they can be readily assessed at the parent sites. I will present the most practiced algorithm **(Fig. 25)** prepared after careful and comprehensive review of guidelines for managing RA patient. Physician should understand the different mechanisms of actions of drugs to control the heterogeneity of rheumatoid arthritis and it often needs cycling and adding drugs to achieve remission or LDA. Currently, five molecular target families are recognized for treatment of RA, viz., tumor necrosis factor (TNF), interleukin 6 (IL-6), CD80/86, CD20, and Janus kinases (JAK) with multiple drugs for several of these molecules. The treatment strategy must be altered based on the disease activity (see above), prognostic factors **(Box 9)**, response **(Fig. 25)**, and economic and social concerns of the patients. Some of the general principles of using DMARDs in rheumatoid patients are mentioned below.

- Optimal care of patients with RA which consists of an integrated approach combining both nonpharmacological and pharmacological treatments initiated as soon as the diagnosis is made, to preserve joint function and quality of life.
- Short-term (<3 months) low-dose corticosteroids (if oral prednisolone is used, the dose should be ≤10 mg OD) may be used as bridging therapy during initial diagnosis and acute flare of RA.
- Methotrexate should be used as the first-line disease modifying antirheumatic drug (DMARD) in all patients with RA unless contraindicated.
- In patients with a contraindication to MTX (or early intolerance), leflunomide or sulfasalazine should be considered as part of the (first) treatment strategy.
- If the treatment target is not achieved with the first csDMARD strategy and poor prognostic factors are present, a bDMARD or a tsDMARD should be added.
- If the treatment target is not achieved with the first csDMARD strategy and poor prognostic factors are present, a bDMARD or a tsDMARD should be added.
- Biologic DMARDs and tsDMARDs should be considered when the treatment target is not achieved with conventional synthetic DMARDs **(Fig. 25)**. Where available, biosimilar DMARDs may be considered as effective alternatives.
- If a bDMARD or tsDMARD has failed, treatment with another bDMARD or a tsDMARD should be considered; if one TNF-inhibitor (TNFi) therapy has failed, patients may receive an agent with another mechanism of action or a second TNFi.
- If a patient is in persistent remission (not defined till now, variably considered as 6–12 months), tapering the csDMARD could be considered.

Conventional Synthetic Disease-modifying Antirheumatic Drugs

Methotrexate

The "anchor" drug for isolated or commonly combination therapies. MTX therapy should always be a part of the first-line treatment strategy (other drugs may be combined) in patients with active RA (low disease activity patients may not need MTX) and in relapse or difficult cases (patients who did not receive MTX initially should receive this). This is one of

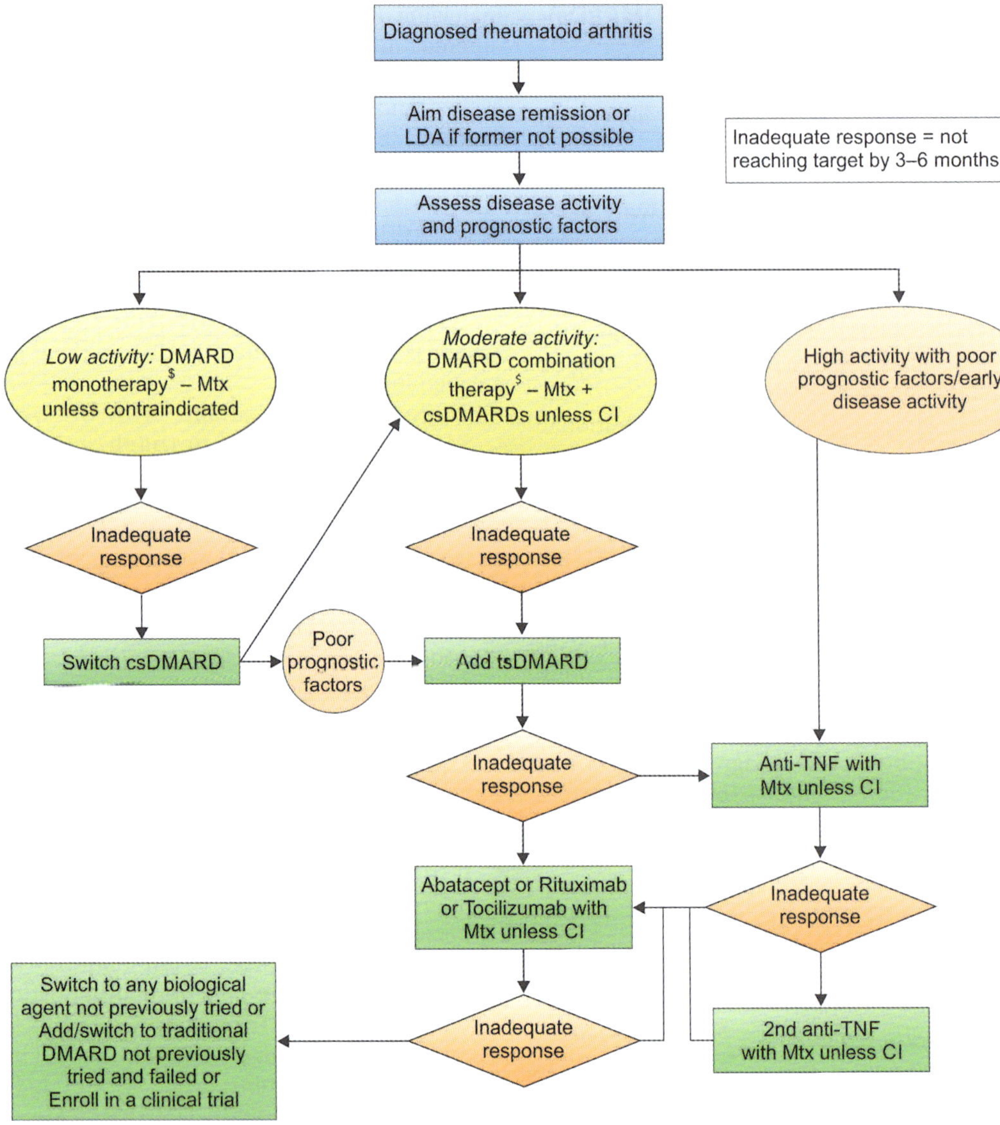

Fig. 25: Algorithm for management of rheumatoid arthritis. (csDMARDs: conventional synthetic disease modifying antirheumatic drugs; LDA: low disease activity; Mtx: methotrexate; ts-DMARDs: targeted synthetic DMARDs)
$Add-on therapy with nonsteroidal anti-inflammatory drugs (NSAIDs) and/or corticosteroid bridge therapy recommended for quick remission.

BOX 9: Poor-prognostic factors for rheumatoid arthritis.

- Persistently moderate or high disease activity despite conventional synthetic DMARD (csDMARD) therapy according to composite measures including joint counts
- High acute phase reactant levels
- High swollen joint count
- Presence of RF and/or ACPA, especially at high levels
- Presence of early erosions
- Failure of two or more csDMARDs

(ACPA: anticitrullinated peptide antibodies; RF: rheumatoid factor; csDMARDs: conventional synthetic disease modifying antirheumatic drugs)

the drugs that has differing actions with different dosage—at low dose it is anti-inflammatory, immunosuppressant, and at higher doses an anticancer drug (the other drug is glucocorticoid). The beginning dose is usually 7.5 mg (three tablets) taken together on 1 day each week. Incremental increases of 2.5 mg/week are made every 4 weeks until either maximum control of joint inflammation or symptoms of toxicity appear. Higher weekly doses (20–30 mg) are more effective than lower doses and take 3–4 weeks for full effect to develop. The efficacy has not been surpassed by any of the available synthetic DMARDs or anti-TNF monotherapy. Stomatitis, anorexia, and nausea or diarrhea often limit increase in dosage that can be partially controlled by twice weekly dosage or injectable preparations. Folic acid should be combined with the dose. Disease suppression is lost within 4 weeks of stopping the drug, but control is regained after restarting the medication within 3–4 weeks. It is recommended to do regular blood counts and LFT every month for first 3 months and 2-monthly thereafter. Bone marrow suppression can result from renal insufficiency, serious systemic infection, and concomitant administration of trimethoprim-sulfamethoxazole. There might be an increase in opportunistic infections in RA patients treated with MTX. Rheumatoid nodules can appear or enlarge in patients taking MTX and it has been suggested that concomitant hydroxychloroquine (HCQ) can control this complication.

Hydroxychloroquine

Very slow-acting (around 3–9 months) low efficacy drug. Commonly prescribed in combination therapy (empirically only) for low toxicity profile and infrequent drug interactions, but the additive efficacy for RA is undocumented. The most common side effects are maculopapular rashes, gastrointestinal disturbances, and nonspecific neurologic complaints; however, the major concern is ocular toxicity due to drug deposition in retinal pigment. Toxicity is reversible if recognised early; however, blindness may result if ignored. Sulfasalazine is a preferable drug compared to HCQ.

Sulfasalazine

It has rapid onset of action (within 3 weeks) and low incidence of serious side effects. It can be used as monotherapy in low disease activity patients. Usually 500 mg twice daily is starting dose increased to 1 g twice daily in the absence of nausea, vomiting, photosensitivity, or skin rash. Because of the rare complications of myelosuppression or hemolytic anemia in individuals with glucose-6-phosphate dehydrogenase enzyme deficiency, monthly blood counts are recommended for first 3 months then 3 monthly.

Leflunomide

It is a pyrimidine inhibitor with good efficacy for RA. The drug has a long half-life hence a loading dose of 80–100 mg is given followed by 20 mg daily. Drug takes 6–8 weeks to take full effect improving arthritis activity and functional status. Diarrhea (managed with reducing dose) and hepatotoxicity (additive with MTX) are the usual side effects. Severe toxicity can be managed by cholestyramine as it enhances leflunomide excretion. This can be used as a primary drug in patients contraindicated for MTX therapy (rare).

Several older drugs like gold compounds (painful intramuscular injections), D-penicillamine (proteinuria, nephrotic syndrome), cyclosporine-A (hypertension and renal insufficiency), cyclophosphamide, chlorambucil (bone marrow suppression, and neoplasms) and azathioprine have either low efficacy or severe side effects or low benefit to risk ratio so they are seldom prescribed anymore. Azathioprine, however, has a mild side effects profile, and is favored by some rheumatologists, especially for lowering the prednisone dose in patients with corticosteroid dependency.

Biological Agents

Biologic agents refer to complex protein molecules produced by using molecular biology methods in prokaryotic or eukaryotic cell cultures. Molecular 3D structure is more important rather than molecular weight and molecules with same molecular weight can have different function so it involves complex assessment methods. Their biological activities can be predefined and are usually directed toward a specific cytokine or cell surface molecule, making it possible to predict a range of activities both in terms of efficacy and toxicity **(Fig. 26)**. There is a marked difference in clinical activity of a drug and its expected theoretical role. Like blockade of IL-1 and IL-17 did not produce that well clinical effects in RA as was antagonism of TNF or IL-6. Also the concept of cytokine cascade should be understood where THF is an upstream cytokine while IL-6 comes later and IL-17 at fag end, so blocking TNF will have additional effects on IL-6 levels (but not always) while blocking IL-17 will spare TNF and IL-6 from their effects so remission is not seen. Also with anti-TNF drugs until IL-6 is blocked complete remission is not obtained.

It is imperative to screen for latent tuberculosis infection (LTBI) in all RA patients being considered for therapy with biologic agents, regardless of the presence of risk factors for LTBI. Clinicians should assess the patient's medical history to identify risk factors for TB (see above). The tuberculin skin test (TST) or interferon-γ–release assays (IGRAs) should be done as the initial test in all RA patients starting biologic agents, regardless of risk factors for LTBI, the latter is preferred in patients who have received BCG vaccination. A positive test mandates chest radiograph and sputum examination to detect active tuberculosis. Screening tests may be negative in RA patients due to immunosuppression. With a negative screening; repeat test should be done in high-risk patients after 1–3 weeks. Biological agents should be started in patients with active TB after completion of antitubercular treatment and after 1 month of latent TB treatment in patients with latent infection. **Table 20** summarizes the commonly used drugs in RA.

Anti-TNF agents improve symptoms while reducing radiographic progression of joint erosions. Five TNF-blocking agents are available and approved for use in RA. Etanercept, adalimumab, and certolizumab have been approved as monotherapy for RA but infliximab and golimumab have been approved only with concomitant use of MTX. MTX in combination has been shown to improve efficiency for prevention of joint structural damage. Etanercept was first agent approved for use in 1998 and bears lower efficacy then infliximab but good response has been demonstrated clinically. It is approved for use in DMARD-naïve patients also. Other approved uses of etanercept are in treatment of PsA and juvenile idiopathic arthritis. Infliximab being a chimeric protein induces antibody response against murine component that is successfully suppressed with MTX. Adalimumab has high specificity for TNF-α and is indicated in patients with moderate to severe RA and persistent disease despite DMARD therapy. Certolizumab pegol is a novel agent containing Fab domain of humanised monoclonal anti-TNF antibody bound to polyethylene glycol. It does not contain the Fc portion so does not activate complement or form immune complexes with TNF.

Seven types of side effects are encountered in different patients: (1) serious infections, including disseminated tuberculosis; (2) hematologic disorders, such as pancytopenia; (3) demyelinating disorders; (4) exacerbation of congestive heart failure; (5) systemic lupus erythematosus-related auto-

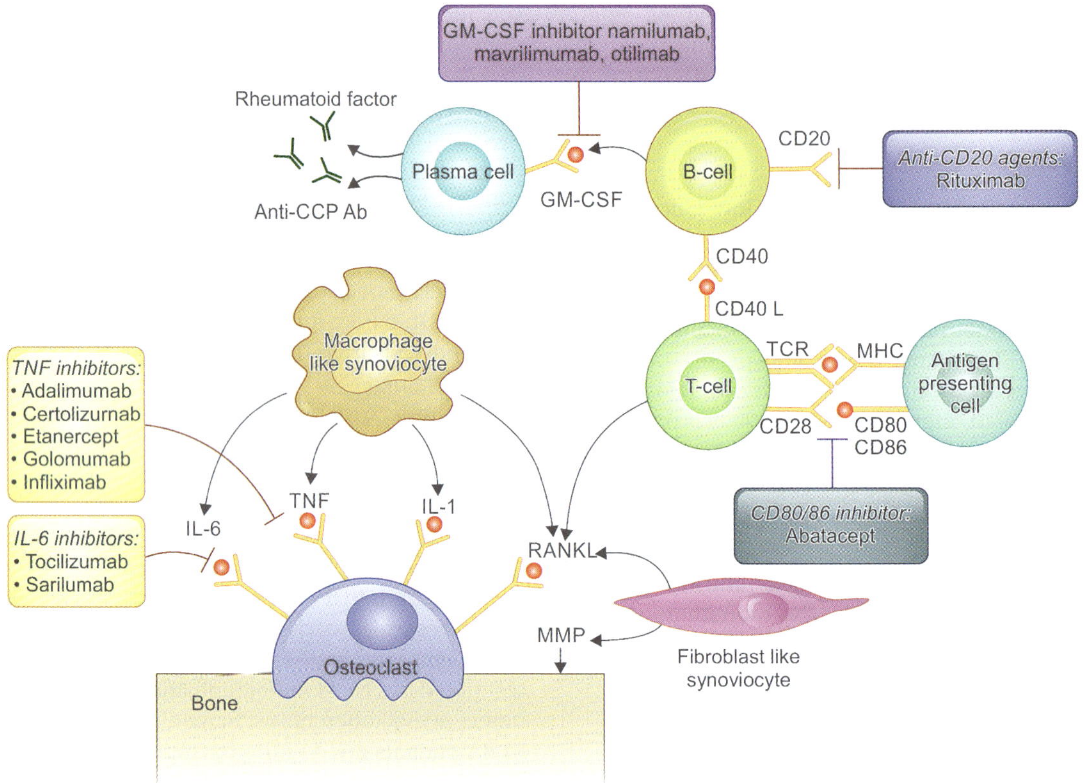

Fig. 26: Biological agents in rheumatoid arthritis and their principal mechanism of action in the cascade of rheumatoid arthritis. (IL-6: interleukin 6; GM-CSF: granulocyte macrophage colony stimulating factor; MMP: matrix metalloproteinase; RANKL: receptor activator of nuclear factor kappa-B ligand; TNF: tumor necrosis factor)

TABLE 20: Commonly used disease modifying antirheumatic drugs (DMARDs) used in management of rheumatoid arthritis.

Medication	***Dosage***	***Adverse effects***
csDMARDs		
Methotrexate	• 5–30 mg weekly (usually 7.5–20 mg) orally, 10–25 mg once weekly IM or SC • Modification with CrCl • <30—contraindicated • 30–59—half dose • ≥60—Full dose	Gastrointestinal intolerance, alopecia, mucositis, photosensitivity, rash, hepatotoxicity (transaminitis), interstitial pneumonia, teratogenic – avoid in pregnancy
Sulfasalazine	500–1,000 mg twice daily	Pruritis, rash, gastrointestinal intolerance , myelosuppression
Hydroxychloroquine	200–400 mg once daily	Retinal damage
Leflunomide	10–20 mg once daily	Alopecia, transaminitis, hypertension, teratogenic. Good alternative to methotrexate if contraindicated.
Minocycline	100 mg twice daily	Nausea, vomiting, anorexia, hepatotoxicity
tsDMARDs		
Tofacitinib (Monotherapy possible)	5 mg twice daily (CrCl 30–60: once daily). Screen as for bDMARDs (see text)	Increased LDL and HDL levels, Herpes Zoster infection, transaminitis, gut perforation, venous thromboembolic events (VTEs) – pulmonary embolism, deep venous thrombosis
Baricitinib (Monotherapy possible)	4 mg once daily	Similar to above
Upadacitinib (Monotherapy possible)	15 mg once daily Contraindicated in patients with absolute lymphocyte count <500 cells/mm^3, absolute neutrophil count <1,000 cells/mm^3	Similar to above

Contd...

Contd...

Medication	***Dosage***	***Adverse effects***
Filgotinib (Monotherapy possible)	200 mg once daily CrCl 30–60—half dose. Precautions as for upadacitinib	Similar to above
bDMARDs		
Infliximab (TNF inhibitor) (with Mtx only)	3 mg/kg IV infusion (weeks 0, 2, and 6 then every 8 weeks). Dose may be increased to 10 mg/kg every 4 weeks in patients who do not respond to lower doses	See text for adverse effects of anti-TNF drugs
Etanercept (TNF inhibitor) Monotherapy possible	50 mg SC; 25 mg SC (weekly; twice weekly)	As above
Adalimumab (TNF inhibitor) Monotherapy possible	40 mg SC every 14 days. May increase dose to 40 mg weekly in patients not on Mtx	As above
Golimumab (TNF inhibitor) (with Mtx only)	50 mg SC monthly	As above
Certolizumab (TNF inhibitor) Monotherapy possible	400 mg SC weeks 0, 2, and 4, followed by 200 mg SC every 2 weeks	As above
Abatacept (CTLA4-Ig, T-cell costimulation modulator, binds to CD80 and CD86 on APC blocking the CD28 interaction between APCs and T-cells) Monotherapy possible	• *IV:* (weeks 0, 2, 4 then monthly) • *<60 kg:* 500 mg • *60–100 kg:* 750 mg • *>1,000 kg:* 1,000 mg • *SC:* 125 mg weekly (may be started without IV loading dose)	Infusion reactions, infections, malignancy
Rituximab (Anti-CD20a) (with Mtx only)	1,000 mg IV at days 1, 15, and may retreat every 24 weeks	• Peripheral edema • Pruritus • Rash, GI intolerance • Infections • Infusion related • Low IgG/IgA/IgM
Tocilizumab (IL-6 receptor antagonist) Monotherapy possible	*SC:* 162 mg weekly *IV:* 4–8 mg/kg every 4 weeks	• Injection site reaction, rash, GI intolerance • Gut perforation (especially in diverticulitis) • Infections (including TB) • Increased LDL level • Elevated liver enzymes
Sarilumab (IL-6 receptor antibody) Monotherapy possible	200 mg subcutaneously every 2 weeks	Hemoptysis, breathlessness, GI perforation, and skin rash
Anakinra (IL-1 blockade) Recombinant IL-1ra binds to IL-1 receptor Not recommended for rheumatoid arthritis treatment	100 mg SC daily	Injection site reactions, infection, and neutropenia
Evolving drugs and their targets	Examples under evaluation/trial	Shown efficacy for:
IL-6 ligand	• Sirukumab • Clazakizumab • Olokizumab • Vobarilizumab	Rheumatoid arthritis
GM-CSF ligand	Namilumab	Rheumatoid arthritis
GM-CSF receptor	Mavrilimumab	Rheumatoid arthritis
IL-12/23 (p40)	Ustekinumab	Preferred for psoriatic arthritis
IL-23 (p19)	• Guselkinumab • Risankinumab • Tildrakizumab • Brazikumab	• Psoriatic arthritis • Psoriatic skin disease
IL-17 ligand	• Ixekizumab • Secukinumab	Spondyloarthropathy, psoriatic arthritis
IL-17 receptor	Brodalumab	
BAFF	• Belimumab • Blisibimod	SLE
IFN-α ligand	Sifalimumab	SLE

Contd...

Contd...

Medication	*Dosage*	*Adverse effects*
IFN-α receptor	Anifrolumab	SLE
Integrin α4/β1	Natalizumab	Inflammatory bowel disease
Integrin α4/β7	• Vedolizumab • Ertolizumab	Crohn's disease

(GI: gastrointestinal; HDL: high-density lipoprotein; IL: interleukin; IM: intramuscular; IV: intravenous; LDL: low-density lipoprotein; Mtx: methotrexate; rcl: creatinine clearance as measured in mL/min/1.7 m^2; SC: subcutaneous; SLE: systemic lupus erythematosus; TNF: tumor necrosis factor)

antibodies and clinical features; (6) hypersensitivity infusion or injection site reactions; and (7) severe liver disease. The increased risk of serious infections particularly tuberculosis especially with anti-TNF agents can be seen with all biological agents. Other significant infections that have been found include *Pneumocystis carinii*, candidiasis, histoplasmosis, listeriosis, nocardiosis, aspergillosis, *Cytomegalovirus*, cryptococcosis and coccidioidomycosis. No cause has been identified though. Higher risk of heart failure has been found so it is better to avoid these agents in risk patients. Malignancy is a matter of debate and no concrete evidence has emerged till now. The presence of demyelinating disease in patients receiving these agents is cause for concern because its incidence seems to be higher than in the general population.

B-cell therapy: The B-cell therapeutic agents target the B-cells. Rituximab is approved for the treatment of moderate to severe forms of RA in patients with inadequate response to at least one TNF-blocking agent or when TNF-blockade is inappropriate. It can also be used as monotherapy or with DMARDs other than MTX. There is, however, no correlation of depletion of CD20+ cells to the clinical response. Other than CD20, other targets have been identified in the B-cell maturation pathway that is project component of future research. These include the B-lymphocyte stimulator (BLyS) also known as B-cell activating factor of TNF family (BAFF) and the related molecule A proliferation inducing ligand (APRIL). Ofatumumab is a fully human anti-CD-20 antibody that binds to a more proximal portion of CD20 closer to B-cell membrane. The ocrelizumab is a humanised monoclonal antibody (instead of the chimeric rituximab) that binds to a different epitope that the rituximab. It increases the antibody dependent cell mediated cytotoxicity (ADCC) and reduced complement dependent cytotoxicity (CDCC). Therapies directed to BLyS or APRIL or their receptors have been developed but are found to be less effective than anti CD-20 therapies. *Belimumab* is a fully human monoclonal antibody that targets BLyS (B-cell stimulator protein) and has been found more effective for SLE. Atacicept binds both the BLyS and APRIL reducing the rheumatoid factors, total immunoglobulin levels and B-cell numbers but the efficacy is not as good as the anti CD-20 agents. *Briobacept* binds only to BLyS.

TABLE 21: The recommendations for perioperative continuation or withholding of various disease modifying antirheumatic drugs (DMARDs).

Medication	*Time withheld before surgery*	*Continuation after surgery*	*Remarks*
csDMARDs			
Methotrexate	None	Yes	Monitor renal function
Leflunomide	None	yes	
Hydroxychloroquine	None	Yes	Monitor renal function
Azathioprine	None	Yes	Monitor renal function
Sulfasalazine	None	Yes	Monitor renal function
bDMARDs	**Stop these medications prior to surgery and reschedule surgery at the end of dosing cycle. Resume medications minimum of 14 days after surgery in absence of wound healing and/or infective complications.**		
Infliximab	6 weeks	No	
Adalimumab	3 weeks	No	
Etanercept	2 weeks	No	
Golimumab	• 6 weeks (for SC dosing) • 9 weeks (for IV)	No	
Certolizumab	6 weeks	No	
Tocilizumab IV	4 weeks	No	May mask signs of inflammation
Tocilizumab SC	3 weeks	No	May mask signs of inflammation
Rituximab	6 months	No	
Abatacept SC	2 weeks	No	
Abatacept IV	4 weeks	No	
Anakinra	2 weeks	No	
Secukinumab	4 weeks	No	
Ustekinumab	12 weeks	No	
Belimumab	4 weeks	No	
Tofacitinib and possibly other tsDMARDs	1 week	No	

Perioperative Management of b-DMARDs

Surgical management of RA patients is challenging as RA is an independent risk factor (twofold to fourfold increased risk) for postoperative orthopedic infection. The concern for additional increased risk of infection caused by immunosuppression from treatment has led some to suggest that perioperative

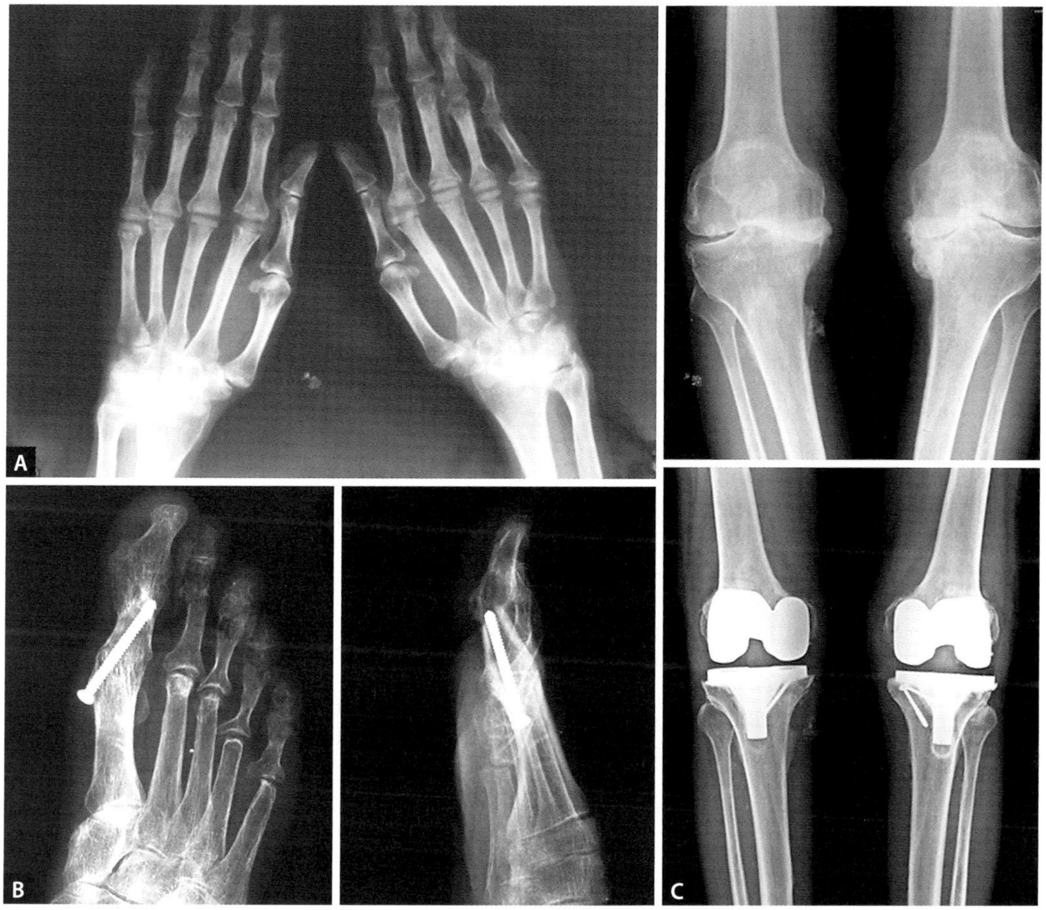

Figs. 27A to C: Various joint reconstruction surgeries performed in rheumatoid arthritis (RA). (A) Metacarpophalangeal (MCP) joint arthroplasty; (B) Arthrodesis of first metatarsophalangeal (MTP) joint; (C) Total knee replacement for advanced RA with secondary degeneration of knee.

treatment be discontinued. However, withholding treatment in some patients could induce a disease flare, complicating wound healing after surgery. Maintaining the balance is a dilemma. Current recommendations for various drugs are presented in **Table 21**.

Abatacept acts earlier in the inflammatory cascade than other biological agents by directly inhibiting T-cells and secondary activation of B-cells and macrophages. It should be considered after inadequate response to one or more nonbiological DMARDs and a failure to at least one TNF-blocking agent. It should not be combined with TNF-blockers due to increased risk of serious infections.

Protein a Immunoabsorption Column

This is a device that has staphylococcal protein that binds IgG and IgG-antigen complexes, removing them from the circulation of patients with severe RA that is not responsive to second-line therapy. The device has been effective in immune thrombocytopenic purpura and has been moderately more effective in RA than a "placebo" that provided sham immunoabsorption. It is costly and time consuming. The trials in RA necessitated a column treatment once a week for 12 weeks. This remains an option only for patients who have failed treatment with traditional DMARDs as well as the newer anticytokine agents.

Surgical Management in Rheumatoid Arthritis Patients

- Surgical, chemical, or radioactive synovectomy can be considered if the synovitis does not adequately respond to medication and there is no structural damage to the joint.
- If structural joint damage exists, and patient symptoms of synovitis do not respond to conventional medical treatment, surgical intervention with arthrodesis or arthroplasty may be indicated **(Figs. 27A to C)**. Patients with multiple joint involvements should receive staged surgical reconstruction to avoid prolonged periods of hospitalization and immobility. The common surgeries performed in cases of RA are:
  - Decompression of the entrapped nerves
  - Reconstructive procedures for joints including arthroplasties
  - Corrective arthrotomies of the metatarsals
  - Stabilization of the cervical spine
  - Tendon transfer and releases
  - Arthrodesis, particularly of ankle joint
- Synovectomy is less frequently performed now although tenosynovectomy for nerve compression is recommended. The results for decompression are quick and the procedure is quite safe.

- Arthroplasties reduce or ameliorate pain and deformity reasonably but functional gain may not be as good when done for other causes like osteoarthrosis.
- Extensive RA involvement of the shoulder, elbow, or wrist may compromise any anticipated postoperative use of crutches or a walker for patients needing lower extremity surgery. Therefore, it is prudent and common to treat the involved joints of the upper extremity before proceeding with lower extremity surgery (for example, wrist arthrodesis may facilitate the use of crutches for lower extremity reconstruction). However, the completion of lower extremity reconstruction before treatment of upper extremity joints may be most appropriate if it is anticipated that the patient's need for a walking device in the postoperative period could overload delicate arthroplasties in the elbow and/or hand.
- Optimally patient should be under remission or should be taking the lowest possible dose for mild active disease.
- *Issue of concurrent medications:* Glucocorticoids can be reduced in the preoperative period, but there is a potential for adrenal suppression in longstanding use. It is currently recommended that most patients taking oral corticosteroids receive stress coverage the day of surgery and for the following 24 hours. If patients are taking low dose steroids or it can be spared then it is better to stop them due to elevated risk of infections. The recommendations for use of various DMARDs are presented in **Table 21**.
- Other foci of infection should be controlled before surgery. For optimal rehabilitation instructing the patient in the use of a walker, crutches, or a cane before surgery may help to facilitate an uneventful transition to these devices.
- Preoperative cervical spine assessment with lateral radiographs is imperative in all RA patients as clinically asymptomatic but significant cervical spine involvement exists in up to 40% of these patients. C1-C2 or subaxial instability might compromise the spinal cord during routine intubation.

SERONEGATIVE SPONDYLOARTHROPATHIES

INTRODUCTION

The term "seronegative spondyloarthritis" encompasses a heterogeneous group of inflammatory diseases characterized by:

- Inflammatory back pain
- Spinal (sacroiliitis) and peripheral joint oligoarthritis
- Enthesitis
- Negative rheumatoid factor
- Young age at onset and familial predisposition and association to MHC Class-I molecule, HLA-B27.

They often have associated asymmetric peripheral arthritis and extra-articular disease (mucocutaneous, ocular, anterior uveitis and/or cardiac manifestations). This family of diseases includes ankylosing spondylitis, juvenile-onset ankylosing spondylitis (juvenile enthesitis-related arthritis), juvenile chronic arthritis, PsA, enteropathic arthritis (associated with inflammatory bowel diseases), reactive arthritis, and undifferentiated spondyloarthropathy (features of many of above but diagnostic to none). There is a controversy over inclusion of other sacroiliitis-associated diseases like Whipple's disease and SAPHO syndrome into the broad banner of spondyloarthropathies.

ANKYLOSING SPONDYLITIS (MARIE–STRUMPELL DISEASE, MORBUS BECHTEREW DISEASE)

The term *ankylosing spondylitis* is derived from the Greek roots ankylos ("bent"), although now it usually implies fusion or adhesions, and spondylos ("vertebral disk"). Ankylosing spondylitis is the most common spondyloarthropathy with strong HLA-B27 association characterized by chronic inflammatory disease of the axial skeleton and manifests as back pain and progressive stiffness of the spine. It is a systemic disease so it not only affects the spine and sacroiliac joints but also causes aortitis and aortic insufficiency late in the disease in about 5–10% of patients, rare upper lobe predominant interstitial restrictive pulmonary disease (1%) and iridocyclitis (25%) or uveitis (20%). About 10% of patients with ankylosing spondylitis will develop secondary amyloidosis. Ankylosing spondylitis characteristically affects young adults (16–45 years), males more than females (clinically; 9:1 but radiologically incidence of 2-3:1); however, 10% may have earlier onset juvenile form of disease.

Clinical Presentation

Patients present with back pain with prolonged morning stiffness (for >1 hour) and progressive loss of motion of the axial spine. The pain should have four or more of these characteristic features (to specify as inflammatory pain): (1) age of onset below 40 years, (2) insidious onset, (3) improvement with exercise, (4) no improvement with rest, and (5) hip and back pain that is worse in the morning on arising up but improves throughout the day ("gel phenomenon"). In addition to the spine, sacroiliac involvement, arthritis of the hips, peripheral arthritis and enthesitis are common. Enthesitis is typically a principal feature, it is the fibrosis and ossification of ligament, tendon, and capsule insertions into bone (the entheses) mainly seen in the region of disks and sacroiliac joints. Typically, ankylosing spondylitis starts in the sacroiliac joints (from inferior to superior with later fusion of the joint) and slowly ascends the spine. The most specific findings involve loss of spinal mobility, with limitation of anterior and lateral flexion and extension of the lumbar spine and of chest expansion. Stress tests for sacroiliac joint (Gaenslen and FABER) are positive. Modified Shober test reasonably assess the spinal flexion. As the disease progresses, increasing flexion of the neck, increased thoracic kyphosis, and loss of normal lumbar lordosis lead to a stooped posture. Disease progression can be estimated clinically from loss of height, limitation of chest expansion and spinal flexion, and occiput-to-wall distance. Onset of ankylosing spondylitis in adolescence and early hip involvement correlate with a worse prognosis. Juvenile onset disease has more frequent peripheral arthritis and delayed axial presentation. Females usually do not go to complete spinal fusion but have increased prevalence of peripheral arthritis and isolated cervical ankylosis. "Bamboo spine" develops in a few patients but in those where it is formed there is significant incidence of collapse of vertebral end-plate and destruction of disk-bone border. This phenomenon leads to sudden increase in pain over dorsal spine with localized tenderness and excruciating pain on movement is a dangerous sign and may represent fracture or tubercular infection or more serious "Andersson's lesion" the latter is a pseudoarthrosis of thoracolumbar bamboo spine that is difficult to treat and represents unstable pattern that can compromise neurology. There are various measures to measure disease activity of which Bath Ankylosing Spondylitis Disease Activity Index (BASDAI) is prominently used. Bath Ankylosing Spondylitis Functional Index (BASFI) is a measure of limitations in activities of daily living **(Box 10)**. The standardized mortality ratio is 1.5 possibly due to cardiac valve, respiratory disease, amyloidosis, and fractures so commonly associated with ankylosing spondylitis. Mortality in ankylosing spondylitis is mainly due to spinal trauma, aortic insufficiency, respiratory failure, amyloid nephropathy, or complications of therapy such as upper gastrointestinal hemorrhage.

Synovitis also occurs in larger peripheral joints (hips and knees in particular). The peripheral joint involvement has been seen in females more so than men. Nearly 50% of patients with ankylosing spondylitis will develop hip arthritis and some of them would need surgery. Ankylosing spondylitis is associated with high rates of job attrition and job changes.

BOX 10: The bath ankylosing spondylitis disease activity index (BASDAI) and bath ankylosing spondylitis functional index (BASFI) indices.

BASDAI Index

The BASDAI consists of a 1 through 10 scale (1 being no problem and 10 being the worst problem) which is used to answer 6 questions pertaining to the major symptoms of AS:

A. Fatigue
B. Spinal pain
C. Joint pain/swelling
D. Areas of localized tenderness (also called enthesitis, or inflammation of tendons and ligaments)
E. Morning stiffness duration
F. Morning stiffness severity

The first five items consist of a visual analog scale 1–10 scale while the sixth item, related to the duration of morning stiffness is scored as 0 for 0 hours, 5 for 1 hour, and 10 for 2 or more hours.

The total score is computed by following formula:

$$BASDAI = \frac{((A + B + C + D) + \left(\frac{E+F}{2}\right))}{5}$$

Scores of 4 or greater suggest suboptimal control of disease, and patients with scores of 4 or greater are usually good candidates for either a change in their medical therapy or for enrollment in clinical trials evaluating new drug therapies.

BASFI Index

The BASFI is a self-administering questionnaire for pain and stiffness control using 10 items evaluated on a scale of 0 (no impairment) to 10 (severe impairment) that can be used for monitoring therapeutic results over time.

1. Putting on your socks or tights without help or aids (e.g., sock aids).
2. Bending forward from the waist to pick up a pen from the floor without an aid.
3. Reaching up to a high shelf without help or aids (e.g., helping hand).
4. Getting up out of an armless dining room chair without using your hands or any other help.
5. Getting up off the floor without any help from lying on your back.
6. Standing unsupported for 10 minutes without discomfort.
7. Climbing 12–15 steps without using a handrail or walking aid (one foot on each step).
8. Looking over your shoulder without turning your body.
9. Doing physically demanding activities (e.g., physiotherapy exercises, gardening, or sports).
10. Doing a full-day activities whether it be at home or work.

There is no cut-off point but higher the score greater is the functional impairment.

Radiographic Features

Sacroiliitis is demonstrable in most. Earliest change includes blurring of the cortical margins of the subchondral bone, followed by erosions and sclerosis of sacroiliac joint. Later there is "pseudowidening" in joint space (**Fig. 28A**, in the lower two-thirds of SI joint which has a synovial lining) due to fibrous ankylosis followed by obliteration of joint space in bony ankylosis **(Figs. 29C and 30)**. The sacroiliitis is graded according to New York criteria as—grade 0 = normal; grade 1 = some blurring of joint margins ("whiskering"); grade 2 = minimal sclerosis with some erosions; grade 3 = definite sclerosis on both sides "or" severe erosions with widening of joint space with or without sclerosis; grade 4 = complete ankylosis.

On plain radiographs of spine, "squaring (or barreling) of the vertebral bodies" as a result of anterior and posterior spondylitis will be seen early along with reactive bone formation in ring apophyses **(Fig. 29A)**. Squaring occurs due to erosion of vertebral corners (Romanus lesions) causing vertebral squaring and eliciting reactive sclerosis appearing as condensation of vertebral corners (shiny corners). These changes are caused by inflammation at the insertion of the annulus fibrosus (enthesitis) at vertebral corners infuriating reactive bone formation. Later "Bamboo spine"—bridging syndesmophytes **(Fig. 29B)**, ankylosis of the facet joints and calcification of the anterior longitudinal ligament occurs with disease progression, anterior atlantoaxial (C1-C2) subluxation can also occur later in the disease process. In advanced disease, the supraspinous and interspinous ligaments may ossify and are visible on frontal radiograph as a slim ossified streak, this single central radiodense streak has been named the "dagger sign". When the ligamentous ossification occurs together with ossification of apophyseal joint capsules, there appear three vertical radiodense lines on frontal radiography called trolley-track sign.

Spinal fractures are life-threatening and should be diagnosed by careful radiography. It is, therefore, mandatory to supplement a negative radiography with CT if fracture is suspected. CT-scan is best for eliciting bony details and fracture evaluation. It is superior to MRI in detecting minor osseous lesions such as erosion and ankylosis of the apophyseal, costovertebral, and costotransversal joints. MRI scan is, however, more successful in detecting active inflammation **(Fig. 28B)** and its sequelae (fatty

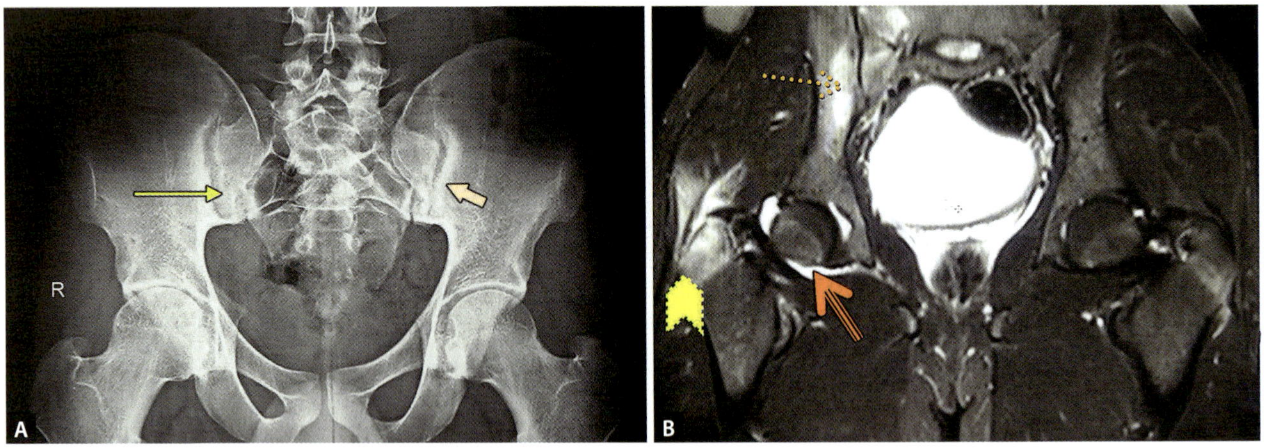

Figs. 28A and B: Typical radiographic appearance of grade 3 sacroiliitis in a patient with ankylosing spondylosis. There is pseudo-widening of the joint (arrow) due to fibrous ankylosis, irregularity of margins with sclerosis (block arrow); that later fuses into bony ankylosis and loss of joint space. There is also reduction of right hip joint space. MRI scan of a patient with radiographic grade 0 sacroiliitis, who presented with fleeting pains in lower lumbar spine and in buttock region without radiation. The MRI scan (B) demonstrated bilateral sacroiliitis (dotted arrow) with bilateral trochanteric region enthesopathy (chevron) and right hip joint significant effusion (patterned arrow). These inflammatory changes are also enough to make a diagnosis of ankylosing spondylosis with clinical correlation.

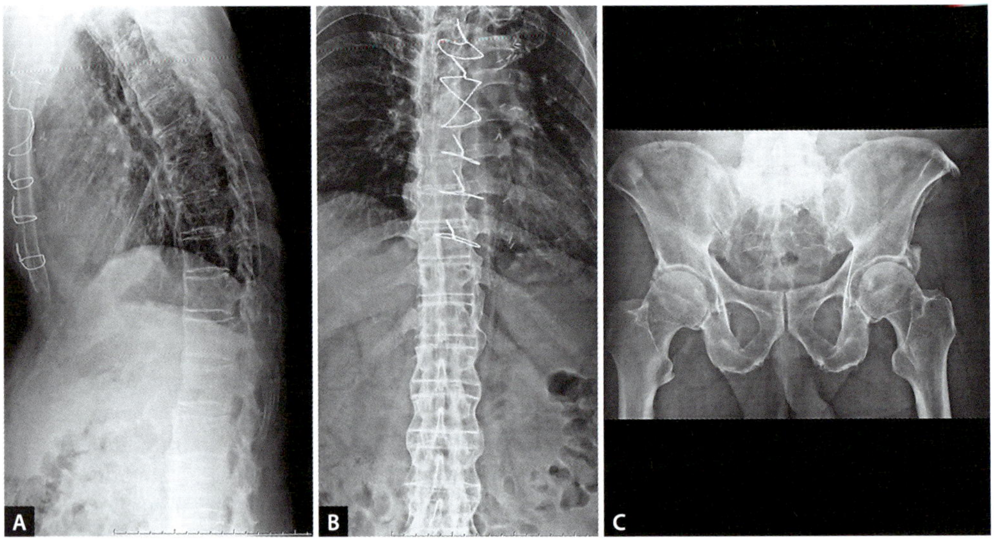

Figs. 29A to C: Ankylosing spondylitis—note the squaring of vertebra seen on (A) lateral projection with classical bamboo spine on (B) anteroposterior radiograph of dorsolumbar spine. (C) The inferior aspects of sacroiliac (SI) joint have started fusing.

deposition in the bone marrow and erosion and fusion of vertebral bodies). MRI demonstration of severe or multiple (≥3) lesions can distinguish ankylosing spondylitis from degenerative changes. Fatty marrow deposition seems to be most important sign of chronicity of ankylosing spondylitis, if radiology is confusing or indicate only early changes. MRI is also an important tool to investigate disease activity especially with biological therapy (like anti-TNF therapy) and can reliably demonstrate treatment success or failure or recurrence of disease later. The dynamic contrast-enhanced MRI is better to static MRI in this regard. To avoid missing the diagnosis and evaluation whole body MR scanning is recommended.

Andersson lesion is a circumscribed, sterile, destructive process involving one vertebral body with its intervertebral disk (diskovertebral) that extends across the three columns of spine **(Box 11)**.

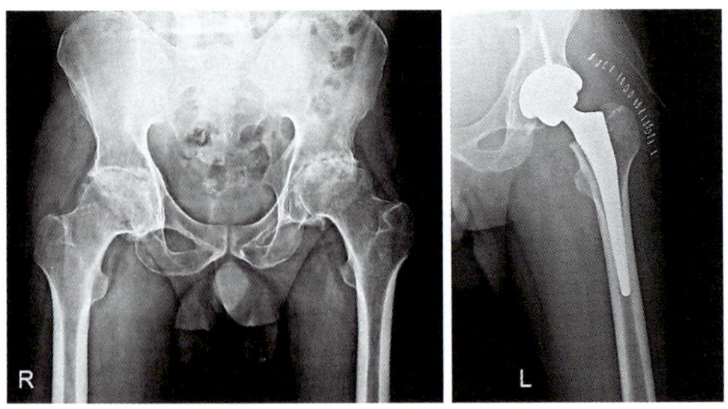

Fig. 30: Total hip arthoplasty (THA) (large head) of left hip in a patient with ankylosing spondylosis and ankylosed hips. Patient was not willing for both hip surgery together.

Laboratory tests add little in the diagnosis of ankylosing spondylitis (AS). *Klebsiella* antigens or infection previously

BOX 11: The Andersson lesion of spine.

The Andersson lesion (rheumatic spondylodiskitis) named after a Swedish radiologist, Olof Andersson (who first described the findings in 1937) refers to an inflammatory involvement of the intervertebral disks by spondyloarthritis.

Epidemiology: It is a noninfectious condition with reported prevalence of 1.5% to over 28%.

Etiopathology: There is a debate about etiology hypothetically varying between **(Figs. 31A to E)**:
- Local delay in the ankylosing process compared to adjacent levels resulting in the last mobile segment **(Fig. 31A)** or stress localization at a specific level in otherwise fused spine
- Spinal (stress) fractures through fused disk **(Fig. 31B)** or vertebral body **(Fig. 31C)**.
- Aseptic inflammation
- Trauma

Whatever the cause maybe it culminates finally into a pseudoarthrosis associated with inflammatory features that is transdiskal or transvertebral and is usually accompanied by fractures or nonfusion of the posterior elements. Cawley et al. divided the Andersson lesion into two groups:
1. *Localized lesion*: Usually seen early in the course of disease and are subdivided according to their exact location:
   a. The diskal surface of the vertebral rim (peripheral)
   b. The cartilaginous part of the vertebral endplate (central)
2. Extensive lesions involve both central and peripheral locations and are exclusively seen in patients with ankylosed spine.

Clinical features: The most common presentation demanding evaluation is a progressive, localized thoracolumbar pain or sharp localized pain that may be preceded by trauma. The lesion may otherwise be asymptomatic and discovered on routine radiographic evaluation. Uncommonly, the patient presents with radiculopathy or neurogenic claudication due to nerve root or cord compression. These symptoms are often aggravated on sitting or standing while getting relieved on lying down. There is localized tenderness and gibbus or short kyphus at the spinal level usually localized to thoracolumbar junction. One should be especially suspicious if a bamboo spine starts to bend. Lesions in cervical or lumbar spine, lesions with thoracic vertebral wedging or those with high disease activity are associated with development of hyperkyphosis. Some patients develop multiple lesions making diagnosis difficult. Fever is not a sign of this lesion.

Radiological features: Plain radiograph depicts irregularities and erosions of the vertebral endplates that are not related to the anterior or posterior edge but rather to the central portion. They are good for localization of the disease visualized as osteolytic destruction with a surrounding zone of reactive sclerosis and vertebral osteophytes. The lesion may be transvertebral, transdiskal, or diskovertebral. Based on variable radiological features, a division into five categories has also been proposed, viz., pseudodystrophic, pseudotuberculous, extensive erosions, bone condensation, and isolated narrowing of the intervertebral spaces. CT scan demonstrates irregular vertebral or diskovertebral osteolysis with surrounding reactive sclerosis with much greater clarity than radiographs, also it accurately demonstrates fractures of posterior elements or nonfusion of facet joints.

MRI depicts disk-related signal intensity abnormalities of one or both vertebral halves of a diskovertebral unit. Andersson lesion appears hyperintense on STIR images and hypointense on T1-weighted images, where they are often hemispherically shaped. MRI also provides a superior view of spondylodiskitis, since the edematous changes in early disease are not visible of plain X-rays. MRI is the standard investigation to evaluate root or cord compression or changes.

Differential diagnosis
- Pott's spine
- Bacterial diskitis
- Neoplasia (malignant fibrous histocytoma or osteosarcoma)
- Spinal neuroarthropathy
- SAPHO syndrome

Treatment: Conservative management with bracing for immobilization of the lesion in thoracic region is usually provided as interim measure till definitive management. This is supported by the partial fixation from rib cage in this region. Immobilization may also be done using Halo-pelvic jacket or plaster jacket. In any case, achieving fusion of the lesion with any immobilization modality is unlikely so surgical fixation for stabilization remains the mainstay of therapy. Symptomatic improvement may be obtained with NSAIDs for pain relief. bDMARDs have not shown any benefit in resolution of the lesion. Rigorous exercise program is contraindicated in Andersson lesion.

Surgical decompression, stabilization, correction of kyphotic deformity, and fusion form the mainstay of treatment. In cervical and lumbar lesions, this should be administered on priority lest development of hyperkyphosis is risky. The indications for surgical fixation are unbearable pain, progression of symptoms, progressive kyphotic deformity, or neurological deficits. The usual practice is instrumented stabilization that may be done through anterior, posterior, or combined approach depending on the location of the lesion, alignment of spine, neurology, and spinal cord compression. The usual thoracolumbar kyphotic deformity is addressed mostly by posterior correction and fixation of Andersson lesion by an anterior opening wedge osteotomy or a transpedicular wedge osteotomy and fixation may be considered.

(bDMARDs: biological disease-modifying antirheumatic drugs; NSAIDs: nonsteroidal anti-inflammatory drugs; STIR: short tau inversion recovery)

implicated have not found to be of any concrete basis. ESR is increased in 80% of patients with active disease. CRP levels may be elevated if ESR is normal. Rheumatoid factor and antinuclear antibody are characteristically absent while serum complement levels are normal or high. Serum IgA levels are high but causative organism in unknown. The only locus definitively linked to the spondyloarthritis is HLA-B27 allele accounting for 20% of the genetic effect. Other important alleles include HLA-B*1:02, HLA-B*40:01, HLA-B47, etc. The most important information deciphered to risk of development of AS is the interaction of ERAP1, the protein endoplasmic reticulum aminopeptidase 1, with the HLA-B27 allele in positive patients. In HLA-B27 negative patients, ERAP1 interacts with HLA-B40 allele. *TLR7* gene is associated with susceptibility of AS in males while it protects females. The presence of HLA-B27 is not needed to confirm a diagnosis of ankylosing spondylitis, but it can be used as a diagnostic test in children and young women who may have normal radiographs and in patients who have an atypical presentation. The presence or absence of B27 greatly increases or decreases, respectively, the probability of AS in patients with equivocal clinical findings lacking radiographic abnormalities (considering Bayes' theorem). It may be useful to assess symptomatic first-degree relatives of HLA-B27 + probands with AS, for whom the risk of developing the disease is nearly 1 in 3. The absence of B27 in a typical case of AS significantly increases the probability of coexistent IBD. A number on interesting observations are seen with the study of HLA-B27:

- HLA-B27 is inherited as an autosomal codominant characteristic: 50% of the first-degree relatives of probands with HLA-B27 possess the antigen.
- Five to ten percent of HLA-B27 positive individuals develop AS over time and 20% individuals with B27 develop a reactive arthropathy after contact with agents like *Chlamydia* or *Salmonella*.
- Only 50% of patients with psoriatic or enteropathic arthritis are HLA-B27 positive.
- Only 50% of non-Caucasians with AS HLA-B27 positive. This is considerably less than the prevalence of HLA-B27 among the Caucasians with AS (95%).
- Relatives of probands with both sacroiliitis and HLA-27 frequently remain disease free.
- Concordance in identical twins is 70% while in nonidentical twins it is 13%.

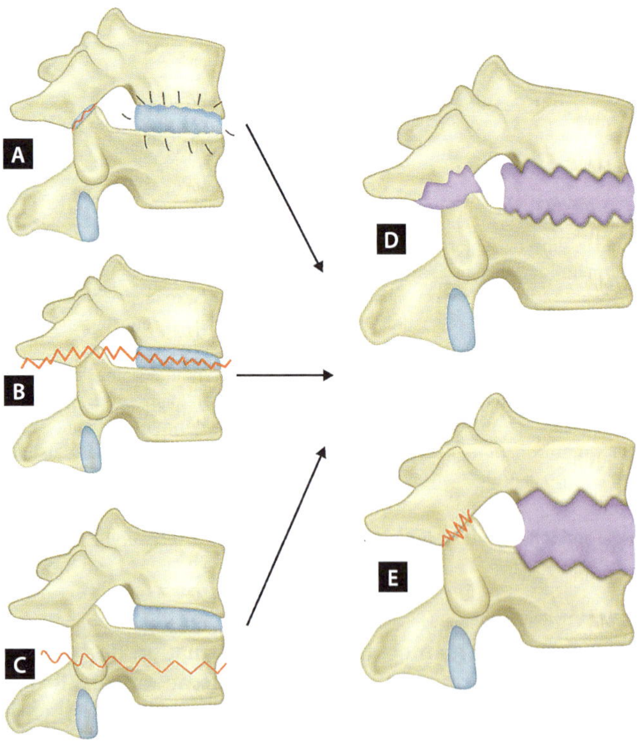

Figs. 31A to E: Pathogenesis of Andersson diskovertebral lesion. Persistent last mobile segment during the course of developing spinal fusion or patchy fusion of the spine (A) with or without inflammation, stress fractures through fused disk (B), or stress fractures through vertebral body (C) that culminates into development of non-kyphotic (D) or kyphotic (E) deformity.

- Uveitis is a common accompaniment of AS. HLA-B27 is found in up to 40% of cases of uveitis, even in absence of underlying rheumatic disease.

Diagnosis

The Assessment of Spondyloarthritis International Society (ASAS) criteria for axial spondyloarthropathy are proposed by ASAS in 2009 for diagnosis of spondyloarthropathy **(Table 22)**. Active inflammation of the sacroiliac (SI) joints as determined by dynamic MRI is considered equivalent to the older criterion of definite radiographic sacroiliitis. Modified New York criteria **(Box 12)** though not sensitive for early disease are more commonly referred to by the clinicians to make a diagnosis for its simplicity.

Differential diagnosis: Ochronosis, diffuse idiopathic skeletal hyperostosis (DISH), metabolic causes of back pain (osteomalacia and osteoporosis), infections (tuberculosis, actinomycosis, and pyogenic), malignancy (myeloma and lymphoma), reactive arthritis, inflammatory bowel disease, SAPHO syndrome, Whipple's disease, and brucellosis. DISH should be differentiated from ankylosing spondylitis specifically. The DISH is seen in patients >50 years of age while ankylosing spondylitis is seen in patients <40 years of

TABLE 22: The ASAS criteria for classification of axial spondyloarthritis (applicable to individuals with ≥3 months of back pain with age of onset <45 years old).

Sacroiliitis on imaging plus ≥1 SpA feature	***or HLA-B27 plus ≥2 other SpA features***
Sacroiliitis on imaging: • Active (acute) inflammation on MRI highly suggestive of SpA-associated sacroiliitis (on short-tau inverted sequence or Gadolinium enhancement) and/or • Definite radiographic sacroiliitis according to modified New York criteria (bilateral Grade 2 or unilateral Grade 3 or 4)	*SpA features:* • Inflammatory back pain • Arthritis • Enthesitis (heel) (tendo-Achilles or plantar fascia pain) • Anterior uveitis (most common extraosseous presentation) • Dactylitis • Psoriasis • Crohn's disease or ulcerative colitis • Good response to NSAIDs (substantial relief for 24–48 hours after full dose of NSAID) • Family history of SpA (first or second degree relative of spondyloarthropathy) • HLA-B27 • Elevated CRP (exclude other causes)

(ASAS: Assessment of Spondyloarthritis International Society; CRP: C-reactive protein; NSAIDs: nonsteroidal anti-inflammatory drugs)

BOX 12: Modified New York criteria.

Definitive sacroiliitis (Grade ≥2 bilateral or unilateral 3–4) and any one of the following (definitive ankylosing spondylitis). Probable ankylosing spondylitis, if three clinical criterion or radiological criterion present but no signs or symptoms to satisfy clinical criteria:

- Low back pain ≥3 months' duration improved by exercise not relieved by rest
- Limitation of lumbar spine movements in sagittal and frontal planes
- Chest expansion decreased relative to normal values for age and sex

age. Increased kyphosis is seen in ankylosing spondylitis but not in DISH. Mobility is reduced in ankylosing spondylitis but not in DISH as is pain which is seen commonly in ankylosing spondylitis but less common with DISH. Chest expansion is characteristically reduced with ankylosing spondylitis but not with DISH. Radiologically, ankylosing spondylitis has sacroiliitis and formation of syndesmophytes with erosive enthesitis. Anterior longitudinal ligament (ALL) and posterior longitudinal ligament (PLL) ossification are seen with DISH but not ankylosing spondylitis.

Treatment

The goals of therapy for patients with ankylosing spondylitis are not only to provide symptomatic relief but, like for the treatment of RA, to prevent permanent irreversible joint damage. The baseline common factor in all therapeutic interventions include exercise program designed to maintain posture and range of motion. Physiotherapy, balneotherapy especially supervised one for maintaining joint mobility has been found highly effective, swimming is a wholesome exercise. NSAIDs are the first-line pharmacologic therapy for ankylosing spondylitis and reduce pain and tenderness and increase mobility in many patients with ankylosing spondylitis. Daily NSAID therapy given continuously (rather than intermittently) is shown to slow radiographic progression but it has significant renal and gastrointestinal side effects. New NSAID, B-D-mannuronic acid produces similar response without these side effects. However, disease progresses in many with incremental deformity and joint ankylosis. Sulfasalazine, in doses of 2–3 g/day, has been shown to be of modest benefit (antibiotic, immunomodulatory or anti-inflammatory effect exactly unknown), primarily for peripheral arthritis. However, updated ASAS/EULAR recommendations for the management of ankylosing spondylitis confirmed that sulfasalazine had no significant effect on BASDAI and pain in patients with established or long-standing ankylosing spondylitis. MTX, gold, azathioprine, cyclophosphamide and glucocorticoids have not been found effective. Moreover steroid may induce osteoporosis a complication of disease itself. Thalidomide by virtue of inhibiting TNF-α has been found to be effective in doses of 200 mg/day but toxicity limits its use. Apremilast (phosphodiesterase-4 inhibitor) has shown improvement in initial studies. Monitoring and response to treatment is assessed by ASAS20 criteria **(Box 13)**.

With increasingly identified role for TNF-α, IL-17, and IL-23 in the pathogenesis of disease (the interested reader is encouraged to read "arthritogenic peptide theory", "unfolded protein response theory", and "HLA-B27 homodimer model" from available literature) the relevance of bDMARD therapy is being increasingly realized. Patients with active disease and persistent symptoms on conventional therapy are candidates for anti-TNF-α therapy. The guidelines for starting the therapy include—two different NSAID should be tested ≥3 months period, active disease for ≥4 weeks (BASDAI >4 at two times, 1 month apart and/or ASDAS ≥2.1) **(Box 14)**, patients with peripheral arthritis who failed to >1 csDMARD (sulfasalazine preferred). Patients with ankylosing spondylitis treated with either infliximab (chimeric human/mouse anti-TNF-α monoclonal antibody), etanercept (soluble p75 TNF-α receptor—IgG fusion protein), or adalimumab or golimumab (human anti-TNF-α monoclonal antibodies) have shown effective, rapid, and sustained reductions in all clinical and laboratory measures of disease activity, other newer agents also have similar efficacy. Half of the patients had reduction in BASDAI score of ≥50% and substantial resolution of bone marrow edema, enthesitis, and joint effusions in the sacroiliac joints, spine, and peripheral joints on MRI. Anti-TNF therapy though does not reduce syndesmophyte formation. Presence of baseline syndesmophyte and cigarette smoking predicts disease progression and limited response to anti-TNF-α therapy with 55% risk of progression. Contraindications for anti-TNF-α therapy include current infection, tuberculosis, multiple sclerosis, lupus, malignancy, pregnancy or lactating mothers. Patients who do not improve for BASDAI score ≥2 units or those with ASDAS ≥2.1 **(Box 14)** persistently over 6–8 weeks should be stopped on treatment and other agent may be considered. Side effects profile has been similar to patients treated for RA, however, malignancy has not been found over 5 years of treatment with these agents. For these complications their use should be restricted to patients with a definite diagnosis and active disease (BASDAI ≥4 out of 10 and ASDAS ≥2.1) that is inadequately responsive to therapy with at least two different NSAIDs. Patients who do not respond to anti-TNF-α agent are considered resistant and other agents may be tried. Anakinra is ineffective and rituximab works in anti-TNF-α naïve patients only not the resistant ones. Abatacept, tocilizumab, and sarilumab (IL-

BOX 13: ASAS improvement criteria in ankylosing spondylitis.

At least 20% improvement AND absolute improvement of ≥10 units in three out of the four following domains, without worsening of 20% or more AND 10 units in the remaining domain:

1. Bath Ankylosing Spondylitis Functional Index (BASFI)
2. Inflammation (the average of BASDAI's last two VAS concerning morning stiffness and duration)
3. Patient global assessment (VAS score)
4. Pain (the average of VAS score and nocturnal pain scores)

ASAS partial remission criteria: A value below 20 units in all four domains

(ASAS: Assessment of Spondyloarthritis International Society; BASDAI: bath ankylosing spondylitis disease activity index; VAS: visual analog scale)

BOX 14: Ankylosing Spondylitis Disease Activity Score (ASDAS).

ASDAS is a lately developed scoring system that is considered better in assessing disease activity and guiding start of bDMARDs. The ASDAS is a data-driven index that combines three BASDAI-PRO-derived questions about spinal pain (1), peripheral joints (2) and duration of morning stiffness (3), as well as the "patient global assessment of disease activity" (4), with either the CRP (ASDAS-CRP) or the erythrocyte sedimentation rate (ESR) (ASDAS-ESR) (5) according to a weighted formula. Using ASDAS-CRP is recommended for clinical practice and trials.

Interpretation of ASDAS:

- ASDAS < 1.3—inactive disease
- ASDAS > 1.3 but <2.1—low disease activity
- ASDAS ≥ 2.1 but ≤3.5—high disease activity
- ASDAS > 3.5—very high disease activity

6 inhibitor) have not been found effective. Ixekizumab and Secukinumab (anti-IL-17A monoclonal antibody) have been shown effective in anti-TNF-α failure patients with maintained reduction of spinal inflammation of MRI. Janus kinase (JAK) inhibitors especially tofacitinib and upadacitinib have also shown good promise in control of the disease and can be administered orally too. IL-23 inhibitors like guselkumab and risankizumab are also being studied that further inhibit downstream production of IL-17.

Surgical Treatment

The indications for surgical treatment in ankylosing spondylitis are—unstable injuries, Andersson's lesion with or without neurological deficit, painful spinal deformity, functionally and/or cosmetically unacceptable deformities. For correction of lumbar and thoracolumbar deformities, a two-stage procedure is uncommonly performed with posterior and anterior osteotomies. Boehm introduced single-stage procedure and a minimally invasive (endoscopically assisted) approach for osteotomy of anterior spine. Similarly, mobile or fixed cervicothoracic region deformities are corrected with osteotomies. Andersson's lesions do not respond to conservative treatment and although posterior, anterior, and combined fusion techniques are described, the combined approach is preferred for high incidence of progressive kyphosis and failure in other techniques. Anterior strut graft or cage is recommended to counter the flexion moments. For hip and knee joint disease, arthroplasty is the usual choice. Patients with ankylosing spondylitis often fail to fully regain the same range of motion after joint reconstruction in comparison with other groups of patients. Although postoperative range of motion may be less, it is still often adequate to significantly improve the patient's ability to perform activities of daily living. Patients with ankylosing spondylitis may have an increased risk of heterotopic ossification. Indomethacin or perioperative radiation may be used to decrease this risk.

It had been always difficult to define the outcome for individual patients in terms of prognosis. The main predictive factors associated with poor prognosis in ankylosing spondylitis appear to be:

- Early hip involvement
- ESR > 30
- Poor initial response to NSAIDs
- Early loss of lumbar spine mobility
- Presence of dactylitis
- Oligoarticular disease
- Onset <16 years
- Low sociological background
- Sporadic disease instead of familial.

PSORIATIC ARTHRITIS

The term "psoriatic arthritis" (PsA) was first used by Wright. PsA is a chronic inflammatory rheumatic disease associated with psoriasis affecting both proximal and distal peripheral joints and, in approximately, one-third of patients, the spine. Although most patients with PsA have a benign course, a subset of patients has a severe, unrelenting, and sometimes mutilating form of arthritis. PsA affects approximately 20–30% of patients with psoriasis equally affecting women and men. The term "psoriatic disease" combines the clinical manifestations of psoriasis (skin disease) and PsA.

Clinical Features

The course of PsA is usually characterized by flares and remissions. The arthritis appears after the onset of a skin lesion in most patients. However, the arthritis can precede the skin disease in approximately 13–17% of patients. There are five distinct patterns of PsA:

1. Arthritis of DIP joints
2. Destructive (mutilans) arthritis
3. Symmetric polyarthritis indistinguishable from RA
4. Asymmetric oligoarthritis (less than five small and/or large joints are affected in an asymmetric distribution)
5. Spondyloarthropathy (including both sacroiliitis and spondylitis)

Most patients with PsA have the classic psoriasis vulgaris pattern of skin lesions. Patients often experience nail pitting and onycholysis as do patients with uncomplicated skin psoriasis **(Figs. 32A to C)**. Other clinical features of PsA include dactylitis (30%, entire digit swollen with DIP, PIP swelling—"Sausage digit"), tenosynovitis, and enthesitis. Spondyloarthropathy alone occurs in only 2–4% of the patients (but is seen in 20–40% of patients in combination). It is now clear that patterns of PsA are not permanent—>60% change from their initial pattern. Also joint damage progresses

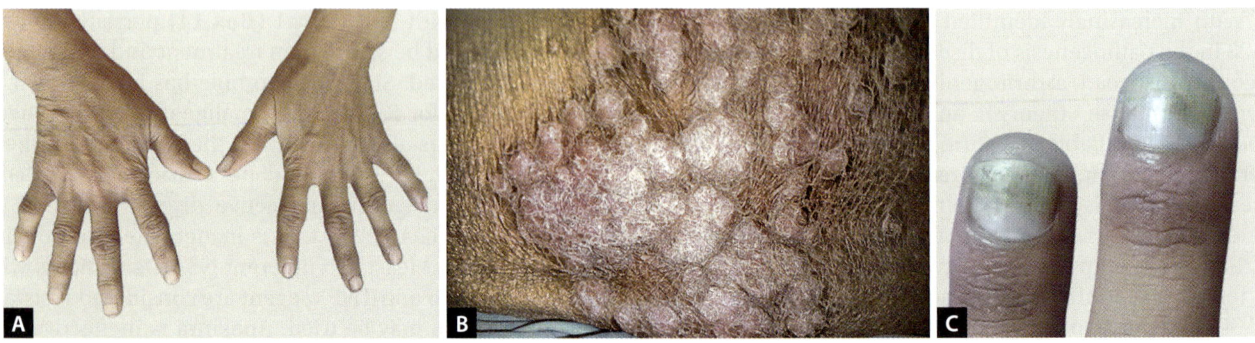

Figs. 32A to C: Psoriatic arthritis: Note the involvement of IP joints (DIP > PIP) and typical skin lesions. Note the fine pitting seen in nail of ring finger. (DIP: distal interphalangeal joints; PIP: proximal interphalangeal joints)

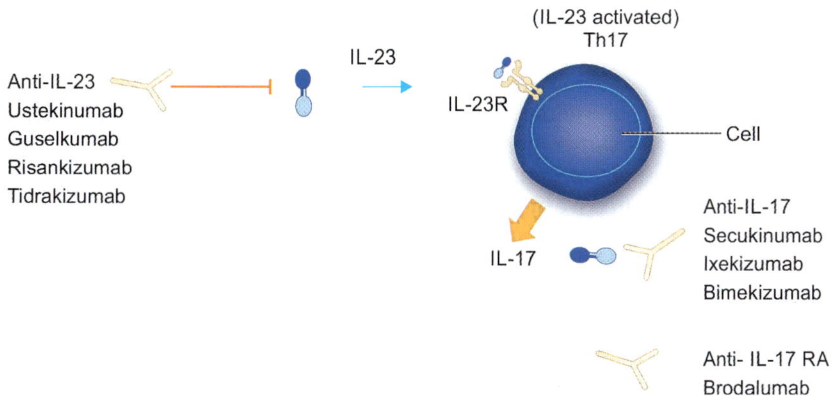

Fig. 33: The cytokines predominantly identified in pathogenesis of psoriasis and psoriatic arthropathy. Newer therapeutic agents are specifically targeted against the IL-17/23 axis. (IL: interleukin)

despite control of the inflammatory process of the disease, and in 5 years of follow-up, the number of patients with five or more damaged joints more than doubles. A younger age at the onset of the arthritis, female gender, and acute onset of arthritis were more common in patients with severe arthritis. Spondyloarthropathy is associated with favorable prognosis. The HLA antigens HLA-B27, in the presence of HLA-DR7 and DQw3, in the absence of HLA-DR7, are predictors of progression through all states of damage, whereas B39 is associated with disease progression in early disease. The presence of HLA-B22 is protective for progression of clinical damage. Interleukin (IL)-17 plays a major role in the development PsA (and also psoriasis). Effects of IL-17 are facilitated and maintained by IL-23. Apprising this fact is important as the IL-17/23 axis now marks major interest in development of targeted therapy **(Fig. 33)**. Some indices are used to measure clinically the response in PsA, one such index is the PsA Response Criteria (PsARC) developed originally to assess the response of sulfasalazine in PsA. The measure includes four items: tender joint count (which must be reduced by at least 30% for response), swollen joint count (must be reduced by 30% for response), physician global assessment (decreased by one point), and patient global assessment (decreased by one point for response) on a visual analog scale. To count as a responder, a patient must demonstrate an improvement in at least two of the four items, one of which must be either the tender or a swollen joint count. In addition, a patient must not demonstrate worsening in any of the items.

The radiographic features characteristic of PsA include asymmetric distribution, involvement of DIP joints, sacroiliitis and spondylitis, bone erosions with new bone formation, bony ankylosis, and resorption of the distal phalanges. The typical change in the peripheral joint is the "pencil-in-cup" picture of marked lysis of the distal end of a phalanx with remodeling of the proximal end of the more distal phalanx.

Diagnosis

Caspar criteria **(Box 15)** are commonly accepted for classifying the disease. The dilemma is differentiating PsA from RA in patients with positive rheumatoid factor and those patients who never had psoriasis. Clinical and radiographic features, including the pattern of the arthritis, the distribution and joints involved, and the presence of a spondyloarthropathy, may facilitate the diagnosis.

BOX 15: The Caspar criteria for psoriatic arthritis.

A patient must have inflammatory articular disease (joint, spine or entheseal) with three points from any of the following five categories:

1. Evidence of current psoriasis (assigned two points) a personal history of psoriasis, or a family history of psoriasis (assigned one point each)
2. Typical psoriatic nail dystrophy
3. Negative rheumatoid factor
4. Either current dactylitis or a history of dactylitis (demonstrated by rheumatologist)
5. Radiographic evidence of juxta-articular new bone formation (excluding osteophytes) in the hand or foot

Treatment

The treatment of PsA is directed at controlling the inflammatory process. Patients are often treated with NSAIDs for PsA, but to date evidence supporting the use of NSAIDs for PsA is scarce. In patients with severe skin inflammation, medications such as MTX, retinoic acid derivatives, or psoralen plus ultraviolet light (PUVA) should be considered which are effective for both skin and joint affections. DMARDs such as sulfasalazine, MTX, and cyclosporine are also commonly used for patients with PsA but the effects are modest. Strong evidence has emerged supporting the use of anti-TNF-α agents for the treatment of PsA and biological agents might be considered first-line therapy. Prompt and dramatic resolution of both arthritis and skin lesions has been with etanercept, infliximab, adalimumab, and golimumab. The clinical response is more dramatic than in RA, and delay of radiographic disease progression has been demonstrated. Paradoxically, rare cases have been reported of exacerbation or de novo appearance of psoriasis precipitated by anti-TNF therapy for a variety of conditions, the therapy can be continued despite. Sustained benefits for patients with skin and joint disease were seen at 1 year in a trial using infliximab. Etanercept was also found to reduce joint symptoms, improve psoriatic lesions, and inhibit radiographic progression of disease at 1 year. Adalimumab showed similar efficacy with significantly improved joint and skin manifestations and a reduction in irreversible structural damage on radiographs. The anti-T-cell biologic agent alefacept, in combination with MTX, has shown benefit in both PsA and psoriasis. Therapeutic agents targeting the IL-23/IL-17 axis have been proven to be very effective in PsA. The available agents include anti-IL-12/IL-23 p40 (ustekinumab, briankizumab), anti-IL-23p19 (guselkumab, tildrakizumab, risankizumab, brazikumab, and mirikizumab), anti-IL-17A (secukinumab and ixekizumab), dual anti-IL-17A and anti-IL-17F (bimekizumab), or anti-IL-17 receptor (brodalumab) monoclonal antibodies. Different agents are available in different countries with specific approval like brodalumab is approved for PsA in Japan but in other countries only for plaque psoriasis, so one needs to refer to country specific pharmacopoeia for availability and approvals. Janus tyrosine kinase (JAK) inhibitors also directly affect IL-23 and, thus, IL-17. Not only the first-generation pan-JAK inhibitors like tofacitinib, and baricitinib but also the newer-generation selective JAK inhibitors like filgotinib and upadacitinib have been studied and discretely approved for treatment of psoriasis and PsA. The surgical treatment is aimed to restore painless mobility of joints, though results are inferior to other groups. Patients with PsA may have skin involvement in the area of the proposed surgical incision. Because local bacterial contamination may increase the risk of infection, it is recommended that the skin be treated aggressively with topical agents or ultraviolet light before any surgical procedure.

ENTEROPATHIC ARTHRITIS (EnA), REACTIVE ARTHRITIS (ReA), AND UNDIFFERENTIATED AND JUVENILE-ONSET SPONDYLOARTHROPATHY

Enteropathic arthritis is the spondyloarthropathy associated with ulcerative colitis (UC) and Crohn's disease (CD). Both ankylosing spondylitis and peripheral arthritis are associated with UC and CD. HLA-B27 is found in up to 70% of patients with IBD and ankylosing spondylitis, but in ≤15% of patients with IBD and peripheral arthritis. This spondyloarthropathy follows a pattern similar to ankylosing spondylitis and runs independently of bowel disease. The spectrum of peripheral arthritis includes acute self-limited attacks of oligoarthritis that often coincide with relapses of IBD, and more chronic and symmetric polyarticular arthritis that runs a course independent of IBD activity. Characteristically, the spinal disease of these individuals progresses independent of activity of bowel lesions. The patients with ankylosing spondylitis and IBD have 30–70% positivity for HLA-B27 while >95% patients of only ankylosing spondylitis are positive for HLA-B27. So, definite or probable ankylosing spondylitis in a B27-negative individual in the absence of psoriasis should prompt a search for occult IBD. Patients with enteropathic arthritis have good responses to the TNF-α inhibitors, infliximab, and adalimumab. Infliximab has been shown to be effective in fistulizing CD.

Reactive arthritis (ReA) is an acute nonpurulent arthritis complicating an infection elsewhere in the body. The term is used primarily to refer to SpA following enteric or urogenital infections. ReA appears to be a clinical syndrome with typical axial disease triggered by specific etiologic agents in a genetically susceptible host (possibly HLA-B27 positive host). The trigger most commonly is an infectious agent such as bowel infection from *Salmonella, Shigella, Yersinia, and Campylobacter* species, by genital infection (sexually transmitted) with *Chlamydia trachomatis*; and by other agents as well [*Salmonella* spp., *Clostridium difficile*, certain toxigenic *E. coli*, even following intravesicular bacillus Calmette-Guérin (BCG) treatment for bladder cancer]. Role of HLA-B27 is not completely understood as the prevalence of B27 in ReA has often been below 50%, and in some instances not elevated at all but HLA-B27-positive patients have shown a worse outcome than B27-negative patients. The organisms well established to be triggers produce lipopolysaccharide (LPS) and share a capacity to attack mucosal surfaces, to invade host cells, and to survive intracellularly. Localization of specific histopathological characteristics has been seen in intestines in postenteric ReA and keratoderma blenorrhagica (skin lesions indistinguishable from psoriasis) associated mainly with venereally acquired ReA. Clinically, the disease has spectrum ranging from isolated, transient monarthritis or enthesitis to severe multisystem disease. Typical features of ReA include asymmetric lower limb oligoarthritis, conjunctivitis, and dysuria. Arthritis typically persists 3–5 months, but courses up to 1 year can occur. Chronic heel pain is often particularly distressing. Low-back pain, sacroiliitis, and frank ankylosing spondylitis are also common sequelae. The dysuria can be either caused by a *Chlamydia* pyuria or by a sterile pyuria that can be triggered by a bowel infection. Approximately 20% of patients with inflammatory bowel disease will develop an inflammatory arthritis with axial and/or peripheral joint involvement. The peripheral joint inflammation often can flare with bowel disease activity, whereas the axial inflammation does not flare in conjunction with the inflammatory bowel disease. Disease patterns mirror those associated with PsA. Indomethacin 75–150 mg is the initial agent of choice. Role of antibiotics to control the inciting infection is logically employed but clinical benefit in ReA is undefined. Therapy used for PsA may be just as effective for reactive arthritis. Anti-TNF-α agents have not been largely studied for ReA but anecdotal reports suggest lack of response. MTX (15–20 mg/week), sulfasalazine (3 g/day), and azathioprine (1–2 mg/kg/day) are the usual agents prescribed.

Patients with *undifferentiated spondyloarthropathy* do not have an adequate number of symptoms or signs to designate them to a specific form. Approximately one-half of the patients with undifferentiated SpA are HLA-B27-positive, and thus the absence of B27 is not useful in establishing or excluding the diagnosis. In familial cases, which are much more frequently B27-positive, there is often eventual progression to classical ankylosing spondylitis.

Juvenile-onset spondyloarthropathy usually begins between 7 and 16 years of age and commonly affects boys. They have asymmetric, lower extremity oligoarthritis and enthesitis without extra-articular features and have been termed seronegative enthesopathy and arthropathy (SEA) syndrome. HLA-B27 is positive in 80% of these individuals and many of them develop ankylosing spondylitis in late adolescence or adulthood. Patients with undifferentiated arthropathy are treated as symptoms dictate until a specific diagnosis is identified. Prolonged treatment with doxycycline has shown some response but there is no concrete evidence.

NEUROPATHIC ARTHROPATHY [CHARCOT'S JOINTS, CHARCOT'S ARTHROPATHY (CA), CHARCOT'S NEUROARTHROPATHY]

Neuropathic arthritis is an extreme form of post-traumatic osteoarthritis. It is a progressive condition of the musculoskeletal system that is characterized by continued bony destruction of a weight bearing joint, joint dislocations, pathologic fractures, and debilitating deformities. It was first reported in 1831 by the American physician John Kearsley Mitchell (tuberculosis induced spinal damage) and more specifically later as denervation-induced joint destruction (as a complication of tertiary syphilis) by Jean-Martin Charcot (French neurologist) in 1868.

Etiology

Diabetes is the most common disorder in modern world etiologically related to development of neuropathic arthropathy. This almost always involves foot; midfoot and ankle are the most commonly affected joints. Involvement of knee, hip, spine, and wrist has also been reported. Type 1 diabetes patients tend to develop the disease at earlier age. The primary disease is usually present for 10–12 years before the onset of Charcot's arthropathy which develops in around 2–8% of diabetics.

Another very common cause for development of Charcot's joint is the Charcot-Marie-Tooth (CMT) disease. It is a hereditary motor and sensory neuropathy (HMSN) that is transmitted most often as an autosomal dominant trait and is characterized by progressive distal wasting and loss of reflexes in the muscles of the legs (and occasionally involving the arms). Onset of CMT is usually in the second to fourth decade of life. This condition has been divided into two subtypes, HMSN Types I and II. HMSN I is also associated with abnormal nerve conduction velocities and nerve hypertrophy, features not seen in HMSN II. Other causes of neuropathic arthropathy include:

- Syringomyelia (in the shoulder)
- Amyloid
- Alcoholic neuropathies
- Leprosy
- Neurosyphilis (in the knee)
- Congenital insensitivity to pain
- Charcot-Marie-Tooth syndrome
- Renal dialysis
- Sensory and autonomic neuropathy
- Spinal cord injury
- Cerebral palsy
- Intra-articular steroid injections
- Traumatic denervation of a limb—spinal cord or peripheral nerve injury

Pathogenesis

Neuropathy and inflammation are the key elements in development of disease. In neuropathic arthropathy, the involved joints lack proprioception and deep sensation. As a result, joint movement is not inhibited and tends to cause unintentional repetitive minor trauma. Ultimately, this constant trauma causes repetitive fracture and fragmentation of the joint and eventually biomechanical instability and severe osteoarthritis. Some theories have been proposed:

Neurotraumatic theory (accumulation of microtrauma in insensate limb): The arthropathy results probably from unperceived trauma (microtrauma) to an insensate limb. Secondary neuropathy renders patient insensate to osseous destruction that occurs with ambulation. The microtrauma accumulates to cause progressive destruction of foot.

"French concept" (Charcot): Damage to central nervous system centers that control the bone and joint nutrition are primarily implicated in joint degeneration.

"German concept" (Volkmann and Virchow): Suggested multiple subclinical trauma in the denervated joint as the precipitating factor.

Neurovascular theory: The underlying condition leads to development of autonomic neuropathy, causing the extremity to receive an increased blood flow. There is mismatch between bone destruction and synthesis leading to osteopenia.

A combination of above mechanisms is possibly present in all **(Fig. 34)**. It is now postulated that minor trauma can stimulate and propagate inflammatory cascade in complex ways although the precipitating event is not clear in majority. There is abnormal joint loading that is disproportionate to pain perception and bones are osteopenic in most disorders. Also neuropathy impairs healing after incidental injury. The resident osteoclasts probably have abnormal reactivity to IL-1, 6 and TNF-α leading to increased expression of NF-$\kappa\beta$ ligand. The increased production of RANKL and TNF-α is mutually enhancing establishing vicious cycle. There could be decreased production of osteoprotegerin that acts as decoy receptor and effectively controls bone loss. The RANKL-NF-κB pathway is implicated in the etiopathogenesis of arterial wall smooth muscle calcification. Monckenberg sclerosis (vascular calcification) is prominently seen in Charcot's joints. In the absence of neuropathy, pain-induced joint immobilization halts the above inflammatory osteolytic process by reducing local blood flow. Baseline blood flow is increased in neuropathic feet as a result of a reduced peripheral vascular resistance and sympathetic denervation, but does not increase in response to warming. Charcot feet retain the capacity to increase vascular flow further, exacerbating the inflammatory process. So immobilization may not halt the destructive process effectively.

Surgical pathology: Pathological findings in neuropathic arthropathy include severe degeneration and fragmentation of the joint surfaces with extensive dendritic synovitis, resulting from particles of bone and cartilage embedded in the synovium.

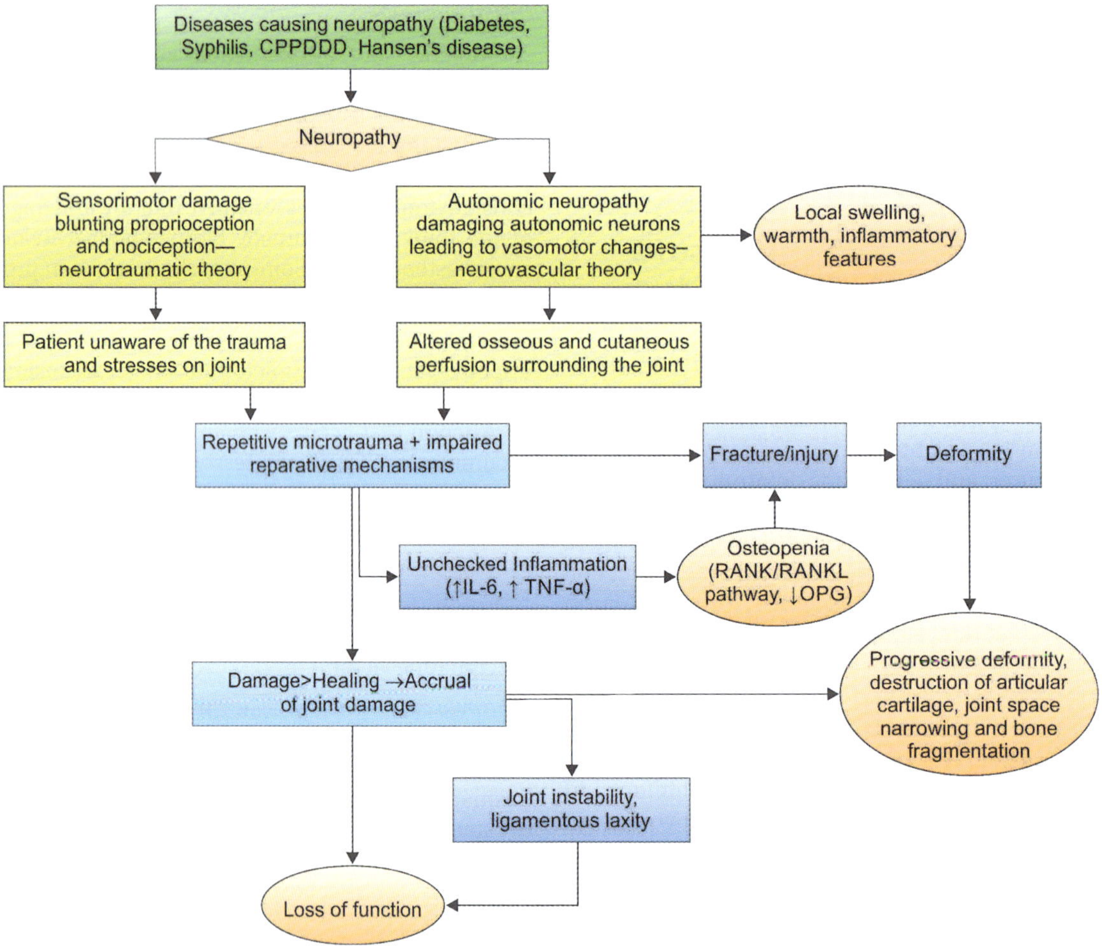

Fig. 34: Pathogenesis of Charcot's arthropathy. (CPPDDD: calcium pyrophosphate dihydrate crystal deposition disease; IL: interleukin; OPG: osteoprotegerin; RANKL: receptor activator of nuclear factor κ-B ligand; TNF: tumor necrosis factor)

Clinical Presentation

Individuals have varied presentations, the onset is usually insidious.

Acute presentation is a common diagnostic dilemma and can present like septic arthritis.

- These individuals almost always present with signs of inflammation.
- Profound unilateral swelling, an increase in local skin temperature (generally, an increase of 3–7° above the unaffected foot's skin temperature), erythema, joint effusion, and bone resorption in an insensate foot are present. These characteristics, in the presence of intact skin and a loss of protective sensation, are often pathognomonic of acute Charcot arthropathy.
- Painless swollen lax and deformed joint is a misconception as pain is present in >75% of patients; however, pain severity is significantly less than expected.
- The joint may reveal erythema, edema, "loose bag of bones" kind of appearance.
- Significant number of patients (40%) has skin ulceration complicating diagnosis to osteomyelitis as primary pathology which is actually incorrect. Bone and synovial biopsy may settle the confusion.

TABLE 23: The staging of Charcot's arthropathy.

Stage	*Description*	*Radiology*	*Clinical presentation*
0	Inflammation	• Radiographs are normal • Bone scan positive for inflammatory features	Edema, erythematous joint and surrounding region
I	Acute presentation	• Joint subluxation/dislocation • Beginning of bony erosions, fragmentation	Features of autonomic neuropathy, swollen and erythematic foot and joints, brawny edema
II	Coalescence (Hypertrophic/subacute phase of Charcot)	Coalesced fragments, Callus formation, bone sclerosis and absorption of bone fragments	Reduced inflammation and edema
III	Phase or consolidation and remodeling	Osseous remodeling, healing, and new bone formation	No features of inflammation but joint deformities persist

Natural History and Staging

It is a progressive disorder and if left untreated can lead to loss of function, even amputation and death. Classically, Eichenholtz described four stages **(Table 23)** of disease progression (stages 2 and 3 are regarded as chronic/ Quiescent stages); however, superinfection modifies the findings in most if not all:

Investigations

- Full blood count (helps distinguish from osteomyelitis), urine examination, creatinine, LFTs, calcium, vitamin B_{12}, folate, VDRL, glucose and glycosylated hemoglobin (HbA1c).
- Joint aspiration may be necessary to exclude septic arthritis.
- MRI can help to distinguish between soft-tissue infection and osteomyelitis

Differential diagnosis: Septic arthritis, osteomyelitis, diabetic foot, leprosy foot, advanced osteoarthritis, monoarticular RA, and crystal deposition disease.

Radiology: The radiographic hallmark of neuropathic arthritis is one of "osteoarthritis with a vengeance". Predominantly there are two types of presentations—the "atrophic form" and "hypertrophic form". In the latter not only will affected joints show narrowing, sclerosis, and osteophytes but they will also show these with such exuberance that the appearance is markedly of marked increased (Yochum and Rowe's 6 "D", **Figs. 35A and B**):

- Density about the joint
- Disorganization of the joint structures
- Debris surrounding and within the joint
- Destruction of the joint surfaces
- Dislocation of the joint
- Distended joint

This collection of "D" word descriptors should bring the diagnosis to mind. Thus, the viewer must be vigilant to make the diagnosis, especially since neuropathic arthritis may have a wide range from the purely productive arthropathy to one that resembles an aggressively destructive process. The atrophic form is less common and has typical radiological appearance of:

- "Licked candy stick" appearance of distal aspect of bones
- Osteopenia
- Osteolysis

Magnetic resonance imaging is not very useful and early images are nonspecific for Charcot's arthropathy (CA) and can be seen in reflex sympathetic dystrophy (RSD), osteomyelitis, etc. There is a significant signal intensity overlap for infection and edema. The greater the signal from marrow in T2-weighted images the more likely the bone is infected. Gadolinium enhancement does not differentiate infection from edema. MRI can be of use possibly in preoperative assessment and monitoring disease progression. PET scan may be better in patients with metallic implants and has been shown to differentiate infection from CA. Bone scan is a sensitive but nonspecific investigation. Three-phase bone scan is positive in all three phases. A four-phase bone scan (taken at 24 hours) can depict woven bone but cannot differentiate CA from fractures, tumors, advanced degeneration. ^{333}In-labelled scan complemented alongside with Tc-nanocolloid marrow scanning can indicate absence of infection if the scan reports are congruent.

Treatment

Charcot's arthropathy should be dealt with as medical emergency to prevent devastating and irreversible consequences. Usually, the surgical measures fail and were cautiously forbidden in many patients, traditionally.

- Upon diagnosis immobilization in total contact casts or brace [Charcot resistant orthotic walker (CROW)] helps to prevent accelerated joint destruction. Patellar tendon-bearing brace is used to transfer weight bearing forces from the orthosis through the patellar tendon, thereby decreasing weight bearing forces through the foot and ankle.
- Joint edema and swelling may take 6–9 months to subside. Average healing times vary from 55 to 97 days depending on location. Up to 1–2 years may be required for complete healing.
- Bisphosphonates have been used in a few patients particularly the injectable ones for possible role of osteoclasts in bone destruction. Though not approved the response to therapy is moderately acceptable with reduction in alkaline phosphatase levels and local temperature accompanied with clinical improvement.
- Calcitonin has also shown improvement (faster healing) in sporadic studies with calcium supplementation.
- Future therapies pointing and attacking the RANKL-TNF-α pathway may provide targeted pharmacotherapy. The role of low intensity ultrasound is controversial.

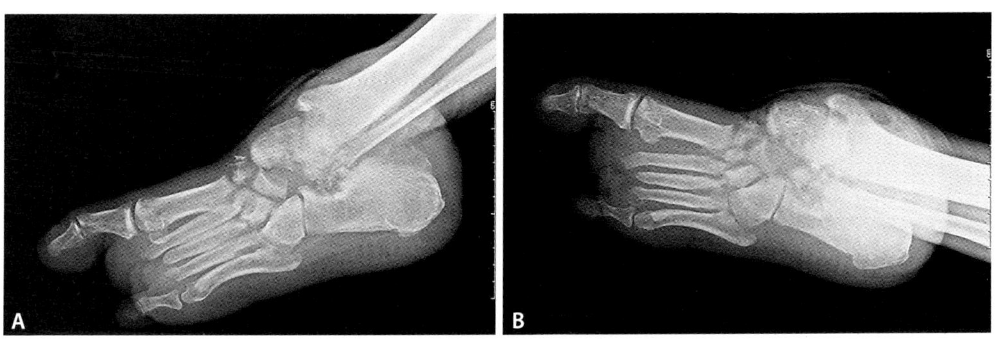

Figs. 35A and B: Charcot's arthropathy: The patient is a known diabetic with multiple surgeries already performed on foot, having lost central three toes. The ankle and subtalar joints are disorganized and dislocated with cystic and sclerotic changes in the bone.

- Surgery is warranted in less than one-fourth of patients and is predominantly preventive. Surgery is specifically contraindicated in active inflammation. It is indicated:
  - If the joint of limb is at extreme risk of ulceration or due to deformity and destruction cannot be placed in accommodative brace or footwear.
  - For malaligned, unstable, or nonreducible fractures or dislocations, as well as for cases in which nonsurgical means fail.

Commonly for foot the aim of surgery is to achieve a stable, plantigrade foot that can be accommodated in protective footwear. Most common techniques employed are:

- Exostectomies
- Reconstruction and tendo achilles lengthening
- Reorientation or stabilization arthrodesis of the joints
- Midtarsus closing wedge osteotomy
- In extremely rare cases has arthroplasty (constrained) been attempted with mixed results and highly selective patient evaluation is required. Revision implants or rotating hinged prosthesis are often required and for preoperative subluxated or dislocated knees cast immobilization for 6 months postoperatively is recommended. Reconstructive surgeries should be attempted only in stage 3 Eichenholtz. The reported benefits of arthroplasty include pain relief, realignment of limb, and functional improvement. Complications include but are not limited to periprosthetic fractures, dislocations, loosening, instability, quadriceps tendon rupture, etc.

SEPTIC ARTHRITIS

INTRODUCTION

Musculoskeletal infections (MSKI) have been reclassified into three-tiered classification system based on severity of infection and degree of dissemination **(Table 24)**. This is done to incorporate infections that involved more than one tissue type and location. The traditional system classified MSKI into superficial abscess, osteomyelitis, septic arthritis, and pyomyositis/deep abscess. The following text deals with septic arthritis and its disabling consequences especially late sequel keeping with the traditional nomenclature of MSKI due to its higher prevalence and common understanding.

Septic arthritis is the pathological microbial invasion of joint space followed by inflammation. Despite the high resistance and isolation of diarthrodial joints, infectious arthritis remains a serious problem. Out of the many pathways for development of septic arthritis **(Box 16)** hematogenous route is the most common facilitated by lack of basement membrane under highly vascular synovium allowing delivery and inoculation of circulating bacteria. It is interesting to note that the transepiphyseal vessels are patent in *children <18 months* and septic arthritis can result by metaphyseal extension of the infective focus. The vessels *again open-up near puberty* to allow free communication predisposing to infection again. The large joints are affected more commonly (hip, shoulder, knee, elbow, and ankle) than the small joints, and monoarticular infection is the rule with polyarticular infection seen in <20% of cases. Some patients are at increased risk for infection **(Box 17)**. The incidence of septic arthritis in the general population is around 2–10 cases per 100,000 but may be as high as 30–70 cases per 100,000 in patients with rheumatoid arthritis. The joint infections are curable in many with the currently available wide range of potent antibiotics and surgical measures but prognosis is poor in patients with underlying RA, the elderly, and patients with multiple comorbidities and those with prosthetic joints. Besides direct involvement of the joint by a pathogen, arthritis may occur by an immune response to a

TABLE 24: Infection severity classification of musculoskeletal infections.

Category	*Definition*	*Example*
Inflammation	All of the following should be true: • Negative blood culture • Negative local culture • The criteria of local or disseminated infection are not met.	• Transient synovitis • Post-streptococcal reactive arthritis
Local infection	One of the following must be true: • Osteomyelitis or pyomyositis in one anatomic site • Local culture positive and/or fluid/tissue consistent with infection • One positive blood culture • The criteria for disseminated infection are not met.	• Brodie's abscess, Garre's osteomyelitis • Isolated osteomyelitis without soft-tissue extension • Isolated septic arthritis
Disseminated infection	Two or more anatomic sites at least one of the following must be true: • Imaging diagnostic for osteomyelitis or pyomyositis • Local culture positive and/or fluid/tissue consistent with infection • Two or more positive blood cultures • Thromboembolic disease	• Septic hip with surrounding muscle pyomyositis • Osteomyelitis with subperiosteal abscess and extension into soft tissue

BOX 16: Potential mechanism of inoculation in patients of septic arthritis.

- Hematogenous (most common, overwhelming infection primary to some other system of the body or in immunocompromised patients)
- *Direct inoculation:*
  - Arthrocentesis
  - Intra-articular injections
  - Animal or human bite
  - Trauma
  - Thorn injury
- Contiguous spread in joints with intra-articular epiphysis (proximal femur, radial head, proximal humerus, and distal fibula)
  - Infants
  - Cellulitis or from septic bursitis
- *Combined:* Joint arthroplasty, tissue allografts

BOX 17: Risk factors for development of septic arthritis.

- Age >80 years
- Diabetes mellitus, rheumatoid arthritis, and gout
- Presence of prosthetic joint (particularly knee and hip)
- Recent joint surgery
- Skin infection
- Sickle-cell disease
- End-stage renal disease
- Advanced hepatic disease
- HIV infection
- Previous septic arthritis
- Intra-articular injection
- Intravenous drug abusers
- Hemophilia with or without AIDS
- Underlying malignancy
- Hypogammaglobulinemia (for mycoplasma infection)
- Late complement-component deficiency (for *Neisseria* infection)

(AIDS: acquired immunodeficiency syndrome)

pathogen causing a reactive arthritis as is seen in chlamydial (Reiters syndrome), some enteric, and sometimes with treponemal and fungal systemic infections. These immune forms of arthritis, however, are excluded from discussion of infectious arthritis here. Prevention is still the best treatment available and with increasing understanding of pathogenesis and biology of periprosthetic infection (probably the most difficult to treat) innovative management is bound to emerge shortly.

Pathophysiology

The basic inflammatory process is marked by synovitis and inflammatory cell infiltrate. The associated exudate may be purulent, serous, or fibrinous depending on infectious agent and reaction. Pyoarthrosis is extremely resistant to antibiotic therapy and requires surgical drainage or repeat arthrocentesis—often emergently. With delayed or inadequate treatment fibrinous adhesions/fibrous ankylosis, articular erosion by pannus (chondrolysis), destruction of the stabilizing ligaments is commonly found sequel. Depending on the degree of erosion of cartilage, the affected joint may develop fibrous or bony ankylosis (erosion to subchondral bone). Chondrolysis is a significant feature of bacterial, mycobacterial, and fungal arthritis but the chronicity of infection and development of intervening pannus in mycobacterial and fungal arthritis leads to development of fibrous ankylosis. The inflammatory cytokines IL-1 and TNF-α, metalloproteinases in concert with granulocytic hydrolytic enzymes, bacterial endotoxins, direct bacterial invasion of synovium, increased intra-articular pressure, and tissue ischemia are responsible for destruction of the articular cartilage. The late sequel of septic arthritis depends on extent of joint damage incurred.

Microbiology

Acute bacterial arthritis is most commonly monoarticular. Polyarticular infection is uncommon (seen in 5–8% of pediatric cases and 10–19% of adult nongonococcal cases). The causative organisms are different for individual forms **(Table 25)**. Acute bacterial arthritis is usually designated gonococcal or nongonococcal. Gonococcal arthritis is a common cause of acute monoarthritis in sexually active young adults typically females (three times as common). In the preantibiotic era, gonococcal arthritis was particularly common in neonates. Gonococcal joint disease has typically two forms. The first (disseminated gonococcal infection, systemic presentation) is characterized by fever, chills, vesiculopustular skin lesions, tenosynovitis, and polyarthralgias. Blood cultures are frequently positive, whereas synovial fluid cultures are rarely positive. *N. gonorrhoeae* can be cultured from genital, rectal, and pharyngeal sites. Tenosynovitis of multiple tendons of the wrist, fingers, and toes is quite characteristic of gonococcal infection and is not seen in other forms of infectious arthritis. In the other form of gonococcal infection, patients have purulent arthritis, most commonly of the knee, wrist or ankle, and more than one joint can be infected simultaneously. *N. gonorrhoeae* can frequently be cultured from the synovial fluid. The classic presentation of nongonococcal septic arthritis is the acute onset of pain and swelling in a single joint. Large joints are affected most commonly. In adults, the knee is involved in >50% of cases, and hip, ankle, and shoulder infections are less common. In infants and small children, hips are more often involved. The type of organism and pattern of joint involvement often depend on the age

TABLE 25: Causative organisms and differentials for various forms of septic arthritis.

Acute monoarticular	*Chronic monoarticular*	*Polyarticular arthritis*
• *Staphylococcus aureus* • *Streptococcus pneumoniae* β-Hemolytic streptococci (adults—mainly groups A, G and B, group A—children ≥5 years, group B—neonates) • *Enterobacteriaceae* (≥60 years or predisposed patients) • *Salmonella spp* (sickle cell disease) • *N. gonorrhoeae* • *Candida* spp. • Coagulase negative staphylococci (prosthetic joint infection)	• *M. tuberculosis* • Nontuberculous mycobacteria • *Borrelia burgdorferi* • *Treponema pallidum* • *Candida* spp. • Fungal arthritis	• *N. meningitides* • *N. gonorrhoeae (sexually active young adults and adolescents)* Nongonococcal bacterial arthritis • Bacterial endocarditis • *Candida* spp. • Hepatitis B virus • Other viral arthritides
Differential diagnosis: • Crystal-induced arthritis (acute flare) • Hemophilic arthritis • Osteoarthritis (acute exacerbation) • Monoarticular RA	*Differential diagnosis:* • Legg-Calvé-Perthes disease • Osteonecrosis • Chronic ligament injuries • Femoro-acetabular impingement • Osteoarthritis	*Differential diagnosis:* • Poncet's rheumatism • Sickle-cell disease flare • Reactive arthritis • Inflammatory bowel disease • Serum sickness • Acute rheumatic fever • SLE • RA

(RA: rheumatoid arthritis; SLE: systemic lupus erythematosus)

(the elderly are at greater risk) of the patient, pre-existing arthropathy, immune status, and habits, particularly intravenous drug abuse **(Table 25)**.

Most septic arthritides are monomicrobial infections, but polymicrobial infections may be seen in patients with direct inoculation of the joint space. In general, *S. aureus* is the most common organism isolated among children of all age groups (followed by group A streptococci and *S. pneumoniae*) and adults. Neonates and younger infants (<2 months age) are predisposed to group B streptococcus and gram-negative enteric bacilli infection. Gram-positive cocci around 80%) are the most common organism causing nongonococcal septic arthritis in adults while rest 20% are caused by gram-negative bacilli. Following staphylococci, streptococci are the next most common organisms (group A, B, G, C, and F in that frequency). Group A streptococcal infections usually occur in immunocompromised while group B streptococcal arthritis is encountered commonly in diabetics and late periprosthetic infections. Gram-negative bacilli infection (*E. coli* and *Pseudomonas*) occur in IV drug abusers, immunocompromised and elderly group. Some uncommon organisms are encountered in special situations like candida and *Pseudomonas* spp. in IV drug abusers, *Salmonella* arthritis in patients with sickle cell anemia, and immunocompromised children are at higher risk for infection with gram-negative bacilli. Anaerobic infections occur in grossly contaminated wounds, joint arthroplasty and immunocompromised adults. *Staphylococcus epidermidis* [coagulase negative *Staphylococcus* (CoNS)] is common in prosthetic joint infections (PJIs). Polyarticular infections occur in imunocompromised, IV drug absures and staphylococci are the commonest organism followed by streptococci group G. Mycobacterial infections should be suspected in patients from endemic areas as in our Indian subcontinent and Africa.

Clinical Features

Hip and shoulder are the most common sites of septic arthritis followed by knee and other joints. The clinical course can be prolonged with staphylococcal arthritis being the most destructive. Most patients with bacterial arthritis are febrile, although chills are unusual. Fever may be absent in the elderly. In children, septic arthritis is usually accompanied by fever, malaise, poor appetite, and irritability, as well as progressive reluctance to use the affected limb. Physical examination typically reveals warmth and tenderness of the affected joint, joint effusion (swollen joint), and limited active and passive range of motion. Painful limitation of joint ROM with swollen joint and high-grade fever with rigors is so characteristic that some physicians label this as diagnostic triad along with elevated ESR for septic arthritis unless proved otherwise. However, individually none of these is highly sensitive or specific for septic arthritis. It has been reported that only 40–60% of patients with septic arthritis may be febrile, only 25–60% had an elevated leukocyte count, and only 60–80% had an erythrocyte sedimentation rate > 50 mm/h.

Septic arthritis manifests as polyarticular arthritis in about 15% of patients especially in patients with prior joint damage, as in rheumatoid arthritis, gout, and systemic connective tissue disorders. Septic arthritis among patients with RA has been a special challenge to clinicians because of the high incidence of infection and the poor outcome. It is well recognized that septic arthritis in patients with RA is associated with poor joint outcome and mortality as high as 56% in those with polyarticular infection. One should take additional pertinent history of immunosuppressive states, intravenous drug abuse, recent steroid injection (as in rheumatoid and other arthritis), history of sexually transmitted disease, and any constitutional symptoms (as for mycobacterial infection).

Imaging

Plain films are nonspecific depicting the effusion and swollen joint **(Figs. 36A and B)** with periarticular osteopenia. Periosteal reaction appear late (after 3–4 weeks as bony reaction is not as prominent as in osteomyelitis), even later joint space reduction can be seen. The characteristic

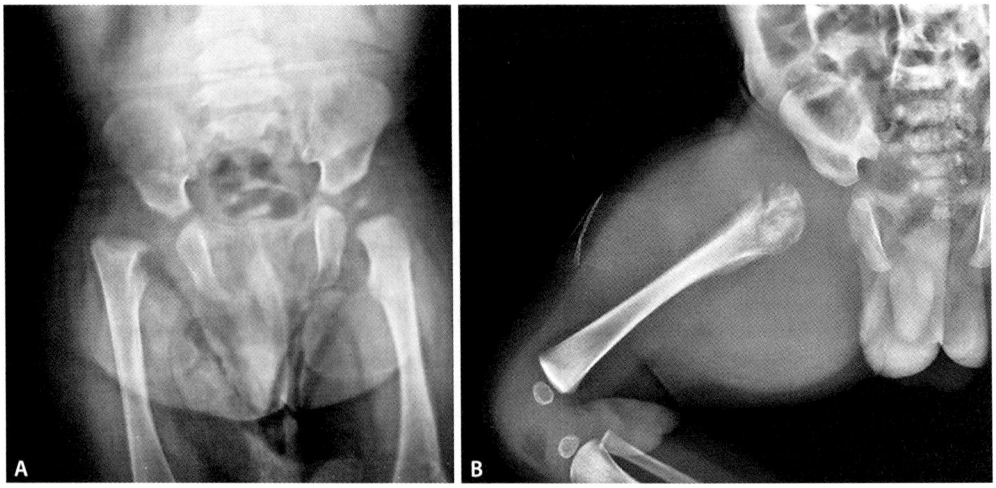

Figs. 36A and B: Septic arthritis: (A) The right hip of this 4-month-old child shows increased joint space and subluxation; (B) 2 months after incision and drainage the proximal physis seems to be missing possibly damaged by the infective process and healing changes appear in the bone.

radiographic feature of septic arthritis is the loss of the white cortical line over a long contiguous segment that differentiates it from inflammatory arthritis that demonstrates segmental disruption. Bacterial septic arthritis often results in rapid joint space loss, with aggressive erosive changes. Ultrasound is helpful to detect effusion and pus in joint with synovial thickening and differentiate from bursitis and cellulitis by identifying the plane of collection. Bone scan demonstrate increased uptake both in early and "blood pool" images at periarticular region, it is particularly the frequent modality used to identify periprosthetic infection in incipient cases. Loosening of endoprosthetic components can occur from a variety of causes (infection, metal reaction, rejection, wear reaction, etc.) and appears late in the course. Separating infection from all the other noninfectious causes is important, since the foreign material acts as a nidus for infection and perpetuates it in a vicious cycle. MRI is sensitive to detect joint effusion however of limited use as it offers no better advantage over clinical judgement. In tuberculous arthritis at axial locations it is the modality of choice.

Diagnosis

The diagnosis is done by a combination of clinical presentation and smear and culture evaluation of synovial fluid (*see* Chapter on "Joints of Skeleton, Synovial Joint Structure and Function"). However, synovial fluid may not always offer a diagnosis especially in partially treated patients. PJIs may be acute (pyogenic and enteric bacteria) or chronic (coagulase negative staphylococci, streptococci or diphtheroids, etc.). The diagnosis in such cases can be difficult, and requires clinical, laboratory and radiological input (*see* prosthetic joint infection later). Ultrasonography is a good tool to identify joint effusion but it fails to differentiate infective from noninfective effusion. It can be more importantly utilized to guide the position of needle during aspiration.

Differential Diagnosis

Acute osteomyelitis, cellulitis, toxic synovitis of hip, reactive arthritis, hemarthrosis, juvenile RA, trauma, malignancy, etc.

Treatment

Objectively assessing the severity of illness **(Table 26)** helps in guiding the antibiotic selection **(Table 27)**. The severity of illness (SOI) score varies from 0 to 10. Patients with mild illness (SOI of 0–2) are unlikely to receive surgery while those with severe illness (SOI of 7–10) will likely require one or more surgical procedure to help resolve infection.

For nongonococcal arthritis, based on aspiration of fluid and Gram stain report empirical antibiotics are started **(Table 27)**; usually the bactericidal agents are used. Direct joint instillation into joint is unnecessary. For negative smears a third generation IV antibiotic is sufficient while IV vancomycin is the choice for gram-positive cocci. In addition, an aminoglycoside should be added for unusual patients (IV drug abusers or suspected *Pseudomonas* infection). Following identification on culture specific drug therapy is started based on the organism and sensitivity

TABLE 26: Severity of illness (SOI) scoring for objective assessment of clinical burden of infection.

Parameter	*Point value*
Initial CRP level (mg/dL)	
<10	0
10–15	1
>15	2
CRP level (mg/dL) 48 hours after presentation	
<5	0
5–10	1
>10	2
CRP level (mg/dL) 96 hours after presentation	
<5	0
5–10	1
>10	2
Band count (cells/μL)	
<1.5	0
≥1.5	1
Febrile days on antibiotic	
<2	0
≥2	1
ICU admission	
No	0
Yes	1
Disseminated musculoskeletal infection	
No	0
Yes	1

pattern. Drainage of pus and necrotic debris (open or arthroscopic) should be done at the initial identification and demonstration of pus by aspiration to prevent joint and cartilage damage. Septic arthritis of hip is best managed with arthrotomy while knee can be adequately dealt with arthroscopy. If clinical and laboratory improvement is not evident in 72–96 hours then repeat surgical debridement and irrigation should be done. Patient with severe illness (SOI of 7–10) at initial presentation is more likely to have osteonecrosis, chondrolysis or bony deformity at 2 years follow-up. High SOI score in patients aged <3 years and MRSA infection predict a severe outcome. These patients should be closely followed up for long duration every 6 months. Joint mobilization and weight bearing should be encouraged early based on pain tolerance following surgical management. Gonococcal arthritis is best managed with intravenous ceftriaxone followed by oral fluroquinolone when symptoms start resolving. For disseminated gonococcal infection treatment should be treated for *Chlamydia trachomatis* infection unless appropriately excluded.

SEPTIC ARTHRITIS OF HIP IN CHILDREN AND ITS SEQUEL

Acute septic arthritis of the hip is a more serious disease in children than in adults and severe complications are

TABLE 27: Commonly recommended empirical antibiotics from Gram staining pattern.

Adults		
Gram-negative diplococci	*Neisseria* spp.	Third generation cephalosporin (ceftriaxone) or fluroquinolone
Gram-positive cocci (clusters)	*Staphylococcus aureus* (methicillin—sensitive)	Third generation cephalosporin (ceftriaxone)
	Staphylococcus aureus (methicillin—resistant)	Vancomycin [or clindamycin (if allergic to vancomycin) or linezolid (allergic to both, restrict use being a reserve drug]
Gram-positive cocci (chains)	*Streptococcus* species	Third generation cephalosporin (ceftriaxone)
Gram-negative bacilli	*Enterobacteriaceae (E. coli, Proteus, Serratia)*	• Third generation cephalosporin (ceftazidime, cefepime) or piperacillin + tazobactam. • Aztreonam (if allergic to penicillin group) or fluoroquinolones
	Pseudomonas species	Ceftazidime + aminoglycoside Or Imlpenam + aminoglycoside
Polymicrobial infection	Staphylococci, streptococci, Gram-negative bacilli	Third generation cephalosporin plus vancomycin (or linezolid, if allergic)
Negative Gram stain	?	Vancomycin + ceftazidime or aminoglycoside
Prosthesis related infection	Coagulase negative staphylococci	Third generation cephalosporin + rifampicin

much more common in children. Normally, epiphyseal plate is a barrier to the passage of bacteria therefore in knee joint where capsule is attached to the area of epiphyseal plate; incidence of septic arthritis is less. But, presence of intrasynovial metaphysis in hip predisposes to infection (other joints so predisposed due to intra-articular location of metaphysis include the shoulder—proximal humerus, elbow—proximal radius, ankle—distal fibula). Also until age of 18 months vessels from metaphysic cross the epiphyseal plate to epiphysis. Hence, septic arthritis following osteomyelitis is more common <18 months of age. In children >18 months of age and less than puberty where transepiphyseal vessels are absent, the infection will not cross the epithelial plate. Coagulase positive hemolytic *S. aureus* remains the most common infecting organism (70%) followed by streptococcus, pneumococcus, *H. influenzae*, *E. coli*, and other gram-negative rods. Rare cases due to *Borellia* and *Brucella* also have been reported. The destructive effect of staphylococcal infection on the articular cartilage and the joint was first detailed by Dallas Phemister in 1924.

The *septic arthritis of infancy* is given specific name of "*Tom-Smith's arthritis*" as first detailed description of the pathology was provided by Thomas smith (an English surgeon) in 1874. For many years this term was used to describe in expanded meaning; the typical affection of hip joint in children not only restricted to infants as he originally described. Infants and premature deliveries are more prone to serious after effects of the disease. Tom Smith's arthritis needs special mention as there is often an associated delay in the diagnosis and inadequate treatment is associated with severe crippling deformities and instability of joint (see below). These infants usually present with irritability, failure to feed or gain weight, muscular spasm, dislike of being handled, occasionally toxemic features such as fever, tachycardia, and anemia. The presence of associated infection should be specifically looked for and localization of disease to hip is suspected with subtle changes in the posture of hip, pain on palpation or passive movement of the joint, unilateral edema or swelling of extremity, asymmetrical buttock folds, lack of active movement (pseudoparalysis), and/or swelling of buttocks or genitalia.

Pathophysiology

The three most important factors that lead to destruction of the hip after septic arthritis are:

1. Increased intra-capsular pressure
2. Direct destructive action of pus on the articular cartilage—Collagen content of the cartilage which is otherwise resistant to all other enzyme (except collagenase produced by *Clostridium welchi* and *histolyticum*) undergoes destruction by proteolysis due to denaturation induced by inflammation. Similarly proteolytic enzymes cause removal of chondromucoprotein from matrix leading to complete chondrolysis later but is not associated with radiological changes due to inevident bone formation.
3. Thrombosis of the vessel on both sides of epiphyseal plate may result in ischemia of the plate. Ischemic damage to growth plate by infection can cause permanent damage to the plate. This may cause early closure of plate or in its complete destruction.

Clinical Features

A. Neonatal period and infancy (Tom Smith's arthritis)—the disease is most common in this age group. Classic signs of fever, chills, rigor, sweat, and prostration are not seen in this age group. Hence, disease becomes difficult to diagnose. Following clinical observation can make physician to suspect septicemia especially with septic arthritis of the hip like:
   - Refusal of feed with regurgitation
   - Cyanosis during feeding
   - Abdominal distention
   - Presence of a focus of infection
   - Edema of lower extremities/buttock/genitalia
   - Crying on handling
   - Child not able to use the lower limb actively
   - Abnormal position of femur in flexion adduction
B. Children—child is unwell, febrile, toxic and has intense pain in the affected leg with restriction of all hip joint movements in particular to rotation. There may be tenderness anteriorly in the Scarpa's triangle.

Establishing diagnosis in infants and small children requires a high degree of suspicion with appropriate clinical findings as listed above. A raised PMN leukocyte count and a raised ESR are usually present. CRP is also positive.

Anti-streptococal and antistaphylococcal titers are positive if they are the causative organisms. Blood culture may also yield the infecting organism in 50% cases. Aspiration of the joint is the most valuable test. High protein and low glucose in synovial fluid is suggestive of septic infection. Radiological features in neonates and children include enlargement of the soft tissue shadows around the hip and increase in the distance and acetabulum and the visualized portion of upper end femur, lateral shift of the upper end femur due to pus under tension within the hip joint, periosteal elevation in upper and femur may be seen and residual deformities in serial follow-up.

Differential diagnosis of septic arthritis hip:

1. Transient synovitis—presents with intense pain, limp, restriction of movements at hip. To differentiate skin traction should be applied in which pain due to toxic synovitis significantly improves within 24 hours. All investigations including nuclear scanning are normal except soft tissue swelling or plain radiograph.
2. Hemathrosis—may be due to hemophilia. In such cases history of hemophilia is known and coagulation profile helps in diagnosis.
3. Iliacus syndrome—occurs in known hemophilia patients who present with severe pain, flexion deformity at hip and a mass in iliac fossa. May also have femoral nerve palsy, with bowel dysfunction and sensory loss in front of thigh can be differentiated. Patient has good range of painless movement at the hip.
4. Retroperitoneal abscess—similarity and clinical symptoms of septic arthritis and retroperitoneal abscess like painful limitation of hip joint movement and painful hip and thigh necessitate development of reliable methods for differentiation. In retroperitoneal abscess—full hip flexion can be achieved by gentle passive movement with slightly restricted internal rotation. In septic arthritis, any movement other than that of external rotation, abduction and flexion causes pain. Rectal examination is valuable in differentiation. Visualization of psoas shadow on plain X-ray and an intravenous pyelogram (IVP) is helpful.
5. Appendicitis—may be associated with psoas spasm but has painless hip movements.
6. Rheumatic fever—characteristically has fleeting joint involvement with investigations pointing to rheumatic fever.
7. Osteomyelitis of the pelvis—difficult to diagnose clinically. Nuclear scanning is of great help in differential diagnosis.
8. Certain conditions more commonly seen in adult may mimic septic arthritis hip like gouty arthritis, avascular necrosis of femoral head, RA, tubercular arthritis, and osteoarthritis.

Treatment of Septic Arthritis Hip Joint

If pus is aspirated, hip joint must be promptly drained to prevent femoral head destruction. Delay of even few hours may result in irreparable damage to cartilaginous head and neck of femur. Anterior approach for drainage is preferred in children to avoid damage to vascular supply of head, to reduce chance of postoperative dislocation. Also the land marks for surgical approach are much clearer in small child in this approach. Some form of immobilization is given until infection is controlled. A long period of immobilization is often required because retarded ossification may delay the appearance of femoral head for many months. Child may become ambulatory on defective hip until a reconstruction hip procedure is planned.

Complication of acute septic arthritis of hip:

1. Pathological dislocation—occurs usually in children **(Figs. 36A and B)**. It needs prompt aggressive treatment as under to prevent any further damage:
   a. When soft-tissue contractures have not formed yet—reduction is accomplished at time of drainage.
   b. If femoral head has been damaged by infection, heavy skeletal traction is used to bring femoral head at level of acetabulum and then is reduced by abduction and gentle rotation.
   c. After reduction, it is immobilized in spica until it is stable or until fibrous or bony ankylosis develops. Sometimes, severe osteopenia may obstruct the view of head and may give false notion of complete destruction.
2. In children <12 year infection may result in complete absorption of femoral head or sometimes may be replaced by new bone if vascularity is restored. In older children, it may remain as a sequestrum and in such cases sequestrum should be removed. Sometimes, osteomyelitis of ilium may complicate septic arthritis of hip in children.
3. Pelvic abscess—this abscess complicating acute septic arthritis of hip is secondary to suppurative iliac lymphadenitis. This retroperitoneal abscess should be drained.
4. Persistent infection—rare and characterized by extensive scarring and draining sinuses. Girdle stone described a radical operation for chronic pyogenic infection about hip where infected area above hip is completely saucerized. A mass of surrounding muscle is also resected to assure drainage. But, this is a poor salvage technique because it results in useless pseudoarthrosis/ankylosis with shortening.
5. Ankylosis of hip
6. Osteomyelitis of femur and persistent infection
7. Myositis ossificans
8. Contractures and various deformities primarily flexion and adduction
9. Coxa breva
10. Coxa magna

LATE SEQUEL OF THE SEPTIC ARTHRITIS HIP IN INFANTS

Septic arthritis of hip (pyogenic or tubercular) results in variable destruction of hip and pathological damage ranging from nearly normal hip to destroyed joint and proximal femur. Besides, intra-articular metaphysis, hip has several other anatomical factors that make it susceptible to severe complications after a septic episode. Transepiphyseal vessels until 18 months of age may make communication of bacteria across epiphyseal plate easy. Intra-articular vessels undergo tamponade effect due to collection of pus in the capsule which results in avascular necrosis and chondrolysis. As mentioned previously that severe SOI (score 7–10) in patients aged <3 years infected with virulent strains (like MRSA) have very high chances for development of late sequel. The prognosis of septic hip is also directly proportional to early diagnosis and adequate treatment with arthrotomy and appropriate antibiotics. In absence of these, the treatment is suboptimal and may result in one of several sequel (see below) described for septic arthritis of the hip joint. The residual deformity remains when diagnosis is not established early and proper treatment is not instituted **(Figs. 37A and B)**. A severe infection and/or delay in treatment also produces this unacceptable outcome **(Figs. 38A and B)**. The spectrum of residual deformities has been included in sequel. Disability usually occurs from pain due to incongruous articular surface/pathological dislocation, stiffness during partial/complete ankylosis or abnormal angulation like coxa vara/shortening and instability resulting from bone destruction and/or pathological dislocation. Gait disturbance occurs due to shortening of the involved extremity (subluxation, dislocation, and contracture), pistoning from instability, abductor insufficiency, soft tissue contracture, and joint ankylosis.

Several authors have attempted to classify the sequel and correlated them with treatment options and outcome. Hunka was the first one to suggest a classification system **(Fig. 39)** based on observation of the patients that he treated **(Table 28)**. Choi et al. modified the Hunka's classification and based their classification on the nature and extent of proximal femoral involvement **(Table 29)**. Besides, these Forlin and Milani suggested a simpler classification based on instability and destruction of proximal femur **(Table 30)**. Recently Johari also classified the sequel depending upon stability of hip joint and presence of capital femoral epiphysis.

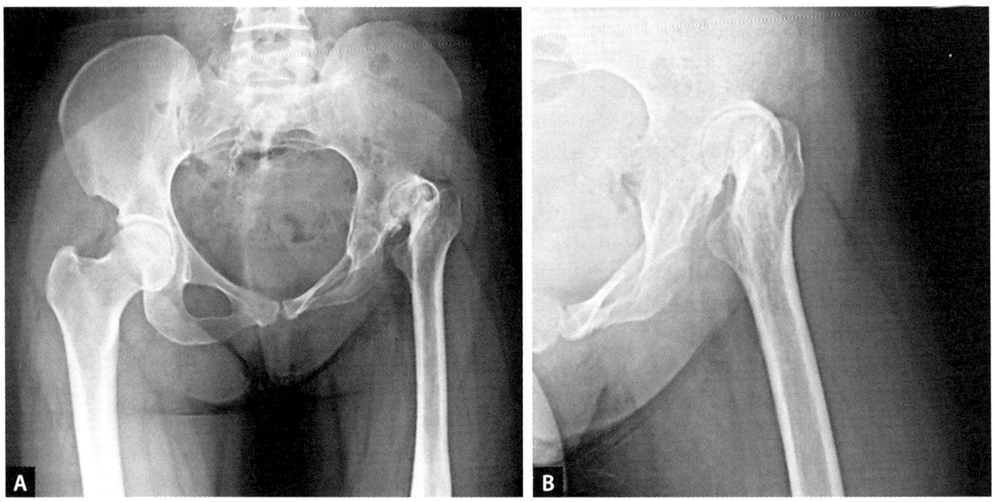

Figs. 37A and B: Sequel of septic arthritis. This is a 23-year-old-female patient who suffered from septic arthritis during infancy but was neglected. The hip possibly got dislocated at that time and a pseudoacetabulum formed over course of time with hypoplasia of the affected extremity and degenerative changes now in the pseudo joint.

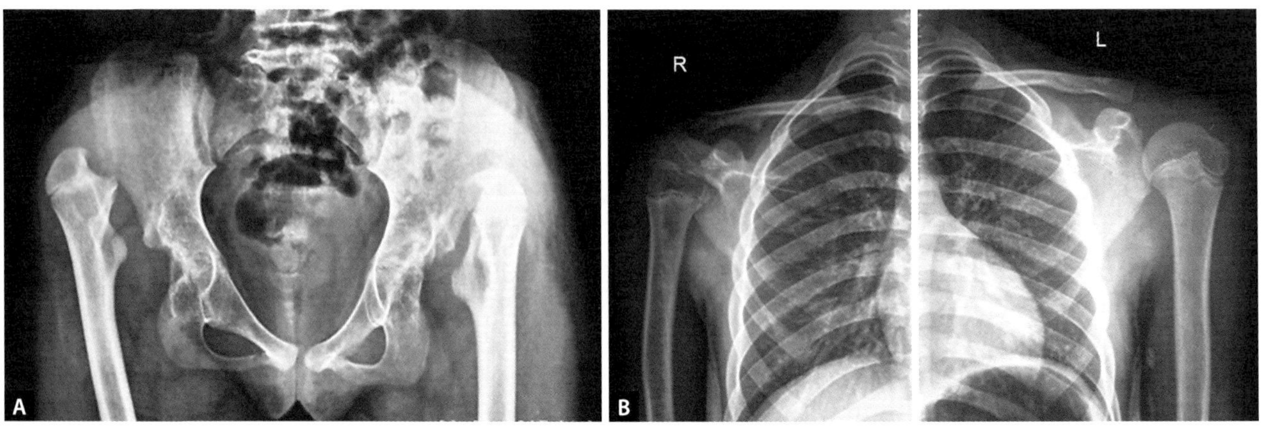

Figs. 38A and B: Hunka type IVB right and type 5 left hip sequel in a patient with multifocal septic arthritis in childhood (A). The patient also had both shoulder sepsis producing deformed right humeral head and absence of left side acromion (B).
Source: Dr Mohinder Singh Chib, Senior Resident, Government Medical College and Hospital, Jammu, Jammu and Kashmir.

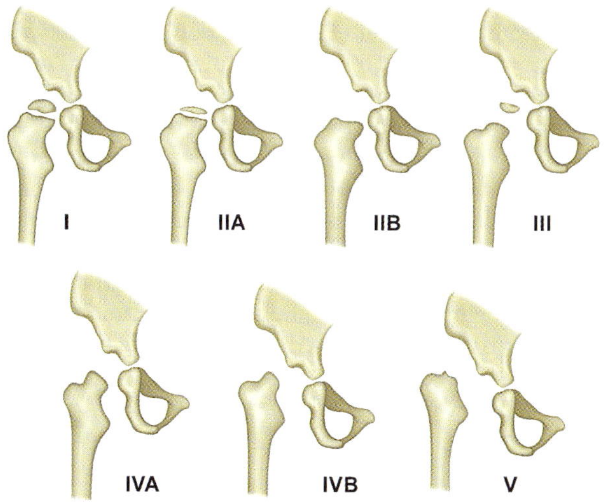

Fig. 39: Hunka classification of sequel of septic arthritis.

TABLE 28: Hunka classification.

Type	*Findings*
I	Minimal or no femoral head changes. The negligible collapse is usually promptly reossified. The course resembles and follows radiologically the pattern of failed Perthes disease.
IIA	Femoral head deformed, but physis intact
IIB	Femoral head deformed, physis fused prematurely so produces deformity of neck as well
III	Femoral neck pseudoarthrosis, the head may or may not be vascular.
IVA	Complete destruction of proximal femoral epiphysis, with a small stable neck segment to maintain articulation
IVB	Complete destruction of proximal femoral epiphysis, with a small neck that fails to maintain stable articulation
V	Complete destruction of head and neck to the inter-trochanteric line with dislocation of the hip

The children with septic sequel of hip generally present with limp, pain, abductor lurch, abnormal hip motion, telescopy, and limb length discrepancy. Degenerative changes set up early in the hip and lumbosacral spine and late reconstruction become difficult. Reconstructive operations to correct bony deformities, however, should be considerably delayed due to following reasons:

1. Danger of reactivating old infection is reduced.
2. Strength and general states of bone improve as necrotic bone is revascularized and abscess cavities are filled.
3. Status of femoral head and proximal femur should be known definitely.

There are various procedures to stabilize/mobilize the affected hip that can be grouped under following categories. In general, the particular procedure used in a patient depends on his age, type of deformity/deficit, residual movements or stability, amount of shortening and previous operations done if any.

A. For loss of movements
   - Soft-tissue release

B. For painful joint degeneration:
   - Interposition/cup arthroplasty—useful in young patients with ankylosed hip

TABLE 29: Choi classification contains four major types and eight subtypes.

Affected region	*Type*	*Disease process*
Proximal femoral Epiphysis and physis	IA (normal radiographic appearance)	Almost normal hip
	IB (early Perthes like osteonecrotic changes)	Mild coxa-magna
Proximal femoral Epiphysis, physis and metaphysis	IIA (symmetric closure of physis)	Coxa breva with no change in neck shaft angle
	IIB (asymmetric closure of physis)	Progressive coxa vara or valga with acetabular dysplasia
Femoral neck	IIIA	Severe anteversion/ retroversion with severe coxa vara/valga
	IIIB	Pseudoarthrosis of femoral neck with slipping of epiphysis
Epiphysis, physis, and metaphysis	IVA	Unstable hip with persistent small remnant of neck
	IVB	Complete loss of femoral head and neck

TABLE 30: Forlin and Milani classification.

Type	*Subtype*	*Criteria*
Grade I (Femoral head within acetabu lum)	A	Total/part of head present
	B	No femoral head present
Grade II (Hip is dislocated)	A	Total or part of head present
	B	No femoral head present

   - THR in old patients.
   - Pelvic support osteotomy
   - Arthrodesis
   - Resection arthroplasty (in social groups where motion is desirable for work, play and ground toilet)

C. For abductor insufficiency.
   - Trochanteric epiphysiodesis (<7 years age)
   - Trochanteric transfer (distal, lateral or both)
   - Pelvic support osteotomy (if there is additional joint instability)
   - Pelvic osteotomy
   - Proximal femoral osteotomy
   - Trochanteric arthroplasty with proximal femoral osteotomy
   - Harmon or L-episcopo reconstruction

D. Operations to correct deformities—deformities should be corrected as soon as infection has subsided:
   - Flexion adduction contracture—treated by transferring the iliac crest
   - Hip ankylosed in flexion and adduction—treated by intertrochanteric osteotomy and fixing hip in 30° flexion, 20–30° of abduction. Various kinds of treatment for osteotomies are Gant operation (transverse open wedge osteotomy), Whitmann's operation (transverse closed wedge osteotomy) and Bracket (ball and socket osteotomy) procedure.

E. Operations to equalize limb lengths:
- Soft-tissue release (abduction and adduction contracture of 10° cause apparent length inequality of 3 cm)
- Osteotomy (if instability of joint exists)
- Epiphysiodesis of other limb (for anticipated discrepancy of 2.5–5 cm)
- Lengthening of involved limb (anticipated discrepancy >5–6 cm).

Principles and Algorithm of Reconstructive Procedures

The reconstructive procedures are done with the aim of:
- Achieving hip stability and concentric reduction of hip subluxation/dislocation
- Correction of limb length discrepancy
- Preservation of the articular cartilage remnants and reorientation of the axis of normal physiological load
- Adequate containment of femoral head
- Correction of other deformities

No surgical intervention is required when the head is contained. However, a procedure to acquire lengthening of femoral neck may be done after Wagner (with three parallel osteotomies in proximal femur, **Fig. 40**) or double opening wedge osteotomy with distal and lateral transfer of the greater trochanter **(Fig. 41)** or double closing wedge osteotomy and distal lateral transfer of trochanter **(Fig. 42)**. In unstable hips with no femoroacetabular articulation with an aim to provide articular stability and reduce limb length discrepancy the previously listed reconstructive procedures are generally performed. Before embarking upon any one of these procedures, however, an MRI or ultrasound should be done to establish absence of cartilaginous proximal femoral physis that may be entirely unossified. The principles of a few are briefed below (for comprehensive discussion however a dedicated text for pediatric orthopedics should be referred).

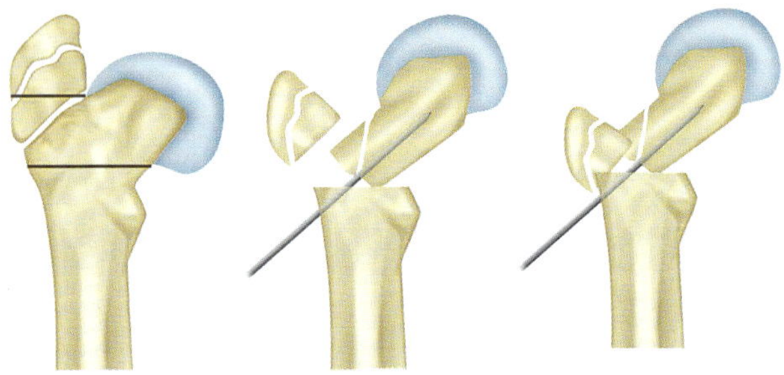

Fig. 41: The double opening wedge osteotomy and distal and lateral transfer of greater trochanter with lengthening of femoral neck.

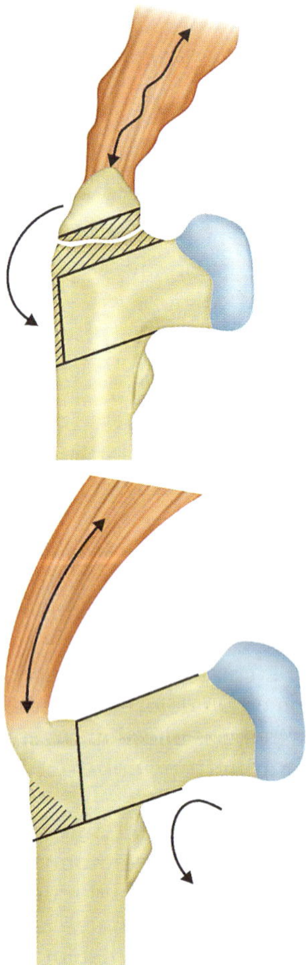

Fig. 40: Double osteotomy with distal and lateral transfer of the greater trochanter and lengthening of the femoral neck.

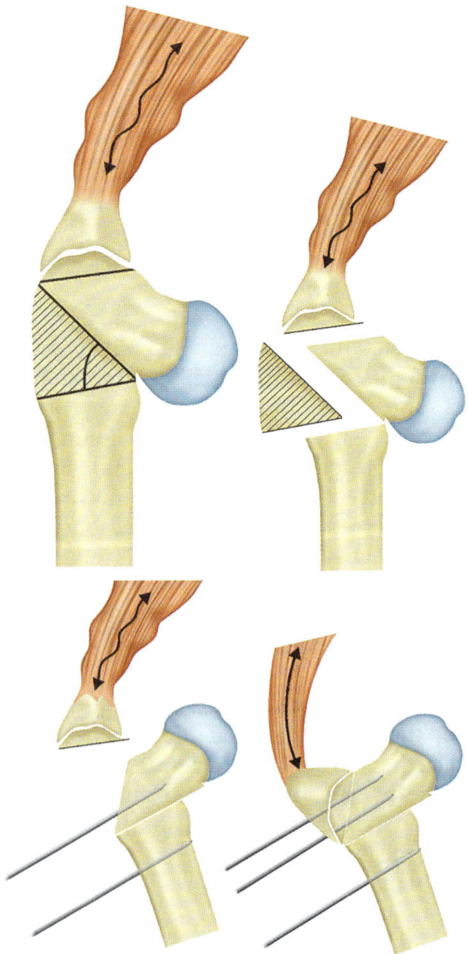

Fig. 42: Double closing wedge osteotomy with distal and lateral transfer of greater trochanter and lengthening of femoral neck.

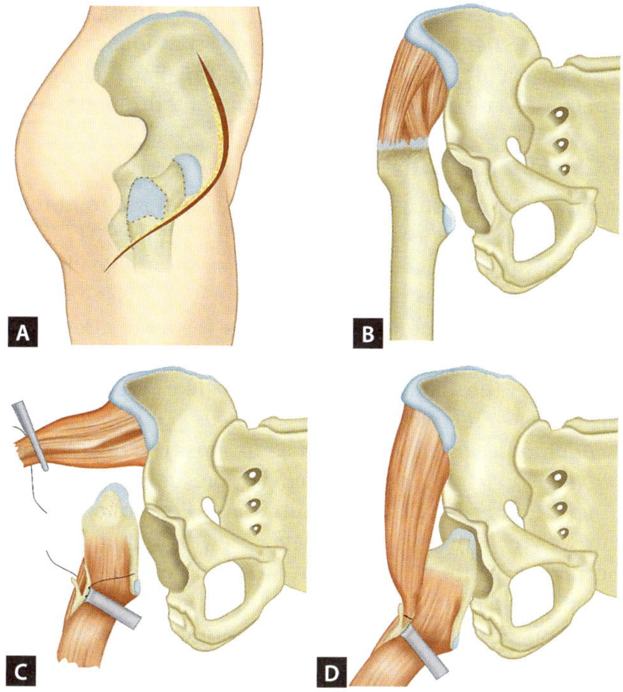

Figs. 43A to D: Trochanteric arthroplasty procedure for reconstruction of hip joint (see text for description).

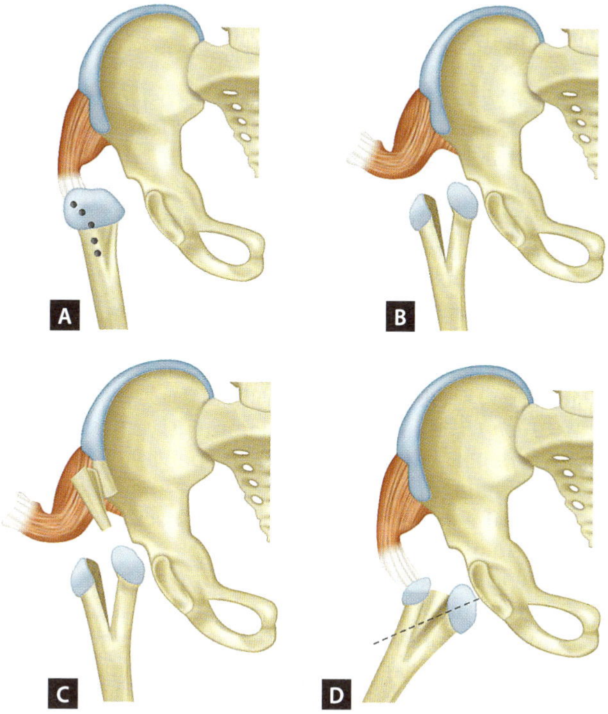

Figs. 44A to D: Harmon neck reconstruction procedure using iliac crest bone graft. The residual proximal femur is split vertically (A) and medial fragment deformed and pushed medially at base into the acetabulum (B). Iliac crest graft is harvested (C) and snugly fitted in the split created in "A" to maintain the medial portion within acetabulum (D).

- Trochanteric arthroplasty includes placement of greater trochanteric physis deep inside acetabulum with distal transfer of abductor muscles accompanied with varus osteotomy of the proximal femur **(Figs. 43A to D)**. This procedure banks upon the growth potential remaining in the uninvolved greater trochanter and remodeling potential which theoretically at least moulds toward the shape of femoral head if subjected to pressure and stresses in acetabulum (Wolff's law). As originally described by Colona, circumferential muscle release is done preserving the periosteum. The neck is removed flush with femoral shaft. The osteotomy is done just below lesser trochanter and medial based wedge is removed. Abductors are sutured distally to a trough in lateral aspect of femur and tensioned at 20° of abduction. Vastus lateralis is reefed over the new glutei insertion. Patient is placed in spica with hip in extension and abduction. In addition, pelvic osteotomy is often needed to improve coverage. The procedure should be performed when the child still has adequate remodeling potential. The most important complication of this procedure includes pain in a formerly painless condition. The complications of the procedure include avascular necrosis of proximal fragment, gradual loss of correction and lateral subluxation due to femoral straightening, abductor weakness, stiffness, degenerative arthritis of hip, and difficult future procedures if required.
- Harmon's neck reconstruction is performed by creating a vertical osteotomy in proximal femur and then pushing the medial remnant into acetabulum by using a fibular graft. This repositions the cartilage remnant attached to neck into acetabulum facilitating remodeling over time. Choi modified it by placing a cartilage graft taken from iliac apophysis into incomplete longitudinal femoral osteotomy that may grow with time and provide a neck lengthening effect **(Figs. 44A to D)**. Additional coverage is required in the form of pelvic osteotomy and limb lengthening may be needed later. The complications include painful stiff hip joint.
- Ilizarov's hip reconstruction includes an acute proximal femoral pelvic support osteotomy with a gradual distraction at distal femoral osteotomy to achieve lengthening. The procedure addresses hip instability, abductor insufficiency, and limb length discrepancy simultaneously. The proximal femoral osteotomy places the greater trochanter distally and laterally thereby improving abductor insufficiency. The valgus osteotomy is overcorrected to eliminate any further adduction that may impinge on pelvis or cause valgus stress at knee. Elimination of further adduction between pelvis and femur prevents pelvic drop in single leg stance please.

Of the various procedures used for reconstruction of hip to manage late sequel of septic arthritis the choice is often difficult, guided usually by surgeon's experience. A simplified algorithm is provided separately for Hunka and Choi classification as follows:

Management algorithm according to Hunka classification:

1. *Type 1:*
   i. Observation.
2. *Type 2:*
   ii. *Type 2A:* Observation or "containment"

iii. *Type 2B:* Containment + greater trochanteric epiphysiodesis
3. *Type 3:*
   i. *Viable head:* Bone grafting + valgus osteotomy
   ii. *Non-viable head:* Removal of head residue followed by trochanteric arthroplasty
4. *Type 4:*
   i. *Type 4A:* Soft release of adductors and/or iliopsoas.
   ii. *Type 4B:* Resection of neck and trochanteric arthroplasty.
5. *Type 5:* Greater trochanteric arthroplasty ± pelvic and femoral osteotomies (usually required).

Management algorithm according to Choi classification:
1. *Type 1A:* Observation.
2. *Type 1B:* Individualize containment.
3. *Type 2A:* Early—containment (pelvic osteotomy) + trochanteric apophysiodesis; Late—may additionally require correction for leg length discrepancy in the form of epiphysiodesis.
4. *Type 2B:* Realignment osteotomy to restore neck shaft angle + growth arrest of proximal femoral physis to prevent recurrence. Later in life additionally manage the leg length inequality by contralateral leg epiphysiodesis.
5. *Type 3A:* Proximal femoral osteotomy as for 2B (add derotation component for excessive anteversion if present).
6. *Type 3B:* Valgus osteotomy + bone grafting the pseudarthrosis.
7. *Type 4A:*
   i. Age <6 years (femoral neck and cartilage head remnant present)—Open reduction by Harmon's osteotomy (Choi modification preferred for possible growth promotion) + distal transfer of greater trochanter and abductors. If this fails then pelvic support osteotomy.
   ii. Age >6 years—Pelvic support osteotomy (Schanz, Lorenz, or Milch-Batchelor).
8. *Type 4B:*
   i. Age <6 years—Trochanteric arthroplasty + varus osteotomy ± pelvic support osteotomy
   ii. Age >6 years—Pelvic support osteotomy.

PROSTHETIC JOINT INFECTION (PJI)

INTRODUCTION

Despite adequate precautions and advances in treatment modalities infection following joint replacement surgery is a major concern with associated morbidities and expenses for treatment. PJIs occur in 0.86–1.1% of knee arthroplasties and in 0.3–1.7% of hip arthroplasties. Elbow, shoulder, and ankle joints have a higher infection rate of up to 6–9%. Incidence is expected to rise due to increasing trend of arthroplasty.

CLASSIFICATION

Based on time to surgery and mechanism of infiltration the PJI is classified as early, delayed or late **(Table 31)**. Early infections (within 12 weeks of index surgery) usually arise from a skin pathogen, most likely a coagulase-negative *Staphylococcus*. Late-onset infections (>1 year after index surgery) in contrast usually result from hematogenous spread of the common organisms like gram-negative organisms—*Escherichia coli*, *Proteus mirabilis*, and *Pseudomonas aeruginosa* and gram-positive organisms—*Staphylococcus epidermidis* being more common than *S. aureus*. Center for Disease Control and Prevention (CDC), however, recognizes only two categories, viz., acute infection (occurring within 90 days from index surgery) and chronic infection (occurring >90 days from index surgery). For acute infections *S. aureus* is the most common isolate while in chronic infections *S. epidermidis* is common with biofilm formation and prolific sessile forms. Another classification system based on symptoms, clinical presentation, and timing of the infection has been proposed. In the detailed system, Type 1 infection has positive cultures after surgical revision, Type 2 has positive cultures 30 days after arthroplasty, Type 3 is by hematogenous spread and with an otherwise well-functioning prosthesis, and Type 4 is known as chronic or late infection. It is, however, common and prudent to follow the system detailed in **Table 31**.

MICROBIOLOGY AND PATHOPHYSIOLOGY

Prosthetic joint infections are usually caused by gram-positive cocci, including coagulase-negative staphylococci and *S. aureus*. Other organisms, such as gram-negative bacilli and mycobacteria, have also been implicated. Polymicrobial infections after hip and knee arthroplasties have been reported in up to 20% of patients. Various conditions predispose a patient to PJI **(Box 18)**. Especially important among these with elevated risk of infection are rheumatoid arthritis, prior joint infection, prolonged surgical time, postoperative bleeding, and urinary tract infection. Various surgery related and microbial factors have also been identified that favor infection at prosthetic sites:

- Prosthetic devices impair opsonic activity and diminish neutrophils' ability to kill bacteria. Especially, the chromium ions impair phagocytosis

TABLE 31: Phases of prosthetic joint infection.

Phase	*Timing after joint replacement*	*Clinical presentation*	*Mode of infection*	*Common pathogens*
Early	<3 months	Erythema, warmth, fever, chills, joint pain, effusion, excessive perioperative drainage	Intraoperative	*Staphylococcus aureus*, Gram-negative bacilli
Delayed	3–24 months	Persistent pain and/or aseptic loosening	Intraoperative	Coagulase-negative staphylococci, *Propionibacterium acnes*
Late	>24 months	Sudden-onset joint pain; fever and leukocytosis less likely	Often hematogenous	*Staphylococcus aureus*

BOX 18: Risk factors for development of prosthetic joint infection.

1. *Preoperative:*
   a. *Local factors:*
      i. Local/locoregional skin infection like pustules, eczema, varicose ulcer, etc.
      ii. Previous local surgery including previous joint arthroplasty (especially for revision cases)
      iii. Deep infection like osteomyelitis or previous septic arthritis (pathogens may hide in osteocytes or necrotic bone tissue)
   b. Distant sources of infection like urinary tract infection, dental infection, osteomyelitis elsewhere, septicemia, etc.
   c. National nosocomial surveillance system risk score of 1 or 2
2. *Postoperative/perioperative:*
   a. Immune-inhibition:
      i. Immunosuppressant medications (bDMARDs, steroids, possibly antimetabolites like leflunomide)
      ii. *Immunosuppressive conditions*
         - Poorly controlled diabetes mellitus (HbA1c > 7)
         - Chronic renal disorder
         - Acute or acute on chronic liver failure
         - Malnutrition (albumin < 3.5, total serum leukocytes <800)
         - HIV (CD4 counts <400)
         - Aplastic anemia
         - Neutropenia
         - Malignancy
      iii. Inflammatory arthropathy like rheumatoid arthritis, psoriatic disease
      iv. *Lifestyle factors*
         - Smoking
         - Excess alcohol consumption
         - Morbid obesity
         - Intravenous drug abuser
         - Poor oral hygiene

- Ineffective and nonspecific neutrophils release lysosomal enzymes and superoxide into the area surrounding the prosthesis, resulting in tissue damage and local devascularization
- Phagocytes are more "focused" to removal of foreign body rather than fighting infection so that fewer cells are available to actually fight infection
- Polymethylmethacrylate bone cement inhibits both neutrophil and complement functions. It also provides an avascular region for bacteria to flourish away from the immunologic defenses of the body. Adherent bacteria form glycocalyx, eventually forming thick biofilms that further impair host defenses. Biofilms have a major role in intractable infections [Kindly vide details in Chapter on "Infections of Bone (Typical and Atypical) and Surgical Site Infection"—under bacteriological factors].
- The heat produced by the polymerization of polymethylmethacrylate result in heat devascularization of bone and necrosis, which is ideal for bacterial growth.
- Prosthetic joints are immediately coated by host proteins after implantation, including albumin, fibrinogen, and fibronectin to which *S. aureus* avidly binds by virtue of possessing a number of host-protein binding receptors (MSCRAMMs).
- Biofilm formation is the biggest defense of bacteria in PJI. A biofilm is defined as *"an assemblage of microbial cells that is irreversibly associated with a surface and enclosed in a matrix of primarily polysaccharide material". S. epidermidis* (found as a commensal on patient's skin or mucous membranes) is particularly adept at attaching to and forming biofilms on foreign bodies such as prosthetic joints. Staphylococcal surface proteins, SSP-1 and SSP-2, are fimbria-like polymers that facilitate adherence of *S. epidermidis* and it also produces a polysaccharide/adhesin (PS/A) substance critical to the formation of critical extracellular matrix known as slime. Organisms in biofilms have three way defenses [*see detailed discussion on Biofilms in* Chapter on "Infections of Bone (Typical and Atypical) and Surgical Site Infection"]. First the antibiotics do not rigorously penetrate the biofilms. Innate defense is also less effective against biofilm. Lastly, the biofilm-associated organisms also grow much more slowly than organisms in suspension so most antibiotics that act on rapidly dividing organisms are ineffective.
- The small colony variants (SCVs) of *S. aureus* or coagulase-negative *Staphylococci* (CoNS) have ability to persist in nonprofessional phagocytes like epithelial cells easily evading them from host defences. Phenotypically, they have slow growth rate and unusual biochemical properties like being auxotrophic for hemin, menadione or thymidine making it difficult for microbiologists to identify. They have been identified in patients with antibiotic-refractory, recurrent, and/or persistent staphylococcal infections.

DIAGNOSIS

History may reveal concomitant or nonconcomitant sepsis locally or at distant site like urinary tract infection. Multiple local surgeries predispose for infection risk. Some invasive procedures like dental work, IV drug abuse, and colonoscopy wound complications predispose for prosthetic joint infection. Pain is usually the first indicator and is present at night or when the patient is taking rest. Pain initially may not be present with activity but gradually weight bearing and movements become painful ultimately crippling till unable to bear weight. Patient may or may not report fever until late. Persistent pain, stiffness and/or wound discharge is also suggestive of infection. Physical examination usually reveals raised local temperature with regional edema that may be associated with erythema and fluctuation if local abscess is formed. Presence of sinus tract communicating with the prosthesis **(Figs. 45A to C)** or exposed prosthesis is definitive sign of prosthetic infection. The movements are usually limited by pain especially weight bearing for which patient seeks medical attention. Blood tests may help to indicate infection like persistently elevated ESR (or continuously rising ESR 48 hours after surgery) and/or CRP though the specificity is very low. Although previously strongly recommended as initial tests to evaluate infection they are now dropped from diagnostic stringency and only have supportive role. IL-6 measurements are being standardized and slowly incorporated in the diagnostic criteria. The levels of IL-6 peaks 8–12 hours after surgery returning to normal in 3 days. It seems to have best correlation with PJI of the available tests having sensitivity of 100% and specificity close to 95%. It may be spuriously positive in patients with rheumatoid arthritis, multiple sclerosis, AIDS, and Paget's disease of bone. Serum procalcitonin levels have till date not proved superiority to diagnose PJI, they specifically serve as biomarkers for bacterial infection than PJI. A list of proposed and studied various biomarkers for PJI is presented in **Table 32**. Simultaneous blood cultures to identify bacteremia are usually obtained.

Apart from the above serological markers, current research is ongoing to study the synovial biomarkers like IL-6, IL-8, CRP, alpha-2 macroglobulins to rapidly diagnose PJI from samples. Alpha-defensin is an emerging and promising marker to this effect. It is an antimicrobial peptide released by neutrophils in the presence of bacteria and has a sensitivity and specificity of 100% and 96% respectively if detected positive. Only deterrent is its high cost. The test is also not influenced by antibiotic treatment. Leukocyte-esterase is an enzyme secreted by neutrophils at the site of infection and inflammation and is simple and cheap to perform. It is available for diagnosing urinary tract infection as a reagent strip test where neutrophils from the sample get lysed and release the esterase causing color change of the dye. The problem is subjectivity in reading color change and also the sample should not at all be mixed with blood else will be false positive. The sensitivity and specificity of the test are lower than alpha-defensin valuing at 84% and 93%. Measurement of synovial fluid CRP is much more sensitive and specific (96% and 91% respectively) than estimation in blood. Newer molecular diagnostic modalities are being increasingly developed that may uniquely help in rapid and possibly specific diagnosis of the PJI, i.e., not only do they identify presence of infection but also reveal the organism. These mainly include nucleic acid amplification tests like PCR amplification (for specific microorganisms such as staphylococci, streptococci, anaerobes or a broad battery covering many organisms) and next-generation sequencing analysis of 16S rRNA (for negative culture of PCR panel), and reverse transcription PCR. Synovial fluid or tissue samples after sonication or bead mill homogenization could be also investigated by these techniques. Enzymatic template

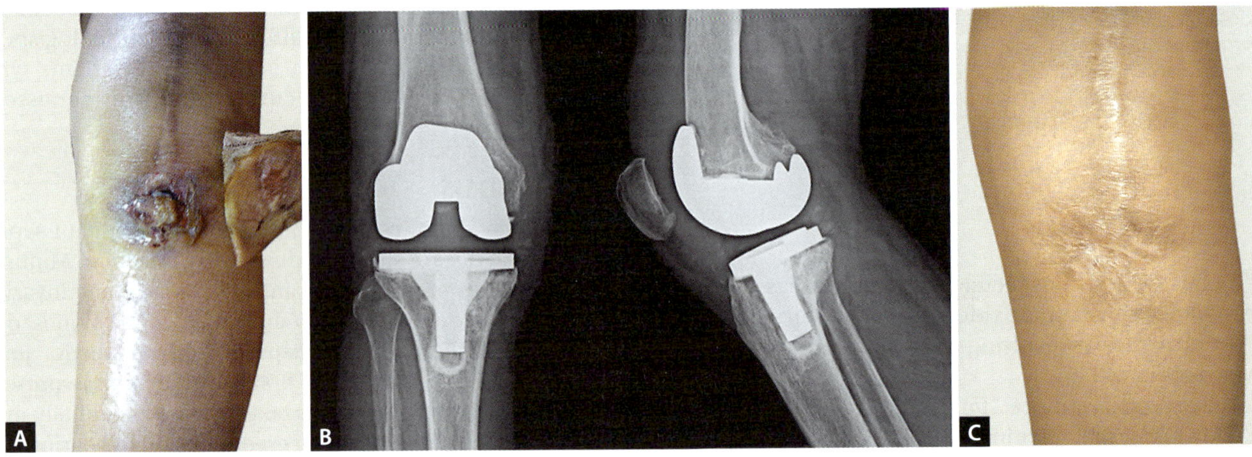

Figs. 45A to C: Infected knee arthroplasty. This patient had total knee replacement surgery done 1 year ago and presented with (A) florid infection of the joint and (B) bony changes. Note the radiolucent lines present on medial aspect of tibia beneath the tibial tray; (C) The infection resolved completely by extensive debridement and managing the defect with antibiotic beads followed by skin flap coverage.

TABLE 32: Utility of various candidate biomarkers other than CRP and ESR for diagnosing PJI.

Candidate biomarker	*Description*	*Sensitivity (SS) and specificity (SP)*	*Positive predictive value (PPV) and negative predictive value (NPV) reported in study(ies)*
IL-6 (>10 pg/mL)	Estimated in serum but normal range itself varies a lot in adults, so difficult to estimate cut-off range	SS ↔ SP ↑	PPV ≈ 75 NPV≈ 80
Serum procalcitonin (>0.3 ng/mL)	Can be performed on routine immunoassay platforms, but its role in localized infections is limited	SS ↓↓ SP ↑↑↑	PPV – 87 NPV – 80
TNF-α (>40 ng/mL)	Studied in synovial tissue, to be done within 1 hour and is laborious	SS ↓↓ SP ↑↑	PPV – 75 NPV – 85
Soluble intercellular adhesion molecule 1 (sICAM-1) (>250 ng/mL)	The gene encoding sICAM-1 can be induced by cytokines and/or bacteria so may distinguish septic from aseptic loosening. Not studied routinely for PJI so insufficient data overall	SS ↑↑↑ SP ↑	PPV and NPV - 65
IgG to short-chain exocellular lipoteichoic acid (sce-LTA)	As this lipid (previously termed lipid-S is produced by coagulase negative staphylococci (CoNS) so the investigation could reveal good marker for implant related biofilm infections	NA	NA
Staphylococcal IgM ELISA (0.35 ELISA units)	Serum IgM antibodies to staphylococcal biofilm polysaccharide antigens may identify delayed PJI. Staphylococcal infections elsewhere in body	SS ↑↑ SP ↑↑	PPV and NPV > 90

TABLE 33: 2018 new definition for prosthetic joint infection (Parvizi et al.)

Major criteria (at least one of the following)				***Decision***
Two positive cultures of the same organism				Infected
Sinus tract with evidence of communication to the joint or visualization of the prosthesis				
Preoperative diagnosis	***Minor criteria***		***Score***	***Decision***
	Serum	Elevated CRP or D-Dimer	2	≥6 Infected 2–5 Possibly infected[$] 0–1 Not infected
		Elevated ESR	1	
	Synovial	Elevated synovial WBC or LE	3	
		Positive alpha-defensin	3	
		Elevated synovial PMN (%)	2	
		Elevated synovial CRP	1	
Intraoperative diagnosis	[$]Inconclusive preoperative score or dry tap		Score	Decision
	Preoperative score		-	≥6 Infected 4–5 Inconclusive[#] ≤3 Not infected
	Positive histology		3	
	Positive purulence		3	
	Single positive culture		2	

Proceed with caution in: Adverse local tissue reaction, crystal deposition disease, slow growing organisms
[$]For patients with inconclusive minor criteria, operative criteria can also be used to fulfill definition for PJI.
[#]Consider further molecular diagnostics such as next-generation sequencing.

generation and amplification can be applied to blood culture bottles to detect microbial DNA polymerase within 3 hours with sensitivity and specificity of 91 and 96% respectively. Matrix-assisted laser desorption ionization time-of-flight mass spectrometry (MALDI-TOF-MS) can rapidly detect staphylococci in patients of PJI with great accuracy. Microcalorimetry is another emerging tool that measures the heat intensity produced by proliferating organisms in relation to their metabolism in real time. This can provide a real time microbiological assay of biofilms. As surgeons are becoming more demanding to not only identify pathogens but also know the virulence factors and drug susceptibility to be delivered rapidly technologies like microarray, phage induced impedance fluctuation analysis, nanomedicine, and metabolomics are under development.

New scoring based definition for PJI had been developed in 2018 **(Table 33)** that was quickly adopted and modified into ICM criteria **(Table 34)** for PJI in the same year and is currently validated in various populations. As of date, these provide the best possibility for defining and diagnosing a PJI with good level of certainty but I expect rapid changes in various criteria with incorporation of more modern methods. The synovial polymorphonuclear (PMN) cell count is a controversial aspect with regard to the cut-off level signifying infection. The current acceptable levels of cell counts and PMN percentages are presented in **Box 19**. Greater than five neutrophils per high-power field in five high-power fields observed (Feldman criteria) from histologic analysis of fresh frozen periprosthetic tissue at 400 times magnification is suggestive of probable PJI. Other criteria such as Mirra [one out of 5 high power field (HPF) showing at least 5 neutrophils], Banit (one out of 5 HPF showing >10 neutrophils), Lonner (all 5 HPF showing at least 10 neutrophils), and Athansou (10 HPF having an average

TABLE 34: 2018 International Consensus Meeting (ICM) criteria for prosthetic joint infection (PJI)—modified version of the 2018 new definition (Shohat et al.).

Major criteria (at least one of the following)				***Decision***
Two positive growth of the same organism using standard culture methods				Infected
Sinus tract with evidence of communication to the joint or visualization of the prosthesis				
Minor criteria	***Threshold***		***Score***	***Decision***
	Acute[&]	Chronic		Combined preoperative and postoperative score: ≥6 Infected 3–5 Inconclusive* <3 Not infected
Elevated CRP (mg/L)	100	10	2	
Or				
D-Dimer (μg/L)	Unknown	860		
Elevated serum ESR (mm/h)	No role	30	1	
Elevated synovial WBC (cells/μL)	10,000	3000	3	
Or				
Leukocyte esterase	++	++		
Or				
Positive alpha-defensin (signal/cut-off)	1.0	1.0		
Elevated Synovial PMN (%)	90	70	2	
Single positive culture			2	
Positive histology			3	
Positive intraoperative purulence[~]			3	

*Consider further molecular diagnostics such as next-generation sequencing
[&]These criteria were never validated on acute infections
[~]No role in suspected adverse local issue reaction
(CRP: C-reactive protein; PMN: polymorphonuclear; WBC: white blood cells)

of >1 neutrophil) are also published but the specificity of Feldman is best—96% nearly always diagnosing infection. It is recommended that microbiology (tissue or fluid) specimens are cultured for at least 5 days. Certain organisms, such as *Propionibacterium* spp. and *Corynebacterium* spp., however, may require longer incubations sometimes up to 2 weeks. Sonication of specimen may improve yield by disrupting the biofilm. A comprehensive though complicated algorithm is presented for diagnosis of PJI using the above advancements and possible future developments **(Flowchart 1)**.

Plain radiography is the most common diagnostic modality employed for its convenience, ready availability and ability to other causes of joint symptoms. Typical signs of a septic process on X-ray films are periprosthetic osteoporosis, periosteal reaction, erosions of the endosteal profile and periprosthetic osteolysis but these have very low sensitivity and the diagnosis is often delayed by 3–6 months. Ultrasonography may demonstrate effusions and synovial hypertrophy and due to high spatial resolution can differentiate abscess in soft tissues from joint pathologies. Ultrasound can guide aspiration also but is limited by user dependence and inability to differentiate hematoma from abscess. Aspiration and tissue biopsy are the ultimate tools to establish diagnosis. MRI is marked by metal artifacts rendering it useless. Radionuclide imaging is very popular and combined leukocyte/marrow imaging with a reported accuracy of 88–98% but it is technically complex and expensive. Bone scan with Tc99m methylene diphosphonate (MDP) is the most common nuclear medicine procedure used but is limited by low specificity especially up to 6 months following surgery. However, a negative scan rules out infection. ^{99m}Tc-hexamethylprophyleneamine oxime (HMPAO) WBS is the currently radionuclide gold standard in the diagnosis of periprosthetic infections in immunocompetent patients. Since neutrophils are used the procedure has accuracy of 90% in septic cases while it is

BOX 19: Joint fluid aspirate white blood cell (WBC) counts and polymorphonuclear (PMN) percentages that suggest infection in prosthetic joint infection (PJI).

Values suggestive of infection/persistent infection:

- Synovial WBC >1,100 cells/μL and PMN >64% in knees
  - Synovial WBC >27,800 cells/μL in the first 6 weeks after TKA suggestive of infection
- WBC >3,000 cells/μL and PMN >80% for hips
- WBC >4,350 cells/μL and PMN >85% for metal-on-metal hips
- WBC >1,166 cells/μL and PMN >64% for hip antibiotic spacers

(TKA: total knee arthroplasty)

Flowchart 1: The workflow for diagnosis of PJI (the text in different color may not be readily available or standardized for routine use).

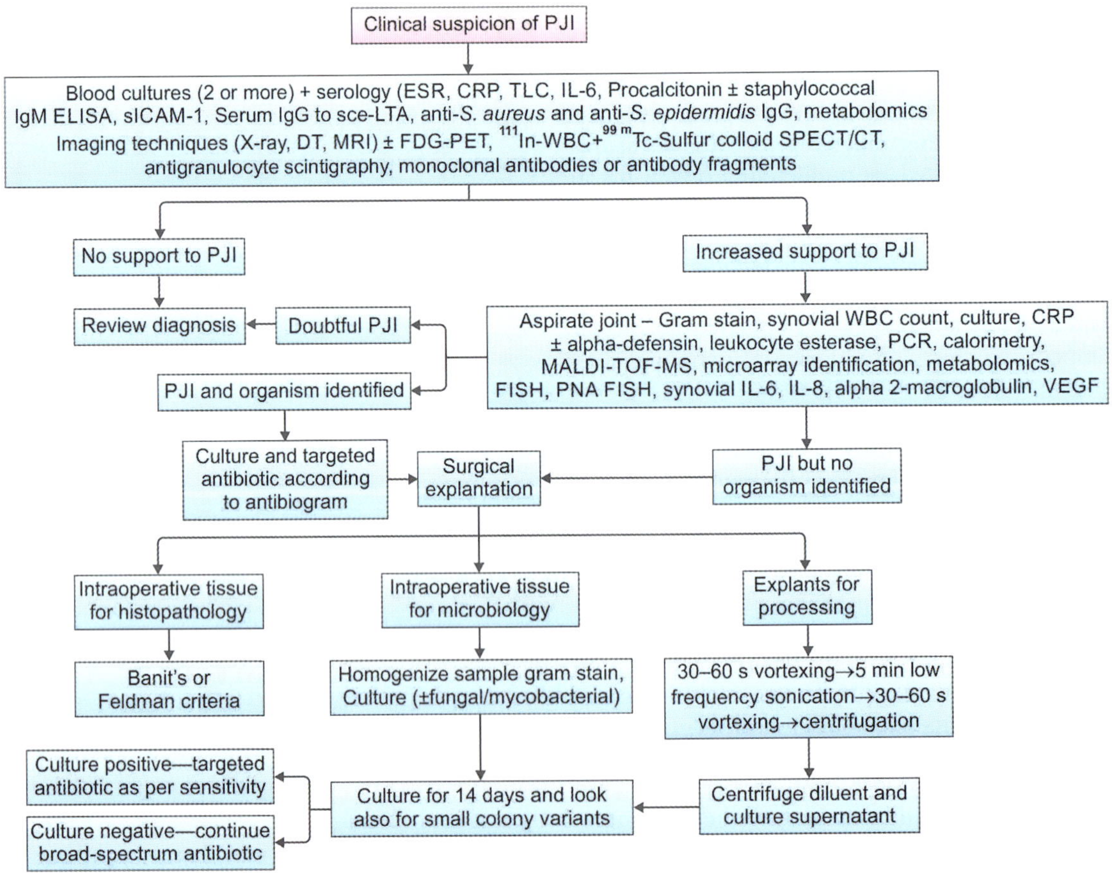

(CRP: C-reactive protein; ELISA: enzyme-linked immunosorbent assay; ESR: erythrocyte sedimentation rate; FDG-PET: fluorodeoxyglucose-positron emission tomography; IL: interleukin; PCR: polymerase chain reaction; PJI: prosthetic joint infection; PNA FISH: peptide nucleic acid fluorescent in situ hybridization; SPECT: single-photon emission computed tomography; TLC: total leukocyte count; VEGF: vascular endothelial growth factor; WBC: white blood cells)

negative in asceptic loosening as the effector cells there are histiocytes, macrophages, and lymphocytes. Antigranulocyte scintigraphy with monoclonal antibodies or antibody fragments is another test that can be done routinely but its variability mars utility. The role of FDG-PET is still unclear as the initial sensitivity and specificity reported of 90% is a bit sobered by finding that scan may be positive even in noninfected patients.

TREATMENT

Dedicated evaluation to limit the obvious consequences on the patient's "*quoad valetudinem*" prognosis should be undertaken to prevent delay in diagnosis and treatment. Multidisciplinary team approach including physician, microbiologist, plastic reconstruction, and occupational therapist should be considered. Options for management include no surgery (with or without antibiotic suppression), amputation, joint fusion or removal, prosthesis retention with debridement and antibiotics, and joint revision in either one or two stages.

Conservative management (no surgery)—For elderly frail patient with multiple comorbidities precluding extensive surgical management (or those who refuse) a functional infected prosthesis may be retained with stoma bag over sinus to collect discharge and/or suppressive antibiotic therapy. Sinus may be deliberately created to facilitate drainage. Proposed guidelines for suppressive antibiotic therapy are presented in **Table 35**. Usually 4–6 weeks sometimes extended to 3 months is used.

Rifampicin 450–600 mg can be combined for CoNS, the usual companion drugs for rifampicin are fluoroquinolones, cotrimoxazole, doxycycline and linezolid. Rifampicin should never be used alone for emergence of resistance. Antibiotic suppression following gram-negative bacillus infection is not recommended.

TABLE 35: Recommended suppressive therapy for PJI (adjust according to renal and hepatic function).

Pathologic organism	*Preferred treatment*	*Alternative treatment*
Staphylococci (MSSA)	Cephalexin 500 mg TDS or QID	Dicloxacillin, clindamycin, amoxicillin + clavulanate
MRSA	Cotrimoxazole 1 DS tablet BD, doxycycline 100 mg BD	Clindamycin, rifampicin + fluroquinolone combination. Glycopeptide + rifampicin + quinolone (resistant infection)
β-hemolytic streptococci	Amoxicillin	Cephalexin
Enterobacteriaceae	Cotrimoxazole 1 DS tablet BD	Oral β-lactam therapy
Enterococcus (penicillin sensitive)	Amoxicillin 500 mg BD or TDS	
Pseudomonas aeruginosa	Ciprofloxacin 250–500 mg BD	
Propionibacterium spp.	Amoxicillin	Cephalexin, doxycycline

(MRSA: methicillin resistant *Staphylococcus aureus*; MSSA: methicillin-susceptible *S. aureus*; PJI: prosthetic joint infection)

Removal of prosthesis alone or with fusion (arthrodesis): Usually in patients with repeated failures to eradicate infection, failed 2-stage revision and factors precluding revision surgery the joint is preferably removed and based on discussion with patient fusion can be attempted though the failure rates are still more than native joint. Also in patients who remain wheel chair bound due to other illnesses attempting revision may be futile so that prosthesis removal for infected joint is appropriate. Prosthesis removal is relatively appropriate for hip and elbow while removal and fusion is common for knee joint.

Repeated debridement, antibiotics and implant retention (DAIR): This is indicated in the acute postoperative time frame. Criteria for this type of surgery include symptoms of <2 weeks duration, gram-positive organisms, no sinus tract or drainage (relative), and no loosening of the prosthesis. Repeated debridement to remove dead infected tissue and reduce disease load is practiced along with exchange of modular liners. Cultures should be always obtained; some people locally inject antibiotics based on sensitivity pattern obtained from aspirate. Sinus tract may need flap cover for reconstruction. Arthroscopic debridement has been found inadequate (compared to open) for inability to exchange liners and limited access to all spaces and ability to debride. Patients having short duration of symptoms with well characterized susceptible organism and well-fixed implant are good candidates for this procedure. Patients with revision surgery, rheumatoid disease, chronic, or gram-negative infection may do less well.

Implant revision: Ideal patients for 2-stage exchange strategy are patients with chronic infections with adequate bone stock, who are medically fit and willing to undergo at least two surgeries. Patients with sinus tracts or with difficult-to-treat organisms such as MRSA, enterococci and *Candida* species would also potentially qualify for this procedure. Obtaining a prerevision sedimentation rate and CRP is recommended to assess the success of treatment prior to reimplantation. More than one 2-stage exchanges can be successful if the first one fails. This procedure is reported to have an overall incidence of success of 87% in a recent review. This strategy involves removal of all infected prosthetic components and cement followed by debridement of infected periprosthetic tissue. Local antimicrobial-impregnated cement with various different concentrations of antibiotics **(Box 20)** and devices are commonly used in the treatment of PJI. Some do not recommend spacers for MRSA infection (though recent studies report successful outcome), infection due to small-colony variants, or fungi as they believe that the use of spacers in these settings may be counterproductive to the eradication of infection. The time from resection arthroplasty to reimplantation varies significantly from 2 weeks to several months. Systemic antimicrobials are administered following resection for 4–6 weeks in many centers. Selected centers use the serum bactericidal test to guide proper dosing of antimicrobial therapy. A new prosthesis is reimplanted in

BOX 20: The various doses of antibiotics available (preloaded cements) or prepared for use in treatment of PJI during two-stage or single-stage revision.

Low-dose antibiotic concentration cements commercially available from various vendors (commonly used in primary high infection risk arthroplasties)

- Cobalt G-HV® (Biomet)
- Palacos R+G® (Zimmer)
- Simplex P® (Stryker)
- SmartSet GMV® (Depuy)
- VersaBone AB® (Smith and Nephew)

High-dose antibiotic-PMMA preparation (used in two-stage revisions where cement spacers are implanted for sterilizing local milieu). High-dose antibiotics damage the cement quality heavily and should not be used for prosthesis implantation. The highest doses of antibiotics that have been used without systemic toxicity are:

- 12.5 g tobramycin: 40 g cement
- 10.5 vancomycin: 40 g cement
- Commonly used/suggested concentrations of antibiotic for use with PMMA in revision arthroplasty
- Use 3 g vancomycin and/or 3.6 g tobramycin in 40 g cement (combination increases elution rate of both antibiotics from cement spacer)
- Use extra liquid monomer (1.5–2 ampules monomer: 1 bag cement)

[PJI: prosthetic joint infection; PMMA: poly(methyl methacrylate)]

delayed second stage. Both cemented and noncemented prostheses are utilized depending on the technical factors. Some prefer reimplantation within 2–6 weeks while systemic antibiotics are being administered. Others prefer delayed implantation after 4–6 weeks of intravenous antibiotics and an antibiotic free period of 2–8 weeks.

A 1-stage or direct exchange strategy for the treatment of PJI may be considered in patients with a THA infection who have a good soft tissue envelope provided that the identity of the pathogens is known preoperatively and is susceptible to oral antimicrobials. There may be a greater risk of failure if bone grafting is required and effective antibiotic impregnated bone cement cannot be utilized. A 1-stage exchange or revision procedure involves excision of all prosthetic components and poly methyl methacrylate cement, debridement of devitalized bone and soft tissues, prosthesis removal, and implantation of a new prosthesis. This procedure is associated with a success rate of 80–90% in patients with THA infection and its success is likely attributable to the extent of the debridement. There are much fewer data for the use of this procedure for prosthetic joints other than a THA or without antibiotic impregnated cement and with bone graft. A relatively healthy patient with adequate bone stock and soft tissues, and patients with an easily treatable organism (streptococci other than enterococci, methicillin-sensitive staphylococci, and nonpseudomonal gram-negative organisms) are preferred candidates for 1-stage exchange. Enterococci and fungal organisms, as well as infection due to small-colony variants, have been thought to be difficult to treat. One-stage exchange is typically not recommended in patients with a sinus tract. Potential advantages of this single exchange procedure result from saving the patient and the healthcare system an additional surgery, and include lower morbidity rate and lower cost.

Amputation: May be required in severe untreatable or unresponding infections or in patients with failed multiple surgeries and mutilated limb. They are also done for associated necrotizing fasciitis or spreading infection, or severe bone loss or inability to achieve tissue cover. It would be appropriate if the deemed functional outcome is better than dragging the infected prosthesis through prolonged and cumbersome treatment.

Antibiotic therapy: Teichoplanin may not be as effective as vancomycin in reducing viable MRSA counts, so can be combined with rifampicin. Linezolid is more effective in initial clearance of MRSA compared to teichoplanin but tolerance is low. In combination therapy glycopeptide + rifampicin + fluroquinolone have been found to generate no resistance. Daptomycin (cyclic lipopeptide antibiotic) has good activity against MRSA and glycopeptide resistant enterococci showing synergy in action with rifampicin. For gram-negative infection concrete evidence for any regimen is lacking though ceftazidime with fluoroquinolone has been found effective.

Prevention of PJI: Few measures are recommended for prevention of PJI as follows:

a. Preoperative evaluation and correction of occult infection, such as periodontal disease or urinary tract infection.
b. *Antibiotic prophylaxis:* Patients with a total joint replacement within 2 years of the implant procedure, and some immunocompromised patients only with total joint replacements who may be at higher risk (comorbidities, immunosuppression, previous infection) for hematogenous infections, should be considered to receive antibiotic prophylaxis before undergoing invasive dental, genitourinary and gastrointestinal procedures with a higher bacteremic risk. Not all patients require antibiotic prophylaxis.
c. Methicillin resistant *Staphylococcus aureus* screening and decolonization for all patients.
d. Patient selection and preparation, surgical technique, theater design, prophylactic antibiotics, and anesthesia should be given due attention.
e. Special precaution to administering antibiotics preoperatively as prophylaxis. Usually short half-life (1–2 hours) antibiotics (ceftriaxone, etc.) are used for orthopedic surgery given within 10–20 minutes before incision. This is acceptable to most surgeries done without tourniquet. It was found that TKA done under tourniquet have higher infection rate. Possible intriguing explanation is that the initial tissue concentration fades during surgery done under ischemia and the bathing tissue fluids have gradually reducing concentration. Most contamination occurs during the surgery however and by the time tourniquet is released the serum concentration of antibiotic has already fallen due to short half-life. So it may be prudent to either do surgery without tourniquet or give boosting dose prior to tourniquet release.

MYCOBACTERIAL ARTHRITIS

INTRODUCTION

About one-third of the world's population is infected with tuberculosis (latent and active), providing a reservoir that will continue to complicate its global control. Despite the emergence of effective chemotherapy for more than 40 years mycobacterial infection remains the single largest infectious disease causing mortality, resulting in approximately 5 deaths every minute. Development of MDR-tuberculosis, XDR-tuberculosis (extensively drug resistant) and spread of HIV infection further ravages the disease control let apart eradication in developing countries. About 3.7% of new cases and 20% of previously treated cases were estimated to have multidrug resistant-TB (MDR-TB). The average proportion of MDR-TB cases with XDR-TB is 9.0%. Almost 80% of TB cases among people living with HIV reside in Africa. "The incidence of tubercular infection seems to be increasing due to coemergence of HIV infection and resulting immunodeficiency". India and China together account for almost 40% of the world's TB cases. Of the global estimate of 9 million (90 lakh) active cases of tuberculosis about 2.6 million reside in India making it harbour the largest number of active cases in world by sheer number. The African Region has 24% of the world's cases and the highest rates of cases and deaths per capita. Skeletal tuberculosis makes up about 1–2% of all cases and about 10% of extrapulmonary "(EPTB)" cases. Osteoarticular tuberculosis most commonly affects the vertebral column and less commonly the hip, knee and sacroiliac joints are affected. In developing countries it is mainly seen in first 3 decades while in developed countries presentation is late ≥60 years due to late exposure. Mycobacterial arthritis and spondylitis deserve separate mention because they usually are diagnosed late and can be extremely destructive.

MICROBIOLOGY

Mycobacterium is a strict aerobe and forms fungus like pellicle in liquid culture medium (hence initially wrongly termed *"Myco-,"* mistaking it for fungus). *M. tuberculosis* is the most common organism isolated from the infected patients while *M. africanum* is common in African subcontinent. In places where pasteurized milk is not used infection with *M. bovis* is prominent. *M. avium* is the most common organism apart from *M. tuberculosis* found in patients with HIV infection. *M. avium* commonly causes tendon sheath infection and secondary wound infections.

PATHOLOGY AND PATHOGENESIS

As for pulmonary tuberculosis, poverty, overcrowding, malnutrition, repeated pregnancies (females) and now the HIV infection remain the major cause of spread of extrapulmonary tuberculosis (EPTB). As previously mentioned, around one-third of world population may be latently infected with dormant mycobacterium bacilli. These patients do not have active disease and are noninfectious (cannot transmit disease) but 10% of them will become infectious at some point in life later (5% in the first 2 years after infection and 0.1% per year thereafter). Osteoarticular tuberculosis (OATB) is usually secondary to primary in:

- Lung
- Lymph nodes
- Kidney
- Bowel
- Other abdominal viscera

Arterial spread with hematogenous seeding is the common mode of infection (except in spine where *venous spread* through Batson's plexus is seen). Pulmonary involvement cannot be detected in two-thirds of cases. When pulmonary findings are present, a miliary pattern is typical. At times, they may be spread contiguously from the bone marrow. Pathologically focus of infection within joint is commonly located primarily in synovium or may arise as extension from bony lesion. The former (synovial primary seeding and proliferation) has a more protracted course and is more commonly seen in knee, shoulder, ankle, wrist while the latter (osseous focus) is seen more commonly in hip and to some extent in elbow.

The *synovial type* demonstrates hypertrophy, congestion and granulation tissue formation. The thickened tissue with inflammatory cell infiltrates spreads as pannus over cartilage and joint surface causing secondary destruction. Joint effusion is prominent and contains "rice bodies" (accumulation of fibrin and articular cartilage). When effective chemotherapy is ensued the synovium transforms into thickened fibrotic tissue and the granulation tissue bridges the pannus regions producing fibrous ankylosis. In spine bony fusion is commonly seen due to extensive cancellous surface and compression from spasmodic muscles.

In *bony extension type* the spread occurs via subperiosteal space, capsule is resistant to spread. Once the cartilage is destroyed the infection reaches joint and cartilage fragments lie free in the joint with exposed subchondral bone. The epiphyseal plate gets involved with spreading infection in opposite direction producing short, deformed extremities. Synovial biopsy is negative in such cases.

CLINICAL TYPES OF TUBERCULAR ARTHRITIS

Granular form (dry form "caries sicca" seen commonly in shoulder): It is more common in adults with a more protracted and indolent course. The bony destruction is less and joint cavity is filled with granulation type tissue and pannus. There is little effusion and infrequent cold abscess formation.

Caseous form (exudative form): Presents with severe constitutional symptoms and is frequently seen in childhood. Joint destruction and abscess formation are common findings with associated deformities and growth stunting.

CLINICAL FEATURES

Tuberculous arthritis is second in frequency to spine (accounts for 50% of the osteoarticular tuberculosis) frequently involving the knee and hip. Other joints commonly involved include the sacroiliac, shoulder, elbow, ankle, carpal and tarsal joints. Tubercular arthritis manifest with chronic indolent localized involvement (monoarticular) with insidious onset of pain and, less often, swelling. Loss of function, muscle spasm, night cries, muscle atrophy, deformity, abscess, and lymphadenopathy are other features observed in various locations. Synovial effusion is often minimal, and the fluid, even if it is obtainable, shows nonspecific inflammation. Synovial fluid findings are variable and do not distinguish this arthropathy from other inflammatory or septic arthritides. The constitutional symptoms of anorexia, evening rise of temperature, weight loss, night sweats, tachycardia, asthenia, and anemia are uncommon. They are conspicuously absent in patients with good nutrition, elderly, and immunocompromised.

Rare and atypical presentation of tuberculosis should also be kept in mind:

- *Poncet's disease (Poncet's rheumatism):* In individuals with active visceral or disseminated tuberculosis, isolated, apparently rare examples of nonsuppurative, symmetric, reactive arthritis are described that are clinically distinct from septic arthritis and resolve with antituberculous chemotherapy (Poncet's disease). They have a similarity to other reactive arthritis and are HLA-B27 positive.
- *BCG associated rheumatic syndrome:* This refers to development of granulomatous bone and joint lesions after immunization or therapy for bladder cancer with "Bacillus Calmette-Guérin" vaccine. Variously reported 0.5–5% of patients treated with "Bacillus Calmette-Guérin" had polyarthralgia and arthritis, typically a self-limited, seronegative, reactive arthritis responsive to nonsteroidal agents. Some patients present with features similar to Reiter's syndrome as well and develop conjunctivitis, fever, urethritis, pericarditis and epididymitis.

RADIOLOGIC FINDINGS

Periarticular osteopenia is the first sign with starkling osteoporosis evident in the joint region. Later with disease evolution "cat bite lesions" on opposing articular surfaces ("kissing lesions") develop. Slowly areas of destruction and joint space reduction occur.

DIAGNOSIS

Misdiagnosis of tuberculosis either false positive or false negative is rampant and detrimental to efforts for controlling the disease. While the former has psychological impact and unnecessarily subjects patient to treatment, the latter has negative impact of patient's and region's health, further denting the disease control efforts. Numerous ineffective methods (interestingly accepted well among physicians due to poor knowledge and urgent need for rapid diagnosis) have been in vogue due to frequent inability to demonstrate acid-fast bacillus (AFB). Traditional methods fail in early diagnosis and either have low sensitivity and specificity (staining for AFB), are protracted in course (culture of *M. tuberculosis*), delay diagnosis (radiology—plain roentgenograms) or are marred by nonpathognomonic findings (MRI—inability to demonstrably differentiate tubercular infection from other chronic infections or neoplasia in every case). Serological diagnosis using antigens or antibody to bacillus is extremely difficult because patients have different antibody response to the mycobacterium infection and antibodies may also develop against other organism (cross-reaction), that share same antigens making it nonspecific. The ELISA for TB against 16-kDa antigen had been found by the World Health Organization (WHO) to yield unacceptable false-positive and false-negative results itself. Accurate diagnosis is needed for disease control at large and prevention of resistant organisms. The following gives a broad outline and current recommendations for diagnosis of tuberculosis including some research molecules.

Definite Case of Tuberculosis

A patient with active *M. tuberculosis* complex is identified in a clinical setting, either by culture (not just by microscopic demonstration—that can be inactive bacillus also) or by a newer method such as molecular or line probe assay. Under ISTC standard-3, for all patients (adults, adolescents, and children) suspected of having EPTB, appropriate specimens from the suspected sites of involvement should be obtained for microscopy and, where facilities and resources are available, for culture and histopathological examination.

Direct Diagnosis

This simply means demonstration of the organism at the lesion. Microbiological detection (staining or culture) of tubercle bacillus or histopathological demonstration of caseous necrosis with typical granuloma formation is diagnostic of tuberculosis (direct diagnosis). As an extended application demonstration using nucleic acid amplification tests (NAAT) in the obtained sample from representative lesion should also be acceptable under proper clinical setup. The following are the strategies that can be used to make a direct diagnosis.

- *Staining* for AFB is usually positive if 10 bacilli/mm^3 are present in specimen while culture requires presence of at least 1,000 bacilli/mm^3, these modalities have sensitivity of around 40% independently. When used together the sensitivity increases to around 60%. OATB is paucibacillary so microbiological demonstration is uncommon (<10% patients), and otherwise also the bacterium may be dormant or inactive. *Culture* is also very slow (requiring up to 45 days) though has the benefit to identify MDR-TB from sensitivity pattern (liquid culture) especially in economically weaker regions unable to afford modern tests.
- Rapid diagnostic methods with centrifugation of specimen to increase yield and analysis by thin layer or gas-liquid chromatography or radioactive labeled DNA probe are expensive.
- *Histopathological demonstration* of caseous necrosis and granuloma formation—conventional diagnosis

relies hence mostly on histopathological demonstration (microbiological demonstration is rather rare) of characteristic features but is invasive and yield is still low in OATB.

- *Molecular diagnosis* using NAAT is gaining popularity for rapid diagnosis (few hours to <1 day), high sensitivity and specificity. The specimens sent to the laboratory are directly subjected to amplification of specific *M. tuberculosis* DNA sequences using one of the many available techniques such as polymerase chain reaction (PCR), real-time PCR or strand displacement amplification. These are highly sensitive and specific to confirm in AFB positive cases and even in AFB negative EPTB cases DNA-PCR is however unable to differentiate between viable and nonviable bacillus and cost is also a prohibiting factor. The mRNA-based reverse transcriptase-PCR (RT-PCR) can differentiate viable from nonviable *M. tuberculosis* and is a rapid diagnostic method for EPTB too. RT-PCR has also been used to monitor drug resistance. Bacterial mRNA has a mean half-life of 3–5 minutes only thus demonstrating positive mRNA signal would indicate viable organisms.
- Newer targets have been studied for differentiation of latent from virulent and active organisms. Alpha-crystallin (α-crystallin, acr) protein encoded by *acr gene* (also known as *hspX*, Rv2031) is such a marker; this protein is synthesized by mycobacterium under stress (reduced oxygen, immune response or treatment by antibiotics) and is associated with increased bacterial wall thickness. Synthesis of acr exponentially increases when bacterium undergoes transition from log phase to stationary mandating that the protein is essential for survival of stationary phase bacteria. Demonstration of acr is, hence, a new tool to identify latent infection, this can be done both in the tissue samples and even in patient serum. In contrast, the early secreted antigenic target-6 (ESAT-6) and culture filtrate 10 protein (CFP-10) act as virulence factors in *M. tuberculosis*, and contribute to pathogenicity. ESAT-6 and CFP-10 are particularly expressed by *M. tuberculosis* but not by bacillus-Calmette-Guérin (BCG) strains so *in vitro* T cell responses to ESAT-6 and CFP-10 appear to be highly sensitive and specific for the detection of infection with *M. tuberculosis* even in those immunized by BCG. Th1 proinflammatory cytokines are expressed at high levels when challenged with CFP-10 and ESAT-6 presentation in patients with active TB. Another method to diagnose active TB due to virulent bacteria expressing CFP-10 and ESAT-6 is to identify the CFP-10/ESAT-6 fusion protein using enzyme-linked immunospot (ELISPOT) assay for diagnosis of active TB either in tissue samples or patient sera.
- The Genexpert test (I personally recommend this test for diagnosis of active infection)—Under the EXPAND-TB (*ex*panding *a*ccess to *n*ew *d*iagnostics for *TB*) project a collaboration between WHO, foundation for innovative new diagnostics (FIND), and STOP-TB partnership's global drug facility (GDF) and global laboratory initiative (GLI) the Xpert MTB/RIF assay was introduced to 6 EXPAND-TB countries (Azerbaijan, Ethiopia, India, Myanmar, Swaziland, and Uzbekistan) in 2012 covering 21 countries in 2013. Xpert MTB/ RIF is a fully automated diagnostic molecular test (applied on the tissue or sputum sample) using the NAAT. It simultaneously detects TB and rifampicin drug resistance (*rpoB gene*) in <2 hours offering treatment opportunity same day. WHO strongly recommends the test to be used as the initial diagnostic test in individuals suspected of MDR-TB or HIV/TB. Conditionally, it is recommended as a follow on test to microscopy in settings where MDR-TB or HIV is of lesser concern especially in smear negative cases (like OATB). Line probe assay (DNA strip test) for first-line drugs (approved by WHO 2008) is recommended (encouraged) for diagnosis of MDR-TB (resistance to H and/or R) and is a good supplement to diagnosis in MDR-TB regions but requires rigorous setup. Still WHO recommends conventional culture methods and DST to determine XDR cases in endemic regions.

Indirect Diagnosis

It is not recommended for relying as a definitive diagnostic measure for discovering presence of TB or refuting it but in setting of strong clinical findings one may resort to these, especially for difficult to approach locations. The diagnosis is mainly based on *immunological tests*—numerous of these are available but *none is diagnostic* of or currently recommended for active tuberculous infection.

- The *tuberculin skin test* (Mantoux skin test, Mendel-Mantoux test, Pirquet test) that detects delayed-type (cell mediated) hypersensitivity (48–72 hours later) against PPD has significant incidence of false positive and negative reaction. Positive reactions (generally considered >20 mm) can develop in previously infected patients while immunodeficient patients might show no reaction despite active infection. Negative reaction in otherwise immunocompetent patient is highly specific to negate tuberculosis as diagnosis.
- As mentioned above the Th1 proinflammatory cytokine release (from T-cells obtained from patient's blood) can be assessed when subject to challenge with ESAT-6/CFP-10 antigen. The ESAT-6/CFP-10 complex is secreted by the ESX-1 secretion also known as RD-1 region. This RD-1 region is absent in BCG, hence presence of activity against it would signify mycobacterial infection other than BCG. The newer higher sensitivity *interferon-γ release assays (IGRAs)* measure the interferon-γ cytokine released by T-cells obtained from a blood sample following restimulation with *M. tuberculosis* antigens (ESAT-6/CFP-10—RD-1 region). These antigens are specific for MTB complex and few other mycobacteria, such as *M. kansasii* and *M. szulgai* and are not found in atypical mycobacteria and in the vaccine strain BCG, which lacks the region of difference 1 (RD1), encoding in MTB complex for these antigens. Cross reactivity to BCG has been but demonstrated by some. IGRAs measure the effector T-cells in the blood against *M.*

tuberculosis that is present only with current infection. So they "indicate" active infection with *M. tuberculosis* but cannot truly differentiate active from latent infection. For improving diagnostic yield in OATB measurement of TNF-α, IL-2 and chemokines IP-10 have been attempted (modified-IGRA) with only partial success. Also IL-10 against Rv2013 (*acr gene* and protein product) can be assayed that indicates latent infection. Also high levels of IFN-γ, TNF-α, and IL-10 against Rv2031 (the *acr gene* and its acr protein product) suggest high level of defense maintained by body against TB and would indicate convalescent form rather than active TB. In any case some individuals recommend IGRA in combination with other tests (microscopy, culture) for OATB. In Pott's disease sensitivity of 84% and specificity of 95% has been found by some. Additionally interferon-γ response clears in patients with effective chemotherapy.

- Serological tests such as ESR and CRP have no definitive role in diagnosis or follow-up of the disease though a lot of people conventionally have a conviction of their role in depicting treatment response (see also spinal infections).

Drug Susceptibility Testing and Line Probe Assay

Due to emergence of drug resistance and wide prevalence of the same it is mandatory to now have knowledge of drug susceptibility testing of the mycobacteria. There are two broad ways to test the drug susceptibility: (1) the phenotypic (observing the characteristics of organism), and (2) the other genotypic (observing the genetic characteristics of organism) method.

- *Phenotypic tests:* These are the conventional methods of detecting drug resistance. There are two models for detecting drug resistance. In the direct drug susceptibility test a set of drug containing and drug free media are inoculated with patient's concentrated specimen. Growth of bacteria indicates drug resistance while inhibition of growth suggests drug susceptibility. In indirect test the drug containing media is inoculated with pure culture grown from original specimen. The indirect test is considered as the "gold standard" for drug susceptibility testing. These tests are complex and time consuming. It takes 4 weeks for bacteria to grow and another 4–6 weeks to detect drug susceptibility using indirect tests. One way to shorten time is to use liquid media for culture and detect early growth by automated BACTEC 320 system.
- *Genotypic tests*: These are molecular tests that aim at directly detecting the gene mutations responsible for drug resistance. These tests have a rapid turnaround time but some may have low sensitivity. There are two main genotypic assays recommended by WHO for use in endemic regions:
    i. *Beacon assay:* The Genexpert test is fully automated, real-time, ultrasensitive PCR that can detect rifampicin resistance. The test has been successfully deployed in many nations but cost and logistics prohibit mass use. Also it has been found by some that the test misses some specific mutations unique to some regions wrongly reporting sensitive bacteria while it is actually resistant. Anyway the test has provided an important landmark in diagnosis and detecting drug resistance.
    ii. *Line probe assays (LPAs):* These tests use PCR and reverse hybridization methods for rapid detection of mutations [single nucleotide polymorphisms (SNPs)] associated with drug resistance (both Rifampicin or/ and Isoniazid). The advantage is that they can be directly applied to the sample revealing the report in as less as 5 hours. The disadvantage of this test could be the use of open tube format susceptible to cross contamination (causing false positive result) and labor intensive requiring skilled personnel. LPAs for second line drugs have also been released that can be combined with tests for first-line drugs to detect XDR-TB.

WHO Recommendations

- Use light emitting diode (LED) microscopy instead of traditional Ziehl-Neelsen staining (2009).
- Interferon gamma release assay (IGRA) and TST are both nondiagnostic and nondiscriminatory for active TB (they mostly detect latent infection) and cannot predict risk of infected individuals developing active TB disease.
- They should also be *not* used in places with routine BCG vaccination, low-middle income group countries having high TB load. IGRA may be useful for detection of latent infection in low-incidence, high-income settings.
- Guidelines for TB—loop-mediated isothermal amplification (LAMP)—have not been developed. The line probe assay for detecting resistance to second-line anti-TB drugs (MTBDRsl) has high specificity but low sensitivity to detect resistance to fluoroquinolones and second-line drugs so cannot replace the conventional phenotypic drug susceptibility testing (DST).
- Use of ELISA for serodiagnosis of active tuberculosis is discouraged (2011).
- Use of nucleic amplification assay Xpert® MTB/RIF rapid and simultaneous detection of rifampicin resistance conferring mutations is encouraged (2010) under EXPAND-TB initiative.

Further Advances in Diagnosis of Tubercular Infection

Due to poor reliability of current tests in immunocompromised patients like concomitant HIV infection and current tedious nature of the available rapid diagnostic tests, efforts are being made to develop test that has following properties:

- Test should be simply able to detect infection in an individual and infectious individual through blood sample.
- Easy to perform and cheaper so that it can be even deployed in rural and remote areas. The appliances could be installed even in regions far away so as to be operable even in absence of regular power supply (hence solar power enabled).

- Removes need to collect sputum or pus.
- Can detect infection in HIV coinfection, latent TB and is not influenced by TB vaccination.
- Should be able to detect infection due to any strain of tubercular bacterium.
- Should be applicable to adults and children equally.
- Test should work even in resistance to antibiotics.

Such a test has been developed at the Stanford University, California that can distinguish active tuberculosis from healthy controls, latent TB and other diseases in a research performed by Dr Purvesh Khatri et al. now called *"Khatri test"*. It is based on the human gene expression in response to tubercular infection that remains constant (out of the hundreds of genes expressed). Three such genes have been identified revealing the presence of active tuberculosis infection serving as a signature for active disease than a latent infection or other disease. This test could also hence identify infectious individuals. The test has been found to have sensitivity of 86% (much more than the WHO recommended level of 66% for an active infection) and a negative predictive value of 99%.

TREATMENT

Chemotherapy is the mainstay of treatment for a diagnosed case of TB. There is no universal consensus on therapeutic guidelines and regimens for osteoarticular antitubercular chemotherapy (ATT). This partially and the issues of monitoring therapeutic response (i.e., to end treatment) in a patient with extrapulmonary tuberculosis (still undefined) the treatment is variably prolonged in endemic areas by treating doctor (though this has no scientific basis). The conventionally described four treatment categories by WHO should be modified or abolished shortly and are mentioned here for historical interest only **(Table 36)**. OATB can be simply classified into drug-susceptible and drug-resistant TB logically for treatment purpose. In WHO categories, OATB is classified in both CAT1 and CAT3 (now correctly removed), where more severe patients (spinal TB with neurological involvement) were placed in CAT1 and others

TABLE 36: WHO categories for treatment category by type of patient (of historical interest now—see text).

Treatment category	*Type of patient*
I	• Sputum smear-positive; new • Sputum smear-negative; seriously ill, new EPTB; seriously ill, new • Others (e.g., TB with HIV infection)
II	• Sputum smear-positive; relapse • Sputum smear-positive; failure • Sputum smear-positive; return after default PTB patients who become smear-positive after 2 months of treatment • Return after default from retreatment • Relapses after retreatment
III	Sputum smear-negative, not seriously ill, new EPTB, not seriously ill, new
IV	Chronic and drug resistant-TB cases (still sputum positive after supervised retreatment)

into CAT3. However, the treatment regimens for these two categories have been unified now by the WHO so there will be no distinction and CAT1 and CAT3 become same. With the promotion of STOP-TB initiative DST is being encouraged and to be universalized by 2015, so WHO treatment CAT2 becomes obsolete. In essence hence only CAT1 and CAT4 (drug-resistant TB) remain. Our recommendation is that cases of diagnosed OATB should be treated as either drug-susceptible or drug-resistant TB. Some definitions are still legible:

- "Drug-resistant TB"—refers to cases of TB caused by an isolate of *M. tuberculosis* that is resistant to one of the first-line anti-TB drugs: isoniazid, rifampin, pyrazinamide, ethambutol or streptomycin.
- "Multidrug-resistant TB"—refers to an isolate of *M. tuberculosis* that is resistant to at least isoniazid and rifampin both, and possibly additional agents.
- The term "extensively drug-resistant TB" (XDR-TB) is defined as TB that is resistant to any fluoroquinolone, and at least one of three injectable second-line drugs (capreomycin, kanamycin and amikacin), in addition to isoniazid and rifampin. It is estimated that 70% of XDR-TB patients die within a month of diagnosis.
- The term "totally drug-resistant TB" (TDR-TB) refers to an isolate of *M. tuberculosis* resistant to all locally tested medications. However, the published studies initially describing TDR-TB did not include susceptibility testing for less frequently used agents with activity against TB, like cycloserine, terizidone, clofazimine, linezolid or carbapenems.
- Primary drug resistance is said to occur in a patient who has never received anti-TB therapy (≈3% of cases, 1 per 10^6 for H, 1 per 10^9 for R, 1 per 10^6 for S, 1 per 10^5 for E, 1 per 10^5 for S).
- Secondary drug resistance refers to the development of resistance during or following chemotherapy in patients who had previously had drug-susceptible TB (≈15% of cases).
- New case is a patient who has never had treatment for TB, or has been on anti-TB treatment for <4 weeks.
- Relapse is a patient who has been declared cured or treatment completed for any form of TB in the past, but who reports back to the health service and is found to be sputum smear-positive or culture positive.
- Treatment failure is a patient who, while on treatment remained sputum smear-positive or became sputum smear-positive at the end of the 5 months or more, after commencing treatment difficult to define for OATB.
- Treatment defaulter is a patient who had previously been recorded as defaulted from treatment or has discontinued treatment for full 2 months in-between and returns to the health service with smear-positive sputum.

For patients with extrapulmonary TB (EPTB), HIV testing is usually recommended as there is increased prevalence of EPTB in them, may be this is less pertinent for OATB. WHO states that pulmonary and extrapulmonary disease (OATB in this case) should be treated with the same regimen. However, some experts do recommend prolonging treatment to

9 months for lack of markers to monitor response to treatment and end therapy. The aims of treatment are:

- To cure the patient and restore quality of life and productivity
- To prevent late effects of osteoarticular TB
- To prevent relapse
- To prevent the development and transmission of drug resistance

The chemotherapy is divided into intensive and continuation phase. Drugs are classified into first-line medications and second-line medications. The first-line medications **(Table 37)** are most effective and used primarily for drug-susceptible TB, the second-line medications are used in drug-resistant TB depending on sensitivity and preference. First-line agents are well absorbed after oral administration, with peak serum levels at 2–4 hours and nearly complete elimination within 24 hours they have high bactericidal activity (rapidly reduce the number of viable organisms and render patients noninfectious), high sterilizing activity (ability to kill all bacilli and thus sterilize the affected tissues and ability to prevent relapses), and low rate of inducing resistance. Standard treatment regimens are prescribed for designated groups of patients. These confer cost reduction, discipline, reproducibility, reducing prescription errors and hence resistance, convenient outcome evaluation. New drug-susceptible patients (no prior history of TB or those receiving <1 month ATT previously) should receive at least 6 months treatment with 2HRZE/4HR (intensive/continuation phase) that can be extended to 9 months (2HRZE/7HR) as by some experts. The combination HE in continuation phase has been withdrawn (high failure rate) similarly omission of ethambutol from intensive phase (previously prescribed for CAT3) is not recommended either. Under DOTS (difficult for all osteoarticular patients as they have difficulty being mobile) thrice weekly intermittent regimens [2HRZE/4(HR)$_3$] and [2(HRZE)$_3$/4(HR)$_3$] extended to 9 months are acceptable provided they are not living in HIV-prevalent setting. Patients living in high isoniazid resistance regions should receive [2HRZE/4HRE] that can be extended to 9 months. For previously treated patients obtaining rapid DST (drug susceptibility testing) is a must and if they are drug-resistant then should be treated as below or if they are drug-susceptible then treat as above. At places where rapid DST is not available then conventional method is acceptable. Till the time results are obtained, a relapsed or defaulter patient could be treated with 2HRZES/1HRZE/5HRE while a treatment failure should be treated with empirical MDR-TB regimen (discussed below) for the region and then individualized based on results.

Multidrug-resistant TB develops due to selection of resistant mutants in the bacterial population, due to killing of susceptible bacilli by anti-TB drugs, inadequate treatment such as direct or indirect monotherapy, slow but constant mutation of *M. tuberculosis*, resulting in resistant mutant organisms and early discontinuation of treatment. The green light committee helps nations to establish drug resistant TB component and integrate into control program. For treatment of MDR-TB the medications are divided into five groups according to efficacy, experience of use and drug class. Group 1 comprises first-line agents except streptomycin which is grouped in group 2. Groups 2–5 are reserve drugs **(Table 38)**. The MDR-regimens are either standardized regimen or tailor made (preferable) where DST is available especially rapid-DST. In India, the MDR-TB patients and those with any rifampicin resistance are referred to the RNTCP designated DOTS-Plus site, with their DST result and request for Category IV treatment form. Under RNTCP the MDR regimen comprises of six drugs—Km, Ofx(Lvx), Eto, Z, E, Cs for 6–9 months of intensive phase and four drugs Ofx (Lvx), Eto, E, Cs for 18 months in continuation phase. PAS is included in the regimen if any bactericidal

TABLE 37: The recommended doses of first-line anti-tuberculosis drugs (adults).

	Recommended dose			
	Daily		Thrice weekly	
Drug	***Dose (range) mg/kg body weight***	***Maximum***	***Dose (range) mg/kg body weight***	***Maximum***
Isoniazid (H)	5 (4–6)	300	10 (8–12)	900
Rifampicin (R)	10 (8–12)	600	10 (8–12)	600
Pyrazinamide (Z)	25 (20–30)	–	35 (30–40)	–
Ethambutol (E)	15 (15–20)	–	30 (25–35)	–
Streptomycin (S) (now not considered first line by ATS, IDSA or CDC)	15 (12–18)	1,000	25 (25–30)	1,500

TABLE 38: Second-line agents for treatment of MDR-TB.

Group	***Drugs (abbreviations)***
1. (First-line oral)	• Pyrazinamide (Z) • Ethambutol (E) • Rifabutin (Rfb) • Rifapentin (Rfp)
2. (Injectable drugs)	• Kanamycin (Km) • Amikacin (Am) • Capreomycin (Cm) • Streptomycin (S)
3. (Fluoroquinolones)	• Levofloxacin (Lfx) • Moxifloxacin (Mfx) • Ofloxacin (Ofx) is less effective and gatifloxacin is too toxic.
4. (Oral bacteriostatic second-line agents)	• Para-aminosalicylic acid (PAS) • Cycloserine (Cs) • Terizidone (Trd) • Ethionamide (Eto) • Prothionamide (Pto)
5. (Agents with unclear role)	• Clofazimine (Cfz) • Linezolid (Lzd) • Amoxicillin/clavulanate (Amx/Clv) • Thiacetazone (Thz) • Imipenem/cilastatin (Ipm/Cln) • High-dose isoniazid (high-dose H) • Clarithromycin (Clr)

(MDR-TB: multidrug-resistant tuberculosis)

drug (K, Ofl, Z, and Eto) or 2 bacteriostatic (E and Cs) drugs are not tolerated. The general principles to design an MDR-TB regimen are as follows:

- Treatment regimens should consist of at least four drugs with either certain, or almost certain, effectiveness.
- More than four drugs may be started if the susceptibility pattern is unknown or the effectiveness of one or more agents is questionable.
- Susceptibility testing for isoniazid, rifampicin, the fluoroquinolones, and the injectable agents is fairly reliable so regimen could be based on the DST pattern for these drugs. For other drugs, the clinical effectiveness of DST cannot be predicted with full surety.
- Each dose in an MDR regimen is given as DOT throughout the treatment.
- Do not use drugs for which possibility of cross-resistance exists.
- Include drugs from groups 1–5 in hierarchical order based on potency. In general, select one of the first-line drug to which add an injectable from Group 2. Use a fluroquinolone and then choose a drug from Group 4 to complete an effective four-drug combination. For a regimen with less than four drugs choose two from Group 5. The total number of drugs often ranges from 5–7 depending on the degree of uncertainty.
- The duration of intensive phase for MDR-TB regimen depends on duration of treatment with injectable agent. The injectable agent should be continued for a minimum of 6 months and for at least 4 months after the patient first becomes and remains smear-negative or culture-negative. Another recommendation is to continue treatment for a minimum of 18 months following culture conversion.

ESSENTIAL FIRST-LINE DRUGS

Isoniazid

It is a hydrazide of isonicotinic acid highly bactericidal against replicating tubercle bacilli.

Pharmacokinetics: It is rapidly absorbed and diffuses into all fluids and tissues. The plasma half-life (genetically determined), varies from less than 1 hour in fast acetylators to more than 3 hours in slow acetylators. Isoniazid is largely excreted in the urine within 24 hours, mostly as inactive metabolites.

Administration: Usually administered orally but intramuscular and intravenous preparations are available for select patients.

Dosage (see Table 37)

Contraindications and precautions: The drug is contraindicated in active unstable hepatic disease or known hypersensitivity. Monitoring should be performed in patients with pre-existing liver disease. Pyridoxine is recommended for patients with risk of peripheral neuropathy (malnutrition, chronic alcohol dependence, HIV infection, pregnancy, breastfeeding, renal failure or diabetes) in a dose of 10 mg daily. Isoniazid can be safely given during pregnancy and breastfeeding along with pyridoxine supplementation.

Adverse effects: Sleepiness, lethargy, systemic or cutaneous hypersensitivity reactions are infrequent. Peripheral neuropathy, optic neuritis, toxic psychosis, and generalized convulsions can develop in susceptible patients. Asymptomatic rise of transaminases is common and of little concern than toxic hepatitis that is infrequent but treatment should be rapidly withdrawn at identification. A lupus-like syndrome, pellagra, anemia, and arthralgias are other rare adverse effects.

Interactions: It inhibits the metabolism of certain drugs [carbamazepine, benzodiazepines metabolized by oxidation (such as triazolam), acetaminophen, valproate, serotonergic antidepressants, disulfiram, warfarin, and theophylline] elevating their plasma levels. Rifampicin has opposite effect on many of these drugs so coadministration has been found to reduce the plasma levels of phenytoin and diazepam.

Over dosage: Nausea, vomiting, blurred vision; occur within half an hour to 3 hours of the over dosage. Massive poisoning leads to respiratory depression, stupor, and coma. Seizures and neurological damage may occur. Gastric lavage, charcoal, and antiepileptics are helpful when administered immediately. Hemodialysis may be considered. Pyridoxine in high doses is administered to prevent seizures and control neurological damage.

Rifampicin

It is a complex macrolide antibiotic semisynthetic derivative of rifamycin that inhibits ribonucleic acid synthesis in a broad range of microbial pathogens. It is bactericidal and has effective intra- and extracellular sterilizing effect. Resistance to drug is fast to develop so it should be coadministered with other drugs.

Pharmacokinetics: The drug is rapidly and completely absorbed following oral administration (especially in empty stomach, food reduces absorption) with good lipid distribution. It easily crosses cellular membranes and body fluid or pus pockets. Significant CSF concentrations with inflamed meninges. Half-life of drug is 2–3 hours and extensive metabolism occurs in the liver with excretion of metabolites (by deacetylation) in the feces.

Administration and dosage: Usually oral administration with intravenous preparation available for critical patients. For dose see **Table 37**.

Contraindications and precautions: The drug is contraindicated in active unstable liver disease and known hypersensitivity to drug. Unusual serious immunological reaction causing renal impairment, hemolysis or thrombocytopenia has been seen in patients resuming treatment after long gap. Permanent withdrawal of drug is recommended. Liver function tests and monitoring is recommended in patients with pre-existing liver disease. Warn patients of reddish orange discoloration of body fluids like saliva, tears, urine, sweat and semen and to avoid contact lens usage for permanent staining. Infants born to mothers taking the drug should be given vitamin K at birth for potential risk of hemorrhage. Women using oral contraceptives should be advised to either increase dose of estrogen or choose a nonhormonal contraceptive.

Adverse effects: Commonly flu-like syndrome (influenza-like) is observed with fever, thrombocytopenia especially with intermittent dosing that usually settles by itself. Abdominal pain, nausea, vomiting and pruritis with or without rash may be observed, exfoliative dermatitis is more frequent in HIV-positive patients. Intermittent dosing has also been observed to result in temporary oliguria, hemolytic anemia and dyspnea that resolve with daily dosing. Rise in transaminase levels is usually temporary but dose-related hepatitis is fatal so maximum dose should not exceed 600 mg.

Drug interactions: Rifampicin is a potent inducer of hepatic enzymes so serum levels of most liver metabolized drugs are reduced with concomitant use. For a comprehensive list pharmacological text should be consulted; however, some common drugs whose dosages need adjustment are as follows:

- Antibiotics (clarithromycin, erythromycin, doxycycline, atovaquone, and chloramphenicol)
- Antimalarial—mefloquine
- Antiviral including antiretroviral drugs
- Azole antifungal agents
- Hormone therapy—HRT, oral contraceptives, tamoxifen, and thyroxine
- Anticonvulsants
- Warfarin
- Cyclosporine
- Cardiovascular drugs—digoxin, digitoxin, verapamil, nifedipine, diltiazem, propranolol, metoprolol, enalapril, losartan, quinidine, mexiletine, and hypolipidemic drugs
- Theophylline
- Sulfonylurea hypoglycemics.

Toxicity: Very large doses may depress central nervous system. Gastric lavage may be helpful, there is no specific antidote.

Pyrazinamide

Pyrazinamide is a synthetic nicotinamide analog and is weakly bactericidal against *M. tuberculosis* but has potent sterilizing activity. It is effective against persisters in the acidic intracellular environment of macrophages. It is highly effective during the acute inflammatory changes in first 2 months. Its use has enabled treatment regimens to be shortened and the risk of relapse to be reduced.

Pharmacokinetics: It is readily absorbed from the GI tract and is rapidly distributed throughout all tissues and fluids. Peak plasma concentrations are attained in 2 hours and the plasma half-life is about 10 hours. It is metabolized mainly in the liver and excreted mostly in the urine.

Administration and dosage: Pyrazinamide is administered orally. For dosage see **Table 37**.

Contraindications and precautions: Contraindications are similar to rifampicin and porphyria. Diabetic patients should be carefully monitored since blood glucose concentrations may become labile. Gout may be exacerbated. Being most hepatotoxic drug liver function tests should be performed during treatment of patients with pre-existing liver disease. In patients with renal failure, pyrazinamide should be administered three times per week. Although detailed teratogenicity data are not available, pyrazinamide can probably be used safely during pregnancy.

Adverse effects: Pyrazinamide may cause gastrointestinal intolerance and rare hypersensitivity reactions, some patients complain of slight flushing of the skin. Sideroblastic anemia and photosensitive dermatitis are very rare. Severe hepatotoxicity is uncommon but needs discontinuation. Hyperuricemia due to inhibition of renal tubular secretion is often asymptomatic, occasional gout may be treated with allopurinol. Arthralgia responds well to NSAIDs. Both hyperuricemia and arthralgia may be reduced by prescribing regimens with intermittent administration of pyrazinamide.

Overdosage: Little is known; acute liver damage and hyperuricemia have been reported. Treatment is essentially symptomatic, no specific antidote exists. Emesis and gastric lavage may be of value if undertaken within a few hours of ingestion.

Streptomycin

Streptomycin is an aminoglycoside antibiotic derived from *Streptomyces griseus* that is also used in the treatment of sensitive gram-negative infections.

Pharmacokinetics: Streptomycin is not absorbed from GI tract but, after intramuscular administration, it diffuses readily into the extracellular component and attains bactericidal concentrations, particularly in tuberculous cavities. CSF concentrations are usually negligible, although penetration increases when the meninges are inflamed. The plasma half-life is normally 2–3 hours; this is considerably extended in the newborn, the elderly and patients with severe renal impairment. Hardly metabolized streptomycin is excreted unchanged in the urine.

Administration and dosage: Streptomycin must be administered by deep intramuscular injection. It is also available for intravenous administration.

For dosage see **Table 37**. Patients aged over 60 years may not be able to tolerate more than 500–750 mg daily, so some guidelines recommend reducing the dose to 10 mg/kg/day for patients in this age group. Patients weighing less than 50 kg may not tolerate doses above 500–750 mg daily.

Contraindications and precautions: The drug is contraindicated in patients with known hypersensitivity, auditory nerve impairment or myasthenia gravis and in pregnancy.

Streptomycin should be withdrawn immediately if hypersensitivity reactions occur (rare). Once fever and skin rash have resolved, desensitization may be attempted.

Dose-related toxic effects resulting from accumulation occur in elderly and patients with renal impairment. There is increased risk of nephrotoxicity and ototoxicity in renal insufficiency patients. The dose should be maintained at 12–15 mg/kg but at a reduced frequency of 2–3 times per week. Where possible, serum levels should be monitored periodically and dosage adjusted appropriately to ensure that plasma concentrations, as measured when the next dose is due, do not exceed 4 μg/mL. The administrator should wear protective gloves to avoid sensitization dermatitis. Streptomycin should not be used in pregnancy: it crosses the placenta and can cause auditory nerve impairment and nephrotoxicity in the fetus.

Adverse effects: Injections are painful and rash, induration, or sterile abscesses can form at injection sites. Numbness and tingling around the mouth occur immediately after injection and patients should be warned. Cutaneous hypersensitivity reactions can occur.

Impairment of vestibular function is uncommon with currently recommended doses.

Manifestations of damage to the 8th cranial (auditory) nerve include ringing in the ears, ataxia, vertigo and deafness; damage usually occurs in the first 2 months of treatment and is reversible if the dosage is reduced or the drug is stopped. Although, less nephrotoxic than other aminoglycoside antibiotics, if urinary output falls, albuminuria occurs or tubular casts are detected in the urine, streptomycin should be stopped and renal function should be evaluated. Hemolytic anemia, aplastic anemia, agranulocytosis, thrombocytopenia and lupoid reactions are rare adverse effects.

Drug interactions: Other ototoxic or nephrotoxic drugs (other aminoglycoside antibiotics, amphotericin B, cephalosporins, ethacrynic acid, cyclosporin, cisplatin, furosemide, NSAIDs, and vancomycin) should not be administered to patients receiving streptomycin. Streptomycin may potentiate the effect of neuromuscular blocking agents administered during anesthesia.

Overdosage: Hemodialysis can be beneficial. Treatment is supportive.

Ethambutol

It is a synthetic congener of 1,2-ethanediamine active against *M. tuberculosis, M. bovis,* and some nonspecific mycobacteria. It is used in combination with other anti-TB drugs to prevent or delay the emergence of resistant strains. *Pharmacokinetics:* It is readily absorbed from the gastrointestinal tract. Plasma concentrations peak in 2–4 hours and have a half-life of 3–4 hours. Ethambutol is excreted in the urine both unchanged and as inactive hepatic metabolites. About 20% is excreted unchanged in the feces.

Administration and dosage: Ethambutol is administered orally.

For dosage see **Table 37**. Dosage must always be carefully calculated on a weight basis to avoid toxicity, and the dose or the dosing interval should be adjusted in patients with impaired renal function (creatinine clearance <70 mL/min). If creatinine clearance is less than 30 mL/min, ethambutol should be administered three times per week.

Contraindications and precautions: The drug is contraindicated in patients with pre-existing optic neuritis and known hypersensitivity. Patients should be advised to discontinue treatment immediately and to report to a clinician if their sight or perception of color deteriorates. Ocular examination is recommended before and during treatment. Whenever possible, renal function should be assessed before treatment. Plasma ethambutol concentration should be monitored if creatinine clearance is less than 30 mL/min. There is no known contraindication except above for use of ethambutol in pregnancy.

Adverse effects: Dose-dependent optic neuritis can result in impairment of visual acuity and color vision (blue vision) in one or both eyes. Early changes are usually reversible and rarely occur at recommended dose, but blindness can occur if treatment is not discontinued promptly. Other rare adverse events include generalized cutaneous reaction, arthralgia and, very rarely, hepatitis.

Overdosage: Emesis and gastric lavage may be of value if undertaken within a few hours of ingestion.

Subsequently, dialysis may be of value. There is no specific antidote and treatment is supportive.

TUBERCULOSIS OF HIP JOINT

In developing countries, the tubercular affection of hip joint usually involves patients <10 years of age and is much more common in males. It is less common than Pott's disease (TB of spine) in a ratio of 10:7. The disease is essentially secondary to TB elsewhere but even could be tertiary involvement from trochanteric bursitis.

Pathology

The initial lesion is usually bony and infrequently only synovial. Bony lesion may arise in:

- Trochanter
- Babcock's triangle (the head side and the neck side distinct foci have been observed)—Babcock's triangle is a weak part of bone that is watershed between obturator and ascending cervical circulation present in the lower half of head and adjoining neck region (near epiphyseal line) below the primary tensile trabeculae medial to primary compressive ones **(Fig. 46)**.
- Acetabular roof (lower aspect of ilium bone)
- Disease may also begin from trochanteric bursitis to involve the joint later.

Natural History of Disease

The disease begins near epiphyseal cartilage with formation of typical granulation tissue and caseous necrosis. This tissue extends beneath the cartilage that gets necrotic due to disrupted circulation from subchondral bone. The nude bone is attacked by pannus forming sequestrate filling the joint cavity. Muscles pull the femoral head upward to continue the acetabular destruction producing wandering acetabulum. In later stage the pus bursts out of capsule spreading along the lines of least resistance often to medial and anterior aspect of thigh. The pus may track along the sartorial canal to point in the lower thigh medially and even up to popliteal fossa **(Fig. 47)**.

Clinical Features

The classical clinical signs of tubercular hip infections are produced by the granulation tissue that results in loss of articular cartilage due to involvement of the subchondral bone, which deprives articular cartilage of its nutrition. Loss of cartilage results in joint instability and later joint destruction and ankylosis. With advanced hip involvement the physeal damage may result in angular deformities or limb length discrepancies.

- The first symptom to appear is stiffness of the limb that is conspicuous on getting up and passes as the day advances, returning next morning. The stiffness is gradually associated with pain to cause limp.
- The limp:
  - In early stages is caused by stiffness and flexion deformity of hip with body bending forward to compensate for inability to extend hip.
  - With disease progression the limp is due to pain from grating of nude bones.
  - Lastly the limp is due to real shortening due to destruction in advanced arthritis.
- Starting pains ("night cries") may wake the patient up due to relaxation of spasm and increasing inflammation and bones rubbing together. Pain in the hip region may be referred to areas distributed by femoral and obturator nerve.
- There is global limitation (limitation in all directions) of movements. Initially, there is FABER deformity (to accommodate the joint inflammation) that changes to FADIR (due to spasm) (see Staging in **Table 39**). With treatment and traction the other noncharacteristic

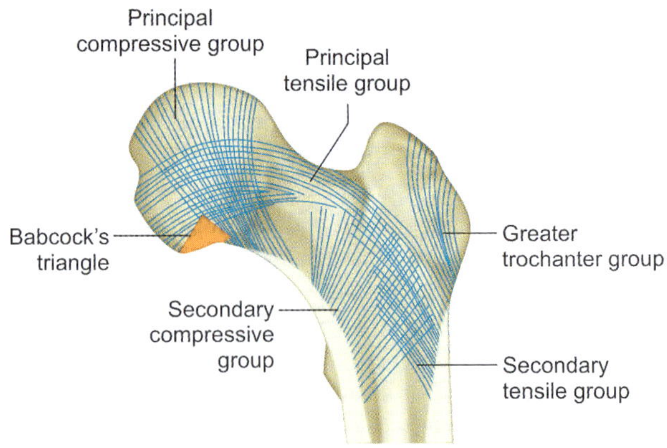

Fig. 46: The Babcock's triangle in femoral neck. It lies in subcapital region of femoral neck bounded by principal compressive trabeculae laterally and principal tensile group superiorly. Inferiorly, it is based on cortical bone of femoral neck. The triangle lies medial to Ward's triangle.

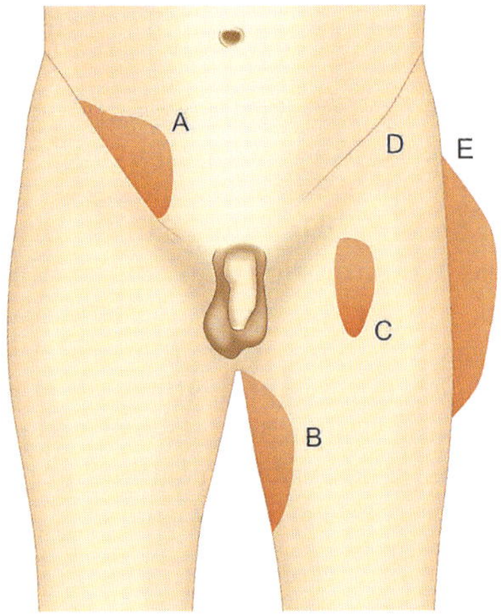

Fig. 47: The cold abscess of hip joint may track in various directions from groin region (A) to medial aspect of thigh (B) or appear in femoral triangle (C). It may track laterally in flank region along the iliac crest or the lumbar region (D) posteriorly (so not drawn here) or in the trochanteric region and below (E) or even in popliteal fossa along the sartorial canal (not shown).

TABLE 39: Clinical stages of tubercular arthritis of hip (modified from Tuli, Babhulkar).

Stage	*Pathology*	*Deformity and attitude of limb*	*Range of movement*	*Radiological features*
I (Stage of apparent lengthening)	Synovitis (Tuli and Babhulkar)	Abduction deformity (pelvic tilt), no true shortening. FABER (flexion, abduction, and external rotation)	>75% preserved	Osteopenia + haziness of articular margins
II (Stage of apparent shortening)	Early arthritis (Tuli and Babhulkar)	Shortening <1 cm, adduction deformity. Flexion, adduction, internal rotation (FADIR)	>50–75% preserved	Osteopenia + haziness of articular margins + marginal erosions
III (Stage of true shortening)	• Arthritis (Babhulkar) • Advanced arthritis (Tuli)	• True shortening >1 cm • FADIR + shortening	Loss of >75% movements	Osteopenia + reduction in joint space + joint destruc tion
IV (Terminal arthritis)	Advanced arthritis (Babhulkar), advanced arthritis ± pathological dislocation or subluxation, wandering acetabulum or ankylosed hip (Tuli)	• Shortening usually >2.5 cm • Usually FADIR. Shortening may be severe in wandering acetabulum or in cases with destruction of femoral head. Some ankylosed hip and partially treated disease may have flexion, adduction and external rotation (FADER) deformity.	Loss of >75% movements. Ankylosed hip will have complete loss of motion or only a jog of movement in fibrous ankylosis. Hips with destroyed femoral head may be hypermobile on the contrary, if pain has subsided, they are only limited by painful muscle spasm.	All above findings with joint disorganization

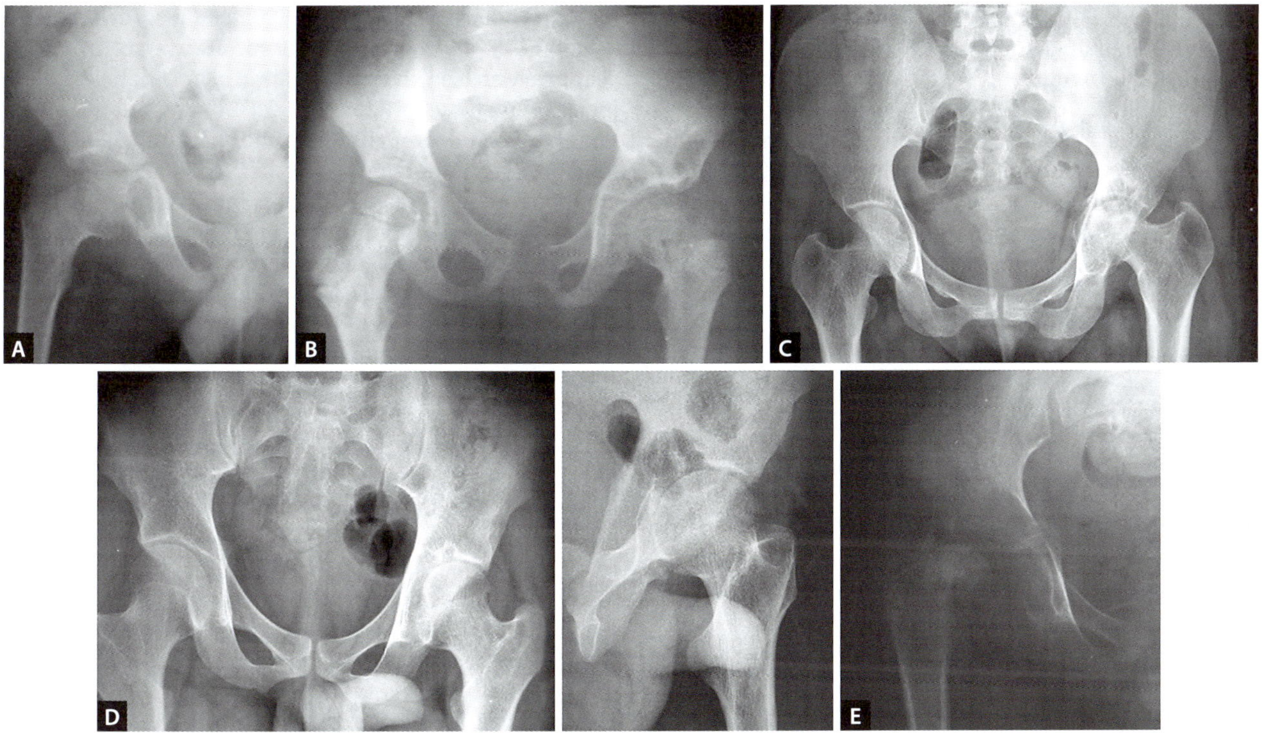

Figs. 48A to E: TB hip—note the different presentations: (A) Predominantly acetabular involvement in TB; (B) Bilateral and femoroacetabular involvement--note the ward's triangle lesion on right side while acetabular changes on left; (C) Protrusio type of TB hip; (D) "Kissing" lesions better depicted on lateral radiograph; (E) Shows the dislocated type with proximal femoral epiphyseal pathological fracture and developing wandering acetabulum.

deformities like FABIR (traction), FADER (spica cast) may appear.

- The cold abscess may be detected in:
  - Femoral triangle
  - Ischiorecteal fossa, lumbar region, flank, and along iliac crest
  - Thigh (anywhere along the subsartorial canal or medially from extension out of inferior capsule)
  - Uncommonly, it may be detected in popliteal fossa.
- Fibrous ankylosis of advanced disease produces fixed deformity.

Radiological Findings

Earliest sign is joint osteopenia that is grossly evident when looked at from a distance. With disease progression reduction of joint space, small erosions—Cat-bite lesions, perthes or osteonecrosis like femoral lesion, kissing lesion (complementary lesion in femoral head and acetabulum), wandering acetabulum, and pencil in cup appearance all develop **(Figs. 48A to E)**.

Shanmugasundaram divided the TB hip into seven clinicoradiological types **(Figs. 49A to G)**:

1. Normal hip—Minimal or initial disease, only synovial involvement minimal if any bony disease, no subchondral bone involvement.
2. Travelling acetabulum—Gradual destruction of bony acetabulum due to preferential location of disease here, weigh bearing part of bone eroded so that femoral head migrates proximally.

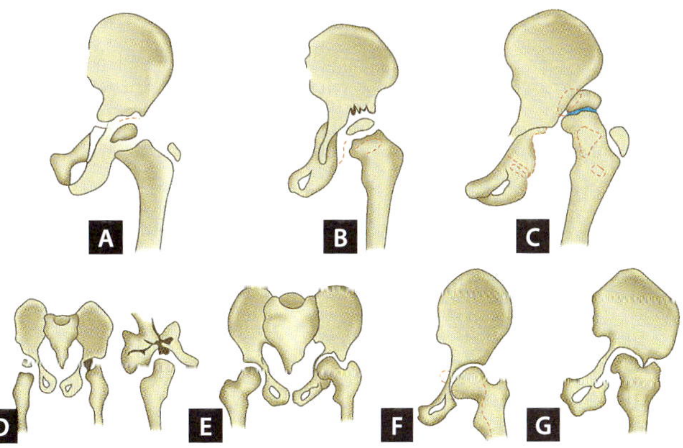

Figs. 49A to G: Clinicoradiological classification of TB hip as described by Shanmugasundaram: (A) Type 1—normal; (B) Type 2—travelling acetabulum; (C) Type 3—dislocating; (D) Type 4— Perthes; (E) Type 5—protrusio acetabuli; (F) Type 6—atrophic; (G) Type 7—mortar and pestle.

3. Dislocating hip—Partially destroyed head and acetabulum with constant adductor and flexor spasm pushing the head posterosuperiorly out of acetabulum. The capsule is also weakened or ruptured by chronic inflammation.
4. Perthes type—Superolateral disease and destruction of head. Sclerosis makes distinguishing the disease from Perthes difficult, presence of cyst and acetabular osteopenia may help in making diagnosis.
5. Mortar and pestle type—Gross destruction of head thin bone left and acetabulum acquiring saucer like shape.

6. Atrophic type—In stage of destruction, the disease burns out due to minimal infection.
7. Protrusio acetabulum—Due to softening of medial wall of acetabulum.

The first four types are commonly seen in children and have better prognosis with the normal type often becoming normal after treatment. The other three are seen in adults and have poor prognosis often needing joint reconstruction or salvage procedures.

Diagnosis and Diagnostic Tests

(See above)

Differential Diagnosis

The diagnosis is clinicoradiological in around 20% cases (not confirmed through microbiology or histopathology or rapid tests). Also in other early presentation the clinical signs are often dramatic to confuse the examiner for other possibilities so discussing the differential diagnosis according to presenting symptoms and elicited signs is better.

1. Limited movements:
   a. Osteonecrosis
   b. Nonunion fracture neck of femur
   c. Irritable hip
   d. Adductor irritation due to lymph nodes or injury
2. Limp:
   a. PIVD, trauma
   b. DDH—certain movements exaggerated
   c. Coxa vara—increased external rotation and deformity
   d. Perthe's disease—decreased wasting, increased bony changes in X-ray, few movements restricted
3. Pain:
   a. SCFE
   b. Septic arthritis
   c. Trauma to hip, secondary osteoarthritis and osteonecrosis
   d. Monoarticular RA
   e. Neoplastic lesion (chondroblastoma)

With complete evaluation of patient the following remain as the common differentials:

- ONFH
- Late onset perthes
- Monoarticular rheumatoid
- Subacute or partially treated septic arthritis
- OM proximal femur with reactive hip arthritis
- Uncommonly:
  - Nonunion fracture neck femur
  - Fracture acetabulum with migration of the femoral head toward pelvis
  - Ankylosing spondylitis

Treatment

Apart from the *antitubercular chemotherapy*, liberal diet education and discipline to restrict weight bearing and movements are important. In acute symptomatic stage give *traction* to the limb. Traction reduces pain, counters, and relaxes spasm by reducing pain, prevents deformity, maintains joint space, minimizes chances of wandering acetabulum, and corrects deformity. A weight of 0.45 kg/year of age is used given bilaterally (to prevent pelvic tilt and increase in abduction deformity). Abduction in the affected limb is given to compensate for the shortening and counter tendency for adduction. *Spica cast* with chemotherapy is cumbersome and disregarded in modern orthopedics for stiffness and painful joint that frequently results. Prognosis for a painless mobile joint with conservative approach is better if the disease is synovial or localized to neck of femur.

Surgery is indicated if there is inadequate response to conservative treatment or outcome of conservative treatment is not good (painful or deformed joint). Also if there is advanced disease with unstable hip joint (stage 4 or 5) surgery will be primarily indicated. In poor response to conservative treatment often the disease load is too high to respond to chemotherapy and joint debridement with excision of focus helps, this is however very infrequently required as an isolated procedure. The advantage is that material for reconfirmation or initial confirmation of diagnosis can be done. With gross joint destruction in healing phase surgical management to provide mobile or fixed painless joint is required. Arthrodesis of hip joint is preferred in a young adult patient with painful hip and doing laborious job for earning his living. In resistant TB cases that fail to respond to chemotherapy multiple debridements to clear disease and sequestra from joint (excision of focus) and obtain tissue for culture sensitivity may be required. It is preferable to do simultaneous arthrodesis in such cases for possible resurgence of disease following joint arthroplasty.

Arthrodesis of hip joint—The following are the various types of hip arthrodesis used in past. It is now a very infrequently done procedure (defunct) if ever. The details are mentioned only for historical interest:

Intra-articular:

- Central dislocation and internal compression arthrodesis of charnley
- Watson-Jones transarticular nail arthrodesis
- Double plating technique of Müller
- Intramedullary arthrodesis of Onji
- Cobra-plate arthrodesis
- Anterior plating technique.

Extra-articular:

- Iliofemoral arthrodesis of Albee
- Ischiofemoral arthrodesis of Brittain

Pararticular (usually done to augment intra-articular procedure): Davis muscle-pedicle arthrodesis.

Indications: Apart from the indications mentioned above for tuberculosis of hip, the following may also be considered for hip arthrodesis:

- Young patient with contraindication for THA like sepsis
- Salvage of multiply operated hip with poor soft-tissue support to provide a mobile joint.

Position of hip arthrodesis: There had been a large variability in recommending optimal position and the outcome based on difficulties in measuring them, choosing a fixed reference point/plane for a position and mobility of spine. The most avid position for arthrodesis of hip appears to be 20–30° of flexion, 5° of adduction and slight external rotation (5–10°). The flexion has always been debated and we feel the amount of required flexion depends on the type of job with more sedentary job requiring higher flexion than a job requiring predominant standing.

Assessment of the Positions of Hip Arthrodesis

Flexion: Due to normally existing lordosis of lumbar spine if the hip is flexed to straighten the lumbar spine (as is done in Thomas test), the angle formed between femoral shaft and the horizontal table explains the angle of flexion. In arthrodesis is done in insufficient flexion it will be uncomfortable while too much flexion will produce shortening. On an operating fracture table the flexion is determined in the last after adjusting for rotation and adduction. Limb is fully lowered to create normal lordosis, then with slowly raising the limb obliteration of lordosis and alignment to thoracic spine is noted (flat of table), fixing the limb in those position.

Rotation: The rotation is always checked with Patella position as there is knee rotation in extended position of the limb and even more rotation at foot giving no useful information of rotation at the hip in extended position on a fracture table. Patella should face slightly externally and not parallel to roof. Inturned foot due to internal rotation at hip will make the patient continually trip during walk while excessive external rotation will load the knee joint markedly in coronal plane during walking.

Frontal plane (abduction and adduction): This is a more complex adjustment. The mechanical axis of femur is perpendicular to the transverse axis through pelvis. The anatomic axis of femoral shaft is aligned 6–7° in adduction to this vertical line. Flexion at hip appears as increased abduction angle. Adduction of 3° creates a shortening of 1 cm while abduction of 3° creates lengthening of 1 cm. The apparent lengthening or shortening is only functional manifesting due to the pelvic obliquity. Adduction improves foot progression and reduces the energy of walking rather than dragging an abducted limb. But correction of limb length deformity might require abducting the limb for compensating for true shortening >1 cm. True shortening of >2 cm can be compensated by the abduction but abduction angles >6° will have negative effect and such patients might require two stage procedure.

Some techniques of arthrodesis of hips:

1. Schneider is credited with developing the *cobraplate technique* for hip arthrodesis. The advantages of this technique are:
   - No need of postoperative cast
   - Reliable fusion rate
   - Easier control of hip arthrodesis position

   The proximal femur is osteotomized to enlarge the area of contact and abductors are stripped off the ilium to accommodate the plate. Beauchamp modification includes avoiding the osteotomy and contouring the plate to match combined contour of new femoroacetabular articulation. Also the gluteus medius was detached as a bony piece and raplaced at the commencement of procedure rather than stripping the abductors.
2. *Anterior plating technique:* This specifically avoids the insult to abductor muscles and hip is approached through Smith-Peterson approach. The technique also facilitates the positioning of hip. Even with osteoporotic bone and bone loss due to various diseases the excellent fixation achieved with placement of plate along the pelvic brim with anteroposterior screws is favorable.
3. Double plating technique is useful for complicated hips, unreduced dislocations, avascularity of bony surfaces and those that have been multiply operated. A broad DCP is applied to the trochanteric bed while a narrow DCP is applied anteriorly.
4. Albee *method:* This technique was restricted only to the hypertrophic arthritis of hip (now almost always managed by arthroplasty). Through an anterior approach the hip was exposed and the upper surface of femoral head and corresponding acetabular region were rawed. Slowly they led to fusion.
5. Brittains *method:* A subtrochanteric osteotomy is performed at the level of ischium and with deeper dissection a trough is made in ischium through osteotomy. Tibial graft is then pushed through osteotomy to effect fusion in spica cast.

Contraindications of hip arthrodesis:

- Uncontrolled active infection—Due to use of indwelling implant one should wait at least 1 year after infection has healed.
- Should not be done if opposite hip and ipsilateral knee already arthrodesed.
- Severe degenerative changes in lumbar spine, opposite hip, ipsilateral knee.

Conversion to hip arthroplasty and performing ipsilateral knee replacement—Conversion of hip arthrodesis to arthroplasty is challenging as localization of hip center and leg-length discrepancies is not easy. The muscle strength is reduced after arthrodesis so the functional results of these hips are often inferior. The results of performing knee arthroplasty in the ipsilateral limb are poor if the hip is arthrodesed in poor position, in such case conversion to hip arthroplasty is recommended. If the hip arthrodesis is in proper position then knee arthroplasty can be cautiously performed.

Complications: Hip arthrodesis is associated with various complications:

- Malposition is the most common complication.
- Due to extensive nature of procedure hemodynamic stability, infection, and other wound complications are quite common
- Nonunion—may be improved with Davis type graft.
- Implant breakage
- Development of secondary degeneration in ipsilateral knee, contralateral hip, and spine

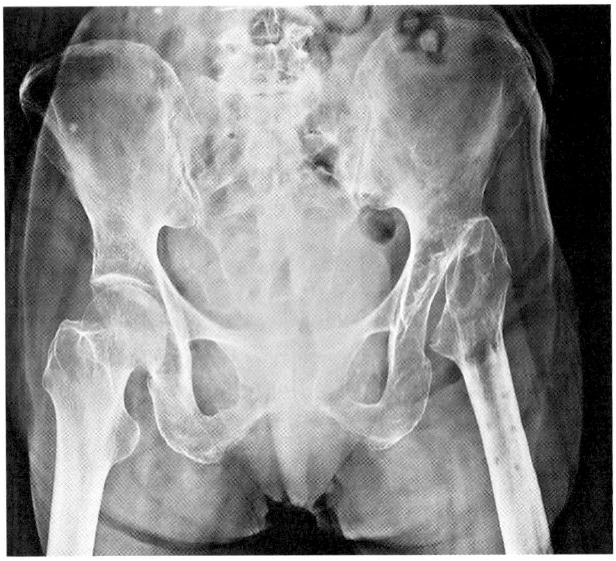

Fig. 50: Girdlestone arthroplasty—not a classical girdlestone indeed but this figure is included here for awareness. This was an infected hip resulting from DHS fixation of fracture intertrochanteric for which the implant and proximal femur were removed.

Girdlestone Arthroplasty

This is not a favorable option for management of hip pathologies. Only in patients needing salvage procedure for failed hip arthroplasty and refusing any further reconstruction does this procedure need to be advocated. Only other situation is in third world countries where patients do not favor a fused hip due to daily routine and habit and requirement of sitting on floor for personal and social reasons, a girdlestone procedure can be done **(Fig. 50)**. Although termed excisional arthroplasty (wrongly termed) the procedure does not deal only with the excision of surfaces rather the surfaces are recreated to provide a pseudo joint formation with intervening fibrous tissue. The concept was first used by A. White and described in detail in literature by G. Girdlestone. The original Girdlestone procedure was essentially a drainage procedure to provide a toilet to the infected hip joint. Transverse cuts were used to debride the joint and the wound was sealed by suturing the peripheral tissue to deep periosteum. The raw healthy exposed tissues were loosely packed with Vaseline gauge to provide drainage. The currently used procedure of preserving the acetabular bone and performing minimal resection is based on various modifications described over time important of which include:

- Taylor—Using the Smith-Peterson approach
- Nelson—Soft tissue interposition to effect pseudoarthrosis
- Nagi et al.—Subcapital osteotomy and reposing the neck into acetabulum with sutured anterior capsule to prevent fusion.

Postoperatively the patient is placed nonweight bearing walk for variable period (6–8 weeks) keeping the joint surfaces distracted to allow for stout fibrous tissue formation.

Complications:

- Infection and other wound complications
- Development of lurch is inevitable and hip is unstable—to stabilize hip a pelvic support osteotomy can be done later (see Section on Hip Osteotomies).
- Reduced power in the limb
- Development of pain after few years in the hip joint
- Degenerative changes in spine

Arthroplasty and joint replacement to provide painless mobile hip is increasing in use for a well-controlled disease but painful hip. Prerequisites for performing replacement include a quiescent joint both clinically and radiologically (increase bone density and thickness of trabeculae) with stable serology (normal ESR and CRP), absence of any pus/abscess cavity in bone or joint and no draining sinus tract. Historical recommendation of 10 years of quiescent disease possibly does not hold true with current treatment regimens and drugs. Antitubercular chemotherapy is given for 4–6 weeks before surgery (minimum 2 weeks) and is continued prophylactically as full course following arthroplasty. Large head prosthesis is preferred but metal on metal implants have been out of favor especially in young patients. The success rate had been high and reactivation is only sparingly reported with antitubercular therapy. The *M. tuberculosis* lesions represent a planktonic form which reproduces slowly, have minimal tendency to adhere to implants and do not produce slime or biofilm but they do have tendency for nidus formation and subsequent proliferation. Few authors have dared to perform total hip arthroplasty even for active disease preceded by antitubercular therapy and thorough debridement during index surgery reporting good outcomes of the approach. The surgery is followed by full course of antitubercular therapy for 9–12 months postoperatively. Both cemented and cementless implants have same successful outcome. Presence of a draining sinus tract suggests superinfection with other bacteria so a two-stage arthroplasty only should be done controlling infection in first-stage similar to revision arthroplasty principles.

HIV-ASSOCIATED MUSCULOSKELETAL CONDITIONS

Bacterial arthritis: There is no concrete evidence to suggest that bacterial infections of bones and joints occur more frequently than usual in HIV-infected individuals though some African studies suggest higher incidence of septic arthritis. This is surprising given the high incidence of staphylococcal bacteremia seen in these patients. When septic arthritis has been reported, it has usually been due to *S. aureus*, systemic fungal infection with *C. neoformans*, *Sporothrix schenckii* or *H. capsulatum* or to systemic mycobacterial infection with *M. tuberculosis*, *M. haemophilum*, *M. avium*, or *M. kansasii.*

Atypical mycobacterial infections: These tend to occur late when the CD4+ T lymphocyte count is <100/μL. Atypical mycobacterial species most commonly implicated in causing septic arthritis or osteomyelitis include *M. avium intracellulare* complex (MAI), *M. kansasii*, *M. haemophilum*, *M. terrae*, and *M. fortuitum*. *M. haemophilum* accounts for more than half of the cases. *M. kansasii* is second accounting for an additional 25%.

Some one-third of HIV-infected individuals experience arthralgias; and, 5–10% have some form of reactive arthritis, such as Reiter's syndrome, PsA or undifferentiated spondyloarthropathy. The frequency of these syndromes increase with disease progression and immunodeficiency possibly related to increase in the number of infections that may trigger reactive arthritis or due to reduced regulatory T-cells. These are managed well with standard treatment; however, therapy with MTX has been associated with an increase in the incidence of opportunistic infections and should be used with caution and only in severe cases.

HIV- or AIDS-associated arthropathy: This syndrome is a subacute oligoarticular arthritis that develops over 1–6 weeks and lasts for 6 weeks to 6 months. The large joints (knees and ankles) are predominantly affected producing only a mild inflammatory response and is nonerosive in nature. Radiographs are inconspicuous. NSAIDs are only marginally helpful; however, intra-articular glucocorticoids give good relief.

Osteonecrosis of distal metaphysis of femur, proximal shoulder, etc. have been associated with HIV infection seen in 4.4% of asymptomatic patients screened with MRI. Symptomatic osteonecrosis is found in 1% of cases. The cause is elusive but may be related to vasculitis, glucocorticoid or alcohol consumption. Some 10% of HIV-infected patients have been found to have symptoms of fibromyalgia.

Painful articular syndrome is another form of arthritis thought to be secondary to HIV infection in as many as 10% of AIDS patients. Patients experience acute, severe, sharp pain in the affected joint primarily involving the knees, elbows, and shoulders; lasting 2–24 hours; and may be severe enough to require narcotic analgesics. The cause of this arthropathy is unclear; however, it is thought to result from a direct effect of HIV on the joint.

Other manifestations: There have been reports of leukocytoclastic vasculitis associated with zidovudine therapy. CNS angiitis and polymyositis have also been reported in HIV-infected individuals.

Spirochetal arthritis: Syphilitic involvement of the joint is important both in congenital syphilis and in adults as also in patients with HIV. Organisms are detected in the early lesions and in paresis, but only rarely in other late lesions. Congenital syphilis may result in stillbirth or neonatal death. The basis of the lesions is an ischemia resulting from an endarteritis, along with a granulomatous reaction often rich in plasma cells (gumma). Characteristically, there is cortical destruction indicating osteomyelitis and nonspecific periostitis as well. Likewise, there may be inflammation of the epiphyseal and articular cartilage of the humerus and tibia. A Clutton's joint is a chronic hydrarthrosis of the knee joints and is a late manifestation of congenital syphilis. In acquired syphilis, bone infection overshadows the joint involvement. In tertiary syphilis, gummatous lesions of para-articular connective tissues may rupture into the joint space, resulting in large painless effusion mimicking neuropathic arthropathy. The synovium will show villous hypertrophy, perivascular lymphoid and plasma cell infiltrate, and endothelial proliferation. Syphilitic polyarthritis is described in patients with AIDS.

GOUT ("PODAGRA") (BIG TOE INVOLVEMENT), RICH MAN'S DISEASE, AND DISEASE OF THE KINGS

INTRODUCTION

Gout is the most common inflammatory arthropathy worldwide and its prevalence is increasing. Gout is also one of the oldest recognized arthropathies and the term "gout" was possibly first used by Randolphus of Bocking, around 1200 AD. Gout is derived from Latin word "gutta" meaning "a drop of liquid (poisonous)" possibly representing the residue left by blood ("dropping") around joints. Hippocrates noted its occurrence in his text especially the conspicuous absence in eunuchs. Galen first described the gouty tophi and Celsus recognized that gout afflicted the rich and powerful, especially those who were most overindulgent. Van Leeuwenhoek, the Dutch microscopist, sketched needle-shaped crystals obtained from a gouty tophus in 1679. In 1683, Thomas Sydenham, an English physician, described its occurrence in the early hours of the morning, and its predilection for older males. Gout was included among the first group of "inborn errors of metabolism" by Sir Archibald Garrod in 1909 who also described the relationship of crystals to gouty inflammation and asymptomatic hyperuricemia but the work was not recognized until monosodium urate (MSU) crystals were specifically identified in the synovial fluid of patients with acute gouty arthritis by McCarty and Hollander in 1961. Today, the term *gout* is used to represent a heterogeneous group of diseases found exclusively in the human species that include:

- An elevated serum urate concentration (hyperuricemia)
- Recurrent attacks of acute arthritis in which MSU crystals are demonstrable in synovial fluid leukocytes.
- Aggregates of MSU crystals (tophi) deposited chiefly in and around joints, which sometimes lead to deformity and crippling.
- Renal disease involving glomerular, tubular, and interstitial tissues and blood vessels
- Uric acid nephrolithiasis

In the present context the term "gout" will refer exclusively to the affliction of joints (the gouty arthritis). Gout roughly affects the same number of patients as RA. Primary gout is predominantly a disease of adult men with a 4:1 male to female ratio making gout as the major cause of inflammatory arthritis in men over the age of 30. In females the onset is less dramatic and often delayed (postmenopausal) secondary to other hyperuricemia-producing conditions.

Relationship of serum urate (uric acid) levels and gouty inflammation: Uric acid is a purine metabolite. Sources include virtually all cells, especially those rich in purine precursors (ATP), such as muscle, whether it is "our" muscles or those we eat. It is continuously synthesized, released and excreted. Its synthesis is accelerated with tissue injury. Uric acid level is lower in females, due to the action of estrogen, on promoting the excretion of uric acid by the kidney.

Hyperuricemia (supersaturation for urate in serum) is the pathogenetic common denominator through which diverse etiologic influences predispose to urate crystal deposition and the potential for the clinical events of gout. Although, hyperuricemia (traditionally defined as serum uric acid levels >6.8 mg/dL) is a necessary underlying feature of gout, it is in most instances insufficient for expression of the disorder. Thus, the distinction between hyperuricemia, a biochemical aberration, and gout, a disease state, is important. Uric acid (urate) crystallizes at a level that exceeds 6.8 mg/dL (with slight variation in temperature and pH). Above this theoretical limit of solubility, increasing risks for gout and urinary tract stones have been documented. In most population groups tested, application of the specific uricase-spectrophotometric serum urate assay has established upper limits of normal [mean + 2 standard deviations (SD)] of about 7 mg/dL in adult men and 6 mg/dL in premenopausal women. Some 10% people with hyperuricemia develop gout. The risk is 0.1% for values < 7 mg/dL, 0.5% when levels are between 7 and 8.9 mg/dL while 4.5% for levels > 9 mg/dL. Values > 9.0 mg/dL have higher (sixfold) predictive value but these patients represent only 20% of the gouty population. Additionally, the incidence of acute gouty flares in subjects at risk is approximately only 3% over a 5-year period. Hence just a diagnosis of hyperuricemia does not confer diagnosis of gout in clinically unrelated patients. Hyperuricemia is also of no clinical importance with respect to renal outcomes until serum urate levels reach at least 13 mg/dL in men and 10 mg/dL in women (uncommon) and even the urolithiasis develops in less than 0.4% patients (annualized risk).

PATHOPHYSIOLOGY (FLOWCHART 2)

Uric acid is the endpoint of purine (adenine, guanine, xanthine, and hypoxanthine) metabolism. The synthesis of purine is by two pathways. One is synthesis from nonpurine precursors that forms the bulk of uric acid component. The other is the salvage of free purine bases derived from the breakdown of nucleic acids of endogenous and exogenous origin. With inefficient salvage mechanism and greater synthesis is from nonpurine precursors, uric acid production is increased and gout may result.

The term *asymptomatic hyperuricemia* is applied to the state in which the serum urate concentration is abnormally high, but symptoms of urate crystal deposition have not occurred. High concentrations of uric acid may result from either underexcretion (90% of primary gout cases) or from overproduction **(Table 40)**. The former is known as primary gout. The function ($C_{urate}/C_{creatinine}$—100) is referred to as fractional urate excretion, or FE_{urate}, expressed as a percentage. Most gouty subjects have a lower FE_{urate} than do nongouty subjects. Gouty subjects require urate levels 2–3 mg/dL higher than nongouty subjects to achieve equivalent uric acid excretion rates. Overproduction (10% of cases) most commonly results from high rates of tissue degradation as one may see in patients on chemotherapy for neoplasms or myeloproliferative diseases or ethanol abuse and now with the use of diuretics extensively in management of hypertension. Excretion of urinary uric acid in excess of 600 mg/day (mean + 2 SD) indicates uric acid overproduction (measured on 2 consecutive days 5 days after initiating isocaloric purine free diet and patient not on any uricosuric agents). Values more than 1,000 mg/day are clearly abnormal. Some rare enzymatic deficiencies result in overproduction of uric acid. These include patients with phosphoribosylpyrophosphate synthetase overactivity, Lesch-Nyhan syndrome (hypoxanthine-guanine phosphoribosyl transferase (HGPRT) deficiency), and Von Gierke's disease (glucose-6-phosphatase deficiency, glycogenosis Type 1). The term *syndrome X* has been applied to a cluster of abnormalities, including resistance to insulin-stimulated glucose uptake, hyperinsulinemia, hypertension, and

Flowchart 2: Gout pathophysiology.

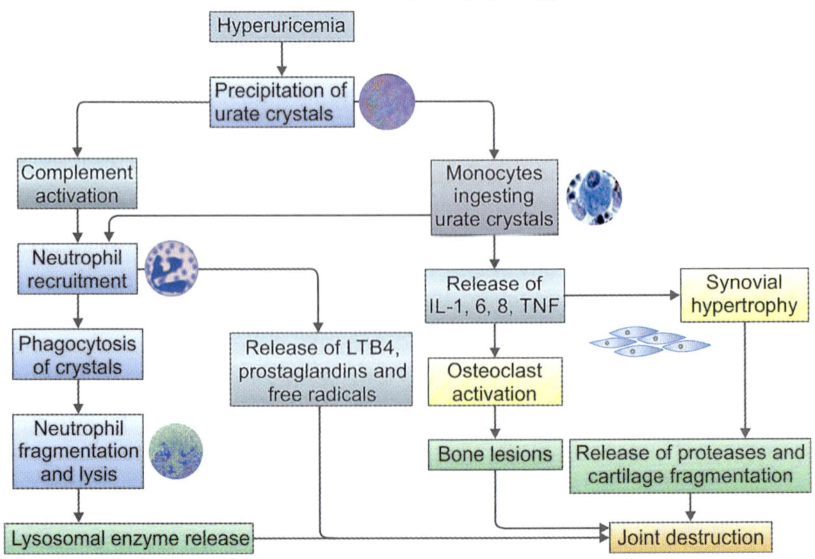

dyslipoproteinemia, that are characterized by high levels of plasma triglycerides and high-density lipoprotein cholesterol. Hyperuricemia closely correlates with the degree of insulin resistance and, therefore, is a likely feature of syndrome X. Factors that may result in the conversion of hyperuricemia into primary gout are as follows:

TABLE 40: Classification of hyperuricemia.

Type	*Metabolic disturbance*	*Inheritance*
Primary:		
Undefined molecular defects, underexcretion (90%) or over production (10%) of uric acid	Not established	Polygenic
PRPP synthetase variants—increased activity	Overproduction of uric acid	X-linked
HGPRT deficiency, partial	Kelley-Seegmiller syndrome	X-linked
Secondary:		
Complete HGPRT	Increased prine and uric acid synthesis; Lesh-Nyhan syndrome	X-linked
Glucose-6-phosphatase deficiency	Overproduction and under excretion of uric acid (glycogen storage disease—Type 1; Von Gierke's disease)	Autosomal recessive
Fructose-1-phosphate aldolase deficiency	Overproduction and under excretion of uric acid	Autosomal recessive
Increased nucleic acid turnover (tumor lysis syndrome, myeloproliferative disorders, hemolytic anemia, psoriasis, trauma, alcohol, cytotoxic drugs, and warfarin)	Overproduction of uric acid	Unknown
Decreased renal excretion of uric acid (alcohol, salicylates, diuretics, laxatives, cyclosporine, ethambutol, pyrazinamide, and levodopa)	Decreased filtration; inhibited tubular secretion or enhanced tubular reabsorption of uric acid	Some autosomal dominant, most unknown
Lead toxicity	Renal impairment and altered purine turnover	

(HGPRT: hypoxanthine-guanine phosphoribosyltransferase)

- Duration of the hyperuricemia (20–30 years)
- *Genetic predisposition:* Enzyme deficiencies as above
- Alcohol and dietary influences
- Obesity
- Thiazide diuretics, low-dose aspirin or chronic renal failure

Synovial fluid has low pH so urate crystals dissolve poorly more so in peripheral joints due to lower temperature there is higher likelihood of crystals to precipitate.

CLINICAL FEATURES

The symptoms of gout arise from precipitation of urate crystals into joint spaces especially feet (1st MTP joint classically called podagra), the marrow and the soft tissues **(Figs. 51A to D)**. The classical features of an acute attack of gout include:

- Pain that suddenly appears in 12–24 hours.
- Usually occurs overnight (metabolic changes).
- Skin over affected joint is red-purplish, tight, and shiny.
- Joints are painful, swelling, and warmth.
- Recurrent attacks in single episode are common.
- Patient may have systemic signs like fever, chills, malaise, and tachycardia.
- One to two joints affected at a time.
- Cooler joints affected more commonly because urate crystals form at cool temperatures.
- Podagra or pain in the first metatarsophalangeal joint is the classic presentation.

In the joints, an inflammatory arthropathy occurs that usually present as recurrent self-limiting attacks of synovitis (gout flare) producing a red, tender, hot, and swollen joint. Deposition in marrow causes intraosseous tophi that may lead to para-articular erosive changes, and the last causes hard, painless soft tissue tophi and inflammatory masses in the soft tissues. The pain in acute flare commonly is felt more at night due to lower temperature. Gout generally passes through four stages:

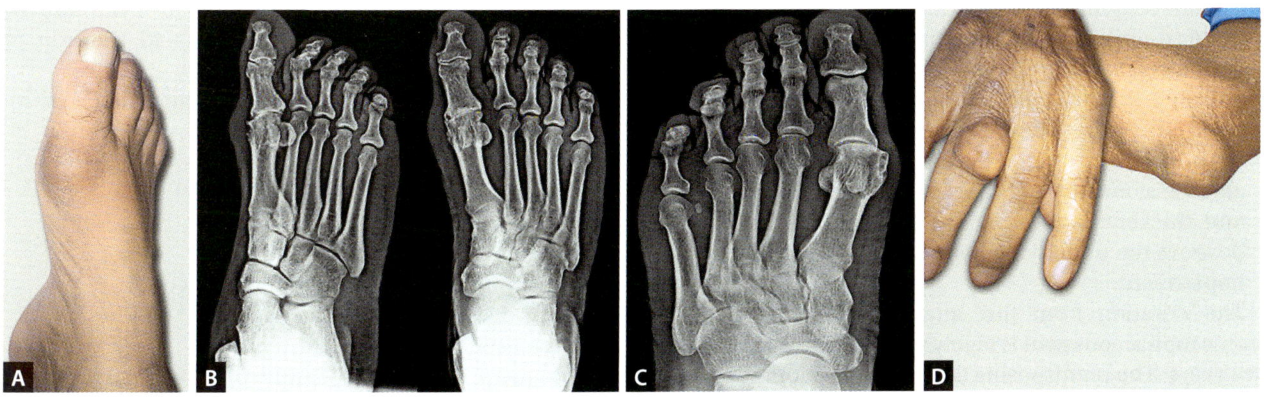

Figs. 51A to D: Gouty arthritis: (A) Typical affection (redness and swelling) of the 1st MTP joint in a patient with gouty arthritis; (B) The AP and oblique radiographs demonstrate arthritic changes in the MTP joint; (C) Note the presence of intraosseous tophus in the metatarsal head of gout patient; (D) The formation of tophi in various regions (PIP and elbow joints). (AP: anteroposterior; MTP: metatarsophalangeal; PIP: proximal interphalangeal)

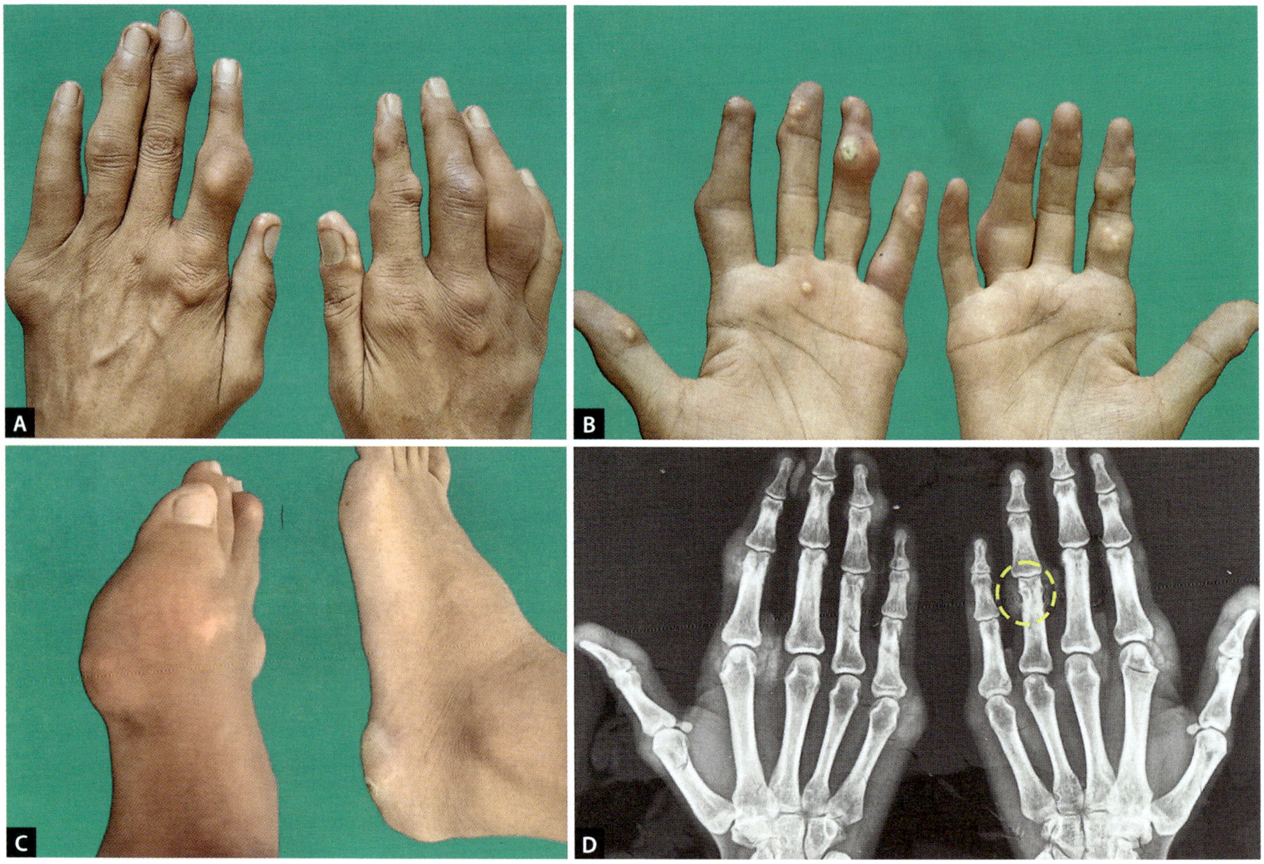

Figs. 52A to D: Clinical appearance of chronic tophaceous gout (A to C) showing ulcerations on the volar skin of hand and heel. The radiographs show erosion of bone from tophi (D, Dotted circle).

1. Asymptomatic hyperuricemia
2. Acute gouty arthritis (the gout flare) lasting few days to weeks
3. Intercritical (or interval) gout is the period when the symptoms resolve fully immaterial of how incapacitation the flare was. This freedom from symptoms during the intercritical period is an important feature in the diagnosis of an episode of acute arthritis as a crystal-induced process, potentially gout, and
4. Lastly chronic tophaceous gout **(Figs. 52A to D)** that is characterized by the identifiable deposition of solid urate (tophi) in connective tissues, including articular structures, with ultimate development of a destructive arthropathy, often with secondary degenerative changes. Here, due to repeated acute attacks monosodium urate crystals precipitate until visible deposits form and the synovium becomes progressively more fibrotic and thickened, with pannus formation. This pannus destroys the underlying bone and associated functional impairment.

The duration from first attack to development into chronic tophaceous gout is highly variable and ranges from 3 to 42 years. The predisposing factors for developing chronic tophaceous gout include:
- Genetic predisposition
- Obesity
- Hypothyroidism
- Cancers and blood disorders
- Alcohol abuse
- Duration of hyperuricemia
- Starvation
- Renal failure
- High intake of purine containing food
- Lead poisoning (moonshine whisky)
- Radiation treatment
- Age
- Pharmacologic agents (thiazides, cyclosporine, pyrazinamide, ethambutol, nicotinic acid, warfarin, and low dose salicylates).

The factors that often trigger an acute attack in such patients include:
- Injury
- Surgery
- Withdrawal of steroids
- Vascular disturbance
- Consumption of large quantities of alcohol
- Disturbed electrolyte imbalance
- Decreased urinary 17-ketosteroid
- Consumption of large quantities of purine rich foods
- Fatigue
- Emotional stress
- Illness

Tophaceous gout is often associated with an early age at onset, a long duration of active but untreated disease, frequent attacks, high serum urate values, and a predilection for upper extremity and polyarticular episodes. For tissue diagnosis the biopsy tissue sample should be fixed in ethanol and not 10% formalin as the crystals then dissolve and nothing is seen in polarizing microscopy.

A *tophus* is an aggregate of monosodium urate crystalline material with its accompanying inflammation and foreign body giant cells. This is the pathognomonic hallmark of this disorder. Tophi can be seen in the articular cartilage, periarticular ligaments, bone and tendons. They are also seen in soft tissue around olecranon and knee (patellar bursae), helix of ear (typical extra-articular site), kidneys, nasal cartilage, skin of the finger tips and soles. They may cause ulceration of the superficial skin infection and secondary septic arthritis.

The definitive diagnosis of gout relies on demonstration of monosodium urate crystals in synovial fluid or tophus; however, clinical diagnosis can be suggested by presence of six or more of the 11 criteria as proposed by American college of rheumatology as follows:

1. More than one attack of active arthritis
2. Maximum inflammation develops within one day
3. Oligoarthritis attack
4. Redness observed over joint
5. First metatarsalophalangeal joint painful or swollen
6. Unilateral first metatarsalophalangeal joint attack
7. Unilateral tarsal joint attack
8. Tophus (proven or suspect)
9. Hyperuricemia
10. Asymmetrical swelling within a joint on radiography
11. Complete termination of an attack

RADIOLOGY

The major role of radiography is to exclude other causes of arthritis during an acute attack. Typical early gout shows deposition of mildly hyperdense material in the soft tissues representing tophi adjacent to joints. The common joints affected are:

- First metatarsophalangeal joint
- Feet
- Tarsal joints
- Ankles
- Fingers
- Wrist
- Elbow

Over time the bones develop sharply punched out round to oval defects situated in the marginal areas of the joint that are surrounded by a sclerotic border. The appearance of clasp-like erosions in a distribution that is typical for gout is nearly pathognomonic. Calcification of tophi is unusual unless renal impairment is associated but some meniscal and cartilage calcification is seen in longstanding cases. Dual energy computed tomography is highly sensitive and specific in visualizing tissue stores of monosodium urate crystals as well as renal uric acid urolithiasis and has the potential to assist in diagnosis of gout in patients with hyperuricemia or joint pain, and to better quantify tophus dissolution in therapy.

DIFFERENTIAL DIAGNOSIS

Calcium pyrophosphate dihydrate disease (pseudogout), BCP arthritis, cellulitis, infectious arthritis, trauma, RA, psoriatic arthritis, erythema nodosum, and reactive arthritis.

TREATMENT

Medicines are the mainstay of treatment both in acute stage and chronic one. Detailed guidelines have been provided by American college of rheumatology **(Box 21),** the practical details are provided below.

- The treatment is aimed primarily at terminating the acute attack as fast and as gently as possible, to reverse or prevent complications of crystal deposition and to prevent recurrences of acute arthritis.
- Nonsteroidal anti-inflammatory drugs are the mainstay for controlling inflammation during acute attack or flare. Few NSAIDs also have uricosuric effect (etodolac and etoricoxib) and can be of clinical value.
- Corticosteroids (through various routes) have been found to be highly effective in controlling the acute flares. Some give injectable long-acting preparation (depot preparations) with oral steroids. Synthetic ACTH is also found useful for treatment.
- For acute severe attack (VAS of ≥7 on scale of 10) initial combination therapy with full dose of either (1) colchicine and NSAIDs, (2) oral corticosteroids and colchicine or (3) intra-articular steroids with all other modalities has been recommended. Colchicine has a low therapeutic index and usually an oral dose of 0.5 or 0.6 mg is taken hourly until one of three things occurs: (1) joint symptoms ease; (2) nausea, vomiting, or diarrhea develops or (3) the patient has taken a maximum of 10 doses. If 10 doses are taken without benefit, the diagnosis should be questioned. Colchicine inhibits E-selectin-mediated adhesiveness for neutrophils and diminishes neutrophil L-selectin expression, random motility, chemotaxis, PLA_2 activation, IL-1 expression, and the chemotactic factors CCF and LTB4. Apart from controlling acute attacks it is not as popular for prophylaxis or control of symptomatic hyperuricemia or intercritical illness.
- For inadequate response in an acute attack to ongoing therapy newer agents like canakinumab or other IL-1 inhibitor may be used. The criteria to define an inadequate response of acute gout to pharmacologic therapy is either <20% improvement in pain score within 24 hours or <50% improvement in pain score ≥ 24 hours after initiating pharmacologic therapy.

For chronic gout the pharmacotherapy is primarily directed to reduce the serum uric acid levels and prophylaxis for acute attack (Details in **Box 21**):

- Reduction of the serum urate concentration is achieved pharmacologically by:
  a. Increasing the renal excretion of uric acid (uricosuric agents) or
  b. By decreasing uric acid synthesis.

BOX 21: The updated 2020 American College of Rheumatology (ACR) guidelines for treatment of gout and urate lowering therapy (ULT).

Indications for Pharmacologic ULT:
- In line with the 2012 ACR guidelines for gout management, ULT is still the preferred treatment for most patients with gout.
- The guidelines subcommittee has included strong evidence to support initiating ULT in patients with gout who have any one of the following signs, including subcutaneous tophi (≥1), evidence of radiographic damage by any modality that appears to be due to gout, and frequent gout flare occurrence (>2 times/year).
- Recommendations for initiation of ULT were noted to be conditional for patients with a previous history of infrequent gout flares (<2 flares/year).
- The subcommittee has conditionally recommended against the initiation of ULT for patients who experience their first gout flare.
- In cases involving urolithiasis, stage ≥3 chronic kidney disease (CKD), and/or serum urate (SU) concentration >9 mg/dL, ULT can be conditionally recommended.
- The subcommittee has conditionally recommended against initiating pharmacologic ULT in patients with asymptomatic hyperuricemia (SU, >6.8 mg/dL and no previous gout flares or subcutaneous tophi), including those with comorbid CKD, cardiovascular disease, urolithiasis, or hypertension.

Choice of Initial ULT:
- Allopurinol has been strongly recommended as the preferred first-line agent for the treatment of all patients with gout, including those with moderate-to-severe CKD.
- Xanthine oxidase inhibitors (XOI) allopurinol or febuxostat have been strongly recommended over probenecid for patients with moderate-to-severe CKD, with pegloticase recommended against as a first-line therapy.
- Allopurinol may be strongly considered at starting doses of ≤100 mg/day, and at lower doses for patients with stage ≥3 CKD.
- For febuxostat, starting doses of ≤40 mg/day with dose escalation to reach optimal dosing has been strongly recommended as the second choice to allopurinol.
- When used as an initial therapy for gout, probenecid has been conditionally recommended at doses of 500 mg 1 to 2 times daily, with titration to higher therapeutic doses.
- The guidelines subcommittee has strongly recommended concomitant prophylaxis anti-inflammatory therapy with colchicine, nonsteroidal anti-inflammatory drugs, or glucocorticoids, such as prednisone or prednisolone, over no prophylactic treatment.
- Continuing anti-inflammatory prophylaxis has been recommended for 3 to 6 months over <3 months, with regular evaluation as long as gout flares persist.

Timing of ULT Initiation:
- Once ULT has been indicated for gout, clinicians may initiate treatment at the time of a flare rather than starting treatment after the flare has been resolved.
- The subcommittee has strongly recommended a treat-to-target strategy with titration to reach target SU over a fixed-dose approach for patients with gout receiving ULT.
- Achieving a stable SU target of <6 mg/dL vs. no target for patients receiving ULT has been strongly recommended.
- Augmenting the ULT treatment protocol with the supplementation of patient education, shared decision-making, and treat-to-target incentives by non-physician providers has been conditionally recommended.

Duration of ULT:
- The guidelines subcommittee has conditionally recommended continuing ULT indefinitely over stopping therapy.

The commonly used drugs and their rationale are discussed below:

- Allopurinol is a popular agent for its broad range of efficacy, safety profile, and easy dosing. Originally designed to be an antitumor agent, its primary biologic activity is to competitively inhibit xanthine oxidase. It is effective in virtually all cases of hyperuricemia but is typically indicated for:
  - Patients with either renal insufficiency or a 24-hour urinary uric acid excretion of >1,000 mg/day
  - Noncompliance or failure to respond to with uricosuric agents
  - A history of renal calculi of any type and a urinary uric acid excretion of >600 mg/24 hours
  - Prophylaxis or treatment of tumor lysis syndrome

  The older traditional approach to start patients on 300 mg/day has fallen into disfavor as most patients normalize with 100–200 mg/day. Also starting all patients at 100 mg/day and gradually increasing the dose every 4 weeks (up to maximum 800 mg/day) until a target serum urate level (<6 mg/dL) is reached, greatly decreases the chances of precipitating an acute gouty attack or of triggering a severe hypersensitivity reaction. The immune mediated allopurinol hypersensitivity syndrome (possibly related to HLA-B58) is rare but could be life-threatening and is characterized by fever, rash, generalized exfoliative erythroderma, marked palmar and plantar hyperkeratosis, Stevens Johnson syndrome, or toxic epidermal necrolysis. The dose needs titration to renal function, e.g., for creatinine clearance of 10–20 mL/min maximum dose is 200 mg/day and for clearance <10 mL/min, it is 100 mg/day. Oxypurinol (not available) is similar to allopurinol.

  Febuxostat (TMX-67) is a new class of uric acid lowering drug. It is a nonpurine, selective inhibitor of xanthine oxidase distinguishing it from allopurinol and oxypurinol that are nonselective inhibitors and inhibit at least five enzymes in the purine and pyrimidine pathway other than xanthine oxidase. Febuxostat is also not reincorporated into nucleotides and does not regulate pyrimidine metabolism. It has been found superior in reducing serum urate levels in stage 2 or 3 chronic kidney disease patients compared to allopurinol. There is recently a labeled warning concerning cardiovascular safety with the use of febuxostat. Feboxostat could be considered primarily in patients with compromised renal function (stage >2 CKD), urolithiasis, inability to increase hydration or identified uric acid production; however, allopurinol remains drug of choice for cardiac patients and otherwise. Tophus size is reduced by 50–80% after 1 year of either febuxostat or allopurinol treatment, with the greatest tophus and gout flare reduction linked to the greatest degree of serum urate-lowering irrespective of drug. All xanthine oxidase inhibitors should be used with great precaution for major interactions in patients receiving azathioprine, 6-mercaptopurine and theophylline.
- Uricase therapy has now found an established role. Expression of uricase enzyme ceased in human during evolution. The therapy is based on premises that the enzyme converts uric acid to allantoin (along with one hydrogen peroxide molecule) which is much more soluble, easily excreted end-product and the fact that rodents that express uricase have uric acid levels

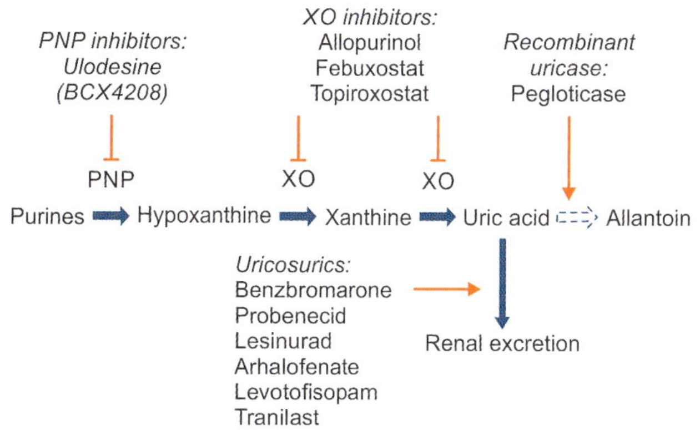

Fig. 53: The pathway of production of uric acid and various drugs that act within to help lower serum uric acid levels. (PNP: purine nucleoside phosphorylase; XO: xanthine oxidase)

less than 1 mg/dL. Rasburicase (the non-PEGylated recombinant fungal enzyme) has gone out of favor due to high antigenicity and plasma half-life of 18–24 hours. The recombinant porcine-baboon uricase (pegloticase) has less antigenicity and longer plasma half-life so that intravenous administration has shown good relief in refractory hyperuricemia and debulking of tophi in weeks to months (compared to years on allopurinol therapy). Pegloticase is a PEG-conjugated uricase produced by genetically engineered *E. coli*. The therapy is associated with oxidative stress (hydrogen peroxide) producing methemoglobinemia and hemolysis that could be substantial in patients with G6-PD deficiency.

- Future strategies and newer drugs for management of gout (also see **Fig. 53**):
  - Lesiunard is a new class of drug called selective uric acid reabsorption inhibitors (SURIs). It acts by inhibiting the urate transporter, URAT1, which is responsible for the majority of the renal reabsorption of uric acid. It also inhibits organic anion transporter 4 (OAT4), a uric acid transporter associated with diuretic-induced hyperuricemia. It is indicated in combination with a xanthine oxidase inhibitor for hyperuricemia associated with gout in patients who have not achieved target serum uric acid levels with a xanthine oxidase inhibitor alone. Adverse effects include renal failure and formation of renal stones. Verinurad is a very promising specific inhibitor of URAT1 with high affinity.
  - Arhalofenate also acts by blocking URAT-1; however, it also blocks the NALP-3 inflammasome providing gout-specific anti-inflammatory effect. Arhalofenate has a weaker urate-lowering effect than lesinurad.
  - IL-1 is a proinflammatory cytokine that has been shown to play an important role in gouty inflammation. MSU crystals activate the NLRP3 inflammasome through a number of pathways one of which causes activation of the important enzyme caspase-1, which leads to the generation of active IL-1β, resulting in an inflammatory response. IL-1 is, therefore, a prospective target for management of gouty inflammation. The drugs currently studied and some being used include canakinumab, anakinra, and rilonacept.
  - Canakinumab is a fully human monoclonal anti-IL-1β antibody. Administered subcutaneously as a single 150 mg dose that may be repeated 12 weeks later if symptoms recur. It has been used for management of flares and flare prophylaxis provided other optimized treatments have failed or there is contraindication to use of NSAIDs, colchicine or steroids. Canakinumab should not be commenced in patients with active or latent tuberculosis or neutropenia, and patients should be monitored for the symptoms of both tuberculosis and the development of neutropenia. Anakinra has similar profile to canakinumab but it is not recommended for treatment of gout for lack of evident literature.
  - Rilonacept acts as a soluble decoy receptor for IL-1α and IL-1β. Its role in flare prevention is being more focused than treatment of flares.
  - Topiroxostat is a novel, nonpurine, and selective xanthine-oxidase inhibitor that bears dual inhibitory effects. Similar to febuxostat, topiroxostat reduces uric acid production through chemical structure-based inhibition of xanthine oxidase. Akin to allopurinol, the drug covalently binds to, and inhibits, molybdenum-pterin, the active center of xanthine oxidase.
  - Pegsiticase provides a potent uricase activity and is aiming to decrease the inherent immunogenicity of recombinant uricases.
  - Ulodesine is a purine nucleoside phosphorylase (PNP) inhibitor being studied for treatment for gout. It acts upstream of xanthine oxidase in the purine metabolism pathway to reduce the production of hypoxanthine and serum uric acid.
  - Tranilast is an anti-inflammatory and immunmodulatory drug for treatment of asthma and atopic dermatitis. It has uricosuric action due to inhibition of both the URAT1 and GLUT9 urate transporters and combined treatment with allopurinol is more effective than either drug.
  - Levotofisopam is the S-isomer of racemic tofisopam (a benzodiazepine) that has been found to lower uric acid levels by increasing its excretion.
  - Bucillamine is an antirheumatic agent developed from tiopronin (derivative of cysteine) having powerful anti-inflammatory and antioxidant effects. It is being studied for controlling acute gout flares.

Lifestyle Modification and Ancillary Therapies

- Restricting dietary purine—the foods rich in purine that should be restricted from diet include:
  - Anchovies
  - Beans
  - Consommé
  - Herring
  - Meat gravies
  - Mussels
  - Sardines

- Shellfish
- Brewer's yeast
- Organ meats (liver, kidney, tongue, and tripe)
- Asparagus
- Broths
- Fish roe
- Lentils
- Mushrooms

- Weight loss in obese and hypertensive patients
- Alcohol restriction (especially beer as in addition to alcohol it is also a high purine rich food) should be emphasized.
- Increased coffee intake is associated with reduction in urate levels. Vitamin C may competitively inhibit the renal excretion of uric acid.
- Increase water intake (restrict in renal patients)—Calculated as a percentage as in 150 lb patient will need 75 oz H_2O/day; 96 oz during attack; 64 oz regularly daily and 30% more than normal overall.

Nondestructive and Nonproductive Arthropathies

These do not actually cause morphological alterations in joint architecture and hence technically are not arthropathies. These include the joint-related abnormalities of systemic lupus erythematosis (SLE), scleroderma, Ehlers Danlos syndrome, rheumatic fever, Jaccoud's arthropathy, etc.

CONCLUSION

- Synovial joints fall prey to both degenerative and inflammatory disorders. The former has gained importance mostly for its successful management by arthroplasty procedures that attract many young trainees to faculty!
- There is no definite medical cure for degenerative synovial joint disorder and mostly medicines are provided for symptomatic pain relief.
- Surgical management is the cornerstone for management of advanced degenerative joint disorder.
- Inflammatory arthritis is an important component of the overall spectrum that is responsible for immense morbidity and functional loss. The disorder is mostly progressive and commonly now taken over by rheumatologists. Orthopedicians should be, however, aware of the commonly used drugs for management of the disorder so that they can incorporate the same as a comprehensive management of deformities in such patients. The advancements are fast in the field and one needs to keep abreast by frequent readings else the flow is bound to quickly get lost and outdated!
- Seronegative arthropathy is an important component of progressive and severe disability to the patient that needs to be managed mostly by surgical measures. One should pay attention to details for procedures as the exposure is difficult and in ankylosed joints often the delineation is unclear, while one has to also compensate for the stiffness and limited mobility at other joints.
- With increased use of arthroplasty procedures for management of patients with advanced arthritis, the problem of periprosthetic infections is fast creeping up and is a common cause of failure of such procedures. It is important to realize the pathogens and pathogenesis of this condition to successfully take the patient out of this very disabling complication. It is important to realize the difference from classical teaching about microorganisms during graduation that there is another subset of organisms that grow and develop slowly and have all different characteristics and sensitivities, so their management is also altogether different.
- Tuberculosis is a rampant disorder in India and lately the diagnosis and management has undergone significant changes compared to the classical teachings prevailing for past 2 decades.

SECTION 3

Basic Sciences

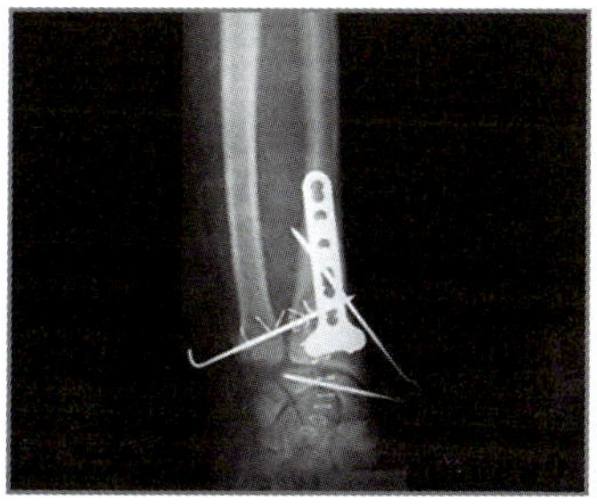

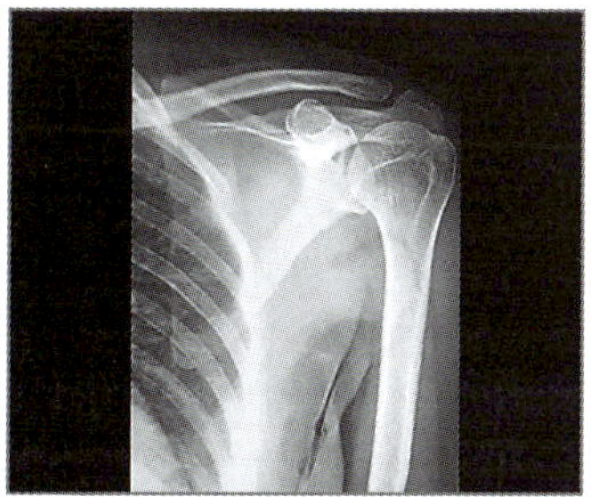

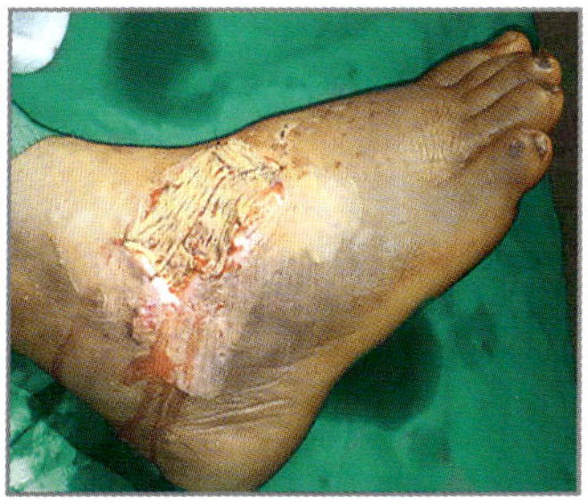

CHAPTER 11

Biostatistics, Ethics, and Research Methods

Manish Kumar Varshney

INTRODUCTION

The literature is ever-growing with continuous reporting of new modalities of treatment, comparison of existing ones with newer ones, comparisons among newer treatment themselves, new techniques of treatment, changed guidelines, and recommendations. These are growing at a fast pace and have variable quality of research involved behind them. The practicing surgeon and researcher both need to understand the relevance of published evidence to apply the appropriate interventions and address the healthcare needs. Nothing is sacrosanct and even best of the current evidence may not be appropriate for a particular situation, especially the "details" of that specific study or recommendation. To understand the criticality, one needs to have basic understanding of biostatistics based on which the evidence was generated. Biostatistics provides the scale in which the information is reviewed, analyzed and generated to decipher strengths and limitations of evidence. The treatment should be based on available evidence but in no way should be copied from it as guidelines/recommendations are meant for population in general while managing an individual patient requires incorporation of specific needs, experience of the treating physician, available options, and then choosing the appropriate treatment based on sound evidence. This practice of evidence-based medicine (EBM) has drastically changed the way disorders and diseases are treated in modern world that involves integration of individual clinical expertise with the best available external clinical evidence from systematic research.

EVIDENCE-BASED MEDICINE

Evidence-based medicine has its philosophical origins from 19th century but was specifically defined by David Sackett in British Medical Journal (BMJ) in 1996 as "conscientious, explicit, and judicious use of current best evidence in making decisions about the care of individual patients". This emphasizes combining individual clinical proficiency gained through experience with externally validated research to guide clinical assessments and treatment. Best available validated evidence/research means clinically relevant literature from the basic sciences of medicine or clinical research into the accuracy and precision of diagnostic tests (including the clinical examination) and/or the power of prognostic markers and/or the efficacy and safety of therapeutic, rehabilitative, and preventive regimens. The practice of EBM essentially involves five steps in sequence **(Fig. 1)**:

1. *Formulating an answerable question:* The diagnostic, prognostic, therapeutic, and other clinical and healthcare issues are converted into answerable questions to gather information.
2. *Gather evidence:* Extensive review of literature is done relevant to the formulated questions to find best evidence usually from level 1 studies, systematic reviews, and meta-analyses.
3. *Appraise the evidence:* Critical appraisal of evidence for its validity (closeness to truth) and usefulness (clinical applicability) is done by asking questions such as "how good is the evidence?" and "is the evidence pertinent to present situation?" One should realize that "perfect evidence" should never be sought as it is impossible.
4. *Implement evidence:* This involves integration of the appraisal with our clinical expertise and apply it in practice.
5. *Evaluate the process:* This involves audit of above and cycling it for other information seeking.

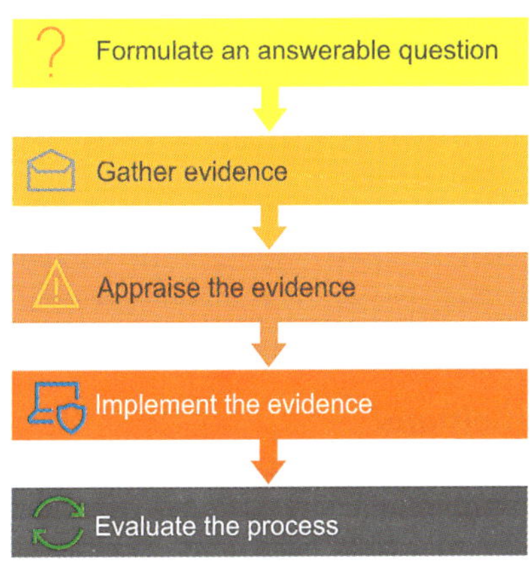

Fig. 1: The steps involved in evidence-based medicine.

BOX 1: The systematic reviews (SyRs) and meta-analyses (MAs).

Systematic review: The aim of a SyR is to use systematic methods to summarize empirical evidence to produce reliable findings that inform decision making (Cochrane, 2021). They are high level summarization of medical reports on a specific clinical question, using explicit methods to search, critically appraise, and synthesize the world literature. Most of available literature reviews and research articles do not involve a systematic search of the literature, but rather authors select the articles reviewed which may result in selection bias. SyR reduces this bias and combines patient outcome to provide a comprehensive synthesis of available evidence on a given topic from various clinical trials. SyR also vary in quality. Robust, reproducible methods for determining eligibility criteria for studies will result in a higher caliber SyR. The creation of a comprehensive and well-conceptualized protocol for study inclusion is an essential component of a strong SyR. The first step for performing SyR is identification of study purpose and an answerable question. Inclusion and exclusion criteria are then determined based on Preferred Reporting Items for Systematic Review and Meta-analysis (PRISMA) flowchart. This enables researcher to focus on dedicated studies, prevents duplication of efforts, and avoids arbitrary review. Extraction of data from standard electronic databases such as Cochrane Library, PubMed, and MEDLINE is done based on checklist provided by Spindler et al. The quality of SyR will be based on choosing studies that have high quality methodology and appropriate grading of evidence and strength of recommendation.

Advantages: SyR provides a comprehensive understanding of the state of the evidence for a specific topic. The knowledge gained through SyRs can provide synthesized empirical support for implementing certain practices or it can suggest areas in need of further research when results suggest practices may be ineffective or lacking support.

Limitations: SyR can be time intensive and require a rigorous methodological approach. They require significant planning and forethought to develop methodology. It is quite challenging to review studies that have been conducted in different ways and incorporate different variables or measures and present a quandary as to how best to capture study methods and appropriately synthesize findings. The approaches are continuously enhancing with the use of multilevel modeling, effect size calculation for single-case design studies, and means for assessing publication bias, all of which require high level understanding of statistical methods.

Meta-analysis: MA is a subtype of SyR. In MA the data from individual studies is pooled quantitatively and reanalyzed using established statistical methods. By quantitatively combining outcomes from all relevant studies, a MA can provide specific estimates of efficacy that are more precise than single studies because they are computed from a larger body of information (Cochrane, 2021). Because the samples of the individual studies are combined, the overall sample size is increased, thereby improving the statistical power of the analysis as well as the precision of the estimates of treatment effects. MA is a two-stage process where first stage involves calculation of a measure of treatment effect with its 95% confidence intervals (CIs) for each individual study using statistics such as odds ratios (OR), relative risks (RR), and risk differences. The second stage of MA focusses on calculating overall treatment effect as a weighted average of individual summary statistics. Greater weights are given to the results from studies that provide more information, because they are likely to be closer to the "true effect". The weights are often the inverse of the variance (the square of the standard error) of the treatment effect, which relates closely to sample size. MA is specifically useful when studies offer conflicting results of varying strengths. The results are typically displayed as a "forest plot" in MA. In SyRs generally, and MAs specifically, a discussion of the way in which the authors reduced their risk of bias is also considered best practice (referred to as publication bias; McClain et al., 2021). Although MAs rely on quantitative data, a different form of SyR called a meta-synthesis summarizes qualitative studies. The differences between SyR and MA are presented below for better comparative understanding.

Systematic review	***Meta-analysis***
More of a qualitative attempt to answer specific question	Objective attempt to synthesize collection of results of similar research studies
Identify and critically analyze relevant research studies	Identify relevant research studies using a defined protocol (weighted average, defining quality of evidence, etc.)
Discuss factors that may explain heterogeneity	Statistical test studies heterogeneity and investigate explanatory variables
Synthesize knowledge	Statistically summarize results to obtain an overall estimate of treatment effect

Despite improving the level of research and improved reliability of evidence it is not without limitations. Ultimately mechanistic logic is applied to deduce and apply large population studies to individual patients. Clinical trials often have underrepresentation of patients due to limitations in funding, resources, geographic location, demographics, comorbidities, confounding, unidentifiable variables, less than perfect understanding of diseases and reliance on statistical significance over clinical significance, etc. EBM continues to evolve to answer various study questions from different locations and aspects so systematic reviews and meta-analyses **(Box 1)** provide the current high level matched evidence. A basic understanding of how this evidence is generated and in turn explaining how the available evidence should be read by a researcher is the core reason of learning biostatistics.

Some Definitions

A *statistic* is a numerical characteristic of a sample.

Data is a set of observations made on one or more chosen variables to define various parameters in study (observational, epidemiological, comparative, and outcome).

A *variable* is a quantity that may vary from one object to another having a particular measurement scale or may vary between presence to absence only (discussed below). A *sample* (or dataset) is a compilation of values of one or more variables.

The *sample space* or *population* is the set of all possible values of a variable.

Each member of the sample is an *element.*

The *size* of a sample is the number of elements in the sample.

An *empirical relative frequency distribution* (ERFD) is an empirical frequency distribution, where the frequencies have been divided by the sample size. Many authors omit the adjective *relative,* so that "frequency distribution" is used in short for "ERFD". The *empirical cumulative distribution* (ECD) of a variable is a listing of values of the variable together with the *proportion* of observations less than or equal to that value (cumulative proportion).

Point estimate is the single number that provides best estimate for a variable.

Confidence interval is the range of values in which the correct value is likely to lay, e.g., 95% confidence interval where there

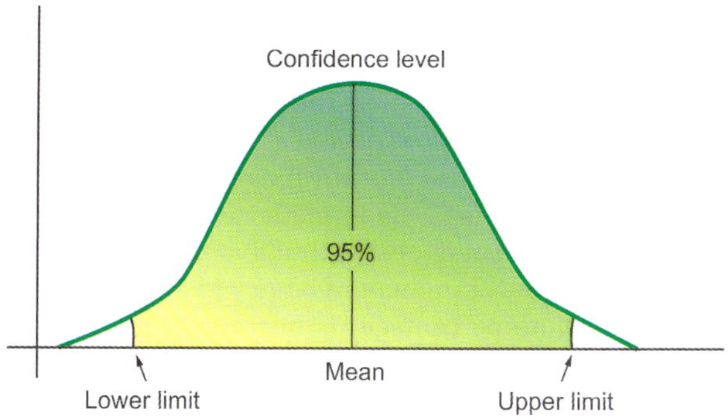

Fig. 2: Confidence interval.

Flowchart 1: Different types of variables.

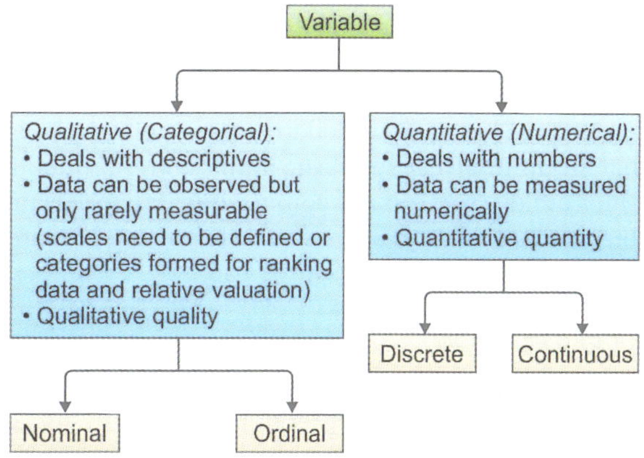

is 5% chance that the correct value lays outside the estimate **(Fig. 2)**.

In *statistical inference,* the investigator tries to find out the population value (true value in whole population) from a sample analysis.

In *hypothesis testing,* the goal is to find out, if the question is true.

In *decision analysis* the results of statistical interference are combined with hypothesis testing with information about outcome to determine the optimal treatment.

THE MEASUREMENT SCALES

Variables for measuring outcomes or observation can be one of the following types **(Flowchart 1)**:

- *Nominal* (text, categorical).
- *Ordinal* (rank order or ordered categories)
- *Interval* (scaled without an absolute zero point)
- *Ratio* (scaled with an absolute zero point)

These scales are often referred to as either *qualitative* (nominal and poorly ordered scales), or *continuous* (well ordered, interval, or ratio).

Qualitative (Categorical) Variables

A *qualitative variable* has values that are intrinsically non-numerical (cannot be expressed in finite numbers (like sex of a person—either male or female but no number), the number represents only relative ranks or a chosen scale).

These variables can be categorized into groups (categorical, like the number of males or females). All qualitative variables are "discrete", that means one is self-explanatory and separate like a female will be an individual entity that another female or male. It must be remembered that not all discrete variables are qualitative though (see below). The values of a qualitative variable can always be put into numerical form (viz. total number of positive response, etc.), but they do not represent the intrinsic value (e.g., weight of a person will be a finite number and will be quantitative, but level of intelligence will be expressed as a qualitative form that can be applied a number to categorize specific level, the number does not measure true intelligence). The simplest numerical form is consecutive labeling of the values of the variable. The values of a qualitative variable are also referred to as *outcomes* or *states.* This involves "counting" of responses. Qualitative variables can often be ordered or ranked that places a set of objects in a sequence according to a specified scale or nominal having distinct categories (gender, success/failure, etc.). There are three types of categorical variables, viz. (1) ordinal, (2) nominal, and (3) binary (dichotomous).

1. Ordinal variable—a categorical variable with some intrinsic order or numeric value, e.g., education (illiterate, high school, graduate, and postgraduate), rating (excellent, good, fair, and poor), or any other scale.
2. Nominal variable—a categorical variable *without* an intrinsic order, e.g., gender (male/female), favorite treatment [conservative, minimally invasive, and open reduction and internal fixation (ORIF)], residence (village, district, town and metro), and nationality.
3. Dichotomous (or binary) variables—a categorical variable with only two levels of categories. The answer to it is "yes" or "no".

Quantitative (Numerical) Variables

A *quantitative variable* has values that are numerically expressed:

- The quantitative variables that have numerical values expressed as pure integers are discrete in true sense. Such variables are called *discrete variables.*
- Other quantitative variables that have values potentially or really associated with real numbers (decimals, fractions, and zero values) will have continuous denominations—such variables are called *continuous variables,* and can be expressed in interval or ratio.

Most quantitative variables are continuous variables. We could refine some measurements to precise values (like say, hours, or even, to minutes or seconds). This refinement can vary between variables and often by experience or by the need of study a reasonable unit is often assumed to serve the purpose. A *pedantic* unit is too refined and is used in studies that do not permit errors in measurements or where such errors are likely to yield unacceptable results (say study on life-saving drugs), on the other hand a *rough* unit does not distinguish between the objects on fine readings and the variable is measured roughly to yield a gross differentiation.

Discrete Variable

Variables that can only take on a finite number of values are called "discrete variables". Some quantitative variables are discrete (expressed in integers), such as performance rated as 1, 2, 3, 4, or 5, or age rounded to years or episodes of acute lumbar strain in a year requiring admission. All qualitative variables are discrete, do not confuse qualitative variable to be equivalent to discrete only as all discrete variables are not qualitative they can be quantitative also.

Continuous Variable

Variables that can take on an infinite number of possible values (decimals fractions, zero values and so on) are called "continuous variables". There is no limitation on the values that the variable can take other than that which restricts us when we make the measurement.

Note: There is a significant overlap in the terms parametric, nonparametric, qualitative, quantitative, continuous, and discrete. A simpler guide is to follow parametric and nonparametric data as explained later (under normal distribution). Discrete variable can be both qualitative (mostly) and quantitative (sometimes) but continuous variable is only quantitative.

DERIVED DATA

Some data are used in medical field as follows:
- Percentages—often the data is measured as percentage of improvement, e.g., percentage improvement of shoulder abduction with physiotherapy. In this case, it is the level of improvement, rather than the absolute value, which is of interest.
- Ratio or quotient—classic examples are international normalized ratio (INR) and body mass index (BMI).
- Rates—sometimes disease events are expressed as those occurring among individuals over a period, e.g., number of pathological fractures in osteoporotic patients occurring over a period.
- Scores—like constant scores and injury severity scores. These are now very commonly used in studies to report outcome or decide management.
- These variables are often statistically analyzed as numerical variables.

CENSORED DATA

This data is mainly unaccounted for in clinical trials. Various laboratory parameters are unable to report values below threshold (say cultures of samples containing few bacteria will be reported sterile but in fact they do contain bacteria). Also patients withdrawing before study ends will not be accounted for in the study, though they may be dissatisfied with the treatment and their outcome will be affecting the overall scores of treatment.

BIAS

Bias is the existence of calculation or interpretation or methodology that deviates from population parameter of interest or any tendency which prevents unprejudiced consideration of a question. Bias introduces systematic unwanted error in the study parameters that influences the outcome and hence the interpretation of results. In statistical term bias refers to a situation in which the statistical method used actually does not estimate the measure which is being thought to be estimated or produces an environment that prevents such a measure thus invalidating the results. Also the test of hypothesis is made ineffective. Bias cannot be interpreted as present or absent, but in a larger perspective some or the other component of large variability of bias (in terms of absolute percentage) is nearly always present in even the best of studies. Unlike random error that arises out of sampling error or study performance bias is independent on sampling size or set level of significance. Bias cannot only alter results, but also even provide exactly opposite results than present in reality. Some common forms of bias in clinical study are as follows:

- ***Bias at inception of study (pretrial bias):*** These are the most dangerous bias and commonly seen in a poorly organized study. They introduce errors that get transmitted or even amplified throughout the study.
  - *Definition bias:* During study design the "patients", disease, inclusion, and exclusion criteria all need to be defined. However, as there is no single standard that has no interobserver variability, there will always be a difference in defining the criteria for a patient, e.g., radiologic grade of osteoarthritis (OA) or chondromalacia. Such variability of expression and gray areas can present immense variability later. Even validation tools have failed to unify the outcome so late in study, the observer variability will also creep in even though the observer in unbiased. The interobserver variability can be minimized though not absolutely eliminated by following standardized protocols for data collection and training the study personnel, especially in studies, where multiple observers are collecting and entering data.
  - *Selection bias:* Here some individuals are more likely to be assigned in a particular group or study unbalancing the comparison groups. This results in biased samples and influences the whole study later. This is also termed *Berksonian bias*. Retrospective cohort and case-control studies are prone to this type of bias in which the outcome and exposure have occurred before the selection of patients. Prospective studies particularly randomized controlled trials (RCTs) are less prone to this.
  - *Attrition bias:* Is said to arise when the elements of sample lost to follow-up in a longitudinal study differ in a systematic way from those *not* lost to follow-up.
  - *Admission rate bias:* Patients may differ from recruiting from different institutions.
  - *Channeling bias:* Occurs when patient prognostic factors dictate the study cohort into which the patients are placed. Younger patients with fracture of wrist are more likely to be operated by surgeons compared to older patients so that younger patients will get "channeled" into the operative arm.

- *Response bias:* Is a randomly introduced error that is caused by difference in characteristics between those who choose or volunteer to participate in a study as opposed to those who do not.

▪ ***Bias during the trial implementation:*** It includes:
  - Spectrum bias arises from evaluation of diagnostic tests performed on this biased sample of patients resulting in altered sensitivity and specificity estimates (usually overestimation).
  - *Interviewer bias:* Occurs due to difference between how information is given, taken, and interpreted. Particularly, if the interviewer knows the disease status of patient the bias creeps in so blinding is a good resort to limit this.
  - *Chronology bias:* Occurs when the comparison groups are from two different time periods like choosing historic controls for present patients. A prospective cohort or RCT will minimize this chronology bias. If this is not possible then it is prudent to use historic controls from only very recent past, so that the effect of time on variables or otherwise is minimized.
  - *Central tendency bias:* Arises when using a Likert scale (comprising a small number of graded alternative responses such as very poor, poor, no opinion, good, and excellent) where responders tend to move toward the midpoint of the scale (usually "no opinion" or "just right").
  - *Recall bias:* Arises in studies particularly following patients with questionnaires or interviewing patient's treated in past. The patient's perceptions get altered by good and bad feelings of the outcome presenting a biased perspective of the treatment. Recall bias in medical studies are most likely when exposure and disease status are known at the time of conduct of study, so that it influences the response systematically. To minimize this bias highly structured questionnaire and methodology (such as used in SF-36) can be used or dummy questions may be introduced as marker.
  - *Estimator bias (observer bias):* Arises from difference in observer expectation and the observed values of parameters. This bias can be readily reduced by blinding the observer.
  - *Lead time bias:* Occurs particularly in studies assessing changes in survival over time where the development of more accurate diagnostic procedures may mean that patients entered later into the study are diagnosed at an earlier stage in their disease, resulting in an apparent increase in survival from the time of diagnosis.
  - *Omitted variable bias (associated with confounding):* Arises when an independent variable is falsely neglected or removed due to faulty study model assuming a particular specification only.
  - *Measurement bias:* Arises when a systematic error is introduced by an inaccurate measurement tool (e.g., a set of poorly calibrated scales); it may also be introduced by digit preference or rounding error.
  - Detection bias is where a characteristic is more likely to be observed or ascribed to or reported for a particular set of study population/subjects. For instance, in older patients surgeons are inclined to look for osteoporosis more often as a cause of back pain.
  - *Transfer bias:* Arises when patients are lost to study due to emigration or unwillingness to participate or change in contact details. It is imperative to define if such patients are different to those being followed as sometimes patients may be averse to respond for bad experiences being part of study.
  - Exclusion bias arises due to the systematic exclusion of certain individuals from the study.
  - *Performance bias:* There being high variability in performing even routine surgeries and "surgeon's choice" for surgical plan, flow of operation and technical maneuvers bias may creep in due to some fine surgeries versus crude surgeries. Same surgeon operating on all patients will reduce the bias greatly.

- ***Post-trial bias:*** Occurs during data analysis or publication.
  - *Citation bias:* Occurs when the investigator conceals particular results (usually the unfavorable ones) and presents a "cooked up" analysis. This may arise in part to prevent negative effect on their personality or from sponsor pressure to suppress the negative aspects. Also "expected" outcomes when differ largely from the "observed" outcomes sometimes discourage the investigator from reporting the "other" events. To reduce this effect the International Committee of Medical Journal Editors (ICMJE) released a consensus statement in 2004 which required all RCTs to be preregistered with an approved clinical trials registry.
  - *Reporting bias (multiple comparisons and data dredging):* When reporting the results often the insignificant data are ignored and significant comparisons are reported to make report "interesting" or significant. This can be done by multiple comparisons to "dredge" the data and even manipulate the p-value especially while testing null hypothesis. With skewed data the reporter may selectively choose to either modulate the p-value by selecting "out of proportion" values for variables.
  - Funding bias is of concern as it may totally mislead the study and its outcome. This bias is introduced by warped selection of outcomes, test samples, or test procedures that specifically favor a study's financial sponsor.
  - *Internal and external validity:* Internal validity is the reliability/accuracy of the results in explanatory trials. This is an indirect measure that ascertains the author's and reviewer's confidence in study. An internally validated study will have optimized study design, implementation, and analysis that have minimized or eliminated bias. Such a study will have findings representative of the true association between exposure and outcome that can be reproduced and concluded with high degree of power. External validity is a measure of research design that

deals with external application of the study based on degree to which outcomes/findings can be accurately generalized to other groups or populations. Pragmatic trials to this end are designed to assess benefits of interventions under real clinical conditions that incorporate as many possible clinical scenarios or population groups encountered. These trials have thus minimal exclusion criteria to incorporate most scenarios and making them very similar to general population, but in this context may reduce internal validity if inclusion criteria are weak.

- *Confounding (hidden variable and lurking variable): Confounding* is occurrence of spurious association between a potential risk factor and a disease or on the contrary missing a real association between them. Confounding can occur by *observed association* due to one of the three factors—the exposure (cause), the outcome (effect), or a third independent factor associated with both effect and the cause but is either unknown to investigator or unaccounted for in the study. This extraneous variable (confounder or confounding variable) could have a positive or negative association with dependent and independent variable, but in any case surely affects the outcome analysis. In analyzing the effect of smoking on coronary heart disease (CHD) alcohol consumption will be an important confounder as it has direct association with CHD and also most of the smoker will also be consuming alcohol. There are instances when this important variable is missed and a relationship between independent and dependent variable is misestimated (spurious relationship) then it is termed omitted variable bias. There are various types of confounding that can be introduced:
- *Confounding by indication:* Various procedures are done for particular indication, however, different prognostic factors [age, chronic obstructive pulmonary disease (COPD), previous myocardial infarction (MI), etc.] have various influences on the outcome. Although attempt is made to account for most of the known prognostic factors still few may get unaccounted for influencing the results.
- *Operational confound*: Here a typical outcome measure chosen to assess a particular construct or question inadvertently measures something else.
- *Person confound:* Here persons from different groups (like k-wire fixation and plating—operated) group are analyzed together for assessing functional outcome of operative fixation of distal radius fractures.
- *Procedural confound:* Here researcher allows one variable to change along with manipulated independent variable [like allowing dual-energy X-ray absorptiometry (DEXA) measurements from different makes of machines to be analyzed to assess fracture risk].

Dealing the issues of confounding: Confounding can be reduced in first instance at the study designing level say by matching (*see* minimization or by randomization) that equally distributes the variable (apparently) in the two groups so possibly nullify the effect.

- Make subgroups by stratifying data based on confounding variable say drinkers and nondrinkers. The problem here is that the subgroups are small and analysis will have reduced power. It will be difficult to combine and pool data from these subgroups that may produce Simpson's paradox though it can be corrected by using Mantel-Haenszel method.
- Identify pairs of individuals that are placed into each category by matching all confounding variables (*see* minimization). The analysis is then performed using the McNemar's test or paired t-test. The problem here is if there are too many confounders minimization will be cumbersome and require a large sample size.
- By performing multiple comparisons at multiple times by independent analysts, peer review, replication of finding in experiments or simply by performing multiple regression analysis (multiple linear, logistic, or Poisson analysis as appropriate) including each confounding factor as explanatory variable.
- Using the propensity score approach—this is a complex method, but in simple words for a binary variable (say smoker and non-smoker) the propensity is calculated for each individual to fall into one of the categories (smoker or nonsmoker) using the logistic regression model. This propensity score is then used (instead of the variable) to generate score in multiple regression analysis or the propensity score is itself used as a stratification variable to randomize the individuals.

BIOSTATISTICS

It is the study of statistics as applied to biological areas (medical research in this context). Best information is obtained from experiments conducted on whole population, but because this is not possible some calculated projections are made estimating the effect on population from smaller experiments. This is made possible by the use of statistics which lets an investigator project his findings, its importance, power of assertion, and possibility of error in a reasonably calculated uncertainty. Biological laboratory experiments, health services, and medical and clinical research all use standardized statistical methods. To answer an identified scientific question many different study "types" may be considered depending on feasibility and logistics **(Fig. 3)**. These may vary from small laboratory experiments to large studies involving humans. Observational studies and experiments on animals prevail in between. A *clinical study* is done in the setting of clinical medicine. Basically, there are two types of clinical studies in medicine realm—observational or experimental, both having differing complexities depending on organization of study.

- In observational studies as the name applies, the investigator simply observes what happens and does

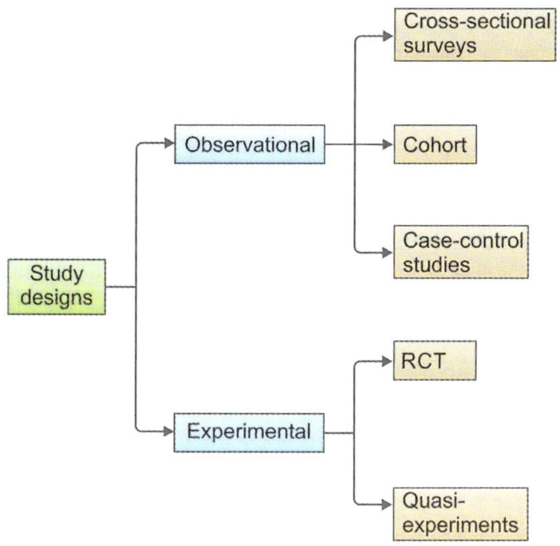

Advantages	Disadvantages
Quick; can cover whole population, giving representative information whether or not people are seeking care	Based mainly on self-report (biases?); diagnostic information usually inaccurate; cannot establish causal sequence
Prospective, so can establish causal sequence; can estimate incidence	Time-consuming; costly; attrition of cohort?
Relatively cheap way of focusing on causal factors	Requires recall of past events (inaccurate?) controls not equivalent to cases
Controls for all main forms of bias; good for both etiological and evaluative research	Ethical concerns in etiological applications; often uses selected populations: issue of generalizability?
May be more practical than RCT: can use "natural experiments"	Allocation bias often significant (experimental and control groups not equivalent)

Fig. 3: Different types of studies performed commonly in medical research (RCT: randomized control trial).

nothing to affect the outcome or intervene to alter the course of the process. Most epidemiological studies are observational. The investigator collects data from an existing population for occurrence of disease or the effect of en masse introduced drug/medication or while studying the natural course of disease without interfering with the existing system. Subjects can however become conscious of the observer and unconscious changes in behavior or practice may get introduced influencing the outcome or observations. This is called the *Hawthorne effect* (act of observation effect). This suggests that humans and animals are not machines or passive elements of the study. These studies are poorer than experimental studies, because it is not always possible to control all of factors, especially confounding ones that significantly affect the outcome.

- Experimental (treatment study) studies in contrast to the observational studies involve the investigator actively intervening in some way or other to affect the outcome. The investigator for example introduces some form of treatment. These studies provide the most effective evidence for any hypothesis as it is performed in a controlled environment and generally predetermined factors can be controlled that may otherwise affect the outcome.

One should have preliminary knowledge to design a relevant study and keep in mind the possible alternatives as more often than not in most cases the first idea for a study is not the best (of course unless it is the only idea). The various types of studies done are detailed below, but some definitions are mentioned for introduction:

- A *cohort* is a group of similar people whose participation in the study is clearly defined based on predetermined criteria (though their selection may be random of course).
- *Baseline variables* are the initial values collected when the study begins (at the element entry into the study).
- An *endpoint* is the most important measure that stands for a clearly defined outcome/event [measurable or determined by presence or absence (qualitative)] associated with the study question and each experimental/study unit. The logical conclusions are derived on the basis of endpoint changes.
- *Unit of observation* is the "individual" or smallest group of "individuals" that can be regarded as independent for determining the outcome variable or ultimate analysis. In a clustered randomized trial, the unit of observation is a group of individuals (e.g., all patients with grade 3 open fracture, all patients with pathological fractures, etc.). In ecological study unit of observation is a community or group of individuals (e.g., breast cancer rates from various countries).
- *Multicenter study:* It may be experimental or observational. It enrolls a number of individuals from two or more centers.
- *Assessing causality:* Most of the medical studies aim at least to establish causation (and it often makes them interesting to publish for even namesake). The best evidence for causation comes from RCTs; however, observational studies may also contribute to same provided strict criteria are met. Hill (1965) provided the most well-known criteria (Hill-criteria) for defining causation as follows:
  - The cause must precede the effect.
  - The association should be plausible, i.e., the results should be biologically sensible.
  - There should be consistent results from a number of studies.

- The association between the cause and the effect should be strong.
- There should be a dose-response relationship with the effect, i.e., higher levels of the effect should lead to more severe disease or more rapid disease onset.
- Removing the factor of interest should reduce the risk of disease.

Observational Studies

In an *experiment,* the investigator deliberately sets one or more factors to a specific level, to act as a measure for studying change. An *experimental unit* in this case is the smallest unit on which an experiment or study is performed and the outcomes are measured for deriving conclusion.

- A *laboratory experiment* is conducted in a created controlled environment (called a *laboratory*) where tight control is possible due to minimal environmental influence for facilitating experimental manipulation and studying its effect. This usually precedes larger or animal based trials for drugs.
- A *comparative experiment* compares two or more techniques or treatments on the study units by dividing them into mutually comparable groups.
- A *crossover experiment* is aimed to further confirm the conclusion derived from initial experiment by eliminating the possibility of error from what is called highly individualistic response. The same experimental unit in this case commonly is crossed to the other group or is investigated under more than one condition of the experiment given. The only factor that cannot be controlled is related to time as the repeat measure is done during nonoverlapping time periods (sequentially often). The main disadvantages of a crossover experiment include: (1) a carryover effect—the effect of initial treatment may get carried to next segment of study when the element is crossed or subjected to some other treatment method/period; (2) changes in the experimental unit over time; (3) introduction of permanent physiological changes in animal or human experiments; (4) waning of enthusiasm of investigator for prolonged experiments; and (5) increased dropouts.
- A *prospective cohort study* is one in which a cohort of people (differing with respect to study variable) is followed over a period of time for the occurrence (or nonoccurrence) of specified endpoints or measurement of impact of occurrences **(Fig. 4)**. Such type of study is helpful to define etiological association of diseases. They are ethically more acceptable, but more expensive than case controlled study.

A ***retrospective study*** is one in which people having a particular disease/outcome/predetermined endpoint are identified and studied backward for defined variables that may have already occurred **(Fig. 4)**. These are simpler and cheap, but have huge potential for bias and misinterpretations unless performed strictly. They provide quick results, and it is easy to obtain large samples. They are useful for investigating *rare treatments or exposures*, but are limited by confounding, selection bias and cannot be blinded.

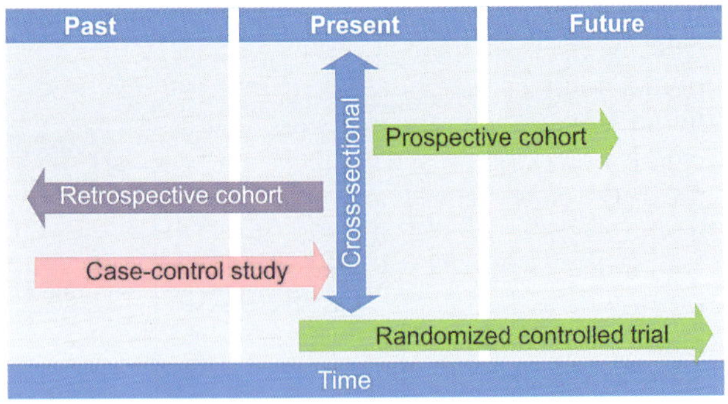

Fig. 4: Studies with respect to time.

BOX 2: Advantages and disadvantages of case control study.

Advantages:
- Relatively quick, cheap, and easier to perform compared to randomized trials, especially where minimization is chosen.
- Particularly suitable for rare disease where randomized trials cannot be designed.
- Allows incorporation of a wide range of risk factors that can be assessed simultaneously.
- There is no attrition.

Disadvantages:
- Recall bias—differential ability of cases and control to remember past events, e.g., patients with lung cancer might remember occasional event long ago while controls might would have forgotten any such event.
- Disease that originated before exposure of risk factor cannot establish causation.
- The study is not suitable when the exposure to risk factor is rare (not that the disease is rare).

A ***case-control study [case-cohort study, retrospective cohort study (misleading)]*** is an observational retrospective study that selects all cases, usually of a disease meeting fixed criteria **(Fig. 4)**. The most important aspect is selection of *control group* that do not have the disease, but are otherwise similar (say as to age/sex/ethnicity/environmental exposure composition). This serves as a comparison for the cases to compare the effects in case, there are not many identified confounding factors or if they cannot be controlled. The cases and controls are further compared with respect to defined outcome variables and set characteristics and protocol. It is a type of observational study and is inferior to RCTs or study. They are cheaper and easier to organize than prospective studies and provide higher statistical power for an argument, if organized properly. Case controlled studies are particularly suited to study *rare diseases* and for preliminary study (pilot study) of associations. The disadvantage is that it gives a narrow picture of risk due to treatment, involves various biases (selection, recall, and confounding) and yield relative estimates than absolute risks **(Box 2)**.

- *Nested case control (NCC) study:* In contrast to a case-control study where all cases are compared to controls; however, in NCC a subset of cases with matched characteristic controls are compared, so that multiple groups defined for particular characteristic (such as age, sex, and exposure) can be studied together. It is less efficient than full case-control study.

- In a *matched case-control study:* These controls are specifically selected to match the defined characteristics of individual cases that commonly involve known confounding variables. The cases and control(s) are hence closely associated with each other and it is believed that the treatment effect will be evenly distributed and absent in the cases and controls respectively that represents "more real" effect free from influence of identified and restricted confounding factors. As it is difficult to exactly match each case to control, there may be more than one control for each case.
- In a *frequency-matched case-control study:* These controls are selected to match individual characteristics of the chosen entire case sample (e.g., age, gender, and year of event), to make the study less cumbersome and easy than a matched study as above. The cases and controls are not individually associated or matched for each identified unit. There is usually more than one control for each case in this scenario that too controls overlap serving for more than one case element.

A ***longitudinal study*** collects information on study elements over a specified period of time. It identifies cases occurring over a period of time. Prospective studies are designed to collect detailed exposure, treatment effect, natural history of disease, and demographic information. They can be blinded to eliminate recall and information bias. They are most useful for investigating rare diseases/treatments and exposures. Prospective observational studies are, however limited by long time to gather meaningful information and often wait for expected exposure to occur by which time the investigator or even the controlled environment may change. Also there is potential confounding due to absence of randomization.

A ***cross-sectional study (cross-sectional analyses, transversal studies, prevalence study, and census)*** collects data on study subjects (of a population, or a representative subset) at a fixed time [ideally point time but usually flash time is used **(Fig. 4)**]. These are also commonly called community survey and are descriptive in nature. They provide a whole lot of data on typically large population (large sample size) rather than a subset of chosen subjects as in case control study. The outcome usually defines relative risk, relative risks and odds ratio, and typically prevalence of a disease (prevalence risk ratio). This study does not (and should not be used also) give answer to any specific study question **(Box 3)**. They may be used, however to find after effect of any treatment of intervention.

- *Survey* is a type of cross-sectional study where, usually, the aim is to describe individuals' beliefs in or attitudes toward a particular issue in a large sample of the population.
- *Census* is a particular type of survey in which the entire target population is investigated.
- The prevalence from cross-sectional study is given by the formula:

$$\text{Point prevalence} = \frac{\text{Number with disease at a single time point}}{\text{Total number studied at the same time}}$$

A ***placebo treatment*** is especially designed to appear similar to comparison treatment (type of drug, dosing method of introduction, etc.), but be devoid of active part of the treatment. This is done to identify or eliminate placebo effect. The *placebo effect* commonly results from the belief and psychological conditioning that one has been treated (despite receiving no treatment really) rather than having experienced actual changes. The cause of placebo effect is thought to arise from neuropsychological changes (endorphins, serotonin, and various transmitters may be released due to the emotional content of the thought to mediate effect) rather than the real physical, physiological, and chemical activities of a treatment.

BOX 3: Limitations of cross-sectional study.

- No causation can be established—investigator can only find an association between the factor of interest and disease and possibly its strength statistically, but never can one establish causative association [or that the factor is likely to have caused disease (as there is no information if and when the events occurred prior to the study)].
- Incidence of the disease cannot be estimated.
- We cannot consider trends over time. We need to do a repeated cross-sectional study to estimate the trends over time. The drawback here is that the study most often will include different individuals (basic measuring unit), so it will be difficult to tell if the changes observed over time reflect the disease trend or changed persons.

Treatment Study

- ***Nonrandomized trial (quasi-experiment):*** Interrupted time series design (repeated measures on a sample from the same population are obtained several times before and after an intervention or exposure)—considered a type of quasi-experiment.
- ***Hybrid designs:*** Some investigators combine different methodologies principally to reduce the drawbacks of different designs. Prospective treatment group can be compared to historical control this eliminates recruiting controls, but there can be chronological bias. Prospective treatment group can be compared with both prospective and historical control that maximizes efficacy minimizing bias, but introduces variability and complicates analysis.
- ***Randomized controlled trials:*** RCTs are considered to be the most reliable form of scientific evidence in the clinical literature that may influence practice. It is considered the gold standard for a clinical trial. These can be of three types depending on the organization of study based on "visibility" of treatment to observer and subjects.
    - *Unblinded:* The interventionist and study subjects are both aware of the treatment given; usually done in surgical trials.
    - *Single blind:* A study is *single blind,* if subjects being treated are unaware of which treatment (including any control) they are receiving.
    - *Double blind:* A study is considered double blind, if in addition to single blinding the investigators of outcome variables are also unaware of type of treatment the subjects are actually receiving.

RANDOMIZED CONTROLLED TRIAL PRINCIPLES AND PROCEDURE

Randomized controlled trials are typically used to test the effectiveness of different medical interventions, especially those having clinical equipoise ("genuine uncertainty within the expert medical community for following or choosing the preferred treatment"). Typically in an RCT, the randomly designed groups (two or more) of subjects are allocated treatment(s) (or no treatment) and followed in exactly the same way differing in terms of primary question variable(s) or intervention (parallel design). A crossover design **(Flowchart 2B)** is better than a parallel design **(Flowchart 2A)** in which the study is repeated on the individual with reversed parameters (if treated early then now made control or vice versa for example). There is usually a washout period between the two periods to allow any residual effect of previous treatment (carry-over) to dissipate. These crossover designs are more precise as the variation within individual is much less than the variation between individuals and they require lesser number of individuals to decipher the effect. Also, if the RCT is performed on a population with large variability having wide variations among the experimental units then complete random design is inefficient and in such cases crossover design helps to limit the impact of variation. Different types of RCT are detailed in **Box 4**.

The term "RCT" is very specific and is used only for trials with a control group. The term *randomized trial* sometimes used synonymously, describe studies that compare multiple treatment groups with each other and there is no control group. Similarly, terms like "randomized clinical trial" or "randomized comparative trial" used to describe "RCT" should be avoided. RCTs have advantage of being the most definitive tool to answer question, eliminate various biases, good question-answer design makes analysis simple. The disadvantage is that long time is taken and various ethical clearances are required before conduct of study.

The *first step* to performing an RCT is to define a relevant *study question*. This requires good literature search and support for various arguments in favor or against. *Second step* is to define the endpoint of study—an outcome variable

BOX 4: Different types of randomized control trials (RCTs).

Based on type of comparison:
- Superiority trials are designed to study superiority of one treatment over other.
- Noninferiority trials are designed to demonstrate that a method is at least not appreciably worse than another. The new treatment is as effective but need not be superior compared to the control. A one-sided test is performed in these studies.
- Equivalence trials are designed to demonstrate that study treatments are equally effective.

Based on type of configuration:
- Parallel-group—each participant is randomly assigned to distinct treatment group, and they receive (or do not receive) an intervention until evaluation.
- Crossover—the participants receive (or does not receive) an intervention for a duration and then are switched over after analysis in a random sequence to re-analyze.
- Cluster—here the elements of study are preexisting groups of participants (viz. cluster of children of particular age group, all alcoholics, school students, factory workers in noisy areas and villages) that are randomly selected to receive the particular intervention.
- Factorial—here each participant is randomly assigned to a group that receives a particular subcombination of interventions or noninterventions (e.g., one group receives antibiotics with probiotics, another group receives antibiotics with vitamins, third group receives antibiotics with placebo, fourth receives placebo and vitamin, fifth receives placebo and probiotics and so on).
- "Explanatory RCTs" are designed in a typical sophisticated research setting with highly selected participants and under highly controlled conditions to determine treatment efficacy.
- Pragmatic RCTs are designed to test effectiveness of interventions in everyday practice. They are conducted under flexible conditions with relatively unselected participants to incorporate as many commonly encountered scenarios as possible and in this way, they can effectively inform decisions about practice.

Flowcharts 2A and B: The concept of parallel and crossover designs.

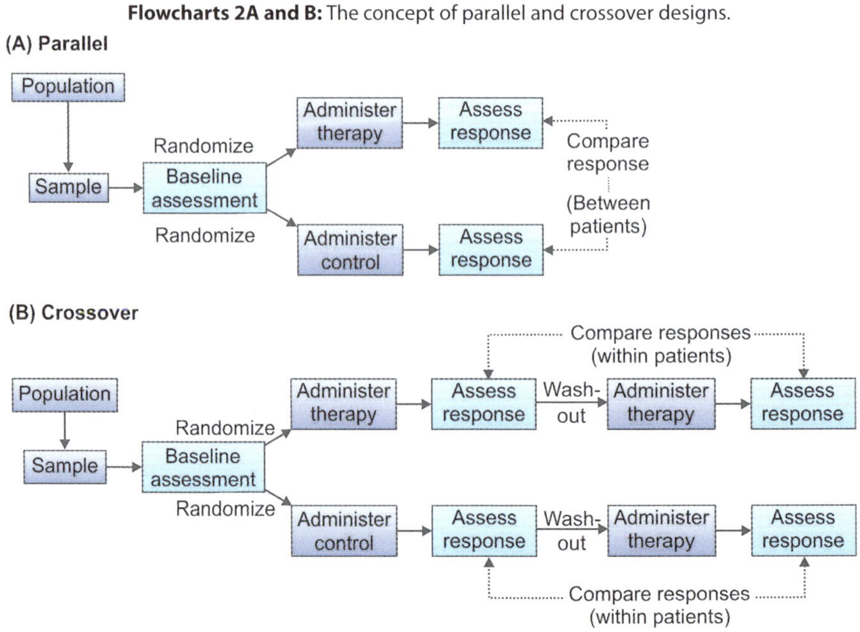

(which can be pragmatically studied) that most accurately reflects the benefit/detrimental effects of therapy. This is the primary endpoint of study often relating to the treatment efficacy. Secondary endpoints often relate to the toxicity or adverse effects (complications in surgery) that should also be considered together. *Next step* is to formulate the suggestion of ambiguity, i.e., to *form a hypothesis* that can be specifically studied and should pose an unbiased question. The *null hypothesis* is setup to be rejected. It is easier to prove a statement is false than to prove it is true. "Alternative hypothesis" that a difference exists is not commonly formulated. Disproving a null hypothesis to find effect is more consolidative than proving alternative hypothesis just like it is easier to disprove that all crows are black just by bringing one white crow. Some errors can arise in null hypothesis analysis out of confounding factors or a poor study:

- *Type I error (α):* When we try to reject a null hypothesis by study there could be a possibility that the hypothesis could be true, but as in real life a researcher has to take chance. Such possibility of *wrongfully rejecting the null hypothesis* (and establishing a real difference) when none really exists is type I error. Such "chance" can be limited to some extent by lowering the "*p*-value" usually set at 0.05 (i.e., 5% chance of a misinterpretation). For serious issues, the value can be lowered to 0.01 or even lower. If we do not want to miss an effect we may even set significance to *p*-value of 0.10.
- *Type II error (β):* Occurs when we *accept null hypothesis when in reality it is false*. The clinical studies are designed to usually reject null hypothesis, so this error should be given due rigorous attention. This is given by *power* of study (type II error), the probability of rejecting null hypothesis when it is false. Though confusing to mind, power by above definition is actually the chance (usually expressed as a percentage) of detecting, as statistically significant, a real treatment effect of a given size. The power usually set at 80 can be escalated for equivocal arguments, but then it requires a higher sample size. Factors influencing power of study are:
    - *Sample size:* Larger the sample greater is the power, i.e., larger sample will have higher ability to detect the clinically important effect. The best way to reduce beta error is by incorporating it in the study, though this increases the sample size significantly. A large sample size can be viewed as a means of decreasing the false negative results rate when a real treatment effect exists. This is also the way to detect the power of study for a given sample size in retrospect.
    - *Variability of the observations:* Variability has inverse relation to power, higher the variability lesser is the power. Thus a wide confidence interval will have less power as arises in smaller samples (this is one way to evaluate the power of a study as a glance, if at all the inferences in a particular study have adequate power or not).
    - *Effect of interest:* Larger effect size has higher power. So, if two treatment methods are markedly different in their outcomes then the power of detecting the particular outcome will be much stronger, conversely if two drugs have nearly similar effects (or treatments have equivocal outcomes) then power will be very less or we will have to choose a large sample to detect the difference.
    - *Significance level:* Higher the significance level greater (higher set *p*-value) is the power. This actually increases the chance of type I error while reducing the chance of a type II error, but it lends us higher chances to detect an effect that exists (kindly also *see* "hypothesis testing—the *p*-value approach" below).

In the next step, all study variables and "*outcome variables*" should be clearly defined that explains the question and the answer in terms of outcome. There are two common ways of determining the outcome—one is called the "hard" outcome variable that can be measured objectively (minimizing bias), can be preserved (radiographs for example), and have dimensions (lengthening, offset, union, and shortening), but they do not necessarily correlate with functional gain/loss of the patient and have weak relation to patient/function related measures that are now in focus. The importance is being given to functional outcome measures in clinical research oriented to the measurement of variables primarily critical to patient and are called "soft" outcome measures. These are more reliable and consistent than the hard measures and are mainly calculated by patient-reported outcomes of symptoms, physical function, and health. This outcome research can also include single or multiple site databases, small area analysis, and meta-analysis (structured reviews of relevant literature), prospective clinical trials and development of guideline. The *outcome instrument* is the tool to measure these variables and is used in conjunction with the clinical measures. The instrument should be clinically relevant and sensible in evaluating the desired parameter. The tools are commonly formed as a questionnaire that should not be too long to respond or cumbersome to calculate in the end. Internal consistency and validity should be judged for appropriateness. The purposes of outcome instruments are common:

- Study of populations in cross sectional studies.
- Determination of impact on health change (improvement/deterioration), function, and satisfaction after index treatment/surgery for specific disease in a patient.
- Measures for prospective clinical trials to determine the effectiveness of intervention (operative versus nonoperative method or comparison of two operative methods).
- Development of disease specific guidelines for delivering effective treatment and care.

Some such commonly used instruments are:

- *General health outcomes:*
    - SF-36/SF-12
    - Health-related quality of life (HRQOL)
    - Nottingham health profile (NHP)
- Patient satisfaction questionnaire (PSQ)
- *Disease-specific instruments:*
    - Oswestry disability index (ODI) for low back pain
    - Quebec back pain disability scale (QBPDS)

- Upper extremity disabilities of the arm, shoulder, and head (DASH)
- Constant shoulder function scoring system
- Western Ontario and McMaster Universities Osteoarthritis Index (WOMAC)
- Harris hip score
- Short Musculoskeletal Function Assessment Questionnaire (SMAF) for trauma

A sample size should be then estimated for studying the outcome variables that have enough power to reject or accept argument.

SAMPLE SIZE ESTIMATION

It is a methodical undertaking that should be done in guidance of a statistician. There are various ways to calculate sample size including general and quick formulae, special tables (exist for special tests such as t-test and chi-square tests), Altman's nomogram, and lastly the computer software of course. The Lehr's formula is the most commonly used "quick formula" for calculation of sample size. For a power of 80% at significance level of 0.05, the sample size in each group is:

$$SS = 16/(standard\ difference)^2$$

The numerator changes to 21 for power of 90%.

Some general detailed guidelines hitherto for sample size estimation are presented:

First set the appropriate α (usually set at two-sided 5%) and β (power is at 80% or 90%) for the predetermined outcome variable(s). Two-sided test (more sample size required) is usually carried out which is more prudent compared to a one-sided test that assumes test therapy to perform clinically better than the standard or control therapy. The effect size specifies the accepted clinical difference between two therapies based on the outcome variable. It needs to be defined before commencing study as it is required to find the sample size. There are usually three ways to get the effect size:

1. The most common is to search from available literature.
2. If the study is novel then literature is obviously not available in that case one can do a small pilot study to determine the estimated effect sizes.
3. Last is by expert clinical expectations based on observations and experience of clinicians frequently encountering/treating such conditions.

In the next step to calculate the sample size, besides knowing the type of design to be used, one has to classify the type of the primary outcome.

- Simply the outcome could be a *qualitative variable,* so that proportion outcomes are observed (yes/no; present/absent; success/failure, etc.). In such studies for a two-sided test of 5%, the formula is as below:

$$m\ (\text{size of each group}) = c \times \frac{\pi_1(1-\pi_2)+\pi_2(1-\pi_2)}{(\pi_1-\pi_2)^2}$$

Here, c = 7.9 for 80% power (10.5 for 90% power), π_1 and π_2 are estimated proportions (sort of effect size). So for a treatment where a group has estimated 25% success rate while for another there is 50% success rate then sample size for each group with 90% power will be 10.5 × [0.25(1 – 0.25) + 0.5(1 – 0.5)]/(0.25 – 0.5)² = 73.5 = 74, so total number of 148 cases will be required (add to this the estimated attrition rate).

Another way of calculating the sample size (m, per group) for tests of difference in proportions using alpha and beta errors is given below:

$$m = \frac{(z_a - z_b)^2 \times 2 \times p(1-p)}{d^2}$$

Here, Z_a = value for α error (1.96 for P = 0.05 in two-tailed test), Z_b = value for β error (0.84 for 20% beta error or 80% power in one-tailed test), p = mean proportion of success, d = smallest clinically important difference to be detected.

- For *continuous variables,* there are two possibilities. In a study where two treatment methods are used in different groups (say group one with plating and the other with nailing), *two independent samples arise* so the primary outcome will be the difference in mean of outcome variable between two groups. Here we should know the possible effect size ($\mu_2 - \mu_1$) from literature [by knowing the mean difference in the outcome variable (say functional outcome for two methods)] or a good expert clinical estimate that is reasonable. Then for a reasonable standard deviation (σ) say 0.5 (or better defined from literature) calculate δ (standardized effect size) as follows:

$$\delta = \frac{(\mu_2 - \mu_1)}{\sigma}$$

The formula for two-sided test of 5% is:

$$m\ (size\ of\ each\ group) = \frac{2 \times c}{\delta^2} + 1$$

Here, c = 7.9 for 80% power (10.5 for 90% power). So, for effect size of 0.6 at 80% power for a two tailed test at 5% of α; the sample size would be 90 patients (45 in each group). The other situation is where we have paired sample (say a pre- and post-treatment group); here the sample size is estimated from the formula:

$$m\ (size\ of\ each\ group) = \frac{2 \times c}{\delta^2} + 1$$

For observational study say with a simple random sampling to study the variable (observe), we cannot chose whole population rather a sample from it which is given by:

$$n = \left[z^2 \times \frac{p \times (1-p)}{d^2}\right]$$

Where n = sample size, z = set confidence interval (1.96 for 2 SD), p = expected prevalence (expressed in fraction of 1), d = relative desired precision (usually taken as 10%).

For cluster design, the sample is given by (do not be frustrated with formulae, these are only for reference and not to be learnt)

$$n = \left[t^2 \times \frac{p \times (1-p)}{d^2}\right] \times DEFF$$

Here all same as above, except that $t = 2$ SD has a value of 2.045 instead of 1.96; DEFF (design effect) is usually taken to be 1.5.

SAMPLING

Since whole population cannot be studied, our only solution while conducting a clinical research is to collect data from a subset of the individuals of interest that we label sample. And researcher would want to know the "truth" about the population so for the selected sample one should mandatorily obtain a representative sample of the population so that correct extrapolations can be drawn. Following are the few commonly practices sampling methods:

- ***Simple random sampling:*** It is the most commonly applied method where every unit in the population has equal chance of being represented in the sample. Sampling for different units is performed separately and is independent of each other, i.e., sample elements do not overlap. A sufficiently large simple random sample (as determined from statistics—see sample size above) will in all circumstances be representative of the population. A smaller sample is likely to miss certain population characteristics (like missing osteoporosis in hip fractures) or misrepresent them (having more females than males).
- ***Systematic sampling:*** The sample is arranged according to some ordering scheme and then the starting point for selecting element is chosen randomly. The sampling then proceeds by counting every Kth element of the sample. This scheme is less accurate than simple random sampling.
- ***Stratified sampling:*** The data is stratified (categorized) to contain a representative from each variable being measured. Each stratum is sampled as an independent subpopulation. This is principally based on minimizing the variability in data within the strata while maximizing the variability between the strata. The advantages of this approach are that it focuses on the specific subpopulations ignoring irrelevant ones, improves accuracy of estimation and permits greater balancing of statistical power of tests of difference between strata. The disadvantages include uselessness when the subgroups are heterogeneous and requirement of relevant stratification variable choosing which can be difficult.
- ***Cluster sampling:*** This is preferred when a large survey is done that requires face-to-face interviews or clinical tests on a given population. Due to the basic nature of study and importance of minimal variation in data it is not feasible to use a simple random sampling that would miss significant data points. In this case, for example, a number of cities (designated as clusters) can be sampled chosen by simple random sampling within the selected geographic regions.
- ***Two-phase sampling:*** This is a specific method used as an adjunct to original study for providing additional important information that adds to knowledge but needs elements from first study. For example, for evaluating smoking characteristic for lung cancer, it is useful to take a large initial sample and then a smaller subsample is taken to measure more expensive or difficult variables (like genetic linkage).

RANDOMIZATION

The patients or study subjects are then randomized into two interventional groups. There are two processes involved in randomizing patients. First is choosing a *randomization procedure* to randomly allocate patients minimizing selection and other bias and second is *allocation concealment*, which prevents revealing the group assignment to treatment introducers prior to definitively allocating patents to their respective groups. There are some crudely, but commonly practiced "systematic" methods of group assignment, such as choosing "odd and even" element entry to define groups, alternating subjects between one group and the other or assigning males to one and females to another. These are unacceptable and can cause "unlimited contamination" by systematically amplifying errors in allocation and other factors and also they cause a breach of allocation concealment.

Types of Randomization

Some commonly used methods of randomization are simple, block, stratified, and covariate adaptive randomization. In addition "minimization" can also be used in select studies. It is notable that alternate allocation (male/female, alternate entry of participant, etc.), using day of week for allocation or odd/even numbers introduce systematic unlimited contamination and are not considered randomization. Moreover, these are open methods so liable to selection bias by the introducer. Flipping a coin or shuffling the sealed envelopes are also subject to bias in case the patient does not have desired characteristics (known to the researcher), coin can be flipped again or envelop seen against strong light to reveal the contents. The later methods (they come under simple randomization) are acceptable only, if adhered to strictly which is often not the case.

Simple Randomization

Here the randomization is done on a single randomly assigned sequence. Each allocation is independent of the others. A random number table found in a statistics book or computer-generated random numbers or online available random number tables can be used. This technique is most commonly practiced and it statistically maintains complete random chance of the assignment of a subject to any particular group. This is simple and easy to implement in most clinical research. In large clinical research, this technique reliably generates similar numbers of subjects with randomly distributed variables among different groups. Random distribution over a large sample size quite reliably distributes the confounding variables equally. However, it can be problematic in relatively small sample size studies where an unequal number of participants or an unequally distributed important confounding variable may get selected in a particular group.

Blocked or Restricted Randomization

The block randomization method is to randomize subjects into groups with equal "sample sizes" and not necessarily according to the participant characteristics. Blocks are kept small for simplicity and speed and are balanced with respect to predetermined group assignments, but paying attention to keeping similar numbers of subjects in each group. In this method, the block size should be always a multiple of the number of groups (i.e., for two treatment groups a block size of 4, 6, or 8, is chosen, similarly for three groups block sizes of 3, 6, and 9 suffice). Blocks are then randomly allocated to each group. It is better to use blocks in smaller increments to control balance. The only advantage of this method is to generate equal size of each group, but the groups may be too heterogeneous to be comparable in terms of certain covariates (e.g., diabetes, multiple sclerosis, cancer, hypertension, etc.) and may not only negatively influence the results of the clinical trial, but also nullify the very purpose of randomization with respect to equidistribution of covariates or confounding factors. Unless the sample need to be equal for statistical purpose, this method is not very appropriate in studies where sample size and covariates must be balanced.

Stratified Randomization

To take care of the problem of blocked randomization, stratified randomization method introduces controls and balances the influence of covariates. The researcher identifies specific covariates by their influence on the research parameter. Stratified randomization is then done by creating separate block for each combination of covariates and assigning subjects to the appropriate block. Subjects are then assigned into one of the groups by simple randomization performed within each block. Stratified randomization is a relatively simple and useful technique (especially for smaller clinical trials). The problem occurs when there are too many covariates, then stratification is complex and often not possible, if they exceed more than four to five. The other big limitation is that it can be done only when all subjects have been identified before group assignment which is not the case in most prospective clinical trials. In most clinical research, subjects are enrolled on a continuous basis often. This problem either needs to be sorted by simple randomization and increasing the sample size or by using minimization for small samples (discussed below).

Cluster Randomization

We randomly allocate a *group* or *cluster* of individuals, rather than each individual, to a treatment. This is usually done when it is not feasible to randomize the individuals separately within each cluster (e.g., fluoride levels in drinking water). This is also preferred in instances where the treatment outcome of one individual affects the outcome of other individuals within the cluster.

Covariate Adaptive Randomization (Minimization)

This is ingenious but cumbersome method where a new participant is sequentially allocated to a particular treatment group by considering specific covariates (as in stratified randomization) and previous assignments of already allocated participants so as to balance the groups appropriately. In simple randomization, there is high likelihood of imbalance between groups with respect to covariates, if the sample size is small. Covariate adaptive randomization uses the method of minimization (minimizing the bias due to unequal distribution of covariates) by assessing and sequentially correcting the imbalance of samples based on covariates by adjusting imbalance by preferential allocation of elements into groups. Covariate adaptive randomization can be used as a valid alternative randomization method for clinical research.

The advantages of proper randomization in RCTs include:
- Eliminates selection bias (subjects in various groups should not differ in any systematic way) and confounding in patient assignment.
- Facilitates blinding (allocation concealment—researchers, subject or patients or participants, and others should not know to which group the subject will be assigned).
- It strengthens the probability theory expressing the higher likelihood that any difference in outcome between treatment groups is by chance.

Blinding/Masking

When the response to be studied is subjective, there is often an introduction of assessment bias when patients/clinicians are aware of the treatment allocation. This background awareness nearly always influences the recording of signs of improvement or even the adverse reactions/complications. Depending on the persons masked from the treatment allocation, a trial can be:
- Unblinded—the interventionist and study subjects are both aware of treatment given; usually done in surgical trials.
- Double-blind—where all participants (clinicians, patients, and assessors) in a trial are blinded to treatment allocation and to randomization list.
- Single-blind trial—where either the treatment provider or the patient is blinded to allocation. As it is easier to blind the treatment provider while for ethical issues not always the patient can be blinded (most of the surgical procedures for example have to be explained to the patient, so he knows which group he would be in) so single blinded trials have often the treatment provider blinded to allocation.

Consolidated Standards of Reporting Trials (CONSORT) statement and guidelines (developed by CONSORT group): It provides guidance for reporting all RCTs **(exemplified in Flowchart 3)**, but focuses on individually randomized, two groups, parallel trials (randomized comparative trials, not RCT). Even though with adequate conduct of randomized comparative trials the lack of adequate reporting (complete descriptions of critical information) fuelled the development of the original CONSORT statement in 1996 that was revised in 2001. Empirical evidence began to accumulate that some poorly conducted or poorly reported aspects of trials

Flowchart 3: A typical way of reporting studies with respect to the Consolidated Standards of Reporting Trials (CONSORT) statement.

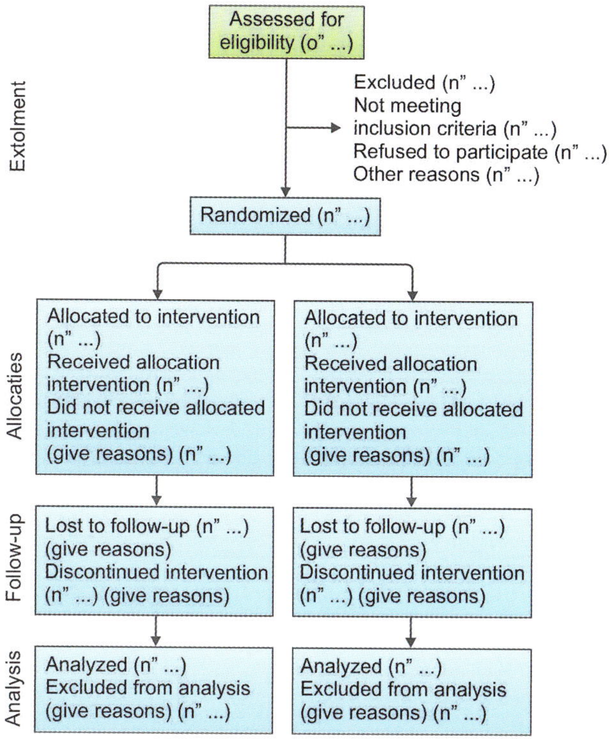

were associated with bias. Despite guidelines many trial reports are still inadequate, furthermore new evidences and experiences have been gained that can improve reporting so revised guidelines were presented in 2010. The CONSORT statement does not give any guidelines on designing or conduct of study; however, it does affect these parameters indirectly. Transparency desired for reporting under CONSORT guidelines makes researcher modify the study to certain standards thus changing the methodology a bit for betterment and uniformity. The CONSORT guidelines being comprehensive do help researcher to design the trial. The CONSORT 2010 guidelines have been adopted to assist authors in writing reports of randomized trials and maintaining uniformity, so that editors and peer reviewers review manuscripts in standard context for publication. This also helps readers in critically understanding the published reports **(Table 1)**.

Simplified steps necessary to perform a study:

- Frame a logical scientific study question or problem area of interest.
- Choose proper study design to answer the question. The design must include the following elements:
    - Identify the study variables, data to be collected including the outcome variables that will be analyzed for conclusion of the study results. Calculate the number of experimental units (sample size) needed for empowering the conclusion to statistical significance.
    - An appropriate analytical model for describing and processing data.
    - What inferences does one hope to make from the study? The conclusions might one draw from the study and to what population(s) is the conclusion applicable?
- The study is carried out with appropriate control of environment, ethics, confidentiality, and the legitimate data are collected (detailed below).
- The data are analyzed according to the standard protocol and statistical analysis and conclusions and inferences are drawn (detailed below).
- Comparing results with existing literature (described below).
- The results are used to initiate change in existing procedures, publishing results, or planning a subsequent study.

DATA COLLECTION

It checks for correctness and meaningfulness of data.

- *Validity checks:* Testing outliers, checking the batch totals, check digits, etc. Longitudinal construct validity is used to evaluate the patient response to questionnaires commonly used to measure health status and HRQOL. A goodness-of-fit test measures whether an observed group of counts matches a theoretical pattern.
- *Consistency checks:* Cronbach's alpha is a coefficient used to estimate the internal consistency. When all test items (say questions in a questionnaire) estimate the same construct (say quality of health) the intercorrelation is maximized. The intercorrelation among test items is determined by Cronbach's alpha, higher the coefficient better is the consistency. Inter-rater reliability (kappa) tests whether two observers looking at the same occurrence (or condition) give consistent ratings in multiple observations.
- *Missing forms*

DESCRIPTIVE STATISTICS

Tabulations and Frequency Distributions

Empirical frequency distribution of a variable relates each possible observation, class of observations (i.e., range of values), or category to its observed *frequency* of occurrence. The observed frequencies of categorical or some numerical data can be depicted by following methods:

- Tables are a concise list of collected data, prepared based on three ingredients: a *collection* of data, a *variable,* and the *frequency* with which values of the variable occur. The tables are a useful method to condense data and derive proper meaning from enormous data gathered in cross-sectional studies.
- *Graphs:* Describe a sample pictorially by plotting on one axis values of the variable (usually the abscissa) and on another axis (usually the ordinate) the frequency of occurrence of a value or a measure related to it. To draw a *histogram* small groups are formed by choosing cut points and the data is tabulated. The relative frequency of observations in each category is divided by the width of the category to obtain the *probability density,* and a bar is drawn with this height. For simplicity and ease

TABLE 1: CONSORT 2010 checklist of information to include when reporting a randomized trial.

Section/Topic	***Checklist item***
1. Title and abstract	
	(A) Identification as a randomized trial in the title (B) Structured summary of trial design, methods, results, and conclusions (for specific guidance see CONSORT for abstracts)
2. Introduction	
Background and objectives	(A) Scientific background and explanation of rationale
	(B) Specific objectives or hypotheses
3. Methods	
(A) Trial design	(i) Description of trial design (such as parallel and factorial) including allocation ratio
	(ii) Important changes to methods after trial commencement (such as eligibility criteria), with reasons
(B) Participants	(i) Eligibility criteria for participants
	(ii) Settings and locations where the data were collected
4. Interventions	The interventions for each group with sufficient details to allow replication, including how and when they were actually administered
5. Outcomes	(A) Completely defined prespecified primary and secondary outcome measures, including how and when they were assessed
	(B) Any changes to trial outcomes after the trial commenced, with reasons
6. Sample size	(A) How sample size was determined
	(B) Interim analysis and stopping guidelines—when applicable, explanation of any interim analyses, and stopping guidelines
7. Randomization	
Sequence generation	(A) Method used to generate the random allocation sequence
	(B) Type of randomization; details of any restriction (such as blocking and block size)
8. Allocation concealment mechanism	Mechanism used to implement the random allocation sequence (such as sequentially numbered containers), describing any steps taken to conceal the sequence until interventions were assigned
9. Implementation	Who generated the random allocation sequence, who enrolled participants and who assigned participants to interventions
10. Blinding	(A) If done, who was blinded after assignment to interventions (for example, participants, care providers, and those assessing outcomes) and how
	(B) If relevant, description of the similarity of interventions
11. Statistical methods	(A) Statistical methods used to compare groups for primary and secondary outcomes
	(B) Methods for additional analyses, such as subgroup analyses and adjusted analyses
12. Results	
Participant flow (a diagram is strongly recommended)	(A) For each group, the numbers of participants who were randomly assigned, received intended treatment and were analyzed for the primary outcome
	(B) For each group, losses and exclusions after randomization, together with reasons
13. Recruitment	(A) Dates defining the periods of recruitment and follow-up
	(B) Why the trial ended or was stopped
14. Baseline data	A table showing baseline demographic and clinical characteristics for each group
15. Numbers analyzed	For each group, number of participants (denominator) included in each analysis and whether the analysis was by original assigned groups
16. Outcomes and estimation	(A) For each primary and secondary outcome, results for each group, and the estimated effect size and its precision (such as 95% confidence interval)
	(B) For binary outcomes, presentation of both absolute and relative effect sizes is recommended
17. Ancillary analyses	Results of any other analyses performed, including subgroup analyses and adjusted analyses, distinguishing prespecified from exploratory
18. Harms	All important harms or unintended effects in each group (for specific guidance see CONSORT for harms)
19. Discussion	
Limitations	Trial limitations, addressing sources of potential bias, imprecision, and, if relevant, multiplicity of analyses
Generalizability	Generalizability (external validity and applicability) of the trial findings
Interpretation	Interpretation consistent with results, balancing benefits and harms, and considering other relevant evidence
20. Other information	
Registration	Registration number and name of trial registry
Protocol	Where the full trial protocol can be accessed, if available
Funding	Sources of funding and other support (such as supply of drugs), role of funders

(CONSORT: Consolidated Standards of Reporting Trials)
Source: CONSORT. CONSORT 2010. [online] Available from http://www.consort-statement.org/checklists [Last accessed December, 2021].

of understanding to common readers histograms are sometimes designed so that on y-axis absolute or relative frequency is plotted rather than the more complicated probability density. The area of a bar is proportional to the frequency of occurrence of values in the interval if probability density is plotted. One can instead choose "pie-charts". A circular "pie" is commonly split into sectors for each category that represents the frequency in that category.

- Though a bit complicated probability density has its advantages than a simple count. The first is that the plotted categories need not have the same width (wider categories can be used for sparsely distributed data). The second advantage is that the height of the bars does not depend systematically on the sample size, so that it is possible to compare on the same graph histograms from two samples of different sizes.
- A *frequency polygon* and *cumulative frequency polygon* emphasize the continuity of the data. A frequency polygon is obtained by joining the tops of the bars of the histogram at their midpoints. More than one variable is often associated with each study element under study. They can be easily plotted as frequency polygons with different colors or lines (dotted, dashed, etc.), where making histograms would be difficult. Such data are called *multivariate data* (most often found in medical research). For multivariate data, the *conditioning* plot examines how the relationship between two variables depends on a third.

Describing the Data

We need to describe the data in a meaningful way that can be reproduced and compared. We need to define a representative value around which rest of the values will be distributed giving us an arbitrary perception. The *average* is a general term for a measure of *location;* it describes a typical measurement.

- *Arithmetic mean:* The *arithmetic mean* of a sample of values of a variable is the simple average of all the observations.

$$\bar{y} = \frac{\Sigma y}{n}$$

  Where, y = observations, n = number of values. The arithmetic mean is more appropriate, if the data is represented by normal or Gaussian frequency distribution that forms the basis for a large part of statistics.
- The *mode* of a sample of values of a variable Y is that value that occurs most frequently in a given dataset. The mode is usually calculated for large sets of discrete data.
- The *median* is the middle value of a data arranged in ascending or descending order of values of variables. The median applies to odd number of dataset, where the median is the $(n + 1)/2$th value. So for a data of 21 values median will be $(21 + 1)/2 = 11$th value of dataset. For even set, there is no true median but we calculate it by taking mean of the middle two values.
- The *geometric mean* of a sample of non-negative values of a variable Y is the nth root of the product of the n-values, where n is the sample size. This is typically suitable for a right skewed data where mean is an inappropriate measure. The data can be made more symmetrical by doing log transformation (to base 10 or *e*) of the data. The geometric mean is usually equal to the median and less than the mean of this right skewed data.
- The average and standard deviation are affected by extreme values in data; however, the median and mode are seemingly unaffected by such occurrences.
- Weighted mean is calculated for values of variable that are more important than other values. Often after defining protocol during study we come across so many data values that are not truly important for final calculations, so these junk values are given less weightage and more important values are calculated.
- The *average deviation* is the arithmetic average of the absolute values of deviations about the sample mean for a sample of values of a variable. The *median absolute deviation* on the other hand represents the median of absolute values of deviations about the sample median. These measures are less affected by extreme values but not commonly used as formulations and understandings are not easily derived based on these measures.

Other than providing the average value, description of data needs "the spread" of data to complete the description in a meaningful way. This spread of data is also called dispersion or variability. The following are the descriptives of data describing the spread:

- Range is simply the difference of highest from lowest value in the dataset. Range provides a misleading measure for spread especially when there are outliers.
- The *standard deviation* (σ) is the square root of the average of the square of the deviations from the sample mean, for a sample of n-values of a variable y the σ is:

$$\sigma = \sqrt{\frac{\Sigma (y - \bar{y})}{(n - 1)}}$$

  Standard deviation can also be calculated by (σ = interquartile range/1.35) equation, but it yields an approximate value only. The standard deviation is measured in same units as that of the variable. Some mathematical properties of standard deviation are as follows:
  - Adding a constant value to each of the observations will not change the value of standard deviation.
  - If the observations are multiplied by a positive value, the standard deviation gets multiplied by the same constant value.
  - Nearly 68% of the observations fall within one standard deviation of the mean.
  - Nearly 95% of the observed values fall within two standard deviations of the mean.

  The square of the standard deviation is called the *variance.*
- *Percentile:* Percentile is a measure of values that defines comparative rank (not exact rank) to a particular value.

They are particularly suitable for ordinal (nonparametric) data. A 75th percentile means that 75% values in the data are less than the given value. Percentile cannot be used in small sample size, for tied values and where unique value (exact rank) is to be derived. The Pth *percentile* of a sample of n observations is that value of the variable with rank (P/100) × (1 + *n*). The 50th percentile is called median, 25th percentile the lower quartile and the 75th percentile is called upper quartile. Interquartile range is the difference between 75th and 25th percentiles and is used to describe the spread out of values of sample. This is a better measure than "range" (difference between largest and smallest values) which is highly sample size dependent. Box plot is a rectangle with upper and lower edges at the 25th and 75th percentiles is drawn with a transverse line in the rectangle at the median (50th percentile). Lines (whiskers) are drawn from the rectangle (box) to the highest and lowest values that are within 1.5 × interquartile range of the median.

- *Variance:* It defines the extent to which each value deviates from the arithmetic mean; the larger the deviations the larger will be variance. The problem with calculating variance simply would be the fact that the positive deviations will cancel out the negative deviations. Thus, we square these values and take the mean of these squared values. The units of variance will hence be the square of variable units (kg², cm², etc.). Variance is hence:

$$S^2 = \frac{\Sigma\,(x - \bar{x})}{n - 1}$$

The divisor is not *n* but "*n* - 1". The reason is that it has been shown for samples the variance is better given by "*n* - 1" divisor than the "*n*", which is suitable for population as a whole.

TYPE OF DISTRIBUTIONS

To understand the types of distributions of the data we need to understand the probability and probability distribution that ascribe the basic theoretical mathematical distribution of the variable.

Probability is the chance of a given event occurring and hence measure the uncertainty (possibility of occurring or not occurring). The value ranges from 0 to 1. Zero means event cannot occur and one means the event must occur. Probability can be conditional meaning the possibility of occurring provided a specified event occurs. Probability calculation can be subjective (personal belief, I would be the richest man by 2020), frequentist (proportion of times event would occur if experiment is repeated, getting a tails if coin is tossed 100 times) or a priori. The latter requires knowledge of theoretical model called the probability distribution, here all possible outcomes of the experiment are taken into account and given a probability value not just a fixed idea about a particular outcome (e.g., probability of a fair, dark or wheatish child being born to a dark father and fair mother). So the probability distribution will give the probabilities of all possible values of the random variable. Depending on the variable type probability distribution can be either discrete or continuous. It is important to realize that this is a theoretical distribution expressed mathematically. They are defined by specific *parameters* (e.g., mean and variance) that characterize the distribution. Only a complete knowledge of them allows the distribution to be fully described. These statistics can be estimated from representative samples.

- *Discrete (binomial and Poisson):* Probabilities corresponding to every possible value of the random variable can be derived. The sum of all such probabilities is one.
- *Continuous (normal, chi-squared, t-distribution, etc.):* Here, only the probability of random variable is derived taking all the measures in certain range (as the values can be infinite). The *total area under the curve* is one representing the probability of all possible events. The probability for a value *x* lying between two limits is equal to the area under the curve between these values. The probability density function (PDF) is the curve that can be drawn from the equation of distribution, if the horizontal axis represents the values of x.

Normal (Gaussian) Distribution

Ideally population is the set of all possible values for a variable, so that any random selection of objects from the population will render a random variable. Such a population is described completely (modeled) if the PDF is specified **(Fig. 5A)**. The PDF is in this case (normal distribution) is completely described by the mean and the variance. The normal distribution is the most widely used distribution in statistics and large number of commonly used statistical methods are based on this distribution. It is sometimes called the "bell curve", by virtue of its shape when plotted. The other name is "Gaussian curve" named after the mathematician Carl Friedrich Gauss although Abraham de Moivre first discovered and described the distribution. The term "*normal*" was coined by Francis Galton. This is just a nominal depiction and it is important to remember that there is nothing abnormal about the normal distribution. Strictly speaking; however, statistically the usage of term "the normal distribution" is incorrect to describe this specific distribution as there are many normal distributions also the term "bell-shaped" distribution is possibly incorrect as other distributions may have similar shape (discussed below). The normal distribution is a subclass of the elliptical distributions that can all differ in their means and standard deviations. Features of normal distributions are listed below:

- They are symmetric around their mean **(Fig. 5B)**, is nonzero over the entire real line, and have inverted bell-shaped curve [though many other distributions are also bell-shaped (such as Cauchy's, Student's, and logistic)].
- The shape characteristics like height; width of Gaussian distribution is determined by mean and standard deviation, so that it represents a family of expression of data with many possible shapes (thin curve, thick curve, etc.).
- Normal distributions are primarily defined by the mean (μ) and standard deviation (σ). A random variable within

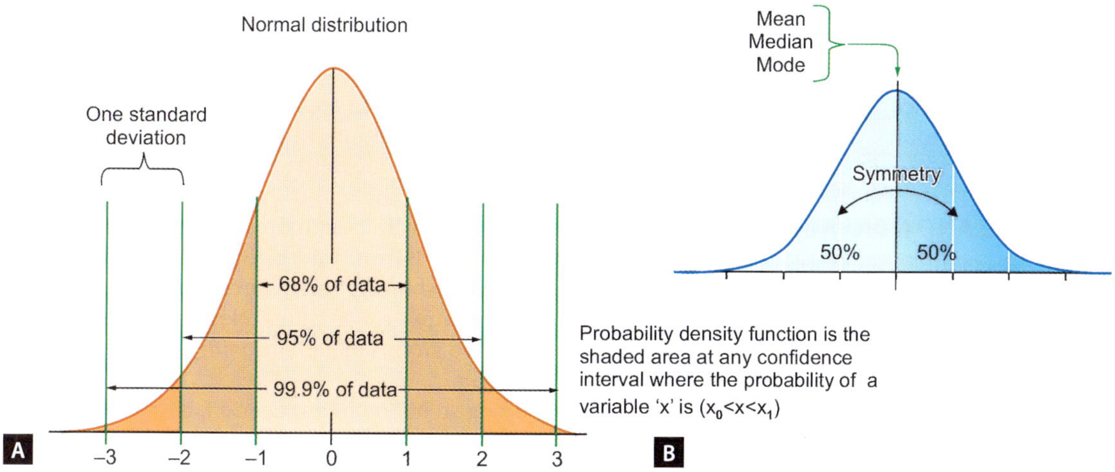

Figs. 5A and B: Normal distribution.

Gaussian distribution is normally distributed and is called a *normal deviate.*

- For such a random variable *x* that is normally distributed with mean μ and variance σ, the *standardized normal deviate* (SND, *z*), will have a standard normal distribution given by

$$z = \frac{x - \mu}{\sigma}$$

- The lesser the standard deviation the lesser the variability of data and narrower the distribution.
- The mean, median, and mode of a normal distribution are equal, a "standardized" normal distribution (unit normal distribution) has mean = 0, variance = 1 and σ = 1.
- The distribution is continuous for all values of a variable *x* between –∞ and +∞ so that each conceivable interval of real numbers has a probability other than zero.
- The area under the normal curve is equal to 1.0.
- Normal distributions are denser in the center and rarer in the tails.
- About 68% of the area of a normal distribution is within one standard deviation (±1σ) of the mean **(Fig. 5A)**, so that for a ±1σ interval, there is almost one out of three chances that the true value is outside these limits. Increasing the standard deviations will increase the confidence interval also and for two standard deviations (±1.96σ), the probability of true value lying outside reduces to only 5%.
- Approximately 95% of the area of a normal distribution is within two standard deviations (precisely it is 1.96σ rounded off to ±2σ) of the mean **(Fig. 5A)**.

Gaussian distribution was first applied to human characteristics by Quetelet who noted that general characteristics such as height, weight, and strength are normally distributed. For characteristics that are not normally distributed, Laplace showed that the means of their repeated measures from the distribution are very nearly normally distributed. This also portended the notion and suggested the now accepted practice that the larger the sample size, the closer is the distribution of means to a normal distribution.

As mentioned previously also most of the statistical procedures and tests for estimating significance of differences between means assume Gaussian distributions. These tests are often based on normal distribution of means which is very close to normal, so that the tests often work well even if the original distribution is only roughly normal. It is interesting to note that the validity of most statistical procedures relies on an assumption of "approximate" normality (taking already into account some amount of error).

Other Distributions

T-distribution: It was described by WS Gossett, who published under the pseudonym "Student"; it is often called Student's t-distribution. Degrees of freedom characterize the t-distribution (unlike the mean and variance for normal distribution). The shape of t-distribution is similar to normal bell-shaped curve, but the tails are longer and it is more spread out. It is more useful to calculate the confidence intervals and testing the null hypothesis about one or two means.

Chi-squared distribution: This is a right-skewed distribution taking positive values, but becomes more symmetrical as the degrees of freedom increases. It is useful for analyzing the categorical data.

F-distribution: This is right skewed distribution and is given by ratio of two estimated variances that is calculated from the normalized data. Unlike Gaussian distribution, f-distribution is characterized by the degrees of freedom of numerator and denominator. F-distribution is most useful for comparing two variances and more than two means using analysis of variance (ANOVA).

Binomial distribution: When there are two possible outcomes or measures then a binomial distribution comes into play. The two parameters that describe the binomial distribution are *n*, the number of individuals in the sample (or repetitions of a trial) and π the true probability of success for each individual (or in each trial). Its *mean* (the value for the random variable that we *expect* if we look at *n* individuals, or repeat the trial n times) is $n\pi$. Its *variance* is $n\pi(1 - \pi)$. Binomial distribution is useful to make inferences about the proportions. The distribution is skewed to right if $\pi < 0.5$ and to the left if $\pi > 0.5$ with a small n. With increase in n the distribution becomes more symmetrical and becomes normal like if both $n\pi$ and $n(1 - \pi)$ are >5.

THE PARAMETRIC AND NONPARAMETRIC TESTS

Means, standard deviations, and proportions are all important values and also called "parameters" when we are referring to a population or large sample in practice. As we do not study the whole population, but only a sample from it, we estimate these quantities for our sample. These quantities for a sample are called "statistics". A statistic estimates a parameter. Parametric statistical procedures as mentioned earlier often assume a normal or near normal distribution in the researched population and hence also the sample. They also assume normality for derived parameters (i.e., mean and standard deviation) of the assumed distribution. This situation was found nonuniversal and in fact for most small sample size studies the parameters and study population is not "normally" distributed. This led to the development of nonparametric tests. Nonparametric statistical procedures rely either on no or few assumptions about the parameters of the population distribution or the studied sample. This gives a liberty to use this test for most studies where population distribution is unknown or cannot be determined or is found to be nonparametric. Just to mention these tests do as well as the parametric tests for normal population when applied in place of the latter, though it is statistically incorrect to do so. The advantages of nonparametric tests are:

- For very small sample sizes (as small as $N = 6$) one has to use a nonparametric test only as no other tests would suit.
- Most nonparametric statistics reveal exact probabilities regardless of the shape of population distribution from which the random sample has been drawn so are best when population type is unknown.
- Nonparametric tests can be used to evaluate samples made up of observations even from several different populations.
- These tests are easier to learn and apply than parametric tests.
- Parametric tests can best handle data which are inherently depicted in ranks and also data which are classificatory.

By above one should not assume that these are the best tests and can be applied everywhere. Although nonparametric tests make few assumptions about the distribution of variables in the population, they have few drawbacks also arising out of this very property of being less exact.

- In general, they are less statistically powerful than parametric tests, especially when the data is normal as they tend to not capture the details of population distribution. "Less powerful" implies a smaller probability that the test will tell us about association of the two variables when they in fact are truly associated.
- *Losing precision/wasteful of data:* For a determinate population a parametric test needs smaller population to tell us the correct outcome while nonparametric test will need slightly larger sample size to have equivalent power thus wasting data.
- Though easier to apply and derive analysis, their results are less easy to interpret for an amateur than parametric tests. This is due to the fact that nonparametric tests use rankings of the values (so a comparative value) in the data rather than actual numerical data. This difference in ranks is less understood in general, for example, analysis showing the difference in mean ranks between two groups of "five" is less clear than knowing that one of the two groups of patients with OA have mean 5 kg more weight.
- Being so liberal in application, they give a false sense of security.
- Higher ordered interactions are not appropriately dealt with.

In short, parametric and nonparametric are basically two broad classifications of statistical procedures. Nonparametric tests can be liberally applied and are useful in many cases though as a matter of fact really needed only in some, if the study is properly organized. One must remember that they are not a perfect solution for their need of less exactness and strictness of criteria. For the application of parametric tests, the biggest worry is deriving incorrect conclusions, if the data deviate significantly from the assumptions made for parametric procedure. Also the assumption of normality of data is particularly challenged for small sample sizes ($n < 30$). Nonparametric tests do well in both these cases. A guide to choosing a test is presented in **Table 2**. It is useful to understand as a rough measure that continuous variables can be both parametric and nonparametric however categorical measures by virtue of being discrete are evaluated by nonparametric analysis.

So, if the data contains categorical variables use nonparametric test, but if the data has continuous variable then first find if the data is normally distributed (and do parametric tests) else if sample size is low or data comes out to be nonparametric then do nonparametric analysis. One can do statistical analysis to determine, if the data is parametric. The methods (called *"normality tests") fall into two broad categories:*

1. Graphical—Q-Q probability plots and cumulative frequency (P-P) plots are the common graphical methods.
2. Statistical methods—Kolmogorov–Smirnov test (and its adaptation Lilliefors test), Shapiro–Wilk test (probably having best power), Anderson–Darling test are few of the common statistical methods to determine the normalcy of distribution.

These test the null hypothesis (H_0) that the observations are distributed normally with unspecified mean and σ^2 (variance) versus the alternative hypothesis (H_a) that the distribution is arbitrary.

ANALYSIS OF CONTINUOUS VARIABLE

Here the situation requires usually the comparison of means of two or more datasets for variables that have intrinsic real number possible infinite values (continuous variable). There

TABLE 2: How to choose a statistical test?

Number of variables in the analysis		*Class of statistics*	
		Nonparametric (nominal; ordinal)	***Parametric (interval; ratio)***
One variable	Categorical	Percentage, chi-square	Impossible
	Continuous	Median, mode and quartile range	Mean, standard deviation, Z-test, and t-test
Two variables	Both categorical	Chi-square (independent) McNemar's test (dependent variables) Contingency coefficient 2 × 2 table Mann–Whitney U (independent rank/ordinal) Wilcoxon matched pairs (dependent ranks) Kruskal–Wallis	Correspondence analysis
	One categorical and the other continuous	Simple logistic regression	Student t-test (dichotomous variable) Simple linear regression One-way ANOVA (multichotomous variable)
	Both continuous	Spearman's rank correlation Kendalls' rank coefficient	Pearson correlation Simple regression T-test (independent sample) Paired t-test (for within group analysis) One-way ANOVA
Three variables	Three categorical	Factorial logistic regression Cross tabulation Chi-square (nominal) Kruskal–Wallis H (rank/ordinal) Friedman's ANOVA (ordinal/rank)	Factorial ANOVA Cochran's Q (nominal)
	Two categorical one continuous	Multiple logistic regression	ANOVA (two way)
	One categorical two continuous	Comparison of proportions	Analysis of covariance (ANOVA) Factorial (two way) ANOVA
	Three continuous	Kendall's W	Multiple regression Multiple correlation one way ANOVA
Four variables	K categorical	Cross tabulation CHAID	Quasi-metric multidimensional scaling Friedman's ANOVA
	One categorical K-continuous		Prohibit analysis (normal probability distribution) Logit analysis (logistic probability distribution) Multiple discriminant analysis
	K-continuous		Multiple regression Multiple correlation Multivariate analysis of variance (MANOVA) Factor analysis
	One continuous and K categorical		CART Multiple regression

are commonly following four situations (simplified, refer **Table 4** for detail) where tests are applied on the basis of whether the data is normally distributed or not:

- For a single patient group (adequate sample size) if comparison is required for pre- and postintervention (or a change over time) then paired sample t-test is used for parametric data else Wilcoxon signed-ranks test is used. For low sample size use nonparametric tests **(Table 2)**.
- If we need to compare the observed values to standard value in literature then test of hypothesis is used for parametric data else sign test is used.
- Comparing means of two different groups of patient with parametric data requires independent sample t-test or Wilcoxon rank sum-test (Mann–Whitney U) for nonparametric data.
- ANOVA is used for multiple comparisons to determine difference of one intervention from several others or where multiple comparisons are required.

When we intend to compare the means of two datasets, it is helpful to understand that larger difference in means makes it more likely that the difference is real (and not emanating from chance observation), smaller standard deviation reduces variability of data and lastly higher sample size will improve the power of the appropriately applied test. The standard error of mean estimates how closely the sample mean resembles true population mean (for a sample undertaking whole population the standard error of mean is zero).

The Student's t-test

The Student's t-test is devised by William Gosset (mathematician) in 1908. He found that if sample is taken from normally distributed population then the sample observations will also be normally distributed and described "t-distribution" which is the probability distribution to evaluate hypothesis regarding means of continuous variables.

The t-distribution is similar to "normal" distribution, distributed symmetrically around mean = 0. But there is a basic difference that the σ of t-distribution varies with the "degrees of freedom". For a data containing "n" observations, the degrees of freedom would be $n - 1$, so whilst there is only one normal distribution there is a separate t-distribution for each possible degree of freedom from one to infinity. T-distribution tables are available from various statistics books. Because of company policy that forbade employee name publishing he forcibly used pseudonym "student" with the t-test. "T" indicates difference of two means (the critical ratio, t-statistic):

$$t = \frac{\bar{y} - \mu}{Standard\ error} = \frac{\bar{y} - \mu}{\frac{\sigma}{\sqrt{n}}}$$

Here, $\bar{y}$ = mean of sample observation, μ = population mean, n = sample size. For a valid t-test the variances of two data should be comparable, the observations should be independent in two groups, median should be equal to mean (normal distribution).

The value of "t" can be obtained from standard t-distribution tables.

Confidence interval should be determined for every mean to determine how confident we are that our sample mean represents true population. Generally the confidence interval extends either side of the estimate by some multiple of the standard error (often taken as 1.96 standard deviation on each side—the confidence limits). If we were to repeat the experiment many times, the range of values determined in this way would contain the true population mean on 95% of occasions, known as 95% confidence interval for the mean. We know that 95% confidence interval = $\bar{y} \pm 2\sigma$. This is an approximate measure however. The exact calculation for a t-distribution can be done as follows:

$$95\%\ \text{confidence interval} = \bar{y} + t \times \text{standard error} = \bar{y} + t \times \frac{\sigma}{\sqrt{n}}$$

For a *proportion* (included here only to complete the discussion on confidence interval. It is not a part of t-distribution) if the sample size is large enough then the sampling distribution is nearly normal with mean π. We estimate π by the proportion in the sample, $p = r/n$ (where r is the number of individuals in the sample with the characteristic of interest), and its standard error is estimated by $\sqrt{p(1p)/n}$. The 95% confidence interval for proportion is estimated by:

$$\left(p - \left|1.96 \times \sqrt{\frac{p(1-p)}{n}}\right. \text{ to } p + \left|1.96 \times \sqrt{\frac{p(1-p)}{n}}\right.\right)$$

The t-test is a commonly used test of hypothesis for normally distributed continuous variables and can be applied from various available software. Where data does not come from normal distribution there are two ways to analyze data, either use nonparametric tests (like the sign test, commonly done) or else transform data to a scale which is normally distributed. Data transformation can be done by taking log of each data point ("logarithmic" method) or using the square root of each data point; these normalize the outliers and reduce the variance. For one sample t-test we assume a normal distribution (or find out by various tests described above) and that the sample size is large enough. If we do not know the population variance then using the t-distribution we can apply t-test else for a known population variance we better use the z-test (though both produce identical result).

For two related samples or for repeated measures paired sample t-test is done, if the sample is normally distributed else Wilcoxon signed-rank test has to be used (this utilizes the sign test as for nonparametric data and also takes into consideration the magnitude of values so is a more powerful test than the sign test). If the samples are unrelated (say from two different groups, in which one outcome of interest) then unpaired t-test (two-sample or independent sample t-test) is used if the samples are from normal population (parametric data). If the samples are not large enough or normality and/or equal variances are not achieved in the samples then nonparametric test like the Wilcoxon rank sum (two-sample) test can be used. Other way to address this is to use Mann–Whitney U test (complicated to do by hand but makes no difference to click in software).

For more than two independent groups that are analyzed for a common numerical or ordinal variable of interest we can perform a simple test to compare the averages in each pair of groups, but this will entail high type I error. So in such instances we use a "global" test ANOVA. One-way ANOVA separates the *between-group variation*—attributed to differences between the individuals from the different groups and *within-group variation*—attributed to the random variation between the individuals within each group. The test statistic for ANOVA is a ratio, F that is the ratio of (between-group variance to the within group variance). This F-statistic follows the F-distribution (discussed above). The nonparametric equivalent test of ANOVA is Kruskal–Wallis test that can be used, if we find that the data is not from normal distribution [finding by Levene's test, Bartlett's test, or others (discussed above)] and do not want to transform the data to make it near normal.

NONPARAMETRIC ANALYSIS (ANALYSIS OF CATEGORICAL VARIABLE)

For simplicity, we recall that independent (explanatory) or dependent (response) variable is categorical that can be nominal or ordinal. Contingency tables represent all combinations of levels of explanatory and response variables [nominal/nominal; nominal/ordinal; ordinal/ordinal simplest being a 2 × 2 table **(Table 3)**]. The numbers in table represent the "counts" of elements. Total number of rows and columns are called marginal counts. A contingency table (cross tabulation; cross tab) analysis is used to examine the relationship between two categorical variables. The following relationships that can be drawn from a contingency table:

- *Sensitivity (true positive rate; recall rate; hit rate):* Sensitivity is the probability of a test reporting positive in a diseased patient. It is a property of a test to measure the proportion of correctly identified cases. A perfect prediction would be 100% sensitive. Sensitivity is measured from the columns as follows:

Sensitivity = true positive count (a)/[total of true positive and false negative (a + c)].

A test with high sensitivity has low type II error. They are considered reliable when "negative" to rule out disease. Screening tests are chosen as to having high sensitivity as they have low false negative rate and are unlikely to miss an affected individual. Sensitive test increases the positive predictive value in low prevalence of disease.

- *Specificity (true negative rate):* Specificity is the probability is a negative test in a person not having disease. It measures the proportion of correctly identified healthy persons (proportion of negative test that is correct). A perfect prediction will again be 100% specific. Specificity is measured as follows:

  Specificity = true negative count (d)/[total of true negative and false positive (b + d)].

  Highly specific test has low type I error. They are considered reliable when positive.

TABLE 3: A 2 × 2 contingency table.

		Disease	
Disease present		***Disease absent***	
Test outcome or 'Exposure'	Positive	True positive (a)	False positive (b) Type I error
	Negative	False negative (c) Type II error	True negative (d)

The common notion of a highly specific test being able to diagnose a disease reliably and a highly sensitive test reliable ruling out a disease, if negative is a misconception. The property of a test to be reliable depends both on sensitivity and specificity. All tests carry some error in measurement so none is 100% specific or sensitive. To avoid missing a diagnosis in population one should choose a sensitive test while for making a correct diagnosis and avoiding overdiagnosis one should choose a specific test. This trade-off can be statistically represented as a receiver operating characteristic (ROC) curve. To draw ROC curve we require true positive rate (sensitivity) and false positive rate (equals to 1 - specificity). The sensitivity defines how many correct positive results occur among all positive samples available during the test. False positive rate (1 - specificity), on the other hand, defines how many incorrect positive results occur among all negative samples available during the test. The sensitivity is plotted on y-axis while (1 - specificity) is plotted on x-axis. The perfect test would come at a point located at (0,1) which represents 100% sensitivity and 100% specificity. A completely random guess would fall at the diagonal line and as sample size approximates population the "random guess" will get located at (0.5, 0.5). The diagonal divides the graph into two portions, tests lying upper left region are "good" tests while lower right region tests are "unacceptable" for characteristics. A good test curve will rise quickly to upper left corner and then continue to rise slowly till end.

- *False positive rate [fall-out, (1-specificity)]:* Represents the possibility of a test reporting positive in absence of a disease (opposite of specificity). False positive rate is given by:

TABLE 4: Oxford Centre for Evidence-based Medicine Levels of Evidence and Journal of Bone and Joint Surgery.

	Therapeutic studies: Investigating the results of treatment	***Prognostic studies: Investigating the outcome of disease***	***Diagnostic studies: Investigating a diagnostic test***	***Economic and decision analysis: Developing an economic or decision model***
Level I	Randomized controlled trial significant difference No significant difference but narrow Confidence interval Systematic review of level I randomized controlled trials (studies were homogeneous)	Prospective study Systematic review of level I studies	Testing of previously developed diagnostic criteria in series of consecutive patients (with universally applied reference "gold" standard") Systematic review of level I studies	Clinically sensible costs and alternatives; values obtained from many studies; multiway sensitivity analyses Systematic review of level I studies
Level II	Prospective cohort study Poor quality randomized controlled trial (e.g., <80% follow-up) Systematic review Level II studies Nonhomogeneous Level I studies	Retrospective study Study of untreated controls from a previous randomized controlled trial Systematic review of level II studies	Development of diagnostic criteria based on basis of consecutive patients (with universally applied reference "gold" standard") Systematic review of level II studies	Clinically sensible costs and alternatives; values obtained from many studies; multiway sensitivity analyses System review of level II studies
Level III	Case-control study Retrospective study Systematic review of Level III studies		Study of nonconsecutive patients (no consistently applied reference "gold" standard") Systematic review of level III studies	Limited alternatives and costs; poor estimates Systematic review of level III studies
Level IV	Case series (no, or historical, control group)	Case series	Case-control study Poor reference standard	No sensitivity analyses
Level V	Expert opinion	Expert opinion	Expert opinion	Expert opinion

False positive count (b)/[total count of disease free individuals (b + d)].

- Accuracy of a test is the probability of a correct test result. It is the percentage correctness of a test (true positive + true negative). This is calculated as follows:
- Accuracy = {correct test result [true positive (a) + true negative (d)]}/total of all positive and negative test result (a + b + c + d).
- *Positive predictive value (PPV, probability of a disease):* This is the probability of having a disease in a subject with positive test result [probability of a test being positive of all positive test results (not truly diseases)]. This is calculated as follows:
  Positive predictive value = true positive (a)/[total number of positive test count (a + b)].
- *Negative predictive value (probability of health):* This is the probability of disease being absent from the individual with a negative test result. This is calculated as follows:
  Negative predictive value = true negative (d)/total negative test count [true negative (d) + false negatives (c)]
- Prevalence of disease is the probability of disease in community given no test information. This is given by the formula:
  Prevalence of disease = (a + c)/(a + b + c + d)
- Prevalence of health is the probability of health in community given no test information is available. This is given by formula:
  Prevalence of health = (b + d)/(a + b + c + d)
- False discovery rate is the probability of a test being wrongly positive (wrongly reporting disease in healthy individuals). This is also equivalent to (1 – PPV). This is given by the formula:
  False discovery rate = false positives (b)/[total positive test counts (a + b)]
- False negative rate = 1 – sensitivity, is the probability of a negative test given the presence of disease. This is calculated as follows:
  False negative rate = false negative (c)/[total count of true cases (a + c)]

Odds ratio and relative risk: Probability is the proportion (expressed in percentage) of times an event would occur if an observation is repeated (this ranges between 0 and 1). "Odds" are specific expression of probability. They are simply the probability of an event happening divided by the probability of event not happening, i.e., probability/(1 – probability). The value can range from 1 to ∞. Odds ratio is the odds of event occurring in a group (exposed to inciting event) divided by odds of same event occurring in another group (not exposed to inciting event). So odds ratio is expressed as follows:

$$\text{Odds ratio} = \frac{\dfrac{p_1}{1-p_1}}{\dfrac{p_2}{1-p_2}}$$

P_1 is the probability of event in group 1 while P_2 is the probability of event in group 2.

Relative risk is easier to understand and is not always same as odds ratio (discussed later). Relative risk is simply a ratio of probability of occurrence of an event in two groups (unlike odds where the ratio of probability to absence of it). From **Table 5**, relative risk will be:

$$\text{Relative risk} = \frac{a/(a+b)}{c/(c+d)}$$

Say for example the probability of another vertebral fracture in a patient with previous osteoporotic vertebral fracture is 807 per 1,000 while the probability of fresh vertebral fracture occurring in osteoporotic patients is 214 per 1,000 then the relative risk = (807/1,000)/(214/1,000) = 4. So, the relative risk of developing a vertebral fracture in a patient who has sustained an osteoporotic fracture is five times. Usually, the calculation of relative risk requires some benchmark for denominator against which the "relative risk" for current procedure in question is being evaluated. If one calculates odds ratio for above example it will come to around 15. This means there is 15-fold increased risk of developing vertebral fracture in patients who have sustained previous vertebral fracture—now considering a baseline risk of 20% for vertebral fractures in females the secondary fractures will come to 300% which is nonsense (as the incidence of secondary fractures should not cross 100%). This is actually what happens when "odds ratio" is used as a "proxy" to relative risk in clinical research. One should be very specific as to when to use one. Odds ratio and relative risk are in agreement till the event is a rare one or at best uncommon (probability < 10%). As the event becomes more common the odds ratio starts exaggerating the event estimates. Also the use and understanding of odds ratio is difficult especially for association to outcome so relative risk is a common measure to apply for better communication. The use of odds ratio is probably restricted to case-control studies and logistic regression analysis for which they are the appropriate measures of association.

To test a hypothesis for categorical variables the following simplified generalization may be applied (*see* also the analysis of continuous variables some tests for nonparametric data are exampled there that apply for categorical variables also):

1. Univariate analysis (gender) for a binary (male/female) variable (i.e., a categorical data with single proportion) can be done by *z*-test.
2. For significance analysis in a 2 × 2 table with small number of samples (<5 in any cell of the table) fisher exact test is appropriate else chi-square is the standard. It should be remembered that the contingency tables should never be built from separate studies or separate subgroups of population. Data pooled from such studies will produce Simpson's paradox. Such pooled data should be analyzed by Mantel-Haenszel procedure or logistic regression.
3. For paired samples (two diseases, two treatments, before and after) McNemar's test is used.
4. Pearson's chi-square test is a commonly applied test to evaluate nominal or ordinal explanatory and response

variables. These variables take up any number of distinct levels or ranks. For a 2 × 2 table with large sample size usually a χ^2 test is used. χ^2 basically tests the distribution/ relation of response variable vis-à-vis each level of the explanatory variable.

5. Though Pearson's χ^2 test can be used to test associations among ordinal variables (as is also commonly used also), there exist more powerful tests to assess the same especially when the association between them is directional (positive or negative). In such cases, "Goodman and Kruskal's gamma" or Kendall's tau are preferred.
6. For multivariate analysis of a binary variable, linear discriminant analysis and multiple regressions will both produce equivalent results. The linear regression analysis is performed to identify the relationship or variability of explanatory variable on the dependent variable. This is best done by linear regression analysis (say the effect of height on blood pressure or the effect of height on development of pilonidal sinus); this is essentially a univariate analysis as we are interested only in one variable. If there are multiple such explanatory variables then multiple linear regression analysis is used, this is a multivariate analysis.
7. Correlation analysis measures the degree of association between two variables. On a scatter diagram a straight line depicts linear correlation. Pearson's correlation coefficient measures the linear relation between variables. The correlation is depicted by symbol *r that can take a value of* −1 to +1.
   - Positive correlation means in general that if one variable increases the other also increases while negative correlation indicates that if one variable increases the other decreases.
   - The magnitude of correlation dictates how close they are to the straight line on a scatter plot. Value of zero depicts no linear correlation. Note that they may still be correlated in other forms like logarithmic or other nonlinear forms.
   - Correlation coefficient has no dimensions, it is just a coefficient.
   - Correlation does not necessarily indicate a "cause and effect" relation.
   - Interchanging the two variables does not affect the coefficient.
   - Correlation should not be calculated when there is a nonlinear relationship, the data includes more than one observation on the individual, one or more outliers are present.

Spearman correlation coefficient:

- PThis is a nonparametric equivalent of the Pearson's correlation coefficient and is calculated if one or more of the following are present:
  - One or both variables are ordinal
  - One or both variables are not normally distributed
  - Sample size is small

HYPOTHESIS TESTING (THE *p*-VALUE APPROACH)

One needs to analyze the outcome variables for testing the hypothesis formulated at the start of study. The most common method is utilizing a calculated *p*-value for rejecting or accepting the null hypothesis. Other methods include E-value and critical value approach that are used in specific circumstances. We will only delve with *p*-value and its significance here.

One should understand the significance and real meaning of *p*-value, so that it can be rationally presented rather than just saying "significant" observation below a certain arbitrary fixed number. The alphabet "*p*" in p-value represents "calculated *p*robability". The *p*-value was first formally introduced by Karl Pearson, in his Pearson's chi-squared test, using the chi-squared distribution and notated as capital *P*, but its role in statistics was popularized by Ronald Fisher where he proposed $p = 0.05$, as the limit for statistical significance applied to normal distribution for a two-tailed test. By definition, the *p*-value represents the probability, under the assumption of hypothesis (usually null hypothesis), of obtaining a result equal to or more extreme than what was actually observed. For naïve investigators, it can be more simply stated that *p*-value defines the probability of obtaining a result equal to or "more extreme" than what was actually observed, when the null hypothesis is true. This probability is calculated by utilizing various tests for parametric or non-parametric analysis (depending on type of variable, study setting and statistic) that will be described below in specific headings. So, for example, if we compare two drugs for pain relief under the null hypothesis that the effect is not different, then p-value tells us the probability of finding a different result. Say drug A and B demonstrate different relief in pain, the investigator will try to determine what is the probability that the difference is falling within the purview of null hypothesis, in other words, what difference in pain relief will tell him that there is difference between the effects of drugs and it exceeds the "null" (no difference) zone. If the *p*-value (probability) is too low then investigator can assume that there is not "no difference" in the effect of drugs, so there must be "some difference" in the drug effects. Now, what is the significance of this difference? To answer the level of significance investigator will set the limits for finding such probability by defining α—usually set at 5% (0.05) or 1% (0.01). Now again, if the drug A was 1.5 times more effective in relieving pain than drug B and on analysis the *p*-value came to be 0.026, then this difference will be considered significant for set *p*-value of 0.05, as the investigator finds that assuming null hypothesis (H_0) the probability is very low to accept the H_0 and the result is actually "extreme", i.e., the probability lies outside the accepted 95% "null" observations. The smaller the *p*-value, the larger is the significance because it tells the investigator that the hypothesis under consideration (null hypothesis, H_0) may not adequately explains the observation. This makes the investigator to reject the null hypothesis and he accepts the alternative hypothesis that there is actual difference between the drugs A and B. A high probability say p-value of 0.35 or 0.66 would have meant that it is highly probable for this difference of 1.5 times to lie very close to the mean within the bell curve of normal distribution based on H_0 where investigator would have accepted the null hypothesis that this 1.5 times difference is actually no difference. For another investigator who has kept significance to 0.01, the found p-value of 0.026 is not significant and he comes to conclusion that the difference is in alignment with H_0 (no difference), as the observation lies within the acceptable 99% of the possible "null values" according to H_0, so he accepts the null hypothesis that there is no difference between drugs A and B. This lays the importance of selecting the significance level. For first investigator, there could be α-error where he would have rejected the H_0 when there was actually no difference as found by second investigator; while for second investigator, it could be β-error. We normally keep α-error low by keeping low significance level (this, however, needs larger sample size). Now we also need to understand that in investigating drugs not always will drug A will be better than B and in fact the drug B could have a better effect than drug A, so we nearly always choose a two-tailed analysis. The only situation in which you should use a *one-sided p* value is when a large change in an unexpected direction would have absolutely no relevance to your study, which is very uncommon. This also prevents us from wrongly assuming only one-sided effect in this random world and we keep open to even reverse possibility.

There are in general four steps in this p-value analysis:

1. Specify the null and alternative hypotheses.
2. Using the sample data and assuming the null hypothesis are true; calculate the value of the test statistic. Again to conduct the hypothesis test for the population mean μ, we use the t-statistic:

$$t = \frac{\bar{y} - \mu}{\frac{\sigma}{\sqrt{n}}}$$

   which follows a t-distribution with $n - 1$ degrees of freedom.
3. Using the known distribution of the test statistic, calculate the p-value—"if the null hypothesis is true, what is the probability that we would observe a more extreme test statistic—(that would reject the H_0 but will more likely align in the direction of the alternative hypothesis) than we did?"
4. Set the significance level, α, the probability of making a type I error to be small—0.01, 0.05, or 0.10. Compare the p-value to α. If the p-value is less than (or equal to) α, reject the null hypothesis in favor of the alternative hypothesis. If the *p-value is greater than α, do not reject the null hypothesis.*

One must understand the significance level is actually the chance investigator is accepting for his observations to be wrong—5% means 1 in 20 chance that his observation is actually incorrect, so low significance level would mean lesser chance of him being wrong say 0.001 indicates 1 in 1,000 chance to be incorrect. Such very low significance cutoff levels need larger and larger sample sizes but reduce the chances of wrongly accepting the difference when there is actually none. No investigator can ever be 100% certain in an analysis unless he has complete population data, so in a sample analysis—we all do that we have to report results with some chance of error incorporated in it. This entails that there are lots of fallacies in use of the p-value, some cautions are mentioned below:

- Beware that even if null hypothesis is rejected one does not know "which" alternative hypothesis is correct unless there is only one alternative possible. For example—if we assumed a null hypothesis with a normal distribution then rejection of the same could imply either—(1) the mean is not zero, or (2) the variance is not unity, or (3) the distribution is not normal all depending on the sampling, randomization, and various study variables. Commonly, we test the means for accepting or rejecting the H_0 assuming normal distribution which is mostly not the case. Also rejecting H_0 means that the zero mean of normal distribution is incorrect, but we would never know which nonzero mean should we adopt as the new mean?
- Also by same corollary, if we cannot reject the null hypothesis by finding that the observed value did not reach the set significance level then this does not mean that the null hypothesis is true and can never be rejected, and may be the study set up was flawed.
- The use of p-value generally applies only to null hypothesis, but it does not allow reasoning for multiple hypothesis or a range of hypothesis where instead Bayesian statistics need to be used.
- Standardization of methodology, introducing blinding, and reducing bias are of utmost importance as it is a known fact that depending on the intentions of the analyst to analyze the data along differing prescriptions (experimental designs and choice of statistic) different results for the same data concerning the same underlying question can be obtained from making the p-value incompatible with the likelihood principle.

LEVELS OF EVIDENCE

For established EBM the levels of evidence are most important that help in making the decision fast and consistently. For best decision, the levels must be easily available and in conformity to universal practice. These are commonly used to produce clinical practice guidelines that are published time and again with evolving evidence. These evidences are classified to minimize therapeutic harm to patients by using evidence that is least likely to be wrong. The Centre for Evidence-Based Medicine (http://cebm.net/levels_of_evidence.asp) has created the categories for levels of evidence (***see* Table 4**) and grades for recommendations **(Table 5)**.

TABLE 5: Oxford Centre for Evidence-Based Medicine Grades of Recommendation.

A	Consistent level I studies
B	Consistent level II or III studies or extrapolations from level I studies
C	Level IV studies or extrapolations from level II or III studies
D	Level V evidence or troublingly inconsistent or inconclusive studies of any level

SOME ESSENTIALS FOR YOUNG INVESTIGATORS AND RESEARCHERS

Ethics

Peer review is an important component for most published researches these days and should be made mandatory. Studies involving humans (or animals) are reviewed by people not concerned or connected with the study or investigators but belong to same realm as that of readers. These reviewers also should not profit directly or even indirectly in any way from the conduct or publication of the study. Usually multiple committees are established to review and analyze the content of study its feasibility, relevance and ethical practice compliance.

Plagiarism (Latin: plagiarius = kidnapper): Plagiarism in simple terms represents copying and/or publishing another author's thoughts, ideas, expression or even language, and representing as one's own original work. Different medical regulatory bodies/councils have their own definitions, but in common all have the common notion that plagiarism involves deliberate appropriation of the works of others represented as one's own. The definitions for various aspects are unclear; however, there are unclear rules and consensus for legal or professional action against the convict. Plagiarism in considered academic dishonesty, a serious breach of ethics of practice and constitutes copyright infringement (that can be possibly legally challenged on this ground). Plagiarism appears similar to copyright violation, but there is a difference that in plagiarism the "gain in author's reputation" ("how much gain" is difficult to quantify in terms of "losses" to the original author—so the legal procedure falls weak) by work done by someone else, so it does not directly come under jurisdiction. In copyright violation, the author use work without consent that is protected by copyright holder and is liable to be directly challenged in court of law. In medical literature, there have been several instances (and are also coming up) where students, professors, and various researchers have used partially or completely the work done by someone else for their publication or thesis work. This amounts to academic fraud and dishonesty. Though difficult to challenge in court of law, there are chances of stringent action and even expulsion of the doer if the authority take cognizance and sincere effort to stop such activities establishing examples for future. The practice of copying gained momentum with the increase in the published literature due to availability of online tools and also partly due to peer pressure for publication and gaining reputation. Some people even resort to self-plagiarism (recycling fraud) where the author publishes one's own work in identical or nearly identical form at various places without acknowledging or citing the original work. These are duplicate or multiple publications, but are difficult to identify because there is a fair acceptance among the fraternity to limited reuse of work. Self-plagiarism embroils dishonesty, but not a theft per se. People argue that the term self-plagiarism in a misnomer as plagiarism involves copying others work so "self" represents oxymoron. Self-plagiarism is thought to represent specific forms of unethical conduct like dual or redundant publication.

INFORMED CONSENT

The principle of informed consent says that a participant should clearly know about the conduct of a study of which he is a part and about any possible harm and/or benefits that may result from his voluntary participation in the study. This disclosure should be full in detail to best of the knowledge of the investigator, made in the best understood language of the participant and best made in writing. It is also important that the participation be voluntary without any force that may invite legal actions, if found so. As regards study of novel method on humans, both the Nuremberg Code and the Helsinki Accords recommend that, as far as possible, animal studies should be done prior to human experimentation.

Informed consent is the procedure of informing the person comprehensively about the complete facts of intervention including future implications and possible alternatives in their best understood language, so as to obtain permission for conducting the intervention. The consent should be "full", "free", and "voluntary" without any boundation or partiality or arising out of ignorance. The consent is also to be obtained before enrolling a patient for a trial that may or may not incur intervention later (placebo treatment group). The consent obtained should be legally valid. A doctor who treats without valid consent will be liable under the offence and criminal laws. Medical practitioners should understand that law presumes the treating doctor/investigator to be in a dominating position who can selectively hide information; hence, the consent should be obtained after providing all the necessary information best in writing. The structure of consent should be guided by the principles of autonomy (of patient's rights), beneficence (treating doctors actions to benefit and consider well-being of patient), nonmaleficence (do no harm), truthfulness, and honesty. A written consent is legible for all major procedures (it is interesting to note that what law demands is mere consent and not written consent and does not prescribe such requirement on a mandatory basis but in medical practice written consent should be practiced for documentary evidence). Informed consent should also be obtained regarding future publication of records and analysis. The Medical Council of India (MCI) has given guidelines for various types of contracts that can be made:

- For routine types of treatment, implied consent would suffice.
- For detailed types of treatment, ideally express oral consent may be needed.
- For complex types of treatment, written express consent is required.

The earliest expression of consent based on autonomy is found in the Nuremberg Code of 1947. The Nuremberg Code was adopted immediately after World War II to curtail medical and experimental atrocities as committed during the period by the then German Nazi regime. Only after the adoption of this code, patients got the right to agree or importantly disagree to offered treatment. It is mandatory to obtain voluntary and informed consent from human subjects according to this code. The "Declaration of Helsinki" adopted by the World Medical Association in 1964 further emphasizes the importance of obtaining freely given consent for medical research after adequately informing the subjects of the study procedure and conduct (including aims, methods, anticipated benefits, potential hazards, and discomforts that the study may entail). The term "informed consent" was first used in a medical malpractice case by Paul G Gebhard. The consent is implied for most of minor procedures (intravenous cannulation, catheterization, etc.) and examination of patient. The basis of obtaining an informed consent is that the patient should have enough information to make a "voluntary decision". A valid consent has following components:

1. Imparting all necessary information for the treatment and planning to the patient (preferably written plan). This is "informed" consent. Also the information should be useful and deciphered and queries of the patient should be satisfactorily explained.
2. "Taking" consent is a part of ongoing discussion not a single interaction. Answer all questions that patient may come up with even later, so that they understand the benefits of treatment, problems of not receiving treatment, other possible treatments, and importantly complications or side effects of the proposed treatment.
3. For practitioners, the charges that will be incurred (including possible complications) should also be disclosed at the time of taking consent as that forms a significant basis for receiving treatment from a place.
4. The patient should be "able" to understand and give "voluntary" decision to undergo procedure.

Ability to Give Consent and Waiver of Informed Consent

Every adult has the right to make one's own decisions and must be assumed to do so unless proved otherwise. For any doubt in understanding of the patient consider whether or not the patient understands and can weigh up the information needed to make decision. For patients seriously ill and either unconscious or incapacitated to understand their illness (say psychiatrically ill) correctly and are not accompanied by responsible relative the consent can be waived off; however, responsible senior or hospital head should be informed regarding the situation and taken into confidence.

Consent from minors: The minors are defined differently in territories. The age of attaining maturity in India is defined as 18 years. The law thus presumes capacity, rationality, autonomy, and freedom if the person has attained the age of so-called maturity. In general, in India minors below 18 years of age cannot give their consent to operative procedures and parents or guardians are required to give voluntary consent for the same; however, this does not take away the right to be informed about the procedure. They can very well refuse treatment and should be explained the intervention in detail. For physical examination, consent (often oral or implied) should be obtained from minor above 12 years of age.

Emergency treatment and consent: Under article 21 Supreme Court stated that there is an obligation on the State to safeguard the right to life of every person. The government hospitals run by the state (and now also included are all private establishments including hospitals, nursing homes, and even clinics) are bound by duty to extend medical assistance for preserving human life in emergent conditions. Failure to render timely medical treatment to any person in need of such treatment results in the violation of his right to life guaranteed under Article 21. To this effect the obligation of a doctor is total, absolute, and paramount, so he is the sole responsible person *prima facie* (others' role needs to be proved). So in such situations under the consonance of Hippocratic Oath the doctor can take decision in the best interest of the patient and proceed with treatment as a lifesaving measure. The problem is deciding what to do if a patient resists treatment in such situations. The law is still unclear.

CONCLUSION

- It is of utmost importance that any new deliberation, view, method, technique, or any procedure that involves deemed use on human beings be supported (or best proven) experimentally. As proving the real worth for human use is not possible in truest of sense, so indirect measure is provided in the form of statistical significance that is kept open for future evaluation. Thus, in the current scenario of "experiment-based medicine" or evidence-based practice, use of statistical methods must be known to the surgeons and physicians so that not only for presenting their evidence but for evaluation of existing evidence in literature they can justify within reasonable limits its worth or superfluous nature.
- The most important aspect for understanding biostatistics is defining variable that has to be studied for providing the answer to research question so defining the variables is the most important step.
- The next step is then determining the methodology that will provide the best answer to deriving the most reasonable answer. This is also, however, compounded by the environment, rarity of the disease being studied and possibility of performing the intervention within a reasonable time frame. This then entails calculating the sample size, defining the method of choosing the sampling technique and creating groups for controlling the outcome and comparing. RCT provide the most reasonable evidence but often it is not possible in all setups so various other methodologies are chosen. The evidence is hence now categorized into "levels" of general strength to make it easier for persons to understand the relevance.
- The next step is using a proper statistic for evaluating the variable and presenting it with the "power" of expression or association or dissociation.
- In any case ethical practice is of utmost importance in any research so that the literature does not get polluted, confusing, or misleading the readers of its utility.

CHAPTER 12

Biomechanics in Orthopedics: General Principles

Manish Kumar Varshney

INTRODUCTION

Biomechanics is considered a branch of biomedical engineering, aimed to solving the problems of physiology and biology with principles and methods from engineering. Musculoskeletal biomechanics is the study of relationships between force and motion as applied to rigid and deformable musculoskeletal systems. The principles of statics and dynamics are utilized to study the rigid body and deformable mechanics. Rigid body mechanics applies to solid body systems like native joints and implants. Joint kinetics follow laws of physics such as summation of forces, moments, and torque that can be explained by free body analysis. Deformable mechanics applies to effects of forces and motions on internal stresses of the body or joint replacement components. Both rigid body and deformable mechanics provide us with the insight into effect of loads on native and non-native structures as they contribute to injury. In day-to-day practice, locomotion is a common task we perform. Locomotion involves muscle pull via tendons (statics) and relative movements of body segments (dynamics) through articulations of joints. Gait is a dynamic process and it is difficult to analyze the joint forces in dynamics because of sheer number of muscles acting in gait cycle. This problem can be simplified by quasi-static approach, which permits the motion to be viewed as a series of static "snapshots". In this approach, only static situations of the body and forces acting on them are considered. This is a simplified approach that at times can be extended to a more complicated dynamic approach. Clinical application and understanding different types of gait patterns with their effect on body are discussed in Chapter on "Gait". Here, we will first describe simple definitions as applied to biomechanics and then would delve into specifics of mechanics of motion as applied to joints or body segments. The considerations of stress and motion on wear and implant mechanics are dealt with separately in Chapter on "Tribology and Bearing Surfaces".

STATICS

Force

Force is the quantity that changes the velocity and/or direction of an object. Its magnitude is equal to the mass of the object multiplied by the acceleration of the object.

$$\text{Force} = \text{Mass} \times \text{Acceleration}$$

The effect of the applying force can be summed up by Newton's three laws:

1. A body (object) is stationary or has a constant velocity unless a net force is applied over it.
2. The acceleration of an object is directly proportional to the net force applied over it and inversely proportional to the mass of the body.
3. For every applied force, there is an equal and opposite reaction force.

Scalars, Vectors, and Tensors

- The concepts in mechanics are mostly demonstrated by scalar or a vector.
- A scalar has only one factor—magnitude, e.g., mass, energy, power, mechanical work, temperature, etc.
- A vector has two factors: (1) Magnitude and (2) direction associated with it, e.g., force, moment, velocity, acceleration, etc.
- Force is described by its magnitude and also by its direction.
- To graphically represent a vector, an arrow is used, whose length indicates the magnitude while its head indicates the direction. There can be more than one vector, if more than one force is being applied.
- "Tensors" are a form of more general category of mechanics. Broadly said, scalars and vectors are forms of "tensors".
- Scalars are "zero-order tensors". Vectors are "first-order tensors". Concepts such as stress and strain are "second-order tensors".

Force Vector

An object deforms or its state of motion is changed, when a force is applied over it. Forces can be classified by their effects on the objects or by their orientation compared to one another. They can be:

- Internal or external
- Perpendicular or tangential
- Tensile, compressive or shear
- Gravitational or frictional

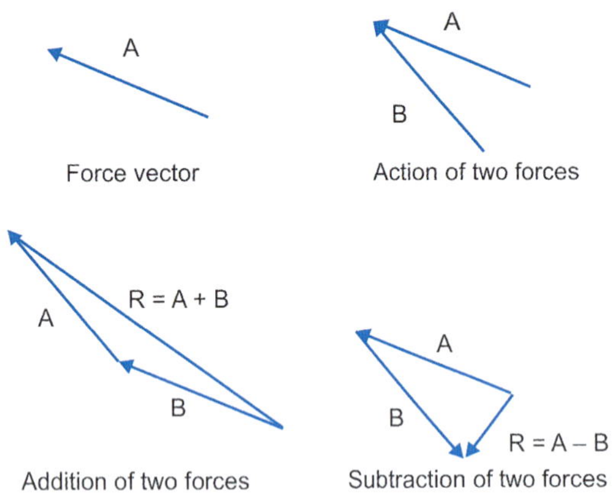

Fig. 1: Illustration of force depicted as vector.

- Coplanar (acting on a two-dimensional plane surface) concurrent (having lines of acting intersecting at a single point)
- Collinear (having common line of action)
- Parallel

Weight is a special form of force. The direction of weight is always vertically downward due to gravitational force of the earth applied on an object.

When two or more forces act, their effect may be represented as net or resultant force **(Fig. 1)**. One force may be in direction of the other, resulting in greater net force, or in the opposite direction, resulting in lesser net force.

Torque and Moment Vectors

The moment of a force at any given point is equal to the magnitude of the applied force multiplied by the perpendicular distance from given point to the line of action of the force.

This perpendicular distance is called the "liver arm".

$$\text{Moment} = \text{Force} \times \text{Distance}$$

Generally, rotational and twisting action of force is described by torque, whereas bending action of force is described by moment. Yet, mathematical definition of the both is same. Moments are called negative when they are clockwise, while they are called positive, if counterclockwise. In the given example **(Figs. 2A and B)**, the tensile force of the flexor muscle applies torque at elbow joint with liver arm being the distance between the elbow joint and the attachment of flexors and the force of pull is equal to tensile force of the flexors. Thus, moment (M) = dF. The direction of the moment here is counterclockwise and that means positive. The units are newton meters or Nm.

Free Body Diagrams (See also Section on Hip)

To help identify the forces acting on different parts of the body with their resulting moments and to ensure the correctness of equations of mechanics in an attempt to analyze the system, free body diagrams are constructed. Free body analysis is typically first applied to distal body segments and joints and then to proximal body segments and joints. For lower extremity joint kinetics are also calculated from distal to proximal, say if the lower extremity is in contact with ground

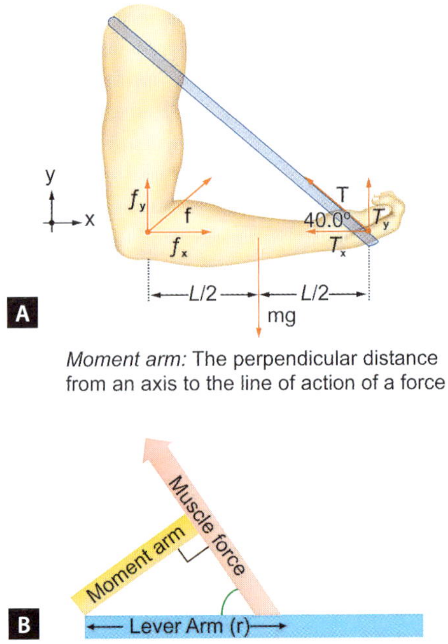

Figs. 2A and B: The moment arm. The yellow column (perpendicular distance from muscle force line to the fulcrum) represents moment arm of flexor muscles of arm. The muscle force counters the weight/downward force acting at the center of forearm {f_x or T_x-component of force/tension along X-axis; f_y or T_y-component of force/tension along Y-axis; f or T-resultant force/tension. The resultant force is generated at the joint due to counter balancing action of muscle tension (T) balancing the weight of the limb (mg). The weight of limb (mg) is considered to roughly act at the center (L/2) of the length (L) of forearm}.

then ground reaction force (GRF) is applied at the known location of foot. This GRF will be used to calculate ankle joint kinetics. Ankle joint kinetics will be used to calculate shank and knee joint kinetics. Finally, free body diagram of the thigh is used to calculate hip kinetics.

How to construct free body diagram: To construct a free body diagram, only the parts in concern are drawn without their surroundings and the effects of surroundings on those parts are replaced by proper forces and moments. Following rules are followed.

Rules to draw a free body diagram:

- According to the desired result, appropriate part or parts of the body are selected.
- Consider all the forces or moments of the forces applied on the concerned body part and draw them on their respective points of application (e.g., weight vector, measured external forces, etc.).
- Also consider all unknown forces and moments directly influencing the free body, especially at points of detachment from the environment or other parts of the body (e.g., at severed joints, ground if no force platform, etc.).
- The internal forces originating and terminating within the free body are avoided (e.g., muscle or joint forces of imbedded joints).

In **Figure 3**, a free body diagram of the forces acting on the forearm is given. The act of holding the weight in the hand

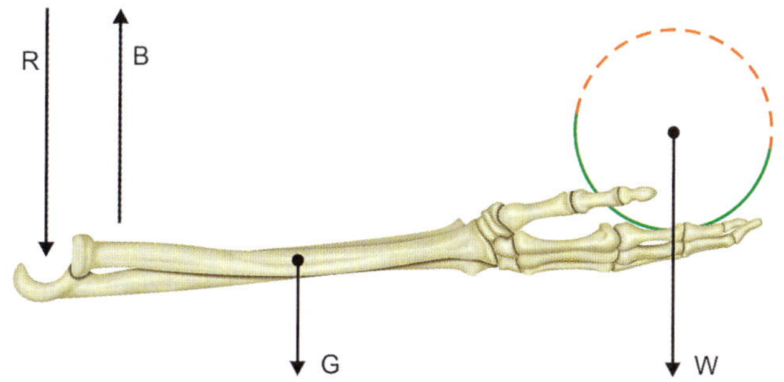

Fig. 3: Free body diagram for forearm with load at hand (W: weight held in hand, G: effect of gravity at center of gravity, B: pull of muscles to counter downward moment from G + W, R: joint reaction forces at elbow due to B).

leads to forces being generated throughout the body. There will be forces acting on the shoulder, along the spine and at other locations, and muscles will be active throughout the body in response to the act of holding the weight. However, here the forces acting on the forearm are being considered, the forces generated elsewhere in the body are of no interest. In fact, the only direct influence of the body is through the humeral-ulna joint and the body can be removed and replaced by the joint reaction force R.

Also, the internal forces are being avoided. Like in this example, it is not necessary to consider the forces acting at the wrist or between the various joints of the hand. This is because these forces are internal and will cancel out by Newton's third law. The influence of rest of the body is summed up by the joint reaction force.

Conditions for Equilibrium

In statics, the study is done for the forces applied on rigid bodies in equilibrium. A rigid body is a body which is assumed to undergo no deformation. When it is said that a body is in equilibrium, it states that it is either at rest or moving with a constant velocity. Both translational and rotational equilibrium must be present for a body to be in equilibrium. When net force acting on a body is zero, it is said to be in transitional equilibrium and it states that linear acceleration of the body is zero and linear velocity of the body is either constant or zero. When net moment acting on body is zero, it is said to be in rotational equilibrium and it states that angular acceleration of the body is zero or the angular velocity of the body is either constant or zero. So, a body in state of equilibrium can be explained by Newton's second law.

$$\Sigma F = 0 \text{ and } \Sigma M = 0$$

Now, forces and moments are vector quantities. So, they have components on x, y, and z directions. So, if the net force acting on the body is zero then the sum of all the forces acting in each direction must be zero.

$$\Sigma Fx = 0, \Sigma Fy = 0, \Sigma Fz = 0.$$

Similarly for moment vectors, $\Sigma Mx = 0, \Sigma My = 0, \Sigma Mz = 0$.

If body is taken as a rigid one then above principles of statics can be applied to various components of the body such as muscles and joint forces involved for various positions of the body. Generally, the forces and their directions are known but the magnitudes of the joint reactions forces and muscle tension are unknown, which states as a static problem. The mechanical analysis of joint requires knowledge of:

- Vector characteristics of tensions in the muscles
- The proper location of muscle attachment
- The weight of body segment
- The locations of the centers of gravity of the body segments

DEFORMABLE MECHANICS

Deformable mechanics is the study of forces and their effects on motion within both rigid and deformable systems. As different from rigid body mechanics the deformable mechanics examines the effect of forces and motion on internal stresses of body. The structural property of tissue determines its ability to resist loads and deformation when considering material and geometry. It is important to distinguish the intrinsic material property which is not influenced by tissue geometry from the extrinsic properties that combines the influence of tissue material and geometry.

Modes of Deformation

If external force is applied on an object, it may translate or rotate or both in the direction of the net force. But, when an object is in state of static equilibrium, some local shape change occurs in the object under the influence of applied force, or in other words, the object deforms under the influence of applied force. This local shape change is known as deformation.

The extent of deformation of an object depends on:

- The magnitude, direction, and duration of the applied forces
- Material properties, size, and shape of an object
- Environmental factors such as heat and humidity

The forces can be distinguished by observing their tendency to deform the object they are applied on. If a body elongates in direction of forces, it is said to be in tension, and if it shrinks in direction of forces, it is said to be in compression.

When collinear forces are applied perpendicular to the areas of an object, tension or compression occurs. When forces are applied in directions tangent to the area resisting the forces, shear occurs. Deformation also occurs in bending or torsion, which is related to the moment action of the applied force.

Normal and Shear Stresses

Whenever any tensile or compressive force is applied to the bone, internal forces are generated in the bone, which are equal in magnitude but opposite in direction to the externally applied force. The intensity of this internal force per unit area of the body is known as stress.

Stress may be:

- *Normal or axial stress* = *F/A:* They may be tensile stresses or compressive stresses. They are measured in newton per square meter (N/m^2) or pascal (Pa).

- *Shear stress:* It is a measure of intensity of internal forces acting tangent (parallel) to the plane of cut surface of a bone. $\tau = F/A$.

Normal and Shear Strain

Strain is a measure of degree of deformation. Two types of strains are possible:

1. *Normal strain:* Ratio of change of length to the original length, denoted by epsilon (ε).
$$\varepsilon = \frac{\Delta l}{l}$$
In tensile strain, the length increases in direction of strain and so strain is positive. In compressive strain, length decreases and strain is negative.
2. *Shear strain:* They are related to distortions caused by shear stresses and denoted by gamma (γ). For example, in a rectangle having height "h", if there is horizontal displacement "d" occurs due to shear stress, strain is calculated by *g*.
$$g = \frac{d}{h}$$

The structural properties of tissue (material + geometry) determine its ability to resist loads. This can be evaluated by plotting the stress-strain curve of the tissue **(Fig. 4)**. The resulting nonlinear elongation of the tissue in response to loading is typical of biological soft tissues. This curve provides information about the pathological and healthy tissues and can be applied when choosing grafts and tissue substitutes. Ligaments and tendons both comprise highly hydrated type I collagen and proteoglycan but ligaments contain more elastin. Both tendons and ligaments are stiffest and strongest when loaded longitudinally in tension along the direction of collagen fibrils. Material properties of bone are anisotropic, varying in different directions, and viscoelastic depending on rate of loading. Cortical bone loaded in longitudinal direction is stiffer and stronger than when loaded in transverse direction. The stress on cortical bone is highest in longitudinal direction. The cortical bone strength is greater in compression than in tension. The cortical bone behaves more stiff if loaded quickly. Tissue composition alters its strength, like in osteoporosis the cancellous bone is weakened in compression and also in tensile strength, the effects are less marked on cortical bone. Antiresorptive therapy improves the risk to fracture by preventing structural change but suppression of bone turnover predisposes to atypical femoral fractures discussed in detail in Chapter on "Metabolic Diseases of Bone".

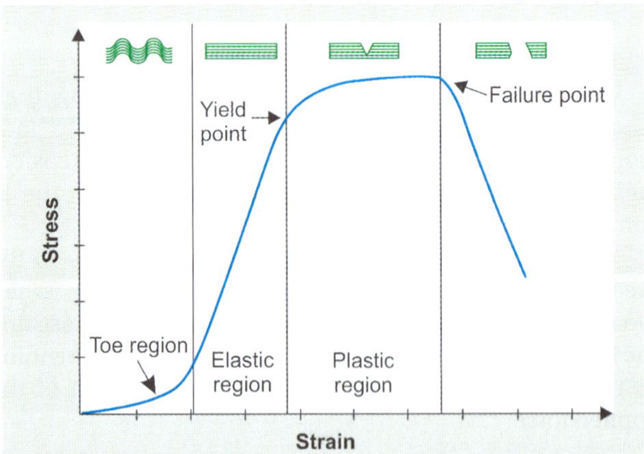

Fig. 4: The typical stress–strain curve for biological tissues like ligaments and tendons. The curve has four major regions: The toe region which results from stretching of the crimp in collagen fibrils; The elastic region depicts the linear variation of strain to stress which results from increased load bearing. Slope of the line determines tangent modulus of the tissue beyond which permanent plastic deformation begins to occur at and beyond "yield point"; The yield region or plastic region refers to microscopic failures where abnormally large levels of strain occur in tissue with only a marginal increase in stress. The tissue does not return to original state in its entirety upon removing the load in this region unlike the elastic region; At failure point and beyond, there is macroscopic failure of tissue with ultimate rupture.

Studies using deformable mechanics have provided insights into how the structural and mechanical properties of tissue change as a result of aging and injury and throughout recovery. Treatments can be improved using these parameters and the effects of treatment solutions like joint replacement on remaining tissues should also be taken into account. Shear wave elastography can be used to evaluate mechanical properties of ligaments and tendons for determining disease status and follow-up to various treatments.

DYNAMICS

The investigation of static equilibrium situations provides the basis for the determination of muscle actions and joint forces. However, most of our day-to-day activities are in dynamic condition and so it is important to consider dynamic aspects of the activity.

A study of dynamic activities includes analysis of joint forces, the motion of the joints and the gait.

Motion of Body Segments

Motion may be linear or angular.

The linear motion is characterized by three quantities:

1. *Displacement:* The liner distance through which the body segment moves. Unit is meter (m).
2. *Velocity:* The rate of change of displacement, or the distance moved in unit time. Unit is meter per second (m/s).
3. *Acceleration:* The rate of change of velocity. Unit is m/s^2.

As per Newton's second law: *Force = Mass × Acceleration.* So, to get acceleration, force must be applied. The acceleration of the body segment will depend upon the magnitude of the agonist muscle forces, the magnitude of antagonist muscle forces and the mass of the body segment. During ambulation, muscles must exert forces both for acceleration and deceleration of leg. The larger the mass of the leg, the larger the force required for acceleration and deceleration. During motion, not only magnitude of muscle actions changes, also there is increase in the joint forces.

The displacement of body segments is not limited to linear movements; there are also angular displacements, e.g., flexion-extension of the knee, which produces relative angular motion between the calf and the thigh. This angular motion is characterized by three quantities:

1. *Angular displacement:* The change in angle between body segments. Unit is radians (rad).
2. *Angular velocity:* The rate of change of angular displacement. Unit is radian per second (rad/s).
3. *Angular acceleration:* The rate of change of angular velocity. Unit is rad/s^2.

For angular motion, Newton's law:

Moment = Mass moment of inertia × Angular acceleration

Angular rotation is derived from a force with a turning tendency—a moment. It is the sum of the moments of the muscle actions and restraint forces about a center of rotation that determines angular acceleration.

Instant Center of Rotation

In the analysis of rotation, it has been assumed that rotation occurs about a single point or center of rotation. However, in many joints, center of rotation changes position during flexion-extension. To completely specify the motion in these joints, it is necessary to find the locus or path of the center of rotation. At any given time, this center of rotation is known as "instant center of rotation".

In **Figure 5A**, there is rotation in a circle about point O. When point A on the circle rotates around center O at the point A' the bisector line passes through middle of the line AA' **(Fig. 5B)**. To find instant center of rotation, another such line BB' is drawn on the circle. Perpendicular bisectors of both the lines AA' and BB' pass through a common center, which shows instant center of rotation **(Fig. 5C)**.

The concept of instant center of rotation has been applied in particular to motion at the knee joint. It has been postulated that the instant center of rotation of the knee joint can be displaced from its normal position because of a meniscal tear, resulting in abnormal surface reaction and leading to excessive joint wear and trauma. In practice, the information on the position of the knee joint can be obtained from successive radiographs taken at varying degree of flexion, with tibia as a reference and the motion of femur in relation to stationary tibia **(Fig. 6)**.

The variation of the position of the instant center of rotation is extremely important when the design of artificial joint replacement is considered. If the design is such that the rotation is constrained about a fixed point, there will be increased forces on the fixation and possible loosening. For knee prosthesis, an attempt to reproduce the locus of the natural instant center of rotation automatically leads to a varying radius of curvature in the femoral component, and to low conformity between femoral and tibial components. This reduces the forces on the tibial and femoral component fixation but increases the contact forces between the tibial and femoral components, which can lead to distortion and possibly to high wear. These are, in fact, the design constraints on a knee prosthesis and compromises must obviously be made.

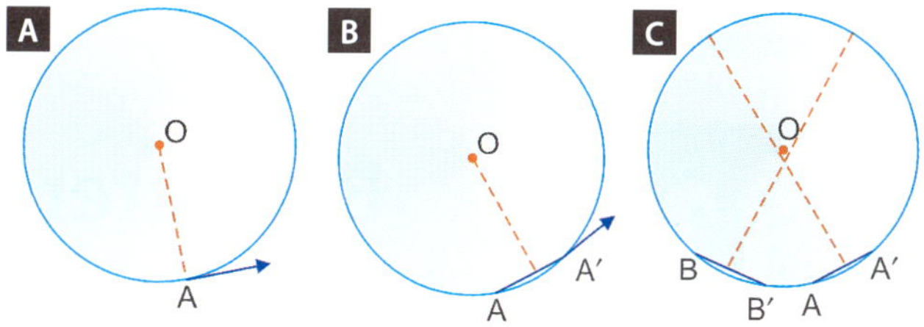

Figs. 5A to C: The concept of instant center of rotation.

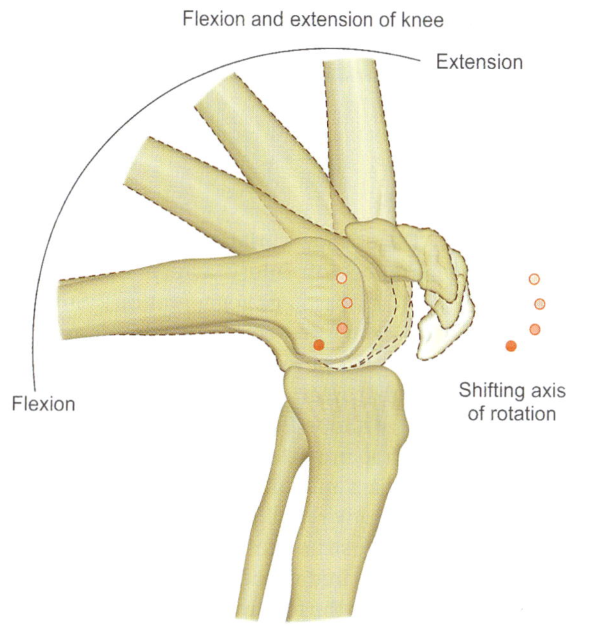

Fig. 6: Instant center of rotation (CORi) exemplified for knee joint. Here, the CORi is not fixed whereas it keeps moving with knee flexion-extension.

CONCLUSION

- Biomechanics makes one understand the principles of force distribution across joints and how the movements occur in a rhythm.
- Understanding the principles of biomechanics helps the surgeon in planning the physiotherapy program for various disorders and also devising muscle strengthening programs. Not only this, one also gets more aware of the use of orthotics, prosthetics, and the rationale of conserving the native anatomy while performing amputations.
- Some principles also help in understanding the principles of making diagnosis especially pertaining to the disorders of hip, shoulder, and foot.
- Biomechanics is a specialized branch for designing the various reconstructive implants commonly used in replacement surgery and people are constantly changing designs to produce as normal mechanics as possible. This makes the young surgeon aware of rationale of newer designs and reasons of failure of the older systems.

CHAPTER 13

Biomaterials and Bioengineering in Orthopedics and their Application

Manish Kumar Varshney

INTRODUCTION

Musculoskeletal tissues show variable regenerative capacity following degeneration of injury which is sometimes extremely limited (e.g., cartilage regeneration). Supportive measures to aid healing are commonly implemented in orthopedic surgery using various biomaterials. Biomaterials are those materials that are implanted in the body to replace or treat tissues. In orthopedics, they are called implants that are used for fracture fixation, ligament and tendon reconstruction or repair, and for replacing articular surfaces. The future of regenerative medicine is the combination of advanced biomaterials, structures, and cues to re-engineer/guide stem cells for desired tissue reconstruction. An ideal biomaterial should have the following properties.

Biological

Biocompatibility: The implanted material must not have any adverse reaction on the host local and systemic environment. Ideally, it should be inert and have no reaction with local tissue.

Corrosion resistance: Corrosion occurs due to electrochemical reaction between metal ions and surrounding biological fluid leading to release of metal ions. Implants are protected from corrosion by coating them with a passivating oxide layer. Factor that accelerate corrosion are:

- Damage to this passivating layer, such as by fretting or wear
- Metal transfer of materials from surgical tool to implant
- Mixing of various metals or various metallurgical states leading to galvanic corrosion
- Surface irregularities such as crevices or pits (the interface of screw and plate).

Resistance to aseptic loosening which is caused by wear and release of small particles that cause tissue reaction and loosening.

Inertness: It should not undergo any degradation inside the body. Factors that affect the degradation of nonmetallic implants are:

- The types of chemical bonds present
- Super molecular structure.

Crosslinking is the process which is used to create larger molecular polyethylene molecules that can be more inert and wear resistant. The higher doses of radiation which produce the greatest amount of crosslinking also causes a degradation in the materials mechanical properties like decrease in fracture toughness and fatigue strength and life. In newer generation of polyethylenes, this is overcome by combining lower dose radiation with postirradiation melting and/or annealing.

Mechanical

The mechanical properties of orthopedic biomaterials can be studied under the following heads.

- *Stress:* This is the force to which the implant is subjected per unit area. It can be normal stress perpendicular to the surface of the implant or shear stress parallel to the surface of implant. Unit: Newton/m^2
- *Strain:* It is the change in dimension that the implant undergoes when it is subjected to stress and is expressed as:

$$\text{Strain} = \frac{\text{Final length} - \text{Original length}}{\text{Original length}} \text{ (No unit)}$$

It is charted as a stress/strain graph and defines how a material will behave when it is subjected to forces **(Fig. 1)**. The following values can be derived from it:

- *Yield strength:* It is the stress level at which a material begins to undergo deformity.
- *Hardness:* It is the property of a material to resist this plastic deformation. It also indicates the tensile strength of the material and its wear properties. Hardness is tested by indentation tests, such as the Rockwell test or the Vickers test. It is measured on Mohs' scale.
- *Ductility:* It is the deformation which a material undergoes before failure.
- *Ultimate strength or yield strength:* It is the stress level at which a material fails or breaks.
- *Fatigue:* Progressive failure of a material due to the application of cyclical stresses below the ultimate stress of the material.

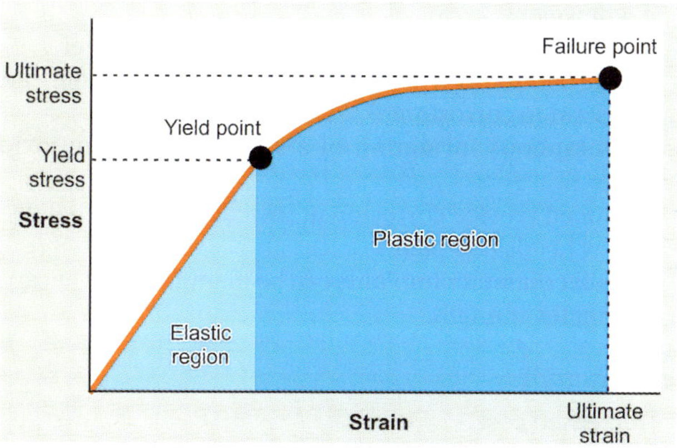

Fig. 1: Stress strain graph.

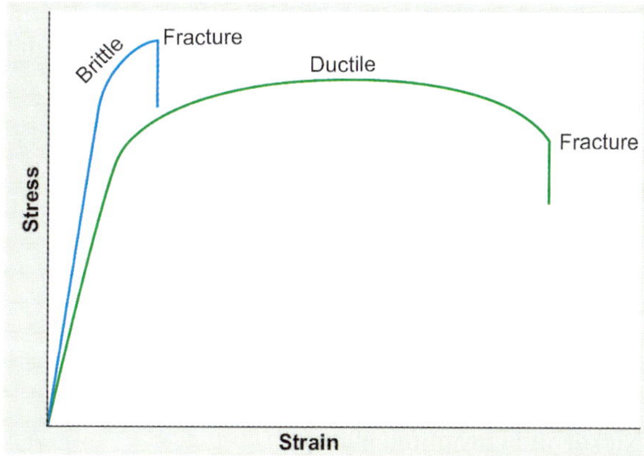

Fig. 2: Brittle and ductile materials.

- *Endurance, fatigue limit:* A stress level below which failure will not occur.
- *Toughness:* It is the energy required for a material to fail and is represented by the area under the stress-strain curve.
- *Young's modulus of elasticity:* It is the linear slope of the materials elastic stress-strain curve before the material undergoes irreversible plastic deformity. It is an intrinsic property of the material and does not vary with thermal or mechanical history.
- *Fatigue:* It is the failure that a material undergoes on repeated or cyclic loading. Fatigue endurance limit is the stress level below which a material does not fail even after cyclic loading (usually must be >10 million cycles) whereas the fatigue life is the number of cycles that a material can withstand at a given stress level. Fatigue strength and life can be significantly improved by heat treatment.
- *Creep:* It is the deformation that occurs under constant load as opposed to cyclic/intermittent load.
- *Isotropy:* Material which properties do not depend on direction of loading. For example, steel and aluminum.
- *Anisotropy:* Material properties depend on the direction of loading. For example, bone, tendons, ligaments, and cement.
- *Galvanic corrosion:* Use of dissimilar metals in contact with each other leads to electrochemical destruction due to setting up of galvanic currents between them. Especially 316L stainless steel and cobalt chromium (Co-Cr) have high risk of galvanic corrosion.
- *Crevice corrosion:* This occurs in fatigue cracks due to differences in oxygen tension 316L stainless steel most prone to crevice corrosion.
- *Fretting corrosion:* This occurs at contact sites between two materials that undergo micromotion common at the head-neck junction in hip arthroplasty or in loosely applied screws.

Based on the above properties, materials can be classified as:

- *Brittle:* These materials exhibit linear stress stain relationship up until the point of failure and undergo elastic deformation only with little to no plastic deformation **(Fig. 2)**. For example, polymethylmethacrylate (PmmA) ceramics.
- *Ductile:* These materials undergo large amount of plastic deformation before failure **(Fig. 2)**. For example, metals.
- *Viscoelastic:* These materials that exhibit a stressstrain relationship that is dependent on the load and the rate at which the load is applied. This is function of the internal friction within the material. For example, ligaments bone.

The mechanical and biological properties of various biomaterials can be modified by making changes in the manufacturing process. These can be at the time of forging by using different techniques for casting, machining and cold working and at the time of finishing with passivation (mainly by acid etching), roughening (shot peening and blasting), and coating with hydroxyapatite (HA) which give the surface greater characteristic of osseous integration.

The following are the major types of biomaterials used in orthopedics:

- First generation includes:
  - Stainless steel and cobalt-chrome-based alloys
  - Titanium and titanium alloys
  - Ceramics, and
  - Polymers
- Second generation includes:
  - Metal implants with biologically active coating inform of HA layer or bioactive glasses (BG)
  - Metal implants with porous coating to encourage bone ingrowth
  - Bioabsorbable polymers such as polyglycolide acid (PGA), polylactide acid (PLA), polydioxanone (Pds)
  - Bioactive ceramics
- Third generation includes:
  - Porous tantalum
  - Ceramics and polymers those are able to stimulate specific cellular responses at the molecular level. They are both bioactive and biodegradable.
  - Development of new three-dimensional scaffolds for bone, cartilage, ligament, meniscus, and intervertebral disk tissue engineering using natural and synthetic polymers.

METALS AND THEIR ALLOYS

Steel

It is one of the most commonly used biomaterials in orthopedics. Most often 316L alloy is used which contains chromium, nickel, and molybdenum. It is the chromium which forms an oxide layer on the outside of the implant that acts as a corrosion resistant layer.

Advantages

- Strong material
- Cheap and easy to manufacture.

Disadvantages

- Stiff material leads to stress shielding **(Table 1)**
- Not as inert as titanium
- Undergoes stress and crevice corrosion
- Nickel and chromium allergy.

Uses: Fracture fixation in form of screws, nails, and plates. Femoral prosthetic stem in hip replacement.

Titanium

Commercially pure titanium (CP Ti) and titanium alloy with aluminum and vanadium (Ti-6Al-4V) are the two most commonly used alloys. Ti-6Al-4V has twice the tensile and yield strength as compared to CP Ti **(Table 1)** and is the major titanium alloy currently in use in orthopedics. The vanadium component in Ti-6Al-4V has the potential to be cytotoxic therefore vanadium free alloys like Ti6Al7Nb and Ti5Al2.5Fe with similar mechanical characteristic to Ti-6Al-4V are under investigation but are not yet available commercially. By using special forging techniques the strength of CP Ti can be improved.

The shape memory effect was discovered in NiTi alloys by Buehler and Wang (1967). This shape memory effect is the ability of a material to recover its shape after undergoing plastic deformity. The ability of such implants to deliver a uniform compressive stress after the recovery of a prestrain makes them useful in applications such as staples for osteotomies, fracture repair, internal fixators for long bone shafts, spinal correctors, vertebral spacers, anchoring of prostheses, and bone distraction devices. But, these alloys have problem of allergy and toxicity with release of Ni ions. The concern of Ni toxicity and potential carcinogenicity has limited the use of NiTi alloys. Niobium (Nb) based titanium alloys with similar shape memory properties are currently under development.

The excellent corrosion resistance of Ti and Ti alloys is due to the formation of an adhesive TiO_2 oxide layer at their surface.

Advantages

- Increased flexibility
- Less stiffness causing less stress shielding
- Light weight
- Greater strength when compared to stainless steel
- Better ability to withstand cyclic loads more inert and resistant to corrosion
- Spontaneous formation of a strong passivating oxide layer
- Reduced crevice corrosion at the contact point between screw heads and plates
- Smaller diameter implants can be manufactured because of greater strength.

TABLE 1: Comparison of various properties of commonly used implant materials with respect to bone.

Material	*Elastic modulus*	*Yield strength*	*Ultimate strength*
Steel (316L)	205–210	170–750	465–950
Titanium	105–110	850–900	960–970
Cobalt	220–230	275–1585	600–1785
Bone	125–184	75–85	110–130

Disadvantages

- Increased cost
- Difficult manufacturing technique
- More brittle as compared to steel therefore cracks occurring from notches in the metal to propagate easily, this limits implant design and makes manufacturing process more exacting.
- Poor resistance to erosion making it unacceptable for bearing surfaces.

Use

Hip and knee prostheses, implants for bone fixation, internal fixator for long bone shafts, spinal correctors, vertebral spacer, anchoring of prostheses and staples.

Cobalt

Commonly used alloy is cast alloy with chromium and molybdenum (Co-Cr-mo). Like in steel implants, the chromium layer forms an oxide layer which resists corrosion. It is a very hard and stiff alloy **(Table 1)** and, therefore, has uses in weight-bearing surface of prosthesis. Because it has higher modulus of elasticity than titanium, it is used extensively in bearing surfaces like head of femoral component where it resists wear and erosion. Titanium, on the other hand, is more suitable for structural applications such as making femoral stem component of hip arthroplasty where its lower elastic modulus provides benefit in load-sharing situations with surrounding bone. Co-Cr-Mo alloy is brittle and not ductile and, therefore, cannot be molded after casting. This limits its use in fracture fixation.

A variant is wrought cobalt-chromium alloy combined with nickel and tungsten. With a working and annealing treatments, its ductility can be improved lending its use as an implant alloy. But, it is more expensive and difficult to manufacture as compared to steel.

Tantalum

Tantalum is a metal which can be fabricated in a highly porous form making it an excellent material to promote bone ingrowth. It acts as a scaffold for bony ingrowth. It is also inert and resistant to corrosion and has modulus of elasticity close to that of bone making it a good material for implants like stem of uncemented prosthesis.

POLYMERS

Polymers are materials that are made up of large chains of carbon, hydrogen, sulfur, and silicone atoms having many repeating units. By varying the length, composition and linkages of these units, polymers can be manufactured with a variety of characteristics to suit various needs.

The commonly used polymers in orthopedics are as follows:

Ultrahigh Molecular Weight Polyethylene

It has low coefficient of friction with metal and this makes it ideal for use as a bearing surface in joints **(Table 1)**.

Ultrahigh molecular weight polyethylene is discussed in detail in Chapter on "Tribology and Bearing Surfaces".

Acrylic Bone Cements

Polymethylmethacrylate is the most common bone cement used in orthopedics. It is an extremely versatile material having the capacity to be molded and polymerized at the time of surgery for tailor-made applications such as for holder or filler material in total-hip and knee arthroplasty.

Bone cements are discussed separately in detail in Chapter on "Poly (Methyl Methacrylate) (PMMA; Plexiglass, Bone Cement, and Acrylic Bone Cement)".

Bioabsorbable Polymers

Polyglycolic acid, Pds, polylevolactic acid (PLLA), and racemic poly (d,L-lactic acid) (PdLLA) are currently the commonly used polymers that are used to make bioabsorbable orthopedic implants. They cannot be contoured intraoperatively and their physical and chemical properties can be modified by changing their chemical composition, manufacturing process and by addition of reinforcing fibers. They undergo biodegradability mainly by hydrolysis of the polymer chain.

Common indications for use of bioabsorbable implants are:

- Fracture fixation like forearm and malleolar fractures
- Fusions osteotomy staples
- As screws and pins for ligament repair and reconstruction
- Fixation of osteochondral lesions.

Advantages

- Gradual load transfer and less stress shielding
- Avoidance of second surgery for hardware removal
- Radiolucency.

Drawbacks

- Rapid loss of strength after implantation
- Uneven rate of absorption in different individuals
- Formation of sinus
- Inflammatory reaction to the degradation products
- Synovitis.

Other less commonly used polymers in orthopedics are:

- *Silicone elastomers:* These are used in the replacement of diseased small joints in rheumatoid arthritis.
- *Polyester and polytetrafluoroethylene (Goretex):* As ligament replacement mainly anterior cruciate.
- *Thermoplastic polyether ether ketone (PEEK):* Cages in spinal fusion.

CERAMICS

Ceramics are a group of polycrystalline materials that have metallic as well as nonmetallic elements. They are extremely hard and brittle and have good resistance to compressive forces and erosion but have poor tensile strength and poor ductility **(Table 1)**. They have low friction and wear coefficient and therefore used mainly in joint replacement.

Their microstructure is dependent on the applied manufacturing process and it has an effect on both the mechanical and biological properties. Generally, a manufacturing process which increases porosity leads to greater bone in growth and osteointegration but reduces strength. Therefore, high density ceramics are used on weight bearing surfaces and porous ceramics like hydroxylapatite are used to coat femoral stem to promote osteoinduction.

The main ceramics used in orthopedic surgery are alumina (Al_2O_3) and zirconia (ZrO_2) for acetabular and femoral components (*see* details in Chapter on "Tribology and Bearing Surfaces"). Hydroxyapatite [$Ca_{10}(PO_4)6(OH)_2$] for coating stem femoral components.

Advantages

- Good wear rates
- High corrosion resistance
- Biocompatibility
- High strength.

Disadvantages

- Low fracture toughness
- Stress shielding due to a very high elastic modulus
- Brittle nature
- Exacting manufacturing process as hip prosthesis components must be perfectly spherical and congruent, making surface finish crucial.

COMPOSITS

These are materials where two or more types of substances are mixed to produce the desired mechanical and biological properties. Composite biomaterials are usually made with a filler or reinforcement which is added to a matrix material in order to obtain improved properties. Biocomposites are now being manufactured using 3D printing that can be used to prepare biomimetic surfaces suitable for stem cell implantation, growth, and regeneration. The same matrix may be combined with different types of fillers for different mechanical and biological properties (details are provided in Chapter on "Regenerative Medicine and Stem Cell Research in Orthopedics").

Some examples of such materials are:

- Polymer matrix reinforced with ceramic particles making them more inert.
- Polyether ether ketone or polysulfone (Ps) reinforced with carbon or glass fibers to make it more rigid for use as fracture fixation device.
- The addition of silicon in biological ceramics and glasses to improve the osteogenesis process.

OSTEOINTEGRATION OF BIOMATERIALS

The anchorage of implants in the surrounding bone depends on its osteointegration. This depends upon the reaction between the implant surface and the surrounding environment.

Roughness, wettability, electrostatic charges, and three-dimensional porous structures that stimulate cells' invasion are some of the factors that affect osteointegration. These properties are modified at the time of manufacturing by treatments like passivation, roughening shot peening blasting, and chemical etching. Some material like tantalum can be manufactured in porous state without loss of strength leading to better integration.

Another method to improve the biointegration of implants is to coat the implant with a bioactive layer. Under ordinary circumstances a layer of fibrous tissue grows on the material surface known as the biofilm. This biofilm is a result of nonspecific cellular response. The bioactive interface elicits a specific biological response and avoids formation of fibrous layer. Instead here is formation of apatite layers on the surface improving the material-bone bonding.

Some of the materials used as bioactive coating are:

- Hydroxyapatite ($Ca_{10}(PO_4)6(OH)_2$)
- β-tricalcium phosphate (β-TCP, $Ca_3(PO_4)_2$)
- Silicone (SiO_2)
- Adhesive proteins like fibronectin
- Peptide sequences that trigger specific cell responses.

Standards for Orthopedic Biomaterials

The Medical Device Rules, 2017 (the Rules) under the Drugs and Cosmetics Act, 1940 (the Act) govern the Indian medical device industry. These rules came into effect on January 1, 2018. In accordance with the notification of February 11, 2020 by the Ministry of Health and Family Welfare (MOH&FW), the definition of medical devices has been amended to mean—any instrument, apparatus, appliance, implant, material or other article, whether used alone or in combination, including software or an accessory, intended by its manufacturer to be used specially for human beings or animals by any pharmacological or immunological or metabolic means, but which may assist in its intended function by such means for one or more of the specific purpose of:

1. Diagnosis, prevention, monitoring, treatment or alleviation of any disease or disorder
2. Diagnosis, monitoring, treatment, alleviation or assistance for any injury or disability
3. Investigation, replacement or modification or support of the anatomy or of a physiological process
4. Supporting or sustaining life
5. Disinfection of medical devices
6. Control of conception.

Orthopedic implants have been classified as drugs. Every device that comes under the purview of this definition is further classified by the Central Drugs Standard Control Organization (CDSCO) on the actual risk; based upon the intended use and purpose:

- Class A—low risk medical devices such as absorbent cotton wools, surgical dressings, alcohol swabs, etc.
- Class B—low moderate risk devices such as thermometer, blood pressure monitoring device, disinfectants, etc.
- Class C—moderate high-risk devices such as implants, hemodialysis, catheter, etc.
- Class D—high-risk devices such as angiographic guide wire, heart valve, etc.

Through the notification dated February 11, 2020 the government has mandated the registration of all devices, except for the notified categories without which marketing of the devices is not permitted. Six advisory committees have been constituted where medical device advisory committee (MDAC)—orthopedics covers the orthopedic implants and materials. The quality control, licensing of products, manufacturing, and marketing—all have to be done as per the laid down rules in the details. The pricing of orthopedic implants is also being reviewed. To this end National Pharmaceutical Pricing Authority (NPPA) has fixed ceiling prices of orthopedic implants (knee replacement) under para 19 of Drugs (Prices Control) Order (DPCO 2013) that are notified from time to time.

In addition to these orthopedic implants, surgeons have the responsibility to identify adverse events related to the use of medical devices and instruments. Adverse events include device packaging or labeling errors; serious adverse events related to medical devices; adverse reactions, systemic toxicities, side effects or injuries from medical device exceeding the expected rates; and excessive chemical or physical deterioration of the medical device or failure. This helps in quality control and improved healthcare standards.

CONCLUSION

- No other faculty in medical science deals with as many implant materials and their variety as orthopedics.
- Biomaterials vary for their usage and application in different reconstruction procedures.
- Increased focus is being laid down on regenerative engineering that involves use of biomimetic scaffolds for tissue regeneration.
- Understanding the implants and biomaterials is imperative to optimize the care of patients.
- Regulation of quality and usage of orthopedic implants is imperative in care to prevent wastage, irrational usage, and exploitation of situation.
- Essential properties of most commonly used biomaterials enable one to plan best for the patient.

CHAPTER 14

Tribology and Bearing Surfaces

Manish Kumar Varshney

INTRODUCTION

Hip arthroplasty involves femoral and acetabular resurfacing with bearing surfaces that may be metallic, polymeric, and/or ceramic components (often a variable combination) mounted/supported upon endoprosthetic component. In view of the extensive diversity of the bearing their individual properties, advantages, and stages of evolution, we need to have a thorough information of the implant to be appropriately used. Also, the concepts of tribology help one to understand the reason why implants fail ultimately and what could possibly be the best implant to choose in a particular patient so that it lasts long enough to satisfaction. The concepts also help to modify the implants and techniques so that better variants are available and the surgeon by understanding the concepts is able to quickly grasp the reason for changes that keep getting introduced time and again.

HISTORICAL PERSPECTIVE

- Metal-on-metal (MOM) total hip replacements (THRs) were developed in the 1950s and 1960s by pioneering surgeons McKee and Ring, though first attempts were made by Wiles in the 1930s.
- Charnley concept of "low-friction arthroplasty" was introduced in 1958. It was based on the principle of a "hard" metallic small femoral component articulating against "soft" polymeric acetabular component that is still being successfully followed as of date.
- Later, Boutin developed the first ceramic-on-ceramic (COC) THR in 1970.

Despite various intermediate developments of hard-on-hard bearing alternatives, Charnley hard-on-soft bearing concept eventually dominated them. Today after all permutations and combinations that have been tried, the most widely accepted and used bearing couple consists of a femoral head (only the size of head remains a matter of discussion/choice) made from cobalt–chromium–molybdenum (cobalt chrome or Co-Cr) alloy articulating against the soft polymeric component made from ultra-high-molecular-weight polyethylene (UHMWPE/UHMPE) and its variations. This Co-Cr/UHMWPE bearing couple has provided consistent results in total hip arthroplasties (THAs) (the ceramic/UHMPE) bearing has not shown any betterment over the large head Co-Cr/UHMPE bearing). The popularity and success of this bearing combination are evident from the fact that overwhelming majority (over 90%) of THAs currently in use world over include an UHMWPE with or without some modifications that are based upon Charnley original concept of hard-on-soft bearing.

Charnley Low-Friction Arthroplasty Concept

All THRs have bearing surfaces that, in addition to providing mobility, also must transmit normal joint loads over a prolonged period of time (ideally lifelong). The term low-friction arthroplasty was used by Sir John Charnley to emphasize two problems of arthroplasty:

1. First, shear forces arising from friction at bearing surfaces increase the risk of loosening. This leads to development of the principle of "low friction-torque" arthroplasty (LFTA).
2. Second important reason for the development of LFTA is that the addition of frictional shear results in the release of wear debris from the surfaces into the surrounding tissue that increases the risk of loosening.

   This is achieved by:
   - *Combining a:*
     - *Small femoral head (22.225 mm = 7/8 inch) diameter:* This has low volumetric wear and allows for a larger poly to be placed **(Figs. 1A and B)**.

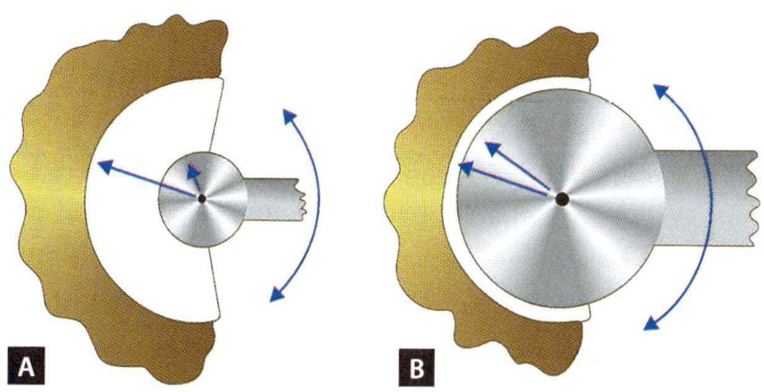

Figs. 1A and B: Charnley concept of LFTA (A). Note as compared to a larger head (B) in LFTA higher poly thickness is possible (difference in the size of arrows). (LFTA: low friction torque arthroplasty)

- *Thick poly:* This provides good support at the acetabular side and favors socket to remain stationary due to larger difference in radii of curvature of the femoral head and the poly. Charnley proposed that with small radius of curvature of the femoral head (11.1125 mm) and long radius of curvature of the poly, movement is more likely to occur at the interface between metal and poly rather than straining the poly-bone interface.
- *Maintain optimal offset for femoral stem*—to optimize the vectorial distribution of forces and avoid undue stress
- *Distributing the load* on a larger surface of bone uniformly by using cement interface between the acetabular cup and bone

PROBLEM STATEMENT

Wear of the UHMWPE component with hard counterpart bearing currently limits the longevity of these reconstructions majorly limiting the universal application. Of concern is the particulate debris generated from rubbing of the hard-on-soft bearing surfaces that initiates biological cascade of adverse tissue response. This results in osteolysis (see later) and ultimately in some cases loosening of the implant components. Thus, the primary research and development is directed to extending the longevity using alternative bearing technologies with improved wear behavior.

- As UHMPE is contested to be the preferred bearing all over the world, primary focus area of research attempts to improve the tribological characteristics of UHMWPE. This is being done primarily by modifying the polymer's structure (cross-linking, highly cross-linked, and carbon fiber-reinforced UHMWPE, etc.)
- The other focus is improving the mechanics of joint by varying the size of femoral head.

TRIBOLOGY OF ARTICULATING SURFACES

Tribology (Greek word, "tribos", meaning "rubbing" or "to rub", coined by H Peter Jost in England) is defined as the science and technology of interacting surfaces in relative motion and all practices related thereto and includes the study of wear, friction, and lubrication.

Friction

Friction is the resistance to relative motion between two bodies in contact. Friction arises from the interaction between moving surfaces in contact. It may prevent surfaces from moving altogether (static friction) or may hinder the continued motion of already moving surfaces (sliding/dynamic friction). Always remember friction is *not* a material property but it is a system property. To begin, one must understand that it requires a greater force to "initiate" sliding than to maintain it, so the latter is generally considered to be 70% of the former. Quantitatively, the friction force is proportional to normal load (i.e., perpendicular to moving/static surfaces) applied to the surface. The friction is also proportional to the coefficient of friction. The coefficient of friction is a property of bearing surface material; different bearings have different coefficients. Also, there are two coefficients of friction—static and dynamic. The contact area (which may vary for surfaces and sometimes the true area is merely 1% of the apparent contact area due to polar contact) determines the frictional force. The direction of friction force is tangential to the interface-resisting motion (bearing movements). At microscopic level, surface irregularities exist in the form of "asperities". Only very small peaks (asperities) from each surface contact each other.

The force of friction is given by Amonton's law equation **(Fig. 2)** as follows:

$$F = \mu N$$

Where, F = frictional force and N is the normal force (perpendicular force across the surfaces). The equation tells that F is proportional to N, so if N increases (compression force) then F also increases for a given surface.

The coefficient of friction μ is a dimensionless number (ratio F/N).

- The kinetic coefficient of friction μk is the coefficient of friction between the two objects when they are under relative motion **(Fig. 3)**.
- Static coefficient of friction μs on the other hand represents the maximum force of friction that must be overcome to initiate macroscopic movement between the two objects **(Fig. 3)**.

The coefficient of friction usually lies in the range from 0 to 1 and is dependent on a multitude of factors:

- Surface roughness
- Presence of lubricant
- Surface chemistry
- Contact stress
- Contact geometry
- Environment
- Temperature
- Sliding speed

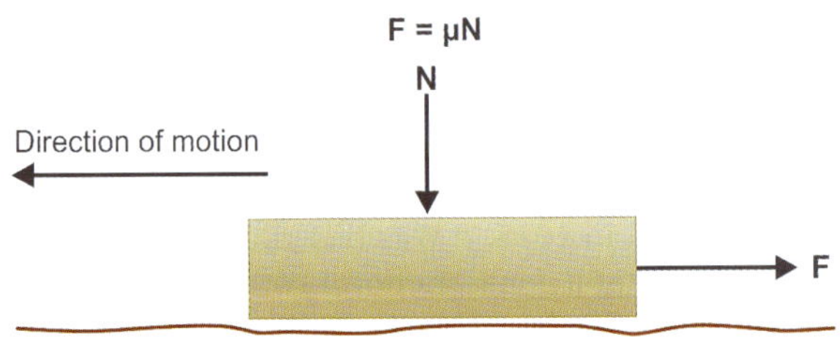

Fig. 2: Amonton's law. (F: force of friction; N: normal reaction)

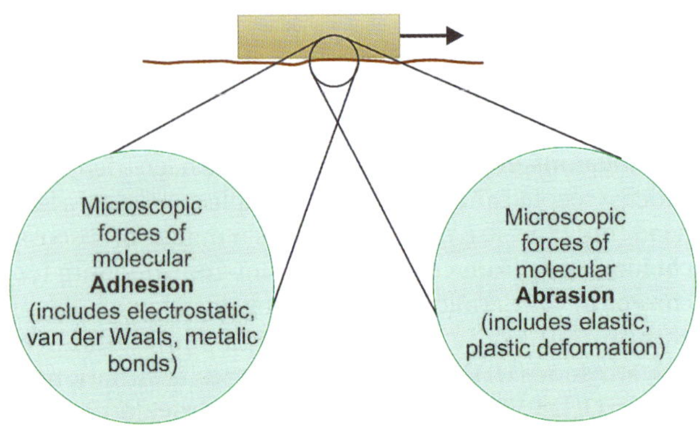

Fig. 3: Friction components. The adhesive component plays role in static friction while abrasive forces play in kinetic friction.

Static coefficient of friction is higher because of the simple reason that to initiate sliding the static bonds between the contact points should be broken so higher force is needed as compared to the force needed to maintain objects in relative motion. The friction has two basic components:

1. *Deformation:* The cyclic elastic or plastic deformation of contact spots (asperities) is transformed into elastic or plastic deformation energy within interlocking surface asperities producing cracks. This deformation is responsible for the generation of particles. Progressive loss of particulate debris from the surface of a solid body due to mechanical action has been defined as wear.
2. *Adhesion:* This is the force between the surface atoms and molecules of two adjacent surfaces that also contribute to friction. This is a combined chemical and physical property of atoms of the surfaces.

The deformation and adhesion can be lowered by surface modifications or coatings as well as by lubrication. Friction leads to loss of 90% of the introduced energy in the form of heat (manifested as average temperature rise and flash temperatures generated). There is an increase of the average temperature within the contact zone. In contrast to average temperature, the flash temperature is dependent only on the relative velocity between two moving points instantly and hence lasts for only a few nanoseconds or milliseconds. 10% of energy is dissipated by storing mechanical energy within lattice defects. These defects are generated by continuous cyclic elastic and plastic deformation, physical phase transformation of crystalline structures, or even chemical reactions.

Wear

Wear is defined as removal (or displacement) of material from one body when subjected to contact and relative motion with another body. Friction is an important factor for production of wear, but represents only a physical property of all moving objects that may not necessarily produce wear. Also to make it clear, "creep" and "plastic deformation" are only dimensional changes of the contacting surfaces and do not represent wear per se; they do not produce wear debris. Similarly, corrosion, though associated with production of debris, is also not directly related to wear because it can take place without any mechanical rubbing/friction at all.

Types of Wear

Wear can be classified based on the nature of the relative motion between the two objects that are responsible for wear and the physical mechanisms by which wear material is removed. In orthopedic practice, the wear mechanisms in bearing surfaces pertaining to arthroplasty are as follows (**Fig. 4**):

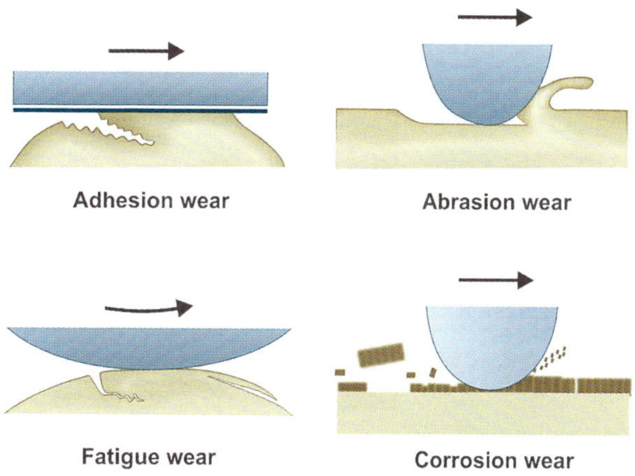

Fig. 4: Types of wear.

- *Adhesive wear (galling, scuffing, and seizing):* Accounts for around 20–30% of wear. By virtue of static friction between two surfaces, the bonds that form between two surfaces need to be broken to allow movement as explained earlier. For obvious reasons, if one of the materials is weaker than the intermolecular bonds, it will break. This may produce free particles or more commonly a layer of the weaker material, which will line the stronger material due to adhesion of molecules. During movements, the microjunctions are torn off and the weaker material gets shredded in the process producing free debris ultimately. The damage is hence marked on the surfaces in the form of flakes and pitting. If the size of generated particles is larger than the clearance of the bearing, they act as abrasive particles causing accelerated damage. They may also be responsible for joint locking. In hip and knee bearings, the wear performance has been related to the flow characteristics of UHMPE that accumulates locally under multiaxial loading conditions until critical strain is reached. The particles then get released into the surrounding and often cause damage in the form of osteolysis.
- *Abrasive wear (erosive wear, scratching, plowing, gouging, and broaching):* Represents around 35–55%, when material is removed from a soft surface by hard surface asperities. So, abrasive wear is seen when two surfaces of different relative hardness are seen. Abrasive wear removes the softer surface, as the harder surface ploughs through it (**Fig. 5**). Third-body wear is an abrasive wear (**Fig. 5**) due to embodiment of hard particles in the soft surface (metallic or bone pieces in the UHMPE). The abrasive particles are mainly released from modular interfaces, metal backing, and/or porous coating. The small cement particles can abrade both UHMPE and the metallic femoral heads. The extent of abrasive wear is proportional to the surface roughness and presence of third-body particles.
- *Surface fatigue wear (spalling, pitting, and brinelling):* Represents around 15%. Repeated loading and unloading induce initiation and propagation of microcracks parallel and orthogonal to the surfaces that result in wear tracks from material-related reasons. Fatigue as a phenomenon occurs during repeated sliding or rolling at the same wear track. This results in shallow pits and filaments (delaminations). In metal on UHMPE articulations as the poly is weak, fatigue wear occurs to it. With repeated cyclic loading, subsurface delaminations and cracking occur. Fatigue fractures in tibial components occur according to the flow characteristics of plastics, i.e., the ultimate stress

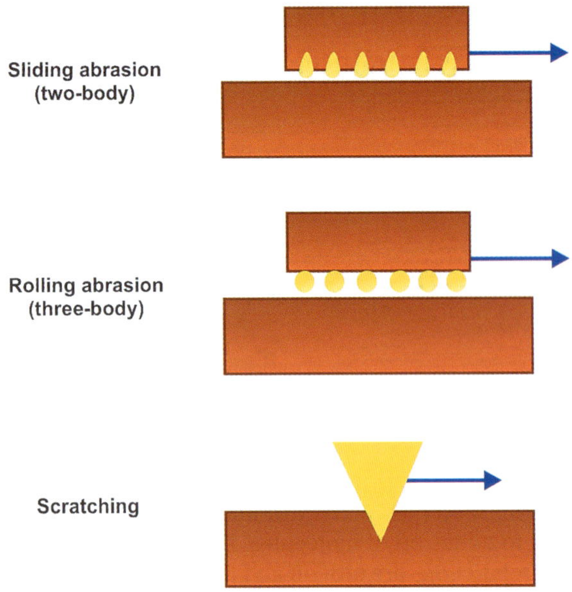

Fig. 5: Types of abrasive wear.

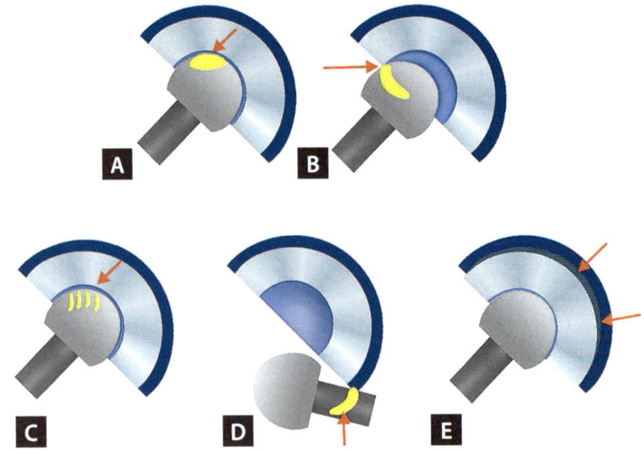

Figs. 6A to E: Modes of surface wear in total hip arthroplasty. (A) Mode 1—normal wear between primary bearing surfaces; (B) Mode 2—subluxation wear from mechanically unstable articulations; (C) Mode 3—third body abrasive wear due to interposition of foreign particles; (D and E) Mode 4—backside wear and impingement abrasion.

and the yield stress. Unconsolidated defects (microscopic voids) in the UHMPE also contribute to fatigue wear. The pitting and delamination are hence contributed to some extent by the fatigue fracture mechanisms. Accelerated fatigue wear, radical rim cracking, cup fracture, and delamination have been associated in part to the oxidative degradation of the polyethylene (PE).

- *Corrosive wear (cavitation corrosion and static corrosion):* Represents around 4–5%, this type of wear occurs by the combination of mechanical wear and chemical reaction. It is an indirect wear mechanism. The material released by corrosion acts as third-body particle causing abrasive wear. Further corrosion exposes more underlying particles that get eroded faster and an accelerated wear might setup. Tribocorrosion can happen with erosion or sliding wear; it is wear in the presence of corrosion causing synergistic increased wear.
- *Fretting wear and corrosion:* Cyclic sliding associated with small oscillating micromotion between two surfaces in contact produces fretting, a special type of fatigue wear. The frictional force between two surfaces produces alternating compression and tension stresses causing surface fatigue. Fretting also disrupts passive lubrication film producing fretting corrosion. This type of corrosion is common at modular connections between hard components in joint arthroplasty such as trunnion and femoral stem of hip arthroplasty—trunnionosis.

Wear Mode

The general mechanical condition under which the bearing is functioning is defined by wear mode. Wear modes are in turn defined by:

- The tribosystem macroscopic element structure and their kinematic interaction
- The combination of different wear mechanisms that is active in the system

Wear mode is a dynamic condition that can change from one form to another based on mechanical conditions and progression of wear itself. This is elegantly exemplified by production of particle-related (third-body) phenomenon from particulate debris generated by two-body abrasion. The commonly referred modes of wear are as follows **(Figs. 6A to E)**:

- *Mode 1 wear* is produced by intended relative motion between two primary bearing surfaces. This would be predominant mode in a newly implanted joint.
- *Mode 2 wear* (subluxation wear) refers to mechanically imperfect moving surfaces that result from either excessive wear in mode 1 or in a subluxating hip (mechanically loose or excessively lateralized hip).
- *Mode 3 wear* refers to mode 1 wear occurring in the presence of third-body particles that are interposed (third-body abrasive wear, may also occur with cement particles not washed out) between surfaces. These unintended particles abrade one or both of the primary bearing surfaces and wear is quite significant cause of early failure of bearings. It is hence emphasized repeatedly to wash away cement and metal debris with copious irrigating solution before closing wound. This wear mode is popularly known as third-body abrasion or wear. The primary bearing surfaces get permanently roughened and produce accelerated mode 1 wear.
- *Mode 4 wear* refers to two secondary surfaces (different from intended primary bearing surfaces/motion segments) rubbing together. These are surfaces not intended to be primarily involved in relative motion (hence secondary). The wear between implant-cement or cement-bone interface (due to poor fixation technique) represents sites for mode 4 wear. Imperfectly fixed uncemented stems are another common example where relative motion of porous coating occurs against bone. Backside wear was lately identified especially in knee large bearings and

BOX 1: Trunnionosis and taperosis—pathophysiology.

Trunnion connections are used in pure rotating environments in mechanical engineering. In hip arthroplasties, these junctions experience not only simple axial and torsional loads but also large bending moments. Micromotion between male and female portions of the modular connections produces fretting wear that removes passive oxide layer predisposing to crevice corrosion. Micromotion between these modular connections and fretting depends on a variety of factors such as implant design (taper angle, surface topography, contact length, and flexural rigidity), patient factors (weight and anatomy), and surgeon factors (implant assembly force). The resulting particulate wear has been associated with adverse local tissue reactions—a common cause of revision surgery. The causes of trunnionosis (head side wear) and taperosis (stem side wear) have been proposed to be one of the following various ways:

1. *Dissimilar materials at the trunnion junction:* Cobalt alloy (head) with titanium (stem/taper) produces more fretting than connections between similar materials.
2. *Flexural rigidity of taper connections:* The flexural rigidity is a function of fourth power of the diameter of taper and its elastic modulus. Small increase in diameter can create large increase in rigidity.
3. Titanium stems undergo oxide-induced stress corrosion leading to gross trunnion failure.

relative motion of the superior surface of a modular PE component against the metal shell in hip also represents mode 4 wear. Trunnionosis (and taperosis) which is fretting and corrosion of modular taper connections between head and stem taper (seen mostly in MOM hips and slightly also in large ceramic on poly articulations) was an important reason for failure of the MOM hips and their retrieval **(Box 1)**. These wear particles may migrate to the bearing surfaces and produce type 3 wear followed by accelerated type 1 wear then.

Factors that Determine Wear

- *Patient factors:*
  - Weight of patient (applied load)
  - Age and activity level
- *Implant factors:*
  - Coefficient of friction
  - Roughness (surface finish)
  - Toughness (abrasive wear)
  - Hardness (scratch resistance, adhesive wear)
  - Surface damage
  - Presence of third bodies

Measurement of Wear

Wear measurement is an important aspect, as it tells us comparatively the "better bearing" and also it indicates the "threshold" level that would result in biological reaction—the functional biological activity (FBA). It is difficult to measure the weight of wear particles being so small and less; there should hence be a reference unit for measuring wear, which is measured in relation to the duration and extent of contact for any tribological system. Measuring volumetric wear is a specific measure to quantify wear rate—this is represented by volume of wear material generated per unit sliding distance (volumetric wear). The volume of wear (w) per unit sliding distance (L) is given by the formula:

$$w = \frac{V_w}{L}$$

Where V_w is the volume of wear from soft surface in the time when sliding distance becomes L, one should note that the dimensions of w are equivalent of area.

Now, the real area of contact (A) of the friction couple for plastically deforming asperities is also dependent on the hardness as they deform during motion, this is hence given by the formula:

$$A = \frac{F}{H}$$

Here, F represents the normal force (acting perpendicular to the asperities causing compression of the surfaces) and H is the hardness of the surface.

The above two equations help us in retrieving the coefficient of friction that objectively estimates the surface properties of bearings. This wear coefficient (K) is given by the ratio of w to A in wear studies, so K is thus a ratio of area over area (ratio of wear area over actual area in contact, units = $mm^3/N\text{-}m$). An important derivation from K is that if we assume that n number of asperities result in actual wear from total number of N asperities then K = n/N, as n will give us the wear volume (w) while N is proportional to the contact area (A), i.e., all asperities present. In reality, the values of K are small, so it indicates that while friction is a surface property causing loss of energy into unproductive pursuits without damage, wear poses a small yet definite chance that a particular contact event results in rupture and real damage. From here, we can derive the possible volume of wear for n contact points. If we assume that there are "n" contact points and for every worn out "n" (asperities), a new "n" (asperities) is created, then number of n will be constant. For a circular contact of radius "a", the possible volume of wear particles generated by sliding distance 2a (diameter), as in THA (head and liner contact), will be nearly half of sphere volume. So, the possible wear volume V for n points of contact after sliding distance L is given by:

$$K = \frac{w}{A} = \frac{V_w / L}{F / H}$$

$$V = n \times \frac{2}{3} \times \pi a^3 \times \frac{L}{2a}$$

As we know that $n\pi a^3$ = the actual area of contact = A, so substituting from above:

$$V = \frac{1}{3} \times \frac{FL}{H}$$

This tells us that the adhesive wear is proportional to the normal load and sliding distance and inversely proportional to the hardness of surface. To increase stability the use of larger bearings will increase L, which will lead to increased wear in turn so harder surfaces have to be chosen (highly cross-linked poly or ceramic). It is found that in MOM bearings, though surface hardness got improved by use of hard bearings, the rate of wear at the trunnion is increased due to high torque and causes excessive wear, metallosis, pseudotumor formation, and failure of the prosthesis.

Another type of wear used by physicians to describe the subsidence of bearing surfaces is the "linear wear", which tells the loss of height of bearing surface and is expressed as mm/year.

Particle Debris and Types of Wear Particles in Various Hip Arthroplasty Systems

Wear generates particulate debris that is the central focus of attention in literature on bearing surfaces. Biologic response to wear debris [manifested as osteolysis, adverse local tissue reaction (ALTR), aseptic lymphocyte-dominant vasculitis-associated lesions (ALVAL), etc., see below] is currently the single most important factor limiting the longevity (other two concerns with bearing surfaces are mechanical strength and oxidative properties especially of poly) of total hip and total knee arthroplasty. Wear particles in joint arthroplasty are generated from various sources and surfaces, and a combination of modes discussed above is as follows:

- Primary articulation surface
- *Secondary articulation surface:*
  - Backside of modular poly insert with metal
  - Screw fretting with the metal shell of acetabular liners
- Cement/prosthesis micromotion
- Cement/bone or prosthesis/bone micromotion
- Third-body wear

The particles may be classified as:

- *Metallic (Co–Cr and titanium):* Metallic particles are gray to black. They show pseudo-birefringence under polarized microscopy but are actually opaque. The shapes vary from globular, irregularly shaped, or elongated with sharp corners. Larger Co–Cr particles may have needle, rod, or splinter shapes. Large Co–Cr particles, from 5 µm to over 1 mm, represent extracellular aggregates or clusters of smaller particles. The majority of titanium particles are blackish-gray material and fine powder.
- *Polymeric:* These are larger than metal but smaller than ceramic. The most common polymer particles encountered are poly(methyl methacrylate) (PMMA) and UHMWPE particles. PMMA is not birefringent. PMMA particles arise from intraoperative debris (most common), mode 4 wear (see earlier), or fatigue failure of cement over long time. Also, poor mixing of PMMA may release very small 25–35 µm "prepolymerized spheres". Irregularly shaped histologic voids are produced during tissue processing due to dissolution of PMMA resembling slivers of glass. When examined under polarized light microscopy, UHMWPE debris is strongly birefringent. The PMMA particles from the femoral area are mostly spherical or globular. They are also associated with fibrillar elongated attachments that may form aggregates of fine particles. UHMPE particles vary according to the type of poly, elongated particles are generated from conventional UHMWPEs that are also more biologically active than globular particles, while wear particles from highly cross-linked UHMPE are much less and also smaller than those from conventional UHMWPE.
- *Ceramic:* Ceramic wear debris is very small ranging mainly into nanometer and submicrometer range most commonly 1–5 µm in size. Ceramic wear debris under microseparation (deliberate loose articulation) is commonly seen in a bimodal distribution of sizes—the larger particles range between 0.05 and 3.2 µm while smaller particles are between 5 and 90 nm (seen through electron microscope). The larger particles possibly develop from microseparation and impaction of the ceramic surfaces as seen in loose hips [so it is recommended that COC bearing hips should be made tighter than conventional metal-on-polyethylene (MOP) hips]. The smaller particles originate from wearing from primary articulation of the bearing surfaces resulting from motion and microfriction (type 1 mode of wear). Under standard conditions, the COC bearing produces insufficient debris (100 times less than highly cross-linked poly) to produce any biological reaction or osteolysis. But, as against the common thought that ceramic is purely bioinert, even ceramic wear debris may generate biologic response (less commonly known or appreciated by arthroplasty surgeons), that may lead to osteolysis and implant loosening. This is especially true of a deliberately loose joint producing microseparation of the articulations that will result in characteristic bimodal ceramic debris (see above). Under microseparation, the ceramic debris is six times less than that produced by highly cross-linked poly articulation surfaces. The inflammatory pattern of biological reaction, however, differs with a predominance of neutrophils in the ceramic–ceramic bearing tissues as compared to macrophages and giant cells in the metal-on-poly group.
- *Particles of corrosion products:* Chromium-ortho-phosphate-hydrate-rich particles are typically seen in trunnionosis/taperosis (at the modular prosthetic head–neck junction) and also identified in the UHMWPE liner and in the membranous pseudocapsule formed around prosthesis in long-term uneventful implantations. They are <5 µm and are noncrystalline, translucent, and colorless. Chromium has been hence regarded as the toxic component of Co–Cr implants and considered to be mainly responsible for most tissue reactions.
- *Anomalous particles:* These are unexpected wear particles not related to implant or PMMA as such and should not be present in common course but due to some artifacts during implant production, surgical procedure, etc., can be imported into tissues.
  - Silica wear particles as artifacts arise from catalysis process in UHMWPE manufacturing or may come from sandblasting of prosthesis. It has been reported in periprosthetic biological membranes in some tissue-processed samples.
  - Iron- and nickel-containing wear particles originate from stainless steel surgical instruments used during surgery.
  - Calcium- and phosphorous-rich artifacts of wear particles arise probably from bone mineral.
  - Aluminum particle has origin similar to silica.

Osteolysis

Osteolysis causes aseptic loosening of the implanted prosthesis and is the biggest cause of revision surgery and failure of arthroplasty. Osteolysis results from resorption of bone as a result of biological reaction to wear particles and is seen more commonly around the acetabular component of hip arthroplasty, though femur is also involved in many cases **(Fig. 7)**. For obvious reasons, osteolysis is seen more commonly in patients with high wear of their implants; thus, it is imperative to improve the wear characteristics of available bearings. As metal-on-poly is the standard bearing for hip arthroplasty, most efforts are directed for improving the wear characteristics of UHMPE. Osteolysis from poly wear has been predicated to FBA or "osteolytic potential" of the UHMPE particles as detailed by Fischer et al. This is defined as the threshold wear level above which osteolysis is most likely to occur. FBA (or osteolytic potential) is obtained by integrating the product of wear volume and specific biological activity over the whole particle size range. Thus, biological reactions are not simply defined by mere wear quantification but comprehensively they are defined by combination of:

- *Size of wear particles:* The size of the wear particles is of equal importance to their number. Nanometer particulate wear debris as seen in ceramic bearings does not appear to affect the osteoblasts or osteoclasts.
- Morphology of wear particles
- Volumetric concentration of wear particles
- Wear volume as such

To clarify, one can refer to the values given for UHMPE wear; a PE linear wear rate of 0.10 mm/year is the threshold for the development of osteolysis that corresponds to 38.8 mm^3/year volumetric wear. As mentioned, COC articulations produce much less wear particles and in microseparation conditions, the wear is still six times less than highly cross-linked poly. On combining the required parameters for identifying osteolysis, COC bearings have fifty times less osteolytic potential as compared to highly cross-linked UHMPE. Conventional UHMPE is probably out and has no role in making implant bearings, so highly cross-linked poly is the standard, which is further improved by varying cross-linking, mechanical integrity, and oxidative properties (see later). Not only this but also the type of resin also has role to play with GUR 1050 being more bioactive than GUR 1020 which is preferred for newer bearings (as in Altrx® poly DePuy).

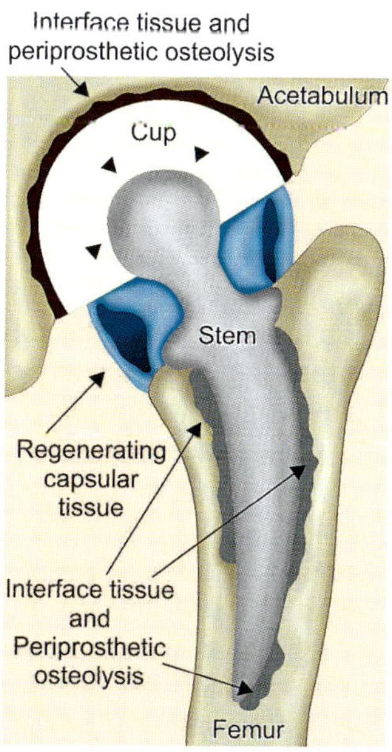

Fig. 7: Osteolysis is seen commonly around the acetabular component of total hip arthroplasty (THA) but perifemoral bone also shows biological reaction to wear particles.

Radiology of Osteolysis

Osteolysis radiologically is seen as lucency around the prosthetic implant and often appears several years after the index procedure. The lysis varies in intensity and extent around the prosthesis with most common areas in acetabulum, located in the superior weight-bearing dome and around screws used to fix an uncemented cup. In femoral regions, the regions of stress such as the calcar are usually the first to show lysis and in advanced cases, areas all around the stem would be osteolytic. The osteolysis around the cemented implants is seen as a uniform gap at the cement–bone interface. Cementless implants typically the acetabular socket show an expansile cavitary pattern of radiolucency. The computed tomography better defines, identifies, and localizes the osteolysis region. In addition, it can also help to measure the lysis volume (less clinically relevant though). The tomography scans show loss of trabecular bone adjacent to the implant and also foci of cavities lined by sclerotic margins. Cortical disruption is seen in 97% of acetabular side osteolysis. The osteolysis in a cementless cup often begins and propagates from the region around holes, especially if screws have been put there. In a cup without holes, the osteolysis is seen around the periphery/rim commonly. Always note eccentric liner wear that is almost always present in these cases. The lesions around acetabulum are recorded with respect to the location [Delee and Charnley zones **(Fig. 8A)** or anterior, posterior, medial, and superior regions involvement]; column involvement is recorded along with the involvement of rami or the ischium. The size and number of cavities may be recorded, if few in number. On the femoral side, lysis is commonly seen in medial, lateral, or circumferential regions. Location of lesions is frequently reported in form of Gruen zones **(Fig. 8B)**.

Biology of Osteolysis

The osteolytic inducing wear particles migrate to the third space (periprosthetic space) by slow convection currents or suction compression mechanisms **(Fig. 9)** and induce biological response locally. The primary cellular mediator is the monocyte/macrophage cell line. They phagocytose the debris particles and produce a number of cytokines and inflammatory mediators [M-CSF, GM-CSF, interleukin-1 (IL-1), IL-6, IL-10, tumor necrosis factor-alpha (TNF-α), NO, macrophage migration inhibitory factor, extracellular matrix metalloproteinase (MMP) inducer

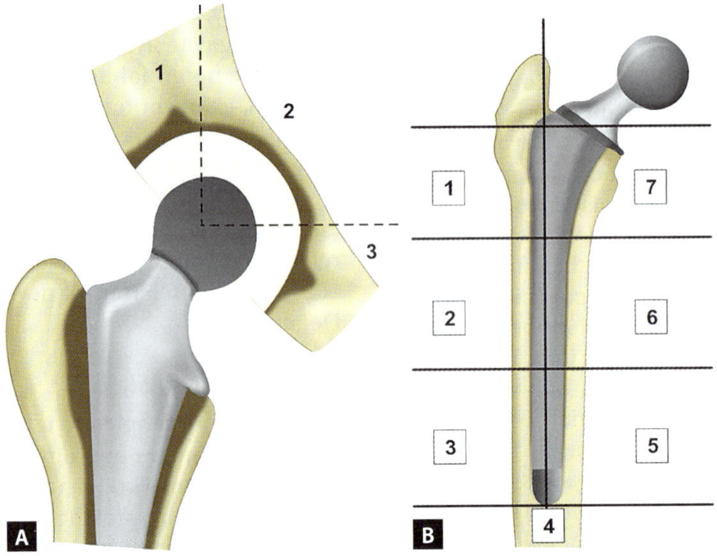

Figs. 8A and B: (A) Charnley zones of acetabular osteolysis; (B) Gruen zones of femoral osteolysis.

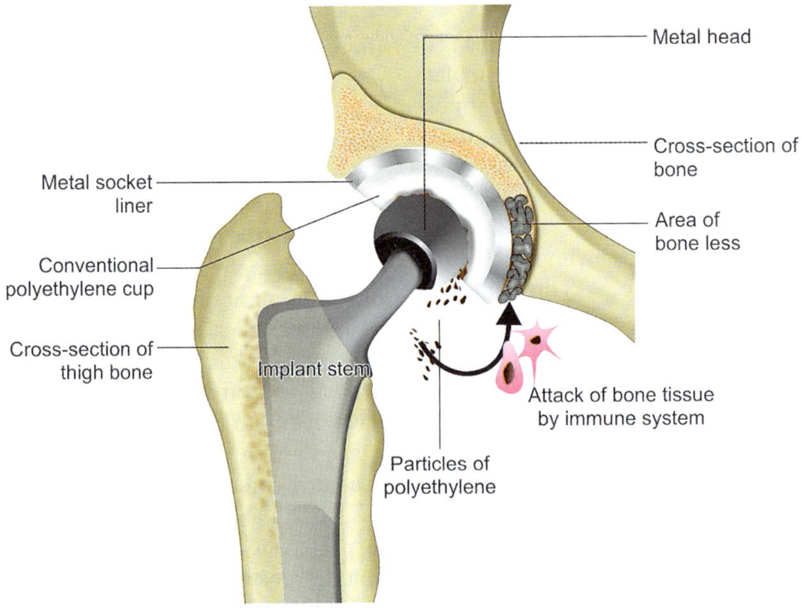

Fig. 9: Migration of wear particles into third space.

(EMMPRIN), and prostaglandin E2] especially in the regenerating interface tissues. These stimulate increased osteoclast activity and differentiation causing excessive bone resorption **(Fig. 10)**. Fibroblasts and lymphocytes mediate the pathological connective tissue modeling in these areas. These are stimulated by transforming growth factor-beta (TGF-β) and acidic (a)-fibroblast growth factor (FGF) and replace the resorbed bone by replacing the bone by pathological connective tissue. Matrix MMPs (especially MMP-1, 2, 9, 13, and 14) are an important mediator of osteolysis. Local tissue tends to counter their effect by increasing production of tissue inhibitor of metalloproteinase (TIMP)-1, 2, and 3. TIMP-2 and 3 are however degraded by the serine proteases seen in increased concentration in the periprosthetic tissues such as the elastase and cathepsin-G. MMP-14/MMP-2/TIMP-2 complex system has been found to degrade all the major periprosthetic intercellular matrix components. Their effect is possibly enhanced in the presence of osteopontin. Erythromycin has been found to reduce the osteolytic effect of wear particles but clinical significance is not yet completely substantiated.

Control of Osteolysis

Possibly complete elimination may not be achieved for osteolysis. There are ways in which it may be reduced or controlled. The primary methods of controlling periprosthetic osteolysis include development of bearing surfaces that reduce wear rate (below the FBA), addition of free radical scavenger in the UHMPE, and improvement in implant designs such as plasma-sprayed surfaces or *hydroxyapatite*

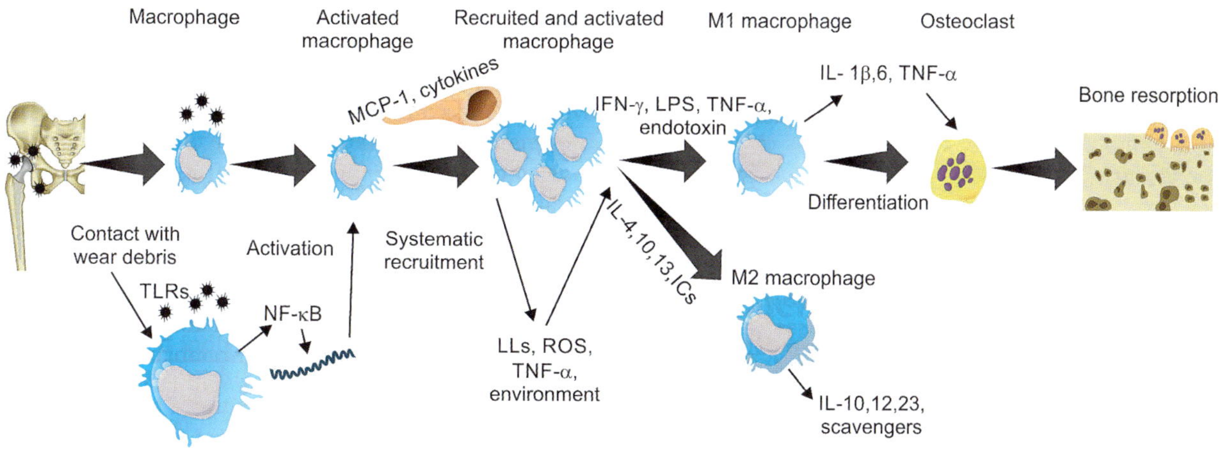

Fig. 10: Biology of osteolysis from wear particles. The principle cells involved is the inflammatory monocyte and macrophage that release various inflammatory cytokines laying down a cascade of inflammatory cells and increasingly detrimental pathway for bone integrity. (IFN-γ: interferon-γ; LPS: lipopolysaccharide; NF-κB: nuclear factor-kappa B; ROS: reactive oxygen species; TNF: tumor necrosis factor)

(HA)-coated surfaces for improved bone integration. Chemotherapy in the form of erythromycin may help to reduce the biological reaction to wear particles. Improved bone quality and implant integration are also portended to be seen with the use of bisphosphonates that are increasingly used following arthroplasty.

Surface Roughness

After a thorough understanding of friction and wear patterns and their clinically deleterious effects, we will continue to understand the tribology and material properties for improving our understanding toward betterment of bearing surfaces in future. The surface roughness of metal femoral heads used commonly in hip arthroplasty is measured as average height using profile view of the surface and defining a mean center line through them. The average height (R_a) usually measures <0.03 µm for very highly polished surfaces to about 0.10 µm **(Fig. 11)**. The center line through the profile is made "average" (arithmetic mean deviation) in the sense that the areas above and below it are equal. Surface roughness evaluation is done by visual comparison of the photomicrographs taken by scanning electron microscope of the surface. The surface roughness of a femoral bearing is dynamic and changes over time after implantation. This is especially true of MOM bearings that smoothen over time. Other changes in surface roughness include:

- Surface abrasions (scratches) result from hard third bodies (PMMA particles, silica particles, etc.) causing increased surface roughness *in vivo*. This also increases the wear rate of PE—a three times increase in femoral head roughness causes nearly tenfold increase in the wear rate of PE.
- As mentioned earlier, if there are little or no hard third bodies ("clean" operating conditions), motion against PE may result in polishing of the metal surface reducing surface roughness; this was also true of MOM bearings (though withdrawn now).
- The decreased hardness of titanium alloy makes it susceptible to increased surface roughness in vivo, especially in presence of third-body particles. In "clean" environment, the wear performance of titanium alloy against UHMPE is comparable to the other metals.
- In general, ceramics are harder than most of the third-body particles than metal so much more resistant to third-body wear.

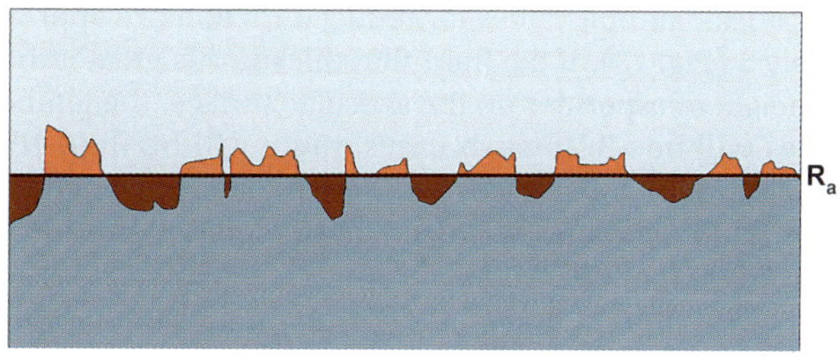

Fig. 11: Surface roughness is given by R_a—made by a mean line that represents arithmetic mean deviation of the crests and troughs as seen for detailed photograph of surface in context.

Lubrication

Now as we know the immense role of friction causing wear due to surface roughness and normal loads, it is a logical idea to reduce friction, which is best dealt by lubrication or by changing physical surface properties. Lubrication interposes a material between two contacting solids to minimize usual interaction between them so that if the interaction was predominantly of friction then it will be reduced. The effectiveness of a lubricant film will depend on the specific film thickness and its uniformity so that it can equally keep the surfaces away. The film thickness is dependent on:

- Lubricant viscosity
- The normal force across the moving surfaces and hence the applied pressure
- The relative velocity between the interface surfaces that determines sliding velocity (velocity at which the fluid is forced into gaps)
- Surface roughness body and counter body

Sommerfeld number (S) incorporates the above parameters determining the thickness of the lubrication film and is given by the formula:

$$S \propto \text{Viscosity} \times \frac{\text{Sliding - Velocity (velocity at which the fluid is forced into gaps)}}{\text{Applied - Stress}}$$

The higher the value of S for a fluid, the thicker will be the lubrication film generated **(Fig. 12)**. This is purely fluid-responsive formula and does not account for the effect of surface roughness. The lambda ratio (λ) given by below formula refers to ratio of fluid-film thickness to the surfaces roughness and indicates that for rough surfaces thicker film is required.

$$1 = \frac{h_{min}}{[(R_{a1})^2 + (R_{a2})^2]\ 0.5}$$

Where h_{min} is the fluid-film thickness, and R_{a1} and R_{a2} are the surface roughness of the two surfaces.

Critical lambda values for reduced friction are approximately 3 **(Fig. 13)**. If the fluid-film thickness is greater than the height of asperities on the articular surface, the lambda values will be >3. In such cases, there will be fluid-film lubrication [MOM surfaces (now abandoned) reached this value]. Lambda values between 1 and 3 represent mixed film lubrication (modern ceramic bearings reach this value), and values <1 represent boundary lubrication. As lambda value increases much >3, the friction starts to increase again. So for any hip-bearing system, a λ value of about 3 is desirable to minimize friction and therefore wear. The lubricating film thickness and λ ratio are also dependent on some specific fundamental properties of various bearing surfaces:

- *Material of bearing, viz., metal, ceramic, and UHMWPE:* Materials amenable to elastic deformation due to softness and complacency can be easily separated by lubricant. The wettability of the materials also plays a part, as it determines the affinity of the bearing surface to lubrication fluid. This parameter is given by wetting angle θ **(Fig. 14)**. In general, metals are more hydrophilic than PE with higher θ. The higher the wetting angle, higher is the affinity to water (wettability) essentially describing how hydrophobic or hydrophilic surfaces are. Of the currently used bearings, ceramics are most wettable surfaces.
- *Radial clearance (half-diametrical mismatch):* Usually, there is an intentionally left mismatch between the cup and head of the bearing surfaces. Even if not, the machining processes are still not so exacting that the cup and fitting convexities will be an exact match. The following scenarios arise:
  - *Head radius/diameter more than cup diameter:* The bearing becomes equatorial, i.e., the load across will be carried at the rim of cup **(Fig. 15)**. Most of the central portion will be left vacant especially the pole will be nearly always empty. This is possibly the most undesirable scenario as the frictional torque is high. Due to equatorial contact, there is poor conformity of the surfaces and almost no lubrication. This also suggests that the head should be always a bit smaller than the cup concavity and never be larger.

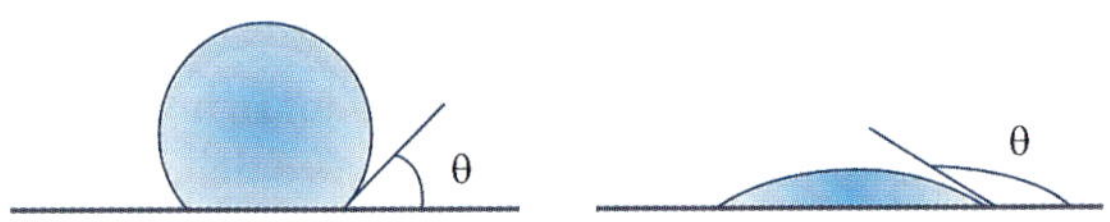

Fig. 12: Wetting angle (theta, "θ") determines the wettability of surface, the higher the angle (right side surface) the higher is the affinity to water and improving lubrication.

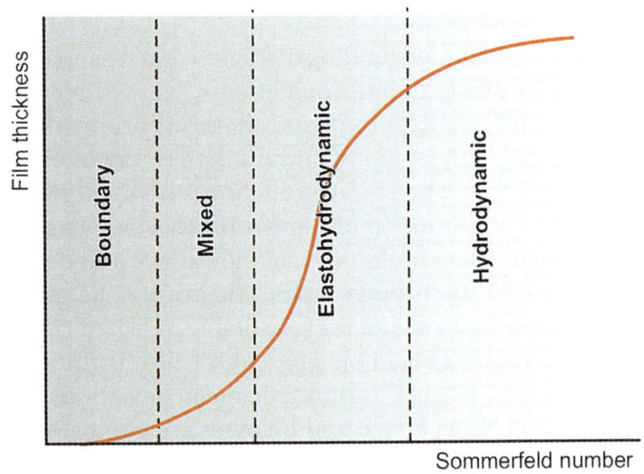

Fig. 13: Sommerfeld number versus type of lubrication.

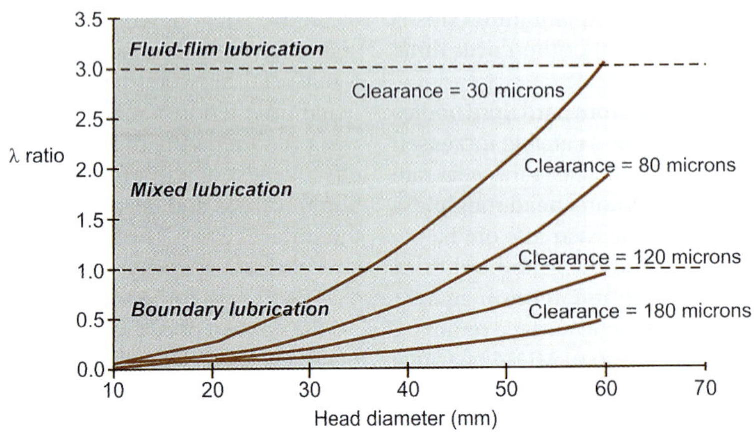

Fig. 14: The role of lambda ratio values on type of lubrication.

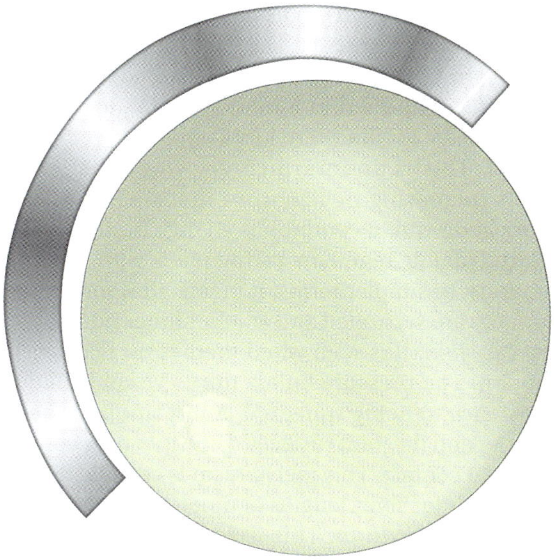

Fig. 15: Equatorial fit results when head diameter exceeds cup diameter resulting in marginal contact only. Most of the region is vacant compromising lubrication.

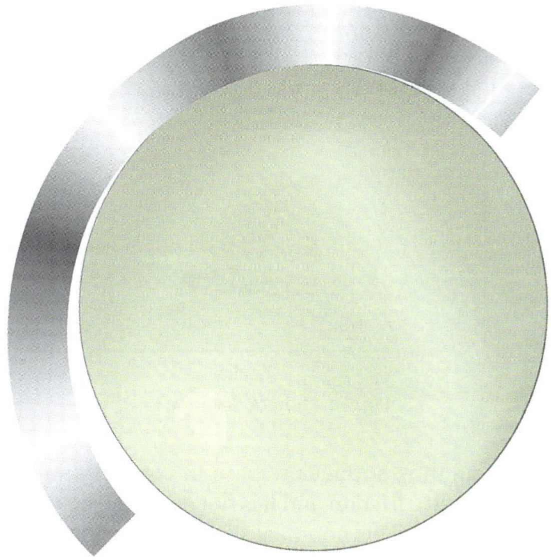

Fig. 16: Polar contact with high conformity.

- *Radius of the head << cup radius:* This again produces low conformity and polar contact. Due to small contact area, higher stress is generated with a thin nearly nonfunctional lubricant film at the contact. This produces high friction at the point contact regions and increased wear.
- *The ideal situation:* Head radius approximately equals to cup radius "and" slightly smaller (never greater). This generates a polar contact with high conformity **(Fig. 16)**. Difference in radius is called radial clearance so the diametrical mismatch (difference in diameters) will be double the radial clearance. But, it is logical that smaller the radial clearance is the larger is the contact area between bearing surfaces and minimal is the stress. Reduced contact areas will increase stress, as stress is equal to force/area (inverse relation). Lower stress allows thicker lubricant film and gives low friction and wear. The fluid is drawn into the moving bearing surface region due to entrainment (term describes drawing-in of lubricant into the sliding contact between closely moving surfaces; **Fig. 17**). The manufacturing has to be exact in the sense that clearance is optimized otherwise if the lubrication is in boundary or even mixed regime then wear will be high.

▪ *Size (diameter):* As the radius of head increases, it aids in lubrication by virtue of reducing contact stresses for a given load and also facilitating "entrainment" due to higher sliding velocity for a given walking frequency. One must be, however, concerned that the larger the diameter, the greater will be the overall sliding distance for a given walking cycle and hence higher the linear and volumetric wear. This especially holds true for soft on hard bearings. Also, the frictional torque will be higher putting stress on trunnion and taper junction possibly causing taperosis/trunnionosis—this was the cause of failure of MOM hips. For newer highly cross-linked poly, some liberty is being taken to increase head size in view of higher wear resistance, one must be cautious, however, that in cemented hips, this changed dynamics may put higher stress on the implant-cement interface and may reduce the success of results compared to smaller head articulations.

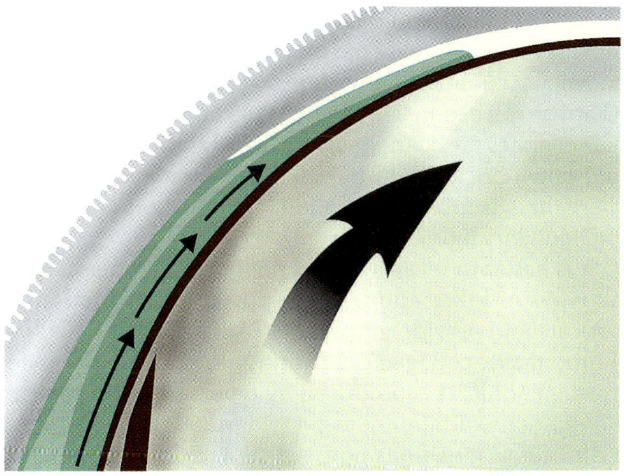

Fig. 17: Entrainment of lubrication fluid (small arrows) between the moving surfaces.

▪ *Sphericity:* It is only theoretically that the bearing surfaces are perfectly spherical. In reality, there is always difference of 5 µm for small heads (22–32 mm) or <10 µm for large heads (40–60 mm). This causes increased stress at the contact points.

Stribeck Diagram

It is used to illustrate the effect of lubrication between the bearing surfaces of hip implants on friction generated between them. The traditionally described Stribeck curve has three phases **(Fig. 18)**. A thickness of the lubrication film less than or equal to the "R_a" of the articulating surfaces will produce boundary lubrication. Contextually in this phase, asperities

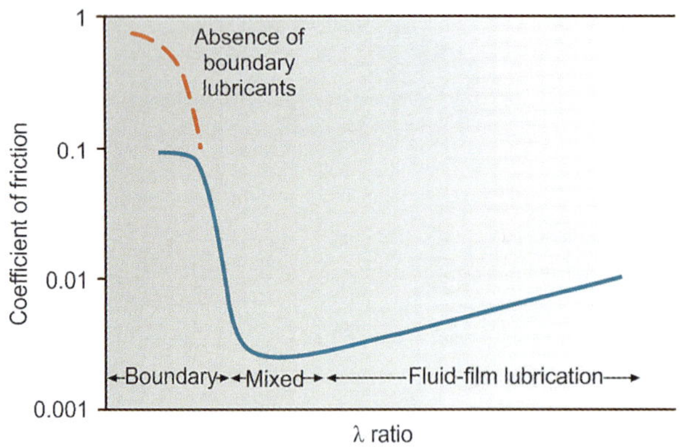

Fig. 18: Stribeck diagram.

of the articulating surfaces remain in contact at all times causing excessive friction and it is not desired proportion for a bearing surface. This nonideal situation develops either in rough-bearing surfaces (poorly manufactured) or otherwise often as a result of third-body interposition or formation (say by lamination of poly or protein deposition). The best way to circumvent this is by improving the surface roughness during manufacture of the bearing surfaces. The longer the implant remain in body the more it is likely to develop this tendency of boundary lubrication that is more specifically true of hard on soft bearings. Increased thickness of the lubrication film separates the bearing surfaces providing hydrodynamic/fluid-film lubrication. In-between, there is a transition stage where there is mixed lubrication (combination of fluid film and boundary lubrication).

It is better to recap synovial fluid before understanding the types of lubrication. The synovial fluid functions to lubricate and provide nutrition to cartilage and is made up of proteinase, collagenase, hyaluronic acid, lubricin, and prostaglandins. It is produced by type 2 synoviocytes and is a dialysate of blood plasma without clotting factors or erythrocytes. It exhibits non-Newtonian flow properties of pseudoplasticity (fall in viscosity as shear rate increases) and thixotropy (time-dependent decrease in viscosity under constant shearing).

The various types of lubrication are:

- *Boundary:* Contact-bearing surfaces separated only by lubricant of molecular thickness. The fluid film is depleted. There is single monolayer lubricant adsorption on each surface. In synovial fluids, glycoprotein is the adsorbed surface molecule and is seen in ceramic bearings. Friction is independent of Sommerfeld number.
- *Fluid film:* The surfaces are separated by a fluid film whose thickness exceeds the surface roughness of bearing. The asperities are effectively separated:
    - *Hydrodynamic:* It is seen in nonparallel rigid bearing surfaces separated by a fluid film that slides tangentially so the fluid film is wedge-shaped. Viscosity within the wedge produces a lifting pressure. There is no contact between surfaces so no wear.
    - *Elastohydrodynamic:* This occurs in nonrigid bearing surfaces. Macroscopic deformation serves to trap pressurized fluid film thus decreasing the shear rate.
    - *Microelastohydrodynamic lubrication:* Assumes asperities of articular cartilage/bearing surfaces are deformed under high loads. This smoothens bearing surfaces and a thin film of synovial fluid is created sufficient for fluid-film lubrication.
- *Mixed:* This is an intermediary when the fluid film starts increasing in size from that seen in boundary lubrication with a continuous change from boundary to hydrodynamic regimens taking place with intermittent motions. In simpler terms, it means that sometimes the surfaces are separated and at other times not.
- *Squeeze film:* It is seen when there is no relative sliding motion. The pressure builds up, as viscous fluid offers resistance to being squeezed. Lubricant layer becomes thinner and the joint surfaces come into near contact but not total contact. This mechanism is capable of carrying high loads for short lengths of time.
- *Boosted lubrication:* This is seen under squeeze film conditions where water and synovial fluid are pressurized into cartilage. This leaves behind a concentrated pool of hyaluronic acid protein that lubricates the joint.
- *Weeping lubrication:* This is the property of articular cartilage that can imbibe and exude lubricating fluid. The cartilage generates tears of lubricant fluid by compression of the bearing surface. The process is thought to contribute to nutrition of the chondrocytes.

Native human body joints demonstrate hydrodynamic lubrication being conforming while artificial joints continuously deform elastically demonstrating elastohydrodynamic lubrication. When we consider realistic loads and lubrication by synovial fluid, a standard MOP hip joint will articulate best in mixed film or mostly under boundary lubrication regime, as the poly surface is too soft and rough ($R_a \approx 0.5$ μm). In the presence of third body, the metal head gets scratched and cause in turn abrasive and fatigue wear of the poly. Hard-on-hard bearings fare much better with predominant elastohydrodynamic and mixed film lubrication regime. The advantage is much promulgated as the head size increases and with femoral head size >28 mm, a shift toward full fluid-film (hydrodynamic) lubrication is observed. Fluid-film lubrication is encouraged, if clearance is reduced and head size is increased as much as possible.

Frictional Torque

This is primarily governed by the size of femoral head and under similar conditions, a 28-mm, a 43-mm, and a 51-mm femoral head will have a frictional torque of 1.3, 2.7, and 3.2 nm, respectively (this substantiated the concepts of low-friction arthroplasty of Charnley using a small head). Though these values are 20–100 times less than static torques needed for failure of cemented acetabular components, given the higher coefficient of friction for the MOM bearing (2–3 times), there is unusual stress concentration at the trunnion and the taper articulation possibly explaining the cause for trunnion wear, metallosis, and other complications resulting in their current withdrawal. The frictional torque is amplified up to 10 times due to the larger diameter of these articulations (usually 40 mm and more). In any case, the frictional torque has never been realized to be an important mechanical event to cause initiation or propagation of aseptic loosening of implanted prosthetic components directly. It is mainly the PE wear particles that have a greater influence on durability of prosthesis fixation. Here also, the Charnley low-friction arthroplasty gets upper hand due to its low volumetric wear generated from the 22 mm bearing and also somewhat from the low frictional torque. Wear is a more important factor in survivorship than frictional torque.

Corrosion

It is the reaction of metal with environment that results in continuous degradation to oxides, hydroxides, and other compounds. Passivation is formation of a protective layer on the metal surface (spontaneously or artificially) that acts as a barrier to prevent corrosion. Oxide layer forms on the alloy surface like Co-Cr (chromium oxide) that is strongly adherent. In spontaneous cases, the later may reform after getting abraded while in cases where it is artificially scaled (as in galvanization), abrasion could be detrimental as the inner metal is exposed for corrosion. The various types of corrosion are:

- Uniform attack—most common that occurs with all metals at all surfaces
- Galvanic—occurs between two electrically dissimilar metals
- Crevice—occurs in crevice/crack in oxygen-depleted environment accelerated in an acidic environment
- Pitting—similar to crevice but a more localized form resulting in pitting or hole formation
- Fretting (combination of wear and crevice corrosion)—combination of wear and crevice corrosion (see above)
- Intergranular—occurs due to granular structure of metals at the boundaries of grains due to included impurities
- Inclusion corrosion—this is due to surface impurities and is similar to galvanic corrosion
- Leaching corrosion this is granular corrosion due to electrochemical difference in the grain patterns
- Stress corrosion—due to repetitive stress and fatigue, the metal is corroded in accelerated fashion and fatigue damage occurs.

Reducing Surface Damage

The risk of surface damage can be decreased by minimizing the stresses or by increasing the strength of the PE. Once the contact stresses are reduced, it significantly reduces the risk of abrasive wear, pitting, and delamination. The geometry/conformity of articulating surfaces and material properties of the PE are to be adjusted to minimize contact stress.

Minimizing contact stress: As mentioned that contact stress is an important factor for bearing surface damage, it is important to know the factors that affect it:

- *Loading:* Of the joint surfaces, eccentric loading increases contact stress. Contact stress increases with increasing load and is greatest where the surface displacement of the bearing is greatest.
- *Conformity of the articulating surfaces:* Higher the conformed surfaces, lesser is the contact stress. In cases of nonconformed surfaces because of design or manufacturing variations, the contact stress gets concentrated at the points of focal contact.
- *Thickness of the PE:* This variable changes according to the material used. For conventional UHMPE, minimum 10 mm was deemed necessary thickness for poly while for highly cross-linked poly, it is now considered that 6 mm represents a reasonable minimum thickness.
- *Stiffness of the material:* A stiff material will not yield to rounded bearing and will not adapt to the curve so point contacts are favored.

Changes in conformity, thickness, and material properties change the contact area and hence contact stress. In general, decrease in contact area increases stress, because the same load must be distributed over a smaller region so the applied force per unit area is more. The contact area should be increased in most bearing surfaces to reduce stress. The contact area is inversely proportional to (directly proportional to contact stress) articulating surfaces conformity, material thickness, and material stiffness.

The structural stiffness of a PE component increases when the elastic modulus of the PE increases and its thickness increases.

BEARING SURFACES FOR TOTAL HIP ARTHROPLASTY

Many different combinations of materials have been explored as candidate bearing surfaces for THA. The results have yielded broadly two classes of bearing couples available **(Figs. 19A to E)**:

1. *Hard-on-soft (see above also):*
   - Femoral head is usually fabricated from cobalt-chromium-molybdenum (Co-Cr) alloy that articulates against highly cross-linked UHMWPE—this is the most widely accepted bearing couple universally
   - Ceramic on UHMPE (highly cross-linked)
2. *Hard-on-hard:*
   - Metal-on-metal (now not favored, withdrawn from most parts of world and no definite indication)
   - Ceramic-on-ceramic (alumina/zirconia/delta ceramic/silicon nitride)
   - Ceramic-on-metal (emerging)

Material Properties

The material properties to consider for bearings in THR include a myriad of factors as follows:

- Corrosion resistance
- Strength
- Hardness
- *Friction properties:* These are further addressed by—
  - Surface roughness
  - Lubrication

The commonly used materials for femoral heads include:

- Metal alloys such as stainless steel and cobalt-chromium alloy
- Ceramic materials (aluminum and zirconium oxide)

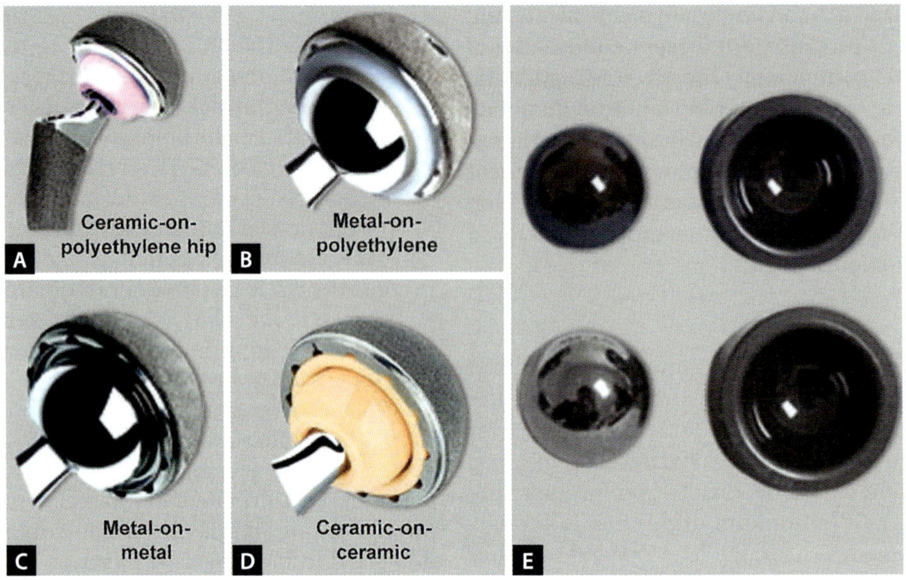

Figs. 19A to E: The different types of bearing surfaces. (A) Ceramic-on-polyethylene hip; (B) Metal-on-polyethylene; (C) Metal-on-metal; (D) Ceramic-on-ceramic; (E) Newer silicon nitride bearings and metal-on-ceramic.

Both these can articulate with poly (highly cross-linked UHMPE) forming MOP or ceramic-on-polyethylene (COP) articulations.

The ideal bearing surface for a THA should have the following properties:

- Low coefficient of friction ideally equal to the native hip (cartilage on cartilage with synovial interface)
- Small volume of wear particle generation
- No tissue reaction to wear particles (biologically inert)
- High resistance to third-body wear, ideally nonscratchable
- Permit adequate fluid-film lubrication

The most widely accepted "choice" of bearing surface is not very difficult to define. This choice can be simplified in the following points:

- Standard 28 mm or large head (32 mm and more) metal femoral head articulating against the highly cross-linked UHMPE is the current gold standard of care for most patients. The large head may be preferred due to improved wear rates of the highly cross-linked poly variants and further improvements available (see below). This large head poly articulation may not be appropriate for cemented hips, however, as the results have not been substantiated and other mechanics as trunnion wear and implant-cement interface motion and failure due to transmission of higher frictional torque may compromise the results compared to 28 mm head on poly articulation.
- *Ceramic-on-ceramic:* This is not a widely preferred bearing though good in many characteristics. It is the preferred bearing surface for replacement in a young female. It may also be preferred in young patients with renal disease or those with renal transplants.
- *Metal-on-metal:* The bearing has been withdrawn but for sure, a surface replacement option is possibly best for patients involved in high-impact activities (such as martial arts). The bearing has advantage in this scenario, as the surface smoothness improves with continued usage.

MATERIALS USED AS BEARING AGAINST POLYETHYLENE

Metal-on-Polyethylene Bearings

The metal bearings used with PE include:

- *Stainless steel*—used if patient is allergic to cobalt or chrome.
- *Cobalt-chromium alloy (in the vast majority)*—most preferred bearing setting gold standard against which other couples are tested. The average wear rate of the cobalt-chrome-poly bearing is 0.1–0.2 mm/year. Improvements in surface characteristics by ion implanting and other surface-hardening techniques have been applied to cobalt-chromium alloy but the clinical effect on wear rate in vivo is undetermined.
- *Titanium alloy*—not much favored due to high wear in presence of third-body particles (run-away wear)

Ceramic-on-Polyethylene Bearings

When envisaged, this was considered a superior counterpart of MOP bearing, but this has not been consistently proven. Alumina and zirconia femoral balls have since introduction been increasingly used as bearing surfaces against poly based on reported substantially lower poly wear rates as compared to metal balls (the wear ratios of 0.25–0.75). Oxidized zirconium (Oxinium®, Smith and Nephew, **Fig. 20**) has been specifically produced for this articulation but wear properties are not very impressive (compared to available materials). The oxinium improves the wear characteristics of zirconium while simultaneously utilizing the hardness and its fracture resistance. This has also allowed the use of large heads as the volumetric wear would be less ultimately while increasing stability. Alumina seems to have outpaced zirconia in the race against wear, as it has reduced wear rates than the latter. The hardness of ceramic renders them highly resistant to scratching even by entrapped (third body) abrasive

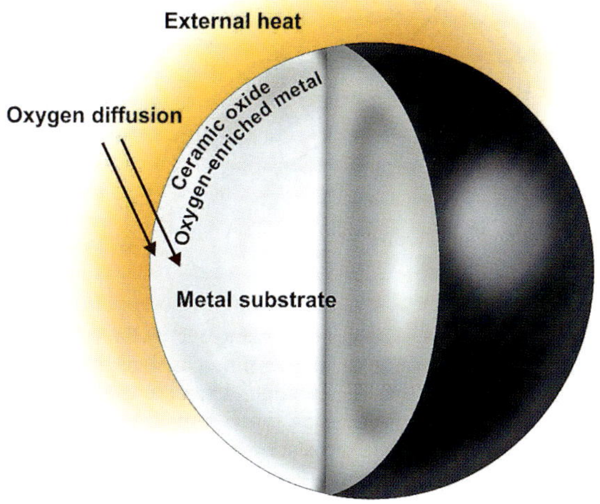

Method of producing oxinium heads

Fig. 20: Oxinium (oxidized zirconium)—contains a highly oxidized ceramic that improves its surface properties.

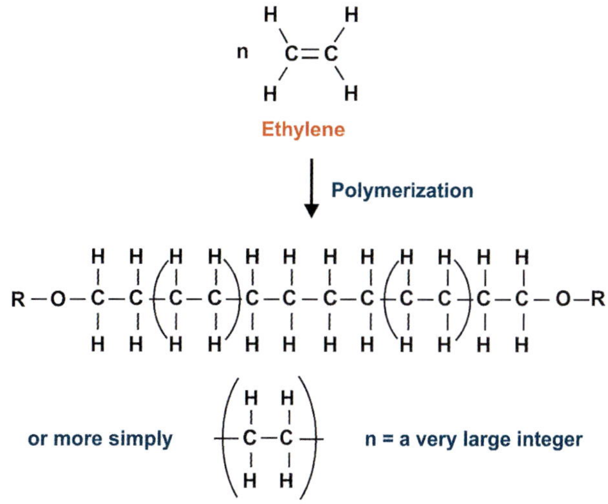

Fig. 21: The ultra-high-molecular-weight polyethylene that is produced from chain elongation of ethylene by unique polymerization process.

contaminants but counterproductively, it can also accelerate the wear of poly (mode 3 wear) and hence increased chances of ultimate implant failure. So, the inconsistent reports of sometimes increased and at other times reduced wear would be explained by presence of third-body wear. This also explains the imperative need of hardened poly as a safety measure to be used against harder femoral head bearings (hence preferring highly cross-linked poly). Also, the need of hard poly is based on the fact that contamination by metal particles in a ceramic ball effectively roughens the ceramic ball because the metal particles can adhere to the surface of the ceramic increasing abrasion of the PE.

POLYETHYLENES

Chemical Structure and Molecular Weight

Polyethylene is a polymer of ethylene. The surgical grade PE is UHMPE **(Fig. 21)**, also known as high-modulus PE or high-performance PE. The older name for UHMWPE was high-density polyethylene (HDPE) or polythene. Clear distinction has been laid now and HDPE refers only to a material with a molecular weight of 100–250,000 Daltons that suits domestic usage in kitchens for water or milk jugs and not joint arthroplasty bearings at all. UHMWPE has been used in orthopedic hip and knee applications from the times of Sir John Charnley since 1962. It has a molecular weight from 2 to 6 million Daltons. It has the goodness of wear and impact resistance combined with ductility and toughness desirable in a bearing surface. The UHMWPEs are fabricated from resin using one of three distinct methods:

1. *Ram extrusion process:* PE powder/resin is driven by a ram through heated nozzle. This high temperature–pressure process fuses the flakes into a continuous bar. The bar can be then machined into specific products.
2. *Compression molding:* The resin is placed in a large mold and heated under pressure. This produces a block or sheet from which the final components can be machined.
3. *Net-shape molding:* This process is a modification of compression molding in the sense that the resin is molded into the desired shape of the implant itself and no final machining is required.

Phases of Ultra-High-Molecular-Weight Polyethylene—Crystallinity and Amorphous Phase

Understanding these phases is important to later address the issues of cross-linking and annealing. Crystallinity is an important attribute imparted to the PE by a natural tendency (driven by thermodynamics) of chains in PE to fold up against themselves in a selective way. The sections of polymer where such organized folded chains are found are known as crystallites, on the other hand, the regions with random organization of polymer chains are called amorphous regions. The crystallites have specific "lamella" shape in the form of twisted, interconnected sheets **(Fig. 22)**. The molecular chains in crystallites are oriented perpendicular to the plane of lamella and may get connected with adjacent lamellae forming primary cross-links that are referred to as "tie molecules". These tie molecules primarily contribute to the inherent wear resistance of UHMPE in a significant manner. Crystallinity of poly determines the elastic modulus and yield stress of PE. Amorphous areas are also equally important. Current UHMPE synthesis process is aimed to "optimize" (the word is carefully chosen as crystalline structure should never be maximized; see below) the crystalline structure. PE typically has a crystalline content of about 50%; the size and shape of crystals are modified by the thermal processing. One must be excited as to why the entire poly is not made into a crystalline structure when it is advantageous. The answer is one has to definitely leave amorphous structure to even better the poly and is not possible in crystalline state (see cross-linking). In short, the properties of cross-linking and

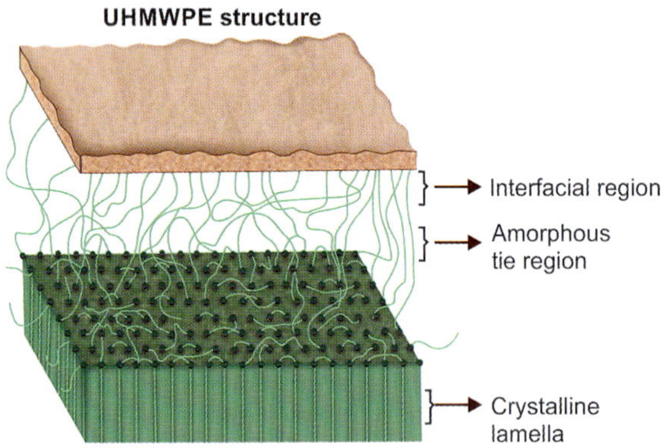

Fig. 22: The crystalline and amorphous structural organization of ultra-high-molecular-weight polyethylene (UHMPE/UHMWPE).

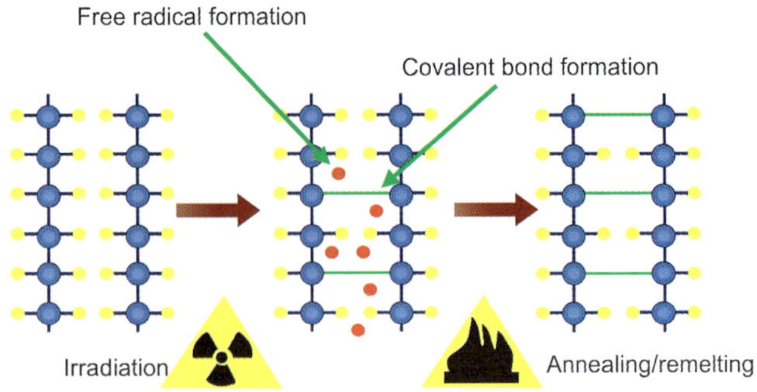

Fig. 23: The process of radiation cross-linking of poly. Radiation produces free radicals, and chain breaks that heal by covalent bond formation in amorphous regions. These are immobile in a crystalline structure so to induce covalent bond formation there, remelting or annealing by heating the poly is done. While radiation only will produce cross-linked poly and reduces amorphous areas, remelting or annealing will induce formation of highly cross-linked poly.

crystallinity in a UHMW poly confer three properties that are most important to a physician:

1. Wear resistance
2. Oxidative stability
3. Mechanical integrity

Cross-hinking

Cross-linking is the most talked about and flaunted characteristic (by different manufacturers) of all modern PE total hip bearings that are marketed under the banner term "highly cross-linked poly", even they have variations of cross-linking quantity. Cross-linking per se refers to the joining of two independent polymer molecules by a chemical covalent bond. In modern practice, radiation cross-linking is the recommended and most practiced method **(Fig. 23)**. This is variably used by different manufacturers to adjust the dose for amount of cross-linking needed in their product and also based on the base resin. Other methods not commonly used for cross-linking include chemical-induced cross-linking by free radical-generating chemical and by use of silane compound cross-linking whereby silane compound is grafted onto the polymer. Once irradiated by a suitable dose (say 2–4 Mrad), a hydrogen-free radical is produced, leaving a so-called "free" radical on the PE molecule. The free radical on the polymer chain that is recently generated has extremely limited mobility due to densely packed adjacent molecules, especially true in crystalline state. For cross-linking to occur, free radicals must be available adjacent and must be mobile. This is facilitated and initiated in the amorphous phase of the polymer where the molecules are available close enough to allow covalent linkage of the inter-chain carbon–carbon, thus inducing cross-linking. The second requirement is generating enough free radicals by irradiating with higher doses (5 Mrad and more) for spontaneous recombination of the free radicals quenching them together else there would be excessive trapped free radicals, if there are few only available at distances. This reunion of the two free radicals produces a covalent bond or cross-link. In the crystalline phase due to increased distance, cross-linking is not favored. The free radicals generated in the crystalline regions become trapped and are the known precursors of oxidation-induced embrittlement secondary to gamma sterilization, so too much retention of crystalline structure in poly is not recommended.

The extent of cross-linking is directly proportional to the absorbed radiation dose, as this determines the amount of free radical generation. PE bearings are commonly "sterilized" by gamma irradiation at a dose of 25–40 kGy. Cross-linking, however, needs higher "absorbed" doses of approximately 100 kGy. Modern cross-linked PEs are hence processed with a total dose ranging from 50 to 105 kGy. The higher the radiation, the higher is the cross-linking of adjacent chains and reduction in the amorphous state. The advantage of cross-linking is that there is a proportional improvement in wear resistance but the effect is seen only till 100 kGy, doses above this show diminished benefits possibly due to excessive trapping of radicals in the new crystalline state, law of diminishing returns, and applies thence. The only way to now improve upon cross-linking is to produce a *highly cross-linked* poly that can be achieved by the following step:

Annealing or remelting (thermal processing): This is the step to produce a highly cross-linked UHMWPE. We know that increasing radiation dose will produce trapped free radicals in the new crystalline state as amorphous areas continuously decrease with radiation. The cross-linked material is hence subjected to a thermal treatment step for reducing the level of free radicals that induce further cross-linking reactions **(Fig. 24)**. Higher temperature increases the mobility of molecules by energy transfer that is true also of UHMPE. This increases the probability of unsettled free radicals on adjacent chains to get excited and hence react with each other forming cross-links. In order to eliminate all free radicals, however, the material must be heated above the melting temperature normally 150°C. This induces another problem that at such high temperatures, the crystallinity is jeopardized and the mechanical properties are lost. A compromise solution commonly followed commercially is to heat the poly to 130–135°C (just below the melting temperature). This method though fails to eliminate "all" free radicals, preserves the original crystal structure, and retains mechanical properties,

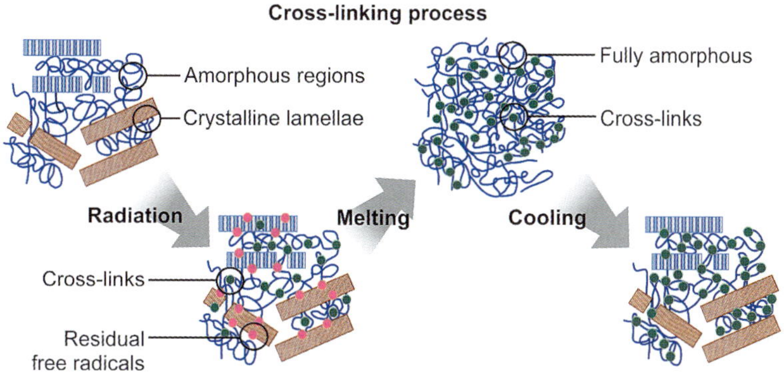

Fig. 24: The process of producing a highly cross-linked poly by thermal processing (remelting or annealing).

while most free radicals still get cross-linked. The number of free radicals is substantially reduced. Some manufacturers have, however, resorted for remelting the poly by heating it above melting temperature (Altrx®, Depuy-Synthes), where the base resin is itself different as persistence of free radicals increases oxidative degradation and reduces shelf-life. Annealing refers to thermal treatment done below the melt transition of 135°C while remelting is done above the melt transition. The former increases crystallinity while the latter decreases it. The other way out to reduce free radicals is by introducing antioxidants such as vitamin E in the poly.

Effect of Cross-linking on Mechanical Properties of Polyethylene

Radiation- and heat-treatment of PE changes the cross-link density and crystallinity, thus altering the mechanical properties. The wear resistance of poly improves by 85% in controlled environment. The greatest reduction in wear per Mrad is seen on increasing dose from 0 to 8 Mrad from where the improvement diminishes (law of diminishing returns) and there is no benefit seen after 15–20 Mrad. The currently accepted best dose of radiation for cross-linking is 7.5 Mrad for GUR 4150 UHMWPE that also does not alter much of the structural integrity [GUR is a registered trademark of Ticona that supplies the GUR resin world over for its UHMWPE grades, GUR stands for "granular", "UHMWPE", and "Ruhrehemie" (older name of Ticona)]. The two most commonly used UHMPEs currently for making bearing surfaces are GUR 1050 and newer GUR 1020 differing in molecular weight and processing method. In a nutshell, GUR 1020 is compression molded with a molecular weight of 4.4×10^6 g/mol while GUR 1050 is produced by ram extrusion process and has a higher molecular weight of 7.3×10^6 g/mL. The crystallinity of PE is a function of the radiation dose level and thermal treatment both. The fine interplay of crystallinity and cross-linking needs to be maintained to increase the longevity of PE bearing.

- *Tensile strength:* If very high doses of radiation are used then cross-linking is facilitated but UHMPE will have reduced ultimate tensile strength that may readily fail by breakage under uniaxial tension.
- *Toughness of the UHMPE:* It is also compromised with increased cross-linking. Cross-linking of chains reduces chain mobility so inhibits the energy-absorbing capacity during impact loading. So, a poly that is too much cross-linked might be highly wear resistant but will fail due to reduced toughness when impact forces are encountered. Amorphous regions have higher energy-absorption mechanisms.
- *Other mechanical properties:* These are also affected by irradiation temperature. Irradiation at elevated temperatures (90°C < T < 135°C) improves large-strain mechanical properties than when it is done at room temperature.

Conventional Polyethylene Surfaces versus Highly Cross-linked Polyethylene Surfaces

Ultra-high-molecular-weight PE has low friction and dampening properties, but has high adhesive and abrasive wear. The thickness of conventional PE should not be <6–8 mm otherwise accelerated wear and poly failure occurs. This causes osteolysis in the short time. Highly cross-linked PE has reduced PE wear rate of 42–100% compared to conventional PE. The newer highly cross-linked PE shows annual linear wear at 45% of conventional UHMPE in prosthesis implanted for 5 years. This indicates that osteolysis may not possibly occur at all. The optimum value of cross-linking is debatable and still undecided, for simple arguments that follow:

- Higher crosslinking reduces some mechanical properties quite significantly, viz., mechanical strength parameters such as ductility and fracture toughness and fatigue strength.
- Non-cross-linked poly will have best values for ultimate strength, elongation, and fracture toughness but will have worst values of linear and volumetric wear values.
- At the other extreme is to irradiate poly with higher (9.5–11 Mrad) than recommended doses to gain additional 5–10% of wear resistance that might avoid osteolysis even in the most active patient but resulting in increased chances of mechanical failure of the poly.
- Moderate doses of 5 Mrad used commonly in various products maintain the benefits of reduction in wear at 85% or below that of a non-cross-linked UHMPE while maintaining the mechanical properties.

So, a surgeon should match his patient according to manufacturer's details of poly cross-linking, an active patient to be matched with higher radiation dose poly, sedentary young patient to non-cross-linked poly!

Sterilization Techniques

Because radiation of PE predisposes to oxidative degradation, there is a growing recommendation to use of ethylene oxide or gas plasma for sterilization of highly cross-linked poly. These methods protect poly from oxidative degradation, as they do not generate free radicals in sterilization process in the material. This gives immediate and long-term advantage in the mechanical properties and wears resistance of highly cross-linked UHMPE. The limitation is, however, inability to produce cross-linking. Most brands still use gamma radiation with the PE protected in low-oxygen environment (vacuum, inert gas, or with an oxygen scavenger). Annealing is preferred to salvage free radicals (by heating them in the nitrogen packaging at 37–50°C for about 6 days).

METAL-ON-METAL BEARINGS

Of note, it is important to note that MOM bearing has been withdrawn world over since around 2010. The description below is more of historical and academic interest as the bearing has interesting history of failures and reintroduction and refailures and possible re-reintroduction in future, who knows?

The first-generation MOM hips [McKee-Farrar (Howmedica, Limerick, Ireland) design, along with the Mueller (Sulzer AG, Winterthur, Switzerland), Ring (Downs, Ltd, Mitcham, England), etc.] were largely superseded by the Charnley prosthesis due to high early failure rates. They were cobalt–chromium alloy bearing. In view of the problem of osteolysis seen in metal on poly bearings (due to unacceptable steady-state wear) in the mid-90s, MOM conventional total hips and surface replacement designs were introduced (actually reintroduced) with refinements. The steady-state wear rates of these designs were very low [only a few micrometers per million cycles (one million cycles is equivalent to nearly 1 year of implant use of moderate physical activity)]. As mentioned above, the MOM bearing implants have ingenious property of "self-healing" by virtue of reduction in asperities. This is the ability to polish-out isolated surface scratches in the MOM bearings. On a wider analysis, the long-term survival had been comparable to metal on poly designs. Laboratory studies suggest that MOM bearings exhibit 10–20 times greater wear during first 1–2 years of use called the "run-in wear" period. These then reduce by virtue of self-heal. However, some MOM hips exhibit extensive surface micropitting due to manufacturing defect and nonstatistical distribution of carbides possibly leading to fatigue corrosion. All Co-Cr alloys contain trace constituents of nickel (maximum 1%), carbon (0.35%), nitrogen (maximum 0.25%), silicon (maximum 1.0%), iron (maximum 0.75%), and manganese (maximum 1.0%). In Co–Cr alloys, the primary cobalt alloy matrix phase is mixed with a secondary metal carbide phase that should be uniformly distributed for optimal effect. The carbide phase of the composite specifically contributes to the hardness and mechanical behavior of the alloy. Thick (8–12 mm) chromium nitride (CrN) and chromium carbon nitride (CrCN) coating reduces the wear rates by 20–30-fold as compared to standard MOM bearings. To note also is the fact that CrN wear particles are much less cytotoxic.

Metal-on-metal bearings are basically constituted by cobalt, chromium, and molybdenum but depending on carbon content, they can be either high carbon (0.20–0.25%) or low carbon (0.05–0.08%). The high carbon bearings have lower in vitro wear rates. MOM hip bearings wear by all the four classic mechanisms (adhesion, abrasion, corrosion, and surface fatigue). The predominant mechanisms are abrasion and surface fatigue. Relatively high wear is seen in running-in phase (first few million cycles) followed by a steady-state phase during which the wear rate is constant and much lower due to self-polishing effect. In the run-in period, surface asperities are polished that reduces contact stress. The improvement in the surface finish facilitates lubricating fluid film (elastohydrodynamic films) by coherence and causing reduction in wear rate. Also, as noticed previously, there is a transition from boundary lubrication (undesirable) to mixed lubrication with increase in diameter of the femoral head as is used for these bearings producing much lower overall wear rates.

The first-generation MOM hips were fabricated by casting, whereas contemporary second-generation implants are manufactured from wrought Co–Cr alloys. This significantly improves the properties of hardness, yield, and ultimate strength of the MOM bearings. Chromium is used specifically in these alloys to enhance mechanical properties; it also promotes the formation of a passive oxide layer. Addition of molybdenum improves its corrosion resistance.

Metal Ions

Metal ions from MOM prosthesis include an array of titanium, chromium, cobalt, vanadium, and molybdenum. On laboratory evaluation, healthy controls were found to have a mean serum cobalt and chromium levels of 0.24 mg/L and 0.28 mg/L [measured by inductively coupled plasma mass spectroscopy (ICP-MS)]. ICP-MS is highly sensitive to detect low levels of metal ions and also allows multielement determinations. Serum/plasma levels of cobalt and chromium ions reflect the true ion levels when using blood to assess systemic ion levels. Relatively higher metal ion concentrations have always been of concern especially in renal impaired patients and females of childbearing age group. Serum chromium ion levels and cobalt ion levels were 22-fold, 23-fold, and 21-fold higher and eightfold, sevenfold, and sixfold higher at 3, 6, and 12 months postoperatively than preoperative levels. There is a corresponding decrease in cytotoxic CD8+ T-lymphocytes. These cells are involved in defense against intracellular pathogens and cancerous cells. In the initial run-in period, volumetric wear rate and average particle size estimation suggested that 6.7×10^{12} – 2.5×10^{14} metal particles are produced per year. This is much higher than standard MOP bearing by 13–50 times and for newer MOP articulation by 500 times approximately. The most important cause of failure leading to a blow on the use of MOM implants in last decade came from systemic dissemination of soluble and particulate corrosion products from modular junctions such as trunnion of head and Morse taper on femoral stem. This is of concern even in MOP hips with large head bearings. The metallic particles have been described in the lymph nodes, liver, and spleen. After the withdrawal of MOM bearings, the present modular total hips with a large head MOP bearing demonstrating moderate or severe corrosion at trunnion/taper junction show that the serum and urine levels of Co average 1.06 ppb and 0.87 ppb respectively, which is similar to long-term values for MOM bearing hips. The values for urine Cr levels of 1.59 ppb also correspond. These higher wear rates have partly been responsible for withdrawal of the MOM bearings.

Unlike an MOP bearing wear that is eccentric and demonstrable on a radiograph, the wear of MOM bearing is generally measured by serum and urine metal ion concentrations. These also indicate the patient activity and tribological performance of these bearings. In a physiologically normal patient, having normal renal function clearance of cobalt and chromium ions is usually adequate to be of any concern however.

Biological Response

Not just higher failure rates of 2–3 fold higher than contemporary THA using MOP bearings, but also the adverse tissue reactions (ARMD—adverse reaction to metal debris; **Fig. 25**) gradually emerged around the hip joint to be an important reason for ultimate withdrawal of MOM bearing.

To understand biology of reaction, one needs to understand the wear particles. The MOM wear particles are very small in the nanometer size range with mostly round to oval structures. Some may be needle shaped as well but constitute a minority. Small size of particles produced in high numbers actually inflates the surface area making them susceptible to corrosion and inducing a quicker and extensive biologic response both locally and systemically. Co–Cr particles have always been known for greater cytotoxicity than PE particles being metallic and reactive. The metal particles show a dose-response effect. In smaller concentrations, they stimulate the release of cytokines from accumulating inflammatory cells (monocyte-macrophage) such as interleukin-1 (IL-1), IL-6, TNF-α, and prostaglandin E1. As mentioned earlier, these are involved in periprosthetic osteolysis and aseptic loosening. Higher concentrations of metallic ions, however, are directly cytotoxic altering the phagocytic activity of macrophages and causing cell death. In all, both the mechanisms cause ALTR.

Metal sensitivity has been characterized by a predominantly lymphocytic immune response and is histologically described as ALVAL that may occur even without excessive metal wear. One should note that this sensitivity is different from the nickel sensitivity as noted for skin allergy. It is yet not proven or shown that skin allergy in any case correlates with deep tissue or bone reaction to the metal ions. The following manifestations of ALTR are seen:

- Effusions
- Soft-tissue masses (pseudotumors)—associated with increased metal ion concentrations and edge loading of the implant
- Early osteolysis and failure
- Late osteolysis

The tissue response can be inflammatory or immunological in nature.

- *The ALVAL reaction:* When comparing tissues surrounding MOP and MOM THAs, more lymphocytes are found histologically in the MOM THAs. This could be due to delayed type hypersensitivity response to the metal wear products but pattern of inflammatory reaction and cellular distribution distinguishes this from classical type IV delayed type hypersensitivity reaction. The presence of B-lymphocytes, plasma cells, and massive fibrin exudation points to a vasculitis-like lesion instead. Thus, descriptive term of ALVAL, viz., lymphocyte-dominated immunologic answer (LYDIA) has been named for the histological finding.
- *Osteolysis:* As noted above, Co and Cr have been shown to induce TNF-α secretion from the local inflammatory cells. They also induce a time- and dose-dependent protein oxidation. Osteolysis following MOM implant could be due to production of potentially osteolytic cytokines rather than recruitment of inflammatory cells (as is common mechanism with MOP bearings). These immunological responses may be triggered by metal ions that act as antigens and stimulate an allergic (hypersensitivity) reaction by forming organometallic complexes with proteins. Hypersensitivity reactions may be mediated by antibodies (type I, II, or III) or type IV delayed type hypersensitivity. The latter cell-mediated process involves activation and expansion of metal-ion-specific major histocompatibility complex (MHC) class

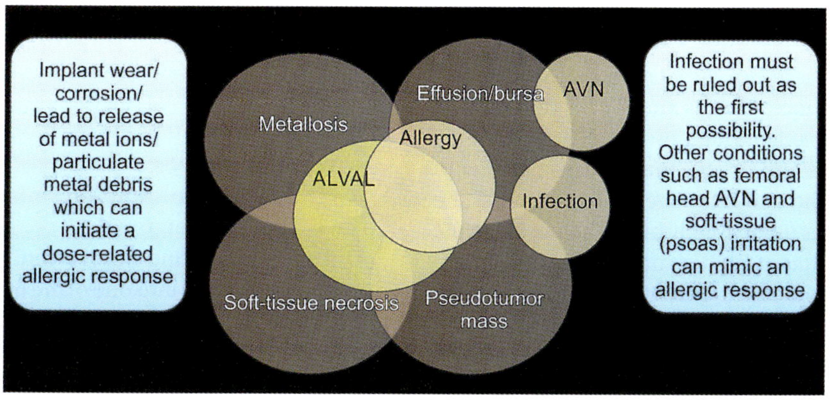

Fig. 25: Adverse reaction to metal debris. (ALVAL: aseptic lymphocyte-dominated vasculitis-associated lesions; AVN: avascular necrosis)

II-restricted T4-lymphocytes. These T4-lymphocytes secrete various cytokines including attracting and activating the inflammatory process mediates by cells that release osteolytic cytokines causing periprosthetic osteolysis.

- *Pseudotumor formation:* Since biopsy of such lesions is difficult to distinguish from necrotic tumor tissue, they were labeled as pseudotumors, but also other descriptions have been used in literature such as bursae, cysts, or inflammatory masses. The pseudotumors are characterized by an extensive necrosis of dense connective tissue, a locally heavy macrophage, and lymphocytic infiltration as well as the presence of plasma cells and eosinophils. Although similar to ALVAL reaction, the pseudotumor formation involves a much more diffuse lymphocyte infiltrate and characteristic presence of connective tissue necrosis. In pseudotumor tissues, tiny metal debris particles have been found and their incidence is accompanied by increased metal ion concentrations in blood serum, which points to excessive wear as possible reason. Pseudotumors may cause severe symptoms that frequently require revision surgery and also compromise the success of revision surgery.

The wear volumes realized with MOM combinations are much lower than those with MOP and COP devices. However, metal debris is much smaller than PE debris and therefore, in spite of drastically reduced wear volumes, in a given time period, the number of metallic particles is much higher than the corresponding number of PE. With first- and second-generation MOM prostheses, no significant osteolysis and aseptic loosening had been observed or reported that was wrongly interpreted as the absence of pathologically relevant toxicity. The high mobility of small metallic debris particles and the damage they may cause were known before they had been classified as nanoparticles (<100 nm) and a lot of research had started in "nanotoxicology". High doses of Co–Cr wear particles could cause cytotoxicity and genotoxicity and were responsible for tissue necrosis in bone marrow, periprosthetic connective tissue, and in lymph nodes. Co–Cr nanoparticles affect the growth of osteoblasts and could therefore interfere with bone formation. It is also possible that nanosized Co–Cr wear debris can induce DNA damage and lead to chromosomal aberrations.

Local and Systemic Effects and Cancer Risk

As mentioned earlier, there is a direct cytotoxicity reaction involving cell death of macrophages and T-cells that may be involved in scavenging cancer initiation. T-cell lymphopenia due to raised levels of Co and Cr ions may be associated with increased cancer risk. The ions have been shown to cross the placental barrier, which is interestingly higher at low maternal metal–ion levels than that at higher maternal levels. There had been lack of complete and demonstrated knowledge regarding the potential effects/maleffects of metal ions on fetal development however. But, ethically MOM THA had been contraindicated in women of childbearing age for possible teratological effects. Cr^{3+} and Cr^{6+} also cause DNA-strand breaks. Cobalt not only causes DNA-strand breaks, but it also inhibits DNA repair, therefore adding to the damage caused by Cr ions. These metal ions hence lead to genomic instability quite similar to ionizing radiation. These findings have been portended to cause mutation by DNA damage during normal cellular function increasing the risk of cancers.

The first well-documented case of cancer associated with total joint replacement was in a patient who developed a malignant fibrous histiocytoma 3.5 years after a MOM THR performed in December, 1969. Few well-documented reports exist in literature for malignancies following MOM THAs, most involving sarcomas. There is also increased risk of hematopoietic cancer [relative risk (RR) of 1.59], which is higher for leukemia (RR: 3.77). Rigorous long-term studies are needed to correctly assess the RR to benefit ratios for total hip bearings. But for ethical reasons, the MOM bearings have been withdrawn as of now. So, it will only be for those patients with still implanted asymptomatic hips that the data can be gathered.

Guidelines for Evaluation of Patients with Implanted Metal-on-Metal Bearings (American Academy of Orthopedic Surgeons)

Patients presenting with painful MOM hip arthroplasty should be evaluated for the following thoroughly [adapted from American Academy of Orthopedic Surgeons (AAOS), available freely at http://www.aaos.org/about/papers/advistmt/1035.asp]:

- *Conditions extrinsic to hip:*
  - *Spine disease:* Stenosis, disk herniation, spondylolysis, or spondylolisthesis
  - Peripheral vascular disease
  - Hernia (femoral and inguinal)
  - Peripheral nerve injury (e.g., sciatic, femoral, and meralgia paresthetica)
  - Malignancy or metastases
  - Metabolic bone disease (e.g., Paget's disease and osteomalacia)
  - Complex regional pain syndrome
  - Psychological disorder
- *Conditions intrinsic to hip:*
  - *Intracapsular/implant-related:*
    - Infection
    - Loosening
    - Instability/subluxation
    - Periprosthetic fracture
    - Adverse soft tissue reaction
  - *Extracapsular:*
    - Trochanteric bursitis
    - Iliopsoas tendonitis

Once identified and other conditions are ruled out, the patient is categorized into one of the three categories **(Table 1)** for further management. Annual follow-up is recommended for low-risk-group patients, while revision is recommended for high-risk patients. For moderate-risk-group patients, consider revision surgery, if symptoms progress, imaging

TABLE 1: Patient stratification for MOM implanted THAs presenting to clinical practice (AAOS).

	MOM "low"-risk group	*MOM "moderate"-risk group*	*MOM "high"-risk group*
Patient factors	Low-activity level patient	• Male or female dysplasia (for hip resurfacing) • Moderate-activity level patient	• Female with dysplasia (for hip resurfacing) • High-activity level patient
Symptoms	Asymptomatic (including no systemic or mechanical symptoms)	• Symptomatic • Mild local hip symptoms (e.g., pain, mechanical symptoms) • No systemic symptoms	• Symptomatic • Severe local hip and/or mechanical symptoms • Systemic symptoms
Clinical examination	• No change in gait (i.e., no limp, no abductor weakness) • No swelling	• Change in gait (i.e., limp) • No abductor weakness • No swelling	• Change in gait (i.e., limp) • Abductor weakness • Swelling
Implant type	Small diameter femoral head (<36 mm) modular MOM THA; hip resurfacing in males <50 with OA	• Large diameter femoral head (≥36 mm) modular or nonmodular MOM THA • Recalled MOM implant • Hip resurfacing with risk factors (female with dysplasia) • Modular neck device	• Large diameter femoral head (≥36 mm) modular or nonmodular MOM THA • Recalled MOM implant
Radiographs (2 views ± serial for comparison when available)	• Optimal acetabular cup orientation • No implant osteolysis/loosening	• Optimal acetabular cup orientation • No implant osteolysis/loosening	• Suboptimal acetabular cup orientation • Implant osteolysis/loosening
Infection work-up (ESR, CRP, ± hip aspiration)	Within normal limits	Within normal limits	Within normal limits
Metal ion level test (if available)	Low (<3 ppb)	Moderately elevated (3–10 ppb)	High (>10 ppb)
• Cross-sectional imaging (if available) These studies include MARS MRI; ultrasound or CT when MRI contraindicated or MARS protocol not available	Within normal limits	• Presence of abnormal tissue reactions without involvement of surrounding muscles and/or bone • Simple cystic lesions or small cystic lesions without thickened wall	• Presence of abnormal tissue reactions with involvement of surrounding muscles and/or bone • Solid lesions • Cystic lesions with thickened wall • Mixed solid and cystic lesions

(AAOS: American Academy of Orthopedic Surgeons; CRP: C-reactive protein; CT: computed tomography; ESR: erythrocyte sedimentation rate; MARS: metal artifact reduction sequence; MOM: metal-on-metal; MRI: magnetic resonance imaging; THA: total hip arthroplasty)

abnormality progresses, and/or rising metal ion levels over 6 months' follow-up.

CERAMIC BEARINGS

Ceramic bearings are among the most exciting bearings of today for their evolution and reported lowest *in vivo* wear rates. This is due to the hydrophilic nature permitting better wettability of the surface by adsorption (see θ angle earlier). These bearings are also scratch resistant due to hardness and the fact that they can be polished to a much lower surface roughness. Ceramic-bearing combination achieves fluid-film lubrication. Importantly, ceramic is highly biocompatible (compared to metal or poly bearings). But all this is not only to cause advantage, the greater hardness of ceramics also make them sensitive to design, manufacturing, and implantation variables. The COC bearings are susceptible to rapid wear, if they are suboptimally positioned in situ. The use of ceramic bearing was historically introduced in April, 1970 by Dr Pierre Boutin, who used alumina-on-alumina bearing. Surgical grade COC bearings are of three types:

1. *Alumina ceramics:* These are inorganic nonmetallic materials formed by compounding of a nonmetal and a metal. In particular, alumina is a monophasic, but polycrystalline structure imparting hardness and stability. Also, it is highly oxidized (gives excellent resistance to corrosion and makes it bioinert) with a high thermal conductivity coefficient (thermodynamic stability). It has low bending stress and low resilience but to make it brittle and may break due to low fracture toughness. The ionic structure of alumina ceramic gives it an advantage of hydrophilic nature making it hydrophilic. This generates fluid-film lubrication resulting from higher wettability, which is quite desirable in moving surfaces. The serum proteins quickly and completely cover the ceramic surface with a monolayer after surgical implantation providing improved lubrication of the joint.
2. *Zirconia ceramics:* Zirconia has comparatively higher fracture toughness than alumina ceramic and is a newer introduction in the field. The bending strength is also higher but pure zirconia is unstable in its phasic structure. It exhibits three crystalline phases—(1) monoclinic, (2) tetragonal, and (3) cubic that result in variations of mechanical properties with loading and temperature changes. Zirconia exhibits large volume changes and decreased mechanical properties because of cracking on cooling. This phase transformation (between the three phases at different temperature and loads) puts pure zirconia at disadvantage by generating internal stresses

within the deformation zone ahead of propagating cracks. Adding oxides [magnesium oxide (MgO) or yttrium oxide (Y_2O_3)] during the tetragonal phase stabilizes zirconia. Best mechanical properties are seen for yttrium-stabilized tetragonal polycrystalline zirconia (Y-TZP) that effectively reduces grain size. The tetragonal phase (unstable, but occupies less volume) tends to transform into the monoclinic phase (stable, but occupies more volume) explaining higher resistance to shock but gives it lower sliding resistance properties. Another concern with Y-TZP is its hydrothermal instability; where during steam sterilization, there may occur slow degradation when the bearing is implanted for long-term.

3. *Alumina-matrix-composite ceramics [AMC, Delta (zirconia)], ceramic-on-alumina [mixture of 75% aluminum oxide, 25% zirconia* **(Fig. 26A)** *with less than 1% chromium and strontium oxides]:* This is the newest generation of COC bearings quite popular nowadays. It incorporates nanosized, yttria-stabilized tetragonal zirconia particles (see earlier) into alumina producing alumina-matrix-composite. For very obvious reasons, one would combine the above two ceramics as both have disadvantages that can be compensated by the other. Alumina is brittle, while zirconia is hydrothermally unstable. Logically combining them into a composite is believed to improve the mechanical properties. These alumina–zirconia nanocomposites have relatively low zirconia content so the hardness is similar to alumina but the susceptibility to hydrothermal instability is drastically reduced. This delta ceramic composite bearing surface has shown high survivorship resulting from improved mechanical properties especially preventing the initiation and propagation of cracks that were significant with previously prevailing alumina ceramics. Oxide additives (see zirconia ceramic) produce "platelet-like" crystals **(Fig. 26B)** that dissipate energy by deflecting cracks. The effect is further augmented by addition of chromium oxide that increases the strength and toughness by composite hardening.

First-generation ceramics were a failure but gradually developments in the production process such as sintering improved material quality. This process reduced the porosity and grain size while increasing density and purity of modern alumina ceramics, increasing its hardness, fracture toughness, and burst strength **(Box 2)**. Specifically, the burst strength improved from 38 to 98 Kilonewtons over a period of 11 years (1977–1988). The new delta ceramic (alumina-matrix-composite) stands still apart with extensive improvements in material properties such as extremely high fracture toughness and resistance to crack propagation. Resistance to crack propagation is imparted by two mechanisms:

1. *Airbag function:* With impact loading, there is dispersion of nanosized, yttria-stabilized tetragonal zirconia particles in a stable, and alumina matrix absorbing the incident forces. These particles get homogeneously distributed producing only local high pressure area at site of crack counteracting propagation of crack, if any simulating vehicle airbag system.

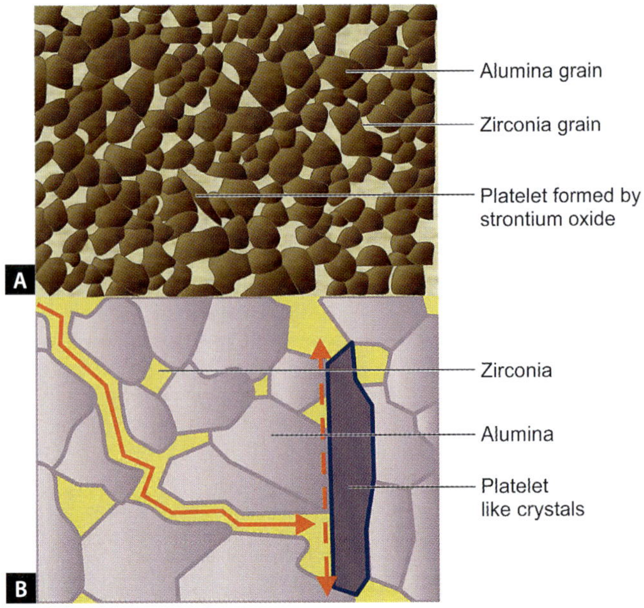

Figs. 26A and B: Delta ceramic: It is a mixture of alumina and zirconia.

BOX 2: The different generations of evolution of alumina ceramic and differences between alumina and zirconia.

Generations of alumina:

1. *First-generation alumina:* This was basically for industrial purpose and not suited for biomedical usage. It had poor microstructure with low density, scarce purity, and large grain size.
2. *Second-generation alumina (BIOLOX®):* This was the alumina used by Boutin in his alumina-on-alumina bearings.
3. *Third-generation alumina (BIOLOX FORTE®):* The improvements and quality control measures were developed by ISO 6474 standard introduced in 1980 to improve raw material, with smaller gain size, low level of impurities, and sintered in air that led to production of third-generation alumina used for a long duration.
4. *Fourth-generation ceramic (BIOLOX DELTA®):* Alumina matrix composite as detailed in text.

It must be realized from above that the generations are for alumina ceramic development and not for zirconia at all.

Alumina	*Zirconia*
Low stress resistance	Stronger than alumina and resist higher degrees of stress
Brittle	Superior mechanical strength and reduced bearing fracture risk
Chemical and hydrothermal stability	Unstable material—tetragonal phase tends to transform into monoclinic phase. It has to be stabilized by yttrium oxide
Harder and higher resistance to wear	Best case scenario hardness is 50% of alumina so lower resistance to wear

2. *Neutralizing crack formation:* The platelet-shaped crystals in the oxide mixture prevent cracking and crack propagation in situ by putting a sudden stop to crack pathway and deflecting it, they also neutralize crack energy.

Advantages of Mechanical Properties of Ceramics

- Minimal wear (COC bearings) and virtually no osteolysis due to inert nature of alumina wear particles. Osteolysis can come through UHMWPE wear particles in hybrid coupling or by silica or metal from wear of modular articulations.

- Because alumina ceramics are highly oxidized, they cannot be further oxidized, so are biologically inert.
- The hardness imparts resistance to surface damage. The hardness of alumina makes it very abrasive and wear resistant increasing its resistance to scratching (the only material capable of scratching alumina is diamond).
- Alumina is extremely strong in compression. Making it a very good bearing on femoral side and less for acetabular liner.

Disadvantages of Mechanical Properties

- Very precise production techniques are needed in order to ensure proper fit of the head within the socket—else accelerated wear would result in COC bearings.
- The lack of ceramic deformation reduces the contact areas between the head and socket increasing contact stress. To counter this disadvantage clearance must be optimized.
- *Incompatibility with cement fixation:* Alumina is >300 times stiffer than cancellous bone and nearly 200 times stiffer than PMMA due to modulus mismatch. So, if ceramic components are cemented, they result in cement fracture and high loosening rates than UHMPE-cemented components.
- *Fracture susceptibility:* Previously used alumina is very brittle and hence susceptible to fracture (now replaced with delta ceramic).

Alumina versus Zirconia

Alumina was the first ceramic acceptable for hip arthroplasty bearings following its introduction in 1970 and was widely used. Medical-grade alumina is produced through a hot isostatic pressing step from high-purity (>99%) alumina powder.

Aluminum oxide (Al_2O_3) could be highly polished reducing its coefficient of friction to extremely low levels. Alumina is not only highly resistant to abrasion but the monocrystalline structure is much more stable than the more recently developed zirconia. While alumina remains the most widely used ceramic and is preferred for COC bearings, zirconia is utilized as a replacement for alumina femoral heads for COP bearings (UHMWPE acetabular liner). This is reasoned on the fact that zirconia is stronger than alumina and therefore, it can resist higher degrees of stress (***see* Box 2**). Zirconium oxide (ZrO_2 or zirconia) was introduced later than alumina as its alternative in 1985. The advantages conferred by zirconia include superior mechanical strength posing a reduction in bearing fracture risk. Smaller femoral head sizes can be made from zirconia while maintaining excellent wear characteristics when coupled with UHMWPE but only in phase-stabilized state else excessive wear is seen. Oxinium (oxidized zirconium) has been specifically designed for the purpose of articulation with UHMWPE but wear characteristics have not been very encouraging in hip arthroplasty. Some features for these ceramic bearings are as follows:

- Volumetric wear for alumina on alumina bearings during run-in phase and "steady-state" phase measure 0.1–0.2 mm^3 per million cycles and <0.02 mm^3 per million cycles respectively that is <5,000 times compared to other bearings.
- Accelerated wear has been reported for alumina on alumina bearing.
    - "Stripe wear" is a specific type of accelerated wear that is localized over a discrete area **(Fig. 27)**. It may be associated with ball and socket separation during the swing phase of gait or when the ball is levered out of the socket by impingement, so it is recommended to keep these bearing joints tight. The femoral head and the acetabular liner when kept loose as in a standard hip can separate by 2 mm during the swing phase of gait cycle.
- Wear rates of alumina on alumina bearing surface range from 0.3 to 5.0 mm/year. Variations occur due to implanted material and design changes while surgical and patient factors contribute minimally. Most catastrophic wear and fracture of bearings were reported with products presiding earlier than 1990.
- A bimodal size range of ceramic wear debris is observed (see earlier) with very small wear particles generated under standard articulating conditions and larger particles generated under microseparation conditions. Microseparation occurs during swing phase (if hip is kept loose) and when load is applied at heel strike, the femoral head is pushed vertically to relocate in the acetabular cup contacting often the rim of liner first resulting in stripe wear.

Ceramic Bearing Complications

Stripe Wear

Stripe wear describes the long, narrow area of damage seen on femoral heads mainly from alumina COC hip bearing couples. This was most common in first- and second-generation bearings and only few, if any third-generation bearings. Stripe wear results from edge loading effects of rigid COC bearings in THA, which are produced during microseparation of the ball from the socket during the swing phase as mentioned earlier. The other mechanism is by impingement of the trunnion on the acetabular rim levering the ball out of the socket. During subluxation, there is an inferior and equatorial stripe created by the rim while during reduction (heel strike), a superior and equatorial stripe is created. Stripe wear **(Fig. 27)** can be quite catastrophic and is of concern because associated volumetric wear with this phenomenon is quite high. This is the reason for not recommending this bearing in individuals with tissue laxity (Marfan's, EDS, etc.) or those that desire excellent range of motion with vigorous lifestyles who perform impact activities. These may place the hip through a provocative range of motion and initiate stripe wear. Surgeon may choose other bearings (best is MOM surface replacement, alas unavailable) for such patients.

Liner Chipping on Insertion

This results from surgeon's failure to seat the ceramic liner fully in the shell before impacting it and causing chipping of the rim.

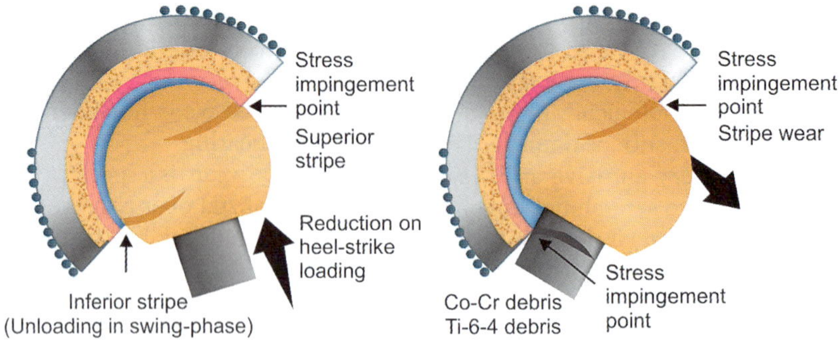

Fig. 27: Stripe wear of ceramic bearing.

Liner Canting or Dissociation

Liner canting also called malseating or dissociation has been reported for surgeries performed in past with first- and second-generation bearings. It usually results from failure to impact the liner with sufficient force. Such dissociated liners would increase the risk of squeaking. Other causes of canting are reduced shell thickness, increased bone stiffness, and increased interference fit.

Edge Loading

This is again mostly a surgeon's failure to correctly position the cup. Poor cup position causes subluxation of the head over the hard posterior edge of the bearing surface during deep flexion. Severe edge loading would result in accelerated wear.

Fracture

This is mainly a drawback from ceramic brittleness, which is still unresolved. The risk factors for fractures are:

- *Short neck femoral heads:* The fracture occurs in the circumferential portion of the head near the edge of the head bore. For 28-mm heads, the distance between the corner/edge of the head bore to the outermost aspect of the ceramic head is smaller for short necks when compared to medium or long neck designs, thus facilitating crack propagation.
- *Long neck femoral heads (less supported):* The increased distance between the edge of the head bore and the outer surface of the head increases the tensile stresses at the taper-bore junction and hence fracture. There is higher chance of impingement-subluxation and edge loading, the effect is intensified in the presence of increased anteversion and increased inclination.
- *Malpositioning the acetabulum*—predisposes for liner fracture. This is also responsible for the chipping of liner during insertion. Poor alignment of the liner during impaction into the acetabular component does significantly increase the risk of liner fractures.
- *Presence of noise*—liner fracture
- Presence of ceramic particles at least 11 ceramic particles smaller than 3 μm or at least one ceramic particle larger than 3 μm per each 90 μm^2 field of observation in synovial fluid examination (100% sensitivity and 88% specificity)—liner fracture
- Trauma and fall
- *Poor surgical technique:* Impaction of the femoral head on the trunnion nonconcentrically or not cleaning and drying it properly by a surgeon in a hurry leads to stress concentrations in the femoral head bearing. The other cause is putting ceramic femoral head on a damaged trunnion causing stress concentration. This compromise burst strength and increased potential for fracture. This raises the concern that trunnion should always be protected during stem implantation.

Improved material processing (purification of alumina powder), laser etching, smaller grain sizes, and proof testing have significantly reduced the risk of catastrophic in vivo fracture in second-generation ceramics (0.014%) and third-generation ceramics (0.004%). Prevention of fractures due to weaker liners during manufacturing involves proof testing that should eliminate weaker components or flawed products that are likely to fail. Theoretically, proof testing should eliminate all bearing components with manufacturing flaws that are likely to clinically fail but no proof test currently available is 100% effective.

Clicking and Squeaking

With third-generation ceramics, wear is not as big a problem as is the noise. Squeaking is a high-pitched noise audible to ears. The squeaking usually occurs in midrange of motion while weight-bearing (viz., stair climbing) and is generally considered a significant issue of concern for the patient. The association of malposition to squeaking is inconclusive and it appears that the squeaking is an isolated phenomenon with no consequence on longevity. Retrieved revised noisy ceramic bearings have not shown any mechanical cause for squeaking and these findings have been inconclusive. Only positive findings in these noisy bearings frequently are a small zone of stripe wear with metallic staining. It has been found that squeaking noise is definitely associated to break in fluid film layer (lubrication) and would disappear if proper lubrication exists between the bearing surfaces. This may result from metal particle transfer (third body) between the COC bearing surfaces and hence also produce metal staining frequently seen. The patients are often worried and commonly perceive this to be a surgical failure, which may prompt litigation for bearing malfunction or even involve the surgeon. Surgeon should reassure patient and obtain informed consent. The recommended flow of evaluation for a squeaking ceramic hip is to rule out ceramic breakage first with a computed tomography scan, which can cause squeaking and it may not be obvious on plain radiographs, only then patient should be reassured. If this fails then injection of viscosupplements can alleviate the noise in many.

If there is noise associated with gross component malposition or impingement is noted with clinically reported pain then revision surgery should be done. It is recommended to use a metal ball and PE socket in revision of COC bearing for noise.

Other noises may still come from this standard bearing and patient should be counseled for this. A thud-like "clicking" sound is observed in MOP bearing. This thud is much more prominent in patients with a COP bearing. "Clicking" sound combined with crepitus is observed for patients having a MOM THA. These patients experience a sound similar to a "rusty door hinge" so in order to avoid any further noise, it is better to revise a COC bearing with Co–Cr on UHMPE (poly) bearing.

Impulse generation and implant vibration: The vibrations that initiate squeaking may come from local intermittent motions propounded by stick-slip friction. This static friction force primarily comes from bearing surface that opposes rotation in static implants. Because of static friction, rotational kinetic force produces local acceleration/deceleration pattern of the magnitude of 450 m/s^2 (45G!). The friction can be increased by ceramic particles in the interface, metal transfer to the head, and reduced lubrication at the interface.

Ceramic-on-Metal Articulation

The wear for alumina ceramic-on-metal (COM) articulations is very favorable, but the articulation should be ceramic femoral heads 28 mm in diameter articulating against acetabular cups manufactured from medical-grade, high-carbon-wrought cobalt–chromium alloy (early catastrophic failure is seen if this pairing is reversed by articulating a metal head against ceramic acetabular component instead). No run-in period is observed with the COM bearings and a volumetric wear rate of 0.01 mm^3 per 1 million cycles is reported. Metal wear particles are of nanometer size (6–30 nm) range small enough to possibly not cause as frequent an osteolysis as with standard or MOM bearings. There is a reduction in serum metal ions in the patients at 6 months postoperatively. In addition, this bearing also appears to produce less stripe wear with edge loading than MOM or COC implants. The potential advantages of this novel COM bearing are thus lower wear and the production of significantly reduced metal particles quantitatively. All said concerns of metal wear particles always remain. This bearing combination possibly will also allow for the use of larger femoral heads (due to low wear) thus improving the stability and jump distance. In addition, larger ceramic heads reduce the fracture risk and an increased number of femoral head options are made available increasing modularity. The clinical performance is unknown.

NEW HORIZONS IN BEARING SURFACES

Silicon Nitride Bearings in Total Hip Arthroplasty

Brittle ceramic bearings are susceptible to failure, so alternative zirconia heads were produced to improve the strength, but it has disadvantage of phase transformation, so the surface of zirconium alloy femoral heads was modified. Though introduced with enthusiasm, the surface hardness, wear reduction, and scratch resistance of oxidized zirconium are less favorable than alumina. Not only this but oxidized zirconium can also not be used in COC articulations. To counter this problem, ceramic material fabricated from silicon nitride (Si_3N_4) powder has been proposed as alternative. On mechanical testing, Si_3N_4 shows good fracture toughness, high-flexural strength, and resistance to hydrothermal degradation (such as alumina). Si_3N_4 is currently used in aerospace bearings and in high-temperature places such as in diesel engines. When studied for THA, the Si_3N_4 cups have been shown to highly reduce the wear rates when used against Co–Cr or Si_3N_4 femoral heads. The Si_3N_4 material demonstrated a near 100% theoretical material density (3.20 g/cm^3) and an organized uniform microstructure of fine elongated grain particles. The Si_3N_4–Si_3N_4 bearings have very low friction coefficient of 0.001 even when compared with COC alumina bearing of 0.08. On note particularly is the toughness of bearing revealed when used against metal head that generated very low wear rates and that Si_3N_4 has been found to withstand high loads even if contact stress-related damage has occurred that may usually fracture a ceramic bearing. The tissue reactions also had not been prominent with these materials and there is indication of acute or chronic toxicity, mutagenicity, allergenicity, carcinogenicity, or localized tissue toxicity.

Carbon Fiber Polymeric Composites

Carbon fiber-reinforced epoxy composites (CFRP) were introduced and showed wear rates similar to highly cross-linked poly. Epoxy resins are thermoset materials and that cannot be machine shaped so they are "set" via chemical reaction in the desired form.

Polyether Ether Ketone

It is an emerging unique thermoplastic high-performance polymer. Polyether ether ketone (PEEK) has gained interest for use as a composite matrix for its high strength, toughness, and tissue biocompatibility.

Preventing retroacetabular stress shielding: Acetabular component is most susceptible to osteolysis, one of the factors for which is stress shielding due to rigid acetabular shells. Few modifications in materials and design have been produced to reduce the stress shielding as follows:

- *Cambridge cup® (Howmedica, Staines, UK):* This is a horseshoe-shaped all polymer acetabular construct of UHMPE liner and carbon fiber reinforced polybutylene terephthalate shell with HA coating to fix to acetabulum. Compete long-term results are awaited.
- *MITCH PCR cup (Stryker SA, Montreux Switzerland):* This is a second-generation horseshoe-shaped cup made of PEEK/carbon fiber composite articulating with alumina femoral head.

Compliant Bearings

This emphasizes a new concept altogether. Hypothetically, it will lead to developing bearing materials that mimic articular cartilage exhibiting friction and wear behavior similar to it. Polyurethanes are one such synthetic polymers and contenders but biocompatibility has been an issue. No further advancements have been concrete but the search is still on!

Sapphire

Sapphire contains 99.99% aluminum oxide. The crystals are placed in a vacuum at 2,100°C to prepare single crystal formations. As a bearing surface, it has many physical and mechanical similarities to alumina, viz., inertness, low friction, high wear resistance, and biologically compatible. They have been explored in a small number of patients with good result, but no large clinical trials are available.

Improvement in Metal Femoral Heads

Various coatings are being tested to increase the surface hardness and improve coefficient of friction of metal alloys and provide a nonmetal interface. This "ceramicization" of femoral head has been attempted with alumina composites, or titanium nitride.

- *Titanium nitride (TiN) coating:* TiN offers scratch resistance with low coefficient of friction that can be used as a coating on metal heads in MOP articulation to reduce poly wear. But, it has been found that if this later is scratched then exposed underlying metal undergoes fast wear, so process of physical vapor deposition used to generate TiN layer needs optimization before commercial use.
- *Silicon nitride (Si_3N_4) coating:* It is harder than titanium alloy and tougher than alumina with reported but unsubstantiated lower wear rates. The alpha phase of Si_3N_4 is soluble in blood and it has bacteriostatic potential against *S. epidermidis*. Si_3N_4 coating on Ti6Al4V generated accelerated wear and noise so was halted. Newer diamond-like carbon (DLC) articulating femoral head against Si_3N_4 acetabular component is being tested for lower wear rates and noise.
- *Diamond-like carbon (DLC) coating of femoral heads:* Hydrogenated amorphous carbon (a-C:H) DLC-coated micro-dimpled prostheses against Si_3N_4 acetabular component is being tested. Some concerns of cytotoxicity of graphite particles have emerged and long-term survivorship has been reported to be inferior to ceramic heads.
- *Nanocrystalline diamond (NCD):* NCD grown on Si_3N_4 by chemical vapor deposition has shown high resistance to wear in testing cycles.
- *Alumina coating:* This combines hardness and scratch resistance of alumina femoral heads with lower fracture risk of metal alloys. Studies are underway but no concrete usage terms have evolved.
- *Copper alloys:* Ti6Al4V5Cu is harder than titanium alloys and has lower coefficient of friction but concerns of copper ion toxicity have possibly precluded their fast integration as bearing surface for clinical usage.

CONCLUSION

- Numerous variations of implants are available in the current orthopedic practice and their number is only expected to rise in future. Continuous evolution and changes in the system are introduced continuously for improvement in implant surfaces or other properties.
- Understanding tribology is essential to grasp the utility of such changes so that they can be utilized to the best of our patients.
- Wear is the predominant mode of failure of most bearing surfaces (except ceramics) that produce undue effects on the implanted system (particularly osteolysis) causing their failure.
- Continuous attempts are directed to reduce the osteolysis due to wear by improving the implant surface or wear characteristics so that longevity can be improved. The methods predominantly have focused to improve the PE characteristics. The other method is to use unique bearing surfaces such as ceramics. The latter of course have their set of unique problems, which have contributed for their modifications.
- Newer bearing materials are bound to develop and will be introduced for improving the design systems so that they can last longer.

CHAPTER 15

Poly (Methyl Methacrylate) (PMMA; Plexiglass, Bone Cement, and Acrylic Bone Cement)

Manish Kumar Varshney

INTRODUCTION

All currently marketed acrylic bone cements are polymers of methyl methacrylate (an ester of methacrylic acid, **Fig. 1**). The bone cement is an integral part of orthopedic surgery. It is used for fixation of artificial joints where it fills the free space between the prosthesis and bone. The cement acts as an elastic zone that because of its stiffness cushions the forces affecting bone, serving as a "grout". So in effect, the term "cement" is a misnomer as cement stands for bonding two surfaces together while poly (methyl methacrylate) (PMMA) serves to transmit the loads uniformly and a space filler to fill the medullary canal. Today, the PMMA finds its use in following procedures enduring orthopedic and dental surgery:

- Synthesis of dentures
- Joint arthroplasty (hip and knee)
- Spine surgery—vertebroplasty and kyphoplasty
- Bone infections—as vehicle/carrier of antibiotics [*see* Chapter on "Infections of Bone (Typical and Atypical) and Surgical Site Infection"]
- Tumor surgery (managing dead space after removal of locally aggressive tumors).

HISTORY OF DEVELOPMENT OF BONE CEMENT

The use of interface material (cement made of plaster and colophony) for fixation of implants was first described by Themistocles Gluck in 1870, so use of "cementing" per se should be credited to him. The identification of the compound PMMA came from the thesis of Otto Rohm's titled "polymerization products of acrylic acid" in Tubingen. Chemical synthesis on industrial scale started in 1920s in laboratories of Rohm and Haas. Denture fabrication was the first clinical biomedical application of the product where exothermic polymerization from heating the methyl methacrylate (MMA) was done.

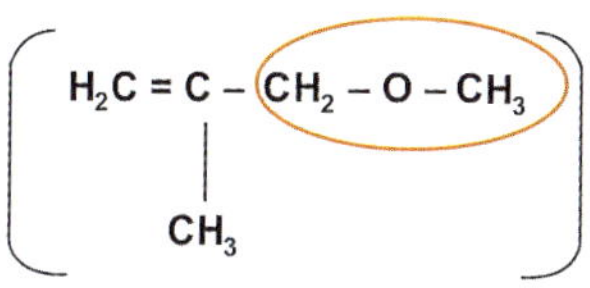

Fig. 1: Ester (circled) of methacrylate.

In 1936, Kulzer (a company) found a dough preparation with grounded PMMA powder and a liquid monomer that hardens with benzoyl peroxide (BPO) when heated to 100°C. This was the first landmark modification in technical usage of PMMA paving the way for widespread use of these raisins for denture and cranioplasties. The first clinical use was to fill/seal cranial defects in monkeys and later only was it used in humans. It was later found that addition of a coinitiator can lead to polymerization at room temperature without heating and is valid till date (cold curing). Fast curing resins were also developed to fill the visceral injuries and some skeletal injuries in 1963 (Rau et al.), but these were quickly abandoned due to bioincompatibility. The biocompatibility of cement (PMMA) was established when the existing bone glue—polyurethanes were shown to produce violent tissue reactions and PMMA acted inert. Judet and Judet in 1956 were the first to introduce arthroplastic surgical technique using the bone cements but it was soon realized that they cannot get integrated in the body. Sir John Charnley was the first to succeed in anchoring femoral prosthesis with the use of bone cement (Nu-Life) and published his report of six cases in Journal of Bone and Joint Surgery (JBJS) British edition. His choice of material was focused on a substance, which could be easily manipulated and which set within a reasonable time and at the same time, the material had to be biologically inert, resistant to body fluids. Most importantly, he discovered the property of PMMA to completely fill the defects/gaps in medullary canal from prosthesis implantation by conforming to bony anatomy. In the 1970s, the United States Food and Drug Administration (FDA) approved bone cement for use in hip and knee prosthetic fixation.

PMMA, Plexiglass (Fig. 2)

When methacrylates are used as bone cements, they must be polymerized. The most important functional bond is C=C covalent double bond. To produce a polymer from MMA is a tedious and long-drawn process that also results in significant shrinkage and uncontrollable heat production. Pure MMA has a shrinkage of 21% (1 L of monomer will produce only 800 cm^3 of polymer) and the heat of production may boil the monomer.

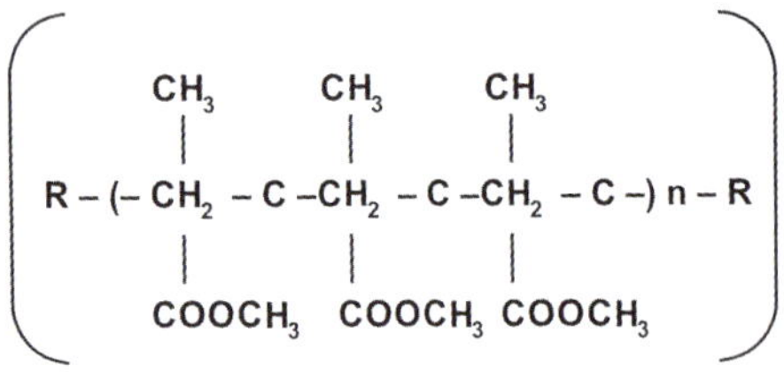

Fig. 2: Poly (methyl methacrylate).

TABLE 1: The typical constituents of the bone cement.	
Powder phase: The powder is the variable part in composition of bone cements among different brands. PMMA beads comprise 83–99% if the component with 8–15% contributed by the opacifier	*Liquid phase:* Ester of methacrylic acid **(Fig. 1)** is a colorless liquid of intense odors. Normally, this liquid is stabilized by hydroquinone derivative that acts as free radical scavenger. The boiling point of the liquid is 100°C
• *Polymer powder:* PMMA/ copolymers • Initiator = Benzoyl peroxide (BPO) (the BPO can be addedas either contained in PMMA balls or added as a separate powder). Other compounds that can be used as initiator include tri-n-butylborane • *Accelerator (optional):* 2,5-di-methylhexane-2,5-hydroperoxide • *Opacifier:* Zirconium dioxide or barium sulfate • Colors like chlorophyllin • *Antibiotics:* Macrolides, amino-glycosides, vancomycin, etc.	• Monomer = Methyl methacrylate/butyl methacrylate • Activator/coinitiator = DMPT (N,N-dimethyl-para-toluidine)—makes 0.4–2.8% of the liquid component • Stabilizer/free radical scavenger = Hydroquinone/ascorbic acid • Coloring agent = Chlorophyllin

[PMMA: poly (methyl methacrylate)]

To avoid the shrinkage during polymerization, the bone cement is supplied in two-component system. Most bone cements have mixing ratio of 2–3 parts powder: 1 part monomer (40 g powder and 20 mL of liquid monomer ampoule), this reduced the heat of polymerization and shrinkage by two-thirds. The other advantage is that the monomer amount is reduced; else, it being a volatile component can produce adverse reactions in the body. The MMA in aqueous suspension is prepolymerized in easily cooled reaction boilers. The polymer obtained as tiny balls (1–125 μm) is easily dissolved in monomeric MMA. This prepolymerization of powder sample avoids shrinkage further while the components are mixed and also the temperature of reaction is considerably reduced. The constituents of two components of a typical bone cement have distinctive characteristics **(Table 1)**.

Without the initiator, the two components when mixed will result in nothing but dough that slowly becomes more viscous. BPO in powder and DMPT [$CH_3C_6H_4N(CH_3)_2$] in liquid react to form free radicals (benzoyl radical and a benzoate anion) at room temperature starting the process of polymerization **(Fig. 3)**. The BPO [$(C_6H_5COO)_2$] is decomposed into benzoyl radical [$C_6H_5COO^*$] and benzoate anion as follows:

$$(C_6H_5COO)_2 + CH_3C_6H_4N(CH_3)_2 \rightarrow C_6H_5COO^* + C_6H_5COO^- + CH_3C_6H_4N(CH_3)_2+ \rightarrow CH_3C_6H_4NCH_3CH_2^* + H^+$$

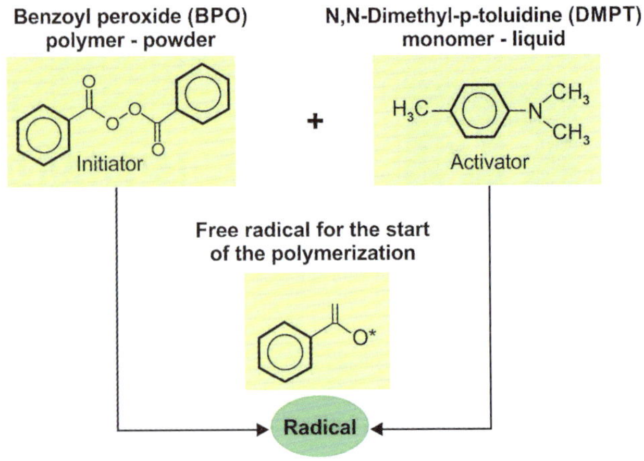

Fig. 3: Benzoyl peroxide (BPO) from the powder and N,N-dimethyl-para-toluidine (DMPT) from the liquid react to form radicals, starting the curing of bone cements.

In the second step, the MMA is polymerized into chain propagation to achieve high molecular weight PMMA of the order of 100,000–1,000,000 g/mol by the reaction of benzoyl radical with MMA [$CH_2 = CCH_3COOCH_3$] as follows:

$$C_6H_5COO^* + CH_2 = CCH_3COOCH_3 \rightarrow C_6H_5COO\text{-}CH_2^- CCH_3COOCH_3 + CH_2 = CCH_3COOCH_3 \rightarrow C_6H_5COO^- CH_2CCH_3COOCH_3\text{-}CH_2CCH_3COOCH_3$$

The chain termination is achieved by either chain coupling or disproportionation via transfer of hydrogen ion. The hardened acrylic bone cement is a polymerized product containing primarily the linear, uncrosslinked, and variable length PMMA macromolecules. The molecular weight of hardened polymerized product depends on:

- The molecular weight of monomer itself (usually MMA, butyl MA can also be used instead)
- The molecular weight of synthesized prepolymerized beads
- The amount and presence of polymerization stabilizers
- The ambient room temperature during polymerization
- The sterilization method used for the raw products.

"Polymerization steps" are divided as follows:

1. *Mixing phase:* Wetting. Some technical points for improving cement handling during mixing, as this is arguably the most important phase:
   i. More powerful and vigorous mixing increases porosity of cement reducing its strength
   ii. Vacuum mixing results in 15–30% improvement of bending strength
   iii. Centrifugation results in approximately equal to 9% improvement of fatigue strength
   iv. Precooling the monomer, polymer, and mixing vessels decreases the number of pores and volume of pores.
2. *Waiting phase/sticky phase:* Swelling + polymerization—
   i. There is increase in viscosity.
   ii. Dough is sticky.
3. *Working phase:* This is the stage of chain propagation—
   i. Reduced mobility
   ii. Increase in viscosity.

For the cement to be in a working phase, the viscosity has to be such that it does not allow the mixing of blood, which may reduce the strength and at the same time, not so high that the interface between the prosthesis and cement is compromised. There is thermal expansion of the cement while simultaneous shrinkage due to polymerization.

4. *Setting/hardening phase:* Chain growth finished, no movability, and high temperature Phase 1 and 2 are together called dough time.

EFFECT OF VARIOUS FACTORS ON CEMENT POLYMERIZATION

Various factors that can alter duration of various phase of polymerization of cement are:

- *Heat of polymerization:* Temperature of cement in body = 43–46°C.
  - Precooling prosthesis will lead to increased and rapid polymerization of cement toward bone leading to shrinkage of material at cement prosthesis interface causing early loosening.
  - Prewarming the prosthesis will reduce the conductive capacity of prosthesis and lead to heat necrosis and early loosening of the implant.

One should hence warm the prosthesis only till body temperature.

- *Viscosity of cement:* It refers to the viscosity of cement during the dough time (i.e., from mixing to the start of working phase). It is largely determined mainly by the chemical composition and the powder to monomer ratio.
  - *High viscosity cement:* They have the smallest sticky phase followed by a long working phase to allow for implantation. Viscosity remains constant till the end of working phase.
  - *Medium viscosity cement:* Sticky period lasts 3 minutes followed by working phase where the viscosity rises slowly. Hardening takes 1½–2½ minutes.
  - *Low viscosity (liquid) cements:* Long wait of 3 minutes or more in sticky phase followed by rapid rise of viscosity in working phase and hardening phase is 1–2 minutes long.
- *Precooling and preheating the cement:* Precooling makes mixing of the cement more comfortable and increases the working time as the heat of polymerization is dissipated. Preheating the cement is done to reduce the operative time.
- *Cement "flaws":* Cement additives or air entrapment produces voids or pores in the polymerized structure referred to as flaws. The causes of flaws include:
  - Air dissolution and their distribution in the powder particles and final product
  - Air entrapment while mixing the two components
  - Persistence of prepolymerized PMMA beads causing their incomplete fusion during setting MMA, commonly resulting from incomplete mixing
  - Evaporation of the volatile monomer due to the heat of reaction during setting causing imbalance in the powder and liquid component resulting in persistence of unmixed powder
  - Air bubble entrapment during transfer of the dough to the gun
  - Air entrapment within the medullary canal during cement pressurization.

When the critical size of the flaw is reached, there is stress concentration causing cement breaks. If critical flaw size is not reached then they act as path deviators while crack propagation. The critical flaw size determined from Griffith criterion for PMMA is 70 μm. If pores are smaller than the critical flaw size then cement fracture strength is not compromised this means that elimination of the macropores in cement (pore diameter > 1 mm) is essential rather than removing the micropores (pore diameter 0.01–1 mm). This is the rationale for vacuum mixing and centrifugation methods.

MIXING TECHNIQUES

Three techniques have been used for mixing of bone cement:

1. *Hand mixing "classical" in air:* Mixing of the liquid and powder components in an open bowl using spatula. Commonly, a speed of 1–2 Hz for a period of 2 minutes is used. This method induces porosity of 7%. Reducing the number of beats and time of beats reduces porosity to 5%. We now mix the two components and wait for 15–20 seconds for the liquid to get imbibed, then beat the mixture five to seven times to wet all the powder and leave it for 2 minutes, then check according to manufactures specification for working time.
2. *Hand mixing followed by centrifugation:* Here, the two components are mixed followed by centrifugation of mixture at a speed of 2,300–4,000 rpm for a duration of 0.5–3 minutes. This reduces porosity to 1% or less. For centrifugation, the cement should be sufficiently liquid and one method for better utilization of the maneuver is to prechill the cement.
3. *Hand mixing in an evacuated mixing device, commonly known as "vacuum mixing":* This method reduces the porosity to <1% and also reduces the exposure to MMA vapors that have been toxicologically proven to be harmful, if inhaled, swallowed, or absorbed through skin. Some studies have found that porosity is not always reduced while very high vacuum can produce cracks and other studies suggest that vacuum mixing merely changes the distribution of pores rather than eliminating them.

Generations of Cementing Techniques

First-generation Cementing Technique (Prior to 1976): Charnley's Original Technique

- Hand mixing of cement in bowls
- Minimal femoral canal preparation and the cancellous bone in the region of neck/trochanter and medullary was left in-situ
- Removing blood and debris from the canal by irrigation with saline and suctioning just prior to the digital application of cement
- Finger pressurization of the cement, no cement plug/restrictor
- The prosthesis was then inserted into the femoral canal, no centralizer used
- Prostheses with sharp corners made of cast metals (no superalloy prostheses).

Second-generation Cementing Technique (1976–1983)

- Meticulous remove all cancellous bone using curette exposing the solid endosteal surface
- Use of distal cement restrictor
- Preparation of femoral canal by femoral brush (no pulsatile lavage), packing the canal by peroxide soaked roller gauge and drying of the femoral canal
- Using a cement gun to introduce the cement in retrograde manner
- The prosthesis is positioned manually without any use of centralizers
- Stem with broad medial border and no sharp corners, frequently collared, made of superalloy metals.

Third-generation Cementing Techniques (Since 1983)

- Use of vacuum centrifugation for cement preparation to reduce porosity
- Pulsatile lavage irrigation of femoral canal and packing with adrenaline-soaked swabs
- Insertion of the cement in a retrograde fashion and cement pressurization using proximal pressurizers
- Adrenaline-soaked sponges for femoral canal
- Prosthesis is inserted using distal and proximal centralizers to ensure optimal position and even cement mantle.

Cartridge Mixing and Delivery

- The system uses a universal power mixer that quickly mixes and then injects nearly all types of bone cement
- The prominent advantage is that it reduces mixing times drastically for obvious reasons fewer steps are needed to load, mix, and transfer the cement
- During mixing of the cement, rotary handpiece of the vacuum mixer maintains consistency of rotation speed and hence allows uniform mixing. This results in consistent mix times and the built-in charcoal filter also reduces harmful fumes exposure to the operating personnel.

Cement mantle is graded according to the system of Barrack and Harris that comprises:

- *Grade A:* Complete filling of medullary canal—complete cement mantle on all views with cement at least 1 mm thick containing no voids, defects, or bubbles. Complete "white-out" of cement-bone interface—unable to distinguish cement from cortical bone in the diaphyseal region. Cement should extend 10 mm from the tip of prosthesis.
- *Grade B:* Mild radiolucency appreciable at the cement-bone interface.
- *Grade C:* Radiolucencies >50% of bone-cement interface or incomplete cement mantles.
- *Grade D:* Gross radiolucencies and/or failure of cement to surround tip of stem.

Optimal cementing technique and improved fixation is provided by:

- Limited cement porosity
- *Using microinterlock technique:* Inject cement after thoroughly cleaning the bone bed and lavage with brush and pulse lavage. Adequate pressurization of cement with cement gun to prevent blood from penetrating the cement
- *Cement mantle >2 mm:* There should be no mantle defect (cement mantle <2 mm at any place) else the chances of cement fracturing are high. Mantle defect is defined as any area where the prosthesis touches cortical bone with no cement between creating areas of stress concentration and increased loosening rates
- Stiff femoral stems (this is the reason why isoelastic stems failed; they put increased stress on cement mantle)
- Centralization of stem.

PHYSICAL PROPERTIES OF CEMENT

Compressive Strength

It is measured according to standards ISO 5833 and ASTM F451. The compressive strength for any material strength is defined as the maximum stress (force applied normally per unit area) a material can withstand before failure in compression. A minimum of 70 MPa is required as a standard for PMMA cement.

Bending Strength

It is measured by a four-point bending test standard of ISO 5833. The minimum requirement for the bending strength is 50 MPa and for the bending modulus, it is 1,800 MPa, respectively, which is achieved by all currently available commercial cements. The elastic modulus of bone cement should be between the prosthesis and the bone. According to Hooke's law, the material stress is directly proportional to the strain when tested within the elastic range. This simply means that the material will regain the original dimensions (show elastic behavior) when the stress is removed. The limit of elastic range is defined by "proportional limit" above which there is some or complete permanent deformation with the applied stress. Cement being a mechanical buffer, its elastic range is an important parameter. Elastic range changes with temperature (higher temperature reduces the modulus), additives to bone cement (antibiotics, radiopacifier, etc. reduce the modulus), still all the current cements meet the standards.

Tensile Strength

It is measured according to the standards ISO 527-1 or ASTM D638. Tensile strength is defined as the maximum stress that a material can withstand before failure in tension. 50–60 MPa is sufficient and is met by most manufacturers. It is not much influenced by additives.

Shear Strength

It is tested by standards ASTM D732. Stem cement interface is an important element identified as responsible for failure. Surface finish of implant has greatest impact on the interface strength. Increasing the roughness increases interface shear strength but also possibly increases the wear at interface due to micromotion. Currently, cement is being used as an interface for transmitting the forces to bone uniformly; hence, subsidence of implant and molding of cement is considered more important.

Fracture Toughness

It is measured by standards ASTM E399 and ISO 13,586: The fracture toughness reduces significantly with γ-irradiation, as it reduces the polymer molecular size. This is the reason why ethylene oxide is preferred for sterilization of cement.

Impact Strength

It measures the energy required to cause permanent damage by inducing fracture in the material when struck by a sudden blow. The impact strength of PMMA bone cement is reduced when radiopacifier and antibiotics are added to it.

In the ascending order of strength under various stresses, the compressive strength of bone cement is greater than the flexural strength, which is still greater than the tensile strength. This property is common to other polymers also. Because bending is a combination of compressive and tensile loading, so for material evaluation, bending test is considered most realistic for stress evaluation.

Fatigue Behavior

It is the ability of PMMA to withstand varying loads and truly determines, if cement will fail or not. Fatigue can be measured in three different ways:

1. Four-point bending arrangement recommended by ISO 5833 standard—similar to bending test measurement ISO 5833.
2. Uniaxial pure tensile test with flat tapered specimens according to ISO 527.
3. Uniaxial compression-tension test with cylindrical tapered specimens according to ASTM F2118.

Fatigue testing is done by sinusoidal cyclic loading of the material under stress control until failure or run-out. The effective test is simple four-point bending test performed under heated (to body temperature) Ringer's lactate solution. As mentioned, irradiation reduces fatigue strength as also the porosity of cement.

Water-uptake

Water absorption has a negative effect on the modulus of elasticity. More the water absorption, lower is the modulus of elasticity eventually resulting in a less stiff material. This reduced stiffness may be advantageous for fracture resistance and long-term stability of the implant. The water uptake of cements is 1–2% for plain cements (higher for antibiotic cements). Cements are completely water saturated at 4–8 weeks. Water absorption also influences the glass transition temperature, which is the transition from a hard and rigid glassy state with a high modulus to a soft rubbery state with a low modulus by heating the polymer (normally around 100°C for PMMA). Water absorption reduces the temperature by 20–30°C. Soft rubbery states are responsible for implant loosening and reduced stability of implant.

Cement Creep Behaviors

Poly (methyl methacrylate) exhibit combination of elastic and viscous behavior called viscoelasticity. There are two physical changes with the applied loads—one is the immediate elastic deformation with the applied load and the other is time dependent, continuous deformation. While the former is instantaneous and time independent, the latter is only partially recoverable. Elastic deformation resulting from stress can be divided into two parts—the primary creep (delayed elastic deformation) that follows application of initial stress and is recoverable. The second part of deformation is mostly permanent and nonrecoverable deformation called secondary creep. Creep is responsible for the subsidence of implant. The degree of creep is dependent on several factors, such as material composition, testing temperature, quantitative load and loading duration, and handling by the surgeon. The last is more important as delayed injection time of the cement increases creep. Practically for prosthesis, the creep is not very significant. The creep behavior is explained by two properties of cement polymer:

1. *Stress relaxation:* This is the change in stress (reducing) with time under constant strain (deformation). The stress relaxation is caused by a change in structure of polymerized cement. Temporal changes in stress are observed by reduction in stress at night that reduces load allowing stress relaxation.
2. *Hysteresis:* The loading and unloading curves for PMMA are not identical. Not all the energy applied to the specimen during loading is recovered on unloading, so some energy is lost/stored in the PMMA possibly responsible for the secondary creep.

ADVERSE EFFECTS/COMPLICATIONS OF BONE CEMENT

Bone Cement Implantation Syndrome

Cardiopulmonary complications associated with PMMA have been reported though rarely. Some mention them to be underreported and hence true incidence is unknown. The syndrome comprises by sudden onset of hypoxia, hypotension, or both that are commonly accompanied with unexpected loss of consciousness. The symptoms appear right at the time of cementation or during prosthesis insertion. Uncommonly, the symptoms appear at the time of performing reduction maneuver of the joint or at tourniquet deflation in a patient undergoing cemented knee arthroplasty. Classically, the observers have postulated that PMMA-associated hypoxia, hypotension, and death possibly result from the direct toxic effects of monomer or anaphylactic reaction. Monomer has been found to be metabolized in Kreb's cycle into carbon dioxide and water in human body. The focus has now shifted to embolization of marrow debris (due to increased intramedullary pressure) and neurogenic reflex (due to release of vasodilatory cannabinoids) following PMMA application thus adversely affecting cardiopulmonary function. Emboli have been demonstrated by various authors using transesophageal echocardiography ("snow flurries" appearance) making it a prominent contender. Pulmonary infarction and death have been reported as a result of embolization of PMMA that was injected in liquid state so cement should be applied only in the working phase.

There is also a significant possibility of hypersensitivity and anaphylactic reaction leading to the syndrome, as type-4 hypersensitivity has been shown in operating surgeons! Complement activation by monomer has been demonstrated that can cause bronchoconstriction and histamine release. Possibly combination of various mechanisms operate. Other acute complications of PMMA application include pulmonary hypertension, pulmonary edema, bronchoconstriction, cardiac dysrhythmia, cardiac arrest, hypothermia, and thrombocytopenia. The risk factors for development of bone cement implantation syndrome (BCIS) have been summarized below (not all have been authenticated and most are possibilities, nevertheless to be kept in mind).

Patient risk factors:

- Poor preexisting physical reserve [New York Heart Association (NYHA) class 3 or 4, Canadian Heart Association class 3 or 4]
- Compromised cardiopulmonary status
- Preexisting pulmonary hypertension
- Poor bone quality
- Presence of skeletal metastases
- Congenital cardiac anomalies such as patent foramen ovale or atrial septal defect (ASD).

Surgical risk factors:

- Although difficult to substantiate, some researchers believe that patients with a virgin femoral canal (no surgery done before) may be at higher risk of manifesting the syndrome
- Presence of pathological fracture
- Development of intertrochanteric fracture intraoperatively
- Using a long-stem prosthesis that pressurizes the cement over a long distance.

Factors that may help in ***prevention of the BCIS*** include (empirical):

- *Intramedullary lavage:* This removes the blood clot plugs from the sinusoids and let the PMMA penetrate and mix to vascular system.
- *Good homeostasis before cement insertion:* Stopping the blood flow by reducing pressure allows cement to occupy spaces that would otherwise have been prevented from its reach.
- *Minimizing length of prosthesis:* Reduces the length of cement mantle over which pressure is applied.
- *Using noncemented prosthesis:* Ideal, if one wants to avoid cement disease and is overly concerned.
- *Providing a vent for medullary pressure:* Quite popular among new surgeons, as it is considered that decompressing the medulla will also prevent fat embolism or at least reduce its chances of occurring.
- Cementing by gun reduces spillage and quick and proper canal fill.
- Retrograde insertion reduces marrow pressurization.
- Vacuum mixing of cement (possibly removes volatile monomer).

Treatment is mainly supportive and 100% O_2 should be continued in postoperative period and patient should be treated as for right-ventricular failure. Aggressive resuscitation helps and is recommended but monitoring should be done with central venous catheter that also guides inotropes [clinical experience is imperative as even central venous pressure (CVP) does not truly reflect pulmonary arterial pressure so resuscitation is decided more by experience]. Choice of inotropes is conflicting with some favoring pure α-adrenergic drugs while other favoring mixed α- and β-receptor agonist. I recommend noninvasive cardiac output monitoring or a pulmonary artery floatation catheter (if facilities exist and merits of patient) to decide between the two drugs.

Teratogenic Effects

Dose-related teratogenic and fetal toxic effects of methacrylic acid have been observed in rats inconsistently. Also, the concern of methacrylic acid vapors in the breast milk is unsettled and possibly overhyped.

Hypersensitivity Reactions

Hypersensitivity to PMMA may be behind a small number of joint replacement cases, which experience early loosening that cannot be explained by polyethylene wear. Allergy to PMMA or its constituents have been reported in dentistry, dermatology, and joint arthroplasty. Hypersensitivity is supported by finding of synovium-like membrane forms, which have the capacity to produce prostaglandin E2, collagenase, and other osteolytic products such as interleukin-1 and tumor necrosis factor. PMMA allergy is very unusual. Direct evidence for allergic reactions to BPO or DMPT has been reported. This delayed hypersensitivity may be produced by a hapten such as BPO that reacts to or conjugates with a body protein producing a neoantigen unrecognized by immune system and in turn generating a sensitivity response. Such body reaction produces symptoms such as insidious pain, systemic inflammatory response (SIRS), and most likely aseptic loosening in long run. This also explains possibly the "denture sore mouth" or the "burning mouth syndrome" sometimes observed in dentistry. After revision to uncemented components in joint arthroplasty, the patient's symptoms have been improved in such cases.

Less regarded complications of using bone cements include:

- Urological complications such as dysuria and formation of bladder fistula
- Neuropathy locally due to involvement of nerves
- Extruded/extravasated cement would cause frictional local vascular erosion, aneurysm formation, or thrombotic occlusion
- Sciatic nerve entrapment is a rare complication if attention is not paid to excessive bone cement extrusion posteriorly that engulfs the nerve then.

Cement Disease

This loose term (and possibly inaccurate) refers to the peri-implant disease that is now referred to as osteolysis. Cement disease pointed to shielding effect of cement and thinning of bone per se. The occurrence of cement disease is difficult to document. The term by itself is a misnomer and originated in past from observation of holes in the bone seen on radiographs that was otherwise unaccounted for so loosely termed "cement disease". The term cement disease originated due to ignorance of the surgeons of the cause of symptoms and weakening of bone. Obviously, the cement was the new foreign material introduced in the region, so it was labeled the culprit. To be precise, it is a conglomerate of periprosthetic infection, osteolysis (septic and aseptic), and cortical thinning (shielding effect or heat necrosis of bone). The name stuck, although it is now known that the cement is not the problem in every case. There are some specific conditions where cement may be a culprit by itself or circumstantially. Cement may act as an interface where bacteria may thrive prohibiting cure. Cement particles have been shown to accelerate the osteolysis induced by poly particles. Shielding is a problem in young active adults where using cemented implants is not universally accepted due to concerns of fatigue strength, longevity, shielding effect on bone, and ultimate loosening due to absence of incorporation of implant. Improved composite cements are being searched for solving this problem at least partially.

IMPROVING CEMENT CHARACTERISTICS

Various substances can be added in cement to improve the properties of cement and interface characteristics producing composite materials (composite cements). The following are some of feature enhancements being sought for:

Fatigue Strength

Poly(methyl methacrylate)-based bone cement has a high modulus but low toughness compared with ductile polymers. Fracture toughness and fatigue strength are improved by fiber reinforcement and incorporation of a low-volume fraction of chopped fibers of approximately 1–2%. The choice of fibers currently includes:

- Carbon fibers as multiwalled carbon nanotubes
- Glass fibers
- Kevlar (used in F1 racing car's petrol tanks)
- Oriented PMMA
- Rubber impregnated PMMA
- Ultrahigh molecular weight polyethylene
- Polyethylene terephthalate
- Aramid
- Graphite
- Nano-sized titanium fibers
- Embedded continuous stainless steel coils
- Zirconia fibers with and without acrylic coating.

The biggest concern for use of any synthetic fiber in the manufacture/integration into PMMA bone cement is biocompatibility, the other is the complication involved in processing that restricting their incorporation.

Integration of Cement and Improving Interface Characteristics

There is a developing interest in manufacturing calcium phosphate bone cements that can integrate in the bone so improving the cement bone interface. However, they have been introduced with rather unsuccessful results due to increased cement viscosity, poor handling, and reduced mechanical performance (no/minimal load bearing capacity so virtually useless). Newer system consists of mixing the 40% w/w calcium phosphate (brushite) into two-solution pseudoplastic system (non-Newtonian material where the viscosity decreases as the shear rate increases) to yield highly viscous, injectable, and bioactive cement with high compressive strength and has shown encouraging results in vitro. Osteoconduction can also be improved by addition of bioactive ceramics. Nearly 60% by weight of ceramic powder needs to be added to PMMA for "Osteoconduction". Also, there is renewed interest in improving the metal–cement interface integrity. Addition of amphiphilic bonder such as glutaraldehyde improves the longevity of cemented metal stems.

Reducing Heat Generation

Heat generation could be responsible for bone necrosis and subsequent cortical thinning contributing to implant loosening. The exothermic reaction is enhanced in the presence of oxygen plasma increasing the peak temperatures. Some agents that have been found to reduce the peak temperatures include:

- 1-dodecyl mercaptan is a chain-stopping agent (lowers peak temperatures by 4–6°C, no clinical significance however)
- Endothermic simultaneous reaction using ammonium nitrate (reduce temperature by approximately 20°C)
- Zeolites in the presence of 1-dodecyl mercaptan or ammonium nitrate further reduce maximal temperatures.
- N-acetylcysteine (1% w/w) significantly reduces the maximum polymerization temperatures.

Opacifying Agents

Zirconium oxide has been found unfavorable in view of increased wear characteristics seen and also adversely influences the mechanical strength. Barium sulfate has been shown to reduce the osteoblast function at cement–bone interface and may affect osteolysis. Higher concentrations reduce mechanical strength and also higher incidence of foreign body reactions with increased barium sulfate concentrations.

- Iodine-containing acrylic bone cement is most similar to the barium sulfate cements in terms of biocompatibility. Also, iodine by itself is radiopaque.
- Nanoceramics such as magnesium oxide improve osteoblast adhesion and also reduce the maximum heat of polymerization. Nanobarium sulfate also improves osteoblast adhesion.
- Organobismuth compound has shown higher opacification at similar concentrations compared to barium sulfate-containing cements and also improved injectability.
- Gadolinium has also been tried for signal-inducing bone cement for magnetic resonance imaging.

Improving Biocompatibility

Free radical polymerization is the essence of PMMA formation. Adding vitamin-E [mixed vitamin E (MVE)] additive (1 part liquid MVE: 1.8 part solid cement) increases cytocompatibility of the cement. This mixture, however, has reduced tensile strength (same compressive strength). 10% vitamin E additive cement reduces the maximal heat of polymerization and also acts as a free radical scavenger while having minimal effect on tensile strength.

Nanoparticle Additives

- Nanoparticles addition in the form of nanotubes and fibers has been tried to improve the tensile strength of cement (see earlier).
- Antibacterial properties of chitosan and quaternary ammonium-derived chitosan nanoparticles have shown encouraging results against *Staphylococcus aureus* and *Staphylococcus epidermidis* with no significant cytotoxicity and pave way for further improvements.
- Silver ions and silver benzoate have been blended to PMMA for inhibiting bacterial enzymes and DNA replication (against *Acinetobacter baumannii, Pseudomonas aeruginosa, Proteus mirabilis,* and *S. aureus*) showing promising results, but the problem is of reduced compression strength. Nanosilver-added cement shows complete inhibition of the methicillin-resistant *Staphylococcus aureus* (MRSA) and methicillin-resistant *Staphylococcus epidermidis* (MRSE) growth.
- The polymer methyl methacrylate-acrylic acid-allyl methacrylate (MMA-AA-AMA) developed in Japan has reduced cement shrinkage problems especially improving the bone-cement interface. This polymer also has improved fracture toughness. The 80:20:10 composition has shown best improvements.

REMOVAL OF BONE CEMENT

This is an essential step in revision arthroplasties unless a cement-in-cement revision has been planned. Only few practical tips are included here and reader is encouraged to refer dedicated text on revision arthroplasty for details.

- The cement should be removed piecemeal from the proximal femur to ensure that bone is not lost during the process and cortex does not get violated.
- Care should be taken particularly while removing bone cement from distal diaphyseal portion of the femur where perforations are likely to occur. If perforations are seen while removing cement from proximal femur region itself then it is best to convert exposure to an "extended trochanteric osteotomy" and directly visualize the bone-cement interface.
- The best method to remove a well-fixed cement plug is by using ultrasonic cement-removing instrumentation.
- Whenever possible, it is better to avoid making small windows for removing distal diaphyseal cement.
- For well-fixed cements and to ease removal, one of the newer systems should be used (provided one has requisite training in its use):
    - Ballistically driven chiselling system
    - Water jet
    - High-energy shock waves
    - *Ultrasonic device:* This is based on change to putty-like consistency of the cement following contact with the ultrasonic waveguide (probe) as the cement absorbs the energy. Bone does not absorb energy as efficiently so is comparatively spared. This technique is, however, prone to superficial bone burns and bone perforations. Pathological fractures and radial nerve palsy have been reported from its use in humerus
    - ROBODOC® system for cement removal may also be used.

CONCLUSION

- Bone cement is a special tool in orthopedic practice that has been in use for a long period.
- The bone cement is put to two main uses commonly—fixation of arthroplasty components and vehicle for antibiotic delivery in management of dead space. The cement is also used for management of vertebral compression fractures (vertebroplasty/kyphoplasty).
- Typical bone cement is provided in two components—the powder phase and the liquid phase—that need to be mixed together in the form of a paste for further use depending on the variable setting characteristics.
- One must be vigilant of the bone-cement implantation syndrome that might occur occasionally and its requisite management.

CHAPTER 16

Regenerative Medicine and Stem Cell Research in Orthopedics

Manish Kumar Varshney

INTRODUCTION

"Regenerative medicine"—as literary constructed by Leland Kaiser in 1992—describes "a new branch of medicine will develop that attempts to change the course of chronic diseases and in many instances, will regenerate tired and failing organ systems". Musculoskeletal problems surmount significant morbidity and reduce the working population that is further escalated by increasing life expectancy and prevailing elderly population, which frequently suffer from them. Some countries have "super-aging society" producing orthopedic disorder endemic regions. Regeneration of degenerating components of musculoskeletal system, viz., bones, muscles, nerves, and joints is expected to benefit such societies and overall human population. This massive potential of regenerative medicine for aiding mankind has been promptly and recently acknowledged by civilization in the form of outstanding distinctions honored as Nobel Prize in Faculty of Medicine and Physiology awarded to John Gurdon and Shinya Yamanaka in 2012. With the reporting of early promising results in international research on regenerative medicine and stem cells for discrete diseases, expectations aroused in society immensely. The interest in orthopedics toward regenerative medicine pertains to those diseases/conditions, which cannot be adequately or satisfactorily addressed by the current treatment methods. These are mostly conditions arising out of degeneration in tissues and associated with wear and tear where treatment modalities meagerly if at all alter the course of disease, sometimes to the extent that patients lose their mobility and autonomy costing dearly to the healthcare systems throughout the world. Specifically, atrophic tendon ruptures, cartilage damage and arthritis, bone defects, and some spinal cord damages have been the main focus of regenerative medicine in orthopedics. The use of stem cells has developed under much expectation and even controversy worldwide, particularly there where human embryonic stem cells (hESCs) are concerned. It is the use of hESCs that has sparked the most controversy calling for strict legislative control and regulations; this, however, will not be the focus of following scientific relevant description.

STEM CELLS

Stem cells are unique undifferentiated cells of a multicellular organism, which are capable of giving rise to indefinitely (theoretically at least) more cells of the same type (self-renewal), and from which certain other kinds of cell arise by differentiation in specific physiological or research controlled conditions. The body is made up of about 200 different kinds of specialized cells, including myocytes, neural cells, adipocytes, etc., all of which are derived from stem cells through differentiation. Stem cells are uniquely different from other cell types, as they possess three distinctive characteristics:

1. *Nonspecialization:* These cells have no tissue-specific structure or function that they would perform in human body. They are "bland" in this sense that they do not produce routine physiological functions such as helping mobility, conducting impulses, and circulating blood, but have one most important function—of replenishing the lost cells in a particular tissue over time (function of tissue-specific stem cell, see below). This repair characteristic is one of the most important distinctions that differentiate living from nonliving.
2. *Self-renewal and theoretical unlimited proliferation:* Stem cells are capable of dividing and renewing themselves for long periods without losing their basic identity and without differentiating. This property is most prominent for embryonic stem cells (ESCs); they can proliferate undifferentiated for months and even to some years; however, the adult stem cells tend to lose their identity (undergo differentiation) and capability of unlimited self-renewal.
3. *Ability to differentiate:* Stem cells can produce specialized cells under specific circumstances (chemokine or physical influence through contact from neighboring cells or microenvironment). Adult stem cells can usually differentiate into cells specific to the tissue in which they reside while ESCs can produce virtually all different cell lines found in the human body. Adult stem cells or tissue stem cells, as they are also called, are however also versatile and show *plasticity* in a sense that experimentally even they have been induced to give rise to cells of completely different tissue.

Types of Stem Cells

1. *Embryonic stem cells:* These are the cells derived from developing embryo during very early stage of its development. James Thompson described the ESCs in 1988. The ESCs are taken usually from the inner cell mass (ICM) of a developing blastocyst [a preimplantation stage of embryo development that consists of a mostly hollow ball (blastocoel) lined by trophoblast (destined to form the placenta later) and an "inner cell mass" of approximately 150–200 cells (source of ESCs)]. Harvesting is done usually on the 5th days of fetal life. These cells have all the properties of stem cells detailed above such as self-renewal and *pluripotency* (can form all cell types found in the body). There is another term called *totipotency*, which implies ability to generate viable embryo including the supporting structures such as placenta and is a higher character than pluripotency. This is mainly a theoretical concept and has not been reproduced in vitro (as none of the studied cell lines has ever produced a viable embryo); however, it has been postulated as a theory for production of twins in vivo. The character of totipotency is seen in cells that form in a fertilized egg within first few divisions (8–16-celled stage), where a cell would be capable of giving rise to another embryo itself. Within few days by the stage of blastocyst, the character is lost and the cells degrade to the level of pluripotency. It is not easy to label the obtained cells from ICM of a blastocyst to "embryonal stem cells", rather this is a tedious process. The human ICM cells are cultured in specialized systems onto feeder layer of mouse embryonal cells on culture dish that forms the "sticky surface" over which the human embryonal cells can attach. When the human embryonal cells proliferate, they are carefully removed and recultured on separate dish into subculture systems. The process of subculture is repeated and is called "passage", only after nearly 6 months of subcultures and passage of 30 cell lines, if the cells retain their undifferentiated characteristics and pluripotency are they termed "ESC line". Fundamental tests are also run on these cell lines to identify the desired characteristics. The first is the maintained potency for self-renewal and maintaining undifferentiated characteristic. Surface markers such as Oct-4 (octamer-binding transcription factor 4) protein are synthesized by these undifferentiated cells that can be mapped. Oct-4 switches off on cell differentiation process. Other tests include injecting the cells in immunocompromised mouse forming teratomas (justifying the capability of these cells to differentiate into multiple cell lines—pluripotency), chromosomal examination and assessing capability of subculturing cells after freezing, thawing, and replating. Why this versatile cell line has remained far from essentially successful is interesting? There are two reasons for it—firstly, the cells can differentiate into every single cell lineage known so controlling their growth is extremely difficult, as all biological processes into cell differentiation are currently unknown. Secondly, the ESCs have huge oncogenic potential among other many logistic limitations currently forbidding their use in patients.
2. *Somatic stem cells or tissue-specific stem cells or adult stem cells:* These are somewhat specialized (included in the "stretched" definition of stem cell); and in specific situations, give rise to some of all of the mature cell types particular to the tissue they are present in. Though these are found in specific organs, they appear "undifferentiated" when compared to the mature cells of that organ. These cells are *multipotent* in the sense that they have the ability to generate multiple, organ-specific cell lines (just for information purpose, *unipotent cells* are the stable mature forms that can replicate into self-type and not differentiate or de-differentiate). Mesenchymal stem cells (MSCs) (bone marrow stromal cells), for example, have the ability to produce bone, cartilage, fat, periosteum, tendon structure, fibrous connective tissue, etc. The primary role of somatic stem cells is to maintain and repair the tissue in which they are found. These stem cells are found in nearly all tissues but are very few in number and located in remote deep-seated places of the tissue often difficult to access, isolate, and grow in laboratory. The most important and common sites for obtaining the somatic stem cells are the umbilical cord of newborn and bone marrow of an adult. Somatic stem cells are different from ESCs in their comparative limited ability to self-renewal on culture systems and higher chances of unwanted differentiation when subcultured. Also, these cells have differentiation capability usually limited to tissue-specific mature cells; however, this limitation can be circumvented by various scientific alterations from which the somatic stem cells start behaving like pluripotent stem cells. Two such alterations are viable as follows:
   a. Induced pluripotent stem (iPS) cells are stem cells made directly from a body cell (a somatic cell) not a somatic stem cell notably. Somatic cells are all the cell types of the human body apart from sperm or egg. Yamanaka et al. discovered induced pluripotent stem cells (iPSCs) and were given Nobel Prize for this in 2012. Takahashi and Yamanaka in 2006 first demonstrated successful dedifferentiation of somatic cells into a pluripotent ESC-like status by transfection with four embryonic transcription factors. These iPSC can differentiate into any type of cell under influence of four reprogramming factors (mostly *oncogenes!*)—*c-Myc*, *Klf4*, *Oct3/4*, and *Sox2*. Skin cells are most commonly used to derive iPS. The iPSC have features very similar to ESCs. An advantage of the iPSC is their ability to make patient-specific cells that can be used for research or clinical translation to treat/prevent disease. Another advantage is immune tolerance, as the cells have the same "self"-markers as the donor nucleus potentially eliminating tissue rejection. The issue is not as simple for clinical application and there are immense safety concerns raised to this calling for strict legislative regulations. Like ESC, these also have huge oncogenic potentially for obviously the inducing transcription factors are themselves oncogenes. Also, the differentiation potential varies widely and mostly does not linearly produce a single cell line (say cartilage or bone) as is

desired and rather teratomas are common! We will not be discussing iPSC any further.

b. *Somatic cell nuclear transfer (SCNT) (therapeutic cloning) stem cells:* This is a reverse strategy for iPSC. The SCNT pluripotent cells are produced by inserting a somatic cell nucleus into an enucleated egg. This synthesis is then stimulated for dividing and developing an embryo. The embryo is harvested in a way similar for obtaining the embryonal stem cells as detailed above. These SCNT stem cells thus resemble ESCs but have the added advantage (similar to the iPSC) that they also have "self" markers as the donor nucleus provides immune tolerance. It seems intriguing and promising; however, technique of producing SCNT stem cells has been successful only in mice and nonhuman primates (monkeys), but it has not yet worked using human cells alas.

The above methodologies are interesting and intriguing; however, for orthopedic relevance, none of them has been *clinically translated* and the use of term "stem cell" per se only pertains to age-old use of bone marrow stromal cells derived from bone marrow aspirate. Literature is quite rich with the use of bone marrow aspirate; however, dedicated comparative and randomized controlled trials (RCTs) are missing; mostly the success and failure have been debated by the proponents based on the case series and their weak outcomes. The most studied and advanced research is available for MSCs and endothelial progenitor cell (EPC), which will be the focus of description; nevertheless, various in vitro researches using iPSC are on and will be incorporated in the discussion below.

Source Cells and Carrier Systems

Endothelial progenitor cell and MSCs are the most commonly used cell types for regenerative medicine in orthopedics. MSCs are the most important in orthopedics, as they have distinctive ability to differentiate into chondrogenic (cartilage formation), osteogenic (bone formation), neurogenic (limited, neuron-like cell formation), myogenic (limited, muscle formation), tendogenic (limited, tendon/ligament formation), and adipogenic (adipose tissue) cell lines. Also, MSCs have low immunoreactivity and high-immunosuppressive properties. MSCs are distinguished by presence of surface markers—CD73, CD90, and CD105 are positive and CD34 and CD45 are negative. Interestingly, the MSCs also can home the injured site by adhesion molecules that help them to direct the target site and proliferate there. The other desirable property is secretion of paracrine factors [insulin-like growth factor 1 (IGF-1), hepatocyte growth factor (HGF), vascular endothelial growth factor (VEGF), IGF-2, and basic fibroblast growth factor (bFGF)] that stimulate host stem cells and possible stimulation of regenerative tissue formation by secretion of exosomes (bilipid membrane vesicles) containing messenger ribonucleic acid (mRNA) and miRNA (micro-RNA). The MSCs not only differentiate into tissue-specific cell lines (cartilage, bone, fat, fibroblast, etc.) replacing the lost cells but also modulate inflammatory process. They have proven to be anti-inflammatory like inhibiting maturation of helper T, cytotoxic T, dendritic, and B-cells and having immunosuppressive properties by secretion of transforming growth factor beta-1 (TGF-β1), NO, prostaglandin-E2, human leukocyte antigen G (HLA-G), HGF, and interleukin 10 (IL-10). The paracrine factors also protect the host cell and facilitate angiogenesis/vasculogenesis, and have been found to enhance lung function in acute respiratory distress syndrome (ARDS) by regulating endothelial and epithelial permeability, reducing inflammation, and inhibiting bacterial growth. This response has invigorated some authors to use the term "injury drug store" for the MSCs.

MSCs can be derived from a number of sources but optimization is lacking and we are in process of identifying the best source for them. The commonly used/ studied sources of stem cells for orthopedic research use are:

- *Bone marrow-derived mesenchymal stem cells (BM-MSCs):* MSCs from the bone marrow were originally described by Friedenstein et al. This has been the most popular source of stem cells, although the yield is small and the procedure is painful. For a long time, BM-MSCs have been used as plain aspirate from iliac crest or greater trochanter for treating nonunions/delayed unions. The cells behave as multipotent cells capable of differentiating into trabecular bone, articular cartilage, ligament, and tendon. Their popularity and utility are, however, been contested now.
- *Bone marrow concentrate:* This is just a centrifuge of bone marrow aspirate from iliac crest containing a higher percentage of BM-MSCs. It has been used particularly for cartilage regeneration in chondral defects.
- *Adipose-derived stem cells (AD-MSCs):* These are recently the emerging popularity group due to their higher reliability and easy harvest (so all the flab is not bad!). AD-MSCs can be easily harvested in good numbers through lipoaspiration and they can resist serum-deprivation-induced apoptosis well.
- *Cortical bone fraction mesenchymal stem cells (CBF-MSCs):* It has been now demonstrated beyond doubt that the matrix dense cortical bone is the more potent compartment of bone than bone marrow as a stromal source for MSCs. Although bone marrow can produce a subset of clonogenic and multilineage cells, they are outnumbered and outperformed by an equivalent harvest of CBF-MSCs. Lineage-depleted CBF-MSCs have shown greater than 150-time enrichment of colony-forming unit-fibroblasts (CFU-F) per cell incidence compared to bone marrow-derived MSCs. They would probably oust the popularity of BM-MSCs for orthopedic research and regenerative medicine. Also, it has been shown that CBF-MSCs retain a greater biosynthetic activity in vitro that has been found increased in hypoxic conditions.
- *Synovial tissue-derived mesenchymal stem cells (ST-MSCs):* The stem cells are scarce, as their availability is limited and has been used for potential regeneration of cartilage.
- *Peripheral blood-derived mesenchymal stem cells (PB-MSCs):* The stem cells are obtained by automated cell separator from peripheral blood. The stem cells have also been used for cartilage regeneration.
- Amnion, tendon, and skin have been also studied as source of stem cells but the usage is limited to specific research.

Development of Carrier System (Also See the Chapter on "Electrospinning, Three-dimensional Printing and Its Application in Orthopedics")

The most pertinent practical problem after homing and proliferation of stem cell is the development of vascularity of the repair region for sustenance. This is a function of patent blood vessels that should carry nutrients and oxygen to the region. As opposed to *angiogenesis* (migration and proliferation of differentiated endothelial cells), which has been commonly considered to be responsible for giving vascularity to a repair region, it is the process of *vasculogenesis* (angioblast-induced vascularization) that produces neovascularization. To affect vasculogenesis, EPC performs the major role. EPC-based cell therapy for ischemic disease (as for myocardial disease) has been promising and could be applied for persistent proliferation of MSC-developed tissue, so the continuous supply of nutrients could be maintained by newer vessels being formed in the region. Such EPCs are obtained from CD34+ and CD133+ hematopoietic stem cells (HSCs) and the hemangioblasts. These cells facilitate tissue repair and regeneration by accelerating neovascularization.

For tissue regeneration, some *scaffolds* are used for three-dimensional proliferation and directional tissue formation. These scaffolds include collagen gels such as type I collagen gel extracted from bovine skin (Atelocollagen®) that has been tried for articular cartilage, muscle, and nerve repair. This gel has also been used for gene silencing by in vivo delivery of embedded small-interfering RNA (siRNA) (*see* Chapter on "Gene Therapy in Orthopedics") or miRNA. Other naturally derived substances such as fibrin, agarose, alginate, gelatin, silk, or hyaluronic acid have also been used but less favored. Synthetic polymers such as polyglycolides or polylactides are quick to produce and have gained lots of interest; however, they suffer from two main problems—one is having unpredictable degradation and the other is lacking bioactivity. Degradation can be controlled by employing hydroxyl acid copolymers, while bioactivity can be imparted by coating or copolymerizing with bioactive materials or functional groups. The other scaffold system in use is hydroxyapatite ceramic that can be modified into interconnecting pores of at least 100-µm diameter (100–400 µm is ideal) for quick early osteoconduction. Substrate materials that have now gone out-of-favor include calcium phosphate, calcium carbonate, and glasses.

PERFORMING REGENERATIVE MEDICINE

It is important to understand how stem cell reaches its target organ/tissue. There are two main strategies used to address this problem. One is to apply the cells directly to the target organ or blood while other one is a bit complex where tissue is engineered using the cell and scaffold created to recreate tissue, the former is called *cell therapy* while the latter is termed *tissue engineering*. Cell therapy had been in use for decades in the faculty of hematology—bone marrow transplantation where the injected HSCs home into the marrow of the recipient. This can be autogenic where patient's own stem cells banked previously can be used for treatment or allogeneic from a donor. Allogeneic stem cell therapy is possible where tissue types match and this is gaining popularity as the HLA matching is not that strict with stem cells—only four of the six HLA class 1 and 2 loci need to be matched. This is further made important as in individual cases having successful cell therapy from relatives with strict HLA-matching requirements is possible in only 30% cases, while widespread use of stem cell banking would make it much more viable. Thus, there arises the need of stem cell banking. The success has been improved further by the double unit cord blood stem cell therapy.

Limited success has also been obtained in patients with myocardial infarction, hepatic intoxication, nephropathy, and lung injury due to irradiation. Beneficial effects of injected mesenchymal cells have been found in patients with osteogenesis imperfecta. Tissue engineering is useful in patients with requirements of replacement of large parts of tissue or organs. Despite advances in tissue engineering and development of three-dimensional scaffolds with synthesis of organ components, the technique is barely available for clinical use primarily for the limitation of the vascularization of the synthesized tissue components—these remain avascular ever. Thus, the technique could be more useful at this moment for tissues not immensely dependent of vascularity like the cartilage or tendons. Typically constructs >400 µm in diameter fare poorly due to limit of critical nutrient diffusion beyond this length. Hollow organs such as trachea and bladder with limited wall diameter thus have been successful by tissue engineering technique.

SPECIFIC ORTHOPEDIC APPLICATIONS

Cartilage Synthesis and Regeneration (*See* also Section on "Joint: Structure, Function, and Related Disorders")

Various standard techniques and advanced methods of articular cartilage reconstruction have been discussed in Chapter on "Articular Cartilage: Structure, Function, Injury, and Management". Most of these techniques are limited by the quality of tissue formed, which is often fragile and nonhyaline cartilage. Techniques that rely on recruitment of subchondral MSCs (drilling and microfracture) still produce lot of fibrocartilage, which is not optimal. Autologous chondrocyte implantation (ACI) and collagen-covered ACI (CACI) have been promising but are restricted by size of defect that can be treated and sometimes cartilage hypertrophy and nongeneration, etc. MACI (autologous cultured chondrocytes on porcine collagen membrane) needs optimization of the extracellular matrix, so that the cells form hyaline cartilage, as the regenerating cells are extremely sensitive to matrix properties for differentiation. Newer techniques of using MSCs in natural matrices hence demand exacting engineering to provide optimal milieu (mechanical stability) for ideal differentiation of the implanted cells into hyaline cartilage. This mechanical stability (protecting from axial and shear stress) imparts important cell-matrix interactions (enough porosity to allow nutrient diffusion while maintaining adequate adhesion), so that functional tissue growth can happen. MSC-based constructs use (as described by various authors) poly(vinyl alcohol)/polycaprolactone (PVA/PCL) nanofibers or alginate or collagen gel/powder covered with periosteum or hyaluronic acid membrane, while free injection of MSCs has also been done. Various studies performed utilizing different combinations claim variable success in obtaining hyaline cartilage. Some of the methods include combining BM-MSCs with Transwell permeable membrane (Murdoch et al.), BM-MSCs with connective tissue growth factor (Zhu et al.), BM-MSCs with TGF-β (Guo et al.), etc. Free injection of MSCs into the knee joint (Vangsness et al.) has been studied in an RCT of partially menisectomized patients that showed improved results, but cellular contents were not specified. None of the techniques has, however, showed complete defect coverage with hyaline cartilage in clinical studies despite producing it in vitro. Further optimization of the techniques in terms of application, cell preparation, and importantly carrier matrix needs to be established before a definite human use can be recommended.

Nonunions and Delayed Unions

This is a common problem in orthopedics, as nearly 5–7% of fractures go into delayed or atrophic nonunion. Treatments have relied on autogenous bone grafting as standard practice with revised fixation as necessary. Bone marrow was used as a means of improving chances of union in such cases by Connolly et al. in 1978, who reported good results in patients with tibial nonunions. MSCs have been used by Libergall et al. [MSC + PRP (platelet-rich plasma) + DBM (demineralized bone matrix)] and Giannotti et al. (iliac crest MSC with induction to osteogenic differentiation in culture). The studies showed good bone formation in the treated patients but as a technical challenge, critics put forward the challenge to prove that the regenerated bone comes from implanted cells. Hernigou et al. demonstrated correlation between callus volume and number of progenitor cells used, thus, quality of bone marrow aspirate would also have bearing when using alone. It has also been shown in animal studies that combining the BM-MSCs with BMP-1-3 increases synthesis of type-1 collagen and osteocalcin at the nonunion sites.

Management of Bone Defects

Bone defects can arise following loss of bone in open injuries and excision of bone for treatment of bone tumors/lesions. Masquelet technique is favored by and large for management of bone defects as is Ilizarov apparatus, the former relying mostly on MSCs in the second stage. It has been postulated that supplementation of bone graft with MSCs may help in enhancing the healing potential of the cancellous bone.

Tendon and Ligament Repair

Various scaffolds such as collagen gel, fibrin gel, 3D solid scaffolds, etc. have been used to reproduce the tendon structure. The scaffolds provide matrix for even distribution of the MSCs that can then be used at repair sites typically the tendon bone interfaces and also be injected into bone tunnels. These techniques currently are meant for improving the tendon to bone healing and not suitable for tendon only reformation. The problem with gel constructs is the issue of stability, as most of these tend to wear away quickly over time. Gulotta et al. have studied such constructs over rotator cuff repair and interestingly have reported good success when used with embryonic transcription factor MT1-MMP and tendon transcription factor scleraxis. Studies have been done to determine the tendon-regenerating capabilities of these techniques but the strength of regenerated tendon has been found to be much low (25% of normal) and complications such as formation of intratendinous bone have been reported in study on reconstructing animal patellar tendon by collagen gel-based MSC composite. Ideal carrier is unknown and inhomogeneous results restrict its clinical translation. For ligament repair, anterior cruciate ligament (ACL) has been the primary contender, as it is commonly injured and has significant morbidity, if not reconstructed. Studies have been done in animals where partially transected ACL showed good recovery and healing in the knees injected with MSCs as compared to controls. Blood supply to ACL is lost in injury reducing the healing potential. This blood supply can be restored in knees possibly by inducing miR-210 in the endothelial cells. Injection of miR-210 mimic has been postulated to improve the biomechanical properties of transected ACL. Repair of Achilles tendon has been attempted with the use of BM-MSCs showing some nonstandardized support to its use. Similar results have also been found in repair of medial collateral ligament of the knee.

Osteonecrosis

For management of osteonecrosis, decompression of a structurally maintained femoral head has been commonly practiced and advised, but the results are often variable with decompression alone and it is difficult to arrest collapse. Often the "forage" is combined with fibular grafting or cancellous grafting depending on the experience of surgeon. Hernigou et al. produced the largest case series of autologous bone marrow concentrate in 2002 and 2009 suggesting that results are very good in early stages and the progenitor cells home well in the transplanted bone. The relation is also proportional to the number of progenitor cells with higher the number of cells higher is the chance of cellular homing. The clinical improvement is in terms of reduced pain and slower progression of the disease.

Spinal Fusion

Surgeries for spinal fusion surely fail, if no fusion occurs or is poor. Bone grafts are a routine for obtaining fusion, however, often along hydroxyapatite-collagen type-1 composite with autologous marrow is tried. If the patient or surgeon is worried of morbidity of autologous bone grafts then bone graft substitutes (say tricalcium phosphate or composites like above) are the best choice for which one would rather tend to combine bone marrow aspirate as source of MSCs with the bone graft substitute. These methods are not, however, systematically studied in large studies and application is based more on the plausible noninferiority to autologous bone graft.

Treating Bone Cysts and Bone Defects

Curettage and bone grafting are the usual gold standard for managing bone cysts especially aneurysmal bone cysts and nonresponding unicameral bone cysts. The patients sometimes need volume of grafts that cannot be supplied by autologous bone; hence, bone graft substitutes are commonly tried. Principally just injecting the bone marrow aspirate into the cavity is not sufficient and yields poor results. Often the aspirate has to be combined to some form of bone either demineralized bone matrix or bone powder to stimulate bone formation in the curetted cavity. For management of traumatic or postsurgical bone defects, it has been found that application of expanded MSCs from marrow on a hydroxyapatite scaffold produces good bone. Combining MSCs with xenografts has also been tried but results have not been compared to autologous grafts in a systemic manner.

Osteogenesis Imperfecta (*See* Disease Description in Chapter on "Congenital, Genetic, Syndromic, and Miscellaneous Disorders")

Stem cell therapy is currently being investigated for dominant negative mutations (a negative dominant mutation occurs when the phenotype determined by the mutant allele predominates over the normal allele). In this approach, normal cells from a normal individual are used to replace the mutant cells of an individual with OI, the object being that enough normal cells will synthesize sufficient normal matrix to have positive effect on tissue function. Bone marrow contains cells with the potential to differentiate into osteoblasts; these stem cells are isolated and then transplanted into the affected individual. Isolated osteoblasts synthesize several proteins localized to bone, including type I collagen, alkaline phosphatase, and osteocalcin. In addition, cultured osteoblasts are capable of mineralizing the extracellular matrix. In order to stem cell therapy to be effective, the most effective and important step is to isolate stem cells with potential to differentiate toward osteoblast lineage that leads to better cell targeting and engraftment.

The fragility of bones in the disease had been considered to be nonmodifiable till the report of improved growth characteristics and improvement in symptoms by the work of Horwitz et al. allogeneic bone marrow transplantation as a source of MSCs improved the bone mass and reduced the incidence of fractures in treated patients. Similar results were reported by Gotherstrom with the use of MSCs harvested from liver and expanded in situ with trilineage differentiation capability CD29+, CD44+, CD73+, CD105+, CD166+, and HLA class I+ but negative for HLA class II antigens, CD14, CD31, CD34, and CD45. There was definite engraftment of the cells as demonstrated at 9 months.

Osteoarthritis

There is a lot of variability in outcome and deemed benefit of use of MSCs in osteoarthritis typically for pain relief or functional improvement. As of date, treatment is symptomatic and ultimately banks on knee arthroplasty for symptomatic relief and functional gain. Wakitani first reported the clinically better results obtained from MSCs injected in osteoarthritic knees and evaluated by arthroscopy/histology. Symptomatic relief at 12 months was obtained in patients with bone marrow-derived MSCs injection directly into the knee that were CD90 and CD166 positive, while negative for CD34, CD45, and HLA-DR as studied by Orozco et al. magnetic resonance imaging (MRI) studies also demonstrated improved cartilage in 11 of the 12 patients; however, the change varied between patients. Wong et al. studied the same in patients treated with additional HTO (high-tibial osteotomy) and microfracture technique but the improvement in this case is difficult to ascribe to MSCs only.

Muscle

Muscle once damaged is only replaced by fibrous tissue. CD133+ MSCs have potential for muscle regeneration in animal models and also possibly hold true for human muscle but the limitation is obtaining such CD133+ cells that are very less in number. Similarly, *miR-1*, *miR-133*, and *miR-206* have been suggested as potent regulators of muscle development and homeostasis locally injecting the same in injured muscle would improve muscle regeneration morphologically and functionally.

Nerves and Spinal Cord Injury

Nerve regeneration has been postulated to improve with the increasing probability of Schwann cell culture and proliferation in situ, but there are a lot of technical hurdles in their application. As a deviation, use of CD133+ cells has been proposed and in rabbits with damaged sciatic nerve, the application of these cells in a closed tube produced promising results, though definite clinical advantage is not proven still. The major limitation is paucity of CD133+ cells in peripheral blood that can be obtained. Intravenously injected CD133+ cells improved angiogenesis and axonal regeneration in spinal cord injury that can be further improved by intrathecal administration and localization using mechanical devices such as magnetic field. One study has demonstrated increased efficacy of BM-MSCs transplanted into rats with spinal cord injury when used in conjunction with propofol.

Miscellaneous

Use of bone marrow-derived MSCs has been described for HTO, femoral, and tibial-lengthening procedures using ilizarov or other distraction systems. Most of these studies have been in combination techniques using bone grafts or platelet-rich plasma.

STEM CELL BANKING

The current requirements of translational orthopedics, regenerative medicine, tissue engineering, and gene therapy all need a limitless supply of stem cells to accomplish their goals. These cells are specialized as described above and cannot be synthesized for practical use by current available method(s). Stem cell banking concept facilitates the above cause by cryogenically preserving stem cells in their most potent state for later usage. As far as therapeutic use of stem cells is concerned (say for treatment of nonunion), allogeneic ESCs fail due to immune surveillance. These allogeneic ESCs though do not have any immune markers on them but their final product does have them and bound to rejection. If one bypasses immune rejection by using iPS cells, problem of teratoma formation still remains. What is then left is to develop the iPS cell lines in a controlled environment to develop the desired tissue and implant or transfer into the body later, but this process is lengthy (>6 months) and defies cost rendering it practically ineffective. This argument strengthens the use of autologous stem cells only presently for all practical clinical usage reinforcing the utility of stem cell banking. Stem cells need to be collected, stored, and processed for two main purposes—one for future use in the person himself when needed and the other for purpose of ongoing research and production of regenerative medicine, tissue engineering, and 3D bioprinting. Umbilical cord blood as a source of HSCs has been in use since 1989 and its banking has been in vogue for more than two decades. There are two major models for cord blood banking—(1) the public and (2) the private cord blood banks. While the former is supported by public funds similar to blood banks and is focused at serving the society at large and supporting regenerative medicine research, the latter is more commercial offering storage of cord blood for use by a child or family later. The evolution of private cord blood banks has also sparked some ethical issues.

Sources of Stem Cells for Banking

It is not easy to obtain stem cells despite their presence in nearly all the tissues of body, primary reason being their scarcity in terms of absolute numbers. The source of stem cells should be easily accessible, should avoid immune rejection issues, should contain sufficient number of stem cells to justify its use [ideally numbers should be large enough, so as to use them clinically directly ($>15 \times 10^6$) without need of prior expansion in culture], and should be economical to utilize. The practical sources for stem cells for banking and brief procedure of banking them are described below:

- *Cord blood:* Nearly 30–120 mL (70–80 mL from a full-term live birth) of cord blood is available for collection in a single case. The limitation of cord blood is that it contains only HSCs and less prominent numbers of MSCs. Studies have also found it to contain pluripotent stem cells capable of producing cells forming ectodermal, mesodermal, and endodermal lineages. The blood is collected within 5 minutes of clamping and sectioning of the cord from umbilical vein. One can also wait for delivery of placenta and collect blood directly from expelled placenta. Collection can be made by use of 50-mL syringes; however, small blood bags (250 mL) are preferred for closed system. The collected blood is rich in red blood cells (RBCs) in which we are not interested while the mononuclear cell (MNC) population is the one that interests scientists in stem cell research, as it contains MSCs. 20% of collected blood is MNC fraction of which 1% is stem cells. Due to high hematocrit, most of the banked collections are RBCs depleted by Hespan sedimentation or density-gradient centrifugation (Ficoll method) or AutoXpress platform® (AXP) method. The last method is automated. While the Hespan and AXP products are all nucleated population of cells, the Ficoll method produces predominant MNC population and the product is 50% less than other two methods (absolute stem cell numbers are similar in all methods). AXP is the Food and Drug Administration (FDA) approved; being a closed system, it is commonly recommended. The cord blood after processing is stored in multiple aliquots, so that they can be further used according to the demand and whole product is not repeatedly subjected to freeze–thaw cycle that is detrimental to stem cell survival. There is significant problem while isolating MSC from cord blood including the limitation of processing the same within 2 hours. Optimal processing occurs with samples of >90 mL of cord blood and even then the MSCs obtained are in the range from few hundreds to thousands of cells. These MSCs are too few to be used immediately and have to be expanded in vitro for further use over weeks-to-months. These problems have shifted the attention to cord tissue as a source of MSCs. HSCs till date could not be expanded in vitro, but by virtue of cord blood containing this (and cord tissue and adipose tissue completely lacking in these cells), it finds unique usage in reconstitution of blood and bone marrow after chemotherapy or radiotherapy. Cord blood can be used to treat >80 hematological malignancies and nonmalignant conditions that need transplant.
- *Cord tissue:* 4–10 inches of cord tissue can be obtained based on gestation period, ethnicity, and maternal factors. It contains primarily mesenchymal stem cells that have wide application. It also additionally contains endothelial and epithelial precursor cells. The umbilical cord is 30–50 cm in length and stem cells can be found in various locations including the amniotic compartment, Wharton's jelly, and perivascular space. The number of MSCs varies from 25,000/cm of the cord tissue to as high as 5×10^6 MSC/cm that may also contain endothelial, epithelial, and hematogenic stem cells depending on the isolation protocol used. Few of the methods for isolation of MSCs include culture of cord tissue explants, culture of amnion explants, digestion of the Wharton's jelly directly, digestion of isolated blood vessels from CT, and isolation and culture of venous epithelial stem cell tissues. Again, depending on the length of cord, the number of MSCs obtained still falls short of any direct clinical application without in vitro culture and expansion. Methods for MSC isolation involve either enzymatic or nonenzymatic digestion of tissues. The cord tissue are collected at the time of birth and banked frozen for later use. Often, 5–10-inch pieces of umbilical cord tissue are cut and cleaned with alcohol and povidone–iodine solution. They are transported in a sterile buffer solution comprising of isotonic saline with 10 U/mL heparin, 1% human serum albumin (HSA), penicillin, streptomycin, gentamicin, and amphotericin. In the laboratory, the sample is again washed with 70% ethanol and given a final sterile saline wash. Ringlets of 5 mm are cut from the cord tissue that are then placed in isotonic saline solution containing 0.1 mol/L sucrose,

20% autologous plasma, and 1.5 mol/L dimethyl sulfoxide (DMSO) for 30 minutes at 4°C. The samples are then kept frozen in 4.5 mL cryovials (using DMSO as cryoprotectant) in a controlled environment and then stored in liquid nitrogen. For use, the samples can be thawed at room temperature for 30 seconds and saline is washed to remove DMSO. The samples are resuspended in 20% plasma for analysis. The tissue for use is minced and placed into a 25 cm^2 culture flask. The pieces are removed after 4–6 days and cultured in a new flask. Colonies of cell are visible after 10–14 days. The cells are harvested from both the flasks using trypsin-ethylenediaminetetraacetic acid (EDTA). Some 25,000 cells are cultured in each subsequent culture flask in alpha minimum essential medium (MEM) expansion medium.

- *Dental pulp:* It contains mesenchymal stem cells but is limited in the absolute numbers.
- *Bone marrow:* Typically, 1,000–1,500 mL can be harvested surgically. It contains both hematopoietic and mesenchymal stem cells, but number and quality of these vary widely based on the age and health of the person. The isolation is painful and has low cell yield. The older the age of patient, the reduced is the proliferative and differentiation capability of the MSCs.
- *Adipose tissue:* This has highest concentration of MSCs and is easily available in large volumes (100–3,000 mL). It has 500 times the number of stem cells compared to bone marrow per gram of tissue. Adipose tissue is currently considered the best alternative source of MSCs. The harvest is done either by syringe harvest or from scheduled liposuction procedures. The aspirates are cryopreserved (controlled rate freezing to –180°C followed by immersion in liquid nitrogen) within 24–36 hours of collection. The lipoaspirate is washed with isotonic saline and kept in a cryobag with equal amount of DMSO solution containing 70% lactated Ringer's buffer, 20% serum or HSA, and 20% DMSO at 4°C. This is then preserved in controlled rate freezer kept at –180°C finally submerging in liquid nitrogen. When needed, the preserved tissue is thawed rapidly in 37°C water bath for 15 minutes. Adipose tissue is commonly removed from slurry by enzymatic digestion. MSCs may be expanded by culture in β-MEM media supplemented with 10% fetal bovine serum (FBS) and 1% solution each of nonessential amino acids, sodium pyruvate, L-glutamine, and streptomycin/penicillin solution. The infranatant from this is centrifuged to obtain "stromal vascular fraction (SVF)". These are plated in 25 cm^2 flasks and after 2 days, nonadherent cells are removed by changing medium.

Religious Aspects of Stem Cell Banking

In our country with a mixture of population, one needs to know the religious guidelines for using and storing cord blood, as this may be a sensitive issue to many. Four major religious populations exist in Indian subcontinent including Hinduism, Islam, Christianity, and Buddhism. Following presents a brief on individual religious belief but in no case should serve as a strict guideline and treating surgeon should respect the patient's belief and expectations.

Hinduism

The exegetical view for or against the use of cord blood may be obtained from ancient written texts. Laws of Manu mention birth rituals as *Jatakarma* but go no beyond severing of the umbilical cord. Indirect acceptance of stem cell therapy may arise from other literary sources such as the *Mahabharata* where birth of Kaurava from a piece of flesh incubated by Rishi Vyas in different containers may liken regenerative medicine. "Bhrunahatya" is condemned in Hindu beliefs, so use of postimplantation embryos for ESCs may not be acceptable, but this also indicates that preimplantation embryos may be utilized, if the technique and intent can enable curative treatment to those already suffering. This also complies with the concept of establishment of "jiva tattva" at the time of conception, and that the singularity of "jiva tattva" would get transferred to other living form only. The soul is said to lie in the umbilical cord according to "Charaka Samhita", so use of cord blood for regenerative medicine would be like transfer of the soul or rebirth. Hinduism is highly absorbing religion and so accommodative that by sheer pragmatism it accepts advances in biotechnology in unaccepted ways and promulgates doctrines, accordingly. Hinduism is unopposed to public or private cord blood banking.

Christianity

Whether Catholics or evangelical Protestants or Anglicans, "nearly" all accept the banking of cord blood cells. Catholics warmly encourage the donation of organs and tissue as a cure of the sick and unless it does not amount to destruction of human (embryonic) life. The life of Jesus is considered so central to the cure of sick that it is broadly accepted to distribute the health resources freely on the basis of sheer need. Why I used the word "nearly" is because some might argue that this distribution should comply with the ideology of "maximum utility", "equality of opportunity", and "provider-consumer choice". Though it is really difficult to justify the ideology but one needs to understand that banking the your cord blood would relieve the use of otherwise banked cells, if you fall sick; that can be deployed for someone else more needy at that time thus maximizing utility to a person who needs it most when you had the chance to improve the opportunity by banking your own cells. Catholics would not however accept private umbilical cord banking. Bible upholds the goodness of relationships and promulgates an expansive view of personhood. So in short, Christianity favors therapies that support people and improve their lives and encourages public umbilical cord blood banking.

Islam

Blood is regarded quite sacred in Islam and use of umbilical cord blood is permissible according to various Fatwas, if no Islamic rule is broken while acquiring the blood (like abortion or maternal damage). The same can be extended to donation, if there is no damage to the donor and acceptability and health improvement benefits are seen in the recipient. Islam would not encourage private cord blood banking.

Buddhism

Buddhists regard birth as a natural process; therefore, there is hardly any significance or rules attached to use of placenta, cord, or its contents. Use of cord blood or banking it would not pose any problem until it is beneficial for human population at large, not harmful for the concerned individuals, and has a social cause. Use of ESCs would be of concern, as this would disrupt their belief of beginning of human life at fertilization and that procuring cells in blastocele stage would interfere with human life. No such reservations apply for use of adult stem cells. Being extensively social in belief and the firm basis of "dana" (generosity), the only concern would be use of the facility of banking for private storage. Buddhism would encourage banking for use of others as a social "giving" (donation) for benefit of the society rather than banking for self-use (private) later. To put to a broader and more generous perspective, however, there seems little resistance to use of stem cell banking, if it is serving a greater social cause than personal one.

CONCLUSION

- Use of MSC and EPC has been studied quite amply and they are being used in the form of bone marrow-derived substrates (either concentrated or in toto).
- Stem cell banking is a rapidly growing model of procuring, storage, and expanding the stem cells for public and private use. This practice is liable to disrupt the conventional orthopedic and medical practice in general in connivance with translational medicine and tissue engineering.
- Availability of iPSCs will make a breakthrough and is expected soon in the next decade. Till then, improvements in MSC and EPC in the form of combination cocktails of labeled MSCs (in vivo or ex vivo expansion) with growth factors are being successfully utilized for various purposes.
- Increased stress is being paid to miRNA/exosome analysis for applying this therapy and for independent clinical usage; so, as a breakthrough expects the miRNA/exosome therapy sooner than iPSC clinical availability in future.

CHAPTER 17

Electrospinning, Three-dimensional Printing, and its Application in Orthopedics

Manish Kumar Varshney

INTRODUCTION

Advances in regenerative medicine and stem cell therapy have enabled us to realize the once considered fantasy of science fictions to replace dead/damaged tissue (or organ in future) with a new one. This new era strategizes on synthesizing biomaterials and scaffolds based on biomimicry of native tissue that involves convergence of advances in material science, stem cell science, physics, and developmental biology. Improved understanding of developmental biology has helped us by incorporation of molecules into scaffolds and biomaterials that promote regeneration of tissues. This regenerative engineering enables us to regenerate complex tissues and organ systems. Current methods of osteosynthesis and reconstruction are limited due to osteoporosis, limited repair capacity of orthopedic tissues (cartilage, bone, and muscles), and inability to fill large gaps following tumor resections. These lacunae in orthopedic care are expected to be filled by regenerative engineering. New tissue synthesis for replacement of diseased part (like cartilage damage) or filling gaps (bone and soft tissue defects following tumor resection) is being primarily focused among other applications of the technology. This basically requires fabrication of nanofibrous scaffolds with desirable characteristics **(Box 1)** for further development of various tissues. This is achieved currently by two specific techniques that are scalable and can be combined also. Electrospinning process is the most versatile and commonly deployed that can be used to process a wide range of materials and composites with controllable mechanical properties through simple and cost-effective operations. The other technique popularly called three-dimensional (3D) printing, as developed for medical field helps in fabrication process with the ability to control bulk geometry and internal structure of tissue scaffolds.

BOX 1: The desirable characteristics of scaffolds.

The scaffolds should have some properties that enable them to be used as graft tissue or substitutes:

1. Biocompatibility—for integration in host tissues and immune tolerance
2. Mechanical stability—to tolerate the local mechanical stresses
3. Biodegradable—with nontoxic degradation products
4. Osteoconductive—to allow cell adhesion, proliferation, neovascularization, and tissue production
5. Ability to integrate with nearby tissues and structures

ELECTROSPINNING

Electrospinning derived from "electrostatic spinning" has been used in tissue regeneration purposes in the late 1990s by Laurencin. It involves application of high electric field to droplet of fluid coming out of tip of die (acting as electrode). The droplet is deformed by electric field and the fluid is ejected as a charged jet toward another counter-electrode forming a continuous fiber. The properties of fiber can be controlled by altering polymer properties, solvent properties, solution flow rate, applied voltage, distance between electrodes, etc. Modifications of the fibers are done by surface modifications and thermal treatment to enhance bioactivity of electrospun scaffolds. Multiaxial structures with desired alignment (radial/wavy/uniaxial) are produced that can be arranged in 3D structure by layer-by-layer stacking, 3D weaving and template deposition. Biomimetic 3D scaffolds have been created by orienting biocompatible polyphosphazene-polyester nanofiber matrices (fiber diameter of 50–500 nm) arranged concentrically with open central cavity to replicate bone marrow cavity and lamellar structure. These biomimetic scaffolds support osteoblast proliferation and differentiation leading to structural organization of native. Electrospun acellular biomaterials/scaffolds may be divided into blended-surface-modified and composite-surface-modified scaffolds. These types can be also combined together in bioengineering.

Blended-surface Modified Electrospun Fibers

The mechanical properties of scaffold have specific impact on cellular behavior. Blending mechanically distinct scaffolds having identical microstructures and surface chemistry improves properties. Combining poly(ether sulfone) core and poly(Σ-caprolactone) sheath improves the modulus of elasticity four times over that of electrospun poly(Σ-caprolactone) alone. The lower modulus scaffold provides an environment suitable for chondrogenesis as evident by upregulation of chondrocyte phenotype gene expression (*Sox9, Type II collagen, and Aggrecan*) while the higher modulus scaffold supports enhanced osteogenesis by promoting osteogenic *Runx2*, alkaline phosphatase, and osteocalcin gene expression. Another example is surface modification of blended electrospun fibers that prevents downregulation of cell differentiation associated with osteoblast lineage. Blended poly-(L)-lactide with collagen and/or Bmp-2 demonstrates enhanced osteoblast differentiation of human mesenchymal stem cells (hMSCs) by upregulation of signal transduction pathways.

Composite-surface Modified Scaffolds

Some human tissues need modification of contemporary bioengineering techniques like synthesis of periosteum. Electrospun nanohydroxyapatite containing fibrous chitosan scaffolds (classical technique) is crosslinked to genipin forming a composite resulting in five times increase in Young's modulus approximating that of periosteum. Similarly, calcium phosphate coating on electrospun scaffolds from a block copolymer-poly(ethylene oxide terephthalate)-poly (butylene terephthalate) improves bioactivity in bone tissue engineering. Such scaffolds when used in combination with mesenchymal stem cells (MSCs) result in bone formation in vivo demonstrating that biomimetic methods can be successfully used to coat electrospun scaffolds with calcium phosphate layer to improve its bioactivity.

THREE-DIMENSIONAL BIOPRINTING

Three-dimensional printing was developed initially by Charles W Hull in 1986 based on techniques of topography assessment and photo sculpture. The objects are built layer-by-layer based on the digital drawings obtained through special imaging tools (usually a 3D scanner) and software, by a process called "additive manufacturing". "Additive manufacturing" differs from "subtractive manufacturing"; as in the latter, shape is obtained by chipping away parts from a large block, while in the former objects are created from bottom-up. A computer-controlled robotic system is used commonly to create 3D objects through layer-by-layer addition of material. In engineering, additive manufacturing typically shortens the design cycle of new products by rapidly producing the desired prototypes—a process called "rapid prototyping". Advances in 3D printing have enabled us in developing custom-made orthopedic implants (replacing the diseased or absent tissue!). This process is termed biofabrication—"process involving automated generation of biologically functional products with structural organization from living cells, bioactive molecules, biomaterials, cell aggregates such as microtissues, or hybrid cell material constructs, through bioprinting or bioassembly and subsequent tissue maturation processes". Further technological advances are helping us to produce complex tissues by depositing bioinks to couture tissue to be repaired. "Bioprinting" or printing of biological tissues has been made possible by advances in automation, miniaturization, and computer-aided designing along with the development of bioinks and cell systems that can survive in there.

In general, 3D bioprinting utilizes a four-step process **(Flowchart 1)** as follows:

1. Imaging and data processing
2. Selection of printing technique
3. Identifying the biomaterials and components
4. Bioprinting

Flowchart 1: Flow of the three-dimensional (3D) bioprinting process.

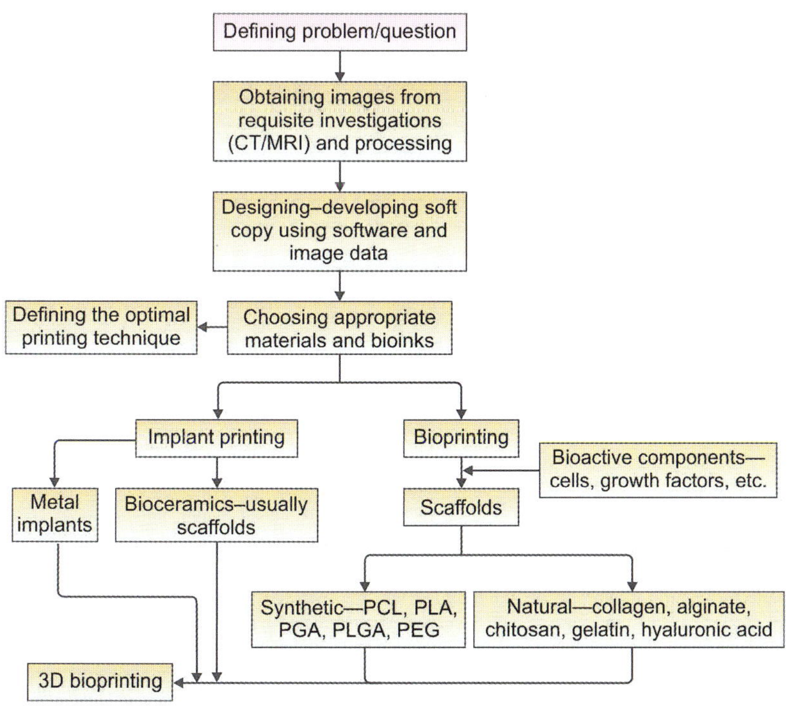

(CT: computed tomography; MRI: magnetic resonance imaging; PCL: polycaprolactone; PEG: polyethylene glycol; PGA: polyglycolic acid; PLGA: polylactic-co-glycolic acid; PLA: polylactic acid)

Imaging and Data Processing

As exampled above with respect to echocardiography and synthesis of cardiac valves, the process can be utilized in orthopedics also. Complicated pathologies such as pelvic bone tumors are being synthesized whereby surgeons can learn about their disposition and plan surgical treatment. This process involves data acquisition from images and synthesis of 3D digital models using software computer-aided design (CAD) followed by 3D printing and postprocessing. Attention is usually paid to obtain high-resolution images for better accuracy; so pertinent X-rays, computed tomography (CT) scans, and magnetic resonance imaging (MRI) are sought for. While the former is used for defining bony pathology and latter is most useful for soft tissue detailing. The region of interest is then marked and the captured data from images is transformed into volumetric data to synthesize 3D digital models by optimizing data at various levels. The architectural design is modified at various levels including macro (gross shape and disposition of the lesion or implant), micro (tissue architecture), and nanoscales (surface structure).

Printing Techniques

Printer and technique are selected based on intended material and resolution of the deemed products. 3D printing uses metals, ceramics, or bioinks to print objects as needed. The various printing techniques include:

- *Fused deposition modeling*—here the heated material is extruded through nozzle that gets hardened gradually after extrusion. Thin multiple layers of the material are deposited to be repeated by the moving print head until the solid 3D object forms.
- *Selective laser sintering*—here laser is used to draw shape of the object by sintering (fusing into solid or porous mass by heating without liquefaction) powdered material. Layers-over-layers are deposited until object is synthesized.
- *Pneumatic extrusion printing*—this process is supposed to be less harmful to cells, here a continuous filament of biomaterial (say a mixture of cells and hydrogel) is extruded (using compressed air) through micron-sized nozzle that dispenses two-dimensional (2D) patterns. The deposition of material and overall architecture can be controlled by differential pressure level, controlling the viscosity of the ink, etc.
- *Inkjet printing*—here thermal, air pressure, electromagnetic, or piezoelectric technology is used to dispense droplets of ink onto a substrate. Droplets of various sizes are created by altering the viscosity, temperature gradient, pressure, and pulse frequency to place a thicker or thinner layer.
- *Stereolithography*—here a 3D object is created by laser coagulation of liquid polymer that hardens on contact with laser light (optical fabrication and photo- solidification).

Depending on the polymer material used for 3D bioprinting, they may be classified as natural, synthetic, natural-composite and synthetic-composite scaffolds **(Box 2)**. Based on the need and availability of printer, versatility, precision, and speed of printers, the techniques have been used for printing the objects for different applications.

ADVANCEMENTS IN THREE-DIMENSIONAL PRINTING TECHNOLOGY

1. *Combining 3D printing scaffolds and electrospinning:* This is specially explored for large osseous defects. Biphasic PCL-hyaluronic acid hydrogel loaded with rhBMP-2 has been developed for vertical bone regeneration.

BOX 2: Different polymers used for three-dimensional (3D) printing of scaffolds (bioinks).

Natural and natural-composite materials: Natural polymers are biodegradable and cellular elements and biofunctional molecules home on their surface somewhat with ease to aid attachment and differentiation. Most of these are used as "hydrogels". Hydrogels are essentially "water-swellable" but "water-insoluble" cross-linked networks that can provide multiple advantages in tissue engineering by incorporating cells, encouraging their growth and proliferation (by retaining water-simulating biological tissues), and acting as carrier system. Polymers-like collagen, chitosan, hyaluronic acid (HA), silk proteins, gelatins, and alginates are all used as hydrogels. These commonly have a common property of inducing a phase change from liquid to semisolid by cross-linking. The primary limitations include poor mechanical properties and pathogenic impurities that may be cytotoxic. Another issue with hydrogels is their inability to maintain uniform 3D structure for long and, hence, they have to be commonly coupled with synthetic biomaterials like polyglycolic acid (PGA), hydroxyapatite (HA), polycaprolactone (PCL), methacrylate, etc.

Alginate is a common bioink that can be used in versatile ways:

- The molecular weight of alginate and choice of ionic cross-linker can be tuned to control mechanical properties like Young's modulus and degradation rate influencing its stiffness and, hence, differentiation of mesenchymal stem cells (MSCs) (stiffer constructs supporting osteogenesis).
- Alginate/gelatin scaffolds can be coated with nanoapatite of varying thickness using amount of phosphate ions in the bioink. The apatite-coated scaffolds demonstrate enhanced proliferation and osteogenic differentiation of MSCs.
- The composite of hydrogel with cells (mature derived cells or stem cells) can act as a bioink to deposit cells or growth factors in a scaffold supported basically by hydrogel.

Synthetic and synthetic-composite materials:

- Metals like titanium that have high biocompatibility which are used mostly for implant synthesis due to favorable mechanical properties.
- Bioceramics like hydroxyapatite, bioglass, and calcium phosphate are good for bone restoration and substitution, as they are osteogenic, porous, maintain shape, and promote cell proliferation on surface.
- Tissue engineering has been utilized to produce composite materials like HA-TCP (hydroxyapatite with tricalcium phosphate), PCL-HA (polycaprolactone with hydroxyapatite) amalgamated to carbon nanotubes, PCL-PLGA (polycaprolactone with poly lactic-co-glycolic acid), PLGA-TCP (poly lactic-co-glycolic acid with tricalcium phosphate), etc. These composites are utilized to prepare scaffolds with optimized architecture, biocompatibility, and manufacturing properties like sintering conditions.
  - Custom built 3D printed PCL scaffolds with anatomic shape and varying internal porosities have been used for craniomaxillofacial bone defects.
  - Implantable scaffolds of poly-(propylene fumarate) coated with calcium phosphate and rhBMP-2 have been developed for substitution of segmental bone defects.

The biphasic scaffold comprises outer shell constructed using 3D printing that mimics cortical bone for mechanical strength while the inner mesh mimicking cancellous bone was electrospun to facilitate hydrogel loading and subsequent osteogenesis and angiogenesis. Hierarchical 3D printed and aligned electrospun fibers of PCL with myoblast-laden scaffold with micro-/nano-topological cues have been developed. The printed myoblasts were viable and expressed myogenic genes that were significantly affected by fiber alignment suggesting this to be a highly promising technique for orthopedic applications.

2. *4D printing (also known as 4D-bioprinting, shape-morphing systems, functional printing, active origami):* Simply speaking 4D printing is 3D printing that transforms over time (4th dimension) when removed from printer. This makes it a type of programmable matter that can change shape and/or function later when desired. The stimulus for the transformation can come from various sources such as light, heat, electricity/ magnetic field, etc. The printed objects change their shape dynamically based on needs and demands of the situation. It is like printing function into the material that will execute once activated. The meta-material structure is created by combining different materials that provide structural responses when activated by external stimuli. The primary matter is produced using principles of 3D printing itself. Differences between 3D and 4D printing are summarized in **Table 1**. The applications of 4D printing:
   a. *Medical and healthcare*—4D printed splints that can automatically expand up to double the size with need—pediatric splints and prosthesis. Development futuristic splints that can be applied on the limb directly and they self-assemble into casts/slabs. Development of foldable molecules that can release drugs as needed (say releasing antipyretics if fever occurs). Development of artificial tissues that can expand or contract or self-assemble on implantation. Targeted drug delivery that would discharge the drug on encountering the target molecule.
   b. Aerospace—shield for spacecraft antennas and spacesuits.
   c. Apparels—developing a shoe that can self-assemble—avoiding cumbersome process.
   d. Automotive—expandable materials in response to air pulses.

CURRENT APPLICATIONS OF THREE-DIMENSIONAL PRINTING IN ORTHOPEDICS

The current and futuristic application of 3D bioprinting in orthopedics offers a range of possibilities to deliver patient-specific therapy. The following are some of the applications which currently used or under development are as follows:

Modeling of Pathological Bone

This is the easiest application where utilizing the images (CT scan or MRI) the bone models are created for further study and use of surgeon. This allows holistic understanding of the pathology such as surgery, approach, excision, and reconstruction can be planned well in advance reducing the amount of intraoperative surprises that would otherwise hamper proper execution of even best of surgeries. Such modeling is quite useful in periarticular regions and anatomically complex regions like scapula and pelvis. Surgeon can study the bioprinted 3D model of the pathological region to plan his procedure.

Patient-specific Surgical Instruments

Though not still very commonly used, but patient-specific instrumentation is available for the precision surgeries like total knee replacement and the use can be extended to ankle, wrist, shoulder, and hip arthroplasty also. Using predecided imaging techniques and protocols, the deemed images are obtained and fed into software that plans and analyzes the optimal treatment for the patient based on standardized protocols. The images are further processed to produce 3D models, customized molds, and surgical guides (patient-specific saw guide/cutting-block) to provide precise cutting of bone. The greatest advantage of this technique is saving the surgical time, as sizing of implants is also done during planning that avoids intraoperative confusion. Most of the planning has already been done outside, so better plans can be made and even changed if needed. Implant fit is better and possibly the morbidity is also low in these cases. Similar application is available for spine surgery where 3D-printed screw-guide system is available to benefit intraoperative pedicle screw fixation. This whole exercise (that usually takes 3 weeks to 1 month) aims to minimize tissue loss, optimize prosthesis, and implant positioning possibly reducing morbidity. Indirectly, this also utilizes other's (other surgeon and planners) experience reducing the dependence on planning on sole surgeon and his limited experience, also this reduces surgical errors due to outliers.

TABLE 1: The differences between three-dimensional (3D) and four-dimensional (4D) printing.

Characteristic	*3D printing*	*4D printing*
Production	Repeating 2D structure layer by layer in a pre-determined print path	Transforming the created 3D printed object over passage of time
Dynamic shape change	Not a feature	Changes color, shape, function, etc.
Materials used	Thermoplastic, metals and alloys, biomaterials, nanoparticles	Smart materials—shape memory alloys and shape memory polymers, hydrophilic polymers, biomaterials, and plant oil
Printing requirements	3D-printer, fused deposition modeling, selective laser sintering	3D printer and multimaterial 3D printers

Patient-specific Implants

This is where interest is being laid down quite immensely but the technology has to encounter various regulatory hurdles. 3D-printed customized axial vertebral body has been implanted in upper cervical spine of one patient; similarly, 3D-printed titanium calcaneal prosthesis has also been implanted in a patient suffering from chondrosarcoma of heel. Another application is synthesizing custom-made cages for significant acetabular defects that cannot be adequately addressed by current available methods.

Cartilage Regeneration

Cartilage regeneration has been the most intriguing aspects and some success has also been encountered regarding the same. Degeneration of cartilage is a common problem limiting joint function with age. Intrinsic healing capabilities of hyaline cartilage are limited due to avascular and alymphatic nature of articular cartilage. Progression of joint degeneration following cartilage damage is relentless and currently remedy is limited. Bioprinting has been envisaged to create or constructs that mimic the architecture of tissues and can be implanted into the body. The deceptively simple appearing morphology of cartilage, in fact masks the heterogeneity, it contains with increasing depth. Not only the cell structure differs with depth but the type of proteins and density also changes within the three layers of cartilage (*see* also Chapter on "Articular Cartilage: Structure, Function, Injury, and Management"). The superficial zone comprising 10% of cartilage depth contains glycosaminoglycans and parallel arrangement of collagen. The proteins here are clusterin, proteoglycan-4 (PRG4) or lubricin, and Del-1. In the middle layer, cartilage intermediate layer protein (CLIP) has the highest density along with haphazardly oriented collagen fibrils. Deeper zone contains primarily cartilage oligomeric matrix protein (COMP) and vertically oriented collagen. This heterogeneity and specialized disposition led researchers to develop strategies based on the use of zonally harvested cells but were found to be too complicated and ineffective. This was changed to use of a single cell source coupled to biomechanical stimulus to encourage zonal differentiation with limited success.

Innovative approach is to use a combination of structures that use "force dissipation pattern" utilizing stem cells or chondroblasts that can be influenced by the mechanical stimuli. "Smart scaffold designs" are created by combining different biomaterials that influence deposition of extracellular matrix by influencing cellular alignment. These constructs have to be, however, grown in a controlled environment in a bioreactor into functional tissue that then matures in the body. The process has been taken a step further by trying to incorporate the functions of tissue into synthesized construct itself. Construct such as cell-laden heterogeneous hydrogel can be produced with 3D printing to be potentially used as osteochondral grafts. Decellularized extracellular matrix (dECM) has been bioprinted that can provide microenvironment to chondrons for induction of cartilage tissue growth by providing crucial signals for cell engraftment, survival, and future functions. To mimic the zonal (three zones of native hyaline cartilage) construct of cartilage combination of polymers have been used like polyethylene glycol (PEG), hyaluronic acid (HA), chondroitin sulfate, and metalloprotease-sensitive peptides that encapsulate single lineage of mesenchymal stem cells.

Bone Regeneration

Bone loss may occur due to trauma, excision of neoplasia, congenital deficiency, etc. whereby there is a need for massive amounts of bone grafts served only through bone-banking currently. These have good osteoconductive properties but are poor in osteoinduction and osteogenesis due to loss of repair capability to a great extent. Donor site morbidity and additional surgeries are major limitations with autograft, while disease transmission and poor graft incorporation encumber use of allograft. Tissue engineering can circumvent the limitations by providing biocompatible porous 3D matrix scaffolds that allow conducive environment for cell attachment, migration, incorporation of growth factors, and encouraging vascular ingrowth. These scaffolds apart from above properties should be sufficiently mechanically stable providing requisite strength at the site of usage. For cellular growth, it has been found that in a hydrogel model (alginate scaffold) addition of peptide like arginine-glycine-aspartic acid increases bone formation. PEG hydrogel as also demonstrated promising results in terms of its properties for supporting cellular growth. 3D printing controls the precise form, architecture, and disposition of scaffold producing clinically optimal combinations. Animal studies using biphasic 3D-printed calcined bone [ceramic composite/polyvinyl alcohol (PVA) gel] have been successful in terms of biocompatibility and allowing growth of bone marrow stromal cells. β-TCP has been a popular material for producing scaffolds, it has been demonstrated that addition of zinc oxide and silica to it instigates osteoinduction in this basically osteoconductive scaffold. Under study are innovative combinations of hMSCs and PEG dimethacrylate with bioactive glass and/or HA. This combination improves collagen synthesis and deposition and also has high-alkaline phosphatase activity promoting osteogenesis.

Animal studies for creation of joints have been done where 3D-printed scaffolds have been used for replacing the native hip joint filled with growth factors and stem cells. The study had got when success new hip joints formed at the site in nearly 4 months and rabbits were able to walk some as early as in the few weeks.

Coverage of Open Wounds

Skin grafts have been attempted to be printed in laboratory from culture of patients own cells. Currently, however, in situ bioprinters are available that spray skin cells, coagulant, and collagen onto the wounds with surprisingly good results. This has got military applications and possibly also for burns patients.

Meniscus Substitution

Polyurethane scaffolds to mimic structural and mechanical properties of menisci have been used that allow interconnective macroporosity facilitating cell ingrowth and differentiation. 3D printing, projection stereolithography, has been used to synthesize scaffolds with seeding of cells from human meniscus allowing cellular growth and meniscal tissue formation. Animal studies using 3D-printed zone-specific matrix phenotypes with spatiotemporally delivered human connective tissue growth factor (TGF) and TGF-β3 has been found to restore meniscal integrity.

Ligament, Tendon, and Muscle Regeneration

Braiding of polymer filaments of 15 μm diameter into circular and rectangular formations is found to mimic the mechanical and structural properties of natural ligament. These synthetic scaffolds can be used for reconstructing ligaments by altering the yarn density and braid shape to match the tensile strength of specific ligament. It has been traditionally deemed that muscle cannot be repaired with native tissue let alone the synthesis and regeneration *in vivo*. Success has, however, been gained in initial stage by seeding the muscle cells onto a scaffold of nanofibers created by electrospinning. There was a favorable muscle cell alignment and myotube formation that has been found compatible for functional muscle tissue implantation.

This can be taken a step further by synthesizing composite muscle–tendon unit. To reproduce functional and biological properties of muscles and tendons, two synthetic polymeric materials with two cell-laden hydrogel-based bioinks have to be used. Ligament scaffold can be created by weaving degummed silk fibers.

Synthesis of Prosthetics and Orthoses

Three-dimensional printing of custom braces, prosthetics, and orthotics is an interesting field where the technique can be easily utilized for patient-specific production. Socket designing and molding is an important part of prosthetic fitting that can be easily achieved by available 3D-printing techniques.

CONCLUSION

Medical field is likely to be most disrupted by the availability of 3D printing and bioprinting. It is the utmost desire of treating surgeons to have available biological replacements for tissue that are damaged by pathologies, so that function can be optimally restored. This is more a fantasy than a reality as of now but steps are being taken in this direction of research and innovation. One such way appears to be bioprinting, though it is in its infantile stage. Significant advances have been made in optimizing bioinks, fabrication time, and biological performance of the constructs, but it will take a lot of time for the technique to be clinically useable in the form of current "fantasy" is imagined. The future of 3D printing lies in combining and advancing tissue engineering (we need to develop more diverse materials for scaffolds), stem cell science (better longevity, preventing dedifferentiation, and improved stability while regenerating), and bioreactor technology. Vascularization is the essence of growth of reconstructed tissue and is the current limiting factor in regenerated tissue implantation; this can be improved by bioreactor science where tissues are incubated with factors that promote angiogenesis and innervation to maintain cell viability. The current utility of 3D-printed metal implants and surgical-assistive instruments need to be optimized to promote the science and encourage further research. In situ bioprinting is an interesting application where the tissues can be printed on the affected areas directly by the printers—such a system is available as a prototype for skin printing but is far from reality for other regions/tissues. Bioprinting is still far from clinical usage but once optimized and technical difficulties overcome, we will soon have laboratory or factory printed tissues.

CHAPTER 18

Gene Therapy in Orthopedics

Manish Kumar Varshney

INTRODUCTION

Orthopedics has seen several breakthrough innovations in the past, particularly with respect to bone stabilization that changed both the quality and possibilities for treatment of orthopedic diseases. But over the past few years, it has become clear that only biomechanical analysis of operative techniques alone does not guarantee surgical success. Additionally, in genetic diseases of primarily orthopedic interest, such as osteogenesis imperfecta (OI) or Duchenne muscular dystrophy (DMD), today's treatment options are purely symptomatic. Even in conditions that have been classically treated operatively, such as osteoarthrosis, bone tumors, ligament and tendon regeneration, and osteoporosis, role of genetics is fast emerging. Curative biological effect of present methods is missing by and large. The direct application of proteins (growth factors or cytokines), though potentially beneficial, is limited by very short half-life and requirement of high doses. Gene therapy could be the potential answer to overcome these problems.

The most important drawback in orthopedic treatment since times immemorial had been protracted recovery times of any treatment (say plaster cast immobilization), so the primary reason for innovations and development of new treatment techniques (say operative stabilization methods) has been primarily directed at reduction of recovery time. The healing response can be improved by the local targeted application of growth factors into the injury site, but they have their own shortcomings. Gene therapy, when successfully applied, provides these growth factors in a sustained manner locally. The following are the potential applications of gene therapy as relevant to orthopedics:

- *Fracture healing:*
  - Nonunion
  - Delayed union
  - Compound fractures
  - Grade 3 open fractures
- *Ligament healing:*
  - Regeneration of ligaments, such as patellar tendon (extensor mechanism), anterior cruciate ligament or improved fixation and incorporation of grafts
  - Meniscal tears
- Chondral (articular cartilage) healing and regeneration
- *Muscular diseases:*
  - Muscular dystrophies
  - Muscle strain
  - Utilization of muscle cells as ex vivo delivery vehicles
- *Osteoarthritis (OA):*
  - Primarily chondral regeneration
  - Alteration of joint milieu to retard joint degeneration
- *Rheumatoid arthritis:* Altering or remitting the inflammatory process

The purposes and structure of gene therapy protocols in acquired or genetic orthopedic diseases are fundamentally different. Gene therapy cannot only be used for management of genetic defects but also to introduce therapeutic agents directly into somatic tissue cells. This somatic gene therapy (as distinct from germline gene therapy) opens up immense possibilities beyond the single gene defect disorders. Somatic gene therapy can be performed locally or systemically, whereas the latter may be advantageous in cardiac or vascular diseases, former is more amenable to orthopedic diseases. Thus, a local gene delivery into the diseased or injured tissue is desirable. Gene therapy is the excellent application to transfer growth factors and to produce them at cell level in a continuous manner. For example, poor strength local tissue scar with reduced mechanical strength can be modified with the application of the growth factors. A gene for a specific growth factor can be transferred to the injured tissue either directly or indirectly. In direct approach, vector with gene is directly injected into the injured tissue. Indirect approach utilizes cells taken by biopsy from the injured tissue, cultured in vitro, and vector is injected into the stabilized cells. This vector can be nonviral (transfection) or viral (transduction).

USE OF DIFFERENT VECTORS AND STRATEGIES FOR GENE TRANSFER IN ORTHOPEDICS

The possible main forms of gene therapy are germline and somatic cell gene therapies. Germline gene therapy has its own technical complexities, ethical issues, and possibility of transmission in future generations. Somatic gene therapy exclusively benefits the individual and cannot be passed to the next generation and is the prototype used today.

Gene therapy has been made possible by carriers or vectors that target specific tissues. These carriers are called vectors and serve as the delivery systems.

Gene delivery systems are categorized as viral-based, nonviral-based, and combined hybrid systems **(Flowchart 1)**.

- *Viral-mediated gene delivery systems* ***(Figs. 1A to C)****:* Commonly used viral vectors consist of adenoviruses **(Fig. 2)**, retroviruses, and *lentiviruses* **(Table 1)**.
- *Nonviral systems are divided into:*
  - *Physical methods:* Microinjection, electroporation, ultrasound, gene gun, and hydrodynamic applications, etc.
  - *Chemical methods:* Polymers, liposomes, dendrimers, and cationic lipid systems, etc.

There are newer viral vectors that have been developed to improve upon the existing delivery systems, such as:

- *Sendai virus (SeV) vectors:* SeV vectors have been developed as a recombinant viral vector. The RNA nature has the advantage as chromosomal integration of exogenous genes can be undesirable (as with DNA virus). They are currently being tested in regenerative medicine to reprogram cell genomes to a pluripotent state and as recombinant viral vaccines for influenza prevention.
- *Lentiviruses:* The most important advantage of lentiviruses compared with other retroviruses is their ability for gene transfer to nondividing cells. Human immunodeficiency virus (HIV)-1 is one of the most widely used lentiviral vectors.

Physical Methods

Gene Gun (Ballistic DNA Delivery or DNA-coated Particle Bombardment)

This method is based on the principle of delivery of DNA-coated heavy metal particles (gold, tungsten or silver microparticles) by crossing them from target tissue at a certain speed. The particles achieve sufficient speed due to a pressurized inert gas (generally helium).

Flowchart 1: Summary of the main methods of gene delivery systems.

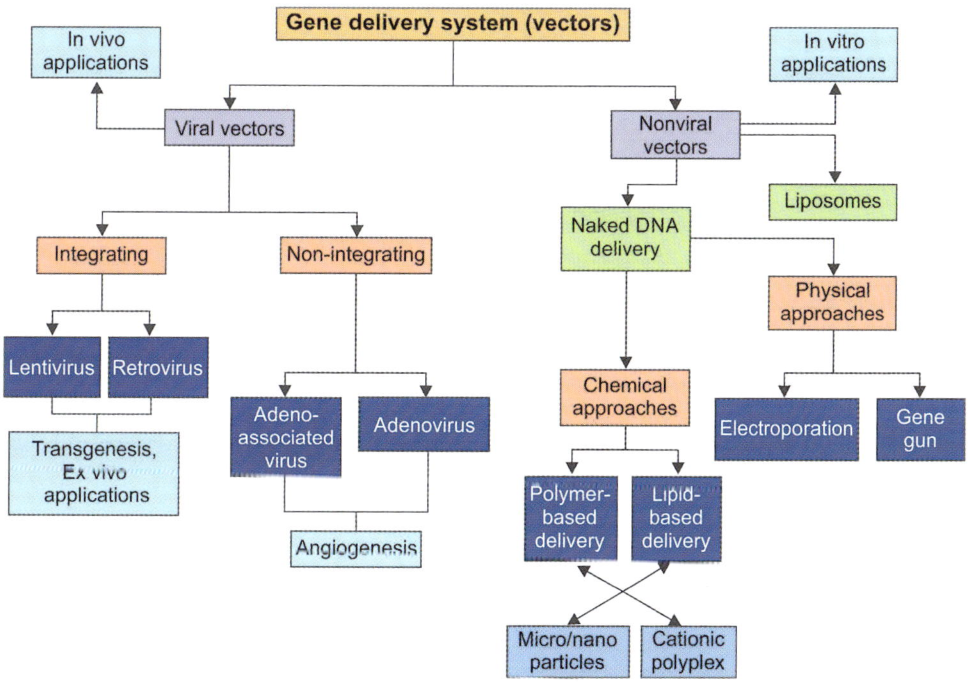

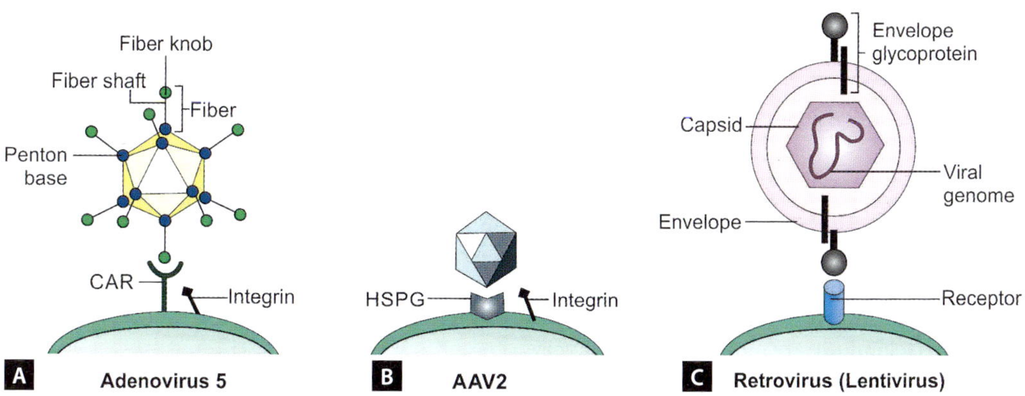

Figs. 1A to C: Some viral-based delivery systems.
(AAV: adeno-associated virus; CAR: coxsackievirus and adenovirus receptor; HSPG: heparin sulfate proteoglycan)

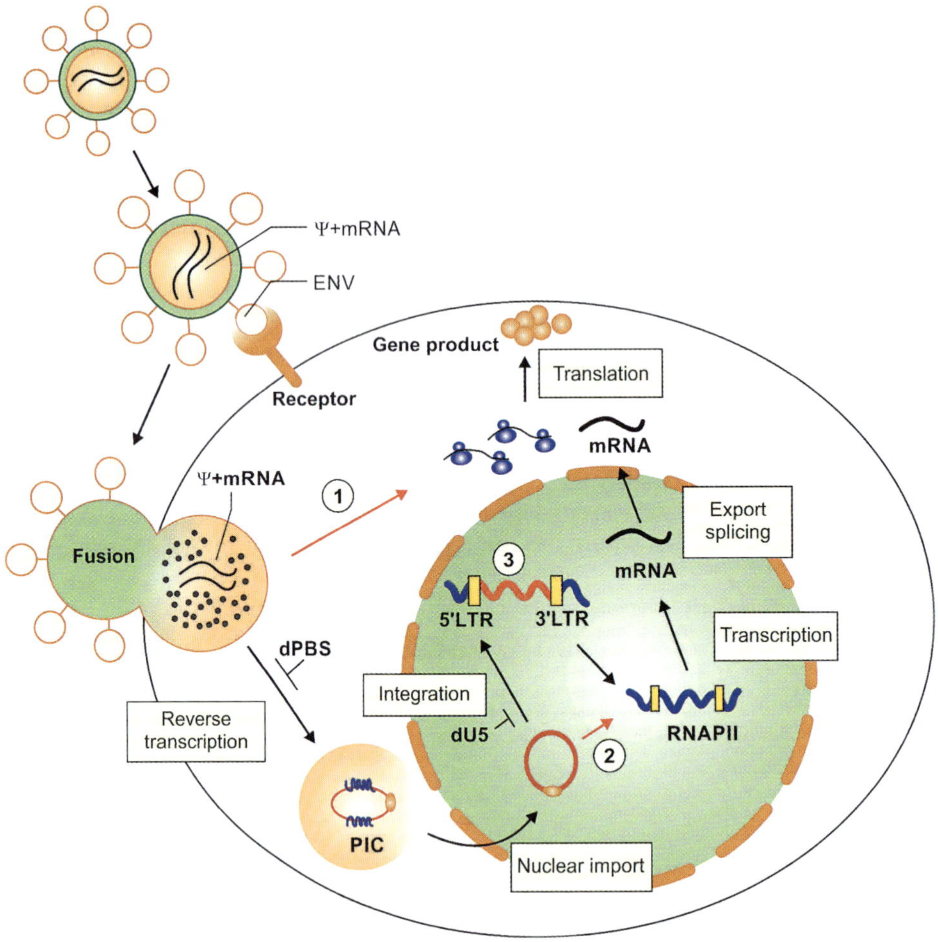

Fig. 2: Adenovirus (recombinant) enters cells via CAR-mediated internalization that involves receptor-mediated endocytosis through clathrin-coated vesicles. The adenoviral vector escapes from the endosomes, followed by disintegration, and its DNA enters the nucleus. In the nucleus, it gains an epichromosomal location and the recombinant protein is synthesized by the native/host cell machinery.

TABLE 1: Characteristics of different vectors used for gene transfer to skeletal muscle.

Vector	**Muscle cell infection capacity**				**Details**
	In vitro		***In vivo***		
	Myoblasts	***Myotubes***	***Newborn muscle fibers***	***Adult muscle fibers***	
Retrovirus	Y	N	N	N	Integrates; low toxicity/immunogenicity but infects mitotically active cells only
Adenovirus	Y	N	Y	N	Does not integrate; infects dividing and newborn cells but not mature ones; low cytotoxicity but suffers from immune rejection problems
Herpes simplex virus (type 1)	Y	Y	Y	N	Nonintegrating but has advantage of large insert capacity. It infects actively dividing cells and newborn cells but suffers from immune rejection problems
Adeno-associated virus	Y	Y	Y	Y	Integrating; low immunogenicity/cytotoxicity with high persistence of gene transfer; infects all types of muscle cells

Electroporation

Electroporation is controlled electric application to increase cell permeability. It introduces foreign genes into the cell by electric pulses. In vivo electroporation has become common in nucleic acid vaccines and improving nonviral gene therapy. The difficulties with this technique are requirement of surgery to implant electrodes in internal organs; high temperature due to high voltage application can cause irreversible tissue damage and can affect the stability of genomic DNA.

Ultrasound

In recent years, it was found that microbubbles applied by ultrasound increased gene expression. The microbubbles were modified with plasmid DNA before the injection and then ultrasound was applied.

Hydrodynamic Therapy

It uses the hydrodynamic pressure created by the injection of the large volume of DNA solution with blood pressure inside veins. The permeability of the capillary endothelium increases and pores form in the plasma membrane. DNA or other related molecules can reach the cell from these pores. Membrane pores later close retaining these molecules within the cell.

Chemical Methods

Polymers

This is a unique application of nanotechnology. Polymeric gene transporters deliver genetic material through electrostatic interactions with nanosized polyplexes for gene therapy. This system of gene delivery is based on three strategies, namely electrostatic interaction, encapsulation, and adsorption.

Some polymeric vectors are as follows:

- *Poly (L-lysine) (PLL)-based gene delivery systems:*
    - Folate-conjugated PLL
    - Sugar-conjugated PLL
    - Antibody-PLL conjugates
    - Arterial-wall binding peptide (AWBP)-conjugated PLL
    - The terplex system
- *Polyethylenimine (PEI)-based gene carriers:*
    - PEI-polyethylene glycol
    - Folate-conjugated PEIs
    - PEI conjugates with targeting moieties

Dendrimers

Dendrimers consist of star-shaped symmetrically branched macromolecules projecting from a central core **(Fig. 3)**. They have highly controllable chemical behaviors and undergo perfect encapsulation capable of carrying material within.

Cationic Lipid Compatible Systems (Lipoplexes)

The complex of DNA with lipids is called lipoplex **(Fig. 4)**. Lipoplexes electrostatically interact with the cell membrane and are then taken up. The most significant disadvantages of cationic lipids are structural instability and heterogeneity, inactivation in blood, low effectiveness due to significant degradation **(Fig. 5)**, and weak target ability when compared to other systems.

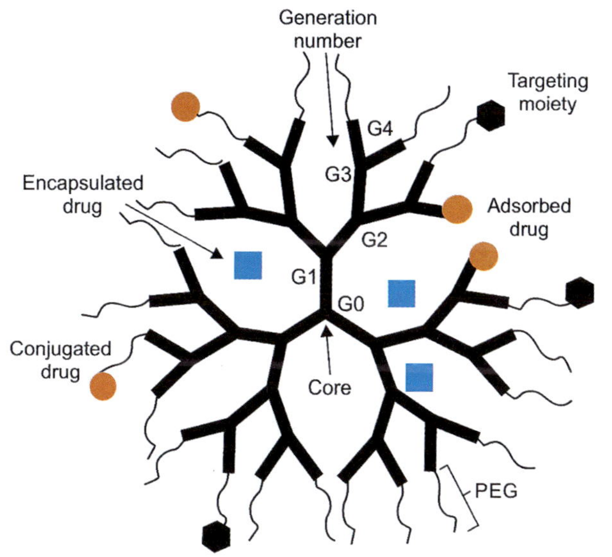

Fig. 3: Dendrimers (G = generation number, G0 = base template/core, G1 = first generation, G2 = second generation, G3 = third generation, G4 = fourth generation). Various ways of attaching the drugs are shown like encapsulation, conjugation, adsorption, etc.

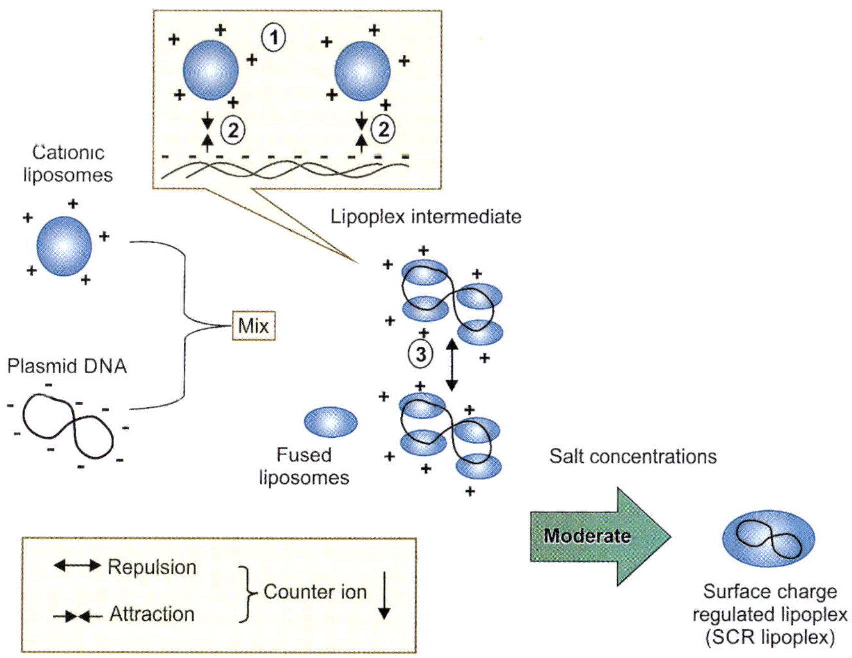

Fig. 4: Surface charge-regulated (SCR) lipoplex formation/synthesis (1—intercationic-liposomal repulsive forces; 2—liposome-plasmid DNA conjugate forces; 3—interlipoplex-conjugate repulsive forces). Forces 1, 2, and 3 are very weak in high salt concentration solutions, while very strong in nonionic solutions so not useful (not shown), only in moderate salt concentrations are SCR lipoplexes formed.

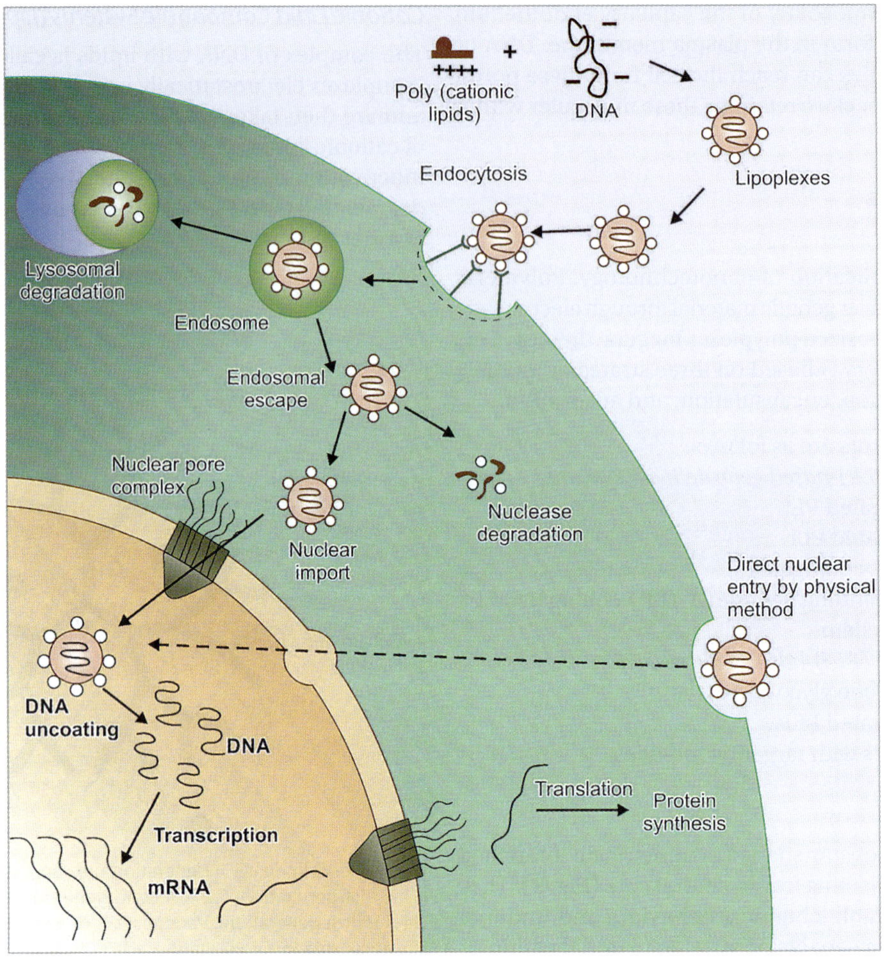

Fig. 5: Nonviral gene delivery using lipoplexes. SCR-lipoplexes are internalized through receptor-mediated endocytosis. Majority of the complexes are degraded and only a small fraction enters into the nucleus providing for desired gene expression.

Cationic Peptides/Cell-penetrating Peptides/ Trojan Peptides

They are capable of delivering therapeutic targets into cellular compartments, so they have been successfully used as efficient tools in vaccine design and gene therapy. In hope of intracellular delivery with possible use in future vaccine design, different cargos have been linked to cell-penetrating peptides (in a way similar to above), such as drugs, peptide/protein, oligonucleotide/DNA/RNA, nanoparticles, liposomes, bacteriophages, fluorescent dyes, and quantum dots.

Novel Nonviral Systems to Achieve Efficient Transgene Integrations

Transposons

Transposons are DNA sequences that work by their enzymes named transposase, with help of which they can move from one chromosomal location to another. There is a potential hope for use of transposons as gene delivery tools [in particular, the sleeping beauty (SB)]. For therapeutic strategies for various diseases, such as junctional epidermolysis bullosa, hemophilia A and B, pulmonary hypertension, glioblastoma, inherited tyrosinemia, mucopolysaccharidosis, lung transplantation-associated complications, and B-lymphoid malignancies, use of SB is the best shot at present.

Hybrid Vectors

The types of hybrid vectors are:
- Virosomes—produced by the fusion of lipoplexes with inactivated HVJ virus (hemagglutinating virus of Japan) or influenza virus
- Hybrids generated by mixing cationic liposomes or polymers with adenoviral vector
- Hybrid viruses—produced by a combination of various types of viral vectors

Bacterial Delivery Systems

The principle of their use lies in the ability of some anaerobic bacteria to selectively colonize hypoxic areas (e.g., tumors) and replicate there. Therefore, it is possible to achieve selective expression of therapeutic genes specifically in tumors.

Two groups:
1. Strictly anaerobic bacteria (*Clostridium* and *Bifidobacterium*)
2. *Salmonella typhimurium*

Eukaryotic Delivery Systems

- *Leishmania tarentolae:* A novel live vector
- *Yeast:* An efficient tool in vaccine development
- *Saccharomyces cerevisiae* (*S. cerevisiae*)
- *Hansenula polymorpha*
- *Pichia pastoris*

NEWER APPROACH: NANOPARTICLES AND NANOTECHNOLOGY

Nanoparticles (size 5–200 nm), mainly maghemite (c-Fe_2O_3) and magnetite (Fe_3O_4) nanoparticles, have emerged as a promising approach to improve the efficacy and the development of new therapies.

Quantum Dots

Quantum dots (QDs) are luminescent nanoparticles typically used for imaging in biological systems. They can also be used as transport vehicles, in photothermal therapy, and also in magnetotransfection.

Magnetic Nanoparticles (Fig. 6)

Magnetofection is a methodology based on the association of magnetic nanoparticles (MNPs) with nonviral or viral vectors in order to optimize gene delivery in the presence of a magnetic field, and to concentrate therapeutic complexes in target areas **(Figs. 7A to C)**.

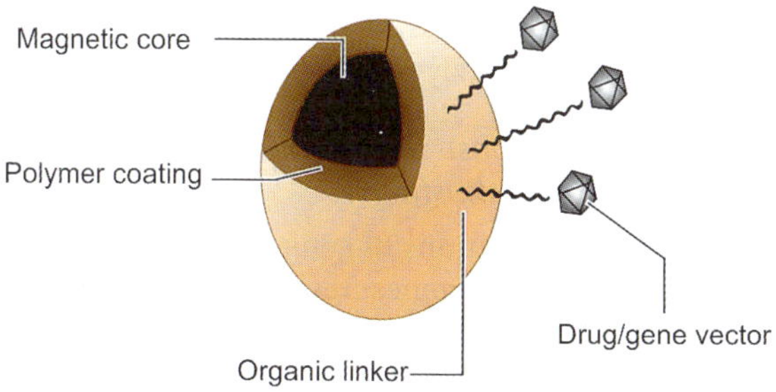

Fig. 6: Magnetic nanoparticle basic structure.

GENE THERAPY USING RNA INTERFERENCE

RNA interference (RNAi) is a phenomenon in which double-stranded RNA (dsRNA) suppresses expression of a target protein by stimulating the specific degradation of the target mRNA. It is well-known that pathological proteins or defective native proteins are responsible for the physical and dynamic malfunction in a cell contributing for many diseases. Gene therapy using RNAi should be effective in ablating protein function. RNAi mechanism eliminates the mRNAs coding for such pathological proteins. It is a form of post-transcriptional gene silencing by which gene expression can be silenced by the targeted destruction of specific mRNA molecules.

RNAi acts through short-interfering RNA (siRNA) sequences. There are various methods to deliver siRNA into the cells, such as:

- Liposome
- Naked siRNA
- Biolistics (gene gun)
- Cationic polymers and polypeptide
- Electroporation
- Microinjection
- Protein transduction domain-mediated siRNA

RNAi is on tenterhooks for:

- Treating HIV infection
- Host protein screening and controlling of viral infection
- Neurodegenerative diseases
- Immune diseases
- Cancer gene therapies

NEW VECTORS OR STRATEGIES FOR STABLE AND SAFE GENE MODIFICATION

Stable gene modification without affecting normal cellular function is a main goal for gene therapy. Currently, there are no methods that satisfy both the criteria simultaneously as either they are very inefficient (homologous recombination) but stable or very genotoxic (retroviral gene transfer) but efficient. New vectors are being preferred and designed for

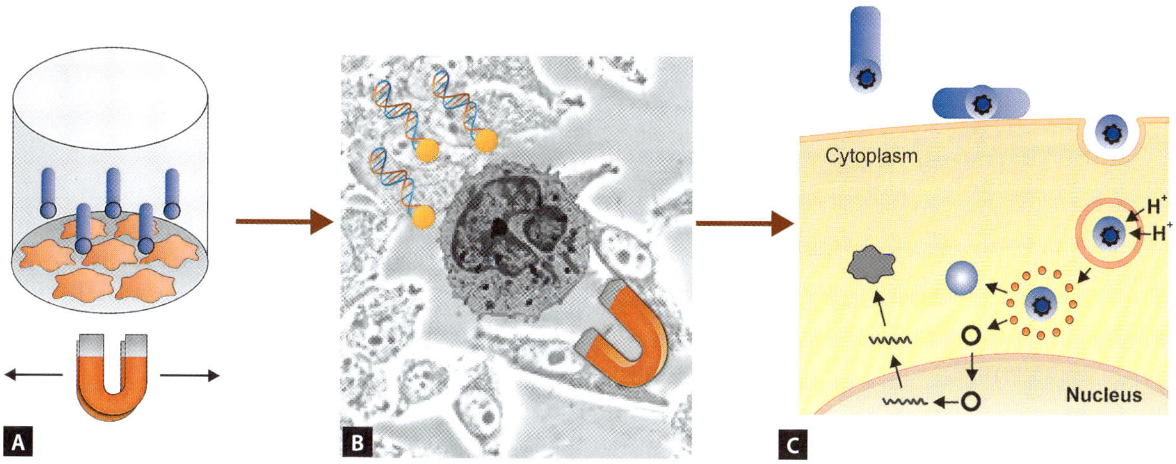

Figs. 7A to C: Oscillating magnetofection. (A) Plasmid DNA or siRNA is attached to magnet nanoparticles and placed with target cell culture system in incubator; (B) These magnetic particles are pulled by an oscillating magnet placed below the cell culture plate. The magnetic particles are endocytosed by mechanical stimulation and the endosomes rupture by proton sponge effect; (C) This releases the DNA free from which target protein is synthesized by translation.

stable expression with increased efficiency versus unregulated expression of the transgene and genotoxicity (genomic alterations due to vector integrations).

Genotoxicity of retroviral-based vectors can be improved by:
- Using alternative retroviruses for vector development
- Improving the properties of existing retroviral vectors

Alternative Retroviral Vectors

Lentiviral-based Vectors

- *HIV-1-based vectors:* HIV-1 is the most commonly used lentiviral vectors. HIV-1-based lentiviral vectors efficiently transduce the most important target cells (neurons, hepatocytes, dendritic cells). They are probably the most efficient vectors for stem cell transduction.
- *Simian immunodeficiency virus (SIV)-based vectors:* They have been used for efficient transduction of human hematopoietic stem cells (HSCs), retinal gene transfer, and the respiratory epithelium (for cystic fibrosis treatment).

Other viruses being studied for the purpose include:
- Equine infectious anemia virus (EIAV)-based vectors
- Feline immunodeficiency virus (FIV)-based vectors
- Bovine immunodeficiency virus (BIV)-based vectors
- The safety profile of various vectors has been improved by few ingenious strategies, such as:
    - Self-inactivating (SIN) vectors
    - Insulators—Genetic elements near chromatin domain boundaries that prevent inappropriate activation of a promoter by nearby heterologous enhancers
    - Improved polyadenylation signal

Gene Correction By Enhanced Homologous Recombination

Gene correction aims to repair a defective gene directly in the cellular genome by gene targeting, a process in which a DNA molecule introduced into a cell replaces the corresponding chromosomal segment by homologous recombination. This is possible now with the development of zinc finger nucleases, which can be considered custom-designed molecular scissors.

Suicide Gene Therapy by Herpes Simplex Virus-1 Thymidine Kinase

Synonyms: Gene directed enzyme/prodrug therapy (GDEPT) and gene prodrug activation therapy (GPAT)

Herpes simplex virus-1 thymidine kinase (HSV-TK) from herpes simplex viruses and cytosine deaminase (CD) from *E. coli* bacteria are the most commonly used suicidal genes at present.

GDEPT acts by either of two ways:
1. *Cell-based therapy (CBT):* Nearby cells (modified to express suicide gene) of the tumor or the tumor itself expresses the suicide gene therapy **(Fig. 8)**.
2. *Viral vectors-based therapy:* Viral vectors themselves carry the suicide gene.

Properties of suicide gene:
- The enzyme produced by the gene should be either absent or present in low concentrations (low expression) in the host.
- The enzyme should have a high catalytic activity (this property is necessary to convert a prodrug even in low substrate concentration to the active one by the tumor cells).

Types of suicide genes for therapy: Among several suicide gene therapies available, HSV1-TK and CD are important.
- HSV1-TK acts mainly through bystander effect mediated by gap junctions, which amplifies the effect of toxic drugs to several folds.
- HSV1-TK suicide gene therapy is used for glioma, prostate cancer, leukemia, and lymphoma.

Effective Transgene Constructs to Enhance Gene Therapy with Trichostatin A

One of the major limitations of gene therapy application is that the introduced transgenes frequently become silenced in the host cells. Trichostatin A (TSA), a histone deacetylase inhibitor (HDACi), enhances several promoter activities, and thereby enhances transgene expression. HDACi regulates the expression of the relevant genes of the tumor cells, by that they

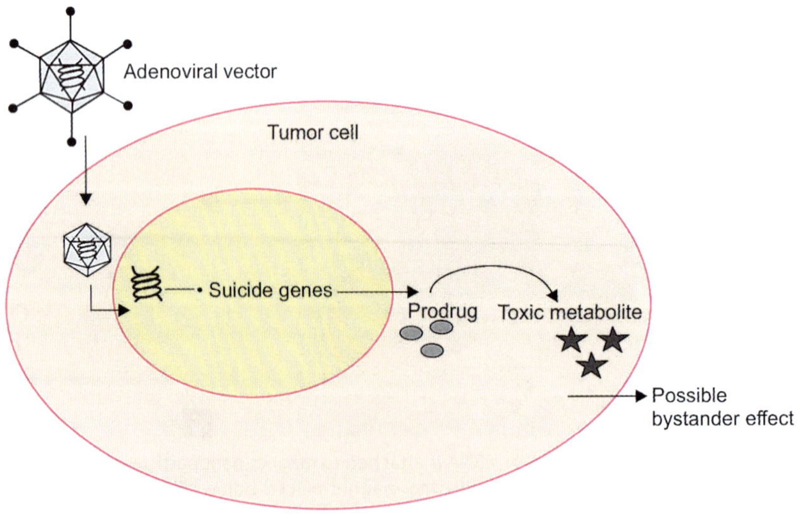

Fig. 8: Suicide gene therapy—basic mechanism.

arrest cell growth of the tumor cells, induce apoptosis, inhibit metastasis, and enhance antitumor immunity. By identifying the TSA-responsive element of the HSV-TK promoter, TSA-inducible killer constructs are developed to enhance the anticancer effects of TSA. With the use of specific delivery systems, these killer constructs can target cancer cells, and they will be beneficial for cancer gene therapy.

TARGETED GENE DELIVERY

In gene therapy, foreign genes are delivered to induce target gene expression. When target cells are distributed throughout the body, various administration routes can be chosen **(Fig. 9)** that have their own advantages and disadvantages **(Table 2)**. The most commonly used target in human body for delivery and propagation of genetic system has been the muscle tissue. Properties that make muscle tissue an appropriate target for gene therapy include:

- Facilitation and long-term expression of introduced genes
- Myogenic precursor cells (satellite cells) can be relatively easily isolated and cultivated in vitro and efficiently transduced using either viral or nonviral vectors.
- The ability of the myogenic cells to fuse with or into myofibers.

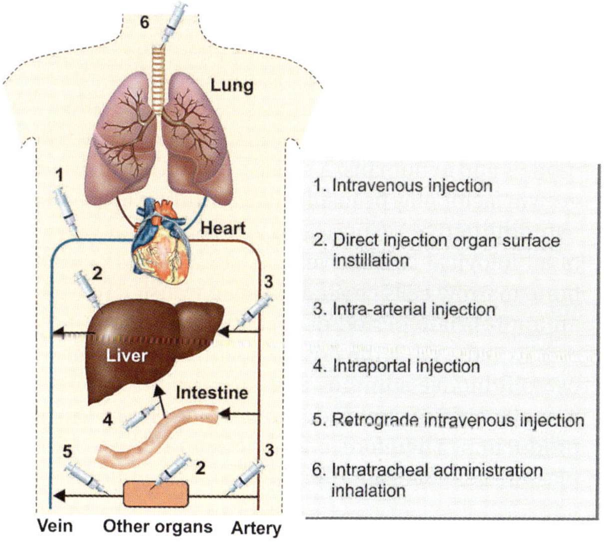

Fig. 9: Various routes of administration for delivering the gene-delivery systems.

- The high level of vascularization of muscle tissue facilitates the systemic delivery of potentially therapeutic proteins, such as growth factors, factor IX, or erythropoietin.

Strategies for Gene Transfer into Muscle

Growth factors can be transferred to the skeletal muscles directly or with the help of the gene transfer methods, including cell therapy, gene therapy or a combination of both techniques in tissue engineering approach.

Direct Injection of Human Recombinant Growth Factor Proteins

During muscle regeneration, trophic substances released by the injured muscle activate the satellite cells. Terminal differentiation of skeletal myoblasts is under control from various growth factors **(Table 3)**, such as basic fibroblast growth factors (bFGF), platelet-derived growth factor BB (PDGF-BB), and insulin-like growth factors (IGF-1 and 2). The latter is mitogenic for myoblasts. Direct injection of the recombinant proteins bFGF, NGF, and IGF-1 displays beneficial effect on muscle healing following injuries (improvement of muscle regeneration and muscle strength), but very high dosages and repeated injections are required because of their short biological half-life and rapid dissemination by the bloodstream. This deficiency can be overcome by various gene transfer methods to deliver high level of growth factors in a continuous manner.

- *Cell therapy:* The transplantation of normal myoblasts or their precursors (satellite cells) improves the muscle strength of injured muscle (laceration, contusion, and strain). However, immune rejection and the poor survival and spread of injected myoblasts after transplantation limit the success of myoblast transplantation. Gene therapy using viral or nonviral vectors to deliver genes to skeletal muscle appears to be the ideal alternative.
- *Tissue engineering based on the ex vivo gene transfer approach:* It combines myoblast transplantation and gene therapy using an autologous myoblast transfer (AMT). The injured myoblasts are cultured ex vivo, transfected or transducted with vectors and then injected into the injured muscles. It leads to persistent expression of marker gene in the injured muscle. This ex vivo technique combines cell and gene therapy. The advantage specific to this strategy

TABLE 2: Routes of administration of various vectors used for gene therapy.

Route of administration	***Advantages***	***Disadvantages***
Direct injection (preferred for skeletal muscle and orthopedic application)	Highly effective gene transfer at the target organ (minimum barriers), high selectivity	Organ trauma, limited region of distribution, frequent dosing not very feasible
Other routes for nonorthopedic applications of gene therapy		
Organ surface	Effective gene transfer, high selectivity	Need surgery and expertise
Oral	Easy administration, multiple dosing possible	Loses efficacy due to multiple barriers (epithelium, digestive fluids), very low selectivity
Intravenous	Easy administration, frequent dosing possible, nearly global distribution	Nonspecific
Intra-arterial, intraportal, retrograde intravenous	Selective delivery	Difficult administration, needs expertise
Peritoneal	Effective gene transfer	Low selectivity

TABLE 3: Effects of growth factors on the musculoskeletal system.

Growth factors	Tissue		
	Skeletal muscle	***Hyaline cartilage***	***Bone***
Insulin-like growth factor (IGF-I)	+	+	+
Basic fibroblast growth factor (bFGF)	+	+	+
Acidic fibroblast growth factor (aFGF)	+/–	ND	ND
Nerve growth factor (NGF)	+	ND	ND
Epidermal growth factor (EGF)	–	+	ND
Transforming growth factor-beta (TGF-β)	+/–	+	+
Bone morphogenetic protein (BMP-2)	ND	+	+
Chondrocyte morphogenetic protein, COMP (1,2)	ND	+	ND

(+ = positive effect; – = no effect; ND: not determinate)

is that the cells can be used as a reservoir of secreting molecules as well as a source of exogenous cells aiding the healing process.

- *Direct gene transfer approach:* The viral vectors are injected directly into the muscle without using myoblasts as intermediates. Muscle cells are successfully transduced in vitro and in vivo using intramuscular inoculation of replication defective Ad, RV or HSV carrying reporter genes. The transducibility is however, inconsistent representing a major limitation associated with AV as a gene delivery vector to skeletal muscle. The use of new generation Ad and AAV is devoid of these shortcomings.
- *Systemic gene therapy:* It is useful when the host tissue is difficult to target by direct injection. The shortcomings, however, are need of higher number of viral particles required, lack of specificity of transduction in the targeted tissue, and loss of viral particles in the reticuloendothelial system. Also, tissues displaying poor vascularity, such as meniscus and cartilage, may not be amenable to this gene therapy approach.
- *Use of magnetic nanoparticles and magnetic fields to enhance viral vector-based gene delivery:* Nowadays, the novel association of nonviral or viral vector-based gene delivery with nanotechnology is possible. Magnetofection is based on the association of MNPs with nonviral or viral vectors in order to optimize gene delivery when exposed to a magnetic field. They are commercially available for biomedical applications, such as cell separation, drug/gene delivery, magnetic resonance imaging (MRI), and hyperthermia. With this technique, manipulation of gene expression in mature skeletal muscle fibers is being made possible.

GENE THERAPY APPLICATIONS FOR THE MUSCULOSKELETAL SYSTEM

Regional Gene Therapy for Hard Tissues

Clinical approaches to a number of different diseases associated with bone and cartilage could benefit from gene therapy, such as treatment of fractures, fracture nonunions, osteoporosis, cartilage defects, OA, and rheumatoid arthritis. The specific application details are as under.

Fracture Healing and Nonunion

Approximately 5–10% of fractures heal slowly (delayed union) or do not heal at all (nonunion). The physiology of bone formation and repair is influenced by growth factors, or proteins that can regulate critical cellular functions including proliferation, differentiation, and matrix synthesis. Therefore, the transfer of the genetic sequence or cDNA for one of these growth factors (i.e., bone morphogenetic protein) could be used to enhance fracture healing or treat nonunions. The growth factors having osteoinductive properties are bone morphogenetic proteins (BMPs), transforming growth factor-beta (TGF-β), PDGF, IGF, and having osteoinductive and angiogenic both properties are FGF. LMP-1 is an osteogenic factor that is a part of the BMP pathway and is a critical regulator of osteoblast differentiation.

- LMP-1 retroviral vectors have been found to enhance fracture healing. Mesenchymal stem cells (MSCs) expressing BMP-2, TGF-β1, LMP-1, IGF-I, and growth and differentiation factor (GDF)-5 have been shown to enhance bone, cartilage, and tendon repair. MSCs can be bone marrow MSCs (BMSCs), adipose-derived stromal cells (ADSCs) or muscle-derived stem cells (MDSCs), with ADSCs having the advantage of being more readily accessible and the harvesting not involving a very painful procedure, such as a bone marrow biopsy.
- The BMPs have been demonstrated to be effective in healing intermediate size bone defects in a variety of animal models and in humans. A single exposure to an exogenous growth factor may be insufficient to stimulate an adequate osteoinductive response. However, the development of a biological cellular vehicle, such as BMP-producing bone marrow cells created via gene transfer, may provide an appropriate period of sustained production of BMP that would enable the host to adequately respond to this osteoinductive stimulus and heal the bone defect. The treatment of a nonunion does not require long-term protein production. Therefore, adenovirus and direct transfer of plasmid genes are appropriate treatment options.

Osteoporosis

The treatment for osteoporosis at this time is to use agents that will enhance bone formation. The formation and resorption of bone is tightly regulated and is partially modulated by systemic hormones. However, local growth factors or cytokines generated in the local bone cell microenvironment should have a significant influence on bone remodeling. The growth factors useful in treatment of osteoporosis are TGF-β, BMP, IGF, PDGP, and FGF. A potential method of the delivery of recombinant growth factors is to use genetically manipulated cells, such as bone marrow cells.

Cartilage Defects

In contrast to bone, chondrocytes do not possess the inherent ability to regenerate themselves. Therefore, the repair of cartilage defects results in fibrocartilage tissue rather than normal cartilage. Presently, treatment of cartilage defects includes autologous chondrocyte, drilling into subchrondral bone to facilitate migration of chondroprogenitor cells into the defect, and osteochondral allografts. However, none of these techniques has been consistently successful in producing normal hyaline articular cartilage. Growth factors known to enhance chondrogenesis are TGF-β and BMP-2. Autologous chondrocytes can be successfully harvested, grown in tissue culture with vectors containing genes for these growth factors, and reimplanted into an articular defect. The proteins secreted by transduced chondrocytes or chondroprogenitor cells could enhance cartilage repair.

Osteoarthritis

Osteoarthritis is a degenerative joint disease characterized by progressive articular cartilage destruction, formation of osseous outgrowths and bony spurs, subchondral sclerosis, and chronic inflammation. There is progressive loss of both tissue architecture and joint functionality leading to painful limited movement, disability, and an inferior quality of life. In the treatment of OA, gene therapy may also play a crucial role. Target cells in the OA joint include chondrocytes, osteocytes, cells of the synovial lining, progenitor cells, or cells of surrounding tissues (muscle, tendons, ligaments, and meniscus).

- As the pathogenesis of OA involves imbalance between normal cartilage degradative and repair mechanisms, native cartilage architecture regeneration is the prime aim to treat OA. To achieve this, the necessities are inhibition of inflammatory and catabolic pathways, which destroy the cartilage, stimulation of anabolic pathways to rebuild the matrix, inhibition of cell senescence, prevention of apoptosis, prevention of osteophyte formation, and/or influencing several of these processes.
- The treatment of OA may also require gene transfer to chondrocytes either to compensate for mutations in structural proteins of the cartilage matrix or to secrete chondroprotective agents. Human chondrocytes have been successfully transduced with an adenovirus containing the cDNA for interleukin-1 receptor antagonist (IL-1Ra) protein. It is hypothesized that IL-1Ra is chondroprotective. Developing a gene therapy strategy to treat OA is obviously more complicated than treating a focal cartilage defect. It must not only provide sustained release of growth factors that enhance matrix synthesis, but also produce cytokines that are chondroprotective and inhibit cartilage degradation. Selective anticatabolic gene products, such as inhibitors of IL-1b, TNF-α, and inhibitors of the metalloproteinases can be overexpressed through the gene therapy. Gene products with anabolic functions will enhance repair of already degraded matrix.

Rheumatoid Arthritis

Apart from disease modifying antirheumatic drugs (DMARDs), steroids, and nonsteroidal anti-inflammatory drugs, biotherapy has also been used as a treatment option for arthritis. Agents used in biotherapy include recombinant proteins, monoclonal antibodies, growth factors, and vaccines. They are but known to have serious side-effects and infrequent persistent remission.

The main purposes of using gene therapy in rheumatoid arthritis are:

- Obtaining therapeutic quantity of useful molecule without side effects that can improve symptoms or alter the course of disease.
- Obtain a prolonged expression of the therapeutic molecule that would ideally not need repeat therapy, i.e., stable expression.
- Targeting joints that are specifically resistant to the usual treatment or those that are vulnerable to fail fast if therapy is not promptly instituted.

Intra-articular gene therapy: Rheumatoid arthritis is a chronic inflammatory disease characterized by hyperplasia of the synovial lining cells with increase in WBCs in synovium and production of various inflammatory molecules, such as TNF-α, IL-1β, IFN-γ. At present, intra-articular corticoids are used to temporary relieve pain and halt the inflammatory process. But as the effect is temporary, frequent injections of corticoids are required. The aim of intra-articular gene therapy is to introduce a therapeutic gene into the articular space by injection to allow a local production of the therapeutic molecule, and thereby reducing the number of injections, the quantity of therapeutic molecules, and to target the joint resisting the usual treatment.

Ex vivo gene therapy: Cells presenting antigen (dendritic cells, macrophages or B-cells) are good candidates to regulate immune response in rheumatoid arthritis. Various cells and strategies used are:

- Dendritic cells transfected with IL-4 using adenovirus encoding FasL or with a siRNA block the production of a pathogenic molecule
- Regulatory T-cells transfected with specific TCR and FOXP3
- *Others:* Mesenchymal cells or autologous fibroblasts can be infected with a retroviral vector encoding IL-1Ra or human-like fibroblasts extract from human joints.

In vitro gene transfer: This method uses viruses to bring a therapeutic gene into the cells developed through culture system.

In vivo gene therapy: This is applied by intramuscular injection of the vectors in arthritic patients. To improve in vivo gene therapy in rheumatoid arthritis, various modalities are used, such as liposomes, electrotransfer, nanoparticle vectors, etc.

Applications of Gene Therapy to the Treatment of Spinal Disorders

Disc degeneration and nonunion/delayed union in spinal fusion are the two critical areas where gene therapy can potentially help.

1. *Applications of gene therapy to the intervertebral disc:* The intervertebral disc is made up of:
    - The nucleus pulposus having chondrocytic cells in an extensive extracellular matrix, such as proteoglycan or collagen.

- Annulus fibrosus
- Endplates connecting adjacent vertebrae

As the disc degenerates, there is loss of water from the nucleus pulposus due to loss of proteoglycans. So, the biomechanical stability of the disc jeopardizes. For degenerative disc disorders, spinal fusion is one of the main surgical treatments at present with good clinical outcomes. However, this surgery is not without problems. Various problems associated are accelerated degeneration in the disc adjacent to the fused segment, breakage of implants, and damage to the nerve tissue during the instrumentation procedure. Gene therapy is a good option to overcome these problems.

Virus vector-mediated intradiscal gene therapy: Adenovirus-mediated transfer of *TGF-β1* gene to the intervertebral disc has shown to improve the proteoglycan synthesis locally suggesting that gene therapy may have potential applications in altering the course of degenerative disc disease—a spinal disorder characterized in part by loss of proteoglycans in the nucleus pulposus. Other viral vectors useful are AAV and baculovirus.

Nonvirus vector-mediated intradiscal gene therapy: "Microbubble-enhanced ultrasound gene therapy" to the disc is a feasible and efficient technique for local gene delivery within the intervertebral disc.

Potential application of RNAi for treatment degenerated disc associated disorders: One approach to treat degenerative spinal disorder is downregulation of gene expressions that are potentially harmful for the physiological condition of the disc, and thus may induce degenerative change in the disc. This kind of approach focuses more on prophylactic treatment of disc degeneration. RNAi is known to be a powerful means of sequence-specific gene silencing and would thus be a good candidate for this new strategy.

2. *Applications of gene therapy to spinal fusion*
   Adenovirus-mediated transfer of *BMP-2* gene to the lumbosacral region has demonstrated that it is possible to produce in vivo endochondral bone formation by using direct adenoviral construct injection into the paraspinal musculature, which suggests that, in the future, gene therapy may be useful for achieving spinal fusion.
   Osteoinductive factors that can be used for gene therapy in spinal fusion are:
   i. *BMPs:* BMP2, BMP7, and BMP9
   ii. *LIM:* LIM mineralization protein-1 (LMP-1)
   iii. *NELL-1*

Consideration of Target Tissues

A consideration of the characteristics of the target tissues is one of the key points for successful gene therapy; for example, being avascular, the intervertebral disc's low oxygen tension, poor nutrition, and low pH create a biologically severe environment, especially within the nucleus pulposus. So, in vivo gene transfer methods offer greater advantages than ex vivo methods as ex vivo transfer of the cells may not survive in the severe environment of the disc. Due to avascularity of the disc, there are less chances of immune reaction, which makes it an attractive site for exogenous genes transfer mediated by adenovirus (which efficiently transduces the cells of the nucleus pulposus) and production of therapeutic growth factor proteins. Long-term gene expression may be possible with this approach.

Approaches Based on Gene Therapy to Improve Muscle Healing Following Injury

Muscle injuries are divided into two types:

1. A shearing injury, in which both the myofibers and the connective tissue framework are torn, includes lacerations, contusions, or strains, depending on the mechanism of injury.
2. An in situ injury, in which only the myofibers are damaged and the basal lamina and connective tissue sheaths are intact.

Orthopedic surgeons face two other challenging muscle conditions: The compartment syndrome and limb lengthening where there is high amount of damage to the muscular tissue and resultant scar formation.

During healing of muscle injury, myofibrils are generated from satellite cells and fibroblasts produce extracellular matrix. In extensive muscle trauma, proliferation of fibroblasts can quickly lead to an excessive formation of dense scar tissue that impedes muscle regeneration and results in an incomplete recovery. Muscle tissue's response to serious injury is thus typically formation of dense fibrotic scar tissue intervening between normal muscle fibers. Gene therapy allows for the continuous local delivery of therapeutic proteins, such as growth factors, and thereby, improving and enhancing muscle healing. The enhancement of muscle growth and regeneration, by continuous and local delivery of specific growth factors by gene therapy, may limit the formation of scar tissue, accelerate muscle recovery, and result in complete healing after severe muscle strain, laceration, and contusion. The enhancement of muscle growth and regeneration might also prevent the occurrence of contracture secondary to limb lengthening and/or compartment syndrome.

The novel approaches in the treatment of muscle injury include:

- Autologous myoblast transplantation
- Growth factors and muscle growth in vitro (the growth factors such as β-FGF, IGF-1, and NGF enhance myoblast proliferation and differentiation)
- Muscle and in vivo growth factors as above

In vivo growth factors have short half-life and their systemic clearance causes rapid clearance of the substances from the desired site. To address these issues, gene therapy may provide an interesting delivery system to the muscle that can be applied as follows. Genetic information encoding for the therapeutic protein is inserted, using nonviral and viral vectors, into living cells (see above). In turn, these genetically modified cells express the protein, encoded by the transferred DNA, in a sustained manner. By using this technology, growth factors can be delivered to the tissue locally on a long-term basis, avoiding the need for repeated injections and systemic administration.

The Potential of Gene Therapy for Osteogenesis Imperfecta

The point mutations (most common mutations in OI) that substitute conserved glycine with a charged amino acid or an amino acid having a bulky side chain that destabilizes the triple helix lead to the abnormal production of ex chains, which associate with normal chains. These are dominant negative mutations. Supplying normal genes in this situation to substitute for the defective gene hence would not correct the defect. In order for the introduced gene to be functional, the expression of the mutant allele would first have to be suppressed. This can be done by antisense therapy, which is designed to suppress the expression of the mutant allele, thus reducing the severity of the disease to that of a milder phenotype. For this approach, short molecules with a sequence complementary to the mutant RNA are employed to bind to the mutant RNA. These sequences can either cleave the target RNA themselves or target the bound site for cleavage by other enzymes. Although bone marrow stromal cells can deliver genes to the bone and that the genes can be expressed in the bone, the number of cells that persist in the bone remains quite small. Better targeting is hence necessary for which bone marrow stromal cells are being transduced with genes that direct the cells toward osteoblastic lineage. Much more progress is needed to make gene therapy for OI a reality.

Limitations of Cell and Gene Therapy: Immune Reactions

Only devising genetically appropriate and competent cells is not enough a challenge for gene therapy; there are much more challenges that limit the effectiveness and success of gene therapy. After transplantation of synthesized "genetically corrected machines", they may still stop working and be rendered useless by the immune system that can identify them as "alien".

Immune Reaction Following Cell Transplantation

Cell transplantation triggers immune responses against xenotransplantation, the major histocompatibility complex (MHC), and minor antigens and against components of the culture medium.

- *Cell xenotransplantation:* The species barrier is the greatest barrier if cells from other species are used. Though easier to obtain, they are easily rejected unless severe combined immunodeficiency is present.
- *Against MHC:* For allotransplantations; MHC incompatible myoblasts are rapidly rejected due to immune reaction, which can be partially controlled by immunosuppression.
- Against minor antigens of the cells which are being transplanted
- *Against components of the culture medium:* Culture medium usually contains animal serum that produces immune reaction. This reaction is like the Rh system sensitization where first transplantation may not be problematic, but it may cause failure of the second and subsequent transplantations.
- *Against the normal gene product introduced by transplantation:* This is most interesting and is like immune reaction to native vitreous. The genes transferred by the cell transplantation produce a normal protein to which immune tolerance has never developed in the individual due to nonexposure. Being a new protein in the body, immune reaction occurs against this protein!

Immune Reaction Following Gene Therapy

Immune responses have been detected against the viral coat, proteins produced by the vector genome itself, the therapeutic gene product, the product of the selection gene, and the marker gene.

- *Against the viral coat:* Every viral vector contains a coat (capsid) made of proteins that represent a new antigenic source. Immune reaction against these proteins usually does not affect the first transplantation, but it reduces the effectiveness of subsequent transplantations. The solution is to ingeniously change the serotype of the vector for the following administration (like the changing serotype of influenza virus in every pandemic).
- *Against the viral vector proteins:* This is the immune response against the viral gene products that are produced by the vector native gene.
- *Against the therapeutic gene product:* Expression of the transgene will lead to the presence of a protein that was either completely absent or truncated in the patient (no immune tolerance), leading to immune reaction against this protein.
- *Against the selection gene:* In bacteria-based gene therapy, the vectors are chosen on the basis of a selection gene usually present in the plasmid. These selection genes may produce new proteins, antigenic to the body, producing immune reaction, which may jeopardize the success of gene therapy.
- *Against the marker gene:* The product of marker gene is usually a new protein that produces immune reaction. The solution (bit difficult) is to introduce a marker gene expressed in a different tissue of the host.

Composite Solution to the Immune Problems

There are two major solutions to these immune problems:
1. Immunosuppression
2. Developing immune tolerance

Immunosuppression:
- Immunosuppression with drugs—cyclosporine and tacrolimus
- Immunosuppression with antibodies against the proteins involved—anti-CD4, anti-CD8, and anti-LFA-1 antibodies
- Immunosuppression with recombinant proteins like one that blocks the interaction between CD28 present on the T-lymphocyte and B7 present on antigen presenting cells
- Introduction of an immunosuppressing gene with a vector

Development of tolerance: Tolerance is the absence of an active rejection against transplanted tissue without any immunosuppressive agent. Different strategies for that are injection of antigen in the thymus, oral antigen presentation, treatments with various antibodies, and recombinant proteins.

- *Injection of antigen or vector in the thymus:* Injection of antigens into the thymus leads to the removal of any new lymphocytes that could react with foreign substances. One needs to destroy existing lymphocytes in the body however (using antilymphocyte serum).
- *Development of oral tolerance:* Oral presentation of antigen induces tolerance or energy (i.e., inactivation) of the lymphocytes that recognize the antigenic substance.
- *Treatments with antibodies:* Monoclonal antibodies are used to block the interactions between antigen-presenting cells (APCs) and helper T-lymphocytes (such as using anti-CD154 treatment following islet transplantation).
- *Treatments with recombinant proteins:* The interaction between APCs and lymphocytes can also be blocked with recombinant proteins that react with the surface proteins involved.
- *Immunoprotection of the transplanted cells:* Cells can be hidden from the immune system by encapsulation. Pore size formed by the polymers are so set that they prevent infiltration by macrophages and lymphocytes but large enough to permit diffusion of the secreted protein.
- *Autologous transplantation of cells:* Transplantation of inducted patients own cells back into them.

Both cell transplantation and gene therapy have barriers of the immune system. Although immunosuppression with drugs provides immediate control, it is not an ideal solution. Development of tolerance toward the new antigens would be an ideal solution as by the use of anti-CD154 antibody that may be a reality soon.

CONCLUSION

- Gene therapy is a newly emerging field that holds promise for future, especially in the management of genetic disorders.
- The success currently is limited in this technique to obtain complete cure; however, introduction of advanced technologies and techniques emerging rapidly has obtained good response in animal models.

CHAPTER

19

Wound Ballistics

Manish Kumar Varshney

INTRODUCTION

Wound ballistics is the science that studies the effects of penetrating projectiles on the body (most of it involved concepts of physics as studied in laboratory-simulated environment). It studies the reaction of the body to projectiles and the interaction of wounding agents (such as bullets and fragments from explosive weapons) with tissue **(Fig. 1)**. Ballistic trauma is the term used to describe the pathophysiological reaction of the body to the physical process and includes blood loss, shock, wound infection, and death. Ballistic trauma is more relevant to a physician, but few terminologies must be understood to grasp the concepts involved.

Projectile: Any object, such as a bullet or fragment that passes through air or tissue. (The use of term in military parlance is different and would include any munition, such as even a shell or a mortar that travels through air and then blast dispersing fragments).

Bullet: Specifically refers to the projectile that accelerates through the barrel, exits the muzzle, and flies through the air to hit target.

Caliber: This is the measured width down to precision of millimeters of the inside of the barrel (and therefore, in most cases, the width of the bullet).

Cartridge: The cartridge case, the propellant (gun powder), and the bullet.

Fragment: This is the term used for part of an explosive munition, which becomes a projectile once munition detonates. The parent weapon may be specifically designed to eject fragments, or else the fragments may result from pieces of the munition generated from blast/detonation and propelled away by sheer force of the explosion.

Twist: The spiral grooves on the inside of the barrel of a gun, which imparts spin on the bullet, so giving it stability in flight.

Twist length: The distance for one turn of the spiral groove. "Low twist" indicates a long twist length.

Wound profile: Conceptual tool for giving a visual impression of the length, shape, and dimensions of the whole track of the bullet or fragment.

Firearm injuries produce damage to the living tissues by two discrete but contiguous mechanisms producing different effects on human body **(Fig. 2)**.

- *Permanent cavitation:* Crush due to rapidly applied pressure surpassing the ability of tissue to expand.
- *Temporary cavitation:* Stretch due to pressure applied at moderately slow speeds on elastic tissues.

Amount of tissue damage and severity of gunshot injuries are due to the energy transmitted by the bullets or projectiles. After a projectile hits the skin, it creates a permanent cavity and small amount of necrosis comparable to the dimensions of the projectile. The tissue around the permanent tract stretches due to its elastic nature and forms a temporary

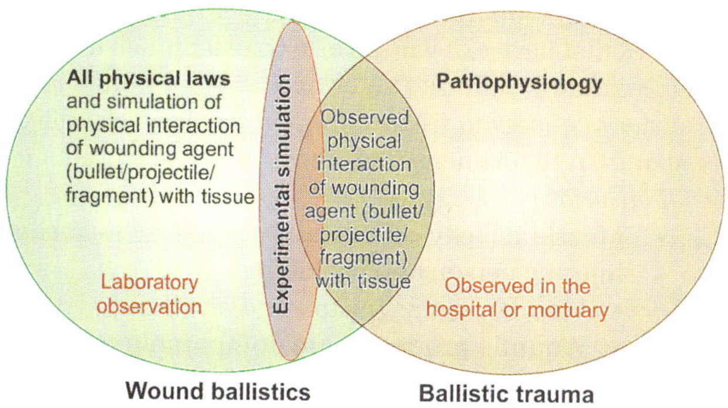

Fig. 1: Wound ballistics versus ballistic trauma.

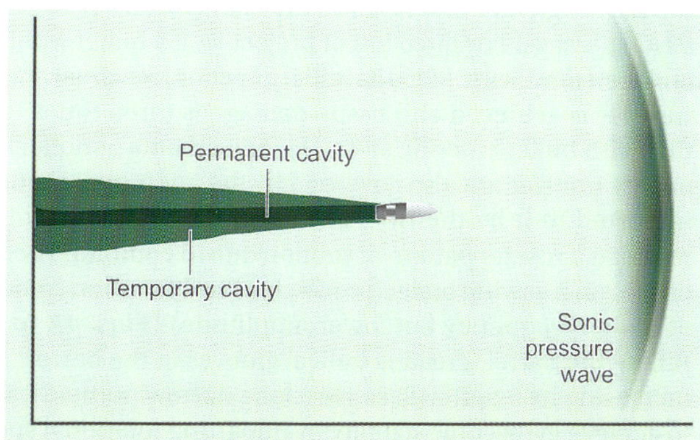

Fig. 2: The two mechanisms of tissue damage by projectiles.

cavity; this area appears grossly as bruised or contused tissue. There is a transient increase in pressure for a few milliseconds; in contrast to soft tissue, the inelastic tissue like the bone may fracture. Preceding the projectile in the tissue, a shock wave of the magnitude of speed of sound, the "sonic wave", hits the tissue and generates enormous pressures **(Fig. 2)**. The sonic pressure wave forms a hemispherical arc ahead of the advancing bullet. The short-lived (2 μm) sonic pressure pulse created may reach pressures of up to 100 atm. This sonic wave has no damaging effect on tissues.

If a bullet fragments, then multiple permanent paths are formed, which along with the stretch of the temporary cavity may increase the effective size of the permanent cavity. If the muzzle of a firearm is in contact with a living body when it is fired, the high-pressure gas that pushes the projectile out of the barrel will pass into the tissues through the hole formed by the projectile—often causing greatly increased tissue displacement and disruption **(Fig. 3)**.

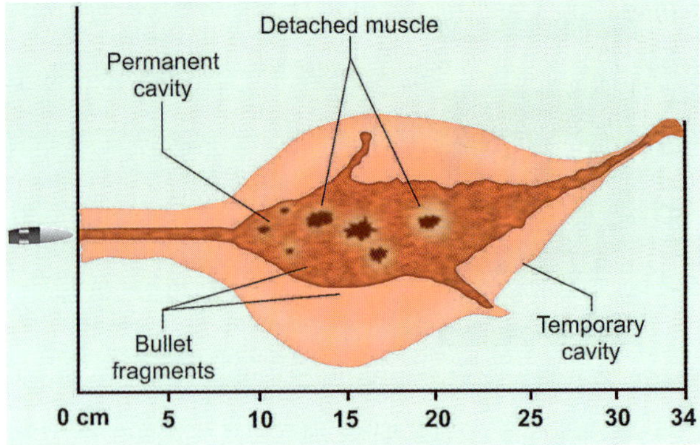

Fig. 3: Cavitation effect of projectile with secondary tracts from fragments.

CLASSIFICATION

When a projectile passes through the tissue, it causes the tissue to move away from the front and sides of the projectile due to pressure wave created by the impact. This causes tissue laceration and injury by crush. The depth to which the projectile penetrates the tissue causing laceration and the amount of crush produced are governed primarily by the kinetic energy available in the projectile to do this work. The amount of kinetic energy is denoted by the well-known equation:

$$E \text{ (joules)} = 1/2\, mv^2$$

(where, m = mass in kg; v = velocity in m/s)

Other theories realize the transfer of energy in the form of momentum (= mv) or power (based again on mv). Now, as the amount of energy is dependent heavily on velocity of the projectile so, injuries have been classically classified on the basis of velocity. The velocity of the M-16 bullet is thrice that of the 0.22 bullet. This explains why although M-16 has almost the same caliber and mass as the 0.22, its kinetic energy is almost 10 times than the 0.22. The energy transfer is also affected by the tissue involved in the projectiles tract (related to the density and rigidity of the tissue), direction of projectile (defined by rotation axis and yaw), and projectile characteristics (regular shape or hollow-point, copper or lead cover, metal or rubber projectile). The higher the rigidity of the tissue, greater and faster is the energy transfer to cause tissue damage. For direction of projectile, if a bullet wobbles and then tumbles to 90° to its initial direction, maximal energy transfer is achieved and tissue damage is three times than that with bullet entering at 0°. The movements of bullet and energy transfer are also governed by the additional motions imparted to it by the rifle. For example, projectiles often rotate in a rosette pattern of motion due to combined action of spin on a yawing bullet (precession) and nutation (motion of higher frequency but lower amplitude) **(Figs. 4A to C)**. Rifling the barrel (creating helical grooves in the barrel) and increasing its length will cause a long narrow pointed bullet to achieve gyroscopic stability by imparting rotational speed

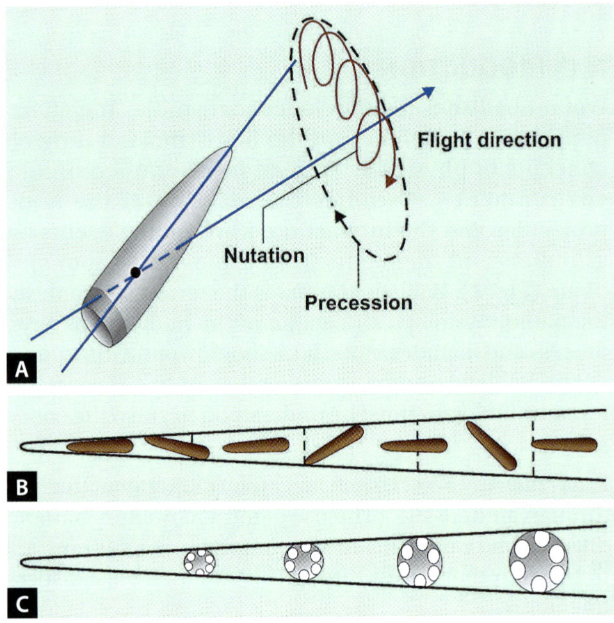

Figs. 4A to C: (A) The direction of bullet and aberrations in it depicting the precession and nutation; (Precession, B) Demonstration of the bullet motion in a rosette pattern due to an action of spin on a yawing bullet; (Nutation, C) Combined with a second complicated motion of higher frequency and lower amplitude.

of 1,500–6,000 rotations per second to the bullet in flight and reducing the tumble. Prescoring bullet so that it fragments at impact (dumdum bullet, declared inhumane now and banned), hollow-tip bullet, etc. have been used to increase energy transfer. Hollow-point or soft-point bullets mushroom upon impact imparting higher energy to the tissues. Bullet injuries that have exit wound also transfer much less energy than retained bullets. The current system hence realizes transfer of energy to tissues from projectile so classification systems based on energy transferred should be used.

- *Low velocity/energy:*
  - Muzzle velocity <350 m/s or <2,000 feet/s—meant for injuring person and not killing:
    - Most handguns (pistols and revolvers)
    - Wounds produced are comparable to Gustillo-Anderson type I or type II due to low energy transfer.

- *Intermediate velocity/energy:*
  - These weapons impart muzzle velocity of 350–500 m/s to the bullet.
  - Shotgun blasts are typical example, magnums also reach this velocity.
    - The wound profile varies according to the firing distance from target.
    - If fired from close range (<21 feet), severe tissue trauma results that reproduces wounding potential of high velocity firearms. Same pattern may result from multiple intermediate-velocity shots fired.
    - Wound contamination is common due to shotgun wadding and causes infection when close ranges are used to fire.
    - Wounding potential of projectile depends on three major factors:
      1. Shot pattern
      2. Load (size of individual pellet)
      3. Distance from target.
- *High muzzle velocity (high kinetic energy):*
  - These are usually military grade weapons having muzzle velocity >600 m/s or >2,000 feet/s
  - Military rifles/assault rifles
  - Due to high energy transfers from the projectile, the wounds produced are comparable to Gustillo-Anderson type III even if the size on superficial inspection is small.
  - They have high risk of infection due primarily to contaminants sucked in during impact and traversal through tissue. Also responsible is the wide zone of injury and tissue necrosis that results from blast effect.

Effect of Projectiles on Various Tissues

The skin around wounding site exhibits vasospasm, which produces blanching; this area usually does not get revascularize for several hours after injury. An impact velocity of only 150 170 feet/s is required to penetrate skin. Cherry-hue appearance is a clue to close-range injury of underlying muscle due to carboxyhemoglobin, formed by carbon monoxide released during combustion. If the loss of blood supply is a criterion for excision, the transitory nature of the blanching shows that viable tissue would be sacrificed in this area if evaluated soon after wounding.

The muscle that is touched by the projectile in the permanent tract has a microscopic rim of tissue that is actually necrotic. If the blood supply to the muscle remains intact, it can heal over time without surgical intervention. The area of cell death sloughs and, as long as the wound can drain, will heal up spontaneously.

Microscopically, there are disrupted skeletal muscle fibers and capillaries. After a period, there is leukocyte infiltration followed by inflammation and healing.

Bony injury: Gunshot injuries to the extremities are usually associated with bony injuries (fracture). There are two mechanisms of fractures occurring, first and commonly when the projectile strikes bone directly or, rarely, indirectly by the temporary cavitation.

1. Direct fractures occur when a projectile strikes the bone. Because of the density and relative inelastic behavior of bone, fracture line propagation may occur well beyond the area crushed by the projectile itself, leading to bone comminution and the production of secondary missiles from the bone itself. Because the secondary missiles of bone disrupt tissue before it is stretched by the temporary cavity, this has the effect of increasing comminution around the bullet path, and might even cause increased soft-tissue disruption, reminiscent of the previously mentioned synergism between bullet fragmentation, and temporary cavity stretch.
2. Indirect fractures may occur when a projectile passes close to the bone in soft tissue and a strain occurs to such a degree as to cause a fracture. Indirect fractures are almost always simple. Clinically, indirect fractures to bone are rare compared with those formed when bone is struck directly by the projectile. They may be of further two types:
   i. *Divot fractures:* These are eccentric perforations of a diaphyseal long bone, they may be occult complete fractures.
   ii. *Drill hole:* It occurs when a bullet or its fragment completely pierces both the cortices, with minimal comminution around the bullet tract. More extensive injury may be present than apparent on plain radiographs, such fractures may be treated as complete fractures unless confirmed by computed tomography (CT).

   The amount of tissue destruction does not depend solely on the muzzle velocity but also on the fragmentation of the bullet; a metal jacketed bullet of same muzzle velocity may cause less tissue damage as compared to a solid lead bullet that may fragment after striking the target.

The possible sources of contamination of wound include:
- Combination of soil, clothing, etc., carried by the projectile. High energy fragments tend to shred the clothes that are then carried into the wound by temporary cavitation
- Skin
- The bullet shell
- The barrel of the gun
- Peripheral material in contact with the wound—although less common, from the exit wound, the vacuum in the temporary cavity pulls foreign material into the wound.

SOFT-TISSUE WOUND MANAGEMENT

Patient Evaluation

Always to emphasize, it should be a thorough history taking and physical examination. The injured extremity should be inspected for both entrance and exit wounds after all clothing has been removed. The limb should also be inspected for swelling, deformity or shortening, and ecchymosis. The limb should be palpated for crepitus. Any neurovascular injury should be ruled out. In an awake patient, assessment should also be done to assess the patient's cognition, motor and sensory status.

Standard radiographs should be taken of the injured limb covering the path of the bullet. Standard long bone radiographs, including both the joint above and below, should be done if included in the bullet's path. If a joint wound is suspected, standard views should be taken of the joint.

Skin Injuries

Gunshot skin wounds have three general patterns:

1. A punctate wound about the size of the penetrating bullet
2. Splits in the skin but has negligible skin loss and can eventually be closed without resorting to more extensive skin grafting or flap coverage
3. Wound in which there is skin loss, which requires the use of partial thickness skin grafting or flap coverage.

Perforating nonarticular wounds without a fracture or vascular injury may be candidates for outpatient treatment. Under controlled circumstances, simple perforating wounds have been shown to heal uneventfully with dressings. Likewise, successful treatment of simple fractures associated with minimal soft-tissue disruption has also been treated with local wound care and fracture stabilization in a cast or splint.

Simple splits in the skin are produced from dilation resulting from the temporary cavity, from a projectile that is traveling sideways and presenting the long axis of the bullet to the skin, or from bone becoming a secondary missile, causing a more extensive wound. The splits produce an exit wound that will allow for free drainage of the wound, preventing the formation of an abscess or a hematoma.

More extensive wounds with skin loss may be produced from shotgun pellets, bullets, or bone fragmentation. Initial treatment of more extensive wounds should be done in the operating room. Longitudinal incisions of the skin and underlying fascia to relieve pressure, remove hematoma and debris, and expose the underlying muscle should be done. Surgical removal of the skin is rarely indicated at the initial surgery, other than trimming irregular edges. As described earlier, blanching may give a false impression of nonviable skin if seen soon after injury and lead the surgeon to excise viable skin.

Skeletal Muscle Injuries

One of the most controversial aspects in caring for gunshot wounds is the treatment of skeletal muscle. Excision of tissue has been recommended for skeletal muscle that would not survive. Viability of the muscle depends on the four "C"s—the color, consistency, contractility, and circulation. A thorough wound debridement and postoperative drainage from the wound will allow it to heal. The wound may be enlarged through use of longitudinal skin incisions. A simple analogy for surgeons is, "muscle that looks like hamburger should be excised, and muscle that looks like steak should stay."

The term débridement is derived from the French verb "*débrider*", which means "to unbridle or release".

Hampton had a similar description: "Debridement of any wound is designed to relieve the area of excessive tension, rid it of dead tissue and massive hematoma, and provide excellent drainage".

Compartment syndrome may occur after a gunshot injury; it may be due to expanding hematoma or displaced fracture, so relieving tension is very important. Diagnosis is primarily clinical. Whenever a compartment syndrome is suspected, fasciotomy may be performed to relieve the compartment pressure.

WOUND INFECTION

Infection has been documented in between 1.5% and 5% for those who sustain gunshot injury. Bullet wounds are contaminated wounds. Bullets themselves, when fired, do not become "sterile" because of the heating and friction encountered in the barrel. Possible sources of contamination are listed in **Box 1**. Wounds from explosive munitions have a higher rate of infection than those from gunshot wounds alone.

Risk factors for fracture site infections were found to be the presence of open drains, amputations, multisystem injury, and a fractured femur.

Proper antibiotic should be used to cover for preliminary contamination. Usually a combination of first-generation cephalosporin and aminoglycoside is prescribed.

JOINT INJURY

Gunshot injuries of the joint are associated with a high morbidity compared with other gunshot wounds. Intra-articular injuries may result in arthritis secondary to trauma as well as through the degenerative effects of lead itself. While elevated serum lead levels may be present with extra-articular gunshot wounds, the most common reports are with intra-articular wounds.

Pathophysiology of Lead Toxicity

Lead is soluble in synovial fluid and has been shown to induce lead synovitis and degenerative arthritis. Retained intra-articular bullets not only cause lead synovitis and arthritis but also can cause systemic lead poisoning. Animal studies have demonstrated significant articular degeneration with implantation of lead into rabbit knees compared with controls. Early changes (1–2 weeks) include synovial hyperplasia, mild inflammation, and articular surface slit formation. Late changes (3–6 weeks) include giant cells and foreign particles (lead and bone fragments) in the synovium, focal chondrocyte proliferation, duplication of the tidemark, and chondrocyte

BOX 1: Possible sources of contamination in a projectile wound.

The possible sources of contamination of wound include:

- Combination of soil, clothing, etc., carried by the projectile. High-energy fragments tend to shred the clothes that then are carried into the wound by temporary cavitation
- Skin
- The bullet shell
- The barrel of the gun
- Peripheral material in contact with the wound—although less common, from the exit wound, the vacuum in the temporary cavity pulls foreign material into the wound

columnar disorganization. Implantation of lead pellets into rabbit knees induces significantly greater degeneration in the femoral and tibial articular surfaces, medial and lateral meniscus, and synovium at 4, 6, 10, and 14 weeks.

Normal blood lead levels for adults are 0–19 µg/dL. Nearly 95% of the lead storage in the body occurs in the bone. The half-life of lead in the bloodstream is <2 months compared with 20–30 years in the bone.

Principles of Management

Lead is still the major component of both rifle and handgun bullets, and it may be a potential source of lead poisoning. Steel shot has replaced lead in many areas of the world in an attempt to reduce the lead burden on wildlife. Bismuth shot is also being used as a lead replacement in Canada. Modern shotguns, therefore, may be firing steel rather than lead shot. Regardless of whether the projectile is known to be lead, trauma from a bullet, pellet, or fragment will still have adverse consequences for the joint. Because of this, all intra-articular projectiles should be removed. Thorough irrigation and debridement of the joint cavity are necessary to remove all the foreign material, including fragments of skin and clothing.

A perforating wound through a joint cavity, even with the absence of fracture, should undergo surgery. Clothing and other debris from the outside may be aspirated into the joint. Also, cartilage damage is common despite the normal radiographic appearance of the joint.

In most cases where articular and periarticular fractures are present, the stabilization of the fractures is carried out initially with spanning external fixation, followed by repeat irrigation and debridement 48–72 hours later and definitive internal fixation once adequate debridement has been achieved.

Arthroscopy has been described as a technique for treating patients with intra-articular bullet injures of the shoulder, elbow, hip, and knee. Advantages of this technique include better visualization of the joint surface and the ability to more easily repair osteochondral fragments, ligaments, or knee meniscus. Disadvantages include increased operative and setup time as well as potential compartment syndrome.

INTERNATIONAL HUMANITARIAN LAW

It is a set of rules expected to be followed worldwide that attempts to limit the effects of armed conflicts that are unfortunately rampant in this world. The guidelines attempt to seek humanitarian reasons for restricting the mutilation and show respect to individuals even during wartimes (though true humanity would lie in peace). The law seeks to preserve and pleads to follow humanity putting forward the guiding principle that even in war there are limits. The law attempts to protect persons not currently engaged or who are no longer in armed conflict directly or indirectly. It also places prohibitions on the use of some weapons and warfare methods that are considered unethical and mutilating in wartimes. International humanitarian law is ideally applied to all parties without any discretion or declaration that engage in armed conflict. There is no location-wise restriction and law applies to any conflicts that may be international (between at least two States) or within a country (like revolts and upsurge). There is also no concern to the causes of the conflict or persons starting it, the law is expected to be followed equally. International humanitarian law is now deemed primary tool available for safeguarding the rights and dignity of people in wartime. Some specific details of the law are as under:

- The law obliges parties involved in armed conflict to give safe passage to medical and healthcare personnel and protect them. It also abides to take care of the wounded and sick. To protect the prisoners of war and civilian population is also the duty of combatants.
- Any armed conflict should refrain from attacking civilians and organizations such as schools and hospitals. There is no reason/justification for doing the same and instead the combatants should provide them with protection. It is required for the combatants to distinguish the civilians and to this effect, the use of any weapon(s) (like biological weapons) or methods of warfare, which have indiscriminate effects and cannot be targeted at specific military objectives, is prohibited.
- The weapons that by virtue of their design cause severe injuries against combatants are prohibited. This is based on the based rationale to prevent "superfluous injury or unnecessary suffering".
    - One of the earliest international humanitarian law treaties dealt with the design-dependent effects of bullets. In the St Petersburg Declaration of 1868, States responded to the development of bullets designed to explode within the human body by renouncing "the use, in time of war, of explosive projectiles under 400 grams weight". The preamble to this Declaration affirms that the only legitimate objective of war is to weaken the military forces of the enemy. It therefore stated that in war it is "sufficient to disable the greatest possible number of men". This objective would be exceeded by the use of weapons, which "uselessly aggravate the sufferings of disabled men, or render their death inevitable."
    - In 1899, States adopted the Hague Declaration Concerning Expanding Bullets. This was "inspired by the sentiments which found expression" in the St Petersburg Declaration. The Declaration prohibited "the use of bullets which expand or flatten easily in the human body, such as bullets with a hard envelope. which does not entirely cover the core or is pierced with incisions (dumdum bullets)".

BLAST INJURIES

In a bomb explosion, the chemical or physical (nuclear) reaction converts solid or fluid explosive material into gas accompanied by high temperature of exothermic reaction that further expands the gas resulting in high pressures. This when let free causes a blast wave that has initial speeds of approximately 6,000–7,000 km/s. The pressure difference between environment's pressure and blast's "overpressure" determines strength of blast and its potential to cause damage. Conventional chemical explosives produce thin (a few millimeters thick) pressure pulse waves that travel at supersonic speed from starting point. These are characteristically short duration positive waves that rapidly ascend in pressure followed by a prolonged negative wave. The pressure then falls below ambient air pressure creating vacuum effect that sucks surrounding debris, contaminating the wound. In controlled environment an open-air explosion, Friedlander waveform describes the blast wave **(Fig. 5)**. Effects are altered if the same explosion happens in an enclosed space magnifying the effects. This is due to reflection of primary waves from the walls and causing secondary damage rather than getting weakened in an open area. In water (or other liquid), the energy transmitted by blast wave is higher as there is little if any attenuation due to incompressible nature of fluid. The pressure wave is transmitted without absorption as it is over a longer distance. The harmful effects of an explosion in water are seen to a much longer distance than the same explosion occurring in air. The potential for damage from explosion depends on:

- The size of the charge/explosive
- Depth of detonation
- Distance from the target.

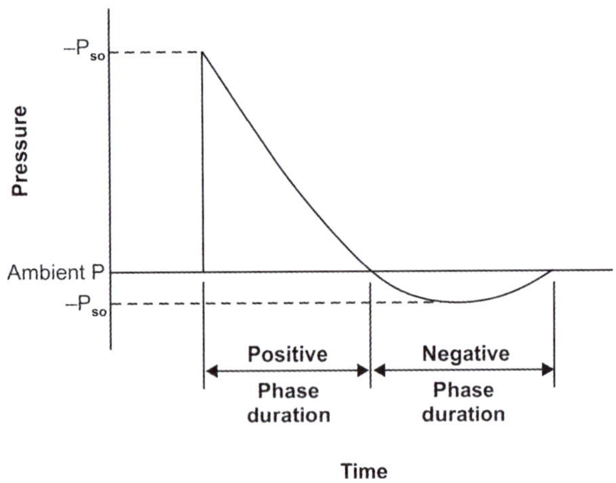

Fig. 5: Friedlander waveform.

The Shrapnel's effect is however diminished in water as the energy of shrapnel is lost prominently in water. Blast injuries mechanisms of tissue damage are categorized into primary, secondary, tertiary, or miscellaneous **(Fig. 6)**.

- The *primary injury mechanism* from blast wave results from direct injury especially to the air-filled organs, viz. lungs, small and large bowels, and auditory system.
  The primary injury results possibly through:
  - Direct compressive effects **(Fig. 7)**
  - Spilling—here the denser tissue fragments migrate into rarer tissue as the blast wave advances
  - Implosion—in implosion, the gas pockets contract momentarily followed by rapid re-expansion
  - Simultaneous development of stress and shear forces because of differential response of tissues to forces causing tissue injury
  - Pathophysiologic alterations, such as elevations in the plasma arachidonic acid metabolites—thromboxane A, prostacyclin, and leukotrienes.

  The primary blast effect decreases inversely ($1/r^3$) to the distance.
- In *secondary mechanism*, the fragments from the bomb (Shrapnel) or the surrounding environment cause blunt and penetrating injury. This causes mild or severe injuries to many of the survivors from the primary blast effect and the span of damage may involve up to two-thirds of the survivors.
- In *tertiary mechanism*, the blast wave propels the subject into another causing injury. The Shrapnel's continues longer to larger perimeter due to kinetic energy ($1/2\ mv^2$) in contrast to the primary blast effect.

Other relative mechanisms of injury are exposure to dust, thermal burns from an explosion, or burns from fires started by the blast, and inhalation of noxious fumes. The perimeter of direct blast injury is much smaller (due to fast attenuation mentioned above) than the shrapnel zone (secondary) injury, which reaches initial velocities of 6,000 m/s **(Fig. 8)**. These bomb fragments/Shrapnel (screws, pins, balls, or from other materials such as rubber, wood, plastics, and ceramics) are

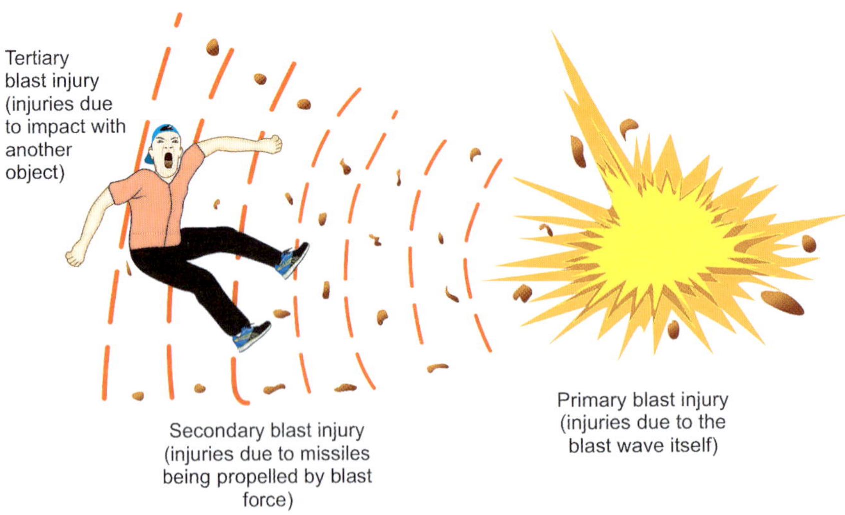

Fig. 6: The three mechanisms of blast injuries.

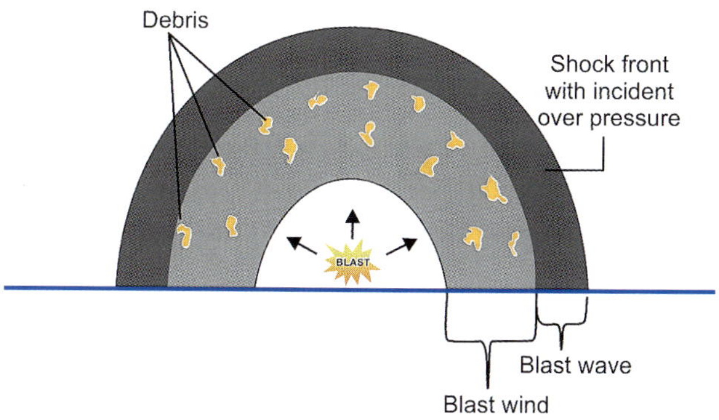

Fig. 7: Blast wave: Air is highly compressed on the leading edge of the blast wave, creating a shock front.

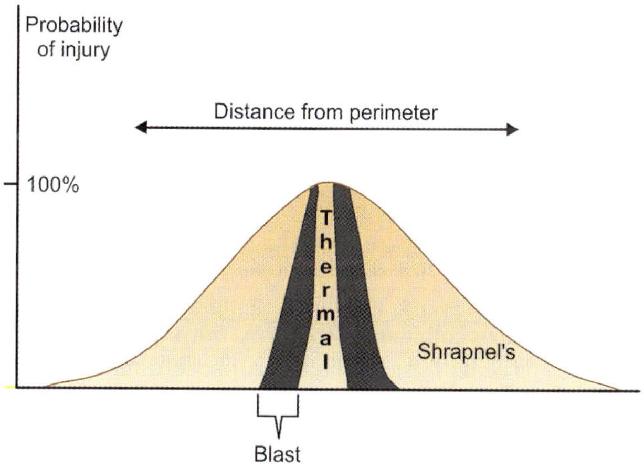

Fig. 8: The difference in the radius of blast effect in accordance to mechanism: thermal, primary blast effect (dark), and secondary (Shrapnel's).

often preplanned to aggravate the damage. The Shrapnel may even contain biologic, chemical, or even radioactive elements that are dispersed by the bomb blast causing other forms of injury.

Blast effects in vehicles have different results that lie intermediate between a completely open area and fully closed space blast effects. For example, in a vehicle, such as a bus, despite being a closed space, it has fewer primary blast injuries as the walls are relatively soft. The secondary or tertiary blast effects are much more prominent and severe because of large number of shrapnel generated in these blasts (secondary injury). The various irregular internal objects, such as the chairs, luggage, etc. cause injury by collision with the human body (tertiary injury). Secondary blast injuries in vehicles involve large fragments (but mainly lower velocity of <600 m/s) that cause direct limb amputation and severe musculoskeletal injuries for their higher momentum. Upon striking tissue, even at a low velocity, these fragments may exhibit a tumbling or so- called "shimmy effect" that can increase the amount of tissue damage by completely transferring the energy. A large, slow projectile can crush a large amount of tissue, and projectile fragmentation that may occur within the body can greatly increase temporary cavity effects. Further damage might be induced by moving environmental debris into the wound.

Most orthopedic blast trauma, however, is caused mainly by the secondary effect that depends on distance of the subject from the point of detonation, the characteristics of the fragments (shape, energy, etc.), and the number of generated foreign bodies that get ultimately implanted in the body. The size and shape of fragments are relevant in the sense that a large flat irregular fragment often transmits its energy quickly causing severe superficial tissue damage as to the muscle and skin; however small objects, such as a bullet, induce less extensive superficial damage due to relatively narrow path but have the ability to penetrate deeper causing possible critical organ damage. The orthopedic injuries from the effects of blast injury are however also ascribed to neurovascular damage, compartment syndrome, and large area soft-tissue damage. The local tissue damage may be less than that in high-velocity injuries.

CONCLUSION

- Projectile injuries and blast injuries are on the rise due to constantly increasing violence in today's world with growing intolerance.
- Surgeons need to keep themselves updated with the principles of ballistic injury so that patients are comprehensively managed.
- Most of the projectile injuries are worse than their superficial appearance. Radical debridement to prevent further complications is the basis of management, but excessive damage to the tissues should not happen by immature extensive removal of even healthy tissues. One should pay attention to the signs of tissue viability to keep the debridement radical.
- Blast injuries are best managed by coordinated care between various faculties in trauma centers with advanced critical care facility.

CHAPTER 20

Wound Healing and Principles of Wound Care

Manish Kumar Varshney

INTRODUCTION

"Wound healing" is a complex reparative process following injury that involves several overlapping cellular and metabolic processes essential for homeostasis. An insight into basic science of wound healing makes us understand possible causes and pathogenic mechanisms of poor healing and complications in otherwise seemingly simple wounds. This would also improve our approach to wound care and restoring the structure and function of the injured tissue.

Though classically segregated into four phases of coagulation (immediate), inflammation (0–7 days), proliferation (4–21 days), and remodeling (14 days to 2 years) the process of wound healing is actually a continuum of processes with considerable overlap in the stages and variability in occurrence and persistence.

Coagulation

Immediately at the site of injury the gap created by injury or surgical procedure is filled by liquid mesenchymal tissue—the blood that has marvelous capacity to coagulate and form a temporary soft tissue bridging the gap. This seal persists unless there is an arterial injury and serves as a base for further processes to occur. This involves vasoconstriction and subsequent platelet plug and clot formation, later there is release of platelet-derived growth factor (PDGF) and transforming growth factor-β (TGF-β) family of cytokines from granules igniting chemotaxis of inflammatory cells.

Inflammatory Phase

The chemokines (histamines and prostaglandins) released at the site of injury produce vasodilation and increased endothelial permeability aiding the migration of polymorphonuclear leukocytes (PMNs) clearing the wound of initial debris and bacteria. Macrophages over the next 2–3 days take place of PMNs and takeover phagocytosis with recruitment of downstream inflammatory and reparative cells mediated by multiple growth factors and cytokines. They comprise the predominant step in wound healing pathway. Gradually, lymphocytes replace macrophages with unclear function.

Proliferative Phase

The basic scaffold of primordial clot is retained while cellular debris is cleared in the inflammatory phase on which the fibroblasts proliferate. Growth factors like vascular endothelial growth factor (VEGF) stimulate angiogenesis. Granulation tissue is formed by the proliferation of fibroblasts and endothelial cells with disorganized capillaries, the former produces collagen which forms the primary structural molecule in scar. Type III collagen predominates initially followed by gradual restoration of the normal adult 4:1 ratio of type I to type III collagen over couple of years.

Remodeling Phase

Nearly 2–3 weeks postinjury only collagen remodeling occurs and there is no further deposition of substrate. The random collagen fibrils are replaced with cross-linked fibrils that organize in a specific pattern. Remodeling may last for up to a year or even more. Despite continuous improvement in strength of scars the ultimate tensile strength of scars only is 70% of normal, achieved years of healing after the original injury/procedure.

EPITHELIALIZATION

The process of epithelialization starts soon after the initial injury where in partial-thickness wounds, the epithelium is derived from saved hair follicles and sweat glands. However, in full-thickness wounds, epithelium slowly propagates from wound edges. This is a time-taking process progressing at the rate of 1–2 mm/day. In large craters, delayed epithelialization causes prolongation of the inflammatory phase and hence delayed wound healing and restoration of structure and function of the integument.

WOUND CONTRACTION

This is an innate property of wounds conferred by myofibroblasts (fibroblasts that contain actin microfilaments). Often it is advantageous as it creates a smaller wound area but wound contraction occurring across a joint would cause joint contractures and functional limitations.

Coverage of Surgical or Injury Wound

Injury to the soft tissues is now considered to be the most important component of injury having its influence on both the initial and the definitive management. With regard to the surgical closure of wound, a surgeon has various methods at disposal **(Fig. 1)**, but we need to understand a few terms commonly used but mostly misinterpreted:

- ***Defining acute and chronic wounds:*** An acute wound is defined as any interruption in the continuity of the body's surface caused by burns, cut, crush or lacerations (Kranke et al., MacLellan). A wound becomes chronic when it requires a prolonged time (exceeding that is considered normal for the site of wound, age of patient, and person's homeostasis) to heal, does not heal, or recurs (Kranke et al., 2003).
- ***Primary closure:*** The surgical closure of a wound (irrespective of number of layers) within hours of its occurrence. The wounds are often washed and cleaned before closure and this is the most common method of closure of surgical incisions and traumatic lacerations. If possible one should do it within golden period of 6 hours, one may undermine wound margins to produce tension-free closure.
- ***Delayed primary closure:*** The surgical closure of a wound is delayed by days to weeks after index procedure or injury. In this procedure, the granulation tissue has to be excised and the edges of the wound are freshened before closure. The typical example is closure of a fasciotomy incision done for management of compartment syndrome. This technique is also done when the primary wound is contaminated or in severely contused wounds with edema and in military practice where one has to observe any progression or development of infection or wound necrosis over first few days/week. In the interval cover wound by commercially available skin covering agents. This is mostly done (recommended) between 5th and 7th day as the edema subsides well by then and bacterial contamination is not yet developed into infection.

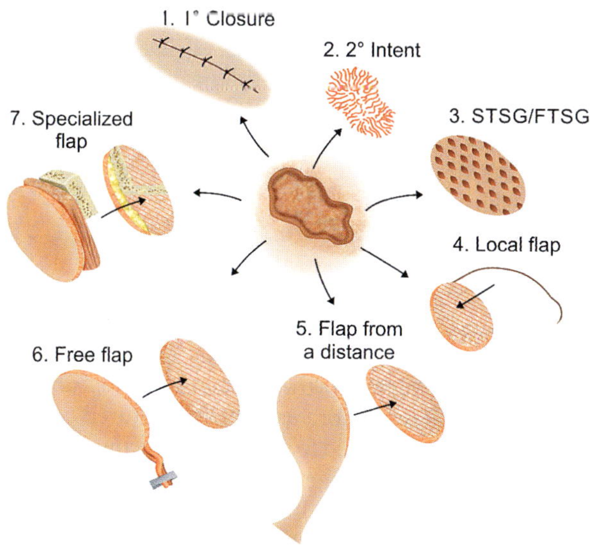

Fig. 1: The "reconstruction toolbox" available to a surgeon for closure of a surgical or injury wound. (STSG: split-thickness skin graft; FTSG: full thickness skin grafts)

- ***Healing by secondary intention (granulation tissue formation):*** It is committed to when a wound cannot be surgically repaired primarily or a wound is too deep that chances of dead space formation are high. The wound needs to granulate and form a healing tissue that fills the space so that skin coverage can be planned. The process is time-taking and daily wound care to minimize bacterial colonization by washing, debridement of necrotic tissue and using local antibiotics is needed. This entails a long-term commitment by the patient and the caregivers so that healthy and stable granulation tissue develops that can epithelialize, wound contraction by myofibroblasts plays an important role in reducing the size of wound and allowing lesser requirement for future procedure. Healing by secondary intention is often not preferred in orthopedic practice for two reasons—this tissue is always inflamed and contaminated posing a risk to the underlying structures (typically bone and more so if implants have been used) to get infected. The second reason is that this tissue contracts and across the flexor creases forms a retracting scar impending the normal excursion of otherwise mobile joints.
- ***Primary skin grafting:*** As mentioned earlier that failure of early epithelization prolongs inflammatory phase; skin grafting is a useful procedure in management of such large defects that cannot be closed primarily, and when creation of flaps is not desirable or feasible. It can also be performed in a delayed manner (2–5 days) in cases where hemostasis is not complete.
- ***Dermal overgrafting (Webster 1958):*** This is a specialized procedure for coverage of defects weight-bearing surfaces (as in heel) and unstable scars of leg. Multiple graftings are done at 3 weeks interval to provide a thick-laminated layer of dermis.
- ***Wound closure by surgical flaps:*** This is a stable method of quick closure of wound by recruitment of local or distant tissue. A flap is best described as a piece of tissue that is moved maintaining its blood supply and is not reliant on the recipient site for its vascularity (Russell and Williams: Bailey and Love's Short practice of surgery, 23rd edition: Arnold 2000). Some other less descriptive definitions of flap are—a piece of tissue partly detached from the surrounding tissue, as for grafting (Webster's new world dictionary), and a tissue transferred from one anatomic site to another (Rockwood and green's: Fractures in adults, 5th edition: Lippincott 2001). Coverage by flaps is often considered for definitive wound coverage when no further procedures for that tissue are being envisaged. Various types of flaps can be harvested—simple random, local rotation axial skin flap (peninsular flaps) local island flaps, distant pedicled flap (like groin flaps), fasciocutaneous flaps, free skin or muscle flaps with vascular anastomosis in situ or flaps revascularized by vascular grafts.

- ***Use of skin substitutes:*** These are a heterogeneous group of wound coverage materials that aid in wound closure by temporarily or permanently replacing the functions of skin. High demands for wound coverage materials in the wounded persons as those with extensive skin loss or burns patients' necessitate the use of alternatives than the native skin. Various synthetic and nonsynthetic (biological) variants are available for wound coverage having distinct characteristics, while the former can be supplied as per demand and affords more control over the scaffold composition; the latter has a more intact extracellular matrix on which natural new dermis can be laid and re-epithelialization would occur. There is no ideal skin substitute available that can provide characteristics of hypoxia tolerance, broad availability, readily synthesizable on demand, rheology identical to native skin, infection resistance, cost-effectiveness, providing both dermal and epidermal components, low antigenicity, easy storage and resistance to shear. The various classes of available components include:
  - *Potato peel* has been used as a biological dressing substitute.
  - *Allograft/alloderm* usually obtained from cadaver or dermis.
  - *Xenograft* obtained from different species like pigs (most commonly) in burn patients. Earliest attempt was using a frog skin in 1,500 BC.
  - *Single layer durable skin substitutes* such as bovine collagen sheet (Kollagen®), porcine collagen sheet (Permacol®), bovine dermal matrix (Matiderm®), and human dermal matrix (Alloderm®)
  - *Amnion* has been used since 1910 as a biological dressing. Amnion forms the innermost semitransparent layer of fetal membrane that has been used for burns patients. It should be collected from placentae of screened donors to limit the transmission of diseases. Membrane is commonly preserved in liquid nitrogen (cryopreservation) while other method includes using silver nitrate, storage in antibiotic solution, glycerol-preservation as sheets, and γ-irradiation. The use had been very popular in partial thickness burns due to cost-effectiveness and minimizing loss of protein, electrolytes and fluids, reduced risk of infection, accelerating wound healing, and versatile handling properties.
  - *Synthetic (bioengineered):*
    - *Acellular skin substitutes:*
      - *Biobrane®:* Nylon mesh as a "dermis" and a silicon membrane as an "epidermis" embedded in porcine collagen—used commonly for temporary coverage of superficial or partial thickness wounds, burns, and congenital diseases such as epidermolysis bullosa.
      - *Integra® (Yannas and Burke):* Bilayered skin substitute composed of a silicone membrane as an epidermis; bovine collagen and shark chondroitin-6-sulfate glycosaminoglycan as dermis. Silicon layer is removed after 2–3 weeks and covered with split-thickness graft.
      - *Alloderm®:* It is derived from cadaveric dermis as an acellular matrix. Epidermis is removed by salt and chemically processed to remove any cellular element. It is supplied freeze-dried containing basement layer.
    - *Cellular allogeneic skin substitute:*
      - *Transcyte®:* Composed of nylon mesh containing embedded allogeneic fibroblasts from neonatal foreskin and a silastic semi-permissible biocompatible layer. In burn cases, it is applied and left to either peel off spontaneously indicating healing or may be removed surgically.
      - *Dermagraft®:* Composed of living neonatal foreskin fibroblasts embedded on biodegradable mesh from polyglycolic acid (Dexon or Vicryl) but lacks silicone layer. It is also supplied cryopreserved at –80°C. It has been used for vestibuloplasty.
      - *Apligraf® (Graftskin®):* It is a composite skin graft ("organotypical skin substitute") by virtue of containing both living dermis and epidermis. It is prepared by mixing living fibroblasts from neonatal foreskin with bovine collagen type I, where the former produces new collagen and matrix and fibrous network over 2–3 weeks on exposure to heat. This is seeded with neonatal keratinocytes that proliferate over 4 days and on exposure to liquid air for further 7–10 days produce stratum corneum. It is United States Food and Drug Administration (FDA) approved for treatment of noninfected partial or full thickness venous ulcers and neuropathic diabetic ulcers, also it has been used for managing wounds in epidermolysis bullosa and surgical excision of skin cancer and burns.
      - *Orcel®:* Human allogeneic skin cells (epidermal keratinocytes and dermal fibroblasts) are cultured in two separate layers into a type I bovine collagen sponge. It is a bilayer tissue matrix used for treatment of chronic wounds and skin graft donor sites.
    - *Cellular autologous skin substitutes:* These provide cultured autologous keratinocytes for permanent skin coverage.
      - *Cultured epidermal autograft (CEA):* The autologous keratinocytes obtained from trypsin treated dermis and subcutaneous tissue taken from biopsy of the patient are cultured on lethally irradiated 3T3 mouse fibroblasts in epidermal growth factor (EGF) enriched medium. Before using these cultured cells, it is recommended to condition the wound bed with cadaveric allogeneic skin for about 4 days that reduces susceptibility to the digestive effects of collagenase enzymes.
      - *Cultured skin substitutes (CSS):* This entails grafting both epidermal and dermal components for permanent coverage. In contrast to

CEA that is susceptible for blister formation due to poor dermal-epidermal junction, CSS is much more stable. Hyaluronic acid derived substitute is used most commonly as the dermal biosynthetic scaffold here.

- ***Fillet approach*:** This is a method in which the parts of body to be discarded are used as a donor tissue for providing skin coverage of the compromised part. Simple split-thickness skin graft (STSG) can be obtained or more complex microvascular free flaps can be harvested in a setting of a B/K amputation where free flap transfer required to salvage the site (ideal choice). Skin of unreimplantable foot harvested either circumferentially based on both dorsalis pedis artery and posterior tibial artery or planter skin alone (fillet of sole) based on posterior tibial artery. Tibial nerve provides potential for sensory innervation. It is recommended to use both the arteries for a better outcome and universal uptake.
- ***Vacuum-assisted closure [VAC®, negative-pressure wound therapy (NPWT)]*:** This is a versatile way of managing chronic wounds especially in the elderly. VAC has improved patient outcomes significantly with respect to the wound care over past 10–15 years. VAC is recommended to be used as a comprehensive treatment plan in indicated acute or chronic wounds especially those that fail (or show delay) to heal normally and are challenging. It incorporates the use of negative pressure to optimize conditions for wound healing and has been found to reduce the need for frequent dressing changes, improve patient comfort, and reduce associated costs. A polyurethane ether sponge is placed/packed into the wound cavity and sealed under an adhesive drape **(Figs. 2A and B)**. Controlled negative pressure (50–125 mm Hg) is applied by an adjustable vacuum pump which reduces interstitial fluid accumulation and edema formation helping to minimize bacterial colonization of the wound and increase proliferation of the granulation tissue by arteriolar dilation in negative pressure. Commercial dressings are very costly so one can improvise inhouse materials for producing a NPWT system also **(Figs. 3A to D)**.

The noted benefits of VAC therapy are:

- Removal of exudate from the wound and reduction in interstitial edema
- Increased local microvascular flow and improved vascularity (arteriolar dilation)
- Increased controlled production of granulation tissue formation by reduction in the exposure to proteolytic enzymes. Vacuum also puts shear force producing cellular hyperplasia.
- Reduce the complexity of wound.
- Wound shrinkage
- Optimization of wound bed reducing the complexity of future surgical procedures
- Reduction in the need of antibiotics

Indications for VAC® therapy (or NPWT): NNPWT is practically indicated now for any wound where surgical closure is not recommended or feasible. It has been found that few wounds would be healed completely by the therapy, however, it is most commonly used as an interim measure for future surgical management of the wound. As an extended indication the therapy has been also utilized after flap surgeries (to increase flap tissue survival) and following skin grafting (increase uptake). The following are some of the *common indications* of NPWT:

- Chronic wounds such as diabetic ulcers, neuropathic ulcers, and pressure sores
- *Traumatic wounds:* There is a recommendation that if it is deemed useful to use NPWT for traumatic wounds then it should be applied as early as possible rather than waiting for some improvement in the condition.
- The best indication for NPWT/VAC® in orthopedics is a large wound that is not considered suitable for skin grafting due to exposed tendons or bone.
- Open abdominal wounds (including burst abdomen)
- Large and deep burn wounds

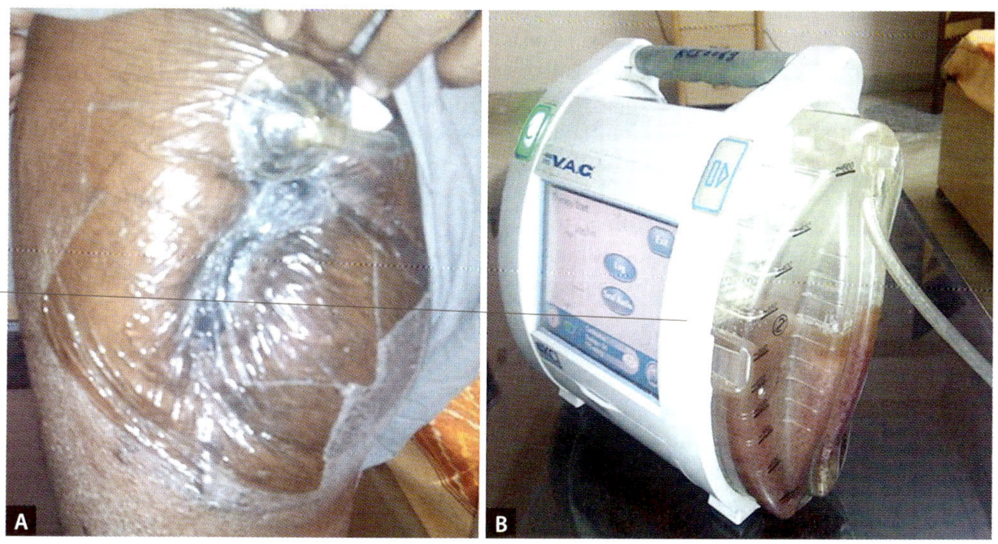

Figs. 2A and B: Commercial negative-pressure wound therapy (NPWT) system and dressing for chronic wounds.

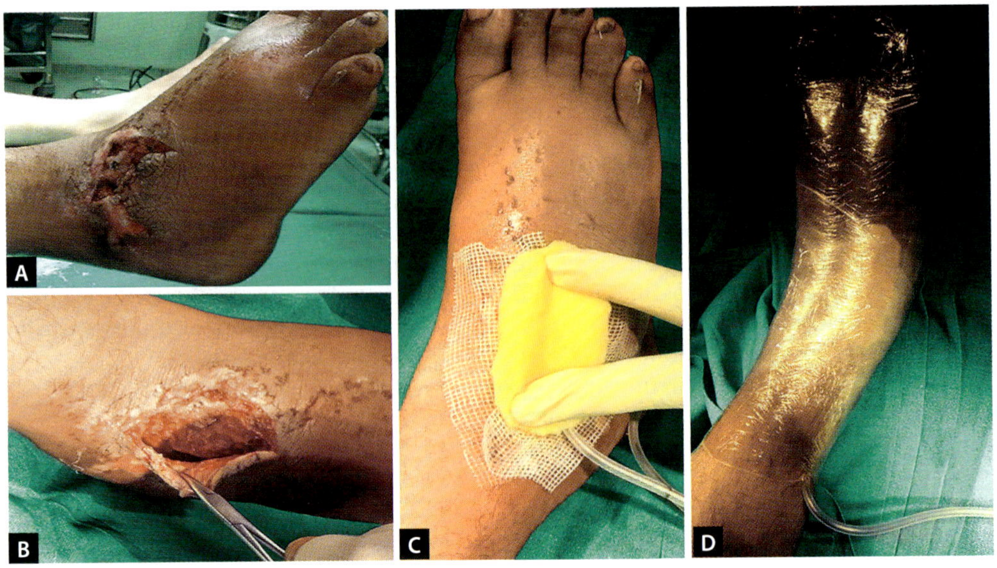

Figs. 3A to D: Improvised negative-pressure wound therapy (NPWT) for deep exudative wound.

- Postflap surgery or skin grafting
- Sternotomy defects

Contraindications for the use of NPWT:
- Local malignancy
- Untreated underlying osteomyelitis or implant-related infection
- Presence of fistulas
- Copious necrotic tissue in the bed
- Active soft-tissue infection
- Exposed viscera (as in abdominal wounds)
- Naked unsupported blood vessel or graft in the wound

Technique of applying NPWT: For an adequate wound perform adequate debridement so that healthy and clean bed and margins are obtained. Clean the surrounding skin and dry it. Cut a polyurethane sponge of size just smaller than the size of wound and cover with an adhesive dressing that seals the wound. Normally, the adhesive dressing overlaps 6 cm of the normal skin to achieve a hermetic seal. Make a puncture in the center and connect a suction tube to this assembly. The suction tube maintains negative pressure in the wound when connected to a pump. Instead of the standard black polyurethane hydrophobic foam white denser foam is also available that is hydrophilic and has nonadherent properties. This can be used in patients who fail to tolerate black foam. The dressings of NPWT need to be changed every 48–72 hours. The white foam requires higher negative pressures, newer foams like silver impregnated foams are also available.

In various circumstances, it is helpful to identify patients who would respond favorably to the VAC® therapy. This would help in prognosticating the patients about the success of treatment and what to expect from it. The following are some of the factors known to improve success of therapy identified over years:
- Adequate blood supply
- Healthy and clean wound bed
- Adequate debridement of the wound
- High exudate discharge from wound
- Wound diameter >2 cm
- Healthy patient with minimal comorbidities
- Compliant patient

CHOICE OF SUTURE MATERIAL

Suturing is the joining of tissues with needle and "thread" (suture in surgical practice) to approximate them for making them heal by primary intention. Sutures of various sizes and materials are available. The sutures are conventionally numbered in zeros (0), the higher the number of zeros the finer is the suture. Beyond "00" the sutures are depicted in whole numbers where higher the number, thicker is the suture. In general, orthopedics practice sutures from number "5" (say large tendon repairs like for tendo-Achilles) to 6–0 (small tendons of hand and neural repair) are commonly used; finer sutures like 9–0 or 10–0 are for vascular or ophthalmological requirements.

In terms of materials, the sutures are broadly classified into absorbable and nonabsorbable **(Table 1)**, however, a number of other factors should also be taken into consideration when choosing suture material:
- Tensile strength of a suture is a property of its material and diameter of the filament (for monofilament) or thread (for braided). Steel sutures are strongest followed by polyester, braided polydiaxanone (PDS)-II, nylon, polypropylene and silk in that order. The diameter of suture is depicted by the USP rating which has "00" as the standard and variations are numbered followed by a "zero", (higher number indicating a thinner suture). In general for surgical the thinnest suture that is of adequate strength should be used to close the wound with adequate strength and minimize tissue reaction.
- ***Monofilament or braided:*** Monofilament sutures have the advantage of passing easily through tissue and causing minimal tissue reactivity. They have least propensity for

TABLE 1: Types of suture materials as a broad classification.

Common name	*Basic component*	*Comments*
Nonabsorbable		
Silk	Silk	Braided suture with low strength but high knot security and high tissue reactivity so that scar is bad.
Prolene	Polypropylene	Monofilament suture with low tissue reactivity and average strength but knot is also insecure so that multiple knots need to be applied. Used for cardiac and vascular surgeries
PVDF	Polyvinylidene fluoride	Monofilament suture with uses similar to prolene but has better knot security and higher strength.
Ethilon®	Nylon monofilament	Monofilament suture with high strength and low reactivity but has poor knot strength. There is high component of memory so that strand is stiffly coiled making suture handling uncomfortable.
Nurolon®	Braided nylon	To improve the suture handling and knot security the monofilament is converted into a braided while retaining the high strength of suture.
Ethibond®	Polyester	This is a braided and coated suture with very high strength and average reactivity, the knot strength is average and decreases with thicker sutures so that for number 5 suture higher number of knots needs to be applied.
Mersilene®	Polyester	This is a specific material available for securing repairs needing high strength like A-C joint reconstruction, ACL reconstruction or for TA reconstruction. The knot strength and tissue reactivity are average.
Steel and titanium wires	• Surgical grade stainless steel (AISI 316 LVM) • Surgical grade titanium	Very tough and truly nonabsorbable monofilament wires. Used especially for bone suturing as for closing sternotomy wound.
Staples	Surgical grade stainless steel	Commercially available sutures preloaded in a device that is used for closure of the skin. The advantage is minimization of time to close wounds but offers no other advantage; in fact, infection and tissue reactivity may be higher.
Dermabond®	Liquid acrylate based compound	Used for closure of simple lacerations without any suture marks. Should be handled carefully else other places especially eyes may get permanently damaged if accidentally falls into it.
Absorbable (absorption here actually refers to reduction of suture strength to half, 50%)		
Plain catgut	Sheep/cattle intestine	This absorbs within a week so that it is useful only for securing fast healing areas like mucous membranes. The tissue reactivity is very high and knot security is poor.
Chromic catgut	This is treated plain catgut.	The suture has high tissue reactivity but less than plain catgut and has higher knot security. The suture absorbs in around 3–4 weeks.
Vicryl	Polygalactin 910	This braided suture has average reactivity and knot security. The suture usually absorbs in 3 weeks (50% reduction in strength).
Vicryl-OS	Treated vicryl with antibacterial coating (blue stained usually), polygalactin 910 and Irgacare MP	This is especially used in orthopedic surgery and has average tissue reactivity. The average half-life of strength in tissue is 3 weeks.
Monocryl	Poliglecaprone 25 and Irgacare MP	It has a good knot security and low tissue reactivity. It is a monofilament suture that absorbs in 1–2 weeks.
Dexon	Polyglycolic acid	It has a good knot security and low tissue reactivity. It is a braided suture that absorbs in 2–3 weeks.
Maxon	Polyglyconate	This suture absorbs in around 2–3 weeks and has average knot security and tissue reactivity.
PDS or PDS-II (Orthocord®)	Polydiaxanone	This has low to minimal tissue reactivity but the knot security is also low. The suture absorbs in nearly 2–3 months.

(ACL: anterior cruciate ligament; PDS: polydiaxanone)

bacterial adhesion. The disadvantages in general are poor handling being stiffer and less secure knot structure requiring multiple closing knots to be thrown.

FACTORS AFFECTING WOUND HEALING

Few factors affect the scar formation and result in poor outcome that may be controlled or averted to produce a better cosmetic scar:

- *Closing the wound in tension (not the surgeon in tension but the wound approximated in tensile strain!):* This causes relative ischemia due to compression of capillaries. This can be controlled by placing incision along the Langer's lines [relaxed skin tension lines (RSTL)] and closing the deeper dermal layers in a separate layer. Undermining or creation of a flap is another way to reduce tension, lastly one may give relaxing incisions to close wound and graft the other site.
- *Infection and abscess formation:* This is more liable to occur in areas of poor vascularity and those exposed for >12 hours. The best way to reduce chances of infection is

by eliminating any dead tissue and using copious lavage to ward off any residing debris. Antibiotic prophylaxis is indicated for all grossly contaminated wounds but performing adequate debridement has no substitute.

- Misaligned wound edges
- *Presence of foreign bodies:* This delays epithelialization (normally an approximated wound epithelializes within 24 hours) and overall wound healing. All contaminated wounds should be explored carefully and foreign bodies removed, if required wound toileting should be done by incising along the edges to expose the hidden areas that may carry foreign bodies. Epithelialization is also delayed with infection. To improve epithelialization moist healing environment is favorable that can be provided by a semipermeable, occlusive dressing for a week or 10 days initially.
- *Relative or absolute ischemia due to microvascular damage or impaired blood flow:* Smoking should be stopped as it causes vasoconstriction. Light bandage should be applied and external pressure should never exceed capillary perfusion pressure (>35 mm Hg).
- Hereditary factors or connective tissue disorders.

Wound Dressings and Dressing Materials

Wound dressings are placed to optimize the healing environment by preventing contamination, reducing edema, and preventing too early drying of the area nor allowing it to macerate either. The specific goals of dressing are as follows:

- Making an optimally moist environment
- Absorbing excessive exudate from the weeping wounds
- Barrier function—against contamination
- Reducing local edema
- Reducing/eliminating dead space—pressure dressings reduce the dead space and they can also be eliminated by packing for irregular cavities.
- Protection of the wound
- Maintaining adequate temperature
- There are a variety of dressing materials available some of which are mentioned in **Table 2** along with specific comments.

Managing a Wound Contracture: Z-plasty

The Z-plasty is commonly deployed to minimize a scar contracture or to treat it once it has developed. Two interdigitating triangular flaps are created and transposed in such a way that **(Fig. 4)**:

1. The oblique limb of Z gets reoriented.
2. The oblique limb gets lengthened in the desired direction.

Point one above can also be used in managing wounds where direct closure is producing undue tension at the suture line or resulting in distortion of nearby structures as is unacceptable in facial region for cosmesis. Increase in length is best used for managing the contractures. The gain in length depends on the angles created for flaps. 45° flaps increase length by 50% while 60° flaps increase length by 75%. Angles more or less than this should not be made. The length of flap limbs depends on the amount of tissue available on either side of the scar—more the tissue is longer the limbs can be designed.

TABLE 2: Types of dressings and dressing materials.

Dressing type	***Composition***	***Comments***
Sterile dry gauze	Treated cotton absorbent gauze	Applied on "closed" wounds. Absorbs the blood and oozing in initial period.
Wet gauze dressing	Saline soaked gauze	Minimally wet gauze dressings are applied on full thickness open wounds where on drying it sticks to dead tissue that gets removed in exchange of dressings. Moist gauze dressings are applied on partial thickness wounds to maintain moist environment and allow epithelialization and provide wick drainage.
Adherent plastic films (Tegaderm®)	Synthetic thin semipermeable (permeable to water vapor but not to water and bacteria) polyurethane or copolyester films (sterile)	Applied to partial thickness superficial wounds it maintains moist environment and an effective barrier to contamination.
Nonadherent dressings (Adaptec®)	Petroleum gauze or nonimpregnated polyurethane films	Used commonly over skin grafts and donor sites with mild exudates, they basically act as nonsticky barrier to contamination.
Hydrogels (Elastogel®)	Polymer of polyethylene oxide or acrylamide or polyvinylpyrrolidone or a combination with 80–90% water. It is available as amorphous dressing or a sheet like dressing	It is applied on a shallow, noninfected wound like pressure sore that maintains moist environment to reduce pain and promote autolytic debridement. Do not use on wounds with heavy exudates.
Hydrocolloids (Duoderm®)	Hydrophilic colloidal substrate like hydroxymethyl cellulose in an adhesive mass like polyisobutylene	These are good for most wounds like partial thickness wounds, pressure sores, wounds with slough or granulation tissue or wounds with minimal exudate. These should not be used for infected wounds or wounds with sinus tract.
Foams (Lyofoam®)	Hydrophilic or phobic nonocclusive foam usually coated with gel	Use on partial- or full-thickness wounds with heavy exudates
Collagen dressings	Bovine of porcine derived collagen as pads, gels or powder	Used for deep cavities and over partial thickness burns to fill dead space and provide moist environment.
Alginates	Natural mannuronic or hyaluronic acid from seaweed	Used over wounds with slough or those with heavy exudates to absorb exudate and fill dead space. Avoid its use over heavily bleeding wounds or dry wounds. It absorbs exudates to become a gel and provides moist environment.
Negative-pressure wound dressings	See text	See text

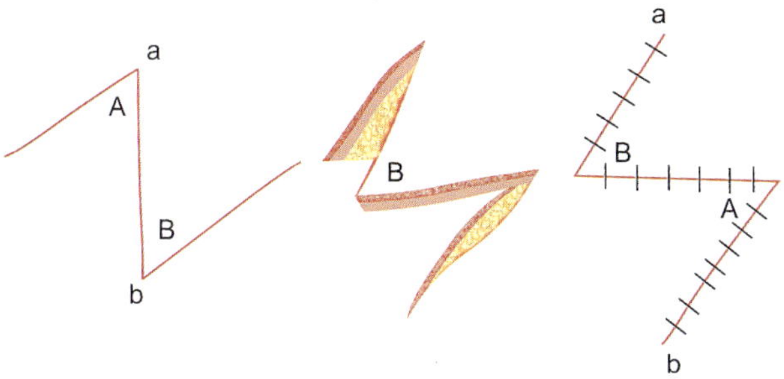

Fig. 4: Z-plasty. The limb A-B is created along the scar and triangular flaps (a and b) are created, over the ends of the limb A–B. The triangular flaps are then rotated so as to change the orientation of scar and its length.

Technique of Making a Z-plasty

Commonly the Z-plasty is made as follows:

1. The oblique limb of the Z should be made parallel to the scar lengthwise. Then draw the transverse limbs at the ends of this at an angle of 60°.
2. Maintain vascularity to the triangular flaps especially their tips during dissection, a broad base of flaps maintains best vascularity in general. The other point is keeping the flap thickness to its maximum.
3. Transposed the created triangles causing reorientation of the scar line and lengthening of the oblique limb.

Factors Affecting Z-plasty

- Z-plasty is ideally performed in patients with good wrinkle pattern on the skin. It is possible to reorient the scar in such patients along the lines of Langers. Children are, hence, not a good candidate for Z-plasty—their skin is more or less wrinkle free.
- Z-plasties perform poorly on hypertrophic scars.
- As a single Z-plasty creates lateral tension chiefly at the apices of each triangle, it is recommended to perform multiple Z-plasties that can provide same amount of scar lengthening with significantly less transverse shortening. This is preferable for long scars that would otherwise require large triangular flaps.

SOFT-TISSUE COVERAGE IN ORTHOPEDICS

Historical Perspective

- 3000 BC: Attempts at flap surgery
- 600 BC: Reporting of specific flap for nose and ear and some facial flaps (*Sushruta Samhita*)
- 1400s: Branca family (Sicily)—delayed pedicle flap
- Early 1500s: Talgliacozzi—arm-pedicled nose flap
- 1552: Pare—first vascular anastomoses
- 1824: Luigi porta—free skin grafting
- 1900s: Gilles—staged pedicle flaps
- 1917: Tansini—latissimus dorsi (LD) flap for breast
- 1951: Zeiss—development of commercial operating microscope
- 1972: McGregor and Jackson—groin flap
- 1975: Free flaps

Soft-tissue coverage or reconstruction is a vast domain that is basically covered under faculty of plastic and reconstructive surgery. We will discuss some of the methods

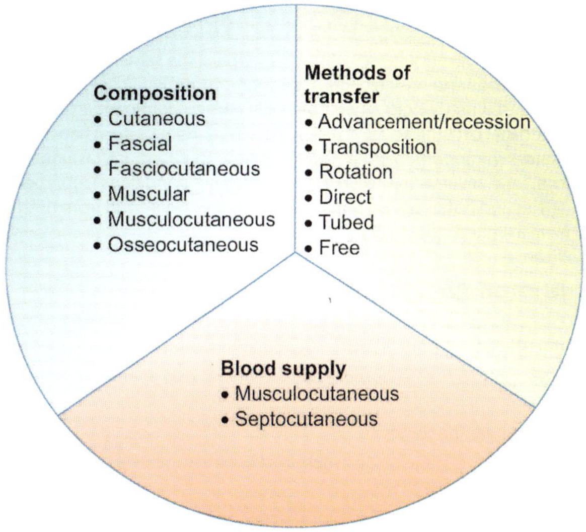

Fig. 5: Categorization of the flap based on key features.

and principles of soft-tissue coverage below as commonly needed in orthopedics. It is hitherto imperative to define and understand some of the terms that would be repetitively used in the text that follows.

A flap is defined variously by different authors. The Webster's New World Dictionary describes a flap as a piece of tissue partly detached from the surrounding tissue, as for grafting. The Bailey and Love's short practice of surgery describes a flap as a piece of tissue that is moved maintaining its blood supply and is not reliant on the recipient site for its vascularity. Similar to varied definitions, flaps can also be classified on the basis of various key features **(Fig. 5)**. A flap has many parts used to describe its structure—a base is the proximal segment of a flap while pivot is a locus around which the flap rotates and can very well be different from base. Distal segment of a flap is the part commonly inserted into the defect and bridge segment of a flap is the central portion of the tissue that caries blood vessels. Vascularity of flap has important implications with respect to its use and survival that should be finely understood by the surgeon **(Box 1)**.

To understand the principles of soft-tissue coverage we can take the example of lower extremity as this is the most vulnerable area an orthopedic surgeon commonly encounters. Various options are available for reconstruction of soft-tissue defects of the lower extremity **(Fig. 6)**. Most of the patients with open wounds have soft-tissue deficits on the lower limb that needs to be covered to prevent future complications and improve outcomes. A common reconstructive ladder for soft-tissue reconstruction of lower extremity below knee is provided in **Flowchart 1**. In general, immediate skin cover is essential and for lower extremity the current recommendation is that it can be best achieved with a muscle flap. Muscle flap is better than a fasciocutaneous flap which is prone to undergo secondary necrosis. Pedicled flaps are traditionally preferred and if there is any doubt use a free muscle flap which are more reliable in Gustilo type IIIB open fractures as significant contusion and devascularization makes local flap unhealthy. Even if local flaps survive the trophic effect is considered minimal to support underlying

BOX 1: Understanding flaps based on vascular blood supply.

The deep and superficial vascular plexus supplies the skin. The deep vascular plexus is also known as the "subdermal plexus" that receives blood supply from septocutaneous and musculocutaneous perforators. Branches from it supply the overlying dermis. The flaps may be classified into axial pattern flaps if they are supplied directly from an anatomically named dominant artery in the longitudinal axis of the flap within the subcutaneous fat (e.g., groin flap based on the superficial circumflex iliac artery); whereas random pattern flaps derive blood supply from subdermal plexus supplied by various unnamed (nondominant) perforators in random manner. Based on how the flaps are fashioned on their blood supply the cutaneous flaps may be one of the four basic types, viz., random, axial, reverse flow axial pattern flaps, and island flaps (subtype of axial flas). Muscle-based flaps may also be axial pattern flaps further classified based on Mathes and Nahai system **(Fig. 7)**. It can be partly inferred from this that the axial pattern flaps will have a robust blood supply where random pattern flaps will have a limited extent to which they can be harvested in size and depth. The differences between random and axial pattern flaps further clarify their clinical significance.

Axial pattern flap	**Random pattern flap**
Blood supply is derived from anatomically named well perfused septocutaneous artery or musculocutaneous perforator	Blood supply is derived from subdermal plexus variably deriving from deep and superficial vascular plexus
Blood supply to the flap is more consistent and sort of guaranteed	Blood supply is precarious and derives from multiple sources so varies with flap design
Large flaps can be designed.	Limits the size of flaps with inconsistent vascularity
Suitable for one-stage reconstruction of large wounds resulting from trauma or mass resections	Suitable for small reconstructions
Can be transferred acutely so quick reconstruction possible	The flaps are harvested typically in delayed manner (delayed fashion flaps) to foster and assure better circulation
Do not need underlying vascular blood as they have their own blood supply	They perform better if the underlying wound has a good vascularized bed
Greater width to length ratio	Smaller transverse span
Better cosmesis due to full thickness skin usage	Cosmesis is not as good as axial pattern flaps
Higher survival rates	Lower survival rates

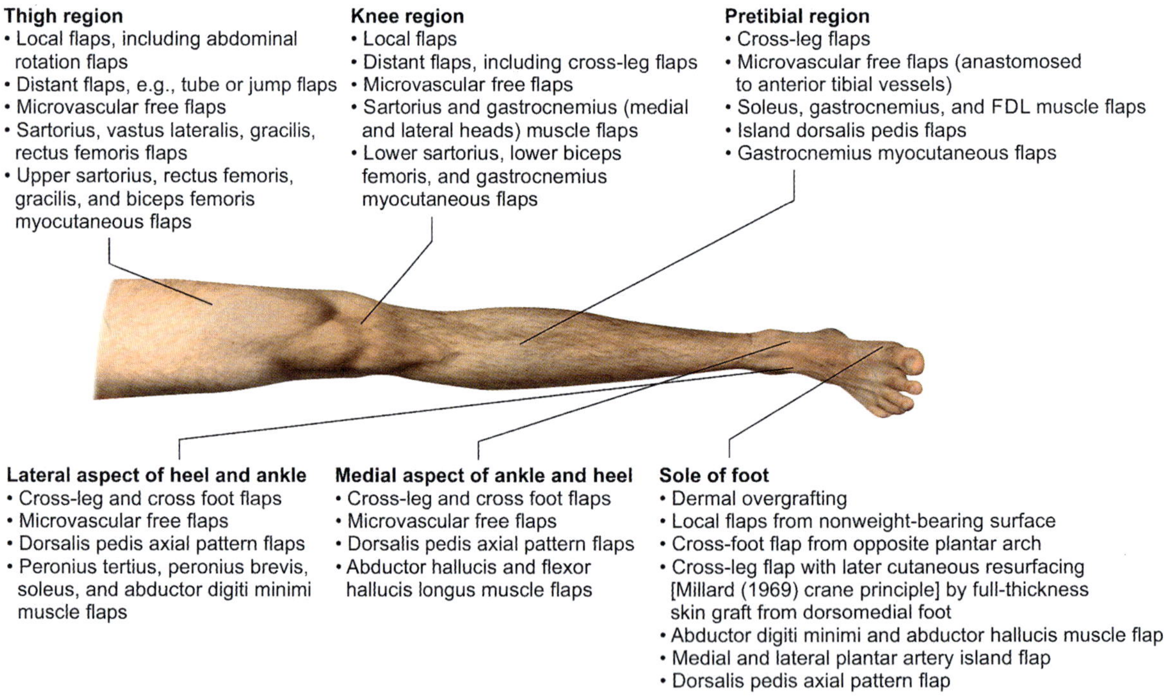

Fig. 6: The various options for wound coverage in different parts of lower limb.

structures to heal. The muscles are classified into various types **(Table 3 and Fig. 7)**. The typical advantages of a muscle or a muscle-based flap include:

- A rigid-walled, deep cavity can be obliterated.
- The vascularity of area is increased:
  - On arterial side promotes healing
  - On venous side, drainage is improved.
- Aids in controlling infection
- Adherence of skin to underlining structures is prevented.
- An ideal recipient site for STSG
- Easy access to muscle locally
- Closure of cavity stops leakage of protein rich exudate, leading to improvement of patient's general condition.

A fasciocutaneous flap instead is classified as:

- *Type A:* Multiple perforators at base (Cross-leg flap and medial thigh flap)

Flowchart 1: Soft-tissue coverage below knee.

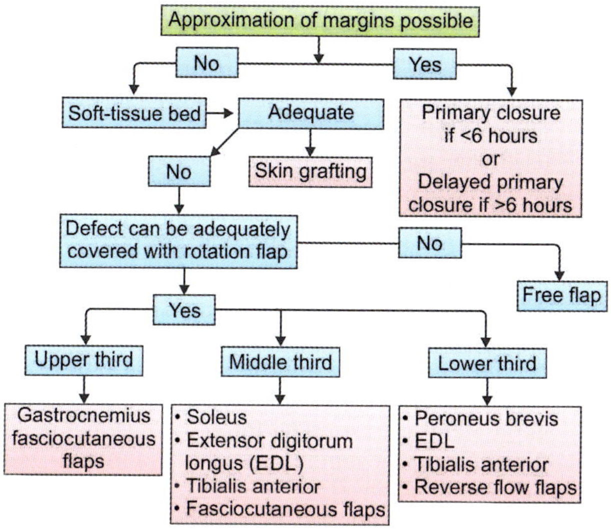

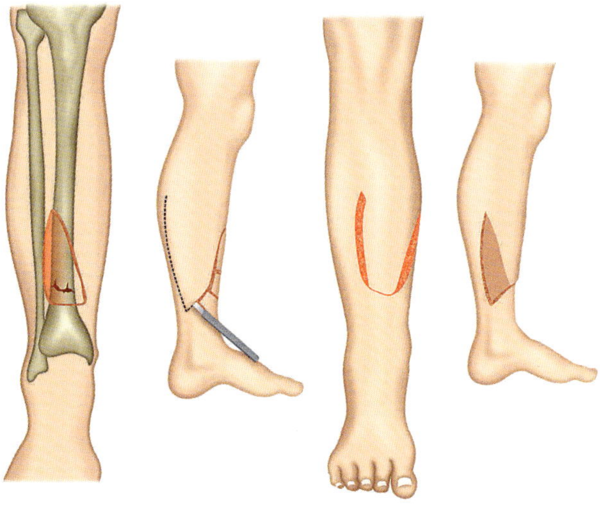

Fig. 8: Fasciocutaneous flaps for leg are to be based on the intermuscular septum.

TABLE 3: Classification of various muscle types.

Type	*Blood supply*	*Muscles*
Type I	Single dominant pedicle	Gastrocnemius, rectus femoris, and tensor fascia lata
Type II	Dominant pedicle and multiple minor pedicles	Biceps femoris, gracilis, peroneus longus, and soleus
Type III	Dual dominant pedicles	Gluteus maximus, rectus abdominis, and serratus anterior
Type IV	Multiple segmental pedicles	EDL, FDL, sartorius, and tibialisanterior
Type V	One dominant and multiple segmental	Pectoralis major, latissimus dorsi

(EDL: extensor digitorum longus; FDL: flexor digitorum longus)

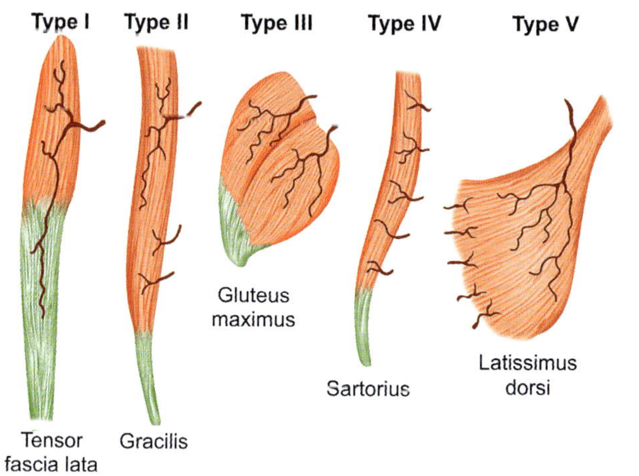

Fig. 7: Classification of muscles based on their blood supply lateral.

- *Type B:* Single vascular pedicle (medial arm flap, antecubital forearm flap, and scapular flap)
- *Type C:* Segmental vascular pedicle (radial forearm flap)
- *Type D:* Single vascular pedicle (radial forearm flap with bone and fibular osseocutaneous flap)

For a fasciocutaneous flap, the feasibility of flap is determined by extent of periosteal damage, location of defect, and available soft tissue. Usually, the tissue over antero-medial tibia is unsuitable so that mostly the flap is based on lateral intermuscular septum or posterior tibial artery **(Fig. 8)** to base flap on fascial perforators. These commonly limit their usefulness in all cases so muscular flaps are preferred over them.

The common methods of reconstruction used in orthopedic practice followed by region-wise options available for soft tissue reconstruction for leg are described here.

Skin Grafting

This is one of the most basics of reconstructive procedures performed for reconstituting the continuity of integument. In simplest terms, the skin or a portion of it is transplanted to a defect for reconstitution of integument integrity. Though appearing innocuous and simple it is prone to failures and complications if not performed well and in a defined manner, so should not be taken lightly anyways. There are three basic modes in which a skin grafting can be done.

1. *Primary skin grafting:* This is done primarily while wound management, it is also done to cover the rotational muscle flaps to seal the skin cover primarily.
2. *Delayed skin grafting:* If the wound is unhealthy with doubtful vascularity of the bed one should let the wound granulate and then skin grafting is done (usually 2–5 days later), it is the most common mode of management for open wound in orthopedics. The other indication is if the hemostasis at the site is incomplete then one should wait for the wound to stabilize before grafting.
3. *Dermal over grafting (Webster 1958):*
   - For coverage of defects weight-bearing surfaces and unstable scars of leg.
   - Multiple graftings done at 3 week interval to provide a thick laminated layer of dermis.

Skin grafts are harvested from a donor site and transferred to the recipient site without carrying its own blood supply.

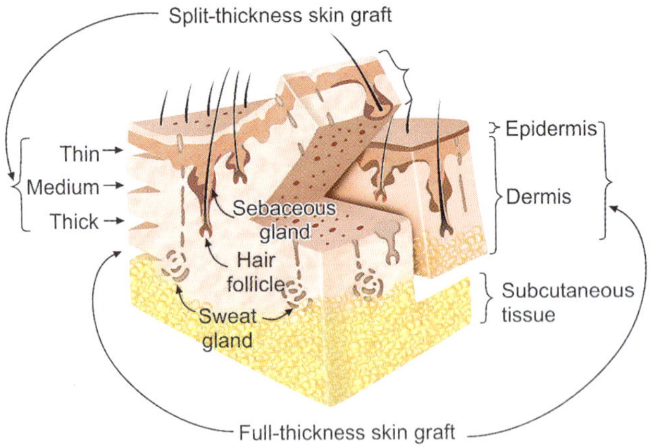

Fig. 9: Classification of the skin grafts based on depth of tissue harvested.

Based on the thickness of the obtained (required) the grafts are classified into:

- *Full-thickness skin grafts (FTSG):* Historically used as pinch grafts by Reverdin in 1869, these consist of entire epidermis and dermis **(Fig. 9)**. Details of FTSG were given by Wolfe and Krause in 1875 and 1893, respectively. These grafts leave no dermal appendages that can reproduce epidermis so the donor site has to be primarily closed. This entails obtaining grafts from places where skin redundancy is abundant to allow closure. Commonly they are obtained using a knife free-hand to create a plain between dermis and subcutaneous fat. Due to requirement of high vascularity and good supply of nutrients these grafts are contraindicated in beds with poor vascularity. They are indicated to resurface smaller defects for limitation of the size. The graft has better color, consistency, and texture serving the better option for coverage of wound on face. Indications of FTSG are as follows:
  - Defects in which the adjacent tissues are immobile or scarce
  - Adjacent tissue has premalignant or malignant lesion precluding the use of flap.
  - When multistaged procedures are precluded.
  - Punch grafting for hair transplantation
- *Split-thickness skin grafts:* STSG comprise epidermis and variable thickness of the underlying dermis **(Fig. 9)** that was initially described by Ollier and Thiersch in 1872 and 1886, respectively. Depending on the thickness of the dermis they can be classified as thin (0.008–0.012 mm), intermediate thickness (0.012–0.018 mm), and thick (0.018–0.030 mm) STSG grafts. The STSG leaves skin adnexa at the donor site (hair follicles/ sweat glands) that allow repopulation of epidermis. The STSG are used to resurface larger defects and when cosmesis is not of much concern. Depending on how much dermis is included they undergo variable contraction of scar (thicker is the graft more is the graft contraction). The graft is harvested using various instruments (depending on surgeon training and preference). Following is a small description of various methods used to harvest a STSG.
  - *Harvesting with the help of dermatome:* Commercial air-powered (Zimmer®) or electric powered dermatomes are available that provide rapid harvest of large areas of graft with uniform thickness. The thickness and width of graft are easily adjustable.
  - *Use of drum dermatomes:* These are uncommonly used now, the oscillating blade is manually powered as the drum rolls over the surface. The device is good for harvesting STSG from irregular and convex or concave surfaces like neck, flank, or buttocks. There may be injury to operating personnel from blade and the device needs adhesive glue for sticking the skin to blade and harvest.
  - *Humby knife:* These are the most typical device in vogue for long **(Figs. 10A to H)**. The device requires good technical expertise for gap adjustments and flow of hand movements to achieve a regular graft. Just as a rough measure for adjustment of gap in the blade passing a number 15 Bard-Parker scalpel blade approximates thickness of 0.015 inches (intermediate-thickness STSG).
  - Finally, STSG may also be obtained from a regular scalpel blade but the method is crude and only small grafts are obtained.

Skin graft survival and adherence to the recipient site: A variety of mechanisms are proposed for graft attachment at the grafted defect that vary with the aging of graft and should occur in a sequence to help in graft survival and complete uptake:

- *Plasma imbibition:* As soon as the graft is applied it is an avascular structure and gains its nutrition from the nutrients in the wound bed that reach it via diffusion. Oxygen is also supplied by diffusion from the thin-walled capillaries in the granulation tissue. This requires a healthy wound bed with healthy granulation tissue.
- *Inosculation:* By day 3 under appropriate environment the cut ends of the vessels in the underside of dermis begin to form connections with those of wound bed, a process called inosculation. The growth factors are provided by the wound bed and surviving skin appendages containing cells.
- *Angiogenesis:* This is the process of growth of blood vessels from the wound bed into the graft and occurs by 5th day to a week. This is the reason often the STSG graft dressings are opened around 5 days or later.
- *Development of lymphatics and bridge vascularity:* After a week, lymphatics develop in the transplanted skin. Reinnervation of the graft is possible but very rare. In small grafts, a special phenomenon called bridge vascularization is seen when there is relatively avascular bed. The vessels migrate from the highly vascular margins crossing across the avascular base.

Technique

- *Preparation of the recipient site:* Maintain vascular structures in the wound bed. Granulation tissue and healthy muscle are best, however, the graft also survives on periosteum, perichondrium, peritenon, perineurium,

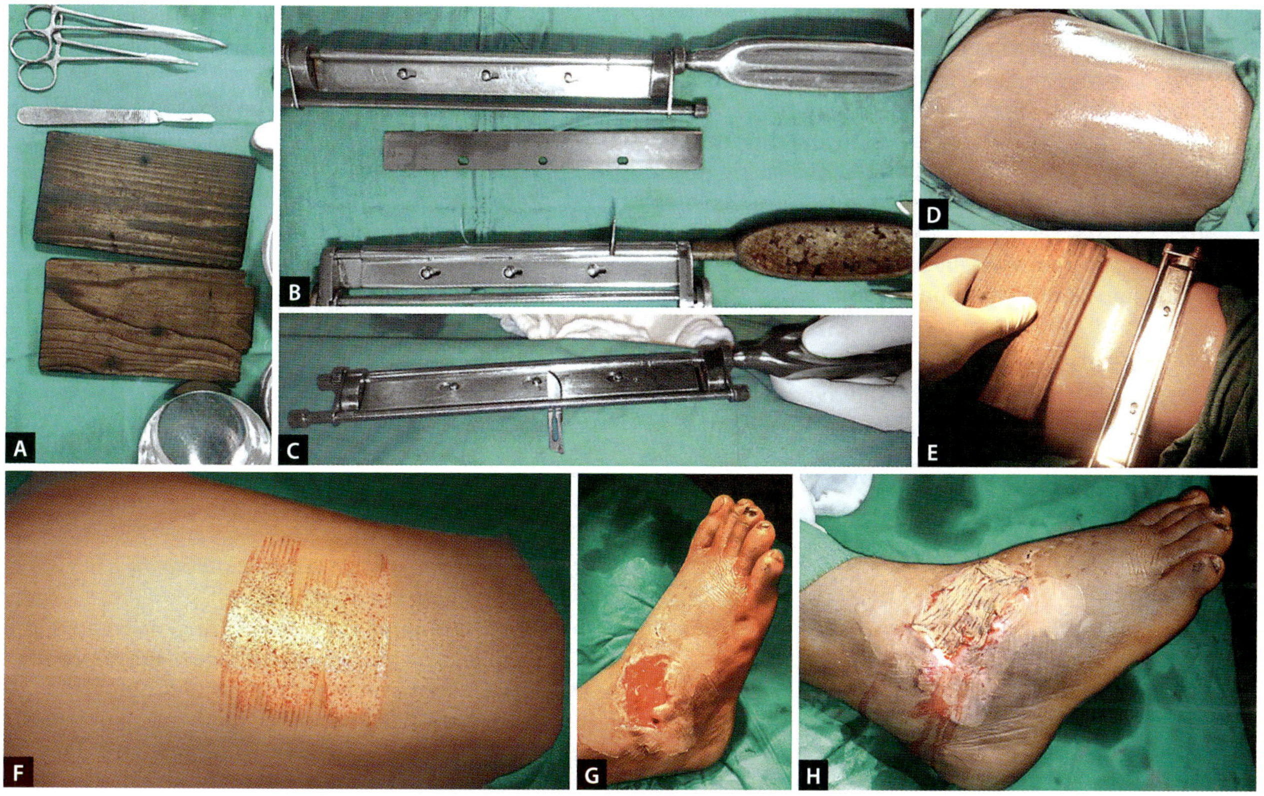

Figs. 10A to H: Common technique of harvesting split-thickness skin graft (STSG). (A) The common tools needed for graft preparation—wooden boards, forceps, knife, and liquid paraffin; (B) The different makes of Humby's knife and the harvesting blade (in middle); (C) Common rough measure for setting the knife to harvest intermediate-thickness skin graft; (D) Preparation of the donor site by applying liquid paraffin; (E) Harvesting the STSG by Humby's knife; (F) Punctate bleeding suggests good intermediate-thickness skin graft; (G) Prepared recipient site—same wound as in **Figure 3** managed with negative pressure wound therapy (NPWT); (H) Applying the prepared STSG and final appearance.

dermis, and fascia. Bare structures such as bone, tendon, ligament, and nerve will not take up the graft. For improved graft uptake postoperative use of NPWT (VAC®) is recommended.

- *Donor site:* Typically for elective cases sites are so chosen that they get hidden under the clothing and are not very obvious. Common sites of STSG are anterolateral thigh portions and buttocks, additional sites are upper inner arm for hand and abdomen when extensive grafts are needed as in burns. Scalp can be used and due to its thickness repetitive grafts can be harvested with minimal risk of alopecia if at all. The obtained grafts are often slit manually or using a mesher for allowing expansion of the graft to cover a larger area and also allow exudate and blood to pass through reducing the chances of graft lift-off.

Complications of Skin Grafting

Graft failure: The skin grafts fail primarily by one of the following four mechanisms:

1. *Poor wound condition:* Grafts put upon avascular structures on the wound bed or structures that are relatively avascular will not let the graft uptake to happen. Tendons, ligaments, and slough or bare bone will not let graft uptake. Fat is relatively avascular and only very thin grafts on a thin fat layer may survive. Periosteum (healthy) or muscle or granulation red beds are best for uptake of the skin graft. Patients who are receiving chemotherapy or graft placed on irradiated tissue also survive poorly.
2. *Sheering movements at graft-bed interface:* Sheer forces separate the graft from wound bed preventing necessary contact and stability for above uptake processes to complete successfully.
3. *Formation of seroma or hematoma that lifts graft above the bed:* Copious exudates or active bleeding will not let the graft attach to the wound bed and hence graft "take" does not happen. If found or any doubt exists one should drain them by 3 days else complete failure of graft would occur.
4. *Infection:* Bacteria produce proteolytic enzymes and the pus accumulation lifts the graft off the bed. This does not allow graft bed bonding and graft fails, if fulminant infections whole graft gets resorbed.

Injury to deeper structures at the donor site: Underlying neural and vascular structures are at risk of damage at the donor site if they are penetrated by an inexperienced person.

Skin Flaps

In few circumstances, it is not possible to close the defect primarily as the skin is either not pliable or the defect is irregular and large. Other indications include:

- Suturing/skin grafting not possible
- Flap over a bare bone may make the difference between viability and sequestration of bone.

The principles or creating local flaps include:

- Carefully map the area on donor tissue with an allowance of 25% excess to compensate for shrinkage of skin after transfer **(Fig. 11)**. Circular defects may be closed by creating tangential cuts in the skin making double opposing semicircular flaps **(Fig. 12A)** or making petal-shaped flaps **(Fig. 12B)**. Various other flaps are shown in **Figures 13A to C**.
- It should not be from a weight-bearing area, also it should not result into an unsightly conspicuous scar.

Distant Skin Flaps

Cross-leg flap (Hamilton 1854): The cross-leg flap is obtained from the other leg (well-leg) and can be of following types:

- Calf-leg flap (preferred, **Fig. 14C**)

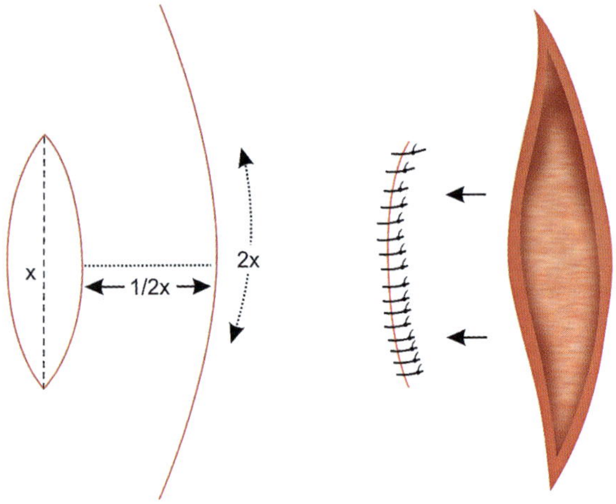

Fig. 11: Creating local flaps for defect coverage.

- *Thigh-leg flap (**Figs. 14A and B**) indicated in:*
  - Female patients wishing to avoid a visible secondary defect
  - Large defects that cannot be closed by opposite calf skin.
- *Principles of cross-leg flap:*
  - Cover defect in every direction
  - Design in a way that the lymphatics are oriented in a direction same as of defect.
  - Delay is indicated if length-to-width ratio exceeds 1½ to 1.
  - Should not undergo even slightest degree of traction.
- *Donor site:*
  - Best-medial calf and anterior aspect of lower one-third of thigh
  - *Alternate sites:* Anterior thigh, posteromedial calf, cross foot flap (Mir-y-Mir)
- *Coverage of raw surface of donor site can be achieved by:*
  - Skin grafting the donor site
  - *Hinge technique (**Fig. 15**):* A hinge is created at the recipient site for proper coverage of the donor site.
- *Postoperative:* As there is propensity for movement the two limbs are fixed by either applying plaster cast or by using an external fixator. One must give deep vein thrombosis (DVT) prophylaxis to these patients.

The "Tube flap": This flap has limited use in reconstructive surgery now. It was first used independently by Filatov, Ganzer, and Gilles. Flap tissue for creating "tube" for lower limb reconstructions is usually removed from anterolateral aspect of abdomen. This is fashioned in the form of a closed tube to restrict infection anchored at both ends. The tube is

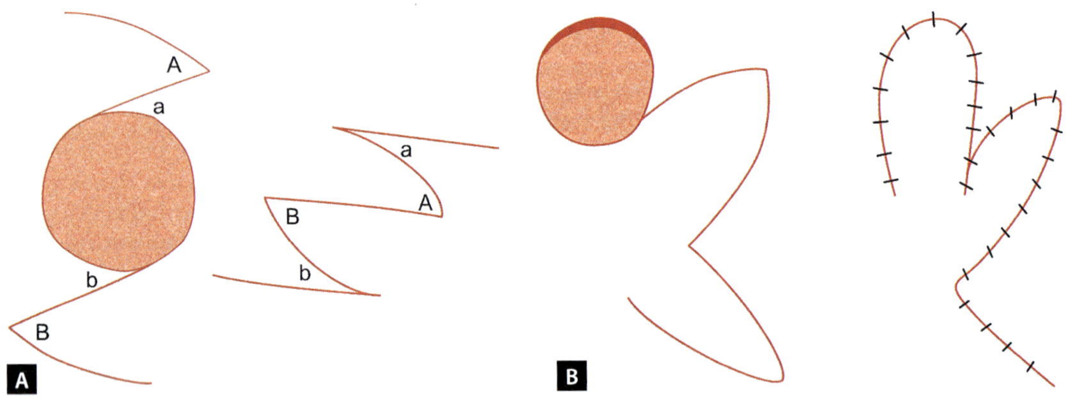

Figs. 12A and B: Closure of circular defect: (A) Using tangential and triangular flaps; (B) Using petal-shaped flaps.

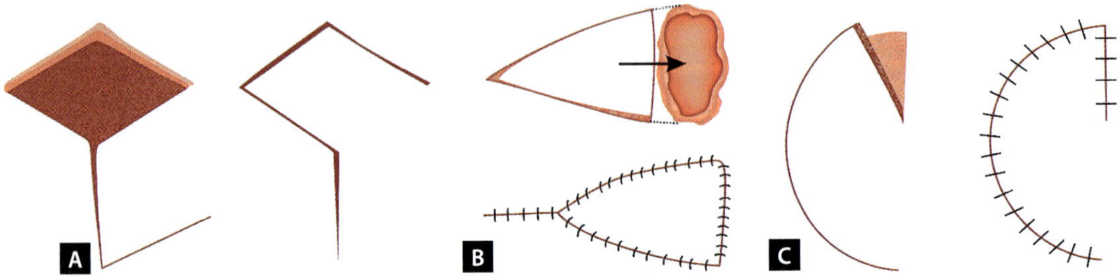

Figs. 13A to C: (A) The Lindberg flap; (B) The V-Y advancement flap; (C) The rotation flap.

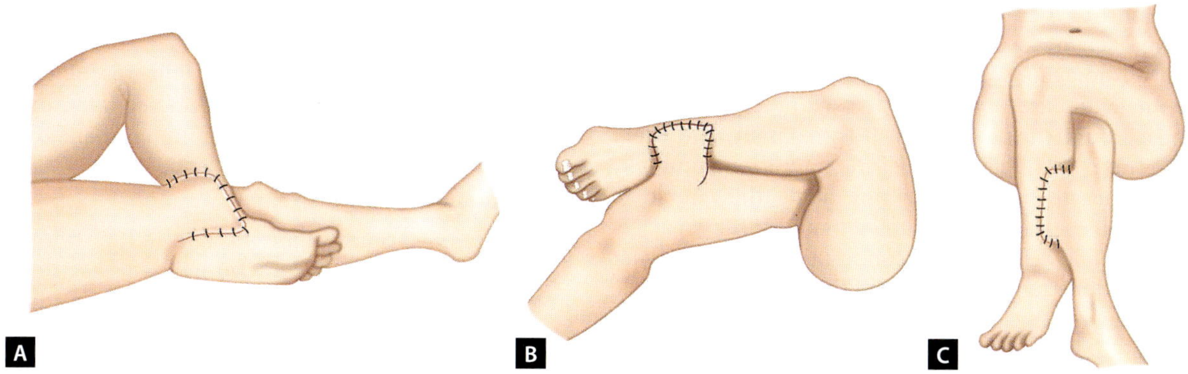

Figs. 14A to C: The cross-leg flap: (A and B) The thigh leg flap; (C) The calf-leg flap.

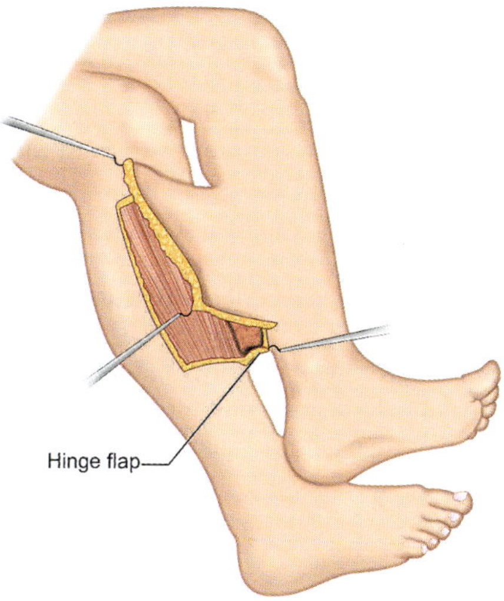

Fig. 15: Hinge technique for cross-leg flaps.

multiply released and progressively anchored till the target tissue is reached.

- *Indication:* Mainly in a female who cannot tolerate position in cross-leg flap or in whom it is not possible due to amputated or disfigured limb.
- *Shortcomings:*
  - Although unlimited in length, but its width is dependent on looseness of tissues to form a tube.
  - Flaps are usually bulky.
  - Excess of fat may constrict circulation.
  - Minimum of fat causes shrinkage.
- *Disadvantage:* Multiple procedures required.

The jump flap: It is typically indicated for coverage of large defects.

- Flap carried from abdominal wall to forearm as an intermediary host and then to fill the defect.
- Success depends upon maintenance of short broad pedicle throughout all stages of transfer.
- Sufficient mobility of leg, shoulder, and body essential
- *Limitations:*
  - Limited to children and young adults
  - Excess of at least one-third of size of defect needed for shrinkage compensation.

Rotational Myocutaneous Flaps

As with rotational skin local flaps, muscle can also be incorporated into the cutaneous flaps.

General principles:

- Pedicled muscle flaps are workhorse for reconstruction .
- Proceed by classifying wounds as acute, subacute, and chronic and by dividing leg into proximal, middle, and distal third.
- Raised flap should be slightly larger than the defect.
- Necessary to have adequate pedicle length
- Choose donor site as per size of flap and its arc of rotation
- Donor site should be out of injury site.
- Prefer free-tissue transfer techniques for complex wounds.

Goals:

- Close the defect with durable tissue
- Esthetically acceptable result
- Minimal donor site morbidity
- Functional result

Contraindications:

- Wounds resulting from high-energy injuries
- Treatment resulting in functional deficit
- Concomitant radiation injury

RECONSTRUCTION OF PROXIMAL THIRD LEG

Options Available

- *Muscle flaps:* Gastrocnemius flap
- *Myocutaneous flaps:* Gastrocnemius flap
- *Fasciocutaneous flaps:* Saphenous flap
  - Sural flap

Gastrocnemius Flap

This is one of the most common flaps used for soft-tissue coverage around the knee and proximal third. It can be used as a muscle flap only or as a musculocutaneous flap. It has been found that the skin overlying the muscle receives much of the supply through perforating vessels originating from the underlying muscle. The skin, hence, can be harvested with the muscle that can then be rotated to cover the soft-tissue defect *in toto*. If only the muscle is used then it has to be covered with a STSG for skin coverage. Gastrocnemius muscle receives most of the blood supply through the sural artery supplying each head (medial and lateral) separately, this is highly advantageous as dissection till the level of pedicle can be made and each head can be used independently by pivoting it around the pedicle that lies proximally. The artery originates from the popliteal vessel and travels longitudinally along the muscle bellies arborizing along the course to supply the muscle. It should be noted that the artery may get damaged in knee dislocation of comminuted supracondylar fractures of the femur limiting use of this flap for soft-tissue coverage in this setting. Perform an arteriogram in such cases.

- The medial flap **(Fig. 16)** has its medial boundary along the long saphenous vein extending till midline posterolaterally (lateral boundary). The distal extent of the flap reaches till 5 cm from medial malleolus where the muscle becomes tendinous.
- The lateral flap **(Fig. 16)** is narrower and shorter than the medial one as the lateral belly of the muscle is smaller.
- The lateral boundary is the fibula and medial boundary is the midline. Distally the flap extends till 10 cm from lateral malleolus. The lateral flap is restricted in mobility due to restriction by lateral popliteal nerve as it crosses over the pedicle.
- *Concerns while using lateral flap:*
  - Lateral head is smaller than medial one.
  - Lateral head has a shorter arc of rotation.
  - Peroneal nerve may get damaged while dissecting lateral head.
  - Smaller defects can be closed with musculocutaneous flap but to close a larger defect use muscle flap and skin graft it to preserve lower limb esthetics.

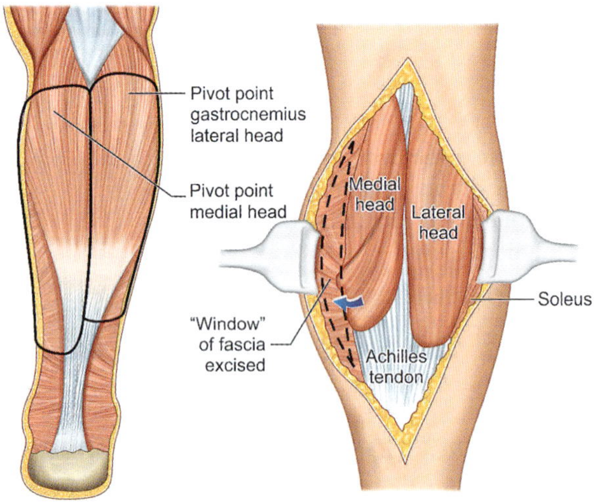

Fig. 16: Gastrocnemius anatomy of medial and lateral heads.

Technique and Some Tricks

- Make a posterior midline incision in the region of calf, make the plane between two heads of gastrocnemius (sural nerve serves as an important landmark in identifying the median raphe if the raphe is not obvious) and then between gastrocnemius and soleus. The tendinous portion is divided distally and skin is usually tacked using a suture to the muscle **(Figs. 17A and B)**. This prevents shearing of the skin away and losing the blood supply. Anterior border along tibia is then incised and flap raised. Proximal dissection is carried out carefully till the vascular pedicle. The defect is then fashioned in the recipient site to fit the flap rather than the flap being adjusted to fit the defect. The skin below the pedicle is then excised as flap is quite successful.
- Excise or score the fascia deep to muscle to increase the length.
- To increase flap's arc of rotation dissect the neurovascular pedicle free and dissect pedicle to its femoral origin—requires expertise of a vascular surgeon.

Complications and Causes of Flap Failure

- Infection
- Injury to flap vascular pedicle
- Venous thrombosis causing impaired viability of the flap. If there is doubt of viability then intravenous fluorescein can be injected and flap observed under ultraviolet light that demonstrates nonviable areas.

Fasciocutaneous Flaps for Proximal Third Leg Region

These are based on the perforators of deep arterial system and include:

- Saphenous flap
- Sural flap

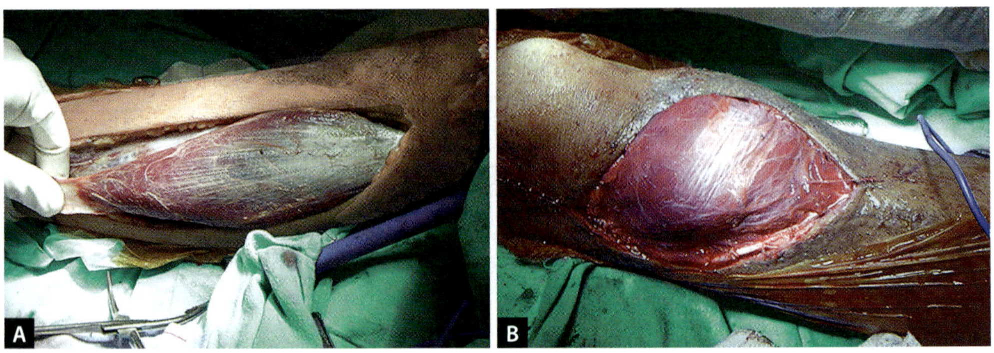

Figs. 17A and B: Gastrocnemius flap for coverage of anterior proximal defect of leg. The flap was covered by a skin graft later.

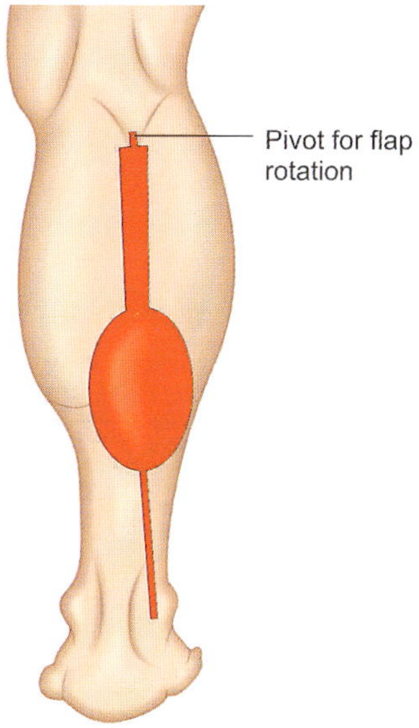

Fig. 18: The sural flap location with pivot point.

Saphenous Fasciocutaneous Flap

- Based on the posteromedial perforators of saphenous artery
- Can be used to close small defects of proximal third of tibia.

Sural flap (This should not be confused with the commonly performed reverse sural fasciocutaneous flap):

- The flap is based on medial superficial sural artery branch of popliteal artery. Mark the course of pedicle from midpoint of the tendo-Achilles and lateral malleolus and midpoint of popliteal crease. The donor site is located along this line. The fasciocutaneous flap is raised as a circular or oval island 15% larger than the recipient defect. The pivot is located proximally 1.5 cm distal to the popliteal crease **(Fig. 18)**. Dissect and ligate the superficial saphenous vein and sural nerve that dips between the two heads of gastrocnemius in midline.
- It has been also employed as a neurosensory flap.
- It must be noted that the *arterial supply of this flap is variable and needs Doppler assessment preoperatively.*
- *Disadvantage:* Leaves posterior aspect of leg anesthetic in the sural nerve distribution.

RECONSTRUCTION OF SOFT-TISSUE DEFECTS IN MIDDLE THIRD REGION OF LEG

Options Available

- *Muscle flaps:*
  - Soleus flap
  - Extensor digitorum longus (EDL)
  - Tibialis anterior
- *Fasciocutaneous flaps:*
  - Lower leg septocutaneous perforator flaps
  - *"Ponten flap"*

Soleus Flap

This is a versatile flap and has been commonly used to reconstitute the soft-tissue defects of middle third region of the leg. The muscle is type II according to the classification of Mathes and Nahai and has a *bipenniform segmental pattern vascular* distribution that receives blood supply from peroneal artery proximally and the posterior tibial artery distally. Soleus occupies posterior two-thirds of the calf region beneath the gastrocnemius so covers a large area. The muscle can be used in various modes and all essentially require additional STSG for coverage as there is no "skin" attached to the muscle.

- Hemisoleus flap (covers soft-tissue defects up to middle-third of leg at a distance >5 cm from medial malleolus)—uses half of the muscle and is the most common way of utilizing this muscle either medially (commonly) or laterally. The muscle can be split into individual halves by virtue of arrangement of its fibers so that half of the muscle is raised free. This flap preserves the plantar flexion power that would otherwise get compromised by complete muscle harvest. The distal tibial perforators need to be ligated to harvest this flap so one must look for necrosis of the distal muscle that may readily occur if the proximal blood supply is inadequate constitutionally or in smokers and elderly due to arteriosclerosis.
- Classical soleus flap—uses whole of the muscle but is limited by restricted rotation and too bulky a soft-tissue prominence at the reconstructed site. This flap also compromises the plantar flexion power as soleus is the most powerful muscle for this movement.
- Distally based flap (can cover distal third defects up to medial malleolus and in some cases at ankle also)—this is an advancement rather modification in the use of this muscle where muscle is used attached distally at the tendo-Achilles while the proximal portion is harvested free. The flap is more in vogue nowadays as this has better mobility and can even cover some defects of distal third. The medial half of the muscle is more consistently supplied by the distal tibial perforators on which the flap is based for its blood supply. The blood supply is, however, tenuous and the flap should be avoided in crush injuries of the leg as then there are high chances of damage to the perforator supply. For assuring the blood supply one may follow the principles of "angiosomes" as detailed by Taylor and Palmer in 1987, which has allowed surgeons to successfully use the flap based even on one or two critical perforators only.
- *Technique:* For harvesting hemisoleus flap make an incision from posteromedial tibial plateau till the medial malleolus and make a plane between soleus and gastrocnemius which is easily identifiable in the middle of muscle bulk **(Fig. 19)**. Separate the soleus from flexor digitorum longus. Split the muscle just lateral to the midline so as to preserve the intermuscular artery and posterior neurovascular bundle is identified. Release the muscle from tendo-Achilles attachment and ligate the distal perforators from posterior tibial artery to mobilize the muscle and transpose it to cover the defect **(Figs. 20A and B)**.

For harvesting the reverse hemisoleus flap—place the incision above 2 cm medial to the medial edge of tibia and split the muscle. The secondary vascular pedicles from

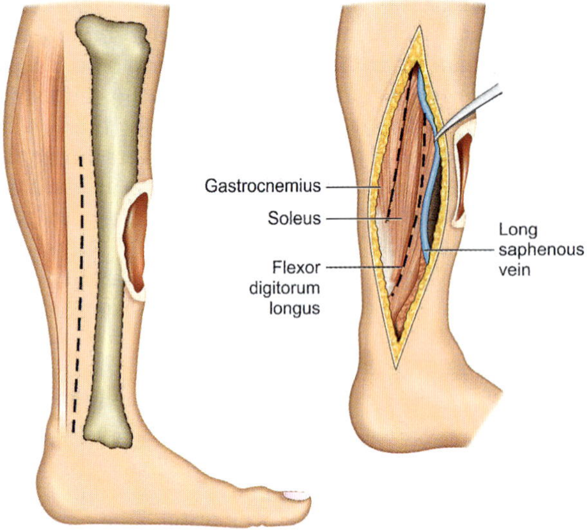

Fig. 19: The soleus flap—incision and creation of planes.

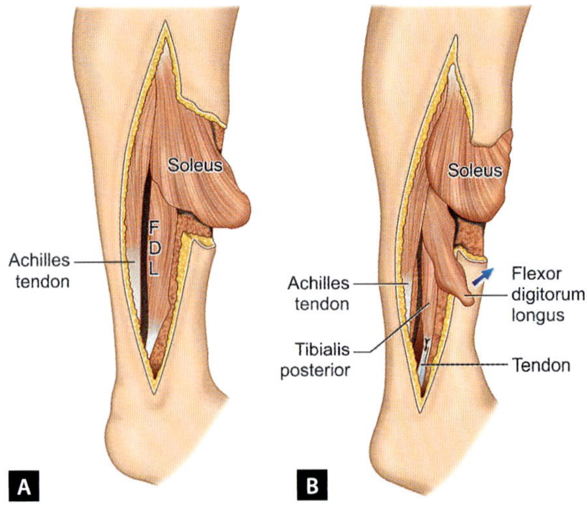

Figs. 20A and B: Hemisoleus muscle flap with rotation of the harvested muscle (proximally based).

perforators are carefully protected in the distal portion. The medial muscle half is separated proximally at the proximal and middle third junction and muscle transposed to the defect. If the perforators permit greater mobilization without undue tension on them the muscle can also be released distally from the tendo-Achilles. Donor area is then primarily closed over drain and skin graft (STSG) is placed on the muscle primarily or as a delayed procedure.

- *Advantages:*
  - Well-vascularized flap
  - Minimal donor site morbidity
  - Minimal functional deficit (hemisoleus flap)

Extensor Digitorum Longus Flap

- Useful for closure of smaller wounds (<5 cm)
- *Blood supply:* Anterior tibial artery that supplies around 9–14 perforators.
- *Disadvantages:*
  - If too many perforators ligated flap may not survive.
  - Close proximity to peroneal nerve—varus deformity if damaged.
  - Permanent loss of toe extension if muscle used in entirety.

Tibialis Anterior Muscle Flap

- Excellent flap to cover long narrow defects
- *Blood supply:* Anterior tibial artery supplies the muscle in a circumpennate distribution that allows the muscle to be split according to the need of surgeon for coverage of different locations of the soft-tissue defects on leg. This makes it a versatile flap for coverage of wide portion of the leg in the middle two-thirds of the leg. The only limitation is the lack of coverage in the width of defect due to small muscle mass.
- Defects of 10–15 cm in length and 2–4 cm in width can be reconstructed.
- Alternatively, partial division of muscle can be used to cover small defects up to 5 cm in diameter.

Fasciocutaneous Flaps for Middle Third Reconstruction

These are based on medial or posterolateral septocutaneous perforators of the lower leg. The greatest limitation is the precarious blood supply and the high likelihood of venous congestion in these flaps due to limited rotation arc and tense closure. The flaps are used only by experienced persons in soft-tissue reconstruction and those with familiarity of the local blood supply. Portable Doppler does come handy in preoperative assessment of the flap harvest.

- *"Ponten flap":* Based upon medial septocutaneous perforators from posterior tibial artery
  - Can cover small defects
- *Random (reticular) pattern flaps:*
  - Pure cutaneous flaps—length to width ratio = 1.5:1
  - Fasciocutaneous flaps—length to width ratio = 3:1

RECONSTRUCTION OF DISTAL THIRD REGION OF THE LEG

Options Available

- *Muscle flaps:* Limitation of all muscle flaps in this region is of providing only a limited small area reconstruction.
  - Soleus flap
  - Extensor digitorum longus
  - Tibialis anterior
  - Peroneus brevis
- *Fasciocutaneous flap:*
  - Reverse flow flaps based on:
    - Anterior tibial artery
    - Posterior tibial artery
    - Peroneal artery
  - Lateral leg fasciocutaneous flap

Soleus Muscle Flap (see also the Reverse Soleus Flap above)

Typically, this is indicated for small wounds. Get preoperative MRI to explore this possibility.

Peroneus Brevis Muscle Flap

Most useful muscle for reconstruction in this region. It is supplied by peroneal artery so there is usually no threat to vascularity of the foot. One must, however, confirm that the patient has adequate vascularity from other sources. To this effect digital subtraction angiography helps.

Fasciocutaneous Flaps

- Vessels in this region perforate fascia in three groups:
  - *Medial:* From posterior tibial vessels
  - *Anterolateral:* From anterior tibial vessels
  - *Posterolateral:* From peroneal vessels
- Medial vessels perforate in four distinct groups between:
  - 4–6 cm
  - 9–12 cm
  - 17–19 cm
  - 22–24 cm from medial malleolar prominence
- Posterolateral perforators lie posterior to fibula clustering at proximal and distal ends of fibula.
- Anterolateral vessels cluster between tibialis anterior and EDL proximally and between EDL and peroneus brevis distally.

Distally-based Fasciocutaneous Rotation Flaps

- The units can be raised from posteromedial aspect of leg from 8 cm below the knee to some 4 cm above the medial malleolus.
- The distally based fasciocutaneous flap is basically an "island flap".
- *Caution:* Foot may go ischemic.

Lateral Leg Fasciocutaneous Flap

- Based on peroneal artery—can be used as a transposition flap or an island flap either to cover tibia proximally or as a reversed flow flap to cover more distal defects.
- Need Doppler angiogram.

MICROVASCULAR FREE FLAPS

These flaps require meticulous preoperative evaluation. Evaluate the needed coverage for size, thickness, durability, and cosmetic appearance of the area to be covered. Ascertain that the recipient site has good availability of and accessibility to adequate size and length of recipient vessels. It should be possible to place anastomoses away from recipient defect if possible. Ideally, the site should be free from infection. Every effort should be made to place the anastomoses away from infection.

Gracilis Muscle Free Flap (Fig. 21)

- Based on medial femoral circumflex vessels
- Motor innervation from obturator nerve (L4–5)
- It can be used as either muscle flap or a myocutaneous flap
- Ideal for small soft-tissue defects

Advantages

- No significant functional deficit
- Donor site scar minimal

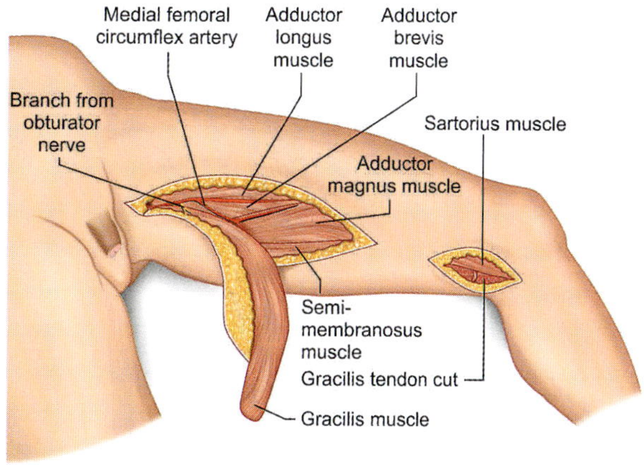

Fig. 21: The anatomy of gracilis muscle free flap.

- Atrophies over a time period of 3–4 months so gives good cosmetic result.

Precautions

- Skin over distal muscle not as well-perfused as on proximal aspect
- Pedicle may be very small.
- Anatomic variations—multiple small pedicles
  - So it is recommended to prepare other potential donor site simultaneously.

Technical Tricks

- For musculocutaneous flap place incision distally over tendon and design skin paddle to ensure its location over muscle.
- For a muscle only flap place incision directly over muscle parallel to and posterior to a line joining pubic tubercle and medial tibial condyle.

Rectus Abdominis Free Flap (Type III Muscle)

- Based on deep inferior epigastric vessels
- Ideal for intermediate sized defect
- Extraordinary geometric versatility due to:
  - Long length of muscle, and
  - Long pedicle
- *Types:* Vertical, transverse rectus abdominis (TRAM), bipedicled, superiorly based, inferiorly based
  - *Advantages of a TRAM flap:*
    - Suprapubic horizontal donor site scar is quite acceptable.
    - Simultaneous abdominoplasty
    - Quality of skin better than LD flap

Latissimus Dorsi Free Flap

- Ideal for covering large soft-tissue defects
- Flap can be based electively on different vessels depending upon required diameter and length of vessels:
  - Usually based on thoracodorsal artery
  - For the need of a small bridging graft—subscapular and medial circumflex scapular artery can be used.

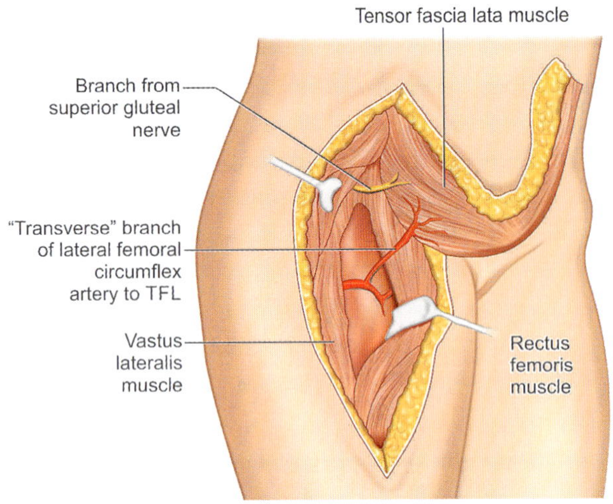

Fig. 22: The tensor fascia muscle flap—anatomy and relations.

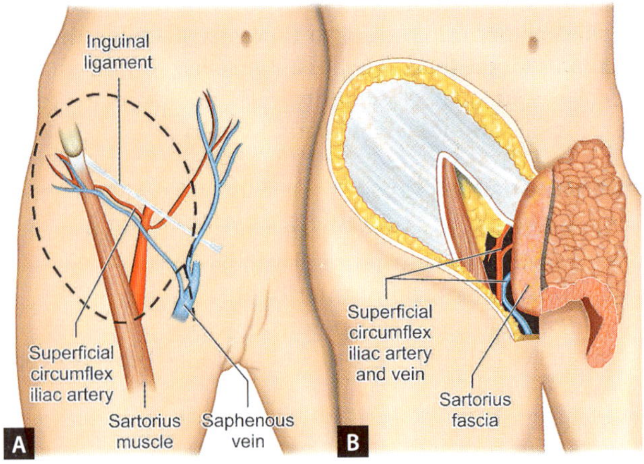

Figs. 23A and B: The groin flap anatomy and relations.

- Also subscapular artery can be used as an interposition graft in lower limb injuries with thoracodorsal artery supplying the flap
- *Advantages:*
  - Latissimus dorsi is a relatively thin muscle.
  - It can also be used in arteriosclerotic vessels when end to side anastomoses is not possible.
  - Muscle atrophies over time to give a pleasing contour.

Tensor Fascia Lata Flap (Fig. 22)

- Provides abundant skin and subcutaneous tissue
- Based on lateral femoral circumflex artery
- Neural innervation—inferior branch of superior gluteal nerve (L4–5, S1)
- Now abandoned due to formidable donor site morbidity.

Groin Flap (McGregor and Jackson, 1972)

The groin flap is a *fasciocutaneous type A* flap supplied by the *superficial circumflex iliac* system that has a variable anatomy. The skin is innervated from T12 segment. The flap can be used either as a rotational flap for coverage of the abdominal or perineal wounds or as a free flap based on its vascular pedicle or even for soft-tissue coverage of hand as a parasite flap (like a cross leg flap, the defect in hand is covered with the harvested flap and kept in place for 3–4 weeks). The flap is then detached to provide skin coverage.

Technique

Mark the flap (Usually made 10–20% larger than defect) and incise the skin down the fascia, elevate the flap distal to proximal superficial to the tensor fascia lata (TFL) which is the distal extent of the flap **(Figs. 23A and B)**. The flap is dissected from the anterior superior iliac spine (ASIS), inguinal ligament, and external oblique fascia. The pedicle of the flap lies in the femoral canal and originates from femoral artery.

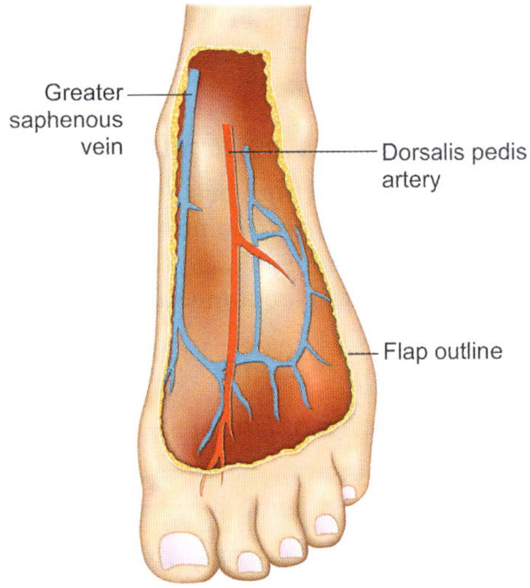

Fig. 24: The dorsalis pedis flap.

Advantages

- Versatile and readily available
- Can be designed into large dimensions.
- Texture and quality of skin are excellent.
- Donor site can be primarily closed.
- Residual defect can be easily concealed.
- Now status relegated to "last resort" flap.

Disadvantages

- Variable arterial anatomy
- Short pedicle
- Unsuitable in obese patient

Dorsalis Pedis Flap (Fig. 24)

- *Based on dorsalis pedis artery:*
  - Accompanies deep peroneal nerve
  - Supplies a mean of 3.8 vertical branches

- *Venous drainage:* Superficial dorsal venous arch medially into great saphenous vein and laterally into short saphenous vein
- Sensory supply—superficial peroneal nerve
- *Advantages:*
  - Thin pliable skin
  - Large pedicle
- *Disadvantages:*
  - Donor site morbidity—simple spilt skin grafting (SSG) required and long-term care
  - Chronic aching foot—obvious disadvantage for footwear

Fasciocutaneous Free Flaps (Description is beyond the Scope of this Book)

- Lateral arm free flap
- Parascapular free flap

Osteocutaneous Free Flaps (Description is beyond the Scope of this Book)

Iliac crest with overlying skin

Osteofasciocutaneous Free Flaps (Description is beyond the scope of this book)

- For coverage of large osseous and skin defects
- Based on fibula with intact lateral septum as vascular supply and variable skin island

PRESSURE SORES (BED SORES, PRESSURE ULCERS)

Pressure ulcers develop at areas where continual pressure exceeds normal capillary pressure (20–32 mm Hg) producing ischemia prolonged enough to cause tissue death. The time duration required for tissue death varies from the tissue type (muscle cells and tissue succumb to 4 hours of ischemia while skin requres 12 hours of complete ischemia to become nonviable). In general, it is believed that continuous pressure for >2 hours is not good and one must keep changing posture for 30 minutes every 2 hours. The pressure sores are mainly of two types:

1. *Insensate ulcers (denervated ulcers):* These patients are suffering from disease or condition where they have lost sensation and are incapable of reporting discomfort due to ischemic damage as in spinal cord injury, transverse myelitis, head injury, etc.
2. *Sensate (innervated ulcers):* Sensate persons too develop ulcers when subjected to prolonged pressure due to lying down on a relatively hard surface where the bony prominence presses the soft tissue relentlessly. These are patients commonly suffering from lower limb trauma and are typically older in age like fracture neck femur and fracture intertrochanteric. Patients needing intensive care are also prone to develop these ulcers.

Pressure sores typically develop over bony prominences that in initial stages appear as erythema and with neglect develop into partial thickness and the complete thickness defects. The most common sites of occurrence of pressure ulcers are over ischium, sacrum, trochanter, calcaneus, and occiput. In late stages, even the bone gets infected and osteomyelitic. The stages of progression of pressure ulcer are as follows:

- Stage I—nonblanchable erythema (skin intact)
- Stage II—epidermis ulcerated and most of the dermis also eroded or nonviable
- Stage III—dermis ulcerated completely with visible deeper subcutaneous tissue
- Stage IV—ulceration extends to underlying bone (usually superficial osteomyelitis)
- Stage V—gross infection with closed large cavities and a small sinus opening

This is Shea's modification of pressure sore classification quite useful to guide treatment. Stage 1 and 2 ulcers often respond to conservative management. Stage 3 ulcers should be evaluated also for osteomyelitis by biopsy. Stage 4 ulcers also need management of bone infection. Stage 5 ulcers should be unrooted.

Management

Conservative management

Strategies for conservative management of pressure sores:

Pressure relieving strategies: Frequent turning, low air-loss beds, and water mattress are commonly employed but turning in bed is the most important measure. For heel ulcers special pressure relieving boots are important. Patients using wheel chairs should be provided with soft cushions.

Dressings and debriding agents: These are the cheapest measures deployed commonly as first line of treatment for ulcer higher than stage 1. Gauze dressings are applied after debriding an eschar. Commonly moist dressings are deployed and repeatedly changed to limit infection and enhance granulation tissue formation. Stage 1 ulcers may be managed by transparent film dressings (see above in dressings). For stage 2 ulcer a moist dressing is best, hydrogels may also be employed. Stage 3 and 4 ulcers need wet-to-dry dressings after a thorough debridement. The dressings dry within the wound and also in turn debride the tissue. The dressing is changed 3–4 times a day. If the wound has a foul smell then use 0.25% Dakins bleach to wetten the dressing. Other enzymatic debriding agents may also be used. If the ulcers are slow to heal or are very large then primary flap coverage may be considered.

Negative-pressure wound therapy (see above): This is a faster way of granulating the wound and healing it.

Hydrotherapy: This is more commonly employed for debridement of the venous stasis ulcer in the lower extremity. Pulsed lavage has now replaced hydrotherapy and provides faster granulation tissue formation and reducing infection.

Surgical Management

Debridement: All necrotic ulcers with slough or eschar are to be debrided for formation of granulation tissue and allow healing. Attempt should be made to preserve as much of bone as possible. The procedure of complete ischiectomy should only be reserved for excessive destruction of bone.

Femoral head excision: It is done if a trochanteric ulcer extends to the joint space and has septic features. One must fill the dead space with a muscle or some soft tissue.

Flap coverage: Most large and deep ulcers will ultimately need a flap coverage. Muscle flaps should be used to fill deep spaces. Commonly the following flaps are used for coverage of a pressure sore:

- Gluteal posterior flap or posterior thigh flap for covering ischial pressure sore
- V-Y advancement gluteal flap for covering sacral pressure sore
- Tensor fascia lata or posterior thigh flap for covering trochanteric pressure sores

For all flap surgeries one must remember that complete healing can only be achieved if appropriate environment is produced. Adequate debridement of the ulcer base to reach the viable tissue and healthy bleeding is a must. The skin margins at the defect should also be viable and bleeding. For all flap surgeries one must protect the site from shear forces postoperatively else the flap will fail. This can be done by using ripple air mattress or water mattress and turning of the patient regularly. This should be followed as a strict regime. In next 1–2 weeks, progressive sitting is done starting 15 minutes twice a day and increased as comfortable. Drains should be used to eliminate dead spaces and use of antibiotics is variable with longer course needed for underlying osteomyelitis.

CONCLUSION

- Proper wound healing is always a concern for deemed successful outcome of surgery and heavily relies on soft-tissue handling.
- Factors that may hamper proper wound healing should be identified and appropriately addressed for all surgical endeavors.
- Loss of soft-tissue cover limits osseous reconstruction options and if not adequate then infection and ultimate failure is common.
- Implant-related surgeries at high risk of deep and superficial infections so soft-tissue coverage gains upper hand in all surgical reconstructions.
- Preliminary knowledge of avenues of soft-tissue reconstructions should be known to an orthopedic surgeon so that appropriate surgical planning and optimal outcome can be provided to the patient. It is especially important in open trauma and mass surgical resections for orthopedic oncology and management of long-standing tissue infections.
- Plastic surgery help should be always sought in planning of soft-tissue coverage but a combined team effort is successful only when the orthopedic surgeon also has knowledge of these reconstructions so that the surgical procedure can be modified and harm is avoided.
- Biology of pressure ulcers should be well understood and in immobilized patients prevention is the best measure that should be always stressed. In unfortunate circumstances, where they develop appropriate care is imperative to prevent catastrophic outcome.

CHAPTER 21

Gait

Manish Kumar Varshney

DEFINITION

Gait is the process of locomotion using lower limbs. It is a rhythmic sequential movement of the lower limbs that moves the body along the required line and maintains stability and conserves energy. Thus, gait needs three components:

1. *Progression:* This is basically the forward fall of the body weight. The primary force for this is generated by the lower limb. Secondary momentum may also be generated by swinging motion of the upper limb.
2. *Stability:* This forward fall is a controlled fall that, at all times, maintains the upright stability of the body. The head, neck, trunk, and upper limb are carried along by the lower limbs and the alignment of various body segments is maintained at all times. The body is most stable during the stance phase when the ankle, knee, and hip are vertically aligned and least stable during the swing phase. The stability during gait is further maintained by strong ligaments at the hip anteriorly and knee posteriorly (tensor fascia lata and iliotibial tract). As the foot length is less posteriorly and more anteriorly, for optimal foot support the body weight line must be anterior to the ankle joint.
   The impact on the joints is reduced at the ankle by pretibial muscles that delays forefoot contact until late in the initial double support period. At the knee, a balance between knee stability and shock absorption is achieved by eccentric quadriceps contractions during loading response and the impact of loading is minimized at the hip through hip abductor muscle contraction. Altered joint motion or absent muscle forces may increase joint reaction forces and lead subsequently to joint pathology.
3. *Energy conservation:* The energy expenditure for walking is calculated as oxygen used per meter traveled. Gait efficiency is improved by reducing the amount of muscular effort required to walk. This can be done in two ways: (a) by substituting momentum for muscle action. This is achieved by smooth swinging movements without jerks and abrupt starts and stops; (b) secondly, by minimizing displacement of the body from the line of progression. This is done by coordinating pelvic, knee, and ankle motion ensuring that the center of gravity of the body displaces only by 5 cm up and down, 5 cm sideways. These optimizations used to minimize the excursion of center of gravity are known as *Saunders' determinants of gait.* Optimum use of energy occurs during one's natural gait velocity. This velocity is determined by age, dimension of limbs, terrain, level of fitness, cadence (the number of steps per minute), etc. Walking slower or faster increases the energy expenditure. Sometimes the critical factor in selecting a wheelchair for mobility is the energy requirement. Patients tend to self-select wheelchair mobility when cost per distance exceeds 300% of normal values.

PHASES OF GAIT (FIG. 1)

- *Stance phase is divided into:*
  - Heel strike
  - Foot flat
  - Midstance
  - Heel off
  - Toe off
- *Swing phase is divided into:*
  - Preswing or initial swing
  - Midswing
  - Late swing or terminal swing

Since the gait cycle blends from one phase to another any event may be taken as the starting point. By convention, heel strike is taken as the first gait phase. While walking when one limb is in stance phase the other limb is in swing phase. With increase in speed, there is an increase in the swing and decrease in the stance phase. Double support is when both limbs are on the ground. During the transition from walking to running, there is elimination of double support period. While running, there is no double stance (double float).

Gait Analysis

Clinically, observational gait analysis is done by making a person walk on smooth surface for a minimum of 15 feet distance. The gait is observed from the front, back, and sides. It is used to assess and treat individuals with conditions affecting their ability to walk. It is also used in sports biomechanics to help athletes and to treat movement-related problems in people with injuries.

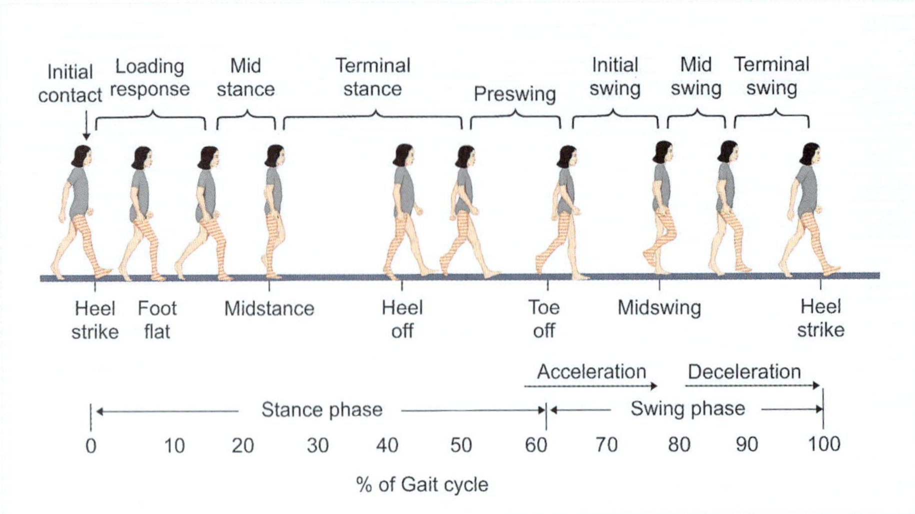

Fig. 1: Gait cycle. The gait cycle is classically divided into two phases—the stance phase (60% of cycle) and the swing phase (40%) involving a combination of open and closed chain activities. The stance phase begins from heel strike and it is further divided into specific instances for point referencing of the describing gait into heel strike, foot flat, midstance, heel-off, and toe-off. The swing phase is a continuum but is separated from stance due to loss of floor contact and is divided into initial swing, midswing, and terminal swing. Because classical descriptions use "point reference" to describe a continuous flow of events so newer descriptions have been used for gait cycle. One such method is gait-cycle phasing (GCP) where it is divided into phases instead of discrete points. The GCP has total of eight phases where five phases comprise the stance phase, viz., initial contact, loading response (from heelstrike till end of foot flat), midstance, terminal stance (ends at heel off), preswing and three phases make the swing phase, viz., initial swing, midswing, and late swing. Both feet are on the ground at the beginning and end of the stance phase comprising 10% duration in each. This is called double support period = 20% of the gait cycle.

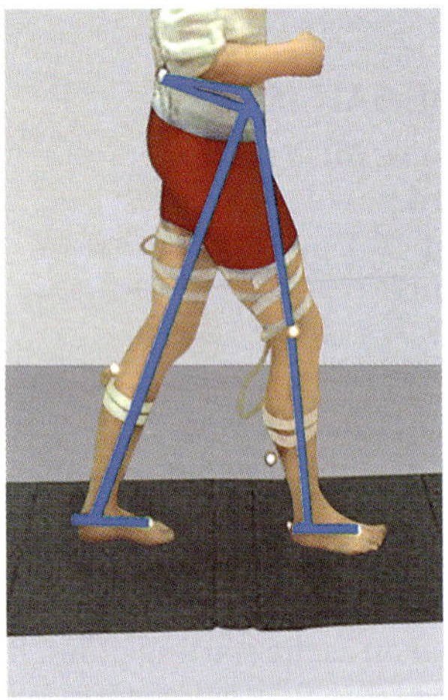

Fig. 2: Gait analysis.

BOX 1: The various terminologies used in describing gait.

- *Step* is one single step while *stride* is whole gait cycle.
- *Stride* is the completion of the gait cycle and stride length is the distance from heel strike of one limb to heel strike of the same limb again.
- *Gait cycle* is composed of two steps, one by each limb.
- *Step length* is distance from heel strike of one limb to heel strike of other limb.
- Stride length is the linear distance covered by one gait cycle. Average stride length for adults is 150–170 cm.
- *Stance time* is the stance phase of one extremity.
- *Stride duration* or gait cycle duration is time taken to complete one stride and, in normal adults, is approximately 1 second.
- *Cadence* is the number of steps taken per minute or per second—average cadence in young adults = 115–120 steps/min.
- *Walking velocity* is the distance traveled per unit time. The preferred walking speed in adults is 1.4 m/s.
- *Step width* is the distance between midpoint of heel of one foot to same point in other foot.

Kinematics is the study of position of the joints during the gait cycle. This can be done by video imaging from the front, back, and sides, by attaching sensors at various points such as iliac spines of the pelvis, ankle malleolus, and the condyles of the knee **(Fig. 2)**. Movements of hip, knee, and ankle can be recorded by a camera with lights strapped to joints (photokinegram). One common method is the Helen Hayes Hospital market set in which a total of 15 markers are attached on the lower body.

Kinetics denotes the forces that act on the body during the gait cycle. These forces are divided into the internal forces due to the action of the muscles and the external forces due to gravity. For kinetic studies of external forces, force plates or pressure pads are used which measure the ground reaction forces and moments including the magnitude, direction, and location of pressure. The spatial distribution of forces is measured with pedobarography equipment. Electromyogram is used to study internal forces.

The following parameters are assessed during gait analysis: Stride length, cadence, dynamic base, foot and hip angle, speed, and progression line. [**Box 1 and Fig. 3:** Ankle, knee, and hip joints go through sequential rhythmic movements enforced by various muscle acting across them **(Table 1)** to produce smooth walking cycle.]

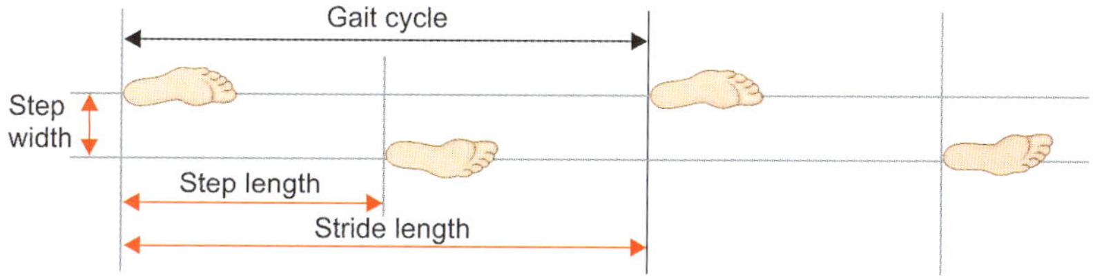

Fig. 3: The various terminologies used in describing gait cycle.

TABLE 1: The common joint positions and activities of muscles during various phases of gait cycle .

Phase of gait cycle	Ankle position	Active leg muscles	Knee position	Active thigh muscles	Hip position	Active pelvic and gluteal muscles
Heel strike	Neutral	Ankle dorsiflexors (tibialis anterior, extensor digitorum longus, and extensor hallucis longus)	Extension (0° flexion)	Eccentric contraction of quadriceps	30° of hip flexion	Gluteus maximus and hamstrings prevent hip flexion beyond 30°. Erector spinae prevents flexion of spine
Foot-flat	15° of plantar flexion	Eccentric contraction of above muscles	20° of flexion	Concentric quadriceps contraction	Movement from flexion to neutral	Same as above
Midstance	3° of dorsiflexion	Plantar flexors of ankle (gastrocnemius, soleus, tibialis posterior, and flexor digitorum longus) control movement of tibia over the foot	15° of flexion	Both quadriceps and hamstrings are inactive. Knee is locked passively (screw-home mechanism)	Neutral position	Hip extensors contraction + gluteus medius and quadratus lumborum maintain pelvic stability
Heel-off	15° plantar flexion	Plantar flexors of foot	Movement from extension to flexion	Gastrocnemius contraction prevents hyperextension	Movement from neutral to hip extension of 20°	Hip extensors and hip abductors to clear the limb away from midline and stabilize pelvis
Toe-off and Push-off	Plantar flexion of 40–60°	Plantar flexors become inactive while toe flexors active (flexor hallucis, flexor digitorum, peronei)	40° of flexion	Hamstring contraction, Vastus intermedius, and rectus femoris activate at the end to prevent excessive flexion at knee	As above	As above
Swing phase	Neutral to slight dorsiflexion	Ankle dorsiflexors and toe extensors	Movement from flexion to extension	Quadriceps active throughout and slow at end, Hamstrings active at end to decelerate swing	Swing from extension to flexion	Gluteus maximus functions to reverse hip flexion to extension

FACTORS AFFECTING GAIT

- *Pathology of muscle function:*
  - *Central causes:* Ataxia and rigidity
  - *Peripheral causes:* Nerve injuries, muscle disease, and disuse atrophy
- *Pathology of joint function:*
  - Excessive movements as in postpolio residual paralysis, Ehlers–Danlos syndrome
  - Restricted movements as in contractures, arthritis
- *Pathology of sensation:* Loss of proprioception, perceptual defects, and ear problems
- Pain
- Psychiatric disorders
- Extrinsic factors such as terrain, footwear, clothing, and weight carried
- Intrinsic factors such as sex, weight, height, age, physique, measurements and body proportions, etc.
- Aging is associated with reduced walk speed and step length with stable cadence. The step width in elderly is 40% larger than younger counterparts (elderly females have approximately 8 cm while elderly men have 10 cm of step width).

CLINICAL EXAMINATION AND TYPES OF PATHOLOGICAL GAIT

The clinical examination of gait starts from evaluation of a standing patient. The patient is inspected from all sides while standing still (preferably with clothes removed) to find asymmetries, postural abnormalities, limb length discrepancies, deformities, etc. Then the patient's walk is evaluated from front and all sides while walking over a distance of several meters. The patient should be made to walk without shoes and unaided (unless totally crippled to walk without). Normal walk is rhythmic, uninhibited, and effortless in a flow of freely swinging legs in an upright posture. It is associated with movements of the trunk and arms swinging opposite to movement of legs. The parameters observed and recorded during evaluation are summarized in **Box 2**. One may also include the "time to up and go (TUG)" test during evaluation. This is measured as the time that a patient needs to stand up from a chair with arm rests, walk 3 meters (walking aids are allowed if used), turn around, walk back, and sit back down. TUG test is a simple assessment used to evaluate the risk of fall in geriatric patients.

Quadriceps Weakness (Fig. 4)

During late swing and early stance phase the knee is maintained in extension by quadriceps muscle. In quadriceps weakness, forces across joints tend to flex the knee. The compensatory mechanisms that prevent knee from buckling are:

- Patients lean forward to bring the body weight anterior to the knee resulting in a straight knee with excessive plantar flexion, hip flexion, and a forward trunk. This results in knee hyperextension where it is stabilized by posterior knee ligaments only. So this is also called "knee hyperextension gait".

BOX 2: The various parameters used to evaluate gait in clinical examination.

- Sitting and standing unaided
- Standing up from a sitting position (unaided and with/without use of upper limbs)
- Posture
- Stance (narrow/wide base)
- Gait initiation (blockage)
- Walking (smooth, stiff, insecure, symmetrical, and limping)
- Step length, lifting of feet, contact with ground, wide/narrow base
- Speed of walk—time taken to walk a specified distance (usually ≤6 m)
- Arm swing
- Freezing
- Turning
- Sitting down (motor recklessness)

- If soleus and hip extensors are strong, premature ankle flexion then is the only sign.
- The knee can be stabilized by using a hand to thigh gait.
- The limb is externally rotated to orient the external force vector medial to the joint axis, reducing the tendency toward knee flexion.
- Hand knee gait is when patient physically pushes anterior thigh to prevent knee from buckling.

Pretibial Muscle Weakness

Weakness of the pretibial muscles causes slapping of the foot during the stance phase at the time of loading response. The compensatory mechanisms that prevent this foot slapping are:

- Ipsilateral circumduction of the limb
- Ipsilateral high stepping gait (*steppage* or *equine gait*) **(Fig. 5)**
- Contralateral hip hiking
- Instead of normal heel strike, there is slapping of whole foot.

Common causes are peroneal nerve palsy and L5 radiculopathy. Bilateral causes are amyotrophic lateral sclerosis, Charcot–Marie–Tooth disease and other peripheral neuropathies.

Antalgic Gait

The patient tries to reduce the weight borne by the painful limb by the following compensatory mechanisms:

- The patient tries to reduce the stance phase of the gait cycle especially the loading response.
- The double support phase is increased and there is decreased single support time.
- There is shortened stride length of the contralateral limb.
- When the hip joint is painful (Coxalgic gait), there is lurch of trunk toward the painful side. This moves the center

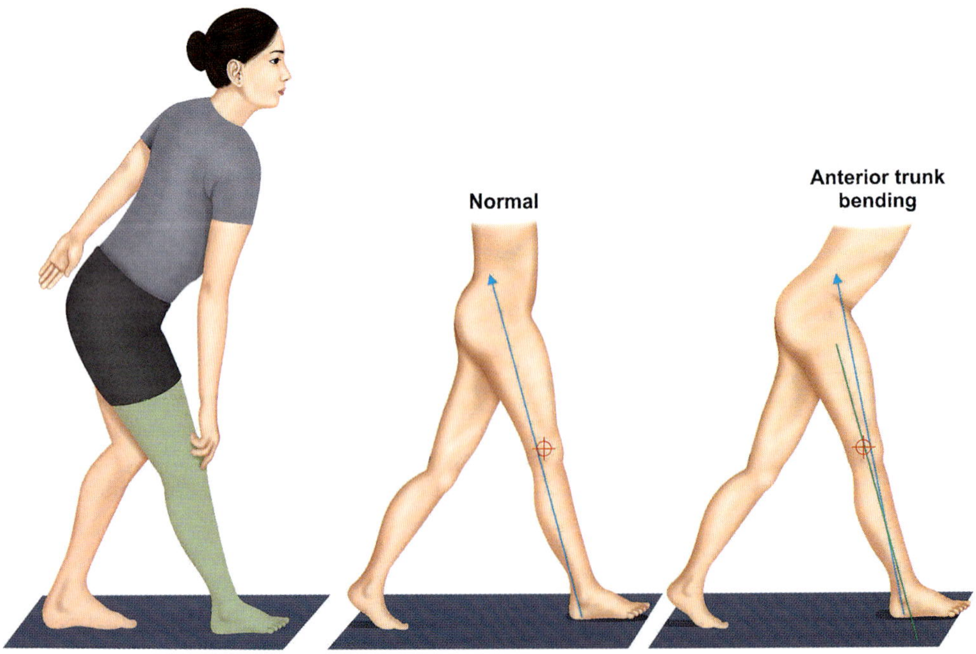

Fig. 4: Quadriceps weakness.

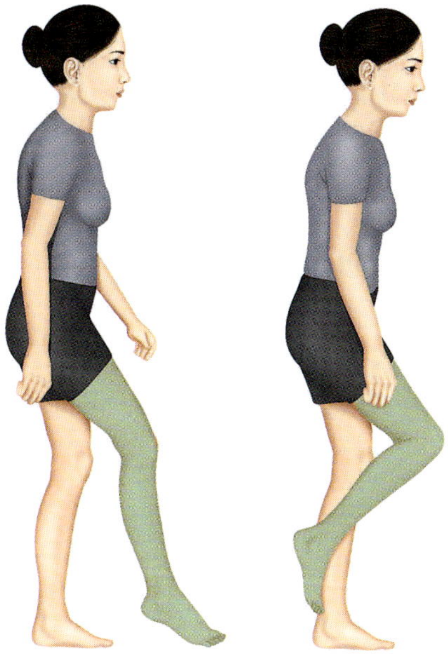

Fig. 5: Steppage or equine gait.

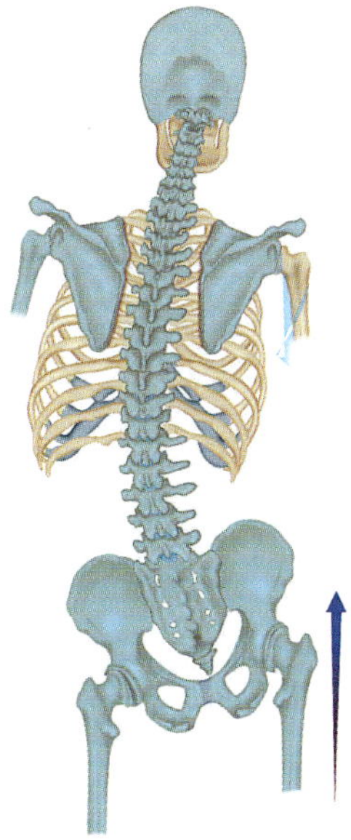

Fig. 6: Hip hiking.

of gravity of body toward the painful hip decreasing the moment arm of body weight to the hip joint and hence, the reaction forces (adaptive maneuver to reduce pain). Unlike the Trendelenburg gait, the lurch is to the same side and the hemipelvis remains level during the stance phase.

Lateral Trunk Bending

In the stance phase, it is seen toward involved side in Trendelenburg, bilaterally in waddling gait. In the swing phase, it is toward unaffected side. Causes include hip abductor weakness, hip dislocation due to dysplasia, coxa vara, hip pain, short limb, fixed flexion deformity, skeletal shortening, discomfort between thigh band and perineum. Long-standing bilateral knee or hip arthrosis also results in duck-like waddling gait because the patient has pain during flexion at these joints due to degenerative synovitis and speed of walk is also reduced.

Hip Hiking (Fig. 6)

In the swing phase, there is elevation of pelvis by quadratus lumborum and abductors to clear the foot.

It is seen in cases of ipsilateral lengthening as in case of hip flexor weakness, ankylosis in extension, extensor spasticity, equinus or foot drop. Contralateral shortness as in hip flexor spasticity, hamstring weakness (knee fails to flex for ground clearance).

Circumduction (Fig. 7)

It is another mechanism to gain ground clearance. It is seen in cases of spasticity, weak hip flexors, weak hamstrings, knee ankylosis, and weak dorsiflexors of foot.

Internal Hip Rotation/In-Toe Stance

It is seen in hip anteversion, biceps femoris weakness, peroneal weakness, and cerebral palsy.

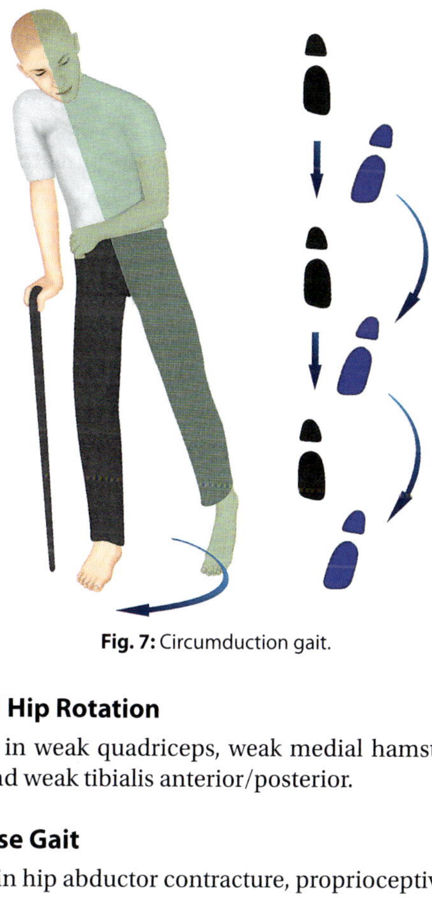

Fig. 7: Circumduction gait.

External Hip Rotation

It is seen in weak quadriceps, weak medial hamstring, pes valgus, and weak tibialis anterior/posterior.

Wide Base Gait

It is seen in hip abductor contracture, proprioceptive deficit, weak lower limbs, and genu valgum.

Narrow Base

It is seen in cerebral palsy (scissor gait), genu varum. In scissoring gait of cerebral palsy the knees and thighs cross like scissors during walk. The person appears crouched due to flexion at pelvis, hip, and knees. The step length is small.

Inverted Foot Stance

It is seen in weak evertors, cerebral palsy, tibialis anterior spasticity, spade foot, tibialis posterior spasticity, invertor contractures, and congenital talipes equinovarus (CTEV).

Everted Foot Stance

It is seen in case of weak invertors, eversion contracture, pes valgus, and genu valgum.

Anterior Trunk Bending

It is seen during midstance late swing in cases of quadriceps weakness **(Fig. 8)**.

Posterior Trunk Bending

It is seen during heel strike midstance initial swing in cases of weak hip extensor, tuberculosis (TB) of spine: Alderman's gait.

Hemiplegic Gait

Arm on affected side is flexed, adducted, and internally rotated with loss of normal arm swing while walking. Affected leg is in extension with plantar flexion of the foot and toes. The affected leg is dragged in a semicircle (circumduction) due to weakness of distal muscles (foot drop) and extensor hypertonia in lower limb. This is most commonly seen in stroke. With mild hemiparesis, loss of normal arm swing, and slight circumduction may be the only abnormalities.

Diplegic Gait

The patient walks with an abnormally narrow base, dragging both legs. This gait is seen in bilateral periventricular lesions, such as those seen in cerebral palsy. There is tightness of hip adductors which can cause legs to cross the midline known as a *scissors gait* **(Fig. 9)**.

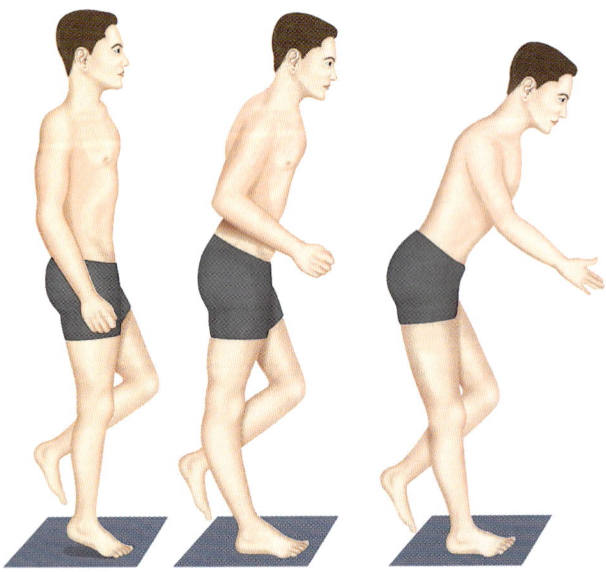

Fig. 8: Anterior trunk bending.

Parkinsonian Gait (Fig. 10)

Also called propulsive or festination gait. The patient has rigidity and bradykinesia. He will stoop forward with flexion at the knees. The patient walks with slow little steps known at *marche à petits pas* (walk of little steps) or *shuffling gait.* Patient also has difficulty in initiating steps. The patient has an involuntary inclination to take accelerating steps and finds it difficult to stop once gait is initiated known as *festination.*

Choreiform (Hyperkinetic) Gait

This is a gait with irregular, jerky, and involuntary movements in all extremities seen with certain basal ganglia disorders including Sydenham's chorea, Huntington's disease and other forms of chorea, and athetosis or dystonia.

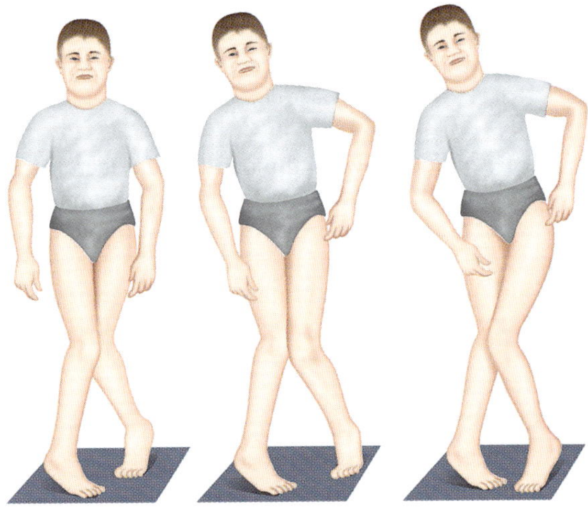

Fig. 9: Scissors gait.

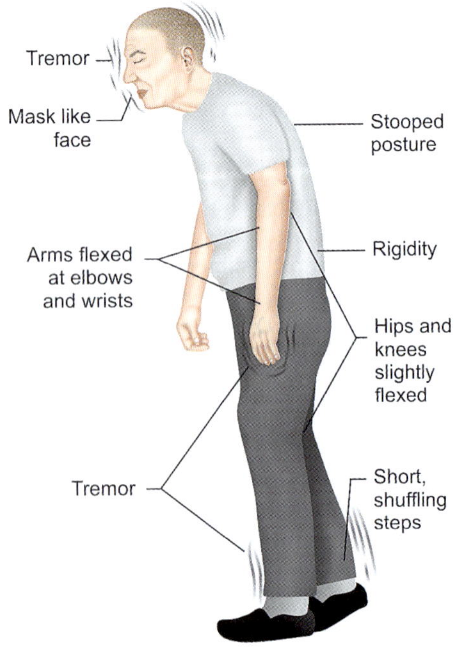

Fig. 10: Parkinsonian gait.

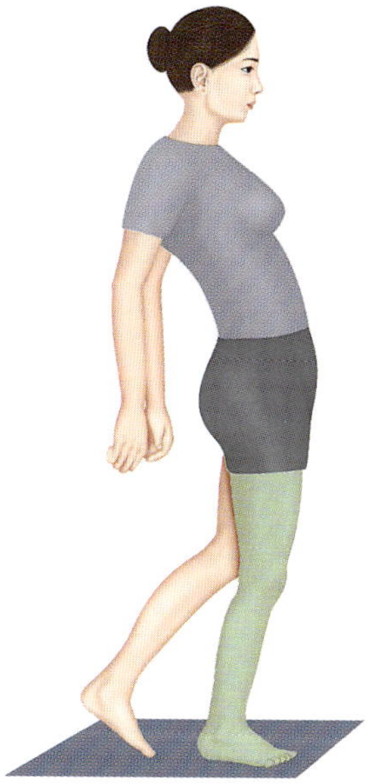

Fig. 11: Rocking horse gait.

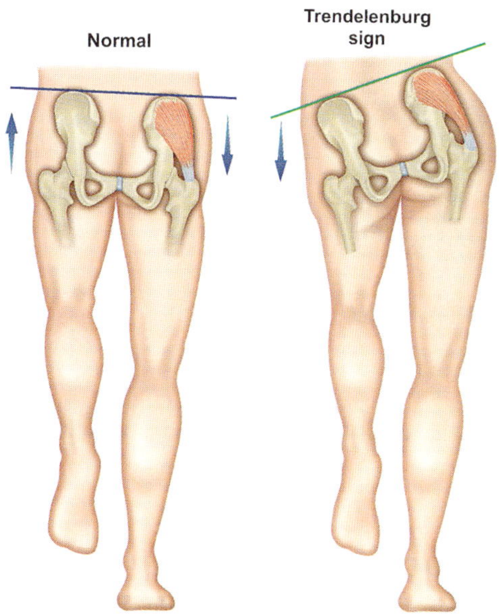

Fig. 12: Trendelenburg gait.

Ataxic (Cerebellar) Gait

Ataxic gait is a clumsy and staggering movement with a wide-based gait. Even while standing still, the patient's body may swagger back and forth and from side to side, known as *titubation*. Patient is not able to walk from heel to toe or in a straight line. It is also known as *reeling gait*.

Sensory Gait

This gait occurs when there is loss of proprioceptive input. The patient will slam the foot hard onto the ground in order to sense it. The gait gets exacerbated when patients cannot see their feet (i.e., in the dark). This gait is also, sometimes referred to as a *stomping gait*. Common causes are disorders of the dorsal columns (vitamin B_{12} deficiency or tabes dorsalis) or in diseases affecting the peripheral nerves (uncontrolled diabetes).

Psoatic Gait

This is seen when psoas bursa is painful. Hip is adducted and externally rotated and knee is slightly bent. This position relieves the tension on the muscle and relieves the pain.

Gluteus Maximus Gait or Rocking Horse Gait

This is seen in gluteus maximus weakness. Here the trunk shifts posteriorly at heel strike to shift the center of gravity posterior to gluteus maximus, thus reducing the effort required by it to keep hip in extension during stance phase. This forward-backward lurching is also known as *rocking horse gait* **(Fig. 11)**.

Gluteus Medius or Trendelenburg Gait

In normal gait during single stance phase when weight of body is on one limb the sag of pelvis to the opposite side is prevented by the ipsilateral gluteus medius. When this muscle is weak, the trunk is shifted the same side to reduce the lever arm of the muscle, thus reducing the effort required by it to hold up the pelvis **(Fig. 12)**. This attempt to counter the dropping of pelvis on swinging side *(Trendelenburg sign)* by bending the trunk on other side which is in stance phase is called *Duchenne sign*. When this is bilateral, it is known as *waddling gait* or *duck gait*. Exaggerated waddling gait is produced in myopathies with increased lumbar lordosis.

Hamstring Gait

During terminal swing, the weak hamstring cannot slow the leg and it snaps into extension.

Unequal Leg Length Gait

In minimal length, difference compensation happens by dropping the pelvis on the affected side (lifting pelvis at lengthier side) and leaning over to the affected side during stance phase. Up to 2–3 inches can be compensated by this.

In case of moderate shortening (3–5 inches) in addition to the pelvic tilt, the affected person walks on the tip of the foot on shorter leg such as in equinus gait.

In severe shortening >5 inches, the knee on the opposite side may, additionally, be flexed.

CONCLUSION

- Evaluation of gait pattern of the patients reveals various useful information and characteristic gait patterns make the diagnosis obvious in many cases.
- Gait evaluation is an essential part of orthopedic examination and to this end one must have complete knowledge of the various parts of gait cycle as various disorders affect particular parts of the gait cycle only.
- Some pathological gait patterns that disable the patients can be also be managed by use of appropriate orthoses only if the evaluating person has a good knowledge of the pathophysiology of the characteristic gait pattern.

CHAPTER 22

Tourniquet in Orthopedics

Manish Kumar Varshney

INTRODUCTION

Operations on the extremities are made easier by the use of a tourniquet as they provide good control over blood spillage and oozing into the surgical wound. In some procedures, a tourniquet is a luxury (as in tibia nailing or percutaneous plating), whereas in others, such as delicate operations on the hand, it is a necessity. The tourniquet is a potentially dangerous instrument and must be used with proper knowledge and care. The following types of tourniquets are in common usage:

- Pneumatic tourniquet:
    - Automatic continuous pressure controlled and regulated
    - Hand pump with pressure gauge
- Esmarch bandage
- Martin rubber sheet

TOURNIQUET SAFETY

A pneumatic tourniquet with a hand pump and an accurate pressure gauge is probably the safest, but an automatic constantly pressure regulated tourniquet is commonly used for ease and dependable technology. These modern tourniquets should be properly checked. A tourniquet should be applied by an experienced individual preferably by the operating surgeon himself. The tourniquet should be safely used and standard rules (Bruner's rules) should be followed **(Table 1)**. Most complications associated with tourniquet usage are due to human errors or equipment failure. These are preventable to a large extent if proper care in clinical practice is taken. Following are a compilation of general recommendations for safer use of tourniquets.

Before applying a tourniquet:

- Regular maintenance checks and marking the date last checked (preferably weekly).
- Aneroid pressure gauges for handheld tourniquets should be checked against calibration devices monthly.
- Check cuff, pipes, and connection for air leaks and do a thorough visual inspection.
- Pressure should remain constant over time.
- Cuff length should exceed the limb circumference by 7–15 cm and be properly chosen for equidistribution of pressure.
- Cuff width should be matched appropriately to the patient's age/size (discussed further).

Use caution while tourniquet and Esmarch bandage application in following patients as they are at high risk at exsanguination:

- Morbidly obese patients (high pressure causes subcutaneous fat amputation).
- Prolonged immobilization prior to surgery—weak osteoporotic bones may fracture during Esmarch application.
- Isolated limb malignancies and infections—infection/pus may migrate and go into circulation during Esmarch exsanguination.

TABLE 1: Braithwaite and Klenerman's modification of Bruner's rules.

Application	*Recommended for healthy limb or follow caution toan unhealthy limb*
Size of cuff	Arm–10 cm; leg–15 cm or wider in large legs
Site of application	Recommended sites—upper arm and mid/upperthigh
Padding	Use two layers of good quality orthopedic wool spread uniformly
Skin preparation	Prevent soaking of wool with preparation solutionsthat may result in chemical burns
Inflation pressure	50–100 mm Hg above systolic for the arm; double systolic for the thigh; or arm 200–250 mm Hg, leg 250–350 mm Hg (large cuffs are recommended forlarger limbs instead of increasing pressure)
Time	Absolute maximum 3 hours (recovers in 5–7 days)generally not to exceed 2 hours
Temperature	Avoid heating (e.g., hot lights), cool if feasible, andkeep tissues moist
Documentation calibration and maintenance	Duration and pressure at least weekly against mercury manometer or test gauge; 3-monthly maintenance

- Patients with left ventricular dysfunction—exsanguinated blood from limb may load the cardiovascular system excessively.
- Patients with deep vein thrombosis (DVT)—embolus may dislodge during exsanguination.

During use:

- Monitor the pressure gauges continuously to check variations.
- Cuffs should be positioned at the level of maximum limb circumference.
- The tourniquet should be adequately padded using cotton or soft foam sheet; newer silicone sheets may also be used.
- After application, do not rotate the cuff.
- Apply an adhesive tape on the distal edge of tourniquet to prevent liquid solutions from seeping under the cuff.
- Regulate the tourniquet inflation time and pressure according to patient's age and comorbidities.
- Surgeons should be kept informed of the inflation times.
- Document the duration and use of tourniquet in patient's notes.

After tourniquet use:

- Thoroughly clean the reusable cuffs to prevent cross infection.
- The limb should be thoroughly inspected for signs of prolonged usage and inadequate pressure transmission in the form of developing blisters at the site of application of tourniquet, distal vascularity should be restored before shifting patient.
- Gently massage the site of application of tourniquet.

For tourniquet application on fingers and toes, rubber ring tourniquet or a tourniquet made from a glove finger that is rolled onto the digit is not recommended. Instances have been noted when it had been inadvertently left in place under a dressing, resulting in loss of the digit. The alternative is application of glove finger or Penrose drain that can be looped around the proximal portion of the digit, stretched, and secured with a hemostat. This is a much safer method for surgery on hand, especially for digits.

SIZE OF TOURNIQUETS AND APPLICATION TECHNIQUE

Several sizes of pneumatic tourniquets are available for the upper and lower extremities. In general:

- The tourniquet should encircle the limb and needs to be 7–15 cm more than the circumference of the limb at the point of application.
- The width of tourniquet should be 20% more than the diameter of the limb at the point of application.

There is no binding evidence that tourniquet should only be applied to upper arm or thigh, any comfortable site can be chosen with equal efficacy. Before application, soft cotton padding should be applied evenly to prevent direct pressure injury and wrinkling of skin during inflation. Krackow maneuver is suitable for conical and bulky thighs with loose soft tissue or fat **(Figs. 1A to C)**. In this, the assistant manually grasps the flesh of the extremity just distal to the level of tourniquet application and firmly pulls this loose tissue distally, while the padding and tourniquet are applied. Traction on the soft tissue is maintained till securing tourniquet. On releasing, the tissue, a fold of soft tissue, forms distally which prevents slippage of tourniquet and gives additional space for surgical exposure if required. All air should be emptied before pneumatic tourniquet application. For firm conical limbs as are found in muscular patients, conical and curved tourniquets should be used for proper fitting and uniform transmittance of pressure (Pedowitz et al.).

Prepare the extremity before inflating the tourniquet to reduce tourniquet application time. The extremity is elevated for 2 minutes, or the blood is expressed by an Esmarch rubber bandage or a cotton elastic (crepe) bandage. Beginning at the fingertips or toes, the extremity is wrapped proximally to within 2.5–5 cm of the tourniquet. Care should

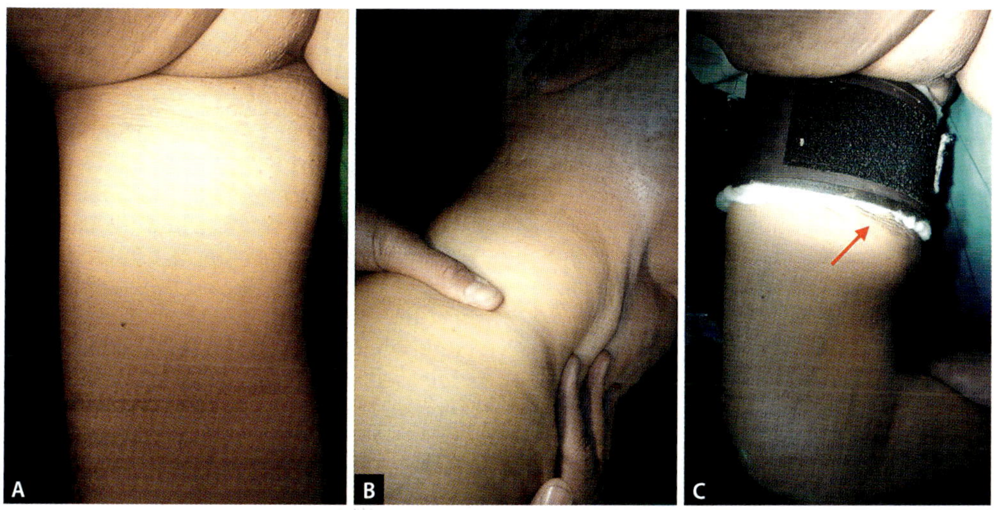

Figs. 1A to C: In patients with fat conical thighs (A) it is better to apply tourniquet by Krackow maneuver. The assistant pulls the skin of the thigh distally (B), and as the tourniquet is applied it does not slip distally due to formation of skin fold (C, arrow).

be taken to prevent slippage of tourniquet at inflation when the Esmarch bandage has been used as the latter thins the limb. An adhesive tape can be applied to additionally secure tourniquet for this purpose if desired during application. The tourniquet should be inflated quickly to prevent filling of the veins again before the arterial blood flow has been occluded. Asymptomatic pulmonary embolism can occur within 1 minute after tourniquet release and their number is directly proportional to duration of inflation.

TOURNIQUET PRESSURE (OCCLUSION PRESSURE) AND SIZE PRESSURE RELATIONSHIP

The exact pressure to which the tourniquet should be inflated has not been determined. The pressure changes occur in limbs during operative trauma and movements of limb to the extent of 50–75 mm Hg. So normally tourniquet pressures higher by this amount from systolic pressure have been used in upper extremity. In the lower extremity due to higher girth of the limb and narrower (than required—discussed above) width of applied tourniquet to provide for surgical exposure, the pressure requirements are higher. Commonly, pressures twice than that for upper extremity have been used (except in children). Evidence indicates that pressures greater than necessary have been used for many years. The correct pressure depends on the age of the patient, the blood pressure, and the size of the extremity and is not easy to determine always. So, often the use of higher pressure is justified. Using a Doppler stethoscope it has been determined that tourniquet pressures of 135–255 mm Hg for the upper extremity and 175–305 mm Hg for the lower extremity were satisfactory for maintaining hemostasis taking care of collateral circulation and pressure changes. Using an automated limb occlusion pressure apparatus (Younger et al.) tourniquet pressures could be reduced by 43%. It is quite easy to understand that wide tourniquet cuffs are more effective at lower inflation pressures than are narrow ones, but they also occupy the usable surgical space so often narrower cuffs are used. The occlusion pressures are inversely proportional to the ratio of tourniquet cuff width to limb circumference (interestingly if the ratio is <0.5 then subsystolic pressures are required). In general, still a cuff that is as wide as possible and is compatible with the surgical exposure should be used. Cuff inflation displaces the tissues underneath. The nerves are the structures most at risk apart from vessels and muscles. The *"displacement effect"* is maximum at the upper and lower edges of tourniquet due to mechanical deformation at acute pressure gradients. It has been suggested to use two tourniquets and alternately inflate and deflate them to minimize this mechanical deformation and resultant damage (Neimkin and Smith).

DURATION OF TOURNIQUET USE (ISCHEMIC TIME)

There is no rule as to how long a tourniquet may be safely inflated. The time varies (1 hour—Bruner, 1951; 2 hours—Boyes, 1964; 3 hours—Parkes, 1973) with the age of the patient and the vascular supply of the extremity. In an average healthy adult younger than 50 years of age, tourniquet use no >2 hours is recommended. If the surgical time exceeds 2 hours, it is better to finish it as rapidly as possible then to deflate the tourniquet for 10 minutes and then reinflate it. However, the practice of deflating the tourniquet for 10 minutes and reinflating is grossly inadequate as it takes 40 minutes for the tissues to return to normal physiology after prolonged use of a tourniquet. The tourniquet time should in no case ever exceed 3 hours as the damage then is surely massive and irreversible by any current method. In fact, the ultrastructural damage to muscles is visible within 30 minutes of application in the form of degenerating fibers and infiltrating phagocytic cells. After 1 hour of application the mitochondria swells and cristae get disorganized. Dissolution of Z-disks is seen after 2-hour application. Tourniquet applied for 5 hours shows complete loss of I-band, A-band, and Z-disks with progressive dissolution of muscle fibers and inflammatory reaction similar to postcompartment syndrome. "Post-tourniquet syndrome" (discussed further under the heading *Complications*) and "no-reflow" phenomenon may occur after prolonged use of tourniquet. The latter is due to microcirculatory obstruction. Muscles ischemic for 1–3 hours successfully reperfuse, while 40–50% cases fail to reperfuse if ischemic for 5 hours or more. Large number of RBCs infiltering and blocking the capillaries are seen obstructing the circulation. Sapega et al. have documented interstitial edema, increased capillary permeability, microvascular congestion, and decreased muscle contractility after 2–3 hours of ischemia.

THE USE OF ESMARCH TOURNIQUET AND MARTIN RUBBER SHEET

Though infrequent the Esmarch tourniquet is still used in some places. It is the most practical and safest of the elastic tourniquets, especially where power supply could be doubtful. The most common site of its use in body is in the middle and upper thirds of the thigh. One of the distinct advantages of this tourniquet is that it may be applied very high on the thigh (near the groin region) where the pneumatic tourniquet is difficult to use, as might be required in some cases of amputation and tumor surgery. The Esmarch tourniquet is applied in layers, one on the top of the other; a narrow band produces less tissue damage than does a wide one. The tourniquet should be applied only after anesthetizing the patient.

For short procedures on the foot Martin rubber sheet bandage is a very safe method for controlling blood flow. Similar to the application of Esmarch bandage, the leg is elevated and exsanguinated by wrapping the Martin rubber sheet up crossing the malleoli and securing it tight with a clamp. The distal third to one-half portion of the bandage is released with knife or scissors to allow exposure of the operative area.

COMPLICATIONS

- *Asymptomatic/symptomatic pulmonary embolism:* The embolus after migration remains static till tourniquet deflation and then quickly travels to lungs causing embolism within 1 minute after tourniquet release. It has been found that the number of small emboli depends on the duration of tourniquet inflation.

- *Chemical burn* from solutions seeping underneath the tourniquet.
- *Superficial slough/abrasion* of the skin usually occurs at the upper margin of the tourniquet near the gluteal fold. It is more pronounced in obese individuals and is commonly seen with use of straight/parallel tourniquet instead of a curved/conical tourniquet.
- *Tourniquet paralysis* (from mechanical effect of tourniquet pressure) is caused by insufficient oxygenation of the tissues and nerves. It may result from one of the following scenarios:
  - Excessive pressure used for inflation
  - Insufficient pressure causing passive congestion of the limb. There occurs hemorrhagic infiltration of the nerve with prolonged usage
  - Prolonged inflation of tourniquet (>3 hours)
  - Tourniquet application without considering local anatomy. The nerves are mechanically displaced and stretched causing local demyelinating block. The nerve is displaced away from the high pressure zone stretching the paranodal myelin and invaginating the same on other side resembling intussusception.
- *Post-tourniquet syndrome* (from ischemic effect of tourniquet application and not mechanical) was first recognized by Bunnell. It is a common reaction to prolonged ischemia seen over too long periods of tourniquet usages. The limb develops edema, joint stiffness, pallor, motor weakness, and subjective numbness without objective anesthesia. This complication is specifically related to duration of ischemia and not to the mechanical effect. Post-tourniquet syndrome usually resolves over time (nearly 1 week) and may result in interference with early motion and increased narcotic requirements.
- *Compartment syndrome* from microvascular occlusion is seen more in previously compromised limbs that go unrecognized.
- *Rhabdomyolysis* from use of tourniquet is extremely rare and few reports exist. In susceptible periods with very long tourniquet inflation periods (>3 hours), reperfusion hyperemia of a swollen and edematous ischemic limb may produce compartment syndrome. Already with prolonged use of tourniquets ischemia develops causing edema and microvascular congestion—"post-tourniquet syndrome" that may be combined with reperfusion oxidative injury.
- *Vascular complications* after tourniquet use occur in predisposed patients like those with severe arteriosclerosis or prosthetic vascular grafts. One should refrain from applying a tourniquet over a prosthetic vascular graft.
- *Intraoperative bleeding:* This develops from venous congestion resulting from poorly fitting tourniquet that improperly distributes pressure or an inadequately inflated cuff that blocks only veins but not arteries. This causes excessive bleeding persisting till tourniquet is readjusted. Incomplete exsanguination of the limb can also increase intraoperative bleeding from venous congestion but that lasts for initial period only. This gets exaggerated by increased intravascular coagulation and fibrinolysis causing excessive bleeding.
- *Reperfusion syndrome:* This is a lately recognized complication. Initially, only ischemia was considered to be the cause of tissue damage. Ischemic injury is understood well in the form of deprivation of cellular energy to maintain ionic gradients and homeostasis, enzymatic failure, and death. Reperfusion injury occurs by the interaction of free radicals (hydroxyl radical), endothelial factors, and neutrophils. These damage proteins, DNA, and lipids. Lipid peroxidation disrupts cell membranes especially the endothelial system, which are composed of polyunsaturated fatty acids and phospholipids. The endothelial disruption induces neutrophil chemotaxis, adherence, and migration inducing systemic injury and local tissue destruction.
  - Accumulation of lactic acid, sodium (associated with water ingress into cell), and calcium (causes mitochondrial disruption) are basic alterations of anaerobic metabolism. The potassium leaks out causing hyperkalemia.
  - Reperfusion removes the accumulated toxic components and replenishes the energy supply to cells. But these produce simultaneously collateral damage by causing systemic toxicity and sensitive organs show depressed function under influence, reoxygenation causes formation of reactive oxygen species.
  - Formation of superoxide radical—this is converted into hydrogen peroxide by superoxide dismutases (SOD) which, in turn, is destroyed by catalase into water as follows:

    $$2O_2 + 2H^+ \rightarrow H_2O_2 + O_2\ (SOD)$$
    $$2H_2O_2 \rightarrow 2H_2O + O_2\ (catalase)$$

    The enzymes are dysfunctional often due to ischemia, so instead the superoxide ions form hydroxyl radicals that are highly reactive as follows:

    $O_2 + H_2O_2 \rightarrow 2OH\cdot + O_2$ (Haber-Weiss reaction—catalyzed by ferrous ions and xanthine oxidase).

    These radicals are not scavenged and cause extensive damage at the site of formation itself. These free radicals produce the thiobarbituric acid reactive substances and diene conjugates causing extensive myocyte damage.
  - Neutrophils release proteolytic enzymes and peroxidases into the circulation.

Pharmacological modification of reperfusion injury: Understanding the pathophysiology as detailed above, some pharmacological agents have been recommended to control reperfusion injury as follows.

- Allopurinol-Xanthine oxidase inhibitor may modify the generation of peroxide radical though relevant clinical effect has not been demonstrated.

- Desferrioxamine chelates iron and may limit the production of toxic hydroxyl free radicals.
- Mannitol has been used to systemically scavenge hydroxyl free radicals.
- Dantrolene controls the release of calcium, limiting the mitochondrial and muscular damage.
- High dose of ascorbic acid and corticosteroids have not shown much of clinical effect.
- Hypothermia has shown to be of benefit in reperfusion injury possibly by reducing the metabolic demand and oxygen requirement itself. This also actually prolongs the ischemia time.

CONTRAINDICATIONS FOR USE OF TOURNIQUETS

No absolute contraindications exist; adequate care needs to be taken in specific group of patients:

- Patients with severe peripheral vascular disease (reduce application time).
- Patients with past history of deep vein thrombosis and pulmonary embolism—avoid tourniquet application or put a prophylactic caval filter.
- Sickle cell disease (reduce application time)/intermittent inflation for prolonged surgeries—intermittent inflation should not be <20 minutes.
- Patients with established diabetic neuropathy— there is ischemia due to arteritis/atherosclerosis.
- Severe crush injury—minimizes usage as already there is relative ischemia.

SYSTEMIC AND LOCAL EFFECTS OF TOURNIQUET USAGE

Inflation and deflation of tourniquets for prolonged periods produce systemic effects while local effects result from limb ischemia or direct mechanical pressure of the inflated tourniquet.

Systemic Adverse Effects

Hemodynamic Changes

These are insignificant clinically in a healthy patient; however, for patients with compromised cardiovascular function the tourniquets can cause detrimental effects. The most significant aspect of this is manifested as *cardiac arrest and circulatory overload* that may occur with use of bilateral thigh tourniquets. Once inflated, blood volume from lower limbs is shifted into the central circulation (15% of circulating blood volume) and it also increases the systemic vascular resistance increasing work of heart. There is transient increase in systolic blood pressure and central venous pressure that quickly settles. There is a second gradual rise in arterial blood pressure and heart rate after 30–60 minutes possibly related to "tourniquet pain". When the tourniquet is deflated there is sudden redistribution of the circulating volume back into the limb which combined with postischemic reactive hyperemia and release of metabolites into the systemic circulation causes sudden drop in blood pressure and reduced central venous pressure. *Cardiac dysrhythmias* rarely occur. It can be prevented by maintaining optimal circulating volume and preloading the patient. There is a suggestion that propofol-based anesthetic may mitigate reperfusion injury due to its property to limit superoxide generation. Emboli are seen in the pulmonary and central circulation peaking at 30 minutes of tourniquet release. This phenomenon persists for 10–15 minutes.

Respiratory System

The effects are minimal and mostly inconsequential. Tourniquet inflation especially has no significant effects; however, deflation causes an immediate increase in end-tidal concentration of carbon dioxide ($FECO_2$) which peaks at 1 minute post deflation. The effect quickly wanes off and $FECO_2$ returns to baseline within 10 minutes. The hypercapnic venous blood from ischemic limb causes the increase in $FECO_2$. The increase in $FECO_2$ is quite significant with the release of lower limb tourniquets than for upper limb. Clinically, there is increase in minute ventilation in spontaneously breathing patients. For patients on controlled ventilation it is recommended to increase minute ventilation for 5 minutes prior to deflation that keeps the increase in CO_2 levels to a minimum.

Central Nervous System

There is an increase in cerebral blood flow due to rapid increase in $FECO_2$ following tourniquet deflation. The increase in cerebral circulation is the result of local circulatory vascular reflex modulation that peaks at around 2 minutes and returns to baseline within 10 minutes. There is a 50% increase in middle cerebral artery blood velocity during this period that may be detrimental in patients of cerebral injury as it may produce secondary brain injury by increasing intracranial pressure.

Hematological System Changes

The effects are complex and can be segregated according to the timing—tourniquet inflation is associated initially with hypercoagulation state whereas this changes to thrombolytic state toward the later stage of inflation and postdeflation.

Hypercoagulable state—postsurgical pain and pain of tourniquet inflation release catecholamines that result in platelet aggregation. Tissue compression and damage from the application of Esmarch bandages also contribute to platelet aggregation. Despite this, tourniquets do not increase the incidence of deep vein thrombosis.

Hypocoagulation—following deflation of the tourniquet there is a transient period of reduced coagulation. Tissue plasminogen activator release due to the hypoxemia and acidosis causes transient increase in fibrinolysis that peaks at 15 minutes after tourniquet release. The thrombolytic effect returns to preoperative levels within 30 minutes. During this transient period of hypocoagulation, increased systemic fibrinolysis results and is also responsible for increased post-tourniquet bleeding.

Temperature Regulation

The body's thermostatic receptors and metabolism tends to maintain body temperature over a broad range. With inflation of tourniquet there is decreased heat transfer from the central to peripheral compartment causing gradual rise in core body temperature. Deflation causes redistribution of body heat resulting in a transient fall in core temperature due to mixing of hypothermic blood from the ischemic limb.

Metabolism Changes

Metabolic changes result primarily from ischemia and will almost always follow tourniquet use exceeding 30 minutes. These changes are fully reversed within 30 minutes. Tourniquet use for 1–2 hours causes significant limb ischemia, and hence plasma potassium and lactate concentrations rise. Metabolic acidosis occurs due to fall in pH mediated by increased lactate and carbon dioxide.

Local Effects

Local effects from tourniquet application are seen as a result of mechanical compression of the tissues beneath the tourniquet and ischemia resulting from ceased circulation in the desired limb.

Nerve

There is a reversible physiological conduction block in motor and sensory nerves seen after 15–45 minutes of tourniquet inflation. Neural ischemia due to loss of blood circulation is the primary cause of conduction block which is supported by the fact that rate of development of conduction block is independent of cuff pressures, some role of cessation of axoplasmic flow might also play role in prolonged tourniquet application (>3 hours). "Tourniquet paralysis" which is seen after prolonged continuous application (>3 hours) results most likely from mechanical block of axoplasmic flow rather than ischemia. This also results in morphological changes and demyelination possibly due to injury to Schwann cells. The changes are more prominent near the proximal and distal edges of tourniquet after 2 hours of inflation. Regeneration and remyelination takes nearly 6 months, permanent deficit is uncommon.

Muscle

Effect of hypoxia is most marked on myocytes as they fail to stage complete recovery once damaged. Fortunately all muscles do have some anaerobic muscle fibers that survive even prolonged cuff inflation times. Muscle cells experience progressive tissue hypoxia after 60 minutes of cuff inflation resulting in depletion of energy stores, reduced intracellular pH, loss of mitochondria and local fiber necrosis (discussed above under the heading Duration of Tourniquet Use). Regaining muscle mass may take more than a year for surgeries prolonged >1 hour.

TOURNIQUET PAIN AND TOURNIQUET-INDUCED HYPERTENSION

A vague and dull-aching pain in the affected limb is experienced in the arms on tourniquet inflation associated with an increased blood pressure. It is not easily controlled and there is no prevention available for it. Increase in heart rate and arterial pressure is noted in patients developing tourniquet pain intraoperatively. The pain possibly arises from cutaneous neural mechanism (unmyelinated, slow C-fibers) while blood pressure rise follows a humoral response to the pain. The large A-δ fibers are blocked early by ischemia that exerts inhibitory influence on C-fibers, loss of this postsynaptic inhibition of C-fibers results in continuous stimulation causing pain. Various drugs have been recommended as adjuncts to the local anesthetic such as morphine, clonidine, epinephrine, low-dose intravenous ketamine, preoperative gabapentin and alkalinization of local anesthetic to reduce the incidence of tourniquet pain though definite success with any method is elusive.

ALTERATION IN DRUG KINETICS DUE TO TOURNIQUET APPLICATION

As drugs administered before tourniquet inflation accumulate in the limb, they will redistribute after deflation while drugs administered after inflation would have changed blood volume of distribution altering concentration. These alterations in pharmacokinetics and pharmacodynamics of the drug suggest that prophylactic antibiotics should be given at least 5 minutes before tourniquet inflation (but within 30 minutes of placing incision) to allow good tissue penetration, and if the surgery lasts >2 hours then another dose of antibiotic should be administered to maintain adequate concentration of the drug in the bathing blood to operative site at release.

CONCLUSION

- Tourniquets are the most common surgical accessory used for most of the orthopedic surgeries.
- Though appearing benign, it is not without complications and the surgeon should be highly vigilant of its correct usage and possible ill-effects or complications. Importantly, it should be realized that young surgeons often keep the tourniquets inflated for long times in the flow of surgery without realizing the possibility of losing the patient's limb.
- Additional effects of alteration of circulatory volume and drug kinetics should be also taken into mind especially in critical patients.

CHAPTER 23

Preoperative Evaluation, Patient Optimization, and Pain Management in Orthopedic Patient

Manish Kumar Varshney

INTRODUCTION

Preoperative assessment (POA) is aimed to identify and quantify medical problems that impact perioperative morbidity and mortality. It helps in delivering high-value, patient-centred surgical care by identifying areas for risk modification. Orthopedic surgery presents specific challenges and, in particular, has a high number of elderly patients. Advanced age, respiratory, renal, hepatic and cardiac disease, malnutrition, obesity, diabetes, and smoking place a patient at increased risk of complications in peri- and postoperative period. Cardiovascular problems are a leading source of mortality needing specific attention. Further evaluation is also done by measuring patient's functional capacity (in terms of metabolic equivalents) to assess patent's ability to meet the surgical and physiological stress. Various risk-scoring systems have been developed to quantify the perioperative risk. Extensive investigations should, however, be ordered only if the results would change the anesthetic technique or help in further risk stratification for patient optimization. POA is also the opportunity to explain the patient about what to expect during hospitalization, the perioperative period, and the expected postoperative course. Functional assessment to determine social support and need for assistance after hospital discharge can also be determined. Despite all these theoretical prophecies, perioperative care of the orthopedic patient remains inconsistent and contradictory. Now, there is need for development of institutional based POA pathways based on sound and up-to-date evidence to minimize unnecessary testing that often delays surgery and wastefully increases healthcare costs.

Identifying specific patient risks helps in optimization of anesthetic plan and change in anesthesia if needed. Surgical plan may also be optimized by choosing a procedure that imposes minimum risk without altering outcome. Identifying medical diseases (such as diabetes, hypertension, renal and hepatic disorders, etc.) and their control/severity gives an opportunity to initiate or optimize the treatment for the time patient is in-house.

Patient and procedure safety is a hospital and surgical team responsibility that requires adequate knowledge of systems and procedures to help to deliver the best care. This requires a combination of trained staff and competent professionals that have requisite experience in handling complications and complex situations rather than just degree holders.

Optimal pain management takes precedence in immediate postoperative period that should include the use of multimodal analgesia and a sensible and balanced approach to pharmacologic treatment. Functional treatment and rehabilitation is provided simultaneously to expedite the recovery and discharge process. The last chapter heading deals with pain management in orthopedic patients including both the postoperative and chronic pain management.

SURGICAL STRESS RESPONSE AND TYPES OF ANESTHESIA

Physiological changes occur in body in response to surgical and anesthetic stimulus that have important bearing on outcome of treatment. Injury and surgery (another type of controlled injury!) stimulates hypothalamus that incites following responses:

- Endocrine response—increases in levels of cortisol, adrenocorticotropic hormone, growth hormone, catecholamines, renin, and antidiuretic hormone (ADH).
- Metabolic changes—catabolism of carbohydrates, fat, and protein to provide for the increased energy demands. There is retention of water and sodium resorption. This lasts nearly for 3–5 days.
- Inflammatory response—driven by cytokines (IL-1,-6, and TNF-α) from leukocytes, fibroblasts, and endothelial cells that spills over to systemic acute-phase response. This lasts nearly for 72 hours.

Perioperative physiology is also altered by type of anesthesia and its duration. The two major types of anesthesia are general and neuraxial anesthesia while peripheral procedures may be also done under regional or local nerve/plexus blocks. General anesthesia (GA) comprises a triad of hypnosis, analgesia, and muscle relaxation and importantly produces hypotension (vasodilatation, ↓ heart rate, and ↓ stroke volume), respiratory impairment (respiratory muscle paralysis, reduced lung volume, and airway closure).

Therefore, patients with impaired cardiac and respiratory functions have elevated risk of such complications with GA. Neuraxial anesthesia (spinal and/or epidural) blocks the sympathetic nervous system causing hypotension and bradycardia that complicates preload dependent cardiac diseases like aortic stenosis and hypertrophic cardiomyopathy. High spinal causes respiratory paralysis requiring requisite support then. Blockade of bladder sensation produces urinary retention. Surgical emergency and urgency status further compromises the care and complicates outcome.

PRE- AND PERIOPERATIVE RISK ASSESSMENT

The American College of Cardiology (ACC)/the American Heart Association (AHA) has provided definitions for formal communication and labeling of the surgical procedures **(Box 1)**. The status of surgery has bearing on postoperative risk and acceptance of the same by surgical team and patients and relatives. Obviously, the urgent need of surgery should have higher bearing than associated risk of procedure on survival of limb/life.

Surgery-specific Risk

The amount of tissue trauma, blood loss, fluid shift, and duration of surgery—all influence the surgical risk. This has primary bearing on cardiovascular events. The risk of major adverse cardiac events was historically separated into low-risk (<1%), intermediate-risk (1–5%), and high-risk (>5%) categories. More recent guidelines recommend a binary approach, using low risk (<1%) and elevated risk (≥1%) for better understanding and decision-making. The evaluation of trauma patients is discussed in detail in Chapter on "Polytrauma, Mass Casualties, and Disaster".

Patient-specific Risk

This is more specific but so deliberate in details that it is nearly impossible to calculate individual risks. Depending on the medical comorbidities and past surgical procedures, the risk factors are identified. Calculation of assessment is then done using various available assessments organ system based tools that preferably incorporate both patient and procedure specific elements. The tools, however, are very nonspecific and not universally applicable because of their development and validation in a small population base.

COMBINED RISK ASSESSMENT

It is better to incorporate the surgical urgency, surgery-specific risk, and patient-specific risk as input for shared surgical decision-making and assessment done for cardiac and pulmonary complications, venous thromboembolism, postoperative nausea-vomiting (PONV), and delirium. Additional risks should be assessed on individual basis.

BOX 1: The American College of Cardiology (ACC)/the American Heart Association (AHA) classification of surgeries.

1. *Emergency surgery:* Life or limb threatened without intervention within 6 hours.
2. *Urgent surgery:* Life- or limb-threatened without intervention within 24 hours.
3. *Time-sensitive surgery:* Medically necessary to operate within 1–6 weeks.
4. *Elective:* It can be deferred for up to 1 year.

Cardiac

Identifying patients with risk of major cardiovascular complication (MCC) is important for surgical decision-making by evaluating patient's surgical candidacy and discussing risk/benefit ratio. The Revised Cardiac Risk Index (RCRI) proposed by Lee et al. and modified by the ACC/AHA Task Force uses a 6-point scale **(Table 1)**.

- Patients with no positive predictors have a perioperative risk of 0.4% of MCC.
- Patients with predictors 1, 2, and ≥3 have a 0.9%, 6.6%, and >11% risk of MCC, respectively.

Although applied at various clinics the RCRI showed significant differences in cardiovascular complications with scores >1 in different cohorts so large databases like national surgery quality improvement program (NSQIP) databases were used for improved calibration. The American College of Surgeons NSQIP myocardial infarction and cardiac arrests (MICA) calculator for calculating cardiac morbidity postoperatively; suggested by Gupta et al. showed that risk factors most predictive of MICA after surgery were American Society of Anesthesiologists (ASA) classification **(Table 2)**, dependent functional status, age, abnormal creatinine (>1.5), and type of surgery. However, MICA does not account for variability within each surgery type. For patients with a risk of <1%, the patient may proceed with surgery. Patients with a risk of >1% better undergo functional capacity assessment. If the functional capacity is ≥4 metabolic equivalent (MET)

TABLE 1: The revised cardiac risk index.

RCRI criteria (1–6)	*Predictors*	*Risk of MCC*
1. History of ischemic heart disease	0	0.4%
2. History of congestive heart failure	1	0.9%
3. History of cerebrovascular disease	2	6.6%
4. History of diabetes	≥3	>11%
5. Chronic kidney disease (creatinine > 2 mg/dL)		
6. Undergoing intermediate/high-risk surgery*		

*Refers to suprainguinal vascular surgery, intraperitoneal surgery, and intrathoracic surgery.

(MCC: major cardiovascular complications, including death, myocardial infarction, and nonfatal cardiac arrest; RCRI: Revised Cardiac Risk Index)

TABLE 2: The American Society of Anesthesiologists Classification of Physical Status.

Grade	*Classification*
I	Healthy
II	Mild systemic disease—no functional limitations
III	Severe systemic disease—definite functional limitation
IV	Severe systemic disease that is a constant threat to life
V	Moribund patient not expected to survive despite surgery

designation **(Table 3)**, the patient may proceed to surgery but if it is <4 METs, pharmacologic stress testing is reasonable if the results would affect management. Medication history especially anticoagulation or anti-platelet therapy should be specifically sought for. Ecosprin is withheld the day before and on the day of surgery while for drugs like clopidogrel a drug holiday of 6–7 days is commonly recommended. The standardization and increased use of oral anticoagulants demand knowledge of interval after which neuraxial anesthesia can be safely given **(Table 4)**.

Pulmonary

Assessment for obstructive sleep apnea (OSA) and hypoventilation syndromes should be done especially for patients undergoing thoracic (scoliosis surgery), head and neck and upper abdominal surgeries due to their direct impact on respiratory mechanics. The common tools used for assessment include use of Gupta respiratory failure, ACS NSQIP, sleep apnea clinical score or STOP-BANG score.

Venous Thromboembolism and Bleeding

Commonly, the American College of Chest Physicians (ACCP) guidelines are followed. All surgical patients should undergo risk assessment for venous thromboembolism with

TABLE 3: The metabolic equivalent (MET) designations.

MET	*Examples*	*Stress testing (Y/N)*
Unknown	Unable to walk because of physical disability or pain	Y
Poor (<4)	Walk 2–3 mph; can perform activities of daily living	Y
Moderate (4–6)	Walk 4 mph, two flight of stairs	N
Good (7–10)	Run a short distance	N
Excellent (>10)	Run a long distance	N

TABLE 4: Time interval guidelines before and after neuraxial block for various oral anticoagulants.

Anticoagulants	*Delaying neuraxial block/ catheter removal after stopping the drug (days)*	*Resuming the medication after catheter removal or neuraxial block (hours)*
Dabigatran	5	6
Rivaroxaban	3	6
Apixaban	3	6
Prasugrel	7–10	6
Ticagrelor	5–7	6

TABLE 5: The commonly performed history and physical examination schema for preoperative assessment.

System	*History*	*Physical examination*
General	-	• Vital signs, body mass index, muscle mass, and cognition • Wounds and pressure ulcers
ENT	• Airway obstruction, neoplasia, past surgery, dental work, smoking/tobacco products • Head or neck irradiation	• Mallampati classification • Dentition • Removable oral appliances
Neck	Rheumatoid arthritis, previous surgery, spondylosis, DISH	• Range of motion • Thyromental distance • Neck circumference
Cardiac	Angina, dyspnea on exertion/nocturnal dyspnea, pedal edema, palpitations, orthopnea, and implanted devices (pacemaker/ stents)	• Auscultation • Jugular venous pressure • Hepatojugular reflex • Peripheral edema
Pulmonary	Breathlessness, snoring, sleep apnea, ILD or COAD, hemoptysis, tuberculosis, COVID, thoracic injury, and scoliosis	Trachea, auscultation, work of breathing, and chest wall abnormalities
Hematologic	• Breathlessness and weakness • Family and past history more indicative for bleeding or venous thromboembolism • Medication—anticoagulation/anti-platelets	• Pallor, anemia, and petechiae • Ecchymosis and peripheral edema
Gastrointestinal	Pain abdomen, altered bowel habits, liver disease, alcoholic, gastritis, tense abdominal swelling, and bleeding per rectum or hematemesis	Signs of cirrhosis, surgical scars, and abdominal distention
Musculoskeletal	Trauma, falls, pains, abnormal posture, deformities, and implanted devices	Findings of rheumatoid arthritis, DISH, ankylosing spondylosis, degenerative arthritis, kyphosis, scoliosis, and gait
Neurological	Seizures (new/old) and hemiparesis/stroke	Higher mental functions, sensory-motor examination, and pupils
Ophthalmologic	Hypertension and altered vision	Retina examination
Urological	Frequency, urgency, burning micturition, and flank pains	Renal angle tenderness and urosepsis
Miscellaneous	Menstrual history, pregnancy, drug abuse, steroid use, detailed medication history, past surgical procedures, and complications	Surgical scars and intravenous access

(COAD: chronic obstructive airway disease; COVID: coronavirus disease; DISH: diffuse idiopathic skeletal hyperostosis; ENT: ear, nose, and throat; ILD: interstitial lung disease)

TABLE 6: Common guideline-directed laboratory tests for elective noncardiac surgery.

Hemoglobin	Expected substantial blood loss, anemia
Total leukocyte counts	Symptoms of infection/sepsis/myeloproliferative disorder/bone marrow suppression/HIV infection/medications impacting marrow
Platelet count	Neuraxial anesthesia, bleeding diathesis
Prothrombin time/INR	Bleeding diathesis, liver disorder, malnutrition, and patient on anticoagulation
Partial thromboplastin time	Heparin use and bleeding disorder
Electrolytes	Renal disorder, altered sensorium, endocrine disorders, and steroid use
Creatinine and renal function tests	Chronic kidney disease (CKD), hypertension, diabetes, major surgery, nephrotoxic medication use/intended use
Serum glucose level	Diabetes, obesity
Liver function test	Liver disease
Urinalysis	Urosepsis, urogenital tract manipulation
ECG	Any patient undergoing intermediate or high-risk surgery (not indicated for low-risk surgery), known cardiac disease, diabetes, uncontrolled hypertension, and CKD
Chest radiograph	No documented support for routine use in patients known to have a pulmonary disorder or those >50 years of age. Done in active pulmonary disease not evaluated recently.
Advanced pulmonary testing	Spirometry may be used in patients with known obstructive or restrictive pulmonary disease especially those recently identified with abnormal chest radiograph or dyspnea of unclear etiology.
Echocardiogram	Unassessed unexplained dyspnea, known cardiac structural abnormalities with worsening symptoms of heart failure or those not evaluated in past year. Not needed in patients evaluated within past year

a specific focus on those with neoplasia, lower limb, and pelvic surgery and those needing immobilization. Caprini risk assessment tool can be applied to several different types of surgery but it is not validated for trauma surgery.

Delirium

Elderly patients are at special risk of delirium especially if it is associated with preoperative cognitive dysfunction. Mini-Cog score of 2 or less is associated with an increased risk of delirium.

Postoperative Nausea and Vomiting

This is commonly seen with prolonged surgeries and ones with greater use of opioids (intrathecal-epidural or intravenous). The Koivuranta score or Apfel score moderately predicts possibility of postoperative nausea and vomiting (PONV).

Geriatric Risk Assessment

Frailty, defined as a decrease in physiologic reserves and accumulation of multisystem impairments separate from the normal process of aging, poses systematic challenge to combined and universal risk assessment. Risk analysis index or modified frailty index is commonly used for assessment. The latter is developed by Canadian study of health and aging to calculate modified frailty index (mFI) based on 11 variables each assigned 1 point. mFI is calculated by adding the total positive score by 11. Value of ≥0.45 independently predicts major postoperative complication.

Total Joint Arthroplasty Cardiac Risk Index

Waterman et al. formulated and tested a cardiac risk index (Total Joint Arthroplasty Cardiac Risk Index, TJA-CRI) specific to TJA patients based on three primary predictors: age ≥80 years, history of hypertension, and a history of cardiac disease. It was shown that each factor independently predicts postoperative MCC and also that patients with all three predictors had the highest MCC risk. It is suggested that TJA-CRI better predicts the occurrence of MCC than RCRI.

PRESURGICAL EVALUATION

The assessment begins with history and physical examination **(Table 5)** that is then extended to metabolic equivalent **(Table 3)** designation and investigations **(Table 6)**.

PATIENT OPTIMIZATION

The role of POA is not only to identify the patient-specific risk factors but also to take appropriate steps for reducing and modifying them to minimize perioperative complications that affect patient outcomes. The common factors that can be optimized for elective surgeries include obesity, malnutrition, diabetes, smoking and drug abuse, psychiatric disorders, rheumatologic diseases, hypertension, etc.

OBESITY

In orthopedic surgery, obesity has the greatest impact on the outcomes of lower limb joint arthroplasty so the following discussion is dedicated to it.

Obesity has been on a rise worldwide lately reaching epidemic proportions now. Morbid obesity [body mass index (BMI) >40 kg/m^2] is also proportionately increasing. It is widely known that obesity accelerates the development of osteoarthritis of the knee and hip possibly through biomechanical alteration and systemic inflammatory changes. Biomechanically, each kilogram of weight rise increases 2–3 N of force across each hip joint and 5–6 N of force across each knee joint. The prevalence of joint pain also increases with increasing BMI. Following higher

TABLE 7: The WHO classification of underweight, normal weight, overweight and obesity.

Class	*Body mass index (kg/m^2)*
Underweight	<18.5
Normal weight	18.5–24.9
Overweight	25–29.9
Obese	
• Class I	30.0–34.9
• Class II	35.0–39.9
• Class III (morbid obesity)	≥40.0

incidence of degenerative joint disorders in obese, they are also subjected to higher incidence of TJA. It is also not infrequent to see younger and heavier patients needing total knee-joint arthroplasty. Obesity predisposes to higher risk of perioperative complications, such as poor wound healing, infection, respiratory complications, venous thromboembolism, need for revision joint surgery, prosthesis loosening, increased total cost of care, and prolonged hospital length of stay. The increased risks and complications preclude the utilization of TJA by surgeons in patients with a BMI of >40 kg/m^2 **(Table 7)**. But, there are patients at extreme spectrum of obesity and joint disease who are so disabled to be unable to mobilize. Medical and noninvasive therapies are unlikely to improve function and quality of life for these patients. These patients are referred to tertiary medical centers. There is growing emphasis on value and outcomes over volume so there will be stringent screening and possibly higher denial rate for obese patients to undergo TJA. The only effective and durable treatment that remains for obesity is bariatric surgery. The patients lose 50–70% of their excess weight and 10–15 BMI points after stapled bariatric procedures. Maximal weight loss is seen 1–2 years after the bariatric procedure, and is usually maintained thereafter in most of the patients.

The safety profile of bariatric surgery has dramatically improved recently. Indications for bariatric surgery are prominently based upon BMI. Obese patients with a BMI ≥ 40 kg/m^2 are generally considered to be candidates for bariatric surgery. Obese patients with a BMI ≥ 35 kg/m^2 are also considered for bariatric surgery when comorbid disease, such as diabetes, hypertension, sleep apnea, or severe osteoarthritis, is present. These patients otherwise also have a higher morbidity profile following TJA.

Alteration in Lower Limb Biomechanics due to Obesity

Loads across the hip and knee joints during normal activities of daily living are proportional to weight with the knee experiencing consistently greater loads than the hip. In nonobese patients, during normal walking (4 km/h) the peak in vivo hip contact forces ranged between 2.1 and 2.9 times body weight (BW) with a mean of 2.4 BW. During stair climbing these loads ranged from 2.3 BW to 2.7 BW (mean ≈2.5 BW). Gait disturbance increase loads across joints while stumbling produces loads in excess of 8.7 BW. The normal tibiofemoral contact loads across the knee during walking and stair-climbing are higher than those measured in the hip. During walking these forces are approximately 3×BW demonstrating large peak tibiofemoral loads after heel-strike and a second peak of smaller magnitude before toe-off. Stair-climbing also results in higher forces with maximum mean forces ranging from 5.09 to 5.88 BW. In obese patients, there are higher loads across the knee and lower loads across the hip compared to normal weight patients. In general, obese individuals exhibit lower self-directed walking velocity, shorter stride lengths, longer times in stance phase, greater step widths measured in the frontal plane, and greater toe-out angles compared with normal weight patients. Lowering walking velocity is assumed to be an adaptive change to increased weight that results in lower joint moments (i.e., torques) in the hip, knee, and ankle. Increased toe-out angle may decrease knee adduction moments in normal gait to lower the load across the knee joint. High knee adduction moments correlate to the development of knee osteoarthritis.

Joint Arthroplasty Outcome in Obese Patients

As the loads transmitted across hip and knee are proportional to the weight so it is quite logical to understand that in patients with TJA these elevated loads will be distributed across the bearing surfaces of the prostheses. The combination of excess load and repetitive joint cycling in obese TJA patients increases the risk for accelerated bearing surfacing wear, early prosthesis failure, and implant loosening compared to patients of normal weight. Obese patients with total hip replacements [total hip arthroplasty (THA)] may have higher risk of prosthesis dislocation arising out of technical difficulties in patients with excessive BMI compared to normal weight patients. Higher number of technical errors has been reported in obese patients. Overall complication rates have been found to increase from 5% in normal weight patients to 22% in obese individuals. Obesity also increases the risk of surgical site infections (including periprosthetic infections, rise from 0.4% in normal weight patients to 4.66% in obese), respiratory complications, thromboembolic events (1.5 times higher for each 5-point increase in BMI), need for revision joint surgery, component malposition, prosthesis loosening, total cost, and hospital length of stay. Comorbid conditions like type II diabetes (doubles periprosthetic infection rates) and obstructive sleep apnea (increases the rate of serious complications and increased length of stay) further increase the perioperative morbidity. Some studies report up to three times increased need of revision of hip prosthesis in obese patients (BMI ≥ 40 kg/m^2) compared to nonobese.

Impact of Arthroplasty on Obesity

It was a misconception or a hyped propaganda for arthroplasty that after TJA increased activity would be helpful in reducing weight and as a consequence produce postoperative weight loss. This is so ingrained among patients too that sometimes they plead for TJA under the misconception that they would be able to lose weight if only they could just be mobile. The reported findings in literature are quite contrary. Patients undergoing either hip or knee replacement that had good orthopedic outcomes actually gained weight afterward. Patients with a normal BMI and obese patients may not lose weight but overweight patients usually gain a significant amount of weight after surgery. The preoperative weight and postoperative weight are tightly correlated. Most studies report that a successful arthroplasty and restoration of a patient's mobility does not necessarily produce subsequent weight loss. The majority of patients instead add on weight, and ultimately there is overall net weight gain despite encouragement to lose weight. Not all report such dismal outcome, in a review by Inacio et al. for 20,060 total knee arthroplasties (TKAs) and 10,572 THAs; the authors found that 69% of TKAs and 64% of THAs maintained their weight (<5% change in BMI) 1 year postoperatively. For TKA patients, 8% gained weight in the year after surgery, 14% lost weight, and the weight change was unknown in 9% of patients. For THA patients, 15% gained weight, 14% lost weight, and the weight change was unknown in 13% of patients. Compared to patients with BMI < 30 kg/m^2, a larger percentage of patients with elevated BMI lost weight after TJA.

Bariatric Surgery and its Relevant Effects

Surgically-induced weight loss not only reduces the quantity of food consumed but also the amount of calories absorbed. Older procedures like jejunoileal bypass were failure as they excessively reduced the surface area for absorption and produced complications such as diarrhea, nephrolithiasis, malabsorption syndrome, and cirrhosis. Presently day bariatric surgeries can be grouped into two broader types—gastroplasty and gastric bypass **(Table 8)**. During inception they were performed open but now both can be laparoscopically performed. Gastroplasty reduces the stomach volume that is commonly achieved by either a silicone ring placed in the cardia creating a 15-mL pouch or by sleeve gastrectomy by stapling along the greater curvature to reduce the volume by 25%. This induces early satiety by reducing the amount of food consumed but nutrients are properly absorbed as distal gastrointestinal tract is in continuity. Despite its ease of doing the results for weight reduction are variable in producing weight loss and failure is not uncommon. Gastric bypass, on the other hand, not only reduces the gastric volume but also limits absorption of nutrients **(Fig. 1)**. The proximal portion of stomach is stapled to create a 20–30 mL pouch and roux loop of jejunum (distal cut end) is anastomosed to the gastric pouch for food passage. The proximal cut end is anastomosed to the Roux loop to provide conduit for biliary and pancreatic juices and prevent blind loop syndrome completing the Roux-en-Y. This system reduces the stomach volume and also induces controlled malabsorption to effect weight reduction. The following are some of the consequences of bariatric surgery that one should be aware of while prescribing the faculty services.

Metabolic Consequences

Malabsorption produces nutritional deficiencies while in restrictive surgeries erratic food consumption also may produce the same. Anemia due to iron and folic acid deficiency is common. Bypass surgery will limit the calcium and vitamin B_{12} absorption to a great extent as most of it is absorbed from duodenum that gets bypassed. Both of these thus need to be replaced in adequate amounts, the effect is though less pronounced after restrictive procedures. Protein deficiency is common after both procedures and produces muscle wasting there is also some amount of protein

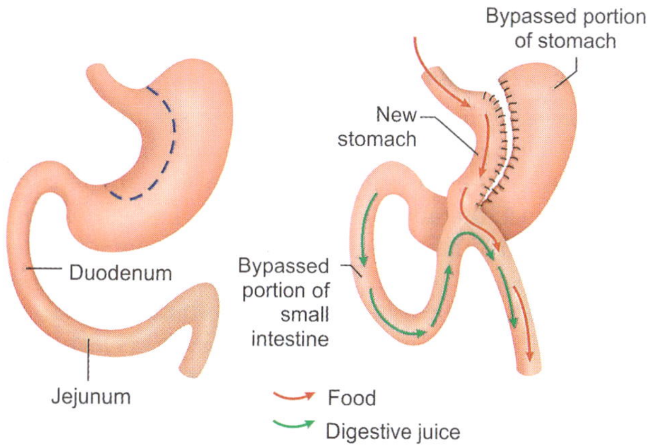

Fig. 1: The mini-gastric bypass in the form of Roux-en-Y. The small gastric pouch is anastomosed to the distal jejunal limb (Roux limb) and proximal is connected to the Roux limb for biliary and pancreatic juices to mix with food. The jejunum forms a Y-configuration deriving its peculiar name.

TABLE 8: Types of bariatric surgery.

	Malabsorptive (Roux-en-Y)	*Restrictive (gastric banding/sleeve gastrectomy)*
Mechanism	• Decreases volume of stomach • Reduces area of absorption	Decreases volume of stomach
Expected weight loss	Quite predictable	Unpredictable
Advantages	Predictable and significant weight reduction	• Ease of performance • Easier to reverse • Less metabolic derangements as the gastrointestinal tract (GIT) is maintained in continuity
Disadvantages	• Malabsorption syndrome and nutrient deficiencies common—deficiency of iron, calcium, vitamin B_{12}, protein and vitamin D is common • Wound healing complications and osteopenia seen frequently • Needs experience to perform surgery and manage complications	• Failure common • Weight loss is very unpredictable • Nutrient deficiency (less common) than malabsorptive procedures—iron, vitamin B_{12}, and protein deficiency

intolerance following both surgeries. Fat-soluble vitamins are also absorbed in limited amount following reduced bile salts.

Effect on Wound Healing

There is reduction in protein absorption and induction of a sort of catabolic state with erratic protein metabolism following bariatric surgery. Based on the studies on abdominal wound healing it has been found that there is significant reduction in the amount of hydroxyproline and other tissue proteins following this surgery. The elastic and collagen fibrils are irregular in structure all resulting in delaying wound healing and suboptimal wound healing (strength).

Effects on Bones and Fracture Repair

The malabsorption reduces bone mineral density (BMD) mediated by several factors such as reduced plasma leptin, ghrelin, and increased adiponectin. There is also reduction of estrogen in females that otherwise is trophic to bones. The reduction in BMD is proportional to weight reduction possibly because osteoporosis is a qualitative disorder that manifests quantitatively and bone quality is reduced in malabsorption and nutrient deficiency. The effect on fracture repair is unknown but hypovitaminosis and mineral deficiency is expected to retard the process.

Effect on Medications

The bioavailability of oral tablet and capsule preparations is expectedly reduced following reduced absorption surface area. Extended release and sustained release preparations may not reach therapeutic plasma levels. The effect is also seen for antibiotics so liquid preparations are preferred. Best is to use intravenous preparations where feasible considering the possibly already compromised renal and hepatic parameters in the obese patients. Nonsteroidal anti-inflammatory drugs (NSAIDs) have a detrimental effect following this procedure so usually centrally acting drugs such as acetaminophen or tramadol or tapentadol are preferred.

Considerations for Faculty Surgery in Bariatric Patients

Thorough preoperative evaluation is needed before embarking on major or even minor surgery in patients who have undergone bariatric surgery as metabolic alterations may compromise the critical functions. Protein deficiency can be estimated by total protein, total lymphocyte count, and albumin and prealbumin levels. Reduced albumin and transferrin levels are correlated with prosthetic joint infection and wound healing complications. Deficiency of vitamin A, B_{12}, C, folate, thiamine, and minerals such as iron, zinc, manganese, and magnesium and calcium would compromise the wound and bone healing. Zinc deficiency has been correlated with poor wound healing. Work-up for osteomalacia (alkaline phosphatase, secondary hyperparathyroidism) with serum vitamin D and calcium levels should be done before orthopedic procedures for optimization, if deficiency is detected.

Timing of Surgery after Bariatric Surgery

This issue is not fully agreed upon and no universal guidelines exist. Maximal weight loss and stabilization is reported at 2 years following bariatric surgery so logically this time-frame is generally mentioned in various studies; however, major orthopedic elective surgeries have been done as early as 6 months without undue complications. Studies specifically looking at 2 years as a time-frame reported higher overall complications for surgeries performed within 2 years but difference may not be significant to reach statistical or practical conclusion.

Impact of Bariatric Surgery on Osteoarthritic Joints

The bariatric surgery has been shown to effect joint pain, function, and osteoarthritis progression in the severely obese patients before arthroplasty. There is a significant reduction of BMI after bariatric surgery reported in different studies beginning within 3 months and stabilizing till 1 year or more. There is also a radiographic improvement of disease and clinically relevant improvement in pain and function. Site-specific pain like for knee and hip reduced both in frequency and intensity. The reduction is other painful musculoskeletal symptoms, particularly concerning the cervical spine, lumbar spine, ankle, and foot is also remarkable. There is also less work-restricting knee and ankle pain overall following improved physical function, reduced knee stiffness, and improved range of motion.

Biomechanics after Bariatric Surgery

Bariatric surgery also affects the kinematics and kinetics of joints following weight loss. Gait analysis to measure both ground reaction forces and three-dimensional kinematics of the lower extremities demonstrate significant decreases in step width in the frontal plane and peak moments (torques) around the hip and knee proportional to the amount of a patient's weight loss. Weight loss resulted in increased stride length and gait speed along with improvement in hip range of motion, maximal knee flexion, and ankle plantar flexion. There is general improvement in self-directed walking speed but no change in the fastest walking velocity. The patients also report subjective improvements in walking and stair climbing ability.

Ground reaction forces are highly correlated to body mass being proportionate to the body weight. The findings, however, revealed that ground reaction forces generally decrease with weight loss at lower gait velocities but they increase to levels beyond baseline measurements as the gait velocity increased. Low velocity and low-impact exercises are hence recommended after weight loss surgery.

Arthroplasty Outcome in Patients Treated with Bariatric Surgery

Quite logically gathering from above that there is increased morbidity in obese patients and improvement following bariatric surgery would follow into recommendation of bariatric surgery before TJA as a strategy. The conclusion is, however, not so straightforward and the reports are mixed in outcome. The following are some of the studies done to look into the matter, however, most of the evidence is retrospective:

- McLawhorn et al. found that bariatric surgery 2 years before TKA can be a cost-effective treatment strategy compared to TKA alone in morbidly obese patients.
- Werner et al. analyzed the 90-day complication rates of TKA, comparing 11,294 morbidly obese patients to 219 morbidly obese patients (using a national database) who had bariatric surgery first. The latter group had half the rate of major complications and 40% fewer minor complications. This improvement, however, did not translate into reduction in complication rate to the level of nonobese controls.
- Parvizi et al. reported improved results after studying 20 patients with a mean BMI of 49 kg/m^2 who underwent bariatric surgery followed by lower extremity TJA. The BMI dropped to a mean of 29 kg/m^2, the cumulative Knee Society Score after TKA improved from 103.6 to 148.9, and the Harris hip score improved from 40 to 67.5 after THA.
- Kulkarni et al. identified 143 obese patients who underwent both bariatric surgery and TJA. Patients with bariatric surgery first were found to have significantly lower wound complications and re-admission rates.
- Severson et al. reported that patients with TJA >2 years after bariatric surgery had an anesthesia time that averaged 28 minutes shorter and operative time that averaged 39 minutes shorter but there were no differences observed in hospital stay or 90-day complication rates.
- Inacio et al. reported that bariatric surgery before TJA did not appear to reduce the frequency of complications, readmissions, deep surgical site infections, or revision following TJA. This study was purely a descriptive study.
- Martin et al. in a retrospective analysis reported that although patients receiving bariatric surgery reduced their BMI before TKA, there was an increased risk of reoperation in the bariatric group compared to the group matched to their prebariatric BMI, and there were no differences in complications, revision, or deep infection. The bariatric group had a higher risk of reoperation and revision TKA compared with patients who underwent TKA at an equivalent BMI, but the risks for complications and periprosthetic joint infection were not different.

The current evidence for supporting bariatric surgery before TJA is gathered from retrospective studies reporting conflicting results. It is unclear as to when the elective surgeries can be done following initial bariatric surgery and one should do a thorough evaluation before taking major surgeries. Perioperative management should also be a team effort including various faculties managing the metabolic parameters and these should be communicated to the patient.

DIABETES

Diabetic patients have shown uniformly poor pooled outcomes following orthopedic surgery. The commonly reported problems are:

- Higher in-hospital complications (wound complications and infections)
- Higher readmission rates (infection and surgical failure)
- Higher infection rates
- Delayed and nonunion
- Poor patient reported outcomes

The outcomes are worse in type 1 diabetes mellitus [insulin-dependent diabetes mellitus (IDDM)] than type 2 diabetes mellitus. Preoperative evaluation of control of blood sugar levels is imperative in stratifying the perioperative risk in elective surgery. This is even more important in patients above 65 years of age. Hemoglobin A1c (HbA1c) is the most widely used biochemistry parameter to gauge control of blood sugar levels several days before. The recommendations for reducing/preventing surgical site infection (SSI) have been blood glucose levels of <200 mg/dL and HbA1c levels < 7% from the Center for Disease Control and Prevention (CDC) and International Consensus Meeting on prosthetic joint infections. HbA1c levels of ≥7.7% are probably associated with higher SSI. Optimization of HbA1c levels would need 3 months before changes can be interpreted so serum fructosamine levels have been proposed that reflect changes over 14–21 days. Patients with fructosamine levels > 292 μmol/L have higher rates of deep infection and revision surgery. Serum fructosamine is a simple and cost-effective test.

MALNUTRITION

The risk of malnutrition is increased with increasing age (especially >55 years of age) and is quite prominent in third world countries. Malnutrition poses problems of SSI, wound healing problems, osseous healing, and higher readmission rates due to postoperative failures and increased mortality. There is no uniformly agreed upon definition of malnutrition but some common parameters that suggest malnutrition include serum albumin < 3.5 mg/dL, serum prealbumin < 15 mg/dL, and serum transferrin < 200 mg/dL. Serum albumin indicates nutrition levels of preceding 14–20 days so it is the most commonly employed measure (and also it is a commonly available inexpensive biochemical test). Transferrin has a shorter half-life (10 days) and is more susceptible to changes in serum level with liver disease or anemia. Serum prealbumin levels have the shortest half-life (2–3 days) and are subjected to acute changes in protein intake. Other measures that can be used are lymphocyte count < 1,500 cells/mm^3 and subjective global assessment (scoring tool). Malnourished patients may benefit from dedicated oral high protein and high calories nutrition supplementation in consultation with a dietician. Parenteral nutritional supplementation is recommended only for those who cannot take oral supplementation in such large quantities (elderly patients in intensive care unit, mentally debilitated, etc.). Elective surgeries may be deferred for the duration of build-up. Surgeries for trauma/infection are not delayed rather nutritional buildup continues in perioperative period. Undernourished underweight patients have high risk of perioperative complications including infection, need of transfusions, readmission, and mortality that should be effectively communicated to them. Wound healing has been variably reported in them, some even reporting lower rates of complications. Arthroplasty patients do have an increased length of stay. In any case, all malnourished patients undergoing elective surgeries should be optimized for nutritional build-up and deficiencies should be treated for better outcome. One such nutritional deficiency now frequently encountered is vitamin D deficiency that is commonly seen in population and patients come with reports of low levels due to common occurrence of the test and awareness. Vitamin D plays an important role in BMD, fracture healing, muscle function, immune function, and various other allied effects. It has been found that patients with peri-periprosthetic joint infections have low vitamin D level but whether it is an independent modifier is unknown. Vitamin D is a modulator if innate and adaptive immune system so it is recommended to optimize 25-hydroxyvitamin D levels above 30 ng/mL especially in patients with darker complexion aged 51 years or more. This should be followed by recommended daily allowance for long periods.

SMOKING

Cigarette smoke has obvious deleterious effects on various systems of body due to its various oxidative and toxic chemicals. Nearly 4,000 chemicals result in vasoconstriction, hypoxia, central nervous system (CNS) effects, autonomic dysreflexia, negative effects on bone and tissue healing, etc. Smokers have high rates of infection, nonunion, wound complications, and higher readmission and reoperation rates. Active smokers can be identified by urine nicotine > 200 ng/mL and urine anabinase > 10 ng/mL (normal values are <17 ng/mL and 2 ng/mL, respectively). Patients should be encouraged to stop smoking and for elective surgeries minimum 4 weeks of cessation period is recommended to have any beneficial effect that should continue for several days/weeks postoperatively (again minimum 4 weeks). Behavior support, nicotine replacement, intensive face-to-face intervention therapy, varenicline, and bupropion may be used to reinforce and aid smoking cessation.

ALCOHOL AND DRUG ABUSE

Alcohol abuse is associated with chronic liver disease and cirrhosis, cardiac dysfunction, hemostatic dysregulation, immune dysfunction, and malnutrition. Heavy drinkers (defined as females consuming >7 drinks/week and males >14 drinks/week) have high complication rates including not following medical advice, prolonged hospital stay, higher re-admission rates, infection, and bone/fracture healing problems. Patients should be counseled for cessation of drinking preoperatively for at least 6–8 weeks (duration unknown) while supplementing with pharmacological therapy (disulfiram, acamprosate, opioid antagonists, and benzodiazepines) for elective surgeries. This should extend for several weeks postoperatively. For trauma and emergency surgeries, preoperative optimization is not possible so postoperative cessation and counseling should be done. The clinical institute withdrawal assessment for alcohol (CIWA) scale can help to guide duration and dosing of withdrawal-preventing medications.

Illicit drug abuse is a growing evil that needs pertinent and strict control. Unfortunately, these patients are unaware of the catastrophic effects of using dirty needles (infections), sharing needles (transmission of various diseases), etc. These patients are at increased risk of pneumonia, endocarditis, soft-tissue and bony infections, hepatitis C virus, and HIV infection. These patients also have greater than normal requirement of opioids, sedatives, relaxants, and analgesic drugs. Blood and urine tests can be done to identify strongly suspected patients. These patients need careful counseling and a programmed approach to de-addiction guided by a psychologist and psychiatrist. The association of psychiatric disorders with substance abuse is called "dual diagnosis". Such patients have increased rates of perioperative complications and optimization should be done in concert with psychiatrist to adequately manage the patients. Patients on lithium pose significant threat to perioperative complications and careful advice with deferring surgery till optimization is imperative.

RHEUMATOLOGICAL DISEASES

Patients on medications for management of various rheumatological diseases [rheumatoid arthritis, systemic lupus erythematosus (SLE), ankylosing spondylitis, psoriatic arthritis, etc.] pose thoughtful challenges to surgical management of orthopedic disorders. Significant number of patients undergoing arthroplasty are suffering from rheumatological diseases that are under pharmacological treatment. Because most of these medications are immunomodulators (mostly suppressors of immune system—general or specific), surgeons tend to withhold them for concerns of wound and osseous healing. A lot of insights have been drawn to the specific recommendation to perioperative use of these drugs. The time duration for which these medications should be stopped preoperatively for rheumatoid arthritis is discussed in Chapter on "Joint Disorders Including Inflammatory and Noninflammatory Arthritis and Infective Arthritides (Including Mycobacterial Infection and Prosthetic Joint Infection)". The other general recommendations are:

- Conventional synthetic disease-modifying antirheumatic drugs (cs-DMARDs) should continue to be used during perioperative period as before with usual dosage and timing.
- Biological disease-modifying antirheumatic drugs (bDMARDs) should be stopped before surgery at the end of their dosing cycle and postoperatively they should be started only 2 weeks after surgery in the absence of wound healing problems, surgical site infections, or systemic infections.
- Medications specific for SLE are discontinued 1 week before surgery if the disease is not severe but, for patients with severe disease and organ involvement, the drugs are continued during perioperative period.

PAIN MANAGEMENT IN ORTHOPEDIC PATIENT

DEFINITION

Pain is a unique subjective experience of an individual, which cannot be adequately defined, identified, or measured by an observer. Pain consists of sensory and motivational-affective and cognitive components. Sensory component describes the quality, quantity, and geography of area involved in pain. The motivational-affective component explains the individuals approach to the pain and cognitive component decides that how much pain that individual is going to feel depending upon past experiences and modulations done by central and peripheral nervous system.

TYPES OF PAIN

Pain is described on the basis of its anatomical origin, intensity, or duration. Somatogenic pain is localized in the body tissue, if causes are inflammatory it is called nociceptive pain and if pain is secondary to sensitization of nervous system (peripheral or central), it is called neuropathic pain. Psychogenic pain is pain for which there is no known physical cause but processing of sensitive information in CNS is disturbed.

Acute and Chronic Pain (Table 9)

Pain with sudden onset called "acute pain" which is protective and alerts the individual to a condition that is immediately harmful to the body. Stimulation of autonomic nervous system can be observed during this type of pain shown by mydriasis, tachycardia, hypertension, tachypnea, sweating, vasoconstriction, and flushing. It also causes rise in blood sugar levels, decreased blood flow to viscera, decreased motility of gut, and occasionally nausea or vomiting. Acute pain also induces psychological and behavioral responses such as anxiety, fear, unease, and general sense of unpleasantness. We can distinguish two types of acute pain: (1) somatic and (2) visceral; they may be localized or referred. Pain arising from the skin or close to the surface of the body is called somatic pain and if it arising from internal organs, abdomen, or chest is visceral pain. If pain is felt away from its origin is known as referred pain. There are many theories to explain the referred pain, like; the area of origin of pain and referred area are supplied by the nerves from the same spinal segment or convergence of impulses occurs from viscera and skin in the CNS. An irritable focus is generated at the level of spinal cord where pain signals from viscera enter and these signals further facilitate the afferent impulses from the skin entering at the same segment resulting in cutaneous pain. Other mechanism for referred pain is the sensitization of dorsal horn (DH) neurons. Painful impulses form viscus stimulate anterior horn motor cells and activate visceromotor reflexes resulting in rigidity of the muscle, muscles ischemia and muscle become a new source of pain. Anterolateral autonomic cells also get stimulated in similar way and cause sympathetic phenomena resulting in pyloerection, vasoconstriction, etc. These mechanisms are also known as positive sympathetic and motor feedback loops.

"Chronic pain" develops insidiously; it is persistent or intermittent in nature and usually defined as lasting at least 6 months. Chronic pain often results in significant behavioral and psychological changes such as helplessness and depression. As soon as the chemical mediators that stimulate the nociceptors are removed, pain relief occurs in acute pain condition, however, chronic pain may persist even long after removal of primary cause of pain due to plasticity of nervous system. If acute pain is not treated timely and adequately it may convert to chronic pain.

Common Chronic Pain Conditions

Persistent low back pain due to degenerative disease of spine, pain due to cancer, neuralgias and causalgia, and reflex sympathetic dystrophies (RSD) which may occur after peripheral nerve injury are few causes of chronic pain. Second most common cause of chronic pain is myofascial pain syndromes which include myositis, fibrositis, myalgia, muscle strain, and injury to the muscle and fascia. This pain is due to muscle spasm which results in tenderness and stiffness in the muscles. A rare condition related to chronic pain is hemiagnosia which may occur after stroke. Affected area shows hypersensitivity to painful stimuli and person is unable to identify the stimulus. Hemiagnosia is also associated with intensified emotional and autonomic responses to the pain. Phantom limb pain is another condition in which individual feels pain in amputated limb.

TABLE 9: Difference between acute and chronic pain.

Characteristics	*Acute pain*	*Chronic pain*
Temporal features	Short history of onset and does not last longer than days or weeks	Long history with often poorly-defined onset; duration unknown
Intensity	Variable	Variable
Associated effects	If pain is severe, anxiety may be prominent and sometimes irritability	Depression and irritability is prominent feature
Associated pain behaviors	When pain is severe pain behaviors (e.g., moaning, rubbing, and splinting) may be prominent features	Specific behavior may or may not be present. If pain is severe and for long duration specific behaviors (e.g., assuming a comfortable position) may occur
Other associated features	Features of sympathetic hyperactivity when pain is severe (e.g., tachycardia, hypertension, sweating, and mydriasis)	Usually have one or more vegetative signs such as lassitude, anorexia, weight loss, insomnia, and loss of libido. Sometimes these signs may be difficult to distinguish from other disease-related effects

PATHWAYS OF PAIN

Afferent pathways, efferent pathways, and CNS are jointly responsible for the sensation and perception of pain. The afferent pathways consist of: pain receptors (nociceptors), afferent nerve fibers, and spinal cord network. Fibers of afferent pathways terminate in the DH of the spinal cord and are called first order afferent neuron, spinal part of afferent system are called second order afferent neuron. Limbic system, reticular formation, thalamus, and hypothalamus and cortex of CNS are responsible for interpretation of the pain signals. The fibers of efferent pathways connect the reticular formation, midbrain, and substantia gelatinosa (SG). Efferent pathway is responsible for modulation of pain sensation. On the perception of first pain sensation by brain, the thalamus and sensitive cortex helps in perceiving describing and localizing the pain. Dull, longer-lasting, and diffuse pain is identified by thalamus, brainstem, and reticular formation. Emotional and affective responses to pain are controlled by the reticular formation and limbic system. The cortex, thalamus, and brainstem are interconnected with the hypothalamus and autonomic nervous system, therefore, the perception of pain is associated with an autonomic response.

Afferent Pathways

Pain sensations from receptors are transmitted by small A-delta (δ) fibers and C-fibers to the DH of spinal cord. A-δ fibers carry well-localized, sharp pain sensation, and the small unmyelinated C-neurons are responsible for the transmission of diffuse burning or aching sensations. Transmission through unmyelinated C fibers is slower than larger, myelinated A-δ fibers where it occurs much more quickly.

Efferent Analgesic System

The main role of efferent system is to inhibit afferent pain signals. Activation of efferent (descendent) antinociceptive pathways occurs when pain afferents stimulate the neurons in periaqueductal-gray (PAG) matter in the midbrain surrounding the cerebral aqueduct.

Role of the Spinal Cord in Pain Processing

All afferent neurons including A-β fibers, some A-δ fibers and small C fibers terminate at the SG in the laminae of DH (first order neurons). Then axons of second afferent neuron from the SG of laminae cross to the other side of the cord either at the same or adjacent spinal segment. In the ventral and lateral horn, impulses are carried through the spinothalamic tract to various areas of brain such as midbrain, thalamus, reticular formation, pons, and limbic system.

GATE CONTROL THEORY (PAIN PRODUCTION AND MODULATION THEORY)

Melzack and Wall gave the theory of gate control to explain the pain modulation production and perception. Although this theory is unable to explain few pain conditions, however, it is still most widely accepted theory about pain perception. According to this theory, large A-δ and small C-fibers carry the nociceptive impulses to the spinal cord through and form synapses in SG. The cells in SG regulate transmission of impulses to CNS depending upon other inputs from other areas of spinal segments or brain and function as a gate.

- "Closed gate" is the situation where stimulation of A-α and A-β (larger nerve fibers) causes decreases stimulation of T-cells (the second afferent neuron) which decreases the transmission of impulses and diminishes pain perception.
- Stimulation of small fiber increases the stimulation of T-cells and inhibits cells in SG. This increased transmission of impulses (open gate) leads to enhance pain perception.
- Other factors in nervous system also influence the functioning of gate control. The CNS may close, partially close, or open the gate through efferent pathways, and modulates pain perception. Naturally occurring opioids like endorphins (ED) also affect the transmission through gate. All ED act by attaching to opiate receptors on the plasma membrane of the afferent neuron. This result is inhibition of release of the neurotransmitter, thus blocking the transmission of the painful stimulus.

POSTOPERATIVE PAIN AND ITS MANAGEMENT

Approximately 80% of patients experience acute pain after surgery. Of these patients, 86% patients suffer from moderate, severe, or extreme pain. Despite an increased focus on pain management programs and the development of new standards for pain management, many patients continue to experience intense pain after surgery. Postsurgical pain is a complex response to tissue injury during surgery and also due to secondary inflammatory response which initiates hypersensitivity of the CNS. If not managed timely and adequately, it may lead to chronic pain. Postoperative pain after orthopedic surgery is usually intense and the goal of postsurgical pain management is to reduce the amount of pain which patient experiences after surgery. Adequate pain control results in better surgical outcome in terms of increased patient satisfaction, early mobilization and shorter hospital stay.

ASSESSMENT OF PAIN

There is no definitive method to measure pain and, only the person, who is experiencing it can accurately indicate its intensity. However, various methods, i.e., charts/questionnaire and other tools have been used to quantify the pain in postoperative period. Accurate pain assessment helps in appropriate treatment by determining the type of pain, its relation with movement (important to assess functional impairment), and also to assess the treatment efficacy.

Three components of pain have to be assessed, intensity, quality, and impact on emotional, social and physical functioning.

Pain Assessment Tools (Scales to Assess Pain Intensity)

Single ratings of pain include the numerical rating scale (NRS), verbal rating scale (VRS), visual analog scale (VAS), and faces rating scale. It is recommended that all the scales should have anchor points such as "no pain" at the lower end and "worst pain possible" at the higher end of the scale.

- *Numerical rating scales (NRS):* The NRS is one of the most convenient ways of determining pain intensity. An 11-point (i.e., 0 = no pain–10 = maximum pain) NRS scale is commonly used. Specific numbers used in these scales are less important than change in ratio during management of pain, i.e., a change from 8 to 4 indicates a reduction in pain which equates to a 50% reduction in pain intensity.
- *Verbal rating scales (VRS):* This scale uses verbal response in form of words to assess severity of pain like no pain, mild pain, moderate pain, or severe pain.
- *Visual analog scales (VAS):* VAS is most popular scale for pain assessment. It usually consists of a line labeled at 0 or no pain at one end and 10 or 100 on other end to express extremes of the feeling to be measured. The patient is asked to make a mark along the scale which best represents their pain intensity. The sole advantage of this scale is that it generates numerical data which can be analyzed easily.
- *Pain measurement by pictures:* The advantage of face pain scale is that the patient does not need to be literate. The faces pain scale-revised (FPS-R) utilizes a six-face scale **(Fig. 2)** from extreme left (pain score 0), through to severe pain on the extreme right (pain score 6). This scale has a strong positive correlation with the VAS and also conforms closely to linear interval scales.
- *Pain assessment by questionnaire:* Qualitative and quantitative experience of pain cannot be assessed by simple single ratings tools described above. More elaborated formats (Questionnaire) are required for such assessment. Two commonly used questionnaires are as follows:
  1. *The McGill pain questionnaire (MPQ):* It is most commonly used questionnaire to assess qualitative and quantitative experience of pain. The MPQ consists of 78 words describing pain in sensory and affective and evaluative terms. Sensory part uses words describing the quality of the pain (e.g., throbbing, burning, or aching) arranged in groups and order of their intensity (more severe first than less severe). Every component of pain (sensory, cognitive, and affective) is evaluated on six-point VRS for pain intensity and sum of various responses gives the total score for severity of pain.
  2. *Brief pain inventory (BPI):* The BPI is more relevant to clinical trials and cancer pain. It includes three items to measure pain, severity, and quality. It also includes seven additional items, e.g., mood, function, sleep, and interpersonal relationships which may be interfered or affected by pain.

Technique to Assess and Measure Postoperative Pain and Evaluate the Treatment Efficacy in Postoperative Patient

Serial measures of pain should be carried out during expected period of pain because a single measurement is like a "snapshot" and may not be true picture of the pain intensity.

- Sum of the pain scores over a time period provides an "area under the pain curve" against the time value. For an example, if VAS is done at interval of 2 hours and scores are 75, 65, 55, 45, and 35 the sum of the VAS (SUMVAS) would be 275 over an 8-hour period.
- Another effective method to measure the pain and efficacy of treatment is the "pain intensity difference (PID)". PID is calculated by subtraction of the current pain score from original pain score over a set time period **(Table 10)** then a correction factor is applied to each PID, to yield corrected "time-weighted" PID.
- The "total pain relief (TOTPAR)" can be calculated **(Table 11)** in a similar manner as PID or SPID were assessed.

SYSTEMIC EFFECTS OF POOR PAIN CONTROL

There are various effects on body, mostly detrimental resulting from poor control of pain.

- Pain results in increased sympathetic response of the body which cause increase in heart rate (tachycardia), cardiac work, and oxygen consumption.
- Increased risk of deep vein thrombosis and consequent pulmonary embolism due to reduced physical activity leading to venous stasis.
- Reduced gastrointestinal (GI) tract and urinary tract motility may lead to postoperative ileus, nausea, vomiting, and urinary retention.
- Inadequate postoperative pain relief may result in psychological changes, increase in the morbidity and mortality as well as the cost of treatment.
- Acute pain if not treated immediately and adequately leads to chronic pain conditions.

BARRIERS TO EFFECTIVE PAIN MANAGEMENT

The common reasons which lead to poor pain management are inadequately trained staff, poor pain assessment either due to lack of knowledge regarding various tools or attitude,

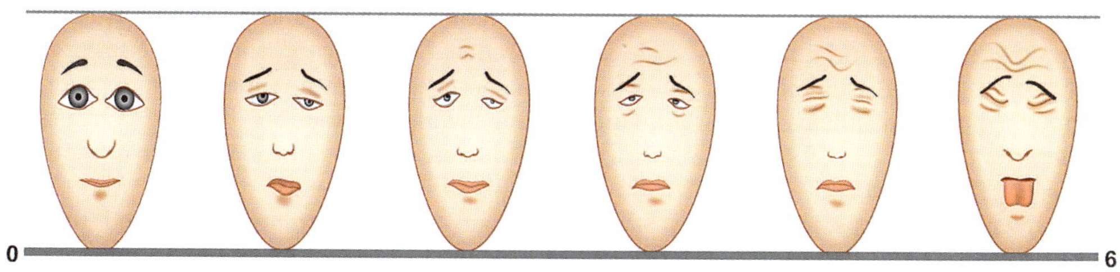

Fig. 2: Extreme left (pain score 0), through to severe pain on the extreme right (pain score 6).

TABLE 10: Serial measurements of pain over a period of time.

Time in hours	*Current pain score (A)*	*Initial pain score (B)*	*Pain intensity difference (PID) = (B – A)*	*Correction factor (time interval between observation)*	*Corrected PID or sum of pain intensity differences*
0.5	2	3	1	0.5	0.5
1	1	3	2	0.5	1
2	1	3	2	1	2
3	2	3	1	1	1
4	3	3	0	1	0

Sum of pain intensity differences (SPID) = 4.5
Maximum possible SPID (MPSPID) = 12 (4 × 3)
(Initial pain rating × number of hours over which ratings were recorded)
Percentage of maximum possible pain intensity difference rating* = 37.5%
(SPID/MPSPID × 100) or (4.5/12 × 100 = 37.5)*

TABLE 11: Calculation of total pain relief.

Time in hours	*Current pain relief (PID)*	*Correction factor*	*Corrected score (SPID)*
0.5	2	0.5	1
1	3	0.5	1.5
2	3	1	3
3	2	1	2
4	1	1	1
Total pain relief (TOPAR)			8.5

TOTPAR = 8.5
Maximum TOTPAR = 12 (maximum relief score × time in hour)
Percentage of maximum TOTPAR = 70.83%
(PID: pain intensity differences; SPID: sum of pain intensity differences)

fear of analgesic side effects, and lack of accountability. These factors are related to nurses, doctors, and patient himself that act as barriers for effective pain control.

- Inadequate assessment of pain by nurses and agreement between nurse and patient about level of pain results in inadequate analgesia being given to the patient.
- Doctors contribute to poor pain control by prescribing inappropriate mode of drug delivery and dosages of drugs. Lack of knowledge about opioid addiction and respiratory depression among doctors is another reason for under treatment with such effective drugs.
- Patent's belief that pain is inevitable and that "good" patients do not complain and made them reluctant to report pain and reluctant to take analgesia.

STRATEGIES FOR ADEQUATE POSTOPERATIVE PAIN CONTROL

- *Prevention of central sensitization:*
  - Treat acute pain adequately and timely.
  - Use drugs that prevent expression of c-fos.
  - Use continuous regional anesthesia in operation and early postoperative period.
- *Management of central sensitization:*
  - If central sensitization develops, treat it early.
  - NSAIDs are not the option to treat it. Use drugs, which stimulate descending inhibitory systems and N-methyl-D-aspartic acid (NMDA) antagonistic actions.
  - Tramadol + Paracetamol ± Tricyclic antidepressants should be ideal to treat central sensitization.

BOX 2: The concept of balanced analgesia.

With the better understanding of pain physiology and application of multitude of drugs that offer analgesia a "balanced" approach to controlling postoperative pain is evolving that replaces overutilization of a single class of drugs (like opioids). This approach integrates use of different class of medications (multimodal analgesia) targeting all the different receptors that activate pain pathway. This integrated approach aims at achieving "equivalent pain control" in postoperative period popularly forming an important pillar of the "enhanced recovery after surgery (ERAS)" pathway. This strategy has improved analgesia while reducing the adverse events and enhancing mobilization and rehabilitation in postoperative period. The interdisciplinary approach to pain management as utilized under various descriptive "terms" is outlined below.

Acute pain

Multimodal analgesia

- Neuraxial analgesia (spinal, epidural, and combined approach)
- Regional analgesia (nerve blocks, plexus blocks, and indwelling catheters)
- Local infiltration (wound/periarticular)

Balanced analgesia

- Pre-emptive analgesia (gabapentin, acetaminophen)
- Nonopioids (NSAIDs, NMDA-antagonists such as ketamine, α-2 agonists like clonidine or dexmedetomidine)
- Long-acting opioids like methadone

Chronic pain

Preprocedure consultation

- History, evaluation of past treatment records, and if possible then consultation with previous physician
- Drug abuse and urine toxicology
- Detailing pain management strategy and clear communication of goals with patient
- Patient education and discussing expectations

Postprocedure follow-up

- Monitoring of symptoms and compliance with prescription
- Scaling down medications
- Interventional procedures for pain
- Opioid detoxification

(NSAIDs: nonsteroidal anti-inflammatory drugs; NMDA: N-methyl-D-aspartate receptor)

METHODS FOR POSTOPERATIVE PAIN CONTROL

There are various methods to manage postoperative pain. For effective postoperative pain management preoperative plan should be made taking into account the type of surgery, patient's profile, and available resources, e.g., infrastructure, medicines, and expertise.

Multimodal Analgesia

No single drug or technique is sufficient to provide complete or near complete pain relief without side effects. Therefore, drugs and techniques are used in combination to maximize the beneficial effects and minimize side effects of an individual approach ["Balanced" analgesia **(Box 2)**]. The multimodal analgesia is a combination of two or more analgesics, each with a different mode of action to improve analgesia and to decrease side effects through a reduction in doses of analgesics, particularly opioids. More than one method of pain management may be used to attain multimodal analgesia approach. By using multiple methods the amount of medications necessary to relieve pain can actually be reduced and thus uncomfortable side-effects are minimized. In principle, "prevention is better than cure" also applies for pain management, therefore, pain management should be started before pain appears rather than in reaction to pain.

Pre-emptive Analgesia

It is now believed that it requires less analgesic to control pain before it starts than after the noxious input has begun.

Mechanism of Action

Surgical incision results in pain signals and nociceptor activation causing discharge of neuropeptides such as neurokinin A, calcitonin gene-related peptide (CGRP), and substance P from peripheral terminals of the primary nerve fibers. At the same time an inflammatory response is provoked by the release of contents from damaged cells. These two processes contribute to the presence of a "sensitizing soup" of inflammatory mediators that includes bradykinin, serotonin, histamine, nitric oxide, and several others. This leads to repetitive stimulation of small-diameter primary afferent fibers causing "sensitization" or "wind-up" of both peripheral and CNS neurons resulting in prolonged pain beyond the duration, which is normally expected with an acute insult. This sensitization can also permanently alter spinal cord function leading to the development of chronic pain following an acute injury. Pre-emptive analgesia decreases postoperative pain by the prevention or attenuation of this wind-up phenomenon.

Methods

A wide variety of drugs have been employed, such as NSAIDs), opioids, α_2-agonists, and NMDA antagonists such as ketamine and dextromethorphan.

Concerns and Current Validity

Pre-emptive analgesia is commonly used to control postoperative pain; however, there is some degree of controversy regarding the validity of pre-emptive analgesia in the clinical setting. Many studies have obtained equivocal results or have failed to clearly demonstrate that pre-emptive analgesia is efficacious.

Preventive Analgesia

Preventive analgesia aims to prevent the effects of other factors which lead to central sensitization throughout the perioperative period, and may be administered at any stage of the perioperative period. Preventive analgesia can be defined as "when postoperative pain and analgesic consumption are reduced relative to another treatment, a placebo treatment, or to no treatment, as long as the effect is observed at a point in time that exceeds the clinical duration of action of the target drug", i.e., 5.5 half-lives). Preventive analgesia is usually given over a longer term, and may be more efficacious, e.g., pre-emptive antineuropathic pain medications have less effect on chronic postsurgical pain (CPSP), compared to preventive regimens.

Locoregional Analgesia for Postoperative Pain Management

Local Wound Infiltration

Local infiltration analgesia (LIA) technique involves infiltration of a large volume dilute solution of a long-acting local anesthetic agent at the time of surgery. Adjuvants (e.g., epinephrine, ketorolac, an opioid) can be mixed with local anesthetic to improve the effect. The duration of analgesia can be prolonged by the placement of a catheter to the surgical site for postoperative administration of further local anesthetic. It is easy to perform and it is very safe procedure with few side effects and low risk for toxicity. Pain relief usually lasts longer than the duration of local anesthetic and the anti-inflammatory effect of local anesthetic drugs could be contributing factor for this prolonged effect. Infiltration carried out at the conclusion of surgery is more effective than preincisional local wound infiltration. Lidocaine 0.5% and bupivacaine 0.25% are commonly used as local anesthetics and recently levobupivacaine 0.25% and ropivacaine 0.2% are being used due to better safety profile.

Periarticular Analgesia

Periarticular injections involve injecting local anesthetic and other agents into joint capsule and subcutaneous tissues postoperatively (commonly done for TKA). It is simple and can be combined with neuraxial analgesia or peripheral nerve blocks (PNB). Ropivacaine is commonly preferred and duration of analgesia can be prolonged by adding epinephrine, ketorolac, and/or morphine in variable combinations. The addition of steroid is controversial but can be done for nondiabetic patients, however, patellar tendon rupture risk should be borne in mind.

Peripheral Nerve Blocks

Peripheral nerve blocks are safe and effective techniques of providing postoperative analgesia that cut down on time to hospital discharge, reduce postoperative pain, and improve overall patient satisfaction. PNB used for postoperative pain can be placed before or after incision and decision is based on the nature of surgery and available resources in recovery or preoperative area. A catheter can be placed to give intermittent boluses or continuous infusion of local analgesia to prolong the duration of analgesia. Bupivacaine 0.125–0.25% and ropivacaine 0.1–0.2% are commonly used for infusion after initial bolus of 0.25–0.5% bupivacaine and 0.5–0.75% ropivacaine. Commonly used PNBs are brachial plexus block (supraclavicular, interscalnae, and axillary) used for upper limb surgeries and sciatic, femoral, three in one block, lumbar plexus block, and fascia illica block for lower limb surgeries **(Table 12)**.

Epidural Analgesia

Epidural analgesia has dual advantage that it provides anesthesia during surgery and extended analgesia to postoperative period by means of a catheter, which provides the potential advantage of an unbroken period of pain control

TABLE 12: Some commonly used peripheral nerve blocks with their indications.

Upper limb	
Interscalene block (root/trunk of brachial plexus)	Shoulder arthroscopy, rotator-cuff repair, shoulder arthroplasty, proximal humerus ORIF
Supraclavicular block of divisions of brachial plexus	Elbow surgeries (joint reconstruction and ligament repair), forearm ORIF, hand surgery
Infraclavicular/axillary block of the cords or terminal branches of brachial plexus	Same as for supraclavicular block
Lower limb	
Lumbar plexus block	Hip surgeries (reconstruction, arthroscopy, hip preservation, and osteotomies), acetabular ORIF, knee arthroplasty, and femur ORIF
Femoral nerve	Knee arthroplasty (adjunctive), ACL and MPFL reconstruction (adjunctive), quadriceps repair. Additional block to sciatic nerve block for foot/ankle surgery
Adductor canal block	As for femoral block
Sciatic nerve block	Foot and ankle surgery, foot amputations, and adjuvant to femoral nerve block for knee arthroplasty

(ACL: anterior cruciate ligament; MPFL: medial patellofemoral ligament; ORIF: open reduction and internal fixation)

from the operating room until the catheter is removed, usually 24–72 hours later. Combinations of local anesthetic, opioids, and other medications (clonidine, tramadol, dexmedetomidine, etc.) can be titrated to patient comfort and allow for an acceptable degree of motor function while effective sensory block. Epidural analgesia helps to reduce opioid use; in addition, other beneficial effects are improved gastric motility, blunted stress response to surgery and reduced thromboembolic complications.

Drugs and Dosage: Diluted solutions of local anesthetics either intermittent boluses or continuous infusions are used for analgesia to avoid motor weakness.

Bolus: Bupivacaine 0.125–0.25%, ropivacaine 0.2% or levobupivacaine 0.25%; 5–10 mL as required can be given. If opioid (morphine 3–5 mg) is mixed with bupivacaine 0.05–0.125%, it gives 8–12 hours of pain relief.

Infusion: This technique is more common than boluses because it provides continuous pain relief and decreases the chances of breakthrough or incidental pain. Bupivacaine 0.05–0.125% with fentanyl 2 μ/mL at 4–6 mL/h provides good analgesia in majority of surgery. Ropivacaine 0.1–0.2% and fentanyl 2 μ/mL is more effective.

Patient-controlled Analgesia

A routine demand analgesia regimen (where patient requests and caregiver gives the drug) results in "roller coaster" effect. It means when patients have pain they request for medicine, they receive analgesics, experience brief periods of relief, followed by repetition of this cycle when the pain returns.

TABLE 13: Intravenous regimens of patient-controlled analgesia (PCA).

Concentration of drug	*Bolus dose*	*Lockout interval (min)*	*Continuous basal infusion*
Morphine (1 mg/mL)	0.5–2 mg	5–10	0–2 mg/h
Fentanyl (0.01 mg/mL)	10–20 μg	5–10	0–60 μg/h
Meperidine (10 mg/mL)	5–25 mg	5–10	0–20 mg/h
Tramadol (4–5 mg/mL)	10–20 mg	6–10	0–20 mg/mL
Sufentanil (0.002 mg/mL)	2–5 μg	4–10	0–8 μg/h

Period of time between request and administration results in increased anxiety and pain in patients. However, where pain control (drug delivery) is given in the hand of patients, [patient-controlled analgesia (PCA)] provides continuous analgesia and leads to higher patient's satisfaction. PCA provides pain medication at the patient's needs. The intravenous and epidural PCAs are commonly used for postoperative pain and represent the philosophy of "patient controlled pain relief but with safety (partly inherent in system and partly provided and controlled by care provider)". There are also other routes of administration for PCA, e.g., oral, inhalation, nasal, and transcutaneous.

Intravenous

Intravenous PCA is provided through an electronically controlled infusion pump that delivers an amount of intravenous analgesic when the patient presses a button. Opioids are commonly used drugs in PCA **(Table 13)**. PCA allows repetitive dosing of small amounts of opioids by the patient on-demand basis, followed by a lockout period during which the machine will not allow any more doses of analgesic. If the patient presses the button earlier than the set time, PCA pump will not give the drug instead; emit a beep telling the patient that dose was *not* delivered. When the patient is too sedated to press the button, unnecessary dose will not be delivered and patient will be prevented from receiving needless doses and thus overdosing.

Minimum Effective Analgesic Concentration

Advances in technology have allowed more flexibility with the PCA systems and PCA can accommodate the widely divergent analgesic requirements of different patients. Bolus doses and background infusion rates can be altered after seeing the patient's pain recording on a specially designed handset which is linked to a computer which can facilitate changes.

Patient-controlled epidural analgesia (PCEA): In this technique, administration of drugs in epidural space is done by infusion pump and dosages are controlled by patients as done in IV PCA. The settings of pump are also similar to IV PCA except, consideration should be given for the onset of drug effect which is marginally longer than IV.

Nasal PCA or patient-controlled intranasal analgesia (PCINA): These PCA devices are in a nasal spray form with inbuilt features to control the number of sprays that can be delivered in a fixed time period.

Transcutaneous PCA: Transcutaneous PCA delivery systems work on the principle of iontophoretic systems. These PCAs are popular for administration of opioids such as fentanyl, or local anesthetics such as lidocaine. "Iontophoretic transdermal system (ITS)" works on the principle of iontophoresis. The drug is absorbed in the tissues by application of low-intensity electrical fields across skin. It is observed that about 40% of the administered drug is absorbed in the first hour and the complete absorption and action may last up to 4 days.

Oral: Self-administration of oral over-the-counter or prescription painkillers by patient may be called as "patient controlled analgesia method" as the administration of drug is under patients control; however, it is not desirable practice because it lacks the control on intake and thus safety.

Inhalational: Ether, chloroform, and mixture of nitrous and oxygen have been used in the past. However, this is more of historical importance and was used commonly for obstetric analgesia. In late 60s, methoxyflurane was used through disposable inhaler "analgizer" and was found to be safe, effective and simple to administer in patients with bone fractures and joint dislocations.

Advantages of Patient-controlled Analgesia

- Self-administration of pain medication and therefore faster relief from pain because there is no delay between pain and its treatment.
- Less amount of drug is required due to adequate and timely control of pain.
- It provides the feeling of self-control, better pain relief with less sedation and enhanced satisfaction.
- Patients can be mobilized early due to less sedation and good pain relief. This results in better respiratory function, less risk of pneumonia and other respiratory complications.
- Reduced length of stay reduces healthcare costs and less chance of nosocomial infections.

Disadvantages

- Possible misuse and abuse of opioid drugs
- Under-dose or overdose of medication, if PCA device is not programmed properly for the patient.
- If patient has learning difficulties and is confused due to any reason, use of PCA is not advisable.
- Critically ill patients and patients with poor manual dexterity may be unable to press the buttons of PCA pump.
- Patient-controlled analgesia may not be appropriate for younger patients (children of <5 years).

Patient-controlled Regional Analgesia

Patient-controlled regional analgesia (PCRA) can be provided by inserting perineural catheter and giving intermittent or continuous infusion of diluted local anesthetic agents through that catheter either manually or by preprogrammed elastomeric or electronic pumps. Adjuvants along with local anesthetics can be mixed for better safety and good results. The indwelling catheter can also be placed in the surgical wound area or intra-articular to obtain the maximum benefit with minimal side effects using very low drug concentrations. On-Q or the "pain relief ball" device is a ball like pump that administers non-narcotic medication to the incision site through a small catheter.

DRUGS USED FOR POSTOPERATIVE PAIN CONTROL

The drugs used for acute surgical pain or postoperative pain management can be divided in three major groups: (1) opioid analgesics, (2) nonopioid analgesic, and (3) adjuvants.

Opioid Analgesics

Opioid analgesics are strong analgesic used for moderate-to-severe pain in the early postoperative period. Opioid analgesics work through opioids receptors which are distributed in the brain, spinal cord, and peripheral nociceptors. The opioid system consists of at least three distinct opioid receptors: (1) mu (μ), (2) kappa (κ), and (3) delta (δ). According to the nature of affinity to receptors opioid drugs are classified as opioid agonists, partial agonist, and agonist antagonist. "Opioid agonist" analgesics bind predominantly to the μ receptor. This group includes morphine, meperidine, fentanyl, sufentanyl, alfentanil, remifentanil, hydromorphone, codeine, oxycodone, oxymorphone, hydrocodone, methadone, and propoxyphene. Mu receptor activation generates desired effects such as analgesia and adverse effects such as constipation. "Opioid agonist–antagonist" analgesics have agonist activity at one receptor and no or low activity on other receptor (antagonist activity). The receptor and drug interaction is very complex for these drugs. Nalbuphine and pentazocine are examples of opioid agonist—antagonist analgesics. "Opioid partial-agonist" analgesics bind to an opioid receptor producing a partial agonist response. These agents are either partial agonist or antagonists at the μ receptor and partial agonist or agonists at the κ receptor. Buprenorphine is an example of a partial agonist at the μ receptor; however, butorphanol is partial agonist and antagonist at the μ opioid receptor, as well as competitive antagonist and partial agonist at the κ receptor. Methadone is a long-acting opioid that is found effective in management of acute pain. It is devoid of "opioid euphoria" and hence has low addictive potential (factually it was used in opioid addiction treatment!), and also it has multireceptor mechanism of action.

Mechanism of action: Activation of receptor results in increased G protein activity which leads to K^+ efflux and inhibition of Ca^{2+} influx into the cell. These events cause hyperpolarization of first- and second-order sensory neurons, with inhibition of synaptic transmission. Opioids also stimulate the supraspinal descending inhibitory system resulting in hyperpolarization of second-order neurons by releasing 5-HT and glycine.

Routes of administration and uses: The most common route of postoperative opioid analgesic administration is intravenous. Other routes of opioid administration are intramuscular, subcutaneous, transmucosal, epidural, intrathecal, and transdermal. Routes such as epidural, intrathecal, and regional techniques should be used in preference to intramuscular opioids to enhance analgesic effect and patient satisfaction. Intrathecal administrations of small doses of opioids are effective to control visceral pain. However, opioids do not have anti-inflammatory property, therefore, are unable to provide effective control of postoperative pain during movement. Extended release epidural morphine (Depodur) is a new addition which can provide a long-lasting pain relief up to 48 hours without producing a higher systemic drug concentration. When administered epidurally, it provides long-lasting analgesic effects in total knee replacements (TKR). The equipotent dose of commonly used opioids are as follows: 10 mg morphine = 100 μg fentanyl = 100 mg pethidine = 0.3 mg buprenorphine = 30 mg pentazocin = 100 mg tramadol.

Side effects: The problem with opioid drugs is the variety of perioperative complications, e.g., drowsiness and sedation, postoperative nausea and vomiting (PONV), pruritus, urinary retention, ileus, constipation, and respiratory depression particularly in elderly patients and hence close monitoring is essential.

Tramadol

Tramadol is a synthetic analgesic that is a racemic mixture of two enantiomers that bind to the μ opiate receptor with low affinity. Tramadol acts by opioid and monoaminergic mechanisms and inhibit pain transmission at the spinal level. Along with activity on μ receptors, tramadol also works through norepinephrine and serotonin reuptake inhibition. After systemic administration, tramadol is metabolized to M1 metabolite in the liver by the enzyme CYP2D6. This metabolite is a potent μ-opioid agonist that contributes to tramadol's analgesic actions. The (–)-enantiomer of tramadol mainly inhibits norepinephrine reuptake whereas the (+)-enantiomer preferentially inhibits serotonin reuptake in the CNS. Reuptake inhibition of norepinephrine and serotonin both augments descending inhibition of pain transmission in the spinal cord. Tramadol is a "weak" opioid analgesic for postoperative pain relief with potency of 10% that of morphine. Like other opioids, it does not produce significant constipation or respiratory depression. Unlike opioids, it has low abuse potential. Tramadol is available for oral, rectal, and parenteral administration.

Nonopioid Analgesics

Nonopioid analgesic drugs have marginalized the use of opioid analgesics in preventing pain after ambulatory surgery due to their ability to reduce postoperative pain with movement. They also reduce opioid analgesic requirement and associated side effects, thereby shortening the duration of the hospital stay. Nonopioid drugs used in postoperative pain management can be classified as:

- NSAIDs and cyclooxygenase (COX)-2 inhibitors
- Acetaminophen
- Paracetamol

Nonsteroidal Anti-inflammatory Drugs

These drugs are known for their anti-inflammatory and analgesic actions.

Mechanisms of action: NSAIDs have ability to decrease prostaglandin formation through inhibition of COX pathways. Surgical insult to tissue results in release of prostaglandins through COX pathways, which sensitize peripheral nociceptors and produce localized hyperalgesia (primary hyperalgesia). If immediate and adequate measures are not taken, this may lead to central sensitization in the postoperative period. NSAIDs inhibit the production of prostaglandins from arachidonic acid, thus decrease peripheral sensitization and the activation of peripheral nociceptors. Recent evidence has suggested that rapid upregulation of COX-2 expression occurs in the CNS following peripheral trauma leading to central sensitization and pain hypersensitivity. Drugs that act on COX-2 in the CNS may play a role in targeting nociceptive pathways.

Indications and routes of administration: The NSAIDs are very effective in increasing efficacy of opioid analgesia as they reduce opioid requirements while providing better pain control postoperatively. If given pre- or intraoperatively COX-2-selective inhibitors provide the additional safety by not affecting platelet function. NSAIDs can be administered orally, intramuscularly, intravenously or by the rectal route. NSAIDs alone are effective analgesic after minor surgical procedures and for major surgical pain t hey work in synergism with other analgesics. They have significant opioid-sparing effect of (20–30%) after major surgery and may reduce the incidence of opioid-related side-effects such as respiratory depression, sedation, nausea and vomiting, ileus and urinary retention, etc. Unless contraindicated, all patients should receive around-the-clock regimen of NSAIDs, COX-2 inhibitors, or acetaminophen during perioperative period.

Concernsandcontraindications: Nonselectiveuse of NSAIDs causes bleeding due to platelet aggregation and gastroduodenal ulcers. Additional toxicity such as reduced bone healing, reduced renal function (in low perfusion states), and rare hepatic toxicity still can occur with both selective COX-2 inhibitors as well as nonselective NSAIDs. NSAIDs should be used with caution in patients of older age group, borderline renal or hematological status, or previous dyspeptic symptoms. Many selective COX-2-inhibitors like celecoxib and rofecoxib are no longer in use due to adverse cardiovascular events.

When to administer NSAIDs: Effective analgesics can be achieved when administered at the conclusion of surgery. Pre-emptive analgesic effect of NSAIDs has also been demonstrated but results are variable. Variability in efficacy or the lack of efficacy of pre-emptive administration of these drugs could be explained by the fact that the COX-2 enzyme which is the primary target of NSAIDs is only inducible and it is not found in damaged tissues until a few hours following the onset of a noxious stimulus.

Acetaminophen: Acetaminophen is a safe antipyretic (action on central COX-2 and COX-3 enzymes), analgesic (due to activation of descending serotonergic inhibitory pathways and inhibition of central nitric oxide synthases) drug with poor anti-inflammatory action. It is marketed under generic name "paracetamol" in Europe and India. Paracetamol/acetaminophen is a good soft-tissue analgesic, but it is poor to manage pain following orthopedic surgery.

It is available in oral form and is used either preoperatively as pre-emptive analgesic or postoperatively as step-down analgesic. Intravenous preparation of acetaminophen is available in 100 mL vial in concentration of 10 mg/mL which requires administration over a period of 15–30 minutes. Sometimes mannitol is mixed which works as stabilizer. Onset of action is within 5–10 minutes, with the peak at 1–2 hours. If optimal analgesia for moderate to severe postoperative pain cannot be achieved with a single agent alone, but when used it can be used in combination with tramadol or nonsteroidal agents, results in up to a 40–50% reduction in opioid requirements.

Adjuvants

In clinical sense, the drugs that do not have an inherent analgesic property but enhance the analgesic potential of known analgesic drug is called an "adjuvant". They play an important role as part of a multimodal analgesic regimen because they can provide beneficial effects when administered in appropriate doses in the perioperative setting.

- Alpha-2 adrenergic agonists:
  - Clonidine
  - Dexmedetomidine

Dexmedetomidine and clonidine: These are selective α2 agonist drugs acts through adrenergic receptors present in the spinal cord and locus coeruleus of CNS. Dexmedetomidine, a potent α2 adrenoceptor agonist, is approximately eight times more selective toward the α2 adrenoceptor than clonidine. Both the drugs do not have any inherent analgesic property, however, work as adjuvants to local anesthetic when used in regional and neuraxial anesthesia and also when used with other analgesics parentally. Usual dose of clonidine is 1–2 µg/kg and dexmedetomidine, 0.5–2 mg/kg IV, or 1 µg/kg slow bolus over 10 minutes followed by infusion 0.2–0.7 µg/kg/h. Both the drugs are known to have excellent anesthetic-sparing and opioid-sparing properties.

- N-methyl-D-aspartate antagonists (antihyperalgesic drugs):
  - Ketamine

Ketamine: Ketamine is an NMDA antagonist. These NMDA receptors are involved in the hyperexcitability of spinal cord nociceptive neurons by C-fiber stimulation. Ketamine inhibits voltage-gated sodium and potassium channels and, in addition, the reuptake of serotonin and dopamine. Use of ketamine (250 µg/kg) with intravenous morphine provides rapid and sustained analgesia in postoperative patients. An excellent analgesia has been achieved by postoperative intravenous PCA using the ratio of morphine and ketamine of 1:1 and a lockout interval of 8 minutes after spine and hip surgery. Commonly available ketamine is a racemic drug [mixture of S (+) and R (–) ketamine]. The S (+) isomer of ketamine is more potent than the R (–) isomer and has less psychological side effects.

- Gabapentin-type drugs:
  - Gabapentin
  - Pregabalin

Gabapentin and pregabalin: Gabapentin is basically an antiepileptic drug. It binds to the α-2 subunit of presynaptic voltage-gated calcium channels of GABA receptors. It works by preventing the release of neurotransmitters responsible for the activation of the pain pathway by preventing the entry of Ca^+ into neurons. Gabapentin has antihyperalgesic property and has shown opioid-sparing effect during 24 hours of the postsurgical period when given orally before surgery. Pregabalin is a derivative of gabapentin and structural analog of GABA, is known to have analgesic, sedative, and antianxiety properties.

- Gluc1corticoids
  - Dexamethasone

Dexamethasone: Steroid adjuvants have been found to prolong the block duration when used in regional blocks. Dexamethasone significantly prolongs duration of analgesia of ropivacaine without affecting the onset of sensory, motor block, and surgical anesthesia during interscalene block (ISB) used for arthroscopic surgeries of shoulder.

- Newer drugs:
  - Capsaicin
  - Tapentadol

Capsaicin: Capsaicin is a non-narcotic alkaloid, TRPV-1 agonist acting peripherally at unmyelinated C-fiber nerve endings. Capsaicin causes a sustained release of substance P at nerve endings and ultimately exhaustion. The use of capsaicin cream with other analgesics has shown opioid-sparing effects. Capsaicin in injectable form is safe and useful for postsurgical pain and chronic long-term pain management, however, should be used with caution in patients with elevated liver enzymes and patients on angiotensin-converting enzyme (ACE) inhibitors.

Tapentadol: It is a new and benzenoid class synthetic centrally acting opioid analgesic (µ-receptor agonist) with 18 times more affinity than morphine and with a dual mode of action as it also inhibits the noradrenaline uptake. Although it has high affinity with opioid receptors still it is two to three times less potent than morphine. Drug can be administered orally every 4–6 hours in divided doses and allowed maximum daily dose is 600–700 mg. Oral intake is well tolerated and can be used safely in patients with renal impairment.

- Liposomal bupivacaine

The formulation of polymer-encapsulated local anesthetics (liposome) provides long duration of action to local anesthetics. The polymer layer is made from a phospholipid which is biodegradable and, hence, can prolong the drug release. This layer is nonimmunogenic, safe, and biofriendly.

Perioperative Plan to Provide Superior Postoperative Analgesia in Special Situations

Arthroplasty of Hip and Knee

Preoperative: Oral paracetamol 10–15 mg/kg 1 hour before surgery provides good pre-emptive analgesia. A preoperative analgesic helps in reducing incidental pain due to movements during positioning of patients for regional blocks. If sitting positioning for spinal/combined spinal-epidural anesthesia (CSEA) is painful, preoperative femoral nerve block or fascia illica block with 20–30 mL local anesthetic (lidocaine 1.0–1.5% or bupivacaine 0.25–0.5% or ropivacaine 0.2–0.5%) is a useful technique.

Intraoperative and postoperative: Combined spinal-epidural anesthesia wherein spinal component provides good operative conditions and epidural analgesia is utilized for anesthetic supplement if surgery is prolonged. It also provides postoperative analgesia through epidural catheter which was inserted at the beginning of the anesthesia (CSEA). If surgery is done under single shot spinal anesthesia, femoral or fascia illica catheter can be inserted after surgery to provide postoperative analgesia. Single shot injection also helps in providing prolonged pain relief following surgery, which can further be prolonged by inserting a catheter and giving intermittent boluses every 4–12 hours. Although, the hip joint has complex innervations where sensory innervation of the hip comes from branches of both lumbar and sacral plexus, lumbar plexus block provides good analgesia after "hip surgery". In addition, if lumbar plexus block is given before surgery it may significantly reduce perioperative pain and blood loss in patients undergoing total hip arthroplasty and reduces intra- and postoperative opioid requirements. The lumbar plexus block, femoral block, fascia iliaca blocks, or the "three-in-one" can all be used to provide anesthesia and perioperative analgesia after knee surgery depending on the extent and type of surgery. These techniques provide unilateral analgesia with less side-effect than epidural analgesia and can be used as an alternative to central neural blockade for patients who are anticoagulated. Pain after TKR is often difficult to control using only IV opioids. PNBs provide better pain scores at rest and morphine consumption if used with PCA and also effective in providing prolonged postoperative analgesia following unilateral TKR without hindering postoperative mobilization.

Foot and Ankle Surgery

Similar anesthetic and analgesia plan of hip and knee surgery can also be used for ankle surgery. In addition, continuous sciatic or popliteal nerve blocks are very simple and effective techniques for pain control after lower extremity surgery. These techniques provide superior pain relief than parenteral opioids. The ankle block is also a safe and simple technique of pain relief for various foot surgeries. However, analgesia with lower extremity blocks lasts significantly longer than do ankle blocks. Sciatic nerve block in the popliteal fossa is an excellent choice for foot and ankle surgery which provides adequate anesthesia and good postoperative analgesia. This is relatively safe technique than neuraxial blockade (spinal or epidural). This block requires a larger volume (30–40 mL) of local anesthetic for blockade of both divisions of the sciatic nerve. In cases of hallux valgus surgery, the tibial nerve block can also be used to treat postoperative pain. And this can be combined with infusion of local anesthetic solution through a perineural catheter of the tibial nerve using 0.25% bupivacaine at a rate of 2.5 mL/h.

Below knee Amputation

Below knee amputation (BKA) patients suffer from severe postoperative pain. Incidence of phantom limb pain is high in such patients and loss of limb causes significant psychological suffering. Cardiovascular disease, uncontrolled diabetes mellitus, decreased pulmonary reserve, sepsis and systemic anticoagulation are common. Coexisting medical problems in patients scheduled for BKA. Low-dose parenteral opioid with nerve blocks and a single shot or continuous sciatic or popliteal block provides an ideal anesthetic/analgesic regimen to this group of patients.

Future lies with procedure-specific, evidence-based, and acute postoperative pain management practices. Use of guidelines may become the routine practice to choose the treatment strategies based on patients comorbid conditions and psychological status.

CONCLUSION

- Preoperative assessment of patient is legible in any surgical planning barring dire emergencies where saving life is the immediate priority. This is a combined surgeon and anesthetists responsibility. The ultimate goal is to minimize the "oops moments" during and after surgery and provide patient the best peri-operative clinically safe environment. This is somewhat similar to "KYC" common in financial sector practice.
- Patient optimization is essential to reducing peri-operative morbidities and complications. No haste should be shown to correcting the identifiable and modifiable factors to their best.
- Medical co-morbidities such as diabetes, hypertension and hepatorenal dysfunctions should be properly corrected before doing planned surgery with appropriate referrals. Malnutrition and morbid obesity have negative influence on outcomes of total joint arthroplasty and other surgical procedures. They should be reasonably evaluated and corrected before joint arthroplasty surgeries. Smoking, drug abuse and alcohol consumption have direct and indirect negative influence on orthopedic surgeries and patient should be counseled to quitting them lest poor outcomes are likely.
- Postoperative pain management has been rapidly improving and multimodal analgesia has become a norm in surgeries that provides adequate and safer pain relief. This has helped in reducing the postoperative complications and morbidities. Further adoption of procedure-specific, evidence based pain management practice has improved the ease of communication between physician-patient-anesthetist and ultimate pain control.

CHAPTER

24 Polytrauma, Mass Casualties, and Disaster

Manish Kumar Varshney

INTRODUCTION

Multiple injuries in a patient push the physiological needs sometimes beyond the body reserves and may threaten the life. The mortality risk in such patients has to be objectively assessed instead of deliberating on vague and arbitrary definitions of polytrauma or major trauma. This helps in universal language communication as the observer and the conversant are clear as to the objective of communication. This also helps in initial management of the patient by classifying the severity level of injury and orthopedicians contribute by reduction and stabilization of fractures promoting pain relief and reducing inflammatory burden. Patients in extremis may benefit by damage control strategies that limit exacerbation of systemic inflammatory response to trauma.

DEFINITIONS

Polytrauma

Polytrauma is the most common cause of death between 15 and 45 years old. It is a product of multisystem injury that induces profound pathophysiological changes and their cumulative effects could be life-threatening. Therefore, a consensus emerged where the word "polytrauma" is used to describe a syndrome of severe multiple injuries associated with systemic traumatic reactions that may lead to dysfunction or failure of remote organs and vital systems not directly injured by the event. This description is good for understanding but lacks any objective criteria to serve as a universal definition. Objective criteria needs both anatomical and physiological parameters to be incorporated to specifically define the condition. Anatomically, the patient with polytrauma should have two or more severe injuries in at least two separate systems of the body. This entails that a patient with multiple fractures will be categorized as multiple injury (i.e., two or more severe injuries in one body area) and not polytrauma. Various societies and expert groups have variably defined polytrauma as:

1. Two major system injury + one major limb injury (only anatomical parameters)
2. One major system injury + two major limb injuries (only anatomical parameters)
3. One major system injury + one open grade 3 skeletal injury (only anatomical parameters)
4. Unstable pelvis fracture with associated visceral injury (only anatomical parameters)
5. Injury severity score (ISS, **Box 1**) > 15, some use ISS > 17 as cut-off (objective anatomical definition and assessment)
6. New injury severity score (NISS)—three highest abbreviated injury scale (AIS) irrespective of anatomic area (better than ISS)
7. Two body regions with AIS > 2 (better than ISS as latter can also indicate monotrauma defying the basic concept)
8. Consensus definition of the American Association for the Surgery of Trauma and the German Trauma Society (2014, both anatomical and physiological parameters incorporated)—two or more injuries having AIS > 2 in different regions + one or more of the following five physiological parameters:
   i. Hypotension [systolic blood pressure (SBP) ≤ 90 mm Hg]
   ii. Consciousness [Glasgow Coma Scale (GCS) ≤ 8]
   iii. Acidosis defined as base excess < –6.0
   iv. Coagulopathy (international normalized ratio) ≥ 1.4
   v. Age >70 years

The above detailed definitions from 1 to 4 are mainly descriptive only and should be only referred for basic

BOX 1: The injury severity score (ISS). [The ISS is calculated by determining three most injured areas and evaluating them on the basis of abbreviated injury scale (AIS). These are then labelled A, B, and C. The ISS = $A^2 + B^2 + C^2$].

AIS body regions:
1. Head and neck
2. Face
3. Abdomen
4. Thorax
5. Extremity
6. Pelvis

AIS severity code:
1 = Minor
2 = Moderate
3 = Severe (non-life-threatening)
4 = Severe (life-threatening)
5 = Critical (survival uncertain)
6 = Fatal

understanding that polytrauma involves two different systems. They are not comprehensive and cannot be used to objectively label polytrauma, they only suggest polytrauma. Only for a negative embracement but importantly the following older vague definitions should *not* be used anymore for description:

- "Polytraumatism"—a broad healthcare and general societal problem area relating to severe associated and multiple injuries (i.e., to polytrauma)
- Simultaneous injury to *several* organs or body systems
- Two or more significant injuries
- Two or more significant injuries that may be life-threatening.
- "Major trauma" or "multiple trauma"
- Injury to several (≥2) physical regions or organ systems, where at least one injury or the combination of several injuries is life-threatening (Tscherne et al.). This was the closest definition to understanding and describe polytrauma and it basically served as primer for newer definitions and has been superseded by other objective definitions.

The use of ISS "only" does not account for the basic tenet of "two" different body systems as score of >15 or 17 may be positive even in single system, alternatively in a patient with bilateral fracture shaft of the femur the "other" femur will be omitted while scoring. This deficiency was partially overcome in NISS and using AIS > 2 in two body regions for defining polytrauma. Both these scores, however, failed to imbibe the physiological parameters now considered in defining "seriousness" of injury. For this reason, the consensus definition (at number 8 above) is more appropriate for defining polytrauma.

Disaster

A disaster occurs when the local resources are unable to meet the needs of the event. The required resources may include additional manpower, heavy rescue equipment, or expertise in dealing with an infectious disease outbreak or weapons of mass destruction. Considering this definition even a single child falling into deep pit would count as disaster. Many disasters are complex and involve large geographical regions. Earthquake, followed by "tsunami" and "nuclear disaster" in Japan, is an example of complex natural disaster.

Mass Casualty Incidents

These are incidents large enough to overwhelm the medical and public health services of the affected community. Mass casualty incidents (MCIs) are traditionally limited to particular geographical location. Incidents in an urban location are liable to extensive damage to lives and infrastructure. The Bhopal gas tragedy (accidental release of methyl isocyanate in 1984) and purposeful release of Sarin gas (1995) in Japan subway are examples of MCIs.

PRINCIPLES OF MANAGEMENT OF POLYTRAUMA

Team approach is essential for the management of different and varied organ systems. The care can be divided into four stages:

1. *Immediate care:* Follow advance trauma life support (ATLS) guidelines. Resuscitate patient and stabilize.
2. *Acute care:* Includes mainly lifesaving procedures to control hemorrhage (embolization, pelvic external fixation, etc.), respiratory support, and circulatory support with revaluation. Practice of damage control orthopedics (DCO) begins here.
3. *Intermediate care:* Skeletal stabilization as a part of DCO, nutritional support and pain control.
4. *Definitive care:* Comprehensive management of injuries and rehabilitation.

It should be borne in mind that there is trimodal peak distribution of trauma mortality:

- Most deaths occur during first hour after injury, mostly due to central nervous system (CNS) injury (approximately 50%), followed by exsanguination (approximately 20%).
- Second peak during 1–4 hours after injury also known as "*golden period*". The most common cause of death in this period is hypovolemic shock.
- Third peak several weeks later. Patient dies of late complications such as sepsis and multiple organ failure.

Early death is caused by severe trauma to vital organs (severe head injury or cardiac insult) or more importantly due to missed opportunity to treat potentially manageable life-threatening injuries. Late death is a result often of multi-organ failure when the compensatory mechanism becomes complicated and down-spiral with improperly managed organal damage. Polytrauma management begins at the injury site itself (prehospital) with raising alarm and informing approachable services, rescue, and transportation of resuscitated patient preferably on spine board supervised by paramedics. To prevent life-threatening complications, a mandatory schema is followed under expert guidance.

Hospital management of polytrauma victim is prioritized to life salvage, limb salvage, and then functional salvage. As stated above, team approach is must to determine the operative plan for the polytrauma patient on immediate basis and to put it in action so the practice of team preparation prior to patient arrival and debriefing following the event must be rigorously followed. Each of the members of the trauma team should be assigned a specific task, so that the patient would be treated as a whole simultaneously and not by treating one injury after another. To this effect, the team leader has following functions:

- Assess the clinical situation
- Gather information
- Direct the setup of the operating room
- Treatment needs from other faculties
- Determine priorities
- Set limits on time and complexity of procedures

As soon as the patient has received cervical stabilization the ABCDEs of trauma management begin. The so-called ABCs of trauma reflect priorities in primary survey for initial trauma management.

- Cx, always assume cervical spine injury in conscious and unconscious patient—always stabilize first (cervical collar—hard) and use backboard. Once evaluation for cervical spine is complete then remove board.
- A—Airway management with protection of the cervical spine

- B—Breathing and ventilation
- C—Circulation with hemorrhage control
- D— *Disability:* Neurologic status
- E—Exposure/environment (remove clothes to evaluate external wounds, but avoid hypothermia)

Each of these areas is addressed simultaneously by the trauma team. The primary survey usually takes no longer than a few minutes, unless procedures are required. Treatment is simultaneously provided, while evaluation is being done.

Airway

- Airway and breathing is handled first and no other procedures are initiated until the airway is secured. Airway compromise is the fastest pathway to death. To check the patency of airway, the simplest way is to ask the patient—how he or she is feeling. If the patient responds verbally—he or she has an intact airway, is breathing, is thinking and, therefore, has a pulse. If unresponsive, airway patency should be checked. Assess the airway by:
  - Listening air movement (nose/mouth and chest movement)—snoring or gurgling suggests partial airway obstruction.
  - Look for intercostal retraction—Look for chest expansion, listen, and feel for air movement.
  - Observe for foreign body obstruction in the oropharynx—stridor.
  - Check for gag reflex—watch for swallowing.
  - Use chin lift or nasopharyngeal airway (Chin-lift maneuver must not be used in confirmed cervical spine injury). Cricothyrotomy may be done in emergent situations if there is obstruction near vocal cords that cannot be immediately removed or bag-mask ventilation is not possible. This achieves three "Ps": (1) airway patency, (2) aspiration protection, and (3) positive pressure ventilation. Any foreign bodies that are seen should be removed. Blind mouth sweep must not be performed. Secretions and blood should be suctioned.

Indications for intubation are:

- Glasgow Coma Scale < 8
- Inability to maintain ventilation
- Apnea
- Severe maxillofacial injury

Management: Seal open pneumothorax

Breathing

For breathing, respiratory rate and depth should be assessed; cyanosis is a late feature. Oxygen at 6–10 L/min via a non-rebreathing face mask should be given. Patient should be ventilated, if needed, with rescue breaths, a bag-valve device (bagging the patient), or a ventilator. Look for trachea and deviation to one side. Chest tube placement may be needed emergently in cases of severe hemothorax or pneumothorax.

Circulation

- To assess circulation—one should look for the level of consciousness, skin temperature, color, nail bed capillary refill time, and rate and quality of the pulses. External bleeding should be controlled with direct pressure without inadvertent use of tourniquet. Blood should be sent for basic laboratory studies. Resuscitation should be done with two large bore (14–16 gauge) intravenous catheters (antecubital—femoral—subclavian or jugular), using warmed fluids (Ringer lactate is the fluid of choice—bolus 2 L crystalloid or in children 20 mL/kg) and packed RBCs, if necessary. Concept of balanced resuscitation has emerged and the initial bolus of 2 L is reduced to 1 L agreeing with concepts of permissive hypotension to avoid disrupting blood clots and preventing dilutional coagulopathy. This also provides space for instituting plasma and platelets to address coagulopathy early. Amount of the fluid to be given is decided by blood pressure monitoring, central venous pressure (CVP) monitoring, urine output monitoring, and the response to initial bolus (sustained, transient, or minimal). The initial aim is to maintain a palpable radial pulse, which will need an SBP of 70–80 mm Hg. If there is any suspicion of head injury, the SBP should be maintained >90 mm Hg in order to maintain cerebral perfusion. No ideal ratio of plasma:platelets:packed red blood cells has been recommended but commonly 1:1:1 is considered to reduce mortality and is frequently followed. Recently goal-directed resuscitation based on thromboelastography (TEG) or rotational thromboelastometry (ROTEM) has been suggested. These techniques promote early diagnosis of coagulopathy and well predict transfusion requirements and mortality. It is imperative to warm the fluids to 39°C to prevent hypothermia:
  - Blood pressure, pulse oximetry, blood gas monitoring, and electrocardiogram (ECG) are used as adjuncts. Urinary catheters and nasogastric tubes may be placed.
  - Upon completion of primary survey response to resuscitation is assessed. Shock should be promptly identified.
  - Hemorrhagic shock is treated with volume replacement. The extent of blood loss is best assessed by the response to initial fluid bolus (lactated Ringer's solution or normal saline: 1–2 L for adults, 20 mL/kg for children). Maintain urine output: 0.5 mL/kg in adults and 1 mL/kg in infants. Assess the response to fluid loading as follows:
    - *Rapid response:* Hemodynamic returning to normal. Usually loss is <20%.
    - *Transient response:* 20–40% loss, need blood transfusion.
    - *No response:* Surgical intervention for blood loss (always look for pericardial effusion).
- If the patient's vital signs are weak or absent, severe blood loss (>40%) is suspected, and additional transfusion with untyped blood is required. If a transient response is noted, but vital signs begin to deteriorate again, moderate blood loss (20–40%) is suspected, and blood should be secured for potential transfusion requirements (type-specific or cross-matched as available). O-negative blood can be used for life-threatening situations or if

type-matched blood is unavailable. Type-matched blood is recommended, however, as O-negative is uncommon and it takes 10 minutes only. Cross-matched blood usually takes 1 hour to prepare and should be ordered electively.

- Being safe with high therapeutic index, tranexamic acid should be used in initial management of all patients having severe injuries. Tranexamic acid should be given within 3 hours of the injury and ideally within 1 hour for maximal benefit. Treatment after 3 hours may increase mortality.
- If vital signs normalize and remain stable after initial fluid bolus, blood loss is minimal then blood transfusion may be avoided.
- If the patient is severely hypotensive (SBP < 70 mm Hg) and not responding to resuscitation in setting of pelvic injury then circumferential sheet at the level of trochanters, dedicated pelvic binder or C-clamp should be immediately used (last two are more effective). Sheet at the level of trochanters provides indirect compression through proximal femur and avoids potential laparotomy incision encroachment. Binding thighs or legs together is also effective adjunct. These patients usually need surgical intervention and retroperitoneal packing because venous bleeding is common in most and stabilization alone does not provide sufficient control. Alternatively, angiography and embolization after pelvic stabilization may be undertaken. Embolization is effective in 85% patients with arterial injury and recently resuscitative endovascular balloon occlusion of the aorta (REBOA) has shown to reduce mortality from exsanguination from major intrapelvic, intra-abdominal, and/or proximal lower extremity injury. Tourniquets should be liberally used to control exsanguination from injury to extremities until definitive control of vascular injury is done.

Management of some specific conditions and evaluation is mentioned below centered to circulation.

For internal bleeding, consider focused abdominal sonography in trauma (FAST) [or diagnostic peritoneal lavage (DPL) if ultrasonography is not available]. Focused assessment sonography in trauma (FAST) is a good adjunct to identify occult hemorrhage. Urgent surgical intervention or embolization of vessel or REBOA (see above) can be planned. Most difficult cavities in which to identify and control hemorrhage is the retroperitoneum. The most common cause of retroperitoneal bleeding from blunt trauma is a pelvic fracture. Manage pelvic fracture aggressively by external fixator and blood and fluid transfusion and these patients would need retroperitoneal packing.

Cardiogenic shock from direct trauma to heart or tamponade needs immediate surgical and medical support. Muffled heart sounds, distended neck veins, low blood pressure, low heartbeat, pulsus paradoxus (decrease blood pressure during inspiration and exceeds by 10). Manage by ECG monitored needle aspiration through xiphisternal approach using a 16-needle—3-way stopcock through xiphisternum cranial toward tip of the left scapula.

Tension pneumothorax should be decompressed, and chest tube inserted. Flail chest is diagnosed by paradoxical movement of the flail segment on the breathing. Multiple segmental fractures of the rib are seen radiologically. Treat by oxygen and intubate if hypoxia persists.

Always assume cervical spine injury in unconscious and also conscious patient needs CT scan for documentation in unconscious patient. Alert; no neurology, no neck pain in conscious patient indicates a stable spine and X-rays are not needed. Five percent head injury is associated with spinal injury. Other sites of spine injury vary in percentage, but in general 55% are cervical, 15% thoracic, 15% thoracolumbar, and 10% multiple levels. A quick neurologic examination should be performed by assessing the patient's level of consciousness, pupillary size and reaction, and gross motor functioning. The GCS is the most commonly used rating system **(Table 1)**. Hypoxia, hypotension, hypothermia or hyperthermia, and hypoglycemia in a polytrauma patient must be suspected and looked for. The patient should be exposed by removing all clothes. Hypothermia should be controlled with adequate warming or blankets. Flaccid paralysis with incontinence suggests spinal shock. Maintain circulation as blood pressure is usually low. Methylprednisolone is controversial.

Adjuncts to the primary survey are:

- *Radiography:* The "trauma triple" is a portable cervical spine lateral view, anteroposterior chest, and anteroposterior pelvis radiographs. By these three X-rays, an idea about the potentially dangerous conditions can be obtained in minimal time.
- *Laboratory studies:* Hemogram, complete blood count including differential count, electrolytes level, assessment of renal function, and urine analysis including toxicology screen should be obtained.
- *Blood preparations:* Blood grouping and typing should be done, and according to severity of trauma and shock, 2–4 units of RBCs should be cross-matched.

TABLE 1: Glasgow Coma Scale (GCS).

Response	*Score*
Eye opening:	
• Spontaneous	4
• Command	3
• Pain	2
• None	1
Verbal:	
• Oriented	5
• Confused	4
• Inappropriate	3
• Nonspecific sounds	2
• None	1
Motor:	
• Follows commands	6
• Localizes pain	5
• Withdraws for pain	4
• Flexion to pain	3
• Extension to pain	2
• None	1

Score < 13 requires CT head while GCS ≤ 8 indication for definite intubation.

Disability

- A—Alert
- V—Vocal response
- P—Responds to pain
- U—Unresponsive to all stimuli

Three causes: Hypoxia, hypovolemia, and head injury.

Secondary survey is said to begin after primary survey; however, practically it is often completed during the process of treating priorities identified in primary survey. There is no specific sequence of trauma patient management and it keeps on changing with the priorities identified by expert from time to time. Some principles, however, apply. Secondary survey is essentially a detailed survey of all anatomic regions from head to toe. Continuous reassessment of patient as in primary survey is an essential part of secondary survey. Focused patient history should be taken. History should include at least following mnemonic "SAMPLE":

- Symptoms—Pain, difficulty in breathing, heaviness in chest, dizziness, and other symptoms
- Allergies to any specific drug/drugs
- Medications regularly taken and taken before the event
- Past history of any surgery/medical diseases
- Last meal timing of last meal is necessary in emergency management to determine the risk of aspiration
- Events responsible for trauma

The survey is postponed till the patient is hemodynamically stable. The more serious injuries are addressed first so as to gradually help the patient recover, e.g., a head injury will get priority over assessment of closed tibial fracture, which can be splinted till head injury is managed. For secondary survey of the head, neck, and trunk, CT scanning has become a necessity and it should be done on urgent basis. Now, it is possible to obtain the scan and the reports within even 30 minutes of patient's arrival in centers of excellence.

- Pelvic injury should be suspected whenever there is pain in the pelvic region or leg length discrepancies. Anteroposterior pelvic radiographs should be taken as soon as the primary survey is completed. Pelvic injuries are serious and marker of high energy injury. Hypovolemic shock in these patients is multifactorial and patients may have blood loss from associated thoracic, intra-abdominal, or extremity injuries.
  - Anterior external fixation frames have been advocated as a method to provide rapid reduction and fixation of pelvic ring injuries. Early fixation limits on-going injury from unstable fracture fragments.
  - Anteroposterior compression fractures, also called open book injuries, with widening of the pelvic ring and increasing pelvic volume, have received particular attention. Reduction of open-book injuries decreases pelvic volume, promoting self-tamponade of retroperitoneal venous bleeding and thus reducing blood loss.
  - Use of pelvic binders, angiography, REBOA or surgical packing is detailed above.
  - Pelvic fractures are frequently associated with urethral injuries, especially the anteroposterior compression injuries. Clinical findings suggestive of urethral injuries are presence of blood at the meatus, perianal hematoma, and history of hematuria:
    - Gentle one attempt of catheterization should be done in patients of pelvic fractures without above findings.
    - Retrograde cystogram must be done if any signs of urethral injury present.
    - In case of positive urethrogram or unable to do catheterization, a senior urologist should be called up on to decide regarding suprapubic catheterization, a Seldinger technique.
- An open fracture is the fracture with open wound reaching the fracture. There are very high chances of infections in an open fracture and they must be treated aggressively. After stabilization of the patient, the initial management of an open fracture includes immobilization of the extremity or part, copious irrigation of the wound, with thorough debridement of devitalized tissue. Prophylactic antibiotics, mostly first generation cephalosporins should be started. Splinting or traction is necessary in case of unstable fracture. The Gustilo and Anderson classification **(Table 2)** is used most commonly to classify open fractures.
  - Soft-tissues and joint injuries should be treated with copious irrigation.
  - Debridement must be done, if any devitalized tissue remains.
  - Open wounds should be covered with saline soaked sterile dressings.

TABLE 2: Classification of open fractures.

Gustilo and Anderson (1976) classification [modified by Gustilo, Mendoza, and Williams (1984)]	***Risk of infection (%)***
Grade I: Clean wound smaller than 1 cm in diameter or puncture wound that appears clean with a simple fracture pattern, no skin crushing or internal degloving	0–12
Grade II: A laceration larger than 1 cm but <10 cm, without significant soft-tissue crushing, including no flaps, degloving or contusion. Fracture pattern may be more complex. High velocity trauma	2–12
Grade III: An open segmental fracture or a single fracture with extensive soft-tissue injury (>10 cm). Injuries older than 8 hours, farm injuries, gunshot injuries, segmental fractures, and fractures with diaphyseal bone loss are also included in this type. Type III injuries are subdivided into three subtypes: 1. *Type IIIA:* Adequate soft-tissue especially periosteal coverage of the fracture despite high-energy trauma or extensive laceration or skin flaps 2. *Type IIIB:* Inadequate soft-tissue coverage with periosteal stripping and bone damage or bone loss. There is often gross contamination. Soft-tissue reconstruction is necessary 3. *Type IIIC:* Any open fracture (irrespective of wound size or bone loss/type of fracture) that is associated with vascular injury that mandates repair	9–55

BOX 2: Some additional general resuscitative measures and medications used in initial management of polytrauma patient.

- The polytrauma patient is hypoxic (low hemoglobin, acidosis causing decreased oxygen carrying capacity, and atelectasis/chest injury/pain reduce oxygenation of blood). Oxygen supplementation is, hence, generally prudent from start.
- The patient is also in catabolic state and has simultaneous high energy requirement thus leads to degradation of lipids and proteins. There is associated altered hepatic metabolism and renal dysfunction, which is primarily prerenal. All these organal functions should be closely monitored and supported.
- Intravenous antibiotics are good prophylaxis for open wounds and must provide broad-spectrum coverage including anaerobic organisms.
- Nutritional support should include balanced amount of fat and protein replacement and prevent neoglucogenesis. Glutamine-based amino acid preparations and omega-3 and omega-4 fatty acids help to restore anabolic state fast and build immunity.
- Pain control is an important aspect to additionally stabilize the sympathetic hyperactivity and drug combinations are usually required. Intravenous paracetamol and continuous infusion techniques are in fashion. Generally, narcotics should be avoided because they cause respiratory depression.

- Flap construction is necessary in case of serious soft-tissue destruction (Gustilo/Anderson type IIIB/IIIC). If patient is stable, immediate free flap construction using latissimus dorsi, serratus anterior, gracilis or rectus abdominis (especially for large wounds) should be done (within 48 hours of trauma). This should be combined with definitive or provisional fixation as soon as is safely possible.

The management should be continuous with collaborative effort of multispecialty expert based on injury analysis, analysis, management protocols, and documentation. Some general "allied measures" in initial management of polytrauma patient are presented in **Box 2**. A thorough understanding of fat embolism, crush syndrome, systemic inflammatory response syndrome (SIRS), acute respiratory distress syndrome (ARDS), and multiple organ dysfunction syndrome (MODS) is essential for prevention of failure of medical treatment and is discussed in other sections of the book.

PRINCIPLES OF MANAGEMENT OF ORTHOPEDIC INJURY

To avoid continuing injury to limb and accelerate inflammation, stabilization of fractures with minimal manipulation should be done with external fixator or plaster of Paris (POP) slabs or splints as appropriate; these also improve nursing and lesser need of analgesia. Practice of DCO should apply at this point. DCO is the stabilization of all life-threatening long bones and pelvic fracture with the intention for definitive treatment later on when the patient has stabilized. Favored tool used in DCO is the external fixator. Indications for "Damage Control Orthopedics" are physiological criteria such as hypothermia, coagulopathy, acidosis (lethal triad), and complex pattern of severe injuries having major blood loss and a prolonged reconstructive procedure in a physiologically unstable patient. Damage control surgery (DCS) intends to control, but not definitively repair the injuries after trauma. It avoids time-consuming reconstructive surgeries in emergency situations. The four key elements of DCS are:

1. Resuscitative surgery for rapid hemorrhage control
2. Decompression of cranium, thorax, pericardium, abdomen, and limb compartments
3. Debridement of the wounds and decontamination of ruptured viscera, and
4. Immobilization of limb to temporarily stabilize the fracture fragments by means of splintage, pelvic binder, and skeletal traction, or casting

The aim is to restore normal physiology, avoiding much damage to the tissues and continued resuscitation of the patients in ICU after their transfer as soon as possible. First 12–24 hours are critical for decision in patients with fracture.

In early care approach [now popularized as "early appropriate care (EAC)"], once the patient is physiologically stable, all the long bone fractures are stabilized within first 36 hours. Full resuscitation of the patient before surgery is the most important aspect.

DAMAGE CONTROL ORTHOPEDICS VERSUS EARLY TOTAL CARE

It was considered the ideal approach to treat orthopedic injuries by doing "definitive fixation" of all fractures in one trip to the operating room. This approach is called early total care (ETC) and was widely used in the 80s to efficiently use the operating theater resources and perform surgeries with one set on investigations and anesthetic exposure. The complications were found higher when this approach was used especially in polytrauma patients. The ETC school emanated from the finding that patients previously managed by conservative methods (say cast or traction for fracture shaft femur) fared worse than the early definitely operated patients. The development of newer methods of osteosynthesis also favored the concept of "early definitive management". These patients were found to have less pulmonary complications (pneumonia, ARDS), reduced length of intensive care unit (ICU), fat embolism syndrome and hospital stay, compared to patients with delayed surgery. Though popular and practiced for more than a decade opposing views came in since 1990s and concept of ETC was challanged. In unstable patients, ETC was associated with an unexpectedly high rate of pulmonary complications. In light of associated risks and benefits of ETC **(Table 3)**, some moderation was needed and concept of "damage control" emerged. The concept of "damage control" comes from US Navy, in reference to keeping afloat a badly damaged ship by procedures to limit flooding, stabilize the vessel, isolate fires and explosions, and avoid their spreading.

There are four phases of DCO:

1. Acute phase—life-saving procedures are performed.
2. Second phase is aimed to control hemorrhage, temporary stabilization of major skeletal fractures, management of soft-tissue injuries, while minimizing the degree of surgical insult to the patient.
3. Phase three consists of a monitoring period in ICU/HDU.
4. Last phase comprises definitive fixation.

TABLE 3: The risks and benefits of early total care (ETC).

It must be emphasized that ETC (previously called early definitive fracture fixation) was deployed uniformly for stable "and" unstable patients especially the concurrent, sequential management of multiple injuries beyond femoral shaft within same anesthesia setting. Just to allay the confusion "early appropriate care" is more scientific application of ETC to "stable" patients but must *not* be generalized to—ETC of stable patients.

Benefits of ETC	*Risks of ETC*
• Promotes control of hemorrhage and further resuscitation of patient • Stable fracture reduces pain and associated sympathetic hyperactivity • Reduced pain also reduces continuing hyperinflammation, improves breathing and oxygenation • Early fracture fixation reduces analgesic requirement and narcotic doses • Pelvic fixation helps in resuscitation • Fixation of unstable thoracolumbar spine, acetabulum helps in early mobilization and upright posture that reduces pulmonary and thrombotic (venous thromboembolism) risks • All above translate into reduced pneumonia, ARDS, fat-embolism, reduced hospital, and ICU stay	• Produces "second-hit" • The second hit further introduces elements of inflammation • Severely injured patients with massive hemorrhage decline further and may go into multiorgan dysfunction and death • Unstable patients (acidosis, coagulopathy, hypotension, hypoxia, etc.) deteriorate very fast and quickly reach irreversible damage with this aggressive approach • Fixation of femoral shaft fractures and reaming was considered particularly deleterious in patients with severe chest trauma

The shift from ETC to DCO comes from better understanding of SIRS followed by a period of recovery mediated by a counter-regulatory anti-inflammatory response (CARS). Initial traumatic injury induces an inflammatory response followed sometimes by an excessive CARS that produces a prolonged and deleterious immunosuppressed state. This initial traumatic injury is called the "first hit" and predisposes the patient to a potential risk of deterioration after surgery (that actually produces a "second hit"). In polytrauma patients, the recognition of high levels of inflammatory markers favors the DCO application in order to prevent the effects of the "second hit" inflammatory reaction. IL-6 is considered the most specific prognostic indicator (discussed later) and early high levels of IL-6 have been associated with the development of organ failure (measuring IL-6 has become a routine in dedicated trauma centers). Thus, the type of initial stabilization and timing of definitive osteosynthesis modulate these adverse events. Initial stabilization came to be highly relied upon external fixation. Simple stabilization with splints and casts, however, is also effective except for lower extremities like shaft femur fractures. For these, skeletal traction has been found to be equal to external fixation in terms of ARDS, MODS, pneumonia, deep venous thromboembolism (DVT), pulmonary embolism (PE) development, as well as ICU stay and death rate. The timing for definitive osteosynthesis has been set at "window of opportunity" between 5th and 10th days. During days 2–4 immunological changes keep occurring along with unsuitable fluid shift and local tissue edema making it unsuitable. After 15 days, the contamination rate around the pins has been found a significant cause of infection. Thus, DCO avoids provoking a severe inflammatory response and while fulfilling the goals of sufficient stabilization of

BOX 3: The guidelines for following early appropriate care (EAC).

- On admission, check ABG, lactate, CBC, platelets, INR
- Repeat above tests every 8 hours until normal then stop
- *Recommend EAC if:*
  - pH ≥ 7.25
  - Base deficit ≥ −5.5 mmol/L
  - Lactate < 4.0 mmol/L
  - And patient is responding to resuscitation without ionotropic support. This may be evaluated with repeat blood tests in presence of persistent bleeding/hypotension.
- If above criteria *are not met* within 12 hours of admission then follow DCS. Continue to reassess the patient until he meets above criteria before proceeding with definitive management.

fractures to prevent further tissue damage and the potential compartment syndrome, while allowing the patient to be mobilized for tests and improved pulmonary care. Newer developments in methods of resuscitation, identification of inflammatory burden, and osteosynthesis challenged this "delay" in definitive fixation based on "days". Treatment plans to expedite definitive fixation of axial, pelvic, and femoral fractures in adequately resuscitated and otherwise stable patient has been found to reduce the complications of delayed fixation of fractures (fat embolism, pneumonia, ARDS, and longer hospital stay). Surprisingly, these benefits have been found to be even more pronounced in early femoral nailing of patients with injury to multiple systems. Emerging literature has increasingly suggested that most patients with femoral shaft fractures may be resuscitated on arrival such that early definitive fixation of femoral shaft fractures can be done instead of damage control. The concept of "early appropriate care (EAC)" has hence developed. EAC involves fixation of fractures within 36 hours of injury in stable patients and it minimizes the risks and costs of staged fixation. EAC consists of definitive fixation of pelvis, acetabulum, spine, proximal, and diaphyseal femoral fractures within 36 hours of injury as long as initial acidosis has improved **(Box 3)** and the patient is otherwise stable. When the parameters listed in **Box 3** are not met then DCS should be preferred. Some controversies in orthopedic management of patient during initial few days of trauma are discussed below.

- Amputation versus limb reconstruction is decided by severity of injury, expertise of the surgeon, available resources, and socioeconomic status of the patient. Reconstruction has advantages like original limb is saved, but having disadvantages of long rehabilitation, prolonged hospital stay, economic burden, repeated operations, and difficulties to family. Amputation has advantages like early return to work, lifesaving procedure sometimes and economical relief, but having disadvantages of loss of limb, and psychological trauma. It is generally decided by Mangled Extremity Severity Score (MESS, **Box 4**). MESS score > 7 means poor limb viability prognosis and limb should be amputated. A diminished pulse, or an ankle-brachial index < 0.9, indicates a high likelihood of an arterial injury.
- *Rule of ten (10):*
  - *10 minutes:* Revive ABC.
  - *10 hours:* Save the limb—early stabilization.

BOX 4: Mangled extremity severity score (Helfet, 1990).

Skeletal/soft-tissue injury:
- Low energy (stab, simple fracture, pistol gunshot wound): 1
- Medium energy (open or multiple fractures, dislocation): 2
- High energy (high speed MVA or rifle GSW): 3
- Very high energy (high speed trauma + gross contamination): 4

Limb ischemia:
- Pulse reduced or absent but perfusion normal: 1*
- Pulseless; paresthesias, diminished capillary refill: 2
- Cool, paralyzed, insensate, numb: 3*

Shock:
- Systolic BP always > 90 mm Hg: 0
- Hypotensive transiently: 1
- Persistent hypotension: 2

Age (years):
- <30: 0
- 30–50: 1
- >50: 2

*Score doubled for ischemia > 6 hours
Score >7 = Correlated well with primary amputation

- *10 days:* Pick up minor injuries and fixation.
- *10 weeks:* Controlled rehabilitation.
- *10 months:* Attempted return to normal life.
- *10 years:* Residual fracture problem.

▪ *Management of extremity injury:* The general principles of management of extremity injury in polytrauma (following EAC) are:
  - *Fractures:* Concomitant injuries to major vessels (supracondylar fractures, femoral fracture with femoral artery, and knee dislocation with popliteal artery injury). "Repair of the artery + Fasciotomy + Stabilize the fracture".
  - *Compartment syndrome:* Fasciotomy.
  - *Open injuries:* Debridement and fixation.
  - *The priority for definitive management of closed shaft fractures is given as follows:* Femur → Tibia → Pelvis or spine → Upper limbs → Complex joint reconstruction.

▪ *In specific situations, the fracture treatment should be deferred (follow DCO):*
  - Head injury with GCS < 8
  - Massive intracranial bleeding
  - Severe thoracic trauma
  - Hemodynamically unstable with uncompensated cardiac function
  - Blood dyscrasias
  - Hypothermia < 32°C

▪ *Role of molecular markers in polytrauma evaluation and management.* Most often just a damage to an organ does not indicate the true decompensation or hemodynamic compensation. The peripheral measures such as blood pressure, pulse rate, and central measures such as cardiac output and CVP are more or less approximations. Such cases are increasingly evaluated by evaluation of the microenvironment and molecular diagnosis. Some of the studied markers are mentioned in **Table 4**. Lipopolysaccharide-binding-protein (LBP) is of hepatic origin and has ability to bind bacterial lipopolysaccharide. LBP level rises during II or III day of trauma or sepsis; SIRS and MODS. LBP is significantly high in-patient with MODS with infection and can be used to differentiate SIRS from nonseptic MODS. CRP has no role in polytrauma. Procalcitonin may indicate sepsis following SIRS. IL-1 (difficult to detect due to short half-life of 6 minutes) appears to be a marker of traumatic insult with significantly elevated levels occurring within 1–4 hours after trauma, and correlates with the severity of illness. IL-6 helps in identifying patients who are less likely to survive. Increased concentrations of IL-6 associated with a poor outcome in patients with ARDS. IL-6 is not predictive of septic complications, but rather correlates with the magnitude of the injury. IL-6 seems to be the most reliable marker systemic inflammation while LBP appears to be an accurate and early marker of infection. The use of these two markers together may offer the ability to detect the onset of SIRS and allows early intervention to prevent MODS.

TABLE 4: The different molecular markers that may help inprognosticating polytrauma patient care.

Acute-phase reactants	LBP, CRP, procalcitonin
Mediator activity	TNF, IL-1, IL-6, IL-10, IL-18
Cellular activity	TNF-RI, TNF-RII, IL-1R-I, IL-1R-II, IL-6-R, mIL-6-R, ICAM-1, E-selectin, CD11b, elastase, HLA-DR class-II

PRINCIPLES OF MANAGING DISASTERS

While the usual medical care aims at doing the greatest good to individual, disaster medical care is based on the principle of doing greatest good to greatest number of patients. A consistent approach to disasters is practiced all over the world and the strategy is called MCI response. MCI response has the primary objective of reducing the morbidity (injury/disease) and mortality associated with disaster. The basic medical concerns related to MCI responses include:

- Search and rescue
- Triage and initial stabilization
- Evacuation
- Definitive care

The public health concerns related to MCI include:

- Water, food, shelter, and sanitation
- Safety and transportation
- Communication
- Disease surveillance
- Later endemic and epidemic disease spread

Incident Command System

Well-developed and managed incident command system (ICS) determines the success and safety of disaster response. The ICS is a standardized all-hazards management approach designed to enhance the ability of multiagency organizations and agencies to work together effectively in response to a disaster. The ICS has a common structure and language and creates a hierarchy of roles and responsibilities to direct the personnel, efforts, and resources. ICS comprises five major functional areas. The individuals in each area have discrete responsibilities. The nature of disaster determines which individuals (functional roles) are necessary and not all may be needed.

- *Incident command:* Sets objectives for disaster response and priorities. Responsible for overall disaster response. Liaison officer assists in coordinating vertically and horizontally with various organizations and support system. The public information officer provides appropriate information to the media and press. Safety officer is responsible for workers safety. Coordinator coordinates with the various teams. Communication officer is responsible for continuous communication with the responding teams and recruitment of personnel (on-call teams). Communication technology should be as reliable as possible taking into consideration the possibility of overload and power failure. Incident commander activates various aspects of response and is informed by these key personnel. The command should stand united and individual responders should report to only one supervisor. An individual should only supervise between three and seven other responders. Specific objectives are laid down to be completed as tasks individually.
- *Operations:* They do main field work and direct the disaster resources.
- *Planning:* Continuous monitoring and developing action plans. Maintains status of resources.
- *Logistics:* Provides resources, personnel, and supplies.
- *Financial/Administrative:* Monitors and regulates expense and redirecting to the priority areas.

The incident commander and key personnel are identified and trained regularly in drills before a disaster occurs not at the time of disaster. ICS is activated before incident gets out of control. The structure of ICS remains the same irrespective of disaster; only the personnel vary, viz., trauma expert for massive railway accidents or infection control expert for biological incident or chemical safety expert for chemical warfare, etc.

Medical Response to Disasters

The primary aim of medical response is to stabilize the victims for definitive medical care. Medical assistance teams are a group of medical personnel identified and trained to deliver rapid response to supplement medical care at disaster site. The teams should be able to deliver medical, surgical, and critical care during disaster. They should be equipped with rapidly deployable and functional field hospital including operating rooms. It is imperative to geographically identify priority areas to set up such medical assistance teams. Proper identification of personnel and regular review of the members should be conducted to maintain preparedness.

Triage

Triage is principally based on providing the greatest good to largest number of patients. This is often the most physically and psychologically challenging mission of medical response team. The primary goal of performing triage is to identify critical patients with the greatest chance of survival with the available facilities and least expenditure of time. Both under-triage and over-triage are common. Under-triage depicts assigning critically, ill patients who are potentially salvageable to "delayed" category. Over-triage is more common and is assignment of noncritical survivors with no life-threatening injuries to "urgent" category. Triage team should comprise triage officer, clerk, and a nurse. The triage officer should be experienced in trauma care but not necessarily the most experienced surgeon or physician. The clerk assigns the color code to all victims as determined by triage officer.

Field Triage (Onsite Triage)

Here, the victims are classified broadly into "acute" and "nonacute". Acute victims are prioritized to receive the arriving help and care. Color coding is useful, if time and finances permit. Local emergency medical personnel are typically assigned for this task.

Medical Triage

This is categorization of victims at casualty collection site or mobile hospital units. This should be performed by experienced personnel (having knowledge of various causes of injuries and medical consequences) to optimize the medical resources and achieve goal of triage. Color coding has been developed that is internationally followed:

- *Red:* These victims require emergent life-saving interventions and are potentially salvageable. Examples are patients having severe bleeding, shock, open chest, or abdominal wounds, emotionally out of control, etc.
- *Yellow:* For them, the treatment can be delayed but need close observation. Sometimes under-triage leads to accumulation of yellow victims, e.g., in bomb blasts a lot of internal injuries are missed that present as compensated patient initially, but actually require emergent stabilization. Examples include patients having burns with no respiratory distress, spinal injuries, moderate blood loss, and conscious with head injuries.
- *Green:* These victims are stable and require no emergent care. Examples include patients having minor fractures, minor bleeding, and minor lacerations.
- *Black:* These are either deceased or so critically damaged that even with the best of utilized resourced chances of survival are bleak and will be wasting precious time of medical services that can be used for other victims. Examples are patients having cardiac arrest, respiratory arrest with a pulse, and massive head injury.

Continuous Triage

Triage errors occur and need correction at medical treatment site with requisite transfers. Also with treatment, the patient's status changes regularly and triage should be conducted at specific intervals by the medical treatment site director. Continuous triage is a part of developing "error tolerant" system to minimize errors that keep occurring.

Evacuation Triage

The victims are prioritized to transfer to higher medical facilities. The closer medical facilities are reserved for potentially unstable and serious patients, while distant facilities are provided to stable patients or lesser injured victims. The casualty collection site should give convenient exit routes for air and land evacuation. Evacuation is necessary to reduce the burden on active services. Various methods of transport including areal evacuation should be considered to send victims for specific needs.

Definitive Medical Care and Hospital Preparedness

Hospitals should be prepared for all hazards and should cover all aspects relevant to such events. Protocols should be predesigned and tested in mock drills anticipating various scenarios. Protocols contain specific series of events to be activated simultaneously or sequentially once MCI is declared (who and how). Declaration of MCI should be confirmed. Standing orders are the detailed sequence of events that are executed by staff members ("what" is to be done). Area specific protocols and standing orders should be clearly notified and readily accessible. Stocks of equipment, drugs, etc., should be prepared and marked in advance. Special training programs should be conducted involving all the defined personnel of hospital regularly.

Once MCI alert is activated, the hospital ICS specified in protocol should be established. Communication should be established using multiple modalities as few may be jammed. The hospital should establish a dedicated receiving area and triage, admitting area, decontamination room, equipment, and stockpiles, etc. The victims should enter from single site for triage and rapid transfers should be established. ICU and operating room should be notified in advance. The treatment sites should be staffed with caregivers according to severity of injury and expertise. The site director is responsible for medical management at different sites. He is a person familiar with all aspects of trauma and mass casualty victims. Minimal acceptable care is the prime method adopted for MCI victims. This is intended to provide lifesaving measures immediately to patients while keeping definitive and comprehensive care for later application. Maintain one directional flow of the patient and perform meticulous tertiary survey prior to discharge of patients. It is better to do minor procedures like suturing at alternative site.

Scene Safety and Personal Protection

Usually with chemical and biological weapons, the victims could carry with them agents that can harm the rescue and medical system. The initial responders should designate a "hot zone" to identify areas of contamination. This should only be accessible to personnel in proper personal protective equipment. Usually no medical care is given to victims in "hot zone". Victims are moved to warm zone for decontamination and emergent lifesaving care by medical personnel in protective gear. Once decontaminated, they can be moved to designated and separate "cold zone".

CONCLUSION

- Polytrauma, mass casualties, and disaster have become a common occurrence due to easy availability and popularity of high-speed vehicles and raging internal and external war like scenarios in various parts of the world respectively.
- Though appearing similar all three have their specific definitions for the purpose of organization of services.
- Evaluation of patients in a polytrauma sitting requires following a set protocol so that emergency care can be delivered at the point to manage critical derangements while thorough examination is also possible to deliver complete care. As regard orthopedic surgeon, it is quite imperative that he should follow the principles of early total care (EAC) and identify patients at risk of developing complications with early care. In the latter circumstance, DCO should be followed.
- Mass casualties and disaster management require organization of services on a wider scale and primarily relying on triage so that efficient use of limited manpower and resources are done.

CHAPTER

25 Role of Radiological Investigations in Orthopedics and Radiation Hazard

Manish Kumar Varshney, Avinash Razdan

INTRODUCTION

Radiology is an essential accompaniment for any orthopedic disorder evaluation. Different modalities are available and the orthopedician should be aware of them and their indications, role, and ability to evaluate the certainty. More importantly, they serve as essential adjuncts to surgical planning, postsurgical evaluation, and follow-up of treatment. The various modalities are discussed below to help understand their specific abilities that would help their usage instead of a blanket prescription of magnetic resonance imaging (MRI) for all disorders that many amateurs do.

CONVENTIONAL RADIOGRAPHY

Radiography is the most frequently used modality for evaluating bone and joint disorders. Despite the increased availability of more advanced imaging modalities, radiographs remain first line for diagnosing fractures; joint dislocations; suspected infection, tumors (benign and malignant); locating foreign objects; and guidance before, during, and after orthopedic procedures. Radiographs are complementary to all imaging modalities and should be routinely available for review when viewing computed tomography (CT), ultrasonography (USG), or MRI.

PHYSICS

Image formation for radiographs depends on the concept of differential absorption, where X-rays are absorbed nonhomogeneously depending on the density of each tissue. Bone, for instance, will absorb much more relative to soft tissue and even more so than fat. This leads to varying levels of radiolucency, such that bone appears white on a radiograph (radiopaque) whereas air, which absorbs the least, appears black (radiolucent). In addition, some X-rays are deflected or scattered as they pass through an object, which contributes to the ionizing radiation dose.

TECHNIQUE

For optimal imaging technique, at least two views of the anatomy of interest at 90° angles are obtained. Generally, this includes standard anteroposterior (AP) and lateral views. Often, oblique views or other specialized views are obtained to help with evaluation of complex joints such as the wrist, elbow, and ankle, to inspect cortical margins in detail, and to assess for joint alignment such as the scapular Y-view for shoulder dislocation **(Figs. 1A and B)**. In pediatric cases, views of the contralateral limb can be helpful to distinguish normal growth variation versus pathology.

Positional views can be helpful to define mechanical pathology that may not manifest at rest. The classic example is cervical or lumbar spine flexion and extension views **(Figs. 2A to C)** to diagnose instability. A weight-bearing view can offer dynamic evaluation of the joint space under body weight.

Trauma Evaluation

Radiographic examination serves as the best initial screening—and often diagnostic—imaging test for nearly all musculoskeletal pathology, as it is cost-effective and easy to obtain. Trauma is a common indication for plain

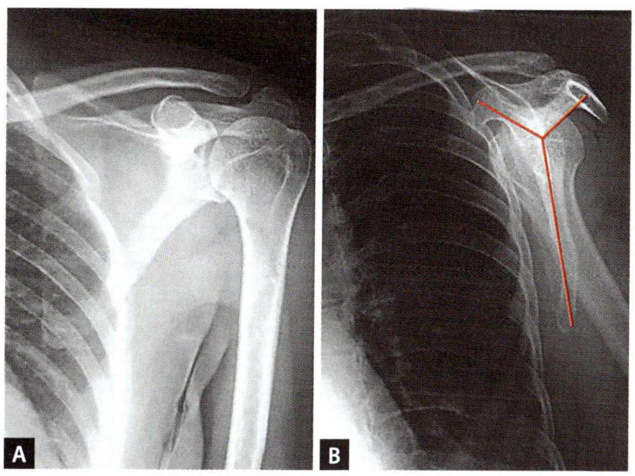

Figs. 1A and B: The radiographs demonstrate the disposition of shoulder joint in anteroposterior (A) and scapular Y-view (B) showing how the humeral head is normally centered at the glenoid which corresponds to the junction of three limbs of "scapular-Y".

radiographs, especially in the acute setting, to evaluate for fracture and joint alignment.

Plain radiographs can provide quick, valuable information on joint alignment prereduction and postreduction in cases of dislocations **(Figs. 3A to E)**. In emergency settings and polytrauma; radiography offers the advantage of portable imaging. Although the imaging quality and positioning is less optimal, it can be extremely helpful for rapidly diagnosing fractures, dislocations, spinal trauma, foreign bodies, and line placements.

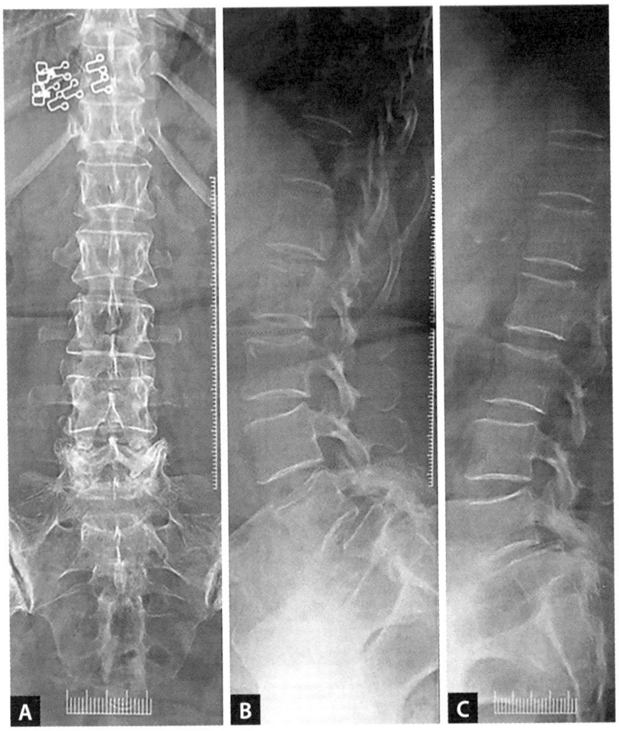

Figs. 2A to C: The stability of spine can be dynamically assessed by performing flexion-extension views where the functional nature of lesion may be more specifically assessed. The spondylolisthesis of lumbar fifth vertebra on sacral first vertebra in this case is not producing overt instability as changing from extension (B) to flexion view (C).

Atraumatic Evaluation

Radiography is also valuable for nontrauma evaluations.

- One of the most common indications for axial or appendicular radiographs is atraumatic pain, and plain radiographs can provide information regarding degenerative changes, impingement syndromes (such as femoroacetabular impingement **(Figs. 4A and B)**, osseous lesions, arthropathies, osteomyelitis **(Fig. 5)**, insufficiency fractures, and osseous mineralization.
- For spinal imaging, radiographs can demonstrate degenerative disk disease **(Figs. 6A and B)** and compression fractures of the spine; however, CT and MRI are better suited for spinal evaluation when indicated.
- Imaging evaluation of arthritis usually requires plain radiographs only **(Figs. 7A and B)**, with clinical and laboratory information helping to narrow the differential. The major findings for arthritis include distribution of the joint alignment, status of the joint space, osseous mineralization, erosive changes, and associated soft tissue pathology—all of which can be adequately and quickly assessed by plain radiograph.

In complex cases, it may be necessary to use more advanced imaging such as MRI to look for synovitis, tenosynovitis, and other potential soft tissue or subtle bone marrow changes.

Neoplasm

Radiographs are extremely useful and often necessary for adequate characterization of a musculoskeletal neoplasm—osseous or soft tissue **(Figs. 8A and B)**. For bony lesions, plain radiographs can evaluate if the lesion is lucent or sclerotic, the location of the lesion within the bone (i.e., metaphyseal and eccentric), and if it has any features suggestive of malignancy such as cortical destruction, periosteal reaction, permeative pattern or wide/one of transition, and a soft tissue component.

These features along with the patient's age and clinical history are usually enough information to narrow the differential diagnosis.

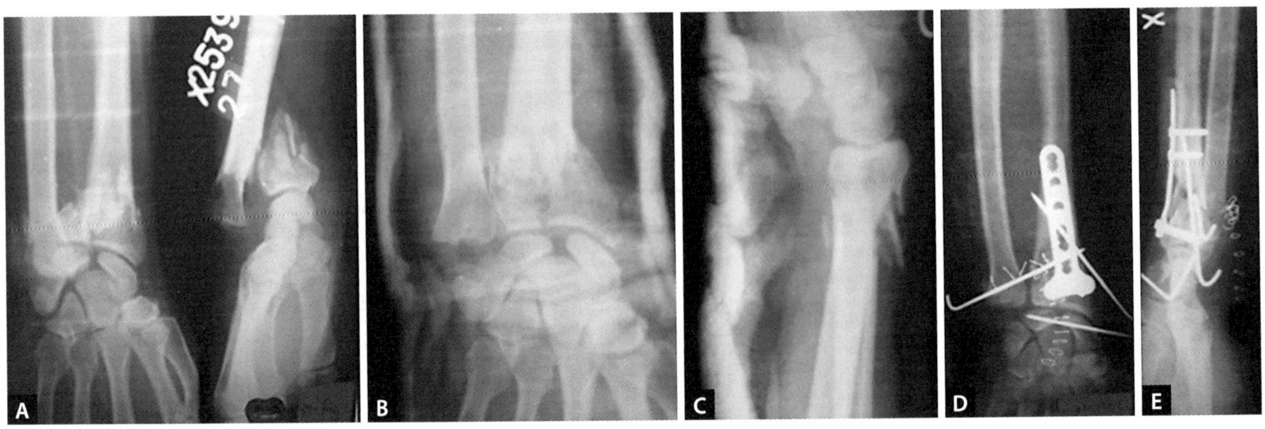

Figs. 3A to E: The anteroposterior (AP) and lateral radiographs of wrist (A) demonstrate comminuted displaced fracture of distal radius with disruption of distal radioulnar ligament complex and volar dislocation of wrist. Reduction and application of cast (B and C) promptly corrected the deformities (partially). The carpal injuries were missed on initial radiographs and there was prominent scapholunate disruption. The injuries have to be managed operatively to restore the anatomy and alignment (D and E).

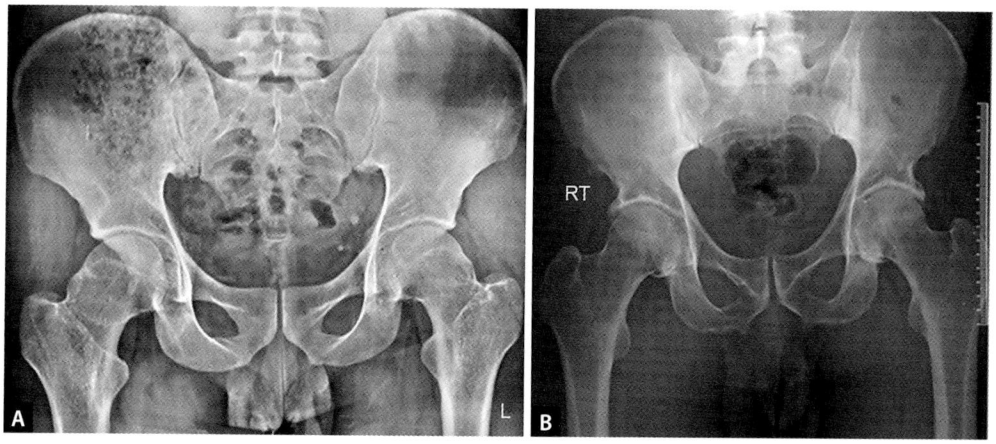

Figs. 4A and B: The anteroposterior radiographs of two patients demonstrating hip pathology. (A) Classical "cam lesion" at femoral head-neck junction bilaterally; (B) Classical "pincer lesion" with developing osteoarthrosis of the hip joint.

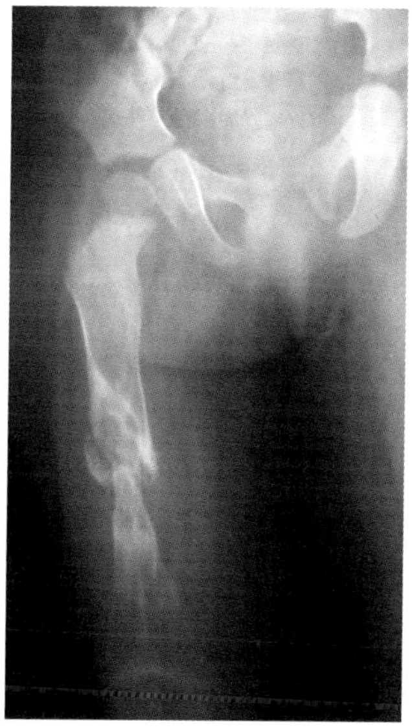

Fig. 5: The radiograph of right thigh demonstrates pathology of femoral shaft with destruction of the bone in middle thirds. There is loss of corticomedullary differentiation of the bone with osteopenia and closure of medullary canal suggestive of nonunion in a pathological fracture of femoral shaft most likely sequel to infectious pathology.

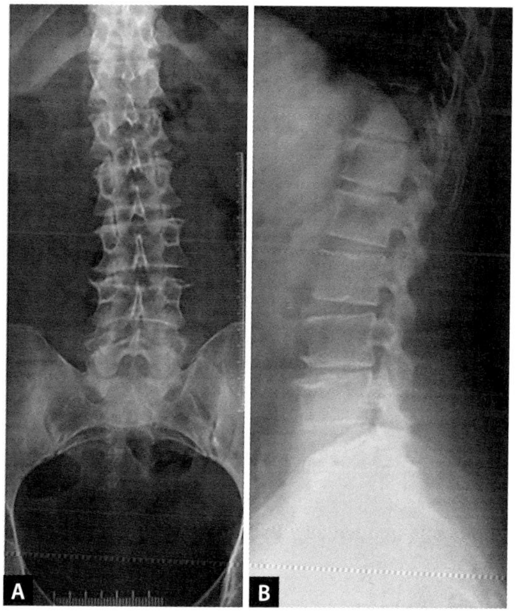

Figs. 6A and B: The anteroposterior (A) and lateral (B) radiographs of lumbosacral spine demonstrate reduces disk height of the lumbar 3–4 space and degenerative changes at the level.

For purely soft tissue lesions, radiography is less robust, but the pattern of calcification or ossification (if present) can still offer valuable diagnostic information, including differentiating between benign myositis ossificans and soft tissue osteosarcoma.

Fluoroscopy

Fluoroscopy passes a continuous X-ray beam through the area of interest, providing real-time imaging evaluation. Although this can be valuable tool to assess anatomy in different positions and under stress, it is most commonly used for image-guided procedures like intraoperative imaging **(Fig. 9)**.

Fluoroscopy is especially useful for arthrograms, joint aspirations, therapeutic joint, and bursal injections and

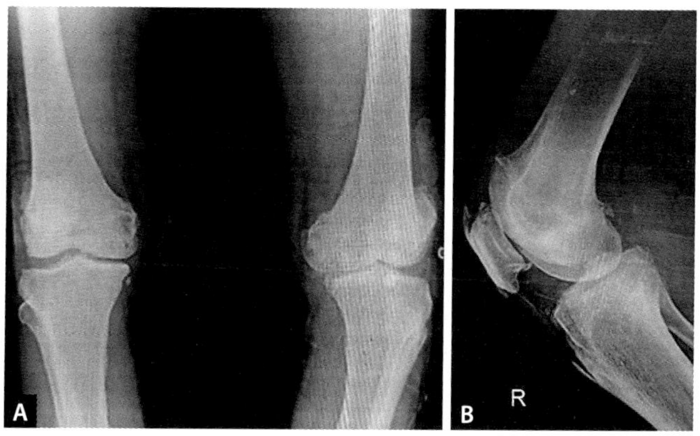

Figs. 7A and B: Anteroposterior (AP) (A) and lateral (B) radiographs of different patient shows degenerative changes in knee joint.

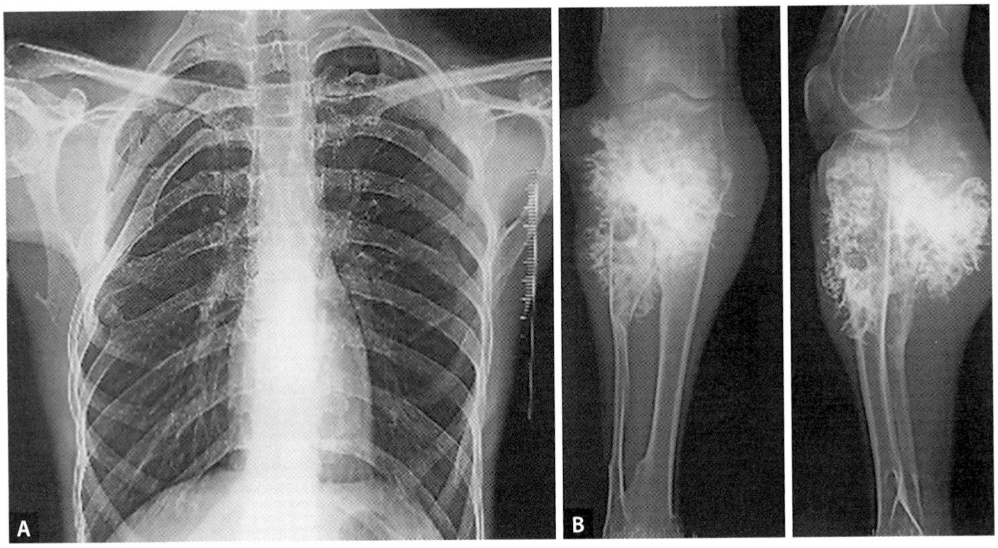

Figs. 8A and B: Posteroanterior (PA) view of chest (A) and anteroposterior/lateral (AP/LAT) view of right knee with leg (B) demonstrate multiple hereditary exostoses with malignant transformation in lesion of the proximal tibia.

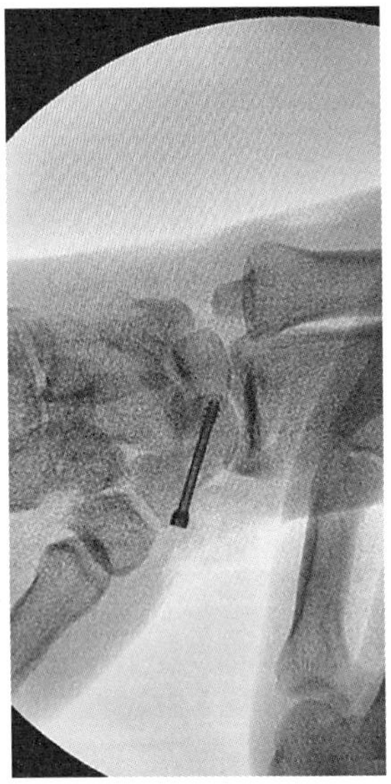

Fig. 9: The intraoperative use of fluoroscopy in a case of percutaneous fixation of fracture scaphoid for evaluation of various aspects of implant related (and allied surgeries) to assess alignment, reduction, and placement of the hardware.

spine interventions. "Plain arthrogram" is performed, but injection for CT and MR arthrography is most commonly done under fluoroscopic or radiographic guidance.

Bone Health Evaluation

X-ray derived technologies are highly accurate in assessing bone, density, and predicting the risk of as future major osteoporotic fracture. Dual-energy X-ray absorptiometry (DXA) is the most widely used and remains the current benchmark. This involves passing two separate, low-dose source beams at distinct energies through the lumbar spine and/or hips. The soft tissue signal is then subtracted and the resultant bone density calculated and scaled against reference values. The World Health Organization Fracture Risk Assessment Tool (FRAX) is a useful adjunct that combines the DXA results with clinical factors and demographics to estimate the 10-year bone fracture risk. The modality and its utility are discussed in detail in Chapter on "Metabolic Diseases of Bone".

Digital X-ray radiogrammetry (DXR) is a peripheral bone mineral density measurement method that uses a standard radiograph. Various measurements are used, frequently the bone width or cortical thickness of the nondominant second metacarpal to provide a computed bone mineral density equivalent. This predominantly automated, software-based method can also accurately predict hip fracture risk in both men and women.

COMPUTED TOMOGRAPHY

Unlike conventional radiography, CT utilizes a motorized X-ray source that rotates within a donut-shaped gantry around the patient. The beams travel through the patient with multiple detectors at the opposite end to acquire the data for that body region. The data are processed and a 2D cross-sectional image ("slice") created. The table then shifts and the process is repeated until the area of interest is fully imaged.

OPERATIVE PLANNING

- Compared with radiography, the three-dimensional data offered by CT allows for better characterization of the fracture and joint alignment **(Figs. 10A to F)**. This is particularly helpful for complex joints such as the elbow, wrist (**Figs. 10A to F**), ankle, and knee joints.
- The CT data can be directly used by 3D printing software, which allows for modeling and preoperative planning for fixation of hardware or prostheses.

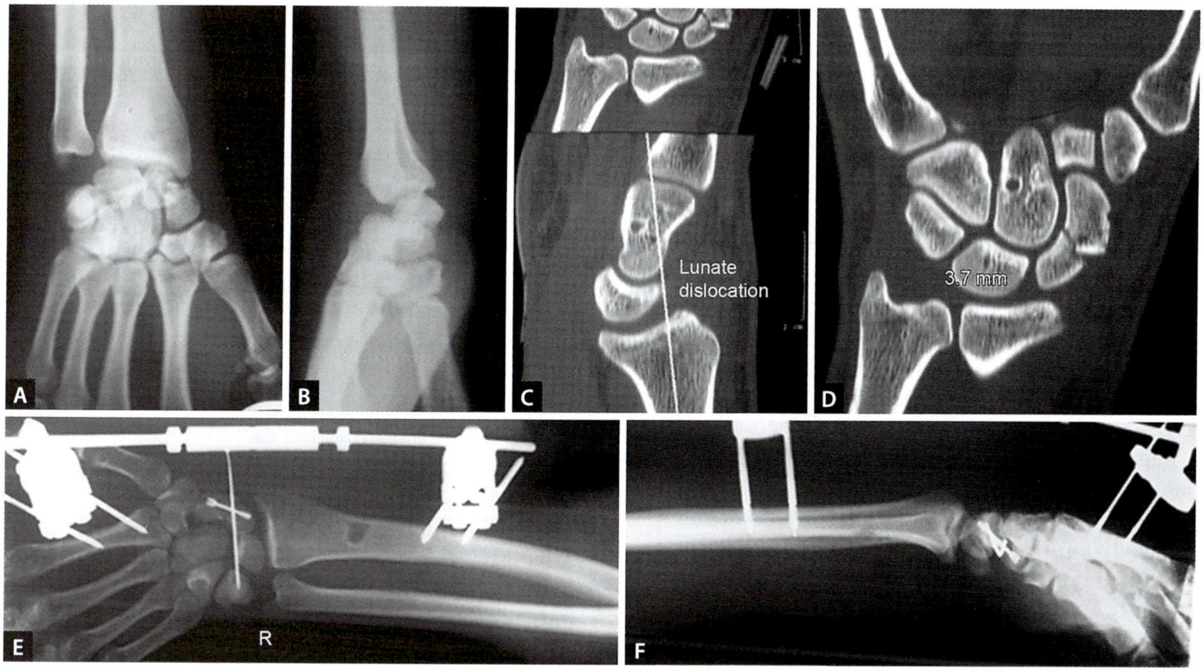

Figs. 10A to F: The anteroposterior (A) and lateral (B) radiographs demonstrate fracture of scaphoid. Only on close examination of the radiographs does one realize that there is excessive overlap of carpal bones with loss of Gilula arcs. The CT scan promptly demonstrates lunate dislocation and scapholunate sprain (C and D). This completes the diagnosis to be trans-scaphoid perilunate injury complex and was hence managed on the standard protocol (E and F).

Trauma Computed Tomography

Given the rapid acquisition time and level of detail, CT is essential for evaluation of spinal fractures in the setting of trauma and has largely replaced radiography for this purpose. MRI is superior in detecting acute fractures, particularly in osteopenic patients or radiographically-negative studies; however, CT can be used if MRI is contraindicated or not readily available.

A CT is excellent for assessing the status of implanted hardware and possible complications such as osteolysis, loosening, or lack of osseous bridging.

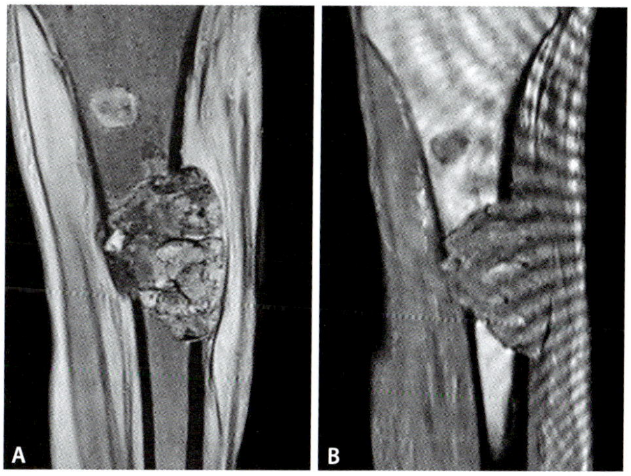

Figs. 11A and B: T1-weighted/proton density (T1W/PD) images (A and B) show soft tissue intensity lesion in proximal shaft. The lesion was abutting the vessels closely and produced segmental defect of tibia needing extensive reconstruction and vascular surgery support.

Neoplasm

- For soft tissue and osseous lesions, MRI is generally preferred because of the superior contrast resolution. However, CT may serve as a complementary tool to MRI particularly to evaluate for ossification and calcification **(Figs. 11A and B)**.
- CT may be the study of choice in contraindications to MRI (pacemakers, vascular clips, ocular implants, and claustrophobia **(Figs. 12A and B)**.

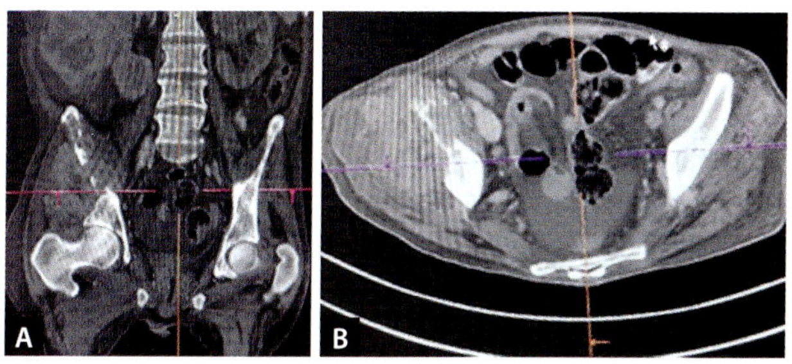

Figs. 12A and B: Coronal and axial CT images of pelvis in a claustrophobic patient show large destructive lytic lesion (metastatic renal cell carcinoma) with associated soft tissue in right iliac bone.

Use of Contrast

- In case where MRI is not available or contraindicated intravenous iodinated contrast can be used with CT to improve detection and characterization of soft tissue lesion. Intravenous contrast generally is not helpful in the evaluation of bone lesions osteomyelitis (unless evaluating for fluid collection) or traumatic injuries.
- Joint evaluation can be significantly enhanced with the administration of intra-articular contrast. CT

arthrography can identify cartilage defects, intra-articular bodies, meniscal tears, and labral tears effectively in patients with contraindications to MRI or MR arthrography.

Image-guided Interventions

- CT guidance is now commonly used for both the diagnosis and treatment of numerous musculoskeletal conditions.
- CT-guided percutaneous biopsies of osseous and soft tissue lesions provide increased safety, decreased cost, decreased time, and reduced pain compared with open biopsies with a high diagnostic accuracy.
- CT guidance can also play a role in injections for pain management, particularly in patients with complex anatomy.
- Other safe and successful minimal invasive therapies included radiofrequency ablation (RFA) for osteoid osteoma and RFA/microwave ablations of tumors.

Bone Health

Quantitative computed tomography (QCT) uses low-dose imaging of the spine and hip to asses bone mineral density. Compared with DXA, QCT is less susceptible to artifact and miscalculation related to degenerative changes, osteophytes, scoliosis, and large body habitus. Additionally, QCT can provide separate assessments of cortical and trabecular bone. Generally, ionizing radiation is a limiting factor but with QCT, low-dose techniques allow for each can to be equivalent to a set of mammograms.

RECENT ADVANCES IN COMPUTED TOMOGRAPHY

- With the advent of multidetector CT, which allows for multiple data streams to be acquired simultaneously, scan times have been cut down to seconds and motion artifact is substantially reduced, which is particularly helpful in the trauma setting. After acquisition, the slices can be viewed in succession and reconstructed in multiple planes (sagittal, coronal, and oblique) as well as in 3D, providing a large amount of cross-sectional information about the osseous and soft tissue structures in that region and serving as an invaluable tool for preoperative planning.
- Newer techniques such as dual-energy CT have shown significant potential in musculoskeletal imaging. Dual-energy CT scanners allow simultaneous acquisition at two different energy levels. This can characterize the chemical composition of material according to the differential attenuation of the structures being examined at the two different energy levels, highly specific in detecting uric acid deposits in gout and in monitoring response to treatment.
- Other applications include minimizing metal prosthesis artifacts, detecting bone marrow edema, and visualizing pathologic tendons and ligaments.

ROLE OF ULTRASONOGRAPHY IN ORTHOPEDICS

INTRODUCTION

Ultrasonography has gained much popularity in musculoskeletal imaging in the past decade and is a powerful tool in the evaluation of musculoskeletal abnormalities. USG is relatively low cost compared with MRI and CT, is fairly quick to perform, has no ionizing radiation, and lends itself to diagnostic evaluation and therapeutic interventions in one visit.

PHYSICS

Ultrasound is sound above the audibly perceptible range of frequencies (20 Hz–20 kHz). Ultrasound waves are produced by piezoelectric crystals. They pass through various interphases and are reflected back based on the variable acoustic impedance produced at tissue interphases. The USG identifies changes in tissue based on physical characteristics rather than MRI scan that discriminates on the basis of changes in chemical structure. Depending on the density of tissue and other variables the reflected waves when correctly interpreted gives information regarding various characteristics of the tissue such as the size, shape, and internal structure, and hence the same can be studied for normal and pathological tissues. The waves in form of electric energy are converted into mechanical energy. Such transfer of energy can be utilized in imparting therapeutic abilities to the modality. The frequency used for therapeutic ultrasound is usually 0.5 MHz [low-intensity pulsed ultrasound (LIPUS)] while those for diagnostic ultrasound range between 2 and 10 MHz. Higher the frequency used, the greater the spatial resolution but the shallower the depth of tissue that can be reached. Higher frequency probes (5–7.5 MHz) are mainly used in pediatric scans and scans of small parts or superficial structures. For adult scans and for deeper structures, the lower frequency probes are preferable (3–5 MHz).

"Piezoelectric effect" was described by, Pierre and Jacques Curie in 1880. It is defined as change in physical dimensions of certain materials, when subjected to an electric field. Such materials are made of innumerable dipoles arranged in a geometric pattern. An electric dipole is a distorted molecule that has a positive charge on one end and a negative charge on other end (much like an ordinary magnet). Positive and negative ends are so arranged that an electric field will cause them to realign, thus changing the dimension of crystal. Sudden burst or pulse of high frequency *alternating current* (AC) voltage causes crystal to vibrate and emit ultrasound waves. Waves travel through the medium and get reflected back from different interphases. The reflected waves carry energy that causes physical compression of the crystal in turn. The dipoles not get reoriented and the reverse phenomenon occurs, i.e., compression produces voltage. This voltage difference between electrodes is amplified producing—ultrasonic signal for display. This compression force and associated voltage are responsible for the name piezoelectricity also called "pressure electricity".

TECHNIQUE

Proper USG evaluation in musculoskeletal imaging requires the use of a high-frequency linear transducer. Higher-frequency transducers produce higher resolution images with the trade-off of lower penetration. However, because most musculoskeletal structures of interest tend to be linear in configuration and superficial, higher frequency transducers are ideal.

Curvilinear transducers can be used to evaluate deeper structures or for deep hip aspirations and soft tissue biopsies. Smaller footprint linear transducers ("hockey stick transducers") are helpful in evaluation of the hands, wrist, and feet where the limited body surfaces prevent use of larger transducers. Correct focal cone location and minimizing depth to include only the region of interest are two additional easily selectable parameters to optimize imaging.

Color Doppler and power Doppler imaging are valuable adjuncts to assess for vascularity within lesions or synovium, with power Doppler being more sensitive and Color Doppler having the ability to provide speed and flow direction. The use of Doppler imaging is very helpful in inflammatory arthropathies to evaluate for synovitis and response to therapy.

In "A" (amplitude) type scanning, the returning echo is displayed as a spike and used to measure the depth of objects in the beam. If there are no returning signals then it indicates a fluid medium. In "B" (brightness) type scanning, the returning echo is seen as a dot which is deciphered on the cathode-ray screen according to the position and impedance of the reflecting tissue. The "hypoechoic" tissues appear black/dark gray while the "hyperechoic" (dense) tissues appear white/light gray. Echogenicity of different tissues are mentioned as under:

- *Air/gas:* Highly reflective and creates characteristics comet tail artefacts.
- *Tendon:* Hyperechoic, consists of interdigitated parallel fibers running in long axis of tendon.
- *Paratenon:* Some tendons do not have a true tendon sheath; instead they are surrounded by a hyperechoic boundary the paratenon, e.g., tendoachilles.
- *Fat:* Hypoechoic, but the echogenicity varies in different anatomy and pathology.
- *Muscle:* Hyperechoic, separated by hypoechoic interfaces.
- *Hyaline cartilage:* Hypoechoic/transonic cartilage, seen against highly reflective cortical bone.
- *Fascia:* Hyperechoic, thin well-marginated soft tissue boundaries.
- *Ligament:* Hyperechoic, similar to tendons fibrillar pattern, may vary in multilayered ligaments.
- *Bone/periosteum:* Highly reflective hyperechoic/ curvilinear line, with acoustic shadowing.
- *Synovium/capsule:* Both appear hypoechoic and similar to joint fluid.
- *Nerve:* Hypoechoic nerve bundles, separated by hyperechoic interphases.

ADVANTAGES OF ULTRASONOGRAPHY

- Safety is the foremost advantage with no known deleterious somatic or genetic effect reported. The examination can be multiply repeated. Most ionizing radiations have effects that are cumulative so there is a drive to keep the amount of radiation as low as reasonably achievable (ALARA) principle, by prescribing only the requisite radiographs. The effects of low-dose radiation are unknown, hence USG plays important role in replacing the modalities where it is equally effective as it is inherently safe (few reports raise the unproven concern of ultrasonics on internal organs and pregnancy, they may be exceptions to this).
- Real-time imaging capability allowing dynamic evaluation. No other technique allows such free examination and analysis of moving parts.
- *Low cost:* Compared to sophisticated CT scans and MRI scans. Also claustrophobia is a deterrent to MRI scans. USG does not generate any magnetic field so there is no risk of various objects becoming projectile and causing injury.
- *Easy accessibility:* It can be installed anywhere and number of centers are there. It can be done on virtually any machine and there is no need for advanced sonography machines.
- Portability.
- Noninvasiveness and no ionizing radiation are imparted to the patient.
- Multiplanar imaging.

USES OF ULTRASONOGRAPHY IN ORTHOPEDICS

Diagnostic

- Tendons
  - Tears
  - Tendinosis, tendinitis, and tenosynovitis
  - Peritendinitis
- Cysts.

Therapeutic (Low-intensity Pulsed Ultrasound)

- Application of USG for different tissues and their associated conditions:
  - Enthesopathy
  - Bursitis
  - Postoperative
  - Interventional
  - Aspiration of cysts, abscess and hematoma, etc.
  - Injection of sclerosant into cysts.

Diagnostic Uses

Antenatal Diagnosis of Musculoskeletal Disorders

Various disorders can be readily identified in the prenatal period at various stages of development:

- Osteochondrodysplasia
- Club foot
- Arthrogryposis
- Limb abnormalities associated with syndromes.

Joints and Tendon Disorders

"Tendon tears" like that of biceps, triceps, rotator cuff, adductor, quadriceps, and posterior tibial tendon can be readily evaluated. The following are the typical findings: *Discontinuity of fibers (complete or incomplete) or focal thinning of tendon (partial tendon tears)* confirmed by tenography (injecting radiopaque dye in tendon sheath and visualizing radiologically).

- *Hematoma of variable size:* Hematoma develops around the whole tendon. The gap between the torn fragments is filled with hypoechoic hemorrhagic fluid (except in Achilles tendon rupture—these ruptures are associated with minimal focal hemorrhage).
- *In case of bone avulsion:* The bone fragments are seen as bright echogenic foci with acoustic shadowing.
- Nonvisualization of tendon commonly indicates retracted tendon (in case of complete tear, e.g., biceps brachii, rotator cuff, and flexor tendons of finger)
- For Achilles tendon tears USG is a good modality if there is pain around the region and no clinical tendon tear. USG can rule out/identify Albert's disease (anterior bursitis of the calcaneal tendon) in this scenario.

Tendinosis

- Degenerative changes in a tendon (no signs of inflammation within the tendon or paratenon)
- *Mostly associated with painful focal or diffuse nodular thickening of tendon* **(Fig. 13)**: Mainly described with patellar tendon and Achilles tendon (achillodynia).
- Hypervascularity is seen on Doppler imaging if performed concomitantly.
- There is decreased echogenicity of enlarged tendon.

Tendinitis

- Thickening of tendon with inflammatory features (edema and blurred margins)
- Decreased echogenicity
- Increased vascularity on Doppler imaging
- Calcification (patellar tendon and rotator cuff predominantly) can be detected in chronic tendinitis.

Tenosynovitis

- Acute tenosynovitis shows fluid in the sheath
- Suppurative tenosynovitis depicts fluid with internal echoes representing debris

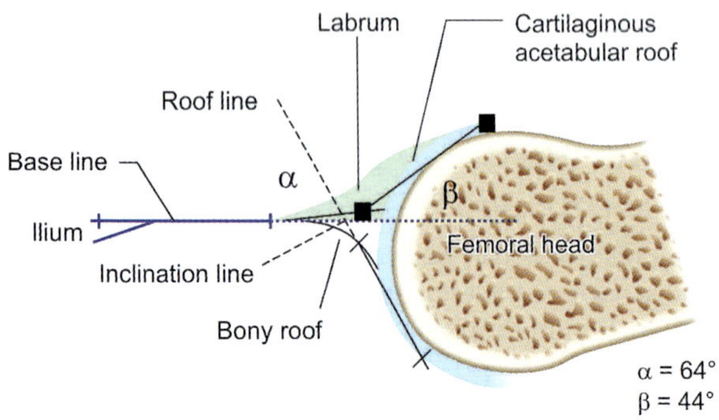

Fig. 13: Developmental dysplasia of hip (DDH) ultrasonography.

- Chronic tenosynovitis reveals hypoechoic thickening of synovial sheath, with little or no fluid
- Rheumatoid tenosynovitis is peculiar as the fluid may be absent and the tendon sheath is involved by pannus that is hypoechoic.

Ultrasonography can also be used for tenography; the needle is directed under sonographic control for injection of contrast medium into the sheath. In a similar way, steroid injection can be done in sonography guidance as else the common mistake is injecting the steroid into the tendon rather than sheath.

Ganglia and Cysts Around Joints

Ganglia around joints and cysts such as popliteal and meniscal cysts are readily identified. They are composed of low echogenic, oval mass adjacent to joint space or anechoic material which surrounds the tendon echo complex; percutaneous drainage can be readily guided. Popliteal cyst is caused by an abnormal distention of the semimembranosus bursa. Chronic cysts may have internal echoes mimicking hypoechoic solid tumor.

Bursitis

- Acute bursitis shows sonolucent and fluid filled collection, with ill-defined margins
- Chronic bursitis depicts a complex sonographic appearance with internal echogenic debris resulting from granulomatous tissue, precipitated fibrin and calcification.

Enthesopathy

Sonographically, the tendon at insertion appears swollen and hypoechoic, with calcification developing in long-standing cases.

Rotator Cuff Tear **(Table 1)**

This is one of the emerging methods in diagnosis that also reveals dynamic motions in the tendon region. Persons need to be thoroughly trained and being highly observer-based, the technique is mastered with a steep curve.

Major criteria for diagnosis of rotator cuff tear are as follows:

- Nonvisualization of the cuff
- Focal nonvisualization or discontinuity
- Abnormal echogenicity.

Minor criteria for diagnosis are as follows:

- Intra- and extra-articular effusions
- Concave subdeltoid bursal contour

TABLE 1: Wiener and Seitz classification of rotator cuff tear visible in ultrasonography.

Tear category	*Imaging features*
Normal	Normal
Partial thickness	Hypoechoic areas
Small full thickness	<1 cm
Large full thickness	1–3 cm
Massive	With or without cuff arthropathy

- Humeral head elevation
- Thickening of subdeltoid bursa.

Other observations are as follows:
- Cuff thickening
- Blood flow characteristic.

Assessment of Muscle and Osseous Structure

Thoroughly performed assessment of the bone and muscle structure helps in assessment of various disorders.
- Quantitative and qualitative assessment of bone can be performed that helps in diagnosing and classifying osteoporosis. Quantitative ultrasound is capable of providing information about the qualities of bone, such as trabecular microarchitecture. Trabecular microarchitecture accounts for up to 50% of total bone strength and is a valid indicator for the risk of pathological fractures.
- Quantitative assessment of structural muscle abnormalities can be easily done.
- Ultrasonography also helps in diagnosis and assessment of fractures, especially stress fractures.
- Ultrasonography has also been utilized to evaluate the progress of healing callus formation and consolidation. Some centers use it to monitor the progress of regenerate formation and adjust the distraction rate according to the quality and quantity of regenerate.

Vascular Complications

It can never be forgotten that USG Doppler is indispensable in diagnosing *deep vein thrombosis* (DVT) which is a frequent complication of many orthopedic surgeries and a frequent cause of otherwise unaccounted for mortality. Other lesions that can be identified are soft tissue hemangiomas (especially differentiating them from ganglion), hemangioendotheliomas, and bone vascular lesions like intraosseous hemangiomas.

Neonatal Conditions

Developmental dysplasia of hip (DDH): Clinical assessment of the neonatal hip is performed routinely in the first day of life, and it has become diagnostic modality of choice for DDH due to its ability to evaluate cartilaginous structures. It is a good idea to perform a USG assessment for doubtful cases before the appearance of femoral head ossification center (4–6 months of age) after which radiographs can be equally useful. During first month of life clinical examination is more relied upon as USG tends to overestimate the incidence of DDH. Graf (1980) described a static nonstress ultrasound measurement technique utilizing the nonossified head as a transmitting material. This is a morphological assessment relying on anatomic landmarks. The transducer is placed on the greater trochanter allowing visualization of the deeper structures. The image includes lateral surface of iliac bone above acetabulum, deepest portion of acetabulum roof, and proximal femoral metaphysis. Draw three lines; one baseline from lateral margin of ilium (intersecting the bony and cartilaginous portions), second line from bony acetabular roof (the acetabular roof line), and third line from lateral aspect of acetabular labrum and cartilage (the inclination line, ***see* Fig. 13**). Measure the alpha (angle between the roof and baseline) and beta (angle between the inclination line and base line) angles. The acetabular angles **(Tables 2 and 3)** are carefully measured on a coronal view of the hip and subcategorized depending on labral echogenicity. Transverse scanning from the lateral aspect of the hip can also be used. Utilizing these techniques and assessing the hip stability by giving the head a push from posterior aspect Harcke and Grissom described dynamic stress sonography where the hip is scanned in transverse and coronal planes. While scanning the posterior lip of the acetabulum, a posterior push is performed to assess joint instability. As the child usually gives little time to examine, a dynamic standard minimum examination (DSME) is commonly done by the physicians succinctly looking for the pathology and diagnosis. Ultrasound examination thus not only establishes static relationship between femoral head and acetabulum but also allows dynamic examination. It is also now a preferred modality for evaluation of children on treatment with Pavlik harness. Role of USG as a screening test is still contested. While in Europe it is done for all newborn babies, in US, it is recommended only for doubtful newborn cases that have been evaluated by standard clinical examination. A good use of USG could be to evaluate infants with risk factors for DDH such as breech position, family history, and torticollis.

TABLE 2: Graf's sonographic classification of developmental dysplasia of hip.

Type	*Alpha angle*	*Beta angle*	*Comment*
1	≥60°	<55°	Normal
2A	50–59°	55–77°	Physiologic immaturity, <3 months old
2B	50–59°	55–77°	Delayed ossification, >3 months old
2C	43–49°	<77°	Labrum not everted
2D	43–49°	>77°	Subluxed, labrum everted
3	<43°	>77°	Dislocated
4	Unmeasurable	Unmeasurable	Dislocated with labrum interposing between femoral head and acetabulum

TABLE 3: Simplified Graf's classification.

Type	*Alpha angle*	*Beta angle*	*Description*
1	>60°	<55°	Normal
2	43–59° (critical angle)	55–77°	Unstable hip
3	<43°	>77°	Lateralization/ subluxated hip
4	Unmeasurable	Unmeasurable	Dislocated

Observations for developmental dysplasia of hip:
- Morphologic evaluation of the location of the femoral head and the degree of acetabulum development.
- Dynamic evaluation of the location of femoral head and degree of hip instability with stress.

- The depth of acetabulum and displacement of femoral head are measured by alpha and beta angles.
- Alpha angle is between body weight base line and acetabular base line.
- Beta angle is measured between body weight base line and acetabular labrum line.

Disadvantages of X-ray: These include:

- The exposure to ionizing radiation
- Lack of ossification of the femoral head in early infancy
- Spinal *lesions:* Various conditions of spine can be readily identified using sonography as it has the advantage of being performed in mild sedation. Investigations like MRI need anesthesia for examination. The conditions that can be identified are:
  - Tethered cord syndrome
  - Low-lying conus medullaris below the l2/l3 level
  - Subcutaneous and epidural masses of the spine
  - Spinal neoplasms like sacrococcygeal teratoma with characterization into cystic, solid (commonly malignant), or mixed types.

Femoral anteversion: Ultrasonography is also emerging as a good careening tool for evaluation of femoral anteversion.

Joint effusions: Plain radiographic films are normal in presence of small joint effusions. In such cases, USG can be used to determine, if effusion is present. USG has been called "orthopedist's stethoscope" very aptly, especially in children. As little as 1 mL of fluid can be detected in the hip and ultrasound can also guide needle aspiration simultaneously. To guide arthrocentesis, saline lavage can be used if fluid cannot be withdrawn. USG can determine the nature of fluid collection—anechoic or hypoechoic fluid is seen in transient synovitis and more echogenic fluid in septic arthritis.

Hematomas and masses: Calcification in the soft tissues, particularly in myositis ossificans, is seen more readily and earlier by ultrasound than by radiography, CT, or MRI. The differentiation between myositis ossificans and a calcified tumor is based on the combination of the ultrasound findings of a mass with highly reflective internal echoes and a characteristic centripetal pattern of development with time.

- Hematomas are more difficult to evaluate due to varying nature of presentation with age of the collection. For first few days they are hypoechoic collection. This is followed by development of complex internal echoes as they start becoming organized and develop variable calcifications. They may dissect through fascial planes and present as diffuse masses.
- Ultrasonography can differentiate tumor mass from hematoma or muscle rupture. Also the tissue can be characterized like fat has high echogenicity, but distinction is poor to differentiate benign from malignant lesion. Benign lesions are often indirectly identified. They have a well-defined margin and have tendency to displace the surrounding tissue rather than invading it. Color Doppler may help evaluate the vascularity that is raised in malignant lesions. USG can also help in guided-biopsy of the lesion.

Septic arthritis:

- May arise *de novo* or may occur secondary to infection in adjacent soft tissue or bone.
- Fluid is seen as anechoic or hypoechoic areas.
- The identification of capsular distension is very nonspecific and is also seen in unrelated disorders such as transient synovitis, Perthes disease, slipped upper femoral epiphysis (SUFE), rheumatoid arthritis and juvenile rheumatoid arthritis (JRA), and tuberculosis. Only a few features may help differentiate septic arthritis else the diagnosis rests only on joint fluid examination for infection. The distension is anechoic in JRA and early Perthes disease while hypoechoic in septic arthritis. In Perthes and SUFE, bone changes can be additionally visualized similarly in JRA and tuberculous affection synovial hypertrophy can be simultaneously seen to help differentiate septic arthritis.
- Doppler can demonstrate increased flow in capsule (infection causes hyperemia), hence power Doppler had been combined with ultrasonological examination to increase specificity but this has not been so fruitful.
- Absence of hyperemia does not exclude septic arthritis.
- Ultrasonography guided-joint fluid aspiration can be done simultaneously.

Infection of soft tissues: Ultrasonography can be used to evaluate infection of soft tissues:

- *Cellulitis:* Heterogeneous soft tissue thickening increase echogenicity in affected area.
- Polymyositis.
- *Abscess:* Usually, hypoechoic can be isoechoic/hyperechoic. Moving internal echoes are quite characteristic. Should be differentiated from hematoma/myositis and necrotic masses.
- In infection of osseous structure, it is used to supplement standard modalities.

Osteomyelitis:

- *Early sign:* Deep soft tissue swelling
- *Late sign:*
  - Fluid along cortex of the bone or subperiosteally
  - Fluid in adjacent joint (sterile or aseptic)
  - Cortical disruption
  - Doppler, increased flow at the margin of elevated periosteum in advanced infection.

Trauma:

- Radiographs are initial diagnostic modality
- Ultrasonography helps when symptoms are present and radiographs are unrevealing
- Growth plate fractures, rib fractures, and soft tissue injury and retained nonopaque foreign body
- Brachial plexus injury from birth trauma can be identified by identifying avulsed nerve roots.

Additional proposed neonatal indications:

- Meningocele and neurogenic tumors
- Congenital musculoskeletal abnormalities
- Proximal femoral focal deficiency
- Congenital joint dislocations

- Teratogenic hip dislocation
- Skeletal dysplasia with "atypical" hip
- Fibromatosis colli.

Interventional Procedures

- Localized aspiration of fluid/abscess
- Injection of drugs into subtle spaces like tenosynovial sheath injection of steroids
- Localization of masses and guided biopsy
- Localization of foreign body for placing incision for extraction. Also the size, site, and nature of foreign body can be identified
- Ultrasonography is now being frequently used for percutaneous needling/tenotomy to promote tendon healing, calcific tendinosis lavage and needling (shoulder), platelet-rich plasma (PRP) injections, and carpal tunnel fenestration and release.

Therapeutic

Aid in fracture healing in fresh fractures or nonunions. Act by upregulating the receptor activity of neurotransmitters at the fracture site like the nitric oxide pathways and the prostaglandin pathways (PGE2). Reports suggest that the effect of application of LIPUS (low-intensity ultrasound of 0.03 W/cm^2 at 1.5 MHz, up to a maximum of 0.1 W/cm^2) on stress fractures, delayed or nonunion or postsurgical intervention is positive. The modality can also be used to diagnose stress fractures effectively. It should be remembered that the therapeutic effect diminishes with the concomitant use of nonsteroidal anti-inflammatory drugs (NSAIDs) and calcium channel blockers. Also high-energy ultrasound (>1 W/cm^2) has inhibitory effect.

- The effect could very well be similar to Wolff's law where the stress generated potential (piezoelectric effect—see above) may play a role similar to stress-related bone remodeling in normal osseous structures as described by Wolff (*see* chapter on "Bone Structure, Physiology, Metabolism, and Associated Disorders").
- Low-intensity pulsed USG has been used for improving regenerate consolidation in distraction osteogenesis, postspinal fusion, and improving the osteogenesis with the use of porous implants.
- Low-intensity ultrasound has a heating effect that prevails superficially and has been utilized in controlling tendinopathies such as the tennis elbow and plantar fasciitis tendoachilles inflammation. This may also help in dispersing the erythema locally and reducing inflammation. The healing fibrous tissue around the lesion is also enhanced.

ROLE OF MAGNETIC RESONANCE IMAGING IN ORTHOPEDICS

This is the mainstay in advanced musculoskeletal imaging. MRI provides a wealth of information on anatomy and tissue composition with unparalleled contrast resolution and no ionizing radiation. After routine roentgenography, MRI has had the greatest effect on the practice of orthopedics. It provides excellent soft tissue contrast and multiplanar capability with resolution approaching that of CT. It has to a certain extent superseded older imaging methods such as myelography, arthrography, and angiography. In areas, such as the knee and shoulder, where soft tissue injuries are common, MRI helps the surgeon to evaluate structures that are otherwise invisible to noninvasive techniques. Continued improvements in both hardware and software are continually expanding the role of MRI in orthopedics and in other fields of medicine as well.

PHYSICS

An MRI is based on the magnetization properties of atomic nuclei. Magnetic resonance images are created by placing the patient in a uniform strong magnetic field ranging from 0.5 Tesla in low-resolution machines to up to 3 Tesla in high-resolution machines. When the tissues are subjected to a strong magnetic field, protons align themselves with respect to the field. This is called the steady state or equilibrium. In this steady state a radiofrequency (RF) pulse is applied, which excites the magnetized protons in the field. After application of this pulse the magnetized protons return back to their steady state and in this process emit a RF signal. This RF signal is captured by a receiver coil or antenna and processed to create the magnetic resonance image. For imaging large areas such as chest abdomen, pelvis, hip, thigh, or legs a main large coil shaped like a hollow tube is used in which the patient lies during the study. For smaller areas like wrist rotator cuff or meniscus special surface coils are used. For adequate MRI, surface coils are necessary because they provide improved spatial resolution. Most surface coils are designed specifically for different areas of the body, such as knee, shoulder, and wrist. Closed magnetic resonance scanners are also being replaced by open varieties that are more patient friendly.

Various changes to the RF pulse sequences and acquisitions such as repetition time (TR) and echo time (TE) create different images with additional information about the tissues of interest. Most musculoskeletal MRI examinations use the spin-echo technique, which produces T1-weighted (T1W), proton (spin) density, and T2-weighted (T2W) images. T1 signal is captured when the protons return to their steady or equilibrium state where as T2 images are captured immediately after the application of the exciting RF. T1 and T2 are tissue-specific characteristics. Fat has a high signal (bright) on T1W images **(Fig. 14)** and fluid has a high signal on T2W images **(Fig. 15)**. Structures with little water or fat, such as cortical bone, tendons, and ligaments, remain dark in all types of sequences.

Some special types of magnetic resonance sequences used for specific conditions are discussed below.

Fast Spin-Echo Technique

This reduces length of T2 sequence by two-thirds. But this produces some blurring artifact that can obscure smaller defects in menisci, labrum, etc.

Gradient-Echo Technique

This is another fast imaging technique that is used selectively for cartilage imaging. It is the most effective method of

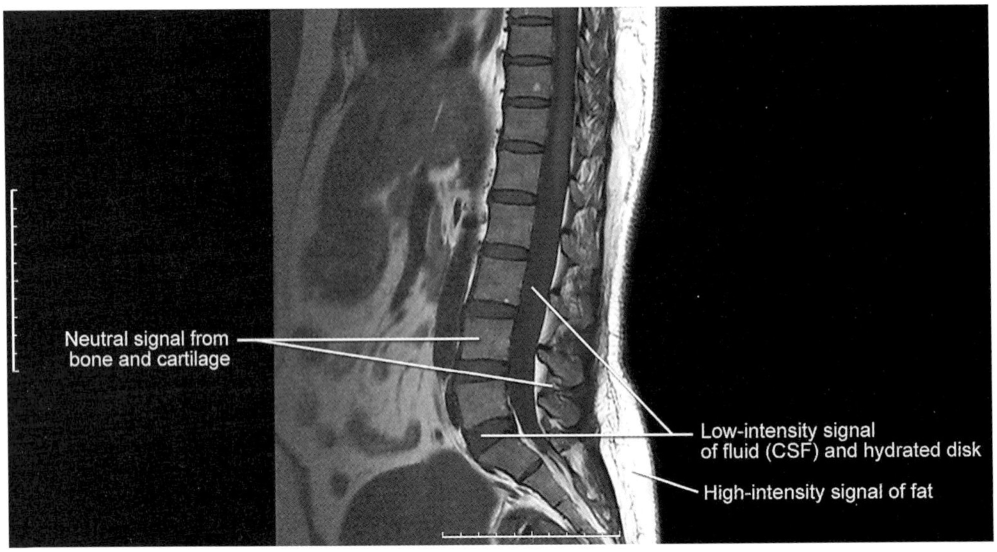

Fig. 14: T1-weighted image of normal spine. (CSF: cerebrospinal fluid)

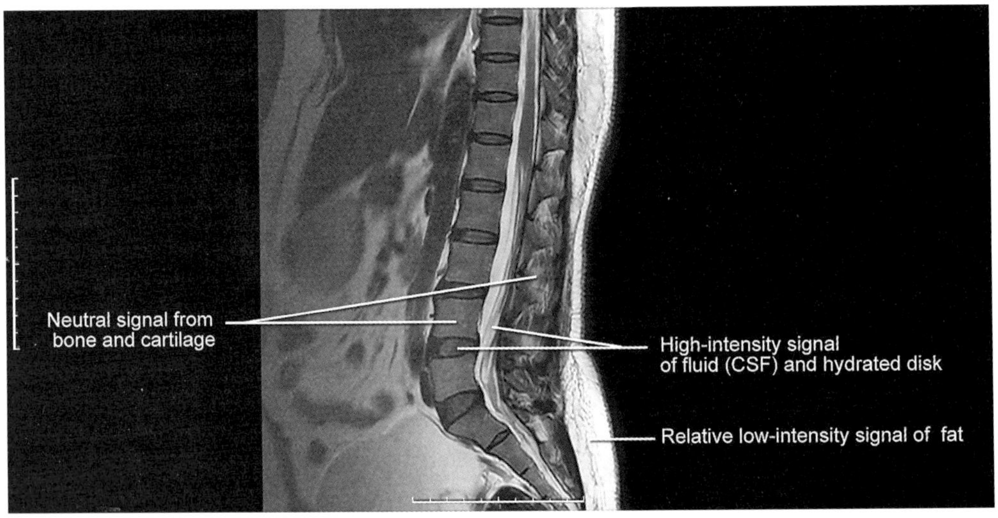

Fig. 15: T2-weighted image of normal spine. (CSF: cerebrospinal fluid)

performing a fast magnetic resonance scan without the blur artifact produced by fast spin-echo technique. A variety of techniques are available all of which rely on reduced flip angle to enhance the signal produced with short TR. Some commonly used acronyms are, fast low-angle shot (FLASH), fast imaging with steady procession (FISP), gradient-recalled acquisition (GRASS), and multiplanar gradient recalled (MPGR).

Short Tau Inversion Recovery Enhanced Images

This technique is short-time inversion recovery (STIR). It causes suppression of signal from fat and is used to detect edema in soft tissues and marrow. This is useful while imaging in cases of trauma and in neoplastic cases **(Fig. 16)**.

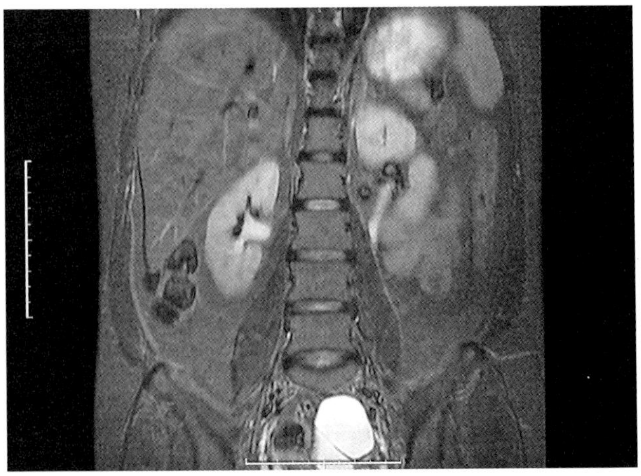

Fig. 16: Short tau inversion recovery enhanced coronal image of spine.

Fluid-sensitive Sequences

T2-weighted sequences are excellent for evaluating pathology, because edema or fluid appears hyperintense. Because fat is also hyperintense on T2W sequences, fat saturation techniques can be used to make the edema and other pathology more apparent.

The most commonly used technique is frequency selective fat saturation, which uses an RF pulse to nullify signal from fat. In MRI of the wrist, for instance, a T2W fat-suppressed sequence provides high-contrast resolution with fluid being hyperintense and the triangular fibrocartilage (TFC) being hypointense. This technique can also be used in postcontrast T1W imaging to assess enhancement patterns. The one pitfall is the possibility of heterogeneous fat suppression, particularly along curved surfaces and adjacent to hardware. An alternative and also commonly used fat suppression technique in musculoskeletal imaging is an STIR sequence. Based on the varying relaxation times of fat and water, signal from far can be markedly reduced. Fat suppression in STIR imaging is less susceptible to heterogeneity and appears more uniform. However, it should not be used for postcontrast imaging, as the relaxation properties of fat and contrast are similar and would cause signal loss of both.

Fluid-attenuated Inversion Recovery

This technique is used to negate or reduce the signal from fluids. It is a T1 image and by changing the inversion time that is the time between inversion and excitation pulses signal arising from fluid can be suppressed. One use of this technique is to highlight hyperintense lesions like multiple sclerosis plaques in the brain by suppressing signals from cerebrospinal fluid (CSF).

Metallic Artifact Reduction Sequence

A variety of techniques exist to image bones and joints with hardware, making MRI useful in the evaluation of postoperative complications or hardware failure. A metal artifacts reduction sequence (MARS) reduces the intensity of the hardware-related susceptibility artifact that results from the magnetic field distortion such sequences allow for evaluation of osteolysis or adverse local tissue reaction with an implant in place.

FUNCTIONAL MAGNETIC RESONANCE IMAGING

This scanning method is able to detect changes in brain due to neuronal activity. Unlike anatomical T1W images this uses a low spatial and high temporal resolution and changes in neuronal activity are seen as changes in the T2 magnetic resonance signal by a blood-oxygen-level-dependent effect (BOLD).

MULTINUCLEAR IMAGING

Magnetic resonance imaging commonly uses hydrogen nuclei for imaging as it is the most abundant nuclei present in all tissues and generates a strong signal due to high gyromagnetic ratio. Other nuclei such as carbon-13, oxygen-17, helium-3, and phosphorus-31 which are naturally present in the body can also be imaged using MRI. Presently, it is a research technique but has potential in imaging of tissues such as lungs and bone that are not well seen on H (Hydrogen-atom based) MRI or as alternative to contrast agents.

CONTRAST MAGNETIC RESONANCE IMAGING

Intravenous contrast for musculoskeletal imaging is generally reserved for problem-solving in noncharacteristic soft tissue lesions and occasionally for osseous lesions. The enhancement pattern can be particularly helpful in discriminating benign versus aggressive lesions, such as a nonenhancing myxoma versus and avidly enhancing sarcoma.

Gadolinium (Paramagnetic)

The most commonly used intravenous contrast agents are based on chelates of gadolinium **(Fig. 17)**. They alter the T1 relaxation times of atoms within body tissues where they are present after oral or intravenous administration. Compared to iodine-based contrast agents used in CT or X-rays, these agents have a lower incidence of anaphylactoid reactions (0.03–0.1%). They are also less nephrotoxic and can be used in presence of renal impairment. Currently, as per US guidelines they can be used in dialysis patients if essential but immediate dialysis should be performed to remove the drug after the imaging. Newer formulations such as gadoxetate, brand name Eovist (US) or Primovist (EU) having dual excretion path have been approved for use.

A variety of routes of administration and a variety of compounds are available depending upon the area that needs scanning. For extracellular fluid ionic agents are Magnevist and Dotarem and neutral agents are Omniscan, Prohance, Gadavist, and optiMARK. Blood pool agents are of two types, those that bind to albumin like ablavar and gadocoletic acid and polymeric complexes like gadomelitol and gadomer-17. Examples of an organ-specific agent are Primovist™ and MultiHance used in hepatobiliary imaging.

Iron Oxide

It is a superparamagnetic contrast agent which acts by reducing the T2 signal of the absorbing tissues. Two types are used; superparamagnetic iron oxide (SPIO) and ultrasmall superparamagnetic iron oxide (USPIO).

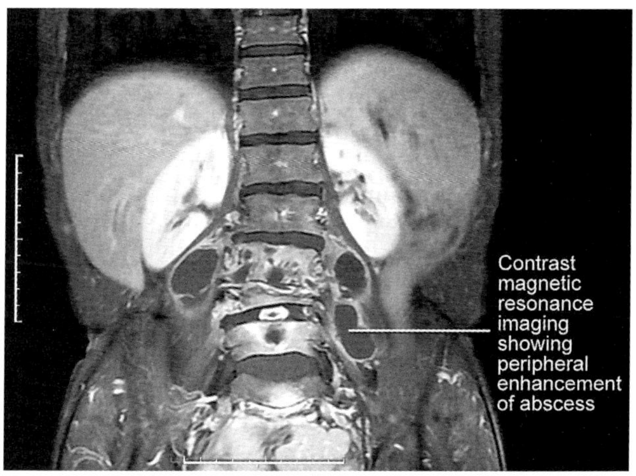

Fig. 17: Contrast magnetic resonance imaging.

Iron Platinum

It is also a superparamagnetic contrast agent that has a better T2 suppressing effect as compared to plain iron oxide and is used in the form of superparamagnetic iron platinum particles (SIPPs). One specialized use of this agent under investigation is to coat it with phospholipids to make multifunctional SIPP stealth immunomicelles that target human prostate cancer cells.

Manganese

Manganese-based nanoparticles chelates (paramagnetic) like mangafodipir trisodium (Mn-DPDP) are under investigation for detection of liver lesions. They act by enhancing the T1 signals.

Perflubron acts a contrast agent by reducing the number of hydrogen ions in a cavity making the cavity appear dark on imaging. It is also used in gastrointestinal imaging in children.

MAGNETIC RESONANCE ARTHROGRAPHY

Magnetic resonance arthrography (MRA) is an excellent tool for evaluation of intra-articular pathology. Direct MRA is most common and involves injection of gadolinium-based contrast into the joint using either fluoroscopic of ultrasonographic guidance. Indirect MRA is less common and involves intravenous injection of contrast followed by delayed MR imaging. All compartments enhance with indirect MRA so abnormal communication of contrast material is absent. Typical imaging sequences include a combination of conventional MRI and fat-saturated T1W sequences to highlight the intra-articular contrast.

The addition of intra-articular contrast causes distention of the joint to highlight structures more clearly and, in present of intra-articular pathology, T1 hyperintense contrast extends into the area involved. Direct MRA is ideal evaluation of labral tears in the shoulder and hip with sensitivity of 92%. MRA can also be used to evaluate for TFC or scapholunate ligament tears in the wrist and ulnar collateral ligament tears in the elbow and for postoperative evaluation of meniscal retears in the knee.

IMAGING QUALITY

In addition to the inherent tissue contrast, several external factors can play a role in the imaging information provided. Magnetic field strengths can vary from 0.2 to 3 T for clinical applications, with 1.5 T being the most common, in the higher the field strength, the higher the signal-to-noise ratio (more signal, less noise artifact), the better the contrast, and higher the resolution, This, in turn improves overall image quality and diagnostic ability.

Magnetic resonance scanners are available in open and closed configurations, with the open scanners generally having a significantly lower field strength and multiple limitations, such as longer scan time (increasing susceptibility to motion artifact), wider field of view, and lack of adequate far suppression. Evaluation of small joints and cartilage is often difficult on low-field-strength, open scanners. Open scanners should only be reserved for claustrophobic patients and obese patients who may not fit satisfactorily into a more robust closed MR scanner. Extremity scanners are available, which only require the patient's arm or leg to be within the bore, minimizing discomfort.

One of the most important and often overlooked decisions in musculoskeletal imaging is coil selection. Given the wide variation in configuration and quality of surface coils for extremities, there is significant potential to produce less than optimal images. In general, the smallest coil possible should be used for imaging to achieve the desired field of view, because the more closely the coil sits against the body part, the better is the imaging quality. Regardless of coil choice, it should be positioned to optimally image the area of interest. When patients are unable to hold a position because of discomfort, sometimes a more comfortable second position should be considered as the original position may cause patient motion and degrade the images.

CONTRAINDICATIONS OF MAGNETIC RESONANCE IMAGING

Absolute

- Presence of intracerebral aneurysm clips
- Implanted cardiac pacemakers and automatic defibrillators
- Biostimulators
- Implanted infusion devices and internal hearing aids
- Metallic orbital foreign bodies
- Metal external fixation devices
- Cochlear implants
- Ferromagnetic foreign bodies like shell shrapnel.

Relative

- First-trimester pregnancy
- Middle-ear prostheses
- Penile prostheses.

Orthopedic implants and prosthetics are safe on MRI. They may become warm during scanning but usually study does not need to be terminated. Presence of metal hardware though creates local artifact that can obscure adjacent tissues.

Clinical Applications

Given the very high contrast resolution, lack of ionizing radiation and ability to assess soft tissues, osseous structures, ligaments, and tendons in detail, MRI is the workhorse of advanced musculoskeletal imaging. MRI is often the study of choice following initial radiography for assessment of joint pathology. The only limitations include longer scan time (relative to CT), potential incompatibilities with implanted nonorthopedic hardware, increased susceptibility to artifact, and cost. In trauma and degenerative joint disease imaging, the primary utility of MRI is in identification of ligamentous sprains, meniscal tears, and tendon or muscle strains that are well visualized on T2W images. Cartilage defects and osteochondral defects are also best seen by MRI. To evaluate for occult fractures, MRI is the best imaging test and an abbreviated protocol can be used for rapid evaluation, such as for femoral neck or scaphoid fractures. This is especially true if the patient is osteopenic, as fractures can be missed on CT in that patient population. Neoplasms have to be specifically evaluated by MRI before any intervention can be planned **(*see* Figs. 11A and B)**. For lesions, fat within a nonaggressive-appearing lesion is identified by MRI and can suggest a benign etiology such and enchondroma or vascular malformation. Hemosiderin, seen as dark signal with blooming on gradient-recalled echo (GRE) sequences, can point toward pigmented villonodular synovitis or giant cell tumor of tendon sheath. Bone marrow replacement on T1W sequences suggests an infiltrative process such as tumor or infection.

The extent of marrow involvement, presence of pathological fracture, muscle on vascular invasion, and soft tissue components can be assessed by MRI for more aggressive lesions.

Now with the help of whole-body MR metastatic disease and multiple myeloma burden can be evaluated **(Figs. 18A and B)**. MRI is also the imaging modality of choice for suspected osteomyelitis, identified by hyperintense signal (bone marrow edema) on T2W imaging and hypointense signal (bone marrow replacement) on T1W imaging. Intraosseous, subperiosteal, and soft tissue abscesses are easily demonstrated by MRI. If MRI is contraindicated, alternative modalities such as triple phase bone scan can be used.

The normal and pathological finding in MRI of various regions of the body of significance in orthopedics is discussed here.

KNEE

Indications

- Meniscal tears
- Degenerative conditions of meniscus
- Ligament tears [anterior cruciate ligament (ACL), posterior cruciate ligament (PCL), and collateral ligaments]
- Patellar or quadriceps tendon tears
- Tendinitis
- Cysts
- Synovial pathology
- Avascular necrosis (AVN)
- Osseous contusion
- Occult fractures
- Popliteal mass
- Physeal injuries in children
- Osteochondritis dissecans
- Evaluation of articular cartilage.

The MRI examination of the knee is obtained in sagittal, coronal, and usually axial planes using spin-echo sequences. The menisci are best evaluated in the sagittal plane. But the chosen plane for scanning is parallel to the ACL and is about 15° internally rotated to the true sagittal plane.

Medial collateral ligament (MCL) and lateral collateral ligaments (LCL) are seen in the coronal plane and the axial plane is used to assess the patellofemoral joint.

The menisci have neither large amount of water nor fat and, therefore, appear as low intensity signals (dark) in both T1 and T2. In the central cuts they are seen as a triangle and in peripheral cuts as a bow tie configuration **(Figs. 19 and 20)**. Lesions are seen as areas of increased signal and are classified as grade 1 which are globular, grade 2 which are linear, and grade 3 which extend to the articular surface. Signals that do not extend to the articular surface of the meniscus do not represent tears and are evidence of mucoid degeneration. A grade 3 signal is a linear abnormality that extends to the superior or inferior articular surface and represents a tear. On further examination in various planes theses tears can further be classified as per their location (anterior horn, body, posterior horn, free edge, and periphery) and orientation (horizontal, vertical, and complex). A bucket handle or complete tear should be suspected when the meniscus appears truncated or small **(Fig. 21)**. The free lying fragment can be seen as a hypotense fragment in the coronal plane. Discoid meniscus is seen as an exaggerated bow tie appearance in more than three slices **(Fig. 22)**. The sensitivity and specificity of MRI in detecting meniscal tears exceed 90%.

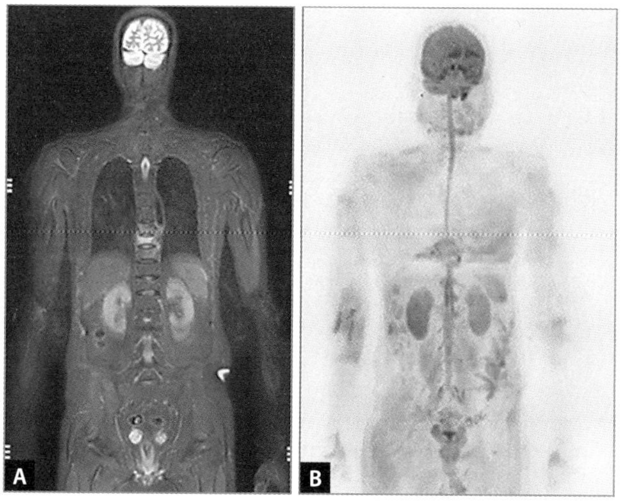

Figs. 18A and B: Whole body MR shows focal altered marrow signal intensity lesion in thoracic vertebral body.

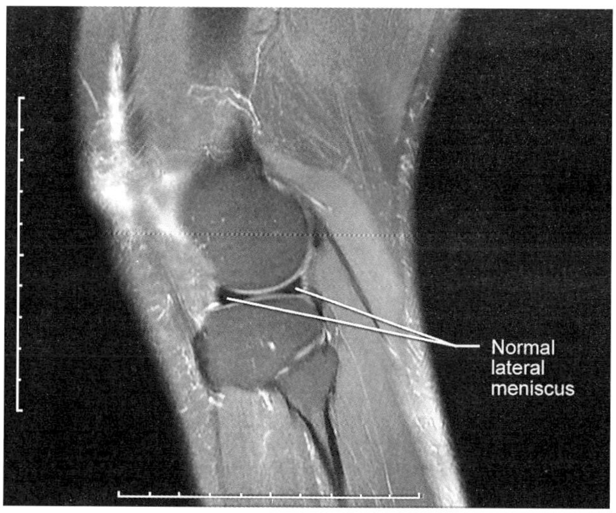

Fig. 19: Normal lateral meniscus.

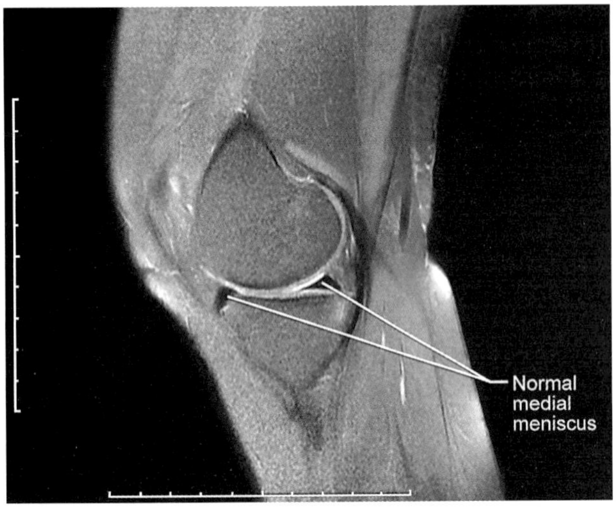

Fig. 20: Normal medial meniscus.

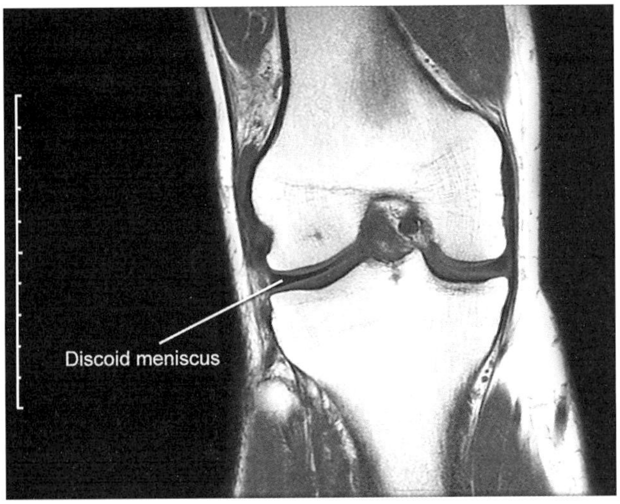

Fig. 22: Discoid meniscus.

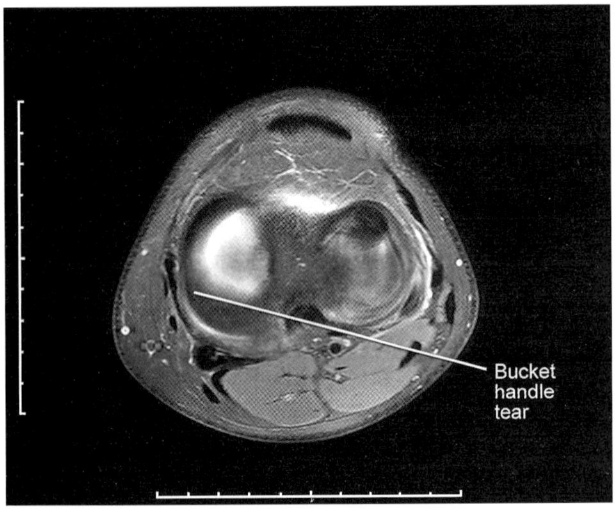

Fig. 21: Bucket handle tear.

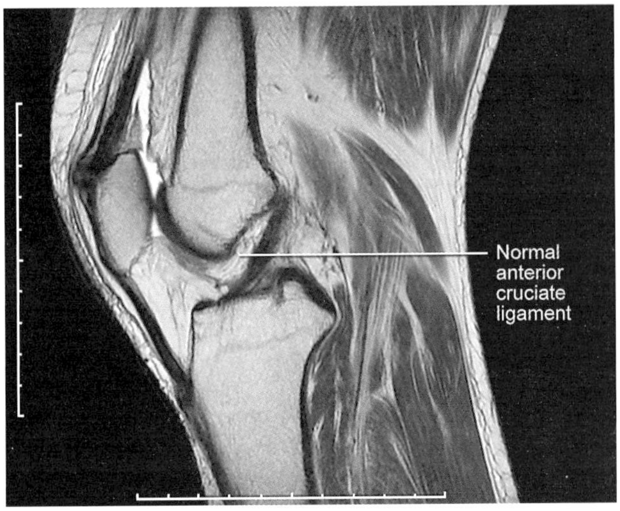

Fig. 23: Anterior cruciate ligament.

Anterior cruciate ligament is best seen in the sagittal plane **(Fig. 23)** but should be examined in the coronal plane for an accurate diagnosis. Signs of ACL rupture include an abnormal horizontal course, a wavy or irregular appearance, or fluid-filled gaps in a discontinuous ligament **(Fig. 24)**. Chronic tears show up as ligamentous thickening without edema or, often, complete atrophy. In cases of ACL, reconstruction a thickened graft or absence of the graft on MRI suggests graft failure. The sensitivity and specificity of knee MRI are in the ranges of 87–94% and 88–93%, respectively.

Posterior cruciate ligament is seen as a curving band of fibrous tissue, appearing homogeneously hypointense on sagittal MRI series **(Fig. 25)**. Discontinuity of the ligament or fluid signal within its substance indicates a tear.

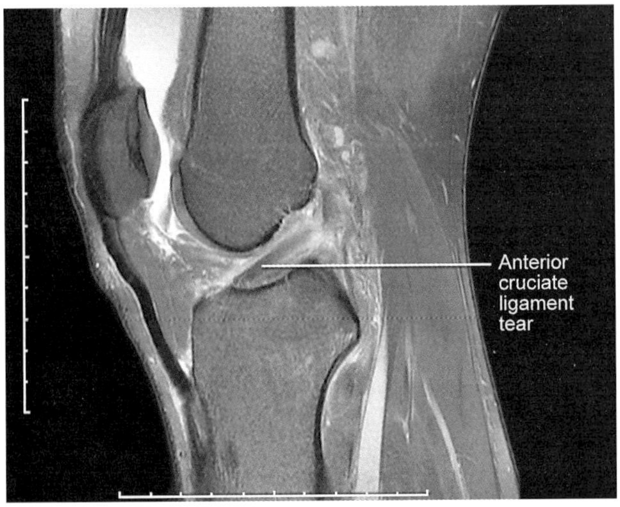

Fig. 24: Anterior cruciate ligament tear.

Pitfalls

- In the central portion of the joint, the meniscofemoral ligament (MFL) and transverse meniscal ligament can create problems.
- Meniscocapsular separation is difficult to detect unless it is complete.
- Elderly patients' exhibit greatly increased intrameniscal signal due to degeneration this can be mistaken for a tear.

- Specificity is also reduced in patients who have undergone previous meniscal repair.
- Partial ACL tears some times are difficult to distinguish from complete tears. Therefore, a decision for ACL reconstruction cannot be based completely on MRI as partial tears can be managed conservatively.

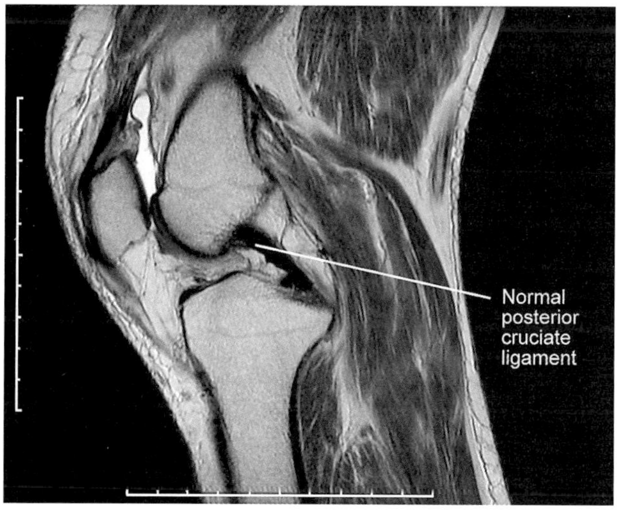

Fig. 25: Posterior cruciate ligament.

SHOULDER

Indications

- Rotator cuff tear
- Impingement syndromes
- Instability
- Evaluation of the labroligamentous complex
- Occult fractures
- Osteonecrosis
- Pathological conditions of the tendon of the long head of the biceps, including rupture, dislocation, or tendinitis
- Suprascapular nerve entrapment.

Magnetic resonance imaging of shoulder is usually done using axial spin-echo or gradient-echo sequences to evaluate the labrum **(Fig. 26)**. The supraspinatus tendon is best seen oblique coronal images with T2 weighting. Further oblique sagittal images confirm abnormalities of the cuff tendons and help evaluate rotator cuff muscles in cross-section.

The tendons of the rotator cuff maintain low signal on all pulse sequences. Tears appear as areas of increased T2W signal, representing fluid within the tendon substance **(Figs. 27 and 28)**. In a full-thickness tear this signal will traverse the entire tendon substance. In partial thickness tears, intact cuff fibers may persist along the articular surface or bursal surface. Fat suppression improves detection of partial thickness tears. In T2 images, fluid is seen in the subacromial-subdeltoid bursa. This may be increased in bursitis. Normally, this fluid does not communicate with the shoulder joint, but in large or chronic tears the cuff may be too atrophied to be visible and the fluid from the bursa communicates with the shoulder joint and the head is migrated upward. MRI has 80–97% sensitivity in detecting full thickness rotator cuff tears and for partial tears, the sensitivity is 67–89%.

Imaging findings that are seen in impingement include narrowing of the subacromial space by spurs or osteophytes, curved or hooked acromial morphology, and signal abnormalities in the cuff indicating tendinosis or tendinopathy. But these need to be correlated clinically as impingement syndrome is primarily a clinical diagnosis.

Labral pathology and the biceps tendon origin are best seen with intra-articular saline or contrast. When saline is used, T2W images are taken showing a hypointense labrum surrounded by bright fluid. When dilute gadolinium is used, T1W images can be taken. These are superior to T2 images because of improved signal-to-noise ratio. Imaging is done on standard position with the arm at the patient's side and also performed with the humerus in abduction and external rotation (ABER) position for assessment of the inferior glenohumeral ligament and its insertion. MRA has

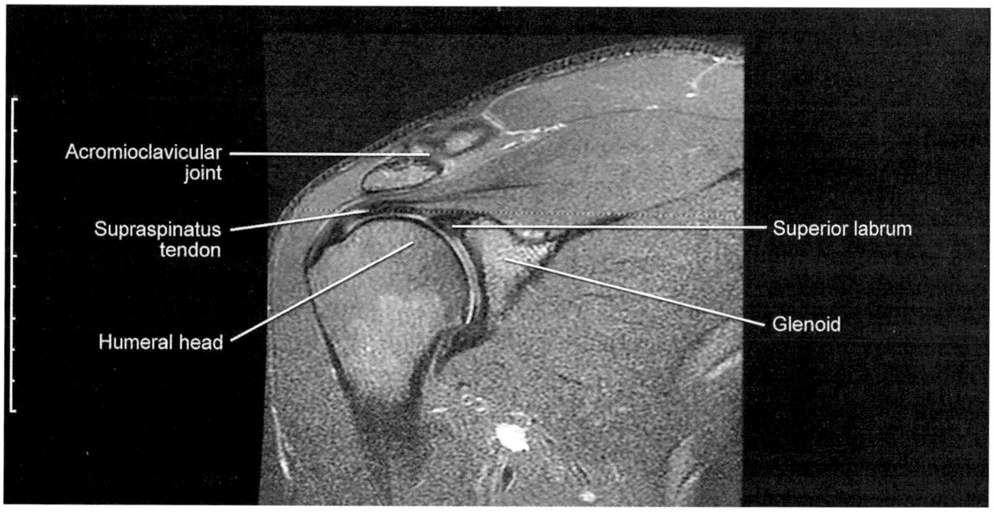

Fig. 26: Normal shoulder.

a sensitivity of 91% and a specificity of 93% for detection of pathological labral conditions.

Pitfalls

- The complex anatomy of the shoulder requires oblique imaging planes and surface-coil technique.
- In patients with large or chronic tears, the cuff may be so atrophied that its identification is impossible.
- In tendinosis or tendinopathy, T1W signal abnormalities may appear in the cuff that diminish or disappear on T2W images. Therefore, in the presence of theses artifacts rotator cuff tears should be diagnosed only if it appears in T2W images.
- In case of old injuries, an increased T2W signal represents healing granulation tissues and should not be confused with partial thickness tears, especially after surgery. But if after surgery large full thickness defects are seen filled with fluid they represent retears or failed repair.

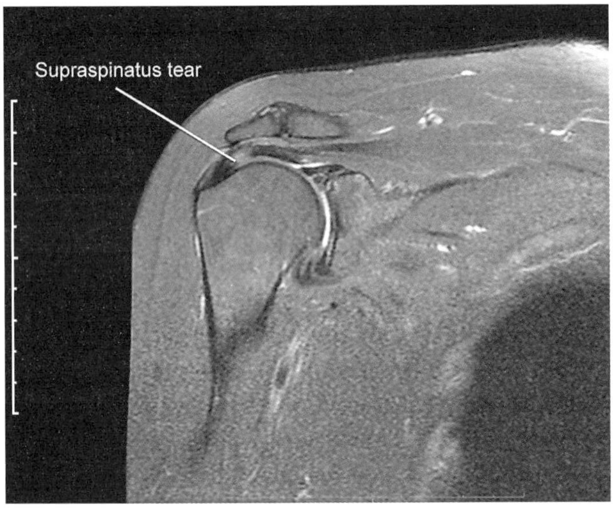

Fig. 27: Supraspinatus tear.

- Seen in cross-section the normal labrum shows many variations and the presence glenohumeral ligaments lead to diagnostic pitfalls.

SPINE

Indications

- Evaluation of intervertebral disk disease
- Evaluation of nerve roots, posterior longitudinal ligament, and intervertebral foramen
- Postoperative back pain (failed-back surgery)
- Discitis
- Pyogenic and tuberculous infections
- Epidural hematoma or abscess
- Primary and metastatic tumors of the vertebral column
- Spinal cord injury
- Spinal cord tumors (extradural and intradural)
- Abnormalities of thecal sac
- Developmental deformities of the spinal cord and vertebral column.

Magnetic resonance imaging of the spine is the most common examinations at most centers. Thoracic and lumbar spine studies can be done with conventional or phased array surface coils but the study of the cervical spine requires a contoured posterior neck coil or a flat "license plate" coil. Routine spinal examinations are done in axial and sagittal planes. Coronal images are needed in patients with scoliosis.

Magnetic resonance imaging of the spine is most commonly done for intervertebral disk disease. In patients with low back or sciatic pain, it is used to see the condition of intervertebral disks, nerve roots, spinal cord, posterior longitudinal ligament, and intervertebral foramen. The intervertebral disks and posterior longitudinal ligament are first seen in the sagittal plane. The normal disk appears as a hyperintense image on T2. This signal is lost as the disk loses its hydration and becomes desiccated. When the disk gets herniated or extruded it is seen as a mass protruding into the epidural space characterized by a signal that is similar to that of the disk **(Fig. 29)**. Because of the bright signal of CSF

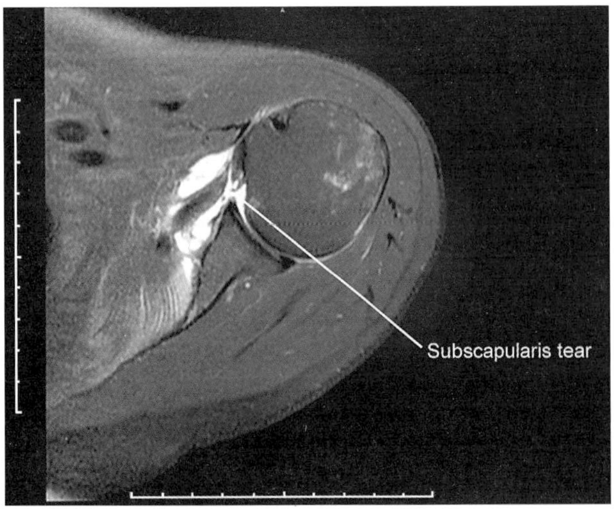

Fig. 28: Subscapularis tear.

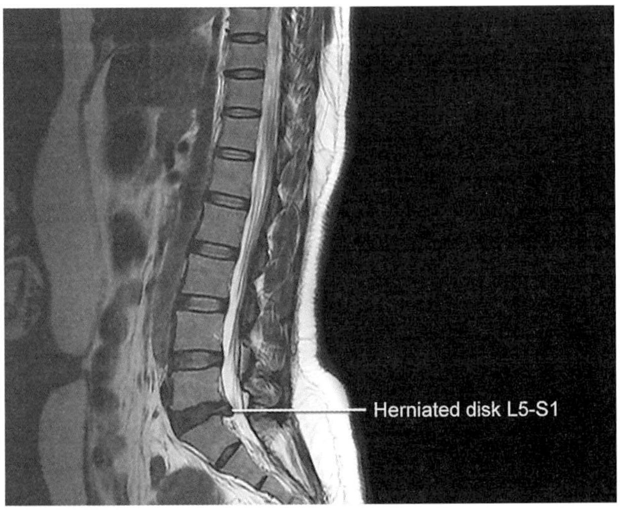

Fig. 29: Prolapsed intervertebral disk.

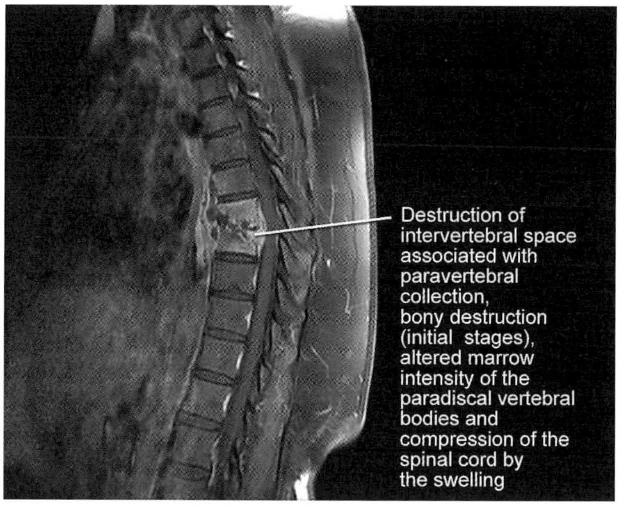

Fig. 30: Potts spine.

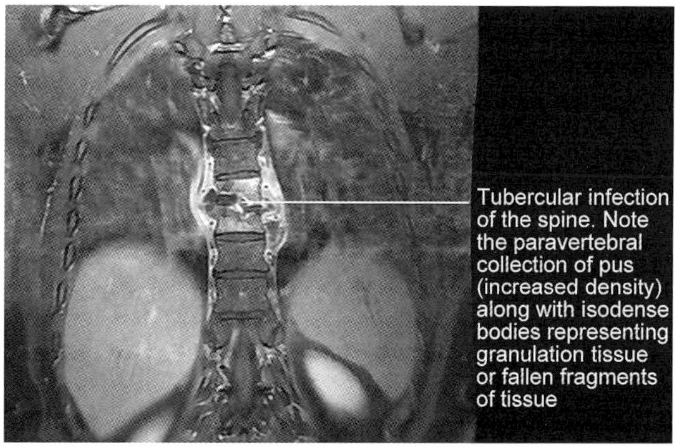

Fig. 31: Potts spine.

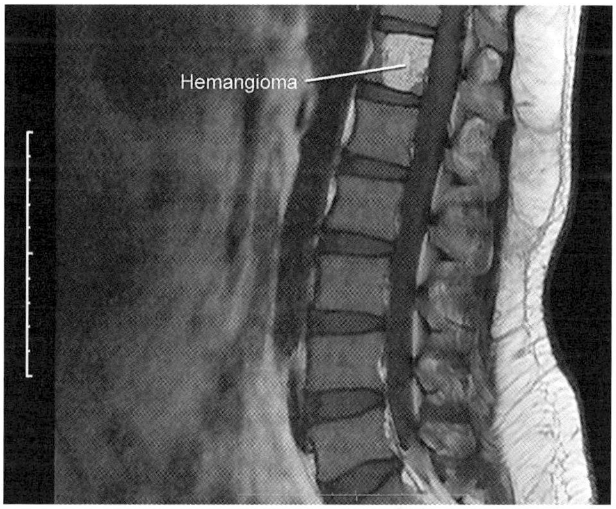

Fig. 32: Hemangioma.

on sagittal T2W a myelography like effect is created which is useful in evaluating compromise of the subarachnoid space. However, narrowing of the neuroforamina is best seen in sagittal T1W images where the bright fat signal in the foramina provides contrast to darker disk material. Lateral disk herniations are best seen on serial axial images, whereas superior and inferior migrated disk material is seen in sagittal and coronal sections. Free disk fragments are discontinuous from the intervertebral disk, and of intermediate T1W signal. Edema within the cord is seen with T2 weighting.

The following terminology is commonly used to describe the appearance of the disk on MRI. Bulge is a circumferential, symmetrical extension of the disk beyond the interspace. Protrusion is a focal or asymmetrical extension of the disk beyond the interspace, with the base broader than any other dimension of the protrusion. Extrusion is a more extreme extension of the disk base of which is narrower than the diameter of the extruding material itself. Sequestration is complete separation of fragment from disk of origin.

Magnetic resonance imaging evaluation of operated spine with intravenous gadolinium contrast agents helps to differentiate between recurrent or residual disk material and scar. After gadolinium administration T1W images show enhancement of scar or fibrosis. Epidural hematomas and abscesses appear as collections within the spinal canal **(Fig. 30)**. The disk material does not enhance with gadolinium on T1W images.

Postoperative discitis can be demonstrated by the triad of vertebral body endplate enhancement, disk space enhancement, and enhancement of the posterior longitudinal ligament after gadolinium contrast. But correlation with the erythrocyte sedimentation rate (ESR), gallium or tagged white blood cells (WBC) radionuclide imaging, and percutaneous aspiration is necessary.

In the lumbar spine, extension of infection into the adjacent psoas muscles is best demonstrated on axial T2W sequences because hyperintense fluid and edema contrast with the normal hypointense musculature even without contrast enhancement **(Fig. 31)**. MRI cannot distinguish between tubercular and pyogenic infection though subligamentous spread of infection with relative sparing of the intervertebral disk is suggestive of tuberculous infection.

Computed tomography is the preferred initial examination in trauma patients as it provides better visualization of the bony structures. MRI helps in evaluating spinal cord injury, epidural hematoma, or traumatic disk herniation. Soft tissue injuries, such as ligamentous tears, can be identified as discontinuity seen on sagittal T2W images. MRI is helpful in the exclusion of underlying pathological condition in nontraumatic compressed vertebrae. Preservation of normal marrow signal is suggestive a benign process, such as osteoporosis. Complete or incomplete marrow replacement with irregular marrow signal is suggestive of infection or metastasis. A follow-up MRI at 6–8 weeks shows reconstitution of normal marrow signal in osteoporotic fractures.

Both primary and metastatic diseases are seen on T1W sequences **(Figs. 32 and 33)**. Normal vertebral body marrow is well-delineated on T1W images. Its signal progressively increases with age because of higher percentage of fatty marrow. In anemia, there is higher percentage of hematopoietic marrow, thus diffusely diminishing this T1W signal.

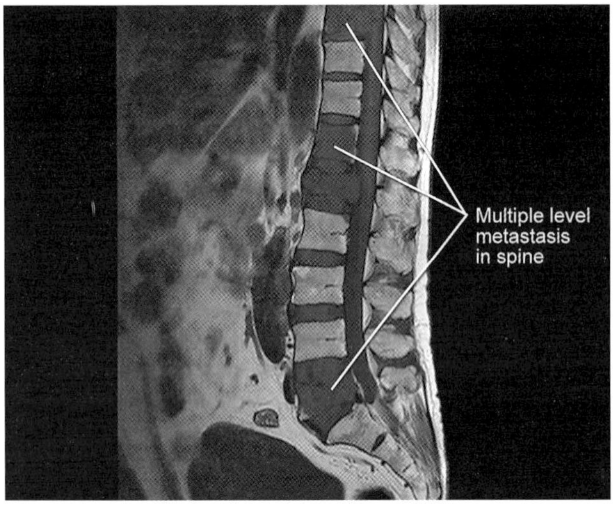

Fig. 33: Metastasis spine.

Vertebral tumor foci appear as discrete areas of diminished T1 signal.

Pitfalls

- The MRI appearance of degenerative disk disease is varied and must be correlated to clinical findings.
- In degenerative disease, vertebral endplate edema and even enhancement can occur in the absence of infection.
- Changes in the disk space and adjacent vertebral endplates are sometimes seen after surgery and can be confused with discitis.
- Neoplasms that diffusely involve vertebral marrow, such as multiple myeloma, are difficult to differentiate from hematopoietic marrow.

FOOT AND ANKLE

Indications

- Tendinopathy
- Articular disorders
- Osseous pathological conditions
- Avascular necrosis
- Fracture
- Osteochondral injuries
- Osteomyelitis
- Tendon injury
- Ligament injury.

Because of the small size of structures to be examined, best images are achieved on a high-field strength (>1.0 T) magnet, and the use of a surface coil. Images can be taken in standard or oblique planes, with combinations of T1W, T2W. and fat-suppressed sequences as per the pathology to be screened.

In chronic tendinitis, the tendons thicken and the enlarged tendon maintains low signal on all sequences. In a partial tear, the tendon shows focal or fusiform thickening with interspersed areas of edema or hemorrhage with bright signal on T2W series. In complete rupture, there is discontinuity of the tendon fibers. Increased fluid in the sheath of the tendon is suggestive of tenosynovitis. Morton neuroma is most often a clinical diagnosis based on the presence of pain on the plantar surface of the foot at this location. This is well-picked up on an MRI and lesion lacks increased signal on T2W sequences. This helps to differentiate it from other tumors.

In diabetic foot, MRI picks up very early marrow edema even before the onset of osteomyelitis. The extent and number of bones involved help to plan the treatment.

Pitfalls

- Though, the ligaments are well-visualized on MRI, the imaging status of ligaments about the ankle does not change the treatment in most patients.
- The sensitivity of MRI for osteomyelitis in foot approaches 100%, but the reported specificity is less.
- In patients with neuropathic disease, the specificity is reduced further because of vascular changes. Therefore, clinical examination and other laboratory test are required to diagnose osteomyelitis. A normal MRI marrow signal excludes osteomyelitis.

HIP

Indications

- Avascular necrosis
- Transient osteoporosis of the hip
- Occult fractures
- Evaluation of the acetabular labrum.

Study of both hips is performed with the main magnetic coil (body coil). This technique allows evaluation of both hips at once. For unilateral evaluation, improved resolution is obtained with the use of surface coils. Torso coils with phased-array design combine improved signal for high-resolution images with large field-of-view coverage. Commonly, spin-echo sequences are performed in axial and coronal planes. Sagittal images are needed while investigating AVN.

Avascular necrosis is the most frequent indication for hip imaging. Even when initial roentgenograms show normal images MRI may be positive for AVN. Between CT and MRI, MRI is more sensitive and better shows the area of necrosis. It also gives the exact location and percentage of involvement of the head which helps to predict the outcome after surgery. The normal fat signal of femoral head which is bright on T1W images is decreased in areas affected by AVN. The surrounding ischemic bone is seen as a low-signal band **(Figs. 34A and B)**. In T2 images, a second inner band of high intensity is seen, which is the "double line" sign diagnostic of AVN. The central area of necrotic bone shows signal patterns that vary through the course of the disease, depending on the degree of hemorrhage, fat, edema, or fibrosis. Flattening of the femoral head, cartilage loss, and effusion are seen in late cases.

Transient osteoporosis is a self-limited process of uncertain etiology related to reflex sympathetic dystrophy and regional migratory osteoporosis. Initial roentgenograms are normal with preservation of the joint space. MRI shows diffuse edema in the femoral head, extending into the intertrochanteric region. This is seen as a low signal area on

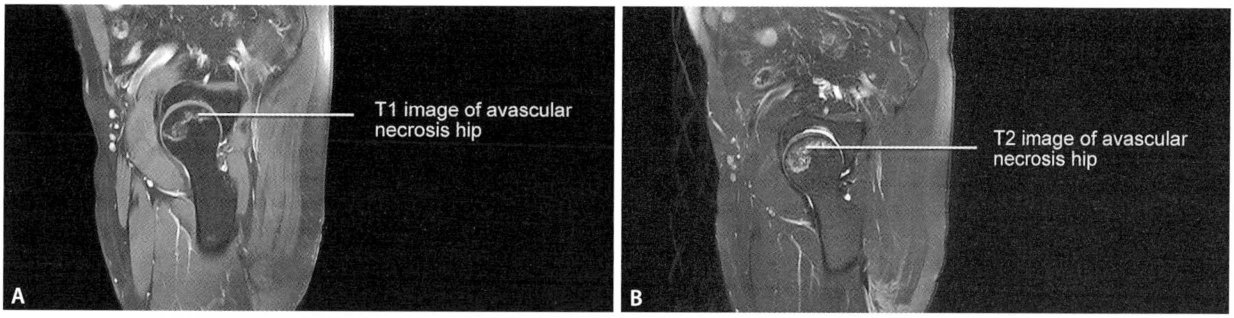

Figs. 34A and B: Avascular necrosis femoral head.

T1 when compared to the normal bone marrow, whereas on T2 it becomes hyperintense. This hyperintensity is further attenuated when fat suppression techniques are used. Focal signal abnormalities, as in AVN, are not present in transient osteoporosis. Sometimes a tiny focal, often linear lesion in the subcortical marrow in the weight-bearing portion of the femoral head may be seen representing insufficiency fracture in the demineralized bone. Transient osteoporosis of the hip generally resolves without treatment within 6 months, and the roentgenograms and MRI appearance return to normal.

Earlier bone scanning was being used to confirm or exclude occult fractures, but this study can be falsely negative in elderly patients in the first 48 hours after injury. The MRI changes are apparent immediately, with linear areas of low signal easily seen in the fatty marrow on T1W images, and surrounding edema seen with T2W images.

Pitfalls

- The pattern seen in transient osteoporosis sometimes may be seen in the earliest phase of AVN. Repeat films 6–8 weeks after the onset of symptoms may be required.
- Though, the advent of MRI arthrography of the hip has greatly improved visualization of the cartilaginous labrum, the geometry of the labrum of the hip displays a wide range of normal variation in asymptomatic individuals. The precise role of this technique in patients with mechanical hip pain is not clear and requires clinical correlation.

WRIST

The most common indication for MRI is evaluation of the intrinsic carpal ligaments and injuries to the triangular fibrocartilaginous complex. Tears in the TFC are seen as linear defects or gaps filled with hyperintense fluid on coronal gradient-echo or T2W pulse sequences. MRI assessment of the extrinsic carpal ligaments has little impact on treatment.

Magnetic resonance imaging has some role in the evaluation of carpal tunnel syndrome although this remains a clinical diagnosis. MRI can show masses within the confines of the carpal tunnel, as well as edema and swelling of the median nerve. MRI is used to detect marrow abnormalities seen in AVN of lunate in Kienböck disease or in the scaphoid after fracture. Like ankle, tenosynovitis and tendon injuries in the wrist and hand can be assessed.

TUMOR IMAGING

Good soft tissue contrast combined with detailed anatomy and multiplanar capability has placed MRI at the forefront of musculoskeletal tumor-imaging methods. MRI is most helpful in defining tumor extent and planning surgical and radiation therapy. It helps in defining aggressive versus indolent processes.

Magnetic resonance imaging examinations are performed after roentgenographic or clinical detection of a lesion. For small lesions (<20 cm), surface coil is used and for larger masses or lesions in the pelvis or thigh body coil or phased-array torso coil is used. The relation of the mass to the surrounding tissue like muscles and neurovascular structures and also the extraosseous extension of bone tumors is best visualized in the axial plane as this plane best shows the anatomy of various compartments. To assess the proximal and distal extent of the lesion the sagittal or coronal images are used. The extent of bone involvement is seen as bone marrow edema on T1W images. In T2W images, most tumors appear hyperintense when compared to surrounding soft tissue such as muscle and fat. Fat-suppression techniques further define smaller foci of tumor or edema. Differentiation between solid and cystic tumors and between active and necrotic tumors is done by contrast enhanced T1W images. With contrast active tumor, tumor edema and granulation tissue all become enhanced and cannot be differentiated. To help separate tumor from surrounding edema dynamic contrast enhancement is used. Routine use of contrast like gadolinium in the initial evaluation of neoplasm is not done. It is more useful in a patient who has undergone surgery to distinguish surgical scar from residual or recurrent tumor nodules. Vascular lesions can be studies with contrast using MRI angiography technique.

The differential diagnosis of bone tumors is derived from routine roentgenograms and later by biopsy and the role of MRI is to define the extent of disease. MRI has replaced CT for the assessment of skeletal tumors except for densely sclerotic lesions, such as osteoid osteoma. Most bone tumors are seen as areas of low or intermediate signal intensity on T1W sequences and high-signal intensity on T2W sequences. MRI reliably identifies the spatial boundaries of tumor masses, encasement and displacement of major neurovascular bundles and the extent of joint involvement. T1W spin-echo images enhance tumor contrast with bone, bone marrow, and fatty tissue and T2W spin-echo images enhance tumor contrast with muscle and accentuate peritumoral edema.

For most soft tissue lesions MRI is not diagnostic for any specific histology. Most soft tissue lesions present a nonspecific MRI appearance, typically isointense to muscle on T1W images and hyperintense to muscle and fat on T2W images. The diagnosis of soft tissue masses is more dependent on history, physical examination, and histopathology.

Certain lesions do exhibit specific signal patterns.

- Lipomas that arise from soft tissue have a homogeneous fat signal on all sequences. The subcutaneous fat makes lipomas in this plane difficult to see. Liposarcomas sometimes show areas of fat and nonfat signal.
- The presence of fat and flowing blood in hemangiomas make them exhibit bright signal on both T1W and T2W studies.
- Hemosiderin present in pigmented villonodular synovitis shows up as a T2W hypointensity.

ROLE OF ISOTOPE BONE SCAN AND PET SCAN IN ORTHOPEDICS

Modern day orthopedic practice demands adequate knowledge of the tools available to investigate a case. Apart from routine cross-sectional imagining, CT, and MRI, nuclear medicine plays a crucial role to provide sensitive functional information in a variety of clinical settings. It is also important for the orthopedic surgeon to be aware of the strengths and limitations of these techniques.

Isotope bone scan or "bone scintigraphy" is an investigative modality which uses radioisotope tagged tracers which are specifically taken up by the bone. These tracers are taken up in areas of increased bone turnover. These isotopes in the tracers undergo radioactive decay and give off gamma radiation. The radiation readings are taken using a gamma camera and the whole body is scanned at the same time. The detected abnormality may consist of decreased uptake (e.g., early stage of osteonecrosis) or increased uptake (e.g., fracture, neoplasm, and focus of osteomyelitis). Some structures under normal conditions may show increased activity (e.g., sacroiliac joints or normal growth plates).

Scintigraphy is the term used for imaging in two dimensions using radionuclides.

Single-photon emission computed tomography (SPECT) uses data collected from a gamma camera from multiple projections to create a 3D image.

Positron emission tomography (PET) is a functional imaging processes. Short half-life radionuclides such as carbon-11, nitrogen-13, oxygen-15, and rubidium-82 are used in PET scanning. They get attached to naturally occurring compounds in the body like glucose, water, ammonia, etc. Of these, the most commonly used molecule is fludeoxyglucose (FDG). It is an analog of glucose and gets selectively taken up in areas of high metabolic activity (see detailed discussion later).

HYBRID SCANNING TECHNIQUES

In hybrid scanning, an imaging modality like MRI or CT is combined with a nuclear scan to provide information on both anatomy and function. This is done either by using software for superimposing the images on each other or by using hybrid cameras. This is also called as image fusion or coregistration. Some examples of such hybrid scan would be SPECT/CT and PET/CT.

Indications

- Bone tumors both malignant and nonmalignant
- For diagnosing metastatic bone disease in cases of primary form breast, lung, or prostate
- *Avascular necrosis* of femoral head
- Infections
- Diagnosis of stress fracture
- Diseases of bone metabolism such as Paget's and osteomalacia
- Fracture of the spine to rule out pathological fracture
- Legg-Perthes disease and sacroiliitis.

Commonly used tracers in orthopedics:

- Technetium methylene diphosphonate (MDP)
- Thallium-201
- Gallium-67
- Indium labeled leukocyte scan.

TECHNETIUM 99 METHYLENE DIPHOSPHONATE

Technetium 99 MDP is the most commonly used scan. After injection of the tracer, the scan is performed in three stages (triphasic bone scan).

The flow phase is the first and consists of images captured 2–5 seconds after injection of isotope. It is indicative of the perfusion of the area and is also called a nuclear angiogram. The second image is captured after 5 minutes and is called the blood pool image. It is indicative of the vascularity of the area. Because the areas of inflammation have dilated blood vessels, such areas get highlighted in this phase. The last phase is the delayed phase and the image is captured 3 hours after the injection. It is indicative of the metabolic bone turnover of an area.

Scintigraphy is a sensitive imaging modality, but it lacks specificity. It is not possible to differentiate between various processes that can cause increased or decreased uptake. However, in some lesions the bone scan may yield very specific information and even suggest the diagnosis.

- In cases of myeloma, there is no significant increase in the uptake of the radiopharmaceutical, but in skeletal metastases, the uptake of the tracer is significantly elevated.
- In osteoid osteoma, there is more increased uptake in the center, due to the nidus and less increased uptake at the periphery, due to the reactive sclerosis surrounding the nidus.
- A three-phase technique can be used to differentiate soft tissue infection (cellulitis) and osseous infection (osteomyelitis).

Thallium-201

Thalium-201 is a potassium analog, and as it is selectively taken up by active tumor cells, its main use is in identifying tumor recurrence and metastatic lesions. It can also be used to identify prosthetic infection from prosthetic loosening in the case of joint replacement surgery.

Gallium-67

67-gallium-citrate is used to diagnose infectious processes in bone and joints. The sensitivity of 67Ga for abscess detection varies from 58 to 100% and specificity from 75 to 99%. The images are usually obtained 6 hours and 24 hours after the injection of 5 mCi. This modality is particularly useful in monitoring response to therapy of chronic osteomyelitis and infectious arthritis. A gallium scan is also used to differentiate sarcomas from benign soft tissue lesions.

Indium-labeled Leukocyte Scan

This technique is specific in the detection of abscesses or acute infectious processes, including osteomyelitis and septic arthritis. The sensitivity varies from 75 to 90% and specificity is approximately 91%. 111In-labeled leukocytes are not incorporated into areas of increased bone turnover; indium imaging reflects inflammatory activity only, thus helping to differentiate from bone reaction. False-negative results often occur for patients with chronic infections due to reduced inflow of circulating leukocytes. False-positive results are seen in patients with inflammatory process without infection (e.g., rheumatoid arthritis mistaken for septic arthritis).

POSITRON EMISSION TOMOGRAPHY AND ITS ROLE IN ORTHOPEDICS

The concept of PET-CT was first proposed by David Townsend and Ronald Hutt that led to production of the first prototype at university of Pittsburg medical center in 1998. It is a state of the art hybrid imaging technique which combines the strengths of structural and functional imaging namely PET-CT. A PET scanner is basically constructed of crystal rings of small scintillation detectors that capture coincidence pattern emerging from positron-electron annihilation. Crystals are made from high density, high atomic number materials such as Lutetium orthosilicate.

Principle: A positron (positrons are emitted from proton enriched nuclei) is a positively charged beta particle which cannot penetrate more than a few millimeters in tissues but when it collides with negatively charged electron, it annihilates and produces two high energy (511 keV) gamma rays that travel essentially in opposite directions. These annihilation patterns can be detected outside the body in a ring of detectors with in a PET scanner. The principle of PET is that radiation emitted from a radiopharmaceutical injected intravenously into a patient is registered by external detectors positioned at different orientations. The isotope distributes within different tissues according to the carrier molecule (isotopic labeling) and emits a positron (a positively charged electron). This positron in turn interacts with a free electron and an annihilation reaction occurs, resulting in the production of two 511-KeV photons emitted at almost 180° to each other.

Then, the distribution of radioactivity is estimated by (filtered) back projection methods. The directionality of the annihilation photons (two 511-keV annihilation photons emitted in opposite directions) provides a mechanism for localizing the origin of the photons and hence, the radioactive decay process that resulted in their emission.

Positron-emitting tracers: There are four positron emitting radiopharmaceuticals available for clinical use, viz. sodium fluoride (Na18F)—for osseous imaging, rubidium chloride (82RbCl)—for myocardial regional perfusion analysis, fluorine-18 deoxyglucose (18FDG)—to detect abnormal glucose metabolism and is the most widely used radiopharmaceutical, and ammonia (13NH). FDG is produced in a cyclotron. It has a half-life of 110 minutes. The most important 18F labeled radiopharmaceutical is 18F-2-fluoro-2-deoxy-glucose (18F-FDG or FDG), which is a nonphysiological analog of glucose. Some other radiotracers using F-18 are F-18-choline (useful in assessing bone metastases), F-18-miso (18) F-fluoromisonidazole] used in oncology to image tumor hypoxia for radiotherapy purpose.

The radiotracer is injected in the body and depending on the metabolic/physiological activity the tracer is accumulated at different sites. Functional imaging involves localizing the tracer activity which tells the metabolic and biochemical activity at the particular region. PET imaging will thus map the functional activity of living tissue; however, it will not be possible to localize it to body parts until we can image the anatomy. This is the reason why CT scanning is simultaneously done. So in effect we have a PET scanner coupled to CT or MR scanner that coregisters the image giving us detailed anatomical location of metabolic differences that can be deciphered further. Newer integrated PET/CT and PET/MR scanners are available worldwide. The diagnostic advantages of a PET-CT involve a CT scan of fairly low radiation dose which is adequate for providing anatomical localization of PET positive functional abnormalities. PET-MR scanners are now available for superior soft tissue discrimination possible with MRI.

Clinical Indications in Orthopedics

Infections

Spinal infections: FDG-PET is superior to MRI for detecting low-grade spondylitis or discitis and is used in association with MRI for differentiating degenerative changes from infections. PET clearly out performs Tc-99m bone and Ga67 imaging. Limitations of FDG-PET are differentiation between infection and tumor.

Diabetic foot infections: Uninfected neuropathic joints show relatively low maximum standardized uptake value. FDG-PET can differentiate osteomyelitis, soft tissue infection from neuropathic disease.

Prosthetic joint infections: Differentiating aseptic loosening from infection is possible with FDG-PET. The correct diagnosis depends on location, pattern, and intensity of perprosthetic uptake.

Tumors

An FDG-PET has an overwhelming role in the evaluation of skeletal metastasis disease **(Fig. 35)**. FDG accumulation in skeletal lesions detect direct uptake by the tumor (increased activity on conventional bone scans reflects new bone formation in response to destruction of bone by tumor).

- Successful treatment assessment on FDG-PET is reflected by decrease in or disappearance of the abnormal uptake. "Burnt out" malignant bone lesion may remain abnormal on CT component of PET-CT but will not demonstrate increased FDG accumulation.
- Advantage of detecting extraskeletal disease remains with PET-CT. PET-CT is more sensitive for detecting bone marrow and lytic lesions than sclerotic lesions.
- FDG-PET is more sensitive than conventional bone scintigraphy for detection of bone metastasis of breast carcinoma, non-small cell lung carcinoma, and lymphoma.
- FDG-PET has a limited role in patients with prostatic carcinoma where F-18 choline may bed preferred.
- Role of FDG-PET in imaging algorithm of primary musculoskeletal malignancies is also limited. It is also not possible to differentiate between benign and malignant lesion. It is useful for monitoring response to neoadjuvant chemotherapy. Accuracy of FDG-PET is affected by therapy. Performing the study within <2 weeks after chemotherapy may result in decreased sensitivity because of metabolic shutdown of tumor cells. Irradiated bone behaves variably and may show increase normal or decrease in activity depending on the time interval between therapy and imaging.
- Treatment with colony-stimulating factors may induce increase FDG uptake in the bone marrow which can mask malignant infiltration or can be misinterpreted as disease.

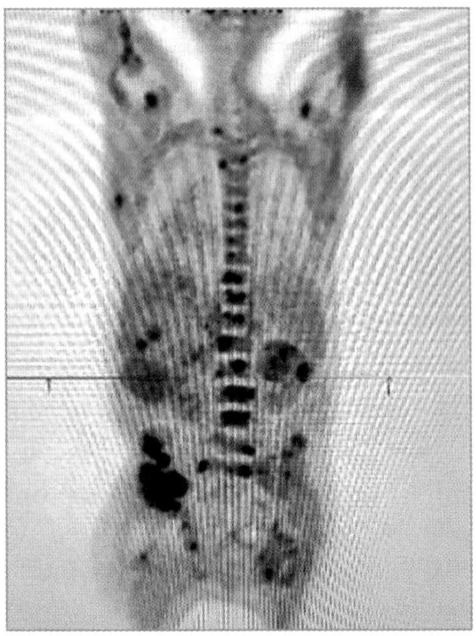

Fig. 35: Coronal positron emission tomography (PET) scan image shows multiple metastatic deposits in bone.

RADIATION HAZARD AND PERSONNEL SAFETY

Radiation hazard in inherent to orthopedic surgeries as the use of fluoroscopy has become a common place. Most of the osteosyntheses for trauma and some planned reconstructions need fluoroscopy assistance to better implant placement and improve anatomy. Fluoroscopy uses X-rays so radiation exposure for the surgeon and staff will be imperative. Certain orthopedic procedures are associated with higher radiation doses; these include open reduction and internal fixation (ORIF) of hip fractures, femoral and tibial intramedullary nailing, and spinal cases. The X-rays passing through the patient interact with bone and soft tissue within the patient resulting in different patterns of X-ray distribution. X-rays are also deflected during the penetration and continue on with lower energy. This pattern of deflection, or scatter, produces a field of radiation that is responsible for the incidental radiation exposure to the surrounding staff.

RADIATION HAZARD

Radiation damage occurs at the cellular level in living tissues. Rapidly replicating cell components such as deoxyribonucleic acid (DNA) and cell membranes are the most susceptible to damage from radiation. This may occur by both direct and indirect mechanisms. Direct damage occurs as energy is absorbed and molecular bonds are broken resulting in cell death or mutations which are the initial step in radiation-induced carcinogenesis. Indirect damage results from ionization of water molecules generating free radicals that disrupt bonds and commonly result into long-term effects of radiation. The thyroid, eyes, hands, and gonads are among the most sensitive organs to radiation exposure. The eyes may exhibit the first effects of chronic radiation exposure in the form of cataracts. 85% of papillary carcinomas of the thyroid are thought to be radiation induced. A surgeon's hands have the greatest exposure risk due to their constant proximity to the radiation beam. Due to these risks, the International Commission on Radiological Protection established dosage limits for radiation exposure. The maximum annual dose limit is 20 mSv for the body, 150 mSv for the thyroid and eyes, and 500 mSv for the hands.

Radiation damage can have deterministic and stochastic effects. Deterministic effects of radiation have a clear relationship between the exposure and the effect. These typically result when very large dosages are received in a short amount of time. The effects are characterized by nonlinear dose responses, with a threshold dose below which the effect is not observed. These effects arise within a few days and may manifest over years. Examples of deterministic effects include erythema, skin and tissue burns, cataract formation, sterility, radiation sickness, and death. Below a certain threshold of exposure there is no increased risk of radiation-induced effects such as cancer or genetic mutation. The deterministic effects can be avoided if the limits are not exceeded. Stochastic effects are those that are expected to occur in populations exposed to ionizing radiation. These effects have no threshold dose and often show up years after exposure, the assumption being that damage from radiation is cumulative over a lifetime.

As the thickness of an area being imaged increases, more X-ray beams will be required in order to achieve an image of similar quality. Therefore, as the size of a patient increases, the dose to the patient's skin and amount of scatter increases as well. Continuous or live fluoroscopy obtains about 30 images per second, which increases the amount of radiation exposure. Pulsed fluoroscopy obtains one to six images per second, which lowers the amount of radiation exposure.

Magnification of the image also greatly increases the dose to both the patient and surgeon, and should be used only when necessary.

METHODS TO REDUCE RADIATION EXPOSURE

Principles

The benefit of obtaining imaging must exceed all risks to the patient and operating room personnel, including radiation exposure.

1. The three basic factors that determine the safety are the time, distance, and shielding. In simple terms; reduce the exposure time, increase the distance from the source, and use appropriate shielding.
2. The as low as reasonably achievable (ALARA) principle refers to reducing the amount of radiation delivered without compromising the integrity of imaging.
3. Radiation should be limited to the permissible radiation exposure limits as prescribed (see above).
4. ***Personal protective equipment (PPE):*** PPE contains lead or similar lightweight materials that attenuate scattered X-rays. There are multiple designs of PPE that may be worn by operating room personnel. Aprons may be one-piece front shielding or offer 360° coverage. A lead-equivalent thickness of at least 0.5 mm is typically required, which attenuates over 95% of scattered X-rays that strike it. Lead aprons must be inspected annually for damage that may cause X-rays to pass through. This may include cracks from improper folding or storage. Another important piece of PPE is thyroid shields.

Image Intensifier

- Keep it as close as possible to reduce the scattering, to reduce the patient dosage and to obtain a larger field of view.
- Personnel should stand on the side of image intensifier to reduce exposure to scatter rays. Laser targeting, floor and draping landmarks, adjusting the size of the aperture, and manipulation of the X-ray beam all reduce the radiation exposure.
- The mini C-arm substantially reduces overall radiation exposure to the surgeon, but may increase dosage to the hands as they can be in the direct path of the X-ray beam.
- An understanding of the terminology used and the ability to effectively communicate with the C-arm technician must be present in order to decrease exposure, reduce frustration and conflict, and avoid wasting valuable operating room time.

Technique

- Use the lowest mA and as large a kVp as possible. Larger kVp increases the penetrability of beam allowing the use of a lower mA.
- Reduce the exposure time to the minimum.
- Use pulse mode than continuous mode.
- When using pulse mode, use a lowest frequency possible.
- Reduce the magnification to the minimum. Dose increases at the rate of square of magnification.

Personnel and Personal Protective Equipment

- Use protective aprons, thyroid shields, and lead goggles. Protective eyewear is commonly used in interventional radiology and is becoming more commonplace in orthopedics. The lens of the eye is a radiosensitive anatomic structure and must be protected from scatter. Leaded eyewear should include lateral protection, as the eyes are susceptible to backscatter from the head and direct scatter when the head is turned. The hands have the greatest exposure to direct radiation during surgical procedures and are the most difficult to protect. Sterile protective gloves are available; however, they do not offer nearly as much protection as aprons or thyroid shields. Hands should not be placed directly in the beam when at all possible. The use of a Kocher forceps or other surgical tool to aid with positioning may help reduce exposure of the hands when obtaining images. Protective gloves should have at least a 0.25 mm Pb equivalency. But remember that these gloves do not protect the hands if placed within the primary beam.
- Exposure from a radiation source decreases by the inverse of the distance squared. Hence, stay as far away as possible from the X-ray source. The X-ray source should be kept as far away from the patient as possible. This is also the reason for keeping the gun beneath the patient to increase the distance from radiosensitive parts.
- Stand on the side of image intensifier as far as possible.
- Use dose monitors.

CONCLUSION

- Use of USG in orthopedic practice is not typical and is under evolution with newer findings constantly introduced in the literature.
- Various pathologies that involve the soft tissue can be amicably diagnosed and evaluated by the sonography, but it is highly user dependent and has steep learning curve.
- Therapeutic use of sonography is controversial and has been favored in specific circumstances but is at best supportive only.
- Future of sonography appears bright; however, with better delineation of the pathologies and greater description the modality is expected to come in the mainstream of diagnostic armamentarium.
- The advent of MRI, its advancements, and acceptance for deemed patient care particularly with respect to diagnosis, clarification of identified pathologies on radiographs, and discerning occult lesions in doubtful cases is beyond question.
- MRI is of particular importance in imaging of spine and neoplasia and some large joints such as knee, shoulder,

and hip where in certain pathologies it can even be diagnostic in itself.

- The imaging modality should be, however, rationally prescribed supported by good clinical evidence and egalitarian thought process.
- With the future bringing advances both in equipment and tracers, nuclear medicine tests providing physiological evaluation can be invaluable. We can expect exponential growth in this field and its applications. Keeping in touch with technology will be necessary to make successful clinicians in future.
- The practice of modern orthopedics is closely associated with various devices that involve variable radiation emission.
- The hazards of ionizing radiation are often neglected and there is callous attitude among the healthcare providers. This predisposes to possible severe complications including development of neoplasia.
- The healthcare workers and providers should be educated and encouraged to follow the relevant practices to minimize radiation exposure risks through use of PPE, vigilance, and regular optimization of the devices emitting radiation.

SECTION 4

Surgical and Medical Complications in Orthopedics

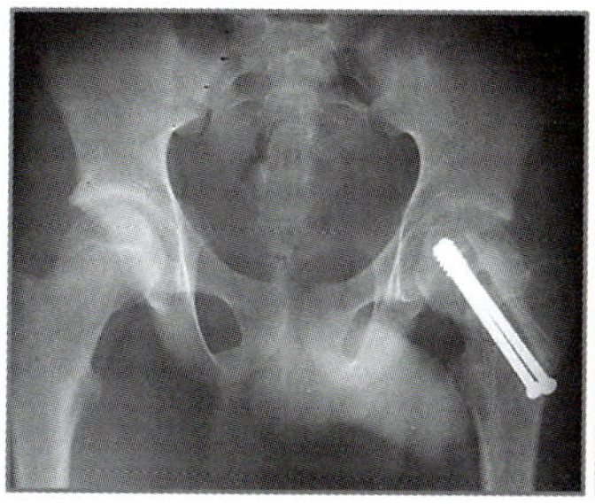

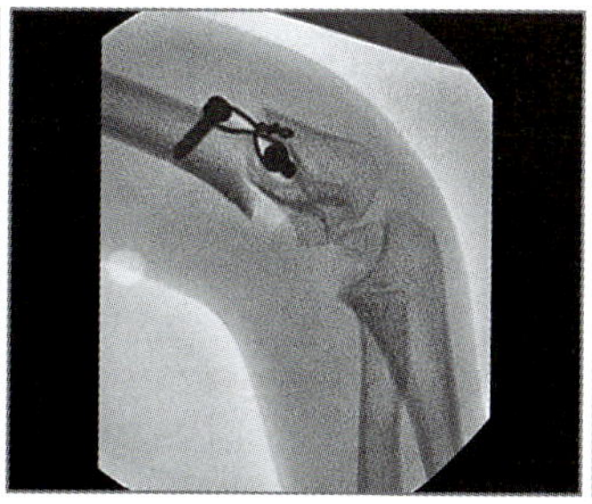

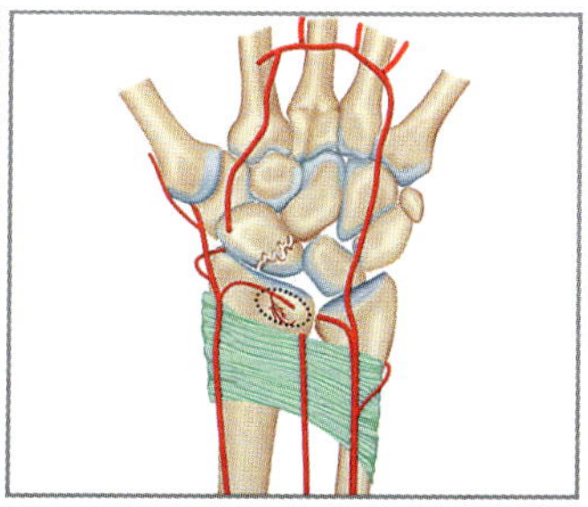

CHAPTER 26

Venous Thromboembolism Prophylaxis and Treatment

Manish Kumar Varshney, Jaydip Patel

INTRODUCTION

Venous thromboembolism (VTE) includes two different clinical entities: (1) deep vein thrombosis (DVT) and (2) pulmonary embolism (PE). The risk for development of DVT and PE increases to a 100-fold in the hospitalized patients. Fatal PE occurs in about quarter of a percent ranging from 0.25 to 0.3%. Orthopedic patients are at high risk due to immobility and direct manipulation of veins in long procedures and hence understanding the disease process, its pathogenesis, prevention, and treatment are paramount to prevent ensuing morbidity and mortality **(see Concept Box)**. Furthermore, it is important to borne in mind the post-thrombotic syndrome (PTS) and chronic venous stasis that may result from inadequate treatment as against to likelihood of bleeding complications that may result from overaggressive treatment.

DEFINITIONS

- ***Deep vein thrombosis:*** It is the presence of coagulated blood or thrombus (obstructing or nonobstructing) in one of the deep venous conduits that return blood to the heart. It occurs most commonly in lower limb veins (distal) or pelvic veins (proximal VTE), but it can occur in other parts of the body also like the arm.
- In ***pulmonary embolism***, some or all of the thrombus becomes detached and moves from the vein through the right side of the heart to lodge in one or more pulmonary arteries.
- ***Acute onset VTE:*** It pertains to sudden and fresh onset of *clinical symptoms* like dyspnea, syncope, pleuritic chest pain in the presence of leg swelling and/or *ultrasound correlation* (vein larger and wider than normal that is not compressible, presence of low-density echogenic thrombus) or *laboratory correlation* (presence of high level of serum D-dimer levels).
- ***Subacute VTE:*** It is labeled when the ultrasound findings suggest a thrombus of intermediate echogenicity with maintained diameter of vein and a D-dimer level that is not extremely high.
- ***Chronic VTE:*** It is defined when one finds chronic venous stasis changes in skin in the presence of chronic leg edema. Ultrasound demonstrates narrowing of vein with thickening of wall and an echogenic thrombus that is adherent to the vessel wall. Venous collaterals commonly develop in this setting and the findings are confirmed on a computed tomography (CT) scan that may additionally show increased bronchial arterial flow in lungs.
- ***Main lobar, segmental or subsegmental PE:*** This defines the anatomical location of enlodgement of migrates embolus into pulmonary arterial system where it can lodge in left or right lobe main artery, segmental arteries or smaller subsegmental branches.

CONCEPT BOX FOR VENOUS THROMBOEMBOLISM

- VTE is an important quality measure for healthcare and is now publically reported.
- DVT and PE are two distinct entities and can occur independently and the terms should be used very carefully. PE can arise even from atrial thrombus in the absence of DVT.!
- Mere occurrence of DVT is not a catastrophe but can lead to serious complications if ignored.
- Immobilized patients and those undergoing major orthopedic surgeries are at an elevated risk for development of DVT.
- Classically taught signs to evaluate DVT (calf tenderness, Homans' sign, swelling, raised temperature, etc.) are very inaccurate and nonspecific. One should instead rely clinically more on newly developed criteria that has better objective relevance.
- Oral anticoagulants have become popular and are now preferred for treatment and prophylaxis of DVT and PE.

HISTORY

First observed by Schenk in 1644, the association between venous thrombosis in the legs and PE was recognized by Virchow in 1846. According to Virchow, for development of VTE, three critically important factors are required **(Fig. 1)**. "The Virchow's triad":

1. *Venous stasis:* Venous stasis (viz., bedridden patient, paralytic patient, etc.) results in an increase in viscosity and the formation of microthrombi which eventually develop into thrombus. Historically Charnley et al. reported very high incidence (3.2%) of fatal PE after total hip arthroplasty (THA); now reasoned to prolonged immobilization (14 days) prevalent at that time.

2. *Activation of blood coagulation:* A hypercoagulable state can occur due to an increase in circulating tissue activation factor, combined with a decrease in circulating plasma antithrombin and fibrinolysins. This may arise from genetic factors (factor V Leiden, protein C or S deficiency), associated disorders [viz., active cancer (pancreatic commonly), renal insufficiency or heart failure], development or presence of complications like sepsis or active infection/inflammation.
3. *Vein damage:* Most commonly due to endothelial (intimal) damage in the blood vessel that may be intrinsic or secondary to external trauma.

EPIDEMIOLOGY

- *Annual incidence:* 80 cases/100,000 population.
- Around 25% of the cases that develop DVT are complicated by PE.
- Most common venous thrombosis is lower extremity DVT (LEDVT) which has prevalence of 1 case/1,000 population.

With improvement in surgical techniques, the incidence of VTE has reduced to 4.3% (2.8% DVT, 1.5% PE) as is seen since 2003. Fatal PE has incidence of 0.25–0.3%.

- Deep venous thrombosis usually affects individuals older than 40 years.
- The male-to-female ratio is 1.2:1. Females have 50% lower risk of recurrent VTE.
- Asian and Hispanic populations have lower risk of VTE, whereas whites and blacks have a higher risk (2.5–4 times higher).

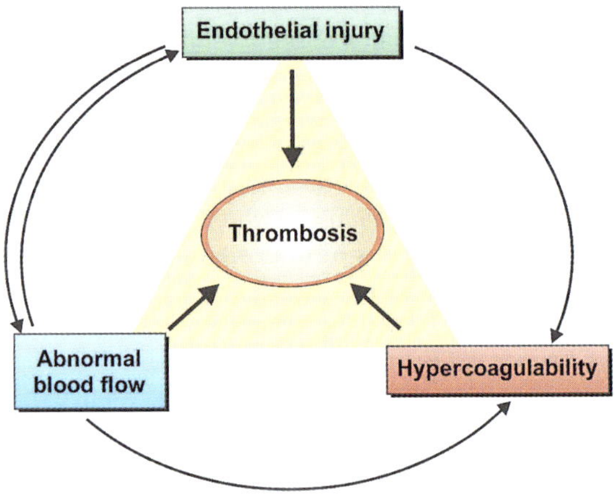

Fig. 1: Virchow's triad.

ANATOMY AND PATHOPHYSIOLOGY

The peripheral venous system has two main functions:
1. It acts as a reservoir to hold extra blood.
2. It acts as a conduit to return blood from the periphery to the central circulation.

The venous system directs blood toward heart through a complex series of valves and pumps. This system is divided into two primary groups of physiologically and anatomically distinct groups:
- Suprafascial (superficial venous system) veins are the primary collecting veins of the lower extremity. They are distensible and dilate to accommodate large volumes of extra blood with little increase in pressure.
- Subfascial (deep venous system) veins have thicker walls that receive inflow from the superficial system.

In lower limb, two separate systems make the deep venous system **(Figs. 2A and B)**:
1. Above the knee
2. Below the knee

In calf, there are three groups of deep veins. These veins are important for the muscle pump function:
1. The anterior tibial veins, which drain the dorsal aspect of the foot.

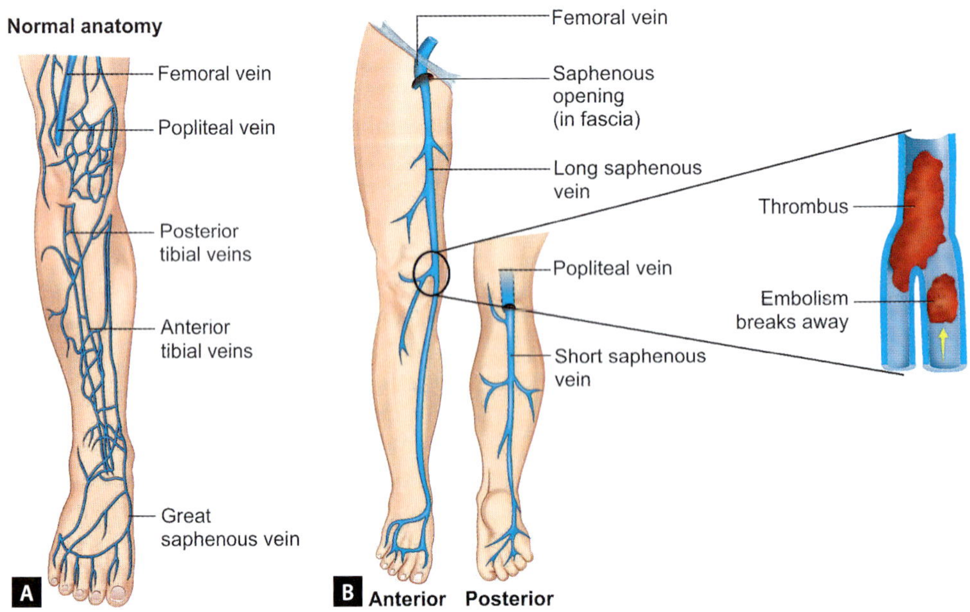

Figs. 2A and B: Elementary anatomy of (A) venous system and (B) venous thrombosis.

2. The posterior tibial veins, which drain the sole of the foot.
3. The peroneal veins, which drain the lateral aspect of the foot.

Together, the calf's muscles and deep vein system are also known as the "peripheral heart" that functions to push blood upward from the feet against gravity.

- With contraction of the calf, proximal migration of the blood occurs due to closure of the feeding perforator vein valves and opening of the outflow valves.
- With relaxation of the calf, superficial venous system refills the veins and sinusoids via perforating veins, and there is closure of outflow valves, resulting in prevention of retrograde flow.
- One contraction of calf drives 40–60% of calf's venous volume proximally.

DEVELOPMENT OF THROMBOSIS AND BALANCING MECHANISMS

There is a well-coordinated mechanism of solidifying the blood (thrombosis) at places of need (as in traumatic leaks from vascular system) in the form of "clot" and then liquefying again when the process is over or no more needed. Thrombosis is the hemostatic mechanism whereby blood coagulates or clots. It may be initiated via several pathways of which the two most common physiological pathways **(Fig. 3)** are:

1. An intrinsic system
2. An extrinsic system

Mechanical injury or trauma causes release of tissue lipoprotein activating the extrinsic pathway of coagulation. The intrinsic pathway is generally activated by circulating plasma factors. The terminal result of both these pathways amalgamates into transformation of fibrinogen to a fibrin clot. Contrary to the above complex process of thrombosis, fibrinolysis **(Fig. 3)**, by lysing the fibrin deposit restores the normal blood flow as soon as fibrin clot completes its function. To prevent inadvertent activation of the clotting process, three anticoagulant mechanisms **(Figs. 3 and 4)** operate with interdependence.

1. Protein C and thrombomodulin protein S system
2. The heparin-antithrombin III (ATIII) system
3. The tissue factor inhibition pathways

These processes physiologically balance each other in a fine tuned system that promote and retard coagulation as needed. Any disturbance in this equilibrium would result in the excessive coagulation or hemorrhage.

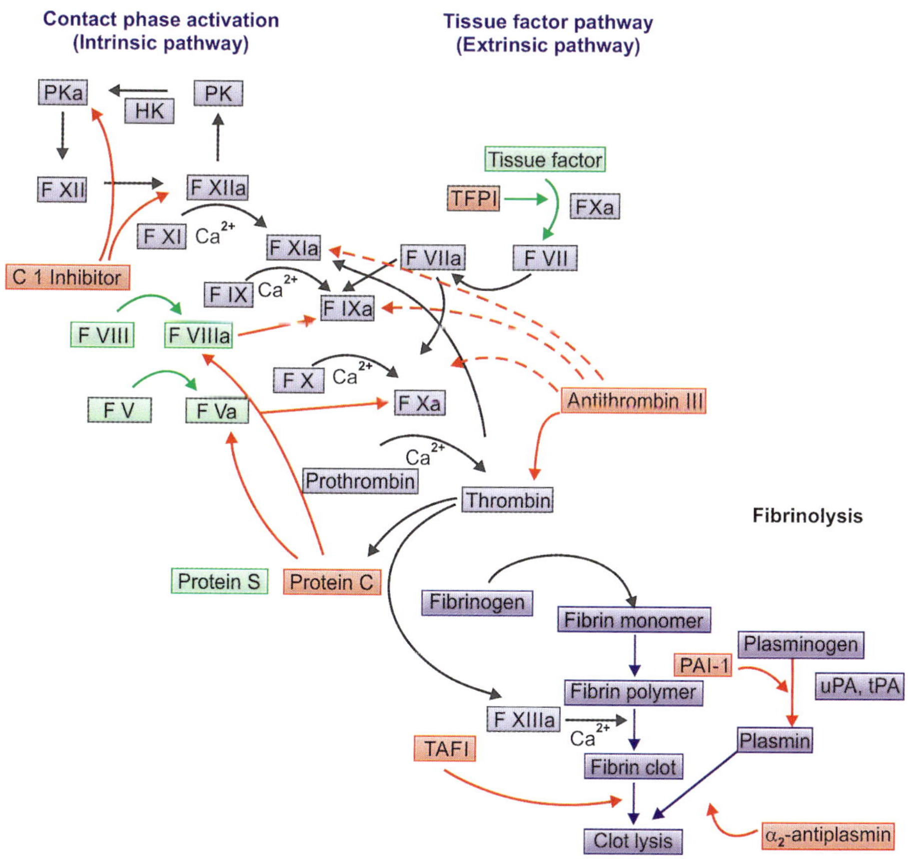

Fig. 3: Thrombosis and anticoagulation (regulatory) mechanisms: the coagulation cascade is divided into an intrinsic and an extrinsic pathway. The fibrinolytic pathway is shown at the lower aspect of figure. Suffix "a" denotes activated coagulation factors. Green boxes denote cofactors while red boxes denote coagulation inhibitors. (F: factor; HK: high-molecular-weight; PAI-1: plasminogen activator inhibitor 1; PK: plasma kallikrein; TAFI: thrombin-activatable fibrinolysis inhibitor; TFPI: tissue factor pathway inhibitor; tPA: tissue plasminogen activator; uPA: urokinase-type plasminogen activator)

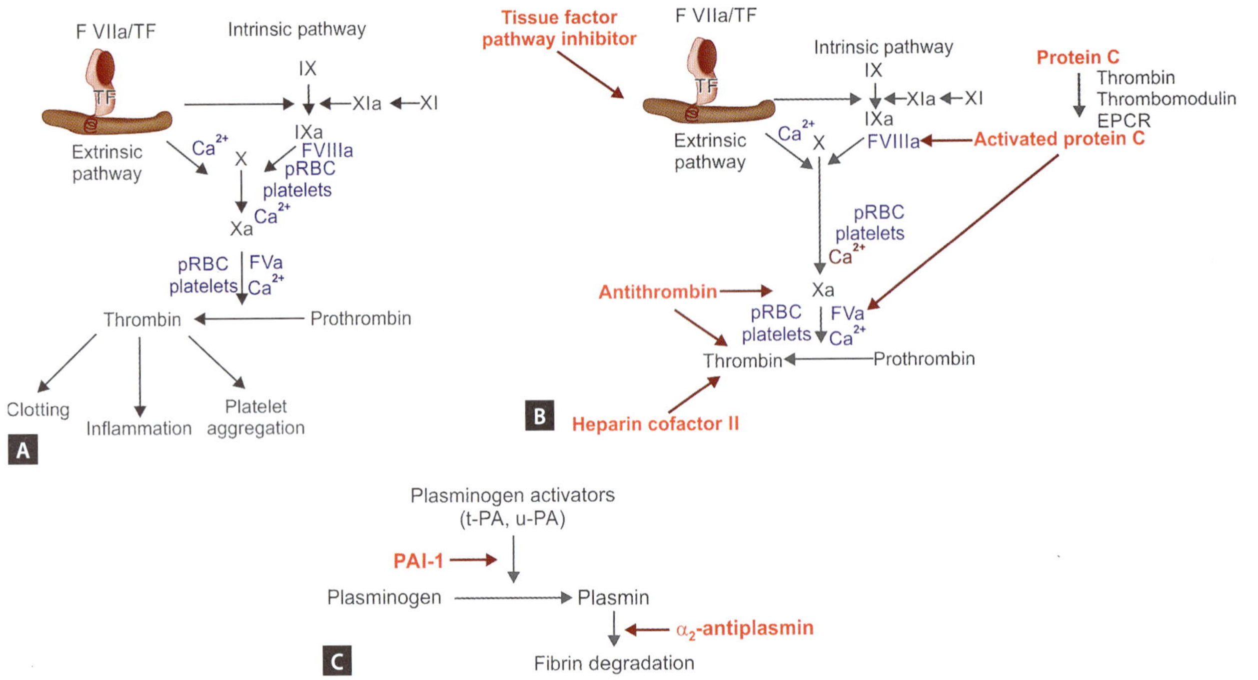

Figs. 4A to C: Summary of (A) procoagulant, (B) anticoagulant, and (C) antifibrinolytic mechanisms.

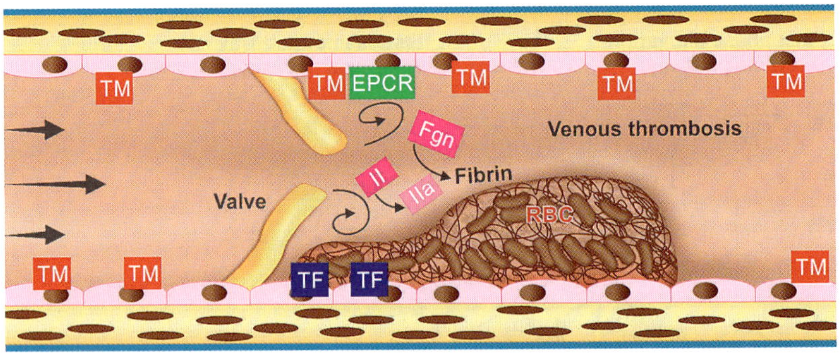

Fig. 5: Development of venous thrombus. The venous thrombosis usually begins behind the valves (see further steps in text). (TM: thrombomodulin; EPCR: endothelial protein C receptor; II: prothrombin; IIa: thrombin; TF: tissue-derived factor; Fgn: fibrinogen; RBC: red blood cells)

PATHOGENESIS OF DEEP VENOUS THROMBOSIS: THE TILT OF BALANCE OF THROMBOSIS

The process of DVT involves distinct processes of thrombus formation and consecutive venous insufficiency, as is detailed for lower limb here.

Evolution of Thrombus (Fig. 5)

- The formation of thrombus usually begins in the calf behind valve cusps or at venous branch points.
- With venodilation, the endothelial cell barrier is disrupted and exposure of the subendothelium occurs.
- Von Willebrand factor or fibrinogen in the vessel wall helps platelets adhere to the subendothelial surface defects.
- Inflammation (due to tissue handling/injury/infection) additionally activates neutrophils and platelets to release procoagulant and inflammatory mediators leading to hypercoagulation and formation of thrombus by the intrinsic pathway.
- The thrombus then migrates proximally along the deep veins due to stasis and activated coagulation pathway, sometimes reaching even the vena cava or right atrium!

Location of Deep Venous Thrombosis

Deep venous thrombosis can occur in any deep venous system but the following are clinically important:

- *Distal DVT:* The clot forms in one or all of the three vessel systems or muscular veins (gastrocnemius and soleus). The clot may propagate or migrate in 23% cases or more commonly resolve without complications. These are less likely to cause PE and hence are one of the benign categories (it is important to note here that Homans' sign or calf pain on foot dorsiflexion assess calf DVT that is actually by itself not much clinically concerning, though in one-fourth of the cases one is likely to catch proximal DVT if the thrombus propagates).

- *Proximal DVT:* The thrombus forms in popliteal vein or higher (femoral, iliac, vena cava veins). The classic presentation of this "isolated" thrombosis site is "phlegmasia cerulea dolens"—painful, swollen blue limb. The characteristic is absent if calf DVT migrates proximally. The condition is more common in left side and in those having femoral lines.
- *Upper extremity DVT (UEDVT):* Most commonly this is due to central venous catheterization. PE may occur in up to 12% cases. Proximal UEDVT is thrombus formation in brachial, axillary, subclavian, brachiocephalic/innominate veins, and superior vena cava (SVC). Distal DVT here is uncommon and is commonly superficial thrombophlebitis.
- *Pelvic vein thrombosis:* This is uncommon but may be devastating. It is commonly missed by the duplex ultrasound and is the site for large friable thrombi that have easy direct access to central venous circulation often causing massive embolism by clogging one of the main pulmonary vessels.
    - *Superficial DVT:* The clot forms in any vein located just under the skin such as lesser saphenous, greater saphenous, basilic, cephalic, and external jugular.
    - *Portomesenteric DVT:* Not of much orthopedic significance.
    - *Cerebral sinus DVT:* The clot forms in sagittal, transverse, sigmoid, or cavernous sinus.

ETIOLOGY AND RISK FACTORS FOR DEEP VEIN THROMBOSIS

Deep vein thrombosis may arise from various factors. Generally, the association of etiology of DVT can be categorized into following causalities:

- *Provoked VTE:* The DVT and/or PE occurs in high-risk setting such as orthopedic surgery of pelvis or lower extremity within previous 3 months, abdominal surgery within preceding 3 months, pregnancy within 6 weeks, trauma or injury with immobilization in previous 3 months or medical hospitalization with variable mobilization within 30–60 days.
- *Idiopathic (unprovoked) VTE:* It occurs in absence of risk factors. It is notable here that prolonged vehicle or plane trip are *not* considered as provocation.
- *Cancer associated:* Cancer is a special category where occurrence of VTE is common especially adenocarcinomas and metastatic disease.

Risk factors which contribute to DVT can be categorized as acquired (e.g., medication, illness) or congenital (e.g., anatomic variant, enzyme deficiency, mutation).

A summary of risk factors is as follows:

- ***Acquired includes:***
    - *Previous DVT:* The single most powerful risk marker (25% patients)
    - Age (the annual incidence of VTE rises with each decade over the age of forty)
    - Obesity
    - Immobilization longer than 3 days
    - Major surgery (especially orthopedic) lasting >2 hours in previous 4 weeks
    - Long plane or car trips (>4 hours) in previous 4 weeks
    - *Mass effect on iliac veins:*
        - Cancer
        - Pregnancy
        - Congenital anomaly
    - Stroke
    - Postpartum period
    - Acute myocardial infarction (AMI)
    - Congestive heart failure (CHF)
    - Sepsis
    - Nephrotic syndrome
    - Ulcerative colitis
    - Multiple trauma
    - Burns
    - *Trauma:* Endothelial injury can convert the normally antithrombogenic endothelium to become prothrombotic:
        - Central nervous system (CNS)/spinal cord injury: Abbreviated Injury Scale (AIS) ≥ head/neck:
            - Mechanical injury to veins: Lower extremity fractures—multiple long bone fractures (≥3)
            - Severe pelvic fracture (posterior elements) + long bone fracture
            - The Glasgow Coma Scale (GCS) ≤ 8
            - Injury Severity Score (ISS) ≥ 15
            - Hip and knee arthroplasty (manipulation of nearby major veins)
            - Inflammation-induced alteration in endothelial function [as in patients with coexisting urinary tract infection (UTI) or respiratory tract infection (RTI)]
    - Oral contraceptives
    - Estrogens
    - Heparin-induced thrombocytopenia (HIT)
    - Intravenous (IV) drug abuse
- ***Congenital includes:***
    - *Antiphospholipid antibody syndrome.* This is defined as clinically documented venous or arterial thrombosis along with presence of antiphospholipid antibodies (must be positive on two separate occasions measured 12 weeks apart). The antibodies include lupus anticoagulant (strong association with DVT, tested using dilute Russell viper venom time); beta-2-glycoprotein I antibody [immunoglobulin G (IgG) and/or immunoglobulin M (IgM) >30 units]; anticardiolipin antibody (low levels insignificant, moderate or high levels > 40 units of IgG or IgM are significant).
    - Behçet syndrome
    - Homocystinuria
    - Polycythemia rubra vera
    - *Genetic mutations in blood coagulation cascade:*
        - Genetic thrombocytosis and thrombophilia
        - Inherited disorders of coagulation/fibrinolysis—altered factor VIII, factor IX, factor XI, and prothrombin, antiphospholipid syndrome

    - Antithrombin III deficiency
    - Protein C deficiency
    - Protein S deficiency
    - Prothrombin 20210A mutation
    - Factor V Leiden
    - Dysfibrinogenemias and disorders of plasminogen activation
  - *Anatomic variants causing venous stasis:*
    - Compression of left common iliac vein at the anatomic crossing of the right common iliac artery, also called **May–Thurner syndrome** or **Cockett syndrome**.
    - Anomalous development of inferior vena cava (IVC) like duplicated IVC, absence of IVC or azygos vein.

CLINICAL FEATURES

The *most common symptoms* and *signs* **(Fig. 6)** of DVT, but *none* of them specific include the following:

- *Edema:* It is the most specific sign. Thrombus that extends above the bifurcation of iliac veins produces bilateral leg edema. Unilateral leg/calf swelling or >3 cm measured 10 cm below tibial tubercle is significant in association with other signs (*see* Wells' criteria).
- *Leg and calf pain:* It occurs in 50% of patients but is nonspecific. Calf pain may be reproduced or provocated on dorsiflexion of the foot (*Homans' sign*, **Fig. 7**).
- *Reddish purple hue of lower limb from venous engorgement and obstruction includes:*
  - Phlegmasia alba dolens (painful white inflammation), which is characterized by pale affected extremity, often having poor or even absent distal pulses—it may be confused with acute arterial occlusion, but the presence of edema, petechiae, and superficial vein distention suggest DVT.
  - Phlegmasia cerulea dolens (painful blue inflammation)—the leg is usually markedly edematous, painful, and cyanotic.
- *Calf tenderness:* It occurs in 75% of patients, it is usually confined to the calf muscles. The tenderness may extend in the medial thigh along with the course of deep veins. The size, location, and extent of the thrombus have no correlation with the pain and tenderness felt.
- Increased temperature or erythema in the area of DVT (may be confused with cellulitis).
- Clinical symptoms of PE as the primary manifestation occur in 10% of patients with confirmed DVT (see **Table 1** for the differentiating clinical features of DVT and PE).
- *Superficial thrombophlebitis:* Palpable, indurated, cordlike, tender subcutaneous venous segment.

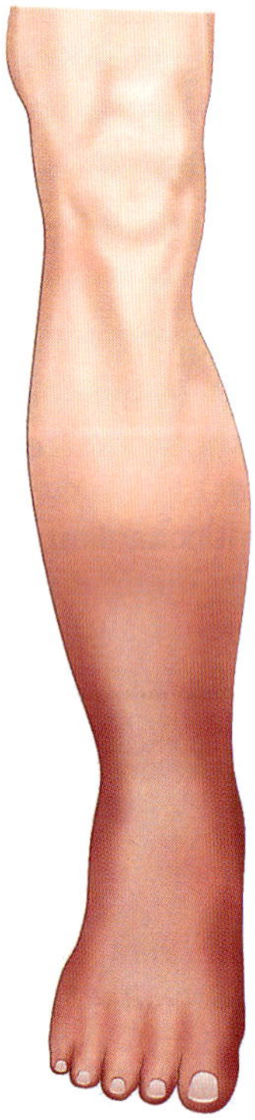

Fig. 6: Clinical features of deep vein thrombosis. The leg is red, swollen and patient might also have fever mimicking cellulitis.

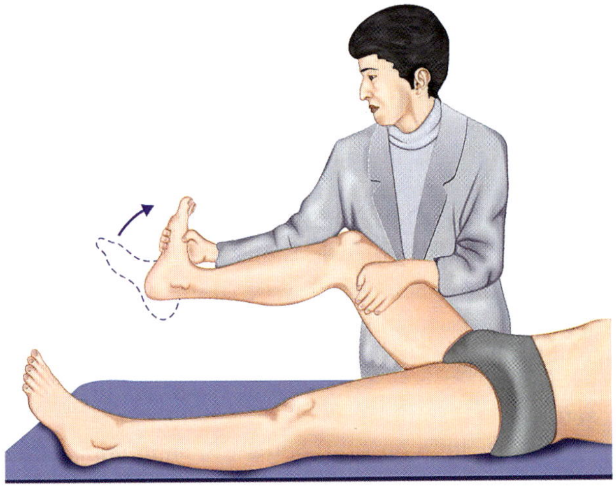

Fig. 7: Homans' sign. Support the patient thigh and leg with knee slightly bent. Give a firm and quick jerk to dorsiflex the foot, this causes deep calf pain and a positive Homans' sign.

TABLE 1: Differentiating clinical features of deep vein thrombosis (DVT) and pulmonary embolism (PE).

DVT	*PE*
Symptoms:	
• Calf and leg pain • Swelling • Raised temperature locally	• Chest pain and tightness • Impending sensation of doom • Cough • Shortness of breath • Palpitations • Hemoptysis • Dizziness
Signs:	
• Calf tenderness • Dilated superficial veins • Palpable cord • Phlegmasia (alba or cerulea) dolens • Homans' sign	• Tachypnea • Tachycardia • Hypotension • Neck vein dilation • Diaphoresis (increased sweating) • Hypoxia

DIAGNOSIS

A clinical practice guideline from the American Academy of Family Physicians and the American College of Physicians (9th edition) provides four recommendations for the workup of patients with probable DVT:

- First, validated clinical prediction rules should be used to estimate the pretest probability of VTE and interpret test results **(Tables 2 and 3)**.
- Second, a moderately sensitive or high-sensitivity D-dimer is obtained in appropriately selected patients with low pretest probability of DVT or PE first, and compression ultrasound (PUSG) of proximal veins later. Venography and whole-leg ultrasound are *not* recommended. A negative result indicates a low likelihood of VTE and no further testing is necessary.
- Third, in patients with intermediate to high pretest probability of LEDVT, proximal vein ultrasonography (PUSG) is recommended. If PUSG is positive then treatment for DVT should be initiated rather than confirmation with venography. If PUSG is negative, there is no need for further testing or repeat sonography. However, if PUSG was chosen as initial modality for diagnosis that came negative it should be followed by D-dimer assay and if it is positive then repeat sonography should be done at 1 week.
- Fourth, diagnostic imaging studies are required in patients with intermediate or high pretest probability of PE. The various options available are a pulmonary angiography, ventilation-perfusion (V/Q) scan, and multidetector helical computed axial tomography. A simplified diagnostic algorithm for PE (not DVT) is presented in **Flowchart 1**.

Because of the significant prevalence of the disease (15–30%) in at risk population, the required screening test should be inexpensive and simple. Venography that remained a gold standard is invasive, expensive and cumbersome also making routine use uncomfortable. Sonography examination is noninvasive but still expensive. Now, the *initial preferred screening test is D-dimer*, which is simpler, cheaper and it reduces the rate of missed diagnosis. Based on pretest probabilities and D-dimer results, algorithms are made. No further evaluation is needed in around 40% of patients whose clinical suspicion is low and D-dimer result is negative.

- Etiological causes should be analyzed by various laboratory tests. When DVT is diagnosed in following situations, these tests are needed:
  - Patients whose age is <50 years
  - Patients having family history of a hypercoagulable state or a familial deficiency
  - Venous thrombosis at atypical sites
  - Warfarin-induced skin necrosis

  The tests commonly performed in these settings are:
  - Serum homocysteine levels
  - Protein S and protein C level estimation
  - Antithrombin III estimation
  - Factor V Leiden determination
  - Detection of prothrombin 20210A mutation
  - Antiphospholipid antibodies detection

The hypercoagulable state is produced by presence of these abnormalities or deficiency of these factors.

- *D-dimer testing:* When cross-linked fibrin is degraded by plasmin, D-dimer generates. In any medical condition which forms clot like in hemorrhage, cancer, trauma,

TABLE 2: Wells' clinical score for deep venous thrombosis (DVT).

Clinical parameter	
Active cancer (treatment ongoing, or within 6 months or palliative)	+1
Calf swelling > 3 cm compared with asymptomatic leg	+1
Collateral superficial veins (nonvaricose)	+1
Entire leg swelling	+1
Localized tenderness along the distribution of the deep venous system (behind the knee and medial anterior thigh to groin and femoral triangle)	+1
Paralysis or recent plaster immobilization of lower extremities	+1
Pitting edema (greater than asymptomatic leg)	+1
Previous DVT documented	+1
Recently bedridden for > 3 days or major surgery < 4 weeks prior	+1
Alternative diagnosis (as likely or greater than that of DVT)	−2

TABLE 3: Wells' score risk stratification grouped in either a 2- or 3-risk group scoring system.

Probability (3-risk group)	*Total score*	*Probability of DVT (%)*
1. Low risk	0	5
2. Moderate risk	1–2	17
3. High risk	>2	53
Probability (2-risk group)	***Total score***	***Probability of DVT (%)***
1. Low risk (DVT unlikely)	<2	6
2. High risk (DVT likely)	2 or more	28

Flowchart 1: Algorithm for diagnosis of PE without shock. In cases with shock, CT is the first investigation to be done. Clinical probability of PE is estimated using Wells' score for PE (see text and **Table 4**).

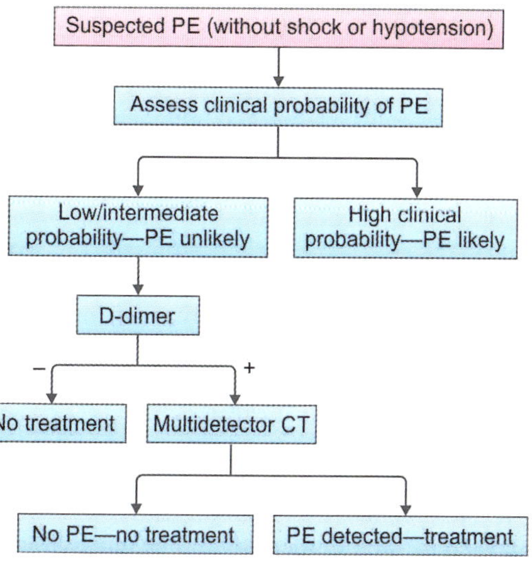

recent surgery, and sepsis, D-dimer level may be elevated. Higher risk of DVT is associated with many of these conditions. Thus, the D-dimer assay has a high sensitivity (up to 97%) but a low specificity (as low as 35%). It may use to rule out DVT, but the diagnosis of DVT must never be confirmed by only D-dimer value. It is now suggested that a cutoff of two times the upper limit may have good negative predictive value for suspected DVT. As D-dimer values rise with age so in patients over 50 years of age with suspected PE it is better to use values equal to and more than patient's age × 10 (so a 70-year old patient will have cutoff of 700 µg/mL). In patients with low-to-moderate risk (Wells' DVT score < 2), a negative D-dimer assay result rules out DVT. Further diagnostic study (e.g., duplex ultrasonography) to support the diagnosis is required in all patients with a positive D-dimer assay result and all patients with a moderate-to-high risk of DVT (Wells' DVT score > 2).

- *Imaging in DVT:* Imaging studies used in DVT include ultrasonography, venography, impedance plethysmography (IPG), angiography, magnetic resonance imaging (MRI), and nuclear imaging.
    - Because of its relative ease of use, absence of irradiation or contrast material, compression ultrasonography with *color Doppler imaging of the blood flow in vessels is the current first-line imaging examination for DVT* with high sensitivity and specificity in institutions with experienced sonographers. It combines real-time B-mode ultrasound with Doppler imaging. The sensitivity and specificity are 95% and is most commonly used modality for infrainguinal DVT. The Doppler imaging allows colored assessment of the blood flow. Whether blood flow assessment is done or not the compression of the vein along the length is key aspect of evaluation of the DVT. Noncompressibility is the primary diagnostic criterion of DVT. Other findings include:
        - Echogenic thrombus within lumen
        - Loss of flow phasicity
        - Loss of Valsalva maneuver augmentation
    - Surveillance ultrasound: Routine weekly surveillance has been done in very high-risk patients to improve the yield of patients with DVT. There is no recommendation for this, however as the cost-effectiveness has not been documented and yield has never been significantly increased.
    - Contrast venography with pedal vein cannulation, IV contrast injection, and serial limb radiographs has been the gold standard for setting the benchmark for other investigations. However, it has many limitations that include its invasive nature, need for contrast with associated complications, etc. It is rarely used now due to increased accuracy and standardization of noninvasive diagnostic tests.
    - CT venography: It uses venous phase contrast to visualize the IVC, pelvic veins, and extremity veins. It is particularly useful for diagnosis of proximal DVT which is often missed on duplex ultrasonography. It can also be combined with pulmonary angiogram though the requirement of contrast agent increases dramatically and may have ill effects.
    - Impedance plethysmography has been shown to be sensitive and specific for proximal vein thrombosis. However, IPG may not detect the calf vein thrombosis and nonoccluding proximal vein thrombus (limitations of IPG).
    - For suspected iliac vein or inferior vena caval thrombosis, MRI is the diagnostic test of choice, especially when CT venography is contraindicated or technically inadequate.

It should be realized that neither the clinical evaluation nor the investigations are of use in half of the patients. As many as 46% with patients with classic symptoms have negative venograms, and as many as 50% of those with image-documented venous thrombosis lack specific symptoms!

POTENTIAL COMPLICATIONS OF DEEP VEIN THROMBOSIS

The potential complications of DVT include the following:

1. *Pulmonary embolism:* PE develops as venous thrombi break off from their location of origin and travel through the right heart into the pulmonary artery. This produces V/Q defect and cardiac strain. As many as 40% of patients have silent PE when symptomatic DVT is diagnosed but most patients (up to 75%) are asymptomatic. Although up to 10% of in-hospital deaths have associated PE but these patients also have compromised cardiopulmonary function at baseline so it is difficult to attribute the deaths only due to PE:
    - Most small thrombi in the lower extremities tend to resolve spontaneously. Calf thrombi usually do not migrate to cause embolism while proximal extension of thrombus and proximal DVT creates loose masses increasing the vulnerability to detach/break and cause embolism.
    - Extension of thrombus to proximal femorocaval venous system occurs in about 15% of cases. Untreated proximal thrombi are a significant source of clinically significant pulmonary emboli. The incidence of PE with untreated proximal thrombi is 29–50%.
    - Although no direct cause of mortality has been affirmatively posited to PE only but it is also a fact that most PEs are first diagnosed at autopsy.
    - Patients have an impending sense of doom, dyspnea, and pleuritic chest pain but these are all nonspecific and may be seen also in chest injury. On examinations, patients have tachypnea, tachycardia, cyanosis, and hypotension (massive embolism).
    - Pulmonary embolism is most often diagnosed by abnormal arterial blood gas (ABG) showing partial pressure of oxygen (PaO_2) < 80 at room air and hypocarbia. The findings are nonspecific and hence Wells' criteria for suspected PE **(Table 4)** have been formulated and now increasingly followed. Chest X-ray (CXR) shows atelectasis, pulmonary infiltrate, and/or pleural effusion. Electrocardiogram (ECG) also shows

TABLE 4: Wells' score for suspected pulmonary embolism (PE).

Criterion	*Points*
Patient has clinically suspected deep venous thrombosis (DVT)	3.0
An alternative diagnosis is less likely than PE	3.0
Tachycardia (heart rate > 100)	1.5
Immobilization (≥3 days) or surgery in previous 4 weeks	1.5
Prior history of DVT or PE	1.5
Hemoptysis	1.0
Malignancy (treatment within 6 months) or palliative	1.0
Traditional interpretation	
High probability (59%) based on pooled data	Score > 6.0
Moderate probability (29%) based on pooled data	Score 2.0–6.0
Low probability based on pooled data	Score < 2.0
Alternative interpretation	
PE is likely, consider diagnostic imaging	Score > 4.0
PE is unlikely, consider D-dimer to rule out PE	Score of 4 or less

abnormalities but that may be present for variety of reasons in trauma patients. CT angiography is currently the gold standard imaging modality for diagnosis of PE (***see* Flowchart 1**). The contrast bolus should be timed so as to maximize the visualization of pulmonary arterial system. Isolated subsegmental filling defects have poor concordance and diagnostic or therapeutic value. It is limited by high radiation exposure (= 130 chest radiographs) and inability to perform in patients with renal insufficiency and patients allergic to contrast. Alternatives in these patients include MRI or nuclear medicine V/Q scanning. Nuclear medicine V/Q scan is primarily indicated in patients unable to undergo CT angiography. Other indication is in patients who have a prior history of PE for which V/Q scan was performed at completion of anticoagulation. This imaging modality is not considered for emergency indications otherwise. The scans are graded as either normal, low probability for PE, intermediate probability for PE or high probability for PE (four grades). The utility is evident only when it is used in association with clinical probability score (Wells' score for PE) and D-dimer testing (***see* Flowchart 1**). Mostly it is considered that at least two of the three modalities (clinical/D-dimer/V-Q scan) should suggest high likelihood of PE to initiate treatment. So in a patient with high clinical probability + positive D-dimer and intermediate or high probability V-Q scan will immediately go on treatment for PE while a patient with unlikely clinical probability, positive D-dimer and normal or low probability V-Q scan would not be treated. Patient with likely clinical probability, normal D-dimer but high probability V-Q scan will also be treated.

- The thrombus may be removed with pharmacomechanical thrombolytic intervention. Treatment options include anticoagulation therapy, thrombolysis [using recombinant tissue plasminogen activator (rtPA)], and suction or surgical embolectomy. Thrombolysis is contraindicated in many injury profiles. It should only be considered in severely hemodynamically compromised patients, and those with right ventricular hypokinesis. There is no documented difference between systemic therapy and catheter-directed therapy. Suction embolectomy may be considered in patients contraindicated for thrombolysis. Surgical embolectomy is associated with various complications. PE prophylaxis is done by placement of an IVC filter and DVT prophylaxis.

2. *Paradoxic emboli (rare)*
3. *Local complications:* Local propagation of thrombus causes phlegmasia cerulea dolens or phlegmasia alba dolens (blanching milk leg) with loss of arterial flow and venous gangrene.
4. *Recurrent DVT:* Without treatment, one half of patients have a recurrent, symptomatic VTE event within 3 months.
5. *Postphlebitic syndrome, post-thrombotic syndrome:* PTS is a chronic complication of DVT that manifests months to many years after the initial event. The venous valves are destroyed due to clot formation and organization. After the clot dissolves, the valvular competence is completely lost. Symptoms are generally exacerbated by standing and relieved by elevation of the extremity. Symptoms include a wide spectrum of mild erythema and localized induration to massive extremity swelling (nonpitting edema) and ulceration. Management includes application of a compression hose and limb elevation. Evolution of venous insufficiency in PTS:
   - Over time, thrombus gets organized with the infiltration of inflammatory cells into the clot.
   - This produces fibroelastic intimal thickening which leads to further valvular dysfunction and wall fibrosis.
   - As deep vein outflow obstruction is present, if adequate collaterals do not develop, dilation of the feeding perforating veins occurs with contraction of the calf muscle. This makes the valves to become nonfunctional and it forces the blood retrograde into the superficial system causing their dilation and hence superficial venous incompetence also.
   - Venous incompetence also occurs because of natural healing process of the thrombotic vein itself. Underlying valves become damaged, incompetent and venous reflux occurs.
   - Over time, the venous damage becomes irreversible. There is no central flow of blood. Venous blood stasis occurs leading to a persistently elevated venous pressure or venous hypertension. As the process progresses, fibrosis occurs leading to compromised tissue oxygenation and lastly, ulcers may form.

DIFFERENTIAL DIAGNOSIS

Deep vein thrombosis is a confusing disease both clinically and even with investigations. Among the patients evaluated for DVT only a quarter of them have it. Numerous patients

with DVT are asymptomatic. The conditions that should be always looked for while making a diagnosis of DVT include:
- Ruptured Baker's cyst
- Budd–Chiari syndrome
- Cellulitis
- Congestive cardiac failure
- Pulmonary embolism
- Septic thrombophlebitis
- Superficial thrombophlebitis

TREATMENT OF DEEP VEIN THROMBOSIS

Deep vein thrombosis treatment falls into the domain of hematologists so only few principles are detailed here. Prophylaxis however is a hot topic and is detailed later. The treatment of DVT is mainly centralized around:
- Prevention of PE
- Decreasing the risk of developing the PTS
- Reduction in morbidity

Anticoagulation Therapy

Anticoagulation (available in various forms) is the mainstay of medical therapy. Contraindications for the use of anti-coagulation include the following:
- *Absolute contraindications:*
  - Ongoing intracranial hemorrhage
  - Malignant hypertension
  - Severe active hemorrhage from wound or in vascular tissues
  - Pregnancy
  - Recent history of brain, eye, or spinal cord surgery
- *Relative contraindications:*
  - History of recent cerebrovascular accident
  - History of recent major surgery
  - Known case of severe thrombocytopenia

The treatment is done usually on outpatient basis but patients have to be hospitalized (contraindications for out patient management) in the following situations:
- Anticoagulation contraindicated
- Pregnancy
- Acute on chronic renal failure (*serum creatinine* level > 2 mg/dL)
- Suspected or proven concomitant PE
- Iliofemoral DVT
- Morbid obesity (>150 kg)
- Familial or inherited disorders of coagulation: ATIII deficiency, protein C or protein S deficiency, prothrombin 20210A, or factor V Leiden
- Familial bleeding disorder
- Significant cardiovascular or pulmonary comorbidity
- Unable to follow instructions
- Close follow-up not possible
  - Homeless
  - No contact telephone
  - Geographic (too far from hospital)
  - Patient or family resistant to outpatient therapy

The immediate symptoms of confirmed DVT often resolve with anticoagulation alone. As anticoagulant therapy is noninvasive and the cure rate is high (approximately 90%) without any immediate demonstrable physical sequelae of DVT and having fewer complications in comparison to invasive methods, it remains the mainstay of medical therapy for DVT. The logical limitation of this therapy however is that it inhibits propagation only and does not remove the thrombus that is deemed to resolve by natural physiological process over time. The other limitation is a variable risk of clinically significant bleeding. In an outpatient setting, low-molecular-weight heparin (LMWH) remains the main mode of treatment for acute DVT. It is continued for 3–12 months depending on site of thrombosis and on the presence of risk factors. Patients should be treated for 3–6 months for the first episode of DVT. If there are recurrent episodes, it should be treated for at least 1 year. Lifetime anticoagulation on the other hand is recommended if:
- DVT recurs.
- Chronic hypercoagulability is identified.
- PE is life threatening.

The following drugs **(Fig. 8)** are commonly used:

Heparin and derivatives: Heparin products used in the treatment of DVT include unfractionated heparin (UFH) and LMWH. Their anticoagulant effect is by interacting with ATIII to inhibit thrombin. The hemorrhagic complications attributed to heparin arise from the larger higher-molecular-weight fragments so LMWH is preferred and is the most popular drug to manage DVT:
- *LMWH:* Exert their anticoagulant effect by inhibiting the activity of activated factor X.
- *UFH:* While the patient is taking IV heparin, every 6 hourly monitoring of activated partial thromboplastin time (aPTT) or heparin activity level must be done and it should be continued until the dose is stabilized in the therapeutic range.

Factor Xa inhibitors:
- *Fondaparinux:* Fondaparinux (direct selective inhibitor of factor Xa) requires only a single-daily subcutaneous dose is required. Fondaparinux is not associated with HIT so therapeutic monitoring of laboratory parameters required for heparin is also not required. Compared to enoxaparin, once-daily fondaparinux is equally effective and safe as twice-daily, weight-adjusted dose of enoxaparin. It is contraindicated in chronic renal failure patients having creatinine clearance < 30 mL/min. No specific antidote to fondaparinux however is available.
- *Rivaroxaban:* Rivaroxaban is an oral factor Xa inhibitor approved by the Food and Drug Administration (FDA) in November 2012 for treatment of DVT or PE and for reduction of the risk of recurrent DVT and PE after initial treatment. Rivaroxaban is as effective in preventing VTE recurrence as enoxaparin. Rivaroxaban can be used in high-risk groups (e.g., fragile patients, cancer patients and patients with a large clot). Advantages include that of being an oral agent, no monitoring needed, can be started without heparin or LMWH. The disadvantages are twice-daily dosing before lowering dose, no instant antidote available should hemorrhagic complications arise and that patient cannot miss a dose.

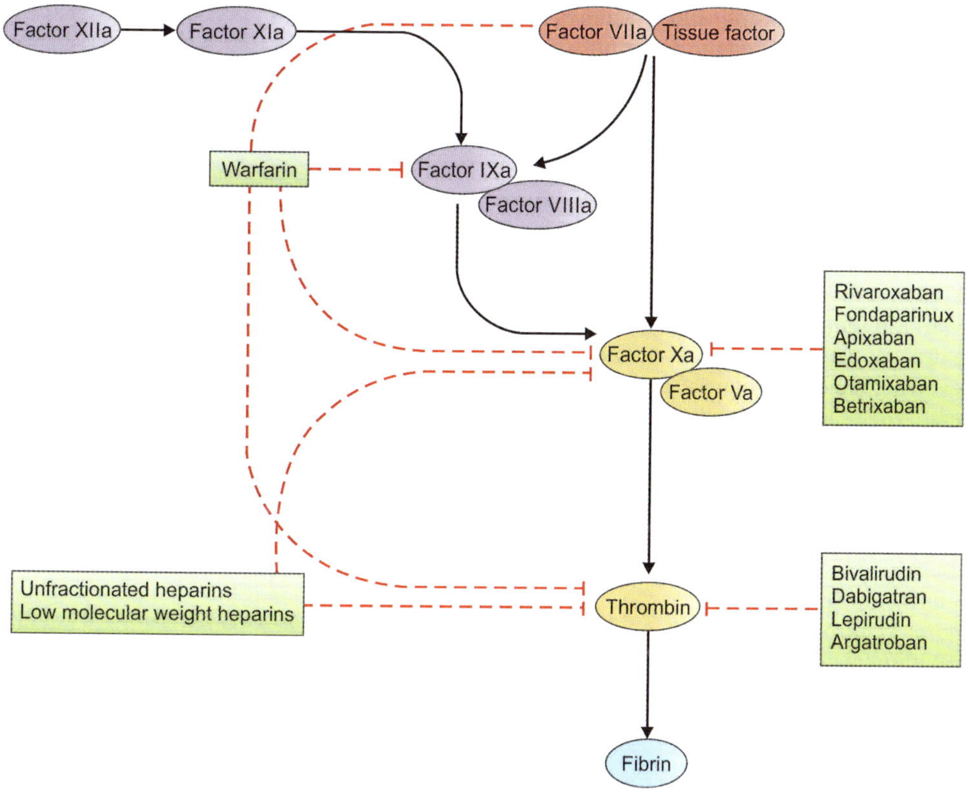

Fig. 8: Sites of action of various groups of prophylactic and therapeutic drugs in the thrombosis pathway.

- *Apixaban:* In March 2014, the FDA-approved apixaban (Eliquis) for the additional indication of prophylaxis of DVT and PE in adults who have undergone hip or knee replacement surgery. In August 2014, apixaban was approved for treatment of DVT and PE. Mechanism of action, advantages, and disadvantages are as for rivaroxaban above.

Direct thrombin inhibitors (dabigatran/ ximelagatran): Dabigatran acts by inhibition of free and clot-bound thrombin and thrombin-induced platelet aggregation (see details in "prophylaxis" here). The advantages include that it is an oral agent, no monitoring is needed and an antidote (idarucizumab) is available should complications arise to reverse the action. Disadvantages include patient cannot miss a dose, significant incidence of gastritis (20%), renal function should be good [glomerular filtration rate (GFR) > 30 mL/min], and need of bridge therapy of 5 days. The goal of therapy is to make international normalized ratio (INR) > 2 for at least 24 hours, for which warfarin 5 mg PO daily (or appropriate dose of LMWH) is initiated and overlapped for about 5 days.

Emerging Anticoagulant Agents

The details and specifications of these agents are out of the scope of this text:

- Razaxaban
- Idraparinux
- Bivalirudin
- Lepirudin
- Ximelagatran (development stopped due to hepatotoxicity)

Patients treated with LMWH or fondaparinux do not require monitoring of the aPTT as for UFH but heparin or LMWH need regular platelet counts and should be discontinued if the platelet count falls below 75,000.

Complications of Anticoagulation Therapy

- Hemorrhagic complications are the most common and most concerning adverse effects of anticoagulant therapy. The complication is especially severe with therapy for 3–6 months. High-risk populations for hemorrhagic complications are:
  - Patients aged > 65 years or 75 years
  - History of previous bleeding including intracranial hemorrhages, gastrointestinal (GI) bleed, etc.
  - Renal insufficiency
  - Diabetes
  - Cancer/metastatic cancer
  - Liver failure
  - Thrombocytopenia
  - Stroke
  - Anemia
  - Antiplatelet therapy
  - Alcohol abuse

  The treatment of hemorrhage while taking heparin depends on the severity of the bleeding and the extent to which the aPTT is elevated above the therapeutic range. The drug should be discontinued and residual effect of the drug can be neutralized by protamine.

Patients having bleeding complications while on oral warfarin are treated by withholding the drug and administering vitamin K. Severe life-threatening hemorrhage in this case require replenishing the coagulation factors by transfusing prothrombin complex concentrate (PCC) as is also done in cases requiring emergency surgery in addition to vitamin K. PCC (Octaplex®) is derived from virally inactivated [though risk of variant Creutzfeldt-Jakob disease (vCFD) still remains] human plasma and contains factors II, VII, IX, X providing immediate reversal of warfarin but the effect wears off in 6–12 hours. Fresh frozen plasma is not recommended for purpose of reversing the effects of warfarin or its toxicity but in centers, where the availability or methods of procuring PCC are unavailable, then may be considered in consultation with hematologist and transfusion medicine specialist. Recombinant factor VIIa is another option especially for CNS hemorrhage.

- Systemic embolism
- Chronic venous insufficiency
- *Post-thrombotic syndrome:* Pain and edema in the affected limb without new thrombosis
- Soft tissue ischemia associated with massive clot and very high venous pressures—phlegmasia cerulea dolens

Pharmacologic Thrombolysis

Use of thrombolytic medications (streptokinase, etc.) to lyse DVT is feared for ensuing intracranial hemorrhage (infrequent side-effect) and death or impairment. The bleeding risk is increased by these thrombolytic agents in patients with recent surgery, stroke, GI or other bleeding, and underlying coagulopathy.

Endovascular Intervention

1. ***Percutaneous transcatheter*** treatment consists of thrombus removal with:
   - Catheter-directed thrombolysis
   - Mechanical thrombectomy
   - Angioplasty and/or
   - Stenting of venous obstructions

   Principles:
   - Venography to guide the anatomy and the particular pathology that must be addressed.
   - The patient must be heparinized before the procedure.
   - Care must be taken to avoid dislodging the clot or breaking it into small fragments else pulmonary embolus will result.

   Specific indications for this intervention include:
   - Phlegmasia
   - Symptomatic IVC thrombosis (it has poor response to anticoagulation alone)
   - Symptomatic iliofemoral DVT (in patients with a low risk of bleeding)

   Absolute contraindications:
   - Cerebrovascular event, trauma or neurosurgery within past 3 months
   - Active internal bleeding
   - Disseminated intravascular coagulation (DIC).

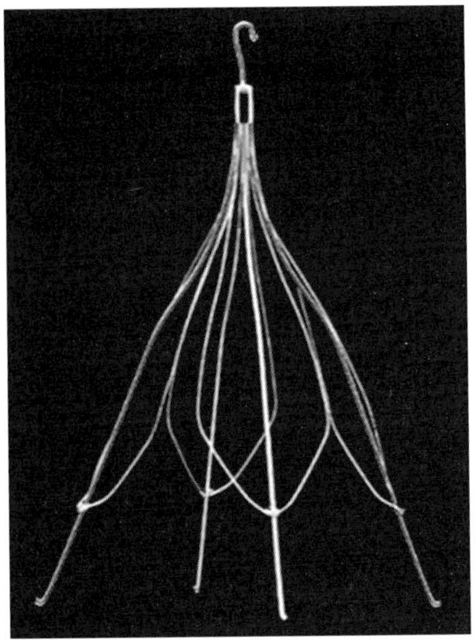

Fig. 9: Retrievable vena caval filter.

2. ***Placement of IVC filters:*** An IVC filter **(Fig. 9)** traps emboli and is a mechanical barrier to the flow of emboli > 4 mm. This option is useful in the setting of:
   - Polytrauma
   - Head injury
   - Hemorrhagic stroke
   - Known VTE
   - Major surgery when PE prophylaxis must be maintained during a short-term contraindication to anticoagulation.

   Filter is useful in the elderly patients who have an increased risk of bleeding, and particularly if the risk of trauma is present. IVC filter provides no survival benefit over standard therapeutic anticoagulation in patients who can be treated so. Of the various designs available, the Greenfield filter is most commonly used filter at present. American Heart Association recommendations for IVC filters include the following:
   - Confirmed acute proximal DVT or acute PE in patient with contraindication for anticoagulation (this remains the most common indication for IVC filter placement)
   - Recurrent thromboembolism while on anticoagulation
   - Active bleeding complications requiring termination of anticoagulation therapy

   Relative contraindications include the following:
   - Large, free-floating iliofemoral thrombus in high-risk patients
   - Propagating iliofemoral thrombus while on anticoagulation
   - Chronic PE in patient with pulmonary hypertension and cor pulmonale
   - Patient with significant fall risk
3. ***Replacement of venous valves:*** These bioprosthetic venous valves are inserted percutaneously. They are still under development. In search of a minimally invasive alternative to the long-term complication of VTE, these valves are a valid choice.

Use of Elastic Compression Stockings

These stockings (especially below-the-knee compression stockings) reduce venous hypertension and venous valvular reflux and assist the calf muscle pump. Leg edema reduces, microcirculation improves, and venous ischemia is prevented. Its regular use with reduces the incidence of PTS by 50% (graduated elastic compression stockings are more useful).

Role of ambulation during the anticoagulation therapy: We recommend full ambulation during anticoagulation therapy. The fear of dislodging clots and precipitating a fatal PE is unfounded.

Duration of Anticoagulation

- *Lower extremity DVT:*
  - *Proximal DVT:* Three months of oral anticoagulation
  - *Distal DVT:* No treatment needed if repeat ultrasonography shows no proximal propagation of clot after initial scan.
- *Upper extremity DVT:*
  - *Catheter-related DVT:* If catheter is removed then full 3 months of anticoagulation is recommended (oral preferred). If catheter is in place then start full dose of anticoagulation (duration of treatment not known currently).
  - *Catheter-related superficial thrombosis:* Remove catheter and treat symptomatically or start full dose of anticoagulation for 4–6 weeks.
  - *Spontaneous DVT:* Treat as for lower extremity.
- *Portal mesenteric:* No definite guidelines available but 3–6 months treatment may be needed.

PROPHYLAXIS OF DEEP VENOUS THROMBOSIS

Rationale for Prophylaxis

- Fatal PE rates range from 0.1 to 0.8% for surgical patients that may be as high as 7% for patients undergoing orthopedic surgery. Though it is difficult to attribute all deaths due to PE solely as nearly all of the reported deaths had other critically compromised vital body function(s) in addition that could have prominently contributed to mortality. Still if we believe that PE could have stressed the body functions further so as to shut them down then prophylaxis from this potential threat is essential. Initiation of therapy especially for LMWH should be done either 12 or more hours preoperatively or postoperatively rather than within 4 hours or less preoperatively or postoperatively [American College of Chest Physicians (ACCP)]. For arthroplasty patients [total knee arthroplasty (TKA)/THA], minimum 10–14 days thromboprophylaxis is needed using any one of the following—LMWH (preferred), fondaparinux, rivaroxaban, apixaban, dabigatran, vitamin K antagonist (VKA), aspirin, low-dose unfractionated heparin (LDUH) or an intermittent pneumatic compression (IPC) device. For hip fracture surgery patients, 10–14 days of prophylaxis is recommended using LMWH, fondaparinux, LDUH, aspirin, IPC device or adjusted-dose VKA. No prophylaxis is needed for arthroscopy patients or isolated lower limb trauma. Patients with increased risk of bleeding should be managed with IPC device only. According to an additional recommendation by the ACCP for extended out-of-hospital prophylaxis, to decrease venous thrombosis rates without major bleeding issues, a total of 35 days of anticoagulation therapy is given.
- As short-term and long-term morbidity and mortality are associated with VTE and associated cost with it, treatment with anticoagulants and a longer hospital stay is required besides diagnostic tests.
- The long-term sequelae of DVT including the chronic venous insufficiency and PTS are highly disabling producing chronic edema, cellulitis, and recurrent venous ulceration. These should be prevented by effectively preventing their cause, i.e., DVT.

There are various methods that can be used to prevent venous thrombosis focusing primarily on one or other component of the Virchow's triad. First we will discuss the various methods used for prevention of DVT followed by the recommendations for their use in various circumstances.

Mechanical Methods

Immobility can lead to the development of DVT as normal venous pump function of skeletal muscles is inhibited causing stasis. Mechanical methods have been a useful adjunct to pharmacological treatment to prevent DVT and focus on reducing venous stasis and blood stagnation by promoting venous blood flow through external compression. Currently they have been recommended as the sole measures to prevent DVT when used along with low-dose aspirin in orthopedic patients by the American Association of Orthopaedic Surgery (AAOS). Other agencies believe that in moderate- or high-risk cases, the use of mechanical means of prophylaxis alone is not effective. The risk of PE or death is not proven to be reduced by any mechanical prophylaxis method. So, with anticoagulant-based prophylaxis, the use of IPC devices (mechanical) is recommended (altering the intrinsic blood properties) by attacking the two components of the Virchow's triad.

Modalities

- *Passive devices such as knee- or thigh-high graduated compression (elastic) stockings (GCSs):* These are least effective measures (**Figs. 10A and B**). Knee- and thigh-high GCSs do not significantly differ in their effectiveness in reducing the incidence of DVT in hospitalized patients.
- *Active (external pneumatic compress or IPC) devices:* They have good efficacy. IPC devices serve as external pumps substituting the function of calf pumps that are inactive in immobilized patients. They reduce venous stasis, improve blood flow velocity, and increase the level of circulating fibrinolysins. Their efficacy is dependent on the time of use the longer the better also asymmetrical devices are found better than circumferential intermittent compression devices. IPC devices do not require monitoring and there is no increase in bleeding complications. It is recommended to use portable, battery-powered devices that can record and report

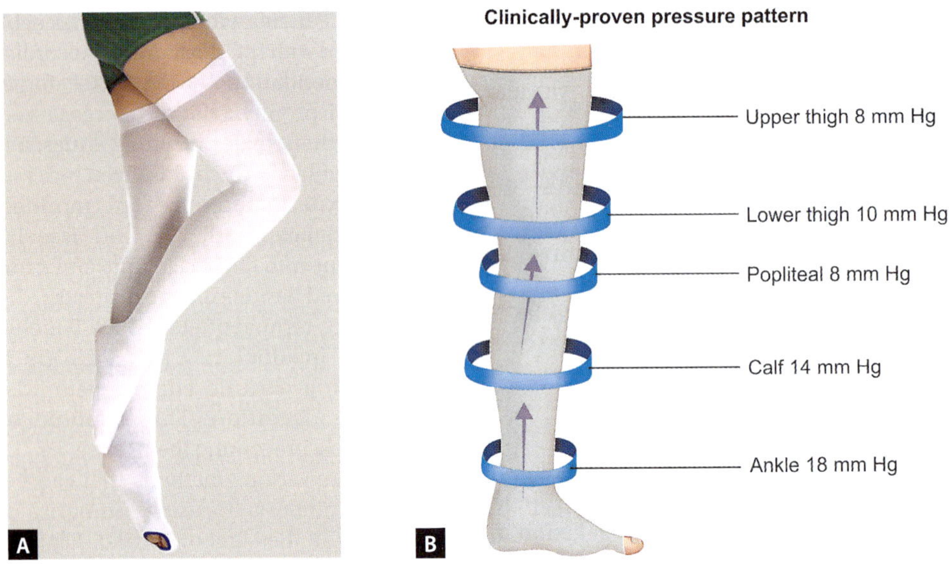

Figs. 10A and B: (A) Graduated compression stockings; (B) These stockings exert graduated pressure over different regions of the legs.

proper wear time on a daily basis for inpatients and outpatients. One should try to achieve minimum 18 hours of daily compliance.

- Venous foot pumps (VFP) which include the foot impulse technology (FIT) and foot impulse devices (FID).

Pharmacologic Methods

To prevent thrombosis, many pharmacologic agents are currently available which can be grouped as follows:

- *Antithrombotic drugs:* They include anticoagulants and antiplatelet drugs as follows:
  - Orally administered VKA, warfarin
  - Orally administered aspirin (antiplatelet drug)
  - Subcutaneously administered pentasaccharide fondaparinux which is a selective inhibitor of activated factor X (Xa)
  - Subcutaneously administered UFH or LMWH
  - Orally administered direct factor Xa inhibitors
  - Orally administered direct thrombin inhibitor—dabigatran etexilate, ximelagatran
- *Thrombolytic drugs* (primary thrombolytic drugs are not used for prophylaxis; however, there are a few drugs that in addition to anticoagulation effect also have antithrombotic action, mentioned in respective drug descriptions).

Antiplatelet Drugs

Platelet-active drugs primarily aspirin have been used to prevent DVT. Aspirin had been known to Neanderthal man for relief of pain and was also used by Hippocrates but its antiplatelet effect at low doses is a more recent discovery. Aspirin (acetylsalicylic acid) is an effective platelet inhibitor at very low doses (50–100 mg/day) that is in contrast to its anti-inflammatory effect at high doses (two other drugs having such differential function are methotrexate that is a immunomodulator at low doses and anticancer drug at high doses, steroids are potent anti-inflammatory at low doses while immunosuppressants at high doses). Surgical Care Improvement Project (SCIP) included aspirin on July 1st, 2013 as acceptable method for TKA and THA. Aspirin is less effective than other options, but it has been recommended by AAOS for DVT prophylaxis after arthroplasty surgeries in association with mechanical methods or even alone.

One should, however, note that the dose used by AAOS in their recommendation is 375 mg given twice daily. Persons using aspirin based on evidence-based medicine for DVT prophylaxis (based on AAOS recommendations) are hence cautioned to use this dose rather than relying on low-dose aspirin as commonly prescribed for cardiac patients. The dosage for aspirin is highly debatable. It is hard to determine the required dose of aspirin for DVT prophylaxis as the numbers needed to treat are very high (approximately 10,000 for each dosage arm if one intends to study). Some facts that may help determine the dosage and rationale of low-dosage are presented as follows. Cyclooxygenase-1 (COX-1 that effects gastroprotection, platelet aggregation, and renal function) is inhibited by aspirin at low doses (<325 mg) while COX-2 (that effects pain, fever, renal function, reproduction, development, and antiplatelet) inhibition requires doses > 325 mg/day. We know that COX activity recovers 10% per day that aspirin not taken. Only 20% COX activity is required for clinically significant platelet coagulation to occur. Factually 100 mg aspirin is needed to achieve platelet inhibition with a single dose. Daily doses of 50–81 mg are required to maintain platelet inhibition. These low-dosage recommendations are designed based on studies for arterial thrombosis and prevention which is mainly a platelet aggregation play (the differences between arterial and venous thrombosis are summarized in **Table 5**). Some dosage guidance provided by orthopedics studies vary tremendously, viz., the Antiplatelet Trialists' Collaborative recommended approximately 1,242 mg/day, PEP trial suggests 160 mg/day while EPCAT trial recommends 81 mg

TABLE 5: Comparison of arterial and venous thrombosis.

	Dissimilarities	
Similarities	***Venous***	***Arterial***
• Thrombus formation depends on presence of platelets and activation of fibrinogen to fibrin • More or less similar risk factors of age, obesity, cigarette smoking, diabetes, hypertension, hyperlipidemia, and metabolic syndrome	• Perpetuated by hypercoagulable state, blood vessel and/or blood flow abnormalities • Thrombosis mainly an activity of coagulation cascade	• Perpetuation more dependent on vessel wall, platelet activity, and/or blood flow abnormalities • Primarily and activity of platelet activation and propagation

after LMWH bridging. It cannot be emphasized anymore that the confusion persists and we are still short of finding answers to aspirin effected thromboprophylaxis for DVT. Users may make an institutional policy in consultation with orthopedic surgeon, hematologist, chest physicians, and transfusion medicine specialists to justify local usage and rationale.

Vitamin K Antagonists

These agents (primarily coumarins/coumadins) inhibit the carboxylation of coagulation factors II, VII, IX, and X which is dependent on vitamin K. Vitamin K acts as a cofactor for their activation while coumarins competitively inhibit this interaction. Prothrombin time (PT) and INR are used to monitor the effect of these drugs (warfarin had been a typical example). The optimal INR to be maintained is between 2 and 3, with a target of 2.5 for DVT prophylaxis. Disadvantages of warfarin include:

- Long onset of action and also long residual activity after discontinuation
- The necessity to monitor INR values frequently
- The long half-life that may require vitamin K reversal in incidents of hemorrhage
- Narrow therapeutic window
- Prominent drug and dietary interactions
- Most unexpected but sure variable patient response
- Hemorrhagic complications are reported in up to 3–5% of patients on warfarin prophylaxis.

"Warfarinization" for orthopedic surgeries is done using adjusted-dose warfarin. It is started the night before surgery and continued postoperatively during the discharge period. At third to fourth postoperative day, INR target levels are reached, so it is not preferred as the need is a fast acting drug with a determined response and immediate therapeutic efficacy.

Heparins

The heparin or "UFH" is both an anticoagulant (prevents the platelet to clot in the vessels) and antithrombotic (lyse the clot formed inside the vessels). It acts in conjunction with ATIII to catalyze the inactivation of factors IIa, Xa, IXa, and XIIa acting as anticoagulant. While by inactivating thrombin, it also inhibits thrombin-induced activation of factor V and factor VIII (acting as antithrombotic).

For DVT prophylaxis, a bolus of 5,000 U is given every 8 hours in low-risk or moderate-risk patients. For high-risk patients, this method is not as effective. The biggest advantage is the prompt reversal of the action of heparin with protamine sulfate but there are a lot of disadvantages of the drug including:

- Variable pharmacokinetics, short half-life and low bioavailability making the consistent dosing difficult.
- Requirement for aPTT monitoring for adjusted-dose regimens due to factors mentioned in above point. It is really an uncomfortable drug in clinical practice.
- Susceptibility to the development of HIT. Benchmark recommendation includes measuring baseline complete blood count (CBC) with platelet count at start of IV therapy then repeating CBC every other day or at least three times a week. Diagnosis of HIT is based on laboratory and clinical features along with antibodies to heparin/platelet factor 4 complexes. One can also use clinical probability tool—the 4T score to estimate probability of HIT.

Low-Molecular-Weight Heparins

Low-molecular-weight heparins are lower molecular-weight moieties that contain the active ATIII-binding site derived from standard heparin by depolymerization of heparin (14–16 kDa) into LMWH product (MW 4–8 kDa). LMWH has differences in both molecular and functional properties. The biggest advantage of LMWHs is that they do not require monitoring of either aPTT or INR, the half-life is longer (compared to UFH) and effect is more consistent so that lesser dose adjustments are needed (in fact standard doses are administered). The hemorrhagic complications are less. LMWHs have gradually replaced heparin for prophylaxis and treatment of DVT (this might change with the increasing use of oral Xa inhibitors).

The LMWHs exhibit their action by anti-IIa and anti-Xa activity. This anti-IIa and anti-Xa potency ratio is used also to characterize the different preparations. The higher the anti-Xa potency higher is the efficacy in general. Several LMWH medications are commercially available in India, most of these LMWHs are sodium salts of depolymerized porcine mucosal heparin (exception: nadroparin, a calcium salt), reviparin has the lowest molecular weight and anti-IIa activity whereas dalteparin has the highest median molecular weight and anti-IIa activity (other LMWHs have values in between dalteparin and reviparin). Nadroparin, dalteparin, certoparin, and reviparin all have a 2,5-anhydro-D-mannose at the reducing terminus whereas enoxaparin and tinzaparin have a 4,5-unsaturated uronic acid at the nonreducing end.

- Enoxaparin (Clexane/Lovenox®)—given 20 mg SC every 12 hours, starting 12–24 hours postoperatively for

low- and moderate-risk patients while 40 mg SC BD for high-risk patients.
- Dalteparin (Fragmin®)—given 5,000 IU SC daily (BD-QID), starting 12–24 hours postoperatively.
- Nadroparin (Fraxiparin®)—given 38 U/kg SC QID, starting 12–24 hours postoperatively.
- Tinzaparin (Innohep/Logiparin®)—given 75 U/kg/day SC, starting 12–24 hours postoperatively.
- Ardeparin (Indeparin/Normiflo®)—knee surgery, dose 50 IU/kg SC every 12 hours, starting 12–24 hours postoperatively.
- Certoparin (Sandoparin®)—3,000 units 1–2 hours before surgery and then 3,000 units every day for 7–10 days.
- Reviparin (Clivarin®)—1750 anti-Xa IU, given 2 hours prior to surgery then continue once daily for moderate-risk patients. For high-risk patients, 4200 anti-Xa IU, given 12 hours before surgery and continued once daily.
- Panaparin (Fluxum®), Bemiparin, etc., are yet to be introduced.

Other identified mechanisms of action of LMWHs:
- Endogenous release of substances such as tissue factor pathway inhibitor (TFPI) and von Willebrand factor.
- Reduced platelet aggregation
- Inhibiting thrombin and its generation by activating thrombin-activatable fibrinolysis inhibitor (TAFI) thus have antithrombotic effects like heparin. Agents with a lower anti-Xa/anti-IIa ratio produce stronger inhibition in comparison to agents with a high anti-Xa/anti-IIa ratio.

During the depolymerization process, LMWH, ultra-LMWH, heparin-derived oligosaccharides such as pentasaccharides are produced that have differential anti-Xa and anti-IIa ratio. Fondaparinux sodium (Arixtra), a synthetic pentasaccharide, selectively binds to ATIII and potentiates neutralization of factor Xa, inhibiting thrombin formation and thrombus development. Fondaparinux is found more effective than enoxaparin in preventing DVT after total knee replacement (TKR), but episodes of major bleeding are more frequent.

Complications with LMWH therapy:
1. Hemorrhage
2. Hematuria
3. Hypersensitivity reactions
4. Urticaria
5. Rash
6. Hematoma
7. Anaphylaxis
8. Prolonged clotting time
9. Thrombocytopenia
10. Irritation
11. Ulceration
12. Hyperkalemia
13. Necrosis
14. Pain
15. Osteoporosis
16. Reversible alopecia

Contraindications for the use of LMWH:
1. Hypersensitivity to drug
2. Hemophilia
3. Severely compromised renal function
4. Severely compromised liver function
5. Bacterial endocarditis
6. Gastric ulcer (active disease)
7. Uncontrolled high blood pressure

Relative contraindications (need special monitoring):
1. Renal impairment
2. Metabolic acidosis
3. Patient on potassium-sparing medications
4. Hypoaldosteronism
5. Diabetes mellitus
6. Spinal or epidural anesthesia

Factor Xa Direct Inhibitors

It was seen with heparin-based drugs that the higher the anti-Xa potency the higher is the effect so the focus shifted to development of drugs that have high or only anti-Xa activity. Rivaroxaban and apixaban are such available direct, selective, reversible factor Xa inhibitors with the biggest advantage of being administered orally and convenient dosing. They have been approved by the FDA for prophylaxis of DVT, which may lead to PE in patients undergoing knee or hip replacement surgery.

These agents are taken orally. Apixaban is excreted 75% through the hepatobiliary system and, 25% renally, having a mean half-life of 12 hours and onset of 3 hours. Half of the administered rivaroxaban eliminated renally and the other half by the fecal route after metabolism of the two-thirds of the dose. Rest one-third is excreted unchanged in urine. Rivaroxaban has a half-life of 5–13 hours. The drugs interact with other drugs having an effect on the CYP3A4 and P-glycoprotein (P-gp) pathway (apixaban is quite safe as it does not induce the CYP pathway but still caution is advised). Drugs inducing this pathway (like rifampicin) reduce the half-life of the drug while there is huge increase in the mean half-life of the administered drug with the CYP3A4 and P-gp inhibitors (like ketoconazole and ritonavir). There is no interaction with concomitant administration of LMWH, nonsteroidal anti-inflammatory drugs (NSAIDs) or aspirin.

Rivaroxaban is administered once daily (10/20 mg) while apixaban needs a twice daily dosing (2.5 mg). For routine administrations, there is no need to monitor the coagulation profile of the patients. The problem with these drugs is that they are highly plasma bound so that in case of rare hemorrhagic complications dialysis will not help reverse the effect of the drug. Also, there is no specific antidote available. Treatment hence relies on replenishing the coagulation factors. The efficacy of these drugs have been comparable to (or better with better compliance and lesser complications) LMWHs.

Edoxaban, darexaban, and betrixaban are other available agents elsewhere.

The *advantages* of these drugs include:
- Rapid onset of action, so no need for bridging therapy
- Short half-life, so easy control of anticoagulant effect
- Little or no food interaction, so no dietary restrictions like warfarin
- Predictability of anticoagulation effect without a need for routine coagulation monitoring

The *disadvantages* of these agents include:
- *Prohibitively* high cost resulting in poor compliance (Apixaban is exception as it is relatively much cheaper)
- *No* monitoring is possible if needed
- *No* specific antidote
- *Serious* bleeding in renal impaired patients and elderly > 80 years. If GFR is 15–30 mL/min prefer warfarin as anticoagulant.

Direct Thrombin Inhibitor and Dabigatran Etexilate (Available as Pradaxa® in India)

Lepirudin, argatroban, and desirudin are expensive parenteral compounds available as reserve drug to treat DVT or PE where heparin is contraindicated. Though available for >6 years, dabigatran (an oral agent) has been approved only in April 2014 for DVT prophylaxis in patients who have been treated with parenteral drugs for 5–10 days (i.e., maintenance therapy). It has also been used and approved to reduce the risk of recurrence of DVT and PE in patients who have been previously treated. Other *indications* for the drug include:
- Treatment of VTE
- Treatment of thromboembolic complications following acute coronary syndromes

Dabigatran belongs to class benzimidazoles and acts on thrombin-mediated conversion of fibrinogen to fibrin which is the final pathway of coagulation so it affects all the pathways. The drug interacts with both the clot-bound thrombin and the thrombin-induced platelet aggregation (***see* Fig. 8**). Recently an antidote (idarucizumab) to dabigatran has been approved for use should serious complications arise.

Contraindications and precautions: The following conditions should raise caution over use of dabigatran and in general should be taken as absolute or relative contraindication:
- Patients with mechanical prosthetic valves
- Presence of pathological bleeding
- Known hypersensitivity reaction
- Dabigatran should be used with caution in elderly patients aged over 75 years and in patients with active peptic ulcer, bleeding, and renal diseases due to risk of bleeding. For same reason, use of alcoholic beverages is prohibited.
- Drug interactions may occur with warfarin, clopidogrel, ticlopidine, streptokinase, urokinase, quinidine, rifampicin, antiarrhythmic drugs, calcium channel blockers, NSAIDs, and antifungal drugs.

In patients undergoing elective THR or TKR, dabigatran etexilate is given once daily (150 mg), and BID for secondary prophylaxis for the treatment of VTE. Dabigatran is the active form of dabigatran etexilate. It is converted to its active form by esterase-catalyzed hydrolysis in the plasma and liver. Mainly it is excreted unchanged renally (~80%) with the remainder eliminated via the bile. The drug does not influence the cytochrome p450 enzymes but concomitant use of P-gp inducers/inhibitors needs alteration of the dosage. Also, the dose is to be altered in patients with renal compromise.

CHOICE OF ANTICOAGULANT

An ideal anticoagulant should be:
- Easy to administer (preferably oral)
- Effect should be promptly reversible
- Effective and safe with a minimum of possible complications or adverse effects
- Have a rapid onset with therapeutic half-life
- Inexpensive
- Predictable dose-dependent action with minimal or no drug or dietary interactions
- Require no monitoring

No single available agent combines all these attributes. Newer oral agents satisfy many of the above requirements but suffer from serious limitation of nonavailability of an antidote if bleeding occurs. These drugs have rapid onset of action, predictable dose response, therapeutic half-life, and do not require aPTT/PT/INR monitoring as for warfarin.

A comparative analysis of the relative efficacies of various agents available for DVT prophylaxis has been done extensively in literature. LMWH is the reference drug against which the anticoagulation efficacy and bleeding complications are assessed. LMWH has been found to reduce the RR of DVT by 50–60% and the same can possibly be extrapolated to PE. Fondaparinux has increased anticoagulation efficacy but that comes with significantly increased risk of major/minor bleeding. LDUH is less efficacious and is associated with increased risk of bleeding. The newer oral anticoagulants are becoming increasingly popular and have replaced LMWH as drug of choice in most circumstances; their comparison is presented in **Table 6**. Most of the oral anticoagulants are costly with the exception of apixaban (Eliquis®).

Other anticoagulants under development include:
- Antithrombin
- Anti-Xa
- Anti-TF

TABLE 6: Relative comparison of the three commonly used newer oral anticoagulants (note the comparison has been done to enoxaparin 30 mg BID given subcutaneously).

Oral agents			
Parameter	***Apixaban (ADVANCE 1, ADVANCE 2, ADVANCE 3)***	***Dabigatran (RE-MODEL, RE-MOBILIZE, RE-NOVATE, RE-NOVATE II)***	***Rivaroxaban (RECORD 1, RECORD 2, RECORD 3, RECORD 4)***
THA—VTE and mortality rates	Proven noninferiority and superiority	Proven noninferiority, failed superiority	Proven noninferiority and superiority
TKA—VTE and mortality rates	Failed noninferiority	Proven noninferiority	Proven noninferiority and superiority
Bleeding risk—THA	Similar rates	Similar rates	Similar rates
Bleeding risk—TKA	Similar major bleeds but fewer nonmajor bleeds	Similar rates	Similar rates

- Heparinoids and hirudin derivatives
- Oral formulations of heparin
- Glycosaminoglycans mixtures
- Activated protein C
- Biotechnology derived serine protease inhibitors (SERPINs) such as the recombinant AT and heparin cofactor II (HCII)

Assessment for Initiating the Prophylaxis

The assessment for the DVT prophylaxis should include the following key points that will decide upon the type of prophylaxis required and duration of prophylaxis:

1. Risk for thromboembolism—the following steps are carefully evaluated for risk assessment:
    - The risk factors listed above (in etiology of DVT)
    - Additional risk for DVT and reasons for hospitalization (surgical procedures, trauma medical illnesses, etc.), the type of surgery (high risk is associated with major joint surgery and curative surgery for cancer), the type of anesthesia, the likely duration of immobility (including duration of surgery)
2. Assess the patient's risk of bleeding (the factors are listed above in complications of anticoagulation)
3. Balance of risks (DVT risk vs. bleeding risk)
4. Select appropriate methods for thromboprophylaxis

Deep Venous Thrombosis Prophylaxis Based on Risk Stratification Levels for Orthopedic Patients

According to severity, the risk factors are grouped and an overall risk factor score is produced, which corresponds to a low through a very high potential for DVT development **(Table 7)**. By using these risk criteria, orthopedic patients can be categorized into four risk groups, ranging from low to very high **(Table 8)**. One should kindly note that the Wells' score detailed above in diagnosis is useful for suspecting DVT clinically and is not established for institution of DVT prophylaxis in a risk stratification model.

In general, the recommendations for cumulative risk assessment for DVT are as follows:

- Patients with a score of 1 or less (low-risk) require early and aggressive mobilization. No specific prophylaxis is required for these patients.
- A patient having a score of 2 or less have the 1–2% risk of developing clinical PE. Successful prevention strategies in this group consist of LMWH (low-dose), GCS or IPC, antiplatelet drugs (alone) or oral agents (direct Xa inhibitors).
- High-risk patients have a score of 3 or 4. The risk of PE occurring is 2–4%. Successful prevention strategies in this group consist of LMWH (higher doses), GCS or IPC with antiplatelet drugs, oral agents (+GCS or IPC or antiplatelet drugs).
- The highest-risk patients have a score of 5 or greater. The estimated risk of clinical PE is 4–10% and fatal PE is 0.2–5%.

Successful prevention strategies include LMWH (higher doses), fondaparinux, and coumarins (to maintain INR 2.5–3). It may be prudent to combine GCS or IPC with LMWHs.

TABLE 7: Grading for various risk factors for cumulative risk of DVT.

One point is assigned to each of the following:	*Two points are assigned to each of the following:*
• Age 41–60 years • History of major surgery within 1 month • Inflammatory bowel disease • Minor surgery • Obesity [body mass index (BMI) >25 kg/m^2] • Oral contraceptives, patch, or hormone replacement therapy • Pregnancy or postpartum within 1 month • Swelling of legs • Varicose veins	• Age older than 60 years • Central venous access for <1 month • Confined to bed longer than 72 hours • Immobilizing cast shorter than 1 month • Laparoscopic surgery (>45 min) • Major surgery (>45 min) • Malignancy or current chemotherapy or radiation therapy • Tourniquet time longer than 45 minutes
Three points are assigned to each of the following:	*Five points are assigned to each of the following risk factors:*
• Age older than 75 years • Congenital or acquired thrombophilia • Factor V Leiden/activated protein C resistance • Family history of thrombosis • History of DVT or pulmonary embolism • Medical patient with risk factors of myocardial infarction, congestive heart failure, or chronic obstructive pulmonary disease	• Acute spinal cord injury with paralysis within 1 month • Hip, pelvis, or leg fracture within 1 month • Major, elective lower extremity arthroplasty, total knee replacement, total hip replacement • Multiple trauma within 1 month • Stroke within 1 month

TABLE 8: Deep venous thrombosis risk factor scores.

Risk factor score	0–1	2	3–4	5+
DVT incidence	2%	10–20%	20–40%	40–80%
Risk level	Low	Moderate	High	Very high

Guidelines have been issued for specific orthopedic procedures as to the initiation of prophylaxis and type of agent that can be used (modified from ACCP, 9th edition and NHMRC, also see above in "Rationale for Prophylaxis"). The guidelines are extensive but in a nutshell the following suffices for arthroplasty in general (details are provided here).

- ACCP recommends minimum 10–14 days thromboprophylaxis is needed using any one of the following (strong recommendation)—LMWH (preferred), fondaparinux, rivaroxaban, apixaban, dabigatran, VKA, aspirin (325 mg/day), LDUH or an IPC device. It further recommends to extend the prophylaxis for 35 days and to preferably use dual prophylaxis (weak recommendations). Prophylaxis should start 12 hours or more after surgery. Use of pharmacological and pharmacological prophylaxis is recommended for all during hospitalization.
- AAOS instead recommends either pharmacologic or IPC device for all THA/TKA without any preference for pharmacologic or mechanical agent. Also, it does not give and guideline for duration of prophylaxis and suggests

a discussion between the treating surgeon and patient to arrive at a time period. Also, AAOS suggests to prefer pharmacologic over IPC device for patients with previous history of DVT/VTE and to prefer mechanical method in patients with bleeding diathesis. For mechanical prophylaxis, AAOS recommends only battery-powered portable IPC device capable of recording.

Elective Total Hip Replacement

Use prophylaxis for all patients. Administer LMWH 12–24 hours before or after surgery followed by a full dose on the next day. Continue for 35 days. Alternatives are:

- Fondaparinux (2.5 mg) started 6–8 hours postoperatively
- Rivaroxaban (10 mg/day)/Apixaban (2.5 mg twice daily)
- Dabigatran etexilate (150 mg or 220 mg/day)
- GCS/IPC ± Aspirin (low-dose) (AAOS recommendation)

Preoperative administration of the drug may be unnecessary. UFH and warfarin are not recommended unless the latter is used as a therapeutic option already.

Hip Fracture Surgery

Use prophylaxis for all patients for a minimum of 10–14 days using one of the following: LMWH, fondaparinux, LDUH, adjusted-dose VKA, aspirin. If pharmacological intervention is contraindicated then IPC or GCS or foot pumps are used till patient gets mobile.

Low-molecular-weight heparins are initiated at the time of admission if the surgery is delayed. They should be discontinued before surgery. Due to their immediate action, reversibility, and short half-life, they are ideal agents for interim prophylaxis during the period between admission and surgery.

Total Knee Replacement

Prophylaxis recommended for all patients. Administering LWMH 12–24 hours postoperatively, and continue for 14 days. Alternative medications are:

- Fondaparinux
- Rivaroxaban/apixaban
- Dabigatran
- GCS/IPC/foot pumps + Aspirin (AAOS)
- Foot pumps or GCS or IPC alone can be used for contraindications to pharmacotherapy.

Aspirin alone is not recommended as is warfarin unless it has been given otherwise for therapeutic measure (as in previous cardiac surgery).

Knee Arthroscopy

Unless the patient has preexisting risk factors for VTE or prolonged tourniquet time is anticipated, thromboprophylaxis is not recommended for these patients. LMWH should be given to the patients with the risk factors.

Lower Leg Injuries

No thromboprophylaxis is recommended for isolated lower leg injury requiring immobilization.

Elective Spine Surgery

Same as for knee arthroscopy. It is recommended to use GCS/IPC/foot pumps instead of pharmacotherapy due to high-risk area and neural compression in case of bleeding.

Impact of Anesthesia on Anticoagulation and Vice Versa

- Regional anesthesia is associated with lower risk of DVT.
- The risk of PE is also much less with regional anesthesia.
- Anticoagulant prophylaxis should be used with caution in patients receiving central neural blockade (spinal or indwelling catheter epidural anesthesia).
- The risk of spinal hematoma is very small (0.0025% with spinal anesthesia and 0.03% with epidural anesthesia) but care should be taken to initiate thromboprophylaxis for at least 2 hours (common practice is to separate the procedures by a minimum of 8 hours). The same guidelines apply for catheter removal. The factors associated with hematoma formation include:
  - Concomitant use of other drugs such as NSAIDs, platelet inhibitors, other anticoagulants
  - Use of indwelling catheters
  - History of traumatic or repeated spinal punctures
- Patients with known bleeding disorders should not receive preoperative prophylaxis if they are to receive spinal anesthesia.

Initiation of Prophylaxis Therapy

Here comes the role of identification of patients at risk of bleeding. For patients with risk of bleeding, preoperative thromboprophylaxis is contraindicated. Postoperative thromboprophylaxis should be monitored in these cases. I would say that preoperative prophylaxis should be given only to very high-risk cases. There is no objective support to this statement from the studies available.

In our practice, we have been using apixaban for all moderate- and high-risk cases undergoing arthroplasty or hip surgeries. We had been using LMWH previously but now have shifted to using only IPC in low-risk patients or combination of IPC with aspirin (low-dose) in moderate-risk to high-risk patients. Our regimen is mainly dependent on cost concern as is throughout most of India and the compliance issues where it is difficult to pursue patients for IPC/GCS. The most significant complication I have observed is ecchymosis near the operative site with the use of thromboprophylaxis and possibly if we were to follow the AAOS regimen then aspirin with IPC should suffice. I strongly suggest that one should develop institutional policy for DVT prophylaxis is association with hematologist (who will rescue, if bleeding occurs) and chest physician (who will come to bail you out in case of PE). There is no alternative to neat and clean surgery performed with as minimal soft tissue manipulation as possible and early mobilization for prevention of DVT.

PERIOPERATIVE MANAGEMENT OF ANTICOAGULATION

Patients already on anticoagulation for associated comorbidities [such as atrial fibrillation (AF), high risk for stroke

(CHADS2 score >4), patients already on treatment for VTE, etc.] are at an increased risk of developing thromboembolic complications. Most orthopedic surgeries cannot be performed with ongoing anticoagulation and commonly perceived "safe" level for surgeries is INR <1.5 (there is however no strong evidence for this value). These high-risk patients are kept on "bridging" therapy (say during perioperative period) to manage anticoagulation between the time chronic anticoagulation is stopped and re-established. This "bridging" only manages the period when INR is subtherapeutic. The following are special scenarios specifically dealt with:

1. *Chronic warfarin therapy:* Stop warfarin for 5 days prior to surgery (for a surgery planned on Monday the last dose should be taken on previous Tuesday not later) for achieving target of 1.3 INR. "Bridge" patients on high risk of VTE by LMWH for 3 days (LMWH administered on Friday, Saturday, and Sunday (not Monday, avoid LMWH within 24 hours of planned surgery)].
2. *High risk for thrombosis patients:* Patients with mechanical mitral valve, older generation aortic valve (tilt-disk, caged-ball), recent history of stroke/transient ischemic attack, AF with CHDS2 score > 4 or AF with rheumatic valve disease, recent VTE event (within 3 months) need full-dose LMWH bridging (1.5 mg/kg of enoxaparin or 200 IU dalteparin once daily in morning).
3. *Intermediate-risk patients* are those with aortic mechanical valve with risk factor like AF or prior stroke or diabetes or hypertension; AF with CHADS2 score of 3 or 4, patient with prior recurrent VTE (last > 3 months) or patient with active malignancy. "Bridge" these patients with prophylactic doses of LMWH or according to institutional policy. Continue anticoagulation in postoperative period.
4. *Low-risk patients* include those with bileaflet mechanical aortic valve only without associated risk factors, AF with CHADS2 score of 0–2, history of VTE > 12 months prior to current event. Consider "bridge" therapy balancing risk of bleeding.
5. *Patients with renal insufficiency/failure:* Maintain high-risk patients on IV heparin (monitor using aPTT monitored) or warfarin (monitor INR). For prophylaxis also these drugs are first choice in patients with renal insufficiency as LMWH, apixaban/rivaroxaban, dabigatran may accumulate if creatinine clearance is <30 cc/min causing excessive anticoagulation.
6. *Liver impairment:* Despite the fact that coagulation factors are synthesized in liver so many physicians consider that patients with advanced liver disease are autoanticoagulated. This perception is *not* true. These patients need anticoagulation with IV heparin (aPTT monitoring or anti-Xa level monitoring) or warfarin (monitor INR).
7. *Thrombocytopenia patients:* Commonly recommended levels of platelet considered "safe" for surgery are >50,000/mL (there is no "documented" level of platelets that is associated with higher bleeding risk). These patients can also clot. Use therapeutic doses of anticoagulants for treating VTE. It is recommended to avoid heparin in these patients as it may cause HIT.

TABLE 9: Guideline for preoperative withholding (in hours) of oral anticoagulants.

Creatinine clearance (cc/min)	*Bleeding risk*	*Rivaroxaban/ Apixaban*	*Dabigatran*
>80	Low	≥24	≥24
	High	≥48	≥48
50–79	Low	≥24	≥36
	High	≥48	≥72
30–49	Low	≥24	≥48
	High	≥48	≥96
15–29	Low	≥36	Patient should not be on this medicine!
	High	≥48	
<15	Patient should not be on these medications!		

8. *Patients on newer (oral) anticoagulant drugs:* Quite frequently patients are found using oral anticoagulants because of their increased popularity and ease of use. Preoperative withholding of these drugs depends on assessment of bleeding risk and creatinine clearance **(Table 9)**. These medications can be restarted 8–12 hours after surgery at a lower dose like rivaroxaban 10 mg, apixaban 2.5 mg, dabigatran 75 mg every 12 hours and escalating to full dose after 2 days.

UPPER EXTREMITY DEEP VEIN THROMBOSIS

INTRODUCTION

Brachial, axillary, and subclavian veins are the deep veins of the upper extremity. Thrombosis of these veins refers to UEDVT. It is an increasingly recognized clinical entity with advancements in upper limb arthroplasty and surgeries. UEDVT accounts for around 10% of overall VTE cases and an incidence of about 3/100,000 has been reported in general population. PE is present in up to one-third of patients with UEDVT.

The lower incidence of UEDVT is possibly related to:

- Fewer and smaller valves in the veins of upper extremity
- Bedridden patients still keep moving upper extremity for activities of daily living (ADL)
- Less hydrostatic pressure in the arms causing less pooling (stasis) or intimal damage
- Increased fibrinolytic activity has been seen in the endothelium of the upper arm as compared to the lower extremity.
- Absence of intramuscular sinusoids (soleal network of veins)
- The UEDVT most commonly involves the subclavian vein (18–67%), followed by axillary (5–25%) and the brachial (4–11%), with predilection for left side. Characteristically UEDVT occurs in more than one segment of the veins at any instance.

PATHOGENESIS AND RISK FACTORS

Causes of Upper Extremity Deep Vein Thrombosis

I. *Primary*
   - Traumatic:
     - Effort thrombosis (Paget-von Schroetter syndrome)
     - Blood vessel injury

- Increased distal venous pressure:
  - Cervical ribs and long transverse processes of cervical spine
  - Musculofascial bands of subclavius muscle and costoclavicular ligament
  - Clavicular or 1st rib anomalies
- Hypercoagulable state:
  - Antiphospholipid antibodies
  - Factor V Leiden
  - Prothrombin gene mutation
  - Antithrombin III deficiency
  - Protein C and S deficiency
  - Homocystinemia
  - Pregnancy and oral contraceptive use

II. *Secondary*

- Central venous catheters: Larger the catheter inserted higher are the chances of a DVT indicating that the peripherally inserted central lines may have a reduced incidence of UEDVT
- Malignant disease includes:
  - Lymphoma/Leukemia
  - Pancreatic cancer
  - Breast cancer and its treatment
  - Pulmonary, pleural, esophageal, and GI tract
- Pacemakers: Patients who had implanted permanent pacemakers with prior use of temporary pacemakers and low left ventricular ejection fractions (<40%) had a much higher incidence of venous thrombosis
- Intravenous drug abuse

III. *Idiopathic*

Primary UEDVT

Primary UEDVT accounts for up to one-third of all thrombosis involving the upper extremities. It mainly includes Paget-von Schroetter syndrome and idiopathic thrombosis.

After strenuous, repetitive or unusual physical activity, such as weight lifting, rowing or playing tennis, Paget-von Schroetter syndrome typically occurs in the dominant arm. The male-to-female ratio is approximately 2:1. It is often associated with thoracic outlet syndrome which is also the most common predisposing factor.

Pathogenesis of effort thrombosis (Paget-von Schroetter syndrome): Repeated microtrauma of the vessel intima causes activation of the coagulation cascade. There may also be perivascular scar tissue formation with persistent vein compression and tethering. The major cause is thoracic outlet obstruction which causes compression of the neurovascular bundle (which includes brachial plexus, subclavian artery, and subclavian vein) as it exits the thoracic inlet. Venous compression typically develops in young athletes with hypertrophied muscles who do heavy labor. Other anatomical factors may also be commonly seen in these patients so chest and cervical spine need thorough evaluation.

Pathogenesis of idiopathic thrombosis: These patients have no known trigger or obvious underlying disease. About one-fourth of patients are associated with occult cancer or developed same within 1 year of follow-up. The prevalence of hypercoagulable states is uncertain. They should be evaluated in idiopathic disease, those with positive family history and recurrent DVT or pregnancy loss, or importantly those having personal history of a prior DVT.

Secondary UEDVT

They have known endogenous or exogenous risk factors. It accounts for about two-thirds of all cases with UEDVT and commonly affects older patients with severe comorbidities unlike the primary/idiopathic form. The most important risk factor for UEDVT is the presence of an indwelling central venous catheter. Catheter characteristics that are associated with an increased risk of UE DVT may include:

- Catheter material (polyethylene, polyvinyl chloride > silicone, polyurethane)
- Catheter tip located proximal to the atriocaval junction
- Catheter-related infection/septicemia
- Multiple attempts for insertion
- Number of lumina (triple lumen > double lumen)
- Prior catheterization at the same puncture site
- Prolonged catheter retention (>2 weeks)
- Use on left extremity

Malignancy is the other main risk factor for secondary UEDVT. Pathogenesis of tumor-related UEDVT is multifactorial:

- Cancer-induced inhibition of natural anticoagulants and fibrinolysis as well as release of prothrombotic factors
- Direct vein compression by the tumor itself
- Endothelial damage caused by indwelling catheters or radiotherapy
- Venous stasis due to immobilization

In the presence of distant metastases, the risk of developing DVT increases. Ovarian carcinoma and lung adenocarcinoma carry a particularly increased risk of UEDVT.

CLINICAL PRESENTATION

Signs and Symptoms of UEDVT

These are nonspecific and vary with the site of obstruction (axillary vs. SVC) **(Table 10)**, also the causal factors for secondary UEDVT should be evaluated.

TABLE 10: Signs and symptoms of upper extremity deep vein thrombosis (UEDVT).

Region of involvement/etiology	*Symptoms*	*Signs*
Axillary or subclavian vein thrombosis	• Vague shoulder or neck discomfort • Arm or hand edema	• Extremity cyanosis • Palpable cord • Arm or hand edema • Catheter blockade
Superior vena cava obstruction	• Arm and head fullness	• Blurred vision • Jugular venous distention, dyspnea
Thoracic outlet syndrome	• Pain radiating to arm/forearm • Hand weakness	• Arm or hand atrophy • Brachial plexus tenderness • Positive Adson's or Wright's maneuver

- Usually the patients of axillary or subclavian vein thrombosis complain of vague shoulder or neck discomfort and arm edema.
- Superior vena cava obstruction causes arm and facial edema, blurred vision, head fullness, vertigo or dyspnea.
- Those patients who have thoracic outlet obstruction may have pain radiating into the fourth and fifth digits via the medial arm and forearm. With hyperabduction of the shoulder or lifting any heavy weight, the pain may worsen.
- Especially for thoracic outlet syndrome, the supraclavicular fossa should be palpated for tenderness (brachial neuritis), the hand and arm should be inspected for atrophy, and provocative tests, such as Adson's and Wright's maneuvers should be performed.

Adson's Maneuver

As the examiner extends the patient's arm on the affected side, the patient is asked to extend neck and rotate head toward the same side. If there is weakening of the radial pulse with deep inspiration, the test is positive and it suggests compression of the subclavian artery.

Wright's Maneuver

The examiner abducts the patient's shoulder and externally rotates the humerus. If symptoms are reproduced and there is weakening of the radial pulse, the test is positive.

Physical Examination

- Fever may indicate thrombosis (low-grade fever) while high-grade fever may suggest septic thrombophlebitis.
- SVC syndrome is associated with sinus tachycardia (reduced venous return to the heart).
- The commonly observed signs in UEDVT though nonspecific include:
  - Arm and hand edema
  - Dilated cutaneous collateral veins over the chest or upper arm
  - Jugular venous distention
  - Mild cyanosis
  - Palpable tender cord
  - Supraclavicular fullness

DIAGNOSIS

Clinical Prediction Score

As for lower limb DVT, the clinical diagnosis and predictability of UEDVT occurrence is essential. The following points help evaluate the same:

- Localized pain — 1 point
- Indwelling venous catheter — 1 point
- Unilateral pitting edema — 1 point
- Other diagnosis at least as plausible — 1 point

Score	*Clinical probability*	*Rate of thrombosis (%)*
≤0	Low	13
1	Intermediate	38
≥2	High	69

This score has sensitivity of 78% and specificity of 64%. Following an intermediate to high clinical probability, further assessment is carried out by one of the following diagnostic imaging:

Duplex Ultrasound

The initial imaging test of choice as for LEDVT. Compression ultrasonography has sensitivity of 97% and specificity of 96%. It has following advantages:

- Noninvasive
- Reproducible technique
- High sensitivity and specificity for assessment of cephalic, axillary, and subclavian veins

The brachiocephalic vein is visible only on venography and magnetic resonance angiography (MRA) so this modality cannot be used.

Diagnostic findings include:

- Noncompressibility of venous segment
- Intraluminal thrombus and flow abnormality (conversion of the normal biphasic flow pattern into a nonpulsatile, continuous flow signal)

Contrast Venography

Venography had been the gold standard but is being gradually replaced by other investigations for the following reasons:

- Technical difficulty in cannulating the vein
- Need of iodinated contrast agent (allergic reaction, nephrotoxicity or a chemical phlebitis)
- Invasive

Venography is ideally indicated now to resolve confusion of a negative ultrasonography scan in a highly suspicious clinical setting. Otherwise venography is a routine before catheter-directed thrombolysis and angioplasty.

Magnetic Resonance Angiography

MRA is investigation of choice for central thoracic veins (SVC and brachiocephalic veins) thrombosis.

Differential diagnosis of UEDVT includes:

- Lymphedema
- Muscle injury
- Cellulitis
- Thrombophlebitis

COMPLICATIONS

Reported complications of UEDVT include:

1. Post-thrombotic syndrome and chronic venous insufficiency: The PTS causes significant functional disability and impaired quality of life especially when occurring in dominant arm. It is associated with symptoms include edema, limb fatigue with exertion, persistent pain or heaviness of the affected arm, skin discoloration and distended collateral veins in the shoulder region.
2. Superior vena cava syndrome
3. Catheter infection
4. Acute and recurrent PE (3–12%) that may cause pulmonary hypertension and/or right-sided heart failure: Acute presentation is more often seen in a setting

of catheter-related DVT with underlying malignancy. Symptoms include dyspnea, visceral or pleuritic chest pain, syncope, low-grade fever, and sinus tachycardia.
5. Venous gangrene
6. Thoracic duct obstruction causing chylous pleural effusion, chylous pericardial effusion
7. Brachial plexopathy

TREATMENT

Various treatment modalities for UEDVT are:
- *Noninterventional measures (preventive):*
  - Limb elevation
  - Graduated compression arm sleeve
  - Anticoagulation
- *Interventional (preventive):* Superior vena cava filter
- *Interventional (therapeutic):*
  - Catheter-directed thrombolysis
  - Suction thrombectomy
  - Vein stenting
  - Surgical thrombectomy
- *Treatment of cause:* Thoracic outlet decompression

Principles of Treatment

- Initiate treatment before the thrombus becomes organized.
- Because the underlying cause of primary UEDVT is usually an anatomic abnormality, surgical decompression of the subclavian vein is essential to prevent recurrent thrombosis.

Anticoagulation

Anticoagulation is the base therapy that is common to all interventions. The goal is to keep INR between 2.0 and 3.0. For which LMWH ("bridge therapy" for warfarinization) followed by warfarin or other antivitamin K agents are typically used for a minimum of 3 months. Therapeutic anticoagulation should not be shortened to fewer than 3 months after catheter removal. This method is more or less ancillary to other measures and possibly definitive for elderly patients. Young patients with UEDVT are managed more aggressively with interventional measures.

Central venous catheter may be retained if the device is functional and needed further for the patient's care. Catheters are removed if patient has any one of the following:
- Infection or thrombophlebitis or line sepsis
- >1-week old thrombus
- >2-cm long thrombus

Guidelines for anticoagulation (ACCP 9th edition):
- Instead of thrombolytic therapy, the use of anticoagulation therapy alone is suggested for UEDVT that involves the axillary or more proximal veins. Length of anticoagulation: at least 3 months.
- UEDVT which is not associated with a central venous catheter: 3 months of anticoagulation is recommended.
- UEDVT which is associated with a central venous catheter:
  - If the catheter is functional and there is an ongoing need for the catheter, it is not removed. As long as the catheter is in place, anticoagulation therapy should be continued.
  - Anticoagulation should continue for 3 months after the removal of the catheter.

Thrombolysis

The treatment is based on the following rationale:
- Quickly restores venous patency
- Prevents long-term damage to the vessel endothelium
- Reduces the risk of PTS

It is preferred for young and healthy UEDVT patients (currently ACCP recommends against thrombolytic therapy). rtPA is currently the agent of choice. The drug is administered through catheter positioned as close to the clot as possible. Thrombolysis is more successful if used within few weeks of the onset of symptoms due to smaller clot size. It is best suited for:
- Young healthy patients having primary UEDVT
- Patients with symptomatic SVC syndrome
- Those who require preservation of a mandatory central venous catheter

Contraindications are common for all thrombolysis patients and include:
- Active hemorrhage
- History of hemorrhagic stroke
- Hypersensitivity to the thrombolytic agent
- Neurosurgery within the past 2 months
- Surgery within the preceding 10 days

Thrombolysis is protected with heparin in postoperative period continued variably.

Suction thrombectomy: Involves percutaneous mechanical thrombectomy. It is often combined with thrombolytics to reduce the dose and duration of thrombolytic therapy.

Surgery: To reduce venous compression evident on venography involves surgical resection of part of the 1st rib or clavicle and lysis of dense adhesions around the subclavian veins. This should be done after initial management to reduce chances of recurrent thrombosis.

Angioplasty and vein stenting: Has to be combined with surgery often to dilate residual venous stricture. The procedure can also follow thrombolysis and is completed by balloon venoplasty and stenting to ensure patency.

Surgical thrombectomy: This is reserved for refractory cases or those who have an infected thrombus as a cause of bacteremia mainly due to high complication rates.

Physical therapy: It is essential in patients with neurological symptoms and otherwise also following surgical procedures rehabilitation is faster with physiotherapy. The plan should also incorporate weight-reduction program to reduce further risk.

Superior vena cava filters: The use is infrequent and is indicated in:
- Patients, in whom anticoagulation is contraindicated, have failed or created complications.
- Those who are poor surgical risk.
- Those who are at definite risk for PE.

PROPHYLAXIS OF UPPER EXTREMITY DEEP VEIN THROMBOSIS

The drug of choice is LMWH (but can be substituted with oral anticoagulants) but for patients having protracted disorders like cancer warfarin had been preferred especially if monitoring can be done. The recommended dose of dalteparin or fondaparinux is 2,500 IU subcutaneously once daily starting 2 hours before catheter insertion. For prophylaxis of patients with liver dysfunction or malnutrition, LMWH is a better choice than warfarin. There is sparse literature on guidelines; the current recommendations from ACCP are as follows:

- Thromboprophylaxis with LMWH or fondaparinux is recommended for:
  - Acutely ill medical patients admitted to hospital with:
    - Congestive cardiac failure or
    - Severe respiratory disease or
    - Who are confined to bed
  - Having one or more additional risk factors, including sepsis, acute neurologic disease or inflammatory bowel disease.
- According to current guidelines of the ACCP, to prevent UEDVT in *cancer patients* with indwelling central venous catheters, the use of LMWHs or VKAs is not recommended. These patients are frequently on other drugs that interact with warfarin and their PT may skyrocket causing intractable bleeding, the risk-to-benefit ratio is too much. As no clear benefit of anticoagulant prophylaxis is observed in *critically ill patients* with indwelling catheters not suffering from cancer, this recommendation also implies for this group.

CONCLUSION

- Venous thrombosis is a common complication in hospitalized patients but occurrence of embolization of the thrombus is quite less.
- Formation of thrombus involves activation of coagulation cascade at site of venous stasis that may involve damage to the venous intima.
- Evaluation of patients that are bedridden should involve regular examination for development of DVT. Use of newer objective scores for suspicion of DVT or PE like Wells' score is recommended over classical signs and symptoms.
- High-risk patients should receive prophylactic therapy. The true incidence of DVT is not documented in Indian patient population due to lack of unified registry but is possibly much less than reported values for western population. The values for embolism are probably even lower.
- LMWHs are commonly prescribed for patients that are being replaced by costly oral formulations but I personally feel that mechanical methods combined with pharmacoprophylaxis with low-dose aspirin would suffice in Indian patients considering low incidence of the disease. More data is awaited for Indian population before any concrete recommendation can be formulated.
- Adequate knowledge of the drugs commonly used for DVT prophylaxis is essential before using them anyhow or prescribing for various patient populations. There is a high chance that unless specifically contraindicated (like renal insufficiency), oral anticoagulants will likely replace injectable heparins (UFH or LMWH) in future.
- UEDVT is another important entity that is commonly missed in patients due to poor awareness. The incidence is possibly on rise due to increase in upper limb surgeries and overall increased interventional procedures as IV access is common to many.

CHAPTER 27

Compartment Syndrome

Manish Kumar Varshney

INTRODUCTION

Compartment syndrome is the emergency condition in which the pressure within an osteofascial compartment rises to a level that exceeds the intramuscular arteriolar pressure, resulting in decreased blood flow to capillaries, reduced oxygen diffusion to the tissues and ultimately cell death. Richard Von Volkmann first described the neural deficit and subsequent contracture from compartment syndrome in 1872 following supracondylar fracture, and in 1881 the conditions of irreversible contractures of flexor muscles attributing both to tight circumferential bandage that finally disrupts muscle blood supply. Later although Jones noted that the condition could arise both from pressure within the limb or from external compression. Hildebrand frost used the term "Volkmann's ischemic contracture" in 1906. Fasciotomy as a prevention for contracture was first suggested by Bardenheuer in 1906 and Murphy in 1914. It was MacGowan who busted the myth of associated pulselessness with development of compartment syndrome and emphasized that compartment syndrome can very well occur even when palpable pulses are present. Compartment syndromes may be acute or chronic (exertional), based on cause and reversibility **(Box 1)**.

- Acute compartment syndrome is also referred to as anterior tibial syndrome, calf hypertension, compartmental syndrome, Volkmann's ischemia, and impending ischemic contracture. It is seen in 7.3 per 100,000 males and 0.7 per 100,000 females. Most of the cases are due to fracture and associated soft-tissue injury. Importantly, incidence of compartment syndrome is same with both high- and low-energy injuries and that open wounds did not decompress the compartments and were not protective.
- The hallmark symptom of chronic compartment syndrome (CCS) is extremity pain induced by exercise or other exertion. This is a commonly overlooked condition and an average delay of around 22 months is seen in diagnosis of CCS. The patient reports recurrent pain that is initiated by exercise over the anterior or lateral compartment of the leg as a feeling of pressure or cramping in the compartment that may be achy, sharp or dull. This could be associated numbness or weakness due to compression on nearby nerve. The majority are young and active women or men with bilateral symptoms that have usually been present for months. The most common compartments involved in CCS are the anterior and/or lateral compartments of the leg. The earliest account of chronic exertional compartment syndrome is documented by Edward Wilson in 1912 for his symptoms on Antarctic expedition. Most of the early reports otherwise were from military recruits described as "march gangrene" by Horn in 1945. Reneman related the symptoms of these recruits to increased compartment pressure and termed "effort-related chronic compartment syndrome". Wilson's symptoms were attributed to increased compartment pressure by French and Price. Mavor described the surgical treatment of CCS in a soccer player.

BOX 1: Concept box for compartment syndrome.

- Acute compartment syndrome is a true medical and surgical emergency. Always keep in mind this possibility in forearm and leg injuries (especially closed ones) while foot, hand, thigh, and upper arm may also be the sites of contention.
- The condition specifically relates to "microvascular ischemia" of the contents within a closed osteofascial or fascial compartment.
- Pulselessness (pulses are a large vessel phenomenon) commonly related by residents to ischemia has *no* concordance in compartment syndrome and should *never* be considered a hallmark. Compartment syndromes very well occur with palpable pulses. Similarly, pallor should not be sought to make the diagnosis at all.
- Pain out-of-proportion to injury is the earliest symptom (but subjected to various fallacies so need evaluation by experienced person) and in children may be indicated by increasing analgesic requirements and anxiety. So, specifically seek and evaluate this abnormality to suspect and detect compartment syndrome early.
- Objective assessment by measuring compartment pressure or intracompartmental pH (if available) "may" supplement diagnosis else clinical suspicion is enough to proceed with treatment (Fasciotomy) to prevent late catastrophe.
- Chronic/exertional compartment syndrome should be suspected in athletes and strenuous workers that do not fit in neuropathic or other bone disorders.

ETIOPATHOGENESIS (FLOWCHARTS 1 AND 2)

Increased intracompartmental pressure due to fluid accumulation and tissue expansion within the confines of a closed, noncompliant, impermeable osteofascial compartment or from decrease in the space available for

Flowchart 1: Etiopathogenesis of acute compartment syndrome.

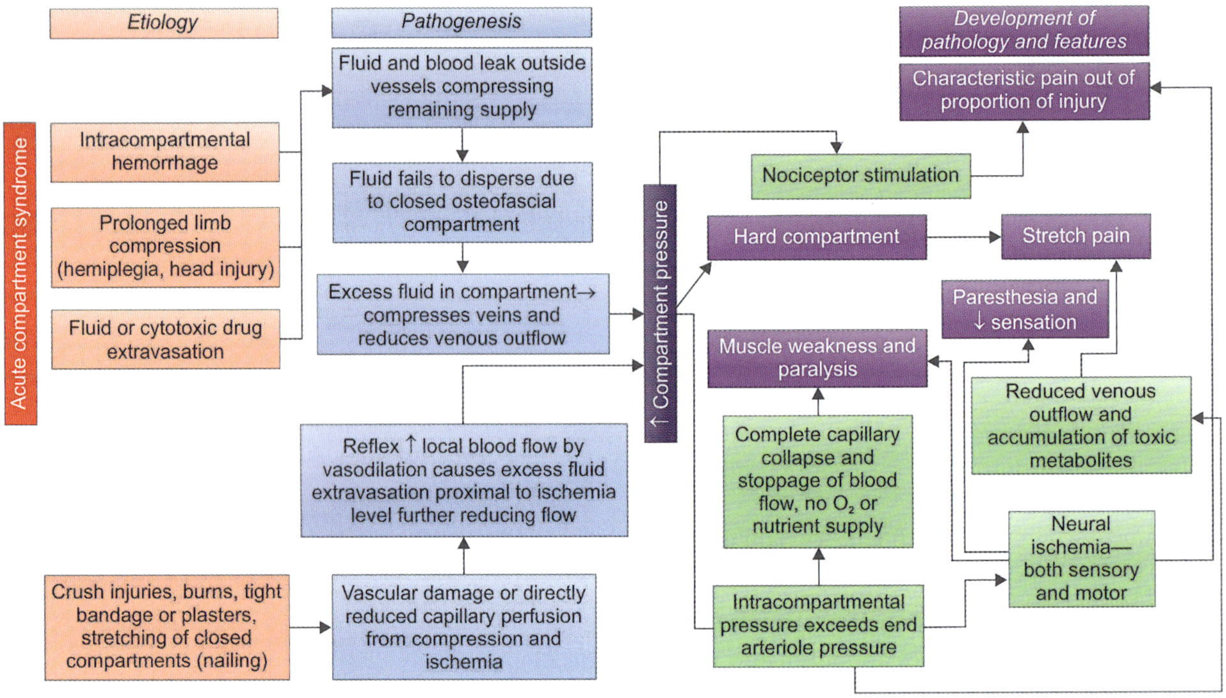

Flowchart 2: Etiopathogenesis of chronic compartment syndrome.

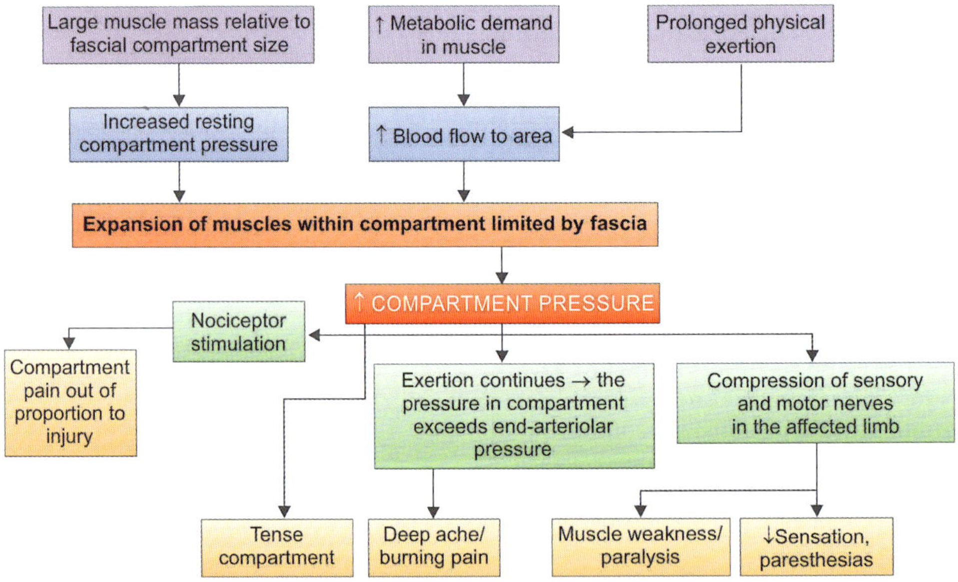

tissues can both result in compartment syndrome as can occur from various causes **(Table 1)**. Fractures are the most common cause followed by blunt trauma to soft tissues. Such closed compartments occur anywhere a skeletal muscle is completely surrounded by fascial sheath, but compartment syndromes are more common in:

- Leg (osteofascial)
- Forearm (osteofascial)
- Hand (osteofascial)—carpal tunnel is a separate compartment.
- Foot (osteofascial)
- Thigh (osteofascial/fascial)—three compartments, the anterior which includes the quadriceps, the posterior which includes the hamstrings, and the adductor groups.
- Upper arm—three compartments, the deltoid, the posterior which contains the triceps, and the anterior (biceps-brachialis)
- Buttock (fascial)—gluteal muscles
- Deltoid (fascial) and upper arm
- Paraspinal muscles (fascial)

The various compartments in different anatomical locations are detailed in **Table 2**. The foot is the most debatable site of all. Three compartments were described for foot in 1920s; however, Myerson later identified four compartments. Later nine compartments were identified in one cadaver study. Only three compartments (medial, lateral, and superficial) run the entire length of the foot. Five compartments (four interossei and adductor) are confined to the forefoot. The calcaneal compartment is separated from the flexor digitorum brevis (superficial compartment) by only a pressure gradient that becomes incompetent at gradient of <10 mm Hg. In high-pressure situations such as calcaneal fractures, the barrier becomes ineffective and FDB also gets involved forming one compartment (with quadratus plantae). This is the cause of claw-toe deformity seen after calcaneal fractures.

TABLE 1: Causes of compartment syndrome.

Increased compartment contents	*Decreased compartment volume*
• Bleeding (fractures, hemangioma, etc.) • Major vascular injury • Coagulation defect • Anticoagulant therapy • Reperfusion after ischemia • Trauma • Contusion • Seizures • Burns • Fluid extravasation • Venous obstruction • Reimplantation • High-pressure injections • Intraosseous fluid transfusion in • children • Reaming in intramedullary nailing • Use of fluid pumps in arthroscopy	• Tight casts, dressings, or air splints • Military anti-shock garments • Tourniquet • Lying on limb (e.g., well leg in lithotomy position) • Entrapment under collapsed weights • Tight closure of facial defects • Excessive traction to fractured limbs • Limb lengthening • Thermal injuries, burn eschar • Intramedullary nailing for long neglected fractures or deformity correction stretching individual muscles

Why a compartment syndrome develops is still unclear? Researchers have not been able to pin-point the microvascular changes/physiology behind compartment syndrome. There are a few explanations, though, for development of acute compartment syndrome:

- *The venous hypertension theory:* The impermeable fascia prevents fluid from leaking out elevating intracompartmental pressure. Elevated pressures beyond a critical limit prevent perfusion of tissues from capillaries (Starling's law) and results in tissue anoxia and death. This is clarified by Rowland and supported by Matsen equating the local blood flow (LBF) and the arteriovenous pressure gradient expressed by following equation:

$$\text{LBF} = (P_a - P_v)/R$$

TABLE 2: Anatomy of compartments of commonly involved regions in acute compartment syndrome.

Compartment region	*Muscles*	*Major vessels*	*Nerves*
Compartments of leg ***(Fig. 1A)***			
Anterior	Tibialis anterior, extensor halluces longus, extensor digitorum longus, peroneus tertius	Anterior tibial	Deep peroneal
Lateral	Peroneus brevis, peroneus longus	None	Superficial and deep peroneal (proximally)
Deep posterior	Tibialis posterior, flexor halluces longus, flexor digitorum longus	Posterior tibial, peroneal	Tibial
Superficial posterior	Gastrocnemius, soleus	None	None
Forearm compartments ***(Fig. 2B)***			
Volar superficial	PT, FCR, FCU, FDS, PL	Ulnar vessels	Ulnar
Volar deep	FPL, FDP	Anterior interosseous, ulnar	Median nerve, anterior interosseous
Extensor	ECRB, brachioradialis, EDC, EDM, ECU, anconeus, supinator, APL, EPL, EPB, EIP	Posterior interosseous	Radial (deep branch)
Lateral (mobile wad of Henry)	ECRL and brachioradialis (ECRB is not a component of this fascial sheath)	Radial vessels	? Superficial radial nerve
Hand **(Fig. 2A)**	Ten separate osteofascial compartments—dorsal interossei (4), palmar interossei (3), thenar and hypothenar (2), adductor pollicis (1)	Deep and superficial arch	None
Foot (ninc) ***(Fig. 1B)***			
Medial	FHB, abductor hallucis		
Lateral	Abductor digiti quinti, flexor digiti minimi		
Superficial	FDB, lumbricals, FDL tendon		Medial plantar nerve
Interossei	Interossei X4		
Adductor	Adductor		
Calcaneal (Manoli and Weber)	Quadratus plantae	Posterior tibial vessels, lateral plantar vessels	Posterior tibial, lateral plantar, medial plantar

(APL: abductor pollicis longus; ECRB: extensor carpi radialis brevis; ECRL: extensor carpi radialis longus; ECU: extensor carpi ulnaris; EDC: extensor digitorum communis; EDM: extensor digiti minimi; EIP: extensor indicis proprius; EPB: extensor pollicis brevis; EPL: extensor pollicis longus; FCR: flexor carpi radialis; FCU: flexor carpi ulnaris; FDS: flexor digitorum superficialis; FPL: flexor pollicis longus; PL: palmaris longus; PT: pronator teres)

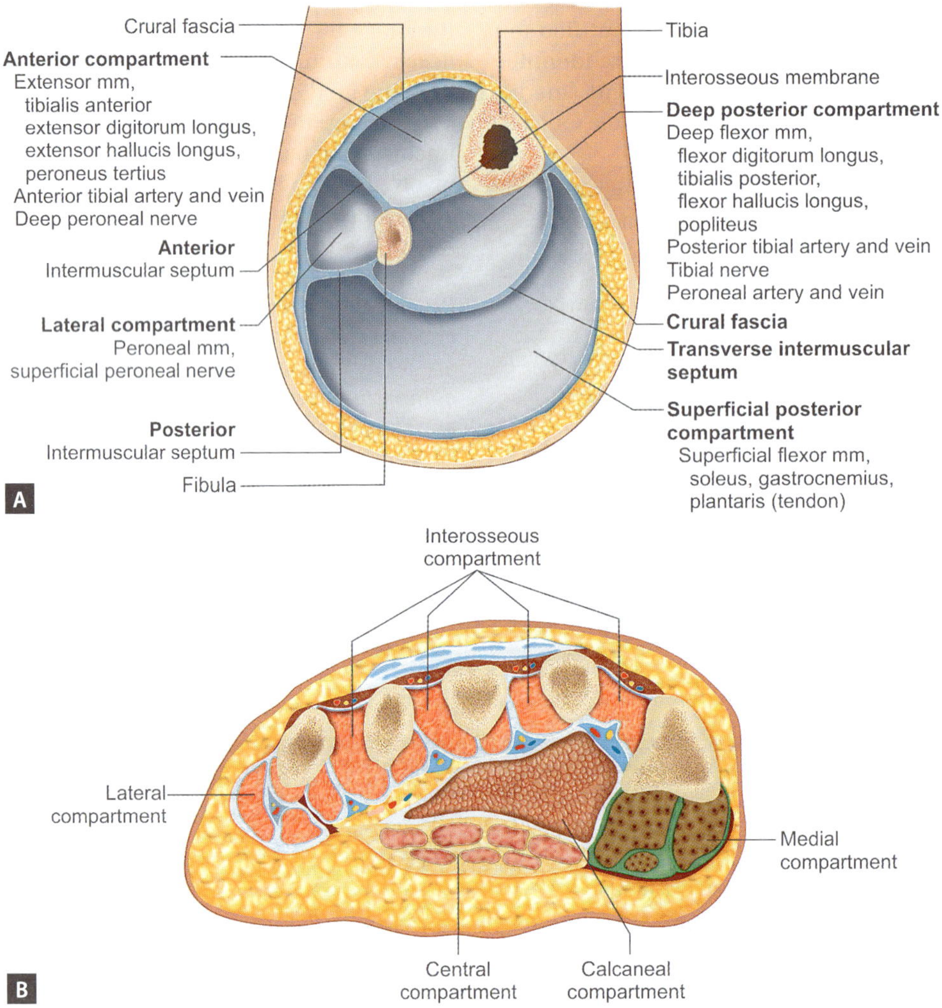

Figs. 1A and B: The various compartments of leg (A) and foot (B).

Where, $(P_a - P_v)$ is the arteriovenous pressure gradient and "R" is the vascular resistance. Raised interstitial pressure proportionately increases venous pressure (P_v) producing local venous hypertension. The gradient (P_a - P_v), thus, reduces and finally LBF = 0, so no capillary perfusion occurs. So it is clear that perfusion within a compartment is only present when the diastolic blood pressure exceeds the intracompartmental pressure. During vasoconstriction or hypotension, perfusion ceases at even lower pressures.

- The other theory suggests *occurrence of arterial spasm* after increased compartment pressure.
- Matsen's unified concept **(Fig. 3)** suggests that compartment syndrome, Volkmann's ischemic contracture, and crush syndrome are a continuum of sequel to raised intracompartmental pressure and a temporal function of the same (develop over time).
- One must also take into account the increase in compartmental pressures due to longitudinal traction and reaming of intramedullary canal. Shakespeare et al. demonstrated increased deep posterior leg compartment pressure by 5% for every 1 kg increase in weight. Ankle position also causes elevated compartment pressures depending on foot position. Intramedullary reaming of bone also causes transient increases in compartment pressures. Although these cannot formulate any consistent theory but do contribute to increased compartment pressure so must be considered into pathogenesis.

With cellular anoxia and death, there is increased intracellular calcium concentration drawing in water into the cells and tissue swells. The cellular toxicity raises capillary permeability further and "leaking capillaries" adds to further increase in the compartment pressure setting vicious "edema-ischemia" cycle. It is important to understand that, despite decreased capillary perfusion from elevated intracompartmental pressure, arterial pressure is almost always adequate to maintain distal flow in the larger vessels. Therefore, distal pulses are usually present and should not be used to rule out the presence of a compartment syndrome. The effect of ischemia on muscle and nerve are temporal; prolonged delay results in greater loss of function. Muscles retain the electrical response up to 3 hours. They can tolerate ischemia up to 4 hours and irreversible damage occurs at 8 hours. Nerves can conduct impulses up to 1 hour. They can survive up to 4 hours (neuropraxia), and at 8 hours irreversible

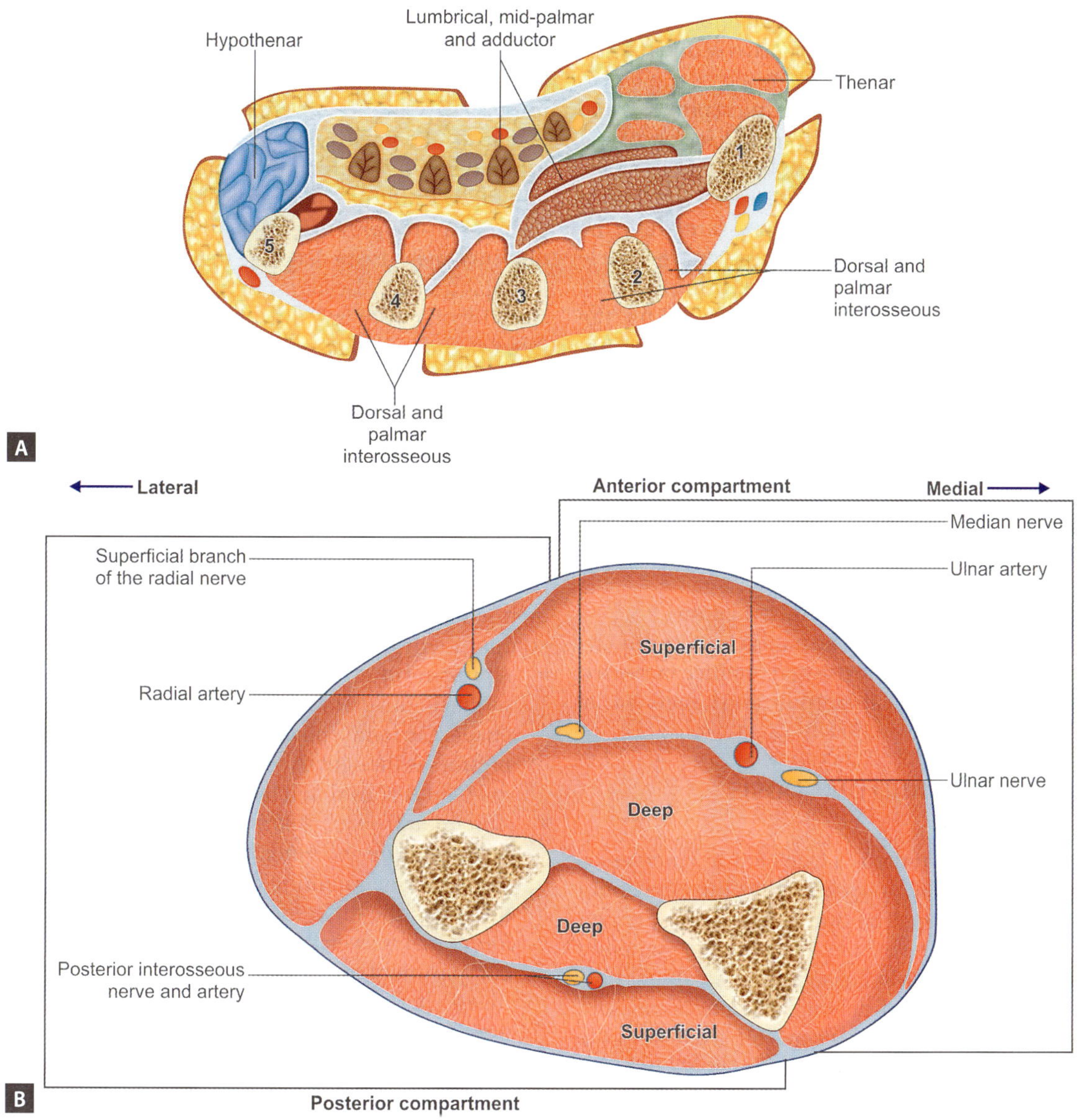

Figs. 2A and B: The various compartments of hand and commonly used incisions to decompress the same (A) and compartments of forearm (B).

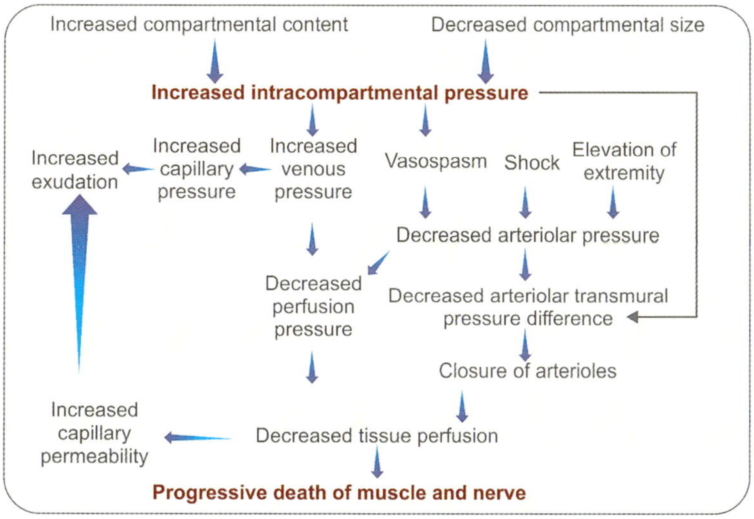

Fig. 3: Matsen's unified concept.

damage occurs. Although these are experimental figures often quoted, in reality muscle necrosis occurs within the first 3 hours for unknown reasons.

Chronic compartment syndrome occurs most probably due to increased muscle mass in a closed fascial space occurring during exercise or exertion. Muscle volume can increase up to 20% of its resting size during exercise. Increased muscle volume causes an increase in the internal pressure within the fascial compartment. Pain occurs due to progressive muscle activity rising intracompartmental pressures causing impaired muscle tissue perfusion. With muscle deoxygenation, the fluid shifts into interstitial space and impairs local capillary circulation and metabolite clearance. The neural ischemia causes pain. Single-photon emission computed tomography (SPECT) findings have, however, found no significant ischemia in CCS patients versus normal controls. So, the pain is now attributed to either of the following possible factors:

- Disproportionate oxygen supply versus demand
- Stimulation of sensory or intramuscular pressure fibers in the fascia from excessive stretch
- Metabolite accumulation and neural irritation

Disproportionate increase in muscle mass is seen in patients on anabolic steroids and creatine use that produce increased muscle mass relative to physical exertion, and hence, fascial stretching.

NATURAL HISTORY AND DIAGNOSIS (FIGS. 4A TO C)

Acute compartment syndrome is a true clinical emergency. Clinically, a missed acute compartment syndrome could be limb or life-threatening. The outcome is dependent on location and time to intervention. Six hours of ischemia (arbitrarily decided time period, also it is nearly impossible to estimate the "real" onset of time of ischemia to measure 6 hours) is currently the upper acceptable limit of tissue viability that may be a little stretchable by a couple of hours for pediatric patients. With prolonged ischemia and muscle necrosis, myoglobin, potassium, and other metabolites are released into circulation. Myoglobinuria can cause acute renal shutdown, hyperkalemia, and metabolic acidosis can cause cardiac arrhythmias and possibly death. Without

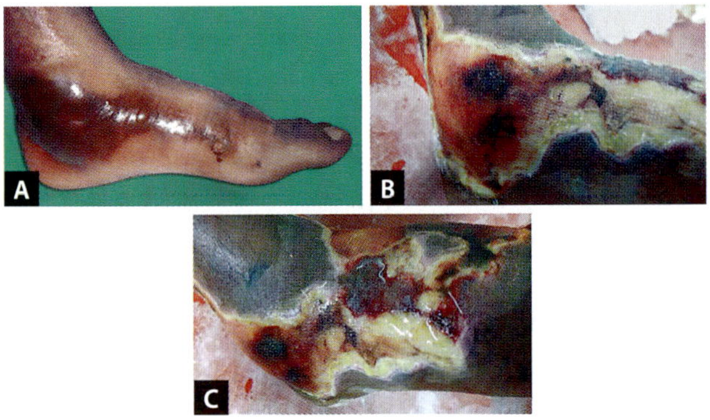

Figs. 4A to C: Natural history of ischemia and compartment syndrome. (A) Patient presented after 14 hours of injury though unremarkable but was missed by resident and developed blisters after 6 hours of presentation; (B and C) This evolved into skin and deep muscle necrosis.

preventive fasciotomy, the muscles undergo atrophy and secondary healing by fibrosis, the myofibroblasts lead to contracture formation and secondary deformities across joints. Polytrauma patients are at high-risk for delay in diagnosis of compartment syndrome as are anesthetized or intubated patients that are so obtunded not to participate in clinical examination or unable to report the symptoms. Compartment pressure measurements remain the only objective measure to diagnose the condition in them.

Diagnosing the compartment syndrome has been traditionally only on clinical suspicion, however, a lot of interest and debates have always occurred regarding some quantitative measure to diagnose compartment syndrome. Nevertheless, the diagnosis of compartment syndrome is still clinical only. The various proposed values, however, serve only as an ancillary guideline for judging when to do compartment release. Nobody, however, knows the exact pressure at which compartment release should be done, the recommended values are clinical and gained through experience. Normal intracompartmental pressure is 0–8 mm Hg. The following are the differently reported measures for diagnosis of acute compartment syndrome:

- A pressure of 30 mm Hg (critical pressure) was reported to be maximum pressure above which muscle necrosis would ensue. Currently, however, *absolute intracompartmental pressure* is thought to convey no meaning and a pressure gradient is considered better reference.
- *Absolute difference of 30 mm Hg between patient's diastolic blood pressure and compartment pressure* is taken as cutoff value for documenting raised compartment syndrome; the lesser the difference the worse it is. Heckman et al. found that irreversible ischemic changes occurred when compartment pressure was elevated within 30 mm Hg of mean arterial pressure and within 20 mm Hg of diastolic pressure. McQueen et al. used cutoff of 30 mm Hg pressure difference from diastolic blood pressure to do fasciotomy and found no patient developing sequel of compartment syndrome above the limit. This reference value should be lowered in hypoxic states and hypotension I feel and would suggest a value close to 20 mm difference between patient's diastolic blood pressure and compartment pressure to diagnose critical perfusion in such cases to guide fasciotomy.
- University of Pennsylvania coined the term *"delta P (ΔP)" referring to the difference between mean arterial pressure and compartment pressure* and found that with ΔP of 20 mm Hg, cellular anoxia and death resulted; however, at ΔP within 40 mm Hg, there was reduced oxygen tension but no anoxia.
- *Intramuscular pH* monitoring has been suggested recently as a better measure for identifying the acute compartment syndrome than measuring absolute pressure or pressure differences as above. An intramuscular pH of <6.38 is 80% specific and 95% sensitive for diagnosing compartment syndrome early and accurately. While comparative values of other measures like absolute pressure > 30 mm Hg or a ΔP < 33 mm Hg were only 30% and 27% specific for 95% sensitivity.

- *Near-infrared spectroscopy (NIRS)* uses differential light absorption properties of oxygenated hemoglobin to measure tissue ischemia. Although the principle is similar to pulse oximetry, NIS can detect changes in tissues as deep as 3 cm below skin. The limitation of the technique is that although poor oxygenation has been demonstrated by various studies, no cut-off value is available to substantiate the diagnosis of compartment syndrome.
- *Metabolic biomarkers* associated with muscle ischemia have been proposed to diagnose compartment syndrome. These are noninvasive but their specificity and sensitivity is poor and temporal association with duration of ischemia is not fully known. Creatine kinase (CK), myoglobin (Mb), and fatty acid-binding protein (FABP) are raised after muscle ischemia and necrosis. Values of >2,000 units/L may be warning sign for impending compartment syndrome in anesthetized patient. The Mb/FABP ratio could serve as a measure to identify skeletal muscle injury. In myocardial injury, the ratio is commonly 5 while for skeletal muscle injury it is nearly four times higher (20 or more). Lactate is the product of anaerobic metabolism in muscle and its measurement could indicate early compartment syndrome. Ischemic modified albumin (IMA) has been identified recently as a biomaker for myocardial infarction and it is transiently decreased with skeletal muscle ischemia. The values get quickly restored with re-establishment of perfusion. CK, Mb, FABP, and lactate or IMA are all, however, not specific as their values are altered in inflammatory conditions and trauma.
- Intra-abdominal pressure of >20 mm Hg leads to failure of one or more organs, and defines abdominal compartment syndrome.

  For CCS, the pressure measurement is the gold standard of course. Compartment pressures are taken prior to exercise and 5 minutes after the patient has exercised. A patient should perform the offending exercise until severe symptoms occur. They are then rested for 5 minutes and compartment pressures are taken.
- One or more of the following criteria are diagnostic of CCS:
  - Rest pressure ≥ 15 mm Hg
  - 1-min and 5-min postexercise pressure >30 mm Hg and >20 mm Hg, respectively. An elevated pressure after 15 minutes is a more reliable cutoff. Often in patients with CCS, the pressure is >25 mm Hg for 30 minutes after exercise.
  - There is also a prolonged period for return to pre-exercise levels.
  - One should keep the ankle and knee joint in uniform position commonly the resting positions.
- MRI is a good evolving test, but cumbersome. Increased T2 signals postexercise correlate well with the increased intracompartmental pressures. Fatty infiltration is associated with chronic ischemia. The sensitivity is good but specificity is lacking. *Pulse-phase-locked-loop (PPLL)* ultrasound detects fascial motion corresponding to arterial pulsation. Decreased micromotion is indicative of raised compartment pressure. Similarly perfusion can be estimated by light backscattering from moving red cells *[laser Doppler flowmetry (LDF)]* as has been used to study chronic exertional compartment syndrome. Radionuclide scintigraphy like *99-tecnitium methoxyisobutilisonitrile (99Tc-MIBI)* scan has good positive and negative predictive values for chronic compartment syndrome but lacks specificity and is limited by time needed for scan and cumbersome repeated studies.
- Near-infrared spectroscopy measures oxygenated and deoxygenated blood in the muscles. Reduction in amount of oxygenated blood is directly proportional to ongoing ischemia so it could serve as a better measure till we arrive at unified "compartment pressure" value for diagnosis of compartment syndrome. Measurements are taken pre-exercise and postexercise. CCS is indicated with delayed return to the level of oxygen at baseline when the muscle is measured postexercise and an increased ratio of deoxygenated to oxygenated muscle postexercise.

MEASUREMENT OF INTRA-COMPARTMENTAL PRESSURE

It has become quite imperative to our understanding that in the setting of a fracture, the pressure is highest at the fracture site and immediately adjacent to it. The pressure decreases the further it is measured from injury site. Thus, pressure measurement should be done at multiple sites especially including area within 5 cm proximal and distal to the fracture. For all forms of intracompartmental pressure measurement, a sterile technique and a small amount of local anesthesia should be used prior to catheter insertion. There are direct and indirect techniques for intracompartmental pressure measurement.

- *Direct techniques:* Here, a miniature pressure transducer is directed at the tissue level. The transducer tip catheters have the advantage of not being affected by variable height of the hydrostatic column (as used for indirect techniques). Good accuracy and dynamic characteristics were reported with the use; however, after exercise, the catheter may underestimate muscle relaxation pressure and muscle rest pressure.
  - Recently advanced solid state transducer-tipped catheter system for the measurement of intracompartmental pressure has been introduced. This method resulted from miniaturization techniques. The advantages of this device are:
    - Easy to use, not needing any calibration
    - It prevents hydrostatic pressure artifacts.
    - It eliminates the need for fluid infusion.
    - Long-term monitoring is possible with this device without any need for manipulation.
    - It can be used to measure compartment pressures intraoperatively.
    - During exercise, this system provides dynamic responses and high-frequency recordings.
- *Indirect techniques:* There is transmission of fluid pressure from the muscle level to a remote transducer.
  - *Wick catheter technique* ***(Figs. 5A and B)****:* Earlier for pressure measurement, fine needles were inserted into

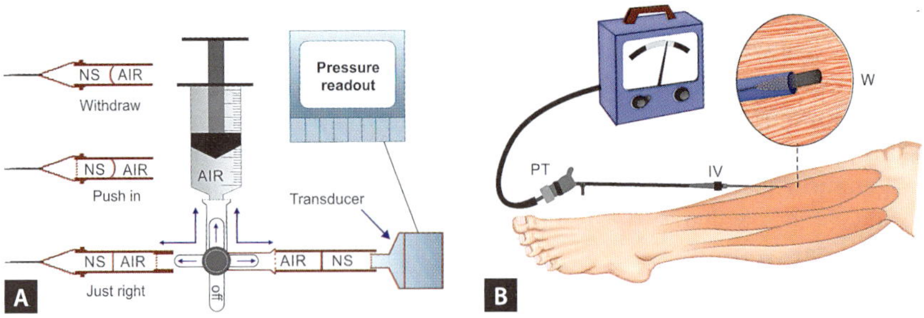

Figs. 5A and B: Wick method using transducer. (A) Technique mechanism; (B) Clinical application.

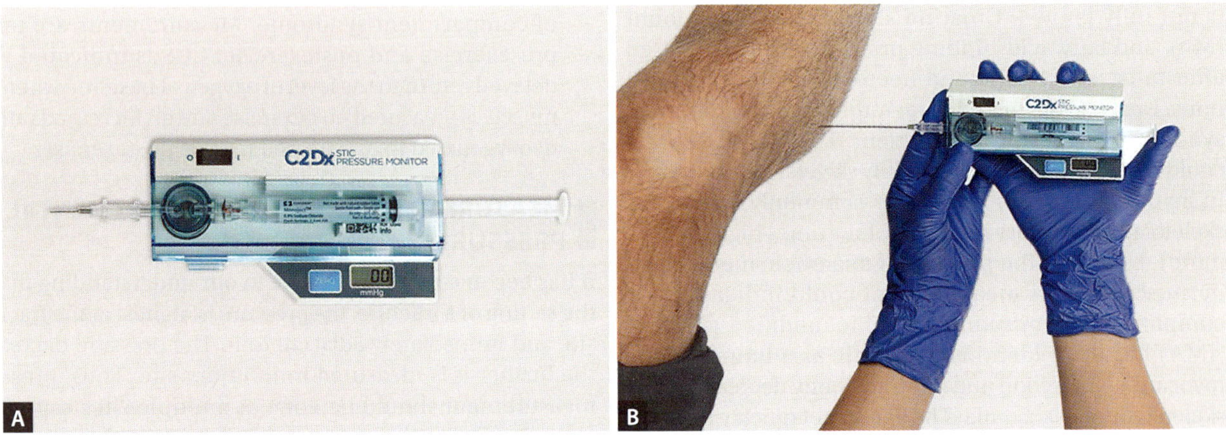

Figs. 6A and B: STIC (Solid-state transducer intracompartmental) Pressure Monitor (A) and its clinical usage (B).
Source: C2Dx (2021), STIC. Intra-Compartmental Pressure Monitor. [online] Available from: https://c2dx.co/products/stic-pressure-monitor/ [Last accessed October, 2021].

the interstitium, and intermittent or continuous fluid injections keep the needle tip from occluding. Excess fluid administration, however, could lead to false readings or even cause acute compartment syndrome in such crude methods. The use of the wick catheter for the clinical assessment of acute compartment syndrome was described by Mubarak et al. To minimize tip occlusion and increase the surface area at the catheter tissue interface, the wick catheter uses Dexon fibers that are fixed at the tip of a fluid-filled polyethylene catheter (in the form of a "wick"). Advancement over this technique came in the form of creation of small slits in the polyethylene tubing catheter—the "slit catheter" that soon replaced the wick catheter. These systems involved transmission of fluid pressure to a remote transducer. This transducer needed to be "zeroed" to the planned level of pressure measurement. The benefits of this catheter included the facts that:
  - It eliminated the risk of retained wick material.
  - It gave a more rapid response.
- *STIC Intra-Compartmental Pressure Monitor (Formerly made by Stryker and now through C2Dx)* ***(Figs. 6A and B):*** The transducer is connected to a needle that has several side ports. These side ports help to eliminate muscle occlusion of the needle. While this device is relatively simple to use, it can produce false readings if it is not applied carefully.
- Sangwan et al. described the effective, safe, and reproducible use of a saline manometer to measure compartment pressures. The benefits of this device include that it is cheap, easy to assemble, and is available to physicians at peripheral hospitals who may not have access to other technology **(Fig. 7)**.
- *Styf and Korner/Uppal et al. technique:* A Teflon catheter is utilized along with constant infusion of 0.2 cc per hour or less. The tip has many side holes which are kept open by the slow constant infusion (IV infusion pump is used for this in Uppal technique). This system has a very high dynamic response for exercise studies. Unfortunately, the changing level of a hydrostatic fluid column causes artifacts that are difficult to control outside of the controlled laboratory condition.

CLINICAL EVALUATION

In patients with CCS, the onset of pain is reproducible for a specific speed and distance. This occurs in athletes in their third or fourth decade, who have exercise-induced pain in the lower leg or foot within 20–30 minutes of beginning to exercise. Often, this occurs after a recent increase in intensity or duration of training or after a change in the training routine.

- It is usually necessary for the patient to discontinue his run and rest for a few minutes (15–30 min). The pain may but persist for hours in few who especially those who try to "push through" the pain.

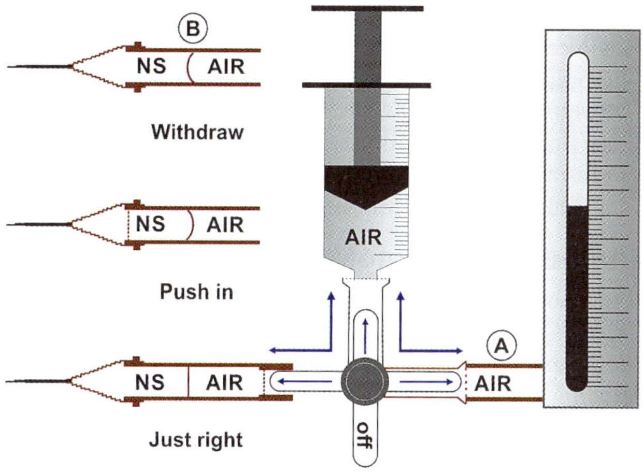

Fig. 7: Sangwan technique: Principles of measurement and technical details of Sangwan technique. Clean the insertion site, if necessary, anesthetize the area locally but be careful not to inject into the suspected compartment. Connect intravenous (IV) tubing to the front and rear ports of the three-way stopcock (as shown in A). Connect a 10 mL syringe, with plunger at 3 mL mark, to the upper port (as in A). One of the IV tubing is connected to sterile 18-gauge needle. Now turn the stopcock so that the other IV tubing is "off" (3 o'clock position on A). Draw up some bacteriostatic saline into needle—IV tubing so as to fill the tubing from tip to a point halfway in the tubing (see A). The other half of the tubing should contain only air. Attach the "off" IV extension tubing to the mercury manometer. Insert the needle into the compartment to be tested. Turn the "off" stopcock to 6 o'clock position so that all three ports are open simultaneously. Push the plunger to increase pressure within the system. The mercury column in the manometer will rise until equilibrium, i.e., the pressure within the system is equivalent to the pressure in the muscle compartment. Once the system pressure exceeds manometer/compartment pressure the saline will start moving; this reading is then recorded. Shape of meniscus is also a good guide, a flat shape represents equilibrium pressure while a convex meniscus (as in B) depicts higher pressure in the system and false high recording.

- The anterior compartment is the most commonly involved, may have diminished sensation in the first dorsal web space.
- Additionally, the patients may report inability to control extremity, extremity weakness, and dysesthesia in sensory distribution of the entrapped nerve. Bilateral involvement is seen in 60–90% patients.
- Muscle herniation through a fascial defect is a common finding (40–60% patients). Most of these defects are located in the lower third of the leg overlying the anterior intermuscular septum between the anterior and lateral compartments. The fascial defect may represent an enlargement of the orifice through which a branch of the superficial peroneal nerve exits the lateral compartment.
- Muscle herniation may cause superficial peroneal nerve irritation and even neuroma formation and hence the sensory symptoms.
- Tense compartment and tenderness is seen in 30–40% cases.
- There should be no changes in the peripheral pulses after exercise [for differential diagnosis of popliteal artery entrapment syndrome (PAES), see below].

For *acute compartment syndrome,* there should be lower threshold for diagnosis in injuries with high-energy mechanism, patients on anticoagulation and those with tight circumferential dressing or plaster. The typical symptoms and signs in a patient are classically briefed into six "ps"; four of which (Pain, Paresthesia, Paresis, and Pain with stretch) were described by Griffiths in 1948, and Pallor and Pulselessness were added later.

1. *Pain:* It is the most sensitive and earliest symptom especially if the pain is out-of-proportion for the injury (symptom) and increases with passive stretch of muscles (sign). Bony injury may cause tremendous pain in a sensitive patient (false positive), or the pain may be absent if compartment syndrome has already set in injuring the nerves or patient has received efficient analgesia/anesthesia (postoperative). Patients under epidural anesthesia are four times more likely to develop compartment syndrome as it blocks the sympathetic system increasing LBF. Also patients under local anesthesia and receiving narcotics are at a higher risk. Other difficult patients to evaluate for pain are those with head injuries, those under influence of ethanol or drugs, those intubated or sedated or any other circumstance that alters patient's ability to accurately sense and communicate pain levels. In pediatric patients, pain is particularly difficult to evaluate as are other signs mentioned below, so instead clinical signs such as anxiety, agitation, and analgesic requirement take prominence.
2. *Paresthesia:* Nerve conduction is altered within few minutes of ischemia. Paresthesia develops early within 2 hours due to early involvement of sensory nerves. Decreased light touch is suggested as the best and first indicator for compartment syndrome as it comes early. It may be better than two-point discrimination as the former represents change in ability of nerves to detect pressure while latter tells the density of nerves in the region that may remain unaltered.
3. *Pulselessness:* Not a reliable sign of compartment syndrome.
4. *Pallor:* Reflects loss of arterial flow and is rarely present ever.
5. *Paralysis* is difficult to interpret and may be caused by ischemia, guarding, pain or a combination of the above. True paralysis develops late (being a function of thicker motor nerves), and till then lot of damage has already occurred.
6. *Pressure:* Just feeling for tight compartments is not enough though they give good indication. Objective of pressure recording is better though not an absolute requirement for considering fasciotomy, which is commonly judged clinically. The indication for pressure evaluation is presence of one or more signs or symptoms in a suspected patient with confounding factor (anesthesia, sedation, and head injury), unreliable examination with firmness of limb, prolonged hypotension in a swollen extremity, and spontaneous increase in pain after adequate analgesia. Handheld systems are best and give quick recordings. Pressure should be recorded within 5 cm of fracture both proximally and distally from all compartments in the affected extremity as suggested by Heckman et al. The highest pressure is compared to diastolic blood pressure for interpretation. The various

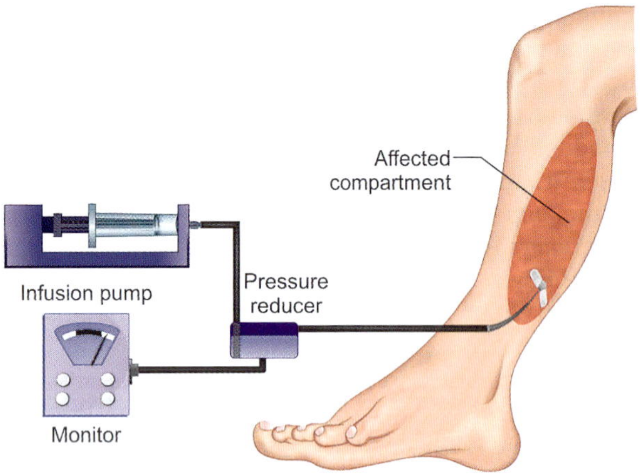

Fig. 8: Infusion technique.

methods of pressure measurement include: Whiteside infusion technique **(Fig. 8)**, solid-state transducer intracompartmental (STIC) catheter technique, Wick catheter technique, slit catheter technique, Camino technique, etc. (see above). If commercial instruments are not available then Whiteside's technique can be used and every orthopedic surgeon should have an idea of it. A simple arterial line setup (16–18 gauge needle) and a mercury manometer are setup to record intracompartmental pressures, but it is important to recognize that this method is considered the least accurate. The values obtained were consistently higher, by an average of 5–19 mm Hg, than those obtained with the other methods. Newer noninvasive methods are becoming popular and standardized and include ultrasonic device (measures submicrometric displacement of fascia by volume expansion), NIRS, tracking variations in the oxygenation of muscle tissue), laser Doppler flowmetry. Rather than measuring intracompartmental pressures, intramuscular pH could serve as a better guide for diagnosis of compartment syndrome.

Leg is the most common location of acute compartment syndromes **(*see* Figs. 1A and B)**. The features of common compartments involvement in leg are detailed below:

- *Anterior compartment syndrome:* Clinical presentation of an acute anterior compartment syndrome includes pain with passive *toe flexion*, some weakness of toe extension and diminished sensation in the first web space because of deep peroneal nerve compression. The extensor hallucis longus usually is the first muscle to show weakness. Anterior compartment syndrome may follow trauma to the extremity, but also can be observed in March gangrene. Local erythema, heat, and brawny edema over the anterior compartment are present.
- *Deep posterior compartment syndrome:* An acute deep posterior compartment syndrome presents as pain and some weakness of toe flexion and ankle inversion. Pain on passive toe/ankle dorsiflexion is referred to the calf. Diminished sensation over the sole of the foot, especially on the medial side is noted, resulting from posterior tibial nerve compression. Foot drop develops because of ischemic contracture of the posterior compartment and is seen if the acute syndrome is not treated.
- *Foot:* There is excessive swelling especially on the plantar aspect obliterating the normal instep fossa. Dorsal intermetatarsal spaces are obliterated and get bulged. Passive dorsiflexion of the toes stretches the intrinsic musculature of the foot increasing the pain out-of-proportion to injury. An absent pulse or complete anesthesia is a late finding in compartment syndrome.

DIFFERENTIAL DIAGNOSIS

Acute compartment syndrome can mimic normal pain response secondary to fracture, muscle rupture, deep venous thrombosis, thrombophlebitis, cellulitis, necrotizing fasciitis, peripheral vascular injury, peripheral nerve injury, and rhabdomyolysis.

The differential diagnosis for CCS includes other causes of exercise-induced extremity pain. These include stress fracture, periostitis, tendinitis, peripheral nerve entrapment, medial tibial stress syndrome (MTSS, shin splints), vascular claudication, venous stasis, PAES, and neurogenic claudication. MTSS represents the periostitis of the posteromedial tibial border. The patient has complained of pain exacerbated by activity and partially relieved with rest. The athlete will have diffuse tenderness of the posteromedial border of the tibia. In PAES, the artery is compressed in the compartment following chronic exercise. Patient has exertional calf pain. The physical examination may reveal diminished dorsalis pedis pulse with passive plantar flexion or active dorsiflexion. Doppler examination helps to confirm the diagnosis.

MANAGEMENT

All patients having suspicious clinical findings and/or increased pressure in a compartment within 30 mm Hg of diastolic blood pressure are commonly considered to have compartment syndrome unless proven otherwise. These patients need emergent management in order to avoid poor outcome. There have been small controversies raised from different experts regarding the timing of intervention that can be logically addressed as follows.

Timing intervention (emerging trends):

- Patients suspected of having acute compartment syndrome by an expert should have emergent fasciotomy.
- Nonoperative treatment (older concept) of this emergency is debatable and is reserved only for patients presenting too late or missed (>24–48 hours) such that the compartment syndrome has fully set in and a fasciotomy will not provide any improvement to the present condition of patient. It is debated that, in such patients, the irreversible damage is complete and fasciotomy might increase the chances of infection and septicemia in the necrosed tissue. Also, there are concerns like extensive scarring and creating more damage than benefit to compromised tissues. It is really difficult to determine how late is too late to perform a fasciotomy after compartment syndrome and in present scenario it is impossible. Duration of 6 hours was classically recommended because there is increased incidence of muscle contractures, weakness, sensory loss, infection, and nonunion of fractures after this time-period.

Some authors, however, take 8 hours as the cut-off while individual studies that compare fasciotomies performed <12 hours and after 12 hours report higher systemic complications (sepsis, shock, and multiorgan dysfunction) and poor function after delayed fasciotomy. I feel that the arguments against delayed fasciotomies are based on fear, unavailability of advanced aggressive reconstruction facilities in basic healthcare steup and not proven, there is always a chance of saving the compromised tissue by performing fasciotomies even in late acute phase (2–10 days following injury). This may improve perfusion of ischemic but not infarcted muscle. It is still advisable that if compartment pressure is within 30 mm Hg of diastolic pressure then a fasciotomy is advisable in any patient as it is difficult to ever know the time of onset of compartment syndrome. Authors have found that if ever one encounters a liquefactive necrosis at this stage, one should debride the tissue and muscle deficit should be reconstructed with free functional muscle transfer. Late transfers are difficult due to poor visualization of the vessels from fibrosis. This optimism for delayed fasciotomy is, however, founded only on the premises of availability of aggressive experienced team with advanced monitoring, reconstructive and resuscitation facilities so caution should be borne in exercising this option.

The crucial steps in management of acute compartment syndrome are identification of high-risk patient (one need not prove that he has compartment syndrome), making a prompt diagnosis, and administering effective treatment.

Immediately provide oxygen by mask, correct any hypotension, and remove the circumferential bandages. Splitting of cast reduces pressure by 30% that increases to 65% if the cast is split and spread. Complete splitting and padding the cast adds 10% to relieve pressure, and complete removal adds another 15%. There could be total of 85–90% reduction if cast is fully removed. Limb should not be elevated as this reduces the mean pressure but not the compartment pressure. Maintain hydration to decrease chances of renal damage from "crush syndrome". Crush syndrome is a sequelae of muscle necrosis (creatine phosphokinase > 20,000 IU) and manifests as nonoliguric renal failure, myoglobinuria, and later oliguria, shock, acidosis, hyperkalemia, and cardiac arrhythmias and may need dialysis. Liu et al. demonstrated in animal model that treatment with phenylephrine and dobutamine can significantly increase muscle oxygenation and viability but till date fasciotomy remains the gold standard of treatment for compartment syndrome. Obtain urgent investigations (viral markers) and send blood sample for complete laboratory panel (do not wait for reports) and do emergent fasciotomy following the universal precautions. Bedside fasciotomies can also be done if theater is not available for any reason or it is not possible to shift the patient.

SURGICAL TECHNIQUE

Forearm Decompression

The volar curvilinear approach of Henry and dorsal approach.

- Begin the skin incision proximal to the antecubital fossa on the ulnar aspect of the arm crossing the antecubital fossa horizontally in the flexion crease **(Figs. 9A to C)**. In the forearm, extend incision in an S-shape to the wrist flexion crease and then cross the crease into the palm to allow release of the carpal tunnel. Release the superficial fascia, and identify the median nerve proximally and release the lacertus fibrosus.

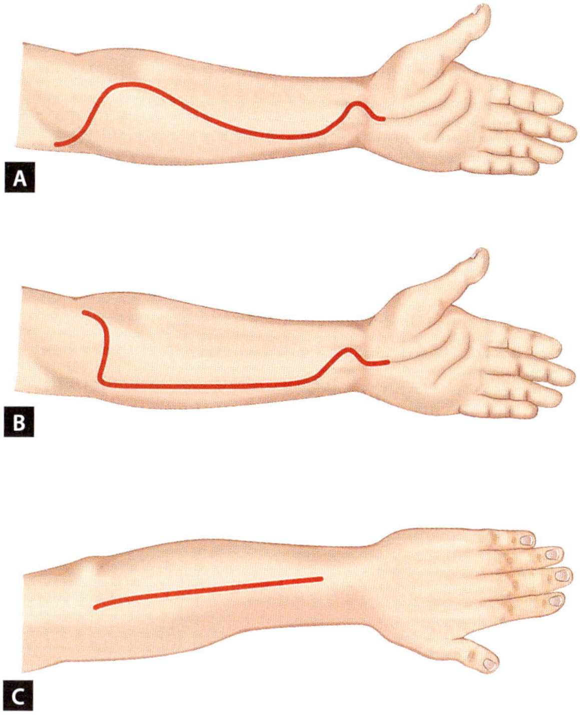

Figs. 9A to C: (A and B) Illustration depicting forearm compartment decompression different incisions for volar decompression, and (C) extensor compartment decompression

- Release the proximal edge of flexor pronator mass from humerus. Follow the median nerve into the forearm between the flexor digitorum superficialis and profundus and decompress it all the way to the carpal tunnel. Identify and preserve the palmar cutaneous branch of the median nerve. Release the carpal tunnel.
- Inspect the deep volar muscles (flexor digitorum profundus, flexor pollicis longus, and pronator quadratus) and release their respective fascial coverings as needed. The mobile wad can also be reached through this approach.
- For dorsal decompression, the incision is similar to that used in the Thompson approach and can extend from the lateral epicondyle to the mid-portion of the wrist. Full incision may not be needed, and fascia of dorsal and mobile wad compartments is easily released.

Decompression of Leg

The two-incision techniques of Mubarak et al.

- *Anterolateral incision:* To approach the anterior and lateral compartments, make an extensive longitudinal skin incision, halfway between the fibular shaft and tibial crest **(Fig. 10)**. Undermine the skin edges to widen exposure of the fascia. Identify the anterior intermuscular septum that separates the anterior compartment from the lateral compartment **(Fig. 10)**. Identify the superficial peroneal nerve, which lies in the lateral compartment next to the septum. Open the anterior compartment fascia. Ensure complete fascial release.

- Make the lateral compartment fasciotomy in line with the fibular shaft. Direct the scissors proximally toward the fibular head and distally toward the lateral malleolus. The fascial incision is posterior to the superficial peroneal nerve.
- *Posteromedial incision:* Make a longitudinal incision 2–3 cm posterior to the posterior tibial margin, and to approach the superficial and deep posterior compartments **(Fig. 10)**. An anterior incision risks injury to the saphenous vein and nerve, which course along the posterior margin of the tibia.
- Retract the saphenous vein and nerve anteriorly. Identify the septum between the deep and superficial posterior compartments **(Fig. 10)**. Identify the tendon of the flexor digitorum longus in the deep posterior compartment and the Achilles tendon in the superficial posterior compartment.
- Decompress the superficial posterior compartment first by releasing fascia proximally as far as possible and then distally behind the medial malleolus. Release the deep posterior compartment distally and then proximally under the soleus bridge. Release the soleus if it attaches to the tibia distally more than halfway. In cases where both the deep and superficial compartments are anchored to the posteromedial edge of the tibia, the deep posterior compartment should be released from within the superficial posterior compartment by retracting soleus.

Single-incision technique of Matsen et al.:

- Make an incision from the head of the fibula to the lateral malleolus. Visualize the posterior edge of the anterior compartment, the lateral compartment, and the anterior edge of the superficial posterior compartment.
- Make a transverse incision in the middle portion of leg through the deep fascia, beginning in the anterior compartment, crossing the lateral compartment, and extending into the posterior compartment. Identify the anterior intermuscular septum running longitudinally between the anterior and lateral compartments, and the posterior intermuscular septum running between the lateral and posterior compartments. Identification of the three compartments can be difficult in the traumatized, distorted, and swollen limb.
- Release the deep fascia of the anterior, lateral, and superficial posterior compartments for the full length of each compartment and decompress all muscle proximally.
- Identify the deep posterior compartment. Dissect the soleus free from its origin on the posterior intermuscular septum in the middle or proximal third of the wound. Release the deep fascia of this compartment throughout its full length, taking care to avoid injury to the neurovascular structures, particularly the common peroneal nerve.

Foot decompression ***(Figs. 11A to D)***:

- Dorsal—two incisions, overlying the second and fourth metatarsals is the gold standard. Maintain the widest skin bridge and bluntly approach the metatarsals.

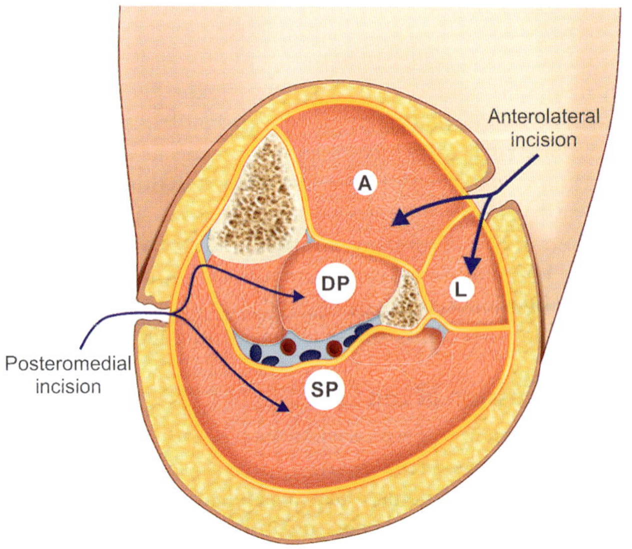

Fig. 10: Illustration depicting decompression of the various compartments of leg using combined two incision technique. (DP: deep posterior; SP: superficial posterior)

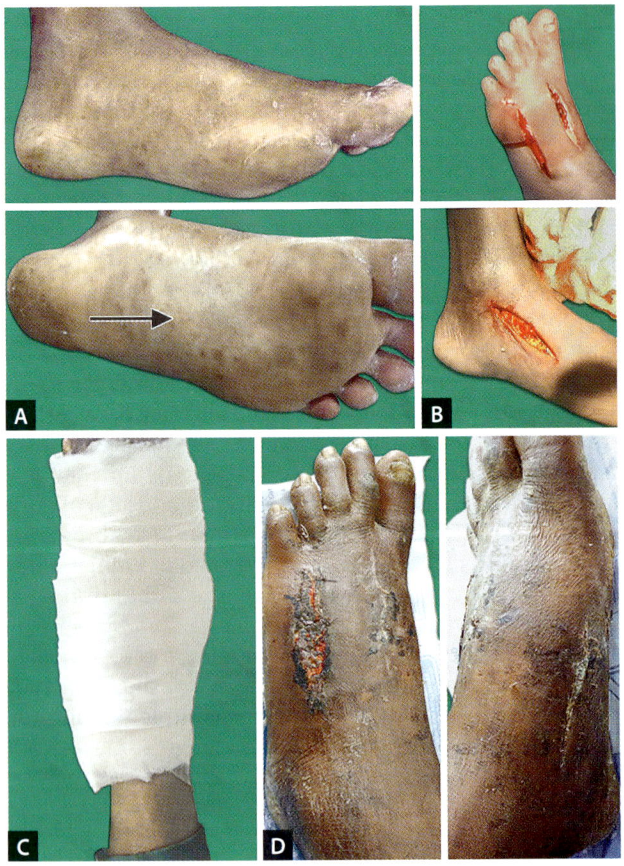

Figs. 11A to D: (A) Compartment syndrome of foot, managed with (B) dorsal and medial fasciotomy and decompression of large hematoma situated in the deep layers of foot muscles; (C) Bulky dressing was applied postoperatively. Note the bulge in plantar aspect of foot in the preoperative photographs (arrow); (D) The fasciotomy wounds were covered by split thickness skin grafts that went to heal uneventfully. Patient regained full function.

Continue blunt dissection into the web spaces, and decompress the hematoma.

- Medial—one incision, along the inferior border of the first metatarsal, but superior to the abductor muscle. Enter the central compartment from superior aspect of abductor muscle.
- Calcaneal (uncommonly used)—one incision, beginning medially, from the inferior border of the posterior tuberosity extending toward the inferior surface of the first metatarsal.

Stabilization of fracture is essential along with compartment decompression. For supracondylar fractures of humerus in children, and metatarsal and metacarpal fractures of hand and feet K-wires are preferred. Forearm fractures are better fixed with compression or locked plates. For femur or tibia fractures, nailing is not a good option as it can worsen an existing compartment syndrome by altering the blood flow from reaming of fragments, even undreamed nails "push" blood and components out of medullary system into surrounding tissues. External fixator is better though there are problems of skin mobilization during delayed primary closure.

CHRONIC COMPARTMENT SYNDROME

Because of the delay in diagnosis (mean 22 months), the conservative measures are often ineffective as they are most useful when deployed early. The most effective nonoperative measure is discontinuing the activity that causes pain (How logical indeed!). It is, but, difficult to pursue for an athlete as his carrier will be ruined. Those who agree may choose a different sport like cycling instead of running. Other less effective measures are decreasing the intensity of training to go into a resting period and slowly increase exercise. This should be aided by ice and nonsteroidal anti-inflammatory drugs (NSAIDs) to reduce symptoms. Arch support orthotics to support the arch in an athlete with planovalgus deformity. Measures like running on hard surfaces, changing footwear, changing the biomechanical techniques of running, deep tissue massage, ultrasound, and stretching before exercise may help variably. The only definitive treatment of CCS, however, is fasciotomy.

Fasciotomy for Chronic Compartment Syndrome

Patients diagnosed with CCS should be explained the need of fascial release and possibility of development of acute compartment syndrome without treatment. The incision and surgery are not as extensive as for acute compartment syndrome and center on releasing the fascia around fascial defect of muscle herniation **(Figs. 12A and B)**. Also carry out prophylactic anterolateral decompression by releasing anterior fascia. Anterior and lateral fasciotomies have the best outcome with a >80% success rate. Deep posterior fasciotomies have a lower success rate of 50%. The fasciotomies can be done open, subcutaneous (two small incisions on either end), or even endoscopic.

Indications for Prophylactic Fasciotomy

- *Suspected compartment syndrome:* Situations like patient with head injury or intubated patients with no facilities available for measuring compartment pressures.
- Patients with arterial ischemia (embolus or arterial injury) persisting for 4–6 hours to prevent reperfusion injury and future risk of compartment syndrome.
- Closely monitor for possibility of compartment syndrome in patients undergoing tibia osteotomies or leg-lengthening procedures, or when the tibia is used as a donor bone graft site. If close monitoring not possible then release anterolateral compartment prophylactically.
- Significant tissue injury in a high-risk patient

POSTOPERATIVE MANAGEMENT AND REHABILITATION

- Pack the wounds loosely open with saline-dampened gauze and apply a bulky dressing after adequate compartment decompression with foot in neutral position. Keep extremity above the level of heart to aid venous drainage. Shoe-lace technique of placing vessel loop suture and skin staple help in gradual closure of skin wound. The sutures can be pulled even at bedside.
- Never close the skin incisions immediately after fasciotomy. Return the patient to the operating room for repeat debridement if necessary and partial or even complete skin closure.
- Most commonly, fasciotomy wounds are not amenable to delayed primary closure due to swollen soft tissues, and split-thickness skin grafting is necessary. With the two-incision technique in the leg, one wound (usually medial) can usually be closed primarily on a delayed basis, and the other wound (lateral) covered with a split-thickness skin graft as it has better soft-tissue bed. Obtain quantitative cultures regularly to provide prophylactic antibiotics and determine the appropriate time for skin grafting.
- Begin active and active-assisted range-of-motion of the adjacent joints on the second day after fasciotomy. After split-thickness skin grafting, immobilize the limb for 3–5 days more.
- Close the wound with an interdermal running stitch after fasciotomy for CCS. Apply a light dressing and allow the patient weight-bearing as tolerated with the use of crutches as needed. After suture removal at 2–3 weeks, initiate light running and progress exercises as tolerated over the next 3–6 weeks according to the patient's abilities and pain tolerance.
- Use of vacuum-assisted closure is highly recommended for immediate postoperative management. Hyperbaric oxygen may help in helping the revitalization of the involved muscles, but only in borderline cases and only after fasciotomies have been performed but concern has been raised about the possibility of reperfusion injury.
- Drugs that may help recovery from metabolic effects of compartment syndrome (by primarily scavenging free radicals) include:
    - Allopurinol
    - Superoxide dismutase
    - Deferoxamine
    - Pentafraction of hydroxyethyl starch

Complications

- In patients treated with fasciotomy altered sensation within margins of wound is the most common complaint.

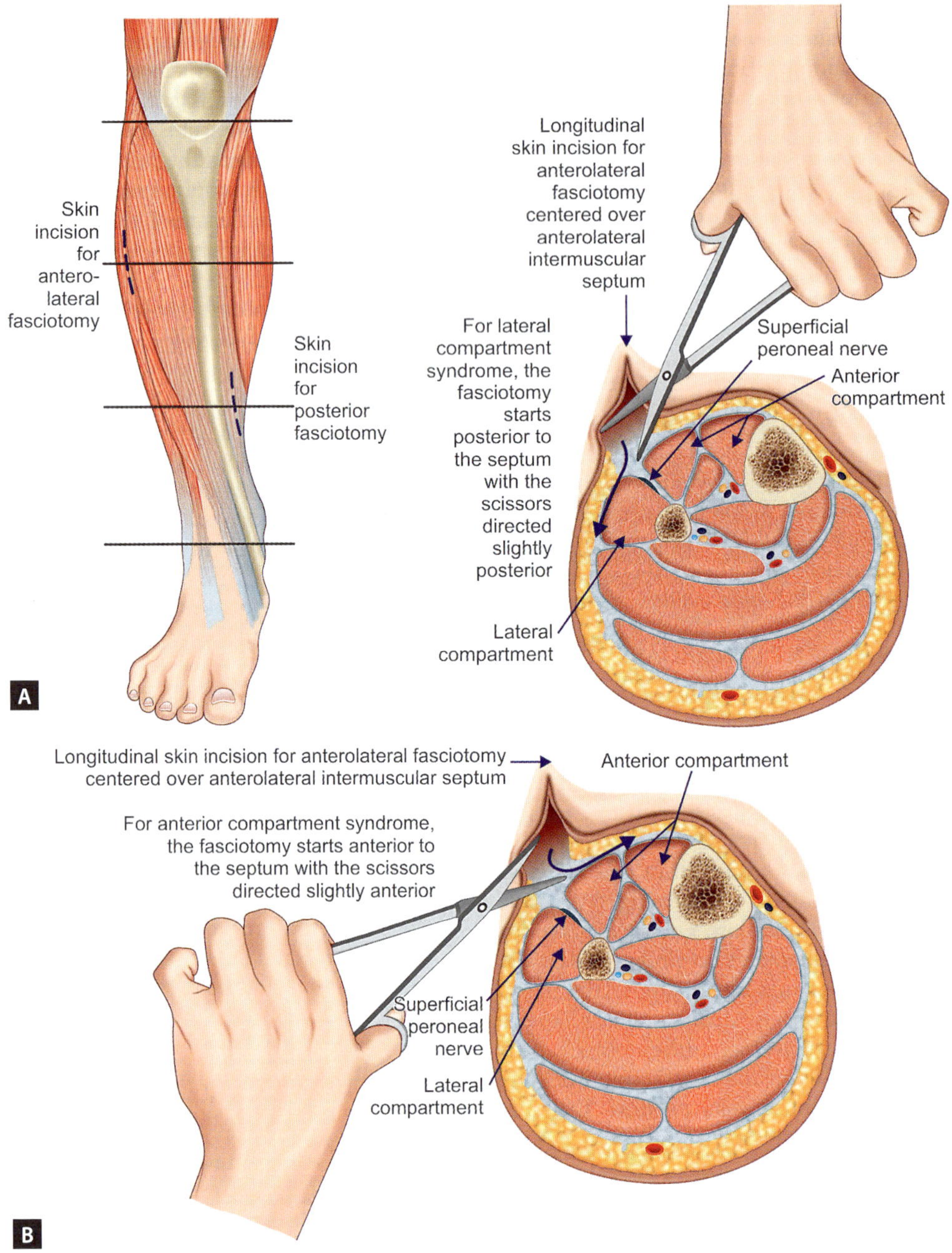

Figs. 12A and B: Fasciotomy for chronic compartment syndrome of leg.

- Dry scaly skin, pruritus, discolored skin, swollen extremity, and tethered skin are found in a third of patients.
- Around 10% have recurrent ulcerations, muscle herniation, and wound pain.
- Late sequelae of compartment syndrome include weak dorsiflexion, claw fingers and toes, and Volkmann's ischemic contracture.
- Delayed fasciotomy after 12 hours has been associated with significant infection rate (around 50%) and amputation in one-third patients. It is therefore recommended that if compartment syndrome has persisted for 24–48 hours and pressure gradient is >30 mm Hg then only supportive treatment for renal failure should be considered. Do not violate skin in such cases and plan for later reconstruction.
- After fasciotomy for CCS:
  - Hemorrhage
  - Skin breakdown
  - Altered sensation over the fasciotomy site
  - Recurrence (6–11%)—more with subcutaneous and endoscopic technique
  - Infection
  - Deep vein thrombosis
  - Vascular injury
  - Nerve damage
  - Lymphocele
  - Nerve entrapment
  - Complex regional pain syndrome

COMPARTMENT SYNDROME IN CHILDREN

Compartment syndrome (CS) in children presents quite differently than in adults and should be vigilantly evaluated. Increased analgesic requirement is often the first sign raising concern for CS in pediatric age group especially young children, as they are too anxious to allow surgeon to evaluate the classic five "*Ps*". Identification of CS is quite delayed in children as most are admitted under pediatric care where the staff is quite untrained in its identification. There are various risk factors for development of CS in children that may be divided into traumatic and nontraumatic ones as are discussed below.

Traumatic Causes of Compartment Syndrome in Children

Supracondylar Fracture of Humerus

Compartment syndrome (of usually the volar forearm region) is a well-described complication of this injury but is rather seen uncommonly, affecting 0.1–0.3% patients only. CS after supracondylar fracture of humerus may be also seen in mobile wad or the anterior arm or the posterior arm compartment apart from the commonly seen volar forearm region. Elbow flexion beyond 90° in cast immobilization for fracture and/or concomitant vascular injury is the risk factor for development of compartment syndrome. After supracondylar fracture, highest pressure is seen in deep volar compartment that gets exaggerated by elbow flexion beyond 90°. In fractures associated with vascular injury, chances of compartment syndrome are significant in pulseless poorly perfused hand rather than a pulseless but well-perfused hand. A reasonable delay of 8–10 hours in treating the fractures (pinning or otherwise) has not been found to increase chances of developing compartment syndrome, however, such delay is *not* recommended. Even in cases with associated neurological or vascular injury treatment, delay is never recommended. Patients who have severe swelling should be closely monitored in preoperative period as nearly all patients who develop compartment syndrome had swollen forearms but the inverse is not true.

Floating Elbow Injury (Ipsilateral Humerus and Forearm Bone Fractures)

This is an uncommon injury but the incidence of compartment syndrome is high especially if circumferential cast is used to treat it. The incidence may be as high as one-third of the cases as reported in study by Blackmore et al. Patients managed with K-wire fixation for humerus fare much better than those treated with plaster of Paris (POP) casts, hence, the latter is not recommended in the management of this injury and one should prefer pinning the fracture(s).

Forearm Fractures

Contrary to the incidence of CS seen in floating elbow managed by casts only, there is a higher incidence of CS developing in forearm fractures managed by closed reduction and pinning especially if performed within 24 hours of the injury and incurs prolonged operative time for obtaining closed reduction or otherwise. Also, the incidence of CS is higher in patients with open forearm fractures. One may resort to putting a small incision to aid reduction, so that manipulation is limited and operative time is reduced. Close monitoring of patients managed by closed reduction and pinning is recommended. This in no way means that POP cast treatment following struggled manipulation is recommended.

Fractures of the Femoral Shaft

Development of CS after femoral shaft fractures is uncommon, however, it has been reported with 90/90 spica casting used to manage some patients. The technique of applying below knee cast followed by traction to obtain reduction of the femoral shaft fracture and completing the cast especially puts pressure on the posterior compartment of the leg increasing the risk for CS.

Tibial Fractures

The risk of developing CS after tibial fractures increases, if the fractures are open injuries and high-energy trauma. Also, avulsion of tibial tubercle indicates some sort of vascular traction and hence concomitant vascular injury and compromise. These patients should be considered high risk for development of CS and closely monitored for emergent fasciotomy, if it is suspected. Distal tibial physeal fractures may predispose for vascular compromise of foot and impending CS of the latter. Prompt release of extensor retinaculum is recommended in these cases along with stabilization of the physeal injury.

Nontraumatic Causes of Compartment Syndrome in Children

Leukemia, hemophilia, renal failure, and liver metabolic failure are some of the causes of CS in children though overall the incidence is quite low. In tropical regions, snake bites are rather a more common cause that previously listed conditions. In these conditions, correction of the primary cause has equal importance as that of compartment release. Correction of coagulation deficit, providing emergent antivenin, and giving supportive care are as important as surgical decompression. In neonates, compartment syndrome of forearm is seen very rarely as a result of birth trauma. The causes possibly link to low-blood pressure and suboptimal homeostasis along with delay in diagnosis in such cases. A "sentinel skin lesion" has been described in these cases of neonatal CS on the forearm. Other uncommon causes of nontraumatic compartment syndrome include fluid extravasation in the compartments in obtunded patients in intensive care unit (ICU), retained tourniquets as is also common in children during play with elastic bands that may get accidently get retained on limb/wrist or even fingers. Sacred threads quite commonly placed on the limbs in Indian subcontinent are another risk factor for development of CS, if it gets tight with growth of the child and left unnoticed.

Clinical Presentation and Diagnosis of Compartment Syndrome in Children

The five "Ps" classically described for diagnosis of CS in general and do not hold true in children as they are difficult to communicate with respect of specific responses required for their evaluation. The children are too anxious and frightened to provide a meaningful response. Increasing use of analgesics has been found to represent abnormality in these children. It is seen that it can indicate development of CS by a mean of 7.3 hours before development of vascular changes. Increased analgesic requirement is now considered to be the first sign of development of CS in children raising alarm for treating physicians. It is, hence, recommended that instead of five "Ps" one may resort to evaluation of three "*As*" as follows in children:

- Increasing Analgesic requirement
- Anxiety
- Agitation

Measurement of compartment pressure may be objectively relied in obtunded child or in a child with severe disability of communication and poor mental status. Few things are important to be noted, however, that normal compartment pressures are higher in children that in adults, while they are <10 mm Hg in adults, the compartment pressure in children average around 15 mm Hg. Compartment pressure must be measured near to the injury site—ideally within 5 cm. The threshold for doing fasciotomy remains debatable but guidelines of ΔP or that of McQueen et al. previously described possibly hold true here too. NIRS or intramuscular pH recordings may be standardized in future for better reference.

Treatment for Compartment Syndrome in Children

Once the diagnosis or strong suspicion of CS is made, the treatment is fasciotomy and decompression of the compartment(s) as described before. In addition, definitive care should be instituted as the case may be, viz., antivenin or correction of coagulopathy.

CONCLUSION

- Compartment syndrome is a surgical emergency that has deleterious consequences if missed as the prognosis is uniformly bad after development of this condition that progresses relentlessly.
- The diagnosis should be promptly made recognizing the condition at earliest and immediately decompressing the compartment—there is no condition as emergent as a compartment syndrome in current orthopedic practice.
- The condition is so emergent that even a mere suspicion by experienced observer qualifies to a surgical decompression. If one is doubtful then compartment pressure measurement serves as a good aid but methods are plagued by subtle inconsistencies.
- Intramuscular pH measurement (cut-off value of 6.38) is possibly the most reliable indicator at the moment but facilities to measure it are not universally available.
- Chronic compartment syndrome is an uncommonly encountered condition in the Indian subcontinent but physicians should be aware of the typical symptomatology and management.

CHAPTER 28

Fat Embolism Syndrome

Manish Kumar Varshney

INTRODUCTION

Fat embolism syndrome (FES) is a common and poorly defined clinical condition comprising a constellation of cardiorespiratory and neurocognitive abnormalities produced as a result of blockage of vascular system by fat droplets. The clinical presentation is variable and it may be either subtle or dramatic and life-threatening. FES mostly occurs with orthopedic trauma and uncommonly with atraumatic conditions. Diagnosis is commonly missed due to its delayed appearance (2–3 days) and subclinical presentation and/or presence of confounding injuries. Presence of fat droplets or fat embolism (FE) does not translate directly to development of FES. Treatment of FES is also ill-defined and is mainly supportive. By and far it is the least understood complication of trauma.

HISTORICAL PERSPECTIVE AND EPIDEMIOLOGY

Presence of fat droplets in the lung capillaries was described by Zenker in 1862 in a railroad worker who sustained a fatal thoracoabdominal crush injury. In 1865, Wagner described the pathologic features of fat embolism. In 1873, von Bergmann, for the first time, clinically diagnosed and used the term FES. The reported incidence varies widely in the reported literature. Retrospective studies have the greatest variability and incidence after long bone fracture has been reported to be 0.9–2.2% while during intramedullary manipulation the incidence tends to be lower. Prospective studies report far higher but consistent rates and the incidence of fat embolism at autopsy is significantly greater. FES due to extensive bone marrow necrosis in sickle cell disease is rare but has a mortality of 64%. High incidences of FE are reported in patients undergoing total knee replacement (46% in unilateral vs. 65% in bilateral) using right atrial blood sampling, however, FES was found only in 2–4%. Presence of pulmonary shunt suggested FES in 11% patients with long bone/pelvic fracture.

CAUSES

Traumatic causes:

- Fractures of long bones—closed and multiple fractures produce more emboli than open fractures
- Major orthopedic surgery such as intramedullary nailing of the long bones, hip or knee replacements
- Extensive soft tissue injury
- Higher degree burns injury
- Bone marrow biopsy
- Hepatic injury
- Cardiopulmonary resuscitation compressions
- Bone marrow transplant
- Lung transplant
- Caisson disease
- Extracorporeal circulation
- Cesarean section
- Tetrachloromethane poisoning

Nontraumatic causes associated with fat embolism include:

- Removal of large volume of adipose tissue in liposuction
- Intravenous lipid infusion
- Collagen vascular disease
- Diabetes mellitus
- Severe infection
- Neoplasm
- Blood transfusion
- Cardiopulmonary bypass
- Hepatic steatosis (fatty liver)
- Long duration corticosteroid therapy
- Acute pancreatitis
- Osteomyelitis
- Medical conditions causing bone infarcts, especially sickle cell disease
- Cyclosporine A solvent

PATHOPHYSIOLOGY

The exact mechanism producing FES is not known; the most widely accepted theories for FES had been proposed years ago and are considered partial explanation while a combined mechanism is more likely.

- *Mechanical theory:* According to Gauss (1924), traumatic injury forces liquified fat droplets from disrupted bone marrow into torn venules facilitated by raised intramedullary pressure. These droplets then enter into the pulmonary capillary beds serving as a primary reservoir and migrate through arteriovenous shunts to the brain, skin. Microvascular deposition of droplets produces local ischemia by occlusion of the vessels and inflammation. The reactive nature of lipid enhances platelet aggregation and fibrin production while capillary occlusion triggers interstitial hemorrhage, edema, and alveolar collapse. This leads to concomitant release of inflammatory mediators as a reaction to both ischemia and ongoing inflammation which proceeds platelet aggregation in the capillaries setting up a vicious loop of ischemia. Ischemia also gets facilitated by simultaneous release of vasoactive amines.

- *Biochemical theory:* Lehman suggested proinflammatory state as a prime cause of FES. Explains nontraumatic forms of FES. A number of biochemical mechanisms are proposed for this theory that are as follows:
  - *Toxic theory:* Baker suggested that local hydrolysis of fat emboli by lung lipase generates chemically toxic free fatty acids, which causes severe inflammatory changes by producing endothelial damage, inactivation of lung surfactant, and increasing lung permeability. They can also enter into systemic circulation causing multiorgan dysfunction. Oleic acid is the most abundant free fatty acid (FFA) in human tissues that provokes alveolar edema and acute respiratory distress syndrome (ARDS) in animal models.
  - *Obstructive theory:* This theory states that hormonal changes caused by trauma and/or sepsis in the patient leads to systemic release of free fatty acids as chylomicrons. Subsequently, chylomicrons coalesce because of elevated acute-phase reactant in these patients, such as C-reactive proteins, which leads to embolization pulmonary epithelium damage and activation of cytokines. Aquaporins form pores in cell membrane. The expression of a specific type of aquaporin1 is increased in FES and it is proportional to pulmonary edema.

PRESENTATION

Fat embolism syndrome is both a clinical diagnosis and diagnosis of exclusion. The principal clinical features are a triad of respiratory failure, cerebral dysfunction, and skin petechiae that generally develop 24–72 hours after trauma, by that time fat droplets become impacted in microvascular beds of lungs, brain, and other organs. Respiratory symptoms and signs are the quickest and most frequent to develop.

Initially, larger fat globules cause mechanical occlusion of multiple blood vessels which is transient and even incomplete as the fat globules are never capable of completely obstructing microcirculation due to their fluidity and deformability. After some time, hydrolysis of fat into more irritable fatty acids occurs, which causes late systemic manifestations of FES.

- *Cardiopulmonary:*
  - Early persistent tachycardia
  - Respiratory signs such as tachypnea, dyspnea, and hypoxemia are the earliest to manifest and seen in 75% of patients. They are liable to progress to respiratory failure in 10% of the cases.
  - Patients have high-grade fever.
- *Dermatologic:*
  - The characteristic petechial rash develops in about 20–60% of cases and may be the last component to develop.
  - The petechial rash develops due to embolization of small dermal capillaries which causes extravasation of erythrocytes.
  - Petechial rashes are seen in mucous membrane (oral), the conjunctiva, and skin folds of the neck, anterior thorax, and axilla. Usually, they appear within first 36 hours and are transient disappearing nearly completely within 7 days. Tachakra suggested that fat droplets aggregate in aortic arch and then embolize to nondependent skin via subclavian and carotid vessels producing this characteristic pattern.
- *Neurologic:*
  - They result from cerebral embolism and are seen in up to 86% of cases.
  - The common presentation is an acute confusional state. Focal neurological signs, such as aphasia, apraxia, hemiplegia, visual field disturbances, anisocoria, seizures, and decorticate posturing, are also sometimes seen.
  - Fundoscopic examination reveals retinal hemorrhages with intra-arterial fat globules.
- *Other miscellaneous findings:*
  - Right heart failure pattern is common on an ECG.
  - Myocardial ischemia causing reduced efficacy of myocardium
  - Macular edema causing scotomata associated with soft fluffy retinal exudates (Purtscher's retinopathy)
  - Coagulation abnormalities similar to disseminated intravascular coagulation
  - Renal symptom presenting as oliguria, lipiduria, proteinuria, or hematuria

DIAGNOSIS

Fat embolism syndrome is clinically diagnosed by grouping of laboratory findings and signs. Several such grouped criteria exist but none has been validated.

1. *Gurd's and Wilson's criteria:* Gurd proposed his original criteria in 1970 and modified it with Wilson in 1974 **(Table 1)**. The criticism of latter is that fat macroglobulinemia is seen in many without evidence of FES.
2. *Schonfeld's criteria:* This is a semi-quantitative means of diagnosing FES and a cumulative score more than five is required for diagnosis **(Table 2)**
3. *Lindeque's criteria* ***(Box 1)****:* According to Lindeque et al., FES can be diagnosed on the basis of respiratory system involvement alone, but it appears to overdiagnose FES and may even capture nonspecific cases of respiratory failure.

TABLE 1: Gurd and Wilson criteria for diagnosis of FES.

Gurd criteria (1970)		***Gurd and Wilson (1970)***	
1 major + 3 minor or 2 major + 2 minor criteria suggest diagnosis of fat embolism syndrome		2 major or 1 major + 4 minor criteria suggest diagnosis	
Major criteria	***Minor criteria***	***Major criteria***	***Minor criteria***
• Petechiae on conjunctiva and upper trunk • $PaO_2 < 60$ at FiO_2 0.2 L with or without pulmonary infiltrate on chest X-ray • Altered mentality with multiple cerebral white matter lesion on brain MRI	• Tachycardia > 100 beats/min • Temperature > 38°C • Platelet < 100 x 10^3/μL • Anemia with coagulopathy or disseminated intravascular coagulation without definite ongoing bleeding site • Anuria or oliguria • Retinal embolism on ophthalmoscopic examination	• Petechiae • Hypoxemia • Altered mentality	• Tachycardia • Fever • Thrombocytopenia • Unexplained anemia • Anuria or oliguria • Retinal embolism • Fat macroglobulinemia (urine or sputum) • Jaundice • High ESR

(ESR: erythrocyte sedimentation rate)

TABLE 2: Schonfeld's criteria.

	Score
Petechiae	5
Chest X-ray changes (diffuse alveolar infiltrates)	4
Hypoxemia ($PaO_2 < 9.3$ kPa)	3
Fever (>38°C)	1
Tachycardia (>120 bpm)	1
Tachypnea (>30 bpm)	1

BOX 1: Lindeque criteria for diagnosing fat embolism syndrome (FES).

- Sustained $PaO_2 < 8$ kPa
- Sustained PCO_2 of >7.3 kPa or a pH < 7.3
- Sustained respiratory rate > 35 breaths/min, despite sedation
- *Increased work of breathing:* Dyspnea, accessory muscle use, tachycardia, and anxiety

LABORATORY STUDIES

Laboratory tests in FES are mostly nonspecific:

- *Arterial blood gas:* Unexplained increase in pulmonary shunt fraction ($P_{alveolar}O_2 - P_{arterial}O_2$) difference is strongly suggestive of the syndrome especially if it occurs immediately after (24–48 hours) a primary event that is clinically most likely associated with fat embolism. It indicates shunting of blood sent to the lungs for oxygenation by heart rendering most of it unoxygenated. Arterial blood gas analysis will reveal hypoxia, with a PaO_2 of <60 mm Hg along with hypocapnia—$PaCO_2 < 30$ mm Hg.
- *Hematocrit, platelet count, and fibrinogen:* Fall in hematocrit occurs within 24–48 hours and is due to intra-alveolar hemorrhage. Coagulation abnormalities (thrombogenesis), thrombocytopenia, and hypofibrogenemia are often seen, but they all are nonspecific. Serum phospholipase A2 (sPLA2) is an important inflammatory mediator that has been shown to be dramatically elevated in acute chest syndrome seen with sickle cell disease. The rise in levels of sPLA2 may be nonspecific and associated with altered lipid metabolism.
- Demonstration of fat globules—staining of urine, blood, sputum, and bronchoalveolar lavage with Sudan or Oil Red O may show fat globules. These may be free or located within macrophages. Sensitivity and negative predictive value of this test is very low to be of any concrete use in diagnosis and is more of academic interest. Fat globules in the urine are as such common after bone injuries or polytrauma.
    - Despite infrequent use studies have found that cytology of pulmonary capillary blood obtained from a wedged pulmonary artery catheter for demonstration of fat globules in patients with FES may be more beneficial in early detection of patients at risk.

IMAGING STUDIES

- *Plain chest radiographs:* Some demonstrable X-ray findings appear within 24–48 hours of onset of clinical findings as follows:
    - Diffusely distributed bilateral pulmonary infiltrates
    - "Snow storm" appearance of fleck-like pulmonary shadows
    - Prominent pulmonary bronchiolar markings
    - Enlargement of the right side of the heart
- *Noncontrast head CT:* Usually it is normal, only in some cases do they show diffuse white matter petechial hemorrhages related to microvascular injury. It is also used to rule out other causes of decreased consciousness.
- *Ventilation/perfusion imaging of the lungs:* This is modality of choice for pulmonary embolus but the findings in FES are usually normal or at most demonstrate a mottled pattern of subsegmental perfusion defects.
- High-resolution CT-chest for pulmonary embolism demonstrates three main patterns described in contemporary literature:
    1. Ground-glass opacities with interlobular septal thickening
    2. Ground-glass opacities in geographic distribution
    3. Nodular opacities

    Filling defects in pulmonary arteries are rarely described in nonfulminant syndromes.
- *Brain MRI:* It is the most useful modality to diagnose cerebral fat embolism early and it correlates well with severity and resolution of symptoms. Findings are typical white matter changes along the boundary zones of major vascular territories. The imaging patterns on brain MRI

vary with the stage of cerebral fat embolism: scattered cytotoxic edema occurs in acute stage, confluent/vasogenic cytotoxic edema occurs in subacute stage and in long-term brain atrophy demyelination can be identified.

- *Other:* These tests are not routinely indicated but may be needed in some special circumstances.
  - Transcranial Doppler sonography
  - Transesophageal echocardiography (TEE)

TREATMENT

No specific treatment is available for FES. Most modalities of management are directed to prevention, early diagnosis and adequate symptomatic relief:

- *Maintain adequate tissue oxygenation and pulmonary ventilation:* To detect desaturations early it is recommended to perform continuous oxygen saturation monitoring in at-risk patients like those with long bone fractures. This would allow early intervention in the form of oxygen therapy and possibly steroids. It also reduces chances of further hypoxic insult.
- Maintain hemodynamic stability
- Blood products should be only instituted as clinically indicated and not irrationally.
- *Adequate fluid balance:* It is better to restrict fluid intake and increase the use of diuretics to minimize fluid accumulation in the lungs provided circulation is not compromised. This latter part of maintenance of intravascular volume is really important otherwise shock can further exacerbate lung injury caused by FES so only "excess fluid" is restricted.
- Institute prophylaxis for DVT according to institutional policy and these patients are also at risk of stress-related gastrointestinal bleeding so adequate prophylaxis should be begun for this also (commonly a PPI).
- Maintain nutrition especially the protein part of it, although a balance is always desirable these patients are at risk of catabolism and hence proteins undergo rapid degradation.
- *Fracture stabilization:* Early immobilization of fractures should be done and operative treatment is more beneficial than the conservative one. Raised intraosseous pressure during orthopedic procedures is quite common so a practice of damage control orthopedics (DCO) would tend to control FES—it is believed. This would reduce the insult from intravasation of intramedullary fat and other debris in a homeostatically unstable patient further compromising his physiology.

MEDICATION

No drug is found completely useful for FES and controversies exist:

1. Steroids:
   - Decrease inflammatory reaction in lungs caused by free fatty acids.
   - Decrease capillary leakage by stabilizing lysosomal and capillary membrane.
   - *Prophylactic dose of methyl prednisolone:* 1.5 mg/kg IV can be administered every 8 hours for six doses.
2. Alcohol, albumin, aprotinin, and hypertonic glucose all are proposed for treatment of FES, but they are found to be of no use.
3. Aliskiren (renin inhibitor) has been found to protect the lungs of rats from gross and histopathological damage of FES. Similar protection to lung parenchyma has been seen with losartan from chronic damage seen in FES. These studies suggest possibility of exploiting renin-angiotensin system in treatment of FES.

Prevention in Orthopedic Surgeries

Some measures (not documented scientifically) can be undertaken to reduce the risk of FES:

- Corticosteroids may be prophylactically used to reduce rates of FES and hypoxia. They have no effect on mortality.
- Immobilization of long bone fractures by temporizing measures like external fixator has been suggested to reduce the incidence of FES. Principles of "Early appropriate care" (*see* Chapter on "Polytrauma, Mass Casualties, and Disaster") should be followed as delayed fracture fixation has been shown to increase incidence of FES. Polytrauma *per se* is not a contraindication of early fracture fixation including femoral nailing.
- Issue of reamed versus unreamed nailing in severe chest injury is unresolved. Logically and also seen in various studies the incidence of FE is higher in classical reaming techniques so chances of FES may be higher (though direct correlation of FE and FES has never been established). Improved systems like vacuum or venting during reaming or using a reaming-irrigation-aspirator system have been found to reduce FE drastically, but whether it translates into reduced incidence of FES is largely unknown.

PROGNOSIS

- Mortality from FES is uncommon (<5–15%). Most cases that fail to recoup result from associated damage to other organs. Even severe pulmonary complication associated with fat embolism seldom leads to death otherwise if managed well.
- Neurological complications such as deficit and coma are often transient and may last for days or sometimes up to weeks. Other complications such as personality changes, memory loss, and cognitive dysfunction may persist longer.
- Pulmonary complications usually resolve completely within a year and are clinically inconsequential despite deficits persistence in residual diffusion capacity.

CONCLUSION

- Fat embolism syndrome is a common occurrence in orthopedics—related both to trauma and treatment.
- It is underrated and ill-identified in most of the mortalities.
- All attempts should be made to minimize its occurrence by gentle handling of bone and tissues and following standardized protocols. One such important SOP involves practicing DCO in polytrauma and multiply injured patients.

CHAPTER 29

Acute Respiratory Distress Syndrome

Manish Kumar Varshney

INTRODUCTION

Inflammatory process in the lungs induces nonhydrostatic protein-rich pulmonary edema that causes profound hypoxemia, decreased lung compliance, and increased intrapulmonary shunt (dead space). There is severe inflammatory injury to the alveolar-capillary barrier, surfactant depletion, and loss of aerated lung tissue. Injury to lungs compromises not only its basic function of gas exchange but also the nonrespiratory immune, acid-base regulation, and humoral functions. Acute lung injury resulting from noncardiogenic causes is also known as acute respiratory distress syndrome, respiratory distress syndrome, wet lung, adult hyaline membrane disease, noncardiogenic pulmonary edema, high-output respiratory failure, congestive atelectasis, hemorrhagic lung syndrome, stiff-lung syndrome, shock lung or white lung but the term "acute respiratory distress syndrome (ARDS)" is most acceptable and will be followed here. ARDS arises from various traumatic and nontraumatic inflammatory causes often complicating critical illness and needs dedicated management else survival is commonly threatened. Decreasing ventilator-induced lung injury (VILI) is of prime importance in managing these patients on supportive therapy.

BACKGROUND AND DEFINITION

It has been seen that some patients with sepsis, severe pancreatitis, nonthoracic injuries, massive transfusion, and other conditions develop diffuse lung infiltrates, respiratory distress leading to respiratory failure. Ashbaugh et al. described 12 such patients in 1967, using the term "adult respiratory distress syndrome" to describe this condition.

The condition was defined in 1994 by the American-European Consensus Conference (AECC) and the term "acute respiratory distress syndrome" was used instead of "adult respiratory distress syndrome" because the syndrome occurs in both adults and children. The AECC defined ARDS as *"An acute condition characterized by bilateral pulmonary infiltrates and severe hypoxemia in the absence of evidence for cardiogenic pulmonary edema."* The more recent Berlin definition proposed by European Society of Intensive Care Medicine provides an objective criteria to define and diagnose ARDS. It needs fulfillment of three criteria, viz.:

1. Acute onset (within 1 week)
2. Bilateral opacities on chest X-ray
3. PaO_2/FiO_2 (arterial to inspired oxygen) ratio of ≤300 on positive end-expiratory pressure (PEEP) or continuous positive airway pressure (CPAP) ≥ 5 cmH_2O.

Acute respiratory distress syndrome is classified as mild, moderate, or severe in Berlin definition based on PaO_2/FiO_2 ratio:

- *Mild:* 200 mm Hg < PaO_2/FiO_2 ratio ≤ 300 mm Hg with positive end-expiratory pressure (PEEP) or continuous positive airway pressure ≥ 5 cmH_2O.
- *Moderate:* 100 mm Hg < PaO_2/FiO_2 ratio ≤ 200 mm Hg with PEEP ≥ 5 cmH_2O.
- *Severe:* PaO_2/FiO_2 ratio ≤ 100 mm Hg with PEEP ≥ 5 cmH_2O.

It has been found that ARDS is missed by primary clinician in nearly 40% cases especially if it is mild. Mortality increases with severity of ARDS that may be as high as 45% in severe ARDS.

PATHOPHYSIOLOGY

Acute respiratory distress syndrome is associated with diffuse alveolar damage (necrosis of type I and II alveolar cells) and lung capillary endothelial injury incited by alveolar macrophage induced inflammation. The disease is usually described in two phases:

1. The early phase which is described as being exudative.
2. The late phase which is fibroproliferative in character.

Early ARDS is characterized by an influx of fluid into the alveoli because of increase in the permeability of the alveolar-capillary barrier. The alveolar-capillary barrier is formed by the vascular endothelium and the epithelium of the alveoli. Hence, insults resulting in damage either to the alveolar epithelium or to the vascular endothelium could result in ARDS.

Neutrophils are thought to play an integral part in the pathogenesis of ARDS, as shown by studies of lung biopsy specimen and bronchoalveolar lavage in early ARDS. The fact that infusion of granulocyte colony-stimulating factor (G-CSF) in patients suffering from ventilator-associated pneumonia (VAP) does not promote the development of ARDS and it may develop in profoundly neutropenic patients also. So in view of this and other evidence it can be rightly said that the neutrophils observed in ARDS may be reactive rather than causative.

The early acute phase of ARDS may resolve completely, which is the usual event (proliferative phase), but sometimes it may progress to pulmonary fibrosis (fibrotic phase). The proliferative phase is a reparative process where type II alveolar cells proliferate and differentiate into type I cells re-establishing the alveolar lining and increasing expression of aquaporins and alveolar ion channels. This removes water from alveoli and shifts it to pulmonary microcirculation and lymphatics. Fibrosis is characterized by neovascularization and extensive damage to basement membrane causing persistent edema, intra-alveolar and interstitial fibrosis, and microvascular damage. Shear forces from mechanical ventilation may also promote this fibrotic phase. Interleukin-1 is the key mediator in the whole process. Pulmonary fibrosis is associated with bas prognosis.

ETIOLOGY

The most common risk factor for ARDS in adults is pneumonia with or without sepsis (60%) or nonpulmonary sepsis (16%) and in approximately 20% of patients with ARDS no identifiable risk factor is found. Risk factors or ARDS can be broadly classified into systemic illnesses, direct lung injury (including aspiration if gastric content) and injuries.

Major risk factors other than sepsis that are associated with the development of ARDS includes:

- Older age
- Trauma, with or without pulmonary contusion
- Burns
- Massive transfusion
- Bacteremia
- Fractures, particularly multiple fractures and long bone fractures
- Pneumonia
- Drug overdose
- Postperfusion injury after cardiopulmonary bypass
- Fat embolism
- Aspiration
- Near drowning
- Pancreatitis

PRESENTATION

Patients developing ARDS are often critically ill associated with the involvement of multisystem organ failure. It usually presents with acute onset of dyspnea with the sensation of rapid shallow breathing and hypoxemia giving the feeling of not able to get enough air to breathe. It is necessary to enquire about any of the risk factor or any event, which possibly can cause ARDS. The event may be sepsis, massive transfusion, acute pancreatitis, aspiration, trauma or any other possible cause. The symptoms usually start within hours to days of an inciting event and typically ARDS develops within 12–48 hours of the event.

PHYSICAL FINDINGS

Physical findings are often nonspecific, and patient has tachypnea and tachycardia owing to the rapid shallow breathing and hypoxemia. The patient may be febrile or hypothermic. Patients on ventilator require high fraction of inspired oxygen and high PEEP. Thorough clinical examination should be done to differentiate ARDS from cardiogenic pulmonary edema by carefully looking for signs of congestive heart failure such as raised jugular venous pressure, murmurs, gallops, and edema of the dependent part.

WORKUP

Acute respiratory distress syndrome is mainly diagnosed clinically and no specific laboratory tests can confirm its diagnosis. Arterial blood gas and chest radiograph can prove useful to support your clinical diagnosis. Arterial blood gas often shows arterial hypoxemia in spite of high fraction of inspired oxygen and chest radiograph shows acute onset of bilateral alveolar or interstitial infiltrates in the absence of any signs indicating cardiogenic pulmonary edema. Although other basic or special workup may be required to find the cause of ARDS along with hemodynamic monitoring to manage a patient with ARDS.

DIFFERENTIAL DIAGNOSIS

Acute respiratory distress syndrome needs to be differentiated from various respiratory, cardiac, infectious and toxic etiologies that may cause acute hypoxia **(Table 1)**. Good examination specific to respiratory and cardiovascular system can help to differentiate ARDS from cardiac causes and pneumonia itself **(Table 2)**.

TREATMENT

First and foremost is identification and treatment of the cause as early as possible. Immediate goals are supportive care and the prevention of complications. The mortality of patients with ARDS is usually not due primarily to respiratory failure. Most patients die from secondary infections, other organ failures, or the complications of prolonged hospitalization.

Mechanical Ventilation

Although mechanical ventilation has the lifesaving potential, it can also aggravate lung injury or VILI. VILI is essentially related to volutrauma (generalized excess stress and strain on the injured lung). Lung stress corresponds to transpulmonary pressure (alveolar pressure-pleural

TABLE 1: The common conditions that should be differentiated from acute respiratory distress syndrome (ARDS).

Common	*Uncommon*
• Asthma • Chronic obstructive pulmonary disease • Congestive cardiac failure • Pneumonia	• Acute eosinophilic pneumonia • Hypersensitivity pneumonitis • Pneumothorax • Salicylate toxicity • Sepsis

TABLE 2: The distinguishing features of acute respiratory distress syndrome (ARDS), pneumonia, and congestive cardiac failure.

Feature	*ARDS*	*Pneumonia*	*Congestive cardiac failure*
Dyspnea/hypoxia/tachypnea/rales on auscultation	Yes	Yes	Yes
Pleuritic chest pain	Usually No	Yes	No
Sputum production	May be	Yes	No
Peripheral edema	No	No	Yes
Fever	Present in many due to sepsis	Yes	No
Raised jugular venous pressure	No	No	Yes
Third heart sound	No	No	Yes
Bilateral infiltrates	Yes	May be (localized infiltrates are characteristic)	Usually
Enlarged cardiac shadow	No	No	Yes
Brain natriuretic peptide levels	Variable	Normal	Elevated
PaO_2/FiO_2 ratio ≤ 300	Present	No	No
Pulmonary wedge pressure ≤ 18 mm Hg	Yes	Yes	No
Response to antibiotics	No	Yes	No
Effect of diuretics	No	No	Yes
Improvement with oxygen by mask	No	Yes	Yes

pressure), and lung strain refers to the change in lung volume indexed to functional residual capacity of the ARDS lung at zero PEEP. Trials show that lung injury occurs because of two processes: (1) recurrent alveolar collapse and (2) repeated alveolar over distention. So to minimize the lung injury, it is recommended to use lung protective ventilator strategy, which includes low tidal volume (6 mL/kg of predicted body weight), limitation of plateau pressure (<28–30 cmH_2O), and appropriate PEEP. Tidal volume should not be increased when the plateau pressure is well below 30 cmH_2O except in cases of marked persistent hypercapnia despite reduction of instrumental dead space and increase of respiratory rate. In ARDS, the presence of alveolar and interstitial fluid and the loss of surfactant can lead to a marked reduction of lung compliance, so a high end-expiratory pressure is required to prevent alveolar collapse at end expiration and to maintain oxygenation. PEEP is usually set to minimize FiO_2 (inspired O_2 percentage) and maximize PaO_2 (arterial partial pressure of O_2). Although high PEEP dose improve lung function but no mortality benefit has been seen. High PEEP should be used in moderate or severe ARDS but not in mild ARDS. High-frequency oscillation ventilation (HFOV) is proposed to improve gas exchange while protecting against VILI using a tidal volume below or equal to the anatomical dead space. Though intuitive the use of HFOV is not recommended in ARDS patients. Instead, prone positioning should be used in ARDS patients with PaO_2/FiO_2 ratio < 150 mm Hg to reduce mortality. Sessions of at least 16 consecutive hours should be performed.

Oxygenation can also be improved by inverse ration ventilation in which inspiration is kept for a longer duration than expiration leading to trapping of more air in the lung causing dynamic hyperinflation, which maintains end-expiratory pressure similar to PEEP.

Recruitment maneuvers that transiently increase PEEP to "recruit" atelectatic lung can also increase oxygenation but a mortality benefit has not been established. Ventilator weaning is recommended as per the American Thoracic Society (ATS) and the American College of Chest Physicians ventilator liberation protocol.

Fluid Management

Fluid management is one of the most difficult measures to manage in septic shock patients with ARDS as vascular and epithelial permeability is increased in ARDS. Conservative fluid management is highly recommended after hemodynamic stabilization in ARDS patients. A conservative fluid management strategy maintains a relatively low central venous pressure which is associated with the need for fewer days of mechanical ventilation.

Neuromuscular Blockade

In ARDS patients, sedation alone is not adequate to maintain synchrony with the mechanical ventilation, so early neuromuscular blockade for at least first 48 hours is recommended with cisatracurium besilate in ARDS patients with a PaO_2/FiO_2 ratio < 150 mm Hg to reduce mortality. This not only increased the rate of survival but also increases ventilator free days.

Extracorporeal Membrane Oxygenation

Venovenous extracorporeal membrane oxygenation (ECMO) should be considered in cases of severe ARDS with PaO_2/FiO_2 < 80 mm Hg and/or when mechanical ventilation becomes dangerous because of the increase in plateau pressure and despite optimization of ARDS management including high PEEP, neuromuscular blocking agents, and prone positioning. Arteriovenous or venovenous low-flow extracorporeal CO_2 removal ($ECCO_2R$) allows so-called "ultraprotective" ventilation strategies (tidal volume < 6 mL/kg PBW and decrease in plateau and driving pressures and in respiratory rate) during ARDS, by controlling hypercapnia induced by the reduction in minute ventilation. The recommendation for $ECCO_2R$ is presently not very strong. Inhaled nitric oxide can be used in cases of ARDS with deep hypoxemia despite the implementation of a protective ventilation strategy and prone positioning, and before envisaging use of venovenous ECMO.

Pharmacotherapy

Initially used to counteract the pulmonary inflammation but recent evidences do not recommend the use of glucocorticoids in ARDS. Similarly, use of surfactant is not recommended in management of ARDS. Patients should receive venous thromboembolism prophylaxis with low-molecular-weight heparin, low-dose unfractionated heparin, or fondaparinux if not contraindicated.

PREVENTION

Although multiple risk factors for ARDS are known, no successful preventive measures have been identified. Careful fluid management in high-risk patients may be helpful. Because aspiration pneumonitis is a risk factor for ARDS, taking appropriate measures to prevent aspiration (e.g., elevating the head of the bed and evaluating swallowing mechanics before feeding high-risk patients) may also prevent some ARDS cases.

CONCLUSION

- Acute respiratory distress syndrome accounts for the most common cause of respiratory failure in intensive care.
- Various etiological factors culminate into development of lung injury that may quickly become irreversible so primary etiological factor identification and its control is the best strategy of management. This epitomizes the dictum "prevention is better than cure".
- Once developed, the management is more or less supportive but involves a tight path with uncertain outcome. Knowledge of supportive ventilation is a must and the most important independent factor in optimal management of these patients and future recovery.

CHAPTER 30

Systemic Inflammatory Response Syndrome and Multiorgan Dysfunction

Manish Kumar Varshney

INTRODUCTION

Systemic inflammatory response syndrome (SIRS) refers to an exaggerated inflammatory state affecting whole body arising out of defense response (cytokine storm) of body to a noxious stimulus. SIRS may arise from various infectious and noninfectious causes. The cytokine storm, if dysregulated, has the potential to produce reversible or irreversible end-organ damage. In 1992, the American College of Chest Physicians (ACCP)/the Society of Critical Care Medicine (SCCM) defined systemic inflammatory response syndrome as two or more of the following variables:

1. Fever > 38°C or <36°C
2. Heart rate > 90 beats/min
3. Respiratory rate > 20 breaths/min or $PaCO_2$ < 32 mm Hg
4. Abnormal white blood cell count (>12,000/mm³ or <4,000/mm³ or >10% bands)

Note:

- Two or more of the above must be present.
- These changes should represent acute alterations from baseline in the absence of other known cause for the abnormalities.

Systemic inflammatory response syndrome is a *clinical response* (not essentially a complication) to a nonspecific insult and in general all septic patients have SIRS but not all SIRS have sepsis. When evaluating a patient with SIRS identifying the initial cause has the greatest impact on outcome. SIRS with a suspected source of infection is called *sepsis*. Sepsis with one or more organ failure (lactic acidosis, systolic BP < 90 mm Hg or systolic BP drop ≥ 40 mm Hg of normal) is termed *severe sepsis*. Presence of hemodynamic instability despite adequate volume repletion is called *septic shock*. Multiple organ dysfunction syndrome (MODS) is the progressive physiological dysfunction of two or more organ systems in acutely ill septic patients such that homeostasis is not maintainable without intervention (discussed later). So SIRS is not an endpoint final diagnosis but it is a pathophysiological change in inflammatory response that produces variable damage in continuum and has the potential to being reversed if adequate initial therapy is given **(Flowchart 1)**. There has been intense debate challenging the criteria used to define SIRS as they are nonspecific (only indicate inflammation and not the cause of it), do not distinguish between beneficial and deleterious host responses that need to be targeted, all criteria have same weightage but not all translate into equivalent risk of organ dysfunction or death. So sepsis has been redefined as "any life-threatening organ dysfunction caused by the dysregulated host response to infection" and it excludes establishment of SIRS criteria. It is recommended to use sequential organ failure assessment (SOFA) for validating sepsis **(Table 1)** instead of SIRS criteria.

PATHOPHYSIOLOGY

The acute insult (initial event and inciting event) leading to SIRS can be an infectious or noninfectious cause **(Table 2)**.

Flowchart 1: The development of systemic inflammatory response syndrome (SIRS) to an inciting event (say sepsis) and then its progression or containment depending on initial Identification. Uncontrolled progression often produces multiorgan dysfunction and damage/death.

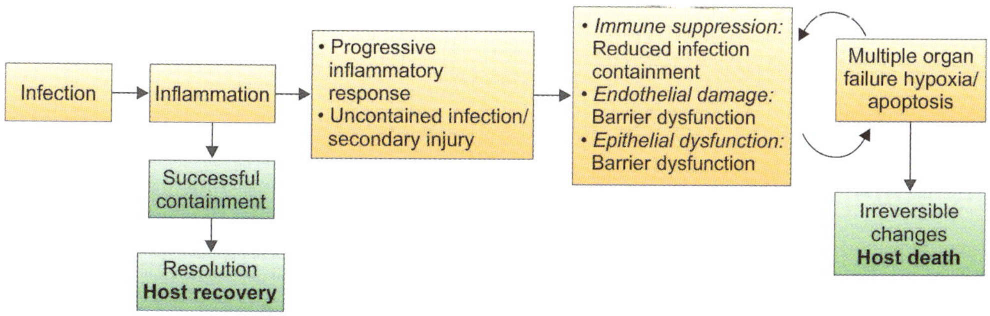

TABLE 1: The sequential organ failure assessment (SOFA) scoring system. The highest daily score is calculated and change in SOFA score of ≥2 points as a consequence of infection increases mortality by 10%.

Respiratory system	
PaO_2/FiO_2 (mm Hg)	*SOFA score*
>400	0
<400	1
<300	2
<200 with respiratory support	3
<100 with respiratory support	4
Nervous system	
Glasgow Coma Scale	*SOFA score*
15	0
13–14	1
10–12	2
6–9	3
<6	4
Cardiovascular system	
Mean arterial pressure (MAP) or administration of vasopressors required	*SOFA score*
MAP > 70 mm Hg	0
MAP < 70 mm Hg	1
Dopamine ≤ 5 μg/kg/min or dobutamine (any dose)	2
Dopamine > 5 μg/kg/min *or* epinephrine ≤ 0.1 μg/kg/min *or* norepinephrine ≤ 0.1 μg/kg/min	3
Dopamine > 15 μg/kg/min *or* epinephrine > 0.1 μg/kg/min *or* norepinephrine > 0.1 μg/kg/min	4
Liver	
Bilirubin (mg/dL) (μmol/L)	*SOFA score*
<1.2 (<20)	0
1.2–1.9 (20–32)	1
2.0–5.9 (33–101)	2
6.0–11.9 (102–204)	3
>12.0 (>204)	4
Coagulation	
Platelets ×10^3/mL	*SOFA score*
>150	0
<150	1
<100	2
<50	3
<20	4
Kidneys	
Creatinine (mg/dL) (μmol/L); urine output	*SOFA score*
<1.2 (<110)	0
1.2–1.9 (110–170)	1
2.0–3.4 (171–299)	2
3.5–4.9 (300–440) (or urine output < 500 mL/day)	3
>5.0 (>440); urine output < 200 mL/day	4

SIRS has a common cascade of development and progression (with minor differences) remaining constant in evolution and is mostly independent of the etiological factors mentioned in **Table 2**. Most probably SIRS is a self-defense mechanism of body that produces consistent predetermined changes involving the inflammatory pathway in response to nonspecific insults/stimuli. Both the humoral and cellular pathways are involved in the production of a "syndrome" of responses that is facilitated by complement and the cytokine cascades. The complex interactions can be divided into three stages (RC bone).

TABLE 2: The common etiological factors inciting the systemic inflammatory response syndrome.

Infectious causes	*Noninfectious causes*
• Bacteremia and bacterial sepsis • Intra-abdominal infections • Meningitis • Septic arthritis • Nosocomial pneumonia • Community-acquired pneumonia • Toxic shock syndrome • Urinary tract infection • Necrotizing fasciitis • Pseudomembranous colitis *(Clostridium difficile)* • Pyelonephritis • Cellulitis • Cholecystitis • Diabetic foot infection • Erysipelas • HIV (acute retroviral syndrome) • Pelvic inflammatory disease	• Hemorrhagic shock • Myocardial infarction • Pancreatitis • Trauma • Pulmonary embolism • Intestinal perforation • Burns • Diabetic ketoacidosis • Malignancy/metastasis • Toxic epidermal necrolysis • Transfusion reactions • Acute mesenteric ischemia • Cirrhosis • Deep venous thrombosis • Alcohol withdrawal • Drug reaction • Electrical injuries • Drug overdose • Gastrointestinal bleeding

- *Stage I:* The initial response is local cytokine production toward an insult/stimuli. This mandates to healing of the damage incurred and promoting wound repair by recruitment of the reticular endothelial system.
- *Stage II:* There is a release of small quantities of local cytokines into the circulation to improve the local response. Following this, there is stimulation of growth factors and the recruitment of macrophages and platelets. This is known as the acute phase response and the goal is homeostasis.
- *Stage III:* If homeostasis is not restored, a significant systemic reaction occurs. The overproduction of cytokines (cytokine storm) causes destruction rather than protection. As a consequence, there is the activation of reticular endothelial system and numerous humoral cascades and subsequent loss of circulatory integrity. This leads to end-organ dysfunction.

MULTI-HIT THEORY

It had been always difficult to digest the connotation that single event/insult/stimulus will produce SIRS. To expand the understanding multi-hit theory has been proposed that bases the concept on "priming the SIRS pump" by initial event/insult. SIRS cascades is caused by each additional event to produce an altered or exaggerated response which leads to progression of illness and pathophysiological changes. Some of the secondary hits that influence resolution/progression of SIRS include:

- Electrolyte abnormalities
- Hyperglycemia

- Intravenous (IV) catheter related bacteremia
- Gastrointestinal (GI) bleeding and stress gastritis
- Deep venous thrombosis
- Anemia

The key to preventing multiple hits is adequate identification of the initial cause/event of SIRS and appropriate resuscitation and therapy. Depending on the inciting factors (and adequate prevention of possible other "hits"), many SIRS states would even resolve without specific intervention. History taking and clinical examination serve as the basic plinth for management of SIRS.

CLINICAL EXAMINATION

There are many triggers for SIRS and patient can present with variety of manners. A detailed history is mandatory and it should be focused around system associated with complaints.

- Typical nonspecific symptoms such as fever with chills and night sweats, that is why infectious causes should be differentiated from noninfectious causes.
- Pain—the duration, site, radiating elsewhere, quality and aggravating factors associated with the pain are useful to help establish a thorough differential diagnosis.
- Medication history of the patient should be asked as it may be the cause of new drug-drug interaction or a new side effect. Also, beta-blockers like drugs prevent important signs like tachycardia.

Initial vital signs should be carefully watched. Vital signs should be repeated at regular intervals initially as multiple other factors such as stress, anxiety, etc., might lead to false diagnosis of SIRS. Any sign of hypoperfusion (delayed capillary refilling, skin mottling, mental status changes, and decreased urine output) should be looked upon. Patients with severe disease who are not able to provide history should also undergo a complete physical examination including a rectal examination to rule out a perirectal abscess or gastrointestinal bleeding.

LABORATORY EVALUATION

In order to completely assess SIRS, complete blood cell count with differential count should be ordered to evaluate for leukocytosis and preliminary diagnosis of type of inflammatory event. In general, a battery of laboratory tests is ordered **(Box 1)**; however, we recommend that they should be individualized based on patient history and physical examination findings.

Acute phase reactants as a rule are not useful in differentiating various causes of SIRS, but their periodic value is useful to monitor response to the treatment.

TREATMENT

There is no drug of choice for the treatment of SIRS. Medications are given according to specific diagnosis. Treatment should be focused on possible/most probable inciting causes of SIRS as identified on clinical examination.

- Patients with hypotension should receive adequate resuscitation with intravenous fluids and if they still remain hypotensive, vasopressor agents, such as norepinephrine and dopamine should be administered with careful monitoring of hemodynamic parameters. All patients should have adequate intravenous access and often require two large bore IV cannulas or a central venous catheter.
- Empirical antibiotics are not indicated for all patients with SIRS. Fever alone is not an indication for antibiotics and there should be specific suspicion/indication of starting them **(Box 2)**. Empiric antibiotic therapy should be guided by knowledge of the local antibiograms. Once a bacteriologic diagnosis is obtained then specific antibiotics is the most appropriate therapy (one may definitely add on the antibiotics pre-emptively for possible complications of the inciting event to prevent additional hit).
    - In high-risk groups (e.g., ventilator-associated pneumonia, infected arthroplasty) where no specific infectious diagnosis is initially identified; broad spectrum antibiotics are started. Due to increased prevalence of methicillin-resistant *Staphylococcus aureus* (MRSA), vancomycin should be considered in initial antibiotic regimen. Third or fourth generation cephalosporin or a fluoroquinolone can be used for gram-negative bacterial coverage. It is recommended to avoid an antibiotic class to which a patient has recently been exposed.
    - Care should be taken to not to use an antibiotic for which the patient is allergic. This may be a "second hit" and lead to worsening SIRS.

BOX 1: Laboratory and imaging studies to consider in a patient with systemic inflammatory response syndrome.

Recommended initial testing:
- Complete blood count with differential
- Chest radiograph
- Urinalysis
- Erect abdominal films
- Metabolic panel including [liver function test (LFT), kidney function test (KFT), electrolytes]

Laboratory testing that may be prescribed based on identified event:
- Urine cultures
- Blood cultures
- Amylase/lipase
- Right upper quadrant ultrasound
- CT of abdomen and pelvis
- Lactic acid level
- CT of chest
- Cardiac enzymes and ECG
- C-reactive protein and erythrocyte sedimentation rate (ESR), D-dimer, serum ferritin, interleukin-6 (IL-6) levels
- Lower extremity ultrasound and Doppler studies
- Spinal fluid analysis
- Sputum culture (if suspecting pneumonia)

BOX 2: Definitive indications for empiric antibiotics in the patient with systemic inflammatory response syndrome.

- Immunocompromised state
- Neutropenia
- Documented or presumed infection [urinary tract infection (UTI), pneumonia, cellulitis, etc.]
- Hemodynamic instability
- Asplenia

- Empirical antifungal therapy (azole group or an echinocandin) may be considered in hemodynamically unstable patients who are neutropenic, or have already been treated with antibiotics, receiving total parenteral nutrition (TPN) or who have long-term central venous access in place.
- No SIRS specific studies have been done to date but role of steroids in sepsis and septic shock has been extensively studied. Their role has always been supportive only and possibly suppressing too aggressive an inflammation.
- Intensive control of blood glucose levels is essential. Controlling the blood glucose levels in physiological range has been shown to:
  - Diminish in-hospital morbidity and mortality in both the surgical and medical intensive care setting.
  - Reduces the need for red blood cell transfusions.
  - Lowers the incidence of critical-illness polyneuropathy.
  - Improve patient outcomes (including renal function and acute renal failure).
  - Reduces the number of days in the ICU.
  - Decreases the need for prolonged mechanical ventilation.

COMPLICATIONS

Potential complications (actually progression of uncontrolled event) of SIRS include:

- Adult respiratory disease syndrome (ARDS)
- Renal failure
- Respiratory failure
- Cardiovascular decompensation
- Disseminated intravascular coagulation (DIC)

MULTIPLE ORGAN DYSFUNCTION SYNDROME (MULTIPLE ORGAN FAILURE AND MULTISYSTEM ORGAN FAILURE)

DEFINITION

The multiple organ dysfunction syndrome (MODS) can be defined as the development of physiologic derangement involving two or more organ systems (such that homeostasis cannot be maintained without intervention), not involved in the disorder that resulted in ICU admission, and arising in the wake of a potentially life-threatening physiologic insult. It is a process rather than a single event.

Usage of the word "failure" is probably inappropriate as normal physiologic function of the failing organ systems can be restored in patients if appropriate treatment is provided early. So the term "dysfunction" is more apt to characterize the process of MODS.

ETIOLOGY

The etiology is an acute factor which causes overactivity of inflammatory response leading to MODS. Sepsis is the most important cause of MODS. MODS is the final stage of continuum of the process: injury → stress reaction → systemic inflammatory response syndrome (SIRS)/compensate anti-inflammation reaction syndrome (CARS) disequilibrium → MODS. Generally, it happens within 24 hours of the triggering episode. The cause can be any of the following:

- Infection
- Trauma
- Ischemia
- Burns
- Cancer
- Pancreatitis
- Transplantation
- Pulmonary embolism
- Ruptured/dissecting aneurysm
- Post-CPB
- Cardiac tamponade
- Anaphylaxis

Major risk factors include sepsis and the SIRS, shock, trauma, bowel infarction and prolonged periods of hypotension, hepatic dysfunction, increased age, and alcohol abuse.

PATHOPHYSIOLOGY

The exact mechanism, which leads to MODS, is not known. Four pathogenic mechanisms (hypoxic hypoxia, cytotoxicity, induction of apoptosis, and immunosuppression) seem to primarily explain the development of MODS but it appears that it is a conglomerate of various other even minor pathophysiologic mechanisms, which may act individually or collectively in the production of organ system dysfunction, as follows:

- *Primary cellular injury:* This is due to histotoxic anoxia, circulating toxins, induction of apoptosis, etc. Apoptosis or programmed cell death removes most of the dysfunctional cells normally. In activated macrophages and neutrophils, the proinflammatory cytokines delay apoptosis, but other tissues (e.g., gut epithelium), on the other hand, undergo accelerated apoptosis.
- *Inadequate tissue/organ perfusion:* This causes hypoxic hypoxia and is due to alteration of metabolic regulation of tissue oxygen delivery caused by septic circulatory lesion. The various mechanisms are:
  - Hypoperfusion
  - *Ischemia/reperfusion:* The reactive oxygen species produced with reperfusion are poorly salvaged in body of such patients and lead to microcirculatory injury.
  - *Microaggregation and/or disseminated intravascular coagulation:* This is induced by microvascular and endothelial abnormalities caused by free radical oxygen species, lytic enzymes, and substances which cause vasodilatation and vasoconstriction (e.g., endothelial growth factors and NO).
- *Diffuse endothelial cell injury:* Caused by endotoxin, TNF-α, and NO that damage transport of electrons in mitochondria and affect energy metabolism causing cytopathic or histotoxic anoxia.
- Circulating humoral factors (viz., myocardial depressant substance)
- Circulating immune/inflammatory mediators
- Immunosuppression caused by:
  - Protein calorie malnutrition
  - Bacterial-toxin translocation

- Defective red blood cells
- Adverse effect of treatment or medication.

Various hypotheses have been proposed by different investigators to explain the development of MODS:

- *Gut hypothesis:* Proposed by Deitch it remains the most popular to explain MODS in critically ill patients. The primary event is thought to be splanchnic hypoperfusion and the subsequent mucosal ischemia that alters cellular function. The gut, hence, becomes leaky and is unable to hold the toxins and pathogenic microorganisms. Simultaneously the ensuing liver dysfunction releases toxins into the systemic circulation and activates immune response escalating the spiral of continuous damage.
- *Endotoxin macrophage hypothesis:* Gram-negative infections in patients with MODS are relatively common. These are known to produce a lot of endotoxins that have hence been the focus for pathogenesis of a shock like state and MODS. With the initial release of cytokines, proinflammatory mediators also get circulated in the system like—tumor necrosis factor-alpha (TNF-α), interleukin-1, interleukin-6, prostacyclin, and thromboxane A2. Prostacyclin and nitric oxide are responsible for further manifestations.
- *Tissue hypoxia-microvascular hypothesis:* With rapid ongoing changes in the vessels and capillaries, oxygen supply is decreased which leads to hypoxemia and in turn causing cell death leading to organ dysfunction.
- *Mitochondrial DNA hypothesis:* Mitochondrial DNA has come into focus by findings of Zsolt Balohh. As mitochondrial DNA resembles bacterial DNA so it is hypothesized that there is leak of large quantity of mitochondrial DNA in the blood, which may lead to severe inflammation triggering, catastrophic immune response.
- Integrated hypothesis—possibly and more likely all above contribute to the pathogenesis.

CLINICAL FEATURES

The following six organ systems characterize MODS and they include:

1. Respiratory
2. Cardiovascular
3. Renal
4. Hepatic
5. Neurologic
6. Hematologic

The signs and symptoms of end-organ dysfunction in the above organ systems consist of:

- Impaired gas exchange manifesting as arterial hypoxemia in respiratory system.
- Hypoperfusion of the vital organs leading to the impairment of the delivery of oxygen causing irreversible injury of the organs.
- Decrease in the urine output even if the intravascular volume is maintained which may later lead to rise in serum creatinine called as acute kidney injury and some patients might require even hemodialysis.
- Hepatocellular injury revealed as rise in bilirubin level or rise in the hepatic enzymes.
- Acute phase reactants such as C-reactive protein, α-1 antitrypsin, or ferritin may be elevated, whereas levels of albumin, a negative acute phase reactant, are depressed.
- Confusion, disorientation, and impaired consciousness are recognizable manifestation of the neurologic dysfunction of MODS.
- Thrombocytopenia, anemia, and leukopenia are also quite common and not so uncommonly patient can develop disseminated intravascular coagulation (DIC).

OTHER SYSTEMS

- *Immunological:* Because of alteration the immunity patient can develop hospital-acquired infections, caused by relatively avirulent organisms.
- *Endocrine/metabolic:* Increase in the blood sugar levels, insulin resistance thyroid abnormalities, and adrenal insufficiency are some of the abnormalities found.

DIAGNOSIS

Diagnosis of MODS is mainly clinical (explained above in clinical features) which is supplemented by laboratory tests and imaging modalities:

- *In hepatic dysfunction:* If ischemic hepatitis: jaundice, increased transaminase, and increased serum bilirubin. If acalculous cholecystitis: right hypochondrial pain and tenderness, abdominal distention, unexplained fever, and loss of bowel sounds.
- *In pulmonary dysfunction:* Symptoms suggestive of acute respiratory distress syndrome (ARDS).
- *In renal dysfunction:* Azotemia, fluid and electrolyte imbalance, decreased creatinine clearance, and fluid volume overload.
- In cardiovascular system (CVS) due to cardiac hypoperfusion, there is decrease in the contractility of the myocardium with fall in cardiac output and stroke volume and inability to maintain the BP without vasopressors.
- *In disseminated intravascular coagulation (DIC):* Microvascular clotting and hemorrhage in organ systems.
- *In central nervous system (CNS) dysfunction:* Impaired mentation, confusion, altered level of consciousness, delirium and psychosis and abnormal bispectral electroencephalogram (EEG) monitoring.
- Muscle wasting, severe weight loss, hyperglycemia, hypertriglyceridemia, increased serum lactate, hypoalbuminemia, decreased prealbumin and serum transferrin, and decreased retinol binding protein.
- *In immune dysfunction:* Nosocomial infection, pyrexia, and decreased lymphocyte anergy.

PREVENTION

The best management of MODS is to prevent it from occurring. The principles of prevention are as follows:

- Decrease the severity of MODS
- Lessen the inflammation
- Appropriate resuscitation
- Control of infection

TABLE 3: The multiple organ dysfunction (MOD) score.

Organ system	*0*	*1*	*2*	*3*	*4*
Respiratory system					
PO_2/FiO_2 ratio without reference to the use or mode of mechanical ventilation, and without reference to the use or level of PEEP	>300	226–300	151–225	76–150	≤75
Renal					
Serum creatinine (µmol/L)	≤100	101–200	201–350	351–500	>500
Liver and biliary system					
Serum bilirubin (µmol/L)	≤20	21–60	61–120	121–240	>240
Cardiovascular system					
Pressure adjusted heart rate (heart rate × RAP/mean BP)	≤10.0	10.1–15.0	15.1–20.0	20.1–30.0	>30.0
Hematology					
Platelet count (per mL 10^{-3})	>120	81–120	51–80	21–50	≤20
Central nervous system					
Glasgow coma score	15	13–14	10–12	7–9	≤6

(PEEP: positive end-expiratory pressure; RAP: right atrial pressure)

- Avoidance for unnecessary interventions and medications
- Maintaining proper nutrition

PROGNOSIS

Several descriptive scales are developed, based on the quantification of organ dysfunction as a numeric scale. Every scale uses all six organ systems to score MODS—the respiratory system, CVS, renal, hepatic, CNS, and hematologic systems. The multiple organ dysfunction (MOD) score **(Table 3)** uses multiple physiologic variables that have been correlated with mortality or shown in **Table 4**.

TABLE 4: The multiple organ dysfunction (MOD) score with mortality.

MODS score	*Mortality*
0	0
9–12	25
13–16	50
17–20	75
>20	100

(MODS: multiple organ dysfunction syndrome)

TREATMENT

At present, there is no specific treatment of MODS. The treatment modality is mainly supportive.

The principles for the treatment of MODS are:
- Early recognition
- Control of infection
    - Incision and drainage of any abscess, antibiotics
    - Sepsis—identification and treatment of the source of infection, volume resuscitation, vasopressors, and inotropes if evidence of hypoperfusion.
- *Maintenance of tissue oxygenation:* Mechanical ventilation and increasing tissue perfusion. Control of bleeding, maintenance of hemoglobin 8–10 g/dL.
- Nutritional/metabolic support

CONCLUSION

- Systemic inflammatory response syndrome represents a continuum of progressive inflammatory changes in the body arising out of defensive recruitment of inflammation against a noxious infectious or noninfectious stimulus.
- Uncontrolled SIRS ultimately causes end-organal damage that may also progress to MODS and death.
- Multiple organ dysfunction syndrome is a complex syndrome and represents multiple pathways that culminate into organ failure.
- Management is mostly supportive and is best instituted at inception of rising inflammation that should be captured by clinical assessment and use of scoring systems regularly to avoid catastrophe.

CHAPTER

31 Shock

Manish Kumar Varshney

INTRODUCTION

Shock is a state of decreased perfusion of the body resulting in inadequate supply of oxygen and nutrients to the tissues leading to dysfunction of the normal cellular milieu, and if not treated promptly resulting in cell death. "Shock" is not synonymous with hypotension, which is often a late manifestation. The defining feature of shock is tissue hypoperfusion, and not a predetermined level of systemic arterial blood pressure. The clinical picture may be overt or subtle. The cardiac output and oxygen delivery may be critically low, even though the blood pressure (BP) remains normal, and the underlying problem should be identified and treated before the BP falls.

If cause of shock is not treated immediately then inadequate tissue oxygenation leads to irreversible cell injury and death **(Flowchart 1)**; timely restoration of perfusion is the only treatment to prevent progression of the shock state, and this forms the fundamental basis for the management of shock. Intervention is aimed to re-expand the intravascular volume and control the inciting process.

Flowchart 1: Common progression pathway of shock and pathogenesis of irreversible injury.

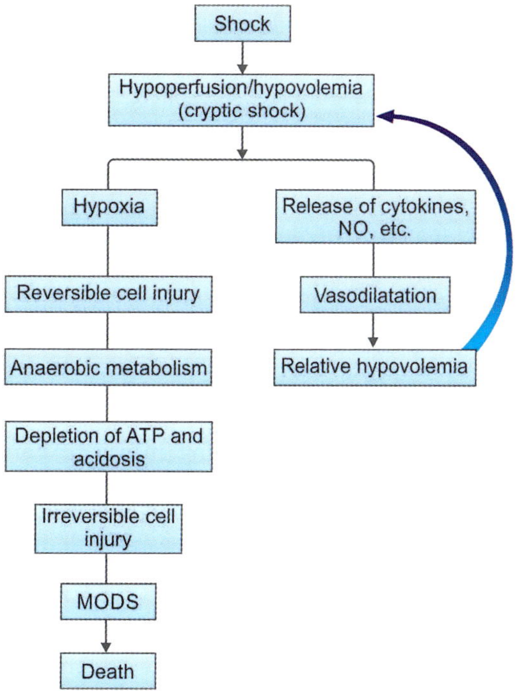

(ATP: adenosine triphosphate; MODS: multiple organ dysfunction syndrome; NO: nitric oxide)

CLASSIFICATION AND CAUSES

- *Hypovolemic and hemorrhagic:* Hypovolemia due to hemorrhage is the most common cause of shock in a trauma patient (hemorrhagic shock). It leads to decreased cardiac output leading to hypoperfusion of the tissues and cell death. "Nonhemorrhagic" hypovolemic shock is usually associated with massive gastrointestinal (GI) fluid or urinary losses leading to severe dehydration (as in diabetic ketoacidosis or diarrhea from cholera). Another form of nonhemorrhagic hypovolemia is caused by diversion of fluid into the extravascular compartments, commonly referred to as "third spacing", and this kind of shock is seen in patients with systemic inflammation, acute pancreatitis, hepatic failure, surgery, burns or intestinal obstruction.
- *Traumatic shock:* In trauma patient, acute blood loss or hypovolemia or direct tissue injury results in release of proinflammatory mediators which causes peripheral vasodilatation leading to global hypoperfusion.
- *Cardiogenic shock:* Cardiogenic shock is caused by decreased capacity of the heart to pump the blood leading to hypoperfusion. Common causes are acute myocardial infarction/ischemia, blunt trauma to the heart, refractory sustained tachyarrhythmias, postcardiac arrest, acute fulminant myocarditis, hypertrophic cardiomyopathy with severe outflow obstruction, pulmonary embolus, severe valvular heart disease, and aortic dissection with aortic insufficiency or tamponade and β-blocker or calcium-channel antagonist overdose. The hemodynamic picture includes sustained systemic hypotension (systolic blood pressure < 90 mm Hg or >30 mm Hg decrease from baseline for >30 minutes),

pulmonary capillary wedge pressure (PCWP) > 18 mm Hg and cardiac index < 2.2 L/min/m^2.

- *Vasogenic shock:* In trauma, acute phase reactions such as anaphylaxis, adrenal crisis, neurogenic shock or later events like sepsis leads to decrease in peripheral vascular resistance. When resistance becomes low enough, perfusion to the tissues fails leading to vasogenic shock.
    - *Septic shock:* It occurs if infection occurs in the trauma patient. Sepsis can be a response to any class of microorganism. It is usually the result of bacteremia, but it is not essential as a simple local infection can lead to multiorgan dysfunction and hypotension. In fact, blood cultures are positive in <20–40% of cases of severe sepsis and 40–70% of cases of septic shock. Primarily, the proinflammatory system of the body becomes systemic leading to profound vasodilation, capillary leak, and loss of intravascular volume. "Septic shock" is defined as severe sepsis with hypotension (systolic blood pressure < 90 mm Hg or a >40 mm Hg decrease from baseline) in spite of fluid resuscitation. Commonly found microbes causing sepsis are gram-negative organisms such as *Escherichia coli, Klebsiella, Proteus,* and *Pseudomonas* and less often can be due to gram-negative anaerobes (e.g., *Bacteroides*), but the incidence of sepsis from gram-positive bacteria (e.g., *Staphylococcus aureus*) and fungal organisms is increasing. Some terms loosely used in place of septic shock need proper definition and usage.

  "Bacteremia" is defined as the growth of bacteria from blood cultures. Sepsis and severe sepsis are defined in Chapter on "Systemic Inflammatory Response Syndrome and Multiorgan Dysfunction".
- *Neurogenic shock:* Following injury to cervical or upper thoracic spine, loss of sympathetic tone occurs which increases vascular capacitance and decreases cardiac output. The other causes include inadvertent cephalad migration of spinal anesthesia, or devastating head injury that result in interruption of sympathetic vasomotor input. However, only about 20% of patients with total high cord transection have neurogenic shock, and patients with incomplete motor or sensory deficits (or both) rarely have hypotension due to neurological causes. Neurogenic shock should be suspected in all hypotensive patients of trauma without any evidence of active hemorrhage.
- *Obstructive shock:* Following decreased venous return or direct cardiac compression due to cardiac tamponade or tension pneumothorax, heart filling decreases leading to decreased cardiac output and shock.

PATHOPHYSIOLOGY

The metabolic rates of brain and heart are high and they have low storage of energy substrate so these organs critically dependent on continuous supply of oxygen and nutrients. To maintain this homeostasis, body has complex physiological response which decreases blood supply to intestine and liver and maintains blood and oxygen supply to brain and heart.

- *Afferent signaling:* Baroreceptors of carotid bodies and aortic arch, volume receptors of atria and chemoreceptors that sense O_2 tension, CO_2, and pO_2, all sense the changes due to hypoperfusion and sent afferent signals to hypothalamic-pituitary-adrenal (HPA) axis-leading to release of vasopressin and autonomic nervous system (ANS) initiating compensatory mechanisms.
- *Cardiovascular:* Activation of ANS results in activation of $\alpha 1$ and $\beta 1$ receptors. Activation of $\alpha 1$ receptors results in vasocompression with selective shunting of blood to brain and heart. Activation of $\beta 1$ receptors causes increase in heart rate (HR) and cardiac output. The result of above cardiogenic mechanisms is twofold:
    - *Hypoperfusion:* It is essential for cellular viability to have adequate delivery and utilization of oxygen and the failure to deliver or utilize oxygen is the most important step in the pathogenesis of shock. Normally, systemic vascular resistance increases to compensate the decreased cardiac output in order to maintain the normal mean arterial pressure (MAP). Despite the near-normal blood pressure, however, the patient is in "cryptic shock" because of tissue hypoperfusion. The metabolic rates of brain and heart are high and they have low storage of energy substrate so these organs are critically dependent on continuous supply of oxygen and nutrients. Blood flow to these organs is carefully regulated and maintained over a wide range of blood pressures. Whereas in other organs, such as the intestine or liver, autoregulation is not as tightly maintained as heart or brain.
    - *Vasodilatation:* Hypoxic vascular endothelial cells activate white blood cells (WBCs), which bind to the endothelium inflammatory mediators [e.g., cytokines, leukotrienes, tumor necrosis factor (TNF)] and release directly damaging substances (e.g., reactive O_2 species). Some of these mediators bind to cell surface receptors and activate nuclear factor kappa B (NF$\kappa\beta$), which leads to production of additional cytokines and nitric oxide (NO), a potent vasodilator. Localized vasodilation increases vascular permeability and may shunt blood past the capillary exchange beds, causing focal hypoperfusion despite normal cardiac output and BP. Blood flow to microvessels including capillaries is reduced even though large-vessel blood flow is preserved in settings of septic shock in order to maintain blood flow to vital organs.
- *Neuroendocrine:* Several hormones are released in response to hypoperfusion. From adrenal medulla, epinephrine, and norepinephrine are released, which increase vasomotor tone. Renin-angiotensin-aldosterone system is activated and vasopressin is released from hypothalamus which increases water reabsorption from kidney. Cortisol and glucagon are released which increase catabolic rate at cellular level.
- *Cellular effects:* Amount of oxygen required by the tissues to avoid anaerobic metabolism is known as the oxygen demand. Normally, systemic oxygen delivery is sufficient to fulfill oxygen demand so that systemic oxygen

consumption is not altered by or dependent on changes in delivery. However, if systemic oxygen delivery drops below a critical value, it is maintained by a compensatory increase in oxygen extraction ratio, which maintains systemic oxygen consumption at an adequate level to meet systemic oxygen demands. When oxygen supply to the cells decreases to critical level, aerobic metabolism is switched to anaerobic one, with decreased production of adenosine triphosphate (ATP) and accumulation of lactate. With depletion of ATP supply, energy dependent mechanisms of the cell such as enzyme synthesis, DNA repair, and signal transduction fails. Na^+/K^+ ATPase fails and cellular swelling with subsequent lysis occurs due to water accumulation. Acidosis leads to changes in local microcirculation, and with activation of neutrophils, proinflammatory damage aggravates.

An oxygen delivery dependency also exists in patients with sepsis, trauma, and acute respiratory distress syndrome (ARDS) and after resuscitation from prolonged cardiac arrest. These patients have systemic oxygen delivery in the normal or elevated range but an impairment of oxygen utilization. This condition of tissue hypoxia is a result of ineffective distribution of blood flow or a defect in the utilization of substrate at the microcirculatory or subcellular level. This process is believed to be an important mechanism of cellular damage in various forms of shock.

SHOCK MANIFESTATIONS

The clinical findings of the patient with shock are primarily the result of hypoperfusion, body's attempt to compensate it, and on the initiating cause. The clinical features depend on the primary pathophysiology and combining the history, clinical picture, and hemodynamic measurements **(Table 1)** one can make the distinction among different types of shock syndromes. Hypotension is a very late sign of shock and patient with normal/near normal blood pressure may have profound hypoperfusion. Hypotension is defined as a systolic blood pressure (SBP) of ≤90 mm Hg or a mean arterial pressure of <60–65 mm Hg but must be evaluated relative to the patient's normal blood pressure. A drop in systolic pressure of >10–20 mm Hg or an increase in pulse of >15 beats/min with positional change suggests depleted intravascular volume. However, blood pressure is often not the best indicator of end-organ perfusion because compensatory mechanisms, such as increased HR, increased cardiac contractility, and vasoconstriction can occur to prevent hypotension. Patients with prolonged hypotension often develop involvement of multiple organs.

The signs of early shock must be thought and recognized as soon as possible to decrease the morbidity and mortality due to shock. On a first look examination of patient under shock, if shock is associated with peripheral vasoconstriction, then the extremities are cool and pale, which is typical of hypovolemic, cardiogenic, and obstructive shock, but with the peripheral vasodilation of septic and anaphylactic shock, they are typically warm and pink.

Clinical findings: Different forms of shock have different clinical findings detailed below:

- *Hypovolemic shock:* Hypovolemic shock produces the "classical" image of shock with cold peripheries, reduced or absent peripheral pulses, weak central pulses, and evidence of a low cardiac output. In early hemorrhagic shock, a narrowed pulse pressure, i.e., a raised diastolic blood pressure (DBP) and reduced SBP, such as 105/95 mm Hg, indicates the combination of hypovolemia (reduced stroke volume, hence SBP) and activation of the sympathetic nervous system, with noradrenaline (norepinephrine) inducing vasoconstriction and so raising the DBP. The clinical features of hemorrhagic shock entirely depend on amount of blood lost which has been classified by the American College of Surgeons **(Table 2)**.
    - *Class I:* Less than or equal to 15% of the blood volume loss (or ≤10 mL/kg). It is usually fully compensated by transcapillary refill. Clinical findings are minimal or absent.
    - *Class II:* About 15–30% of the blood volume loss (or 10–20 mL/kg). This represents the compensated phase of hypovolemia, where BP is maintained by systemic vasoconstriction. Postural changes in pulse rate and BP may be evident, but these findings are inconsistent, and the hypovolemia can be clinically silent.
    - *Class III:* Loss of 30–40% of the blood volume (or 20–30 mL/kg). This marks the onset of decompensated phase of hypovolemia, where the vasoconstrictor response is no longer able to sustain blood pressure and organ perfusion. The clinical consequences can include evidence of impaired organ perfusion (e.g., cool extremities, oliguria, and depressed consciousness), supine hypotension and evidence of anaerobic metabolism (i.e., lactate accumulation in blood).

TABLE 1: Hemodynamic characteristics of various forms of shock.

Type of shock	*CVP and PCWP*	*Cardiac output*	*Systemic vascular resistance*	*Venous O_2 saturation*
Hypovolemic	↓	↓	↑	↓
Cardiogenic	↑	↓	↑	↓
Septic (hyperdynamic)	↓↑	↑	↓	↑
Septic (hypodynamic)	↓↑	↓	↑	↓↑
Neurogenic	↓	↓	↓	↓

(CVP: central venous pressure; PCWP: pulmonary capillary wedge pressure)

TABLE 2: Classification of hemorrhagic shock (for a 70-kg patient).

Characteristic	*Class I*	*Class II*	*Class III*	*Class IV*
Blood loss (mL)	Up to 750	750–1,500	1,500–2,000	>2,000
% volume	Up to 15	15–30	30–40	>40
Pulse rate (per minute)	<100	>100	>120	>140
Blood pressure	Normal	Normal	Decreased	Decreased
Pulse pressure	Normal or increased	Decreased	Decreased	Decreased
Respiratory rate (per minute)	14–20	20–30	30–40	>35
Urine output (mL/h)	>30	20–30	5–15	Negligible
Mental status	Slightly anxious	Mildly anxious	Anxious and confused	Confused and lethargic
Fluid replacement	Crystalloid	Crystalloid	Crystalloid and blood	Crystalloid and blood

TABLE 3: Manifestations of cardiac involvement in shock.

General CVS	Neck vein distention (e.g., heart failure, pericardial tamponade) or flattening (e.g., hypovolemia), ischemia due to decreased coronary perfusion, decreased ventricular compliance and increased LV diastolic pressure
HR	Usually elevated. However, in case of pre-existing cardiac disease and severe hemorrhage paradoxical bradycardia can be seen. Heart rate variability is associated with poor outcomes
SBP	In early shock it may actually increase slightly when cardiac contractility increases and then fall as shock advances
DBP	Correlates with arteriolar vasoconstriction and sometimes rise early in shock, then fall when compensatory mechanism fails
Pulse pressure (SBP–DBP)	Related to stroke volume and the rigidity of the aorta. Increases early in shock and decreases before systolic pressure decreases
Mean arterial blood pressure	DBP + (pulse pressure/3)
Shock index (HR/SBP) normal = 0.5–0.7	A persistent value of shock index > 1.0 indicates impaired LV function which is associated with increased mortality

(CVS: cardiovascular system; DBP: diastolic blood pressure; HR: heart rate; LV: left ventricular; SBP: systolic blood pressure)

- *Class IV:* Loss of >40% of the blood volume (or >30 mL/kg). This degree of blood loss results in profound hypovolemic shock, which may be irreversible. Clinical manifestations include multiorgan failure and severe metabolic (lactic) acidosis. Perfusion of the CNS is well maintained until shock becomes severe. Hence, mental obtundation is an ominous clinical sign.

- *Cardiogenic shock:* Many of the clinically apparent manifestations of "cardiac involvement" in shock result from sympathetic and adrenal stimulation, with tachycardia being the most sensitive indicator that shock is present. Other features are presented in **Table 3**. The diagnosis of cardiogenic shock mainly clinical which includes hypotension combined with signs of poor tissue perfusion, including oliguria, altered sensorium, and cold extremities, all in the setting of myocardial dysfunction. To make the diagnosis, it is important to document myocardial dysfunction. In these patients, peripheral vasoconstriction, tachycardia/dysrhythmias and depressed mental status are present along with some new ECG changes like bundle block and T wave abnormalities. History of pre-existing cardiac disease or chest trauma is present. Chest X-ray should be obtained. Echocardiography is test of choice to confirm heart failure or other cardiac dysfunction.
- *Vasogenic shock:* There is hyperdynamic response with increased cardiac output and tachycardia. Vasodilatation leads to warm extremities, which are falsely thought of well-perfused one. The BP pattern is distinctive (e.g., 115/42 mm Hg), with a low DBP in the early stages due to peripheral vasodilatation, but a normal SBP, as the left ventricular (LV) afterload is reduced and stroke volume thus maintained. If sepsis occurs, fever and leukocytosis become evident but there is no specific diagnostic test to diagnose septic response. Common findings include—leukocytosis with a left shift (although leukopenia is also seen in case of severe sepsis), thrombocytopenia, hyperbilirubinemia, and proteinuria. The neutrophils may contain toxic granulations, Döhle bodies, or cytoplasmic vacuoles.
- *Neurogenic shock:* Similar to vasogenic shock, warm extremities and hypotension are present, but patients mainly have bradycardia and some motor or sensory deficits due to spinal injury are present. Interruption of sympathetic vasomotor input results in loss of sympathetic tone with a reduction in systemic vascular resistance and hypotension without a compensatory tachycardia. Sometimes reflex vagal parasympathetic stimulation evoked by pain, gastric dilation, or fright may produce hypotension, bradycardia, and syncope leading to neurogenic shock.
- *Obstructive shock:* It may occur due to tension pneumothorax or cardiac tamponade. In patients with tension pneumothorax, there will be tachycardia, hypotension, and cool extremities along with decreased or absent breath sound on affected side. Jugular venous distention and tracheal deviation are not reliable signs and they are late findings. In patients with cardiac tamponade, Beck's triad of hypotension, distended jugular veins, and muffled or distant heart sound is present, although one or more finding may absent.

It is acuity in the development of cardiac tamponade which is more important rather than volume of hemopericardium to decide degree of clinical derangement. Focused ultrasonography is the investigation of choice.

The general manifestations in addition to above are:

- *Neurologic manifestations:* Alteration in the level of consciousness with restlessness, agitation, confusion, lethargy or patient may even become comatose, although mentation may remain normal in some patients.
- *Respiratory manifestations:* Tachypnea, increased dead space, increased minute ventilation, bronchospasm, hypocapnia with progression to respiratory failure, acute lung injury, and finally adult respiratory distress syndrome (ARDS) which causes increased work of breathing, respiratory muscle fatigue, impaired gas exchange, and ventilatory failure.
- *Renal manifestations:* Oliguria, although polyuria may be seen in early shock. Paradoxical polyuria in sepsis may be confused with adequate hydration.
- *Gastrointestinal system related manifestations:* Abdominal pain, pancreatitis, acalculous cholecystitis, ileus, erosive gastritis, and submucosal hemorrhage. Bacteria and their toxins can reach into the bloodstream when the integrity of the gut barrier is compromised. The most common manifestation of liver involvement in shock is a mild increase in serum levels of aminotransferases and lactate dehydrogenase. Shock liver may manifest with massive aminotransferase elevations and extensive hepatocellular damage if there is severe and prolonged hypoperfusion.
- *Metabolic manifestations:* Respiratory alkalosis is the first acid-base abnormality, but metabolic acidosis occurs as shock progresses. Hyperglycemia, hypoglycemia, and hyperkalemia may variably develop.

MANAGEMENT

Assessment of Blood Volume

The importance of an accurate assessment of the intravascular volume is matched by the difficulties encountered and the clinical evaluation of intravascular volume is so flawed that it has been called a "comedy of errors".

- *Vital signs:* Increase in pulse rate, decrease in blood pressure, and sometimes bradycardia also occurs with acute blood loss. Supine tachycardia and hypotension are absent in patients with blood loss up to 25% (i.e., 1 liter).
- *Postural changes:* On moving from supine to standing, there is shift of 7 mL/kg blood to lower extremities causing increase in HR of 10 beats/min and fall in blood pressure of 4 mm Hg. Increase in pulse rate of 30 beats/min and fall in blood pressure of ≥20 mm Hg. It is sensitive and specific marker of moderate to severe acute blood loss. Sensitivity and specificity is up to 98% in severe acute blood loss.
- *Hematocrit:* Change in hematocrit shows a poor correlation with blood volume deficit and erythrocyte deficit in acute blood loss as it involves the loss of whole blood. An initial normal hematocrit does not disprove the presence of significant blood loss. In the absence of volume resuscitation, the activation of renin-angiotensin system leads to retention of sodium and water that follows will have dilutional effect on hematocrit. This change takes 8–12 hours to begin after acute blood loss.

Quantification of Hypoperfusion

- *Oxygen debt:* Its direct measurement is difficult, so other measures of hypoperfusion are necessary.
- *Lactate and base deficit:* Compared to cardiac output, blood pressure and volume loss, lactate levels (chemical marker of impaired tissue perfusion), and arterial base deficits are better indicators of oxygen debt and to decide therapy. Elevated serum lactate in setting of acute blood loss is presumptive evidence of hemorrhagic shock. Lactate level of >4 mM/L is usually life-threatening (normal up to 2 mM/L).

Management Proper

The injured patient with shock is assumed to have hypovolemic shock until proven otherwise.

- *Airway, breathing, and circulations (ABCs):* In initial approach, always look and correct ABCs and prevent hypothermia with adequate warming and warm intravenous (IV) fluids (discussed in detail in Chapter on "Polytrauma, Mass Casualties, and Disaster"). If severe metabolic acidosis is present in association with shock then ventilatory failure should be anticipated. Mechanical ventilation along with sedation can decrease the oxygen demand of the respiratory muscles and allow improved oxygen delivery to other hypoperfused tissues although sedatives might decrease the peripheral vascular resistance, cortisol levels and catecholamine levels, which can result in hypotension. Because the Trendelenburg position may impair gas exchange and promote aspiration, an alternative is to elevate the legs to 45° above the horizontal plane while in the supine position that will move 150–750 mL of blood out of the legs and toward the heart, thereby serving as a built in fluid challenge. Cardiac monitoring can detect myocardial ischemia or malignant arrhythmias, which can be treated by standard advanced cardiac life support (ACLS) protocols. Unresponsive or minimally responsive patients should have their glucose checked immediately and if their glucose level is low, 1 ampule of 50% dextrose intravenously should be given. An arterial line should be placed for continuous blood pressure measurement, and a Foley catheter should be inserted to monitor urinary output.
- *Hypovolemic and hemorrhagic shock:* Detailed discussion on resuscitation, its markers, and guidelines is provided in Chapter on "Polytrauma, Mass Casualties, and Disaster" under advanced trauma life support (ATLS), while role of vasopressors is detailed here.
    - *Role of vasopressors:* If the patient remains hypotensive even after administration of appropriate amount

of fluid, vasopressors such as norepinephrine, dopamine, should be administered to restore adequate systemic arterial pressure while the diagnostic evaluation is ongoing but only after blood volume has been restored. Increases in peripheral vasoconstriction with inadequate resuscitation leads to tissue loss and organ failure. However, vasopressors may also mask hypovolemia when they increase blood pressure.

- If the volume status cannot be defined or the hemodynamic condition requires repeated fluid challenges or vasopressor treatment, a central venous catheter should be placed to determine ventricular filling pressure, intravascular volume status, and central venous oxygen saturation.
- Based on these data, patients can usually be classified and managed according to their hemodynamic and oxygen transport patterns.
- These catheters had previously been used in critically ill patients to guide response to volume and vasopressor therapy, but data emerged suggesting that pulmonary artery catheters (PACs) increased mortality, prompting further studies. Thus, the routine use of PACs cannot be recommended. However, in some complex situations, PACs may be useful in distinguishing between cardiogenic and septic shock.

- *Cardiogenic shock:* As these patients have pretraumatic intrinsic heart disease, continuous cardiac monitoring is mandatory for these patients, which is efficiently done by invasive measures such as central venous and arterial line placement for adjusting volume status to a level that ensures optimum LV filling pressure. Even after fluid replacement, if hypotension persists, inotropic drugs like dobutamine should be started with a low threshold to do so. Aortic balloon pump is used in case of refractory shock. In case of vessel-based disease, coronary revascularization is useful. Cardiogenic shock is mainly treated by supportive measures until heart recovers from the insult. It is essential to distinguish between hypovolemic and cardiogenic shock because, while both may respond to volume initially, definitive therapy differs significantly. Both forms are associated with a compensatory sympathetic-mediated response characterized by tachycardia and elevated systemic vascular resistance and a reduced cardiac output. However, the findings in cardiogenic shock of jugular venous distention, rales, and an S_3 gallop help in distinguishing it from hypovolemic shock, signifying that ongoing volume expansion is undesirable and may cause further organ dysfunction.
- *Vasogenic shock:*
  - *Septic shock:* Septic shock is present in trauma patient in late cases or when infection is prevalent. The first step is to correct hypoperfusion by giving IV fluids typically beginning with 1–2 L of normal saline over 1–2 hours. To avoid pulmonary edema, the central venous pressure should be maintained at 8–12 cmH_2O. Vasopressors such as epinephrine and norepinephrine are used when hypotension persists after fluid resuscitation.
    - Underlying infection must be treated on prompt basis. Source of infection should be identified and treated accordingly whether medically or surgically. Thorough debridement is done and broad spectrum antibiotics are started. Pus should be drained and any devitalized tissues should be removed. Pus should be sent for culture and antibiotic sensitivity testing.
    - As soon as culture and sensitivity report become available, antibiotics should be changed to sensitive one. If no organisms are found, empiric antibiotic therapy should be stopped and close follow-up should be started.
    - Mechanical ventilation is required in majority of patients who have septic shock because acute lung injury is the most common complication. Lung-protective ventilation, as discussed in Chapter on "Acute Respiratory Distress Syndrome" should be followed.
    - Immunomodulatory therapy and use of protein C are under experiment at present in treatment of septic shock.
    - For a successful outcome, early goal directed therapy is recommended, these measures should be initiated within 1 hour of the patient's presentation with severe sepsis or septic shock (the physician should be prompt in diagnosing hence!).
  - *Neurogenic shock:* As common with other forms of shock, fluid resuscitation is the initial treatment of choice. Excessive volumes of fluid may be required to retain normal hemodynamic functions if given alone. In persistent hypotensive patients once hemorrhage has been ruled out, vasopressors (to augment vascular resistance) like adrenaline or phenylephrine may be used. The latter is preferred because of its pure alpha agonistic activity. Generally, patients recover well within 48 hours of the initial treatment.
- *Obstructive shock:* These patients present with rapidly deteriorating condition requiring emergent steps to save the patient. Tension pneumothorax should be treated promptly by needle thoracostomy and chest tube insertion. Cardiac tamponade may require thoracotomy in extreme conditions, but if the patient is stable, cardiac window should be made.

Endpoints of Resuscitation

When oxygen debt and acidosis are eliminated and aerobic metabolism restored, treatment of the shock becomes successful. But, it is difficult to measure when this has been achieved. Normalization of BP, HR, and urine output may occur in the face of ongoing hypoperfusion as measured by lactate levels or base deficit. Various methods to measure these parameters (along with some reference values) are:

- *Stabilized cardiac output:* Cardiac index above 3 L/min/m^2, mean arterial pressure higher than or equal to 65 mm Hg, urine output > 0.5 mL/kg/h, optimized right ventricular end-diastolic volume index (RVEDI—to above 90 mL/m^2 to a maximum of 138 mL/m^2).
- *Lactate and base deficit:* Serum lactate < 2 mM/L within 24 hours, minimizing base deficit to a value of 2–5 mmol/L. Higher serum lactate and higher base deficits predicts multiple organ dysfunction syndrome (MODS).
- *Restoration of aerobic metabolism:* Systemic O_2 consumption > 100 mL/min/m^2, mixed venous O_2 saturation > 70%.
- Tissue pH (7.3 ± 0.1)
- *Optimized oxygen delivery:* Systemic O_2 delivery > 500 mL/min/m^2, SaO_2 > 90%, Hb > 7–9 g/dL.
- *Gastric tonometry:* Measured by placing a special semipermeable balloon in the stomach inflated by CO_2 and continuously measuring intramucosal pH (pHi). The difference between intragastric pCO_2 and arterial pCO_2 (the pCO_2 gap) or pHi correlates with the degree of gastric ischemia.
- *Near-infrared spectroscopy:* It better measures the skeletal muscle oxyhemoglobin levels that correlate with hemorrhagic shock and response to resuscitation parameters noninvasively in terms of normalizing tissue oxygenation.
- *Restored hemostasis:* INR < 1.5, aPTT < 1.5 × control, platelet count > 50 × 10^9/L.

CONCLUSION

- Shock is a catastrophic situation where somehow the body is unable to maintain the circulatory system optimized threatening other vital body functions.
- The window of opportunity is quite small so systematic approach to identification of type of shock should be initiated urgently.
- Once identified one can better identify the cause of failure to maintain circulation and initiate appropriate corrective measures and save patient's life.
- Also important is not to over-resuscitate the patient and convert one catastrophe into another one by monitoring the patient continuously and following endpoints of resuscitation.

CHAPTER 32

Transfusion Medicine

Manish Kumar Varshney

INTRODUCTION

Blood transfusion is one of the important components in the management of patients with hemorrhage, polytrauma, severe anemia, thrombocytopenia, and coagulation disorders. Routine blood bank procedures, including ABO typing, antibody screening and compatibility testing, identify most patients at risk for serious immune-mediated red-cell transfusion reactions. It has improved the transfusion therapy and also has reduced the transfusion-related reaction. Red blood cell (RBC) antigen-antibodies study forms the basis of transfusion medicine. Antigens to a blood group are based on the structure and its composition; it may be made up of carbohydrate or protein, e.g., ABO blood groups are sugars **(Figs. 1 and 2)**, Rh blood groups are proteins.

BLOOD GROUP SYSTEMS

There are >250 antigens present on the RBC surface. In 1900, ABO was the first blood group antigens system discovered. ABO blood group is the most important blood group system in transfusion medicine. There are four principal types: A, B, AB, and O. There are two antigens and two antibodies that are mostly responsible for the ABO types. Gene for antigens A and B located on chromosome number 9 and expressed codominantly. Antigens A and B are attached to the precursor antigen called H antigen. O blood group is the antigen where both A and B antigen are absent but precursor antigen H is present. While individuals who inherit both A and B antigens are typed as AB.

Rarely, individuals lack precursor antigen H; these individuals are homozygous for "h" allele, i.e., hh. Blood group of these individuals is typed as "Bombay phenotype" (Oh) **(Figs. 1 and 2)**.

The AB antigens are of critical importance because individuals who lack the A and/or B antigens form immunoglobulin M (IgM) and immunoglobulin G (IgG) antibodies directed against the missing antigen(s). AB phenotype individuals are called as universal recipients because neither anti-A and anti-B isoagglutinin found in AB individuals, similarly O phenotype individuals called as universal donor as they have both anti-A and anti-B isoagglutinin **(Table 1)**.

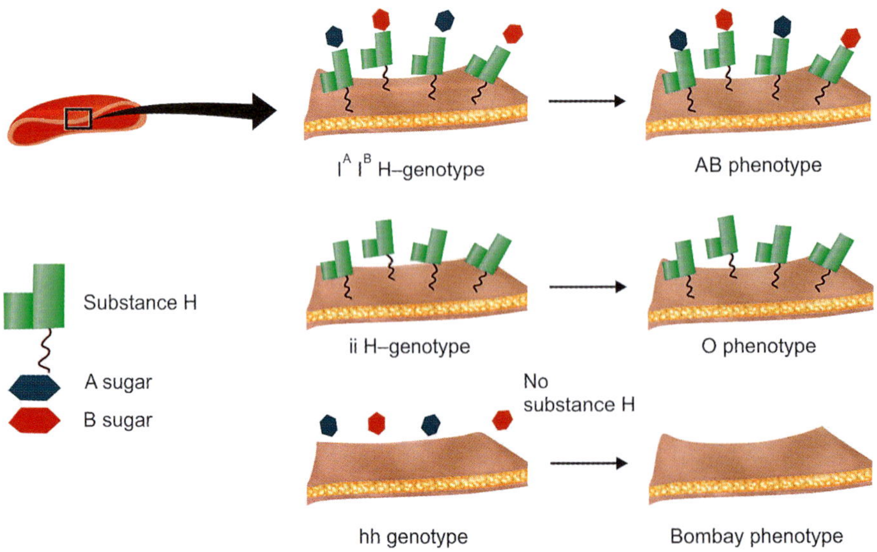

Fig. 1: The genesis of different ABO blood groups.

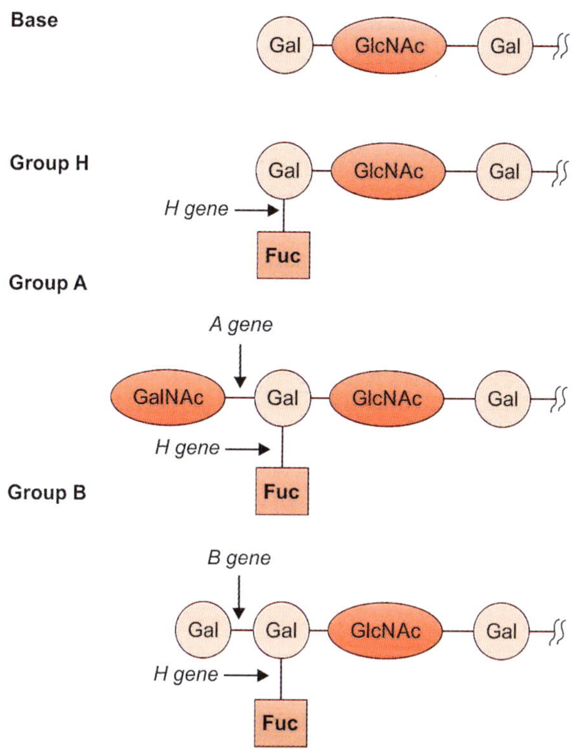

Fig. 2: The functioning and site action of *A, B,* and *H* gene.
(Gal: galactose; Fuc: fucose; GlcNAc: N-acetyl glucosamine; GalNAc: N-acetyl galactosamine)

TABLE 1: The ABO system—antigen and antibody distribution.

ABO blood type	Antigen A	Antigen B	Anti-A antibody	Anti-B antibody
A	Yes	No	No	Yes
B	No	Yes	Yes	No
O	No	No	Yes	Yes
AB	Yes	Yes	No	No

Rh System

It is one of the most complex blood grouping systems in human; it is the second most important blood group after ABO blood grouping in transfusion medicine. It has 49 antigens, out of them five (D, C, E, c, and e) are among the most significant. Rh-positive blood group contains D antigen on RBC while those who lack are Rh-negative blood group.

These five antigens are mainly responsible for majority type of Rh-related transfusion reaction and hemolytic disease of newborn (HDN).

Anti-D, anti-C, anti-E, and anti-e are involved in hemolytic transfusion reactions that are mostly of delayed type of hemolytic reactions. Nowadays because of increased use of pretransfusion typing for RhD status of donor and recipients, the incidence of transfusion reaction has significantly reduced due to this discrepancy. Typing for RhD status is quite not helpful for patients with sickle-cell anemia as these patients are likely to express variants of Rh e antigens rather than RhD antigens.

Hemolytic disease of the newborn: Rh-negative women most commonly produce anti-D following exposure to D-positive red cells during pregnancy, a miscarriage or abortion. The anti-D formed is of the IgG class and therefore can cross the placenta where it may cause a potentially fatal intrauterine HDN in a Rh-positive fetus.

DETECTION OF BLOOD GROUP ANTIBODIES

Antibody Screening and Antibody Identification

Prior to receiving a blood transfusion, patient's red cells are typed for ABO and Rh status using commercially available reagents.

- During *front typing or forward typing,* the donor's red cells are reacted with antibodies directed against the A, B and D antigens.
- Blood grouping is confirmed during *back typing* in which donor serum is tested for the presence of anti-A and anti-B antibodies.
- Cross-matching is used to make sure that the specific donor blood that will be used during a transfusion does not react with a patient's blood. It is basically a transfusion done in a test tube. The process may take 45 minutes to an hour and should be done ideally at least 3 days prior to the transfusion to be accurate. The tests are also used on pregnant women in order to prevent HDN.

It is also indicated when planning to transfuse packed RBC (PRBC). It is done to rule out minor antigens and to be done once major typing mismatch are ruled out (ABO incompatibility).

BLOOD AND BLOOD PRODUCTS

Blood can be separated into various major useful components **(Flowchart 1)**.

Other useful blood products are:

- *Single donor apheresis platelets (SDAP):* By apheresis technique, multiple units of platelets are collected from single donor. It is equivalent to six units of random donor (RD) platelets.
- Plasma-derived albumin, immunoglobulin and antithrombin coagulation factors—prepared from pooled plasma and treated for elimination of infectious agents.

CLINICAL USE OF BLOOD AND BLOOD COMPONENTS

By the slow centrifugation, whole blood is first separated into PRBCs and platelet-rich plasma. The platelet-rich plasma is then centrifuged at high speed to yield one unit of RD platelets and one unit of *fresh frozen plasma* (FFP). Cryoprecipitate is produced by thawing FFP to precipitate the plasma proteins, then separated by centrifugation **(Flowchart 1)**. The clinical use of various blood components has been summarized in **Table 2**.

Packed Red Blood Cells

It is indicated in acute hemorrhage and chronic anemia. RBC storage is done in solution containing citrate, dextrose, and phosphate buffers. Addition of adenine in storage solution increases the shelf-life of RBC by increasing the intracellular

Flowchart 1: The processing of blood and its blood components.

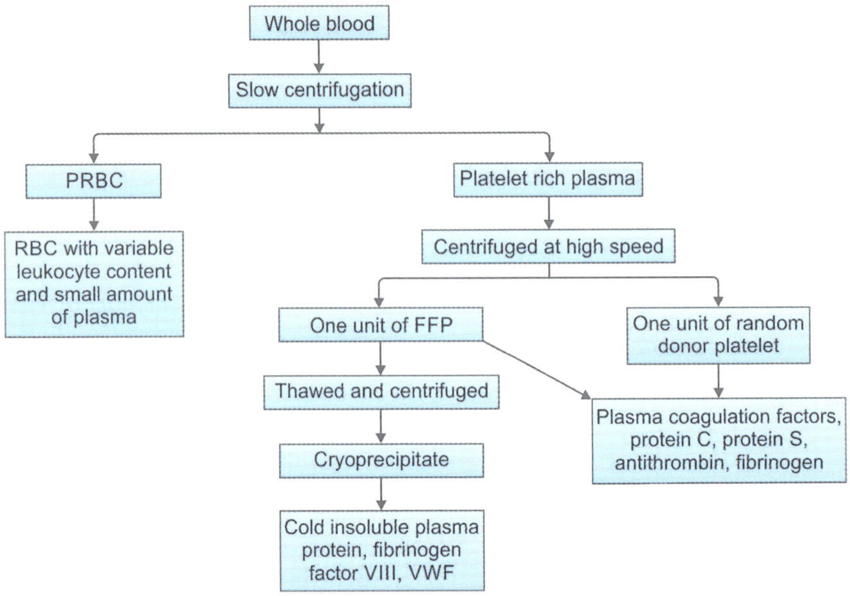

(FFP: fresh frozen plasma; PRBC: packed red blood cells; VWF: von Willebrand factor)

TABLE 2: Commonly used blood product.

Components	*Volume (mL)*	*Content*	*Clinical significance*
PRBC	180–200	RBC with variable content of WBC and platelets	Increase hemoglobin 10 g/L and hematocrit 3%
PCV with leukocyte-reduced components		Packed cell blood containing RBC and platelets without WBC	Symptomatic anemia, reduce febrile reactions from leukocyte antibodies, alternative to CMV seronegative components
Platelets	50–70	5.5×10^{10}/RD units	Increase platelet count 5,000–10,000/µL
	200–400	3.0×10^{11} SDAP units	CCI ≥ 10×10^9/L within 1 hour
FFP	200–250	Plasma proteins—coagulation factors, proteins C and S, antithrombin	Replacement of labile and stable plasma coagulation factors for which specific factor concentrates are not available, liver disease, DIC, hypofibrinogenemia, TTP
Cryoprecipitate	10–15	Fibrinogen, factor VIII, vWF	Fibrinogen and factor XIII replacement, factor VIII and vWF replacement, topical fibrin glue

(PRBC: packed red blood cell; FFP: fresh frozen plasma; RBC: red blood cell; WBC: white blood cell; DIC: disseminated intravascular coagulation; CMV: cytomegalovirus; TTP: thrombotic thrombocytopenic purpura; CCI: corrected count increment; RD: random donor; SDAP: single donor apheresis platelets)

adenosine triphosphate (ATP). Shelf-life varies from 35 to 42 days depending upon type of buffer used. During storage, the following changes are observed in red cell units:

- Fall in pH
- Decrease in red cell ATP and 2,3-diphosphoglycerate
- Increased supernatant potassium
- Decreased supernatant glucose

Decrease in 2,3-diphosphoglycerates leads to an increase in the oxygen affinity of the hemoglobin and a decreased capacity to deliver oxygen to the tissues, a problem with all red cell storage. Citrate contained in blood preservatives binds calcium to inhibit clotting and may cause hypocalcemia and alkalosis in neonates and massively transfused patients. Leukocytes can be removed from the product at the blood center collection site (prestorage leukodepletion), in the hospital blood bank prior to release, or at the patient's bedside using leukoreduction filters. Prestorage leukocyte reduction is better. Leukocyte-reduced PRBC contains white blood cells (WBC) < 5×10^6. Their use lowers the incidence of post-transfusion fever, cytomegalovirus (CMV) infections, and alloimmunization.

One unit of PRBC is 180–200 mL and it increases the hemoglobin (Hb) by 1 g/dL or hematocrit by 3% in the absence of active RBC destruction. Transfusion is rarely indicated when the Hb is >10 g/dL and is often not considered until the Hb is <7 g/dL. This also holds true for postoperative cases. The notion of better tissue healing at Hb levels ≥ 10 g/dL is not supported in literature for an otherwise normal patient without cardiovascular/pulmonary comorbidities. A patient's cardiac and pulmonary status must be considered when determining transfusion thresholds. Patients with coronary artery disease may require transfusion when the Hb is <10 g/dL. Similarly, various surgeons find it comfortable to maintain Hb above 10 g/dL in postoperative period for better wound healing, however, there is no rationale and it has been found that at Hb of 7 or more there is no difference in wound healing unless there are other comorbidities. It may be prudent to maintain higher Hb (>10) in patients with chronic obstructive pulmonary disease (COPD) and cardiac disease to maintain higher oxygen carrying capacity but this needs to be determined in large dedicated studies.

Platelets

Threshold for prophylactic platelet transfusion is platelet count < 10,000/μL, in case of sepsis < 5,000/μL while for invasive procedure it is <50,000/μL.

Each unit of RD platelets (volume 50–70 mL) contains at least 5.5×10^{10} platelets/RD. And two units of RD/m^2 increases platelet levels by 5,000–10,000/μL. Single donor apheresis platelets typical volume 200–400 mL contains ≥3×10^{11}/SDAP unit.

Platelets stored at 20–24°C in plastic containers have shelf life of 5 days. Whenever possible, ABO type specific platelets transfusion should be done but it is not necessary because uncross-matched platelets provide 10–20% less increment than expected increase in platelet. Rh-positive platelet concentrate may be given to Rh-negative patients with administration of Rh immune globulin within 72 hours of transfusion.

Platelet Refractoriness

It is a major problem in patients who require multiple platelets transfusion. It is evaluated by corrected count increment (CCI). The CCI is calculated as follows:

$$\text{CCI} = [\text{Post-transfusion count (per } \mu\text{L)} - \text{Pretransfusion count (per } \mu\text{L)}]/(\text{Number of platelet transfused} \times 10^{11}) \times \text{BSA } (m^2)$$

Suboptimal response is considered when platelet count after 1 hour is <10×10^9/mL or increase is <7.5×10^9/mL after 18–24 hours. Likely causes of suboptimal response in most of the patients are multiple transfusion and formation of antibodies against the class I human leukocyte antigens (HLA). So in this case, ABO identical and HLA-matched SDAP will provide good response (crossed matched platelets). Other causes of a platelet refractory state include disseminated intravascular coagulation (DIC), sepsis, and circulating immune complexes.

Fresh Frozen Plasma

Fresh frozen plasma contains stable coagulation factors, plasma proteins, albumin, fibrinogen, and antithrombin. FFP should not be transfused for volume expansion because of the risk of transfusion-transmitted disease and the availability of other, safer nonplasma substitutes. The primary indications for FFP transfusion include deficiency of multiple coagulation factors as seen in liver disease, DIC, reversal of warfarin toxicity [prefer prothrombin complex concentrate (PCC) as this is the standard (*see* Chapter on "Venous Thromboembolism Prophylaxis and Treatment"], thrombotic thrombocytopenic purpura (TTP). It does not transmit the intracellular infection like CMV as it is acellular component. Immunoglobulin A (IgA) deficient patients should get FFP from the IgA deficient donor. Typical volume of FFP is 200–250 mL and it increases the coagulation factors by 2%.

Cryoprecipitate

Cryoprecipitate is prepared by thawing FFP between 1°C and 6°C from FFP. Each 10–20 mL unit contains 100–350 mg fibrinogen/unit, at least 80 IU/unit factor VIII and some von Willebrand's factor.

- Use of cryoprecipitate is generally reserved for patients with von Willebrand's disease (types 1 and 2) or those with severe hypofibrinogenemia (<100 mg/dL).
- Cryoprecipitate and thrombin are combined to make fibrin glue. This biological sealant works well but exposes the recipient to the risks of transfusion-transmitted disease due to the use of cryoprecipitate.

Albumin

Available as a 5% or 25% solution and is used to treat hypovolemia and hypoalbuminemia, primarily in surgical settings. Properly processed albumin is not considered to transmit viral disease.

Intravenous Immunoglobulin

It is used to treat patients with immune thrombocytopenia (ITP), Guillain-Barré syndrome, and autoimmune hemolytic anemia.

ADVERSE REACTIONS TO BLOOD TRANSFUSION

There are three types of blood transfusion-related reactions:

1. Immune-mediated reactions are often due to preformed donor or recipient antibody; however, cellular elements may also cause adverse effects.
2. Nonimmune causes of reactions are due to the chemical and physical properties of the stored blood component and its additives. Transfusion-transmitted viral infections are increasingly rare due to improved screening and testing.
3. *Infections:* It includes viral infections such as hepatitis C virus (HCV), human immunodeficiency virus type 1 (HIV-1), hepatitis B virus (HBV), and parvovirus. Bacterial infections such as *Yersinia*, *Pseudomonas*, *Serratia*, etc.

The various immunological and nonimmunological reactions are summarized in **Table 3**.

Immune-mediated Transfusion Reactions

Acute hemolytic transfusion reactions: Incidence 1:12,000 units of transfusions. Recipients have preformed antibodies to donor RBC antigens. Mainly these ABO isoagglutinins and only rarely Rh, Duffy and Kell antibodies are also involved.

- *Clinical features:* Hypotension, sudden onset back pain, fever with chills, diaphoresis, and dyspnea; chest pain may occur.
- Laboratory results may show unconjugated hyperbilirubinemia, increased lactate dehydrogenase (LDH) and decreased haptoglobin. Sometime patients may develop DIC.

Treatment

Maintain airway. Stop blood transfusions → Maintain intravenous (IV) line → Inform blood bank → Label the

TABLE 3: Various immunological and nonimmunological reactions of blood transfusions.

Immune complications	*Nonimmune complications*
Acute hemolytic transfusion reactions	Transfusion-associated bacterial sepsis
Delayed extravascular hemolytic reaction	Circulatory overload, cardiac failure
Febrile transfusion reaction	Viral transmission (hepatitis A, B, C, cytomegalovirus, and parvovirus)
Allergic transfusion reaction (urticaria and anaphylaxis)	Iron overload
Transfusion-associated sepsis	Hypocalcemia
Alloimmunization	Hypothermia
Transfusion-associated graft-versus-host disease	Dilutional coagulopathy due to factor depletion, thrombocytopenia
Transfusion-associated acute lung injury	

post-transfused blood sample and untransfused blood → Send back to blood bank for repeat typing, direct antiglobulin typing, direct Coombs test, and other clerical work. Lysis of RBC may result in renal damage, so diuretics (furosemide) and mannitol may be given. Monitor prothrombin time (PT) and activated partial thromboplastin time (aPTT), as patient may develop DIC.

Febrile Nonhemolytic Reactions

It is the most common transfusion-associated reaction. Incidence is 1–4 per 100 transfusions. There are antibodies that cross-react with donor's leukocyte and HLA antigens. Risk factors for febrile nonhemolytic transfusion reactions (FNHTR) include multiparous women, multiple transfusions.

Clinical Features

- Fever with chills and rigors
- Other cause of fever with chills must be ruled out.

Treatment

Prestorage leukocyte reduced blood product. Supportive measures include corticosteroids, premedication with acetaminophen and intramuscular or subcutaneous meperidine for rigors.

Transfusion-related Acute Lung Injury

It is the most common cause of transfusion-related mortality.

Clinical Features

- Dyspnea, tachycardia, cyanosis and hypotension
- Hypoxemia, i.e., $PaO_2/FiO_2 < 300$
- Patients may develop noncardiogenic pulmonary edema during or within 6 hours of transfusion.

Mechanism

Donor plasma containing high titer of anti-HLA class II antibodies binds with the recipient's WBC causing clumping of WBC in pulmonary vessels leading to cytokine release, increased capillary permeability, and development of pulmonary edema.

Risk Factors

Multiparous female donor, smoker, alcoholic, shock, and mechanical ventilation with positive pressure ventilation >30 cm of water.

Diagnosis

Laboratory testing of donor plasma for HLA antibodies and/or granulocyte antibodies in either donor or recipient serum and corresponding antigens on recipients or donor leukocytes.

Treatment

- Supportive care and treatment of noncardiogenic pulmonary edema with ventilator support and oxygen
- Leukoreduced blood product, corticosteroid, and diuretics

Anaphylactic Reactions

It presents with severe reaction just after starting of blood transfusion (milliliters of blood product) exposure.

Clinically, patient presents with breathing difficulty, coughing, hypotension, bronchospasm, loss of consciousness, respiratory arrest, and shock.

Risk Factors

Immunoglobulin A deficient individuals.

Treatment

- Stop transfusion, maintain IV line, 0.5–1 mL of epinephrine (1:1,000 dilution) subcutaneous epinephrine
- IgA deficient plasma for IgA-deficient patients

Graft-versus-Host Disease

- It is caused by donor T-lymphocytes that recognize the host HLA antigen as foreign and mount the immune reaction causing the cutaneous eruption, fever, diarrhea, and abnormal liver function test. It manifests 8–10 days after transfusion and death occurs at 3–4 weeks after transfusion. In case of immune-deficient recipients, it causes bone marrow aplasia and pancytopenia.
- Treatment resistant to immunosuppressive therapy
- Prevented by irradiation of cellular component of donor blood

Septic Reactions

- It is seen highest with platelets transfusion as it is stored at room temperature.
- *Staphylococcus, Enterobacter,* and *Pseudomonas* are the common bacteria implicated.
- Management includes obtaining the blood culture, and sensitivity treatment includes initial broad-spectrum antibiotics and then sensitivity directed antibiotics, fluids, and cardiopulmonary support.

NONIMMUNOLOGIC REACTIONS

Hypothermia

It occurs when refrigerated blood product (4°C) is transfused soon after removed from refrigerator. Hypothermia can result in cardiac dysrhythmias due to exposure of sinoatrial (SA) node to cold fluid.

Prevention

- Keep blood product at room temperature for adequate time.
- Transfusion rate in adults 5 mL/min or less so that transfused cold blood gets completely mixed with patient's body temperature blood.

Electrolyte Disturbance

This occurs during massive blood transfusion; it is a concern of pediatrics and neonates. It is associated with increased level of potassium, ammonia, hypocalcemia (citrate is used as anticoagulant), and acidosis.

Hypocalcemia may manifest as tingling, numbness, and circumoral numbness.

Fluid Overload/Circulatory Overload

- It was seen when whole blood was used and is concern in patients with compromised cardiac reserve and massive blood due to trauma. Nowadays removal of plasma from the whole blood has reduced the risk until and unless massive blood transfusion is required.
- Prevention involves monitoring the volume and rate of transfusion.
- Use of diuretics simultaneously also reduces the risk.

Iron Overload

This is seen mainly in patients of thalassemia and to less extent in sickle cell anemia patients, where chronic blood transfusion is required. 200–250 mg of iron is present in each unit of RBC. These patients develop iatrogenic hemochromatosis. Treatment is deferoxamine and deferasirox. Use of erythropoietin is alternative of blood transfusion in such cases at high risk of iron overload.

Infections

Even after major improvements in blood safety during the past >20 years, there still remains a relatively small risk of transfusion-transmitted disease.

The use of volunteer donors and predonation screening questionnaires, advent of enzyme immunoassays in the 1970s, and more recent nucleotide testing nucleic acid test (NAT) have decreased the risk of transfusion-transmitted diseases. Pretransfusion testing typically includes screening for HBV, HCV, HIV-1 and 2, human T-cell lymphotropic virus, and syphilis. NAT testing is expected to reduce the transfusion-related HCV by decreasing the window period from approximately 60–80 to 10–20 days. Other pathogens, such as CMV and parvovirus B19, are common in the general donor population and may pose a serious threat in immunocompromised patients. More than 50% of the general population is exposed to CMV and is transmitted by the infected WBCs found in transfused PRBCs or platelet components. Malaria, Chagas disease, leishmaniasis, babesiosis, toxoplasmosis, and Lyme disease are the major parasitic diseases that are either known or are suspected to be transmitted by transfusion.

ALTERNATIVES TO BLOOD COMPONENT THERAPY

Autologous Transfusion

It is collection of patients own blood cells. In an attempt to reduce the incidence of allogenic blood transfusion reactions various ways have been determined to use patient's own blood. Preoperative blood donation can be utilized in elderly patients, although there is higher risk of iatrogenic preoperative anemia and more serious cardiovascular complication. However, it decreases risk of viral infections; the risk of bacterial contamination still remains.

There are four methods of autologous transfusion:

1. *Intraoperative cell salvage (ICS; **Fig. 3**):* Blood is collected from suction, surgical drains, or both and retransfused back to the patient after filtration or washing. The common indications for use of ICS are summarized in **Table 4** for various faculties.
2. *Preoperative autologous donation (PAD):* Blood is collected in advance of an elective procedure, stored in the blood bank, and transfused back to the patient when required. Some have used erythropoietin to increase the hemoglobin preoperatively to improve the yield.
3. *Acute normovolemic hemodilution (ANH):* Blood is collected immediately prior to surgery and blood volume restored by crystalloid or colloid. The blood is then retransfused toward the end of surgery once hemostasis is achieved. It is mainly used in cardiac bypass surgery.
4. *Postoperative cell salvage (PCS):* It is a rarely used system and not recommended except in rarest of circumstances. Here, the blood from wound drains of total hip arthroplasty or total knee arthroplasty is filtered or processed in an automated system, then reinfused to patient.

Indications of Autologous Blood Transfusion

- Major elective orthopedic surgery, cardiovascular surgery, obstetrics surgery, and gastrointestinal surgery.
- When anticipated, blood loss is >20% in any surgery.
- Blood collected in abdominal cavity due to organ rupture or during surgery.
- Jehovah's witness who is not willing to accept allogeneic blood.

The British Committee for Standards in Hematology (BCSH) gives a comprehensive and practical recommendation for use of autologous blood transfusion in exceptional circumstances as follows:

- Patients having either rare blood group or having multiple blood group antibodies where compatible allogeneic (donor) blood is not available or very difficult to obtain—use PAD.

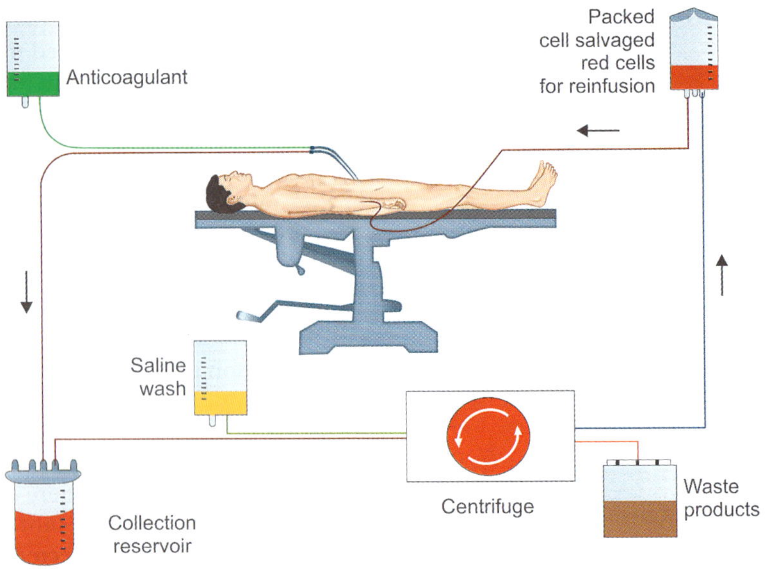

Fig. 3: Intraoperative cell salvage and transfusion system. Salvaged blood is collected separately and is then centrifuged and washed to produce red blood cells (RBC) suspended in normal saline (NS) for reinfusion to the patient. The discarded products (plasma, platelets, anticoagulant, etc.) are removed during processing.

TABLE 4: Common surgical indications for use of intraoperative cell salvage (ICS).

Surgical faculty	*Surgical procedure*
Orthopedic surgery	• Extensive spine surgery like osteotomies or combined instrumentation for large scoliotic curve correction • Simultaneous or concurrent bilateral knee replacement • Revision arthroplasty of hip • Excision of large tumors say from pelvis extensive acetabular surgery needing combined anterior and posterior pelvic fixation
Cardiac	• Valvular replacement • Revision bypass grafting
Urology	• Radical retropubic prostatectomy • Cystectomy • Nephrectomy
Liver transplant	
Vascular	• Thoracoabdominal aortic aneurysm repair • Abdominal aortic aneurysm repair

- Psychiatric patient with serious risk of acute precipitation of psychological attack because of anxiety about exposure to donor blood—use PAD
- Patients refusing to give consent for donor transfusion —PAD
- Children undergoing scoliosis surgery—use PAD
- Surgery where anticipated blood loss >20% of patients estimated blood volume **(Table 4)**—use ICS
- Elective or emergency surgery in patients with risk factors for bleeding (high-risk cesarean section)—use ICS
- Major hemorrhage—ICS
- *Jehovah's witnesses:* The patient is unwilling to accept allogeneic blood but will give consent to receive blood from intraoperative blood salvage—use PAD for elective surgeries/ICS in case of emergency).

Advantages of Autologous Transfusion especially the Intraoperative Blood Salvage

- The patient's own fresh RBCs are reinfused and have higher levels of 2,3-diphosphoglycerate than allogeneic blood. These become immediately active and have no lag period for oxygen carrying capacity compared to allogeneic transfusion.
- Readily supplies blood in proportion to the losses that are occurring.
- Reduces exposure to allogeneic transfusion and hence reduces transfusion-associated risks.
- There is no error like "wrong type" of blood transfused.
- Acceptable to patients who otherwise refuse allogeneic transfusion.

Contraindications to Autologous Blood Transfusion

- Use of substances in the surgical field that is not licensed for IV use:
  - Iodine, antibiotics not licensed for IV use, topical clotting agents (likely to cause derangement in coagulation system)
  - Orthopedic surgeries using polymethyl methacrylate (PMMA) cement wherc some solvent may be temporarily released.
  - Irrigation solutions that are difficult to separate or causing direct damage to the blood/components (alcohol, bleach, hydrogen peroxide, and hypertonic/hypotonic solutions).
  - Use of solutions incompatible with action of citrate-based anticoagulants acid-citrate-dextrose (ACD) like lactated Ringer's.
  - Extensive bone reaming fragments that contaminate the blood indiscriminately.

- Aspiration of body fluids and potentially contaminated fluids into the wound site:
    - Gastric or pancreatic secretions
    - Pleural effusions
    - Urine
    - Fat
    - Bowel contents
    - Amniotic fluid
    - Malignancy
    - Catecholamines (pheochromocytoma)
- Unknown significance:
    - Thalassemia
    - Sickle cell disease
- Cautions to ICS use:
    - Do not combine the ACD and leukocyte depletion filters (LDF) as incidence of hypotension has been reported though the cause is unclear.
    - In instances of heparin-induced thrombocytopenia, heparin should not be used as anticoagulant.

BLOOD SUBSTITUTES

Red cell substitutes currently in development include hemoglobin-based oxygen carriers (HBOCs), perfluorocarbon emulsions (PFCs), and liposome-encapsulated hemoglobin. The two major types of blood substitutes, HBOCs and PFCs, are in phase II and III clinical trials. HBOCs though targeting oxygen delivery may interfere with other functions causing system imbalance and producing unwanted reactions. PFCs use in the future is based on the concept of augmented acute normovolemic hemodilution that is useful in augmenting tissue oxygen delivery where low endogenous hemoglobin levels are expected during surgery. Other uses for PFCs are in potential treatment of diseases with compromised tissue oxygenation as in cerebral/myocardial ischemia, emergency trauma surgery till allogeneic blood is awaited, air embolism, etc. Hematopoietic growth factors used in transfusion therapy are designed to limit the exposure of patients to allogeneic blood. Recombinant erythropoietin is one of the most important advances in decreasing red cell transfusions. Use of recombinant erythropoietin has dramatically reduced the transfusion needs of patients with renal failure and various anemias. Granulocyte colony-stimulating factor (G-CSF) has been shown to decrease infection rates in neutropenic patients undergoing chemotherapy, replacing marginally effective granulocyte transfusions. Thrombopoietin (TPO), a natural physiologic regulator of platelet production, has been used for improving platelet count. It works on megakaryocyte precursor cells activating antiapoptotic and cell maturation pathways. "First-generation" recombinant TPOs were found to increase platelet count in patients undergoing nonmyeloablative chemotherapy for immune thrombocytopenic purpura (ITP) and myelodysplasia. "Second-generation" TPO romiplostim (injectable peptide TPO) and eltrombopag (oral nonpeptide TPO) are now the United States Food and Drug Administration (US FDA) approved for the second-line treatment of patients with ITP. Adverse events have been few but long-term assessment for reticulin formation and development of thromboembolism is still evaluated in various researches.

CONCLUSION

- Blood transfusion is a common requirement in surgical and medical fields.
- It is an important science that should be utilized rationally and for proper indications.
- There are quite frequent instances of overutilization of the blood products that are commonly advised irrationally especially the use of packed RBC for increasing the patient's hemoglobin levels pre- and/or postoperatively. Uniform policy should be formulated to this end in every hospital so that the use of blood products is rationalized.
- To this end every hospital must have dedicated blood bank and a transfusion medicine specialist, who can vouch for the rationale use, development of hospital policy, and for time-to-time audit.
- Transfusion is fraught with frequent complications and can also be life-threatening so must be prescribed in definite indications only and under proper care. One must be aware of various immunological or nonimmunological reactions so that healthcare providers can identify them fast and render proper care.
- Surgeries that are expected to have large intraoperative blood loss must utilize organized and standardized cell saver systems to reduce load on blood banks that can better serve to provide blood products for emergency care.
- Blood substitutes have a definite role in special conditions like Jehovah's witnesses.

CHAPTER 33

Complex Regional Pain Syndrome

Manish Kumar Varshney, Mohinder Singh Chib

INTRODUCTION

Complex regional pain syndrome (CRPS) is a syndrome of regional pain where pain is usually disproportionate to the precipitating event in both duration and intensity and is associated with vasomotor changes, trophic, and skin changes, regional osteoporosis and functiolesia (functional impairment). CRPS may occur with or without injury, and severity of trauma has no relationship with occurrence of CRPS. Upper limbs are most commonly affected. It usually occurs in one limb but may sometimes involve the other limb. Rarely, pain may also spread from upper limb to lower limb and vice versa. CRPS is a multifactorial disorder clinically manifesting with:

- Neurogenic inflammation
- Changed nociceptive mechanism (abnormal response to sensations like hyperalgesia or allodynia)
- Abnormal vasomotor response
- Neuroplasticity [caused by an aberrant response of peripheral and central nervous system (CNS) to tissue injury].

About 30% of patients with limb trauma suffer from CRPS. It is either due to the abnormal response of pain receptors to catecholamine (neuronal messengers) in the affected part of the body or to the deregulation of the CNS and autonomic nervous system. Although a genetic predisposition is unknown but there is increased prevalence of *HLA-DQ1* in patients. Usually adults are affected but it may also be seen in children.

DEFINITION

According to the International Association for Study of Pain (IASP), CRPS describes an array of painful conditions that are characterized by a continuing (spontaneous and/or evoked) regional pain that is seemingly disproportionate in time or degree to the usual course of any known trauma or other lesion. The pain is regional (not in a specific nerve territory or dermatome) and usually has a distal predominance of abnormal sensory, motor, sudomotor, vasomotor, and/or trophic findings, including osteoporosis. The syndrome shows variable progression over time.

The term "CRPS" has a specific relevance and each word describes an aspect of the disease:

- *Complex:* Variable clinical presentation
- *Regional:* Symptoms affect particular region
- *Pain:* Disproportionate to the severity of injury
- *Syndrome:* A cluster of symptoms and signs

HISTORY AND NOMENCLATURE

Silas Weir Mitchell (founding father of American neurology) with Morehouse and Keen observed a chronic pain syndrome in soldiers who suffered traumatic nerve injuries during the American Civil War (1864) and first time used the term "causalgia" to describe it, which is derived from two Greek words "kausis" (heat) and "algos" (pain). This condition was also known as *reflex sympathetic dystrophy* (RSD) due to the hypothesis that sympathetic hyperactivity might be the cause of this condition. The name "complex regional pain syndrome" along with causalgia and RSD as its subtypes was given in a special consensus workshop held at Orlando, Florida in 1993.

Alternative Terms for Complex Regional Pain Syndrome

- Reflex sympathetic dystrophy—introduced by Evans in 1946 and promoted by John Bonica, the founder of IASP
- Causalgia
- Sudeck's atrophy (this term applies to the radiological appearance of osteoporosis)
- Reflex neurovascular dystrophy (RND)
- Amplified musculoskeletal pain syndrome
- Algoneurodystrophy
- Minor causalgia
- Mimo-causalgia
- Algodystrophy
- Post-traumatic pain syndrome
- Painful post-traumatic dystrophy
- Painful post-traumatic osteoporosis
- Transient migratory osteoporosis
- Shoulder–hand syndrome
- Sympathetically maintained pain

EPIDEMIOLOGY

The incidence of CRPS in India is unclear. Incidence of CRPS is 26 per 100,000 person-years in Europe, 5.5 cases per 100,000 persons/years in the United States of America and 2 per 100,000 person/years in the Netherlands. Most common in people aged 9–85 years, dominantly affecting the persons toward the median. Cases occur even in children. Incidence of CRPS possibly increases with age. Females are affected more than males with ratio of 3.5:1 and the age group 60–70 years is the most susceptible, in children the ratio broadens to 9:1. The arm is affected in about 60% of cases and the leg in about 40% (lower limbs are more commonly affected in children). The disease resolves spontaneously in 74% cases in the first year and 23–36% within 6 years of treatment. This data may be inconsistent due to heterogeneous study population and nonuniform diagnostic criteria.

TYPES OF COMPLEX REGIONAL PAIN SYNDROME

Basically, it was divided into two types based on the presence of nerve lesion; now, a third group has been included where CRPS criteria are partially fulfilled.

1. *Type I:* When there is no evidence of nerve injury. RSD, Sudeck's atrophy, RND or algoneurodystrophy all come under this category.
2. *Type II (causalgia):* When there is obvious nerve damage (partial or complete). The differences between type I and II are summarized in **Table 1**.
3. *Complex regional pain syndrome-NOS (not otherwise specified):* When the criteria for CRPS are partially met and the condition (sign and symptoms) cannot be explained by any other disease.

Patterns of Spread

It has been observed that CRPS (type I) can spread from the initial site of presentation to other area or limb. The risk of spread is increased with the number of limbs affected. If multiple limbs are affected, spread occurs on the same side of limbs (ipsilateral) or opposite side (contralateral). Diagonal spread (one upper limb to contralateral lower limb and vice versa) is rare however. Chance of spread is more in younger age group and more severely affected phenotype. Interestingly, single photon emission computed tomography (SPECT) in patients with CRPS has shown involvement of contralateral thalamus and the perfusion first increases then decreases over time, explaining the adaptive changes in CNS and features:

- *Contiguous spread:* Gradual increase within the affected area.
- *Independent spread:* CRPS appears in distant areas.
- *Mirror-image spread:* Symptoms appear on opposite side in an area that is almost similar in location of original side.
- *Diagonal spread (not well accepted):* Symptoms appear on diagonally opposite region that closely matches size and location of original side.

TABLE 1: The differences in type I and type II complex regional pain syndrome (CRPS).

CRPS I	*CRPS II*
Older name—reflex sympathetic dystrophy (RSD)	Older name—causalgia
Circumferential, nondermatomal/ myotomal distribution	Follows discrete nerve distribution
Good response to sympathetic blocks	Variable response
No response to nerve blocks	Responds well to nerve blocks
Both mechanical and thermal allodynia	Mechanical allodynia

PATHOPHYSIOLOGY

Some individuals are more susceptible than others to develop CRPS. The definitive factors responsible for the occurrence and final course of CRPS are not known; however, history of asthma, migraine, and angiotensin-converting enzyme (ACE) inhibitors group of antihypertensive drugs which increase the availability of substance P and bradykinin have been identified as risk factors for CRPS. Everolimus has been associated with CRPS and adenosine is associated with recurrence of disease in studies. There is evidence that supraspinal mechanisms are involved in the pathophysiology of CRPS. After injury, activated cutaneous nociceptors induce retrograde depolarization of small-diameter primary afferents through axon reflex. This causes the release of neuropeptides such as substance P and calcitonin-gene-related peptide (CGRP) from sensory terminals in the skin. These neuropeptides are primarily responsible for CRPS. Few hypotheses have been proposed to elaborate understanding, viz.:

- Induced neurogenic inflammation
- Autonomic dysfunction
- Neuroplasticity within CNS

Induced Neurogenic Inflammation (The Inflammatory Theory of Complex Regional Pain Syndrome)

Classical signs of inflammation are present in CRPS, i.e., pain, swelling, erythema, hyperthermia, and impaired function. The neurogenic inflammation is facilitated by a special group of C-fibers called "mechanoheat insensitive C-fibers". The afferent C-fibers mediate pain and itch, and the efferents have a neurosecretory function releasing neuropeptides via "axon reflex". The action potentials generated in these fibers can be conducted retrograde to terminal branches via axon collaterals. Substance P leads to extravasation of plasma protein and osteoclastic activity.

Autonomic Dysfunction (The Autonomic Dysfunction Theory of Complex Regional Pain Syndrome)

The adrenergic receptor sensitivity (mainly alpha-2 receptors) developed due to pathological sympathoafferent coupling of peripheral nociceptors leads to tonic sympathetic efferent activity on their activation. Painful impulses maintain the CNS in sensitized state via these nociceptors and result in hyperalgesia and allodynia to painful and nonpainful stimuli, respectively. However, it is seen that catecholamine levels are actually lower in the affected extremity; thus, it is not a problem of excessive sympathetic nerve output. The traditional use of selective sympatholytic blocks (e.g., stellate ganglion or lumbar sympathetic block) for pain and symptom relief in CRPS patients was based on assumption that autonomic features of CRPS were the result of excessive sympathetic nervous system (SNS) outflow and the pain in CRPS was sympathetically maintained. Vasoconstriction to cold challenge is absent in patients with acute CRPS (warm CRPS), but it is exaggerated in patients with chronic CRPS (cold CRPS). Although there is no evidence to support the traditional three sequential stages of CRPS, a transition from a warm, red CRPS presentation to a cold, bluish CRPS presentation is common as CRPS moves from the acute to the chronic state.

Neuroplastic Changes within the Central Nervous System

Functional brain imaging of patients with CRPS has shown a significant degree of cortical reorganization in the sensory and motor cortex and the pain intensity correlates with the amount of reorganization. There is a reduction in size of the representation of the CRPS-affected limb in the somatosensory cortex compared with the unaffected side. These changes may reflect brain plasticity occurring as a part of CRPS development because alterations return to normal after successful CRPS treatment.

SYMPTOMS/CLINICAL PRESENTATION

Reflex sympathetic dystrophy can have predominantly inflammatory features, sympathetic features or could be a mix of the two. Apart from the varied features, there is a temporal evolution of the disease (see staging below). The symptoms usually initially manifest near the site of injury and are often minor. Patient complains of spontaneous pain described as simple aching or burning to throbbing shooting or stabbing. Moving or touching the limb is often painful. Patients may also present with muscle spasms, local swelling, and sensitivity to air, water, touch, and vibrations with abnormally increased sweating. On examination, there may be change in skin temperature (usually hot but sometimes cold) and color (reddish violet) along with joint tenderness or stiffness and or restricted/painful movements. The motor changes include weakness, distal tremors, dystonia, and myoclonus. Radiologically, softening and thinning of bones (osteoporosis) especially periarticular but usually "cat bite" lesions are seen **(Figs. 1A and B)**. Over a period of time loss of function, muscle and limb atrophy become evident with trophic changes like reduced and abnormal nail growth, thin and glossy skin associated with reduced elasticity and ulceration. Over prolonged period of immobility, contractures and fibrosis develop in the nearby joints. Due to long-standing and progressive nature of disease, patients often have associated psychological and psychiatric disturbances. Various features that may be associated with RSD and pain are presented in **Box 1**.

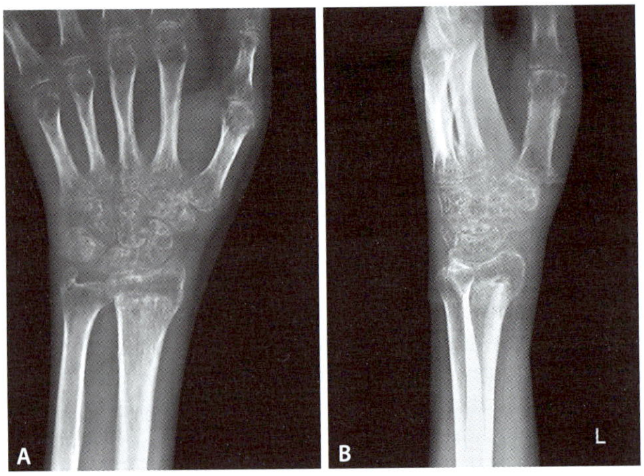

Figs. 1A and B: The characteristic radiographic appearance of CRPS type 1. There is periarticular osteopenia masquerading as cat-bite lesions and thinning of cortices.

BOX 1: Compiled features that may be associated with complex regional pain syndrome.

- *Pain:* Allodynia, hyperalgesia, hyperpathia, hyperesthesia, dysesthesia, and hypoesthesia
- *Sweating:* Excessive, reduced or absent
- *Skin color:* Reddish or bluish, pale or blotchy
- *Skin temperature:* Inappropriate warmth or coldness, poikilothermia
- *Skin appearance:* Swelling, atrophy or pigmented
- *Skin texture:* Loss of skin wrinkles or glossiness, subcutaneous atrophy or thickening
- *Skin appendages:*
  - Excess or loss of hair
  - Nails ridged, curved, thin, brittle or clubbed
- Skin contractures
- *Joint:* Stiffness similar to acute or chronic arthritis
- *Bones:* Localized or diffuse osteoporosis
- *Muscles:* Weakness or evident wasting
- Involuntary movements such as tremors, muscle spasms or dystonia
- Urinary sphincter dysfunction

The symptoms of CRPS and its evolution can be divided into three stages (Bonica's) that have limited therapeutic and prognostic relevance:

1. *Stage 1—Acute (it begins immediately after injury for up to 3 months):* This stage has a good prognosis and it is reversible. Severe burning pain at the site of injury, associated muscle spasm, joint stiffness, and restricted mobility are characteristics of this stage. Increased hair **(Fig. 2)** and nail growth and changes in skin (red, warm, swollen, dry, and inflamed) may be seen due to vasodilatation. At later stage, color may change to mottled with marked hyperhidrosis. This is the most definitive stage as appropriate treatment.
2. *Stage 2—Subacute or dystrophic (6 weeks to 1 year):* The pain intensity increases. Swelling spreads; hair growth diminishes; nails become cracked, brittle, grooved and spotty (mainly due to vasospasm); osteoporosis becomes severe and diffuse; joints thicken, and muscles get atrophied.
3. *Stage 3—Atrophic (6 months to may be forever):* With the progression of disease, irreversible changes in the skin and bones occur and unresolved pain may involve the

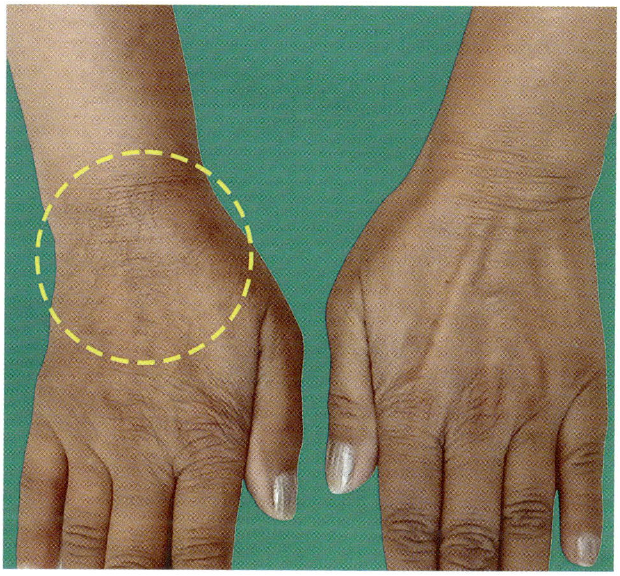

Fig. 2: Excessive hair growth on the dorsum of right wrist of this 43-year-old female who suffered from complex regional pain syndrome (CRPS) type 1 due to elbow injury managed conservatively. Most of the other signs of CRPS have vanished in her barring this excess hair growth.

entire limb along with marked muscle atrophy, flexion contractures, atrophy of skin, and brittle nails. The limb has "woody" feel on examination. Severe osteoporosis with washed-out appearance of bone is seen in radiographs (***see* Figs. 1A and B**).

DIAGNOSIS

The diagnosis of CRPS is mainly clinical and rests on identification of specific clinical features with typical developmental history and evolution of symptomatic disease. Few groups and investigators have proposed criteria for objectively diagnosing CRPS and are presented below.

International Association for Study of Pain Diagnostic Criteria ***(Box 2)****:* They were introduced in 1994, though a formal validation before introduction was not done. These have high sensitivity but low specificity. Current IASP diagnostic criteria may lead to overdiagnosis of CRPS due to low specificity.

Budapest diagnostic criteria ***(Box 3)*** *(Harden et al., 1999):* The Budapest clinical criteria is a better clinical tool as it has greatly improved specificity due to inclusion of four distinct CRPS components and also maintains the sensitivity of IASP criteria.

BOX 2: International Association for Study of Pain Diagnostic Criteria.

- The presence of an initiating noxious event or a cause of immobilization may or may not be present.
- Pain is disproportionate to any known inciting event.
- Presence of edema, changes in the skin blood flow or abnormal sudomotor activity in the region of pain (can be sign or symptom)
- The diagnosis of CRPS is by exclusion (no other conditions that would otherwise account for the degree of pain and dysfunction).

BOX 3: Budapest diagnostic criteria.

- Presence of continuous pain which is disproportionate to any inciting event.
- Complaints of at least one symptom in three (clinical diagnostic criteria) or four (research diagnostic criteria) of the following categories:
  - *Sensory:* Hyperesthesia or allodynia
  - *Vasomotor:* Temperature asymmetry and/or skin color changes and/or skin color asymmetry
  - *Sudomotor or edema:* Edema and/or sweating changes, or sweating asymmetry
  - *Motor or trophic:* Decreased range of motion and/or motor dysfunction (weakness, tremor, or dystonia), and/or trophic changes (hair, nails, or skin)
- Presence of at least one sign at time of diagnosis in two or moreof the following categories:
  - *Sensory:* Hyperalgesia to pinprick and/or allodynia to light touch, deep somatic pressure or joint movement (usually nonpainful)
  - *Vasomotor:* Asymmetry of temperature and/or skin color changes
  - *Sudomotor or edema:* Edema and/or sweating changes and/ or asymmetrical sweating
  - *Motor or trophic:* Decreased range of motion and/or motor dysfunction, i.e., muscle weakness, tremors, or dystonia and/ or trophic changes (hair, nails, or skin)
- No other condition or diagnosis that could better explain the signs and symptoms.

Note: The diagnosis of CRPS is by exclusion and it should be differentiated with diseases of similar clinical sign and symptoms. As a diagnostic rule, there should be at least one symptom in *all four* symptom categories and at least one sign (observed at evaluation) in two or more sign categories.

Investigations and Diagnostic Tests

Sympathetic Blockade

- Stellate ganglion block (upper extremity)
- Lumbar paravertebral ganglia (lower extremity)

A successful block that results in pain relief helps to confirm a diagnosis of CRPS in the presence of other consistent clinical findings. The success of the block needs to be thoroughly evaluated by effects of the block on sudomotor and vasoconstrictor function by assessing skin blood flow and temperature and also by assessing a positive (pain relief) or negative response (no relief in pain) to the block. False positive response may be seen if:

- Somatic nerve block occurs due to local anesthetic spread to nearby nerve roots affecting the patient's pain. Ascertain locally by clinical examination.
- Pain relief occurs due to systemic uptake of local anesthetic (if large dose is used).
- Placebo effect of the invasive procedure itself.
- Visceral sensory afferent fibers that are traveling with the sympathetic chain may get blocked by local anesthetic and result in pain relief.
- Regional intravenous blockade with guanethidine: Injected guanethidine is taken up by postganglionic sympathetic nerves. There it depletes norepinephrine stores and prevents further release of norepinephrine for 1–2 days. The initial depletion of norepinephrine stores can cause short-term excitation of nociceptors due to the increased norepinephrine release leading to increased pain during the procedure.

Other Diagnostic Tests

Thermography: It is not a reliable test for diagnosis of CRPS.

Sweat testing: Qualitative assessment can be done by color changing dyes that indicate sweating on coming in contact with water. Two quantitative tests that may be used are quantitative sudomotor axon reflex test and the resting sweat output test. They also correlate well with clinical signs of CRPS.

Quantitative sensory testing and autonomic testing:

- Quantitative sensory testing demonstrates a decrease of cold pain thresholds and an increase in warm perception thresholds in patients with CRPS types I and II.
- Quantitative sudomotor axon reflex test shows an increase in sweating on the affected side due to abnormal sudomotor function in patients with acute CRPS.

Radiography: The radiological features were first recognized by Sudeck. Patchy osteoporosis (post-traumatic osteoporosis) which may be due to disuse of the affected extremity commonly expands to periarticular osteopenia. Conventional radiographs may be normal (30%) or may show severe osteopenia in about 2–3 weeks after the onset of the disease. Classically, it has a socks and glove-like distribution affecting distal tibia, distal forearm, wrist, hand, and foot but sparing remainder of the forearm or leg. It is not sensitive or specific for CRPS.

Three-phase bone scintigraphy: Three-phase radionuclide bone imaging is done to make differential diagnosis and exclude other lesions like infection for which information about the perfusion to the extremity (phase I) or relative vascularity of the extremity (phase II) is helpful.

For regional RSD of the hand or foot, the classical findings on the radionuclide angiogram (RNA; phase I) is diffuse increased perfusion to the entire extremity. Similarly, increased vascularity with diffuse increased tracer accumulation on blood pool or tissue-phase images (phase II) and juxta-articular accentuation may be seen. Fifty percent of blood-pool findings and 40% RNA shows some abnormality with clinical stage I or II of the disease. Delayed images also demonstrate diffuse and increased tracer uptake throughout the hand or foot including the wrist or ankle, with juxta-articular accentuation. Significant uptake in the metacarpophalangeal or metacarpal bones has high sensitivity and specificity for CRPS. The best timing for this study is in the subacute phase of the condition, i.e., up to 1 year. It is suggestive of CRPS but it is not diagnostic.

Electrodiagnostic testing: These tests are helpful to distinguish between CRPS I and II.

DIFFERENTIAL DIAGNOSIS OF COMPLEX REGIONAL PAIN

- *Inflammation:*
  - Erysipelas
  - Seronegative arthritis
  - Rheumatologic diseases
- *Vascular diseases:*
  - Thrombosis
  - Acrocyanosis
  - Atherosclerosis
  - Raynaud's disease
- *Neuropathic pain:*
  - Peripheral (poly) neuropathy
  - Plexopathy
  - Nerve entrapment
  - Radiculopathy
  - Postherpetic neuralgia
  - Deafferentation pain after cerebrovascular accident (CVA)
- *Myofascial pain:*
  - Overuse or disuse of muscles
  - Tennis elbow
  - Injury due to repetitive strain
  - Fibromyalgia syndrome
- *Psychiatric problems:*
  - Malingering and Münchhausen syndrome
  - Somatoform pain disorders

TREATMENT

Physical and Occupational Therapy

In the acute stage, physical therapy is the most important factor in reversing the syndrome. In subacute and chronic stages, it works to improve pain and function and helps to prevent joint stiffness and contractures. Always combine this with aggressive pain relief with or without sympathetic and/or somatic blockade. To avoid atrophy and contractures of the affected limb, early physical therapy is essential. Early physical therapy reduces pain, motor impairment, and improves function and coordination ability of the limb. Physical and occupational therapy act primarily by desensitizing the affected body part, restoring motion, and improving function.

Specific modalities used are progressive weight-bearing, transcutaneous electrical nerve stimulation (no documented benefit), tactile desensitization, massage, compressive garments to control edema, and contrast bath therapy. These interventions are tailored for individual needs.

Due to intolerable symptoms and hyperalgesia, some people may not accept physical therapy. In such situation, graded motor imagery and mirror therapy (see below) are particularly helpful.

People suffering with CRPS may develop guarding behaviors and avoid using or touching the affected limb which perpetuates the pain cycle. To improve function of affected part pain exposure physical therapy (PEPT) is utilized. This involves the use of progressive loading (i.e., loading extremities beyond limit of pain) with pain-avoidance behavior management. These passive and active exercises and muscle stretching mobilize the joints and are believed to reduce sensitization (may also restore autonomic deregulation and cortical representation).

Drugs

There is some evidence that vitamin C 500–1,000 mg daily for 50 days reduces CRPS after wrist fractures and limb surgery. Innumerable drugs have been successfully tried in treatment of CRPS **(Table 2)** and many are still being investigated.

TABLE 2: Drugs used in common management of complex regional pain syndrome.

Drug	*Proposed mechanism ofaction*	*Route of administration*
Prednisone	Anti-inflammatory and neural membrane stabilizer	Oral
Vitamin C	Antioxidant	Oral
Alendronate	Osteoclast inhibitor	Intravenous
Bretylium	Autonomic ganglion blocker	
Ketanserin	Serotonin and alpha-adrenoceptor antagonist	
Phentolamine	Alpha-1-adrenoceptorantagonist	
Lidocaine	Sodium channel blocker	
DMSO	Free radical scavenger	Topical
Calcitonin	Osteoclast inhibitor	Intranasal
Clonidine	Alpha-2-adrenoceptor agonist	Epidural/intrathecal
Baclofen	GABA-B receptor agonist	Intrathecal

(DMSO: dimethyl sulfoxide; GABA: gamma-aminobutyric acid)

Some nonspecific drugs include antidepressants, anti-inflammatory drugs, bisphosphonates, vasodilators, gamma-aminobutyric acid (GABA) analogs such as gabapentin and pregabalin, alpha- or beta-adrenergic-blocking compounds, and the opioids.

- *Corticosteroids:* For anti-inflammatory and neuronal membrane stabilizer effect.
- *Vitamin C (oral):* Acts as an antioxidant and has increased tissue healing potential.
- *Bretylium:* Acts as autonomic ganglia blocker.
- *Ketanserin:* It is serotonin and alpha-receptor antagonist.
- *Phentolamine:* Works on alpha-1 receptor as antagonist.
- *Lidocaine:* Membrane stabilizer through sodium-channel blockade.
- *Dimethyl sulfoxide (DMSO, used as 50% topical ointment):* It is a free radical scavenger. This can be combined with topical ketamine and anti-inflammatory ointments.
- *Baclofen (intrathecal):* GABA-B receptor agonist to treat CRPS-related dystonia, tremor or myoclonus.
- *Ketamine:* Ketamine, a dissociative anesthetic, has reported some anecdotal success. The hypothesis is that ketamine blocks N-methyl-D-aspartate (NMDA) receptors that might reboot aberrant brain activity.
- *Calcitonin:* The antinociceptive effects of calcitonin might be attributed to its catecholaminergic and serotoninergic mechanisms or action on opioid receptors.
- *Bisphosphonates:* The antinociceptive effect of bisphosphonates is primarily due to their effect on osteoclasts and control of regional osteoporosis. They also inhibit prostaglandin E2, proteolytic enzymes, and lactic acid contributing to positive effects. Neridronic acid is a newer bisphosphonate that has shown promising results.
- Tadalafil is a PDE5 inhibitor and promising treatment in patients with chronic cold CRPS.

Mirror Box Therapy

Mirror box therapy confuses the patient to assume that his affected limb is actually functional and may reinforce the effect of other therapies. It uses a mirror box to create a reflection of the normal limb such that the patient thinks they are looking at the affected limb. Movement of this reflected normal limb appears as if they are being performed with the affected limb. Mirror box therapy may benefit in early CRPS. It appears to be mainly psychotherapy and brain retuning as the precise neural mechanisms of action are unknown.

Tactile Discrimination Training

This training was originally developed for phantom limb pain. Sensory discrimination training reduces pain, increases sensory acuity, and helps in normalization of cortical reorganization.

Intravenous Regional Sympathetic Blockade

The guanethidine was the first drug used for intravenous regional sympathetic blockade in patients with CRPS. It works through ganglion blockade. However, due to potential side effects and its failure to prove its superiority to even placebo, it is not used nowadays. Many other medications have been subsequently used which include sympatholytics such as reserpine, bretylium, and clonidine; local anesthetics such as prilocaine or lidocaine. Few other drugs such as ketanserin (serotonin antagonist), methylprednisolone, and droperidol have also been tried with variable and inconsistent success.

Local Anesthetic Sympathetic Blockade

Sympathetic blocks are given when other conservative treatments such as drugs and physical therapy are insufficient to control the symptoms. However, use of these blocks at early stage of disease not only helps in diagnosis but also in controlling the severity of pain and other symptoms. A local anesthetic solution can be injected by placing a needle tip in the proximity of sympathetic structures such as the stellate ganglion or lumbar sympathetic chain (LASB) under fluoroscopic or computed tomographic guidance. These blocks provide effective pain treatment of patients with CRPS. Although the relief is of short duration, they can be used to improve mobility, range of motion, and motor strength by physiotherapy. If pain relief is 50% or more, this procedure can be repeated a few times with local anesthetic. Repeated blocks are beneficial in selected patients to help to facilitate participation in physiotherapy, particularly when signs of continued improvement are observed. Phenol neurolysis can be used for prolonged block of sympathetic ganglia. However, for a more prolonged sympathetic block radiofrequency treatment is preferred over phenol neurolysis because effects are comparable and the risk for side effects is lower. For patients suffering from CRPS refractory to conventional treatment and sympathetic blocks, continuous brachial plexus block or continuous epidural infusion analgesia coupled with exercise therapy may be tried.

Spinal Cord Stimulation

The system comprises stimulating electrodes inserted in epidural space. These electrodes are connected to a source which generates electrical impulses similar to a pacemaker.

The level of electrode placement depends upon the site of CRPS. The factors like intensity and nature of stimulation can be programmed and manipulated through a wireless remote. Stimulator can also be implanted surgically to reduce the pain by directly stimulating the spinal cord. The mechanism of relief is very complex and poorly understood; however, it may involve restoring normal GABA levels in the dorsal horn and effect the release of adenosine, thus reducing neuropathic pain.

Neuraxial Techniques

These are complicated and considered last resort measures to treat CRPS. Epidural local anesthetics, clonidine, or opioids have been studied in the management of CRPS. Use of these agents has reduced as other techniques are available. Morphine, bupivacaine, clonidine or baclofen can also be delivered intrathecally via an implanted pump producing relief.

Sympathetic Denervation

Diagnostic sympathetic block is the first step for any denervation procedure. Patients who show good response to initial diagnostic sympathetic blocks respond better to radiofrequency denervation, chemical destruction of the sympathetic innervation or surgical sympathectomy. The results of such procedures may not be permanent and, in fact, the analgesic effects persist only in two-thirds at 2 years and one-third at 5 years for unknown reasons. Minimally invasive procedure like videoscopic lumbar sympathectomy has been proven to be as effective as an open surgical intervention and is less aggressive. Rare but serious complications can result from these neurodestructive procedures which include postsympathectomy sympathalgia, compensatory hyperhidrosis, Horner's syndrome, myelitis, and spinal cord injury. However, compared to percutaneous approach surgical sympathectomy (both videoscopic and open) is better in precision.

Intramuscular Botox Injections

In patients of CRPS when symptoms are localized to one extremity, intramuscular botulinum injections have shown beneficial effects. These injections may reduce the muscle spasm and also decrease the inflammation which is caused by CRPS. The limitation of this treatment is that it may need to be repeated after a few months and there is reduced efficacy after repeated use.

Neuropathic Pain Medication

Pharmacological treatment with tricyclic antidepressants, gabapentin, and pregabalin, centrally acting medications such as tramadol, opioids, and clonidine is an important ancillary to controlling inflammation by conventional medications [nonsteroidal anti-inflammatory drugs (NSAIDs) and opioids].

Adjunctive Treatment

Of unknown utility but commonly prescribed as a comprehensive curative program at dedicated centers are electroencephalographic (EEG) biofeedback, various forms of psychotherapy, relaxation techniques, and hypnosis that probably facilitate maintain compliance of patient than actually having any curative effect.

Miscellaneous and Newer Therapeutic Options

Various novel and innovative therapeutic options are being designed and explored for control of CRPS in view of limited success gained from the prevailing measures. Graded imagery, repetitive transcranial magnetic simulation, hirudotherapy, ozone therapy, polarized polychromatic light therapy (Bioptron), fluidotherapy, hyperbaric oxygen, intravenous infusion of iloprost and immunoglobulin, subanesthetic infusion of ketamine are a few. Interestingly, it has been found that the incidence of CRPS is significantly reduced with use of axillary block or intravenous regional anesthesia with clonidine (and lidocaine) and use of vitamin C in postoperative period.

Amputation

Not very well accepted among the fraternity but this remains the ultimate option for intractable symptoms of a debilitating limb affected by CRPS. It should be borne in mind that mere absence of limb created by amputation may still fail to eradicate the symptoms if central neurocircuitry gets established. So, late amputations may not be beneficial at all.

Treatments to be Avoided

Deep brain stimulation is ineffective in CRPS. High-dose opioid should be avoided due to risk of opioid-induced hyperalgesia. Opioids also have potential risk of addiction, diversion risk (the transfer of a prescription drug from a lawful to unlawful channel of distribution or use) and overdosage.

Treatment Algorithm

Overall treatment algorithm is shown in **Flowchart 1**. This algorithm has suggested that all patients with CRPS should have access to medications and/or psychotherapy and/or injections, as and when indicated. If the patient fails to progress (poor response to advised treatment) at any step or in any regard, the clinical team should consider starting or adding stronger medications and/or more intensive psychotherapies **(Flowchart 2)** and/or different interventions **(Flowchart 3)**. The algorithm also guides about treatment approach to the CRPS patients. Poor response (inadequate or partial response) to any given therapy should lead to a stepwise progression through various modalities (moving from less to more invasive) in conjunction with other noninterventional treatments.

PROGNOSIS

If treatment of CRPS is instituted early in the course of disease (within 3 months of the first symptoms), prognosis is usually good. If treatment is delayed, the disorder can quickly spread to the entire limb and irreversible changes can occur in bones, nerves, and muscles. Patients with cold

Flowchart 1: Overall treatment algorithm.

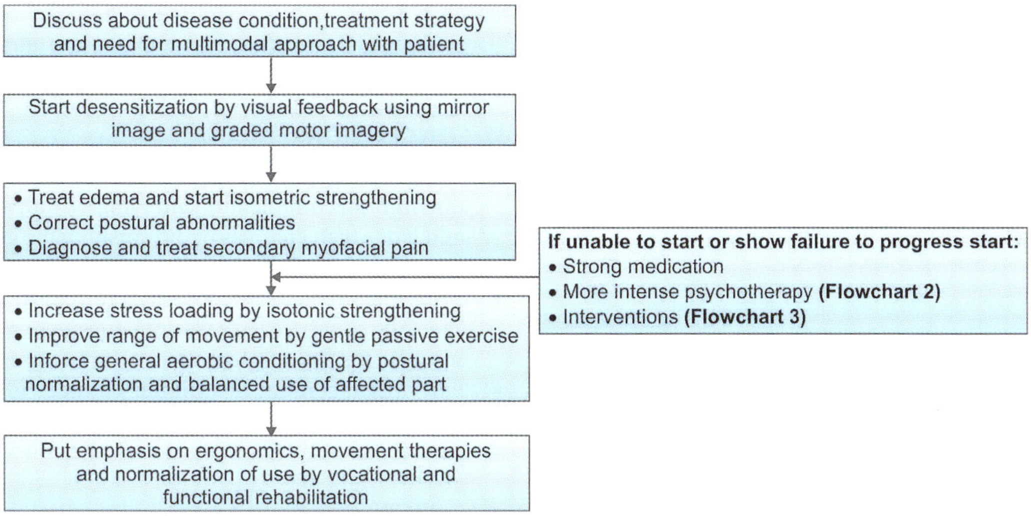

Source: Modified from Harden et al. Complex Regional Pain Syndrome: Practical Diagnostic and Treatment Guidelines; 2013.

Flowchart 2: Algorithm for psychological intervention and treatment.

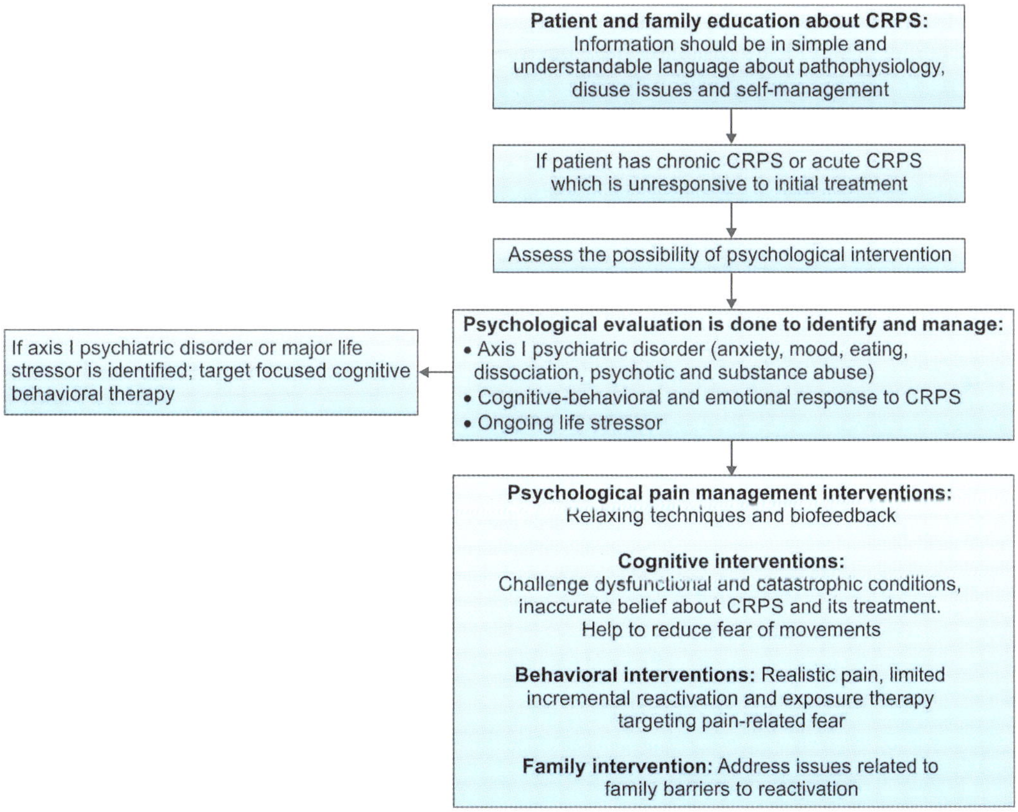

Source: Modified from Harden et al. Complex Regional Pain Syndrome: Practical Diagnostic and Treatment Guidelines; 2013.

CRPS have a worse prognosis than those with warm CRPS. Left untreated, the limb can experience muscle atrophy, loss of use and functions and may require amputation. CRPS is usually not a self-limiting disease and will not "burn itself out"; if treated early, it is likely to go into remission. Early intervention through adequate pain relief and interventional pain procedures as well as psychological support are important to reduce the suffering.

COMPLEX REGIONAL PAIN SYNDROME IN CHILDREN

In addition to features of CRPS in adults, symptom migration can also be observed in children affected with CRPS. The techniques which are used for diagnosis of CRPS in adults can also be utilized in children. Lower limbs are commonly affected by CRPS in children unlike adults. Trophic changes are less commonly seen than sensory, motor, and autonomic

Flowchart 3: Algorithm of interventional pain treatment in complex regional pain syndrome.

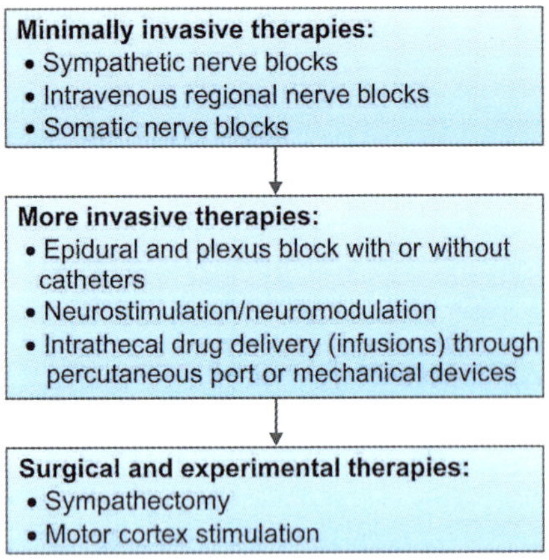

Source: Modified from Harden et al. Complex Regional Pain Syndrome: Practical Diagnostic and Treatment Guidelines; 2013.

disturbances. Similar to adult population, response to sympathetic blocks is variable. Prognosis (chances of recovery) is better in children although recurrence rate is higher (~30%). Refractory cases resulting in significant disability have been reported. Interventional approaches are rarely needed but familial issues and psychological need to be addressed. Psychological dysfunction has a high association with CRPS in children.

CONCLUSION

- Complex regional pain syndrome (CRPS) is not an uncommon complication after limb orthopedic surgeries and it has high chances of diminishing the good outcome of primary treatment/surgery.
- Diagnosis of CRPS is purely clinical and should be specially sought for in cases of persistent pain or burning sensation at the surgical site.
- Early management has higher chances of quicker and complete remission. Delay in treatment gives time for central brain circuit changes making control or treatment of CRPS difficult.
- Cold CRPS is difficult to treat due to central reorganization.
- Primary prevention by aggressive postoperative pain control is currently the favored approach to minimize development of CRPS even in susceptible population.
- Once CRPS develops combination therapy is the only way to control the disease as no specific therapy is known.

CHAPTER 34

Neurogenic Bladder

Manish Kumar Varshney

INTRODUCTION

Neurological injury to bladder results in significant disability. The neurogenic bladder may arise from spinal cord injury, nerve root/cord compression, or central nervous system (CNS) disorders. Recognizing the type of neurological involvement helps in appropriate management of the condition.

DEFINITION

A dysfunctional urinary bladder caused by an injury to the central or peripheral nerves controlling urination is called a "neurogenic bladder".

ANATOMY OF THE BLADDER

Urinary bladder can be broadly divided into: body and neck regions. Body is made up of detrusor muscle and neck has of two sphincters: (1) internal urethral sphincter and (2) external urethral sphincter **(Fig. 1)**. The urinary bladder functions to store and expel urine in a coordinated and controlled fashion. The central and peripheral nervous systems work in coordination to control this. Parasympathetic fibers arising from S2 to S4 cord segments innervate the urinary bladder via pelvic splanchnic nerves and the inferior hypogastric and vesical plexuses **(Fig. 1)**. They are motor to the detrusor muscle and inhibitory to the internal urethral sphincter. Sympathetic fibers arising from the T11 to L3 cord segments innervate the neck and trigone via lumbar splanchnic nerves **(Fig. 1)**. Their stimulation allows for bladder neck closure required for bladder filling. The external urethral sphincter is controlled by somatic fibers arising from motor neurons in the S2–S4 cord segments via the pudendal nerve. When micturition is initiated via cortical signals and the internal sphincter opens, the external sphincter relaxes reflexively but still can be contracted voluntarily **(Fig. 1)**.

NEUROANATOMY OF THE BLADDER

A spinal reflex controlled by the CNS (brain and spinal cord) causes normal voiding. This is controlled by three sets of peripheral nerves arising from the autonomic nervous system (ANS) and somatic nervous system.

Brain

The brain is the master control of the entire urinary system. In its frontal lobe, micturition center is located which sends inhibitory signals to detrusor muscles to prevent voiding until socially acceptable space to urinate is available.

Brainstem

The pons via the pontine micturition center (PMC) coordinates the activities of the urinary sphincters and the bladder. The stimulation of this center causes the urethral sphincters to open and contracts the detrusor to void the urine. The stretching of the receptors in the detrusor muscle signals the pons, which stimulates the brain to create a sensation of a full bladder and a sudden desire to go to the bathroom. The brain inhibits the pons and prevents the bladder from contracting until a bathroom is found.

Spinal Cord

In sacral spinal cord, there is sacral reflex center which is primitive voiding center, and it is responsible for bladder contractions. Spinal cord injury causes detrusor sphincter dyssynergia with detrusor hyperreflexia (DSD-DH) in which the urinary bladder and sphincter are both overactive. In severe spinal cord injury, detrusor areflexia and urinary retention occur.

Peripheral Nerves

It includes ANS—sympathetic and parasympathetic nerves and somatic nerves. Under normal conditions, bladder is under influence of sympathetic nervous system, which causes detrusor relaxation and internal sphincter contraction and also inhibits parasympathetic nervous system, so urinary accommodation occurs and micturition reflex is inhibited. The parasympathetic nerves cause detrusor contraction and so voiding occurs. Somatic innervation of bladder is through pudendal nerve which originates from the nucleus of Onuf and regulates the actions of external urinary sphincter and pelvic diaphragm. Its activation prevents voiding to occur.

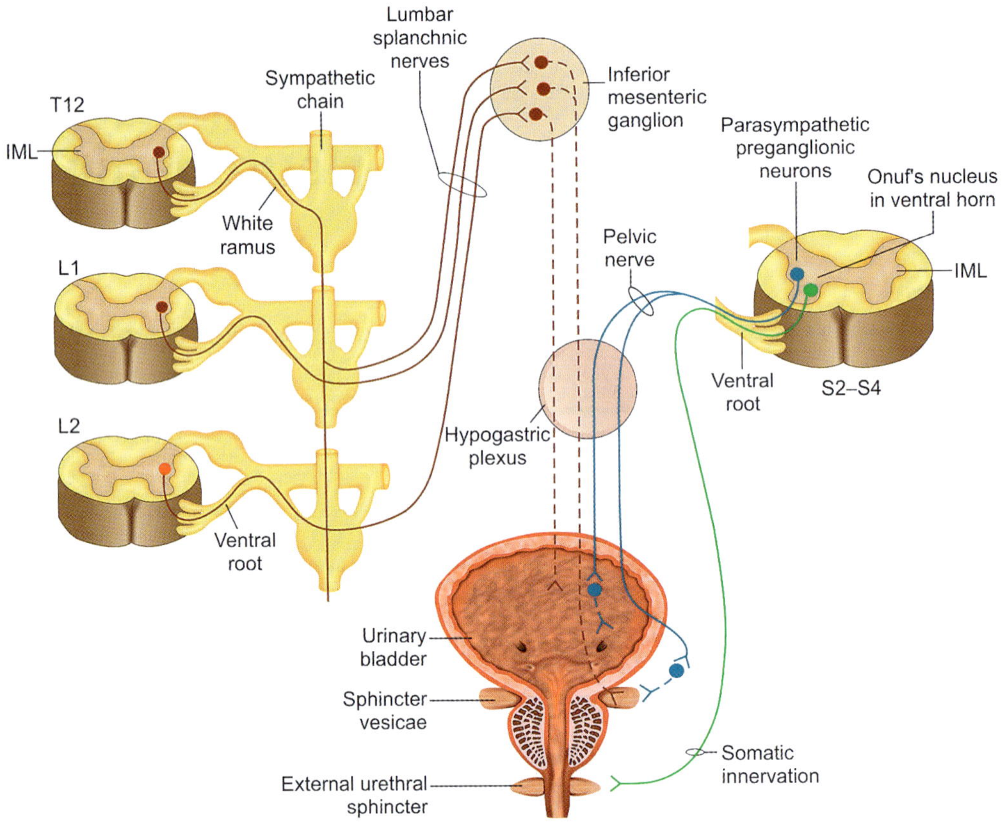

Fig. 1: Neurology of micturition. The sympathetic innervation (red) causes bladder inhibition by inhibiting the parasympathetic fibers, causes bladder relaxation directly (β-adrenergic), and causes bladder neck and urethral contraction (α-adrenergic). The parasympathetic supply is the motor supply to bladder muscle (blue). It also inhibits the bladder neck contraction. Voluntary (somatic, depicted by green) causes contraction of pelvic floor muscles through pudendal nerves. (IML: intermediolateral)

PATHOPHYSIOLOGY AND ETIOLOGY

Voiding cycle is affected when any part of the nervous system is affected. The common causes are spinal cord injury, cauda equina syndrome, stroke complications, multiple sclerosis, Parkinson's disease, and paralytic syndrome **(Box 1)**. It may result in overactive bladder (spastic bladder) or urinary retention or a combination of both. Bladder overactivity is associated with stress incontinence while sphincter underactivity is associated with urge incontinence **(Fig. 1)**. A combination of both may also occur.

BOX 1: Common causes of neurogenic bladder.

Congenital:
- Sacral agenesis
- Myelomeningocele
- Cerebral palsy

Acquired:
- Cerebrovascular accident (stroke)
- Spinal cord involvement
  - Injury
  - Spinal surgeries
  - Cord/root compression
  - Cauda equina
- Head injury
- Central nervous system tumors
- Multiple sclerosis
- Erectile dysfunction
- Heavy metal poisoning
- Parkinson's disease
- Pelvic trauma
- Sacral neoplasia

Brain Lesions

Lesions above the pons destroy the master control center and entire control over the voiding is lost. Patients develop urge incontinence, the bladder empties too quickly and too often (spastic overactive bladder). They rush to bathroom and can leak urine on their way to the bathroom. Some common causes are stroke, hydrocephalus, brain tumor, Parkinson's disease, cerebral palsy, and Shy-Drager syndrome.

Spinal Cord Lesions

Diseases or injuries to the spinal cord result in spastic bladder and patients develop urge incontinence. It differs from the brain lesions in that the external sphincter may have paradoxical contractions as well, patients develop urge for voiding simultaneously with urinary retention, the condition known as "DSD-DH". The bladder would keep filling until the detrusor muscle stretch reflex gets activated and causes emptying of bladder by its contraction making the bladder "automatic". The cerebral control is lost and the bladder more or less becomes like that of an infant.

Examples:
- Traumatic spinal cord injury
- Multiple sclerosis
- Myelomeningocele
- Spinal cord tumors

Sacral Cord Injury

Sacral cord injury can cause a sensory neurogenic bladder where the patient cannot sense that the bladder is full, or motor neurogenic bladder where the patient senses the bladder is full but detrusor does not contract (flaccid bladder), a condition known as "detrusor areflexia" causing overflow incontinence (autonomous bladder).

Examples:
- Sacral cord tumors
- Herniated disk
- Pelvic crush injuries
- Radical hysterectomy or abdominal perineal resection
- Tethered cord syndrome in teenagers

Peripheral Nerve Injury

Destruction of the nerves to the bladder results in silent and painless distention of bladder with urinary retention. Causes are diabetes mellitus, Guillain-Barré syndrome, herpes in genital area, acquired immunodeficiency syndrome (AIDS) and poliomyelitis, neurosyphilis (Tabes dorsalis).

CLASSIFICATION

The Lapides classification is the most commonly used classification.
- The *sensory neurogenic bladder* with lesion in posterior columns of the spinal cord or in the afferent tracts leading from the bladder
- The *motor paralytic bladder* with damage to motor neurons of the bladder
- The *uninhibited neurogenic bladder* in which there is an incomplete spinal cord lesion above S2 or a cerebral cortex or cerebropontine axis lesion.
- The *reflex neurogenic bladder* with a complete spinal cord lesions above S2 showing a pine cone bladder on cystogram.
- The *autonomous neurogenic bladder* seen in cauda equina or conus lesions.

INVESTIGATIONS

Laboratory Studies

Urinalysis and urine culture: For urinary tract infection which may cause urge incontinence and irritative voiding.

Urine cytology: To rule out bladder carcinoma which may also cause urinary frequency and urgency.

Chemical profile: Blood urea nitrogen (BUN) and creatinine for renal function.

Other Tests

Voiding diary: It is used to keep track of patient's incontinent episodes, voiding pattern, and inciting events.

Pad test: To document and quantify the urine loss. It can be used to assess severity of incontinence and it uses methylene blue or phenazopyridine that changes color on coming in contact with urine.

Diagnostic Procedures

Postvoid residual urine (PVR): Used for basic evaluation for urinary incontinence. If it is high, the bladder is not contracting enough or the outlet is obstructed.

Uroflow rate: It is volume of urine voided per unit of time. Low uroflow rate may be due to weak detrusor or outflow obstruction or a combination of both. It cannot be differentiated by this test.

Filling cystometrogram: Used to estimate the bladder capacity, phasic contractions (detrusor instability) and bladder compliance.

Voiding cystometrogram (Pressure flow study): The voiding detrusor pressure and the rate of urinary flow are recorded in this test. It enables clinician to assess bladder contractility and the extent of bladder outlet obstruction.

Cystogram: It may be static or voiding. Static cystogram diagnoses stress incontinence, the degree of urethral motion, internal sphincter deficiency, presence of cystocele, bladder diverticulum or vesicovaginal fistula. Voiding cystogram diagnoses urethral obstruction, urethral diverticulum, and vesicoureteral reflux.

Electromyography: It allows diagnosis of DSD-DH seen in spinal cord injuries.

Cystoscopy: Identifies causes of bladder over activity such as stone, cystitis, and tumor.

Videourodynamics: It is a combination of voiding cystourethrogram and multichannel urodynamics. Used to diagnose the functional pressure-flow relationship between the bladder and the urethra, vesicoureteral reflux, and bladder diverticulum.

TREATMENT AND MANAGEMENT

Treatment may be nonsurgical or surgical. Nonsurgical treatment measures include medications and other measures.

Treatment of urinary incontinence varies by types, such as:
- Treatment of urge incontinence is done with behavioral modification or with bladder-relaxing agents.
- Treatment of stress incontinence is done with surgical and nonsurgical means (see below).
- Mixed incontinence also requires a combination of medications as well as surgery.
- Catheter regimen is used for overflow incontinence.

- Functional incontinence is treated by correcting the underlying cause (e.g., urinary tract infection, constipation) or changing medications.

Nonsurgical Treatment Measures

They include medications and nonmedical measures.

Nonmedical Measures

Absorbent products: These are temporary means to keep the patient dry. Various types of pads or garments designed to absorb urine to protect skin and clothing.

Urethral occlusive devices: For an active woman with incontinence who does not desire surgery devices are inserted into the urethra or placed over the urethral meatus to leakage.

Catheters: These various types are used as a temporary measure or a permanent solution for urinary incontinence. There are various types of urinary catheters:

- *Indwelling urethral catheters:* It is like Foley catheter. Its use should be restricted as a permanent measure in terminally ill patient, patients with bed sores to prevent contamination, inoperable urethral obstruction, in acutely ill patients requiring accurate monitoring of fluid balance.
- *Suprapubic catheters:* It is an attractive alternative to long-term urethral catheter use. It is mainly used for long term in patients with spinal cord injuries and a malfunctioning bladder.
- *Intermittent catheterization:* It is used to decompress the bladder in a motivated individual without any physically handicap or mental impairment.

Diet

Foods that should be avoided are foods containing hot spices such as curry, chili powder, and dry mustard. Citrus fruits such as grapefruits and oranges should be avoided. Chocolates and caffeine-containing products should be avoided.

Pelvic Floor Exercises (Kegel Exercises)

These exercises are used to tighten and tone the pelvic floor muscles. They strengthen the external urinary sphincter and prevent stress incontinence and also avert impending pelvic prolapse. They also eliminate urge incontinence and induce reflex bladder relaxation. They can be used to decrease the frequency of incontinence episodes.

Vaginal weights: In premenopausal women with stress incontinence, vaginal weight training is used for strengthening the pelvic floor.

Biofeedback: Biofeedback therapy is used for patients who are having difficulty in identifying levator ani muscles. It uses an electronic device to provide biofeedback about the status of pelvic muscle activity which is relayed via auditory or visual means to the patient. This allows the patient to receive feedback on the activity of the pelvic floor muscles. It can be used to treat urge incontinence, stress incontinence, and mixed incontinence.

Electrical stimulation: It involves stimulation of levator ani muscles using painless electric shocks. It contracts external urethral sphincter and inhibits bladder contraction.

Bladder training: It consists of self-education, scheduled voiding with conscious delay of voiding up to certain predefined time and positive reinforcement.

Medications

Incontinence may be either stress incontinence, which is due to weak urinary sphincter or urge incontinence, which is due to overactive bladder. Internal sphincter has high concentration of α-adrenergic neurons and bladder has parasympathetic supply. So, α-adrenergic drugs are used in treatment of stress incontinence and anticholinergic drugs are used to treat urge incontinence.

Anticholinergic Drugs

They are the first-line drugs in females with urge incontinence. They work by inhibiting involuntary bladder contractions. Contraindications are ulcerative colitis, severe heart diseases, narrow-angled glaucoma, urinary retention, bowel obstruction, and myasthenia gravis. It can cause side effects such as blurred vision, facial flushing, heart palpitations, dry mouth, and drowsiness.

- Propantheline bromide
- Dicyclomine hydrochloride
- Hyoscyamine sulfate

Estrogen Derivatives

They are used in postmenopausal women with mild-to-moderate incontinence. They work by stimulating the α-adrenergic neurons and increasing the tone of the urethral muscles to improve mucosal seal effect, which is required for proper urethral function.

Antispasmodic Drugs

These drugs decrease urge incontinence and increase the bladder capacity. They work by relaxing the smooth muscles of the urinary bladder.

- Solifenacin succinate
- Darifenacin
- Oxybutynin chloride
- Tolterodine L-tartrate
- Trospium
- Fesoterodine

Tricyclic Antidepressant Drugs

They increase norepinephrine and serotonin level and are anticholinergic and direct muscle relaxants to the urinary bladder, e.g., imipramine hydrochloride, amitriptyline hydrochloride.

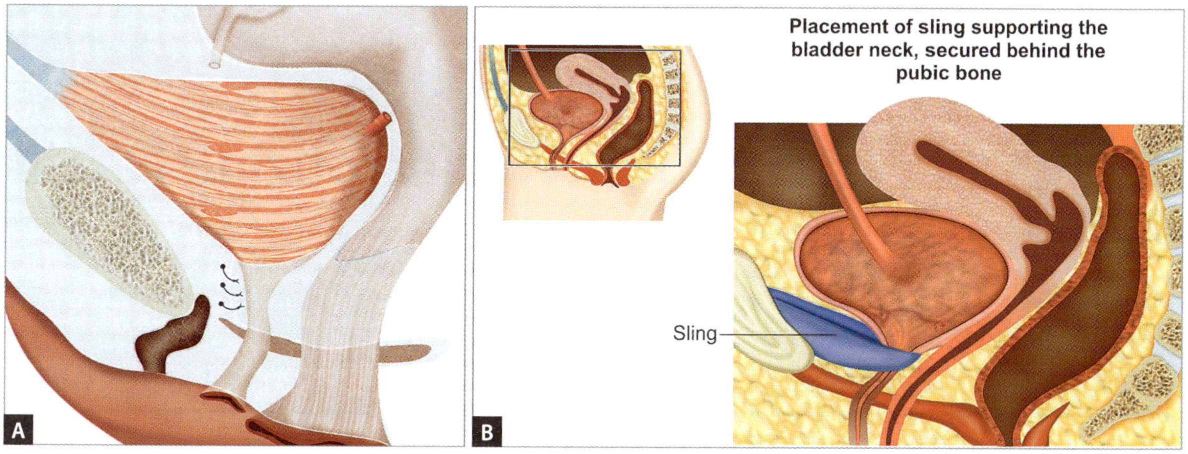

Figs. 2A and B: Retropubic suspension (A) and sling procedure (B) for stress incontinence.

Surgical Measures

Surgical care for stress incontinence involves procedures which improve urethral outlet resistance. Some such procedures are bladder neck suspension, sling procedures **(Figs. 2A and B)**, periurethral bulking therapy, and artificial urinary sphincter.

Some surgical procedures work by improving bladder compliance or bladder capacity such as sacral neuromodulation, bladder augmentation, botulinum toxin injections, and detrusor myomectomy.

CONCLUSION

- Urinary bladder is involved in various spinal and central nervous disorders and spino-pelvic trauma.
- Understanding the pathophysiology of neurogenic bladder helps in appropriate management.
- Supportive treatment and clean intermittent catheterization form the backbone of management aimed to reduce morbidity.
- Patient should be managed in expert association with urologist and nursing care and rehabilitation should be properly explained and supervised.

CHAPTER 35

Necrotizing Fasciitis

Manish Kumar Varshney

INTRODUCTION

Necrotizing fasciitis (NF) is a serious soft tissue infection characterized by rapid spread along the fascial planes and dissolution and necrosis of fascia by enzymes released by the infecting organism. In the later stages, it involves the skin and underlying muscles. Wilson, in 1952, used the term "necrotizing fasciitis" for infection of subcutaneous tissue and fascia mostly sparing the underlying muscles. NF has average mortality of 21% and is a surgical emergency, despite this misdiagnosis in early stages is common. It is a potential life- and limb-threating infection if not recognized and treated early. It is also known as hemolytic streptococcal gangrene, acute dermal gangrene, hospital gangrene, synergistic necrotizing cellulitis, suppurative fasciitis, "flesh-eating disease", and Meleney ulcer. Fournier gangrene is a variant involving the scrotum and perineal area.

ETIOLOGY

The most identified pathogen is group A *Streptococcus* (*S. pyogenes*) which is seen in nearly one-third of the cases overall. Other types of bacteria that can cause NF include *Klebsiella*, *Clostridium*, and *Escherichia coli*. Approximately one-half of NF cases caused by streptococcal bacteria occurs in young and otherwise healthy individuals. Morgan et al. classified NF into four types:

1. Type 1 is polymicrobial where a mix of aerobic and anaerobic organisms is seen. This is seen in 70–80% cases.
2. This is seen in 20–30% cases and in monomicrobial mostly caused by *S. pyogenes* or sometimes by *Staphylococcus aureus*.
3. Type 3 is seen in Asian population caused by gram-negative marine-related organisms.
4. Fungal NF caused by candida in immunocompromised patients or *Mucor/Rhizopus* in zygomatic NF.

Apart from the bacterial and fungal causes, NF may also result from use of sodium-glucose cotransporter-2 (SGLT2) inhibitors in diabetic patients and there is also a suggestion of NF from use of nonsteroidal anti-inflammatory drugs (NSAIDs) during varicella infections.

The common bacteria isolated in various reports are: Group A *Streptococcus* (*Streptococcus pyogenes*), *Staphylococcus aureus*, *Bacteroides fragilis*, *Clostridium perfringens*, Zygomycetes, *Pseudomonas*, *Aeromonas hydrophila*, *Escherichia coli*, *Neisseria meningitidis*, *Klebsiella pneumoniae*, *Serratia marcescens*, *Eikenella corrodens*, *Haemophilus aphrophilus*, and *Saksenaea vasiformis*.

There is initial trauma that may be trivial such as lacerations, contusions, injections, insect bites, and sometimes there is no history of trauma. Major trauma such as open fractures, cutaneous abscesses, burns, frostbite, or surgical procedure may also lead to NF.

Comorbid factors that reduce immunity predispose to NF such as diabetes, peripheral vascular disease, alcoholism, liver disease, hepatitis C infection, smoking, morbid obesity, intravenous drug abuse, multiple myeloma, human immunodeficiency virus (HIV), and chemotherapy.

PATHOPHYSIOLOGY

The infection is characterized by rapid spread along the fascial planes rapidly involving the whole limb and even invading the chest wall if left untreated. This spread is facilitated by enzymes released by the bacteria which dissolve the fat and fascia and form a watery gray pus known as "dishwater pus". The necrotic tissue undergoes secondary aerobic and anaerobic infection leading to mixed cultures in most cases. This rapid spread characteristically spares the muscles but in some fulminant cases, myonecrosis may occur. The vascular supply to the overlying skin gets occluded leading to ischemia and necrosis of skin **(Fig. 1)**. There is severe systemic toxicity and sepsis leading to multiorgan failure and death if left untreated.

CLINICAL FEATURES

There is usually a history of minor trauma followed by swelling and pain in the limb. In the earliest presentations, the patient has a triad of pain, swelling, and erythema that is commonly passed as cellulitis or abscess. Erythema is the most common sign. The toxicity and pain are usually more than can be seen on clinical examination of the limb and this

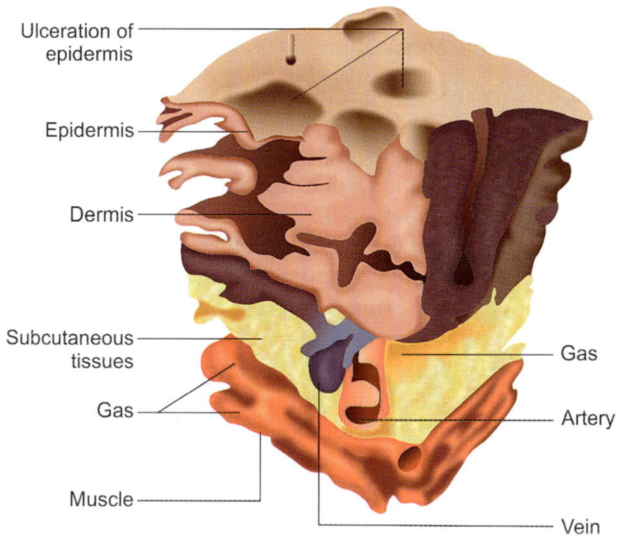

Fig. 1: Necrotizing fasciitis (ischemia and necrosis of skin).

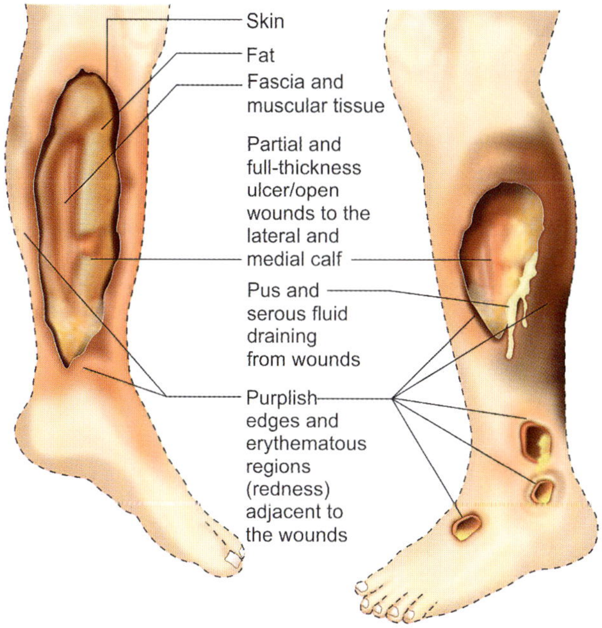

Fig. 2: Necrotizing fasciitis (patches of gangrene).

should be used as first pointer to NF instead of labeling it as other simpler infections. One should, hence, also look for other distinctive features of NF, viz., extension of tenderness beyond the apparent involved area, indistinct margins, absent or minimal lymphangitis as the infection is in deep fascia and lastly rapid progression despite use of antibiotics. There is minimal redness initially which rapidly spreads. The overlying skin undergoes ischemia as its blood supply is occluded and appears bluish. Patches of gangrene appear **(Fig. 2)**. Development of clear fluid blisters (bullae) in the skin marks the intermediary stage between early (without skin necrosis) and late (with skin necrosis) NF **(*see* Table 1)**. Local crepitation develops in case of infection by gas forming organism. The skin gets detached from the underlying tissues and appears loose and in case open wound can be

TABLE 1: The clinical evolution of necrotizing fasciitis.

Early stage	***Intermediate stage***	***Late stage***
• Local warmth • Erythema • Local tenderness beyond the region of apparent skin involvement • Swelling	• Bullae formation • Skin fluctuation • Skin induration	• Hemorrhagic bullae • Skin anesthesia • Crepitus • Dusky skin, discoloration, and frank gangrene

easily lifted off. The underlying muscle layer usually remains red and viable but, in later stages, it also undergoes necrosis.

Patient is toxic and shows signs of sepsis even though external signs may be minimal. Untreated it progresses to severe sepsis and shock (see definitions of these terms from Chapter on "Acute Respiratory Distress Syndrome").

Laboratory investigations are suggestive of infection with leukocytosis, raised erythrocyte sedimentation rate (ESR), and C-reactive protein. A complete workup consists of complete blood count, serum chemistry studies, arterial blood gas analysis, urinalysis, blood, and tissue cultures.

As the clinical and laboratory findings are usually deceptive till later stages, a high index of clinical suspicion is needed to diagnose NF at an early stage. The probability of cellulitis developing into NF can be estimated based on laboratory finding. It is called the laboratory risk indicator for necrotizing fasciitis (LRINEC) score.

The scoring is done as follows:
- *C-reactive protein (CRP) (mg/L):* ≥150:4 points
- *White blood cell count (WBC) count (×10^3/mm^3):*
  - <15:0 points
  - 15–25:1 points
  - >25:2 points
- *Hemoglobin (g/dL):*
  - >13.5:0 points
  - 11 13.5:1 points
  - <11:2 points
- *Sodium (mmol/L):* <135:2 points
- *Creatinine (umol/L):* >141:2 points
- *Glucose (mmol/L):* >10:1 points

A score of equal to or greater than six indicates a high probability of NF.

Skin and superficial tissue cultures are inaccurate and can be misleading. Deep tissue samples obtained at the time of surgery are more accurate in identifying the correct organism and are needed to obtain proper cultures for microorganisms. Performing a "finger test" helps in making bedside diagnosis (incising the suspected area under local anesthetic infiltration 2 cm long and deep to fascia, insinuating finger along the subcutaneous plane to see if it easily dissects through indicating a positive test). Presence of dish water pus is also suggestive of NF. Excisional deep skin biopsy can be used to obtain specimen from deeper tissues before surgery. Ultrasound-guided aspiration for culture from deep collections is also used. Advanced studies such as polymerase chain reaction (PCR) and gene typing further help to pinpoint the exact strain.

Imaging studies such as ultrasound, computed tomography (CT), magnetic resonance imaging (MRI), and Doppler studies help to evaluate the extent of the disease and plan the surgical debridement. They may help in distinguishing between cases that require urgent surgical debridement and those that may respond to antibiotic therapy. Plain radiographs may show gas in the subcutaneous plane.

NF is a medical and surgical emergency and the use of all the above-mentioned investigations should not delay treatment and surgical intervention if infection spreads rapidly.

TREATMENT

Necrotizing fasciitis is an emergency and should be treated in a referral center, which has access to a good surgical and reconstructive team and good intensive care.

The treatment consists of general supportive measures to control sepsis, prevent organ failure and to maintain electrolytes, start of wide spectrum antibiotic until culture reports are obtained, and radical surgical debridement followed by reconstruction.

Antibiotic therapy should be started immediately consisting of penicillin/clindamycin and an aminoglycoside, or third-generation cephalosporin and metronidazole for anaerobic organism. The second-line antibiotic consists of imipenem and vancomycin.

Surgical debridement is the mainstay of treatment and should be undertaken as soon as condition of patient permits and as soon as extent of disease has been determined. The emergency of surgical intervention is also guided by quick sequential organ failure assessment (qSOFA) score > 1.

The following are certain principles of surgical debridement in NF:

- The superficial signs are usually misleading, therefore, proximal extension of debridement should be done till fully healthy tissues are obtained.
- Finger test can be used to determine the extent of proximal spread. In this, the incision is given over skin and finger is inserted into the wound. If it can easily be passed between the skin and underlying fascia that means that the spread is till the skin can be lifted off.
- Wound should be kept open.
- Inspection and debridement should be done in the operation theater (OT) on a daily basis.
- Amputations sometimes can be lifesaving if the spread is into the deeper tissues.
- Coverage and reconstruction should be started only after complete control of infection.

CONCLUSION

Necrotizing fasciitis is a rapidly developing and progressing infection, which, if not recognized early, would threaten the limb and even life of patient. One should look for the pointers to NF in cases presenting with "apparent" simpler infections such as abscess and cellulitis. Emergent extensive debridement and antibiotic therapy along with supportive measures should be rapidly instituted to provide the best chance of protecting the limb and life of the patient.

CHAPTER

36 Thoracic Outlet Syndrome

Manish Kumar Varshney

INTRODUCTION

Thoracic outlet syndrome (TOS) is a complex constellation of varied symptoms that result from the compression of neurovascular structures at the thoracic outlet. Identification of the syndrome requires careful differentiation of the symptoms from various allied disorders in history taking and examination. A casual patient interaction often misses the real diagnosis. It should be strongly suspected in a patient who frequently visits the treating physician complaining no relief from treatment instituted for common disorders such as spondylosis or shoulder disorders. Identification of TOS and then finding out the exact cause of it helps in timely institution of therapy for appropriate treatment.

HISTORY

In 1821, Cooper first described arterial thoracic outlet syndrome (TOS) in a young woman with arm ischemia. Paget in 1875 and Schroetter in 1884 independently described spontaneous thrombosis of subclavian vein. Although Galen described "cervical rib" in 150 AD but it was not until 1861 when Coote resected it for treatment of arterial TOS was its pathological importance recognized. Murphy then used cervical rib resection in 1905 to treat patient with subclavian artery aneurysm. In 1919, Stopford and Telford described compression of the brachial plexus by a normal first rib and improvement following its resection. In 1929, Naffziger and Grant introduced the concept of neurovascular compression due to scalene muscle anomalies in TOS. All these and advancements in diagnostics led to build up of current knowledge of TOS.

Various names for this condition are proposed, which are now clubbed under one term "thoracic outlet syndrome" by Peet in 1956:

- Acroparesthesia
- Brachiocephalic syndrome
- Cervical rib syndrome
- Cervicobrachial neurovascular compression syndrome
- Cervicothoracic outlet syndrome
- Costoclavicular syndrome
- Effort vein thrombosis
- First thoracic rib syndrome
- Fractured clavicle syndrome
- Humeral head syndrome
- Hyperabduction syndrome
- Naffziger's syndrome
- Nocturnal paresthetic brachialgia
- Paget–Schroetter syndrome
- Pectoralis minor syndrome
- Pneumatic hammer syndrome
- Rucksack paralysis
- Scalenus anterior syndrome
- Scalenus medius band syndrome
- Scalenus minimus syndrome
- Shoulder-hand syndrome
- Subcoracoid syndrome
- Syndrome of the scalenus

DEFINITION

Thoracic outlet syndrome is a collection of various signs and symptoms in neck, shoulder, and upper limbs arising from compression of neurovascular bundle in the thoracic outlet region. The compression results from various osseous or muscular or soft tissue disorders or a combination of these.

ANATOMY

In the upper most part of the thorax, the brachial plexus (C5-T1) and the subclavian vessels pass through cervicoaxillary canal to reach the upper limb. First rib divides this cervicoaxillary canal into two parts: The proximal part consists of the interscalene and the costoclavicular triangle and the distal part consists of the axilla **(Fig. 1)**. Mainly TOS occurs due to compression of neurovascular bundle in the proximal part. More specifically, the cervicoaxillary canal includes three compartments:

1. *Interscalene triangle:* Anatomically limited anteriorly by anterior scalene muscle, posteriorly by middle scalene muscle and inferiorly by medial surface of the first rib. Brachial plexus and subclavian artery pass through this triangle. Spasm, hypertrophy, or shortness of the scalene muscles can cause compression of the brachial plexus in this triangle.

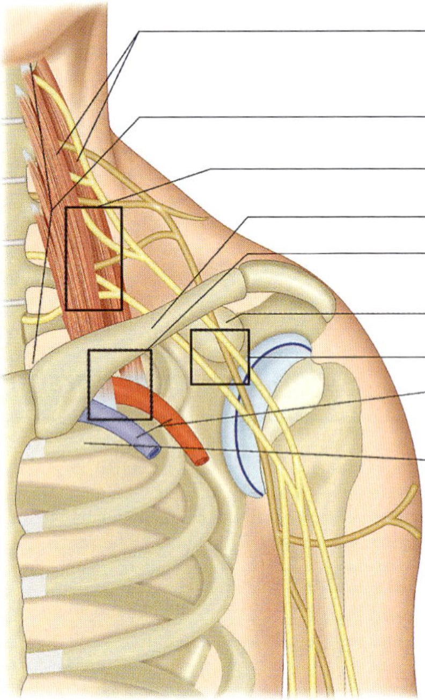

Fig. 1: Understanding the anatomy of cervicoaxillary canal and thoracic outlet.

2. *The costoclavicular triangle:* It is bounded by middle third of the clavicle anteriorly, the first rib posteromedially and by upper border of the scapula posterolaterally.
   Brachial plexus along with subclavian artery and vein pass through this space.
   These both the triangles are, in fact, thoracic inlet and not the thoracic outlet.
3. *Subcoracoid or pectoralis minor space or thoraco-coraco-pectoral space:* It is bounded superiorly by coracoid process, anteriorly by pectoralis minor muscles, and posteriorly by 2–4 ribs. Brachial plexus along with subclavian artery and vein pass through this space.
   Presence of a cervical rib, congenital soft tissue bands, hypomobility of clavicle, and functionally acquired anatomical changes such as upper limb dysfunction or muscle imbalance of the neck and shoulder region compromise the thoracic outlet predisposing to TOS.

EPIDEMIOLOGY

Incidence and Prevalence

It is assumed that TOS affects around 8% of the general population and is more common in females. Cervical ribs are found in about 0.5–0.6% of general population, 80% of these cases are bilateral but <10% of the cases produce symptoms of TOS. Depending on the structure compressed TOS may be classified into neurological TOS (nTOS), arterial TOS (aTOS), or venous TOS (vTOS).

- *nTOS* accounts for the majority occurring in 95–98% of cases and mostly affects 20–60-year-old population. Female to male ratio is 3.5:1.
- *vTOS* is the second most common affecting 2–5% population especially in 20–35 years age group. Males are more commonly affected.
- *aTOS* is the least common (<1%) affecting young adults and persons over 50 years old. There is no sex predilection.

BOX 1: List of causes of thoracic outlet syndrome (TOS).

Congenital:
- Cervical rib
- Elongated transverse process
- Fibrous bands (transversosostal/costocostal)
- Anomalus insertion of scalene muscles
- Exostosis of first rib
- Cervicodorsal scoliosis
- Sprengel deformity
- Arteriovenous malformation

Acquired:
- Postural disorders
- Drooping shoulder
- Oversized breasts
- Trauma—ribs and/or clavicle
- Hyperextension neck injury
- Repetitive motion/injury
- Overuse injury

Muscular:
- Naffziger syndrome (Scalenus anticus syndrome)—hypertrophy of scalene muscles
- Short scalene muscles, trapezius or levator scapulae
- Reduced tone of trapezius, levator scapulae, rhomboids

ETIOLOGY

Thoracic outlet syndrome can occur due to various reasons (listed in **Box 1**) that can be grouped into four major groups as follows; more than one cause may affect the patient simultaneously.

1. *Congenital anomalies:* It may be bone anomalies like presence of cervical rib, prolonged transverse process of C7 cervical vertebra, elevation of the scapula, fibrous anomalies like presence of transversocostal and costocostal fibrous bands, muscular anomalies like abnormal insertion of scalenus anterior muscle or sickle-shaped scalenus medius muscle.
2. *Post-traumatic causes:* Like fracture of middle-third clavicle or upper ribs, hyperextension neck injuries and shoulder injuries (whiplash injury), injuries to the scalene muscle with their subsequent fibrosis.
3. *Functional acquired causes:* They are thought to be the most common causes of TOS. It includes adoption of abnormal postural habits, drooping shoulder conditions, heavy breasts, hypertrophy of the scalene muscles, decreased tone of trapezius and rhomboids, rapid weight loss due to vigorous physical activity, etc. Repetitive movements and overuse injury are increasingly recognized cause of TOS. Paget–Schroetter disease (effort thrombosis) is caused by strenuous repetitive activity of arms causing axillary or subclavian venous thrombosis.
4. *Other acquired causes:* Tumors such as Pancoast tumor, osteomyelitis, and exostosis of the first rib are rare causes.

CLINICAL PRESENTATION

The various clinical presentations of TOS depending on the structure being compressed are presented in **Table 1**. The following gives detailed description and explanation.

TABLE 1: Grouping of characteristic symptoms in different clinical forms of thoracic outlet syndrome (TOS).

True nTOS	*Mimicking nTOS*	*vTOS*	*aTOS*
• History of neck or shoulder girdle trauma/chest trauma • Paresthesia, neck pain, and/or weakness • Occipital headache • Symptoms present all throughout day and night • Loss of fine motor skills • Cold intolerance (possible Raynaud's phenomenon) • Demonstrable motor weakness • Compression of thoracic outlet aggravates symptoms usually in day. Activities include head forward + protracted shoulder posture, overhead activities, depressed shoulders	• History of neck trauma • Pain, paresthesia, and "feeling" of weakness • Occipital headaches • Nocturnal paresthesias awakening patient • Loss of fine motor skills • Cold intolerance • No demonstrable motor weakness • Release of tension or compression on thoracic outlet in night wakes up the patient—possible explanation is restoration of blood supply to the perineural region signaling return of normal sensation	• Young men with vigorous arm activity • Cyanosis • Feeling of heaviness of arm • Edema • Paresthesia in fingers and hand	• Overuse of extremity • Pain in hand • Claudication • Pallor • Cold intolerance • Paresthesias • Symptoms appear spontaneously

(nTOS: neurologic TOS; vTOS: venous TOS; aTOS: arterial TOS)

Neurological Symptoms

Most of the patients present with one of the neurological symptoms (95–98%). They may range from mild pain and sensory changes to limb- or life-threatening complications. Neurological TOS can be divided into two groups—true neurological thoracic outlet syndrome, associated with true neurological deficits (mainly muscular atrophy) and symptomatic TOS associated with symptoms of TOS without any neurological, radiological or electrophysical abnormalities. Most of the patients belong to latter group. The main symptoms are paresthesia (most common symptom), neck pain, numbness and/or weakness. The symptoms of the neurological TOS do not follow dermatomal or myotomal pattern. They can be categorized according to area or roots of the brachial plexus involved. If the upper plexus (C5–C7) is involved, the patient presents with ipsilateral neck or ear pain, pain over the face, mandible and occipital region, headache, pain over the clavicular and pectoral region moving toward trapezius and deltoid down lateral arm. If the lower plexus (C8–T1) is involved, patient presents with pain over anteroposterior aspect of shoulder radiating down to the medial side of arm, forearm and hand in the fourth and fifth fingers. Mostly, the symptoms are seen in all five fingers, but they are more pronounced in fourth and fifth digits. Atrophy of the abductor pollicis brevis results in deformity of the hand known as "Gilliatt-Sumner hand". The general features of neurological TOS includes headache with pain in the occiput area, exacerbation of pain with overhead activities or carrying heavy objects, numbness, and paresthesia in the upper limbs. The patient may develop progressive weakness and dysfunction of the hands. The timing of the symptoms is also important. Some patients may awake in the night because of paresthesia in the upper limb, the reason is thought as return of normal sensation after release of compression of the perineural blood supply to the brachial plexus (known as "release phenomenon"). Other patients have pain throughout the daytime because of using prolonged posture resulting in increased tension or compression on the brachial plexus (known as "compressors"). In trauma cases, the brachial plexus injury leading to nTOS results in Erb-Duchenne like palsy if the upper plexus is involved, and Klumpke's palsy if the lower plexus is involved. nTOS must be differentiated from other pathologies of the upper arm like carpal tunnel syndrome and cervical radiculopathy. In carpal tunnel syndrome, the symptoms originate in the hand and travel up in the forearm, while symptoms of the nTOS radiate from neck downward toward arm, forearm, and hand. The pain of cervical radiculopathy because of herniation of disk or stenosis is generally constant in nature instead of intermittent pain of nTOS, follows dermatomal pattern and most of the time, more severe and sharp than nTOS pain.

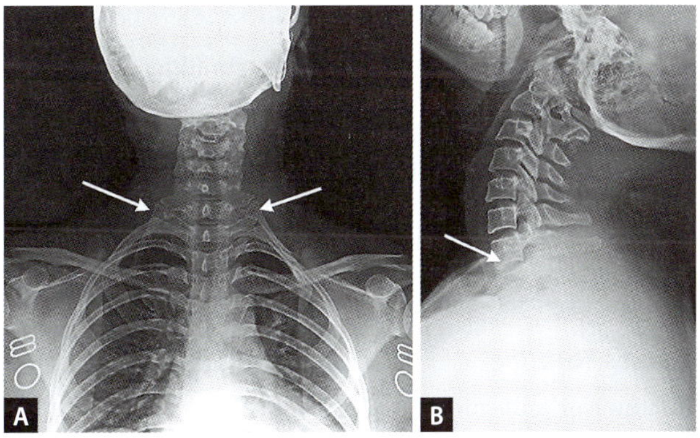

Figs. 2A and B: The radiographs of a 33-year-old female showing well-developed bilateral cervical rib (arrows) attached to the cervical 7th vertebra.

Arterial Symptoms

The symptoms are due to compression of the subclavian artery or its branches, mainly by the cervical rib **(Figs. 2A and B)**. The compression of the subclavian artery results in "poststenotic" arterial aneurysm. Thromboembolization may occur and dislodgment of clot results in distal ischemia and arm fatigue. With overhead activities, pallor, weak or absent pulses and coolness of the upper extremity result. All these symptoms worsen by exposure to cold. If vertebral artery is compressed, postural vertigo, balance difficulties, falls and drop attacks, diplopia, syncope, etc., may be present. Blood pressure difference between affected and nonaffected arm of >20 mm Hg is sometimes noted which indicates arterial involvement.

Venous Symptoms

This is also known as "effort thrombosis" or "Paget-Schroetter syndrome". Symptoms are due to compression of subclavian and axillary vein between clavicle and the first rib, mainly seen in young athletes involved with sports requiring frequent overhead activities like in swimmers, water polo, baseball players, etc. The symptoms include sudden spontaneous swelling of the upper limb, cyanosis of the arm, feeling of heaviness in arm, hand, and fingers, and pain in the upper extremity. Distended veins in the shoulder or chest are noted. Rarely, pulmonary embolism may occur.

PHYSICAL EXAMINATION

In inspection, asymmetry of the shoulders, drooping shoulders, large breasts should be noted.

During palpation, supraclavicular fossa for tenderness and scalene muscles for increased tone should be palpated.

The base of the examination is formed by stress tests or provocative tests, though it should be noted that they have low specificity, sensitivity, and predictive value.

Adson's Test

The anterior and middle scalene muscles are tensed in this test to see their compressive effects over axillary artery. The arm is abducted, externally rotated, and extended while the examiner locates the radial pulse. Patient is asked to turn the head toward the affected side, take a deep breath and hyperextend the neck. If the pulse is diminished or obliterated, it indicates compression of the axillary artery by the anterior scalene muscle. The patient now turns the head to the opposite side (reverse Adson's test); if the pulse is obliterated, it is due to middle scalene muscle. This test has high false-positive results.

Halstead Maneuver

The examiner continuously palpates patient's radial pulse applying downward traction on the tested arm while the patient rotates the head toward opposite side and hyperextend the neck. Disappearance of radial pulse indicates the compression of the neurovascular bundle by the cervical rib and the test is positive.

Wright's Hyperabduction Test

Patient's arm is passively abducted up to 180° and then extended; disappearance of the radial pulse indicates the compression of the neurovascular bundle between pectoralis minor and the rib cage in the subcoracoid space and the test is positive.

Roos Test

This is also called elevated arm stress test (EAST). Patient first keeps both the shoulders abducted and externally rotated to 90° with elbow flexed to 90°. Patients then rapidly open and close both the hands for 3 minutes. In case of arterial compromise, patient experiences cold sensation or fatigue in the involved extremity. Patient of TOS may not be able to keep both the arms in elevated position because of ischemic, vascular type of pain and the test is positive.

Retroclavicular Spurling's Test

Examiner compresses the brachial plexus and vascular structure by placing the thumb behind the clavicle in the retroclavicular space and depressing the thumb. Tingling or numbness in the tested limb indicates the positive test.

DIFFERENTIAL DIAGNOSES FOR THORACIC OUTLET SYNDROME

- Apical pulmonary neoplasm
- Brachial plexus neuritis
- Bursitis
- Cervical arthritis
- Cervical radiculopathy
- Cervical spondylosis
- Complex regional pain syndromes
- Fibrositis
- Glenohumeral joint instability
- Myositis
- Neoplasm of the peripheral nerve
- Peripheral nerve compression (cubital and carpal tunnels)
- Raynaud's disease
- Shoulder impingement syndrome
- Spinal metastasis
- Thromboangiitis
- Traumatic peripheral nerve lesions

DIAGNOSTIC STUDIES

- *X-rays:* Radiographs of chest and cervical spine should be obtained to find any underlying congenital or acquired bony abnormality such as presence of cervical rib, elongated process of C7 vertebra, Pancoast tumor, healed old fracture, etc.
- *Arteriography:* It demonstrates the extrinsic arterial compression and whether there is subclavian artery aneurysm. It is especially indicated in patients with ischemic upper extremity symptoms.
- *Venography:* Ascending brachial venography is the most definitive examination if venous thrombosis is suspected. It is generally indicated when duplex ultrasonography suggestive of venous abnormalities or if definitive symptoms of venous obstruction are present.
- *Electromyography:* In patients of TOS, these studies are usually negative. They are mainly indicated to rule out other pathologies with similar clinical features in which these tests are positive such as cervical radiculopathy, carpal tunnel and cubital tunnel syndrome.

- *MRI:* MRI, being a noninvasive and nonionizing study, is an attractive tool for soft tissue imaging. Findings suggestive of TOS are significantly smaller distance between the rib and the clavicle and compression of the brachial plexus in abduction images. Arterial and venous compressions can also be diagnosed by MRI.
- *Duplex ultrasonography:* It is the most dominant noninvasive test for vascular TOS. In neutral position and in abduction of the arm, velocities and waveforms are obtained, reduction of which in the abducted position is diagnostic of vascular TOS. In arterial TOS, the waveforms are reduced, but the velocities are either increased like in stenosis or absent like in complete occlusion.

TREATMENT

Nonoperative

Conservative treatment including nonsteroidal anti-inflammatory drugs (NSAIDs), strengthening and stretching exercises, ultrasound, transcutaneous nerve stimulation, occupational therapy, and biofeedback is sufficient for most of the patients and it must be the initial treating approach for the patient of TOS. If the symptoms do not respond to conservative treatment or worsens while the treatment, surgical intervention becomes necessary.

Treatment of Neurogenic Thoracic Outlet Syndrome

- *Physical therapy:* Physical therapy relieves the pressure on the thoracic outlet by correcting postural abnormalities and improving muscle imbalance. It will help in overcoming the shortening and tightness of the scalene muscles, weakness of the cervical flexor muscles, and poor diaphragmatic breathing. Various modalities used are deep heat or superficial heat therapy, ultrasound, stretching exercises, postural correction, and strengthening exercises. Most of the patients respond to this physical therapy, trial of which should be given for at least 3–12 months before going for surgical procedures.
- *Medications:* Nonsteroidal anti-inflammatory drugs such as aspirin, ibuprofen, and naproxen are used to reduce pain and inflammation of TOS.
- *Surgery:* If the symptoms persist despite the conservative therapy and interferes with activities of daily living, surgical decompression of the thoracic outlet becomes necessary.

Treatment of Venous Thoracic Outlet Syndrome

Thrombolytic and anticoagulation medicines are started to reduce the risk of blood clot formation, to dissolve the already formed clot, and to reduce the risk of pulmonary embolism. In patients with compression of the vein, surgical correction becomes necessary depending on the severity of the compression.

- *Thrombolytic medications:* They are used to promote lysis of the already formed clot and the thrombus in the occluded vessels. Angioplasty may be needed to open the occluded vein and to prevent further clot formation. Best results can be achieved with combination of thrombolytic and surgical decompression.
- *Anticoagulant medications:* This group includes drugs such as warfarin, heparin, low-molecular-weight heparin and fondaparinux. They are used to treat acute arterial and venous occlusion. If surgical procedures are done for venous TOS, anticoagulation must be continued for 3 months after the surgery.
- *Surgery:* As stated above, surgery may be necessary along with medications to correct the symptoms. The venous stenosis is corrected with angioplasty (<2 cm long lesion) or venous bypass surgery (>2 cm long lesion).

Treatment of Arterial Thoracic Outlet Syndrome

- *Surgery:* As the subclavian artery is obstructed in narrowed thoracic outlet, surgery may be required to decompress the space, like with removal of the first rib or with lysis of the abnormal fibrous bands. If the artery is injured, surgery may be necessary to repair the artery.
- *Thrombolytic medications:* It is given as the same way as described above for venous TOS.

Other medications: Other temporary treatment modalities are intra-articular or intramuscular cortisone injections and "scalene block" with the Botox injections that may provide relief for 3–4 months.

Operative Treatment

Only few of the patients with neurological TOS require surgical treatment, but most of the patients with venous or arterial TOS eventually need surgical decompression. If the conservative measures fail and the symptoms persist, surgical treatment may become necessary. It is mainly done to decompress the thoracic outlet. The procedure can be performed by either transaxillary approach, supraclavicular approach or by infraclavicular approach. With any of the approach, the goal of the surgery may involve:

- Partial or complete removal of the scalene muscles
- Removal of the first thoracic rib
- Removal of any supernumerary abnormal rib
- Removal of the fibrous band causing compression of the neurovascular bundle
- Removal of the subclavian artery aneurysm, if present, and reconstruction of the artery.

In surgical correction for all the three forms of TOS, the first rib and the anterior scalene muscles are removed. As the underlying brachial plexus is revealed, any fibrous scar tissue causing compression is searched and removed if found. Medial scalene muscle behind the brachial plexus is also removed. Now, the first rib is exposed and it is divided and removed. With an infraclavicular approach, pectoralis minor tendon may be removed if found necessary. For neurological TOS, this much decompression generally results in improvement of the patient's symptoms.

If the patient has arterial TOS, the extra cervical rib is also removed. Repair of the subclavian artery is done along with removal of the aneurysm and grafting with artificial vascular prosthesis to repair the artery.

If the patient has venous TOS, the entire first rib may need to be resected, subclavian vein needs to be freed from any scar tissue and if the vein remains occluded, angioplasty or bypass grafting becomes necessary.

Physical therapy is often used before and after the operation to decrease recovery time and improve outcomes.

COMPLICATIONS

Immediate Complications

- Pneumothorax
- Injury to thoracic duct
- Injury to subclavian artery
- Injury to subclavian vein
- Apical hematoma
- Injury to brachial plexus
- Injury to long thoracic nerve
- Intercostobrachial nerve injury
- Injury to phrenic nerve
- Rib fracture
- Lymphorrhea

Late Complications

- Intercostal neuralgia
- Causalgia in the surgical wound
- Development of new fibrous bands

CONCLUSION

Thoracic outlet syndrome is a complex constellation of neurological and vascular symptoms that complicated upon compression at thoracic outlet of passing neurovascular structures. It mimics various degenerative neurological conditions and in a precursory examination is bound to be missed. High index of suspicion should be borne in clinical examination if the presentation deviates from classical presentation of other contemporary common compressive or neurological conditions. Good understanding of varied presentation is necessary to correctly diagnose TOS. Early identification and treatment resolves the symptomatology quite appropriately.

CHAPTER 37

Nonunions and Malunions

Manish Kumar Varshney

INTRODUCTION

Standard orthopedic treatment (surgical or otherwise) is aimed at correcting bone alignment, primarily, but there is an increased perception among the patients and their relatives that it also "improves" or hastens healing. Failure of bone to unite is disheartening to patient and challenging to the surgeon due to involved complexities. Failure to unite can manifest in many ways and specific term should be used with diligence. The following are commonly used terms and are defined for most acceptable perception. The reader hitherto is encouraged to read also the fracture repair biology elsewhere in the text.

Slow Union

The term is used to refer "slow start" of the union process radiologically and clinically. There is, however, no biological or mechanical intrinsic deficit that will hamper process of healing in future. So the process of healing once kicks off; takes its normal course in terms of time to union and quality of united bone. The fracture takes ultimately longer than usual time to repair (union occurs finally) but passes through all the healing stages without departure from normal, both clinically and radiologically. It manifests as delayed callus formation radiologically. Most of the fixations done using open reduction and plate fixation tend to fall here as the bone healing process is "stunned" by stripping of periosteum and additional vascular compromise. This is also the reason why stress is put on periosteum sparing implants (like locked plates), biological fixation, minimally invasive procedures, and soft tissue protection. Some cases of tibial fractures managed with interlocked nail may also fall into this category; here, the cause is however the critical blood supply to bone itself that may be compromised to threshold level in few patients.

Delayed Union

Here the union process is normal to start with but somehow due to biological or more commonly mechanical inadequacies the process is partially interrupted and misses its original trajectory and timeline for fracture repair. Delayed union is defined as "the temporary failure of a fracture to heal in usual period of time, depending on the type and site of fracture and on the bone and soft tissue damage". It manifests as normal duration for callus formation that then somehow fails to consolidate into healing bone visible as persistent fracture line even after months. The progress is very slow and interruption of healing process is not complete but indicates surgeon to incorporate additional measures supporting it. Indeed with small measures such as stabilization by cast application, immobilization, traction, dynamization, or bone grafting the bone ultimately heals well. It is important to understand that "delayed union" can progress to nonunion or complete union depending on biology and the course taken by the treating surgeon with warning signs.

Clinical Warning Signs

- Persistent tenderness at the fracture site
- Mild persistent movement (in case not fixed)
- Presence of persistent nonresolving edema at the fracture and distally
- Discomfort and pain on using the limb for moderate activities

Radiological Warning Signs

- Persistent radiolucent line at the fracture site
- Persistent nonremodeling external or internal or both callus(es) at the fracture site
- Diminishing cortical thickness, somewhat increased medullary density
- Beginning of marginal rounding of fracture ends—"woolly" bone ends

Nonunion

This is the most confusing and most abused term to describe a failure of union. Though it indicates a specific entity of clinical, radiological **(Figs. 1A and B)** and biological permanent failure of fracture to unite (the term dictates endpoint and not merely an ongoing process); it is most difficult to describe and even interpret once the case is intermediary for differentiating delayed and nonunions.

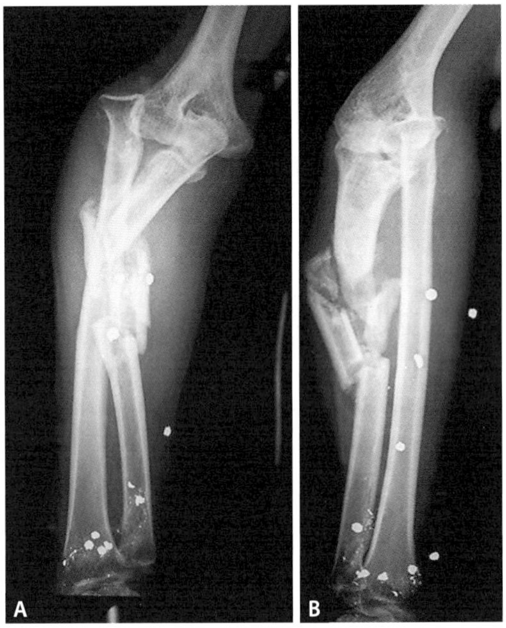

Figs. 1A and B: Nonunion of ulna. The proximal fragment of ulna shows sclerosis of the canal and obliteration. Note that the pattern is a Monteggia fracture dislocation with old unreduced radial head dislocation also.

Various definitions exist to understand nonunion, comprehensively are mentioned here.

- The failure of a fracture to heal in twice the usual period of time (at least 6 months after trauma) for type, site, and fracture pattern, this tends to define nonunion temporally in a generalized fashion. The greatest criticism is for use of "time duration" itself as it neither guides treatment nor can it be generalized for all fractures like tibial shaft and distal third fractures are seen to unite even at 8–9 months.
- Nonunion is a permanent failure of the fracture to heal—most succinct definition but useless as it provides no guide whatsoever to diagnose or treat itself. It is just an expansion of the term.
- Brinker defined nonunion of a fracture as a permanent end situation where the treating physician feels that the fracture will not heal unless some radical change in intervention is applied. This definition is completely subjective and opinions will vary depending on experience of treating surgeons.
- Nonunion of fracture is said to exist when the fracture shows clinically, radiologically, and biologically no signs of progression to repair itself after prolonged duration [United States Food and Drug Administration (US FDA) considers this as 9 months following injury with failure of progression for three consecutive months] for the type, site, and pattern of fracture and will not unite unless radical alteration in management is undertaken—comprehensive and most acceptable definition but quite speculative for future events "will not unite". This definition was basically developed for defining specific time-period to proceed for bone growth stimulator and adjunctive healing methods. It has been unanimously agreed that 9-months is excessive and hence FDA has dropped "9 months following injury" from definition.

Clinical signs include inability to bear weight due to instability, pain on bearing weight (impingement on surrounding tissues), abnormal mobility at nonunion site in various planes (with maintained implant in situ abnormal mobility cannot be elicited), pain at the site on stress examination, and warning signs of inflammation at the pathological site. Radiologically one does not see callus formation, persistent fracture line, resorption of the fracture ends, thinning of cortices, increased intramedullary density sometimes obliterating the canal completely, CT confirmation of lack of cortical continuity, and additionally implant failure may be seen in the form of broken implant or loosening of screws.

Pseudoarthrosis (Synovial Pseudoarthrosis)

This is defined as a fracture that has undergone nonunion and a cleft develops between the bone ends resembling joint formation with one end becoming convex and the other concave. Both the ends are completely closed from medullary cavity. The cleft or cavity gets filled with fluid and is lined by a membrane and pseudocapsule. The structure is hypermobile and has no restraints. Radiographically, the characteristic appearance is that of "mortar and pestle".

Ununited Fracture

This is a general term and very nonspecific that indicates the persistence of fracture line. It can indicate a uniting fracture in early stages, delayed union or nonunion. It should not be used in any parlance.

EPIDEMIOLOGY

Nonunion is not a very frequent problem. Only a small percentage of fractures (between 2 and 7%) undergo nonunion. Older reported distribution of nonunion among the long bones showed similar distribution among the tibia, femur, humerus, and forearm (Boyd). Newer reports demonstrate predominance of tibial nonunions (Connolly and Weizel, et al.). Incidence of delayed union and nonunion is higher in open diaphyseal fractures. For open tibial diaphyseal fractures, the nonunion rates increased from 40 to 90% with higher grade of open tibial shaft fractures. Cost analysis indicates significantly increased cost of treatment of nonunion that is highest with simplest (and mutilating) surgery, viz. amputation as the long-term cost of prosthesis fabrication and usage is quite high. Limb reconstruction with ring external fixators possibly is cheap and dependable methods for treating nonunion.

CLASSIFICATION

For clinical evaluation and mobility at nonunion site, the nonunions have been classified into:

- *Mobile (or lax) nonunion:* The arc of motion >7° with radiological defect >1 cm. This should be differentiated from pseudarthrosis (see above), CT scan or bone scan may help in differentiation.

- *Short-stiff (nonmobile) nonunions:* The arc of motion ≤7° (classically <1 cm defect radiologically) at nonunion site that is quite adequately bridged by fibrocartilage to resist movements grossly. Often only micromotion can be elicited; even the patient may bear weight partially in such cases.

 For practical purpose, the nonunion can be simply classified into:
 - Infected nonunion (with active or quiescent infection)
 - Noninfected nonunions

Noninfected Nonunions

The noninfected nonunions have been classified variedly by different authors. The most popular system is the modified Müller and Judet and Judet classification given by *Weber and Cech*. The system is based on radiographic, scintigraphic (strontium-83) and histologic appearance, according to the viability of bone ends **(Figs. 2A to G)**. Scintigraphic studies show a rich blood supply in the hypertrophic types (hypervascular nonunion) and a poor blood supply in the ends of fragments in the atrophic types (avascular nonunions).

Hypervascular Nonunion

- *Elephant foot:* They have hypertrophic callus formation and result from either inadequate fixation/immobilization or premature weight-bearing. This is commonly seen in closed treatment of diaphyseal fractures with poor stability. Increasing mechanical stability will usually permit union.
- *Horse hoof:* The ends are mildly bulbous exceeding the thickness of bone with lesser callus formation. Commonly this is seen in mildly unstable plate osteosynthesis or moderately unstable intramedullary fixation/plaster cast. Also it is seen in metabolic bone diseases.
- *Oligotrophic:* The ends are not hypertrophic but callus is also absent and result from inadequate apposition, displaced fracture, and distracted fragments with adequate vascularity. As it is difficult to differentiate from atrophic nonunions—scintigraphy may help by demonstrating vascularized ends.

Avascular Nonunion

- *Torsion wedge (dystrophic) nonunion:* The intermediate butterfly (wedge) fragment has compromised blood supply that heals to one main fragment of bone but not to other. It is termed dystrophic as there is still some viability remaining evident in partial healing.
- *Comminuted (necrotic) nonunion:* Has one or more necrotic fragments in between that fails to unite to any fragment and remains isolated disrupting the continuity of the repair process. Commonly seen after open plating of a comminuted fracture.
- *Defect (gap) nonunion:* In open fractures or sequestration process of long-standing osteomyelitis, the intermediate fragment or a part of bone is lost in full circumference (differentiating from torsion wedge or necrotic non-union). These often need intercalary graft or staged grafting (like membrane inducing technique) with or without antibiotic spacers.
- *Atrophic:* The ends of bone are osteoporotic and atrophic due to lack of trophic factors and loss of blood supply.

Paley classification of nonunion specifically deals with legs bones and is based on bone loss, fracture laxity, deformity, and shortening **(Figs. 3A and B)**.

- *Type A (<1 cm bone loss):*
  - A1: Mobile deformity
  - A2: Fixed deformity
    - A2-I: Stiff nonunion without deformity
    - A2-II: Stiff nonunion with fixed deformity
- *Type B (>1 cm bone loss):*
  - B1: Bony defect no shortening
  - B2: Shortening but no defect
  - B3: Both (shortening with defect)

Infected Nonunion

Presence of infection completely changes the perspective and management plan. One should take detailed history and perform directed investigations to determine if nonunion is septic. Usually the history of open fracture, presence of local drain for longer duration, prolonged antibiotic usage, history of pus discharge, recent infections in other parts of body, dental hygiene, etc. Additionally total leukocyte counts

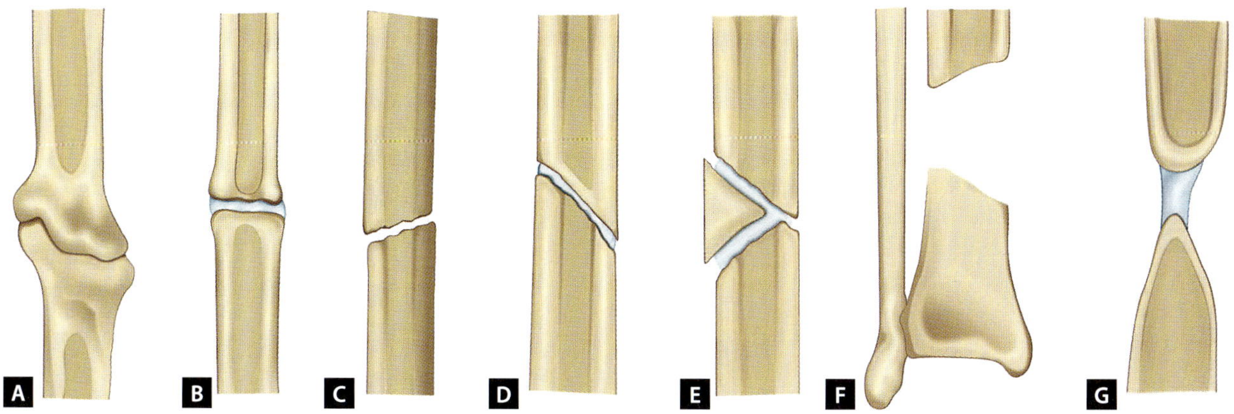

Figs. 2A to G: Weber and Cech classification of nonunion. (A) Elephant foot; (B) Horse hoof; (C) Oligotrophic; (D) Torsion wedge; (E) Comminuted; (F) Gap; and (G) Atrophic nonunions.

(TLCs) (with differential counts), erythrocyte sedimentation rate (ESR), C-reactive protein (CRP), and procalcitonin (>0.4 ng/mL, good indicator of pyogenic infection) should be assessed. *Infected nonunions* are also classified by various authors. As infection is the prominent component that needs to be addressed the *Cierny and Madar* classification is quite useful [*see* Chapter on "Infections of Bone (Typical and Atypical) and Surgical Site Infection"]. *Umiarov* divided infected nonunions into four types based on the viability of bone ends, the presence of limb shortening, the presence of bone and soft tissue defect.

- *Type I:* Normotrophic without shortening
- *Type II:* Hypertrophic with shortening
- *Type III:* Atrophic with shortening
- *Type IV:* Atrophic with bone and soft tissue defect usually with shortening

May and Jupiter classification for post-traumatic osteomyelitis of tibia also describes infected nonunion in types III, IV, and V.

- *Type I:* Intact tibia and fibula capable of withstanding functional loads
- *Type II:* Intact tibia needing bone graft for only structural support
- *Type III:* There is tibial defect 6 cm or less with intact fibula
- *Type IV:* The tibial defect is >6 cm with intact fibula
- *Type V:* The tibial defect is >6 cm with no usable fibula

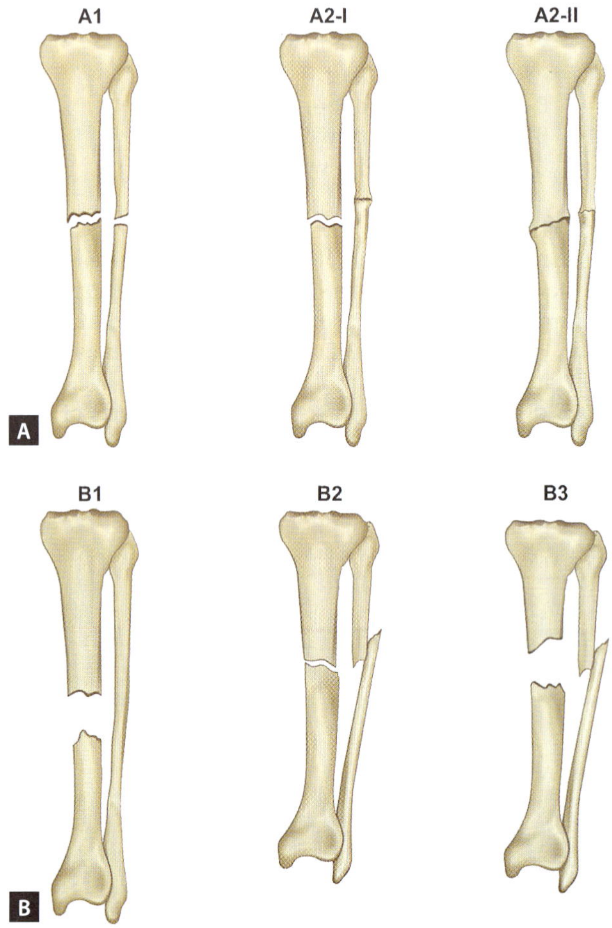

Figs. 3A and B: Paley classification of nonunion of leg bones.

PATHOGENESIS

There are a number of identified and possible *risk factors* that may be responsible for development of nonunion **(Table 1)**. The bone commonly fails to unite due to organizational defect in callus or its formation. The connective tissue in the interior of *the callus undergoes fibrinoid degeneration* similar to chronic adventitious bursitis. The degeneration is primarily due to lack of bone trophic factors and reduced vascularity resulting from extensive trauma, inadequate immobilization (preventing neovascularization and consolidation), and infection. The fibrocartilage continues to degenerate into fibrinoid tissue with uncontrolled motion and friction at the fracture site and may result in pseudoarthrosis formation if not controlled. The fibrinoid unlike fibrocartilage has no propensity to bone formation and does not support osteogenesis by induction. The surrounding tissue with continued excessive motion develops into fibrous capsule and adventitious bursa like tissue containing fluid. This is lined by pseudoendothelium forming a false joint called pseudoarthrosis.

In open fractures and fractures reduced by open methods a larger amount of bone needs to be resorbed before repair. The fracture personality is such that the bone may not unite in such cases. The bone derives significant portion of blood supply from the surrounding soft tissue that gets lost in open fractures. Often with high energy injuries bone-loss frequently accompanies.

Infection per se does not directly inhibit union but has some bearing on repair process as follows:

- Elevation of periosteum by pus that devascularizes the ends

TABLE 1: Possible factors responsible for development of nonunion.

Systemic factors	*Local factors*
• Age (elderly) • Malnutrition (albumin <3.4 g/dL; lymphocyte count <1,500/mm^3) or malabsorption syndrome including bypass procedures (Roux-en-Y, etc.) • Corticosteroid therapy • Immunosuppressive treatment • Systemic disease (hepatic and renal) • Diabetes mellitus (secondary to neurovascular compromise) • Metabolic bone disease, hyperparathyroidism, hypothyroidism, vitamin D deficiency, testosterone deficiency • Anticoagulants • Nonsteroidal anti-inflammatory drug (NSAID) therapy • Burns • Smoking, narcotic, or tobacco abuse • Alcohol • Radiation	*Fracture related* • Site (fracture neck of femur, scaphoid, capitellum, fracture neck of talus, lateral condyle of humerus fractures, and diaphyseal fractures of distal third tibia) • Open • Infected • Comminuted • Segmental • Fractures of irradiated bone • Intra-articular fractures *Treatment related* • Inadequate reduction • Inadequate immobilization • Inadequate fixation • Inadequate blood supply • Inadequate soft tissue cover • Interposition of soft tissue • Inadequate apposition "distraction"

- Dissolution of fracture hematoma
- Alteration of the cytokine milieu by inflammatory mediators that promote fibrous tissue formation
- Implant gets loosened by reduced purchase on the poor and osteoporotic bone which destabilizes the fracture and causes gross movements
- There is increased catabolic activity at the fracture ends than the required anabolic activity for fracture repair.

Smoking decreases peripheral oxygen tension (increased carbon monoxide levels forming carboxyhemoglobin) and reduces the blood flow possibly through vasoconstriction, arteritis, or atherosclerosis. Thrombus formation and microembolization via platelet aggregation also potentially limit tissue perfusion. There is also a possible inhibition of osteoblasts and inflammatory cells directly. Smoking has been associated with nonunion of scaphoid fracture and ulnar osteotomies and increases risk of nonunion, infection, and wound complications in open tibia fractures. Alcohol abuse has been closely linked to problems of fracture healing primarily by inducing malnutrition (vitamin, mineral, protein, and calorie malnutrition). It is recommended that an adult with a fracture receive *two times* the amount of daily recommended intake of calcium for age. Beneficial role has been shown in proximal humerus fractures. Surgeon should however note that intake is not same as absorption so history of malabsorption (light-colored bulky soft stools, hair loss, bloating, flatulence, history of gastric bypass, celiac disease, short bowel syndrome, inflammatory bowel disease, etc.) should be obtained. Calorie requirement for a polytrauma patient has been similarly estimated to *three times* the normal of active adult.

Osteoporotic bones show altered pattern of fracture repair and may be predisposed to delayed/nonunion. There are two aspects to it; one is the possible biological inferiority of the osteoblastic cells or bone matrix in these bones to respond to the fracture. This may be due to the reduced number or intrinsic qualitative defect of the cells or/and reduced matrix content to form callus. The other is the reduced fixation strength of the implants used and hence the not-so-stable mechanical construct (plate/nail, etc.) to support fracture repair. Patients with poliomyelitis have no bony pathology that would preclude fracture union but due to deficient muscle mass remodeling would be delayed or inadequate (vide Wolff's law in Chapter on "Fracture Repair, Bone Grafting, and Bone Banking").

Patients with diabetes, neuropathy, peripheral vascular disease, and renal dysfunction have higher rates of infection following surgery and bones take longer time to unite. The initial inflammatory response to fracture in disorganized and results in hyperemia, osteopenia, and excessive bone resorption.

Fixation method and soft tissue handling are important factors influencing fracture repair:

- Inadequate immobilization + adequate blood supply—there is attempt by body at extensive callus formation to stabilize the bone but it ultimately fails leading to hypertrophic nonunion (failed endochondral ossification).

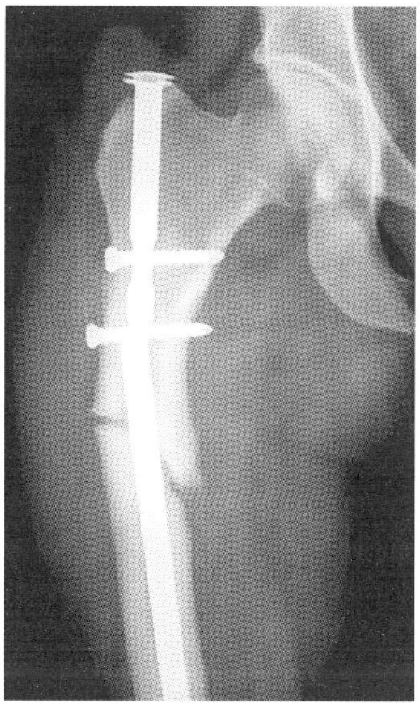

Fig. 4: Nonunion subtrochanteric fracture. This patient was operated 7 months ago and now presents with nonunion and nail breakage. The case exemplifies poor choice of implant (inadequate fixation) and possibly also inadequate apposition of the fragments that were fixed in distraction.

- Poor blood supply + inadequately immobilized bone—will produce atrophic (avascular) nonunion **(Fig. 4)**.
- Adequate blood supply + displaced fracture fragments (inadequate reduction)—oligotrophic nonunion.

DIAGNOSIS

The diagnosis rests on clinical examination supplemented with radiological investigations. History specifically concerning the nutritional status, systemic diseases, weight, and fracture history (damage to soft tissues, type and duration of previous treatment, pain, motion at the fracture site, soft tissue swelling, neurovascular limb compromise, and presence of infection). Physical examination demonstrates classical findings. On inspection, look for signs of active (discharging sinus) or past [scar, tethered skin, discoloration (dressing material and hyperpigmentation), and irregular bone due to periosteal reaction] infection. At the nonunion site, there can be angular or rotational deformity, swelling due to hypervascular nonunion or pseudoarthrosis, and bayoneting of fragments can be seen in subcutaneous location. Wasting and shortening are other common findings. On palpation check for raised local temperature due to infection, palpate the defect, and elicit tenderness with nail of thumb. The hallmark of nonunion is presence of abnormal painless mobility at the nonunion that is present in two perpendicular planes and also on axial rotation. Also with axial rotation, there is loss of transmitted movements proximally. Painless crepitus (differentiating from acute fracture) is also a characteristic. Telescopy and distraction of fragments are found in lax nonunion. Always end examination with evaluating the range of motion (ROM) of nearby joints as stiffness due to previous treatment and disuse is common and has a bearing on treatment and prognosis.

Although painless mobility at fracture site is characteristic but nonunion can also be painful in certain circumstances especially, if:

- There is an infection at the nonunion (inflamed tissues)
- Implant is present that can irritate the periosteum due to loose screws
- Periosteum, muscle, or neural tissues are interposed between fracture ends
- There is nearby adventitious bursa formation that has got inflamed
- Bayonet fragments that impinge the surrounding tissues
- Intra-articular nonunion with secondary osteoarthritis (OA)

INVESTIGATIONS

Radiographs

Radiographs should be obtained always in two perpendicular planes and oblique views are also helpful sometimes. Stress views for demonstration of deformation at fracture site objectively demonstrate nonunion. Typically, the varus-valgus and anteroposterior (AP) stress is employed. Radiographs show some characteristic features:

- *Delayed union:*
  - Slight resorption of bone ends with "woolly" appearance (no evidence of sclerosis or very slight)
  - Medullary canal is open at both ends
  - Fracture line is clearly visible
  - External and internal callus are minimal
- *Nonunion:*
  - Marked sclerosis of ends with rounding off appearance **(Figs. 5A to E)**
  - Medullary canal closed
  - Diffuse osteoporosis of both fragments
  - Fracture gap persists and widened due to unsuccessful bridging
  - Proximal end convex and distal end concave (pseudoarthrosis)

Computed Tomography

Any doubt for cortical continuity can be readily evaluated with high-resolution CT and three-dimensional (3D) reconstruction. It is especially useful for oblique and spiral fracture.

Magnetic Resonance Imaging

Magnetic resonance imaging (MRI) can be used for evaluation of vascularity of the fragments and small bones. Especially, bones susceptible for osteonecrosis due to fracture (scaphoid, talus, and head of femur) should be evaluated using MRI.

Bone Scan

- Used to detect the presence of synovial pseudoarthrosis—a cold cleft is seen between two areas of high uptake.
- Scintigraphy is employed to assess nonunion biological activity and infection.
- Scintigraphy is a particularly useful technique to distinguish hypervascular active nonunion and non-responsive avascular nonunions.
- Indium scans are more sensitive and specific for diagnosing infections.

Positron Emission Tomography Scan

Positron emission tomography scan increases the sensitivity and specificity when combined with bone scan and MRI for diagnosing infection and vascularity but cost is a prohibiting factor.

Laboratory investigations are aimed to find infection at the nonunion site and include ESR, CRP, and TLC. Renal and liver functions are other investigations that can be done to find risk factors. For choosing surgical treatment nutritional status of the patient should also be evaluated.

Bone biopsy is rarely if ever employed to diagnose non-union.

TREATMENT

The treatment of nonunion is aimed to achieve a durable union of the fracture ends allowing patient to regain reasonable function of the limb. The objectives include obtaining proper alignment, correcting the shortening, improving muscle strength, and neurovascular status along with achieving union. The treatment in infected nonunions

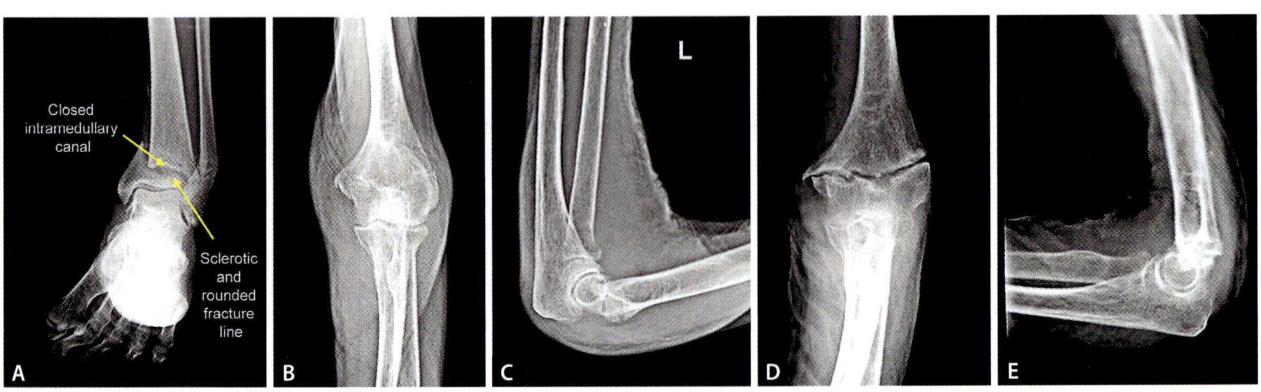

Figs. 5A to E: Typical radiographic features of nonunion. (A) The fracture line is sclerotic with closed intramedullary canal; (B and C) Even innocuous looking fractures managed conservatively may go into nonunion (D and E).

is aimed at healing and eradication of infection to gain a functional limb.

The various options can be grouped into following approaches (*see* also Chapter on "Fracture Repair, Bone Grafting, and Bone Banking")

Nonsurgical Measures

There are some specific situations where reconstruction of nonunion should either not be offered at all or at least delayed. Surgeon should balance the burden of reconstruction compared to possible deficit or functional gain envisaged. At nonunions of clavicle, fibula, pubic or ischial rami and sometimes humerus that patient has merely presence of radiographic nonunion which is clinically stiff, aseptic, functionally aligned, and with minimal pain. Other situation is where patient is medically unfit for extensive surgical procedures like class "C" host in Cierny-Mader classification. These need no treatment possibly. Some patients have unrealistic pain and functional gain expectations that need thorough moderation before adventurous multiple or single procedure(s) are undertaken, as dissatisfaction is bound to occur later. Delay the procedure in these situations, counsel the patient and bring them to realistic expectation. The following nonsurgical measures are most viable in these patients taken on an individualized basis.

- Continuation of cast immobilization (Watson-Jones additionally recommended traction)—occasional nonunion heals by these measures **(Figs. 6A to F)**.

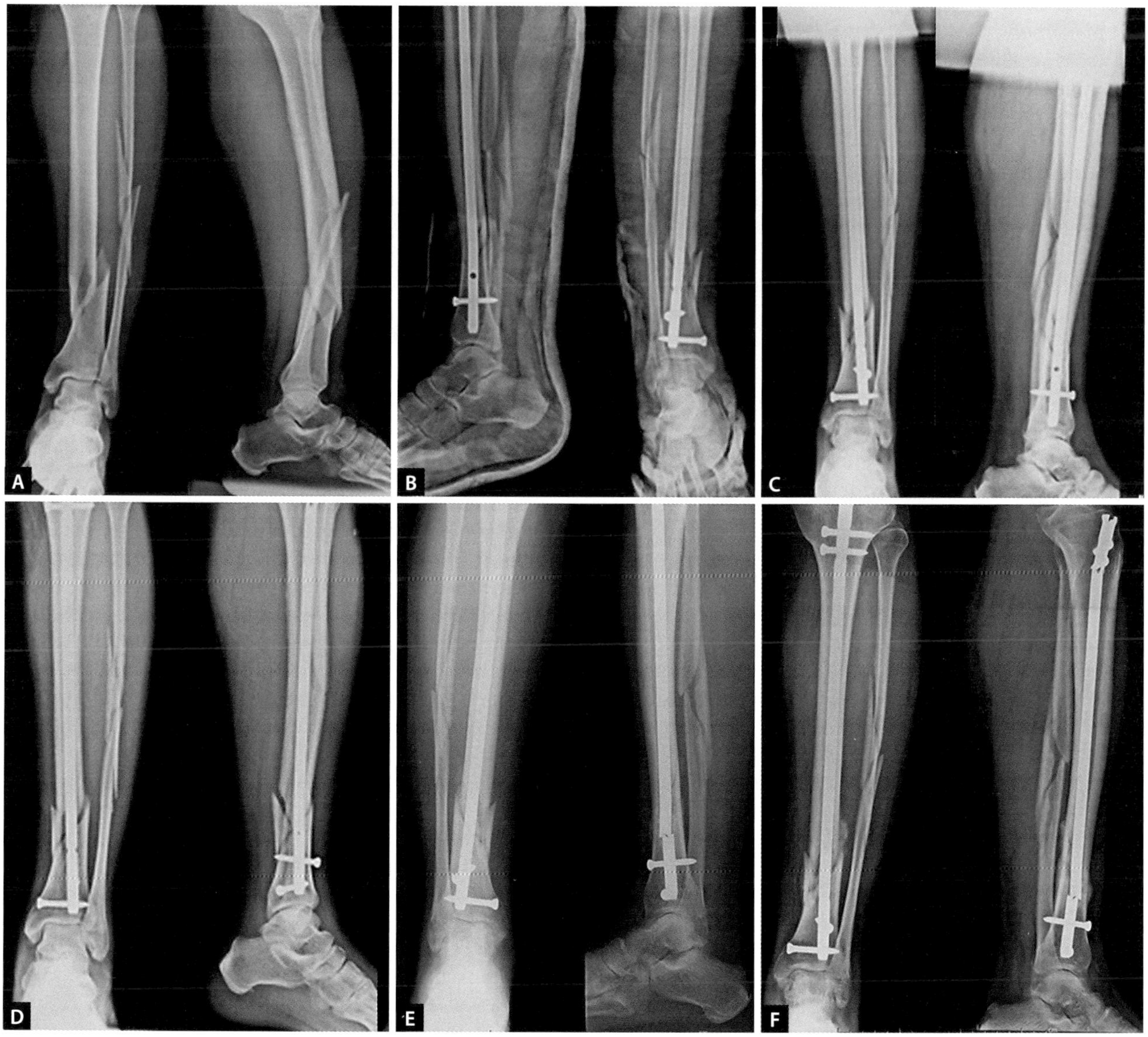

Figs. 6A to F: The patient suffered from high velocity motor vehicle accident sustaining fracture of both tibia and fibula (A), he may manage with locked intramedullary nail but due to less than satisfactory fixation was put on plaster of Paris (POP) slab immobilization for 3 weeks (B). Patient was mobilized toe-touch walk with walker but fracture still did not show any signs of healing by 4 months (C). Status quo was maintained still at 6 months (D). The patient presented to us and was managed with full weight-bearing walk in Sarmiento type brace—though the nail broke the fracture did show signs of healing (E) and progressed rapidly with good healing at 8 months (F)

- Pharmacotherapy—vitamin D has been found useful in animals. Bisphosphonates have been tried but results are equivocal. Various unconventional drugs such as arginine, collagen specific amino acids, *Cissus quadrangularis*, boron, and magnesium have been sporadically mentioned but no definitive study is available to this effect. There is a possible likelihood of the use of teriparatide (an anabolic drug used in osteoporosis management) for treatment of delayed union, especially in atypical fractures or osteoporotic fractures.

Biophysical stimulation (see also Chapter on "Fracture Repair, Bone Grafting, and Bone Banking" for detailed description of the methods):
- Extracorporeal shockwave
- Ultrasound stimulation
- Electrical stimulation

Surgical methods:
- Osteosynthesis by external and internal fixation
- Compression-distraction osteogenesis (DO)
- Bone grafts
- Bone graft substitutes
- Adjunctive measures such as bone marrow injection, platelet rich plasma and bone growth supporting molecules.

Treatment Principles for Surgical Management of Nonunion

The indications for surgical treatment of nonunion in eligible patients include the following:
- Presence of objective functional deficits that can be improved
- Failed hardware with concerns of migration and additional tissue damage with nonunion of fracture
- Presence of uncontrolled infection with nonunion that needs treatment
- Complaints of pain on loading the nonunion precluding mobilization

Nonunions with retained implants (broken or intact): Prevalent usage of operative orthopedics for management of fractures has made it a common place to see nonunions with retained hardware. There are a few dictums and procedures one should always keep in mind, as follows:
- Implants once failed can fail again! Removal of retained implant is imperative in case they have failed (broken). Now the first issue is whether to use the same type of implant again—common sense says NO! One should switch implants preferably using intramedullary for a failed extramedullary implant but failed intramedullary implants are commonly retreated with intramedullary implants. Second issue is whether to retain an intact implant. For this I would state that every implant has a run-through strength for given number of loading cycles and it is impossible to determine how many loading cycles has the implant gone through and it may be at critical point of giving away so one should better consider replacing it with a newer one (individualize in each case).

Implant removal is always tricky and more difficult than putting in implants during primary osteosynthesis. Plan your best thoroughly and communicate to your team but expect the worst. Things get weird and harder quickly, take time in each step and try not to spoil the already challenged implant. Have a full gamut of implant removal tools and also think out-of-box, some tools meant for other purpose might become suddenly useful for a different situation. Be open to suggestions, be patient and do expect to break some common tools in the "stuck-up" situations. Some commonly practiced and recommended methods (with experience) to remove implants are presented below.

- *Failed intramedullary nails:* The nails commonly break or may bend (uncommon). Broken proximal portion can be removed by engaging the locking bolt of jig or universal locking bolt from nail removal set—ensure not to damage the threads of nail. Removal of distal broken portion is challenging—one can use a long guidewire with tip hook from nail removal set or one may custom make a guidewire with bent tip (say from Ilizarov wires, etc.). Other method is to use a ball tipped guidewire slightly bent at the tip. Negotiate it through the nail and once crossed the nail tip, stack the cannulated nail with other wires/pins so as to get an interference fit. Attach a T-handle to the first guidewire that negotiated the tip and extract the portion. If it is not possible to approach the nail antegrade then one can make a small bone window in the retained nail portion and try pushing the nail proximally (make a hole in nail and push back up). Femoral nail broken distal portion can also be pushed up through knee (as for making entry hole of distal femoral nails) should the nail be not approachable antegrade. Nails that are bent and not broken often need cutting them at the bend using metal cutting burs or disc and then removing the fragments. Sometimes the nail bend is only mild and it can be extracted like an unbent nail (take care not to shatter bone in the process). All this is possible once the locking bolts have been removed successfully!—very often one sees broken locked bolts itself. Remove the head portion in usual manner. The far end of bolt can often be pushed/tapped across other cortex using sturdy pins through the nail holes, else if the far end is protruding enough from the other cortex then one can twist remove the portion from other end using counter-incision and vise-grip pliers. In very extreme cases the far end broken bolts and/or broken distal fragment of nail may be left in place (extraction impossible) if a reconstruction procedure is planned that would bypass the fragment.
- *Failed plate and screw constructs:* This presents a myriad of possibilities but some principles are common. Always loosen all the screws first before removing them sequentially, screws may fail anywhere and may compromise implant removal anytime. Often it is recommended to tighten the screw gently to break contact with bone (I do not recommend it for locked screw-plate implants mostly). Screw-head recess (where

screw-driver fits into the head) failure is most common, especially with substandard implants. Always completely visualize the screw-head-recess before engaging the driver and derotating it manually (power drives are not good for this purpose). Use good quality screw drivers (keep them separate for this purpose only!) in the first go because once the recess is stripped removal becomes very hard. Once stripped one may try filling the irregularity in recess with a lap and then use a screw-driver or use different screw-driver (say a start shaped driver for a hexagonal recess). One can use reverse thread cutting conical bolts to dig into the recess and remove the screw. One may instead use a vise-grip plier to hold the screw head and derotate it (some bone removal may be needed in this case along the screw head to gain purchase). If all fails one may drill/burr-off the screw head and remove plate followed by removal of the retained shaft. Screw-run-out failure is the breakage of screw at neck portion (beneath the undersurface of screw head and first screw-thread)—it is similar to burred-off screw head. The shaft portion can be removed using hollow-mill reamer that drills a hole in the bone around the screw-shaft and helps removal *en masse* else one can use an extraction bolt that has reverse threads and gets locked into the screw shaft providing necessary torque force. Jammed locking screws (or cold wedded locking screws) are a special situation that need metal cutting implants to burr away the plate screw interface or in rarer circumstances whole screw head. Broken or intact plates often need separation from integrated soft tissue or bone before removal. Then they can be removed by gentle twisting movements.

Some general principles involved in managing the various common scenarios pertaining to nonunions are presented below.

- Infected and noninfected nonunions can both be managed with compression distraction method commonly provided with Ilizarov method (see here).
- For infected nonunion with active infection and discharging pus initially thorough debridement should be done followed by second stage stabilization ± bone grafting when the infection settles.
- For infected nonunion with quiescent infection single stage debridement with Ilizarov fixation ± bone grafting may suffice.
- For *hypervascular nonunions* in thigh and upper extremity, Ilizarov method is cumbersome so other surgical techniques are commonly employed:
  - Long bone nonunion (femur, tibia, and humerus) that has been treated with nailing can be very well managed with *exchange nailing* using a larger diameter nail **(Figs. 7A to C)**. This has following advantages:
    - Better stabilization of the nonunion due to larger nail diameter
    - Providing bone graft (autograft) from reaming at the endosteal side
    - Stimulation of bone formation by reaming process that alters blood flow making it centripetal from the usual centrifugal one. There is increased vascularity at the periosteal side and surrounding soft tissue that enhance the migration and maturation of multipotent cells in the cambium layer of periosteum.
    - The nonunion site is grossly untouched surgically so preventing additional loss of vascularity from periosteal stripping or soft tissue trauma.
    - The reaming process also debrides the fibrous tissue formed at the nonunion site giving way to formation of newer callus and fibrocartilaginous tissue capable of healing the bone.
    - Sometimes for a distracted fracture compression can be achieved by backslapping the new nail.
  - If the cause of nonunion is torsional instability following nailing, then it is advisable to use *augmentative/auxiliary unicortical plate fixation* (preferably locked plate) ± bone grafting (usually not necessary as it is a mechanical failure).
  - *Plate fixation and bone grafting:* Exchange plating is a viable option for stable nonunions that can be loaded without excessive shortening especially in metaphyseal regions or juxta-articular nonunions. For femoral metaphyseal nonunions, if site permits the application of locked distal femoral plates with bone grafting is preferred for distal nonunions. For proximal femoral nonunion, proximal femoral nail with bone grafting is a better option. If the nonunion is too near the trochanteric region, then dynamic condylar screw with plate construct or condylar blade plate with bone grafting is preferred. Shortening is a concern in lower limb though up to 4 cm can be managed with shoe raise. Shortening more than this may need secondary procedure to improve limb length (say by Ilizarov method or monolateral distractors). In upper limb, shortening is not that much of concern though excessive shortening does impair function. For humerus 4–5 cm of shortening is acceptable. For forearm bones up to 4 cm of shortening will not impair function, if needed to achieve union.
  - *Arthroplasty:* If the site of nonunion is too near the joint, then hinge prosthetic replacement could be an option in less active population (in active population allograft and plate fixation is desirable). In distal humerus as the longevity of arthroplasty and functional results are somewhat subdued, reconstructing using bone and onlay bone grafting with dual plate fixation can be done in select cases.

THE PRINCIPLE OF DISTRACTION OSTEOGENESIS AND ITS APPLICATION TO NONUNION OF LONG BONES

Distraction osteogenesis is a surgical technique in which the intrinsic capacity of bone to regenerate is being harnessed for various purposes. Controlled stress to a biologically created bone defect is utilized to this effect. The method emanated from the observation that hypertrophic callus

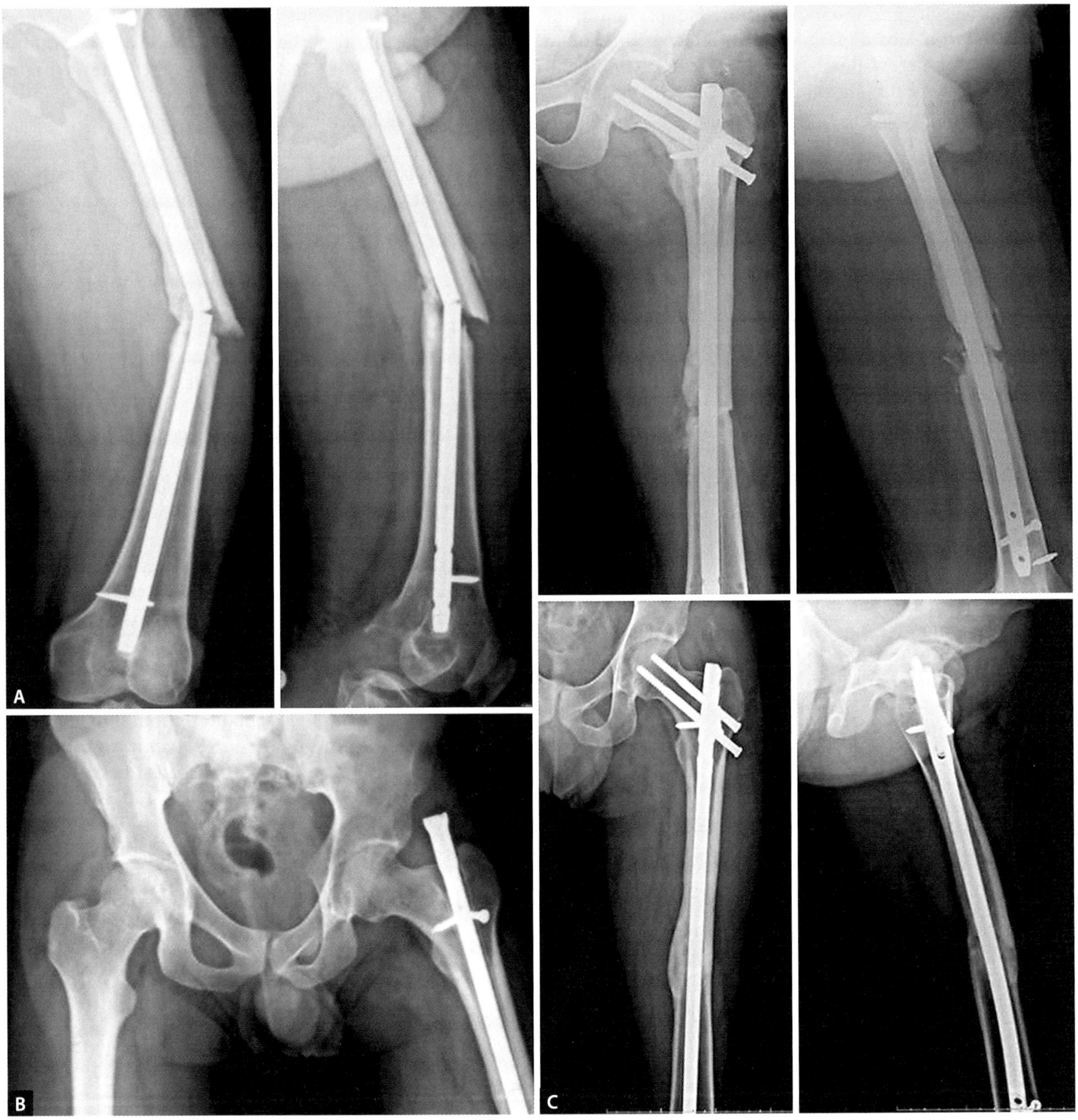

Figs. 7A to C: Exchange nailing for treating nonunion diaphyseal fractures. The patient was managed for fracture of left femur diaphysis by an intramedullary nail. (A) The implant choice was bad with a longer nail causing fracture distraction and inability to lock distally (the metallic piece is a broken drill bit in the anterior muscles!). (B) The patient was managed with exchange nailing using a recon nail of larger diameter and (C) fracture united completely in 7 months.

when subjected to "tension-stress" ossifies and forms new bone. The principle was highlighted by Professor Gavril Abramovich Ilizarov (propagated as law of tension-stress) from Kurgan in Western Siberia in early 1950s. The "hidden technique" of his practice was highlighted and brought to the modern world by an Italian explorer "Carlo Mauri" who was treated of resistant nonunion by GA Ilizarov. The underlying principle is that "living tissues when subjected to slow, steady traction (distortional strain), under appropriate conditions (of vascularity and alignment) become metabolically active and regenerate indefinitely". So, this principle is not restricted to bone only, any living tissue can be indefinitely regenerated (including soft tissues). The term "appropriate conditions" in the statement above should be properly understood as it underlies the biological principles essential for success of the method, these can be summarized as:

- Minimal disturbance of bone—use of corticotomy (see below)
- Delay before distraction—this provides sort of conditioning effect for distraction. The bone prepares healing and *osteogenesis* (or new bone formation) begins that can then be utilized for progressively increasing bone

formation in the form of "regenerate". This new tissue is just a regenerative tissue (so better called "distraction neohistogenesis") that under adequate conditions will form bone so the term "regenerate" was originally chosen instead of callus. Duration of delay varies (5 days in a child to 7 days, in adult and even more in elderly—nearly 10 days). *Callotasis* as a concept was introduced by DeBastiani in 1980s. This depends on increasingly organization of callus tissue for reliable bone formation. As callus takes minimum 2 weeks so here the delay or priming period was kept at 2 weeks.

- Rate of distraction—Ilizarov recommended a rate of distraction of 1 mm/day by his various experiments and he proposed motorized distraction for continuous distraction throughout the day. However, for sake of convenience, it is divided into four equal periods as 6 hourly intervals where 0.25 mm distraction is done at each siting (0.25 × 4 = 1 mm). Faster distractions commonly cause poor regenerate formation and "shark-bite" lesions which usually fail to form new bone and are prone to nonunion. A rate of 1.5 mm/day may be still acceptable in children but in no case in adults should it ever exceed 2 mm/day. Slower distraction rates 0.5 mm/day or less are prone to premature consolidation.
- Rhythm of distraction—the higher the frequency of distraction the better is the quality of regenerate. So Ilizarov himself recommended motorized distraction throughout the day.
- Site of the osteotomy—metaphyseal corticotomy is the best place for optimal result as it has larger surface area and good quality osteogenic cells in high numbers. Also the nutritional artery has already branched so chances of arterial injury are minimal. Soft tissue in metaphyseal region are better adapted for changes in length (effect of growth plate in the region) and have intimate bony insertions providing additional vascular feeding in case the endosteal supply inevitably gets disrupted. Diaphyseal osteotomy (cortical bone) is, however, required in certain cases but should be based on the principles of corticotomy. This diaphyseal corticotomy is called "compactotomy" to distinguish the counterpart at metaphysis.
- Number of lengthening sites should be physiologically determined—the physiological limit of number of lengthening sites probably varies with the type of bone. For tibia lengthening at two sites is common (bifocal), some even perform trifocal lengthening (rare), instead the common variant is bifocal lengthening and compression at the third site. Femur is less tolerant to multiple site osteotomies and nonunion is commonly seen in bifocal procedures here.

Physiological Aspects of Distraction Osteogenesis

Molecular and Cellular Events in Distraction Osteogenesis

Regenerate and bone formation is basically a physiological process closely resembling fracture healing. Hematoma formation followed by fibrous and fibrocartilaginous tissue formation in a longitudinal pattern along the direction of distraction is seen with progressive distraction. New bone is formed from periosteum, cortex, and spongiosa that proceeds from the osteotomy cuts toward the center supported by a fibrous "radiolucent interzone" located at the center of regenerate. As one proceeds from center of regenerate to cut bone ends the bone maturation increases. A process of mechanotransduction underplays at the regenerate—mechanical tension-stress forces due to distraction of the bony segments stimulate molecular signals and cytokines [bone morphogenetic protein (BMP), fibroblast growth factor (FGF), insulin-like growth factor (IGF), platelet-derived growth factor (PDGF), transforming growth factor-beta (TGF-β), and vascular endothelial growth factor (VEGF)] that activate cellular events like differentiation and proliferation forming bone ultimately.

Angiogenesis

It is a well-known fact the DO is associated with increased vascularity of the region. There is 330% increased vascularity of the limb as demonstrated in specific studies. Neoangiogenesis and neovascularity is mediated by increased expression of numerous vascular growth factors in the distracted zone including VEGF, FGF, and angiopoietin.

There is an Ongoing Debate on the Type of Bone Formed in Distraction Osteogenesis

Most early and recent studies confirmed intramembranous bone formation. Few studies reported predominant endochondral bone formation. Ilizarov himself described intramembranous bone formation with groups of cartilage in between. A third type of bone formation has been described by Yasui who called it "transchondroid" bone formation.

Indications of Ilizarov Frame Fixation

- Tibial/femoral lengthening (limb lengthening, **Fig. 8**)—say for dwarfism or post-traumatic or pathological (infection/neoplasia—surgery) or congenital short limb.
- Long bone deformity correction—the following deformities are usually addressed by Ilizarov method.
  - Mechanical axis deviation (MAD)
  - Rotational malalignment
  - Translation
  - Leg length discrepancy
  - Angular and multiplanar deformities
  - Combined deformity and shortening
- Open fractures—as a minimally invasive stabilization method
- Nonunion **(Figs. 9A to F)** and malunion management/correction
- Slow correction of joint contractures
- Correction of congenital deformities of foot (clubfoot)
- Reconstruction of bone defects [trauma/neoplasia/infection/congenital (pseudoarthrosis of tibia)]—bone transport
- Vascular insufficiency (Berger's disease)

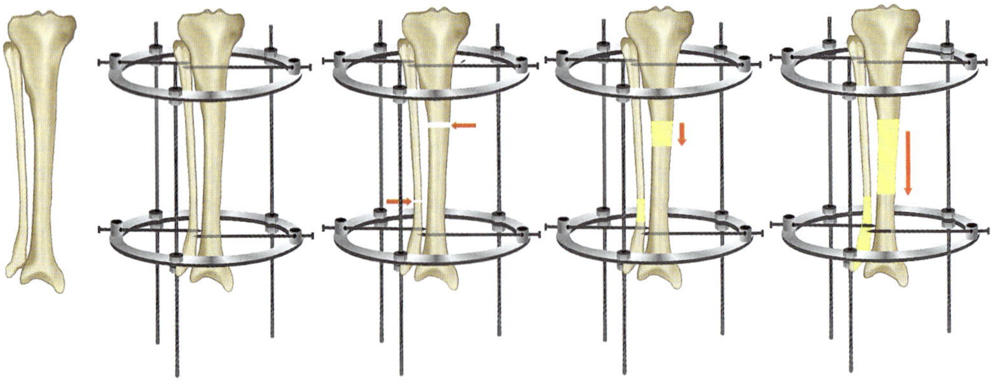

Fig. 8: Lengthening of bone using Ilizarov method. Low energy corticotomy is performed in metaphyseal or metaphyseal-diaphyseal region of tibia with a complementary osteotomy of fibula performed usually at same or different level (arrows). The frame is gradually distracted at suitable rate (see text) until desired limb length is obtained. The frame is then kept in situ for equal duration for consolidation of regenerate.

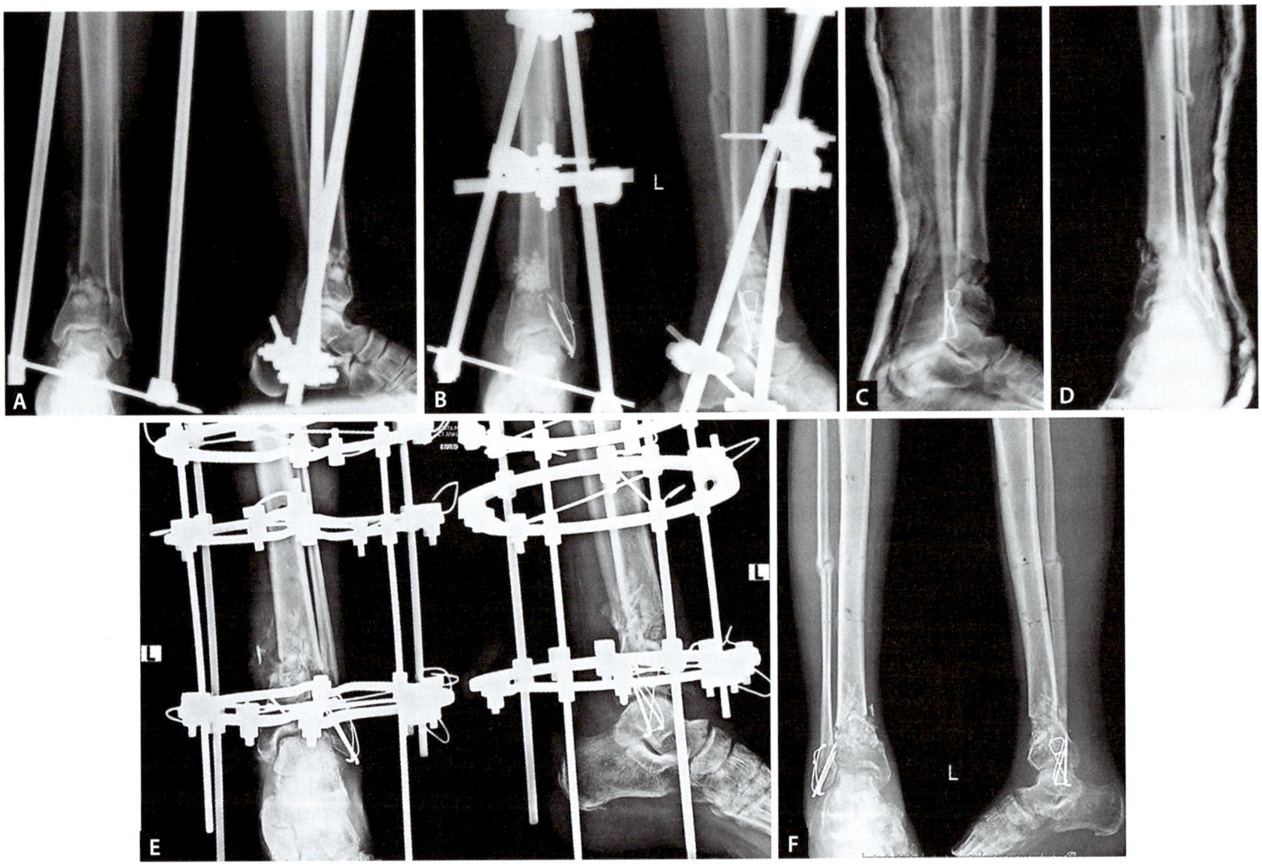

Figs. 9A to F: Example of Ilizarov management of nonunion. (A) The patient with compound fracture distal tibia was poorly managed by an inexperienced surgeon initially by external fixation; (B) The fixator was revised and fibula grafting was undertaken for poor stabilization and unacceptable radiology by him; (C) To top it up, he removed the fixator early and put patient in a below knee slab after 6 weeks; (C and D) Patient came with this nonunion of distal tibia at 8 months; (E) The patient was managed with bone grafting and calcium phosphate cement combination and Ilizarov fixator for stabilization and (F) united at 3 months.

Prerequisites for Distraction Osteogenesis

- Patient willing for a prolonged treatment and ready to carry the frame
- Stability—the fixation and frame construct should be stable and provide good stability to the corticotomy site else nonunion will ensue with a floppy frame.
- Maintenance of adequate blood supply (maintaining the periosteal and endosteal blood supply to maximal)
- Likelihood of obtaining a functional limb and not compromising the current function by the method.

Basic Methods or Modifications of Ilizarov Technique Employed for Various Types of Nonunion

- *Small segment nonunions (short stiff nonunions):* These can be crushed by pressure effect in compression and then growth of fibrocartilage ensues which slowly ossifies due to trampoline effect, if patient is bearing weight.

- *Gap nonunions (<4 cm):* Diseased or malunited segments can be removed for relatively longer nonunions, and if the resulting gap <4 cm, then acute docking in compression followed by lengthening can be done.
- *For long and atrophic nonunions where the gap will be/is >4 cm:* It is better to hold out the extremity to its length and do bone transport (internal/external/ combined) in various modes, else there is risk of kinking of neurovascular bundle:
  - Monofocal
  - Bifocal
  - Trifocal

It is commonly accepted that lengthening of limb is needed if the shortening or expected shortening is ≥5 cm.

Principles and Types of Osteotomy Performed for "Excising" Nonunion

The osteotomies performed in the management of non-unions can be classified into three types:

1. Intrafocal osteotomy (performed at the nonunion site: It consists essentially of the resection of the entire area around the nonunion).
2. Transfocal osteotomy (performed through the nonunion site to reshape the bone ends: It is indicated for nonunions with a longitudinal or oblique fracture line).
3. Parafocal osteotomy (Paltrinieri's osteotomy, performed some centimeters from the nonunion site).

Corticotomy

This is defined as an open, subperiosteal, and low-energy partial osteotomy of bone cortex, followed by manual osteoclasis of the remainder of cortical circumference maximally preserving the periosteum, endosteum, and bone marrow with its blood supply as well as the muscle and soft tissue surrounding the bone. Usually the corticotomy is done in cancellous metaphyseal regions; a corticotomy done in diaphyseal cortical bone is called compactotomy. Ilizarov preferred rotational osteoclasis of the created defect that was made by externally rotating the distal fragment. External rotation protects the neurovascular structures from tension and stretching. In essence, the steps of performing corticotomy are:

- Low energy—use only as much injuring force as necessary for inflicting bone scar
- Minimal incision only slightly larger than the width of corticotome or osteotome
- Periosteum incised longitudinally and preserved all around the corticotomy site
- A row of holes are predrilled using saline for continuous cooling. This technique allows low heat generation, reducing corticotomy site bone necrosis
- An osteotome or corticotome is used to join holes, with a twist to break the posterior cortex.

Various types of corticotomy as needed in different indications are:

- *Transverse:* Lengthening, correction of deformity, and bone transport

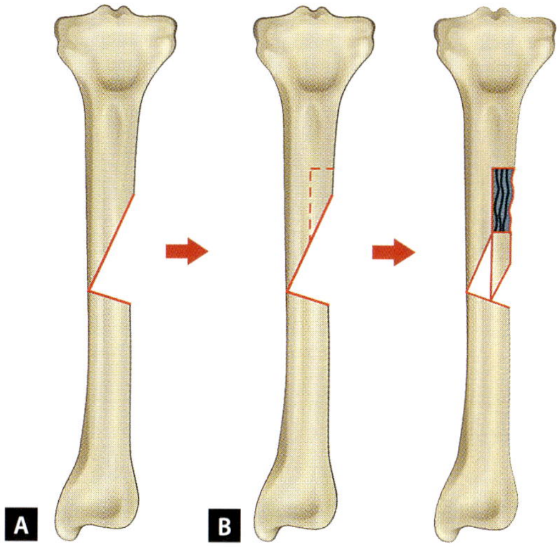

Figs. 10A and B: Splinter corticotomy to bridge the nonunion site.

- *Longitudinal:* To widen bone (overcoming defect in one of two bones), improve shape of a thin atrophic limb
- *Splinter:* Splints off a piece of bone with attached periosteum, soft tissue and skin—bridging nonunion site **(Figs. 10A and B)**, eliminate partial bony defects
- *S-shaped corticotomy:* Chronic osteomyelitis
- Complete
- *Partial:* To correct bow/curved defect in bones, e.g., osteogenesis imperfecta

If not properly performed or stabilized then the cortico-tomy may well be associated with various complications like:

- Vascular damage
- Displacement of corticotomy
- Incomplete corticotomy
- Premature consolidation

Phases of Distraction Osteogenesis

After a corticotomy is done, the typical management of patient is commonly grouped into four phases:

1. Latency phase—see above in delay before distraction.
2. *Distraction phase:* The cut ends are distracted at given rate and rhythm for a predetermined period. The period is equal to the desired lengthening in millimeters. For 60 mm, lengthening distraction will continue for 60 days.
3. *Consolidation phase:* This phase involves ossification of regenerate and bone consolidation to gain strength enough to bear weight. This is the most cumbersome to patient as it is typically double that of distraction phase in duration. The other common formula is 1 month per cm of lengthening which is even lengthier.
4. *Fixator removal:* After completion of regenerate formation the fixator is removed once the quality and strength is ascertained using various methods (commonly radiography).

Modes commonly employed for Ilizarov fixator application: Ring fixators (Ilizarov used full rings that were then modified into half rings later) can be applied in following modes:

- *Monofocal distraction* ***(Fig. 11A)****:* Appropriate for hypertrophic nonunion. Distraction is considered "bad" for fractures and is true for fresh fractures where it causes

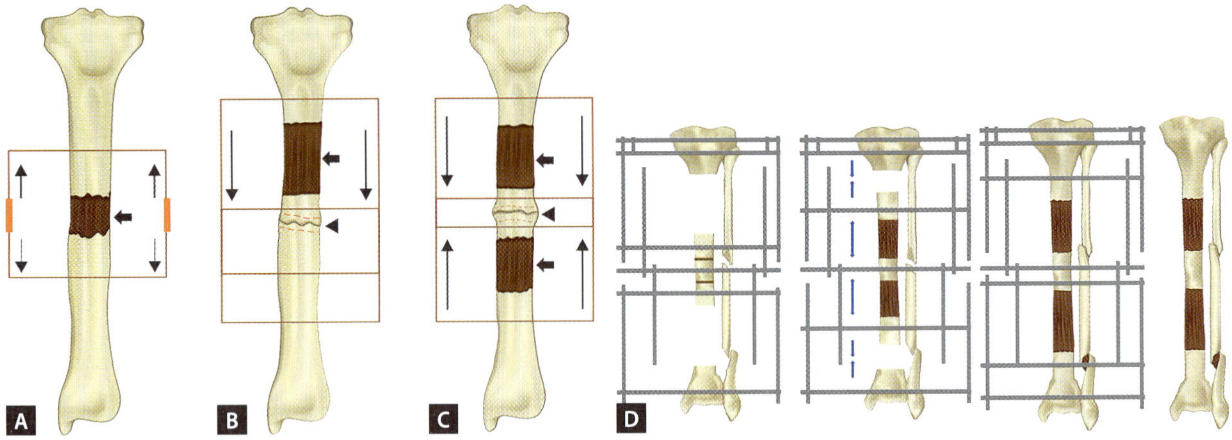

Figs. 11A to D: Various modes of application of Ilizarov. (A) Monofocal distraction; (B) Monofocal distraction and monofocal compression; (C) Bifocal distraction and monofocal compression; (D) Bifocal distraction and bifocal compression.

nonunion. However, for an established nonunion, it acts as an antidote and heals the fracture, if principles laid down by professor Ilizarov are properly followed. He established that for hypertrophic nonunion gradual distraction applied to the fibrocartilage or fibrous tissue produces intense osteogenesis. Here the cartilage acts as an "interzone" similar to the one seen at corticotomy site done for lengthening.

- Monofocal compression-distraction **(Fig. 11B)**
- Bifocal compression distraction **(Fig. 11C)** replacement (up to 5–7 cm)
- Trifocal [bifocal distraction and monofocal/bifocal compression **(Fig. 11D)**]

Types of Bone Transport

- *External bone transport:* External bone transport is easier and can simultaneously correct deformity and shortening but produces more skin scarring and is inadequate for major bone loss. It is done for bone loss replacement (up to 5–7 cm) or when correction of deformities and limb lengthening is needed together. It can be monofocal (single corticotomy) or bifocal (dual site corticotomy and movement in opposite directions toward each other). For larger bone defects, there is a problem of invagination of skin into the bone defect, needing multiple readjustments (prefer internal bone transport).
- *Internal bone transport using olive/hooked wires:* For defects 7–10 cm and larger. Internal bone transport is better for larger bone defects and easier for patient as fewer wires are involved and that skin invagination is not seen but it is difficult to apply and does not have enough "compression effect" at docking site.
- *Combined bone transport:* For larger defects due to major bone loss (resection of malignant bone tumors) associated with limb deformities, deep soft tissue scars and local blood supply insufficiency.

Complications of Ilizarov Method

- Pin site infection
- Pain at the corticotomy site and during lengthening procedure (usually initial period only)
- Vascular complication—direct arterial/venous injury by the Ilizarov wires. Aneurysm formation is a reported complication that commonly occurs with partial damage to the arterial walls, as may occur when the Ilizarov wire brushes the artery. The weakened wall then gradually distends forming aneurysm.
- Neurological damage—usually direct injury to nerves while passing wires. Traction injury is less common, can be reduced or minimized by reducing the rate of distraction and early identification by clinical examination during follow-up.
- Soft tissue contractures and joint stiffness—when the frame spans joints—common in knee, elbow, and ankle (Achilles tendon contracture is common). One should hence incorporate foot plate in cases of frame fixation near to ankle joint else equinus deformity develops.
- Osteoporosis
- Reflex sympathetic dystrophy (RSD)
- Progression of angular deformity or creation of new one after fixator is removed. Pathological fracture may also ensue, if the regenerate is not strong enough.
- Swelling of limb—usually due to immobilization, the venous tone is reduced causing edema and may progress to lymphedema—manage with passive mobilization, massage and physiotherapy.
- Lengthening site—nonunion and premature consolidation (requires redo procedure)

Some Technical Pearls

One of the prerequisites for a successful Ilizarov frame application is maintaining or improving stability of the construct. There are various ways by which this can be achieved:

- *Wire:*
    - Increase diameter (1.8 mm for adult, 1.5 mm for child)
    - Increase tension (130 Nm for adult, 110 Nm for child)
    - Increase crossing angles—the wires should cross each other at the largest possible separating angles (perpendicularly placed wires have highest stability)
    - Use opposing "olive" wires

- Increase number of wires
- Use "slotted" bolts—increases surface area for frictional resistance

- *Half-pins:*
  - Use larger diameter pins
  - Hydroxyapatite coating—improves bone integration (problematic while removal) and possibly also reduce infection (silver-coated pins also reduce infection rate)
  - Increase crossing angles and use multiplanar construct, if possible
  - Decrease distance of external construct to bone
  - Increase number of pins
- *Ring:*
  - Decrease diameter (allow at least 2 cm clearance for swelling)
  - Fix bone in middle
  - Near and far positions of rings
  - Increase number (including "dummy" rings)

Period of consolidation of regenerate is too lengthy. Attempts have been made to reduce the period by using various modalities, some of which are listed here:

- *Mechanical:* This enhances the process of mechano-transduction by mechanically stimulating cells to mature and hasten bone formation.
  - Loading, axial compression, and dynamization of frame
  - Accordion maneuver—this consists of alternating cycles of compression and distraction (daily/weekly cycles)
  - Trampoline effect—vibrations applied by way of plates improve the bone formation
- *Physical methods:*
  - Ultrasound application to regenerate
  - Extracorporeal shock wave—too cumbersome and only theoretical
  - Electrical stimulation (*see* Chapter on "Fracture Repair, Bone Grafting, and Bone Banking")
- *Medications:*
  - Calcitonin
  - Bisphosphonates
  - Sparsely reported and untested—locally applied vitamin E, adiponectin, inhibin A, nerve growth factor, thrombin peptide 508, calcium sulfate cement/ injection, NEL-like-molecule-1, bone marrow, platelet-rich plasma, autografts, demineralized bone matrix, etc.
  - Growth factors—BMP, NEL-1, TGF-β, IGF, FGF, and PDGF.

SCAPHOID FRACTURE AND NONUNION

Fracture of scaphoid was first identified by Destot in 1905, and these fractures quickly caught interest of surgeons for troublesome healing. Nonunion in fracture scaphoid is quite common despite good and early management. For an overall understanding of the condition, we will discuss fractures of scaphoid also. The fractures of scaphoid account for 2–7% of all fractures, 10% of all hand fractures, and 60–90% (average of 71%) of all carpal bone fractures. The incidence reported in literature is highly variable ranging from 29 to 43/100,000/ year and surprisingly in the newer literature after 2005, the reported incidence is reducing. The mean reported age is around 25 years and males (80%) outnumber females (20%) largely. Fractures in males commonly occur in the age group of 15–29 years while in females, the reported age is lower between 10 and 14 years. There is a seasonal variation where more fractures are seen in summers and autumn and much less in winters. For daily trends, the fracture seems to occur more on weekends but mostly present on Monday for care. This may be related to increase in outdoor activity of youngsters sustaining falls on weekends. Socially deprived population is more susceptible to scaphoid fractures but no such relation exists to occurrence of nonunion. Fractures through waist are much more common compared to fracture of tubercle or proximal pole fracture. Horizontally-oriented fractures heal much better than transverse (along width of bone) or vertical shear ones. Proximal fractures take even longer to heal. Most common associated injury is scapholunate ligament disruption that is seen in 20% of displaced scaphoid fractures and 31% of undisplaced ones (due to incomplete dissipation of energy).

Anatomy

Scaphoid derives its name from the Greek word "scaphe" meaning boat. The bone has been anatomically studied into four parts—(1) the tubercle, (2) distal pole, (3) waist, and (4) the proximal pole **(Fig. 12)**. The scaphoid bone represents primary link in the proximal carpal row effecting carpal and wrist functions. More than two-thirds of the surface of the scaphoid is covered by articular cartilage rest providing attachment to various ligaments, thus the blood supply is mostly limited and being devoid of periosteum callus formation is also restricted. The primary blood supply is derived from palmar and dorsal branches of the radial artery **(Fig. 13)** where the proximal segment of the scaphoid receives mainly retrograde blood flow only. All of the proximal pole and about 70–80% of the internal vascularity of the scaphoid are supplied by dorsal vessels that enter scaphoid through dorsal ridge. Thus, untreated scaphoid

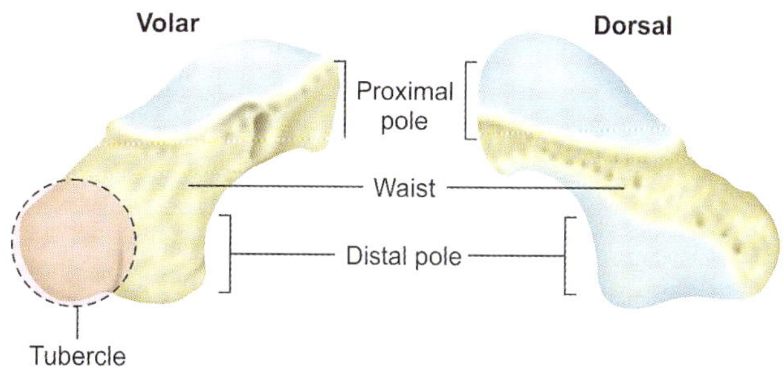

Fig. 12: Bony anatomy of scaphoid—mainly four parts of scaphoid are identified the proximal and distal poles with central waist and the tubercle on the volar distal pole. Note that the major part of bone is covered by articular cartilage and the vascular supply enters only through narrow strips in the waist region visible here as tiny pores.

fractures of the proximal pole are prone to nonunion and osteonecrosis. The distal pole and remaining 20–30% of scaphoid are supplied by volar vessels.

Diagnosis

Most fractures occur due to fall on outstretched hand (FOOSH) with dorsiflexion of scaphoid where it hits the dorsal edge of radius **(Figs. 14A and B)**. The classically described Chauffer's/crank handle injury does not result in fractures of scaphoid (at least now). There is local snuffbox swelling and pain on wrist movements. Examination reveals anatomical snuffbox tenderness (sensitivity 90% and specificity 40%) ± swelling, scaphoid tubercle tenderness (good sign, specificity 57%, and sensitivity 87%), and loss

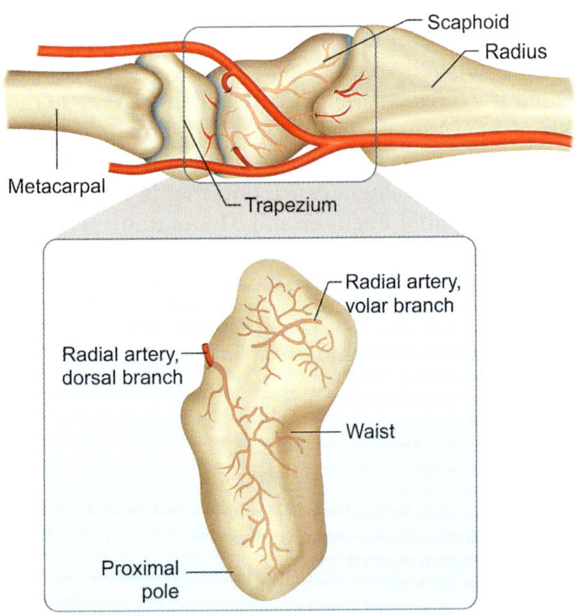

Fig. 13: The blood supply arises from dorsal and volar branches of radial artery. Note the precarious blood supply of proximal pole that receives retrograde blood supply and may be even very limited in 15% cases. In a fracture of scaphoid, the blood supply will be completely interrupted.

of grip strength. Axial compression along the first or second metacarpal producing pain at wrist is possibly the best sign (compression test, specificity 92%, and sensitivity 94%).

Radiographs have a 70–90% detection rate for fracture scaphoid. The standard views include posteroanterior (PA), lateral, and ulnar deviation oblique view (Stecher's view, **Fig. 15**). The Stecher's view is best for detection of scaphoid fractures. Clenched fist view can also be taken that distracts the fracture scaphoid by pushing in the capitate but may displace fracture, if done overzealously. For occult fractures (not seen on plain radiographs), the fracture line is usually evident by 6 weeks and classical teaching of repeating the radiograph at 2 weeks has no logical/literature support. Waiting for 2 weeks adds only 4–5% sensitivity for detection of scaphoid fractures by radiographs. One must additionally appreciate associated injuries like S-L disruption (scapholunate interval up to 9 mm at 7 years of age and 3 mm at 15 years of age is considered normal), trans-scaphoid perilunate dislocation, other carpal bone injuries, distal radius injuries, etc. Intrascaphoid angle is normally 40° in coronal plane and 30° in sagittal plane (>35—humpback deformity). Ultrasonography may reveal effusion around scaphoid (sensitivity 50% and specificity 91%). Tomosynthesis is a technology available in some countries based on mammography that increases the sensitivity to detect fractures without significantly increasing radiation risk, and it is relatively quick and is cheaper than noncontrast computerized tomography (NCCT). *MRI* is the preferred (gold standard) modality for early diagnosis of scaphoid fractures with sensitivity of nearly 100%. In comparison **(Table 2)** to NCCT of wrist, the MRI has higher cost but it has been calculated that MRI becomes cost effective, if its sensitivity is >5% of that of CT and that is exactly the case. It is undoubtedly the preferred modality for diagnosing *occult* fractures of scaphoid (so also called "clinical" fracture scaphoid). An algorithm for radiological diagnosis of fracture scaphoid is presented in **Flowchart 1**. *NCCT wrist* (carpal bones) is a very good modality for diagnosis of fracture line and classification of fracture scaphoid but has

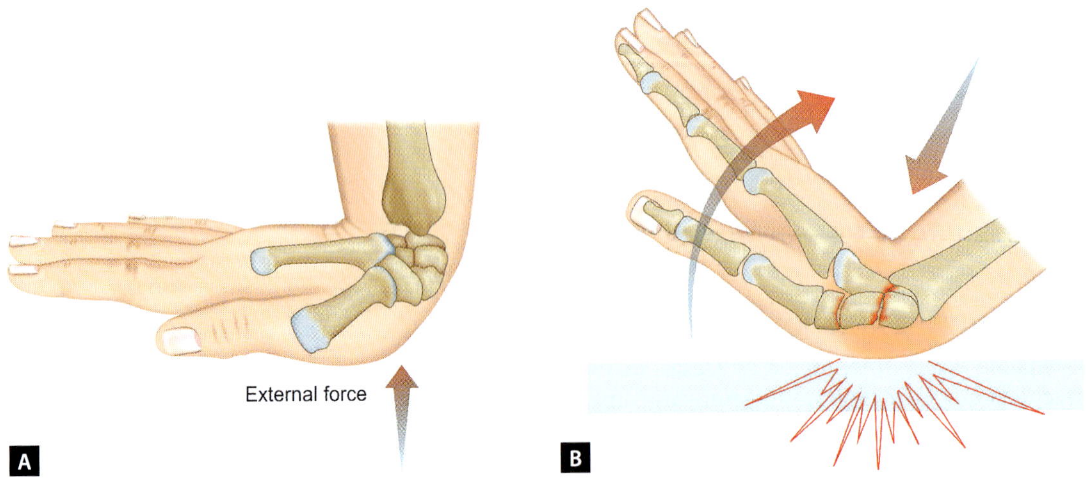

Figs. 14A and B: The scaphoid fracture results commonly from fall on outstretched hand (A) resulting in levering of the bone against dorsal lip of radius due to forced dorsiflexion (B).

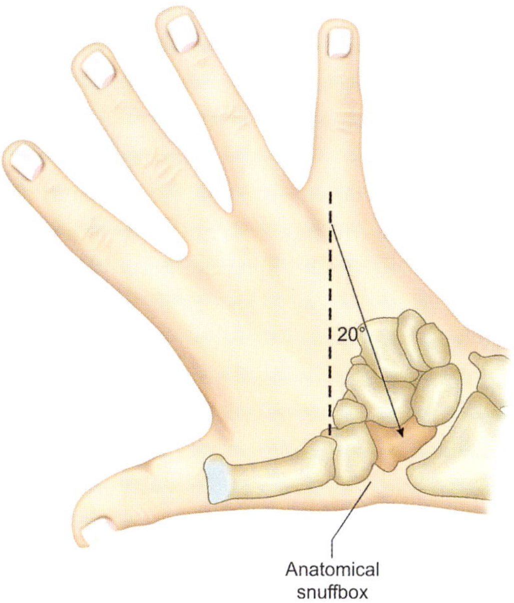

Fig. 15: Stecher's view—the wrist is placed in ulnar deviation and slight extension with the tube beam directed at 20°. Perpendicular beam results in foreshortened scaphoid while increasing angle beyond 30° results in lengthening of scaphoid image.

TABLE 2: The relative comparison between bone scan, computed tomography (CT), and magnetic resonance imaging (MRI) for diagnosing clinical scaphoid fractures. The numbers of + or – indicate the relative advantage or disadvantage.

Bone scan	*CT scan*	*MRI*
Sensitivity (+++)	Specificity (+++)	Specificity (+++)
Specificity (--)	Quickness (++)	Ligament injury (+++)
Radiation (---)	Availability (++)	Sensitivity (±)
Invasive (--)	Radiation (--)	Availability (--)
Time consuming (---)	Sensitivity (--)	Time consuming (-)
Delays diagnosis by 3–5 days (---)		

Flowchart 1: Radiological fracture diagnosis.

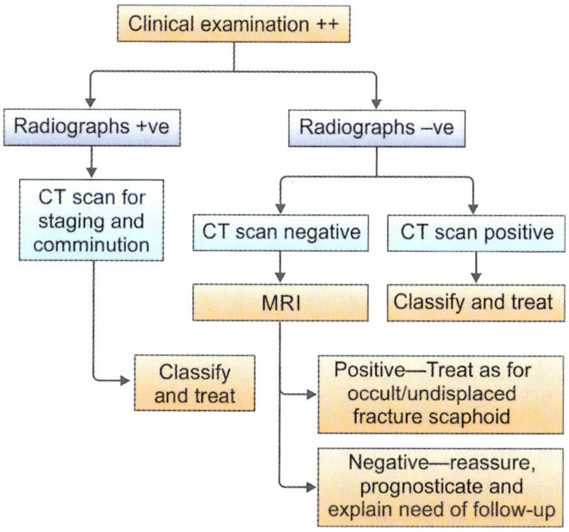

the drawback of increased ionizing radiation. Also, NCCT still misses significant numbers of undisplaced fractures of scaphoid. For displaced fractures of scaphoid, 3D CT reconstruction is the best guide detailing the fractures into two types:

1. *Humpback deformity* **(Figs. 16A to C)**:
    - Fracture through waist
    - It has been generally considered that the humpback deformity is due to pronation, flexion, and ulnar deviation of distal fragment but now it has been shown that in fact the proximal fragment is extended and supinated with lunate producing the characteristic deformity. The distal fragment more or less remains in place.
2. *Ad latus dislocation:*
    - These are proximal third fractures of scaphoid.
    - The fracture line runs parallel to forearm.
    - It encompasses lateral dislocation of the distal fragment.

Classifications of Scaphoid Fracture

Fractures of scaphoid receive many classifications by different researchers. Broadly, they can be divided into two groups as follows:

1. *Classifications based on fracture position/plane orientation:*
    - Bohler's (1954) and Russe (1960, **Fig. 17**)
    - Compson—1998 [1—transverse waist (surgical waist), 2—oblique waist (dorsal sulcus), 3—proximal pole]
    - Schernberg—1984 **(Fig. 18)**
    - Prosser—1988 **(Fig. 19)**
    - AO/OTA—2007 (scaphoid is given number 72 and is divided into noncomminuted (A) and comminuted (B, more than three fragments). There are three subtypes—(1) proximal pole, (2) waist, and (3) distal pole, so 72-B2 will be comminuted waist fracture.

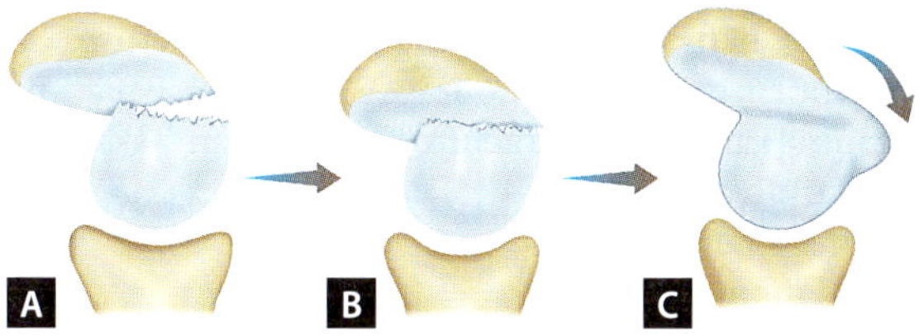

Figs. 16A to C: Development of humpback deformity of scaphoid. Extension of proximal fragment with lunate and flexion of distal fragment (A) increases the intrascaphoid angle beyond 35° (B) that consolidates to form a dorsal hump and foreshortened scaphoid (C).

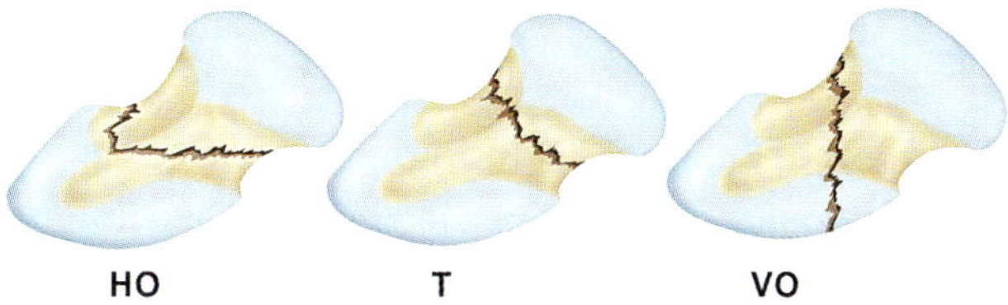

Fig. 17: Russe classification of fracture scaphoid. VO induces shear stress across fracture line causing displacement (HO: horizontal oblique; T: transverse; VO: vertical oblique).

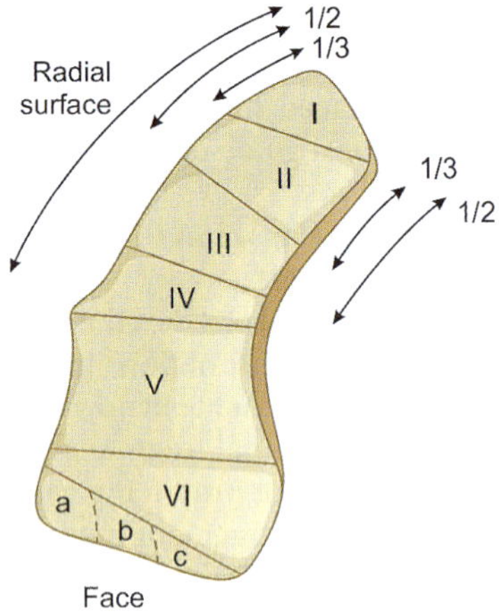

Fig. 18: Schernberg classified six fracture type (I–VI) from proximal pole to distal tubercle. Distal tubercle fractures (type VI) are further divided into small (a), intermediate (b), or large (c) fragments.

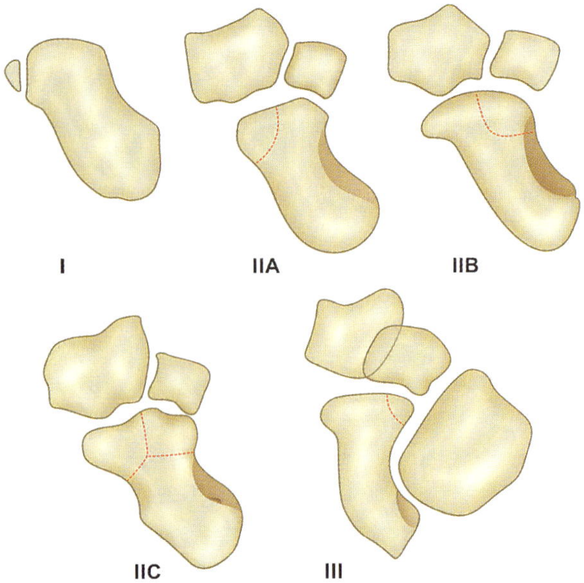

Fig. 19: Prosser classified distal fractures into tuberosity fractures (I), intra-articular fractures of scaphotrapezial joint involving radial half (IIA), ulnar half (IIB), or combined (IIC), and osteochondral fractures at capitate border (III).

2. *Classifications based on displacement and/or stability:*
    - McLaughlin and Parkes—1969 (A—incomplete, B—undisplaced and stable, C—displaced and unstable)
    - Cooney (Mayo)—1980 (**Fig. 20**, further subdivided into nondisplaced/stable or displaced/stable)
    - Weber—1980 (1—undisplaced, 2—angulated, 3— displaced)
    - Herbert and Fisher (1984)—modified by Herbert in 1996, further modified by Herbert, Krimmer, and Schmitt in 2000 to use CT scan for classification of fracture—category B5 has been added to include comminuted fractures of scaphoid. Fractures presenting after 6 weeks are classified as type C or D (see below) (**Fig. 21**).
    - Garcia-Elias and Lluch—2001 (1—stable proximal to S-L ligament, 2—unstable, distal to S-L ligament)

Unstable fracture scaphoid has been described by a combination of radiological findings, though it is not very frequently applied in radiological or general assessment but it does help in defining an unstable fracture. Young orthopedic surgeons are encouraged to use these parameters for defining an unstable fracture scaphoid and for research and descriptive purposes.

- Displacement >1 mm
- *Angulation at fracture:*
    - Intrascaphoid >35° **(Fig. 22A)**
- Rotational displacement [dorsal intercalated segment instability (DISI) angle] **(Figs. 22A to C)**
    - Capitolunate angle >15°
    - Scapholunate angle >60°
- Bone loss or comminution at fracture site
- Perilunate dislocation

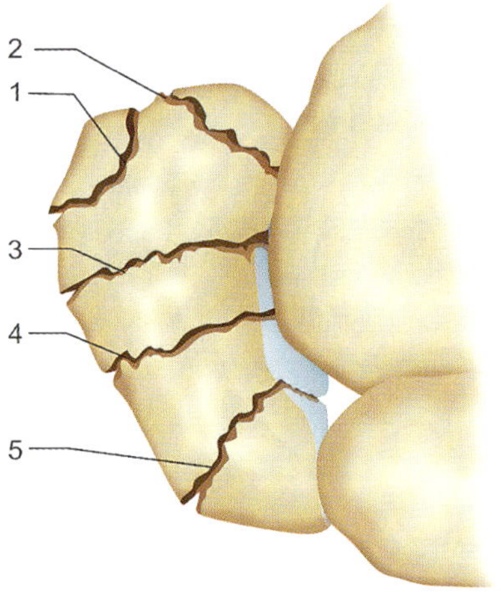

Fig. 20: Cooney (Mayo) divides scaphoid fractures into: (1) distal tubercle, (2) distal intra-articular, (3) distal third, (4) waist, and (5) proximal pole.

Treatment of Scaphoid Nonunion

The management of diagnosed fracture scaphoid is accurate reduction and fixation of the fracture. An algorithm for management is provided in **Figure 23**. Tuberosity fractures are mostly managed in short-arm plaster of Paris (POP) cast for 4–6 weeks. There is no role for long-arm POP cast, as they do not offer any advantage in preventing interfragmentary motion. There is little controversy if any to fix a displaced fracture scaphoid, however, when it comes to management of undisplaced fracture scaphoid, the world seems divided with the balance tilting toward percutaneous fixation now, especially when return to work is used as a criterion to assess endpoint. Union percentage is also higher in surgically managed undisplaced fractures. Proponents of POP cast management cite increased complications and morbidity of surgical management, especially open reduction, percutaneous fixation limits these although to a large extent. Below-elbow cast immobilization incorporating thumb metacarpophalangeal (MCP) joint for 6–8 weeks is largely accepted but limits the activity of daily living (ADL) and time

A1	Stable	# tubercle
A2	Stable	Non-displaced transverse–waist/distal 1/3rd
B1	Unstable	Extended oblique #s
B2	Unstable	Dislocated or gaping transverse #s
B3	Unstable	Proximal 1/3rd #s
B4	Unstable	Trans-scapho-perilunate fracture dislocation
C	Delayed union	After 6 weeks of immobilization
D	Nonunion	Type D1 – stable (fibrotic) Type D2 – unstable (sclerotic, pseudoarthrosis) Type D3 – nonunion with fixed DISI Type D4 – nonunion with AVN

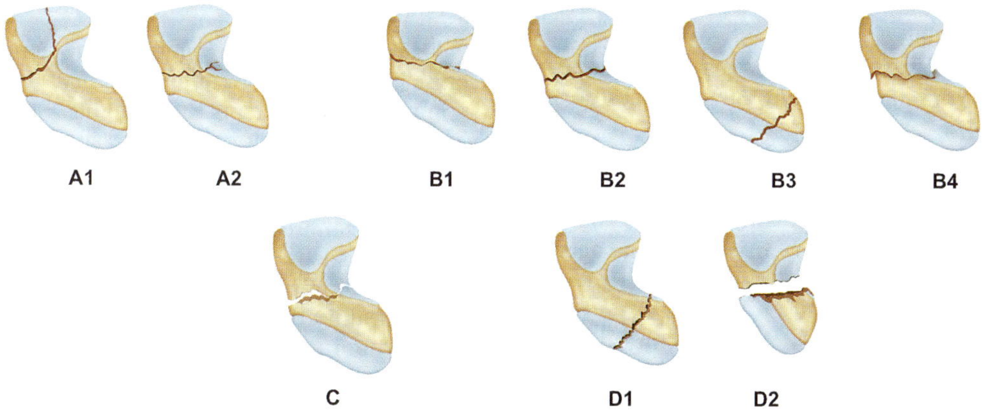

Fig. 21: Herbert and Fisher classification for fractures of scaphoid.

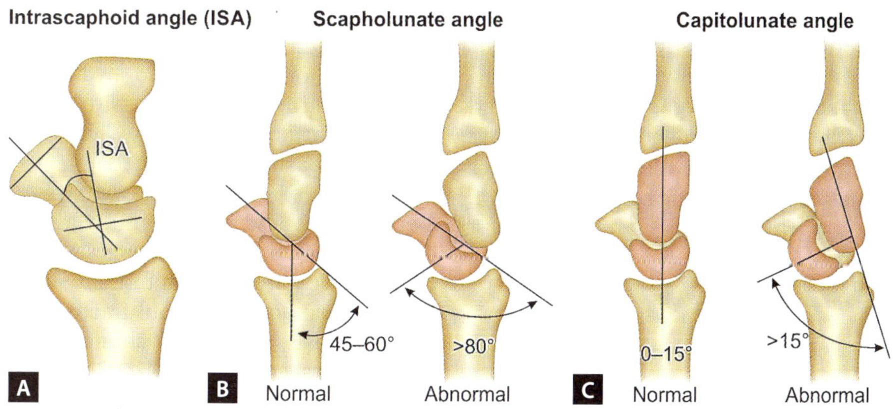

Figs. 22A to C: Schematic representation of the various radiological parameters for identifying unstable fracture of scaphoid.

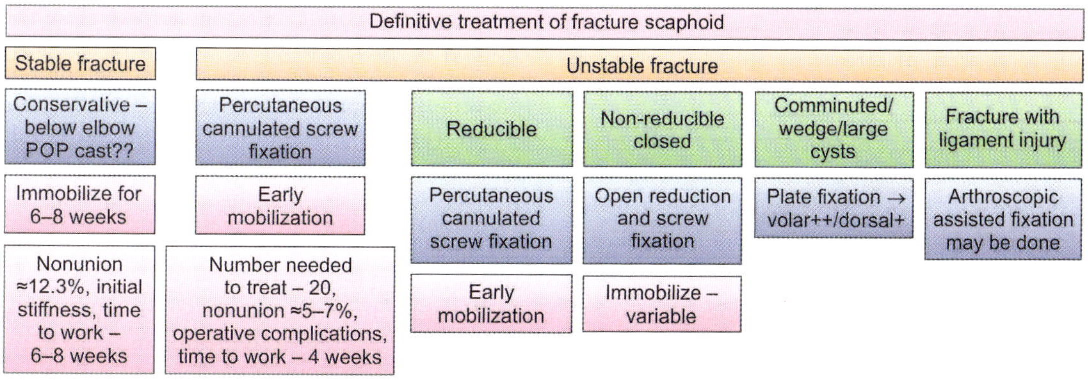

Fig. 23: Simplistic treatment algorithm for fracture scaphoid (POP: plaster of Paris).

to return to work. Around 90–95% of the undisplaced fractures of scaphoid heal in POP cast but studies report 1.5–37% of nonunion rate and otherwise also patients that develop nonunion and scaphoid nonunion advanced collapse (SNAC) wrist often report a prolonged period of cast immobilization in their history. Nonunion after POP cast treatment is more difficult to heal by treatment modalities than those after surgical fixation. This then entails that undisplaced fracture scaphoid are better managed by percutaneous fixation when compared to nonoperative management or open reduction. Proximal pole undisplaced scaphoid fractures should be possibly fixed without controversy. Poor outcome following scaphoid fracture is related to:

- Smoking
- Volar comminution
- Accuracy of fracture reduction
- More than 3 mm displacement (50% chances of going into nonunion)
- No consolidation at 4 weeks (CT scan)

All these are, hence, indications of operative management as conservative management fails in these conditions. To complete the list of indications for surgical management comprehensive, one can include:

- Unstable fractures
- Associated carpal injury/distal radius fractures
- Delayed presentation (>3 weeks)

Screw fixation is the main work-horse for stabilization of the scaphoid fracture. Headed cannulated screw was first used for fixation of scaphoid by Streli in Germany. With various developments in designing screw, a variety of screws have been produced but mostly the preference is for a headless central threadless screw with variable pitch-threaded portion at either end or a conical fully threaded screw **(Figs. 24A to C)**. Conical screw provides better compression at the fracture site making the construct stiffer and less prone to failure even in eccentric screw placement.

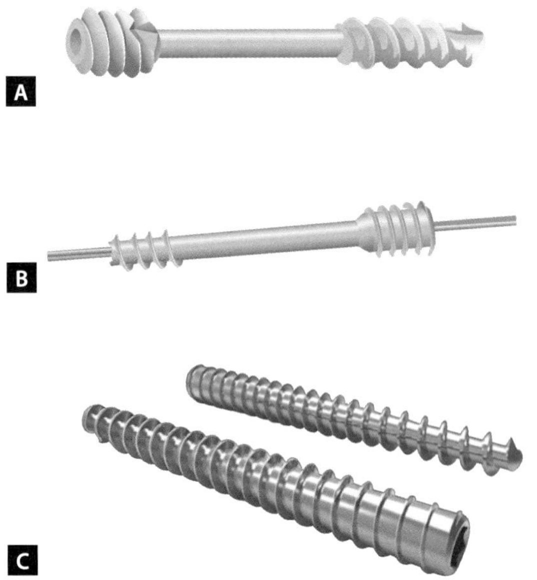

Figs. 24A to C: Different types of screws used for fixation of fracture scaphoid: Herbert (A); Herbert–Whipple (B); Conical screw (C).

Headless screws come in noncannulated (Herbert, **Fig. 24A**) and cannulated variants (Herbert/Whipple, etc.) but require central placement. With advancements in developing implants, 3D-printed screws have come across though their availability and usage is limited. For 3D-printed screws, detailed CT scan images are obtained in 0.625 mm cuts and exported digital imaging and communications in medicine (DICOM) format that are then reconstructed and analyzed by dedicated software developing volar and dorsal templates. Patient-specific guiding tubing screw system is developed using Boolean calculation and 3D printed. Commonly, wrist arthroscopy is used for assistance in screw placement. Arthroscopic-assisted fixation provides additional advantage of treating associated carpal ligament injury in the same sitting.

Fixation strength using either a conical screw or a central threadless screw appears similar as there are studies supporting both in comparative studies. Both the designs try to achieve compression at fracture site by virtue of variable linear progression velocity of the screw with rotation. Due to nonsynchronous progression of the screw through two portions a compression effect is generated between fracture fragments usually the distal fragment travels faster toward fracture compressing it against the proximal. Positioning of screw within the bone and its orientation to the fracture is an important determinant of outcome. The screw should be positioned in as central a position as possible (not always necessary) but more importantly should be perpendicular to fracture line. Shortened time to union is correlated with higher sum-of-smaller-angles (SSA). SSA is calculated by adding smaller screw fracture angle in three different radiographic projections (PA, supination oblique, and pronation oblique) and a value of ≥190° is considered optimal. Normally the screws are placed 2–3 mm below the articular cartilage and screw length should be 4 mm less than the measured scaphoid length.

Percutaneous approach for screw insertion has been standardized and proponents claim it to be better than open approach, as it preserves ligaments and vascularity. Contraindications for minimally invasive screw fixation include displaced scaphoid fractures, scaphoid nonunions with sclerosis, and cystic changes. Both volar and dorsal approaches have been utilized for this purpose where the former is especially useful for fractures running through waist while the latter is most suitable for proximal pole fractures. Haddad and Goddard first described the volar percutaneous approach placing the wrist in ulnar deviation and extension **(Fig. 25)**. The guidewire is placed from distal to proximal. Slade et al. described percutaneous dorsal (proximal) approach where wrist is held in pronation and flexion **(Fig. 26)**. Anatomically, the proximal approach allows for more accurate guidewire and screw placement. In the volar approach, trapezium tends to block more central placement of guidewire but is technically less demanding and allows for greater ease of guidewire insertion. It has been proposed by some to use two screws for improving the fixation strength or to additionally use antirotation wire with one screw in a quest to reduce nonunion rate. There is no definite literature support to this view and also placing two screws can be very challenging.

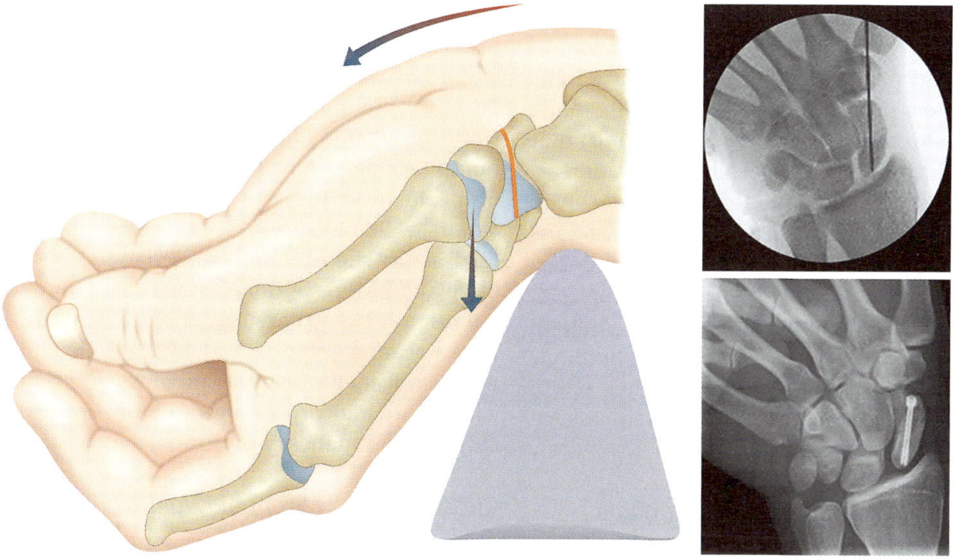

Fig. 25: The volar percutaneous approach to fix scaphoid fractures. In supine position, traction is given along the first metacarpal with wrist extended to reduce the fracture. Under fluoroscopy identify and mark scaphotrapeziotrapezoid (STT) joint. Put the guidewire through a longitudinal stab incision 1 cm distal to STT joint toward the center of proximal pole aiming at Lister's tubercle.

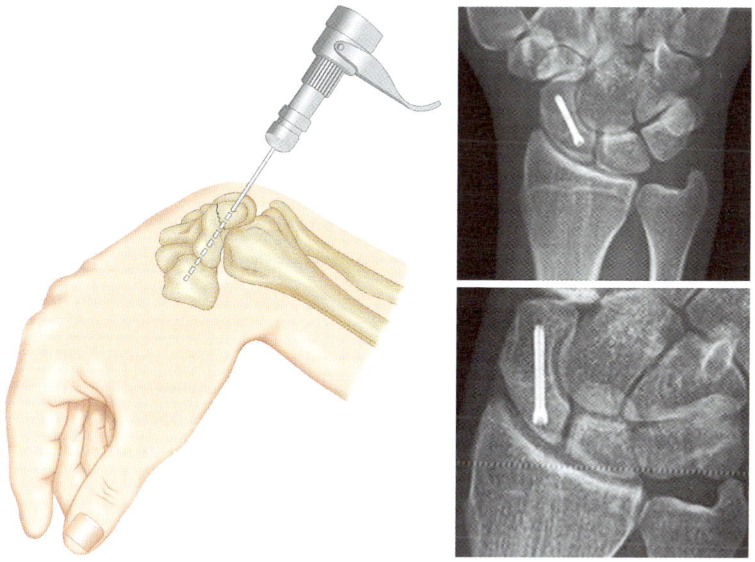

Fig. 26: Dorsal percutaneous approach to fix fractures of scaphoid. With forearm pronated mark scapholunate interval at wrist. Pronate and flex the wrist to 45° till the scaphoid is seen as a circle with overlap of proximal and distal poles. Give a stab incision at the center of circle and dissect up to the bone. Pass a guidewire through center of the circle starting 3 mm radial to the attachment of S-L ligament aiming toward a point 5 mm distal to scaphoid tuberosity. Drive wire out volarly to clear the scaphoradial joint and confirm the position in anteroposterior (AP), lateral, and oblique views. Then push the wire back and place screw after drilling.

Open reduction: For fracture that cannot be reduced by closed methods as in comminuted fractures or old fractures with humpback deformity or nonunions of scaphoid; open reduction is done utilizing again either a volar (palmar) or a dorsal approach. The palmar approach has been proclaimed to preserve blood supply but tends to disrupt ligaments that commonly attach to volar aspect. Dorsal open approach is preferred by surgeons due to easier screw placement but may damage blood supply. One needs to balance the risk associated with these approaches and usually training and comfort decides the approach used by a specific surgeon. Reduction is commonly achieved by longitudinal traction given to index and middle fingers or may also be achieved by inserting K-wires into individual fragments manipulating them as joysticks. Fixation can then be achieved by screw (detailed above)/plate or staple.

Two contemporary methods have evolved in an attempt to improve fixation of scaphoid fractures. *Staple fixation* provides good strength and union rates but there are concerns with degenerative changes due to hardware impingement. *Plate fixation* was introduced by Ender in 1977. It is especially useful when screw osteosynthesis is not possible as in wedge and multifragmentary fractures or fractures with large preexisting intraosseous cysts or in cases of scaphoid nonunion with extensive deformity. Edner's was a dorsally applied beaked plate hooked to proximal scaphoid and fixed to distal fragment by screw. An especially designed precontoured volar locking plate has been developed (Medartis AG, Basel, Switzerland) that is applied to nonarticulating area. Dorsal plate fixation is biomechanically sounder, as it is applied to tension side of the bone; however, in cases of volar comminution, it functions only as neutralization plate and is prone to fail, also dorsal plate may violate the precarious blood supply of scaphoid. I feel plate fixation is an option only for particularly difficult cases as a backup procedure or for difficult nonunions. One must remember that hardware removal after union is commonly needed due to mechanical and biological disturbances caused by hardware prominence.

Complications of Management of Fracture Scaphoid

Despite optimal management and best of the surgical hands complications are common following operative management of fracture scaphoid. Pain at the incision site and wrist pain persisting till a year are common. General complications include infection, RSD, implant penetration into the joint, osteosynthesis failure, and implant failure. Specific complications in management of fracture scaphoid that interest surgeon are:

- Nonunion of fracture scaphoid that is seen in 1–45% of the cases (operated or managed conservatively) with a mean rate of 10% that is quite high.
  - Humpback deformity
  - DISI
  - Progress to SNAC or SNAC *plus*.
- Malunion—usually the classical humpback deformity but is usually well tolerated. Malunion after treated nonunion significantly impairs function for variable reasons.
- Osteonecrosis of proximal pole of scaphoid—seen in 5% of cases. It may be discernible in radiographs after 12 weeks but gadolinium contrast MRI is the best investigation to outline the extent of necrotic region. Bone scans are sensitive but inaccurate in localization and difficult to quantitate.

Scaphoid Nonunion

Nonunion of fracture scaphoid is said to have established, if fracture fails to unite after 6 months, before this time period (but after 6 weeks of immobilization) it is called delayed union. The overall incidence of scaphoid fracture progressing to nonunion is around 10% while it is 30% for proximal pole fragments due to precarious blood supply. The predisposing factors that commonly lead to nonunion are:

- Proximal pole fractures
- Displaced unstable fractures inadequately immobilized
- Vertical oblique fracture pattern
- Comminuted fractures
- Associated carpal injury
- Delayed diagnosis
- Osteonecrosis
- Smoking

Nonunion is commonly associated with DISI carpal instability pattern because of dorsal displacement of proximal scaphoid (humpback deformity) as mentioned before. Proximal nonunions are associated with crescentic defects while distal nonunions have large triangular defects with humpback deformity. Patients usually have variable amount of pain in the wrist, loss of grip strength, and on and off swelling at the site. Radiologically there is discernible gap in the bone at the fracture site with rounded sclerotic fracture margins. The bone may be foreshortened or may have humpback deformity (commonly called flexed scaphoid). In advanced cases, there is radiocarpal arthritis and may develop into SNAC wrist where advanced arthritis progress from radial styloid to extend into midcarpal arthritis. If the arthritis extends into all carpal bones (pancarpal arthritis) then it is called SNAC *plus*.

Classifications of Scaphoid Nonunion

Scaphoid nonunion is commonly classified using Ikeda classification **(Figs. 27A to C)**, which is simple to remember and guides treatment. The system divided the nonunion into three types namely:

1. Linear type
2. Cystic type
3. Sclerotic or displaced type

The other system is ***classification of Herbert and Fisher*** where fractures presenting after 6 weeks (nonunion, type D) or after 6 weeks of immobilization (type C, delayed union) are also classified. Type D fractures are further classified as:

- Type C—delayed union after 6 weeks of immobilization—manage like type D1/D2
- Type D1—stable (fibrotic)
- Type D2—unstable (sclerotic, pseudarthrosis)
- Type D3—nonunion with fixed DISI
- Type D4—nonunion with avascular necrosis (AVN)

Another elaborate system for classification of nonunion is described by Slade and Dodds **(Table 3)**. The system is quite elaborate and useful for dedicated hand surgeons for practice but difficult to remember for general orthopedic surgeon. Types 1 to 3 and some type 4 can be treated with rigid fixation alone. Higher grades need elaborate management modifying also on the basis of subtypes.

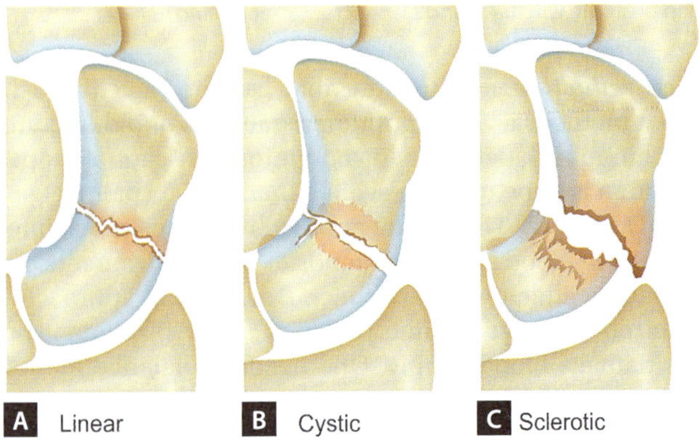

Fig. 27A to C: Ikeda classification of scaphoid nonunion.

TABLE 3: Slade and Dodds system for classification of scaphoid nonunions.

Grade	Category	Characteristics
I	Delayed presentation	Delayed presentation of fractures (408 weeks)
II	Fibrous nonunion	Cartilaginous envelop intact and minimal fracture line at nonunion interface no cyst/sclerosis
III	Minimal sclerosis	Minimal sclerosis at nonunion and resorption <1 mm
IV	Cyst formation and sclerosis	Bone resorption <5 mm, cyst formation maintained alignment
V	Cyst formation and sclerosis	Bone resorption >5 mm but <10 mm, cyst formation but maintained alignment
VI	Pseudarthrosis	Separate bone fragments, extensive bone resorption. Unstable due to gross fragment motion and deformity
Subtype		**Characteristics**
A	Proximal pole nonunion	Higher chances of ultimately failed union
B	Osteonecrosis	Osteonecrosis confirmed by MRI/absence of intraoperative punctate bleeding
C	Associated ligament injury	Static or dynamic imaging or arthroscopic evidence of ligament injury
D	Deformity	Needs strut grafting and rigid fixation

Treatment of Scaphoid Nonunion

Goals of treatment are to achieve stable union, restoration of shape, avoid carpal instability, and ultimately avert arthritis. There are various options that developed over a period of time with modifications of technique as none of them were perfect in true sense of achieving all the goals completely. At the most basic level one can leave the nonunion as it is and immobilize using cast/brace waiting for biology to ultimately prevail and achieve union (masterly inactivity) or may combine with electrical or ultrasonological stimulation (not encouraged). But this approach I feel is merely extending the vagaries of patient and would lead to stiff wrist; however, for an uncooperative patient or an uninterested patient who does not want an operative intervention may be managed with this approach as is also true for a rare patient who is medically unfit to undergo any surgery. The management otherwise relies on operative reconstruction of the bone and stimulation to achieve stable bony union. Adams and Leonard (1928) first described operative treatment of the scaphoid nonunion by bone grafting. Traditionally, bone grafting was suggested for all nonunions but type D1 and Ikeda's linear and cystic types have been successfully managed solely by compression screw fixation but Ikeda recommended conical Acutrak screw due to its more compression capability. I still keep a low threshold to bone graft these nonunions as repeat surgery, if needed, will be complicated. Type D2/D3/D4 and Ikeda type sclerotic nonunions are usually due to delay in receiving treatment. Depending on the delay in presentation the operative management options are divided into two groups. In the first group where no degenerative changes have set in, one tries to achieve union by either of the following methods:

- *Nonvascularized bone grafting (NVBG):*
  - *Cancellous inlay (Matti–Russe):* Indicated in type D1 or cystic type Ikeda.
  - *Wedge (Fisk–Fernandez):* Indicated in nonunion with deformity as in some unstable D2 and D3 type nonunion.
  - *Arthroscopic-assisted bone grafting*—not very popular but may be indicated for addressing associated injuries together like triangular fibrocartilage complex (TFCC) injury or SL ligament or other ligament(s) injuries. It may additionally facilitate guidewire placement. Indications are similar to cancellous inlay bone grafting.
- *Vascularized bone grafting (VBG):* This may be preferred for most type D2 and D4 where there is high suspicion of osteonecrosis.
- *Ilizarov fixation of scaphoid nonunion:* Using three-stage compression-distraction technique Marko Bumbaširević successfully treated 20 scaphoid nonunions without opening the nonunion site or bone grafting. The frame is applied to forearm and metacarpal bones and not to scaphoid or its fragments. The biology tends to result from tension stress at the nonunion that stimulates angiogenesis and bone formation.
- Use of BMP—not a standard or established method but sporadic reports appear in literature to its use. The nonunion is curetted and 50 mg BMP is implanted without any bone grafting or screw fixation resulting in complete healing. Also, researchers have tried various bone graft analogs, injectable bone substitutes, and demineralized bone matrix individually.

For patients who present late to the treating surgeon so that some form of degeneration has set in, only salvage procedures can be proposed as just achieving union will not treat the patient completely. These options include one of the following depending on the extent of degeneration that has set in:

- Distal scaphoid resection—indicated in cases with failed chronic nonunions with overgrown distal scaphoid pole ± arthritic changes at radioscaphoid joint
- Limited intercarpal fusion
- Proximal row carpectomy
- Scaphoid excision + four-corner fusion
- Scaphoid allograft and fixation for proximal pole nonunions and fragmentation
- Proximal pole reconstruction using rib osteochondral autograft in unsalvageable proximal poles
- Proximal pole excision and filling by fascial/tendon spacer
- Wrist arthroplasty
- Wrist arthrodesis

We will discuss the typical techniques and their relative advantages and disadvantages in the following discussion:

Nonvascularized bone grafting: This has been for long the preferred technique for achieving union, as they are less

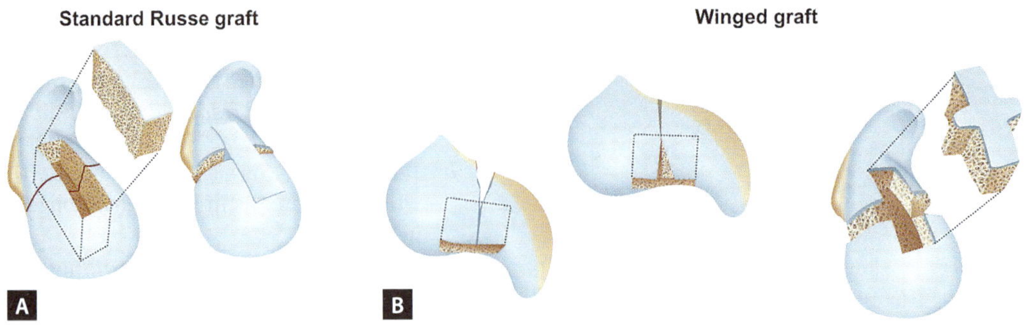

Figs. 28A and B: The Matti–Russe procedure (modified). The corticocancellous wedge of bone is placed after making an oval cavity across the nonunion (A). The graft can be straight (A) or winged (cross-shaped) to improve contact areas for better healing (B).

demanding surgically. NVBG is preferred for simple and undisplaced nonunions. The procedure involves filling the excised nonunion by some form of bone graft obtained from iliac crest or distal radius or other suitable source (ribs also described). The Matti–Russe technique **(Figs. 28A and B)** is the typical procedure describing NVBG for treating scaphoid nonunion. In the original description (Matti, 1936) cancellous iliac crest bone graft was filled into an egg-shaped cavity created across nonunion site extending into the fragments. Nonvascular bone was excised at the nonunion but no deformity correction was achieved. The technique was then modified to using corticocancellous bone graft to provide additional strength (Russe, 1960) using volar approach. Screw (Verdan, 1968; Fisk, 1970) or K-wire (Russe, 1960) is used to stabilize the construct. The disadvantage of the technique is that it does not address osteonecrosis if that is concomitantly present and also leaves the deformity uncorrected as no attempt is made to excise the nonunion for correcting deformity. For correcting the deformity, other techniques have been used like wedge bone grafting (Fisk–Fernandez) where a tricortical wedge graft carved from iliac crest that matches the defect created after nonunion excision and correcting the deformity **(Figs. 29A to D)**. Fisk (1980) described that wedge graft restores the anatomy and establishes the tension in volar radiocarpal ligaments. Fernandez (1984) modified the technique by using opposite wrist X-ray as template, using a palmar approach [between flexor carpi radialis (FCR) and radial artery], complete resection of the nonunion and use of internal fixation. Screw fixation and K-wires have been both used for fixation of the tricortical wedge into place where it was proposed that screw provides better fixation strength and support to the construct but recent literature suggests that screws tend to disrupt the intraosseous blood supply and may limit the benefits of the technique favoring use of smooth K-pins. In the recent literature, there has been a shift from iliac crest bone graft to increasing use of distal radius bone graft and similarly preference of K-wires over screw fixation. It has been argued that the bone graft quality and quantity from distal radius are inadequate to sufficiently fill the nonunion (Wong and Ho) as compared to iliac crest. Aguilella and Garcia-Elias presented an ipsilateral distal radius metaphyseal graft taken from anterolateral

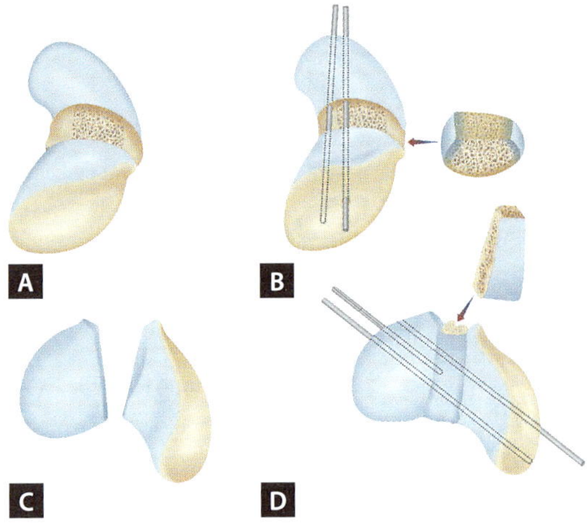

Figs. 29A to D: The Fisk–Fernandez procedure. Wedge of bone graft is placed after excising the nonunion (A and B). Note the wedge is shaped in contour to maintain the shape of scaphoid bone and fixed with K-wires (C and D) or screws.

corner. This technique has the advantage of providing good subchondral bone and allows graft to be harvested from same incision and not requiring GA. Because of the need to design an accurately sized wedge for correction of humpback deformity, which is often inaccurate, Stark developed a technique where after excising the nonunion; deformity is corrected by forceful extension of the wrist opening up the space and fixing temporarily in position by K-wires and cancellous chips are impacted into the defect.

Vascularized bone grafting: There are two types of vascularized bone grafts in use—(1) the pedicled vascularized bone grafts and (2) the free vascularized bone grafts. There came extreme interest in the use of vascularized bone graft for treating scaphoid nonunion for two sound arguments. One vascularized bone tends to incorporate faster (as they do not need creeping substitution) and will bring in the blood supply that is "possibly" deficient locally to cause nonunion and second that this will be a remedy for two common complications—(1) nonunion and (2) osteonecrosis. This lead to descriptions of various techniques by different authors and researchers as listed below:

- Pronator quadratus pedicled bone graft (Kawai and Yamamoto 1988)

- Pedicled grafts based on the ulnar artery from the distal ulnar aspect of ulnar head
- The palmar carpal artery (branch of radial artery) based graft from distal radius (described by Kullman in 1989 and popularized by Mathoulin, **Fig. 30**)—the radial styloid fasciosteal graft
- Pedicled grafts from the index finger (2nd) metacarpal (Sawaizumi et al.) and the thumb metacarpal (Bertelli et al.)
- Iliac crest-free VBG—Pechlaner et al. (1987), based on deep iliac circumflex artery
- Microsurgical-free medial femoral condyle periosteal VBG **(Fig. 31)**—usually based on descending genicular artery and vein but may also be based on superomedial genicular artery. The arteries are located by Doppler and can be found by retracting the vastus medialis. The graft is harvested free based on one of the pedicles depending on better caliber and sutured end-to-side to radial artery.
- Dorsal capsular vascularized bone grafts based on fourth extensor compartmental artery of dorsal carpal arch.
- 2,3-ICSRA (intercompartmental supraretinacular artery) and 4,5-intercompartmental retinacular artery **(Figs. 32A and B)**—they have longer pedicle than Zaidemberg.
- Zaidemberg technique [1,2 intercompartmental supraretinacular artery (1,2 ICSRA)]—this involves

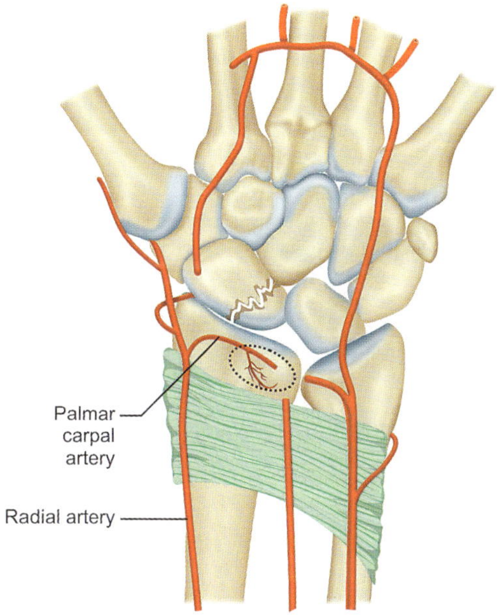

Fig. 30: The Mathoulin–Kullman palmar carpal artery based pedicle graft from distal radius.

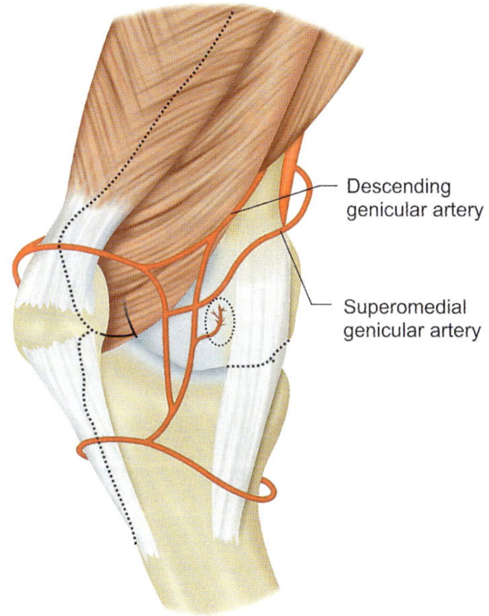

Fig. 31: Microsurgical free medial femoral condyle periosteal vascularized bone graft.

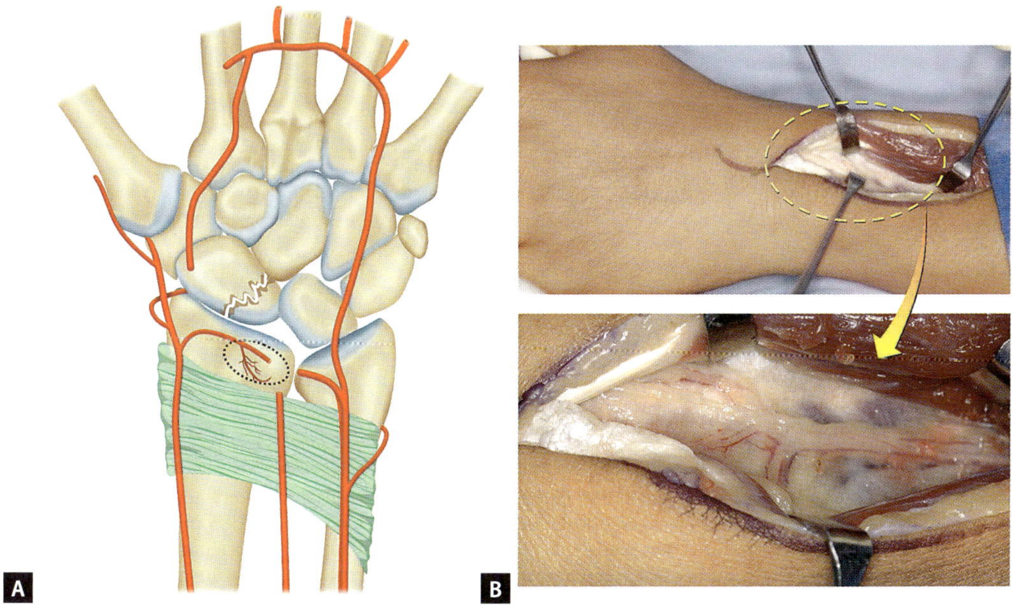

Figs. 32A and B: The dorsal 4,5-intercompartmental retinacular artery based pedicle bone graft. Schematic diagram (A) and intraoperative photographs depicting the retinacular vessels entering bone to be harvested (B).

harvesting bone graft from dorsal distal radius from the 1,2 ICSRA territory as a vascularized pedicle graft **(Figs. 33A to K)**. Good union rates have been reported but disadvantage includes kinking of vascular pedicle while rotation and need of radial styloidectomy for correction of humpback deformity. This is the method I commonly

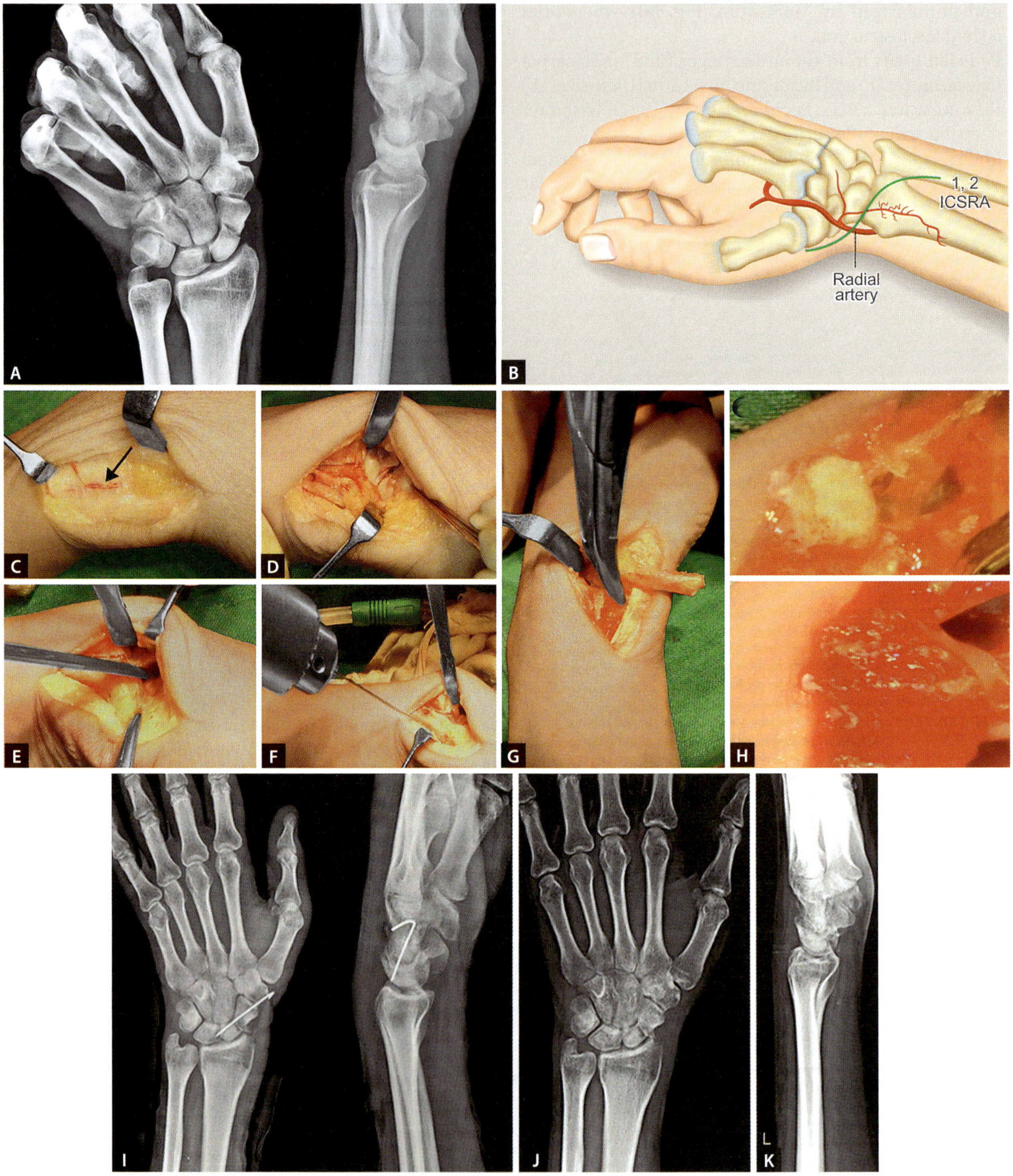

Figs. 33A to K: (A) Nonunion of fracture of scaphoid; (B) Illustration of the 1,2 intercompartmental supraretinacular artery (1,2 ICSRA). This patient though does not have any overt carpal instability as he was diagnosed early. Long-standing nonunions become unstable and often present with dorsal intercalated segment instability (DISI). The patient was managed by Zaidemberg vascularized graft technique for correction of nonunion and deformity. That went into uneventful union; (C) Exposure of the intercompartmental vessels (arrow); (D) Exposure of the nonunion site; (E) Preparation of the nonunion site and measuring the required graft size; (F) Marking the bone graft size by drill holes using K-wire; (G) Elevating the graft and performing partial radial styloidectomy; (H) Ensuring the vascularity of graft by deflating tourniquet; (I) Placement of the graft and fixing with smooth pin; (J and K) Radiograph of patient at 3 months showing well-placed graft and ensuing start of union, also note the partial radial styloidectomy.

used for revascularization of osteonecrotic scaphoid and for nonunions but it seems to form the current literature that 1,2 ICSRA lost the battle (as it has worse union rates) to microsurgical free periosteal vascularized bone grafts from the femoral medial condyle. The latter seems to have nearly 100% union rates but there are some drawbacks for medial femoral condyle periosteal VBG:

- Needs GA
- Needs two surgical teams
- Microvascular anastomosis
- Ectopic bone formation

Comparison of vascularized versus nonvascular bone graft for scaphoid nonunion: When a pooled head-to-head comparison is made for use of VBG to NVBG, it is found that there is no difference in union rates after both techniques (87% for both) but a definite shift to increasing use of VBG was seen in current literature. The lack of difference could definitely be real but one should consider that commonly surgeons tend to use VBG for more complicated cases and also VBG has a learning curve that is greater than NVBG, so initial cases may be failing. It is recommended to prefer VBG in proximal pole nonunions, established osteonecrosis, long-standing pseudarthrosis, failed prior surgery, and nonunions with humpback deformity. I feel free microvascular medial femoral condyle grafts would be superior for failed previous surgeries, if facilities are available. Also, free VBG are good if a large wedge is needed for deformity correction. VBG are contraindicated in patients with arthritic changes and those with unsalvageable proximal pole (egg-shell cartilage remnant devoid of any significant bone). The results of VBG are also not good in smokers.

Despite best of the treatments, it has been seen that nonunion persists in 10% of initially ununited cases. Nonunions after nonoperative treatment of the acute fracture in a plaster cast appear to have a lower ultimate union rate than when primary fixation had failed and was revised. Other prognostic factors for these resistant cases appear to be:

- Time since initial injury to nonunion surgery (≥5 years)
- Proximal pole nonunion
- Osteonecrosis
- Smoking
- Previous surgery

FEMORAL NECK NONUNION

Femoral neck fractures are a common occurrence in elderly population, which is at risk for prevalent osteoporosis. Only 2–3% occur in younger patients (<50 years) as a result of high-energy trauma. Due to increased outdoor activity and road traffic accidents, the incidence seems to be increasing in younger population. In elderly patients, females have a higher incidence of fractures; but in younger population, males suffer more from fracture neck femur. Prognosis is worse in younger patients, as extreme force is required to produce fracture, which explains the increased incidence of AVN and nonunion. It is considered that this is the most expensive fracture to treat when calculated on per person basis. The primary reason is prevalence of complications, especially osteonecrosis of femoral head and fracture

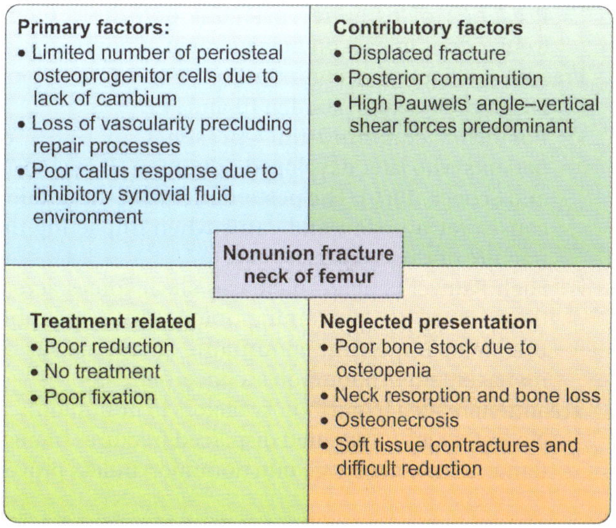

Fig. 34: Pathogenesis of development of nonunion fracture neck of femur.

nonunion despite adequate management for the fracture in younger patients. In elderly, mortality is quite high which ranges from 25 to 30% at 1 year that is double in patients with renal compromise. Nonunion has been reported to occur in 10–34% of patients while osteonecrosis seemingly is seen in 25–40% of the patients. Early fixation of fractures seems to influence osteonecrosis primarily, but may also help in somewhat preventing nonunion. The factors that are responsible for development of nonunion include **(Fig. 34)**:

- Compromised biology of the fracture (primary factors leading to nonunion):
  - Poorly developed cambium layer of periosteum, so there is very limited supply of osteoprogenitor cells at the fracture, if any (Phemister, 1939).
  - Poor callus formation due to continuous bathing of the fracture in synovial fluid washing away the healing factors and lysis of hematoma. The synovial milieu is chondrogenic and is tilted to maintain the chondrogenic surfaces, so it also prevents osteogenesis.
  - Loss of vascularity preventing biological stimulation to occur at fracture instead the ends go into atrophic nonunion. Hulth (1961) postulated that as healing callus comes from the neck shaft side of the fracture so due to injury to vascularity, the osteogenesis suffers. The femoral head is hypovolemic structure (Nakamura et al.) as seen in hemodynamic studies and it has been postulated by Konishiki that almost all displaced femoral neck fractures are avascular, which regain vascularity slowly after adequate treatment. For similar reasons, osteonecrosis is seen accompanying nonunion. Interestingly, patients with good bone stock are at higher risk of osteonecrosis (Portzman and Burkhalter, 1976) probably because higher forces are required to disrupt the bone causing much higher or complete damage to vascularity. One must bear in mind, however, that not every nonunion has associated osteonecrosis and nonunion is not always a certainty in avascular heads (Marti, 1993).

Presence of osteonecrosis but definitely has a tremendous impact on management of nonunion.

- Fracture configuration (contributory factors to nonunion):
  - Displaced fracture (Garden III and IV)
  - Posterior comminution—presents in >60% of patients who later developed nonunion (Banks, 1974 and Scheck, 1980). The posteroinferior comminution causes retroversion and varus when impacting the fracture during fixation.
  - High Pauwel's angle—increases shear forces across the fracture line preventing union. This is possibly the most important modifiable factor as far as management of nonunion is concerned.
- Treatment related (contributory factors to nonunion):
  - No treatment—untreated displaced fractures of neck femur almost always go into nonunion unless proved otherwise
  - Poor reduction
  - Poor fixation
- Neglected presentation—this is a common occurrence in developing countries due to poverty, ignorance, and lack of facilities that complicates the already compromised state by:
  - Osteopenia
  - Neck resorption
  - Osteonecrosis
  - Development of contractures and in some cases damage to acetabular cartilage

Delayed presentation as mentioned above is quite common in Asian subcontinent due to various reasons such as lack of awareness, remote location of adequate facilities, dominance of quacks in the remote villages, illiteracy, and poverty. The late presenters have been classified who seek medical attention after 3 weeks to 3 months. They present unique challenges in management of fracture neck of femur and are prone to develop further complications.

Definition of nonunion: For fracture neck of femur, the temporal definition usually agreed upon is a fracture that fails to unite (or present) after 3 months of occurrence. Biologically, it is the time when reparative process has halted (Cave, 1958). The FDA panel definition of 9 months cannot be applied here as the morbidity is too high and any chance of improvement reduces to negligible after 3 months. Classifications of femoral neck nonunion are not very helpful in decision making as regards the treatment and not even prognosticating the outcome. The followings are the attempts made to classify femoral neck nonunion by some authors.

1. *Sandhu et al.*—based on the various parameters evaluated on plain radiographs, MRI, and computed tomography (CT) scan, the fractures are allocated into one of the three stages (no validation of classification system available). They have also suggested treatments based on the classification system **(Box 1)**.
   i *Stage I:*
      a. Irregular fracture surfaces (fresh)
      b. Size of proximal fragment (measured from upper margin of fovea centralis to the midpoint of fracture margin) ≥2.5 cm
      c. Gap between the fragments ≤1 cm
      d. Viable femoral head—no sign of osteonecrosis on MRI/CT

   ii. *Stage II:*
      a. Smoothened fracture surfaces
      b. Proximal fragment ≥2.5 cm
      c. Gap between fragments >1 cm, but <2.5 cm
      d. Viable femoral head

      If either of features a or c is present, the nonunion is classified as stage II.

   iii. *Stage III:*
      a. Smoothened fracture surfaces
      b. Proximal fragment size <2.5 cm
      c. Gap between fragments >2.5 cm
      d. Head shows signs of osteonecrosis

      If any of the features of b, c, or d is present, it is classified as stage III.
2. *Leighton classification*—this is a system of classification based on the cause of the nonunion and clarifies treatment options to maintain the femoral head and produce union of the femoral neck.
   i. Type I—nonunion resulting from inadequate fixation or nonanatomic reduction
   ii. Type II—nonunion due to loss of fixation with displacement
   iii. Type III—fibrous nonunion with no displacement and intact fixation

BOX 1: Sandhu classification based treatment options for various stages of ununited fracture neck of femur as proposed same authors.

Stage I:
- Closed reduction with fibular graft/closed reduction with muscle pedicle bone graft
- Valgus osteotomy
- McMurray's osteotomy with plaster of Paris (POP) spica

Stage II:
- Closed reduction and internal fixation (CRIF) with screw + fibula
- Open reduction freshening of nonunion and screw fixation with fibula
- Open reduction and internal fixation (ORIF) with muscle pedicle bone grafting
- McMurray's osteotomy
- Bachelor's procedure
- Girdlestone procedure

Stage III:
- Hip arthroplasty
- McMurray's osteotomy
- Subtrochanteric osteotomy with internal fixation
- Girdlestone procedure or Bachelor procedure

Investigation

Plain X-rays are the initial modality to assess and diagnose fracture nonunion. One can estimate the nonunion angle (very crudely), assess osteopenia (Singh's index), bone loss and resorption **(Fig. 35)**, length of remaining proximal fragment, presence of osteonecrosis (discernible by 2 months but evident clearly by 6 months), calcar comminution, and angulation at nonunion. Radiographs of contralateral hips with proximal femur are also needed to plan the treatment, especially calculation of wedge size in case of osteotomy and estimation of neck resorption ratio (NRR, see below). ^{99m}Tc methylene diphosphonate (MDP) bone scan had been quite popular in past to assess vascularity of the proximal fragment and to look for infection if suspected; but with wide availability of MRI at comparable cost, MRI has become the investigation of choice for assessing osteonecrosis. NCCT hip may be ordered, if the size of proximal fragment is not evident on radiographs and/or the angle of nonunion is difficult to calculate.

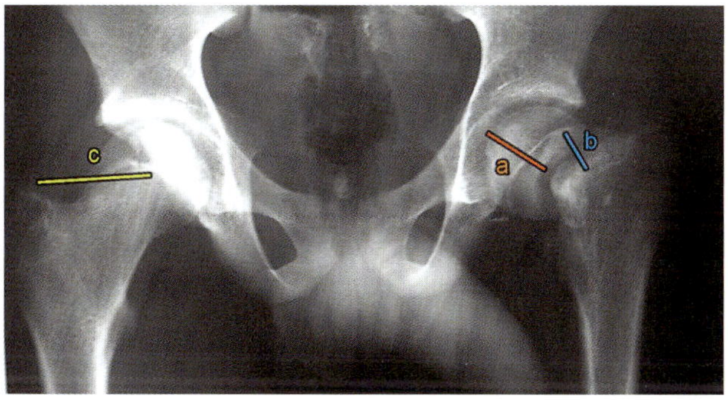

Fig. 35: Nonunion fracture neck of right femur in a 20-year-old male. Plain radiographs help in estimating some of the parameters useful for planning of treatment. "a" is the size of proximal fragment, "b" is the gap between fragments and represents neck resorption, and "c" is neck length on uninvolved side. The ratio a/c is the neck resorption ratio helpful in prognostication of treatment.

Treatment

The treatment of nonunion is highly influenced by the age at presentation, presence of osteonecrosis, and functional demands of patient. Other factors that may have additional bearing on planning treatment include presence of degenerative joint disease (tilt to arthroplasty), smoking, liver, or renal disease (reduces chances of success of union). An algorithm is presented in **Flowchart 2** incorporating these decision-making factors and available options. While prosthetic replacement is considered best choice for the treatment of displaced fractures in patients above 60 years of age or even in some younger patients with physiologically higher age or whose life expectancy is limited by associated comorbidities, efforts are focused on preserving the femoral head in physiologically younger patients. Chronologically, patients aged <60 years should be offered femoral head-preserving surgery. This means that we have three broad categories of surgical options.

Flowchart 2: Decision making in management of nonunion fracture neck of femur.

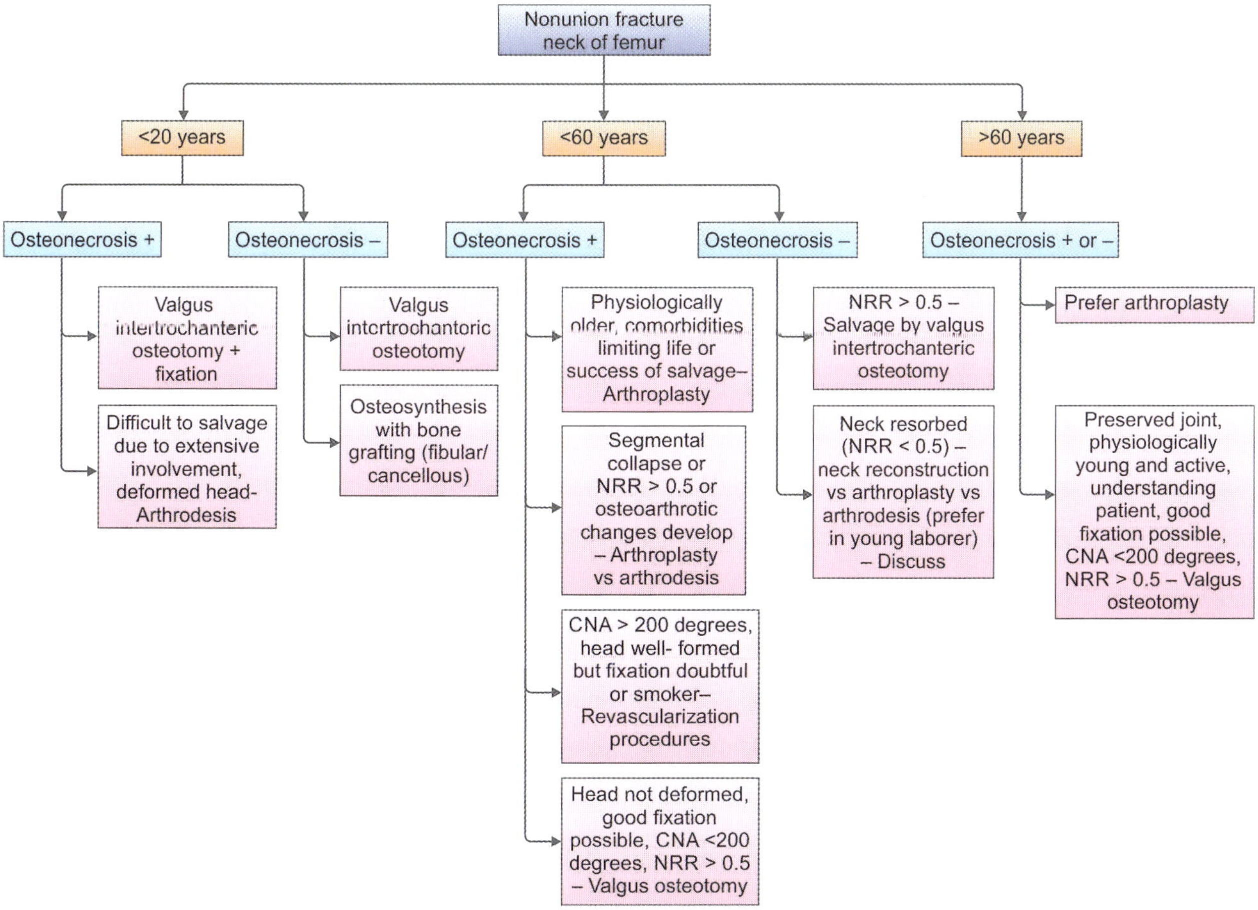

[+: present; –: absent; CNA: combined necrotic angle of Kerboul (*see* Chapter on "Osteonecrosis and Osteochondrosis"); NRR: neck resorption ratio (see text)]

Head-preserving Procedures

These are most suitable for patients aged <60 years and physiologically younger patients, if femoral head is viable and adequate neck length is left over. If the head is congruous then radiographic presence of osteonecrosis is not an absolute contraindication for performing osteotomy.

One needs to choose appropriate option from the many available as detailed below:

- *Fixation alone*—this is *not at all* a treatment modality of established nonunion, it is mentioned here only for late presenters or untreated fractures that report within 3 weeks of injury, which are undisplaced or are reducible.
- Open reduction and internal fixation (ORIF) with cortical (fibular) or corticocancellous bone grafting—ORIF or closed reduction and internal fixation (CRIF) with fibular grafting has been reported by various authors from India with limited to moderate success in achieving union **(Figs. 36A and B)** and is individually popular among believers. Inserting fibula along with two to three partially threaded cancellous screws has been portended to initiate or hasten osteogenesis by somehow modifying vascularity but defies logic of how the biological factors really change by just inserting fibula across the nonunion, which also is a weak mechanical fixation.
- Open reduction and internal fixation with cancellous bone grafting—(Deyerly, 1980 and Dickson, 1953)—the nonunion site is grafted anteriorly by carving out a window across the nonunion. The method is similar to bone grafting as done for any other nonunion and had moderately acceptable results.
- "Triple attack technique" for femoral neck nonunion—here three techniques are combined to reduce the chances of femoral neck shortening. Iliac autogenous cancellous bone grafting is done after excising nonunion using open technique combined with static fixation across nonunion, followed by valgus intertrochanteric osteotomy. I am unsure of the reliability or advantage of this extensive procedure as literature is sparse.
- Open reduction and internal fixation with various revascularization procedures (for an exhaustive list and details of the various revascularization procedures including vascularized fibular grafting kindly refer to Chapter on "Osteonecrosis and Osteochondrosis" under treatment for osteonecrosis of femoral head). These are popular methods, especially in the Indian subcontinent where neglected fractures are a common occurrence. The procedure additionally addresses the issue of osteonecrosis as revascularization is deemed not only to hasten osteogenesis at the fracture but also provide vascularity to the femoral head. It is interesting to note in this instance that revascularization after femoral neck fractures usually stops at the anterosuperior portion, so vascularized grafts may improve this aspect of healing as well.
- Proximal femoral osteotomy ± fixation—orientation of the fracture line is possibly the most important contributory factor for development of nonunion apart from the primary biological factors. Reorientation of this nonunion line to more horizontal has been intrigued by various surgeons in turn developing their methods of achieving the same. The proximal femoral osteotomies work on the principle of converting shearing displacing forces to compressive forces by realigning the fracture site.
    - *Pauwels' osteotomy*—this is by far the most popular method. The valgus intertrochanteric osteotomy was initially described by Pauwels and subsequently modified by Müller for management of Coxa Vara and associated limb length discrepancy (LLD). It was later popularized by Marti et al. in management of nonunion fracture neck of femur. The advantages of this procedure are that it preserves the native head and patient can sit cross-legged as is commonly needed in Indian population for various functions and practices. It is not a panacea and around 80–85% of nonunions unite by the procedure. One must also look at the contraindications or pitfalls of the procedure as it has been described in detail below.

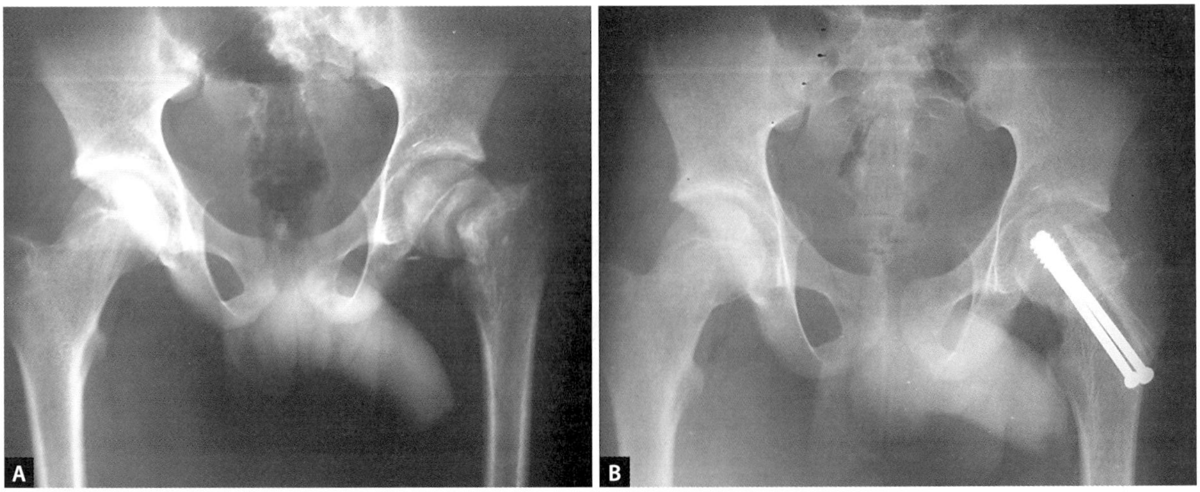

Figs. 36A and B: Fracture left femoral neck nonunion successfully treated in a 20-year-old male using screw osteosynthesis (A) and fibular grafting (B).

- *Dickson high geometric osteotomy*—similar to Pauwels osteotomy; but after osteotomy, the distal fragment is abducted to 60°. Thus with weight-bearing the femoral head gets abducted and fracture line would become horizontal.
- *McMurray's osteotomy*—this was an agreeable method of managing nonunion fracture neck of femur in patients with associated osteonecrosis that would limit the success of salvage procedure (say osteonecrosis >50% or 75% of the head volume). The weight-bearing line got shifted medially decreasing abductor efficiency by changing the lever arm and predisposing to early OA of hip joint. Also the distortion created by this medially displacing osteotomy in the anatomy of proximal femur precluded future arthroplasty. These drawbacks pulled this procedure out-of-favor now.
- *Schanz angulation osteotomy*—the osteotomy is done below lesser trochanter and produces excessive valgus at the angulation to produce apparent lengthening. No longer popular nowadays.

- Combination of osteotomy and bone grafting.
- *Neck reconstruction*—where most of the above methods do not address the issue of resorption at fracture site leading to shortened femoral neck in case union is achieved, neck reconstruction was proposed by a small group of surgeons creating a trough by carving anterior, posterior, and inferior walls in the resorbed space and filling it with cancellous bone. Later, the method was modified by using a titanium cage filled with bone graft to provide length to femoral neck and improve offset. Very limited quality literature is available for this unproven method, however.

Head-sacrificing Procedures

These are indicated in patients with chronological age >60 years, physiologically older patients, and those with comorbidities limiting the success of head salvage procedures or reducing life expectancy itself. The procedure is also indicated in patients where the head is deformed due to osteonecrosis or in whom signs of osteoarthrosis have developed or were present from beginning. Lastly, patients who do not accept the 15–20% failure rate of head salvage procedures may also be offered arthroplasty as an option explaining that they may need revision, if they outlast the life of the implanted prosthesis. The various options for head sacrificing are:

- *Hemiarthroplasty:*
  - *Unipolar prosthesis*—hardly used ever now (older versions included Thompson cemented collared and Austin-Moore prosthesis).
  - *Bipolar*—cemented/uncemented bipolar prosthesis is used in patients with limited life expectancy or associated comorbidities that would make total hip arthroplasty high-risk surgery.
- *Total hip arthroplasty*—this is the preferred option in the head-sacrificing group. Cemented and uncemented with partial options of hybrid and reverse hybrid are all used depending on indication, training, and preference. Good success rates and immediate mobility are the advantages of this surgery but one should also understand the high morbidity of a failed or infected procedure.

Salvage Procedures

These are rarely offered but have their own specific place in the management of nonunion fracture neck femur. There are two ultimate salvage procedures:

1. *Arthrodesis of hip*—this option is specifically indicated for young patients who either do not want head salvage or in whom there is high concern of fixation/procedure failure due to osteopenia or osteonecrosis of the femoral head. The option is also specifically proposed for patients younger than 20 years of age where osteotomy or vascularization procedures are somehow not feasible.
2. *Girdlestone arthroplasty*—this is a mutilating procedure and I personally feel has no role in initial management of nonunion neck femur. This may be an option in case of failed hemiarthroplasty or failed total hip arthroplasty or a head salvage surgery that had failed due to infection where secondary arthroplasty procedure is not possible or not desired. It may be combined with Milch-Bachelor type pelvic support osteotomy to improve some of the drawbacks like shortening and instability associated with Girdlestone procedure.

Valgus Intertrochanteric Osteotomy for Nonunion Neck of Femur

(kindly also refer to Chapter on "Osteotomies Around the Hip Joint" for Additional Details and Comparison with Contemporary Techniques)

The following is a concise description of the procedure as modified from Müller. The primary aim of the procedure is reorientation of the nonunion line to a more horizontal plane, so that the displacing forces are converted into compression ones. The secondary effect is apparent limb lengthening by the procedure. The procedure is not without contraindications and it must be carefully chosen in patients. Patients having small proximal fragment are prone to failure. The appropriate guideline has still not be elucidated but Sandhu et al. suggested that patients with <2.5 cm of head size have worst outcome so are possibly not amenable to salvage by this method, but this classification has its own drawbacks. Some authors suggested that absolute head volume of ≤43 mm^3 (measured by NCCT) is associated with high-failure rates; however, it is debatable and inconsistent. Measuring head size is not possibly appropriate, as it varies with the stature, ethnicity, and sex. Better measure is the NRR, which is given by the formula:

$$\text{NRR} = \frac{\text{Size of femoral head remnant}}{\text{Size of femoral neck on the sound side}}$$

This measure of NRR is hence a ratio depending on the individual. A ratio of <0.5 indicates high chances of failure from the valgus intertrochanteric osteotomy. Following are the steps of the procedure:

- *Step 1*—template the other hip for determining the position of the osteotomy and implant placement.
  - Measure the nonunion angle (angle the fracture line makes with horizontal), which is difficult to calculate on a radiograph due to spiral orientation of fracture. Say for example, it comes 65°.
  - Then calculate the angle of correction. It is important to orient the fracture (nonunion) line to ≤30° (25° to be exact) for physiological force transmission causing compression else still the shear forces remain and preclude the aim of doing osteotomy. Body forces subtend an angle of 16° at hip joint. The anatomical axis is at an angle of 8–10° to body forces, so the pseudarthrosis site should be oriented to forces at around 25° (9° + 16°). Now, if the fracture angle was 65° and correction till 25° is needed then angle of correction will be 65° – 25° = 40°. This is the angle of correction.
  - Now calculate the size of wedge needed. There are two ways of calculating the size of wedge:
    1. *Approximation method:* It is generally considered that 1° of angle corresponds to 1 mm of wedge size (which is really crude but very easy). This means that for angle of correction of 40°, we need a wedge of 40 mm. The approximation method is often incorrect, but if one sees practically up to 3–4 mm, error in the correct direction will not make much difference, if still performed meticulously.
    2. *Geometric method:* This relies on the tangent to the angle of correction and diameter of the bone at osteotomy site. The size of wedge is given by the formula:

       Wedge in mm = Tangent to angle of correction × angle of correction × diameter of bone

       This is a bit difficult for general calculation purposes, so a simpler version is as follows:

       Wedge in mm = 0.02 × angle of correction × diameter of bone at the osteotomy

- *Step 2*—reduction and stabilization—closed reduction is attempted on fracture table without much traction, as this may damage the retinacular vessels. If closed, reduction is not possible then open reduction is needed commonly to excise the inferior spike of the proximal fragment. The reduction is maintained with a K-wire or Guide pin passed through center of the head and as perpendicular to the femoral shaft as possible. The fracture is then fixed with an osteotomy blade plate commonly or as some may prefer a screw plate construct. The osteotomy blade plate is commonly passed perpendicular to the femoral shaft to aid in achieving the correction. So, if 130° angle blade plate was chosen as fixation method then when it is brought down parallel to shaft (placed at 90°) for fixation **(Figs. 37A and B)**; the rotation of proximal fragment to bring down the plate will be 130° – 90° = 40°. This was the desired angle of correction.
- *Step 3*—osteotomy at the deemed site is performed and shaft pulled up and fixed to the osteotomy blade plate. Dynamic hip screw is now commonly preferred as some compression can also be given at the nonunion site.

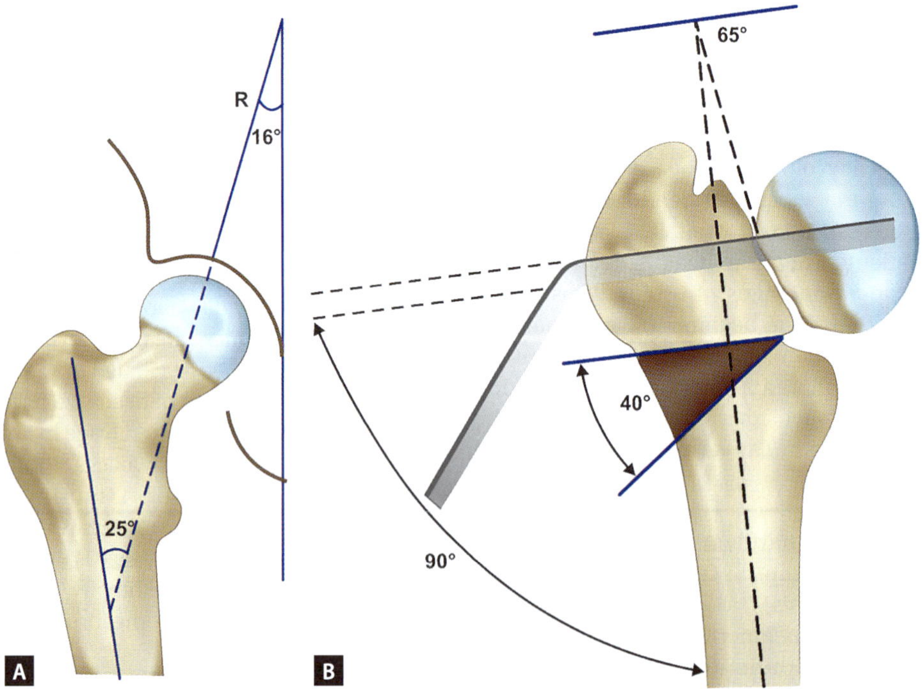

Figs. 37A and B: The resultant of forces across hip form an angle of 25° to the anatomical axis of femoral shaft and 16° to the vertical. For valgus intertrochanteric osteotomy, the osteotomy angle is calculated as the angle of fracture line –25°. This is due to the fact that if the fracture line/plane is oriented at 25° then the forces will pass perpendicular to the fracture producing maximal compression and minimal shear. In this example the osteotomy angle hence is 65° – 25° = 40°

Pitfalls of Intertrochanteric Valgus Intertrochanteric Osteotomy of Müller (Modified Pauwels)

- Large wedge >30–35 mm produces excessive valgus. This causes increased tension in the muscles across the joint increasing joint reaction forces and may cause early OA. Also, the excessive stretch placed on the retinacular vessels this way may predispose to osteonecrosis. Large wedge >40 mm reaches the subtrochanteric regions distorting the canal anatomy (abduction and external rotation deformity) of femur compromising future procedures. It has been reported that valgus of >15° compared to the normal hip results in poorer functional outcome.
- Appropriate blade length should be chosen as longer blade would cause distraction at the nonunion while smaller blade may not adequately fix the proximal fragment getting prone to failure.
- There is a finite chance of developing osteonecrosis after valgus intertrochanteric osteotomy in patients who did not have it before. This possibility is seen in 20–32% patients and should be kept in mind explaining also to the patient that if secondary changes occur, this may be the cause of late failure of procedure.

Complications of Valgus Intertrochanteric Osteotomy

- Osteonecrosis of femoral head (20–32% chance)
- Persistent nonunion
- Implant failure and cut out
- Infection
- Increased joint reaction forces causing persistent pain and development of osteoarthrosis
- Shortening of lever arm presenting as persistent limp in walking
- Altered femoral canal anatomy making future total hip arthroplasty difficult (especially, if wedge size is larger than 35–40 mm).

MALUNION

Definition

Osseous union in nonanatomical position is considered malunion. This is purely an anatomical or radiological definition that considers any deviation however large or small from normal as a malunion. Functional, esthetic, or mechanical problems are not typically addressed by this definition. Small malunions (<10° of angulation, <2 cm shortening in lower limb bones, or <30% translations) usually do not pose any functional deficits. Larger deviations variably pose functional deficits and mechanical problems altering movements and weight-bearing significantly. The variability in functional expression of malunion differs from bone to bone, upper limb versus lower limb, and the type of function of the bone (e.g., childbearing for pelvic bones will affect only females of childbearing age while a malunited calcaneum will cause problems to all age groups). Thus, it is important to specify malunion/deformity for individual bones and a generalized definition that is universally applicable is impossible.

Etiology of Malunion

Conservative management with plaster cast, traction, or splints commonly produces malunion. Unacceptable conservative management may be deliberate (far reaching places, quack treatment) or enforced. Pandemic situations like Coronavirus disease (COVID) overwhelm medical services that get restricted to lifesaving procedures only. Fractures are commonly hence treated with conservative and classical methods increasing the incidence of malunion. Inadequate reduction during fixation or loss of reduction after fixation also produces malunion. Shortening may result from fixation of comminuted fractures where acute docking is done to achieve union.

Defining Deformity

Bones can have angulatory, translatory, rotational, or overriding malunion that produces specific deformity and have discrete bearing on the extremity/limb function.

- *Angulatory malunion:* Angulation is a displacement pattern in which all the reference points on distal segment of bone rotate around a stationary point (located at deformity site). This point is called center of rotation of angulation (CORA, **Fig. 38**). Angulatory malunion is usually described along coronal plane (mediolateral) or sagittal plane (AP) because the radiographs are taken in these two perpendicular projections. Sagittal plane malalignment produces procurvatum or recurvatum deformity having anterior or posterior angulation, respectively. Coronal plane malalignment produces varus or valgus deformity having lateral and medial angulations. Commonly, however, angulation is a point that does not fall in either of

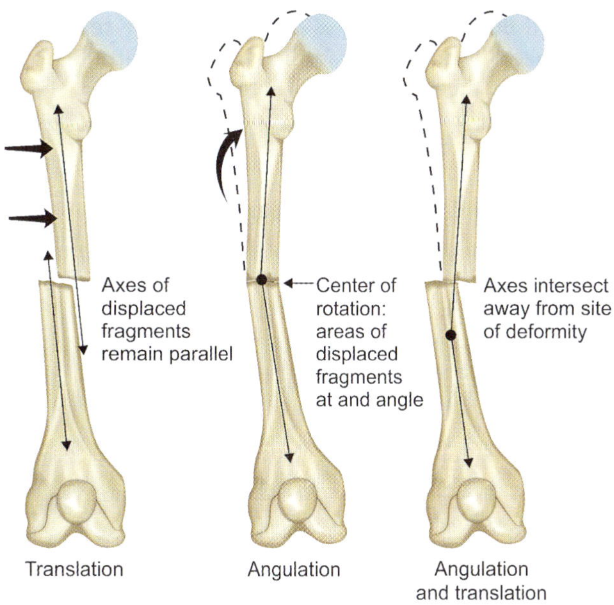

Fig. 38: Translation, angulation, and combined deformities. In translation, the anatomical axes of the two fragments do not intersect. In pure angulation, the anatomic axes of the fragments intersect at the obvious deformity transverse plane. If the deformities are combined then anatomical axes intersect at a point away from deformity.

these planes and this can be currently evaluated only on a CT scan to describe it fully. Such descriptions are however useful only if correction is planned using 3D modeling and specific instruments that would provide correction in x-, y-, and z-coordinates together. Most of conventional surgical procedures are based on two-dimensional projection of the angulation deformity. On a radiograph, angulation is easily identified by drawing central axial lines [anatomic axis (AA), see below] of the two segments that meet at some point on the transverse plane of deformity site (obvious location of deformity). If they meet distally or proximally then translatory component is additionally present, if the lines do not intersect at all then there is pure translation **(Fig. 38)**.

- *Translatory malunion:* All points on distal segment of bone are displaced for equal distance in same direction. There is transverse plane displacement of the distal fragment. If anatomical axes are drawn for the fragments then the lines will not intersect at all **(Fig. 38)**.
- *Rotational malunion:* All the points on distal segment are rotated along axial plane when seen in reference to proximal segment. It produces torsional malalignment. This cannot be seen on conventional radiographs and need axial imaging techniques (computed tomography scanning) to describe them. The distal segment can be externally or internally rotated.
- *Overriding malunion:* Here the segments override and produce shortening of variable magnitude. It can be considered as translation along axial axis.

Recording Deformity

Malunions generally produce a combination of above deformities and displacements; finding pure deformity is unusual. So, we need to have a universal template on which all the components of deformity can be recorded. I recommend using Maurice Müller devised deformity matrix for recording the displacements in malunion **(Table 4)**. This is based on radiographic evaluation on two perpendicular planes.

Approach to Patient with Malunion

After the malunions, deformities and displacements are ascertained and recorded. One needs to understand the clinical and functional significance and the limitations they produce. The following points represent the common thought process while evaluating and prescribing treatment for malunion.

TABLE 4: The Maurice Müller deformity matrix for recording the various displacements in a malunion.

Deformity	*Coronal plane*	*Sagittal plane*	*Axial plane*
Translation	Medial	Anterior	Shortening
	Lateral	Posterior	Lengthening
Angulation	Varus	Apex anterior (procurvatum)	Internal rotation
	Valgus	Apex posterior (recurvatum)	External rotation

- Record a good, detailed history to know the cause of malunion—surgical/circumstantial (polytrauma/open trauma)/implant related/soft tissue contractures/secondary gain and no real functional limitation. Take appropriate surgical/medical/psychiatric/addiction and medication history. Some patients may have started unsolicited walking like psychiatric patients or drug addicts that would have led to implant and osteosynthesis failure.
- Ascertain the level of functional deficit/limitation. One may take the help of scoring systems such as lower extremity functional score (LEFS), disability of the arm, shoulder, and hand (DASH), SF-36 (for quality of life), and constant score for quantification of the current disability.
- Correlate the functional disability with radiological findings—if correlation is not substantiated then look for additional modifiers such as pelvic obliquity, scoliosis, or soft tissue contractures and then compensate for correlation.
- Once correlation is established, the most important aspect is aligning the surgeon and patient expectations/needs/demands and possibility of fulfilling them. Not always a malunion is a surgical candidate and many can be compensated by nonsurgical means if disability or limitation is minimal.
- Surgical correction of malunion needs careful planning and replanning with expert consultation and discussion. The following are necessary points to ponder in a surgical plan:
  - Surgical approach
  - Osteotomy type + additional methods such as bone grafting, lengthening of bone, and addressing soft tissue conditions/complications
  - Fixation technique and correction method (single stage/gradual)
- Discussing the complications of surgery—nonunion, under/overcorrection, nerve injury, skin and soft tissue complications, infection, and compartment syndrome

Evaluation

The first step is obviously detailed trauma (initial), treatment (logic, soft tissue, and bony management), surgical, relevant medical, drug addiction, and psychiatry history recording. The functional deficit and limitation is documented and is better objectively recorded using various function scoring systems as detailed above. This is followed by dedicated physical examination as follows:

- Measure coronal and sagittal plane deviations viz. varus/valgus angulations, adduction/abduction deformity, procurvatum, and recurvatum deformity
- Evaluate nearby joints for movements/stiffness, limitation in mobility, deformity, and ligament laxity. Contractures across joints has significant bearing on the correction of deformity planning.
- Record leg length inequality:
  - Indirect technique using measured block method **(Fig. 39)**—subjective as one person's understanding of squaring of pelvis may be different from other's. In

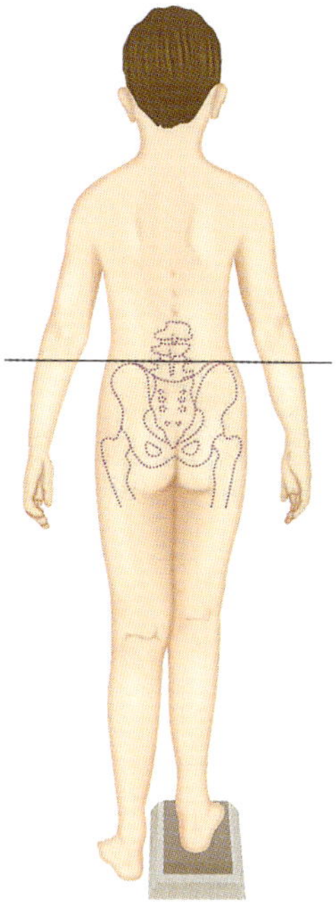

Fig. 39: The measured block method for assessment of limb shortening. Measured blocks of fixed height are placed under short limb and squaring of pelvis noted manually. The block at which pelvis gets squared reveals the magnitude of shortening.

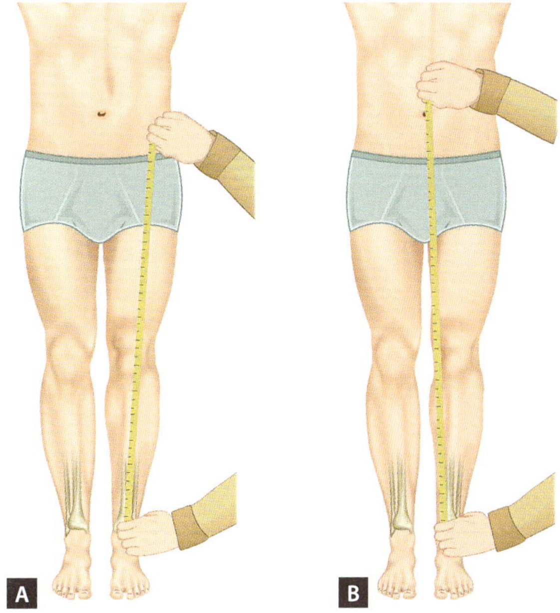

Figs. 40A and B: Assessment of true and apparent lengths for calculating shortening of lower limb. The values are compared from uninvolved limb to determine change in values (shortening/lengthening). The difference between true and apparent shortening tells about the compensation done by body.

between measures not possible so it is not precise. Cannot be done for upper limb.

- Direct method—measure length from anterior superior iliac spine to medial malleolus (lower limb) or angle of scapula to radial styloid for upper limb **(Figs. 40A and B)**. Overall assessment and ignores specific bone. It can, however identify intrinsic compensation done by pelvic obliquity and spinal compensation.
- Segmental length measurement—humeral/arm length, ulnar/forearm length, thigh/femoral length, and leg/tibial length can be measured individually. This method is more specific to identify individual bone shortening but may miss some bones and those that do not have definite superficial palpation points.
- Evaluate rotational deformities:
  - Femoral torsion—Craig test helps in identifying femoral torsional abnormalities **(Fig. 41)**. Utility is limited in patients with joint disease and painful contractures where free movements are not possible.
  - Tibial torsion—thigh foot axis evaluation (with patient seated and knee flexed 90° identify intermalleolar axis and compare from other side). It can be performed in prone position also with knees flexed to 90° **(Figs. 42A to C)**. The test cannot be performed if knee flexion is not possible.
- Gait analysis is done to reveal overall function of the lower limb for lower limb malunions and its impact on walking (*see* Chapter on "Gait" for details on assessment).

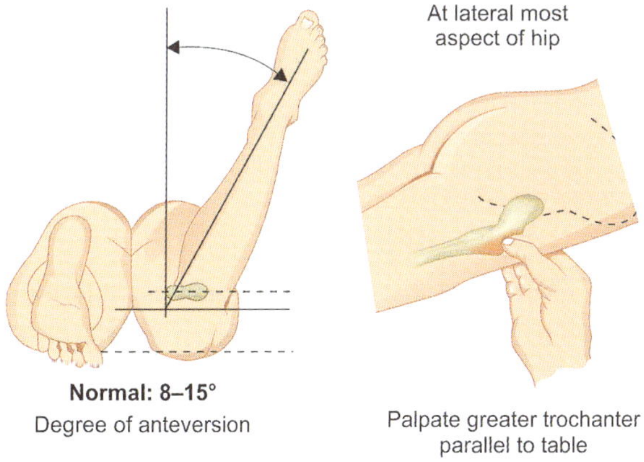

Fig. 41: The Craig test helps in assessing hip anteversion clinically. The patient lies prone and leg is flexed to 90° at knee. Move the leg while simultaneously palpating the greater trochanter for prominence. The trochanter is most prominent when neck of femur is in horizontal plane. The angle tibia makes with vertical gives the angle of anteversion. Comparison from opposite side will reveal the rotational malalignment due to femoral malunion. If deformity is present in both limbs then subtract normal femoral anteversion that will give rotational malalignment.

Imaging and Radiology

This provides the most important information about malunion and is quite precise. Ideally full-length radiographs should be obtained on large single film cassettes (51-inch cassettes). Because these are not commonly available, CT scanograms with scaled magnification are more commonly obtained **(Fig. 43)**. The radiographs should be obtained in optimal rotation for the bone in focus like 15° internal

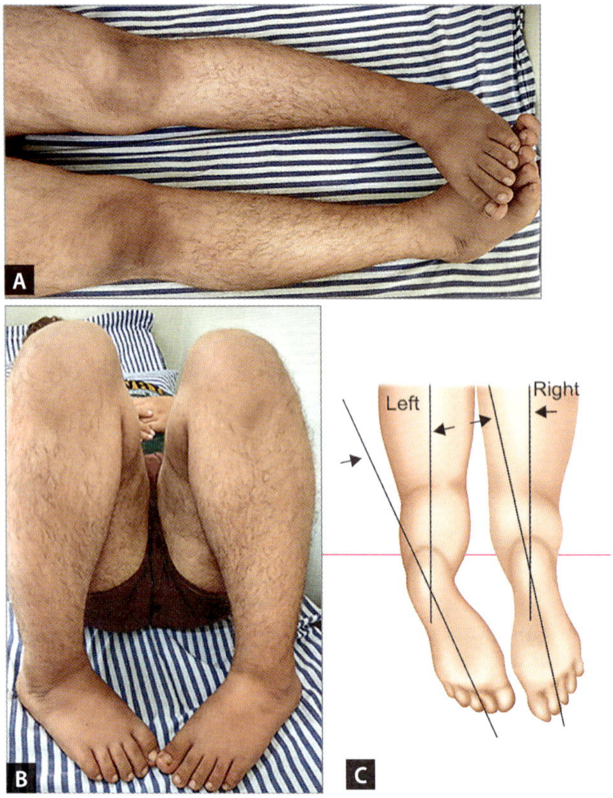

Figs. 42A to C: Clinical presentation of tibial intorsion. In supine position (A) the feet are internally rotated with patella pointing to roof. The patient has severe intorsion of tibia as seen with knee flexed (B) demonstrating some 60° of deformity (provisional estimation only). The thigh foot angle measurement gives much accurate assessment of tibial torsional malalignment (C). It is to be done in prone position (as illustrated) or with patient seated on a couch with legs hanging.

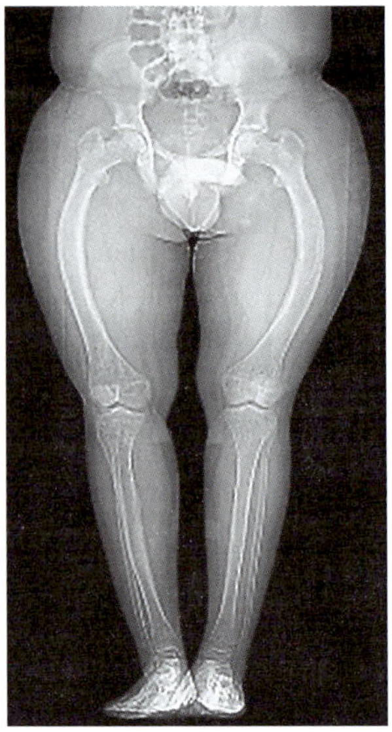

Fig. 43: The full length radiograph on large cassettes is difficult to obtain so CT scanograms are commonly ordered. They have the ease of single shot, single film radiography and also provide measures of length alterations, angulations, etc., in the same sitting using appropriate software. The scale used for compression of image should be strictly adhered to for extrapolation to real deformities, especially length changes.

rotation for true coronal plane placement of the tibia/femur. Radiographs are obtained in two orthogonal planes. Special views may be ordered if needed for a particular bone. True lateral view should be obtained by ascertaining overlapping femoral condyles so that correct malunion deformities are revealed. Images of contralateral limb are indispensable for comparison. The deformities are evaluated as follows:

- Determine and draw the mechanical axis of bones and the limb. This is usually done in frontal/coronal plane **(Figs. 44A and B)**. Limb mechanical axis are also defined in sagittal planes but uncommonly used.
- *Mechanical axis deviation:* This is the frontal/coronal plane deviation of current limb axis from standard measures. For example, for lower limb the line joining the center of femoral head to center of ankle joint passes within 6–7 mm medial to center of tibial spines (the correct reference is 4.1 mm ± 4 mm). If it deviates by any measure more than this on compensated measurements (for magnification, etc.) then MAD is said to be present **(Figs. 45A and B)**. Detailed discussion is also done in Chapter on "Anomalies of Pediatric Lower Limb". Upper limb mechanical axis is drawn as a straight line connecting the center of the humeral bone head and the center of the ulna head **(Fig. 44)**. MAD tells grossly how much the deformity impacts mechanical orientation of the limb. Because of weight-bearing profile of lower limb in humans, MAD is commonly not stressed for upper limbs. MAD does not reveal true measure of actual deformity. Deformity is calculated in coronal and sagittal planes or oblique plane (see below) by drawing the anatomical axes and CORA. MAD only tells the deviation in mechanical axis from normal and that the larger it is the more will be the impact on mechanical properties and biomechanics of the limb.
- *Drawing AA is the next step:* For a long bone, AA is the mid-diaphyseal line **(Fig. 46)**. It can also be called "longitudinal axis". AA is drawn for all fragments of deformity in coronal and sagittal planes. Intersection of these AA lines reveal the angular deformity and CORA. Oblique plane of complex deformities can be calculated by trigonometric or graphical method (see below). The deformity is corrected along the bisector of CORA such that the MAD ultimately disappears. In simple deformities correction of angular deformity usually aligns the MAD but in multifragment malunions there may be many CORAs. In such scenario, individual AA may not be restored and ultimate aim is alignment of joint plane and MAD. The restoration is done taking into account the adjacent joints and choosing suitable place for correction of deformity so that MAD is corrected, and joints reoriented. So, one needs to also draw and refer joint orientation lines and angle.
- *Joint orientation angle:* This is created by drawing a line tangential to subchondral shadow of the joint surface **(Fig. 47)** and an intersecting line drawn along the mechanical axis (mechanical angle) or AA (anatomical

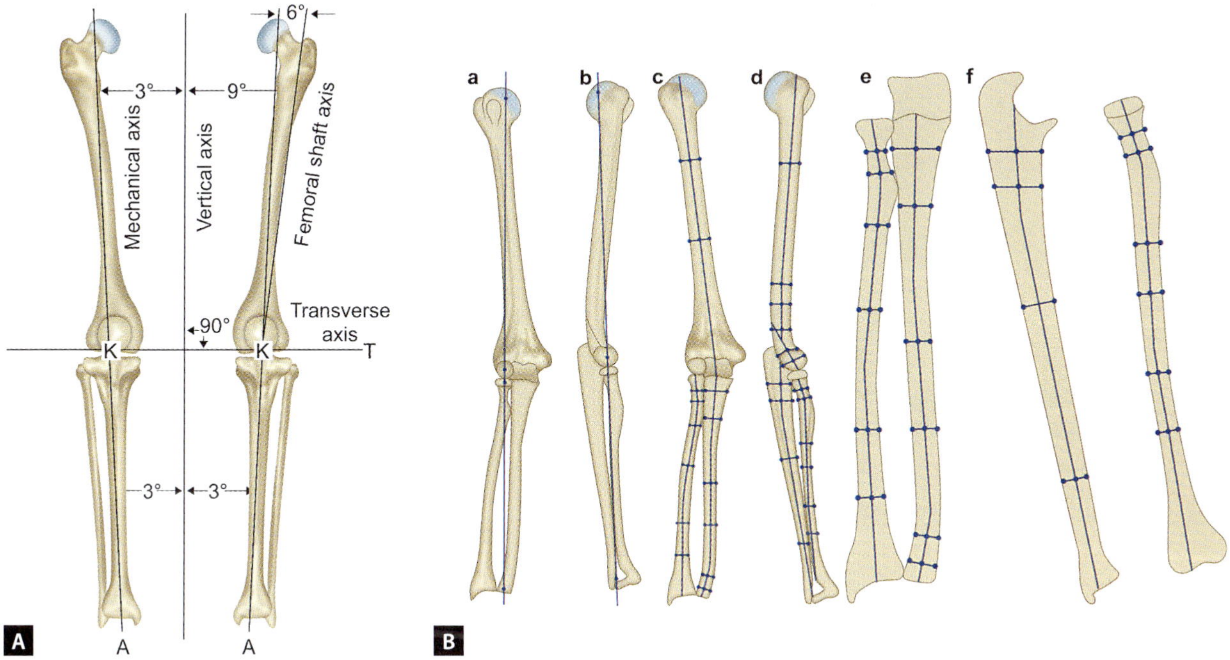

Figs. 44A and B: (A) Illustration showing the drawing of mechanical (left) and anatomical axis (right) of lower limb. (B) Upper limb mechanical axis in frontal and sagittal plane is illustrated in (a) and (b), respectively while the anatomical axis in frontal and sagittal plane are represented in (c) and (d). Also shown are the anatomical axes of radius and ulna in frontal (e) and sagittal (f) planes. (A—anatomical axis, T—transverse axis, and K—knee center).

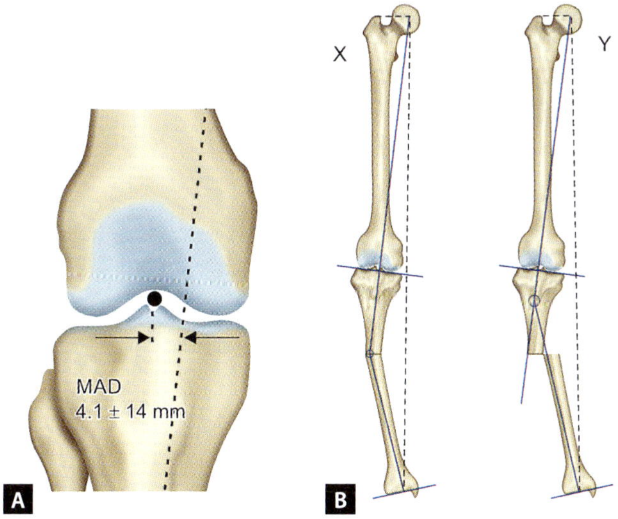

Figs. 45A and B: Mechanical axis deviation (MAD). (A) The illustration depicts the normal relation of mechanical axis of lower limb to knee center (see text for details). (B) Drawing the mechanical axis (dotted line) in various deformities, (X) there is pure angulation deformity of tibia and the mechanical axis passes medially. The magnitude of angulation is assessed by drawing anatomical axes that meet at center of rotation of angulation (CORA) which lies at the deformity in this case because it is pure angulation in corona l plane, (Y). There is combined angulation and translation deformity so the CORA lies far away proximally in tibia. Bisector to the CORA would determine the plane of correction of deformity.

angle). The anatomical and mechanical angles differ for bones so one should be careful in choosing them and reproducing the measures. These angles can be drawn medially or laterally across the joint **(Figs. 48A to D)**. Joint orientation angle is very important and possibly the only one that can be used for calculation of juxta-articular deformity. The AA line of the short juxta-articular fragment is constructed using one of three methods:

1. Drawing and extrapolating AA of adjacent, intact bone small segment if its anatomy is normal
2. Comparing the joint orientation angle of the abnormal side with the opposite intact side
3. Drawing a line that creates the population normal angle formed by the intersection with the joint orientation line **(Figs. 48A to D)**

- *Assessing axial plane deformities:* Standard radiography is not of much help in measuring torsional malalignment however shortening (axial translation) can be measured on it. So, first record the shortening/LLD and proceed with axial imaging like CT scan for rotational/torsional malalignments.
  1. *Femoral torsion:* Two level cuts are taken one at the level of femoral neck and the other at the level of femoral condyles without altering the limb position. The proximal femoral axis is the line connecting center of femoral head and midpoint of femoral neck. Distal condylar axis is formed by tangential line drawn from posterior aspects of the femoral condyles. The angle formed between the two axes is the femoral torsion angle **(Fig. 49A)**.
  2. *Tibial torsion estimation:* It is done by bimalleolar method. Proximal cut is made just distal to femorotibial joint space and a line drawn tangential to posterior plateau is taken as the axis. Distal cut is taken just distal to distal tibia where posterior malleolus is not visible, line bisecting tibial plafond is

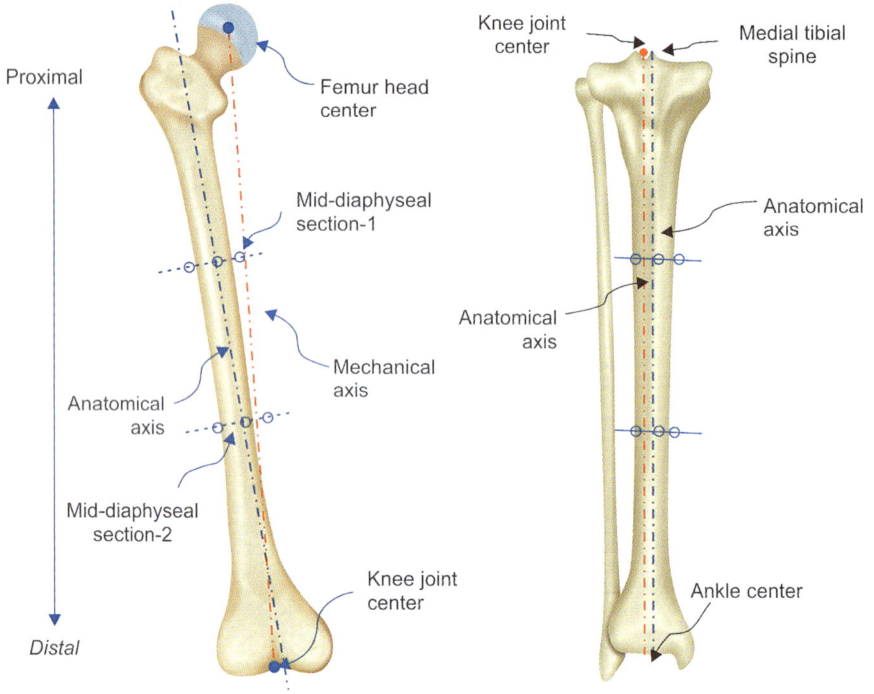

Fig. 46: Illustration detailing the drawing of mechanical axis (MA) and anatomical axes (AA) of femur and tibia. In some bones, the MA and AA do not coincide, e.g., femur (shown on left). One should realize that MA is not bone specific; it is the axis of the limb overall projected on the bone so MA is not drawn for bone specifically but AA is bone specific and is drawn along its longitudinal axis. For drawing AA first find two points on the bone along the longitudinal axis. This is done by drawing two lines exactly transverse to the bone length on diaphyseal region of bone [it can be less commonly also done for metaphyseal region (see the markings in **Fig. 44** for upper limb bones)]. Find the center of these lines and join them. Extrapolate the line to represent the longitudinal or anatomical axis of bone.

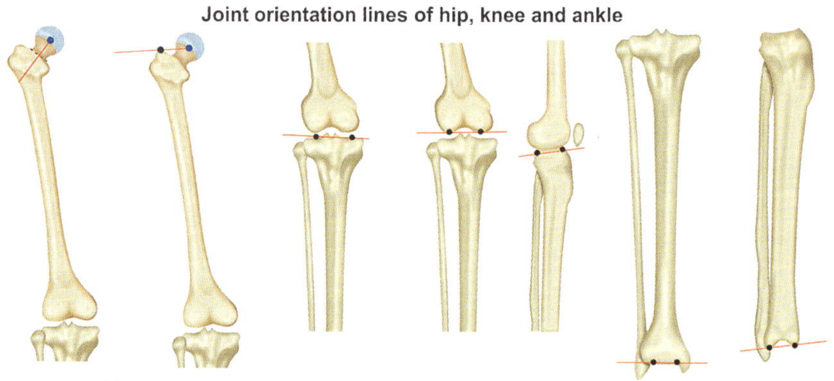

Fig. 47: The various joint orientation lines for bones of lower limb. These lines are indispensable for doing correction at juxta-articular deformities.

taken as the axis. Angle between these two lines is the tibial torsion angle **(Fig. 49B)**.

3. *Assessing humeral torsion:* It can be done by radiographs using the Kronberg method which is crude and inconsistent. CT scan measure uses defining three axes, first is humeral head axis formed by a line perpendicular to plane created by humeral head articular surface, second is interepicondylar axis formed by joining most medial and most lateral extensions of distal humerus, third is the elbow trochlear tangent axis defined as the line tangent to the anterior border of trochlea and lateral condyle. Superposition of first line over 2nd or 3rd gives the rotational axis of humerus **(Fig. 49C)**. Another way of assessing proximal axis is joining the peaks of the mounts of bicipital groove.
4. *Rotational deformity assessment of distal radius:* This is done using CT scan imaging and method described by Frahm et al. and Prommersberger et al. First the "distal angle" is calculated on axial image taken just proximal to radiocarpal joint. The midpoint of the sigmoid notch is identified, and a line is drawn

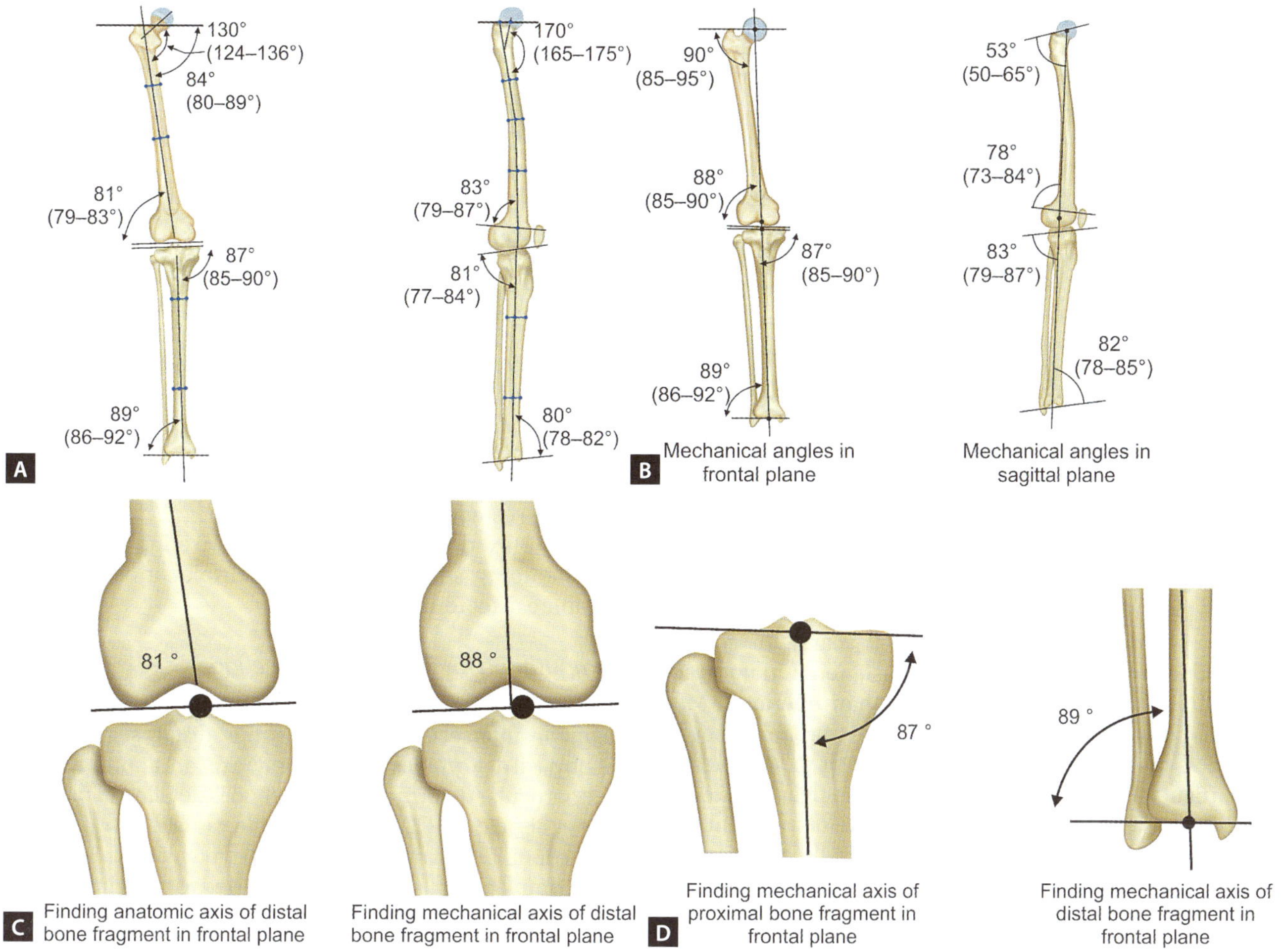

Figs. 48A to D: Illustration showing the various anatomic (A) and mechanical angles (B) in frontal and sagittal planes (here depicted for lower limb) serving as population reference. (C) The illustration demonstrates how these angles can be used using joint orientation line to draw reference lines for correction of juxta-articular deformity of distal femur if the remaining bone fragment is too small for drawing anatomic axis. First draw the joint orientation line and then through the center point of line draw another line at an angle equal to the anatomical reference angle (see from "A"), this will represent the anatomical axis of bone. Same step can be done using mechanical angle to draw mechanical axis (as shown on right). (D) For tibia the anatomical and mechanical axis coincide so any one can be used for drawing the mechanical/anatomical axis of bone in proximal (left) or distal (right) juxta-articular deformities.

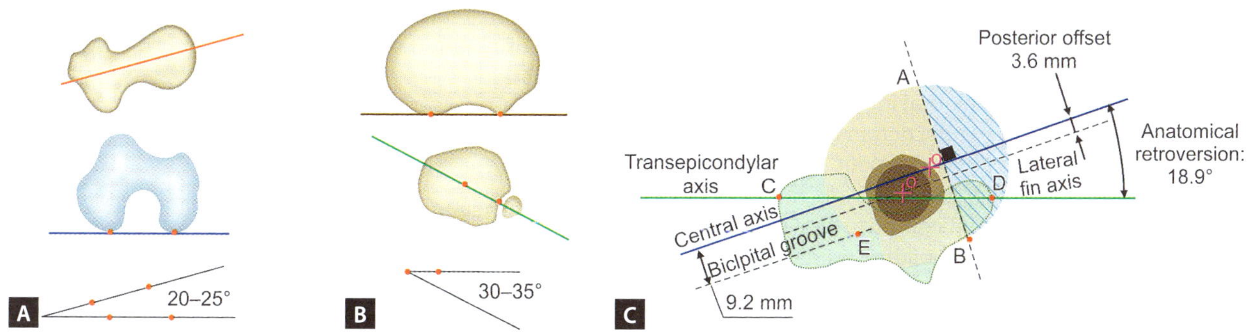

Figs. 49A to C: Assessment of rotational alignment of various bones. This is done by CT scan axial imaging as detailed in text. The drawing is described below. (A) For femur find the proximal femoral axis (red line) and distal femoral condylar axis (blue line). Angle between the two is the femoral torsional index (it will be equal to femoral anteversion for a normal femur). (B) For tibial torsion draw the posterior tibial plateau axis (brown line) proximally and the tibial plafond axis (green line) distally. Angle between these lines determines the reference tibial rotation that can be compared on both sides. (C) For humerus it is a bit tricky, proximal humeral central axis drawing requires some estimation. First find the limits of the articular surface (cartilage) of humeral head on largest axial cut, mark these two points (A and B) and join them—this forms the articular plane. Perpendicular line passing through the center of it forms the central proximal humeral axis. Next draw the transepicondylar axis and angle between these two lines represent the anatomical retroversion.

between this and the most radial cortex of the distal radius (radial styloid). A second line is then drawn horizontally across the image and the angle between the two lines is determined. This is the distal angle. Then "proximal angle" is calculated. Proximal axial images are scanned till an image demonstrating flattening of the volar surface of radius is identified. This level lies somewhere 2–3 cm proximal to proximal end of distal radial ulnar joint (DRUJ). A line tangential to the flattened volar cortical surface of radius is drawn. A horizontal reference line is the drawn for the image. The angle between these two lines forms the proximal angle. The difference between proximal and distal angles is called the "radial rotation angle".

Treatment Decision-making

Observation

The deformity in children is usually observed and not immediately operated, especially if enough growth period and bone modeling time is left (>1-2 years). In general, lesser degrees of angular and translational deformities and younger age are best observed than operated. Most of these deformities get modeled and the tendency to corrective modeling is highest the closer it is to joint surface (periarticular). Even overriding deformities shortening get compensated by physeal growth acceleration but to a lesser extent. Shortening <2 cm is very well compensated. Rotational deformities however do not get modeled and persist forever. In adults, observation is exercised till solid union is obtained so that bone is strong enough to hold the fixation implants. Presence of complex regional pain syndrome type 1 (CRPS and RSD) is also a contraindication to surgical management so the deformities are merely observed till resolution of CRPS.

Nonoperative Management

Supportive treatment is prescribed for patients unwilling/unfit for surgery or those who do not align with the deemed goals of surgical correction or if there is expectation mismatch. Measures such as shoe raise, exoskeleton extension prosthesis for shortening, and aided walk are prescribed for axial translations. Pain control, bracing is recommended for patients having pain due to angular or translational malunion. Joints are supported to prevent ligament laxity developing in these patients. Physiotherapy and joint mobilization is instituted for joint stiffness and contractures if present along with strengthening and muscle building exercises.

Operative Treatment

The indications for surgical management of malunion can be summarized as follows:

- Functional limitation
- Possible future damage or complications (such as joint arthrosis, ligament laxity, degenerative spine disease, and complications in childbearing) due to altered limb alignment and mechanics, intra-articular malunions altering joint function
- Cosmetic demands
- Gait abnormality
- Inability to do daily activities such as wearing clothes and combing hair
- Inability to place the foot flat ton ground (plantigrade)

Usually osteotomy is the most important surgical technique that is used to correct deformities **(Table 5)**. The following indicates a simplified choice of osteotomy for correction of different displacements/deformities:

- Correcting leg length discrepancy—transverse osteotomy/corticotomy
- Rotational deformity correction—transverse osteotomy in a plane perpendicular to axis
- Angular deformity correction—oblique osteotomy or wedge osteotomy
- Complex deformity correction—wedge or step-cut osteotomy, sometimes biplanar/triplanar osteotomy or dome osteotomy may be used.

Computation for Deformity Correction

The CORA is the point at which the axis of the proximal segment intersects the axis of the distal segment. For diaphyseal deformities, the anatomic axes are appropriate. For juxta-articular deformities the method is detailed in radiology above. Bisector to CORA provides the yardstick for deformity correction. If deformity(ies) are corrected along this bisector then complete correction will be achieved without introducing any translation or angular deformity in other plane. Simple single plane angular deformities can be corrected this way. Usually the deformities are in oblique plane where both sagittal and coronal plane deformities exist. In these patients computation of real magnitude of deformity is done by either graphical or trigonometric method as follows:

Graphic method:

$$\text{Magnitude of oblique plane deformity} = \sqrt{(CD)^2 + (SD)^2}$$

Where, CD = coronal deformity in degrees, SD = sagittal deformity in degrees

The orientation of corrective osteotomy plane is given by the equation:

$$\tan^{-1}\left(\frac{SD}{CD}\right)$$

Trigonometric method:

$$\text{Magnitude of oblique plane deformity} = \sqrt{tan^2(CD) + tan^2(SD)}$$

The orientation of corrective osteotomy plane is given by equation:

$$\tan^{-1}\frac{\tan(SD)}{\tan(CD)}$$

Translation deformities also need to be calculated in magnitude and direction. The magnitude of translation is measures in millimeters and is the perpendicular distance between AA of two fragments at deformity **(Fig. 50)**. If

TABLE 5: The different types of osteotomies used in management of malunion.

Osteotomy	*Comment*
Closing wedge osteotomy: The triangular wedge is removed from the convex side of angulation and fragments closed and compressed onto each other	Advantages: Intrinsically stable, compression produces better chances of unto union, large corrections possible, translation of fragments can be done if needed, easier, and more reliable. Disadvantages: Produces shortening and bone loss, cut cannot be reversed once made.
Open wedge osteotomy: Done on the concave side of deformity by producing a cut and opening it to required correction. The defect created is filled with bone graft.	Advantages: Produces lengthening, can be intraoperatively adjusted to change the requisite correction, more forgiving in providing correction. Disadvantages: Needs another surgery to obtain filler bone, unstable, nonunion possible due to absence of compression, no rotation or translation possible, small degree of correction only.
Neutral wedge/double wedge osteotomy: Here a closed and open wedge osteotomy is combined. Closed wedge is made on the convex side on deformity and the obtained wedge is used as filler bone wedge that is inserted on the same level opposite open wedge osteotomy cut.	Advantages: Length neutral, stable, compression obtained, allows translation, greater angular correction. Disadvantages: Difficult procedure, needs careful planning preoperatively, concave side open wedge osteotomy remains gaped and may not compress well—chances of nonunion.
Dome osteotomy: Dome-shaped cut is made centered around the CORA and distal fragment rotated to obtain desired correction in metaphyseal region.	Advantages: Stable, large angular corrections possible because centered on CORA, good union, some degree of other perpendicular plane angulation correction also possible. Disadvantages: Needs precise planning and execution, other plane angular/translation correction is limited, not useful for diaphyseal malunions.
Single cut: There are two indications for this: 1. Limb lengthening by corticotomy or compactotomy and correction of rotational deformity. 2. The deformity is assessed in 3D and CORA is mathematically derived using dedicated software and protocol. The plane of osteotomy is revealed based on the calculation along which all the deformities/displacements can be corrected using appropriate computer guided frame placement.	Advantages: Compressible, quite accurate, single bone cut needed, all deformities corrected in a single procedure. Disadvantages: Requires dedicated evaluation protocol and software for calculation of correction, needs precision cut.
Clamshell osteotomy: The bone is split osteotomized at the deformity site in the form of two shells and correction of deformity done by manipulating distal fragment. The shells are created retaining all soft tissue attachments and periosteal blood supply so that union is not compromised. The osteotomy is done in diaphyseal region.	Advantages: Minimal preoperative planning (just create clam shells and do correction and fix—straightforward), large corrections possible, allows translation. Disadvantages: Unstable, needs direct approach to osteotomy.
Step-cut and intra-articular osteotomies: These are complex procedures done for correction of specific malunions. Intra-articular malunions need to be elevated in part and not universally so a step cut of the depressed or malunited fragment is done and elevated with bone grafts.	Advantages: Treats specific malunion, aligns the cartilage line/plane so that joint function is properly restored. Disadvantages: Complex planning, expertise needed, joint stiffness may result, excess pressure on damaged cartilage may lead to chondrolysis and function may not be restored, painful resulting joint.

(CORA: center of rotation for angulation)

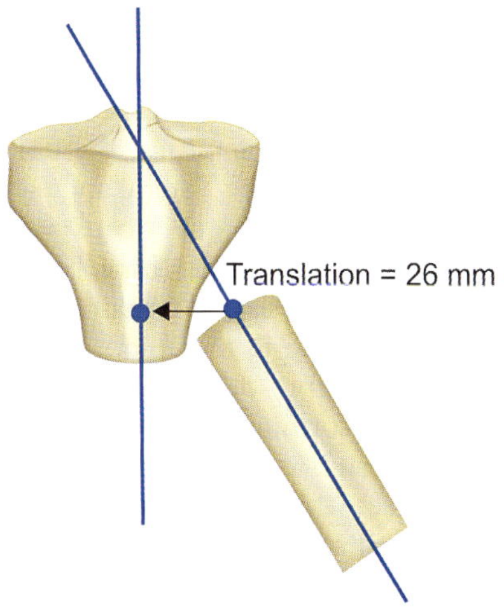

Fig. 50: Finding and measuring the translation between fragments.

combined angulation and translation exist, then CORA will be away from obvious deformity site **(Figs. 51A and B)**. In such cases, translation is measured at the level of proximal end of distal fragment **(Fig. 50)**.

Also radiographically assess the compensatory deformities in adjacent joints (like subtalar varus in tibial valgus deformity and vice versa) or regions (pelvis/spine) that should be addressed during correction planning.

The concepts can be well summarized in discussion on specific malunions as follows.

MALUNITED FEMORAL SHAFT FRACTURE

Femoral shaft fractures are the result of high-energy injury in adults (osteoporotic fractures in elderly may occur with lesser grade of trauma). Malunions of the femoral shaft are not uncommon. They frequently result from:

- *Inappropriate treatment:* Cast, brace, and traction

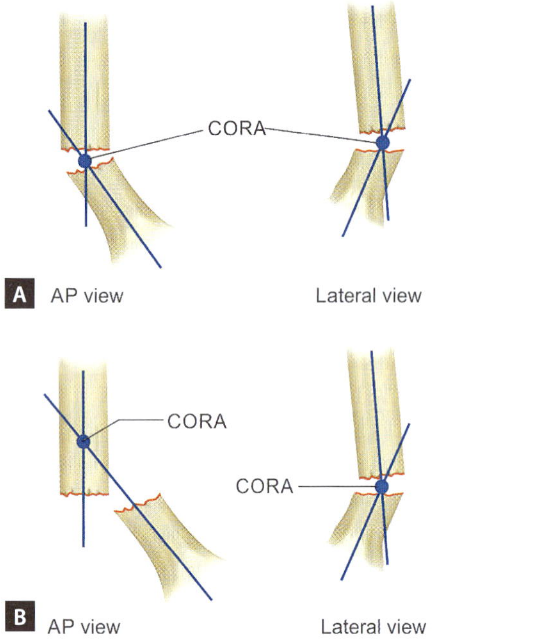

Figs. 51A and B: Center of rotation for angulation (CORA) may be located at the deformity site in cases of pure angulation (A), but in cases where angulation and translation coexist the CORA lies away from site of obvious deformity (B). (AP: anteroposterior)

- *Inadequate treatment:*
  - Smaller diameter nails that do not hold fracture well and give way due to poor strength and flexible nailing in patients above 16 years of age
  - Inadequate plating of the fracture
  - A mentally unstable patient who mobilized too early and implants gave way
  - Use of older K-nail that have poor bending strength
- Open fractures that were managed with external fixators and could not be converted to better reduction in want of soft tissue complications.
- Practice of damage control orthopedics in head injury patients using external fixators that healed too fast without giving surgeon the time for undertaking osteosynthesis because of overall poor patient medical condition.

The fracture may be transverse, spiral, oblique, segmental, or comminuted depending on the bending moment and mechanism of injury. The site of fracture also varies depending on the force concentration of impact. The deformities that result in a femoral shaft fracture are the result of differential pull of muscles on different fracture fragments.

- *Proximal fragment:*
  - Abducted—gluteus medius and minimus abduct as they insert on greater trochanter
  - Flexed—iliopsoas flexes fragment as it inserts on lesser trochanter
- *Distal segment:*
  - Varus—adductors inserting on medial aspect of distal femur
  - Extension—gastrocnemius attaches on distal aspect of posterior femur

The usual displacements of femoral shaft fracture **(Figs. 52A to C)** that may translate into malunion deformities later can be summarized as follows:

- *Fracture at isthmus level:* The proximal fragment is flexed, abducted, and externally rotated. Distal fragment is adducted and proximally pilled (shortening). This produces a varus and procurvatum deformity at fracture site with anterior + lateral angulation. Additionally, there is shortening and rotational malalignment. Although, it appears to be external rotational deformity, but in a malunited fracture, the distal fragment is in fact internally rotated with respect to the proximal fragment.
- *Midshaft femoral fractures:* The adduction-abduction forces usually balance each other for the proximal fragment, but the distal fragment is adducted and pulled proximally causing axial shortening or overriding of variable magnitude and medial angulation. The proximal fragment is flexed and externally rotated. Fascia lata restrains any length change laterally but there is unrestricted pull of adductors medially producing medial angulation and a valgus deformity in some cases. In others, if the fracture lies a bit higher than middle thirds then adductor magnus may still pull the whole distal fragment into adduction resulting in lateral angulation at the fracture site.
- *Distal fractures:* The proximal fragment is pulled into adduction by unrestricted and powerful adductors attaching medially producing medial angulation and distal fragment goes into hyperextension due to pull of gastrocnemius muscles producing posterior angulation. It should be noted that some confuse posterior angulation of distal fragment to be "flexion" but in reality it is "hyperextension" in relation to knee joint and not flexion.

Rotational malalignment of variable degrees is added to these. The acceptable limits of deformity that can be managed conservatively are detailed in **(Box 2)**. Beyond these limits the malunion needs surgical correction as they result in poor function of the extremity.

Clinical Features

The patients usually present with short limb gait and depending on angulation of deformity there may be added circumduction (varus deformity/lateral angulation) component. If there is associated quadriceps weakness then quadriceps weakness gait may be there. The walk may be painful if knee or hip arthrosis has developed or pathological ligament laxity occurs due to malunion. The patients have problem in running and other sport-related activities. External rotation deformity produces grasshopper eye patella. Excessive posterior angulation may result in flexion contracture at knee while excessive anterior angulation would result in recurvatum knee. Patellar instability and lateral knee ligament laxity may result in varus (lateral angulation) malunions. The ankle joint may have equinus deformity in long-standing cases.

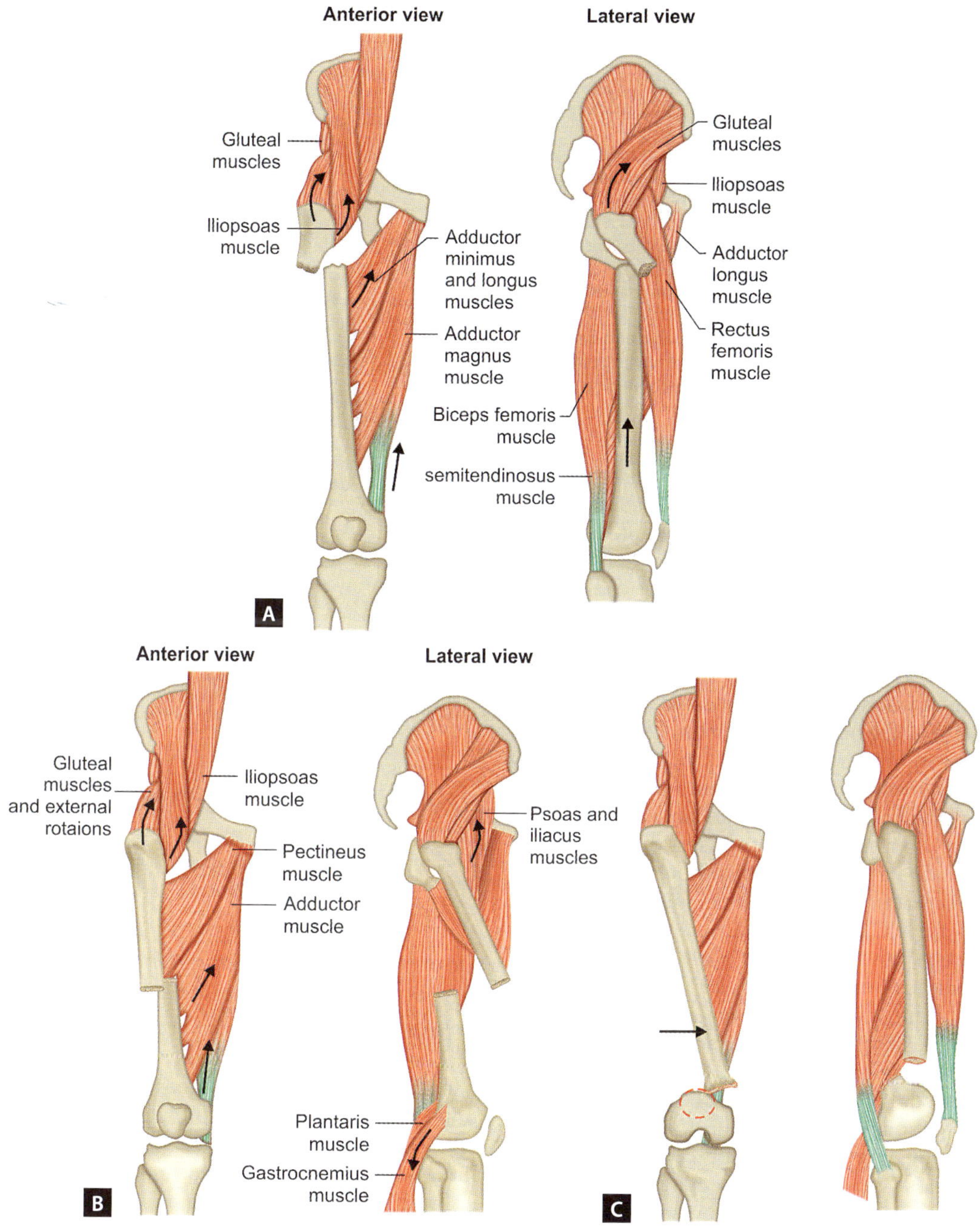

Figs. 52A to C: Illustration demonstrating the various displacements of femoral shaft fragments in proximal third (A), middle third (B), and distal third (C) fractures.

Surgical Correction

The type of surgical corrective procedure for malunited femur depends on the degree of deformity (angular), the alignment of the medullary canal (translation deformity), shortening, and the location of the deformity. It is indicated only in patients with disabling pain and significant functional disability. Cosmetic appearance is only a relative indication. It should be considered usually when 6–12 months have elapsed from injury. The operative procedures range from open corrective procedures to closed intramedullary osteotomy and Ilizarov method. Age of patient, socioeconomic status, adjacent joint function, bone stock, and degree of osteoporosis, and status of surrounding soft tissues should all be considered when planning the surgical procedure.

Closed Intramedullary Osteotomy

Closed intramedullary osteotomy is a specialized technique for correcting malrotations and shortening <5 cm without opening the deformity site. It can be done only if the offset of medullary canal is <25% so that intramedullary instruments can pass across the deformity. It is especially suited for malunions of middle third of femoral shaft while some cases

BOX 2: The variably acceptable limits of deformity in malunited fracture shaft of femur.

- Malrotation is better tolerated in external rotation than in internal rotation. Mostly 10° of internal and 15° external malrotation rarely produce functional problems. Beyond this gait abnormalities arise.
- In general, angulation of <10° rarely produces significant functional or cosmetic impairment. Angulation of 15–20° or more will create problems for the patient. Lesser values of angulation will be more significant in taller patients because of trigonometric malposition of foot. Coronal plane malalignment would stress the knee, foot, and ankle joints and produce late arthritic changes. Preexisting varus or valgus deformity will have additive or subtractive effect that needs to be counted before offering correction.
- Shortening of 2 cm is adequately compensated by pelvis and spine. 5–10 mm additional shortening may be well managed by shoe raise, but beyond this the shortening is mostly not accepted and patients seek equalization.

of proximal third can also be corrected by this method. The procedure is greatly simplified if an intramedullary nail is already in place as the medullary canal would be patent in these cases and instruments can be introduced easily once nail is removed. Otherwise the medullary canal at the fracture site is often blocked by callus needs to be reopened by sharp canal openers or drill bits or hand reamers. Pass the guidewire and ream the proximal fragment till desired size (for later nail insertion). Then pass the canal opening instrument to break the blockage and ream distal fragment. If the blockage is too large then it is better to perform open osteotomy instead of wasting time and landing in complications like cortical perforation and creating false tracts. For correction of malrotation insert two unicortical Steinmann pins laterally one above and below the level of osteotomy each. With closed technique, insert the Pearson intramedullary saw **(Fig. 53)** and transect the femur at the appropriate level. This site is usually slightly proximal or distal to the fracture site in normal bone. Due to irregularity of canal and bone at deformity site the osteotomy is often incomplete and needs osteoclasis or may damage soft tissues at deficient site. Slight angular deformities are automatically corrected once nail is passed. Rotate the distal pin to achieve desired correction in axial plane and maintain it till nail is locked. Smaller shortenings like <5 cm can be corrected by acute distraction at osteotomy and ample bone grafting the site. One can use reamings and bone marrow to augment bone graft. Closed bone grafting is recommended **(Figs. 54A to E)**. Place a chest tube over the intramedullary guidewire till the level of osteotomy under fluoroscopy and push morselized graft through the tube till the distraction gap. The graft can be pushed using flexible reamers or solid rod. Overfill the defect site with graft. The distraction at osteotomy site is best achieved using AO femoral distractor and should be done gradually over 15–20 minutes. Sensory-evoked potentials to monitor function in the sciatic nerve during lengthening can also be used. Use a statically locked nail to fix the construct. A separate lengthening procedure with an external fixator is usually necessary when the discrepancy is >5 cm. In such cases, the nail is not locked distally and external fixator is applied to gradually distract the osteotomy site as done for railroad lengthening of long bones (the so-called two stage procedure for correction of shortening).

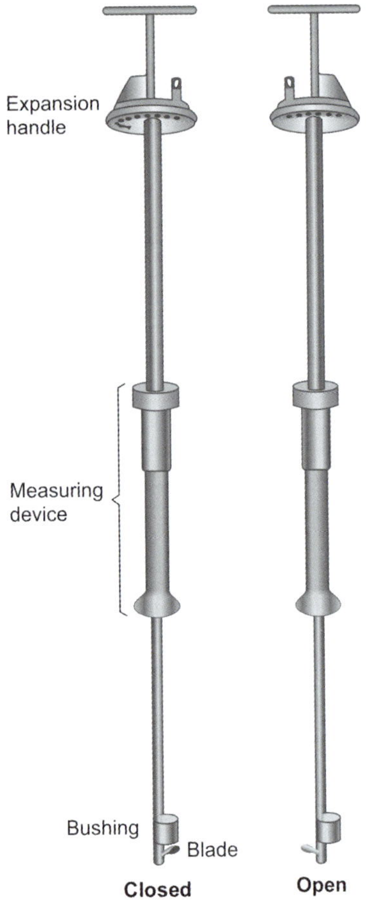

Fig. 53: The Pearson saw for intramedullary osteotomy of femoral diaphysis.

Closed Intramedullary Shortening of the Contralateral Femur

In patients, with moderate shortening of 5–8 cm, lengthening of bone is cumbersome and time-consuming process as above. In such cases, acute lengthening of 2.5–4 cm can be done on the affected site and closed intramedullary shortening of opposite femur by 2.5–4 cm can be done to equalize limb lengths, although it shortens the overall stature. Shortening the contralateral femur is technically much easier and safer than gradual lengthening. Closed intramedullary shortening was originally described by Küntscher but practical popularity was achieved by work of Winquist et al. It offers the advantages of immediate weight-bearing, early union, and early return to function. It is best performed in lateral decubitus position on a fracture table. Make entry point and pass the guidewire and ream femoral canal to desired size. Insert the appropriate size intramedullary saw (guided by the size or reamer last used) and set it for the most distal cut first as identified under fluoroscopy **(Figs. 55A to E)**. Make the cut and if needed complete it either by osteoclasis or by placing a 5 mm osteotome percutaneously from lateral approach. Carefully set the measuring device on the saw for proximal osteotomy. Again insert the saw, and verify correct position by fluoroscopy. Complete the osteotomy as neat as possible so that no spikes remain.

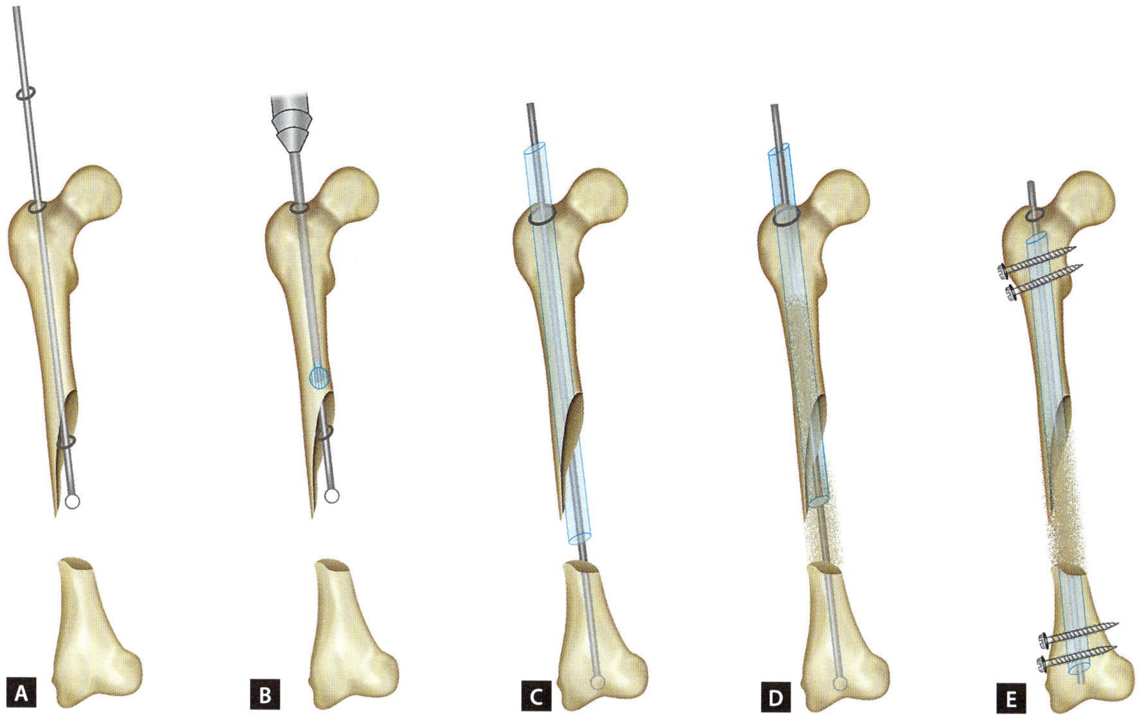

Figs. 54A to E: The method of closed bone grafting in case of distraction for correction of shortening. (A) Pass the guidewire; (B) Ream proximal fragment; (C) Pass a chest tube over guidewire till the level of defect; (D) Push the bone graft into the defect; (E) Remove chest tube and insert nail.

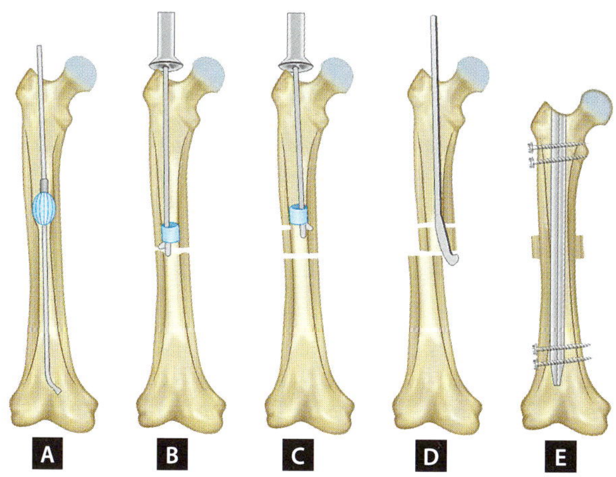

Figs. 55A to E: Method of closed intramedullary shortening of femur. (A) Ream the intramedullary canal; (B) Make distal cut; (C) Make proximal cut and separate the fragment; (D) Split the fragment into clamshell; (E) Impact the fragments and fix with intramedullary nail.

This will allow complete docking of the fragments and approximation. Next, split the intercalary fragment using the back-cutting osteotome. Under fluoroscopic control, insert the back-cutting osteotome and pull it firmly against the distal surface of the intercalary segment at the linea aspera. Hold it firmly in position and gently tap the handle of the saw with the slotted mallet to split the fragment into two halves producing clamshell **(Figs. 55A to E).** Displace the split intercalary fragments away from osteotomy site. Insert the intramedullary nail and lock it distally first. Gently impact the osteotomy to close it and then lock proximally.

Open Osteotomy with Osteosynthesis

This is the preferred method for correction of angular femur malunion and otherwise preferred for correction of all femoral deformities by most surgeons. Open osteotomy is technically much simpler than closed osteotomy. Preoperative planning for determining the degree of angular correction is a must. Place the patient on fracture table and expose the deformity site using direct lateral approach. For closed wedge osteotomy, pass a K-wire transversely across the femoral shaft just proximal to the deformity. Place another K-wire distally at the desired angle of correction from first wire. Intraoperatively this angle is difficult to draw so preoperatively prepare a template by bending K-wire and send it for autoclave with the instrumentation the day before. Alternatively, a thin metal sheet or foil can be cut in the shape of a triangle with desired corrective angle that can be used intraoperatively. Simpler procedure is to perform an open wedge osteotomy. Here a single cut is made in the femoral shaft and the deformity site is split open. Intramedullary preparation for nailing is done in a standard fashion and reamings are saved for bone grafting of the open wedge void. Additional cancellous graft can be harvested from ilium and mixed with reamings and bone marrow. Nail is passed across the osteotomy site fixing it. There should be cortical contact at the apex of the wedge for pure angular corrections **(Figs. 56A to D)**. The rest of void is overfilled with prepared bone graft. If lengthening is desired to correct additional shortening then distraction at osteotomy is maintained using femoral distractor. Ample grafting is the key and one should note that nail should be inserted in neutral rotation that needs careful maintenance during insertion and final locking.

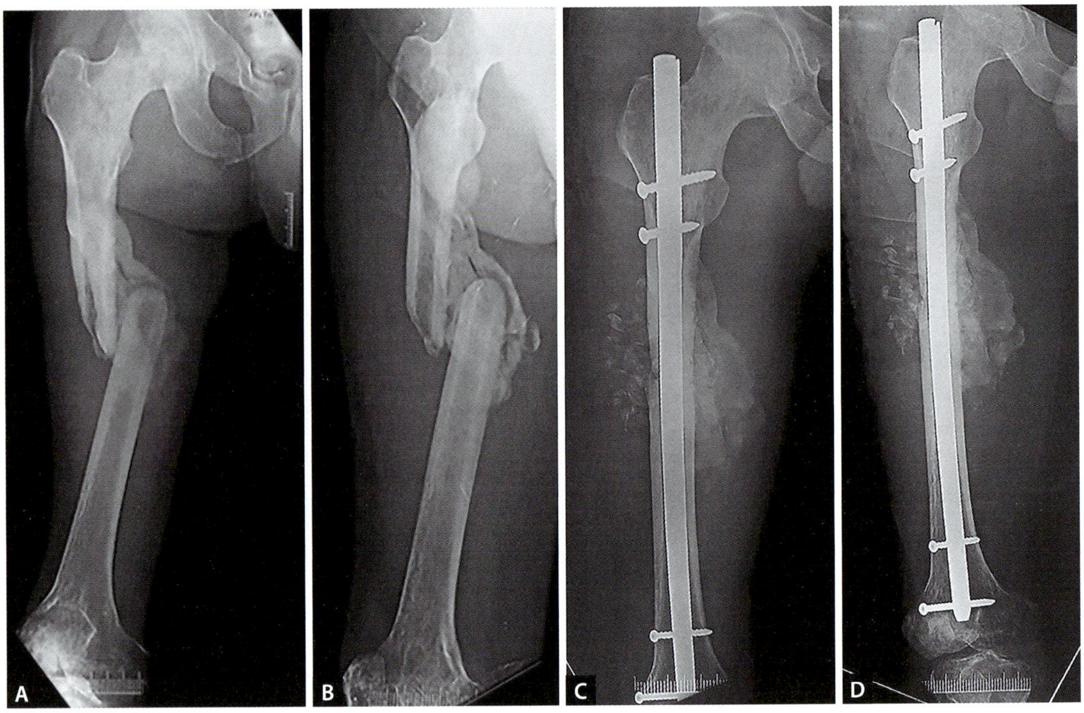

Figs. 56A to D: Malunited fracture right femur shaft with translation, shortening, medial and posterior angulation, and external rotation deformity of nearly 70° (A and B). The malunion was treated with corrective osteotomy for angulation, rotation, and translation correction and fixation by intramedullary nail + bone grafting (C and D). The shortening was partially overcome by realignment. There was 3 cm shortening postoperatively that was managed with shoe raise.

For rotational deformity correction in open approach, step-cut osteotomies were used to gain rotational control and stability in plating era. With locked nails, a step-cut osteotomy is not necessary and a transverse osteotomy does the job well.

Ilizarov Distraction Osteogenesis and External Fixators

The Ilizarov method of bone lengthening allows surgeon to perform complex lengthening and deformity correction. The technique is difficult for femur and time consuming. Multiplanar deformities need precise planning and frequent follow-up lest they may deviate from corrective path. Principles of maximal preservation of marrow and periosteal blood supply, stable external fixation preventing torsion and bending forces but maintaining axial micromotion and gradual distraction is essential for optimal result. It is more suitable for congenital shortening rather than post traumatic ones. It may also be used as a last resort measure for multiple failed attempts at deformity correction but needs expert hands. Complications of pin tract infection, mental trauma, soft tissue, and bony complications mar the outcome. A simpler technique is application of Taylor multiaxial deformity correction frame that provides precise planning for deformity correction in six degrees of freedom and is comparatively simpler to manage.

Complications of Corrective Osteotomy for Malunion of Femur Shaft

The corrective osteotomy of the femur is not without complications. There is significant blood loss in both closed and open methods so a good preoperative hematocrit is a prerequisite. Usually postoperative blood transfusion is not needed in most but substantial blood loss may need it. The other complications are listed in **Box 3**.

BOX 3: The complications associated with corrective osteotomy of malunited femoral shaft fracture.

- Infection
- Nonunion (higher with plate fixation)
- Undercorrection/overcorrection of deformity (less with use of nail for angular deformity)
- Nerve paralysis (acute lengthening >4 cm)
- Hardware failure
- Blood loss
- Fat embolism

MALUNION DISTAL RADIUS FRACTURE

Distal radius fracture is the most common fracture of upper extremity. Malunion of distal radius fracture is the most common long-term complication which is seen in 10% of surgically treated patients and its rate increases to as high as 25% in conservatively managed fractures. The incidence of nascent malunion may be still higher than the above figures. Nascent malunion is used for fractures that show deviation from acceptable radiological alignment **(Box 4)** but may not necessarily have functional limitations. Patients with functional problems in a malunited fracture may be called mature malunion or malunion with functional deficits. It is a good practice to document the functional limitation by QuickDASH or other dedicated scores. Malunited distal radius fractures (MDRFs) in age group of 18–65 years are

BOX 4: The acceptability criteria for distal radius fracture reduction.

1. Radial length shortening ≤2 mm [in relation to ulnar head or from contralateral distal radius, normal ulnar variance is ±2 mm (mean = −0.9 mm)]
2. Radial height loss <5 mm from contralateral normal radius (this is the height of radial styloid from articular surface/ulnar head, normal is 13 mm)
3. Palmar tilt change up to neutral is acceptable, (some consider >5° of dorsal tilt or >20° from contralateral normal palmar tilt as unacceptable, normal palmar tilt is 10°)
4. Change in radial inclination <5° (normal radial inclination is 23°). This is considered too strict by some so some consider maintaining radial inclination to >10° as acceptable.
5. Intra-articular step-off/gap <2 mm

more likely to produce adverse clinical outcomes in terms of activity limitation and pain. There are various patterns of distal radius fracture ranging from extra-articular to complex intra-articular varieties and all of them may have some or a variable combination of persistent deformities. Rotational deformities are also common but not very well addressed in literature. They are best appreciated and calculated on CT scans (*see* radiology above). Biomechanical different deformities produce discrete functional loss viz.:

- Overall, all of the malunions result in altered mechanics across the wrist joint so can result in joint arthrosis, pain, and limited mobility in long run.
- Decreased radial inclination can result in a change in the direction of the flexor tendons, leading to a decreased mechanical advantage, and can cause hand weakness.
- Loss of palmar tilt produces loss of forearm rotation due to incongruity of the DRUJ and tightening of the interosseous membrane. It also limits flexion and supination. Increased palmar tilt would similarly result in reduced wrist extension and pronation.
- Presence of dorsal tilt results in:
  - Dorsal radial subluxation and/or
  - Adaptive midcarpal DISI (*see* Chapter on "Carpal Instability")
- Intra-articular step predisposes to joint arthrosis
- Reduced radial height results in ulna impaction syndrome and stress on DRUJ
- Stress on DRUJ would result in:
  - Limited forearm pronation and supination
  - Strain on TFCC
  - Increased loading of ulnocarpal joint

Clinical Features

The patients most commonly present with pain variably located at wrist, ulnar head, or radial aspect. There may be obvious deformity (in conservatively managed fractures) or often subtle deformity in operated patients. Pain in aggravated on supination/pronation movements due to incongruity of sigmoid notch or it may be present with wrist flexion/extension if there is articular step-off or loss of radial length/angulation. Associated tendinosis or capsulitis and contractures also contribute to pain and loss of movements.

Radiological Evaluation

Detailed assessment is imperative before planning treatment. The following radiographs are commonly recommended for initial assessment:

1. Neutral rotation PA view
2. Pronated oblique
3. Strict lateral view
4. Anatomic/tilted lateral view for articular surface and lunate fossa

A CT scan is additionally important for intra-articular step-off quantification and assessment of the fracture line. It is also needed for assessment of rotational malunions. MRI may be done for assessment of TFCC and wrist and intercarpal ligaments.

Surgical Management

Corrective surgery is indicated in patients that have functional limitations and/or pain with documentable correlative radiological features predictive of them. Most often the radiological features do not match the functional limitations as the acceptability criteria are too strict in my opinion. This requires a clever and experienced orthopedician who can give a balanced opinion. Timing of surgery has not been documented but according to Jupiter and Ring, the grip strength is higher in those reconstructed within 14 weeks after injury than in delayed reconstructions.

Malunited Distal Radius Fracture with Volar Angulation

This is the most common malunion where the distal fragment is tilted dorsally producing volar angulation. Inquisitively these malunions are best approached dorsally (between the second and fourth extensor compartments) and open wedge osteotomy with fixation would be expected to correct the deformity **(Figs. 57A to F)**. The only concern is tendon attrition resulting from implant prominence that may cause tendinosis and frictional tendon rupture. Newer low proflle implants with sunken screws delimit this concern. Open wedge is filled with wedge corticocancellous graft that can be harvested from iliac crest. In addition, the implants can be removed after osseous healing if concerns of tendon complications remain. Introduction of robust volar implants have attracted surgeons to use volar approach in correcting this MDRF. Osteotomy is done using extended volar approach or carpal tunnel approach. It has additional advantage of direct visualization of volar angle and maintaining volar cortical continuity as anatomically as possible. Using dorsal approach, the distal fragment may become unstable and difficult to control if the osteotomy gets inadvertently completed making anatomical reduction bit difficult. However, this can be overcome by distal fixation of plate before osteotomy is made to maintain control on the distal fragment (it also helps in reduction). Also, some suggest that close anatomical contact of volar cortex in volar approach would avoid the need of bone graft but this is debatable. Tendon irritation concerns still remain with volar approach as dorsal screw penetration can still irritate the tendons while volar fixation adds to volar tendon complications.

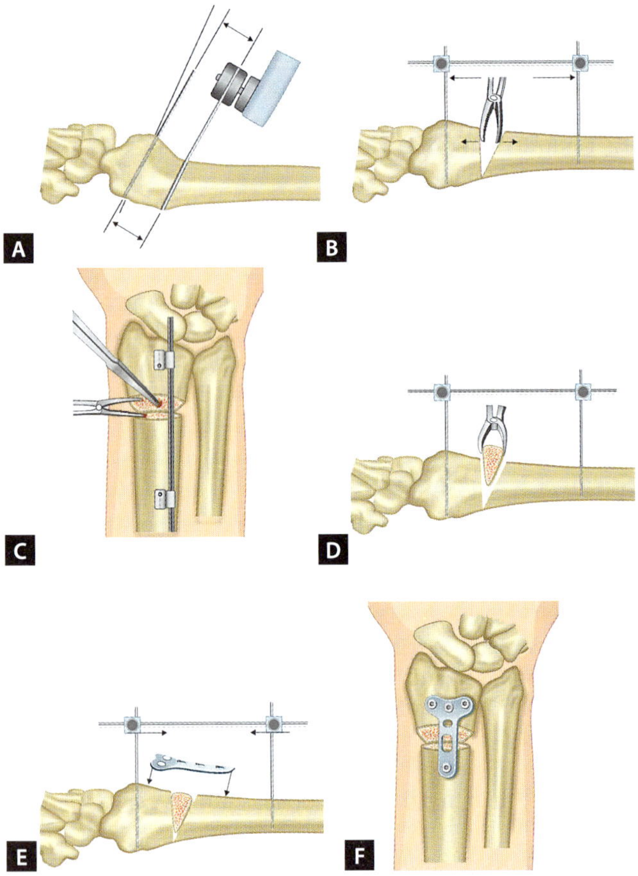

Figs. 57A to F: The illustration demonstrating dorsal open wedge corrective osteotomy for MDRF with volar angulation. Reference wire is placed in bone parallel to the articular surface and osteotomy cut made with saw blade (A) parallel to the reference wire, correction of palmar ± radial tilt is done and maintained with distractor (B and C), wedge bone graft usually structural corticocancellous graft harvested from ilium is impacted in the void (D), plate fixation with preferably a locked fixed angle low-profile implant is done dorsally (E). Alternatively, the plate can be fixed to distal fragment in (F) itself and then osteotomy cut made, this provides better control to the fragment during reduction and intraoperative manipulation.

Open wedge osteotomies theoretically have higher chances of nonunion and implant failure due to graft subsidence. Volar closed wedge osteotomy offer better osteotomy site stability and compression averting this complication. Making a double wedge would also correct radial inclination. This also fulfills the need of direct volar visualization and correction of angulation. Doing a closed wedge correction would lead to shortening (increased ulnar variance and subsequent ulnar impaction) so, additionally ulnar head resection or ulnar shortening is needed.

Malunited Distal Radius Fracture with Dorsal Angulation

This is a less common type of malunion but managing this malunion is much straightforward. Using a volar open double wedge osteotomy to correct palmar tilt and inclination would address even the radial length and fixation implants are robust for volar approach. The created open wedge is usually filled with iliac crest bone graft.

Malunited Distal Radius Fracture and Intra-articular Step

This is a challenging malunion and needs dedicated CT scan evaluation to visualize and reconstruct the anatomy. Here timing of surgery seems to be more important that other MDRFs as after 3 months the articular cartilage health may not be good enough to prevent late arthrosis. Dorsal approach and capsulotomy is the best approach for intra-articular MDRF with dorsal subluxation and vice versa. People have used arthroscopy-assisted correction of articular deformity and step with good results.

Additional Concerns

Bone graft is classically used to fill the void created by open wedge osteotomies. The void may be filled with nonstructural (such as chips) or structural (contoured wedge) iliac crest bone graft. Synthetic bone graft substitutes like calcium hydroxyapatite has also been successfully used with volar approach. Use of calcium phosphate bone cement may not be appropriate as it does not offer requisite compressive strength. There has been suggestion that if the volar cortex is well aligned then there is no need for using a bone graft.

Ulnar-sided wrist pain indicates presence of additional pathology beyond MDRF. It may arise from TFCC tearing, posttraumatic arthritis of the DRUJ, or symptomatic ulnar styloid nonunion or ulnar abutment syndrome. Abutment syndrome commonly resolves with anatomical correction of distal radius deformity or ulnar shortening. Repairing TFCC primarily may be explored with corrective osteotomy if surgery is planned early (within 3 months). This usually stabilizes DRUJ also. Unstable DRUJ and late cases usually need ligament reconstruction of peripheral tears. Posttraumatic symptomatic DRUJ arthritis would need one of the reconstructive options such as distal ulna resection, hemiresection arthroplasty, Sauvé-Kapandji, or implant arthroplasty (*see* Chapter on "Distal Radioulnar Joint Disorders and Ulnar Wrist Pain"). Nonunion of ulnar styloid is usually inconsequential but in some cases with tendon irritation from the fragment may need excision (if small) or fixation with headless compression screw (if large).

Use of 3D printing and cutting jigs has been described for precise cutting of the malunion and correction. 3D surface rendered CT images (stereolithography) are translated into cutting jigs using dedicated software that can be used to intraoperatively cut the bone at precise site as determined in preoperative planning on console. These can be custom set for type of implant being used so that fixation points are also not violated and completed correction is achieved as close to osseous anatomy as possible. The technique is similar to customized jig development for total knee arthroplasty.

Complications

Corrective osteotomy for MDRF is not without complications **(Box 5)**. The surgery is more complex than primary fixation of distal radius fracture so complication rates are also high (as much as 50%). These quite substantially limit the outcome of corrective osteotomy for MDRF.

BOX 5: Complications after corrective osteotomy for treating malunited distal radius fractures.

- Overcorrection
- Undercorrection
- Infection
- Nonunion
- Loss of reduction
- Implant failure
- Nerve injury
- Tendon injury
- Tendon irritation
- Tendon rupture (extensor pollicis longus)
- Complex regional pain syndrome type 1

CUBITUS VARUS DEFORMITY

Malunion of pediatric displaced supracondylar humerus fracture commonly results in cubitus varus deformity, which is the most common long-term complication (incidence ranging from 3 to 57%). Cubitus varus is said to exist if the carrying angle of the limb is reduced compared to the other limb **(Figs. 58A to G)**, if both the limbs are involved then cubitus varus is labeled if the carrying reduces to <5°. The malunion results from impacted type 1 fractures, rotationally unstable type 2 fractures that lose reduction later or are inaccurately reduction in plaster cast, comminuted fractures that cannot maintain reduction or type 3 fractures that are not appropriately reduced during surgery or present late precluding surgery. Other causes of cubitus varus are AVN of trochlea **(Figs. 59A and B)**, growth arrest of medial distal humeral physis, congenital epiphyseal dysplasia, malunited lateral condyle fracture, malunited intercondylar fracture, malunited medial condyle fracture, and exostosis in the region of lateral humeral condyle. The exostosis may not produce true cubitus varus but it is only the appearance of limb that suggests so. The deformity that arises from malunion of supracondylar fractures of humerus has four main components that should be carefully recorded and evaluated as follows:

- *Lateral angulation* resulting from *medial tilt* of distal fragment towards the midline of body producing "varus" component of the deformity. In early cases, *medial shift* (translation) also exists making this a complex deformity but in late cases due to modeling of the fracture translation mostly gets obliterated and only angulation is appreciable.
- *Anterior angulation* resulting from *extension of distal fragment (posterior tilt)* producing "recurvatum" in sagittal plane. There is also associated *posterior shift* but in united fractures this component commonly regresses. This lies in the plane of motion so it remodels fastest however, large deformities may not completely remodel until osseous maturity.
- *Internal rotation* of the distal fragment causing torsional malunion component. This does not remodel but is fairly compensated by shoulder joint movements.
- *Shortening (proximal migration)* is variable and quite insignificant, more appreciable medially (upriding of medial epicondyle).

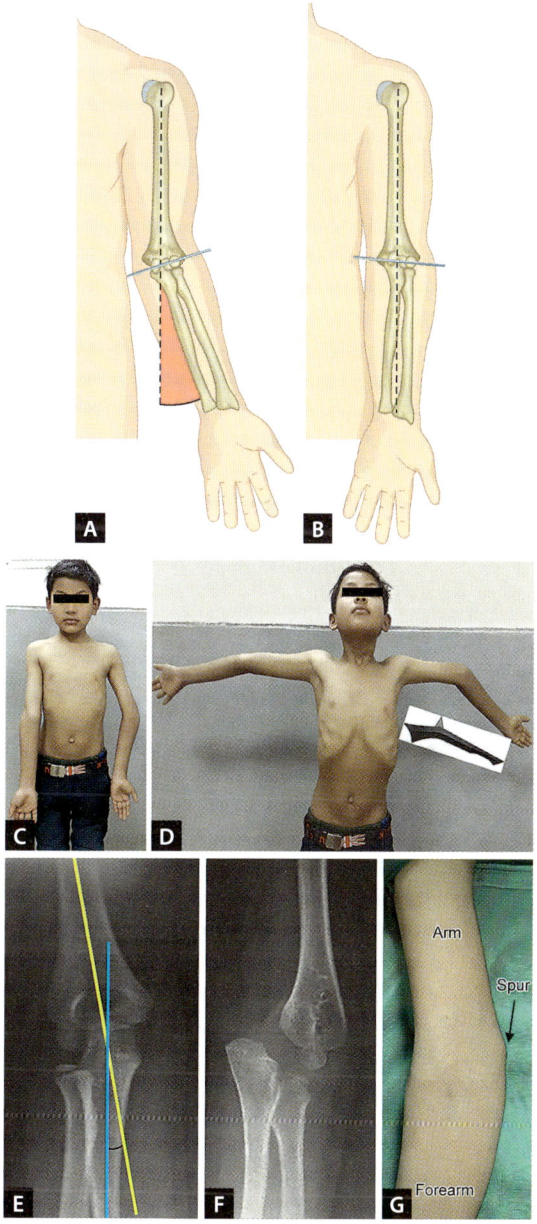

Figs. 58A to G: Normal carrying angle and cubitus varus. (A) The normal carrying angle ranges from 5–15° of valgus at elbow. It is somewhat less in males (mean of 11°) than females (mean 14°). The angle is also less on the dominant arm than nondominant arm so a comparison within the individual may also not be accurate! (B) The carrying angle is reduced in cubitus varus deformity as compared to normal side. If both sides are abnormal then absolute reduction below 5° is called cubitus varus; (C) The child has distinctive varus deformity of the left elbow (cubitus varus) visible obviously as compared to the right upper limb; (D) Same child demonstrates associated hyperextension with the deformity and better appreciation of cubitus varus. The deformity resembles stock of old guns (inset picture) so it has got this colloquial name of "Gun-Stock deformity"; (E) Radiographically the mechanical axis deviation can be assessed by humero-ulnar angle on AP radiograph while quantification of cubitus varus is done using Baumann angle. The lateral radiograph (F) demonstrates gross hyperextension at elbow due to maluniting fracture (the radial physis is in line with capitellum so the elbow is not dislocated as may appear on cursory examination initially!). In some cases the cubitus varus deformity may be exaggerated by the presence of lateral spur at the malunion site (G). This spur needs smoothening/excision to provide aesthetic result.

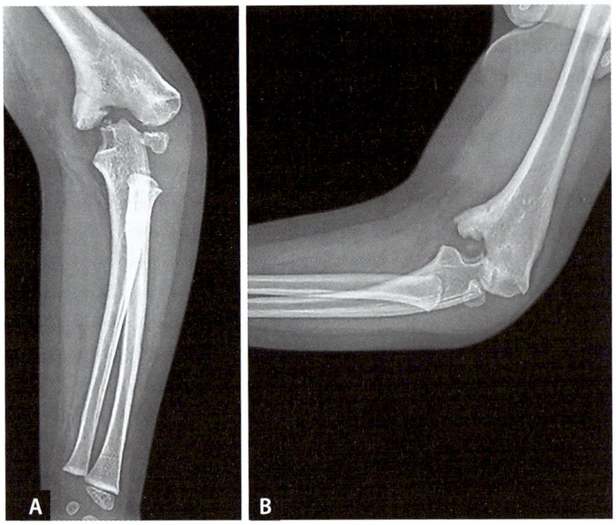

Figs. 59A and B: Trochlear osteonecrosis producing cubitus varus deformity.

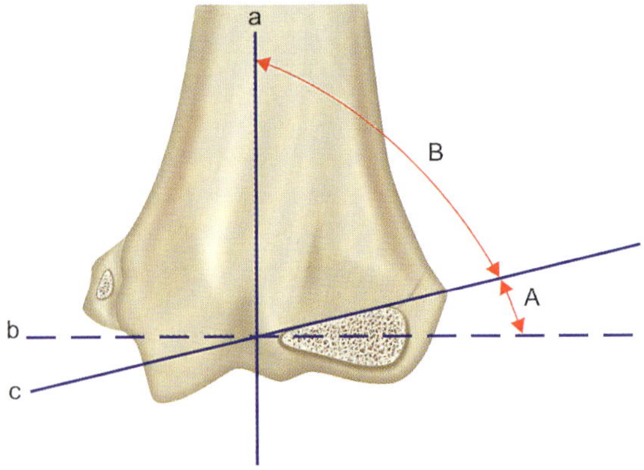

Fig. 60: The Baumann's angle has two values. Baumann calculated angle A for his radiological assessment but over a period of time angle B is considered a better measure that can be more reliably calculated. Normal value is approximately 72° (range 64–81°). Change in Baumann's angle of 5° correlates with 2° of corona l plane angular variation. In any case value of >81 would indicate cubitus varus. Difference in value of >10° from uninvolved limb would be significant.

BOX 6: Long-term complications/problems of cubitus varus deformity.

- Cosmetic appearance (gunstock deformity)
- Posterolateral instability
- Increased risk of secondary fractures
- Tardy ulna nerve palsy
- Snapping elbow

- There may be *hypoplasia of medial humeral condyle* in patients with medial physeal injury or epiphyseal dysplasia.

The cubitus varus deformity mainly produces cosmetic problem but some long-term consequences have been also reported **(Box 6)**.

Clinical Features

The most common presentation of cosmetically unsightly deformity due to altered carrying angle with mostly preserved functional ROM at the elbow. Carrying angle is altered solely due to medial tilt and angulation. The patients have asymmetrical flexion arcs when comparing both elbows with limitation of elbow flexion range on affected side. Flexion is limited only due to procurvatum deformity that causes bony block at terminal ROM. There is also flexion contracture of variable degree in some patients who were managed by plaster cast immobilization or were managed by unstable fixation that needed plaster cast and could not regain complete movements. Due to altered mechanics, there are increased chances of lateral condyle fractures or other secondary fractures, posterolateral elbow pain, and instability. Tardy ulnar nerve palsy (high type ulnar nerve palsy) may also develop in some patients due to compression from chronic malposition of triceps. Morphological alteration and abnormal alignment of the elbow joint in cubitus varus has not shown to produce arthrosis of the elbow joint so the deformity is mostly painless. The deformity due to malunion is static but if it arises from medial physeal defect or trochlea osteonecrosis then deformity may progress till osseous maturation and physeal fusion. On examination there is thickening and irregularity of lateral supracondylar ridge, prominent lateral condyle. Maintain three-point relationship with olecranon. The carrying angle is reduced and flexion ROM is variably reduced. In a few patients, there is hyperextension at elbow and flexion arc of motion may be overall same to that of uninvolved side where the loss of terminal flexion is compensated by hyperextension at elbow. Look for previous scar of surgery and note flexion contracture, if present. The coronal plane deformity is graded by some authors into four grades:

1. Grade 1—loss of physiological valgus (cubitus rectus)
2. Grade 2—0–10° of varus deformity
3. Grade 3—11–20° of varus deformity in coronal plane
4. Grade 4—>20° of cubitus varus

Radiology

Obtain standard AP of the straight elbow and a lateral view of the flexed elbow. Identify the bony landmarks and secondary centers of ossification. The order of appearance of secondary centers of ossification are specified in the mnemonic C-R-I-T-O-E (Capitellum - Radius - Internal or medial epicondyle - Trochlea - Olecranon - External or lateral epicondyle). The usual ages of appearance of these are 1, 3, 5, 7, 9, and 11 years, respectively. The varus deformity is evaluated on AP projection. Because the bony anatomy is not fully developed so use of joint orientation line is futile for varus calculation. Instead, Baumann angle is used for calculating coronal plane deformity. On AP view, draw a line parallel to the longitudinal axis of the humeral shaft and an intersecting line along the lateral condylar physis. The angle between them is the Baumann's angle **(Fig. 60)**. Compare it with the opposite uninvolved limb (See also Annexure 1 of upper limb trauma for details) for measuring the radiological varus deformity. Draw MAD on a full-length radiograph and compare from opposite side. The metaphyseo-diaphyseal angle described by Kleb-Sherman

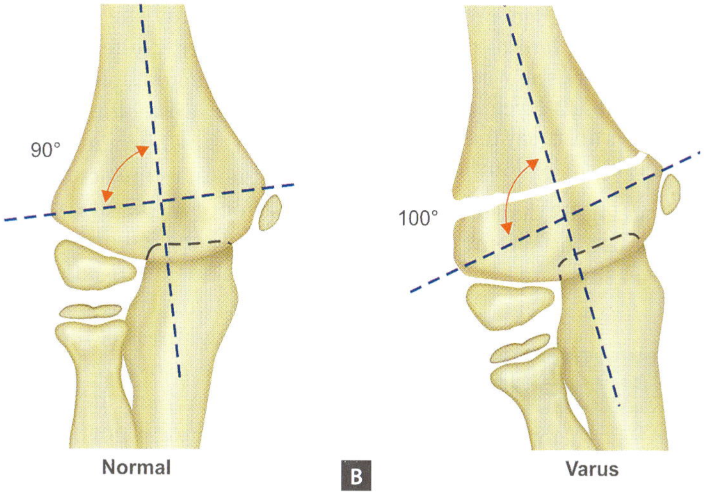

Figs. 61A and B: The metaphyseal-diaphyseal angle of O'Brien. Normal value is 90° measured on the lateral side (A). Values >90° indicate varus deformity (B) while valgus would reduce the value below 90°.

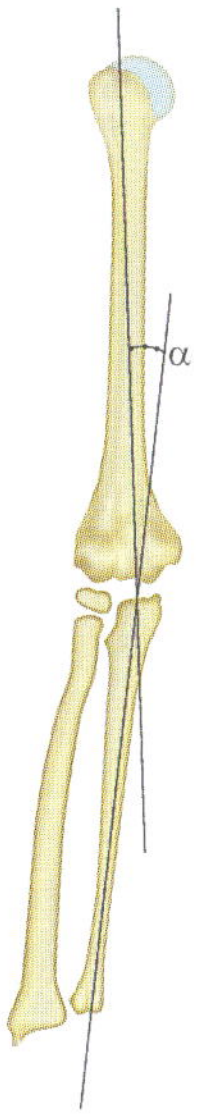

Fig. 62: The humeroulnar angle of Oppenheim. This correlates better with the carrying angle. Reduction of the angle indicates cubitus varus while the angle is increased in valgus deformity.

is normally 90° **(Figs. 61A and B)**. This is increased in varus deformity. The humeroulnar angle of Oppenheim **(Fig. 62)** is quite accurate in delineating varus deformity as other angles rely on measures that can be inaccurately marked on radiographs depending on the observer. On the lateral projection of elbow, anterior humeral line (AHL) identifies sagittal plane deformity. AHL should intersect the middle third of the capitellum in children ≥5 years old, and touches the capitellum in children in children <5 years old. Line passing posterior to capitellum indicates flexion deformity.

Treatment

The treatment option that can be offered for correcting the varus deformity is surgical only if detailed discussion with parents for expectations and outcomes is successful. Observation for expected remodeling should not be offered by an experienced surgeon because the varus does not improve with natural modeling of bone. Only some correction of hyperextension deformity may occur that has no bearing on cubitus varus per se. The physis is normal in a patient with malunited cubitus varus so growth modulation by hemiphysiodesis will not work. It may be suitable only in rare cases where deformity results from medial physeal growth arrest. Apart from correction of deformity if the patient has developed tardy ulnar nerve palsy, it should be also managed (discussed in Chapter on Peripheral Nerve Injuries).

Surgical Options

Osteotomy is the best option for correcting the cubitus varus deformity. Various types, modifications, and methods have been described for performing and fixing the osteotomy **(Box 7)**. The aim of all corrective osteotomy is restoration of mechanical axis and carrying angle symmetrical to uninvolved side by correcting the cubitus varus. There are general prerequisites before performing corrective osteotomy as follows:

- Bone should be mature enough to hold fixation implants—usually an arbitrary period of 1 year following injury is chosen expecting major completion of bone modeling and tissue equilibrium. It can be partly judged by radiologist on radiographs.
- Patient and parents understanding the outcome which is predominantly correction of cosmetic deformity and minimal effect of functional profile. Late complications may be prevented by restoration of anatomy. ROM is not improved by this osteotomy *per se*.
- The corrective osteotomy is best performed between 6 and 11 years of age. By 6 years the bone is strong enough to hold implants and before 11 years there is enough modeling potential left to correct the lateral prominence that may appear after unequal limb corrective wedge osteotomy producing Z-correction. Some osteotomy

designs (like simple lateral closing wedge) produce larger base of distal wedge that causes lateral prominence appearing as uncorrected or persistent cubitus varus (Z-correction). It models over time 2–3 years. So 11 years is an optimal upper limit. This is not to say that osteotomy cannot be done after this age, it can be done at any age.

Lateral closing wedge osteotomy **(Fig. 63)** had been the most popular and commonly performed osteotomy to correct cubitus varus deformity. However, there are a few limitations of this standard approach:

BOX 7: Types of corrective osteotomies used and described for surgical correction of cubitus varus.

1. Lateral closing wedge osteotomy of Siris—using K-wires or Steinman pins does not offer good stability
   a. French and modified French ± rotatory correction—used screws and figure of 8 loop of stainless steel wire but persistence of lateral prominence following surgery (Z-correction) made correction appear suboptimal in immediate postoperative period. Although this regresses with time.
   b. Lateral equal limb osteotomy of Oppenheim **(Figs. 64A and B)**—this osteotomy is done at a higher level than conventional osteotomy to equalize the limbs of bone cut. This however produces more translation.
   c. Oblique Lateral closing wedge osteotomy **(Figs. 65A and B)**—this reduces the Z-correction by creating two cuts that have equal lengths and no lateral prominence occurs in postcorrection. Both osteotomy arms slant proximally from the medial epicondyle in such a way that the contact lengths are approximately same opposing completely without any step/lateral projection.
2. Medial opening wedge osteotomy
3. Special osteotomies:
   a. Dome osteotomy **(Fig. 66)**
   b. Pentalateral/triplanar osteotomy/3D osteotomy for correcting deformities in all three planes **(Fig. 67)**—requires complex planning and posterior approach
   c. Oblique osteotomy with derotation (Amspacher and Messenbaugh)
   d. Step-cut osteotomy of DeRosa and Graziano **(Fig. 68)** using posterior approach
4. Distraction osteogenesis following corticotomy
5. Callotasis following osteotomy

- Osteotomy site is more proximal than malunion site; therefore, it often is difficult to cross the fixation pins at the osteotomy site for rigid fixation.
- Because osteotomy is proximal to CORA so the osteotomy works by introducing another deformity in a direction other than the actual deformity. This produces a zigzag effect (valgus at osteotomy and varus at malunion). Thus, the Z-correction leads to lateralization of the distal malunion site (instead of correcting it) commonly producing lateral prominence.
- The tightness of the medial soft tissue after the closing wedge osteotomy tends to produce a strong varus moment that can lead to loss of fixation if rigid fixation like plating is not used.
- The osteotomy is not suitable for correcting deformities >25–30°.

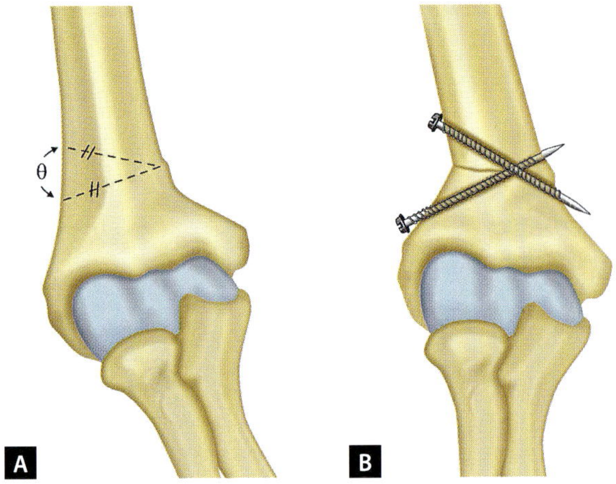

Figs. 64A and B: The lateral equal limb closing osteotomy of Oppenheim.

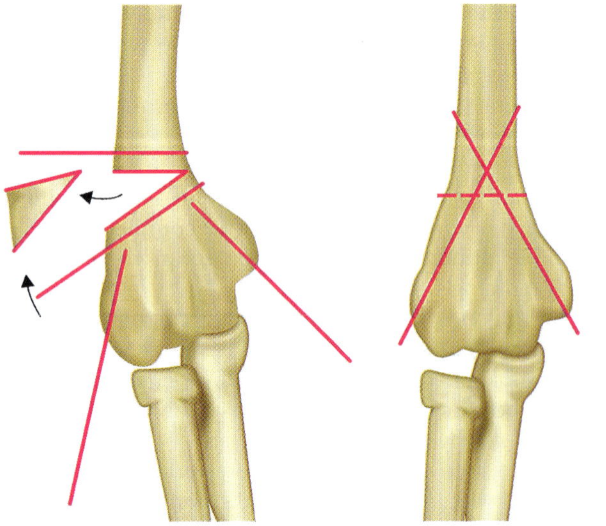

Fig. 63: The lateral closing wedge osteotomy for cubitus varus deformity correction. The osteotomy correction is premarked by K-wires and the wedge is sawed off. Osteotomy is fixed with K-wires or threaded K-wires or Steinmann pins.

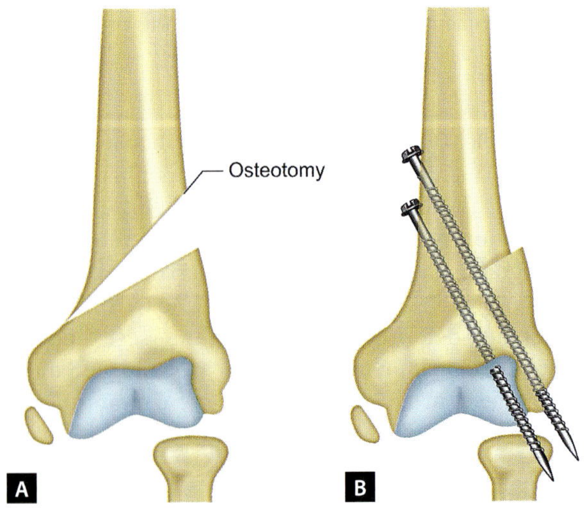

Figs. 65A and B: The oblique lateral closing wedge osteotomy. The obliquity allows apex of the osteotomy to be as close to center of rotation of angulation (CORA) as possible while proximal and distal limbs of osteotomy are more or less equal in length minimizing lateral prominence.

Medial opening wedge osteotomy has been recommended by some for correction of large varus deformities (>30°). This is based on the premised that such large deformities medialize triceps muscle and thus the dynamic pull on the olecranon shifts it medially over a period of time. The repeated pull of the triceps during each flexion movement also smoothens the medial ridge of trochlea. Both these effects combine to shift the olecranon medially that may virtually override the

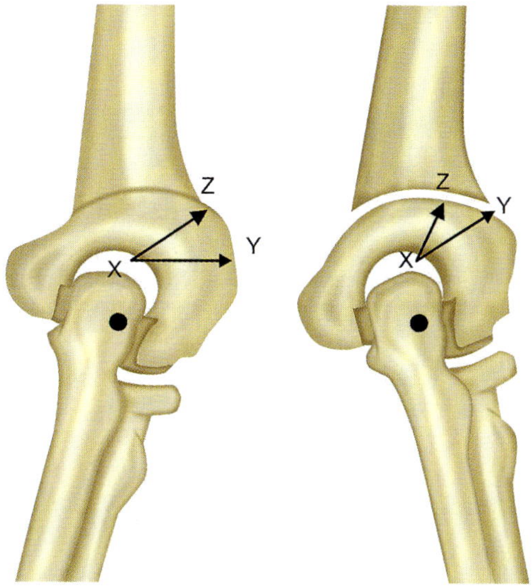

Fig. 66: The dome osteotomy for cubitus varus correction. Posterior triceps splitting approach is used. Intraoperatively point "X" is marked either at the highest point of olecranon fossa in midline or tip of olecranon is used. Point "Y" is marked horizontally on the lateral ridge. The line AY is used to mark angle YXZ equal to the calculated correction angle preoperatively. Metal foil template or a K-wire bent to desired correction angle preoperatively can be used to assist in marking the point Z. Dome-shaped semicircular cut pivoted at point "X" is completed by drilling holes and small osteotome from lateral to medial. The distal fragment is rotated in position so that point "Y" now meets lateral cortex. Before rotation the anterior and posterior cortical spikes should be trimmed and segment "YZ" also need some trimming so that it can fit in the proximal osteotomy arc. Fix the osteotomy with plate or threaded K-wires.

medial epicondyle in full flexion. Medially-based correction will release the tight medial structures and correct alignment of triceps, in fact the triceps was medially detached and stitched to the lateral part to correct line of pull. This approach is associated with high incidence of nerve palsy and stretch on nerve. The real benefit of triceps partial transfer has not been documented and appears futile for just correcting cosmetic deformity. Another procedure for harvesting bone grafting is needed and results have not been reproduced by other authors.

Dome osteotomy for correction of cubitus varus **(Fig. 66)** has gained popularity due to its potential to correct large varus deformities without lateral prominence. It reduces lateral prominence directly and may also correct internal rotation deformity simultaneously using modification.

Correction of malrotation simultaneously is debated. Some consider it useless for various reasons such as compensation by shoulder movements and regression over time (debatable as rotational malunions do not model). Malrotation has minimal bearing on varus deformity, 30° internal rotation produces 6° loss of carrying angle and 45° produce 8° loss of carrying angle. Arguments in favor include simple technique for correcting internal rotation (placing distal screw more anterior in French method reduces the osteotomy in external rotation). Also, correction of malrotation places lateral epicondyle more posterior reducing the lateral prominence so improves cosmesis. I personally correct malrotation in majority of the corrective osteotomies but opinions differ.

Methods for stabilization of osteotomy **(Table 6)** vary from simple above elbow cast (Watson-Jones, now abandoned), K-wires, single or double cortical screw, screws with tension wire loops, plates, and external fixators. Smooth K-wires may back out with loss of fixation and have additional pin tract issues. Threaded wire or Steinmann pin have better fixation but pin tract infection remains an issue. Single or crossed screws have been used but holding the osteotomy reduction while passing screw is a must and inadvertent translation has been reported. Use of screws

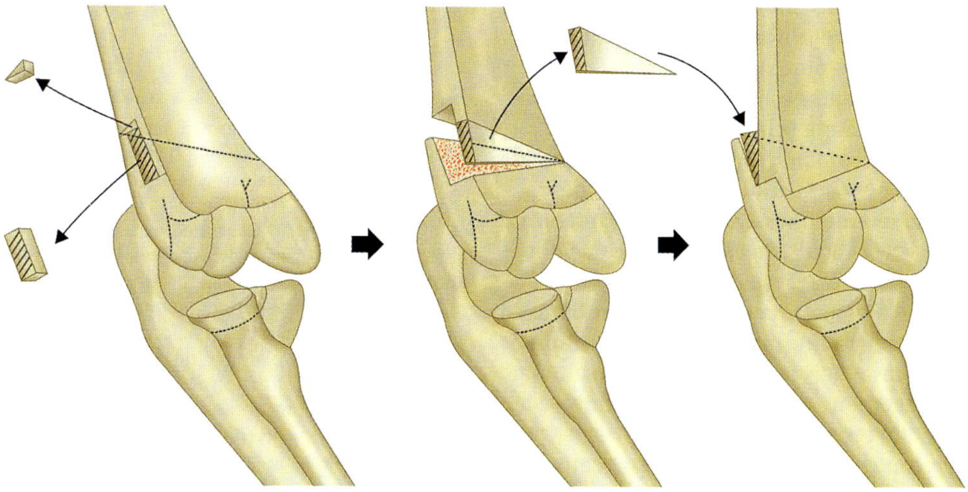

Fig. 67: The triplanar pentalateral osteotomy complex corrective osteotomy for cubitus varus.

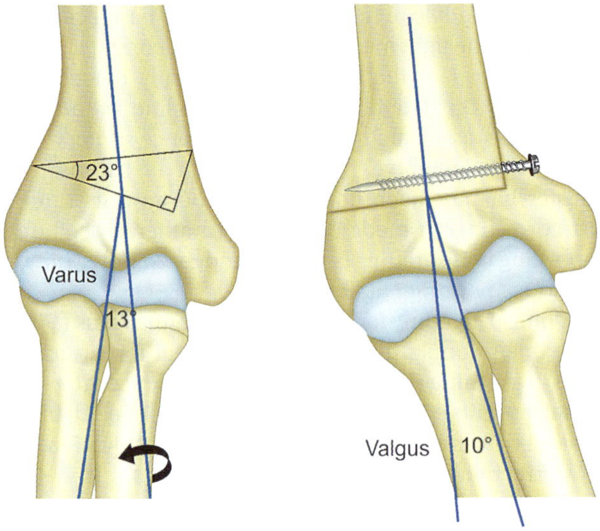

Fig. 68: The step-cut osteotomy of DeRosa and Graziano.

with tension band wire loop as proposed by French should only be used when the medial cortical hinge and periosteal integrity is maintained **(Fig. 69A to G)**. Osteotomies in older children are better stabilized with one-third tubular plate or reconstruction plate. This gives rigid stable fixation with less chances of loss of fixation. Early mobilization can be done. External fixation has been used by some authors but it requires larger distal fragment to hold pins. Appears cumbersome and pin tract issue remain.

Complications

As with all surgeries the corrective osteotomy for cubitus varus deformity is also associated with a myriad of complications that vary with the technique used and fixation device deployed for stabilization of osteotomy. The list of complications is provided in **Box 8**.

CONCLUSION

- Nonunion of fractures is a disabling complication that critically limits the functionality of the patients. Fracture nonunion prolongs the morbidity and treatment duration causing multiple hospital visits and mostly several therapeutic procedures are needed.
- It is important to differentiate infected from noninfected nonunions as the treatment principles usually differ.
- Most of the treatment principles are aimed at enhancing the fracture union by stimulation of the repair process. Biological stimulation methods are commonly preferred as they have consistent success rates. Biophysical methods are more ancillary to use.
- Ilizarov method is a discrete method that can be used more or less universally in the management of nonunions even the complex cases. It is often thought as the ultimate method in management of nonunion that have even failed to heal by other methods.
- Malunions commonly arise from conservative or inadequate reduction of fractures. COVID pandemic has

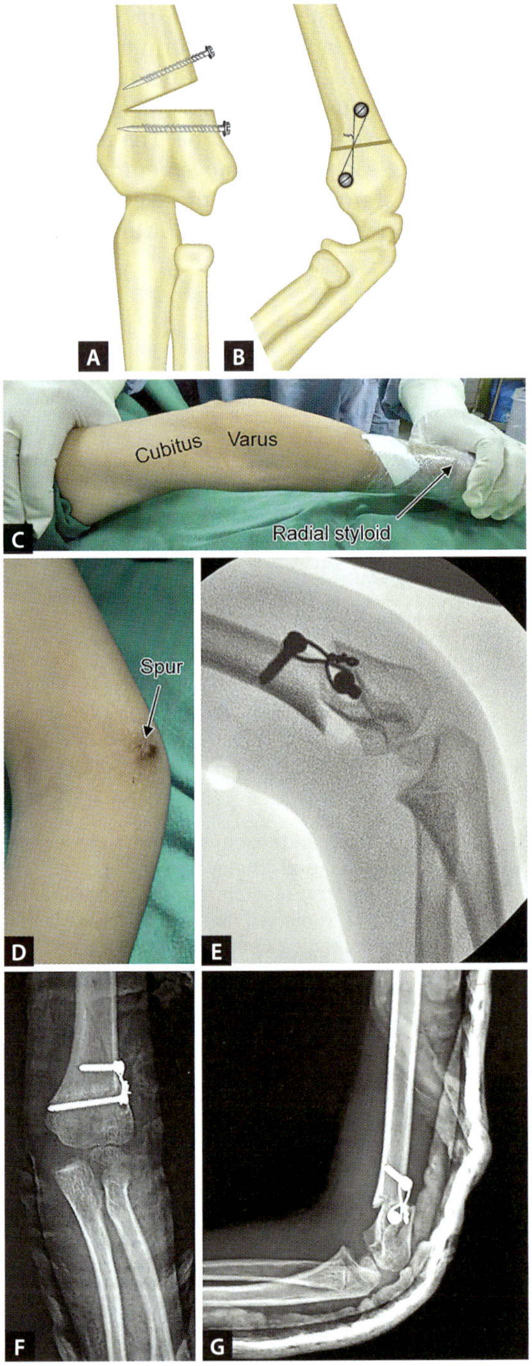

Fig. 69A to G: The use of cortical screws and metal wire figure of 8 loop as advocated by French should be used only if medial cortical hinge is intact (A). Note the distal screw is anterior to coronal line that may help in some correction of internal rotation (B); (C) The cubitus varus deformity of left elbow. There is associated excessive internal rotation deformity of forearm as visualized by prominent radial styloid nearing anterior midline. The cubitus varus deformity is exaggerated by the presence of lateral spur (D); The correction entailed excision of the spur and also correction of internal rotation deformity by externally rotating the distal fragment (E); The halo around distal screw is the site of excision of spur. External rotation correction was achieved in this case by placing the distal screw anteriorly and on tightening of the stainless steel wire the fragment got into external rotation; medial hinge was kept intact in this patient. Final radiographic correction (F and G) demonstrates good correction of varus, excised lateral spur (seen as a halo around distal screw).

TABLE 6: The various methods of fixation used to stabilize osteotomized fragments.

Method of fixation	*Comments*
Plate osteosynthesis. One can use the conventional low contact dynamic compression plates or newer locked plate osteosynthesis. Periarticular implants are used for correction of intra-articular or periarticular malunions. Specialized plates like Puddu plate or high tibial osteotomy plate may be used in specific situations.	*Advantages:* Age old method, surgeons well versed, direct approach so fixation under direct vision, acute correction possible, contouring possible, compression at osteotomy and precision control. *Disadvantages:* Loss of vascularity due to approach, moment arm of fixation away from neutral axis, immobilization till union needed, correction once done cannot be changed or modified later, does not address shortening.
Intramedullary fixation	*Advantages:* Fixation along neutral axis, preserves vascularity, fixation along neutral axis, ideal moment of inertia. *Disadvantages:* Suitable for diaphyseal malunions only, minimal compression achievable, correction once achieved cannot be redone or changed, can be used for simultaneous lengthening of railroad fixation done.
Ilizarov technique	*Advantages:* Preserves vascularity, versatile—applicable to wide variety of malunions at different sites, limited metal in bone, quite assured union if properly done, simultaneous lengthening and translatory correction possible. *Disadvantages:* Needs expertise, pin tract issues.
Computer aided frames for deformity correction like hexapod/ Taylor spatial frame	*Advantages:* Computerized calculation of deformity and its correction axis, simultaneous correction of all deformities, minimal implant load. *Disadvantages:* Cost, needs dedicated software, familiarity with usage, needs dedicated evaluation as per protocol.
K-wires and Steinmann pins	These are used to fix relatively smaller bones in children such as correction of supracondylar humeral malunion (cubitus varus). Fixation of periarticular malunion correction in skeletally immature patients where other methods of fixation would damage growth plate.
Condylar blade plate and osteotomy blade plate (sometimes dynamic lag screw-plate construct is used like the dynamic condylar screw)	These are specialized implants used (or having improvised usage) in correction of proximal femoral deformity/malunion. They also have extended and successful usage in distal femoral malunions.

BOX 8: The complications following corrective surgery for cubitus varus deformity.

- Z-correction producing lateral prominence
- Undercorrection
- Overcorrection
- Loss of correction
- Loss of elbow movements (stiffness)
- Myositis ossificans
- Delayed union/nonunion (flimsy fixation and stability)
- Nerve injury/palsy—more with medial opening wedge and dome osteotomies. (It may also be compounded by the fact that these osteotomies are done in large deformities that need big corrections stretching the nerves)
- Pin tract issues
- Osteomyelitis
- Unsightly scar
- Pseudo-varus formation: Sometimes lateral spur forms from lateral humeral condyle due to ossification in elevated periosteum. This produces lateral bulge that appears as cubitus varus deformity; however, the carrying angle is normal.

seen resurgence of malunions due to limited accessibility of operative reduction.

- Malunions alter mechanical disposition producing abnormal stresses around joints and may produce accelerated degeneration.
- Unacceptable malunions need proper clinical, radiological, geometrical assessment, and correction based on principles of deformity correction.
- Limb length may also be altered that need simultaneous correction in many.
- Improved operative techniques and fixation methods have bettered the outcome of correction of deformity but surgery for malunion is a different ball-game all together compared to primary fixation. The pros and cons, along with expectations and possibilities should be properly balanced before embarking on this usually prolonged path of deformity correction.

SECTION

5

Pediatric Orthopedics

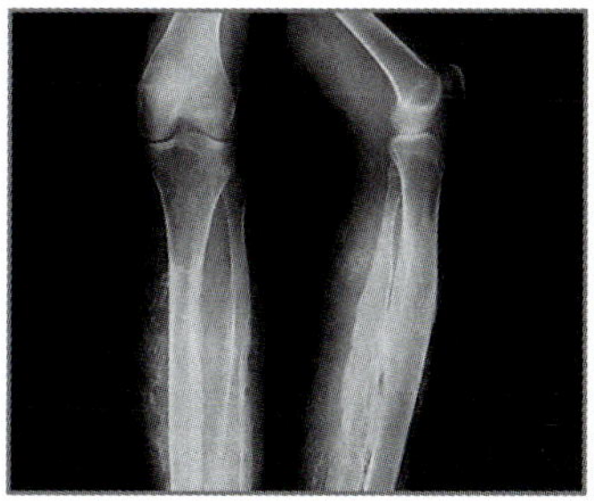

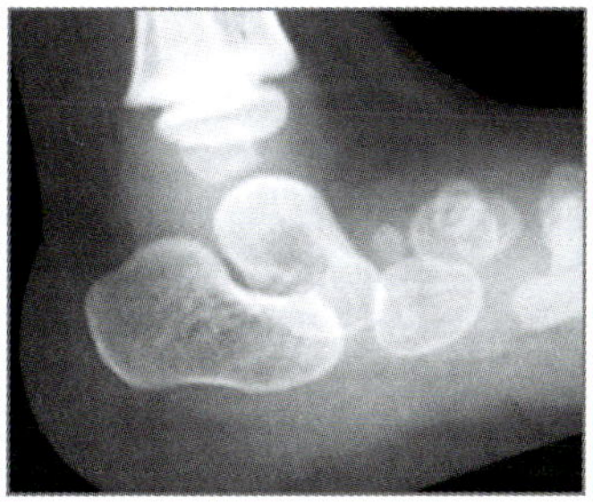

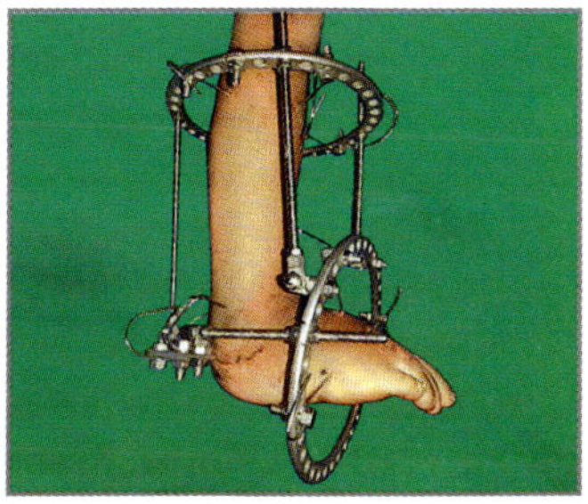

CHAPTER

38 Congenital, Genetic, Syndromic, and Miscellaneous Disorders

Manish Kumar Varshney

INTRODUCTION

Defining "normal" is very difficult as many perceived abnormalities in form and function represent a variant or extreme spectrum of deemed normal. This entails putting stop at the extremes of the spectrum of abnormality that can be accepted as normal. This has been arbitrarily put as 95% of population that usually falls within 2 standard deviations (SDs) from mean for any measurement. With this wide variation one should understand that this definition of statistically normal in no way equates with "ideal" for any person. For descriptive purpose various terms are used to define common deviations from normal.

The term "congenital" refers to any anomaly that is present or apparent at birth while the term "developmental" refers to deviation that occurs over time and may not be present or apparent at birth. "Deformity" refers to alteration in the shape of body part that falls outside the normal range. A *congenital disorder* describes a condition existing at or before birth. One that clearly and evidently develops during first month of life is considered neonatal disease (they are countable only if any orthopedic disease comes under this category).

An *anomaly* is abnormality of the structure (usually refers to morphological terms) of a body part. An anomaly may not be necessarily perceived as a problem or disease that requires treatment (like, clinodactyly of the fifth finger so common) and it may be congenital or developmental or even acquired (say, a malunited fracture producing deformity).

Birth defect is a loosely used term for congenital anomaly that can be recognized at birth and often refers to pathological conditions (but most common usage is as a layman's term for any defect), usually they are the result of a complex mix of genetic and environmental factors.

Congenital malformation is a structural defect that is deleterious and is associated with a *disorder of tissue* development. It is defined as a single localized poor development of tissue that initiates a chain of subsequent defects. The fetal growth and development did not proceed normally due to underlying genetic, epigenetic, or environmental factors that altered the development of a particular structure. Further the growth will take a pathological route to produce unique constellation of signs and symptoms characteristic of a particular disease, e.g., anencephaly. There can be associated malformations in other parts of body whence it can become a malformation syndrome.

Sequence is a group of related anomalies that generally stem from a *single initial major anomaly* that alters the development of other surrounding or related tissues or structures, e.g., Potter sequence. *Disruption* is an abnormality where a fetal structure is growing normally and then growth is arrested due to something which disrupts the process, e.g., amniotic band syndrome.

Dysplasia specifically refers to *anomalous intrinsic cellular architecture* of a tissue that is not normally maintained throughout growth and development. Here the primary defect is a *lack of normal organization of cells into tissue* and describes the malformation at organ or tissue level, e.g., achondroplasia.

A *deformation* is a result of extrinsic mechanical forces on otherwise normal tissue, like postural clubfoot in primigravida or oligohydramnios.

The word *"syndrome"* (Greek) means to "run together". When several relatively uncommon anomalies occur in the same individual, it is highly likely to arise from coincidence. However, there are conditions that result from the same cause or occur in the same pattern. This well-recognized combination of major or minor birth or genetic or developmental anomalies that occur together in a predictable fashion characterizing a specific disorder or like is called a syndrome. In medical genetics, the term is specifically used to define a condition that is pathogenetically related to identify genetic cause. Most of the pediatric syndromes are genetic (most of the specific gene alterations are, however, undefined or not substantially linked). Certain conditions are not genetically linked but have characteristic features and are termed *"associations"* like the toxic shock syndrome or acquired immune deficiency syndrome. Association is a group of anomalies that occur more frequently together than would be expected by chance alone but that do not have a predictable pattern of recognition and/or a suspected unified underlying etiology (like the VATER association). Suspicion of a syndrome should clinically arise when:

- A known component of syndromic manifestation (e.g., radial club hand) is encountered
- If the limb deformities are symmetric
- If all the four extremities are affected
- If there is a familiar dysmorphic face
- If there are several associated nonorthopedic anomalies

There is often a dictum that the children who have syndromes look more like each other than they do to their parents.

TORTICOLLIS

The term *torticollis* semantically stands for "twisted neck" originating from Latin words "*tortus*" meaning twisted and "*collum*" meaning neck. Historical descriptions of the deformity have been found in the writings of Plutarch's written references describing the features of thence emperor Alexander the great [ruler of the kingdom of Macedonia (aka-Macedon), believed to have this deformity]. The typical components of deformity grossly include lateral inclination of the head to the ipsilateral shoulder combined with torsion of the neck and deviation of the chin to other side **(Fig. 1)** as first defined by Tubby in 1912 for congenital muscular torticollis (CMT). Torticollis can be seen in adult or in pediatric patients **(Table 1)**.

Adult form is commonly neurodegenerative disease seen commonly in females aged 40 years or more, resulting in cervical dystonia arising from some thalamic lesion (underactivity of D2 dopamine receptors in the indirect pallidal outflow pathway). This is also referred to as idiopathic spasmodic torticollis. The dystonia results in dynamic or fixed position of the head and neck in tilt, rotation, or flexion due to spasm in one or combination of sternocleidomastoid, trapezius, or other neck muscles. Depending on position of head the tilt can be lateral (laterocollis due to increased tone of ipsilateral cervical muscles), torsional (partial rotation or rotation of the head), anterior (anterocollis, increased tone of anterior cervical muscles), or posterior (retrocollis, neck hyperextension due to increased tone of posterior cervical muscles). The basic pathophysiology is that the normal rhythmic horizontal (as if to say "no") or vertical movements (as if to say "yes") of head and neck become unequal due to dystonia producing characteristic tonic head tilt/rotation. The other variety of adult torticollis is due to sudden spasm of sternocleidomastoid muscle (SCM) due to sleeping in awkward position or irritation of its nerve supply. These adult forms will not be discussed any further as they are dealt within faculty of neurology.

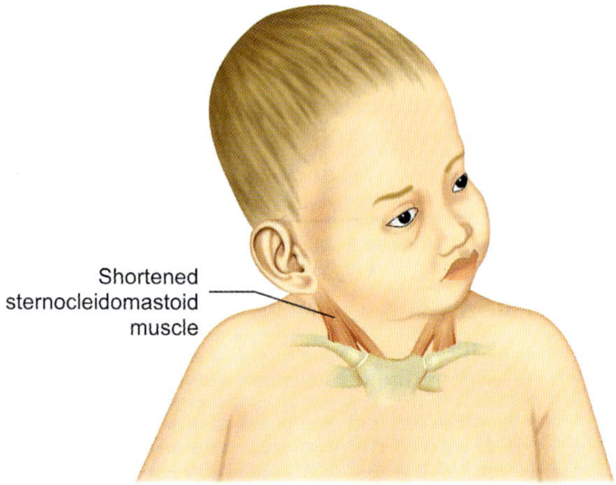

Fig. 1: Illustration of child with torticollis due to shortened sternocleidomastoid muscle, note the head tilt to ipsilateral side and chin pointing to contralateral side.

Pediatric variety of torticollis can be congenital or acquired **(Table 1)**. The congenital form is further divided into muscular (CMT) and nonmuscular [previously referred to as "postural" form wrongly as there are various known causes for it **(Table 1)**]. MacDonald further divided CMT into sternocleidomastoid (SCM) tumor group (20% of infants with torticollis and 35% of patients with CMT) and those with tight SCM but no identifiable tumor, this classification is more arbitrary and possibly superfluous from treatment perspective. CMT is a painless condition caused due to unilateral shortening of the SCM usually presenting during infancy. Shortening of the SCM results in lateral inclination of the neck combined with contralateral torsion. It is seen in 0.3–1.9% of all live births with slight preponderance of male patients (M:F = 3:2). CMT is recorded as is the third most common congenital musculoskeletal anomaly after dislocation of the hip and clubfoot. There is a preponderance of involvement on the right side (>80%) as compared to left side (~15%) in patients with CMT.

Pathoanatomy

The SCM comprises of four distinct anatomical elements, comprising of two origins and two insertions supplied by spinal accessory nerve and cervical plexus roots (C1 and C2). The sternal origin rotates the head while the clavicular origin is responsible for lateral tilt of the head. Insertion is still broad onto mastoid and over superior nuchal line of occiput. Depending on the predominant part of affected muscle a clinical spectrum of disease is produced. The typical description is of a shortened SCM with a firm mass sized between 1 and 3 cm. The mass is commonly palpable between 1 and 4 weeks of age. Previously considered to be hematoma due to birth trauma and muscle strain, the absence of hemosiderin in pathological specimens does not support the view. Also ultrasonography and magnetic resonance imaging (MRI) often record isoechoic or homogeneous findings devoid of any iron rich signals. The basic abnormality of CMT is now believed to be endomysial fibrosis (resulting most likely from some ischemic process—traumatic or atraumatic) associated with deposition of collagen and the aggregation of fibroblasts around muscle fibers. This is followed by atrophy of the involved region and contraction occurs by activity of myofibroblasts over resolution phase.

Etiology

Till now no concrete documentation has been obtained for the exact cause of SCM shortening in patients with CMT. It is

TABLE 1: Etiology and differential diagnosis of torticollis.

Type		***Comments***
Adult-onset variety		Not related to sternocleidomastoid muscle (SCM), mainly neurological
	Cervical dystonia	
	Acute spasm of SCM	
	Acute cervical disk calcification	
	Bone tumors	Eosinophilic granuloma, osteoid osteoma, and osteoblastoma of upper cervical spine
Pediatric variety		
Congenital		Torticollis present since birth and due most commonly to SCM involvement but other rare causes also found
	Congenital muscular torticollis	SCM tumor, shortening due to fibrosis
	Congenital absence of SCM of one side	
	Pterygium colli	
	Klippel–Feil syndrome	
	Unilateral atlanto-occipital fusion	
	Vertebral anomalies	The anomalies mostly present as developmental torticollis due to progression of the curve on one side rather than at birth, though the underlying cause in true sense congenital
	congenital positional torticollis (CPT)	
Acquired		
	Infectious or inflammatory	Cervical lymphadenitis, upper respiratory tract/pharyngeal infections, otogenic torticollis, cervical discitis (commonly tuberculosis in India) or vertebral osteomyelitis, Grisel syndrome (nontraumatic rotatory subluxation of the atlantoaxial joint due to inflammation in upper respiratory tract), upper lobe pneumonia, and juvenile rheumatoid arthritis
	Traumatic	Atlanto-occipital or atlantoaxial subluxations, cervical 2nd to 3rd vertebral subluxation, fractures of C1, and muscular injury to neck muscles
	Neurological	Cervical cord tumor, syringomyelia, posterior fossa brain tumor, acoustic neuroma, Wilson disease, dystonia musculorum deformans, and irritation of accessory nerve
	Ocular torticollis	Nystagmus, paresis of muscles supplied by abducent (lateral rectus) or trochlear nerves (superior oblique), Duane's syndrome, and Brown's syndrome
	Medications	Phenothiazines, metoclopramide, haloperidol, etc.
	Psychogenic	
	Postural	Playing video games in abnormal head posture for prolonged periods
	Sandifer syndrome	Spasmodic torsional dystonia associated with gastroesophageal reflux, esophagitis, and hiatal hernia
	Benign paroxysmal torticollis	Also known as paroxysmal torticollis of infancy mostly due to some vestibular dysfunction. The deformity may last from minutes to days and may also alternate on side of involvement. No specific treatment is needed other than treating the underlying cause.

postulated that a variety of causes may be responsible for the development of fibrosis, important of which are:

- Fetal malposition in the womb
- Intrauterine or perinatal compartment syndrome due to difficult labor
- Breech birth and ensuing birth trauma
- Hereditary venous or arterial occlusion which may create fibrous tissue within the sternocleidomastoid
- Hematoma formation in the SCM from an intrauterine vascular disturbance
- Intrauterine infections and congenital SCM cysts have also been discussed sparingly.
- Congenital (apart from CMT) or acquired pediatric torticollis may also result from uncommon causes like congenital postural torticollis (CPT, there is no SCM lesion or shortening and resolves very fast within 3 months, it may also arise in children in the habit of playing prolonged video games in a tilted head posture), pterygium colli (webbed neck), spina bifida, vertebral anomalies, odontoid hyperplasia, cervical musculature

abnormalities, and Arnold–Chiari syndrome. It can also be seen with clavicular fractures, especially in neonates secondary to birth trauma and various neurogenic causes like ocular tumors or paresis of lateral rectus (trochlear nerve) or superior oblique muscles (abducent nerve), Sandifer syndrome (gastrointestinal reflux with cerebral palsy), posterior fossa tumors, syringomyelia, and spinal cord tumors. Infections of upper respiratory tract, pharynx, and inflamed lymph nodes in the posterior triangle of neck and irritation of spinal accessory nerve may also uncommonly produce torticollis. Atlantoaxial subluxation in cases of juvenile rheumatoid arthritis (JRA) must also be kept in mind.

Signs

Appearance of CMT is characteristic with tilt of the head toward the same side while chin points to the contralateral side due to torsional deformity of neck consequent upon shortened SCM. The other characteristic signs of torticollis include:

- Orbital dystopia (the eye on the unaffected side is higher up)
- Restricted rotation of the neck
- Dental malocclusion (the lower midline is deviated to the affected side, causing a unilateral crossbite, postnormal Class II molar relation on the affected side, and prenormal Class III molar occlusion on the unaffected side)
- Anteriorly shifted ear contralateral to the shortened SCM
- Secondary plagiocephaly (flattened parieto-occipital surface on the same side), frontal flattening (ipsilateral), and facial asymmetry
- Compensatory postures include shoulder elevation and side bending of the trunk on the ipsilateral side
- In late and neglected cases of CMT craniofacial asymmetry are seen that include:
    - Posterior displacement of ipsilateral ear (94%)
    - Posterior regression of ipsilateral zygoma (87%)
    - Posterior regression of ipsilateral forehead (81%)
    - Inferior positioning of the affected eye (31%)
    - Mandibular deviation toward affected side (44%)
    - Deviation of nasal tip toward affected side (31%)
    - Rhomboidal shape skull

Associations of Torticollis

Congenital muscular torticollis is often associated with other congenital deformities such as developmental dysplasia of the hip (DDH) with a coexistence rate estimated as high as 15–20%. Other coincident lesions less frequently recorded include tibial torsion, clubfoot, calcaneovalgus foot, flexible pes planus, metatarsus adductus, and hallux valgus.

Evaluation and Diagnosis

The diagnosis of CMT is based on the clinical appearance and signs as mentioned above along with finding of a firm mass (firm painless not tender pseudotumor is commonly palpable within first few weeks of birth) or fibrous band (endomysial mass of fibrotic tissue due to deposition of collagen) within SCM. One should record past medical history and perform clinical examination of the child **(Flowchart 1)**. The points to be specifically noted in the history include:

- Antenatal history for oligohydramnios, complicated labor, and the coexistence of previous birth trauma such as clavicular fracture.
- Evaluation of perinatal records for asphyxia, jaundice, seizures, medication, gastroesophageal reflux disease (GERD), or Sandifer syndrome.
- Fever, stridor, increased drooling, sore throat, respiratory discomfort, and dysphagia suggest an infective cause most likely retropharyngeal abscess that may be life threatening.

Flowchart 1: Algorithm showing evaluation of a patient presenting with torticollis.

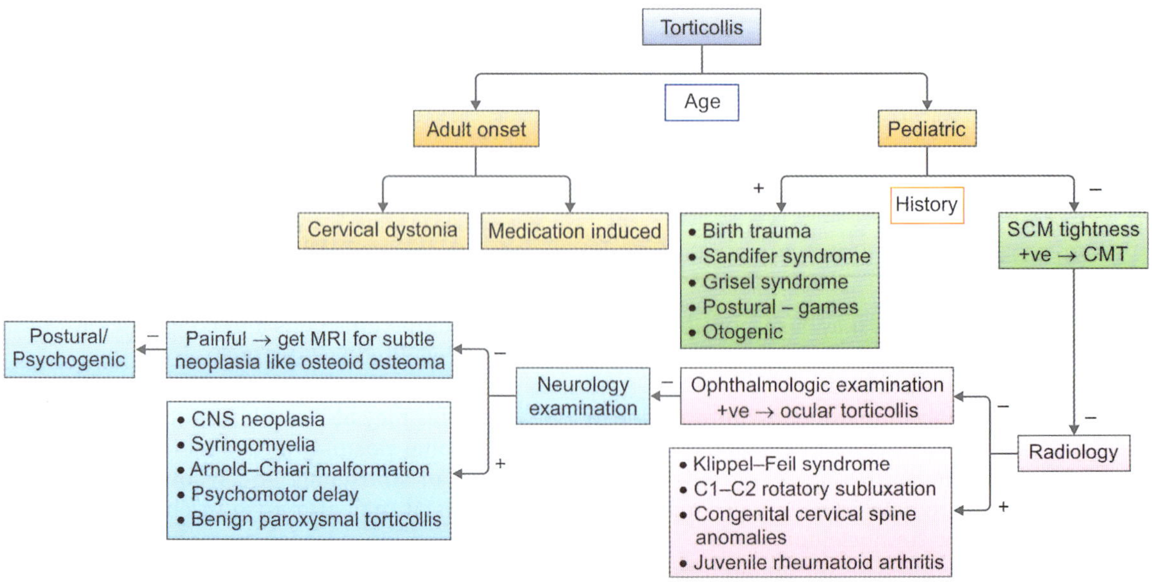

(CMT: congenital muscular torticollis; CNS: central nervous system; SCM: sternocleidomastoid muscle)

- Neurological symptoms, e.g., headache, strabismus, diplopia, photophobia, ataxia, and seizures.
- Recent head and neck surgery.
- Medications that may cause dystonia such as metoclopramide, haloperidol, phenytoin, and phenothiazine therapy.

Clinical examination

- Evaluation of neck for palpable nontender firm mass in sternal or clavicular portion of SCM, lymphadenopathy, abscess formation, and any midline tenderness. The type of deformity should be evaluated in detail to record the combination of flexion and rotation (separate assessment should also be made in individual cases), whether the deformation is rigid or flexible, and whether it can be corrected by the child itself (postural torticollis). Assess range of motion (ROM) of neck that is commonly done by electrogoniometer in sitting position or alternatively strap-on goniometer can be used. In infants the same is done in supine position.
- Thorough neurological assessment along with assessment of spine for signs of spina bifida (tuft of hair/dimple).
- Ear, nose, and throat (ENT) examination—upper respiratory and ontological infections.
- Ophthalmology examination for extraocular muscle imbalance.
- Note and assessment of associated musculoskeletal conditions should be made and never ignored, especially the developmental hip dysplasia. One may consider performing ultrasonological examination (preferred) in these patients for hip joint at 4 weeks of age or a pelvic radiograph (if facilities for ultrasonography not available) at 1 months, repeated at 4–6 months of age. Ophthalmological examination may reveal the causing factor of torticollis.

Imaging and Investigations

Radiographs of cervical spine should be obtained to identify bony abnormalities, especially unilateral fusions (not very helpful in infancy) and identification of atlantoaxial subluxations in JRA. Radiographs are especially ordered if there is cervical spine tenderness that persists following short course of analgesics, severe pain, JRA, ligamentous laxity, or persistently restricted ROM. Ultrasonographic imaging has high sensitivity and specificity of 96% and 83%, respectively and has good diagnostic and prognostic value. It is considered investigation of choice though findings vary in accordance with different CMT stages. MRI has limited role in CMT diagnosis with evident clinical features though the radiological findings have high concordance with histopathological findings.

Differential Diagnosis of Congenital Muscular Torticollis

As mentioned in the **Table 1** differential diagnosis includes a myriad of nosocomial conditions including (but not limited to) Klippel–Feil syndrome, Grisel syndrome, various osseous, neurological and functional causes of torticollis, otogenic torticollis, ocular torticollis, neoplasms, infections, and systemic diseases such as rheumatoid arthritis **(Table 1)**.

Treatment

Initial management of CMT is always conservative manipulation to stretch the SCM. This can be done by parents or dedicated physiotherapists. Some other modalities may be combined but exquisite details to their use have not been described.

Physical Therapy

Manual passive stretching of the SCM is recommended to be done for two to four times a day till the age of 12 months. Stretching is done by one hand lying between child's head and the ipsilateral shoulder to reduce lateral flexion (side-to-side stretch), while the other is applied on the face and chin to derotate the neck (ear-to-shoulder stretch, **Fig. 2**). Ten to fifteen stretches of 30 seconds each are performed in one sitting. This is considered the most effective form of therapy with >90% patients showing positive response when performed correctly. Recurrence rate is estimated to be nearly 2% with physical therapy mainly due to carelessness. Higher recurrence rate and incomplete response is seen when the initial rotation of the head from the neutral position is >15°, there is well palpable sternomastoid tumor, and initiation of the treatment done after first year of life. In between revaluation of the stretching program is done at the age of 4 months where if head tilt of the infant is found to be ≥6° then a cervical collar or brace [tubular orthosis for torticollis (TOT)] is added to the program during waking hours. With the increasing use of botulinum toxin it has been proposed that earlier injection of the toxin in less than optimally progressing or refractory cases of CMT at 3 months of age may improve the outcome significantly. This has also been found to be effective in cases of adult onset torticollis (cervical dystonia). Other forms of physical therapy have also

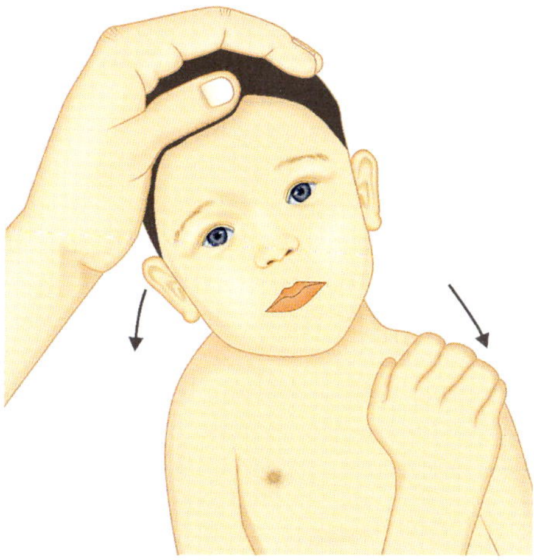

Fig. 2: The manipulation and stretching for correcting torticollis. The derotatory "ear-to-shoulder stretch" for tight left sternocleidomastoid muscle of the child.

been tried but their use is not prevalent as briefly mentioned here.

- Heat application using paraffin therapy and thermotherapy
- Iontophoresis from 2 to 3 weeks of life (possibly for resorption, organization, and resolution the endomysial mass)
- Microcurrent therapy (may improve head tilt at supine and neck rotation ROM to the affected side)
- Massage of tight neck muscles and subcutaneous tissues to improve pain-free ROM
- Kinesiology taping to improve muscular imbalance

Patients with suspected rotatory subluxation of atlantoaxial joint due to Grisel syndrome, postsurgery, or trauma need to be evaluated by dynamic rotational computed tomography with neck in right and left lateral rotations. For symptoms last few days, treatment with anti-inflammatory and cervical spine immobilization would suffice. Symptoms lasting more than a week would need admission for injectable analgesics, traction and muscle relaxants, failing which 6 weeks halo-vest traction would be needed. Patients presenting late or with fixed deformity would need posterior atlantoaxial fusion.

Surgical Treatment

Failure of conservative and physical therapy would necessitate surgical release of the tight SCM or neurotomy. Surgery is highly recommended when a restriction of movement up to 30° is present, as well in cases complicated with deformities of facial bones. Timing of surgical intervention is contested for by authors. In general, surgical release may be considered in children with CMT between 1 and 4 years of age (Chandler and Altenberg) resistant to conservative treatment. Manual stretching is not as effective after 1 year of age. For children aged >6 years of age Chen and Ko recommended bipolar release. With the reporting of safe surgical release by Coventry and Harris the age for providing surgical treatment has been extended to 12 years. Cranial base and cranium deformities occur early in uncorrected torticollis while facial deformity develops in childhood. After puberty the remodeling potential of bones decreases tremendously so surgery may not be very effective when the disease with deformity has fully settled. In these cases the crooked appearance may be improved along with improved ROM of cervical spine and elimination of head tilt to better their quality of life. All considerations and recommendations taken into account it has been believed that age at the time of release is an important determinant of outcome and that most favorable results are seen in children aged between 1 year and 4 years. This does not mean that surgery done within first few weeks of birth would be more successful. Rationale is that as most cases (>90%) resolve with stretching program with or without bracing and that there is a high tendency for surgical hematoma formation in infants, it is better to restrict use of knife in them. Also this does not mean that patients be deprived of surgery if they cross 4 years of age as then proper release will help prevent development of (or progression of) complications of torticollis such as facial asymmetry, plagiocephaly, strabismus, blinding, cervical scoliosis, etc.

Surgical lengthening of the contracted SCM is needed in only 3% of the cases. Two types of surgical procedures may be performed.

1. *Classical surgical division of the SCM:* Here various options include endoscopic release, unipolar release at the sternoclavicular origin **(Figs. 3A and B)**, bipolar open tenotomy (bipolar release), transection of the middle of the muscle, Z-plasties on the attachments of the sternal portion of SCM, and complete excision of the muscle. A section/release of the clavicular insertion of the SCM along with elongation in a Z-shape of its sternal insertion is commonly recommended and practiced. This provides adequate release and maintains normal outline of the SCM. Bipolar release intends release of the mastoid insertion as may be needed in neglected cases (generally it is considered in children over age of 6 years as reported by excellent results of Arslan et al). Once developed, facial asymmetry is difficult to correct and should be explained to the family and child that surgical release may not have any significant role in improving the facial discrepancies that have already set-in. An important practical guide to perform bipolar release is when unipolar release is unable to give satisfactory correction irrespective of age. Transaxillary endoscopic release of the fibrotic bands has been described by few authors to provide neck scar free method. The advantages include quick and direct access with prevention of injury to neurovascular structures and cosmesis.
2. Surgical resection of the spinal accessory nerve and/or the anterior and posterior divisions of the first three cervical motor roots.

Postoperative immobilization of the head and neck in an overcorrected position is commonly recommended to prevent recurrence and improve outcome. This can be done by the use of a cast brace along with early exercise or molded PVC braces.

Complications of surgical procedure (lengthening/release of SCM): Though mostly unipolar release is innocuous if

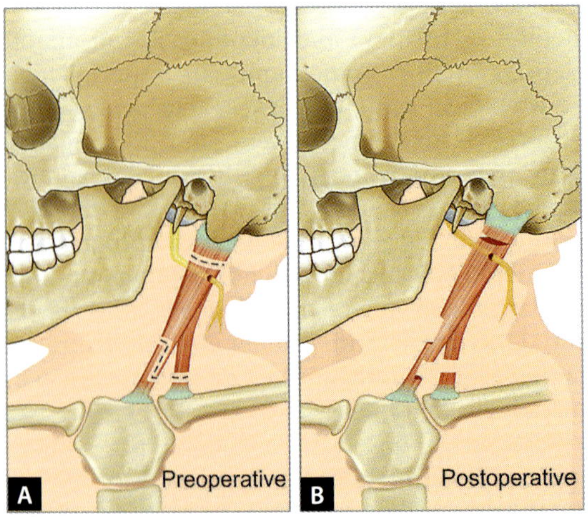

Figs. 3A and B: The unipolar release of sternocleidomastoid muscle from the sternal end (A) marking the site and releasing, (B) correction and gaping after release. This can also be done endoscopically nowadays.

performed well with care, bipolar release is commonly fraught with complications.

- Injury to the spinal accessory nerve particularly in bipolar release, injury to facial nerve
- Reported relapse of up to 1.2%
- Infection
- Hematoma formation
- Injury to underlying vascular structures—carotid vessels and anterior and external jugular vein

The satisfaction rate also varies in different study with an overall reported acceptability to surgical release of above 80%.

Conclusion

Torticollis is not an uncommon finding in the pediatric and pediatric orthopedic clinics. Most common presentation is with CMT with the typical findings of shortened SCM. One should, however, bear in mind the uncommon causes for evaluation of nonmuscular causes of torticollis and providing appropriate treatment. CMT is commonly managed quite successfully by conservative approach and manipulations. Only a minority of patients fail to respond to the physical therapy and they can be then treated by surgical release for the tight muscle. Role of unconventional physical therapy and botulinum toxin injections needs further evaluation with respect to superiority and added advantage, before mass use in management of torticollis.

EHLERS–DANLOS SYNDROME

Ehlers–Danlos syndrome (EDS) is a group of the most common heritable disorders of the connective tissue with considerable diversity, largely caused by extensive genetic heterogeneity. Although all heterogenic subgroups have following unifying features:

- Skin and joint hypermobility-generalized laxity for EDS has been defined as Beighton score **(Table 2)** of 6 or more in prepubertal and adolescents or 5 or more in pubertal males and females up to age 50 years. For those above 50 years score of 4 or more is enough for classifying as hypermobile EDS.
- Easy bruisability
- Dystrophic scarring

TABLE 2: The Beighton score. The total maximum possible score is 9.

Criteria	*Score*
Hyperextension of the fifth finger metacarpophalangeal (MCP) joint 90° or more. The patient is evaluated with palm and forearm resting on a flat surface with elbow flexed at 90°.	1 point for each hand
Thumb can be passively moved to touch the forearm. Arms are outstretched and hands kept pronated.	1 point for each hand
Extension of elbow >10°. The upper limb rests on side of body and hands are kept supine.	1 point for each elbow
Knees extend >10°. Patient standing and knees locked in extension.	1 point for each knee
Patient standing and knees locked straight, feet together. The patient is asked to bend forward at waist and place the total palm of both hands flat on the floor.	1 point

- Increased joint mobility
- Abnormal tissue fragility

As is common for most of the medical diseases the features of EDS were first described by Hippocrates in 400 BC. This syndrome is named after two physicians, Edvard Ehlers (Denmark) and Henri-Alexandre Danlos (France). The combined prevalence of all types of this condition is about 1 in 5,000. The previous classification system of 11 different types has been reduced to 6 in the present Villefranche classification system (1997) on the basis of phenotypic and inheritance characteristics **(Table 3)**. EDS is presently classified based on genetic transmission, biochemical anomaly, and major and minor clinical findings. Classic EDS (cEDS) and hypermobile EDS (hEDS) are most common types encountered clinically. cEDS is transmitted in an autosomal dominant (AD) fashion and is associated with the mutations in collagen gene described below in genetics. hEDS is also similarly transmitted but no genetic mutation is definitely identified. Biochemical studies have demonstrated considerable heterogeneity within individual types. Among the various heterogeneous groups, chronic joint discomfort debilitating and disabling are common orthopedically and these patients are susceptible to osteoarthritis (OA). Internal manifestations, such as rupture of great vessels, diverticula of the gastrointestinal and genitourinary tracts, hiatal hernia, spontaneous rupture of the bowel, spontaneous pneumothorax, etc., tend to occur only in specific types of EDS.

The classic type combined with hypermobility and vascular types are by far the most common, comprising >90% of all types of EDS. The hypermobility type affects around 1 in 10,000–15,000 people, while the classic type probably involves 1 in 20,000–40,000 people. The extensive phenotypic and biochemical characterization **(Table 3)** is of limited use to a clinician prompting search for EDS genes.

Genetics

Mutations in the *ADAMTS2*, *COL1A1*, *COL1A2*, *COL3A1*, *COL5A1*, *COL5A2*, *PLOD1*, and *TNXB* genes cause EDS. Some of these genes (*COL1A1*, *COL1A2*, *COL3A1*, *COL5A1*, and *COL5A2*) provide instructions for making proteins that are used to assemble different types of collagen. Collagens as described previously (*see* Chapter on "Bone Structure, Physiology, Metabolism, and Associated Disorders") are molecules that give structure and strength to connective tissues throughout the body. Other genes (*ADAMTS2*, *PLOD1*, and *TNXB*) provide instructions for making proteins that process or interact with collagen. Mutations that cause the different forms of EDS disrupt the structure, production, or processing of collagen, preventing these molecules from being assembled properly. These defects weaken connective tissues in the skin, bones, and other parts of the body, resulting in the characteristic features of this condition.

Clinical Features

Classic

- Classic EDS includes the type I (gravis) and type II (mitis) subsets described in past.

TABLE 3: Classification of Ehlers–Danlos syndrome (EDS).

Name	Type	Clinical features	Molecular defect	Inheritance
Classic	EDS type I and II	Joint hypermobility; skin hyperextensibility; atrophic scars; velvety skin; subcutaneous spheroids	Structure of type V collagen *COL5A1, COL5A2(AD), COL1A1 (AD), COL1A2(AD, AR)*	AD, AR (minor)
Hypermobility	EDS III	Joint hypermobility; some skin hyperextensibility; ± smooth and velvety skin	*COL3A1* in some *TNXB* in some (tenascin X protein deficient)	AD
Vascular	EDS IV	Thin skin; easy bruising; pinched nose; acrogeria; rupture of large and medium caliber arteries; uterus and large bowel	Deficient type III collagen *COL3A1*	AD
Ocular-scoliotic (kyphoscoliotic)	EDS VIA and VIB	Joint hypermobility; congenital, progressive scoliosis; scleral fragility with globe rupture; tissue fragility; aortic dilatation; MVP	Deficient procollagen-lysine, 2-oxoglutarate 5-dioxygenase (*PLOD*)	AR
Arthrochalasia	EDS VII A + B	Joint hypermobility, severe, with subluxations; congenital hip dislocation; skin hyperextensibility; tissue fragility	No cleavage of N-terminus of type I procollagen 2α mutations in *COL1A1* or *COL1A2*	AD
Dermatosparaxis	EDS VIIC	Severe skin fragility; decreased skin elasticity, easy bruising; hernias, premature rupture of fetal membranes	No cleavage of N-terminus of type I procollagen due to deficiency of peptidase *ADAMTS-2* in some	AR
Unclassified types	EDS V	Classic features	Unknown	X-linked
Periodontic	EDS VIII	Classic features and periodontal disease	Unknown, but linkage to 12p13	AD
	EDS X	Mild classic features, MVP	Deficient in fibronectin	
	EDS XI	Joint instability		AD
	EDS IX	Classic features; occipital horn syndrome	Allelic to Menkes syndrome	X-linked
EDS-like syndrome tenascin X deficiency	Similar to EDS II	Hyperelastic skin; hypermobile joints; fragile tissue with easy bruising; atrophic scars and delayed wound healing *NOT* prominent	Deficient in tenascin X	AR
Progeroid form of EDS	-	Deficiency of β-galactosyltransferase 7 (defective synthesis of dermatan sulfate proteoglycans)	*B4GALT7*	AR

(AD: autosomal dominant; AR: autosomal recessive; MVP: mitral valve prolapse)

- The classic type is characterized by hyperextensibility of joints and increased stretchability of skin along with widened atrophic scars, and joint hypermobility. Other minor criteria for identification includes the following:
  - Velvety skin
  - Spheroids
  - Hypotonia
  - Tissue fragility
- The patients can be identified early in life due to various manifestations of loose joints like:
  - Congenital dislocation of the hips
  - Habitual dislocation of selected joints in later life
  - Joint effusions
  - Clubfoot deformity of the feet
  - Spondylolisthesis
- Up to 33% of patients will have aortic root dilatations (echocardiography for workup should be done).
- Nearly 30% of patients will have scoliosis (predominantly the thoracic or thoracolumbar type).
  - Tower vertebra may be a feature.
- More than 50% of these patients may have chronic musculoskeletal pain that responds to most common analgesics and better managed with physiotherapy (muscle conditioning).
- *Management* of the classic type includes stress on prevention of trauma and great care in treating wounds. Most of the management resides on conservative lines and support.
  - Young athletes benefit from wearing shin guards to avoid frequent hemorrhage, unsightly scars and absence from school.
  - Patient's should be discouraged from demonstrating their joint laxity as entertainment for their friends.
  - Joint stability can be improved only by developing the muscles in view of lax ligaments.
  - Rigorous endurance exercises should be restricted and supervised due to fragility of tendons. A small number of case reports describing aortic root dilatation in patients with EDS is another reason for avoiding vigorous exercise in some patients.

Hypermobility Type

- This is the most debilitating of all forms of EDS orthopedically, and the most likely to require orthopedic surgical intervention.
- The molecular basis is unknown, so no diagnostic test presently exists. The unifying defect being abnormal production of type III collagen.
- Clinically these patients have soft skin and both small and large joint hypermobility.
  - Recurrent and/or chronic dislocations are also common. Multidirectional instability of the shoulder,

patella subluxation, and chronic ankle instability are common.

- Up to 20% of patients may have aortic root anomalies.
- A snapping of the iliotibial band is often misinterpreted as a dislocated hip, although true dislocations can occur (albeit rarely) even in the presence of radiographically normal bony architecture.
- Surgical interventions such as capsular shift or plication should be undertaken only if physical therapy is ineffective. Results and prognosis are often reserved. Bracing is frequently used, especially of the hands because for finger instability.
- Nearly 90% of patients with hypermobility type have debilitating pain (often accompanying abnormal gait) that needs assistive devices.

Vascular

- Though less disabling this is the most serious type because of a propensity for spontaneous rupture of arteries and bowel. Bruisability is typically very striking and hence the term *ecchymotic type* is used as a synonym for vascular type.
- Hypermobility of the small joints and clubfoot are a less prominent feature.
- These patients have thin, translucent skin, and may experience spontaneous rupture of the bowel, uterus also apart from large arteries.
- Aortic root dilatation is present in >75% of patients. 25% of women die during pregnancy because of complications, most often uterine rupture.
- Life expectancy is 45–50 years.

Kyphoscoliosis (Previously Type VI)

- This rare subtype is an autosomal recessive (AR) disorder with a biochemical deficiency in lysyl hydroxylase, an enzyme that modifies collagen.
- In addition to the skin and joint involvement seen in EDS classic form, the hallmarks of the kyphoscoliotic form are fragility of the ocular globe and a propensity to severe scoliosis. The major diagnostic criteria include:
  - Muscle hypotonia at birth and a progressive scoliosis
  - Scoliosis of spine (double thoracic curves common)
  - There is generalized joint laxity.
  - Ocular findings such as, scleral fragility and globe rupture are found in 50% of patients.
- Minor criteria include bruising, tissue fragility, osteopenia, and arterial rupture.
- Kyphoscoliosis EDS may be confused with Marfan syndrome as patients have scoliotic, cardiac, and ocular involvement and often a tall and thin body habitus.

Arthrochalasis

- The patients with arthrochalasia type of EDS have predominantly loose-jointedness with congenital dislocations.
- This is extremely rare form of EDS. The basic abnormality includes an inability to convert type I procollagen to mature collagen, by cleavage of the N-propeptide which is uniformly seen in all patients who have been studied. Deficiency of procollagen N-peptidase, the enzyme that cleaves the propeptide from the amino terminal end of type I procollagen, is deficient in fibroblasts from a minority of patients while most have had normal N-peptidase activity but instead had an amino acid sequence alteration around the site of the procollagen molecule where cleavage ordinarily occurs.
- Patients are moderately short of stature. The children with arthrochalasis type EDS have bilateral (DDH; recalcitrant to surgical intervention).
- They may also have skin hyperextensibility, osteopenia, muscle hypotonia, and kyphoscoliosis.

Dermatosparaxis (Formally Known as Type VII-C)

Dermatosparaxis (tearing of skin) is a rare and AR form of EDS notable for a deficiency of procollagen I N-terminal peptidase (defect as described above). The features are more severe in the skin for unknown reasons. This may be due to the possibility that N-propeptidase could have other molecules besides type I procollagen as substrate. Patients have redundant, severely fragile, and often sagging skin. Premature rupture of fetal membranes and large hernias can be seen.

Other Forms

In addition to the six major forms of the Villefranche classification, other rare forms of EDS exist that include the previously described types V, VIII, and X. These forms are those with periodontal friability (type VIII) and the poor clotting/fibronectin deficient (type X). In addition, a form of EDS described in only one family with symptoms similar to the classic form exists that specifically has an X-linked inheritance pattern (formerly type V EDS).

OSTEOGENESIS IMPERFECTA

(Synonyms and other uncommon terms used—brittle bone disease, Lobstein's disease, Vrolik disease, Van der Hoeve disease, fragilitas ossium, osteomalacia congenita, and osteoporosis fetalis)

Osteogenesis imperfecta (OI) is a series of syndromes (not just a disease as previously thought) representing classes of molecular defects, each with a reasonably well-defined clinical pattern. It is the most common genetic cause of osteoporosis due to generalized disorder of connective tissue. By its etymology it simply means "imperfect development of bones" and the description is quite apt. OI is a hereditary condition resulting from an abnormality in type I collagen that is manifested by an increased fragility of bones and low bone mass (osteopenia). The spectrum of disorder is so broad that it ranges from perinatally lethal forms to barely recognizable disease in adulthood. The disorder was probably first described by Malebranche in 1674, and since then it has been discussed under at least 40 different names or eponyms.

Sillence classification system as modified by Cole is the most accepted **(Table 4)** by the geneticists and researchers but Shapiro might be more helpful from a pediatric orthopedist's point of view where one is asked the questions regarding the management and the prognosis of fractures occurring at different age **(Table 5)**. This classification has excellent practical application for the orthopedic surgeon in regard to prognosis for survival and ambulation. The distinction between the two congenita types is based on the timing of the fracture and radiographic features of the affected bones. Patients with congenita A sustain fractures in utero or at birth, with the additional radiographic features of crumpled long bones, crumpled ribs with rib cage deformity, and a fragile skull **(Figs. 4A to C)**. These features are incompatible with life, and the patients are almost always stillborn or die shortly after birth from intracranial hemorrhage or respiratory insufficiency. Patients with congenita B have fractures at birth but are radiographically distinct from congenital-A patients in that the long bones, as typified by the femur, are more tubular and have more normal funnelization in the metaphysis, the ribs are more normally formed and there is no rib cage deformity. These patients are severely affected, but this type is compatible with survival. Patients with tarda A have an onset of fractures before walking. The age at onset of fractures was not prognostic for ambulation within this group in Shapiro's study. Patients with tarda B suffer their first fracture after walking age **(Figs. 5A to E)**; all these patients were ambulatory in Shapiro's study. Older classification systems divided the disease into "congenita" and "tarda" (Looser)—based on when the first fractures occurred, applying congenita only to intrauterine fractures. Seedorff used this definition of congenita but divided tarda into *gravis* (i.e., fractures occurring at birth or within the first year of life) and *levis* (fractures occurring after 1 year). About 80–90% of patients with OI can be grouped into the Sillence type I to IV categories and have mutations of one of the two type I collagen genes **(Table 4)**. The *COL1A* gene encodes the pro-1α(I) protein chain and the *COL2A* gene encodes pro-2α(I) protein chain of type I procollagen. The etiologies of the remaining 10–20% remain unclear. With further identification of >280 locations of disruptions in the genetic coding for type 1 collagen and finding of noncollagen mutations causing OI the classification system is continuously expanding. A newer classification has been proposed that placed the various Sillence types into five groups **(Table 6).**

Pathoanatomy and Pathophysiology

There are characteristic histological changes in bones of body but they are seldom used to make a diagnosis. These changes, however, throw an insight into the development of the disease. Iliac crest biopsies of patients with OI show a decrease in cortical widths and cancellous bone volume, with increased bone remodeling. There is a direct relationship between the increase in bone turnover and the severity of the disease.

In normal bones, the collagen is almost entirely type I, although, in fetal tissues and in very young infants, some of the collagen is in the form of type III or V. The collagen types III and V decrease with age and in older children, only type I collagen can be recognized. In lethal OI, a considerable increase in the concentration of types III and V and a marked variation in cross-linking are found. Other changes described in the various types of OI include:

- An increase in collagen hydroxylysine residues in bone
- A decrease in hydroxylysine or leucine in skin collagen
- Abnormalities of a1- and a2-polypeptides of type I collagen in cultured skin fibroblasts.

Qualitative defects (e.g., an abnormal collagen I molecule) and quantitative defects (e.g., decreased production of normal collagen I molecules) describe the full clinical spectrum of OI types I–IV. The quantitative defects can cause very severe (even lethal) syndromes resembling OI. Type I collagen is a heterotrimer formed of two alpha 1(I) chains and one alpha 2 chain arranged in the form of helical domain which in turn is composed of uninterrupted repeats of Gly-X-Y [glycine-proline (or lysine)-hydroxyproline (or hydroxylysine)] sequence commonly. Presence of glycine is essential for the helical arrangement. The prolyl and the lysyl residues in the helical chains are hydroxylated by respective hydroxylases. Collagen defects are mostly of two types—commonly (80%) point mutations result in substitution of glycine or other critical residues by other amino acids; less commonly (20%) single exon splicing defects are found. Substitution of glycine in the two types of alpha chains has distinct result. One-third of the mutations in alpha 1(I) chains are lethal while those of alpha 2 are commonly not life-threatening.

Recently the focus has shifted to *CRTAP*, *LEPRE1*, and *PPIB* genes predominating the AR forms of the disease. The newly described types of OI constitute 10–15% of patients and are caused by genetic defects whose protein products interact with type I collagen. Cartilage-associated protein (CRTAP) is a protein required for prolyl 3-hydroxylation, and with the protein products of the *LEPRE1* and *PPIB* genes, forms a heterotrimeric protein that is crucial for proper post-translational modification of collagen I. OI caused by mutations in CRTAP have been designated type VII disease, whereas OI caused by mutations in *LEPRE1* and *PPIB* are designated type VIII and type IX disease, respectively **(Table 4)**. The disorder due to defects in these three genes result in "overmodified collagen" due to abnormal activity of propyl-3-hydroxylase (encoded by *LEPRE1* gene) or associated protein of propyl-3-hydroxylation complex (CRTA protein) or cyclophilin B (CyPB, encoded by *PPIB* gene). The AR forms of the disease account for <10% of the OI. OI types V and VI arise due to defects in mineralization due to defects in IFITM5 and SERPINF1. Mutations in *FKBP10* encoding peptidyl-propyl-cis-trans isomerase and mutations of *SERPINH1* encoding collagen chaperone HSP47 result in OI types XI and X, respectively.

Clinical Features

The clinical features of nonlethal forms of OI are osteopenia dominated by bone fragility and fractures. General features include the characteristic fragility of bone, short stature,

TABLE 4: Cole's modification of osteogenesis imperfecta classification modified from Sillence and Danks. The original Sillence classification (1979) included only four types: types I and IV were autosomal dominant while types 2 and 3 were autosomal recessive.

Type	*Transmission*	*Biochemistry/genetic mutation*	*Orthopedic manifestation*	*Other features*
IA IB	AD	Quantitatively they have half the amount of type I collagen of age-matched individuals	Mild-to-moderate bone fragility, osteoporosis, late fractures. Normal height	High pain tolerance but poor exercise tolerance and muscle strength. Blue sclerae, hearing loss, easy bruising, normal life expectancy. IB—More severe than IA with dentinogenesis imperfecta, slightly decreased life expectancy
IIA IIB IIC IID	AD, AR and mosaic	Unstable triple helix	Perinatally lethal. Skeleton is extremely weak and patients have multiple intra-uterine fractures (crumbled bones, accordion femora), beaded ribs, broad bones, and platyspondyly. The disease is usually lethal in infancy. They may have a small nose, micrognathia. Severely osteopenic with generally well-formed skeleton, normally shaped vertebrae and pelvis	Usually (not necessarily) lethal in perinatal period due to extreme fragility of the ribs, pulmonary hypoplasia, and malformations or hemorrhages of the CNS. There is delayed ossification of skull.
III	AD and AR	Abnormal type I collagen	Severe progressive deforming phenotype, severe bone fragility with fractures at birth (in utero fractures are common), "popcorn" epiphyses/metaphyses, scoliosis and platyspondyly, severe osteoporosis, extreme short stature. There is usually joint hyperlaxity, muscle weakness, chronic unremitting bone pain in the survivors. Limb deformities limit function	Hearing loss, blue sclerae becoming less blue with age, shortened life expectancy, dentinogenesis imperfecta, relative macrocephaly with triangular faces. Presence of dentinogenesis imperfecta is independent of the severity of the OI. Basilar invagination, if present, is lethal. Vertigo is common. Hypercalciuria is seen in one-third of the cases. Respiratory complications arise from kyphoscoliosis. Constipation and hernias are also common due to abdominal muscle weakness
IVA IVB	AD AD	Shortened pro-α1 chain	Mild-moderate bone fragility, bowing of long bones, scoliosis	Blue sclerae, normal hearing, normal dentition. Fractures reduce after puberty IVB—same as IVA plus dentinogenesis imperfecta present, slight decreased life expectancy
V	AD	Mutation in the 5′-untranslated region of a gene encoding interferon-induced transmembrane protein 5 (*IFITM5*)	Three classic features: 1. A radiodense band adjacent to the physis of long bone 2. Hypertrophic callus after fractures 3. Calcification of interosseous membrane between the radius and ulna restricts forearm rotation (may cause radial head dislocation)	Represents 5% of moderate-to-severe OI cases. Sclera is white and patients have radial head dislocation. Irregular mesh-like lamellar bone, lack of parallel organization of collagen fibers. Women with OI type V anticipating pregnancy should be screened for hypertrophic callus in the iliac bone
VI	AR	SERPINF1, which encodes pigment epithelium-derived factor (PEDF), has been identified as the causative gene. Mineralization defect, abundance of osteoid	Hyperosteoidosis phenotype (mineralization defect). Low BMD, frequent fractures, vertebral compressions, long bone deformities	Fish-scale organization of lamellae. Normal vitamin D levels, absence of hypocalcemia and hypophosphatemia
VII	AR	Recessive inheritance of a mutation in the *CRTAP* gene. Partial (10%) absence of *CRTAP* produces moderate bone dysplasia while total absence of *CRTAP* is lethal in all cases	Some cases resemble type IV disease while others resemble type II with rhizomelic limb shortening. Coxa vara is common	
VIII	AR	Extreme under-mineralization of the skeleton. Absence or severe deficiency of prolyl 3-hydroxylase activity due to mutations in the *LEPRE1* gene	Severe growth deficiency. Similar to OI type II or III in appearance and symptoms	White sclerae
IX	AR	*PPIB* gene mutation encoding components of cyclophilin B (needed for triple helix formation) and components of a RER protein complex	–	No rhizomelia

Contd...

Contd...

Type	Transmission	Biochemistry/genetic mutation	Orthopedic manifestation	Other features
X	AR	Mutations in *SERPINH1*	Severe bone dysplasia, blue sclera, dentinogenesis imperfecta	Transient skin bullae, pyloric stenosis, and renal stones
XI	AR	Mutations in *FKBP10*. The product of *FKBP10*, *FKBP65*, is localized to RER having collagen chaperone functions	Bone dysplasia, ligamentous laxity, platyspondyly, and scoliosis	Normal sclerae and teeth
XII	AR	Mutations in the bone morphogenetic protein 1 gene (*BMP1*)		
XIII	AR	Frameshift mutation in SP7	High bone mass OI	Short stature, scoliosis, and bone deformity
XIV	AR	Mutations in *TMEM38B*	Variable degree of severity of multiple fractures and osteopenia	
XV		Mutations in *WNT1*	Moderately severe to progressive form of OI	

(AD: autosomal dominant; AR: autosomal recessive; BMD: bone mineral density; CNS: central nervous system; OI: osteogenesis imperfecta)

TABLE 5: Shapiro classification for osteogenesis imperfecta.

Type	Features	Prognosis
Congenita A	Fractures in utero/at birth, crumpled femur and ribs	Mortality rate, 94%
Congenita B	Fractures in utero/at birth, normal contour of bones	Mortality rate, 8%; Wheelchair-bound, 59%; Ambulatory, 33%
Tarda A	Fractures before walking age	Wheelchair-bound, 33%; Ambulatory, 67%
Tarda B	Fractures after walking age	Ambulatory, 100%

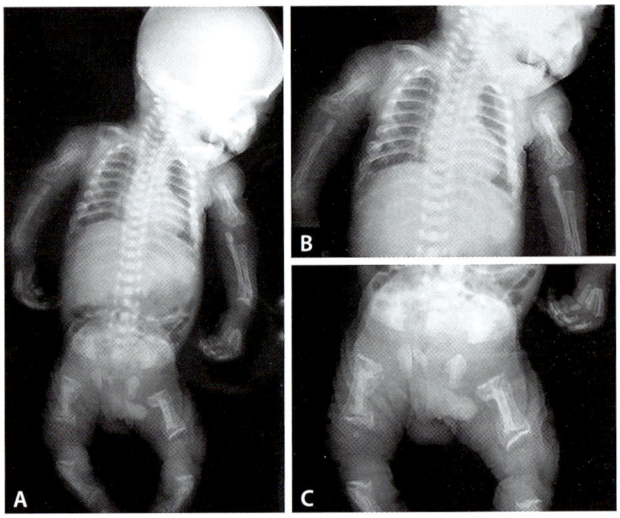

Figs. 4A to C: Osteogenesis imperfecta. Severe variety with various fractures of long bones that occurred intrauterine and are healing aggressively showing bone within bone appearance.

defective dentinogenesis of deciduous or permanent teeth or both, premature middle ear deafness, laxity of ligaments, and blue tympanic membranes. Other features may include some or all of those listed in **Box 1**.

It is believed that repeated microfractures in OI bone combined with healing and remodeling is responsible for the "soft" bones. Bone fragility or "soft bones" are responsible for:

- Producing deformities such as protrusio acetabuli in the pelvis.
  - Basilar invagination at the craniovertebral junction. Symptoms of basilar invagination in OI typically occur in the third and fourth decades but may be present during the teenage years. These symptoms include brainstem dysfunction such as apnea, altered consciousness, lower cranial nerve deficits, myelopathy, and ataxia.
- Pelvis in OI often develops a trefoil shape presumably because of repeated fractures.
- The forearm may be in pronation, and its rotation is often severely limited. Angulation is generally greater in the upper part of both bones of the forearm.
- Coxa vara deformity of proximal femur.
- The forehead is broad, with prominent parietal and temporal bones and an overhanging occiput. The bulging calvaria cause facial-cranial disproportion, which gives the face a triangular, elfin shape. Ears are displaced down and the configuration is likened to soldier's helmet (helmet head).
- The long bones have narrow diaphyses and bowing (saber shin), and fractures are common. Bowing results from multiple transverse fractures of the long bones and muscle contraction across the weakened diaphysis.
- The fracture-healing process is undisturbed in terms of sequence of events, but the new bone has the same deficient biomechanical characteristics. Fractures may occur at any age, and the age of occurrence is one basis for classification (*see* above).
- Fracture callus is wispy but may be occasionally hypertrophic.
- The frequency of fractures declines sharply after adolescence.

Diagnosis

Skin biopsies and fibroblast cultures may be helpful, but are only positive in 80% of patients with type IV OI (the most commonly confused with nonaccidental trauma). Prenatal deoxyribonucleic acid (DNA) mutation analysis can be performed in pregnancies with risk of OI to analyze uncultured chorionic villus cells. Severe OI can also be detected by level II ultrasonography as early as 16th week.

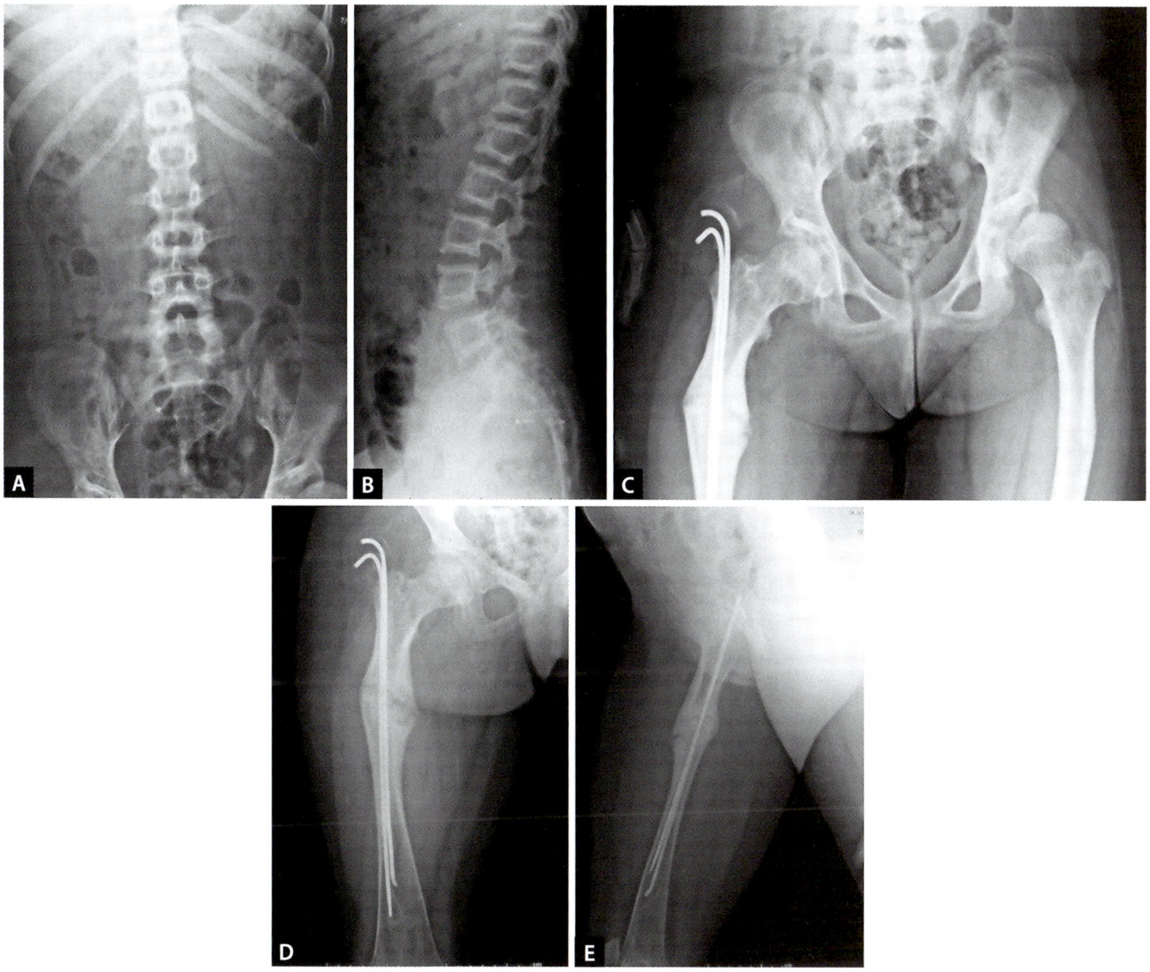

Figs. 5A to E: Osteogenesis imperfecta in a grown-up female with typical vertebral changes (picture frame vertebra and bone within bone appearance of ilium). The fracture in femur was managed with elastic intramedullary nails.

TABLE 6: Newer proposed classification of osteogenesis imperfecta.

Group	*Mechanism*	*Included Sillence types*
Group A	Defects in collagen synthesis, structure, or processing	Types I, II, III, IV, XIII
Group B	Post-translational modification of collagen	Types VII, VIII, IX, XIV
Group C	Collagen folding or cross-linking	Types X, XI
Group D	Defects in bone mineralization	Types V, VI
Group E	Defects in osteoblast differentiation	Types XII, XV, XVI

BOX 1: The common features of osteogenesis imperfecta.

- Gracile and diffusely osteopenic bones with thin cortices and an attenuated trabecular pattern.
- *Gray-blue sclerae:* The blueness of sclerae is inversely proportional to the severity of disease with most patients with milder forms having blue or gray-blue sclerae. "Saturn ring" is caused by white sclera immediately surrounding the cornea. Embryotoxon or "arcus juvenilis" may be seen.
- Dentinogenesis imperfecta
- Kyphoscoliosis
- Many patients have misshapen skulls with wide intertemporal measurements and small, triangular faces.
- Neurologic abnormalities are consequences of direct neural compression, altered cerebrospinal fluid flow, or vascular compromise.
- Inguinal, umbilical, and diaphragmatic hernias are common. The skin is thin, translucent, and easily distensible. Although increased vascular fragility is common, major arterial or aortic aneurysms are rarely encountered.
- Basilar invagination (prolapse of the upper cervical spine into the base of the skull)

Raised alkaline phosphatase in neonatal period would distinguish OI from hypophosphatasia.

Differential Diagnosis

- Juvenile osteoporosis
- Nonaccidental injury (multiple fractures at different stages of healing, posterior rib fractures, and metaphyseal corner fractures are highly specific for nonaccidental injury). Although it may be difficult, determining the clinical distinction between children with OI and those with has obviously important implications. A patient with Menkes kinky hair syndrome can present with metaphyseal corner fractures.
- A malignancy such as leukemia
- Blue sclera may also occur in other disorders, such as progeria, cleidocranial dysplasia, Menkes syndrome, cutis laxa, Hajdu–Cheney syndrome, and pyknodysostosis.

Nonsurgical Treatment

Treatment depends on the type of OI. Type I osteogenesis, at least in its milder forms, may have little impact on the patient, and the role of the pediatric orthopedic surgeon may be limited to conventional fracture care. Patients with severe disease die before the intervention of pediatric orthopedic surgeon is ever sought. Types III and IV remain the greatest challenge for orthopedic surgeon. With the recent advances in understanding of genetic basis of the disease, for patients with OI, advances in the pharmacologic treatment has and will continue to lead to decreased pain, increased ease of drug administration, and a reduction in fractures and deformity.

The medical treatment of OI involves strategies to improve bone mass.

- Sex hormones, sodium fluoride, calcitonin, calcium, growth hormone, magnesium oxide, and vitamin D and C have shown no consistent results.
- Recombinant human growth hormone has been used in the past because of its anabolic effects on bone; however, clinical studies showed no increase in bone mass or change in natural history.
- Cyclic administration of bisphosphonates has been used to treat patients with types III and IV OI quite extensively. Bisphosphonates decrease the resorption of bone by suppressing the activity of osteoclasts. Pamidronate, alendronate, risedronate, neridronate, and olpadronate have all been tried with improvement in bone density but translation into improved bone strength and fracture risk mitigation has been variable. There is concern, however, that bisphosphonates may make bone more brittle and in any case the disease is not cured with persistent type 1 collagen defect.
- Denosumab may improve the bone quality similar to cyclic bisphosphonates. Use of teriparatide for improving bone density has been successful in sporadic study with improved fracture risk reported. Sclerostin inhibitor setrusumab has been studied for improvement in bone density and detailed results are being reported. Fresolimumab a transforming growth factor-beta (TGF-β) inhibitor is also a potential contender under study for improving bone strength and fracture risk.
- Bone marrow transplantation, which introduces normal marrow stem cells that could potentially differentiate into normal osteoblasts, has been used with some success for severely affected patients with OI. Problems of graft rejection and graft versus host reactions limit this approach.
- Hematogenous infusion of mesenchymal stem cells (MSCs) has been tried with success in these patients. The MSCs are infused from bone marrow that home the bone to produce YY normalized collagen. However, the technique requires prior bone marrow transplant from same individual so has not been widely adopted. Gene therapy is being explored for providing treatment of OI or at least reduces the morbidity and mortality (*see* Chapter on "Gene Therapy" for details).
- Orthotic devices are indicated to stabilize lax joints, prevent progression of deformity and fractures, and allow early weight bearing following surgical intervention.

Surgical Treatment

Principally, the orthopedic surgery is advised to decrease the risk of fracture, allow for early weight-bearing, and to achieve union. The mainstay of orthopedic surgical treatment of patients with OI is realignment osteotomy. This is performed to improve the mechanical axis of appendicular bones, which in turn, also helps in balancing and reducing morbidity by reducing stress on other parts of bone and other bones. Other surgical interventions include management of basilar invagination and correction of scoliosis.

- The realignment osteotomies should be performed through small incisions to preserve the blood supply, some prefer closed osteoclasis. Sofield-Millar procedure entails multiple diaphyseal osteotomies (fragmentation) with intramedullary fixation for long bone deformities that preclude orthotic fitting, good function, and are susceptible to repeated fractures. Intramedullary devices are preferred for stabilization including the telescopic (Sheffield rod and Fassier-Duval rod) and nontelescopic forms (Rush rods and Williams rods). Telescopic rods appear to decrease the incidence of re-rodding to accommodate for growth and therefore are preferred for use when possible.
- The treatment of spinal deformities in OI can be challenging. It is partly due to the fact that one cannot effectively push on the spine through the ribs because of the fragility of the rib cage and the possibility of further aggravating the thoracic deformity.
  - When the curves approach 45° in the mild forms of OI and 30–35° in the severe forms, a posterior spinal fusion with segmental instrumentation to prevent progression of the curve should be considered.
  - Because of bone fragility, it is often necessary to reinforce the upper and lower hook claws with bone cement or use Mersilene tape instead of sublaminar wires.
  - Because of the paucity of bone in the iliac crest, allograft bone should be used.
  - Anterior spinal fusion may be considered in the very young patient to prevent crankshafting of the spine.
- Surgery for basilar invagination is indicated for patients with radiographic progression or with neurologic deficits resulting from brainstem and high cervical cord compression. The recommended treatment of basilar invagination in OI consists of extensive removal of bony compression by a transoral approach followed by a posterior fusion and posterior rigid fixation that transfers the weight of the head to the thoracic spine.

Complications

Few complications from annoying to dreaded ones have been seen in OI including:

- Hyperplastic callus formation
- *Basilar invagination:* Usually seen in OI types III and IV, best detected by CT scan of craniovertebral junction.

- Osteogenic sarcoma
- Formation of aneurysmal bone cyst (ABC) and unicameral bone cysts (UBC)

MARFAN SYNDROME

Marfan syndrome is an inherited multisystem disorder of connective tissue that primarily affects the skeleton, the cardiovascular system, and the eyes, is usually transmitted as an AD trait. The incidence is roughly 1:10,000. There is no ethnic or gender predilection. The genetic mutation of Marfan syndrome is on the fibrillin-1 (*FBN1*) gene located on chromosome *15q21* which encodes fibrillin-1, a large extracellular matrix protein that provides stretch and elasticity to connective tissues and is also involved in regulating the bioavailability of TGF-β family members. Approximately 25% of cases arise from new mutations. More than 135 mutations in the *FBN1* gene have been identified. The genetic heterogenicity explains the pleiotropic manifestations of Marfan syndrome with variable phenotypic expression.

Clinical Features

Males and females are equally affected. Historically the disease was identified using a triad of:

1. *Skeletal changes:* Long, thin extremities, and frequently associated with loose joints
2. Reduced vision as a result of dislocations of the lenses (ectopia lentis)
3. Aortic aneurysms

Revised Ghent criteria are now used to characterize the disease (see below). The general features of the disease as appraised on clinical examination are as follows **(Fig. 6A)**:

- Increased height
- Disproportionately long, gracile limbs (dolichostenomelia)
- Generalized ligamentous laxity
- Ratio of the upper segment (top of the head to the top of the pubic ramus) to the lower segment (top of the pubic ramus to the floor) is usually 2 SDs below the mean for age, race, and sex.
- An arm span greater than height (span to height ratio >1.05) **(Fig. 6D)**
- Arachnodactyly with a positive wrist (Walker-Murdoch) and thumb (Steinberg) sign **(Figs. 6B and C)**
- Severe planovalgus and/or long thin feet with a disproportionately long great toe
- Scoliosis is seen in 60–70% of patients (right thoracic lordotic curves are the most common).
- Anterior chest wall deformity (pectus excavatum >pectus carinatum)
- Spontaneous pneumothorax may occur secondary to lung bullae.
- A high arched palate

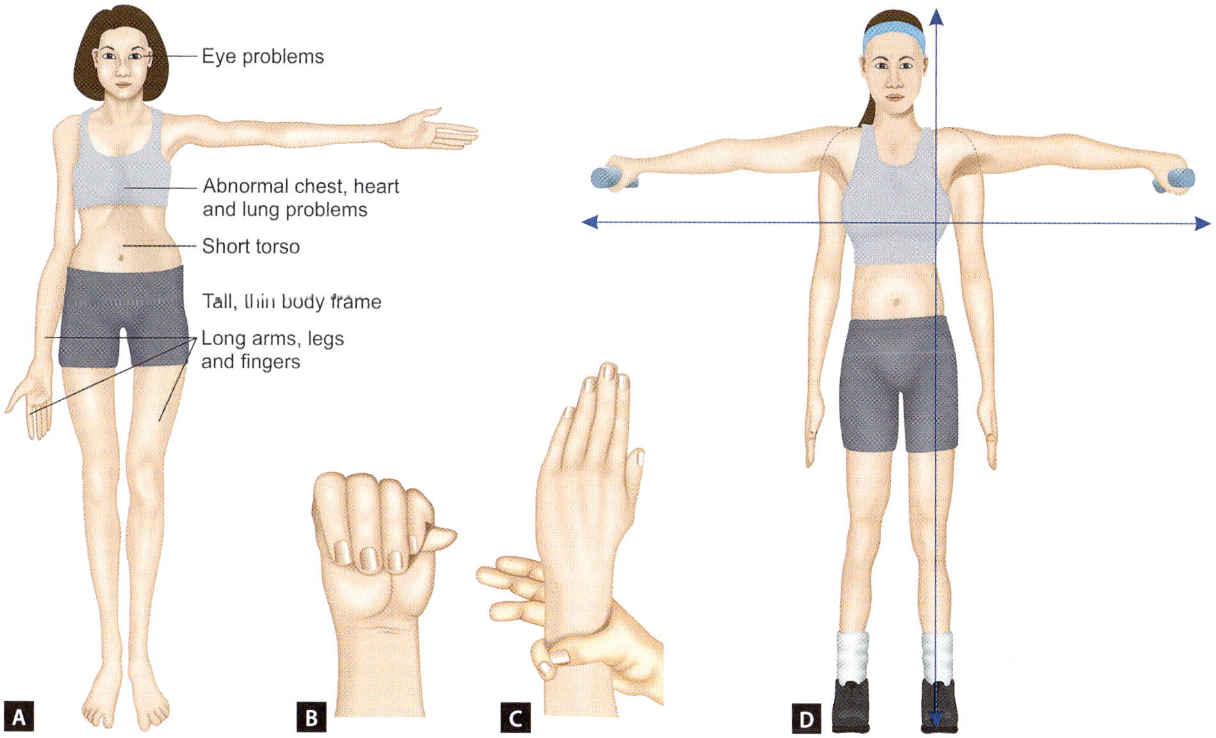

Figs. 6A to D: Marfan syndrome. (A) Illustration of the bodily features that are typical of Marfan syndrome, the cardiac anomaly commonly found is mitral valve prolapse. Hand signs are another useful evaluation feature, the Steinberg sign is positive if the thumb tip projects easily out of the palm in a closed fist (B) is due both to long digits and hypermobility of joints (joint motorics). (C) The Walker-Murdoch sign denotes significant overlap between pinkie finger over thumb when the wrist is gripped with these two digits; (D) In anthropometric measures the arm span exceeds the patient's height. For adults, a ratio of arm span to height >1.05 is abnormal. The upper segment to lower segment ratio is also an important anthropometric measure; this is reduced in Marfan syndrome. Cut-off for abnormal values include—for white adults, an upper segment to lower segment ratio of <0.85; for black adults, <0.78; for children, <1 at 0–5 years, <0.95 at 6–7 years, <0.9 at 8–9 years, and <0.85 at >10 years.

- Ocular examination reveals myopia, corneal flatness, dislocation of lenses (ectopia lentis), and iridodonesis (tremor of the iris secondary to lens dislocation).
- Cardiac manifestations include mitral valve prolapse, mitral regurgitation, dilatation of aortic root, aortic regurgitation, aortic dissection, and aortic aneurysm (abdominal).
- Striae distensae (shoulder and buttocks) are seen in the skin.
- Severe neonatal Marfan syndrome. This is an uncommon form where within the first few months of life, children are found suffering from serious cardiac abnormalities and congenital contractures. It is believed to result from a spontaneous mutation in the *FBN1* gene.

Diagnosis

Revised diagnostic criteria (revised Ghent criteria, **Fig. 7**) have been proposed for Marfan syndrome that helps differentiation of Marfan syndrome from marfanoid phenotype. More than 90% patients classified using Ghent criteria have *FBN1* mutation. 10–15% of remaining patients have *TGFBR2* or *TGFBR1* mutations. In this modified diagnostic process **(Fig. 7)**, the focus has shifted from the musculoskeletal signs to the cardiovascular and ocular abnormalities. Thus, the presence of a dilated aorta plus ectopia lentis is now sufficient to give an unequivocal diagnosis of Marfan syndrome. In the revised criteria, skeletal, skin, lung, facial, other ocular, and other cardiovascular signs have been included in a new scoring system, which resolves some difficulties encountered with the earlier criteria **(Fig. 7 and Table 7)**. Any form of *pectus excavatum* or chest wall asymmetry is allocated one point, regardless of severity, while pectus carinatum is allocated two points since it is less common in the general population and is more frequently associated with Marfan syndrome **(Figs. 8A and B)**.

Investigations

- There are no specific laboratory investigations for Marfan syndrome, although genetic testing is now available. Prenatal molecular diagnosis is possible only if the family's mutation is known or several affected family members are available for genetic linkage analysis. DNA testing for *FBN1* mutations has been difficult because of the large size of the gene. It is among the largest in

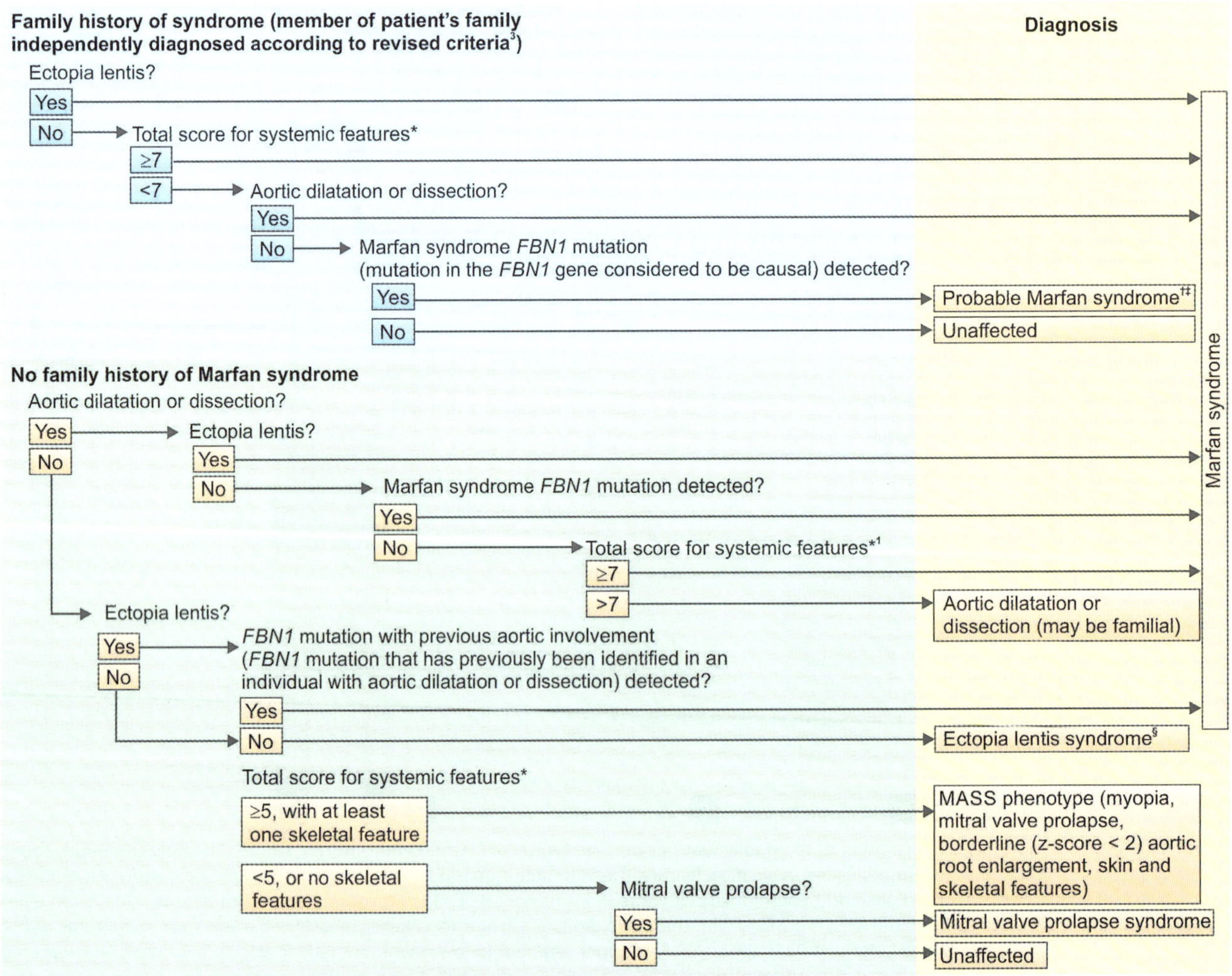

Fig. 7: Diagnostic algorithm for Marfan syndrome. (FBN1: fibrillin-1)

TABLE 7: Revised diagnostic clinical features of Marfan syndrome.

Feature	*Score*
Wrist or thumb sign†	1
Wrist and thumb sign†	3
Pectus carinatum deformity	2
Hindfoot deformity	2
Plain pes planus	1
Pectus excavatum or chest asymmetry	1
Pneumothorax	2
Dural ectasia	2
Protrusio acetabuli	2
Reduced upper segment to lower segment ratio,‡ and increased ratio of arm span to height§ and no severe scoliosis	1
Scoliosis or thoracolumbar kyphosis	1
Reduced elbow extension	1
Three of the five typical facial features (dolichocephaly, enophthalmos, downward slanting palpebral fissures, malar hypoplasia, and retrognathia)	1
Skin striae	1
Myopia of >3 diopters	1
Mitral valve prolapse	1

† See **Figures 4A to C**.
‡ For white adults, an upper segment to lower segment ratio of <0.85; for black adults, <0.78; and for children, <1 at 0–5 years, <0.95 at 6–7 years, <0.9 at 8–9 years, and <0.85 at >10 years.
§ For adults, a ratio of arm span to height >1.05.

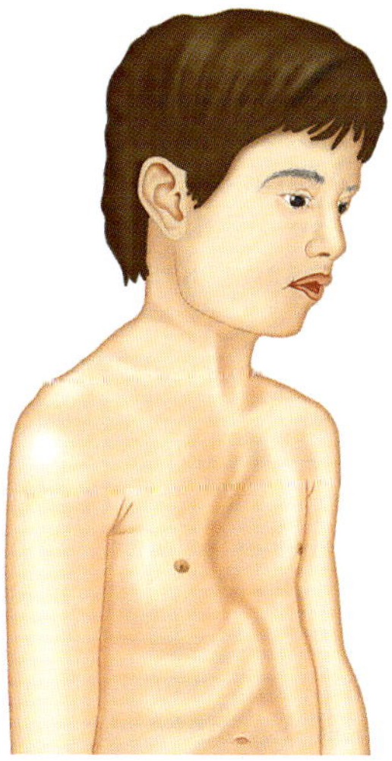

A Indented breastbone (pectus excavatum)

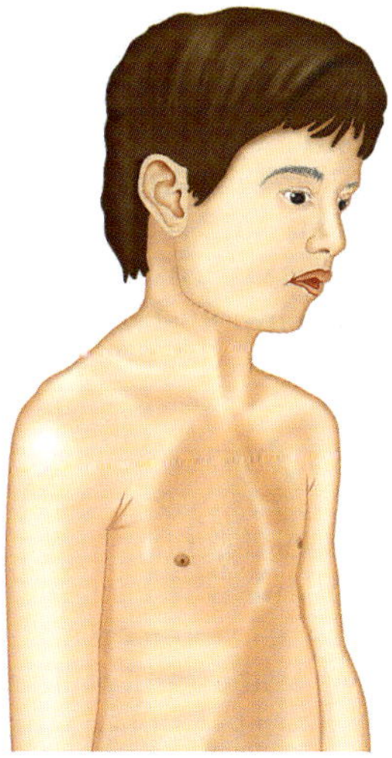

B Protruding breastbone (pectus carinatum)

Figs. 8A and B: The sternal deformity in Marfan syndrome. The bone may be pushed inside the rib cage (A) forming the pectus excavatum deformity or it may protrude forward (B) forming pectus carinatum deformity.

the human genome at over 200,000 bases and 65 exons and some 550 different mutations have been described already. More importantly, there are few, if any recurrent mutations of *FBN1*, it is difficult to diagnose the disease by mutation analysis as most are fairly new. It is now possible to sequence the exons of all human genes in a single reaction (exome sequencing). This approach may be utilized in future for Marfan syndrome.

- Radiographic analysis of Marfan syndrome may reveal the presence of scoliosis, protrusio acetabuli, chondrolysis, and high-grade spondylolisthesis. MRI reveals dural ectasia in >60% of patients.
- Other important investigations include transesophageal echocardiogram, electrocardiogram, slit-lamp examination, and keratometry to diagnose the associated abnormalities and offer treatment.

Differential Diagnosis

- Marfan syndrome must be differentiated from the MASS phenotype. MASS is an acronym assigned to the following clinical features:
  - Mitral valve prolapses
  - Aortic root diameter at the upper limits of normal; the aortic root diameter may be at the upper limits of normal for body size but there is no progression to aneurysm or predisposition to dissection as in Marfan syndrome.
  - Stretch marks
  - Skeletal features of Marfan syndrome (including scoliosis, pectus excavatum or pectus carinatum, and joint hypermobility)

  Ectopia lentis does not occur in MASS phenotype. MASS patients therefore have a better prognosis than those with classic Marfan syndrome. This condition can be inherited within families and has been shown to result from mutations in the *FBN1* gene.
- In addition to the MASS phenotype, the differential diagnosis of Marfan syndrome includes congenital contractural arachnodactyly (Beals syndrome), Loeys-Dietz syndrome (due to TGF-β receptor gene mutations), Stickler's syndrome (arthrochalasia type EDS), hypermobility syndrome, and homocystinuria.

Treatment

- The medical treatment of Marfan syndrome includes the use of β-blockers to slow the progression of aortic dissection and lower the blood pressure.
- Aortic replacement is indicated if aortic diameter is >5 cm; pregnant women with aortic dilatation should have a cesarean section at 38 weeks.
- The success rate for bracing of spinal deformities is much lower than in adolescent idiopathic scoliosis. Curves >25° in children with Risser grade II skeletal maturity will likely require surgery despite bracing. Preoperative imaging of the spine with MRI to identify dural ectasia and CT to assess fixation points are essential.
- Preoperative cardiopulmonary evaluation is mandatory.
- There is an increased incidence of pseudarthrosis in posterior spinal fusion.
- Closure of the triradiate cartilage to treat protrusio acetabuli also has been proposed.

If untreated, the life expectancy of a patient with Marfan syndrome is 30–40 years, with death resulting from aortic dissection, aortic rupture, or valvular-induced cardiac failure. With modern cardiovascular treatment regimens, the average life span is now 70 years. It is important to remember that the tall, agile, and athletic patient with Marfan syndrome is at risk for aortic dissection and sudden death. It is imperative to educate patients about the signs and symptoms of aortic and cardiac disease, and to counsel them on activity restriction and the possibility of genetic transmission.

Newer Trends in Treatment of Marfan Syndrome

- Losartan (angiotensin II receptor antagonist) blocks *TGFB* signaling and has demonstrated significant reduction in cardiovascular and lung abnormalities in mouse *FBN1* mutant strain. Similar benefits have been seen with the use of beta-blockers in clinical study.
- Losartan has no effect on the skeletal phenotype whereas alendronate was effective in reducing these signs.
- Advanced understanding of the genetic basis will potentially allow for intervention at a molecular level with gene therapy. Although a safe mode of introducing genetically modified collagen for patients with EDS, osteoblasts for those with OI, or fibrillin-1 for those with Marfan syndrome is presently elusive, it should become a reality. Several new strains of Marfan mice have recently been developed with mutant fibrillin-1 proteins to further clarify the mechanism of disease and eventually its treatment. For patients with Marfan syndrome, advances in cardiothoracic surgery have doubled the lifespan, and new drugs such as doxycycline and losartan may decrease the incidence of aortic aneurysms. Ophthalmologic interventions and rigorous slit-lamp screening have decreased the incidence of blindness. As the knowledge of the genetics and biochemical anomalies of connective tissue disorders expands, patient care improves.

TRISOMY 21 (DOWN SYNDROME)

Trisomy 21 or Down syndrome (DS) is the most common chromosomal abnormality. DS is caused by trisomy of chromosome 21 (*Hsa21*) and is associated with a number of deleterious phenotypes, including learning disability, heart defects, early-onset Alzheimer's disease, and childhood leukemia. The imbalance in expression of *Hsa21* and non-*Hsa21* genes is hypothesized to result in the many phenotypes that characterize DS. The risk of having DS increases with maternal age; it is 1 in 1,500 for mothers of 15–29 years of age and 1 in 50 for mothers older than 45 years of age. The increase in expression of some *Hsa21* genes caused by trisomy of *Hsa21* has been shown to lie within the range of natural variations in the phenotypic expression of these genes in the normal population. Trisomy of *Hsa21* is associated with a small number of conserved features, occurring in all individuals, including mild-to-moderate learning disability, craniofacial abnormalities and hypotonia in early infancy as also with a reduction in brain volume, the size of the hippocampus and cerebellum being particularly affected. This can be partly controlled at least by treatment with the antidepressant fluoxetine, which is a selective serotonin reuptake inhibitor.

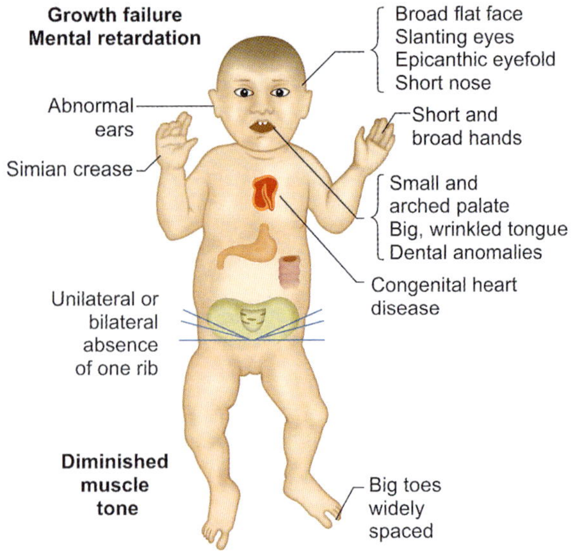

Fig. 9: Down syndrome. Illustration showing the clinical features of Down syndrome.

Clinical Features

The general clinical features with stress on diagnostic features and orthopedic relevance are as follows **(Fig. 9)**:

- Characteristic facial features [upward-slanting eyes, epicanthal folds, and a flattened nose base profile (Mongolian facies)], a single transverse flexion crease in the palm (the simian crease), and clinodactyly of little finger help in diagnosis at birth.
- Achievement of developmental milestones is delayed and most children do not walk until they are 2–3 years of age. They have a classic broad based, toed out, and waddling gait pattern.
- Short stature is characteristic and a cardinal feature.
- In pelvis, the bony changes are characterized by flat acetabula and flared iliac wings (being characteristic these were used previously to make diagnosis rather than the chromosomal analysis).
- Patients may have hip instability, characterized by subluxation secondary to the degree of ligamentous laxity. Acetabular dysplasia may develop in late childhood and progress into maturity.
- Slipped capital (upper) femoral epiphysis also occurs in patients with trisomy 21; it is associated with an increased risk of osteonecrosis.
- Marked joint hypermobility is commonly seen possibly related to subtle change in shapes of bone and partly only due to ligamentous laxity.
- Patellofemoral instability can occur as a result of ligamentous laxity.
- Lower extremity alignment often is characterized by genu valgum.
- Scoliosis is more common (five times) in severely retarded institutionalized patients than ambulatory patients.
- Polyarticular arthropathy occurs in approximately 10% of patients.
- Feet manifestations include pes planovalgus with an increased space between the great and second toes and hallux varus.

- Polyarticular arthropathy occurs in approximately 10%.
- Other manifestations of trisomy 21 syndrome include mental retardation, duodenal atresia, hypothyroidism, leukemia, and congenital heart disease, which affect 50% of patients, typically as a septal defect.
- C1–C2 instability occurs in approximately 10% of patients.

Diagnosis

Amniocentesis can be used for prenatal diagnosis if screening laboratory tests are positive.

Management

Chronic treatment with picrotoxin or pentylenetetrazole has been found to improve hippocampal-based learning in animal models.

- For hip instability and DDH, the treatment is controversial. Some authors recommend bracing for 6–8 months if the patient is younger than 6 years. Surgery has been associated with a high failure rate.
- It is important to address cervical spine instability. In the presence of myelopathy, fusion is indicated for an atlanto-dens interval >10 mm (the associated complications with surgery are, however high).
- In general, patients with an atlanto-dens interval of 4.5–10 mm and no neurologic findings are advised to avoid high-risk sports such as football and diving.

TURNER SYNDROME

Turner syndrome is present only in girls and can be defined as a combination of characteristic physical features and complete or partial absence of one of the X chromosomes (the XO genotype). This is relatively common chromosome disorder affecting 1 of 2,500 live births and accompanied by cell mosaicism (one-third cases). The effects of the single X chromosome depend (due to imprinting) on whether it was derived from the father or mother. The general *manifestations* include:

- Short stature (growth retardation is cardinal feature with lack of skeleton maturation and absent secondary sex characteristics)
- Cubitus valgus
- Genu valgum
- Scoliosis (idiopathic scoliosis progresses with growth hormone administration so caution should be exercised)
- Webbed neck (similar to Klippel–Feil syndrome)
- Low hairline
- High incidence of fractures secondary to underlying osteoporosis

Treatment

Treatment with exogenous estrogen allows affected females to pass through puberty and develop secondary sexual characteristics. Growth hormone treatment can increase height. The treatment of scoliosis in Turner syndrome is similar to that of idiopathic scoliosis, although delayed skeletal maturation allows for a long period of scoliosis curve progression. Genu valgum can be corrected with osteotomies and cubitus valgus does not need any treatment.

DISORDERS CAUSED BY ABNORMALITIES IN TUMOR-RELATED GENES

Disorders that are caused by mutations of tumor-related genes and have orthopedic manifestations include neurofibromatosis (NF) and hereditary multiple exostoses [*see* Chapter on "Orthopedic Oncology (Bone Tumors and Metastasis) and Heterotopic Ossification"].

Neurofibromatosis (Von Recklinghausen's Disease)

The disease was first described by German pathologist Von Recklinghausen. NF is divided into three types (first two are most common):

1. NF1 (Von Recklinghausen's disease)
2. NF2 (central NF, familial acoustic neuroma, and associated with bilateral vestibular schwannomas)
3. Segmental NF (with the features of NF1 but involving a single body segment)

Also described is NF4 which is similar to NF1 except the absence of Lisch nodules.

Neurofibromatosis type 1 is the most common single gene disorder and occurs in 1 in 3,000 live births. The gene-encoding neurofibromin is responsible in most of the cases. The inheritance pattern is AD. Though inheritable in many, 30–50% arise from de novo mutations. Neurofibromin helps regulate cell growth through the *RAS-dependent* and phosphatidylinositol 3-kinase (PI3K) dependent hyperactivation of mammalian target of rapamycin (mTOR) signaling pathway. Though the neurofibromas comprise of various cell types, the Schwann cells are the principle tumor cell type. Neurofibromin is expressed at higher levels in the neural crest during development. Cells from the neural crest migrate to become pigmented cells of the skin, parts of the brain, spinal cord, peripheral nerves, and adrenals, thus explaining the common sites of abnormalities in the disorder. Both the *NF1* gene copies need to be inactive for the production of the disease (complying with Knudson's two-hit hypothesis).

Diagnosis

The diagnostic criteria for a conclusive diagnosis of NF1 were established by the National Institutes of Health Consensus Development Conference. Two of the major criteria **(Box 2)** at least need to be present to make the diagnosis.

Orthopedic Manifestations

Orthopedic manifestations of the disease include:

- Abnormal skeletal development (seen in 15–20% patients). These comprise of bony dysplasia, bony erosion (scalloping), demineralizing osteoporosis, nonossifying fibroma, and scoliosis. Patients might exhibit mild anisomelia to massive gigantism and overgrowth is commonly seen that may range from single digit to entire limb.

- Fractures and bony deformities are present in 5–10% patients (especially boys).
- Pseudarthrosis is common even after fracture treatment.
- Radiographs of pelvis demonstrate coxa valga of various degrees and may also show protrusio acetabuli.
- Patients with NF1 may develop cystic lesions in long bones and congenital tibial dysplasia. Congenital tibial dysplasia includes a spectrum from anterolateral tibial bowing to pseudarthrosis. Congenital pseudarthrosis (distal tibia and/or fibula) is difficult to treat in such cases.
- Osteoporosis has been reported in around 50% cases. This metabolic bone disease is similar to hypophosphatemic rickets/osteomalacia.
- Short, sharp, single thoracic, and angular scoliosis is seen in 15–20% cases though other forms of scoliosis are also seen making overall percentage of the scoliosis even higher. The typical curve is associated with distortion of the ribs and vertebrae. The onset is early in childhood, and it is relentlessly progressive.

BOX 2: The major criteria for diagnosis of neurofibromatosis (NF).

Presence of two or more of the following is needed to make a diagnosis of neurofibromatosis:
- Six or more café-au-lait spots (CALS) >1 cm in size—appear by 1 year of age. They have smooth edge, often described as similar to the coast of California, as opposed to the ragged edge of spots associated with fibrous dysplasia, which are described as similar to the coast of Maine.
- Axillary or inguinal freckling appears by 1 year of age.
- Two or more cutaneous neurofibromas **(Figs. 10A to C)** may appear till first decade and increase rapidly with puberty.
- One plexiform neurofibroma usually present at birth.
- Characteristic bony defects (see below).
- Optic glioma, acoustic neuroma, or astrocytoma [in central nervous system (CNS)] appears by first decade.
- Two or more iris Lisch nodules are characteristic for disease (hamartomas of iris) and appear by 5–10 years of age.
- First-degree relative with NF1.

The risk of malignancy is increased in a patient with NF1 and includes a 10% lifetime risk of a malignant peripheral nerve sheath tumor, which typically arises within a plexiform neurofibroma. Pheochromocytoma, astrocytoma, and brainstem glioma also occur. Hypertension may develop due to renal artery stenosis or pheochromocytoma.

Management

Management of orthopedic manifestations is as follows:
- *Long bone pseudarthrosis (see also congenital pseudarthrosis of tibia):* To prevent fracture, prophylactic application of a total contact ankle-foot orthosis is indicated before a child reaches walking age. After the child begins walking, a knee-ankle-foot orthosis is needed. The definitive treatment consists of pseudarthrosis excision, bone grafting, intramedullary fixation, or Ilizarov reconstruction. Vascularized bone grafting, typically from the contralateral fibula has been attempted in a limited fashion.
- Scoliosis occurs in approximately 20% of patients with NF1. The curves are classified as dystrophic or nondystrophic. Nondystrophic curves have radiographic features similar to those of idiopathic scoliosis and are treated similarly. Nondystrophic curves can evolve into dystrophic curves (70% chance) which are:
  - Short (fewer than six segments)
  - Sharp
  - Enlarged neural foramina

These dystrophic curves typically occur in patients who are:
- Younger than 6 years
- Have an apical vertebra with associated scalloped end plates
- Radiological rib penciling
- High Cobb angle
- Curve located in middle to lower thoracic region

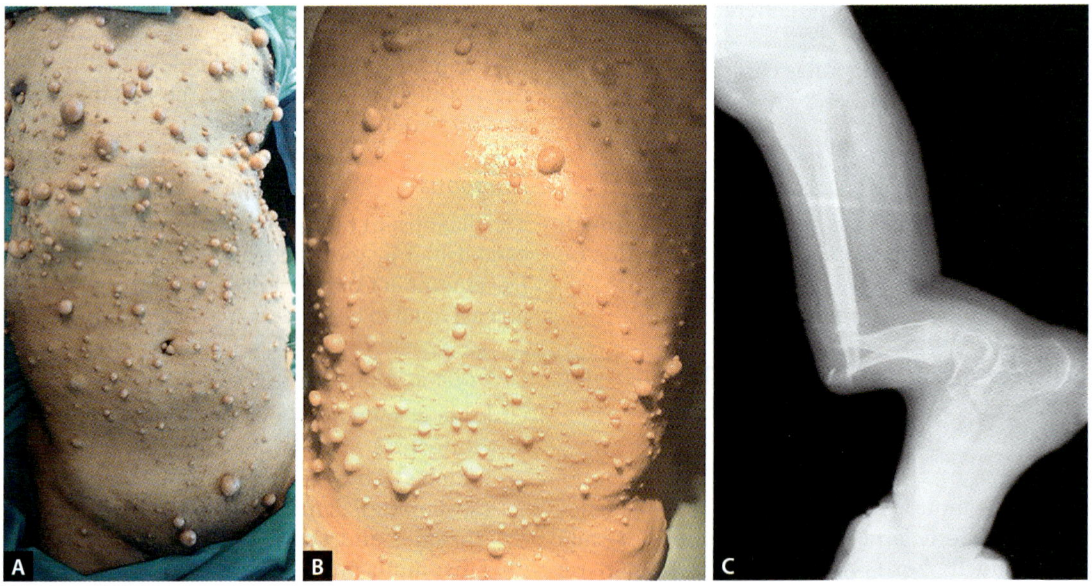

Figs. 10A to C: Von Recklinghausen's disease. (A and B) Note the multiple neurofibromas spread all over the body prominently on the torso; (C) Pseudarthrosis of tibia and fibula in a patient with neurofibromatosis.

The curves are dangerous as they progress rapidly, are resistant to bracing, and may have an associated sagittal plane deformity. Surgical treatment is done using growing rod instrumentation in younger children or combined anterior and posterior fusion in older children. The risk of pseudarthrosis after spine surgery is higher in NF than idiopathic scoliosis. It is preferable to do circumferential fusion to prevent this. Preoperative CT and MRI are helpful to identify defective pedicles and dural ectasias. One should be also vigilant of the developing anterolateral meningoceles due to outpouching of the dura that can erode the pedicle and may lead to weakening (they may also cause dislocations in cervical spine).

ACHONDROPLASIA AND RELATED DISORDERS

Achondroplasia is the most common nonlethal skeletal dysplasia and the most common cause of diastrophic dwarfism [diastrophic means "to grow twisted", campomelic means "bent limbs", and chondrodysplasia punctata refers to stippled cartilage; these terms describe the appearance of skeleton, other eponyms used are Kniest (*see* below), Morquio, and McKusick type dwarfism]. Its clinical phenotype has been recognized for centuries and the notion that it reflects a disturbance of cartilage-mediated (endochondral) bone growth has existed for about 100 years until *FGF3* mutations were recognized. The gene for achondroplasia was assigned to chromosome 4 at locus p16.3 by linkage analysis. Mutations in the fibroblast growth factor receptor-3 (*FGFR-3*) gene can result in several skeletal dysplasias of different severity, including achondroplasia, hypochondroplasia, and thanatophoric dysplasia. The risk of having a child with achondroplasia is associated with increased *paternal* age.

Achondroplasia has an incidence of 1 in 30,000 persons, inherited as an AD trait. It is characterized by rhizomelic shortening [short-limbs especially the proximal portion ("rhizo" meaning "root") compared to truncal height]. The term "mesomelic", refers to shortening of the middle segment, and "acromelic", to the distal segment. The inheritance pattern is AD, although the condition results from sporadic mutations in >90% of patients. All patients with the classical features of achondroplasia have the same glycine to arginine substitution at position 380 (G380R), which maps to the transmembrane domain of the receptor A. This single amino acid substitution results in stabilization of the FGFR receptor dimer, with accumulation on the cell surface (due to decreased internalization) and uncontrolled activation on the receptor. The FGFR negatively regulates endochondral ossification. This sustained FGFR activity results in growth retardation in the proliferative zone of the physis.

Clinical Features

Achondroplasia is characterized by the following clinical examination findings:

- Short limbs compared to normal trunk length
- Upper and lower limbs are rhizomelic (short proximal portions) with abnormal bony anatomy **(Figs. 11A to C)**.
- Frontal bossing and midface hypoplasia
- *Trident hands:* Characterized by a persistent space between the long and ring fingers when approximation of the fingers is attempted in full extension.
- Spinal deformities (e.g., thoracolumbar kyphosis, lordosis, and scoliosis). Thoracolumbar kyphosis can occur when the child begins to sit, and the risk of kyphosis can be decreased by not forcing or encouraging the child to sit upright until he or she is ready to do so. The kyphosis typically resolves when the child begins to walk at 18–24 months of age.
- Spinal stenosis (intervertebral foramen and interpedicular narrowing due to short thick pedicles) anterior wedging of vertebral bodies. The achondroplastic spine is characterized by cranial-to-caudal narrowing of the lumbar interpedicular distance and shortened pedicles

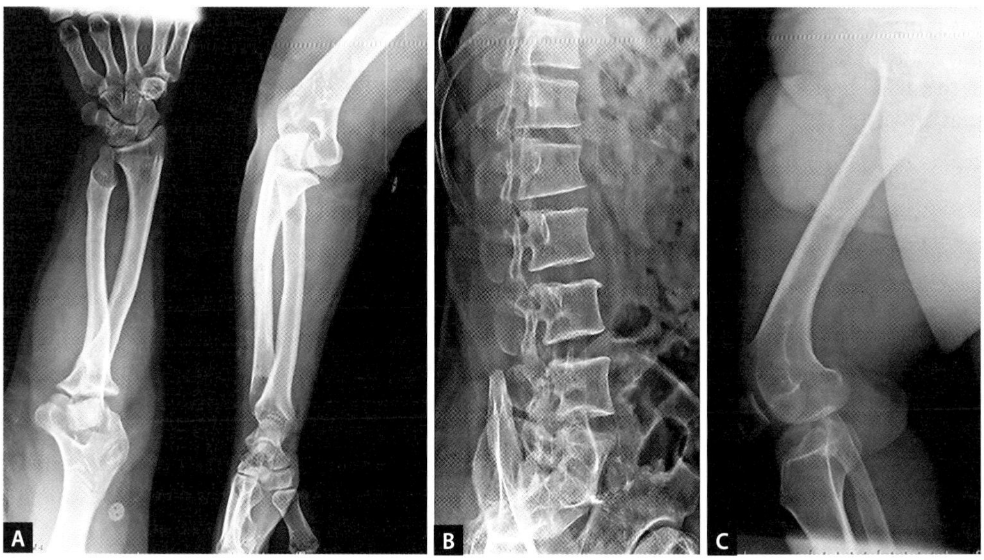

Figs. 11A to C: Achondroplasia. (A) Note the various osseous abnormalities like, poorly developed ulna; (B) Short pedicles; (C) Short and terminally bwed femora.

BOX 3: The nonorthopedic manifestations of achondroplasia.

- Recurrent otitis media (eustachian tube malfunction)
- Maxillary hypoplasia leads to dental crowding and malocclusion
- Obstructive sleep apnea (75% patients)
- Decreased respiratory drive and pulmonary function, hydrocephalus, and lifetime difficulty with weight control
- Hearing loss (60% patients)

(Fig. 11C). Lumbar spinal stenosis usually occurs in the adult patient, but it can begin as early as the second decade of life.

- Waddling gait and circumduction motion at hips on brisk walking or running
- Macrocephaly (triventricular enlargement)
- *Genu varum:* The cause of genu varum in patients with achondroplasia is controversial.
    - Foramen magnum and upper cervical stenosis can occur during the first 2 years of life. Stenosis may result in cervicomedullary cord compression, which is manifested by hypotonia, delayed development, weakness, and apnea; the diagnosis is confirmed through a sleep study and MRI.
    - Other orthopedic manifestations of achondroplasia include:
        - Flexion contractures of the elbows
        - Subluxation of the radial heads
        - Ligamentous laxity
    - The nonorthopedic manifestations causing increased morbidity are provided in **Box 3**.

Radiological Features

The radiological features of achondroplasia include:

- Squared iliac wings
- Flaring of the metaphyses of long bones
- The diaphyses of all long bones are thick owing to subperiosteal bone apposition
- *Genu varum:* Angulation at both the distal femoral and the proximal tibial metaphyses contribute to it. Growth of the fibula is typically greater than that of the tibia that may also contribute to the varus in some cases.
- The shape of the distal femoral physis is an exaggeration of the normal inverted "V" in the midline (chevron physis).

Diagnosis

The condition is diagnosed via prenatal ultrasonography or at birth. Later the clinical features are quite characteristic to make diagnosis.

Management

- *Foramen magnum stenosis:* Surgical decompression of the brainstem and spinal cord alleviates symptoms.
- *Thoracolumbar kyphosis:* Bracing (extension-type thoracolumbosacral orthosis) is indicated for progressive kyphosis with apical wedging. Spinal fusion is indicated if severe kyphosis (greater than 30° at 5 years of age) persists despite bracing but the specific indications, including the child's age and the degree of kyphosis, remain unclear.
- *Lumbar canal stenosis:* Symptomatic stenosis requires wide decompression (usually extends from the lower thoracic spine to the sacrum) and extradural removal of herniated disk material to avoid an early recurrence. Because wide decompression in the skeletally immature patient with achondroplasia has been associated with early postlaminectomy kyphosis so concurrent spinal fusion is recommended. The extent of the laminectomies should be 3 levels cephalad to the proximal extent of compression, distal to the second sacral level, and lateral to the facet joints.
- *Genu varum:* Surgical treatment is indicated for symptoms such as pain or fibular thrust or progressive deformity. Osteotomies are performed at the site of the deformity (proximal tibiofibular osteotomy). Associated tibial torsion should be corrected concurrently.
- Limb lengthening though intriguing is a long-term investment for these cases. They need to be explained that the two femora, two tibia, and the two humeri (six segment) lengthening will need lot of time devotion and dedication. The period usually exceeds 2 years. Humeri need lengthening to improve personal care.

Targeted medical therapy includes strategies to interfere with FGFR-3 synthesis, block its activation, inhibit its tyrosine kinase activity, promote its degradation, and antagonize its downstream signals and are under evaluation particularly the role of atrial natriuretic peptide (ANP), brain natriuretic peptide (BNP), C-type natriuretic peptide (CNP), and MEK inhibitor.

Hypochondroplasia

Hypochondroplasia (achondroplasia tarda and atypical achondroplasia) is a milder form of achondroplasia characterized by short stature; stocky build; disproportionately short arms and legs; broad, short hands and feet; mild joint laxity; and macrocephaly. Lamy and Maroteaux in 1961 suggested the term hypochondroplasia. In contrast to achondroplasia, however, intellectual disability and epilepsy is more prevalent in hypochondroplasia. The disorder genetically is similar to achondroplasia and about 70% of affected individuals are heterozygous for a mutation in *FGFR-3*. More phenotypic heterogeneity is seen in hypochondroplasia, probably because of mutations arising in different portions of the *FGFR-3* gene. The inheritance pattern of hypochondroplasia is AD.

Clinical Features

Common findings: Stocky build; short stature; shortening of the proximal (rhizomelia) or middle (mesomelia) segments of the extremities; broad and short hands and feet (brachydactyly); limitation of elbow extension; mild joint laxity that is generalized; and macrocephaly with relatively normal facies.

Uncommon features seen in some patients only: Mild genu varum; lumbar lordosis with protruding abdomen; learning disabilities; adult-onset OA; scoliosis; mild-to-moderate intellectual disability; and temporal lobe epilepsy.

Radiological Features

These include shortening of long bones with mild metaphyseal flare; narrowing of the inferior lumbar interpedicular distances; short, broad femoral neck; and squared, shortened ilia albeit less prominent than achondroplasia.

Diagnosis

If one defines hypochondroplasia as a mild allelic form of achondroplasia with *FGFR-3* gene mutation then there is high likelihood of overdiagnosis and false-positive diagnosis when it is checked against a complete mutation search of the *FGFR-3* gene. The diagnosis is difficult to make in children <3 years of age as the clinical features are late to develop. Genetic mutation identification is done by targeted mutation analysis (for two common mutations) and sequence analysis (if there is high clinical suspicion but normal targeted mutation analysis).

Treatment

Most of the treatments are based on standard guidelines to address the manifestations of disease. The concerns of dwarfism are better allayed in parents than trying any treatment. Laminectomy relieves symptoms of stenosis. Epilepsy is treated in standard fashion.

Thanatophoric Dysplasia

It is a short-limb dwarfism syndrome that is usually lethal in the perinatal period. It is divided into:

- *Type I,* characterized by micromelia with bowed femurs and, uncommonly, the presence of cloverleaf skull deformity (Kleeblattschädel) of varying severity.
- *Type II,* characterized by micromelia with straight femurs and uniform presence of moderate-to-severe cloverleaf skull deformity.

Other features common to type I and type II include:

- Short ribs
- Narrow thorax
- Macrocephaly
- Distinctive facial features
- Brachydactyly
- Hypotonia
- Redundant skin folds along the limbs

  Most affected infants die of respiratory insufficiency before the patient reaches 2 years of age.

Other rare phenotypes associated with FGFR mutation include:

- FGFR-related craniosynostosis and its related eight disorders [Pfeiffer syndrome, Apert syndrome, Crouzon syndrome, Beare–Stevenson syndrome, FGFR 2-related isolated coronal synostosis, Jackson–Weiss syndrome, Crouzon syndrome with acanthosis nigricans (AN), and Muenke syndrome.
- SADDAN (**s**evere **a**chondroplasia with **d**evelopmental **d**elay and **a**canthosis **n**igricans).

DISORDERS RELATED TO TYPE II COLLAGEN ABNORMALITIES

These disorders include spondyloepiphyseal dysplasia (SED) congenita, SED tarda, and Kniest dysplasia.

Spondyloepiphyseal Dysplasia Congenita

Spondyloepiphyseal dysplasia congenita is an inherited disorder (first described by Spranger and Wiedemann in 1966) of bone growth that results in short stature (dwarfism), skeletal abnormalities, and problems with vision and hearing. This condition affects the bones of the spine (spondylo-) and the ends (epiphyses) of long bones in the arms and legs. Congenita indicates that the condition is present from birth. Dwarfing conditions are frequently referred to as short-limb or short-trunk types, according to whether the limbs or trunk is more extensively involved. SED, metatropic dysplasia, and Kniest syndrome are short-trunk type dwarfing conditions.

Genetics

It is caused by mutations in the collagen type II α-1 chain (*COL2A1),* which encodes type II collagen. The inheritance pattern is AD, but most patients acquire the disease through new mutations.

Clinical Features

This extremely rare dysplasia is characterized by:

- Short stature (very short trunk, neck, and shortened limbs)
- Abnormal formation of the long bone epiphyses with variable metaphyseal involvement.
- Abnormal curvature of the spine (kyphoscoliosis and lordosis) becomes more severe during childhood and can cause problems with breathing.
- Flattened vertebrae (platyspondyly)
- Lower extremity malalignment can be caused by coxa vara, genu valgum, or distal tibia valgus.
- Odontoid hypoplasia or ligamentous laxity can result in atlantoaxial instability, which can progress to cervical myelopathy. Instability should be evaluated during infancy and continuously monitored.
- *Coxa vara:* The evaluation of coxa vara is complicated by delayed ossification of the femoral capital epiphysis **(Fig. 12)**.
- Other manifestations include retinal detachment, severe myopia, and sensorineural hearing loss.

Management

- Abnormal epiphyseal development typically results in early degenerative joint disease, which may require total joint arthroplasty during young adulthood.
- Symptomatic or excessive cervical spine (measuring 8 mm or more or myelopathy) instability requires fusion with decompression if stenosis is present.
- Scoliosis should be initially treated with bracing which is often difficult due to rigid small trunk. Patients with

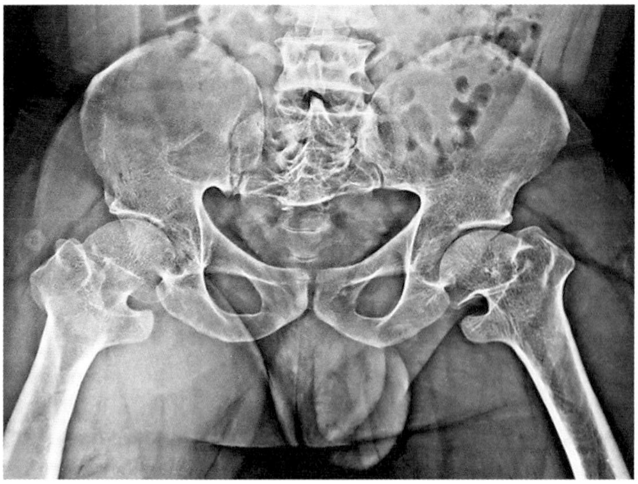

Fig. 12: Spondyloepiphyseal dysplasia. Note the abnormal pelvic inlet and short femoral neck.

curves that progress despite brace treatment or that measure >50° should be considered candidates for a posterior spinal fusion.
- Coxa vara should be corrected to 140° or more.
- Varus supracondylar osteotomy is required for correction of symptomatic knee or valgus deformity.
- Clubfeet if present need surgical correction being often recalcitrant to manipulation.

Spondyloepiphyseal Tarda

Spondyloepiphyseal tarda is milder than SED congenita and occurs almost exclusively in males. It may not be diagnosed until school age, unlike SED congenital, which may be diagnosed at birth. "Tarda" indicates that signs and symptoms of this condition are not present at birth, but appear later in childhood, typically between ages 6 and 10 years.

Spondyloepiphyseal tarda can result from a mutation in type II collagen, but the mechanism has not been shown. Several patterns of transmission have been reported, of which X-linked transmission is the most common. Mutations in the *TRAPPC2* gene (often called the *SEDL* gene) cause X-linked SED tarda. The *TRAPPC2* gene provides instructions for producing the protein Sedlin, the functions of which remain unclear.

The manifestations include odontoid hypoplasia, scoliosis, and OA. They have a short trunk and neck, and their arms appear disproportionately long. Impaired growth of the spinal bones (vertebrae) causes the short stature seen in this disorder.

Management

Similar to the congenital form these patients also need management of scoliosis. OA needs reconstructive procedures. Hip arthroscopy has been used for the management of intra-articular pathologies, such as labral tears, chondral flaps, and loose bodies.

Kniest Dysplasia

(Kniest Chondrodystrophy, Metatropic Dysplasia/Dwarfism Type II)

Kniest dysplasia is an AD disorder caused by mutations in the *COL2A1* gene.
- It is characterized by a trunk that is disproportionately shorter than the limbs (truncal dwarfism) and dumbbell-shaped long bones with broad metaphyses and irregular dysplastic epiphyses.
- Affected individuals have abnormally large joints that can cause pain and restrict movement, limiting physical activity.
- These joint problems can also lead to arthritis.
- Other manifestations include odontoid hypoplasia, kyphosis, mild scoliosis, platyspondyly, clubfoot, joint contractures, and limb malalignment.
- Characteristic facies includes a round, flat face with bulging and wide-set eyes.
- Other characteristics include myopia, retinal detachment, and deafness. Type II collagen mostly forms the vitreous and articular cartilage which get prominently affected.
- Degenerative arthritis can develop as early as the second decade of life and needs reconstructive procedures in the form of joint replacement.

DISORDERS CAUSED BY ABNORMALITIES IN GENES IMPORTANT IN NORMAL SKELETAL DEVELOPMENT

This spectrum of disorders includes cleidocranial dysostosis and nail-patella syndrome.

Cleidocranial Dysostosis

Cleidocranial dysplasia is a condition that primarily affects the development of the bones and teeth. It is caused by a mutation of the core-binding factor α-1 (*CBFA1*) gene (also called *RUNX2*), a transcription factor that activates osteoblast differentiation. *RUNX2* gene (*CBFA1*) provides instructions for making a protein that is involved in bone and cartilage development and maintenance. *RUNX2* protein acts as a "master switch", regulating a number of other genes involved in the development of cells that build bones (osteoblasts). Due to mutational shortage of functional *RUNX2* protein the normal bone and cartilage development is interfered, resulting in the signs and symptoms of cleidocranial dysplasia. Although it should be remembered that one-third of the patients do not have a mutation of the gene and the cause of disease in these patients is unknown. The inheritance pattern is AD. Incidence is nearly 1 per million individuals.

Clinical Features

The affected individuals characteristically have the following features:
- *Clavicle hypoplasia or aplasia:* Their shoulders are narrow and sloping with an increased ability to oppose the shoulders **(Fig. 13)**.
- Widening of the symphysis pubis

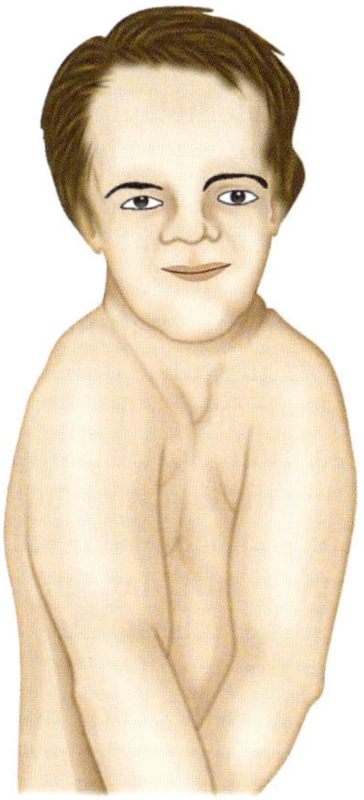

Fig. 13: Cleidocranial dysostosis. The patients are able to bring their shoulders together anteriorly.

- Delayed closing of fontanels (may persist up to adulthood)
- Coxa vara
- Short stature (3–6 inches shorter than family members)
- They may also have short, tapered fingers and broad thumbs; shortened middle phalanges of the third, fourth, and fifth fingers; short forearms; flat feet; knock knees; and an abnormal curvature of the spine (scoliosis).
- Characteristic facies may include a wide, short skull (brachycephaly); a prominent forehead; wide-set eyes (hypertelorism); a flat nose; and a small upper jaw.
- In females due to abnormal shape of pelvis the rate of cesarean section is quite high.
- Dental abnormalities in these individuals are characterized by:
    - Delayed loss of the primary (baby) teeth
    - Delayed appearance of the secondary (adult) teeth, often they are supernumerary and unless get absorbed, crowding of teeth occurs in adults requiring removal.
    - Unusually shaped and peg-like teeth
    - Misalignment of the teeth and jaws (malocclusion)
    - Extra teeth are sometimes accompanied by cysts in the gums.
- The individuals are also predisposed to ear and sinus infections have hearing loss. Some children have delayed motor functions and development, but intelligence is normal.

Treatment

- Clavicle hypoplasia does not require treatment unless there is irritation of brachial plexus in which case the clavicular fragments need excision.
- Valgus osteotomy is indicated for coxa vara with a neck shaft angle <100° and an associated Trendelenburg gait, usually by 5 years of age, also prevent the worsening of deformity.
- Oral checkups should be done regularly and otologist referral should be done for hearing problems.
- Craniofacial surgery may be needed in uncommon cases to correct skull defects.

Nail–Patella Syndrome

Nail-patella syndrome is caused by mutations of the LIM homeobox transcription factor 1-β gene (*LMX1B*), which is involved in determining dorsoventral patterning of the limb bud and renal formation (so mutations are associated with nephropathy also). The syndrome derives its name from the predominant involvement of the knee (patella) and the nails. The inheritance pattern is AD.

Clinical Features

The manifestations of nail-patella syndrome have a quartet of findings:

- Nail dysplasia—most prominent feature. They may be completely absent, hypoplastic, or show grooves and distortions in its surface. The thumb is more involved than the small finger, and the ulnar border more involved than the radial. The hands are often very symmetric, and fingernails are more involved than toenails.
- Patellar hypoplasia—quite small and may even be absent.
- Elbow dysplasia—abnormal lateral humeral condyle. The trochlea is large and the capitellum hypoplastic, creating an asymmetric shape that may predispose the radial head to dislocation.
- Iliac horns—bony exostoses on the posterior surface of the ilium.

Other features in knee include a spectrum of femoral condyle dysplasia (hypoplastic lateral femoral condyle with genu valgum) and a septum running from the patella to the intercondylar groove (septum interarticularis), dividing the knee into two compartments. In elbow, posterior dislocation of radial head is quite prominent. Patients have short stature and associated shoulder girdle dysplasia although the functional deficit is minimal. The foot deformities include variations of stiff calcaneal valgus, metatarsus adductus, and clubfeet. Joint contractures at knee and feet are peculiar in some often confused with arthrogryposis.

Treatment

- The knee disability is variable and related to the magnitude of quadriceps dysfunction and the dislocated patella. Knee deformity and patellar realignment require soft-tissue releases and osteotomies, limited soft tissue or capsular releases are however ineffective.
- Quadricepsplasty is indicated along with the patella realignment due to associated quadriceps contracture.
- Combined proximal and classically described distal realignments have to be performed as the patellar stability is compromised by the hypoplastic femoral condyles.
- Knee flexion contracture may need to be release by capsulotomy and hamstring release. Intra-articular septum may be released arthroscopically.
- Symptomatic radial head dislocation may also require surgical treatment by removing the radial head but movements seldom improve.

- Clubfeet are managed as idiopathic clubfeet.
- The medical complications like renal failure due to nephropathy need early identification and often require long-term nephrology management.

DISORDERS CAUSED BY ABNORMALITIES IN GENES THAT PLAY A ROLE IN THE PROCESSING OF PROTEINS

This group of disorders includes diastrophic dysplasia and the mucopolysaccharidoses (*see* Chapter on "Metabolic Diseases of Bone").

Diastrophic Dysplasia [Previously Called "Achondroplasia with Clubfeet" (Wrongly)]

This is associated with the most severe skeletal abnormalities. The term "diastrophic" comes from a Greek root meaning "distorted", which aptly describes the ears, spine, long bones, and feet. Diastrophic dysplasia is caused by mutations in the sulfate transporter gene located on chromosome 5. It primarily affects cartilage, because of the presence of negatively charged sulfate groups in proteoglycan molecules. The defective gene causes undersulfation of the proteoglycan in the cartilage matrix. This dysplasia is extremely rare, except that in Finland 1–2% of the population are carriers. The inheritance pattern is AR. The manifestations include:

- Cauliflower ear
- Flattened nose bridge and cleft palate
- Marked short stature with rhizomelic shortening (previously called "cherub dwarf")
- *Cervical kyphosis:* Often resolves but may develop into quadriparesis and increasing deformity in some
- *Scoliosis:* Idiopathic like or sharply angular
- *Hitchhiker thumbs:* Due to short proximal first metacarpals
- Severe clubfeet
- *Genu valgum and recurrent subluxation of patella:* The fibula is typically shorter in these cases
- Skew foot
- Joint contractures
- Severe OA

Management

Surgery for cervical kyphosis is required if myelopathy or progressive kyphosis or kyphoscoliosis occurs. If the kyphosis exceeds 60° and/or the apex vertebra is round or triangular and totally displaced posteriorly, then progression is likely. The clubfoot in diastrophic dysplasia is typically rigid and often recurs after complete release. Hip and knee flexion contractures may require releases with or without osteotomies. End-stage OA can be treated with total joint arthroplasty.

OTHER SKELETAL DYSPLASIAS

Metaphyseal Chondrodysplasia

This is a group of disorders characterized by metaphyseal involvement with epiphyseal preservation, short stature, and genu varum.

- *The Schmid type* [Schmid metaphyseal dysostosis, metaphyseal chondrodysplasia type Schmid (MCDS), and Japanese type spondylometaphyseal dysplasia], which is most common type of metaphyseal chondrodysplasia, is caused by α-1 chain of type X collagen (*COL10A1*) mutation. The inheritance pattern is AD. Bone maturation is always normal. It is milder form as compared to the Jansen type. The manifestations are mild, including moderate short stature, disproportionately short limbs, enlarged capital femoral epiphysis in childhood, coxa vara, waddling gait, anterior rib changes, and genu varum (often confused with tibia vara, but the distal femoral metaphysis is predominantly affected).
- *The Jansen type* (Murk Jansen type metaphyseal chondrodysplasia) is caused by a mutation in the parathyroid receptor gene (*PTHR1*) that regulates the differentiation of growth plate chondrocytes. *PTHR1/PTHrP* being predominantly located in the bones and renal tissue, disease manifestations are related to the mineral homeostasis and growth plate development. Inheritance is AD. It is characterized by short stature with extremity malalignment, "bell-shaped" thorax, bowed legs, and some patients have choanal atresia and micrognathia. The radiological features include rachitiform metaphyseal changes (widening, fraying, and cupping of physis) due to altered mineral metabolism. The base of skull and calvaria are sclerotic. Spine is normal. The ends of most bones remain expanded and the large calcified metaphyseal masses form bone.
- *The McKusick type* (cartilage-hair hypoplasia) is caused by a mutation of the *RMRP* gene (ribosomal nucleic acid component of mitochondrial ribosomal nucleic acid processing endoribonuclease). The common manifestations include fine sparse, unpigmented hair, atlantoaxial instability, genu varum, ligamentous laxity, pectus abnormalities, and increased risk of viral infection and malignancy. The skull is normal unlike achondroplasia as also is absence of spinal stenosis.

Pseudoachondroplasia

It is an inherited disorder of bone growth that was previously considered similar to achondroplasia but without characteristic facial features. Now pseudoachondroplasia is considered a separate disorder.

It is caused by a mutation in the cartilage oligomeric matrix protein (*COMP*) gene. COMP is an extracellular matrix glycoprotein found in the space between chondrocytes where it interacts with other proteins. With COMP mutation the produced defective protein cannot be transported out of the cell. The inheritance pattern is AD.

All people with pseudoachondroplasia have short stature. Pseudoachondroplasia is characterized by involvement of the spine, metaphyses, and epiphyses; facial features may be normal or delicate. The manifestations include a short trunk and rhizomelic or mesomelic shortness, waddling gait, ligamentous laxity, odontoid hypoplasia, scoliosis, platyspondyly, hip subluxation, and varus or valgus malalignment at knee (commonly it is the windswept deformity).

Surgery is required for symptomatic atlantoaxial instability. Scoliosis is managed by bracing for curves between 25° and 45° while spinal fusion is indicated for larger curves. Femoral and iliac osteotomies often are needed for hip subluxation. Windswept knees are corrected with femoral and tibial osteotomies.

Multiple Epiphyseal Dysplasia

Multiple epiphyseal dysplasia (MED) includes a spectrum of disorders resulting from different mutations and is thus heterogeneous. It is one of the most widely known and commonly occurring skeletal dysplasia. Mutations have been identified in the *COMP* gene (as in pseudoachondroplasia), *COL9A2* (collagen, type IX, α-2), and *COL9A3* (collagen, type IX, α-3). The genetic mutation identification has resulted in reducing the use of terms historically used to describe the two forms of the disease eponymously called Ribbing's dysplasia (mild involvement) or Fairbank's dysplasia (more severe type). The inheritance pattern usually is AD.

Clinical Features

The disease predominantly affects the weight-bearing epiphysis. The typical features of patients with MED include:

- Short stature with epiphyseal dysplasia
- Delayed ossification
- Genu valgum
- Early OA
- Hip osteonecrosis
- Radiological features include:
  - Flattening of the femoral condyles **(Fig. 14)**
  - An ovoid femoral head
  - Decreased sphericity of the humeral head (hatchet head appearance in adults)
  - Squaring of the talus
  - Premature OA in the hips

Differential Diagnosis

Perthes disease (in MED, the acetabulum is predominantly affected, with symmetrical involvement). The radiographs of knee, ankles, and shoulders should be obtained to evaluate epiphysis.

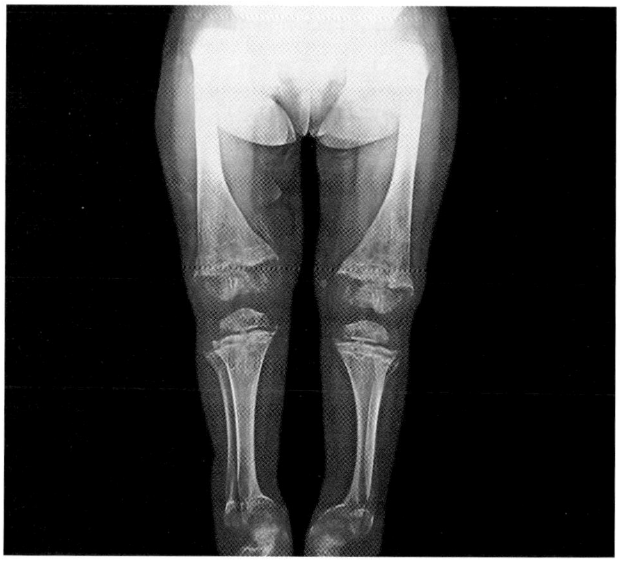

Fig. 14: Multiple epiphyseal dysplasia.

Management

Treatment modalities for the hip are similar to the containment methods used for Legg-Calvé-Perthes disease, and realignment osteotomies may be required for genu valgum. Progressive hip or shoulder arthritis can require arthroplasty.

Chondroectodermal Dysplasia

Chondroectodermal dysplasia is also known as Ellis-van Creveld syndrome. It is a generalized defect of maturation of endochondral ossification characterized by disproportionately short stature and abnormalities in the mouth, teeth, limbs, and heart. It is caused by mutation in the Ellis-van Creveld gene localized to the short arm of the fourth chromosome, the function of which is unknown. The inheritance pattern is AR.

Clinical Features

Neonates are most severely affected and around one-third dies within this period. The manifestations include:

- Short stature with mesoacromelic shortening (opposite to achondroplasia where rhizomelic shortening is seen)
- Medial and lateral spikes from the acetabular margins
- Genu valgum
- Hypoplasia of the lateral femoral epiphysis
- External rotation of femur and internal rotation of tibia
- Narrow chest with small ribs
- Postaxial hand polydactyly
- Wrists show fused capitate and hamate
- Proximal femoral physis ossify early and the greater trochanter is prominent
- *Cardiac defects:* Atrial septal defect (ASD) and single atrium
- Teeth appears and are lost early, the nails are hypoplastic
- Sparse and thin hair

Management

Osteotomies or hemiepiphysiodesis can be required to correct genu valgum. Syndactyly or polydactyly needs to be addressed when the cardiac status is favorable.

SOME MISCELLANEOUS SYNDROMES

ARTHROGRYPOSIS

Arthrogryposis refers to a physical finding (not a diagnosis) of having joint contractures present at birth seen in large group of disorders. Arthrogryposis is defined as multiple congenital contractures affecting two or more areas of the body. Isolated congenital contractures affect only one part like the classic talipes equinovarus deformity [congenital talipes equinovarus (CTEV)]; in contrast, arthrogryposis would affect multiple regions. This term finds varied uses as a noun to describe specific diseases [arthrogryposis

Flowchart 2: The classification of contracture syndromes.

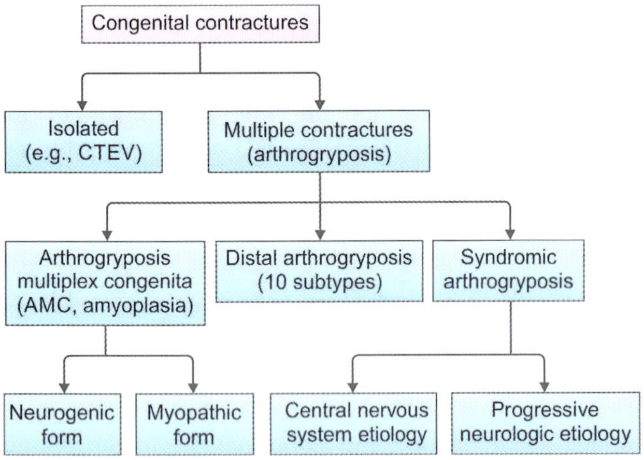

(CTEV: congenital talipes equinovarus)

multiplex congenita (AMC)], and as an adjective, "arthrogrypotic", to refer to rigid joint contractures. Some 65 distinct syndromes and 300 disorders can be grouped under the broad term "arthrogryposis" [conditions caused by environmental agents, single gene defects (AD, AR, and X-linked recessive), chromosomal abnormalities, known syndromes, or unknown conditions]. Some experts believe that it is clinically and descriptively simpler to group these into broader term contracture syndromes **(Flowchart 2)** all of which include arthrogryposis also as its component.

Contracture Syndrome Groups

- Those involving all four extremities arthrogryposis—multiplex congenita **(Fig. 15)** and Larsen syndrome.
- Those predominantly or exclusively involve the hands and feet—distal arthrogryposis and facial involvement can occur with some of these syndromes (Freeman-Sheldon syndrome; **Fig. 16**). The distal arthrogryposis has been subclassified into 10 different subtypes **(Table 8)**.
- Syndromic forms

There is an alternative (less commonly followed) way of classifying the condition into three groups. Group I disorders involve only the limbs and it includes classic AMC and distal arthrogryposis. Distal arthrogryposis is further classified into 10 subtypes **(Table 8)**. Group II disorders involve both the limbs and other body areas (like the associated craniofacial, vertebral, or cardiac abnormalities). Examples of group II include pterygium syndrome and Larsen syndrome. The group III disorders involve both, the limbs and the CNS as in myelomeningocele, sacral agenesis, and congenital muscular dystrophy.

Contracture Syndromes Involving All Four Extremities

Arthrogryposis multiplex congenita (multiple congenital contractures, amyoplasia, and human wonder with curved limbs) *AMC* comprises nonprogressive conditions characterized by multiple joint ("multiplex") contractures ("arthro-

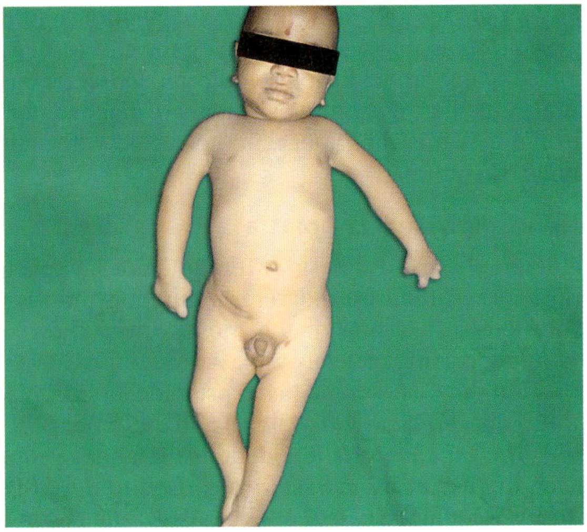

Fig. 15: Arthrogryposis multiplex congenita. Note the smooth skin and absent creases at places where the flexion-extension creases are normally found. All four extremities are involved.

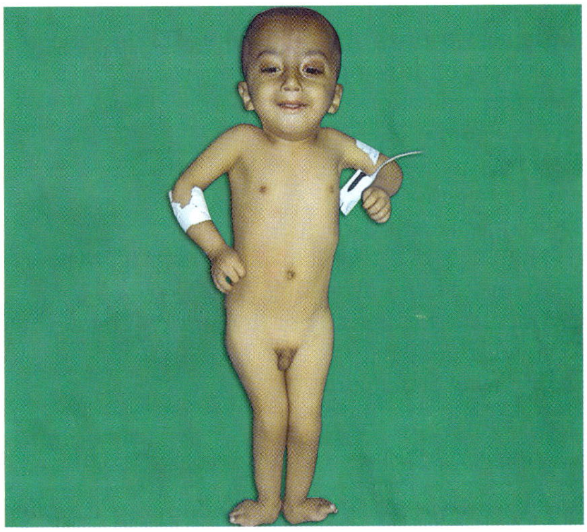

Fig. 16: Freeman–Sheldon syndrome. Note the whistling facies with prominent cheeks and pursed lips. The elbow and knee have flexion contractures along with vertical talus deformity of the foot.

TABLE 8: The classified different subtypes of distal arthrogryposis.

Type	*Remarks/older description*
DA1	Distal arthrogryposis type 1
DA2	
• DA2A	Freeman–Sheldon syndrome
• DA2B	Sheldon–Hall syndrome
DA3	Gordon syndrome
DA4	Scoliosis
DA5	Ophthalmoplegia, ptosis
DA6	Sensorineural hearing loss
DA7	Trismus pseudocamptodactyly
DA8	Autosomal dominant multiple pterygium syndrome
DA9	Congenital contractural arachnodactyly
DA10	Congenital plantar contractures

gryposis") found throughout the body at birth ("congenita"). The disorder is sporadic with affected individuals having reproduced only normal children. Worldwide incidence is 1 in 3,000 live births but is more common in Finland and Israel. Males and females are equally affected except in X-linked recessive disorders where males are predominantly affected.

Etiopathogenesis

Etiopathogenesis is essentially unknown. The following have been proposed as a possible cause:

- It is now commonly believed that the development of arthrogryposis may be influenced by an adverse intrauterine factor. Fetal akinesia is the predominant factor leading to development of the joint and soft tissue abnormalities. This may arise out of fetal abnormalities such as neurogenic, muscle, or connective tissue abnormalities or mechanical limitations to movement or maternal disorders such as infection (rubella, rubeola, coxsackievirus, and enterovirus), drugs and trauma. During early embryogenesis the joints are normal only with poor intrauterine fetal movements do the joints and periarticular structures fail to develop/mature as the movements are essential for joint molding (Wolff's law). Generalized fetal akinesia is also responsible for polyhydramnios, pulmonary hypoplasia, micrognathia, ocular hypertelorism, and short umbilical cord. The relationship to fetal akinesia is also supported by the finding of a more severe disease in those diagnosed early. Though explaining most of the features this theory does not fully explain the histological findings of primary neurological involvement (see below).
- Some mothers of children with arthrogryposis have serum antibodies that inhibit fetal acetylcholine receptor function. One possibility is that maternal antibodies to these fetal antigens cause the disorder (possibly by reducing the uterine functions).
- Teratogens (drugs, alcohol, curare, methocarbamol, and phenytoin) have been suggested, but none are proven, despite various animal models shown to have similar disease development.
- Molecular basis has been recognized in very rare AR forms of AMC using linkage analysis:
    - Pena-Shokeir phenotype lethal congenital contracture syndrome (LCCS) (9q34)
    - Neurogenic type of AMC (5q35)
    - Arthrogryposis-renal dysfunction-cholestasis syndrome (15q1)
    - LCCS type 2 (12q13) and LCCS type 3 (19p13, mutation of PIP5K1C)

Types of Arthrogryposis Multiplex Congenita

Neurogenic types of AMC: These include

- Dysgenesis of the motor nuclei of the spinal cord and brainstem. There is replacement of fasciculi of muscle fibers by small muscle fibers and adipose tissue, e.g., Pierre-Robin syndrome and Möbius syndrome.
- Disorganization of neurons and a decrease in neurons of the cortex and motor nuclei of the brain stem and spinal cord, e.g., partial deletion of the long arm of chromosome 18 syndrome and Zellweger syndrome.
- Dysgenesis of the anterior horn cells, e.g., Meckel-Gruber syndrome and anencephaly.

Myopathic forms of AMC: These include

- Central core disease
- Congenital myasthenia gravis
- Nemaline myopathy and its subtypes
- Congenital muscular dystrophy

The pathoanatomical features of AMC are summarized in **Box 4**.

History and Clinical Examination

Mothers affected with myotonic dystrophy, myasthenia gravis, or multiple scleroses are at risk. Maternal infections (see above) can lead to CNS or peripheral nerve destruction with secondary congenital contractures. Maternal fever of >39°C for an extended period or maternal hyperthermia can cause contractures due to abnormal nerve growth or migration. Other causes that may possibly restrict fetal movements include oligohydramnios, chronic amniotic fluid leak, large fibroids, or bicornuate uterus.

In two-thirds of the patients, all four limbs are affected equally, but in one-third, lower-limb deformities predominate, and only on rare occasions do the upper extremities predominate. Deformities tend to be more severe and more rigid distally.

- The limbs are striking in appearance and position. They are featureless and tubular and deformities distributed symmetrically.
- Normal skin creases are lacking, but there may be deep dimples over the joints.
- Muscle mass is reduced, although, in infancy, there is often abundant subcutaneous tissue.

BOX 4: The pathoanatomical features of arthrogryposis multiplex congenital.

- Connective tissue abnormalities in tendon, bone, joint, or joint lining restricts fetal movements, resulting in congenital contractures.
- Joint abnormalities include synostosis, lack of joint development, and aberrant fixation of joints that restrict fetal movements.
- In some distal arthrogryposis types, the tendon develops normally but attach abnormally.
- Histologically there is a small muscle mass with fibrosis and fat between the muscle fibers.
- Myopathic and neuropathic features are seen in the same muscle biopsy specimen.
- Neurological abnormalities are the most common associations and possibly also the cause of arthrogryposis. Abnormalities include meningomyelocele, anencephaly, hydranencephaly, holoprosencephaly, spinal muscular atrophy, cerebro-oculo-facial-skeletal syndrome, and Marden-Walker syndrome.
- The periarticular soft tissues are fibrotic resembling (fibrous ankylosis).
- The number of anterior horn cells in the spinal cord is decreased.
- The pattern of motor neuron loss in specific spinal cord segments correlates with the peripheral deformities and the affected muscles. This finding actually points to primary central nervous system disorder being an important cause in pathogenesis of the disease.

- Typically, the shoulders are adducted and internally rotated, the elbow more often extended than flexed, and the wrist flexed severely, with ulnar deviation.
- The fingers are flexed, clutching the thumb.
- In the lower extremities:
  - The hips are flexed, abducted, and externally rotated.
  - The hips may be dislocated, unilaterally or bilaterally.
  - The knees are typically in extension, although flexion is possible.
  - Clubfeet
- Joint motion is restricted. The condition is pain free, with a firm, inelastic block to movement beyond a very limited range.
- Absent deep tendon reflexes or very sluggish.
- The visceral malformations are minimal. Some cases have been reported to have gastroschisis. Inguinal hernia is seen due to abdominal muscle weakness.
- Feeding difficulties arise due to a stiff jaw and an immobile tongue. There may be respiratory infections and failure to thrive.
- The facial features may include a small jaw, frontal midline hemangioma, narrowing of the face, hypertelorism, cleft palate, and occasionally, limited upward gaze (secondary to ocular muscle involvement).
- Radiographically the joints are normal at birth but adaptive changes occur over time as a consequence of fixed position.

Natural History of Disease

Some contractures seem to worsen with age, and the joint becomes stiffer. No new joints become involved. At least 25% of affected patients are nonambulators, and many others are limited household walkers. As a rule, those with arthrogryposis, who are very weak as infants stay weak, and those who appear stronger as infants stay strong. Adult interdependency seems to be related to education and coping skills, more than to the magnitude of joint contractures.

Diagnosis

Electromyograms and muscle biopsies do not help in diagnosis. However, they can be used to differentiate primary myopathies and neuropathies. Skin biopsy should be performed for culture of fibroblasts to be used for chromosome analysis. Prenatal ultrasound gives an indirect indication if fetal movements are absent and the earlier it is detected the worse is the disease and prognosis. The findings gain significance in presence of polyhydramnios. The common findings on an ultrasound are:

- Fetal immobility
- Increased nuchal translucency
- Joint contracture of all the extremities with clinched hands, clubfeet
- Cystic hygroma associated with pleural effusion (lethal types)
- Micrognathia, polyhydramnios, hypoechogenicity, and hypomineralization of the long bones.

Treatment

Early gentle manipulation soon after birth improves passive and active ROM. Early motion and avoidance of prolonged casing may increase joint motion, improving function. Vigorous physical therapy to stretch contractures is very important in improving joint motion and avoiding muscle atrophy. Patients with amyoplasia or distal arthrogryposis respond well to physical therapy with excellent functional outcome. However, physical therapy may actually be harmful in patients with diastrophic dysplasia, because it may lead to joint ankylosis.

Joint problems should be addressed individually. The overall goals are lower-limb alignment and stability for ambulation, and upper extremity motion for self-care. In general, the outcomes are better if joint surgery is done early, before adaptive intra-articular changes develop. Osteotomies are usually performed closer to the growth completion. Distal to proximal joint stabilization or reconstruction and correction of deformities is executed so that the foot followed by knee and lastly hip deformities are addressed in that order.

Foot deformity: This includes:

- A severe and resistant clubfoot is characteristic. It is rare for the arthrogrypotic clubfoot to become plantigrade, braceable foot by physical therapy and casts.
- Ponseti manipulation should be done to make foot supple enough to reduce extensive surgical dissection and morbidity.
- Surgical intervention is usually necessary as recurrence is quite common. It is difficult to generalize the outcomes and benefit in patients as there is a wide range of severity. Some feet, therefore, respond better to surgery than others.
- Surgery for clubfoot is sometimes delayed until 1 year of age or later and bony procedures like lateral column shortening may be needed. Neglected cases into teenage group or into adulthood need triple arthrodesis.
- There has been a trend recently to perform combined procedures, with minimal immobilization earlier in life. Primary talectomy has been recommended by few because of the high incidence of failed soft tissue surgery; however, we feel that Ponseti followed by circumferential release yields satisfactory outcome if performed before 1 year of age. Talectomy can always be performed later, if necessary.
- A vertical talus is an unusual foot deformity in AMC, and, if encountered, the physician must think of the distal arthrogryposis or pterygia syndromes.

Knee deformity: This includes:

- Although classically described as hyperextension deformity at knee with anterior dimples most knees are in flexion. The goal of treatment is an extended knee for ambulation. This is more easily accomplished in an extension or hyperextension deformity than in a flexion deformity.
- Physical therapy may result in medial lateral instability. Hyperextension deformity responds better to physical therapy and splinting than do flexion deformities.

- Residual flexion deformity of >30° needs surgical management as ambulation is precluded. The quadriceps and gluteus maximus are itself weak to support knee in flexion providing less than required power for proper ambulation.
- Surgery should be performed before 2 years of age and soft tissue release including posterior capsulotomy is commonly necessary in moderate contractures up to 60°. Deformities are usually kept slightly undercorrected initially, and posterior soft tissue procedures are often repeated later in life to aggressive full correction, as most often even if initially corrected repeat surgeries are a rule. Initial aggressive surgery will carry surgical morbidity and possible stiffness. Deformities of >60° need femoral shortening to relieve the tension on the neurovascular structures.
- Supracondylar osteotomies of the femur are recommended for severe contractures toward the end of growth to correct residual deformity. Femoral shortening may need to be added to the osteotomies.
- Many hyperextension deformities of the knee can be treated without surgery, but quadricepsplasty may be needed in some cases with residual lack of motion.
- Regarding the timing of surgery vis-à-vis other deformity correction, traditional teaching is to correct knee deformity before treating a dislocated hip and is especially true for a flexed knee deformity. This has been proposed to allow stretching of the muscles, which cross both joints because it is impossible to appropriately immobilize the hip with the knee held extended. Currently both hip and the extension knee deformities can be corrected simultaneously with improved understanding and methods that require a short period of immobilization. Hip spica cast as a short-term measure for immobilization allows flexion at the knee (the hamstring muscles are relaxed by procedures at both joints).
- An alternative technique of correction of the knee deformity is using an external fixator, with gradual correction; however, this also entails the use of at least a limited release in most hands. We consider an open procedure to release the contracted structures more appropriate though results of gradual correction may be comparable at dedicated centers.
- Late OA seems more common in those with persistent hyperextension contracture and needs treatment later mostly arthrodesis or arthroplasty in select cases.

Hip: This includes:

- Two-thirds of patients have DDH and/or Frank dislocation. Closed reduction is rarely successful. Flexion contractures of hip are more difficult to treat.
- Operative reduction of such hips is needed to improve function or decrease pain. Assessment of function is tricky due to wide variability in function in these individuals as per the underlying severity of the disease. ROM at hips is crudely taken as a measure for functional assessment as often better movements entail good function. Stability, however, is as important we think to maintain gait and proper ambulation. Relocation procedures that improve stability carry a necessary risk of possible reduction of movements at hip and are deemed by many as reduced functionality so individualization is necessary.
- In general, considering the balance between movements and stability it is considered that for bilateral dislocation, physiotherapy, and rehabilitation improves function. The determinant in them of poor function is involvement of all four extremities.
- Those with unilateral dislocations have progressive scoliosis due to limb length inequality and fare poorly. To balance gait, surgical reduction of the hip at 1 year is more logical.
- Early open reduction and relocation of hips (by 6 months of age) is now purported to improve function even in bilateral dislocations. The only argument against this concept is that the surgery will be futile for nonambulators, but it is impossible to predict which child will be a nonambulator. This balance is hence shifting to early relocation of the hip explaining the parents that this will possibly improve function (even in bilateral dislocations) provided the child will be an ambulator due to limited effect from the disease else the surgery will have no effect in improving function in a nonambulator.
- Flexion contractures of >30° need surgical release.

Upper extremity: This includes:

In contrast to the lower extremities, the reconstruction of upper limb is performed from above to lower joints addressing the elbow, wrist, and then fingers in that order.

- The goals of surgical correction of upper extremity deformity are to help develop self-help skills (feeding and toileting) and mobility skills. Most patients do not require upper extremity surgical procedures and the function of whole arm should be considered while prescribing the treatment. Also both hands should be evaluated as a unit to understand the functional effectiveness together. For this reason the surgical procedures are usually delayed until the children are old enough to make such an assessment.
- The shoulder has minimal effect on overall functionality and the residual function is difficult to improve upon so no surgical correction is advised if ever.
- Elbow flexion is important and should be aimed for at least 90° for feeding and toileting. When both elbows are involved, surgery to increase flexion should only be done on one side. Such cases have fibrotic joint capsule and weak muscles that make the prospect of achieving active elbow flexion unlikely. Elbow joint capsulotomy, triceps lengthening along with a Steindler flexorplasty, a triceps transfer, or a pectoralis major transfer (to provide motor power) is commonly done. Due to extensive nature of surgery correction of only one side is recommended. The prerequisites for this procedure still are quite stringent:
  - Passive elbow flexion to a right angle
  - Transferred motor should have at least grade four strength power.
- To improve the hand-to-mouth function a distal humeral osteotomy that places the elbow into flexion and corrects

some of the shoulder internal rotation deformity may be performed toward the end of the first decade.

- In the characteristic deformity, the hand and wrist is usually flexed and ulnar deviated and the ulna-side digits are more involved. Early stretching should begin but proximal interphalangeal flexion deformities rarely respond to physical therapy or even surgery for that matter. Proximal row carpectomy may be done for flexed wrists some though prefer a dorsal wedge excision.
- Scoliosis in AMC responds poorly to bracing. The curves usually have a C-shaped, neuromuscular pattern and respond poorly to orthoses. Surgery (spinal fusion and instrumentation) is indicated for progressive curves interfering with balance or function that are generally >50°.

Larsen Syndrome

Larsen syndrome affects the development of bones throughout the body resulting in multiple joint problems present since birth. The signs and symptoms of Larsen syndrome vary widely even within the same family. Larsen syndrome occurs in approximately 1 in 100,000 newborns.

Genetics

This condition is inherited in an AD pattern. AR pattern has also been described with more severe phenotype but is less common. Uncommon sporadic mutations are also reported. Heterozygous mutations in the *FLNB* gene located on chromosome 3p14 cause Larsen syndrome. The *FLNB* gene provides instructions for making a protein called filamin B. This protein helps build the cytoskeleton that gives structure to cells and allows them to change shape and move. Filamin B binds to another protein called actin and also links it to many other proteins to perform various functions culminating ultimately to cell signaling that helps determine how the cytoskeleton will change as tissues grow and take shape during development. It thus plays an important role in vertebral segmentation, joint formation and endochondral ossification and is also seen mutated in atelosteogenesis types I and III, and in spondylocarpotarsal syndromes. Filamin B is especially important in the development of the skeleton before birth. It is expressed in the cell membranes of chondrocytes where it is involved in cell proliferation and differentiation, and ossification of cartilage. *FLNB* gene mutations produce an abnormal filamin B protein that interferes with the proliferation or differentiation of chondrocytes, impairing ossification, and producing characteristics of Larsen syndrome.

Clinical Features and Manifestations

The essential features of Larsen syndrome are:

- Congenital dislocations of multiple large joints—dislocations of the hip, knee, and elbow joint often bilateral. Knee dislocation should always raise the suspicion of Larsen syndrome. The tibia is dislocated anteriorly over femur.
- Craniofacial abnormalities and a characteristic flat face—hypertelorism, prominence of the forehead, micrognathia, a depressed nasal bridge, and a flattened midface. Cleft palate and short stature are often associated features.
- Ligamentous laxity, hypermobility, and short stature
- Equinovarus or equinovalgus bilateral foot deformities
- Scoliosis
- Cervical kyphosis that may be fatal if apex compresses the cord.
- The tips of their fingers, especially the thumbs, are typically blunt and square shaped (spatulate) with short terminal phalanx and pseudoclubbing.
- Hearing loss is caused by malformations in the tiny bones in the ears (ossicles).
- Supernumerary bones in wrist and ankle on radiographs
- Some patients have respiratory problems as a result of weakness of the airways that can lead to their partial closing, short pauses in breathing (apnea), and frequent respiratory infections.

BOX 5: The radiographic features of Larsen syndrome.

- Knees are dislocated with tibia lying anterior to femur.
- Elbows have complex radial-humeral, ulnar-humeral, and radial-ulnar dislocations.
- Radioulnar synostosis
- A spheroid ossicle anterior to the elbow joint (of unknown significance)
- There are an increased number of carpal centers of ossification
- *Foot:* Extra ossification centers in the foot and a curious double ossification pattern of the calcaneus.
- Abnormal cervical spine segmentation, with instability, is typical, and kyphosis a complication often associated with myelopathy.
- Arthrograms demonstrate:
  - Small or absent suprapatellar pouch
  - Absent cruciate ligaments
  - Misaligned patella

The radiographic features of Larsen syndrome are listed in **Box 5**.

Differential Diagnosis

- Otopalatodigital syndrome type 1 characterized by pugilistic facies, hearing loss, paddle-shaped metatarsal bones, no juxtacalcaneal bones, and no supernumerary carpal bones.
- *Natural history of disease:* The prognosis is generally good with aggressive orthopedic treatment, if the child survives the first year of life. The mortality in first year may be as high as 40%.

Treatment

Knee dislocation: The following are general guidelines and techniques used:

- The knee is usually reduced before the hips, although simultaneous procedures are possible.
- Although most knees do not respond to manipulation and cast correction, it is commonly ingrained in the minds of physicians to try this approach. Success is bleak and is associated with physeal fractures so we do not recommend manipulation for knee dislocation in Larsen syndrome.
- Reduction nearly always requires surgery but the knee may remain unstable even after reduction because of

the lack of major stabilizing ligaments. Surgery may be undertaken as early as 3–4 months of age. Long-term orthoses are often needed to guard against redislocation.

- Anterior cruciate ligament reconstruction has not been reported.

Hip joint: The following are general recommendations:

- The hips are dislocated (without acetabular dysplasia). Reduction of hip is surgically necessary and as for AMC there is trend towards earlier treatment. Reduction of the hip is, however, associated with a high redislocation rate and revision surgery. It is commonly agreed for this reason that pelvic osteotomies should be combined with open reduction when managing bilateral dislocations and is usually done after 1 year. For unilateral dislocation like AMC both knee and hip deformities are addressed together as the hyperextension deformity comes to advantage by restoring the flexion at knee and simultaneously reducing hip and applying spica cast that relaxes hamstrings. If required secondary osteotomy of the pelvis and femur can be performed later.

Clubfeet: The following is the commonly recommended approach:

- Till hip and knee are managed the feet are manipulated by Ponseti method and maintained in the best possible correction. Residual deformities can be surgically addressed after hip and knee deformities are corrected. The foot may need to be braced to control ankle instability.

Cervical kyphosis and dislocation: The common management is as follows:

- Kyphosis is often due to hypoplasia of the vertebral bodies. Early posterior stabilization (within the first 18 months of life) may avoid myelopathy and allow for correction of kyphotic deformity with growth.

Some anesthetic concerns: These include:

The mobile infolding arytenoid cartilage creates airway difficulties. The associated tracheomalacia can be especially problematic in the newborn. Cervical kyphosis should be properly addressed before giving general anesthesia. Congenital cardiac septal defects and acquired lesions of the mitral valve and aorta also complicate anesthesia management.

Freeman–Sheldon Syndrome (Distal Arthrogryposis Type II, Craniocarpotarsal Dystrophy; see Fig. 16)

This syndrome is usually sporadic, although some cases have AD and AR inheritance.

- It is recognized by its most characteristic feature, a "whistling face". The eyes are deeply set. The cheeks are fleshy, and pursed lips simulate whistling. There is a small mouth and a curious H-shaped dimple in the chin. The cause is unknown, but the buccinator muscle is hypoplastic histologically, there are similarities to AMC.
- Half of the patients have thoracic scoliosis that is more rigid than idiopathic curves and not always favorably respond to bracing.
- The hands demonstrate the classic distal arthrogryposis pattern described earlier. Other upper limb abnormalities include elbow contractures and decreased shoulder ROM.
- There is decreased neck ROM.
- Flexion deformity at knee is seen as are dislocated hips in some cases.
- Clubfoot is the most common foot deformity, with vertical talus being second most common.
- Dysphagia and aspiration lead to failure to thrive, and to death.

Treatment

- Upper limb is managed similar to that in AMC.
- The clubfoot and vertical talus deformities are resistant to nonoperative manipulation and surgical releases are necessary.
- During infancy, surgery to permit adequate mouth opening for feeding may be necessary.

PTERYGIA SYNDROME

"Pterygium" (Greek, means "little wing") is a web seen at the flexion creases commonly. Following forms are commonly seen:

- As an isolated malformation like the pterygium colli in the neck of patients with Klippel-Feil syndrome
- Multiple pterygium syndrome (AR)
- Popliteal pterygia syndrome (AD)

Lethal form (AR): The affected patient dies in utero or immediately after birth. It can be ultrasonologically diagnosed prenatally by detecting hydrops and cystic hygroma colli.

Multiple Pterygia Syndrome (Escobar Syndrome; Figs. 17A and B)

This is characterized by a web across every flexion crease in the extremities. The most common sites of pterygium formation are:

- Popliteal space
- Elbow
- Axilla
- Finger spaces are webbed
    - Across the neck laterally
    - Anterior midline pterygium extending from sternum to the chin drawing the face down.

Mobility is restricted by the lower extremity pterygium and respiratory compromise may arise out of lordoscoliosis. Adaptive changes in the joints occur over time. Radiographically, the patella becomes elongated, and the femoral condyles flattened, as a result of knee flexion deformity. Though the changes are restricted to lower extremities in

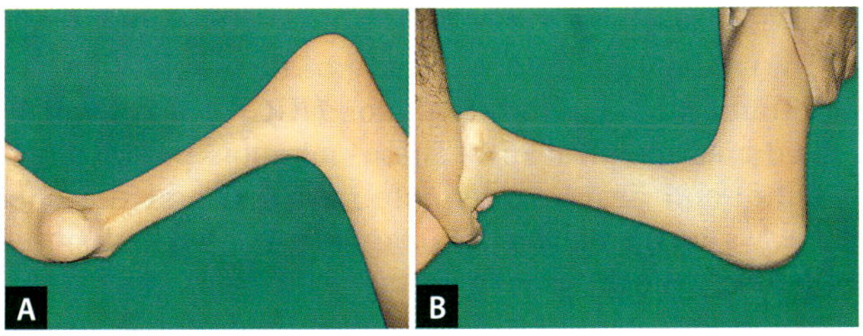

Figs. 17A and B: Pterygia syndrome.

popliteal pterygium syndrome, mild webs in joints of the upper extremity may be found in these patients also.

Differential Diagnosis

Arthrogryposis multiplex congenita (particularly if the web spaces are not well formed). Presence of vertical talus and congenital spine deformity (multiple segmentation abnormalities and a lordoscoliosis) differentiate the Escobar syndrome from AMC.

Treatment

- Surgery is rarely needed for the upper extremities.
- Preoperative evaluation of intraspinal contents by MRI and ultrasound of the kidney should be done. The thoracic vertebral dysplasia, thoracic lordosis, and the small chest impair lung development, resulting in death in the first years of life in those with multiple pterygium syndrome. For the longer-term survivor the spine deformity is managed in a way similar to those with nonsyndromic congenital scoliosis.
- As mobility is primarily restricted by knee pterygia it is commonly aggressively addressed. Treatment of the knee though begins with physical therapy, early popliteal web surgery is recommended before the onset of adaptive changes in the articular surfaces, and before further vascular shortening. The nerve is usually located just deep to the skin and web requiring careful dissection. The web is resected, and Z-plasty of the skin is performed. High recurrence rates are seen despite braces.
- Femoral shortening and extension osteotomy are usually postponed until near or after maturity. However, this is not to be strictly followed and if almost full knee extension cannot be achieved at surgery during infancy or childhood femoral shortening should be considered.
- Gradual distraction techniques have also been described. Posterior soft tissue procedures can be combined with distraction techniques to gradually extend the knee.

FETAL ALCOHOL SYNDROME

Fetal alcohol syndrome is a pattern of malformations seen in children born to alcoholic mothers. Lesser manifestations of the syndrome, known as fetal alcohol effects, may be related to more moderate alcohol ingestion. The full-blown syndrome is only seen if mother drink throughout pregnancy. The overall incidence of full-blown fetal alcohol syndrome is 0.33 per 1,000 live births. For an alcoholic mother, there is a 30% risk for fetal alcohol syndrome in her child.

Features

- The cardinal feature is reduced growth; the children have intrauterine growth retardation (IUGR), small weight, and small length at birth. These limitations persist during childhood despite adequate nutrition and the child always looks small for age. The patients often look similar to those who are growth hormone deficient.
- The second cardinal feature is disturbed central nervous system development (similar to cerebral palsy). The typical child has a small head, a small brain, and delayed motor milestones. Hypotonia is present early but many develop spasticity later.
- The face has three typical characteristics:
  1. Short palpebral fissures (small eyes)
  2. Flat philtrum (no groove below the nose)
  3. Thin upper lip.
- Orthopedic manifestations:
  - At birth, the ROM of the hands and feet is restricted. The contractures respond well to physical therapy.
  - Clubfoot is common and DDH is seen in few patients. The clubfoot is commonly easily treated by manipulation.
  - Cervical spine fusions (especially C2 and C3) are incidentally discovered on radiographs (similar to Klippel–Feil syndrome).
  - Synostoses are common in the upper extremity (commonly the radioulnar and the carpal bones).
  - Stippled epiphyses may be seen in the lower extremities.

Treatment and Prognosis

The orthopedic problems are managed in a standard way. The future for children with fetal alcohol is bleak. Intellect remains retarded and future development is often dicey due to social factors also.

PRADER–WILLI SYNDROME

Prader–Willi syndrome represents an example of genetic imprinting arising out of the loss of chromosome 15 from paternal origin. The syndrome is characterized by hypotonia, obesity, hypogonadism, short stature, small hands and feet, and mental deficiency and it may be remembered with an "H" mnemonic:

- **H**ypotonia
- **H**ypogonadism
- **H**yperphagia
- **H**ypomentation
- Small **h**ands

All probably based on a **h**ypothalamic disorder.

The incidence is 1 in 5,000 births, with a prevalence in the population of 1 in 16,000–25,000.

Clinical Features and Natural History of Disease

- As newborns these patients are floppy babies, having hypotonia, poor feeding, and delayed milestones. Some may have DDH.
- After 1 or 2 years of age characteristic face of upward slanting, almond-shaped eyes appear, obesity begins, and there is voracious eating disorder suggesting the diagnosis. Often the patient has an insatiable appetite. Obesity has a central distribution, sparing the distal limbs.
- The patient has short stature, below the 10th percentile, with an ultimate height of not more than 150 cm (59 inches).
- There is no adolescent growth spurt. The genitalia are hypoplastic and the patient has small hands and feet.

- Patients have variable grade of mental retardation and skills for independent living are nonexistent.

Treatment

Dedicated behavioral modification programs are occasionally effective, and fenfluramine can be tried to control appetite.

ANGELMAN SYNDROME (HAPPY PUPPET SYNDROME)

Angelman syndrome is the counterpart of Prader–Willi syndrome that arises from absence of *maternal* chromosome 15.

- These patients are small and mentally retarded, and they have athetosis and seizures.
- About 50–90% have juvenile-onset scoliosis.
- The legs are malaligned, with genu valgum and pes planus.

Treatment

Scoliosis is difficult to control with an orthosis due to obesity; anesthesia risk is also similarly high. Growth hormone may improve body composition, fat utilization, physical strength, and growth but large trials are unavailable.

BECKWITH–WIEDEMANN SYNDROME

Beckwith–Wiedemann (BW) syndrome is presented by a triad of:

1. Organomegaly
2. Omphalocele
3. A large tongue

The incidence is 1 in 14,000 with AD trait of variable expression. BW syndrome is linked to chromosome *11p15*, which is near the Wilms' tumor gene (*11p13*) and the insulin-like growth factor gene (*11p15.5*) with paternal genomic imprinting.

- Patients are large for age (as against the fetal alcohol syndrome). It is a true hemihypertrophy but the growth is asymmetric in 20% which can be significant if the spastic hemiplegia affects the smaller side.
- The tongue is gigantic at birth and although it tends to regress, hemiglossectomy is sometimes needed.
- Omphalocele is common, helps identification of disease at birth (around 15% of cases).
- The abdominal viscera are enlarged due to single cell hypertrophy.
  - In the adrenals, giant cortical cells.
  - In the gonads, increased number of interstitial cells.
  - In the pancreas, islet cell hyperplasia causes hypoglycemia and seizures by day 2 or 3 and should be identified early to prevent consequences. If there is CNS damage then cerebral palsy like picture appears.
- For an orthopedist two features suggest the diagnosis: (1) spastic cerebral palsy and (2) hemihypertrophy. The former is due possibly to neonatal hypoglycemia but spastic hemiplegia is most commonly seen. The patients with cerebral palsy are small while those with BW syndrome are large so can be differentiated. Scoliosis is common, mostly idiopathic type with similar management. Cavus feet, dislocated radial heads, and occasional cases of polydactyly can also be seen.

There is 10% risk of developing benign or malignant tumors. Wilms' tumor is the most common. The proximity of the BW gene locus and the embryonal tumor gene loci accounts for the higher incidence of tumors seen in this syndrome. Abdominal ultrasounds at regular intervals (4 months) until the age of 6 years, to screen for Wilms' tumor, are advocated.

TRICHORHINOPHALANGEAL SYNDROME

There are two basic types: types I and II with significant overlap. Both trichorhinophalangeal (TRP) I and TRP II are due to mutation or loss of the *TRPS1* gene. However, TRP II is due to a larger loss of the chromosomal region, with loss of the adjacent gene, *EXT-1*, as well. The *EXT-1* gene is one of the genes responsible for hereditary exostoses, explaining the associated exostoses. Larger loss of *TRPS1* gene leads to mental retardation.

- Patients with TRP I have a pear-shaped, bulbous nose, prominent ears, sparse hair, and cone epiphyses (seen after 3 or 4 years of age). The thumbs are broad, and the fingers are often angled at the distal interphalangeal and proximal interphalangeal joints. Radiographically, the hand in a patient with TRP I or TRP II shows short fourth and fifth metacarpals. The function of hand is but not or mildly compromised. The hips mimic a Perthes-like disease unilaterally or bilaterally that progresses to MED like changes and then precocious arthritis. They have mild growth retardation. There may be lax ligaments.
- Patients with TRP II (Langer–Giedion syndrome) have multiple exostoses, especially involving the lower extremities. There is a higher chance of mental retardation in TRP II. In infancy, the skin is redundant and loose, which may be severe enough to mimic EDS. Marked ligamentous laxity may further support this error in diagnosis. There is a tendency toward fractures. The features that are similar to type I include the typical facial features and cone epiphyses, microcephaly, large and protruding ears, and sparse scalp hair. Also they have the Perthes-like picture and the hand anomalies similar to TRP I.

Treatment

Osteotomy of the thumb may be needed. Perthes disease should be managed like standard radiological changes and classic Perthes disease. A large exostosis may require excision.

PROGERIA (HUTCHINSON–GILFORD SYNDROME)

Progeria is characterized by premature aging but is exceedingly rare. AD and recessive inheritance patterns have been proposed, but a sporadic mutation is more likely. Instead of true aging or accelerated aging process the normal tissues undergo a degenerative change that mimics normal aging. The principal tissues involved include the skin, subcutaneous tissue, bone, and cardiovascular system. There are no cataracts; there is no senility.

These individuals have abnormally low levels of growth hormones (hormone supplementation increases growth velocity, but not result in improved survival). The cause is unknown but fibroblasts from these individuals have a variety of abnormalities, including a deficient ability to clear free radicals. There is severe growth retardation and an inability to gain weight. Those surviving to adolescence show no pubertal growth spurt. Alopecia and a loss of subcutaneous fat cause the appearance of a skinny old man or woman. These patients have periarticular fibrosis. Osteolysis occurs in the fingertips, clavicle, and proximal humerus. The vertebrae may become quickly osteoporotic with classical fish-mouth appearance, radiographically. Fractures due to bone weakness are common with compromised healing process and delayed union. There is late DDH and coxa valga. The children do not live long enough to develop arthritis. Atherosclerosis with myocardial infarction by 10 years of age is the rule, and life expectancy rarely exceeds 20 years.

Treatment

Treatment is still not available primarily due to lack of understanding of the disorder. One should not increase suffering by surgery. Hip surgery is indicated only if there is a documented functional impairment; one should refrain from it.

RUBINSTEIN–TAYBI SYNDROME

The Rubinstein–Taybi syndrome is characterized by the following:

- Mental retardation
- *Digital changes:* Consisting mainly of broad thumbs (broad terminal phalanges) and large toes. Great toes are affected in all cases. Radial angulation of thumb is seen in half of patients and hallux varus is seen in many.
- *Characteristic facies:* Comical face with a Cyrano de Bergerac-like nose and the nasal septum extending below the nostrils. The facial changes improve with time and are not reliable for diagnosis.

Genetics

Patients with Rubinstein–Taybi syndrome have microdeletions of chromosome 16p13.3. This region contains gene for CREB-binding protein, a nuclear protein participating as a coactivator in cyclic adenosine monophosphate (AMP) regulated gene expression. This protein plays an important role in the development of CNS, head, and neck. Clinical features are thus explained by mutation. It is relatively common in the mentally retarded population, with an incidence of 1 in 500 in this population.

Clinical Features

Apart from the above there is microcephaly, patellar dislocation, visual disturbances, congenital heart disease, and gastrointestinal abnormalities. There is no true pubertal growth spurt and severe dental caries are common. There is some predisposition to certain types of central nervous system, head, and neck tumors.

Radiologically, the thumb shows a wide distal phalanx and a triangular proximal phalanx (i.e., delta phalanx) that accounts for the radial deviation. The toe may have a duplicated or broad distal phalanx, but true polydactyly is not seen.

Treatment

The thumb is treated to correct radial deviation by osteotomy of the proximal phalanx. The deformity is progressive and recurrence is common. The toe rarely requires treatment except for hallux varus. Patellar dislocation is treated in standard way but additionally needs extensive quadriceps mobilization to decrease the revision rate. Anesthetic risk is increased due to conductive heart defects and these patients are sensitive to neuromuscular blocking agents, which tend to induce arrhythmias and prolong awakening from anesthesia.

CONGENITAL CONSTRICTION BAND SYNDROME

[Amniotic band syndrome, Streeter dysplasia, Amniotic deformity, adhesions, mutilations (ADAM) complex, Amniotic band constriction, Ring constriction syndrome, Amniotic band sequence, and Pseudoainhum]

This is a common cause of terminal congenital malformation of limbs, with a reported incidence of 1 in 15,000 and believed to be the cause of 178 in 10,000 miscarriages. It affects both sexes equally. The three main components include:

1. Acrosyndactyly
2. Superficial or deep constriction bands involving a digit or extremity
3. Intrauterine amputation

Etiology

Despite many theories (developmental problems in the formation of limb connective tissues, germ plasma defect, histology, and maternal trauma leading to a rupture of the amniotic membrane), the etiopathogenesis of constriction band syndrome remains unclear. There are two main and conflicting theories that portend intrinsic or extrinsic initiation to the embryo or fetus. The disorder may be more heterogeneous than considered in the past.

- The *intrinsic theory* by George Streeter (Director of Embryology at Carnegie Institute, in 1930) proposed that a defect of the subcutaneous germplasm caused soft tissue necrosis and subsequent healing, with the formation of constriction bands. His theory consisted of a disrupting event occurring during blastogenesis which leads to soft tissue sloughing off without formation of amniotic bands. Then, external healing of the slough begins leading to the constricting rings resulting in local developmental defects. There is evidence that in utero vascular disruption from the death of a co-twin, or from placentally derived embolic infarcts, can cause constriction band syndrome and that the infant affected is born with the amnion intact. The support also comes from finding that renal and cardiac abnormalities occur in 37% cases where amniotic bands cannot reach. He explained the ring constrictions as areas of defectively formed tissue due to defective germ plasma areas. In these children, there was no ultrasound evidence of amniotic bands. It appears this syndrome may result from factors other than amniotic entanglement. This theory lends the eponym "Streeter's dysplasia" to the entity.

- The *extrinsic theory* has the widest acceptance. Richard Torpin (Obstetrician, in 1965) has proposed that entanglement of the limbs in defects or free strands of amnion result in constriction band syndrome from which the other eponyms have risen **(Fig. 18)**. His theory was first suggested by Hippocrates that maternal trauma lead to rupture of the amniotic membrane. Proceeding rupture, the amniotic sac stops growing properly and eventually separates from the chorion. The chorionic side of the amnion emanates numerous mesoblastic fibrous strings which entrap and catch the fetal parts. This then leads to the constriction of the body part stopping blood flow to that area leading to fetal amputations as one of many consequences. Similar explanation has been given by Michael Harrison who explains that amniotic band syndrome occurs when the inner membrane ruptures, or tears, without injury to the outer membrane. The developing fetus is still floating in fluid but is then exposed to the floating tissue from the ruptured amnion. This floating tissue can become entangled around the fetus. Supportive evidence includes the lack of hereditary factors, the ultrasonographic demonstration of prenatal amniotic bands, the involvement of the longer digits and the histologic demonstration of amnion in constriction bands. Experimentally amniocentesis in animals produces fetal malformations that resemble constriction band syndrome in humans. Kino demonstrated in rats that these malformations result from subcutaneous hemorrhages that are caused by excessive uterine contractions after amniocentesis.

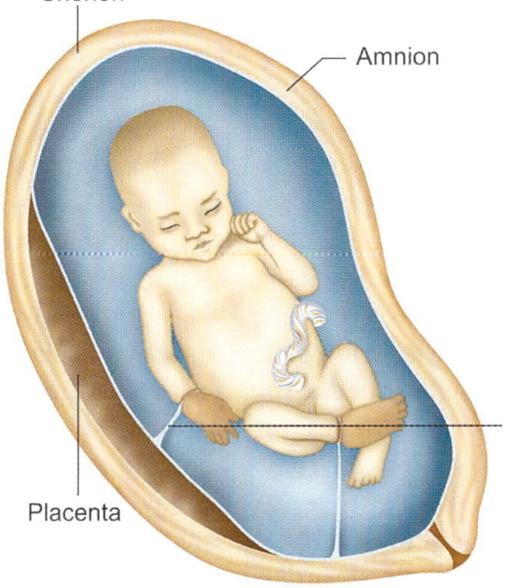

Fig. 18: Congenital constriction band syndrome.

Clinical Features

The clinical presentation is quite variable. The severity of the problem depends on the location and the tension of the band and if severe can be life-threatening for the fetus. For example, a band becoming wrapped around areas such as the head or umbilical cord might get fatal. The bands may be superficial and incomplete or extend deeply to the underlying bone, and be circumferential. Indentations occur when the fibrous bands were not tight enough to cause amputation of the limb. However, after the fetus is born this could lead to edema if not surgically corrected. Amputations are prevalent when the limbs of the fetus were not able to grow due to the band entirely preventing blood flow to the area causing necrosis, or cell death. Two bands may be present in one extremity. Distal to the band, there may be significant neurovascular impairment. Impaired venous and lymphatic drainage causes swelling of the limb distal to the constriction. With growth, the constriction band occasionally gets more severe and becomes symptomatic. If these bands cross the body, congenital fissure of the chest wall can happen, this is called thoracoschisis. Upper extremity involvement is more frequent than the lower extremity. Head, neck, or trunk constriction bands are very uncommon. Constriction bands across the face and head however may possibly lead to facial clefts, and if extended into the cranium encephaloceles can occur. The distal aspect of the limb, particularly the longest digits (index, long, and ring fingers, and great, second, and third toes) are most frequently affected. In some cases these bands act as thread threading digits together resulting in a condition called acrosyndactylization. Acrosyndactylization can vary in severity from a few digits being bound together to multidigit.

Patterson developed a classification system based on the severity of the syndrome:

- Simple constriction rings
- Constriction rings associated with deformity of the distal part, with or without lymphedema
- Constriction rings associated with syndactyly and intrauterine amputation

The orthopedically important features of constriction band syndrome are the following:

- *Amputations and syndactyly* are seen in more than one-half of affected children—transverse, terminal, and digital amputations. The proximal skeletal development is normal. Simple syndactyly is commonly compared to complex syndactyly with bony fusions. Acrosyndactyly or fenestrated syndactyly can also be seen. Hypoplastic or absent nails are consistently present.
- *Clubfoot:* The incidence of clubfoot in constriction band syndrome is variable (12–56%). These feet are often rigid and more difficult to treat. Most of these feet have weakness of the peroneal muscles (paralytic form) and are always associated with ipsilateral constriction bands. They are caused by deep constriction bands that may press upon peroneal nerve to cause compression neuropathy, direct muscle injury, or even a compartment syndrome. The nonparalytic clubfeet usually are devoid

of constriction bands and are considered to be idiopathic clubfeet or resulting from oligohydramnios.
- *Angular deformity, bone dysplasia, and pseudarthrosis* can occur deep to constriction bands in the upper and lower extremities. The anterolateral tibial bowing appears similar to that seen in congenital pseudarthrosis of the tibia associated with NF. They, however, differ by bone healing, and remodeling following realignment osteotomies. Zionts et al. prefer the term "discontinuity", rather than "pseudarthrosis", because they spontaneously heal.
- *Leg-length discrepancy* is seen in fourth of the patients. Surgical management is needed in some depending on the predicted discrepancy at skeletal maturity.

Differential Diagnosis

- "Michelin tire baby syndrome" (multiple benign circumferential skin creases, disappear by 5 years, transmitted autosomal dominantly).
- Hair-thread constriction (occur in infants, usually younger than 2 years of age from hair or thread wrapped around the fingers or toes and cause circulatory compromise).
- Ainhum (mainly seen in Africa) is a disorder characterized by ulceration at the base of the fifth toe on the plantar surface, which progresses to a circumferential constriction ring with autoamputation.

Treatment

- For deep constrictions (extending beneath subcutaneous fat and fascia) excision of the band and closure with multiple Z-plasties is done. This is highly indicated especially if there is edema distal to the band, in the presence of vascular insufficiency or neurologic deficit, and if the band is increasing in severity. It is originally done in a staged manner releasing one-half of the bands at a time with a 6–12 weeks interval. This is due to the concern that impaired venous or lymphatic flow and skin-flap necrosis could result in complete single-stage release. Single-stage releases of constriction bands have been found safe however.
- The constriction band and underlying fibrous tissue in the subcutaneous tissue, fascia, and muscle are completely excised with an adjacent 1–2 mm cuff of normal tissue. To avoid injury to already compressed, damaged and often inconspicuous neurovascular structures, they should be exposed proximally or distally and followed under the band. The wound is closed with Z-plasties fashioned with large flaps at a 60° angle. In children with ischemia of the distal limb, a fasciotomy may be required.
- Nonparalytic clubfeet in neonates with an ipsilateral constriction band can be treated by serial manipulation and casting, however, resection of the constriction band should be done prior to surgical release of the clubfoot. In paralytic clubfoot, nonoperative management is rarely successful if ever. Muscle imbalance of the foot, resulting from peroneal weakness, should be managed by a split transfer of the tibialis anterior tendon (*see* Chapter on "Clubfoot—Congenital Talipes Equinovarus").
- Surgical intervention in children with acrosyndactyly is generally done between the ages of 6 months and 1 year because of the severity of the deformity and to allow for longitudinal growth and function.

MELORHEOSTOSIS

(Also known as Leri disease, melos meaning "limb" and rhein meaning "to flow", as in wax)

Melorheostosis was first described by Leri and Joanny in 1922. It is a nonhereditary mesenchymal dysplasia. The distinguishing feature from other forms of sclerosing bone disease is association with soft tissue contractures in childhood overlying slowly evolving dysplastic linear hyperostosis (dripping wax or flowing candle wax appearance radiologically).

Clinical Features

Both sexes are equally affected. The prevalence of the disease is 0.9 per million and half the cases are diagnosed before 20 years of age. They are typically painless, asymmetric joint contractures developing quite early (by 6 years of age) in lower extremities. A significant number of cases have a benign appearance of the disease with symptoms occurring only later in life. Upper extremities are less frequently involved. Melorheostosis may involve only one bone (monostotic), one limb (monomelic), or multiple bones (polyostotic). It is almost always unilateral. The underlying hyperostosis develops slowly and progresses with age, usually more rapidly in childhood. Intra-articular extension of disease occurs in 35% of patients. The overlying soft tissues show thickening that may arise from the following:
- Fibrolipoma
- Lymphedema
- Osteoid or chondral elements that are unossified
- Sclerodermatous skin changes (thickening and fibrosis)
- Vascular malformations

The muscles are atrophied. Periarticular fibrosis with flexion contractures at the knee, hip, finger, ankle equinus, and patellar dislocation are the most common joint deformities. Valgus and varus deformities around the knee and ankle develop due to fibrosis and physeal abnormalities. Limb lengthening or shortening can both be seen.

Etiology

The etiology is unknown but the lesions are distributed along sclerotomes. So a popular hypothesis is that it is caused by an infection analogous to herpes zoster that spread along the distribution of affected nerve roots with associated scarring and osseous changes. Mixed sclerosing bone dysplasia is comprised of melorheostosis, osteopoikilosis and/or osteopathia striata in the same individual. There is a high likelihood of common etiopathogenesis of the three diseases arising from mutations in the *LEMD3* gene. These three rare bone dysplasias are thus postulated to have a close association but the clinical features vary in individuals as is frustratingly common in genetic diseases. Mutation of the *LEMD3* gene may produce a segmental sensory nerve disorder to cause sclerotomal distribution typically seen (Murray and McCredie).

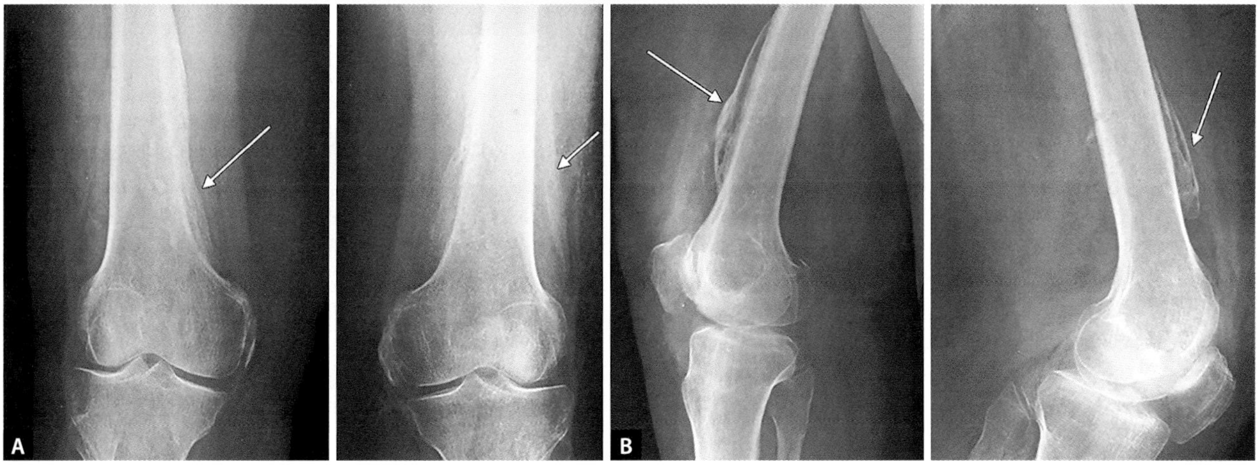

Figs. 19A and B: The characteristic radiographic appearance of melorheostosis as viewed on anteroposterior (AP) and lateral radiographs of both femora (arrows). The extra bone formation usually involves the diaphyseal and diaphyseal-metaphyseal region appearing like flowing molten wax.

Radiographic Features

The classic appearance on an X-ray is asymmetrical bands of sclerosis in an irregular, linear pattern colloquially described as molten wax flowing down the side of a candle. There is difference in the location of hyperostosis in children and adults whereby it is endosteal in the former while extracortical, subperiosteal hyperostosis is seen in adults. Five patterns of hyperostosis are described:

1. Classic
2. Osteoma like
3. Myositis ossificans like
4. Osteopathia striata like
5. Mixed

The hyperostosis is seen typically on one side of the diaphysis of long bones **(Figs. 19A and B)** and may flow across the joints to other side bone. The ribs, skull, and spine are affected least. In the carpal and tarsal bones patches of hyperostosis, rather than a linear pattern are seen (similar to osteopoikilosis). Increased uptake is noted in involved areas on bone scan.

Histologically, the hyperostosis consists of woven or nonlamellar dense bone with thickened, sclerotic, and irregular laminae.

Differential Diagnosis

The differential diagnosis includes osteomyelitis, osteopetrosis, osteopoikilosis, and osteopathia striata, all of which can have similar radiographic findings. Osteoma, osteoid osteoma, and myositis are other differentials. The transient periosteal reaction in infantile cortical hyperostosis is less dense and is found in different locations. Focal scleroderma may cause soft tissue fibrosis and contractures but the bones are radiologically normal.

Treatment

Most patients are asymptomatic. In symptomatic patients the soft tissue contractures are primary concern. These contractures are resistant to manipulation or casting. Nonsteroidal anti-inflammatory medications can control pain. Surgical treatment is often indicated for soft tissue contracture releases and capsulotomies. Bone deformities and osteotomies are difficult and incomplete correction or rapid recurrence of the deformity is common. Extreme deformities that have been uncorrected after multiple surgical treatments may need amputation. Gradual corrections have been attempted with Ilizarov technique, distal limb ischemia can occur when the chronically contracted and flexed joint is extended. Bone shortening osteotomies can be a good salvage and avoid this complication. The Ilizarov technique can also be used for realignment of angular deformities.

OSTEOPOIKILOSIS (OSTEOPATHIA CONDENSANS DISSEMINATA)

This disorder is characterized by numerous small foci of increased radiodensity in the periarticular regions.

These enostoses represent sclerosing bone dysplasia. It develops during childhood, without any gender predilection, and persists throughout the life. Often it is asymptomatic but some may have mild articular discomfort with a joint effusion. There is no evidence for predisposition to malignancy. Osteopoikilosis is frequently seen in association with a hereditary dermatologic condition: dermatofibrosis lenticularis disseminata or Buschke-Ollendorff syndrome, where the skin has papular fibromas. This syndrome is usually asymptomatic but soft tissue fibrosis and joint contractures can occur in these children that appear clinically similar to that seen in melorheostosis.

Diagnosis

The diagnosis is often an incidental radiological finding. Bone function is unhampered, fractures heal uneventfully and pathological fractures have not been reported.

Radiographic Features

The osteosclerotic nodules are well defined, homogeneous, bilateral, circular to ovoid-shaped from 1–15 mm, located in the metaphyses and epiphyses of long bones, the carpus, the tarsus, the pelvis **(Figs. 20A and B)**, and the scapulae. The

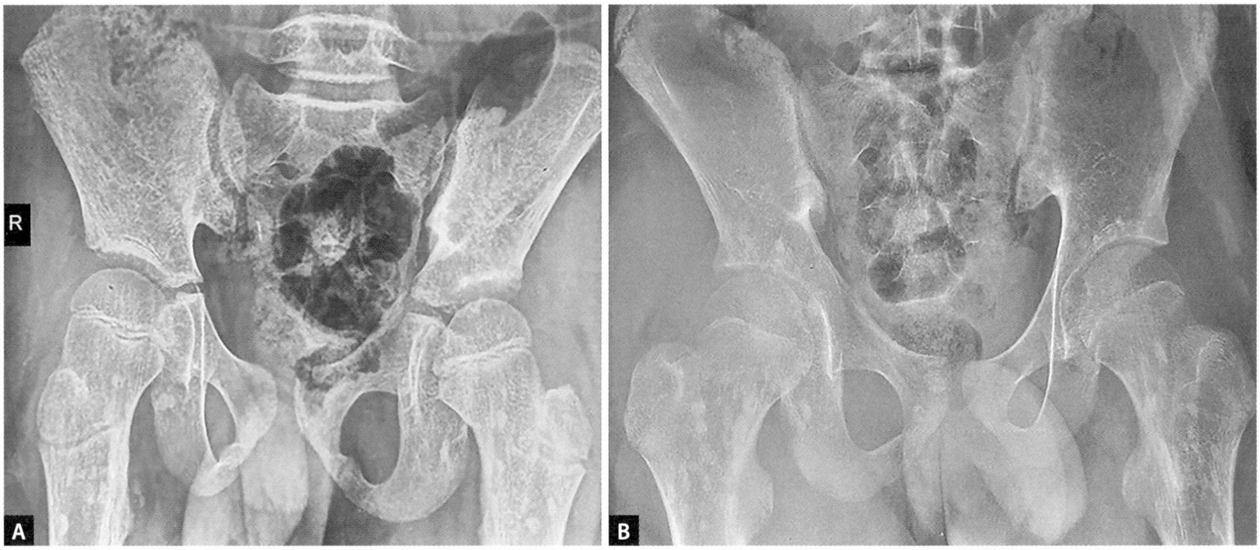

Figs. 20A and B: The radiographs of a child with osteopoikilosis. The round to oval bone lesions involve epiphysis and metaphyseal regions of the proximal femora (A) and have started to appear in the pelvic bones (see acetabular rim, B) with passing age.

sclerotic areas consist of focal condensations of compact lamellar bone within the spongiosa. The ribs, clavicle, and skull are not involved. The lesions may increase or decrease in size or number. The bone scan usually does not demonstrate increased uptake in the lesions suggesting inactivity and it helps to differentiate this condition from metastatic breast or prostate carcinoma.

It also has sclerotomal distribution and is associated with abnormalities of mesodermal tissues suggesting a relationship with osteosclerotic disorders.

Treatment

There is no treatment for this benign disorder. In the rare cases of associated fibrosis and joint contracture, the management is the same as for melorheostosis.

PYKNODYSOSTOSIS

Pyknodysostosis ["pucnos" (dense), "dys" (defective), and "ostosis" (bone condition)] is a rare AR disorder of bones and is called osteopetrosis acro-osteolytica or Toulouse-Lautrec syndrome. The name Toulouse-Lautrec syndrome is derived from the French impressionist, Henri Marie Raymond de Toulouse-Lautrec-Monfa who was a victim of this unusual disorder.

Clinical Features

- Shortness of stature (prominently acromelia)
- Short broad hands with stubby fingers
- Onychodysplasia (hypoplasia of nails)
- Nasal beaking and relative proptosis on observing face from side
- Delayed closure of fontanels causing frontal and occipital bossing
- Underdevelopment of the mandible (with relative prognathism) and abnormal dentition (persistence of primary teeth)

The presence of blue sclerae and propensity to fracture may cause confusion with osteogenesis imperfecta. The condition is caused by a lysosomal disorder due to genetic deficiency in cathepsin K (essential for normal osteoclast function) which has been mapped to chromosome 1q21 and is inherited as an AR trait.

Radiologically, the bones are dense (osteosclerosis) with narrowed medullary canal in a generalized fashion; the skull is enlarged, with wide suture lines, calvarial thickening and open fontanels, but the facial bones and mandible are hypoplastic, thus accounting for the typical "triangular" facies. Mandible has prominent obtuse angle. There may be partial agenesis of terminal phalanges of fingers appearing as acro-osteolysis. There is delayed bone age radiologically. Spine demonstrates increased lumbar lordosis, vertebral body sclerosis, and vertebral segmentation abnormalities in upper cervical and lower lumbar region. The most important radiological differential is osteopetrosis.

Management

Despite appearances, it causes little trouble (apart from the odd pathological fracture) and needs no treatment.

OSTEOPATHIA STRIATA

Osteopathia striata, or Voorhoeve disease, is characterized by dense linear striations in bone. This is a rare, AD disorder with the diagnosis usually made on an incidental radiograph.

Radiographic Features

Hallmark is dense linear striations seen in tubular and flat bones with the exception of the skull and clavicles. These lesions do not change with time. In the long bones, the striations are parallel to the long axis and affect principally the metaphyses and sometimes the epiphyses. A fan-shaped pattern of linear striations can be seen in the iliac wings. The

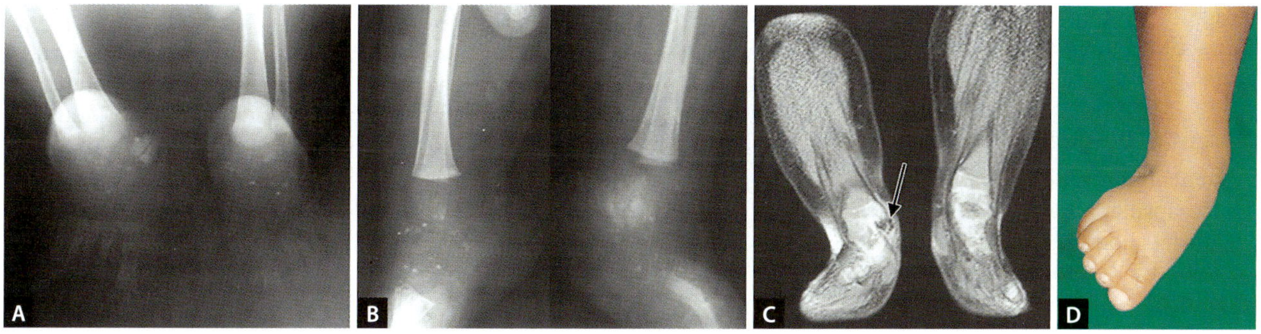

Figs. 21A to D: Trevor disease. (A and B) Note the dysplastic tarsal bones and tibial physis distally; (C) The MRI demonstrates dysplastic changes in the ankle mortise, tarsal bones, and metatarsal complex on right side. The foci of fine calcifications at medial malleolus (arrow) are suggestive more of Trevor disease; (D) Forefoot valgus is also more prominent at the right side.

lesions are metabolically inactive and do not predispose to malignancy. Bone scan does not show increased uptake.

Osteopathia striata, occasionally, is a component of osteopathia striata with cranial sclerosis and mixed sclerosing bone dysplasia.

Treatment

Treatment is not required for asymptomatic isolated osteopathia striata.

DYSPLASIA EPIPHYSEALIS HEMIMELICA

[Fairbank's disease, Tarsoepiphyseal aclasia, Epiphyseal chondrodystrophy, Dysplasia epiphysealis hemimelica (DEH), Epiphyseal osteochondroma, Tarsomegaly, and Trevor disease]

Dysplasia epiphysealis hemimelica is a rare nonhereditary, developmental disorder of localized epiphyseal osteochondral overgrowth, involving single or multiple epiphyses. It was termed "tarsomegalie" by Mouchet and Belot but later described by Trevor, who termed the disorder "tarsoepiphysial aclasis". Fairbank later suggested the currently accepted term "dysplasia epiphysealis hemimelica". This term describes the predilection for unilateral involvement of the medial or lateral aspect of one or more epiphyses. The medial aspect of the epiphysis is commonly affected (twice as common as lateral). When multiple sites are affected the disease is usually unilateral, and the lesion can present on both sides of an affected joint.

Etiology

Trevor considered it to be a congenital error of skeletal development with an altered process of cell division at the superficial zone of articular cartilage (now considered to be from perichondrial ring of LaCroix). This allows for persistent proliferation and production of a large cartilaginous mass like an exostosis. Fairbank considered it to be a localized disturbance of the pre- or postaxial part of the apical cap of the limb bud in early fetal development.

Clinical Features

The disorder affects 1 per million population, with a predilection for males. Presentation is usually in childhood or early adolescence. Patients typically complain of painless swelling or a mass on one side of a joint (commonly the knee or ankle), limitation of motion, and occasionally locking, angular deformity, limp, regional muscle wasting, or limb-length discrepancy. The lower limbs are commonly affected with the distal ends of the limb developing the disorder more frequently. Distal femur is one of the most common sites. In cases of multiple sites of involvement, the lesions are characteristically unilateral, although rare bilateral cases are reported. Three forms of disease affection have been described (Azouz et al.):

1. *Classic form (involving more than one bone in a single limb):* This is the most common form. It has characteristic hemimelic distribution involving more than one bone or epiphysis within a single lower extremity.
2. *Localized form (involving only one epiphysis):* Single bone affection, unilateral or bilateral.
3. *Generalized form (involving an entire lower extremity from the pelvis to foot):* Involving whole limb from pelvis to foot.

Apart from knee (femur) and ankle (talus, **Figs. 21A to D**), other reported sites include the capital femoral epiphysis and acetabulum, sacroiliac joint, metacarpophalangeal joint, wrist, shoulder, and subtalar joint.

Radiographic Features

Typically the lesion is an irregular often multicentric lobulated mass protruding directly from one side of the affected epiphysis or tarsal bone. The affected ossification center appears prematurely, and may be larger than the contralateral side. Modeling abnormalities of the adjacent metaphysis have also been reported. Early lesions present with only joint space enlargement, small foci of irregular calcification appears with some maturation. With further maturation, the lesion enlarges and ossifies, and becomes confluent with the underlying epiphyseal bone.

MRI demonstrates the extent of the lesion better and also depicts the cleavage plane between the lesion and the underlying epiphysis.

Histopathology

The lesion resembles an osteochondroma without discrete stalk (sessile). Microscopically there is a boundary of cartilage separating the lesion from the underlying bony epiphysis. Malignant degeneration of the lesion has not been reported.

Differential Diagnosis

- Osteochondroma
- Intracapsular para-articular chondroma
- Synovial chondromatosis

Treatment

If the cartilaginous overgrowth is not on the weight-bearing surface of the joint (i.e., juxta-articular lesions), excision is advisable to relieve pain and improve function. Recurrence of the lesion prior to skeletal maturity has been reported. Associated angular deformities often correct after excision.

The treatment of articular lesions in weight-bearing region is somewhat controversial. Excision is followed by pain and degeneration in most and results are not satisfactory. Corrective osteotomies to correct the angular deformity without excision of mass is preferred if an arthrogram demonstrates a smooth joint surface.

CONCLUSION

- Birth defects and anomalies comprise an important aspect of pediatric orthopedic practice apart from trauma.
- It is important to recognize them well and identify the associated abnormalities to provide a comprehensive treatment. This entails that the orthopedic surgeon should be well versed with the important and related aspects of the various congenital and syndromic anomalies.
- Although an orthopedic surgeon is more concerned about the surgical aspects of management, he should also have updated information on the medical management of the disorders that can be thoroughly incorporated in the overall management of the patients. It is also important to realize that medical and orthotic management often comprise a majority part in the preoperative and postoperative management of these patients, surgical management is mostly limited to deformity correction and is often a point event in the management protocols.
- One must also realize that with increasing knowledge and reporting of subtle variants the classification systems are constantly changing, to keep updated with the evolving changes is hence essential.

CHAPTER 39

Poliomyelitis

Manish Kumar Varshney

INTRODUCTION

The success of polio eradication programs has substantially reduced the number of patients suffering from paralytic complications of the disease. New cases have literally reduced to nil while only older patients suffering from the postpolio residual paralysis (PPRP) come as follow-up cases. This, however, does not undermine the importance of principles of deformity correction that evolved over years for managing PPRP limb because the same can be applied to other congenital and paralytic neuromuscular deformity correction. Thus, the chapter is still maintained but discussion will be restricted to main and practical principles only.

PATHOLOGY

Poliomyelitis is an infectious disease caused by a neurotropic virus which initially invades gastrointestinal (GI) and respiratory tracts and subsequently spreads to central nervous system (CNS). Poliovirus 1 (PV1, Mahoney or Brunenders), PV2 (PV2, MEF-1/Lansing), and PV3 (PV3, Saukett/Leon) belong to enterovirus (RNA virus) group (which also includes coxsackie and echovirus) and are a member of picornaviridae family. The virus multiplies in alimentary tract wall and its lymph nodes causing viremia. This results in minor illness in most of the patients characterized by fever, malaise, sore throat, and GI upset. One patient in 500 develops CNS symptoms during its invasion. Motor neuron cells of the anterior horn of spinal cord and brainstem are either destroyed or rendered temporarily functionless. Within 48 hours of being attacked, some cells are completely destroyed (and never replaced) while others show changes short of complete chromatolysis in a ring of Nissl's substance which forms at periphery of cells (such a cell may recover in a subsequent week). A number of cells show no histological changes but still are functionless during inflammation. These will recover within a few days.

Histological Changes

The specific histological changes seen in acute and recovery stages of polio attack are as follows:

- Acute stage shows extensive nonspecific inflammatory reaction with polymorphonuclear (PMN) leukocytes and edema surrounding the disintegrating nerve cells. The spinal cord destruction occurs focally. At the center of destruction is the involved motor neuron and sometimes internuncial cells of Clarke's column. Toward the periphery of focus, some motor cells show prechromatolytic changes and some show no histological changes at all. Axons of affected motor neurons show Wallerian degeneration within 3 days, and atrophic changes subsequently develop in muscles innervated by them.
- Recovery stage shows areas of gliosis and lymphocytic cell collections occupy the sites of destroyed motor neuron cell. Any remaining neurological cells show little or no histological abnormality. Peripheral trauma during the first 2 weeks preceding the onset of paralysis can affect the localization of the paralysis in anatomically related segments of the spinal cord. Such trauma includes intramuscular injection, excessive physical activity, or an operation.

The paralyzed muscles depend upon the neurological lesion **(Fig. 1)** and the development of PPRP is a gradual process **(Fig. 2)**.

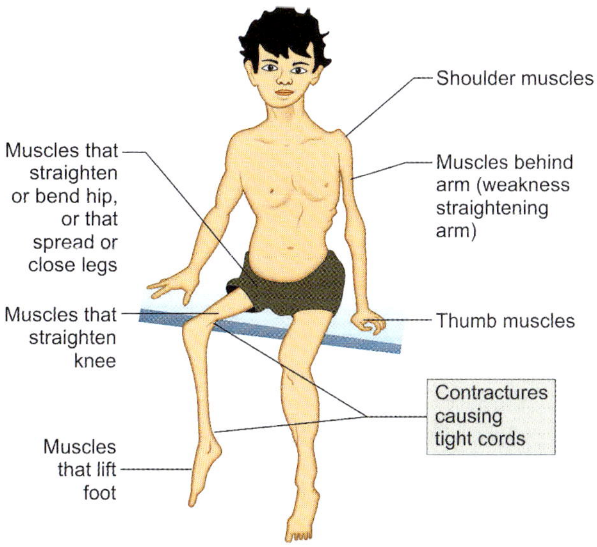

Fig. 1: Muscles affected in postpolio residual paralysis.

- In terms of segmental innervation, second and third lumbar and fifth and sixth cervical segmental show the greatest involvement.
- Lower limbs are affected twice as frequently as upper limbs.
- Muscles with the highest incidence of involvement are quadriceps, tibialis anterior, hip abductors, medial hamstrings in the lower limb and deltoid, and triceps and pectoralis major in the upper limbs.
- Certain muscles like intrinsic muscles of foot and long finger flexors of hand have the lowest incidence of involvement.
- Certain muscles are notoriously prone to complete paralysis, e.g., tibialis anterior, tibialis posterior, long flexor and extensor muscles of toes in lower limbs and intrinsic muscles of hands, deltoid and triceps in upper limbs. Hence, a muscle which has a high susceptibility of involvement may not necessarily have complete paralysis. For example, quadriceps has a high incidence of involvement, but may not necessarily be completely paralyzed. Such pattern of paralysis may be explained by the fact that motor neuron cells of the normal human spinal cord are disposed in columns of varying length.

Some of them are short column such as tibialis anterior, tibialis posterior and long toe flexors, while others are long columns, e.g., the hip flexors and adductors and quadriceps. Hence, muscles supplied by long columns are more often paretic than paralyzed while muscles supplied by short column are more often paralytic than paretic. Cells disposed ventrally in anterior horn supply proximal muscles while those lying dorsally supply more distal muscles. Columns supplying flexor muscles are situated medial and caudal to those supplying extensor muscles.

More frequent involvement of upper lumbar segments and sparing of the sacral segments accounts for the frequency with which hip flexors, quadriceps, and gluteal muscles are involved and intrinsic muscles of foot are spared.

The amount of residual neurons in a segment determines the residual strength **(Table 1 and Fig. 3)**.

Clinically, detectable weakness is only present when at least 60% of motor nerve cells supplying a muscle have been destroyed.

Mechanism of Neuronal Recovery

Significant clinical recovery occurs during first 2 weeks following acute stage. Spontaneous improvement occurs during first 4 months and slowly thereafter. Muscles with >80% of normal strength recover spontaneously without specific therapy. An individual muscle with <30% of normal strength at 3 months should be considered permanently paralyzed **(Fig. 4)**. All significant neural recovery is complete by the end of 6th month which occurs by sprouting of axons from intact cells to re-innervate the paralyzed muscle, reorganization of functional pathways of spinal cord and recovery of neuropraxia.

CLINICAL FEATURES OF AN ACUTE ATTACK OF POLIO

The incubation period is 6–20 days. Acute stage lasts for 7–10 days with symptoms ranging from malaise to general encephalomyelitis with paralysis. The child may present with minor illness characterized by sore throat, listlessness, and temperature elevation (influenza-like). These symptoms precede major illness by a few days. Major illness presents with

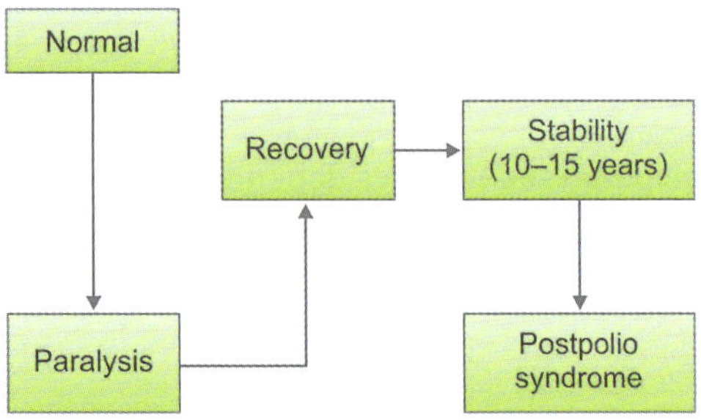

Fig. 2: Polio to postpolio residual paralysis (PPRP) syndrome.

TABLE 1: Clinical power as determined by remaining motor neuron cells.

Remaining motor neuron cells	*Clinical power*
Total loss	0/5
5–10% of residual cells	3/5
10–20% of residual cells	4/5

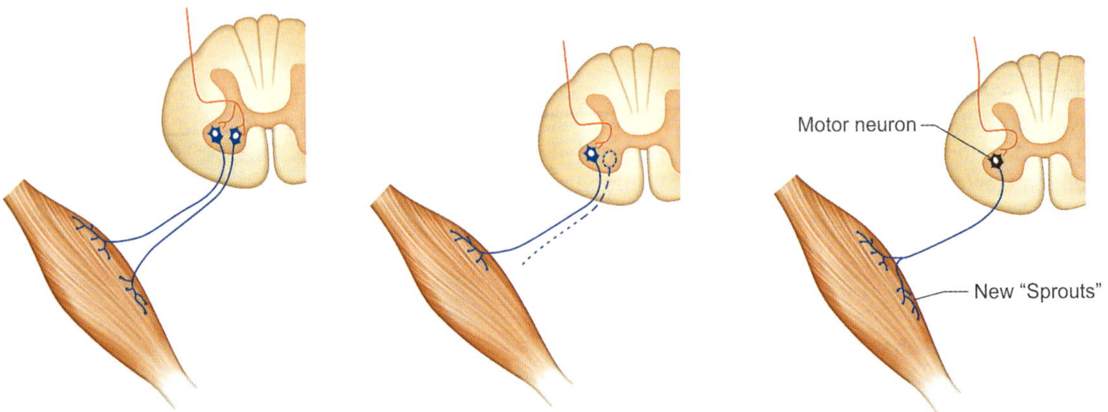

Fig. 3: Pathogenesis of motor unit loss in acute poliomyelitis.

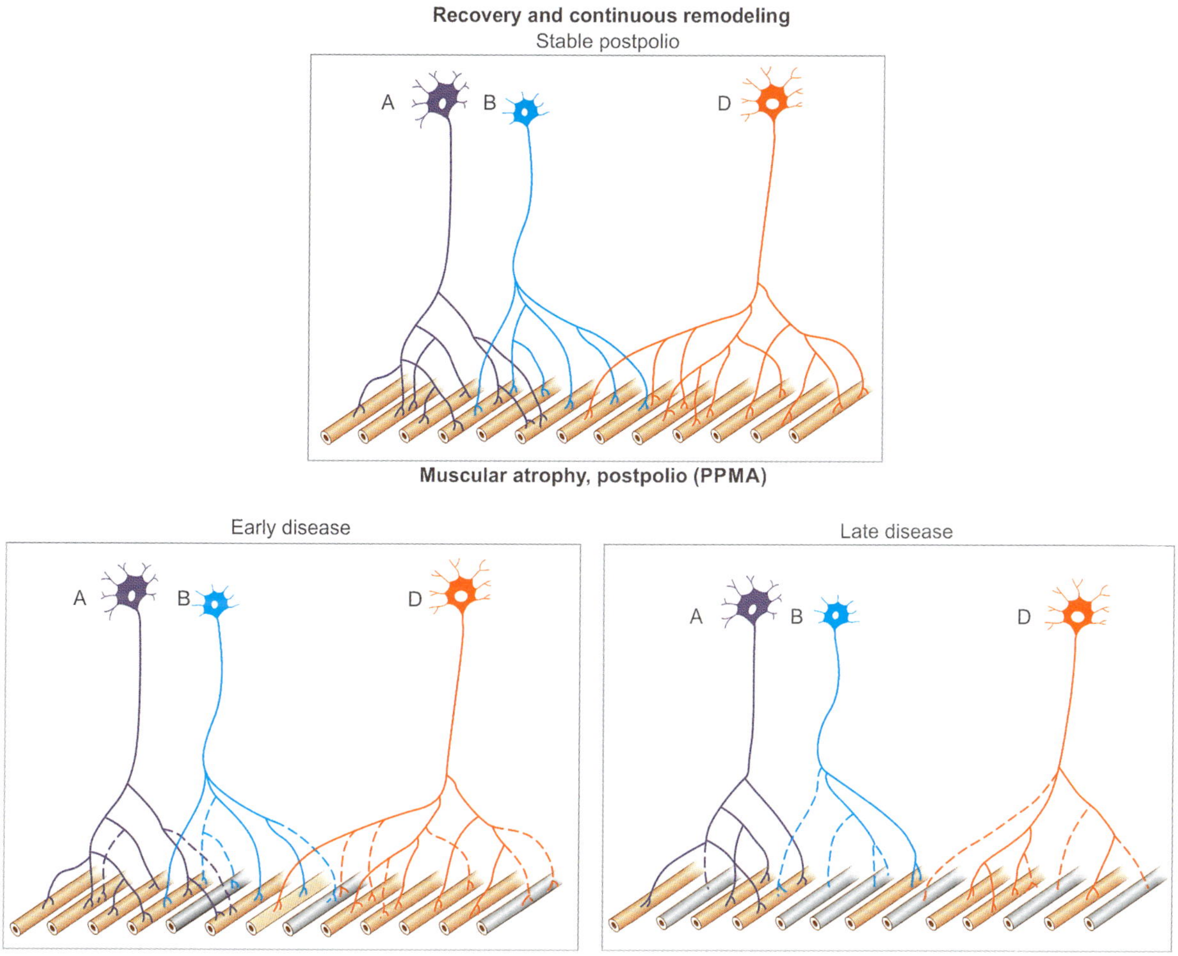

Fig. 4: Loss of muscle fibers in polio. (PPMA: postpolio muscle atrophy)

severe headache, vomiting, hyperesthesia and paresthesia, nuchal rigidity, backache, and limitation of straight leg rise. Muscle tenderness is conspicuously present. The paralysis usually occurs on 3rd or 4th day after commencement of the major illness. This is heralded by tremors of the affected muscle and the first sign is diminution or loss of tendon reflex in the affected limb. Bulbar paralysis is indicated by progressively nasal speech; difficulty in swallowing or early embarrassment of respiration. Paralysis may cease within 24 hours or may progress for several days. Live virus continues to be excreted for as long as 6 weeks; therefore, an over-vigorous assumption of activities at an early stage may result in recrudescence of infection. Meningism causes peculiar posture adaptation by limbs, i.e., adduction of upper arms, flexion at elbow, flexion at hip and knee and plantar flexion at ankles.

The acute stage of disease (within first 2–3 weeks following it) is characterized by a tendency to develop rapid fibrous contractures in the tendons, muscle sheath, and fascia especially in the iliotibial band (ITB), hamstring tendons, tendons and fasciae of the calf, and flexors of the elbow. These contractures occur independently of the level of paralysis. The cause of acute stage contracture is not understood.

The cerebrospinal fluid (CSF) examination shows PMN leukocytosis with slightly raised proteins and is under high pressure when tapped. The diagnosis is confirmed by virus culture from throat swab/excreta.

MANAGEMENT

Acute Stage

The child is put on bed rest under isolation. Analgesics, hot water packs, and sedatives are used to relieve anxiety. Supportive nutrition is given to improve immunity. The child is turned frequently to prevent formation of pressure sores. Correct posture is important to prevent contractures. The upper limbs are best held by simple slings with shoulders abducted, elbows moderately flexed and wrists neutral or slightly dorsiflexed and fingers semiflexed. In lower limbs, the hip and knees are kept in slight flexion with pillows to prevent any lateral rotation and splints are given to maintain ankles in dorsiflexion.

Gentle passive range-of-motion (ROM) exercises across affected joints several times a day prevent contracture formation. Bulbar symptoms may require a tracheostomy/mechanical ventilation.

Convalescent/Recovery Stage

Convalescent/recovery stage begins 2 days after temperature returns to normal and continues for 2 years. Muscle power improves spontaneously during this stage. Clinical examination reveals paresis/paralysis of the affected muscles, absence/diminution of the tendon reflexes with no sensory loss or bladder/bowel dysfunction. By 4th week, obvious muscle atrophy is seen. Muscle power increases rapidly from 1st to 4th month and slowly thereafter. At end of first year, 14/15th of the total recovery has occurred.

Ultimate grade of power may be estimated as follows:

In lower limb:

- +2 to original grade at 1 month
- +1.5 to original grade at 2 months
- +1 to original grade at 4 months
- +0.75 to original grade at 6 months

In upper limbs:

- +2.5 to original grade at 1 month
- + 2 to original grade at 2 months
- +1.5 to original grade at 4 months
- +1 to original grade at 6 months

The above is not true for a completely paralyzed muscle. After 6 months, any muscle, which is still paralyzed, will remain so permanently. Deformities secondary to muscle imbalance do not develop until after the end of first year. Fixed deformities at 4th month are usually due to fibrotic contracture which had developed during acute stage. Muscle strength should be serially assessed each month for 6 months and then every 3 months till 2 years. Passive ROM at each joint should be recorded at each clinical examination. In involvement of trunk and hip muscles, periodic radiological examination of the spine is done for scoliotic deformity or hip subluxation.

Treatment in this stage is directed toward:

- Correction of any deformity left over from acute stage
- Avoidance of any new deformity
- Enhancement of recovery of paretic muscle by graduated exercises
- Resumption of normal activity as early as possible.

Early Deformity

Early deformity is managed by manipulation at each joint through full ROM at least once a day. If progressive limitation of passive ROM is seen then passive movement should be supplemented by splint at night. Joints in which movements have become limited during acute stage should be managed by passive movements carried more frequently for shorter periods, but within tolerance of pain. It should be possible to discard any splint by end of 3rd to 4th week. Special attention must be paid for the correction of flexion-abduction deformity of hip, and flexion deformity of knee and equinus deformity of the ankle.

Stretching should always be gentle because overintensive stretching results in tearing of muscle fibers/tendons leading to fibrosis and ultimate reduction in the ROM. If full movement is not achieved by 6th month then simple operative division of tight/short fascia and elongation of short muscles/tendons should be done. For example:

- At hip, shortness of ITB is corrected by division of ITB at iliac crest and below inguinal ligament (Ober's release) or by division of ITB and lateral intermuscular septum in lower thirds of thigh (Yount's release).
- Elongation of hamstrings to correct knee-flexion deformity if wedging casts fail.
- Active ankle elongation of tendocalcaneus for equinus. Division and mobilization of plantar fascia may be needed.
- In upper limb, division of shortened pectoral fascia and sometimes division of shortened fascia which limits elbow extension.

Activity of individual muscle groups initially and functional activity of the limb, later as a whole aids in muscle recovery. Thus, spontaneous recovery can be accelerated by measures to encourage efficiency and hypertrophy of surviving muscles and neuron. Paretic muscles should be given a program of graded activity.

Two types of exercise regimes are employed.

1. Specific exercises, where the individual muscle/muscle groups are made to act to the maximum of their capacity for up to 10 contractions per day. The load against which contraction occurs is increased gradually.
2. General exercises are prescribed after 4 months in form of rolling, crawling, swimming, walking in water, sitting up and lying down, movements with sling suspension, cycling, etc.

Walking: Complete paralysis of trunk/lower limbs with moderate to severe involvement of the upper limbs may preclude walking even with crutches. Severe paralysis of trunk/lower limbs associated with moderately strong upper limbs may allow crutch walking. When paralysis is limited to lower limbs, walking with crutches or leg appliances can begin at 3rd to 4th month in water and then on dry land. Various orthoses are required according to functional requirement of the child.

Chronic Stage

Chronic stage begins 24 months after acute illness. In a growing child, important sequelae can still arise. Progressive deformity can arise which is directly related to the pattern of original muscle paralysis even 2–3 years after acute illness. The causes include maintenance of a particular posture by gravity or unopposed muscle action. Failure of muscle/tendon growth due to lack of growth stimulation from their weak/paralyzed opponents, so that stronger muscles become shorter relative to the length of the bone. Thus, the deforming muscles produce a bow stringing effect, which puts the opponent muscles in a mechanical disadvantage resulting in its stretching and eventually loss of any effective action. Therefore, greater the disparity and opposing muscles, greater is the deformity produced. Hence, all patients after 2 years of acute illness must be examined every 6 months to detect any developing deformity. Once paralytic deformity starts to develop, it continues to worsen until growth ceases.

Goals of treatment in chronic stage are to obtain muscle balance and to prevent or correct soft tissue or bony deformities.

Deformities around Foot and Ankle

The following are the commonly encountered deformities around ankle and foot in chronic stage of disease with PPRP **(Fig. 5)**.

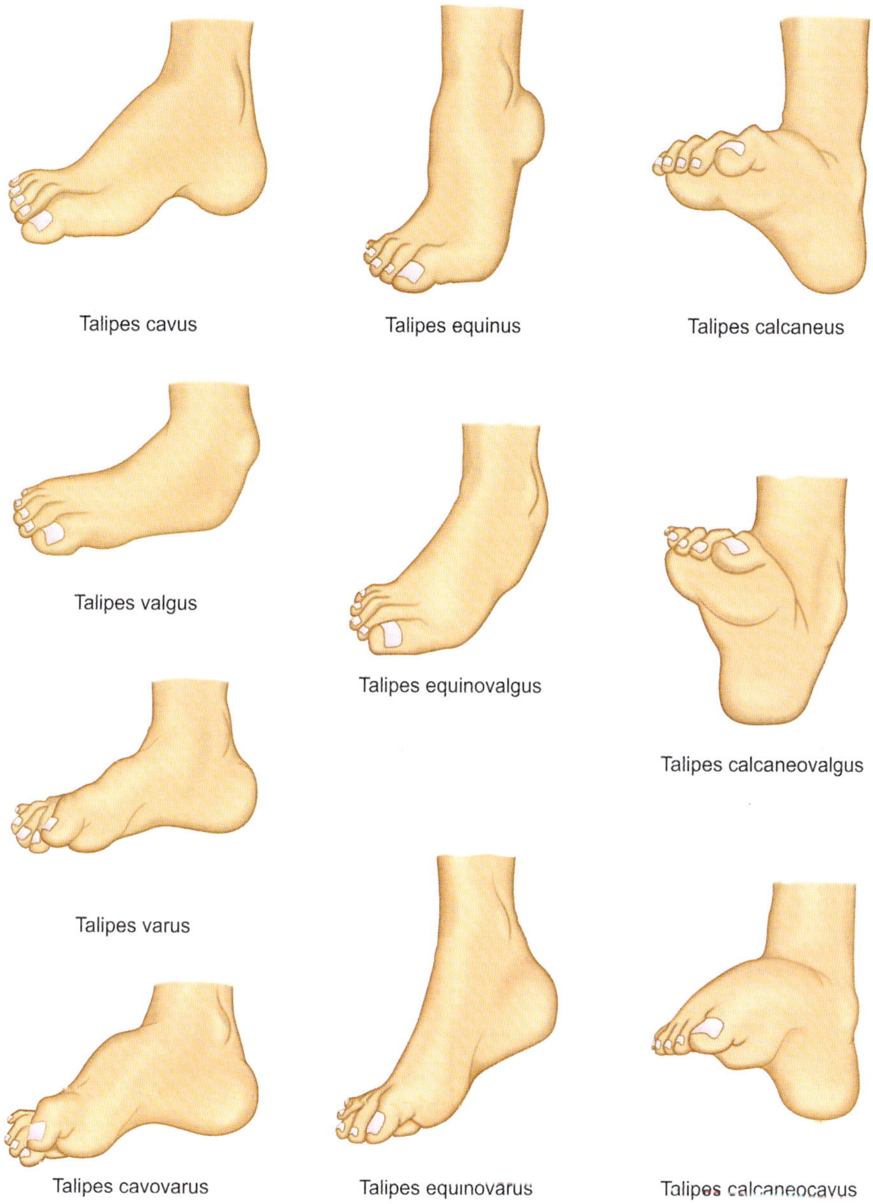

Fig. 5: Deformities of ankle and foot.

- *Talipes equinus:* Fixed plantar flexion deformity that arises when the dorsiflexors of the ankle and foot are weak and calf muscles are strong. Gravity aggravates the liability to deformity.
- *Talipes calcaneus:* Fixed dorsiflexion deformity that arises when the triceps surae is weak or paralyzed and the dorsiflexor muscles have remained strong. Calcaneum tilts so that its posterior surface becomes the weight-bearing surface.
- *Talipes calcaneocavus:* Talipes calcaneus with cavus as the forefoot plantar flexes through the action of long toe flexors.
- *Talipes calcaneocavovarus:* When calcaneocavus is combined with the varus deformity.

In addition, claw toes, claw toes with cavus, dorsal bunion, valgus deformity **(Fig. 6)** and equinovalgus and varus deformity, and equinovarus are commonly seen in postpolio residual contracture.

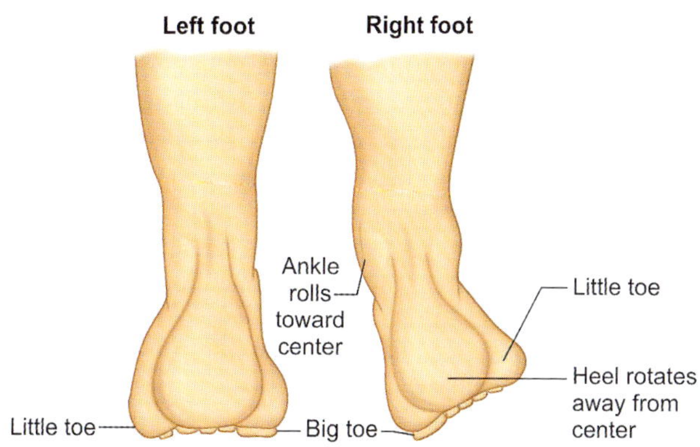

Fig. 6: Development of valgus deformity of the foot (pronation).

When the paralysis is of short duration, the deformities are dynamic and not fixed and may become evident only on contraction of unopposed muscles or on weight bearing. Later a permanent deformity is established from soft-tissue contracture and distortion of normal contour of the bones which occurs as a result of muscle imbalance, habitually faulty posture, growth and abnormal weight-bearing alignment. Foot and ankle are especially susceptible to deformity because they bear weight of the body.

The requirements for a satisfactory function of foot are stability, plantigrade weight bearing, absence of fixed deformity and power sufficient to allow toes to clear the ground and allow push off for forward propulsion of body. There are a few repeated terms while understanding the principles of treatment and need to be clarified before:

- *Stability* implies that ankle and hindfoot will not roll into valgus and varus on bearing weight.
- *Plantigrade posture* implies that weight will be reasonably, evenly distributed at heel, midfoot, and forefoot.
- *Adequate muscle power* indicates general dorsiflexor and plantar flexor power at ankle and foot of grade 3 or more. If ideal power is not available then a supportive splint/sling will be required to give additional stability.

The operative management should be considered 1.5 years after paralytic attack and falls under following headings:

- Procedures that correct and prevent deformity and achieve balanced muscle power.
- Procedures that obtain stability.

In general, for operative procedures, the broad understanding has been that:

- Tendon transfer done in skeletally immature
- Extra-articular arthrodesis done usually between 3 years and 8 years
- Tendon transfer around ankle and foot after 10 years of age can be supplemented by arthrodesis to correct the deformity.
- Triple arthrodesis should be done in children over 10 years.
- Ankle arthrodesis should be done in children after 18 years of age.

The aim of muscle balancing operations is to achieve a balanced power of dorsiflexors, plantar flexors, and invertors and evertors of forefoot and hindfoot. Function of invertors or evertors might be sacrificed to obtain active dorsiflexion or plantar flexion. The primary muscle balancing procedures are tendon transfers. The objectives of tendon transfer in poliomyelitis are:

- To provide active motor power.
- To eliminate the deforming effect of muscle.
- To improve stability by improving muscle balance.

GENERAL RULES FOR TENDON TRANSFER IN FOOT

- Results with tendon transfer are better in patients who are >10 years of age.
- Tendon transfers about foot and ankle after the age of 10 or 11 years are usually supplemented by stabilizing procedures to correct fixed deformities, to establish enough mediolateral stability on weight bearing, and to compensate in part for loss of abductor-evertor and adductor-inverter muscles.
- When tendons are transferred to the dorsum of foot, to be used as active dorsiflexors, a bone block operation to limit plantar flexion is necessary to prevent overstretching of the transferred tendon.
- When tendon transfer and stabilization procedure are to be done together, then latter is done first.
- When there is any significant imbalance, then transfer of even a single tendon should be preceded/accompanied by stabilization of foot.
- In a child, even a slightest imbalance will lead to significant deformity over a long period of growth. However, in adults where the onset of paralysis is after skeletal maturity, significant deformity is rare.
- After stabilization of foot, only dorsiflexion and plantar flexion remain and since these are the motions at ankle joint, restoration of muscle power on medial and lateral sides of the ankle is unnecessary. Hence, inverters/evertors should be transferred into midline either anteriorly or posteriorly into calcaneum/tendocalcaneus.
- Tendon transfer is usually preferable to excision, not only to restore function but also to prevent further atrophy of leg.
- In rare instances where muscle function has to be discarded, 7–10 cm of its tendon should be excised to prevent reunion of the tendon ends by fibrous tissues.
- After tendon transfer, other deformities of the leg should be corrected like excessive tibial torsion, knock knees or bowlegs.

PARALYSIS OF SPECIFIC MUSCLE AND MUSCLE GROUPS AND FUNCTIOLESIA (MODIFIED FROM PEABODY)

- Limited paralysis of inversion
  - Isolated paralysis of tibialis anterior
  - Isolated paralysis of tibialis anterior and tibialis posterior
  - Isolated paralysis of tibialis posterior.
- Paralysis of dorsiflexion and inversion (i.e., paralysis of tibialis anterior, tibialis posterior, and toe extensors)
  - Type A—Paralysis of tibialis anterior and toe extensors
  - Type B—Paralysis of tibialis anterior, tibialis posterior, and toe extensors.
- Paralysis of dorsiflexion, inversion, and eversion (i.e., paralysis of tibialis anterior, toe extensors, and peroneal muscles).
- Paralysis of eversion (paralysis of peroneals alone and paralysis of peroneals with toe extensors).
- Paralysis of plantar flexion (paralysis of triceps surae muscles).

  The Peabody classification of paralysis of muscles of foot and ankle is provided for reference as it had been used for long by the reconstructive surgeons.
- Limited exterior inverter insufficiency—only tibialis anterior.

- Gross exterior invertor insufficiency
  - Type A—tibialis anterior + long toe extensors
  - Type B—tibialis anterior, tibialis posterior and toe extensors.
- Evertor insufficiency.
- Triceps surae insufficiency.

We will discuss the management of each type as mentioned in the modified classification of foot and ankle muscle paralysis.

PARALYSIS OF INVERSION

The most common manifestation of paralysis in foot is paralysis of inversion in form of an isolated paralysis of tibialis anterior or both tibialis anterior and tibialis posterior.

Isolated Paralysis of Tibialis Anterior

If tibialis anterior alone is paralyzed in the presence of other normal muscles, first metatarsal head tends to be depressed by combined action of peroneus longus (PL) and extensor hallucis longus (EHL). Extensor of the long toe, which normally assists in dorsiflexion, becomes overactive in an attempt to replace the paralyzed muscle resulting in hyperextension of proximal phalanx and depression of metatarsal head. Thus, deformities which may occur include equinus (due to loss of dorsiflexors), cavus (due to depression of first metatarsal head), varying degrees of planovalgus which is first seen in swing phase (due to unopposed activity of evertors), clawing of great toe (due to hyperextension of proximal phalanx by overactive EHL) and cavovarus, which occurs occasionally (due to unopposed activity of PL with active tibialis posterior).

Treatment

- *Equinus:* Passive stretching and serial casting is done to correct equinus contracture. Tendocalcaneus lengthening and posterior ankle capsulotomy may be required in resistant cases.
- *Cavus:* Anterior transfer of PL to the base of second metatarsal corrects cavus deformity. To prevent dorsal bunion (occurring as a result of detachment of PL), the tendon of peroneus brevis (PB) is sutured to the stump of PL.
- Extensor hallucis longus may be transferred to the neck of first metatarsal with arthrodesis of interphalangeal (IP) joint of great toe and suturing of the remaining stump of the EHL to extensor hallucis brevis (EHB) to prevent its re-growth. If this fails to lift metatarsal head then this procedure is combined with division of plantar ligaments and capsulotomy of cuneiform—first metatarsal joint. As an alternative, extensor digitorum longus (EDL) may be transferred to midfoot to supply active dorsiflexion.
- Claw toe may be corrected by transfer of long toe extensor to metatarsal neck.
- Cavovarus is dealt with plantar fasciotomy and release of intrinsic muscles of foot accompanied with PL transfer to base of second and EHL transfer to neck of first metatarsal. When peroneus tertius is functioning, it may be used to reinforce EHL function.

Paralysis of Tibialis Anterior and Tibialis Posterior

Paralysis of tibialis anterior and tibialis posterior in the presence of active peronei results in rapid development of equinovalgus at hindfoot and forefoot. Initially, valgus deformity occurs only on standing but later peroneal tendons become short and deformity becomes fixed. The deformity may be similar to congenital vertical talus on a standing lateral film.

Treatment

- Equinus is dealt with passive stretching and serial casting or tendocalcaneus lengthening as above.
- For valgus, one of the peroneal muscles is transferred. Because of its greater excursion, PL may be transferred to base of second metatarsal to replace tibialis anterior and one of the long toe flexors is used to replace tibialis posterior. PB is sutured to distal stump of PL.
- Sometimes PB may be transferred to tibialis posterior insertion by passing through the space between triceps surae and deep muscle layer. If the foot is in marked fixed eversion, then it may be necessary to perform lengthening of PL and PB before any transfer.

Paralysis of tibialis posterior alone is rare but may result in hindfoot and forefoot eversion.

Treatment of Isolated Tibialis Posterior Paralysis

- Flexor hallucis longus (FHL) or flexor digitorum longus (FDL) may be used for tendon transfer. The tendon is dissected and re-routed through sheath of tibialis posterior to attach to navicular. Rarely EHL may be transferred posteriorly through interosseous membrane and then through tibialis posterior tunnel to attach to navicular.
- For children 3–6 years of age, Axer recommends bringing the conjoined tendon of EDL and peroneus tertius through a transverse channel in talar neck and suturing the tendon on itself.
- For severe valgus, he recommends transfer of PL into medial side of the neck of talus and PB to the lateral side of the neck of talus. However, an isolated transfer of PB should not be done to avoid forefoot inversion.
- For fixed equinus deformity, passive stretching and casting with tendocalcaneus lengthening may be considered.

PARALYSIS OF DORSIFLEXION AND INVERSION (TIBIALIS ANTERIOR, TIBIALIS POSTERIOR AND TOE EXTENSORS)

Type A (with spared tibialis posterior) may be treated with transfer of PL to dorsum of first cuneiform bone or talonavicular arthrodesis is combined if deformity is fixed. Paralysis of all of these muscles in the presence of active peronei and triceps surae results in equinovalgus deformity.

Treatment

- When the deformity is not fixed then below-knee iron with toe raising spring and a valgus insole helps in its progression. However, progressive limitation of dorsiflexion and inversion is an indication for the correction of deformity surgically.

- Transfer of PB to dorsum of foot over base of second metatarsal/intermediate cuneiform or alternatively to neck of talus (Axer) may be performed. The latter method is used when preoperative X-ray shows plantar flexion of talus, which is likely to develop in equinovalgus deformity.
- If peroneus tertius helps in increasing valgus, it may be transferred medially to the base of second metatarsus or intermediate cuneiform. However, transfer of PL is not recommended because it may result in varus and forefoot instability. Any instability of hindfoot resulting from above-mentioned tendon transfer may be dealt with extra-articular subtalar arthrodesis.
- For less severe paralysis of dorsiflexion and inversion, transfer of long toe flexor tendon/PB tendon to the insertion of tibialis posterior with EHL to neck of first metatarsal and EDL to bases of second, third, and fourth metatarsals may be performed.
- Correction of any equinovalgus deformity may require a preliminary period of passive splinting or possible plaster cast for 3 weeks with foot in inversion and dorsiflexion. If this fails to allow passive dorsiflexion beyond right angle and passive inversion beyond neutral, then tendocalcaneus lengthening must be performed at the same sitting.

PARALYSIS OF DORSIFLEXION, INVERSION, AND EVERSION

Paralysis of dorsiflexion, inversion, and eversion may present in two forms.

1. In the first form, tibialis anterior, toe extensors, and peronei are paralyzed but tibialis posterior and triceps surae are normal resulting in progressive equinovarus deformity. Equinovarus results from unopposed tibialis posterior and contracture of triceps surae, which acts as a fixed point against which all intrinsic muscles pull and increase the forefoot adduction. The cavus and shortening of the medial arch of foot occur due to depression of the head of first metatarsal by tibialis posterior. Initial treatment is by serial casting and gentle passive stretching. Tendocalcaneus lengthening may be required in some cases. Radical soft tissue release for forefoot cavus and transfer of tibialis posterior to the base of third metatarsal or middle cuneiform supplemented anteriorly by anterior transfer of long toe flexors may be required in severe cases.
2. In the second type, tibialis anterior, tibialis posterior, toe extensors, and peronei are all paralyzed in the presence of intact triceps surae and intrinsic muscles. This combination is uncommon in poliomyelitis but when present gives rise to severe equinovarus deformity. Stretching and casting have no role in its correction. It may recur even after tendocalcaneus lengthening. A plantar flexor power of three and more in absence of any other muscle activity at ankle is an indication for hemitransfer of tendocalcaneus. First, the lengthening of tendocalcaneus is obtained by Z-plasty in coronal plane. After 6 weeks, the lateral half of tendocalcaneus with muscle originating from later femoral condyle is transferred to the lateral side of foot to be inserted on cuboid. Although no independent activity is expected from such a transfer, recurrent deformity is prevented and an orthosis may be discarded.

Paralysis of Eversion

Paralysis of eversion may occur due to paralysis of peroneals alone or peroneals with long toe extensors. Paralysis of peroneals alone is rare in poliomyelitis, but when present may cause severe hindfoot varus deformity because of unopposed tibialis posterior. Hence, various deformities include hindfoot varus, inversion of calcaneus, and adduction of forefoot due to unopposed activity of tibialis posterior and dorsal bunion due to unopposed tibialis anterior.

Treatment is by transfer of tibialis posterior to cuboid. For dorsal bunion, tibialis anterior is transferred laterally to the base of second metatarsal. However, isolated transfer of tibialis anterior may lead to EHL overactivity resulting in hyperextension of hallux and painful callus under first metatarsal head. Thus, in children below 5 years, EHL lengthening is required, whereas in children above 5 years, EHL transfer to neck of first metatarsal is recommended.

Paralysis of peroneal muscles with long toe extensors causes a less severe equinovarus, which is treated by transfer of tibialis anterior to the base of third metatarsal or middle cuneiform.

PARALYSIS OF PLANTAR FLEXION (TRICEPS SURAE)

Triceps surae paralysis leads to calcaneus deformity due to unopposed dorsiflexion. When activity is retained with secondary plantar flexors of the ankle (i.e., tibialis posterior, peronei, and long toe flexors) then initial loss of function may be misleadingly slight. However within 2–3 years, calcaneocavus deformity develops insidiously. Other causes of calcaneocavus deformity include myelomeningocele and hereditary neuropathies.

The deformity begins by downward tilting of calcaneus coinciding with the long axes of tibia and calcaneus negating any residual power in the triceps. Tibialis posterior, peroneals, and long toe flexors cannot effectively plantar flex the hindfoot in absence of a strong triceps surae. However, they depress the metatarsal heads and cause equinus. Shortening of intrinsics and plantar fascia draws the metatarsal heads and calcaneus together like a bowstring. Thus, the lever arm of calcaneum (represented by distance between tibia and posterior end of calcaneum) is much diminished relative to the distance between ankle joint and bottom of calcaneum.

Treatment

The aim of treatment is to prevent overstretching of triceps by keeping foot in slight equinus during acute stage of poliomyelitis. If triceps is weak, walking is delayed in convalescent stage. Serial standing X-rays in children below 5 years may be performed to recognize the deformity early. Surgical correction is required to prevent development of calcaneus deformity and to restore hindfoot plantar flexion;

thereby preventing retrograde displacement of tibia, providing a more stable base for stance and gait and creating a counter thrust against which the remaining muscles can act. In acute stage, the only indication for surgery in children below 5 years of age is progressive calcaneal deformity.

Principles

The combination of muscles transferred posteriorly for triceps surae depends upon its residual strength and pattern of remaining muscles. If motor strength of triceps is fair, 2–3 muscles may be sufficient. However, as many muscles should be transferred as available (at least 3) if the motor strength is zero. Tibialis anterior should be reserved for possible transfer to dorsum of the midfoot. Plantar fasciotomy and release of intrinsics of foot is required prior to tendon transfer.

- *Procedures done when triceps power is fair:* Transfer of FHL and FDL to calcaneum/tendocalcaneus may be sufficient to prevent the deformity if power in triceps surae is three or more. Transfer of the tendon of tibialis anterior alone may give good result if triceps is not completely paralyzed and tibialis anterior is strong (particularly in presence of calcaneocavovarus deformity). This may be done as an isolated procedure if lateral stabilizers are balanced. After transfer of tibialis anterior, toe extensors may be used for dorsiflexion of midfoot. It is better to transfer the toe extensors to metatarsal heads and fuse the IP joints to prevent claw toe deformity developing later.
  - If triceps strength is fair and invertors and evertors are well balanced then transfer of one group of muscles causes instability and deformity. In such cases, transfer of PB and tibialis posterior to heel is sufficient to control the calcaneus deformity.
  - If lateral imbalance is present due to loss of one of the lateral stabilizers in presence of fair strength in triceps then both peroneals may be transferred to heel for calcaneovalgus deformity or tibialis posterior and FHL may be transferred to heel for cavovarus deformity. In addition for calcaneovalgus, tenodesis of tendocalcaneus to fibula may be done. For mobile calcaneal deformities, transfer of PL tendon to a groove on the plantar surface of calcaneum without disturbing its origin and insertion, maintains the foot in plantar flexion.
- *Procedures done when triceps power is poor (0/5):* Transfer of FHL, FDL, PB, and tibialis posterior to heel is an ideal transfer provided the muscles have power 4/5 or more. Use of tibialis posterior and PB for triceps may result in subtalar instability requiring an extra-articular subtalar arthrodesis.
  - When no evertors or invertors are available for transfer, then hamstrings may be used for tendon transfer. Prerequisites include complete paralysis of triceps surae, strong medial hamstrings/biceps femoris with strong ankle dorsiflexion and quadriceps. If early correction of muscle imbalance by tendon transfer to calcaneus is successful, this deformity may correct itself. However if left uncorrected, a posterior displacement calcaneum osteotomy may be required in addition to muscle transfer, especially in children between 7 years and 12 years. Paralysis of triceps with both tibialis anterior and posterior may be treated by transfer of both PL and brevis, supplemented by long toe flexors.

STABILIZATION OF JOINTS OF FOOT AND ANKLE

The main objective of these procedures is to reduce the number of fits (joints/functions) a weakened or paralyzed muscles must control.

Foot stabilization is indicated only when a deformity of the foot is accompanied by lateral stability of the talus in ankle mortise. Lateral instability can be detected by taking X-rays in varus/valgus. When talus is unstable in mortise then ankle arthrodesis with stabilization of foot is indicated.

- Anterior subluxation of ankle often results following stabilization of foot for equinus deformity. Tendon transfer to restore dorsiflexion of ankle therefore should be accompanied with stabilization procedure.
  Following stabilization underlying goals should be met with:
- Medial border of foot should be straight.
- Heel, first and fifth metatarsal heads should be in exactly same plane.
- Heel should be neutral or valgus but never varus.
  Muscle balance of the foot and ankle determines how much the foot should be displaced posteriorly. Whenever posterior displacement of foot is required Hike/Dunn procedure is preferred. Posterior displacement of foot helps in following ways.
- Transfer the fulcrum (ankle) posteriorly near the center.
- Lengthen the posterior lever arm, which is of advantage when triceps is weak.

When dorsiflexion and plantarflexion are equally strong Ryerson's triple arthrodesis may be done.

During stabilization of foot, it must be placed in correct relationship to ankle joint without regard to other deformities such as knock knee and those corrections must be done later. While stabilizing foot in adults no attempt should be made to change the weight bearing alignment. Avascular necrosis of talar body may occur after triple arthrodesis or pantalar arthrodesis. The complication more commonly occurs in adolescents and adults. As revascularization in adolescents occurs in 6–9 months, the complication may be avoided by not bearing weight for 6–9 months.

Stabilizing procedure for foot and ankle is of five kinds.

1. Calcaneal osteotomy
2. Extra-articular subtalar arthrodesis
3. Triple arthrodesis
4. Ankle arthrodesis
5. Bone blocks to limit motion at ankle fit

Causes of recurrence of deformity after stabilization of foot:

- Muscle imbalance is the most common because muscle balance should always be achieved with arthrodesis
- Insufficient immobilization
- Failure to align foot with the ankle mortise
- Loss of position at time of cast change

- Pseudarthrosis most commonly seen in talonavicular ligament
- Operation done on immature bones.

Out of various studies, following conclusions were made.

- Hoke arthrodesis can correct any foot deformity.
- However, it should not be relied upon alone for correction of foot drop when good muscle is available for transfer to dorsum of foot.
- Triple arthrodesis does not allow posterior displacement of foot and hence many deformities cannot be corrected by this method alone.
- Lambrinudi is best for correcting equinus. But, this is not indicated to correct foot drop if muscles are available for transfer.

CLAW TOES

This deformity is characterized by hyperextension of metatarsophalangeal (MTP) joint and flexion of the IP joint **(Fig. 7)**.

Causes

- Neuropathic clawfoot
- Talipes cavus

In poliomyelitis, they occur in two scenarios ***(Fig. 8)****:*

1. When long toe extensors are used to substitute for weak ankle dorsiflexors. Here, the clawing is more marked when tendocalcaneus is contracted. Gait analysis shows increased deformity in the swing phase and disappearance in stance phase. Treatment is correction of equinus contracture and transferring suitable tendons to restore active dorsiflexion of ankle.
2. When long toe flexors are used to substitute for a severely weak triceps surae group in propulsive/push off phase. Gait analysis shows clawing only when propulsion/push off is attempted. Treatment is by correcting any foot deformity and tendon transfer to restore ankle plantar flexion.

Clinical findings include clawing, irritation at flexed proximal interphalangeal (PIP) joints by shoes, and painful callosities at metatarsal heads. Eventually, clawing becomes permanent.

1. *Surgical management for clawing of lateral toes* ***(Fig. 9)****:* Expose and completely resect dorsal capsule of MTP joint and achieve forcible plantar flexion in an overcorrected position at MTP joint. Divide the EDL tendon or lengthen them. Divide the FDL tendon at its insertion at distal

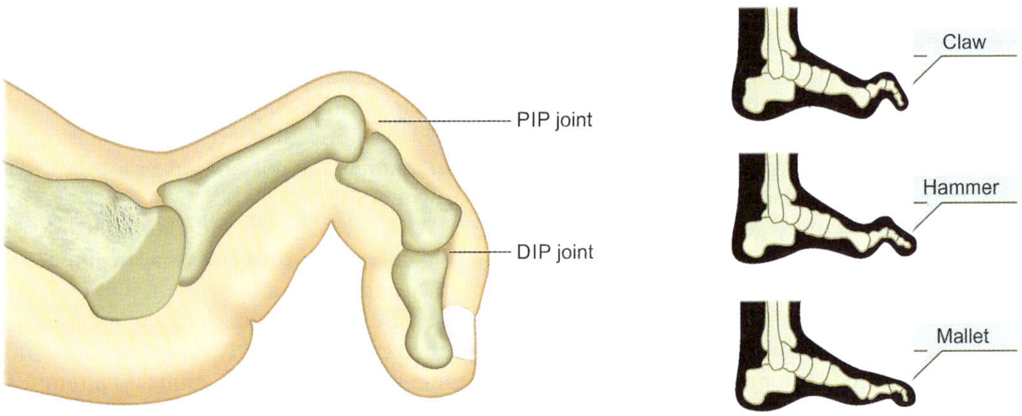

Fig. 7: Claw toes and differentiating the deformity from hammer toe and mallet toe. (DIP: distal interphalangeal; PIP: proximal interphalangeal)

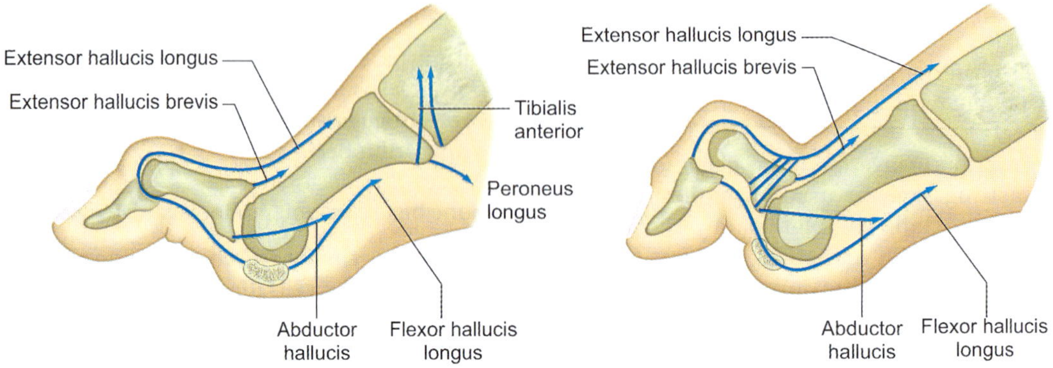

Fig. 8: Pathogenesis of claw toes. The dorsal subluxation or dislocation of metatarsophalangeal (MTP) joint causes flexion at the interphalangeal (IP) joint by various mechanisms.

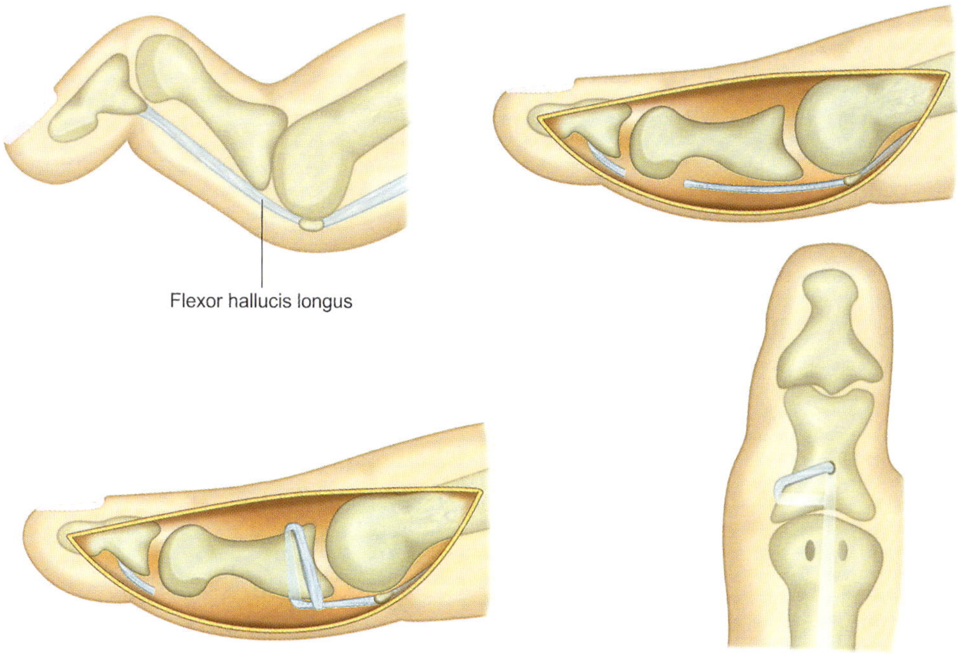

Fig. 9: Claw toes correction.

phalanx. Correct clawing deformity of IP joint by capsulotomy. Re-attach the FDL tendon to plantar aspect of the proximal phalanx. One can also perform Girdlestone-Taylor procedure.

2. *Surgical correction for clawing of great toe:* When clawing is caused by insufficiency of plantar flexors at ankle and persists even after appropriate foot stabilization and tendon transfer (to restore plantar flexion at ankle), the treatment is done by transfer of FHL from distal to proximal phalanx and arthrodesis of the IP. When clawing is due to insufficiency of dorsiflexors of ankle and contracture of tendocalcaneus, then modified Jones operation is preferred.

- *Principles of Jones operation* ***(Fig. 10)****:* Extensor hallucis longus is divided proximal to IP joint, its proximal segment is attached to the neck of first metatarsal and its distal stump is secured to soft tissue. IP joint is fused.

Modifications of Robert Jones procedure ***(Fig. 10)****:*

- Hypertrophic scar that forms in dorsal incision is minimized by preserving a bridge of intact skin by "L-shaped" incision.
- Pseudarthrosis is minimized by using medullary fixation with "k" wire and accessory cancellous bone.
- Regeneration of tendon of EHL is less likely when tendon sheath is completely excised for 5 cm in proximal segment.

DORSAL BUNION

- Shaft of first metatarsal is dorsiflexed and great toe is plantar flexed.
- Causes:
  - Muscle imbalance is the most common cause.
  - Hallux rigidus where dorsiflexion of first MTP joint is painful **(Fig. 11)**, later the bone on dorsum of first metatarsal becomes pronounced and blocks dorsiflexion of the joint.
  - Severe congenital flat foot with rocker bottom deformity.

Pathological Anatomy

Usually only the MTP joint of the great toe is flexed, and on weight bearing, the first metatarsal head is displaced upward. The longitudinal axis of the metatarsal shaft may be horizontal or its distal end may be directed upward. First cuneiform may also be tilted upward. When flexion of great toe is severe enough, the MTP joint may subluxate and dorsal part of the cartilage of metatarsal head may degenerate. A small exostosis may form on dorsum of metatarsal head. Plantar aspect of joint capsule and flexor hallucis brevis (FHB) will eventually contract.

Two types of muscle imbalance are known to cause bunion.

1. Muscle imbalance that causes dorsiflexion of first metatarsus with secondary flexion of the great toe. This is caused commonly by imbalance between tibialis anterior and PL. Tibialis anterior normally raises the first cuneiform and base of first metatarsal. PL opposes this action. Hence, when PL is weak/paralyzed/transferred somewhere else, then unopposed action of tibialis anterior leads to dorsiflexion of first metatarsus which in turn leads to active plantar flexion of the great toe to establish contact with the ground on weight bearing and to assist in push off. Weakness of the dorsiflexors of great toe may also favor this position. The most common cause of such muscular

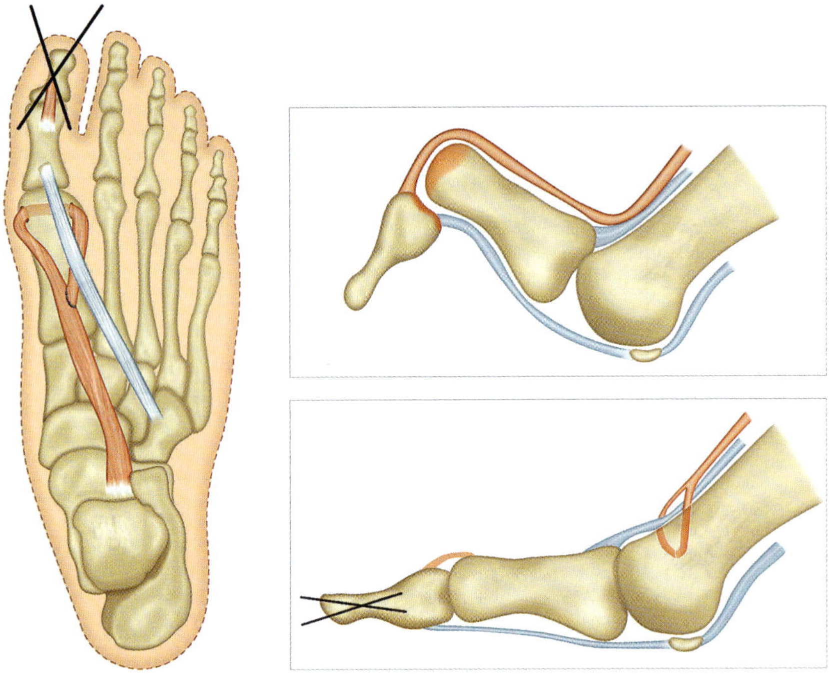

Fig. 10: Modified Jones procedure.

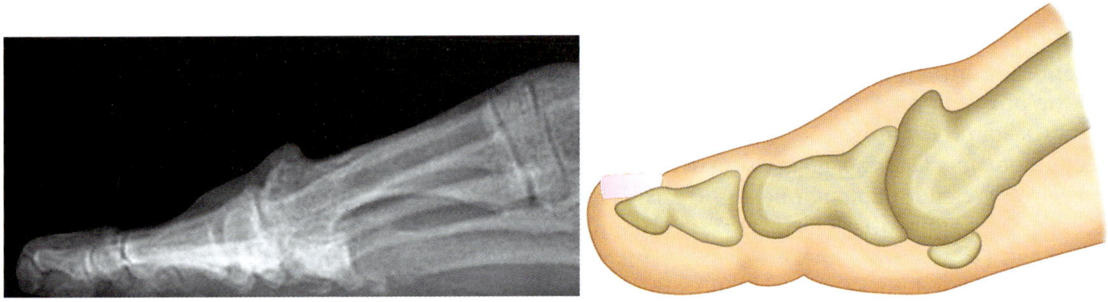

Fig. 11: Hallux rigidus.

imbalance is ill-advised tendon transfer. To prevent this situation, following precautions should be taken:

- When tibialis anterior is paralyzed, PL/PB should be transferred to third cuneiform rather than to insertion of tibialis anterior. Transfer of PB should be preferred, leaving PL intact.
- For weak triceps (with strong PL and tibialis anterior), PL should not be transferred to calcaneus unless tibialis anterior has been transferred to midline, to avoid muscle imbalance.

Treatment—for progressive deformity—transfer tibialis anterior (or previously transferred PL) to third cuneiform. For fixed deformity, correct the flexed deformity in addition to muscle transfer (see below).

2. The second less common muscle imbalance causes plantar flexion of the great toe primarily and dorsiflexion of first metatarsal is only secondary. The dorsal bunion—results from paralysis of all muscles controlling foot except triceps and long toe flexors. The long toe flexors help in steadying foot in weight bearing and to sustain a push off. Thus, active use of FHL may lead to constant plantar flexion of the great toe and upward displacement of first metatarsal head. A stray FHB may also produce such a deformity.

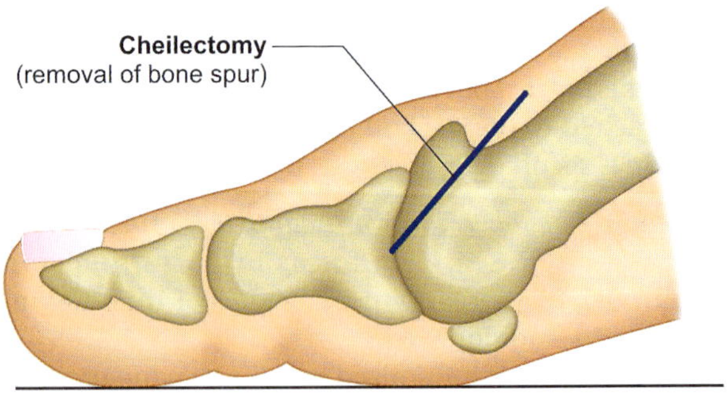

Fig. 12: Cheilectomy.

Lapidus repair for dorsal bunion:

- Open capsule of MTP joint and remove any abnormal bone from the dorsum of metatarsal head (cheilectomy) **(Fig. 12)**.

- If tibialis anterior is overactive, detach its tendon from its insertion and transfer it on second or third cuneiform on dorsum of foot or into the navicular.
- Wedge of bone is removed from first metatarsocuneiform joint and first naviculocuneiform joint with bases inferior.
- Detach FHL from its insertion to distal phalangeal base and bring it through an oblique tunnel in the shaft of first metatarsus from its proximal plantar aspect to distal dorsal aspect and insert it at capsule of MTP joint. This converts FHL into plantar flexor of first metatarsal and eliminates its action as plantar flexor of the great toe.

After treatment:
- Below-knee cast is given for 2 weeks.
- Walking cast after 2 weeks with gradual weight bearing
- This cast removed after 8–10 weeks

CAVUS DEFORMITY AND CLAW TOES

Cavus foot is one with abnormally high longitudinal arch that results from an equinus position **(Figs. 13A and B)** of the forefoot in relation to the hindfoot. In skeletally immature feet, spinal dysraphism, cerebral palsy, primary cerebellar disease, arthrogryposis or severe club feet may cause cavus. Neuromuscular (Charcot-Marie-Tooth disease, poliomyelitis, etc.) is the most common cause in skeletally mature patients. Other causes include traumatic episodes such as deep posterior compartment syndrome after fracture of tibia and fibula, malunions of midfoot fracture or other fracture dislocations of the foot. Fibrosis and contracture of tibialis posterior, FHL and FDL following ischemia, increased compartment pressure or laceration of the muscle tendon units may also lead to cavus deformity.

Etiology

Etiologically cavus foot may be divided as follows:
- Idiopathic—occurs after 3 years of age, male and female equally affected, often associated with spina bifida occulta.
- Secondary—caused by following:
    - Neurological diseases
        - Charcot-Marie-Tooth disease
        - Poliomyelitis
        - Cerebral palsy
        - Spina bifida
        - Disorder of conus medullaris (e.g., diastematomyelia and cauda equina syndrome)
        - Friedreich's ataxia
        - Spinocerebellar hereditary degeneration of Mollaret
    - Direct trauma to foot/leg
    - Myopathies (e.g., muscular dystrophy)
    - Plantar fibromatosis
    - Congenital talipes equinovarus

Pathogenesis

- Unknown mechanism in idiopathic cavus foot.
- Post-traumatic cavus deformity is a hindfoot–midfoot deformity caused by malunion of a fracture such as talar neck.
- In patients with neuromuscular diseases, the cause is believed to be an imbalance between extrinsic and intrinsic muscles of the foot. Normally intrinsic muscles flex the MTP joints and extend the IP joints. Hence, any weakness of intrinsic muscles causes imbalance with extrinsic muscles. However, this theory is untenable as paralysis of the intrinsic muscles produces a planovalgus foot. Still, overactivity of intrinsic muscles in an otherwise flail foot does result in cavovarus deformity.
- In patients with muscle imbalance, following pathogenesis may be given:
    - Weak tibialis anterior with normal PL results in plantar flexed and pronated first metatarsal. Long toe extensors try to substitute for weak tibialis anterior and produce extension at MTP joint concomitantly. Hindfoot inverts to compensate for forefoot eversion producing a cavus deformity. The tibialis posterior exacerbates the forefoot equinus and causes inversion at mid-tarsal joint. Further action of tibialis posterior results in varus at heel. This sequence of events results in cavus and contracture of the plantar fascia.
    - Weakness of gastrosoleus leads to calcaneus deformity and push off by long toe flexors forcing forefoot into equinus. A hindfoot deformity follows forefoot equinus. The rigid plantarflexed first ray forces heel into varus and eventually the deformity become fixed.

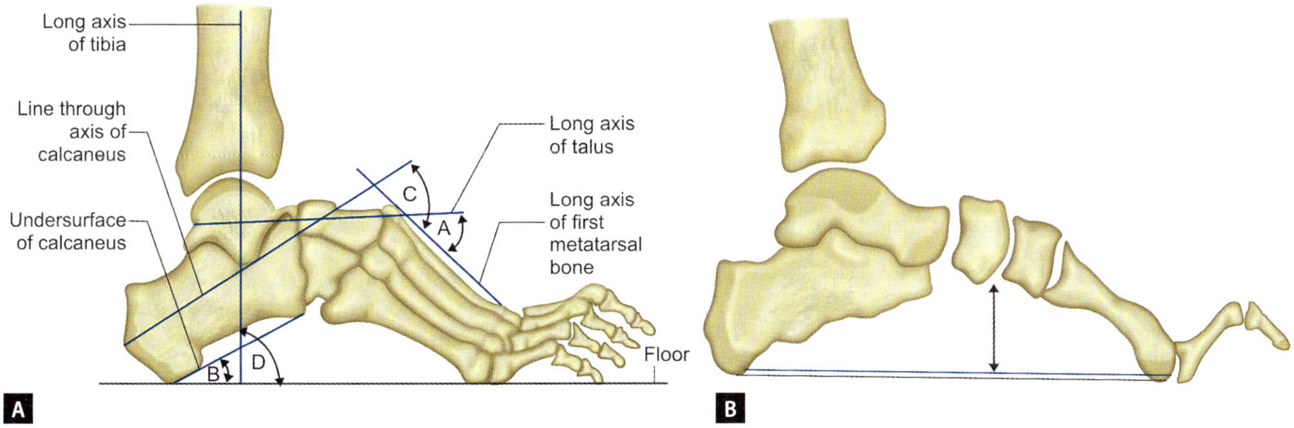

Figs. 13A and B: (A) Cavus foot; (B) Development of clawing in cavus foot.

Pathological Anatomy

The high arch of cavus foot is accompanied by a number of deformities:

- Hyperextension of MTP joint and hyperflexion at IP joint (claw toes) (***see* Figs. 13A and B**)
- Pronation and adduction of forefoot
- The skin on dorsum of midfoot is thin revealing bony prominence with wrinkled skin folds on medial plantar aspect
- Lengthened lateral border of foot and shortened medial border
- Callosities beneath metatarsal heads
- Varied stiffness of subtalar joint
- Varus deformity of heel
- Tightness of tendocalcaneus with/without equinus contracture

Sequence of Events

Dropping of forefoot (initially at first metatarsus) → eversion of forefoot → contracture of plantar fascia → varus of heel (to balance forefoot eversion so that all metatarsals can be placed evenly on the ground) → clawing of toes.

Clinical Findings

- Idiopathic, nonprogressive cavus deformities, where claw toes correct by weight bearing have no symptoms except metatarsalgia.
- Those with fixed claw toe deformities experience metatarsalgia, fixed pronation of forefoot, and painful callosities.
- In patients with progressive cavus, with normal sensory and proprioceptive feedback, response to treatment is good.
- Charcot-Marie-Tooth disease has profound sensory loss, which ultimately may result in amputation. They carry worst prognosis than poliomyelitis due to sensory impairment. These feet do not have hindfoot calcaneus deformity.
- Cavus feet due to poliomyelitis have both anterior and posterior components, i.e., a forefoot equinus and a hindfoot calcaneus (this combination of deformity is produced by strong gastro-soleus + tibialis posterior but weak toe extensors and tibialis anterior) and carry better prognosis due to intact sensations. Recurrence of deformity, nonunion, and degenerative arthritis of adjacent and distant joints are less likely complications of postpolio residual deformity.

Coleman/Chestnut's block test (described elsewhere) is excellent for determining the hindfoot relation in pes cavus and to determine whether hindfoot varus is flexible or fixed.

Types of Deformity

- Simple pes cavus has evenly distributed forefoot where all metatarsals bear weight equally and heel is in neutral or slight valgus position.
- Pes cavovarus is characterized by plantar flexion of medial column alone, which resists dorsiflexion. Lateral toes can be dorsiflexed. Forefoot is pronated with a neutral hindfoot. In stance position, the hindfoot inverts producing heel varus to place all metatarsals evenly on ground.
- Calcaneocavus occurs due to paralysis of triceps surae producing a heel calcaneus (vertical heel) and forefoot in equinus to produce a plantigrade foot.
- Equinocavovarus is a typical deformity of an uncorrected clubfoot.

X-ray Findings

Weight-bearing anteroposterior and lateral views are taken:

- Lateral view (standing) is taken to show **(Figs. 13A and B)**:
  - Position of ankle joint
  - Calcaneus pitch (normal 30°)—line drawn as a tangent from the inferior cortex of the calcaneum. Angle between this and the horizontal is the calcaneus pitch—reduced in planus and increased in cavus
  - Midfoot and forefoot position
  - Degree of plantar flexion of first ray
  - Angle of cavus, i.e., angle between intersection of axis of first metatarsal and axis of talus or calcaneus
  - This also allows the estimation of the hindfoot (talus + calcaneus), midfoot (navicular, cuboid, and cuneiform), and forefoot (Lisfranc) contribution to cavus deformity.
- Anteroposterior view is taken with hindfoot in as neutral position as possible to help corroborate any metatarsus adductus component.
  - Talocalcaneal angle (Kite's angle) is reduced when heel is fixed.
  - Other changes include degenerative changes in ankle and foot joint, and rotation of talus in ankle mortise. Dystrophic ossification in soft tissue suggests a tendon or ligament injury.

Degrees of Cavus Foot

First degree:

- Relatively normal
- Deformity appears when foot is relatively relaxed
- Flexible cavus which disappears on pushing the first metatarsal bone dorsally
- Heel may be easily manipulated into neutral/valgus.

Second degree:

- Equinus and pronation of first ray becomes irreducible
- Early contracture of plantar fascia
- Clawing of big toe

Third degree:

- In addition of dropping of first ray, the other metatarsals also participate in equinus.
- Calcaneus is inverted and resists passive manipulation.
- No bony structural deformity is present.

Fourth degree:

Various components become pronounced and resist a passive correction.

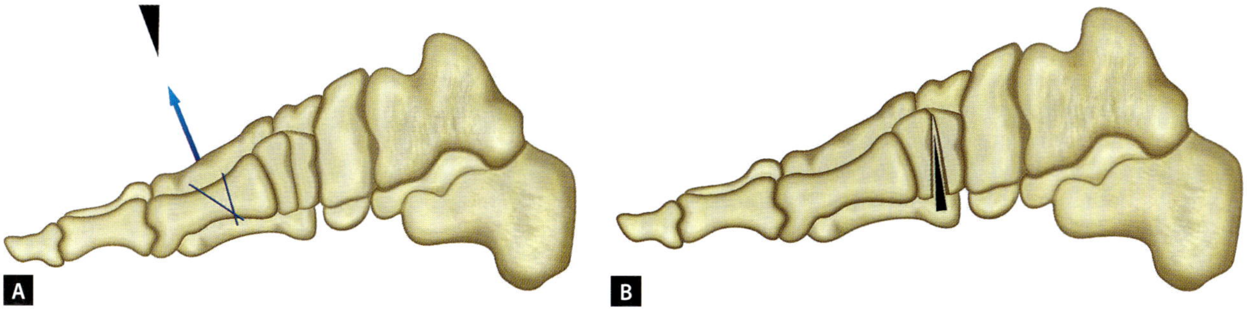

Figs. 14A and B: Jahss truncated wedge osteotomy. (A) To correct the cavus, the dorsal wedge osteotomy is made in the metatarsal; (B) Same can be reinserted in a reverse (open) osteotomy made into the tarsal bone.

Fifth degree:
- All components firmly fixed.
- Structural bony deformities pronounced.
- Toe dislocated dorsally.
- Painful calluses at metatarsal heads and dorsally over PIP joints.
- Plantar fascia is severely contracted

Principles of treatment are directed toward correcting the primary deformity. In skeletally immature foot, when deformity is recognized early, stretching should be used. Transverse lift under metatarsal heads and lateral sole wedge to counteract inversion can also be used.

Treatment of Cavus Foot according to Degrees

First degree:
- Gentle manipulation
- Physiotherapy to exercise dorsiflexors without cocking of toes
- Anterior arch bar in shoes
- Night splint

Second degree:
- Modified Jones procedure
- Steindler's fascial stripping if pleural structures are contracted.

Third degree:
- Hibbs procedure/modified Jones procedure in immature foot
- Dwyer's osteotomy in older child or young adult

Fourth degree:
- Japas osteotomy
- Anterior tarsal wedge osteotomy
- Fusion of first metatarsocuneiform joint

Fifth degree:
- Tendon transfer for muscle imbalance
- Triple arthrodesis
- Jones procedure for the great toe

Specific Surgical Treatment for Various Components of Cavus Foot

- *Claw toes:*
  - Supple deformities—metatarsal bar with insole and care for calluses
  - *Rigid deformities:*
    - Lengthening of EHL and EDL
    - Tenotomy of extensor digitorum brevis and EHB
    - Dorsal capsulotomy of MTP joints
    - Resection of head and neck of proximal phalanges
    - Release of plantar fascia
    - Arthrodesis of IP joint of hallux or release of plantar plate with sectioning of collateral ligaments at IP joint of hallux
    - Tendon suspension of first metatarsal with arthrodesis of IP joint (Jones)
- *Forefoot equinus:*
  - Proximal metatarsal osteotomy with plantar fasciotomy (Gould) with/without Jones procedure (i.e., double plantar fasciotomy and closing wedge, green stick dorsal proximal metatarsal osteotomy)
  - *Hibbs technique:* Transfer of EDL to middle cuneiform
  - Tarsometatarsal truncated-wedge arthrodesis (by Jahss) **(Figs. 14A and B)**.
- *Midfoot cavus:*
  - Anterior tarsal wedge osteotomy (Cole)
  - "V" osteotomy of tarsus (Japas) **(Fig. 15)**
- *Calcaneocavus:*
  - Dwyer's osteotomy of calcaneum which corrects both varus and calcaneus of the hindfoot
  - Crescentic calcaneal osteotomy (Samilson)
- *Calcaneocavovarus and cavovarus:*
  - Triple arthrodesis (Siffert, Forster, and Nachamie)
  - Dunn's technique
  - Hobs-Kite technique
  - Lambrinudi procedure

TALIPES EQUINUS

Caused by the following:
- Muscle imbalance at ankle in which plantar flexors are stronger than dorsiflexors.
- A completely flail foot may develop a fixed equinus deformity of ankle with contracture of the tendocalcaneus and posterior capsular structures (caused by gravity and posture).
- With appearance of medial/lateral instability, equinovalgus or equinovarus deformities will develop.

Conservative treatment includes gentle passive stretching **(Fig. 16)** and serial casting. Surgical treatment includes

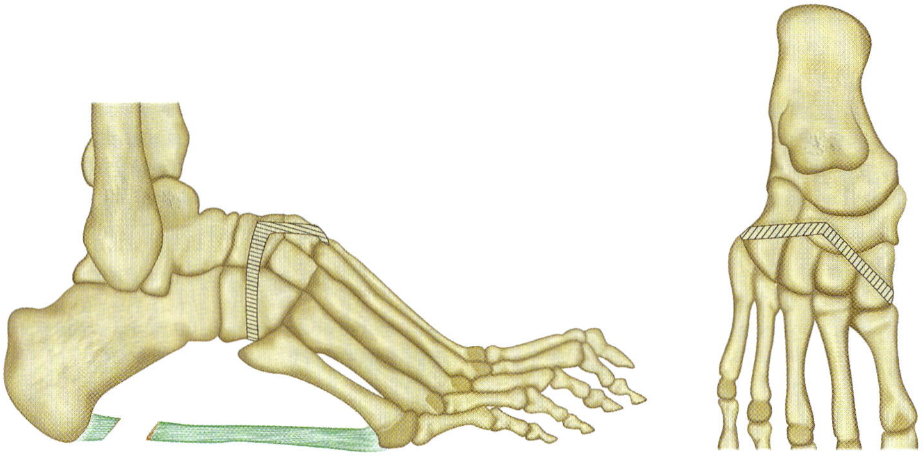

Fig. 15: Japas osteotomy.

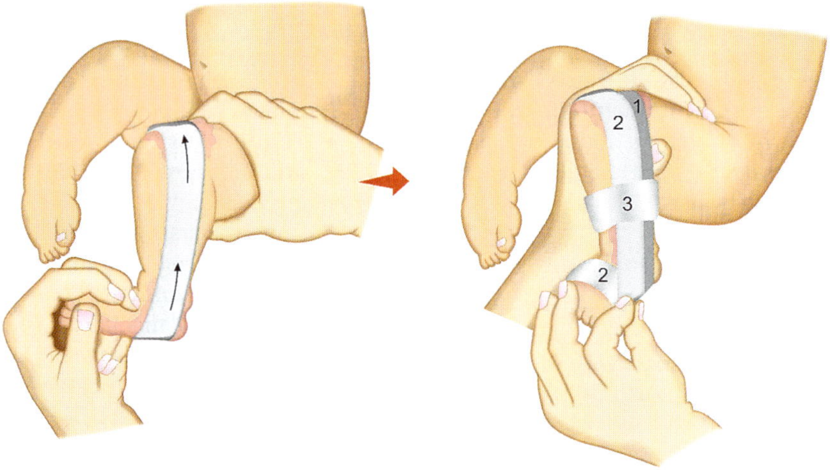

Fig. 16: Manipulation for gentle stretching of equinus deformity.

tendocalcaneus lengthening with or without posterior capsulotomy of ankle joint in long-standing cases. After correction of equinus deformity, one of the following procedures is done to prevent its recurrence:

- Posterior bone block
- Lambrinudi procedure
- Pantalar arthrodesis
- Arthrodesis of the ankle joint

Techniques of Tendocalcaneous Lengthening

- *Tendocalcaneus lengthening by incomplete tenotomy: White's method* based on the observation that tendocalcaneus rotates ~90° between its origin and insertion in its longitudinal axis. Rotation from the posterior view is from medial to lateral. Tendocalcaneus is exposed through a 10-cm long posteromedial incision. Divide its anterior two-thirds near insertion and its medial two-thirds 5–8 cm proximal to site of first division. Passive dorsiflexion of the foot results in lengthening the tendon. There is no need to suture.
- *After treatment:*
  - Above-knee cast is applied from mid-thigh to toes with knee in 30° flexion and ankle in desired degree of dorsiflexion.
  - However if skin is taut on forced dorsiflexion, then deformity should only be partially corrected to prevent sloughing of skin and tendon which will ultimately result in increased deformity by fibrosis. Foot should be held in partial correction until acute reaction has subsided.
  - Cast is removed at 6 weeks and active and passive ROM is begun.
  - Walking with a brace that allows dorsiflexion but prevents plantar flexion.
  - A repeated surgery for recurrence might lead to a recurrence again. When recurrent deformity is severe, excising the superficial scar tissue and replacing it with full thickness skin grafts may be advised before surgery for equinus correction.
- *Hauser's method* based on the observations that calcaneal tendon undergoes varying degrees of rotations between

origin and insertion. Three types of rotations are generally seen:

- Least rotation (52%)—Soleus composed posterior one-third surface and the gastrocnemius anterior two-thirds.
- Moderate rotation (35%)—Soleus composed one-half of the surface and gastrocnemius the other half.
- Extreme rotation (13%)—Soleus composed the posterior two-thirds of surface and gastrocnemius the anterior one-third.

Rotation begins 12–15 cm proximal to the insertion of the tendon, which correlates to level when soleus begins to contribute fibers to the tendon. The tendon is exposed through a posteromedial longitudinal incision. The tendon is incised transversely 8–12 cm proximal to the insertion depending upon amount of correction desired as follows. Insert blade into tendon in coronal plane, so that two-thirds of tendon is posterior to blade, then turn the sharp edge posteriorly to incise tendon till its posterior surface. Now incise the tendon 1.2 cm proximal to its tendon insertion by inserting the curved tenotome anterior to the medial two-thirds of the tendon and drawing it posteriorly and medially to divide the tendon at this point. Tendon lengthens as the foot dorsiflexes. After-treatment remains the same.

- *Stewart technique* is the Z-plastic tenotomy **(Fig. 17)** of tendocalcaneus with/without posterior capsulotomy. The White and Hauser's procedures are usually done when the tendocalcaneus has not been lengthened previously. Z-plastic tenotomy may be done in two planes. The anteroposterior plane is preferred for correction of equinovarus deformity of the clubfoot, while the lateral plane is preferred for tendocalcaneus contracture in poliomyelitis.
- *Technique (lateral plane):* The patient is placed on unaffected side/prone. A posteromedial longitudinal incision measuring 8–10 cm is given. The tendon is divided longitudinally from side to side beginning proximally and continuing distally. The division is completed posteriorly in the proximal part and anteriorly in the distal part. Thus, posterior flap remains attached to calcaneus and anterior remains attached to gastrosoleus. When held in dorsiflexion, the only raw area is in superior part of wound which can be closed by closing tendon sheath above it; thereby, decreasing the chances of skin adhesions. In anteroposterior plane, the tendon is incised longitudinally in the midline. Severe one-half laterally at the proximal end and the other half medially at the distal end **(Fig. 18)**. A lateral plane lengthening is preferred to preserve total width of tendon and reduce the amount of exposed anterior surface except in clubfoot where a tendocalcaneus lengthening in anteroposterior plane is preferred because tendon is often inserted medially and if

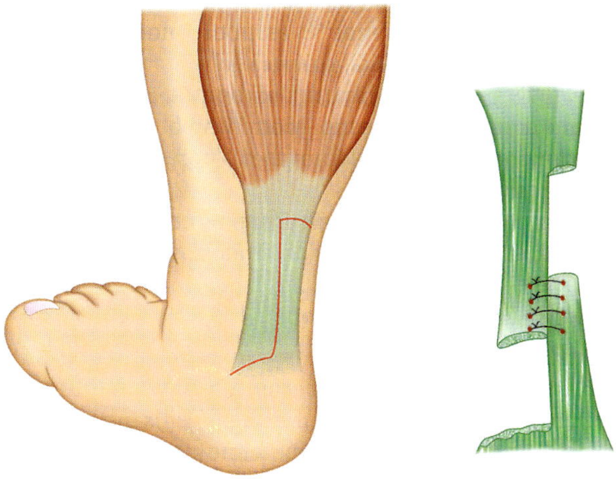

Fig. 17: Achilles tendon lengthening.

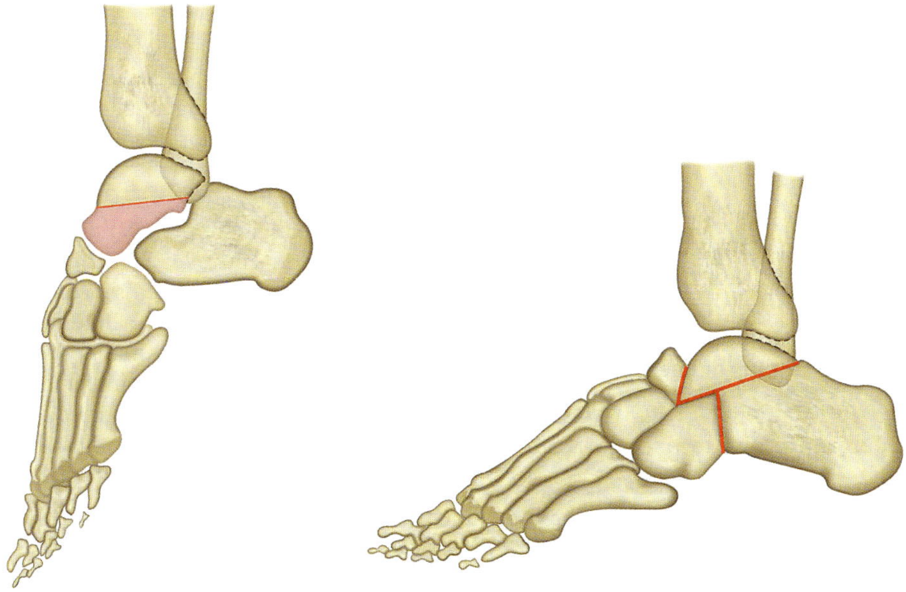

Fig. 18: Lambrinudi arthrodesis.

not detached favors formation of hindfoot varus deformity. After-treatment remains the same.

Posterior ankle capsulotomy and lengthening of tendon of tibialis posterior should be considered in long-standing cases.

Posterior bone block operation (Campbell) is usually combined with triple arthrodesis for preservation of dorsiflexion and prevention of plantar flexion contracture. This is done by construction of a bony buttress on the posterior aspect of talus and superior surface of calcaneus that impinges upon the posterior lip of tibia to prevent ankle plantar flexion.

- Gill modified the Campbell's procedure by lifting a thin layer of bone from posterior surface of talus and opposing it to the posterior lip of tibia. A wedge of bone was then driven into the space thus formed thereby preventing plantar flexion.
- Irwin modified Gill's procedure by using a bone peg to support the osteocartilaginous flap of the talus.
- Inclan used talar head (excised while performing a triple arthrodesis) as a wedge so as to use smooth articular surface for tendon gliding posteriorly.

Recurrence of deformity, fibrous/bony ankylosis of ankle, degenerative arthritis, and flattening of talus are some of the complications of Campbell's posterior bone block procedure.

This technique is rarely indicated now because of effective tendon transfers and other arthrodeses.

Lambrinudi Procedure

Lambrinudi operation is indicated in correction of isolated fixed equinus deformity in patients >10 years of age for conditions when residual dorsiflexor power is insufficient to make reasonable walking possible without toe raising spring. A wedge of bone is removed from plantar and distal part of talus, so that talus remain in completed equinus at the ankle joint, while rest of the foot is in desired degree of corrected plantar flexion **(Fig. 18)**.

The prerequisites to perform a Lambrinudi's procedure include:

- Intact anterior ankle ligaments
- Good power in dorsiflexors. If dorsiflexors are absent then tendon transfer should be done before doing Lambrinudi's procedure.

Good result depends upon strong dorsal ankle ligaments because if ligaments are not strong then recurrence of deformity might occur. If these are weak then equinus position should be slightly overcorrected. Contraindications include flail foot and paralysis in remainder of the limb so that an orthosis will still be required for hip or knee instability.

Complications include:

- Recurrence of deformity due to pseudarthrosis of talonavicular joint
- Stretching of anterior ligaments of the ankle
- Residual deformity of foot (either valgus or varus caused by muscle imbalance)
- Tarsal arthritis
- Pseudarthrosis of talonavicular joint
- Ankle arthritis
- Instability and flattening of superior surface of talus

Pantalar Arthrodesis

Pantalar arthrodesis is surgical fusion of:

- Tibiotalar
- Talonavicular
- Subtalar and calcaneocuboid joint

It is indicated in patients with:

- Calcaneus or equinus deformity combined with lateral instability of foot whose leg muscles are not strong enough to control foot or ankle when the foot is stabilized (flail foot).
- In patients whose deformity has recurred after a posterior bone block/Lambrinudi's procedure.
- For patients with unstable knee occurring from paralysis of quadriceps.

For the last indication, the braces required for stability of knee and foot may be discarded after pantalar arthrodesis and gait becomes easier, less fatiguing. The prerequisites to pantalar arthrodesis include:

- Ability of the knee joint to fully extend or even hyperextend
- A strong gluteus maximum for toe off
- Strong hamstrings or triceps surae are desirable to prevent genu recurvatum.

Postoperatively, the foot should be stabilized in good weight-bearing position after pantalar arthrodesis. Heel should be neutral/valgus, but not in varus. Ankle should be fused in slight equinus (5–10°) to produce a backward thrust on knee joint for a stable weight bearing (acceptable plantar flexion should be confirmed by a weight bearing lateral film with shoes). Excessive plantar flexion may lead to pain and increased pressure under metatarsal heads. A compensatory increase in forefoot motion occurs in patients after pantalar arthrodesis that assists in stance and gait.

When pantalar arthrodesis is being done to stabilize knee after quadriceps weakness, heel should be just high to stabilize knee in extension or hyperextension. Effectiveness of pantalar arthrodesis in stabilizing a flail foot with unstable knee can be determined by a short leg walking cast with foot in 10° of equinus preoperatively. If the knee is stable on walking, it will be stable even after surgery.

An ideal patient for pantalar arthrodesis has flail foot and ankle with normal muscles about hip and the knee. In patients with flail limb, stability of knee is increased by genu recurvatum when foot has been placed in a little more plantar flexion than normal. Pantalar arthrodesis may be done in single stage fusing all the joints in one sitting (Steindler) or in two stages (Leibolt and King), where the foot is stabilized by Hoke's method in the first step followed by ankle arthrodesis in the second step. Two stage operation is better as it is difficult to achieve and maintain the proper positions of foot and ankle simultaneously. Also there is danger of avascular necrosis of talus and failure of fusion in a single stage operation.

Complications (apart from infection, skin necrosis, etc.) include:

- Pseudarthrosis and avascular necrosis of talus
- Painful plantar callosities due to unequal weight distribution and excessive head equinus causing increased pressure on the forefoot.

Ankle arthrodesis is rarely indicated for talipes equinus deformity except in adults where muscle function is too weak to allow tendon transfer or stabilization of foot aimed at restoring dorsiflexion of the ankle.

TALIPES EQUINOVARUS

Talipes equinovarus in poliomyelitis has following characteristic deformities:

- Equinus deformity at ankle
- Inversion of heel
- Adduction at mid-tarsal joint
- Supination at forefoot

Equinovarus deformity of long-standing duration may develop a cavus deformity of foot or claw toes additionally.

Pathogenesis

- Peronei are paralyzed or severely weak.
- Tibialis posterior is usually normal and stronger than peroneals.
- Tibialis anterior is weak or normal.
- Triceps surae is comparatively strong.

A strong triceps surae leads to equinus due to motor imbalance. Disproportionate growth, gravity, and posture increase chances for development of equinus. The equinus position increases the advantage of tibialis posterior, which increases hindfoot inversion and forefoot adduction and supination. Toe extensors substitute for a weak tibialis anterior to dorsiflex the ankle resulting in cavus and clawing of the toes. Clawing is aggravated by triceps surae contracture. A brace may also contribute to equinovarus deformity in case of external tibial torsion unless this torsion is taken care off during brace construction.

Treatment depends upon age of patient, forces causing the deformity, severity of deformity, and the rate of progression.

Treatment in Skeletally Immature Foot

Conservative treatment consists of gentle passive stretching of plantar fascia and posterior ankle structure and application of a brace. The brace is given to help to prevent the deformity. Double bar with 90° ankle stop and an outside T-strap is constructed. When there is external tibial torsion, the shoe is attached to brace in an externally rotated position. If equinus has become fixed then a raised heel is given.

If deformity increases despite above measures then gradual correction with wedging cast technique is done. This is usually successful if the deformity is not too severe.

Surgical management consists of Steindler's fascial stripping, tendocalcaneus lengthening and posterior capsulotomy may be necessary.

After correction of deformity, surgery is indicated to prevent its recurrence. Tibialis posterior is usually strong and deformity will recur unless its influence is removed. It may be transferred anteriorly through interosseous membrane to anterolateral tarsal area (Barr and Blount) or it may be transferred to triceps surae if it is weak. Tibialis anterior when strong can be transferred to dorsum of foot over fourth ray to replace peronei. If weak, it can be transferred to second or third ray. When tibialis posterior is weak, with strong tibialis anterior, then the latter should be split and a portion transferred to the insertion of PB (Hoefer) to substitute for evertors.

External tibial torsion of 30° or more should be corrected by derotation osteotomy of tibia and fibula.

Treatment in Skeletally Mature Foot

Foot is stabilized by triple arthrodesis and cavus is corrected at same time by Steindler's fascial stripping. If this does not correct the foot completely, then manipulation is tried under anesthesia after 10 days and a long leg cast is given. Residual deformity is corrected by wedging at 3–5 days intervals until deformity has corrected clinically and on X-rays.

Tendocalcaneus is lengthened 4–6 weeks after Steindler's procedure. EHL is transferred to neck of first metatarsal. Tendon of tibialis posterior is transferred anteriorly through interosseous membrane to anterolateral tarsal area. This removes the dynamic deformity force and aids in active dorsiflexion of foot. However, when no other dorsiflexor is available, the transfer of tibialis anterior should be combined with triple arthrodesis and a posterior bone block of the ankle. When tibialis posterior is weak, tibialis anterior is transferred to a point slightly lateral to the midline on dorsum of foot. External tibial torsion is corrected by derotation osteotomy of tibia and fibula.

Ankle arthrodesis for equinovarus deformity is done only when no suitable muscle for transfer is available for foot stabilization. Ankle arthrodesis is usually followed by subcutaneous plantar fasciotomy and tendocalcaneus lengthening.

TALIPES CAVOVARUS

Paralytic talipes cavovarus is caused by an imbalance of extrinsic muscles (as described earlier in talipes equinovarus) or by persistent action of intrinsic muscles like short toe flexors when rest of the foot is flail.

Treatment

Excising short flexor muscles and a block of plantar flexion with neurectomy of motor branches of medial and lateral plantar nerves. The sensory branches of plantar nerves should be preserved. However, neurectomy should not be done in cavovarus foot of arthrogryposis multiplex congenita. Best results are obtained in skeletally immature foot (Discussed in Chapter on "Osteonecrosis and Osteochondrosis").

TALIPES EQUINOVALGUS

The deformity arises from:

- Weak tibialis anterior and tibialis posterior
- Strong PL and PB
- Strong and contracted triceps surae

Strong triceps surae and peronei pull the foot into equinovalgus especially when EDL and peroneus tertius are also strong. Such a child walks with foot in valgus position. Eventually, plantar calcaneonavicular ligament becomes stretched and attenuated as weight-bearing thrust shifts to medial border of the foot. Forefoot abducts and pronates, and head and neck of talus get depressed and prominent on the medial and inferior side of foot.

Treatment in Skeletally Immature Feet

Conservative management consists of gentle passive stretching and braces with double bar, 90° ankle stop, inside T-strap, shoe with an arch support and medial heel wedge. Wedging casts may be applied if above regimen does not help.

Surgical treatment involves tendocalcaneus lengthening as described above. After correction of deformity, surgery to prevent recurrence is necessary. One of the following procedures helps in prevention of a recurrence.

- Subtalar arthrodesis (Grice and Green) **(Figs. 19A and B)**
- Anterior transfer of PL and PB
- Triple arthrodesis if necessary (in case of failure of treatment)
- *Axer's procedure:* Axer described an operation for children between 3 years and 6 years of age, where talonavicular and subtalar joints are opened; talus, calcaneus, and navicular are placed in normal position to each other and one or more of the deforming evertor muscle is transferred to the neck of talus. Tendocalcaneus lengthening may be done when necessary.

Dynamic valgus is caused by paralysis of tibialis anterior/tibialis posterior or both. Paralysis of tibialis anterior causes moderate valgus which increases on dorsiflexion but may disappear on plantar flexion. Long toe extensor (EDL) substitutes for the dorsiflexion of the foot resulting in claw toes. Because of anterolateral anchorage of EDL and its insertion at lateral toes, it acts as an evertor in dorsiflexion. Hence, this is treated by transferring PL/EDL to first cuneiform or by Jones' operation. Clawing of lateral toes will disappear after tarsal reconstruction, tendocalcaneus lengthening and peroneal tendon transfer, but clawing of great toe is corrected by Jones operation.

Normally, tibialis posterior inverts during plantar flexion and supports the longitudinal arch. Paralysis of tibialis posterior alone causes a planovalgus deformity by collapse of the arch resulting in planovalgus.

Treatment is transferring the tendon of PL/FHL/FDL/EDL to navicular through sheath of tibialis posterior. Paralysis of both tibialis anterior and posterior results in severe convex per planus, deformity similar to rocker bottom or long convex planus. Treatment is done by tendon transfer for tibialis posterior and later for tibialis anterior if required.

Treatment in Skeletally Mature Foot

Tendocalcaneus lengthening is performed with triple arthrodesis. This is followed by anterior transfer of PL or PB/modified Jones operation after 4–6 weeks.

A valgus deformity without equinus/calcaneus occasionally occurs in patients where PPRP after growth is complete. Tibialis anterior, tibialis posterior, and triceps surae are usually weak in such cases. Triple arthrodesis and Jones operation followed by posterior transfer of peroneals to triceps after 6 weeks is the desired treatment.

TALIPES CALCANEUS

It is caused by paralysis of triceps surae, and other extrinsic foot muscles, which plantar flex the toes. Those muscles that dorsiflex the ankle remain functional.

Pathogenesis

Severely weak/paralyzed triceps surae is unable to stabilize calcaneum and results in loss of push off in walking. Unopposed dorsiflexors result in thin and elongated triceps. On attempting walking, the calcaneus rotates, because its posterior end is pulled plantar ward by long and short toe flexors and other intrinsic muscles resulting in cavus. Gravity assists in development of forefoot equinus. Peronei and tibialis aggravate the deformity. Plantar fascia gradually becomes

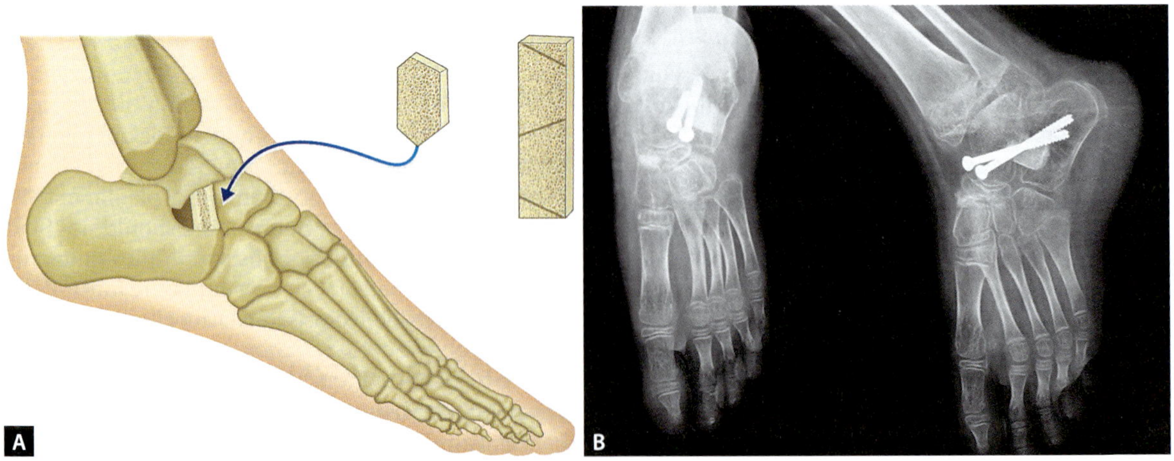

Figs. 19A and B: The extra-articular arthrodesis of Grice-Green: (A) Illustration showing the insertion of bone graft in the sinus tarsi after clearing the tissues there and roughening the bone surfaces; (B) Kite's view and oblique radiographs of the procedure.

contracted. On gait analysis, normal push off is lost at the end of stance phase and instead of heel raise, ankle rotates into dorsiflexion and ultimately into subluxation. Such ankles have valgus deformity, thinning of wedging of distal tibial epiphysis, and decrease in rate of growth of fibula. The calcaneotibial angle (normal 70–80°) is measured at the intersection of long axis of tibia and a line drawn along the plantar aspect of calcaneum. Values < 70° denote calcaneus deformity and those >80° equinus deformity.

Treatment

In a skeletally immature foot when the deformity is mild, a brace with elevated and posteriorly extended heel with limited ankle motion and an elastic posterior ankle strap will help in checking the progression of the deformity. Exercises are prescribed for normal alignment of foot and ankle and to restore power in triceps surae. Early tendon transfer is recommended when the deformity in progressing rapidly especially in a young child. The purpose of surgery in a skeletally immature foot is to prevent deformity from increasing or to correct a severe one already present without damaging the bones.

However, foot stabilization is necessary after skeletal maturity. Plantar fasciotomy is followed by tibialis posterior, PL, and PB transfer to calcaneus. If these muscles are weak then post-transfer of tibialis anterior is recommended. When EHL and EDL have good strength, both tibials and both peroneals may be transferred to calcaneus but EHL and EDL must be transferred proximally to prevent any equinus deformity. For talipes calcaneocavus, posterior transfer of tibialis anterior to calcaneus is recommended to prevent excessive dorsiflexion at ankle. For talipes calcaneovalgus, transfer of PL and PB to calcaneus as far posteriorly and immediately lateral to its midline is recommended.

If adequate muscles are not available then tenodesis of tendocalcaneus to fibula prevents calcaneus hitch (Westin).

Treatment in a skeletally mature foot includes plantar fasciotomy with Hoke stabilization. Any foot stabilization procedure used for calcaneocavus deformity should displace the foot as posteriorly as possible to increase the posterior lever arm (calcaneum) requiring less muscle power to provide push-off force. Beak's triple arthrodesis is designed to preserve the circulation of talar head, to correct the calcaneus deformity, and to make the shape of foot normal by lengthening its plantar surface. If deformity is not corrected satisfactorily at operation then Knowles pin partially threaded cancellous screw is inserted through long axis of calcaneum and incorporated in a cast. Subsequent wedging then corrects the deformity.

Four to six weeks after stabilization, one of the following tendon transfers may be done to prevent recurrence:

- Peroneus longus, PB, and tibialis posterior to calcaneum.
- Extensor digitorum longus to cuneiform.
- Tibialis anterior to cuneiform. The results are good if its power is between 4/5 and 5/5, the transfer is carried before deformity becomes fixed and the tendon is transferred along the interosseous membrane through a window rather than a hole.
- Posterior transfer of tibialis posterior, PL, and FHL to calcaneus.

In a skeletally mature foot, Hoke's stabilization preceded by fusion of the IP joint of great toe and excision of a block of plantar fascia (2–3 cm) is recommended (Irwin). This is followed 4-week later by transfer of EHL to first metatarsal neck and one of the tendon transfers as listed above. Pantalar arthrodesis may be done when no useful muscle is available for transfer. Talectomy, done in past, has become obsolete now for this deformity.

In calcaneovalgus deformity, medial border of the foot is longer than lateral (opposite to equinovarus deformity where vice versa is true). Evans described osteotomy and lengthening of calcaneus for calcaneovalgus (flat foot). This technique consists of transverse osteotomy of calcaneus 1.5 cm posterior and parallel to calcaneocuboid joint and insertion of a bone graft to open a wedge thereby increasing the length of lateral border.

CONCLUSION

- The incidence of new cases of poliomyelitis has reduced drastically to near nonexisting levels.
- Older cases of polio still present with significant morbidity due to muscle paralysis and instability at the joints. Secondary deformities develop in the joints that need correction for improving the function of patients.
- It is important to evaluate the muscle groups affected and those spared so that proper motors can be provided for lost function. Also stability at the various joints need to be provided so that patients can be made ambulatory without support.

CHAPTER 40

Cerebral Palsy and Inherited Neuromuscular Disorders

Manish Kumar Varshney

INTRODUCTION

Cerebral palsy (CP) and other inherited neuromuscular disorders encompass a broad range of disorders origination either in brain or at muscle fiber. These disorders may be static or progressive due to varied etiology but share many similarities among themselves in terms of musculoskeletal manifestations. Muscular weakness causing decreased function temporally translates into contractures, deformity, gait disturbances, and scoliosis in many. Nevertheless the differences among disorders should be well appreciated because subtle variants of many present late and even in adulthood. There has been increasing shift in transitioning care to adult care. No cure exists for these disorders but advances in genetic engineering, gene therapy may soon make it possible. Growth sparing implants offer more physiological options for managing spinal deformity. Continuous updation is necessary to provide optimal treatment to these patients and improve their function.

CEREBRAL PALSY

Cerebral palsy describes a group of permanent disorders of the development of movement and posture, causing activity limitation, that are attributed to nonprogressive disturbance that occurred in the developing fetal or infant brain. The motor disorders of CP are often accompanied by disturbances of sensation, perception, cognition, communication, and behavior by epilepsy, and by secondary musculoskeletal problems. It has been estimated that about 80% of children with CP have some type of movement disorder. CP is most often classified as either spastic, dyskinetic, or ataxic **(Fig. 1)**. Although spasticity is often the dominant disorder, many children with CP have mixed spasticity and dystonia. When more than one type of movement disorder is present in patients, experts recommend classifying patients by the predominant disorder.

- ***Hypertonia*** is defined as "abnormally increased resistance to externally imposed movement about a joint". Hypertonicity can be caused by spasticity, dystonia, or rigidity (though rigidity is rare in children and not associated with CP).
- ***Spasticity*** is hypertonia in which resistance to passive movement increases with increasing velocity of movement (or exhibits a spastic catch), and "varies with direction of the movement, and/or rises rapidly above a threshold speed or joint angle". Spasticity is often a component of upper motor neuron syndrome, along with hyperreflexia, clonus, reflex overflow, positive Babinski sign, and pyramidal distribution weakness (upper extremity extensors and lower extremity flexors). Spasticity is caused by a hyperactive stretch reflex mechanism, and is amenable to treatments, such as botulinum toxin, baclofen, selective dorsal rhizotomy, and orthopedic surgery.
- ***Dystonia*** is defined as "a movement disorder in which involuntary sustained or intermittent muscle contractions cause twisting and repetitive movements, abnormal postures, or both". Dystonic hypertonia is present in cases where the resistance to passive movement does not change with changes in speed of passive movement or joint angle, may be associated with simultaneous agonist and antagonist contraction (equal resistance when the direction of passive movement is reversed). Dystonia is not associated with hyperreflexia and often disappears when the child is asleep. Because myelination is needed for development of dystonia, it typically occurs later in life than spasticity (around 5–10 years of age). Dystonia is associated with disruption of the basal ganglia and therefore is not improved by selective dorsal rhizotomy. It is generally accepted that tendon lengthening and transfer procedures are contraindicated

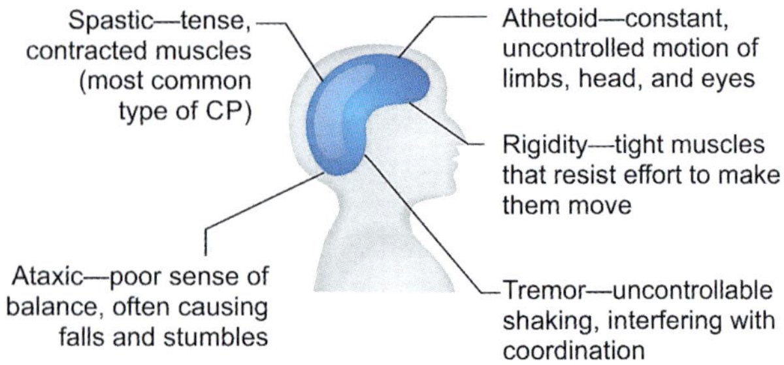

Fig. 1: Types of cerebral palsy (CP).

in cases of dystonia, because of the risk for recurrence of deformity or development of reverse deformities. Dystonic hypertonia is responsive to botulinum toxin as well as intrathecal baclofen, which generally weaken overactive muscles or muscle groups.

- ***Hyperkinetic movements*** are defined as "any unwanted excess movement" that is performed voluntarily or involuntarily by the patient, and represent what have traditionally been referred to as extrapyramidal symptoms. The hyperkinetic movements most commonly seen in CP, include dystonia, chorea, athetosis, and tremors. Hyperkinetic dystonia is characterized by "abnormal postures that are superimposed upon or substitute for voluntary movements". Orthopedic surgery in cases of predominantly hyperkinetic movement disorders associated with CP is most often limited to bony procedures, as fixed contractures are rare because of the often nearly continuous movements of the extremities and joints. Such patients should be referred to a movement disorders specialist for management. Tendon lengthening in patients with hyperkinetic movement disorders is unreliable and may result in a reverse deformity. It should be remembered that split tendon transfers are more successful in patients with dystonia than are whole tendon transfers.
- ***Chorea*** is defined as "an ongoing random appearing sequence of one or more discrete involuntary movements or movement fragments". Choreiform movements are also random, can appear continuous and jerky, and can be difficult for patients to relax. Athetosis is defined as "a slow, continuous, involuntary writhing movement that prevents maintenance of a stable posture". It usually involves the hands or feet and perioral muscles. Athetosis is not common as an isolated movement disorder in CP and is most often found in combination with chorea.

Hypertonia in CP is most often rated using the Modified Ashworth Scale (MAS) **(Table 1)**. The Tardieu Scale **(Table 2)** is preferred by some clinicians and researchers, because it assesses resistance to both fast and slow stretches, the angle at which resistance is felt initially (R1), as well as the end of passively available range of motion (ROM) (R2). Neither test is able to distinguish spasticity from hypertonic dystonia (or contracture, in the case of the MAS). Hypertonicity and dyskinetic movements actually constitute positive motor signs of increased activity.

TABLE 1: Modified Ashworth Scale for assessment of hypertonia.

0	No increase in muscle tone
1	Slight increase in muscle tone, manifested by a catch and release or by minimal resistance at the end of the range of motion (ROM) when the affected part(s) is moved in flexion or extension
1+	Slight increase in muscle tone, manifested by a catch, followed by minimal resistance throughout the remainder (less than half) of the ROM
2	More marked increase in muscle tone through most of the ROM, but affected part(s) easily moved
3	Considerable increase in muscle tone, passive movement difficult
4	Affected part(s) rigid in flexion or extension

Negative signs include characteristics that are decreased or insufficient and include weakness (insufficient muscle activation), poor selective motor control (inability to activate a specific pattern of muscles in an isolated fashion), ataxia (inability to activate the correct pattern of muscles during a movement), and apraxia/developmental dyspraxia (inability to activate the correct pattern of muscles to perform a specific task, either because of loss of ability or lack of acquisition of the skill). Negative signs should be recognized because

TABLE 2: Tardieu Scale for assessment of hypertonia.

For each muscle group, reaction to stretch is rated at a specified stretch velocity with two parameters x and y.

Velocity to stretch (V)
- V1: As slow as possible
- V2: Speed of the limb segment falling
- V3: As fast as possible (> natural drop)

V1 is used to measure the passive range of motion (PROM). Only V2 and V3 are used to rate spasticity.

Quality of muscle reaction (X)		*Angle of muscle reaction (Y):*
0	No resistance throughout passive movement	Measure relative to the position of minimal stretch of the muscle (corresponding at angle) *Spasticity angle:* R1: Angle of catch seen at velocity V2 or V3 R2: Full range of motion achieved when muscle is at rest and tested at V1 velocity
1	Slight resistance throughout	
2	Clear catch at a precise angle, followed by release	
3	Fatigable clonus (<10 sec) occurring at a precise angle	
4	Unfatigable clonus (>10 sec) occurring at a precise angle	
5	Joint immobile	

Upper limb (to be tested in a sitting position, elbow flexed by 90° at the recommended joint positions and velocities)

Shoulder	Horizontal adductors	V3	
	Vertical adductors	V3	
	Internal rotators	V3	
Elbow	Flexors	V2	Shoulder adducted
	Extensors	V3	Shoulder abducted
	Pronators	V3	Shoulder adducted
	Supinators	V3	Shoulder adducted
Wrist	Flexors	V3	
	Extensors	V3	
	Fingers		Angle PII of digit III-MCP
	Palmar interossei + FDS	V3	Wrist resting position

Lower limb (to be tested in supine position, at recommended joint positions and velocities)

Hip	Extensors	V3	Knee extended
	Adductors	V3	Knee extended
	External rotators	V3	Knee flexed by 90°
	Internal rotators	V3	Knee flexed by 90°
Knee	Extensors	V2	Hip flexed by 30°
	Flexors	V3	Hip flexed
Ankle	Plantar flexors	V3	Knee flexed by 30°

(FDS: flexor digitorum superficialis; MCP: metacarpophalangeal)

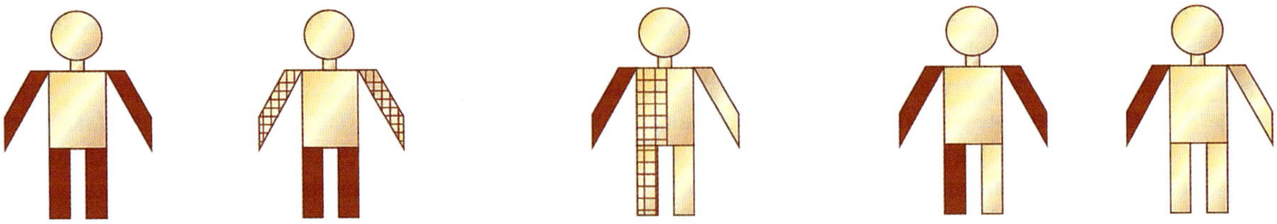

Quadriplegia
All four limbs are involved.
Diplegia
All four limbs are involved. Both legs are more severely affected than the arms.
Hemiplegia
One side of the body is affected. The arm is usually more involved than the leg.
Triplegia
Three limbs are involved, usually both arms and a leg.
Monoplegia
Only one limb is affected, usually an arm.

Fig. 2: Distribution of primary spastic form of cerebral palsy.

their presence may contribute to poor surgical outcomes. These problems are best addressed through physical and occupational therapy.

The traditional classifications of limb distribution for the hypertonic (primarily spastic) form of CP, hemiplegia, diplegia, and quadriplegia/tetraplegia (and occasionally triplegia) continue to be used clinically **(Fig. 2)**. Inconsistencies arise because of lack of definition of how much upper extremity impairment is needed to classify patients as quadriplegic versus diplegic. In addition, children with hemiplegia often have some motor signs on the contralateral side.

CLASSIFICATION OF ACTIVITY LIMITATION AND ASSESSMENT

This system rates patients' ambulatory function, including use of mobility aids and performance in sitting, standing and walking activities. The Gross Motor Function Classification System (GMFCS)—expanded and revised (ER)—includes children up to 18 years of age.

The GMFCS-ER **(Box 1)** provides a method for communicating about gross motor function, based on the use of mobility aids and performance in sitting, standing, and walking activities. It is intended to classify a patient's level of gross motor function based on his or her typical performance, rather than his/her best capability. It classifies gross motor function on a 5-point ordinal scale with descriptions of skills provided for five age groups <2 years of age, 2–4 years of age, 4–6 years of age, 6–12 years of age, and finally 12–18 years of age. In general, the levels are as follows:

- Level I—Walks without limitations
- Level II—Walks with limitations
- Level III—Walks using a hand-held mobility device
- Level IV—Self-mobility with limitations; may use powered mobility
- Level V—Transported in a manual wheelchair

The GMFCS has also been used to study and document the age at which peak gross motor function is achieved for each level (approximately 5 years of age for GMFCS Levels I and II, 8 years of age for Level III and 7 years of age for Levels IV and V), and to document the stability or decline in gross motor skills through adolescence. Further, the GMFCS has been useful in categorizing patients for orthopedic prognostic and experimental studies, both short and long term. Hip surveillance data in children with CP have shown that the incidence of hip dislocation increases linearly with GMFCS classification from Level I (0% incidence) to Level V (>90% incidence).

BOX 1: Gross Motor Function Classification System (GMFCS) for cerebral palsy.

GMFCS- expanded and revised (ER) between 6th and 12th birthday:

- *GMFCS Level I:* Children walk at home, school, outdoors, and in the community. They can climb stairs without the use of a railing. Children perform gross motor skills such as running and jumping, but speed, balance, and coordination are limited.
- *GMFCS Level II:* Children walk in most settings and climb stairs holding onto a railing. They may experience difficulty walking long distances and balancing on uneven terrain, inclines, in crowded areas or confined spaces. Children may walk with physical assistance, a hand-held mobility device or used wheeled mobility over long distances. Children have only minimal ability to perform gross motor skills such as running and jumping.
- *GMFCS Level III:* Children walk using a hand-held mobility device in most indoor settings. They may climb stairs holding onto a railing with supervision or assistance. Children use wheeled mobility when traveling long distances and may self-propel for shorter distances.
- *GMFCS Level IV:* Children use methods of mobility that require physical assistance or powered mobility in most settings. They may walk for short distances at home with physical assistance or use powered mobility or a body support walker when positioned. At school, outdoors and in the community children are transported in a manual wheelchair or use powered mobility.
- *GMFCS Level V:* Children are transported in a manual wheelchair in all settings. Children are limited in their ability to maintain antigravity head and trunk postures and control level and arm movements.

GMFCS-ER between 12th and 18th birthday:

- *GMFCS Level I:* Youth walk at home, school, outdoors, and in the community. Youth are able to climb curbs and stairs without physical assistance or a railing. They perform gross motor skills such as running and jumping but speed, balance and coordination are limited.
- *GMFCS Level II:* Youth walk in most settings but environmental factors and personal choice influence mobility choices. At school or work, they may require a hand-held mobility device for safety and climb stairs holding onto a railing. Outdoors and in the community, youth may use wheeled mobility when traveling long distances.
- *GMFCS Level III:* Youth are capable of walking using a hand held mobility device. Youth may climb stairs holding onto a railing with supervision or assistance. At school, they self-propel a manual wheelchair or use powered mobility. Outdoors and in the community, youth are transported in a wheelchair or use powered mobility.
- *GMFCS Level IV:* Youth use wheeled mobility in most settings. Physical assistance of 1–2 people is required for transfers. Indoors, youth may walk short distances with physical assistance, use wheeled mobility or a body support walker when positioned. They may operate a powered chair, otherwise are transported in a manual wheelchair.
- *GMFCS Level V:* Youth are transported in a manual wheelchair in all settings. Youth are limited in their ability to maintain antigravity head and trunk postures and control leg and arm movements. Self-mobility is severely limited, even with the use of assistive technology.

(For additional details, the eager reader is referred to http://motorgrowth.canchild.ca/en/gmfcs/resources/gmfcs_english.pdf)

BOX 2: Functional Mobility Scale (FMS) rating system.

- *Rating 6*
  Independent on all surfaces:
  Does not use any walking aids or need any help from another person when walking over all surfaces including uneven ground, curbs, etc., and in a crowded environment.
- *Rating 5*
  Independent on level surfaces:
  Does not use walking aids or need help from another person. Requires a rail for stairs.
- *Rating 4*
  Uses sticks (one or two):
  Without help from another person
- *Rating 3*
  Uses crutches:
  Without help from another person
- *Rating 2*
  Uses a walker or frame:
  Without help from another person
- *Rating 1*
  Uses wheelchair
  May stand for transfers, may do some stepping supported by another person or using a walker/frame.
- *Rating C*
  Crawling: Child crawls for mobility at home (5 mL).
- *Rating N*
  N–does not apply [for example child does not complete the distance (500 m)]

Gross Motor Function Classification System level observed around 12 years of age is highly predictive of adult gross motor function. Children who use a wheelchair as their primary mode of mobility have a 96% chance that they will continue to use the wheelchair into adulthood.

The Functional Mobility Scale (FMS) was designed by Graham and colleagues as a measure of ambulatory performance in children with CP **(Box 2)**. The FMS is administered via parent/patient interview and categorizes the assistance needed (none, canes, crutches, walker, and wheelchair) or a child to walk three distances (5, 50, and 500 yards, or 5, 50, and 500 m). The distances are not specifically measured, but are used as estimates to represent household, school, and community ambulation. Ratings are given for each distance category: 1 uses wheelchair, 2 uses walker or frame; 3 uses crutches; 4 uses sticks (canes); 5 independent on level surfaces; 6 independent on all surfaces. A rating of C is given if the child crawls the designated distance and an N is given if the child is unable to move through a given distance. A child who ambulates independently for all distances and on all types of surfaces would be given a rating of 6, 6, and 6. A child, who ambulates independently on level surfaces in the home, uses crutches at school and a wheelchair for shopping trips and family outings would be given a rating of 5, 3, and 1. The FMS specifically addresses ambulation and, therefore, is not intended to substitute for the GMFCS, which assesses mobility on a more general level. The FMS should be used as a companion rating scale to the GMFCS.

Manual Ability Classification System

The Manual Ability Classification System (MACS) was designed to describe upper extremity performance in activities of daily living for children with CP. It reports on performance of upper limb tasks in daily living, regardless of how they are accomplished, and the collaboration of both hands together (bimanual tasks).

The MACS is also desired as a five-category scale:

- Level I—Handles objects easily and successfully
- Level II—Handles most objects but with somewhat reduced quality or speed of achievement
- Level III—Handles objects with difficulty; needs help to prepare or modify activities
- Level IV—Handles a limited selection of easily managed objects in adapted situations
- Level V—Does not handle objects and has severely limited ability to perform even simple actions
- It should be noted that neither the GMFCS-ER nor the MACS is intended to identify the cause of activity limitation (neurologic or musculoskeletal impairments, cognitive, or attention deficits), but is simply intended to categorize a child's ability to function in daily life.

CLINICAL ASSESSMENT OF A CEREBRAL PALSY CHILD

Medical history, birth history, developmental milestones, and treatment history provide important insight in the management of CP. Functional Assessment Questionnaire (FAQ), the Pediatric Orthopedic Society of North America Outcomes Data Collection Instruments (PODCI), and FMS are some of the currently used tools to measure functional outcome in children with CP after invasive procedures. The FAQ is 10-level report of ambulation. The child who is able to keep up with peers is marked at Level 10. The score decreases with decreasing ability to perform community ambulation. PODCI includes measures for upper and lower extremity motor skills, relief of pain, and restoration of activity. FMS is a measure of functional mobility in children with CP aged 4–18 years. FMS also includes use of assistive devices. All have been shown to have changes after orthopedic interventions.

The standard physical assessment form used at Gillette Children Specialty Healthcare is a useful reference to comprehensive physical examination.

The physical examination consists of seven broad parts:

1. Strength and selective motor control of isolated muscle group
2. Degree and type of muscle tone
3. Degree of static muscle and joint contracture
4. Torsional and other bone deformities
5. Fixed mobile foot deformities
6. Balance, equilibrium responses and standing posture
7. Gait by observation

The information collected by static physical examination and gait analysis provides the information that is important in management of ambulation problems in children with CP.

The 5-point Kendall Scale is a time honored easy way to assess for muscle strength. To increase objectivity, the hand-held dynamometer has been used increasingly. Assessment of selective motor control involves isolating movements on request. Typical muscle selectivity reports three grades of control: 0—no ability, 1—partial ability, and 2—complete ability to isolate movements. Muscle tone may be differently perceived on separate occasions by some on different practitioners. To standardize the examination, the muscle is first palpated to determine contracture at rest. The limb is then moved slowly to assess available passive ROM.

Next, the limb is moved through the available ROM at different speeds to assess the presence of spasticity or rigidity. Lastly, the limb or joint is observed while asking the patient to move the same joint on contralateral side. Ashworth scale; MAS; Tardieu Scale, and Isokinetic dynamometer can be used to assess severity of hypertonia. Static and dynamic deformities are best differentiated under general anesthesia. Dynamic contractures disappear under anesthesia.

Thomas test is used to measure the degree of flexor tightness of the hip joint. The pelvic position during test is important. The anterior-superior iliac spine (ASIS) and posterior-superior iliac spine (PSIS) should be aligned vertically.

The cause of *limited range of abduction* can be found by measuring hip abduction in different positions of knee. One joint adductors (adductor longus, adductor brevis, and adductor magnus) are isolated (active) with knee flexed. Two joint adductor (gracilis) is relaxed in this position. Hence, if hip abduction is limited with knee fully extended, the responsible muscle should be gracilis.

While assessing knee joint, it is necessary to differentiate between the *knee joint contracture* and *hamstring contracture*. The knee joint contracture true can be identified if knee extension is limited with hip extended and ankle plantar flexed. This position relaxes hamstrings and gastrocnemius. The hamstring contracture is identified if knee extension is limited with hip flexed to 90° (the popliteal angle). This is measured by flexing the ipsilateral hip to 90° with contralateral hip fully extended. The knee is now fully extended. The unilateral popliteal angle is measured as degrees lacking from full extension of the knee. The bilateral popliteal angle is measured by flexing the contralateral hip till ASIS and PSIS are vertically aligned.

Hamstring shift is the difference between unilateral popliteal angle measured in neural pelvis (with ASIS and PSIS vertically aligned) and that measured with lordosis present. The former measures the true hamstring contracture and the latter measures the functional hamstring contracture. A hamstring shift greater than 20° usually indicates excessive anterior tilt. Normal popliteal angle measurement between 5 and 18 years old vary from 0° to 49°.

Femoral anteversion can be estimated clinically in prone position by rotating hip externally and internally until greater trochanter is palpated to be maximally prominent, with tibia perpendicular to posterior aspect of the femoral condyles (when the knee is flexed to 90°). Femoral anteversion at birth is 45° with normal remodeling; adult values are reached by the age of 8 years (10° for men and 15° for women). *Tibial torsion* may be measured by thigh foot angle and is commonly present in patients with CP. *Patella alta* is also common in CP children due to excessive knee extensor forces of rectus femoris, spasticity, and crouch gait. Patella alta may lead to extensor leg, which is measured as difference between the active and passive ranging motion at the knee joint. The top of patella is palpated with knee fully extended in supine position. The superior pole of patella is typically one finger width proximal to adductor tubercle.

Pronation and supination are triplanar motions *of the foot and ankle* which occur along an oblique axis passing through the subtalar joint. The neutral subtalar joint axis helps to evaluate the rear foot (varus, neutral, and valgus) and forefoot (forefoot varus and valgus) deformities of the foot.

Observational gait analysis is an extremely important part of examination, which consists of observing the gait without use of formal computerized gait analysis. The observational gait scale and the Edinburgh visual gait score are validated scales for outcome measures. The interpretation can be enhanced by viewing the video recording of the gait. The consistency of observation is markedly improved on reviewing slow motion videos. The observational gait analysis comprises keen observation of feet, knee, hip, trunk, and upper limbs while the child is ambulating. Beginning with feet, following points must be considered:

- Position of foot at the end of terminal swing (whether it is neutral, varus, or in valgus position)
- Position of ankle (neural or equinus); portion of the foot that first comes in contact with the floor)
- Foot progression angle during stance and swing; position of foot in stance phase (whether plantigrade or not).
- Alignment of forefoot with hindfoot; arch of the foot; point of gait cycle where deviation from normal occurs; any deviations in normal phases of foot position during gait (e.g., premature plantar-flexion in midstance or prolonged dorsiflexion in terminal stance) and finally position of toes in the swing and stance phase.
- At knee, the points to be observed include position of knee in terminal swing and initial contact; loading response (normal loading in slight flexion followed by extension in early stance, as the limb is loaded); extension of knee at any point in stance; maximum degree of knee flexion in swing; foot and knee alignment; shank thigh alignment and finally varus/valgus motion during stance.

Observational gait analysis is more difficult proximally where large muscles obscure hips and pelvis. Computerized gait analysis is helpful in determining any deviations in these joints of the body. However, an observational gait analysis following points must be noted for pelvis:

- Hip and trunk alignment of thigh (knee) to the line of progression (neutral, external, or internal rotation)
- Hip extension in terminal stance; excessive abduction (circumduction) or excessive adduction (scissoring) in swing phase; pelvis position (normal, anterior, or posterior); any pelvis obliquity
- Trunk movements in each plane, movement of arms (symmetrical and reciprocal or postured) and whether child elevates his/her arms to maintain balance.

The importance of instrumental gait analysis (IGA) cannot be overemphasized. It enhances the understanding of gait abnormality by providing real-time objective data that cannot be comprehended by observational gait analysis. However, IGA is not a substitute for clinical examination and experience. The combination of both provides a sound basis for charting out a treatment plan for the patient.

The *normal gait cycle in human beings* is different from animals. As bipeds, the most efficient way for forward propulsion is to alternate support from one leg to another consecutively.

- Normal gait pattern is cyclical and symmetrical and associated with minimal body movements.
- One complete gait cycle or stride begins when one foot makes contact with the ground (initial contact) and ends when the same foot makes contact again.
- The gait cycle may be divided into stance and swing phases. In general, stance phase occupies 60% of the gait cycle and swing phase occupies 40% of it.
- The step frequency of the gait cycle is called cadence and distance traveled by each foot with each step is called step length.
- The graphic representation of the patterns of gait cycle showing joint angles at different time of the gait cycle is called motion kinematics.
- The most easily observed angular displacements occur in sagittal plane. Small and less obvious displacements occur in transverse and coronal plane. The sagittal plane pattern shows hip flexion to extension of back to flexion in mid-swing and knee flexion and extension. The sagittal curve at ankle shows three rockers. The first (heel rocker) is associated with controlled plantar flexion of foot for weight acceptance. The second (ankle rocker) is associated with controlled tibial advancement and increasing ankle dorsiflexion in the midstance phase. The third (toe rocker) is associated with rapid ankle plantar flexion for push off.

The graphic representation of individual with CP is thus compared with the graph of normal individuals to detect abnormalities in gait pattern.

Some common gait patterns in spastic diplegia CP include **(Figs. 3A to D)**:

- Jump knee gait
- Toe-toe gait pattern in which differentiation between apparent equinus and true equinus must be made
- Crouch knee gait
- Stiff knee gait
- Rotational deformities that affect gait.

The *jump knee gait* is characterized by increased hip and knee flexion, with slight dorsiflexion of ankle at initial contact followed by rapid knee extension and ankle plantar flexion during midstance. The initial forefoot contact with the ground is followed by stretch of ankle plantar flexors leading to rapid plantar flexion of the ankle. This causes heel rise and prevents second rocker at the ankle that normally levels to tibial advancement anteriorly. The resultant proximal joint reactions include knee and hip extension as the plantar flexors of ankle contact giving any appearance of the patient jumping from one knee to another. This occurrence is caused by normal quadriceps and gastrocnemius-soleus strength with spasticity of hamstring and hip flexors. This gait is most commonly seen in patients with diplegia and hemiplegia with GMFCS Levels II and III. A younger patient with jump knee gait may change his pattern with increase in age and weight.

Equinus deformity is one of the most common deformities present in CP. It is characterized by excessive plantar flexion of calcaneus relative to the tibia. This may be associated with planovalgus or cavovarus deformities. The equinus deformity results in forefoot making an initial contact that persists through the stance phase resulting in *toe-toe gait*. This should be differentiated from the apparent equinus deformity, where the initial contact of forefoot occurs because of excessive hip and knee flexion and not because of plantar flexion at the ankle as in true equinus. In true equinus gait pattern, the calf spasticity is dominant resulting in plantar flexion of ankle with hips and knees either extended or minimally deviated from normal one the gait cycle. This may ultimately result in genu recurvatum with increased hamstring length and gradual stretching of the posterior capsule of knee joint. By contrast, the apparent equinus is dominated by hip and knee flexion throughout the stance period with almost normal ROM at the ankle joint. For

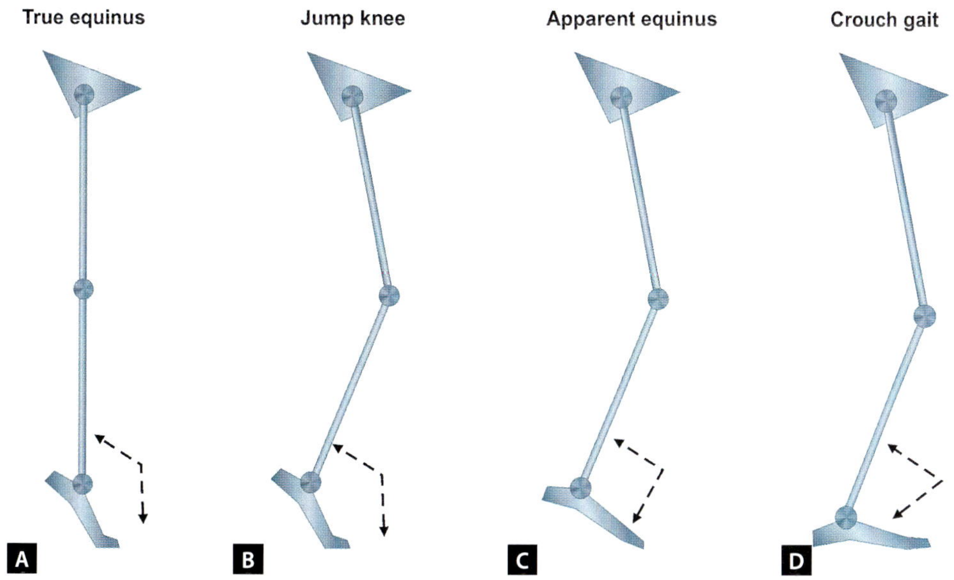

Figs. 3A to D: Common gait patterns in spastic diplegia.

a child with apparent equinus, any procedure that weakens the calf will result in a crouch gait pattern and should be strictly avoided. Failure to recognize apparent equinus is one of the most common errors made on observational gait analysis. The appropriate treatment depends upon recognition of the true nature of toe-toe gait. Children smaller than 8 years having true equinus due to calf muscle spasticity respond very well to Botox injection. However, in older children where calf muscle spasticity continues to produce true equinus, an intermuscular lengthening of gastrocnemius (Vulpius/Silfverskiöld) may be required. For children with apparent equinus, the treatment should be directed toward hamstring and iliopsoas recession, which are the cause of an apparent equinus. Postoperatively, a solid or ground reaction ankle-foot orthosis (AFO) helps to direct the ground reaction force vector in front of the knee encouraging knee extension.

Crouch gait comprises increased hip and knee flexion with excessive ankle dorsiflexion. This gait pattern is generally seen in weaker patients with diplegia. The cause may be dynamic muscle contraction, spasticity, lever arm dysfunction, bony deformity and/or fixed joint contractures. Another significant cause is iatrogenic, where the calf muscle weakness is produced by lengthening of the calf muscles in the absence of a true equinus. The crouch pattern is usually seen in GMFCS Levels II, III and IV patients. In sagittal plane, the body's center of mass falls behind the already flexed knee, providing and increasingly larger deforming force as the child grows and increases his weight. Such body forces place quadriceps mechanism into disadvantage and increase all three components of the crouch gait. The excessive knee flexion gradually becomes fixed with overstretching and lengthening of the quadriceps resulting in patella alta, anterior knee pain, and sometimes avulsion fracture of the patella. The muscles responsible for the gait pattern include an overactive or spastic iliopsoas and rectus femoris at the hip and spastic hamstrings at the knee. Rectus femoris is especially responsible for the hip flexion deformity. Excessive ankle dorsiflexion results from uncontrolled tibial advancement in the second rocker during midstance due to weak or over-lengthened calf muscles.

Stiff knee gait is one of the most common gait patterns to limit gait performance in children with spastic CP. The cause of stiff knee gait is believed to be spastic/shortened biarticular rectus femoris whose inappropriate activity during swing phase results in a decrease of the magnitude of knee flexion causing foot clearance and limb advancement difficult. The compensation is done by circumduction of the involved limb, external rotation of the foot, pelvic elevation, or a trunk lean away from affected side. On the normal or less affected side, compensatory mechanism includes early heel rise and reduces knee flexion to aid in foot clearance on the affected side. The physical examination of such patients usually includes a position Duncan-Ely test. However, all patients with positive Duncan-Ely test may not have positive outcome with lengthening or transfer of rectus femoris.

The most common *rotational abnormalities (and* gait resulting from them) of the lower extremities in spastic CP include femoral anteversion and tibial (in) torsion. These deformities progress with age until skeletal maturity. Usually more severe rotational deformities are seen in eight higher GMFCS levels. The IGA can visualize the dynamic position of pelvis, femur and tibia more clearly and accurately as compared to naked eye. Femoral anteversion is best measured as a CT scan. When the distal femur is internally rotated with relation to proximal femur, it is femoral anteversion. The reverse is called femoral retroversion. Increased femoral anteversion is the most common cause of intoeing gait. This is best corrected after/near skeletal maturity to avoid recurrence. Excessive tibial (internal/external) torsion is common in individuals with CP. Typically the tibia and foot deformities occur in the same direction, such as external tibial torsion is coupled with planovalgus foot deformity and internal tibial torsion with equinovarus foot. The treatment of tibial torsion is thus linked to foot deformities. However, its treatment should be delayed till skeletal maturity to avoid recurrence.

PRINCIPLES OF MANAGEMENT OF CHILD WITH CEREBRAL PALSY

A child with CP has to be looked upon globally and parents need to be counseled for slow progress of the treatment effectiveness. In any case, the treatment is directed at reducing disabilities only and improving the learning, self-dependency of child, and socialization. Parents should be clearly counseled that the treatment is not for controlling or curing disease but to achieve the above goals only. The medical and surgical treatments have to be combined together to achieve improved functionality on a logical and predetermined basis. CP is primarily a central nervous system (CNS) disorder where musculoskeletal and movement disorders develop as secondary manifestations. These include joint malpositioning, muscular imbalance, and functional impairment. If untreated these evolve further into fixed skeletal deformities over time. Hence in a broad overview the treatment is directed accordingly **(Table 3)**.

TABLE 3: General approach to treatment of cerebral palsy according to disease evolution and functional impairment.

Degree of impairment	*Remarks*	*Management*
Primary	Movement disorder and postural defect arising from lesion of immature central nervous system (CNS)	None specifically
Secondary	Joint malpositioning, muscle imbalance, and loss of function	Tone-reducing medications, physical therapy, splints, and surgical correction (detailed in text under specific anomaly)
Tertiary	Development of fixed bony deformities, joint contractures, and muscular contractures	Prevention is better by performing early correction. Salvage procedures (described specifically in each section in the chapter)

The surgical treatment for most deformities fall into one of the three categories: (1) Lengthening (or releasing) of spastic muscles that cause deformity; (2) Tendon transfers to supplement weak muscle(s) or replace lost muscle function; (3) Stabilization of unstable joints.

TREATMENT FOR SPASTICITY IN CEREBRAL PALSY

The spasticity may be treated in many ways. The chosen treatment generally depends upon the magnitude of involvement (trunk and number of limbs) and the magnitude of spasticity. Passive stretching followed by splinting is commonly used method to treat spasticity. There is limited evidence of the benefit of this technique in certain situation in the peripheral joints, especially ankle equinus in younger children.

Spasticity may also be treated by oral medications. Benzodiazepines (e.g., diazepam), baclofen, dantrolene sodium, and tizanidine have been used in the past. Benzodiazepines act by facilitating transmission at the inhibitory synopsis in the central nervous system called the γ-aminobutyric acid type A gamma-aminobutyric acid (GABA) receptors. Facilitated transmission reduces mono-synaptic and polysynaptic reflexes resulting in increased inhibition, thereby reducing spasticity. Benzodiazepines can act in the brain as well as spinal cord. Sedation is one of the most common side effects. In addition, there is a risk of developing tolerance or dependence. The pediatric dose ranges from 0.12 to 0.8 mg/kg/day. The drug should never be stopped abruptly as withdrawal symptoms may include agitation, irritability, tremor, muscle fasciculation, nausea, hyperreflexia, and seizures.

- Baclofen is a structural analog of GABA and binds to GABA-B receptors resulting in inhibition of mono- and polysynaptic reflexes. It also reduces release of excitatory neurotransmitters and substance peptide (P). It primarily acts at the spinal cord, thus offering an excellent treatment for patients with CP. It reduces spasticity, hyperreflexia, and clonus. It can often cause sedation. The pediatric dosing starts between 2.5 and 10 mg/day and may increase up to 40 mg a day in divided doses. Withdrawal symptoms can occur when the drug is stopped suddenly after an extended period. These include intense spasticity, hallucination, compression, and seizures.
- Dantrolene sodium acts at the site of skeletal muscle as opposed to other drugs which act on the neurotransmitter system. It acts by inhibiting the release of calcium ions from sarcoplasmic reticulum during muscle contraction. The drug reduces clonus and muscle spasm. It is usually preferred in hemiplegia, traumatic brain injury, spinal cord injury, and spasticity due to CP. The pediatric dose is 6–8 mg/day is divided doses. The most important side effect is hepatotoxicity for which regular monitoring with liver function test is required.
- Tizanidine has also been used for treatment of spasticity. It is an 2-adrenergic agent which reduces the tone through hyperpolarization of motor neurons. The drug has not been used extensively for the pediatric patient and common side effects include hepatotoxicity, sedation, dizziness, and dry mouth.

Neuromuscular/chemodenervation with extramuscular injection is an extremely effective method of controlling spasticity selectively in a single muscle/joint. Injection of phenol and ethyl alcohol perineurally results in decrease of spasticity by axonal degeneration. However, the effect is reversible with reinnervation occurring over months to years. The side effects include muscle necrosis and vascular complications. The advantage is their cost-effectiveness and their use in spasticity in large powerful muscles which cannot be treated with recommended dose of botulinum toxin.

- Botulinum toxin is an effective synaptic blocker which acts by inhibiting the release of acetylcholine at the presynaptic junction **(Fig. 4)**. This toxin produced by *Clostridium botulinum*. Effects are reversible; hence the injection is required every 3–4 months. Dosing is usually 10–12 U/kg but should never exceed 400 units in a single sitting. Two serotypes are available in the international market—A and B. Botulinum toxin type A is commonly marked at BOTOX®. Type B is generally available as MYOBLOC®. The most appropriate candidate for botulinum toxin is a patient where reduction of spasticity in a limited number of muscles can provide a meaningful benefit in care, comfort, and activity of the child. It acts by reducing spasticity in focally affected muscles. Thus the affected muscles can be stretched, antagonists can be rebuild by physiotherapy helping improve balance around joints and also surgeon can assess the possible effects of surgery, if needed. It can also be used in conjunction with orthopedic surgery or in combination with serial casting and splinting.
- Neurosurgical treatment of spasticity includes selective dorsal rhinotomy (SDR) and intrathecal baclofen therapy (IBT). SDR, first started by Warrick Peacock, is performed through laminoplasty. The dura is opened and dorsal rootlets are identified from T12 through S1. Each rootlet is stimulated and the response is recorded

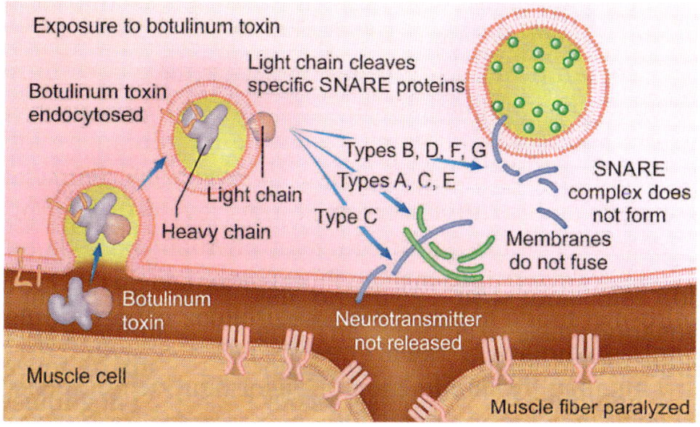

Fig. 4: Mechanism of action of botulinum toxin. SNARE → SNAP (Soluble *NSF* Attachment Protein) *Receptor*. This mediates vesicle fusion to cell membrane and exocytosis.
Source: Arnon SS, Schechter R, Inglesby TV, Henderson DA, Bartlett JG, Ascher MS, et al. Botulinum toxin as a biological weapon: medical and public health management. JAMA. 2001;285:1059-70.

electromyographically. Those with abnormal or generalized response are severed. About 40–60% of nerve rootlets are sacrificed. The procedure helps by cutting of the aberrant afferent activity from muscle spindles which are normally conveyed by dorsal nerves. This reduces the spasticity profoundly, so that the patient has significant amount of weakness postoperatively. Extensive physiotherapy is required afterward to treat the weakness. SDR should not be done with underlying dystonia.

- Intrathecal baclofen pump uses just 1% of the dose that is required orally to produce reduction of spasticity. It is an excellent method for patients with multisegmental/extensive spasticity with limited side effects. The pump placement is done subcutaneously or intramuscularly and the catheter is inserted intrathecally at the levels of T11–T12. Dose adjustments are done through telemetry with a remote. Refills which are required every 2–6 months are usually delivered through needle which passes through the skin into the part of the pump. Refills should not be missed to avoid dangerous withdrawal symptoms such as itching, paresthesia, rebound spasticity, seizures, and change in mental status.

The drug treatment and neurosurgical treatment of dystonia are limited. Dystonia due to CP may be dopamine (DOPA)-responsive or DOPA-resistant. The carbidopa/levodopa is highly effective in the former. In the latter, anticholinergic drugs can be tried. Trihexyphenidyl is usually given in such cases. The limiting factors being side effects such as confusion, memory loss, dry mouth, blurred vision, and urinary retention. Intramuscular injection with botulinum toxin may be successful in focal dystonia. Those refractory to above treatments may benefit by intrathecal baclofen pump or deep brain stimulation (pallidal stimulation).

MANAGEMENT OF HIP DEFORMITIES IN CEREBRAL PALSY

The children with CP are born with normal hips. If subjected to abnormal forces by spastic muscles, they develop changes which are characteristic of CP.

The pathogenesis of hip deformity in CP is as follows:

The deforming muscles in CP usually include the adductors, hip flexors, and the hamstrings. Besides these, the ability to ambulate has immense repercussions on the fate of hip.

- Children who start ambulating by 5 years of age usually have a stable hip, though they may develop acetabular dysplasia and femoral head deformities.
- Children who ambulate with aids may develop silent or painless subluxation, while nonambulators may develop dislocation by the age of 7 years.
- This may be due to continuous sitting or lying down position which has very little containment for posterior or lateral surfaces of the femoral head. In addition, increased femoral anteversion redirects head away from the depth of the acetabulum toward the rim. Once the hip dislocates, the acetabulum and femoral head undergo deformation.
- In cases of asymmetrical spasticity, windblown deformities develop with intrapelvic obliquity, where the higher side usually dislocates. As femoral head subluxates, it presses upon the lateral edge of acetabulum resulting in flattening and loss of sphericity. The femoral head typically becomes triangular and the articular cartilage is slowly denuded.

On *clinical examination* contribution of adductors, hip flexors, and hamstrings may be tested for development of hip dislocation. Passive adduction <40° with hip in flexion and abduction may raise suspicion of instability. Crouch gait, scissoring, and rotational abnormalities besides spinal deformities and pelvic obliquity are usually associated with the hip joint instability. As noted earlier, age at ambulation is one of the most important prognostic factors for hip joint instability:

- Any child who could walk by 30 months does not develop any hip joint instability, while those walking between 30 months and 5 years have 15% incidence of developing hip joint instability.

Radiological evaluation is invaluable in assessment of instability.

Anteroposterior (AP) and frog leg lateral images are the mainstay of radiological assessment. Out of all parameters, acetabular index **(Fig. 5)** and Reimer's migration index (percentage of head that is not covered by acetabulum—calculated by dividing the width of uncovered femoral head by the total width of the femoral head) are the most helpful. Combined hip abduction angle is not as reliable a measure as compared to Reimer's migration index.

- The acetabular index may vary with pelvic obliquity, rotational malposition. It decreases with lordosis and increases with flexion at the hip. Still the ease of measurement and low interobserver variability has led

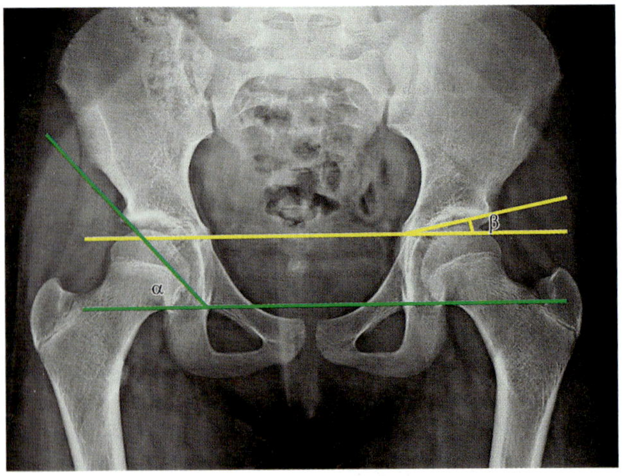

Fig. 5: Acetabular index: The angle (β) is formed by a horizontal line connecting both triradiate cartilages (Hilgenreiner line) and a second line which extends along the acetabular roof, the angle β should be <28°. In the adult, the inferior margin of the pelvic tear drop is used instead to make the horizontal line though this changes the value of the angle (α). The α angle above 47° indicates dysplasia and is normal between 33° and 38°. 39–46° in indeterminate.

to its universal use. Acetabular index >30° is generally associated with instability.

- Assessment of Reimer's migration index (most useful index) over a time period is helpful in predicting subluxation **(Fig. 6)**. In a normal child, the progression is <1%. In children with CP who are unlikely to walk, the index may increase by 7.7%. In all circumstances, a Reimer's migration index of 30% is considered to be abnormal.

An increased neck shaft angle and persistent anteversion are associated with spastic hips. The acetabular deformity is most commonly present in its superolateral part. Frequent clinical evaluation and radiological surveillance can reduce potential of hip joint instability. For GMFS III to V levels, radiology should be conducted every 6 months using acetabular index and migration index, until skeletal maturity.

Nonsurgical treatment includes pharmacological agents like baclofen which reduce spasticity of the muscles, followed by physical therapy and bracing in abduction. However, no conclusive report exists that has identified usefulness of both physical therapy as well as bracing. Use of botulinum toxin in hip has been more difficult than in gastrocnemius-soleus complex. Dose/weight limitation and the number of spastic muscles limit the effectiveness of botulinum injection. Also the muscles around hip joint are more difficult to inject with the botulinum toxin.

Surgical treatment of hip abnormalities in CP can be divided into four levels:

1. Level one consists of soft tissue release intended to prevent hip instability (managing the hips at risk).
2. Level two addresses management of hip subluxation/dislocation/acetabular and femoral dysplasia by bony procedures and soft tissue balancing.
3. Level three involves palliative/salvage procedures for painful, dislocated, and arthritic spastic hip.
4. Windswept deformity of hip is managed as for abduction at one hip and adduction at the other.

The procedures commonly done to address hip deformity in CP include the following:

Adductor Tenotomy (± Flexor Release)

It is one of the most common procedures performed as adductors are the main disabling force on hip in CP **(Fig. 7)**. The indications include:

- A ROM of <30° abduction with hips and knee flexed.
- A migration index of 20% or more on progression of >10% annually is also an indication. Contractures of iliopsoas and hamstrings are also dealt with in comprehensive manner.

A medial approach is used. Adductor longus is released in the tendinous portion followed by adductor brevis and gracilis, both of which require myotomy on account of smaller tendon. Muscles are released until 50° of symmetric abduction is obtained in flexion of hip and knee. Obturator neurectomy is no longer used because of propensity to produce an abduction contracture. The abductor tenotomy is generally combined with release of hip flexors. The recession of iliopsoas at the level of pelvic brim is generally done for patients who are ambulatory. For nonambulatory patients, an iliopsoas tenotomy is done at lesser trochanter. The improvement of extension parameters is seen better in those where iliopsoas tenotomy is done. However, recession at pelvic brim is not associated with any flexion deficit on doing stairs and hence recommended by most authors. Combined adductor tenotomy and iliopsoas recession lead to good clinical and radiological results.

Correction of Rotational Deformities

The rotational deformities of the hip need to be corrected if they interfere in the gait. The internal rotation deformities are generally caused by overactive/spastic medial hamstrings and week gluteus medius. Persistent femoral anteversion contributes to the deformity especially in hemiplegics and diplegics with crouch gait.

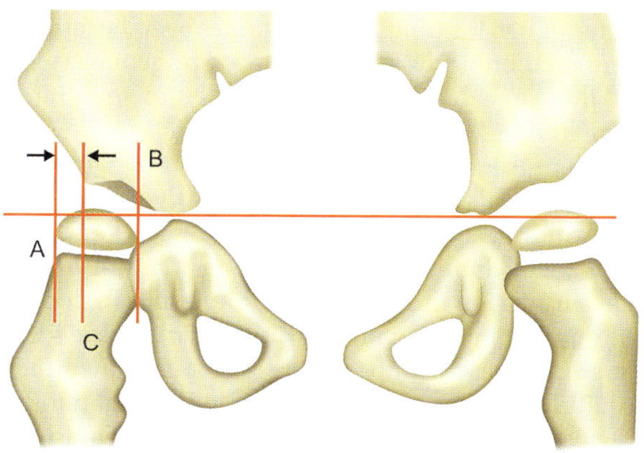

Fig. 6: Reimer's migration index = AC/AB expressed in percentage. A = outer limit of the epiphysis, C = Perkin's line, and B = inner limit of the epiphysis.

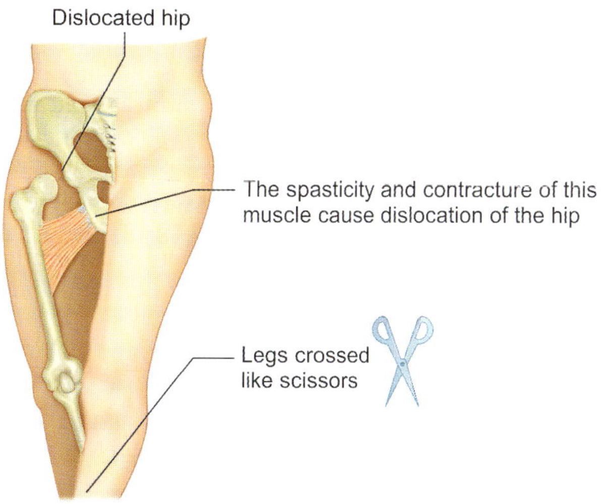

Fig. 7: Adductor tightness causing scissoring.

- Soft tissue procedures have not led to satisfactory outcomes in rotational deformities, hence a derotation osteotomy is the procedure of choice. The indication includes internal rotation greater than 60° and a femoral anteversion of 40–45° besides frequent tripping or catching of involved leg. The goal is to retain about 30° of passive internal rotation.
- If hip subluxation or coxa valga is present a varus derotation osteotomy (VDRO) is preferred. The osteotomy is generally done toward skeletal maturity to cut the risk of recurrence. Use of rigid fixation methods is preferred to produce early ambulation and less pain. The goal of surgery is to redirect femoral head into the deepest part of acetabulum so as to eliminate forces on the superolateral part of acetabulum and femoral head. In addition to correction of the rotational deformities, a VDRO shortens the limb thereby relaxing the spastic musculotendon units.

Management of Dislocated Hip

- A child who presents with a dislocated hip benefits best on *single stage* intervention consisting of open reduction of the hip joint; soft tissue lengthening; femoral osteotomy with shortening and pelvic osteotomy. Of all pelvic osteotomies, periacetabular osteotomies relying on the hinge of triradiate cartilage are preferred to allow effective treatment of superolateral acetabular deficiency. The bone graft left from VDRO may be used to redirect the acetabulum. A Dega osteotomy is the prototype of such periacetabular osteotomies. For children, in whom the triradiate cartilage has closed, Chiari osteotomy or slotted augmented shelf procedure is beneficial.
- The painful dislocated hip in an older child is a challenge to treat. The options include valgus redirectional osteotomy, hip arthrodesis, femoral head resection, interpositional arthroplasty, and total hip arthroplasty. Valgus redirectional osteotomy redirects hip away from the acetabulum and allows transfer of load through the subtrochanteric region indirectly. This relieves pain as head is redirected away from the acetabulum during abduction. Hip arthrodesis is a good option in individuals who have unilateral/asymmetric involvement. Resection of the femoral head, although easy and apparently logical, is not of benefit and is often associated with complications such as persistent pain and heterotrophic ossification. Postoperative immobilization may be associated with pressure sores, infection, and pneumonia. Usually total joint replacement is not used in hemiplegic or diplegic patient due to potential complication of dislocation, infection, heterotrophic, ossification, loosening, stiffness, and persistent pain.

MANAGEMENT OF THE KNEE IN SPASTIC DIPLEGIA

There are four sagittal knee patterns prevalent in spastic diplegia:

1. Jump knee (increased knee flexion in early stance followed by near normal knee extension in later stance)
2. Crouch knee (increased knee flexion and ankle dorsiflexion in stance phase)
3. Stiff knee (decreased knee flexion and reduced knee rom during swing/resulting in inefficient foot clearance)
4. Recurvatum knee (hyperextension deformity in mid-to-late stance)

As described earlier, four major gait patterns affect the sagittal plane of the body including: (1) pelvis, (2) hip, (3) knee, and (4) ankle. These are true equinus, jump gait, apparent equinus, and crouch gait. Each group has progressively less ankle equinus, increasing proximal contractures, a shift of the ground reaction force from in front of the knee to behind the knee and decreasing plantar flexion/knee extension coupling. Dynamics of these gait patterns have been already described earlier. The crouch gait, which has increased hip and knee flexion with calcaneus at ankle can include a pelvis which is titled posteriorly, is neutral or is tilted anteriorly. The hamstring length is short in the posterior tilting, normal in neutral tilting, and longer in anterior tilting. Hence, distal hamstring lengthening may help only in first case and may increase anterior pelvis tilt in the third case.

Management

- The nonoperative treatment for knee in spastic diplegics includes selective botulinum toxin injections and oral medication like baclofen followed by physical therapy for strengthening exercises. Surgical treatment remains the mainstay for managing the knee deformities in these individuals. The surgeons need to consider GMFCS levels, age of the patient, and severity of knee dysfunction besides sagittal gait pattern before commencing upon surgical procedure.
- Hamstring lengthening in the distal part remains the most common surgical procedures for management of knee deformities even in the absence of precise indications. In GMFCS IV or V individuals, proximal hamstring lengthening with adductor lengthening provides case of perineal care and aids in the sitting posture. Distal lengthening is preferred in ambulatory children. Generally, medial hamstrings are lengthened alone leaving lateral hamstrings intact to prevent anterior pelvic fitting. Circular stripes over the fascia over semimembranosus suffice, followed by gentle extension of the knee leading to intramuscular lengthening. Gracilis and semitendinosus may be lengthened by "Z" lengthening or intramuscular tendon recession. However, this method is used only when fixed flexion deformity at knee is not present.
- The distal hamstring lengthening may improve the knee extension in stance phase, but results in decreased flexion during swing phase. The child may have stiffness in swing phase with problems of foot clearance and toe scuffing. Such cases are best treated by distal transfer of rectus femoris to semitendinosus. The prerequisites are spasticity of rectus femoris confirmed by Duncan-Ely prone rectus test in children with GMFCS Levels I and II. Dynamic electromyography (EMG) shows prolonged

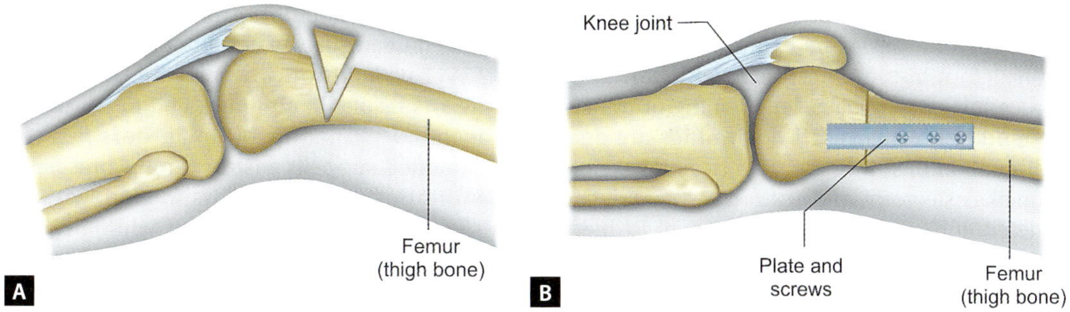

Figs. 8A and B: Extension supracondylar osteotomy.

rectus firing in swing phase. The proximal part of semitendinosus is cross-sutured to semimembranosus after transfer of rectus femoris to the stump of semitendinosus tendons. For fixed flexion deformity between 5° and 20° medial hamstring lengthening is combined by transfer for semitendinosus to adductor tubercle at the tendon of adductor magnus. An anterior growth plate surgery may be used to deal with residual fixed flexion deformity.

- Another effective method to deal with flexion deformity at knee with crouch gait includes supracondylar extension osteotomy **(Figs. 8A and B)** with patellar tendon shortening. The supracondylar osteotomy is performed by removing a trapezoidal piece of zone (broader anteriorly) from the distal femur and then fixed the osteotomy rigidly. The patellar tendon shortening is combined with this by resecting the tendon in the midsubstance and then repairing it in double breast fashion. This procedure is generally performed in children near skeletal maturity. Anterior growth plates are an effective method for children with at least 2 years of growth left.

MANAGEMENT OF FOOT AND ANKLE IN CEREBRAL PALSY

The most common complaints in individual with CP who are ambulatory are pain, tripping, and in-/out-toeing. Most of disruptions in the ankle foot function in CP can be picked as careful clinical radiological examination and observation IGA. The foot deformities can be best identified and classified by dividing the foot into three segments (hindfoot, midfoot, and forefoot) and two columns (medial and lateral). The relative length of each column and alignment of each segment is then analyzed to determine the foot deformity.

The foot deformities in children with CP are a result of a dynamic muscle imbalance which may be a consequence of spasticity, abnormal motor control, and/or impaired balance. These imbalances are progressive with growth and development and hence may be classified into three levels:

- *Level I:* It includes dynamic soft tissue imbalance.
- *Level II:* It is characterized by fixed deformities where the muscle length is fixed but skeletal changes are yet not seen.
- *Level III:* Its deformities are characterized by structural skeletal deformities.

The three most common malalignment patterns that occur in CP include:

1. Equinus
2. Equinoplanovalgus
3. Equinocavovarus

Typically in spastic CP, the ankle plantar flexor muscles are overactive and dorsiflexors are ineffective leading to equinus deformity.

Equinoplanovalgus deformities are characterized by equinus of the hindfoot coupled with pronation of midfoot and forefoot. The lateral column of the foot is structurally and functionally shorter than medial column. Ankle valgus and hallux valgus are frequently seen to be associated with equinoplanovalgus.

Equinocavovarus is characterized by equinus of hindfoot coupled with supination of the midfoot and forefoot. The lateral column is structurally and functionally longer than the medial column. Compensatory ankle valgus deformities may be seen in equinocavovarus. These deformities are usually supple (Level I) but may exacerbate to Level II/III with age and suboptimal treatment. The foot and ankle malalignment may disrupt the function in both stance and swing phase. The heel strike does not occur in any of the deformities.

Equinus and equinocavovarus pattern disrupt the ankle rocker (see gait analysis discussed earlier) by blocking ankle dorsiflexion resulting in compromised stability in midstance. Equinoplanovalgus deformity maintains the midfoot and forefoot in segments in unlocked alignment resulting in excessive loading of medial plantar aspect of the midfoot. Interventions to correct foot deformities are performed to improve cosmesis and function. It is presumed that improved foot shape can restore the stability and function by restoring the relative length of columns. However, increased stiffness of the foot by surgical procedures such as arthrodesis may result in reduction of the shock absorption function of the foot.

- For Level I (*equinus deformity*), the interventions are designed to reduce muscle tone and spasticity. This is accomplished by pharmaceutical methods (oral baclofen and botulinum toxin injection), neurosurgical methods (selective dorsal rhizotomy and intrathecal baclofen), or orthotic interventions. Split or complete muscle transfer may also be performed to produce balance. The Level II deformities are best dealt with soft tissue surgical procedures like release, lengthening or transfer of muscle tendon unit. Level III deformities are dealt with a combination of soft tissue surgeries and skeletal intervention like osteotomy and arthrodesis.

The true equinus deformity may be Level I (due to overactivity) or Level II (tightness of ankle plantar flexors). As discussed earlier, true equinus must be differentiated from the apparent equinus. Intervention done for ankle plantar flexors in apparent equinus may result in hindfoot calcaneus leading to severe crouch. Level I equinus deformity in young children (<5 years) is an ideal candidate for botulinum toxin injection in each head of gastrocnemius, where equinus deformities are due to isolated overactivity of gastrocnemius. Silfverskiöld test, as described in clinical examination, helps in identifying the causative muscle. A short course of lasting, use of ankle foot orthosis and physiotherapy may help to prolong the time limited effect of botulinum toxin.

- Level II deformities where the shortening of plantar flexors results in equinus need to be surgically treated. Isolated limitation of ankle dorsiflexion with knee extended suggests gastrocnemius muscle involvement; limitation of ankle dorsiflexion with knee flexed suggests soleus involvement while limitation in both positions suggests involvement of both muscles. A selective fractional lengthening of gastrocnemius (Baumann/Strayer) is required for the first instance; which is done in the muscle belly (called Zone I). This will achieve 5% or less of ankle dorsiflexion. When both muscles are involved; selective fractional lengthening at myotendinous junction (Zone II, Vulpius/Baker) or formal lengthening of tendo-Achilles (Zone III, White/Hoke) may be required **(Fig. 9)**. Of course, tendo-Achilles lengthening gives more dorsiflexion (Zone 3) at the cost of weakness of ankle plantar flexors.

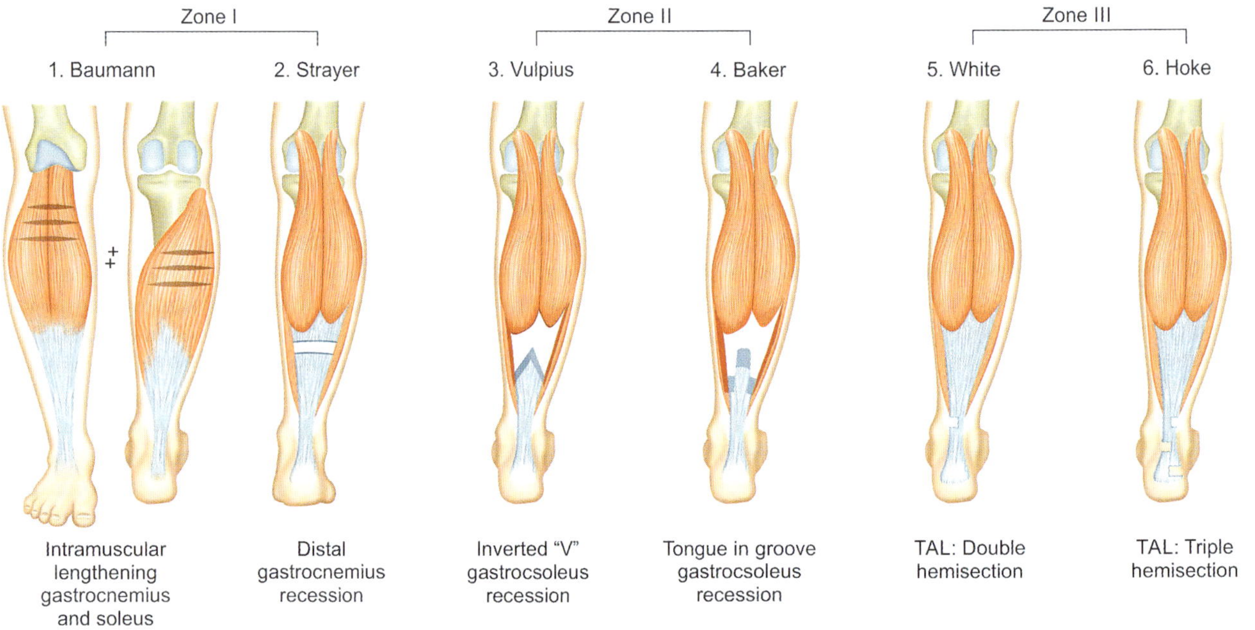

Fig. 9: Correction of limitation of ankle dorsiflexion.

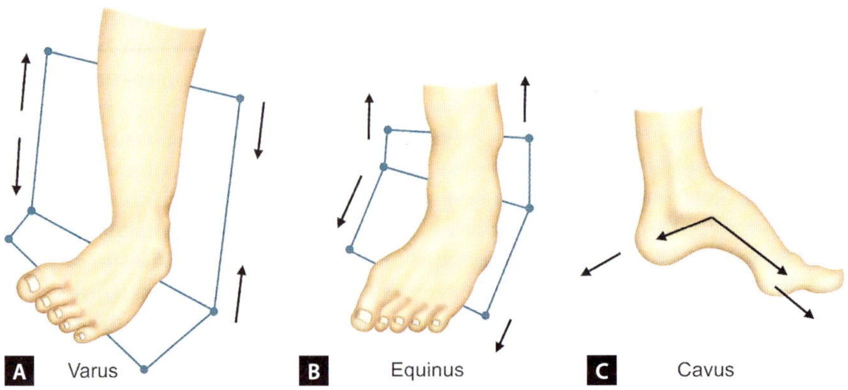

Figs. 10A to C: Equinocavovarus deformity.

Equinocavovarus deformity is a consequence of overactivity (Level I) or tightness (Level II) of ankle plantar flexors and invertors **(Figs. 10A to C)**. Physical examination not only differentiates between dynamic (Level I) and static (Level II) deformities, but can also pinpoint the inverter muscle responsible for varus foot in majority of cases. Confusion test is done by asking the child to flex hip against resistance applied to knee in sitting position (hip and knee flexed to 90°). When the flexion is accompanied by dorsiflexion and inversion of ankle, tibialis anterior is the overactive muscle. This can be confirmed by dynamic EMG and pedobarography. The ankle dorsiflexion in midstance generally occurs due to tibialis anterior overactivity.

- Level I equinocavovarus deformities in young children (<5 years) may be treated with intramuscular injection in plantar flexors and inverters; requiring general anesthesia and ultrasonic or EMG guidance for the latter.
- Level II deformities may be managed by fractional lengthening of the ankle plantar flexors. Split transfer of tibialis anterior is considered when this muscle is found to be overactive in physical examination/EMG. In cases of doubt or when EMG assessments are not available, dynamic varus deformity may be treated by simultaneous split transfer of tibialis anterior and fractional lengthening of the tibialis posterior. Level II deformities may require further fractional lengthening of flexor hallucis longus and flexor digitorum longus muscles; abductor hallucis muscle on the medial border of foot and sequential release of plantar fascia and intrinsic muscles of the foot. Peroperative reassessment (clinical as well as radiological) of the foot after soft tissue release is necessary to plan any bony procedures. Gross alignment and dynamic loading of the foot may improve by sequential osteotomies. Lateral closing wedge osteotomy of calcaneus is used to correct heel varus. Lateral column shortening through cuboid using a dorsolateral closing wedge osteotomy is used to correct midfoot supination deformity.
- Dorsally based closing wedge osteotomies of medial cuneiform or first metatarsal when the physis has closed, may be used to treat residual forefoot inversion and varus.
- Triple arthrodesis (see details of procedure in section on foot) is used in older patients with very stiff feet **(Fig. 11A)**.
- Subtalar arthrodesis (see details of procedure in section on foot) is used to correct hindfoot varus; calcaneocuboid arthrodesis corrects midfoot supination and talonavicular arthrodesis corrects forefoot inversion **(Fig. 11B)**.

Equinoplanovalgus deformity is a consequence of over activity (Level I) or tightness (Level II) of ankle plantar flexors and evertor group of muscles.

- Level I deformities in younger children (<5 years) may be treated with selective botulinum toxin injection in the muscle belly of gastrocnemius and, sometimes, peroneus brevis. Static deformities are usually seen in children between 6 and 8 years of age and will require fractional lengthening of ankle plantar flexors with transfer of peroneus brevis to peroneus longer muscle distal to the lateral malleolus.
- Level II deformities where skeletal changes have started to appear require lengthening of the lateral column. The procedure may be performed at the neck of calcaneus; calcaneocuboid joint or in the body of cuboid, with the help of a tricortical iliac graft. A lengthening of 1–2 cm usually corrects deformities of all these segments of the foot.
- If there is residual forefoot varus deformity due to shortening of medial column (after surgical lengthening of lateral column), then a plantar-based closing osteotomy may be performed through the medial cuneiform or at the base of the great toe metatarsal.
- A triple arthrodesis is required, if lateral column lengthening fails to correct the deformity. It may be combined with lateral column lengthening through calcaneocuboid joint.

Ankle valgus may result due to tightness of the ankle plantar flexors. Overall hindfoot valgus alignment is a contribution from both subtalar and ankle joint. Ankle valgus is best seen on drawing tibiotalar angle on an AP view of ankle in standing position. Narrowing of lateral part of distal tibial epiphysis and shortening of distal fibula (called high fibular station) are frequently associated with it.

- Ankle valgus should be corrected when it contributes to overall hindfoot valgus alignment. It is not treated when

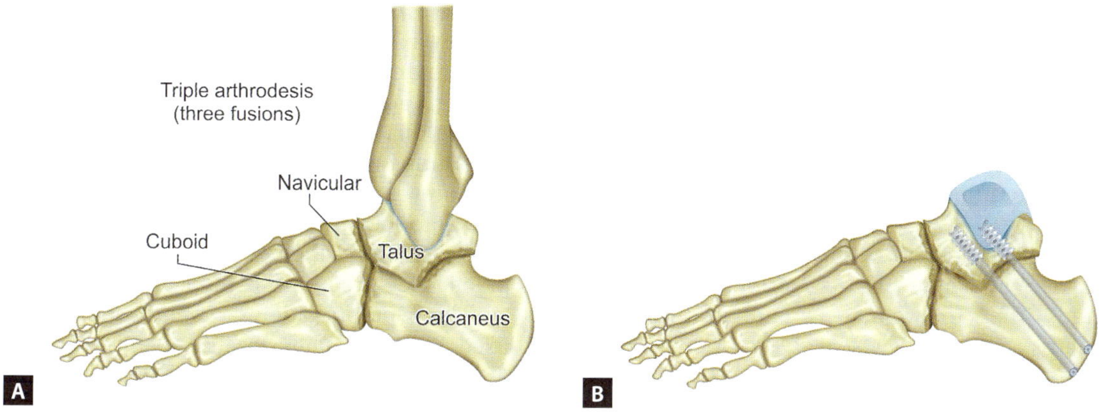

Figs. 11A and B: Triple arthrodesis (A) and subtalar arthrodesis (B).

ankle valgus is due to compensation for equinocavovarus deformity.

- Growth modulation is one of the best methods available to treat ankle valgus sufficient (>2 years) remaining growth. Reversible/temporarily hemiepiphysiodesis can be performed on the medial side of distal tibial epiphysis using a single fully threaded medial malleolar screw placed percutaneously under image guidance. The screw is removed after an overcorrection of approximately 5° has been achieved. The screw is preferred over a figure of eight plate on staples to minimize unintentional joint penetration by the distal screw.
- Supramalleolar osteotomy may be done in children when epiphysis has closed or has insufficient remaining growth potential.

Hallux valgus deformity in children with CP may be a consequence of intrinsic and/or extrinsic muscle imbalance. For example, imbalance between the abductor and adductor hallucis muscles and extensor hallucis longus muscle may result in hallux valgus and metatarsus varus alignments. The correction of the deformity is indicated to:

- Address pain
- Facilitate footwear
- Promote hygiene in between the first and second phalanges

Soft tissue balancing usually has poor results in individuals with CP. The preferred treatment for this deformity is metatarsophalangeal (MTP) arthrodesis after alignment of the MTP joint. Slight overcorrection is effective to compensate for associated hallux valgus interphalangeal deformity. Associate metatarsus varus deformity generally corrects with time after MTP arthrodesis.

MANAGEMENT OF THE UPPER EXTREMITY IN CEREBRAL PALSY

Surgical options in the upper limb are aimed to improve:

- Function
- Appearance
- Self-esteem

Conservative methods as discussed before such as physiotherapy, casting, splinting, electrical stimulation, oral baclofen, and local intramuscular botulinum toxin injections may also be used when indicated. These methods are primarily used to preserve normal ROM at the joints, to delay tendon muscle contractures and to prevent upper extremity deformities. A passive stretch of at least 6 hours out of 24 hours may be required to prevent development of fixed joint contracture where the antagonist muscles are incompetent. However, physiotherapy with splinting/casting, cannot accomplish long-term reduction of spasm in the overactive muscles.

Good clinical examination should precede surgical intervention. The patient is observed during ambulation, standing, and sitting to evaluate certain posturing and motion patterns. Preoperative sensory testing including evaluation of proprioception, stereognosis, and 2-point discrimination is also tested. Functional classification systems such as Melbourne Assessment of unilateral upper limb function; the Upper Extremity Rating Scale (UERS) and Jebsen–Taylor Hand Function test may be used to find impact of surgical intervention. The passive and active ROM at each should also be carefully noted. Dynamic EMG; assessment of a video recording of patient's function and selective motor blockade produced by botulinum toxin before surgery may serve as the diagnostic tools to select proper surgical interventions. Generally, the aims of surgical intervention include improved function, facilitation of oral and perineal care, pain-reduction and enhancement of confidence and esteem.

The most common *deformity around shoulder* is adduction and internal rotation due to overactivity/spasticity of internal rotators (pectoralis major, latissimus dorsi, subscapularis, and teres major). The surgical treatment for these deformities is typically rare. The dynamic deformities can be addressed by lengthening of the tendon of pectoralis major and subscapularis. Latissimus dorsi and teres major may be transferred so as to augment active external rotation. In fixed deformities or when the soft tissue surgery fails, an osteotomy (proximal/distal humeral) may correct excessive internal rotation deformity. Osteotomy is also indicated in dysplastic/subluxed or arthritic shoulder joint.

The most common *elbow deformity* is flexion produced by overactive/spastic biceps-brachii, brachialis and brachioradialis. The flexion deformity not only produces functional discrepancy but also results in cosmetic disability with low self-esteem. The reach of hand is severely restricted by lack of extensor. Secondary fixed contractures of the capsule and adjacent flexor pronator muscles contribute to elbow flexion deformability with pronation of the forearm. Long-standing flexion and hyper pronation may be accompanied with radial head subluxation/dysplasia. The radial head subluxation is usually posterior and is present in almost one-fourth of the children with flexion-pronation deformity. This must be carefully looked for in children before carrying out a soft tissue procedure. Operative treatment for dynamic elbow flexion deformity is indicated only when the extension loss exceeds 30°.

- For elbow flexion deformities between 30° and 60°, soft tissue release like excision of lacertus fibrosus, Z-lengthening of biceps brachii, and fractional lengthening of brachialis aponeurosis are indicated.
- For deformities exceeding 60°, flexor-pronator origin slide (Max Page procedure) with/without anterior elbow capsulotomy may be indicated.
- Z-lengthening of biceps tendon may increase the hyperpronation deformity due to pronator overactivity.
- Rerouting or lengthening of the pronator teres tendon may prevent increased pronation deformity associated with anterior elbow release.
- Elbow fusion is a theoretical option which is, sometimes, practiced in dysplastic, painful, and subluxed elbow.

The hyperpronation of *forearm* may be dynamic or fixed and is usually because of overactivity/spasticity of pronator teres and/or pronator quadratus. Inability to produce supination in the absence of compensation at shoulder may interfere with day-to-day activities. In dynamic deformities, the predominant muscle can be identified by examining pronation in flexion, when the pronator teres is relaxed. If pronation deformity persists in flexion, the deformity is largely due to overactive pronator quadratus. The surgical intervention may be classified into two groups:

1. Group 1 procedures improve functions such as wrist dorsiflexion, elbow motion, and hand grasp release. The flexor pronator release not only improves supination but also relieves elbow flexion deformity. Transfer of flexor carpi ulnaris (FCU) to a wrist extensor [extensor carpi radialis brevis (ERCB)/longus] to augment wrist extension creates a supination moment when the muscle is transferred from ulnar to radial side.
2. Group 2 procedures tackle the pronation deformity exclusively. These include fractional release, Z-lengthening, and pronator teres rerouting. Rerouting of brachioradialis has also been described to improve supination ROM. In severe cases, radial osteotomy and distal radioulnar fusion may be indicated rarely.

Flexion deformity of *wrist* restricts grasp/release function of the head. The deformity is produced due to overactive wrist-flexors with weak extensors.

- Dynamic wrist flexion deformities may be managed by fractional lengthening of the flexors of the wrist. If flexor carpi radialis is functionally sufficient, transfer of FCU to ECRB/extensor carpi radialis longus (ECRL) may be preferred.
- Alternatively, transfer for FCU may be done to extensor digitorum communis (EDC), which improves extension of wrist and fingers.
- Static, wrist deformities will require flexor release along with bony procedures such as proximal row carpectomy or wrist arthrodesis. Before considering arthrodesis, finger flexion and extension capabilities should be evaluated. While extension is required for effective grasp, active wrist flexion will be necessary for effective release. Therefore, arthrodesis should be used when effective grasp release function exists.

The *finger deformities* are generally due to spasticity of flexor digitorum superficialis (FDS) and/or flexor digitorum profundus (FDP) in the presence of weak digital extensors. Nonsurgical treatment includes injection of botulinum toxin in the affected muscles followed by muscle stretching and splinting.

- The surgical treatment consists of fractional lengthening of FDS alone or combined with FDP fractional lengthening in selected cases.
- A flexor-pronator muscle slide may be recommended in severe cases.
- Swan neck deformity (resulting due to hyperextended position at proximal interphalangeal joint) may adversely affect the grasp. Central slip tenotomy or lateral band translocation can correct the deformity effectively.

Thumb-in-palm deformity consists of static (contracture) or dynamic shortening of adductor pollicis, first dorsal interosseous and flexor pollicis longus (FPL). Various progressive types **(Figs. 12A and B)** are found depending on the severity of metacarpal adduction and phalanx flexion into the palm. The muscles responsible for active thumb abduction and extension, extensor pollicis brevis and longus (EPB and EPL), and abductor pollicis longus (APL) are weak and overstretched. This may be associated with instability of the metacarpophalangeal (MCP) joint, fixed contracture of the skin and soft tissue of the first well space and flexion deformity of the thumb. Surgical intervention helps to hold the thumb out of the palm during grasp.

The deformity may be corrected by release of adductor pollicis (from its origin on the 3rd metacarpal) and first dorsal interosseous from the 2nd metacarpal. This is accompanied with z-plasty of skin and soft tissue of the first webspace.

- Active abduction is reinforced by transfer of brachioradialis to the APL.
- Rerouting of the tendon of EPL lateral to Lister's tubercle may also augment thumb abduction.
- The flexion deformity is addressed with fractional lengthening of plaster of FPL. This may be followed by extensor reinforcement with transfer of brachioradialis or FDS tendon to ring finger to the EPL.
- Alternatively, EPL tendon may be sectioned and rerouted through first dorsal compartment, plicated, and reattached to EPB at MCP joint.
- Instability of the MCP joint in hyperextension may be addressed with volar plate capsulodesis or MCP joint arthrodesis. In case of failure of tendon transfer, MCP joint arthrodesis holds a good chance of giving better results.

MANAGEMENT OF SPINAL DEFORMITY IN CEREBRAL PALSY

Overall incidence of scoliosis in CP is around 20–25%. The rate is highest in spastic CP (about 70%) and lowest in athetoid CP (6–50%). The incidence of scoliosis is related to the severity of neurological involvement. Patients with subluxated or dislocated hips have higher incidence of scoliosis. The incidence of scoliosis is also related to GMFCS levels. Ambulatory patients have lower incidence than those who are unable to walk. The cause is thought to be combination of muscle weakness, tropical imbalance, and asymmetric tone in paraspinous and intercostal muscles. The scoliosis in CP tends to occur at an earlier age as compared to adolescent idiopathic scoliosis (AIS), the curves being larger and stiffer. The curves may also progress even after maturity, rate being 1–4° every year in curves that are greater than 50%. The skeletal maturity may also be delayed in individuals with CP. The characteristic "C" shaped curves are typical of neuromuscular scoliosis and are found in about two-thirds of CP individuals who are bed-ridden. Curve progression is seen more in quadriplegics, nonambulatory patients with apex at thoracolumbar region. The treatment of scoliosis in CP is done with the aim of maintaining balance in sitting and standing, to allow functional use of the upper extremities.

In addition, untreated patients may develop cardiopulmonary complications. Bracing in CP individuals may not check the curve progression as in AIS, but helps

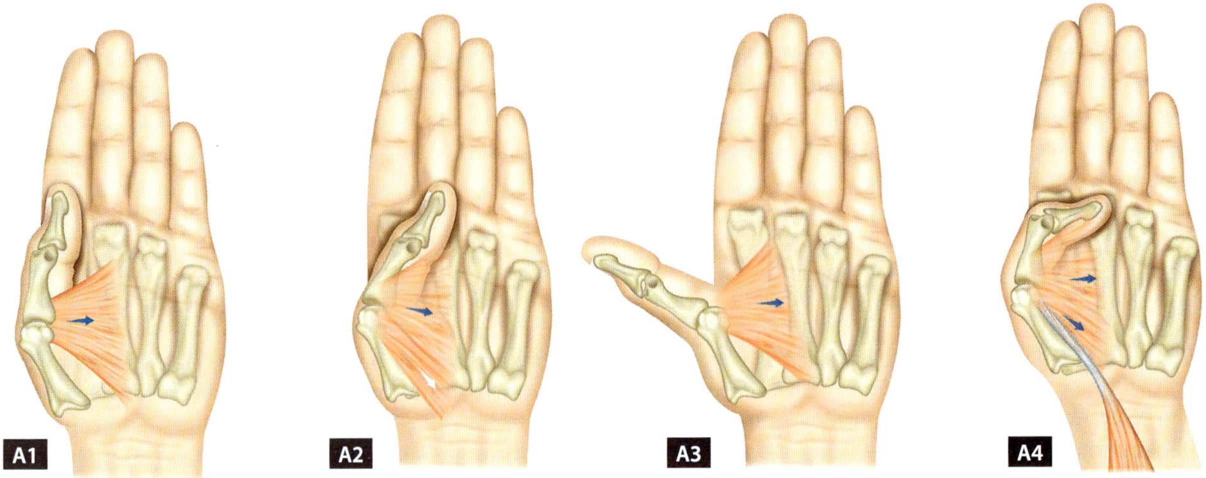

The type 1 thumb-in-palm deformity. Spasticity in the adductor pollicis causes significant adduction of the first metacarpal, narrowing the first web and limiting grasp. The adductor pollicis is the primary deforming force.

Type 2: In addition to the thumb metacarpal adduction deformity from the adductor pollicis muscle spasticity, the type 2 thumb-in-palm deformity additionally has a thumb metacarpophalangeal joint flexion deformity due to flexor pollicis brevis spasticity.

The type 3 thumb-in-palm deformity. With prolonged adductor pollicis spasticity, the thumb will extend and abduct through the metacarpophalangeal (MCP) joint (i.e., secondary MCP joint instability, subluxation, and dislocation). The MCP joint becomes dorsally unstable with an incompetent volar plate.

The type 4 thumb-in-palm deformity. In addition to the thumb metacarpal adduction deformity due to adductor pollicis spasticity and the metacarpophalangeal joint flexion due to flexor pollicis brevis spasticity, the type 4 thumb-in-palm deformity has interphalangeal joint flexion deformity due to flexor pollicis longus spasticity.

A

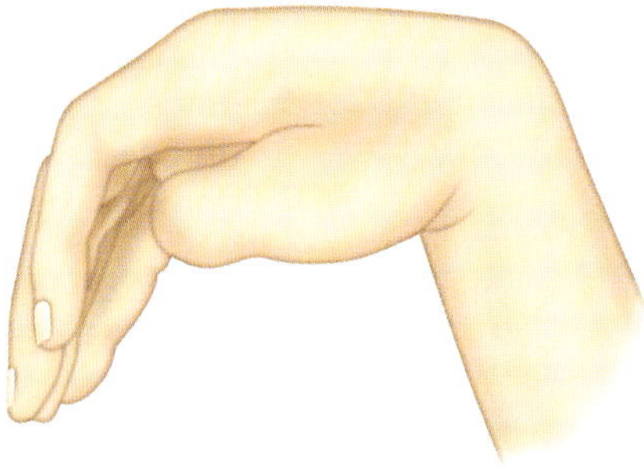

B

Figs. 12A and B: (A) Thumb-in-palm deformity types (A1-4); Side view of the deformity (B).

in maintaining an upright position while sitting. Seating modification can also be carried out in the wheelchair for an upright posture in patients who do not tolerate brace very well. Physical therapy, electrical stimulation and botulinum toxin have not been reported to be effective in controlling the curve progression. The definitive treatment for progressive, debilitating scoliosis patients with CP is surgical fusion with instrumentation. The general indication for surgical intervention is curve magnitude of 50° or above which leads to deterioration in sitting function.

However, surgical intervention in CP is different from AIS and is associated with a much higher complications. The scoliosis correction in CP may lead to worsening of hip deformities. Subluxation or dislocation may appear necessitating surgical intervention in the hip. Hip asymmetry, pelvic obliquity, and scoliosis are interrelated and corrective force on one aspect may worsen the others. Fixed flexion deformity at hips may predispose to hyperlumbar lordosis after instrumentation. Antiseizure drugs such as phenytoin and valproic acid alter vitamin D metabolism leading to poor bone quality. These patients may also have prolonged bleeding time requiring more blood and blood products. Intrathecal baclofen pump if used must be turned off to prevent faulty intraoperative neuromonitoring. These patients are also prone to develop severe pulmonary injections in the postoperative period due to prolonged immobilization. The pulmonary function is as it is compromised due to large curve and weak cough reflex. Patients at increased risk of aspiration may benefit from gastrostomy. This not only controls gastroesophageal reflux disease (GERD), but also plays important role in correcting malnutrition. Malnutrition is shown to increase postoperative complications such as infection, longer length of intubation, and a larger hospital stay. For most CP curves, pedicle instrumentation has been shown to increase fusion rates and to reduce chances of pseudoarthrosis. Early ambulation following this instrumentation reduces pulmonary complications and morbidity. The proximal level of fusion generally extends till T2 vertebrae to reduce chances of junctional kyphosis and pullout of instrumentation. Distally the fusion may end at L5. However, those patients with significant pelvic obliquity should include sacrum in the fusion.

SINGLE-EVENT MULTILEVEL SURGERY

Single event multilevel surgery (SEMLS) has become standard of care in management of ambulatory children with CP, spina bifida, and spastic diplegia. It is also sometimes called multilevel surgery (MLS). The movement disorder and gait is significantly improved in pediatric patients undergoing SEMLS. Multiple corrections for addressing muscle imbalance, contractures, and bone problems are done in single surgical sitting targeting the musculoskeletal system at ≥2 levels (feet, ankles, knees, and hips). SEMLS hence minimizes the number of surgeries and just one phase of rehabilitation is sufficient to manage the patients. Procedures include tendon/tissue lengthening to correct contractures, tendon transfers for muscle imbalance, rotational osteotomies for torsional deformities, and stabilization of the hip and foot. The standardization of indications has not been done for SEMLS and it is more of a physician preference and experience that culminates into SEMLS. It is less commonly performed in adult population. The greatest contention to using SEMLS is the popularity of baclofen pump and dorsal rhizotomy for some spastic conditions that control the spasticity so well that some of the components of SEMLS may not be needed if proper classical corrective and rehabilitation program is instituted. Moreover the rate of subsequent surgery and implant removal is not negligible and is nearly 30–40% so parents should be properly counseled for same. In any case SEMLS has shown better maintenance of GPS scores due to enhanced walking abilities, increased mobility skills, reduced need of oxygen, maintained joint mobility, and improved limb alignment.

INHERITED NEUROMUSCULAR DISORDERS

There are many inherited disorders involving the neurological and musculoskeletal system. The focus here will be on the commoner ones **(Table 4)** with orthopedic implications so that proper identification and management can be instituted. The rarer ones may not be encountered in the entire life of a practicing orthopedic surgeon and are mostly domain of pediatrician or neurologist.

TABLE 4: The common inherited neuromuscular conditions.

Disorder	*Inheritance/protein involved*	*System affected*
Duchenne muscular dystrophy	X-linked recessive [Duchenne muscular dystrophy (*DMD*)] Dystrophin protein	Skeletal and cardiac muscle
Spinal muscular atrophy	Autosomal recessive (*SMN 1-5q*) Survival motor neuron 1	Motor neurons
Friedreich ataxia	Autosomal recessive (*FXN-9q*) Frataxin	Cerebellum
Charcot–Marie–Tooth disease	Autosomal dominant (*PMP22*) Peripheral myelin protein 22	Peripheral nerves

TABLE 5: The common types of muscle dystrophies (from the most common to rarer).

Type	*Characteristics*
Duchenne muscular dystrophy	See text
Facioscapulohumeral muscular dystrophy	Unable to close eyes even with effort, sleeps with eyelids slightly open, and unable to purse lips
Myotonic dystrophy	Stiff muscles, clouding of lens, excessive sleeping, swallowing difficulty, behavior and learning disability, and cardiac rhythm abnormality
Becker muscular dystrophy	Delayed walking and muscle cramps in strenuous tasks
Limb-girdle muscle dystrophy	Weak girdle muscles (hips, thigh, and arm), loss of muscle mass in these regions, back pain, abnormal cardiac rhythm, and palpitations
Oculopharyngeal muscular dystrophy	Delayed onset of symptoms >50 years, drooping eyelids, difficult swallowing, restricted eye movements, and shoulder and hip weakness
Emery–Dreifuss muscular dystrophy	Symptoms in childhood and adolescence, muscle weakness, difficulty climbing stairs, frequent falls, and slow irregular heartbeat

DUCHENNE MUSCULAR DYSTROPHY

Duchenne muscular dystrophy (DMD) is the most common type of inherited pediatric muscle dystrophy out of more than 20 described types (commoner ones summarized in **Table 5**. It was first described by French neurologist Guillaume-Benjamin-Amand Duchenne in the 1860s. DMD is characterized by severe, progressive, skeletal, and cardiac muscle-wasting caused by deletions, nonsense or frame-shift mutations in *DMD* gene located at Xp21 (encodes dystrophin) so that dystrophin protein (Dp427m) is absent in the basement membrane of muscles. Weakening of basement membrane causes release of myofiber content into extracellular matrix causing inflammation, fibrosis, dysfunction and eventual degeneration resulting in weakness, inability to walk, deformities, respiratory insufficiency, cardiomyopathy, and death. Lack of dystrophin produces group of disorders called "dystrophinopathies" that include four disorders. DMD is one of them and other three are Becker muscle dystrophy, an intermediate form between Becker's and DMD and the last one is DMD associated with dilated cardiomyopathy without skeletal muscle involvement. Dystrophinopathies including DMD inherited as X-linked recessive disorder so that boys are mostly affected (they have just one X chromosome so mutated gene will cause disease expression). Girls will have disease if both the "X chromosomes" are affected (rare) or in Turner's syndrome, they are mostly carriers. A few cases of translocation of involving *DMD* have been reported that produce the disease in both males and females.

Pathophysiology

Duchenne muscular dystrophy results from sarcolemmal damage due to defect in subsarcolemmal dystrophin protein. The damages produced by lack of dystrophin protein are varied some of them are cytosolic calcium overload, free radical damage, functional ischemia, sarcolemma weakening, and regeneration failure. Dysfunctional muscle tissue and loss of regeneration replaces the native tissue by fat and fibrous tissue. Pathological tissue produces muscle stiffness and weakness of skeletal and cardiac muscles and joint contractures and scoliosis. Muscle breakdown causes elevation in creatine kinase (CK). Small amounts of dystrophin is also produced by nerve cells in hippocampus, lack of it there produces nonprogressive memory and learning problems.

Clinical Features

Duchenne muscular dystrophy is overt till the age of 2–3 years when symptoms start appearing. The muscle weakness is first to appear that too it involves the proximal muscles near trunk and hips and shoulders **(Fig. 13)**. The weakness then gradually starts moving distally. Weakness in upper limbs appear later than lower limbs so fine movements of hands and fingers are much less affected than body balance and gait disturbances **(Fig. 14)**. The list of symptoms is provided in **Table 3**. The disease progresses through early ambulatory, late ambulatory, early nonambulatory, and late nonambulatory phases.

Diagnosis

Classic clinical feature and history **(Box 3)** raise strong suspicion of DMD. Diagnosis is made by getting CK blood levels. CK is raised to 10–100 times normal in DMD, normal levels rule-out diagnosis of DMD. Raised CK can be seen in other conditions including trauma to skeletal muscles so it is nonspecific so muscle biopsy and genetic tests are undertaken.

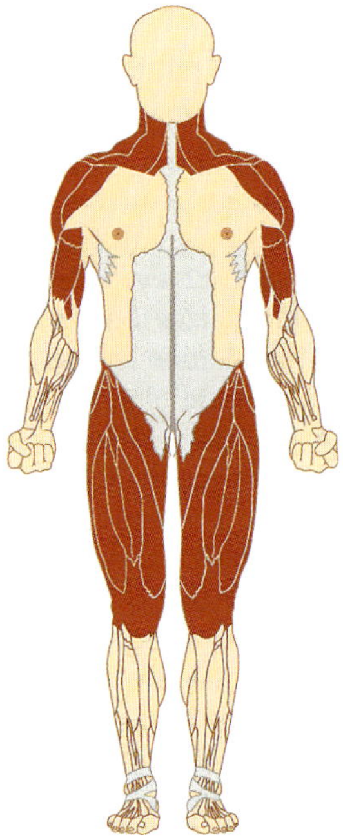

Fig. 14: The typical proximal muscle involvement (colored dark red) early in the course of Duchenne muscular dystrophy.

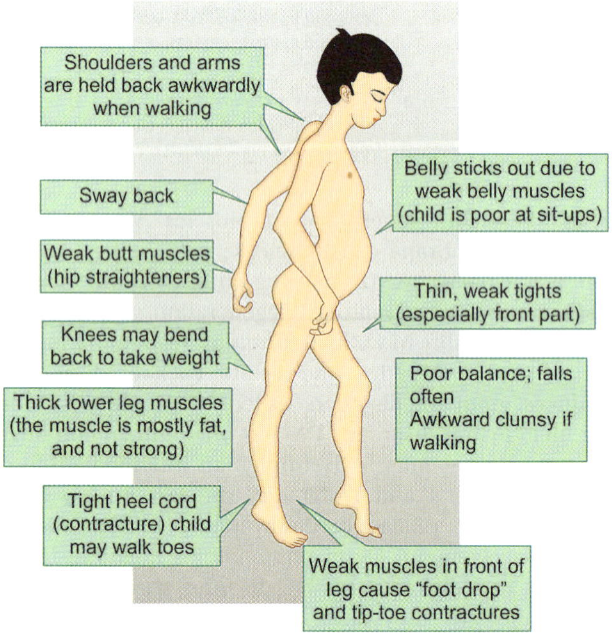

Fig. 13: The gait pattern and various abnormal components in a patient with Duchene muscular dystrophy.

BOX 3: The symptoms and presenting features of Duchenne muscle dystrophy.

- Proximal muscle weakness (more marked in lower limbs)
- Delayed walking
- Short stature due to slower growth
- Difficulty with walking, running, jumping, and climbing stairs
- Waddling gait due to weak abductor
- Toe-walking and wide-based gait with an increased curve in the lower back
- Because of loose shoulder muscles child appears sloppy when picking up into lap
- Frequent falls
- In adolescents the calf muscles may look bulky (pseudohypertrophy), although they are not strong. Thigh muscles may also be hypertrophied.
- "Gower's sign"—as the child gets older and disease progresses, he uses his hands to help him get up sort of "climbing up his legs".
- Positive Trendelenburg test
- Some children have a learning difficulty (usually not severe).
- Developmental delay and delay in speech may be first symptom (nonspecific).
- Joint contractures
- Progressive enlargement of heart
- Difficult coughing and weakness of respiratory muscles—absolute breathing difficulty may not be a symptom but other symptoms such as headaches, mental dullness, difficulty in concentrating or staying awake, and nightmare. Pulmonary function is poor.
- Increased risk of respiratory infection

Exome sequencing or next-generation sequencing of Sanger is the most definitive evaluation but expensive so preferably multiplex ligation-dependent probe amplification (MLPA) or alternatively array comparative genome hybridization (array CGH). In remote locations only multiplex polymerase chain reaction (PCR) may be available and is commonly used in third-world countries but not recommended for DMD diagnosis. Muscle biopsy is not needed if genetic diagnosis is made. It is needed only if no mutations are detected in MLPA or Sanger sequencing. It assesses assess whether dystrophin is properly localized (using immunofluorescence analysis) or absent/reduced (using Western blotting and immunofluorescence, absent levels are diagnostic of DMD) or has an altered size (using Western blotting, an altered size is diagnostic of BMD). Prenatal diagnosis can be made by analyzing cell-free deoxyribonucleic acid (DNA) in maternal serum. This technique reveals fetal aneuploidies (trisomy 21, 13, and 18) and maternal copy number variations (CNVs). Maternal CNVs are common in DMD and genotype-phenotype correlations with frameshift rule applied to CNVs allow differentiation of DMD from Becker muscular dystrophy.

Management

Medical management beyond the use of corticosteroids is not available. Steroid therapy alters the natural history of disease by delaying the decline in walking, scoliosis progression, cardiomyopathy, and pulmonary function. It prolongs the duration of independent immobilization but side effects are many including cataracts, weight gain, short stature, delayed puberty, and osteoporosis. Stem cell therapy and gene therapy are under development. Gene therapy with adenovirus is attractive as it can infect the skeletal muscles and deliver the gene. The loading capacity of AAV is low (≈4.3 kb) whereas the dystrophin gene *DMD* needs ≈11.4 kb complementary DNA (cDNA). Partly functional mini- and microdystrophin constructs are being deployed. Because majority of DMD involves frame shift mutation so antisense oligonucleotides (ASOs) that restore the reading frames of dystrophin transcripts is being utilized. These ASOs bind to target exon during pre-messenger ribonucleic acid (mRNA) splicing and prevents the inclusion of exon into mRNA (exon skipping). Exon skipping using ASO is mutation specific and exon 51 (using eteplirsen), 45, 53 (using golodirsen and viltolarsen) and 44 are being currently targeted. Similarly nonsense mutation read through is being attempted. Goals of orthopedic management in DMD can be grouped under the various phases of disease progression.

Ambulatory Phase

The chief role of orthopedist in this phase is counseling the family members for prevention of joint contractures as the disease progresses. This is accomplished by passive stretching that needs to be done frequently but not-at-all very aggressively. Damage to myofibrils will not heal and instead change to fibrosis. Night-time orthosis are an important addendum, especially if dorsiflexion is <10°. Knee-ankle-foot orthosis is the most commonly use brace with locked knee joints that preserve lower limb function and walking. Brace fitting may need surgical release of some contractures. One should always remember that surgical release always leads to some weakness in the muscle group. Disuse and steroid-induced osteopenia commonly weakens bone and is an important cause or premature loss of ambulation. Surgical fixation of fractures is important in such cases to immediately mobilize the patient and delay the eventuality. Also the already compromised cardiorespiratory function predisposes these patients to fat embolism syndrome and respiratory complications postoperatively and death.

Nonambulatory Phase

By the time of reaching adolescence most DMD patients are already wheel-chair bound. Contractures progress rapidly in these patients. Devices and use of walking aids to help them stand is an option in only a few where severe contractures have not developed. Severe contracture of upper or lower limb that limit position is compromising to skin needs surgical release. Surgical releases designed to correct lower extremity contractures have mostly not shown to improve walking ability so surgery for scoliosis is commonly resorted to. Scoliotic curves progress very fast in this phase and surgery is recommended, if the curves measure >30°. Scoliotic corrective surgery improves quality of life, reduce pain, and improve sitting balance. This is however a high-risk endeavor and it needs optimization of cardiorespiratory status and vigilance for postoperative rhabdomyolysis and hyperkalemia by anesthetist.

SPINAL MUSCULAR ATROPHY

Spinal muscular atrophy (SMA) is an autosomal recessive disease resulting from mutation in *SMN1* gene located at 5q chromosome. It is the second most common inherited neuromuscular disorder. The mutations cause degeneration of anterior motor neurons due to absence/abnormality in survival motor neuron (SMN) protein. The number of remaining functional SMN proteins produced from *SMN2* gene determines disease severity representing a spectrum of disorder classified into 4 subtypes **(Table 6)**.

TABLE 6: The subtypes of spinal muscular atrophy.

Subtype	*Age of onset*	*Characteristics*
SMA type I (Werdnig–Hoffmann disease)	At birth or infancy	Low tone, loss of deep tendon reflexes, tongue fasciculations, intercostal muscle weakness, atelectasis, pneumonia, respiratory failure and death by 2 years of age
SMA type II	6 months to 2 years	Milder course of muscle weakness and loss of ambulation
SMA type III (Kugelberg–Welander disease)	Late toddler to early adolescence	Maintain ambulation and normal life expectancies
SMA type IV	Adult onset	Mild disease course

Patients with SMA have more prominent motor weakness of the lower limbs compared to upper limbs. Motor weakness arises due to degeneration and involvement of alpha motor neurons of the spinal cord anterior horn cells. The weakness is predominantly in the proximal muscle groups accompanied with hypotonia and hyporeflexia. The major orthopedic manifestations include joint contracture (flexion, abduction and external rotation of hip, knee flexion contracture, and ankle equinus), hip dysplasia, pathologic fractures, and scoliosis. Lower extremity is more commonly affected, contracture of elbow may be associated with hypermobile wrist joint. Cranial nerves V-XII may also be involved affecting speech, breathing, and feeding.

Treatment

There is no available cure for SMA. Nusinersen is an ASO drug that is administered intrathecally and it alters the *SMN2* gene to produce more functional SMN protein improving motor function in SMA type I disease. The orthopedic management is based on current functional status of the child viz. nonsitters, sitters, or walkers. The contractures are surgically released if they are painful or limit function/bracing. This should be aimed at improving the ambulatory status. Hip dislocation is commonly left as it is because it is mostly intermittent and asymptomatic. Relocation is usually associated with redislocation. Modern methods and techniques may have better relocation rates.

Scoliosis occurs in three-fourths of the patients with SMA. This is the most common orthopedic manifestation that is surgically managed. Scoliosis in SMA is rapidly progressing compromising respiratory function. Dependent sitters do not benefit from surgery and are managed with custom-molded lightweight orthoses to improve sitting balance. Any improvement in curves or pulmonary function is not usually seen. For dependent sitters bracing is recommended for curves between 20 and 50° to improve truncal support. Surgery is recommended for curves >50° and those with rapid progression. It is prudent to delay surgery till 4 years of age and one should utilize growth sparing instruments to achieve trunk height.

CHARCOT–MARIE–TOOTH DISEASE

Charcot-Marie-Tooth (CMT) disease is the most common type of hereditary sensorimotor neuropathy. It is subdivided into two subgroups—demyelinating and axonal neuropathy. Next-generation sequencing has identified more than 80 genes responsible for the disease but peripheral myelin protein 22 gene duplication on chromosome 17p11.2 is identified with CMT type 1 phenotype and mitofusin 2 gene is responsible for CMT type 2. The clinical features seem to be similar in different subgroups of described CMT and include distal sensory loss, distal lower followed by upper extremity amyotrophy, loss of deep tendon reflexes, and gait disturbances. Three characteristic gait patterns are identified—flail foot, cavovarus foot, and toe walking gait. Other common orthopedic manifestations of CMT include hand and foot deformity, ankle instability, hip dysplasia, and scoliosis.

Treatment

The management is directed to improve gait and correct various deformities. Patients with flail foot are commonly supported with orthosis and surgery helps in them to keep the foot in braceable position. Cavovarus foot is painful in walking and need surgical correction like plantar fasciotomy, midtarsal osteotomy, extensor hallucis longus tendon transfer to first metatarsal, and dorsiflexion osteotomy of first metatarsal in variable combinations. Recurrence of deformity is prevented by transfer of peroneus longus tendon to brevis and tibialis anterior tendon to lateral cuneiform. Toe walking may be secondary to plantar flexor contracture and/or cavus. The plantar flexors may themselves be weak actually and cautious lengthening of plantar flexors should be done else further weakness ensues. The most common foot deformity occurring with CMT is pes cavus followed by hammer toes and pes planus in that order. The goal of surgical treatment is to obtain a plantigrade stable painless foot that would need a variable combination of soft tissue procedures and muscle transfers, osteotomies to correct fixed deformities, and fusion for salvage. The details of management of these deformities are discussed in Chapter on "Poliomyelitis". Hip dysplasia in CMT is more severe than seen in dysplastic development of hip. There is severe acetabular dysplasia, hip subluxation, acetabular anteversion, coxa valga, and earlier development of hip arthritis. The pathogenesis involves selective hip abductor and extensor weakness causing progressive subluxation. It is recommended that all patients with CMT be screened with radiographs of pelvis. The treatment and surgical principles are same as for DDH but periacetabular osteotomies are more frequently needed. The results are worse in treatment of CMT than those with classical DDH. Scoliosis occurs in 15% of the patients with CMT most of which are progressive and one-third eventually need surgery. Bracing is not effective in halting curve progression. The correction is performed on the principles of AIS with similar success and complication rates. Intraoperative neurological monitoring is difficult due to demyelinating polyneuropathy.

FRIEDREICH ATAXIA

This is the most common spinocerebellar degenerative disorder characterized by progressive limb and trunk ataxia, muscle weakness, gait disturbance, areflexia, dysarthria, and loss of vibratory sense and proprioception. The disease is due to mutation of *FXN* gene on chromosomal 9 that results in loss of mitochondrial protein frataxin. The loss of frataxin results in iron accumulation in mitochondria and pathologically alters muscle and neural tissue causing dysfunction. The patients typically present with slowly progressive ataxia, weakness, and areflexia that begins in adolescence. These get gradually associated with dysphagia, hand clumsiness, upgoing plantar response, and peripheral sensory neuropathy. Orthopedic manifestations such as pes cavus and scoliosis develop along with cardiomyopathy and disorderly glucose metabolism. Patients become wheelchair bound by 50 years of age and the most common cause of death is cardiac failure. Presently, there is no cure for the disease while strategies for treatment include reducing iron accumulation in mitochondria, reducing oxidative and inflammatory stress, enhancing mitochondrial function, and modulating frataxin production.

Scoliosis is seen in all patients with Friedreich ataxia. The recommendation is bracing to delay surgical treatment, if it does not interfere with compensatory trunk movements needed for walking. It does not prevent surgery or reduce curves. Surgery is indicated for curves >40° if the cardiopulmonary status can be optimized accordingly and surgical benefits of halting curve progression, restoring balance outweigh the surgical risks, and life expectancy. Foot cavovarus deformity is stretched initially by gradual manipulation—Ponseti method commonly utilized. Once the foot is supple tendon transfer may be considered to prevent recurrence.

CONCLUSION

- Although the incidence of CP and inherited neuromuscular disorders is more or less static, improved orthopedic care is providing better function to these patients. The diseases remain incurable till date.
- Cerebral palsy patients require a specialized approach much different from the conventional orthopedic training principles.
- The patients should be evaluated as a whole for providing holistic treatment.
- Development of deformities is quite fast if proper care is not begun initially. Botulinum toxin is a marvelous tool for controlling the spasticity and allowing movements at the joints to prevent development of contractures and joint stiffness.
- Still in late cases limited releases have to be done to improve function of the patients.
- Orthopedic management should always be combined and supplemented by dedicated counselors, physiotherapists, rehabilitation experts, and pediatricians so that comprehensive care is delivered at source.
- Fusionless and growing rod implants are being increasingly used for management of neuromuscular scoliosis.
- Steroid treatment prolongs ambulation and decrease the onset of scoliosis in DMD.
- Scoliosis surgery in DMD is associated with improved quality of life.
- Nusinersen has shown promising results in patients with SMA.
- Proactive orthopedic intervention for managing hip, spine, and foot deformity improves patient remarkably with CP and CMT disease.

CHAPTER 41

Anomalies of Pediatric Lower Limb

Manish Kumar Varshney

INTRODUCTION

Pediatric lower limb conditions are frequently identified in pediatric orthopedic clinic. Understanding the pathological and anatomical change helps identify and scale the functional limitations and future deficiencies. The orthopedic surgeon must be well aware of growth-related changes and age-appropriate differences so that the anomalies can be optimally corrected. Angular and rotational abnormalities and limb-length discrepancies should be evaluated for the possible correctable cause and if need surgery then appropriately planned and executed. Foot deformities may be intrinsic or part of syndromic or neurological anomaly. They require dedicated specialty precision correction and handling to prevent long-term morbidity and improve function.

DEVELOPMENT OF LOWER LIMB

- Lower limb bud develops during fourth week as elevations of the ventrolateral body wall **(Figs. 1A and B)**. The lower limb buds form opposite the lumbar and upper sacral segments.
- Fibroblast growth factors from the apical ectodermal ridge activate the zone of polarizing activity, which causes expression of the sonic hedgehog (*Shh*) genes. It has been suggested that *Shh* secretions (morphogens) control the patterning of the limb along the anterior-posterior axis (see also cleft foot below).
    - The intervening regions of mesenchyme break-down due to apoptosis separating digits (fingers and toes) by the end of the eighth week. This is probably mediated by bone morphogenetic proteins [β-transforming growth factor (TGF) family].
- Osteogenesis of long bones begins in the seventh week from primary ossification centers in the middle of the cartilaginous models of the long bones. Ossification centers are present in all long bones by the 12th week.
- During 5–7th week, limb bud rotates medially through almost 90° to bring the hallux into the midline **(Fig. 1C)**. The knees come to face ventrally and the extensor muscles lie on the anterior aspect of the lower limb. Rotation continues in the sixth week (14–16 mm), leading to nearly 90° of inward rotation.
- During the eighth week, the thigh continues to internally rotate producing femoral anteversion of around 40° at birth. This reduces to 15° at maturity. Tibia increases its lateral rotation from approximately 5° at birth to 15° at maturity **(Fig. 1C)**.
- The development of the foot occurs in following progressive stages:
    - The foot is in 90° equinus and adducted during second month of development.
    - During the middle of third month foot dorsiflexes at the ankle, but a mild degree of equinus persists. The marked supination is still present.
    - During beginning of fourth month, the foot pronates and reaches a position of midsupination. Equinus vanishes. The pronation continues during the remainder of fetal development.

CONGENITAL FEMORAL DEFICIENCY

Congenital anomalies of the femur occur in about 1 in 10,000 live births. The broad term "congenital abnormalities of the femur" encompasses spectrum from hypoplasia to complete absence of femur and includes following entities:

- Congenital short femur
- Proximal femoral focal dysplasia (PFFD)
- Femoral hypoplasia
- Mini femur
- Congenital coxa vara

Bilateral abnormalities are found in approximately 15% of patients. The milder forms of femoral anomalies (short femur and femur hypoplasia) are associated with coxa vara while the PFFD is associated with subtrochanteric bowing. Femoral hypoplasia is a commonly seen deficiency that may be variably associated with other anomalies **(Box 1)**.

BOX 1: Anomalies associated with femoral hypoplasia.

- Proximal femoral retroversion
- Coxa vara
- Lateral femoral condyle hypoplasia
- Patellar subluxation
- Congenital absence of cruciate ligaments

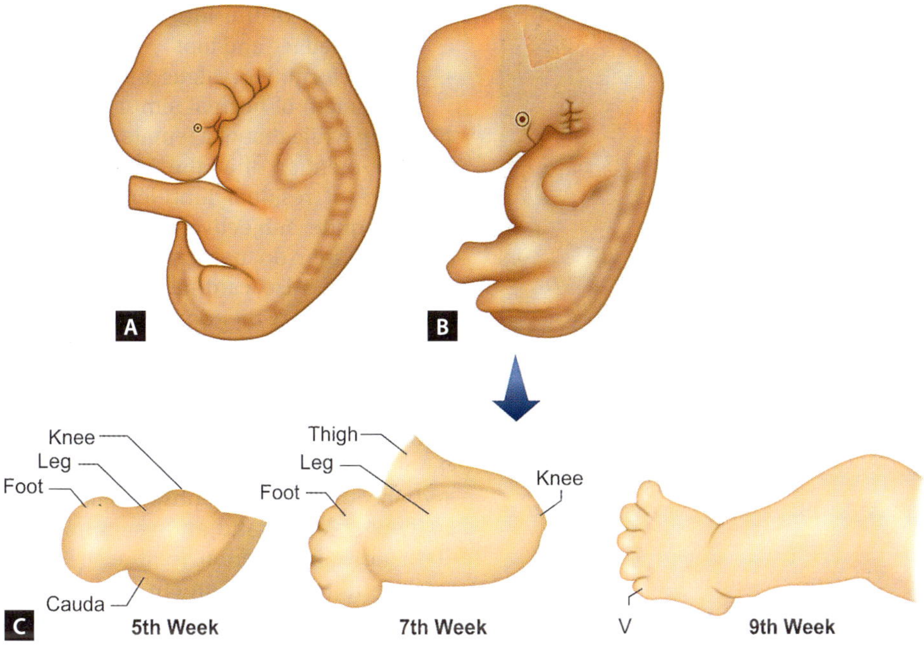

Figs. 1A to C: Development of lower limb. (A) The development at 5 weeks and (B) at 7th week; (C) The development and differentiation into individual parts then follows.

Similarly, patients with congenital short femur are found to have:

- Fibular hemimelia
- Congenital absence of foot rays
- Ball-in-socket ankle
- Tarsal coalition

The treatment of femoral hypoplasia or congenital short femur is basically guided by the prediction of the limb-length discrepancy at skeletal maturity and associated abnormalities. The options are:

- *Limb lengthening* for projected discrepancy at skeletal maturity of <17 cm and who have a stable hip and knee with good foot and ankle function
- *Amputation* and early prosthetic fitting (predicted discrepancy >17 cm)
- *Limb reconstruction* by rotationplasty with or without hip fusion. This option can be an alternative to amputation if facilities exist.

Proximal Femoral Focal Deficiency or Dysplasia

Proximal femoral focal deficiency or dysplasia is a characteristic abnormality of the proximal femur (focal as the distal part is grossly normal whatever size is left!) that has typical changes at the hip. This has led most of the classification system focus on hip anatomy rendering them meaningless in terms of management of the condition that is guided nevertheless by expected residual shortening at skeletal maturity. Some classifications are radiologic, some functional, and others merely designed to adapt authors' preferred treatment! None, however, cumulatively include shortening, radiographic, and muscle abnormalities together, to guide treatment. Aitken's is the most widely used classification that divides the true PFFD into four categories based on the radiographic findings. Being radiographic, the classification should be used reasonably on sufficient bony ossification and is more of a material for reporting cases in medical literature rather than collectively helping framing treatment.

- *Class A:*
  - Femur is short, with its proximal end at or slightly above the acetabulum.
  - There is a defect in the subtrochanteric region with lateral bowing causing varus deformity (different from coxa vara)—subtrochanteric defect eventually ossifies, establishing bony continuity.
  - The femoral head may be absent but will later ossify, and its presence is indicated by a well-developed acetabulum.
- *Class B:*
  - More extensive defect or absence of the proximal femur
  - The femoral head is present, although its ossification may be delayed.
  - There is usually a bony tuft on the proximal end of the femoral shaft. The defect does not heal spontaneously, and the proximal end of the femur will be above the acetabulum.
- *Class C:*
  - Femoral head is absent and will never ossify.
  - The acetabulum is severely dysplastic.
  - The femoral shaft is shorter than in class B, and the entire proximal portion of the femur, including the trochanters, will not appear **(Figs. 2A and B)**.
- *Class D:*
  - Femoral shaft is extremely short, often with only a tuft of irregularly ossified bone proximal to the distal femoral epiphysis.

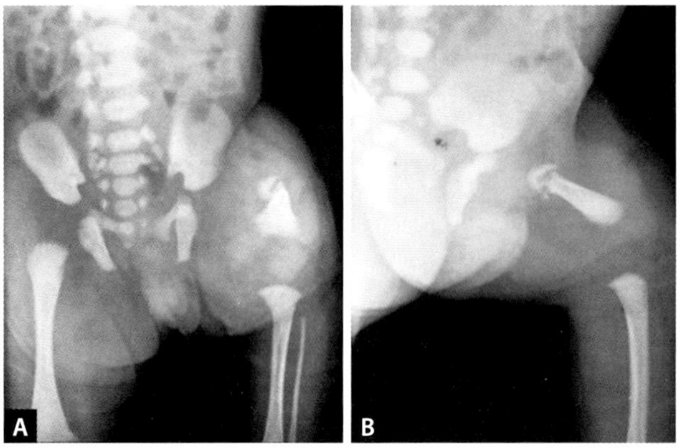

Figs. 2A and B: Radiographs of a patient with class "C" Atkins PFFD (see text for details).

- The lateral pelvic wall is flat, without hint of an acetabulum.

The classification by Gillespie divides femoral deficiencies into three groups for purposes of treatment quite usefully:

1. *Group A (short femur) has congenital short femur and clinical hip stability:* There is no significant knee flexion contracture, and the foot of the affected extremity lying at or below the mid-point of the opposite tibia. These patients may be candidates for limb-lengthening.
2. Group B patients include the Aitken class A, B, and C as above.
3. Group C (very short femur) represents the Aitken class D patients.

Clinical Features

- Proximal femoral focal dysplasia is bilateral in 15% of the cases.
- The femoral segment is short, flexed, abducted, and externally rotated.
- Hip and knee joint commonly have flexion contractures. The hip (globally—all directions) and knee [in anteroposterior (AP) direction] are unstable.
- The proximal thigh is bulbous and rapidly tapers to the knee joint (inverted conical shape).
- Fibular deficiencies (fibular hemimelia) are associated with PFFD in 70% cases with valgus foot and other characteristics of fibular deficiency.

Management

Decide if:

- Child has a useful extremity that can be lengthened.
- *Dictum:* The length of the short leg compared to the normal leg at infancy remains in the same proportion at maturity (Amstutz)—helping calculate the residual length at skeletal maturity.

Gillespie recommended lengthening for his group A patients, and prosthetic treatment for his group B and C patients.

The functional deficits that need reconstruction include:

- The shortening of the limb
- Hip stability (especially the lurch)
- Alignment of the limb—knee flexion, and anteriorly positioned leg and foot
- Foot deformities (valgus and fibular hemimelia)

The length of normal femur of an adult male is around 43–46 cm while that of a female is 41–43 cm. It is reasonable here to mention that the absolute values mentioned in literature of residual limb-length deficit of 17 cm or 20 cm are quite subjective and are based on the fact that these children do not gain functionally even if the limb is preserved. Also cardinal values of "percentage of limb-length deficit" are mentioned in the literature that precludes surgical reconstruction. We feel that a limb that will be 40–50% shorter than the other limb or deemed normal length at maturity (for bilateral deficiency), then it is better to counsel the parents avgainst limb savage. A child with PFFD should receive extension prosthesis to equalize the limbs and encourage normal physiological development as soon as he is able to stand and walk incorporating the flexion, abduction and external rotation of the proximal segment into the prosthetic alignment.

The options available with surgeon for management of various types of PFFD include:

- *Limb-lengthening rather lengthening of femur:* The easier option of lengthening the femur is available in fewer children with PFFD. Hip should be stable before the procedure. The knee is also frequently unstable and lengthening in this instance often produces anterior subluxation of femur on tibia.
- *Knee arthrodesis:*
  - Creates a single longer and more efficient lever arm for prosthetic fitting.
  - The fusion is done in full knee extension. The abduction and flexion deformity at the hip joint will correct, thus aligning the limb under the axis of the body.
  - One should anticipate the limb length in advance and remove one, both or none of the growth plates around the knee else the limb may be too long or short for prosthetic fitting.
  - Syme's amputation can be done at same sitting or delayed by 6 weeks.
- Shortening the limb and prosthetic fitting—can be done in two forms:
  1. Syme's amputation and fitting as extralong below knee prosthesis. This is less cosmetic option as the knee height difference is remarkable when the child sits.
  2. Knee arthrodesis and fitting with above-knee prosthesis as mentioned previously.
- *Rotationplasty:* The Van Nes procedure used the function at ankle to benefit the child. The limb is rotated by 180° bringing the ankle to substitute for knee and the original knee is fused. Three prerequisites for performing this procedure should be carefully examined and communicated:
  1. Ankle should be sufficiently functional.
  2. Obtainable length should be appropriate.
  3. Psychosocial acceptance to the procedure and "weird looking" limb should be there.

Management of hip instability: Most patients have unstable hips due both to bony anatomy and deficient musculature. In Aitken class B, the pseudoarthrosis is corrected. Acetabular procedures are often required in class B to provide additional coverage to the femoral head and also in class A. For class C and D, the previously described surgical options for PFFD are undertaken. Some authors described iliofemoral arthrodesis previously but it does not find any useful way to address the problem. Two potentially useful procedures need mention:

1. *Steel procedure:* The distal femur is fused to the ilium in 90° flexion. This makes knee extension to substitute hip extension and *vice versa*; however, as the growth of distal femur fragment is not restricted the knee often becomes off-centric to serve this purpose.
2. *Brown rotationplasty:* Here, the distal femur is rotated 180° before being fused to ilium.

Reduction of thigh: It can be achieved by liposuction or surgical reduction to aid prosthetic fitting.

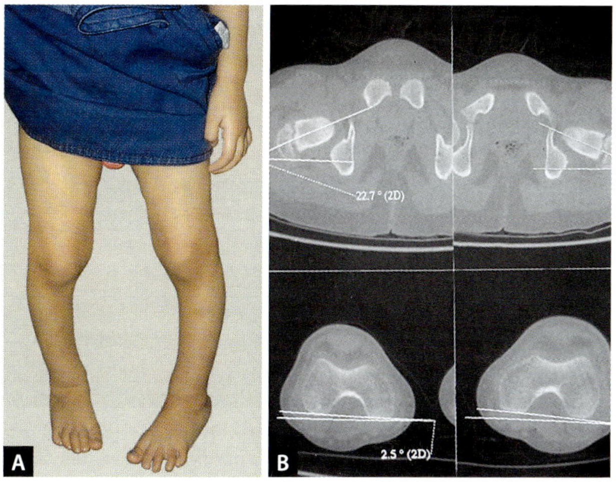

Figs. 3A and B: In-toeing gait (A) in a patient with increased femoral anteversion. The anteversion can be measured using computed tomography scan (different patient) as depicted here (B) or by using dedicated software (available commercially) that superimpose the images.

ROTATIONAL AND ANGULAR ALIGNMENT OF LOWER LIMB, COMMON PATHOLOGIES AND PRINCIPLES OF CORRECTION OF DEFORMITY IN CHILDREN

The normal spectrum of rotational alignment is difficult to quantify in children. This is because the foot progression angle can vary with gait in children <5 years and that rotational profiles vary widely. The term "version" refers to tilt or inclination around the longitudinal axis of a long bone while the term "torsion" is pathological and represents a range of more than two standard deviation (2SD) errors from version. Most infants have external hip rotation because of residual muscle contractures from intrauterine positioning. Due to fetal position in praying position at 8th week of gestation, there is internal rotation of the limb for the foot to be in plantigrade position. Additional uterus pressing effect results in outward rotation of the femur and inward rotation of tibia. At the time of birth, the femur anteversion is as high as 30–40°, and the tibia is neutral. Later, during the growing age, both the femur shaft and tibia tend to rotate outward; thus, the femur anteversion reaches to 10–15° and the tibia gains version to 15°. So, toddlers begin to walk with an out-toeing gait. Out-toeing and in-toeing **(Figs. 3A and B)** commonly depict the rotational malalignment in a child when he walks.

- ***Persistent in-toeing gait*** is pathological and can result from:
  - Residual metatarsus adductus
  - *Persistent internal tibial torsion:* An infant's tibia is rotated 5° internally while this changes to 10° of external rotation in an average 10-year-old child. Internal tibial torsion can also be seen with physiologic genu varum (bow-leg deformity). Most cases of internal tibial torsion resolve by 18–24 months. Persistence beyond 8 years is pathological.
  - *Excessive femoral anteversion:* Transverse plane rotation of the femoral neck axis lies anteriorly relative to the transcondylar axis. Excessive femoral anteversion typically is seen in children 3 years of age or older. Although fetal anteversion can be as much as 50°, by maturity the anteversion reduces to approximately 20° and, therefore, the incidence of in-toeing is reduced. In most cases, it resolves with time (95%). Compensatory lateral tibial torsion may develop after age 4–5 years. There is little functional disability, however, >50% of patients with persistent femoral anteversion achieve normal gait. Interestingly, this mechanical malalignment does not predispose to osteoarthritis (OA). The children walk with "squinting patellae". They sit in typical "W" position **(Figs. 4A and B)** and have increased internal rotation at hip (>60% of the total ROM at hip) than external rotation. In severe cases, the external rotation may be absent!
  - *Neuromuscular disorders (usually unilateral, asymmetrical and progressive):*
    - Cerebral palsy (CP)
    - Myelomeningocele
    - Iliotibial band (ITB) contractures
  - *Protective in-toeing:*
    - Genu valgum
    - Flexible pes planus
- *Out-toeing gait* is due to:
  - External tibial torsion
  - Pronation/abduction of the feet
  - Physiological persistence as mentioned above: This is more prolonged in premature births due to lack of uterine molding effect on inward rotation of legs
  - Femoral retroversion: The children walk with "frog eye" patella (outpointing) and prefer to sit in "Buddha position" **(Figs. 4A and B)**.
  - Congenital vertical talus (CVT)
  - Fibular hemimelia
  - Developmental coxa vara
  - Tarsal coalition

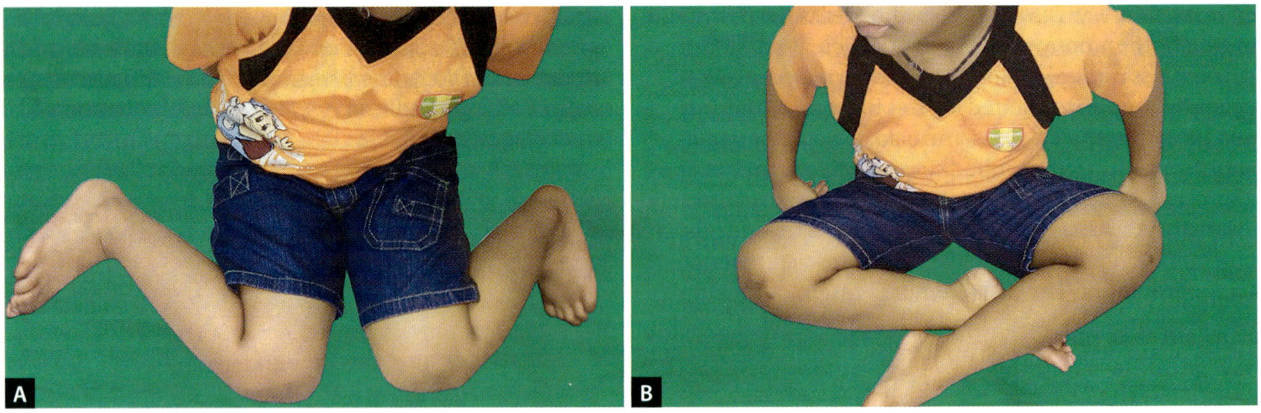

Figs. 4A and B: (A) In this patient with increased femoral anteversion and in-toeing gait, he used to prefer sitting in "W-position"; (B) Sitting in Buddha position was very uncomfortable and could not touch his knees to the couch at all.

Measurement of Rotational Alignment of Limb

The rotational alignment can be measured radiologically and clinically.

- ***Tibial version:***
  - *Clinical measurement:* It can be variously done.
    - *Thigh-foot angle measurement* ***(Fig. 5)****:* With the child in prone position, the knee is flexed 90°. Foot and ankle are held in neutral position so that the plantar surface is parallel with the ceiling. The angle between the line along the thigh and the line along the foot sole is the thigh-foot angle indicating the tibial torsion. The normal range for thigh foot angle is -5–30° by 8 years of age that remains constant thereafter. In infants, the angle is negative that gradually corrects to mature range.
    - The child is made to sit on the edge of the examining table with the legs dangling free. The leg firmly pressed to the table edge. By putting the thumb and index fingers on the medial and lateral malleoli, the transmalleolar axis is identified. The angle between this transmalleolar axis and the table edge shows tibial version.
    - The child sits on the edge of the examining table, with his foot held at a 90° angle relative to the leg. A perpendicular line drawn from tibial tubercle (TT) should cross the second metatarsal or second web **(Fig. 6)**. The degree of deviation from second metatarsal indicates the tibial version.
  - *Radiological measurement:* On tomogram axial cuts, the horizontal line is determined proximally by joining the most posterior aspect of tibial condyles. Distal axis is obtained by joining the two malleoli. These are superimposed to determine any torsion. Normal is around +20° (external tibial torsion) by and after 8 years of age.
- ***Femoral torsion:***
  - *Clinical measurement:* This is done indirectly by assessing the internal and external rotation of the hip measured in prone position. With knee flexed at 90°, the legs are made to fall under gravity, when they are moved away they indicate hip internal rotation. If one of the legs falls more than the other then it indicates increased anteversion of the femur; magnitude can be measured by the difference of passive internal rotation. Similarly, legs falling toward each other and

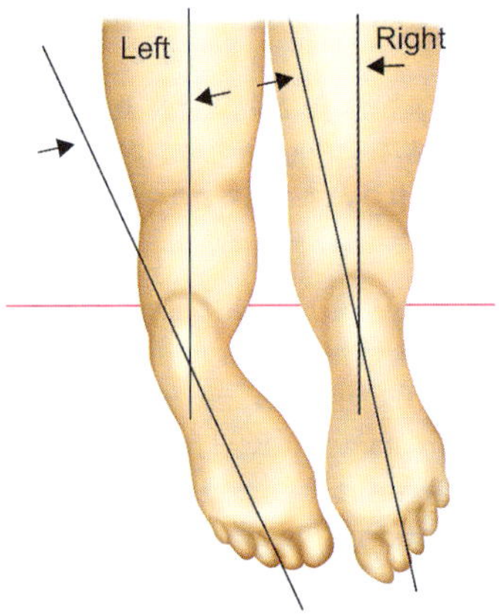

Fig. 5: Thigh-foot angle measurement (see technique in text)—the left side shows tibial intorsion.

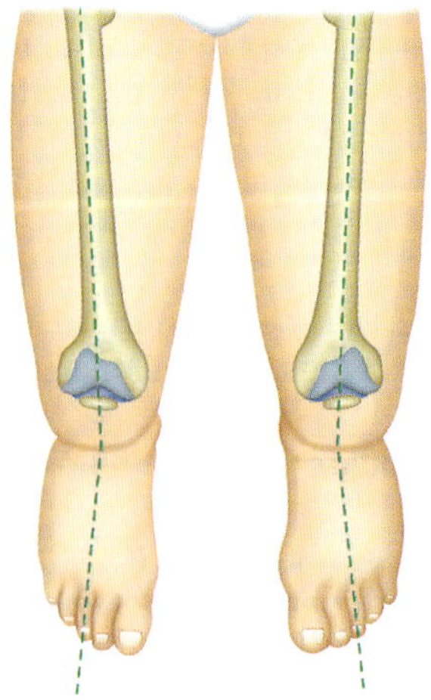

Fig. 6: Tibia foot axis as determined from line passing through tibial tuberosity.

crossing indicate femoral external rotation deformity and if excessive then pathological retroversion or reduced anteversion of the femur is suggested.

- *Radiological measurement:* Radiologically, the femoral version is determined by tomography. One image is taken to determine the axis of femoral neck-head proximally while other is drawn distally at the level of femoral condyles. The distal horizontal line is obtained by joining the most distal aspects of femoral condyles while the anteversion is measured by superimposed head-neck angle on this line **(Fig. 3)**. The normal value is <25° at the age of 8 or older for both male and female.

Evaluation and Treatment of Rotational Deformity

History

Prematurity, child's walking attitude, hand dominance, health of previous child, and process of evolution should be generously enquired. The most common cause of in-toeing varies according to the age of child:

- *In the first year of life:* Metatarsus adducts
- *In the second year of life:* Internal tibial torsion
- *In the third year and later:* Internal femoral torsion

In internal tibial torsion, the transmalleolar axis is medial and there may be compensatory foot abduction and pronation.

The rotational malalignment of the limb could be of various types depending on the disposition of various individual components:

- *Simple:* When the rotational malalignment is present in one bone.
- *Additive:* If there is rotational malalignment present in both or all of the components of the limb that adds to deformity (increased femoral anteversion plus tibial intorsion).
- *Compensatory:* The malalignment in one bone is compensated by the reverse malalignment of other bone.

Examination

Apart from the measurement of rotation, also measure:

- *Foot progression angle* ***(Figs. 7A and B)****:* The line along the foot sole during walking and movement direction. Foot movement outward from the movement line is marked "+" while foot line pointing toward the movement line is marked "–". The normal foot progression angle is +10° with a range of -3° to +20°. Grading is done as:
  - *Mild:* "-5° to -10°"
  - *Moderate:* "-10° to -15°"
  - *Severe:* More than -15°
- Measure the foot deformities like metatarsus adductus (see below).

Treatment

Most of the rotational deformities correct by 8–10 years of age and <1% need surgical correction. Orthotics are proven to be of no therapeutic or preventive value still very frequently prescribed (instead they confuse the young graduates to wrongly assume that rotational malalignment is pathological and should be quickly intervened!). External rotator muscle contracture resolves spontaneously as is out-toeing. Hallux adductus is often a dynamic deformity secondary to overstrain of abductor pollicis longus. This resolves with increasing age and nervous system maturity. Metatarsus adductus if flexible resolves spontaneously while rigid type needs treatment (see below). Tibial intorsion if uncorrected by 8–10 years and if transmalleolar axis lying >3 standard deviations from the mean (< -10° or >35°) causing significant gait abnormalities need correction by supramalleolar tibial derotation osteotomy. The osteotomy is fixed with K-wires and a cast.

Excessive femoral anteversion is the most common cause of in-toeing after three years of age. These children often have habit of sitting in "W-posture". Their internal rotation at hip is >75° and external rotation is often limited below 25°. Waiting for spontaneous correction is futile and

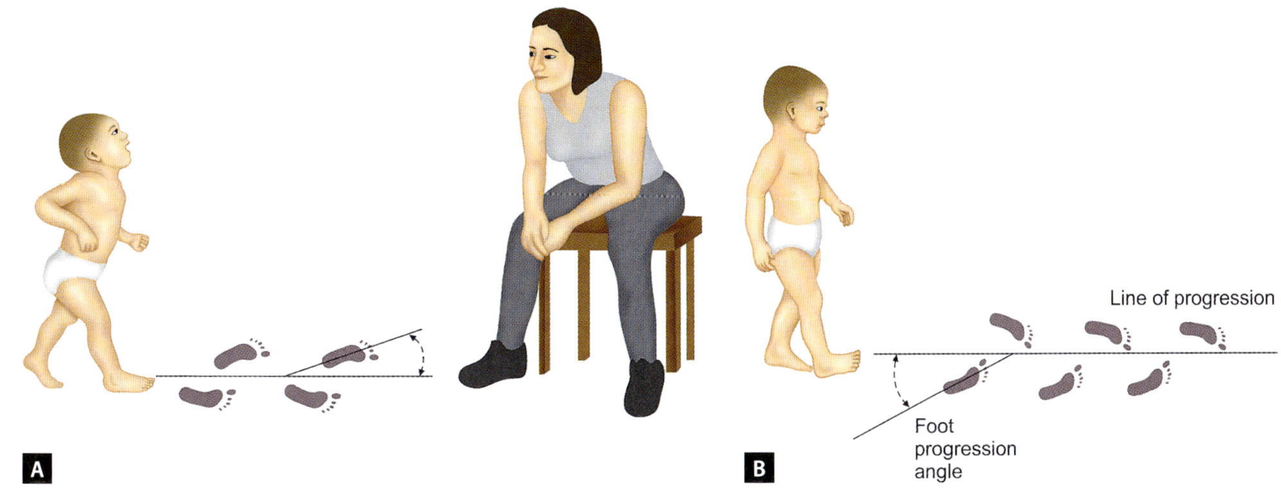

Figs. 7A and B: (A) Foot progression angle is measured along a straight line of walk and is arbitrarily observed. Normally, the feet are directed outward (away) from the central line of walk; (B) While in the in-toeing gait, they are either parallel or in more severe cases turn inward toward the midline.

primary corrective osteotomy should be done. Children should be encouraged to sit in Buddha position though waiting for prolonged periods may produce genu valgum or foot abduction. Derotation osteotomy of proximal femur is the preferred treatment that should be performed after 8 years of age. Typical indications include anteversion >45°, internal rotation at hip >80° and external rotation <20° with gait disturbance. The proximal intertrochanteric osteotomy is judged intraoperatively for correction by equal resulting internal and external rotations. Osteotomy performed at other places (shaft or distal aspect) is neither cosmetic and may produce knee stiffness, respectively. Proximal osteotomies heal well due to wide opposing cancellous surfaces.

ANGULAR DEFORMITIES OF LOWER LIMB

Angular deformity can increase the likelihood that degenerative arthritis eventually develops. So, angular deformities are to be corrected if they are beyond the acceptable physiological range. Treatment is basically done by realigning via osteotomy or by altering the forces within the growth plate to correct the deformity via asymmetric growth (guided growth method). To understand the correction of deformity, basic anatomical disposition and principles need to be understood that are described in detail here.

Angular Alignment of Knee

Normal Evolution of Angular Alignment of Knee

- Infants are born with a varus alignment at birth due to molding effect of the uterus resulting into tight posterior capsule of the hip (external rotation) and internal tibial torsion. This physiological alignment corrects only after the child starts walking.
- Correction to a neutral position usually occurs by age 18 months (may take up to 36 months in some cases).
- Interestingly, the corrective realignment overshoots and progresses to valgus (10–15°) by age 3–4 years which is true genu valgum (no rotational components) but physiological as this also slowly remodels to a physiologic valgus of 6–7° during the next 5–8 years (mean 7 years). Girls due to physiological habitus have a persistent genu valgum attained at 5–8 years while boys tend to have persistent slow correction of the valgus till 16 years of age.

Assessment and Principles of Correction of Angular Deformities

Assessment should include a good medical history, physical examination, and, for some patients, detailed standard radiographs. These assessments are aimed to differentiate:

- Progressive versus stable
- Painful versus painless deformity
- Associated abnormalities like neurologic and circulatory disturbances that may require special modifications in the treatment.
- Deformities of spine like scoliosis and foot abnormalities that may contribute to the angular deformity and may make them appear worse. These actually change the prognosis of treatment.
- Leg-length discrepancy (LLD) that may need to be simultaneously corrected during the index surgery.

History should note the time when the deformity was noticed first, any change or improvement with walking or time, the time when child started walking (children with Blount's disease walk early). Take nutritional history, history of vitamin or other deficiency (PEM), treatment received, allergy to milk, history of trauma, infections, metal intoxication (lead, aluminum, fluoride, and zinc). Family history of bowlegs or other limb deformity, short stature (bone dysplasia or generalized growth disorder, vitamin D resistant rickets, and renal osteodystrophy) should also be obtained.

Clinical Examination for Angular Deformities

- ***Measure the intercondylar and intermalleolar distance*** for genu varum and valgum, respectively **(Figs. 8A and B)** expressed in centimeters for bilateral deformities. For unilateral deformities, measure the same from midline. Intercondylar distance of ≥5 cm indicates tibia vara. A distance of >7.5 cm is an indication for surgery. Intermalleolar distance of >10 cm indicates genu valgum.
- ***Measure the femorotibial alignment (Figs. 9A and B):*** Measure the angle formed between lines joining anterior superior iliac spine to center of patella and another line joining center of intermalleolar line to center of patella. Subtract normal valgus from the measured alignment (7° for males, 8° for females >7 years of age) for estimating valgus malalignment and add the same for varus. This gives the clinical magnitude of angular deformity (in degrees). It should be, however, noted that varum or valgum is said to exist if the measured angle is outside 2 standard deviations (SD) from the normal for males and females for that age. This 2SD is variable but a ball-park figure of 5° is generally taken beyond which the deformity

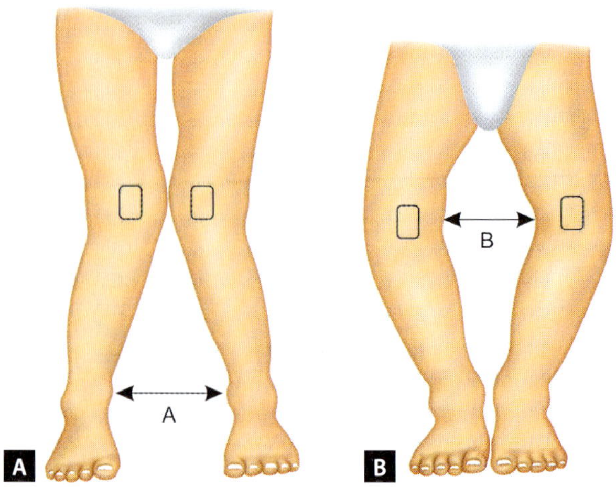

Figs. 8A and B: Illustration depiction method to measure (A) intermalleolar and (B) intercondylar distance measurement.

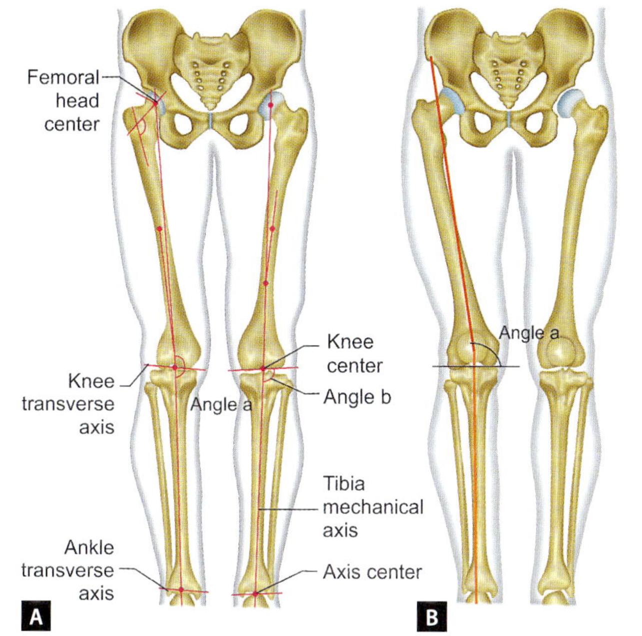

Figs. 9A and B: (A) Measuring the mechanical femorotibial alignment. The mechanical axis of femur and tibia are straight and coincide very nearly (there is average 2° or so varus variation which can be ignored for practical purposes). Angle a: Femorotibial angle is generally hence construed to be 180° for all practical purposes but is not actually so (medially it would be nearly 181–182°, while laterally it would be 179–178°). Angle b is medial obliquity of the knee joint (normally 0–2°). Because of angle b, the value of medial proximal tibial angle (MPTA) reduces to 87°. (B) Measuring the alignment clinically, here the angle is measured from ASIS and not femoral head center.

is considered pathological (see the details in discussion on genu varum and valgum).

- ***Measure the Q-angle (Figs. 10A and B):***
  - Determine and note femoral or tibial bow and obvious bony angulations.
  - Determine if the deformity of knee joint is due to femoral or tibial component by flexing the leg-knee varus/valgus deformity due to primary femoral involvement will get corrected on full flexion of knee while deformity due to tibial involvement will persist in flexion and extension both.
- Look for features of ligament laxity and fibular overgrowth (seen in Blount's disease, achondroplasia, and longitudinal deficiency of tibia)
- ***Look for tight structures*** (ITB in polio, etc.)
- ***Look for features of neurological causes*** (CP, polio, metabolic bone disease, toxicity, etc., as mentioned above in history)

Special examination that needs to be done includes:

- An observational gait analysis to:
  - Document foot progression angle
  - Lateral thrust (shifting of proximal tibia and fibula laterally due to capsular and ligament laxity—seen in pathological varum)
  - Antalgic gait
  - Rule out global pathologic conditions such as limb scissoring and hyperlordotic gait (spastic conditions)

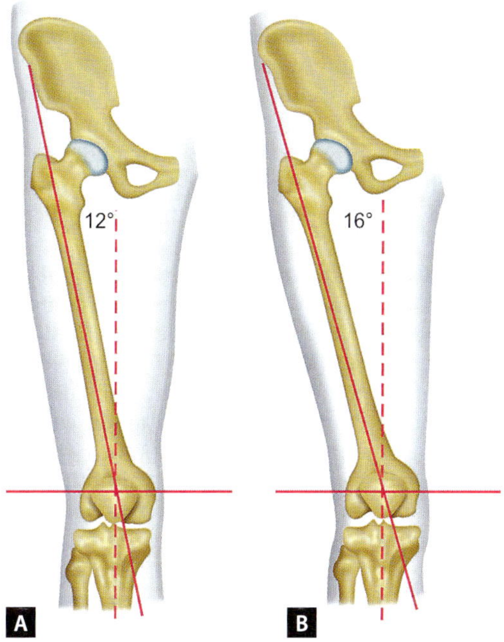

Figs. 10A and B: The Q-angle (quadriceps angle) is more in females (A) than males (B).

  - A Trendelenburg gait
- Examination for rotational alignment of the limb is done as above.

Radiology

A standing alignment radiograph (orthoradiogram) is obtained to document the direction and magnitude of the deformity. A teloradiogram allows assessment of angular deformity, using a single exposure of both lower extremities; the patient is standing, and a radiopaque ruler often positioned to give "scale" to figure and aid limb-length assessment. Mostly, this is not possible, so commonly a computed tomography (CT) scanogram is ordered. A scanogram is helpful in accurately assessing total limb lengths and has the advantage of using a relatively short film. CT also can be used to assess lengths, rotational deformity, and is especially useful if the deformity is in the sagittal plane. To take this view, the patella, not the foot should point forward (standing) or ceiling (supine). Standing lateral radiographs of the femur and tibia are taken to confirm a sagittal plane deformity and tibial slope. Radiographs are indicated in:

- Children above 3-years of age with progressive or unimproving varus deformity
- Asymmetric (unilateral) deformity
- Angulation just below the knee
- Pathological or associated deformities or malformations present on clinical examination (see above)

Commonly, the radiographs are taken for the following two purposes:

1. Measure the femorotibial angle, mechanical and anatomical axis, and the metaphyseodiaphyseal angle. In physiological genu varum, the metaphyseodiaphyseal angle is <11°.

2. Apart from measurement of deformity, it is also important to assess a patient's current *level of skeletal maturity* by radiology (see below in genu varum).

Radiological analysis of deformity is very important and has been detailed by specialty authors. In simpler method, the analysis of a deformity can be done in following steps:

1. Assess the radiographs to document any obvious anatomic coronal or sagittal limb deformities (step 1, bowing or angulation of bones).
   - *Draw the coronal mechanical axis of the limb* on a full-length film. This is drawn by joining the center of head of femur to center of the ankle [mechanical axis—lower extremity (MALE); **(Fig. 11)**]. Center of ankle is defined as a point midway across the tibial metaphysis (this point coincides with the ankle center). The coronal mechanical axis line passes within close to mid-point of the tibial spines in both knees. Any deviation from this is the **mechanical axis deviation (MAD),** which is measured as the perpendicular distance from the mechanical axis line. Normally, the line is no > 6–7 mm medial to the knee **center.** In varus deformity, the MAD would increase while in valgus deformity, the MAD would decrease or turn negative. It is argued that tibial spine center as reference should not be taken because tibial subluxation in coronal plane is common causing unwanted errors in measurement. In varus knees for example, the tibia often subluxates laterally so that the MAD is exaggerated. Given a choice femur center would represent a better landmark but has not been defined well in literature. Commonly center of femur is represented by the midpoint at superior aspect of intercondylar sulcus.
   - *Draw the individual axis of femur and tibia* (truly speaking, these are not the "axis" per se but somehow the nomenclature is fixed in literature). *For femur,* determine the:
     - Mechanical axis of femur [line from the center of the femoral head to the center of the distal femur or center of the knee; **(Figs. 12A and B)**].
     - *Femoral shaft axis:* Line drawn from the center of the proximal femur to the center of the distal femur or center of the knee. The difference between femoral shaft axis and mechanical axis of femur is 6°. The femoral shaft axis exits from the piriformis fossa superiorly.
     - *Mechanical axis of tibia and tibial shaft axis* ***(see Figs. 12A and B)****:* These two coincide in normal tibia, a line extending from the center of the proximal tibia to the center of the ankle.
     - *Anatomic tibiofemoral angle* ***(Figs. 13A and B)****:* Angle formed between tibial and femoral shaft axis; this indicates the anatomic misalignment. This is usually an average of 6° of valgus in normal adult population.
     - *Mechanical tibiofemoral angle* ***(Figs 14A and B)****:* The angle formed between the mechanical axis of femur and mechanical axis of tibia, indicates the mechanical misalignment (it averages to 180° in normal population). This is typically used to determine the amount of varus or the valgus deformity referred to commonly in literature. Now a measured mechanical tibiofemoral axis of 15° will be called 15° of valgus, but if anatomical axis was used then the same would indicate 21° of valgus. This may seem a discrepancy but strictly it is not the case as anatomical valgus of 6° has to be subtracted from the measured anatomical tibiofemoral angle of 21° giving 15° of valgus again! Anatomic tibiofemoral angle measurement is done only in cases where the mechanical axis angle cannot be measured say in femoral head deficiency, else as a rule all deformities are expressed in relation to mechanical axes. Remember to subtract 6° in such cases (God has somehow simplified the calculation of deformities by equalizing (and hence canceling) the difference between femoral shaft axis and mechanical axis of

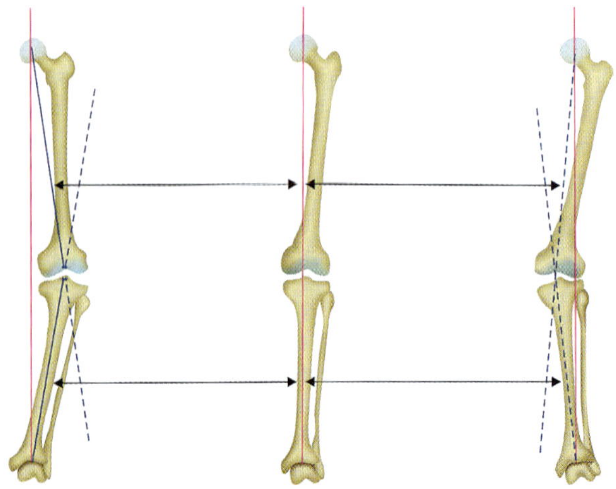

Fig. 11: Normal femorotibial mechanical alignment (center) and genu varum (left) and valgum (right). The distance of red line from knee center is the mechanical axis deviation (MAD)—positive for genu varum and zero to negative for valgum deformity.

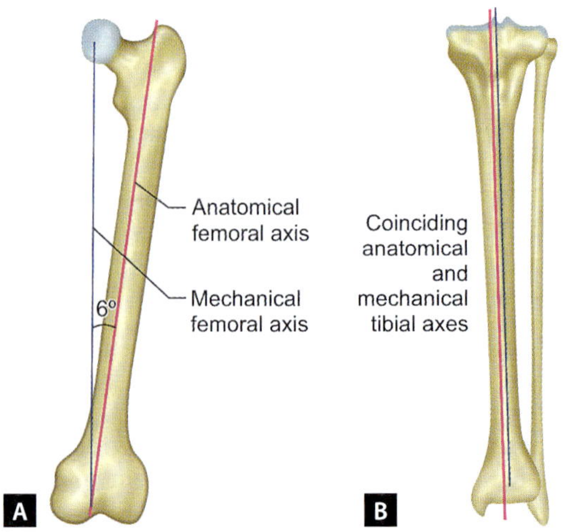

Figs. 12A and B: Illustration depicting drawing the femoral shaft and tibial–anatomical plus mechanical axis. (A) The anatomical and mechanical femoral axis are discrepant by 6–7°; (B) while they coincide exactly for tibia.

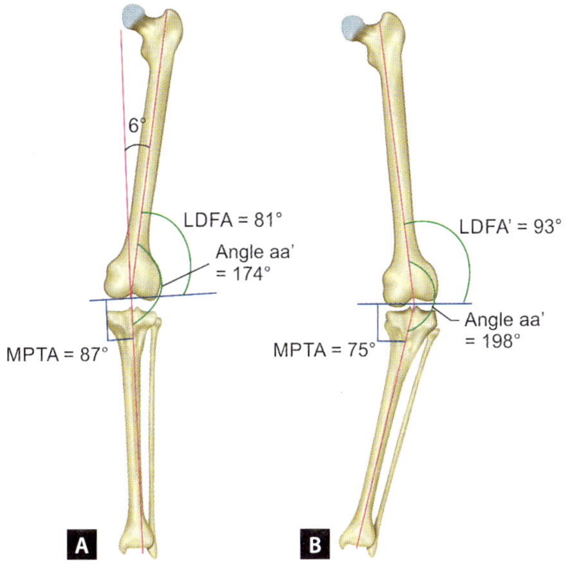

Figs. 13A and B: Anatomical tibiofemoral angle (A) is drawn between anatomical axes of femur and tibia—this angle is 6° less when measured laterally (so, here it will be 174°, angle aa'). The angle is reduced in genu varum (B). The lateral distal femoral angle (LDFA) is complementary to MPTA when mechanical axes are drawn so in that case will be 87° (see next **Figs. 14A and B**), but when anatomical axes are drawn, it will be reduced to 81° due to 6° tilt of anatomical axis. In this example of genu varum, the femur is also tilted so LDFA increased to 93° and there is varus at tibia of 12° reducing the MPTA to 75°. The anatomical femorotibial angle is hence 198° (angle aa'). The varus alignment is 24° (198–174°).

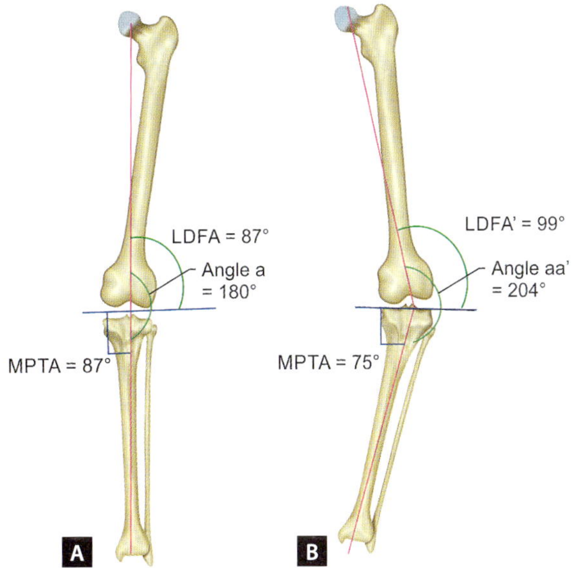

Figs. 14A and B: (A) The mechanical tibiofemoral angle. This is drawn between the mechanical axes of femur and tibia (angle a). The angle is reduced in genu varum. One should thoroughly note here importantly that if we mention genu varum as an absolute angle then mechanical tibiofemoral measurements will be higher than anatomical tibiofemoral angle measurements for genu varum in the same patient (the difference is nearly 6°) when measured laterally. For example, in this case as carried from previous figure, the mechanical tibiofemoral angle laterally is 204° compared to 198° in previous figure; (B) The varus angle, however, remains 24° here also (204–180°). To resolve confusion of various angles, I suggest using only mechanical alignments radiologically. The easier way to determine varus is mentioned in the following figures, but this complicated description was necessary to acquaint the reader with the finer details of various measurements involved so that one will make necessary adjustments in some uncommon cases.

6° to average valgus at knee—again 6°, else it would have been very difficult and quite uncomfortable to explain the deformities!). Thus the mechanical axis is very near to 180° due to cancelation of 6° of femoral varus by 6–7° of valgus at knee. One should understand that the valgus is incorporated within this mechanical femorotibial alignment. However, if one refers to anatomical femorotibial alignment then it will be 173–174° measured on lateral side.

2. After first step where one identifies if there is any deformity (MAD) and the direction of the deformity (varus/valgus), next *determine the bone containing the deformity* (step 2)—it should be determined if the deformity is in femur or tibia, or both bones. There are two ways to do this.
   - If the deformity is in one limb then the other limb serves as reference for determination of magnitude of true deformity. The mechanical axes of the normal-side leg, affected-side leg and individual mechanical axis of femur and tibia are constructed and compared.
   - If the disease is bilateral, the comparison is made with established norms. The mechanical axis of the femur drawn from the center of the hip to the center of the knee normally intersects the articular surface of the distal femur to produce a lateral distal-femoral angle of 87°; this will be 81° if angle is calculated from the anatomical femoral (femoral shaft) axis **(Figs. 13 and 14)**. Similarly, tibial mechanical axis is drawn as a line from the center of the knee to the center of the ankle that normally intersects the articular surface of the proximal tibia to produce a medial proximal

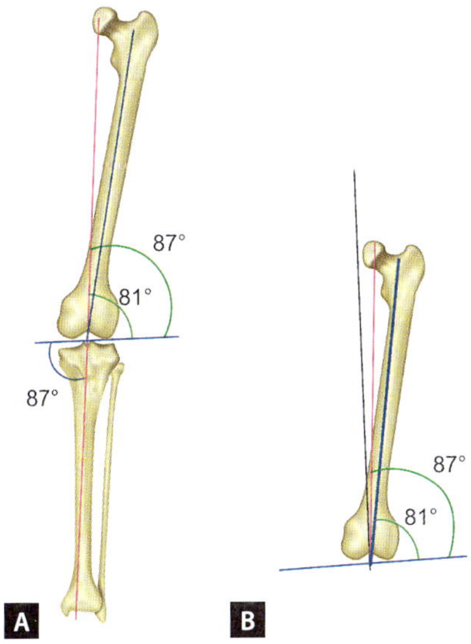

Figs. 15A and B: (A) Illustration detailing the effect of medial joint line obliquity (angle b) on LDFA and MPTA and the role of anatomical versus mechanical femoral axis. Note that due to angle b or oblique knee joint line (≈2°), the LDFA and MTPA reduce to 87° from 90° when measured from mechanical axis; (B) The 3° discrepancy is partially also contributed by 1–2° obliquity of mechanical axis from the normal drawn to horizontal, i.e., even the mechanical femoral axis is not perpendicular to horizontal and is 1–2° varus tilted so LDFA = 90 – 2 – 1 = 87°. The normal tibial joint angle is similarly 2–3° varus to the mechanical axis of tibia.

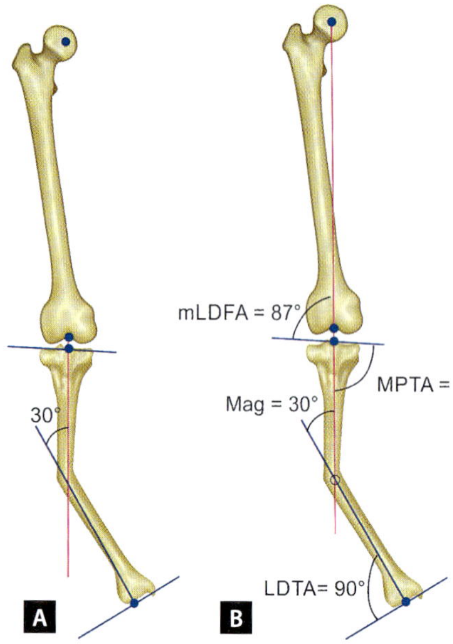

Figs. 16A and B: Determining pure extra-articular deformity. If the deformity is purely extra-articular, then the measurement is pretty simple. (A) The deformity is determined by drawing the shaft axes of the parts proximal and distal to the deformity. The angle at the intersection gives the anatomical deformity (30° in this case); (B) Draw also the LDFA and MPTA to find, if there is deformity at the joint as that may coexist.

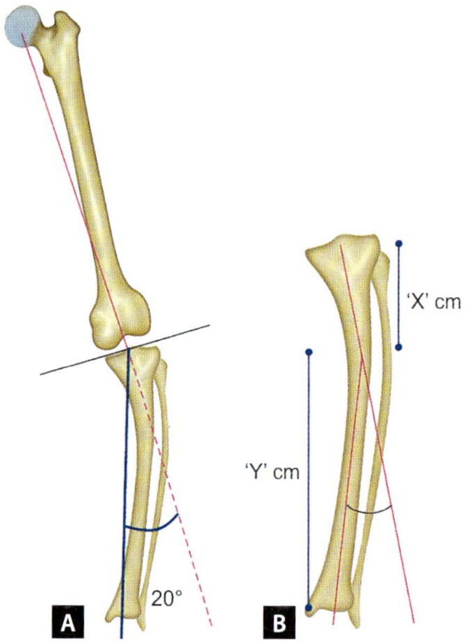

Figs. 17A and B: Measuring extra-articular deformity. In compound deformities where there is extra-articular deformity contribution to total angular deformity, one needs to calculate the percentage contribution of extra-articular deformity. In this example, the varus angle is 20° as calculated from mechanical axes (A). The extra-articular deformity contribution seems to be 15° as done from anatomical axes drawing (B), but this is an apparent measurement only. Suppose the deformity exists 'y' cm from the ankle, then the proportional distance is calculated as {y/(y + x) × 100) = Z%. Now calculate the Z% of 15° (say 'E') and this will give the real contribution of the extra-articular deformity for knee malalignment.

tibia angle of 87° **(Figs. 15A and B)**. The distal tibial articular surface normally is 90° with the mechanical axis of the tibia.

- Extra-articular deformities are determined by drawing the anatomical axes from proximal and distal bone fragments **(Figs. 16A and B)**. The point of intersection of these two lines is considered the site of deformity's or technically the center of rotation of angulation (CORA). Percentage contribution of the extra-articular deformity to deformity at the knee is calculated by multiplying the proportion of length deformity is away from the joint **(Figs. 17A and B)**.
- Degenerative deformities are common in the joint itself due to asymmetric wear of the cartilage. To determine this, draw lines along the articular surface of femoral and tibial condyles **(Figs. 18A to I)**. If these are not parallel then deformity at knee is confirmed. The femoral line is drawn by connecting the center points of two distal femoral condyles and the tibial articular line is similarly drawn by connecting two center points from medial and lateral plateau.

3. After the existence of a bony deformity has been confirmed then its exact location within bone is determined by drawing the normal mechanical axes of the proximal and distal ends of the bone in coronal plane. Similar approach is applied on lateral radiographs and can be used for assessment of sagittal plane deformity—sagittal CORA (*see* also Chapter on "Nonunions and Malunions").

Magnitude of deformity: For this in a typical case use mechanical axis alignments as reference to determine the magnitude of deformity. The following steps are used:

1. Determine the overall deformity by drawing the mechanical axes of femur and tibia (the clinically apparent or "revealed" deformity) **(Fig. 19)**.
2. Draw the femoral joint angle (FJA) and compare to standard (2–3° valgus).
3. Draw the tibial joint angle (TJA) and compare to standard (2–3° varus).
4. Draw the intra-articular angle (IAA) and compare to standard (0°).
5. Measure the deformity magnitude due to shaft angulation **(Figs. 20A and B)**:
   i. Measure angulation in the shaft.
   ii. Determine its proportional distance away from the hip or ankle.
   iii. Multiply the proportion with the shaft angulation and compare to the deformity angles obtained during FJA, TJA, and IAA comparisons.

Steps 1, 2, and 3 are the typical steps for calculation of deformity and magnitude (not CORA, it is determined as mentioned above). Step 4 is seen in degenerative knees where contribution of the joint malalignment additionally contributes to the overall deformity. This is a complex situation as correction of deformity inside the joint is not possible except in knee replacement. This step can be often omitted in congenital anomalies unless one sees hypoplasia of condyles! In any case, the correction is attempted as near to joint as possible [as by doing high tibial osteotomy (HTO) for medial compartment OA]. Now details of step 5—often

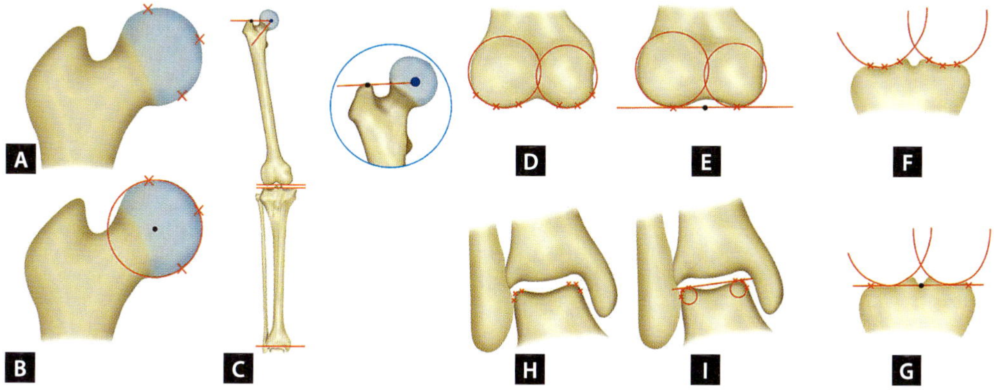

Figs. 18A to I: There are often situations where due to intra-articular fractures or intra-articular pathology the joint surfaces no longer remain parallel and a deformity develops within the joint. In this case, the assumption that the joint surfaces are parallel does not hold true and lines drawn through them itself intersects at an angle and the concept of "joint center" fails. For finding if there is intra-articular deformity, first one must meticulously locate the landmarks. (A and B) Femoral head center is located by drawing three points on the femur head corners and drawing a circle to fit the three points, center of circle gives femoral head center; (C) The center of femoral head coincides with the tip of trochanter and joining them will yield a straight line. For distal femoral line, draw three points on periphery of each condyle and draw circles fitting these points. Tangent drawn to the circles gives distal femoral reference line; (D and E) The center of this line is the center of distal femoral reference point. Similarly, draw three points in the lateral and medial parts of tibial plateau and draw circles. Tangent to the circles gives proximal tibial reference line; (F and G) Center of this line is the proximal tibial reference point for tibial mechanical axis line; (H and I) Similarly, for ankle place three points at each corner of talar dome and draw two circles; tangent to the circles drawn through the circles of these three points give talar reference line. Tibial plateau reference can be drawn similarly and angle between these lines would give talar tilt and intra-articular deformity.

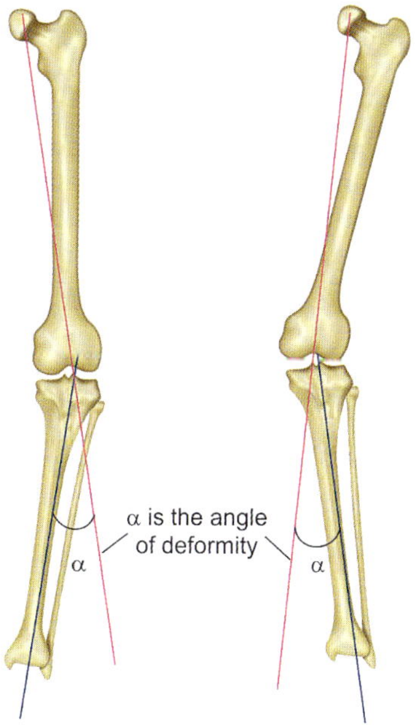

Fig. 19: Measuring the varus or valgus angle is pretty easy and not a cumbersome as detailed in previous figures. Just draw the mechanical axis of femur and project it beyond the knee joint. Draw the tibial axis and at its intersection with femoral axis will give the varus or valgus deformity. Adjust the 6° valgus from measured deformity and we get the true magnitude of deformity.

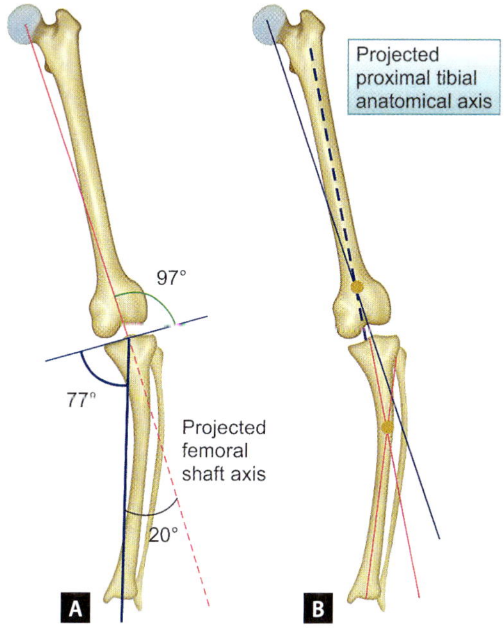

Figs. 20A and B: Finding CORA. We take forward the example from **Figure 18** above. Considering there is no intra-articular deformity measure the total varus deformity. Calculate the extra-articular deformity as detailed in **Figure 18**. Now draw the LDFA and MPTA. Here, the LDFA is 97° and MPTA is 77°. The Z% was actually 65%. 65% of 15° is 10° so the contribution of extra-articular anatomical deformity of 15° at the knee joint is 10°. (A) We describe the complete deformity as—there is a 20° overall varus at knee alignment. 10° of the deformity is located at the femur (97–87°), and 10° is found within the tibia. The 10° at the proximal tibia is due to the extra-articular tibial deformity, which is 15° at its apex and contributes 10° at the joint level. So, there are two CORA; (B) One at the extra-articular deformity site in tibia, its apex being determined by drawing anatomical axes of shaft lines. The other deformity is at the joint which needs to be corrected distally at femur.

the post-traumatic angulations have CORA at the malunion site that can be simply calculated **(Figs. 20A and B)**. In congenital and complicated deformities, the extra-articular deformity partially contributes to the overall deformity and should be assessed separately to determine the exact contribution which needs separate correction. Also this

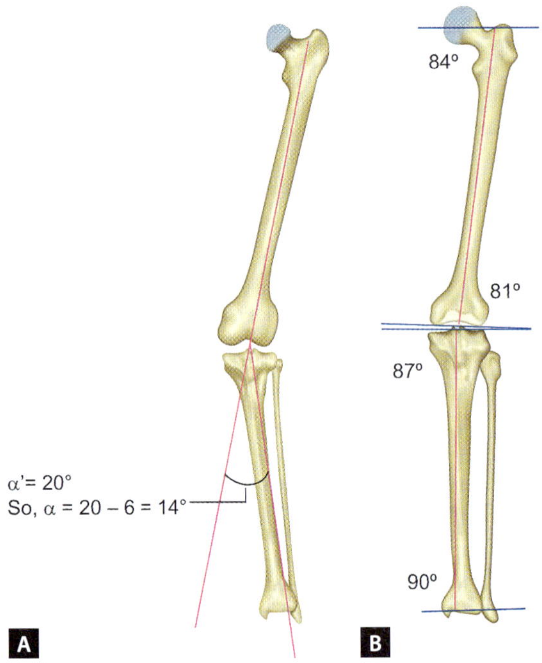

Figs. 21A and B: (A) Finding deformity from anatomical axis; if the angle of deformity is measured from anatomical femoral axis then one needs to subtract 6° of normal valgus to yield the correct valgus deformity; (B) The LDFA is different when measured from anatomical axis, so proper calculation must be done from that aspect also.

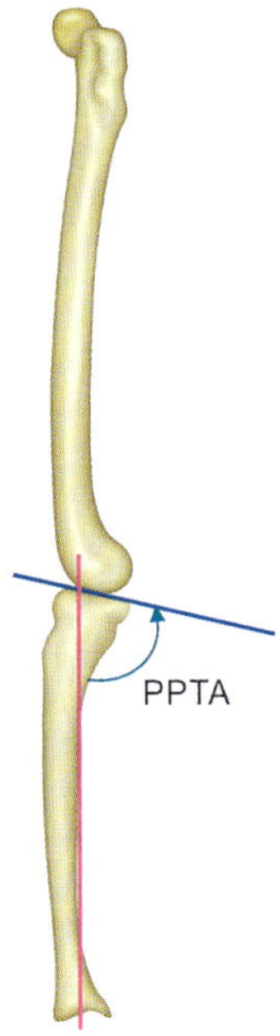

Fig. 22: Sagittal deformity and its assessment for CORA in this plane. The PPTA (proximal plateau tibial angle) is usually 80°.

entails finding another CORA in the same bone or different bone contributing to the overall deformity. This is a typical situation where multiple CORAs exist.

Finding CORA by anatomical axis: Anatomical axes of femur and tibia can also be used to determine the deformity as follows:

- The normal proximal femoral angle is 84° (6° varus from mechanical axis) but as it is difficult to construct instead a neck-shaft angle of 130° is used.
- The lateral distal-femoral anatomic angle is 81°, the medial proximal tibial anatomic angle is 87°. The distal tibial articular surface is at 90° angle from the tibial shaft **(Figs. 21A and B)**.
- In the lateral plane, the angle subtended by the femoral shaft and Blumensaat line is normally 83°.
- The tibial plateau is sloped posteriorly at 80° to the shaft of the tibia **(Fig. 22)**, and the tibial plafond is sloped anteriorly at 80°.
- If abnormal articular angles are found, then it can be concluded that a deformity exists within that bone.
- Constructing the normal anatomic axis of the proximal and distal ends of the bone in both the coronal and sagittal planes reveals the location of the CORA.

Important conclusions that can be drawn from both these methods to understand the geometry of deformity are as follows:

- If the standing alignment radiograph reveals an obvious anatomic deformity, although the mechanical axis line is intact, a compensatory deformity must exist.
- If proximal and distal constructed axes do not intersect, as outlined above, or do not intersect at an obvious deformity, another deformity must be present. This situation arises principally in two unique cases, first there may be associated translation (usually post-traumatic deformities) or second there may be multiple centers of rotation and angulation (mCORA) as shown in **Figures 20A and B**. mCORA is more readily derived **(Figs. 20A and B)** and is clinically more useful than just the anatomical axis deformity assessment. Although the deformity is best corrected at the centers of rotation and angulation, doing so may not be feasible because of anatomic constraints. In such instances, an osteotomy followed by multiplane correction is needed. This osteotomy is usually performed at a location away from the CORA for simplicity but in turn produces translatory deformity that has to be compensated during the correction. The other situation where a translatory deformity coexists with angulation is uncommon in congenital or developmental situations and its calculation/correction is described in Chapter on "Nonunions and Malunions".

Using Growth Modulation for Correction of Periarticular Angulatory Deformities

Calculation of CORA and principles of correction of angulatory deformities by osteotomy are described above. Correcting deformity at CORA in congenital/developmental joint deformity where it lies close to joint line is a bit challenging using these methods. Although osteotomy can be done even in these cases, there is another versatile method to achieve correction in such cases. Periarticular angulatory deformities in children can be corrected by modulating the osseous growth. The bones in children keep growing till physeal fusion. This bony growth can be in fact utilized to guide the future growth of bone in order to produce a reverse "compensatory deformity" which would either reduce or fully correct the original deformity depending on the time available. This method of treatment is called "**guided growth method**" detailed as follows:

The continuous growth of physis can be modulated by principles laid down by Hueter-Volkmann (*See* Section on Bone Anatomy, Physiology, Pathology, and Related Diseases). This is principally based on the fact that restricting the growth by "clamping" physis increases physeal pressure which inhibits the growth temporarily in that region but the other side of bone will continue to grow. If performed correctly, the deformity slowly corrects, and the inhibition can be removed (temporary methods) or if growth charts are properly utilized, then permanent inhibition of the physis can be done to utilize the remaining growth potential by performing ablation at predetermined age.

Hemiepiphysiodesis is a well-accepted method of correcting long bone deformity, especially in children who have significant remaining bone growth. This method has been found to be associated with lesser morbidity than the osteotomy method.

Control of physeal growth can also be done globally which is suitable for correction of LLD. Here it is called physiodesis as whole of the physis is being stopped from growing rather than one half as is done for correction of angular deformities. It is a compensatory method for correcting LLD and not a corrective operation as the longer leg is treated in this manner to equalize limb length, thus making normal limb abnormal. Phemister described the first physiodesis in a girl with dyschondroplasia. The method for correction of LLD will be discussed in detail in section on LLD.

There are various **methods of performing hemiepiphysiodesis:**

- *Temporary:* Here in any method, care should be taken to remain outside periosteum and not damaging the same. One should avoid directly exposing the growth plate for the sake of preventing injury to physis.
    - *Staples* ***(Figs. 23A and B)****:*
        - *Blount's staples:* One staple usually breaks; two staples often bend, so three staples are recommended.
        - Vitallium staples
- *Two-hole plate and screws* ***(Figs. 23A and B)****:* The screws are placed above (epiphysis) and below (metaphysis) the growth plate fixed to a two-hole plate shaped like "8" on one side of the physis. This causes unilateral tethering of the physis to control the growth on that side. It is very easy and has lesser morbidity than stapling. This can be done with hand itself rather than using power instruments in smaller children due to soft bones.
- *Permanent:* These procedures should be done only after logical and thorough judgment of the deformity and remaining growth (Bowen's tables). As the growth on the side of hemiepiphysiodesis will be halted permanently, the patient will have residual deformity if the growth period was too short or deformity was too much. Else the patient will have overcorrection and even reverse deformity if the deformity was too small compared to remaining growth.
    - Removal, rotation, and reinsertion of bone piece (Phemister, White's, and Blount's methods)
    - Bone grafting
    - Dowel grafts
    - Physeal curettage—done with a curette, should remove 50% of the central and peripheral region of the physis on that side
    - Percutaneous physeal curettage using burr

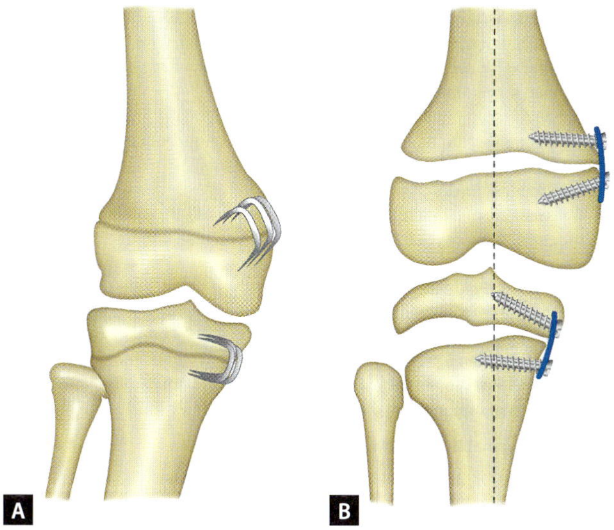

Figs. 23A and B: (A) Hemiepiphysiodesis can be done using staples (B) or using figure-of-eight plate.

Complications of temporary method:

- Complete arrest
- Breakage and bending of staples
- Intra-articular protrusion
- Extrusion
- Overlying bursitis
- Asymmetric physeal arrest
- Need of second surgery to remove staples
- Infection

Complications of permanent methods:

- Unsightly scar
- Infection
- Incomplete arrest
- Hematoma formation
- Donor site morbidity in cases of bone grafting

GENU VARUM

Genu varum [bow legs, bandiness, bandy legs (for tibia vara specifically)] is the lateral angulation (outward protrusion) at knee in coronal plane with inward bending of the legs. In terms of definition, it is a true coronal plane deformity, where the leg is shifted toward midline and the knees

BOX 2: Causes of genu varum.

- Nutritional rickets (the most common cause in India)
- Tibia vara (Blount's disease)
- Traumatic physeal injury
- *Tumors:*
  - Direct affection of physis by tumors (ABC, chondroblastoma, etc.)
  - Mechanical effect of the neoplasm (exostosis)
  - Iatrogenic injury to physis
  - Alteration of bone anatomy (fibrous dysplasia)
- Infection (osteomyelitis–acute, chronic, tubercular, and treatment-related injury)
- Renal osteodystrophy
- Osteogenesis imperfecta
- Hypophosphatemic rickets
- Skeletal dysplasia (achondroplasia, enchondromatosis, metaphyseal chondrodysplasia, and focal fibrocartilaginous dysplasia)
- Osteogenesis imperfect

(ABC: aneurysmal bone cyst)

drifted away. However, some rotational components are always found particularly in severe deformities (increased femoral anteversion and tibial internal torsion). This is more common angular malalignment than valgum because of the high incidence of physiologic varus seen in early years of life. The patients are brought for medical care due to undesirable cosmetic appearance and the perception of diminished function by parents. The cosmetic appearance is made worse by accompanying internal tibial torsion. The pathologic causes of genu varum are mentioned in **Box 2**.

As there is a gradual realignment of the lower limb till 7–8 years and as the normal limb alignment of 7° of valgus at knee for boys or 8° for girls, there is confusion as to when should a limb be labeled pathological. It is quite logical but to call genu varum pathological at and after 3 years of age as by this time according to natural history of disease the limb should be in valgus. So finding a varus alignment after 3 years of age is pathological. Secondly, the measured value if exceeds the normal alignment of limb by >2SD for that age (Bowen's charts), then only is considered significant. The 2SD value is 5° beyond normal. So even a genu rectus (0° alignment of femorotibial axis) is a genu varum and abnormal.

Clinical Examination and Assessment (See above also)

Along with the measurement of deformity, clinically one should also try and look for the etiological cause of the deformity.

- Children with metabolic bone disease are usually short and the bones are gradually bowed rather than angulated throughout their length **(Fig. 24)**. The features of physeal changes (clinical widening) due to metabolic cause are evident clinically and radiologically (cupping and flaring of the metaphysis). Pathologic varus deformities of the limb usually result from congenital or early-onset disease else if the nutritional deficiency sets in after establishment of physiological valgus, then genu valgum results. Latter is often the case with acquired renal deficiency or following a transplant where valgus deformity is common while with nutritional and genetic hypophosphatemic rickets, the varum is the most common.

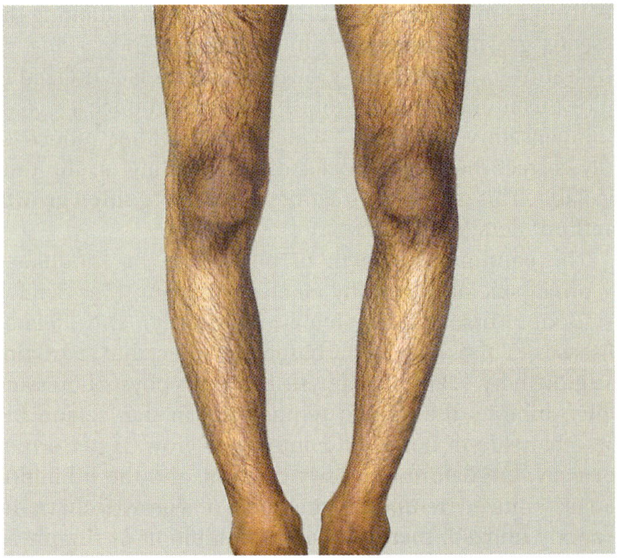

Fig. 24: Clinical appearance of genu varum.

- Systemic features of fluoride toxicity, skeletal dysplasia, neoplasms (skin lesions of fibrous dysplasia), and osteogenesis imperfecta should be examined. Secondary affection of the foot like pes planovalgus and associated deformities like femoral anteversion and tibial intorsion should be measured and recorded as they have bearing on management.
- Blount's disease is often diagnosed in endemic regions (African descent) children with apparent physiologic genu varum that fails to improve within 2–3 years. Children with infantile Blount's disease are typically large for their age and walk relatively early. The posteromedial physis gets damaged due to the combination of large size and excessive pressure and early walking compresses the "soft" immature physis on the medial side of the tibia affecting the tibia bilaterally in 80% cases. This form predominates in females and anatomically is characterized by medial metaphyseal beak. Late-onset tibia vara occurs in boys predominantly and can be classified as juvenile (4–10 years of age) or adolescent (in a child age 11 years or older). There is no medial metaphyseal beak but often medial collateral ligament (MCL) laxity is seen. These patients have progressive deformity and may have pain on walking due to joint degeneration. Patients may also have a limb-length discrepancy because of long-standing growth retardation. The juvenile form may represent a continuation of infantile tibia vara that did not improve. Patients with adolescent tibia vara are also usually overweight but have unilateral involvement in contrast to the infantile form. Bilateral involvement if seen is usually asymmetric.

Laboratory Investigations

The serum and urine levels of electrolytes, calcium, phosphorus, and alkaline phosphatase are done to evaluate metabolic bone disease—activity, progression, and remission. Otherwise they are of value only for anesthetic workup and do not append any surgical help.

Radiological Evaluation

The radiological features of physiological genu varum include:

- Medially tilted knee and ankle joint lines
- Lateral bow of tibia, especially in proximal half and lateral femoral bow in distal half
- Thickening of medial cortices of the tibia and femur (commonly seen in physiological genu varum)
- Symmetrical involvement of bones on both sides

Radiologically, the deformity magnitude should be determined on a full-leg radiogram (orthoradiogram). Measure MAD, CORA, and template for corrective osteotomy if planned **(Figs. 25 and 26)**. Generally, it is considered that deformities up to 25° are mild, 25–40° are moderate and >40° are severe. Measure the individual contribution from femur and tibia to deformity as they guide if correction is needed in both bones **(Figs. 25 and 26)**. For tibia vara apart from the standard evaluation described above and done in **Figures 27A to D**, measure the metaphyseal-diaphyseal and metaphyseal-epiphyseal angles as described by Levine and Drennan. Radiographs of a child with infantile tibia vara show sloping of the medial metaphysis and fragmentation of the epiphysis. The metaphyseal-diaphyseal **(Fig. 27E)** and metaphyseal-epiphyseal angles are helpful in predicting further progression and eventual diagnosis of infantile Blount's disease (see below). A metaphyseal-diaphyseal angle (MDA) >16° or both a MDA >10° and a metaphyseal-epiphyseal angle >20° are suggestive of Blount's disease. Conversely, patients with physiologic genu vara are likely to have a MDA <9° or both a MDA <10° and a metaphyseal-epiphyseal angle <20°. These angles help in early diagnosis of Blount's disease and guide the orthotic management.

Apart from the measurement of deformity, the radiographs are also obtained to assess the skeletal maturity so that the treatment can be appropriately planned. Boys generally stop growing at age 16 years and girls generally stop growing at 14 years. A PA radiograph of the left hand can be compared with data in the Greulich and Pyle atlas of normal standards to estimate the child's bone age which though has lot of inter- and intraobserver variability is commonly used. The charts are much less accurate for smaller ages.

Treatment Principles and Methods

- *Physiological bowing:* Successful management of physiologic bowing usually begins by recording the deformity and mentioning it. Further educate the family

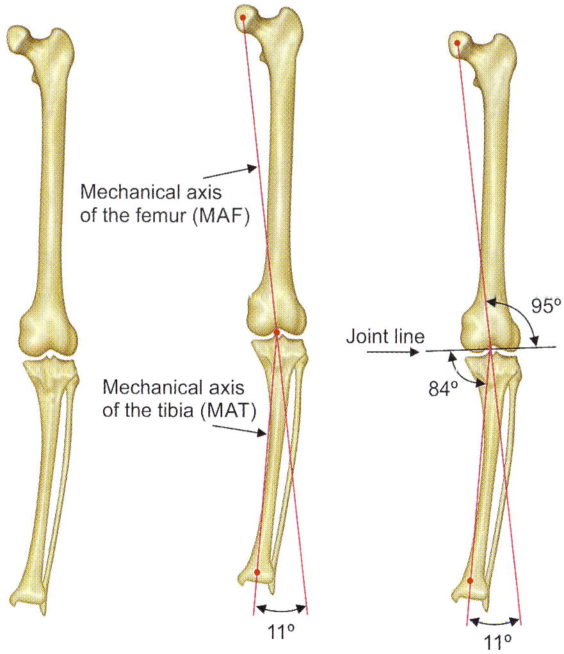

Fig. 25: Genu varum deformity assessment. The terms femoral and tibial joint angles are commonly used. The femoral joint angle (FJA) is nothing else but the LDFA and the tibial joint angle (TJA) is nothing else but the MPTA. Measure these angles and compare from normal of 87°. The overall deformity is calculated by drawing the mechanical axis of femur and tibia which is 11° varus here. The femoral joint angle (FJA) is normally 87°. Since the femoral joint angle (or LDFA) here is 95°, there is an "error", or deviation of 8° depicting 8° varus deformity at the femur. The tibial joint angle (TJA or MPTA) is normally 87° and as it is 84° here, the deviation is 3° of varus at tibia. To double check the deformities add the error in LDFA and MPTA (8 + 3 = 11°). So, here there is 11° overall varus deformity of which 8° is contributed by femur and rest by tibia.

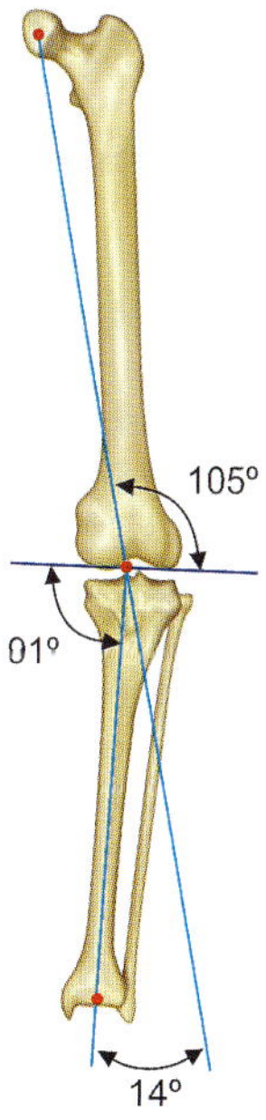

Fig. 26: Special and some complicated scenario arise when compensatory deformities develop in the other bones. Tibial compensation of varus deformity in femur. The first step as detailed above is finding the overall deformity by mechanical axis of femur and mechanical axis of tibia. Here, the deformity is 14° of varus. Now to determine the region that contributes to deformity draw LDFA and MPTA. We see that the LDFA is 106° and LDFA is 89°. So, there is (105 – 87 = 18°) of varus contributed by femur. But this is more than the overall deformity, so some compensation must exist to reduce the overall varus! We see that MPTA is 91°, so in effect, there is 91–87 = 4° of valgus in tibia; this compensates the varus at femur and commonly develops in young patients due to remodeling. So, the varus deformity = LDFA + MPTA = 18 + (–4) = 14°. We describe this scenario as there is overall varus of 14° of which 18° is the femoral component that gets partially compensated by the 4° of valgus at tibia. Next step will be to identify CORA that can be done by drawing anatomical axes as detailed previously.

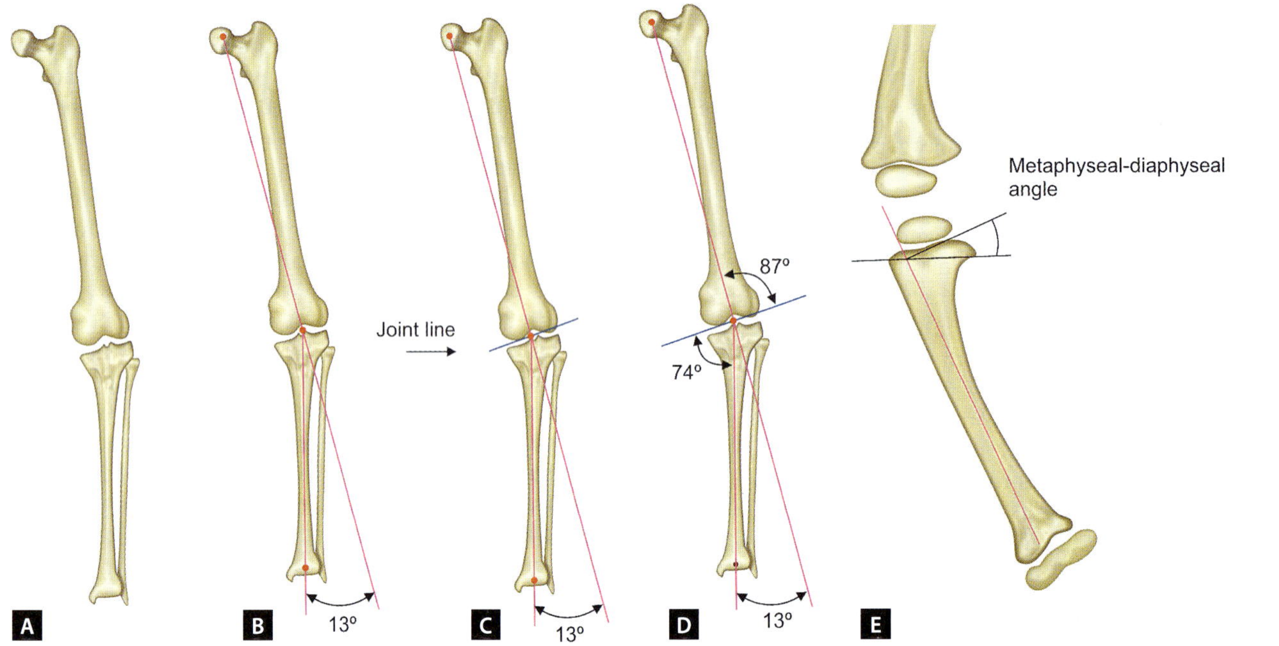

Figs. 27A to E: (A) Tibia vara is a special form of genu varum where (B) deformity is intra-articular with tilted joint line; (C) The overall deformity is determined by femoral and tibial mechanical axes intersection; (D) The LDFA is normal while all of the deformity lies on tibial side with reduction in the MPTA; (E) Metaphyseal-diaphyseal angle is an important in patients with genu varum as it helps in early identification of tibia vara and also guides treatment. Angle more than 16° indicate presence of Blount's disease quite accurately.

about its benign natural history. Clear understanding to the family should be given that nonsurgical treatment methods to correct torsional or angular deformities are futile but aggressive management should be done only for progressive pathological deformities. Patients should hence be kept under surveillance and they need to return for treatment if the deformity progresses.

- *Pathological or progressive deformity:* A progressive or painful or pathological varus deformity (caused by metabolic abnormality or other causes mentioned in **Box 2**) should be corrected with surgery. There are no written guidelines for magnitude of deformity that should be corrected but it is generally believed that any amount of varus at knee produced malalignment of the forces acting on the joint and lead to early arthritis. Varus deformity is commonly due to tibial side deformity, so most of corrective modalities apply for tibia in the text below unless specified otherwise. Generally, a cosmetically and functionally unacceptable deformity is considered for surgical correction which is >10° or if the intercondylar distance exceeds 7.5 cm (some consider 6 cm). There are some prerequisites for performing surgical correction:
  - Underlying disease should be medically controlled.
  - Center of rotation of angulation should be established and templating done before proceeding.
  - Osteotomy should be done near skeletal maturity else undercorrection or overcorrection will get magnified with remaining growth.

The *goals* of surgical correction include:

- Correction of deformity in the coronal, sagittal, and axial plane producing normal alignment of the knee:
  - Treatment done at skeletal maturity (usually osteotomy) should aim at complete correction of the deformity.
  - Treatment done at earlier stage (say in tibia vara) or by guided growth methods should aim to bit overcorrect the deformity (say 5°) as progression (and recurrence) in the pathological direction (varum) is quite common.
- Correcting limb-length discrepancy (and significant rotational malalignment if any)
- Maintaining the alignment with good function of the knee

The two feasible and currently practiced *surgical options* include:

1. *Valgus producing osteotomy around the CORA:* Osteotomy is needed for a patient with a considerable deformity who has reached skeletal maturity and thus is not suitable for guided growth via hemiepiphysiodesis. There are a lot of options for doing osteotomy and that to they can be done in tibia or femur. Variously practiced and historical methods include closed wedge lateral distal femur osteotomy, opening wedge medial tibial osteotomy, opening wedge medial oblique tibial osteotomy, barrel vault (dome) tibial osteotomy with fibular osteotomy, and chevron osteotomy. Opening wedge osteotomies can be fixed with Puddu plates (has prebuilt metallic wedge of different sizes) or synthetic bone graft wedges and locked plate. Methods of fixing closed wedge and dome osteotomy include pins, screws, plaster of Paris (POP) casts or even plates, and screws depending on desired stability. Some general guidelines for osteotomy can be summarized as below.

- The osteotomy should be done around CORA and also rotated around it correcting along the angle bisector. The derotation component should be planned in the calculated wedge. Closed-wedge osteotomies are often preferred for better healing potential and stability. They can be easily fixed and do not require a bone graft. Open-wedge osteotomies though maintain limb length require a bone graft and sturdy fixation. Severe deformities are difficult to correct by open wedge due to stretching and possible damage to neurovascular structures. Osteotomy in tibia should be accompanied with diaphyseal fibular osteotomy.
- The decision to perform an osteotomy and correction above and below the knee depends on the magnitude of the femoral deformity. Mild deformities (<25°) can be corrected by single stage closed wedge osteotomy at CORA. The ensuing shortening is well acceptable and may get compensated with growth or pelvic tilt. Moderate deformities need to be managed ingeniously by opening wedge method and gradual distraction using distractors or ilizarov apparatus (this also allows for multiplane correction of deformity and also addresses the rotational malalignment). These distractors are but placed medially and are cumbersome. Surgeons for these reasons recommend a staged surgery or simultaneous femoral and matching counter tibial osteotomy (viz. an opening wedge tibial and closed wedge femoral osteotomy). Such a procedure but may distort the joint line so should be carefully planned.
- Children with a distal femoral varus deformity of 8° or greater should undergo osteotomy or guided growth at this level, in addition to tibia correction. Failure to correct for excessive distal femoral deformity and overcorrection of the tibia leads to shear stresses at the knee and degenerative changes.

2. *Guided growth (lateral hemiepiphysiodesis or physeal stapling of femur or tibia or both):* For a growing patient with a varus deformity can be performed above and below the knee joint, with expected resolution of the deformity but is more popular for a valgus deformity. It has been generally seen that the varus deformity predominates in tibia and valgus predominates in femur. Proximal tibial stapling laterally is hindered by presence of fibular head laterally so not favored for varus correction while distal femoral stapling is easily done on medial side in valgus knees. Guided growth cannot be expected to correct internal rotational deformities and is of limited use in patients with extreme deformity and little remaining growth.

The treatment of Blount's disease is discussed separately.

Other Methods for Correction of Genu Varum (Not Commonly Practiced)

- *Hemichondrodiastasis (physeal lengthening):* This utilizes the Hueter-Volkmann law and is aimed to reverse the mechanism of production of genu varum. Constant or gradually progressive distractive force is expected to enhance the physeal growth according to the law so a distractor is applied on both sides of growth plate and gradual distraction done. Over time, there is physiological overgrowth on the medial side that gradually corrects the deformity.
- *Callotasis:* This is distraction of the callus and done with the help of external fixator. Osteotomy is done at the desired site (CORA) and the fixator distracts the healing tissue formed at the site. It differs from ilizarov as callus forms and not regenerates, and osteotomy is done rather than corticotomy.
- *Ilizarov correction:* This is frequently done at dedicated institutions and has the capability of addressing coronal, sagittal, and rotational deformities together in a single apparatus with minimal modification. The bone formed is near physiological and morbidity is minimal in terms of scarring. The patient can also remain weight-bearing with the fixator on. Major drawback is that it is cumbersome to carry the apparatus.

TIBIA VARA

Tibia vara is being rediscussed as a special case as it has distinct etiopathogenesis and specific treatment guidance. Growth retardation at the medial (specifically posteromedial) aspect of proximal tibial epiphysis, physis, and metaphysis resulting in persistent bow legs is called tibia vara. This varus deformity at the upper end of the tibia was initially reported by Erlacher (1922) and Lulsdorf (1931), who considered it to be a type of osteochondritis. The term "tibia vara" was suggested by Blount (1937) and also stipulated the use of term osteochondroses instead of osteochondritis. Langenskiold stated that "tibia vara is a disturbance of growth, maturation, and ossification". This conclusion is however not fully correct as physeal disturbance is only partially responsible for development of deformity, additional mechanical factors have significant contributory role like the higher incidence of knee hyperextension and posterior ligament laxity in Negros. Also, the Negro child stands and walks earlier than European child possibly stressing the posteromedial physis at a time when physiological varus dominates. These factors indicate contributory role of mechanical and environmental factors in development of tibia vara (Hueter-Volkmann law). The mechanical forces, hence cause weight-bearing line to pass from the medial physis and produce growth disturbance. This further stalls the physeal growth in this region and the cycle continues. Correction with osteotomy reverses the growth-related changes at physis indicating that the notion of Langenskiold that physis is primarily responsible for tibia vara is not fully correct. The disease is common in West Indies and African blacks. It appears early and progresses rapidly in them needing early correction. The involvement of posteromedial part of proximal tibial physis produces three deformities, viz. varus, internal tibial torsion and variable flexion of diaphysis on upper tibial epiphysis (procurvatum).

Two types are commonly seen as initially described by Blount:

1. Infantile tibia vara (early onset) where the onset is before 3 years of age.

2. Adolescent tibia vara (late onset) where the onset is at or after 10 years of age. The late onset variety usually has associated distal femoral varus also.

Alternatively, it can also be classified as infantile (<3 years), juvenile (4–10 years), and adolescent (>10 years).

Infantile Tibia Vara (Blount's Disease)

Blount classically described the deformity as an abrupt angulation just below the proximal tibial physis, an irregular physeal line and a wedge-shaped epiphysis with beaking of the medial metaphysis. The etiology may be multifactorial with several reports of a familial occurrence. However, the condition is largely considered a developmental disorder and not a congenital one as it never occurs in children below 1 year of age. The deformity occurs essentially as a result of defective ossification on the medial side so that growth continues laterally resulting in the characteristic deformity. In later stages, an actual bony bridge may be found tethering the medial physeal plate. Unossified fibrocartilage is present on the medial side which produces the appearance of a defect on an X-ray. Apart from lateral angulation and medial deviation of the distal leg, there is also a significant internal tibial torsion deformity that constitutes an important part of tibia vara.

Clinically, the child has exaggerated genu varum with a clinically apparent lateral thrust of the knee during stance phase of the gait. This is because of varus instability due to ligamentous laxity that frequently develops on the lateral side of the knee. The typical child is obese and often exceeds 95th percentile for weight. Indeed increased weight produces sufficient compressive forces to retard the physeal growth by Hueter-Volkmann principle.

Radiology

Standard AP view of lower limbs in standing position from hip to knee is obtained. The characteristic findings include sharp varus angulation and prominent beaking of the medial metaphysis with radiolucent areas denoting cartilage islands; irregular and wide medial physeal line; and irregularly ossified and medially sloping epiphysis. The entire ossific zone of metaphysis shows irregularity. Little lateral islands of calcified tissue may appear that are separated from metaphysis by clear zones. These features are usually not seen before 18 months of age, but when appear are progressive. Beaking is due to sloping away from joint line distally. Attempts have been made to diagnose the condition before pathognomonic radiographic signs appear. Tibial MDA of Drennan >11° and tibial epiphyseal-metaphyseal angle >20° identify the *toddlers at risk* of developing Blount's disease. The MDA values of 16° or more have 95% chance of progression so are considered diagnostic of infantile tibia vara (MDA of >15° is possibly more appropriate reference). MDA of <10° is associated with resolution of deformity in 95% cases. A child without the characteristic metaphyseal lesion (also called the Blount's lesion) cannot be labeled as infantile tibia vara. Magnetic resonance imaging (MRI) is a useful modality for diagnosis in these children.

BOX 3: The characteristic magnetic resonance imaging (MRI) findings in Blount's disease.

- *Physis:*
  - Widening of physis
  - Down sloping/irregularity medially
  - Physeal bridge
  - Lateral physis is wide and irregular
  - Perichondral membrane is thickened
- *Epiphysis:*
  - Medial and posterior down sloping
  - Epiphyseal cartilage is thick far medially
  - Epiphyseal cartilage is thin in central medial region increasing the joint space
  - Perichondral membrane is thickened

Anterior cruciate ligament (ACL) laxity:
- Medial meniscus—thickened ± abnormal signal
- Nonspecific femoral epiphysis and metaphysis changes

The characteristic findings of MRI in Blount's disease are listed in **Box 3**.

Differential Diagnosis

The *differential diagnosis* includes physiological genu varum (beaking of medial tibial physis palpable clinically and visible radiologically differentiates tibia vara) and other nonphysiological causes like skeletal dysplasias (multiple epiphyseal dysplasia and spondyloepiphyseal dysplasia), metabolic diseases (vitamin-D resistant rickets), postinfective and post-traumatic causes, and proximal focal fibrocartilaginous dysplasia.

Classification

Langenskiold is classified infantile tibia vara into six stages **(Table 1 and Figs. 28A to F)**, the severity increasing with stage. Simple osteotomy may be effective up to stage IV before 8 years of age, beyond which osteotomies are likely to fail. However, the child must be treated as soon as the diagnosis is confirmed so that substantial articular damage can be effectively prevented. Epiphysiolysis (removal of physeal ossification bar) and medial epiphyseal elevation may be needed in types V and VI.

Treatment

Lot of treatment options have been described for the management of infantile tibia vara including observation, orthotic treatment, corrective osteotomy (acute or gradual correction), elevation of medial tibial condyle, resection of physeal bar, lateral hemiepiphysiodesis, and guided growth of proximal tibial physis (inhibiting lateral growth and promoting medial physeal growth).

Bracing: A child younger than 3 years especially in stage I and II can be effectively treated by orthoses. A KAFO may be used to correct the mechanical axis using the principle of three-point fixation. To be effective, it should be applied during the day time for a period of at least 1 year. Night application is also recommended by some. The orthoses must be used till there are radiological signs for healing of the metaphyseal lesion. Usually, children above 4 years of

TABLE 1: The Langenskiold classification of infantile tibia vara.

Stage 1	Mediodistal beaking of the upper proximal tibial metaphysis.
Stage 2	Wedging of the medial part of the upper tibial epiphyseal secondary ossification center plus a saucer-shaped defect of the upper surface of the metaphyseal beak due to its dissolution, fragmentation and collapse.
Stage 3	Stepping of the inferomedial border of the secondary os sification center but without extending distal to the physeal plate level plus deeping of the metaphyseal saucer into a step in the medial metaphysis.
Stage 4	The epiphyseal secondary ossification center passes more distally and cross distal to the physeal level to fill the meta-physeal step.
Stage 5	Separation of the most medial part of the ossification center from the bulk of the secondary ossification center and resides now in the depth of the metaphyseal step below the physis. This is radiologically expressed as either a horizontal cleft (double epiphysis) or complete absence of the medial secondary ossification center as it will be overshadowed by the upper medial tibial metaphysis.
Stage 6	Medial epiphyseal plate closure with a bony bridge

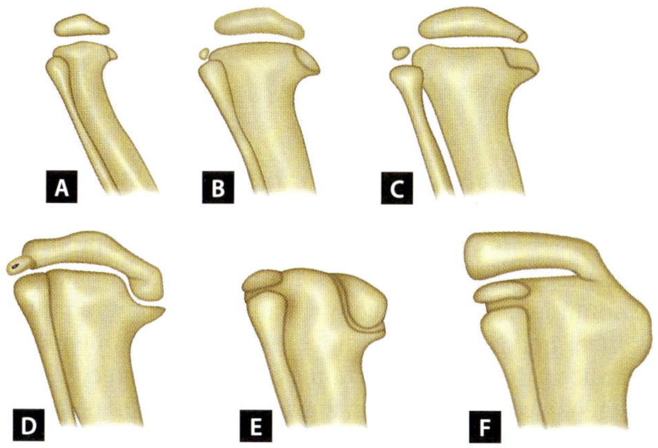

Figs. 28A to F: Langenskiold classification of tibia vara.

age do not respond to this treatment and therefore should be treated by osteotomy. Brace treatment is more effective for patients with initial low MDA and those who are not obese.

Hemiepiphyseal stapling: Surgically guided growth is a good option for a patient with infantile Blount's disease because they have good remaining growth period but the deformity should have minimal rotational component disease must be only stage I or II. Guided growth is chosen for patients who show early Langenskiold changes and has several years of remaining bone growth, to permit correction of the deformity. It is also often done in combination with osteotomy for advanced disease with bony bar formation that is prone to recur after osteotomy (see below).

Corrective osteotomy of tibia and fibula: Patients with stage I and II deformity who do not respond to bracing should be taken up for corrective osteotomy (closing/opening wedge or dome) of the proximal tibia. *Surgical overcorrection of the mechanical axis to at least 5° with lateral translation* of the distal fragment reduces the rate of recurrence. The level of osteotomy is just below the patellar tendon insertion. Some external rotation should be added to the distal fragment to compensate the internal rotation deformity. A fibular osteotomy in the proximal third is routinely added through a separate incision. Prophylactic fasciotomy is recommended for impending compartment syndrome. Postoperative weakness of flexor hallucis longus may denote partial peroneal nerve palsy. Stage III deformities should be treated aggressively because delay in surgery after 4 years of age increases the chances of recurrence. Osteotomy should also address the internal rotation deformity by appropriate external rotation correction otherwise the negative foot-progression angle would persist. Surgeon should also make additional compensation for out of plane correction as the CORA lies at epiphysis but corrective osteotomy is often done distally. So, in summary the indications for surgical correction of deformity by osteotomy are:

- Langenskiold stage 3 and above all ages
- Age 4 and above any Langenskiold stage
- Stage 1 and 2 in children >4 years
- Failure of brace treatment with progressive deformity
- Metaphyseodiaphyseal angle >20

Lesions greater than stage III (stage IV and V) cannot be treated satisfactorily by simple corrective osteotomy alone due to the physiological physeal arrest that occurs on the medial side. There are very high chances of recurrence following simple osteotomies alone and therefore these should be accompanied by lateral epiphysiodesis or medial epiphysiolysis or both. The former, however, is not preferred due to unacceptable limb shortening that it is likely to produce. Thus, treatment of choice is realignment osteotomy with the excision of the medial bridge and lesion consisting of abnormal fibrocartilaginous structures and use of an interposition substance (usually methylmethacrylate) to prevent the rebridging.

Stage VI lesions are difficult to treat due to established bony bridge across the medial physis. If the child has <2 years of growth potential, realignment may be accompanied by lateral epiphysiodesis which reduces the chances of recurrence. This may be followed by limb-lengthening procedures when indicated. External fixators can be planned for realignment osteotomy and lengthening together. The osteotomy can be carried through the physis itself in the older children. If significant incongruity and depression of the joint surface exist, an intra-articular osteotomy may be performed to elevate the medial tibial plateau which corrects the instability and restores alignment.

Recurrence of the deformity is the most common complication of proximal tibial osteotomy. An osteotomy done at the level of TT may result in proximal tibial recurvatum. Prophylactic fasciotomies should be done in all to prevent compartment syndrome. Other complications include injury to anterior tibial artery and peroneal nerve palsy.

Adolescent Tibia Vara

The adolescent tibia vara is less common than the infantile variety **(Table 2)**. It is a distinct entity on account of later

TABLE 2: Differences between infantile and adolescent tibia vara.

Characteristic		*Infantile tibia vara*	*Adolescent tibia vara*
Age		0–3 years of age (by definition)	>10 years of age (by definition) 4–10 age group is sometimes called juvenile tibia vara Juvenile + adolescent tibia vara = late-onset tibia vara
Bilateral occurrence		Yes—nearly half of cases	Not so—it is mostly unilateral
Epidemiology (risk factors and incidence)			
	Early walking	++	–
	Large stature	++	±
	Obesity	++	+
	Occurrence	More common	Less common
Disease progression and staging		Common and classified into 6 stages by Langenskiold	No regression and no classification
Physis/epiphysis		Growth and structural abnormalities seen in physis	No structural abnormality seen
Deformity severity		Severe due to physeal involvement	Less severe
Deformity location		Physeal epiphyseal CORA	Metaphyseal
Deformity components		Proximal posteromedial tibial physis abnormality producing varus, flexion (procurvatum), internal rotation, lateral tibial subluxation and sometimes distal femoral compensatory valgus	Proximal tibia physeal abnormal growth causing varus, may be associated with distal femoral *varus* and distal tibial valgus compensation
Natural history		Early stages with mild Langenskiold grades may resolve spontaneously (grade I and II)	No spontaneous resolution
Treatment		Bracing (early stage I and II) and surgery	Surgical correction only

age of onset and consequently more mature and rigid physis which is more resistant to mechanical compression and disruption. The etiology could be already existing mild degree of physiological genu varum that failed to resolve to neutral alignment or physiological genu valgum. When such children, especially those who are male and obese, undergo adolescent growth spurt, a gradual varus of the proximal tibia develops due to mechanical suppression of the growth. True bony bridges are rarely seen.

Clinically, a typical patient is an obese, black male whose body weight is usually 2SD more than the mean. The disease is frequently unilateral. There may be tenderness along the medial joint line. Some of these may also have slipped upper femoral epiphyses.

Radiological features lack the characteristic metaphyseal lesion and beaking of the infantile tibia vara. The shape of the tibial epiphysis is normal and without any depression. This demonstrates that the proximal tibial physis formed and ossified normally before undergoing mechanical compression later on. There is widening of the proximal medial physeal plate which sometimes extends to the entire width of the plate. In addition, there may be widening of the lateral distal femoral physis on the same side. This may be accompanied by distal femoral varus and a compensatory distal tibial valgus deformity.

Bracing is ineffective to treat such patients due to obesity and maturity of age. The treatment is therefore surgical with a goal to correct the mechanical axis. This can be achieved most successfully by a valgus producing HTO with rigid internal fixation. *Overcorrection in adolescent tibia vara is contraindicated.* Even neutral correction in these patients may result in apparent excessive valgus with thighs rubbing against each other while walking. Some authors therefore recommend an undercorrection so as to produce a femorotibial angle of 0–5° varus. The common complications are nonunion, malunion, compartment syndrome, common peroneal nerve palsy, infection, and sometimes deep vein thrombosis due to obesity. Some authors have recently felt the need to correct the distal femoral varus simultaneously.

External fixators give the advantage of postoperative adjustability but may be very difficult to apply and maintain in these obese patients and are therefore best avoided. Lateral epiphysiodesis is an attractive alternative procedure provided at least 2 years of growth potential is left. Proximal fibular epiphysiodesis is not necessary. The main disadvantage of lateral epiphysiodesis is that rotational deformity cannot be corrected. The advantages are significantly simpler technique, minimal morbidity and subsequent correction can be carried out without added complications if the final correction is inadequate.

Tibia vara secondary to focal fibrocartilaginous dysplasia is a distinct entity and should be differentiated from infantile tibia vara. It is frequently unilateral with deformity appearing distal to the knee joint. Hyperextension may be noted in a walking child. Radiographs are characteristic: Abrupt varus at the metaphyseal-diaphyseal junction of tibia without physeal involvement. Sclerosis may be present at the area of abrupt varus. This may be accompanied by an area of radiolucency just proximal to sclerosis. It is important to recognize this condition and differentiate it from infantile tibia vara because it usually resolves on its own without any treatment.

GENU VALGUM (KNOCK-KNEES)

This is outward deviation of legs so that there is medial angulation at the knee. The ankles are shifted outward while the knee is deviated toward each other **(Figs. 29A and B)**. Though commonly the overshooting corrective valgus recorrects by 4 years of age but in normal variation, it is deemed that normal limb alignment is produced by 7 years of age only (see above on the description of angular alignment of limb). Genu valgum is a physiological deformity so not considered a serious deformity by parents or even physicians. Also this does not readily result in knee degeneration or excess abnormal stress distribution as seen with genu varum, so the acceptability to this deformity is a bit higher. In general, the more medial is the weight-bearing line across the knee joint, higher are the chances of arthritis [one should, however, never assume that lateral displacement of weight-bearing axis would protect from arthritis, this is also a malalignment that would produce arthritis **(Figs. 30A and B)** but usually the deformities in the direction of normal disposition are more forgiving]. Genu valgum is definitely pathological, if the deformity is >2 SD from normal for the age. Now a normal limb alignment of 7° valgus at knee for males and 8° for females plus 2 SD of 5° comes to around 12–13° of acceptable upper limit of valgus at knee. It is deemed that valgus (anatomical femorotibial alignment not MAD) of >15° (taking into consideration the measuring error) above 8 years of age is pathological (if we take mechanical axis then angle of >5° from normal mechanical axis would also qualify for genu valgum). In the clinics, however, the parents are quite concerned about the valgus disposition of the limb even in younger children. We recommend using Bowden's charts for determining if the valgus disposition is pathological or excessive. Excessive valgus deformity (say >20°) in a child >4 years may be associated with numerous conditions, including idiopathic genu valgum, skeletal dysplasia, metabolic bone disease, and renal abnormalities **(Box 4)**. Unilateral, progressive valgus deformity at the tibia, known as Cozen's phenomenon,

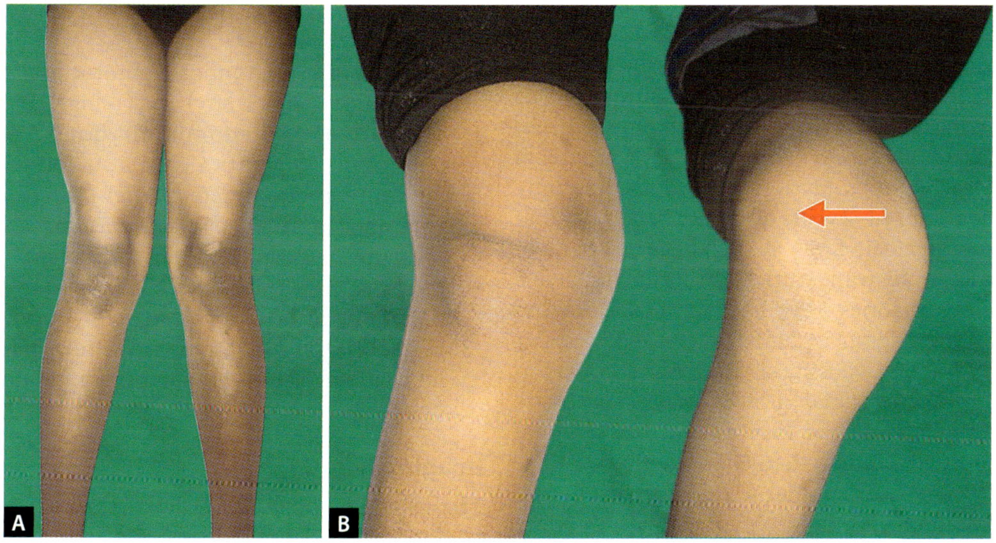

Figs. 29A and B: Genu valgum clinical features. (A) The medial angulation at knees with outward deviation of both legs; (B) Patellofemoral instability of right knee; the patella subluxates laterally on flexing the knee (arrow).

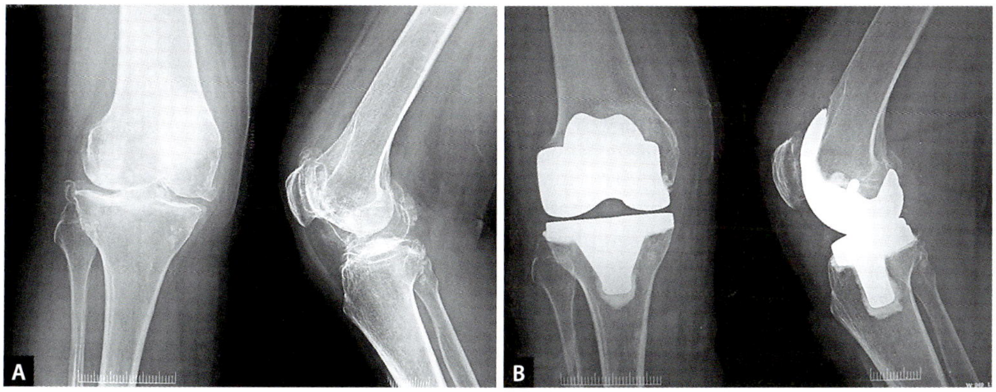

Figs. 30A and B: This patient developed genu valgum deformity following a partial attack of poliomyelitis with weakness in the lower limb in 1970. (A) By the age of 55 years, she developed crippling pain in the knee with degenerative arthritis and (B) restricted ROM requiring TKA. The other knee had grade 2 Kellgren-Lawrence arthritis.

BOX 4: Causes of genu valgum.

- Developmental or physiological (till 8 years of age)
- *Idiopathic:* There is no intrinsic bone disease or congenital anomaly
- Metabolic bone disease especially that develops after valgus disposition is gained during development
- Congenital—fibular hemimelia
- *Trauma:*
  - Malunion
  - Growth stimulation by greenstick fracture of the proximal tibial metaphysis (Cozen's phenomenon) or periarticular hyperemia from osteomyelitis or arthritis
  - Asymmetric growth arrest due to physeal injury
- Iliotibial band contracture (poliomyelitis)
- Infection—causing asymmetric growth disturbance
- Arthritis of knee—rheumatoid, hemophilia
- Bone dysplasia—Morquio's syndrome, multiple hereditary exostosis, Ollier's disease (multiple enchondromatosis), Ellis-Van Creveld syndrome, metaphyseal dysplasia, and multiple epiphyseal dysplasia
- Osteogenesis imperfect

may follow a greenstick fracture of the proximal tibia metaphysis. Cozen's phenomenon (initially described by Dr Cozen in 1953) is described as the late-onset post-traumatic valgus deformity associated with proximal tibial medial metaphyseal fractures in children usually aged 3–6 years. It is an uncommon complication and is seen associated with innocuous looking green stick (buckle or fissure type) or torus fractures commonly occurring as trampoline injuries. The fractures were classically described as incomplete medial metaphyseal injuries. Mysteriously valgus deformity develops in patients after 1–2 years of the original injury that had been successfully treated. Not all such fractures go on to develop valgus deformity with a variably reported incidence of 10–25%. Various theories have been proposed for the developing of genu valgum including increased vascular response to the fracture causing asymmetric stimulation of the medial proximal tibial growth plate, soft-tissue interposition at the fracture site, loss of reduction or initial malreduction of the fracture, tethering by the fibula or the ITB, and early weight-bearing after fracture superimposed on native valgus angulation before rigid callus formation. None of these have been substantiated anywhere. The issue related to treatment is also not settled. Many authors have suggested willful observation because the deformity tends to model with time while some found residual significant deformity after the age of 5–6 years that needs surgical correction. Limb-length discrepancy of as much as 1 cm has been reported in as many as 70% of adult patients. The causes of limb-length discrepancy include changes in bone length, such as those following fracture malunion, changes in growth rate, or a combination of these factors. Traumatic injury to the growth plate can lead to osseous bar formation and limb-length discrepancy. Trauma in the metaphyseal region can lead to angular deformities, such as tibia valgus or overgrowth, and a longer limb.

Clinical Features

- Pain in the thigh and/or calf and easy fatigability
- Child walks with his knees rubbing together and one leg swinging around the other
- Unstable patellofemoral joint and recurrent lateral subluxation of patella. This is due to exaggerated Q-angle of quadriceps extensor mechanism **(Fig. 29B)**.
- Pronated feet and toeing-in to shift the alignment medially
- Laxity of MCL
- Genu recurvatum (genu varum, there is usually FFD at knee)
- Lateral knee pain, patellar facet tenderness due to recurrent patellar subluxation and increased patella-femoral pressure syndrome.

Assessment

- *Look for etiological cause of genu valgum:*
  - Short stature [multiple epiphyseal dysplasia, multiple metaphyseal dysplasia, multiple enchondromatosis (Ollier's disease), multiple hereditary exostosis, and Ellis-van Creveld syndrome]
  - Swollen hot knees for rheumatoid arthritis
  - Fibular hemimelia
  - Iliotibial band contracture—Ober's test
  - Tibia valga is usually associated with tibial external torsion.
- Measure the anatomical femorotibial alignment (for magnitude of deformity) and Q-angle
- Measure the predominant bone contributing to deformity—in genu valgum, it is the femur where the deformity predominates rather than tibia which is the common culprit bone in genu varum.
- Measure the sitting and standing height
- *Measure any limb-length discrepancy:* Limb-length discrepancy is associated with conditions such as congenital short femur, infection, paralysis, tumor, mechanical factors, vascular inflammation, and skeletal dysplasia.

Imaging (Fig. 31)

The criteria for obtaining radiographs include:

- Progressive deformity (above 4 years of age)
- All pathological cases of genu valgum
- Asymmetric deformity
- Looking for proximal tibia valga following a fracture (greenstick) and ensuing progressive genu valgum (Cozen's phenomenon).

Additional radiological assessment includes:

- Obtaining the patella views for assessment of patellar instability
- Full-length radiographs or scanogram **(Fig. 32)** for radiological assessment of deformity, MAD, CORA, and templating the osteotomy **(Figs. 33 and 34)**
- Assessment of skeletal maturity (see *genu varum*)

Treatment

Orthosis and special shoes are ineffective for preventing progression or correcting the deformity. However, University of California Biomechanics Laboratory (UCBL) orthotics helps the child during walk by supporting the foot.

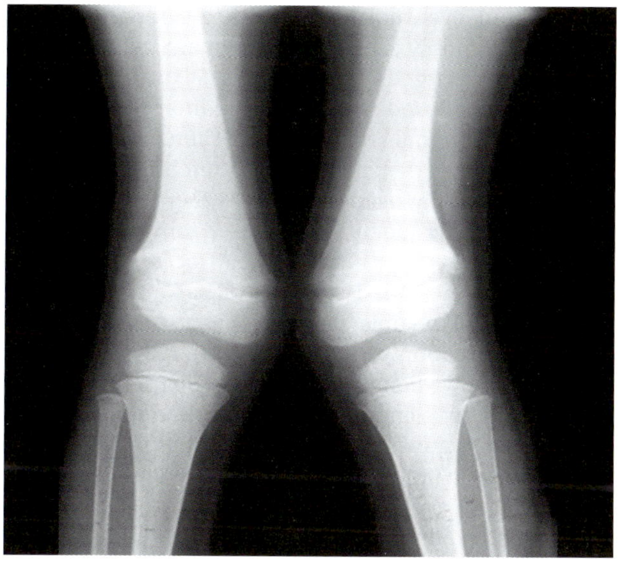

Fig. 31: Radiographic deformity in bilateral genu valgum.

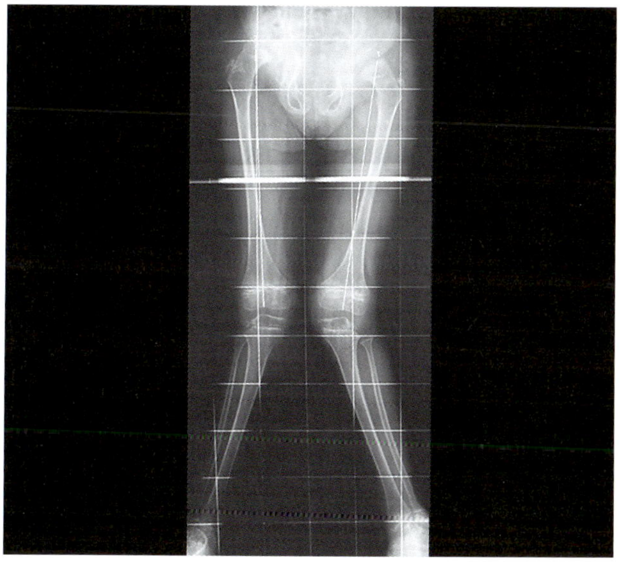

Fig. 32: Scanogram of both legs with genu valgum deformity.

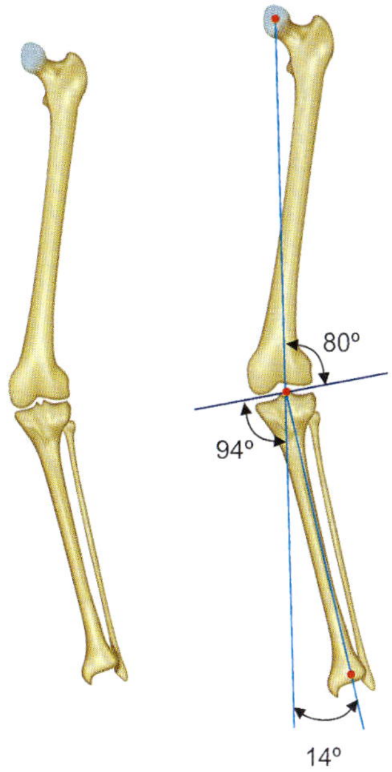

Fig. 33: The example here is of valgus deformity of the knee joint (genu valgum). The overall valgus deformity here is 14° measured by drawing the mechanical axes of femur and tibia. The femoral joint angle (LDFA) is 80° while tibial joint angle is 94° suggesting that equal amount (7°) of valgus deformity is contributed by both femur and tibia.

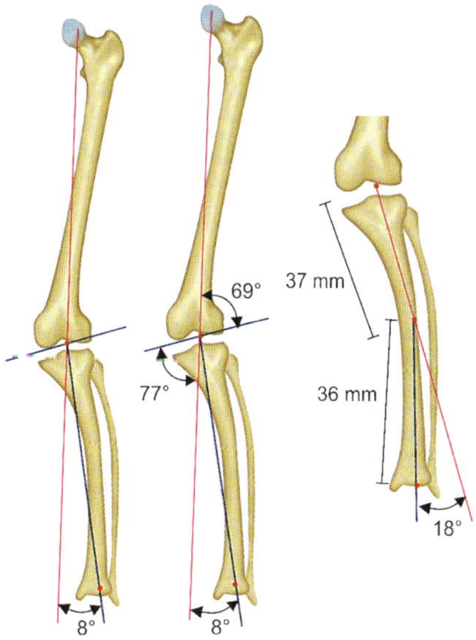

Fig. 34: In unique situations such as trauma, there can be genu valgum associated with extra-articular varus at tibia, though latter may also very rarely arise out of compensation. As a first step, the overall deformity is determined that comes to 8° of valgus at knee. Intra-articular deformity is captured by drawing the joint line where the joint line itself is tilted suggesting that both tibial and femoral articular surfaces are parallel still. In the next step, the femoral and tibial joint angles are calculated (LDFA and MPTA) that comes out to be 69° and 77° suggesting that there is 18° of valgus due to femoral deformity while 10° of varus at tibia compensates for the valgus reducing the overall deformity to 8°. The anatomical deformity at tibial angulation is measured to be 18°. Though one may assume that this anatomical tibial varus should fully compensate the femoral valgus deformity but as detailed above we need to calculate the percentage contribution of this deformity at the knee joint. According to calculation of parts, there is 50% contribution {37/(36 + 37)} of this deformity at joint = 9°. So, of the 10° proximal tibial varus 9° is due to angular deformity of shaft.

They relieve foot strain, easy fatigability, and foot-calf pain. Orthotics may somehow help in preventing the developing ligament laxity in unrestricted cases that are not being operated. Children with a discrepancy >2 cm can compensate by walking on their toes or, as they grow older, vaulting over the short leg.

Deformities >15° need surgical management. The treatment of these deformities includes one of the two options used according to their merits and requirement:

- *Guided growth (see also the genu varum for details):* Hemiepiphysiodesis is done by stapling or fusing the medial part of the distal femoral and/or proximal tibial growth plates. Timing is crucial for permanent methods and should be judged from remaining skeletal growth (assessed by radiological skeletal maturity) and the magnitude of deformity. Stapling is more forgiving and flexible to be used as a growth control method. After hemiepiphysiodesis, the physis is weak and protected in knee immobilizer for 2 weeks. This also allows for skin and soft tissue healing.

- *Osteotomy with deformity correction:* All the methods as discussed in genu varum can be used. Principles of osteotomy correction remain the same. The gradual correction of deformity by a progressive gradual opening osteotomy of lateral aspect of tibia or femur is more feasible done laterally. As the deformity commonly lies in the femur, distal femur osteotomy is commonly done. This also corrects the lateral tilt to joint line usually associated with the deformity. Medially, the vascular structures are located so, commonly the osteotomy is done from lateral aspect; hence, lateral opening wedge osteotomy is preferred. Puddu plates if available are often handy here else a synthetic bone graft block or autogenous iliac crest bone graft with locking plate can be used. Attention should be given to the fact that for moderate-to-severe deformities (>25°) the nerve may get stretched so gradual correcting methods or doing osteotomy in both distal femur and complementary osteotomy in proximal tibia may be better. By no way are medial femoral osteotomies contraindicated if properly done. Dome osteotomies are better avoided in distal femur as they are difficult in this region. If the deformity is present in proximal tibia, then closing wedge option is a common and easier option. There is often external torsion of these bone associated with deformity which should be simultaneously corrected and given priority. Correcting the rotational deformity first often reduces the magnitude of valgus deformity which is then corrected. Partial fibular diaphyseal osteotomy has to be done, if the method chosen for correction is acute else for gradual correction no surgery to fibular aspect is needed. Healing takes 4–6 weeks, till then the osteotomy should be protected. Knee bending and exercises are gradually begun thereafter with night brace for first 2 weeks and without protection later.

Additionally, correct the limb-length discrepancy: Here, it is important to predict the extent of limb-length discrepancy at skeletal maturity and management is done as discussed in limb length discrepancy. Ilizarov method of correction is useful in cases where the deformity is associated with significant limb-length discrepancy (shortening >2.5 cm). Limb-lengthening may also be needed for patients where the deformity is corrected by closing wedge osteotomy with a wedge size of >2.5 cm producing significant shortening.

CONGENITAL ANGULAR DEFORMITIES OF TIBIA AND FIBULA

Angular deformities of tibia are rare but do occasionally occur. The deformity can be:

- Anterior angulation or bow—seen commonly with fibular hemimelia.
- Posteromedial angulation or bow—seen commonly with calcaneovalgus foot deformity. It is a benign congenital anomaly without fracture or pseudoarthrosis. The foot deformity usually corrects itself within the first year of life but eventual limb-length discrepancy of 2–5 cm is commonly seen that is the main reason why an orthopedic surgeon is consulted. At birth, the foot is grossly dorsiflexed with limited plantar flexion. Tibial bow is evident only on palpation. There may be a small skin dimple at the site of bow. Stretching and casting are occasionally used to improve the deformity, and, rarely, an ankle-foot orthosis is used for weight-bearing. Gradual correction is expected to occur over several years until the tibia is straight or has a mild S shape. Treatment of the tibial deformity consists of observation versus correction of the limb-length discrepancy and residual bow. Lengthening of the extremity may be done with distraction osteosynthesis and bow corrected with guided growth. Contralateral physiodesis may be considered in individuals with a limb-length discrepancy but no residual tibial bow.
- Anterolateral angulation or bow—seen commonly with pseudoarthrosis of tibia as discussed below.

The former two have excellent prognosis following correction; the last one is often complicated and associated with multiple failures even after best of dedicated surgery.

Anterolateral Bowing of Tibia

This refers to the angular deformity seen in lower third of tibia and fibula and may or may not be associated with fibular deformity. The anterolateral bowing of tibia is commonly seen in few congenital disorders apart from malunion resulting from trauma:

- Congenital pseudoarthrosis of tibia
- *Congenital anterolateral bowing of tibia with polydactyly:* Here, the bowing resolves spontaneously often. There may be associated duplication of great toe, clinodactyly, tibial shortening, and carpal or metacarpal anomaly.
- *Neurofibromatosis type 1:* This is associated in 50% of anterolateral bowing cases with or with congenital pseudoarthrosis of tibia. It may be unilateral. Fibula may or may not be hypoplastic. The stigmata of neurofibromatosis including the skin and other osseous lesions are present.
- Tibial hemimelia (congenital longitudinal deficiency of tibia)
- Fibular hemimelia (congenital longitudinal deficiency of fibula)
- Nonunion or malunion following osteomyelitis
- *Fibrous dysplasia:* The bone is of poor quality due to geographic defect in bone quality. There may be associated skin lesions.
- Amniotic band syndrome

Congenital Pseudoarthrosis of Tibia

This is a congenital condition of unknown origin associated with bone pathology and angulation seen at the junction of middle and lower thirds of the tibia first described by Hatzoecher in 1708. The deformity is present since birth and does not resolve spontaneously but pseudoarthrosis may not be present from birth and is not essentially congenital. The bone discontinuity usually develops later during growth period permitting persistent movement characteristic of pseudoarthrosis. Once established, the natural history is that of persistent instability and progressive deformity. The incidence has been estimated to be 1 in 190,000 live births. Left side is affected slightly more often than the right. Bilateral involvement is rare and seen in familial association.

Pathophysiology

The etiology is intriguing with frequent association of neurofibromatosis (40–80%) first described by Barbar and fibrous dysplasia (20% around) but still the bony changes are segregate and unresolving. The tissue at the pseudoarthrosis site demonstrates cellular fibrous connective tissue with areas of variable cartilage formation. Electron microscopically, the cells lack basement membrane and resemble fibroblasts rather than Schwann cells (even in neurofibromatosis). The bone defect being referred to as pseudoarthrosis is incorrect as the tissue in gap is filled with fibrocartilage and fibrous connective tissue that extends to the bone ends and surrounding periosteum and the soft tissues possibly also around the nerve and vascular supply to the region! It more closely represents a local hamartoma that somehow involves bone.

Clinical Examination

- There is congenital anterolateral bowing of tibia (**Figs. 35A and B**; often without abnormal mobility).
- The swelling and angulation are painless and nontender.
- Café-au-lait spots are seen in patients with associated neurofibromatosis—to label the disease neurofibromatosis criteria laid down by Crawford should be followed (*see* Chapter on "Congenital, Genetic, Syndromic, and Miscellaneous Disorders"). Café-au-lait spots are typically smooth-edged (coast of California). The presence of at least five spots measuring >0.5 cm in diameter is considered diagnostic.
- Other features of neurofibromatosis, viz., the short, sharp angular spinal deformity, or hemihypertrophy may be present.
- The skin lesions of fibrous dysplasia are marked by rugged edges (coast of Maine appearance) and are fewer in number. Examine other limbs for deformity in fibrous dysplasia (polyostotic type).
- Foot deformity in type VI disease

Classification of Congenital Pseudoarthrosis of Tibia

The dysplasia at apex of deformity ranges from fracture with atrophy of the fracture ends to failure of tubulation of the diaphysis, with a sclerotic or cystic appearance that eventually develops into a pseudarthrosis. Various classification systems described by Crawford, Boyd's, and Anderson **(Table 3)** attempt to classify the deformity incorporating these components; however, none succeed in guiding the treatment or prognosticating the disease exactly and did not consider fibula deformity. Paley classification (2019) emphasizes importance of fibular deformity **(Fig. 36)** and may serve as a better guide for treatment and prognosis.

Treatment

The cases are difficult to treat and the prognosis is not very encouraging for these patients as the attempt to bony union often fails. A lot of methods are described in literature itself supporting the notion that failure rates are high. The employed methods also can be grouped into prefracture management and those used to treat fracture/pseudoarthrosis. Prefracture management aims at preventing fracture from occurring till skeletal maturity and is usually supportive. Surgical methods such as prophylactic bypass grafting have been described but are not very popular. Usually, surgery is deployed for management of fracture/nonunion/pseudoarthrosis.

Conservative management: This is the initial preferred treatment for all cases, especially for patients without fracture or pseudoarthrosis (prepseudoarthrosis). Total contact plastic clamshell orthosis, AFO (prior to walking), and KAFO (after they start walking) are commonly employed methods as they are easier to manage than plaster casts. These are worn indefinitely full time; if fracture does not occur, tibial

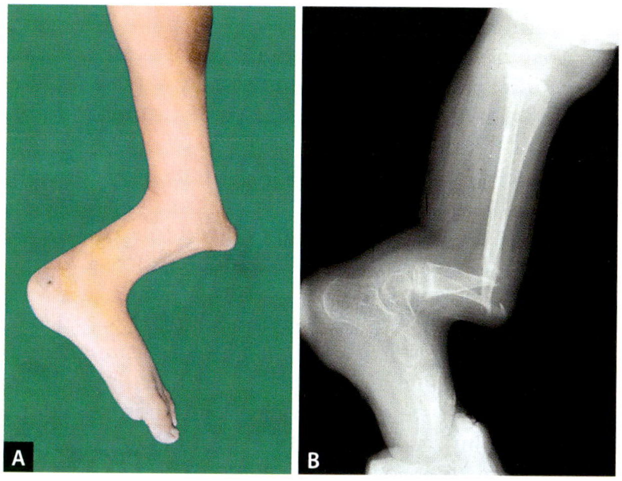

Figs. 35A and B: Congenital pseudoarthrosis of tibia.

TABLE 3: Classification of congenital pseudoarthrosis of tibia.

Boyd	Description	Anderson equivalent
I	Patients born with anterior bowing and tibial defect	
II	Anterior bowing + hourglass contracture (# by 2 years) associated with neurofibromatosis (worse prognosis)	Dysplastic type
III	Bone cyst	Cystic type
IV	Sclerotic segment of tibia (no narrowing), usually develops stress type fracture—nonunion	Late/sclerotic type
V	Also have dysplastic fibula	Fibular type
VI	• Intraosseous neurofibroma/Schwannoma (rarest type) • Foot deformity (CTEV/Streeter's band associated)	Clubfoot/congenital band type

(CTEV: congenital talipes equinovarus)

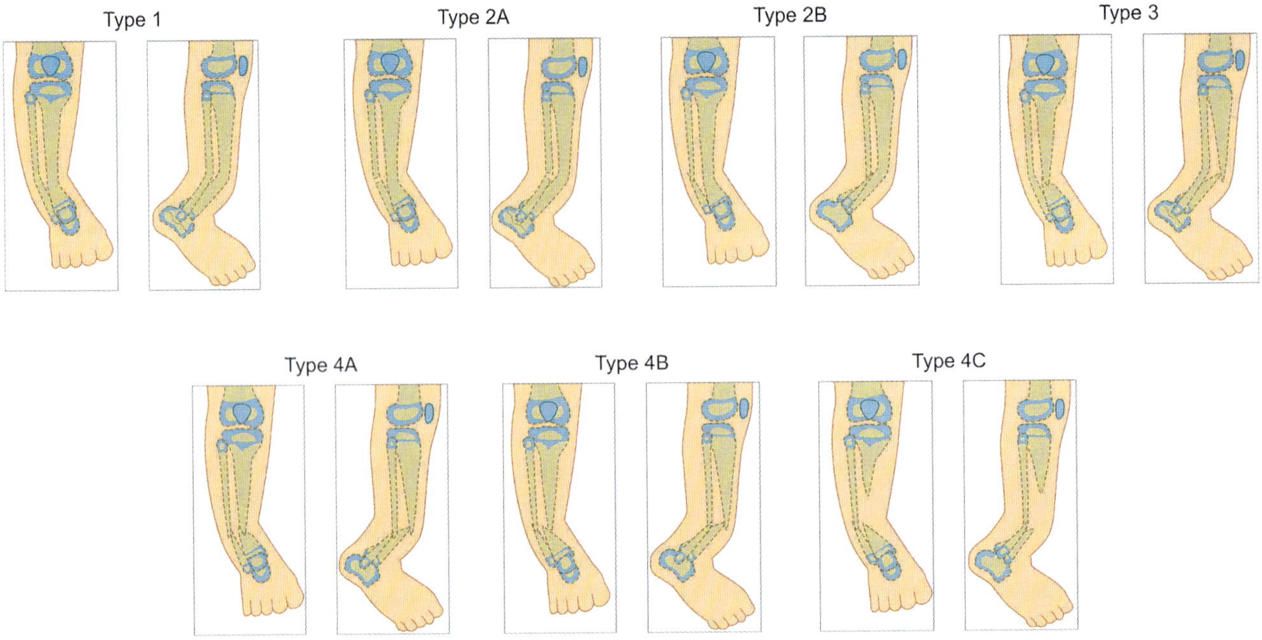

Fig. 36: The Paley classification of congenital pseudoarthrosis of tibia. Type 1 = No fracture; Type 2A = No tibia fracture, fracture in fibula but bone in place; Type 2B = No tibia fracture, fibula fractured and proximally migrated; Type 3 = Fractured tibia but fibula maintained-no fracture; Type 4A = Tibia and fibula both fractured; Type 4B = Tibia and fibula fracture and fibula migrated proximally; Type 4C = Bone defect in tibia + fibula migrated proximally.

bowing usually gradually improves, particularly in Boyd's type 4 and reformation of medullary canal may occur requiring up to 5–10 years. Even in cases where a fracture is visible before age of 4 years, the bracing is done to stimulate the tibia to hypertrophy based on Wolf's law, so that later reconstruction is stable. The bracing is discontinued if:

- There is sufficient straightening of tibia.
- Medullary canal is reformed.
- Adequate cortical thickness is achieved.

Parents should be counseled that there are chances of recurring disease and definitive treatment is surgical. The type 4 CPT patients respond well to onlay bone grafting.

Surgical treatment: Goals of surgical treatment include:

- Lasting union at fracture site
- Maintaining alignment to avoid undue stress at the pseudoarthrosis site
- Obtaining acceptable limb length

Treatment options: Better surgical outcomes are seen in children older than 3 years. Between 3 and 5 years intramedullary nailing and bone grafting has shown good results while Ilizarov method is particularly recommended for children older than 5 years. Fibula is commonly left untreated but addressing pseudoarthrosis of fibula may protect against development of late ankle valgus and tibia refracture. The following are commonly described surgical treatment options mentioned here in decreasing order of popularity.

- Intramedullary (IM) nailing with iliac crest bone graft and transfixation of ankle (Charnley). It involves extraperiosteal pseudarthrosis excision and IM stabilization of the tibia and fibula. An autogenous bone graft, with or without iliac crest periosteum, is used at the resection site. The success rate for IM nailing and bone grafting approaches 80–90%, although the pseudoarthrosis may recur and necessitate repeated bone grafting, with or without bone stimulation units. This technique is generally practiced with variously described modifications from different authors:
    - *Intramedullary bone graft with vascularized fibula and iliac crest cancellous graft:* Transfixes ankle and subtalar joint (retrograde insertion of rod). Masquelet technique of induced membrane technique (stages resection + cement spacer --> delayed bone grafting) may also be used.
    - Intramedullary nailing with two part solid Peter Williams rod, pseudoarthrosis excision and iliac crest bone grafting. The rod is advanced into the talus and calcaneus correcting the calcaneovalgus deformity of the foot simultaneously and then the rod is advanced retrograde into the proximal fragment. The gap at osteotomy site is filled with bone graft obtained from iliac crest. Another osteotomy may be required proximally in case of extensive deformity and tibial bow.
    - Adding bone morphogenetic protein-7 has not shown to improve outcomes.
    - After surgery, children are placed in a cast for 3–4 months and then in an ankle-foot orthosis, with the ankle locked.
- *Microvascular fibular graft (contralateral,* ***Figs. 37A to D****), rib, and iliac crest with excision of tibial pseudoarthrosis:* The microvascular procedures are particularly useful and have shown better healing rates than other procedures, especially in cases with severe atrophied bones at the ends of fracture. For this procedure to be successful, the pathological region should be excised extraperiosteally.

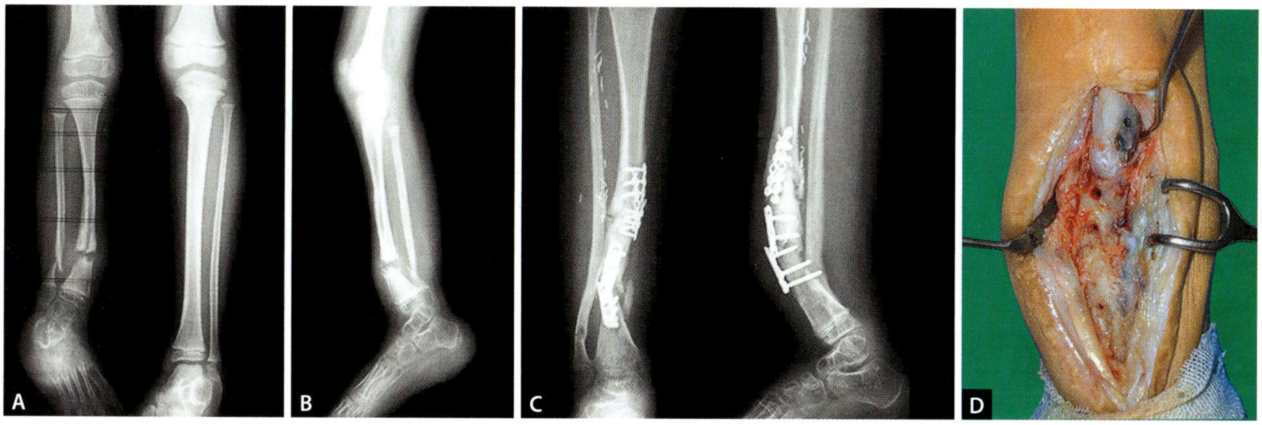

Figs. 37A to D: Case of congenital pseudoarthrosis of tibia. (A) The AP radiographs of both legs; (B) Lateral radiograph of the involved leg; (C) Patient managed with vascularized fibular graft that failed after 3 years; (D) Implant removal was done and pseudoarthrosis site demonstrated bone formation so managed with cast immobilization.
Source: Professor PP Kotwal, Chairman, Institute of Orthopedics and Joint Replacement, Pushpavati Singhania Research Institute, New Delhi, India.

The graft bone is then fitted in a dowel-like manner and protected with plate osteosynthesis or external fixator. Subsequent additional surgical procedures are, however, required due to inadequate consolidation of the grafted bone in the form of secondary bone grafting commonly.

- *Ilizarov method:* The method is versatile in producing consolidation at the fracture site and simultaneous correction of the deformity. It can be applied in various forms including compression only, compression plus tibial lengthening, compression followed by distraction, and distraction alone for hypertrophic nonunion. This method can also be used in children who were not successfully treated using the previous method or those who are older or in patients with atrophic bone ends at the fracture site. The pseudarthrosis is resected, and the two bone ends are impacted. A proximal corticotomy allows for bone transport to make up for the tibial shortening. The bone is compressed distally. As in other techniques, autogenous bone graft and bone morphogenetic protein are used to facilitate union at the distal site. The success rate of this method is 70–90%. Variations include implantation of an IM nail throughout the distraction-compression process (SCONE—slow compression over nail using external fixator) or after union has been obtained. Compression using an external fixator often leads to deformation at the pseudoarthrosis site while placing an IM nail will prevent deformation in sagittal or coronal plane but allow axial compression to occur. Atrophic type (Boyd type II) poses special challenge as the contact areas are very small and bone apposition may not be appropriate. 4-in-1 osteosynthesis places all the four segments (proximal and distal tibia and proximal and distal fibula) in one healing mass creating cross-union, thus improving the chances to union. This strategy is effective for moderate deformity but for severe forms distal tibiofibular fusion is additionally needed.
- *Methods of historical importance:*
  - *Electric current stimulation of osteogenesis:* These have been used primarily as adjuncts to bone grafting. Brighton used insertion of cathode into the site while Bassett used the pulsed electromagnetic field (PEMF) for bone formation.
  - McFarland type posterior bypass onlay graft from opposite tibia (this is prophylactic grafting done in imminent fracture cases, inadequate bone structure, and child whose activity cannot be controlled!). The method is suitable for type 4 Boyd classification where chances of consolidation of disease are better.
  - Boyd's dual onlay cortical bone grafting with bicortical screw fixation (bone of parents/allograft): Early success but much ultimate failure.
  - *Sofield and Millar's double proximal and distal osteotomy followed by reversal of tibial shaft with IM nailing:* Reversing healthy bone to involved site may stimulate osteogenesis.
  - Eyre-Brook's delayed bone grafting (older the patient with presentation > are the chances of success)
  - Moore's staged bone grafting and external fixation
  - *Farmar's cross-legged vascularized pedicle bone grafting from opposite tibia:* Problematic as it is cumbersome and potential for infecting uninvolved tibia.
- *Amputation (McCarthy); Boyd/Symes type to produce end-bearing stump:* This is a mutilating surgery but may need to be employed judiciously in some cases.
  - Failed three surgical attempts
  - Shortening > 5 cm
  - Deformed foot
  - Prolonged hospitalization
  - Pseudoarthrosis <2.5 cm from ankle joint

Prognostic factors: The following factors are associated with poor prognosis of surgical treatment apart from those mentioned in indications for amputation.

- Boyd's type 2 is difficult to consolidate.
- Disease associated with neurofibromatosis is likely to progress and has higher chances of treatment failure.

Complications of surgical treatment:
- Refracture
- Limb-length discrepancy
- Ankle and subtalar stiffness
- Progressive anterior angulation
- Ankle valgus
- Donor site morbidity

CONGENITAL DEFICIENCIES OF THE TIBIA

These are extremely rare with incidence of 1 in 1 million but tibial deficiency is associated with high likelihood for deformities in later generations. Tibial hemimelia was first described by Otto in 1941. Tibial hemimelia is characterized by deficiency of the tibia with relatively intact fibula **(Figs. 38A and B)**. Tibial hemimelia is also known as congenital longitudinal deficiency of the tibia, congenital dysplasia of the tibia, paraxial tibial hemimelia, tibial dysplasia, and congenital deficiency or absence of the tibia. The deficiency is bilateral in 30% of patients. Most of the affected children (60% and 70%) have concurrent musculoskeletal disorders that include:
- Equinovarus foot
- Congenital short femur
- Congenital dislocation of the hip
- Cleft hand

The associated syndromes with tibial hemimelia include:
- Tibial hemimelia diplopodia
- Polydactyly triphalangeal thumb syndrome (Werner syndrome)
- Tibial hemimelia-split-hand/foot syndrome
- Tibial hemimelia-micromelia-trigonal brachycephaly syndrome

Tibial deficiency is classified based on the presence of a proximal tibia (and hence a functional quadriceps mechanism). The jones classification divides tibial hemimelia into four groups:
1. *Type 1 deficiency:* No tibia is seen on radiographs. Cartilage tibia anlage may appear on ultrasonography or MRI which ossifies later.

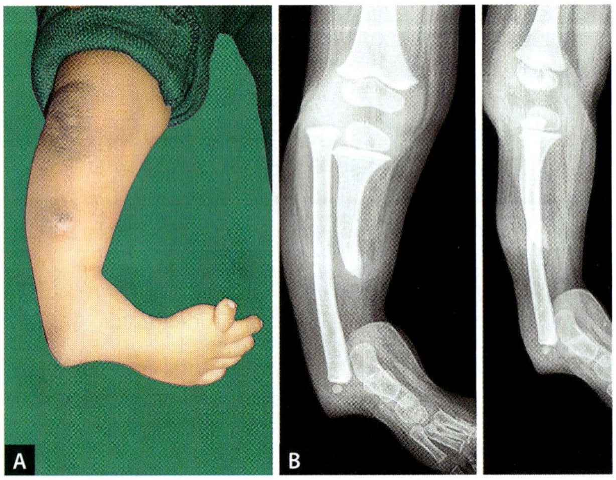

Figs. 38A and B: Tibial hemimelia. (A) Clinical presentation; (B) Radiographic characteristics with partial absence of tibia distally.

   - In type 1 A, fibula is dislocated proximally, tibia is not radiographically evident and distal femoral epiphysis is smaller than on normal side.
   - In type 1 B, fibula is dislocated proximally and proximal tibial cartilaginous anlage may be visible at birth on ultrasound or MRI, but not on plain radiographs that may ossify later.
3. Type 2 deficiency has proximal dislocation of fibula and radiographically visible proximal tibia with normal-appearing knee joint.
4. In type 3 deficiency, fibula is dislocated proximally, distal tibia is radiographically visible, but proximal tibia is not seen.
5. In rare type 4 deformity, fibula has migrated proximally, with congenital diastasis of the ankle joint (tibiofibular joint).

Clinical Features

There is shortening of the involved leg. The fibular head is palpable and foot is held in severe equinovarus. The knee generally has flexion contracture and in more severe deformities quadriceps insufficiency causes lack of knee extension. The superficial peroneal nerve may extend up to ankle. The anterior tibial artery is absent, and the plantar arterial arch is incomplete. Tendons of leg muscles that insert on the plantar surface of the foot often fuse into single mass. The talus and calcaneus are often fused.

Treatment

The type of surgical treatment depends on the radiographic classification and clinical appearance. Type 1A deficiency is usually treated with transarticular amputation (knee disarticulation) followed by prosthetic fitting. Fibular centralization is not considered unless an intact functional quadriceps mechanism is present that can be reconstructed to provide active knee extension. Type 1B deficiencies can be reconstructed to give a functional knee joint. The foot and sometimes distal leg are amputated to be fitted later with a prosthesis. A type 2 or even the type 1B deficiency is treated with Syme amputation of the dysfunctional foot and a proximal tibial-fibular synostosis is created to produce a functioning below-knee amputation. Type 3 deficiencies are extremely rare to occur and are managed with foot amputation (Syme or Chopart) and prosthetic fitting. Patients with type 4 deficiencies need individualized treatment after explaining the options. Easiest and quite reliable method is to do a Syme amputation and prosthetic fitting. Exquisite procedures like customized reconstruction of the ankle joint to retain the foot and ankle by combinations of distal tibiofibular synostosis and distal fibular epiphysiodesis have been described but require multiple surgeries followed by soft tissue releases for equinovarus deformities of the foot.

FIBULAR HEMIMELIA

This is complete or partial absence of the fibula which can occur either proximally or distally. It is the most common congenital long bone deficiency. The boys are affected twice

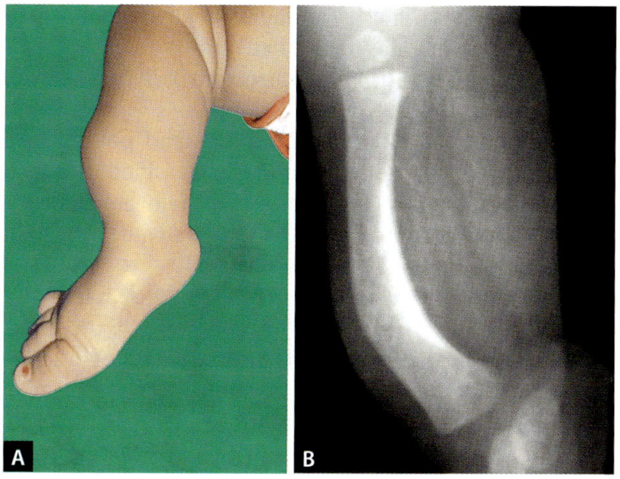

Figs. 39A and B: Fibular hemimelia. (A) Clinical presentation with anteromedial bow and valgus at ankle; (B) Radiograph shows complete absence of fibula and a ball in socket ankle. Also note the bow in tibia.

as often as girls. Affected individuals may have a normal-appearing but short foot and leg, or the limb may be severely deformed and nonfunctional. The tibia is shorter than normal and may be anteriorly bowed **(Figs. 39A and B)**. Associated skeletal abnormalities include:

- Congenital deficiency of the femur
- Genu valgum
- Absence of the lateral rays of the feet
- Tarsal coalitions
- Ball-in-socket ankle
- Valgus positioning of the ankle

The classification systems are mainly descriptive based on the extent of fibular deficiency, the amount of shortening and the presence of any concurrent foot abnormalities.

Treatment

Fibular hemimelia is treated with amputation and prosthetic fitting or limb reconstruction and lengthening.

Amputation and Prosthetic Fitting

- Syme or Boyd amputation is considered for patients who have a nonfunctional foot with severe valgus positioning or fewer than three rays, as well as a projected limb-length discrepancy >30% compared with the contralateral side.
- Amputation and prosthetic fitting are also strongly indicated for a patient with bilateral fibular hemimelia who has normal upper extremity function.
- Children treated with amputation and prosthetic fitting have good function, and long-term studies found athletic and psychological function similar to that of unaffected children.

Limb Reconstruction

Limb lengthening is considered for children who have a projected length discrepancy of <10%, compared with the contralateral side, as well as the potential for good foot function after ankle and foot reconstruction.

Children with a discrepancy of between 10% and 30% can be managed with either amputation and prosthetic fitting or limb reconstruction and lengthening. The decision is based on the preference of the treating physician and the family.

CONGENITAL DISLOCATION OF THE KNEE

Definition and Epidemiology

This is a rare deformity of knee that varies from simple hyperextension to anterior dislocation of tibia on the femur. The spectrum varies from recurvatum to subluxation, and dislocation. Unilateral or bilateral congenital dislocation of the knee (CDK) occurs in approximately 1 in 100,000 live births. Most of the cases are sporadic. Females are more commonly affected than males. There is a 50% incidence of hip dysplasia, clubfoot deformity, or CVT in these patients. Bilateral deformity is associated with other conditions, such as spina bifida, arthrogryposis, or Larsen syndrome. CDK is classified as hyperextension, subluxation, or knee joint dislocation but in comparison to hip joint pathology the incidence of CDK is 10 times less than DDH. In any case, a true CDK is always associated with significant quadriceps contracture.

Etiology

- Familial cases may have a genetic basis. This could be especially true when one considers the association with DDH and congenital foot abnormalities (clubfoot and vertical talus) that have polygenic inheritance.
- Bilateral cases **(Figs. 40A and B)** are almost always syndromic and associated with either:
  - Larsen syndrome, Beal's syndrome
  - Ipsilateral hip dislocation and clubfoot
  - Gastrointestinal and genitourinary anomalies
- Milder varieties of CDK such as the hyperextension deformities (passive flexion past 45°) occur in patients with a history of breech birth or oligohydramnios and may represent positional deformities that are not truly pathological.
- Severe CDK often occurs in the presence of muscle imbalance as in myelodysplasia, arthrogryposis, or Larsen syndrome.

Pathophysiology and Pathogenesis

- Fetal malpositioning in utero is the major factor in development of CDK. These infants typically have severe hyperextension in utero, and presumably decreased fetal mobility.
- Imbalance about the knee is further created by a relatively strong or contracted quadriceps muscle, along with deficient hamstrings. The chronic knee hyperextension gradually leads to anterior subluxation of the hamstrings, making them "perverted" knee extensors.
- Once the abnormal position occurs, deformity is propagated by persistent hyperextension and reduced fetal movements due to arthrogryposis, etc.; the lack of trophic factors to nearby structures further leads to hypoplastic changes and production of characteristic deformity.

Pathoanatomy

- The quadriceps muscle is short and contracted.
- There is early fibrosis of the quadriceps, absence of the suprapatellar pouch, and incomplete patellofemoral cavitation. These findings are intrinsic to the extensor mechanism and are the primary cause of knee subluxation, rather than being secondary to some other extrinsic cause.
- Elongated, absent, or insufficient cruciate ligaments
- Global ligament laxity
- Hamstring tendons positioned anteriorly
- Iliotibial band contracture with lateral septum tightness
- Hypoplastic or absent patella
- Atrophy and fibrosis of vastus lateralis muscle
- Collateral ligaments are placed anteriorly from their usual attachment.

Clinical Features

- Hyperextension deformity of the knee with inability to actively or passively flex the knee **(Figs. 40A and B)**
- Quadriceps tendon is contracted palpable as a tethering cord over anterior aspect of thigh.
- There is associated valgus rotatory instability in severe cases.
- A dimple or deep crease may be present over the anterior aspect of the knee.
- The patella is difficult to palpate, and often laterally displaced.
- The severe forms have associated congenital abnormalities of hip and foot as mentioned above.
- Milder forms have usually recurvatum or hyperextension abnormality only.

Clinically, based on the movements and possibility of passive corrections, the CDK has been classified into three grades. These grades are important to help elucidate the extent of knee deformity **(Figs. 41A to C)** and guide the treatment initially.

1. ***Grade 1 (hyperextended knee):*** The knee has hyperextension deformity (>15°) but reduces with gentle stretching of the quadriceps and passive knee flexion goes past 45°. Radiologically, the tibia is seen reduced on femur but knee is hyperextended.
2. ***Grade 2 (subluxated knee)*:** The knee does not flex beyond 45° and in most cases not beyond neutral. Tibial and femoral epiphysis are in contact and do not subluxate on attempted flexion. Anterior subluxation of the tibia onto the distal aspect of the femur can be seen on radiographs **(Figs. 40A and B)**.
3. ***Grade 3 (dislocated irreducible knee)*:** Knee flexion is not possible and anteriorly subluxated or translated, tibia further translates laterally over femur on attempted flexion. There is significant anterior quadriceps contracture. The tibia is dislocated anterior to femur and proximally migrated with absent suprapatellar pouch (knee in reverse position appearance). Hamstring tendons can be palpated anterior to femur.

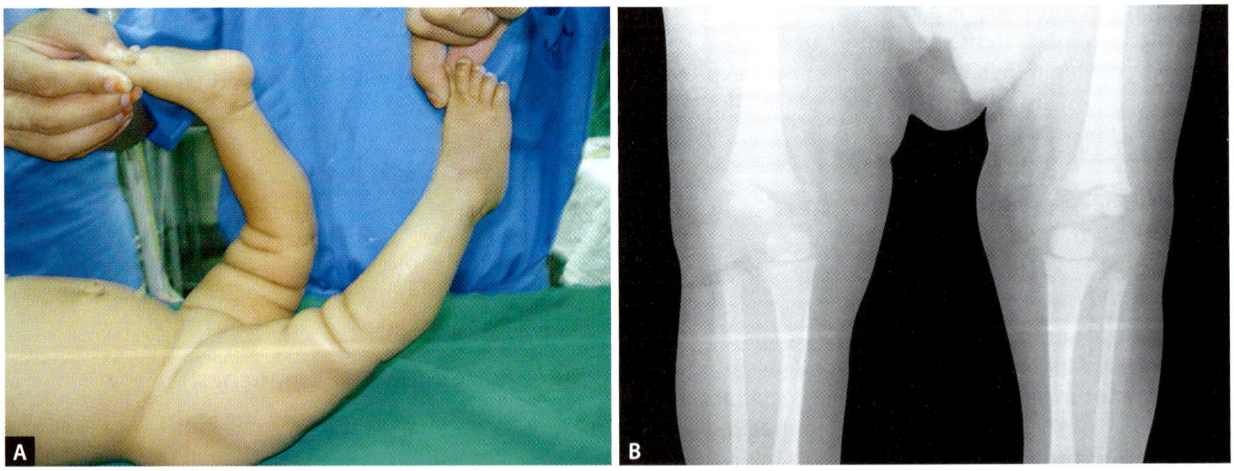

Figs. 40A and B: Congenital dislocation of the knee. (A) Clinical picture; (B) Radiographic presentation.

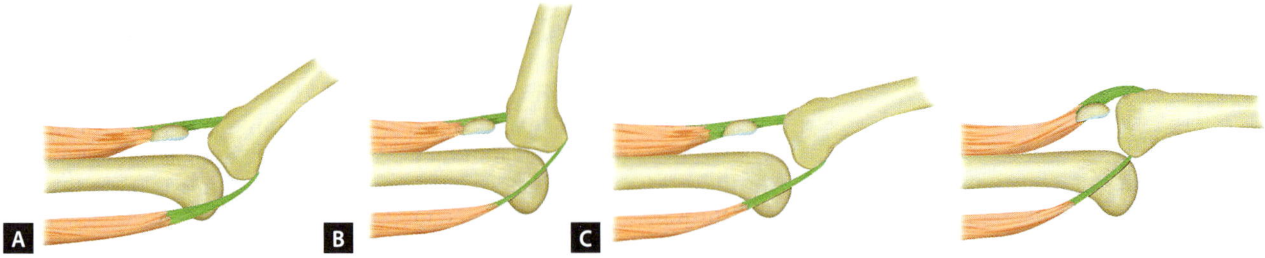

Figs. 41A to C: Illustration of the three grades of knee instability in CDK. (A) Recurvatum; (B) Subluxation; (C) Congenital knee dislocation.

Management

The management begins with identification of associated congenital abnormalities (like foot and hip dysplasia) so that they can be addressed simultaneously.

Initial treatment consists of gentle stretching, casting, and use of an orthotic device such as a Pavlik harness that should begin as soon as possible. The treatment is aimed at stretching the quadriceps contracture to improve flexibility. Apply longitudinal traction on tibia and push the tibia posteriorly to reduce and establish contact with femoral condyles in anatomical alignment. Maintain position in a cast or slab reinforced anteriorly so that it does not give way under pathological forces. The casts are changed every 2–3 weeks. Once stable flexion to 30° is obtained (for grade 2 or 3 knee), manipulation is done to force knee up to 90°. There after a removable splint is used. Beyond 90°, the flexion at knee is not required. Successful conservative treatment according to Richard includes knee bending till 90° and radiological alignment of the limb. It is imperative to document the restoration of a normal relationship of the femur to the tibia by obtaining a lateral knee radiograph. For severe deformities, the tibia is brought down by longitudinal traction or even a distractor at times to stretch the contracted tissues. Gradual reduction, realignment, and flexion are then attempted as before. One should be gentle enough in these cases not to damage the distal femoral physis that is soft and liable to separate on attempted flexion. In these severe cases, femoral nerve block or botulinum toxin has been suggested as a measure to improve quadriceps contracture and allow better relaxation of the structures and deformity.

Surgical Treatment

Surgical treatment is considered for patients who have:

- Fixed knee dislocation
- Knee subluxation that has not improved and inability to obtain >60° knee flexion using nonoperative method detailed above.

Two surgical approaches have been described:

1. For children younger than 3 months, a percutaneous section of the quadriceps tendon and suprapatellar retinaculum is performed, followed by early serial casting and motion. Performing extensive bilateral surgeries may not be a feasible option due to general health of the child.
2. For older children, a VY quadricepsplasty (advancement) is performed, with release of the contracted structures of the suprapatellar pouch and the quadriceps tendon. For severe cases, the Z-plasty of whole extensor mechanism can be performed to obtain better length. The anterior knee joint is transversely released till the level of collateral ligaments which should be reflected forward or released if required. The medial hamstrings, ITB, and the lateral intermuscular spectrum may need to be released to correct valgus and external rotational deformity. The quadriceps mechanism is sutured in 30° of knee flexion to protect the repair and prevent necrosis of the anterior knee skin. Postoperatively, the knee is immobilized in spica cast for 3–4 weeks. This is then followed by long-term physical therapy and splinting. Long leg brace is usually given for up to 1 year to prevent hyperextension of knee.

Management of Difficult and Recurrent Cases

- For very severe cases where after extensive release if knee flexion to 60° is not obtained then femoral shortening may be done.
- Patients with hyperlaxity may be managed with ACL reconstruction and posterior capsulorrhaphy.
- Ipsilateral hip dislocation is managed after management of CDK with spica cast for milder forms or staged surgical procedure as needed for severe cases.

Outcome

Conservatively, managed cases have good outcome with nearly normal radiographs and function. Complicated and severe cases managed surgically also do well with 80–120° of knee movements albeit hyperlaxity persists in many.

Bilateral and syndromic cases have poorer outcome with knee stiffness but they do not develop hyperextension deformity as often. They may later require femoral shortening.

Complications of Surgical Management

- Knee stiffness
- Anterior knee skin necrosis

LEG-LENGTH DISCREPANCY

Discrepancies in lower limb length of up to 2 cm are commonly seen. In fact, differences of 1 cm (prevalence as high as 25% in general population) are often considered a normal occurrence among individuals. The main discomfort with unequal lower limbs is gait asymmetry that puts the child into self-consciousness, psychological regression, and social attention. Physiologically, this demands increased energy expenditure needed for ambulation. It is logical to expect abnormal lumbar curvature of spine resulting from unequal limb lengths but it is unproven as to if it causes structural scoliosis or degenerative arthritis. There are various factors that can result in unequal limb lengths due to shortening or lengthening of the extremity ranging from congenital to acquired causes.

Causes: There are various causes of discrepancies in the leg length. Not only can they be due to shortening of the limb (interference in length or interference in growth) but they may also arise from lengthening in some cases **(Table 4)**.

Another way to classify the leg-length discrepancy is dividing them into congenital-syndromic and acquired causes that may both include inhibition or stimulation of growth. While typically the PFFD, tibial or fibular hemimelia account for shortening; Klippel–Trénaunay–Weber and Sturge–Weber syndrome **(Figs. 42A to C)** cause limb lengthening. Among traumatic causes physeal injuries often cause shortening but healing juxtaphyseal fractures of tumors may cause lengthening. Various causes can be referred from **Table 4**. It is important to know the underlying cause and get a wholesome assessment of the patient as many would also have underlying visceral and other musculoskeletal abnormalities that should be addressed simultaneously during management of LLD.

TABLE 4: Causes of leg-length discrepancy.

Conditions causing shortening of the affected extremity	*Conditions causing lengthening of affected extremity*
Congenital: • Femoral deficiencies • Tibial hemimelia • Fibular hemimelia • Pseudoarthrosis of tibia	*Reactive overgrowth:* • Post-traumatic overgrowth • Osteomyelitis • Inflammatory arthritis
Neurological disorder: • Poliomyelitis • Hemimyelomeningocele • Peripheral neuropathy	*Overgrowth syndromes:* • Gigantism with neurofibromatosis • Klippel-Trenaunay-Weber syndrome—typical and atypical forms • Beckwith-Wiedemann syndrome • Proteus syndrome • Idiopathic hemihypertrophy
Trauma: • Malunion • Physeal growth disturbance following epiphyseal injuries	
Developmental: • Infantile Blount's disease • Adolescent Blount's disease • LCPD • DDH	
General: • Idiopathic nonsyndromic hemiatrophy • Russell-Silver syndrome • Infection • Neoplasia • Irradiation • Iatrogenic following treatment of lesions around physis	

(LCPD: Legg-Calve-Perthes disease; DDH: developmental dysplasia of the hip)

Assessment of Leg-length Discrepancy

History

Assess the cause, magnitude of discrepancy, and previous treatment received. Family history is important for genetic diseases and dysplasias. Assess for unstable joints and/or weakness in limb. These help in future limb reconstructions and guide treatment. The unstable joints need to be stabilized and weaker limbs are left a bit short for ground clearance. Femoral lengthening is contraindicated with an unstable hip.

Assessment of Leg Length

Assess the real length, apparent length, and pelvic obliquity **(Figs. 43A and B)**. Abduction and adduction contractures of hip commonly cause apparent LLD. Approximately 10° of coronal plane contractures would produce 2–3 cm of LLD. Flexion contracture of hip would produce limb shortening while an equinus deformity of ankle would produce limb lengthening. Structural scoliosis similarly produces suprapelvic LLD. Measure the segmental length individually. Measurement by block method [keeping premeasured blocks below the short limb **(Fig. 44)**] reveals quite reproducible measure of limb length. In this method, blocks of premeasured sizes are placed under the short limb until the pelvis is squared. It can also guide the feasibility and

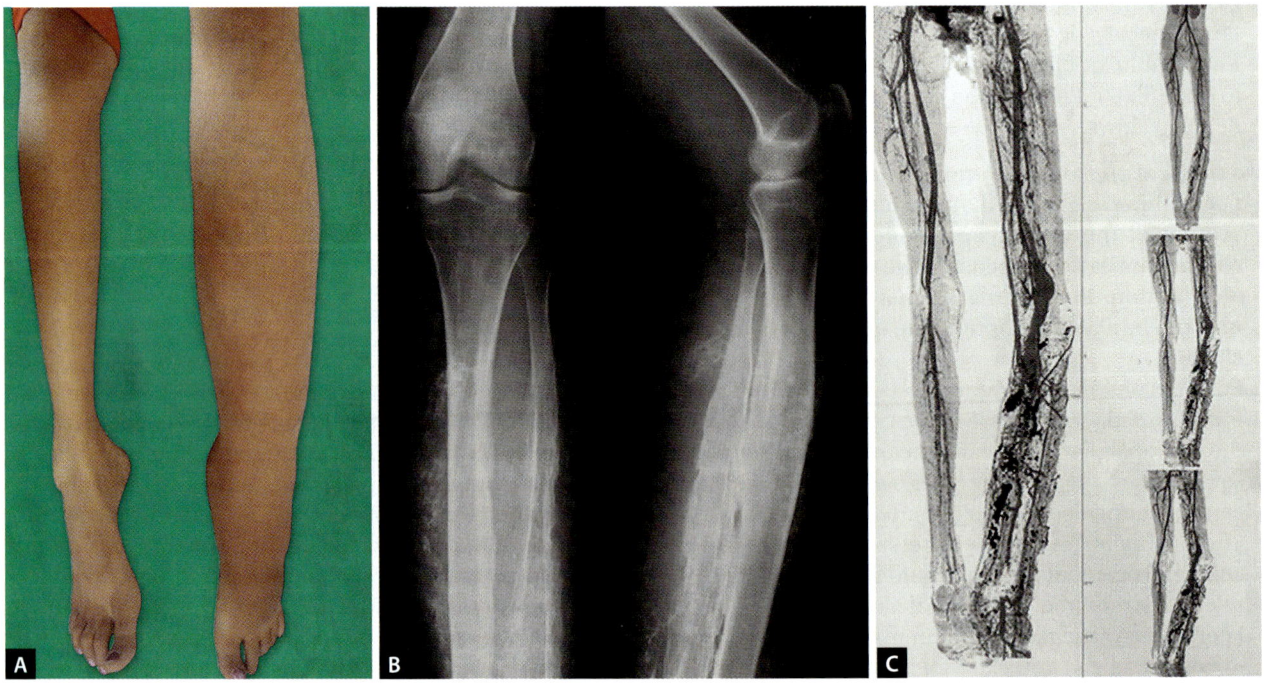

Figs. 42A to C: (A) Klippel–Trenaunay–Weber syndrome showing hypertrophy and lengthening of left lower limb; (B) The radiographs show numerous phleboliths and osteoperiosteal changes more marked in fibula; (C) The digital subtraction angiogram depicts the extensive vascular malformations.

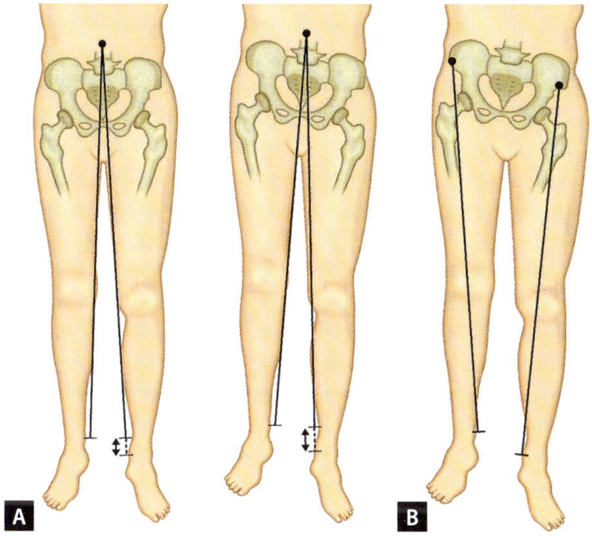

Figs. 43A and B: The assessment of (A) Apparent length and (B) real length.

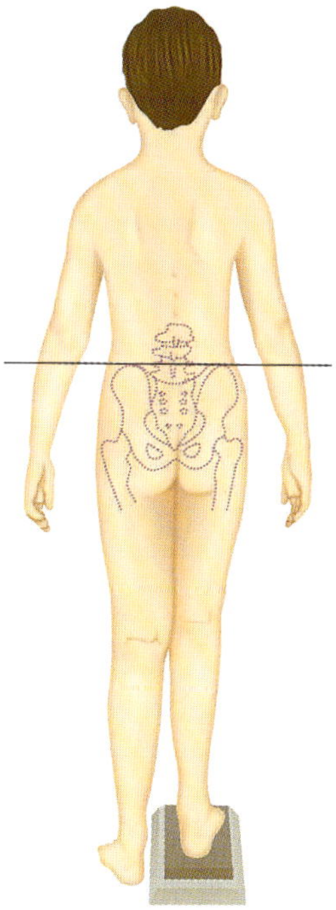

Fig. 44: The estimation of limb-length discrepancy (LLD) by block method. Measured blocks of wood or other suitable material are placed under the short limb (in the illustration right lower limb) until the ASIS (or iliac) crest becomes leveled. The total height of blocks gives the estimate of LLD.

adequacy of correction by giving a similar amount of shoe raise to the patient that will help physician to understand if the lengthening will "suit" the patient. Other crude and less reliable methods include the Allis test and Galeazzi test (*see* Chapter on "Pediatric Hip Joint Disorders"). Angular deformities such as valgus and varus at knee or congenital osseous malformations should also be assessed for other cause of possible limb shortening.

Radiographic Assessment of Limb Length

These methods are more accurate than clinical methods. There are five radiologic techniques that measure leg lengths directly. For any technique, it is essential that the limbs are kept straight with patellae pointing the roof and importantly same technique should be used for sequential measurements. In case of sagittal plane (flexion or extension) deformities each bone should be radiographed individually with a ruler with beam perpendicular and ruler parallel to the bone. The terminology is confusing, because names used for these techniques are inconsistent in the literature. What we call a scanogram today was actually a tightly collimated X-ray beam in the form of a slit used to expose the affected extremity.

- The ***teleradiograph*** **(Fig. 45A)** is a single exposure of both legs on a long, 35 × 90 cm (14 × 36 in) film. It is taken from 6-feet distance, usually with the patient standing and a radiopaque ruler placed on the cassette. Teleradiograph has the advantage of showing comparative angular deformities using a single exposure, but the large film is inconvenient to handle. The measurements are subject to magnification and cumbersome in assessment.
- The ***orthoradiograph*** **(Fig. 45B)** avoids magnification factor as here separate exposures of the hip, knee, and ankle are taken so that the central X-ray beam passes through the joints, giving true readings from the reference scale. The stitched film is still cumbersome and additionally an error may get introduced from the multiple exposures taken by moving the gun.
- The ***conventional scanogram*** **(Fig. 45C)** avoids magnification in the same way, but reduces the size of the resulting film by moving the film cassette beneath the patient between exposures. It is again plagued by the error from moving the cassette and cumbersome film. The patient has to remain still for three exposures and quite prominently the angular deformities cannot be measured.
- ***CT scanogram*** **(Fig. 46)** is a standard today for the readily available scale with the film, single exposure, known contraction/reduction scale, and demonstration of comparative deformities. Additionally, detailed study of the affected part can be taken simultaneously.
- Another technique similar to CT scanogram but bit more sophisticated called EOS® (low-dose biplanar radiography, slow, and fast) deploys a 3D scanner. The technique has the advantage of providing much less radiation amounting to <1/7–1/10 of that needed for CT scanogram but needs a skilled radiologist to align limbs for correct measurement of the limb lengths. Other advantages include true to size imaging without magnification (as wide 45 cm X-ray beams are used instead of divergent X-ray in conventional radiography), imaging during weight bearing in standing position and microdose protocol reducing the delivered dose still further.

Determining the skeletal age: Using radiography is in part a cumbersome and at best a rough method for assigning skeletal age to a patient, using available standards. All

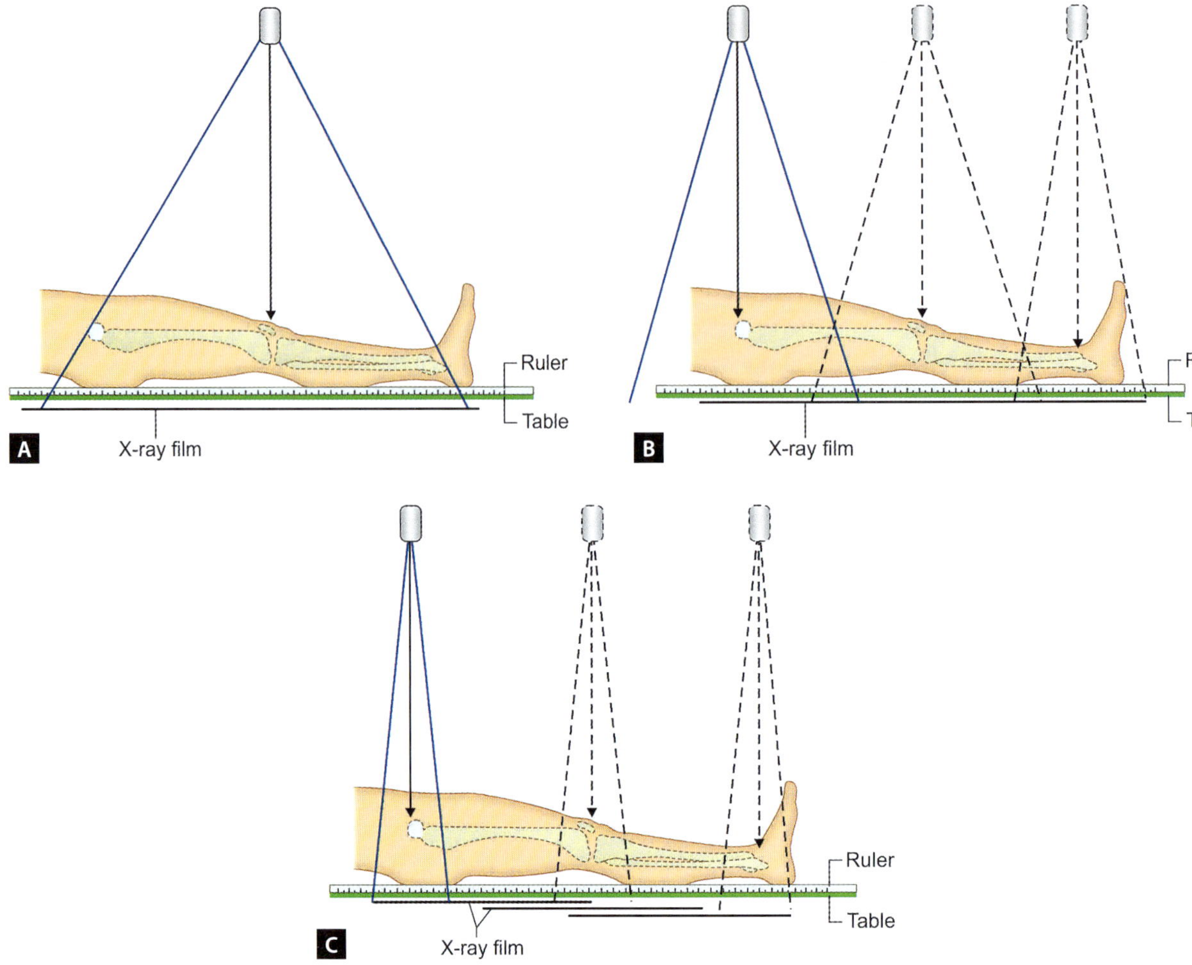

Figs. 45A to C: (A) Obtaining a teleradiogram; (B) An orthoradiogram; (C) A scanogram.

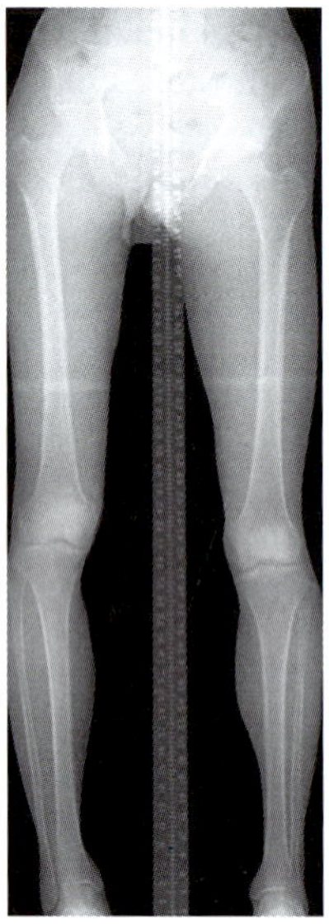

Fig. 46: Use of computed tomography for obtaining a scanogram is in fashion today due to ease of obtaining the same and quick imaging with ready scale for measurement assuring accuracy.

the standards are flawed by errors of assignment and capture, cannot exactly reproduce the variation in skeletal development and are difficult to extrapolate into accurate LLD resulting at maturity. The Greulich and Pyle method and the Tanner-Whitehouse method are commonly available for predicting the skeletal age. While in the former, a radiograph of the left hand and wrist is taken according to the technique described in the atlas, and this film is then compared with the standard radiographs of the appropriate gender, according to qualitative and quantitative criteria; the latter is a complicated system of assessment of 20 specific bony landmarks the scores of which are added after assignment to reveal a score telling the skeletal age. There is a high degree of interobserver and intraobserver variability associated with the use of these charts aside from the cumbersome procedure. It is interesting to note that using the Greulich and Pyle method Green and Anderson published data and charts of growth of boys and girls. It became clear from these studies that the *lower limb grows in length predominantly by the physis near knee (distal femur and proximal tibia) while the upper limb grows by the prominent activity from physis away from elbow (proximal humerus, distal radius).*

Estimating the Leg-length Discrepancy at Maturity

The treatment goal is chosen with respect to the discrepancy that would be present at maturity for most patients so analyzing the leg-length data is important with respect to LLD at skeletal maturity. For this purpose, these methods are commonly used:

- The growth-remaining method
- The arithmetic method
- The multiplier method
- The straight-line graph of Moseley

All three methods differ considerably in procedural details but have common principles. All have three stages comprising of estimation of the past growth followed by estimation of the future growth and lastly the prediction of effects of corrective surgery.

The growth-remaining method (Fig. 47): This is based on the published data from Green and Anderson studies. It relates leg lengths to chronologic and skeletal age. Their graphs describe the lengths of the legs of boys and girls related to age and can be used to determine the growth percentile of the child and the future growth of the long leg **(Fig. 47)**. This can be easily extrapolated to understand the effects of successful epiphysiodesis in distal femur or proximal tibia.

Advantages:

Based on skeletal age and describes the growth pattern well:

- It takes into account the child's growth percentile in predicting future growth.

Disadvantages:

- The inherent error in the Greulich and Pyle method of skeletal age estimation will be confounding to the charts (see above).
- Needs two sets of charts

Arithmetic method: This method is purely described to estimate the effect of epiphysiodesis and determine the timing of epiphysiodesis. The method was first described by White. It is a simple tool to use but has many small flaws that preclude accurate estimation. Also there are a lot of conditions that need to be satisfied before depending on the measured effect from this method.

- Firstly, this method is based on chronological age rather than skeletal age and assumes these critical growth-related statements:
  - Girls stop growing at the age of 14 years.
  - Boys stop growing at the age of 16 years.
  - The distal femoral plate grows 10 mm (3/8 in) per year.
  - The proximal tibial plate grows 6 mm (1/4 in) per year.
  - The discrepancy increases by 3 mm (1/8 in) per year.
- Secondly, these assumptions are fairly accurate only in children nearing growth completion so may be out of clinical range for epiphysiodesis as it requires some growth period to have significant effect.

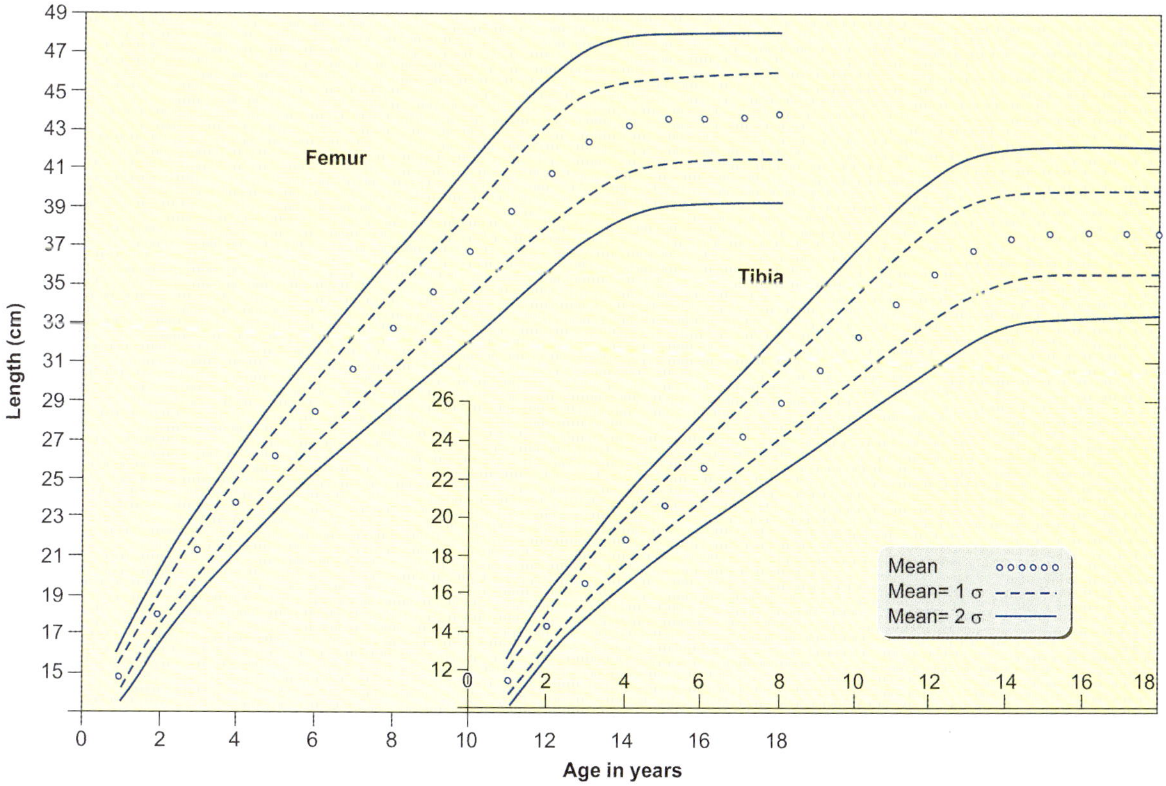

Girls Length of femur and tibia (including epiphyses)

Charts prepared in the growth study of the Children's Hospital Medical Center, Boston from data compiled in the Department of Maternal and Child Health, Harvard School of Public Health.
Further details are described in the following:
1. Harold BS, Robert BR, et al. Pediatrics. 1959;24(5, pt II):875-974.
2. Anderson M, Mussner MB, Green WT. Journal of Bone and Joint Surgery. 1964;46A:11997-1202.

Contd...

Contd...

Growth remaining in normal distal femur and proximal tibia following consecutive skeletal age levels

Means and standard deviations derived from Longitudinal series 50 Girls and 50 Boys

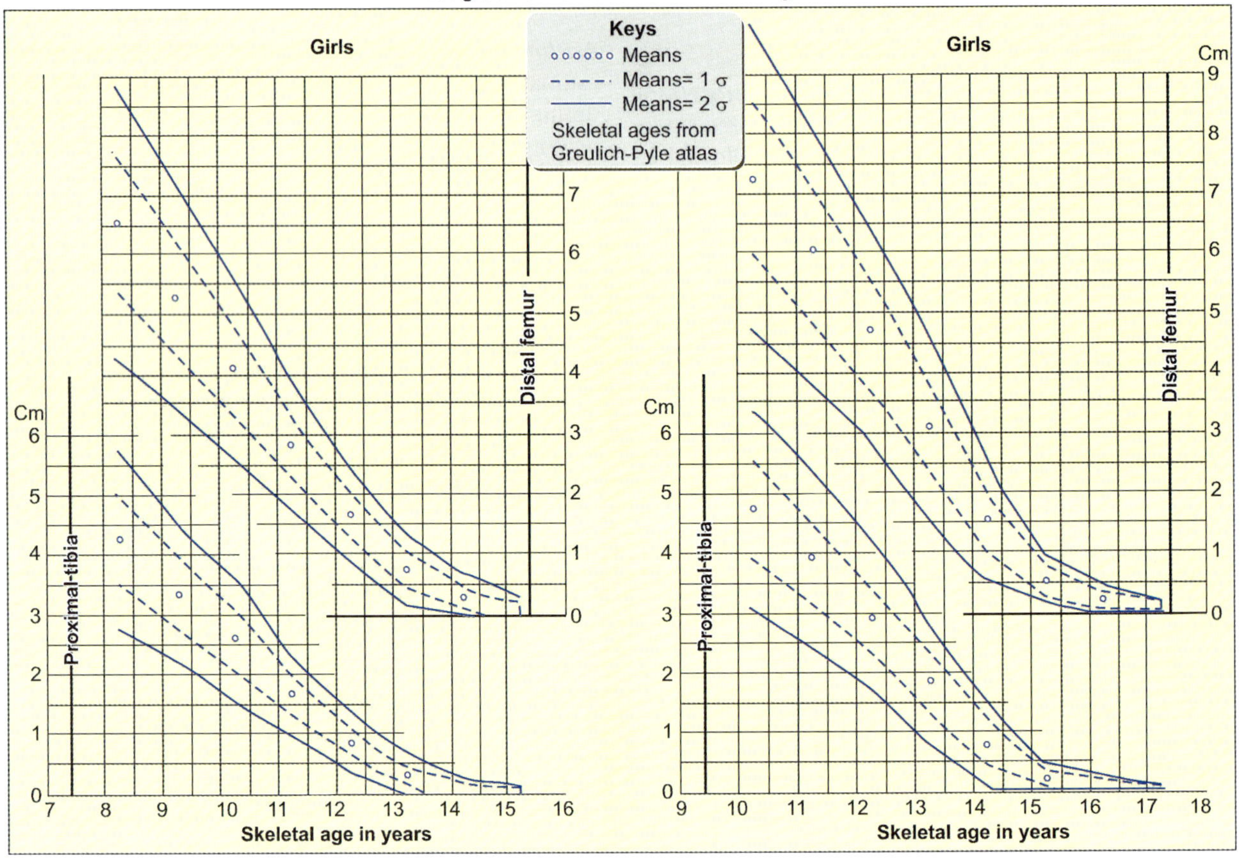

Assessment of past growth	**Prediction of future growth** (see charts adjacent to this table for predicting future growth)
1. Growth of both legs = Present length–first length 2. Present discrepancy = Length of long leg–length of short leg 3. Growth inhibition (growth of long leg–growth of short leg) / Growth of long leg	1. Plot present length of long leg on Green-Anderson leg length graph for appropriate sex 2. Project to right parallel to standard deviation lines until maturity to determine mature length of long leg 3. Future growth of long leg = Mature length – present length 4. Future increase in discrepancy = Future growth long × inhibition 5. Predicted discrepancy at maturity = Present discrepancy + future increase
Prediction of effect of surgery 1. The effect of epiphysiodesis of the distal femoral and proximal tibial plates for a given sex and skeletal age can be determined by the Green-Anderson growth = remaining graph 2. The effect of lengthening is not affected by growth	

Fig. 47: Growth-remaining method.
Source: The Children Medical Center, Boston, Massachusetts.

Thus, the method is limited for use in those children who are in the last few years of growth, whose discrepancies began at birth, whose maturation is not significantly advanced or delayed relative to their chronologic ages, and whose discrepancies are within the clinical range for epiphysiodesis.

Paley multiplier method: This method is based on Green and Anderson's growth graph. Multipliers for each age and sex are available as charts **(Table 5)** that can be used to calculate the possible discrepancy at maturity by the following formula:

$$Dm = \Delta \times M$$

where, Dm = LLD at skeletal maturity, Δ is the current LLD, M is the multiplier.

So for 2 cm of LLD at 4 years in a male child the estimated LLD at maturity will be 2 × 2 = 4 cm. The above formula

TABLE 5: The multiplier chart for lower limb.

Age (in Years + Months)	Boys	Girls
0 + 0 (at birth)	5.080	4.630
0 + 3	4.550	4.155
0 + 6	4.050	3.725
0 + 9	3.600	3.300
1 + 0	3.240	2.970
1 + 3	2.975	2.750
1 + 6	2.825	2.600
1 + 9	2.700	2.490
2 + 0	2.590	2.390
2 + 3	2.480	2.295
2 + 6	2.385	2.200
2 + 9	2.300	2.125
3 + 0	2.230	2.050
3 + 6	2.110	1.925
4 + 0	2.000	1.830
4 + 6	1.890	1.740
5 + 0	1.820	1.660
5 + 6	1.740	1.580
6 + 0	1.670	1.510
6 + 6	1.620	1.460
7 + 0	1.570	1.430
7 + 6	1.520	1.370
8 + 0	1.470	1.330
8 + 6	1.420	1.290
9 + 0	1.380	1.260
9 + 6	1.340	1.220
10 + 0	1.310	1.190
10 + 6	1.280	1.160
11 + 0	1.240	1.130
11 + 6	1.220	1.100
12 + 0	1.180	1.070
12 + 6	1.160	1.050
13 + 0	1.130	1.030
13 + 6	1.100	1.010
14 + 0	1.080	1.000
14 + 6	1.060	NA
15 + 0	1.040	NA
15 + 6	1.020	NA
16 + 0	1.010	NA
16 + 6	1.010	NA
17 + 0	1.000	NA

stands true for congenital anomalies producing LLD. For developmental conditions, i.e., postnatal LLD the following formula is used instead:

$$\Delta m = \Delta + I \times G$$

where, G is the growth remaining obtained from following equation—

$$G = L(M - 1)$$

and, I is Inhibition of growth obtained from following equation—

$$I = 1 - [(S - S')/(L - L')]$$

S and L are the current length of short and long legs.

S′ and L′ are the lengths of legs at any other date since LLD began.

Straight-line graph: With evolution of the technique, this has become a good tool for recording, analyzing, and predicting growth though it was initially designed only for presenting relative growth of legs in a simple graphical fashion. The principles for this method are:

- The growth of the legs can be shown graphically by straight lines.
- A nomogram can be used to determine the growth percentile from the skeletal age and leg length (Green and Anderson charts).

The straight line is nothing but the Green and Anderson growth curves manipulated by scaling the X-axis to make it in a linear equation **(Figs. 48A to C)**. The graphs are as accurate as the original curves. In the absence of active disease, a short leg will also grow in a straight line and the difference between the well leg and the short leg represents the growth inhibition (in other words can be translated as the effect of physiodesis if done on well leg). The growth rate is represented by the slope of straight line. Nomogram of skeletal age plotted for long limb depicts the growth percentile. The straight-line graph predicts the effect of physiodesis. Alteration in length is represented by vertical shift in growth line, shortening being represented by downward shift and vice versa. The slope is also decreased by a growth inhibitory procedure like physiodesis. The method is preferred over other methods for various advantages:

- It uses skeletal age and the actual growth pattern (Green and Anderson).
- The growth percentile is referred to predict future growth and the effect of surgery.
- It minimizes errors of skeletal age estimation.
- It can be used in children with large discrepancies, extreme growth percentiles, and marked alteration in pattern of maturation.

Goals of Treatment

The chief goal is obtaining the functional length of the limb LLD of <2–2.5 cm so that patient gains function maximally. If the LLD is a discrete problem then equalizing the limbs is primary aim while for a short limb associated with paralysis then often undercorrection by 1–2 cm is done. This is to clear floor by the weak short leg during the swing phase of gait. It should also be borne in mind that the spine should remain vertical after equalizing the limb lengths to prevent stress at spine. Sometimes, the deformities are too large to be corrected by limb lengthening or shortening—in such

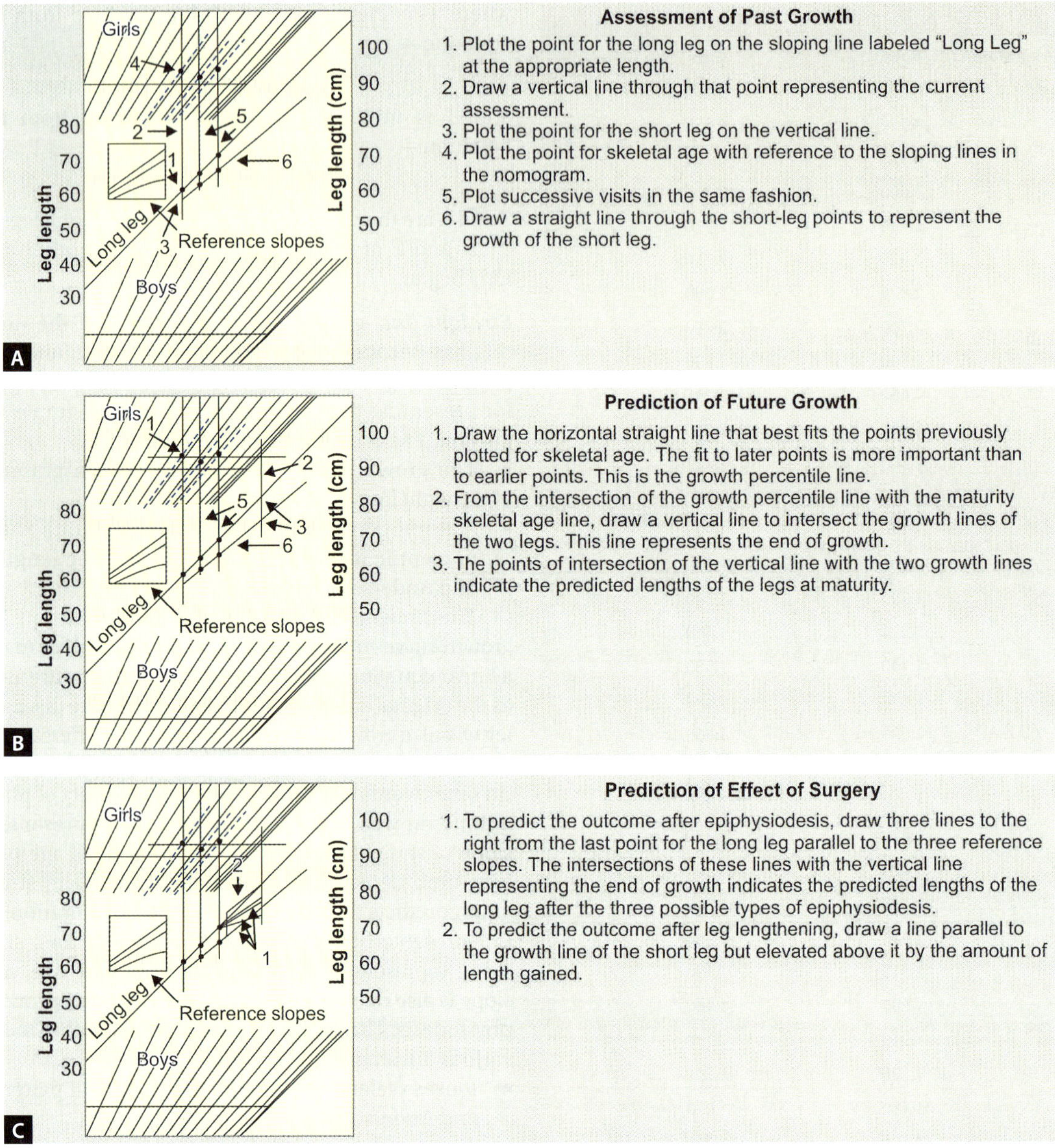

Figs. 48A to C: Straight-line graph.

cases, amputation and prosthetic fitting are reasonable and less morbid procedures, e.g., in PFFD. In a nutshell, the procedures for limb balancing fall into one of the broad categories, viz., observation and use of supportive methods (shoe lift/orthosis), limb-shortening procedure (acute shortening and fixation or gradual shortening by physiodesis), and limb-lengthening procedures.

General Principles of Treatment

- The decision to treat limb-length discrepancy depends on the predicted discrepancy at skeletal maturity.
- A patient with a predicted discrepancy of <2 cm requires no treatment, although a 1–2 cm shoe-lift can be used inside the shoe; sometimes a wedge is placed on the bottom of the shoe.
- For LLD between 2 and 6 cm, the reasonable treatment options are:
  - A shoe-lift **(Fig. 49)**
  - Epiphysiodesis
  - Skeletal shortening

  Lengthening is socially favored over shortening for advantages of height. Hence, shortening procedures are usually not appropriate for correction of >6 cm, because a disproportionate appearance results (smaller lower limbs compared to the body height) which may not be pleasing to the patient. It is better to leave the decision of shortening versus lengthening on the patient at LLD of 5–6 cm as this is a gray zone.
- Limb-lengthening should be performed for a patient with a predicted discrepancy between 6 and 17 cm at skeletal

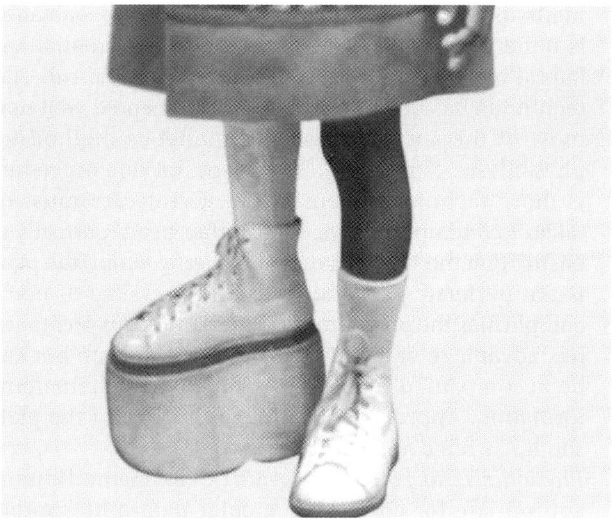

Fig. 49: Shoe lifts can be used for patients who do not wish for surgery; also it can be used in patients who are inappropriate for surgical correction. It should be, however, remembered that shoe lifts >5 cm are poorly tolerated.

maturity. This is commonly performed by osteotomy of the short bone and gradual lengthening with internal or external devices.

- A predicted discrepancy >17 cm often requires amputation and prosthetic fitting (see below).

Though intriguing one major limitation to limb-lengthening is the long period of external fixator required for the bone to consolidate. Two recent methods developed to circumvent this problem include:

1. Bone-lengthening using external fixation over an IM nail
2. Bone-lengthening from within, using IM nails

The use of lengthening IM nails offers the benefit of decreased pin tract complications and elimination of exposed hardware. These newer methods are particularly useful for patients with minimal growth potential or closed growth plates and are discussed later in detail below.

Prerequisites for Balancing the Limb Lengths

- Estimating the limb-length discrepancy correctly, growth remaining, skeletal age, and percentile of growth
- Correcting the associated deformities that have bearing on functional outcome prior to balancing the limb lengths.
- *Choose the site of correction:* A site that will leave the patient as symmetric as possible should be chosen particularly with respect to balancing the knee height [though maintaining the same is neither necessary (functionally or cosmetically) nor absolute, and the rule is freely flaunted in limb-balancing protocols].

The ***various methods*** used for height balancing or limb balancing are as follows:

Nonoperative/Ancillary Methods

Shoe lift: Shoe lift is the best option for those patients who do not agree or are not good candidates for surgical correction. The shoe lift is given only for walking patients for logical reasons. Cosmetically, up to 2 cm of the lift can be put inside the shoe to hide it and the remainder on the outside. It should be borne in mind that infinite shoe lift is not possible and lifts higher than 5 cm result in frequent ankle sprains (**Fig. 49**; you see ladies walking with high heels have unstable gaits and is not recommended; this is only one of the drawbacks of high heels!). This is due to the fact that muscles controlling the subtalar joint are not strong enough to resist inversion stress. For higher lift, an orthotic extension up the posterior is added for stability.

Prosthetic fitting: This is considered a treatment of last resort but is useful for patients with very large discrepancies (PFFD) and those with deformed and functionally useless feet (tibial, fibular hemimelia). The methods are detailed specifically in the respective headings elsewhere.

Limb-shortening Procedures

Epiphysiodesis: Better called physiodesis (as it is done to control the growth of physis and not epiphysis). This is a popular method and considered treatment of choice for the surgical correction of LLD. The major limitation is need for early capture of patient and consistent follow-up so that enough data is available for accuracy of the procedure. It is only suitable for children who have sufficient growth remaining and have sufficient leg-length data to enable a confident prediction of the discrepancy at maturity. Also corrections of 2–6 cm are favored with these methods and not more. One should recollect that distal femur and tibia contribute for 65% of the growth of lower extremity. The average contribution for distal femur is nearly 9 mm/year accounting for 37% while that of tibia is nearly 6 mm/year accounting for 28%. Also one should remember that males would typically grow till 16 years of age and females till around 14 years of age, so if there is 3 years of remaining growth then some 4.5 cm of correction can be achieved by combined physiodesis of distal femur and proximal tibia *The methods used for physiodesis can be either temporary or permanent*, the latter being preferred for correction of LLD often.

Temporary physiodesis: This was proposed by Blount's (dissuaded by the cumbersome methodology for permanent methods) to control the growth of physis temporarily so that:

- It can be done any time before achieving a particular age for permanent procedure.
- There is no need for accurate predictions of future growth from the charts.
- Growth would resume following later removal of the staples and both limbs would proportionately grow.

However, the method went into disfavor due to:

- Permanent fusion of the physis was quite common due to ensuing physeal damage from the operative procedure itself (periosteal elevation and stapling) and from the compression of physis due to increasing pressure.
- Extrusion, intra-articular migration of staples, and superficial bursitis caused by the staples commonly
- Asymmetrical growth arrest by the procedure
- Compensatory overgrowth occurred after removal of staples recurring the limb-length discrepancy.

The arrest of physis was done by placing three staples on each side till equalization of limb length is achieved (one staple breaks, two bend, or extrude). The staples are then removed requiring another surgery. Proponents have refined the procedure by placing the staples extraperiosteally so that intraoperative injury to physis does not occur and growth resumes after removing the staples, though other complications still can occur. Also the staples have changed from steel to vitallium for better strength and fixation so that they do not break or extrude.

Permanent physiodesis: For its more extensive use, detailed procedure and predictable growth alteration, it is the preferred method by most surgeons. The prerequisite for performing the procedure is accurate determination of remaining growth and hence the gain from the procedure if done. Permanent method is an all-or-nothing procedure that completely and permanently arrests physeal growth. It is imperative that the exact amount of desired shortening can be achieved only by performing the surgery at exactly the correct time. Performing the operation too late results in undercorrection otherwise performing it too early results in overcorrection. Because there is an advantage to being tall, it is better to err on the side of undercorrection than overcorrection. Slight discrepancies are well tolerated in population so commonly undercorrection of 0.5–1.0 cm is aimed for (commonly done by delaying surgery a bit). In general, the following points should be realized:

- The loss from proximal tibial physiodesis is 27%.
- Loss of growth from distal femur physeal arrest is 38%.
- If both the plates are fused, then there is 65% loss of remaining growth.

Tibial epiphysiodesis should be accompanied by concomitant proximal fibular physeal arrest, if the tibial shortening is >2.5 cm. The objective of the surgery is to produce a symmetric bony bridge that tethers the physis and prevents future growth. Permanent fusion can be achieved in two ways. Basically, the second method is an alteration of the first one to reduce cosmetic problem.

1. Conventional physiodesis—done through open method on both sides of growth plate. Incisions are placed on both the medial and lateral aspects of the knee so a total of four incisions are needed if both tibial and femoral epiphysiodeses are performed. A block of bone from both sides is removed and plate extirpated (curette or burr). The block is then replaced distorting the disposition of growth plate. This produces a bony bridge precluding the growth. Phemister removed a rectangular block **(Figs. 50A and B)**, two-thirds on the metaphyseal side and one-third on the epiphyseal side of the plate, and reversed it while replacing. White and Stubbins used a special chisel to remove a square block that is rotated 90° at replacement. Blount used a circular trephine to remove a cylindrical block that is also rotated 90° before replacing.
2. Physiodesis using Blount's staples **(Figs. 50C and D)**
3. *Percutaneous physiodesis* ***(Figs. 50E to G)***: Due to cosmetic dissidence of the open procedure, percutaneous methods were proposed. Percutaneous physeal ablation is done with a drill or burr, through small medial and lateral incisions, under image intensifier control. This technique has become popular and accepted well now most of the surgeons use percutaneous method for physiodesis, especially in tibia, femoral side procedure is more technically demanding. Great care must be taken to line up the image intensifier beam perfectly to ensure that the tool is in the plate. In the femur, the plate is not perfectly perpendicular and presence of notch complicates the procedure. The percutaneous technique has advantage of a wider excision of the plate but can be accompanied by excessive bleeding or hematoma formation. Approximately 50% of the area of the plate should be removed.
4. *Physiodesis using 8-plate* **(Fig. 50H)**: This method is more appropriate for correcting angular deformities rather than doing growth arrest.

The disadvantages of physiodesis in general include:

- Unsightly scar is the primary concern with the open procedure.
- As such it is a compensatory, and not a corrective operation. Well leg is being disturbed rather than correcting the affected leg; it makes the normal leg abnormal.
- Infection causing local growth disturbances and hypertrophic bone formation.
- Compared to lengthening, it results in a decrease in the patient's stature that may be undesirable.

Femoral or tibial shortening (Figs. 51A to D): Shortening of the femur has the same indications as physiodesis, but is preferred for patients who cannot be managed by physiodesis, either because they are too old or if confident prediction of their discrepancy at maturity cannot be made. It should be done in the mature patient when the discrepancy is known and unchanging, and the desired degree of correction can be obtained precisely. Shortening of the tibia also has been performed, but is very rarely done in cases where the femur cannot be shortened. The problems associated with tibial shortening are:

- The risk of neurovascular complications is higher in the tibia (proximity and tethering of neurovascular structures)
- The risk of delayed and nonunion
- Because of closed compartments, concomitant fasciotomy is advisable (scarring is a concern for this not really necessary surgery for deformity correction!) to reduce the risk of compartment syndrome.
- *Internal fixation is more difficult in the tibia:* Closed techniques cannot be used, because the bone is subcutaneous, and the muscles of the leg are slower to recover strength than those of the thigh (fibers of soleus are oriented obliquely and are short so unable to adjust to short length as well as long fibers of thigh muscles).

Functionally, shortening of up to 7.5 cm in femur and 5 cm in tibia are acceptable but practically femur is not shortened >5 cm and tibia not >3 cm.

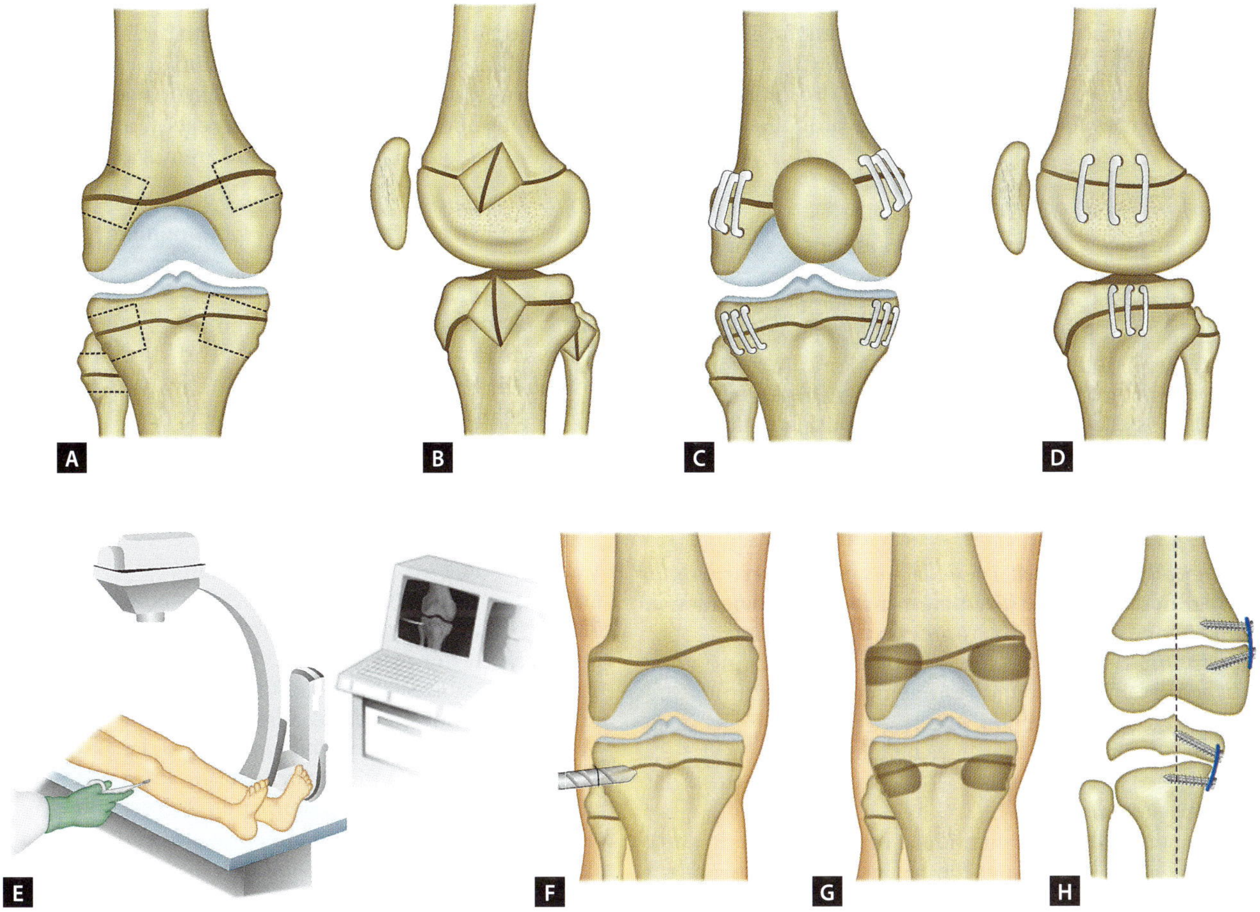

Figs. 50A to H: Various techniques of physiodesis. (A and B) The Phemister type technique; (C and D) The Blount staple technique; (E to G) The percutaneous method of physiodesis; (H) Physiodesis using 8-plate.

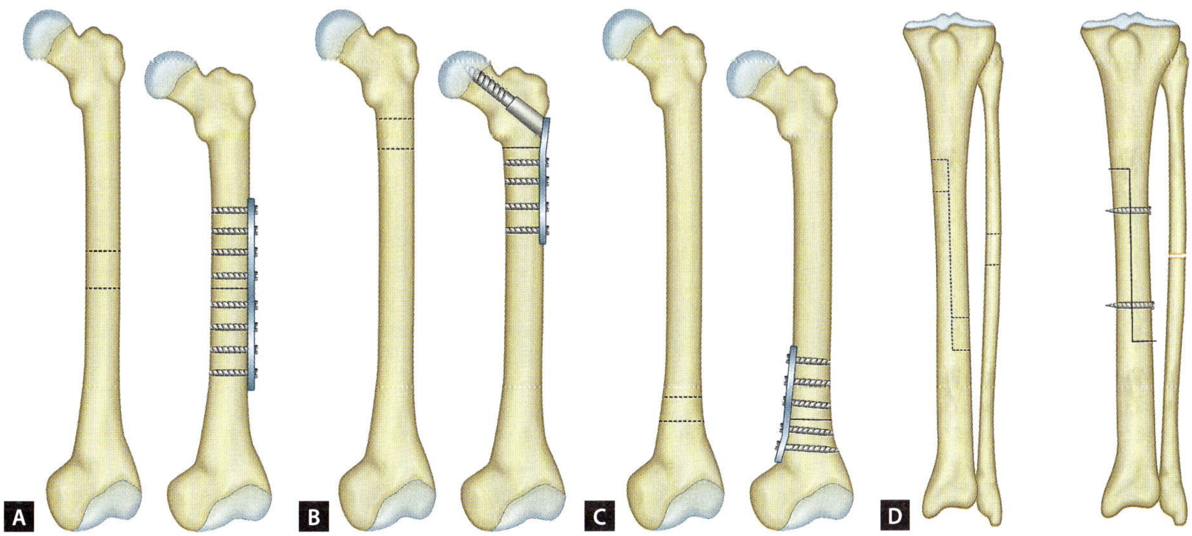

Figs. 51A to D: Various shortening procedures and sites for bones of lower limb.

Proximal femoral shortening: Shortening through the proximal femur is done at the level of the lesser trochanter. The fragments are fixed with blade plate fixation. Isthmus is proximal to most of the quadriceps origin, and therefore does not disadvantage the knee to the same extent as shortening done in the midshaft. Patients recover function better, fuller, and quicker. Scaring of lateral thigh and a second procedure to remove implant are the disadvantages. Closed femoral shortening as a special technique has been described using special set of instruments that cut the femoral shaft from within (IM approach) and then later fixed with a locked IM nail (*see* Chapter on "Nonunions and Malunions"). This method is not available apart from the proponents so not done.

Leg Lengthening Procedures

For the purpose of comprehensiveness, the inconsistent, experimental, and predominantly inadequate procedures of *growth stimulation* of bone are being mentioned initially. They have never been found to be adequately successful to excite surgeons, but they expand the thinking horizon out-of-box beyond conventional techniques to derive meaningful methods possibly in future by understanding of the bone physiology.

- *Implanting foreign materials next to the growth plate:* Irritation of growth plate leads to increased activity and growth of the physis.
- *Surgically constructed arteriovenous fistulae to stimulate:* This increases local circulation providing hyperactive and hypermetabolic environment to growth plate.
- *Stripping and lifting the periosteum by packing bone beneath it:* Periosteum has been considered to be the biggest tether preventing excess growth of the physis so disrupting the same may have benefit in this regard.
- *Electrical stimulation:* Most intriguing but most inconsistent reports.

Lengthening was first mentioned in the 18th century and next detailed by Codivilla at the beginning of the twentieth century. Though sounding logical and "socially acceptable" notion of a taller guy, lengthening procedures are cumbersome to patient and associated with many surgical complications. Instant lengthening procedures for femur and tibia have been described but they are limited by the extent of length gain and are not favored. Gradual lengthening methods are most commonly preferred using different constructs.

General principles for gradual limb-lengthening:

- These procedures should not be done for shortening <6 cm as the morbidity of procedures for leg-shortening procedures is much less than lengthening procedures.
- Femur can be lengthened up to 10 cm and tibia up to 7 cm after which the risks outweigh the benefits. >15–20 cm lengthening (total) is never advisable and if required then can be better combined with shortening of other leg.
- Gradual lengthening is not recommended if there is <60° of flexion at knee (Wagner). In general, it is believed that lengthening of the femur should be discontinued if there is a knee flexion contracture >10°, or knee flexion <30° at any time even during the distraction process itself. Lengthening can be started again, if movements are gained and contracture stretched, before consolidation of the regenerate prevents it. It has been found that patients regain flexion in the first year after lengthening if >30° of flexion is maintained throughout the lengthening. Maintaining extension is more important.
- Distraction is discontinued, either when the goal has been achieved or an unresolvable complication (usually loss of motion) supervenes.
- In the consolidation period, dynamization of the device should be done to subject the bone to cyclic longitudinal loading and stimulate bone formation.
- Corticalization (three cortices visible on two radiographs and the appearance of a medullary cavity) are considered signs of adequate strength, to guide removal of the device.

Surgical methods of lengthening: Wagner technique: Wagner's device **(Fig. 52A)** is a development over older devices like Anderson's device and was first used in North America in 1973.

- It is unilateral.
- It uses half-pins (not through-and-through pins, so useful in femur).
- It is small and light and allows ambulation.
- Lengthening is easy to do by just turning the knob at one end.
- It is adjustable in varus-valgus and AP angulation but not rotation.

Lengthening using Wagner frame is a three-step surgical procedure. The first involves osteotomy, releasing soft tissues, and applying the device. Lengthening is then continued. At the end of the lengthening phase, a second procedure involves bone-grafting the lengthening gap, and fixator removal is done. Plating the bone at this stage is advised by and performed by Wagner. Later when the bone has achieved sufficient strength, a third procedure is done to remove the plate. The plating is not recommended following fixator removal due to contaminated pintracts, so newer methods that involve neither plating nor grafting were searched.

Orthofix technique ***(Fig. 52A)****:* De Bastiani and colleagues developed the Orthofix device applied to bone with two sets of conical screws. The pin blocks move along a rail placed beside the pins. It is technically similar in operation to the Wagner device, but it offers more stability. The disadvantage is that it has a more cumbersome method of elongation and is not easily adjustable once in place.

Distraction physiolysis: Distraction physiolysis was pioneered by Ring. It is achieved by applying a distraction force across the physis until it fractures. Lengthening is then done by gradual distraction. This major disadvantage is that the lysis is sudden and painful, and not well tolerated. In the process of physiolysis, the physis can be injured, thus further compounding LLD. Due to higher complication rate, it should be done by surgeons versed in procedural detail and should be done very near the end of growth, to minimize the LLD if physeal damage occurs.

Ilizarov technique using ring fixators ***(Fig. 52B)****:* They are technically more complex than the Wagner and Orthofix devices but are highly versatile. Ilizarov method can not only lengthen limb but also correct the deformity in coronal, sagittal, and axial planes if required simultaneously including translation of fragments. They allow intermediate adjustments and have been consistent in success. Also they can be fixed in trifocal manner controlling more than two segments and can extend across joints. Frame assembly is applied to the bone using the tensioned through-and-

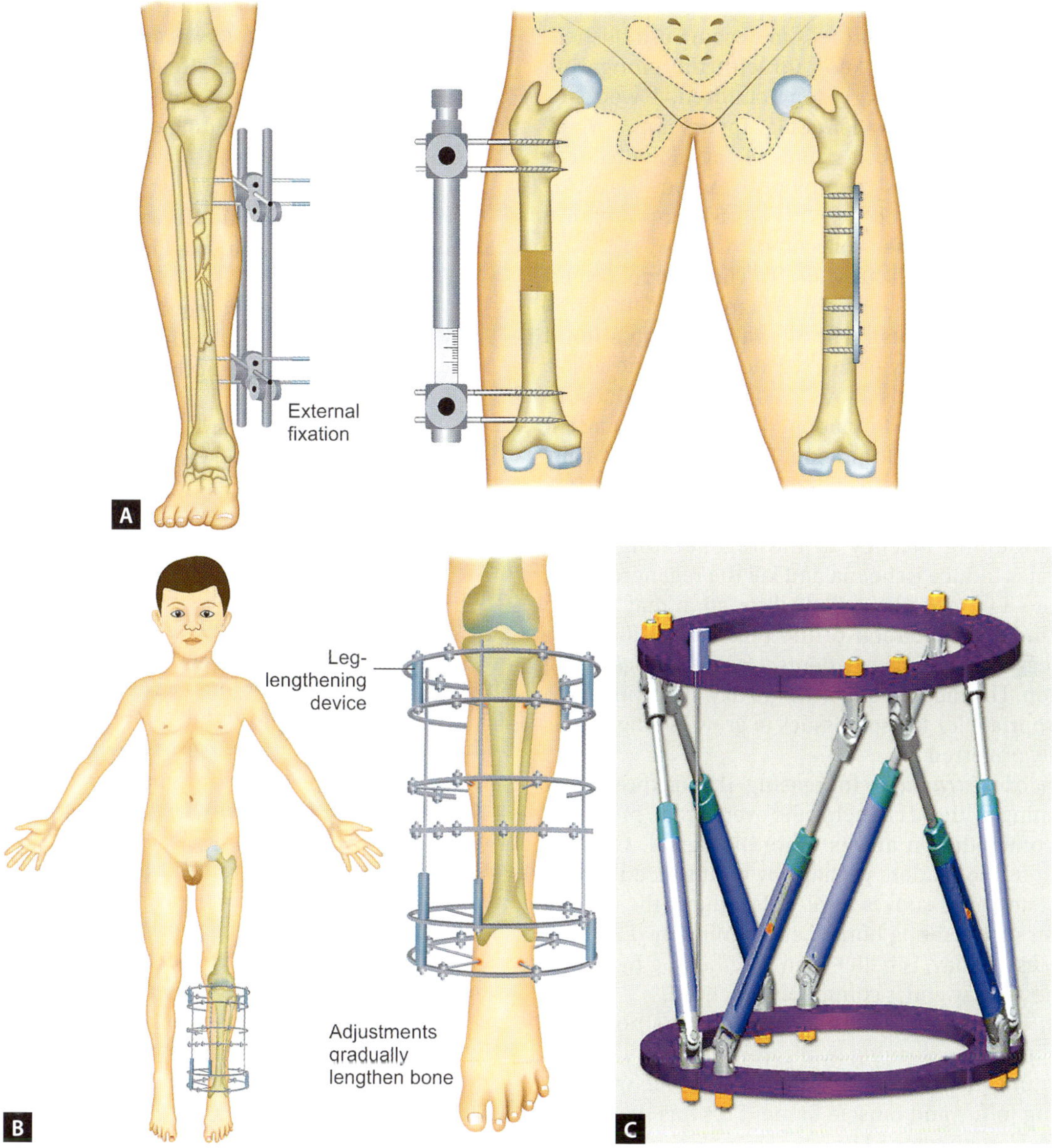

Figs. 52A to C: Some of the surgical limb lengthening methods. (A) Wagner type lengthening device or Orthofix device (shown here) which is more appropriate for femur as other methods are not so appropriate for this bone; (B) Ilizarov ring fixators are more appropriate for leg bones. (C) The other method is to use a Taylor spatial frame that can correct deformities in many planes also along with lengthening of the limb.

through wires attached to rings. Rancho modification evolved to provide unilateral fixation possibility using half-pins.

Principles of Ilizarov method:

- *Biological:*
  - *Distraction histogenesis:* Controlled biological distraction of tissues in a vascular environment can lengthen the tissues indefinitely according to Ilizarov.
  - *Tissue modeling:* Allowing physiological stress on tissues favors modeling and tissue development in consolidation phase.
- *Minimal disturbance of the bone:* Ilizarov recommended corticotomy—a low-energy osteotomy in which the cortex only is cut taking care not to disturb the medullary contents and the periosteum is maintained in continuity. The idea is to prevent any osteonecrosis (thermal or vascular damage) and allow for quick formation of regenerative tissue.
- *Location of lengthening site:* The lengthening is preferably done in the metaphysis, where the bone is metabolically more active. Here, there are greater numbers of active osteoblasts to participate in the process of regeneration. Also, larger diameter gives greater stability to fixation pins or wires.
- *Number of lengthening sites:* The frame can be applied in monofocal, bifocal, or trifocal manner. The lengthening can be isolated or combined with compression at the docking site. Dual lengthening by creation and fixation of more than two segments of the same bone make it possible to lengthen a single bone both proximally and distally at the same time **(Fig. 52C)**.

- *Delay before distraction (latency period):* This is done to allow the osteogenic process to become established. Osteogenesis can then keep up with the elongating gap. Delays of 5 days for young children, 1 week for adolescents, and 10 days for adults appear appropriate. The delay is increased by a couple of days if inadvertent injury to IM contents (complete osteotomy) and/or injury to periosteum occur; without risking premature consolidation of deemed corticotomy.
- *Rate of distraction:* Ilizarov and Deviatov recommend a distraction rate of 1 mm/day (Wagner used 1.5 mm/day for his apparatus). The distraction rate should just exceed the ability of the regenerating bone in the gap to form bone. This allows a continuous process of lengthening and bone formation. If the rate is too fast, it will inhibit regenerate formation. The rate is periodically adjusted based on the quality of the regenerate; it is slowed if radiographs show inadequate regeneration and a widening lucency in the regenerating bone. Faster rates induce ischemia and kill the regenerate that turns into a fibrous tissue. Slow distraction may lead to premature consolidation of the regenerate. Rate can be increased in younger patients with good regenerate formation. Distraction rate of 1 mm/day also appears to be appropriate for the soft tissues to grow in length so is generally preferred.
- *Rhythm of distraction:* Increasing the frequency of lengthening, without changing the overall rate, promotes faster consolidation and is more biological. Gradual continuous elongation, perhaps by a motorized device as suggested by Ilizarov is ideal. This reduces the tension stress on regenerating bone. Lengthening by 0.25 mm, four times per day, is better than lengthening by 1 mm, one time per day and is commonly practiced.
- *Amount of lengthening:* Principally, there is no upper limit to tissue lengthening by ilizarov method but it has been found that permanent changes do occur in the adjoining joints and muscle tissue. This has been seen with tibial lengthening >11%.
- *Dynamization:* Cyclic loading of the regenerate promotes osteogenesis. The ring fixators have the advantage of allowing dynamic loading of the lengthening gap throughout the period of fixation. This is produced through the trampoline effect of the tensioned wires that elastically compress and distract regenerate with movements and axial loading of the limb and assembly. The Ilizarov construct of thin wires and circumferential rings provides rigidity against bending in the sagittal and coronal planes, but allows flexibility in the axial direction, allowing slight axial movement in response to applied loads.
- *Consolidation:* A period equal to that for lengthening has to be used for allowing regenerated bone to develop adequate strength and then the fixator is removed.
- *Lengthening index:* This is the number of months of external fixation required per centimeter of lengthening. It is generally between 1 and 1.5 months per centimeter, and tends to be greater for lesser lengthening.

Lengthening over an intramedullary rod **(Figs. 53A to G)**: Using any of the external fixator-based systems for lengthening numerous unsightly scars result, because of the multiple percutaneous pins or wires used to achieve sufficient stability. They are also kept for long periods so are cumbersome. It is possible to use an IM rod to maintain alignment during both the distraction and consolidation phases, and the external device only during the lengthening phase (GLONE, gradual lengthening over nail using external fixator). In this way, the number of percutaneous tracts can be reduced; the external device can be removed at the conclusion of lengthening itself. Lengthening over the rod has the disadvantage that commonly the axis cannot be changed during the lengthening process which is often required in case of femoral lengthening. Because the anatomic axes of the femur and tibia are not collinear, elongation in this manner increases valgus of the mechanical axis of the leg. An implanted nail with fixation into proximal and distal epiphysis and gradual lengthening is a novel concept. Usually, the lengthening is achieved by mechanical lengthening of the nail, however, newer implants using less cumbersome methods have been developed.

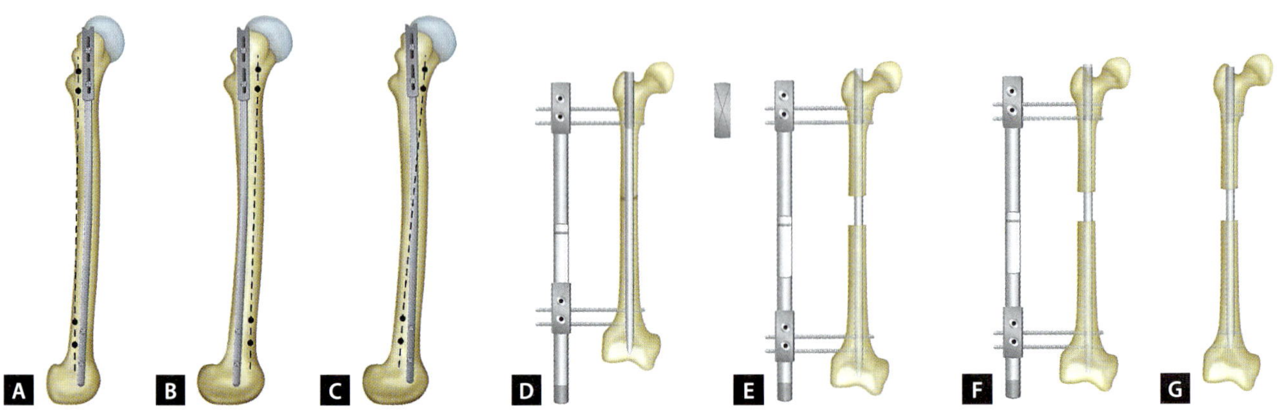

Figs. 53A to G: Combined method of lengthening of limb using external fixator and intramedullary nail. The latter acts to prevent losing the track and causing malformation of bone.

Complications of lengthening:

- Deformity and bowing at lengthening site due to soft tissue tension
- Pin tract infection
- *Mechanical failure:*
    - Pins breakage
    - Pin loosening
    - Bending of ring loss of tension in wires
- Fracture through the lengthening gap may occur due to increased compressive forces across from the tensioned soft tissue.
- Hypertension may be seen during lengthening—the mechanism is not clear, but it resolves with shortening of the gap and may not recur when lengthening is resumed.
- Subluxation of the knee may occur during femoral lengthening.
- Dislocation of the hip may be seen particularly in pathological conditions at hip or operated hips. Hamstring tightness is the main cause.
- *Delayed union:* It is common to see the delayed consolidation of the regenerate, understanding the cause, and defining it as delayed are both difficult.
- Femoral lengthenings are more prone to complications than tibial lengthening. The complication rate increases with lengthening exceeding 25% of the initial bone length.
- Lengthening the tibia >14% slows its growth—though the effect is inconsistent and not very clinically significant, but is sure a complication of lengthening of bone.

PATELLAR INSTABILITY

Pain secondary to patellofemoral dysfunction is a common disorder of the knee. The various forms of patellar instabilities seen are:

- *Traumatic:*
    - Seen commonly in sports injuries usually due to direct blow
- *Chronic patellar instability (dislocation):*
    - Often follows primary traumatic event
    - Associated with malalignment and other predisposing factors.
- Habitual dislocation of patella—often a congenital form of patellar instability.

Acute Traumatic Patellar Dislocation

This is the second most common cause of traumatic hemarthrosis of the knee. In a subluxation, the patella slips but immediately goes back into trochlear groove (TG); there is never an instance of complete separation of articular surfaces that lock the knee. In a true patellar dislocation, the patella locks the knee following complete separation of articular surfaces and reduces with some maneuver (usually when the knee is straightened). Though, in recurrent episodes later, the patella may spontaneously reduce after a dislocation. When a patella dislocates, the chance of another dislocation is around 45%. This is especially greater if there are associated predisposing factors (see recurrent patellar instability). After two dislocations, the risk of further episodes of dislocation is even higher nearing 70-80%. Recurrent episodes are usually not associated with hemarthrosis (may have reactive joint effusion). Women are more likely to sustain a patellar dislocation injury than men and are also more likely to become chronic dislocators. The dislocation is seen highest in the young adults in second to third decades.

Mechanism of Injury

Knee flexion and valgus have been noted as the leading mechanism of injury associated with patellar dislocation along with a lateral force directly on patella. Sports and dance are the two most common gross mechanisms for patellar dislocation. Isolated direct blows on patella causing dislocations are less common.

Pathoanatomy: The following are commonly observed with patellar dislocation:

- Hemarthrosis
- Medial patellofemoral ligament (MPFL) tear
- Medial retinacular tear
- Capsular injury
- Osteochondral injuries

Clinical Evaluation

Evaluate prior history of a dislocation in same knee or the contralateral knee (six times chances of becoming chronic), the family history of patellar dislocation. Examine for hyperlaxity, knee alignment, rotational malalignment of the limb, muscle mass, injury to capsule and medial retinaculum, and locking due to osteoarticular fragment. Patellar apprehension and hypermobility may be painful unless local anesthetic is injected in the joint. Local skin contusion on the medial side indicates medial structure rupture and if this extends distally examine for MCL rupture also.

Radiology

Obtain plain radiographs of the knee in:

- Anteroposterior projection for articular injuries to tibia
- Lateral—condylar hypoplasia screening, patella alta or baja, hemarthrosis, and osteochondral fracture
- Mercer-Merchant view—patellar tilt, osteochondral fragment, and patellar malalignment

Computed tomography scan: To evaluate the various predisposing factors (see below). CT scan gives a clearer picture of patellofemoral alignment, the presence of osteochondral defects, patellar tilt, translation, tibial tuberosity (TT): TG distance, and trochlear dysplasia.

Magnetic resonance imaging may help in evaluating the ligaments (MPFL, retinaculum) but provides no further information than this.

Natural History of Acute Patellar Dislocation

The patellar dislocation is associated with various problems in the knee over ensuing period in a significant number of patients (>50%).

- Some level of osteoarthrosis of the patellofemoral joint
- Recurrent patellar dislocations in 40% patients

- Recurrent patellar subluxation (milder form of recurrent patellar instability)
- Anterior knee pain
- Long-standing muscle dysfunction

Treatment

Because the prognosis of untreated disease is not so favorable so guided and aggressive treatment is commonly favored. Nonsurgical treatment is commonly recommended initially.

- Acute phase management should apply the PRICE principle (protection, rest, ice, compression, and limb elevation). They help in a number of ways to tackle the initial inflammation that causes tissue weakening and delays the healing process. Weakened tissue is difficult to reconstruct if planned, also if there is active inflammation surgery is associated with significant incidence of arthrofibrosis. A period of immobilization is beneficial as it gives time to heal the disrupted medial structures. The best outcomes have been seen in patients treated with splint for 3 weeks. Posterior splint and plaster cast are both recommended while the latter may be used for longer periods of immobilization. Indications for longer immobilization (>3 weeks) are few and include MCL injury or associated condylar fracture. Also, immobilization for only 3 weeks only avoids muscle atrophy, knee joint restrictions, and retropatellar crepitation.
- Quadriceps strengthening is initiated during the acute phase. The static exercises are initiated during the period of immobilization. Quadriceps electrical stimulation [transcutaneous electrical nerve stimulation (TENS)] is introduced later or for those unable to pursue the exercises due to pain. Electrical stimulation may also help reduce the knee joint effusion.
- McConnell taping may be done after 2–3 weeks to restore proper alignment and also control pain. With proper alignment, vastus medialis oblique (VMO) retraining is initiated. Successful taping reduces pain while performing painful activities such as stepping down from a stool. The goal of taping is to optimize patellar positioning and facilitate better activation of the medial patellar stabilizers (especially the dynamic stabilizer VMO).
- The overall emphasis of nonsurgical treatment then is to build up the quadriceps muscle on the front of the thigh and in particular the VMO muscle. Stretching of the structures on the outside of the knee (ITB and the lateral retinaculum) may be simultaneously attempted.
- Orthotics may be prescribed in rehabilitation period to improve the alignment of the foot and ankle (as for pes planus, etc.).

Surgical management: This is indicated in the following situations:

- Osteochondral fracture fragment requiring removal—often done arthroscopically
- Fracture of lateral tibial condyle (from valgus injury) requiring elevation and stabilization
- *Disruption of MPFL-VMO complex requiring reconstruction:* The rationale is less clear as it has been found that with MPFL tear the incidence of recurrent patellar instability is less compared to those who have intact ligament (possibly the latter group has lateral femoral condylar hypoplasia causing recurrence than a primary ligament injury)
- Subsequent redislocation
- Patient that fails to improve on conservative treatment and has symptoms of instability.
- The two most common surgical options are arthroscopic retrieval of osteochondral fracture fragment ± medial plication and reconstruction of the MPFL.

Recurrent Dislocation of Patella

When patella dislocates more than once it is termed "recurrent" (older definition of >3 episodes is a mere confirmation that dislocation is truly recurrent and patient is not just a chance dislocator!) as far as the management perspective is concerned. "Recurrent" specifically denotes the traumatic etiology while the term habitual dislocation refers to congenital condition where the patella dislocates every time knee flexes and is associated with quadriceps contracture. Recurrent patellar dislocation is a common sequel to acute patellar dislocation as noted above and is associated with quite significant disability. Both come under the spectrum of chronic patellar instability. Patellofemoral arthritis is ultimately frequent sequelae to recurrent and also acute patellar dislocation.

Pathophysiology and Pathoanatomy

The first episode of patella dislocation usually goes uneventful if proper management is done and no predisposing factors are present. The degree of trauma associated with the first dislocation is an important indicator of subsequent dislocation. As against to the common belief (and the so called hype created for the role of MPFL in patellar stabilization), in patients who have MRI-documented disruption of the medial retinaculum and the MPFL, the incidence of subsequent patellar dislocation was found to be lower than in patients without retinacular injury. This finding may be concurred by the fact that patellar dislocation in the absence of MPFL trauma is indicative of coexisting patellofemoral dysplasia. The following are the common predisposing factors identified in recurrent dislocators:

- Previous patellar dislocation
- *Soft tissue factors:*
    - Ligamentous laxity (Ehlers-Danlos syndrome)
    - Dysplastic VMO muscle
    - Medial patellofemoral ligament insufficiency
    - Lateral retinacular contracture or/and ITB contracture
- *Alignment of the limb and relation of patella to femur:*
    - Familial lateral disposition of patella
    - Patella alta
    - Genu valgum
    - Increased Q-angle

- Increased TT:TG distance
- Excessive lateral patellar tilt
- Femoral anteversion
- "Miserable malalignment syndrome" (James, et al.)—all three increase Q-angle:
  1. Femoral anteversion (Squinting patella)
  2. Genu valgum ± medial femoral torsion
  3. External tibial torsion ± pronated feet
- *Bony deformity/dysplasia/hypoplasia:*
  - Trochlear dysplasia
  - Lateral femoral condyle hypoplasia
  - Small patella—may be caused by partial patellectomy.

Biomechanics

The stabilizing mechanisms for patella: Patellar motion and stability (the so called patellar tracking) is affected by the complex interaction of muscles, ligaments, bone morphology, and lower extremity alignment. The position of patella in trochlea is maintained by the ligaments and bony conformity (the static stabilizers) while the tracking and mobility in guided path is mainly a function of the dynamic stabilizers and the compressive effect of extensor mechanism. Following are the studied stabilizers of patella:

- *Passive stability:*
  - Medial patellofemoral ligament (*see* detailed anatomy in Chapter on "Sports Medicine: Knee"): The MPFL is the primary soft-tissue restraint to lateral translation of the patella during the initial 20–30° of knee flexion. MPFL has been identified as the essential lesion for recurrent dislocations of patella; however, recently it has been found that less than half of the patients with torn MPFL become recurrent dislocators. This ligament is most taut in full extension, with the quadriceps contracted, and assists in guiding the patella into the trochlea during the early stages of flexion. MPFL has femoral origin between medial epicondyle and adductor tubercle and attaches to the upper third of the medial surface of patella. The fibers of ligament blend variably with the fibers of VMO providing a dynamic component of stability to it. Femoral attachment is the usual site of MPFL avulsion.
  - Medial inferior stability is conferred partially by the medial patellotibial and patellomeniscal (attaches to inferior pole and anterior horn of medial meniscus) ligaments.
  - Lateral ITB and the retinaculum, lateral patellofemoral ligament (a thickening of retinaculum)
  - Bony conformity—TG morphology, patella height, and tracking
- *Dynamic stability* ***(Figs. 54A and B)****:*
  - *Vastus medialis obliquus:* Pulls the patella in a direction around 55° medially providing the necessary medial tug to patella during tracking in the TG in extension. It counters the Q-angle lateral force vector on patella.
  - *Compression dynamic force:* Once engaged in the trochlea and with neutralizing lateral and medial tug forces the main patellofemoral joint force remains that of compression provided by the increasing force vectors of the quadriceps and patellar tendons.

Clinical Features

Patient has symptoms of recurrent instability at knee, particularly during pitching activities and movements that require rotation at the knee, like turning. Also patient complains of instability while stair climbing and general activities that involve tracking of patella in compression. Patient often complains of knee hurting all of the time and often giving way; sometimes, it slips out and causes a lot of pain.

- The gait of patient changes due to adaptive changes to avoid the recurring episodes. There may be hyperpronation of feet and valgus thrust at knee while walking.

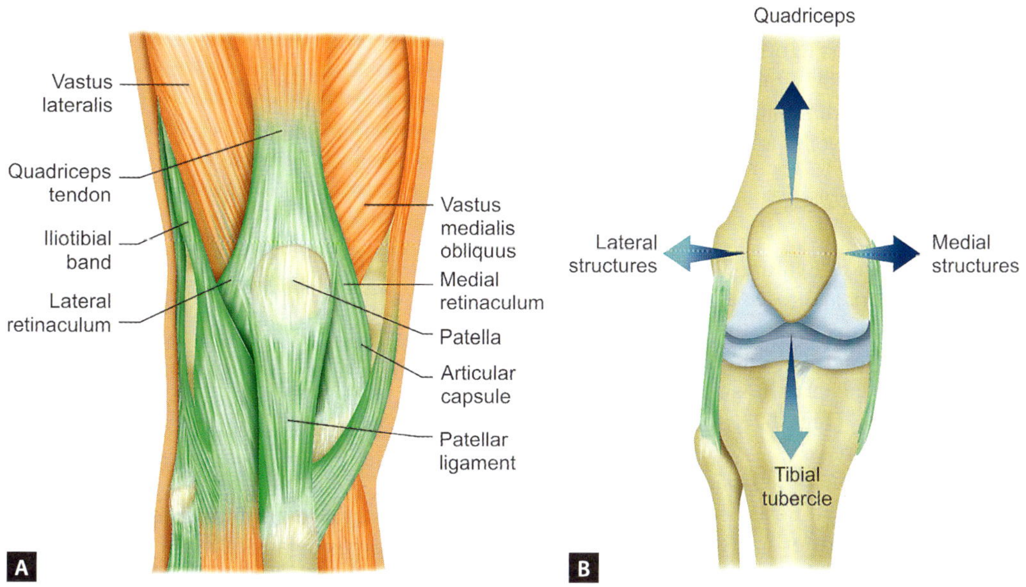

Figs. 54A and B: Dynamic stability of patellofemoral joint. (A) Muscles attached to patella; (B) Forces applied by various muscles on patella.

- Examine for patella baja, Q-angle, extensor lag, patellofemoral crepitus, and apprehension by Fulkerson's relocation test.
- Evaluate the quadriceps mass by thigh and leg girth measurements and signs of generalized laxity.
- Look for signs of damage in extensor apparatus particularly medially in retinaculum and for MPFL tear. Palpate for articular cartilage damage and facet tenderness.
    - Medial-sided patellar tenderness over retinaculum (over MPFL)
    - *Increase in passive patellar lateral translation (hypermobility of patella;* ***Fig. 55****):* Divide patella hypothetically into four equal quadrants mediolaterally and translate the patella by firm thrust laterally. The translation is measured in quadrants of translation (midline of patella is considered "0"), and also should be compared to contralateral side.
        - *Normal motion is <2 quadrants of patellar translation:* Lateral translation of medial border of patella to lateral edge of TG is considered abnormal amount of translation.
    - ***Fulkerson relocation test:*** The knee is passively supported in extension, and the patella is gently subluxated laterally. Then the knee is gently flexed while resisting the patella to relocate. If this maneuver results in sudden pain or apprehension and especially if the patient relates the sensation to his or her presenting symptoms test is considered positive. It is further reinforced if the symptoms subside by manually pulling the patella medially and repeating the test.
    - *J sign* indicates poor patellar tracking (**Fig. 56**; characteristically seen with patella alta)
        - There is excessive lateral translation of patella in extension which slips back ("pops") into femoral groove as the patella engages the trochlea early in flexion.
    - In prone position, examine for rotational malalignment, Ely's test (for rectus tightness).
    - Examine for tight ITB by Ober's test in side lying position. Iatrogenic medial patellar subluxation can also be examined (Nonweiler and DeLee).

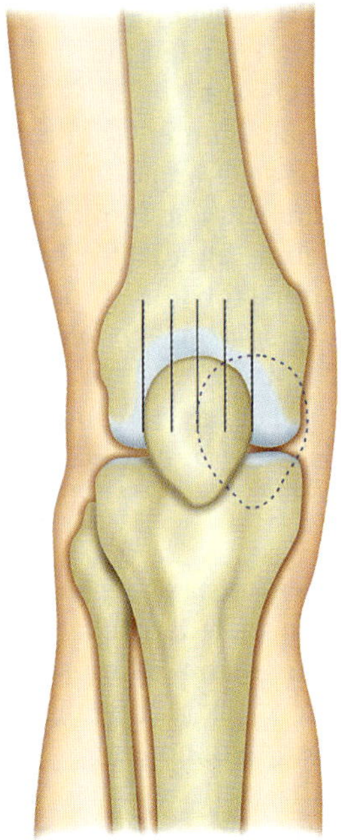

Fig. 55: Patellar glide test: Shift of patella "quadrants"—for right knee (as shown here), the patella is grasped in the resting position and pushed/translated medially. The displacement is measured in terms of arbitrary equal quadrants drawn across the width of patella. If patella displaces less than one quadrant medially, it indicates tight lateral structures. Displacement of more than three quadrants is considered hypermobile. The same test is repeated using lateral pushing thrust. Translation of patella laterally by two quadrants is normal but translation by four quadrants (medial patellar border reaching lateral edge of TG) is abnormal and indicates hypermobile patella.

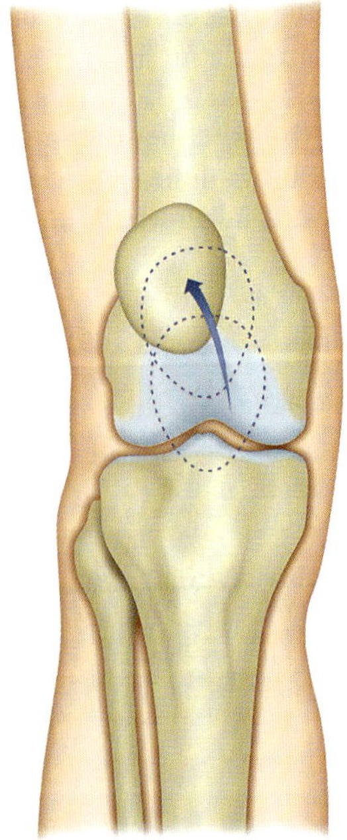

Fig. 56: J-sign.

Radiology of Patellar Dislocations

- *Standard radiographs:*
    - *Anteroposterior views:* Evaluate lower extremity alignment and version, arthrosis.
    - *Lateral views:*
        - Look for articular fracture (femoral lateral condyle or medial patellar facet) or loose body
        - Patellar subluxation **(Figs. 57A and B)**
        - Patella femoral arthrosis
        - *Trochlear dysplasia:* The "crossing sign" (X-sign) is formed by the line represented by deepest part of TG, crossing the anterior aspect of condyles. **"**Double contour sign**" (parallel lines)** is a double line seen if medial condyle is hypoplastic.
        - **Evaluate patellar height (Fig. 58A)** [patella alta versus baja]:
            - *Bernageau length (distance between inferior part of patellar articular surface and superior*

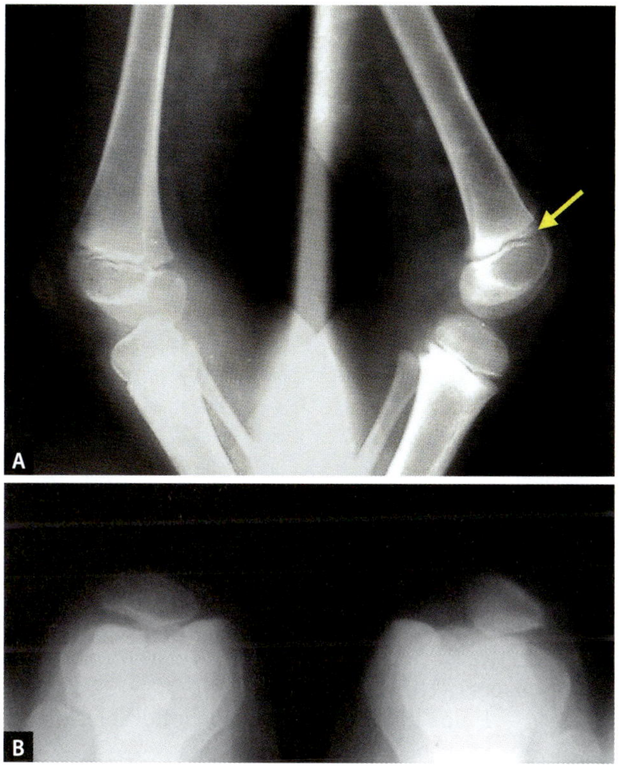

Figs. 57A and B: Recurrent dislocation of patella. Radiology lateral and skyline views. (A) Note the type 3 trochlear dysplasia (arrow) of left femur on lateral radiograph; (B) Subluxation of left patella laterally on skyline radiographs.

part of trochlea on a lateral knee radiograph): ranges between +6 to -6 mm. If > -6 mm then patella baja **(Fig. 58B)**, if > +6 mm then patella alta.

- Blumensaat's line should extend to inferior pole of the patella at 30° of knee flexion.
- *Insall-Salvati method **(Fig. 58A)**:* Ratio of length of patellar tendon to length of patella—normal between 0.8 (baja if less) and 1.2 (alta if more).
- *Modified Insall-Salvati ratio **(Fig. 58A)**:* Ratio of length of patellar tendon to length of articular surface of patella—normal is <2 (alta if more).
- Blackburne-Peel method **[(Fig. 58A)**, ratio of vertical distance between a tangent line to tibial plateau and the inferior point of patellar articular surface and length of articular surface of patella]—normal between 0.5 (baja if less) and 1.0 (alta if more)
- *Caton-Deschamps method **(Fig. 58A)**:* Ratio of distance between upper part of tibia and inferior part of patella and length of articular surface of patella—normal between 0.6 (baja if less) and 1.3 (alta if more).
- Patellar nose ratio is the ratio of length of patellar nose to length of patella, normally >0.25.

- *Sunrise/merchant views **(Figs. 57A and B)**:*
    - *Assess lateral patellar tilt:* Patellar tilt was supposed to be due to quadriceps weakness (VMO) or

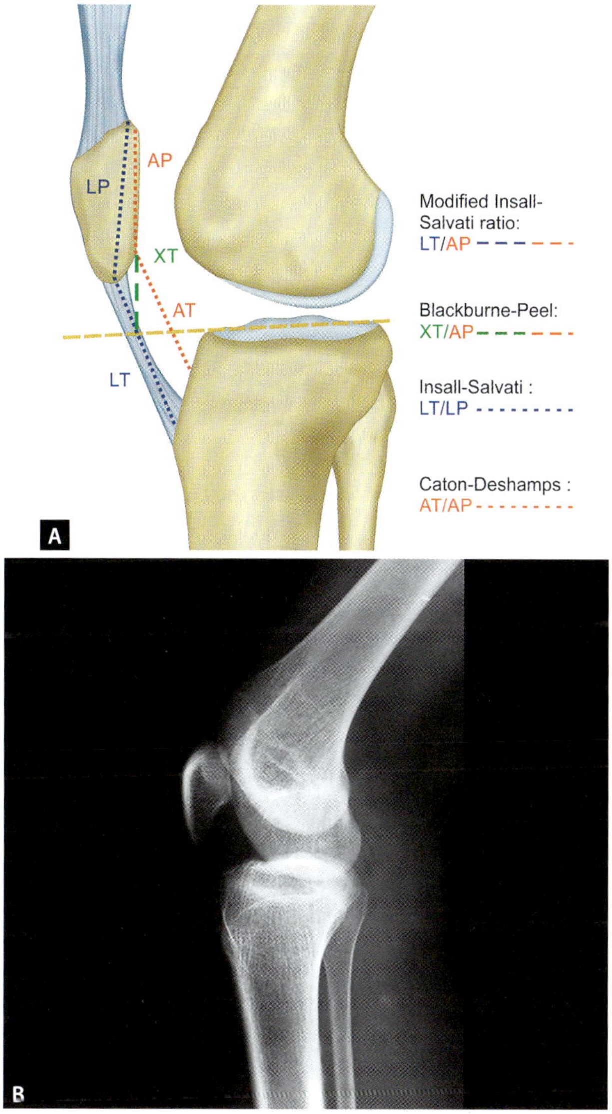

Figs. 58A and B: (A) The various indices used to evaluate patellar height; (B) Lateral radiograph of knee demonstrating patella baja.

dysplasia (Dejour) but others have related this to MPFL insufficiency (Beasley and Vidal).
    - Depth of femoral intercondylar sulcus >5 mm.
    - *Patellar tilt **(Fig. 59)**:* Angle between axis of patella and bicondylar femoral line. Normal is <20°.
    - Femoropatellar joint space should be <5 mm. Distance more than this indicates effusion.
    - Congruence angle **(Fig. 60**; normal is -6°)
    - Patellofemoral index is the ratio of medial patellofemoral joint space to lateral patellofemoral joint space; normal is <1.6.
    - Lateral trochlear inclination
    - Bisect offset **(Fig. 59)**
    - *Sulcus angle **(Fig. 60)**:* Angle between lateral and medial condylar femoral lines; normal range is 126–150°. Trochlear dysplasia present in this angle is >150°.

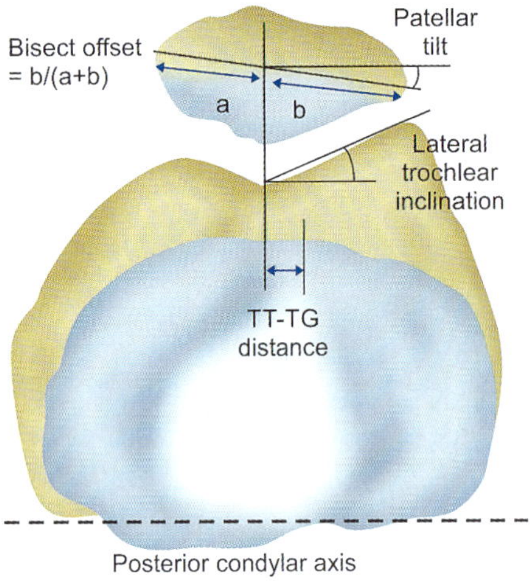

Fig. 59: Various radiological parameters used to assess the patellar stability and tracking (*see* text for details).

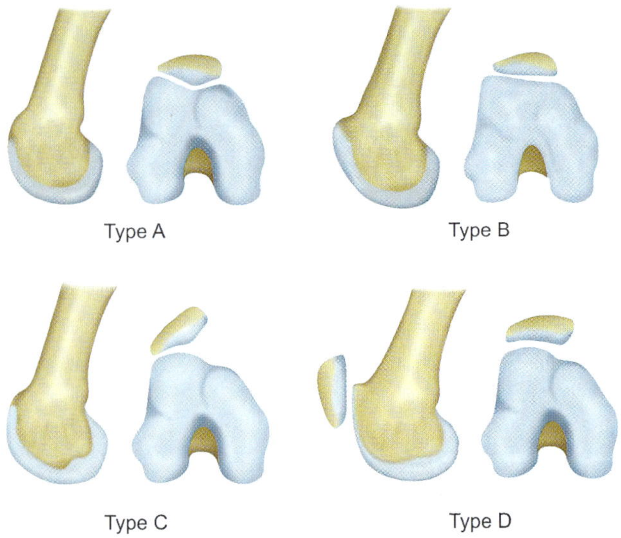

Fig. 61: Trochlear dysplasia (*see* text for description).

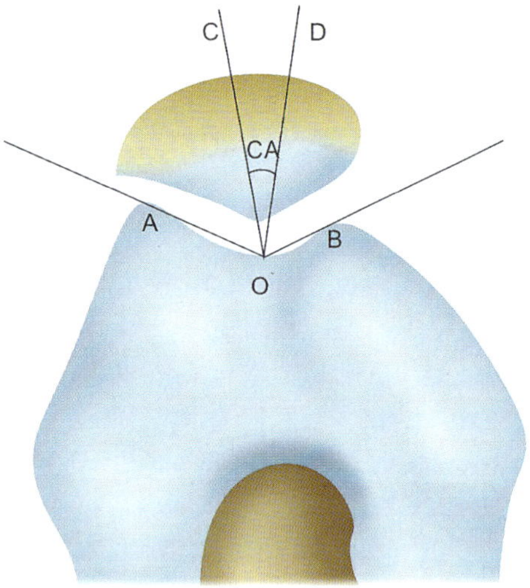

Fig. 60: The sulcus angle is a measure of trochlear depth (angle AOB here). OC is the bisector of this angle. OD is a line that passes through the lowest point on the median ridge of patella forming angle COD which is the congruence angle. Toward the medial femoral condyle, the congruence angle is denoted negative (–) while if it crosses toward lateral femoral condyle, the angle will gain a positive (+) sign. (CA: congruence angle)

- *Computed tomography scan:*
  - *Tibial tubercle*-TG *distance* ***(Fig. 59)****:* It measures the distance between 2 perpendicular lines from the posterior cortex to the TT and the TG, >20 mm usually considered abnormal.
- *Magnetic resonance imaging:*
  - Estimation of trochlear dysplasia and classification **(Fig. 61)**:
    - *Type A:* Normal shape but shallow TG
    - *Type B:* Flattened or even convex trochlea
    - *Type C:* Trochlear facet asymmetry—too high lateral facet, and hypoplastic medial facet
    - *Type D:* Above along with vertical link between facets ("cliff pattern")
      - Helps in identifying osteochondral lesion and loose bodies.
      - Identifies tear of MPFL also.

Management

The commonly practiced methods can be divided into nonsurgical and surgical methods. Nonsurgical conservative management is to be done in only infrequent dislocators or isolated dislocations and if the surgeon feels that the patellar mechanics are able to accommodate the rehabilitation process. VMO training, pelvifemoral rehabilitation, and orthotic support can be tried with experience. Truly speaking these measures often serve only as an interim measure till some surgical intervention is undertaken.

Surgical management: Since 1960, the literature is replete with innumerable procedures and their modifications described to contain recurrent dislocation of patella. Most are, however, incomplete in addressing the versatile nature of presentations and do not encompass all the features of patients with the disorder. This has led to combining the procedures to optimize the results. There are few things that are essential before prescribing a particular procedure to the patient. Assess the skeletal maturity, the Q-angle, retinacular tightness, patellar tilt, TT-TG distance, trochlear dysplasia, and patellar height specifically for each patient. It is not that other clinical and radiological parameters described previously are not useful but these primarily decide the choice of surgery commonly. The classical description of various proximal realignment, distal realignment, or combination of the two procedures can be read from various standard operative books. The proximal realignment procedures (Madigan's quadricepsplasty, arthroscopic medial imbrication, MPFL reconstruction, etc.) have been classically advocated in skeletally immature patients or those skeletally mature patients in whom TT-TG distance, Q-angle, medial patellar facet, and patellar height are normal with or without trochlear dysplasia. Distal realignment procedures (Elmslie–Trillat, Fulkerson, Hauser, etc.) on the other hand are performed in patients who have an increased TT-TG distance or where Insall-Salvati ratio is >1.2 (patella alta). The degree of anteriorization, distalization, and/or medialization to be achieved depends on associated arthrosis of the lateral patellar facet and the presence of patella alta (usually to correct Insall-Salvati ratio to 1.0). Associated medial or proximal patellar cartilage damage is a contraindication to distal realignment as there is potential to overload tissues that have already undergone degeneration. In general, the algorithm commonly followed is presented in **Flowchart 1**. With the growing dissatisfaction and poorer results in following the classical guidelines of proximal/distal realignment; the philosophy is currently biased more toward correcting the identified pathology. Based on this emerging ideology, the following recommendations are made.

- Arthroscopic debridement is indicated only for removal of loose body or in some cases for intra-articular lateral release may be in a first time dislocator or infrequent one.
- Medial patellofemoral ligament repair is commonly done in first-time dislocation with bony fragment who presents early giving a chance for acute management. Most of the avulsions occur from the femoral side so the native MPFL should be plicated or retensioned at its femoral attachment. As this is often associated with retinacular injury so commonly acute medial repair is done rather than just a MPFL repair.
- Medial patellofemoral ligament reconstruction **(Figs. 62A to I)** with autograft versus allograft is commonly done for recurrent instability due primarily to MPFL insufficiency ± medial structure deficiency. More specifically MPFL reconstruction is indicated in a patient with recurrent instability, who has a normal TT-TG distance and a normal patellar height with or without trochlear dysplasia. It may or may not be combined with limited lateral retinacular release. Care should be taken not to overtighten the MPFL else loss of motion and increased patellofemoral loads result causing arthrosis. This method is also useful in patients with hyperlaxity syndromes as MPFL guides the motion of patella in TG and these patients have more of medial tissue insufficiency.
- Vastus medialis oblique advancement and quadriceps balancing (proximal quadricepsplasty) are more difficult and complex procedures. The procedure involves release of tight lateral structures and simultaneous advancement of the VMO insertion distally and laterally on the patellar surface. This sort of medial imbrication tightens the medial soft tissue restraints and reestablishes a medially-directed force. The philosophy is to balance the excessive vastus lateralis pull by advancing the VMO. Arguments against the procedure are that it is a nonanatomic procedure and has limited utility. As suggested by Sallay, it appears that the MPFL and VMO heal in a more superior and lateral position reducing the obliquity of VMO thus the pull is not truly medializing.
- *Lateral release:* Some people disfavor release to a lateral lengthening. The rationale is that the lateral retinaculum contributes to lateral and medial patellar stability. Lateral release risks further destabilization of an unstable joint. Lateral retinacular lengthening could be a better but more cumbersome option. Lateral retinacular release is easier to perform provided excessive medial laxity is not created. Isolated releases are no longer done except if lateral patellar tilt or tightness is the sole cause of instability. It is often combined with medial tightening procedures as a safe vent for excessive tight extensor mechanism created by medial imbrication.

Flowchart 1: Simplified algorithm for management of recurrent dislocation of patella.

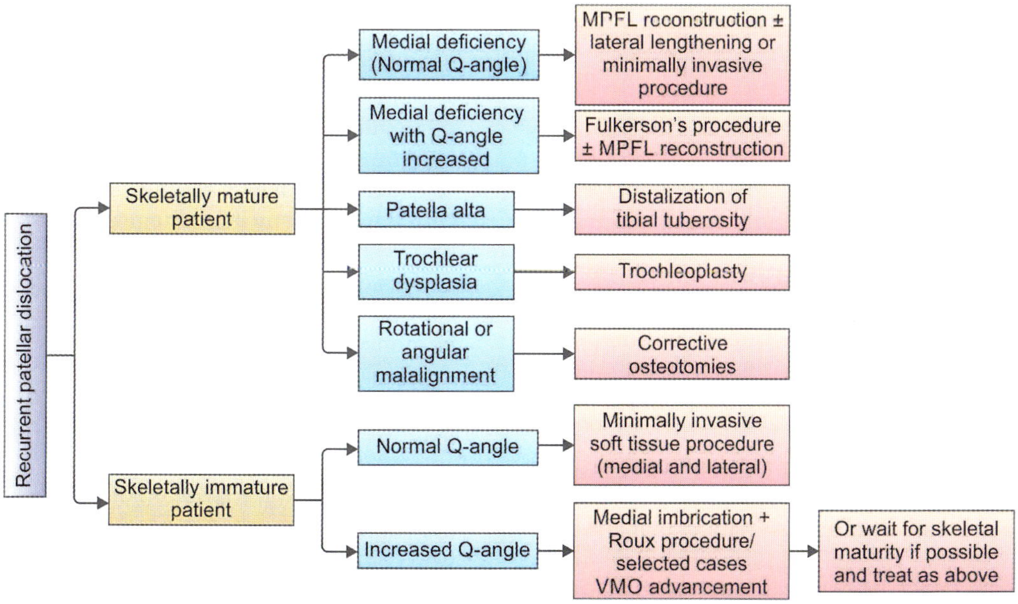

(MPFL: medial patellofemoral ligament; VMO: vastus medialis oblique)

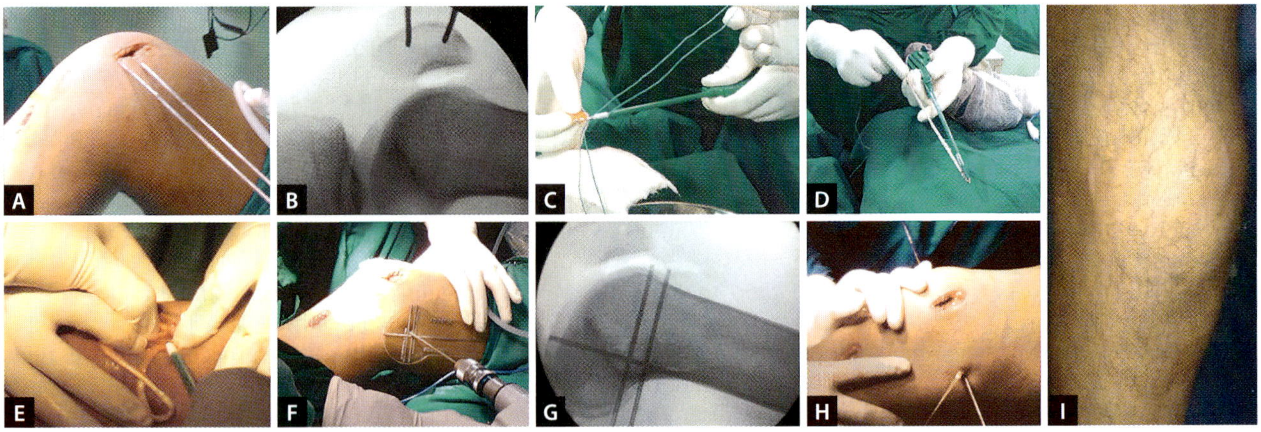

Figs. 62A to I: Anatomical medial patellofemoral ligament (MPFL) reconstruction using gracilis tendon autograft. (A) Placing the guidewires for patellar tunnel insertion sites for MPFL; (B) Checking the placement under C-arm; (C) Loading the suture anchors; (D) Loading the graft and placing it in one of the tunnels fixed with suture anchor; (E) Placing the other end of graft similarly into the other tunnel; this forms a loop which is to be fixed to the femoral attachment of MPFL; (F) Marking and placing guidewire into femur using a prefabricated guide; (G) Checking the correct placement of guide under C-arm; (H) Passing the loop of tendon graft through a subcutaneous supracapsular tunnel delivering it through the femoral attachment site and fixing using bioabsorbable 6 mm interference screw; (I) Follow-up of the patient after 3 months.

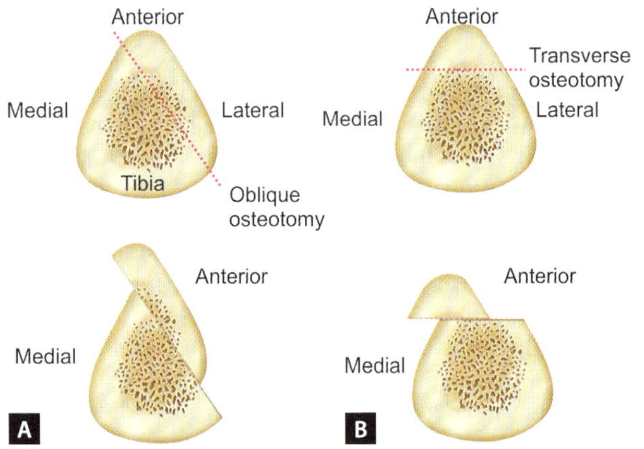

Figs. 63A and B: The different tibial tubercle osteotomies for distal realignment. (A) Fulkerson type anteromedialization of tuberosity involves anterior and medial shift of the patellar tendon attachment by performing a sliding type osteotomy at an angle of 45°; (B) Direct medialization osteotomy of Elmslie-Trillat involves shifting the tibial tuberosity transversely medially.

- Distalization of TT is indicated for patella alta specifically. This may be combined with soft-tissue imbrication of patellar tendon.
- *Fulkerson-type osteotomy* ***(Figs. 63A and B****, anterior and medial TT transfer):* This is indicated for TT-TG >20 mm on CT scans and is often combined with MPFL reconstruction due to frequent occurrence of MPFL insufficiency simultaneously. This procedure is a combination of Elmslie–Trillat procedure and Maquet procedure. It involves anteriorization and medialization of the TT correcting both the Q-angle and unloading the patellofemoral joint. The osteotomy is made from medial to lateral at an angle of 45° leaving a periosteal hinge distally to rotate and translate the TT. The aim should be to correct TT-TG to 10–15 mm (never <10 mm).

  The classic Hauser procedure of transferring the TT medially and posteriorly is discredited due to accelerated patellofemoral degeneration in the long run though immediate results are satisfactory. The TT medialization of Elmslie–Trillat procedure involves direct medial transfer of the tubercle (as an improvement over Hauser procedure) and is done with lateral release. A transverse plane osteotomy is made from lateral to medial leaving a periosteal hinge intact distally, about which the tubercle is rotated medially, approximately 1–1.5 cm. The tubercle is then fixed anteroposteriorly with bicortical screws. This is also but contraindicated if there is patellar medial facet condrosis and there is a higher chance of nonunion. These distal realignment procedures, however, do not address an incompetent MPFL and are obviously contraindicated in skeletally immature patients besides having the potential for nonunion and neurovascular complications.
- Trochleoplasty is a less common and more complex procedure to do that involves deepening the anterior femoral sulcus to provide a congruous patellofemoral articulation. Albee osteotomy is preferable for trochlea with a hypoplastic lateral femoral condyle. For convex trochlear dysplasia (type 3), a Dejour type osteotomy is preferred but is a highly specialized surgery.
- Derotation osteotomies of femur and leg bones can be done for rotational malalignment and have been mentioned elsewhere.
- *Minimally invasive realignment procedures:* These have become popular as a general method of so-called proximal realignment based on the conventional philosophy of tight lateral and lax medial structures. Medial plication is done with sutures or thermal wands whereas the lateral release can be done with small lateral incision or arthroscopically. Long-term success needs to be substantiated for these.

CONGENITAL VERTICAL TALUS (CONVEX PES VALGUS, RIGID ROCKER BOTTOM FLATFOOT)

Congenital vertical talus is a rare foot deformity consisting of an irreducible dorsal dislocation of the navicular on the talus, producing a rigid flatfoot deformity **(Fig. 64)**. Patients with reducible navicular dislocation that realigns on stretched plantar flexion, lateral films are termed congenital oblique talus **(Fig. 65)**. One-fifth of the cases of CVT are familial (genetic) and around half of the patients have associated neuromuscular anomalies commonly:

- Myelodysplasia (spina bifida)
- Sacral agenesis
- Arthrogryposis
- Diastematomyelia
- Genetic and chromosomal abnormalities

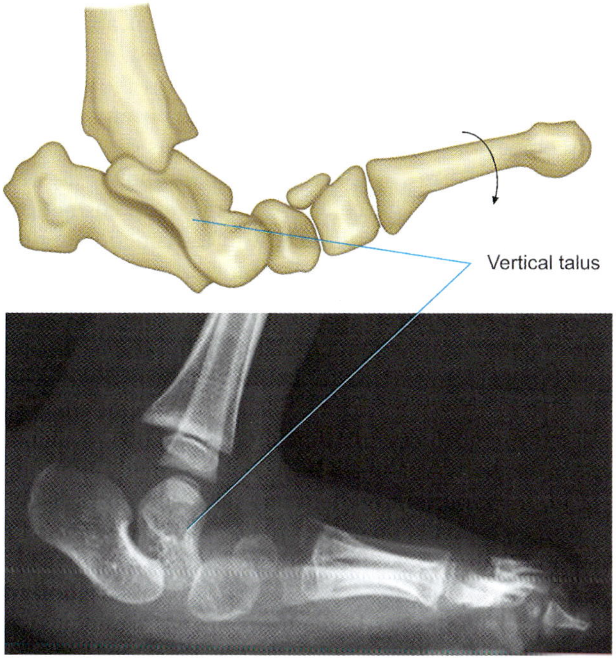

Fig. 64: Radiograph and illustration of congenital vertical talus.

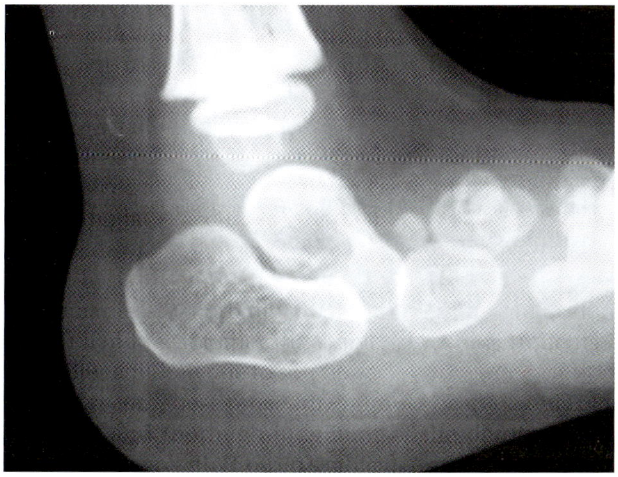

Fig. 65: Radiograph of congenital oblique talus.

Because of the common association of neurological anatomical anomalies if no association is clinically apparent, a MRI evaluation of the spine and pelvis is indicated to ascertain normal spine or other anomalies of the lumbosacral plexus.

Pathoanatomy

The equinus and valgus position results from posterolateral contracture of tendo-Achilles and peroneal tendons. The midfoot is dorsiflexed on the hindfoot (rocker bottom foot) as a result of anterior contracture of the extensor hallucis longus (EHL), the tibialis anterior and the extensor digitorum longus (EDL), and anterolateral contracture of peroneus tertius and inferior retinaculum of ankle. This contracture leads to a dorsal dislocation of navicular and a prominent talus head on the plantar aspect of the foot; in severe cases, there is also a concurrent dorsal cuboid dislocation (*See* Coleman classification below).

Components of deformity thus can be understood in three specific headings:

1. Fixed hindfoot equinovalgus—due to contracture of the Achilles and peroneal tendons
2. Rigid midfoot dorsiflexion—secondary to the dislocated navicular
3. Forefoot abducted and dorsiflexed—due to contractures of the EDL, EHL, and tibialis anterior tendons

Coleman divided the CVT into two types:

1. *Type 1:* Associated with calcaneocuboid dislocation. These are rigid and stubborn foot that are difficult to treat and require calcaneocuboid joint release.
2. *Type 2:* Without calcaneocuboid dislocation

Radiographic Evaluation

The films are obtained in AP and lateral projections in forced plantar flexion and dorsiflexion.

- The *forced plantar flexion lateral view* confirms rigid dorsal displacement of the first metatarsal axis to the longitudinal axis of the talus [Meary's angle > 20° (*see* Chapter on "Anatomy of Ankle and Foot"), also called TAMBA—talar axis 1st metatarsal base axis]. There is persistent dislocation of the talonavicular joint [reduced joint will come under the category of *oblique talus* **(Fig. 65)**]. In patients with oblique talus, the forced plantar flexion lateral radiograph shows colinearity of the first metatarsal and the longitudinal axis of the talus, suggesting that the primary disorder is a posterior lateral contracture and not true CVT.
- Forced dorsiflexion lateral radiograph is needed to confirm and demonstrate the equinus deformity of the ankle.
- Anteroposterior view shows the midfoot valgus and a talocalcaneal angle >40° (normal range 20–40°).
- Mostly as the foot bones are not ossified in infants, an ultrasonographic evaluation is needed to demonstrate and document the vertical position of talus. Forced plantarflexion should be done while sonography also.

Differential Diagnosis of Congenital Vertical Talus

- Congenital oblique talus **(*see* Fig. 65)**
- Tarsal coalition
- Pes valgus deformity either congenital, paralytic, or pes planovalgus

Treatment

Manipulation of the deformity: Serial casting was thought to be an unsuccessful method of correction while lately described "reverse Ponseti" method of reducing navicular over talus has been found satisfactory. It is indicated in a child with mild or oblique CVT and is getting popular as initial treatment for CVT.

Dobb's method: Manipulation is done to stretch the foot in plantar flexion to elongate anterior structures and achieve inversion while applying counterpressure to the medial aspect of the talus. This prevents compression of the navicular. Dobbs used to fix the navicular to talus once satisfactory correction was obtained. To correct the equinus, an additional Achilles tendon tenotomy is always necessary.

Surgical Treatment

This has been the standard method of correcting the deformity. Coleman and others described two-stage two-incision procedure but this method had higher complication rate. In this procedure, lengthening of EDL, EHL, and tibialis anterior is done along with anterior capsular releases (talonavicular and calcaneocuboid joints). The second stage consists of tendo-Achilles release and posterior release (ankle and subtalar capsulotomies). Single-stage approach has become popular as described by Seimon and others. Here, the EHL and peroneus tendons are tenotomized and talonavicular joint reduced by open reduction and K-wire fixation. Achilles tenotomy is mandatory as usual. In children 2 years of age or younger, surgical reconstruction involves lengthening the Achilles, peroneus longus and peroneus brevis tendons, and performing a posterolateral subtalar release. Talonavicular joint is then reduced and pinned. The tibialis anterior, EHL, and EDL tendons are lengthened. The above procedure can be done in children up to 4 years of age with less severe deformities.

Older children with residual deformities may require a salvage procedure, such as a naviculectomy, talectomy, triple arthrodesis, or subtalar fusion. Children 3 years or older often require navicular excision at the time of open reduction. Children 4–8 years of age often require open reduction and soft-tissue procedures along with extra-articular subtalar arthrodesis. Neglected cases presenting after 12 years of age often have developing arthrosis and deformities so rigid that cannot be corrected. They are best treated by triple arthrodesis for correction of the deformity.

POLYDACTYLY

Toe polydactyly most commonly presents as an isolated trait with an autosomal dominant inheritance pattern and variable expression but may occur in established genetic syndromes. It is the most common toe abnormality with an overall incidence of approximately 2 cases per 1,000 live births. Surgical treatment of polydactyly is amputation of the accessory digit or ray amputation if any extrametatarsal is present that articulates with the digit. A combined polydactyly-syndactyly deformity requires resection of the more peripheral digit. The skin of excised digit is used as fillet graft for coverage of syndactyly wound. In preaxial polydactyly, the most medial great toe is excised taking care to carefully repair the capsule and soft tissues to prevent hallux varus. These cases are stabilized with K-wires for 3–6 weeks.

MACRODACTYLY (BANANA TOES)

Macrodactyly is the hypertrophy and increases in size of toes due to increase in size of all elements (tendons, nerves, vessels, phalanges, subcutaneous fat, nails, and skin) except the metatarsal. It is a rare congenital abnormality but the cause is not known. Some suggest irritation of nerves and deposition of fibrofatty tissue in the digit with trophic influence due to neural stimulation and resulting enlargement of the same. Few associations are seen with macrodactyly like syndactyly, neurofibromatosis, and hemangiomatosis. The condition is not only cosmetically unacceptable but also interferes with the function of digits **(Figs. 66A to F)**. Writing and fine functions are impaired in hand while in foot fitting foot wear is difficult to customize. The deformity as such needs surgical correction to improve function and fitting the toes. Secondary goal is to improve cosmesis of the toes to achieve a foot similar in size to the opposite foot. Total reduction is unusual and should be communicated to the patients beforehand to correct the expectations.

The various surgical options mentioned in literature are as follows:

- Bulk reduction procedures
- Above with osteotomy and/or physiodesis
- Toe amputation/ray amputation
- Neural stripping
- Neurectomy
- *Kotwal and Farooque procedure* ***(Figs. 66A to F)****:* Staged procedure of defatting on one side of the digit (convex side) followed by phalangeal resection and reduction in the length of the toe three months later. Initial defatting is done on the convex side to straighten the toe. In the second stage with the resection of phalanx, the extensor tendon is shortened but flexor tendon is left to adjust in length later, the capsule is repaired and toe stabilized with K-wire.

LESSER TOE ABNORMALITIES

Congenital curly toe deformity is common but its true incidence and natural history are unknown. The deformity frequently is bilateral involving typically the third or fourth toes. It commonly corrects itself with time. Stretching and taping early may benefit in mild deformity. Surgical treatment is indicated in symptomatic patients who have pain or a nail

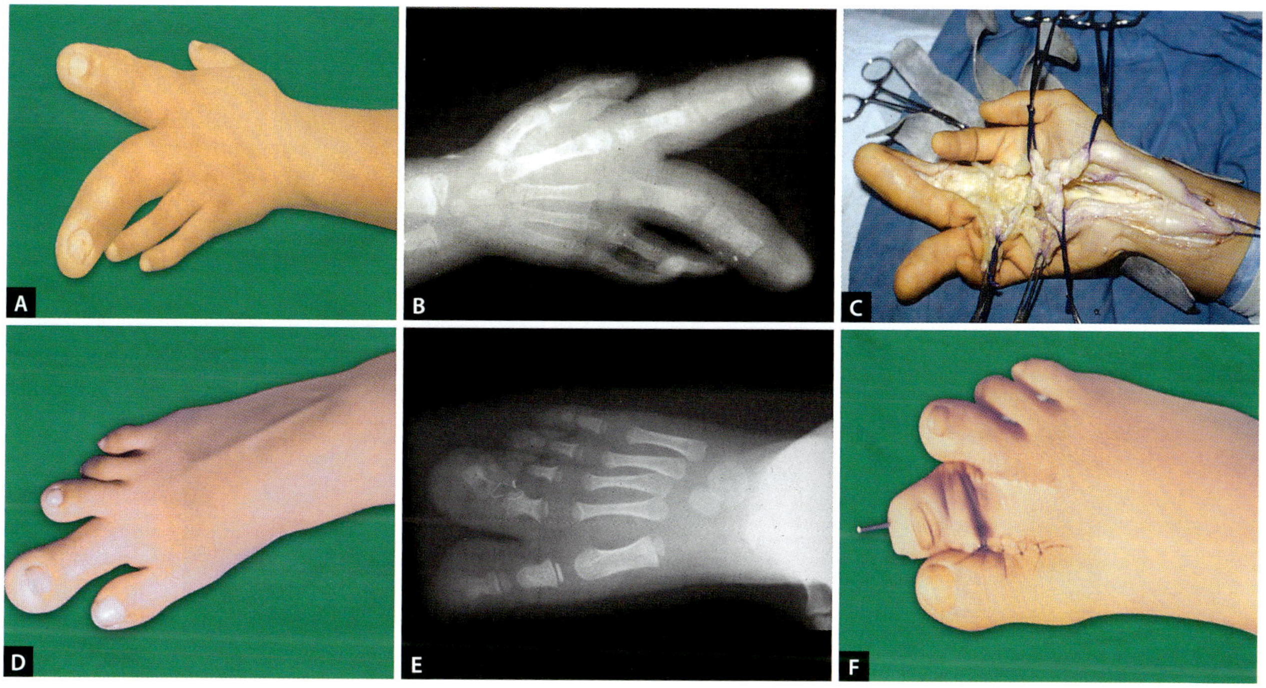

Figs. 66A to F: (A to C) Macrodactyly of hand and (D to F) foot showing the clinical presentation, radiographs, and operative correction.
Source: Professor PP Kotwal, Chairman, Institute of Orthopedics and Joint Replacement, Pushpavati Singhania Research Institute, New Delhi, India.

bed deformity resulting from pathologic positioning. Surgical release of the long toe flexor at the distal interphalangeal joint is effective in persistent cases. Congenital *overriding fifth toe* is an adducted and dorsiflexed malpositioning of the lesser toe. It is bilateral in one-third patients. There is subluxation or dislocation of the fifth metatarsophalangeal joint without clawing of the IP joint. Mild cases may get relieved by taping while others require capsular reconstruction and relocation, to correct painful shoe wear problems.

CLEFT FOOT (ECTRODACTYLY, LOBSTER FOOT, PARTIAL ADACTYLY)

Cleft foot (lobster foot) is a central ray anomaly that presents as a single central cleft in the forefoot that may extend proximally into the midfoot **(Figs. 67A to G)**. They represent terminal longitudinal limb anomalies. The term ectrodactyly though literally means "missing digits" but over a period of usage, it is now used to describe a central ray anomaly and should specifically be limited to describe split-hand split-foot syndrome. The deformity was earliest depicted by Pare. Cleft foot is rare and has an incidence of approximately 0.7 per 10,000 live births and there is predilection in affected sons of affected fathers. Genetically focus for deformity has been laid onto the 7q21.2-q21.3 region. This association is, however, not complete and is seen with mild anomalies to ectromelia and fatal anomalies. Homeobox genes (*HOX D, HOX 7, MSX1, HOX A,* and *D*) are the most probable candidates. Sonic hedgehog is another candidate as it is involved in establishing polarizing activity in the developing limb bud and hence AP patterning.

Associations:

- Split-hand split-foot syndrome
- Cornelia de Lange syndrome
- Ectodermal dysplasia, ectrodactyly, and clefting syndrome (EEC syndrome)
- Acrorenal syndrome
- Ectrodactyly and cleft palate syndrome
- Focal dermal hypoplasia
- Ectrodactyly and macular dystrophy
- Ectrodactyly/mandibulofacial dysostosis

Clinical Features

Absence of the central digits is the major feature with varying association of both bony and soft tissue syndactyly. Disease is bilateral in half of the cases and there is no sex predilection. Presentation ranges from skin cleft to several ray deficiencies of the central region of the forefoot up to midfoot. Two additional forms have been identified: cleft foot with central polydactyly, called polydactylous type, and monodactylous foot with the lower-leg diastasis or tibial aplasia or both, described as diastatic type. The deformity is more cosmetic than functional except in uncommon cases with a single metatarsal (coexisting preaxial anomaly; monodactyly) where balancing the limb is a problem. These functional problems are more common with wide and deep clefts, especially with respect to foot wear. Generally, one or more central toes and parts of their metatarsals are absent but as a rule if a metatarsal is partially or completely absent, its respective toe is always absent. Often the tarsals are abnormal. Except in cases with monodactyly (rare), the first and fifth rays are usually present. Involvement may be seen in one limb to all four limbs.

Classification

Based on the number of metatarsals present Blauth and Borisch classified the deformities into six types. The

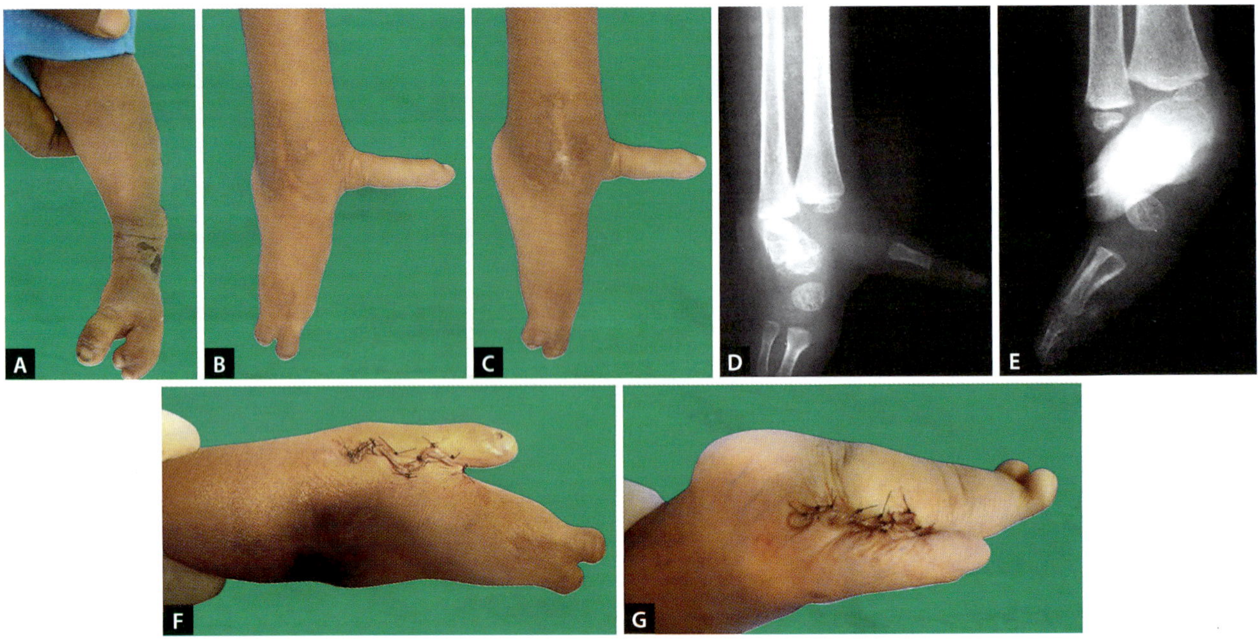

Figs. 67A to G: Cleft foot deformity. (A) The infant has been managed conservatively for associated equinovarus deformity; (B to G) Operative management of cleft foot deformity.
Source: Professor PP Kotwal, Chairman, Institute of Orthopedics and Joint Replacement, Pushpavati Singhania Research Institute, New Delhi.

BOX 5: The types of cleft foot based on number of metatarsals. It is not very practical for clinical use.

- Type 1 and type 2 are (minor deficiencies) all metatarsals present. The metatarsals are normal in type 1 and hypoplastic in type 2. There may be cross bone present between metatarsals.
- Type 3 has four metatarsals.
- Type 4 has three metatarsals.
- Type 5 has two metatarsals.
- Type 6 has one metatarsal.

number of identifiable metatarsals decreases progressively **(Box 5)**:

Abraham et al. gave a simplified clinical classification with treatment recommendation:

- Type 1 has deficiency of usually second or third rays or both extending up to midmetatarsal level without splaying of medial or lateral rays. These feet are corrected with soft tissue syndactylism ± partial hallux valgus correction.
- Type 2 has a deep cleft up to tarsal bones without forefoot splaying—best treated with soft tissue syndactylism ± first-ray osteotomy.
- Type 3 has a complete absence of the first through third or fourth rays; no treatment is recommended.

Management

Surgery for cleft foot is aimed to improve shoe wear and appearance. In Blauth and Borisch types 1 and 2 and Abraham's type 1, simple closure of the cleft is appropriate. If present, the cross bone may need to be excised simultaneously. Till first 3 years, the forefoot is supple and syndactylism (cleft closure) by triangular or rectangular flaps or double opposing Z-plasty is a reasonable method especially for Abraham's type 2 (Blauth and Borisch types 3, 4, and 5). Hallux valgus correction may be needed simultaneously. For cleft closure of deep clefts, the skin of the opposing surfaces within the cleft is excised and the two parts are sutured together **(*see* Figs. 63A and B)**. It is imperative to preserve the dorsal and plantar flaps for closure of the gap. If a metatarsal has no corresponding toe, it is resected before closure. Bony or joint deformity of the first or fifth ray should be corrected at the time of surgery and fixed with a pin. In severe deformities (type 5 and 6), heel-cord lengthening, osteotomies of the navicular and cuboid, excision of prominent bony masses, or even tendon transfers may be necessary.

CONGENITAL METATARSUS ADDUCTUS (METATARSUS VARUS, METATARSUS ADDUCTOVARUS)

Metatarsus adductus is the most common foot deformity commonly seen in newborn infants with incidence approaching 1 in 1,000–1,500 live births. There is adduction of forefoot with normal hindfoot alignment or minimal valgus. Half of patients have bilateral involvement and there is no sex predilection. The exact cause of metatarsus adductus is not known, although intrauterine positioning (packaging defect) is commonly implicated. Not very popular theories include trapezoid-shaped medial cuneiform (may be a developmental bone form), contracture of tibialis anterior tendon, etc. There is increased incidence in:

- First pregnancy
- Twin pregnancy
- Oligohydramnios

Metatarsus adductus may be associated with few conditions like:

- Clubfoot
- Torticollis

- Developmental dysplasia of the hip (1–5%, recent studies have not confirmed this theory)

Clinical Features

Metatarsus adductus is a common cause of in-toeing gait. The forefoot is deviated medially with respect to the hindfoot that may show some valgus (higher valgus equates to skewfoot). Lateral border is convex **(Fig. 68)** with variable medial crease depending on severity (see below). The hindfoot and subtalar motion are usually normal. Metatarsus adductus may be seen as a residual deformity in patients previously treated surgically or nonsurgically for congenital clubfoot. This residual metatarsus adductus is often rigid (fixed positioning of the forefoot on the midfoot and hindfoot) but can be dynamic also, caused by imbalance of the anterior tibial tendon during gait. The rigidity or flexibility of the forefoot should be determined before undertaking any surgical correction in an older child. Late sequelae of metatarsus adductus may include an increased risk of stress fractures of the lateral metatarsal bones, due to altered biomechanics.

Classification

The deformity is classified by its magnitude and the stiffness of the metatarsus adductus (Bleck, **Fig. 69**):

- *The mild form:* The forefoot can be clinically abducted to the midline of the foot and beyond. This can be clinically tested by gently stroking the lateral border of foot that elicits spontaneous movements and active correction. The heel bisector line passes through third toe (in a normal foot, it passes through second webspace).
- *The moderate form:* Heel bisector line passes through third and fourth toe webspace. There is enough flexibility to allow abduction of the forefoot to the midline, but usually not beyond.
- *Rigid metatarsus adductus:* Heel bisector line passes through fourth and fifth toe webspace. The forefoot cannot be abducted at all. There is often a transverse crease on the medial border of the foot or an enlargement of the webspace between the great and second toes.

The other classification (Berg) incorporates the metatarsus adductus and skewfoot together:

- Simple metatarsus adductus
- *Complex metatarsus adductus:* Metatarsus adductus with lateral shift of midfoot
- *Skewfoot:* Metatarsus adductus with valgus hindfoot
- *Complex skew foot:* Metatarsus adductus along with abducted midfoot and valgus hindfoot

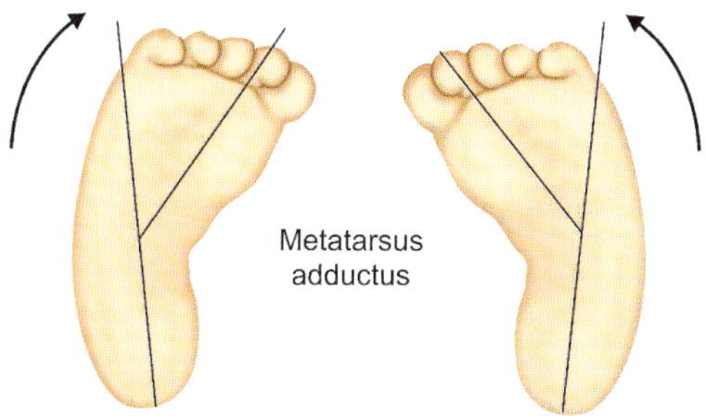

Fig. 68: The metatarsus adductus deformity.

RADIOLOGY

Metatarsus adductus is best viewed on a dorsoplantar view and diagnosed with metatarsus adductus angle >21°. This angle is made by intersection of two lines **(Fig. 70)**, one bisecting the second metatarsal and the other perpendicular

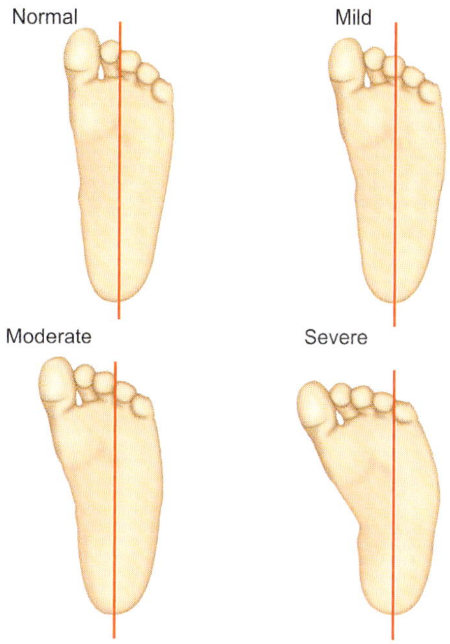

Fig. 69: The various grades of metatarsus adductus (see text for description).

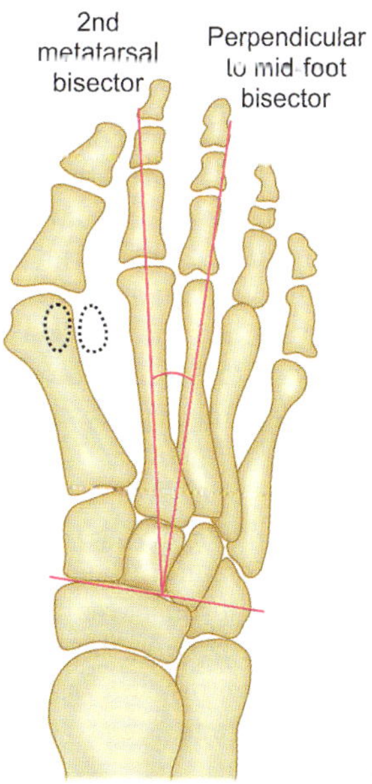

Fig. 70: The radiological definition of metatarsus adductus. Normally, the bisector of second metatarsal is parallel to a line perpendicular to midfoot bisector. If the angle is >21°, then it is metatarsus adductus.

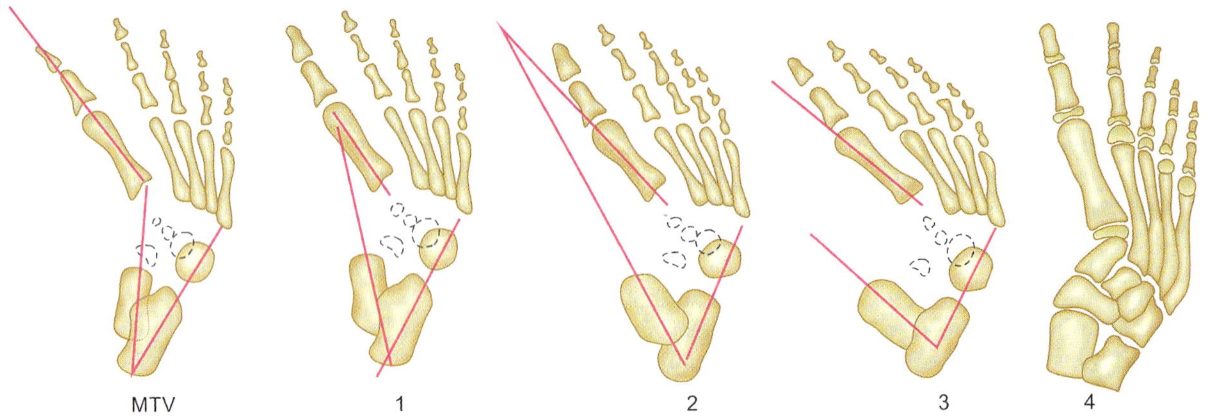

Fig. 71: Metatarsus adductus according to Berg's criteria and its various grades. In an isolated metatarsus varus (MTV), the talus bisector meets the 1st metatarsal at its base with normal talocalcaneal divergence. In increasing deformities, the talus bisector crosses the shaft of 1st metatarsal (grade 1), goes beyond the 1st metatarsal (grade 2), or becomes parallel to 1st metatarsal (grade 3). In Z-deformity [serpentine foot (4)], there is fixed metatarsus adductus with abduction of anterior tarsal bone and exaggerated talocalcaneal divergence.

to the midfoot bisector (one can also use a perpendicular to second cuneiform bisector instead).

When using the cuneiform bisector upper limit of angle is taken as 24°.

Berg considered metatarsus adductus to be present, if the bisector of first metatarsal was medial to the bisection line of talus **(Fig. 71)**.

Differential Diagnosis

- Clubfoot
- Skewfoot
- Congenital hallux varus (atavistic great toe)

Treatment

The primary treatment of mild flexible metatarsus adductus is observation. Most of the patients have a benign natural history (>90% cases) with good correction of the deformity by age 4–5 years. Mild residual deformity is rarely if ever a problem to patient or parents. Most of the deformity corrects in walking age group with corrective footwear. Patients with moderate or rigid, severe metatarsus adductus can be treated with manipulation and serial casting before the age of 6 months. Manipulation involves abduction of the forefoot against counterpressure placed over the calcaneal cuboid joint. To maintain the correction after manipulation, children are placed in a long leg plaster cast, and the cast is changed every 2 weeks for three or four sessions. Serial stretching and casting is done for 6–12 weeks or until the foot is clinically flexible. Medial release is described for resistant rigid foot that can then be manipulated. After the deformity is fully corrected, the child must wear a Denis Browne bar and shoes to prevent a recurrence. Surgical intervention can be used for the rare child with severe, stiff residual deformity and is done after 3 years of age.

Surgical indications include:
- Pain
- Objectionable appearance
- Difficulty in fitting shoes 2–4 years

The common surgical technique involves medial column opening and lateral column shortening:
- Medial column opening consists of medial tarsometatarsal capsular release, abductor hallucis recession (recession only as a procedure is done in young patients with rigid resistant feet), and release of intermetatarsal ligaments. Soft tissue only procedures are helpful in younger patients. Medial cuneiform opening osteotomy is done in older patients to change its shape from trapezoid to rectangular. This also improves the 1st metatarsocuneiform relationship.
- Lateral column shortening involves cuboid closing wedge osteotomy which can be combined with medial cuneiform osteotomy in severe deformities (double osteotomy).
- In children >5-year-old, multiple metatarsal osteotomies (Berman and Gartland), medial cuneiform, and lateral cuboid double osteotomy can be done to correct deformity. In Berman and Gartland osteotomy, all five metatarsal bases are exposed dorsally. A small power drill is used to make a dome-shaped osteotomy in each with the apex of the dome proximally. Forefoot is the rotated in corrected position and foot transfixed using small Steinman pins through the shafts of the first and fifth metatarsals across the osteotomies.

Complications of surgical procedures:
- Skin slough
- Recurrence of deformity
- Osteonecrosis of second and third cuneiforms
- Dorsal prominence of first metatarsal cuneiform joint
- Early degenerative arthrosis of released joints

TARSAL COALITION

A tarsal coalition is an abnormal connection/union between two bones (tarsal bones) in the hindfoot or midfoot producing rigid flatfoot. This is the result of congenital failure of differentiation and segmentation of primitive mesenchyme. As against its name, the bones do not "coalesce" always

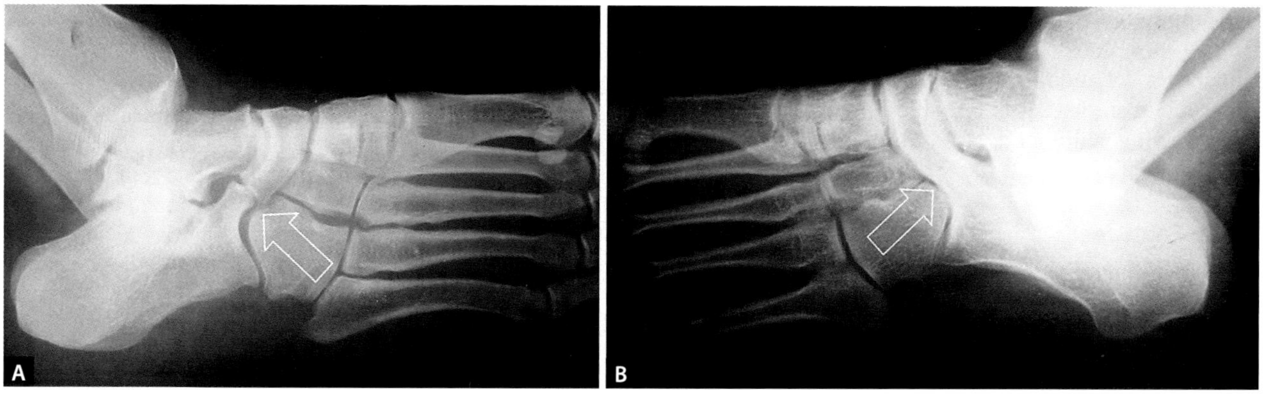

Figs. 72A and B: Incomplete (A) and complete (B) calcaneonavicular coalition.

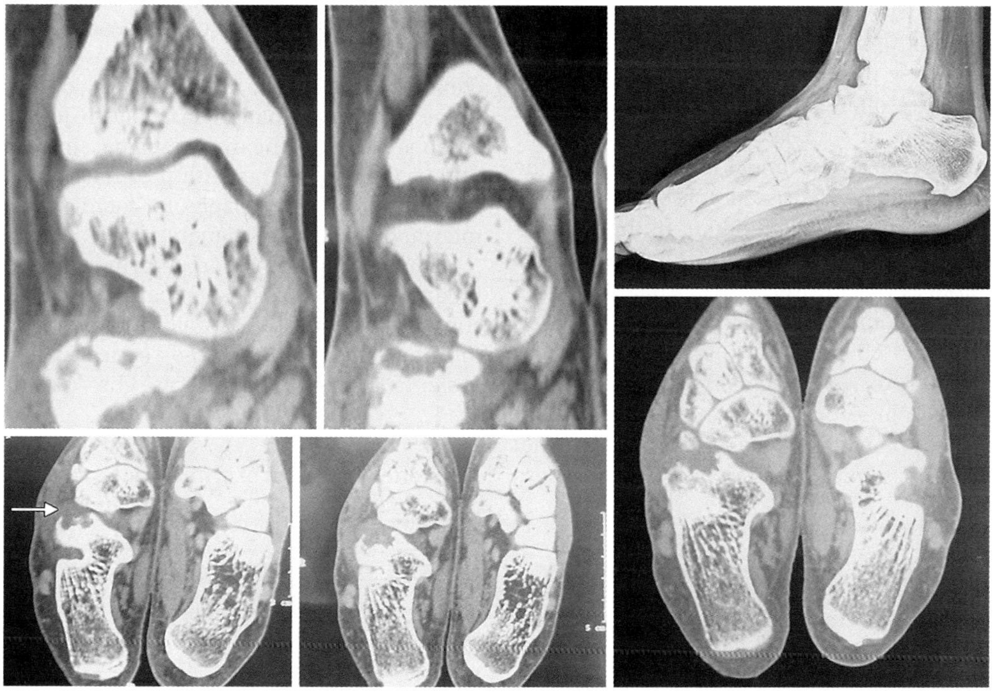

Fig. 73: Talocalcaneal incomplete (fibrous) coalition (arrow).

but actually have only a nonanatomical, nonphysiological connection. Also the coalition can be fibrous (syndesmosis), cartilaginous (synchondrosis), or bony (synostosis). Other ways of categorizing the coalition are by classifying it according to the development into congenital or acquired, according to completeness of coalition into complete or incomplete. The coalitions are classified according to the bones they connect. The two most common types (comprise the majority, >90%) are:

1. Calcaneonavicular (most common; **Figs. 72A and B**)
2. Middle facet of talocalcaneal articulation (second most common; **Figs. 73 and 76**).

The calcaneocuboid, talonavicular, cubonavicular, or navicular-first cuneiform tarsal fusions comprise 10% of the remaining. The term "bar" refers to complete bony connection between the two bones. The association of peroneal spastic flatfoot to the calcaneonavicular coalition or talocalcaneal coalition was established late in 1921 and 1948 specifically by Solomann and Harris and Beath, respectively. Rare tibialis spastic varus or cavovarus foot has also been linked to tarsal coalition. Other recognized associations of the tarsal coalition are as follows:

- Fibular hemimelia
- Hand-foot-uterus syndrome
- Carpal coalition
- Clubfoot
- Symphalangism
- Arthrogryposis
- Apert syndrome
- Nievergelt-Pearlman syndrome

Pathogenesis

Coalitions are bilateral in 50–60% of patients, and they can be inherited in an autosomal dominant pattern. Congenital or developmental, coalition appears to represent a failure of primitive mesenchymal differentiation, while the acquired form occurs secondary to trauma, infection, and surgery or articular disorders. It is possible for some coalitions to resolve during childhood, as a result of weight-bearing biomechanical activity.

Clinical Features

Tarsal coalitions are seen in 1–6% of population with slight male preponderance and interestingly majority are asymptomatic (around 80%). Commonly they are discovered incidentally and are not of any clinical significance. The calcaneonavicular coalition, if present becomes symptomatic by 8–12 years of age while talocalcaneal coalitions become symptomatic later by 12–15 years of age. Approximately, 25% of patients report activity-related pain on the dorsolateral and occasionally, the posteromedial aspect of the ankle and hindfoot, and they may have spasm of the peroneal muscles. The children often report tired or fatigue legs. In case of involvement of subtalar joint, the distal joints overcompensate and typical deformities result including the flattening of arch, hindfoot valgus, and peroneal spasticity. It is important to realize that inflammation of the subtalar joint from infection or inflammatory arthropathy can also produce peroneal spasm. The onset of pain usually occurs in children with a calcaneonavicular coalition between 8 and 12 years of age and in children with a subtalar coalition occurring after 12 years of age. The child may have a history of inversion ankle injuries caused by limited subtalar motion. The hindfoot mobility is decreased and it does not invert as it normally does during toe standing. Also heel cord contractures could be found.

Investigations and Radiology

For clear documentation AP, lateral and oblique views should be obtained; the last is particularly useful for calcaneonavicular coalition viewing. The calcaneonavicular coalition is best seen on 45° oblique radiographic views. On a lateral radiograph, a long anterior process of the calcaneus, called the "anteater sign" **(Fig. 73)**, may also be noted. Subtalar (talocalcaneal) coalitions is seen on a lateral radiograph as a condensation underneath the medial facet of the calcaneus, called the "C sign" **(Fig. 74A)**. A traction spur on the talus neck (talar beak sign) may appear, most likely as a stress reaction from increased movement of the talonavicular joint. Harris-Beath axial radiographic view may help to visualize some of the cases of talocalcaneal coalitions that focus upon the posterior and medial facets. CT (though not preferred over MR) can be used to confirm the diagnosis and rule out the presence of other coalitions **(Figs. 74A to F)**.

Magnetic resonance imaging is the investigation of choice to document the presence of abnormal fibrous tissue and inflammation in adjacent joints and bones. In osseous coalition, the marrow signal shows continuity while fibrous union presents with proximity of surfaces with loss of fat plane. The cartilaginous coalitions have in addition intermediate T2/STIR signal.

A bone scan and blood work may be needed to rule out inflammatory processes in patients who have significant subtalar loss of motion, pain, inflammation, and negative imaging studies. Increased bone scan uptake in the sustentaculum tali may indicate fibrous coalition.

Treatment

The initial treatment of symptomatic coalition is nonsurgical and includes activity modification, anti-inflammatory

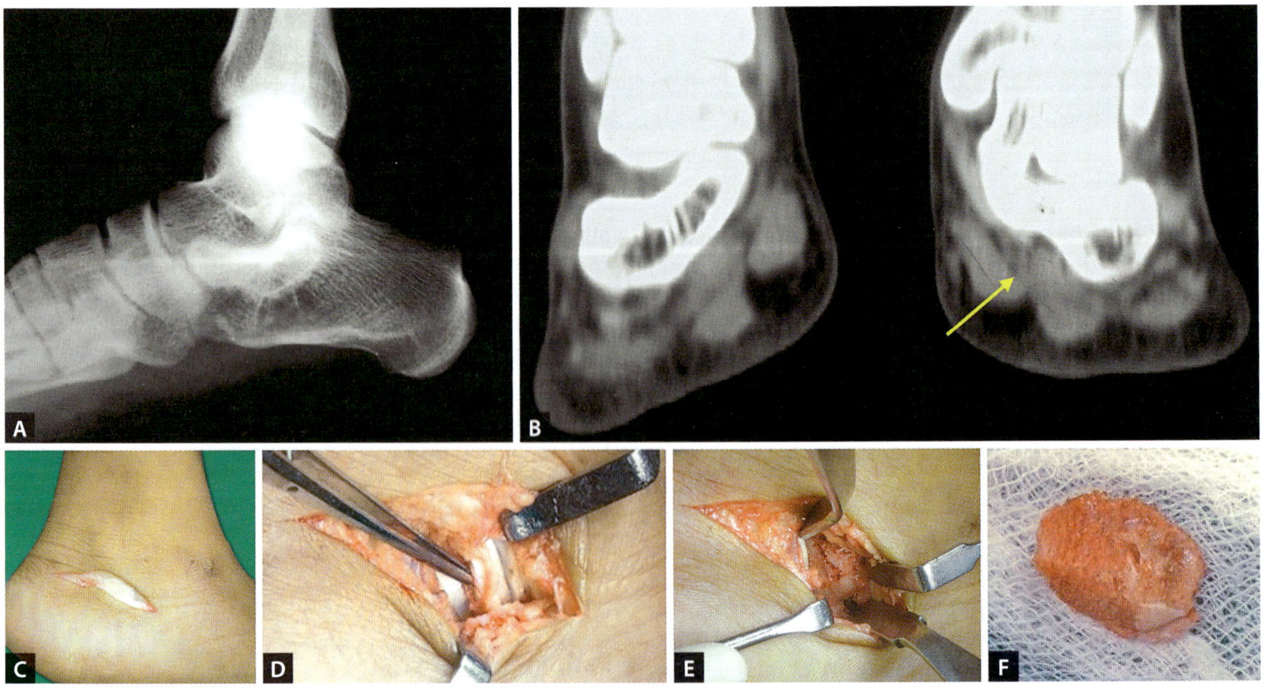

Figs. 74A to F: (A) The radiograph demonstrates the classic "C" sign as a prominent condensation of bone beneath the medial calcaneal facet; (B) Complete (arrow) talocalcaneal coalition of the left foot as demonstrated in the CT scan; (C to F) Managed by excision of the bony mass.

drugs, an orthotic device, or a short-leg walking cast. The goal of nonsurgical treatment of tarsal coalition is to relieve the symptoms and reduce the motion at the affected joint. Physical therapy in the form of massage, range-of-motion exercises, and ultrasound therapy may additionally be offered. This regimen is successful in approximately one-third of patients. In patients with inflammatory component to the subtalar joint, an injection of cortisone into the affected joint reduces the inflammation and pain. Patients who are to be put in plaster cast may be relieved of pain and spasm by an injection of local anesthetic into the region.

Surgical Treatment

Surgery for tarsal coalition falls into following categories:
- *To remove or excise the bar (calcaneonavicular or talocalcaneal as the case may be) and attempt to restore normal motion between the two bones:* With successful resection of bony bar and interposition of fat or extensor digitorum brevis muscle, patients with calcaneal-navicular coalitions do well **(Figs. 74A to F)**. Resection of a subtalar coalition may be indicated if the total area is <50% of the subtalar joint. The results of subtalar resection (for talocalcaneal coalition) and interposition of fat or split flexor hallucis tendon are less predictable than the results of calcaneal-navicular coalition, possibly because of the large coalition size or excessive valgus deformity.
- *To fuse the affected joints together solidly (subtalar/ triple arthrodesis):* This may also be used as a salvage surgery for previous failed resections.
- Osteotomy to correct residual valgus positioning.

SKEWFOOT (Z-FOOT, SERPENTINE FOOT, METATARSUS ADDUCTOVARUS, AND CONGENITAL METATARSUS VARUS)

The term skewfoot was first coined in 1949 by Blount and McCormick. It basically represents a metatarsus adductus foot type with congenital calcaneovalgus hindfoot deformity. Skewfoot is a rare deformity characterized by:
- Medial deviation of the forefoot
- Lateral translation of the midfoot with a trapezoidal medial cuneiform
- Valgus positioning of the hindfoot

The pathogenesis and natural history of deformity that develops idiopathically is unknown; however, it may be seen developing:
- Iatrogenically in overtreated clubfoot (see also clubfoot).
- Untreated metatarsus adductus that is compensated by excessive subtalar joint pronation.

In a young child because of the unossified midfoot bones, it is difficult to distinguish skewfoot from metatarsus adductus. With maturation, the metatarsus along with the collapsing pes valgo planus deformity becomes evident. The base of fifth metatarsal is prominent. There is a large space between the hallux and second digit. There is talar bulging or ptosis, low medial arch, abducted midfoot position, and internal rotation of malleoli. With growth and ossification of the bones as the midfoot develops, radiographs reveal the characteristic Z-deformity and an uncovering of the talus because of lateral translation of the navicular and a lateral offset of the first metatarsal axis in line with the longitudinal axis of the talus. The skew foot has been classified as proposed by Berg (see metatarsus adductus).

Treatment

Initially, the foot is manipulated to obtain proper shape that if fails is an indication for surgical correction (relative indication only). Other indications include:
- Foot too old for correction by conservative means
- Progressive deformity despite conservative treatment
- Deformity not manageable by conservative methods
- Development of secondary deformities and callosities
- Patient having pain during ambulation due to incomplete or nonphysiological compensation
- Inability to wear footwear or uncomfortable to wear footwear

The common surgical procedures include:
- Achilles tendon stretching and a soft orthotic device to support the talus head.
- Achilles fascial lengthening and gastrocnemius recession (Fulp and McGlamry)
- Evans calcaneal lengthening osteotomy and medial arch tendosuspension (for collapsing pes valgo planus correction)
- First cuneiform opening wedge osteotomies with or without talonavicular joint reefing.
- The modified Berman-Gartland procedure and the Lepird procedure that shift the metatarsals laterally by lesser metatarsal osteotomy.

CAVOVARUS FOOT

The cavovarus deformity is a complex three-dimensional combination of forefoot, midfoot, and hindfoot deformities. The components of deformity include:
1. Plantar flexion of first ray (forefoot)
2. Elevated medial longitudinal arch (mid-foot)
3. Hindfoot varus

The deformity is common in various disorders **(Box 6)** that result in progressive deformity which becomes rigid over time. Clinical examination reveals plantar callosities under first and fifth metatarsal heads, intrinsic muscle wasting, elevation of medial longitudinal arch, heel varus (inversion) as seen from behind. The flexibility of deformity should be carefully judged as it impacts management. Many tests have been described including Coleman block test, oblique block test, and prone Price and Mubarak test. In Coleman block test, patient stands with a block of wood under the

BOX 6: The etiological association of cavovarus deformity.
- Congenital
- Infection and osteomyelitis
- Post-traumatic deformity
- Charcot-Marie-Tooth (CMT) disease
- Tethered cord syndrome

lateral side of hindfoot, midfoot, and forefoot. In a flexible deformity, the heel varus corrects into valgus because the hind foot varus is driven by first metatarsal plantar flexion, the fixed contractures have not developed yet. This indicates that hindfoot deformity will correct if midfoot/forefoot plantar flexion is corrected. Because of association of spinal involvement in many, it is imperative to perform spinal cord examination in these patients. Radiographic assessment of all the three segmental deformities should be done. Forefoot supination is assessed by metatarsal overlap, midfoot cavus is assessed in lateral projection and quantified by talar-first metatarsal angle, hindfoot varus is quantified by talocalcaneal angle in anteroposterior projection.

The treatment of cavovarus deformity is aimed at symptomatic relief, increased forefoot contact, and alignment of forefoot and hindfoot. Nonsurgical management options include bracing and orthosis for patients with mild, nonprogressive flexible deformities. The braces/orthosis recesses the first metatarsal and elevates the whole lateral part of foot. Surgical treatment is decided based on flexibility of hindfoot. In flexible deformities, options include soft tissue release, tendon transfers, and small joint fusion. Mostly plantar or medioplantar soft tissue release is done. Only in uncommon cases calf muscle lengthening is needed. Peroneus longus muscle when transferred to brevis removes plantar flexion force on first ray and aids correction of peroneal tendon dysfunction. Posterior tibialis tendon is transferred to dorsum of foot to alleviate weak dorsiflexion associated with Charcot-Marie-Tooth (CMT) disease. Claw toes can be corrected by rebalancing flexor-extensor tendon transfer often combined with proximal interphalangeal joint fusion. In rigid deformities typically the joint sparing osteotomy like medial tarsometatarsal ray and realigning calcaneal osteotomies are first choice. Naviculocuneiform arthrodesis for correction of severe cavus component and hindfoot fusion at the Chopart line, or Lambrinudi triple fusion for advanced rigid deformities. Severe deformities would need supramalleolar rotational osteotomy.

FLEXIBLE FLATFOOT

This is a planovalgus deformity of foot present in half of the newborns that corrects itself quite promptly. "Flatfoot" describes a weight-bearing foot shape in which the hindfoot is in valgus, the midfoot sags in a plantar direction touching the floor, and the forefoot is supinated in relation to the hindfoot. <10% have it in early adolescence. The condition, its development, resolution all remains poorly understood largely due to conflicting and poorly conducted research. The shape of foot is common, often familial, rarely painful, and even more rarely disabling so it should be considered normal in most. The definition and magnitude of medial arch height are itself undefined.

Flatfoot deformities can be rigid or flexible, depending on the mobility of the hindfoot. In a flexible flatfoot, the valgus position of hindfoot corrects itself to a varus alignment when the patient is standing on the toes **(Fig. 75A and B)**. A rigid hindfoot does not have subtalar motion, either with toe standing or manipulation (as defined by defined by Harris and Beath). These later patients should be suspected of having a tarsal coalition or subtalar pathology. Three types of flatfoot have been classified by Harris and Beath but they are not very popular. The flexible (hypermobile) type has good mobility of joints and tendons. Flexible flatfoot with short Achilles tendon has contracted tendon and is often painful due to poor adaptation. The last is rigid type as detailed above.

Pathogenesis and Hypotheses

- Normal arch but presence of fat pad that obscures it (Morley)
- *Subclinical muscle weakness (Duchenne):* Coordinated and normal function of the muscles of the foot and ankle was responsible for the maintenance of the longitudinal arch and that subclinical muscle weakness was responsible for the flexible flatfoot.
- *Bone-ligament theory (Basmajian et al.):* Height of the longitudinal arch is determined by features of the

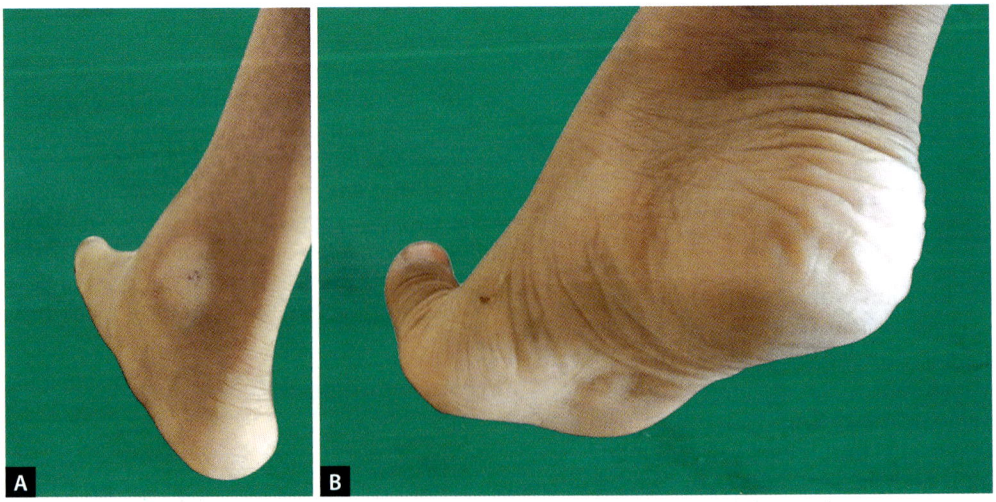

Figs. 75A and B: Flexible flatfoot. In children, (A) the feet may appear flat with an absent curved instep due to delayed development of the same but when asked to lift the heel; (B) Normal arch appears. This is a normal foot in which development of arch takes some time.

bone-ligament complex, and that the muscles maintain balance, accommodate the foot to uneven terrain, protect the ligaments from unusual stresses, and propel the body forward. They concluded that excessive ligamentous laxity is the primary abnormality and that muscles are necessary for function and balance, but not for structural integrity.

Pathoanatomy and Pathomechanics

- There is hindfoot valgus and a compensatory forefoot supination deformity.
- A tight Achilles tendon may be a component for patients with painful callosities over the head of the talus (flexible flatfoot with short tendo-Achilles).
- Some intrinsic ligamentous laxity with external tibial torsion
- Biomechanically in a normal foot tibia and talus internally rotate during the first half of the stance phase while the subtalar joint complex everts. Talar head plantar flexes unlocking the foot making it supple and hence the foot flattens. During the latter part of the stance phase, the tibia and talus externally rotate, while the subtalar joint complex inverts, so that the acetabulum pedis once again supports the head of the talus that dorsiflexes and foot regains its arch and becomes more rigid. The flexible flatfoot begins stance in an unlocked, everted position, and does not completely convert to a rigid, inverted lever during the latter portion of stance.

Clinical Features

There is a straight or convex plantar-medial border of the foot. The lateral border is straight or concave. The midfoot sags and touches the ground in weight-bearing. The foot appears externally rotated in relation to the leg and the weight-bearing axis of the lower extremity passes medial to the mid-axis of the hindfoot. The hindfoot is in valgus alignment.

The flexibility of flatfoot is a more important feature than the static shape. The subtalar joint will invert from valgus to neutral and a longitudinal arch will be observed in a flexible flatfoot that is not supporting body weight. A longitudinal arch can also be created by dorsiflexing the great toe—toe-raising test of Jack and Hicks. This is due to the "windlass action" of the plantar fascia. Dorsiflexion of the toes shortens the plantar fascia around the heads of the metatarsals and thus elevates the medial longitudinal arch. The same effect can be produced by standing on toes (Jacks toe-raising test, **Figs. 75A and B**).

Supination deformity of the forefoot on the hindfoot is revealed when the valgus hindfoot is passively inverted to neutral. The flexible flatfoot with short tendo-Achilles will have limitation of ankle dorsiflexion additionally.

Treatment

- Strengthening, stretching, and a soft accommodating shoe insert are often helpful to relieve symptoms.
- Surgical intervention to correct a painful flatfoot is rarely necessary and generally involves a combination of osteotomies and Achilles tendon lengthening. Isolated soft tissue procedures are not very reliable.
- Pseudoarthrodesis (arthroereisis literally means that limits but not eliminates movement) procedures were introduced between 1946 and 1977 to restrict subtalar motion (eversion) without creating arthrodesis have fallen into disfavor as either the graft resorbs recreating the deformity or else it remains there creating unique problems like pain. Arthroereisis using implants (like Maxwell-Brancheau arthroereisis implant) has also been described but not very popular.
- A sliding calcaneal osteotomy of Gleich (or Dwyer's lateral opening wedge osteotomy) can correct the hindfoot valgus along with a plantar base closing wedge osteotomy of the first cuneiform to correct the supination deformity. Dwyer's osteotomy though does not correct the deformity fully. Lateral column lengthening by Evans calcaneal osteotomy is a quite favorable option and can be combined with dorsolateral talar reefing and metatarsal osteotomies.
- Hoke's limited midtarsal arthrodesis is another feasible option commonly followed.

ACCESSORY NAVICULAR (OS TIBIALE EXTERNUM, NAVICULAR SECUNDUM AND PREHALLUX)

Approximately 10–15% of the general population have an accessory navicular. The term is applied to plantar and medial enlargement of the tarsal navicular bone beyond its normal size. It is often bilateral and is more often symptomatic in girls (and also common) than boys.

Pathogenesis

The navicular bone ossifies at age 3 in girls and 5 in boys. The accessory navicular does not begin to ossify prior to age 8. Accessory navicular represents a malformation of tarsal navicular and was considered by McKusick to be inherited as an autosomal dominant trait.

Clinical Features

A prominence is noted on the plantar medial aspect of the foot at the base of the navicular, within the substance or the insertion of the posterior tibialis tendon. Flatfoot as a deformity may coexist but is neither related nor the pathogenic event. Three types have been described **(Figs. 76A to D)**:

1. *Type I:* A small sesamoid bone in the substance of the posterior tibialis tendon itself.
2. *Type II:* A large wedge-shaped bone fragment that attaches to the navicular either through a synchondrosis or synovial joint. The gap histopathologically often contains proliferating vascular mesenchymal tissue, cartilage proliferation, and osteoblastic, and osteoclastic activity. This supports the hypothesis of microfractures from repetitive stress.
3. *Type III:* A large horn-shaped navicular resulting from fusion of a type II deformity.

Commonly an adolescent female presents with medial arch pain that gets worse with overuse. The pain may start

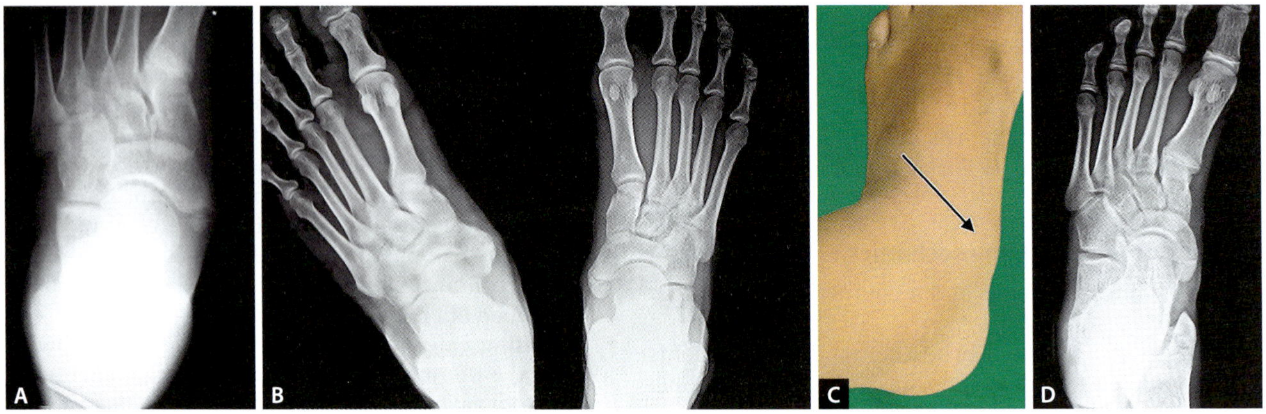

Figs. 76A to D: Accessory navicular (A) Type 1; (B) Type 2; (C) Clinical picture (arrow); (D) Type 3.

after a traumatic event or insidiously. There is usually tenderness over the prominent aspect of the accessory bone that may be accompanied with redness and swelling. Mere presence of accessory navicular should not be ascribed to the cause of symptoms for its common radiological presence.

Treatment

The nonsurgical options include rest, anti-inflammatory medicines, and a shoe-insert or padding with good arch support to decrease the strain of the posterior tibialis tendon. This should always be tried as most patients become symptom-free at skeletal maturity and for symptomatic flare-ups, the pain should be relieved conservatively. Good padding provides relief by diminishing direct pressure over the bony prominence. A period of cast immobilization can be used to decrease inflammation in patients getting less than complete relief or those who are unable to restrict strenuous activity.

For recalcitrant cases that fail even extended conservative trials simple excision of the accessory bone and reattachment of any disturbed posterior tibialis tendon, may be needed. The bone should be excised flush with medial cuneiform through a dorsomedial incision to prevent painful scar. There is no need to advance posterior tibialis tendon (Kidner procedure) as this does not play any role in the formation of medial arch but should be surely reattached. Management of flatfoot can be done as described above.

CONCLUSION

- The lower limb anomalies generate quite a lot of worry amongst parents with respect to ambulation of the child in future.
- Angular anomalies are commonly encountered, the pathophysiology of which should be clear to the treating surgeon. One should be able to find the exact location of deformity, how to measure it and importantly plan and time the correction well. Poor planning or execution would lead to unsatisfactory results and may even invite litigation as parents are quite sensitive with respect to the children.
- Congenital anomalies produce significant morbidity and mostly the results are unsatisfactory and compromised. The best part, however, is that the children are able to cope-up well with the deformity and compensate for them quite well over time.

CHAPTER 42

Pediatric Hip Joint Disorders

Manish Kumar Varshney

INTRODUCTION

Hip joint anomalies are common in pediatric orthopedic disorders. They form a range of spectrum from abnormalities in individual part of bone (coxa vara) to abnormalities in development of hip joint (dysplastic development of hip). Slippage of the femoral epiphysis and osteonecrosis of epiphysis will be the other two intermediary disorders of this range that will be discussed here. Therapeutic time window is quite short for many of these disorders. The associated morbidity is quite high and unacceptable, if no or suboptimal treatment is done. It is imperative to understand and optimally manage the disorders to mitigate complications and provide maximum long-term benefit.

COXA VARA

Coxa vara is defined as any decrease below the normal values of the neck-shaft angle of the proximal femur **(Fig. 1)** that can arise from various conditions:

- *Congenital:* Due to embryonic limb bud abnormality. The deformity is present at birth itself and is seen associated with proximal femoral focal deficiency (PFFD), congenital short femur and congenital bowed femur, and fibular hemimelia.
- *Acquired:*
    - Metabolic (rickets)
    - Neoplastic (fibrous dysplasia)
    - Traumatic **(Fig. 2)**
    - Slipped upper femoral epiphysis (SUFE)
    - Inflammatory
    - Perthes
    - Infective (tuberculosis)
- *Developmental [infantile coxa vara (ICV)]:* This is a progressive coxa vara with associated neck lesion that makes it characteristic. Usually, there are no other associated musculoskeletal abnormalities. This lesion is discussed below.

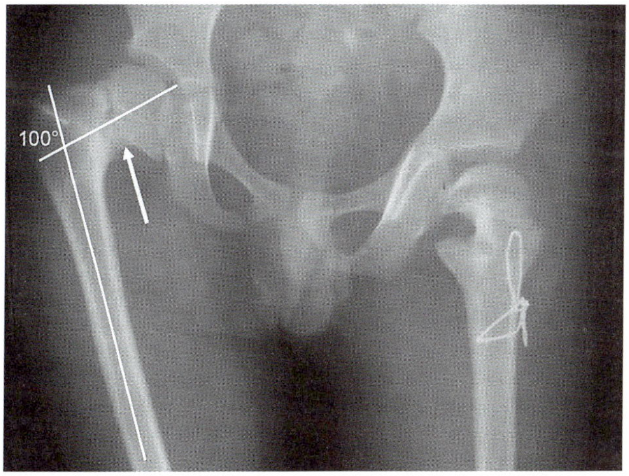

Fig. 1: Infantile coxa vara; left side has been operated elsewhere, right side disease still persists. The neck lesion in the form of Fairbank's triangle (arrow) can be characteristically seen.

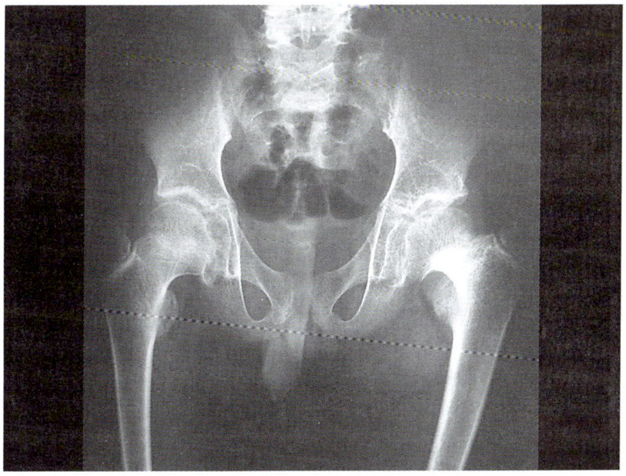

Fig. 2: Acquired (traumatic) coxa vara of left hip.

INFANTILE COXA VARA

Infantile coxa vara (some call this congenital coxa vara but should be finely differentiated as detailed above) has been described in literature for a long time **(Box 1)**. ICV is an autosomal-dominant disorder that occurs in 1 in 25,000 live births [around 20 times less than developmental dysplasia of the hip (DDH)]. There is no sex or side predominance and bilateral involvement is seen in 30–50% cases. It occurs

BOX 1: Historical perspective of coxa vara and infantile coxa vara.

- *1881:* Fiorani described "bending of the femoral neck" in adult patients.
- *1894:* First radiographic description of decreased neck-shaft angle given by Hofmeister and also used the term "coxa vara"
- *1896:* Kredel described coxa vara occurring during childhood and proposed "congenital origin" (corrected later by others).
- *1907:* Elmslie used the term "infantile coxa vara".
- *1928:* Progressive nature of deformity was described by Fairbank and also differentiated this from congenital form. He used the term developmental coxa vara. This developmental (termed infantile to differentiate from congenital) form has been supported by Amstutz that separates congenital from acquired form (developmental/infantile).

perinatally and is characterized by a decreased femoral neck shaft angle in association with a primary femoral neck defect.

Etiology and Pathophysiology

The progressive deformity is possibly the result of fatigue of dystrophic bone resulting from poor endochondral ossification under physiological stress. The physiological stress then becomes pathological due to increased neck-shaft angle and the vicious circle keeps progressing (Pylkkanen's theory).

As for most disorders, the exact etiology is unknown but there have been a lot of hypotheses projected to explain the disorder:

- *Defective endochondral ossification:* Metabolic abnormality causing a deficient production of (or delayed) normal ossification process of the proximal end of the femur.
- *Mechanical abnormality occurring during hip development:* Excessive intrauterine pressure on the developing hip results in a depression in the neck of the femur (Hoffa and Alsberg).
- *Partial vascular insult*, causing an arrest in the early development of the femoral head and neck (Nillsone).
- Secondary to a developmental error, resulting in faulty maturation of the cartilage and metaphyseal bone of the femoral neck (Duncan).
- Variant of metaphyseal chondrodysplasia (Schmidt type) localized to hip joint (similar to Blount's disease at knee).

Pathoanatomy

Grossly, the "Y-shaped" defect involves both the inferior portion of the capital physis and the adjacent metaphysis. Histopathologically, there are:

- Increase in the width of the growth plate—typically seen in the inferior portion of the femoral neck and radiologically evident as "fairbank triangle"
- Irregularly distributed germinal cells in the resting zone of physis
- Absence of normal orderly progression of the cartilage columns
- Poorly defined zone of provisional calcification
- Increased vascularity and predominance of fibrous element between bony spicules

Clinical Features

- *Progressive Trendelenburg gait:* This results from the reduced length-tension relationship of the hip abductors from tucked-up greater trochanter
- Decrease in hip abduction, internal rotation (progressive decrease in anteversion), and later global restriction (painless)
- Flexion contracture of hip
- Limb-length discrepancy (unilateral)
- Lumbar lordosis
- Prominent trochanters palpable on affected side
- Positive Trendelenburg sign

Radiology

There is decreased neck-shaft angle that keeps progressing on sequential films. The proximal femoral physis is vertically oriented with a triangular metaphyseal fragment in the form of inverted radiolucent "Y". This fragment is often called the "Fairbank fragment" and the triangle as "Fairbank triangle". There is reduced femoral anteversion that may actually become retroversion. There are usually associated coxa breva and mild acetabular dysplasia. The vertical position of the physis is the cause of progression of pathology due to nonphysiological transmission of forces. This position on a radiograph is quantifiable and also a guide for treatment.

- *Hilgenreiner physeal angle (HPA, used to quantify the verticality of proximal femoral capital physis):* HPA is defined by the angle subtended by intersection planes of the physeal plate and the Hilgenreiner line. This angle is normally 25° or less, but in developmental coxa vara, it is usually in the range of 40–70°.
- *Neck-shaft angle:* This is another method to guide surgery and commonly used. Angles >110° have possibility for better resolution of the disease, while those <90° should always be operated. Angles between 90 and 110° should be observed for progression or resolution of disease.

Natural History of Disease

If untreated, the deformity keeps progressing similar to stress fracture-related nonunion of the femoral neck. There is prominent premature development of degenerative arthritis in the hip joint causing pain and disability. The changes are marked in patients with HPA >60°. While patients with lesser angles (<45°) often show spontaneous healing due to compressive vector in the transmitted forces. Children with angles between 45 and 60° have a variable course and should be closely observed to determine signs of progression.

Treatment

The treatment is guided primarily by HPA or neck-shaft angle as given below:

- Neck-shaft angle of <90° + limp should be operated
- Hilgenreiner physeal angle >60° should be operated, especially if associated with limp.
- Children with HPA between 45 and 60° (at risk cases) and progression of deformity should be considered for surgery after proper counseling.

Conservative Treatment

It is done for patients with HPA <45° and patients under observation (at risk) of progression. These patients are taught range of motion (ROM) exercises and strengthening exercises to retain good muscle power and unload hip. Spica cast immobilization and skeletal traction with bed rest are not favored in modern orthopedics anymore due to lack of literature support.

Surgical Treatment

It is commonly recommended for indicated patients >2 years of age to prevent further damage to the region (dysplasia at femoral head, neck, and acetabulum). The bones are softer at this tender age, but adequate fixation can be achieved with modern implants. Some surgeons are concerned that physeal closure will produce shortening. Physeal growth at the capital physis does not significantly contribute to femoral length (at most providing 2–3 cm overall length to lower limb). Delaying surgery for better skeletal growth and fixation and gaining as much length before surgery may thus not be a wise recommendation. Goals of surgical treatment are to:

- Restore a more anatomic alignment—creation of neck-shaft angle that permits normalization of the femoral head and acetabulum.
- Repositioning of the femoral head in acetabulum so that the upper pole of femoral heads points up rather than medially.
- Gradual lengthening of the abductors. Often, however, the length gain is done acutely with osteotomy. This can be done with Ilizarov method.
- Creation of leverage to increase the efficiency of abductors eliminating the Trendelenburg sign
- Eliminate the knee deformity and correct shortening.
- Improve the hip ROM and mechanics.

Corrective intertrochanteric or subtrochanteric valgus osteotomy [Pauwel's "Y" shaped or Langenskiold type **(Fig. 3)**] is the preferred method to restore the proximal alignment. The osteotomy is done to overcorrect the neck-shaft angle to 150–160° (HPA < 30°). Because of reduced anteversion or actual retroversion in these cases, a rotational corrective option (*derotation*) needs to be added to the osteotomy. This is done by internally rotating the distal fragment during fixation. The physis must be protected from the fixation implant. Additional *adductor tenotomy* and/or *proximal femoral shortening* can be done to unload the femoral head and ease valgus correction.

- These convert the angulatory forces to compressive forces.
- Mechanical redirection of forces to improve acetabular dysplasia (dysplasia does not improve if the angle is <140°)

Brackett's procedure has high morbidity and is not done anymore considering the favorable outcome of valgus plus derotational osteotomy. In Brackett's procedure, the pathological portion of neck is resected followed by insertion of the remaining shaft into femoral head and advancing the greater trochanter.

After surgery, it is seen that when the desired valgus correction has been obtained, the triangular fragment heals spontaneously in 3–6 months. Unfortunately, in many of these patients (>90%), the physis also closes at 12–24 months postoperatively.

Complications of surgical treatment:

- Violation of the physis and closure
- Premature spontaneous closure of the physis
- Recurrent varus deformity consequent upon the premature capital physeal closure but continued trochanteric growth—treat with trochanteric apophysiodesis or advancement.
- Development of limb-length inequality

SLIPPED CAPITAL FEMORAL EPIPHYSIS (SLIPPED UPPER FEMORAL EPIPHYSIS)

Though uncommon as such, slipped capital femoral epiphysis (SCFE) is the most common hip disorder in adolescents of predisposed population (African American, Polynesian). The condition is defined as rotational deformity of capital femoral epiphysis in relation to metaphysis **(Fig. 4)** where there are posterior and inferior slippages of the proximal femoral epiphysis on the metaphysis (femoral neck) through the epiphyseal growth plate (physis). This injury is similar to Salter-Harris type I physeal separations, but it differs in features such as slower displacement, maintained periosteum, and presence of antecedent epiphysiolysis. It is often missed

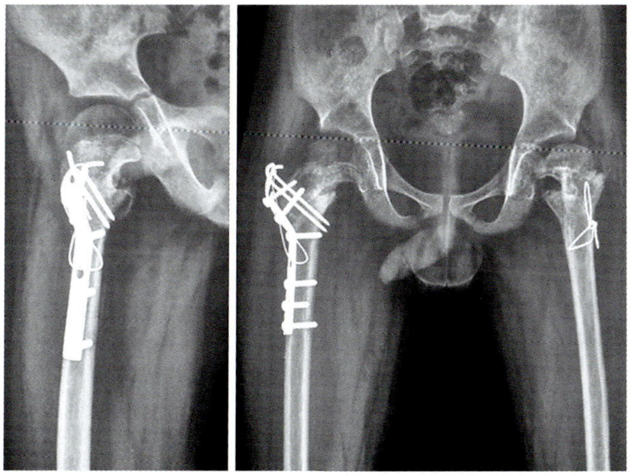

Fig. 3: Correction of coxa vara in patient shown in **Figure 1** with a subtrochanteric valgus osteotomy.

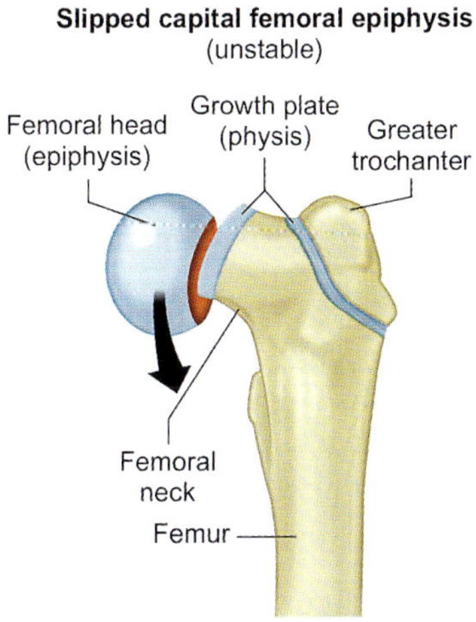

Fig. 4: Illustration of rotational displacement of epiphysis in relation to metaphysis in slipped capital femoral epiphysis (SCFE).

TABLE 1: Causes of limping child.

Infants and toddlers (up to 3 years old)	*Walking age group and adolescents*
• Septic arthritis (including Tom–Smith arthritis) • Osteomyelitis • Tubercular arthritis • Developmental dysplasia of the hip • Clubfoot • Leg-length discrepancy including proximal focal femoral deficiency • Toddlers' fracture • Trauma • Stress fracture or overuse syndromes • Cerebral palsy • Meningitis • Osteoid osteoma • Neuroblastoma • Leukemia • Transient synovitis • Child abuse • Foreign body	• Slipped capital femoral epiphysis • Tubercular arthritis of hip • Psoas abscess • Transient synovitis often viral • Perthes' disease • Trauma • Osgood–Schlatter disease • Sever disease • Ewing's sarcoma • Chondromalacia patellae • Juvenile idiopathic arthritis • Hemarthrosis • Osteonecrosis of femoral head • Stress fracture • Muscular dystrophy • Cerebral palsy • Chondromalacia • Myelomeningocele • Discitis and TB spine • Vertebral osteomyelitis • Diastematomyelia • Osteosarcoma • Sickle cell disease • Gonococcal septic arthritis • Sever disease

due to possible vague symptoms pointing to referral regions (medial thigh/knee). Dire consequences of missing the diagnosis and complicating outcome mandate that good prognosis is directly related to how quickly the condition is diagnosed and treated. SCFE should be considered in children who present with limping and pain in the hip, groin, or thigh. Other causes of a limping child are tabulated in **Table 1**.

EPIDEMIOLOGY

The prevalence of SCFE is 2 per 100,000 children (ranging from 0.2 per 100,000 in eastern Japan to 10.8 cases per 100,000 children in predisposed regions). Seasonal predilection for SCFE during the summer months has been reported (late summer and falls in patients who reside north of 40° latitude, US). It is more common in boys (2:1.4) and in blacks and Pacific Islanders (possibly because of increased prevalence of overweight population here). The average age at diagnosis is 13.5 years for boys (range 10–16 years) and 12.1 years for girls (range 9–15 years). SCFE presents bilaterally in 18–50% of patients; half of these are simultaneous and other half develop it sequentially (metachronous SCFE) within 18 months. The characteristics related to high risk of developing SCFE include:

- Obesity
- Race (African-American)
- Short stature (<10th percentile)
- Medical problems such as endocrinopathy, craniopharyngioma, Down's syndrome, renal osteodystrophy, pituitary tumors, and adiposogenital syndrome.

ETIOLOGY

The etiology is thought to be multifactorial and following factors have been forwarded as possible causes/theories for pathogenesis:

- *Obesity:* Weight in the 90th percentile or higher. Obesity is associated with metabolic and endocrine abnormalities and it causes mechanical overload of the inclined femoral epiphysis predisposing to slip.
- *Hormonal influence* (should be considered in SCFE with unusual presentations, including patients who are younger than 8 years, older than 15 years, or underweight):
  - ↑ Estrogen, ↓ growth hormone—decreases growth plate strength as in puberty.
  - Endocrinopathy—hypothyroidism, panhypopituitarism, hyperparathyroidism, and hypogonadism. Increased leptin levels are associated with SCFE regardless of obesity.
- Mechanical factors such as trauma
- *Inflammatory cells:* Presence of some inflammatory cells in joint such as round cells and plasma cells that cause physeal weakness.
- *Genetic influence:*
  - About 2–5% incidence in immediate family members
  - Association with human leukocyte antigen (HLA)-DR4 antigen
- *Hip joint morphology:* Acetabular retroversion causes shear stress across epiphyseal plate in SCFE; this is further aggravated by femoral retroversion, posterior epiphyseal inclination, and reduced head–neck offset common in SCFE. The epiphyseal plate morphology is an interesting topic in contention. Epiphyseal cupping and extension are protective against physeal instability. The epiphysis peripherally expands around the metaphysis (extension) producing cupping and increasing engagement **(Fig. 5A)**. Second feature is the presence of epiphyseal tubercle, which is a bony prominence located over the posterosuperior surface of epiphysis and insinuated into metaphysis **(Figs. 5B and C)**. It is not seen after skeletal maturity. In rotational theory of SCFE, the physeal slip and rotation occur about epiphyseal tubercle as fulcrum where the epiphysis rotates over metaphysis. In chronic SCFE, metaphysis progressively rotates externally around the tubercle. It also suggests that if screw is placed around such a pivot point then postoperative slip progression would likely occur and treatment would fail, so such a placement should be altogether avoided. In adolescence, there is thinning of perichondrial ring and unlocking of mammillary process would contribute to physeal instability.

PATHOANATOMY

The physis is already in strain due to external rotation of the femoral shaft with posterior counterforce on the femoral head. The head thus moves posteriorly, while neck moves cephalad. Also, the position of physis changes from horizontal to oblique in preadolescence and adolescence changing the direction of force from horizontal to oblique increasing vertical strain. The separation in SCFE results from the hypertrophic zone of physis that may occupy up to 80% of the width of the physis in affected patients. There are abnormal cartilage maturation, endochondral ossification, and perichondral ring instability. The physis is wide and undergoes disruption with reduced numbers of cartilage cells and disorganization.

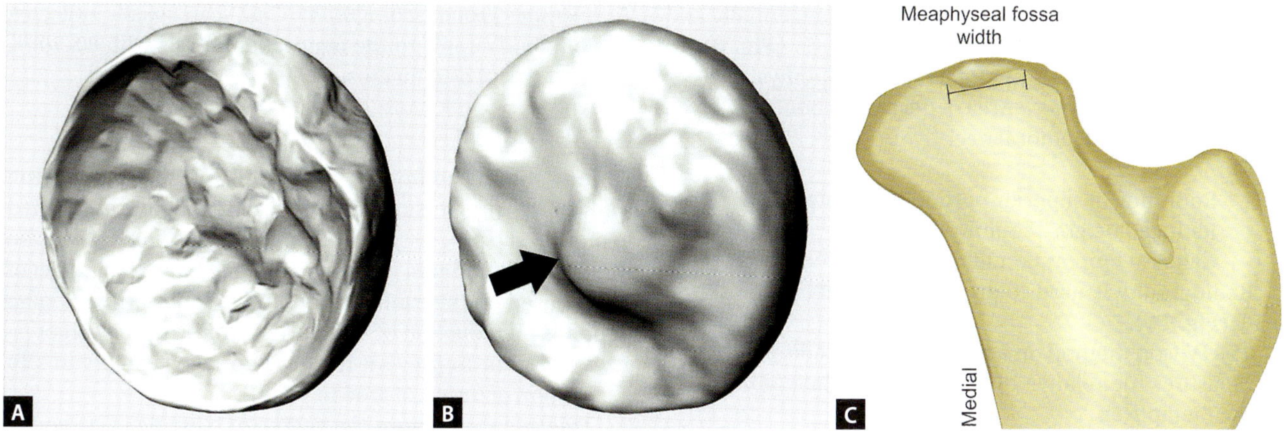

Figs. 5A to C: (A) The cupping of epiphysis provides stability from slip as the epiphysis sits over femoral neck (metaphysis). (B) The epiphyseal tubercle (arrow) is a prominence in the epiphysis posterosuperiorly towards the physeal plate that insinuates into femoral neck metaphysis (C) in the marked fossa region. It regresses with age and rotation around this tubercle has been proposed to cause slip in slipped capital femoral epiphysis (SCFE). Peritubercle lucency is considered predisposing factor for slip.

CLASSIFICATION

Slipped capital femoral epiphysis is clinically classified based on the stability of the physis or duration of symptoms or anatomic displacement. The classification based on stability (Loder et al.) has prognostic value as most stable SCFEs have better prognosis.

- *Stable SCFE (90% of all slips):* The patient is able to ambulate with or without crutches.
- *Unstable SCFE:* The patient is unable to ambulate even with crutches and there is higher rate of complications.

Based on duration of symptoms, the slip could be:

- Preslip (prodromal stage)
- *Acute:* Symptoms for <3 weeks
- *Chronic:* Symptoms present for >3 weeks
- *Acute-on-chronic:* Chronic slip with sudden failure at physis and exacerbation of symptoms

This classification suffers from problems of recall (exact duration is usually unknown) and is hence not very reliable. Also, it is worth noting that neither all acute slips are unstable nor all chronic slips are stable (this correlation though deemed logical is untrue and should be taken off mind).

Anatomic classification:

- *Linear displacement:* Wilson method (see below)
- *Angular displacement:* Southwick angles (see below)

HISTORY AND PHYSICAL EXAMINATION

Patients with SCFE present with limp and pain in the hip, groin, thigh, or knee. Knee or distal thigh pain is the initial presenting symptom in 46% of patients with the condition. This pain is usually disregarded as muscle pull, making it prone to misdiagnosis and missing the condition. History of trauma is uncommon.

There are four typical clinical presentations. The first and most common is the chronic SCFE that presents in above manner and the pain and external rotation deformity progress over several weeks or months. The patient is overweight and has features of early puberty in general. He may be unable to bear weight with a severe slip or else walks with an abductor lurch/antalgic gait. On examination, the patient has variable loss of internal rotation and flexion at hip due to synovitis and mechanical blockade of displaced metaphysis, respectively. Attempted hip flexion beyond the limit results in abduction and external rotation deviation of the lower limb (Drehmann sign). Unless the patient has bilateral SCFE, it is helpful to compare ROM with the uninvolved hip. The other common presentation is sudden onset of severe pain in the hip due to acute dissociation of epiphysis from metaphysis—characteristic of acute SCFE. It may also be acute or chronic presentation where the child has features of previous chronic slip that suddenly get aggravated into acute presentation. The third variety is presence of hip pain but no radiographical abnormality defining a preslip stage. Magnetic resonance imaging (MRI) may be helpful in such cases. The last presentation of disease remains completely asymptomatic without any significant progression (subclinical slip) that heals itself over time. It is recognized in later life as femoroacetabular impingement.

DIFFERENTIAL DIAGNOSIS

The differential diagnoses are apophyseal avulsion fracture, fracture, transient synovitis, Perthes' disease, septic arthritis, and hip apophysitis.

RADIOGRAPHY

Anteroposterior and true (cross-table) lateral radiographs are obtained for patients aged 8–15 years of age with new-onset limping and/or pain in the hip, groin, thigh, or knee.

- *Early mild SCFE:* The lateral radiographs are more sensitive in identifying SCFE in early cases by demonstrating periosteal elevation, loss of anterior concavity at head-neck junction, and sharpening of metaphyseal border of head.
    - Widening and irregularity of physeal plate
    - *Trethowan's sign:* It is failure of Klein's line to intersect with the femoral head. The Klein's line is drawn along

the superior aspect of femoral neck tangentially and extended proximally toward epiphysis **(Fig. 6)**. In normal hips, it always intersects the epiphysis.
  - *Blanch sign of steel:* Area of decreased bone density in the proximal femoral neck
- *Chronic SCFE:*
  - Rounding of superior portion of femoral neck
  - Reduced height of epiphysis
  - Callus at epiphyseometaphyseal junction

Radiography is used to grade the severity of the slip in SCFE **(Fig. 7A)**.

- The Wilson method on a frog-leg lateral radiograph. Measures the relative displacement of the epiphysis on the metaphysis.
  - *Mild slip:* Epiphysis displacement less than one-third of the width (the radiograph in **Figure 7A** shows a moderate slip, though the radiograph is not taken on a frog-leg lateral view, so this assumption could be wrong as shown by Southwick method that revealed severe slip) of the metaphysis.
  - *Moderate slip:* Displacement between one-third and one-half of the width
  - *Severe slip:* Displacement greater than one-half of the width.
- The Southwick method measures angular displacement between the epiphysis and shaft on lateral radiograph **(Fig. 8)**. The angular displacement is calculated by the difference between affected and unaffected sides.
  - Mild slip is <30°.
  - Moderate slip is angular displacement between 30 and 50°.
  - Severe slip is >50° **(Fig. 7A)**.

Ultrasonography (USG):
- Hip effusion—indicates acute event or infection
- Metaphyseal remodeling—chronic slips

Computed tomography (CT) scan and MRI: Three-dimensional imaging may be done in cases of unclear cases and to confirm the status of growth plate. In preslip stage, physeal asymmetry may be better judged by CT scan. Peritubercle radiolucency representing micromotion is also suggestive of SCFE. MRI is recommended for preslip status, as it demonstrates juxtaphyseal edema in metaphysis.

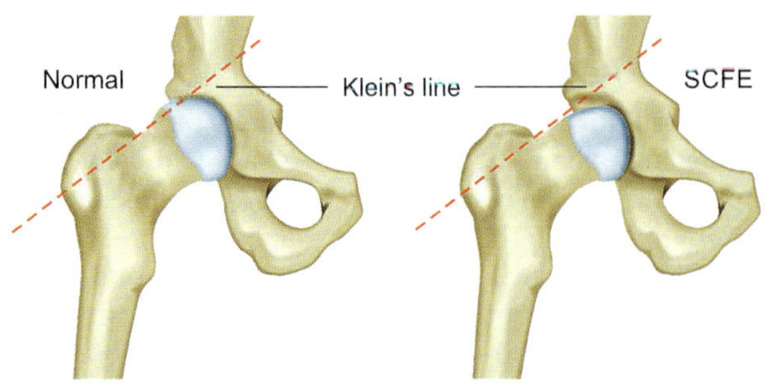

Fig. 6: The Klein's line is drawn along the superior aspect of femoral neck and its proximal extension intersects epiphysis normally. If the line passes above epiphysis without intersecting then it indicates epiphyseal slippage. (SCFE: slipped capital femoral epiphysis)

Technetium-99 bone scintigraphy: Cold scan usually indicates loss of blood supply to the femoral epiphysis with 80–100% incident risk of osteonecrosis.

TREATMENT

Patient should be immediately kept nonweight-bearing (prevent slip progression) and surgical treatment is also aimed to prevent slip progression and avoid complications. There are three broad treatment methods available for management of SCFE based on the evolving notion that long-term outcome depends on reduction of original deformity during surgery:

1. Treatment to prevent further slippage (usually in situ fixation of fusion of growth plate)
2. *Treatment to reduce the degree of slippage:* Corrective osteotomies to correct the deformities and reduce the severity of slip from moderate and severe to mild or anatomical levels
3. Salvage procedure

Prophylactic treatment of the contralateral hip in patients with SCFE is controversial, but it is not recommended in most patients. Prophylactic pinning may be indicated in patients at high risk of subsequent slips. Radiological presence of posterior sloping angle >14° and/or peritubercle lucency (CT scan) in a patient with open triradiate cartilage or modified Oxford bone age score of 18 or less or stage 0 to 3 calcaneal apophysis ossification is predictive of metachronous slip needing prophylactic fixation. This is further strengthened, if patient is obese and has a low likelihood of follow-up.

Unstable Slipped Capital Femoral Epiphysis

Unstable SCFE is a severe injury than stable SCFE with rate of osteonecrosis is as high as 20–50%. The acceptable treatment recommendations include in situ percutaneous fixation or open epiphysiodesis with bone graft. There is controversy as to the timing of surgery, preoperative reduction, and role of traction, if any. In situ percutaneous screw fixation is the most common method of fixation **(Figs. 7A to C)**; the screw must not penetrate joint (high chances of chondrolysis) but provide adequate stability and must not disturb the vascularity of head. I am not averse to trying reduction and one single gentle attempt at the same can be given relying on clinical evidence of acute slips that have higher chance of reduction. The screw is so placed that the screw tip is central in femoral head in all views and the screw crosses the growth plate perpendicularly. This often requires an anterior starting point in high-grade slips going posterior through or out of the femoral neck and placing the screw centrally in the head. The starting point should, however, never go medial to intertrochanteric line, as this would cause impingement against acetabular rim. Reduction of slip also reduces the kink in posterosuperior epiphyseal vessels that may be responsible for osteonecrosis.

The other reason why I prefer reduction of the slip before fixation is the documented evidence that femoroacetabular impingement (FAI) is associated with development of chondral damage and late osteoarthritis. Unsatisfactory outcomes of in situ pinning (10–20% failures/complications) have resulted in advocating other surgical procedures.

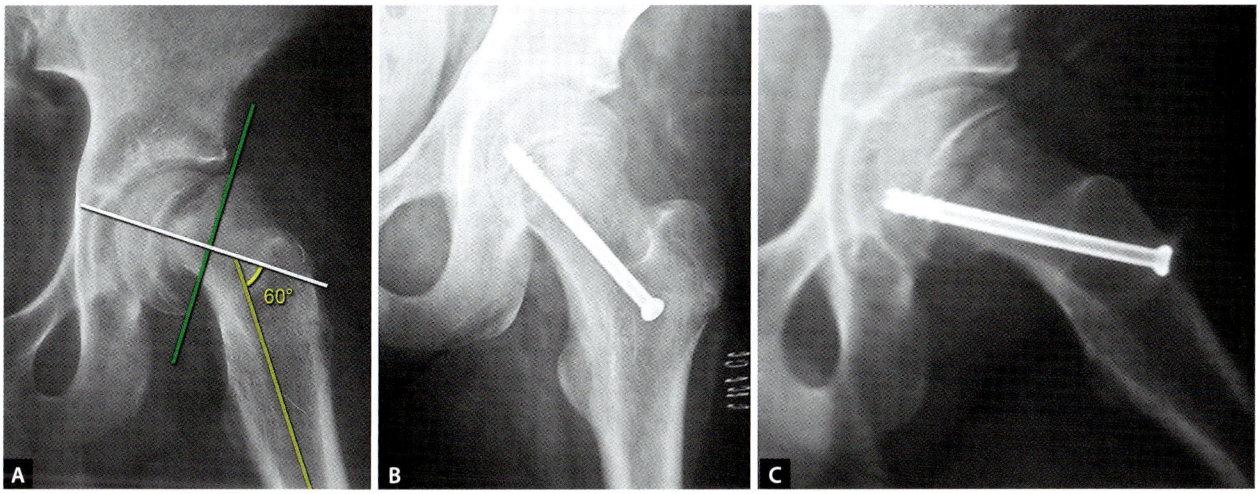

Figs. 7A to C: Slipped capital femoral epiphysis. Radiograph showing typical displacement of the proximal femoral epiphysis in a patient who complained of pain in thigh and knee for 2 months with acute nontraumatic exacerbation (A). The slip was managed by a single attempt at reduction and fixation with a single cannulated cancellous screw (B and C).

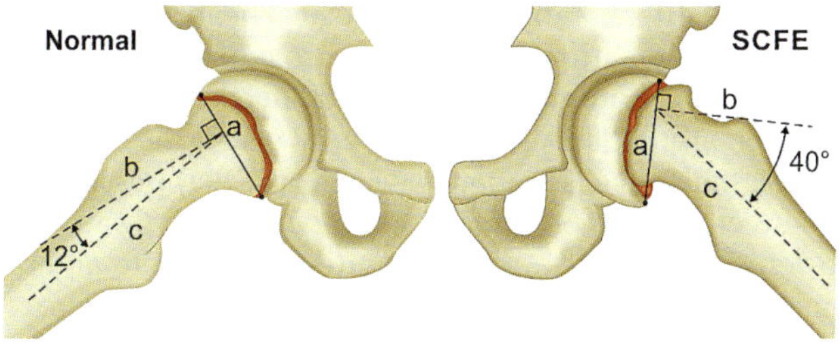

Fig. 8: The Southwick method of grading slipped capital femoral epiphysis (SCFE) severity (see text for details).

Open reduction through anterior or anterolateral approach (Parsch et al.) may be advantageous in achieving intraoperative reduction held by digital pressure and simultaneous decompression of the intracapsular hematoma. Performing modified Dunn procedure acutely in management of unstable SCFE is associated with high rates of osteonecrosis. In patients with persistent deformity, capital realignment performed at the level of epiphyseal plate (Fish/Dunn procedure) produces optimal results (see osteotomies later). Other methods to deal with FAI later include surgical dislocation, limited anterior approach, or arthroscopic femoral head-neck osteochondroplasty.

Stable Slipped Capital Femoral Epiphysis

The standard acceptable treatment of stable SCFE is in situ fixation with a single screw. Other methods include hip spica cast, open epiphysiodesis with bone grafting, open reduction internal fixation (ORIF) with cuneiform osteotomy, intertrochanteric osteotomy with internal fixation, and base of neck osteotomy with in situ stabilization. Screw fixation is a simple technique that is preferred for its low rates of recurrence and complications. After closure of the growth plate, progression of athletic activities may be allowed, including running and, eventually, participating in contact sports. Most patients have good to excellent long-term outcomes with in situ screw fixation. For larger slips (grade 3), it is better to perform neck osteotomy and place in situ screw to reduce the deformity. Persistence of deformity will cause late-onset arthritis.

Correction by osteotomy: Correction of femoral neck deformity by performing osteotomy allows good anatomical realignment of epiphysis and improves the chances of future functioning hip. This also reduces the chances of development of FAI and degenerative hip disease in future. Osteotomies at various levels have been described, some close to physis and some away from it. The closer the osteotomy is to physis, the greater are chances of correction of deformity while it risks the vascularity more. The osteotomies done away from physis will result in lesser amount of correction but reduce the risk of complications.

- *Fish and Dunn osteotomy:* These are performed close to physis; the fish's cuneiform osteotomy differs from Dunn in the fact that it involves complete removal of physis so that there is good bone-to-bone apposition and revascularization. These are contraindicated, if the physis is fused.
- Osteotomy at the base of neck.
- *Intertrochanteric osteotomy:* This is preferably done for residual deformity. Though the complication rates are low, it may be associated with difficult future total hip arthroplasty (THA).

Salvage procedure: Arthrodesis of hip joint

COMPLICATIONS

Early

- Joint penetration of screw
- Pathological fracture
- Continued slippage
- Infection
- *Osteonecrosis:* Up to 60% in patients with unstable slip. The incidence was 10–15% with older treatment methods while 0–5% with in situ fixation.

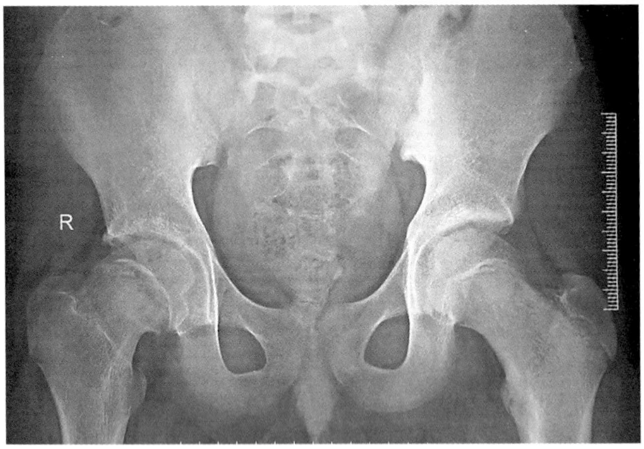

Fig. 9: Slipped upper femoral epiphysis (SUFE) managed conservatively in a patient presenting after 8 months of development of pain in right hip. Development of such deformity is liable to evolve into "cam type" femoroacetabular impingement and would ultimately need treatment, as remodeling potential for a varus hip deformity is minimal.

- *Chondrolysis:* This is acute loss of articular cartilage causing joint effusion and pain usually occurring with unrecognized pin penetration. The chance of occurrence of chondrolysis is high even with cast treatment rather than other modalities.

Late

- Residual deformity **(Fig. 9)**
- Osteoarthritis

PERTHES' DISEASE

Manish Kumar Varshney

Synonyms: Morbus Legg-Calvé-Perthes, Legg-Calvé-Perthes' disease, LCP disease, LCPD, Legg-Calvé-Perthes-Waldenstrom disease, Coxa plana (Waldenstrom), pseudocoxalgia (Calve), Ischemic necrosis of the hip, Juvenile/idiopathic avascular necrosis of the head of the femur, Osteochondropathia deformans coxae juvenilis (Perthes), precoxalgia (Soudart), Coxa vara capitalis (Levy), Osteochondritis coxae juvenilis.

INTRODUCTION

Legg-Calvé-Perthes (LCP) disease is a self-limiting disease of hip in children produced by varying degrees of idiopathic osteonecrosis of the capital femoral epiphysis and often the most proximal part of the metaphysis. It is also recognized as osteochondritis that was independently identified by AT Legg (United States), J Calvé (France), and GC Perthes (Germany) at the beginning of the 19th century (1910). The disease was described by Waldenstorm in 1909, Fragenheim gave pathological description in 1909, while first pictures were given by Alban Kohler's atlas in 1905 itself. It is interesting to note that the word "creeping substitution" used to describe cancellous bone healing actually originated from Phemister's observation (and use of the phrase) of bone healing in Perthes disease in 1921. Only Legg, however, attributed it to vascular disruption, while Calve thought it to arise from rickets and Perthes' thought this to be secondary to degenerative arthritis possibly infective in nature. Some important historical dates and investigators for Perthes' disease are as follows:

- With simultaneous description of the disease by the three investigators, choosing a name for the disease became an issue for which Perthes (1920) wrote—"What's in a name? That which we call rose, by any other name would smell as sweet".
- 1909: Waldenstrom used the term "der obere tuberkulose collumherd"
- 1910: Legg described this as "an obscure affection of the hip joint"
- 1910: Calve described "pseudocoxalgia"
- 1910: Perthes described "arthritis deformans juvenilis"
- 1910: Soudart used term "precoxalgia"
- 1911: Levy used term "coxa vara capitalis"
- 1915: Taylor used term "quiet hip disease"
- 1920: Waldenstrom gave the term "coxa plana"
- 1922: Waldenstrom gave classification of the disease
- 1971: Catterall proposed radiological head at risk signs
  1984: Salter stressed pathogenic role of stress fractures.

It is not an uncommon disorder and affects 5–15 in 100,000 children around the age group of 2–12 years (mean age of 7 years). Incidence is higher in whites (1:1,200) possibly due to late establishment of foveolar blood supply. The male-to-female ratio is 4–5:1 due to often incomplete anterior anastomosis in boys. Onset of disease in Indians is often late. The disease is bilateral in only 10% patients that too affects the hips sequentially and not simultaneously. It is more common in children with relatively short stature, exposure to second hand smoke, delayed bone age, disproportionate growth, and *hyperactivity disorder*. The hyperactivity may account for higher incidence of injury in affected individuals (especially females) compared to unaffected population. The disproportionate growth may explain relative lack of vascularity in the fast-growing femoral heads causing ischemia. Children of lower socioeconomic status are also at increased risk of LCP disease. The disease is rare among African-American children. The association with abnormal clotting factors has not been fully established.

ETIOLOGY AND PATHOGENESIS

Although the etiology remains unknown, the disease is associated with following factors:

- *Deprived populations:* It is much more common in deprived white population as compared to Asians and Africans.
- Global growth disorder characterized by delayed and disproportionate growth (see above). Some investigators found a "standstill phenomenon" where new carpal bones did not ossify while the existing ones kept growing; this relationship of delayed bone age was more prominent in patients with bilateral Perthes. Disproportionate growth pattern has been recognized in the form of subtle dysmorphic pattern called "rostral sparing". Often, there is finding of a foot that is short relative to tibia and forearm and hand short relative to arm. An Ockham's razor for this

concept with differential distribution could be that young children from all social class with delayed development or disproportionate growth are at risk of developing Perthes' disease, but only those with some systemic factor will develop the disease. To support the hypothesis is the fact that there is abnormally low urinary deoxypyridinoline/creatinine quotient during the condensation phase of the disease, suggesting low skeletal metabolism.

- Hormones—it is difficult to establish relationship and even the levels of thyroid hormones have been found to be normal, but the age of occurrence of Perthes is similar to hypothyroidism.
- Third born or later child of older than average parents
- Exposure to smoke (particularly cigarette smoke but also *chulah* smoke)
- Role of intravascular mechanisms—any role of heritable thrombophilic factor is unproven but some reports suggest factor V Leiden deficiency.
- Local anatomical abnormalities—there is finding of increased anteversion at the affected hip.
- Developmental anomaly—this theory is promulgated based on finding of nongenetic associations of inguinal hernia, undescended testis, renal abnormalities (females with bilateral affection), pyloric stenosis, congenital heart disease, etc. in some cases.
- Focally identified but unproved factors—?skeletal dysplasia (acromesomelic dwarfism), ?genetic (autosomal dominant??), malnutrition, and manganese deficiency?

It is difficult to attribute any systemic factor to causation of disease, as the affection is mostly unilateral. The most popular assumption of some sort of vascular disruption as the underlying cause of disease originates from Legg's work that attributed development of disease to trauma while the often-quoted Trueta hypothesis was described as "epiphyseal anemia" due to precarious blood supply of femoral head and possible finding of deficient anterior vascular network. Caffey proposed intraepiphyseal compression of blood supply that compromises the oxygenation.

PATHOPHYSIOLOGY AND PATHOANATOMY

Disruption of the normal blood supply and, hence, the nutrients and oxygen to the femoral head are the key pathogenic events that affect the articular cartilage, bony epiphysis, and, in some patients, the metaphysis and physis. The compromise of blood supply may arise from tamponade effect on retinacular vessels or transient synovitis temporarily causing obstruction to retinacular blood flow from tense intra-articular effusion in a hip with borderline blood supply (no foveolar supply). Characteristic changes in the blood supply of femoral head in children may be partially responsible for development of disease:

- Children <3 years have two major arteries supplying the head—the metaphyseal and retinacular system
- From 4 to 8 years—the metaphyseal supply is obliterated with development of capital physis, so only the retinacular system is the predominant blood supply that enters the head as lateral epiphyseal artery. The lateral epiphyseal system is divided into posterosuperior and posterior-inferior systems. Obliteration of the former is responsible for osteonecrosis of anterolateral aspect of femoral head.
- After 8 years, the development of foveolar system gives the head a dual supply again (foveolar and retinacular).
- From 16 to 18 years, as the growth plate disappears, all three groups become re-established to supply the femoral head.

The "Caffey hypothesis" proposes osteonecrosis to result from *intraepiphyseal compression* of the blood vessels and interruption of supply to ossification center. The compression somehow occurs from the pressure from acetabular roof.

The necrotic changes in Perthes' disease are mainly observed in the deeper layer of the cartilage, which is responsible for the circumferential growth of the bony epiphysis. Due to ischemia, there is cessation of the endochondral ossification at cartilage-subchondral bone junction. Separation of the cartilage from underlying bone followed by vascular invasion of the cartilage and accessory ossification centers occurs leading to bone resorption and deposition of reactive fibrous tissue. The bony epiphysis shows necrotic changes followed by fracture of the trabeculae and subsequent thickening of trabeculae due to fracture healing. The deposition of fibrous tissue and formation of immature bone are responsible for future deformation of femoral head due to biological plasticity of the tissue. "Biological plasticity" implies that though head is not physically soft, but can be molded into round or flat surfaces depending on containment. With subluxation, later capital deformity and true Perthes' disease develop.

The physis (growth plate) continues to function normally in most of the patients.

Osteonecrosis causes mechanical weakening of the femoral head, so that it begins to deform under the load of normal activities, which the normal head is able to resist easily. In the early stages of vascular insult, the brittleness induced by increased calcium content makes it more prone to fractures. However, these fractures remain unrepaired due to absence of cells (osteocytes, osteoblasts, and osteoclasts) due to necrosis.

Nonspecific changes occur in the metaphysis (part of bone below physis). These include formation of columns of normal/degenerated cartilage cells and fibrosis in the metaphysis. Although the cause of metaphyseal changes is not clear, the presence of radiolucent changes is generally associated with poor prognosis.

The cumulative microdamage in various portions of proximal femur thus results in subchondral fracture in the superior region of the bony epiphysis. Subsequent resorption of the necrotic bone, associated with vascular invasion, further weakens the bone. There is an imbalance between bony resorption and formation, with resorption far exceeding the new bone formation. This results in further mechanical weakening adding to femoral head deformity. Substantial forces act on the femoral head with weight-bearing activities. These forces may become tremendous in children who are usually very active in case of Perthes' disease. The remodeling potential associated with age <8 years imparts a good prognosis in younger children. The change in the relative size of bony epiphysis and cartilage with age also affects the prognosis in older children. The disease process can be classified according to the stage of disease. Waldenstrom's classification **(Table 2)** defines four radiographic stages of the Perthes' disease. Each radiographic stage is variable. For example, the stage of fragmentation may last for 1 year while that of reossification lasts for around 3–5 years. Modification to this classification is proposed in 2015 that seems to have better interobserver variability. The first three stages are subclassified into two (A and B) subgroups **(Table 2)**.

TABLE 2: Waldenstrom stages of natural progression of Perthes [the modifications (2015) are detailed under radiographic features].

Stages	***Radiographic feature***
Initial (stage of increased radiodensity)	Smaller ossific nucleus, increased radiodensity of the nucleus, widening of medial joint space, subchondral fracture in some, metaphyseal cyst in some, and mild flattening of the ossific nucleus *Stage 1A:* All or part of epiphysis is sclerotic, there is no loss of height of epiphysis *Stage 1B:* There is sclerosis and loss of height of epiphysis but no fragmentation
Fragmentation stage (resorptive stage)	Appearance of radiolucencies in the ossific nucleus, fragmented appearance of the ossific nucleus, flattening and lateralization of the head. The central radiodense fragment (sequestrum) may demarcate from the medial or lateral pillars. *Stage 2A:* Early fragmentation seen as 1 or 2 vertical fissures in AP or Lauenstein frog-lateral view. *Stage 2B:* Advanced fragmentation seen but no new bone lateral to the fragmented epiphysis.
Reossification stage (healing/repair stage)	Appearance of new bone on the medial and lateral aspects of femoral head, disappearance of radiodense fragment. The head may show further flattening or some may show improvement in the head shape. *Stage 3A:* Early new bone lateral to fragmented epiphysis seen. It covers less than one-third of the width of epiphysis. *Stage 3B:* New bone covers more than one-third of the width of epiphysis.
Residual stage (healed stage)	Femoral head regains normal radiodensity. The shape may change according to remodeling potential left

Morphological Changes

Some distinct morphological changes that can be appreciated in Perthes' disease are as follows **(Figs. 10A and B)**:

- Small capital femoral physis
- Loss of sphericity of femoral head
- Increased width of epiphysis
- Lateral extrusion of physis
- Broadening and shortening of femoral neck
- Decreased neck shaft angle
- Increased anteversion on both sides
- Convex proximal femoral growth plate
- Step-like irregularities in growth plate and bony epiphysis
- Increased width of articular cartilage
- Overgrowth of greater trochanter
- Increased radius of acetabulum flattened lateral lip of acetabulum
- Coxa magna
- Tear of acetabular labrum
- Short stature and delayed bone age, as mentioned above

CLINICAL FEATURES

Perthes' disease is mostly unilateral; bilateral affection should trigger a search for dysplasias, metabolic, endocrine, or syndromic causes (see differential diagnosis). The stereotyped patient is a very active male who is short of stature for his age, presenting with limp or pain or both. The common presenting features are described below.

- Limp while walking is the earliest common notable finding. The limp is initially painless and appears later.
- Pain is typically present in the groin region and aggravates during activity. The pain may also radiate to the thigh and knee (anteromedial aspect). Some cases may have only knee pain without any symptom referring to the hip. In such cases, the diagnosis is often delayed. Most

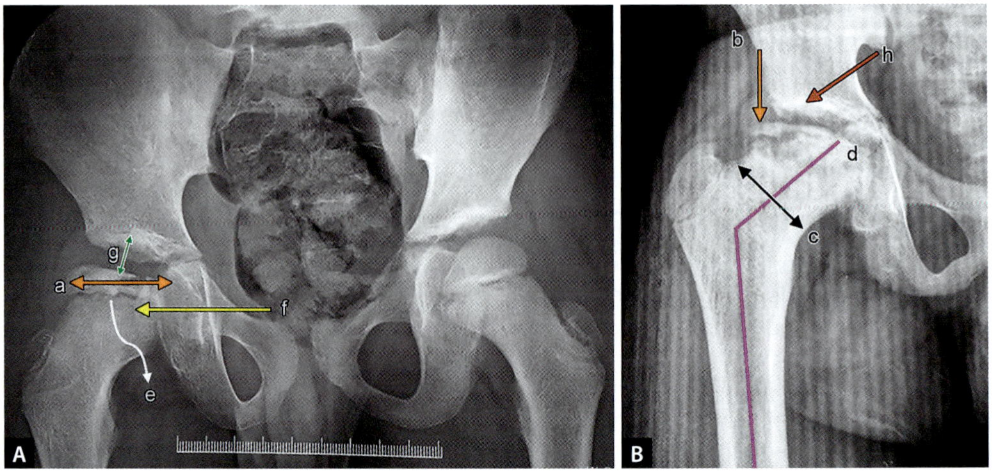

Figs. 10A and B: The radiology of Perthes' disease. (a) Increased width of epiphysis; (b) Lateral extrusion of epiphysis; (c) Broadening and shortening of femoral neck; (d) Decreased neck shaft angle; (e) Convex proximal femoral growth plate; (f) Step-like irregularities in growth plate and bony epiphysis (Gage's sign); (g) Increased width of unossified articular cartilage; (h) Increased radius of acetabulum, flattened lateral lip of acetabulum.

TABLE 3: Differentiating features between Perthes' disease and irritable hip.

Legg–Calvé–Perthes disease	*Irritable hip*
Male:female ratio = 4:1	Male:female ratio = 2:1
Mean age of occurrence is around 7 years	Mean age of occurrence is around 3 years
Average duration of symptoms is 6 weeks	Average duration is 6 days
There is synovial thickening	Synovitis with capsular distension
Bony changes and necrosis	No bony changes

common differential diagnosis is the irritable hip that can be differentiated by specific clinical features **(Table 3)**.

- On examination, there is frequent limitation of internal rotation and abduction (especially in flexion) and in advanced stages, the leg-length discrepancy may be observed. Limitation of abduction in flexion is the *earliest clinical sign* present, if carefully elucidated.
- Mild to moderate atrophy of the thigh
- Gait is antalgic that also develops Trendelenburg component later.
- In bilateral cases, the disease is characteristically asymmetric and begins 1 year prior to other hip.
- Hernias and undescended testis should be ruled out during examination especially in bilateral cases.

DIFFERENTIAL DIAGNOSIS

The differential diagnoses are coxitis fugax, Juvenile idiopathic arthritis, osteomyelitis, multiple epiphyseal dysplasia, Meyer's dysplasia, (bilateral disease with mild involvement of epiphysis and delayed ossification or granular fragmentation) spondyloepiphyseal dysplasia, metachondromatosis, Schwartz–Jampel syndrome, chondroblastoma, and steroid-induced osteonecrosis. Symptomatic differentials include thalassemia, sickle-cell anemia, trisomy 21, trichorhinophalangeal syndrome, achondroplasia, Gaucher's disease, Martsolf syndrome, Maroteaux–Lamy syndrome, hypothyroidism, and hemophilia.

RADIOLOGICAL WORKUP

Radiographs are obtained in two perpendicular views: a pelvic survey film and the lateral of involved hip. Plain radiography remains the mainstay in treatment and prognostication. Radiography is also used to evaluate possible methods of treatment. Radiological classifications are commonly used to assess severity and prognosticate the patients. Ultrasonography can be used to investigate the differentials of Perthes-like effusion in coxitis fugax or osteomyelitis. MRI can be used to diagnose the disease early (identification of necrotic areas and assessment of femoral head for shape changes) and dynamic MRI can be used to assess "hinged abduction" that is often difficult to identify in the unossified epiphysis of young children on radiographs. MRI is, however, not prognostic so not a standard investigation and its use should be selective. The characteristic radiographic signs observed in Perthes' disease and their possible explanation(s) are as follows **(Figs. 10A and B)**:

- Smaller size of ossific nucleus of capital femoral epiphysis along with widened joint space (this is the "earliest radiological sign" that can be appreciated in patients of Perthes' disease).
  - Due to temporary cessation of endochondral ossification
  - The articular cartilage continues to grow as it derives nutrition from synovial fluid.
- Subchondral fracture (Caffey sign, crescent sign, **Fig. 11C**) is a radiolucent line seen in the anterolateral region of femoral head best visualized in Frog-leg lateral (Lauenstein) view:
  - Requirement for true Perthes' disease
  - Heralds clinical onset of disease
  - Minimal extension of fracture or this line is seen after initial visualization
  - Transient finding early in course of disease with average of 2–9 months
  - The anterolateral region is affected due to:
    - Maximum weight-bearing stresses
    - Maximum bone resorption seen here due to area supplied by posterosuperior vessel distribution
- Increased radiopacity of femoral head **(Fig. 11A)** due to:
  - New appositional bone deposition (creeping substitution)
  - Calcification of necrotic marrow
  - Crushing and collapse of trabeculae
- Radiolucent areas in head **(Figs. 11A and C)** due to:
  - Resorption of loose necrotic bone
  - Reactive fibrous tissue formation
  - Formation of immature bone
- Metaphyseal changes appreciated include:
  - Ill-defined juxtaphyseal lucent band
  - Metaphyseal cysts
  - Metaphyseal expansion:
    - The radiolucency is due to adipose tissue in early stages and fibrocartilage in later stages
    - Larger metaphyseal lucency is possibly related to poorer prognosis.
    - Involvement of anterolateral cortex of femoral head is also associated with possible poor prognosis.
- *Gage's sign:*
  - This is a V-shaped defect in the lateral part of epiphysis and adjoining metaphysis **[Figs. 10A and B(a to f)]**
  - It indicates excess growth of cartilage laterally that causes rarefaction in the adjoining epiphysis and metaphysis.
- *Lateral subluxation:*
  - It is denoted by center edge (CE) angle if Wisberg of >20°
  - Or the distance between two vertical lines (one from outer edge of acetabulum and other from lateral edge of femoral head) of >3 mm compared to normal side.
- Lateral calcification—these are specks of calcification lateral to epiphysis
  - They represent the extruded cartilage and degenerative calcification of the same.

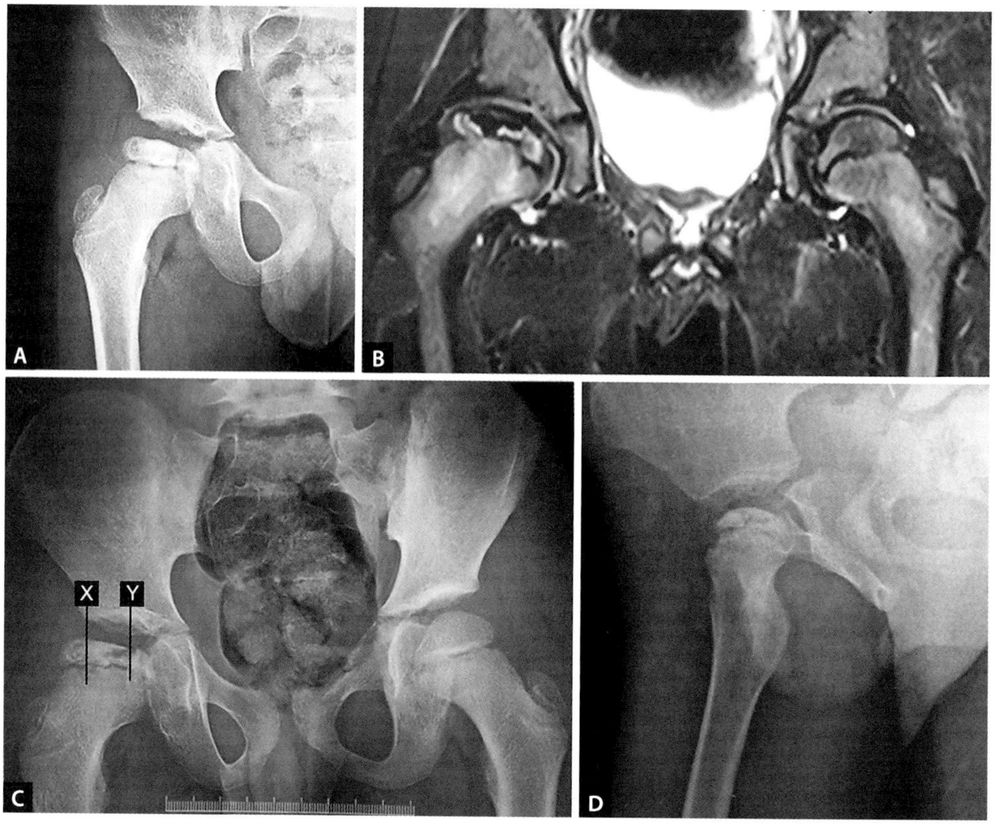

Figs. 11A to D: (A) Radiograph of a 10-year-old patient with late-onset Perthes' disease showing radiodense femoral head developing fragmentation with central lucency (C) after 4 months of conservative management The femoral physis is divided into three equal parts called "pillars" along its length using two geometrical vertical lines. This is used for Herring classification where the height of epiphysis lateral to "x" (the lateral pillar height) is used to grade the disease. The corresponding width of epiphysis for these three pillars is different as the head is a globular structure; (D) There is characteristic crescent sign seen on lateral projection; (B) MRI of the same hip rules out infection as differential while demonstrating large flattened epiphysis with central necrotic region.

- *Head within head appearance:* Deposition of immature woven bone in cartilage matrix and sclerosis of the necrotic nucleus produces this characteristic appearance.

Bone Scan

The indications have diminished for its use. It shows marked reduction in the radionucleide uptake at the site of osteonecrosis and has good sensitivity and specificity that presents the osteonecrosis earlier than radiographs, but utility is not translated into clinical practice. The four stages seen on a typical bone scan for Perthes' disease are:

1. Total lack of uptake
2. Lateral column uptake indicating vascularization
3. Gradual filling of anterolateral part of epiphysis
4. Base filling in epiphysis adjacent to physis

Arthrography

Arthrography offers an opportunity to evaluate coverage and mobility under direct vision. It should be performed prior to surgery to help in determining the best position for femoral head containment and demonstrate absence of hinged abduction before containment procedures are performed. Laredo classified hips into five types depending upon arthrographic findings.

1. Type 1 hips are normal
2. Type 2 hips have spherical femoral head, which is larger than normal
3. Type 3 hips have ovoid femoral head
4. Type 4 has large and flattened femoral head, with straight and elevated labrum, hinged abduction may be present
5. Type 5 hips show a femoral head larger than normal and saddle-shaped, the labrum is straight and elevated.

All hips froms Type 2 to Type 5 show femoral head extrusion in neutral position and normal coverage at about 30° of abduction with some internal rotation.

STAGING AND CLASSIFICATION OF DISEASE

Classification systems help us in understanding the natural history of disease, staging them, planning treatment, and prognosticating the disease. Waldenstrom classification describes the Perthes' disease into four stages and it has been modified for better interobserver reliability **(Table 2)**. "Salter-Thompson" is a two-category classification system based on the necrosis and subchondral fracture on lateral radiographic view—Group A denotes involvement of less than half of femoral head and Group B denotes involvement of more than half of the femoral head. The extent of head involvement is based on the subchondral fracture (Crescent sign), because of which this system can be applied at an earlier stage than stage of fragmentation.

"Catterall classification" emphasizes the relationship between the extent of head involvement and outcome. It classifies the disease in four stages: I (25% involvement), II (50% involvement), III (75% involvement), and IV (100% involvement). It is generally applied during the stage of fragmentation when the necrotic sequestrum becomes well demarcated. However, this classification has low interobserver reliability. The detailed classification is presented in **Box 2**.

The "lateral pillar classification" introduced by Herring is a four-category system based on the height of lateral pillar (defined as the lateral 15–30% of epiphysis, ***see* Figures 11C and 13**). The head is simply divided into three sectors or pillars **(*see* Fig. 13)**. The lateral pillar occupies the lateral 15–30% of the width of head, 50% of width is occupied by the middle or central pillar, while medial pillar forms 20–35% of the width of head. Group A represents no loss of lateral pillar height **(Figs. 12A to D)**; B represents <50% loss of height and group C represents >50% loss of height. Category B and C ("border group"—recently added by Herring) represents loss of height in-between group B and C. In group B/C1, the lateral pillar has >50% of its original height but is <2–3-mm wide; group B/C2 has >50% of its original height, but minimal ossification; group B/C3 has exactly 50% of its original height but is depressed relative to the central pillar **(Fig. 13)**. This classification has better inter-observer reliability and also has been reported to be a better predictor of Stulberg radiographic outcome. In the fragmentation stage, the system has greater

BOX 2: Catterall system of classification of Perthes' disease radiologically.

Group 1:
- Affects the anterior aspect of femoral head
- No sequestrum
- No subchondral fracture
- No metaphyseal rarefaction
- Maintained epiphyseal height

Group 2:
- Affects anterolateral one-third to one-half of femoral head
- Sequestrum formation with clear junction
- Subchondral formation with clear junction
- Subchondral fracture does not extend into posterior half of femoralhead
- Anterolateral metaphyseal rarefaction
- Lateral pillar is preserved

Group 2½: These cases have intact lateral pillar, but a radiolucency is present in thelateral column

Group 3:
- Affects three-fourth of femoral head
- Sequestrum is large and junction is sclerotic
- Subchondral fracture extends into posterior half
- Diffuse metaphyseal rarefaction
- Lateral pillar is not preserved

Reverse group 3: Affects three-fourths of femoral head but in anteromedial aspect of femoralhead rather than anterolateral aspect

Group 4:
- Affects entire femoral head
- Dense well-marked sequestrum
- Subchondral fracture extends throughout the head
- Diffuse or central metaphyseal rarefaction
- Posterior remodeling seen

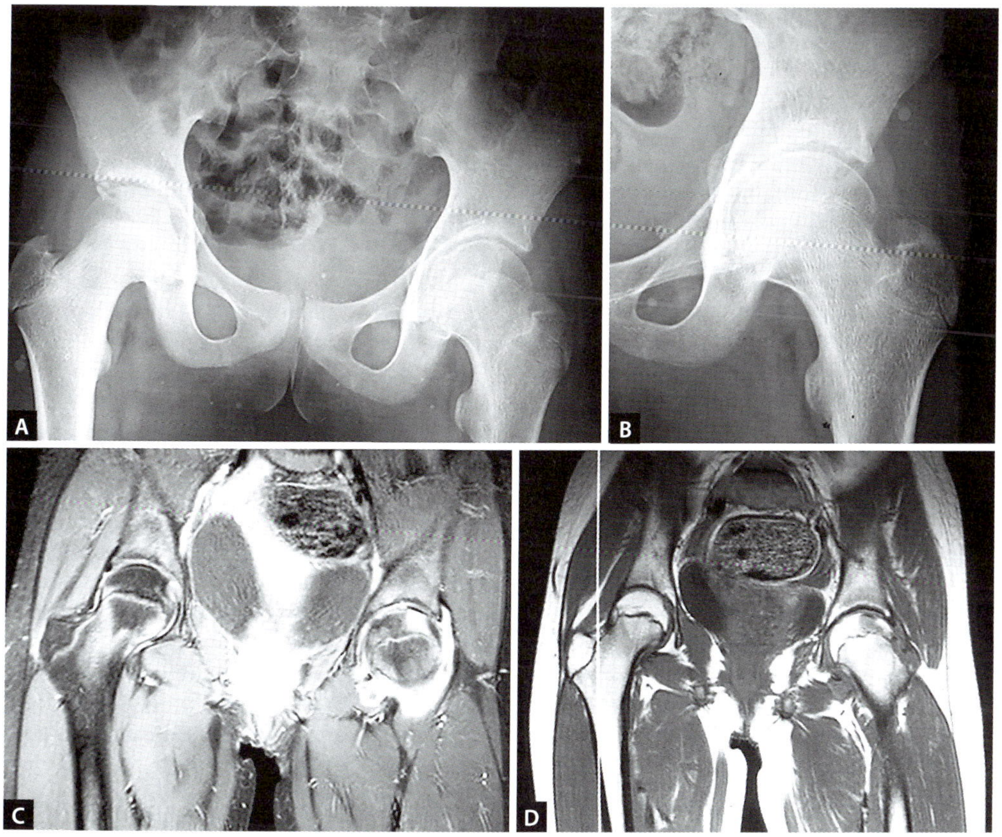

Figs. 12A to D: This patient presented with pain in left hip for 3 months and the radiograph demonstrated a small lucent lesion in the lateral part of femoral epiphysis. The MRI scan demonstrated a small hyperintense lesion on T2-weighted images and hypointense lesion on T1-weighted images that were suggestive of necrotic lesion in the epiphysis and later healed with conservative management.

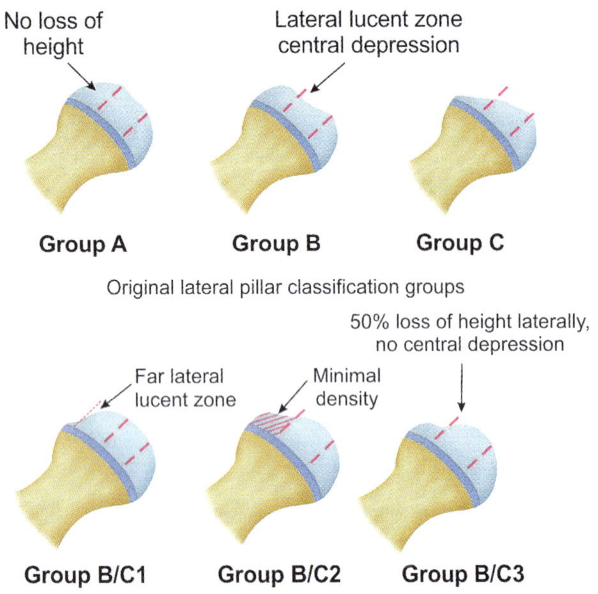

Fig. 13: The lateral pillar classification of Herring.

prognostic value. The predictive value increases when age of patient is taken into account simultaneously. Lateral extrusion of epiphysis is an important prognosticating feature beyond the extent of involvement as predicted by above classifications. Lateral extrusion of >20% indicates worse prognosis.

Though intriguing, but the "limitation of these classification systems" is that they should be ideally applied in the stage of fragmentation when the femoral head is at its peak deformation. If the child presents at an earlier stage, the classification may be wrong and may proceed to a higher grade later on. In such cases, the child needs to be seen repeatedly to observe the pathogenesis of the disease process. Such an approach is called "wait and classify" and may prevent unnecessary treatment and surgery in unwarranted cases. On the other hand, it may lead to wastage of precious time in cases where the onset is late, because the older child may lose the remodeling potential quickly. MRI may be developed to guide the treatment in future.

The *Stulberg classification* **(Table 4)** of the radiographic outcome is applied at skeletal maturity to prognosticate long-term outcome based on residual sphericity of femoral head after disease healing. This system classifies disease at final stage thereby enabling better assessment of disease. Low intra- and interobserver reliability and the necessity to wait till skeletal maturity are limitations of this classification system. It has been generally observed that the hip with flattening will have more chances of developing osteoarthritis and will require arthroplasty. However, a typical patient will have minimal limp, mild pain, and minimum to no functional impairment.

PROGNOSTIC FACTORS

The long-term outcome is affected by shape and size of the femoral head. The shape of femoral head can be assessed by Mose's circles or separate circular disks of different sizes. The head is considered spherical when the articular margin

TABLE 4: Stulberg system of classification of Perthes' disease.

Stulberg class	*Descriptive feature*	*Radiographic sign of OA at mean follow-up of 40 years*	*Radiographic evidence of joint space narrowing at mean follow-up of 40 years*
I	Normal hip joint	0	0
II	Spherical enlarged head short neck or sleep acetabulum	16%	0
III	Nonspherical head (ovoid, mushroom, or umbrella shaped)	58%	47%
IV	Flat head	75%	53%
V	Flat head with incongruent hip joint	78%	61%

of the femoral head perfectly matches the arc of the circle of the same radius on both anteroposterior and frog-leg lateral radiographs. The head is regarded ovoid, if the margin of femoral head matches the arc of a circle in both views, but the radius of femoral head differs in both views by 2 mm or less. If the femoral head does not match any arc or if femoral head matches to arc of circles in both views, with differences in the radius of femoral head of >2 mm, it is called flattened or irregular.

It is imperative here to realize that most factors are predetermined and do not alter by treatment or surgery, except lateral extrusion of the femoral head. This can be prevented and can be corrected if it develops. There had been various prognostic factors that were outlined previously and portended to determine the clinical outcome but real significance of all or some is unknown and not documented **(Box 3)**.

Cause and Assessment of Lateral Extrusion

The necrosis of the epiphysis triggers synovitis, articular cartilage hypertrophy, and hypertrophy of ligamentum teres. These changes along with muscle spasm cause the femoral head to extrude beyond the acetabular margin. When the weight-bearing stresses, the damaged epiphysis, and forces generated by muscle contraction are transmitted from acetabular margin to the extruded part of femoral head, it begins to get deformed. If >20% of the width of epiphysis extrudes outside the acetabular margin, there is very high risk of femoral head deformity. The femoral head is maximally prone to deformation forces when it is soft—in stage of fragmentation (when the necrotic bone is being actively resorbed) or in the stage of early reconstitution (when the trabeculae of newly laid woven bone are vulnerable to collapse). Hence, the aim of treatment in early part of the disease is to prevent femoral head deformation by forces transmitted across the hip joint.

TREATMENT PRINCIPLES AND METHODS

The goals of treatment are to prevent deformity of femoral head and any incongruence of the affected joint to avoid any late onset arthritis and improve mobility.

BOX 3: The variously identified head at risk signs.*

Clinical head at risk signs:

- Children aged 5 years or younger have the best prognosis. The outcome is especially dismal when the onset of disease is in adolescence (>8 years).
  - Younger patients have more time to remodel
  - Acetabulum in older patients loses remodeling potential
  - Older patients are heavier and more likely to damage the epiphysis
- Contrary to popular belief, there is no strong evidence to suggest a worst prognosis in girls. Most of the other important prognostic signs can be identified on plain radiographs. It was proposed that the girls achieve skeletal maturity early, so get less time for bone remodeling. Age for age, however, the girls seem to be more severely affected for unknown reason(s).
- Extent of epiphyseal involvement (as classified by Catterall and Salter–Thompson) and extent of epiphyseal collapse (Herring's lateral pillar) do determine the prognosis. More involvement is expected with extrusion of the epiphysis. This can be measured by assessing the femoral head coverage by acetabulum. Center-edge angle of Wiberg is usually not used because it is generally impossible to ascertain the center of the femoral head, which is deformed. Reimer's migration index and acetabular head index are much more commonly used.
- Obese patient has more stress at the epiphysis compromising the blood supply and rapid collapse of the head.
- Patient with limited range of motion—flexion <80° and abduction <30°
- Increasing abduction contracture—increases the tendency of hip to subluxate laterally
- Subluxating hips on clinical examination

Radiological head at risk signs:

- The metaphyseal abnormalities such as osteoporosis, metaphyseal cyst, and widening of the central femoral metaphysis have been identified as poor prognosticators.
- Altered centers of acetabulum (bicompartmentalization) are also associated with poor outcome. In this, the central femoral head articulates with the lateral part of the acetabulum and the lateral part of femoral head extrudes out. Lateral extrusion of >20% indicates poor prognosis.
- Catterall in addition mentioned some head at risk signs, the utility of which is debatable:
  - Diffuse metaphyseal reaction
  - Calcification lateral to the epiphysis
  - Gage's sign—a V-shaped defect in lateral bony epiphysis indicating cartilage overgrowth without ossification
  - Horizontal alignment of the femoral epiphysis and lateral extrusion of the epiphysis. This lateral subluxation of femoral head is the most important prognosticator as mentioned earlier.

Scintigraphic head at risk signs (now rarely used to assess the Perthes' disease):

- Failure of revascularization of lateral column
- Decreased activity of physis
- Anterolateral extrusion of epiphysis
- Disappearance of previously present lateral column
- Intense metaphyseal activity

*Though mentioned for comprehensiveness, the exact and priority-wise significance of individual signs is unknown and not established.

The principles of treatment to achieve above goals are—containment (concentrically reduce the femoral head into acetabulum), preventing lateral subluxation of the head, regaining a spherical femoral head, and resumption of weight bearing. The treatment should also reduce stress on femoral head.

As the lateral extrusion of epiphysis is the most important modifiable determinant of clinical outcome on a long-term basis, the focus of treatment is realized on this pathology. Historically, this has been achieved by two methods:

1. The first approach attempts to save the affected part of femoral head from bearing these transmitted forces by preventing or reversing the extrusion of head.

Conservative

- Physiotherapy exercises, mobilization under anesthesia, botox injections
- Abduction splint, braces and casts

Operative

- Improving range of motion by soft tissue procedures (tenotomies, etc.)
- Femoral side osteotomies (valgus or varus trochanteric)
- Pelvis [pelvic side (salter, dega or pemberton, triple, Chiari, etc.)]
- Combination of above

Fig. 14: Methods of containment of hip in Perthes' disease with subluxation.

2. The second approach is to reduce transmitted forces by minimizing the stress on femoral head by weight-sharing or weight-bearing braces. This method is uncommonly used due to high patient noncompliance and being itself cumbersome in the modern orthopedic practice.

The first approach is called "containment" which ensures that the anterolateral part of the epiphysis is positioned within the acetabulum, so that edge of acetabulum does not transmit any force on to this part of femoral epiphysis. This may be achieved by abduction and internal rotation or abduction and flexion through either casting or bracing but more reliably through surgery **(*see* Fig. 14)**. Adductor tenotomy can be combined with any treatment depending on adduction contracture. A simplistic treatment algorithm is presented in **Flowchart 1**. For containment to work, it is imperative that it is carried out before the stage of fragmentation. If done at right time, containment will prevent femoral head deformation and produce a spherical and congruent head on healing. *Good ROM is a prerequisite for achieving containment. Status of the lateral pillar and the extent of extrusion* are *not used* widely for decision making to perform containment because this procedure needs to be done before stage of fragmentation. Patients aged <4 years with small involvement of femoral head necrosis <50% (Salter-Thompson I), mild involvement of lateral pillar (Herring A), no femoral head extrusion, and no subluxation can be treated with home-based exercise program and physical therapy for preserving abduction. Surgical procedures have not shown to improve outcomes in patients <8 years of age at onset of Perthes' disease with lateral pillar A and B groups. Patients >6 years benefit from surgical containment. If the head can be concentrically reduced within acetabulum by abduction and internal rotation (as assessed by arthrogram under general anesthesia) then release of abduction contracture + extensive casting/bracing treatment program can be instituted. Abduction casts are applied serially increasing range of abduction every 2 weeks or in tight hips, they can be applied every 6 weeks under general anesthesia. If the head cannot be concentrically reduced under anesthesia (arthrogram) or the patient has gradual loss of abduction during treatment then femoral and/or pelvic osteotomy should be resorted to. Loss of abduction is a very important risk factor for worse prognosis and is associated with femoral head extrusion and development of hinged abduction (see management of severe disease below). Also, it has been reported that patients >6 years with lateral pillar B or lateral pillar B/C and/or >50% head necrosis benefit from femoral and/or pelvic osteotomy.

Flowchart 1: General treatment algorithm for management of Perthes' disease in different age groups.

Age < 6 years
- Mild disease
  - Conservative treatment
- Severe disease
  - Intertrochanteric osteotomy

Age 6–10 years
- Head contained
  - Conservative (mobilization, weight relieving calipers, physiotherapy maintain ROM)
- Uncontained or at high-risk for subluxation
  - Surgical containment – femoral (preferred) or pelvic

Age > 10 years
- Contained head
  - Trochanteric apophysiodesis (for coxa magna)
  - Valgus osteotomy (for coxa vara)
  - Lengthening of femoral neck (for coxa vara et magna)
- Uncontained head no hinge abduction
  - Femoral varus osteotomy (should not reduce neck shaft angle below 105°)
  - + pelvic osteotomy for additional coverage if unable to centralize by femoral osteotomy alone or if coxa vara present)
  - + trochanter transposition (for coxa vara)
  - + femoral neck lengthening (for coxa magna)
- Uncontained head with hinge abduction
  - Selective and cautious soft tissue release + manipulative reduction and cast immobilization (see text)
  - Femoral valgus osteotomy and secondary coverage by triple pelvic osteotomy (preferred)
  - Garcieu chielectomy
  - Chiari osteotomy for large mushroom head

- Cast or brace if used **(Box 4)** as method for containment should be continued for 12–13 months and should be worn for most of day. Ambulatory brace treatment has declined in use due to noncompliance especially in older children. Bracing is done as an attempt to prevent deformity of femoral head by prolonged mechanical unloading and immobilization of femoral head. It was assumed that such prolonged bed rest and immobilization reduce hip joint pressure but on investigation, it was found that it actually raised intra-articular pressure. Further immobilization is associated with muscle atrophy, contractures, weight gain, and social exclusion. So, these measures have been replaced by active joint motion and physiotherapy. Strict mechanical unloading is not required and also patients can be allowed to participate in lighter sporting activities such as swimming and cycling strictly avoiding jumping and activities associated with extreme stress. Along with physiotherapy, the use of prostacyclins as vasoactive analogs is investigational. Pain control should be done with adequate use of analgesics.

Surgical containment procedures are most widely used to provide containment. Surgical procedures should be done with proper prerequisites and reasonable patient selection **(Box 5)**. Preoperative arthrogram is a must for containment procedures to understand the extent of cartilaginous femoral head and congruency and adequacy of reduction. Various modern authors prefer varus derotation osteotomy (VDRO) of proximal femur to contain the femoral head and do it as a standard procedure. Staheli, however, suggested the combination of VDRO and pelvic procedure to enhance the containment while limiting the complications of VDRO (abductor weakness, shortening, and coxa vara).

- *Femoral side surgical procedure:* The most popular method has been the proximal femoral varus osteotomy. The advantages of this relatively simple procedure are that this method can be undertaken even when there is moderate restriction of motion
- Relocates the femur in normal attitude of limb
- It shortens the femur so in turn reducing joint reaction forces and mediation the direction of such forces
- Surgically is simpler to perform.

  The acetabular remodeling capacity drastically reduces after 8 years of age, so this procedure is less reliable in children >9 years. Major disadvantage of the procedure is potential for residual shortening with coxa breva and trochanteric prominence. This may be associated with early abductor lurch. Usually, not >20° of varus is required

BOX 4: Use of cast or braces for containment of the hip.

Types of braces:
- Nonambulatory weight relieving:
  - Abduction broomstick plaster casts
  - Bivalved hip spica cast
  - Milgram hip abduction orthosis
- Ambulatory static applied to affected limb only:
  - Harrison hip containment splint
- Ambulatory dynamic applied to both limbs:
  - Petrie cast
  - Scottish rite orthosis
- Ambulatory unilateral orthosis:
  - Trilateral socket orthosis

Prerequisites of bracing:
- Range of motion at hip should be preserved
- Entire femoral head should be containable
- Motor strength and balance should be adequate
- *Arthrography:* Essential to judge congruency throughout range of motion, rule out hinge abduction

BOX 5: Prerequisites for surgical procedures.

- Good range of motion at hip, abduction should be at least 30°
- Child should be in early stage of disease for containment surgery
- Stable hip without any signs of synovitis, etc.
- Possible concentric reduction of the femoral head

to produce containment. Open wedge varus reduces the limb length shortening. Derotation is generally not added because this leads to an externally rotated gait. Trochanteric apophysiodesis may be added in an older child to reduce trochanteric prominence.

- *Pelvic osteotomies:* Anterolateral coverage can also be improved by Salter's osteotomy. A 30° wedge of bone graft can improve anterior coverage by 25° and lateral coverage by 15°. The prerequisite for this procedure is a completely round or almost round head. Shelf procedures and Chiari's osteotomy may also be utilized for increasing the coverage of anterolateral hips especially in coxa magna (large deformed heads). However, containment with triple pelvic osteotomy allows greater amount of coverage. The *triple pelvic osteotomy* basically combines the transverse osteotomy of Salter with complete osteotomies of superior pelvic ramus and ischium. This allows acetabulum to be redirectioned over femoral head without interfering with the growth of triradiate cartilage.

Treatment of Severe Disease or Delayed Presentation

Some children with severe Perthes' disease present later in the course, when the head has already collapsed and deformed. In such patients, abnormal hinge movement of the hip joint, so called "hinge-abduction", occurs due to extrusion of the femoral head. It is a phenomenon of impingement of the outer part of the femoral head on the lateral lip of acetabulum, typically showing widening of medial joint space by levering of inferomedial part of femoral head against the lateral edge of acetabulum. *Hinge abduction is thought to be presented, if there is lateralization of femoral head by >2 mm on an abduction radiograph.* The hinged abduction may be **reducible** when the soft extruded part can be gently reduced inside acetabulum as in transitional phase of disease; or it may be **irreducible** when the head cannot be reduced. Arthrography forms an important part of investigation to deduce the type of hinged abduction.

- The treatment in reducible hinge abduction (early stages) includes: *Closed reduction after adductor and psoas tenotomy:* It may be augmented by medial capsular release through medial approach. This is followed by Petrie's cast for 3–6 weeks followed by ROM exercises. At the end of this period, appropriate containment procedure may be performed.
- The surgical treatment for irreducible hinged abduction aims to improve the joint congruity by reducing femoroacetabular impingement. Proximal femoral valgus osteotomy alleviates abnormal hinge movement. This may be later augmented by acetabular procedures to improve coverage of the femoral head, which may provide hyaline cartilage to hyaline cartilage of acetabular osteotomy (triple pelvic or peri acetabular) or hyaline cartilage to fibrocartilage salvage procedure (Chiari or shelf procedure). Other procedures, which may be done in irreducible hinge abduction, include acetabular enlarging procedures, hip joint distraction, osteochondroplasty, and femoral head reshaping (Garceau's cheilectomy). Soft tissue releases should not be done with cheilectomy, as it increases the tendency to hinged abduction by proximal migration.
- Treatment of residual deformity after Perthes' disease (Stulberg class III and further) needs surgical dislocation of the hip and osteochondroplasty + relative neck lengthening with or without periacetabular osteotomy. This is specialty surgery and management of FAI is discussed in respective chapter. Higher class Stulberg patients usually present with osteoarthrosis early (in third decade itself) needing arthroplasty. Higher incidence of intraoperative fractures is reported in these patients.

SOME NOTES ON SURGICAL CONTAINMENT PROCEDURE

Salter's Innominate Osteotomy (Elizabethtown Osteotomy)

See also the Section on Dysplastic Development of Hip for technique details.

Indications

- Patients above 6 years of age
- Less than 20% femoral head extrusion. Extrusion more than this and an attempt to reduce it would incur excessive pressure of femoral head to possibly cause disease progression and fragmentation of head.

Prerequisites

- Absence of hip irritability
- Normal or near-normal ROM
- Absence or minimal deformity of femoral head
- Concentric containment possible on arthrography

Contraindications

- Persistent limitation of hip ROM
- Grossly deformed femoral head
- Age ≤5 years

Advantages of Salter's Osteotomy

- Lengthening of extremity
- Anterolateral coverage
- Avoidance of second operation for plate removal

Disadvantages

- Postoperative stiffness of hip joint
- Osteotomy requires skills and dedicates center
- Increased length may cause compensatory adduction deformity and uncoverage of the femoral head
- Increased hip joint pressure
- Inability to obtain adequate coverage of femoral head particularly in patients >8 years of age due to stiffness in symphysis pubis (prefer triple innominate osteotomy).

Femoral Varus Derotation Osteotomy (Figs. 15A and B)

Indications

- All at risk cases
- Patients > 6 years of age with lateral extrusion and head fragmentation

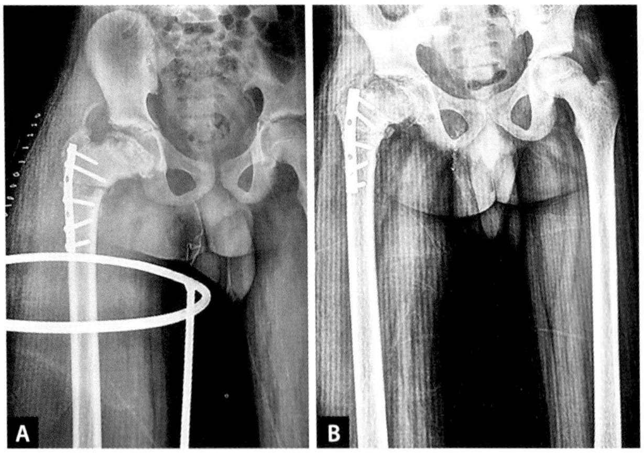

Figs. 15A and B: Proximal femoral varus osteotomy for Perthes. (A) Immediate postoperative radiograph; (B) After healing of the osteotomy and good coverage.

- Reducible head with abduction and internal rotation on arthrogram

Contraindications

- Age <5 and >10 years
- Severe flattening of femoral head that is unlikely to remodel
- Avoid if neck shaft angle <110° or >20° of axial rotation needed for containment

Advantages

- Decompresses the femoral head
- Suitable for bilateral cases
- Decreases stress across the hip joint
- Tends to enhance remodeling process
- Ability to simultaneously correct the anteversion
- Ability to obtain maximum coverage and put the fragmented region of head away

Disadvantages

- Elevation of greater trochanter
- Coxa vara that may persist throughout the life
- Abductor weakness and Trendelenburg gait
- Shortening
- Nonunion
- Requirement of second surgery for implant removal

DYSPLASTIC DEVELOPMENT OF HIP (DEVELOPMENTAL DYSPLASIA OF HIP, CONGENITAL DYSPLASIA OF HIP, AND CONGENITAL DISLOCATION OF HIP)

Manish Kumar Varshney

INTRODUCTION

The term congenital dislocation of hip (CDH) indicates partial or complete displacement of the femoral head from acetabulum because of inadequacy. The inherent problem to term CDH is that it does not give an indication of dysplasia, so the terms congenital dysplasia or better developmental dysplasia of hip (DDH) (Klisic, 1989) should be used that better refer to the basic pathology. The process is not limited only to congenital abnormalities of the hip but also includes some hips that were normal at birth and subsequently became abnormal. Hence, the term DDH is preferred and used throughout this text. The term DDH as an entity *per se* includes following distinct clinically recognizable increasingly severe spectrum of conditions:

- Dislocatable hips
- Partial dislocation (subluxation) of the femoral head
- Acetabular dysplasia (deficient development of acetabulum)
- Complete dislocation of the femoral head

Usage and understanding of some commonly used terms with reference to DDH are clarified as follows:

"Instability" of hip is defined by Ortolani's and Barlow's test classically.

"Dysplasia" is a radiographic finding of increased obliquity and loss of acetabular concavity.

"Dislocation" means complete displacement of the articular surfaces with no remaining contact or congruity of the joint **(Fig. 16)**.

"Subluxation" refers to partial displacement with some contact remaining **(Fig. 16)**.

The incidence of *congenital dysplasia* has been found to vary between studies, type of evaluation method used, and ethnic population (0% in African and Chinese newborn to 75 per thousand in Yugoslavia to 188.5 per 1,000 in a district in Manitoba, Canada). Historically, it has been estimated around 1/1,000 live births. However, the incidence varies as:

- 8.6 per 1,000 live births on physical examination by pediatricians
- 11.5 per 1,000 live births by dedicated orthopedic screening
- 25 per 1,000 live births by ultrasonographic examination. This is probably an overestimation.

Most of the hips, which are diagnosed to have congenital dysplasia on ultrasound, stabilize and become normal on physical examination by 6 weeks of age. There are a few descriptive secondary forms of hips with dysplasia that should not be clubbed with the term DDH. Use of term DDH strictly refers to idiopathic form of developmental dysplasia.

Klisic introduced subgroups of DDH, their clinical relevance and addition to current knowledge of DDH are unknown. They are mentioned only for detailed evaluation and description done by Klisic and his contribution for encouraging the use of term "developmental". Possibly, they represent different clinical forms of DDH with varying presentation but hardly contribute to the prognosis or treatment.

- DDH at risk—family history positive, breech presentation, female child, etc. (see below in risk factors for DDH)
- "Hypoplastic" DDH with limited abduction
- DDH—reducible with click of entry
- DDH—reducible with click of exit
- DDH—subluxation and limited abduction
- DDH—dislocation with limited abduction, femoral shortening, and telescopy

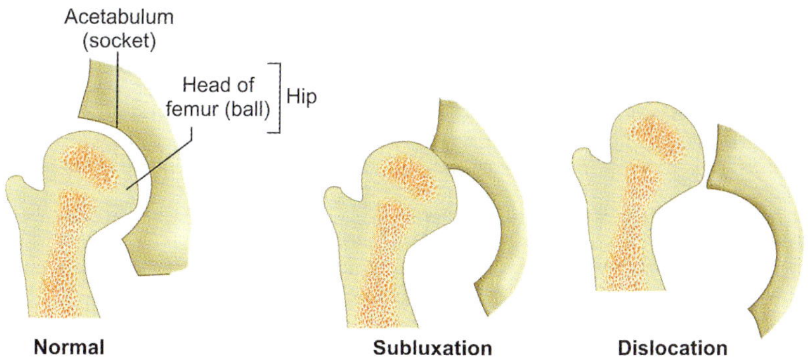

Fig. 16: Difference between a subluxated and a dislocated hip.

RISK FACTORS

Certain risk factors are associated with acetabular dysplasia that have been found to be increasingly associated with DDH but not proven to be the cause for same:

- Female sex—due to greater susceptibility maternal hormones such as relaxin-inducing greater joint laxity.
- *Breech presentation:* Children delivered by cesarean section have lower chances of developing DDH (shown by Lowry et al.) than those delivered vaginally.
- *Intrauterine crowding phenomenon:* Conditions producing tighter intrauterine space such as oligohydramnios, large birth weight, and first born child provides for less room to fetal movements predisposing to less than optimal development of hip and predisposing to DDH. This theory of "crowding phenomenon" is supported by frequent association of DDH with other "intrauterine molding abnormalities" such as torticollis and metatarsus adductus.
- Family history (increases the incidence by approximately 10%)
- White children have a higher incidence than black children.
- Chinese have a lower incidence while Navajo Indians have higher incidence.

Protective Factors

Like the risk factors, certain protective factors have been identified that protect the child from developing DDH such as:

- Preterm baby <2 kg weight
- Premature babies
- Population where the ladies are in the habit of carrying child by the side against their bodies in a shawl. This habit of Asian and African caregivers places the child's hip in flexed and abducted posture, free to move providing optimal position for hip molding and development of acetabular cartilage anlage against the femoral template.

Associations

Lot of musculoskeletal abnormalities have been strongly associated with congenital dysplasia of the hip (most of these results from tight packaging say in primigravida) that includes:

- *Congenital torticollis:* The coexistence rate of congenital torticollis and congenital dysplasia is about 8%.
- Metatarsus adductus
- Genu recurvatum
- Talipes calcaneovalgus deformity
- The association with clubfoot deformity is controversial with conflicting reports.

ETIOPATHOGENESIS

Several theories exist regarding pathogenesis of congenital dysplasia. The actual cause appears to be a combination of more than one factor. The causes include mechanical factors, primary acetabular dysplasia, hormone-induced joint laxity, and genetic inheritance that ultimately fail to maintain a stable femoroacetabular articulation. Apart from the classical congenital/developmental forms described here, DDH may also arise in specific situations associated with or following certain situations like paralysis, etc. These forms are described in **Box 6**. Following are the various etiopathogenetic processes involved in development of classical DDH.

- *Mechanical:*
  - *In-utero position:* The most common intrauterine position of the fetus places left hip against maternal sacrum forcing it into a position of adduction resulting in dislocation. In fact, left hip dislocation and dysplasia are the most common, followed by both hip involvement and right hip involvement alone.
  - Breech delivery is also an important mechanical factor for predisposing dislocation of the hip. The incidence of DDH in infants born in breech presentation is as high as 16–25%.
- *Positional:* An increased incidence is also seen in communities that swaddle infants (Americans and Swedish) with the hips lying in constant adduction and extension. "This position increases tension in the psoas muscle and predisposes for dislocation of the hip laterally and superiorly." In India, the incidence is low due to the habit of carrying the children by side.
- *Hormonal:* Maternal hormones such as relaxin may produce ligamentous laxity thereby increasing chances of dislocation. This hormone can cross placental barrier.
- *Genetic:* Finally, there may be familial occurrence of a shallow/dysplastic acetabulum, which may predispose dislocation. The risk of genetic influence was observed by Ortolam who reported a 70% incidence of a positive family history in children with congenital dysplasia of the hip.

BOX 6: The secondary descriptive forms of developmental dysplasia of hip (DDH).

- A teratologic dislocation is commonly used to describe complex and "resistant-to-treat" forms of dislocations. Actually, it is associated with other disorders that make the reduction difficult such as "genetic syndromes, arthrogryposis, or myelodysplasia. The hips in these forms are dislocated before birth and early intrauterine life with limited range of motion (ROM), complete acetabular malformation, and marked displacement of femoral head and they are not reducible on examination (Barlow's test) due to short and tight soft tissues producing sort of fixed deformities.
- Paralytic dislocation of hip is associated with disorders such as spina bifida or absent vertebral segments and primarily needs management of paralytic limbs with secondary stabilization.
- Diastrophic dysplasia is due to intrauterine defects of bone and cartilage development as in mucopolysaccharidosis. These hips are prone to recurrence due to muscle imbalance and often develop ischemic necrosis of the femoral head.
- *Adolescent DDH:* Acetabular dysplasia may be diagnosed for the first-time during adolescence or in later age group. It is commonly bilateral and the issue is unsettled whether it represents a unique entity or represents residual deformity of DDH in childhood.

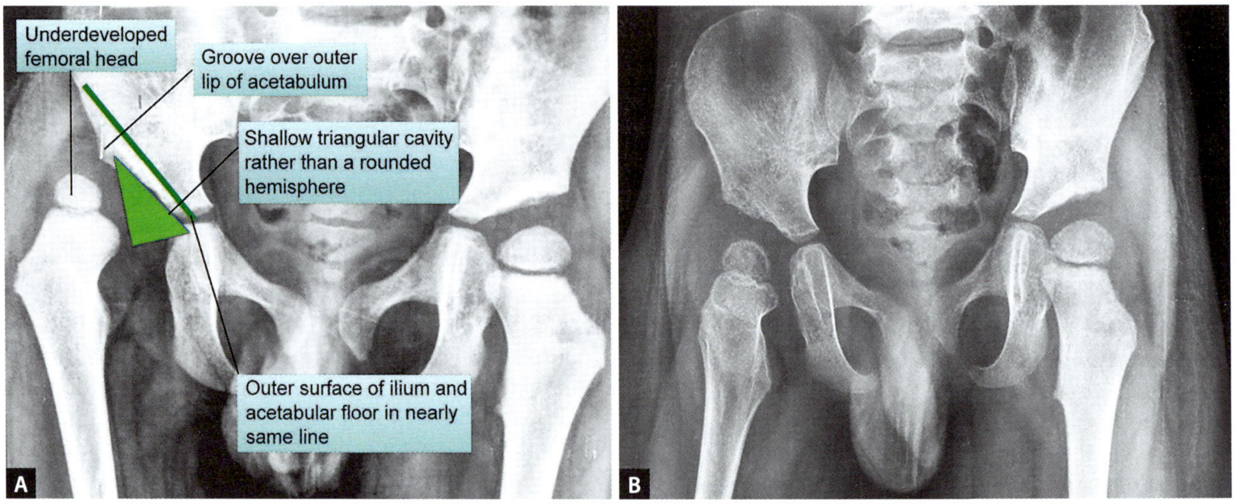

Figs. 17A and B: Radiograph of developmental dysplasia of hip (DDH). (A) The head of femur is dislocated high; (B) Reduction of femoral head and molding of acetabulum around the head.

- *Anatomical:* Lax joint capsule fails to correct the neonatal anteversion of femoral neck.
- *Physiological:* Iliopsoas and glutei paralysis—the former causes lateral torsion while the latter causes increased femoral anteversion.

PATHOANATOMY

Before understanding pathological anatomy of the structures, it is better to understand few important points in hip developmental anatomy:

- Acetabulum appears as a mesodermal condensation at the end of 4th week of intrauterine life.
- The concavity develops due to pressure from the developing cartilaginous femoral head (molding effect, **Figs. 17A and B**).
- The triradiate cartilage is the basic structure occupying a rotated "Y" position having lower vertical segment, anterosuperior limb, and a horizontal posterior limb.
- Triradiate cartilage ossifies to ilium, ischium, and pubic bones during further development.
- Labrum lies at the edge of acetabulum and capsule inserts above its rim; some consider the hypoplastic development of labrum to cause DDH and hip subluxation. This deficient form is also found in some lower vertebrates where the hindlimbs serve no useful purpose.
- At birth, both the hips are in flexion contracture of 15–20° that is stretched by the infant's activity in the first 6 weeks.

Bone Pathology

Acetabulum: It is mainly amalgamation of malformation of the anatomical structures that have developed normally during the embryological period. The following changes are seen:

- Dysplastic acetabulum is shallower than normal **(Figs. 17A and B)**
- Gap/groove in posterosuperior part [over which the head subluxates **(Figs. 17A and B)**]
- Triangular depressed cavity with lack of rounded concavity **(Figs. 17A and B)**
- Outer surface of ilium and acetabular floor in a straight line (**Figs. 17A and B**)
- Overgrowth and hypertrophy of the fibrocartilage in acetabulum (pulvinar) and hypertrophic remains of ligamentum teres prevent relocation of the femoral head **(Fig. 18)**
- A ridge of thick articular cartilage forms over posterosuperior wall—termed "neolimbus" by Ortolani that remains inverted **(Fig. 18)**. It is over this that the femoral head slides in and out with a "clunk" or "scatto", the latter term used by Ortolani.

Uhthoff identified that the acetabular roof is well developed but the posterior wall is made of only little cartilage, mainly a fibrous labrum.

Femoral head: It develops into a conical shape or buffer shape if resting on ilium. The ossification is delayed and flattening is seen on both posterior and medial aspects. Cartilage portion is larger than acetabular space.

Neck of femur: It is anteverted (up to 90°) and shortened.

Pelvis and lower spine:
- Pelvis tilts forward
- Deformation in pelvis seen in the form of approximated ilia and separated ischium (bilateral cases). For unilateral DDH, the inlet is obliquely ovoid.
- Increased lumbar lordosis.

Soft Tissue Pathology

Capsule

- Hourglass shape (iliopsoas-induced constriction of the capsule between head and acetabulum)
- Adherent to acetabular floor

Muscles:
- Pelvifemoral muscles [adductors, hamstrings, gracilis, sartorius, tensor fasciae latae (TFL), pectineus, and rectus femoris] shorten and serve as most formidable obstacle to reduction.
- Pelvitrochanteric group (obturator, quadratus, and iliopsoas) becomes stretched and functionally incompetent.
- Gluteal muscles (medius, minimus, and maximus) reduce power due to shortened lever.

Pathoanatomy of a Subluxatable Hip

- Loose hyperelastic capsule
- Elongated ligamentum teres
- Slightly everted hypertrophied acetabular rim
- Excess femoral and acetabular antetorsion
- Normal shape of femoral head

Pathoanatomy of Dislocatable Hip

- Stretched out and loose capsule
- Marked elongation of ligamentum teres
- Everted labrum
- Neolimbus formation
- Normal femoral head

Pathoanatomy of Irreducible Hip

Intra-articular obstructions prevent hip relocation **(Fig. 18)**.
- Pericephalic insertion of capsule (33%)—hourglass configuration of capsule with dislocated hips, the central constriction is augmented by iliopsoas tendon.
- Ligamentum teres hypertrophied and elongated (32%)
- Inverted limbus (31%)
- Iliopsoas tendon (25%)
- Capsular adhesions (16%)
- Thick pulvinar deposition in acetabulum
- Transverse acetabular ligament pulled upward

CLINICAL PRESENTATION

The clinical presentation varies with the age. A small child <6 months with congenital dysplasia may go unnoticed by the parents. Such cases may even be ill diagnosed by physician. "Ilfeld phenomenon" refers to poor clinical examination of infants due to crying/hungry/tense baby or a hurried/inexperienced doctor using too tight a grip (white knuckle sign of Ortolani). The radiographs may not be reliable, as the epiphyseal ossification center may be delayed in appearance. Such cases may be diagnosed by good and careful clinical examination. Hart mentioned that the classic signs for diagnosis of hip dysplasia include limited hip abduction with 90° knee flexion, positive Ortolani sign found up to 3 months, and apparent shortening of thigh. The prominent findings are:
- Upriding trochanter riding above Nelaton's line, shortening of the limb **(Fig. 19)**
- Adduction contracture
- Absent femoral pulse (due to lack of support from underlying femoral head in a dislocation)—the Narath sign for femoral pulsations. Often, the pulsations are less marked than totally absent to an experienced finger.
- Asymmetric thigh folds—increased in number on the side of dislocation **(Fig. 20)**
- Higher buttock fold on side of dislocation
- Widened perineum in bilateral dislocation
- Galeazzi sign positive **(Fig. 21)**
- Range of motion—restricted abduction and increased internal rotation

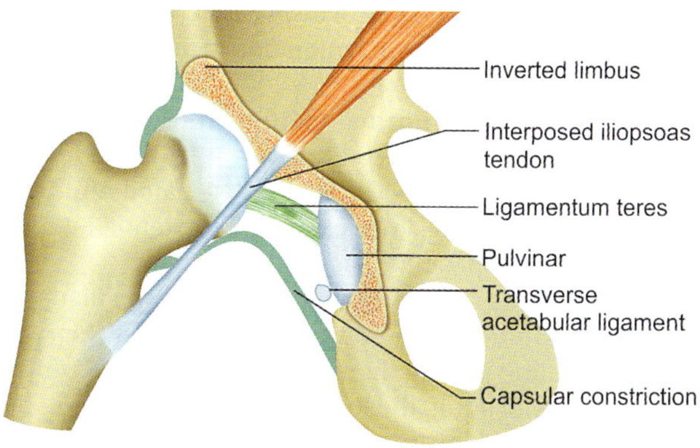

Fig. 18: Pathological changes in developmental dysplasia of hip.

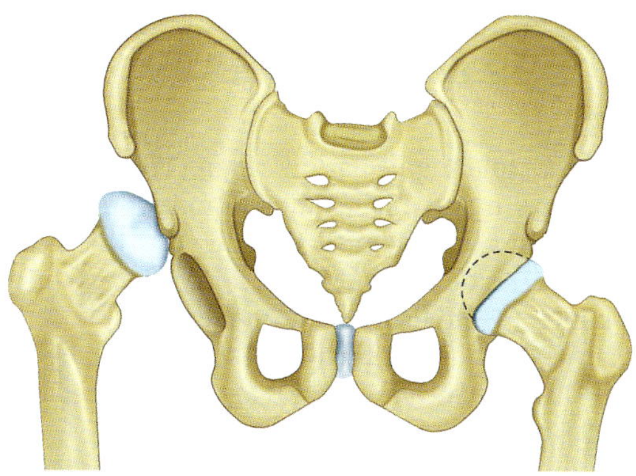

Fig. 19: Upriding of the greater trochanter and limb shortening.

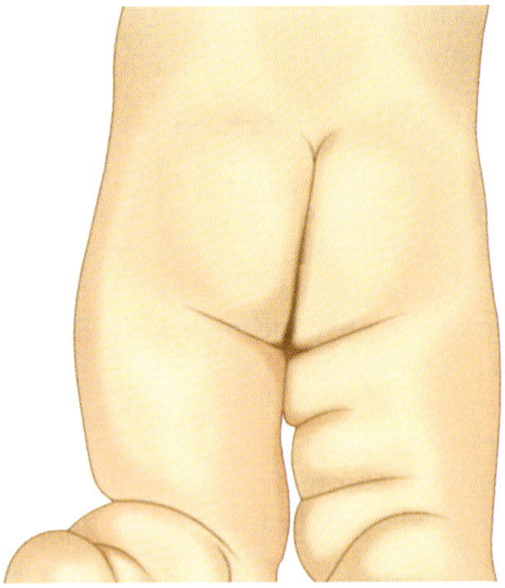

Fig. 20: Extra and asymmetrical thigh folds.

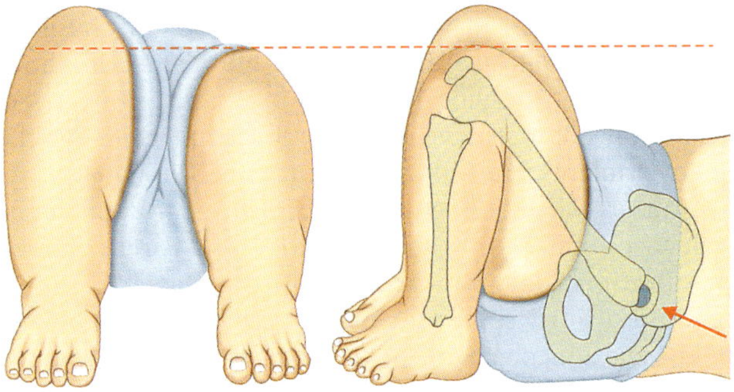

Fig. 21: Galeazzi sign. Lesser knee height on affected side (shown by dotted lines).

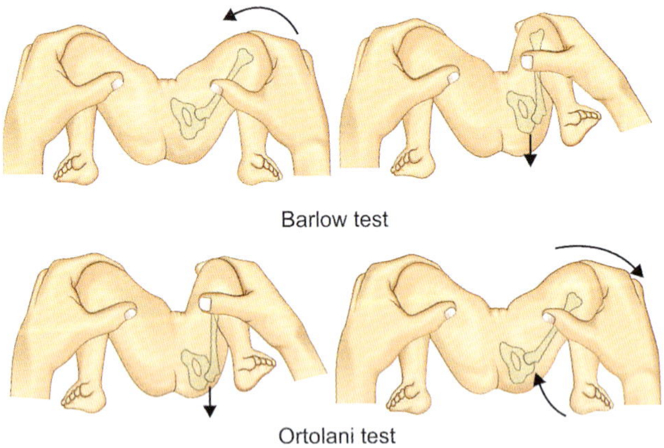

Fig. 22: The Ortolani and Barlow test.

- Positive Ortolani and Barlow's sign **(Fig. 22)**: Once the infant is calm and pacified, the examiner places his/her hand around the infant's knee such that the thumb lies on the inner side and index and long finger at the greater trochanter (avoid Ilfeld phenomenon).
    - Now, Ortolani (1937) test [described also by Froelich (1911) and LeDamanu (1912)] is performed by gently abducting the initially adducted and flexed hip through 90° arc while applying an anteromedial force to the greater trochanter (from fingers) to detect any reduction of the femoral head into acetabulum. If one of the hips is dislocated then a clunk or "scatto" of entry is produced in 90° arc somewhere along. In patients of arthrogryposis multiplex congenita (AMC) or meningomyelocele, limited abduction reduces the ability of test to detect a clunk/jerk/scatto of entry.
        - False positive—fascia lata snapping over greater trochanter or iliopsoas tendon over femoral head
        - False negative—markedly lax capsule produces a smooth reduction without clunk
    - On the other hand, Barlow's test (modification of Ortolani test) is a provocative measure, which detects the potential of hip joint instability. The first part of the test is similar to Ortolani test, while the second part is the provocative maneuver. For the first part with the knees fully flexed and both hips adducted the normal hip kept in 90° of flexion, the affected hip is placed in 45–60° of flexion (in this position, it is likely to be more unstable). The thighs are carried into mid abduction and pressure exerted by middle finger onto greater trochanter toward pubis to reduce the hip. For second part of the test (Barlow's test for dislocatable hips), outward pressure is exerted by the thumb onto inner aspect of thigh and pushing the shaft of femur along longitudinal axis posteriorly, the clunk/jerk of exit is felt as the head slips out over the posterosuperior lip of acetabulum. This indicates a dislocatable hip and not a dislocated one.

As the child grows and reaches between 6 and 18 months of age, it is usually not possible to abduct the hip and reduce it on clinical examination. The following are the findings in a walking child:

- Limitation of abduction and asymmetric thigh and gluteal folds are the most common clinical findings in such children.
- The Galeazzi sign may be positive when the femoral head is displaced laterally as well as proximally causing an apparent shortening of the femur.
- A child in walking age may walk with Trendelenburg gait (unilateral dislocation) described as waddling by parents with exaggerated lumbar lordosis. For bilateral cases, the child has a duck-like or Sailors gait.
- Increased lumbar lordosis **(Fig. 23)**
- *Positive Trendelenburg sign:* Amount of hip drop is proportional to the degree of displacement. The glutei are inefficient due to proximal migration of head and absent/unstable fulcrum.
- *Ludloff's sign:* In a normal child with hips fully flexed and abducted, the knee cannot be fully extended due to hamstring tightness while in a dislocated hip due to proximal shortening, knee can be fully extended.
- Galeazzi sign is positive (see above)
- *Klisic test:* Keep index finger on anterosuperior iliac spine (ASIS) and middle finger on greater trochanter **(Figs. 24A and B)**. A line joining them meets at umbilicus while in bilateral dislocation, the lines meet below it.

In unilateral dislocation, a line drawn in a similar way would pass beneath the umbilicus.

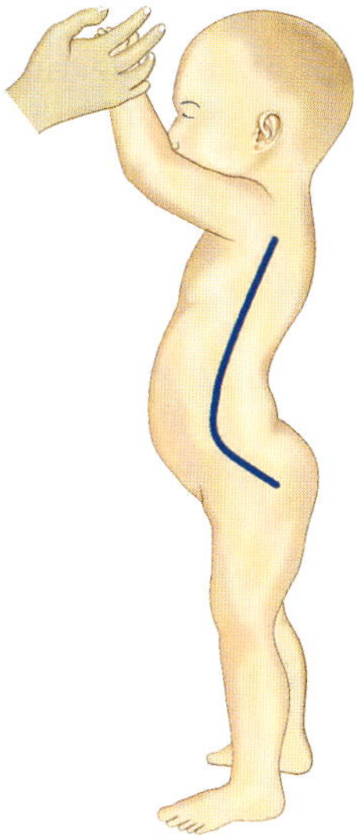

Fig. 23: Excess lumbar lordosis in toddler especially with bilateral dislocation.

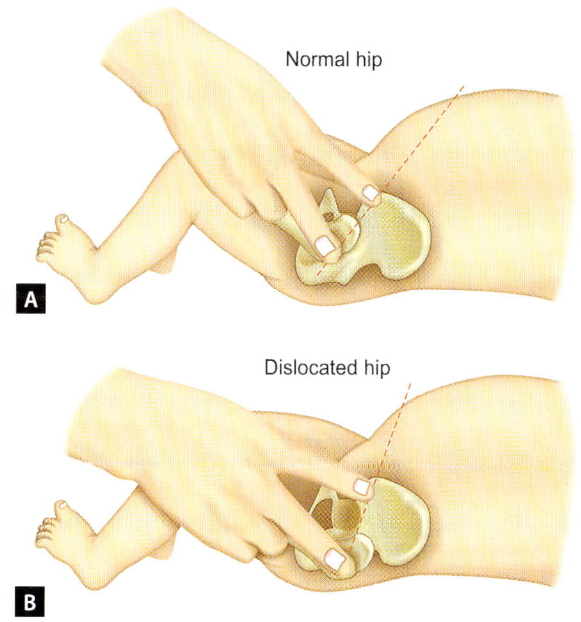

Figs. 24A and B: Line joining anterosuperior iliac spine (ASIS) and tip of trochanter represented by index finger tip and middle finger tip respectively normally passes through or just above umbilicus (A) while in a dislocated hip, the line passes inferior to the umbilicus (B).

IMAGING STUDIES

Radiography

- Obliquity of the acetabulum depends on the ossification of the outer third.
- Upriding of trochanter and limb shortening **(*see* Fig. 19)**.
- Proximal femoral epiphysis begins to ossify around 4–6 months of age and is delayed in DDH. In these cases, the line drawn up the femoral long axis with radiograph taken in 45° of abduction (Andren-Von-Rosen line) should transect the triradiate cartilage and is true irrespective of the position of hip joint **(Figs. 25A and B)**.

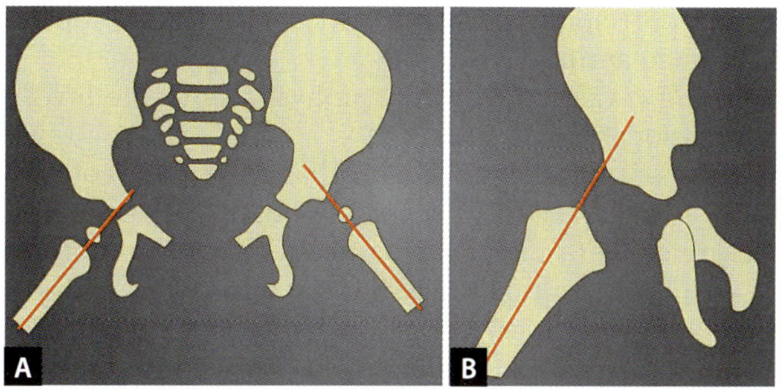

Figs. 25A and B: Andren–Von–Rosen line. The line normally bisects or ends just above the triradiate cartilage (A, right hip, i.e., on your left side). In a subluxed or dislocated hip, the line bisects or goes above the anteroinferior iliac spine (A; left hip, i.e., on your right side and B).

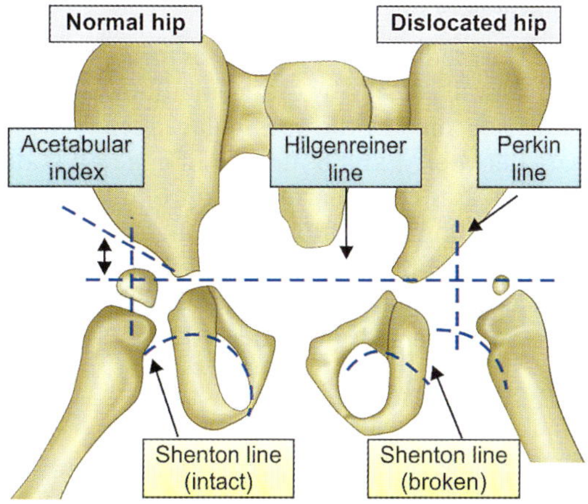

Fig. 26: Radiographic lines and depictions used to describe developmental dysplasia of the hip (DDH) on X-ray. The Shenton–Menard arc is broken on the dislocated side (left hip), which is dislocated (low dislocation, Grade 3 Tonnis).

- *Hilgenreiner's line:* It is the horizontal line drawn joining the uppermost aspect of triradiate cartilage of both sides **(Fig. 26)**
- *Perkin's line (Ombredanne's line):* It is the line perpendicular to Hilgenreiner's line drawn at lateral margin of acetabulum. It divides the hip into four quadrants **(Figs. 27 and 28)**:
  1. Normal hip—femoral epiphysis lies in the lower inner quadrant
  2. Subluxated hip—femoral epiphysis lies in the upper medial quadrant
  3. Dislocated hip—epiphysis in the lower outer quadrant
  4. High dislocation—epiphysis in the upper outer quadrant

Quite often, a grading system is used for DDH to evaluate hips in research papers and studies based on this "quadrant position of the femoral head". The system gave rise to the classification of hip dysplasia by Tonnis (one should note that both systems are not exactly identical, and I feel that the Tonnis system is correct to follow) as follows:

1. *Grade 1:* Capital femoral epiphysis medial to Perkins line
2. *Grade 2:* Capital femoral epiphysis lateral to Perkins line but below the level of the superior acetabular rim

3. *Grade 3:* Capital femoral epiphysis at the level of superior acetabular rim
4. *Grade 4:* Capital femoral epiphysis above the level of superior acetabular rim

Tonnis evaluated the position of "capital femoral epiphysis (CFE)" in reference to the quadrants but ossific nucleus and CFE are absent in younger patients, so the international hip dysplasia institute suggested use of superior midpoint of metaphysis **(Fig. 27)**. Also, the inferolateral quadrant is divided into two through a 45° line.

Shenton–Minard line (see Fig. 26): It is a curved line that begins at lesser trochanter and joins the upper border of obturator foramen passing along the lower border of femoral neck as an even curve. In fractures and DDH, the neck portion is not congruent to the curve.

Teardrop: The medial wall of teardrop is formed by the lesser pelvis, lateral wall is made by the acetabulum, and the lower curved line is formed by the acetabular notch **(*see* Fig. 19)**. It appears between 4 and 6 months of age and is delayed in DDH. Appearance of teardrop after 6 months of age is pathological. With DDH, it loses its convexity and is wider from superior to inferior—"U" shaped, due to eccentric position of femoral head. Other pathological forms are open, closed, crossed/reversed, and v-shaped.

Acetabular index (see Fig. 26):

- Normal = 27.5° (mean in newborns)
- 6 months = 23.5°
- 2 years—decreases to <20°

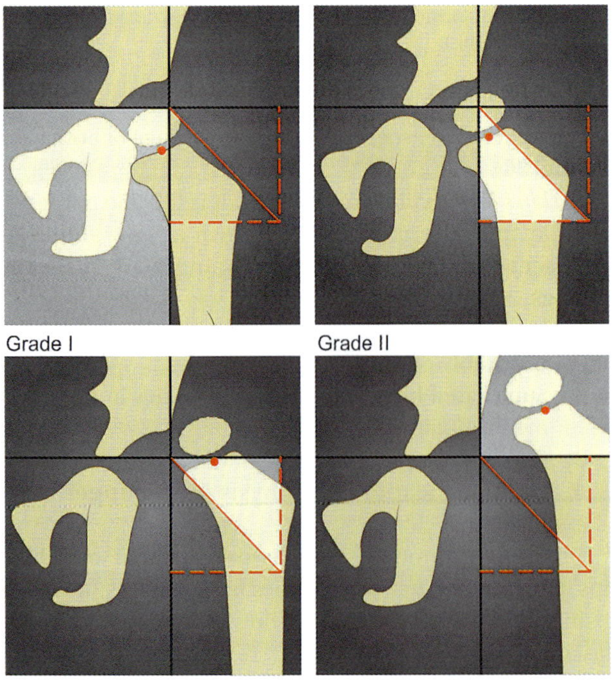

Fig. 27: Perkin's line and international hip dysplasia institute revised quadrants. Perkin's line is a vertical line drawn perpendicular to the Hilgenreiner line drawn at the lateral margin of acetabulum on anteroposterior (AP) view. In a normal hip, the femoral epiphysis is located in the lower inner quadrant.

- 30° is the upper limit of normal hence for any age
- Anteroinferior zone of weightbearing or sourcil is <15° of the curve.

Medial gap (Fig. 28): This is the distance between the ossified proximal portion of the femur and lateral wall of teardrop. Normal is < 4 mm, 5 mm is suspicious and ≥6 mm is dislocation.

- Dimension "H" is the distance from top of ossified proximal portion of femoral head to Hilgenreiner line.
- Dimension "D" is the distance from middle of the proximal ossified femur to the inner border of teardrop. These measures are useful in unossified or absent femoral head to grade the dislocation or displacement of femoral head.

Central edge angle of Wiberg **(Figs. 29A to C)**:

- 6–13 years; >19° is normal
- 14 years and more; >25° is normal
- Acetabular depth and femoral head extrusion index are other measures used to describe severity of DDH **(Figs. 29A to C)**.

Ultrasound

Ultrasound screening is increasingly being used for the diagnosis and follow-up of treated cases of congenital dysplasia of the hip (*see* Chapter on "Role of Radiological Investigations in Orthopedics and Radiation Hazard"). Although it is noninvasive and easy to use, its interpretation is observer-dependent and may pick up several false-positive cases resulting in overdiagnosis and tendency toward overtreatment. Nevertheless, ultrasonic examination is a useful adjunct to the physical examination. It has a useful role in documenting the response of hip to closed reduction in Pavlik harness or spica. There are two distinct methods used for ultrasonological evaluation of hip. One is by the static technique of Graf and the other by dynamic stress testing of Harcke. Based on the measured α and β angles, Graf has distinguished various ultrasonographic hip types **(Table 5)**.

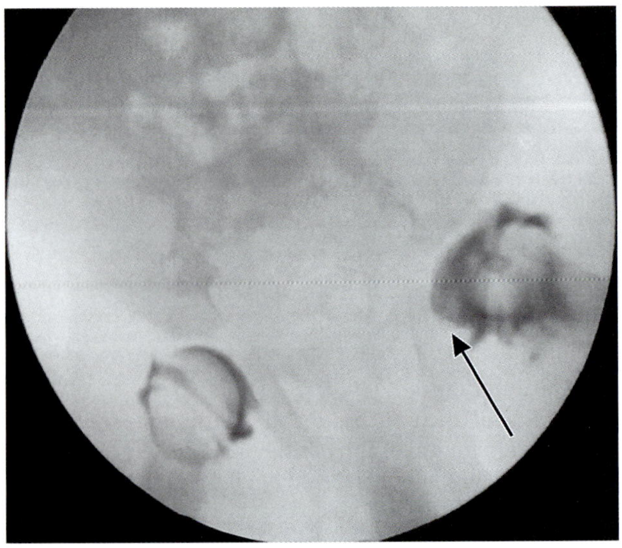

Fig. 28: Arthrogram with acceptable reduction on the right hip while increased medial space on the left side (arrow) that needs repositioning or better an open reduction, if closed reduction is unsuccessful.

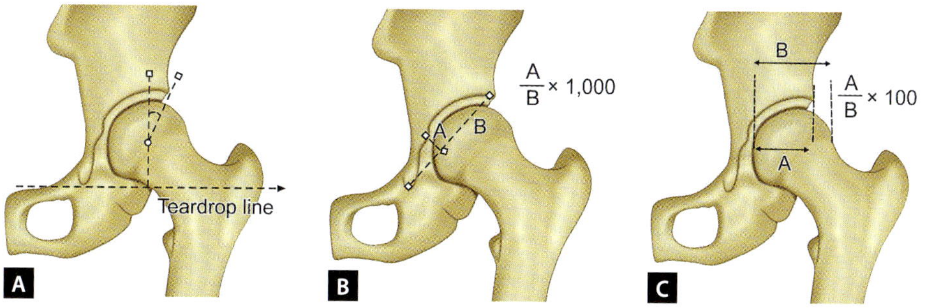

Figs. 29A to C: (A) The central edge (CE) angle of Wiberg is the angle between a line drawn perpendicular to the horizontal (inter-teardrop line) passing through the femoral head center and a line from the femoral head center to the lateral edge of the acetabulum; (B) The acetabular depth ratio is a line drawn as follows. First a line is drawn from the teardrop shadow to the lateral edge of the acetabulum. A second line perpendicular to above is drawn to intersect the medial corner of the superior weight-bearing surface of acetabulum. The length of this line denotes acetabular depth; (C) The femoral head extrusion index indicates the percentage of the femoral head diameter that is uncovered by the acetabulum. This part lies lateral to Perkin's line.

TABLE 5: Ultrasonographic hip types according to Graf technique.

Hip type	*Osseous roof contour*	*Superior osseous rim*	*Cartilaginous rim*	*α-angle*	*β-angle*
Fully mature (any age)–Ia	Good	Angular	Narrow; triangular; covers femoral head	≥60°	<55°
Ib	Good	Blunt (usually slight roundishness)	Wide-based; short; covers femoral head	≥60°	>55°
IIa+: Physiological delay of ossification appropriate for age (<3 months)	Adequate	Round	Wide; covers femoral head	50–59	>55
IIa: Physiological delay of ossification with maturity deficit (<3 months)	Deficient	Round	Wide; covers femoral head	50–59	
IIb: Delay of ossification after age of 3 months	Deficient	Round	Wide; covers femoral head	50–59	>55
IIc: Critical range (any age)		Round to flat	Wide; still covers femoral head	43–49 (critical range)	70–77
IId: Decentering (any age)	Severely deficient	Round to flat	Displaced	43–49 (critical range)	>77 (decentering range)
Eccentric					
IIIa	Poor	Flat	Displaced, without structural alteration	<43	>77
IIIb	Poor	Flat	Displaced, without structural alteration	<43	>77
IV	Poor	Flat	Displaced inferomedially	<43	>77

The Graf's angles are highly user dependent, so other measures are also described. Percentage of femoral head coverage is a good indicator of reduction. Values > 50% are considered normal but again the positions of probe and limb are compounding variables. The pubofemoral distance is a better measure and has good reliability even in hands of inexperienced ultrasonologist. The upper cut-off values are 6.0 mm in hip flexion and adduction, 4.9 mm in hip flexion, and 4.6 mm in neutral position. The values reduce with successful head coverage and reduction. USG is recommended at 1–2 weeks in patients with clinically unstable hips (positive Barlow and Ortolani signs). In patients with clinically reduced stable hips but with risk factors, USG should be postponed to 6 weeks of life avoiding false positives.

Arthrography

It is a wonderful tool to assess the reduction (closed reduction), depth of acetabulum, and stability of reduction. The width of medial dye-pool indicates the likely stability of reduction. Fair reduction is indicated by 5–6 mm of medial dye pool. Medial space >6 mm indicates poor reduction, which is difficult to hold (***see* Fig. 28**).

Magnetic Resonance Imaging

Magnetic resonance imaging is not a routine due to availability, cost, and logistics of performing the lengthy investigation in a child (requires short anesthesia).

Kashiwagi classification of acetabular dysplasia based on MRI:

- Group 1—sharp acetabular rim, reducible with pavlik harness
- Group 2—rounded rim, almost all reducible with harness
- Group 3—inverted acetabular rim; none reducible with harness

CT Scan

It is rarely indicated for cases with doubtful nonconcentric reduction, difficult to evaluate on radiographs (say in spica cast), and bilateral dislocations for evaluation of bony acetabulum.

Radiological Screening

Ultrasonography screening is currently indicated in female infants delivered by breech and/or positive family history of DDH. Other plausible indications for screening of hip include:

- Family history
- Breech presentation
- Torticollis
- Metatarsus adductus
- Oligohydramnios

DIFFERENTIAL DIAGNOSIS (CLINICAL AND RADIOLOGICAL)

Coxa vara, pathological dislocation, paralytic dislocation, cerebral palsy, septic arthritis, and its sequel are commonly confused with DDH and should be specifically sought for and differentiated.

TREATMENT

Primarily, the treatment in DDH is aimed at obtaining and maintaining a concentric reduction of hip with femoral head positioned within the acetabular cartilage anlage so that reciprocal development of both can occur into stable hip. The later the diagnosis of DDH is made the difficult is to achieve this goal due to reduced potential of molding and remodeling. Also with delayed diagnosis and treatment, the treatment options become complex. The treatment of DDH is age related, i.e., the age at presentation for treatment. Generally, the age-related treatment groups have been divided into five types:

1. Newborn (birth to 6 months)
2. Infant (6–18 months)
3. Toddler (18–26 months)
4. Child (3–8 years)
5. Adolescents (>8 years)

Treatment in Newborn (Birth to 6 Months)

The aim of treatment in this age group is to stabilize hip in reduced position and to allow flexion and abduction movements simultaneously. Although various splints such as "Von Rosen splint", "Tubingen splint", "Ilfeld splint", and "Pavlik harness" are available with indigenous variants; the last one has been most effective and popular. A success rate approaching 95% has been found with **Pavlik Harness** that should be applied as soon as the diagnosis is made. The treatment is most effective in all reducible dislocations (positive Ortolani), located hips with positive Barlow test (i.e., dislocatable), and hips that are normal to clinical examination but sonologically abnormal. It is unclear if newborns <4 weeks of age should be treated; as significant number of these become normal by 4 weeks, especially if the diagnosis had been made by USG. Also, no difference in outcome at 6 years has been noted, if the treatment is initiated at 4 weeks or at birth by observers. Pavlik harness is a "dynamic flexion-abduction orthosis", which has a chest strap, two shoulder straps, and two stirrups **(Figs. 30A and B)**. The harness is applied with the child in supine position (the most effective position for the harness to work).

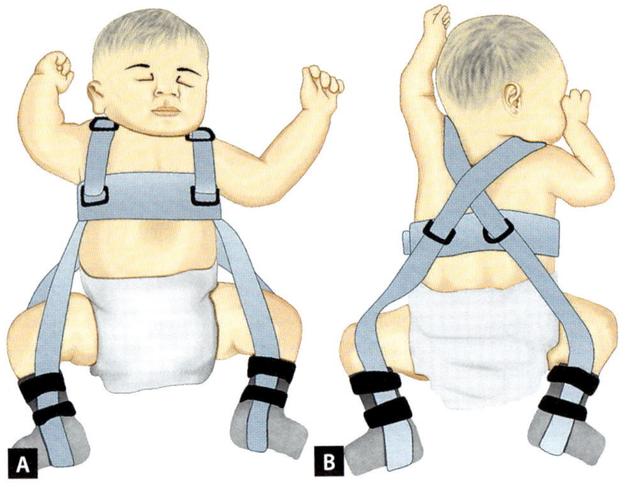

Figs. 30A and B: Pavlik harness. (A) Brace components and (B) acceptability of application.

- Each stirrup has an anteromedial flexion strap and posterolateral abduction strap.
- The chest strap is applied first allowing enough space between skin and the strap.
- The shoulder straps are adjusted to keep the chest strap at the nipple line.
- The feet are placed in stirrup one by one.
- The hip is placed in 90–110° of flexion and anterior flexion strap is tightened.
- Lastly, the lateral abduction strap is tightened to limit adduction and not produce forced abduction.
- At full adduction, the knees should be 3–5 cm apart. An X-ray may be made on the harness, which should show femoral neck directed toward the triradiate cartilage.
- An ultrasound evaluation is a good means to follow-up patients on a Pavlik harness after closed reduction.

The harness works on the mechanism of "dynamic flexion-abduction of hip". In supine position, the hip goes into abduction giving relief to the child when a reduction is affected. This further relaxes adductors (that are also relieved by sleep) further maintaining the reduced position and abducts the hip still more. The harness treatment cannot be applied to an older child where soft tissue contracture has started to form or the child has started crawling.

The Pavlik harness should be worn full-time until stability is achieved, which takes about 8 weeks (some recommend 12 weeks especially in hips that were dislocated at presentation). During this time, the child is examined clinically (range of abduction movement, Barlow's, and Ortolani's test) at a period of 1–2 weeks. Ultrasonographic examination should be done at least once at the end of 3–4 weeks (if reduction is not achieved by 6 weeks, it is better to stop use of harness and switch to other treatment). This may be followed by radiographs at 6 months and then at 1 year of age. Brace changes are required to take care of the growth every 3–4 weeks. Once a stable hip has been achieved, the harness is weaned off allowing more harness-free time in the day. However, the harness is applied during night and gradually transitioned to night-time abduction orthosis for few weeks or months. The guidelines for weaning are not clearly defined and may depend upon experience of the physician, degree of instability, and age of the child at presentation.

Potential Complications

Potential complications of treatment in harness include:

- Avascular necrosis (<1%)
- *Persistent dislocation:* It is generally seen in superior, inferior, lateral, or posterior directions in decreasing order of frequency. Further, flexion may be added in superior dislocation and flexion may be reduced in inferior dislocations. Lateral dislocations may be just observed as long as the femoral neck is directed in the direction of triradiate cartilage. This hip may gradually reduce into the acetabulum on follow-up. A posterior dislocation is generally difficult to treat on a Pavlik harness. Such patients have tight adductor muscles. If signs of persistent dislocation remain for >3–6 weeks of treatment, then Pavlik harness should be discontinued and child should be taken up for closed reduction under general anesthesia followed by spica casting. The risk factors for failure of Pavlik harness include high-grade dislocations (Graf type IV), male sex, and age >4 month.
- *Femoral nerve palsy:* Femoral nerve palsy may occur due to acute flexion (>90°) required to apply the Pavlik harness. The physician should look for active knee extension after removal of the harness on each visit. If femoral nerve palsy develops, the harness treatment should be discontinued for minimum of 2 weeks. Abduction bracing may be used in these cases when the nerve function returns.

Failure of Treatment

Failure of treatment on a Pavlik harness (reduction not achieved by 6 weeks maximum) may occur in the following situations (risk factors):

- Absent Ortolani sign at initial evaluation (irreducible dislocation)
- Bilateral hip dislocation
- Development of femoral nerve palsy during treatment leading to discontinuation of treatment
- Acetabular index of 36° or more on an X-ray
- Initial coverage of <20% as determined on ultrasonographic examination
- Inability to treat beyond 7 months of age

In these cases, if the dislocation is reducible, the child should be taken up for closed reduction under general anesthesia (see below for details). A forced reduction should never be attempted, as it increases chances of avascular necrosis. Continued use of Pavlik harness beyond 6 weeks in hips, which are not concentrically reduced with its use, can lead to development of "Pavlik harness disease". This involves wearing away of the posterior wall and column of acetabulum or its hypoplasia due to pressure effect and it makes the ultimate reduction by other methods less stable.

Contraindications

Contraindications for Pavlik harness:

- Older child in walking stage
- If the hip cannot be centered toward triradiate cartilage in 90–110° of flexion
- Dislocations developing several weeks after birth
- Dislocations associated with muscle imbalance:
  - Meningomyelocele
  - Stiff-extended knee
  - Down syndrome
  - Marfan syndrome
  - Osteogenesis imperfecta

Of note, there are other harnesses also available that can be variably used and have good success (especially the first two); these include:

- Ilfeld splint
- Von Rosen splint
- Tubingen splint

Also, one should note that "Frejka pillow" is no longer used due to its poor outcome and high risk of osteonecrosis with its use. "Triple diapers" should be abandoned, as they have been totally ineffective and give a false sense of relief to the surgeon and parents that something is being done.

Treatment in an Infant (6–18 Months)

A Pavlik harness usually fails once the soft tissue contractures have developed and the child begins to crawl, the success rates drop to <50% with its use in children >6 months of age. In this age group, the infant will require a closed or open reduction followed by a hip spica. The abduction is usually limited and a positive Galeazzi sign (lower knee height of the flexed limb with child lying supine) is seen. A Trendelenburg gait may be seen in an ambulatory child. Once the child begins to walk, the femoral head displaces superiorly and laterally.

Pathology-anatomical changes in the hip are conspicuous:

- The capsule becomes thick and elongated.
- The ligamentum teres becomes hypertrophied.
- The limbus may hypertrophy around the rim of the acetabulum and the psoas tendon may obstruct reduction of the femoral head by producing an hour-glass constriction in the capsule anteriorly.
- The true acetabulum is characteristically shallow.
- The volume of true acetabulum during surgery appears low due to anterior capsular constriction, hypertrophied limbus, and constriction of the deep acetabular ligaments.

Some authors advocate use of *skin traction* before considering closed reduction to reduce chances of avascular necrosis. Its role is controversial and advantages are not fully established. It increases the time of hospitalization and home-based traction programs may not be suitable for developing countries such as India. Secondly, a primary femoral shortening is routinely done in an older child to bring a proximally displaced femoral head down to the level of acetabulum so as to allow a more gentle reduction. This obviates the need for preparation traction. Bryant's traction was a popular modality in past but not used nowadays.

A percutaneous or open "adductor tenotomy" may be performed for adductor contracture. This improves the range of abduction and helps in the case of reduction.

Closed Reduction

The closed reduction is generally preceded by *arthrography* because a plain radiograph or an ultrasound is unable to provide all the desired information. An arthrogram may help in determining the acetabular dysplasia, degree of femoral head dislocation, extent of soft tissue obstruction to closed reduction, condition of the limbus, and the quality of reduction. A "concentric initial reduction" is the most important factor that determines the outcome of treatment of a congenital dysplasia of the hip. The criteria for accepting closed reduction include a medial dye pool of 5 mm or less and maintenance of reduction in a "safe zone". The safe zone concept of Ramsey is used to determine the zone of adduction and abduction in which the femoral head remains reduced in the acetabulum. While a wide safe zone (20–45°) is desirable, a narrow safe zone indicates an unstable/unacceptable reduction. It is imperative to make clinical judgment regarding stability of reduction before an arthrogram is performed, because clinical examination becomes difficult when the capsule is distended by the fluid.

- To perform an arthrogram (***see* Fig. 28**), the child is laid supine under general anesthesia.
- The fingertip locates hip joint immediately beneath the middle of inguinal ligament and a finger breath lateral to the femoral artery pulsation.
- A 22gauge spinal needle is inserted into the hip joint under image intensifier.
- Alternatively, the needle may be inserted medially, anterior to the adductor musculature.
- Resistance is met as needle passes through the hip joint capsule followed by sudden give-way feel.
- Now, saline solution is injected into capsule.
- If the joint has been successfully entered, the saline solution under pressure will reverse the plunger of the syringe.
- The saline is now aspirated and 1–3 mL of 25% hypaque solution is injected into the capsule.
- The needle is quickly removed and an arthrogram is made in unreduced position in adduction and extension.
- Further arthrograms are made after reducing the hip in flexion and abduction.
- Best position for concentric reduction and safe zone are noted carefully.

A frog-leg lateral view in flexion and abduction is also made; once a stable reduction has been achieved and confirmed, a spica cast is applied in 90–100° of flexion and 40–45° of abduction (**Figs. 31A and B**). This position has been described as "human position" by Salter and reduces chances of avascular necrosis. However, generally, the hips are always flexed less than they appear and are abducted more than they appear. A gentle mold at the greater trochanter can aid in reduction. The spica cast immobilization is continued for 3–4 months. The spica may be changed at 6–8 weeks. A radiography following spica cast may be difficult to interpret. Hence, a CT scan or MRI may help in the assessment of a concentric reduction. A CT scan takes less time, approximately 3 minutes but is less specific. The MRI takes more time (approximately 10 minutes) but is more specific. Failure to obtain stable concentric reduction by closed method is an indication for open reduction.

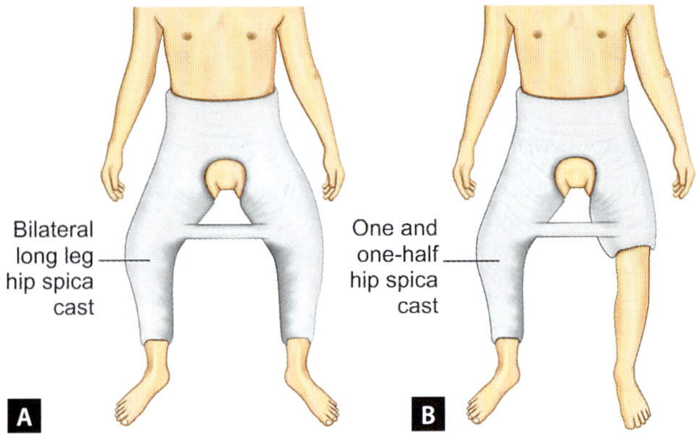

Figs. 31A and B: Spica cast for developmental dysplasia of the hip (DDH). (A) The spica can be applied for both legs in case of bilateral DDH, while often for (B) unilateral case, the one-half hip spica is applied. See text for details of position, etc.

Open Reduction

When gentle reduction without force is not possible, an open reduction may be indicated. Other indications for open reduction are:

- Femoral head lying persistently above the triradiate cartilage. be applied for both legs in case of bilateral DDH, while often for (B) unilateral case, the one-half hip spica is applied.
- Arc of reduction or "safe zone" of <25°, i.e., redislocation occurs with hip adducted within 25° of the reduced position
- Previous failed reduction
- Femoral head remains laterally displaced at 6 weeks (most likely due to hour-glass constriction of the capsule).

Aim: The aim of open reduction is to achieve concentric reduction of the femoral head in the acetabulum after correcting the soft tissue interposition. However, open reduction is not always age specific. A child <6 months may require open reduction and a child >18 months may occasionally respond to closed reduction.

The open reduction may be performed through an anterior, anteromedial, or medial approach. I perform the open reduction utilizing the *anterior approach* (**Figs. 32A to D**). The following are the usual steps:

- An anterior approach utilizes the interval between sartorius and tensor fascia lata muscles.
- The lateral cutaneous nerve of the thigh is protected with proper retraction.
- The iliac apophysis is detached from ilium beginning from ASIS and extending 4 cm posteriorly along the crest of ilium.
- The tensor fasciae latae is lifted subperiosteally to expose the lateral surface of ilium and the anterolateral aspect of capsule of the hip joint.
- The sartorius is detached from the ASIS.
- Now, tendon of iliopsoas muscle is identified medially in its groove on the superior pubic ramus.
- The tendon of the iliopsoas muscle is separated from the neurovascular bundle and a recession tenotomy is performed.

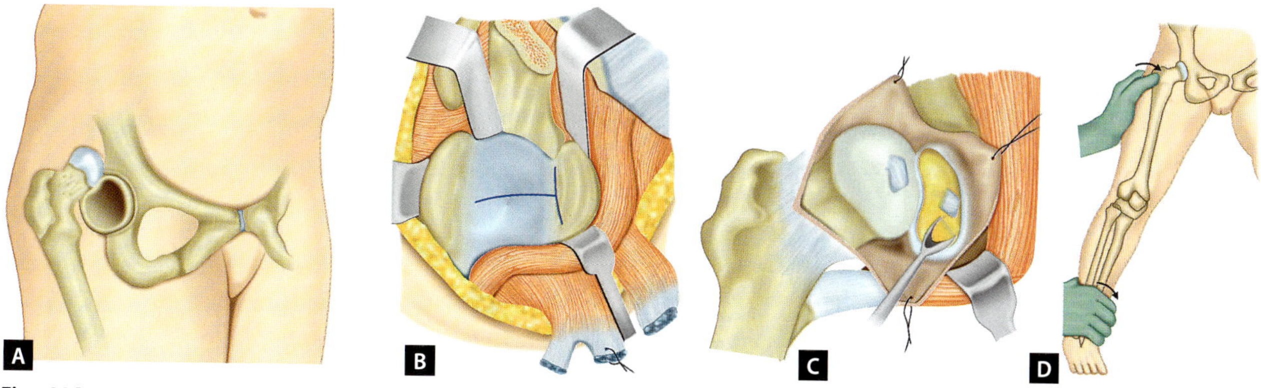

Figs. 32A to D: Open reduction for developmental dysplasia of the hip (DDH). (A) Dislocated hip joint; (B) Capsulotomy for exposure of the joint; (C) Bringing the hip down by removing the restraints; (D) Finally reducing it and fixing with smooth pins.

- The tendon of rectus femoris (both direct and oblique heads) is identified and tenotomy is done approximately 1 cm distal to the attachment.
- This exposes the hip capsule laterally anteriorly and medially.
- A "T" shape is made in capsule from the most medial aspect of the capsule to the most lateral. This exposes the head with hypertrophied ligamentum teres.
- The ligamentum teres is detached from the femoral head and traced proximally to the acetabulum.
- The acetabulum is cleared of any pulvinar with sharp dissection.
- The hip is reduced and then moved through complete ROM (including flexion, extension, adduction, and abduction) to know the "safe zone" of reduction.
- A capsulorrhaphy is performed suturing the lateral flap of "T"-shaped incision as far medially as possible, after serving a concentric reduction.
- After repair of the tendons and deep and superficial closure, a double-spica cast is applied with hips in 90–100° flexion and 40–55° of abduction.

The cast is changed 5–6 weeks afterward under general anesthesia. The spica is continued for 10–12 weeks followed by abduction brace for 4–8 weeks in the night. The major advantages with anterior approach include greater versatility, and that pelvic osteotomy, if necessary, can be done through the same approach.

The *anteromedial approach* described by Ponseti and Weinstein is actually an anterior approach to the hip through an anteromedial incision. The hip is approached between pectineus muscle and the neurovascular bundle. It is recommended for bilateral hip dislocation that can be simultaneously operated. The *medial (Ludloff's) approach* utilizes the interval between iliopsoas and pectineus. However, it is associated with a higher risk of osteonecrosis because it places medial circumflex vessels at a higher risk. The disadvantages of both these approaches are inability to allow a capsulorrhaphy.

Also, if pelvis osteotomy has to accompany, then a separate incision is required.

Additional Procedures

Usually, an additional femoral or acetabular procedure is not needed in children <2 years of age. Additional procedures may be needed for stable reduction of the hip in the still dysplastic shallow acetabular cup.

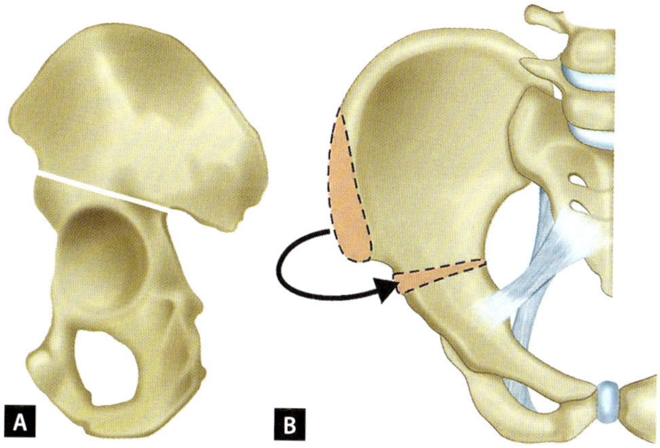

Figs. 33A and B: Salter's osteotomy. (A) Site of osteotomy from anterior inferior iliac spine (AIIS) to greater sciatic notch; (B) Displacement of distal fragment downward, outward, and laterally.

- As a rough guide, if >30% of head is visible after open reduction then additional procedures are needed to improve stability. Other signs that indicate an inadequate or eccentric reduction are moderate or pronounced limitation of abduction and instability of reduction with easy dislocation.
- Also, acetabular side osteotomies are needed, if there is progressive subluxation after either conservative or operative treatment.
- The third indication for ancillary procedure is uncommon cases where the acetabulum fails to remodel after open reduction.

In addition to open reduction and capsulorrhaphy, concomitant bony procedures may increase the stability of reduction as follows:

- *Innominate osteotomy (like Salter's,* ***Figs. 33A and B****):* Generally, when the hip is stable in neutral position in child <18 months, no osteotomy is required. When the hip is stable only in flexion and abduction but dislocates posteriorly on adduction, an innominate osteotomy may be required to reposition the acetabulum for better coverage. Choose Salter when rotational stability is required (for an abnormally oriented acetabulum) and capsular reefing is essential. See technical details below.

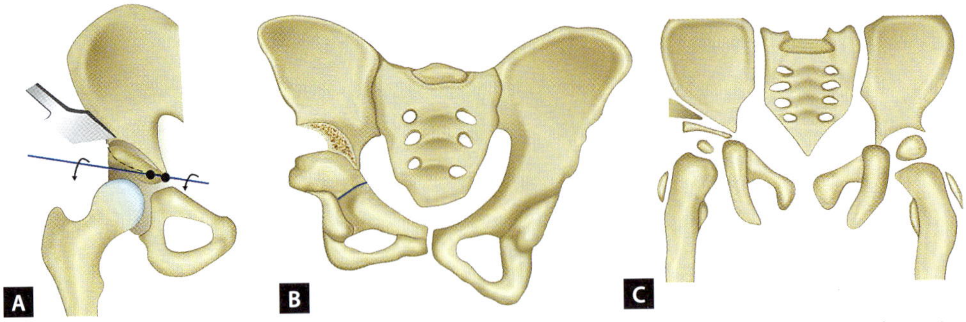

Figs. 34A to C: Pemberton osteotomy. (A) Site of osteotomy—curvilinear from a point between anterosuperior iliac spine (ASIS) and anterior inferior iliac spine (AIIS) (usually just above AIIS) to the triradiate cartilage. The osteotomy is done along the full curve above acetabulum cutting the lateral and medial cortices but trying to protect the inner wall at anterior column of the pelvis where the osteotomy ends at the triradiate cartilage; (B) displacing the osteotomy using a large osteotome downward and laterally to improve the coverage; (C) stabilizing the osteotomy using a bone graft commonly harvested from iliac crest.

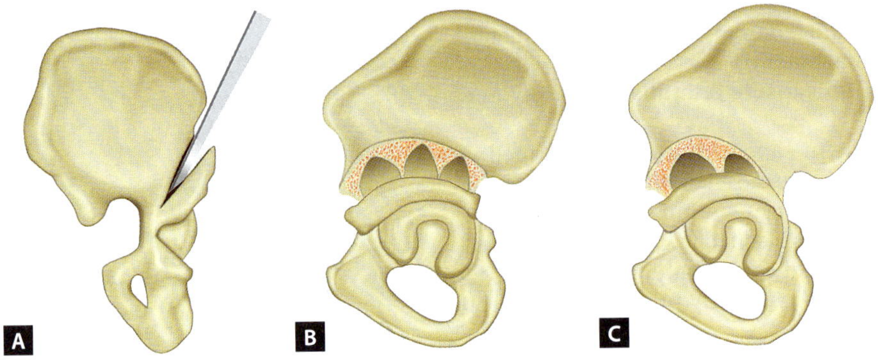

Figs. 35A to C: Dega osteotomy. (A) The osteotomy cut begins from a point lower than that of Pemberton and finishes near middle of the horizontal limb of triradiate cartilage at the inner aspect (depth). The osteotomy is hence more curved in depths than Pemberton, the anteroposterior extent is same but obviously being more near to acetabular roof, it gives better remodeling and plastic modeling. Strong and thick inner-wall hinge due to farther endpoint (from the inner wall/column) gives the osteotomy better stability; (B) The osteotomy is stabilized using contoured fibular struts and cancellous grafts. Placing the struts more posteriorly gives additional posterior coverage.

- *Acetabuloplasty (like Pemberton or Dega):* When the acetabulum is larger with undue anterolateral insufficiency—a Pemberton type osteotomy **(Figs. 34A to C)** will help in providing better cover that helps by improving acetabular dysplasia. Concomitant osteotomy may be combined with open reduction to maintain a safe and stable reduction. Choose Pemberton/Dega **(Figs. 35A to C)**, if the shape of acetabulum is abnormal. See technical details below.
- *Proximal femoral VDRO:* Proximal femoral VDRO may be required when hip is stable in internal rotation and abduction.
- *Femoral shortening osteotomy:* This is often an integral component of most ancillary procedures that help to reduce incidence of osteonecrosis, chondrolysis, and redislocation. This is especially considered for a child who has started walking.

In a younger child, however, these procedures may not be required due to high potential for acetabular remodeling.

Teratologic Dislocations

Teratologic dislocations in this age group represent a challenge, not that they are easy to manage even if identified early but with the success of other methods in this age group, their management is really frustrating for orthopedic surgeon.

- They are associated with significant anatomical changes in acetabulum and femoral head. The acetabulum is small, oblique, and flat and the femoral head is of variable size and may be flattened on the medial side.
- Typically the hip is stiff and irreducible with superolateral displacement of the head.
- These dislocations often accompany arthrogryposis, Larsen's syndrome, myelomeningocele, and diastrophic dysraphism.
- While unilateral dislocations are treated aggressively, bilateral dislocation may be left as such. This is because of high complication rates associated with open reduction for teratologic dislocation. Redislocation or subluxation may be as high as 40% and rate of osteonecrosis may approach 70%. Typically, closed reduction is impossible and open reduction should be accompanied with primary femoral shortening.

Toddler (18–36 Months)

Such cases are commonly seen in the outpatient departments of developing countries due to lack of screening programs in most pediatric set-ups. These patients characteristically have:
- A wide perineum
- Short extremity
- Hyperlordosis of the lower spine due to femoropelvic instability

Management

It is though manageable but extensive procedures in combination are often needed with less successful results than for previous groups. Often, an "open reduction and capsulorrhaphy" is accompanied by a "femoral or pelvic osteotomy or both".

- When the primary dysplasia exists in acetabulum, a pelvic redirectional osteotomy will be more appropriate. Generally, pelvic osteotomies are indicated only after the femoral head has been concentrically reduced, but the acetabulum is dysplastic, or the joint has failed to develop satisfactorily or the growth potential for acetabulum no longer exists. An upper age limit of 8 years is generally assumed, after which acetabular dysplasia does not remodel even with open reduction.
- The femoral osteotomy for correcting rotation/anteversion is generally associated with shortening of femoral length to decrease pressure on the reduced femoral head, thereby diminishing the chances of avascular necrosis.

After exposing the proximal femur through lateral incision, a transverse line is marked with an osteotome at the level of or just distal to the lesser trochanter. A longitudinal mark is also made on the anterior femoral cortex to determine correct rotation. After making an osteotomy at the transverse mark, the proximal femur is internally rotated by 15–30° to correct excessive anteversion. An appropriate wedge of bone is now removed from the medial cortex to achieve a neck-shaft angle of 120–135°. The osteotomy is fixed with an appropriate device followed by spica cast application, which is worn for 8–12 weeks. The fixation device is removed after 12–24 months.

Child (3–8 Years)

These are categorized as basically neglected DDH. Untreated or neglected congenital dislocations after 3 years are difficult to treat due to adaptive changes in the soft tissue, pelvis, and femoral head. The treatment is also hence directed to correct the identified adaptive pathology that is unique to individual case. Preoperative traction is not used due to high chances of osteonecrosis (54%) associated with it.

- In such cases, primary femoral shortening should accompany the open reduction and capsulorrhaphy with or without pelvic osteotomy.
- Younger children may be treated with femoral shortening when the dislocation is teratologic or severe enough to form a false acetabulum.
- It is important to identify the soft tissue abnormalities in an older child to produce a reduction which does not redislocate.
    - In older children, the capsule may become enlarged, sometimes double the size of the normal capsule.
    - Ligamentum teres becomes hypertrophied and sometimes may avulse from its femoral attachment on weight-bearing. In such cases, it forms a mass of tissue impeding reduction of the femoral head.
    - The fibrous cartilaginous labrum is flattened superolaterally. The femoral head protrudes superolaterally into the abductor muscle with adhesion between the muscle mass and the capsule. The middle and inferior portions of the capsule are constricted by the tendon of iliopsoas. The transverse acetabular ligament crossing the base of true acetabulum is also thickened and contracted.
- Hence, the capsular dissection is necessary to produce lasting results; rarely, tendon of piriformis muscles and gluteus medius may have to be released to bring the femoral head down to the level of acetabulum.
- Open reduction is then followed by femoral shortening at the level of or just distal to lesser trochanter. The amount of shortening is measured from most proximal aspect of femoral head to the triradiate cartilage. Usually, the required shortening ranges from 1–3 cm. Alternatively, an osteotomy is produced at the level of lesser trochanter and the femoral head is gently reduced. The overlapping distal shaft is removed.
- A varus angulation may be produced in the distal shaft additionally, if required. Once the osteotomy has been fixed, a pelvic osteotomy may be added to correct acetabular dysplasia, thorough capsulorrhaphy is essential to prevent redislocation.

Adolescents and Young Adults

More than 8 years with unreduced hip dislocation may be treated with palliative salvaging surgeries. Even if this hip is reduced with pelvic and femoral osteotomies, it is rare to expect a normal hip in the rest of lifetime. Despite this, a unilateral hip dislocation must be attempted to reduce. Bilateral dislocations in this age group should be left and total hip arthroplasty may be done during adulthood.

SOME PROCEDURAL DESCRIPTIONS

Pelvic Osteotomy

The operations on the pelvic side are done to ensure or increase the stability of the hip joint. The operation may belong to one of the following five categories:

1. Innominate osteotomy (Salter)
2. Acetabuloplasty (Pemberton)
3. Osteotomies that free the acetabulum (steel triple innominate or Ganz acetabular osteotomy)
4. Shelf operation (Staheli), and
5. Innominate osteotomy with medial displacement of the acetabulum (Chiari)

Salter Osteotomy (1961)

Osteotomy of innominate bone (devised by Salter) can be done in a child from 18 months to 7 years of age for unilateral cases (not recommended above 5 years of age for bilateral cases) to provide coverage to femoral head anteriorly and laterally. The osteotomy is not done below 18 years, as iliac wings cannot support the bone graft and fixation. The osteotomy is recommended in the prescribed age limit for:

- Primary treatment of congenital subluxation in early childhood
- Secondary treatment of any residual or recurrent dislocation persisting after primary treatment

- Persistent subluxation along with other methods of treatment (with inadequate coverage after closed/open reduction)
- Failure of acetabular angle to improve within 2 years following reduction or persistent dysplasia at 3–5 years (neglected cases)

The prerequisites include:
- Concentric and congruent reduction of femoral head inside the acetabulum
- The femoral head must be seated into the depth of acetabulum completely
- Ability to bring down the head to a position opposite acetabulum—the contractures of iliopsoas and adductor should be released
- The ROM of the hip must be good, especially abduction, internal rotation, and flexion.
- Mild (preferable) to moderate (upper limit) dysplasia of acetabulum

The *level of osteotomy* is just above the acetabulum at the anteroinferior iliac spine through the sciatic notch done in a transverse direction **(*see* Fig. 33A)**, completed using a Gigli saw. Entire acetabulum together with pubis and ischium is rotated forward, downward, and outward **(*see* Fig. 33B)** as a unit with symphysis pubic acting as a hinge. The osteotomy is then held open anterolaterally by a wedge of bone fixed by K-wire, which shifts the roof of acetabulum anteriorly and laterally. Patient is kept in a hip spica for 6 weeks after the procedure. Strict subperiosteal dissection is recommended to reduce bleeding and minimize nerve and vessel injury.

Complications:
- The sciatic nerve may be crushed or irritated by wrong placement of bone retractors in the sciatic notch.
- Prolonged retraction on iliopsoas may cause femoral nerve compression.
- Inadequate subperiosteal application of bone retractor medially may compress the obturator nerve.
- The anterior approach may endanger the lateral cutaneous nerve of thigh.
- The approach also risks the nutrient vessels of the tensor fascia lata muscle, if retraction is prolonged.
- Posterior displacement of the distal fragment

Disadvantages:
- Unstable osteotomy and requires internal fixation
- Correction is limited by the size of graft and length of pubic ramus
- "Defect" (pseudo) is created in the posterior acetabulum (due to repositioning) with narrowing of joint space
- Limb lengthening ≈ 1 cm is created

Acetabuloplasties of Pemberton and Dega

Pemberton osteotomy (1955, Pemberton incomplete pericapsular osteotomy): The term acetabuloplasty denotes redirection of the inclination of the acetabular roof by an osteotomy of the ilium superior to the acetabulum followed by leveling the roof inferiorly. Pemberton described a pericapsular approach, which is made through full thickness (cf-Dega osteotomy done through outer cortex only) of ilium using the triradiate cartilage as hinge around which the acetabular roof is rotated anteriorly and laterally. The osteotomy is curvilinear beginning between ASIS and anterior inferior iliac spine (AIIS) ending at the posterior limb of triradiate cartilage near the inner wall of acetabulum (*cf-Dega*). Stability is achieved by forward, lateral, and downward rotation of the anterosuperior acetabulum over femoral head improving coverage **(*see* Figs. 34A to C)**. The osteotomy is performed in several steps: the medial and lateral cortices are resected separately, and then the cancellous zone is resected using a curved osteotome. If lateral tipping is to be increased, the resection of the medial cortex must be more distal than the lateral cortical section. Posterior limb is deemed to remain intact at the inner wall of ilium but it often fractures due to thin support. The deeper extent of osteotomy toward inner wall (posterior hinge/limb) is farther than in Dega osteotomy so that the hinge is thinner in Pemberton osteotomy.

The advantages over innominate osteotomy include:
- Absence of internal fixation and thus need of a second operation to remove the implants
- Also, a greater degree of correction can be achieved by acetabuloplasty as the fulcrum of rotation; the triradiate cartilage is near the site of desired correction.

The operation is recommended for dysplastic hip between 1 year and the age when triradiate cartilage loses its flexibility totally generally 12 or 14 years in girls and boys respectively for moderate acetabular dysplasia. For severe dysplasia, however, the osteotomy does not have good results when done above 8 years of age, as the acetabulum does not remodel after that.

The prerequisites include concentric reduction of any existing subluxation or dislocation.

The disadvantages include technical difficulty and alteration in the configuration and capacity of acetabulum which may result in incongruous relationship between femoral head and acetabulum and that it reduces the diameter of acetabulum (though overall volume is increased). The osteotomy fails to improve the coverage of posterior part of acetabulum, as the posterior most point remains untouched in the repositioning maneuver.

Dega osteotomy:
It comprises a transiliac osteotomy designed for treatment of residual acetabular dysplasia secondary to congenital hip dysplasia and subluxation.
- It consists of an incomplete transiliac osteotomy involving the anterior and middle portions of ilium leaving a posterior hinge (inner wall) intact.
- The osteotomy is placed just above acetabulum (closer than Pemberton) and ends at the triradiate cartilage.
- The osteotomy line is located 15 mm above the acetabular rim, following the contour of the acetabulum **(*see* Figs. 35A to C)**.
- It extends from the anteroinferior iliac spine to the greater ischiatic incisura (greater sciatic notch).
- The procedure begins at the two extremities (ASIS and greater ischiatic incisura) with bicortical resection for a few millimeters.

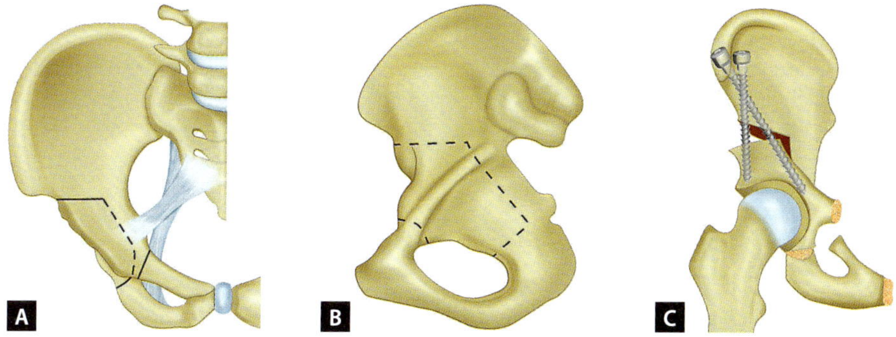

Figs. 36A to C: Ganz osteotomy is a periacetabular osteotomy that is aimed to release the acetabular component from the pelvis and reorient into a place more conducive for the stability and coverage of the hip and femoral head, respectively. These osteotomies are easily shown in picture that performed. The biplanar roof-shaped osteotomy is complex (A) with the anterior cuts shown by straight line and posterior cuts by dotted lines. The cuts actually meet on the inner aspect of the pelvis for completion of the osteotomy (B). This separates an irregular-shaped piece of bone containing the acetabulum that can now be reoriented (C). Proximal pubic ramus cut is made for separating the fragment completely (A) shown by a straight line.

- It passes toward the triradiate cartilage and stops just above it. The medial cortex is not resected **(*see* Figs. 35A to C)**.
- The osteotomy is levered open with a lamina spreader or/and cortical graft is inserted anteriorly and posteriorly to open up the osteotomy.
- The graft insertion can change the direction of coverage. Larger graft placement posteriorly may lead to posterior coverage, vice versa resulting in an anterior coverage.

The osteotomy can be done before or after closure of triradiate cartilage. The osteotomy reaches the triradiate cartilage closer to acetabulum than in Pemberton osteotomy.

Osteotomies that Free Acetabulum

The Salter's innominate osteotomy and Pemberton's pericapsular osteotomy are limited by flexibility of the triradiate cartilage and symphysis pubis. Although, former may be done in older children, its potential for femoral head coverage is limited. The osteotomies that free the acetabulum devised by Steel, Eppright, and Ganz **(Figs. 36A to C)** can provide much more correction and improve femoral head coverage. These operations free the part of pelvis that contains acetabulum, which can be placed in desirable position. These surgeries are indicated in adolescents and adults with residual dysplasia or subluxation where potential to remodel has been lost.

The triple innominate osteotomy developed by Steel involves division of the ischium, the superior pubic ramus, and the ilium superior to the acetabulum. Now, the acetabulum is repositioned over femoral head and stabilized by bone grafts and pins. The articular surfaces must be congruous or become congruous after acetabular redirection for the operation to yield successful results.

The complications include excessive external rotation of the acetabulum, posterior coverage, and nonunion of the ischial and pubic osteotomies. The pericapsular dial osteotomy of the acetabulum described by Eppright consists of freeing the acetabulum superiorly, posteriorly, inferiorly, and anteriorly as a single segment and redirecting it to cover the acetabulum.

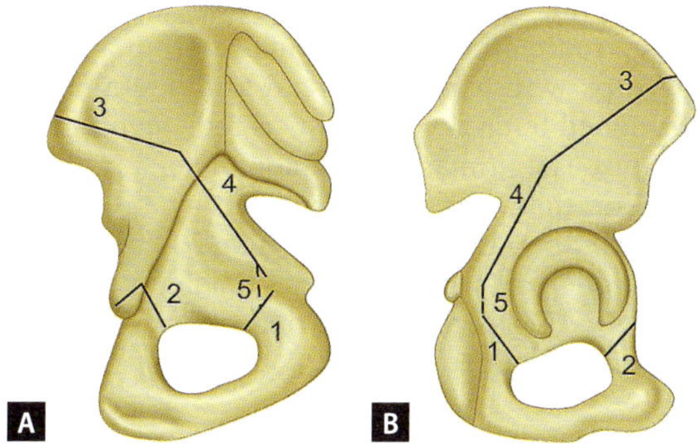

Figs. 37A and B: The Bernese periacetabular osteotomy (PAO) is a modification of Ganz osteotomy with the cuts as shown in the two figures (A) anterior aspect and (B) posterior aspect.

The Bernese periacetabular osteotomy (Ganz) has been developed for adolescent and adults with dysplastic hips which achieving congruency and containment are desirable **(Figs. 37A and B)**. The advantages include:

- Use of single approach to create all osteotomies
- Achieving larger amount of correction in all directions
- Preservation of blood supply to acetabulum
- No change in the shape of pelvis
- The intact posterior column of hemipelvis, which allows immediate weight bearing.

Shelf Procedures

The shelf procedures have been used to enlarge the volume of acetabulum. The shelf procedure of Staheli involves extension of the acetabular roof laterally, anteriorly, or posteriorly by a graft or by turning part of the lateral cortex of ilium distally superior to the femoral head. It can be combined with other reconstructive or osteotomy procedures but is commonly done in a young adolescent with mild symptoms and well-positioned head (sort of preventive procedure). The procedure is performed extracapsularly and the superior capsule dedifferentiates into fibrocartilage over time getting incorporated into acetabulum with growth of child. This procedure is used when no other osteotomy can establish a

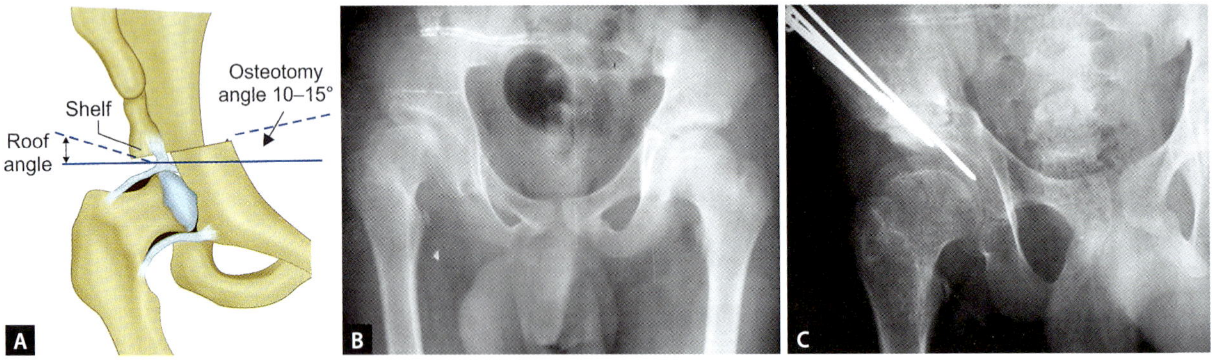

Figs. 38A to C: Chiari osteotomy: (A) the osteotomy is made in a slanting cut (reverse to that of Salter), the cut goes upwards medially at an angle of 10–15° from just below anterior inferior iliac spine (AIIS) to the greater sciatic notch. The acetabulum is displaced medially with the remaining ilium acting as a shelf to provide added coverage to the head. Capsule undergoes metaplasia into fibrocartilage over time and gets incorporated into the newly remodeling acetabulum, if the reduction is maintained congruent. Radiograph of patient treated using Chiari osteotomy (B and C).

congruous joint with apposition of acetabulum and femoral head. The redirectional osteotomies are not appropriate for the hips where femoral head and acetabulum are malpositioned but still congruent, as redirection can cause incongruity. The primary indication for shelf is a deficient acetabulum that cannot be corrected by a redirectional pelvic osteotomy. The contraindications include hips with spherical congruity, which makes it suitable for redirectional osteotomy and hips requiring open reduction that should have supplementary stability.

Innominate Osteotomy

Innominate osteotomy with medial displacement of the acetabulum, devised by *Chiari*, is a modification of shelf procedure. This is suitable for hips in which concentric reduction is not possible due to various reasons. It should be remembered that the procedure is for subluxated hips and not dislocated ones.

- The osteotomy of the innominate bone is performed at the superior margin of the acetabulum, and the part inferior to the osteotomy along with femur is displaced medially (deepens acetabulum). Osteotomy proceeds in a direction medially upward from just below AIIS to the greater sciatic notch. The starting point is important, as higher starting point fails to provide support. The superior fragment of osteotomy then becomes a shelf and the capsule is interposed between it and femoral head **(Figs. 38A to C)**. Hence, it is also called a capsular interposition arthroplasty.
- This procedure is recommended where other reconstructions are not possible as in situations when femoral head cannot be centered adequately.
- The Trendelenburg's limp generally improves due to displacement of head medially.
- Chiari recommended this procedure for:
  - Congenital subluxation in patients between 4 and 6 years or above
  - For untreated CDH in patients >4 years soon after open or closed reduction
  - For dysplastic hip with osteoarthritis
  - For paralytic dislocation caused by muscle weakness or spasticity
  - For coxa magna following Perthes' disease or osteonecrosis of head following treatment of congenital dysplasia

However, today in most cases, it is not used for subluxations or dislocation that can be reduced surgically or conservatively or in situations that can be dealt better with Salter's osteotomy. Acetabuloplasty or redirectional osteotomies are preferred especially when the age is <10 years.

Chiari procedure should be ideally reserved for patients older than 10 years who have subluxation of hip with severe acetabular dysplasia, which cannot be treated by other pelvic osteotomies.

CONCLUSION

- Coxa vara produces abnormal hip dynamics. Early identification and reorientation of the proximal femur by corrective osteotomy restore the hip joint offset and biomechanics.
- Slipped capital femoral epiphysis is not a very common disorder in Indian subcontinent, but if identified then treatment has to be precisely formulated to minimize damage and optimize function. Acute slips are mostly emergencies and should be emergently managed. Chronic slips should be prevented from progressing by appropriate management. Long-term management is very important considering the high incidence of development of FAI that compromises long-term outcome.
- Physeal softness due to some growth delay in a hyperactive child with global growth disorder possibly related to some intrinsic genetic factors and underprivileged populations is forerunner for explaining pathogenesis of Perthes' disease.
- Children are affected usually in the later part of first decade of age with variability of expression and symptoms.
- Extrusion of the femoral epiphysis is a troublesome complication and >20% extrusion demands coverage of the epiphysis by surgical or nonsurgical measures that are decided on a case-to-case basis.

- Developmental dysplasia of hip is not an uncommon condition and produces significant morbidity, if missed.
- Lots of subtypes of the disorder and many pathogenic mechanisms are proposed but none is definite. The most consistent finding is hip dislocation with inadequacy of the acetabulum that secondarily delays or restricts femoral head development.
- Radiography gives preliminary information of level of dislocation (Tonnis system is preferable), which should be ascertained clinically and also associated malformation should be taken into account for overall management. An arthrogram is more revealing than plain radiographs. Also, use of USG elicits good information in experienced hands; its use should be encouraged. For follow-up of management of DDH by harness, USG is an excellent tool.
- The management of DDH at different age groups is quite different and mostly relies on whether the hip is reducible that can be maintained by conservative measures or the dysplasia is so advanced that reduction cannot be stably maintained (this can be partly identified on arthrogram). Threshold for open reduction should be low in older ages and if reduction cannot be obtained gently.
- Ancillary procedures are often needed in patients with severe dysplasia and in whom 30% or more of head is visible after reduction. Mostly, acetabular osteotomies are done to increase the head coverage and are of various types with discrete indications, advantages, and disadvantages.

CHAPTER 43

Clubfoot—Congenital Talipes Equinovarus

Manish Kumar Varshney

DEFINITION AND PROBLEM STATEMENT

The word "talipes" is a *portmanteau* of two Latin words referring to ankle (talus) and foot (pes). The vernacular term "clubfoot" should be restricted to congenital variety of talipes equinovarus deformity only and not the paralytic forms. The term "talipes" by itself has also been applied to other congenital abnormalities of the foot such as talipes varus, talipes calcaneovalgus and calcaneovarus, and talipes equinovalgus in which the patient does not in any strict sense have typical congenital talipes equinovarus (CTEV) deformities. The clubfoot was defined as congenital subluxation of talocalcaneonavicular (TCN) joint by Scarpa. Brockman defined it as congenital atresia of the astragalo-calcaneal scaphoid joint (TCN joint). CTEV is a *nonembryonal* deformity in which foot is turned inward to varying degrees. Nonembryonal in the sense that the deformity develops during second trimester of pregnancy and is not possibly genetic at least always, so it can safely be classified to the best of current knowledge as a developmental deformity similar to congenital scoliosis or dysplastic development of hip. Clubfoot is one of the most common musculoskeletal birth defects and around 1 newborn is affected in every 1,000 live births though the incidence varies (0.5–5%) in different geographic locations and among ethnicities (more common in Hawaii, Middle East, and Mediterranean Coast of North Africa). Up to half of the cases are bilateral and males are more commonly affected than females with a ratio of 2.5:1. Though less common in females they have a greater proportion of relatives with clubfoot abnormality compared to males. The incidence in first-degree relatives is around 2%. The incidence of occurrence of CTEV in second monozygotic twin if the first one has deformity is 32%, this supports multifactorial inheritance rather than a purely genetic one. Pathoanatomically, it is defined as rotatory subluxation of TCN joint complex (subtalar complex) with talus in plantar flexion and subtalar complex in medial rotation and inversion. In its most characteristic forms, the deformities are a combination of the following components **(Figs. 1A to C)** that vary in severity in different pathological feet:

- Equinus at ankle
- Varus and internal rotation of heel (*varus of heel is equivalent to inversion at subtalar joint*)
- Adduction + Supination of forefoot (some people refer to this combination as varus of forefoot—but this is more confusing as a uniplanar deformity of hindfoot described by term "varus" becomes multiplanar for forefoot. I feel the term "forefoot varus" should be dropped for this inconsistency).
- Cavus of midfoot
- Internal tibial torsion

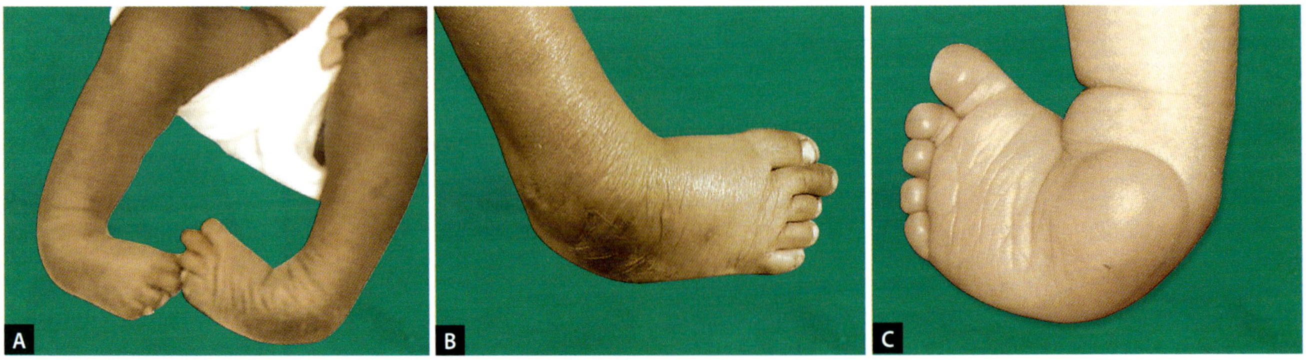

Figs. 1A to C: Clinical pictures of a clubfoot—look at the remarkable deformity that can be never misdiagnosed. The disposition of foot in Figure A gives it the classical name of "clubfoot"; (B) The appearance of foot from lateral (outer) aspect; (C) Look at the prominent medial crease and the heel varus. The medial column of leg is also shortened producing the medial skin fold while lateral aspect is normal.

Equinus is composite of ankle joint plantar flexion, inversion of TCN joint, and plantar flexion of forefoot. Varus primarily occurs at TCN joint when the whole tarsus is rotated inward except talus. Adduction occurs when the foot is rotated inward. It occurs at talonavicular, anterior subtalar joint, and tarsometatarsal area. Cavus occurs due to relative pronation of the forefoot as compared to hindfoot which is supinated. This causes plantar flexion of the first metatarsal resulting in cavus. There is no differential diagnosis to CTEV—it is a classical presentation. Deformity may be mild—slight exaggeration of normal equinovarus position or severe—when foot lies almost in contact with medial border of tibia. A rigid clubfoot usually refers to short, stubby foot with short first metatarsal ray, and very little change is visible after manipulation. On the other hand, a supple foot refers to less rigid; more pliable foot on manipulation which is usually longer. Other abnormal findings often present at the affected limb include atrophy of calf muscles and a smaller foot. Deformities (apparently presenting as CTEV) that can be fully corrected on initial manipulation should not be considered true idiopathic clubfeet.

HISTORICAL PERSPECTIVE

Chinese Tradition of Binding Feet

For thousands of years, Chinese girls had their feet bound in a stiff iron shoe. This was considered to make them look sexy but was a mutilating procedure wherein few children also died! The original idea was to make a "bonsai foot" with metatarsals approximated to the calcaneum and telescoped toes. Instead of arousing any sexual dignity, this leads the females with a small unstable painful foot and possibly the tradition was supported by males for the chauvinistic myth of female helplessness. The relative historical perspective of CTEV is enlisted below.

- 2000 BC—pictures of clubfeet in Egyptian tombs were painted.
- 400 BC—Hippocrates ascribed clubfeet to intrauterine pressure changes.
- 1740 AD—manipulative correction done with egg white and flour bandages.
- 1500–1800 AD—use of various braces described by Jean-Andre Venel, Scarpa, Dieffenbach, Pare's iron boot (1564), and foot manipulative procedures were popular.
- 1784 AD—surgical releases begin with Thilenius, Petit, and others.
- Mid-1800s—controversy between surgical and manipulative correction of clubfeet. Proponents of each debated often vehemently.
- 1900s—new organized methods of foot manipulation along with surgical correction became popular due to less than satisfactory results of manipulation. Surgery had an upper hand here.
- 1990s–Present—upper hand of manipulative correction of clubfeet due to better understanding of reasons for failure of previous manipulative methods.

ETIOLOGY

The true etiology of CTEV is still elusive. There has been no "definite" identifiable genetic, syndromal, or extrinsic cause. The genetic linkage is partially supported by some relation in progenies being affected in a family. If a male child is affected then next male child has 1 in 42 chance of being affected while for a first female affected child next male will have 1 in 16 chances and otherwise next female will have 1 in 40 chance of having the deformity. These incidences are higher than normal population but far from identifying the disease truly genetic one.

Extrinsic and intrinsic associations for CTEV (>200) have been identified in 10–11% of clubfoot patients and range from chromosomal deletions to syndromic to use of teratologic agents **(Box 1)**. The present notion is that idiopathic CTEV in otherwise healthy infants is the result of a multifactorial system of inheritance. Various theories have been proposed for pathogenesis of clubfoot and are as follows:

- *Heredity: Polygenic multifactorial trait:* Quite envisaging and as it is always said, may come true with exponential exploration of human genome and linkages. It could provide molecular insight too. Currently, the focus is on PITX1-TBX4 transcriptional pathway that is uniquely expressed in hind limbs.

BOX 1: Common associated anomalies with clubfeet.

- Chromosomal anomalies (3–22% incidence):
  - Deletion of chromosome 2 (2q 31-33) related to *Caspase-10* gene
  - 4p and 18q deletion syndrome
  - Trisomy 13, 18, and 21
  - Wolf-Hirschhorn syndrome
- Malformations:
  - Cleft lip and palate
  - Micrognathia
  - Congenital heart disease
  - Hip dislocation
  - Inguinal hernia
  - Tibial hemimelia
  - Polydactyly
- Renal anomalies:
  - Prune-belly syndrome
  - Renal agenesis
- Connective tissue disorders:
  - Marfan syndrome
  - Ehlers–Danlos syndrome
- Spinal anomalies:
  - Caudal regression syndrome
  - Diastematomyelia
  - Spina bifida/meningomyelocele
- Syndromic associations:
  - Arthrogryposis multiplex congenita (AMC)
  - Larsen syndrome (autosomal recessive) and Down syndrome—the ligament laxity in these syndromes lends good prognosis.
  - Freeman–Sheldon syndrome
  - Prune-belly syndrome
  - Nail-patella syndrome
  - Mobius syndrome
  - Gordon syndrome (autosomal dominant—camptodactyly, cleft palate, clubfoot)
  - Meckel–Gruber syndrome
  - Opitz syndrome
  - Roberts syndrome
  - Pierre–Robin syndrome (X-linked recessive)
- Skeletal dysplasias:
  - Diastrophic dwarfism
  - Muscular dystrophy
- Lead poisoning
- Fetal alcohol syndrome

- Germplasm defect (manufacturing defect of feet bones and ligaments)
- *Defective cartilage anlage of talus (Irani Sterman):* Quite popular but fails to explain why only the proximal tarsals are affected (around talus) as they do not seem to have any separate origin.
- *Intrauterine packaging defect [Hippocrates, Dennis-Brown (1937)]:* Excessive packing in a tight uterus of a primigravida or a large baby with oligohydramnios that causes initially postural and then later permanent tight clubfoot deformity.
- *Seasonal variations (Robertson):* Interesting hypothesis to explain the seasonal variations in epidemiologic studies in developing countries. This could have been very well be compounded by seasonal alteration in sexual habits in developing countries but the finding of polio-like seasonal variation and additional finding of motor neuron changes in the CTEV patients has made it more interesting. There is a proposal that CTEV could be a prenatal polio-like condition (limited polio!).
- *Neuromuscular defect (Isaacs):* Spina bifida; arthrogryposis multiplex congenita (AMC)—this is based on the histopathological findings of soft tissues around the ankle and foot. It is postulated that innervation changes due to altered neurology leads to secondary tightening and fibrosis of the muscle fibers. Supported by 35% incidence of the disease in spina bifida but challenged by the possibility of secondary muscular changes due to primary foot abnormality.
- Fetal developmental arrest in fibular stage (Bohm)
- Congenital atresia of talonavicular joint (Brockman, 1930)
- Retracting fibrosis "Crimp" (Ippolito and Ponseti)—due to increased fibrous tissue in muscles and surrounding tissues there is excessive deposition of collagen with wavy fibrillar structure (crimp). The collagen is particularly tight in the tendo-Achilles where the sheets of fibrillar collagen are arranged more complexly than parallel structures and resistant to stretch. The crimp of other tissues, however, is more supple and liable to stretching and restoring the length.
- Three-dimensional developmental bony deformity of subtalar complex (McKay)
- *Infective pathogens (Carney et al.):* Enteroviruses—conflicting evidence.
- *Anomalous tendon insertion (Inclan):* Possibly a misunderstanding arising out of examining the pathological feet. Deformity is primary with apparent shifting of tendinous insertion later.
- *Myoblast in medial fascia (Zimny et al.) on microscopy:* May cause the medial contracture by progressive lying down of the fibrous tissue and retraction. Electromagnetic radiation, toxins (maternal and/or paternal smoking, drugs, "ecstasy" use during pregnancy), elevated maternal homocysteine levels, and methylene tetrahydrofolate reductase polymorphisms have been implicated but none pinpointed as a single cause, again supporting multifactorial causation.
- *Vascular theory:* Absent; anterior tibial artery in patients or posterior tibial artery in parents!
- *Obsolete but worth mentioning for its mentors:*
  - Nerve lesion (1839, Little, Adams, and Chapman)
  - Spinal cord theory of clubfeet (1897, Courtillier)
  - Genetic etiology (1928, Aschner and Engelmann)
  - Lateral popliteal nerve lesion (1929, White)
  - Primary muscular disease (1932, Middleton)
  - Medial mesenchymal dysplasia (1940, Keith)

BIOLOGY OF DEVELOPING CLUBFOOT

As described by Ponseti in detail the deformities are a combination of soft-tissue contractures and possibly secondary bony changes.

- There is excessive pull of the tibialis posterior reinforced by the gastrosoleus, the tibialis anterior (TA), and the long toe flexors. These muscles are also smaller and shorter than the normal foot. The size of the leg muscles is inversely proportional to the severity of deformity.
- The "crimp collagen" arises from gastrosoleus and spreads to whole tendo-Achilles and the deep fascia tightening the structure. The bundles of collagen fibers display a wavy appearance known as *crimp*.
- The ligaments of the posterior and medial aspect of the ankle and tarsal joints are very thick and taut, thereby severely restraining the foot in equinus and the navicular and calcaneus in adduction and inversion. The tautness is partially related to excess disorganized collagen synthesis. Excessive collagen synthesis (and crimp) may persist until the child is 3 or 4 years of age and can cause relapses. This crimp allows the ligaments to be stretched and, hence, explains the utility of manipulative maneuvers for treatment. The crimp reappears a few days of stretching, allowing for further stretching.

CLINICAL EXAMINATION AND CHARACTERISTIC FINDINGS

Pathognomonic signs of idiopathic clubfoot include absence of dorsiflexion even on application of strong pressure (dorsiflexion test!). Normal foot of newborn will usually touch or reach out anterior aspect of leg. On clinical examination:

- The characteristic CTEV deformity will have an equinus that is accompanied by inversion of heel, adduction and varus of foot **(Figs. 1 and 2)**.
- The medial border is concave, elevated, and its plantar surface faces upward **(Figs. 1 and 2)**.
- The lateral border is convex and depressed downward **(Figs. 1 and 2)**.
- The posterior tuberosity of heel is pulled upward, difficult to palpate, and less visible.
- An older child in addition may have callous on the dorsal aspect of fifth metatarsal.
- Bony prominence over dorsolateral aspect of foot represents head and neck of talus which are partially uncovered. Skin on the dorsolateral aspect the foot is usually stretched out and atrophied.
- In clubfoot, the skin over posterior tuberosity of calcaneum is smooth and lacks usual wrinkles. Normal

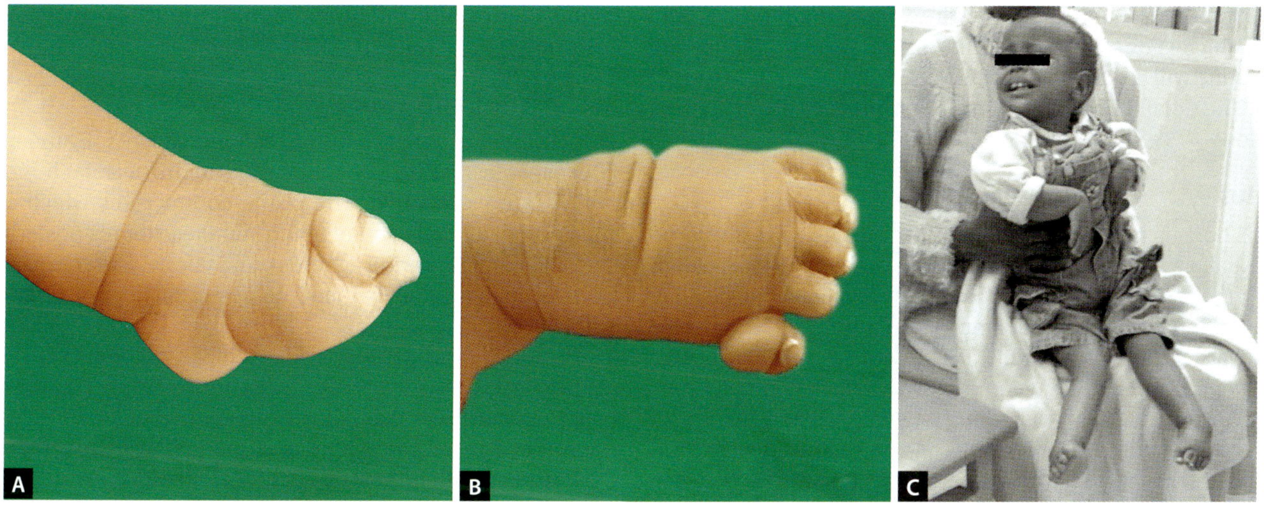

Figs. 2A to C: Severe clubfoot (Intrinsic variety)—look at the deep medial crease, chubby feet with toe deformity (A and B). The heel is tucked up indicating severe posterior contractures (A). (C) Syndromic clubfoot difficult to correct. Functional results in such syndromic cases are often poor due to associated limitations. Note the genu valgum, knee hyperextension, and shiny skin (absent wrinkles). The legs are cylindrical. There is associated ulnar clubhand.

foot has skin creases over tendo-Achilles insertion on the post-tuberosity of calcaneus. This is because a fixed equinus prevents normal upward and downward excursion of the posterior tuberosity **(Figs. 1 and 2)**.

- Skin over dorsolateral aspect of foot is atrophied, stretched, and thin.
- There is a deep cleft over medial plantar surface (usually accompanied with severe cavus with a forefoot flexion contracture). Some feet with severe cavus and equinus may have cleft on medial plantar surface and a cleft above heel **(Figs. 1 and 2)**.
- The knee shows hyperextension deformity due to fixed equinus of foot. Genu valgum and external rotation at ankle joint may result on child's attempt to walk on a plantigrade foot.
- Increased external rotations of ankle mortise occur due to repeated attempts to dorsiflex and evert the deformed foot to compensate varus adduction deformity of foot by rotating the leg externally on weight bearing.
- The underdeveloped medial malleolus is slightly anterior to its normal position while lateral malleolus is palpable slightly posterior.
- The overall limb length is decreased. The atrophy of lower leg becomes prominent after child grows.
- *Plumb-line test (to detect tibial torsion):* A line drawn from center of patella to tibial tubercle, when extended down, will pass normally through first web space. In CTEV due to medial rotation of tibia, it passes through third web space.
- Scars and callosities are features of patient walking on the deformity and are seen in neglected clubfoot.
- Pain in clubfeet, if present, may be caused by peroneal spasm, trauma, and callosities.
- Patients with severe deformities have a "stumbling" gait.
- Patients should be examined for movements at knee and hip that may be restricted in AMC. Significant number has developmental dysplasia of the hip (DDH) and may have hypermobile hips. Iliotibial band (ITB) contracture may be seen in polio cases (Ober's test) and should be specifically looked for.
- Other examination includes identification of syndromes and skeletal dysplasias that have significant bearing on treatment outcome.

CHARACTERISTIC BONY CHANGES AND RADIOLOGICAL EXAMINATION

There are two basic components of CTEV deformity:

1. Malposition of tarsal bones and joints which are in extreme position of flexion, inversion, and adduction producing the primary deformity.
2. Ligaments and muscles on the posterior and medial aspect of ankle and tarsal joints are very thick and taut, thereby severely retaining and maintaining the foot in equinus, inversion, and adduction.

Bean-shaped deformity of clubfoot is due to varus and adduction of heel, medial displacement of navicular on the medially angulated head and neck of the talus and forefoot adduction. Overall size of tarsals is reduced. Talus is the least displaced and shows most severe and consistent changes in form. Since no muscle attachment occurs at talus, it is passively forced into equinus by calcaneus and navicular. Deformity in clubfoot, hence, is due to abnormal relationship of tarsal bones, i.e., navicular and calcaneus are displaced medially around the talus. Severity of deformity depends upon degree of bony displacement. Resistance of deformity is determined by rigidity of soft-tissue contractures.

- Adapted alteration in shape of tarsal bones is acquired in accordance with *Wolff's law* which states that every change in the use of static functions of a bone causes changes in its internal form and architecture, external formation, and function according to mathematical law.

- Soft-tissue contractures are explained by *Davis law*, which states that ligaments and soft tissues in loose/lax state will gradually shorten.

The detailed bony and soft-tissue changes are described below.

Talus

This bone is in severe plantar flexion with its head displaced medially and deflected plantarward. Due to persistent equinus, the anterior wider part of body never enters the ankle joint, therefore, this part may become relatively broad. There may be outward flaring of the facet which articulates with fibula. This prevents full dorsiflexion and causes persistent equinus.

- Normal angle between long axis of neck and head with body is 150°. But, in clubfoot, the medial deviation is increased so that angle (angle of declination) is between 115° and 135° (i.e., more acute). Hence, neck is medially deviated and foreshortened.
- Normal constriction at neck which accommodates anterior lip of tibial plafond on dorsiflexion is absent, which decreases the dorsiflexion.
- Head and facet for navicular face medially instead of facing forward. It is broader with varying degree of flattening. In severe cases, it may be wedge-shaped.
- Posterior facet on the inferior surface of talus is underdeveloped and shallow. The three plantar facets on head appear as a single surface.
- Medial borders of talus and calcaneus are congruent and underdeveloped.

Calcaneum

The calcaneus is involved in all three components of the deformity, i.e., (1) equinus, (2) varus, and (3) adduction.

- Its posterior tuberosity is displaced upward and laterally.
- The anterior end is displaced downward, medially, and is inverted.
- Sustentaculum tali is medially displaced, underdeveloped and fails to provide usual pulley for flexor hallucis longus (FHL) tendon.

Navicular

The navicular is usually medially displaced. Its articular surface faces laterally to articulate with medially deviated head and neck of talus. In severe deformities, dorsomedial subluxation of navicular is present. Normal concavity of the proximal articular process is flattened. The navicular tuberosity is elongated and in close proximity to medial malleolus.

Cuboid Bone

Cuboid bridges the midtarsal and tarsometatarsal joint and as it occupies a position in both rows of tarsal bones, hence, significant medial displacement of cuboid is obstructed by navicular. Minimal changes occur in calcaneocuboid joint.

Metatarsals

Medial migration and inversion of all five metatarsals cause forefoot adduction which contributes to the convexity of the lateral border of the foot and composite varus adduction deformity.

Soft-tissue Contractures

This involves muscles, tendons, tendon sheaths, ligaments, joint capsule, and skin. Posterior tibial neurovascular bundle may also be shortened. The prime contractures which are common to all patients are tendo-Achilles, tibialis posterior, deltoid ligament, spring ligament, and talonavicular capsule. Contractures may be divided into posterior, medial, plantar, and subtalar.

- Posterior contractures (tendo-Achilles, tibiotalar capsule, talocalcaneus capsule, post-talofibular ligament, calcaneofibular ligament) resist equinus deformity and correction of calcaneus and ankle joint. Contracted tendo-Achilles, posterior talocalcaneal capsule, and the calcaneofibular ligament are the structures which maximally resist correction by preventing downward excursions of the postcalcaneal tuberosity. Contracted tibiotalar capsule and posterior talofibular ligament resist dorsiflexion of talus by preventing the downward exit of posterior part of trochlea out of the mortise. Of the two capsules talocalcaneous joint capsule is more contracted. TA tendon in clubfoot is broader and inserts distally on medial surface of calcaneus because tendon attaches itself to the deviated posterior end of calcaneus.
- Medial plantar contractures [tibialis posterior (TP) tendon and sheath, tendon of FHL and flexor digitorum longus (FDL), deltoid ligament, talonavicular capsule, and spring ligament] form an indistinguishable scar, which maintain navicular tuberosity and sustentaculum in close proximity with medial malleolus causing atresia of "acetabulum" of TCN joint. They prevent forward and lateral migration of navicular and prevent eversion and lateral movement of anterior end of calcaneus. The tendons of TP, FDL, and FHL do not contribute to the deformity but may increase resistance to correction. The contracted Henry's knot (annular ligament for two tendons) restricts mobility of navicular because of its attachment.
- Subtalar contractures comprise talocalcaneal interosseous ligament and bifurcate Y-ligament. These are usually seen in older children.
- Plantar contractures consist of abductor hallucis, intrinsic toe flexors, quadratus plantae, and plantar aponeurosis. Plantar aponeurosis is palpable as a tight band along medial plantar surface and is less prominent in children <4 years. Abductor hallucis has an abnormal attachment to TP tendon sheaths, the sheaths of FDL and FHL, and to the navicular tuberosity. Intrinsic toe flexors are short and the first metatarsal is plantarflexed. The TA tendon may be attached till mid-shaft of first metatarsal.

RADIOLOGY

The ossification center for calcaneus and talus appear at 5–6th month and 8th month respectively in the intrauterine period. The ossification centers for the metatarsals appear between 9th and 10th week of gestation. Thus, ossification centers for talus, calcaneus, and shaft of metatarsals have already appeared before birth. The ossification center for the cuboid appears at birth and those for medial, intermediate, and lateral cuneiforms appear at second, third, and the first year, respectively. As a rule, navicular is the last to appear among tarsus at 3–4 years of age. The skeletal maturity of foot appears at 12 years of age. There is delayed appearance of ossification centers for tarsal bones in CTEV.

First radiographs of CTEV were taken and described by Charles Morton in 1897. The radiographs are taken in CTEV to correlate with clinical findings, to assess effect of treatment, to rule out any other bony anomaly and to keep a record. The X-rays give a fair idea of the talocalcaneal relationship. The basic radiographic examination in evaluating any foot deformity consists of weight-bearing AP and lateral views. In infants or nonambulatory patients, simulated weight-bearing views must be obtained by applying plantar pressure with a plastic board. The AP projection is obtained with the tibia perpendicular to the film plane. The central ray is angled approximately 15° toward the heel to minimize overlap between the lower leg and the posterior foot. The lateral radiograph should also be taken with the child standing and tibia perpendicular to the cassette.

Normal Foot Radiology

In a normal foot on an AP view, long axes of talus and calcaneus have a divergent angle (30–55°). The talo-first metatarsal angle is measured by drawing lines through the long axis of the talus and along the long axis of the first metatarsal **(Fig. 3A)**. The normal range is 0–20°. On a stress limit lateral view, long axis of talus looks downward and that of calcaneus upward. The talocalcaneal angle in lateral view increases with dorsiflexion and decreases with plantar flexion, (normal 25–50°) **(Fig. 3B)**.

Radiology of Congenital Talipes Equinovarus Foot

- On an AP view, the divergent angle between talus and calcaneus decreases because calcaneus is inverted and its anterior end is adducted under talus **(Fig. 3C)**. Angle of <20° indicates hindfoot varus.
- The continuation of long axis of talus falls lateral to the first metatarsal due to inversion-adduction of heel and forefoot adduction making talo-first metatarsal angle positive. This is well-appreciated in Kite's view (foot plantarflexed 30° and X-ray tube angled 30° anteriorly in sagittal plane). Navicular is medially displaced (talonavicular subluxation).
- Lateral view shows talonavicular parallelism. The talocalcaneal angle is markedly reduced and the lines may become parallel in severe cases. On a lateral view with foot in maximum dorsiflexion three signs of persistent equinovarus deformity include:
    - No dorsiflexion of heel in relation to ankle joint
    - Parallelism of talus and calcaneus (decrease in talocalcaneal angle)
    - No overlap of anterior ends of calcaneus and talus (open sinus tarsi)
- The tibiocalcaneal angle (normal 10–40°) assessment is considered most reliable method for evaluating correction.
- Talocalcaneal index = Combined talocalcaneal angle on AP and lateral views. This should be >40° normally but is less in CTEV foot.

Flat top talus is an apparent deformity **(Figs. 4A and B)** when talus is deformed due to forcible correction in CTEV. Longer duration of casts treatment (>3 months) is also associated with flat-top talus deformity.

Some Definitions

The following definitions are used in relation to foot disorders and varieties of CTEV:

Hindfoot: It refers to the talus and calcaneus.

Forefoot: It is composed of the metatarsals and phalanges.

Midfoot: It comprises cuboid, navicular, and cuneiform bones.

Untreated clubfoot: A patient presenting for first time with CTEV <2 years of age who has not received any treatment.

Neglected clubfoot: A patient remaining untreated after 2 years.

Corrected clubfoot: All deformities corrected by manipulative or other method on defined parameters

Recurrent clubfoot: Some (supination, equinus, or usually both) or all deformities developing after initial good

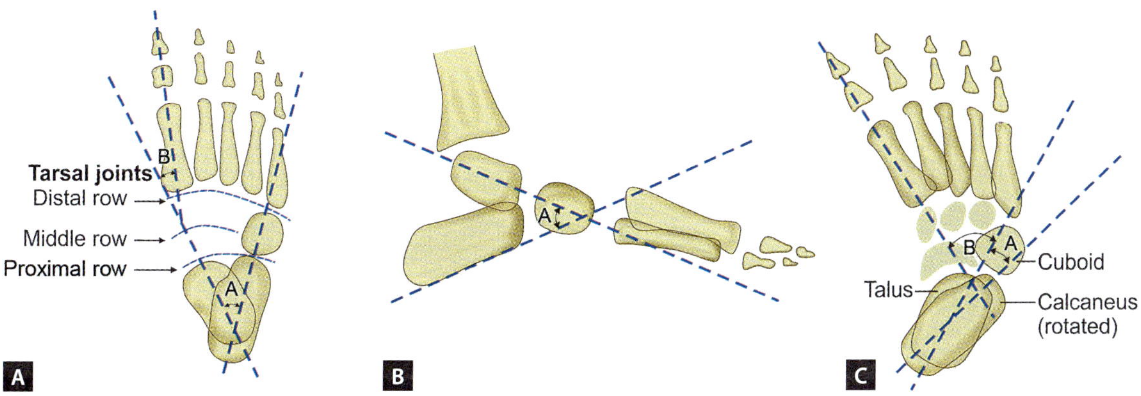

Figs. 3A to C: Illustration of radiological parameters of clubfoot.

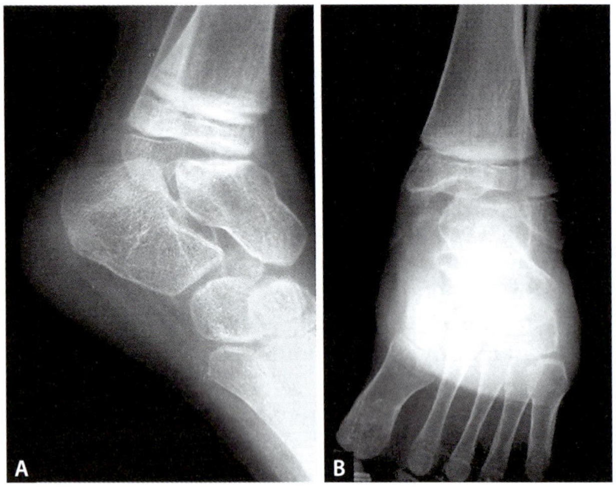

Figs. 4A and B: Flat top talus.

correction during continuing treatment. Due to ambiguity with the usage of term relapsed clubfoot a better definition for recurrent clubfoot is one where deformity worsens after incomplete correction.

Relapsed clubfoot: Some (usually equinus) or a combination or all of deformities developing after the foot has been declared corrected. It should be noted that continuing treatment nowadays with Ponseti method is very short (older manipulation methods entailed treatment for 2–3 years and further maintenance for 7–8 years of age), so often the foot develops deformities after being fully corrected so the distinction between words recurrent and relapse is difficult as most will fall under the term "relapsed".

Resistant clubfoot: Stiff clubfoot resistant to manipulative correction often seen in association with syndromes such as AMC. The resistant clubfoot shows no evidence of further improvement with manipulation (after 3 weeks) and radiological and clinical examination confirms the persistence of equinovarus deformity. In such cases, forced manipulation should be avoided to prevent Rocker bottom feet.

Complex clubfoot: This term specifically applies to foot deformities that have been complicated (bean foot, skewed foot, etc.) by treatment methods other than Ponseti management or simply a foot initially treated by a method other than Ponseti management is termed complex foot. So, this term is used by proponents of Ponseti management only.

Atypical foot: This term applies to certain feet that are difficult to treat than others. The atypical features in a foot are any one or a combination of the following (though their presence is never a certainty that the feet will really be difficult to treat):

- Short, fat, and swollen foot
- Great toe pointing outward
- Sole crease deep and running from side to side
- Rigidly inturned heel
- Tugged-up heel with emptiness felt at the heel point
- Rigid and fixed equinus with downward flexion. The heel cord is small and very tight.
- Deep crease in the skin above heel
- Calf muscle is small and bunched up high in the calf.

TYPES OF CONGENITAL TALIPES EQUINOVARUS

The primary or classical differentiation of CTEV that was used to prognosticate the outcome of manipulative treatment was by dividing the foot into intrinsic and extrinsic clubfoot as follows:

"Intrinsic clubfeet" (type 1 or "Rigid") were thought to arise from abnormalities of the structures within foot primarily (teratologic changes possibly) leading to severe variety that was difficult to manipulate and was expected to fail with this management (now the concept is less well-recognized as they also manipulate well with Ponseti management). The feet are small with marked varus of the heel. The heel cord is very tight and the heel is tucked-up feeling soft when the tip of heel is insinuated with finger. There is deep medial and a posterior crease. The foot can be translated on anterior drawer test.

"Extrinsic clubfeet" were thought to arise secondarily from the intrauterine posture or otherwise (spinal/sensorimotor disorders) where the changes in feet were ascribed secondarily to the postural habitus of the foot. The feet were considered an extension of this postural abnormality that became variably rigid with time and development of the foot. The feet are normal size with variable degree of varus but a firm heel and palpable heel cord with calcaneus bone at the tip of heel. The deep creases are absent from the feet.

Some surgeons mention clinical types of CTEV as idiopathic (primary clubfoot) and secondary types [muscular type—AMC; osseous type—tibial hemimelia; neuromuscular—cerebral palsy (CP), polio; traumatic; teratologic, etc.], but these carry no relevance except being descriptive. They do not indicate treatment or guide planning or prognostication so can be dropped from frequent use.

CLASSIFICATION OF CONGENITAL TALIPES EQUINOVARUS

Most of the classification systems are based on either assessing the severity of deformity or for assessment of correction of deformity after treatment. Individual assessors have used different classifications so that there are too many of them without clarity on which one to use. The following are the commonly referred classifications:

Harrold Walker classified the CTEV based on ability to correct the deformity **(Table 1)** at first examination with firm pressure insufficient to cause pain.

Catterall described the system based on evolution of deformity based on several clinical parameters **(Table 2)**.

TABLE 1: Harrold–Walker classification of congenital talipes equinovarus.

Grade	Definition
I	Foot correctable beyond neutral
II	Pushed to neutral, but with fixed equinus or heel varus < 20°
III	Fixed equinus or heel varus > 20°

TABLE 2: Catterall system of classification of congenital talipes equinovarus.

Characteristic	*Resolving pattern*	*Tendon contracture*	*Joint contracture*	*False correction*
Hindfoot				
Lateral malleolus	Mobile	Posterior	Posterior	Posterior
Equinus	No	Yes	Yes	Yes
Medial crease	No	No	Yes	No
Posterior	No	Yes	Yes	Yes
Anterior	Yes	No	No	Yes
Forefoot				
Lateral border	Straight	Straight	Curved	Straight
Mobile	Yes	Yes	No	Yes
Cavus	±	±	±	No
Supination	No	No	Yes	No

TABLE 3: Dimeglio system for classification of congenital talipes equinovarus.

Grade	*Type*	*Score*	*Reducibility*
I	Benign	<5	>90% soft-soft, resolving
II	Moderate	5 ≤ 10	>50% soft-stiff, reducible, partly resistant
III	Severe	>10 ≤ 15	<50% stiff-soft, resistant, partly reducible
IV	Very severe	>15 ≤ 20	<10% stiff-stiff, resistant

TABLE 4: The Ponseti and Smoley system of classification of congenital talipes equinovarus.

Ankle dorsiflexion (degrees)	*Heel varus (degrees)*	*Adduction of forefoot (degrees)*	*Tibial torsion (degrees)*	*Grade*
>10	0	0–10	0	Good
0–10	0–10	10–20	Moderate	Acceptable
0	>10	>20	Severe	Poor

The system of Dimeglio is based on four parameters with intrinsic details. These include equinus in sagittal plane, varus deviation in frontal plane, derotation around the talus, and adduction of forefoot on hindfoot **(Table 3)**. Four additional parameters include the presence of medial crease, posterior crease, cavus, and poor calf musculature. The system requires dedicated understanding and practice.

The Ponseti and Smoley system is based on assessment of deformity correction following treatment and classifies them into good acceptable and poor **(Table 4)**.

The Pirani system of scoring foot **(Fig. 5)** has been widely accepted and applied for assessment of the progress of deformity correction with the Ponseti method of manipulative correction of CTEV deformities. The system is based on clinical assessment of deformities and grading them from mild (or normal)—0, moderate—0.5, and severe—1. The scores are added for midfoot (midfoot contracture score—MFCS) and hindfoot (hindfoot contracture score—HFCS) individually. The clinical criteria used for MFCS include curved lateral border, medial crease, and talar head prominence while for

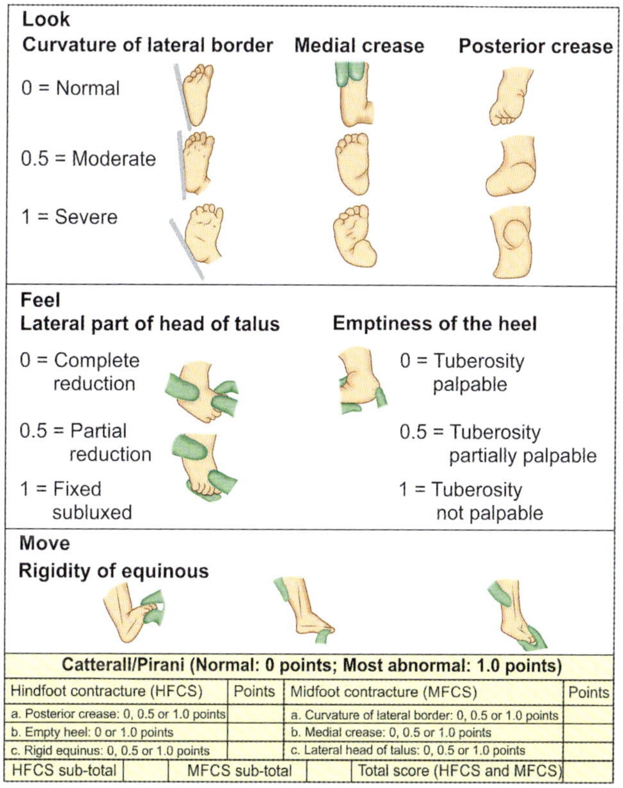

Fig. 5: The Pirani scoring system for evaluation/follow-up of clubfoot.

HFCS includes posterior crease, rigid equinus, and empty heel. Tendo-Achilles tenotomy is required if HFCS is >1 and MFCS is <1 with the head of talus covered.

TREATMENT

The goal of treatment is to achieve:

- A plantigrade, pliable, functional, and cosmetically acceptable foot in the shortest treatment time with least disruption of the family life.
- A lasting correction.

The objectives are:

- To obtain concentric reduction of TCN joint and ankle joint—the forefoot deformity should be corrected so that it points outward 20° then the keystone hindfoot deformity should be addressed to realign vertically with the leg instead of inversion. Lastly, the equinus is corrected.
- To maintain the reduction.
- To establish balanced muscular activity.
- To produce normal function and movements.

On first visit, parents should be reassured and explained that they are not responsible for deformity. They should also be told about nature of deformity, course of treatment, unpredictability of response to the treatment, and propensity for recurrence.

Nonsurgical Treatment

The initial management of clubfoot is nonsurgical treatment that should be started as soon as possible. A common saying is that "given a clubfoot deformity an orthopedician will apply cast to the foot before the child is born if it is a breech delivery". As such the first 3 months of life are best for manipulative correction of foot. Different methods of nonoperative treatment include manipulation of serial plaster casts, stretching and adhesive strapping and continuous passive motion (CPM). The first casts used for manipulative correction were made from egg-white and flour (Cheselden, 1740). The use of plaster of Paris (POP) for bandaging the clubfeet was described by Mathijsen in 1854.

Thomas Wrench (1834–1891): This involved forceful correction of the deformity using device developed by HO Thomas. This often led to iatrogenic introduction of complex deformities and incomplete corrections. The acute corrections often lead to uncontrolled failure of important structures that often healed with stiffness.

The "French method" of treatment by adhesive strapping + CPM (Bensahel/Dimeglio regime): It works on a principle to apply an eversion corrective force (eversion tug) on feet by knee's motion. Daily manipulation is done by a physiotherapist and maintenance is done by elastic or nonelastic adhesive taping. CPM machine is used in sleep hours. The improvement is seen by first 3 months and if successful the regime is continued till the child starts walking. Irritation of skin and blister formation are its limiting factors.

Manipulative Treatment

The manipulative treatment is based on the inherent properties of the young connective tissue, cartilage, and bone which respond to the appropriate mechanical stimuli created by the gradual reduction of the deformity. The ligaments, joint capsules, and tendons gradually stretch to accommodate reduction of the TCN joint. The displaced bones are gradually brought into normal relationship with serial casts. The casts must be applied with "eversion tug" principle, i.e., with each application of the layer of the cast an eversion force is gently applied to the foot. Correction must be maintained until tarsal bones remold to a stable articular surface. Recurrence occurs due to failure to attain a complete correction or maintain a correction.

Kite's Method of Manipulation and Kite's Error

Kite's method of manipulation (1939) for sequential correction of deformities (as opposed to simultaneous correction done in Ponseti): The classical method described by Kite included correction of adduction and varus components first (adduction → inversion → varus → equinus). The foot is grasped by both hands so that thumb tips press over the lateral bony prominence formed by cuboid and base fifth metatarsal (some mention that the site of fulcrum was calcaneocuboid joint as originally described by Kite, but it was possibly a mistake as the prominence is formed by cuboid-metatarsal joint). This acts as a fulcrum while fingers about heel and metatarsals pull these structures into abduction and eversion. The cast is applied in corrected position and changed every week. The cavus is corrected next by pressing the foot on a glass plate. Equinus deformity is corrected last after varus and adduction have been corrected. However, the results were not very encouraging with this method as there were a large number of children who had either unsatisfactory results or relapsed feet. The rate of surgical intervention was also very high. The primary "error" (commonly now called as "Kite's error") with this method is premature or initial correction attempted by direct abduction of forefoot that actually locks the calcaneum beneath the talus (the subtalar joint is rendered immobile). Secondly, it should be remembered that the relative pronation of forefoot in relation to hindfoot is the *cause* of cavus deformity. The attempted pronation of apparently supinated forefoot (as the deformity appears to any untrained eye) tilts the forefoot into further pronation, thereby increasing the cavus and pressing the adducted calcaneus against the talus. The anterior portion of calcaneus underlies talar head in CTEV. Forceful pronation pushes the anterior aspect of calcaneum into talus rather than abducting the calcaneus. This dorsiflexion and fixation of subtalar joint prevents correction of heel varus at all. Heel varus will not correct unless the calcaneus is abducted while Kite thought that the heel varus would correct by simply everting the calcaneum. The second error was choosing the lateral prominence (calcaneocuboid joint or the cuboido-fifth metatarsal joint) instead of talar head for counter pressure. Thus, the method often leads to prolonged cast treatment up to 2 years and often had to be surgically corrected.

Ponseti Method of Simultaneous Correction of Congenital Talipes Equinovarus Deformities

Ponseti method of simultaneous correction of CTEV deformities was described by Ponseti in 1948, but became popular only recently. The results with this method have been consistently satisfactory and produce very low rates of relapse. The rate of surgery has also reduced significantly. The method has been found to be effective even in neglected, resistant, and syndromic feet. The "principle" of the method is based on relative and interdependent intertarsal motion. The movement of each tarsal bone involves simultaneous shifts in the adjacent bones. These are determined by the opposing joint surfaces, their curvature, and ligamentous anatomy. Individual joints have its own specific motion pattern but that influences the adjacent joint by producing requisite shift. Therefore, it is logical that correction of the medial displacement and inversion of the tarsal bones will require a simultaneous gradual lateral shift of the navicular, cuboid, and calcaneus into proper apposition (by correcting cavus, **Figs. 6A and B**) before they can be everted into a neutral position **(Fig. 7)**. These displacements can be achieved by gradual correction utilizing the creep in ligaments (see above). There are three stages to Ponseti method of correction:

The *first stage* is manipulative correction to stretch out the tendons and straightening of the foot. This is gradually achieved as follows:

- The first deformity to be corrected is cavus which is because of excessive plantar flexion of the first ray **(Fig. 8, cast 1)**. The fifth ray, in contrast, is well-aligned with the cuboid. Consequently, although the entire foot is supinated, the forefoot is pronated as compared to the hindfoot resulting in the cavus deformity. Therefore, the

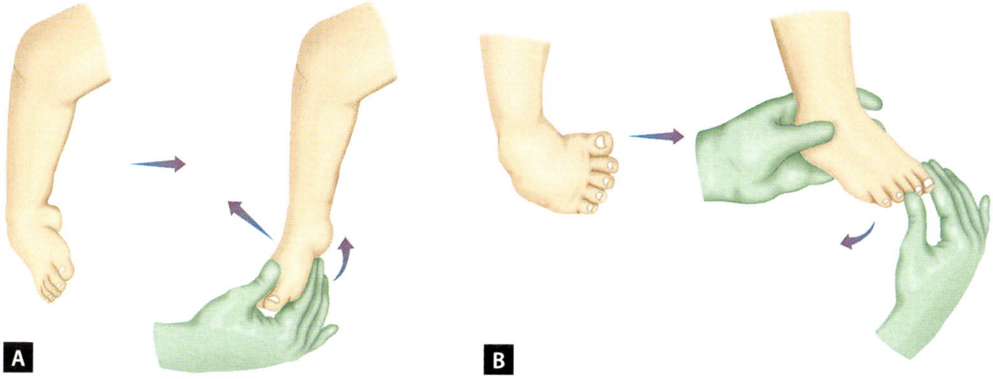

Figs. 6A and B: (A) The principles of Ponseti method for correction of clubfoot. Note is made of first aligning the forefoot with rest of foot by correcting the cavus; (B) This is done by correcting the"relative" pronation of forefoot by supinating it. Cavus correction is then followed by correction of adduction and varus deformity using talar head as fulcrum.

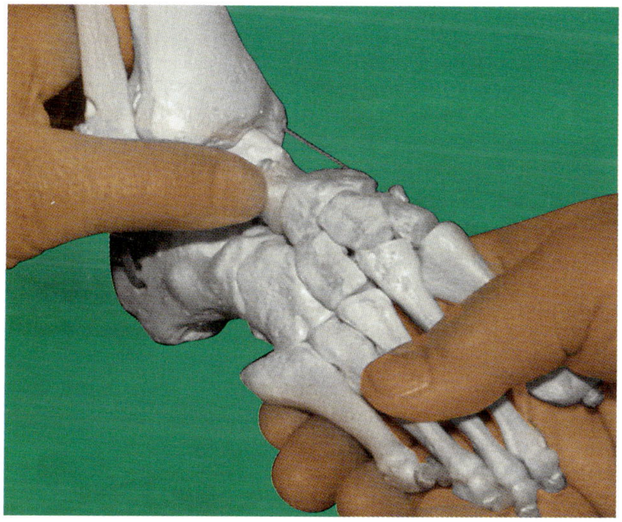

Fig. 7: Reduction of clubfoot deformity by Ponseti method of correction. Note that the forefoot is first supinated to correct the cavus and then abducted with fulcrum at talar head.

cavus deformity is corrected by supinating the forefoot gently, thereby placing the first metatarsal in alignment with the rest of metatarsals. Although the foot now may seem to be more deformed, it actually corrects the cavus. An attempt to correct the supination of the foot by forcibly pronating will only increase the cavus deformity by producing further plantar flexion of the foot.

- The varus and adduction deformity are corrected next **(Fig. 8, cast 2)**. The inverted and adducted calcaneus and medially displaced navicular and cuboid produce a severe heel varus and forefoot adduction deformity respectively. The correction of cavus brings all the metatarsals, cuneiforms, and navicular and cuboid in the same plane of supination. This provides the necessary lever arm to displace the navicular and cuboid laterally and slightly downward. This manipulation includes stretching the tight medial structures by abducting the foot held in flexion and supination while counter-pressure is applied by thumb to the lateral aspect of head of the talus.
- The abduction is gradually increased with each consecutive cast to achieve reduction of navicular on the head of talus **(Fig. 8, cast 3)**. At least 60–70° of abduction is

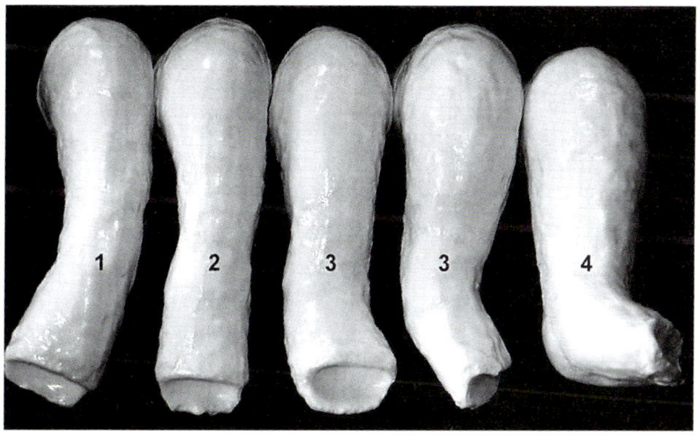

Fig. 8: Ponseti casts for correction of congenital talipes equinovarus (CTEV) deformity by manipulation.

achieved at the end of treatment to reduce rate of relapse. *Under no circumstance, the foot is everted which locks the clacaneus under talus and prevents further correction.* On the other hand, gradual abduction of forefoot in flexion and supination unlocks the calcaneus from underneath the talus producing eversion of the heel.
- The equinus is corrected by stretching the tight posterior structures **(Fig. 8, cast 4)**. The foot is extended by placing the flat of the hand under entire sole and pulling the heel down with the other hand. The above knee cast applied weekly from toe to groin produces correction in an average of five casts when treatment is begun in the first month of life. Cast may slip due to cylindrical tapering calf, significant equinus, extremely small inverted heel, chubby legs, short rigid feet and considerable subcutaneous fat of baby foot.

The *second stage* comprises quickened correction of equinus by percutaneous TA tenotomy and casting: The correction of the equines can be hastened by percutaneous tenotomy of the tendo-Achilles. The last plaster after tenotomy is generally applied for 3 weeks following which foot abduction brace (FAB) is given.

The *third stage* involves bracing of the feet. The FAB consists of comfortable sandals with a molded sole with a bar attached in between. The width of the bar matches the width of the shoulders and the feet are maintained in approximately 70°

of abduction and 10–15° of dorsiflexion (bilateral deformity). For unilateral deformity, the normal foot is kept in 30–50° of abduction and neutral dorsiflexion. The FAB is applied 23 hours a day initially for the first 3 months. The 1 hour out of the brace is used for hygiene and toilet. After 3 months weaning is begun by reducing wearing time @2 hours/month until FAB is applied only during sleeping time for a minimum of 4 years. Bracing is discussed in detail below. Noncompliance with the FAB is the most common reason of recurrence especially the equinus deformity. Specific precautions must be explained to the parents for successful outcome **(Box 2)**.

Pirani's method has been widely used for assessing, measuring, and recording the clubfoot deformity. This is necessary to know severity and stage of treatment, to know when to move on the next treatment stage and when treatment is finished, to identify a relapse and to maintain accurate records. The scoring system developed by Dr Shafique Pirani, tests six different components of deformity, and assigns each a severity score of 0, 0.5, or 1. It is a valid and reliable method of measuring and recording deformity with good intra-observer reliability. It comprises the midfoot contracture score (MCFS) consisting of curved lateral border (CLB), medial crease (MC), and lateral head of talus (LHT); the hindfoot contracture score (HFCS) consisting of the posterior crease (PC), rigid equines (RE), and empty heel (EH) **(Fig. 9)**. The Pirani score should be measured and recorded at each visit including bracing and general check-ups. It is best done with the child in a comfortable position, sitting on its mother's lap.

Evaluation of Deformity Correction and Prognostic Factors

The correction of deformity can be clinically evaluated by following features:

- Plantigrade foot
- Cosmetically acceptable foot with pliable subtalar motion
- Dorsiflexion equal to that of normal side (or above right angle in bilateral cases)

BOX 2: The precautions and general information that should be explained to the parents of congenital talipes equinovarus (CTEV) patients.

- Children grow fast so frequent changes of shoe and brace are needed.
- Bracing has to be done continuously without any bracing holidays in between. Even few days of holiday cause loss of many months of correction.
- Follow instruction for securing braces every time. Daily correction is needed for optimal outcome.
  - After wearing the brace always check that the heel touches the floor of the shoe orthosis.
  - The shoe should be laced tightly but not so much so as to stop blood flow.
  - Look for clawing of toes and report to surgeon if found.
- Examine braces weekly for loosening of screws, straps and laces, and foot structure. Replace damaged braces.
- Protect the child's feet by cotton socks while donning brace as the child's feet are insensitive (stunned) following cast treatment for first few days.
- Watch for pressure signs/early pressure sores. Areas of redness or dimpling should be thoroughly reported so that proper care/modification is done.

Patient name:__________ Patient #__________ Clinic location:__________

CCK Patient Treatment Record

Appt. Date																
Age																
Visit	1		2		3		4		5		6		7		8	
	R	L	R	L	R	L	R	L	R	L	R	L	R	L	R	L
PC																
EH																
RE																
HFCS																
MC																
LHT																
CLB																
MFCS																
TS																
Treatment																
Staff initials																

Complications

Date	Week	Description of complication	Treatment of complication	Results

Fig. 9: Example of scoring sheet that can be used for congenital talipes equinovarus (CTEV) patient follow-up managed by Ponseti method. (CLB: curved lateral border; EH: empty heel; HFCS: hindfoot contracture score; LHT: lateral head of talus; MC: medial crease; MFCS: midfoot contracture score; PC: posterior crease; RE: rigid equines; TS: total score)

Source: Cure Clubfoot Worldwide.

- Active eversion
- Good gait and strong push-off

Overcorrection may result in severe pes planus, heel valgus with metatarsus adductus (skewfoot), increased dorsiflexion, limited plantar flexion, and limited subtalar motion. The uncorrected feet will show no dorsiflexion of calcaneus in lateral view of stress dorsiflexion and anterior ends of talus and calcaneus will show no overlap in an AP view. Radiological parameters of corrected foot can be read above.

The factors that have been associated with the poor prognosis in CTEV management are:

- Female child
- Late presentation
- Severe deformity
- Rigid foot
- Associated cavus
- Clawing of toes
- Small heel

Bracing for Congenital Talipes Equinovarus

Bracing the foot is an important part of clubfoot management specifically the maintenance of correction and improving the modeling of foot. Importantly, this part should be emphasized by the treating physician else parents often consider casting as the end of treatment and land up with recurrent deformities and loss of correction.

Currently, three major groups of braces are available:

1. Ankle foot orthosis
2. Wheaton brace or Wheaton's type brace
3. Foot abduction brace

Ankle Foot Orthosis

It is similar to historically used tin rectangular night shoe covering the ankle and foot fully with neutral position at ankle. There is correction of plantar flexion only, while abduction is not provided by the brace so metatarsus adductus may not be corrected. Its use is also associated with calf-muscle atrophy. In cases of arthrogryposis or peroneal nerve palsy, this brace may be used as an adjunct to the abduction orthosis. The Phelps brace is used for children between 6 and 18 months of age. This is fitted with an inside bar and outside T-strap on a high top shoe. Simple ankle foot orthoses can also be used for holding correction after soft-tissue release.

Wheaton's Type Braces (Knee-ankle-foot Orthosis)

They provide reasonable abduction to the foot and medial stretching force pushing the forefoot in abduction if applied properly. Velcro strap is tightened against the apex of deformity to provide direct force for correction of deformity. The brace comes in two forms one in plantigrade position (foot in 15° dorsiflexion and the other with ankle in neutral position (0° plantar flexion). The brace being tied to the thigh may produce thigh muscle atrophy also along with the calf atrophy.

Adjustable Length Foot Abduction Brace

Ponseti advised abduction and dorsiflexion of the foot for proper maintenance of the correction. Both these are optimally met with the use of foot abduction *brace* (also called though wrongly Denis-Browne shoe/bar/splint or "wobbly shoes", it is a brace not a splint/shoe.). The brace comprises two shoes connected by an abduction bar, the length of bar being guided by the distance between shoulders and changed with the growth of child. Feet are typically placed in 60–70° of external rotation/abduction or in case of unilateral deformity the normal foot is placed in 30–50° of external rotation. The Denis-Browne brace utilizes an L-shaped bracket to hold the foot in significant dorsiflexion and is connected to open-toe boots. The active kicking movement of each leg exerts a counter-corrective force in other foot. For concerns of cost, Steenbeeck braces (**Figs. 10 and 11**, developed in Uganda by Michiel Steenbeek and David Okello) have been developed that can be made from locally available cheap material while following the recommendations of Dr Ponseti. Various modifications have been added to the standard brace for improving the comfort and pliability of use:

- Flexible connecting bar (Kessler brace)—this facilitates the dorsiflexion twist provided by child's kicking action.
- Horton's click brace—here the shoe can be easily changed by just attaching the shoe through a clicking mechanism. The shoe size changes fast in a growing infant and needs frequent changes. This is facilitated by the brace.
- Dobb's dynamic clubfoot brace—to improve compliance this brace allows independent movement of the legs and thus allows movements at knee and hips.
- ALFA-Flex shoe produced in Europe has nontoxic biocompatible materials and has "intelligent' foam (having both viscous and elastic components) allowing close fit to the child's foot and equidistribution of pressure.

Commonly followed bracing protocol:

- After correction, wear brace for 22–23 hours a day for first 3 months.
- Weaning schedule involves reducing the wearing time of brace by 2 hours every month for next 4 months.
- Maintain night-time bracing for 12–14 hours as child grows along with using CTEV shoe for during day till the age of 4–5 years.

Maintenance of the FAB and general instructions should be given to the parents (***see* Box 2**).

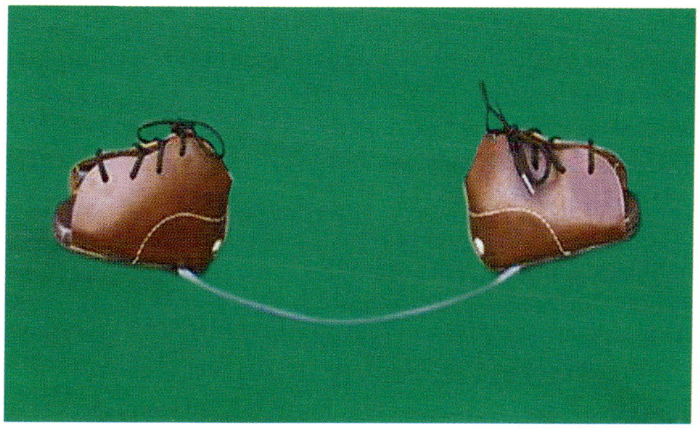

Fig. 10: A Steenbeek brace for maintenance of correction after Ponseti technique.

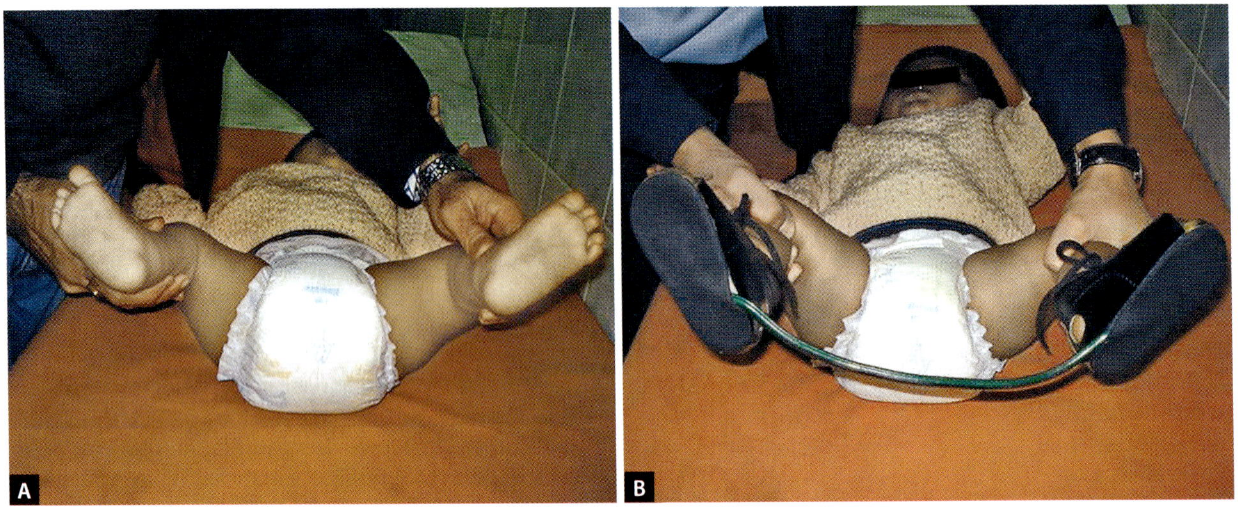

Figs. 11A and B: Use of congenital talipes equinovarus (CTEV) brace during follow-up.

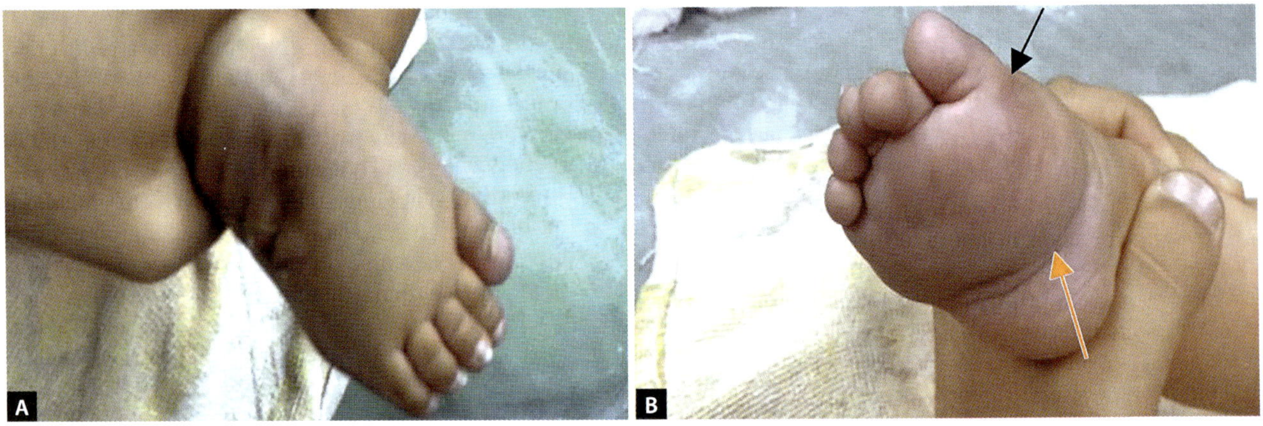

Figs. 12A and B: The photographs show a 3.5-month-old infant with atypical clubfoot. Atypical clubfeet have a characteristic rigid equinus and a short and hyperextended first toe (black arrow), transverse crease in the sole of the foot (orange arrow) and another deep crease above the heel.

MODIFIED PONSETI MANIPULATION FOR ATYPICAL CONGENITAL TALIPES EQUINOVARUS

Orthopedicians have been treating idiopathic CTEV successfully using Ponseti technique. However, there is a small subset of clubfoot which does not correct or shows resistance to correction by standard Ponseti method. Over the course of treatment of idiopathic clubfoot by Ponseti technique, some feet show resistance to treatment. The common clinical features of these resistant (to manipulation)/atypical clubfeet are:

- Short and stubby feet
- Deep medial crease present over sole of foot **(Figs. 12A and B)**
- Deep crease above the heel
- Severe equinus and supination
- Forefoot in adduction and plantarflexion of all metatarsals except great toe which is short and hyperextended **(Figs. 12A and B)**.

These feet are not usually identified by orthopedicians initially but over the course of treatment these features become more apparent. Turco (1994) advised against surgery in these feet. He classified them as atypical clubfeet. Ponseti et al. (2006) advised about change in his standard treatment in these feet. Standard Ponseti method of correction in these feet produces secondary unacceptable deformities in these cases. It leads to hyperabduction of forefoot at tarso-metatarsal joint but cavus and equinus do not get corrected. Frequent slippage of cast causes sores over bony prominences and edema of the foot.

This type of clubfoot is difficult to treat and requires modification of standard Ponseti technique.

- Adduction of forefeet should not be corrected beyond 40° to prevent hyperabduction at tarso-metatarsal joint.
- Adduction should be corrected by keeping thumb on lateral aspect of talar head and index finger of same hand behind lateral malleolus **(Fig. 13)**. This also corrects heel varus.
- Once the heel varus is corrected, the plantarflexed forefoot and the equinus are corrected simultaneously by forcefully dorsiflexing the metatarsals with both thumbs while keeping index fingers of both hands on dorsal aspect of talar head **(Fig. 14)**.

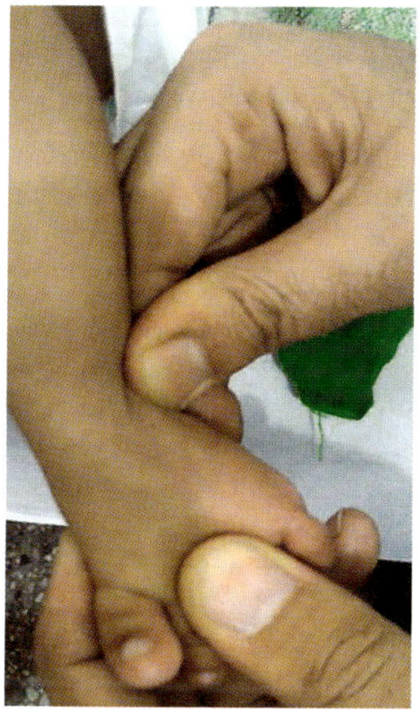

Fig. 13: The photograph shows position of hand for manipulating and holding an atypical clubfoot. The index finger should rest over the posterior aspect of the lateral malleolus while the thumb of the same hand applies counterpressure over the lateral aspect of the head of the talus.

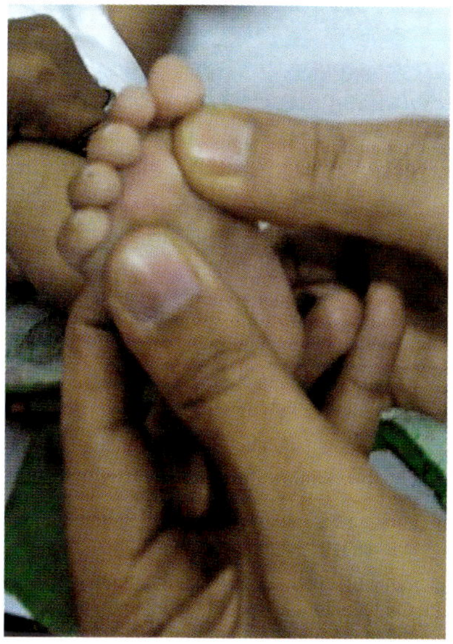

Fig. 14: Clinical photograph showing modification of Ponseti method for correction of plantarflexed metatarsals and ankle equinus. Metatarsals are being extended by two thumbs over heads of first and fifth metatarsals. Heel is also being dorsiflexed.

- The cast is re-enforced by applying a posterior slab behind the ankle.
- To prevent the cast from slipping, knee is immobilized at 110° of flexion and it is re-enforced with a slab applied anteriorly over the knee.
- A tenotomy is performed before applying the last plaster cast to facilitate correction of a non-yielding equinus.

Correct identification of talar head is paramount. In these cases, anterior process calcaneum is prominent and can be mistaken for head of talus which lies above the anterior process of calcaneum. Talar head is identified by moving index finger and thumb of one hand down medial and lateral malleoli respectively and then grasping the head of talus. With the other hand, forefoot is abducted which causes movement at talo-calcaneo-navicular joint and thus helps in the precise identification of talar head. To correct forefoot adduction, abduction is done by putting thumb on lateral aspect of head of talus. Index finger of same hand is put behind lateral malleolus **(Fig. 13)**. Using thumb and index finger of other hand forefoot is abducted. Abduction is done up to 20–40° only. Standard abduction of 70° is not done. Abduction is always kept <40°. Abduction beyond 40° leads to excessive abduction at tarsometatarsal joints and thus disruption of this joint. While abduction is being done, the foot usually comes into alignment with the long axis of the leg. This usually leads to slippage of cast which may cause foot edema and skin excoriation. To prevent this, the cast is applied with the knee bent to 110°. Proper molding of the cast is also imperative. To prevent bunching of excessive cast behind the knee, slab is applied anteriorly to strengthen the cast instead or wrapping too many bandages. A similar short slab is applied behind ankle.

When desired forefoot abduction is obtained, it is common to see severe persistent plantar flexion of the metatarsals. Here, another modification in corrective manipulation is needed. Thumbs of both hands are placed under the heads of first and fifth metatarsals. Index fingers of both hands are placed dorsally over the talar head and dorsiflexion of metatarsals and ankle is performed **(Fig. 14)**. Percutaneous tenotomy of tendo-Achilles is performed in all cases above the posterior deep crease. Post-tenotomy additional correction in plantar flexion of 5–10° is usually obtained. The cast is applied for 3 weeks if overall ankle dorsiflexion of 5–10° is achieved by this maneuver. If ankle dorsiflexion is not obtained post-tenotomy then cast is applied weekly with increasing dorsiflexion till 10° of dorsiflexion at ankle correcting equinus is obtained. Following cast removal Dennis–Brown brace is applied. Feet are kept at 40° abduction on both normal and affected sides **(Fig. 15)** unlike standard Ponseti protocol, where feet are kept at 70° abduction on affected side and 30–50° abduction on normal side. Brace is applied for 23 hours for first 3 months. During the hour when the brace was removed, two exercises were performed. One, the child is made to squat for 10 minutes. Second, the parents passively dorsiflex the affected foot for 10 minutes. Following initial 3 months in brace, weaning from brace was done with 2 hours of bracing time reduced every month until night-time bracing (12 hours) remains and is advised to be kept for 3–4 years.

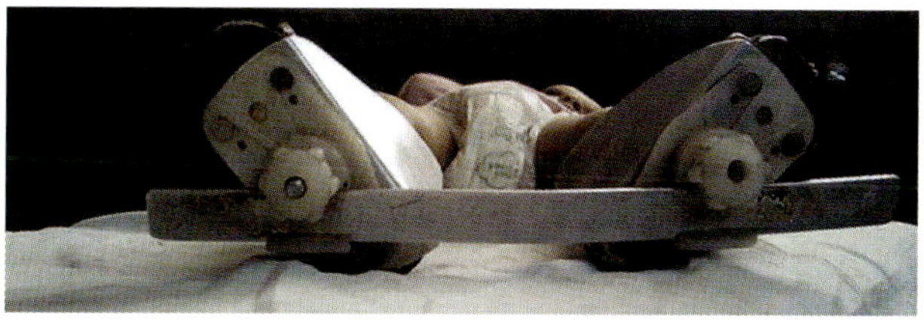

Fig. 15: Clinical photograph showing Dennis Brown brace applied with both feet in 40° abduction.

SURGICAL MANAGEMENT OF CLUBFOOT

When proper treatment of clubfeet is started shortly after birth a good clinical correction is a rule. After advent of the Ponseti's treatment, there has been a worldwide decline in the surgical intervention. The classical operations like posteromedial release and complete subtalar release are no longer required where Ponseti's method is being practiced correctly. Still surgery might be mainstay in rigid, relapsed, and neglected clubfeet in developing countries where Ponseti method is not practiced. The kind of surgeries done for a clubfoot may be classified as:

1. Soft-tissue surgery
2. Bony surgery
3. Combined soft tissue and bony surgery
4. Correction of deformities by external fixation application

Soft-tissue Surgery

The soft-tissue surgeries which are commonly required even after Ponseti's method include percutaneous tenotomy **(Fig. 16)**, tendo-Achilles lengthening, and lateral transfer of the TA tendon. The historical releases of 1800s were crude and based on observation rather than any science. Ogston described the removal of ossific nucleus of talus to correct deformity in 1902! Surgery in current era is performed as need arises—*ale carte* approach.

Percutaneous tenotomy of the tendo-Achilles: It is an OPD procedure done under local anesthesia (it should be known that tenotomy was first used and described by Delpech in 1816 and Stromeyer in 1836 itself and is not something of a modern era!). A 15-number blade is introduced on the medial side of the tendon about 2 cm above its calcaneum insertion **(Fig. 16)**. The blade is introduced in the front of the tendon which is severed from front to back. The angle of dorsiflexion increases suddenly to about 10–15°, following which the final cast is given in about 70° of abduction and 10° of dorsiflexion for 3 weeks. A preliminary tendo-Achilles lengthening can also be done before manipulation to allow talus to enter ankle mortice. *Tendo-Achilles lengthening and posterior capsulotomy* of the ankle joint is indicated in children between 6 and 12 months of age who have obtained adequate correction for forefoot adduction and hindfoot varus, but equinus is still persisting.

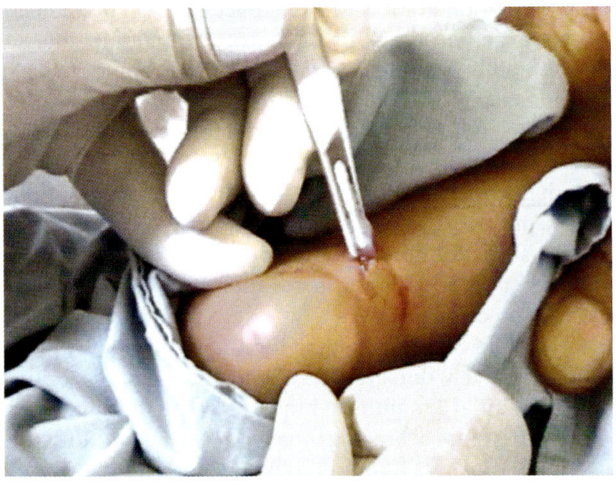

Fig. 16: Surgical treatment.

Open Z-lengthening of the tendo-Achilles: It may still be rarely indicated in an older child. Percutaneous tenotomy has been done even in an older child with complete regeneration of the tendon thereby precluding use of Z-lengthening.

Tendon transfers: Various types of motor power balancing may be needed in patients during or after correction of deformity. Some of the common procedures done are:

- *Tibialis anterior transfer of Peabody:* It is usually indicated after relapse in a child older than 3 years of age where the tendon has significant supination pull or in patients with a relative "evertor insufficiency". In both the conditions, the patients walk on lateral border of foot. TA transferred to lateral aspect prevents further relapses, corrects the AP talocalcanean angle, and reduces the need for medial release operations. The transfer can be done as split anterior tibialis transfer (SPLATT) or whole tendon transfer. In SPLATT, the tendon is exposed by 4–5 cm long incision from just below ankle to medial cuneiform. Another incision is made over the lateral cuneiform. The split half of tendon is now anchored subcutaneously in a drill hole in the lateral cuneiform with a pull-out suture. To prevent bow stringing, the tendon is left under the superior retinaculum. Some people prefer to transfer entire tendon into a position just lateral to midline of foot into a tarsal bone for sake of simplicity. There is loss of power by one grade in such cases.
- *Peroneus transfer:* Sometimes excessive lengthening of tendo-Achilles is done for aggressive correction of equinus deformity. This produces weakness of the gastro-soleus complex due to lengthened tendon. Most commonly the peroneus brevis is used to provide plantar flexion power by rerouting it into calcaneal tuberosity. Eversion insufficiency is prevented by tenodesing the distal cut stump to peroneus longus.
- Tibialis posterior transfer is usually done in older children (>8 years of age) where the muscle is transferred anteriorly through the interosseous space on middle cuneiform. It is indicated in children with severe in-toeing, weak peroneals, cavus, and forefoot equinus. The principle is to eliminate the deforming force and use it as a corrective force.

Soft-tissue releases: The following surgical operations are of more or less academic interest only as their utility for the management of clubfoot is no longer or rarely required. These posteromedial soft-tissue releases (PMSTR) were frequent previously with inadequate manipulation of the feet. However, they may still be useful for correction of teratologic and neglected clubfoot or in a more limited manner in association with external fixation. The classical age for performing the release has been debated. French recommendation is doing the release as early as possible (few weeks to months) due to the higher potential for remodeling in a relatively immature foot. The biggest problems here are that smaller feet have indistinct structures and under- or overcorrection will get magnified as the foot grows. Simon recommended a foot size of at least 8 cm for doing the PMSTR. Turco favored doing PMSTR, after 1 year but within 2 years, for better identification of structures while correcting them in a reasonable time-frame so as to prevent development of rigid deformities and also not hamper ambulation for long.

One-stage posteromedial release (PMR) (Turco): This is indicated in mild deformity with no severe internal rotation deformity of the calcaneus. The operation is based upon the concept that the deformity is due to congenital subluxation of the TCN joint. Correction of abnormal tarsal relationship is prevented by a rigid soft-tissue contracture. For a lasting correction, complete surgical correction must be obtained and must be maintained while tarsal bone remolds to form stable articular surfaces. It is impossible to correct any one component completely without simultaneously eliminating others. Optimal age for surgery is considered to be 1–2 years because structures can be recognized easily. In addition, a walking child can take advantage of physiological stimulus for tarsal remodeling. Under 1 year, it is difficult to maintain foot in correction after internal fixation has been removed. Delayed surgery minimizes operating on an unrecognized neuromuscular deformity. Minimal error of overcorrection in infancy represents a greater overcorrection than some degree of overcorrection in older children. Long-term result does not show any increased advantage of operating under 1 year. In selected cases, age may be extended till 8 years of age. Surgery should be delayed in a deformity due to myopathy, neurologic deficit or a genetic syndrome, and should be carried only when it is mandatory. The technique involves a release of posterior, medial plantar, and subtalar soft-tissue contractures in one stage. The following structures are released:

- *Medial release:*
  - Posterior and medial subtalar joint capsule (preserve interosseous ligament)
  - Talonavicular joint capsule
  - Spring ligament
  - Y-ligament
  - Medial calcaneocuboid joint capsule
  - Knot of Henry
  - Abductor hallucis
  - Lengthening of posterior tibial tendon, FHL, FDL
  - Plantar fascia, quadrates plantae origin
- *Posterior release:*
  - Ankle joint capsule
  - Subtalar joint capsule
  - Achilles tendon Z-lengthening
  - Posterior talofibular ligament
- *Lateral release:*
  - Lateral subtalar joint capsule
  - Peroneal tendon sheath
  - Calcaneofibular ligament
  - Lateral talocalcaneal ligament
  - Extensor digitorum brevis origin, calcaneocuboid ligament, inferior extensor retinaculum, and cubonavicular ligament may be released in resistant cases.

Structures that should be preserved include dorsal structures, medial neurovascular bundle, deep deltoid ligament, and interosseous ligament.

- After the contractures are released, the navicular and calcaneus are restored to their normal relationship with talus and the surgical correction is temporarily stabilized by temporarily transfixing the talonavicular and talocalcaneal joints with K-wires.
- A Steindler's release may be required in older patients (See below in correction of cavus foot).
- Postoperatively, the cast is changed under general anesthesia after 3 weeks of operation. A new above knee cast is applied after proper skin care and foot in more dorsiflexion. The cast is changed again at 6 weeks in OPD. The wires are removed at 6 weeks if full dorsiflexion is possible and there is no danger of causing severe heel valgus or dorsal subluxation of navicular as the foot is dorsiflexed. However, the wires should be left in place for several weeks longer if:
  - The dorsiflexion is limited because of impingement of talus upon anterior lip of the tibial plafond.
  - The talus is markedly plantarflexed (as these feet are more prone to develop planovalgus).
  - There is danger of dorsal subluxation of navicular on dorsiflexion of the foot.
  - In chubby feet and fat legs where it is difficult to retain correction after removal of internal fixation and in cases of talocalcaneal synchondrosis. Once K-wires are removed, a long above knee cast in 90° of knee flexion is given to retain correction and to discourage child from walking. The cast should be well-molded above heels in corrected position. The last cast is below knee to allow walking for physiological stimulus for tarsal molding stretches the heel cord and prevents disease atrophy.

The advantages of one-stage PMR include correction of the deformity in a single sitting, mobilization of both ends of calcaneus and navicular to permit restoration of normal anatomy. A posterior release alone does not change relationship between calcaneus and talus, therefore, calcaneus remains locked under talus in varus. The internal fixation ensures maintenance of surgical correction which is maintained without cast pressure or hyperdorsiflexion of the foot. This reduces incidence of skin necrosis and tension on the wound. The talus-calcaneus-navicular relationship remains constant as dorsiflexion is increased. Dorsal subluxation of navicular and increased inversion of calcaneus is prevented when dorsiflexion is increased. Wire fixation is especially helpful in small feet and in cases where previous surgery has been done. Undercorrection, overcorrection, osteonecrosis of the talus or navicular and development of sinus tarsi syndrome due to acute correction of the deformity and reduction of space are some of the complications (**Box 3**). Some specific interesting complications are discussed below.

Overcorrection may lead to rocker bottom clubfoot. It is more prone to develop in a child with hyperflexible joints. The rocker bottom deformity occurs when the navicular is overreduced in a lateral position and when complete resection of interosseous talocalcaneal ligament occurs. Only that much of talocalcaneal interosseous ligament should be excised which is necessary to unlock calcaneus from locked varus position. Calf atrophy and weakness may occur due to excessive or repeated tendo-Achilles lengthening.

BOX 3: Complications of soft-tissue releases [especially posteromedial soft-tissue releases (PMSTR) and complete subtalar release].

- *Loss of correction*: This is common if K-wires are not used to stabilize bones in recorrected position.
- Skewfoot
- Neurovascular damage, bone damage, physical injury, and wound complications **(Figs. 17A to D)**
- Osteonecrosis of talus and or navicular bones
- *Overcorrection:*
  - Hindfoot valgus—should be prevented by preserving the interosseous ligament. Also aggressive casting should be avoided as it causes subtalar break in the foot.
  - Forefoot abduction
  - Calcaneus
  - Pes planus
- *Undercorrection*:
  - Equinus
  - Heel varus
  - Adduction of forefoot
  - Medial spin
  - Cavus
- Sinus tarsi syndrome
- Dorsal subluxation of navicular—due to failure to release the tibionavicular ligament and dorsolateral talonavicular ligament release. There is failure to accurately reduce navicular over talus. This can be prevented by beginning midfoot release from lateral side (calcaneocuboid, cubonavicular → lateral → dorsal → medial talonavicular joint).
- Dorsal bunion—in clubfoot occurs due to persistent overpull of long and short great toe flexors with weak plantar flexors (calcaneus gait). Treatment requires release of flexed metatarsophalangeal (MTP) joint by volar, medial, and lateral capsulotomy, lengthening of FHL tendon, and dorsal transfer of FHB.

(FHB: flexor hallucis brevis; FHL: flexor hallucis longus)

Excessive one-time correction may lead to wound problems like skin necrosis. Rocker bottom deformity may also occur iatrogenically from persistent vigorous attempts to dorsiflex and evert the foot in presence of unyielding soft-tissue contractures (during manipulative correction of CTEV). Rigid contractures at midtarsal and subtalar joints prevent deemed correction. In contrast, the contractures at tarsometatarsal joints are pliable. Hence, the force applied to forefoot is more effective. Also, it can be gripped firmly. Repeated manipulation causes breech at tarsometatarsal joint which result is dorsiflexion, abduction of the forefoot, and convex plantar surface with hypermobility at tarsometatarsal joint. Clinically, the foot appears to be spuriously corrected because of forefoot abduction that obscures the dorsolateral prominence of uncovered head of talus. Forefoot dorsiflexion obscures equinus and a heel pad that is displaced laterally causing an apparent correction of heel varus. An AP radiographic view shows apparent divergence of hindfoot. Continuation of a line drawn along the lateral border of calcaneus and cuboid crosses the mid-tarsal area (instead of falling on the fifth metatarsal). Lateral view shows no dorsiflexion of calcaneus and more than usual plantar flexion of talus. It should be differentially diagnosed from congenital plantarflexed talus which is differentiated by taking an X-ray in plantar flexion. In rocker bottom foot the dorsal concavity disappears, but in plantarflexed talus, this does not disappear.

Varying degree of *toe-in gait* may be seen the after surgical correction (Pigeon-toe gait). Improvement occurs with growth with the remodeling of talus. The abnormal medial angulation of the neck and head of talus gradually decreases. Increase in the peroneal muscle strength also contributes to improvement.

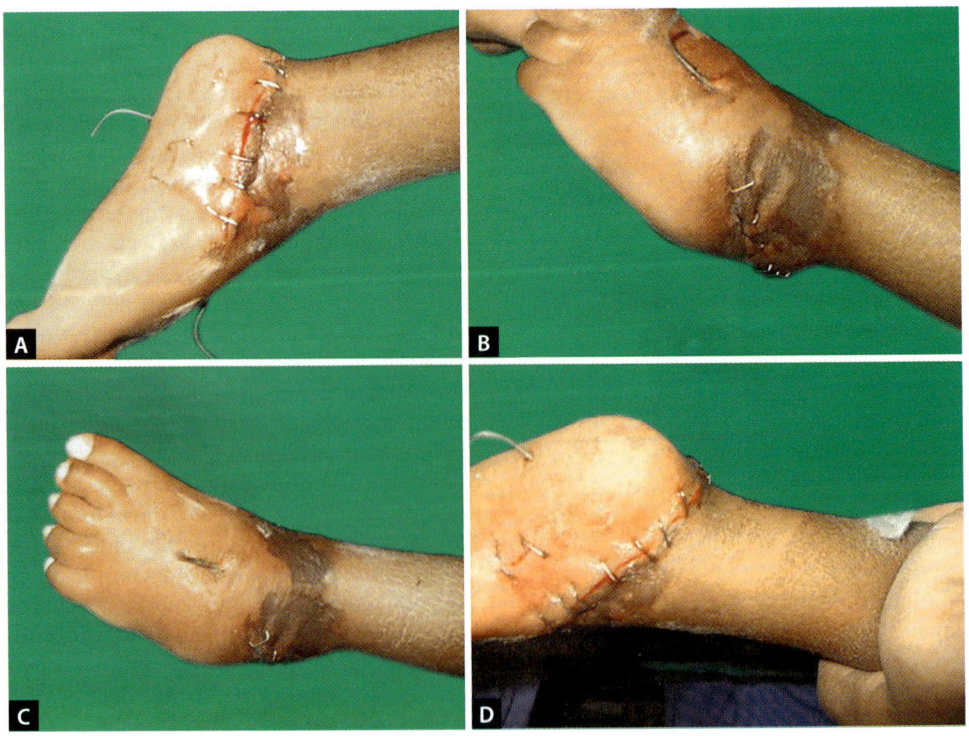

Figs. 17A to D: Wound complications following soft-tissue release.

In *"skewfoot "* marked metatarsus adductus (forefoot adduction) is seen with marked overcorrection of navicular (lateral translation of midfoot) and valgus angulation of heel (hindfoot valgus). This deformity is also called Z-foot or serpentine foot. Exaggerated plantar flexion of the talus and spina-bifida occulta is associated with increased chances of developing skewfoot. In congenital cases, the skewfoot deformity is difficult to differentiate from metatarsus adductus. With growth the midfoot starts ossifying and an uncovering of head of talus is revealed. This is due to lateral translation of navicular and lateral offset of first metatarsal axis in line with talar axis. Skewfoot is treated with manipulation and serial cast to invert heel, abduct forefoot, and stretch the tendo-Achilles. After a course of casts, child is allowed to wear soft padded (if callosities present) scaphoid pad or Thomas heel. Corrected position may be maintained at night by a bivalve cast. Surgery in the resistant cases consists of medial and lateral soft-tissue release with internal reefing and fixation for TCN joint along with Achilles fascia lengthening. Calcaneal lengthening osteotomy with or without first cuneiform opening wedge osteotomy may be additionally needed. Grice Green procedure is recommended for older feet.

Hallux valgus may be present in severe clubfeet with multiple prior surgeries.

Other described soft-tissue releases: *Modified McKay's procedure* (complete subtalar release of McKay and Simon) is done through transverse Cincinnati approach, for severe deformities which require extensive release including posterolateral ligament complex. They envisaged that results of clubfoot release without subtalar release indicate more of undercorrection and these children have residual internal foot progression angle. Caroll's procedure utilizes the posteromedial incision similar to Turco's and a small lateral incision over subtalar joint.

Surgical correction of cavus deformity: Cavus deformity is recognized in a lateral view by plantar flexion of first metatarsal. The cavus deformity of a clubfoot is distinguished from idiopathic/neuromuscular cavus by position of calcaneus. In clubfoot, the calcaneus is plantarflexed where as in idiopathic cavus, the calcaneus is dorsiflexed. Other features of idiopathic/neuromuscular cavus are normal talus shape, high longitudinal arch, well-aligned metatarsals, and clawed toes. In children with severe cavus, Stiendler's plantar fascia stripping may be done in the same sitting. First, the plantar fascia is stripped followed by the origin of abductor hallucis and intrinsic toe flexors subperiosteally from the plantar surface of calcaneus. This is the only time when a periosteal elevator is used in PMR. Remaining attachment of TA on shaft of first metatarsal and abnormal attachment of abductor hallucis is incised. Causes of cavus in clubfoot are contracted plantar aponeurosis, insertion of the tendon of TA more distally on shaft of first metatarsus and more dorsal origin of abductor hallucis with abnormal attachments to tibialis posterior tendon sheath and navicular tuberosity.

Bony Procedures

Bony procedures are generally done in children above 5 years of age in addition to soft-tissue release. The following are the commonly described bony procedures as in literature. Very uncommonly will even a practicing pediatric orthopedic surgeon ever use them, however:

Osteotomy of calcaneus (Dwyer's osteotomy, **Figs. 18A and B**) is used for persistent varus deformity of heel without affecting the subtalar joint function. The original description of medial opening wedge osteotomy though capable of restoring length fell into disfavor due to high rate of wound dehiscence, development of equinus deformity, and problems of bone healing. The present practice of lateral closing wedge osteotomy (modified Dwyer) is well-accepted for improved union rates and avoiding complications.

Resection and arthrodesis of calcaneocuboid (Dillwyn Evans procedure) joint may be carried alone or with soft-tissue release, it often produces hindfoot stiffness. But, this is preferred for so-called short medial column CTEV where soft-tissue release is the essential surgery rather than correcting the lateral aspect of foot.

Medial release and osteotomy of distal calcaneus (Lichtblau's) is used for persistent varus deformity of the hindfoot. This is done for the "long lateral column" CTEV,

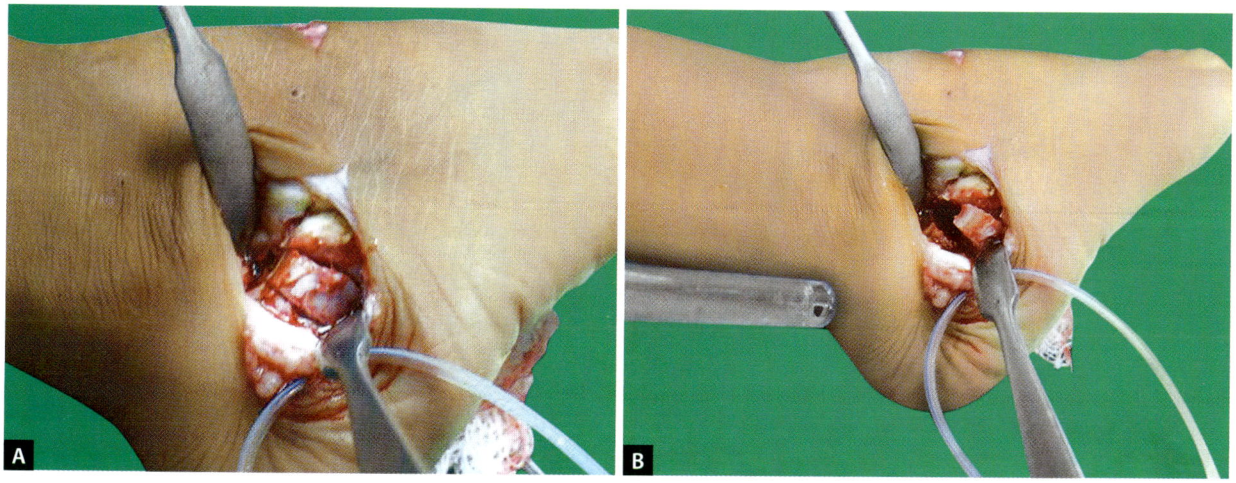

Figs. 18A and B: (A) Intraoperative picture of Dwyer osteotomy being performed; (B) The wedge removed.

The lateral column is shortened by resecting the anterior process of calcaneum or a shortening osteotomy.

Enucleation of the cuboid, anterior part of the calcaneus and head of the talus may be used for more resistant and syndromic feet in older children. Talectomy has also been used for the same indications with variable results. *Supramalleolar osteotomy* (for persistent intoeing gait) and osteotomies of the bases of metatarsals are used to correct residual deformities. The *triple arthrodesis* is used for the correction of equines and varus in adolescents and adults (neglected clubfoot) and also for varus or valgus overcorrected feet. The talonavicular joint is most difficult to fuse in triple arthrodesis.

External Distraction Devices for Clubfoot

They have been popular for short periods when there was a shift from Kite to Ponseti method of manipulation and also previously when a lot of cases of resistant and recurrent deformities were found due to unsuccessful manipulation. The prolonged period of manipulation also led investigators to search for methods other than open releases (due to inherent complications) that could serve to correct deformities. At few centers, these methods continue to be preferred over manipulation and surgical methods for correction of deformity as the correction is usually more reliable easily observed and the foot length is also restored. These methods can be used with or without osteotomy. The correction of clubfoot in a child >8 years is generally done with an osteotomy. Three types of external fixators have been used in clubfoot:

1. Wagner's device
2. Joshi's device
3. Ilizarov apparatus

Wagner's apparatus was used to lengthen medial column of foot to correct extensive medial scarring resulting from previous surgery.

Controlled differential distraction, Joshi's external stabilization system (JESS, **Figs. 19A and B**), method has been widely used in Indian subcontinent due to advantages like minimal surgery avoidance of surgical scar, and correction of all deformities either simultaneously (commonly) or sequentially (correction of forefoot adduction then correction of equinus). Foot length can also be gained. The tarsal joints are realigned by distraction at medial border of foot at rate of 1 mm/day. Lateral border is distracted at the rate of 0.5 mm/day (differential distraction), thus preventing crushing of cartilage of lateral border. The distractors along tibial and calcaneal pins allow correction of hindfoot equinus and heel varus. Correction of deformity by manipulation takes 3–6 weeks that has to be further maintained in POP cast for further 6 weeks. The procedure involves two major steps:

1. Insertion of K-wires
2. Formation of hold and connection between the hold

Insertion of K-wires: These include:

- Two tibial K-wires are placed one finger breadth distal to tibial tuberosity parallel to each other and to the knee joint line. The wires are placed 3–4 cm apart inserted from lateral to medial side. In older children, three wires can be passed to increase the stability.
- Two parallel calcaneal K-wires are passed into the tuberosity of calcaneum from medial to lateral side around 1–1.5 cm apart protecting the neurovascular structures. One additional half K-wire is passed from the posterior aspect of the calcaneum axially.
- *Metatarsal K-wire placement:* One transfixing K-wire is passed through the necks of first and fifth metatarsal from lateral to medial side. Additional wires are passed parallel to and 10–12 mm apart from either side engaging three metatarsals each. The third metatarsal will have engaging pins from either side.

Creation of Holds and Connecting between the Holds: Two "Z" bars are attached to the tibial pins one on either side.

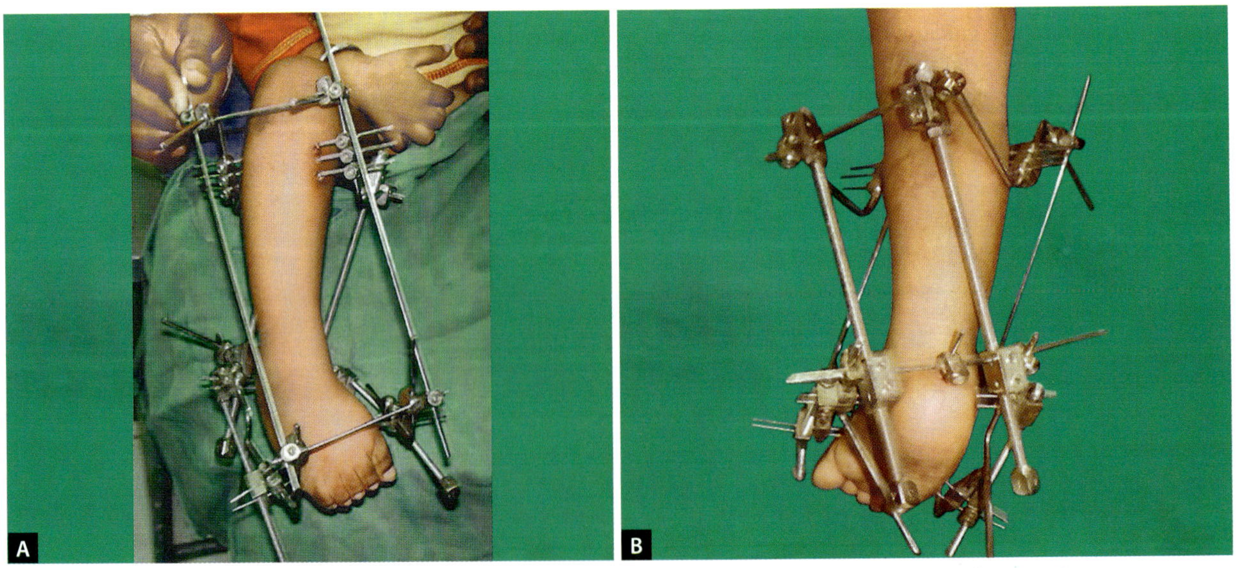

Figs. 19A and B: The Joshi external stabilization system (JESS) for clubfoot deformity correction.

Transverse bars are attached to the "Z" rods anteriorly and posteriorly each. Calacaneometatarsal distractors are then attached to K-wires. "L" rods are then attached to calcaneal and the metatarsal K-wires on either side. A transverse bar is placed connecting the posterior calcaneal half-pin and the posterior limbs of "L" rods.

Tibiocalcaneal distractors are applied, one on each side connecting the corresponding transverse rods. Toe sling can be attached to L-rods to prevent toe clawing and anterior static tibiometatarsal bar may be additionally used to improve glide of talus during equinus correction. All the pins are put pretensioned and the four distractors are distracted at the end of procedure till resistance is felt. Avoid any skin tethering at pin sites, achieve good hemostasis before closure.

Distraction schedule: Fractional calcaneo-metatarsal distraction is begun from third postoperative day to correct forefoot adduction at tarsometatarsal joint, reducing talus and calcaneocuboid joint. Differential distraction on medial side is performed twice as fast as on the lateral side (0.25 mm every 6 hours medially and 0.25 mm every 12 hours laterally).

The tibiocalcaneal distraction is first carried out parallel to the leg and just posterior to the transfixing calcaneal wires at the rate of 0.25 mm every 6 hours medially and 0.25 mm every 12 hours laterally to correct varus of the hindfoot and equinus. The distractors are then shifted posteriorly to stretch posterior structures and correct hindfood equinus at the ankle and subtalar joints @0.25 mm every 6 hours.

Radiological record keeping may be done pre- and postcorrection. Apparatus is maintained for 3–6 weeks in situ after correction for soft-tissue maturation and further maintenance is done in ambulatory below knee POP cast changed two to three times every 15 days.

The advantages of JESS methods are:

- Semi-invasive nature
- Bony procedures often not required
- Bloodless surgery
- Controlled correction of deformity
- Avoids fibrous tissue formation
- Actual lengthening and neohistiogenesis avoiding pressure on growing epiphysis

"Correction with Ilizarov's apparatus" (**Figs. 20A and B**, principled on distraction histioneogenesis) may be done with or without osteotomies. The correction is based on two principles elucidated by Ilizarov himself:

- *Tension-stress principle*—Gradual traction on living tissue stimulates the genesis of tissue and growth throughout the distraction period.
- *Shape-forming process* acting upon bone tissue depending on the magnitude of applied load and vascularity. Increased load with accompanied adequate blood supply will lead to increased bone tissue while without good supply same load leads to reduction in bone volume.

The added advantages include simultaneous correction of leg shortening. This method is a viable alternative to major operations such as triple arthodesis, V osteotomy, or wedge osteotomy in an adult. However, it is a complex operation that is technically demanding and may produce stiffness of subtalar and tarsal joints. The forefoot adduction is corrected by simultaneous distraction of 1 mm/day on medial side and 0.5 mm/day on lateral side. Equinus deformity is corrected by distraction with tibial and calcaneal rings and shortening of connecting bars between tibial and metatarsal rings until foot is 10° dorsiflexed. By virtue of its location lateral to center of metatarsal ring, the anterior bar also corrects supination. After full correction a fixed device is kept for 8–10 weeks after which it is removed and a long leg cast in corrected position is applied for 3 months. For children above 8 years, usually distraction with osteotomy will be required otherwise there are increased chances of recurrence. Various osteotomies that can be combined with Ilizarov's apparatus include supramalleolar osteotomy, U osteotomy, V osteotomy, posterior calcanean osteotomy, talocalcaneal osteotomy, midfoot osteotomy, and metatarsal osteotomy.

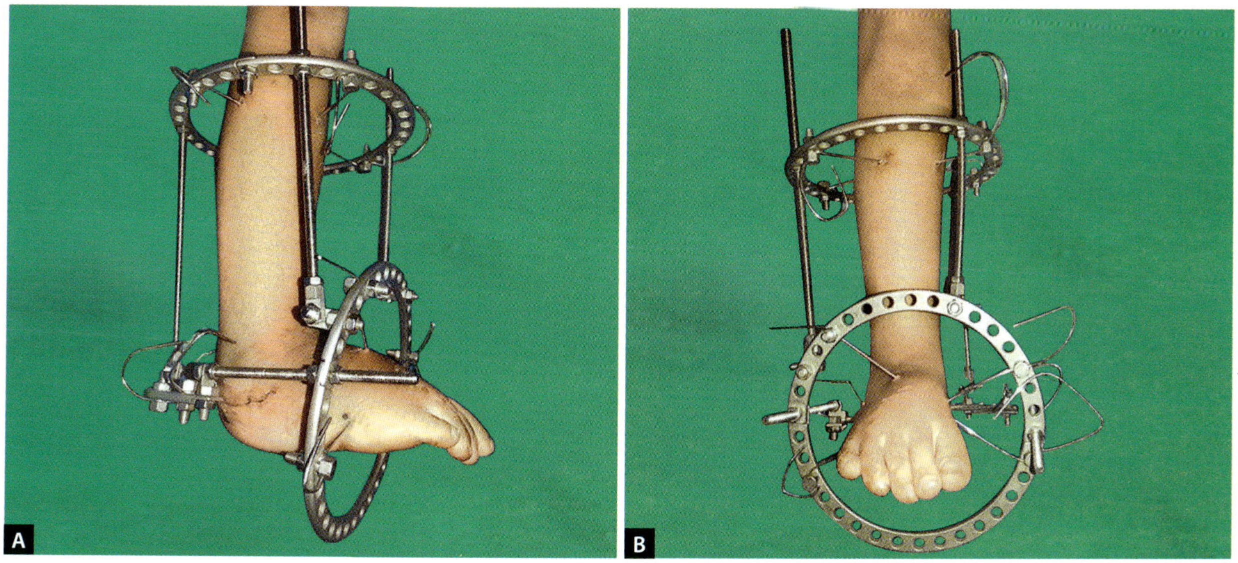

Figs. 20A and B: The use of Ilizarov apparatus for correction of congenital talipes equinovarus (CTEV).

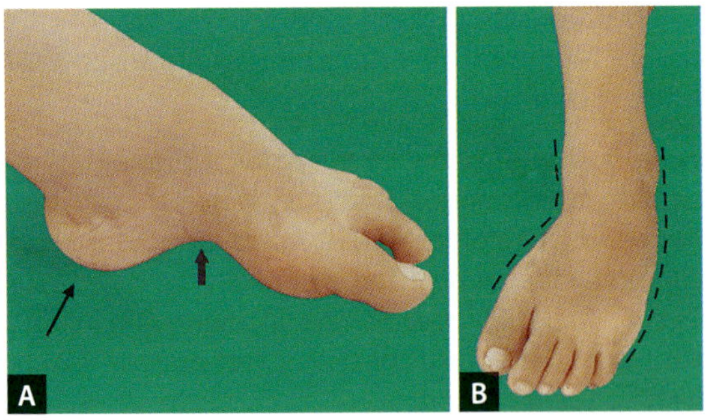

Figs. 21A and B: The clinical features of resistant clubfoot in a 4-year-old child. The foot has been operated thrice but still the equinus [solid arrow (A)], cavus [black arrow (A)] and forefoot adduction deformities persist with long lateral and small medial border of the foot (B).

TREATMENT OF RESISTANT DEFORMITY AND RELAPSED CONGENITAL TALIPES EQUINOVARUS

Common components of a resistant deformity **(Figs. 21A and B)** are:

- Adduction of forefoot
- Short medial column or long lateral column
- Varus of calcaneum
- Equinus of the ankle

Correction of forefoot adduction deformity is preferably done by metatarsal osteotomies. Hindfoot deformity may be due to isolated heel varus with long lateral column of foot or short medial column of foot. In children <3 years a residual heel varus may be corrected by modified Mckay's procedure. For isolated heel varus with mild supination of forefoot a Dwyre osteotomy or a lateral closing wedge osteotomy of calcaneum may be performed. Persistent hindfoot deformity constituting heel varus and internal rotation of calcaneus with a long lateral column of foot a Dillwyn Evans or Lichtblau's procedure is of choice. Residual heel equinus correction is done by TA lengthening with posterior ankle and subtalar capsulotomies. Rarely an isolated fixed equinus in an older child will require a Lambrinudi's procedure. Presence of all three deformities in a child of age above 12 years may require triple arthrodesis or an Ilizarov's external fixator. Preliminary TA tenotomy in small, markedly inverted/plantarflexed feel is helpful. This is done at musculotendinous junction. After this, feet may be held in Dennis-Brown brace.

CONCLUSION

- Clubfoot is a common lower extremity deformity. The deformity is quite characteristic and the diagnosis is quite obvious on inspection but evaluation entails going into much finer details to comprehensively manage the patient and follow-up.
- The components of the deformity should be carefully laid down so that they can be thoroughly corrected without missing any. It is better to use a standard classification system for organizational purposes, research, and later evaluation.
- The management of clubfoot has in a sense regressed from operative to conservative manipulation of the deformity—mostly followed that of Ponseti. In fact, this shift is unique to CTEV and has begun with the widespread use of Ponseti cast correction technique.
- Bracing is an important component of management of the patients for maintenance of correction so that deformity does not recur and for this parents should be counseled and prepared before beginning correction itself else the compliance is usually low.
- I recommend that specialized CTEV clinics should capture patients from newborn nursery and hospitals should make it a regular practice for evaluation of all newborns suspected to have foot deformity by preliminary training the staff.
- Neglected and long-standing cases that fail to respond to manipulation and cast treatment (rare) need surgical correction that may also be assisted by external fixation techniques if needed.
- External fixators (various forms, JESS, Ilizarov, etc.) may be used solely for correction of deformity in many cases.
- Other soft-tissue procedures such as tendon transfers, various bony procedures are reserved for specific cases judged on a case-to-case basis by experts dealing with CTEV deformity on a regular basis.

CHAPTER

44 Anomalies of Pediatric Upper Limb

Manish Kumar Varshney

INTRODUCTION

Congenital anomalies of the upper extremity are not uncommon and arise from either genetic or developmental factors in approximately two infants per 1,000 live births. The congenital anomalies of the upper extremity have been categorized by the American Society for Surgery of the Hand (ASSH) and International Federation of Societies for Surgery of the Hand (IFSSH) **(Table 1)**. About 40–50% of these infants also have other associated anomaly; bilateral affection is seen in more than 50% of these patients. Overall, boys are affected more than girls by a ratio of 3:2. Advanced maternal age is a significant factor for development of congenital upper extremity malformations.

DEVELOPMENT OF UPPER LIMB (FIGS. 1A AND B)

- The upper limb bud appears 26 days after fertilization (24 hours before appearance of the leg bud)
- It grows distally and the development is guided by apical ectodermal ridge inducing the mesoderm that is also responsible for interdigital necrosis. Other signaling centers include the zone of polarizing activity that guides radioulnar development, and the Wnt signaling center that guides dorsoventral development. Homeobox, or *HOX*, genes regulate the development of the limb by controlling the timing and extent of growth.
- The upper limb anlage elongates to a hand paddle by day 31.
- The digital rays then develop (day 36) with fissuring of the hand paddle. Fissuring appears first in the central rays followed by the border digits.
- Mesenchymal differentiation and tissue development (bone, joint, muscle and vascular development) also occurs in proximal-to-distal manner.
- Joint formation and digital separation both require apoptosis. In utero, joint motion is also required for development of the joints.
- The entire process completes by 8 weeks after fertilization.

TABLE 1: ASSH and IFSSH categorization of congenital anomalies of upper extremity.

Category	*Example*
Failure of formation • Transverse arrest • Longitudinal arrest	• Congenital below-elbow amputation (transverse) • Radial dysplasia (longitudinal)
Failure of differentiation (separation)	Syndactyly
Duplication	Preaxial polydactyly, postaxial polydactyly
Overgrowth	Macrodactyly
Undergrowth	Poland syndrome
Congenital constriction ring syndrome	Constriction band syndrome
Generalized skeletal abnormalities	Arthrogryposis

(ASSH: American Society for Surgery of the Hand; IFSSH: International Federation of Societies for Surgery of the Hand)

BIRTH-RELATED BRACHIAL PLEXUS PALSY

Perinatal brachial plexus palsy (PBPP) also called obstetric brachial plexus palsy is a flaccid paralysis of the arm at birth that affects different nerves of the brachial plexus supplied by C5 to T1. There are ***various described causes*** for the involvement of brachial plexus causing paresis or palsy of specific or all of components, these include:

- Obstetrical brachial plexus palsy—resulting during the process of birth itself
- Maternal uterine malformation
- Infection of the cervical vertebral bodies
- Osteomyelitis involving the proximal head of the humerus
- Tumors
- Familial congenital brachial plexus palsy
- Intrauterine maladaptation
- Congenital varicella syndrome
- Vascular lesions (hemangioma) in the region of the brachial plexus
- Exostosis of the first rib
- Kaiser Wilhelm syndrome

We will restrict the following discussion to obstetrical brachial plexus palsy that is the most common alleged cause of PBPP. This is a misnomer as it refers to causality from obstetric causes but as it is becoming bit clearer that in

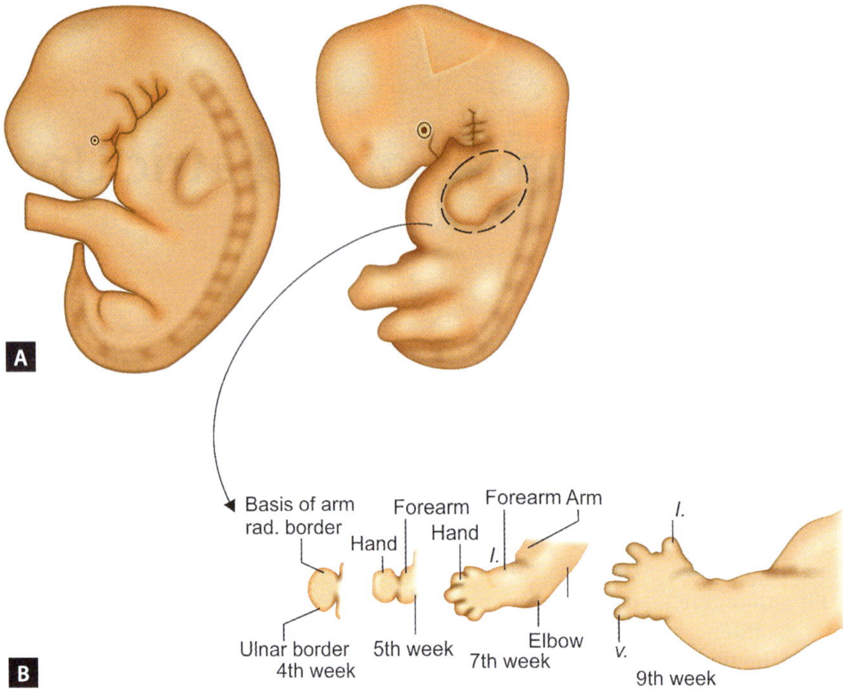

Figs. 1A and B: Development of upper limb. By 4th week distinctive upper limb bud is visible that slowly grows into discrete morphological parts by 2–3 months.

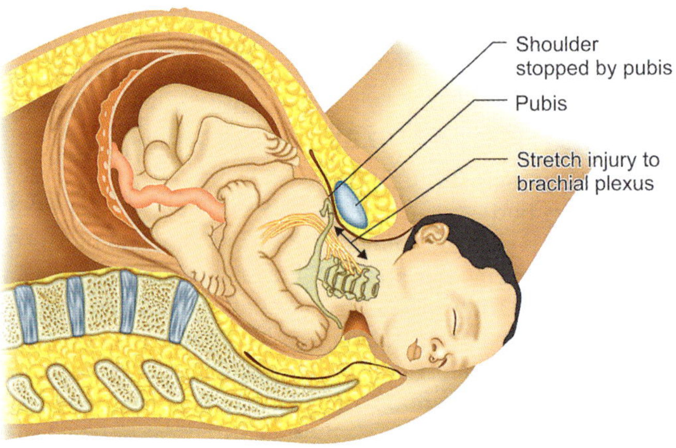

Fig. 2: Brachial plexus injury due to lateral traction force generated in shoulder dystocia.

utero and birth-related causes may itself be responsible in some rather than strict involvement of obstetric intervention only so, a better term is birth-related brachial plexus palsy (BRBPP). The most common conception of BRBPP is that the traction forces during labor stretch the brachial plexus beyond its resistance **(Fig. 2)** and the damage is augmentatively modified by hypoxemia, pressure, infiltration or compression injury simultaneously. The probability of BRBPP is proposed directly proportional to the magnitude, acceleration and cosine of the angle formed by the direction of the vector of the stretching force and the axis of the most vulnerable brachial plexus bundle, and inversely proportional to the resistance of the most vulnerable brachial plexus bundle and of the shoulder girdle muscles, joints and bones. This has been represented by the following formula:

$$p = \frac{F \times a \times cas\ \phi}{R}$$

- Probability (p) of BRBPP
- Traction force (F), a = acceleration, ϕ = angle of the stretching force and the axis of the most vulnerable brachial plexus nerve bundle
- R = combined resistance of the most vulnerable brachial plexus nerve bundle, muscles, joints (j) and bones (b)

The risk factors for brachial plexus palsy have been debated and mostly proposed based on certain observations but none is solely proven. ***Predisposing factors*** for BRBPP can be divided into maternal, labor-related and fetal.

- *Maternal factors:*
  - Diabetic disease of pregnancy [odds ratio (OR) 3.2; 95% confidence interval (CI) 1.6–6.2]
  - Excessive weight gain during pregnancy
  - Primiparity (possibly increased compressive forces)
  - Grand multiparity (possibly through precipitous second stage of labor)
- *Labor-related factors:*
  - Shoulder dystocia (OR 340; 95% CI 47–897)
  - Instrumented delivery (OR 18.3; 95% CI 5.7–59.3)
  - Vacuum delivery (OR 17.2; 95% CI 5.1–58.2)
  - A short second stage of labor
  - Prolonged second stage of labor (possibly due more to shoulder dystocia) (OR 8.3; 95% CI 4.0–17.3)
- *Fetal risk factors:*
  - Macrosomia (OR 17.9; 95% CI 10.3–31.3)
  - Decreased fetal arm movements
  - The presence of a first cervical rib
  - Clavicular fracture
  - Previous sibling with BRBPP (220 times increased risk)

Cesarean section has a significant protective effect on BRBPP. Increased rates of cesarean sections globally and reduction in shoulder dystocia could not reduce the incidence of BRBPP because the improvememt is mitigated by an increase in the fetal macrosomia these days.

Epidemiology, Pathogenesis and Classification

Birth-related brachial plexus palsy is seen in 0.42–5.1 infants per 1,000 live births. BRBPP can be classified as upper, middle, lower or complete **(Table 2)**.

The BRBPP can also be classified depending on grades of nerve injury as:

- ***Neurapraxia*** is a temporary conduction block due to damage to the myelin sheath at the site of injury, and function usually returns within weeks.
- ***Axonotmesis***, nerve fibers are disrupted, but the myelin sheath remains intact. The function often returns within months, although the recovery may not be complete.
- ***Neurotmesis***, the nerves have been totally disrupted no chance for spontaneous recovery.

TABLE 2: Different types of birth-related brachial plexus palsy (BRBPP).

Primary involvement of brachial plexus	*Roots involved*	*Narakas group*	*Description*
Upper	C5, C6	I–Erb/ Duchenne	Weakness of shoulder external rotation or abduction of arm and elbow flexion/supination
Middle	C5, C6, C7	II–Erb/ Duchenne	Along with the findings for upper there is also elbow flexion/supination paralysis and loss of wrist extension
Lower	C8, T1	Klumpke's	Floppy hand with claw deformity
Complete	C5, C6, C7, C8, T1	III–IV = III + Horner's	Flail arm

The pathogenic mechanisms have been commonly stated into:

- *Excessive lateral traction on the brachial plexus at the time of delivery:* This mechanism is considered central to development of BRBPP as it also explains the concomitant presence of facial nerve palsy, fracture clavicle and humerus and torticollis. The common cause is traction on the anterior shoulder in shoulder dystocia when pressed against symphysis pubis. The theory is challenged by the finding that one-third of shoulder dystocia had BRBPP in the posterior arm whereas the dystocia occurred in anterior shoulder. This is partially explained by impaction of the posterior shoulder on the maternal sacral promontory.
- *The process of labor itself:* Maternal propulsive forces possibly are responsible for BRBPP in the absence of shoulder dystocia, macrosomia, any predisposing traction forces against promontory, compression from contracting uterus, etc.
- *In utero insult:* McFarland et al. noted that cesarean section did not totally eliminate the risk for PBPP and only 63% of BRBPP from vaginal delivery had shoulder dystocia. In infants with BRBPP, the characteristics are a bit different. They are normal or low birth weight, the rate of persistence of BRBPP at 1 year of age is significantly higher (i.e., 41.2% vs. 8.7%) and the posterior shoulder is more commonly affected. This has led to an in utero mechanism possibly resulting in BRBPP (compression, infiltration, ischemia, etc.). These may explain the bilateral occurrence of palsy in 10–20% cases.

Other less commonly accepted mechanisms for BRBPP include:

- Clavicular compression
- Fracture of the proximal humerus
- Neurotoxic effects of effusions escaping from the torn capsule of an injured glenohumeral joint (possibly absurd).

Pathoanatomy

The rupture of the C5 through T1 roots from a traction force is a graduated, rostral-to-caudal pattern of injury. Upper plexus lesions are usually ruptures of the spinal nerves or the upper trunk while the C8 and T1 roots typically avulse. Isolated avulsions of the upper roots are uncommon and seen only with breech deliveries, if any. C5-7 nerve roots rupture due to their adherence to the periosteal lining of troughs of the transverse processes through which they pass. The traction forces get concentrated at this tether causing rupture. The lower cervical and T1 are not so protected so often avulse. Nerve rupture is a favorable for a surgeon because it can be repaired with a graft. The mechanism of root avulsion can be central or peripheral.

In the peripheral mechanism, traction through limb on the spinal nerve pulls the root with dura mater sheath from the spinal cord. This produces an irreparable damage to the root. With a central mechanism the cervical spine and cord are pushed to the opposite side transmitting traction force to the ipsilateral spinal root and not the dural sheath. This leads to a disruption of the nerve and not the dura. Root avulsion can be further differentiated into pre- and postganglionic lesions where the former occur proximal to the dorsal root ganglion.

Natural History

There is extensive heterogeneity of plexus injuries, and variable use of evaluation measures. The natural history of BRBPP is not very favorable. Recovery to "normal or near normal" levels occurs in only around 55% patients. Patients destined to complete recovery have good antigravity strength in the deltoid and biceps by the end of the second month and in the external rotators by the end of the third month. Patients with near normal recovery on the other hand have perceptible contractions in the biceps and deltoids by the end of the third month and if antigravity strength has returned by the end of the fifth month. About 10–15% benefit from brachial plexus surgery undertaken within 3 months of age. More than one-third require surgical correction of a secondary upper extremity deformity. Poor functional outcome is seen in patients who fail to show any recovery by 3 months. Those who show no progressive recovery by 3–6 months will not have any spontaneous recovery later. Those who do not show any antigravity muscle strength by 6 months will have persistent severe weakness in the muscles. Children with total plexus injuries have developmental apraxia or agnosia so are prone to accidental contact burns and self-mutilation. Developmental and behavioral problems develop in children with BRBPP. A high level of dissatisfaction has been reported among parents of children with BRBPP also.

Mallet system has been developed and commonly referred to prognosticate the BRBPP. Mallet test categorizes the upper limb with respect to five natural actions (predominantly a function of upper plexus) **(Fig. 3)**. Mallet terminology helps prognosticate the parents:

- If the biceps and deltoids reach the M3 grade in the second month, recovery should be complete
- If the above muscles reach the M1 grade in the third month and the M3 grade in the fifth month, recovery to a Mallet class IV shoulder can be anticipated
- If there are perceptible biceps contractions only even after the third month then a Mallet class III or II shoulder is expected.

Clinical Findings

The clinical features depend on the part of plexus involved:

The upper trunk of the brachial plexus (C5 and C6) is most frequently injured, resulting in Erb palsy, which is characterized by the "waiter's tip" posture **(Fig. 4)**. Erb's palsy is the most common form of BRBPP. It has following components:

- Weak abductors and external rotators of the shoulder + weak flexors and supinators of the elbow + weak radial extensors
- Good power in internal rotators and adductors of shoulder + elbow extensors and wrist flexors (all supplied by the middle trunk and C7)
- Sensory loss occurs over the outer aspect of the arm and forearm.
- *Associated phrenic nerve damage* may cause diaphragmatic paralysis. Erb palsy carries the best prognosis of recovery.

Total plexus palsy (C5–T1) presents with total paralysis of the upper limb and is often associated with Horner's syndrome. Horner's syndrome reflects injury to the preganglionic fibers serving the hand and neck region and is a valuable sign in severe traction injuries to the brachial plexus. The eye is examined for the presence of ptosis, loss of ciliospinal reflex, enophthalmos, miosis and anhidrosis. If present, it indicates injury to the white rami of the T1 root to the stellate ganglion and signifies a partial or complete avulsion of the T1 root and other neighboring roots as well. The prognosis is poor.

Pure lower plexus injuries: Klumpke's palsy (C8 to T1), involving only the lower trunk, is most uncommon, accounting for only 0.6% of all BRBPP.

These injuries may cause claw hands, drop wrists and severe loss of hand function. Sensation is lost in the ulnar forearm and hand. There may be unilateral Horner's syndrome.

Preganglionic and postganglionic injuries should be also differentiated for prognostication and management purpose. The preganglionic lesions (root avulsions) are irreparable and have worst prognosis while postganglionic lesions may either recover or can be surgically helped. The features that point to a preganglionic lesion (root avulsion) are:

- Presence of Horner's syndrome (see above)
- Burning pain or excessive pain out of proportion in an anesthetic hand
- Associated major vascular injury and/or fractures of the cervical spine
- Accompanying paralysis of scapular muscles or diaphragm
- Spinal cord dysfunction due to traction injury of the cord
- To diagnose root avulsions the function of muscles innervated by the branches from the root level should also be assessed. Presence of function in this muscle group denotes an intact root with a good surgical prognosis.
    - *Serratus anterior:* The long thoracic nerve (C5–C7)
    - The levator scapulae and the rhomboid muscles: The dorsal scapular nerve (C5–C6)
    - Phrenic nerve (C4–C5)
    - Nerve to the subclavius muscle
- Histamine test has been proposed to help diagnose a root or near root avulsion. Following the intradermal histamine injection if flare reaction (triple response) persist then the lesion is a root avulsion as the ganglion is in continuity with the injured root. Ganglion is needed for flare response. If the flare was absent then ganglion is discontinuous with the injured root (a postganglionic lesion).

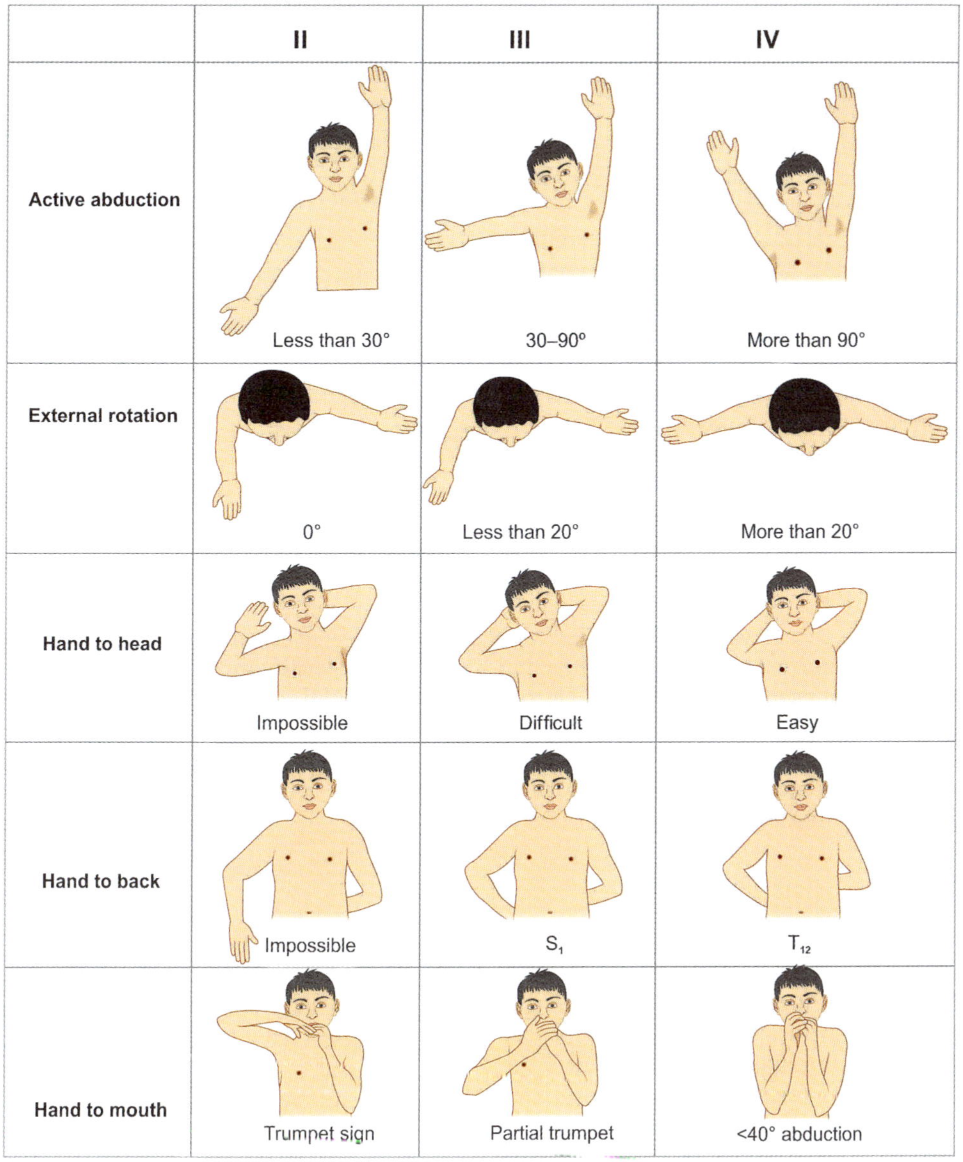

Fig. 3: Mallet system for prognosticating birth-related brachial plexus palsy (a score of 0 is assigned for no movement in the plane, and a score of 5 is assigned for full movement. Trumpet sign is abduction of ipsilateral shoulder while making an attempt to bring hand to mouth).

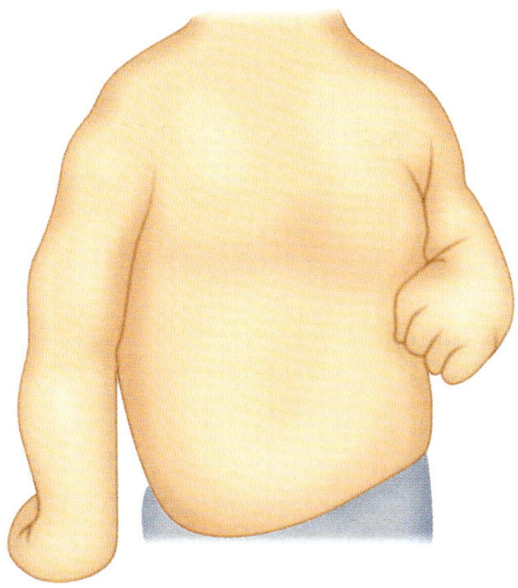

Fig. 4: The characteristic waiter's tip posture in Erb's palsy.

Evaluation

The initial evaluation of the neonate with suspected BRBPP should include a thorough history and physical examination as above with particular emphasis on signs of concurrent injuries.

- Observe for signs of respiratory compromise, suggesting phrenic nerve injury
- Inspect upper extremities for asymmetry in size, temperature, position and posture
- Look for fractures of the clavicles, humeri and ribs, or shoulder dislocation
- Assess range of motion (ROM), spontaneous motor activity and presence and symmetry of deep tendon and motor reflexes
- Response to sensory stimulation is evaluated (touch, pain, static, two-point discrimination, joint position and

vibration). The head and neck should be examined for Horner's syndrome, signs suggesting damage to other regional nerves and the presence of torticollis.

Ancillary Diagnostic Aids

- Chest X-ray and ultrasound of the diaphragm may reveal evidence of phrenic nerve palsy.
- X-rays of the cervical spine, clavicle and upper extremity can assist in identifying fractures and congenital malformations.
- Electromyography (EMG) helps in determining the functional status of muscle. About 4–6 weeks after injury before fibrillation potentials appear on EMGs. Sensory conduction studies are also done to ascertain the functional status of afferent fibers along the median ulnar and radial nerves. Nerve conduction studies should only be performed after 4–6 weeks post-injury.
- Magnetic resonance imaging (MRI) helps in distinguishing the tissues and detailing the level and extent of injury. If a lesion of the central nervous system is suspected, it can also be evaluated with MRI. The MRI is especially advantages for imaging the distal brachial plexus injury. Presence of pseudomeningoceles, i.e., out pouching of the dura at the level of roots is an indication of root avulsion. MRI only demonstrates the side of extraforaminal nerve damage without detailing further. Magnetic resonance neurography better demonstrates extraforaminal nerve root pathology, and also its correlation with clinical examination is better.
- CT scan: Posterior humeral head subluxation and glenoid version are commonly measured using CT scan. Glenoid version (normally 0°) is measured using axial CT/MRI images **(Fig. 5)**. Scapular line connecting the mid-glenoid to the medial spine of the scapula is constructed. The angle formed between the scapular line and a line drawn tangential to the glenoid surface interacting closely with the humeral head is calculated and 90° is subtracted from it to measure the glenoscapular angle. Posterior subluxation of the humeral head **(Fig. 5)** is expressed as percentage of humeral head anterior to the glenoid (PHHA, normal value = 50). PHHA is calculated from the ratio of the distance between scapular line to the anterior aspect of humeral head and the greatest diameter of the head, multiplied by 100.

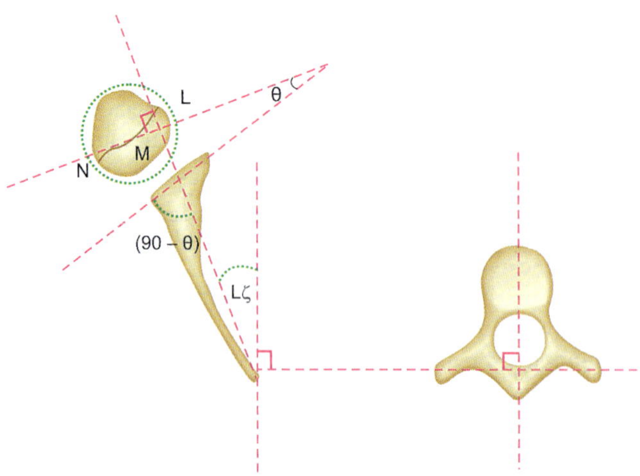

Fig. 5: The method of calculating glenoscapular angle (glenoid version θ), posterior subluxation of the humeral head [(LM/LN) × 100] and spinoscapular angle (ζ).

Differential Diagnosis

The differential diagnosis of BRBPP includes:

- Pseudoparalysis from
  - Fracture of the clavicle or humerus
  - Vitamin C deficiency: Scurvy
- Osteomyelitis
- Sepsis of the glenohumeral joint
- Arthrogryposis
- Brachial neuropathy secondary to sepsis
- Lesions of the spinal cord and cerebral palsy

Treatment

Prevention

Shoulder dystocia continues to represent a largely unpredictable obstetric emergency. Cesarean section has been associated with a lower risk for BRBPP. With the estimated relative risk, it has been predicted that 3695 elective cesarean sections would be needed [number needed to treat (NNT)] to prevent one permanent case of BRBPP among those non-diabetic mothers who carry a fetus with an estimated weight of greater than 4.5 kg. Because there is currently no accepted method to objectively quantify "excessive" lateral traction, the mere occurrence of BRBPP should not be taken as clear evidence of medical negligence.

Management Decision-making

The principle task of surgeon is to identify patients who will have benefit from surgery vis-s-vis conservative management. Based on the above explanation of prognostication and natural history of disease, the following decision-making points are obvious:

- The patient with early full recovery does not need surgical exploration and repair.
- Those with Horner's syndrome and total palsy will most often require some sort of surgical intervention.
- Children with incomplete recovery are the more difficult ones to predict, if they will benefit from primary surgery. Not only is it difficult but the time period is also constrained and an early decision needs to be made for optimal outcome, if repair is desired.
- Prognosis and outcome of early surgical decision- making is multifaceted and depends on:
- Clinical examination
- Electrodiagnostics
- Radiographic studies

Gilbert et al. in his reviews suggested the role of biceps and deltoid function in predictive value that is used for most close relevance still today. Narakas divided patients into three groups:

1. Those who started recovery before 3 weeks did fine

2. Those who started recovery between 3 weeks and 2 months often required secondary surgeries
3. Those who began recovery after two months required early exploration.

The modified Mallet classification (see above) and Toronto Test Score are other reliable instruments for assessing upper extremity function in patients with BRBPP. Active movement scale (devised by hospital for sick children) scores; elbow flexion and extension, wrist extension, and finger and thumb extension. If children do not reach a preset score by 3 months of age, surgery is generally advised. Children who pass "the test" at 3 months are followed conservatively and retested at 9 months for improvement of elbow flexion using the "cookie test". With the child sitting, a cookie is given. If the child can get the cookie to his or her mouth with the elbow held at the side and less than 45° of neck flexion, the elbow flexion is deemed adequate and surgery is not indicated. Failure to get the cookie to the mouth is an indication for primary exploration and repair of the brachial plexus.

The role of electrodiagnosis and needle electromyography is more controversial. They tend to overestimate recovery. Similarly, the role of MRI in surgical planning is controversial. Clinical examination remains the most valuable means of assessing the severity and location of injury.

Nonoperative Management

The goals of conservative therapy are to:

- Prevent soft tissue contractures and joint dislocations
- Correct muscular imbalance
- Prevent development of maladaptive patterns of movement
- Maintain ROM
- Optimizing functional use of the affected extremity.

Strengthening exercises with ROM training at joints is initiated for functional improvement along with sensory awareness program to prevent agnosia. Parents are taught and encouraged to carry out exercises at home as the more the time is spent, the more is functional gain. Parents should be instructed to take care of the affected arm with respect to minimizing discomfort and prevent further injuries so that the program progresses well. Additional therapies are often used on institutional basis as follows:

- Botulinum toxin to weaken the overpowering antagonist muscles
- Neuromuscular electrical stimulation to strengthen recovering muscles.

Primary Surgical Exploration of the Brachial Plexus

Primary reconstructive techniques are to be done before 6 months of age and can be basically divided into three groups depending on the need:

- ***Primary repair:*** It involves excision of neuroma and repair of the ends using cable graft or direct suturing. Primary repair can be done for transected brachial plexus structures. Ruptured and retracted roots do not allow good primary repair. End-to-end suturing of roots is done only if there is no tension at the repair site. There is long latency for functional recovery after repair.
- ***Secondary repair*** (usually done within 8–12 weeks)
  - Neurolysis is not an independent procedure. It is usually an accompaniment to other procedures and not performed in isolation alone. Neurolysis is basically freeing the nerve of scar tissue and can be:
    - *Extraneural neurolysis:* Resecting scar tissue from around the nerve
    - *Intraneural neurolysis:* Resecting scars and tissue within the nerve.
  - *Nerve grafting (Fig. 6):* Anatomical reconstruction of the plexus is attempted through a nerve graft commonly in the form of cable using donor from sural, intercostal or spinal accessory nerves. Plexus is explored through extended supraclavicular approach. Nerve grafting is also preferred if primary repair without tension cannot be achieved. The reconstruction involves neuroma resection and interpositional cable nerve grafting. The nerves are often anastomosed using fibrin glue to shorten the operating time. This procedure is best suited for upper plexus injury (C5 and C6).
- ***Neurotization:*** In multilevel injuries, the roots may be nonanatomically reconstructed to best available motors ignoring the plexus anatomy (intraplexal neurotization). If C5 root is available then it should be grafted to lateral cord and if both C5 and C6 are available then C5 to lateral and C6 to posterior cord should be transferred. If intraplexal donors are unavailable then extraplexal neurotization using expendable nerves like the spinal accessory nerve, phrenic nerve, intercostal nerves, contralateral C7 and hypoglossal nerves. Spinal accessory nerve is commonly used to neurotize suprascapular nerve or musculocutaneous nerve (to restore shoulder external rotation and elbow flexion). Intercostal nerves may be alternatively used for musculocutaneous nerve. These can also be combined together. In complete palsy the contralateral C7 nerve is extended across by cable grafts to provide a transfer source for the plexus. The deficit on

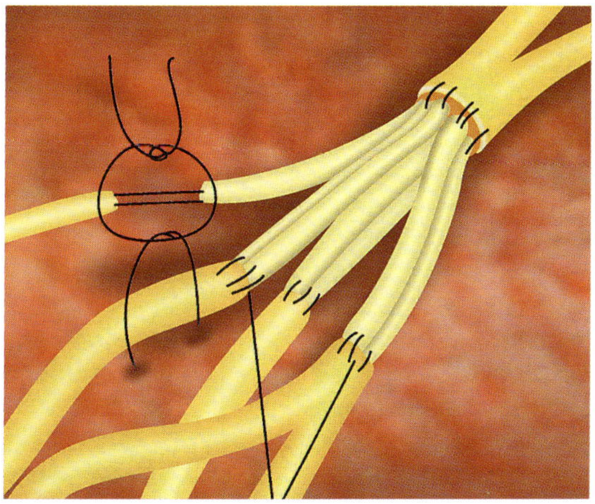

Fig. 6: Surgical repair of brachial plexus by sural nerve grafts.

the donor side is minimal. These result in 60–70% success with reasonable gain in power.

There has been no conclusive evidence to prove that surgery for brachial plexus injury is better compared to conservative management in BRBPP.

Secondary Reconstructive Surgery

Secondary reconstructions are inferior to proper primary intervention. They are aimed at augmenting the function. The clinician should ensure that these intervention(s) improves the overall functions of daily living for the patient. Internal rotation contracture with weakness of shoulder abduction and external rotation is the most common secondary reconstruction needed even in patients who underwent primary plexus reconstruction. The various treatment methods commonly practiced are detailed here.

Internal rotation contracture and glenohumeral dysplasia: Unresolved upper trunk palsy is associated with internal rotation contracture of shoulder, glenohumeral dysplasia, subluxation and dislocation. Internal rotation contracture may develop by two mechanisms. Posterior shoulder subluxation/dislocation causes rapid loss of passive external rotation, asymmetric axillary skin folds and apparently shortened humeral segment. This can be felt as a palpable clunk during shoulder manipulation. Additionally the imbalance between functional internal rotators and paralyzed external rotators causes further posterior subluxation of humeral head and eventually dislocation. The other mechanism may involve development of scapular hypoplasia, elevation, and rotation (SHEAR) bony deformity caused by elevation and extrusion of the affected scapula beyond the clavicle. This produces abnormal anterior rotation of the clavicle + protracted scapula producing forward tilt of acromioclavicular plane. The acromion impinges upon the humeral head pushing it posterior producing posterior subluxation of humeral head and prevents external rotation evolving into internal rotation contracture. SHEAR can be measured in 3D reconstruction of upper chest CT scan. The percentage area of scapula migrating above clavicle divided by the total area of scapula gives measure of SHEAR deformity. The different surgical options for correction of internal rotation contracture include glenohumeral capsulorrhaphy, biceps tendon lengthening, tendon transfers, muscle releases, axillary nerve decompression, humeral osteotomy, anterior capsule release or a combination of these.

- Posterior glenohumeral capsulorrhaphy tightens the posterior capsule surrounding the humeral head and repositions it anteriorly, addressing the posterior subluxation temporarily atleast.
- For C5-C7 asymmetric nerve injury biceps tendon lengthening or the Z-lengthening is an option to overpower triceps and add length to straighten elbow.
- Internal rotation contracture release involves sectioning internal rotators (the subscapularis and/or pectoralis major) and transferring functioning muscles (latissimus dorsi and/or teres major) to the posterior or posterosuperior rotator cuff augmenting external rotation and abduction. Shoulder function improves initially but gradually deteriorates over time. This procedure apparently only halts the development of dysplasia but does not prevent it. One must be vigilant enough to not create external rotation contracture else that would need correction then.
- Because of the deteriorating results of contracture release and muscle transfer some tend to combine procedures such as neurolysis and decompression of the axillary nerve with an untethering release of soft tissue contractures (modified Quad procedure, **Fig. 7**). The four components of modified quad procedure include transfer of the latissimus dorsi muscle to give external rotation and abduction, transfer of the teres major muscle to stabilize

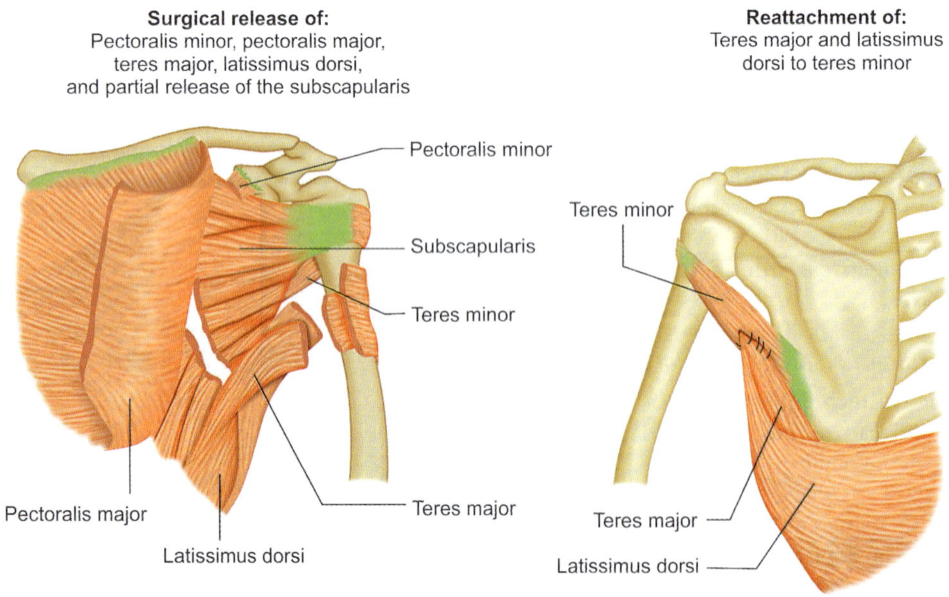

Fig. 7: The modified Quad procedure for correction of internal shoulder contracture.

the scapula, release of the subscapularis, pectoralis major and minor contractures and decompression and neurolysis of the axillary nerve.

- The modified quad extensive procedure still fails to address glenohumeral dysplasia so a bony surgical procedure known as triangle tilt has been advocated by select surgeons (Nath RK and Somasundaram C). This procedure consists of osteotomy of the clavicle at the junction of the middle and distal thirds, osteotomy of the acromion process at its junction with the spine of the scapula, ostectomy of the superomedial angle of the scapula to reduce scapular winging and splinting of the extremity in adduction, external rotation and forearm supination. By virtue of tilting the plane of AC joint posteriorly the impingement on humeral head is relieved and it can be repositioned in a neutral position in the glenoid cavity.
- Humerus external osteotomy is not a very popular method for correction of internal rotation contracture but may be indicated in a child who has advanced glenohumeral dysplasia or insufficient power in the muscles needed for transfer. The only controversy here is determining the level of dysplasia that precludes osteotomy to give way to osteotomy. The results of humeral osteotomy also deteriorate over time.
- If the muscles have fibrosed due to long standing degenerative changes in end-plates then motor plate units can be transferred like that of gracilis transfer.

Reconstruction for elbow problems requires improving the flexion weakness, static flexion contracture and weakness of extension. Pectoralis major (Clarke's transfer) or Steindler's transfer help regain elbow flexion. The latissimus dorsi flap is another good method to provide elbow flexion power. Free muscle transfer (gracilis or rectus femoris) innervated through intercostal nerves are other ways to regain elbow flexion and wrist extension.

Supination contracture is especially seen in lower trunk/complete injury. They are usually associated with late onset pronation weakness also. Impaired supination can be restored by tendon transfer but supination contracture correction needs forearm osteotomy. Usually distal ulna and mid-shaft radius osteotomies are done while some advocate only radius osteotomy. Pronation deformity can be treated by pronator teres rerouting or release of pronator quadratus or both.

For the wrist, the most common problem is weakness of extension (wrist drop) and grasp and pinch of hand. Splinting followed by stabilization of wrist in extension using arthrodesis or tenodesis usually helps. Providing sensation in hand is of utmost importance and hence lower trunk reconstruction should be attempted at priority early. Finger flexion is difficult to provide but some success has been achieved by augmentation of flexor digitorum profundus function using free gracilis.

Postoperative Therapy

Postoperative rehabilitation is very important and demanding. The reinnervation is slow progressing at 1 mm/day approximately and may even be incomplete. Contractures, dislocations and other deformities, as well as sensory agnosia, need to be prevented during this period by a rehabilitation program aimed at maintaining ROM, and strengthening and promoting age-related functional skills. Rehabilitation also is important to maximize the functional recovery following secondary reconstructive surgery.

SPRENGEL DEFORMITY (CONGENITAL ELEVATION OF SCAPULA)

The superior border of scapula is situated normally at the seventh cervical vertebra and its inferior angle is at the level of the sixth rib. During embryonic development scapular anlage is situated opposite the fifth cervical vertebra. Sprengel deformity results from failure of scapular descent during embryologic development. The scapula remains hypoplastic, high-riding with varying degrees of reduced scapulothoracic movement.

Epidemiology

The disease affects girls slightly more commonly than boys. The right and left scapulae are affected with equal frequency, and the condition is bilateral in 10–30% of patients. Associated conditions with congenital elevation of scapula include:

- *Omovertebral bar:* About up to 50% of patients have an abnormal fibrous, cartilaginous or bony connection between the superior scapular angle and the cervical spine
- Omoclavicular bars
- Klippel-Feil syndrome
- Abnormal musculature
- Scoliosis
- Spina bifida
- Torticollis
- Rib anomalies (fused or absent ribs)
- Facial asymmetry
- Vertebral anomalies, anal atresia, cardiac defects, tracheoesophageal fistula and/or esophageal atresia, renal and radial anomalies and limb defects (VATER) association
- Foot deformities
- Pulmonary and kidney disorders

Diagnosis

Primarily, the condition is identified on physical examination where the affected scapula appears small and high riding into the cervical spine **(Fig. 8)**. There is increased scapular width to height ratio. The inferior pole is rotated medially with the glenoid pointing inferiorly (downward rotation of scapula). Due to weakening of periscapular muscles there could be scapular winging. Other findings include presence of webbed neck and a variable loss of ROM. Usually, the deformity is painless.

Differential Diagnosis

Brachial plexus birth palsy, scoliosis, Turner syndrome.

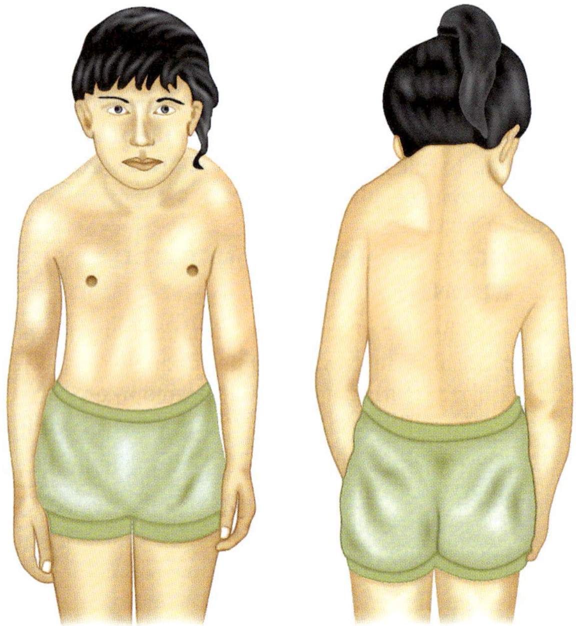

Fig. 8: Sprengel shoulder. Clinical presentation with raised shoulder due to high riding scapula on left.

TABLE 3: Classification of Sprengel deformity.

Grade	*Characteristic findings*	*Treatment*
Grade 1	Glenohumeral joints are level and no deformity is visible with the dressed-up patient	No treatment required
Grade 2	The glenohumeral joints are level but a prominence in neck is visible with the patient dressed-up	Extraperiosteal resection of scapular prominence and the tethering omovertebral bar. Caution patients that the lump will be replaced with scar that may be even hypertrophic
Grade 3	Moderate deformity with 2–5 cm elevation of glenohumeral joint	Excision of the superior margin of the scapula and the anomalous omovertebral connection, with derotation and caudal repositioning of the scapula (see text)
Grade 4	Severe deformity with the scapula situated near occiput	As for grade 3

Investigations

Anteroposterior radiographs of shoulder confirm the diagnosis and a bony omovertebral bar may also be visualized. The condition can also be diagnosed prenatally by ultrasonography.

Treatment

The treatment is primarily surgical for conspicuous deformities with disability. Treatment is guided primarily based on Cavendish classification **(Table 3)**. The age of surgical intervention is of primary concern and often debated. Early intervention has chances of maximal correction during further growth before adaptive movements and restrictions develop. But the child may not bear the extensive nature of intervention and may succumb. So, the age of at least 3 years is considered by most as the optimal time for intervention. Surgical treatment involves primarily releasing the scapular tethers by resection of the superior angle of the scapula and the tethering omovertebral bar. Additionally, the scapula is derotated and relocated to a more caudal position. The greatest challenge put with caudal repositioning of the scapula, is the risk of compressive injury to the brachial plexus and it increases with age. This risk is greatest in children older than 8 years. Concomitant clavicular osteotomy may reduce the risk. Surgical techniques described for scapular relocation include:

- The *Woodward procedure* relocates the scapula by detachment and caudal relocation of the midline origin of the parascapular muscle (shifting the trapezius and rhomboids caudally along the spine). In addition, the superomedial scapular prominence may also be resected (Borges modification to Woodward procedure). Clavicular osteotomy allows additional scapular descent. It is the most common surgical technique used for correction of a moderate or severe Sprengel deformity with good cosmetic and functional improvement. The outcome of procedure is independent of the age of the patient or the presence of an omovertebral bone. Cervical spine anomalies, however, affect the outcome negatively.
- *The Green procedure:* Here scapula is derotated by extraperiosteal detachment of scapular muscles at their scapular insertion and scapula is laid free. After caudal relocation of the scapula and fixation using scapular traction cables, the parascapular detached muscles are reattached.
- *Vertical scapular osteotomy* ***(Fig. 9)****:* The lateral half of scapula is brought down caudally with concomitant clavicular osteotomy or morcellization. The clavicular osteotomy is recommended to reduce the risk of neurovascular injury and to provide anterior release. The correction achieved is limited, however, compared to other procedures.

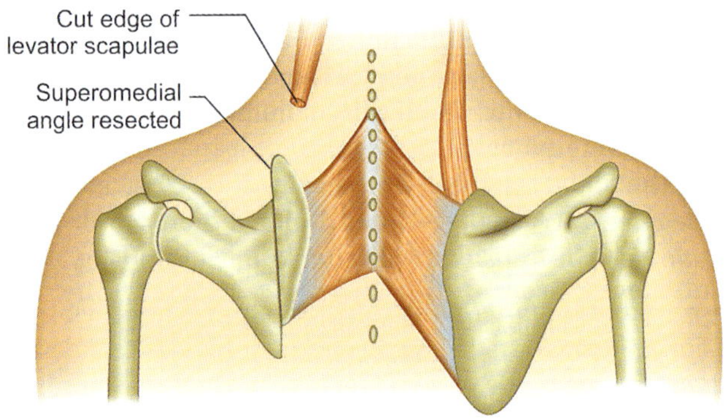

Fig. 9: Vertical scapular osteotomy for Sprengel shoulder.

GLENOID HYPOPLASIA

The normal concave glenoid develops from consolidation of the secondary centers of ossification of the superior glenoid, inferior glenoid and coracoid that develop between 9 and 16 years of age. Glenoid hypoplasia occurs from failure of the inferior glenoid to ossify. The condition is typically bilateral and symmetric. This rare condition can occur in isolation or in association with other conditions such as:

- Skeletal dysplasia
- Mucopolysaccharidoses
- Cornelia de Lange's syndrome
- Holt-Oram syndrome
- Apert syndrome

Clinical Features

The patient has limited shoulder abduction and forward flexion, mild axillary webbing and multidirectional instability of shoulder joint. However, most patients have minimal functional limitations.

Investigations

Plain radiographs or noncontrast spiral CT scan confirms the diagnosis.

Treatment

Most patients are managed by conservative methods only and counseling. Symptoms can be controlled with physical therapy and strengthening exercises.

CONGENITAL PSEUDARTHROSIS OF THE CLAVICLE

This is a rare anomaly that results from failure of normal clavicular ossification. There are three predominant hypotheses to explain the malformation:

1. Congenital pseudarthrosis of the clavicle may result from failure of medial and lateral primary centers of ossification to unite during development. The biggest contradiction to this theory is the fact that normal clavicle developing in an embryo has only one ossification center.
2. Vascular pulsations of the subclavian artery may cause the failure of coalescence is interesting and explains the clinical observation that congenital pseudarthrosis of the clavicle occurs on the right side predominantly (>90% of patients). The right subclavian artery is more cephalad as it courses over the first rib so, may affect the right clavicle predominantly. Also supporting the view is the finding of left-side involvement seen in patients with dextrocardia and the condition is very rarely if ever bilateral.
3. Genetic (*see* also the Chapter on "Congenital, Genetic, Syndromic, and Miscellaneous Disorders"): The disease may be inherited in an autosomal recessive pattern though the exact chromosomal anomaly and linkage is not identified.

Clinical Presentation

The diagnosis is usually made at or shortly after birth. The children have a prominence at the middle third of clavicle that may increase with age but is rarely painful. The movements at adjacent joints are full and unhindered.

Investigations

Radiography confirms the diagnosis. The ends of clavicle are large and rounded with missing intermediate bone or the appearance of short fibrous nonunion.

Differential Diagnosis

- Birth-related fracture but there is no fracture callus.
- Neurofibromatosis cleidocranial dysplasia, or another skeletal dysplasia—clavicle pseudarthrosis has never been linked with any dysplasia or syndrome.

Treatment

The condition is benign and few long-term follow-up studies have reiterated this fact. There is no functional limitation or any symptomatic involvement due to the pseudarthrosis in majority though spontaneous ossification does not occur. Cosmetic concern is primary in most of the patients and they may seek surgical help. Other rare indications for surgery are:

- Development of thoracic outlet syndrome
- Shoulder asymmetry or reduced ROM
- Pain at the site of pseudarthrosis

Surgical Procedure

For a skeletally immature patient between 7 months and 6 years the recommended procedure excision of pseudarthrosis, preservation of periosteum approximation of the ends and plate fixation.

For older children (older than 6 years), the initially performed procedure of excision of prominence without any other intervention seems to be an under treatment and it is better to do bone grafting and rigid internal fixation after excision of prominence and pseudarthrosis.

Complications

Surgical intervention is met with multiple and serious complications with high frequency so often the surgical intervention is not preferred. The complications include:

- Hypertrophic scar formation
- Nonunion
- Infection
- Brachial plexus palsy
- Bone graft donor site morbidity
- Neurovascular injury
- Migration of k-wires or pins if used (now their use is contraindicated for frequent complications).

CONGENITAL RADIAL HEAD DISLOCATION

Congenital radial head dislocation (CRHD) is the most common congenital anomaly of the elbow that often gets unrecognized until late childhood or adolescence, because most patients are asymptomatic and have no functional limitations. The condition is commonly bilateral (differential from traumatic dislocation of radial head) though isolated and sporadic forms are also seen. Also, progressive subluxation of radial head finally dislocating has been reported that were not dislocated at birth. CRHD has been commonly seen to be associated with other conditions like:

- Congenital proximal radioulnar synostosis (CPRUS), developmental dysplasia of the hip (DDH), club feet, brachydactyly, clinodactyly, tibiofibular synostosis, congenital below-elbow amputation and radial or ulnar clubhand **(Figs. 10A and B)**
- Capitellar hypoplasia
- Silver's syndrome
- Arthrogryposis
- Larsen syndrome
- Cornelia de Lange
- Klippel-Feil
- Klinefelter's
- Nail-patella syndrome

Acquired form of radial head dislocation may be found with:

- Madelung deformity (MD)
- Osteochondromatosis

Clinical Features

Patients may have a bony prominence on the posterolateral aspect of the elbow, with limitations in elbow flexion extension or forearm rotation. Identification usually escapes in infancy and especially unilateral cases. Pain is an uncommon feature (differential from traumatic dislocation) until adolescence which may be accompanied with popping sensation of elbow. The dislocation may be posterior, anterior, or lateral though posterior or posterolateral is the most common followed by anterior. The head can be palpated as a bony prominence just distal to cubital fossa. Movement restrictions are more prominent with anterior dislocation that blocks flexion. Forearm rotations are restricted with supination restricted more than pronation.

Investigations

Plain films **(Figs. 11A to E)** reveal the dislocated head with capitellar hypoplasia or flattening (differential from traumatic

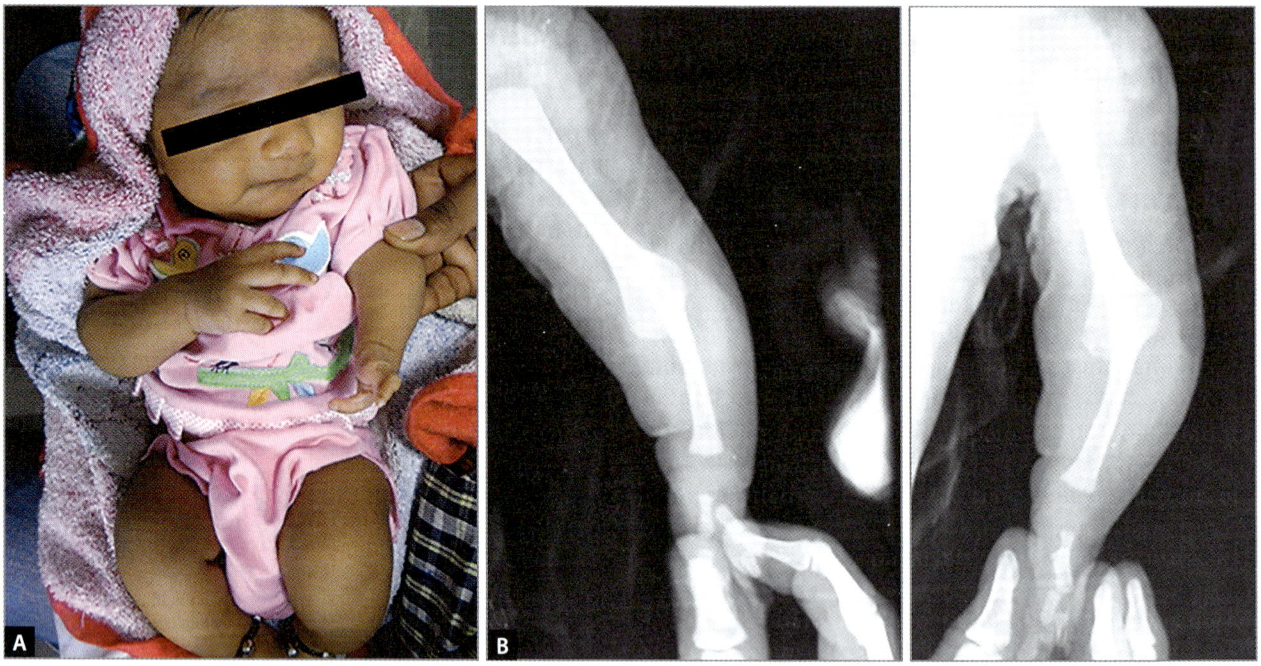

Figs. 10A and B: Ulnar clubhand. (A) Clinical presentation; (B) Radiographical appearance.

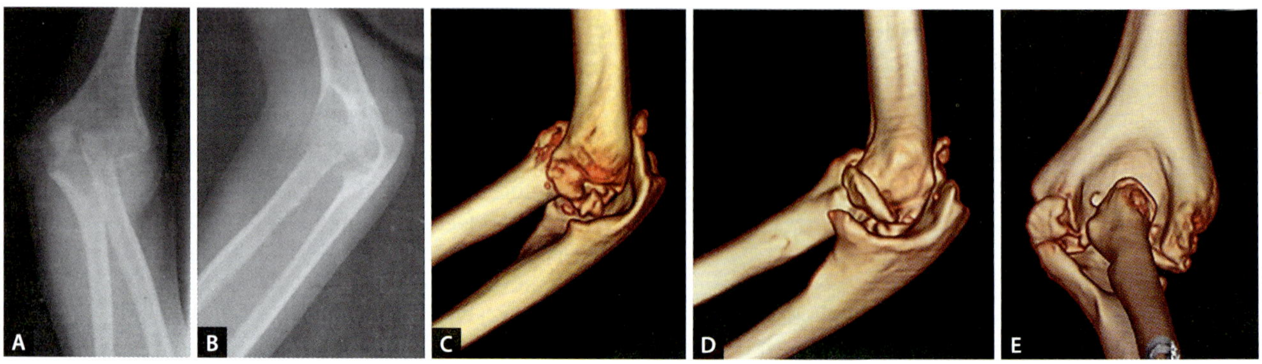

Figs. 11A to E: Congenital anterior radial head dislocation. (A and B) Plain radiographs; (C to E) Noncontrast computed tomography scans of left elbow.

dislocation). The longitudinal axis of radius does not bisect capitellum. The radial head is dome shaped or convex rather than normal concave shape (differential from traumatic dislocation of radial head). The ulna is also bowed proximally (differential from traumatic dislocation), the bow is volar in anterior dislocation and dorsal in posterior dislocation. In an infant, due to absence of radial epiphysis diagnosis has to be made by ultrasonography. Radiological diagnostic criteria have been proposed by McFarland that include:

- Absent or hypoplastic and flattened capitellum
- Prominent ulna epicondyle of humerus
- Partially abnormal trochlea
- Domed radial head with a long neck and negative ulnar variance at wrist.

Differential Diagnosis

Traumatic dislocation of radial head **(*see* Table 4)**, Old unreduced Monteggia fracture dislocation.

Treatment

Long-term complications of severe deformity include loss of motion and development of osteochondral loose bodies. For a symptomatic patient at or near skeletal maturity, radial head excision is recommended. Before skeletal maturity an older child say >5 years of age, the complications are too many to recommend surgical intervention, except removal of osteochondral loose bodies. These loose bodies may cause mechanical blocking to movements or arthrosis later on. So this means that observation is the first-line treatment in these children. This is logical because attempts at restoring proximal radioulnar and radiocapitellar joint anatomy by remodeling has not been surgically successful and it also does not improve movements at the elbow. Restriction of elbow movements are of little concern in this disease so improving it surgically is futile and also the patients present late mostly after 5-6 years of age when the anatomy is so much disturbed and remodeling potential lost that restoring it is not possible. Still, some people have tried open radial head reduction along with ulna lengthening or radial shortening + annular ligament reconstruction and radial or ulnar osteotomies with lengthening device for gradual radial head reduction but the results have been discouraging if done in children >2–3 years of age. Annular ligament reconstruction and radial head relocation may be done early in life (<2 years). Early identification of the disease by ultrasonography is mandatory for this to be successful, but the disease is not so common that advising routine ultrasound for diagnosis in infancy (like DDH) is recommendable. Still recurrent dislocations, failure of reconstructed annular ligament, elbow stiffness, etc., are common so balancing risk to benefits is a must. The complications of radial head resection include:

- Painful bony regrowth of the proximal radius
- Wrist pain
- Radioulnar synostosis
- Proximal migration of the radius and radiocapitellar impingement
- Cubitus valgus deformity and tardy ulnar nerve palsy
- Posterior interosseous nerve injury

These complications, however, arise after resection of traumatic conditions and possibly do not hold true for congenital conditions. Bony regrowth and radiocapitellar impingement are the most troublesome aspects here.

TABLE 4: The differences between congenital and traumatic radial head dislocation.

Congenital radial head dislocation	*Traumatic radial head dislocation*
Commonly bilateral	Mostly unilateral
No history of trauma	History of injury to elbow present May be associated with Monteggia fracture
Mostly painless	Painful
Mild functional limitations such as restricted rotations at elbow and terminal restriction of extension	• Functional limitation is significant and is mostly due to pain • Painless limitation of rotations at elbow may be due to radioulnar synostosis
Radial head loses its concave depression and instead becomes convex	Maintained concavity of radial head
Hypoplastic capitellum	Normal capitellum
Malformed trochlea	Normal trochlea
Prominent ulnar epicondyle of humerus	Not so
Associated smooth ulnar bow	Uncommon unless associated with old neglected monteggia fracture dislocation
Associated other congenital anomalies	Not typical

CONGENITAL PROXIMAL RADIOULNAR SYNOSTOSIS

Congenital proximal radioulnar synostosis (CPRUS) results from failure of normal prenatal separation of the radius and ulna. During the embryonic period of fetal development, the humerus, radius and ulna are conjoined. Longitudinal segmentation begins distally. For some time, the proximal ends are united and share a common perichondrium that then separate gradually. Genetic or teratogenic factors can disrupt this separation and radioulnar joint development, leading to bony synostosis. In most instances, radioulnar synostosis is bilateral and affects males and females with equal frequency with the synostosis being almost always proximal (distal congenital synostosis has been rarely described). The radioulnar junction is initially cartilaginous but eventually ossifies. The radial head may be dislocated or absent, and the forearm is typically fixed in pronation (fetal position). Disease is bilateral in 60–80% of cases. The malformation occurs in isolation but uncommon associations have been described in literature as follows:

- Apert syndrome (acrocephalosyndactyly)
- Carpenter syndrome (acropolysyndactyly)
- Klinefelter syndrome
- Arthrogryposis
- Acrofacial dysostoses of Nager and mandibulofacial dysostosis
- Symphalangism

- Clubfoot
- Thumb hypoplasia
- Carpal coalition
- Fetal alcohol syndrome
- Cardiovascular (tetralogy of Fallot and ventricular septal defects) and thoracic (hypoplasia of the first and second ribs) anomalies

The cause is unknown but autosomal dominant inheritance has been reported.

Clinical Presentation

The children usually present during 3–6 years of age or are often neglected until adolescence when they seek medical help themselves. Parents or teachers realize the inability of the child to perform activities with an open hand (supinated) and has to catch the ball or any object in hyperpronation. The children usually have a forearm fixed in pronation of varying degrees. Pronation more than 60° causes greater morbidity. About 10–20° of elbow contracture is noticeable though the ROM at elbow is free and painless. Shortening of the forearm is more apparent in unilateral cases. There is compensatory hypermobility of wrist and shoulder in older children. The functional limitations in all are not great and children are not really concerned with the deficit. There are two forms of presentation:

- *Type 1* with a bony synostosis between the bones due to complete failure of separation of the proximal region.
- *Type 2* is a less severe form with a rudimentary joint developing before developmental arrest, a rudimentary radial head will develop in such cases.

Radiology

Plain radiographs depict the synostosis **(Fig. 12)**. In type 2 form, there is presence of rudimentary radial head but it is often posteriorly or posterolaterally subluxated. In complete synostosis, the radial head is absent and there is always an increased anterior bow of the radius. Occasionally, there will be a patient with limited forearm rotation and normal radiographs. MRI in such cases reveals a cartilaginous synostosis that has yet to ossify or a fibrous tether.

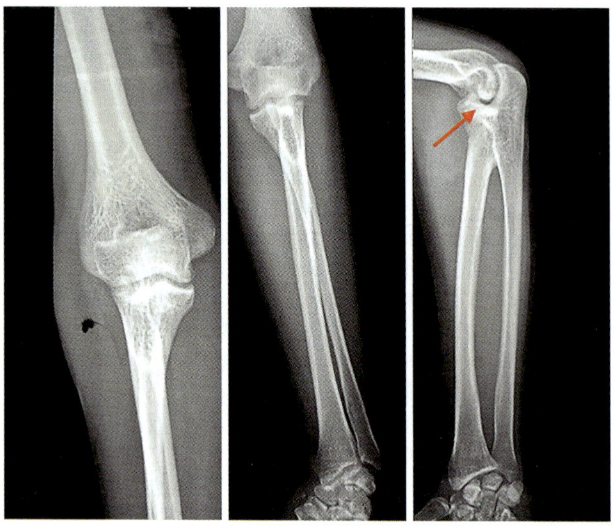

Fig. 12: Proximal radioulnar synostosis. The radiodense bar connects the radius and ulna proximally (arrow).

Treatment

For patients with severe fixed pronation (more than 60° and/or bilateral disease) and functional limitations (e.g., children with fetal alcohol syndrome), an osteotomy through the bony synostosis or distal radius can be performed to rotate the forearm into a more functional position. The functional position is, however, debatable. Functional use and need of supination varies with the region and social needs. Western recommendation is placing the nondominant forearm in neutral rotation and dominant forearm in 10–20° of pronation for bilateral disease. However, 0–15° of pronation has been found sufficient for unilateral disease. In developing countries and the need of ablution surgeons advocate placing the nondominant forearm in 20–35° of supination and the dominant forearm in 10–30° pronation for bilateral disease.

Surgery to regain function and successfully remove synostosis has been uniformly a failure. Reported procedures include resection of the synostotic proximal radius saving the bicipital tuberosity with and without muscle interposition; division of the interosseous membrane and muscle, fat, fascia or silastic interposition after synostosis excision. Synostosis excision followed by free vascularized fascio-fat graft interposition has been reported to separate the radius and ulna, restore motion, and prevent reformation of the synostosis but is technically demanding. Most surgeons prefer derotation osteotomy through fusion mass and fixation with pins. Few have attempted gradual correction with Ilizarov apparatus following osteotomy.

Complications of Surgical Procedure

- *Vascular compromise and compartment syndrome (rotational osteotomy):* Commonly occur with more than 80° of rotational correction. The increasing analgesia requirement and a high level of anxiety, are the most diagnostic clinical signs of compartment syndrome in children. Routine measurement of compartment pressures is recommended. Immediately the oblique k-wire should be removed while maintaining the longitudinal ulnar k-wire to possibly gradually achieve the correction later. If there is no improvement then emergent fascial release is required
- Neurovascular injury (Ilizarov method)
- Infection
- Loss of correction
- Nonunion

RADIAL LONGITUDINAL DEFICIENCY

Radial longitudinal deficiency represents a spectrum of upper limb hypoplasia (dysplasia) that may range from mild hypoplasia of thumb to absence of radius or even proximal humerus. Radial clubhand (RCH) or radial dysplasia is a preaxial (occurring on the radial side, postaxial occurs on the ulnar side) longitudinal failure of formation. In 1733, Petit first described RCH on an autopsy specimen. Being preaxial, the radius aplasia is associated with thumb hypoplasia, or anomaly of the radial aspect of the carpus. The incidence is between 1 in 30,000 and 1 in 100,000 live births varying according to the region and ethnicity. It is bilateral in 50% of cases and is seen slightly more commonly in males than in females (3:2).

Pathogenesis

Earlier, it was thought to be either a congenital absence or an acquired defect secondary to syphilis. Later Kummel theorized abnormal pressure upon the embryo along the radial bud between the third and seventh week of gestation to cause RCH. It can be inherited as an autosomal dominant or recessive disorder while some cases are sporadic. The exact pathogenesis of RCH is unknown though it has been postulated that injury to the apical ectodermal ridge during upper limb development is the cause. The injury can occur from factors such as:

- Intrauterine compression
- Irradiation
- Vascular insult
- Inflammatory process
- Maternal drug exposure (thalidomide, insulin)

There is no specific genetic cause attributable to RCH except when it is associated with other congenital abnormalities. In such cases, the pattern of inheritance can be autosomal dominant or recessive, depending on the syndrome. There are many associated congenital syndromes **(Box 1)** and chromosomal anomalies. These are most often sporadic, however still. About 40% of patients with unilateral radial clubhand, and 27% of patients with bilateral radial clubhand, have associated malformations. These organ system malformations may present in a nonsyndromic pattern and may be associated with variable anomalies of the cardiac, craniofacial, hematopoietic, musculoskeletal, gastrointestinal and renal organ systems.

Natural History of Radial Clubhand

Generally the central nervous system of patients with radial clubhand (RCH) is normal. Children with higher grade anomalies use adaptive mechanisms. These generally include a spherical grip, chest arm grip and lateral pinch to compensate for the absence of opposition. Children with unilateral disease adapt so well that no functional impairment is seen in these patients. Individuals with bilateral involvement have more difficulty. In patients with bilateral disease, activities of daily living, such as hygiene, eating and dressing, are affected. Kotwal et al. found that patients without surgical correction were more limited than surgically treated patients even with well-developed adaptations. Also, the issue of the cosmetic and psychologic impact of radial dysplasia (peer-comparison) is difficult to quantify and definitely plays a role in development and functional aspect of patients.

BOX 1: Syndromic associations of radial clubhand.

- *VACTERRLS:* VATER (vertebral anomalies, anal atresia, tracheoesophageal fistula and renal anomalies) + cardiac abnormalities + radial longitudinal deficiency + lower limb anomalies + single umbilical artery.
- *Holt-Oram syndrome:* Upper-limb malformations and major cardiac malformations inherited in an autosomal dominant fashion. Unusual presentation of RCH are common in this syndrome that include presence of atypical radio-ulnar synostosis extending distally into forearm or first web-space syndactyly. Such patients should be evaluated in genetic clinic and pediatric cardiologist consultation obtained.
- *Fanconi anemia:* Characteristic facial features (microphthalmos, strabismus, hearing deficits), pancytopenia, progressive bone marrow failure inherited in an autosomal recessive fashion. This can be diagnosed with the mitomycin-C chromosomal challenge test.
- *Thrombocytopenia with absent radius (TAR syndrome):* Thrombocytopenia is present at birth that usually improves with growth.
- *Chromosomal anomalies:* Trisomy 13, 18 and 21.

Pathoanatomy

Radial dysplasia involves various skeletal malformations from the most proximal parts of limb to distally but all on the radial (preaxial) side. These are paralleled by soft-tissue deficiencies of the hand, wrist, and forearm. The severity of the soft-tissue loss also parallels the skeletal deficiency. Associated skeletal anomalies with radial longitudinal deficiency include:

- Small scapula
- Short clavicle with an increased curvature
- The humerus may be short with deficiencies of the capitellum and trochlea.
- Elbow movements are usually diminished (more restriction of flexion than extension).
- The forearm is always reduced in length.
- The ulna is approximately 60% of the normal length at the time of birth. This discrepancy persists throughout the growth period.
- True forearm rotation is absent in patients with partial or complete aplasia of the radius.
- The articulation between the carpus and ulna is usually fibrous and abnormal.
- Wrist motion is primarily in the radial or ulnar plane with limited flexion or extension.
- Ossification of the carpal bones is delayed.
- The scaphoid and trapezium are often absent or hypoplastic.
- The capitate, hamate and triquetrum ossify late.

Muscular anomalies include:

- The preaxial muscles arising from the lateral epicondyle (radial wrist extensors and brachioradialis) are often absent or deficient (normally innervated by the radial nerve) along with pronator quadratus. These structures are replaced by a fibrous tissue (radial anlage) that maintains or worsens wrist deformity during growth.
- The deltoid or pectoralis major muscle can be hypoplastic or partially absent.
- The biceps may be absent or fused to the underlying brachialis muscle.
- The extrinsic flexors and extensors of the fingers are usually adherent.
- The abnormalities of the thumb muscles are related to the degree of thumb hypoplasia.

Neurovascular structures include:

- The radial nerve often terminates at the elbow and interosseous sensory nerve is absen.t
- An enlarged median nerve substitutes for the absence of the radial nerve and supplies a dorsal branch for dorsoradial sensibility.
- The radial artery is often absent, and the interosseous arteries usually remain patent.
- The blood supply to the hand comes through the ulnar artery, and possibly the interosseous vessels or a persistent median artery.

Clinical Features

These depend on the severity of involvement and associated anomalies present. The clinical features of radial longitudinal deficiency typically include elbow flexion contracture, variably shortened and bowed forearms, radial wrist deviation **(Figs. 13A and B)**, and variable thumb hypoplasia or aplasia. Parallel deficiencies appear in radial soft-tissue structures (see below). The RCH has been classified usually according to the Bayne system **(Table 5)**, the types represent incremental deficiency of the radius. Type I deformity has a defective distal radial physis causing foreshortening of the radius and a prominent distal ulna. Despite radial deviation and radial shortening, problems arising from radioulnar incongruity such as triangular fibrocartilage tears, ulnocarpal impaction syndrome, and distal radioulnar joint pain usually do not occur. Thumb hypoplasia with opposition weakness is the major disabling feature here. Type II deficiency involves limited proximal and distal radial physeal growth and the ulna bows. The thumb hypoplasia is usually more significant, with more deficiency of the radial carpus. Type III deficiency is the absence of the distal two-thirds of the radius. Deformities are more severe and there are associated thumb and finger abnormalities of hypoplasia **(Figs. 13A and B)** and camptodactyly. Type IV deficiency involves complete absence of the radius with marked ulnar bow. The thumb is usually absent or rudimentary (pouce flottans). The index, long and even ring rays are often involved. The function at elbow, hand, wrist and forearm are compromised. Global classification of RCH **(Table 6)** has been also proposed that additionally takes into account the thumb and carpal anomalies, and proximal radius deficiency in addition to the distal radius deficiency. Conventionally, the thumb hypoplasia associated with RCH is classified on the basis of modified Blauth system **(Table 7)**. Usually orthopedic surgeon is the first medical contact for these children because of the obvious deformity and consultation being sought for it. A thorough evaluation of associated abnormalities **(*see* Box 1)** and if possible correction to optimization surgical risk is needed. Commonly prescribed "battery" of tests for evaluation of these children include complete blood count, echocardiogram, abdominal ultrasonography and diepoxybutane testing (for Fanconi anemia).

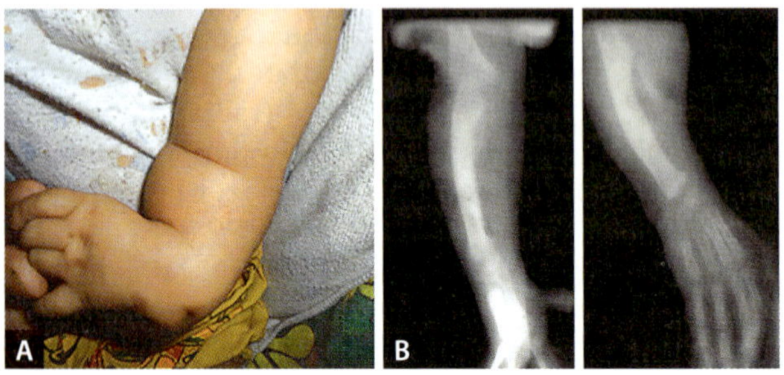

Figs. 13A and B: Radial clubhand. (A) Clinical deformity with the appearance of a "golf club" giving it the characteristic name; (B) Radiograph showing small radial bone enlarge (Type 4, Bayne).

TABLE 5: Radial clubhand is classified into the following four types (Bayne), based on the amount of radius present.

Type I deficiency	*Mildest form:* There is mild shortening of the radius (distal) without considerable bowing. Minor radial deviation of the hand is apparent, although considerable thumb hypoplasia may be evident. Ulna straight.
Type II deficiency	*Small radius with shortening from both ends:* There are distal and proximal physeal abnormalities and moderate radial deviation ofthe wrist. Ulna bows.
Type III deficiency	*Partial radius absent:* Significant part of the radius is absent (most commonly the distal portion) and there is severe wrist radialdeviation.
Type IV deficiency	*Complete absence of radius:* It is the most common variant characterized by a complete absence of the radius. The hand acquires aperpendicular relationship to the forearm.

TABLE 6: Global classification of radial longitudinal deficiency.

Type	*Thumb anomaly*	*Carpal anomaly**	*Distal radius*	*Proximal radius*
N	Absence or hypoplasia	Normal	Normal	Normal
0	Absence or hypoplasia	Absence, hypoplasia, or coalition	Normal	Normal, radioulnar synostosis or radial head dislocation
1	Absence or hypoplasia	Absence, hypoplasia, or coalition	>2 mm shorter than ulna	Normal, radioulnar synostosis or radial head dislocation
2	Absence or hypoplasia	Absence, hypoplasia, or coalition	Hypoplasia	Hypoplasia
3	Absence or hypoplasia	Absence, hypoplasia, or coalition	Physis absent	Variable hypoplasia
4	Absence or hypoplasia	Absence, hypoplasia, or coalition	Absence	Absence

*Carpal anomaly includes hypoplasia, coalition, absence or bipartite carpal bones. Hypoplasia and absence are more common on the radial side of the carpus, and coalitions are more frequent on the ulnar side.

TABLE 7: Classification of thumb hypoplasia (after Buck-Gramcko's and Manske's modification of the Blauth's classification).

Type I	Mild underdevelopment
Type II	Thenar hypoplasia, abduction contracture, MCP laxity
Type III	• Thenar hypoplasia, abduction contracture, MCP instability, extrinsic tendon hypoplasia, metacarpal underdevelopment • Stable carpometacarpal joint
AB	• Unstable carpometacarpal joint
Type IV	Pouce flottant
Type V	Complete absence of thumb

(MCP: metacarpophalangeal)

Treatment

The goals of treatment are:

- To correct basic deformity (radial deviation of the wrist) - although this is the contention of all corrective surgeries done for treating congenital anomalies but it has been found that in adult patients with RCH grip strength, key pinch, forearm length and elbow and finger motion is more important than radial angulation.
- Balance the wrist on the forearm
- Maintain wrist and hand position and function (particularly finger weakness)
- Improve opposition by recreating thumb function—this has a significant bearing on the acceptance of results and overall outcome of treatment.
- Improve social and emotional aspect of patients.

Nonsurgical Intervention

Corrective casting, bracing and physical therapy are used in infancy to achieve passive correction of the radial deviation. Simultaneously the elbow extension contracture is also corrected to improve function. It is recommended that all patients undergo passive stretching to improve suppleness whether planned for future surgery or not. In mild cases, a home-based exercise program of wrist ulnar deviation and distraction stretching is taught whilst in more severe cases it involves serial corrective casting or splinting to gradually stretch the contracted soft tissues. Splinting is difficult in a newborn due to rapidly changing size so is commonly reserved for maintenance phase. For failed attempts to passively correct the radial deviation contracture by 6–12 weeks of vigorous conservative treatment, external fixation with gradual distraction of soft tissues and obtaining musculoskeletal alignment is considered. Maintenance of correction is done using night-time corrective splinting program till surgical stable correction is done. In patients with grade 1 or sometimes grade 2 deformity, this conservative treatment itself may suffice. Children with greater deformity are candidates for operative correction generally undertaken at 10–12 months of age.

Surgical Treatment

Surgery is usually undertaken at around 1 year of age that allows maturation and formation of anatomical structures to be identified distinctly and improvement in forearm length. Also by this time discrete fixed motor learned skills of the patient have not fully developed so they can be easily retrained. Correcting deformity around this time will give the child adequate time for better adaption to motor functions and avoid trick movements. To the surgeon this allows enough time for additional reconstruction for thumb hypoplasia in a staged manner (or sometimes even simultaneously). Children with bilateral deficiencies that affect both the forearm and thumb require staged treatment. It was shown by Kotwal et al. that surgical intervention of RCH (centralization or radialization) improves cosmesis, function and ease of performance of activities in comparison to nonoperative management especially in Bayne type 3 or 4. There are, however, instances where surgery is contraindicated for specific reasons that include:

- Medically unfit patient or limited life expectancy in a child
- Mild deformity with acceptable carpus support
- An elbow extension contracture that prevents the hand from reaching the mouth
- Development of adaptive movements for grip and pinch (older children)
- Severe index finger deformity and weakness that will result in failed pollicization.

The surgical intervention for RCH is commonly divided into two aspects:

1. To correct the wrist deformity and
2. To correct the functionally limiting thumb deficiency (See also the detailed discussion on thumb hypoplasia and aplasia later in the chapter).

The various surgical options for the wrist deformity correction and stabilization include:

- Centralization of carpus over ulna **(Figs. 14A and B)**
- Radialization
- Wrist fusion

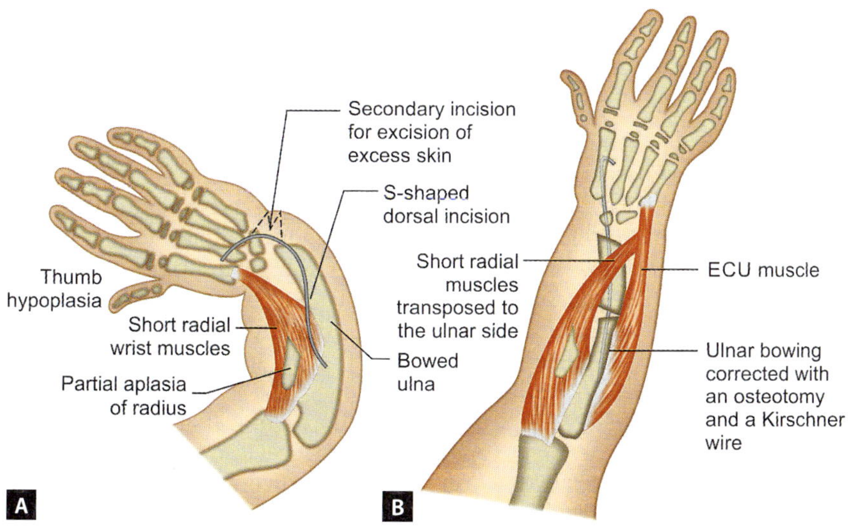

Figs. 14A and B: Radial clubhand. Illustration depicting centralization of carpus over ulna. (ECU: Extensor carpi ulnaris)

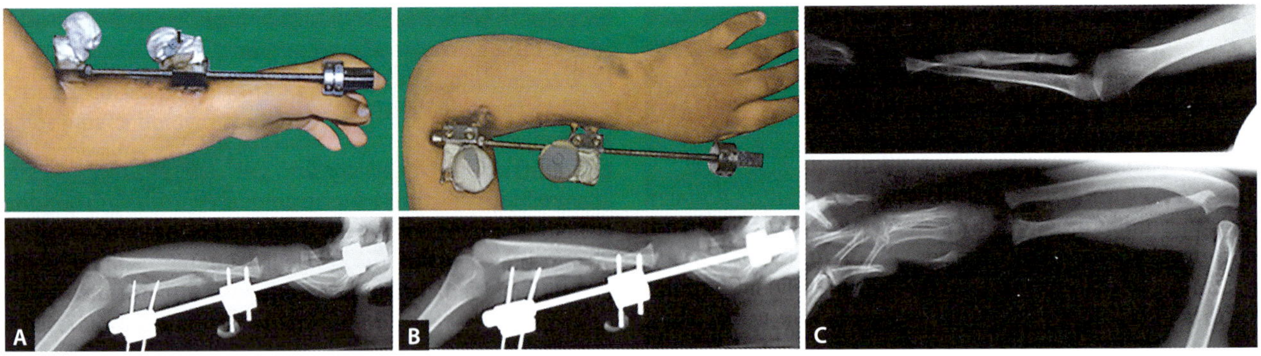

Figs. 15A to C: Radial clubhand distraction lengthening of radius using Joshi's external stabilization system distractor. Regular distraction and follow-up of patient (A and B) and final follow-up radiographs (C) with corrected deformity.

- Lengthening of radius by distractors **(Figs. 15A to C)**
- Bone graft procedures to the ulna.
- Release of radial soft tissue and volar bilobed flap transposition.

Centralization or radialization is indicated in RCH types III and IV, in which there is severe deformity and insufficient support to the carpus. Controlled lengthening of radius by a distractor can be performed after osteotomy in patients with radius shortening (type 2) to rebalance the wrist.

Surgical options for thumb anomalies are more limited and include:

- Recreating first-web space, opponensplasty
- Pollicization
- Microvascular toe-to-thumb transfer.

A hypoplastic thumb may be surgically corrected with first web space deepening, metacarpophalangeal (MCP) joint stabilization, and opponensplasty tendon transfer while pollicization is required for aplasia.

Bone grafting of ulna was the earliest form of surgical correction for RCH. This was aimed to reconstruct distal radius. Various authors described the use of nonvascularized bone grafts from the proximal fibula to the ulna in Y-configuration to support the carpus and hand. These procedures gave short-term improvement but ultimately failed due to absent growth of the graft and recurrent deformity resulting from continued ulna growth. Vascularized bone grafting has been again advocated recently but is tedious and requires expertise. This finds limited usage in the current management of RCH.

Centralization of the carpus over the third metacarpal has been a standard treatment for long period practiced by surgeons world over. The typical steps of centralization include:

- Transverse ulnar incision and removal of ellipse of skin
- Preserving the enlarged median nerve after identification in the skinfold
- Ulnar capsulotomy
- Soft tissue release of the radial contracture and notching the carpus to accept ulna.
- Contouring of the ulna to match the carpal notch
- Capsular reefing
- Extensor carpi ulnaris (ECU) tendon advancement
- Aligning the third metacarpal on ulna and stabilization with pin fixation until healing
- *Modifications:*
  - Lamb (166) advocated modifying the technique by notching the carpus to inset the distal ulna. This lessened recurrence, but also decreased wrist motion and increased early ulnar physeal closure postoperatively. Function is but impaired when there is less than 30° of wrist motion postoperatively.
  - Transfer of flexor carpi ulnaris (FCU) to ECU
  - Transfer of index and long finger flexor digitorum superficialis (FDS) to dorsal side
  - Using a zig-zag dorsal incision to do plasty later
  - Evans flap to avoid skin buckling on ulnar aspect.

Buck-Gramcko introduced ***radialization*** for anatomical redirection of distractive forces during the thalidomide crisis. The carpals are overcorrected and preserved (no notching) and wrist is balanced by tendon transfers of the radial wrist motors (extensor carpi radialis, flexor carpi radialis) to the dorsal ulnar wrist. Tendon transfer are required to balance the carpals over small ulna. Here, the ulna is aligned with the second (index finger) metacarpal and fixed with a pin. If there is a concomitant ulnar bow of greater than 30°, ulnar osteotomy should also be performed after centralization or radialization. This usually involves a multiple-level open osteotomy and intramedullary fixation that can be done with the same k-wire used for fixation of carpus.

Wrist fusion is not performed in young patients. This leads to loss of wrist motion and potential loss of ulnar physeal growth. People have tried concomitant lengthening of ulna with wrist fusion but as mentioned before loss of wrist movements produces poor functional results.

Thumb reconstruction should be done before 18 months of age as a staged (higher grade RCH deformity) or a concomitant procedure (milder forms) to better develop the pinch grip. In the mild forms of radial dysplasia, the thumb hypoplasia can be corrected by deepening the first web space with Z-plasties or rotation flaps. Additional release of adductor and first dorsal interosseous fascia is often necessary. The MCP joint should be stabilized by one of the following methods:

- Using local fascia or extra FDS tendon length for ligament reconstruction.
- MCP joint chondrodesis (fusion of the proximal phalanx epiphysis to the metacarpal head) or arthrodesis.

Opponensplasty is performed simultaneously with the use of the abductor digiti quinti or ring-finger FDS, or accessory digital extensors with equal success.

Thumb aplasia is best addressed with pollicization of index finger. Toe-to-thumb microvascular transfers have been reported, but the results of index-finger pollicization are fantastic. For microvascular transfer, the quality of index-finger donor determines reconstructed thumb function. The commonly reported unacceptable complications are stiff and weak thumb due to camptodactyly. Frequent development of compensatory lateral pinch between adjacent digits. The results of pollicization are better only if additional opponensplasty are done else there are high chances of developing a weak and just structural thumb.

Complications of Various Surgical Procedures

The commonly reported complications of corrective surgeries for radial clubhand are listed below:
- *Recurrent deformity:* More common with radialization procedures, if the balancing fails.
- *Premature closure of the distal ulnar physis:* More common with centralization and leads to gross cosmetic and functional limitation
- Pin tract irritation and infection
- Transient loss of finger movements
- Incomplete correction

MADELUNG'S DEFORMITY

{Also known as Carpus curvus, radius curvus, progressive subluxation of the wrist, manus valgus, manus furca and idiopathic progressive curvature of the radius.}

History

Dupuytren (1834) attributed the deformity to a repetitive occupational injury. Nelaton (1847) superficially and uncharacteristically described an anatomic specimen possibly similar to Madelung's deformity. The term Madelung's deformity (MD) was coined after the German surgeon named Otto W Madelung in 1878 at the Seventh German Surgical Congress of 1878 as "Die spontane subluxation der hand nocte vorne" for the characteristic "spontaneous forward subluxation of the hand". He was the first to accurately describe the anatomic differences and possible causes of this rare congenital wrist deformity which was similar to other pediatric growth deformities such as genu varum.

Introduction

Madelung's deformity is a rare congenital, characteristic anatomic abnormality of distal radial growth caused by disturbance of the volar and ulnar distal radial physis leading to asymmetric growth. The deformity is characterized by ulnar and palmar curvature of the distal radius, positive ulnar variance and proximal subsidence of the lunate.
- True incidence in unknown
- There is no racial distribution.
- Females are affected more than males (4:1).
- Bilateral disease (>50% cases) is much more common.
- Deformity can accompany syndromes such as mesomelic dwarfism, mucopolysaccharidoses, etc.

There is typical presence of a thick volar ligament (called Vicker's ligament) that tethers the lunate to the distal radius. It is fibrous or fibrocartilaginous, 5–7 mm thick band like structure that inserts into the anterior surface of the lunate and the anterior radioulnar ligament portion of the triangular fibrocartilage complex (TFCC). It is a secondary pathologic structure rather than a primary abnormality. It may be arising from coalescence of normal structures. This ligament, however, causes the wrist to deform even more due to tension it creates between the structures and even myofibroblasts have been identified that may further lead to shortening of the ligament. MD often has a genetic etiology commonly localized to a mutation on the X chromosome. The deformity has to be treated surgically by correcting bony deformity and ligamentous lesions, correcting the abnormal position of the radial articular surface, and equalizing the longitudinal levels of the distal radius and ulna.

Etiology

On the basis of etiology, MD is classified into four different groups by Henry and Thorburn which are as follows:
1. Post-traumatic
2. Dysplastic
3. Chromosomal or genetic (Turner syndrome)
4. Idiopathic or primary

The post-traumatic deformity has been found following repetitive trauma or following a single event that disrupts growth of the distal radial ulnar-volar physis. Secondary causes of wrist deformity that may mimic MD include sickle-cell disease, infection, tumor and rickets. Bone dysplasias associated with MD include:
- Multiple hereditary osteochondromatosis
- Ollier disease
- Achondroplasia
- Multiple epiphyseal dysplasias
- Mucopolysaccharidoses (e.g., Hurler and Morquio syndromes)
- Dyschondrosteosis (Leri-Weill syndrome-mesomelic dwarfism inherited as autosomal dominant trait)

Genetics

The pattern of inheritance varies, with some cases following a pseudoautosomal pattern and many others lacking a clear family history. MD is transmitted in an autosomal dominant fashion in one-third of cases with variable expression and 50% penetrance.

A primary chromosomal association with Madelung's deformity has been observed in patients with Turner syndrome (karyotype XO). The idea that an X chromosomal translocation causing dyschondrosteosis was first proposed in 1985. An X chromosomal translocation also was found to be associated with MD in 1997. Molecular genetic studies have clarified the association of the female predominant MD, dyschondrosteosis, and the missing X chromosome in Turner syndrome.

A marker has been identified in the pseudoautosomal region (PAR1) of the X and Y chromosomes. Within families affected by a short stature dysplasia, there are some deletions and a premature stop codon (exon 4) in the short stature homeobox (*SHOX*)-containing gene, SHOX that segregated the marker in band Xp22. The *SHOX* gene mutation has been found in patients with dyschondrosteosis and MD. Families with this mutation and individuals with Turner syndrome (both essentially hemizygous individuals for the *SHOX* gene) and families with a history of MD have been shown to exhibit a variable expression of MD and dyschondrosteosis. The variability in expression indicates that a modifier gene on another area of the X chromosome or on an autosomal gene is also. The *SHOX* mutation is under study for association.

Presentation

Symptoms usually begin during adolescence only and most commonly in girls aged 10–14 years. MD is observed very rarely in males. Patients experience increasing deformity and pain in the wrist with decreased ROM. On physical examination, the deformity varies in degree from a slight protrusion of the lower end of the ulna abutting the carpus and becomes prominent dorsally relative to the carpus and hand. There is complete dislocation of the inferior radioulnar joint in advanced disease with marked radial deviation of the hand. The hand is translated volarly to the long axis of the forearm. ROM is decreased, with a limitation of supination, dorsiflexion and radial deviation. Pronation and flexion usually are normal.

Investigation

Radiographs

Posteroanterior (PA) and lateral plain radiographs of the forearm and wrist usually suffice as standard radiological investigation, it is better to obtain marked films to estimate the length of future wedge correction. Carter and Ezaki protocol for obtaining the PA view of forearm in patients with MD. Both right and left forearm images are placed on the same radiographic plate for comparison. The true PA radiograph is obtained with the forearm in neutral rotation, the elbow at 90° of flexion, and the shoulder abducted to 90°. According to them, this method of analysis is useful in preoperative planning. A lateral radiograph is obtained by rotating the shoulder to the side of the patient and laying the ulnar border of the forearm on the plate.

There are several distinct radiographic features of MD.

Dannenberg et al. described elements of radiographic diagnosis after their review of 172 cases. The diagnostic criteria included are (*see* **Figs. 16A and B** for most of the radiographic features are seen here):

- Lateral and dorsal curvature of the radius
- Widened interosseous space
- True shortening of the total length of the radius
- Premature fusion of the ulnar half of the distal radial physis
- Focal osteopenia in the area of the ulnar portion of the distal radius appearing as a "flame-like" lesion corresponding to the attachment of ligament of Vickers
- Exostosis at the distal ulnar border of the radius
- Triangularization of the distal radial epiphysis
- Ulnar and palmar facing distal radial articular surface
- Relative dorsal subluxation of the ulna
- Increased radiodensity of the ulnar head
- Carpal wedging with the lunate at the apex of the wedge
- An arched curvature of the carpal bones in direct continuation of the dorsal bowing of the radius on the lateral radiograph
- An increased radial tilt on the PA radiograph and the radial epiphysis becomes teardrop shaped. On the lateral view, the radius tilts volarward and the ulna appears dislocated from its normal articulation with the radius. The ulna lies dorsal to the proximal carpal row. The distal ulna does not actually sublux dorsally **(Figs. 16A and B)**. Rather, the hand and radius are translated palmarward, resulting in incongruence of the distal radioulnar joint (DRUJ) injuries. The unaffected ulna continues to grow, ultimately becoming longer than the ulnar aspect of the radius.

Vickers and Nielsen used a physeal measurement for preoperative and postoperative assessment of severity and correction, respectively. PA radiographs are used for measurement, as lateral views have too much variation to be of value. The longitudinal and transverse axes of the radius are difficult to determine due to the considerable bowing of the radius. The ulna usually is straight, which provides a reliable longitudinal axis. Therefore, a perpendicular

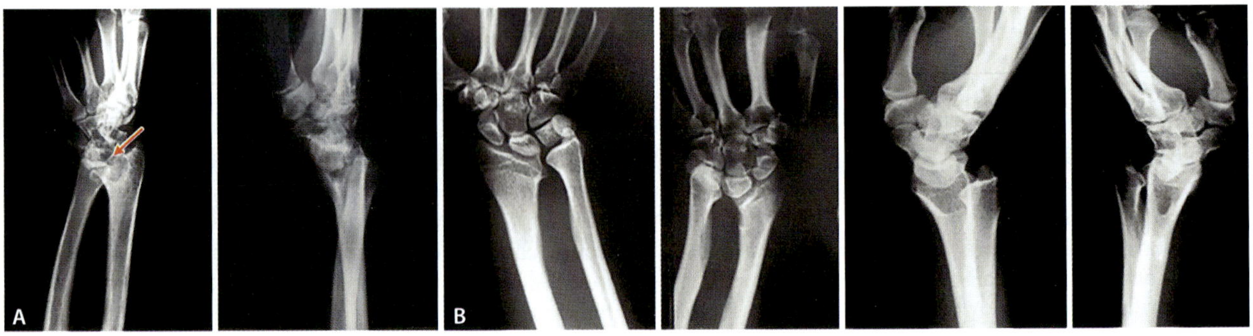

Figs. 16A and B: Madelung's deformity: Classic radiographic appearance with volar ulnar translation of carpals over radius. (A) Note the flame-shaped defect in distal radius corresponding to the "ligament if Vickers"(arrow); (B) Bilateral Madelung's deformity in a patient, more severe at left wrist, note the volar ulnar physeal defect and apparent dorsal subluxation of ulna with widened interosseous space.

line to the long axis of the ulna can be passed through the most radial extent of the radial physis. A line joining the most radial and ulnar extents of the physis is drawn. The angle subtended by the transverse line and the physeal line is termed the physeal angle. With increasing severity, the lunate follows the ulnar-volar corner and eventually becomes interposed between the radius and ulna. The relative position of the proximal aspect of the lunate can be measured from the transverse line.

CT Scan or Tomogram

For better understanding, computed tomography scans should be done as the deformity is three-dimensional. These studies help in precise visualization of physeal and articular morphology. They are not a part of standard work- up of the patient.

Treatment

Nonsurgical

Rest and nonsteroidal anti-inflammatory drugs (NSAIDs) are the treatments initially offered usually as interim measure till definite surgery is planned. If no improvement is made, a splint or brace can be used to keep the deviated arm straight. If pain is predominantly DRUJ pain, then a sugar-tong-type splint is used to prevent joint irritation from over activity. If pain is radiocarpal, then a volar splint should be used. Often the conservative measures fail as the malformation is progressive with a continuous conspicuous increase in deformity with growth and surgical intervention is designated. The acceptability to deformity and disability should be, however, always assessed individually (as we all differ) before pushing surgery.

Surgical

In general physiolysis with release of Vicker's ligament is proposed for treating younger skeletally immature patients. In older, skeletally mature patients, combinations of epiphyseodesis, lateral closing wedge osteotomy or dome osteotomy, and ulnar shortening osteotomy may be performed.

- *Physiolysis (Vickers and Nielsen):* Here removal of the epiphyseal band is done that causes the abnormal growth of the wrist. The region of defective physis is approached through volar-radial incision (ulnar to classic Henry's approach) going between flexor pollicis longus (FPL) and palmaris longus leaving the median nerve and radial artery protected. The pronator quadratus muscle is identified and detached from the radius. The abnormal epiphysis is identified and released carefully to prevent formation of bone bar. Fat or silastic material interposition can also be done. This procedure is always combined with the Vickers ligament release.
- *Correction of radius deformity by dome osteotomy* ***(Fig. 17)****:* This osteotomy has the advantage to straighten the abnormal radius by three dimensional correction of the deformity while maintaining adequate bony contact.

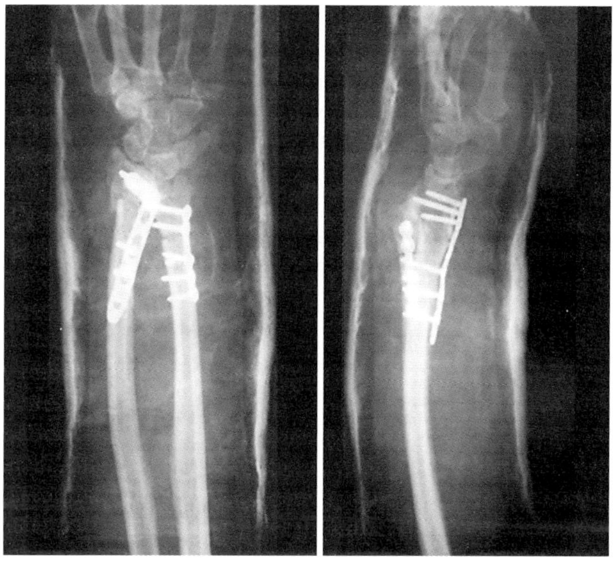

Fig. 17: Osteotomy for correction of Madelung's deformity.

- *Vicker's ligament release:* The Vicker's ligament originates on the radius in a fossa that is seen radiographically as a flame-shaped radiolucency distal to a bone spur on the ulnar aspect of the distal metaphysis. The purpose of its release is to remove the tension and leave the wrist straight for further growth.
- *Ulna shortening:* Adults with MD may suffer from ulnar-sided wrist pain. Apart from the usual treatment by distal radial osteotomy if patients have a positive ulnar variance and focal wrist pathology, ulnar-shortening osteotomy is helpful. In these patients, the radial deformity may or may not be simultaneously treated.
- *Distal radioulnar joint replacement:* An alternative treatment for patients with ulnar-sided wrist pain is a total replacement of the distal radioulnar joint. The prosthesis helps in managing the pain and may also improve ROM of wrist.
- *Radioulnar length adjustment:* There is relative dorsal subluxation of growing ulna on the volar radius in MD. This disparity can be addressed by ulnar shortening, ulnar head resection or a Sauve-Kapandji-type (Lauenstein) DRUJ arthrodesis.

Complications of Operative Treatment

- Postoperative wound infections
- Reflex sympathetic dystrophy
- Recurrent deformity after continued growth

CENTRAL DEFICIENCY

Central deficiency, also called cleft hand, is rare with estimated incidence of 1 in every 90,000–150,000 live births. It was previously classified as typical or atypical deficiency but now the standard terms are "cleft hand" and "symbrachydactyly," respectively **(Fig. 18)**. Symbrachydactyly has unilateral central digital deficiencies and simple syndactylies. It is a sporadic event without genetic inheritance and comprises of multiple absent digital rays. There are often finger nubbins

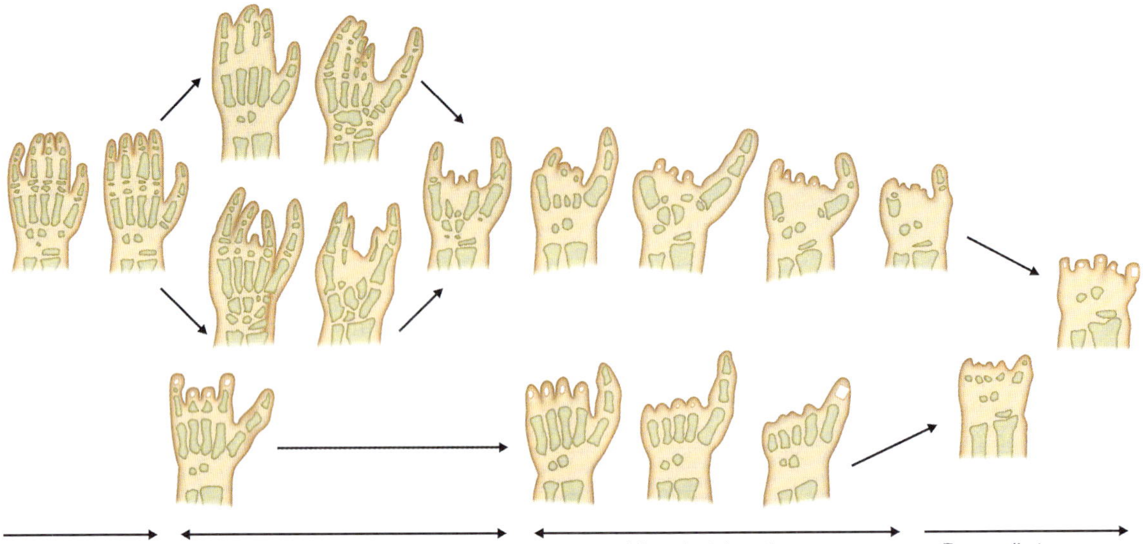

Fig. 18: Classification of central deficiency of hand.

present (not seen with cleft hand). Symbrachydactyly is a transverse deficiency and may represent an advanced form of transverse absence of digits. Cleft hand on the other hand represents basically a longitudinal deficiency in the center of hand. Although, most instances of this central deficiency are unilateral and sporadic, it may sometimes be inherited in an autosomal dominant pattern where it is often associated with cleft feet. There are often radial and ulnar syndactylies or digital hypoplasia. Other associated anomalies with cleft hand include:

- Cleft palate or lip (ectrodactyly, ectodermal dysplasia, cleft syndrome)
- Cleft foot (see above)
- Syndactyly and polydactyly
- Cornelia de lange syndrome
- Deafness
- Ocular malformations
- Heart defects
- Anal atresia

Treatment

The cleft hand though looks weird has excellent function and in fact there is a functional gain of the grasp, releases and pinch functions. Surgical treatment typically involves closure of the central deficiency with appropriate reconstitution of a functional thumb and first web space. Typically transverse bone separating the cleft if any should be removed and the carpals may need closing wedge osteotomy to close the cleft. Index and ring finger MCP joints should be stabilized along with the separation of syndactylies (z-plasties, etc., see below). If the first web space is narrowed then deepening can be done with z-plasty. Adduction contracture of thumb should be simultaneously released with ulnar transposition of the index finger. For marked syndactyly of first web space flaps should be used (Snow-Littler, Miura and Ueba flaps) from the redundant skin of cleft closure to reconstruct.

The treatment of symbrachydactyly is more complicated and indecisive. Primary goal is to achieve pinch that depends largely on the quality of remaining digits. For adequate soft tissue pockets in between rays a vascularized toe transfer will give lateral pinch but not digital length. With a functional thumb lengthening of digits can be attempted.

SYNDACTYLY

Syn (together) + dactylos (digits) is the result of failure of apoptosis. Normal digital separation occurs during fifth to eighth week of gestation. Syndactyly occurs due to failure of interdigital necrosis of the developing hand paddle in utero and is one of the most common congenital differences occurring in 1/2,000 and 1/2,500 live births. The condition is inherited in an autosomal dominant pattern with variable penetrance in approximately 40% of patients and is bilateral and symmetric in up to 50% of patients. It is more common in boys than in girls. Syndactyly can occur in isolation or associated with other disorders. Associated conditions include:

- Poland syndrome (absent sternocostal head of the pectoralis major, upper limb hypoplasia and symbrachydactyly)
- Apert syndrome (acrocephalosyndactyly)
- Carpenter syndrome (acrocephalopolysyndactyly)

Syndactyly is classified (***see also*** **Figs. 19A to E**) by the extent of interdigital webbing (incomplete or complete) and the character of the conjoined tissue (simple, complex, or complicated). The separation of digits starts distally and progresses proximally. Normal commissure extends to 30–35% of the length of proximal phalanx. The third web space being the most distal web space is most commonly affected as any residual separation that is incomplete will affect it. Syndactyly then occurs with reducing frequency in the fourth, second and first web spaces.

- *Incomplete syndactyly:* The separation fails at intermediary stage so that the connection is incomplete throughout the length and the web is more distal than normal.

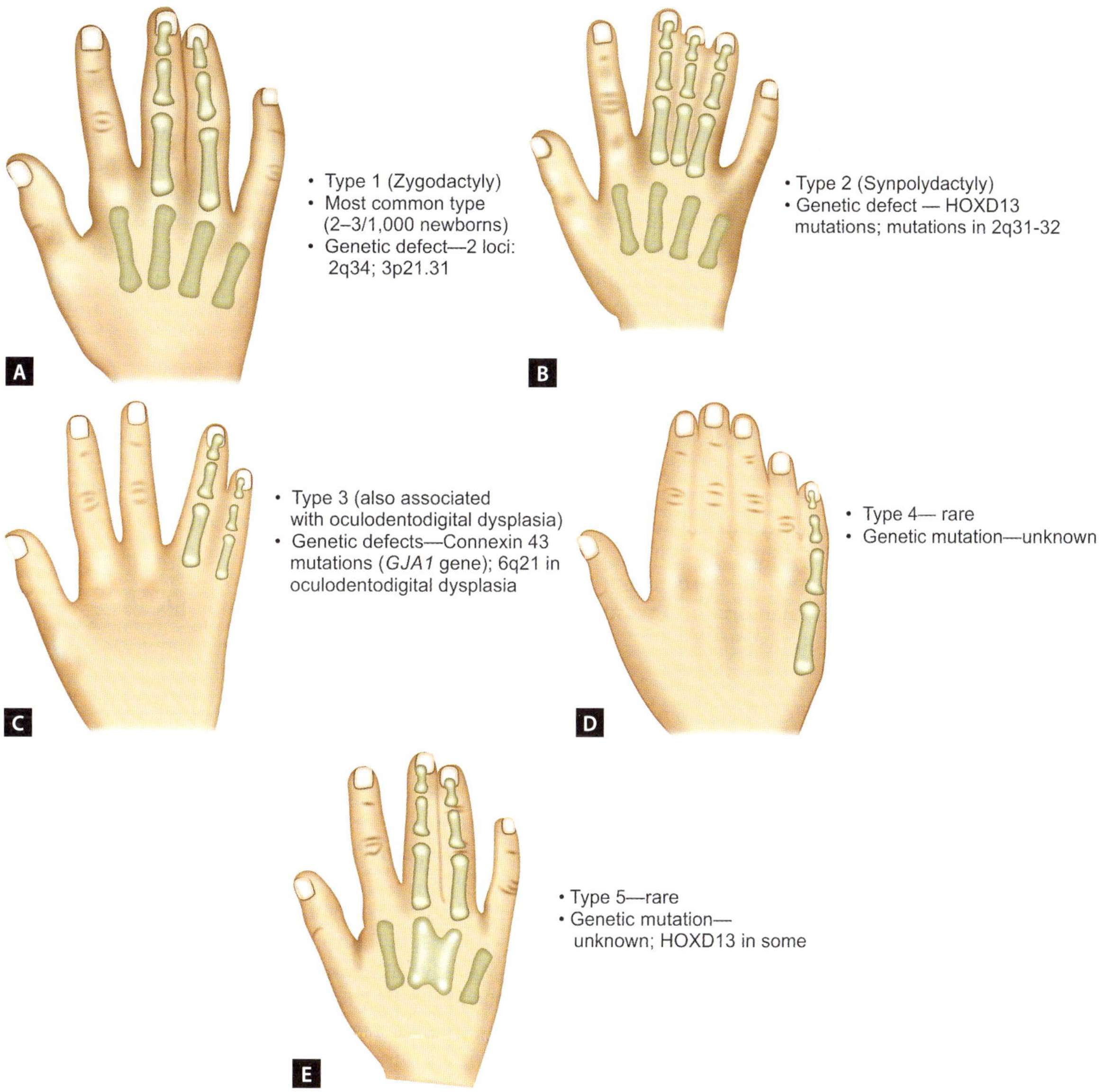

Figs. 19A to E: Classification of syndactyly.

- *Complete syndactyly:* Connection between involved fingers extends over the entire length of the phalanges.
- *Simple syndactyly:* When the digits are joined by skin only.
- *Complex syndactyly:* When there is osseous connection between the digits.
- *Acrosyndactyly* involves webbing of the tips of all the digits.
- *Complicated syndactyly:* Syndactyly occurring in association with other major developmental problems in the hand that affect hand function, such as brachydactyly, camptodactyly, clinodactyly, symphalangism or polydactyly.

Clinical Features

Syndactyly may be associated with the syndactyly of toes. Syndromic associations mentioned above should be evaluated and the hand needs to be evaluated for type of syndactyly. The patients in simple syndactyly have good function and are disabled only by the absence of independent digital function. Some degree of bony malalignment and joint contracture occurs in the border digit syndactylies (first and fourth web spaces) due to discrepancy in the lengths of the adjacent digit's asymmetric pattern of growth.

Evaluation

Radiographs of hand should be obtained to evaluate complex syndactyly involving bony connection. Malalignment, stiffness should be evaluated for prognosticating functional outcome. MRI and arteriography are used only in very complex situations to define digital anatomy preoperatively.

Treatment

Most patients require surgery for functional (independent digital motion) and cosmetic reasons. The surgery is performed usually around the age of 12 months considering the anesthesia risk (after 6 months anesthesia risk is same throughout childhood) and development of skills versus visibility of structures. Surgical release is made easy with the help of loop. There is some concern of skin scarring when operated in neonatal age so some recommend operating at 18 months but developed functional skills may be difficult to modify. Contraindications to surgical release may be:

- Syndromic and chromosomal conditions
- The overall medical condition or mental capacity of the patient precluding surgical separation
- Complex syndactyly in which the affected digits are too hypoplastic, malaligned or stiff to warrant separation.

Principles of surgical release:

- It is often imperative to counsel parents that the separation is not usually as easy as they think of cutting the intermediary skin linearly. This leads to long-term joint contractures, digital malalignment, and loss of motion and function.
- Early surgical release is advocated when the syndactyly affects digits of different sizes (the first and fourth web spaces) to avoid deformity and growth disturbance.
- Only one side of the digit is operated on during a single procedure to avoid vascular embarrassment.

Surgical release comprises:

- *Zig-zag incisions for reconstruction of skin coverage* ***(Figs. 20A and B)****:* To avoid linear scar and later complications
- Avoiding the interdigital creases to prevent scar contractures.
- Dividing Grayson's and Cleland's ligaments and removing any synostosis or synchondrosis union of the distal phalanges.
- *Local rotation flap coverage for the commissure:* Dorsal skin is used as a local advancement flap to reconstitute the interdigital commissure and avoid web space contracture. In incomplete syndactyly surgery usually involves the use of local flaps such as double-opposing z-plasties and "stickman" flaps. An incomplete syndactyly extending to the middle phalangeal region requires full-thickness skin grafting. Graftless techniques of syndactyly release (as some parents might prefer) use extended dorsal metacarpal island flaps as v-y advancement flaps to reconstitute the web commissure and facilitate direct skin closure.
- Split or better full-thickness skin grafts to cover all uncovered areas of the digits.
- *Eponychial reconstruction:* Conjoined nails are divided, and the exposed eponychial and paronychial regions are reconstructed with local flaps or composite grafts.

The depth of the reconstructed web space may be limited by a distal digital artery bifurcation where one needs to be ligated. In complex syndactilies joint instability may require ligamentous reconstruction and joint stiffness, camptodactyly or symphalangism for complicated syndactyly may need to be dealt with later. Acrosyndactyly should be separated early in life where the first and third webs are separated together followed by the second and fourth webs together later (3–6 months).

Complications

- *An avascular digit:* Theoretically most dreaded but practically almost never encountered unless one is too careless (avoid releasing both sides of digits together)
- Flap necrosis and scar contracture
- Skin graft failure
- Infection
- Nail deformity and poor eponychial coverage
- Web space creep
- Angular deformity
- Joint stiffness

POLYDACTYLY

Polydactyly is a common congenital malformation that is grouped into:

- Radial (preaxial)
- Central
- Ulnar (postaxial) portion of the hand.

Preaxial (radial, thumb polydactyly or thumb duplication) polydactyly has been reported to occur in 1 infant per 1,000–10,000 live births. The term thumb duplication should not be used as there are two hypoplastic thumbs and not two normal thumbs as the term applies. Males are more commonly affected than females as are the Asian and white children more often than black children. Occurrence is usually sporadic, and associated congenital anomalies are rare [acrocephalopolysyndactyly (Nocack and Carpenter types), Holt-Oram or Robinow syndromes]. Autosomal dominant inheritance is seen with triphalangeal thumb. The Wassel classification is used to categorize preaxial polydactyly on

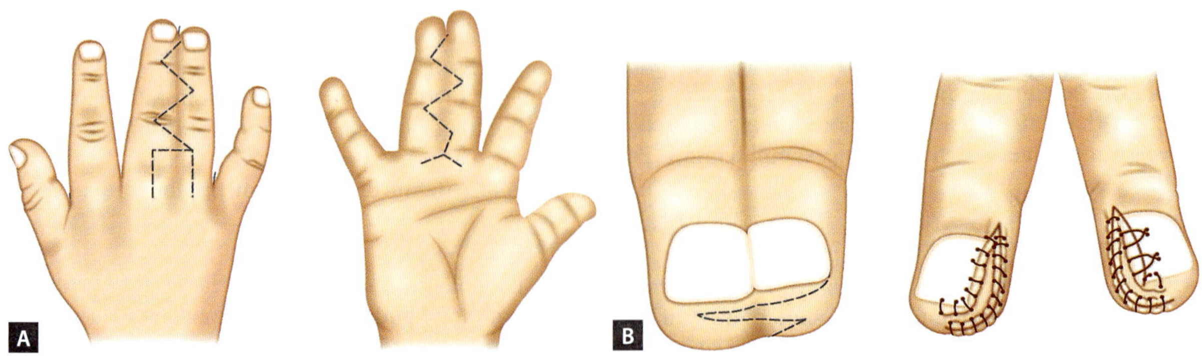

Figs. 20A and B: Syndactyly surgical release. (A) Illustration of standard flaps made during syndactyly release; (B) Shows the flaps for release of nails.

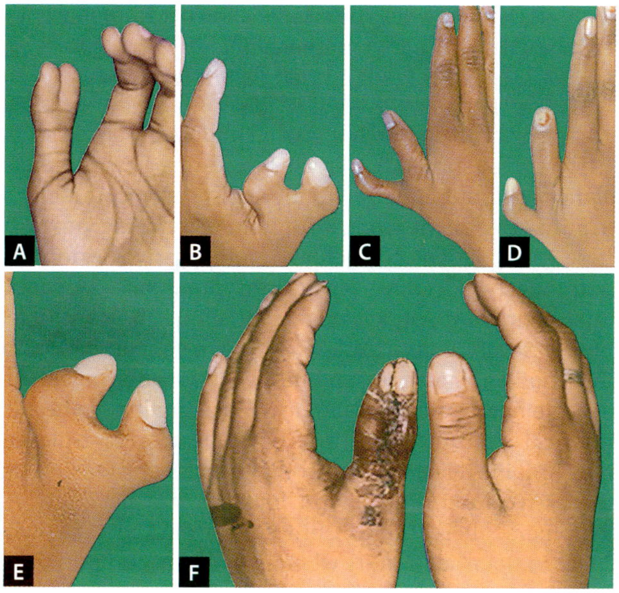

Figs. 21A to F: Various types of radial polydactyly (A to D, see text); (E and F) Surgical correction of type 4 anomaly.
Source: Professor PP Kotwal, Chairman, Institute of Orthopedics and Joint Replacement, Pushpawati Singhania Research Institute, New Delhi, India.

the number of bifid or duplicated phalanges or metacarpals, from distal to proximal **(Figs. 21A to F)**.

- *Type 1:* Bifid distal phalanx
- *Type 2:* A duplicated distal phalanx
- *Type 3:* Duplicated distal phalanx with a bifid proximal phalanx
- *Type 4:* Duplicated proximal and distal phalanges (most common type)
- *Type 5:* Duplicated proximal and distal phalanges with a bifid metacarpal
- *Type 6:* Duplication of all phalanges and metacarpals
- *Type 7:* Any duplication with a triphalangeal thumb.

Wassel type 4 (40%) and type 2, and type 7 (20% each) are the most common. In triphalangeal thumb, the extra phalanx is the middle phalanx that may be wedge-shaped or rectangular. The thumb may be in a position of opposition, or in the plane of motion of the other fingers. The latter situation represents index finger duplication with an absent thumb. Triphalangeal thumbs may be associated with Holt-Oram syndrome, Fanconi and Blackfan-Diamond syndromes. Triphalangism of thumb is classified as:

- *Type 1:* Delta phalanx with radial deviation deformity
- *Type 2:* Normal middle phalanx with opposable thumb
- *Type 3:* Index finger duplication.

Types 1 and 2 have normal first web space with available thenar muscles. Type 3 is a five-fingered hand with contracted first web space and lacks thenar muscles. Treatment is surgical reconstruction. For type 1 thumb, the delta phalanx is excised in infancy preferably to produce good interphalangeal (IP) joint. Later in life shortening and corrective osteotomy with arthrodesis is done. For type 2 web space deepening, excision of the extra phalanx, opposition transfer procedure is done. Type 3 requires a modified pollicization and deepening of first web space.

Treatment

Surgical reconstruction is the treatment of choice. Both hypoplastic thumbs contain structures that must be preserved and reconstructed to provide a single, stable, mobile and functional thumb so simple excision of one thumbs is absolutely contraindicated **(Figs. 21A to F)**. The radial thumb is usually more hypoplastic and excised. Surgery consists of ablation of the radial thumb with reconstruction of the radial collateral ligament and transfer of other soft tissues to the ulnar digit. Bifid proximal digit or metacarpal (types 2 and 4) need to be excised. Chondroplasties or corrective osteotomies of the metacarpals or phalanges are needed to reproduce longitudinal axis. First web space needs to be deepened by z-plasties. A late deformity develops in approximately 15–20% of patients due either to:

- Failure to recognize a pollex abductus
- Inadequate correction of the longitudinal thumb alignment
- Inadequate reconstruction of the collateral ligament
- Failure to centralize the extensor or flexor tendons.

Postaxial polydactyly refers to duplication of the ulnarmost digit (small finger polydactyly). Inheritance is autosomal dominant, and the condition affects black children more often (1 in 300) than white children (1 in 3,000). In black children, postaxial polydactyly is usually an isolated condition but in affected white children one- third will have and associated organ system disorder. The duplicated digit can be fully developed (type A) or rudimentary and pedunculated (type B). Polydactyly has also been classified by Stelling and Turek into three types:

- Type 1 involves soft tissue alone (very common in the black population)
- Type 2 involves only phalangeal duplication that articulates with a single or bifid metacarpal head
- Type 3 involves complete ulnar ray duplication, including the metacarpal.

Only postaxial soft-tissue polydactyly (type I or rudimentary) or type B can be treated by excision alone. All other forms require reconstruction. Type B can be treated with suture ligation in the newborn nursery. The reported complications of this treatment still are:

- Infection
- Bleeding
- Incomplete removal.

Type A postaxial polydactyly (or type 1 and 2) may require collateral ligament and hypothenar muscle transfer (abductor digiti quinti, flexor digiti quinti) from the sixth to fifth digit are necessary. Bifid metacarpal excision and reconstruction of collateral ligament are necessary. It is imperative here to preserve the physis in these situations. In type 3, polydactyly entire ray is resected and the basilar joint is stabilized.

Central Polydactyly

Central polydactyly is very rare. It is usually bilateral, associated with syndactyly and the underlying digits are rarely normal (usually hypoplastic and associated with osseous and soft tissue malformations). It may be inherited in an autosomal dominant manner and girls are more commonly affected than boys. To treat major decision is taken based on feasibility of obtaining an independently functioning digit. The choices here are to leave the digits conjoined to attempt reconstruction to a five-digit hand, or to perform ray resections of part or all of the synpolydactyly. Often the involved digits have osseous malalignment, hypoplasia, and poor neurovascular supply. The reconstructed digit is usually smaller, stiffer, weaker, and malaligned and mostly cosmetically distinct often acceptable that should be conveyed to the family from beginning.

CAMPTODACTYLY (BENT FINGER)

Camptodactyly refers to flexion contracture [usually of proximal interphalangeal (PIP joint)] and deformity of a finger (typically the small finger). Although, the true incidence is unknown, it is estimated that less than 1% of the general population is affected. Most cases appear in infancy with equal male to female occurrence. Uncommonly, initial occurrence may be seen in girls during adolescence. Camptodactyly is usually sporadic, but some patients have an autosomal dominance inheritance. Bilateral affection is seen in around 60% cases. Pathogenically, the deformity results from imbalance between flexor and extensor mechanisms. Abnormal insertion of lumbricals, FDS or anatomically abnormal retinacular ligaments are seen most commonly and cited the most common cause. Other minor defects that have been identified in these cases cited also as potential etiologies are skin contracture (volar aspect), volar plate anomalies, absent extensor tendon function and articular incongruity. Articular incongruity is possibly developmental and develops over growth period due to abnormal position, head of proximal phalanx becomes narrowed volarly and flattened dorsally along with notching of the base of proximal phalanx. The patient compensates for the PIP flexion deformity by MCP and distal interphalangeal (DIP) hyperextension. Compensation usually fails if contracture exceeds 30°. The deformity usually progresses with growth. The classification of camptodactyly is partly based on the age at presentation.

- Type 1 occurs in infancy **(Figs. 22A to C)**.
- Type 2 occurs during adolescence.
- Type 3 occurs in the setting of an underlying syndrome.

Treatment should be directed to restore flexor extensor balance. Splinting and stretching exercises are recommended for initial treatment along with home stretching program. These are aimed to achieve full passive extension. Camptodactyly rarely results in profound functional impairment, and surgical treatment should be considered only for severe contractures (>45°) with functional loss or those not amenable to splinting. Proponents of surgery advocate nearly universal surgical repositioning of aberrant lumbrical (and/or FDS) insertion along with z-plasties and PIP joint release. For incomplete active extension but full passive extension tendon transfers can be done. We recommend these surgical procedures only in cases with "finger in palm" deformity where the fingers curl into palm. The results of surgery have not been very encouraging in the past and result merely in change of arc of motion rather than normalization of abnormal balance. This also results from osseous changes at the PIP that preclude any restoration of normal alignment or motion. Other problems like incomplete correction and recurrent deformity are also common and concerning with surgery.

CLINODACTYLY

Clinodactyly is abnormal angular deformity of digit (>10°) in the radioulnar plane. It is typically bilateral, and the small finger (pinkie finger) is most commonly affected (just check most of you will be having borderline clinodactyly). The deformity arises mainly from middle phalanx trapezoidal deformity. The vertical height on radial side is less than ulnar cortex **(Fig. 23)**. In severe cases, the middle phalanx may be a delta phalanx (more aptly called longitudinal epiphyseal bracket). In delta phalanx, the proximal physis of the phalanx

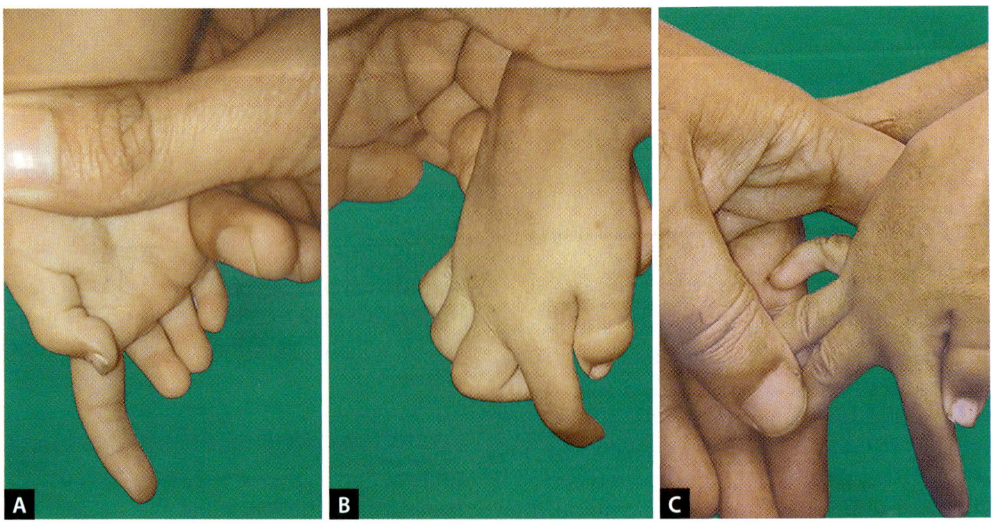

Figs. 22A to C: Camptodactyly. (A and B) Note the flexion deformity at proximal interphalangeal of 3rd to 5th finger and it is passively correctible (C) in the 2-year-old child.

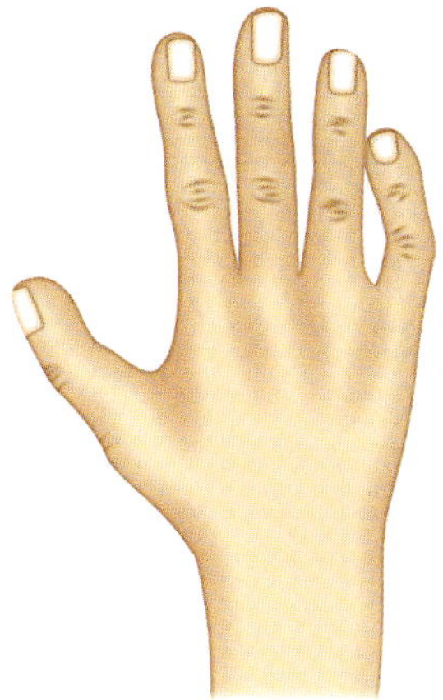

Fig. 23: Clinodactyly clinical appearance.

is not perpendicular to the long axis of the bone resulting in a triangular or trapezoidal-shaped bone. This is a non-progressive deformity unless associated with bracket delta phalanx. Inheritance is believed to be autosomal dominant but there are many associated syndromes including:

- Trisomy 21 and 18
- Holt-Oram syndrome
- Silver syndrome
- Rubenstein-Taybi syndrome (clinodactyly of thumb)
- Diastrophic dwarfism (clinodactyly of thumb)
- Cornelia de Lange syndrome

Clinodactyly is classified as:

- Simple (bony deformity alone) or complex (soft-tissue involvement)
- Uncomplicated (<45° angulation) or complicated (>45° angulation, with rotation).

Treatment

Splinting and stretching exercises can be implemented, although they are not always successful. Clinodactyly is more of a cosmetic rather than a functional problem. Surgery is indicated only for severe deformity with functional compromise as with delta phalanx. The shortened side of the phalanx contains the epiphyseal bracket. Treatment includes:

- Bracket resection and surgical realignment (opening-wedge, closing-wedge, and reverse-wedge osteotomies) or
- Physeal bar resection and fat graft interposition (Vicker's) to restore longitudinal growth and provide correction.

Osteotomy is generally delayed until sufficient ossification of the middle phalanx to allow for precise cuts. The complications of surgical procedure include:

- Persistent deformity (undercorrection)
- Loss of interphalangeal motion: This is dreaded and unacceptable to patients and parents for an initially functional finger that becomes stiff.

THUMB HYPOPLASIA OR APLASIA

Thumb hypoplasia or aplasia (see RCH above also) lies within the spectrum of radial longitudinal deficiency universally but is classified as undergrowth because it can occur in isolation also. Apart from radial deficiency syndromes (Holt-Oram, Fanconi syndromes, TAR, VACTERRLS) it can be seen associated with other congenital anomalies or malformations including:

- Malformations of the cardiac, craniofacial, musculoskeletal, renal, gastrointestinal and hematopoietic systems
- Hypoplasia of the metacarpals (Cornelia de Lange syndrome, diastrophic dwarfism)
- Hypoplasia of phalanges (Rubinstein-Taybi and Apert syndromes).

The term thumb hypoplasia is not a simple reduction in size of thumb and in fact encompasses:

- A contracted first web space
- Unstable MCP joint
- Thenar weakness
- Interphalangeal joint stiffness or instability

The condition is often bilateral occurring in 1 infant per 30,000–100,000 live births. It affects males and females equally.

The condition is classified using Buck-Gramcko and Manske modification of the Blauth classification into five types **(Fig. 24)** that guides the choice of treatment also ***(see* Table 7)**.

- Blauth type I thumbs are slightly smaller than normal.
- Blauth type II thumbs are characterized by the absence of thenar muscles.
- Blauth type III thumbs lack both intrinsic and extrinsic motor function, and the thumb metacarpal is underdeveloped. They are subdivided into:
    - Type IIIA, in which the carpometacarpal (CMC) joint is stable.
    - Type IIIB, in which the CMC joint is unstable or absent.
- Floating thumbs (pouce flottant) are classified as type IV.
- Type V refers to an absent thumb.

Pathoanatomy depends on the severity of the thumb hypoplasia.

- The thumb ray bones are smaller and narrower with stiffness at interphalangeal joint.
- The first web space is contracted in all except the rare type I thumb.
- The MCP joint usually has ulnar collateral ligament insufficiency. Global instability is less common.
- The thenar intrinsics are progressively deficient in higher grades and are completely absent in type 4 or 5 often.
- The thumb extrinsic musculature are also similarly progressively deficient.
- Reconstruction for higher grades is guided by the condition of CMC joint that is absent in type IIIB and IV thumbs (no basilar joints).

Plain radiographs are obtained to clarify the osseous anatomy and delineate skeletal development, of carpus and distal radius. Type II and type IIIA thumbs are characterized by a tight first web space, interphalangeal joint stiffness, MCP joint instability and thenar weakness. They are best treated with web space deepening, MCP joint stabilization and opponensplasty. For type IIIB, IV and V, thumb ablation and index finger pollicization is recommended.

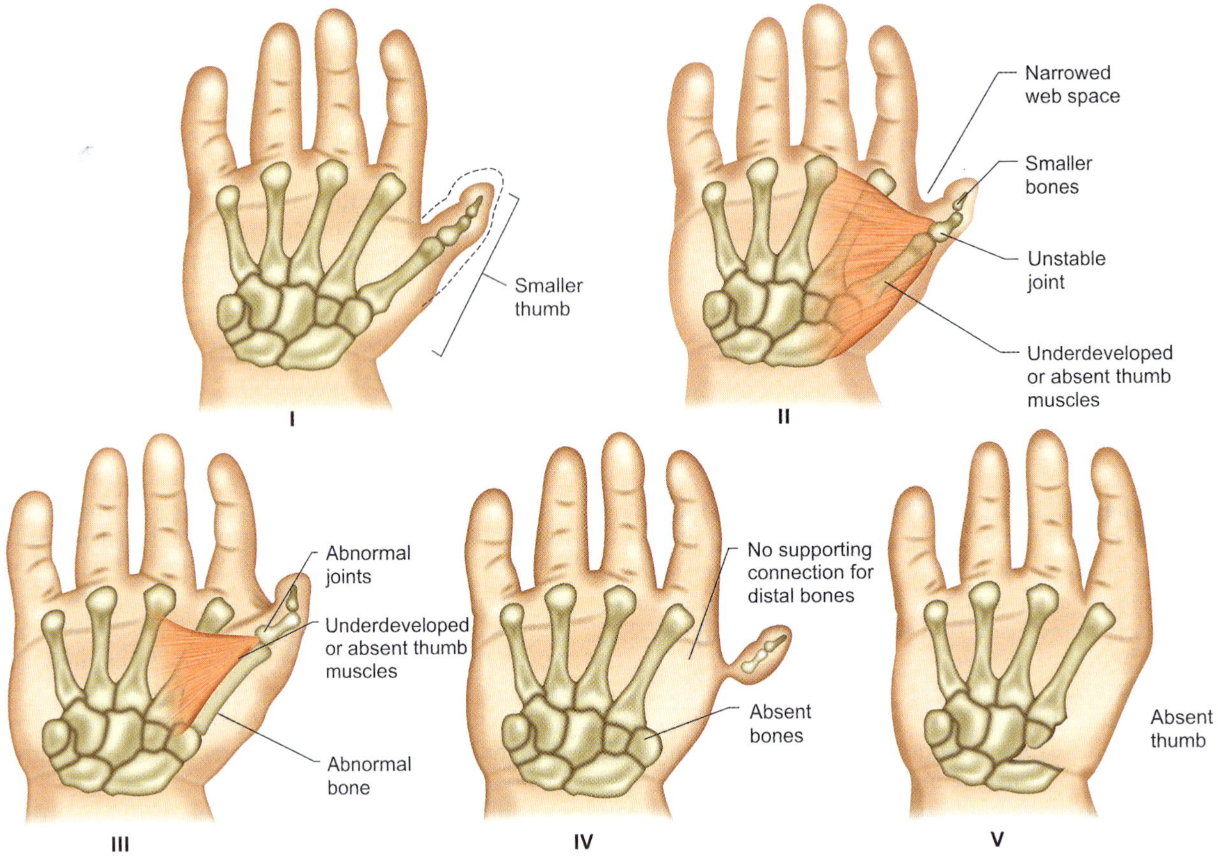

Fig. 24: Classification of thumb hypoplasia.

Treatment

Adaptation to nonphysiologic movements and pinch in children is fast if not operated. They use lateral pinch between the long and index fingers. Still, the deficiencies in pinch, grasp and fine motor activities remain significant. Surgical reconstruction can improve function and cosmesis so should be recommended strongly.

- For Blauth types I to IIIA: Reconstruction of the hypoplastic thumb includes first web space deepening, opponensplasty (with either the abductor digiti quinti or the ring-finger FDS tendon) and MCP joint stabilization.
  - The MCP stabilization is done with either ligamentous reconstruction (using FDS or local fascia) or arthrodesis. For arthrodesis, the physis of the proximal phalanx should be preserved to maximize growth of the thumb ray. Chondrodesis of the metacarpal head to the epiphysis of the proximal phalanx is desired.
  - The choice of first web space deepening procedure includes two-part and four-part Z-plasties or the use of dorsal rotation flaps from the index finger, thumb or hand.
  - The abductor digiti quinti transfer for opposition can be used in the infant with a relatively stable MCP joint. In older children or patients with marked instability of the MCP joint, the ring finger FDS is used for opposition. As an advantage the additional tendon length can be used for ligamentous reconstruction.

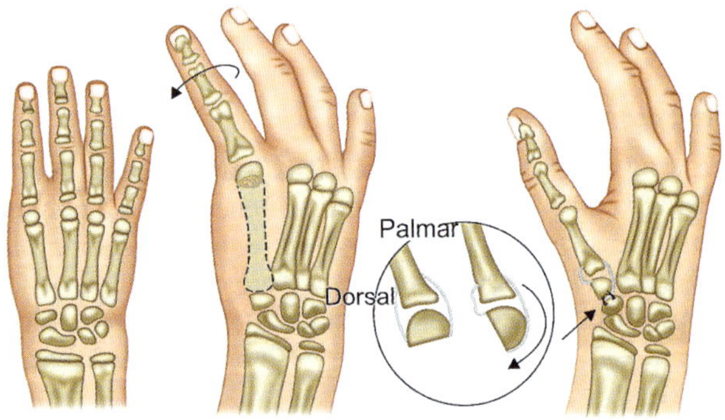

Fig. 25: Pollicization of index finger for thumb aplasia or severe hypoplasia (Type IIIB to Type V).

- Type IIIB, pouce flottant (type IV), or aplasia of the thumb (type V) need pollicization **(Fig. 25)**. Counseling parents for pollicization in type IIIB thumb is a task in itself as they see a thumb in their child that we are asking for sacrifice. A sincere effort in explaining the poor results of reconstruction in absence of basilar joint should go through. These children will continue to use lateral pinch even after reconstruction and the thumb is mere cosmetic. Microvascular transfer of a toe metatarsophalangeal joint can be performed but needs expertise and is rarely if ever indicated against wonderful results of simpler pollicization. Pollicization involves the conversion of the triphalangeal index finger to a biphalangeal thumb with a

CMC joint and a deep first web space. Index metacarpal epiphysis is used as the trapezium. Pollicization is generally performed between 6 months and 18 months of age. Results depend on the quality of the original index finger, in terms of tendon function and joint motion. Patients with thumb aplasia and radial dysplasia generally have poorer prognosis because the involved index finger has deficient soft tissues.

CONGENITAL TRIGGER THUMB OR DIGITS

Trigger thumb is actually an acquired (as opposed to congenital) abnormality of the FPL tendon and its sheath at the A1 pulley. This is a relatively common condition having an estimated incidence of 3 infants per 1,000 live births that is acquired in first two years of life. There is a palpable mass, a nodule called Notta's nodule **(Figs. 26A and B)** that represents the FPL constriction at the A1 pulley. The condition is caused by a size mismatch or a differential growth of the tendon and its pulley leading to progressive constriction. There is no inflammatory component involved (as opposed to adult form). The condition has been found to spontaneously resolve by 9 months of age in 30–50% of patients, but the chances of such favorable outcome diminish as the child grows older (<10% after 1 year). It occurs sporadically and as many as 30% of patients have bilateral involvement.

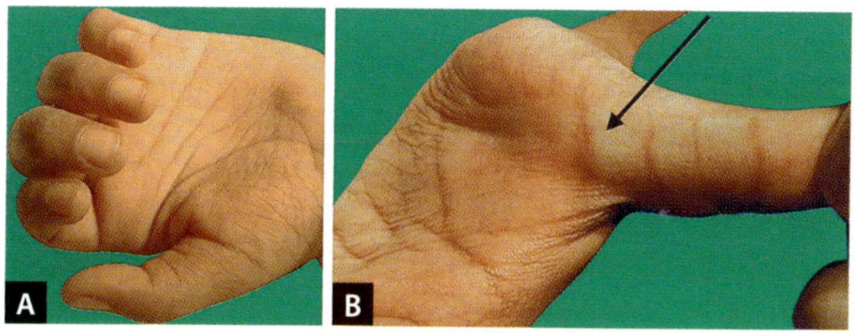

Figs. 26A and B: Congenital trigger digit. Note the flexed thumb (A) and Notta's nodule (B, arrow).

Clinical Examination

It reveals a palpable nodule of the FPL tendon at A1 pulley with either triggering (less common) or a fixed flexion contracture (more common) of the interphalangeal joint. Longstanding trigger presents as compensatory hyperextension at MCP joint in an effort to bring the thumb out of palm.

Treatment

Surgical release of the A1 pulley is the treatment of choice and is almost always successful. It is recommended for patients who are older than 1 year and fail to resolve spontaneously or those presenting after 1 year of age with fixed PIP. Care should be taken to preserve neurovascular bundle and the oblique pulley (and hence avoid bowstringing). Transverse incision is much more cosmetic. Recurrence is extremely rare.

Trigger fingers are much less common than trigger thumbs but when present are often multiple. Unlike trigger thumbs they are often associated with central nervous system disorders and syndromes (trisomy 18, mucopolysaccharidoses, diabetes and juvenile rheumatoid arthritis). They result from anomalous anatomy, such as abnormal lumbrical insertion or proximal decussation of the FDS tendon at the A2 pulley (not at A1 as in trigger thumb). The triggering appears to occur as the flexor digitorum profundus passes through the chiasm of the FDS. The treatment of trigger fingers is more complicated than the trigger thumb and just release of the A1 pulley alone leads to frequent recurrence (as high as 50%). Additional surgical release has to be obtained in the form of lumbrical, A1 pulley, and A3 pulley releases as well as excision of the slip of the FDS tendon.

CONCLUSION

- Upper limb congenital anomalies are not uncommon to find in children.
- Lot of these are neglected due to various social and financial factors in Indian subcontinent. The other major reason is lack of expertise to deal with these disorders so elusion amongst the practitioners as to where to refer the patients. Middle-class and lower middle-class population cannot afford the prolonged treatment often due to migrating nature of population. With improvement in the available expertise there is better management of these conditions that is gradually refining.
- It is of utmost importance to the orthopedic surgeons to realize the importance of early treatment of most of these conditions as children develop quick adaptation to the absence of normal function and once that develops it is difficult to rehabilitate the patient even with corrected anomaly.

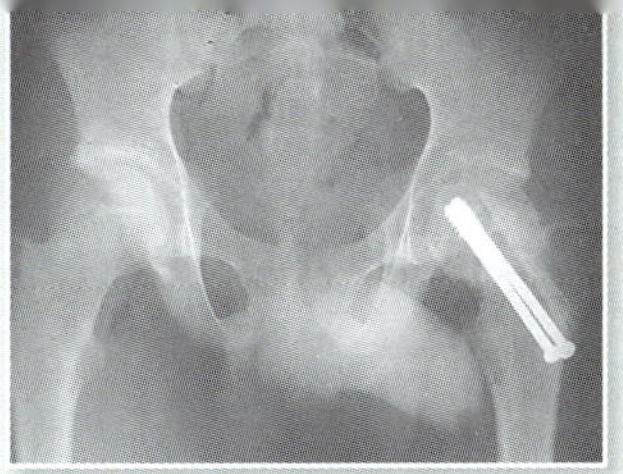
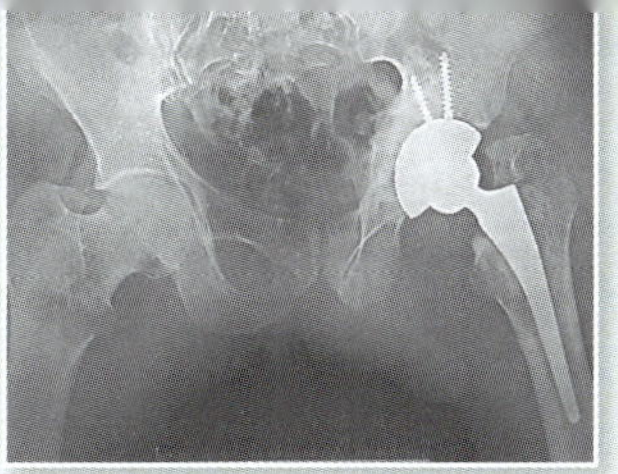
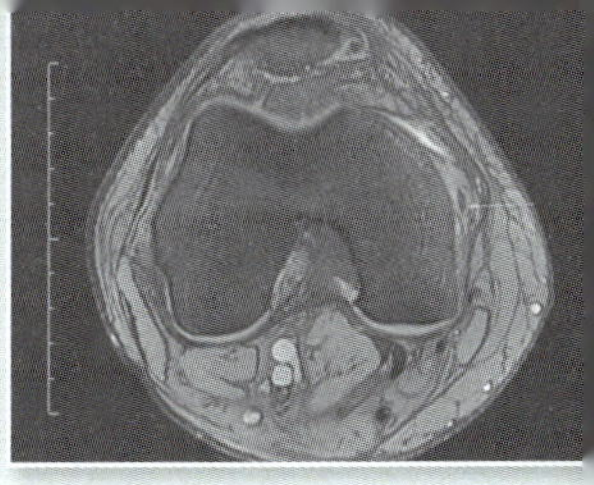

Essential ORTHOPEDICS Principles and Practice

VOLUME 2

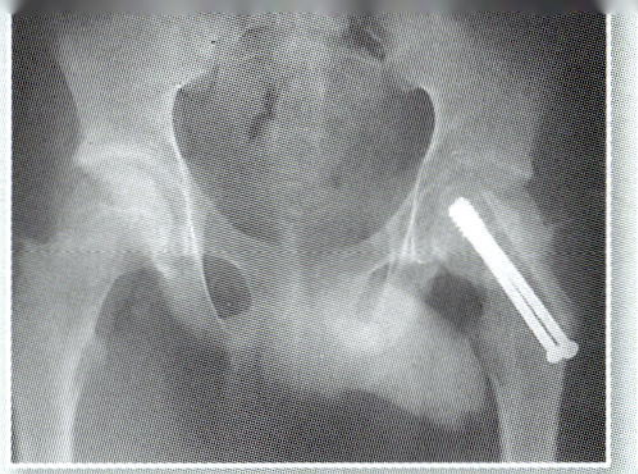
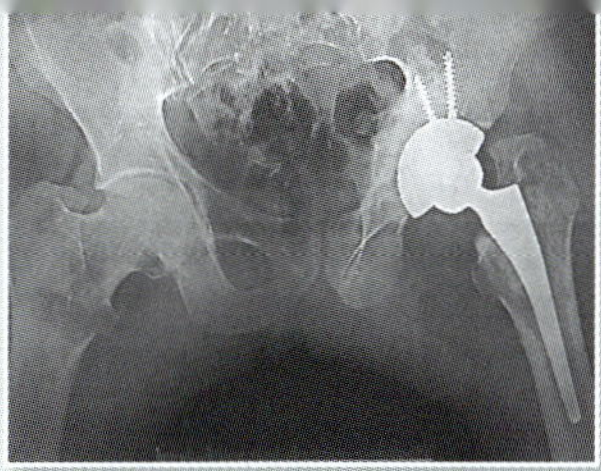
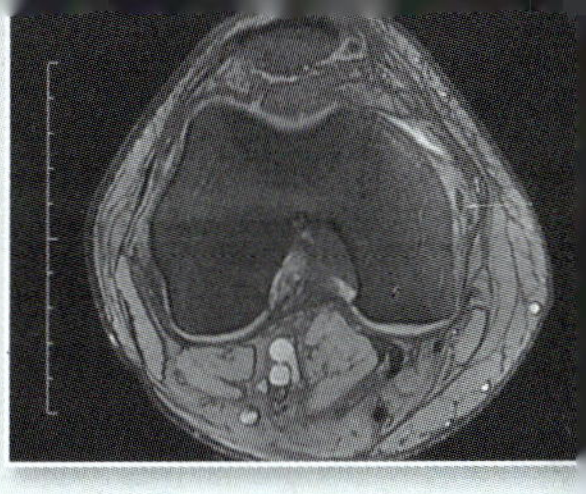

Essential ORTHOPEDICS Principles and Practice

THIRD EDITION

Manish Kumar Varshney
MS (Orth) DNB (Orth) MNAMS MRCS (Glasgow)
Senior Consultant Orthopedic Surgeon
SMVD Narayana Superspeciality Hospital
Reasi, Jammu and Kashmir, India

JAYPEE

JAYPEE BROTHERS MEDICAL PUBLISHERS
The Health Sciences Publisher
New Delhi | London

Jaypee Brothers Medical Publishers (P) Ltd.

Headquarters
EMCA House
23/23-B, Ansari Road, Daryaganj
New Delhi 110 002, India
Landline: +91-11-23272143, +91-11-23272703
+91-11-23282021, +91-11-23245672
Email: jaypee@jaypeebrothers.com

Corporate Office
4838/24, Ansari Road, Daryaganj
New Delhi 110 002, India
Phone: +91-11-43574357
Fax: +91-11-43574314
Email: jaypee@jaypeebrothers.com

Overseas Office
J.P. Medical Ltd
83 Victoria Street, London
SW1H 0HW (UK)
Phone: +44 20 3170 8910
Email: info@jpmedpub.com

EU GPSR Authorised Representative
Logos Europe, 9 rue Nicolas Poussin
17000, La Rochelle, France
Phone: +33 (0) 6 67 93 73 78
E-mail: Contact@logoseurope.eu

Website: www.jaypeebrothers.com
Website: www.jaypeedigital.com

Essential Orthopedics: Principles and Practice (Volumes 1 and 2)

First Edition: 2016

Second Edition: 2018

Third Edition: 2022, ***Reprint:*** **2025**

ISBN: 978-93-5465-105-2

Printed at: Samrat Offset Pvt. Ltd.

Dedicated to

All my students, my teachers from
whom I learned Orthopedics,
both my sons—Siddhant and Mrigank
who taught me how to teach,
and my loving wife—Neeta
who spared me from my homely duties
while being engaged in preparing this book.

Contributors

Avinash Razdan
DMRD DMB (Radio Diagnosis)
Associate Consultant
SMVD Narayana Superspeciality Hospital
Reasi, Jammu and Kashmir, India
avinash.razdan@gmail.com

Jaydip Patel
DNB FIAS FISS
Director
Trinay Hospital
Ahmedabad, Gujarat, India
jaydipshyani.js@gmail.com

Manish Kumar Varshney
MS (Orth) DNB (Orth) MNAMS MRCS (Glasgow)
Senior Consultant Orthopedic Surgeon
SMVD Narayana Superspeciality Hospital
Reasi, Jammu and Kashmir, India
drmkvarshney@gmail.com

Mohinder Singh Chib
MBBS MS FIAS FIAP
Consultant Orthopedics and Trauma
Gupta Hospital
Kathua, Jammu and Kashmir, India
drmohindersinghchib@gmail.com

S Pavan MS
Chief Consultant and Head
Department of Orthopedics
Tata Motors Hospital
Jamshedpur, Jharkhand, India
pavan.sudarshan@tatamotors.com

Shafiq Hackla
MS (Orth) DNB FNB (Sports Medicine)
Attending Consultant
Artemis Hospital
Gurugram, Haryana, India
hacklashafiq17@gmail.com

Shalinder Kumar Sharma MS (Orth)
Associate Professor
Government Medical College
Rajouri, Jammu and Kashmir, India
drshalinder@gmail.com

Preface to the Third Edition

In a nutshell, the third edition of *Essential Orthopedics: Principles and Practice* is a thoroughly revised edition. I am glad that readers pointed to some critical mistakes in the previous editions, and the same have also been included. The revision and upgradation do not involve only the clinical text but even the grammatical and spelling mistakes are thoroughly corrected. The book has been revised literally word by word. Upgradation of clinical knowledge involves incorporation of the latest developments that have made a significant impact on orthopedics (leaving behind the investigational approaches/methods to minimize cluttering and confusion). The clinical and core text changes significantly involve:

- General orthopedics as lots of changes have been made in the diagnosis for diseases, tools used (e.g., for slipped upper femoral epiphysis, etc.), and therapies based on molecular targets (rheumatoid arthritis, osteoporosis, etc.).
- Various new diseases (scurvy, chronic renal disease, etc.) and techniques (electrospinning, etc.) have been added that were omitted in previous editions. Annexure 1 for Upper Limb Trauma is revised for newer treatment methods and expanded to include small bone injuries of wrist and hand.
- Regional orthopedics have also undergone changes with respect to better understanding of diseases and their management (viz. Shoulder Instability, Imaging of Shoulder Joint, Total Hip Replacement, etc.). Certain previously omitted conditions (patellar tendon rupture, etc.) have been added or expanded.
- Totally new additions include chapters on Musculoskeletal Imaging, Preoperative Planning, Nanotechnology, Orthopedics in Digital Renaissance, Neglected Trauma to Bones and Joints (Annexure 4), expansion on Malunions, etc.
- Addition of lots of relevant figures and photographs along with tabulation and compression of details in text considered too descriptive to be of any use.

Most importantly the *chapter organization of the book has massively changed* as there was discontinuity in previous presentation and mis-positioning of related topics. Various chapters have been merged to maintain comprehensiveness and provide space for adding newer chapters without increasing overall numbers of chapters! The total number of chapters have been in fact reduced compared to previous edition (to partly reduce scare amongst the readers). I hope the current text will meet the comprehensive need of readers to learn and repair orthopedic knowledge.

Happy reading!

Manish Kumar Varshney

Preface to the First Edition

Orthopedics like other medical faculties is a growing branch. The growth is, however, much faster than other fields. Till the beginning of the last century, the orthopedics as a discrete was nonexistent to this world but the efforts of pioneers in the field gave birth to the baby that boomed possibly the fastest to become one of the most favored surgical branches to new entrants in the postgraduation. Orthopedics is the most glamorous and preferred surgical faculty for all youngsters aspiring to quickly gain sort of "superspecialization" as not much is available or required after one does his postgraduation in orthopedics, the regionwise faculty development into knee, shoulder, hip, pediatric orthopedics, orthopedic oncology and spine surgery are mostly fellowship dependent.

The scenario in orthopedics was not similar when the faculty started and in the beginning most of the evidences were mere "possibilities" as propounded in the replete literature of the older times written by the eminent persons in the field. Soon it came to be realized that opinions do not count and are often deleterious to general practice that may be true only for certain circumstances, so the era of "evidence-based practice" gradually evolved. With a few hitches then dawned the time where evidence was sought for most of the prevailing practices that were repeatedly questioned by surgeons around the world. This was pioneered by efforts of Association for Osteosynthesis (AO) Foundation and others and did help to some extent. In the beginning, however, the evidence was more of confusion rather than leading and the laid down facts had to be constantly changed and adjusted more due to poverty in exactness of the previously laid principles and less also to the emerging evidence as is evident from changing AO philosophy and the glaring failure of metal-on-metal hips. As a postgraduate, it became difficult for me to comprehend the historical errors and practice, changing philosophy and emerging new evidence and importantly remember them all. It was even more difficult to be accurate in orthopedic examinations to rationalize my understanding and teachings to that of the senior examiners who had started the practice even in a more bleak and confused environment prevailing at their time. However, I did realize during the course that some fundamentals were constantly getting lost in these times of evolution that could not be passed on to the youngsters and clinical examination has by now become a mere formality due to higher dependence/pervasiveness on advanced imaging and some illicit activities. The beginning of this century was marked by two major developments I feel—the development of improved implants and instrumentation (particularly the locked plate-screw constructs) and higher importance laid down for minimally invasive surgery. It became quickly evident to me that we need a text that encompasses all these facts so that the student gets a "One Stop" text where he can refer to most of his queries. This encouraged me to write down the current text and incorporate the most significant of previous practices and the current developments, some attempts have been made to incorporate the futuristic techniques but it is limited by unavailability of "evidence-based practice", so I have personally restricted that.

I feel that the future of orthopedics lies in correct and prudent diagnosis (aided solidly by sound knowledge and clinical examination) and ethical practice (not just money making as is considered an important practice nowadays); the basis of which should be correct and true literature and not polluted one. I found that some youngsters in the race of just publishing even resort to unethical practice and publish skewed and incorrect findings that pollute the sacred literature which has access to all and even amateur people who may not be able to rationalize and fall prey to wrong practice. This, I feel, also is the reason that newer meta-analysis and even systematic reviews are unable to yield evidence in favor of one or the other method rather often end in saying "no statistically significant different in practice".

The current text will help a practicing surgeon to acquaint himself with the alternatives available for a particular condition. I have tried to integrate most of the methods that are in practice or known currently for different orthopedic conditions and also organize the text in the form of answers to common theory questions for use to a postgraduate student. I tried to make a sincere effort in producing a text that can give an orthopedic surgeon insight into the orthopedic practice importantly the basic sciences and how diseases are based on faults in them. The textbook has been organized in the form of regional disposition to capture the region-specific conditions. There is vast emerging evidence and will keep emerging even at the time of this writing in the form of modern and new molecular markers that aim to diagnose disorders correctly and fast. The future for treatment of some of these disorders might also lie in the molecular level by using microinstruments such as nanotechnology and gene therapy, so I tried to cover that topic also comprehensively.

I would like to thank from my heart to all those who have contributed to the text. Particularly, Professor Alok Sud from Lady Hardinge Medical College and Associated Hospitals, New Delhi, India, who stood by the commitment once made and put constant efforts in providing me the text in pediatric orthopedics and helped till end in organizing some photographs despite ourselves being only formally introduced and worked for a short duration together. The other person who has helped in preparing the text is Dr S Pavan, who stood always by my side whenever required and also relieved me of my duties often at even hectic times to prepare the text. My juniors Dr Jaydip Patel, Dr Amit Singh and Dr Swapnil Sharma have provided help at difficult times when I needed them for text correction and improvement despite some of them being engaged in their own academic work. Especially, I would thank Dr Jaydip, who even woke-up untiringly at nights despite his duties to correct the text and add to the base work done by others and Dr Swapnil, who provided support regardless of his examinations going on. The contribution of others is not nevertheless small and Dr Ashok Jadon, Dr Sanjay L Srivastav, Dr Ankit Data and Dr Sachin Bharti have contributed thoroughly to the nonorthopedic topics and Dr Aditya Soral, Dr Ram Kinkar Jha and Dr S Dutta, without their help the text could never be completed. My family had been very supportive in displaying immense courage to face social restrictions and my untimely absence from home due to writing work, sometimes when my kids needed me most to play, read, learn and enjoy and my wife missing me sometimes altogether in important festivals and ceremonies. There are, however, some sour memories also and it is also important to mention that the writing had not been easy at all, with minimal help coming from persons I thought would contribute the most. The most respected and dear ones from my earlier relations in the field got too busy or otherwise to provide any help but this was to my best use and possibly advantage that it made me write all the topics by myself, which gave me further knowledge and confidence in areas where I was lacking in my training.

Lastly, I am highly thankful to Shri Jitendar P Vij (Group Chairman), Mr Ankit Vij (Group President), Ms Sunita Katla (PA to Group Chairman and Publishing Manager), Ms Samina Khan (Executive Assistant to Director–Publishing), the artists and all the team members who untiringly worked to bring out this wonderful text despite various delays and hitches from my end. It is only with the help of the publishing team at M/s Jaypee Brothers Medical Publishers (P) Ltd, New Delhi, India, that I could produce the text with confidence. Especially Shri Jitendar P Vij has grown in respect and stature in my thoughts who gave me the opportunity and initiated me for writing giving timely broad outlines, similarly production team has constantly assisted me in sorting out nitty-gritty problems that an author would usually encounter.

Providing an updated and correct text is always a challenge and some concepts would keep changing over time—is a fact. To this end, I reiterate all the readers of this text to kindly keep posting me in case, they find fundamental errors in the text or some critical updates that should be incorporated so that we can help all others in their future reading. I am open to all the criticism as they are bound to arise by difference of opinion that should be freely communicated to me at my e-mail—drmkvarshney@gmail.com. One may also reach me at the so-called in fashion social sites such as Facebook® or WhatsApp. In the name of Almighty, I present the text as an endeavor to promote the proficiency of both the neophyte and experienced orthopedic surgeon, bearing in mind to the truest of an attempt to present contradictory accumulation of discernment into logical concepts and the fact that condensing the mountain of knowledge may not be possible in the lifetime with ever-evolving concepts.

Manish Kumar Varshney

Acknowledgments

I am extremely thankful to Shri Jitendar P Vij (Group Chairman), Mr Ankit Vij (Managing Director), Mr MS Mani (Group President), Ms Chetna Malhotra Vohra (Associate Director—Content Strategy), Ms Pooja Bhandari (Production Head), and Ms Nikita Chauhan (Senior Development Editor) of M/s Jaypee Brothers Medical Publishers (P) Ltd, New Delhi, India, for giving the go-ahead at the very beginning and helping us in every way possible to bring out this book.

Contents

VOLUME 1

VOLUME 2

SECTION 6 Sports Medicine

SECTION 7 Regional Orthopedics: Shoulder

SECTION 8 Regional Orthopedics: Hip

SECTION

6

Sports Medicine

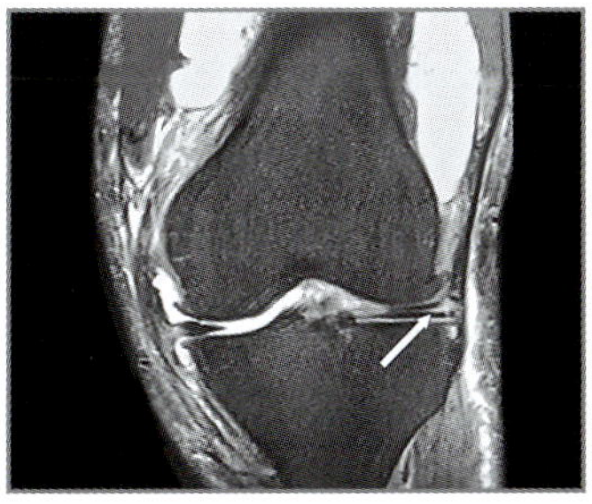

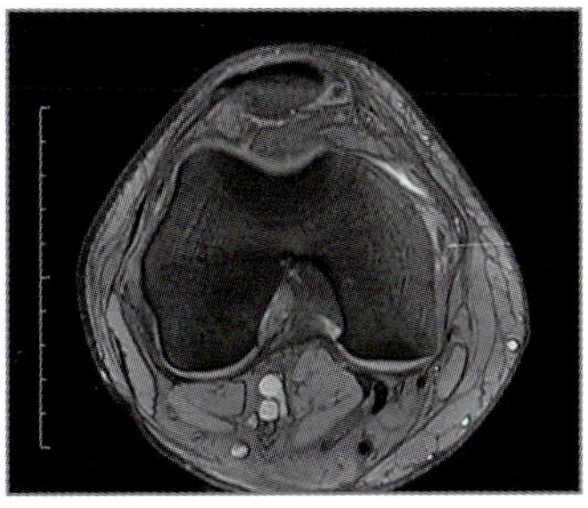

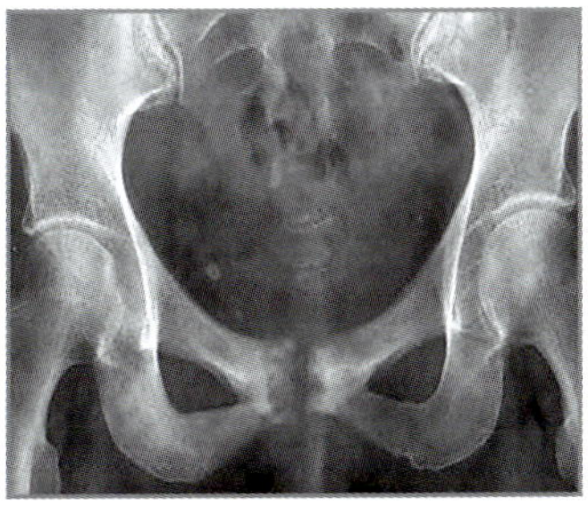

CHAPTER 45

Sports Medicine: Knee

Manish Kumar Varshney

INTRODUCTION

The knee is anatomically a very complex joint. Though there are only three bones articulating, the articulation is so big that there are numerous stabilizing structures maintaining smooth function and movements superimposed on stability. The joint has also to bear the excessive forces transmitted due to long lever arms. These stress are responsible for number of injuries in contact and noncontact sports. To understand the pathomechanics of knee disorders hence a good understanding of the anatomical structures, their disposition, and intricate relationship is important. The information on anatomy has evolved more into biomechanical and functional significance of the structures rather than mere description of their origins and insertions. This is described in detail in nearly first one-third of the chapter here. This helps understanding their role in the joint mechanics and prioritization of importance of repair/reconstruction following injury. Latter the principles dealing with injury to collateral ligaments, cruciate ligaments, patellofemoral articulation and menisci are described. Sports persons also suffer from various other wear and tear problems of structures surrounding the joint like the disorders of extensor mechanisms, bursae (bursitis, Baker's cyst), fad-pad syndromes (Hoffa's disease), patellofemoral pain and iliotibial band friction pain syndrome, etc., young athletes may additionally suffer from osteochondrosis like Osgood-Schlatter disease.

FUNCTIONAL ANATOMY

The knee has simplistic disposition of three bones **(Fig. 1)**, but a complex design to maintain simplicity in movements and ability to withstand immense forces. There are two distinct articulations that makeup the joint:

1. Tibiofemoral (this is a modified hinge joint)—participates in transmission of body weight from the femur to tibia and provides for sagittal plane joint rotation along with mild tibial axial rotation.
2. Patellofemoral (saddle joint)—provides the extensor mechanism. Eccentric contraction of quadriceps provides extension of the joint through transmission of the force along patella. The mechanism may be damaged in open injuries and patellar fractures.

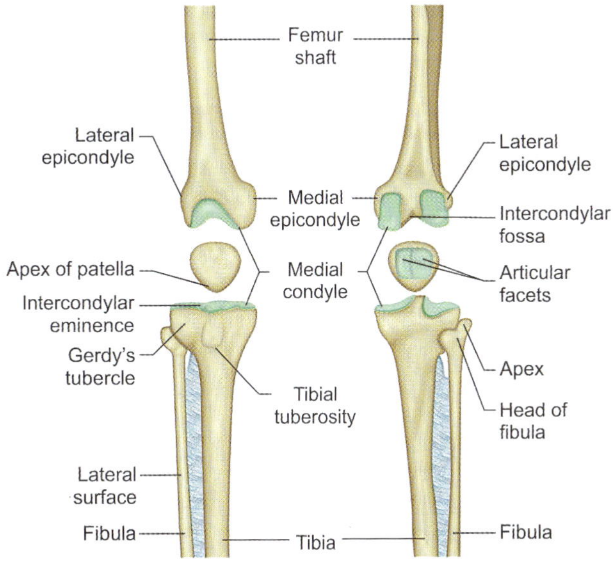

Fig. 1: Bones forming the knee joint: three bones form the knee joint that are placed quite simply, but the articulations are complex in dynamics.

TIBIOFEMORAL ARTICULATION

The tibiofemoral joint **(Fig. 2)** is the largest articulation of human body (surface area of contact) and is minimally constrained by bony anatomy (at least laterally). Due to versatile movements of such a large joint also having to bear weight of the body, various structures provide static and dynamic stability in different directions **(Table 1)**.

Static stability is due to interplay of:

- Tibiofemoral collateral ligaments **(Figs. 3A to C)**
- Medial and lateral meniscus **(*see* Figs. 2, 3, and 6)**
- Topography of the articular surfaces **(*see* Fig. 5)**
- Loads across the articular surfaces

Knee ligaments provide <30% of all the stability across the joint (majority being provided by muscles), however, being most amenable to surgical reconstruction they have

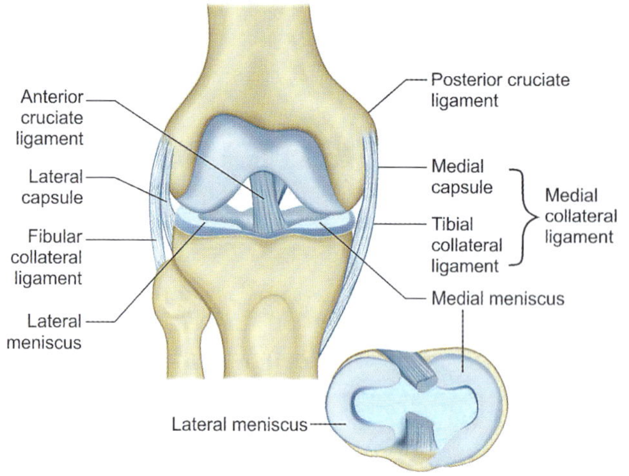

Fig. 2: Tibiofemoral articulation is the largest articulation of body. It also homes maximum articular cartilage and needs the strongest conjunction of intra-articular ligaments for stability. It is a modified (in the sense that it permits some axial rotation also) hinge joint.

TABLE 1: Various structures providing stability to knee.

Stability	***Ligaments***	***Muscles***
Medial	TCL	Semimembranosus
Lateral	LCL	Popliteus and ITB
Anterior	ACL	Quadriceps and patella
Posterior	PCL	Biceps femoris and popliteus
Anteromedial	TCL and ACL	Quadriceps
Anterolateral	LCL and PCL	
Posterior medial	Oblique popliteal ligament	Semimembranosus
Posterior lateral	Arcuate popliteal	Popliteus

[ACL: anterior cruciate ligament; ITB: iliotibial band; LCL: lateral collateral ligament; PCL: posterior cruciate ligament; TCL: tibial collateral ligament (also known as medial collateral ligament)]

been emphasized often as the most important mechanisms, devising treatment protocols and algorithms.

Dynamic stability is provided by muscles around the knee joint which acts on or across it **(Figs. 4A to C)**.

- Quadriceps acts as the main eccentric decelerator of the knee. The action of the quadriceps besides producing knee extension also causes anterior tibial translation and prevents posterior subluxation of the tibia, an action which is antagonistic to anterior cruciate ligament (ACL), but synergistic to posterior cruciate ligament (PCL). The hamstrings that produce knee flexion are antagonizers of PCL (tend to cause posterior subluxation) and are synergistic to ACL (reducing anterior subluxation).
- Hamstrings by the virtue of their tensioning effect on the capsular ligaments reduce the laxity present in the joint, increasing the articular surface load and congruency (dynamic constraint action). Thus, hamstrings provide dynamic stability of tibiofemoral joint more than quadriceps, which provide more for knee extension movement (and stability of patellofemoral joint). This way they augment the static mechanism of stability.
- Gastrocnemius and popliteus also provide dynamic stability by their tensing action on capsular and other structures.

Osseous Anatomy

Tibiofemoral Articulation

- The medial femoral condyle and medial tibial plateau as compared to the lateral compartments (more circular and smaller) are more elongated (ovoid) and larger **(Fig. 5)**.
- The lateral tibial plateau articular surface is convex anteroposteriorly as compared to the concave medial tibial plateau. This topography accounts for two significant events in knee mechanics and trauma:
    - Screw-home mechanism (internal rotation of the femur on the fixed tibia as the knee approaches extension) (discussed below)
    - The medial tibial condyle fractures are less common due to larger, concordant weight-bearing surface and if they occur, are shear type providing larger fragments, while lateral tibial plateau fractures are more common and are often comminuted due to small area of contact (convex femoral condyle articulating against flattish lateral tibial plateau) "resulting in" higher force transmission per unit area.
- Weight-bearing occurs in a saddle-shaped fashion between the tibiofemoral condyle—weight is transmitted both centrally and also in a cephalad sloping area in the medial and lateral tibial eminences similar to horseback rider bearing weight in a saddle.
- The tibial articular surface gives attachment to menisci and cruciate ligaments. Their order is different in the anterior and posterior aspect. Anteriorly the sequence of attachment of structures from anterior to posterior is medial meniscus, ACL, and lateral meniscus **(Fig. 5)**. On the posterior aspect, the structures are lateral meniscus, medial meniscus, and PCL.

Menisci

The menisci are two oval (semilunar) fibrocartilages, one on each side of a knee **(Fig. 6)**. The Greek word *meniskos* (meaning crescent), a diminutive of *mene* meaning *moon* is the parent word of meniscus. Originally considered to be embryological remnants their phylogeny has been traced back to 300 million years, and they are now considered to be important developed structures specific to bipedal gait. Medial meniscus is also seen in primates; however, the lateral meniscus with two tibial attachments is characteristic of hominids and bipedalism. The menisci develop between 8th and 10th week of gestation with blood supply to "whole meniscus". Gradually, the collagen content increases and with weight-bearing and reduction of cellularity the blood supply also gets restricted to lateral one-third.

Microanatomy

The cells of the menisci are fibrochondrocytes (mixture of fibroblasts and chondrocytes) where the superficial cells

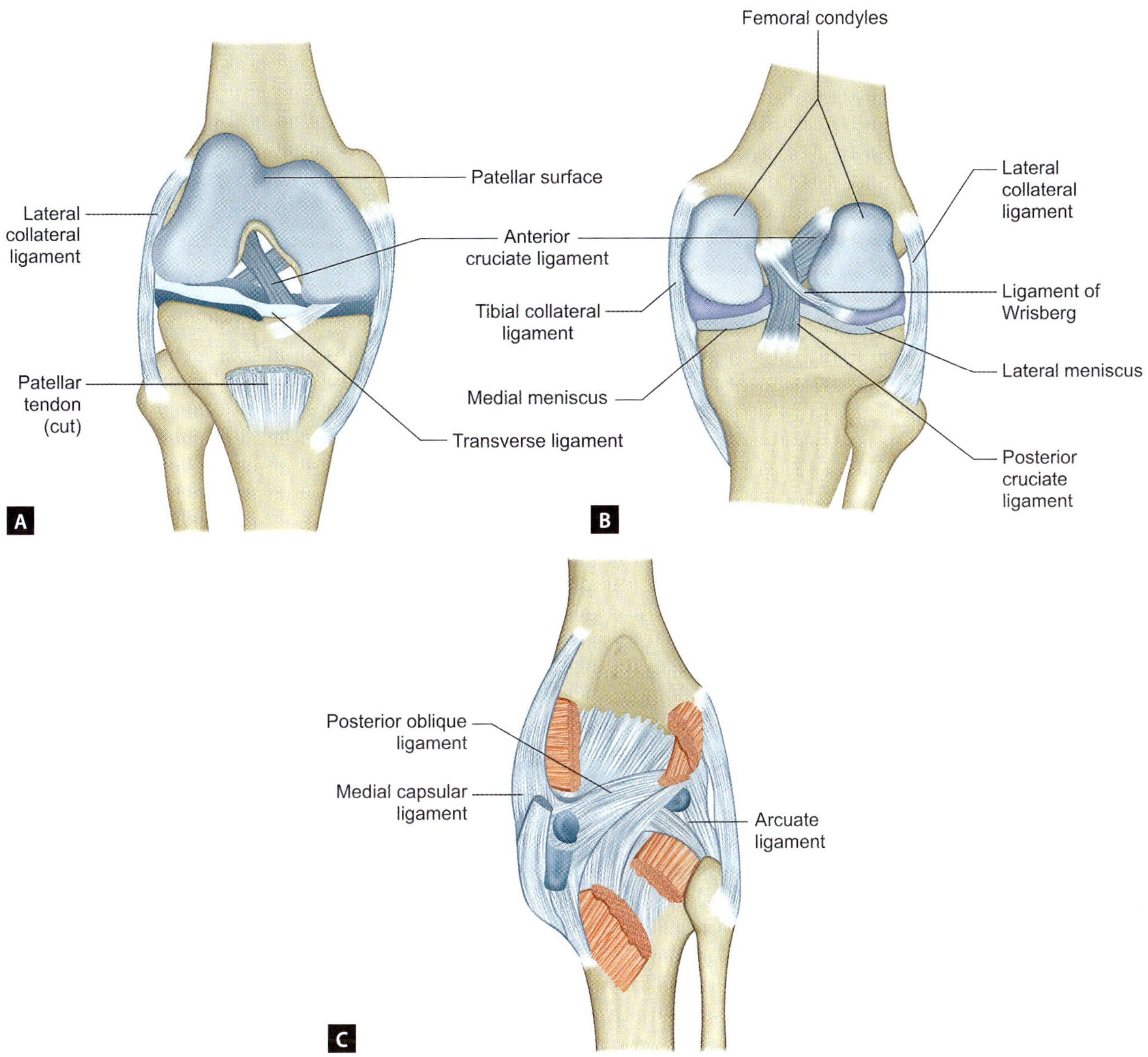

Figs. 3A to C: Ligaments of knee: (A) Anterior overview; (B) Posterior overview; (C) Ligaments of the knee as seen from posterior aspect.

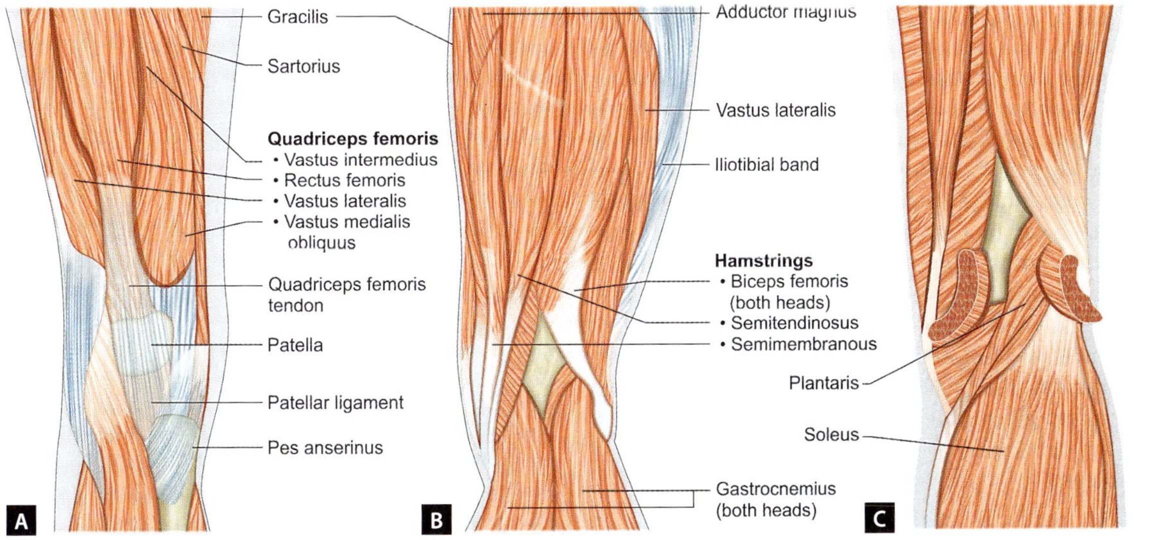

Figs. 4A to C: Dynamic stabilizers of knee joint. Muscles crossing the knee joint provide dynamic stability: (A) Muscles as seen from anterior aspect; (B) Muscles as seen from posterior aspect; (C) After removal of gastrocnemius.

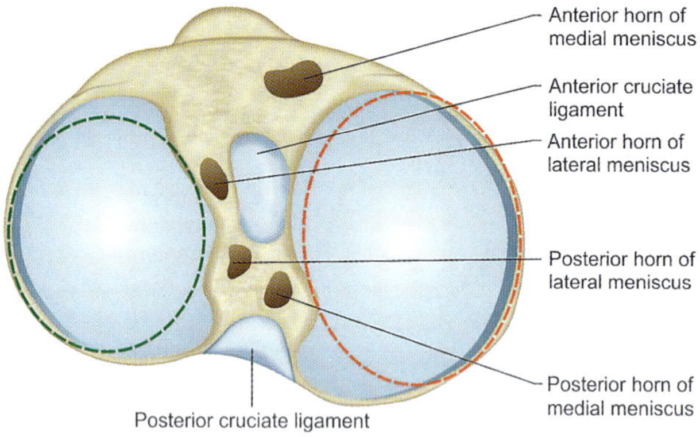

Fig. 5: Superior topography of tibial plateau of tight knee. The medial plateau is ovoid and longer (red circle) than the lateral (green circle).

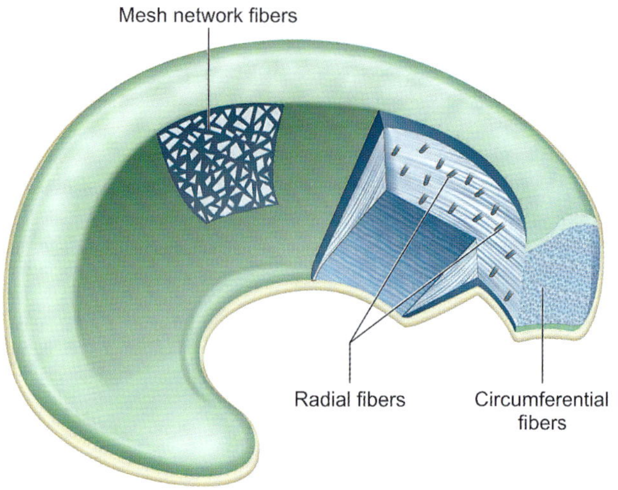

Fig. 7: Organization of collagen fibers in meniscus.

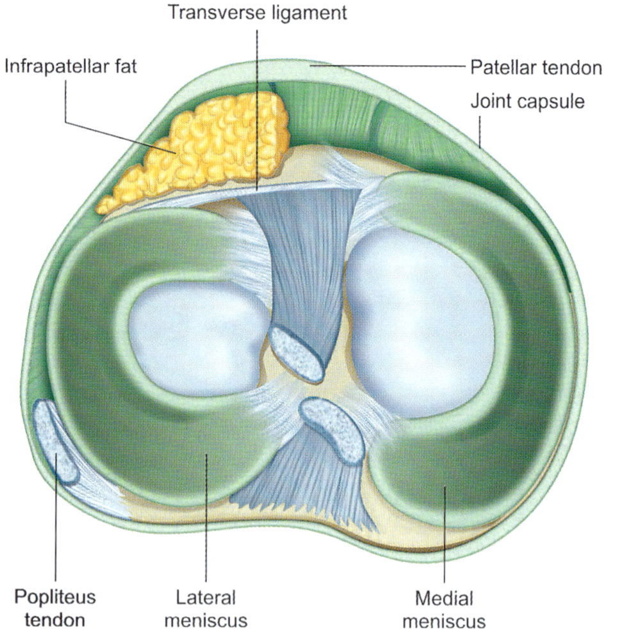

Fig. 6: The menisci of left knee as seen from above and structures in relation to them. Note the lateral meniscus is smaller and more circular "O"-shaped while medial meniscus is more like "C" shape.

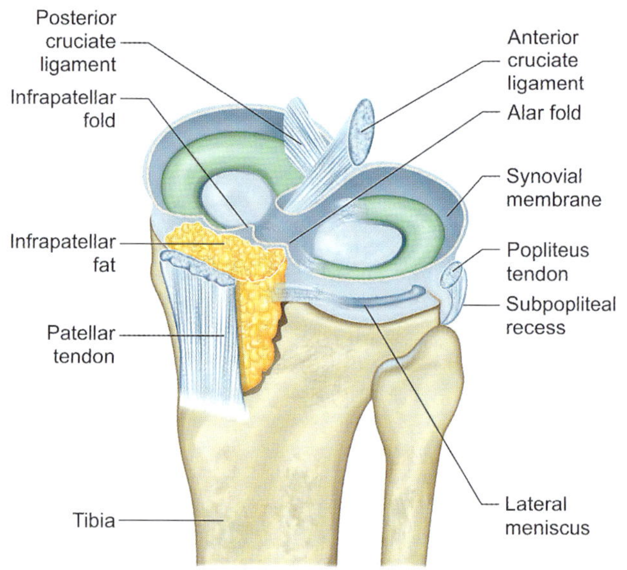

Fig. 8: Disposition of the menisci and relationship to nearby structures.

are spindle-shaped resembling fibroblasts, while the deeper ones are polygonal resembling chondrocytes. As opposed to hyaline cartilage the menisci contain predominantly the type I collagen (similar to bone) with variable amount of type II, type III, type V, and type VI collagens. The collagens are highly cross-linked by hydroxylpyridinium aldehydes. The unique arrangement of collagen fibers in menisci transfers the vertical compressive loads (weight-bearing) into circumferential "hoop stresses". The superficial fibers are radially oriented, while the deeper fibers are oriented circumferentially. Deeper fibers are also "tied" by some radially oriented fibers **(Fig. 7)**. Proteoglycans (aggrecan) and other matrix glycoproteins are found in smaller amounts.

Gross Anatomy

The lateral meniscus is more circular "O-shaped" and smaller while the medial one is longer and C-shaped **(Fig. 6)**. The medial meniscus is broader, but thinner than the lateral meniscus with a flat under surface. Medial meniscus is much broader posteriorly than in anterior aspect and is around 35 mm in anteroposterior diameter **(Fig. 8)**. Medial meniscus with the help of coronary ligaments (meniscotibial segment of capsular ligaments) at circumference is attached firmly to the medial articular surface of the tibia and to the joint capsule and tibial collateral ligament (TCL) at the circumference. Posteriorly, it is attached to the fibers of semimembranosus muscle **(Figs. 9A and B)** and anchored onto tibial surface near the fovea centralis (posterocentral area of the intercondylar spine). The lateral meniscus is loosely attached to the superior articular surface of tibia and lateral joint capsule. Posteriorly, it is attached to popliteus tendon **(Fig. 8)**. The lateral meniscus is more saucer-shaped superiorly and inferiorly develops a slanting shape to accommodate the convex architecture of the lateral tibial plateau. This makes it more triangular shaped in coronal cross-section as compared to the wedge-shaped medial

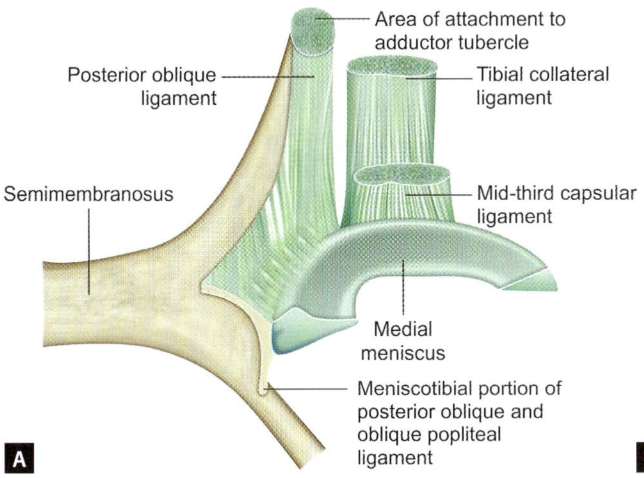

Figs. 9A and B: Contraction of the semimembranosus (arrow) retracts the posterior horn of the medial meniscus and bowstrings the capsule increasing joint contact pressure.

meniscus. In sagittal section the shape resembles a bow-tie [as seen commonly on magnetic resonance imaging (MRI)]. Its anterocentral attachment merges with the insertion of the ACL.

The ligament of Wrisberg [posterior meniscofemoral ligament (MFL)] is a continuation of lateral meniscus posteriorly projecting upward close to the attachment of the PCL **(*see* Fig. 3B)**. The anterior band on MFL is termed ligament of Humphrey (seen in approximately 60% individuals). The MFLs span between the posterior aspect of posterior horn of lateral meniscus and the lateral femoral condyle. Anteriorly, the two menisci are connected by transverse ligament in front of ACL by the anterior intermeniscal ligament.

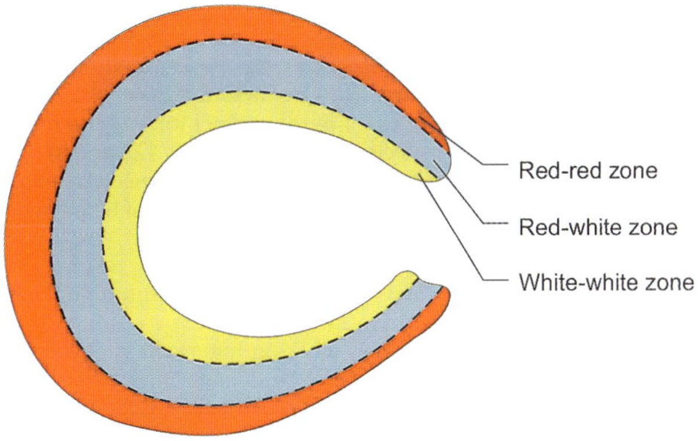

Fig. 10: The vascular zones of meniscus (*see* text for details).

Vascular and Neural Anatomy

The menisci are supplied by the medial, lateral, and middle genicular arteries via a network of premeniscal capillary network. Depending on the depth of blood vessel penetration three circumferential zones are identified **(Fig. 10)**:

1. Red-red zone is the outer peripheral one-third zone has good blood supply. Quantitatively, it is peripheral 20–30% for medial meniscus and 10–25% for lateral meniscus.
2. Red-white zone is the middle one-third has minimal blood supply.
3. White-white zone is the inner one-third with no blood supply. This region receives nutrition and oxygen through diffusion.

Articular branch of posterior tibial nerve, terminal branches of femoral and obturator nerves, and recurrent peroneal branch of common peroneal nerve provide the necessary innervation to both menisci. Outer third is more densely innervated than middle third. Menisci contain various mechanoreceptors predominantly of three types: (1) the Ruffini endings, (2) Pacinian corpuscles, and (3) Golgi tendon organs. Mechanoreceptors are in highest concentration in posterior horns.

Biomechanics and Dynamics of Menisci

The menisci are not static structures and actually move with knee flexion and extension. Medial meniscus moves 2–3 mm during full range of flexion-extension, while the lateral meniscus is much more mobile and moves 8–10 mm **(Fig. 11)**. The medial meniscus is limited by its fixation to extracapsular structures and capsule itself as discussed above.

The biomechanical functions of the menisci are detailed in **Box 1**.

Capsular and Collateral Ligaments

They are divided into the medial and lateral complexes **(Fig. 14)**. It is easier to understand their anatomy by dividing them into thirds **(Fig. 15)**.

- The posteromedial or posterolateral corner (PLC) of the knee—these are formed by large aponeurotic expansion of the medial or lateral hamstrings respectively. Capsular ligaments form the central portion of this expansion and help in tibiofemoral stability. This expansion spans from the muscle belly to (and including) the meniscus (the meniscocapsular ligament-musculotendinous unit complex—coined by Terry and Hughston).

- Posterior aspects of the femoral condyles are buttressed by these structures and at the same time accommodate their increased volume in extension and decreasing volume in flexion.

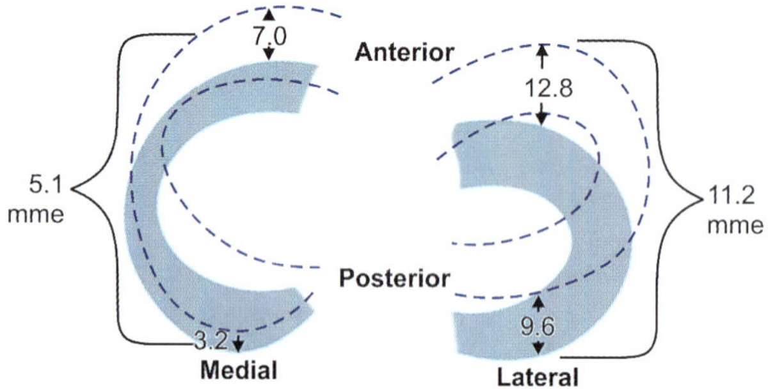

Fig. 11: Movement of menisci with knee movements (dynamic menisci movements). Movement in each meniscus is depicted in shaded in flexion and dotted (extension). The lateral meniscus is more mobile. (mme: mean meniscal excursion)

BOX 1: The functions of menisci.

- Load bearing—transmit one-half of the contact force in the medial compartment and more in lateral compartment **(Figs. 12A and B)**
- *Joint stability:* Stabilize the knee in flexion—function of medial meniscus at 90° knee flexion that prevents anterior translation of tibia (wedge effect, **Figs. 12A and B**)
- Shock absorber
- Guiding rotation of femoral condyle over tibia and terminal axial rotation during extension
- Spreading the lubrication evenly and distributing the synovial fluid across the joint (for nutrition)
- *Joint congruity:* Filling the voids in knee joint between the femur and tibial, giving static stability
- Limiting extremes of flexion and extension
- Increasing surface area of contact reducing the stress per unit contact area **(Figs. 13A and B)**
- Proprioception
- Protecting collateral and capsular ligaments from getting caught between the articular surfaces

- They allow anterior tibial translation, but prevent the posterior subluxation of the femoral condyles.
- The semimembranosus provides expanded insertion into posteromedial corner and gives dynamic stability. Its insertion has five components **(Fig. 16)**:

1. The anterior arm, the tibial arm, or pars reflexa insert on the tibial condyle at the TCL insertion. It courses distally and anteriorly from the muscle belly.
2. The direct arm inserts into the posterior tibial tubercle.
3. The posterior arm forms the inferior border of the oblique popliteal ligament.
4. The capsular arm becomes confluent with the posterior oblique ligament (POL) and the proximal border of the oblique popliteal ligament.
5. The inferior arm courses directly distally and forms a broad distal attachment along the posteromedial corner of the proximal tibia.

Medial knee ligament complex—this is a complex organization divided into layers:

- *Layer 1:* The sartorial fascia is the most superficial layer. An aponeurotic extension of the sartorius tendon merges into the fascia of the vastus medialis obliquus (VMO) and the anteromedial retinaculum and continues along the anterior aspect of the knee as the arciform layer of the extensor mechanism [the gracilis, semitendinosus, and saphenous nerve run between the layers 1 and 2]
- *Layer 2:* The tibial (medial) collateral ligament, structures of posteromedial corner (including the musculotendinous attachments of the semimembranosus) and the medial patellofemoral ligament (MPFL) are included in layer 2.

Note: Medial collateral ligament (MCL) is not a recognized term in "Nomina Anatomica" so should not be used, instead the correct nomenclature is TCL.

- The TCL originates near medial epicondyle (3.2 mm proximal and 4.8 mm posterior) and inserts on the tibia deep to the anterior border of the sartorius and pes

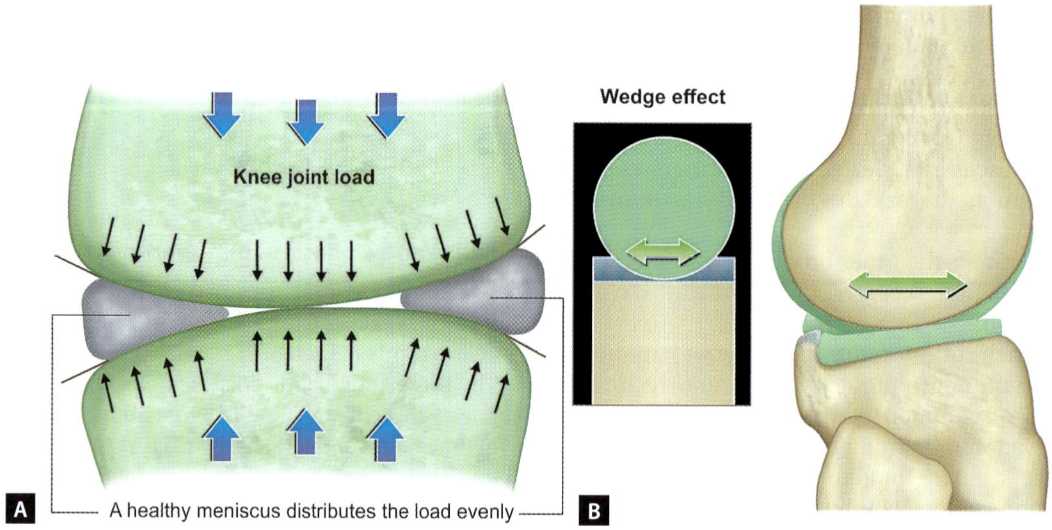

Figs. 12A and B: The menisci play an important role in evenly distributing the force across the knee joint. (A) Wedge effect of meniscus in improving knee joint stability; (B) The meniscus blocks the anteroposterior glide in a static knee despite rounded shape of femoral condyles—akin to use of blocks under tyres to prevent vehicles from moving by themselves on sloping surfaces.

anserinus distally. It is divided into superficial and deep structures by bursa. The superficial component is hence extracapsular. Middle third of the medial meniscus is attached to the capsule through the deep component of the TCL. The deep component inserts just distal to the articular margin. It has two segments formed by intermediate insertion to meniscus. The meniscofemoral segment extends from its femoral bony origin to the meniscus and the meniscotibial segment extends from the meniscus to the tibial insertion **(Fig. 17)**. The size of the meniscotibial segment at the mid-third portion of the capsule is maximum 5 mm in length. A void greater than this indicates tear of the tibial insertion. Superficial part of the TCL has two distinct insertion—one (less prominent) is to the soft tissue over the termination of the anterior arm of the semimembranosus tendon and is 12 mm distal to the tibial joint line, other insertion is more important and is ≈61 mm below the tibial joint line slightly anterior to posteromedial tibial crest.

- *Layer 3 (true joint capsule and the deep medial capsular ligaments):* They attach the meniscus to the femur and allow tibia to move on the menisci inferiorly. Deep medial capsular ligaments **(Fig. 18)** are divided into three parts:
  1. The anterior capsular ligament connects with the extensor mechanism and the medial meniscus through the coronary ligaments. It relaxes during knee extension and tightens during knee flexion.
  2. Middle portion is the deep component of TCL (discussed above).
  3. Two capsular ligaments originating from the adductor tubercle are enclosed in the posterior-third capsule.
     - The oblique popliteal ligament:
       - Courses obliquely across the popliteal surface of the posterior capsule.
       - Becomes confluent with the medial aponeurotic extensions of the posterior arcuate ligament.
     - The posterior oblique ligament (POL, studied in detail by Hughston and Eilers) originates just anterior to the oblique popliteal ligament. It is an extension off the distal aspect of the semimembranosus that blends with and reinforces the posteromedial capsule. It has three arms the capsular, tibial, and superficial **(Fig. 18)**. The capsular arm of the POL provides attachment to the posterior horn of medial meniscus.
- During range of motion, the TCL gets taut at full extension, relaxes at 20–30° of flexion and again begins to tighten between 60 and 70° of knee flexion. Functionally, it has been found by studies of Hughston and Eilers that the knee should be immobilized in 60° of flexion for optimal healing without placing excessive tension on the medial ligament complex.

The superficial ligament acts as the primary stabilizer to valgus stress at all angles of knee flexion as well external rotation stress, while the deep component is the secondary stabilizer. Secondary stability against external rotation is provided by both the deep component and at 30° of flexion by the POL. POL, superficial, and deep portions of TCL jointly resist internal rotation. The different portions of the ligaments share the stress at different angles of knee flexion in this case also.

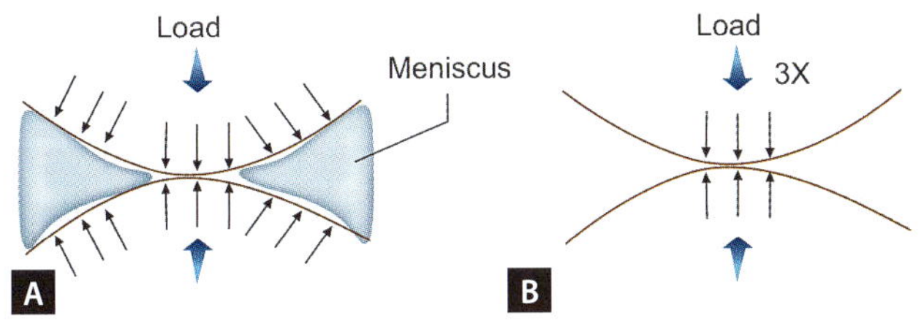

Figs. 13A and B: Meniscus helps in reducing contact forces: (A) Load transmission with meniscus; (B) Without meniscus the load gets concentrated.

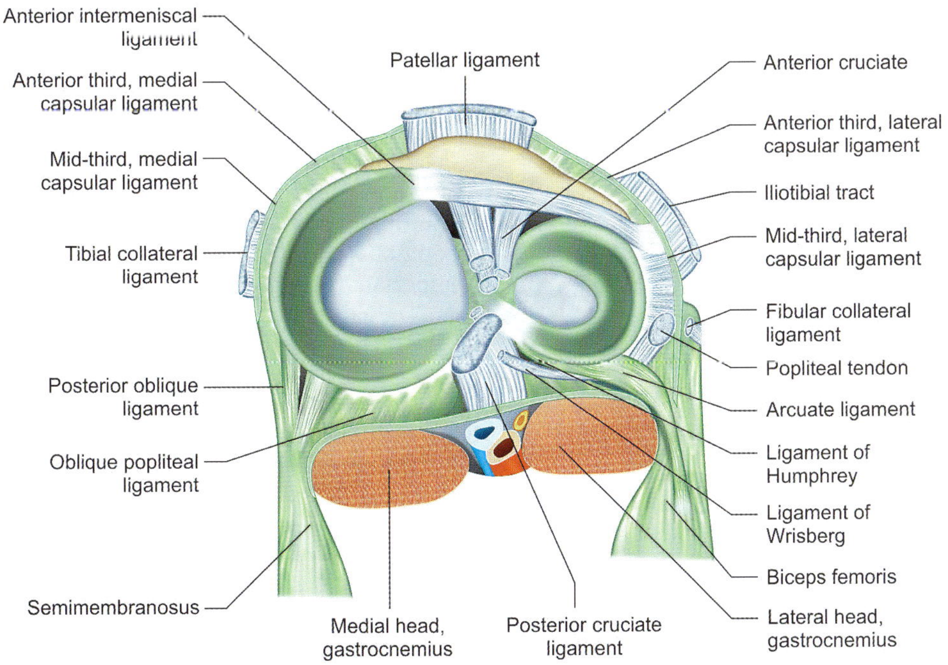

Fig. 14: The medial and lateral ligamentous structures.

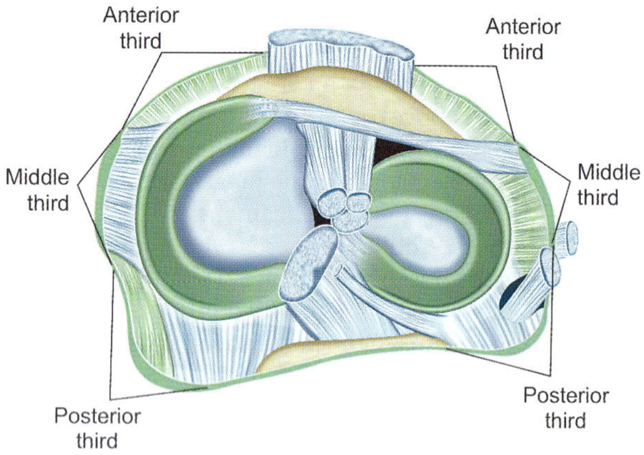

Fig. 15: Capsular ligaments of right knee—the medial and lateral complexes can be divided into thirds for anatomical description.

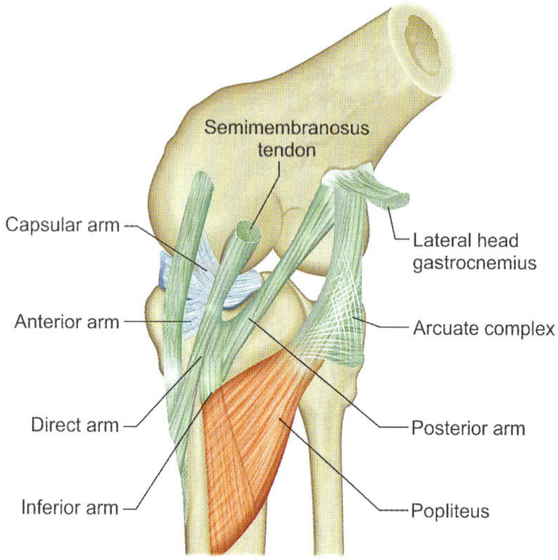

Fig. 16: The five insertions of the semimembranosus (*see* text for details).

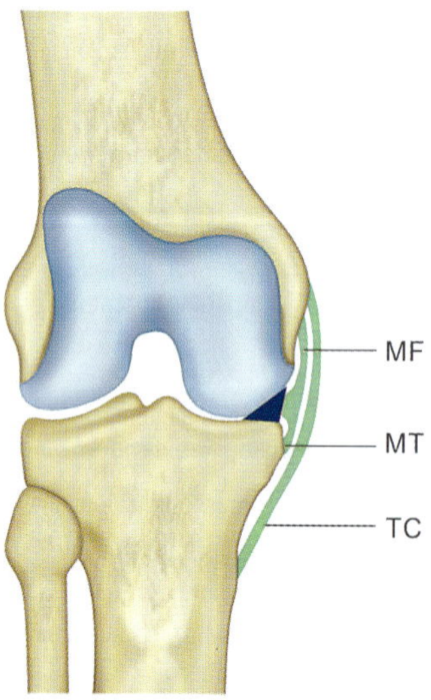

Fig. 17: The mid-third capsular ligament (deep portion of tibial collateral ligament) is divided into a proximal longer meniscofemoral (MF) segment in a span from the medial epicondyle to the meniscus and a distal shorter meniscotibial (MT) segment.
(TC: tibial collateral ligament)

Lateral ligament complex are arranged into three layers **(Fig. 19)** as follows:

- *Layer 1:* Iliotibial tract and biceps femoris
- *Layer 2:* Patellar retinaculum and patellofemoral ligament (the common peroneal nerve lies between layers 1 and 2)
- *Layer 3:* Divided into superficial and deep layers:
  - *Superficial:* Fibular collateral ligament and fabellofibular ligament
  - *Deep:* Arcuate ligament, coronary ligament, popliteus tendon and popliteofibular ligament (PFL) (lateral geniculate artery runs between deep and superficial layers).

These are much better described by dividing into anterolateral and posterolateral structures that are clinically important.

Anterolateral side: The iliotibial band (ITB) is the most prominent and most superficial structure. Proximally, part of gluteus maximus and the tensor fasciae latae (TFL) insert on the ITB. ITB inserts on Gerdy's tubercle on the proximal—lateral tibia and acts as an accessory anterolateral ligament. With flexion—ITB moves posteriorly exerting external rotation and posterior force on lateral tibia. With extension varus stress and posterolateral rotation. It is controlled by TFL muscle proximally to control the exerted tension. The ITB consists of two functional divisions **(Fig. 20)**:

1. The iliopatellar ligament, which is a functional component of the extensor mechanism.
2. The iliotibial tract (encompassing the posterior 2 cm of the ITB)—provides functional component to the tibiofemoral joint. Distally, the iliotibial tract has deep aponeurotic expansions—the middle, deep, and capsulo-osseous layers. The capsulo-osseous layer is partially confluent with the fabellofibular ligament and wraps anteriorly and distally to insert on the lateral tibial (Gerdy's) tubercle. Rupture of this component is responsible for rotatory component of pivot shift or "jerk test".

Posterior to ITB are the aponeurotic insertions of the biceps femoris muscle. Though the origins are two the insertions are six for short head and two for long head. It is a powerful dynamic external rotation of the tibia and contributes as a lateral stabilizer. Out of the six terminal arms of the short head of the biceps femoris muscle only three are important **(Figs. 21A to C)**:

1. The capsular arm attaches to:
   - The posterolateral capsule
   - Fabella
   - Lateral gastrocnemius complex
2. The direct arm attaches to fibula just lateral to the styloid.
3. The anterior arm inserts on the tibia just at or just lateral to the Gerdy's tubercle and is responsible for the lateral avulsion fracture or the lateral capsular sign (better known as the Segond sign for ACL avulsion).

The long head of the biceps femoris has two arms **(Fig. 21C)**:

- While the direct arm inserts on the fibula in front of the short head of the biceps the anterior arm inserts

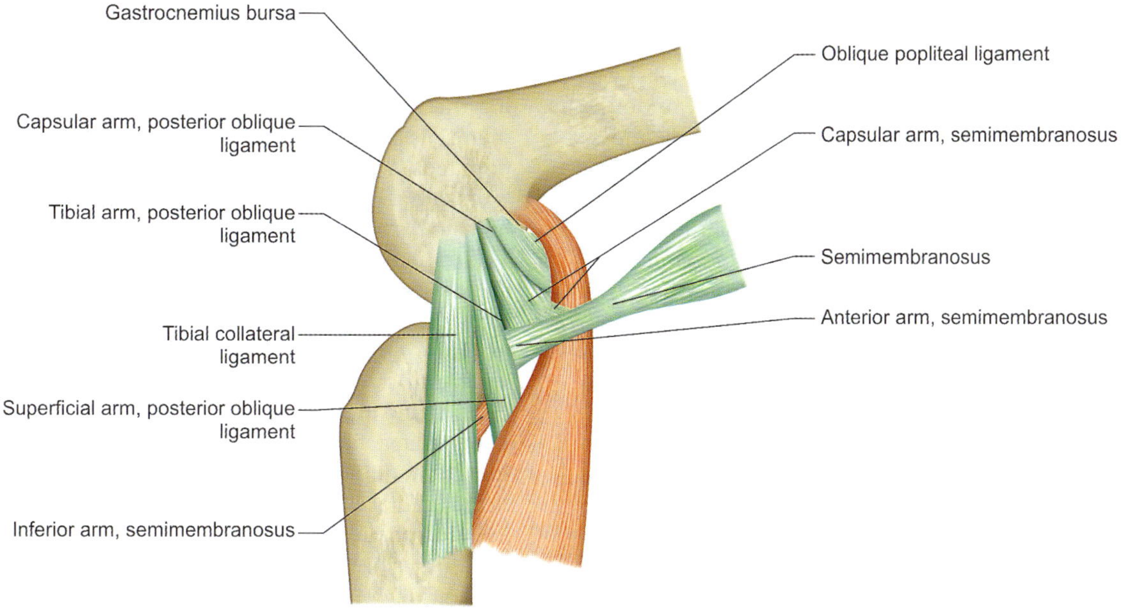

Fig. 18: The anatomy of deep capsular structures on medial side. The posterior oblique ligament and its three arms are shown with related structures (deep portion of tibial collateral ligament is not shown here).

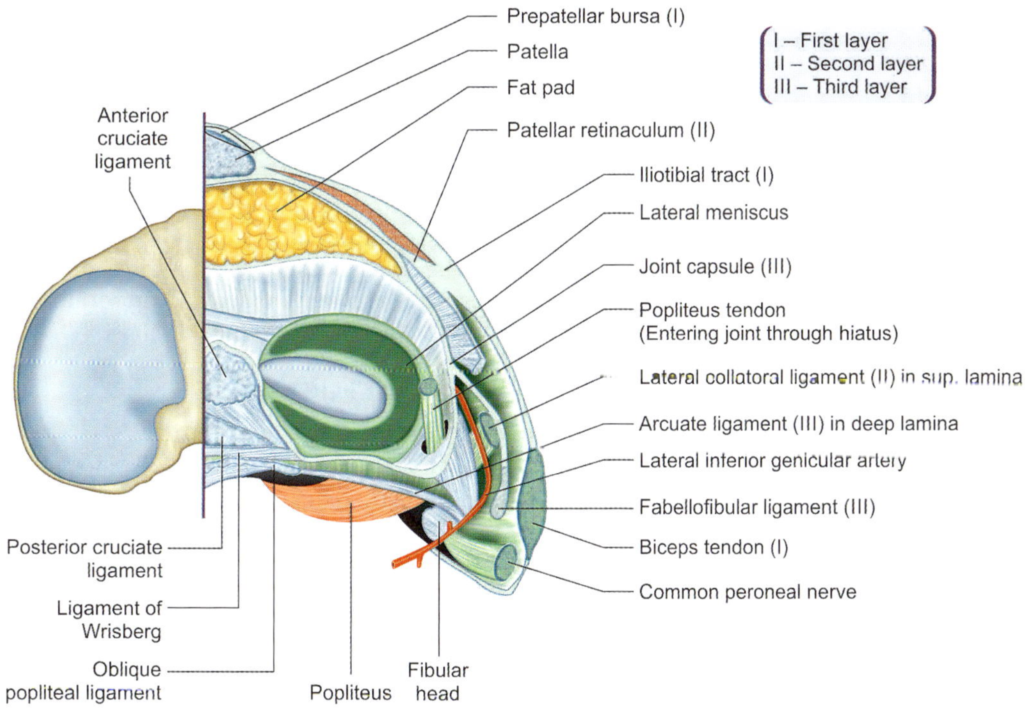

Fig. 19: The three layers of lateral ligament complex.

on the lateral tibia distal to short head insertion. The fibular collateral ligament and distal biceps tendon are separated by a bursa.

Posterolateral Side

- The anterolateral ligament (ALL, Vieira, and Vincent) or mid-third lateral capsular ligament of Houghston and Johnson **(Fig. 22A)** has recently caught the interest of anatomists and orthopedic surgeons (while intriguing the less than complete results of ACL reconstruction). It is also known as "capsulo-osseous layer of the iliotibial band (*see* above in discussion of iliotibial tract)", "anterior oblique ligament", etc. It was first described by French surgeon Paul Segond in 1879 as a "pearly, resistant, fibrous band" at the anterolateral aspect of the human knee that resists tibial internal rotation and is attached to the eponymous Segond fracture. The Segond's fracture was consistently located just behind the Gerdy's tubercle and its association with knee instability (ACL tear) was demonstrated by Woods et al. based on the work of Dr Jack Hughston. ALL originates from lateral epicondyle coursing deep to both the iliotibial tract and iliopatellar ligament and provides an attachment for the lateral meniscus. It inserts just distal to the articular margin on the lateral tibia midway between Gerdy's tubercle and the tip of the fibular head separate from ITB insertion. The popliteal tendon and fibular collateral ligament lie deep to the lateral mid-third capsular ligament **(Fig. 19)**. Its clinical significance lies in resisting the internal rotation of tibia and hence contributes to pivot shift test. Orthopedicians have found incompetence of the ALL to negatively influence the results of ACL reconstruction and recommend simultaneous reconstruction of ALL to optimize the results.

- The popliteal tendon inserts at lateral epicondyle slightly anterior to the origin of fibular collateral ligament **(Fig. 22B)**. The popliteal muscle belly takes its origin from the proximal posterior fibula coursing obliquely and proximally continuing with the tendon. It is attached to the lateral meniscus through anteroinferior, posterosuperior and posteroinferior popliteal meniscal fascicles. The functions of the popliteus muscle include stabilizing the knee during flexion and protecting the lateral meniscus by pulling it posteriorly while contracting. The popliteus is also a secondary restraint to posterior tibial translation. It also plays an important role in screw-home mechanism.

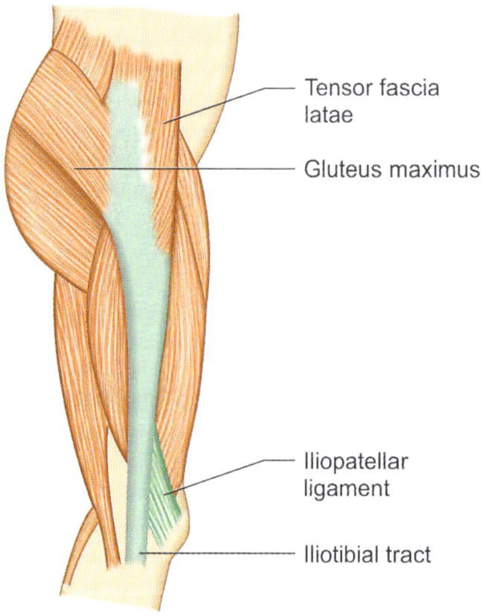

Fig. 20: Iliotibial band.

- The fibular collateral ligament is a round, fibrous cord and courses distally to insert just anterior to the lateral aspect of the fibular head **(Fig. 22C)**. It is taut during knee extension, but relaxed during flexion. It is the primary static varus restraint for the knee (especially at 30° of flexion) and limits external rotation at 30° of flexion.
- The popliteal fibular ligament originates at the popliteal-musculotendinous junction and courses distally to attach to the medial aspect of the fibular styloid **(Fig. 22C)**.
- Both the popliteus and popliteal fibular ligament provide restraint against tibial external rotation at higher flexion angles (≈60° of flexion).
- The fabellofibular ligament originates from the lateral aspect of fabella and inserts lateral to the tip of the fibular styloid just lateral to the insertion of the popliteal fibular ligament.
- The arcuate ligament **(*see* Fig. 19)** is formed by thickening in the posterior joint capsule and has three components.
  1. The lateral portion borders mid-third capsular ligament.
  2. The medial portion lies deep to the lateral gastrocnemius head.
  3. Posterior component merges with the oblique popliteal ligament.

The arcuate complex comprises the fibular collateral ligament, popliteus, lateral head of the gastrocnemius muscle, and arcuate ligament.

CRUCIATE LIGAMENTS

Anterior Cruciate Ligament

The ACL origin spans from posterolateral surface of the intercondylar notch (medial surface of the lateral femoral condyle) and courses distally and anteriorly to insert on the intercondylar eminence. ACL ranges from 22 mm to 41 mm in length (average 32 mm) and 10 mm to 12 mm in

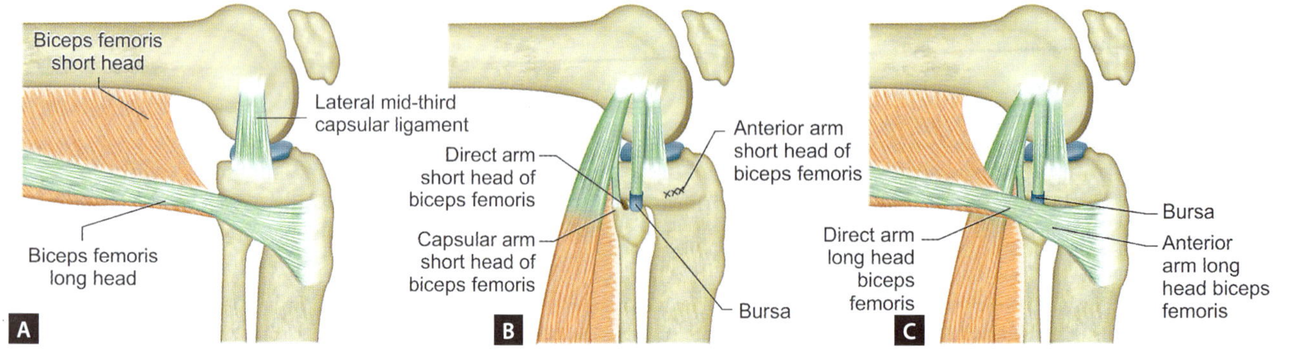

Figs. 21A to C: Biceps femoris muscle: the two heads. (A) Have different prominent insertions over proximal tibiofibular region important of which are, three for short head: The direct arm, the anterior arm, and the capsular arm; (B) The long head has two arms: a direct arm and (C) an anterior arm.

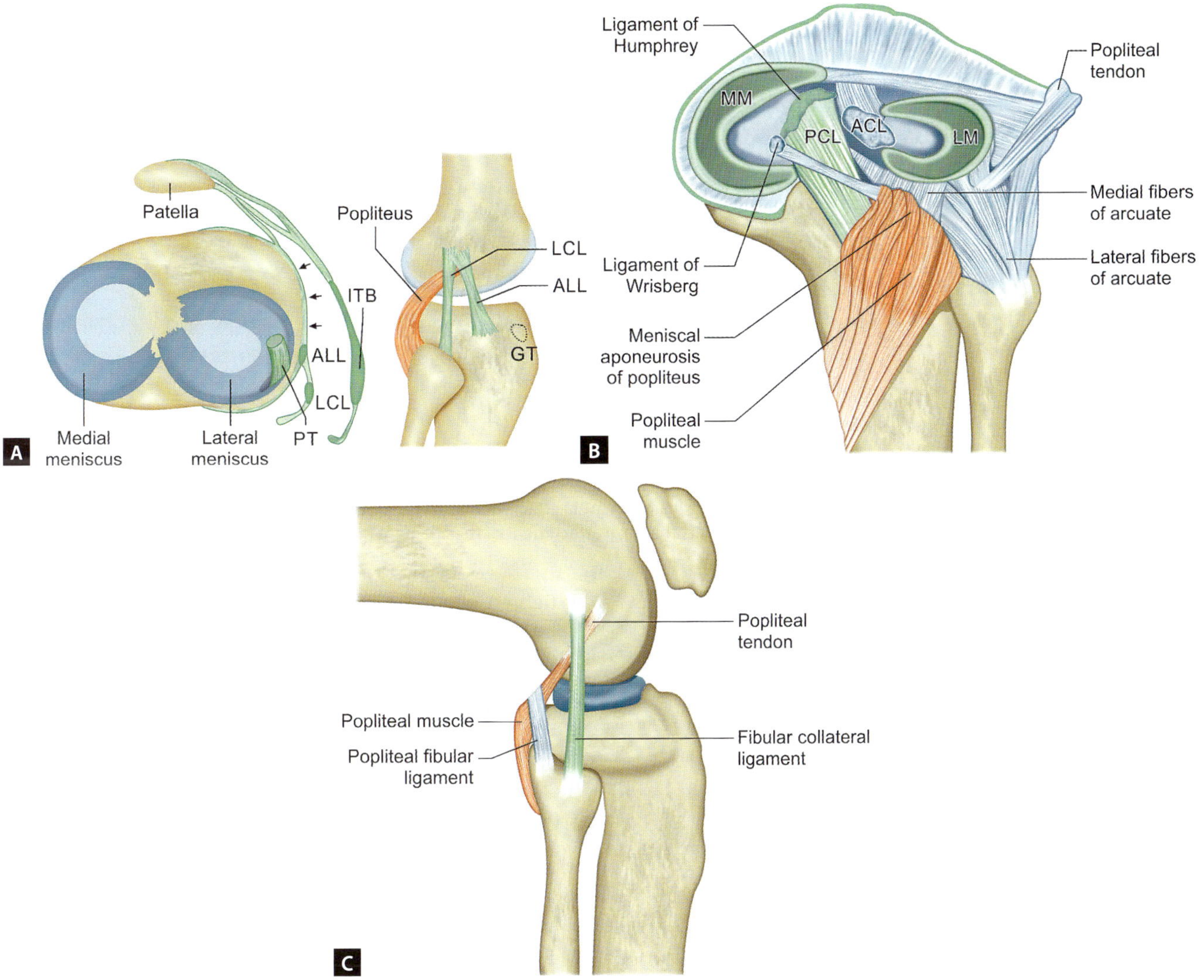

Figs. 22A to C: The lateral capsuloligamentous anatomy. (A) Illustration of the anterolateral ligament (ALL) in the axial and lateral disposition showing its relationship to the iliotibial band (ITB), lateral collateral ligament (LCL), Gerdy's tubercle (GT) and popliteus tendon (PT); (B) The posterolateral ligament complex; (C) The popliteofibular ligament originates at popliteal musculotendinous junction and inserts on to medial aspect of the fibular styloid. (PCL: posterior cruciate ligament; ACL: anterior cruciate ligament; LM: lateral meniscus; MM: medial meniscus)

width. The tibial attachment of ACL is around 30–32 mm wide **(Fig. 23B)** and has four organized histological zones that help in transmitting the loads from hard to soft tissue; these are ligament, uncalcified fibrocartilage, calcified fibrocartilage, and bone. The femoral attachment is around 21–23 mm in diameter **(Fig. 23A)**. The ligament comprises fibroblasts surrounded by type I and type III collagen (some amount of type III and IV collagens are present at insertion). The blood supply to the ACL comes through the fat pad by an anastomosis between the medial and the lateral genicular arteries and also through the middle geniculate artery which branches off the posterior capsule (at right angles from popliteal artery). In ACL tear **(Fig. 24)** the blood supply is permanently disrupted partially explaining poor healing of the ligament after tear. The nerve supply is from posterior articular nerve a branch of tibial nerve. The ligament is extrasynovial, but intracapsular. After complete tear it also becomes intrasynovial and the synoviocytes line the torn ends that ultimately form an obstructive synovial layer precluding healing. The innervation of ACL consists of mechanoreceptors derived from the tibial nerve and contributes to proprioception, there are no pain fibers.

- Anterior cruciate ligament contains two bundles **(Figs. 25A to C)**—an anteromedial and a posterolateral bundle (mnemonic AMPL), an intermediate bundle is also proposed by some. The bundles are named after their disposition at the tibial end. 26% knees have single bundle. The anteromedial bundle on average measures 6–7 mm in width, while the posterolateral bundle measures 5–6 mm. The lateral intercondylar ridge (sometimes referred to as resident's ridge) and the lateral bifurcate ridge (also known as the cruciate ridge) are utilized to identify the femoral footprint of bundles (while doing anatomical double bundle ACL reconstruction). The anteromedial bundle is tighter in extension and the posterolateral bundle is tighter in flexion. The bundles have a spiral configuration where the bundles wrap on themselves in a lateral to medial fashion and they

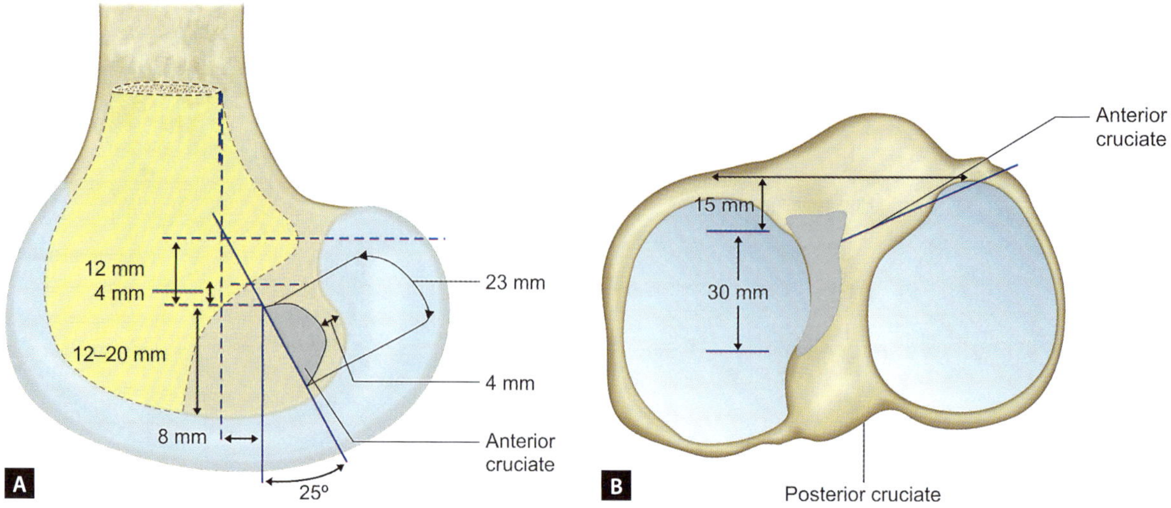

Figs. 23A and B: Anatomy of anterior cruciate ligament (ACL) attachments: (A) The details of femoral attachment (origin) of the ACL; (B) Depicts the tibial attachment of the ligament (insertion).

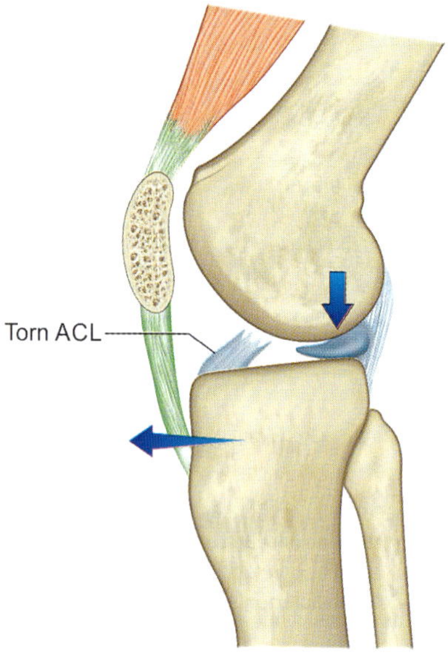

Fig. 24: Anterior cruciate ligament (ACL) tear with anterior tibial subluxation partially restricted by posterior horns of menisci.

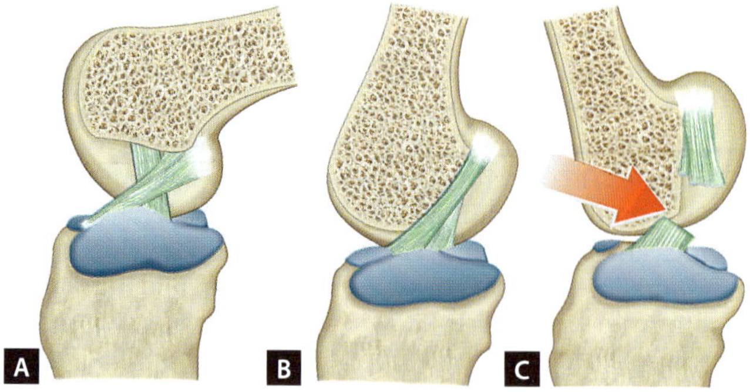

Figs. 25A to C: Anterior cruciate ligament (ACL) physioanatomy: (A) During knee flexion anteromedial bundle is lax and posterolateral bundle is taut resisting anterior tibial translation; (B) During knee extension both bundles are taut and resist coronal plane forces; and (C) During knee hyperextension the bundles are torn by the femur.

tighten when the tibia internally rotates. Anteromedial bundle resists anterior translation of tibia in flexion, but the posterolateral bundle is the primary restraint to anterior tibial translation in extension and contributing to rotatory stability.

- The functions of ACL are:
  - The ACL primarily resists anterior translation of tibia on femur especially at approximately 20° of knee flexion.
  - In full extension, the anterior surface of the ACL lies against the intercondylar notch preventing hyperextension.
  - It is a secondary stabilizer of knee against rotational forces (tibial rotation) and varus and valgus stress.
  - The ACL together with PCL guides the instantaneous center of rotation of the knee (helicoid knee action) preventing meniscal injury.
  - It pivots during the screw-home mechanism for tibial rotation as the knee extends.
  - Couples translation to tibial axial rotation.

Posterior Cruciate Ligament

The posterior cruciate ligament (PCL) is also intra-articular and extrasynovial. The PCL originates from the medial surface of the intercondylar notch in its anterior part and extends distally to insert on the proximal tibia in the fovea centralis posteriorly, inferior to the articular surface **(Figs. 26A and B)**. Distal part of PCL is covered by its synovial sheath medially, laterally, and anteriorly while posteriorly PCL blends with posterior capsule and periosteum. The PCL is longer and thicker than ACL, the average length is around 38 mm while width is 13 mm with cross-sectional area 50% greater at the femoral end and 20% greater at the tibial end. The femoral footprint for the PCL on average measures 209 mm^2 while the tibial footprint measures 244 mm^2. The proximal origin of PCL represents the center of axial rotation of the knee as it is in line with the epicondylar axis of the femur. The blood

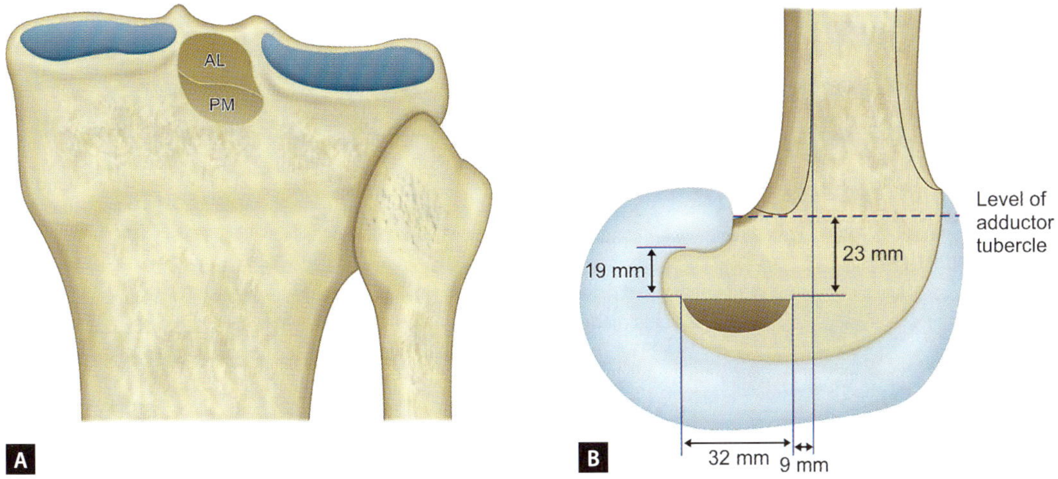

Figs. 26A and B: Posterior cruciate ligament (PCL) anatomy: its attachment on (A) tibial and (B) femoral surfaces. Note that in the femoral region PCL has a semicircular origin.

supply to PCL is maintained even in substance tear of PCL due to close association with the posterior capsule where the blood supply is derived from middle genicular artery. Neural innervation is mainly through the tibial and obturator nerves via popliteal plexus. Ruffini corpuscles (type I, pressure receptors), Vater-Pacini corpuscles (type II, velocity receptors) and free nerve endings (type IV, pain receptors) are found in PCL along with some Golgi tendon organs for proprioception.

- The PCL has two bundles **(Fig. 27)**—a posteromedial and an anterolateral bundle (nomenclature based on femoral insertion). Anterolateral bundle is larger than posteromedial bundle. The posteromedial bundle is tauter in extension and the anterolateral bundle is tauter in flexion. These bundles tighten during the internal rotation of tibia as they wrap around each other as occurs in 90° anteroposterior drawer tests in internal rotation as a test of PCL competency. Though thinner than anterolateral bundle the posteromedial bundle has higher stiffness and ultimate strength to failure.
- The ligaments of Wrisberg and Humphrey comprise 22% of the entire cross-sectional area of PCL.
- Functions of PCL:
  - In full extension, the PCL is the primary restraint to posterior translation of tibia on femur at all flexion angles >30°. At 90° this restraining effect is maximum. Posteromedial and posterolateral capsule, MCL (TCL), lateral collateral ligament (LCL), arcuate, meniscofemoral and fabellofibular ligaments provide the primary restraint from 0 to 30°.
  - Tibial external rotation and abduction or adduction stress at 0° as PCL acts as a secondary restraint for them.
  - Resists extremes of flexion.

PATELLOFEMORAL ARTICULATION

The patellofemoral articulation is a part of the larger extensor mechanism of knee **(Figs. 28A and B)**. The joint

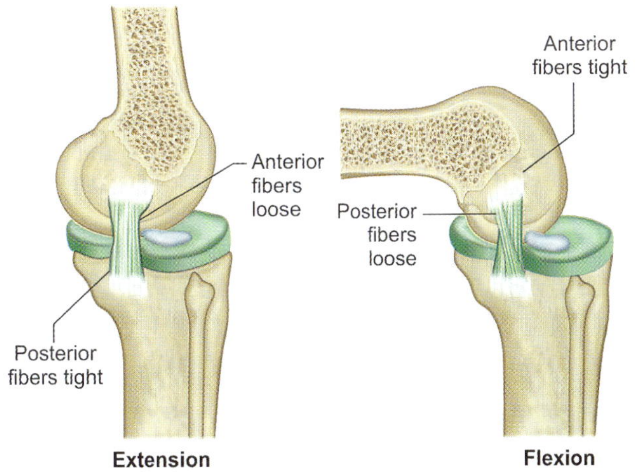

Fig. 27: Posterior cruciate ligament (PCL) bundles: the bundles of PCL have been named after femoral attachment distribution. They are differentially taut in different positions of knee.

is motored by the quadriceps that acts eccentrically during gait, running or jumping. The joint has gained attention due to high prevalence of patellofemoral arthritis and is often a precursor of arthritis of the knee joint as a whole. Commonly the joint is first involved in females and the degeneration extends to the whole joint later. It is also a common site of anterior knee pain in females and athletes.

Osseous Anatomy

Femoral trochlea:

- Trochlear groove consists of a shallow depression (5–6 mm) bound by the medial and the lateral femoral articular surfaces.
- Prominent lateral surface of trochlear groove projects anteriorly **(Fig. 29)**.
- Variation in the structural anatomy of the trochlear groove predispose to maltracking (normal groove angle is 130°).

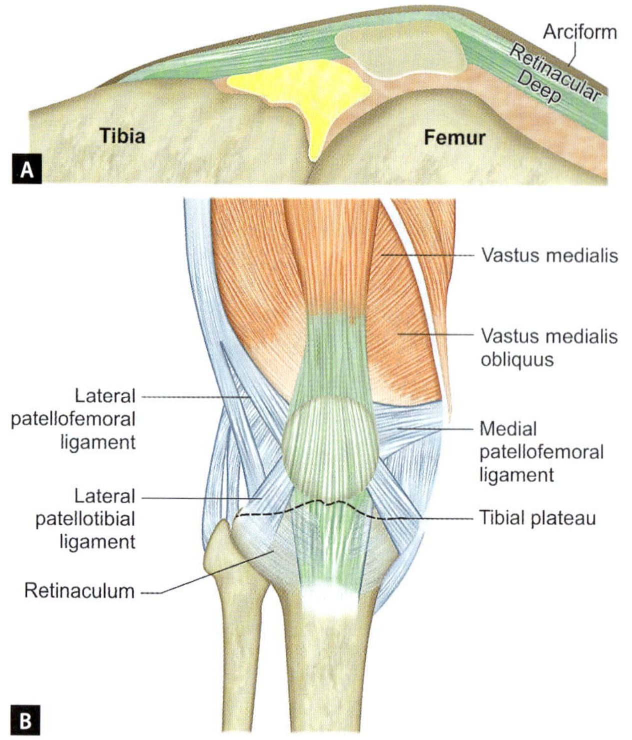

Figs. 28A and B: (A) The patellofemoral joint anatomy and extensor mechanism; (B) Primary motor of the extensor mechanism the quadriceps and its components.

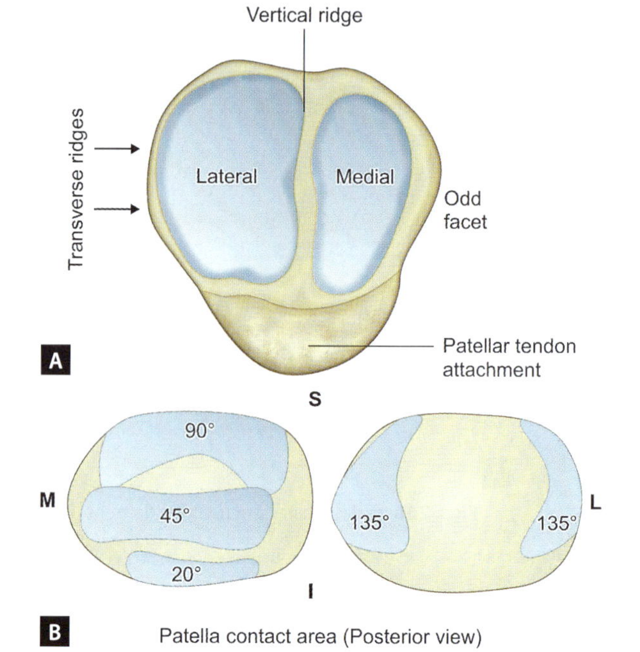

Figs. 30A and B: The facets of patella: (A) Separated by vertical and transverse ridges; (B) Its contact surfaces at different angles of knee flexion.

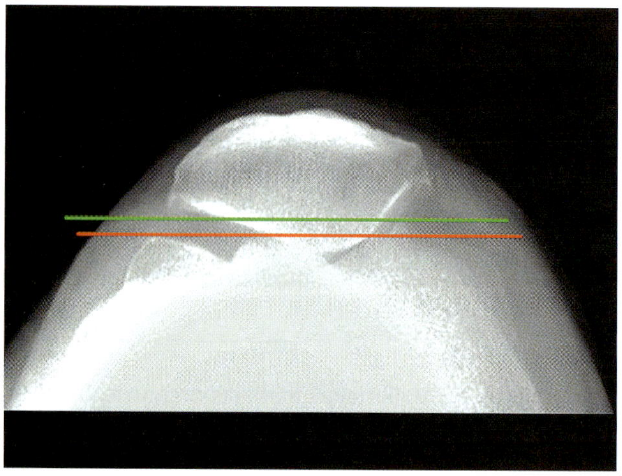

Fig. 29: Radiograph of skyline view showing anterior projection of the lateral trochlear groove (the green line is superior to the red line).

Patella (knee cap):

- It is the largest sesamoid (triangular and circular in shape) bone in the body with the thickest articular cartilage in the human body.
- The patella develops in the retinacular layer of the extensor mechanism.
- It serves as insertion to vastus intermedius proximally and as origin of the deeper layer of the patellar tendon distally.
- The articular surface of the patella contains a broader lateral facet (larger), a medial facet (smaller) and a still smaller, more medial "odd" facet (far medial) separated by a vertical central ridge. The medial and the lateral facets are further subdivided by indistinct transverse ridges into superior, middle, and inferior facets **(Figs. 30A and B)**:
  - At 10–20° of flexion, the contact between patella and femur is minimal. The contact is mainly between lateral patellar facet and lateral femoral condyle. The contact area gradually increases with flexion so that by 30° knee of flexion the contact is evenly distributed between both femoral condyles and is estimated to be 2 cm^2.
  - By 90° of flexion all aspects of facets have contacted the femur except the odd facet.
  - At 135° knee flexion, the odd and lateral facets contact the femur.
- The patella articulates with the femoral trochlea or anterior articular surface of the distal femur. By the virtue of its anatomy (broader lateral portion and a higher ridge than the medial potion), the joint is stabilized at an angle of approximately 45° of knee flexion **(Fig. 30B)**. The dynamics and contact congruence of patellofemoral articulation is as follows:
  - No contact between the femur and patella in full extension (patella lies against the supratrochlear tubercle).
  - From extension to flexion, the patella follows a gentle S-shaped curve, beginning laterally and then moves medially following the grove until the knee has flexed to 90° when the patella again moves laterally until it covers the lateral condyle at 135°. This S-shaped track of patella has been copied by few total knee designs with S-shaped groove in the femoral component.
  - Seats in the trochlea at ≈20°; at this point **(Fig. 30B)**, the congruence and compressive forces provide stability along with anatomic topography of patellofemoral joint.
  - Before 20° the stability is provided by soft tissues only.

- Three types of patella have been described (Wiberg):
  - *Type 1:* Roughly symmetrical facets, concave facets, equally sized facets, and 10% population.
  - *Type 2:* Slightly smaller size of medial facet; concave lateral facet.
  - *Type 3:* Markedly smaller size of medial facet, more vertical orientation of medial facet.
- The functions of patella:
  - Increase the force production of the quadriceps by pulley action (fulcrum), redirecting the forces at varying flexion moments of knee by increasing the distance of line of action of extensor mechanism from center of rotation of the knee **(Fig. 31)**. Patella increases lever arm of extensor mechanism enhancing forces of quadriceps by 30%.
  - Reducing patellofemoral forces
  - Protection of femur from direct impact
  - Unifying the force of diverging quadriceps

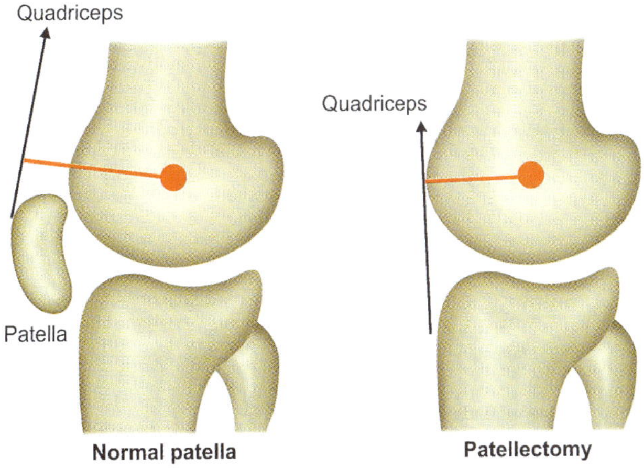

Fig. 31: Function of patella as a pulley (to improve mechanical leverage): as a pulley changes the direction of force of application, similarly, the patella improves the direction of action of quadriceps force across the knee and improves lever arm.

Capsular Ligaments

The capsular ligaments spanning patellofemoral joint are studied by dividing them into thirds:

- The anterior-third capsular ligaments are formed by the medial and lateral retinacular ligaments of the extensor mechanism that form a sling action **(*see* Figs. 28A and B)**. They also attach to the anterior horns of the menisci but are devoid of femoral attachments.
- The extensor mechanism, tendinous and capsular structures also provide dynamic stability to the patellofemoral joint **(Fig. 32)** and are organized into following layers:
  - A thin peritendinous membrane, the arciform layer (superficial) spans from the sartorial fascia medially and the biceps fascia laterally and embrace along the patella and patellar tendon anteriorly. They serve a proprioceptive role.
  - The retinacular (intermediate) layer is made up of:
    - Anterior-third capsule and its condensations
    - Iliopatellar ligament laterally is a condensation of retinaculum lying on the anterolateral aspect of the knee. It has surgical significance in stabilizing the patella.
- Patellofemoral ligaments course along the distal and deep border of the VMO and vastus lateralis obliquus. The muscles have a dynamic role in stabilizing patella in the region **(Fig. 33)**. The patellofemoral ligaments originate from medial or lateral isometric points on femur and insert on the corresponding superior poles of the patella:
  - The lateral patellofemoral ligament courses from the proximal lateral epicondyle to the vastus lateralis tendon insertion on the patella.
  - The medial patellofemoral ligament or MPFL (quite prominently signified recently in recurrent patellar instability) courses from the adductor tubercle to the VMO insertion on the patella **(Figs. 34A and B)**. MPFL was first described by Warren and Marshall in 1979. It is 4.5–6.4 cm long and 1.9 cm wide at the widest point (attachment to patella) situated outside

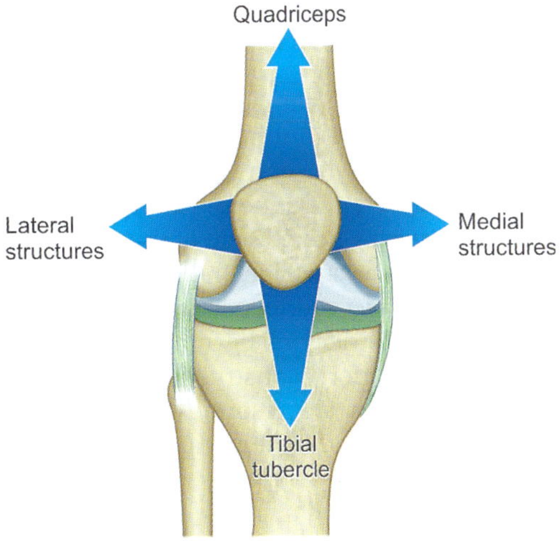

Fig. 32: Dynamic stability of patellofemoral joint.

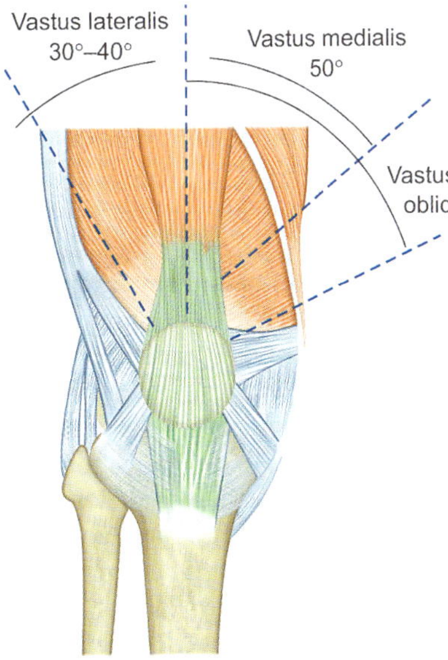

Fig. 33: Q-angle dynamic balancing by the counter pull of vastus lateralis and vastus medialis oblique (VMO) and secondary static balancing by the patellofemoral ligaments.

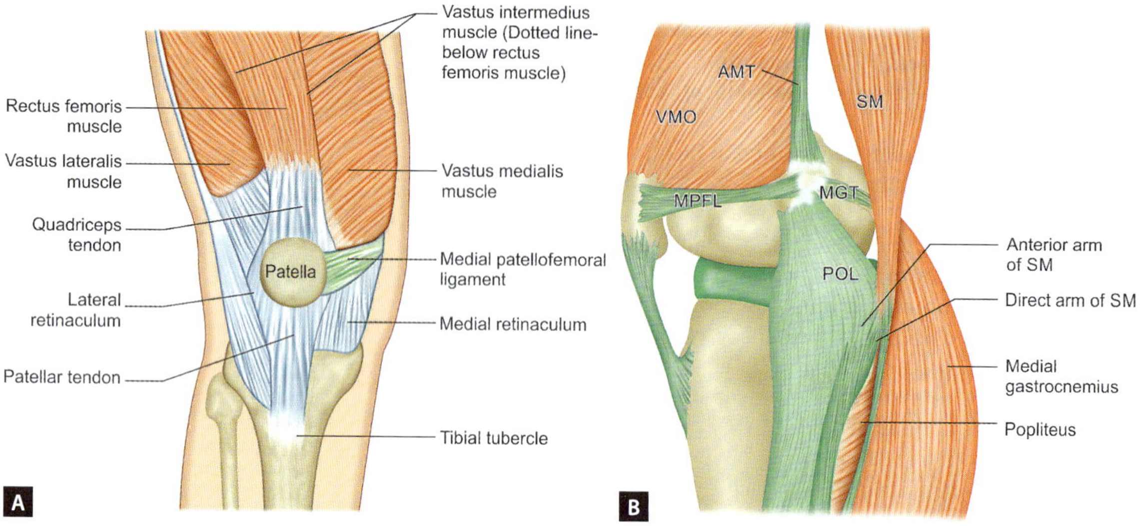

Figs. 34A and B: The medial patellofemoral ligament: (A) Anterior and (B) Lateral views.
(AMT: adductor magnus tendon; MGT: medial head gastrocnemius; MPFL: medial patellofemoral ligament; POL: popliteal oblique ligament; SM: semimembranosus; TCL: tibial collateral ligament; VMO: vastus medialis obliquus)

the knee capsule but beneath the deep fascia. It originates from a 10.6-mm transverse groove between medial epicondyle and adductor tubercle. The insertion is onto the superomedial aspect of medial patella spanning nearly 3 cm of the ventral edge just near to articular cartilage. Insertion may sometimes be in the VMO/quadriceps instead of patellar bone directly. Isometricity of ligament is not completely established but for reconstruction purposes assorted isometric points are resorted to. Determining the isometric point for the femoral attachment of MPFL is most important in reconstruction techniques of the ligament in cases on recurrent patellar instability. Smirk and Morris determined the most isometric points on the femur to be 1 cm distal to the adductor tubercle and 5 mm posterior to it. Points slightly distal or slightly posterior to this point are also acceptable. The MPFL provides 50–60% restraint to lateral patellar translation. Nomura has classified the chronic MPFL injury into three grades—(1) type I is a loose femoral attachment, (2) type II is an elongated scar posteriorly (29/49), and (3) type III is complete absence of the ligament.

- The tibial counterparts of patellar ligaments have no muscular attachments and hence are purely static.
  - The medial patellotibial ligament extends from the inferomedial patella to the anteromedial physeal scar of the proximal tibia. The ligament can be tightened in recurrent patellar instabilities where Q angle is excessive especially in skeletally immature patients as bony procedures are avoided.
  - The lateral patellotibial ligament courses from the inferolateral patella to the lateral tibial tubercle deep to the iliopatellar ligament. Though uncommon but development of medial instability of the patella after lateral release is due to insufficiency of this ligament.

Quadriceps

The quadriceps muscle group consists of seven discrete heads **(*see* Fig. 4)** that is responsible not only for extension at the knee but also stabilizing the patellofemoral joint dynamically:

- Articularis genu (deepest head) is the only muscle that does not insert directly into the patella. The muscle prevents impingement of the superior synovial plica between patella and femoral sulcus by dynamically raising it.
- The vastus intermedius originates through a broad origin on the anterior femoral shaft and inserts into the superior pole of the patella.
- The rectus femoris (two heads) parallel originates on the anteroinferior iliac spine (AIIS) and blends into the central tendon of the quadriceps.
  - The rectus femoris tendon is 8–10 cm in length, triangular in shape with insertion 3–5 cm in width at the superior pole of patella. A bursa separates the rectus tendon from the intermedius tendon along the entire length. It crosses two joints and causes flexion at hip while extension at the knee.
- The vastus lateralis originates from the anterolateral aspect of the femur and lateral intermuscular septum:
  - It makes up approximately 50% of the bulk of the entire quadriceps muscle group. Its angle of insertion is approximately 22–45° laterally off the axis of the femur (producing lateral displacing moment at patella).
- The vastus medialis originates from the anteromedial aspect of the femur and medial intermuscular septum. Its angle of insertion is approximately 50° medially off the axis of the femur (producing medial displacing moment at patella, balancing lateral displacement partially). It is responsible for last 10–15° of knee extension.
- The VMO originates from the adductor tubercle and distal medial intermuscular septum. Its angle of insertion

at superomedial border of patella is oriented obliquely 55–70° medially off the axis of the femur (producing medial displacing moment at patella—its primary function is in balancing patella dynamically against the force of vastus lateralis).

- The rectus femoris, along with the VMO, vastus medialis and vastus lateralis terminates in an aponeurosis that merges into the anterior-third joint capsule forming the retinacular layer:
  - The retinacular layer is a continuous layer on the superficial aspect of patella. Distally, it extends to the tibial periosteum and invests the superficial portion of the patellar tendon.

Patellar Tendon

- The patellar tendon extends from the inferior pole of the patella and inserts on the tibial tubercle.
- The infrapatellar tendon bursa and fat pad separates the patellar tendon from the underlying tibia.
- The patellar tendon comprises a superficial layer (continuous with the retinacular layer) and a deeper layer—the deep layer of the extensor mechanism. While operating on patella these layers are more or less confluent and inseparable.
- The infrapatellar fat pad (IFP) (Hoffa's fat pad) is attached to ligamentum mucosum (a persistent plica—discussed below). The pad is often inflamed by mechanical misalignment (females), injury, microtrauma (Hoffa's disease) and may also undergo ankylosis causing extension block and secondary contracture of the patellar tendon producing limitation in flexion.

Synovial Structures

Plica: Synovial plicae are membranous infolds that are part of the synovial lining of knee capsule (Latin "plica" = "fold"). These are remnant of embryologic development and are found variably. Large persistent plica may septate suprapatellar pouch or may persist as a mild synovial band that is clinically insignificant at the other extreme. Ligamentum mucosum **(Fig. 35)** is the most common plica. Suprapatellar plica **(Fig. 35)** is the second most common and may divide the quadriceps bursa into two parts or even the compartment into two. It may also tether the quadriceps tendon, limiting movements.

Medial plica syndrome (9–50% cases)—medial plica are least common, but most symptomatic if present. It runs distally along the medial aspect of the knee from the level of the superior pole of the patella to insert into the medial fat pad.

Development of plicae can be understood by detailing the embryological formation of the knee. There are two theories regarding the formation of knee joint:

1. The knee is formed by the fusion of three synovial compartments (medial, lateral, and suprapatellar) that are divided by membranes of mesenchymal tissue and the intervening synovial tissues are resorbed over time (9–12 weeks of gestation). Persistence presents as plica.

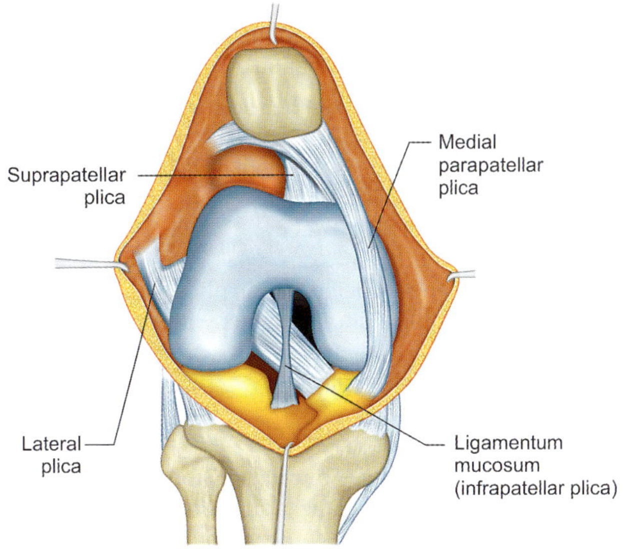

Fig. 35: Plica system demonstrated for right knee (patella is reflected open to depict the various plica).

2. At 8 weeks, the mesenchymal tissue fills space between femur and tibia. The tissue then undergoes condensation to form menisci, cruciate ligaments while at other regions the tissue is resorbed to form the joint cavity. Incomplete resorption produces incomplete cavitation and formation of plica.

There are four distinctly identifiable plicae in knee of normal population: (1) medial (plica synovialis mediopatellaris, mediopatellar plica, medial shelf, Lino's band, Aoki's ledge and plica alaris elongate), (2) superior (plica synovialis suprapatellaris), (3) inferior (ligamentum mucosum), and (4) rare lateral. Medial plica syndrome is defined by Ewing as "a painful impairment of knee function which cannot be explained by any other structure except the presence of a thick hypertrophic medial plica". Medial plica is symptomatic only in 4–6% patients although its presence is reported in 20–80% population.

Anatomy of medial plica is seen in medial gutter under the VMO muscle. It runs obliquely downward and parallel to medial patella edge inserting into the IFP and covering it. On arthroscopy it should be differentiated from superomedial plica (transverse and lies well above the patella), plica alaris elongate (longitudinal fold medial to patella), transverse arcuate folds and anteromedial small synovial fold covering medial meniscus.

The medial plica is classified morphologically into four types (Lino types rearranged by Sakakibara):

1. *Type A:* A *cord-like*, thin elevation of the synovial wall, under the retinaculum.
2. *Type B:* A *narrow* synovium, with a *shelf-like* appearance not covering the anterior surface of the medial femoral condyle.
3. *Type C:* A *larger* synovium, with a *shelf-like* appearance, which partially covers the medial femoral condyle.
4. *Type D:* A type C plica that is fenestrated, creating tags or a plica with double insertions into medial wall with central defect.

Types C and D are likely to become entrapped and impinged causing symptoms (Munzinger classification is a modification of above classification).

Dandy classification based on the width of plica:
- Type A—no plica
- Type B—narrow ridge at the medial wall of the knee joint
- Type C—width of plica <1 cm
- Type D—width of plica 1–2 cm
- Type E—width of plica >2 cm
- Type F—presence of defect within plica
- Type G—high plica not in contact with medial femoral condyle
- Type H—reduplicated plica.

Etiopathogenesis of the Medial Plica Syndrome

The pathological plica are thickened, fibrosed, and histologically demonstrate hyalinization and calcification. The impingement results in secondary mechanical synovitis (inflammation and progressive fibrosis) and a change in the patellofemoral joint mechanism. These changes further produce chondromalacia. The plica shows a mediolateral translatory motion across the medial femoral condyle during flexion and extension movement. This also causes cartilage damage and further increase in symptoms. Following are the common causes for plica to become pathological:
- Trauma
- Twisting injuries
- Repetitive activities requiring vigorous flexion-extension
- Increased activity levels
- Altered knee mechanics due to osteochondritis dissecans, torn meniscus, patella subluxation, etc.

On passive knee flexion in the range of 30–60° this plica slides over the medial femoral condyle beneath the patella. Wedging and impingement of the plica between the medial facet and the anteromedial femoral condyle can be reproduced by external rotation of the tibia. It has been commonly envisaged that as plica gets inflamed (due to above etiologies) it thickens into a cord-like structure that further gets impinged during normal knee movements establishing a vicious cycle. With evolution the structure gets tightened by shortening and the band rubs against femur eroding the cartilage and causing secondary changes in the knee.

Clinical Features

The disease usually becomes symptomatic in younger population affecting both sexes equally. The common symptoms are as follows:
- *Anteromedial knee pain:* Intermittent dull aching pain in the area medial to the patella area above joint line.
- *Positive cinema theater sign:* There is increased pain when the knee is flexed for a long time which is relieved by extension of the knee.
- Pain increases with knee flexion and squatting.
- *Positive duvet test:* Pain eased by using a duvet between the knees to ease pain in bed.
- Other nonspecific complaints include clicking, catching, pseudolocking, snapping, giving way, and tightness around knee.

Physical Examination

- Tender, palpable thickened cord-like plica that pops and rolls under the fingers in the medial parapatellar area [Rovere positive TARP sign (taut, articular band, and reproduces pain)]
- Crepitus during knee flexion-extension
- Knee effusion
- *Pipkin's sign:* Popping sound on extension of the knee from 90° of flexion, combined with internal rotation and medial gliding of the patella. Popping can be felt by examiner between 60° and 45° of knee extension arc.
- *Holding test:* The patient holds the knee in extension while the examiner tries to flex the knee and pushes the patella medially—produces pain ± clicking.
- *Magee test:* In 30° knee flexion the patella is moved medially, provoking pain as the edge of the plica is pinched between the patella and the femur.
- *Active extension test (Irha and Vrdoljak):* Lying supine with the knee flexed at 90°, quick extension of the tibia is performed, imitating a football kick. Pain is produced due to pulling of quadriceps on plica abruptly.
- *The flexion test (Irha and Vrdoljak):* Patient lies supine with the tibia extending out of the couch or examining table. He is asked to quickly flex knee and the quick swing of knee flexion is stopped at between 30° and 60° of flexion = "blocking of the swing". The plica is pulled by quadriceps in an eccentric contraction producing pain.
- *Rotation valgus test of Koshino and Okamoto:* The knee is flexed and valgus force is applied. The tibia is then rotated internally and externally while a simultaneous attempt is made to displace patella medially, pain is elicited pain due to plica impingement.
- *Kim's medial patella plica (MPP) test:* Applying a manual force to the inferomedial portion of the patellofemoral joint and flexing the knee to 90°. Positive test is indicated by pain at extension and eliminated at flexion.
- Wasting of muscles around knee (inhibitory effect of pain).

Shetty's diagnostic criteria for presence of medial plica syndrome (diagnostic accuracy of 91.7%, sensitivity 100% and positive predictive value of 91.7%).
- Essential criteria:
  - History of anteromedial knee pain
  - Pain primarily over medial femoral condyle
  - Visible or palpable plica
  - Tenderness over palpable plica
  - Exclusion of other causes of anteromedial knee pain.
- Desirable criteria:
  - Onset blunt or trivial trauma
  - Duvet test (discussed above)
  - Audible snap during active range of motion
  - Palpable snap during flexion

Differential diagnosis: TCL sprain, medial meniscus tear, osteochondritis dissecans, patellar maltracking, medial joint arthritis, pes anserinus bursitis, bipartite patella, etc.

Investigations

- Plain radiographs are needed to rule out other pathologies (differentials).

- Ultrasonography enables dynamic examination, but is user dependent.
- *Magnetic resonance imaging is possibly the best investigation:* Abnormal medial patellar plica may be seen as a thickened band of low signal intensity. Chondromalacia of femoral or patellar or both bone cartilage may be seen. The plica is seen to extend to the Hoffa's fat pad on sagittal images.
- Arthroscopy gives the definitive diagnosis and plica can also be treated successfully, if symptomatic and nonresponsive to conservative measures.

Treatment

- *Conservative treatment is preferred initially:* NSAIDs, rest, ice, and physiotherapy in the form of quadriceps, hamstring and gastrocnemius stretching, and quadriceps isometric strengthening exercises. The measures are recommended for 6–8 weeks. Intra-articular or localized injections of depot steroids also help a lot if the results with above are suboptimal.
- Surgical excision of plica is indicated in patients not responding to these measures. The most common reason of excision is plica causing friction on medial femoral condyle or getting pinched between the patella and medial femoral condyle. Arthroscopic approach is the most popular and plica is readily seen with an anterolateral portal, but best excised or resected through superolateral portal. In addition, synovial pannus and synovitis should be excised. Intra-articular steroid can be instilled at the end of procedure if significant synovitis is there. The treatment is successful in around 75–90% patients. Secondary lesions—chondromalacia, etc. are a frequent cause of persistent pain and need to be addressed by cartilage regenerative techniques (*see* Chapter on "Articular Cartilage: Structure, Function, Injury, and Management").

Joint Reaction Forces across Patellofemoral Joint

- The forces are generated by the quadriceps primarily, but manipulated by disposition and orientation of various structures, position of which changes constantly with knee movements **(Figs. 36 and 37)**.
- The forces increase with knee flexion. The magnitude of various forces at the joint are:
  - Walking—half body weight = 850 N
  - Riding bike—half body weight = 850 N
  - Open chain—half body weight (full extension) → 1.4 body weight at 36° flexion → 0 body weight at 90° flexion at rest

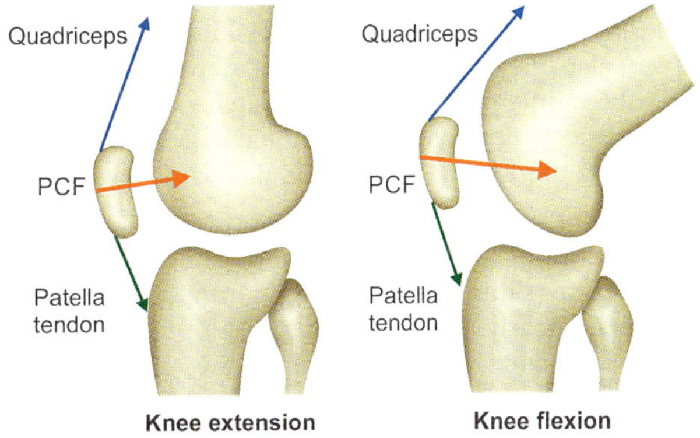

Fig. 36: Patellofemoral joint reaction forces. The active pull of quadriceps is countered by static patellar ligament. By simple vector analysis pull in a straight line, i.e., along the patellar ligament orientation (180°) would have net zero resultant; however, force oriented at some other angle would result in a force couple that produces compression force directed at femoral trochlea which maintains the bone in place. In the figure direction of compression (resultant force) is depicted by the red line vector and its magnitude is represented by length of red line (PCF—patellar compression force = joint reaction force).

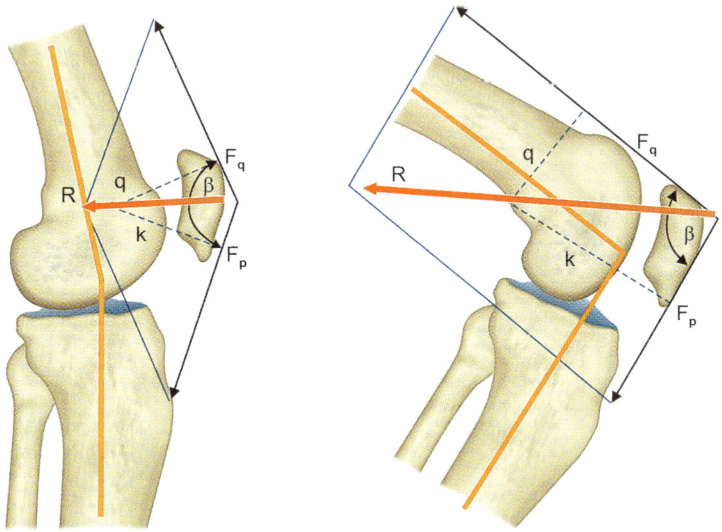

Fig. 37: The patellofemoral joint reaction forces—vectorial representation. Compressive force at patellofemoral joint is one half the body weight during walking. The forces, however, increase to three times when knee is flexed 90° or during stair climbing. Simply speaking compressive forces increase with increasing flexion angle and thus will be highest in squatting.
(Fq and Fp: represent quadriceps pull and patellar tendon reaction forces; β: angle of knee flexion; q and k: represent the perpendiculars to force vectors and their intersection determine direction of compressive force generated; R: resultant compressive force)

- Isokinetic exercise—at 70°–75° of knee flexion → 5.1 body weight at 60°/sec and 4.9 body weight at 180°/sec
- Stair climbing—3.3 body weight = 1,500 N **(Fig. 37)**
- Stair descending—5 body weight = 4,000 N
- Jogging—7 body weight = 5,000 N
- Squatting—7 body weight = 5,000 N
- Full squatting (Indian toilet)—20 body weight = 20,000 N
- Impact of abnormal tracking—results in higher forces/unit area. Minor lateral shift of the patella decreases the contact area by 60% and increase stress by 2.5 times.

▪ *Impact of surgical procedures:*
  - The joint reaction force can be reduced by up to 50% at 45° angle by elevating the tibial tuberosity by 2 cm. It also increases the quadriceps moment arm.
  - By reducing the Q angle, patellar stress can be reduced. For example, by reducing the angle from 15° to 5°, there is 50% decrease in patellar stress.

Kinematics of patellofemoral joint:

▪ Motion of patella occurs in two planes—frontal and transverse (sliding articulation). In frontal plane, patella traverses nearly 7 cm of distance.
▪ Due to poor bony congruity the patellofemoral articulation is primarily supported by dynamic forces of muscles **(*see* Fig. 32)**:
  - *Laterally:* Lateral retinaculum, vastus lateralis and iliotibial tract.
  - *Medially:* Medial retinaculum and vastus medialis.
  - *Superior:* Quadriceps via quadriceps tendon.
  - *Inferior:* Patellar tendon.
▪ The mean directional force vector across patella acts toward the knee joint pushing the bone into trochlear groove of femur. This patellofemoral compression force varies with the flexion of knee joint and primarily maintains the patella in the groove.

BIOMECHANICS OF KNEE JOINT

The biomechanical functions of knee joint are:

▪ Locomotion with:
  - As little energy requirements from the muscles as possible
  - Stability while performing activity on different terrains.
▪ To transmit, absorb, and redistribute forces caused during the activities of daily life:
  - Support during weight-bearing
  - Mobility during nonweight-bearing.

The knee is a combination of ginglymus (hinge) and arthrodial (pivot and gliding) joint permitting gliding, sliding, and rotational movements in 6° of freedom **(Fig. 38)**:

▪ *Three rotations:* Flexion-extension, internal and external rotation, and varus and valgus rotation.
▪ *Three translations:* Anteroposterior, mediolateral, and compression—distraction.

Movements at knee joint:

▪ Rotation:
  - Flexion-extension: Up to 160° of flexion (from 5° of hyperextension)
  - Varus-valgus: 6–8° in extension
  - Internal-external rotation: 25–30° in 90° of flexion (in full extension internal rotation or external rotation is not possible as it is a "locked", closed pack position).
▪ *Translation:*
  - Anteroposterior: 5–10 mm
  - Compression: 2–5 mm
  - Mediolateral: 1–2 mm
▪ Instantaneous center of rotation:
  - The center of rotation for different rotations **(Fig. 39)** are different and for flexion it is in the form of a spiral or semicircle **(Fig. 40)** due to different radii of curvature of the femoral condyles and posteriorly **(Figs. 41A and B)** and also due to coupled gliding movement.

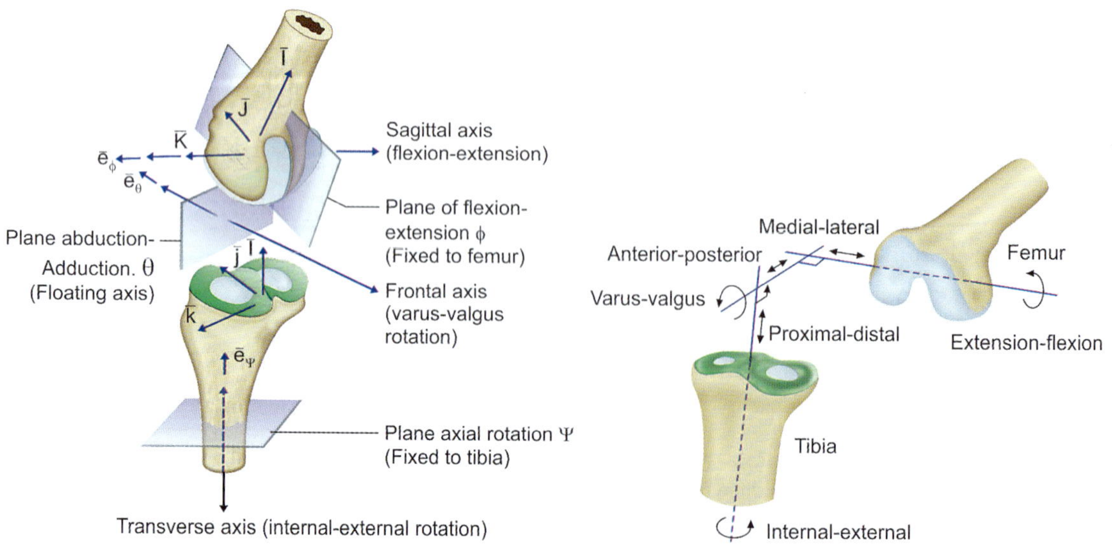

Fig. 38: Knee joint: movement planes and the six degrees of freedom of human knee joint.

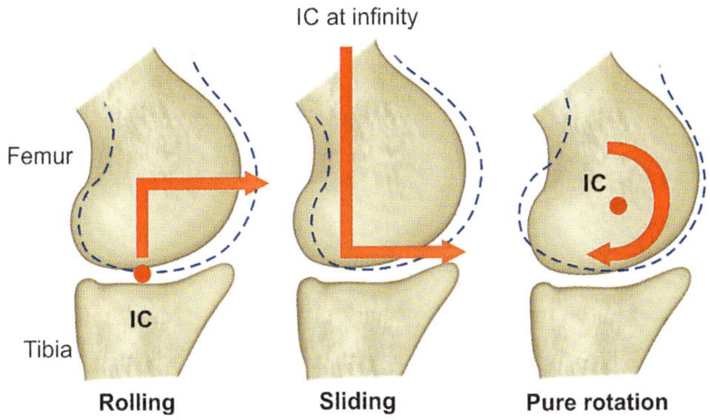

Fig. 39: Movements at knee joint and respective instant center (IC) of rotations for femur motion during flexion or extension.

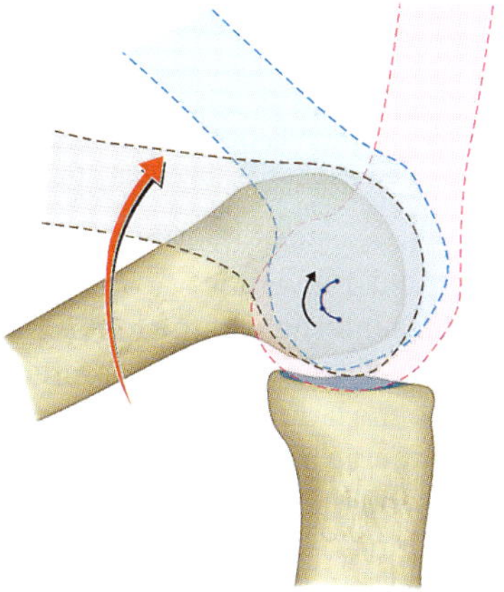

Fig. 40: Instant center of rotation.

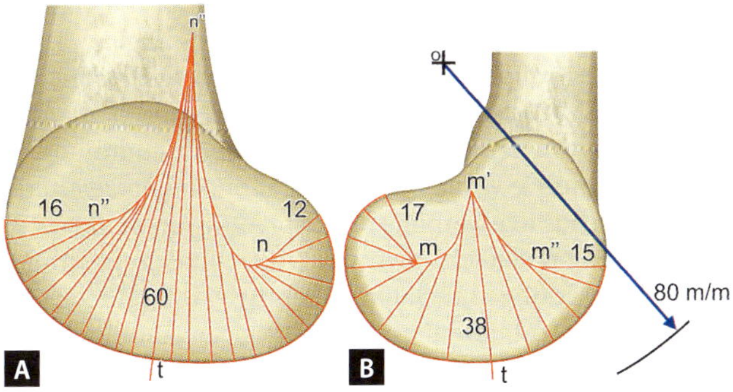

Figs. 41A and B: Different radii of curvature of medial and lateral femoral condyles and either of the condyles have a larger radius of curvature for the anterior two-thirds as compared to the posterior third which is more circular also.

Functional range of motion of knee required for different activities are different and they also produce different compressive loads on the joint **(Table 2)**.

The compressive loads at patellofemoral joint are more important from biomechanical standpoint and have been discussed previously tibiofemoral compression loads are only for reference to clinicians to help patients during physiotherapy and rehabilitation. We will elaborate and understand the tibiofemoral movements further, however.

The movements at knee are peculiar. The most predominant movement at knee joint the flexion-extension

TABLE 2: Functional range of motion of knee and compressive loads on the joint.

Activity	*Knee joint flexion (degrees)*	*Compressive loads across the joint (times body weight)*
Walking on level surface	15–20	3.0
Cycling	60–100	1.2
Stair climbing	45	3.8
Stair descending	85	4.3
Rising from chair	90	4.5
Rising from closet seat	115	4.8
Rising from squat	130–140	5.0
Squatting down	140	5.6

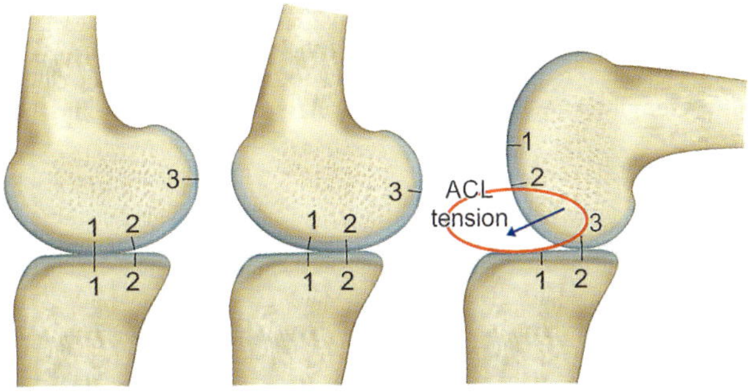

Fig. 42: Complex flexion movement at knee is a combination of roll and slide—in the first 20–25° of flexion, only rolling occurs causing shifting of contact points posteriorly. After 25° gliding movement predominates while roll is also seen to some extent. In extreme flexion, like squatting only sliding occurs terminally to prevent joint dislocation.

occurs through 5° of hyperextension to 160° of flexion. But the movement is not simply a roll and occurs through a combination of gliding and rolling. In early flexion, up to 20°, there occurs a rolling movement for first 10° followed by rocking movement till 20° that translates the point of tibiofemoral contact posteriorly **(Fig. 42)**. With further flexion there is a gliding movement, with a greater posterior translation of the lateral tibiofemoral contact point in relation to the medial contact point. Pure rolling movement will only lead to femoral condyle falling off the posterior edge **(Figs. 43A and B)** before even 50% of condyle has rolled over tibia so glide is important (though this incurs wear and possibly osteoarthritis seen with bipedal gait). This is affected by the roller shape of two femoral condyles and the flattened plateau shape of tibial condyles over which "roll-back" of femoral condyles can occur on flattened tibial plateau while also gliding can occur on the flat tibial plateau. "Femoral roll-back" is an ingenious way of allowing increased ranges of knee flexion. The four-bar link mechanism **(Fig. 44)** produced by the two cruciate ligaments along with the femur and tibia articular surfaces contribute to posterior femoral roll-back by causing a posterior translation of the instantaneous center of rotation of knee joint with increasing flexion, preventing soft tissue impingement posteriorly while also decreasing patellar load. As compared to the

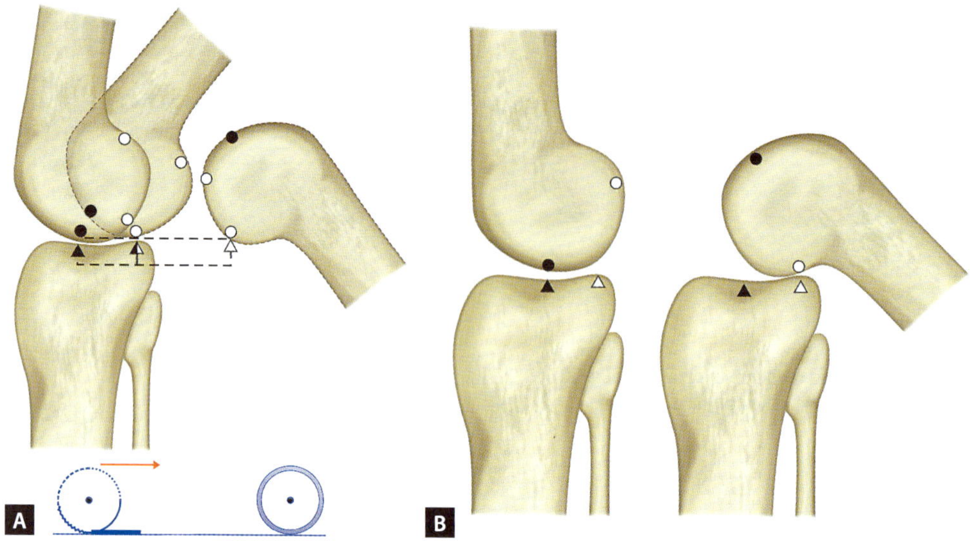

Figs. 43A and B: Importance of combined roll and glide—the circumference of femoral condyles is much larger than the anteroposterior length of tibial plateau. If rolling movement only occurs: (A) The femur will fall posteriorly of the posterior edge of tibia; (B) Gliding hence is mandatory to maintain femur within limits of tibial articular surface and maintain the joint.

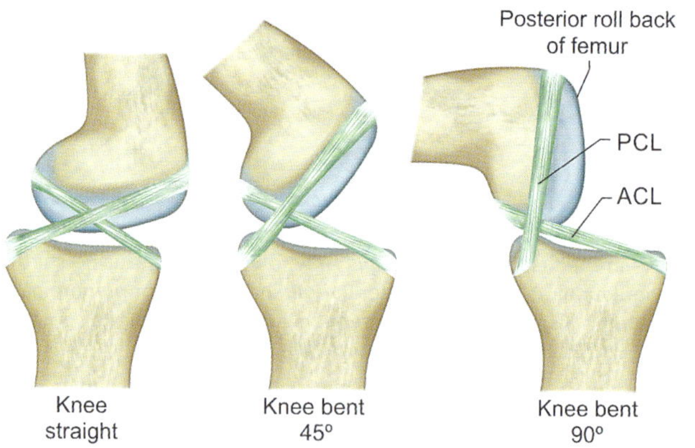

Fig. 44: Four-bar linkage mechanism of cruciate ligaments: femoral roll is made possible by the fixed length of anterior cruciate ligament (ACL) and posterior cruciate ligament (PCL).

medial femoral condyles, during the initial 20° of flexion, the larger lateral femoral condyles roll a greater distance (so also during terminal 20° of extension). At full extension there is hence coupled external rotation of tibia with knee extension and the knee is locked by screw-home mechanism.

Screw-home Mechanism

It refers to the "homing action" of tibia in the last 15° of extension. The tibia has to "home" itself on the femur by a screwing action of external rotation at the end of knee extension, so it externally rotates 5° in the last 15° of extension **(Figs. 45A and B)**.

Effectors of the mechanism:

- The mechanism is primarily due to bony topography, the medial tibial plateau is much longer than the lateral so a longer distance is to be covered medially for same amount of knee extension than laterally requiring an asymmetrical condylar tracking which is not possible. Due to continued movement at medial tibial plateau the femur rotates internally if the foot is planted (or tibia rotates externally if the foot is free) producing a rotatory movement. Also the lateral femoral condyle is larger than the medial producing a net external rotation of tibia with knee extension and internal rotation with knee flexion.
- Posterolateral bundle of ACL takes part in acting as a pivot for the mechanism.
- *Relative lengths of the cruciates:* Van Dommelen and Fowler suggested that the PCL plays an important role in the screw-home mechanism because of the variable region of tautness at different flexion angles. There is anterior rolling of tibia during knee extension, this elongates PCL. PCL's pull on tibia causes it to glide anteriorly on femur. This anterior glide continues on medial condyle while on the lateral one it gets restricted and tibia has to externally rotate pivoting on ACL.

Thus, when weight-bearing; the tibia must rotate externally pivoting on lateral condyle to achieve full extension. The rotational component gives stability to the knee in full extension and sort of locks the knee preventing its buckling even when no muscular contraction is there. This is effected by tensioning of the collateral ligaments. Thus, it relaxes the quadriceps during standing.

At the beginning of knee flexion, the femur rotates externally to unlock the knee. This action is brought about by the contraction of the popliteus muscle. Tibia now begins to roll posteriorly, but in this case the ACL gets elongated. The pull of ACL causes it to glide posterior that begins at medial condyle (it being longer). So during the first 0–20° of knee flexion, the tibia in effect internally rotates reversing the screw-home mechanism.

KNEE INSTABILITY

The American Orthopedic Society for Sports Medicine Classification of knee laxity into either a straight or a rotatory

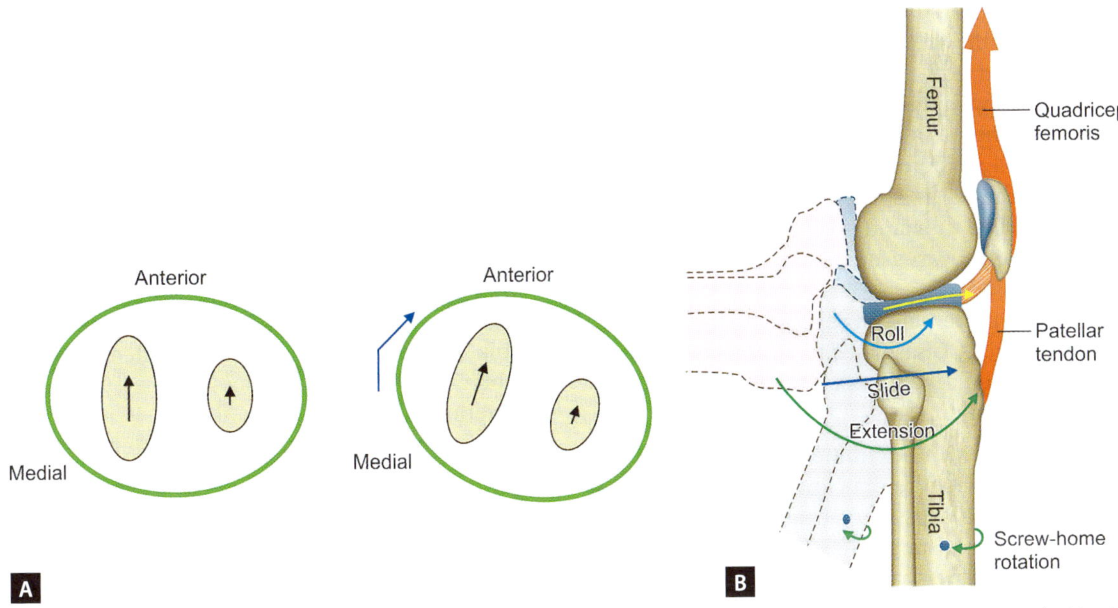

Figs. 45A and B: Screw-home mechanism—simply stating it is the external rotation of tibia during last 15–20° of knee extension, locking it for stability and muscular rest: (A) Viewing the right tibial plateau from top; (B) The different movements at knee during extension and relation with screw home mechanism.

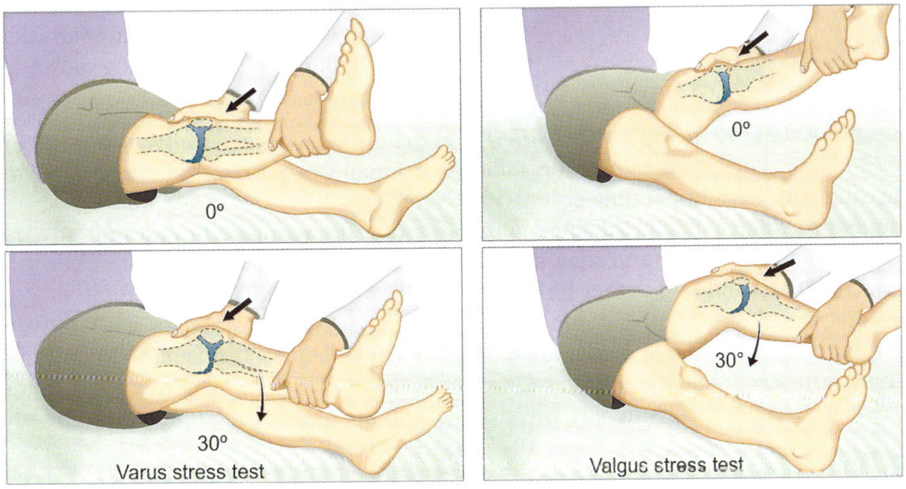

Fig. 46: Varus and valgus stress test for evaluation of collateral ligaments. The tests are performed at full extension and 30° of knee flexion.

instability is most favored and followed, that also in a sense defines knee instability.

- *Straight instability* implies uniplanar or unidirectional instability—medial, lateral, anterior, or posterior.
- *Rotatory instability* is said to be present when there is abnormal rotation of the tibial plateau in relation to the femoral condyles. It is identified as anterolateral, anteromedial, posterolateral or, rarely, posteromedial. Combined instabilities are much more common and they are the direct derivative of the number of structures that have been injured, defeating the very purpose of this classification, however, this classification is considered basic to understand the principles of various injury patterns and management. To add to the above patterns, concept of tibial translation has been introduced to make the classification more complete.
- *Translation* refers to the degree of excessive gliding that occur at the medial tibial plateau (this being longer) as compared with the lateral tibial plateau relative to the femoral condyles. These translations take part in rotatory instabilities. The amount of anterior translation is inversely proportional to the integrity of the anatomical restraints that normally restrict excessive translation. Anterior tibial lateral plateau translation increases in anterolateral instability.

Testing Knee Instability

***Valgus and varus stress test (Fig. 46)**:* Though considered to test the collateral ligaments primarily these also test the additional stabilizing structures (secondary restraints) for varus and valgus stability including even the cruciates.

Method: The patient lies supine with the leg extended. To test the medial side, hold the ankle firmly with one hand while placing the other hand over the head of the fibula gripping the knee firmly. Push with an inward force in an attempt to open the side of the knee at 0° and at 30° of flexion.

- At 0° it tests the TCL, posteromedial capsule and cruciates.
- At 30° of flexion, the TCL is isolated for testing its integrity.

For varus instability, the hand positions are reversed to test the lateral side with a varus force at 0° and then with 30° of flexion.

- At 0° the LCL and posterolateral capsule are tested.
- At 30° of flexion, the LCL is isolated for testing its integrity.

The lower limb should be in a neutral position with no internal or external rotation.

Apley's distraction test: The examiner applies distraction force to the leg to separate the tibia and femur and moves it back and forth. If the capsule or ligaments are injured pain will occur. This test distinguishes if the pain in knee is coming from meniscus injury or extra-articular structures. Torn meniscus pain will be relieved in distraction test. Next the examiner applies compression and repeats the maneuver if the pain is due to meniscus tear then distraction test will be negative while pain will occur on compression test **(Figs. 47A and B)**.

Tests for Anterior Cruciate Ligament

The following tests help to evaluate ACL tear:

Anterior drawer test at (Fig. 48A) 90° of flexion (sensitivity of 90–93%, mean 62%): The patient lies supine on table with knee flexed. The examiner holds upper tibia or leg with both hands encircling it immediately below the knee joint. Fingers are placed in the popliteal space and they ensure that the hamstrings are adequately relaxed as they lie on the tendons. The thumbs are placed on the medial and lateral joint lines. Examiner tries to pull the tibia forward if the tibia slides forward from under the femur and there is no sudden "hard or firm" stop to translation this is considered a positive anterior drawer sign (the stop in ACL tears is often "mushy or soft").

- Grade 1 = translation of half inch (1.25 cm)
- Grade 2 = translation of half to three-fourths inch (1.25–1.9 cm)
- Grade 3 = translation of three-fourths inch or more (1.9 cm or more)

  Slocum anterior rotary drawer test is basically anterior drawer test performed in both external as well as internal rotation of 30°.
- Excessive anterior translation with externally rotated tibia indicates—injury to posteromedial aspect of the joint capsule, the ACL or possibly the TCL.
- Anterior translation when the leg is internally rotated indicates that the ACL and posterolateral capsule may be torn.

Feagin modification—performing the test in sitting position with the legs hanging down the edge of table (relaxed muscles) avoids the effect of meniscus.

Weatherwax modification **(Fig. 48B)**—placing the lower leg in examiner's axilla.

The drawer test can be negative (false negative) if:

- There is hamstring tightness (prevent anterior subluxation).
- *Hemarthrosis:* The knee cannot be flexed to 90°.
- Door stopper effect of the posterior horn of medial meniscus.

Lachman test (sensitivity of 60–100%; mean 84%): The Lachman test is preferred over drawer test. The advantages are:

- Can be performed in an injured knee without eliciting too much pain.
- Eliminates the hamstring tightness.
- No restriction from menisci.

  The Lachman test is done in approximately 30° of knee flexion **(Fig. 49)**. An attempt is made at translating the tibia anteriorly by holding on the proximal end of tibia

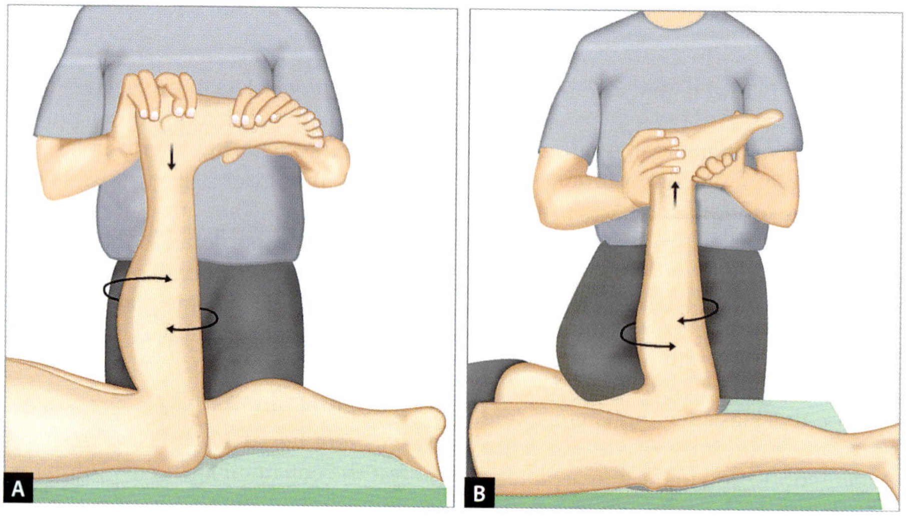

Figs. 47A and B: Apley's compression and distraction test.

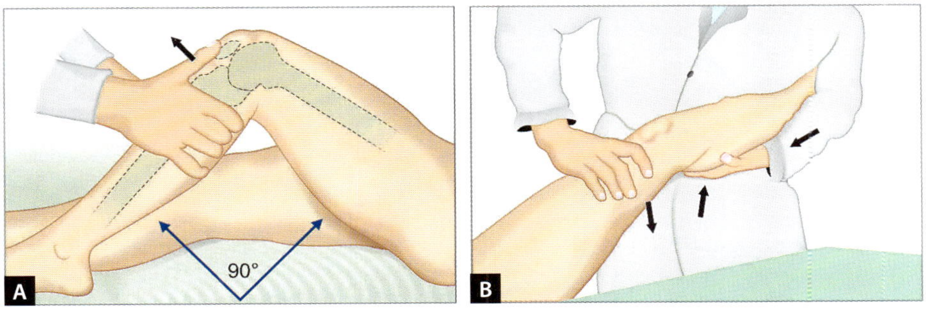

Figs. 48A and B: (A) Anterior drawer test classical; (B) Weatherwax modification.

with one hand and at the same time stabilizing the distal thigh by the other hand. For large thighs or small examiner hands following alternatives help:

- Place a tightly rolled towel or other support under the femur and use one hand to stabilize the femur and the other to anteriorly translate the tibia.
- Slide the lower leg off the edge of the examining table with the knee and femur supported by the edge of the table. Now stabilize the femur with one hand and use the other to anteriorly translate the tibia.
- *Prone Lachman test:* The patient lies prone with the knee and lower leg just off the edge of the table. This position minimizes any posterior sag of the tibia that can mask a positive test. Examiner then tries to translate the tibia.

The grading for Lachman test is performed as follows:

- Grade 1+ has 0–5 mm displacement with a firm end point.
- Grade 2+ has 5–10 mm displacement with no end point.
- Grade 3+ has >10 mm displacement.

Pivot shift test of MacIntosh (sensitivity of 27–95%, mean 62%, specificity of 35–99% in chronic tears): The pivot shift test specifically elicits anterolateral rotary instability of which ACL injury is a part. It is used in chronic conditions and is a sensitive test when the ACL has been torn. Even in an ACL deficient knee the capsule maintains reduction of tibia on femur in extension. This phenomenon is possibly attributed to anterolateral ligament (ALL) of Segond (*see* anatomy). Loss or deficiency of ALL is supposed to produce higher grades of pivot shift test. With the patient lying supine, the hip of the patient is flexed to 30°, knee is flexed to 20°, and the leg is internally rotated by holding at the ankle to unlock knee. Internal rotation of tibial condyle is necessary to reverse the screw home mechanism (*see* earlier) and begin knee flexion. Unlocking the tibia this way relaxes the collaterals so that examiner can then flex knee. Examiner also keeps thumb of one hand over fibular head (pivot) while supporting the knee by fingers from behind. The knee is then further flexed and a simultaneous valgus force is applied by one hand at the level of proximal fibula (pivot) and an axial force is applied by the other hand holding ankle **(Fig. 50)**. In patients with damaged ACL and lateral knee structures **(Fig. 51)**, the lateral tibial plateau subluxates anteriorly producing a palpable shift of pivot (fibular head) or clunk when the knee is in 20–40° of flexion. With further flexion the knee is again reduced by the iliotibial band that pulls back the tibia posteriorly.

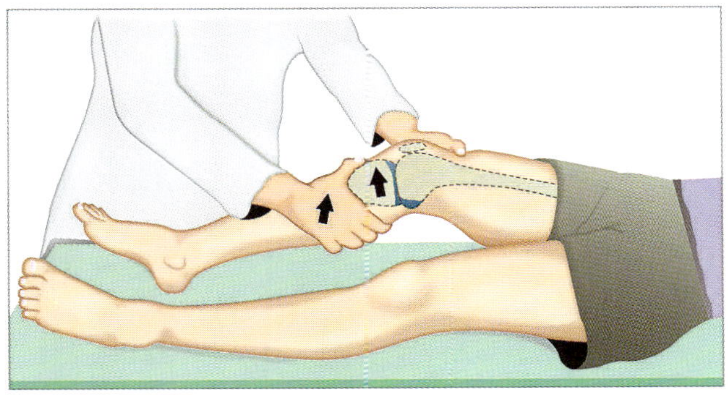

Fig. 49: Lachman test.

The pivot shift is graded subjectively:

- Grade 1+ is a pivot glide.
- Grade 2+ is a pivot shift.
- Grade 3+ is a gross pivot shift with feeling that the condyles will dislocate. With grade 3+ pivot shift test it is assumed that the ALL is also torn/deficient so it should also be reconstructed.

Jerk test: The jerk test is a pivot shift test begun in flexion and the knee is then extended. If there is anterior cruciate insufficiency, the tibia will subluxate at about 20° of flexion as the knee moves into extension; producing a palpable shift or clunk.

Flexion-rotation drawer test of Noyes: Here the lower leg is held with the knee flexed between 15° and 30°. At 15°, the tibia is subluxated anteriorly with the femur externally rotated in an ACL deficient knee. As the knee is flexed to 30°, the tibia reduces posteriorly and the femur rotates internally.

- Losee test is similar to the flexion-rotation drawer test, but it is done in a sidelying position.

Posterior Cruciate Ligament Tests

Posterior drawer test (Fig. 52): The posterior drawer test is performed in a position similar to the anterior drawer test, but in this test instead of anteriorly directed force, the proximal tibial plateau is pushed posteriorly. A positive posterior drawer test is indicated by posterior tibial translation and is due to damage to the PCL.

External rotation recurvatum test (Fig. 53): The athletic trainer grasps the great toe and lifts the leg off the table. In a PCL deficient knee the tibia externally rotates and slides posteriorly, an associated injury to the posterolateral joint capsule makes the test more conspicuous, due to posterolateral instability.

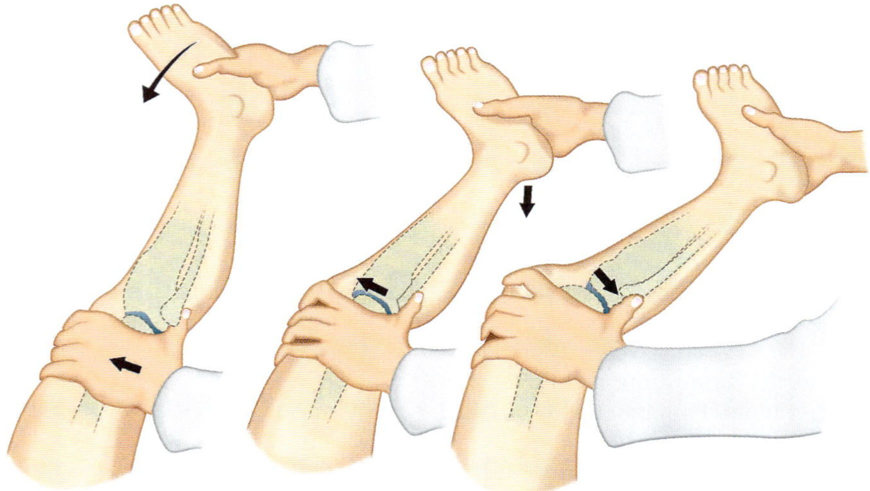

Fig. 50: The pivot shift test (*see* text).

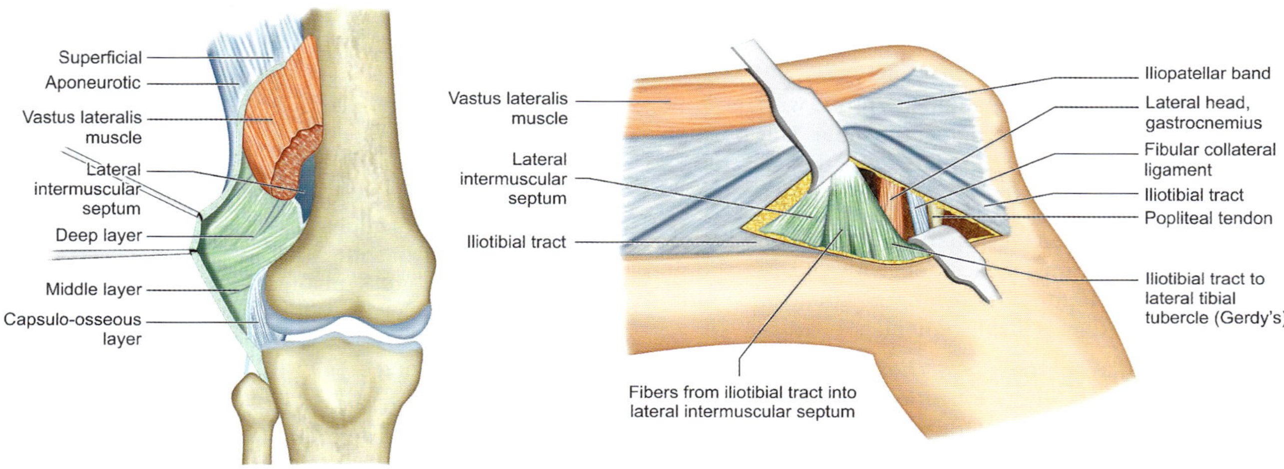

Fig. 51: Pathomechanism of pivot shift test: Deeper layers of the iliotibial tract. Rupture of the layers deep to iliotibial band (ITB) (the superficial layer) allows anterolateral rotatory subluxation of the lateral tibial plateau on the fibula. They must be ruptured for the pivot shift to occur.

Posterior sag test of Godfrey: An apparent posterior sag in the PCL deficient knee when both the knees which are placed in 90° flexion with the patient lying supine are observed from the lateral aspect **(*see* Fig. 68A)**.

Instrument assessment of cruciate laxity: Ligament testing devices (arthrometers) reduce the subjectivity involved in the above-mentioned tests by objectively quantifying the amount of anterior and posterior translation. The KT-2000 knee arthrometer, the Stryker knee laxity tester, and the Genucom are such testing devices. They can be used to follow patients after surgery and to evaluate the effectiveness of the treatment program objectively.

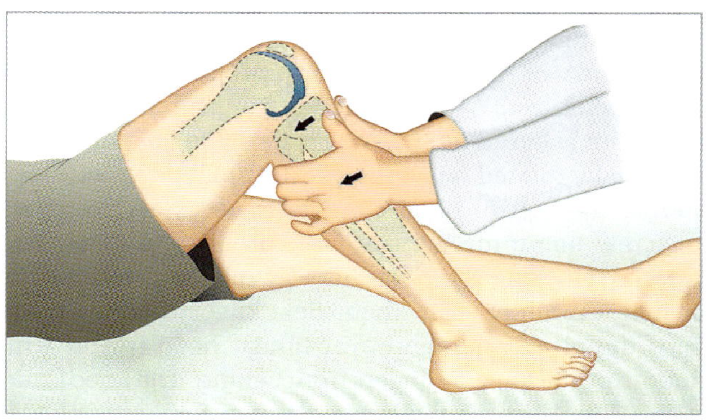

Fig. 52: Posterior drawer test.

Girth measurement: Muscles around knee quickly loose mass and atrophy due to pain or reduced activity (firing of neurons is reduced in an injured or misaligned knee). Girth measurement detects former injuries or determines the extent of exercise rehabilitation. Five sites have been suggested for girth measurement **(Fig. 54)**:

1. The joint line (tibial plateau)
2. From 8 to 10 cm above the tibial plateau
3. The level of the tibial tubercle
4. The belly of the gastrocnemius muscle measured in centimeters, always maintain the level of this measurement as fixed distance from the tibial tubercle.

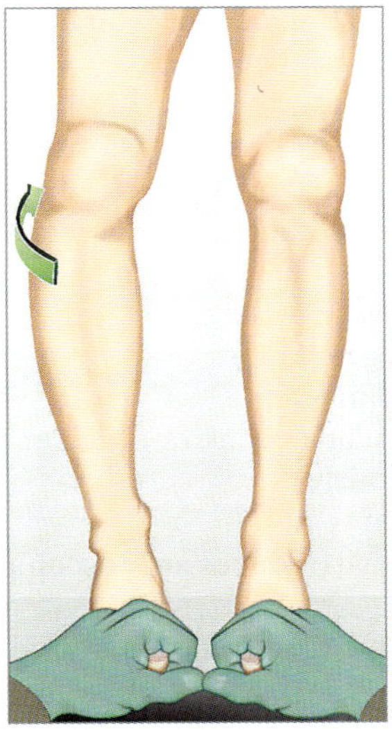

Fig. 53: External rotation recurvatum test. The great toes are held by the examiner as both legs are raised simultaneously. A positive test results in hyperextension, external rotation of the tibia, and apparent tibia vara of the affected limb.

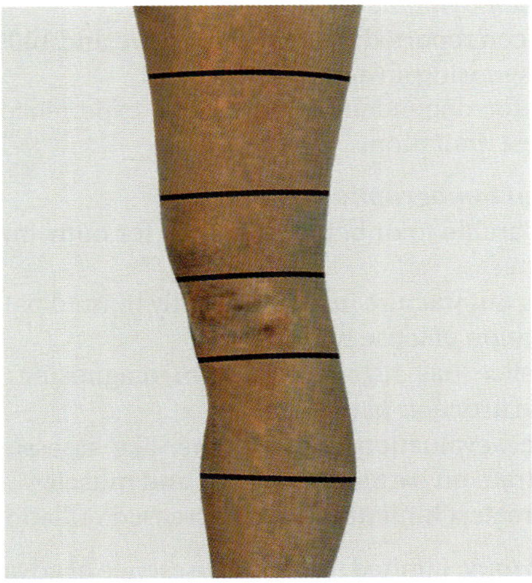

Fig. 54: Girth measurement.

5. 10 cm above the superior border of the patella—this measures the thigh girth irrespective of the effusions seen commonly in suprapatellar pouch that may falsely alter measurement.

Examining the Patella

The Q (quadriceps) angle: The Q angle gives a measure of the angle of pull of quadriceps muscle group. The angle is created at the intersection of lines drawn from the middle of the patella to the anterosuperior spine and from the tubercle of the tibia through the center of the patella **(Fig. 55)**. It should be measured with the knee fully extended and with the knee flexed at 30°. The normal Q angle is 10° for males and 15° for females. Q angles >20° (in extension) are considered excessive and could lead to a pathological condition associated with improper patellar tracking in the femoral groove.

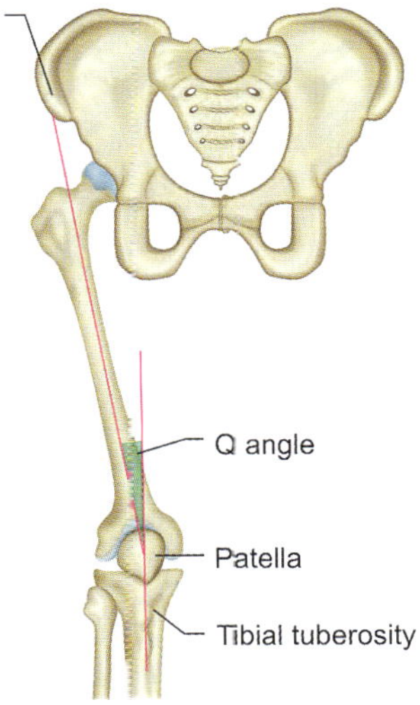

Fig. 55: Q angle.

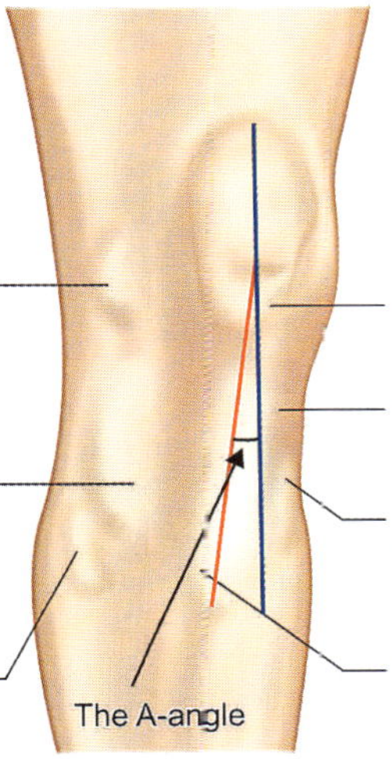

Fig. 56: The A angle.

The A angle: The A angle is a less often used measure of relative orientation of patella to tibial tubercle. It serves as a quantitative measure of patellar realignment after intervention. It is the angle sustained at the intersection of a line bisecting the patella longitudinally (vertical line perpendicular to floor) and a line from the tibial tubercle to the inferior pole of the patella **(Fig. 56)**. An A angle of 35° or greater is pathological and correlates with patellofemoral pathomechanics causing pain at the articulation.

Patellar compression, patellar grinding, and apprehension tests: Aims at eliciting pain or grating sound when the patella is compressed on the femur and moved forward and backward with the knee in approximately 20° of flexion, the patella is compressed downward into the femoral groove and moved forward and backward. A positive grind test indicates a patellofemoral joint pathology **(Fig. 57)**.

- *Clarke's sign:* With the knee still flexed, the patella is forced forward and is held in this position as the athlete extends the knee. A positive test is indicated by presence of pain.

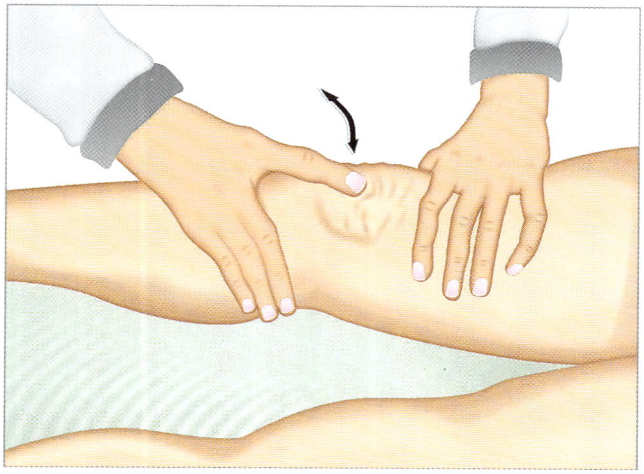

Fig. 57: Patellar compression test.

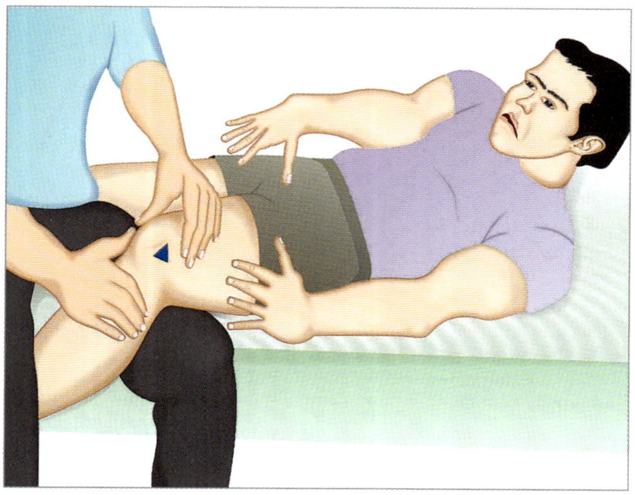

Fig. 58: Apprehension test for patellar instability.

- *Apprehension test **(Fig. 58)**:* With the knee in 20–30° of flexion and patella in a relaxed position, the examiner pushes the patella laterally manually. The patient will express sudden apprehension and a feeling of giving way at the point at which the patella begins to dislocate.

Diagnostic Investigations Used for Evaluating Knee Instability

One should know the basis for prescribing the investigations as a part of evaluation of patients sustaining sports injury to knee and its various parts. Below is mentioned briefly the utility of various modalities for knee evaluation.

Plain radiograph: This is the initial investigation of choice for evaluation of post-traumatic knee pain and instability. The primary utility of this investigation is to:

- Identify fractures
- Detect indirect signs of instability like "Segond sign"—this cortical avulsion fracture of the proximal tibia is commonly associated with ACL injury.
- Evaluate direction of dislocation.

Magnetic resonance imaging: It is the definitive study of choice for post-traumatic knee pain and instability.

- It is the investigation of choice for evaluation of:
  - Meniscal tears
  - Ligament tears
  - Pain caused by bone contusions
  - Osteochondral defects
  - Uncommon pathologies or associated pathologies
- Advantages:
  - Noninvasive
  - No ionizing radiation
  - Soft tissue imaging
  - Intra-articular and extra-articular tissues evaluated simultaneously
  - Multiplanar
  - Cost effective (reduces arthroscopic evaluation)
- Limitations:
  - Unidentified diagnostic ability with multiple knee injuries
  - High cost and lack of universal availability

Sonography: It is a very good investigation for evaluation of soft tissue injuries or even chronic lesions in experienced hands. Most of the pathologies can be identified and tested even in their dynamic environment.

- Has been reported to be 91% sensitive and 100% specific for diagnosing an acute ACL tear.
- Operator dependency and lack of experience serve as greatest limitation.

Computed tomography scan:

- Comparable to or better than MRI for bony injuries and fractures
- Ruling out fracture in a significantly injured patient
- Evaluation of loose bodies
- Multislice has high accuracy in diagnosing ACL and related articular pathology.
- Limited evaluation of soft tissue, like assessing edema and strain on cartilage, menisci, and muscles
- The greatest limitation is the increased radiation risk.

Arthrography: Limited role in the presence of advanced and newer imaging techniques. Limited by contrast sensitivity, ionizing radiation, and no further details compared to other noninvasive investigations.

Tc-99m bone scan: Not a preferred modality for acute injuries, no current indication exists for such evaluation.

- Can detect radiographically occult injuries or lesions.
- Useful in chronic knee pathology only as acute injuries are nonspecifically reported and details are not furnished.
- Focal increased uptake at sites of bone repair: fractures, avulsions, torn menisci or infarctions.
- Limitations:
  - Very low specificity
  - Inferior anatomic definition

Single-photon emission computed tomography (SPECT): Proposed for diagnosing meniscal injuries, but fares inferior to MRI: A specific crescentic uptake pattern on transaxial view has sensitivity of 77% and specificity of 74% for identifying meniscal tear.

Computed tomography or magnetic resonance angiography: Used mainly for assessing injury to the vascular structures, like in hyperextension blunt and penetrating trauma to the knee.

Arteriography: Useful for evaluation of vascular injury, but adds little information if any ahead of noninvasive computed tomography or magnetic resonance angiography.

The ACR appropriateness criteria of radiological evaluation for acute knee trauma in sports trauma (according to the first to last choice) is as below:

- Plain radiograph of knee—quickest, high exclusion reliability, and minimal radiation.
- Magnetic resonance imaging knee (noncontrast)—high yield possible over diagnosis and no radiation.
- Tc-99m bone scan with SPECT of lower extremity—low yield and nonspecific, but can locate the focal lesion and medium radiation risk.
- Computed tomography scan knee (noncontrast)—locates the bony pathology with great detail, poor soft-tissue details so limited utility in sports medicine and low to medium radiation.
- Ultrasonography—unclear visualization in subacute lesions due to edema, highly user dependent so yield is directly proportional to the observer experience, no radiation.
- Magnetic resonance angiogram knee—indicated only in suspected vascular injury, false negative is a concern as distal flow is highlighted even if minimal, no radiation.

TIBIAL COLLATERAL LIGAMENT INJURY

This is the most common ligament injury. Most of the isolated tibial collateral ligament (TCL) injuries are sports related and the incidence is 14 times that of LCL. Primary restraint to valgus stress is provided by TCL while the deep component giving secondary restraint. Dynamic stability is provided by the pes anserinus muscles, semimembranosus, VMO, and medial head of gastrocnemius.

Pathomechanism and Classification

- Most common mechanism is a contact injury at the lateral or posterolateral knee imparting a valgus stress to the knee **(Fig. 59)**.
- External tibial rotation as occurs in skiing or other sports where the foot is caught and the knee collapses medially over it also causes ligament disruption. These are much more likely to be associated with ACL and occasionally PCL tears.
- Overuse injuries are seen in certain sports, like breaststroke swimmers repetitively stretch their TCL.
- The risk factors for injury to the ligament are:
  - Contact sports and sports requiring pivoting or cutting maneuvers
  - Poor muscle strength and muscle mass

The impact of injury is much more on the knee from medial sprains than from lateral sprains because of closely associated articular capsule and medial meniscus. The position of knee at the time of injury is important in establishing its vulnerability to traumatic sprains. However, irrespective of the knee position, if the force is sufficient, it can injure the TCL. Position of foot is also very important and TCL sprains result often from adduction and internal rotation. A TCL deficient knee is rendered prone to further internal derangements and associated meniscal tears are common. The force and angle of the trauma usually determine the extent of injury that takes place in an acute setting, but is difficult even on witnessing the event. Knee examination soon after injury before the effusion yields the maximum result.

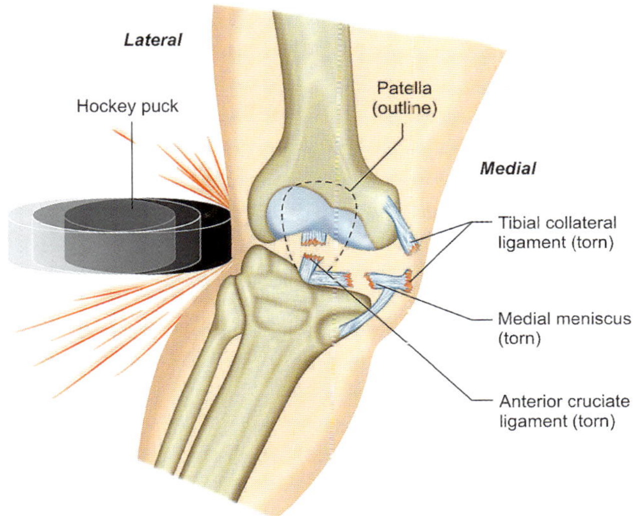

Fig. 59: Tibial collateral ligament injury basic pathomechanism.

The TCL injuries are classified into three grades (McCue; **Figs. 60A and B**):

- *Grade I:* Microscopic (intrasubstance) tearing with no measurable loss of function; no laxity.
- *Grade II:* Partial disruption or stretching of the ligament with some loss of function (one-third to two-thirds tear); 0–5 mm opening with good endpoint.
- *Grade II+:* 6–10 mm opening with soft endpoint.
- *Grade III:* Two-thirds to complete tearing of the ligament without any continuity with >10 mm opening.
- *Grade III+:* Complete failure with loss of continuity.

Clinical Features

These are presented with description of grades of injury and management below, additionally however the following may be noted.

The patient complains of pain and tenderness on the inner side of the knee and notes a popping, tearing or pulling sensation at injury. Swelling and bruising at inner aspect of knee is noted with variable knee stiffness and limp on walking.

Valgus stress test: As described earlier.

Dial test: Primary used for evaluation of posterolateral structures and PCL, but pain at medial aspect of knee on external rotation of tibia during the test suggests injury to this area.

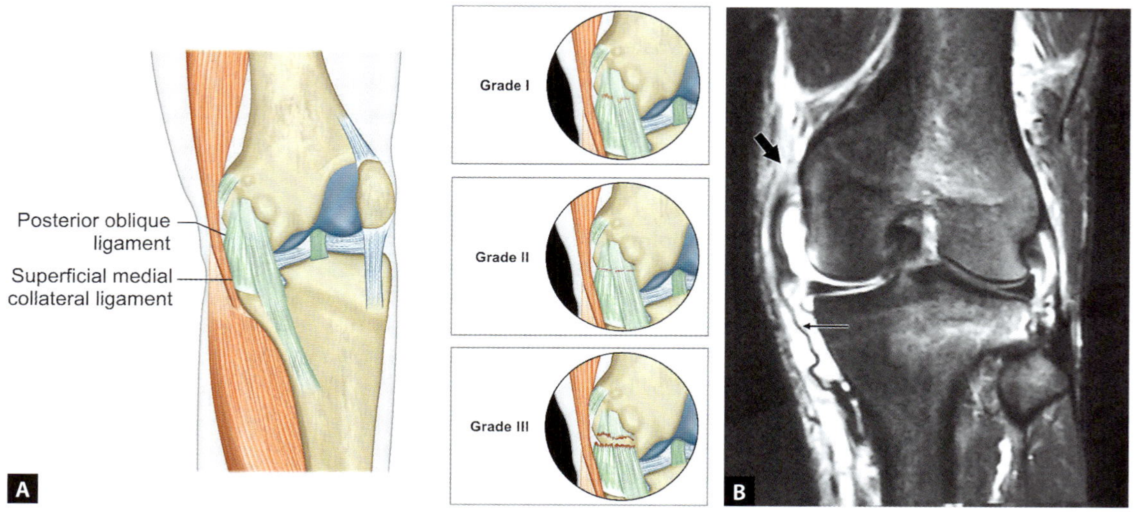

Figs. 60A and B: Injury of the tibial collateral ligament and the three grades of deficiency. (A) Grade I injuries: localized tenderness, but no gross laxity, the fibers are stretched mostly and minimal disruption in continuity. Grade II injuries broader area of tenderness as the fibers are partially torn. Grade III injuries have complete disruption of the fibers and there is gross laxity when tested with valgus stress; (B) MRI of knee coronal section T2-weighted image depicting complete TCL avulsion injury (thick arrow) with slump in the ligament and wavy structure (thin arrow) that is otherwise a taut straight line.

Perform additional tests to evaluate injury to ACL, PCL, MPFL, etc.

Radiology

Radiographs are important to determine associated injuries to bone and other structures. Obtain knee radiographs if any of the following five criteria is met (Ottawa knee rules):

1. Patient aged ≥55 years
2. Isolated tenderness of the patella (no other bone tenderness)
3. Tenderness at the head of fibula
4. Inability to flex knee to 90°
5. Inability to bear weight both immediately and in emergency department for four steps.

Stress radiographs have been used, but caution should be exercised as under anesthesia the radiographs may perform poorly, mislead diagnosis and inexperienced examiner may make the injury complete. For a stress radiographs, the following are some commonly used grading measures:

- Isolated injury of superficial MCL:
  - Medial knee joint opening of 1.7 mm at 0° of knee flexion, and
  - 3.2 mm at 20° of knee flexion
- Complete medial knee injury (superficial MCL, POL, and deep MCL):
  - Medial joint gap of 6.5 mm at 0° knee flexion, and
  - 9.8 mm at 20° flexion

Differential diagnosis: Medial meniscus tear, pes anserine bursitis, medial plica syndrome, and femoral chondral damage.

Management According to Grades of Injury

The historical literature of management of collateral ligament injuries is mixed with surgical and nonoperative treatment. In any case there is often a bias toward conservative management presently and that the literature does not support initial choice of surgery as a treatment modality. The other general rule is that remobilization of six times the duration of immobilization is needed for complete recovery, so one should minimize immobilization. For grade I injuries return to work or play is made as short as 5–7 days while for grade III injuries it may need 4–8 weeks depending on recovery. In football players especially linemen use of functional knee brace has been proposed to prevent injury.

Grade I MCL sprain has the following characteristics:

- Ligamentous fibers are torn and stretched, but ligament is in continuity.
- The joint is stable during valgus stress tests.
- Little or no joint effusion
- Joint stiffness (mild to moderate)
- Point tenderness just below the medial joint line
- Almost full passive and active range of motion

Management: Immediately—PRICE (protection, rest, ice, immobilization, compression, elevation for at least 24 hours) prescribe:

- Crutches for 2 weeks.
- Cryokinetics (20 minutes of ice pack treatment before exercise or a combination of cold and compression or pulsed ultrasound) to begin within 2–3 days.
- Isometrics and straight leg exercises until the knee can be moved without pain. Introduce stationary bicycling slowly with pain tolerance.
- Strengthening exercises and range of motion (ROM) exercises to regain neuromuscular function by 2–3 weeks until knee regains normal power.

The patient returns to full participation when the knee has regained normal strength, flexibility, and endurance which takes 2–3 weeks. Brace may be required for a short period, mostly less than a week.

Grade II MCL sprain is both microscopic and gross disruption of fibers of the TCL and also the medial capsular structures. Grade II sprain is characterized by:

- A complete tear of the deep capsular ligament and partial tear of the superficial portion (grade II+) or partial tear of both (grade II).
- No or minimum laxity at full extension. Instability is greater at 30° of flexion when valgus stress test is performed.
- *Mild to moderate swelling:* Swelling mainly is determined by additional damage to the knee say ACL tear, subluxated or dislocated patella or an osteochondral fracture, that result in excess swelling and hemarthrosis.
- Moderate to severe joint stiffness—the person is unable to fully extend the knee actively.
- Patient is unable to place the heel flat on the ground.
- Loss of passive range of motion
- General weakness and instability

Management: Conservative care, mostly grade II sprains can be managed conservatively because other structures are there to act as secondary constraint.

- Immediately—PRICE, continued for 2–3 days. Provide crutches to patient.
    - I prefer a universal knee brace with ROM control applied immediately and kept in extension locked at 0 degree for 2–5 days.
- Range of motion exercises are begun at 4–7 days and passive knee flexion is set to pain tolerance limit.
- Analgesics and anti-inflammatory medications are prescribed for initial 3–5 days followed by SOS basis.
- Along with passive knee flexion isometric quadriceps to improve the strength should be done as soon as the pain is tolerable with >90° of knee flexion.
- The above is supplemented with closed chain exercises—stationary cycling, stair climbing, and resisted flexion and extension.
- Early functional progression is now a part of the rehabilitation program.
- The hinged universal brace is continued till functional rehabilitation is complete.
- As other structures of the knee, like ACL can also protect the knee against valgus and rotatory motion, it is possible for the spontaneous ligament and capsular healing. Studies have validated this finding.

Grade III MCL sprain is a complete tear of the supporting ligaments (primary and often the secondary restraints also). The features are:

- Complete loss of medial stability
- Immediate severe pain
- Dull ache after the initial episode
- Swelling
- Hamstring guarding
- Valgus stress test that reveals medial instability to valgus stress—joint opening in full extension with a significant opening at 30° of flexion.

Management: For grade III injury is primarily guided by presence of associated ACL tears.

In isolated TCL tears, conservative management may suffice. I have personally found that femoral side avulsions do better with conservative management, but tibial side or mid-substance tears do poorly and knee remain lax afterward. Mid-substance tears are actually the worst and do not heal—I would recommend ligament reconstruction for them. Rest, ice, compression, and elevation (RICE) should be used for at least 72 hours. The knee should be immobilized in a hinged brace which allows the knee to move between 30 and 90° of motion. Progressive weight-bearing for 2–3 weeks, with gradually increasing movements to 0–90° for another 2–3 weeks as described above suffice for femoral side tears or avulsions.

Surgical treatment: Indicated for:

- Collateral ligament tears with ACL or PCL tears
- Midsubstance TCL tears [often iatrogenic say while doing total knee arthoplasty (TKA)]
- Tibial side avulsions of TCL. Stener lesions where the torn end of the TCL gets trapped in medial compartment are especially amneable to acute repairs.

Repair of acute injuries (up to 3 weeks) is done by various methods including use of spiked washers, suture anchors, heavy braided sutures or their combination. The results are good, if there is bony avulsion then the repairs even fare better with reattachment of bony fragment and can be done even up to 6–8 weeks.

The following text gives a brief detail of technique for surgical reconstruction of medial knee ligament structures:

For complete TCL and POL ruptures anatomical reconstruction of both should be carried out. Two grafts and four reconstruction tunnels are used **(Fig. 61)**. Graft for TCL (superficial one is reconstructed) should be tightened at 30° of knee flexion, while the one for POL should be tightened at 0° of knee flexion. The patient is allowed to move the knee joint in a closed chain fashion for up to 90°. Simultaneously quadriceps strengthening exercises are begun. Initially, the aim is to prevent adhesion formation while permitting improvement in strength, later stress is mainly on improving muscle strength and initiating weight-bearing (after 6 weeks). Once patient starts walking gait mechanics is improved gradually.

Reconstruction of chronic tears is still a difficult problem. Associated ACL or PCL tears if repaired are bound to fail. For these chronic injuries reconstruction involves advancement of TCL attachment on femur or recession of femoral epicondyle,

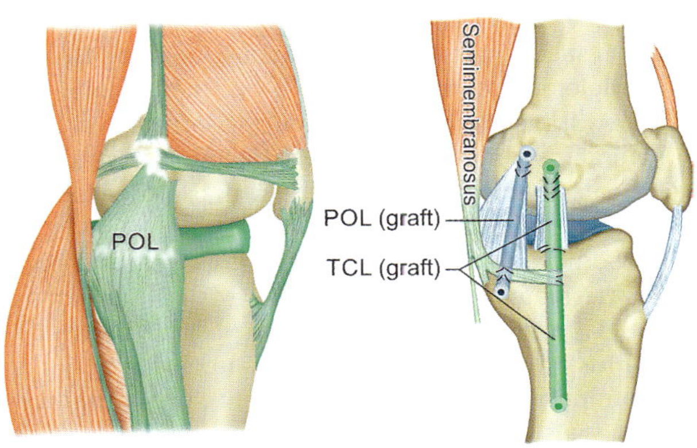

Fig. 61: Tibial collateral ligament reconstruction.
(POL: popliteal oblique ligament; TCL: tibial collateral ligament)

the latter is preferred. Posterior capsule and POL are plicated to posterior aspect of tightened ligament. The results of isolated TCL injury treatment massively deteriorate if it is associated with ACL injury. Weak and thin TCL can be reconstructed using hamstring autograft or tendo-Achilles allograft.

Complications of nonoperative management (Natural history of immobilization and its effects on body):

- Immobilization for 9 weeks results in a clear disruption of the deep fibers; the ligament is much more prone to avulsion at the tibial insertion following immobilization should injury recur.
- Decrease in the tensile strength of the ligaments is observed. Histologically, the changes include widely spaced irregular collagen fascicles, glycosaminoglycan degradation, decreased cytoplasmic, and mitochondrial enzymatic activity.
    - Such ligaments are inferior structurally as well as mechanically. The ultimate load and energy absorbed at failure is just 80% of normal.

LATERAL COLLATERAL LIGAMENT INJURY

Incidence is much less as compared to TCL injuries. Lateral collateral ligament along with PFL and ITB are primary restraints to varus producing force. ACL and to a lesser extent PCL provide secondary restraint. The lateral head of gastrocnemius, tendon of biceps femoris, and vastus lateralis are dynamic stabilizers against varus producing force.

Pathomechanism

Varus force is the primary mechanism of injury often applied in hyperextended knee. The force is more prone to cause LCL damage, if it is associated with internal rotation of tibia. Position of foot is also important; the most prevalent mechanism involves the knee being forced laterally into the varus position with the foot in an everted position. In skiing the LCL gets injured when the unstable skier crosses his tips throwing the body weight to the outside edge of the ski and loses support of snow plough. Such injuries are severe if occurring at good speed injuring lateral structures along with PCL and ACL—equivalent to knee dislocation. Even peroneal nerve may get injured.

Clinical Features

- Pain especially in grade I or II tears [in grade III injuries (complete ruptures)—pain will be intense initially and then will become a dull ache] and tenderness over the LCL.
- Lateral instability and gap may be found in grade II and III tears respectively, especially with the knee flexed and internally rotated:
    - Some joint laxity with a varus stress test at 30° is seen in isolated LCL injury. If laxity exists in full extension, ACL and possibly PCL are also possibly injured.
- Contusion and swelling over LCL attachment
- Examine the peroneal nerve as in severe injuries the nerve gets stretched. The injury may be palsy or complete injury and needs specialty management especial in complete cases.

Management

Management of the grade I and II LCL sprains are along the lines of management of TCL injuries. The grade III LCL injury—a complete rupture of the ligament has to be managed by operative treatment as the results of conservative management are dismal and results in persistent functional disability which may progress. Acute injuries, sleeve avulsions, or best the bony avulsions should be repaired. Late injuries >3 weeks are better reconstructed as the ligament ends are friable enough to have poor holding strength of sutures. Bony avulsions can be repaired till even 2 months if significant retractions have not occurred. Isolated injuries of LCL especially the grade III injuries are uncommon and occur in association with PLC injury. Reconstruction can be done as a single-stranded graft or fibular-based reconstruction (Larson technique), etc. (see PLC injuries).

ANTERIOR CRUCIATE LIGAMENT INJURY

The ACL injury is one of the most common serious ligament injury in the knee due to its primary stabilizing role and importance in knee biomechanics (anteromedial knee instability). The incidence is estimated to be about 32–40 injuries per 100,000 person years or 1 in 1,750 active people. The injury is common in athletic population; however, young athletes often escape ligament injury as the force leads to avulsion fractures often. Otherwise the risk factors for ACL injury can be summarized as below:

- Extrinsic factors (somewhat controllable):
    - Uneven playing field
    - Level of conditioning
    - Higher intensity of play than usual—as in championships rather than training sessions
    - Skill acquisition
    - Rainy weather with slippery and muddy surfaces
    - Aggressive playing attitude
- Intrinsic factors (physiological and psychological factors that are more difficult to control):
    - Higher flexibility (ligament laxity), reduced muscle strength and poor reaction time
    - Hormonal fluctuation in females (increased incidence during ovulatory and postovulatory phase)
    - Low trunk, hip, and knee flexion angles
    - Increased Q angle and valgus knee
    - Narrow intercondylar notch of femur
    - Increased recurvatum
    - Quadriceps dominance (reduced hamstring power or dominance compared to quadriceps)
    - Small ACL size
    - Increased external tibial torsion
    - High dorsiflexion of ankle
    - Increased pelvic width (as in females)
    - Neuromuscular factors (muscle activation latencies, electromechanical delay, and muscle recruitment patterns) are also important contributors to the increased risk of ACL injuries in females.

Pathophysiology

The ACL is most vulnerable to injury when the knee is in a valgus position and the tibia is internally rotated (with respect to femur). This is the reason why females are 4–10 times more prone to ACL injury (higher valgus angle at knee): other possible factors are mentioned above. The ACL can sustain injury from a direct blow to the knee (30%) or more commonly by a noncontact single-plane force (70%) typically called as noncontact pivoting injury. Noncontact injury occurs when the lower leg is rotated while the foot is fixed. In this situation, the ACL becomes taut and vulnerable to sprain. This scenario is seen in:

- Skiers or skateboarders whose ankles are locked when they fall backward.
- Phantom foot mechanism in skiers—the foot gets internally rotated due to tibial internal rotation and knee flexed fully—landing in this position will rupture ACL for sure. In such cases the ligament tend to avulse from the femoral attachment and is amneable to acute repair.
- Soccer players who do sudden cutting maneuvers, pivoting in full knee extension.
- Basketball players that land on internally rotated knee without full flexion.
- Increased knee valgus while landing especially with foot flat.

These *noncontact injuries* are decelerating injuries where quadriceps is maximally contracted and the knee is near full extension making ACL taut causing an isolated tear of the ACL. Rotatory instabilities occur when besides ACL, other supporting structures are also injured.

- *Anterolateral rotatory instability—Associated injury to the anterolateral joint capsule and the LCL:* PCL and structures in the PLC may also be injured.
- *Anteromedial rotatory instability—Associated injury to the anteromedial capsule and the TCL:* Again the PCL and posteromedial corner may also be injured.
- With continued valgus stress on internally rotated tibia the TCL ruptures and lateral meniscus gets injured along with ACL injury (O'Donoghue's triad). The O'Donoghue's triad is also known as horrible triangle, unhappy triad or blown knee and was described by O'Donoghue (American orthopedic surgeon) in 1950. The classical description included medial knee structures as an injury complex that was difficult to manage and produced dismal results; it included TCL, ACL, and medial meniscus. This injury complex is, however, uncommon and atypical as it has been found that the lateral meniscus is commonly injured with acute ACL disruptions and not the medial meniscus. For practical purposes and descriptions of the O'Donoghue's triad lateral meniscus should be included in the injury complex (needs concrete modification in literature), however, one tends to mention medial meniscus keeping with the original description or O'Donoghue's triad per se. The injury pattern is seen from lateral blow to the knee as seen in football and rugby games. Involvement of medial meniscus is indirect as the valgus stress would produce medial joint opening so that the medial meniscus would be unloaded, but being tethered to the TCL the meniscus gets shearing force and is torn. Lateral meniscus gets trapped between the two bones and is directly injured in most of the cases so its injury is much more frequent. In chronic ACL and TCL combined injuries the medial meniscus is injured due to repetitive unbalanced mechanics of the meniscus movement catching it often between the two bones. "Terrible triad" emphasizes the difficulty in treatment that entails, and frequent failure if only ACL is reconstructed. Even after ACL and TCL reconstruction the meniscal injury commonly causes locking and other symptoms in the knee causing early degenerative arthritis.

Other mechanism is a contact injury: When the knee is struck in front by a hyperextension force with the foot planted which can tear the ACL and in severe cases, even the TCL.

Apart from the noncontact and contact injuries; the *third mechanism* of ACL injury is external rotation of the tibia relative to the femur with varus stress leading to impaction and bone edema medially and distraction laterally producing Segond fracture.

Biomechanical factors are important to consider when eliciting the mechanism of ACL injuries. The biomechanical factors in many noncontact ACL injuries include:

- Impact on the foot or heel during landing or changing directions suddenly while running instead of toes.
- Deceleration with valgus stress and rotation.

Pathoanatomy

Anterior cruciate ligament tears may be partial or complete:

- Partial tears (20%) can be minor ranging from a tear of few fibers to a high grade near complete tear which damages almost all of the ACL fibers. Also either of the two bundles could be involved, the anteromedial being the more common one.
- Sometimes, ACL laxity and insufficiency can be caused only by plastic deformation.
- Most ACL tears (approximately 80%) are complete. Location wise, middle one-third is the most common site (90%).

Clinical Features

Symptoms and Signs

- The patient with a torn ACL experiences a popping sound followed quickly by swelling over knee over a few hours. The swelling usually appears by a couple of hours and becomes significant by 6 hours.
- Pain is variable and is often not intense unless there is bone contusion or meniscal tear.
- "Double fist sign" is often used by the patient to describe instability. Patient uses fists facing each other, rotating in a grinding manner to describe knee feeling of "shifting".
- Patients often do not have full extension due to either torn ACL stump lying between the femur and tibia or torn meniscus preventing tibial extension.

On examination there is (see above for tests of ACL):

- Positive anterior drawer sign
- Positive Lachman sign (most accurate test)
- Positive pivot shift test—more sensitive for rotatory instability.

Jerk test and flexion-rotation drawer test may also be positive even with an isolated ACL tear.

Investigations

Radiograph

Obtain standing anteroposterior radiograph of both knees in full extension along with lateral and merchant's views. A 45° posteroanterior views is helpful to evaluate for condylar lesions and loose bodies.

- Capsular avulsions (Segond fracture, **Figs. 62A to C**) are identified on standard anteroposterior views. It is a cortical avulsion fracture of the proximal tibia, located just below the level of the lateral plateau and superior and posterior to the Gerdy's tubercle. The fracture results from excessive medial rotation and varus stress and is associated with injury to ACL and thus anterolateral rotatory instability. The Segond fracture is considered pathognomonic of ACL injury. The fracture is readily evident on AP projections of the knee and presence of one indicates higher grade injury. It is considered that to optimize the results of ACL reconstruction in such cases this fracture and ALL needs to be fixed or reconstructed.
- Calcification at the femoral origin of TCL (Pellegrini-Stieda lesion, **Figs. 62A to C**) indicates previous injury.
- Lateral femoral notch sign (also called deep sulcus sign)—Osteochondral impaction fracture in the condylopatellar sulcus of the lateral femoral condyle. A sulcus deeper than 1.5 mm is a fairly specific though very insensitive indirect radiographic sign of a torn ACL.
- Hemarthrosis is seen as opacity in suprapatellar pouch, fluid level may be seen with lipohemarthrosis.
- Anterior cruciate ligament avulsion fractures **(Figs. 62A to C)** can be seen in younger patients.

Magnetic Resonance Imaging

Anterior cruciate ligament is best visualized on two-dimensional (2D) turbo spin echo (TSE) sequences with or without fat suppression. TSE sagittal intermediate-weighted sequences and T2 coronal TSE and TSE axial intermediate-weighted sequences with fat suppression are good enough to evaluate ACL integrity. T1-weighted sequences are used for suspected fracture or characterizing loose bodies within the knee. Small field of view (FOV) is helpful at delineating peripheral pathology around the knee. Three-dimensional (3D) fast spin echo reduces imaging time and reduces volume averaging artifacts, but have same diagnostic accuracy.

- Normal ACL—appears as a taut structure with continuous fibers visible in all planes and sequences. It appears as a low to intermediate signal intensity structure running parallel to intercondylar line (Blumensaat's line). The posterolateral bundle has higher signal intensity than anteromedial bundle.
- ACL tear—the primary sign is fiber discontinuity visible in oblique sagittal plane.
  - In complete ACL tear "empty notch sign" is seen. Thickening of ACL due to edema is observed along with increased signal intensity on T2 or intermediate weighted sequences **(Figs. 63A and B)**. In chronic lesions, the fibers are completely absorbed and may be adherent to PCL. MRI has >90% accuracy in diagnosing ACL tear. Oblique plane imaging is much better than conventional plane imaging.
  - Partial tears are identified by altered intensity and heterogenicity within the substance of ACL and increased concavity (bowing) of ACL. The sensitivity and specificity are low for diagnosing partial tears. 3T imaging improves the resolution and hence the sensitivity and specificity of imaging. High-grade tear is defined by tear of >50% fibers, while medium grade tear has injury to 10–50% fibers.
  - *Indirect signs:* Bony contusion in the posterolateral tibial plateau + middle third of lateral femoral condyle, deep lateral femoral notch sign, Segond

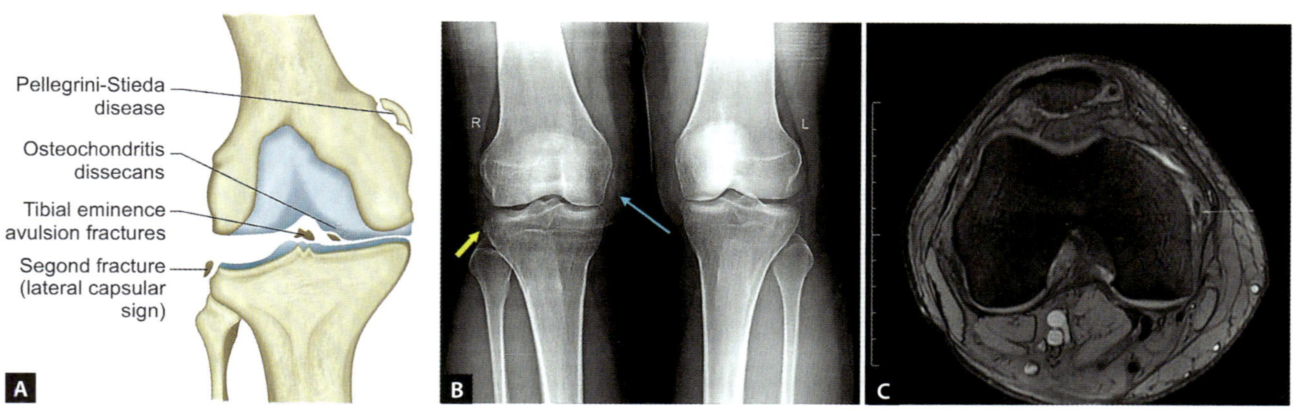

Figs. 62A to C: Radiographic evaluation. (A) For anterior cruciate ligament (ACL) tear illustrating various findings associated with acute and chronic ACL injury; (B) Radiograph demonstrating the calcification near medial femoral condyle of right knee (arrow) in a patient with Pellegrini–Stieda disease that can also be appreciated in the T2-weighted axial MR scan (arrow, C). Also visible in plain radiograph (B) is the old healed Segond injury (block arrow) over lateral tibial plateau of right knee often seen in association with ACL injury.
Source: Dr Nittin Vermani, Consultant Radiologist, Shri Mata Vaishno Devi Narayana Superspecialty Hospital, Kakryal, Katra, Jammu and Kashmir.

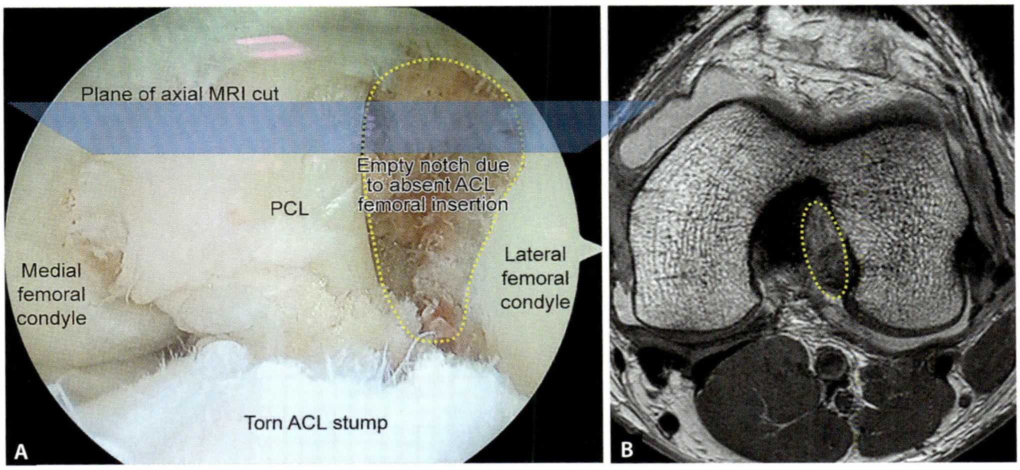

Figs. 63A and B: The absence of anterior cruciate ligament (ACL) from the lateral femoral condyle attachment site (A) vacates the notch in the region (dotted closed curve). The region is filled with fibrofatty tissue or synovial fluid that can be easily visualized (dotted arrow) on MRI axial (B) or coronal images.

fracture, Bosch-Bock bump (bony excrescence located 2–5 mm below the lateral articular margin of the tibia—indicates chronic tear of ACL), anterior tibial translation (≥5 mm anterior translation of tibia relative to femur indicates tear, >7 mm is diagnostic of ACL tear), buckling of PCL, uncovered posterior horn of medial or lateral meniscus, shearing fat pad injury, etc.

- *Associated injuries:*
  - *Meniscal tear:* PLC tear of the lateral meniscus which appears as a peripheral vertical tear in posterior horn of lateral meniscus is commonly associated with ACL tear.
  - In chronic ACL tear posterior horn of the medial meniscus can also show a peripheral vertical tear.
  - PLC injury—it includes injury to fibular collateral ligament, popliteus tendon, PFL, lateral and postero-lateral capsule, and biceps femoris tendon injury. This should be identified and reported as ACL reconstruction in this circumstance is likely to fail and result in retear.

Management

Conservative Management

A trial of conservative management may be considered if the patient has:

- Few giving-way episodes
- Near normal range of motion on knee extension
- Minimal or no meniscal damage on MRI
- Strong quadriceps femoris
- No difficulty performing the crossover hop test. The patient is made to jump as far as possible three consecutive times on a single leg. In-between the hops the patient has to cross midline for each hop needing side to side stability. For a negative test, the patient should land firmly on ground without buckling of falling.

Balance training and hamstring strengthening are introduced to minimize anterior tibial translation with activity.

Operative Treatment

In patients with anterior cruciate ligamentous injury and overt knee instability; high performance activity invariably requires an intact ACL. This is especially important in patients who play jumping sports and have high agility activities. Controversy exists about how best to treat an acute anterior cruciate ligamentous rupture and when to operate. ACL repair (repair of native ACL to bone) is an uncommon practice and followed in only a few select centers across the world. This method is amenable more-so rather, I would say it is limited to injuries in skiers as here the ligament commonly comes off its femoral attachment and majority of it is structurally preserved. Internal support to ligament (suture braiding/scaffold) is commonly needed for improving the outcome of repair. After intraligament braiding with strong suture the construct is fixed using specialized device to femur, personally I have no experience with this uncommon technique. Use of platelets rich plasma or bone marrow access through drill holes with repair have undefined role. Intra-articular ACL reconstruction is considered the best way to manage ACL tears. Acute reconstruction (within 3 weeks) is feared with development of arthrofibrosis and is often discouraged though strong supportive literature to this thought is missing. In any case an unsatisfactorily treated or untreated ACL tear will eventually lead to major joint degeneration. Therefore, decision to operate, its timing and type of surgery are based not only on the patient's age and the type of stress applied to the knee, but also upon the amount of instability present and the techniques available to the surgeon.

Arthroscopic ACL reconstruction using different graft choices have become the standard of care, the controversy here though is to choose between conventional versus anatomic; single-bundle reconstruction versus double-bundle reconstruction **(Figs. 64A and B)**. The latter requires higher level of training and experience but the results demonstrate better stability and revision rates than single bundle reconstructions. Also the anatomic single

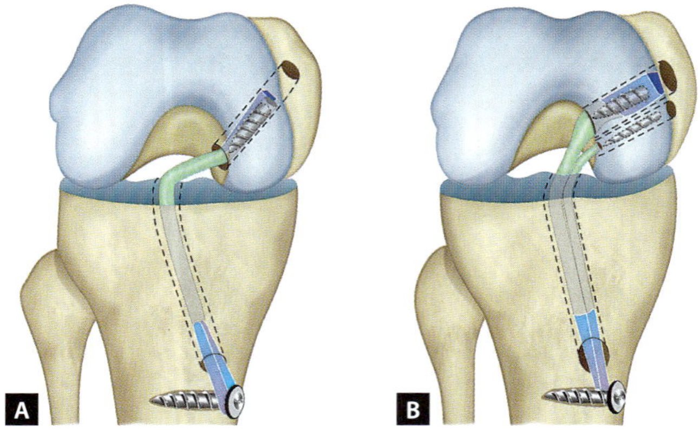

Figs. 64A and B: Posterior cruciate ligament (PCL) reconstruction: (A) Single bundle; (B) Double bundle.

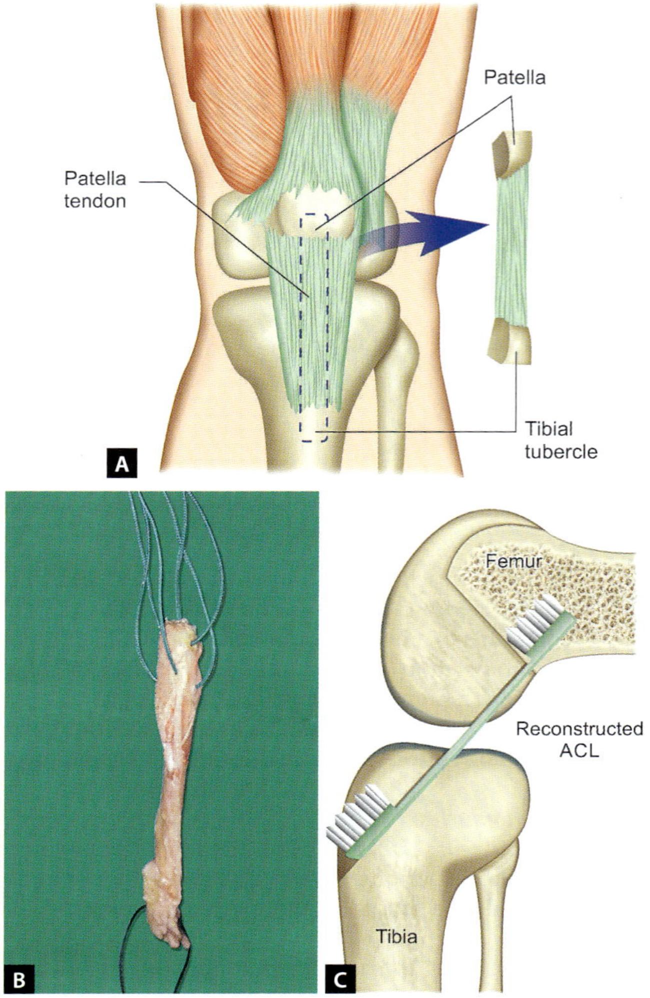

Figs. 65A to C: Anterior cruciate ligament (ACL) reconstruction using bone patellar tendon bone (BPTB) graft. (A) Harvesting the graft; (B) A typical BPTB graft preparation; (C) Fixation of graft in the tunnels of femur and tibia.

bundle reconstruction appears to have better survival than nonanatomic single bindle ACL reconstruction. Due to recent concerns raised for suboptimal results after ACL reconstruction it has been proposed that one should also carefully evaluate anterolateral ligament (ALL) patency especially in high-grade pivot shift positive patients and those with anteromedial rotatory instability. There is often an ALL deficiency that negatively influences the results of ACL reconstruction so ALL should be additionally reconstructed in such cases. A lot of grafts have been proposed in the literature, however, the commonly used grafts for ACL reconstruction involve:

- Autograft tissue
  - Bone–patellar tendon–bone graft **(Figs. 65A to C)**—described by Jones in 1960, popularized by Erickson in 1970s.
  - Four-strand (quadruple) hamstring tendon (semitendinosus and gracilis)
  - Quadriceps tendon
- Allograft tissue
  - Patellar tendon
  - Achilles tendon
  - Tibialis anterior tendon
  - Posterior tibialis tendon
- Synthetic—high failure rates and difficult revision so not used mostly (GoreTex, Leeds-Keho, LARS, etc.). These synthetic ligaments are now into their third generation having a knitted extra-articular portion with intra-articular free longitudinal fibers. The intra-articular fibers resist elongation and also are devoid of synovitis causing braided portion. First generation ligaments were knitted, woven or braided that were prone to early breakage and also tended to elongate. To overcome problem of elongation the second generation ligaments incorporated additional longitudinal and transverse fibers into the braid or knit. Polyethylene terephthalate or Dacron was used as an improvement to act as a permanent replacement and allow fibroblastic ingrowth. Still these ligaments suffered from wear, fraying and had low abrasion resistance. The wear debris so created additionally caused catastrophic synovitis. Third generation ligaments such as the ligament advanced reinforcement system (LARS) retain polyethylene terephthalate as material advancement while design changes have been done to remove any braids to cause intra-articular wear and production of biologically active wear debris.

Goals of surgical reconstruction: Restore knee stability, maintain normal knee motion, minimum donor site complications, and return of patient to desired level of activity.

Addressing some controversies:

- *Autograft versus allograft:* Autograft is associated with donor site morbidity, and bone patellar tendon bone is associated with anterior knee pain. Quadruple hamstring graft has less fixation strength than patellar tendon graft, but clinically has comparable results. Allograft is free of donor site morbidity but carries risk of poor tissue strength and infectious disease transmission.

I personally favor quadruple hamstring graft to minimize postoperative morbidity, better cosmesis and comparable results, also soft-tissue allografts are not accessible easily in our country. Allografts also have higher failure rates in young athletes. The most important advantage of patellar tendon graft is that unlike hamstring grafts, which can be of variable diameter, the patellar tendon offers a graft of consistent size and shape. Obtaining full extension after patellar tendon graft is a task, so if the surgeon is unsure of rehabilitation program then hamstring graft is preferable. Hamstring grafts leave permanent weakness in flexion knee power which by itself is a risk factor for graft rupture.

- *Graft placement:* The correct position of tibial and femoral tunnels is most important. Poor placement of tunnels is the most common cause of ACL graft failure. Femoral and tibial footprints of native ACL are the best sites for graft placement. Following points usually surmise acceptable tunnel positioning otherwise:
  - Tibial tunnel should be centered in the posteromedial aspect of the tibial footprint or 5–7 mm in front of PCL. This point is along the line drawn from the posterior edge of anterior horn of lateral meniscus to the medial tibial eminence.
  - Center of native ACL femoral footprint appears to be the best site for single bundle ACL femoral tunnel. Femoral tunnel placement should be at 10:30 position for right knee or 1:30 for left knee.
  - The femoral tunnel should embrace the posterior cortex that can be achieved by 7 mm offset drill guide.
  - It is better to widen the femoral notch **(Figs. 66A to C)** so that it looks like a smooth inverted U "roman arch" rather than a pointed "gothic arch".
- Though double-bundle technique has been envisaged to provide better rotational control, the clinical differences are yet to be proven. Single-bundle technique by using anteromedial portal to create femoral tunnel more anatomically possibly yields similar results.
- *Graft fixation:* Depending on the graft choice fixation methods mainly involve fixing soft tissue (tendon) to bone or fixing bone to bone (as in bone patellar tendon graft or one side of Achilles tendon allograft). The fixation sites are located either in the distal femur or the proximal tibia. Tibial fixation has been since long considered to be the precarious one with a higher chance of failure/slippage. The reconstruction graft may be fixed within a bony tunnel or located some distance away from it (suspensory fixation). Happa has classified the graft fixation methods into four types:
  1. Tissue fixation in the femoral site
  2. Tissue fixation in the tibial site
  3. Bone fixation in the femoral site
  4. Bone fixation in the tibial site.

  Innumerous devices have been described for graft fixation on either side and they are still under constant evolution to finding a universal system. For purpose of general understanding of how devices achieve fixation of the graft a better way is to divide the ***femoral fixation devices***/methods into:
- Compressive fixation (these produce compressive forces to the longitudinal axis of the graft pushing them against the bony tunnel). The commercial devices for such fixation are various interference screws that may be metallic (steel or titanium), bioabsorbable screws (polyglycolic acid, poly-L-lactic acid, poly-D, L-lactic acid, polyglycolic acid with trimethylene carbonate, poly-L-lactic acid with hydroxyapatite and poly-L-lactic acid with tricalcium phosphate). The metallic screws have been available since >30 years (introduced in 1983) and have good initial fixation strength and easy usage but often they cut the graft tissue complicating the fixation and have MRI compatibility issues. In revision surgery they need to be removed as an added procedure. Bioabsorbable screws (available since 1995) instead are more compatible with ligament fixation and get absorbed in the body over a period but are susceptible to breakage and foreign body reactions. The Aperfix® system uses PEEK cage to provide strong fixation of soft tissue grafts with circumferential aperture compression.
- Expansive fixation (these devices produce a bulging effect of the graft again compressing it against the bony tunnel). The cross pin (Rigidfix) system has been a popular technique among expansion mechanisms that utilizes two bioabsorbable (poly-L-lactide) cross pins inserted across the graft through two parallel drill holes from the lateral femoral condyle perpendicular to the femoral

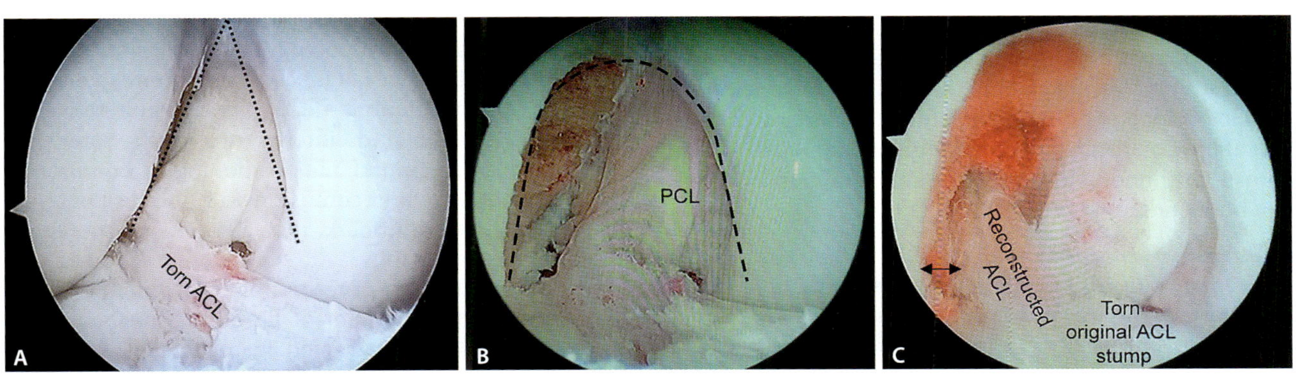

Figs. 66A to C: The arthroscopic view of a "gothic arch" notch seen as inverted "V" shape (A). The anterior cruciate ligament (ACL) fibers are torn and thinned out seen running obliquely in the lower half of the photograph. The reason for tear also may be linked to their impingement and friction over the medial edge of the lateral femoral condyle. The notch plasty is done using small 3–5 mm osteotomes and arthroscopic burr (preferred) widening it into inverted 'U' shape (B). Intact posterior cruciate ligament (PCL) is seen attached to the lateral aspect of medial femoral condyle. Completed ACL reconstruction using quadrupled hamstring tendon graft running comfortable away from the medial wall of femoral condyle (C).

socket made by a guide. The system has good stability and a high failure load, easier revision surgery, and overall lower complication rate. The problem, however, is higher cost and guide misfire after prolonged usage. Expansion bolt is another expansive fixation device.

- Suspension of the graft (suspending the graft into the femoral tunnel). The suspension mechanism may be located within the graft bone interface (as in transfix) or may be located more or less far away from the knee joint. Depending on the type of bone the fixation system latches into three divisions can be made:
  - *Cortical:* This system is most common in practices and utilizes buttons (endobutton®, endobutton-CL®, flip-button®, retrobutton®, tightrope®, XO button®, ToggleLoc® etc.), Swing Bridge, or Ligament Plate as fixation device.
  - *Cortical-cancellous:* These suspension devices consist of cross pin (Transfix), cross pin (Sling Shot) and bone mulch screw.
  - *Cancellous:* Cancellous fixation is very near to or just abutting the graft as is used with Linx-HT, PEEK cage fixation device or TLS® screw system.

The tibial fixation is more precarious as mentioned above and commonly a combination approach is used to secure the graft here. Two broad categories of fixation methods are utilized for fixation of graft on tibial side:

- *Intratunnel fixation:* These are the primary methods of fixation deployed in most reconstructions and comprise mainly of interference screw (metallic or bioabsorbable) providing fixation by compression. Evolgate® system utilizes titanium-based components for fixation of graft on tibial side by reinforcing the tunnel wall with a coil while metallic screw provides interference fit and a washer gives stable cortical fixation. Xenogenic spongiosa cylinders have also been used as bone plugs to provide interference fit. Intrafix system (compressive fixation) provides relatively more secure fixation, while cross pins and CentraLoc® have also been used for expansive fixation. TLS® system or PEEK cage fixation suspends the graft within the tunnel.
- *Extratunnel fixation:* Most surgeons use this as a supplementary fixation method to intratunnel fixation. Common methods are using a cancellous/cortical screw as a post, staples, or ligament washers. My personal choice is closed loop endobutton at femur end and interference fit at the tibial end with or without augmented fixation of post. The bone-patellar tendon-bone graft I fix by screws at both ends.

Postoperative rehabilitation:

- *For first 2 weeks:* Continuous passive motion (CPM) is started the next day and done for 5–10 hours/day. Dressing is done after 2 days and replaced with disposable or waterproof dressings. Cryotherapy should be given and continued for 5–7 days. Braces are often prescribed though there is no rationale to its use. They are used as protective methods and support to knee initially making the patient deliberately conscious and follow the mandatory precautions. Movements should be gained fast following surgery to allow 90° knee flexion by 5–7 days and full knee movements should be gained by 2–3 weeks. It is imperative to gain full extension by 7–10 days. For patellar tendon graft full weight-bearing is allowed immediately, but some physicians prescribe partial weight-bearing walk for hamstring graft. I, however, allow full weight-bearing even with hamstring graft. Exercises are kept closed chain.
- *2–6 weeks:* Brace is continued to protect the knee but movements should be gained fully by 3 weeks. Usually knee brace is locked in full extension for 6 weeks while weight-bearing if meniscus is also repaired concomitantly. Stationary bicycle is started for 5–7 days/weeks. Strengthening exercises are prescribed for quadriceps training and hamstring rehabilitation. Exercises remain closed chain.
- *6–12 weeks:* The braces are discontinued. Additional hip or trunk exercises are begun. Wall slides and chair squats to stretch the quadriceps are allowed. Open chain exercises are begun. Running, jumping, pivoting and knee extension with weight lifting machine are prohibited.
- *12–16 weeks:* Continue above exercises. Begin cardiovascular conditioning. Jump and plyometric training is begun. Progressive knee strengthening program is begun. Sports specific training is begun at 20–24 weeks.

Complications

- Arthrofibrosis—refers to loss of knee ROM due to extensive fibrous tissue growth postsurgically. This may develop, intra-articularly, extra-articularly, or globally. Risk factors for development of arthrofibrosis include:
  - Acute ACL reconstruction
  - Repair of concomitant injuries to secondary restraints (collateral ligaments, ITB and meniscus)
  - Prolonged immobilization or rehabilitation
  - Complex regional pain syndrome (CRPS)
  - Infection
  - Allograft reconstruction
  - Open ACL reconstruction

  Arthrofibrosis should be managed by progressive active and passive rehabilitation, pain management, intra-articular steroids, arthroscopic lysis of adhesions and open arthrotomy and release if it is severe and nonresponsive.
- Graft malpositioning—leads to postoperative loss of movements and interference with screw-home mechanism. Femoral malpositioning is common due to inexperience and confusion with the resident's ridge (raised bony landmark just anterior to the femoral attachment of ACL):
  - Cyclops lesion—anterior tibial placement of the graft causes development of fibrotic tissue between the notch and reconstructed ligament **(Figs. 67A and B)**. The ligament continuously impinges into the notch during extension causing irritation of tissue and development of the fibrocartilage. The tissue causes loss of extension and pain. Further the graft may get ruptured later.

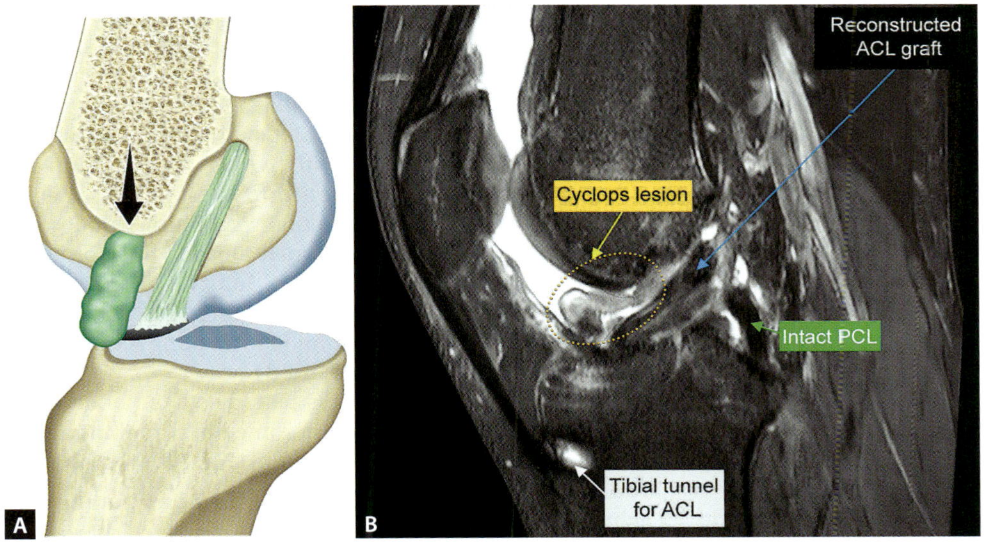

Figs. 67A and B: Cyclops lesion: (A) Development of fibrocartilaginous tissue in front of anterior cruciate ligament (ACL) causes loss of knee extension; (B) The MRI appearance of cyclops lesion demonstrating edematous soft-tissue lesion in front of the reconstructed ACL partially engulfing it. (PCL: posterior cruciate ligament)

- Patellar fracture—for bone-patellar tendon-bone grafts.
- Infection—intra-articular sampling and analysis of synovial fluid is necessary to diagnose them as the presentation is unusual. The treatment includes lavage, graft retention and antibiotics. In recalcitrant cases graft removal may be necessary.
- Early graft failure—often due to poorly tensioned and lax fixation. There have been reports of persistently positive pivot shift test despite adequate ACL reconstruction. In such cases one must look for anterolateral ligament (ALL) laxity/deficiency that may additionally need reconstruction.

Contraindications of ACL reconstruction: In some situations, ACL reconstruction should not be done like:

- Established arthritis
- Infection in the joint
- Patient unable to comply well with the postoperative protocol
- For double bundle technique—skeletally immature patient, multiple ligament injuries and significant chondral injuries.
- Restricted knee movements

POSTERIOR CRUCIATE LIGAMENT INJURY

The PCL being the central axis of rotation of the knee is now considered as the most important knee ligament. Due to subtle changes, finding and reporting exact incidence of PCL tears is not possible but reported incidence varies from 3 to 37% depending on the clinical setting. This is because functionally crippling knee instability is much less common with isolated PCL injury. In general, two types of patients suffer from PCL tear: (1) athletes involved in contact sports and (2) individuals involved in high energy trauma, like vehicular trauma.

Natural History

- It has been classically considered that functional deficit or long-term impact on knee after PCL injury is minimal. The outcome following PCL reconstruction or a conservative management is comparable.
- But long follow-up studies later revealed significant impact on knee function. Nearly 80% of patients have significant pain that worsens with time. Joint deterioration is seen in 80–90% patients after 4 years. Significant knee osteoarthritis develops in majority after a mean duration of 25 years. These changes are accompanied by abnormal cartilage wear (as in tires of malaligned car wheels) and meniscal tears.
- Medial femoral condyle lesions were common, and stress on patellofemoral compartment is abnormally raised.

Pathophysiology

The PCL is most at risk to injury at 90° knee flexion.

- In contact sports:
  - Fall with full weight on the anterior aspect of the bent knee with the foot in plantar flexion tenses the ligament which then gives way. Rotation forces as seen in PLC injuries can also lead to PCL injuries.
  - Direct posterior blow to the upper leg is second mechanism with the knee in flexion and ankle plantarflexed.
  - The third mechanism is hyperflexion (less commonly hyperextension) of the knee joint.
- In vehicular accidents:
  - PCL injury occurs when the car occupant's knee hits the dashboard and there is a posteriorly directed force pushing the tibia posteriorly. This mechanism is the same as that for posterior dislocation of the hip and therefore the name "dashboard injury".

Clinical Features

The patient reports feeling a pop in the back of the knee. Hemarthrosis, inability to bear weight, instability, and decreased ROM are common. Knee dislocation should be ruled out as a differential and all attempts should be made to identify associated neurovascular injury. In chronic tears, the most common complaint is pain with long walks and descending stairs. The patient feels unsteadiness in descending stairs and the pain is felt during mid-flexion stance. Athletes have problem in rapidly changing the direction.

On examination: The popliteal fossa may show tenderness or minimal swelling.

Tests for laxity: These include:

- Sag test demonstrates posterior laxity (Godfrey, **Fig. 68A**). Normally the tibial plateau is a bit anterior to femoral condyles. The normal relationship of tibial plateau to the femoral condyle gets reversed in posterior laxity. One must also remember this anterior position of tibial condyle as normal else in a PCL injury with posteriorly subluxated tibia the anterior drawer test would come falsely positive as will be a pseudopositive Lachman test **(Fig. 68B)**.
- The posterior drawer test (discussed above) is most reliable for identifying PCL injury, but definite diagnosis of a torn PCL is made by an abduction stress test that is positive both at 30° and in full extension.
    - Posterior translation of tibia at 30° but not at 90° indicate PLC injury while in both positions indicate combined injury.

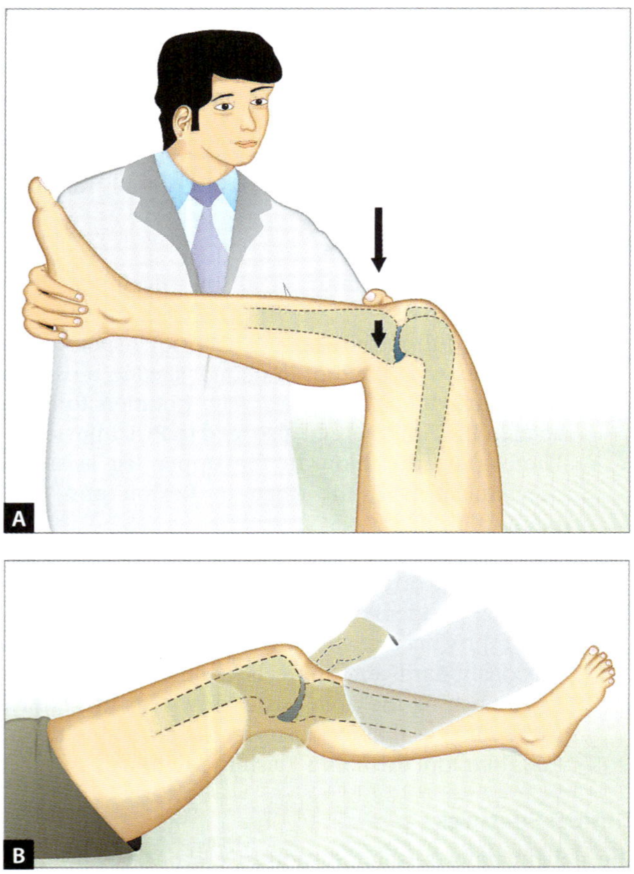

Figs. 68A and B: Physical examination for posterior cruciate ligament (PCL) injuries. (A) Posterior sag test; (B) Lachman test.

- *Quadriceps active test* ***(Fig. 69):*** When the patient who is lying supine on the bed with knee in 90° of flexion is asked to extend the knee against resistance provided to the foot, the tibia shifts anteriorly in PCL deficient knee (>2 mm translation is considered positive for PCL tear).
- *Posterolateral corner evaluation:* External rotation force is applied to the foot with knee in 30 or 90° knee flexion. External rotation of 10° more than contralateral limb at 30° knee flexion (but not at 90°) is considered positive for PLC injury. Increased external rotation at 90° indicates associated PCL injury. Tibial rotation test is also helpful in evaluating-associated ligament injuries **(Figs. 70A and B)**.
- Valgus stress test (discussed above) should be done to evaluate posteromedial corner injury.
- Reverse pivot shift (**Fig. 71**, discussed above).

Classification: The PCL injury can be classified based on the whether the injury is isolated or seen in combination to other ligaments. Acute injuries are defined as within 3 weeks of injury.

- *Type I (PCL stretched):* Laxity on posterior drawer test of <5 mm
- *Type II (PCL torn; MFLs stretched):* Laxity 5–9 mm
- *Type III (PCL torn; MF ligaments torn):* Laxity >10 mm
- *Type IVA (PCL and LCL; posterolateral injury):* Laxity >12 mm
- *Type IVB (PCL and TCL; posteromedial injury):* Laxity >12 mm
- *Type IVC (PCL and ACL):* Laxity >15 mm.

Investigations

Radiography: Same views as described for ACL tear are obtained. Radiographs reveal posterior sag of tibia

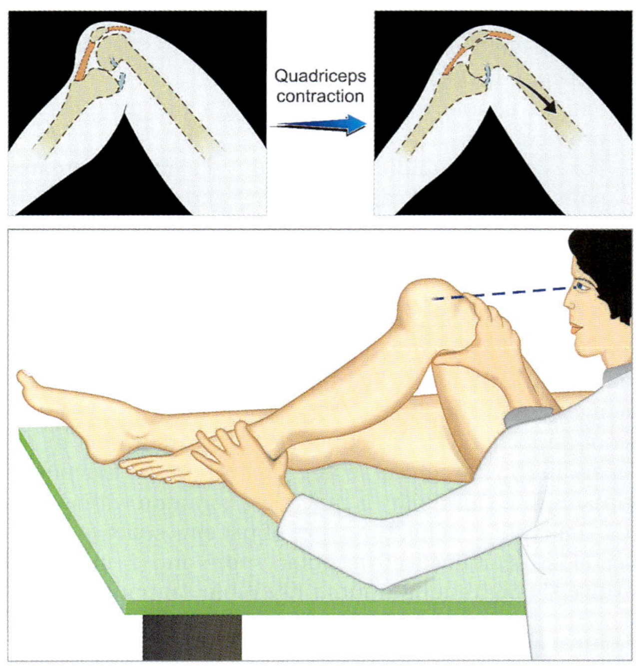

Fig. 69: Quadriceps active test. Contraction of the quadriceps causes reduction of the posteriorly subluxed tibia.

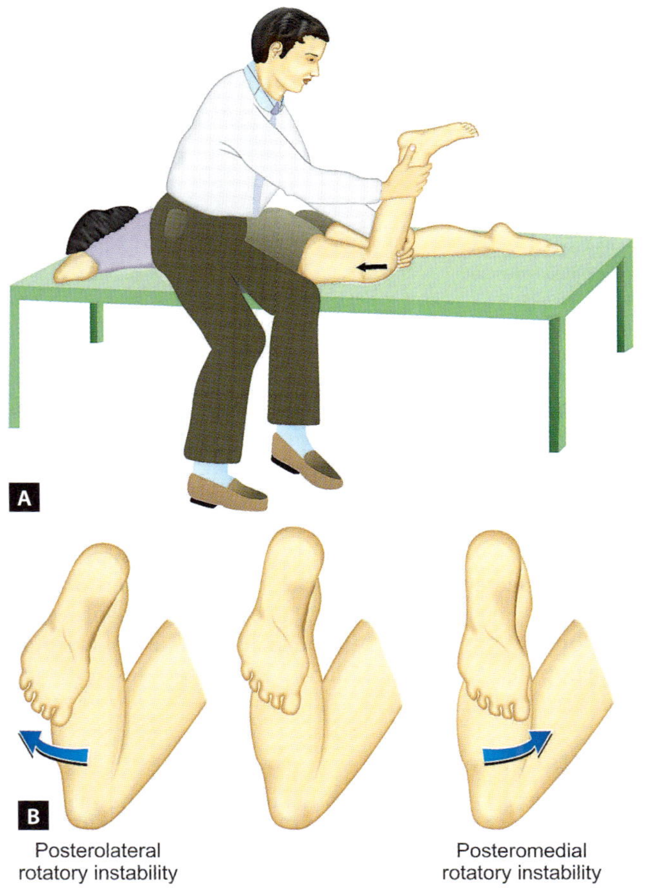

Figs. 70A and B: Tibial rotation test: (A) Patient in prone position; (A) Degree of external rotation (posterolateral corner instability) and internal rotation (for posteromedial rotatory instability) from neutral position is compared with the uninvolved side.

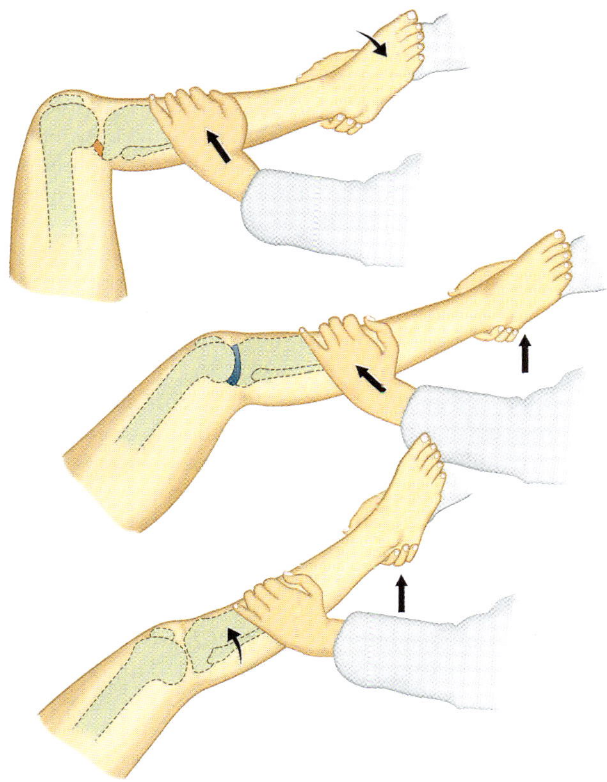

Fig. 71: Reverse pivot shift test.

[displacement >8 mm is diagnostic of PCL injury and >12 mm suggests injury to additional restraints of the knee (posterolateral corner injury)], long-standing tears may reveal degenerative changes in the knee. To objectively define the posterior displacement stress radiography can be obtained. In acute injuries fibular head fracture and LCL avulsion may be seen. Also lateral radiographs may demonstrate isolated avulsion of the PCL.

Magnetic resonance imaging: It is the most accurate non-invasive investigation to diagnose PCL tear if examination is dubious or difficult to perform. Actually, PCL injuries can be so accurately diagnosed by examination that MRI is not needed routinely. MRI is useful as it can also assess menisci, articular surfaces and other ligaments.

Management

Acute trauma setting: RICE should be initiated immediately. Diagnostic arthroscopic evaluation may be performed for inconclusive acute settings.

Nonoperative management is practiced for grade I and grade II injuries—the focus is on quadriceps strengthening, protected weight-bearing and early range of motion. Once movements are full and quadriceps regain 90% of initial (or contralateral) strength sports activities are begun.

Immobilization in extension for 3–4 weeks is recommended for grade III injuries. Isometric quadriceps and hamstring exercises are continued during immobilization. Functional exercises, like cycling and swimming are then begun.

Operative treatment: This is prescribed for symptomatic grade III and combined ligament injuries (grade IV).

- For combined injuries repair or reconstruction should be done within 10–14 days to avoid capsular contracture development of fixed posterior tibial translation. Delay can also lead to scarring of capsular structures and atrophy of collateral ligaments. Open reduction and internal fixation is done for isolated avulsion injuries. This can be done using cancellous screw + washer or staple fixation.
- Reconstruction simulating the anterolateral bundle of PCL is most important. Arthroscopic or open is surgeon's choice and training. PCL does not demonstrate isometric behavior along the ROM and therefore for a single bundle PCL reconstruction, the graft placement should be nonisometric. So for single bundle PCL reconstructions nonisometric anterolateral bundle reconstruction should be done. While tensioning the graft it has been found that tensioning the graft on femoral side produces overstrain on the intra-articular portions compared to tensioning the graft on tibial side. Also the PCL graft

should be tensioned in flexion and not in extension which otherwise produces overstraining on the intra-articular graft and reduces ROM at knee. Double bundle reconstruction of PCL injuries has become popular, but there is no documented clinical difference between the outcomes of these methods. It has also been found that single bundle technique better reproduced the normal PCL force profile following reconstruction:

- In single-bundle technique graft is passed through a tibial tunnel that exits through the PCL footprint and enters a femoral tunnel placed in the position of the anterolateral bundle of the native PCL on the medial femoral condyle.
- Open posterior tibial inlay technique provides theoretical advantage by obviating the acute angular turn (killer turn) that is encountered with passage of a graft through a tibial inlay technique (arthroscopic tibial tunnel reconstruction). The killer turn has been proposed to result in graft wear and elongation but the findings have not been substantiated.
- In double-bundle technique—the anterolateral and posteromedial bundles of the PCL are reconstructed through two grafts or a split graft. The grafts pass through the tibial tunnel and are fixed to separate femoral tunnels.

▪ Associated lesions should be appropriately addressed in the same sitting like the TCL reconstruction or repair, fixation of proximal fibular fractures, etc.
▪ In patients with malalignment, proximal tibial osteotomy is often resorted to for treating functional disability arising from chronic PCL tear. This osteotomy corrects both the varus malalignment and increased tibial slope to control posterior tibial sag from deficient PCL.

Rehabilitation after surgery generally involves 2 weeks of immobilization in extension locked brace with partial or full weight-bearing (isolated PCL vs. combined ligament injuries respectively). Isometric quadriceps and ankle pump exercises are begun. Patients tend to loose terminal flexion that can be regained by manipulation under anesthesia at 2 months. Passive range of motion exercises are begun at 4 weeks, while active-assisted exercises are begun at 8 weeks along with closed chain and dynamic quadriceps exercises.

POSTEROLATERAL CORNER INJURIES

Posterolateral corner of the knee is a complex structure formed from various static and dynamic components **(Box 2)** providing stability against valgus and rotatory stress/instability. Injuries of the PLC produce considerable disability and can be difficult to diagnose. In the past PLC injuries were often missed due to less importance given to the region and complex anatomy of the PLC. In 1980, Hughston correctly mentioned the obscurity in diagnosing PLC injuries—"presentation of this instability may be subtle and diagnosis requires a keen awareness and astute observation on the part of the examiner and the meticulous performance of specific tests for knee stability. The examiner requires all information as to the mechanism of injury, symptoms and physical examination to establish a diagnosis". Injuries of the PLC are far less common than collateral or cruciate ligament damage, but they rarely occur isolated also. Isolated PLC injuries account for only 1.6% of all knee ligament injuries. Associated ligamentous injuries are common ranging from 43 to 80% of cases. ACL or PCL injury is most commonly associated. PLC injuries are seen in association with tibial plateau fractures significantly (68%). Neglected PLC injury can render isolated anterior or posterior cruciate reconstructive surgery unsuccessful. Additionally, a significant number of patients also have injury to the popliteal artery for which appropriate assessment and management is needed.

BOX 2: Structural components of posterolateral corner of the knee.

Primary structures:
1. Lateral collateral ligament
2. Popliteus tendon
3. Popliteofibular ligament

Accessory structures:
1. Posterolateral capsule
2. Arcuate ligament
3. Fabellofibular ligament
4. Biceps femoris tendon and muscle
5. Popliteus muscle
6. Iliotibial band
7. Lateral head of gastrocnemius

Etiopathogenesis

Posterolateral corner injuries occur with trauma in sports (most common), motor vehicle accidents, and falls from height landing on feet with knees flexed and internally rotated. Sports injuries account for up to 40% PLC injuries.

▪ The most common mechanism of injury is a blow to the anteromedial knee, hyperextension or varus forces causing direct propulsion of the PLC causing stretching and sprain of the involved ligaments.
▪ Noncontact hyperextension, external tibial rotation, and varus stresses can also cause PLC injury.

The static stabilizers of the PLC prevent the convex surfaces of the lateral femoral condyle and lateral tibial plateau from opening up laterally with weight-bearing and a varus thrust gait. PLC injuries thus result in lateral instability and gait abnormalities.

Clinical Features

After acute event patients have pain in posterolateral aspect of the knee and anteromedial direct impact region.

Patients with chronic instability have activity limitation secondary to instability. Running is difficult because of a varus thrust gait.

Knee gives-way during extension maneuvers requiring absolute stability posteriorly (preventing posterior subluxation of femur) as in climbing stairs.

Pivoting maneuvers cause the lateral tibial plateau to rotate externally and this produces symptoms of instability—especially in football.

Examination:

▪ *Acute:* Knee swelling and ecchymosis, contusion and abrasions on anteromedial tibia, and antalgic gait.

- *Chronic:* Asymmetric, pathologic varus alignment on standing, and varus thrust gait.
- Asymmetric hyperextension suggests PLC injury
- *Motor and sensory deficits (peroneal nerve injury):* Rule out common peroneal nerve injuries. The peroneal nerve injury is not uncommon and with possible knee dislocation vascular injury can also occur.
- *Special tests:*
    - *External rotation recurvatum test (Hughston and Norwood, discussed above):* The examiner holds onto both of the patient's great toes with knee in extension and lifts their heels off of the examination table at the same time. The affected knee hyperextends and the tibia rotates externally.
    - *Posterolateral drawer test (Hughston and Norwood, **Figs. 72A and B**):* With the knee in 90° of flexion the foot is rotated externally by 15°. Posteriorly directed force is applied to the proximal tibia and degree of subluxation is compared to normal leg. A positive posterolateral drawer test usually indicates a popliteal tendon or PFL injury.
    - Varus stress testing (discussed above).
    - *Dial test **(Fig. 73)**:* Performed at 30 and 90° of knee flexion. Positive test at 30° knee flexion suggest PLC injury, while at 90° knee flexion indicates combined PCL and PLC injury.
    - *Reverse pivot shift test (Jakob, 1981):* With knee at 70–80° of flexion and foot externally rotated, posterior sag of tibia is noted due to posterior subluxation. The leg is then slowly brought into full extension as a valgus force is applied. With this maneuver performed slowly the knee is felt to reduce at about 20° of flexion.

Grading PLC injury (this is arbitrary grading based on varus stress test and posterolateral drawer test, not validated, it helps in differentiating severe injuries from milder ones):

- Grade I injuries have minimal instability (either varus 0–5 mm opening or rotational instability 0–5°).
- Grade II injuries have moderate instability (6–10 mm or 6–10°).
- Grade III injuries have significant instability (>10 mm or >10°).

Investigations

Radiographs: May show a variable combination of:

- Segond lateral capsular avulsion fracture (seen also with ACL injuries).
- Medial Segond fracture (usually with combined PCL and PLC injuries).
- Arcuate sign (fibular styloid fracture)—pathognomonic sign for PLC injury. It is better seen in lateral radiographs in slight external rotation **(Fig. 74)**.
- Gerdy tubercle avulsion fracture
- Abnormal widening of lateral joint space

Magnetic resonance imaging: Grade 1 injuries are visualized as increased signal intensity on T2-weighted images superficial to ligament; grade 2 injuries are seen as increased signal intensity within the ligament, but ligament is in continuity; grade 3 injuries are visualized as complete disruption of the ligament with deep and superficial edema.

For patients with suspected popliteal artery injury or ankle-brachial index <0.9 a CT-angiogram should be done.

Treatment

Nonoperative: For milder grade 1 injuries and minimal disability to patient:

- Hinged knee brace × 6 weeks
- Locked in extension for ambulation
- Progressive ROM, weight-bearing (WB) and strengthening with return to activity at 3–4 months.

Operative care is acceptable in avulsion fractures, multiligament injuries and grade 3 injuries. For grade 2 injuries meticulous reconstruction gives good results particularly in active individuals and sports persons.

- Acute ligament repair (<3–4 weeks) is indicated with sutures and anchors or bioscrews fixing the avulsed fragments with attached ligamentous structures. Acute repair is always better than late reconstruction.

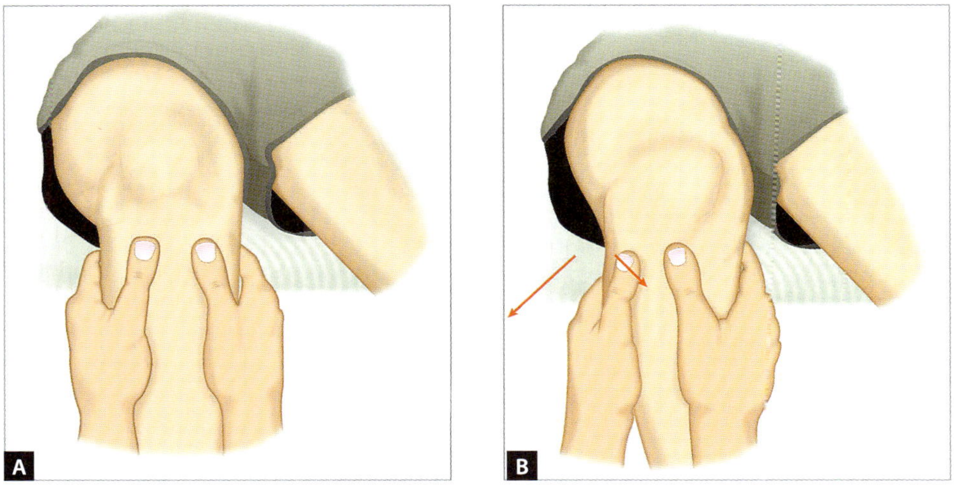

Figs. 72A and B: Posterolateral drawer test. A significant increase in posterior translation compared with the contralateral knee denotes a posterolateral corner injury.

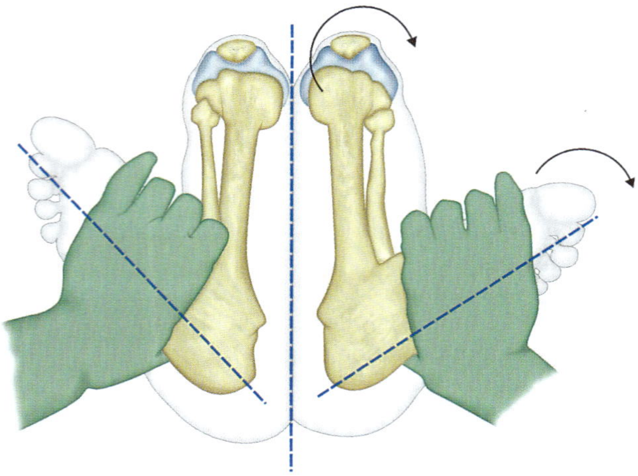

Fig. 73: Dial test is performed either prone or supine. The rotation is noted by the thigh-foot angle. Increased rotation at 90° of knee flexion indicates additional PCL injury.

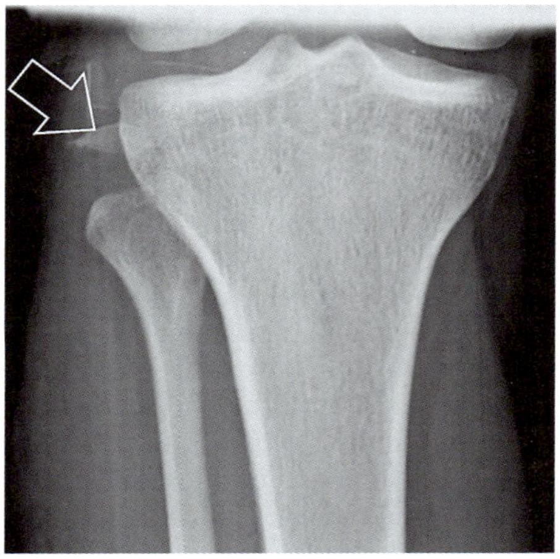

Fig. 74: The pathognomonic arc sign of posterolateral corner injury seen as fracture of fibular styloid (block arrow) here in anteroposterior view of knee with leg.

- *Reconstruction of the PLC* (**Figs. 75A to C**): Mainly following techniques are used:
  - *Nonanatomical:* Biceps tenodesis, proximal bone block advancements, extracapsular ITB sling, and arcuate complex reconstruction.
  - Anatomical reconstructions of prominent ligaments, like the Laprade style anatomic reconstruction or fibular-based larson type reconstruction, are commonly preferred. These aim to reconstruct the functionally predominant components of PLC like, the fibular collateral ligament, popliteofibular ligament (PFL) and popliteus tendon.
  - Larson procedure aimed at reconstructing the LCL and PFL with distal insertion sites located at the fibula. It was one of the first fibular-based techniques. It is less technically demanding with good clinical results. The anatomical reconstructions are more cumbersome and detailed with potential for over constraining PLC if force distribution between LCL and PFL is not balanced.

COMBINED LIGAMENT INJURIES AND KNEE DISLOCATION

Brief description and principles for management only are mentioned here.

- Injury to ACL and PCL classifies as knee dislocation or else whenever combined ligament injuries are seen (ACL + PCL and any combination of other ligaments) it results from knee dislocation until proved otherwise.
- These are the result of severe forces incurred onto joint especially in vehicular accidents. Commonly a violent force to proximal tibia or knee is the mechanism in a particular direction causing dislocation of knee. In hyperextension injury (posteriorly directed force on tibia) posterior capsule gives way first followed by cruciates and at 50° of hyperextension the popliteal artery also fails. Posterolateral knee dislocation results in

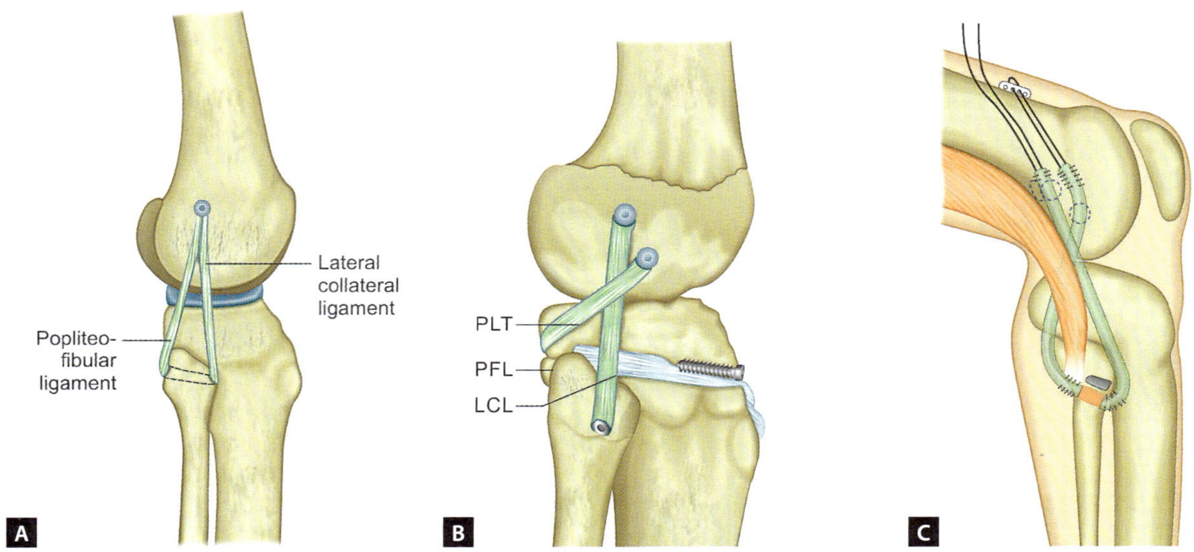

Figs. 75A to C: Posterolateral corner (PLC) reconstruction methods: (A) Larson's; (B) Laprade; (C) Modified Larson's.

a flexed knee subjected to a rapid abduction and internal rotation force moment.

- The dislocations often reduce spontaneously so are commonly missed by the time they are seen in emergency room on a casual examination.
- Posterolateral corner injury is the most common association and should always be repaired, reconstructed or augmented with autograft or allograft.
- The dislocation is classified according to either:
  - *Direction:* Anterior (most common), posterior (second most common), anterolateral, posteromedial, and posterolateral.
  - Open dislocation (one-third of the injuries) or closed dislocation
  - High-energy or low-energy
  - *Schenck classification:*
    - *Knee dislocation 1:* Intact PCL with variable injury to collateral ligaments.
    - *Knee dislocation 2:* Injury to both cruciates with intact collaterals.
    - *Knee dislocation 3:* Complete injury to both cruciates with one collateral ligament disrupted.
    - *Knee dislocation 4:* Both cruciates and collateral ligament disrupted.
    - *Knee dislocation 5:* Dislocation with periarticular fracture.
- Vascular and neurological injuries are common, should be looked for and comprehensively dealt with. Popliteal artery injury (30–50% cases) due to intimal injury and stretch (anterior dislocations or hyperextension injuries) should be suspected in most cases to mandate vascular evaluation for 6–8 hours even after injury. Less than optimal stabilization may lead to even further injury if reduction is not maintained. Direct contusion of the vessel results from posterior dislocations. Compartment syndrome is likelihood if vascular injury persists for more than 6 hours (duration is never an absolute guide), rely on clinical examination. Duplex ultrasonography is the investigation of choice that may be supplanted by arteriography (little added information).
- Neural injury is seen in 20–30% cases and although stretch neuropraxia is most common mechanism no recovery has been reported in more than 50% cases suggesting most are complete injuries (grade 3 and more Sunderland).
- Evaluate the patient by thorough history regarding position of knee at injury, mechanism, associated injuries, etc.
- Procure radiographs before manipulation if the knee is not spontaneously reduced to decipher the mechanism that will aid in planning, manipulation and reduction, and legal aspects.
- *Acute management comprises:* RICE, analgesics, medications to reduce swelling, evacuation of hematoma if it is tense and management of vascular injury (emergent vascular reconstruction with reverse saphenous vein graft). If on exploration nerve injury is seen as a transaction then acute repair may be attempted immediately. After acute management obtain MRI to confirm and aid in planning reconstruction of the ligamentous structures. Maintain the patient in long leg brace for 3–4 weeks, if there is associated TCL and or LCL injury.
- For critically ill patients or those with sedentary lifestyle or patients with grossly contaminated wounds immobilization in long leg cast may suffice. External fixators may also be used as a definitive management in such cases especially open injuries.
- For active individuals the management is often a staged or single sitting reconstruction. Arthroscopic reconstruction for intra-articular ligaments is preferred; however, due to associated capsular injury the reconstruction should be delayed by 3–6 weeks. Also they have often associated chondral injuries that need to be taken care of. Delay in reconstruction also helps reduce chances of arthrofibrosis. Nerve injuries are managed after reconstruction procedures. Electromyography (EMG) or nerve conduction velocity (NCV) if do not show any progress then neurolysis or nerve grafting is done as indicated.
- Fracture dislocations (associated tibial or femoral fractures, term coined by Moore) need simultaneous fixation of the fracture element. These indicate high-energy injury and result in marked instability along with associated neurovascular compromise.

MENISCAL LESIONS

Meniscal injuries are common. In older patients with degenerated knees the meniscal tears are common. These degenerative meniscal lesions are universal occurring in 3rd, 4th, or 5th decade and will not be discussed here. Sport-related injuries to meniscus are common in football, soccer, and basketball. The incidence is 60–70 per 100,000 with a higher incidence in males than females (male:female = 2.5:1–4:1). The meniscal injuries occur in males mostly between 31 and 40 years of age while the incidence is constant in females after 20 years. Posterior horn tears are most common. The medial meniscus by the virtue of its peripheral capsular attachment and attachment to TCL making it fixed in place has a much higher incidence of injury than does the lateral meniscus. The medial meniscus is hence tethered and is unable to escape the abnormally applied valgus and torsional forces. The lateral meniscus is freer and moves with the knee movements, this helps it to escape injuries and forces applied across the joint. With respect to location and type, peripheral tears are seen in 26%, flap tears in 21%, horizontal cleavage in 12% and radial tears in 9%, while most tears are combination or irregular making them complex tears as seen in 30% patients.

Historical perspective: Bland-Sutton first described meniscus as "functionless remnants of intra-articular leg muscles" that has now been proven wide of the mark. Annandale in 1885 first reported meniscal repair. Smillie, in 1944, believed in meniscal regeneration so advised and practiced total excision even with a suspicion of meniscal injury. Arthroscopic repair was first reported by Ikeuchi in 1981.

PATHOPHYSIOLOGY AND PATHOANATOMY

A valgus force applied medially at knee adducts the knee and twists the medial meniscus outward via TCL. Repeated sprains reduce the strength of ligament and its capacity to pullout the meniscus which at some course of time gets entrapped between the femur and tibia. This serves as one of the basic failure of safety mechanism that protects meniscus normally. Most of the injuries are noncontact injuries followed by contact injuries.

Noncontact Injuries

- The most common mechanism is rotatory force at the knee in either extended or flexed position when it is bearing weight. Sudden strong internal rotation of the femur with the foot planted on the ground and knee in partially flexed position is responsible for the maximum number of medial meniscus tears. This force moment pulls the meniscus out of its normal bed while the inner mass is pinched between the femoral condyles. The lesion produced is of variable morphology (e.g., radial, **Figs. 76A to F**) depending on the direction of resultant force.
- The second common mechanism is deceleration or acceleration with direction change as in a cutting motion while running. This primarily distorts the medial meniscus.
  - Vertical longitudinal or "bucket handle" tear (complete vertical longitudinal tear) results from forceful stretching of anterior and posterior horns as in translatory movements. Longitudinal medial meniscus tear also results when internally-rotated femur pinches the fibrocartilage while a forceful extension of knee is done.
  - "Parrot beak" tears occur in the inner periphery of the meniscus and are commonly seen in lateral meniscus. These are produced by forceful knee extension that pulls the meniscus back while the femur is externally rotated.
- The third mechanism is hyperextension or hyperflexion (one of the functions of meniscus is preventing these movements). These mechanisms often produce root avulsion and peripheral tears.

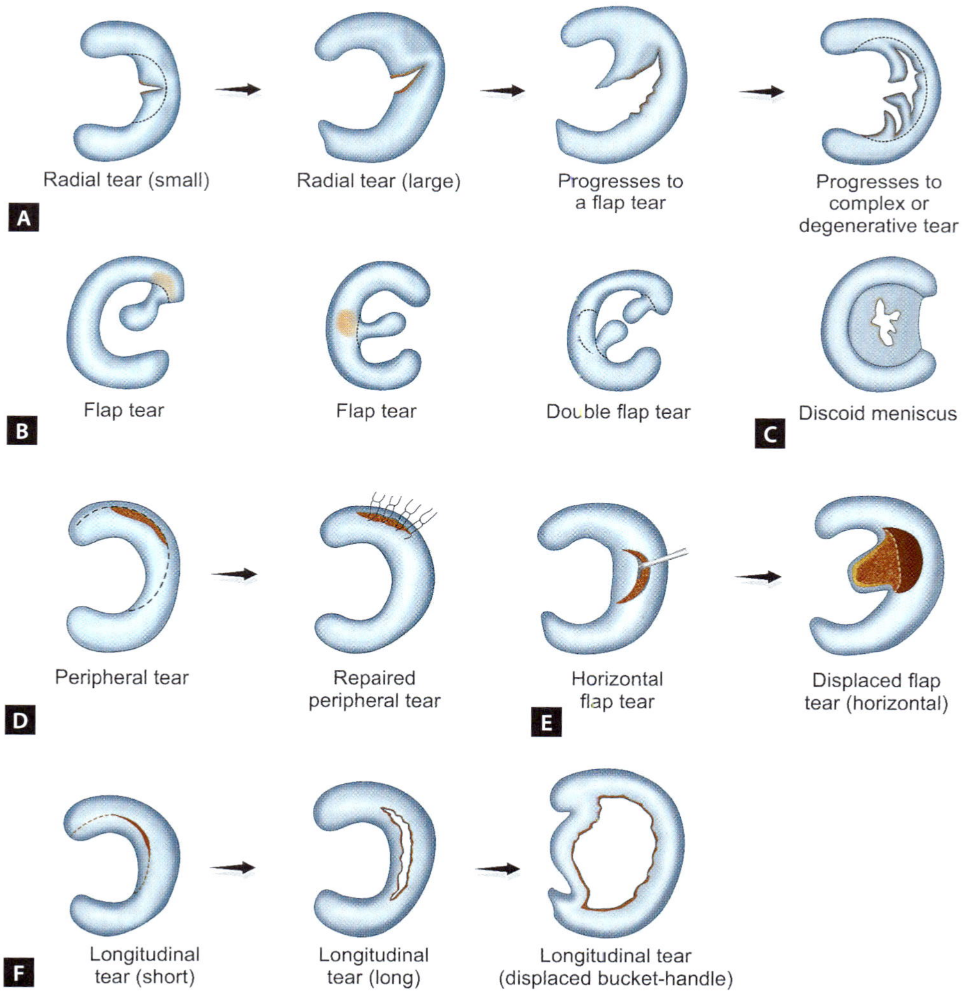

Figs. 76A to F: Types (patterns) of meniscal tears.

Contact Injuries

Lateral or anterolateral blow causing valgus, varus or hyperextension, respectively and commonly result in meniscal tears. These produce injury complexes often associated with ACL tears.

Associated other injuries with meniscal tears: Tibial plateau fractures, and ACL tears.

Unlike the tears in the outer one-third of the meniscus which heal overtime if the region is unloaded, the midsubstance and inner margin tears fail to heal primarily due to poor blood supply.

Clinical Presentation

Though with meticulous examination and appropriate diagnostic tests diagnosis of meniscal injury can be made, but an absolute diagnosis of meniscal injury just by history and physical findings is difficult. The following points in history help in suspecting meniscal injury:

- Twisting injury or hyperflexion event
- Catching or locking episodes (may also occur with chondral injuries or loose bodies)—this is due to wedging of the torn piece of meniscus between the articulating femoral and tibial surfaces.
- *Giving way of the knee:* Sudden collapsing sensation or a sensation of knee popping.
- Inability to fully extend knee or pain with full extension/flexion or squatting (displaced bucket handle tear).
- Inability to change direction quickly without pain when running.

Physical examination: To evaluate and identify meniscal tear clinically; examination should be done immediately after the injury otherwise the ensuing swelling and pain will prevent any logical evaluation of the joint. However, it can still be done sometimes after instilling local anesthetic into the joint.

There may or may not be:

- Muscle atrophy—usually seen with chronic painful lesions or lesions with associated cartilage injury.
- Effusion (develops gradually over 48–72 hours)—they are often recurrent in chronic tears.
- Joint line tenderness (74% sensitivity and 50% positive predictive value).
- Loss of motion—commonly result from flap tears that get caught in the femorotibial movements. Everted flaps at the poles prevent completion of movement producing loss of terminal movements.
- Positive McMurray and/or Apley's grinding test—finding of medially-based thud with flexion and rotation correlated closely with meniscal tear in McMurray test. In McMurray test, the patient lies supine and knee is maximally flexed. Left hand stabilizes the knee and palpates along the joint line from above while the right hand holds the sole of foot. For medial meniscus, the leg is externally rotated by right hand and leg extended gradually till 90° of knee flexion while the left hand palpates for pop, click or thud. Same maneuver is repeated with leg internally rotated for lateral meniscus. It is used to assess posterior horn tear of menisci. Commonly examiners add varus and valgus stress to the knee while testing for lateral and medial menisci and also extend the leg fully to find tears in middle and even anterior regions. These are modifications of original test. The test is much less sensitive for tears of middle and anterior thirds of menisci.
- Inability to perform a full squat.

Investigations

Radiography: To identify bony pathology, evaluate degenerative changes and joint space narrowing.

Magnetic resonance imaging: They have sensitivity of 95%, specificity of 91% and accuracy of 93% (false positives are common in posterior horn). Normal appearance of meniscus is of uniform low-signal structure **(Fig. 77)**. Increased signal is seen in children and with increasing age normally. The reported grading system for meniscal tear involves classifying them into grades 0, 1, 2, and 3 of which only grade 3 (linear intensity change in meniscus that abuts periphery or communicates with joint or capsule) is consistent with meniscal tear **(Fig. 78)**, others are intrasubstance changes of varying intensity and extent that may represent varied pathology and not just tear. In case of bucket-handle tear of medial meniscus the torn segment may get displaced medially toward the center lying anterior to the PCL. This is seen as "double PCL sign" on posterior aspect of sagittal MRI images **(Fig. 79)**. The displaced fragment is usually of medial meniscus (80% cases). Similarly a "double-anterior horn" sign is seen anteriorly.

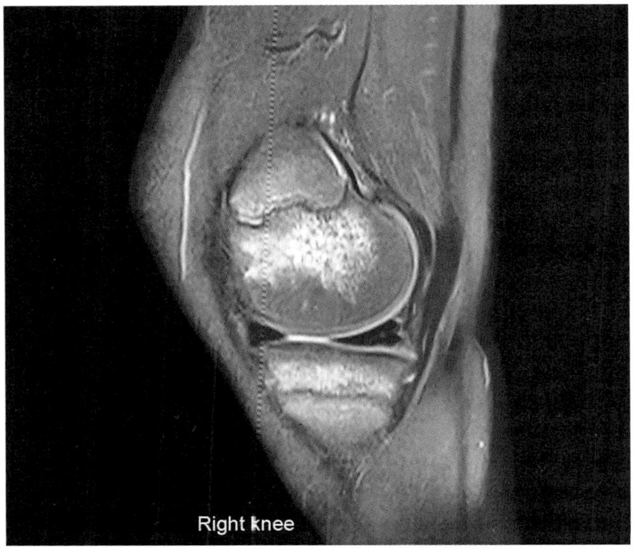

Fig. 77: The normal MR appearance of meniscus as uniformly low signal intensity wedge between femur and tibia in sagittal images remarkably improving the joint congruity and functioning as "door stopper". The linear hyperintensity in the posterior horn is often reported as grade I tear and is responsible for false positive reporting as tear on MRI scans.

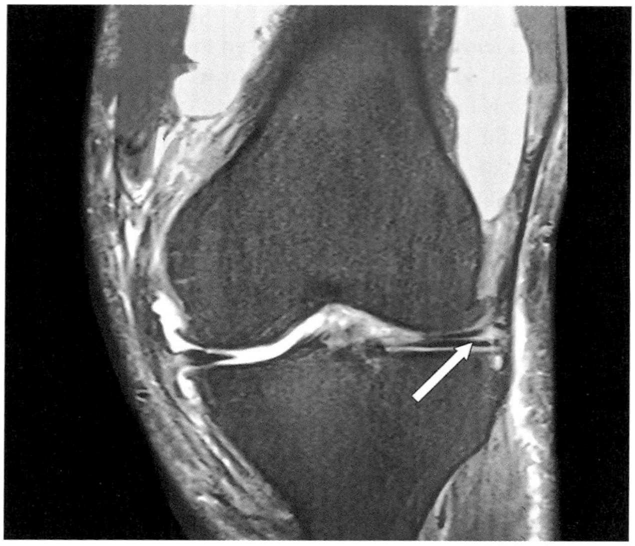

Fig. 78: T2 STIR coronal image of knee showing grade III tear of lateral meniscus extending and involving the articular surface (arrow). There is associated moderate knee joint effusion.

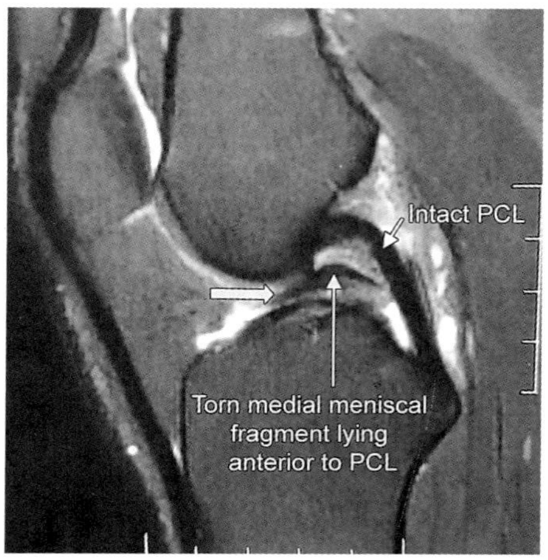

Fig. 79: The double posterior cruciate ligament (PCL) sign seen due to medial displacement of the torn meniscal fragment (block arrow).

Management

Symptomatic meniscal tears can eventually lead to serious articular degeneration with major impairment and disability necessitating surgical intervention.

Anesthesia may be needed to either examine a patient in nonconcluding situations or more necessarily to unlock a locked knee. Diagnostic arthroscopy commonly reveals tear that can be addressed even in the same sitting. The indications of surgery (including diagnostic arthroscopy) in meniscal tear include:

- Symptoms of meniscal injury that affect routine activities and/or sports.
- Positive physical findings, like joint line tenderness, joint effusion, limitation of motion and provocative signs, such as pain with squatting.
- Positive flexion McMurray or Apley's grind test
- No response to conservative management: Medications and physiotherapy.
- Absence of other causes of knee pain identified on plain radiographs or other imaging studies.

The goal of surgical treatment is to remove the offending piece of torn meniscus, relieve obstruction and smoothening the edges while minimizing loss of any portion of the meniscus.

The common methods used for management of meniscal injuries are:

1. *Partial meniscectomy:* This is indicated in tears that cannot be repaired or cannot be stimulated to heal. The unstable fragments are removed to eliminate catching and locking. This is also done to reduce pain associated with unstable fragments. The menisci are critical in preventing degenerative joint disease. Total meniscectomy has been abandoned and is no longer indicated except possibly in extremes of unavoidable circumstances in rarest of the patients. Degenerative joint changes occur quickly following total meniscectomy and include (elucidated by Fairbank in 1948): formation of marginal femoral osteophytic ridge, flattening of medial femoral condyle, narrowing of joint space, pain and articular cartilage changes. Even partial meniscectomy is associated with development of degenerative changes that correlate with the amount of meniscus removed.
   - Peak local stress increase by 65% after 10% removal of meniscus
   - Peak local stress increase by 235% when contact area reduces by 75%.
2. *Meniscal repair:* The criteria for meniscal repair include:
   - Symptomatic tears preferably seen in acute setting
   - Vertical longitudinal tear >10 mm long which are complete.
   - Tear within peripheral 10–30% (red-red or red-white region) of meniscus or within 3–4 mm of menisco-capsular junction
   - Unstable tear (displaceable on probing): >3 mm excursion
   - No degenerative changes in the joint and no deformity
   - Viable clean tissue and nondeformed overall structure
   - Tear in active patient
   - Concomitant ligament surgery

Both open and arthroscopic techniques are available for meniscal repair and results are comparable. Open repairs as popularized by DeHaven (who made a marked shift from meniscectomy to meniscal repair) is less preferred today with advancement in arthroscopic techniques. Only in cases where simultaneous capsular reefing or cartilage repair is needed, open technique is utilized. Arthroscopic techniques are many and could be divided into:

- *Inside-out technique (**Fig. 80A**, Henning, Scot, Cannon, etc.):* Considered the "gold standard" method of meniscal repair. The technique requires arthroscopic cannulae that are contoured for side and site of tears. Extra-long suture needles are passed through the cannula across the tear that are captured through posteromedial or posterolateral accessory incisions. Using a double lumen tube can help in repairing by multiple patterns, like horizontal, vertical or oblique. After the bites are taken sutures are tied over the capsule. For medial meniscus tear the sutures are tied at 20° of knee flexion, while for lateral meniscus they are tied at 90° of knee flexion. The advantages of the technique are:

- Good strength of repair
- Compression and approximation of the tear is good.
- Vertical suture patterns are possible.
- Good experience

The disadvantages are as below:

- Time consuming and needs assistance
- Accessory incision so not truly arthroscopic rather arthroscopy assisted
- Arthrofibrosis is a possibility.
- Pain from added dissection

▪ *Outside-in technique (**Fig. 80B**, Warren):* Used for repairing anterior horn and mid-third body tears. Series of 18-gauge spinal needles are placed from outside inferior tibial sites directed to inside superior femoral aspect of meniscus. Nonabsorbable suture material is passed through them and withdrawn from arthroscopic portals. "Mulberry" knots are tied at the ends and sutures withdrawn into the joint pushing the inner limb of torn meniscus against the outer limb. The sutures are tensed from outside to maintain approximation. The other method involves passing two needles as above and the suture is passed from one and retrieved from other using loop and the ends are tied outside the joint.

▪ *All-inside technique (**Fig. 80C**, all arthroscopic fixator technique):* Various meniscal repair devices that can be placed arthroscopically across the tear and tethering the same. The technique is truly arthroscopic, easier, quicker, and needs minimal assistance. Many of the devices are based on reverse-barbed fish-hook design using bioabsorbable polylactic or polyglycolic acid copolymers. The tears are freshened and its distance from periphery is measured. Appropriate sized fixator device is chosen and passed perpendicular to the tear so vertical longitudinal tears are most amenable to this method. The fixators are best utilized for peripheral capsular detachments and meniscal allografts tethering. The head should be countersunk so that articular cartilage is not damaged. The various fixator devices available are either first-generation (meniscus arrow, staple, SD sorb staple, biostinger, fastener, dart, creafix screw, etc.) or second-generation (RapidLoc, FasT-Fix, etc.). The advantages of all-inside repair technique are:

- Quick
- Easy insertion
- Minimal or no assistance
- All arthroscopic
- Bioresorbable

The disadvantages of technique are:

- Limited compression, reduced strength
- Hydrolysis of implant is undefined and has variable course.
- Breakage
- Chondral injury from prominent implant

▪ *Fibrin clot technique:* This is designed to promote the healing of repair by introducing blood-associated biological factors including platelets that have been used at other parts of body for enhancing healing. From 30 to 50 cm^3 of intravenous blood is retrieved and transferred to glass vessel. Clot is formed, blot dried and it is transferred under arthroscopic visualization using a grasper and inserted on the tibial surface (undersurface) of the repair. Sutures are not necessary to secure the clot.

3. *Stimulation of healing:* For meniscal tears that cannot be repaired, but have potential to heal by virtue of their location or otherwise can be managed by rasping or trephining to stimulate formation of tissue helping them to heal. These tears (in red-red or red-white zones) include:
   - Short tears (<10 mm)
   - Stable vertical longitudinal tears
   - Stable partial thickness tears (<50% of meniscal depth)
   - Small (<3 mm) radial tears

   Techniques for delivering growth factors, like platelet-derived growth factor (PDGF), epidermal growth factor (EGF), transforming growth factor-beta (TGF-β) and vascular endothelial growth factor (VEGF), by delivering concentrated platelets into repair site or in native tears at avascular zone is being developed by investigators.

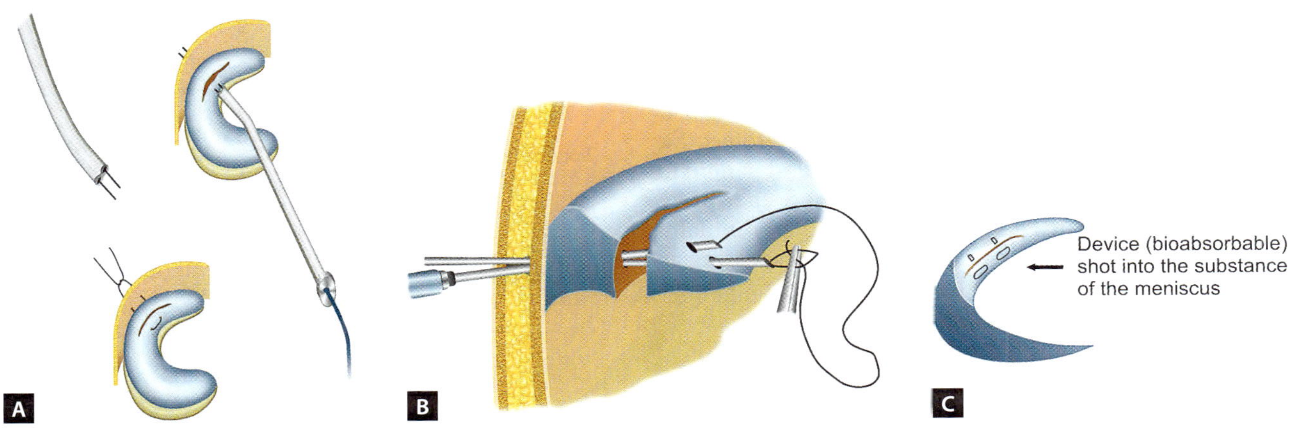

Figs. 80A to C: Techniques of meniscus repair: (A) Inside-out; (B) Outside-in; (C) All inside.

Platelet-rich gels are introduced to the tear sites and promising results are found in animal studies.

4. *Meniscal allograft transplantation:* This is an option if there is total meniscal deficiency or in cases of failed repair, extensive complex tears, retears or tears of remaining tissue. It is a viable option only in a limited number of patients and the following conditions should be met:
   - Stable knee
   - Young patient <50 years of age
   - Compartment specific pain (e.g., "postmenisectomy syndrome")

The general opinion is that partial meniscectomy is beneficial in managing degenerative knee with pre-existing arthritis (early or late) and mechanical symptoms. In younger patients also this technique provides earlier return to play, lower revision surgery rate and equal long-term symptom relief when compared with meniscal repair though it is associated with earlier development of osteoarthritis. Also meniscal repair is available for selected patients with peripheral tears in red-red zone including bucket-handle or vertical/longitudinal tears and root avulsions. The various meniscal repair techniques though seem simple are not without complications and one should take formal training before attempting them. The complications of meniscal repair techniques include:

- Common peroneal, tibial, and saphenous nerve injuries—inside-out and outside in techniques
- Popliteal artery and vein injuries
- Deep infection
- Postoperative septic arthritis
- Arthrofibrosis
- Complex regional pain syndromes
- Chondral injury
- Deep vein thrombosis (DVT) and pulmonary embolism
- *Failure of procedure:* Pain, swelling, and mechanical symptoms are considered major complications.
- Pull-out and pull-through device failure—all inside technique
- Migration and breakage of device—all inside technique
- Cystic hematoma
- Foreign body reaction

For very poor results meniscal transplant is contraindicated in patients with inflammatory arthritis, instability, obesity, malalignment, significant cartilage damage in that compartment or diffuse knee arthritis.

Postoperative rehabilitation: Brace immobilization for 5–6 weeks is required in the postoperative period to protect the repaired meniscus. ROM exercises are begun and patient is made to do exercises to maintain quadriceps tone (quad drills or isometric exercises). The patient uses crutches initially progressing gradually from partial to full weight-bearing at 6 weeks. Progressive impact loading, functional progression, and endurance training are begun after 6 weeks.

SPORTS-RELATED PERONEAL NERVE INJURY

It is a common complication of sports injuries reported to occur as commonly as in 50% of sports-related injuries. These are commonly seen in association with severe ligament injuries. Although a majority have stretch or contusion, but some do have serious damage to the nerve requiring specialty treatment. Past descriptions and reports mentioned higher incidence of peroneal nerve injury related to vehicular accidents while increasing interest in competitive sports have made sports injury of peroneal nerve to be the most common cause of peroneal nerve damage nowadays in the developed world. In sports injuries they are found commonly associated with the PLC injuries due to close proximity to the structures **(Fig. 81)**.

Pathophysiology of Nerve Injury

The mechanism of nerve damage includes laceration, stretch or contusion, entrapments, iatrogenic, compression or gunshot wounds. The primary mechanisms can be divided into three types for nerve damage:

1. Direct blow as occurs in skiing or football causing compression of the peroneal nerve as it crosses directly behind the underlying neck of the fibula.
2. Repeated usage of muscles in low intensity sports making the nerve vulnerable to injury or compression.
3. As mentioned previously in discussion for PLC injuries, stretch or contusion of the nerve are the most common mechanisms of injury to peroneal nerve in sports injuries **(Figs. 82A to D)**.

Pathoanatomy and risk factors responsible for higher incidence of common peroneal nerve injury:

- Superficial location along the fibular neck
- Relative fixity of the nerve to soft tissues
- Proximity to the lateral ligament structures making the nerve fall into focus of the injury and bear maximum brunt of damage.

Symptoms and Signs

- The patient reports local pain from the contusion
- Skin abrasions or ecchymosis
- Tenderness of the underlying peroneal nerve

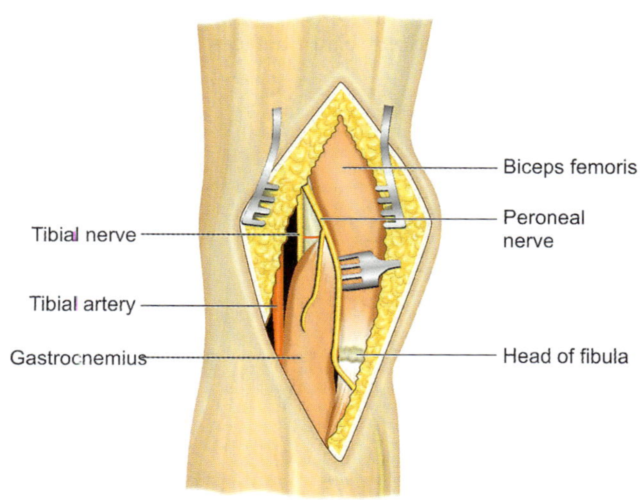

Fig. 81: Proximity of peroneal nerve to posterolateral structures.

A B C D
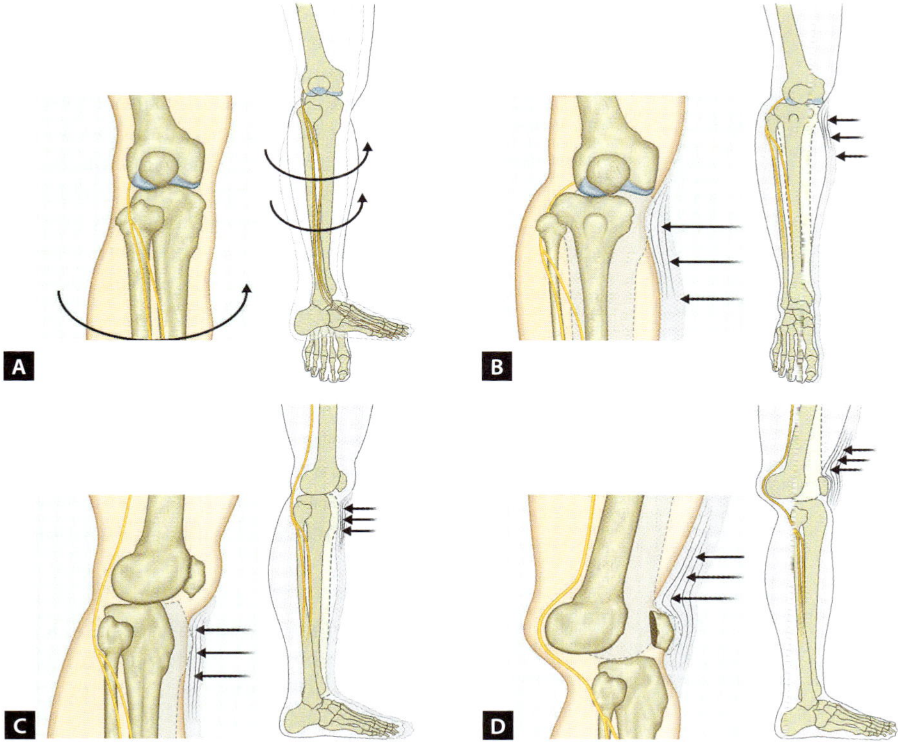

Figs. 82A to D: Peroneal nerve injury mechanism(s).

- There is sensation of an electric shock like paresthesia radiating to the dorsum of the foot down from the anterior leg at the time of injury.
- Numbness and paresthesia are felt in the cutaneous distribution of the nerve in moderately severe injuries. Local pressure further exacerbates the tingling.
- For severe injury, the hypoesthesia and weakness of the peroneals and ankle dorsiflexors (tibialis anterior and peroneus tertius) persist producing foot drop.
- Damage to deep branch produces numbness in the first web space of foot while superficial branch damage results sensory disturbance in the region of anterolateral calf and dorsum of foot.
- As local vascular damage is seen in 4–20% cases so pertinent examination should be done.

Management

Immediately the injury is managed with RICE. The patient is managed conservatively if there is only transient sensory damage and no motor damage. The symptoms abate usually within few hours or a few days and there is no weakness of the peroneals or ankle dorsiflexors. Patients with persistent sensory or motor symptoms should invite specialized treatment including surgical exploration, repair, reconstruction and/or tendon transfers depending on duration of injury and delay in presentation. In general the regenerative capacity of the nerve is poor compared to other peripheral nerves.

Neurolysis ± graft repair is common treatment option. Amount of nerve damage and length of the graft determines the outcome of grafting. Poor rates are reported for graft lengths longer than 6 cm. The common cause of failure is due to continued traction force in the region and friction across the fibular head.

Tibialis posterior tendon transfer is commonly preferred and recommended to patients with injury at the common peroneal level as the chances of recovery following repair are bleak.

Prevention

Fibular head area should be padded to protect the nerve for a few week. Most of the times there is no need for an orthosis for foot drop.

BURSITIS

Bursa is a fluid-filled structure which reduces friction between adjacent moving structures. Normally, it is present between the skin and tendon or tendon and bone **(Fig. 83)**. A number of bursae are found around the knee joint. Inflammation of bursa is called bursitis. Bursitis in the knee can be:

- *Acute:* Trauma, infection, and hemorrhage.
- *Chronic:* Overuse, collagen vascular disease, and rheumatoid arthritis.
- *Recurrent:* Crystal arthropathies, rheumatoid arthritis, and occupational [Housemaid's knee (prepatellar bursitis) and Clergyman's knee (infrapatellar bursitis)].

Anteriorly the prepatellar, deep infrapatellar, and suprapatellar bursae have the highest incidence of irritation and inflammation.

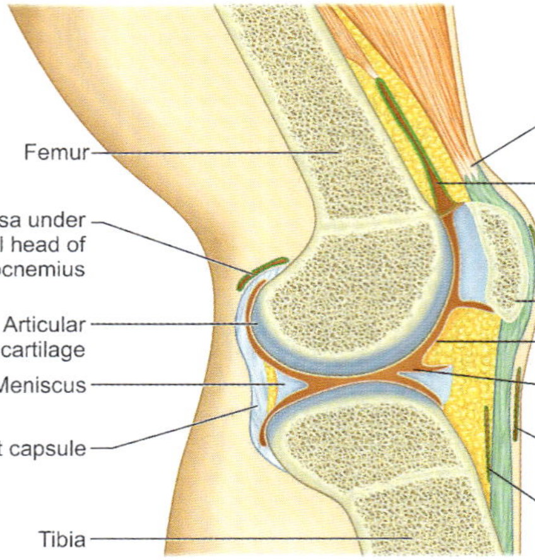

Fig. 83: Bursae and synovial membranes around the knee joint.

Prepatellar Bursitis

This is usually chronic (but may also be acute) inflammation of the prepatellar bursa. It is also known as housemaid's knee. The bursa is present between the patella and the overlying subcutaneous tissue.

Etiology

Prolonged and repeated kneeling causing repeated pressure on the bursa inflames it, leading to inflammation and hemorrhagic bursitis. The deep infrapatellar bursa becomes irritated from overuse of the patellar tendon.

Symptoms and Signs

It presents as localized swelling of variable size over the patella. The swelling is ballotable, extra-articular and may be associated with some redness and raised local temperature.

Magnetic resonance imaging: Not routinely indicated, only in indecisive cases (very rare cases) one may recommend MRI. The bursa appears as an oval fluid signal intensity lesion between the subcutaneous tissue and the patella.

Hemorrhagic lesions show T2 shortening on gradient-echo (GRE) images.

Management

- Cold compresses (elastic compression bandage) for acute cases supplemented with analgesics or anti-inflammatory.
- Aspirate fluid and send for routine fluid examination and bacteriological examination (staining and culture).
- Blood investigations to substantiate inflammation [erythrocyte sedimentation rate (ESR) and C-reactive protein (CRP)] and infection [total leukocyte count (TLC) and differential leukocyte count (DLC)] are obtained along with preanesthetic workup. Uric acid levels should also be obtained in suspected crystal arthropathy.
- Noninfected cases should be managed conservatively for up to 3 weeks.
- In cases with thickened synovium and chronic or recurrent bursitis, the use of aspiration and a steroid injection may be warranted.
- For infective cases incision and drainage with curettage of the cavity is indicated, the wound should always be closed over drain else seroma forms separating the two layers again. I prefer bursal arthroscopy to debride the lesion and it also allows continuous lavage. I also tend to put approximating sutures (one or two) to bring the two layers together with polyglactin threads. Compression bandage is then applied.

Infrapatellar Bursitis

There are two infrapatellar bursae: (1) Superficial and (2) deep. The superficial bursa lies between the tibial tuberosity and skin. On the other hand, the deep bursa lies between the patellar tendon and tibia. The inflammation of superficial infrapatellar bursa is called Clergyman's knee.

Clinical Features

The swelling is just inferior to patella in front of the patellar tendon, fluctuant, tender or nontender depending on amount of inflammation. Local temperature may be raised in infected cases.

Magnetic resonance imaging: The swelling is often lobulated projecting exophytically anterior to the patellar tendon forming a swelling. The swelling is localized differentiating it from subcutaneous edema. Deep infrapatellar bursitis appears as a triangular fluid collection posterior to the patellar tendon.

Differential diagnosis: Superficial infrapatellar bursitis—cellulitis and subcutaneous edema. Deep infrapatellar bursitis—Osgood-Schlatter disease (OSD).

Management: As discussed above.

Pes Anserine Bursitis

The bursa separates the pes anserine tendons (sartorius, gracilis and semitendinosus) from the TCL and it also separates the tendons from each other. The bursitis results from overuse as in runner's presenting as a tender swollen area medially in the proximal 6 cm tibial region over posteromedial aspect. The region may be inflamed and fluctuant in long standing cases (rare).

Magnetic resonance imaging: The bursitis appears as an oblong multiloculated fluid collection on the posteromedial aspect of knee.

Differential diagnosis: Popliteal cyst or Baker's cyst (located more centrally in midline posteriorly often larger than pes bursa may extend to thigh and communicates with the knee joint).

BAKER'S CYST

Inflammation and collection of fluid involving the gastrocnemius-semimembranosus bursa located between the medial femoral condyle, semimembranosus tendon and the medial head of the gastrocnemius is known as Baker's cyst (also known as the popliteal cyst). It was originally described by Adams in 1840 though it bears the name of Baker who described it in 1877. Baker's cyst occurs commonly under the medial head of the gastrocnemius muscle (gastrocnemius bursa) or may involve the semimembranosus bursa also. The latter is a double bursa located between the semimembranosus tendon and the medial tibial condyle and between the semimembranosus tendon and the medial head of the gastrocnemius. The cyst is connected directly to the joint in most cases but not all. This is commonly associated with degenerative knee joint disease in adults and it swells primarily due to problem in the joint and only uncommonly (if at all) because of bursitis itself. The cyst may also develop as a direct outpouching of the synovial membrane in a degenerated knee especially in rheumatoid arthritis **(Figs. 84A to C)**.

Clinical Features

One-third to one-half of the cysts are seen in children, second most common is the elderly people with degenerative knee disease. The most common presentation is an annoying cosmetic swelling of variable size in the popliteal region often seen off midline (most commonly medially in the popliteal fossa) due to displacement by nearby structures. A Baker's cyst is commonly painless, causing no discomfort or disability. Some inflamed bursae may be painful and disabling because of the swelling (giant synovial cyst or rheumatoid arthritis). Giant popliteal cysts are seen on rheumatoid arthritis that communicate with the joint cavity. These cysts can rupture and extend inferiorly or superiorly along the gastrocnemius muscle or semimembranosus muscle respectively. When it extends or ruptures into the calf the symptoms could be severe enough to mimic DVT or even compartment syndrome. Compartment syndrome may also be produced by hemorrhage into cyst in patients on strong anticoagulants. These latter complications should be excluded by thorough investigations. Popliteal vein thrombosis may coexist in such cases.

Investigations

Radiography: This is used to demonstrate the intra-articular pathology (osteoarthrosis and rheumatoid arthritis) and not the cyst primarily.

Ultrasonography: Most handy investigation that can give a quick diagnosis of cystic lesion in the popliteal fossa. It is noninvasive, user dependent and needs experience to differentiate other diseases.

Magnetic resonance imaging: Imaging shows a well-defined hyperintense lesions on T2-weighted images at the characteristic location localized and identified best on axial images. They also demonstrate the characteristic location occupying the space between the semimembranosus tendon and medial head of gastrocnemius **(Fig. 84C)**. Ruptured cyst appears as fluid dissecting into the gastrocnemius muscle. Demonstration of neck of the Baker's cyst and communication with joint fluid is the best imaging finding to differentiate other diseases.

Differential diagnosis: Popliteal artery aneurysm, tumors (lipoma, xanthoma, and fibrosarcoma), meniscal cysts, and pyogenic abscess. Ruptured cyst—deep vein thrombosis (DVT) and compartment syndrome.

Management

- In children, benign neglect usually works well and some cysts may even regress. Aspiration may be done in chronic cysts after diagnosis.
- The posterior horn of medial meniscus acts as a valve to prevent fluid from migrating back into joint in some cases. Arthroscopic shaving of the posterior horn helps in such cases.
- Cyst may be resected by posterior portals arthroscopically or by open technique (Henderson posteromedial

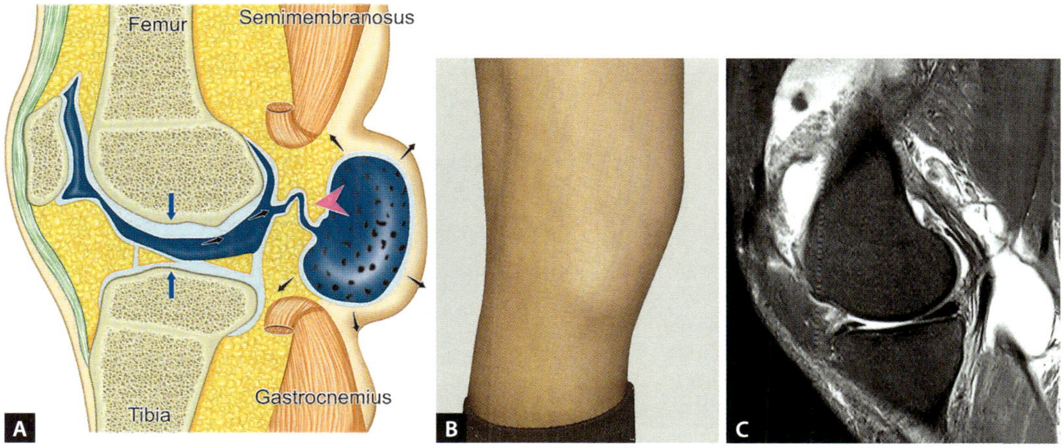

Figs. 84A to C: Baker's cyst—the cyst is an outpouching from the capsule posteriorly connected still to the synovial cavity by a tube pedicle. (A) The tortuous route of the pedicle acts like a valve through which the fluid reaches cyst when intra-articular pressure rises, but does not escape back into the joint; (B) Clinical photograph showing the eccentric location of the Baker's cyst as a typical swelling along the inferior medial margin or medial angle of popliteal fossa; T2 STIR sagittal MR image of knee showing muscular planes. Mild knee joint effusion is also seen.

incision) in disabling cases or if the patient demands so for cosmetic reasons. In arthroscopic procedures intra-articular pathology should always be addressed like treating synovitis by excision, managing chondromalacia or degenerative meniscus tears. Study the cyst anatomy well before arthroscopic removal as a closely lying popliteal artery may get damaged. In such cases, leave the lateral wall of the cyst untouched. Arthroscopy is contraindicated if the cyst opening cannot be identified.

- Giant synovial cysts need to be excised, but simultaneous intra-articular synovectomy should be done (arthroscopic or open).
- Compartment syndrome due to rupture of Baker's cyst should be managed accordingly (fasciotomy).

INFRAPATELLAR FAT PAD SYNDROME (HOFFA'S DISEASE, HOFFA'S FAT PAD SYNDROME, AND LIPOSYNOVITIS PREPATELLARIS)

There are two most important fat pads of the knee one located beneath the patellar tendon—the infrapatellar pad (IFP, **Fig. 85A**) and the other one above it—the suprapatellar fat pad. The IFP separates the synovial membrane from the patellar tendon. Due to its large size and predilection for activity related injury the IFP is more often injured and is also subjected to frictional wear chronically (Hoffa's disease). Fat pad irritation (Hoffa's syndrome or disease) is a common cause of anterior knee pain and is often mistaken for patellofemoral pain syndrome (PFPS) or knee osteoarthritis.

Etiology and Pathophysiology

The IFP can get involved in various ways as follows:

- Direct trauma to anterior aspect of knee joint.
- Chronically, it may get wedged between the tibia and the patella (due to excessive posterior tilt of inferior pole of patella, **Fig. 85B**) or get irritated by chronic kneeling pressures.
- Knee hyperextension causing excessive anterior pressure on patella due to buckling and consequent impingement, exacerbated by internal femoral rotation.
- Consequent to impingement there is fat pad edema that produces swelling making the pad further prone to impingement and catching between the two bones.

Anatomy and Pathoanatomy

The IFP is extrasynovial, but intracapsular limited anteriorly by patellar tendon and capsule, superiorly it is bordered by inferior pole of patella and inferiorly by the deep infrapatellar bursa and proximal tibia. Posteriorly, it is separated from joint synovium. The fat pad is suspended by ligamentum mucosae (infrapatellar synovial plica). The fat pad is also attached to the anterior horns of menisci and the periosteum. The transverse geniculate ligament courses through the fat pad directly. Fat pad receives blood supply from superior and inferior geniculate arterial vertical branches that intercommunicate above and below tibial plateau.

Infrapatellar fat pad contains multipotent cells capable of changing into chondrocyte, osteoblast, and adipocyte cells. Repeated injury to the fat pad produces capillary hemorrhages and swelling of the fatty tissue; continued irritation causes scarring and calcification. Calcified IFP is called by various names—acquired intra-articular osteochondroma, IFP ossification, para-articular chondroma or osteochondroma capsular osteoma, etc. The calcification and chondral metaplasia could also be due to the recently identified endocrine function of IFP. Cytokines involved in chondrocyte metabolism are produced in IFP, such as the basic fibroblast growth factor, VEGF, TNF-α, and interleukin-6. This may also explain the development of osteochondroma in the IFP.

Risk Factors for Hoffa's Disease

- Sports requiring repeated, forceful straightening or bending of the knee (judo, taekwondo, football, etc.)

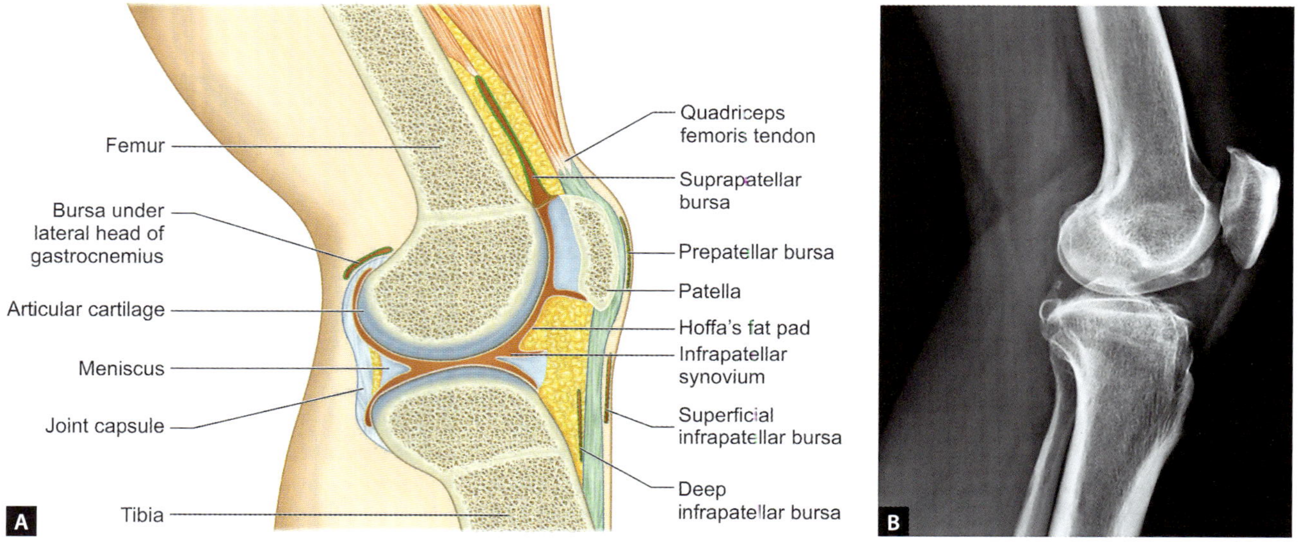

Figs. 85A and B: Hoffa's disease: (A) Impingement of the fat pad and subsequent inflammation; (B) Inferiorly tilted patella impinging the fat pad.

- Repeated injuries of knee due to ligament imbalance or deficiency.
- Violent sports causing repetitive injury—volleyball, rugby, etc.

Symptoms and Signs

- Pain beneath the patellar ligament especially during knee extension.
- Pain getting worse with physical activity and sports.
- Frog eye deformity with pain may be seen in chronic cases with protrusion of the fat pad on either side of tendon anteriorly. Do not label females with hypertrophied fat pads as having Hoffa's disease.
- The knee may display weakness and stiffness during movement.
- Pressing on the inferior pole of patella increases symptoms.
- Tipping patella away from inferior pole relaxes the symptoms and pain.
- Hoffa's test—palpate the tenderness in IFP and ask the patient to contract quadriceps to tense the quadriceps tendon. This pulls patellar tendon and limits the access to IFP. The pain reduces with this maneuver in Hoffa's disease. If the pain increases then pathology is more likely in the patellar tendon.

Imaging: There is usually no finding on plain radiographs unless there is ossification or calcification. MRI shows increased T2 sequence signal due to edema and hemorrhage (acute phase). The fibrin and hemosiderin buildup in chronic phase produce low signal intensity on both T1- and T2-weighted magnetic resonance images. Ossification also produces low signal intensity so radiographs should be readily referred.

Differential diagnosis:

- *Intrinsic abnormalities*—Hoffa's disease, intracapsular chondroma, localized nodular synovitis, postarthroscopy and postsurgery fibrosis, and shear injury.
- *Extrinsic abnormalities:*
  - Articular disorders (joint effusion, intra-articular bodies, meniscal cyst, ganglion cyst, and cyclops lesion)
  - Synovial diseases [pigmented villonodular synovitis (PVNS); hemophilia; synovial hemangioma; primary synovial chondromatosis; chondrosarcoma; lipoma arborescens; rheumatoid, seronegative, septic arthritis, and synovitis associated with primary osteoarthritis].

Management

Conservative management consists of:

- *Management of swelling:* Ice application 2–3 times a day for 15–20 minutes. Local ultrasonic therapy. Rest from irritating activities until inflammation has subsided.
- Heel elevation of ½–1 inch (1.25–2.5 cm). Heel elevation prevents added irritation during full extension.
- *Stretching exercises:* This is done to stretch the rectus femoris especially.
- Taping to lift the inferior pole of patella and prevent impingement. Taping may also be done to prevent knee hyperextension.
- *Strengthening exercises:* Quadriceps strengthening and improvement in muscle coordination.
- *Biomechanics:* Avoid heels.

Surgical option: If the above conservative measures fail then release of tight fascial bands, inflamed synovium, and ligamentum mucosae is required. The bands that tether the lower pole of patella need to be selectively released during arthroscopy. Fat pad may be debulked to avoid further impingement.

PATELLOFEMORAL PAIN SYNDROME AND ANTERIOR KNEE PAIN

Patellofemoral disorders are likely the most common knee pathology in sports persons. *Patellofemoral arthralgia* or patellofemoral pain syndrome (PFPS) is basically a basket term encompassing any type of pain occurring in or around the patellofemoral joint. Anterior knee pain is a much broader term encompassing pain occurring even outside the patelofemoral joint **(Box 3)**. So in effect PFPS is a part of anterior knee pain that involves the patella and retinaculum excluding other intra-articular and peripatellar pathologies. Also "runner's knee" and "chondromalacia patellae (described later)" are discrete terms clinically and anatomically distinct from PFPS, but commonly included as components of anterior knee pain. PFPS should not be, hence, used interchangeably to any of the other terms used above. Patellofemoral maltracking (PFM) is one of the most important causes of PFPS in sports persons and is described in detail below. PFM refers to abnormal deviation of patella during gliding movement along the femoral trochlea, the patella shifts out laterally or tilts laterally or both during extension, but often reduces with knee flexion. Patellofemoral stress syndrome (PFSS) (or excessive lateral

BOX 3: Various causes of anterior knee pain (in order of frequency).

- Patellofemoral pain syndrome (PFPS)
- Osgood–Schlatter disease (OSD)
- Patellar instability/subluxation
- Hoffa's disease
- Chondromalacia patella
- Articular cartilage injury
- Prepatellar bursitis
- Patellofemoral arthritis
- ITB syndrome
- Loose bodies
- Pes anserine bursitis
- Referred pain from spine or hip pathology
- Patellar tendinopathy
- SLJ syndrome
- Plica syndrome
- Osteochondritis dissecans (patella)
- Quadriceps tendinopathy
- Bone tumors
- Patellar stress fracture
- Symptomatic bipartite patella
- Saphenous neuritis P

(ITB: iliotibial band; SLJ: Sinding-Larsen-Johansson)

pressure syndrome, also called "overuse injury") is a term used to describe anterior knee pain due to excessive pressure between the patella and femur, it is a subcomponent of patellar maltraking and hence PFPS also.

Considering the strict definition of PFPS as mentioned above we will restrict ourselves to the description of patella and patellofemoral joint (with intervening retinaculum). PFPS affects females commonly.

Stabilizers of patella and patellofemoral joint:

- *Static:* Patellofemoral articulation (trochlea and patellar shape), medial and lateral retinaculum, patellofemoral ligaments, quadriceps tendon, patellar tendon, and ITB.
- *Dynamic:* Quadriceps and VMO.

Pathophysiology and Theories of Development of Patellofemoral Pain Syndrome

There are various factors that predispose to development of patellofemoral pain syndrome **(Box 4)**. The subtle or gross abnormalities either increase the patellofemoral joint forces or cause patellar maltracking or both. These factors ultimately involve one of the many mechanisms described below to produce pain.

- *Patellofemoral malalignment versus tissue homeostasis theory:* Two factors that cause pain are PFM and PFSS. PFM reduces contact area causing overload and PFSS. PFM represents the loss of tissue homeostasis (reduced envelop of function) causing perception of patellofemoral pain when the "envelop of function" is exceeded by overuse, training error, patterns of faulty sports or trauma. PFM can coexist with reduced envelop of function till it remains within the threshold limit. The goals of surgical realignments in such cases are to restore the retinacular and osseous structures without creating other harmful effects.
- *Neural model:* Lateral retinaculum is involved in production of pain in most cases as this structure is shortened in patients with PFM. Displacement of patella into trochlear groove with knee flexion causes recurrent stretching of the structures and may produce nerve changes such as neuromas and neural myxoid degeneration. Morton's neuroma like changes are observed in lateral retinaculum as supported by studies of Fulkerson and Mori et al. Hyperinnervation into the lateral retinaculum by nociceptive myelinated and nonmyelinated fibers could be another cause of PFPS along with neurological changes. There is also increased vascular infiltration associated with myelinated fibers akin to that seen in osteoid osteoma.
- *Loss of vascular homeostasis "role of ischemia":* Chronic changes of ischemia have been demonstrated in the vascular supply of the retinaculum. There is an increase in the number of vessels possibly due to production of VEGF following tissue ischemia. Ischemia also produces secondary neural changes. The ischemia is possibly produced by vascular torsion or bending following medial traction over retracted retinaculum.

BOX 4: Risk factors for development of patellofemoral pain syndrome.

- *Lower extremity malalignment:*
  - Increased Q angle—genu valgum, external tibial torsion, internal femoral torsion, and coxa vara
  - Pes planus
  - Subtalar pronation
  - Dynamic malalignment—altered mechanics during motion, altered firing of VMO and quadriceps, and quadriceps weakness
- *Anatomical abnormalities:*
  - Small patella
  - Hypoplastic lateral femoral condyle
  - Hypoplastic trochlea
  - Patella alta
  - Hypoplastic medial patellar facet
- *Muscle dysfunction:* VMO weakness or weakness of hip adductors to which VMO is attached
- *Tight lateral structures:* ITB tightness and tight lateral retinaculum
- Hamstring or gastrocnemius tightness
- Patellar hypermobility
- Overuse of patella
- Pronation of foot
- Trauma

Clinical Features

Pain around or beneath patella is commonly reported. Patients often report stiffness or pain after prolonged sitting as in movie theater "theater sign". Patients often indicate achy dull pain making a circle around patella using index finger—"circle sign". Feeling of giving way especially in walks on uneven surfaces or climbing downstairs (dynamic instability of patella).

On examination: The following signs indicate PFPS due to either patellar maltracking or increased patellofemoral joint surface forces.

- "J-sign": Lateral patellar tracking as the patella leaves the trochlea **(Fig. 86)**
- VMO atrophy
- Medial or lateral retinaculum tenderness
- Medial or lateral patellar facet tenderness
- Abnormal swelling patella on superolateral region
- ITB tenderness or tightness: Ober's test.
- Patellofemoral crepitus
- *Increased lateral patellar glide **(Fig. 87)**:* Less than one quadrant slide medially indicates tight lateral structures. More than three quadrant glide laterally indicate lax medial structures.
- *Patellar tilt **(Fig. 88)**:* If patella cannot be tilted to horizontal plane laterally then it indicates tight lateral structures.
- *Patellar grind test:* Pain on pressure and movement of the joint.
- Positive apprehension test
- Assess motor power of muscles around knee and hip.

Investigations

Standard (weight-bearing anteroposterior and weight-bearing true lateral) and skyline views are done to evaluate various causes of PFPS or to rule out other diseases—patellofemoral osteoarthritis in elderly, osteochondritis dissecans, physeal injury, bone tumors, loose bodies, etc. malalignment is best evaluated on orthoradiogram or computed tomography scanogram. Computed tomography scan is not

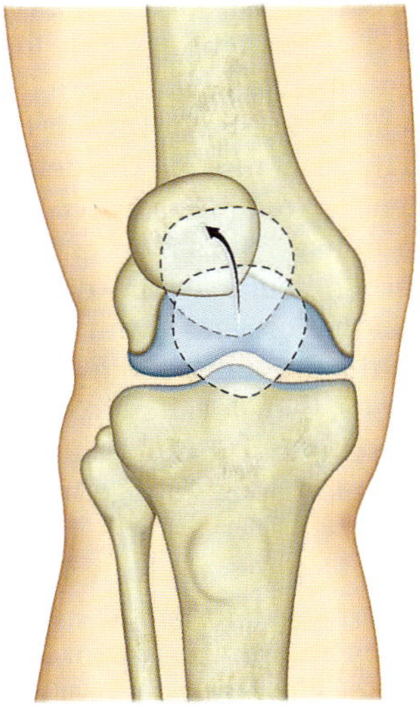

Fig. 86: J-sign.

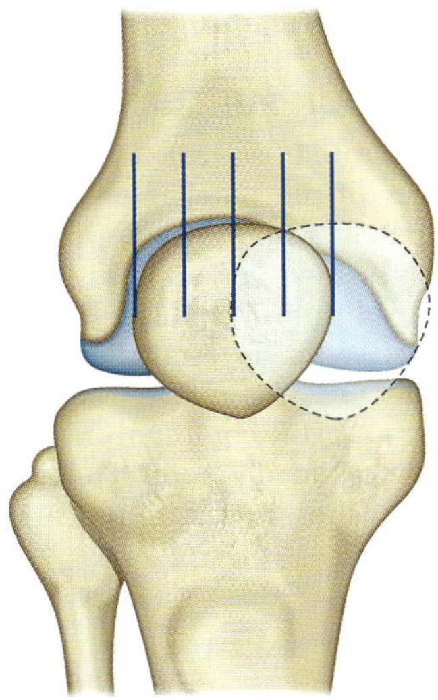

Fig. 87: Patellar glide test. Shift of patella "quadrants": for right knee (as shown here) the patella is grasped in the resting position and pushed or translated medially. The displacement is measured in terms of arbitrary equal quadrants drawn across the width of patella. If patella displaces less than one quadrant medially it indicates tight lateral structures. Displacement of more than three quadrants is considered hypermobile.

routinely indicated unless femoral or patellar hypoplasia is to be quantified. MRI is indicated to evaluate cartilage injury, chondromalacia, loose bodies, patellofemoral ligament injuries, etc.

Management

Rest: Reduce the activities that have been found to aggravate pain (distance running, squats, lunges, etc.)

Physical therapy: Exercise program aimed at strengthening of adductor muscles and biofeedback techniques to reduce imbalance between VMO and vastus lateralis are quite useful.

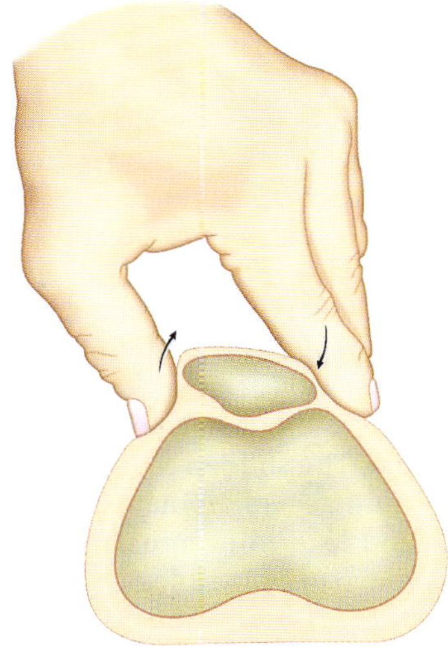

Fig. 88: Patellar tilt test: with the knee in full extension the patella is grasped examiners thumb and forefinger. Examiner tries to lift the patella from lateral aspect while pushing it down medially. Normally itself the patella slants down laterally, if the examiner is unable raise patella to at least the horizontal position (0°), it indicates tight lateral structures.

Stretching exercises for the hamstrings, gastrocnemius, and ITB.

Bracing, taping, and correction of deformity: Foot pronation and other deformities may be corrected by use of orthotics, but their role is not substantiated. McConnell taping helps in patellar alignment and subsequently allows for more symmetrical loading of the patella-femoral joint. Taping corrects the orientation of the patella. It was invented by Jenny McConnell a physiotherapist from Australia. These tapes are rigid and applied for 18 hours or less depending on patient comfort. These tapes are usually applied after warm up and before strengthening exercises. By centralizing the patella, the force is distributed to a larger area and hence reduces cartilage damage. The advantages of taping include:

- Decrease pain at activity
- Healing cartilage injuries
- Corrects patellar alignment
- Earlier return to activity
- Prevents dislocation of patella

Surgical management: Indicated for poor response to conservative management for 6–12 months. The procedures often used are:

- Lateral retinacular release
- Articular cartilage reconstruction
- *Patellar realignment procedures:* Distal realignment with anteromedialization of the tibial tubercle (Fulkerson type tibial tubercle osteotomy; see recurrent patellar dislocation in Chapter on "Anomalies of Pediatric Lower Limb") benefits patients with lateral compression and cartilage injury.

PATELLAR TENDINITIS (JUMPER'S KNEE)

The term jumper's knee (patellar tendinopathy, patellar tendinosis, and patellar tendinitis) was use for the first time in 1973 by Blazina et al. to describe an insertional tendinopathy seen in skeletally mature athletes. This condition is seen in both young and skeletally mature jumping athletes gathering its name "jumper's knee". The condition is though not uncommon in nonjumpers. Around 20% of jumping athletes sustain jumper's knee with twice as much incidence in males than females. Basketballers and volleyballers are particularly affected. Jumping, kicking or running put extreme tension on the knee extensor muscle complex. These repetitive extreme activities injure and cause patellar tendinitis occurs in susceptible persons. With continued activity the patellar tendon may completely fail and even rupture. The sudden repetitive forceful extensions of the knee initiate inflammatory process by inciting microtrauma and lead to eventually tendon degeneration. Due to common pathophysiology (jumping) of tendinitis of quadriceps tendon attachment at patella, the quadriceps tendinitis has been also included in the definition by some. Overtraining, tall athletes, landing on hard surfaces and male sex are some of the risk factors for development of jumper's knee apart from jumping sports.

Symptoms and Signs

The patient reports pain and tenderness at the *inferior pole of the patella* commonly on the posterior aspect. Tenderness or occasionally swelling is noted on the proximal part of patellar tendon. The pain is reproduced on landing from a jump. Night pain after provocative activity may be noted. Patellar tendinitis commonly progresses through three stages of pain **(Box 5)**.

Investigation: Ultrasonography is the best investigation and helps not only to diagnose but also to exclude and identify partial tears. There is only a limited correlation between the findings and symptoms however.

Differential diagnosis:
- Osteochondritis dissecans
- Meniscus injuries
- Osgood-Schlatter disease (OSD)
- Patellar injury and dislocations
- Patellofemoral pain syndrome

Management

Rest: Patients with patellar tendon pain should avoid sudden and explosive knee joint movements. No running or jumping is allowed till pain subsides fully. Ice, topical application of ointments or gel, and anti-inflammatory should be used as additional measures. Phonophoresis, iontophoresis, ultrasound, and various forms of superficial heat modalities, such as whirlpool are used in specialty centers though documented role is missing from literature. Progressive concentric and eccentric strengthening exercise training is begun around 3–4 weeks. Though considered a tendinosis it has been demonstrated that there is a predominant degenerative change in the involved tendon, so actual improvement in the structure may be delayed for months.

BOX 5: The stages of patellar tendinitis.

Stage 1—pain after activity
Stage 2—pain during and after activity (the patient is able to perform in sports at his level)
Stage 3—pain during activity and prolonged after activity (performance is hampered); may progress to constant pain and complete rupture later

A patellar tendon tenodesis brace may also be used in stage 2. Deep transverse friction massage at the inferior patellar pole perpendicular to the direction of the fibers accelerates inflammation and eventually induces healing by progressing to the fibroblastic phase. If there is too much pain and worsening then local steroid infiltration may be done. Still, if the symptoms do not subside then either the athlete has to abandon sports altogether or surgical option can be tried.

When these modalities fail to reduce symptoms or a partial tear fails to heal then surgical debridement should be done followed by immobilization for 3 weeks and gradual mobilization as above. In addition, the lower pole of patella may be drilled to increase vascularity though the benefits have not been documented. If more than half of the tendon is involved it is preferable to excise the inferior pole of patella, freshen the surfaces and reattach the tendon.

PATELLAR TENDON RUPTURE

Patellar tendon rupture (also called patellar tendon strain) is a complete tear of the patellar tendon that can occur anywhere from patella's inferior pole to the tibial tubercle where the tendon has weakened. It is a crippling injury as this disrupts the extensor mechanism of knee which is very important for our day-to-day activities and obviously the sports related activities. It is mostly seen in males in their third or fourth decade of life commonly resulting from tensile forces straining a weakened tendon. These tendon ruptures are mostly acute but chronic tears may also be seen.

Etiology

Direct anterior blow or a sharp trauma can directly injury patellar tendon, otherwise conditions that cause weakening of the tendon predispose to its rupture. These range from chronic inflammation to medical conditions can lead to an overall weakened tendon. The various risk factors are tabulated in **Box 6**.

Epidemiology

Males are more commonly affected than females possibly due to higher activity levels and greater physical strength while females also have lax ligaments and tissue strength varies with hormonal changes of the menstrual cycle.

Pathophysiology and Pathoanatomy

Apart from direct trauma (less frequent) the most common mechanism otherwise for patellar tendon rupture is tensile overload on the extensor mechanism on a flexed knee. The rupture becomes more so common in long-standing chronic tendon degeneration and other predisposing factors weakening patellar tendon. Normal patellar tendon commonly bears stress equivalent to three times the body

BOX 6: The risk factors predisposing to patellar tendon rupture.

- Diabetes mellitus—advanced glycation end-product accumulation
- Corticosteroid overuse
- Local corticosteroid injections
- Inflammatory disorders:
  - Systemic lupus erythematosus
  - Rheumatoid arthritis
- Chronic renal disease:
  - Dialysis leading to accumulation of β_2-microglobulin in bones and soft tissue causing dialysis related amyloidosis
- Fluoroquinolone antibiotics
- Patellar tendinitis
- Patellar tendon degeneration
- Patellar tendon graft harvest (for ACL reconstruction)
- Iatrogenic—total knee replacement (the blade may skive off causing tear of patellar tendon), anterior midline knee arthrotomy for various reasons (infection and pus drainage, cartilage reconstruction, etc.)
- Previous injury
- Overuse injury

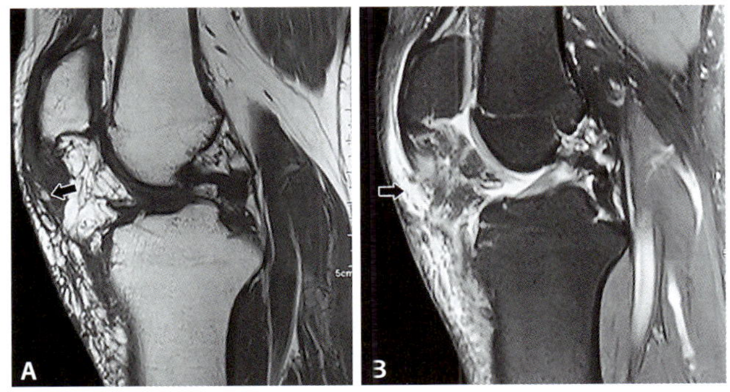

Figs. 89A and B: The T1 (A) and T2 (B) sagittal images demonstrate complete mid-substance tear of patellar tendon at lower third mid-third junction (block arrows). There is also altered anterior cruciate ligament signal intensity and tear noted on T2 images. MRI is the most sensitive investigation for evaluation of patellar tendon ruptures.

weight in day-to-day activities and will not rupture until forces cross 17 times the body weight. Eccentric quadriceps contraction with the knee in a flexed position as in landing from a jump, suddenly stopping to change directions impart great forces on the patellar tendon. Forces are greatest when the knee is flexed more than 60°. Pathoanatomically, the tear can occur at three distinct locations:

1. Proximal avulsion of the tendon at its lower pole (with or without bone) is most common because strain at this region is three to four times higher than at the mid-substance of the tendon.
2. Mid-substance of the tendon
3. Avulsion of the patellar tendon from the tibial tubercle

History and Clinical Examination

Patients present with inability to straighten the knee and bear weight on the limb with infrapatellar knee pain and swelling. They commonly report an audible "pop" or the sensation of their knee giving way during the activity. A thorough history of predisposing factors is legible. Most are acute tears but some tear present 6 weeks after injury (chronic tendon rupture).

Inspect the surrounding skin for signs of direct trauma. Look for associated swelling or knee effusion. Large hemarthrosis and surrounding ecchymosis are common. Patella is usually pulled proximally compared to other uninjured knee. Palpate the patellar tendon for tenderness, obvious gap, and localize the site of injury. Also evaluate the extensor retinaculum and its other components like patellar tendon and quadriceps tendon and muscle. The knee range of motion is reduced in acute setting due to pain and disruption of the extensor mechanism and there is loss or lag of active knee extension depending on severity of injury. Usually there is extensor lag in isolated patellar tendon injury but with retinacular disruption there is loss of extension. Patients are unable to perform active straight leg raise or hold a passively extended knee.

Investigations

The anteroposterior and lateral views of the affected knee demonstrate patella alta (superiorly displaced patella). The Insall–Salvati ratio greater than 1.2 or a Blackburne-Peel ratio >1.0 signify patella alta. Additional information like avulsion fractures or other concomitant knee injuries may be revealed. Ultrasonography is a good aid in confirming diagnosis, viz., acute versus chronic tear and localization of lesion. MRI of the knee **(Figs. 89A and B)** best demonstrates the completeness of the injury and associated lesions (degeneration/intra-articular changes).

Differential Diagnosis

- Quadriceps tendon rupture
- Patella fracture
- Tibial tubercle avulsion fracture

Treatment

Partial patellar tendon ruptures with an intact retinaculum and other components of knee extensor mechanism can be managed conservatively by immobilization with the knee in full extension with a progressive weight-bearing exercise and range of motion program. Otherwise, the treatment for complete patellar tendon ruptures involves surgical repair. The two surgical options are repair of the tear and tendon reconstruction. Primary tendon repair is favored in acute setting where the tendon ends can be approximated. For the common proximal tears, a transosseous tendon repair using bone tunnels drilled through the patella is commonly used but a repair using suture anchors may have better outcomes (re-rupture rates and improved mechanical strength). A suture anchor tendon repair is preferred for distal avulsion. End-to-end repair is used for midsubstance tendon tears; however, it is weak and commonly needs augmentation with allograft or autograft (preferred). Hamstring tendon graft is imbricated through the torn fragments of patellar tendon. The grafts may also be passed through tibial and patella in an encirclage fashion to protect the primary end-to-end repair as is done for patellar tendon reconstruction. Acute repairs perform better than chronic repairs. Postoperatively, the limb is immobilized in extension for 3–4 weeks while full weight-bearing is immediately allowed. Gradual movements at knee are begun focusing on active flexion and passive extension with muscle building and strengthening program. The usual time to recovery and return to sport activities is 6 months from acute repair. If the patellar tendon quality is poor due to degeneration then it is preferrable to do primary tendon reconstruction. For patellar tendon reconstruction, various surgical techniques and graft options have been described including autograft and allografts (Semitendinosus, Gracilis, Ipsilateral or contralateral central quadriceps tendon-patellar bone, and Achilles tendon with a bone block). If reconstruction is done for chronic tears then patellar retraction would need release of scar tissue and/or quadricepsplasty.

Prognosis

Good to excellent outcomes are reported for acute tendon repairs than chronic repairs. Poor outcomes, complications, and failures are typically associated with missed/delayed diagnosis, delayed treatment or surgical errors.

Complications

- Re-rupture
- Residual extensor mechanism weakness/lag
- Knee stiffness
- Quadriceps atrophy
- Infection

QUADRICEPS TENDON DISORDERS

Quadriceps Tendinitis

Quadiceps tendinitis is the inflammation of the distal quadriceps tendon at its attachment to superior pole of patella. The quadriceps tendon is a three-layered structure:

1. Anterior layer receives fibers form rectus femoris.
2. Middle layer receives fibers from vastus medialis and lateralis.
3. Deep layer is formed from the tendinous insertion of vastus intermedius.

The tendon receives its blood supply from medial, lateral, and peripatellar arcades and is innervated by femoral nerve.

Etiology

The most common mechanism is repetitive injury to the tendon at its insertion from quadriceps contracture inn adult athletes. The eccentric contracture of quadriceps pulls the tendon causing microtears that induce inflammation and cause pain. This is common in jumping sports like basketball, long jump, high jump, etc. Males are specifically predisposed (eight times more common) to development of quadriceps tendinitis. The injury is typically common in demanding scenarios near to competitive sport activity and it is often a recurring complaint.

Clinical Examination

The patient quite specifically points to the superior pole of patella for pain and there may be swelling in acute setting. The area is locally tender and in late neglected cases there may also be gap signifying local tear in the tendon. The knee range of motion is painful as is also the straight leg raising and resisted open-chain knee extension. All these activities localize pain to superior pole of patella.

Investigations

Plain radiographs may show localized calcific tendinitis in chronic cases. If there is patella baja then it indicates quadriceps tendon rupture. Ultrasonography and/or MRI are used to diagnose tendinitis and define extent of disease. While the former is more cost effective latter has more sensitivity and can simultaneously assess other intra-articular pathologies.

Treatment

The treatment is mostly conservative comprising activity modification, anti-inflammatory pain medication, and physical therapy. Rest from activities is prescribed until complete pain resolution followed by graduated range of motion improvement and strengthening exercises. Local ultrasonics, gentle massage, topical anti-inflammatory ointments, and cold fomentation are useful accessories. Local corticosteroid injections are contraindicated as they may lead to tendon rupture. Recalcitrant and resistant cases may need surgical debridement of affected tendon/lesion (**Figs. 90A to D**).

Quadriceps Tendon Rupture

Quadriceps is a very important component of extensor mechanism. Quadriceps tendon rupture is twice as common as patellar tendon rupture (1.37/100,000 vs. 0.68/100,000). Incidence increases with increasing age. The tendon usually gets torn in individuals over 40 years of age due to intrinsic weakness and degeneration (comparatively patellar tendon rupture is common in individuals <40 years old). In younger individuals, the quadriceps tendon most commonly is ruptured from direct trauma. Risk factors causing weakness of quadriceps tendon include:

- Renal failure and dialysis related amyloidosis
- Diabetes mellitus
- Inflammatory disorders like rheumatoid arthritis and enteropathy
- Hyperparathyroidism
- Connective tissue disorders
- Steroid overuse
- Local corticosteroid injections
- Intra-articular steroid injections

Weak tendon gives way when sudden eccentric quadriceps contraction loads the tendon with foot planted and slightly flexed. This happens in athletic injuries (jump and land or sudden change in direction) or eccentric quadriceps contraction in a flexed or flexing knee. The tendon rupture occurs commonly at the myotendinous junction. The tears may be classified as partial or complete tears.

Clinical Features

The patients report pain at superior pole of patella and difficulty in walking on the affected limb. There is tenderness at the affected site and a palpable defect. The person is

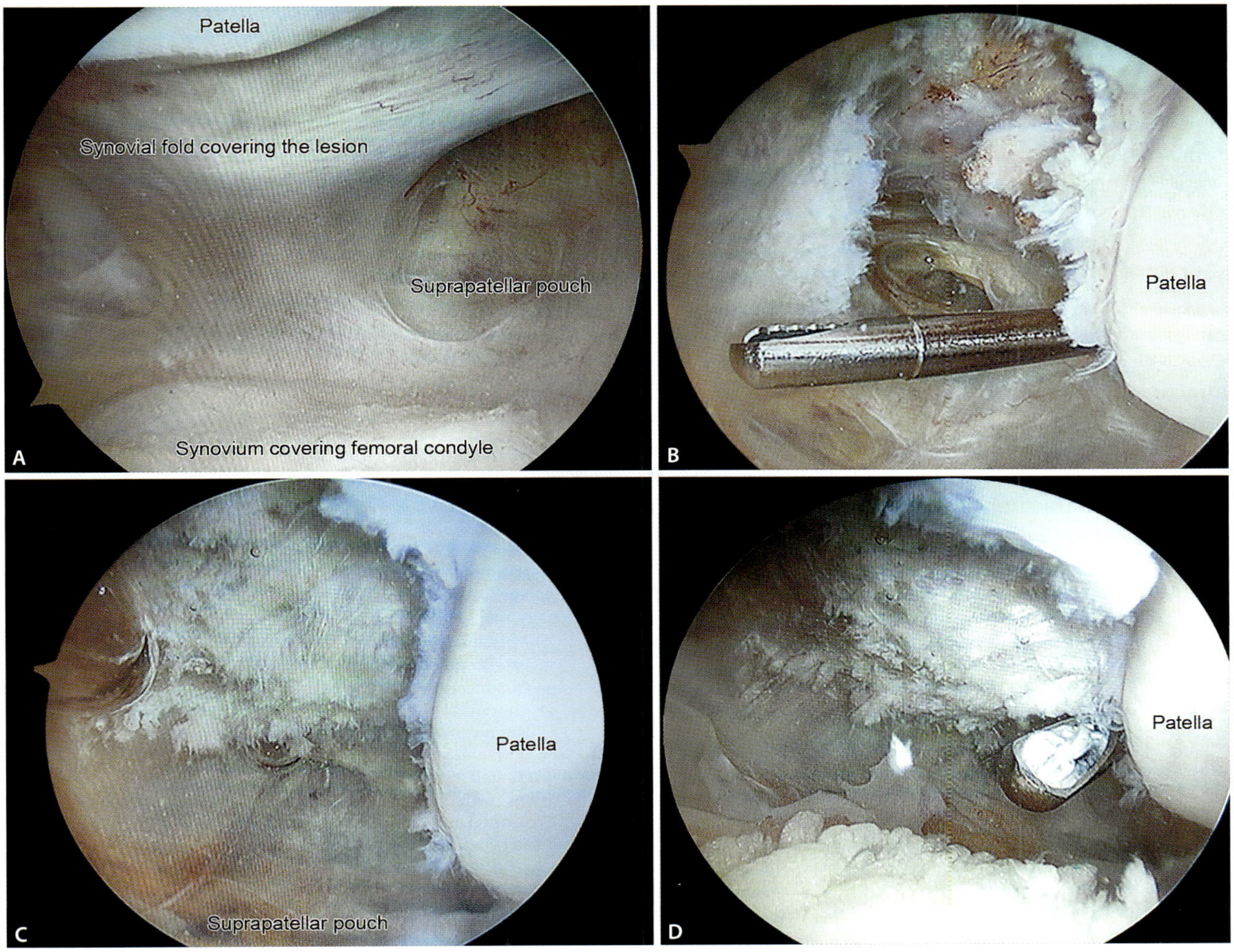

Figs. 90A to D: Articular side involvement of quadriceps tendon that progressed in symptoms despite conservative treatment. The lesion as viewed from standard arthroscopic portals was seen covered with synovial fold just superior to patella producing intra-articular bump (A). Deroofing of the synovial roof as viewed from superolateral portal exposing the lesion made up of fibrofatty degenerated tissue and increased vascularity (B). Excision of the lesion till base (C). Completion of the lesion removing its infiltration into the tendon fibers exposing some fibers of tendon (D).

unable to perform straight leg raising and maintain the limb in extended position. Patients may complain of past episodes of pain in the region indicating underlying tendinopathy and tendinitis.

Investigations

Plain radiographs demonstrate patella baja which in association with clinical findings is sufficient to make a diagnosis with utmost certainty. MRI is not needed typically unless other concomitant pathologies are suspected.

Treatment

Nonsurgical conservative management is indicated only for partial tears without any functional deficit in individuals not demanding any further care or are too frail for treatment. Surgery is the treatment of choice for restoration of completely torn quadriceps tendon and it should be done early (within 72 hours). The principle is to restore continuity of extensor mechanism by reattaching the quadriceps tendon to the patella superiorly. This is done usually by midline anterior approach where the tendon is braided in a locked fashion using strong nonabsorbable suture. These are then passed through patellar osseous tunnel and tied at the other end. Additional retinacular repair is commonly needed. Intraosseous tunnels are now replaced with suture anchor repair technique that also needs a smaller incision. For retracted tendons, direct repair will lead to quadriceps contracture and loss of extension causing knee stiffness. In these cases, quadriceps lengthening using V-Y plasty or allograft augmentation is needed. Postoperative knee immobilization is done in extension for 4–6 weeks using brace/cast/splint (bias toward early mobilization growing). The movements are begun for improving knee range of motion from 0 to 45° protected in range of motion knee brace initially and it is progressed 10–15°/week thereafter. This is combined with quadriceps strengthening program. Early aggressive mobilization program may be associated with failure of repair and higher reoperation rates. Unfortunately, 50% patients never reach their preactivity levels and have to abandon the sports. Competitive level sports are usually banned for lifetime in most of the degenerative tears. Complications of surgical repair include:

- Arthrofibrosis
- Loss of quadriceps strength
- Functional impairment
- Knee stiffness due to quadriceps tendon contracture
- Rerupture

Quadriceps and Extension Contracture of Knee

Extension contracture of knee limiting flexion movement is a common complication of various surgical procedures as well as a well-known entity in pediatric patients—the quadriceps contracture. The flexion movement is limited for variable degrees and in extreme cases it produces stiff extended knee. The pediatric quadriceps contracture has been reducing in incidence due to better injection techniques and care. In extension contracture the extensor mechanism and/or quadriceps muscle fails to elongate for providing required flexion at knee. This results in crippling disability where squatting and movements needing knee flexion like kneeling and sitting cross-legged is not possible. The various causes of extension contracture have been summarized in **Box 7**. The primary responsibility of a surgeon is to obtain functional flexion at knee or regain it fully without impairing the quadriceps power and minimal/zero extensor lag.

BOX 7: The various causes of extension contracture.

- *Quadriceps contracture (pediatric):*
  - Congenital/dysplastic quadriceps (Hnevkovsky, Fairbank, and Barrett)
  - Intramuscular injections (especially penicillin and those injections that are given frequently over a long period of time and have high volume of injectate)
  - Pentaceps femoris—the fifth component of quadriceps the "tensor vastus intermedius or accessory quinticeps femoris" often produces progressive limitation of knee flexion
  - Trauma to quadriceps mechanism
  - Infection of soft tissue of thigh
  - Femur osteomyelitis and/or surgery for the same
  - Arthrogryposis
  - Spastic conditions like cerebral palsy, myelomeningomyelocele, head injury
- *Extension contracture (all ages):*
  - Scarring after trauma (including iatrogenic trauma—surgery through or over quadriceps)
  - Femoral lengthening (ilizarov or external fixator over nail)
  - Incarceration of quadriceps in fracture callus
  - Postpolio residual paralysis
  - Arthrofibrosis
    - Intra-articular knee surgery
    - Hemophilic arthropathy
    - Intra-articular fractures of knee
    - Septic arthritis of knee and post-treated tuberculosis
    - Tibial eminence fracture fixation
    - Patellar tendon injuries
    - Quadriceps tendon injury treatment
    - Rheumatoid arthritis and other inflammatory arthropathies like juvenile chronic arthritis, mixed connective tissue disorders, untreated urate arthropathy, etc.
  - Malunited fractures of femur
  - Burns-related extensor knee stiffness
  - Prolonged immobilization in extension following trauma/surgery/ head injury

Pathoanatomy

Intramuscular injections induce fibrotic response in the muscle due to infiltration of high volume of drugs frequently in the tissues. Repetitive injections are a known cause of muscle contracture as also seen in gluteus maximus contracture. The muscle cells cannot regenerate and heal by fibrosis that contracts as a natural process producing contracture. The only limitation in this understanding is why a longitudinal band forms in the whole muscle. Possible explanation is spread of the drug intrafascially into the whole muscle and extension of inflammatory response in the tissue. Also localized increased sympathetic response may be responsible.

Progressive limited knee flexion without intrinsic pathology in pediatric patients is commonly due to presence of a fifth component to quadriceps femoris muscle the quinticeps femoris or tensor of vastus intermedius. This muscle often is nonfunctional and fibrotic restricting the flexion movements at knee.

Arthrofibrosis of knee due to various causes **(Box 7)** prevents knee flexion and secondarily produces contracture of quadriceps by limiting the muscle length as time passes. Muscle length limitation is also in congenitally short limbs that are then lengthened by surgery causing relative shortening of quadriceps. Surgery around thigh causes scarring of quadriceps muscle. Large open wounds or irresponsible dissection would damage the muscle producing long scars causing muscle contracture. Treatment of femoral fractures by open methods may also incarcerate the muscle fibers in healing callus tissue. Lastly spastic conditions prevent regular lengthening of the muscle fibers as is also the case with immobilization of the limb in extension causing limitation in muscle fiber length and muscle contractures. Cerebral palsy and arthrogryposis are dealt in appropriate chapters elsewhere. Post-traumatic immobilization may also reduce fiber length due to component of reflex sympathetic dystrophy and negative feedback from pain pathways limiting fiber elongation.

Clinical Features

The patients have present mostly with painless limitation of knee flexion range of movements. The quadriceps contracture mostly involves vastus intermedius and rectus femoris muscle although vastus lateralis is also involved in significant number of patients. There is wasting of thigh muscle and patient may have a palpable band of fibrotic tissue. Involvement of rectus femoris muscle would be indicated clinically by occurrence of hip flexion if knee is progressively flexed (examined in prone position). The knee range of motion is variably limited and there is a sudden stop to further movement. The stop is at a fixed point beyond which knee flexion is not possible. Painful knee flexion often indicates knee joint pathology (inflammatory arthropathy or degeneration following intra-articular fracture). It may also occur in uniting fractures of femoral shaft.

Radiology and Investigations

Plain radiographs are of no use in pediatric quadriceps contracture. They may reveal healing or healed fractures in other cases or intra-articular knee pathology (intra-articular fractures/inflammatory pathology). MRI is indicated in patients with progressive knee flexion movement limitation due to quinticeps femoris or it may also be done in preoperative planning of injection-related quadriceps contracture for distal versus proximal release. Blood investigations are important only mostly for preoperative workup; however, in patients with rheumatoid arthritis and juvenile chronic arthritis appropriate workup may be done to substantiate the disease. In hemophilic arthropathy, determining the deficient factor levels is very important if later any surgical intervention is planned.

Treatment

The management of quadriceps contracture depends on the severity of limitation of the knee flexion. Movements up to and above 90° of knee flexion need no surgical intervention. These patients have enough functional movements at knee that daily activities are not hampered at all. Passive knee flexion and stretching exercises may further help in young patients to stretch the contracture. Patients with no progression in gaining movements with physiotherapy and those with long-standing contractures restricting knee flexion below 90° are candidates for surgical release and lengthening of quadriceps muscle or muscle-tendon unit. The technique of releasing adhesion and contractures of quadriceps muscle is known as quadricepsplasty. Various methods have been proposed by different authors and depending on the predominant site of release and technique used can be summarized as below:

1. *Distal quadricepsplasty:*
   a. Thompson-Payr quadricepsplasty—this is done primarily for contractures of the vastus intermedius although extensive releases can be done simultaneously. The thigh is exposed from proximal third to distal pole of patella. The rectus femoris is isolated from vastus lateralis and medialis along with the knee joint capsule distally on both sides. The vastus intermedius contracture is excised completely which is usually in the form of a fibrotic band. The knee flexion is regained by bending the knee and releasing any other intra-articular adhesions. If the vasti medialis and lateralis are relatively spared then they are sutured back to rectus femoris else soft-tissue interposition is needed for improving coverage. The wound is then closed and continuous passive motion of knee is begun.
   b. Bennet's rectus femoris V-Y plasty—the rectus femoris is isolated and identified in distal quadriceps region using anterolateral approach. The musculotendinous junction is incised in a long inverted "V" and knee forced into flexion to distract the cut tendon limbs as desired. Any intra-articular adhesions or other adhesions hampering the knee range of motion are released. Limbs are sutured back in an inverted "Y" fashion.
2. *Proximal release:*
   a. Judet proximal muscle slide—this is a combined approach where the intra-articular adhesions and suprapatellar space is freed using an anteromedial incision at knee. The other major incision is placed posterolaterally from just distal to greater trochanter to all the way to lateral aspect of patella. Using this incision, the vastus lateralis is released proximally from greater trochanter and linea aspera vastus intermedius is elevated extraperiosteally in toto. The vastus medialis and rectus femoris is untouched.
   b. Sengupta proximal release—this combines proximal rectus femoris origin release with Judet procedure.
   c. Lenart-Kullmann rectus femoris contracture release—the origin of rectus femoris is exposed at the anteroinferior iliac spine and at acetabulum and released.
3. *Miscellaneous procedures:*
   a. Pie crusting of quadriceps tendon—for isolated contractures of quadriceps that restrict knee flexion mildly pie crusting can be done by selectively releasing the taut fibers using no. 11 blade. This is done usually as an ancillary procedure for knee reconstructive surgeries like total knee replacement or osteotomies around knee.
   b. Arthroscopic arthrolysis—this is a favorable approach to release intra-articular adhesions following infective or inflammatory arthropathy. In addition, this can also be used to release the intra-articular component in various procedures described above instead of doing open release.
   c. Z-lengthening of quadriceps—this is an option in adult patients with limitation of knee flexion due to inflammatory knee conditions (such as rheumatoid arthritis) or following prolonged immobilization of limb in extension. It is often combined with arthroscopic arthrolysis for this purpose. In pediatric patients isolated Z-lengthening may be done in patients with spastic conditions (cerebral palsy) or in patients where there is associated patellar instability it can be done in association with lateral release.
   d. Fractional lengthening of quadriceps—this may be done for isolated rectus femoris contracture where the fraction of tendon formed by rectus femoris muscle is lengthened. Identify the component of quadriceps tendon formed by rectus femoris and release it distally. Flex the knee so that this component retracts and suture it to the remaining quadriceps tendon proximally.

Postoperative care: The principle is regaining and maintaining movement at knee and preventing contracture to reform by combined passive and active methods. Some surgeons tend to apply spica cast after major releases to maintain the correction. This is followed by passive knee mobilization and bending. Improved mobilization protocols include continuous passive mobilization (CPM) of the knee. I prefer earliest possible CPM of the knee and intense analgesia control using femoral and adductor canal blocks. In noncompliant cases, manipulation under anesthesia and cast immobilization may be done.

Complications

Complications of various quadriceps lengthening and plasty approaches: There are various complications reported following the above procedures, chief amongst them are—

- Loss of gained flexion movement and even increase in stiffness at knee—this is commonly due to recurrence of adhesions and reformation of contractures.
- Wound dehiscence—this is seen in extensive releases.
- Extensor lag—this is common after the procedure and some of it resolves with strengthening exercises over time.
- Quadriceps tendon rupture—seen with Z-plasty and V-Y release due to weakening of tendon and sometimes devascularization.
- Infection, development of reflex sympathetic dystrophy or complex regional pain syndrome type 1, muscle wasting, etc. are common surgery-related complications.

RUNNER'S KNEE (ILIOTIBIAL BAND FRICTION SYNDROME AND PES ANSERINUS TENDINITIS OR BURSITIS)

At the outset it must be made clear that runner's knee is not in any case related to patellofemoral pain syndrome (PFPS) as is mentioned by many if one searches on internet. Though *Runner's knee* is a general expression for many repetitive and overuse conditions that may be attributed to malalignment and structural asymmetries of the foot and lower leg, including leg length discrepancy it is better to keep the PFPS separate and not mix up with conditions more prevalent in runner's or joggers. Two conditions that are prevalent among joggers, marathon runners, and some cyclists are ITB friction syndrome and pes anserine tendinitis or bursitis.

Iliotibial band friction syndrome is an overuse condition occurring due to the inflammation of the ITB insertion due to repeated friction over the lateral femoral condyle. It commonly manifests as lateral knee pain in people who are involved in running activities like runners, military personnel, and cyclists. The contact stress and friction is greatest at 20–30° of knee flexion when the band is excessively tight or stressed, so downhill running that reduces knee angle aggravate pain while sprinting and fast running that increase flexion angle reduce pain. The friction is most prominent at the foot strike. The risk factors for development of ITBFS are:

- Genu varum
- Pronated feet
- Limb length discrepancy
- Abductor weakness

Clinical Features

- Pain and tenderness localized to lateral knee. Crepitus is felt at 30° of knee flexion at the posterior border of ITB. Restriction in hip adduction is common due to tightness of ITB.
- Ober's test will cause pain at the point of irritation.
- *Noble test:* With the patient supine and knee at 90° of flexion the examiner applies firm digital pressure around the lateral femoral condyle. Knee is passively extended eliciting pain at approximately 30° of flexion.
- *Thomas test:* The patient lies supine on the edge of table holding the knees bent to chest. This flattens the lumbar spine. The affected limb is released and slowly the foot brought down to floor. Test is positive if the patient is unable to flex the knee to 90°.
- *Renee creak test:* Pain is produced at the posterior border of ITB when patient flexes knee to 30–40° while applying pressure on the femoral condyle (Renne test), creak test is reproduction of pain without applying pressure.

Investigations

Radiographs rule out bony pathology and joint arthritis.

Magnetic resonance imaging demonstrates increased signal intensity deep to the ITB and lateral synovial recess. In chronic cases in addition thickened fascia may be seen.

Ultrasonography may allow dynamic examination of the ITB.

Treatment

Treatment mainly relies on conservative treatment that is effective in nearly all of the patients. Anti-inflammatory medications reduce edema and pain providing good relief. Rest is needed to reduce ongoing trauma. Local ice is an important adjunct that helps to reduce swelling, pain, and local vascularity. Using local electrical stimulation with topical steroid (iontophoresis) or ultrasonics (phonophoresis) also helps to control inflammation.

Stretching the ITB by dedicated exercises should begin with reduction of pain. This is also aimed to restore hip movements especially abduction. In the end, strengthening exercises should begin to successfully rehabilitate the patient that takes around 6 weeks–2 months in all.

Patients not responding to conservative management need to be managed surgically by either excision of a small triangular portion of ITB from posterior aspect of the band at the level of lateral femoral condyle and/or arthroscopically resecting or debriding lateral synovial recess.

SINDING-LARSEN-JOHANSSON DISEASE (LARSEN-JOHANSSON SYNDROME AND SINDING-LARSEN DISEASE)

Sinding-Larsen-Johansson disease (SLJ) affects the proximal end of the patellar tendon as it inserts into the inferior pole of the patella in adolescents (10–14 years). It is the traction apophysitis of lower cartilaginous pole of patella and called by some as a pediatric version of "jumpers knee". It is essentially a chronic stress injury with overuse of the patella-patellar tendon junction, where the tendon cells die at the junction and fail to heal. There is eventually fragmentation of lower pole of patella and associated inflammation of fat pad and bursitis. SLJ was first described by the Norwegian physician Christian Magnus Falsen Sinding-Larsen (1866–1930) in 1921. Sven Christian Johansson described it independently in 1922.

Clinical Features

Patients have activity related anterior knee pain especially straight leg raising test (SLRT) against resistance. There is slightly swollen, warm, and tender bump below the patella. On examination, there is point tenderness at the inferior pole of the patella associated with focal swelling.

Risk factors:
- Overzealous sporting activity in young age
- Overweight
- Boys between 10 and 14 years of age
- Cerebral palsy
- Rapid skeletal growth
- Poor physical activity and flexibility

Investigations

Radiographs: Thickening of the proximal patellar tendon shadow adjacent to the Hoffa's fat pad. Dystrophic calcification or ossification may occur in chronic and late cases. Eventually they heal with lengthening of lower pole of patella as seen in footballers.

Ultrasound: Investigation of choice in dedicated centers or in experienced hands. There is thickening and heterogeneity of the proximal patellar tendon, especially involving the posterior fibers that attach to patella. Also focal regions of hypoechogenicity may be seen that represent small tears.

Magnetic resonance imaging: Demonstrates proximal and posterior part of the patellar tendon thickening with high T2/STIR signal. Patellar edema is seen as high T2/STIR signal in the inferior pole and in the adjacent fat.

Differential diagnosis: Osgood-Schlatter disease, jumper's knee, patellar sleeve fracture, and infrapatellar bursitis.

Management

Acute phase: RICE, abstaining from sports activity for at least 1–2 months. Sports that exert less strain on tendon like swimming may be tolerated. NSAIDs may help to reduce pain additionally. Physiotherapy to improve quadriceps strength is begun at 6–8 weeks till full strength. The disease is self-limiting and surgery has no role.

In moderate to severe cases, immobilization may be needed in a cast or brace. If untreated there is risk of complete rupture of patellar tendon. There is often persistence of ossicle at inferior pole of patella or a persisting bump below patella in suboptimally treated cases. Later in adult period the region may remain less than optimal in strength so may even fracture.

OSGOOD-SCHLATTER DISEASE

Repeated microtrauma at the insertion of the patellar tendon at tibial tuberosity causes traction apophysitis. In active adolescents, the disease normally presents as avulsion fracture of the tibial tubercle and occurs usually in patients who jump or kick, often boys as compared to girls. It is bilateral in 25–50% cases and is seen at 12–15 years of age in boys; the onset in girls may be slightly earlier (8–12 years). Paget originally described in 1891 the clinical symptoms, which later came to be known as Osgood-Schlatter disease. The condition was separately described (1903) by Robert B Osgood (a Boston orthopedic surgeon) and Carl Schlatter (a Swiss professor of surgery).

Pathophysiology and Natural History

The tibial tuberosity fragment is cartilaginous initially and with continued traction a bony callus forms and the tuberosity enlarges with growth. This condition usually resolves when the patient reaches approximately at the age of 18 years. The only remnant is an enlarged tibial tubercle. Repeated irritation causes swelling, hemorrhage, and gradual degeneration of the apophysis as a result of impaired circulation (osteochondrosis). Complete avulsion of the patellar tendon is a major complication of OSD seen in extremely rare and neglected circumstances **(Figs. 91A and B)** else the condition spontaneously resolves once the physis closes by 16–18 years. These avulsion fractures need closed or open pinning. Only in severe cases patients may have continued symptoms despite physeal fusion. The symptoms in such cases probably mount due to enlarged tuberosity or ossicle formation within the tendon insertion.

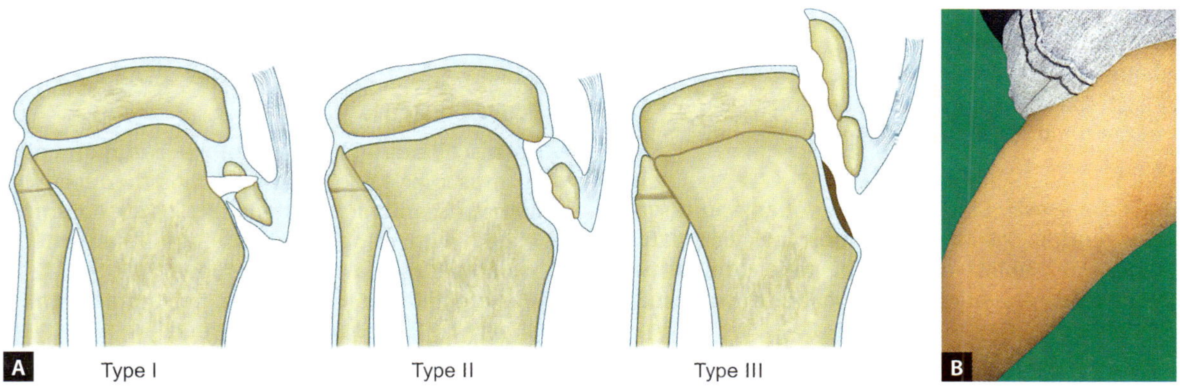

Figs. 91A and B: (A) Types of avulsion fractures in Osgood-Schlatter disease; (B) Clinical photograph of type 1 Osgood-Schlatter disease.

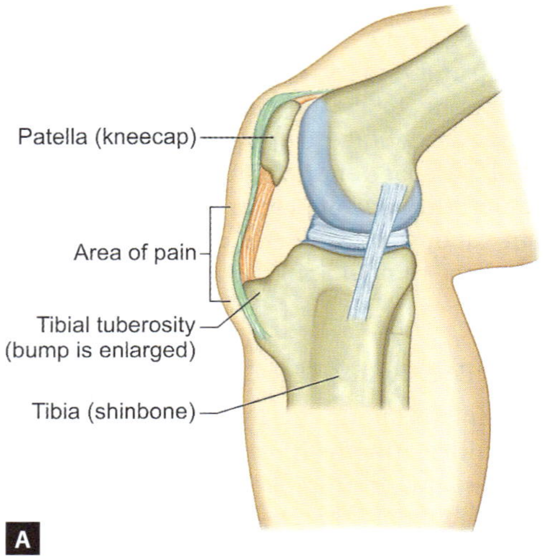

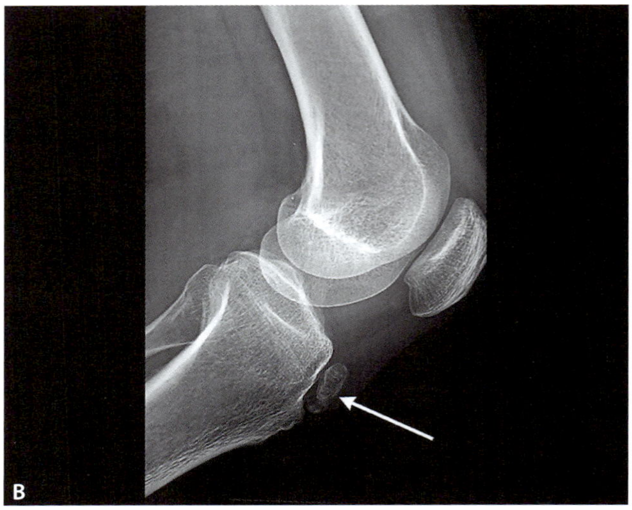

Figs. 92A and B: Neglected Osgood–Schlatter disease persists in an adult as a bump if healed (A) or as accessory ossicle(s) around the patellar tendon attachment on tibial tuberosity (arrow, B).

Clinical Features

Patient complains of pain and swelling over the tibial tuberosity, exacerbated with exercise. The pain increases with kneeling, jumping, and running. There is point tenderness over the anterior proximal tibial tubercle which is enlarged. Pain aggravates with resisted knee extension. The knee has full range of motion but may have hamstring tightness.

Investigations

Radiographs: Fragmentation of the tuberosity, calcification within the patellar tendon, ossicle formation within the tendon, etc. may be seen on a lateral view of knee especially taken in 10–20° of internal rotation.

Ultrasound: This is the investigation of choice, the chief findings are:

- Swelling of the unossified tibial tuberosity cartilage and overlying soft tissues
- Fragmentation and irregularity of the ossification center with reduced internal echogenicity
- Thickening of the distal patellar tendon
- Infrapatellar bursitis

Magnetic resonance imaging: It is not indicated routinely but may demonstrate—thickening and edema of infrapatellar tendon, loss of sharp inferior angle of IFP, soft-tissue swelling anterior to the tibial tuberosity and sometimes infrapatellar bursitis.

Differential diagnosis: Sinding-Larson-Johansson disease, quadriceps tendon avulsion, chondromalacia patella, Hoffa's syndrome, tibial tubercle fracture, tumor, plica syndrome, pes anserine bursitis, osteochondritis dissecans, etc.

Management

As the disease is self-limiting and the disorder stops progression with rest the management is usually conservative and includes the following:

RICE in acute phase with strict immobilization for 2–4 weeks. Anti-inflammatory medications reduce pain and swelling. Counsel patients that rest is the best medicine. Also explain that reduction in stressful activities until the epiphyseal closure will prevent any aggravations.

Use a cylindrical cast in severe and noncompliant cases.

Perform isometric strengthening of the quadriceps and hamstring muscles once pain subsides.

Steroid injections are totally discouraged as they may in fact cause tendon weakness and are also responsible for atrophy of the subcutaneous tissue over the tuberosity. Surgery is not commonly indicated. In skeletally immature patient, in fact, surgery is contraindicated as it may cause premature fusion of tibial physis. The only indication of surgery in children could be avulsion of tibial tuberosity that may be fixed in place by pins (preferably bioabsorbable ones). The other indication of surgery is in adults where ossicle formation or prominence **(Figs. 92A and B)** causes undue irritation at the site locally. This is treated by removal of ossicle, bursa, and any prominence if any, but carefully protecting the patellar tendon.

CONCLUSION

- Meniscal injury is the most common reason for arthroscopic knee surgery. TCL is the most commonly injured ligament. Ligament injuries are commonly associated with crippling disabilities if untreated (except isolated PCL injuries sometimes).
- Posterolateral corner injuries are commonly missed and should be thoroughly investigated.

- The patellofemoral articulation is important in itself as it forms the chief extensor mechanism of the joint. The articulation is inherently unstable requiring various static and dynamic structures, injury to any of which would produce significant disability.
- Understanding the biomechanics of knee joint is important as injuries to the anatomico-biomechanical structures alter the biomechanics and secondary damage to the joint so primary aim of reconstruction should be restoring the joint biomechanics.
- Instability of the knee joint arises from injuries to various important ligaments all of which are important in their own end. Thorough clinical examination to identify combination injuries is essential which needs simultaneous reconstruction/repair. Injuries to collateral and cruciate ligaments are most common that need usually surgical management. It must be noted that there is a growing shift in understanding from isolated ligament injury to "ligament complex" injuries that should be comprehensively addressed.
- Meniscus injuries are very common but often neglected or undertreated. On the other hand, for financial inconsistencies and insurance claims some innocuous injuries are overtreated. It is ethically important to understand and realize which injuries need surgical management and which can be treated conservatively.
- Chronic PCL deficiency results in altered joint contact forces producing medial compartment and patellofemoral arthrosis in longer term. The importance of chronic PCL injuries is being increasingly recognized.

CHAPTER 46

Sports Medicine: Foot, Ankle, and Leg

Manish Kumar Varshney

ACHILLES TENDON

Achilles tendon disorders account for a small percentage of sports-related tendon disorders. The frequency had been increasing with the introduction and enthusiasm for running-related sports and is also seen in the nonathletic population with blue-collar jobs mandating the use of heavy shoes. Most disorders result from overuse, ultimately resulting in a diseased tendon that is both symptomatic and biomechanically inferior. This makes tendon susceptible to rupture (*see* Chapter on "Tendo-Achilles Rupture").

Anatomy

Achilles tendon is formed by merging of the insertions of the gastrocnemius and the soleus **(Figs. 1A and B)**. The soleus component is small (varies from 3 cm to 11 cm) while the gastrocnemius is the prominent contribution for formation of the tendon (varies from 11 cm to 26 cm). The tendon inserts on the calcaneus posterior and inferior to the superior calcaneal tuberosity **(Figs. 1A and B)** and is protected from friction by retrocalcaneal and posterior subcutaneous bursae **(Figs. 1A and B)**. The Achilles tendon rotates 30–150° before insertion. This makes possible elongation and elastic recoil within the tendon permitting to the need of adjustment during activities. The anatomy has been detailed in the Section on "Disorders of Foot and Ankle".

Achilles Tendon Biomechanics

Peak forces of 3,786 N are applied to the Achilles tendon, which corresponds to a force six to eight times body weight. However, strain in tendon is <4% for a force applied five times the body weight.

Achilles Tendinitis

It is easier to categorize them under:

- Insertional tendinitis **(Fig. 2)** involving the tendon-bone junction. This may be further subdivided into:
    - Insertional calcific tendinitis
    - Haglund's deformity (referring to a prominent posterior superior tuberosity of the calcaneus)
    - Retrocalcaneal bursitis
    - Precalcaneal bursitis
    - Calcaneal exostosis "pump bump" or "skaters heel"

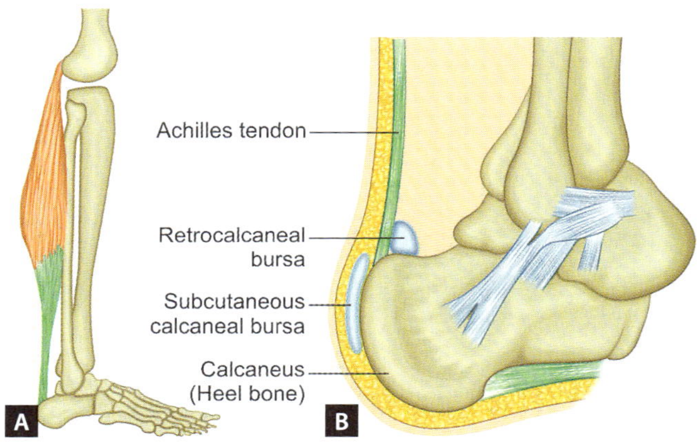

Figs. 1A and B: Anatomy of Achilles tendon. (A) It is formed from the conjunction of gastrocnemius and soleus tendon, so it is a conjoint tendon at least in the proximal most portion, then becomes a single mass; (B) The tendon inserts on the posteroinferior aspect of calcaneum. Note the two prominent bursae in relation to the tendon that gets frequently inflamed.

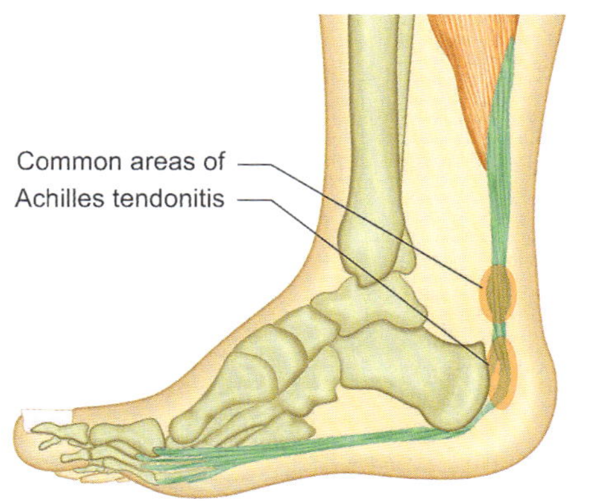

Fig. 2: The two common sites of Achilles tendinitis—"insertional" at the calcaneus bone and noninsertional tendinitis usually just below the midpoint.

- Noninsertional tendinitis **(Fig. 2)** involving the tendon proximal to its insertion—this involves the paratenon and/or the tendon itself.
  However, these may also occur simultaneously.

History and Physical Examination

In the early phases, patients have mild-to-moderate pain following strenuous activities that usually progress quickly to pain with regular activities in the absence of rest/ treatment. It is common for the patient to report of pain and stiffness, worse in the morning or after inactivity typical of "start-up pain" that quickly resolves with a few steps taken through pain. This start-up pain is due to the paratendinitis adhesions. Other points that should be noted in history to identify underlying pathology include:

- Onset of symptoms paying particular attention to an episode of trauma
- Changes in activity level to better delineate the repetitive overuse
- For athletes, gather information regarding warm-up, mileage, intensity, running surface, and shoe wear
- Ask for other joint pains concomitantly or in sequence.

Physical Examination

- Inspection of the patient's shoe wear
- Lower limb weight-bearing alignment (anterior, posterior, and lateral)
- Observe gait
- Quite significantly one finds excessive hindfoot varus or valgus that actually shortens the Achilles enroute its insertion point. One should move the subtalar joint while flexing and extending the knee to assess the extent of Achilles contracture.
- Localized findings are quite obvious in the form of gastrocnemius or soleus wasting or localized swelling bruising or defect about the Achilles in long-standing cases. Wasting of the gastrocnemius soleus complex is suggestive of severe affliction.
- Neurovascular examination
- Detailed assessment of strength and range-of-motion is needed; an inability to tip-toe walk may suggest chronic rupture or neurological problems.
- Examine the patient in prone position and feet hanging off the end of the examining table for a systematic assessment of mechanical alignment, palpation of areas of tenderness, nodules, defects in the tendon and crepitus.

Laboratory Investigations

The only role for laboratory investigation is for investigating underlying diseases:

- Crystal arthropathy—uric acid levels
- Inflammatory arthropathy—erythrocyte sedimentation rate (ESR), C-reactive protein (CRP), rheumatoid factor
- Enthesopathy—human leukocyte antigen B27 (HLA-B27)

Imaging Studies

- An exostosis growing into the Achilles tendon is visualized best on true lateral view of the heel as a proximally extending posterior prominence **(Fig. 3)**.

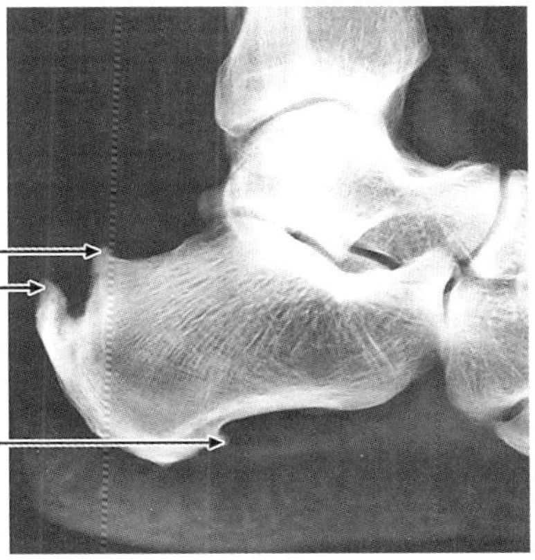

Fig. 3: The Haglund's deformity and the bony excrescence (exostosis) into tendo-Achillis. Also appreciate the calcaneal spur seen all in a single radiograph.

- Haglund's deformity **(Fig. 3)** is also easily depicted on the lateral view using the parallel pitch lines where the tuberosity projects above the upper parallel pitch line and a Phillip and Fowler angle > 69°.
- Distal calcification is easily identified near the Achilles insertion.
- Signs of Achilles tendon rupture (*see* Section on "Disorders of Foot and Ankle")
- Ultrasound is useful for demonstrating bursal inflammation and any tendon degeneration. Some also use this for making the diagnosis of tendon rupture.
- MRI is the gold standard for imaging musculoskeletal soft tissues yielding detailed information about the mid-substance of the tendons and surrounding structures.

Nonoperative Treatment

Nonsteroidal anti-inflammatory drugs (NSAIDs) may help additionally but the effect is moderate only.

Intratendinous injections of steroids are best avoided and not recommended.

- Rest from excessive stress is foremost introduced but should be done only for short periods (2–4 weeks) because prolonged immobilization is detrimental to tendon and muscle strength, articular cartilage, and worsens joint stiffness if present.
- Customized orthotics to correct flexible hindfoot malalignment in the coronal plain relieves symptoms and provides a more biomechanical favorable condition to halt or reverse progression.
- Shoe modification with a good sole and solid heel counter should be recommended to prevent excessive heel movement:
  - Pump bump spacers may be utilized to unload pressure areas in the heel posteriorly.
  - A heel lift may unload the Achilles to some extent through decreased dorsiflexion angle at the ankle.
- Stretching is very useful for pain relief. If bearable night splints will provide one with a continuous minor stretch that reduces morning pain and stiffness.
- Once the acute painful and inflammatory period settles one should concentrate more on a strengthening

program, especially the eccentric strengthening exercises that cause a greater overall reduction in pain than the traditional concentric exercises.

Operative Treatment

One should be aware of negative prognostic patient factors specifically for outcomes in Achilles tendon surgery including diabetes mellitus, smoking, malnourishment, and generalized poor medical condition.

Noninsertional Achilles tendon disease that fails nonoperative treatment and Achilles rupture are the most common indications for surgical treatment. For an intact tendon with disease in the mid-substance, Achilles tendon debridement that includes excision of areas of tendon degeneration through a longitudinal incision should be done.

For insertional Achilles tendon disease, the surgery is directed at removal of the bony prominence if present and resection of calcification and inflamed bursal tissues. With Haglund's deformity, the posterosuperior calcaneal prominence must be completely removed and a second lateral incision in addition to the medial one is sometimes necessary to assure complete resection. Prolonged recovery period is needed sometimes taking 6–12 months for resolution of symptoms. For simple posterolateral calcaneal exostosis (pump bump), only a small lateral approach is necessary for limited resection of the exostosis alone.

TIBIALIS POSTERIOR TENDON DISEASE/ INSUFFICIENCY

This is one of the most common reasons for midfoot pain and the associated disability. It is commonly misdiagnosed. Posterior tibial tendon insufficiency is discussed in detail in Chapter on "Acquired Flatfoot (Pes Planus) and Posterior Tibial Tendon Dysfunction".

Differential Diagnosis

Accessory navicular and navicular tuberosity fractures; these clinical conditions may progress to full blown posterior tibial tendon (PTT) disease and medial arch collapse if not diagnosed and treated early.

Anatomy

The posterior tibial muscle originates from the posterior aspect of the proximal one-third of the tibia, fibula, and interosseous membrane forming the deep posterior compartment of the leg. The tendon courses posterior to medial malleolus to insert principally on the navicular tuberosity but also on cuneiforms and bases of the second, third, and fourth metatarsals. The innervation to muscle arises from the tibial nerve while the blood supply is derived from the branches from the posterior tibial artery, periosteal vessels from the medial plantar artery of the posterior tibial artery or the medial tarsal artery from the dorsalis pedis artery (*see* also the Section on "Disorders of Foot and Ankle").

Tibialis Posterior Tendon Biomechanics

The primary function of the PTT is inversion and plantarflexion of the foot. This results in locking of the midfoot transverse tarsal joints (talonavicular and calcaneocuboid). It is also a secondary adductor of the forefoot at the midtarsal joint apposing the action of the peroneus brevis and provides support for the longitudinal arch of the foot.

Clinical Implications

The common presentation is of:

- Medial ankle pain and swelling
- Tenderness localized directly over the navicular tuberosity or accessory navicular
- Lateral sinus tarsi pain due to medial arch collapse and forefoot abduction.

Physical examination:

- Forefoot abduction (too many toes)
- Midfoot pes planus (flat foot)
- Hindfoot valgus
- On heel rising test, the normal heel inversion is absent if the PTT is dysfunctional. Single foot heel rising on the symptomatic limb is usually not possible or at least painful and weak.

Classification of PTT dysfunction [Johnson and Strom, kindly also see the Chapter on "Acquired Flatfoot (Pes Planus) and Posterior Tibial Tendon Dysfunction"]:

The pathology is divided according to deformity and whether or not it is correctable.

- *Stage 1* involves pain localized along the course of the PTT.
- *Stage 2* represents a situation in which the PTT is diseased as in stage 1 with the tendon being functionally incompetent (PTT tear) resulting in medial arch collapse.
- *Stage 3* has all the features of stages 1 and 2 but the deformities are rigid and not passively correctable.
- *Stage 4* includes the features of stage 3 plus ankle joint incongruency.

Investigations and Imaging

Laboratory investigation would rule out/identify underlying diseases or predisposing conditions (i.e., infection, inflammatory disease, etc.). Imaging studies are needed for objective assessment of the alignment of foot to identify pes planus. Accessory navicular or tuberosity fracture is easily identified. MRI is reserved for accessing PTT synovitis or intrasubstance tendon disease or PTT tear.

Treatment

Early nonoperative treatment includes activity modification, anti-inflammatory medication, physiotherapy, and medial arch support orthotics. If not relieved then POP cast for 2–4 weeks reduces inflammation and even treats accessory navicular pain or tuberosity fracture.

Surgical options for resistant cases can be discussed based on stage of disease:

- *Stage 1* with tendon debridement with or without a bony procedure such as a medial weight-bearing axis shifting calcaneal osteotomy or lateral column lengthening procedure.

- *Stage 2:* The passively correctable flatfoot is treated with a combination of soft-tissue reconstruction of the tendon in an attempt to restore a functional PTT with a bony procedure (above) to reverse deformity. The other choices for reconstruction of the tendon include transfer of the flexor digitorum longus or flexor hallucis longus (FHL).
- *Stages 3 and 4:* Posterior tibial tendon results in fixed deformity, thus necessitating tarsal arthrodesis such as subtalar, talonavicular, and calcaneocuboid.
- *Stage 4:* Needs even ankle (tibial calcaneal) arthrodesis.

PERONEAL TENDON DISEASE

Peroneal tendon disease secondary to trauma or stenosis is very common. Traumatic includes overuse with micro-rupture or calcification, dislocation or subluxation, lateral malleolar fractures, calcaneal fractures, and inversion ankle injuries. Nontraumatic entities include inflammatory arthritis, infection, os peroneum, congenital enlarged peroneal tubercle, or very rarely local tumors.

Anatomy and Biomechanics

The peroneus longus inserts on the lateral tubercle of the first metatarsal and the first cuneiform while the peroneus brevis inserts on the base of the fifth metatarsal. The superior peroneal retinaculum serves as the primary restraint to peroneal tendon subluxation partly also enhanced by fibrocartilaginous ridge of the lateral malleolus and the retromalleolar sulcus. The primary function of the peroneal tendons is eversion and plantarflexion of the foot. The peroneus longus is also responsible for plantar flexion of the first metatarsal.

Clinical Features of Peroneal Tendinitis

Inflammation in the area posterior to the fibula with swelling and tenderness. Pain is exacerbated by resisted stretching of the tendons with a plantar flexion inversion force. There is also a decrease in subtalar motion and subsequent difficulty with walking on uneven ground.

Treatment

- Activity modification (cast immobilization for a short period if necessary), protection, rest, ice, compression and elevation (PRICE), and NSAIDs
- Orthotics and shoe wear modifications (decreasing calcaneal fibular impingement with a medial heel wedge)
- Physiotherapy directed at muscle strengthening and improving mobility should be instituted.
- Surgery is reserved for resistant cases and mostly comprises debridement of the diseased tendon. Often peroneal instability contributes to the diseased peroneals (see below), and therefore strong consideration should be given to a peroneal stabilization procedure concurrent with a debridement. An acute rupture may benefit from early surgical intervention to promote rehabilitation and prevent re-rupture as with other tendons. With respect to partial or chronic tears, a debridement and repair or reconstruction of the tendon is indicated.

Peroneal Instability

Peroneal tendon instability often coexists with peroneal tendon disease and partial tears. Instability may range from frank traumatic dislocation at one end to subluxation within the peroneal groove at the other end. Traumatic dislocation is associated with sports, such as skiing, soccer, football, and gymnastics, and is also associated with weak restrains of the peroneal tendons. The weak restraints include abnormal superior peroneal retinaculum, shallow fibular groove, and calcaneal varus.

Apart from the symptoms of tendinitis patients also have complain of a click or audible snap with or without pain. The click/snap may be reproducible with resisted eversion and dorsiflexion while palpating the tendons.

Nonoperative treatment—immobilization or/and bracing effective only in acute scenario that too partially. More often the treatment fails and a persistence of symptoms needs surgical procedure. The various surgical options for subluxation include:

- Direct repair of retinaculum
- Rerouting procedures of the peroneal tendons
- Fibular sliding osteotomies
- Fibular groove deepening procedures

STRESS FRACTURES

A stress fracture is the accumulation of microtrauma that ultimately leads to the macrofracture of bone. Stress fractures were originally recorded by Breithaupt (a Prussian military physician in 1855) on soldiers with swollen and painful feet. He called them "march fractures", although Aristotle had described them earlier in 200 BC. While military personnel are more prone to stress fractures of the calcaneus and metatarsals, sports personnel have more of tibial stress fractures. Stress fractures are seen in 10–15% of sports medicine patients. Stress fractures are most common in running sports as vertical ground reaction forces are three times greater compared to walking. Stress fractures are different from insufficiency fractures that occur in abnormal bone which has been subjected to normal stress. Fatigue/stress fractures occur when normal bone is subjected to abnormal stress.

Risk Factors for Developing Stress Fractures of Feet Leg

- Pronated feet—tarsal and tibial stress fractures
- Talocalcaneal and calcaneonavicular coalitions—stress fracture of neck of talus
- Leg-length inequality and excessive forefoot varus
- Rigid cavus foot

Pathogenesis

The most common mechanism *is repetitive injury* due to continuous excessive activity. *Other mechanisms* that result in higher strain could be:

- Fatigue of muscles around the joints that result in diminished shielding effect and transmittance of all of the compressive and tensile forces across bones. Muscle contraction converts tensile forces into compressive

TABLE 1: The classification of stress fractures.

	High risk	*Low risk*
Stress type	Tension	Compression
Natural history	Poor	Good
Management	• *Aggressive complete fracture:* Surgery • *Incomplete fracture:* Strict nonweight-bearing (NWB)	• *Conservative symptomatic:* Activity modification ± Immobilization • *Asymptomatic:* No treatment needed

forces; a phenomenon referred to as stress shielding. This protects the bone and prevents injury. This mechanism fails with muscle fatigue.

- Also muscle fatigue results in gait alteration and instability which may also alter the forces on bone.
- In nonweight-bearing bones, repetitive pull of overworked contracting muscles can produce microfractures that propagate to produce stress fracture.

Based on the likelihood of displacement and complications that stress fractures may undergo, they are classified as high-risk and low-risk fractures **(Table 1)**. The common high-risk lower extremity fractures (in order of their potential to displace) include:

- Femoral neck–superolateral (tension side)
- Patella
- Anterior tibial diaphysis
- Talus
- Tarsal navicular
- Fifth metatarsal
- Medial malleolus
- Femoral neck—inferomedial
- Sesamoids

Pathophysiology

Based on the Wolff's law of transformation, bone remains in a state of dynamic activity due to cyclical stress and rest. This process is affected by remodeling of the bony architecture to optimally withstand its environment. The stress induced failure in osteons of microstructure is cemented and continuously modified by osteoclastic resorption (that "erase" the defect by a larger organized defect) at the level of the osteon followed by filling of cavities promptly by the osteoblasts (construction work—restoring the architecture). Bone loss (resorption activity) peaks at 3 weeks while the whole cycle takes 3 months to complete. An imbalance of resorption and bone deposition leads to weakening of bone as is produced by more than tolerable activity. On the tensile side of bone, osteons debond at the cement lines causing microfractures. Oblique cracks and longitudinal splitting occurs through canalicular defects and the Haversian canals on the compression side. In cancellous bone, stress forms trabecular microfractures producing microcallus. These thickened trabeculae then appear as sclerosis on radiographs. It is not that there is no bone restoration activity going on the stress fractures but simply the activity lags behind the damage being incurred. In this dynamic process, if the stress continues, the fatigue fracture may become complete and ultimately get displaced.

History

- Insidious onset of pain that persists from weeks to months in a localized area. Onset could be related to changes in distance, intensity or frequency of workout. There may also be change in the running surface or shoes. Inadequate footwear can contribute to development of stress fractures.
- The pain is exacerbated by repetitive activity and relieved by rest.
- As the injury progresses, the pain will occur earlier and with greater intensity during activity.

Physical Examination

Point tenderness over the affected bone along with some subtle soft-tissue swelling. No signs of inflammation (osteomyelitis/periostitis). Joints and surrounding muscles are normal. Neurovascular examination is also normal.

Imaging

- Classically, the radiographs will initially be negative. After several weeks, long bones such as the metatarsals or tibia will show periosteal new bone formation or frank but incomplete cortical break.
- Cancellous bones such as the calcaneus show medullary sclerosis.
- A Tc-99m bone scan is the investigation of choice, and it will be positive as early as 3 days after injury. The bone scan will be positive in all three phases with a focal intense area of uptake, even in the setting of normal X-ray findings. The bone scan is virtually 100% sensitive in diagnosing stress fractures, but its specificity is less than X-ray. Bone scan also cannot distinguish stress fracture from neoplasm or infection.
- Ultrasonography is an important tool that can be used in case of normal radiology; for metatarsal fractures, the USG scan has been found to have 83% sensitivity, 76% specificity; 59% positive predictive value, and 92% negative predictive value.
- Computed tomography (CT) scans may be ordered for strongly suspected navicular, calcaneal, tibial, and pediatric fatigue fractures.
- MRI can be a useful adjunct in cases with negative radiographs and equivocal bone scan. It can now be considered investigation of choice as it has marked specificity and is able to differentiate other lesions remarkably well.

The important stress fractures of foot and leg are being described below ***(Figs. 4A and B)***.

Sesamoids

Stress fractures of the sesamoids are uncommon. The sesamoids are subject to continuous stress as up to 50% of body weight is borne through the great toe complex. The sesamoids impart mechanical advantage to the flexor

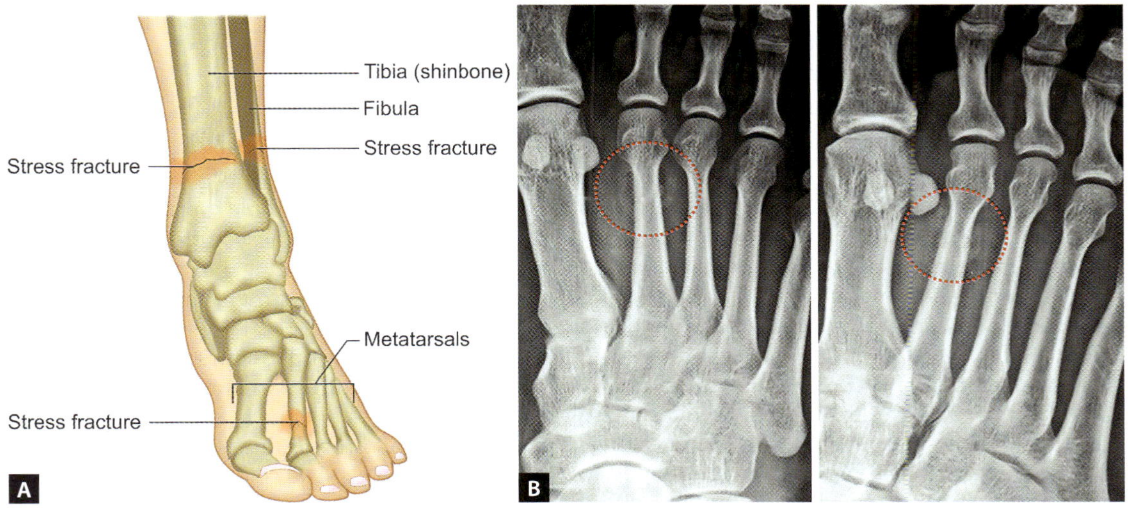

Figs. 4A and B: (A) Illustration depicting various sites for stress fracture in the foot and leg; (B) Radiographs depicting the stress fracture of second metatarsal bone common in soldiers and ballet dancers.

hallucis brevis tendons by acting as a fulcrum. The medial sesamoid is more frequently injured, although in one study the medial and lateral sesamoids were found to be equally involved.

Patients have pain while standing on their toes or with dorsiflexion of the first toe.

Differential diagnosis: Sesamoiditis, chondromalacia, osteochondritis, turf toe, hallux valgus, medial plantar digital proper nerve syndrome and bursitis.

Radiographs will show a bipartite or multipartite sesamoid or a normal bone. Bone scan is the best investigation that will show increased uptake with a stress fracture.

Treatment of a stress fracture of sesamoid involves 6 weeks of immobilization in a cast or walker boot or K-wire fixation in flexion. After 6 weeks, the foot is re-examined and radiographs taken. If symptoms persist and the site is unhealed, surgery may be considered.

Surgical excision of one sesamoid is adequate, if the sesamoid is fragmented. Excision of both sesamoids will produce an unacceptable cock-up-toe deformity and is highly discouraged. Partial excision of the smaller fragment can also be performed. If there is a fracture, nonunion bone grafting is recommended, especially for nonmobile nonunions else for a mobile nonunion, it is better to excise the bone.

Metatarsals

These are most commonly seen in the second and third metatarsal shafts. The second and third metatarsals are relatively fixed in position within the foot; the first, fourth, and fifth metatarsals are relatively mobile placing more stress on the former, and hence increased incidence. Stress fractures of the first metatarsal are uncommon (1% of foot and 10% of metatarsal stress fractures). They are predominantly seen in the cancellous proximal end of the bone. Stress fractures of the second metatarsal in ballet dancers occur at base as they are routinely in the en pointe position. With the foot plantar flexed and the weight borne on the first and second phalanges, the leg forms a long lever arm with the forces concentrated at the second tarsometatarsal junction being directly transmitted by the cuneiform bone. The typical described "march fracture" was located in the second metatarsal bone in distal thirds **(Fig. 4B)**. This is due to prolonged impact walking (marching) common in military recruits. Jones originally described the stress fracture of fifth metatarsal in dancers, but it can be seen in a wide variety of athletes, especially basketball and football players. In the athlete, this fracture may be seen acutely or in a chronic course. A stress fracture occurs 1.5 cm distal to the tuberosity of the fifth metatarsal in the metaphyseal-diaphyseal junction. [The pseudo-Jones fracture should not be confused with the dancer's fracture, which is an avulsion of the tuberosity of the fifth metatarsal; also Jones fracture (fracture in the metadiaphyseal junction of the fifth metatarsal) is a distinct entity.] The risk factors for metatarsal stress fractures include:

- Hypermobile first ray
- Short first ray
- Gastrocnemius equinus contracture
- Morton foot, which has a second metatarsal longer than the first metatarsal (controversial as a predisposing factor).

Clinical findings: Localized pain and tenderness over the metatarsal with subtle swelling. Initially, radiographs are inconclusive. Bone scan diagnoses the condition well and early. This is imperative as with early treatment patients will simply respond well to cessation of training/activity. A delay in treatment beginning with visible findings on radiographs will necessitate nonweight-bearing immobilization until callus is seen and the patient is asymptomatic. For fifth metatarsal base stress fractures, breaking and sclerosis is seen at the lateral cortex on radiographs.

Differential diagnosis of metatarsal stress fracture: Synovitis of Lisfranc joint, extensor digitorum brevis tendinitis, Morton's neuralgia, metatarsalgia, and turf toe.

Treatment: Immobilization is the primary treatment for all stress fractures only the duration of immobilization varies with the location and type of fractures. The duration of treatment is also dependent on the delay in diagnosis with most fractures diagnosed on radiographs needing longer immobilization. The treatment for first metatarsal stress fracture is activity and shoe modification for 4–6 weeks. Dancers with second metatarsal fractures will require a fracture shoe or walking cast.

The fifth metatarsal stress fractures in dancers are a tricky problem with their predisposition to nonunion as these fractures occur at a watershed area for the blood supply, and thus take a particularly long time to heal compared to the other metatarsals. If it is associated with a cavus foot position then excess load on the lateral border of the foot results in slow healing or refracture. Treatment, hence, involves 6–8 weeks of nonweight-bearing. As it is prone to refracture, some surgeons consider early operative fixation to allow quicker return to competition and decreased risk of refracture. The most common method is compression screw fixation and if possible then simultaneous bone grafting. It is recommended that the underlying cavus foot should also be corrected. The patient is placed in a short leg cast for 2 weeks and then in a walking boot walker with progressively increasing weight-bearing for 3–4 weeks. The patient may progress to full activity 8 weeks postoperatively.

Navicular

Stress fractures in the navicular were first described in 1970 by Towne et al. and are quite common in basketball, football, and track and field athletes. They are difficult to diagnose and treat as the patient will complain of diffuse midfoot pain. The physical examination sign described by Khan is the "N" spot which is pain with direct pressure on the dorsal talonavicular articulation. To reproduce the pain, patient can be made to hop on the affected foot in a plantar flexed position. Plain films are normal initially so diagnosis relies on bone scan or better a CT scan that defines the anatomy and displacement of the fracture quite comprehensively. The most common fracture pattern is a linear sagittal fracture at the junction of the middle and lateral one-third of the navicular which occurs in the vascular watershed area.

Treatment: Conservative therapy is preferred initially with 6 weeks of a nonweight-bearing cast. After cast removal re-examination of foot is performed. If the "N" spot is still tender treatment is extended for 2 weeks. When asymptomatic, a gradual return to activity is initiated.

Surgical intervention is contemplated in acute complete displaced fracture, delayed union, and nonunion. Open reduction and internal fixation with a lag screw across the fracture, preferably from lateral to medial, is performed. In the acute setting, this is sufficient. In delayed or nonunion, autologous bone grafting is recommended in addition to the lag screw fixation. Postoperatively, the patient is kept nonweight-bearing for 4 weeks, with gradual return to full-weight-bearing over next 4 weeks. Return to full activity needs at least 3 months.

Leg

Fibula

Stress fractures of the fibula were originally described by Burrows who classified these injuries into two groups.

- The first is seen in young male runners with the fractures occurring 6 cm proximal to the distal tip of the lateral malleolus **(Fig. 5)**
- The second group occurs in middle-aged females sustaining fractures 3 cm proximal to the distal tip (most common)
- Occasional high fibula stress fractures are seen in runners.

Treatment is nonweight-bearing until asymptomatic. Displaced fractures should be treated with open reduction and internal fixation.

Medial Malleolus

Stress fracture of the medial malleolus as described by Devas and Shelbourne is an injury occurring at the junction of the medial malleolus and tibial plafond. There is point tenderness over medial malleolus. Radiographs show a vertical fissure at the junction of the medial malleolus and the tibial plafond in later stages. If fracture is seen on X-ray, an open reduction and internal fixation (ORIF) is recommended while for radiologically occult fractures (bone scan positive) conservative therapy is warranted. In the case of nonunion, ORIF with bone grafting is indicated.

Tibial Shaft

This is the most common site for stress fractures in athletes (two-thirds to three-fourths of all stress fractures). Based on

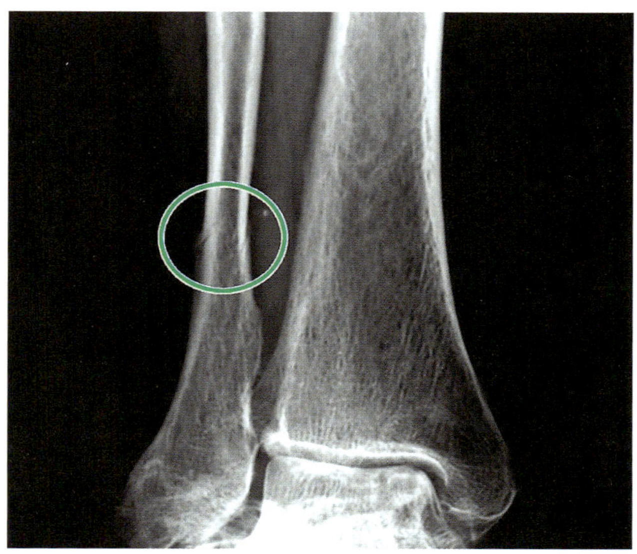

Fig. 5: Stress fracture of fibula.

the pathogenesis and impact on treatment, the tibial stress fractures are classified into two types:

1. *Fractures of posterior tibia (usually posteromedial):* These are more common and are caused by compressive forces. Runners typically injure the posterior aspect at middle and distal third junction.
2. *Fractures of anterior tibia:* Anterior fractures are caused by tensile forces and are harder to treat. These are seen in jumping athletes such as dancers, volleyball and basketball players. The anterior diaphysis is the tension side of the tibia and is a high-risk zone that is more prone to nonunion and displacement. Poor blood supply and musculotendinous support in addition to tensile loads contribute to the delayed healing of this injury.

A proximal type of stress fracture is rarely seen in elderly patients with varus deformity of knee and associated metabolic bone disorder (osteomalacia). This occurs in proximal metaphyseo-diaphyseal junction and is prone to nonunion if the mechanical alignment is not restored **(Figs. 6 and 7)**.

Most of these fractures have transverse and oblique patterns although longitudinal and spiral patterns also occur occasionally.

Differential diagnosis: Medial tibial stress syndrome, peripheral nerve compression, and chronic compartment syndrome.

Radiology: Usually, the radiographs are normal but in late anterior stress fractures the "dreaded black line" represents a cortical break and may progress to a complete fracture if left untreated. If the solitary anterior cortical fracture is surrounded by sclerosis; this is representative of a nonunion that will progress to complete fracture and requires operative fixation.

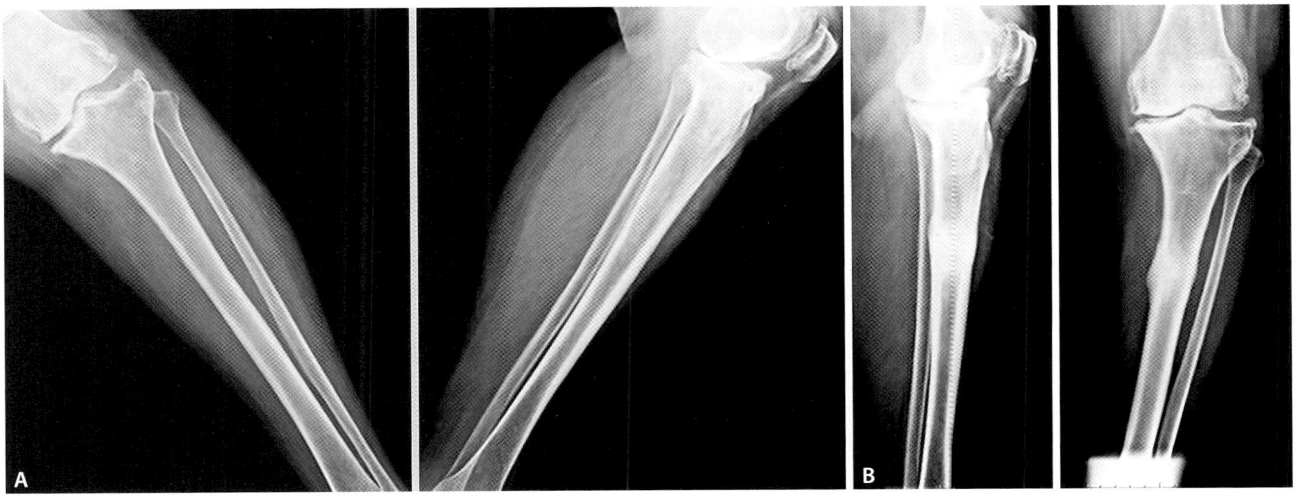

Figs. 6A and B: (A) Proximal stress fracture of tibia; (B) Healed with conservative management.

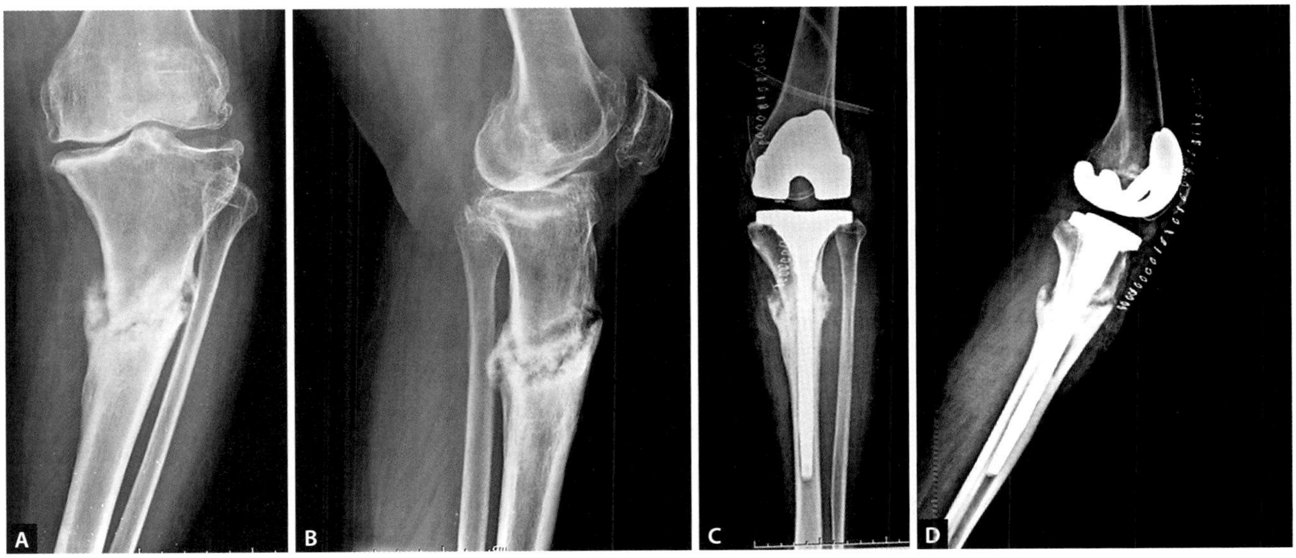

Figs. 7A to D: Stress fracture of proximal tibia that had to be operated due to failure at the fracture site.

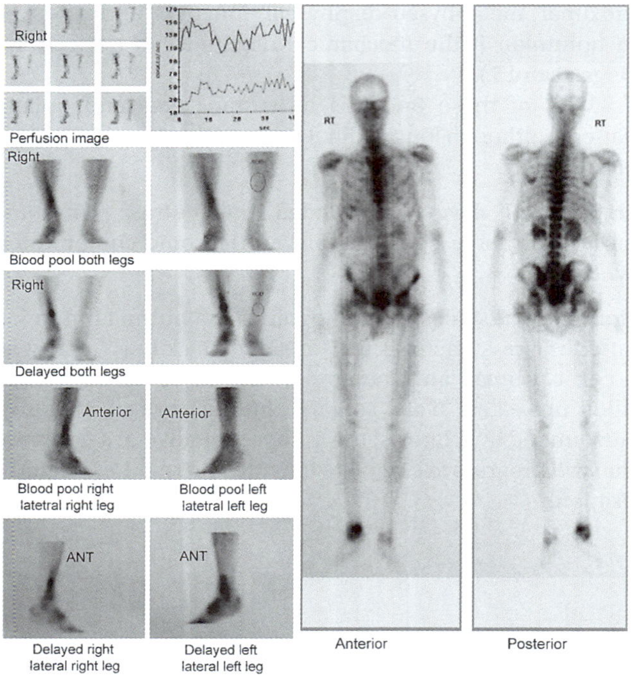

Fig. 8: Bone scan is an effective modality to diagnose stress fractures. This patient had normal X-rays (not shown) but an increased uptake on Tc-99m bone scan in the lower right tibial region. He was symptomatic for 1 month previously for which various analgesics were tried.

Bone scan of posterior fractures initially shows a diffuse uptake pattern and later shows a sharply marginated fusiform uptake pattern **(Fig. 8)**.

MRI is a preferred investigation to comprehensively locate the region of stress fracture (anterior versus posterior) as the spatial differentiation in bone scan is poor.

Treatment: Posterior stress fractures of the tibial shaft are treated with nonweight-bearing cast immobilization of 8–12 weeks. Anterior stress fractures of the tibia present a very difficult rehabilitation problem. These fractures are more likely to progress to complete fracture or go on to nonunion compared to posterior tibial stress fractures. Conservative therapy needs 6 months of activity cessation with graduated return to sport. Electrical stimulation may be beneficial to healing. As the period of recuperation is long, some surgeons primarily treat patients with surgical methods. For undisplaced fractures, the cortex is drilled to stimulate bone growth or better perform an intramedullary locked nail fixation. Delayed or nonunions should be primarily surgically treated with intramedullary locked nail fixation and bone grafting. Bone grafting may be avoided as reamings graft the fracture and site quite adequately, and this will also prevent an additional incision. Still the fracture takes approximately 9 months to heal.

PLANTAR FASCIITIS (PLANTAR FASCIOSIS, CALCANEAL PLANTAR ENTHESOPATHY)

This is a self-limited condition and a common cause of heel pain **(Fig. 9)** in adults and adolescents. It is the most

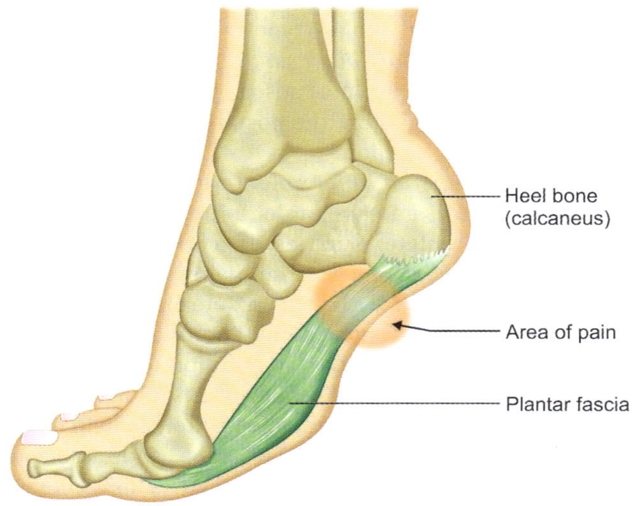

Fig. 9: Illustration of the classical site for pathology and pain in plantar fasciitis.

common foot condition for which a patient seeks attention of podiatrist. Plantar fasciitis affects as much as 10% of the population over the course of a lifetime. Plantar fasciitis is thought to be caused by biomechanical overuse from prolonged standing or running, thus creating microtears at the calcaneal enthesis. There is a suggestion that the term should be modified to "plantar fasciosis" as it represents more of a degenerative process rather than acute inflammation.

Anatomy and Pathoanatomy

The plantar aponeurosis consists of three bands: (1) lateral, (2) medial, and (3) central. The central band originates from the medial tubercle on the plantar surface of the calcaneus and travels toward the toes as a tight band of tissue. Just proximal to crossing the metatarsal heads, it divides into five slips. Each slip further divides into half to insert on the proximal phalanx of each toe. The plantar fascia gets functionally shortened when the toes are extended (as it wraps around each metatarsal head) producing the characteristic "windlass effect" (described by Hicks, **Fig. 10**). The windlass effect assists in supinating the foot during the latter portion of the stance phase and provides stability to the toes. The plantar fascia is a continuum of Achilles tendon fibers (similar to attachment of gluteus medius and vastus lateralis on greater trochanter).

Muscles and nerves in the vicinity play an important role in clinical assessment of pain. Three muscles: the flexor digitorum brevis, abductor hallucis, and quadratus plantae have the same origin and insertions as that of plantar aponeurosis so could be the source of origin of pain. The tibial nerve divides into the medial and lateral plantar nerves while traveling through the tarsal tunnel; these and their branches (including the second branch of the lateral plantar nerve, also referred to as "Baxter's nerve") can get entrapped causing "tarsal tunnel syndrome." The plantar heel pad is supplied by medial calcaneal branches of tibial nerve.

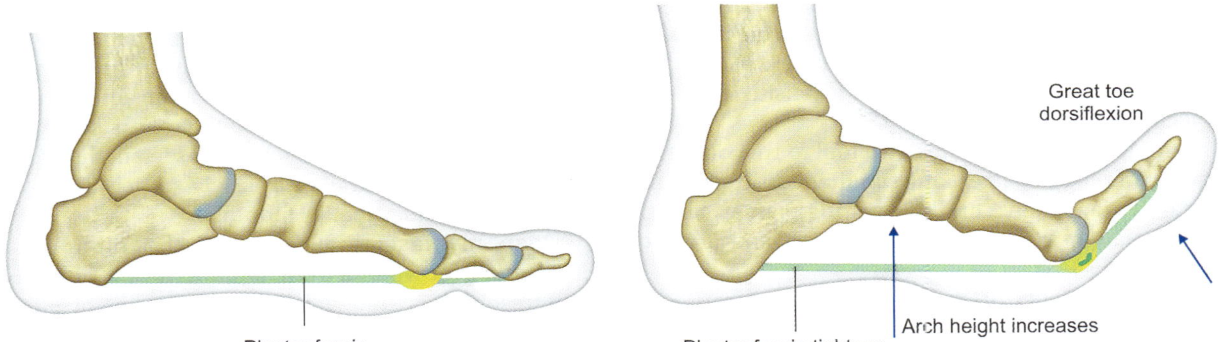

Fig. 10: Windlass effect of plantar fascia. Stretch on fascia increases the arch as in a bow.

The most common site of abnormality in patients with plantar fasciitis is near the origin or enthesis of the central band of the plantar aponeurosis at the medial plantar tubercle of the calcaneus. Occasionally, the pain could be located at the mid-portion of the central band, just prior to it splitting into the five slips. Plantar fasciitis occurs as an enthesopathy in patients with a seronegative arthropathy (Reiter's syndrome, psoriatic arthropathy, ankylosing spondylitis, and enteropathic spondyloarthropathy).

Risk Factors for Plantar Fasciitis

The etiology of condition is poorly understood, however, some patient population seems to be predisposed for development of the plantar fasciitis related heel pain. Few of the associated risk factors reported by various investigators are as follows:

- Decreased dorsiflexion ankle range-of-motion
- Excessive foot pronation (pes planus)
- High arch (pes cavus)
- Obesity (body-mass index of 30 kg/m^2 or more)
- Calcaneal spur on radiographs
- Prolonged standing/walking occupation (military personnel/surgeons)
- Excessive running
- Leg-length discrepancy
- Sedentary lifestyle
- Intrinsic foot muscle tightness

Clinical Features

Most patients report heel pain and tightness after standing up and taking first step from bed in the morning ("start-up" pains) or after they have been seated for a prolonged time (as in movie theaters). The heel pain commonly improves within a few steps if they walk through the pain but in a few, the pain could intensify by day's end if the patient continues to walk or stand for a long time.

Physical Examination

Patients may walk with equinus gait to avoid placing pressure on the painful heel. Tenderness on medial plantar calcaneal region is commonly reported as a sharp stabbing pain. Passive ankle or first-toe dorsiflexion (windlass test) elicits pain.

Clinicians should use validated self-report questionnaires, such as the Foot Function Index (FFI), Foot Health Status Questionnaire (FHSQ), or the Foot and Ankle Ability Measure (FAAM), before and after interventions.

Diagnosis

The diagnosis is quite easily made by the following characteristic findings:

- Morning start-up pains that relieve by few steps of ambulation, pain reappears after prolonged sitting (watching TV).
- No history of trauma but a history of recent changed activities (starting walking or running)
- Pain localized to plantar heel more on the medial aspect with absence of paresthesias.

Differential Diagnosis

As stated earlier, the vicinity of muscles and nerves makes it imperative to rule out pain emanating from these sources. The following are the common differentials:

- Heel contusion
- Plantar fascia rupture
- Bone bruise
- Posterior tibial tendinitis
- Achilles tendinitis
- Retrocalcaneal bursitis
- S1 radiculopathy and referred pain
- Calcaneal stress fracture
- Fat pad atrophy
- Medial calcaneal and abductor digiti quinti nerve entrapment
- Tarsal tunnel syndrome
- Neuropathy
- Sever's disease
- Calcaneal neoplasia
- Systemic arthritis including rheumatoid arthritis
- Metastasis
- Paget's disease of bone

Imaging

Plain radiography is useful in patients with recalcitrant disease to rule out other pathologies especially. Calcaneal spur is not at all a diagnostic feature but mere contributory in a symptomatic patient. Instead soft-tissue radiographs are more sensitive and informative. Plantar fascia thickness and fat pad abnormalities are the two best factors for differentiation of plantar fasciitis, with a sensitivity of 85% and a specificity of 95%.

Ultrasonography is an inexpensive tool to rule out other soft-tissue pathology of heel and simultaneously evaluate the plantar fascia. Positive finding favoring plantar fasciitis is proximal plantar fascia thickness > 4 mm and areas of hypoechogenicity.

MRI is the modality of choice for assessing causes of recalcitrant heel pain. Diagnosis relies on finding thickened plantar fascia with increased signal intensity on T2-weighted and short tau inversion recovery images.

Treatment

Plantar fasciitis usually improves within 1 year regardless of treatment. The disabling heel pain, however, is a concern and cause of morbidity. The treatment options vary a lot and often are used empirically in different combinations without much evidence attached to them. Conservative treatment is the first choice for nearly all patients that should be impressed with an explanation that the condition is chronic and needs time to respond. Within 6 weeks to 2 months, 90% of patients will improve with conservative therapies. If a patient's symptoms persist 6 months or longer, further invasive procedures may be resorted too.

Rest and Analgesics

Nonsteroidal anti-inflammatory drugs comprise the primary modality of treatment to reduce pain and swelling associated with acute exacerbation of symptoms. This is combined with activity modification, ice massage, or contrast water bath (alternate hot and cold fomentation). NSAIDs have been found to give short-term improvement in pain relief and disability when accompanied by other conservative treatments. They may be, however, not so effective when used alone.

Stretching and Physical Therapy Modalities

- Eccentric calf stretches, defined as exercises performed under load while the muscle is slowly lengthened, have supportive evidence in improving various tendinopathies and can be prescribed for lengthening the Achilles tendon. The plantar fascia tissue-specific stretch is performed while patient is sitting, with the patient placing the fingers of one hand across the toes of the involved foot, then pulling the toes back (extension) toward the shin until stretching was felt in the arch of the foot. Both calf and plantar fascia stretch improve pain symptomatology for 2–4 months.
- Deep myofascial massage of the plantar fascia, manually or with instrumentation (locally administered ultrasonics) is thought to promote healing by increasing the blood flow to the injured fascia. Most evidence is, however, anecdotal.
- *Manual therapy:* Talocrural joint posterior glides, subtalar joint lateral glides, anterior/posterior glides of the first tarsometatarsal joint and subtalar joint distraction manipulations have been shown to be effective in relieving pain by modulating the restricted dorsiflexion and excessive pronation of feet. So patients having these clinical findings can be definitely subjected to manual therapy. The effect is again short term (1–3 months).
- Iontophoresis uses electrical pulses to cause absorption of topical medication (5% acetic acid or 0.4% dexamethasone) into the soft-tissue beneath the skin. Iontophoresis had some effectiveness in treating plantar fasciitis; results need to be fully substantiated. The use of iontophoresis does not have an effect on long-term pain or function, however, and hence this modality should be considered for those patients who need an immediate reduction in pain symptoms.

Arch Supports, Silicone Soft Soles (Figs. 11A and B), and Night Splints

- Foot orthotics aid in preventing overpronation of the foot and to unload tensile forces on the plantar fascia. The following are the commonly used orthotics:
  - Night splints prevent plantar fascia contracture by keeping the foot and ankle in a neutral 90° position, preventing foot plantar flexion during sleep. Night splints used alone have been shown to improve plantar fasciitis pain. The problem is compliance due to cumbersome use (anterior night splints have better compliance).

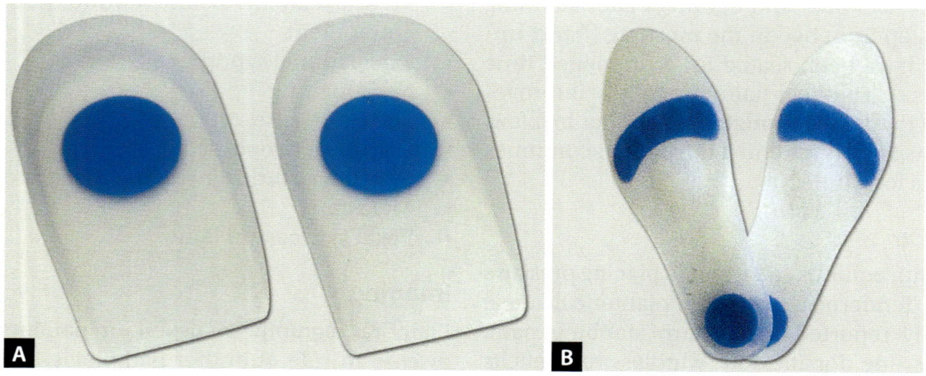

Figs. 11A and B: Silicone heel cups and foot insoles.

- Medial arch supports are not used in isolation but are commonly combined with silicone soft soles. They disable the tendency of feet to go into pronation.
- Silicone full length soft soles or heel cups provide good pain relief and prefabricated ones are no inferior to custom made ones. Foot orthoses can reduce the strain in the plantar fascia during static loading, reduce the collapse of the medial longitudinal arch, and reduce elongation of the foot associated with pronation. The compliance is also good.
- Supportive arch taping (low-dye taping or calcaneal taping) may provide relief in first-step heel pain, but is inconsistent for long-term plantar fascia pain.

Injections

Corticosteroid injections have proven effective. Possible risks associated with corticosteroid injection include fat pad atrophy and plantar fascia rupture. The incidence of latter complication is too low to be really clinically significant, even if so then it produces fasciotomy (a method used for recalcitrant cases).

In recent years, other injectable options have also been used to treat plantar fasciitis.

- Percutaneous fenestration (dry needling) has been shown to reduce pain in as early as 4 weeks.
- Hyperosmolar dextrose (prolotherapy) using 25% dextrose/lidocaine solution
- Whole blood—Intralesional whole blood injections do not appear to be as effective as corticosteroid injections.
- Platelet-rich plasma—Platelet-rich plasma is produced via centrifuged autologous blood. The plasma collected is rich with platelets that release growth factors to stimulate healing in degenerative tissue. Currently, the use is at best controversial.
- Botulinum toxin-A (Botox) shown to relieve pain for as long as 14 weeks after injection.

Chronic Recalcitrant Plantar Fasciitis Treatment

After exhausting all options if the patients still do not respond for 6 months then the following alternative methods can be deployed as final salvage.

Extracorporeal Shock Wave Therapy

Extracorporeal shock wave therapy promotes neovascularization to aid in healing degenerative tissue found in plantar fasciitis. The result is, however, conflicting. Benefits are that it is noninvasive and offers the hope for a faster recovery time. The adverse effects of extracorporeal shock wave therapy are pain during and after the procedure, local swelling/ecchymosis and numbness with dysesthesia.

Plantar Fasciotomy

Plantar fasciotomy can be performed when all conservative measures have been ineffective. Both open and endoscopic methods (preferred by me) have been used. Disadvantages of surgery include incision care, immobilization, and potential complications (e.g., arch flattening, nerve injury, calcaneal fracture, and long recovery time).

POSTERIOR ANKLE IMPINGEMENT SYNDROME

(Posterior Block of Ankle, Posterior Triangle Pain, Talar Compression Syndrome, Os Trigonum Syndrome, Os Trigonum Impingement, Posterior Tibiotalar Impingement, Nut-cracker Type Syndrome)

Definition

A clinical disorder characterized by posterior ankle pain that occurs in forced plantar flexion due to a conglomerate of bony and soft-tissue pathologies. The condition is common as it incorporates a lot of etiologies so the incidence could be as high as 15–20% in clinical practice; however, due to lack of awareness, posterior ankle impingement syndrome (PAIS) is often misdiagnosed.

Etiology

The following conditions have been put into etiological classification of PAIS:

- Pathologies of talar posterolateral (trigonal) process **(Figs. 12A and B)**—acute fracture, chronic stress fracture, synchondrosis, true compression, impingement of the os trigonum against the posterior tibial plafond.
- Flexor hallucis longus tenosynovitis

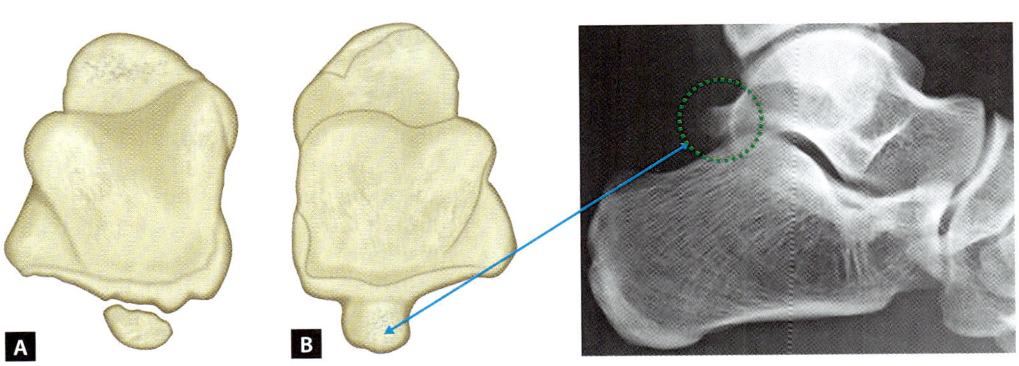

Figs. 12A and B: (A) Os trigonum fractured or separated and (B) fused as a process to talus (trigonal process). Radiograph depicting fused os trigonal process as seen in lateral view.

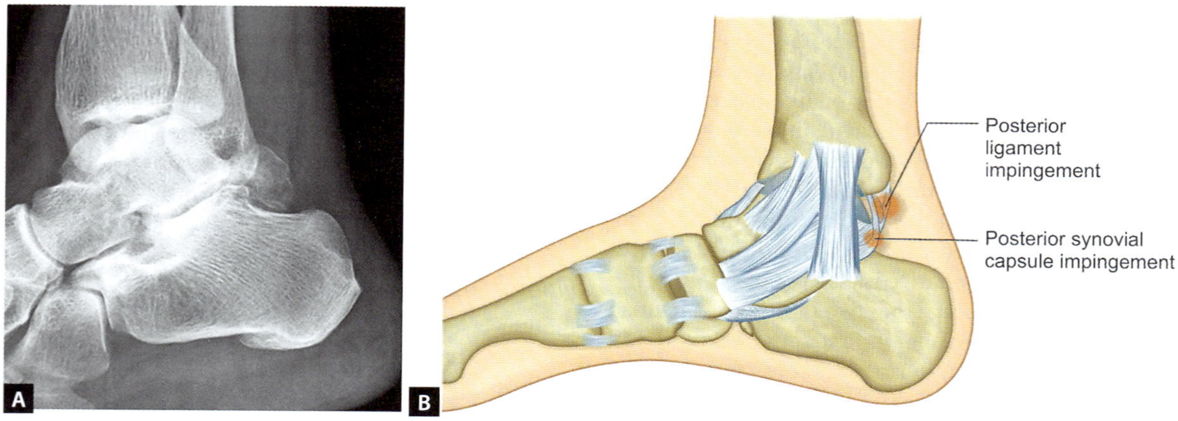

Figs. 13A and B: Other causes of PAIS. (A) Bone exostosis from the posterior talus; (B) Soft-tissue impingements and inflammation.

- Tibiotalar pathology—posterior capsuloligamentous injury/impingement **(Figs. 13A and B)**, osteochondritis, and fracture
- Subtalar pathology—osteochondritis and arthritis
- Calcified inflammatory tissue, prominent calcaneus posterior process
- Combination—FHL tenosynovitis and synchondrosis injury

Anatomy

The most important impact on the PAIS comes from posterior talar anatomy. Soft tissues behind the talus extending 4 cm above and below (in a curved line) the tip of lateral malleolus are mostly involved in the pathogenesis of PAIS. The posterior talar process protrudes posterior to the articular surface of the ankle joint. Extending both posteriorly and medially from the talus are the posteromedial process and posterolateral process. The posterolateral process is also named the trigonal process **(Figs. 12A and B**, most common cause of PAIS). A groove containing the FHL tendon divides these processes. If the posterolateral process remains as an ossicle separate from the talus, it is called the os trigonum. The os trigonum is a secondary ossification center of the talus that mineralizes between 7 and 13 years of age and fuses within 1 year, forming the Stieda process. The os trigonum may remain separate in 7–14% of patients **(Figs. 12A and B**, often bilaterally). The FHL tendon then runs in a sulcus medial to os trigonum.

Clinical Features

- The patient usually reports chronic or recurrent posterior ankle pain exacerbated by forced plantar flexion or push-off activities. Such activities include dancing, kicking, downhill running, and sliding and walking in shoes with high heels.
- Pathology of the trigonal process and os trigonum usually affects young, athletic individuals, such as ballet dancers, javelin throwers, and soccer players, whose activities involve forceful plantar flexion. It is characterized by pain and tenderness deep toward the Achilles tendon with symptoms exacerbated by forced plantar flexion of the foot.
- Dancers due to pain in the plantar flexion tend to assume a more inverted en pointe (sickling) position to decrease impingement. This increases loads on the anterior tibiofibular ligament, which thus predisposes the dancers to frequent ankle sprains.
- Symptoms of FHL tenosynovitis typically begin insidiously with pain and tenderness at the posteromedial ankle that may radiate distally along the medial arch. Swelling and crepitus may be present in acute cases. Osteochondral lesions of the talus produce nonspecific symptoms such as swelling, pain, catching, and locking.

Imaging Studies

- Lateral radiographs of ankle may show trigonal process fracture appearing as a triangular jagged structure. Old fractures will reveal fragment with smoothened edges. The impingement can be demonstrated on forced plantar flexed views.
- Bone scan always depicts increased uptake if the trigonal process has pathology. Normal bone scan virtually rules out trigonal process pathology.
- MRI is *the investigation of choice* for PAIS with its ability to differentiate bony and soft-tissue pathologies and its characterization **(Fig. 14)**.
- Osteochondral lesions of talus are best delineated by CT scans of the joint.

Treatment

- Initial treatment of the trigonal process disease includes rest, ice, compression, and elevation (RICE) and NSAIDs, and occasionally, casting for 4–6 weeks for patients who fail to respond to these conservative means. With subsidence of pain, physical therapy such as progressive resistive exercises and strengthening is begun. I prefer corticosteroid injection in patients who fail to respond within 1 week of beginning treatment or those who are virtually limping from day 1. This effectively provides temporary pain relief.

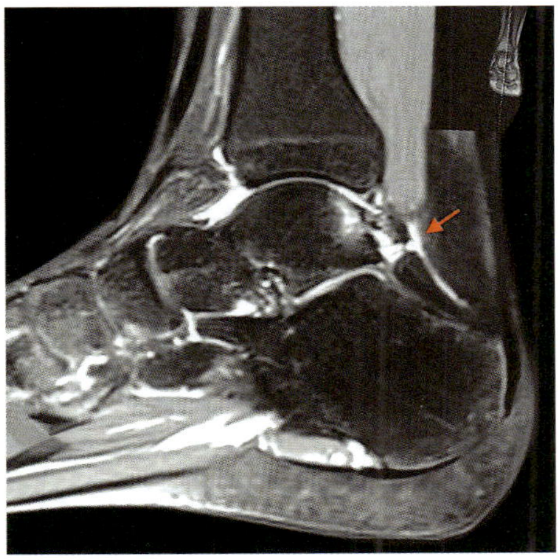

Fig. 14: MRI of a 17-year-old male with posterior ankle impingement syndrome revealing posterior talar process and partial body contusion with surrounding soft-tissue edema (arrow). There is also mild joint effusion.

- Treatment for FHL tenosynovitis consists of RICE and strapping of the foot supplemented with longitudinal arch supports placed in firm-sole shoes. The patient is better immobilized in a cast for 3 weeks if he/she has crepitus on palpation.
- With rigorous but failed conservative treatment, surgical excision of the fractured trigonal process or os trigonum is indicated. This can be done arthroscopically also.
- In patients with a concomitant or isolated nonresponsive FHL tenosynovitis, tendon sheath release is indicated. Stenosis of the fibro-osseous tunnel is released to relieve pain and/or triggering.

CONCLUSION

- Foot and ankle injuries are quite common in athletes.
- Achilles tendon is a frequent site of injury that may present as tendinosis or frank rupture/avulsion. Repair is imperative else the morbidity is unacceptable.
- Peroneal tendon dysfunction is another important aspect that should be suspected in all cases of lateral side leg and chronic calf pain.
- Bony injuries commonly present as pain from stress fractures that may occur at various sites though tibia is most commonly involved in athletes (dancers and military personnel have commonly stress fractures of less mobile second or third metatarsal bones).
- Plantar fasciitis is a common disorder that is usually managed conservatively.
- Posterior ankle impingement syndrome is an often missed finding in athletes complaining of posterior ankle pain during ankle movements. One needs to have proper knowledge of the disorder and high suspicion in order to make the diagnosis and treat the patients well.

CHAPTER 47

Sports Medicine: Hip and Thigh

Manish Kumar Varshney

INTRODUCTION

Involvement of the hip joint in sports persons is being increasingly recognized and specialty to treat the same effectively is fast evolving. The frame shift in recognizing hip pathologies emerging from sport injuries has come from increasing recognition of femoroacetabular impingement and its progression into osteoarthrosis primarily. The focus has also expanded to periarticular pathologies such as tendon pathologies, bursitis, periarticular impingement and nerve entrapments. Arthroscopy of hip joint has emerged as an important tool in managing hip pathologies now.

HIP ARTHROSCOPY: INDICATIONS AND PRINCIPLES

- Hip arthroscopy is the most expanding minimally invasive procedure in orthopedic practice. Among all arthroscopic procedures, hip arthroscopy developed latest in its indications and sophistication. The prime reasons for late development of the technique include:
    - Hip joint is enclosed in a compact soft tissue envelope unlike knee that limits the ease of introducing arthroscopic instruments.
    - The constrained nature of joint and depth of ball and socket's bony architecture are big impediments to an easy access and maneuverability of instrumentation.
- The capsule is quite tight and comparatively non-compliant resisting adequate distraction of the joint.
- The disorders of hip were not so finely recognized, and pathophysiology of most disorders treatable by arthroscopy has only recently been detailed.
- The procedure is cumbersome requiring fracture table and changeover of operating room (OR) setup rather than simpler open procedures that can be performed in side lateral positions.
- The instrumentations have to be extra-long, so discrete inventory is needed.

Brief Procedural Details

The procedure is usually done as an outpatient procedure and can be done in supine (preferred) or lateral position.

- *Supine* **(*Fig. 1*)**: Use a fracture table with lateralized perineal post to provide a transverse component to traction. Abduct hip 25° for proper traction vector **(Fig. 2)**. Adduction is used to improve path for screw fixation if needed. Flexion of hip is avoided as it brings sciatic nerve near and vulnerable to injury. Vacuum effect is seen in the joint with distraction that gets released with fluid insufflation.
- *Lateral position:* Here, the standard table is used with a custom distractor attached. Necessary changes are made in the position of monitor and instrument table to accommodate for this position.

Some Procedural Cautions

- Traction should be used for less than 2 hours, if more than that is needed then better time-out.

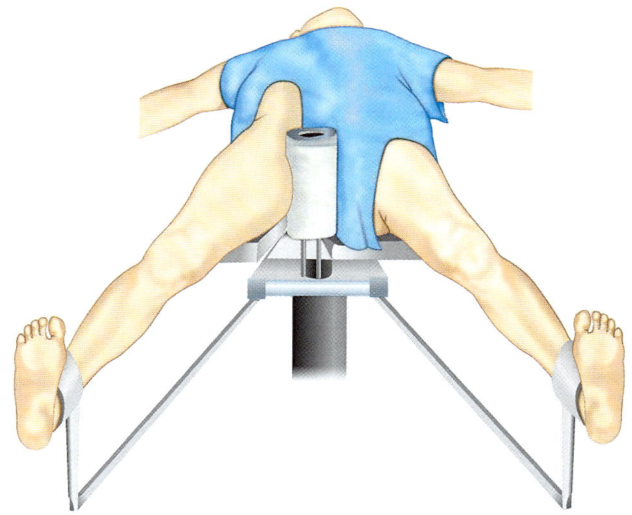

Fig. 1: Supine position: The peroneal post is lateralized to the operative side. The operative hip is placed in extension, approximately 25° abduction and neutral rotation.

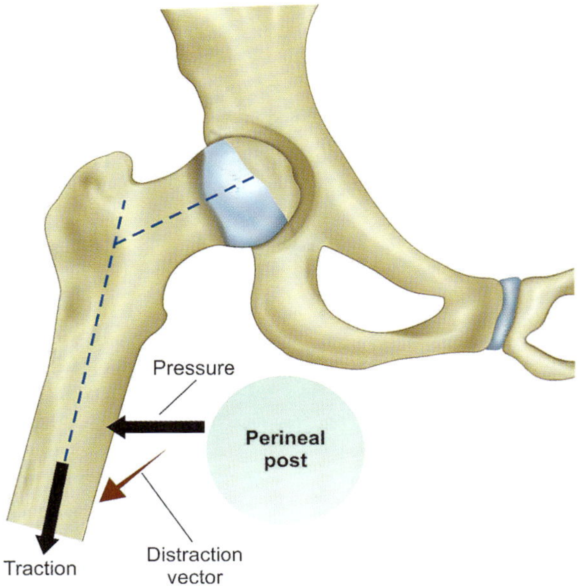

Fig. 2: Distraction of hip joint should be done obliquely that is partially aided by hip abduction and the small transverse component achieved by lateralizing the peroneal post.

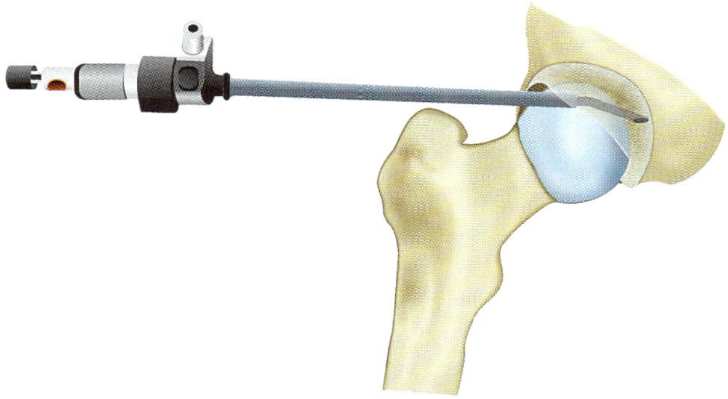

Fig. 3: Extra-length flexible cannula and extra-length curved shaver blade are essential for hip arthroscopy.

- Portals should be made lateral to anterior superior iliac spine (ASIS) sagittal line.
- Fluid pressure management should be a pressure between 40 and 60 mm Hg in a high-flow system.

Equipment

Equipment needed for hip arthroscopy include but is not limited to the following:

- 30° and 70° arthroscopes
- Fluid management system
- Extra-length cannulas **(Fig. 3)**
- Cannulated obturators and a sharp obturator
- Curved shaver blades passed through flexible cannulas **(Fig. 3)**
- Hand instruments for hip arthroscopy (laparoscopic instruments are fragile and break easily if ever used in hip arthroscopy).

Portals (Figs. 4 and 5)

Commonly for hip joint, two standard portals are enough if the distraction is adequate else three portals are needed; special portals for extra-articular procedures are not described here and the reader can refer dedicated text:

1. ***Anterior portal:*** Made at intersection of vertical line through ASIS and horizontal line across proximal margin of greater trochanter (skin incision is 4–6 cm distal to the ASIS). It passes through sartorius and rectus femoris. Protect lateral femoral cutaneous nerve (LFCN) and femoral nerve **(Fig. 6)**.
2. ***Anterolateral portal:*** The skin incision for this portal lies about 2 cm anterior to the anterosuperior edge of the greater trochanter. The path of this portal is not straight but instead the needle is directed about 10–20° cranially

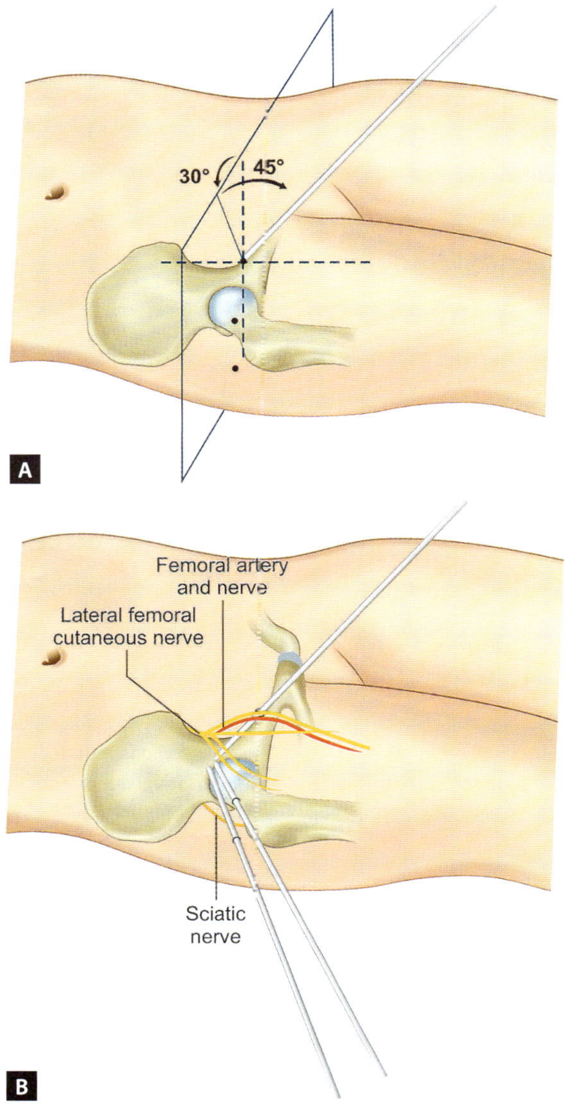

Figs. 4A and B: Anatomical landmarks guide portal positioning: The site of the anterior portal coincides with the intersection of a sagittal line drawn distally from the anterior-superior iliac spine and a transverse line across the superior margin of the greater trochanter. The anterolateral and posterolateral portals are placed as marked below (see text) with a distance of around an inch between them.

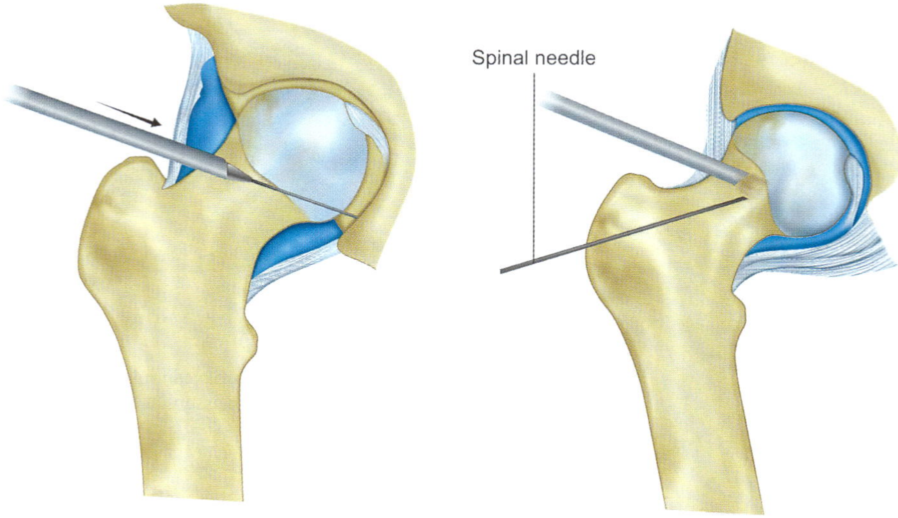

Fig. 5: Anterior and other portals are made over a spinal needle passed under guidance from arthroscope placed in the joint through the anterolateral portal.

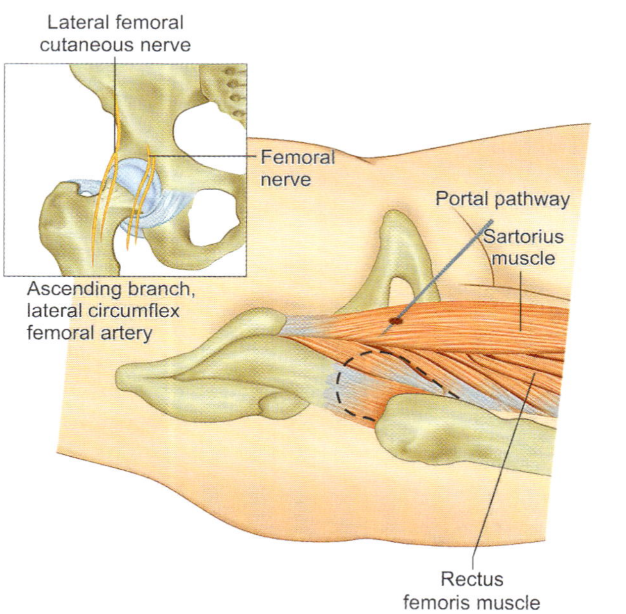

Fig. 6: Anterior portal pathway/relationship to lateral femoral cutaneous nerve, femoral nerve and lateral circumflex femoral artery.

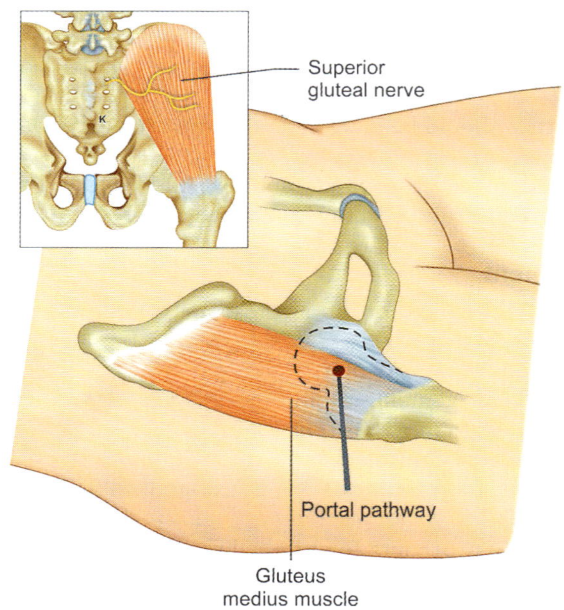

Fig. 7: Anterolateral portal pathway/relationship to superior gluteal nerve.

and 20-30° posteriorly. The portal is thus made through the gluteus medius and then at the anterior margin if femoral head. Protect the superior gluteal nerve **(Fig. 7)**. This is the first portal to be made as it lies in the "safe zone" and usually homes the scope.

3. ***Posterolateral portal:*** Penetrates gluteus medius and minimus anterosuperior to piriformis tendon. Protect the sciatic nerve **(Fig. 8)**.

Usually, the camera is placed through the anterolateral portal and other instruments are switched through the other portals **(Fig. 9)**.

Despite the limitations and procedural sophistications needed, advancements have now been made in the procedure and a lot of diseases are now amenable to be treated by arthroscopy. The current ***indications*** for hip arthroscopy include:

- *Loose bodies and osteochondromatosis:* This is probably the best indication as arthrotomy for same has significant morbidity and limited exposure.
- *Labral tears and femoroacetabular impingement:* Both cam and pincer type. Labral tears are often elusive and not fully characterized on even advanced diagnostic investigations. Arthroscopy serves in localization, debridement, confirming and repairing the tears. In addition, the chondral injuries can also be simultaneously addressed.

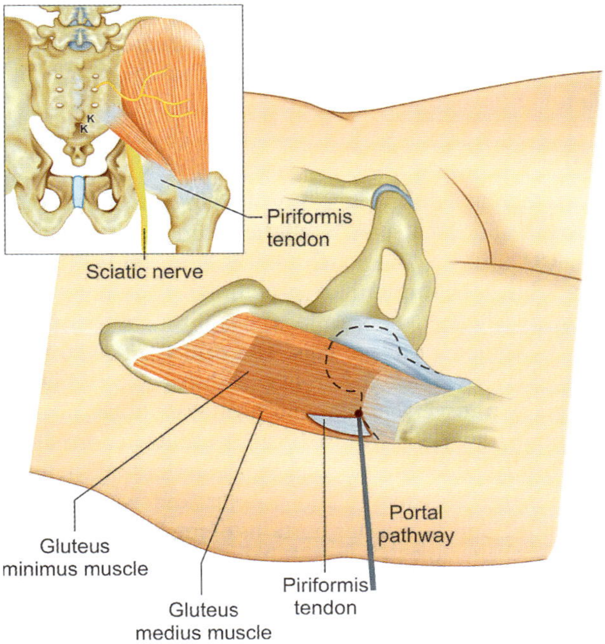

Fig. 8: Posterolateral portal pathway/relationship to sciatic nerve and superior gluteal nerve.

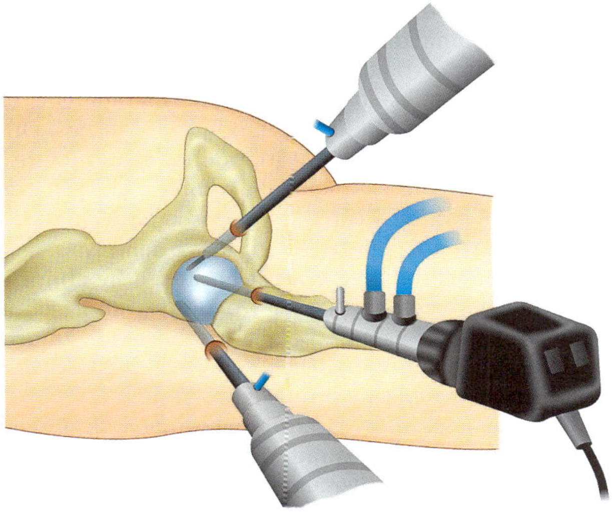

Fig. 9: Usual placement of instruments. The anterolateral is the common viewing portal.

- *Chondral injuries:* For a badly damaged surface that is bound to still damage more of the articular surface, it is better to remove the cartilage by debridement.

Other options for improving the viability are microfracture and repair. The last option is being developed and current modalities only serve to act as scaffolds as of now.

- *Synovial disease:* Synovial debridement is quite adequately performed arthroscopically.
- Joint sepsis
- Osteonecrosis
- *Early osteoarthritis [one may call this as advanced femoroacetabular impingement (FAI)]:* The pathology involves thickened labrum synovitis, labral degeneration, osteophytes, articular cartilage damage, geodes formation, loose bodies in the joint, etc.; arthroscopy in this context may at best be considered an interim measure (bridge technique). Patients undergoing this procedure must have 50% range of motion (ROM) and must have greater than 50% normal cartilage. The arthroscopic procedure comprises of partial capsulectomy (T-type along neck and rim for most patients or H-type for capsular plication) or capsulotomy only, acetabular rim trimming and cystectomy, notch osteophytectomy, labral refixation or grafting, microfracture for cartilage regeneration, head-neck osteoplasty, bone grafting defects and capsular repair or plication.
- Ruptured ligamentum teres
- Unresolved hip pain
- *Greater trochanteric pain syndrome (GTPS):* This involves a mix of unrelated entities like external hip snapping, trochanteric bursitis (arthroscopy is indicated for refractory cases not responding to medical treatment), gluteus medius or/and minimus tears. Release of the iliotibial band (ITB) endoscopically is an effective procedure for management of external snapping and trochanteric bursitis causing resolution in nearly 100% cases.
- *Deep gluteal syndrome:* This is due to sciatic nerve entrapment from any of the structures in the gluteal region (including piriformis—part of piriformis syndrome). The deep gluteal space is defined anteriorly by posterior acetabular column, capsule of hip joint and proximal femur, posteriorly by the gluteus maximus muscle, medially by sacrotuberous ligament and falciform fascia, laterally by lateral lip of linea aspera and gluteal tuberosity. Superiorly, it is bounded by inferior margin of the greater sciatic notch and inferiorly it extends to the attachments of hamstrings at ischial tuberosity. The four common sources of pain around the region include:
  1. Pain at the ischium is mostly due to hamstring problem or uncommonly by ischitis.
  2. Pain lateral and superior at the level of the external rotators or piriformis muscle along the sciatic tract—due to sciatic nerve entrapment.
  3. Pain lateral to the ischium is produced mostly from ischiofemoral impingement (see later) but also uncommonly from ischial tunnel syndrome.
  4. *Pain medial to the ischium (pudendal nerve entrapment):* The *pudendal nerve entrapment* is diagnosed by the diagnostic criteria laid down by Nantes as:
     - Pain is localized to the anatomical territory of pudendal nerve.
     - The pain is worsened by sitting.
     - Pain is *not* intense enough at night to wake the patient up.
     - There is no objective sensory impairment with pain.
     - Importantly, the pain is relieved by diagnostic pudendal nerve block.

The most common cause of deep gluteal syndrome is blunt trauma to buttock causing hematoma formation followed by scarring around the involved nerve(s) in the region of short external rotators and entrapment. This may also involve the region around hamstrings. Other causes of syndrome include irritation of the structures of the obturator internus/gemellus complex. The piriformis syndrome can be treated by endoscopic technique to release the tendon and or sciatic nerve neurolysis.

- *Ischiofemoral impingement:* It is caused by abnormal contact between the lesser trochanter and ischium causing compression of the quadriceps femoris muscle. There is groin pain or pain in buttock that radiates distally along the leg typically produced by combination of hip extension, adduction and external rotation. Endoscopic debridement of the quadratus femoris tendon with removal of the impingement lesion can be done.
- *Internal snapping:* Internal snapping of iliopsoas can be managed by endoscopic partial or complete iliopsoas release ± subtendinous bursectomy.
- Arthroscopically assisted computer-guided pelvic-acetabular osteotomy (PAO) is another option in future.

Contraindications

- Ankylosis or advanced arthrofibrosis
- Soft tissue compromise
- Bony compromise—either those precluding arthroscopy itself or those that prevent application of adequate distraction forces across the joint.
- Severe obesity
- Advanced destruction of hip.

ACETABULAR LABRAL TEARS

Traumatic tears of labrum were described first by Peterson in 1957 (associated with posterior dislocation of hip). Altenberg in 1977 reported first nontraumatic tears of the acetabular labrum and was the first one to describe torn labrum as a cause of pain. The improved awareness and role of the acetabular labrum in role hip pathologies have made their identification frequent.

Anatomy

The acetabular labrum is a rim of triangular fibrocartilage (in cross-section) that attaches to the perimeter of acetabulum **(Figs. 10A and B)**. The attachment is either direct (in outer thirds—direct continuum of structures) or indirect (inner two-thirds where the labrum attaches through intermediate zone of calcified cartilage; **Figs. 10A and B**). The labrum is absent inferiorly in the region of acetabular fossa where it is replaced by transverse acetabular ligament. Round, irregular and flattened shapes have also been identified in normal hips. The labrum is 2–3 mm thick with the posterior portion thicker and narrow compared to the thinner and wider anterior labrum. The anterosuperior portions of the labrum are richly innervated with pain, pressure, and deep touch sensitive fibers [Vater-Pacini corpuscles, Golgi-Mazzoni corpuscles, Ruffini corpuscles and articular (Krause) corpuscles]. The vascular supply is predominantly located in the outer thirds of the base of labrum that has dense connective tissue and is connected to joint capsule while the rest of it (inner two-thirds) in contact with intra-articular cartilage is largely avascular. The vascular supply is provided by superior, inferior gluteal and obturator vessels. The functions of acetabular labrum are:

- Provides structural resistance to lateral motion of the femoral head within the acetabulum
- Shock absorption
- Enhances joint stability—deepens the acetabulum for femoral head coverage by 21%
- Preserves joint congruity
- Distributes synovial fluid
- Pressure distribution—increases surface of acetabulum by 28% reducing point contact forces

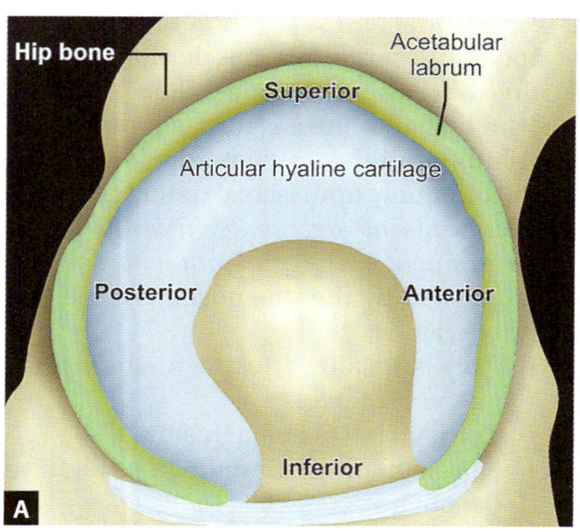

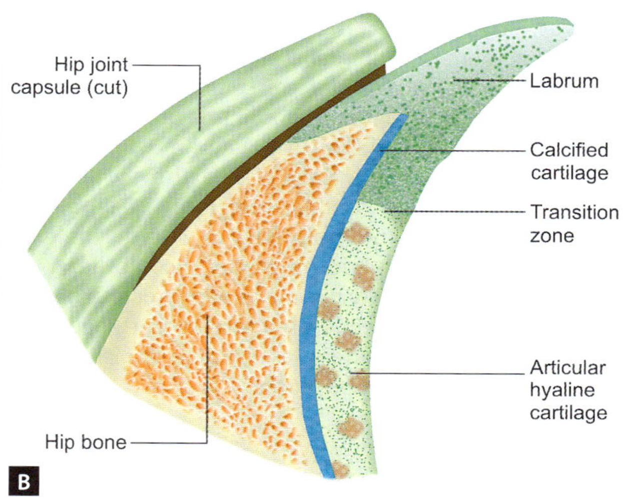

Figs. 10A and B: (A) Acetabular labrum is attached at the rim of acetabulum and is deficient in the inferior portion at the region of transverse acetabular ligament; (B) Cross-section of acetabular labrum and its attachment. On the nonarticular side of the bone, the labrum attaches directly to bone. On the articular side, the labrum attaches indirectly via zone of calcified cartilage. It also merges with the articular hyaline cartilage through a transition zone.

- *Maintaining seal around the femoral head (like a washer):* This increases the hydrostatic pressure of synovial fluid inside the joint preventing direct contact of femoral head and acetabulum at most places. Removing the labrum increases contact pressures by 92%.
- Proprioceptive feedback.

Pathophysiology

Tears in labrum leads to various biomechanical and physiological alterations in the hip joint:

- Loss of joint seal
- Altered pressure distribution causing increased load on cartilage—initiating degenerative process
- Altered femoral head movement in the hip joint causing aberrant movements and erosion of the cartilage
- Pain due to movements cause inhibition of the muscles around and weakness and increased instability.

Mechanism of Labral Tears and Classification

The mechanism of labral tearing can be either:

- ***Traumatic and acute:*** These are localized to one quadrant depending on the direction and extent of the trauma. Anterior tears are caused mostly by externally applied force to a hyperextended and *externally rotated* hip. External rotation activities or position of hip compromises the anterior capsular region causing impingement. Posterior labral tears occur in patients with a known posterior subluxation or dislocations. If a bone fragment is avulsed as a result of injury, it not only radiologically helps in identifying a dislocation, but also indicates that the lesion is often an isolated one occurring on capsular or peripheral region of the labrum. This tear is amenable to arthroscopic repair.
- ***Repetitive trauma-induced chronic damage:*** Repetitive loading of the hip as is seen in sports can cause labral damage by putting alternative tensile and compressive forces. This is especially seen in sports needing pivoting or twisting activities like football, basketball or ballet dancing.
- ***Chronic degenerative tears:*** Hip impingement is a harbinger for chronically loading anterosuperior labrum and producing degenerative tears in the labrum and underlying acetabular cartilage of that region. Femoroacetabular impingement causes minor repetitive trauma producing these anterior and more central tears.

Classification of Tears

The tears can be classified based on their morphology, etiology or location.

Tear ***classification by location*** is commonly used. The tear can be anterior, posterior or superior (some call it lateral also). The tear location can be better communicated in the form of clock face description **(Fig. 11)**. Fifty-five percent tears occur just between 3 o'clock and 12 o'clock position. Interestingly, the location of labral tears varies based on different regions. Americans have vast majority of tears located anteriorly caused by sudden pivoting or twisting motions while the Asian populations have tears located posteriorly caused by hyperflexion or squatting. The common anterior lesion is a "watershed lesion" (McCarthy) which is a combined anterior tear and anterior acetabular chondral injury.

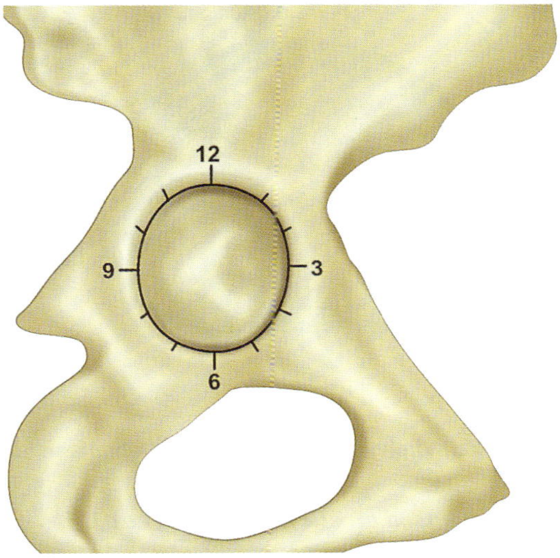

Fig. 11: Describing labral tears in terms of face of clock.

Cause of increased incidence of anterior labral tears:

- Reduced blood supply
- Mechanically weaker tissue for sudden forces Some patients have been found to have areolar tissue (weak tissue) at the inner aspect of the labrum (this might reflect a degenerative tissue due to pathological tears in long run)
- Higher prevalence of stress in this region than other parts of labrum due to less coverage of the femoral head in anterior compared to posterior region transferring loads on the labrum
- The chondrolabral transition is abrupt in anterior segment of labrum compared to posterior region making it more susceptible to tearing ("watershed" region of McCarthy).
- Cause of higher posterior location in Asian population is possibly due to habit of squatting and sitting on floor transferring loads posteriorly.

Classification by morphology (arthroscopic classification of Lage et al.; **Fig. 12**) is based on the knee meniscal injuries and following patterns (four) can be identified:

1. *Radial flap (smooth torn edges):* This is the most common type of tear that involves the free margins of labrum. Discrete contrast cleft is seen extending through the meniscus partially or wholly through the substance.
2. *Radial fibrillated (irregular torn edges):* There is irregularity of the labrum outline but no distinct cleft.
3. *Longitudinal peripheral:* They involve the acetabulum-labral junction and are of variable lengths. The contrast extends through the labrum at the junction between labrum and acetabulum.
4. Unstable (mobile) tears have no fixed pattern but frequently cause mechanical symptoms of buckling, clicking, catching or locking.

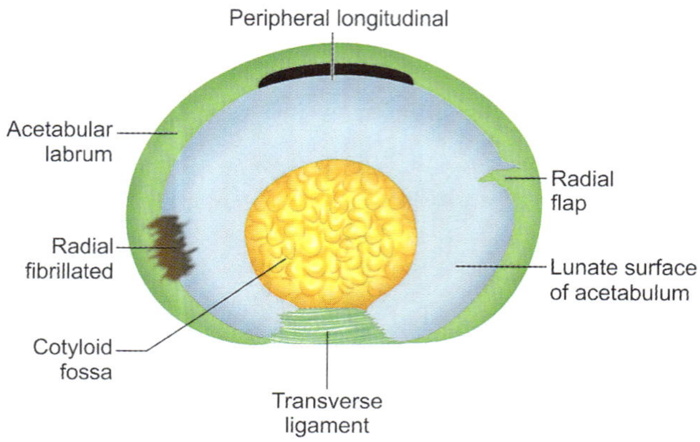

Fig. 12: Morphological classification of labral tears.

Classification based on etiology (Lage et al.):
- *Traumatic:* Clear history of trauma
- Congenital (acetabular dysplasia): Center-edge (CE) angle less than 25° or Tonnis angle greater than 10°
- *Degenerative:* The degenerative tears are further classified based on location and the extent of the tear. The extent of the labral degenerative tear correlates with the degree of degenerative changes in hip joint similar to meniscal changes seen in knee joint. Higher stage of degenerative labral tears (according to classification) correlates with erosive changes of hip joint cartilage.

  When examined arthroscopically or during open exploration of the hip, these lesions are often located adjacent to labral tear at the labrochondral junction supporting the theory that labral tears may initiate degenerative changes in the joint. The classification of degenerative tears is as follows:
  1. *Stage I:* The degenerative tears are localized to one of the segment in an anatomic region, anterior or posterior.
  2. *Stage II:* The degenerative tears involve an entire anatomic region.
  3. *Stage III:* The degenerative tears are diffuse and involve more than one anatomic region.
- Idiopathic

Histological classification of labral tears describes them into following types:
- *Type 1:* Labrum is detached from articular cartilage surface (at the cartilage labral transition zone). The tear can extend to even subchondral bone.
- *Type 2:* Variable depth cleavages of labrum extending within the substance of labrum.

Czerny classification (Fig. 13): This MRI based classification has high correlation with arthroscopic findings. It is based on a combination of labrum morphology, intralabral signals on imaging, presence of labral tear or labral detachment and the presence or absence of an adjacent perilabral recess on MRI. The labrum is graded as:
- *Stage 0:* Normal
- *Stage 1A:* Increased signal in the substance that does not extend to surface. Triangular shape is maintained with perilabral recess.

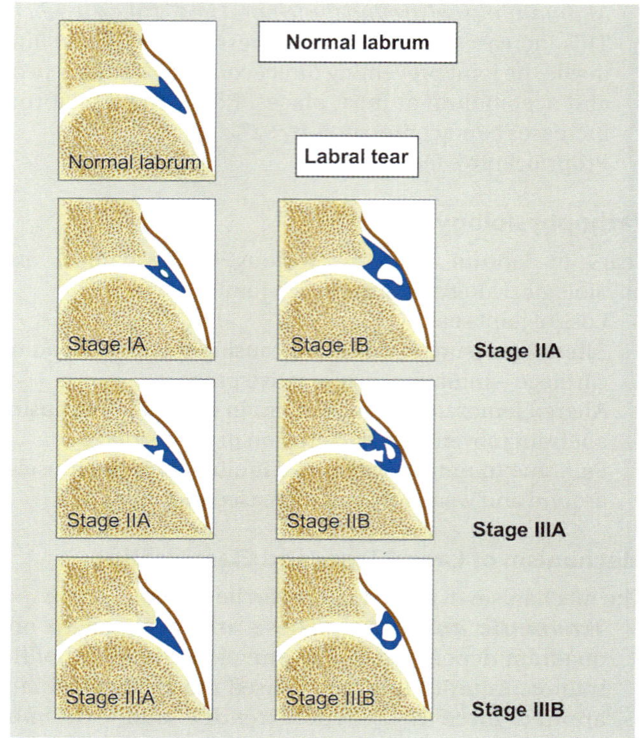

Fig. 13: MRI classification of labral tears (Czerny et al., 1996).

- *Stage 1B:* In addition to stage 1A, there is thickening of labrum and absent recess.
- *Stage 2A:* Contrast extends into labrum but no detachment is seen. Normal shape and recess.
- *Stage 2B:* As for 2A but with thickened labrum and absent recess
- *Stage 3A:* Detachment of labrum; normal shape
- *Stage 3B:* Detached and thickened labrum.

Etiology

Labral pathology is frequently associated with osseous pathology in most of the cases. The etiological factors can be grouped into following types:
- *Trauma:* High-velocity motor vehicle injuries, subluxation, dislocation, falls.
- *Capsular laxity:* Redundant capsules, hypermobility syndromes, hormonal influence, etc.
- *Biomechanical imbalance:* For instance, the "lower crossed syndrome". This is a tightness of hip flexors and lumbar erector spinae associated with weak gluteal and abdominal muscles. These cause muscular imbalance leading to anterior pelvic tilt and hip flexion posture with a hyperlordosis of the lumbar spine. There is increased stress concentration on the anterior acetabulum/labrum causing respective tear.
- *Dysplasia [**Figs. 14A and B**; shallow acetabulum (CE angle <25°; **Fig. 15**), increased femoral anteversion, acetabular retroversion, reduced femoral offset **(Fig. 15)**]:* Slipped upper femoral epiphysis (SUFE), Legg-Calvé-Perthes disease (LCPD), developmental dysplasia of the hip (DDH).
- Age-related degeneration

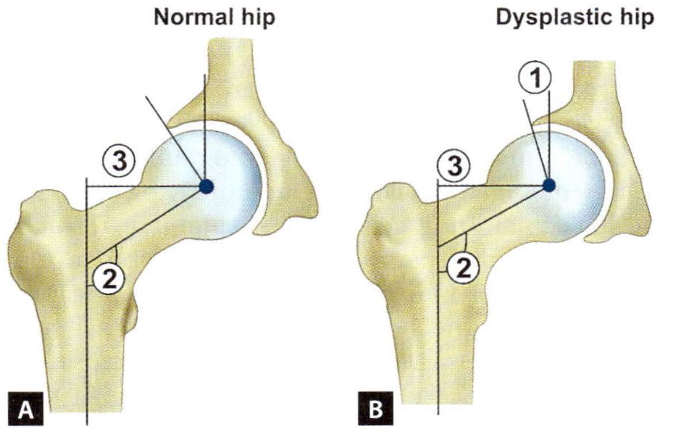

Figs. 14A and B: (A) Normal hip; (B) Dysplastic hip. (1) Center- edge angle of Wiberg (see text) the angle reduces in dysplasia and angle of less than 30° is seen in undercoverage of hip, e.g. developmental dysplasia of hip; (2) Neck-shaft angle or the angle of inclination is reduced in coxa vara and increases in coxa valga; and (3) Head center offset—the distance between center of femoral head and the shaft. It is decreased in coxa breva and dysplastic small neck.

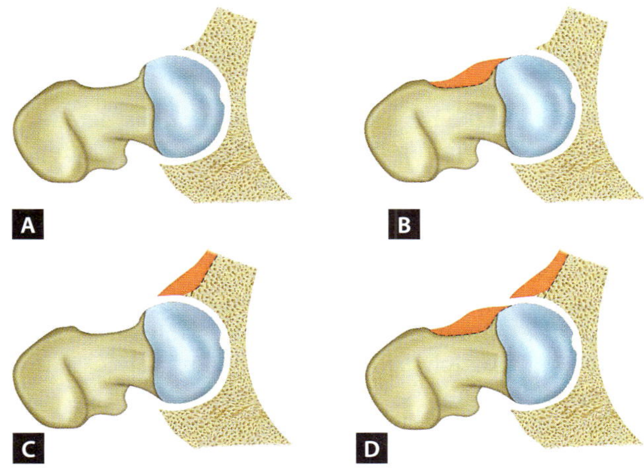

Figs. 16A to D: Femoroacetabular impingement (FAI) morphology. (A) A normal hip; (B) Cam-type impingement; (C) Excessive anterior overcoverage of the femoral head (pincer-type impingement); (D) Combination of cam and pincer types of impingement.

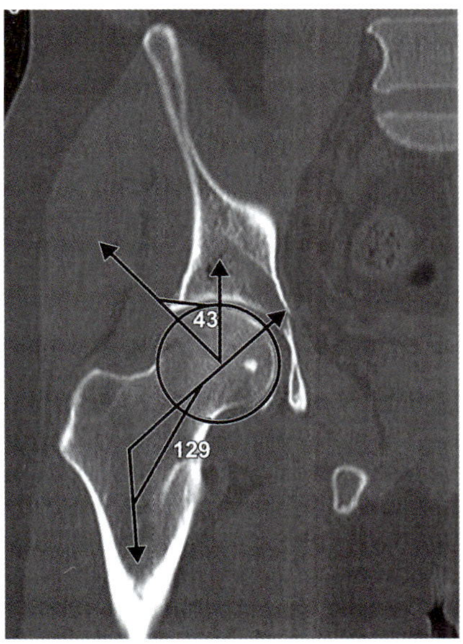

Fig. 15: Demonstration of method of measuring the CE angle and the angle of inclination of the neck (neck-shaft angle), both normal in this case.

- *Femoroacetabular impingement:* Most common in younger population, especially the cam type **(Figs. 16A to D)** causes anterosuperior lesions and pincer type **(Figs. 16A to D)** causes peripheral or circumferential lesions.
- *Idiopathic:* Often in athletes (though they have some or other cause that we are unable to identify still). Most of these have FAI indeed.

Natural History

Due to minimal penetration of vessels in labral tissue, the healing potential is minimal. No area has the potential for spontaneous repair, but some authors have found potential for neovascularization coming from capsule and hence possible healing. Vascularity is seen in the peripheral one-third of the labrum similar to knee meniscus "red zone". The inner two-thirds of the labrum are hitherto avascular (again akin to knee meniscus "white zone"). Logically for acetabular labrum also peripheral tears will have potential to heal and debridement of the tear and repairs should be considered; the problem only is finding such rare tears! McCarthy et al. strongly suggested that labral tears are harbinger of degenerative disease of the hip in the long run. An association between progression of labral lesions to progression of anterior acetabular articular cartilage lesions has been found but causal relationship is not fully established still. Currently, the labral disruptions and degenerative joint disease are considered to represent a continuum.

Clinical Features

Tears have been reported in patients as young as 8 years to as old as 75 years.

The patients present often with nonspecific findings like dull pain that is often induced by activity seen in particular positions (that might impinge the damaged cartilage) and commonly fails to respond to rest. Trigger for these symptoms or a definite inciting event is not commonly identified, so there is a history of patients being seen by multiple healthcare workers for groin pulls, muscle strains or hip contusions before being finally diagnosed as having labral tear ultimately. The average delay in diagnosis is around 2 years.

Most patients have anterior hip or groin pain. Symptomatic labral tears occur more frequently in women than in men. Less common sites of pain are deep buttock region, lateral pain, pain radiating to knee. Buttock pain is common with posterior tears while groin pain is more consistent with anterior tears. Pain is usually constant and dull aching with intermittent sharp episodes that worsen with activity. Walking, pivoting, prolonged sitting, and impact activities aggravate symptoms. Rest does not fully relieve pain and three-fourths patients describe night pain interfering sleep.

Other symptoms are clicking (most common), locking or catching, or giving way. Hip instability is also reported.

Physical Examination

The findings of various tests are inconsistent due to variable location of the tears.

- Rotations of the hip are commonly found restricted.
- *Positive anterior hip impingement sign:* This is often the most consistent finding. With the patient supine and the hip and knee in 90° flexion, the hip is internally rotated along with and adducting the thigh. This maneuver produces anterior groin pain.
- *Posterior impingement test:* Patient is positioned prone and the examiner extends, externally rotates and adducts the thigh which produces posterior pelvic pain or anterior hip pain.
- *Thomas test:* Here, both hips are put in flexion, followed by maneuver of abduction and extension of the involved hip. A palpable or audible click along with pain is felt/heard in a positive Thomas test.
- *McCarthy test:* Here again, both hips are flexed as for Thomas test above. The affected hip is then extended, first in external rotation followed by extension in internal rotation. Hip extension in internal rotation typically puts the anterior labrum at stress while hip extension in external rotation will similarly stress the posterior labral pathology causing pain in respective maneuvers.
- Resisted straight leg raise test (SLRT) (Stinchfield test)
- Patrick test/flexion, abduction and external rotation (FABER) test
- Log-Roll test
- Apprehension test

Investigations

Radiographs are often unremarkable and serve as a screening tool for hip dysplasia (DDH, LCPD). Both anteroposterior (AP) and cross-table lateral views (or Dunn view) should be obtained. Findings that suggest FAI include:

- Signs of dysplasia **(*see* Fig. 14)**
- Subtle irregularities in superior aspect of femoral neck **(Figs. 17A and B)**
- Small femoral head-neck offset **(Figs. 17A and B)**—cam type impingement
- Decreased neck concavity compared to the contralateral side which would suggest impingement.

Other abnormalities found on radiographs include: coxa profunda (medial wall of the acetabulum lying on, or medial to the ilioischial line), coxa valga, acetabular retroversion and presence of degenerative changes. Acetabular retroversion is identified on radiographs from the following findings:

- The anterior and posterior walls of the acetabulum are seen to cross over the femoral head ("crossover" or "figure-of-eight" sign; **Fig. 18**)—pincer type FAI
- *The ischial sign:* Ischial spine is visible on the AP pelvic radiograph **(Fig. 18)**.
- *The posterior wall sign:* Posterior acetabular wall shadow is medial to the center of the femoral head **(Fig. 18)**.

Computed tomography scans are limited in their utility to diagnose or identify the labral tears and should not be prescribed. *MRI* themselves are also limited in diagnostic

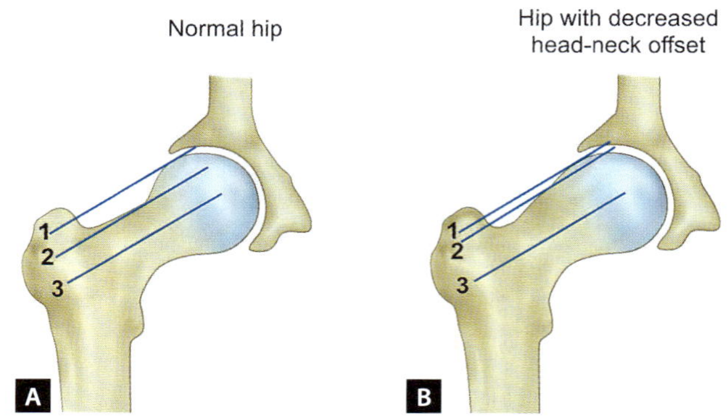

Figs. 17A and B: Femoral head-neck offset. This offset represents the distance between the tangent to most superior aspect of the femoral head (line 1) and the tangent to femoral neck (line 2). Line 2 is drawn parallel to a line across the center of femoral neck (line 3). The distance between line 1 and line 2 is the femoral head neck offset. Reduced head neck offset reduces the clearance of femoral head from acetabular neck.

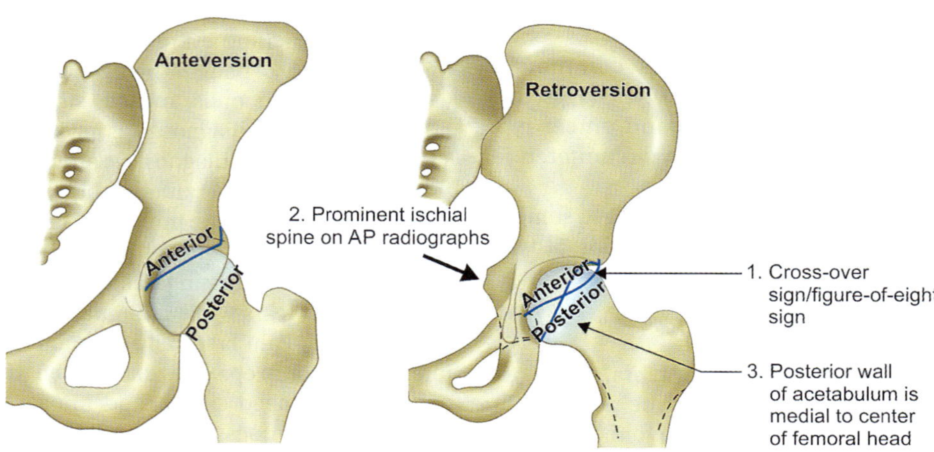

Fig. 18: The three signs of acetabular retroversion. (1) The anterior and posterior walls cross forming a figure-of-eight; (2) The ischial spine is prominent on AP film; (3) The posterior acetabular wall is medial to femoral head center. Schematic diagram of AP radiograph is provided on the left side for reference.

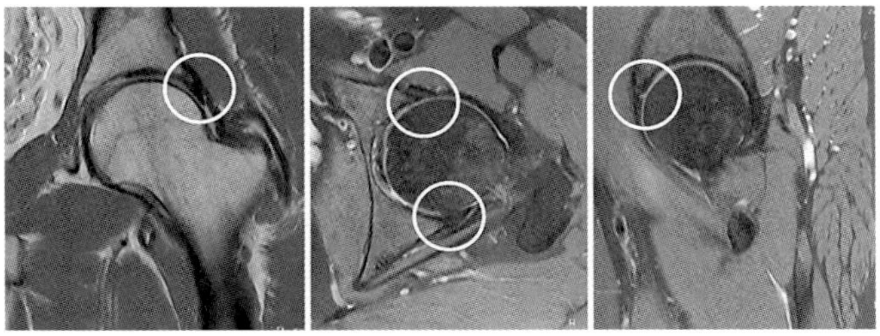

Fig. 19: MRI morphology of normal labrum (circled).

capability for labral tears and have only 30% sensitivity and 36% diagnostic accuracy. The normal appearances of labrum on MRI are depicted in **Figure 19**.

Contrast-enhanced ***MR arthrography*** is more sensitive than standard MRI at detecting intra-articular lesions of the hip with 95% and 88% sensitivity and specificity. Posterior tears are less effectively identified; the diagnostic accuracy increases after joint distension that causes the contrast to fill and outline tears more definitely. The procedure is performed in two stages: First, fluoroscopically guided hip arthrography performed through anterior approach. The joint is distended using diluted (2.5 nM) gadopentetate dimeglumine (by mixing 0.1 mL of contrast to 20 mL saline). The hip joint space is around 8–20 mL and is completely distended. In the second stage, MRI is performed using recommended protocols. The diagnostic criteria for identifying the labral tears are intrasubstance contrast material, labra with irregular margins with and without labral detachments. Labral detachment is identified by contrast material interposed at the labral-acetabular interface with or without displacement. Cartilage lesions are identified by the contrast material filling the area normally occupied by articular cartilage.

Magnetic resonance arthrograms, however also have 8% false-negative rate and a 20% false-positive interpretation for all types of intra-articular pathology of the hip, so a cautious interpretation is advised. False positives can be avoided by knowing the anatomical location of sulci in the labrum that are often reported wrongly as tears:

- Perilabral sulci/recess, which are located at the labrocapsular junction on the capsular surface of the labrum.
- Labroligamentous sulcus—sulcus created by the junction of the transverse ligament and the labrum
- Sulcus located at the posteroinferior aspect of the joint which is a normal variant.

"Acetabular rim syndrome" has been defined for DDH where two types of anatomical abnormalities are identified.

- In type 1, the acetabulum is shallow and the femoral head and acetabulum are incongruent.
- In type 2, the acetabular roof is short but the acetabulum and femoral heads are congruent.

In type 1, there is increased abnormal stress distribution on the labrum causing hypertrophy and separation. In type 2, the acetabular rim is stressed and fails with fatigue fracture forming os acetabuli.

Newer MR imaging modalities such as fast spin echo have improved the imaging capability of articular cartilage and may obviate the need for intra-articular arthrogram.

Tc-99 bone scintigraphy and single photon emission tomography (SPECT) have been reported to be of value in interpreting the labral tears. The patients show a characteristic pattern of increased uptake in the superior aspect of the acetabulum. The modality still needs full evaluation before concrete application.

Diagnostic hip injections are most reliable minimally invasive method for clearing a doubt with regards intra-articular origin of pain. These injections have 88% sensitivity and 100% specificity for localizing any groin pain emanating from hip joint structures.

Hip arthroscopy is the new gold standard for not only diagnosing but also treating patients with hip pain due to intra-articular pathology and mechanical symptoms. This is favored in many dedicated centers due to the additional advantage of treating various pathologies simultaneously.

Management

There should always be a trial of conservative therapy directed at unloading the tear, improving hip stability and muscle mass along with symptomatic relief to the patient. The therapy should be given for 6–10 weeks before labeling it ineffective. The general course includes rest, anti-inflammatory medications and focused physiotherapy (PT) protocol. Acute flares can be managed by intra-articular steroids. Intra-articular steroids are more effectively advised in patients with degenerative changes. Focused PT consists of:

- Reducing anteriorly directed forces on the hip
- Controlling abnormal patterns of recruitment of muscles
- Limiting pivoting motions
- Strengthening the identified inhibited muscles by weight-bearing exercises, proprioception enhancement, etc.

Surgical Intervention

The decision to proceed with operative intervention should be heavily weighted on refractory, mechanical symptoms not responding to aggressive, directed PT.

Excision of labrum is now abandoned unless the tear is extensively damaged beyond repair and causing symptoms. It can be done as an additional procedure in patients with acetabular dysplasia where some containment procedure is planned for improving coverage of the head of femur simultaneously.

The majority of labral tears are treated by ***debridement***; however, some tears are amenable to arthroscopic repair. Debridement is relied upon to remove the unstable flap tears, free fragments, loose bodies and microfracture of chondral lesions to relieve symptoms. Debridement of the joint has its rationale, labral tears, idiopathic, traumatic or degenerative in nature, can progress to articular cartilage delamination beside the labral lesions and further chondral damage and joint degeneration (see natural history earlier).

Therefore, treatment of patients with underlying labral pathology not only relieves the symptoms but its proponents also advocate additional possibility of preventing or limiting the possibility development of degenerative joint disease (at least potentially postpone it) that may develop from the mechanical effect.

Debridement can be performed open or arthroscopically.

For arthroscopic approach, the following points should be noted:

- Use a large peroneal post with good soft padding to minimize injury to pudendal nerve
- Adequate distraction of the femoral head from acetabulum helps in fully visualizing the articular surfaces
- Anterior portal is preferably made under fluoroscopic guidance to avoid injury to cartilage or labrum
- Labrum and labrocapsular junction should be probed (and not just inspected) to rule out detachment to the acetabular rim
- Additional procedures that can be performed with standard arthroscopic debridement include:
    - Capsulorrhaphy for redundant capsule
    - Debriding the ligamentum teres in cases of hypertrophy or identified tears
    - Synovectomy
    - Femoral or acetabular osteoplasty in FAI
    - Iliopsoas release
    - ITB release
    - Bursectomy
    - Addressing gluteus medius tendonitis
- The centrally based articular tears and degenerative tears of femoral head or acetabulum are debrided with the prime goal of relieving pain and associated mechanical symptoms while simultaneously preserving healthy portions of the cartilage and labrum.
- The patient outcomes are better for isolated labral lesions without concomitant degenerative (cartilage) joint disease.

Postoperative protocol includes the same focused protocol mentioned above beginning as soon as the patient can bear pain. Weight-bearing is also recommended to begin as early as possible after debridement. Prophylaxis for deep vein thrombosis (DVT) and heterotopic ossification should be begun and given for 2 weeks. The physiotherapy is continued for a minimum of 6 weeks. Active hip flexion is usually limited for 3–4 weeks to prevent tendonitis. The following activities should be restricted:

- Walking with knee or hip in hyperextension—increases anterior joint forces
- Recumbent bicycling—entails too much of hip flexion than permitted
- *Avoid sitting:*
    - With knee lower than hips
    - Cross-legged
    - On the floor
    - On the edge of seat
- Avoid pushing or rotating the pelvis on a loaded femur while getting off car seat or getting up from chair.

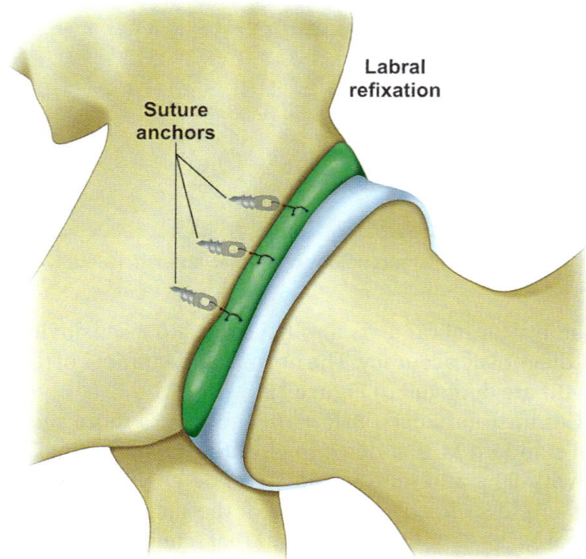

Fig. 20: Fixation of labrum using suture anchors.

In general, whether open or arthroscopic, the treatment is effective in a majority of patients. ***Repair of labrum*** is amenable only in the peripheral tears **(Fig. 20)** where potential vascularity exists. However, such tears are rarely found. To repair labrum, first determine if there is adequate substance. Then detach the labrum with an arthroscopic knife (no need in small tears). Next trim the acetabular rim to create smooth surface for seating labrum and improve vascularity. One must take care for resecting the margin as too much trimming would reduce the CE angle. The change in CE angle due to arthroscopic trimming can be estimated from the formula:

$$\textit{Change in CE angle} = 1.8 + (0.64 \times \text{rim reduction in mm})$$

Unstable rim fragments are removed. Anchor is placed 2–3 mm below the articular cartilage. Determine the rim angle at this point to safely place the anchors. Loop the suture around the torn labrum or pierce it through (if there is adequate tissue); the latter tends to invert the labrum while loop sutures tend to evert the labrum rebalancing the suction mechanism. Once the whole labrum is stabilized on the rim, judge the impingement. If there is impingement from a cam mechanism, then it also should be resected. Capsulotomy is closed. Some surgeons tend to inject PRP-plasma both in the joint and repaired tissue to prevent arthrofibrosis and enhance repair healing respectively.

Labral avulsions are common and refixation should be promptly considered to maintain the femoral head coverage. Suture anchors are used to refix the labrum if the labrum is detached from its extra-articular osseous insertion. Acetabular retroversion can be corrected by either trimming the acetabular rim (absence of posterior wall sign; see radiology above) or reverse periacetabular osteotomy (positive posterior wall sign).

Complications of Hip Arthroscopy

- *Hip derangements (often transient):* Pain, nonspecific swelling and inflammation, joint stiffness or heaviness sensation, reduced muscle strength and endurance and altered position sense (proprioception)

- Deep vein thrombosis
- *Neurovascular damage:* These are uncommon but result from neglecting attention to detail. The at-risk bundles are superior gluteal neurovascular bundle and the femoral neurovascular bundle while the most commonly reported nerve injured is LFCN. Sciatic and pudendal bundles may be injured indirectly due to traction.
- Articular cartilage damage

FEMOROACETABULAR IMPINGEMENT (ACETABULAR RIM SYNDROME, CERVICOACETABULAR IMPINGEMENT)

Definition

The term is itself descriptive of an early pathological contact between the bony prominences of the acetabulum and femur that mechanically limits the physiologic movements of hip producing pain at the extremes of hip range of motion. The most readily identifiable FAI is the pathological early contact of anterior acetabular rim with femoral neck causing "anterior impingement" that typically restricts hip flexion and internal rotation movements. This has been the commonly taught form of hip impingement to students. In fact, there are various other forms of impingement that can be also appraised from definition which does not limit itself to only the anterior impingement. So, anteroinferior FAI is commonly seen in a valgus hip, superior impingement is seen in varus hip, likewise global impingement results in protrusio hip and so on. This entails the fact that FAI is by itself not an entity (it is a disorder of hip movements) rather a conglomerate of various "modes" that restrict the complete hip range of movement ultimately leading to painful arthritis in a common pathomechanism. For FAI to occur two requirements need to be fulfilled—motion at the hip and pathomorphology (i.e., altered morphology). First requirement is imperative as without movement impingement would not occur and it is seen that in some circumstances even without and altered morphology of the hip joint, impingement would occur if the demands of hip movements are in extremes as would occur in ballet dancers. Otherwise in common practice, the commonly encountered forms of impingement are due to altered morphology of the hip. The most discretely recognizable forms of hip pathomorphology are the *cam*-type and the *pincer*-type that will be discussed in detail here.

Impingement of the hip is not at all a new concept with estimated prevalence of 10–15%. Open cheilectomy of the femoral head has long been done as a salvage procedure for painful restricted motion associated with the late sequel of Legg-Calvé-Perthes disease and slipped capital femoral epiphysis (SCFE). The concept of FAI has been proposed by Ganz and others, so it was quite known to the orthopedic population. Per se, the phenomenon of impingement was first recognized as an iatrogenic complication seen with overcorrection of aggressive periacetabular osteotomy (PAO) performed for dysplasia. Only the disorder (FAI) as a native cause of osteoarthritis was linked later and is quite in vogue now. This may yield as a significant percentage of patients previously categorized as idiopathic. As mentioned earlier femoral neck impingement against the acetabular labrum results from structural abnormality of either or both of the opposing surfaces coming "early" in contact that produces chronic hip pain and subsequent acetabular labral degenerative tears. Repetitive microtrauma resulting from impingement of femoral neck against acetabular labrum produces initially traumatic lesions of labrum that degenerate later presenting as degenerative joint disease. Clinically and radiologically, two types of FAI have been classified **(Figs. 21A to C)** though most patients have a mixture of both:

- *Cam FAI impingement* is due to femoral cause and is due to an aspherical portion of the femoral head-neck junction. This asphericity of femoral head may arise from various causes like growth disturbance, LCPD (Legg-Calve-Perthes disease), missed SUFE (Slipped upper femoral epiphysis) or subsequent to trauma. There are two prominent morphological features of femoral head that can produce a cam impingement:
  1. Commonly cam impingement is due to a "pistol grip" deformity (decreased femoral head-neck offset on the

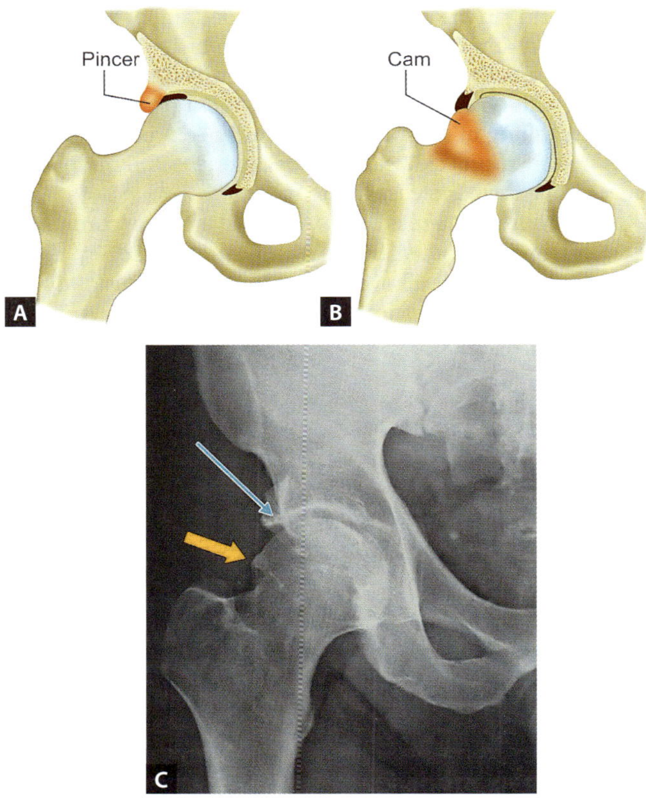

Figs. 21A to C: Two types of femoroacetabular impingement (FAI). Pincer lesion is seen over the lips of acetabulum (A) while the cam lesion is seen as a bump in femoral neck (B). Radiograph showing the cam lesion in femoral neck (bold arrow) and pincer lesion (small arrow) in the acetabulum (C).

superior or anterolateral region; **Fig. 22**) of the femoral neck. The reduced offset of head-neck junction in the anterolateral region hampers joint clearance; this is marked especially in hip joint adduction and flexion range of movements. Impingement causes repetitive abutment of superior femoral neck along the acetabular rim in flexion, exaggerated in variable degree of adduction and internal rotation causing damage to the labrum in anterosuperior quadrant.

2. The other significant cause of cam impingement is due to bony abnormalities of the anterior and lateral femoral head/neck junction. Commonly, this morphological aberration expresses itself as a variable thickness "bump" or exuberant bone that arises in the anterosuperior region of the femoral neck producing the classic anterior impingement but lateral femoral neck and rarely posterior "bumps" are also seen. Bony prominence in these area results in a "nonspherical" femoral head. A cam effect occurs with flexion, as this nonspherical head is forced into the acetabulum. As this aspherical portion squeezes itself in the acetabulum the motion is slowed and hence a subtle stop is appreciated clinically. The pathological bump stretches out and pushes the labrum peripherally while the articular cartilage is pushed centrally producing "chondrolaberal separation". The resultant pathology is selective articular breakdown with lesser degrees of associated labral tearing in the anterior-superior quadrant of the labrum in an anterior impingement. The articular surface is essentially peeled away from its articulolabral junction by this bony prominence as it pushes up inside the joint resulting in delamination of cartilage producing flaps. The femoral side cartilage degenerates and underlying bone there increases in density.

- *Pincer impingement* is due to acetabular cause (commonly a retroverted acetabulum)—characterized by focal (anterior) or general overcoverage (as in protrusio hip) of the femoral head as in retroverted acetabulum. Anterior pincer impingement is attributed to a bony lip of the anterior acetabulum. With flexion of the hip, the labrum becomes entrapped between the acetabular lip and the anterior neck of the femur. This impingement produces a sudden stop in hip range of motion testing appreciated clinically as opposed to gentle stop of cam FAI. If the anterior stop occurs too early there could be a tendency for the posterior subluxation and posteroinferior cartilage to delaminate producing "contrecoup lesion". The principal lesion is labral tear and deterioration with secondary articular breakdown.

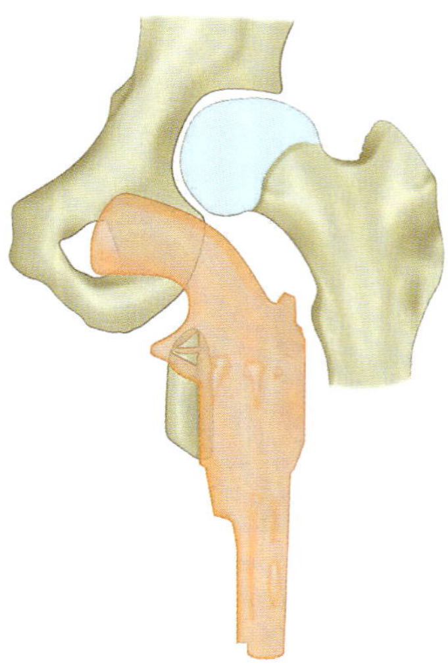

Fig. 22: The pistol-grip neck deformity.

Etiology, Pathophysiology and Natural History of Disease

Several theories exist to explain FAI but the inciting event is elusive.

- *Cam impingement:* The pistol-grip neck deformity could represent a form of mild or subclinical SUFE/SCFE or Perthes disease. Nonspherical head with a wide neck result from growth disturbance of the proximal femur. These patients have increased physeal extension into the cranial hemisphere of the femoral head neck suggesting that growth abnormality of the femoral head physis possibly results in decreased head-neck offset developmentally in anterolateral FAI. The cam impingement can be mechanically understood by mismatch between the radius of curvature of the femoral head/neck and the acetabulum where the former exceeds the latter. This discrepancy may be also compounded by reduced head–neck offset further intensifying the effect. The cam deformity is radiologically quantified by measurements of offset-ratio, alpha and beta angles on X-ray or MRI **(Fig. 23)**. With the rotation of higher profile head-neck portion into acetabulum, the labrum is displaced outward tearing the chondrolabral junction and producing type 1 tear at the watershed (See labral tears earlier). This traction force produces flap tears or carpet lesions in the cartilage. Further rotation and migration of the head-neck region into acetabulum causes chondral damage and producing the "wave sign" seen at arthroscopy.
- Pincer impingement may be due to deep socket [coxa profunda, protrusio acetabuli **(Figs. 24A to C)**; *See* Chapter on "Protrusio Acetabuli" for details], bony build-up

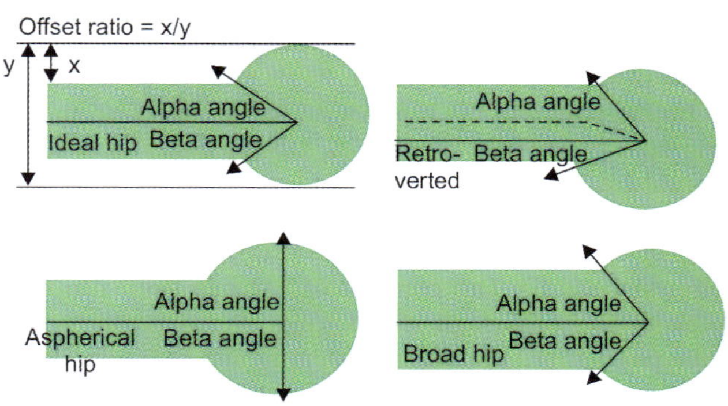

Fig. 23: Measures of cam impingement on MRI.

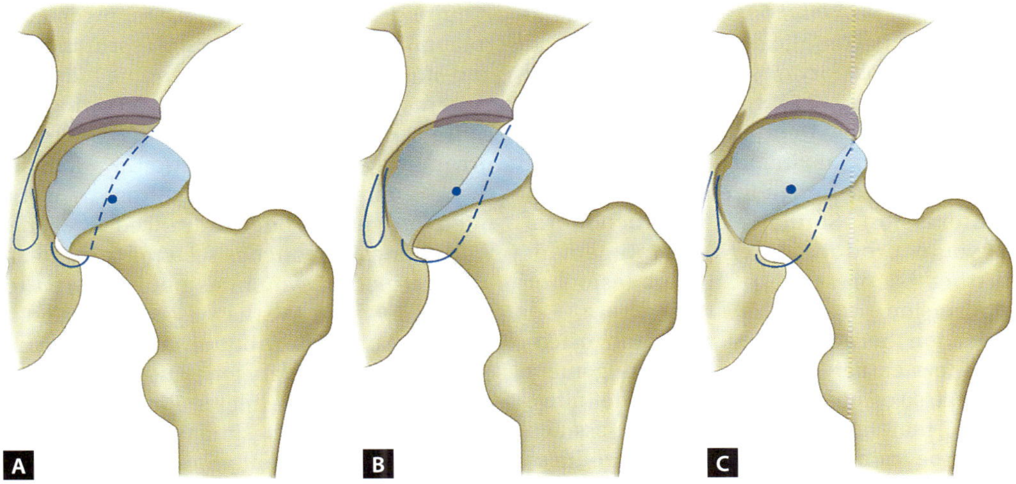

Figs. 24A to C: In a normal hip (A), the acetabulum sufficiently covers the femoral head and the acetabular floor is medial to femoral head, and the ilioischial line is further medial; (B) Coxa profunda, the head is more medial and the acetabular fossa just touches but is medial to the ilioischial line, does not cross it. In protrusio (C), the femoral head is medial to the ilioischial line crossing it and the acetabular roof over covers the head (negative tonnis angle). This can also be ascertained by the finding that center of the femoral head goes medial to the anterior and posterior acetabular walls.

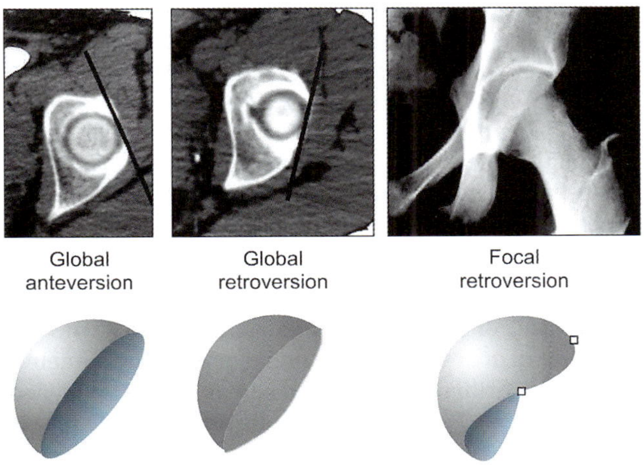

Fig. 25: Abnormalities of acetabular version.

of the anterior acetabular rim, high CE angle, low sourcil angle or a more complex acetabular retroversion **(Fig. 25)** seen constitutionally in some individuals. Dynamic pincer impingement occurs in dancers and gymnasts where the ROM at hip is high **(Figs. 26A to C)**. These mainly produce labral damage with development of patulous labrum and blunting of labral edge with cystic changes and in extreme cases, the labrum might disappear. Countercoup lesions produce additional cartilage damage in the part opposite the impingement causing early osteoarthritic changes **(Figs. 26A to C)**.

Apart from the two classical described forms of FAI above some additional morphological abnormalities of the proximal femur are being increasingly considered as causes of FAI. Prominent amongst these are the sagittal plane and torsional deformities of femur.

- *Sagittal plane deformities* of proximal femur produce coxa valga or vara. These morphological alterations lead to static overload of the hip joint laterally in valgus deformity and medially in varus hip. In full flexion, a valgus hip will produce anteroinferior impingement due to low lateral femoral offset, while a varus femur (reduced neck-shaft angle) would aggravate a superior pincer-type FAI though by itself it is unlikely to cause FAI.

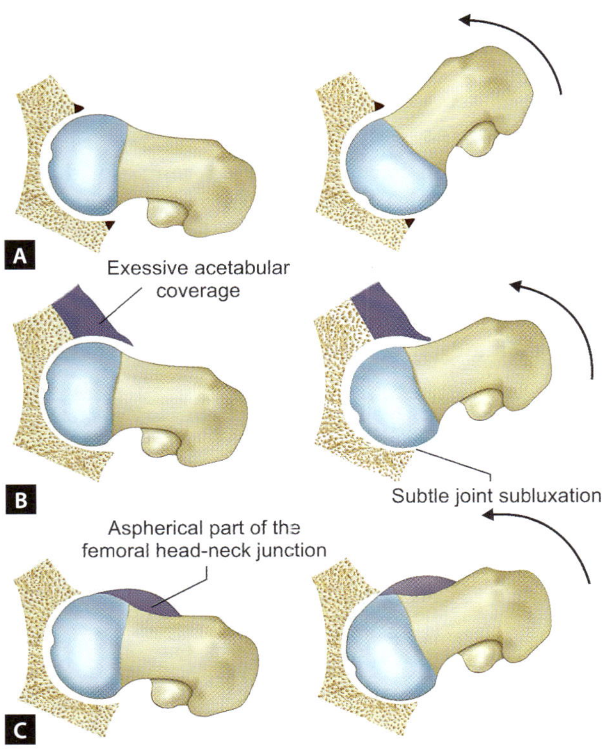

Figs. 26A to C: Normal configuration of hip with sufficient joint clearance (A). Excessive acetabular overcoverage leads to early linear contact between femoral head-neck junction and acetabular rim, resulting in pincer impingement, labrum degeneration and secondary changes. Contrecoup lesions are produced in posteroinferior portion due to subtle subluxations (B). Irregularities in femoral neck produce early impingement of head-neck junction into acetabulum (C).

- *Torsional deformity of proximal femur:* The FAI due to torsional deformities is complicated to understand at least due to the compensatory or supplementary effect of acetabular torsion **(Fig. 27)**. In general increased femoral anteversion is liable to produce posteroinferior impingement if the person maintains a normal gait not in-toeing gait, this is further prejudiced by an increased acetabular anteversion. Similarly reduced femoral anteversion would produce anterior impingement worsened further by presence of a cam lesion or acetabular retroversion.

There is association between labral tears and osteoarthritis (see labral tear earlier). Pincer type impingement produces labral defect, so osteoarthritis could be a definitive possibility from FAI that had been previously classified as idiopathic. Also the cam-type impingement produces direct articular cartilage damage causing osteoarthritis. Impingement occurs in extreme ranges of motion. The repetitive trauma not only damages the labrum, but also the adjacent cartilage (See labral tears earlier). Currently, some evidence points to development of future osteoarthritis from FAI in patients with structural proximal femoral head-neck abnormalities, especially in younger and more physically active adults.

Clinical Features

The patients often have a protracted course of diagnosis and seen by multiple physicians previously labeling various diagnosis like sports hernia, tendonitis or synovitis. FAI usually affects patient in active middle years and is more commonly seen in athletic individuals. The usual complaint is a deep groin pain often accompanying activity appearing with or after it. Typically, the pain is exacerbated by activities requiring hip flexion (cam impingement) and internal rotation. Initially, the sporting (sprinting or kicking sports) and strenuous activities (ascending hills or stairs) requiring large movements of hip (prolonged sitting in low lying chairs) cause symptoms, but later even simple acts like walking, driving or getting in and out of low vehicles may produce them. Symptoms could range from mild to severe and are often intermittent but in advanced cases may also come up with sitting. Pain often is seen radiating to anterior thigh, or in the region of symphysis pubis or even to the ipsilateral testicle in men. We have seen radiation to trochanteric region in an oval distribution covering proximal lateral thigh, especially in sedentary job patients. The groin pain could be activity limiting for athletes. Pincer impingement anteriorly presents complaints similar to cam impingement while posterior impingement produces buttock or sacroiliac pain. Posterior impingement produces pain in hyperextension activities like fast walking and walking downhill and during intercourse. Pincer impingement is more common in middle-aged women, occurring at an average age of 40 years, and can occur with various disorders. Labral tears additionally produces catching, clicking and a feeling of giving way. The differentiating features for the two types of impingement syndrome are presented in **Table 1**.

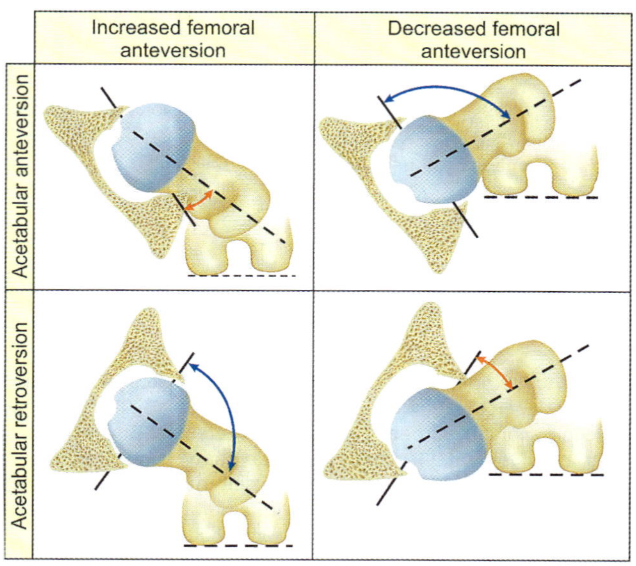

Fig. 27: The possibility of FAI with alteration of femoral and acetabular torsion. Increased femoral anteversion would produce posterior FAI while reduced femoral anteversion would produce early anterior contact of femoral neck/head-neck junction with acetabular lip. The deformity has additional impact of compensation or jeopardizing effect from acetabular torsional deformity and/or presence of cam/pincer lesion(s) (see text).

On examination, patients have characteristic finding of reduced internal rotation and adduction both while the hip is positioned in flexion. This maneuver exacerbates pain, if already present or produces pain, if asymptomatic during presentation.

Impingement test (See also labral tears above, Figs. 28A to C): Passively flexing the adducted hip and gradually internally rotating will often elicit anterior groin pain. For cam impingement or anterior pincer impingement, the maneuver places the proximal and anterior part of the femoral neck (deformed in cam) into contact with the rim of the acetabulum (prominent in cam) causing pathological contact. As impingement can occur in various places so to locate the site of the same, the hip is progressively rotated from external to internal rotation while moving from abduction to adduction **(Fig. 28A)**. This locates the most-likely area of impingement and acetabular region injury. Positive impingement tests usually correlate with labral tears on MR arthrograms. The problem of test is however its nonspecificity as it can elicit pain in various joint pathologies like bursitis, nerve entrapments, and referred pain. “Drehmann’s sign” is passive external rotation of the hip while performing hip flexion **(Fig. 28B)**. Pain on painful forced external rotation and extension indicates posterior impingement **(Fig. 28C)**.

Fitzgerald’s acetabular labral tests: The test has been described to identify anterior or posterior labral tear. In the first maneuver, test is performed by flexing, adducting and externally rotating the patient’s hip followed by extending and abducting it in internal rotation. Anterior labral tear is possibly present if there is perception of pain with or without clicking sound. For a possible posterior labral tear, this maneuver is performed in reverse order by first placing the hip in extended, abducted, and internally rotating position

TABLE 1: The characteristics and differentiating features of the two types of femoroacetabular impingement syndrome.

Feature	*Pincer impingement*	*Cam impingement*
Pathoanatomy	Acetabular focal or global overcoverage or retroversion	Aspherical head-neck interface or reduced offset
Mechanism	Repetitive trauma due to contact between theovercovering rim and head-neck junction	Jamming of the aspherical component into acetabulum
M:F ratio	1:3	14:1
Average age at presentation	Late middle age (40–57)	Early middle age (21–51)
Location of cartilage damage	Usually peripheral few millimeter near the rim	Extends up to 10–12 mm deep into the acetabulum
Distribution of cartilage damage	Circumferential	10–3 o'clock position (anterosuperior) region of acetabulum
Associated disorders	• PFFD • Post-traumatic malunion • Pelvic abnormalities like in bladder extrophy, rickets, etc. • DDH • LCPD • Iatrogenic as in corrective reorientation surgeries for acetabular dysplasia in children • Retroverted acetabulum	• SUFE/SCFE • LCPD • Retrotorsion of femoral neck (malunion) • Coxa vara • Pistol-grip deformity • Femoral retroversion • Femoral epiphysis growth abnormalities
Radiographic features	• Coxa profunda • Protrusio acetabuli • Figure-of-eight configuration (focal acetabular retroversion) • CE angle >39° • Acetabular index ≤0° • Posterior wall sign • Linear indentation sign • Ossification of labrum • Os acetabuli • Loss of joint space on posterior inferior aspect(faux profile of Lequesne radiographs)	• Horizontal growth plate • Head-neck angle <125° • Pistol-grip deformity • α-angle > 50° • Femoral head-neck offset <8 mm • Offset ration <0.18 • Femoral retrotorsion

(DDH: developmental dysplasia of the hip; SUFE: slipped upper femoral epiphysis; SCFE: slipped capital femoral epiphysis; LCPD:Legg–Calvé–Perthes disease; PFFD: proximal focal femoral deficiency)

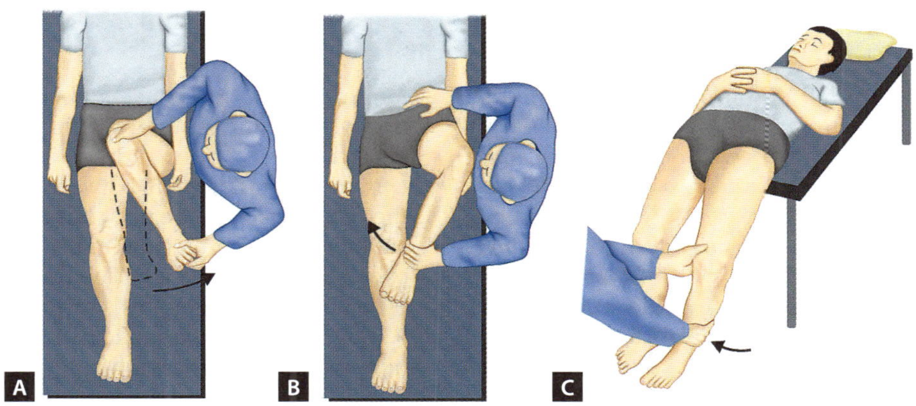

Figs. 28A to C: Anterior impingement sign (A) is positive, with painful forced internal rotation in 90° of flexion. In extreme forms, there is unavoidable passive external rotation of hip during hip flexion ("Drehmann's" sign; B). "Posterior impingement" sign is positive when there is painful forced external rotation in maximal extension (C).

and then gradually bringing it into a flexion, adduction and external rotation.

Investigations

Plain hip radiographs are usually normal, but subtle abnormalities could be present that should be suspected, especially for symptomatic patients. These are better detailed by AP radiograph of pelvis with both legs in 15° of internal rotation that gives a gross comparison of both proximal femurs, with particular attention to head-neck offset. Avoid gonadal shielding. Some characteristic features are seen in radiographs that indicate cam-type or pincer-type impingement **(Table 2)**, kindly also see the radiographic features described above for acetabular labral tears.

Cam Impingement

The usually described findings of Cam impingement are totally nonspecific and often also observed in patients with

TABLE 2: Some radiographic features discernible in cases of femoroacetabular impingement (FAI).

Impingement type and broad group of reference	***Radiographic feature***	***Comment***
Cam-type impingement, sphericity of femoral head	Alpha angle	Normal is less than 50°, angle more than 50° is pathological
Cam-type impingement, sphericity of femoral head	Anterior offset	Normal is more than 10 mm, values less than 8 mm are definitely pathological
Cam-type impingement, sphericity of femoral head	Offset ratio	Should be more than 0.20, value less than 0.18 is pathological
Pincer-type impingement, acetabular coverage	Lateral CE angle of Wiberg	Normal range is 25–39°, value less than 25° indicates dysplasia while values >39° indicate over-coverage and possible pincer impingement
Pincer-type impingement, acetabular coverage	Acetabular index	Normal range is between 33 and 38°, in *pincer* FAI values are much lower—usually less than 15°. Exact value for labeling hip as pincer based on acetabular index has not been defined. Negative values are seen in protrusio hip
Pincer-type impingement, acetabular coverage	Extrusion index	Normally around one-fourth (25%) of the femoral head is uncovered (range 17–27%). Values less than 15% are pathological indicating pincer impingement.
Pincer-type impingement, acetabular orientation	Crossover sign (figure-of-8 sign)	Not seen in normal hip, presence indicates excessive anterior over-coverage
Pincer-type impingement, acetabular orientation	Retroversion index (%)	Less than 5% is normal, more than 5% indicates acetabular retroversion
Pincer-type impingement, acetabular orientation	Posterior wall sign	Normally, it runs very near to femoral head center, if the posterior wall is medial to head center then it indicates retroversion of acetabulum. Wall running lateral to femoral head center indicates protrusio acetabuli.
Pincer-type impingement, acetabular orientation	Anterior acetabular wall index—this is the ratio of anterior acetabular wall width to the "radius" of femoral head	Normal is 0.41 (range, 0.30–0.51), values above 0.61 are pathological indicating increased anterior coverage
Pincer-type impingement, acetabular orientation	Posterior acetabular wall index—this is the ratio of width of posterior acetabular wall to femoral head radius	Normal value is 0.91 that may range between 0.81 and 1.14, values more than 1.15 are pathological
Pincer-type impingement, acetabular orientation	Ischial sign	Spine projects medial to pelvic brim in acetabular retroversion

no hip symptoms. In anatomically normal hips, the superior femoral neck has a distinctive concave contour in the form of a regular arc which also matches with pelvic side (reverse Shenton's line). The concavity takes off exactly at the head-neck junction and ends at neck-greater trochanter junction in the form of a uniform arc. This is constant in all rotational views. Cross-table lateral radiograph (Dunn/Rippstein view) illustrates the anterolateral appearance of the femoral neck and it is exactly where the cam lesions are located as a bump disrupting the concave arc **(Fig. 29A)**. This bump makes the head appearing aspherical in Dunn/Rippstein views and may be missed on a standard AR projection. Quantification of the amount of asphericity is commonly done by:

- *Measuring the angle* α*:* Angle α is the angle between the femoral neck axis and a line connecting the head center with the point of beginning asphericity of the head-neck contour **(Figs. 29B and C)**. It can be measured on radiographs but better done on a CT film **(Figs. 29B and C)**. Angle α exceeding 500 indicates an abnormally shaped femoral head-neck junction most commonly a cam lesion.
- *Anterior offset:* It is the difference in radius between the anterior femoral head and the anterior femoral neck on a Dunn/Rippstein projection of the proximal femur. Normal hips have anterior offset of 11.6 ± 0.7 mm while value less than 10 mm strongly indicates cam lesion.
- *Offset ratio:* It is the ratio between the anterior offset and the diameter of the head. It has been observed that for smaller hips, the measurement of anterior offset may overestimate cam lesion. The problem can be resolved by taking head of femur as a reference. The offset ratio is 0.21 ± 0.03 in asymptomatic patients and ≤0.13 ± 0.05 in hips with cam impingement.

The cam impingement can also arise from femoral retrotorsion that may be constitutional **(Figs. 30A and B)** or may arise out of malunion from congenital trauma.

Pincer Impingement

Acetabular features for *pincer impingement* on the AP film include the presence of a deep (coxa profunda, protrusio) or shallow socket (dysplasia) and an alteration of acetabular version (anteverted or retroverted that may be focal or global). For diagnosing pincer lesion, a properly centered AP radiograph (see acetabular labral tears earlier) of the pelvis should be obtained. One should also look for presence of both femoral and acetabular lesions present simultaneously in many individuals—the "kissing lesions".

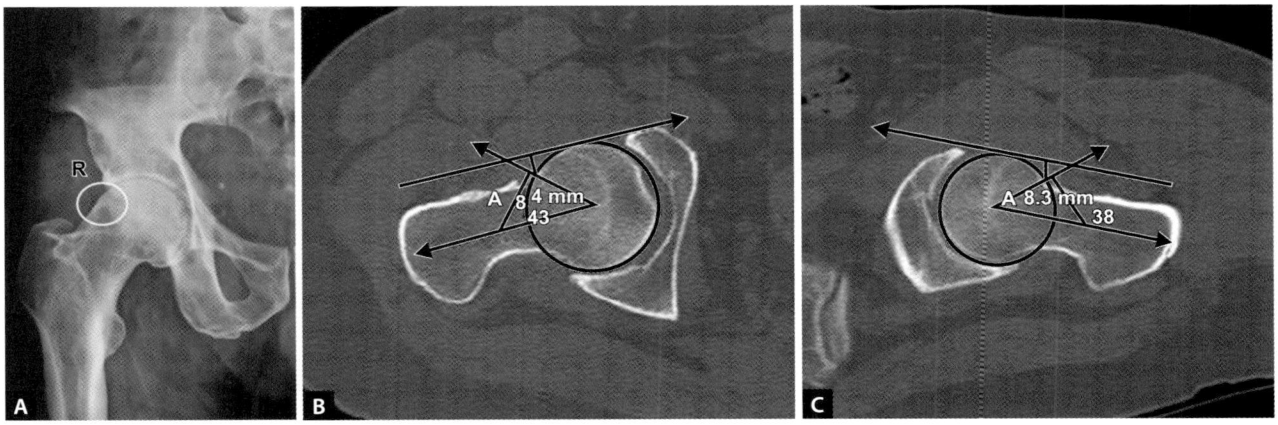

Figs. 29A to C: (A) The radiograph depicting typical "bump" seen at the femoral head neck junction in a Cam lesion (encircled); (B and C) The proximal femur appears to have the typical pistol grip deformity enhanced by the bump; Measuring the radiological parameters to determine impingement syndrome. This patient has a normal hip and the angle α is normal as is also the head-neck offset in both hips.

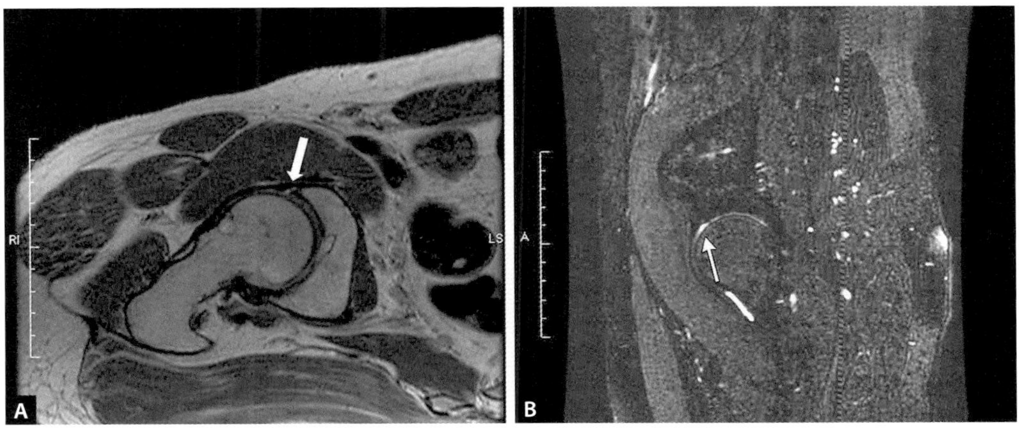

Figs. 30A and B: The T2 axial (A) and sagittal STIR (B) images of hip joint showing CAM type impingement secondary to femoral head retrotorsion (conspicuous on axial image in A); showing anterior labral tear (block arrow, A), and focal hyperintensity in the acetabular cartilage (arrow) representative of chondral wear (B).
Source: Dr Nittin Vermani, Consultant Radiologist, Shri Mata Vaishno Devi Narayana Superspeciality Hospital, Kakryal, Katra, Jammu and Kashmir.

Pincer Lesion Radiographic Findings

General acetabular overcoverage: Observe the depth of acetabular fossa by one or more of the following findings:

- The acetabular fossa line lies in a normal hip lateral to the ilioischial line on AP pelvic radiograph.
- *In coxa profunda:* The floor of the acetabular fossa touches or just overlaps the ilioischial line medially **(*see* Fig. 24).**
- *In a higher grade of deformity:* The protrusio acetabuli **(*see* Fig. 24)**; the femoral head itself overlaps the ilioischial line medially, obviously the floor of acetabular fossa lies medially.
- Femoral head overcoverage is quantified by:
  - *Lateral CE angle:* The lateral CE angle is formed by a vertical line and a line connecting the femoral head center with the lateral edge of the acetabular roof. A normal lateral CE angle varies from 25° (angle less than this defines dysplasia) and 39° (angle more than this indicates acetabular overcoverage; **Fig. 15**).
  - *The acetabular index "acetabular roof angle":* The acetabular index is the angle formed by a horizontal line (Hilgenreiner line in children and lower border of tear drop in adults) and a second line extending across the acetabular roof. It is less than 28° at birth and normal range is between 33 and 38°. In hips with coxa profunda or protrusio acetabuli, it is typically 0° or even negative. Values above 47° indicate dysplasia (DDH) of acetabulum.
- If the AP radiograph is centered over the hip then the depth of acetabulum is falsely increased resulting in so called pseudodeep acetabulum, so these views are not relied upon.
- *Femoral coverage can also be quantified by femoral head extrusion index:* This is the percentage of femoral head that is uncovered from the width of femoral head, measured along a horizontal line. The extruded portion of femoral head is identified by a line drawn perpendicular to the horizontal from lateral acetabular margin. A normal extrusion index is less than 25%.
  - *Focal femoral head overcoverage:* This can be either anterior (cranial acetabular retroversion, anterior focal acetabular retroversion, the classic type) or posterior.

The following should be observed in the radiographs:

- *Cross-over sign* ***(see Fig. 18)***: The anterior and posterior walls form a figure of eight configuration. The cross-over sign (*See* acetabular labral tears above) is indicative of overcoverage of the anterior acetabulum, while the posterior wall sign reflects the presence of acetabular retroversion.
- Posterior wall sign (See acetabular labral tears; **Fig. 18**)
- Impingement between the posteroinferior acetabulum and posteromedial aspect of femoral head due to posteroinferoinferior subluxation from anterior impingement. This produces loss of joint space on a faux profile and indicates bad prognosis.

- Computed tomography, with 3D reconstructions, can be especially helpful for mapping the bony morphology in preparation for surgery. MR arthrography is very useful to detect labral pathology. MRI (radial cuts) may also help in assessing the alpha and beta angles.

Management

Hip impingement is not only a difficult diagnosis, but also a difficult disease to treat. It needs to be differentiated from various more common clinical conditions **(Box 1)**. For this mechanical problem, the conservative methods often fail. Indeed physical therapy might exacerbate the problem in many. Activity modification gives relief but takes away the professional excellence of the athletes and their passion. Analgesics give only temporary relief. Hence, any patient put on conservative treatment should be counseled with the understanding that a *structural abnormality* often does not improve with *conservative treatment* (like osteoarthritis is only symptomatically treated).

Nearly all patients failed on conservative management have to be operated and the modality is determined by the location of the pathology that dictates the ultimate treatment plan. The deformity has to be corrected surgically and both hip arthroscopy and open surgery have their proponents. The *operative management* of these lesions gives two prime benefits:

1. Pain relief by virtue of removal of the structural abnormality
2. Early recognition and addressal of this entity may curb or halt the unfortunate progression to osteoarthritis in these younger patients.

The technical goals of surgery for FAI are:

- Precise deformity correction (intra-articular and extra-articular)
- Consistent deformity correction
- Comprehensive deformity correction
- Treatment of soft tissue abnormalities (labrum, articular cartilage, etc.)
- Dynamic examination to assess all potential sources of FAI.

A general simplified guideline for management of FAI is presented in **Flowchart 1**. The various surgical tools for management of FAI include:

- Femoral osteochondroplasty **(Fig. 31)**
- Proximal femoral osteotomy

BOX 1: The differential diagnosis of femoroacetabular impingement.

- Sacroiliitis
- Osteonecrosis hip
- Early osteoarthritis of hip joint
- Transient osteoporosis of hip
- Bursitis
- Piriformis syndrome
- Iliopsoas tendonitis
- Stress fracture femoral neck
- Fatigue fracture femoral head
- Groin pain (athletic pubalgia, sports hernia)
- Apophysitis
- "Growing pains"
- *Uncommon:*
  - Neoplasia
  - Infectious arthritis
  - Intra-articular loose bodies
  - T12-L2 spine pathology with radiation of pain
  - Groin muscle strain
  - Pelvic pathologies like endometriosis, ovarian mass, etc.

Flowchart 1: Simplified algorithm for management of a case of femoroacetabular impingement (FAI).

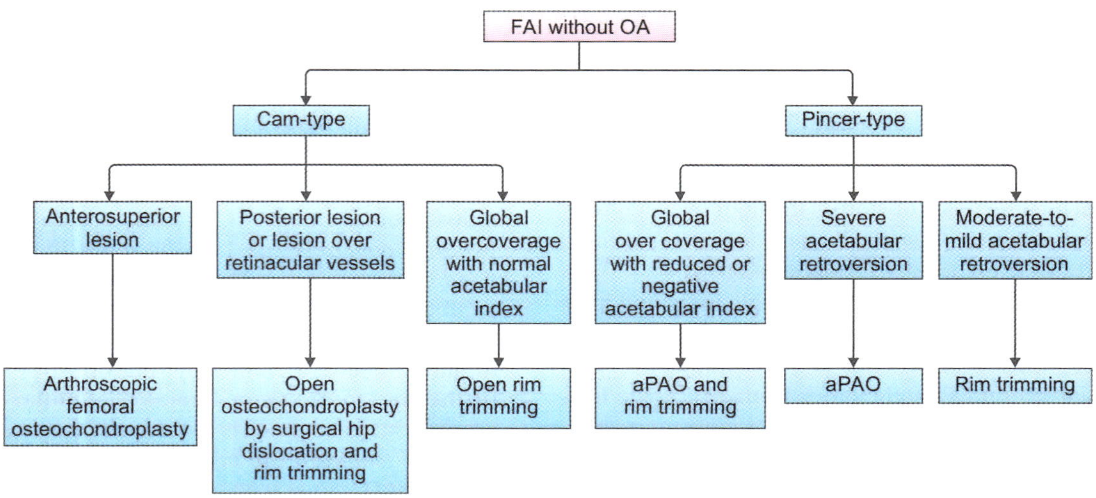

(aPAO: anteverting periacetabular osteotomy)

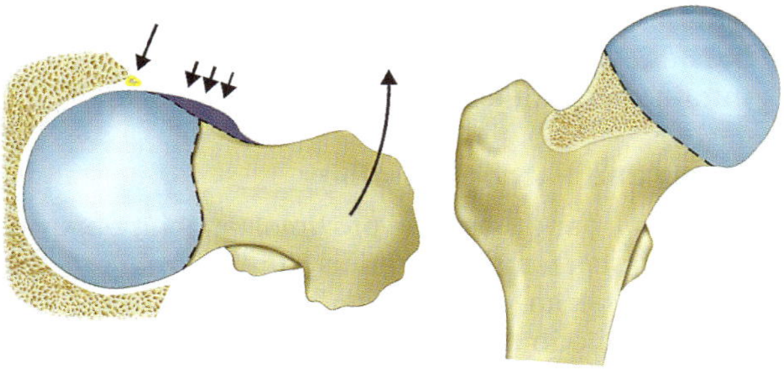

Fig. 31: Femoral osteochondroplasty. The irregularity at the femoral head-neck junction is recontoured.

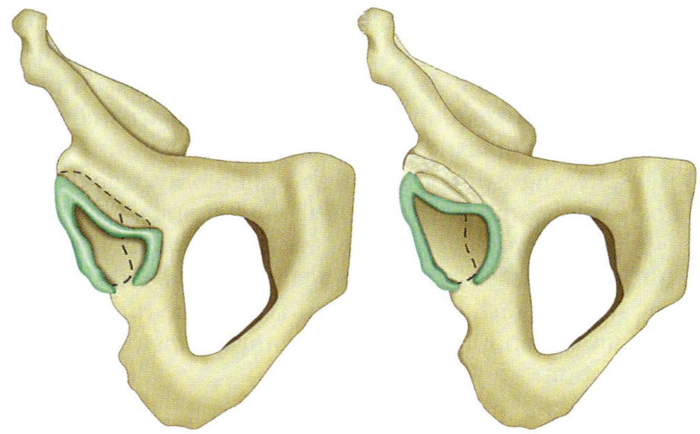

Fig. 32: For overcoverage (pincer lesion), the acetabular rim is shaved and labrum reattached.

- Labral repair/refixation, resection or replacement
- Reshaping of the acetabular rim **(Fig. 32)**
- Acetabular chondral debridement
- Acetabular realignment (periacetabular osteotomy)

Cam impingement due to aberrations in femoral neck anatomy is usually amenable to arthroscopic debridement/correction **(Figs. 30A and B)**. Once corrected and if the head-neck offset is correct, then repetitive impingement will not occur. Open techniques (and modifications like surgical dislocation of hip–Ganz osteotomy, etc.) have been the traditional approach to address most of FAI abnormalities that can be used to treat nearly all abnormalities whether femoral or acetabular. Arthroscopy has only recently been introduced as a method of treating hip impingement mostly of the abnormalities of the anterolateral neck. The peripheral compartment is entered and the neck is debrided and contoured under fluoroscopy control. The central or intra-articular region is then explored and concomitant labral and chondral pathology corrected. Recontouring of the proximal femur (femoral osteoplasty) is also best accomplished with open surgical dislocation. Open approach provides not only excellent visualization of the bony lesion but also to assess the adequacy of the chondro-osteoplasty. Arthroscopy has the advantage of significantly less morbidity but is technically demanding and should be only done by surgeons after gaining considerable experience in hip arthroscopy.

For pincer impingement: The anterior acetabulum is simply recontoured ("acetabuloplasty") to eliminate the impingement in "focal retroversions". The retroversion may be severe and global needing correction with reverse PAO **(Fig. 33)**, but the risk of destabilizing the joint is very high. For acetabular retroversion or generalized overcoverage; reverse/anteverting periacetabular osteotomy (r/aPAO) is needed as most of the acetabular retroversion emanates from malrotation of hemipelvis. The anterior column is approached through Smith-Peterson approach where the Sartorius and anterior abdominal wall muscles are detached from anterior third of iliac crest. Hueter interval is then entered preserving the rectus origin. The iliopsoas and iliocapsularis are medially mobilized to expose infra-articular ischium which is then osteotomized. Osteotomies are also performed in the pubic bone, supra- and retroacetabular area. The acetabular fragment is controlled for rotation by a Schanz screw that acts like a joystick to reorient the acetabulum. The fragment is then fixed with long 3.5 mm

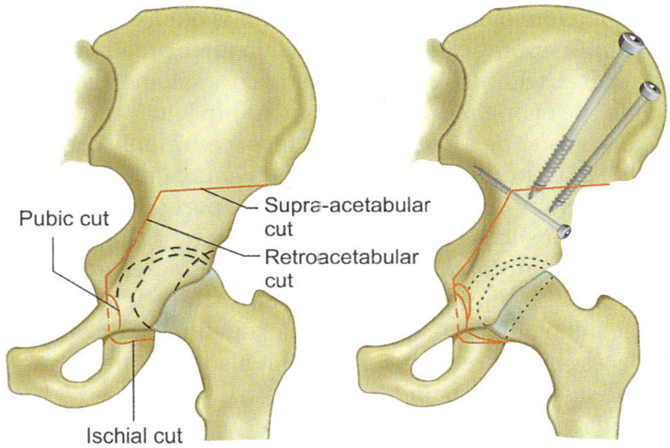

Fig. 33: "Periacetabular" osteotomy to correct acetabular retroversion.

cortical screws. Patient has to be partial weight-bearing for 6–8 weeks till union of osteotomies. Acetabuloplasty is traditionally been performed via surgical dislocation of the hip (Beck et al.). Focal rim corrections (acetabuloplasty) can be arthroscopically performed with success approaching the open methods but need expertise. There is often more difficulty in establishing the anterior portal as the impinging lip may hinder access, making this technically more challenging. The impinging lip is excised with a burr after removing the labrum which is then attached later.

Some complex disease patterns currently need complete open procedures and may be corrected as follows:

- *Perthes' disease:* The head is aspherical with wide varus neck and high trochanter. There is associated acetabular dysplasia and retroversion making a combination of "cam" and "pincer" type. After thorough dynamic examination intraoperatively, the surgical correction includes repair of intra-articular soft tissue abnormalities, acetabular osteoplasty, femoral osteoplasty, femoral head reduction, relative neck lengthening ± proximal femoral osteotomy, trochanteric osteoplasty and trochanteric advancement. PAO will be additionally needed to correct the acetabular version and make hip stable in severe cases.
- *Slipped capital femoral epiphysis:* Residual SCFE has slip angle greater than 30°, complex head and neck

malformations, reduced internal rotation in flexion and increased external rotation ± shortening. Surgical dislocation of hip is done followed by repair of intra-articular soft tissue abnormalities, acetabular osteoplasty, femoral osteoplasty, femoral neck osteotomy and/or neck lengthening ± proximal femoral osteotomy, trochanteric osteoplasty and trochanteric advancement.

- *Protrusio acetabuli and posterolateral lesions:* These are difficult to assess arthroscopically and are best accessed by surgical dislocation of hip. This procedure requires circumferential osteoplasty for comprehensive deformity correction.

SNAPPING HIP (COXA SALTANS)

This is an audible snapping seen with flexion and extension of the hip during exercise or with normal activities. As such most snappings are painless but coxa saltans is often accompanied by pain. Snapping can be classified into three broad categories (Allen et al. who also coined the term coxa saltans) depending on the site of origin with relation to the hip joint:

1. *External:* The external type is most commonly caused by the ITB (and rarely by the gluteus maximus tendon). A thickening develops in the posterior part of iliotibial tract where it slides over the greater trochanter **(Fig. 34)**. The band anatomically lies posterior to greater trochanter while the hip is in extension and slides forward with flexion causing snap of the thickened posterior portion facing higher resistance. This may also cause trochanteric bursitis adding pain component to it.
2. *Internal:* Produced by musculotendinous iliopsoas moving over bony structures behind it commonly the femoral head **(Figs. 35A and B)**. This may cause psoas bursitis causing pain.
3. Intra-articular due to loose bodies or labral tears.

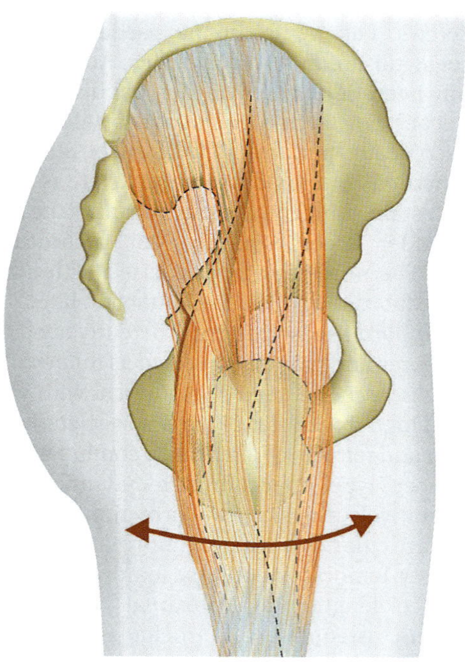

Fig. 34: During normal hip activities and flexion, the iliotibial band snaps back and forth across the greater trochanter. This flipping of the tendinous portion over the moving trochanter underneath may thicken the posterior part that may produce snapping during rotations.

Anatomy and Pathophysiology

The iliotibial band has two proximal attachments one to the tensor fascia femoris anteriorly and the other to gluteus maximus posteriorly. The latter actually inserts into the band. As the iliotibial tract remains taut throughout motion of the hip, any small anatomic change can cause snapping over the trochanter. The snapping occurs as the ITB flips back and forth across the greater trochanter (remember the trochanter is mobile and not the band) and is accompanied by thickening of the posterior part of the iliotibial tract or anterior border of the gluteus maximus. Reduced offset as in coxa vara or excessive tightness of the ITB as in reduced biiliac width have been proposed as predisposing anatomic factors. Some patients can demonstrate this phenomenon as an incidental asymptomatic maneuver. Symptomatic cases are mostly those indulging in repetitive activities and pain is especially described in the downside leg of joggers/runners typically while countering a sloped surface. Snapping may also occur following trauma and has also been reported as a postsurgical iatrogenic process.

The musculotendinous junction of the confluence of the iliacus and psoas muscles occurs at the level of a groove between the iliopectineal eminence and the anterior inferior iliac spine (AIIS). The tendon moves throughout this groove during movements; however, with rotation, the tendon translates across the femoral head while fixed in the groove, thus causing the snapping. Also the tendon may snap against osteophytes, lesser trochanter or an exostosis of the lesser trochanter or may have anomalous tendon slips. Snapping due to the iliopsoas involvement commonly occurs when the tendon subluxates from lateral to medial when it is moved from flexion, abduction and external rotation to extension and internal rotation. The tendon possibly snaps it is considered, backward and forward across the anterior aspect of the prominence of femoral head and capsule. The other more plausible explanation is that it jumps across the pectineal eminence at the pelvic brim.

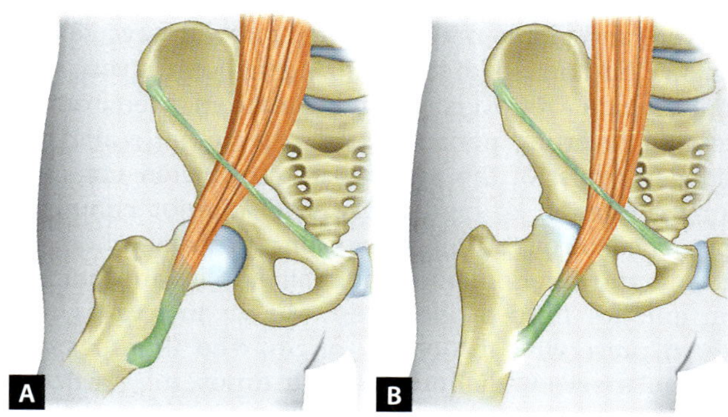

Figs. 35A and B: Internal snapping is produced commonly by iliopsoas tendon flipping back and forth across the anterior hip and pectineal eminence. (A) In flexion, the iliopsoas tendon lies lateral to the center of the femoral head; (B) In extension, the iliopsoas shifts medial to the center of the femoral head.

Clinical Examination

The history of snapping is characteristic and does not need description. The vast majority of snapping hips are asymptomatic (painless) but definitely arouse curiosity in patients. In few patients, the attention is attracted with the start of snapping with some new activity that may exacerbate the problem. In such cases, simple avoidance of the activity relieves the snapping also. It can be difficult to isolate and differentiate the various types mentioned earlier. The physical examination should be in supine position and having him or her demonstrate the characteristic sound. Usually, the flexion and extension of the hip produces the symptoms. Snapping of the ITB is visually evident itself though patient may describe it as a sense of the hip subluxing or dislocating. The symptoms and findings are located laterally in external snapping and the patient can usually produce this best while standing. The Ober test evaluates associated tightness of the ITB.

Patient with internal snapping describes a painful clicking sensation emanating from deep within the groin. Though often audible, it may also just be a sensation experienced by the patient rather than what the examiner can objectively observe. It is uncommon for patients to describe sensation of ache in the region of flank, buttock or sacroiliac region attributed to irritation of the iliacus and psoas muscle origins. Internal snapping is made more prominent when the hip is brought into adduction, internal rotation and extension from abduction, external rotation and flexion. The snapping can often be eliminated or significantly lessened by applying pressure over the iliopsoas tendon at the level of the femoral head in internal snapping or by applying manual pressure over the greater trochanter to prevent tendon subluxation in external snapping. Unlike internal snapping, the external type of snapping is often painful usually secondary to trochanteric bursitis.

Investigations

Radiographs are usually obtained to rule out coexisting bony pathologies in the external variety; the diagnosis is usually straightforward. Intra-articular snapping needs to be characterized by MRI or MR arthrogram or simply an arthrogram of the hip. But as the pathology may be dynamic in nature, no anatomical abnormalities may be elicited with even advanced investigations.

The dynamic studies that are useful in snapping syndrome are ultrasound and iliopsoas bursography. Abrupt movements of the ITB or the gluteus maximus muscle picked up by the transducer at the posterior side of trochanter mostly correlate with the painful click reported by the patients. With bursography, the psoas tendon is usually seen as a filling defect adjacent to the opacified psoas bursa; moving the hip through ROM produces a sudden jerk diagnostic of the snapping.

Differential Diagnosis

- *Intra-articular:* Loose bodies, FAI, lax capsule, ligamentum teres rupture, chondral injuries
- *Extra-articular:* Iliopsoas tendinitis, trochanteric bursitis, gluteus medius/minimus tear, stress fracture, piriformis syndrome, sacroiliac stress syndrome

Treatment

Conservative Treatment

Conservative treatment yields good result in many. The measures include modification of activities, nonsteroidal anti-inflammatory drugs (NSAIDs), physical therapy and a gentle stretching and conditioning program directed specifically at the ITB or iliopsoas tendon. For less than optimal responders corticosteroid injection in the bursa may alleviate pain though snapping persists.

Surgical Treatment

Patients who have severe symptoms or those who do not improve (uncommon) may benefit from surgical treatment. The results of surgical intervention for recalcitrant snapping of the ITB are inconsistent. Most surgical methods aim at relaxing the ITB. One should carefully exclude persons having secondary gain from snapping and voluntary snapping syndrome—they will uniformly fail. The patient should be counseled for possibility of similar or different pain or dysfunction. ITB can be lengthened by the Z-plasty technique popularized by Brignall and Stainsby and its modifications **(Fig. 36)**. The other procedure involves excision of an ellipsoid-shaped segment of the ITB over the greater trochanter as described by Zoltan et al. **(Fig. 37)**.

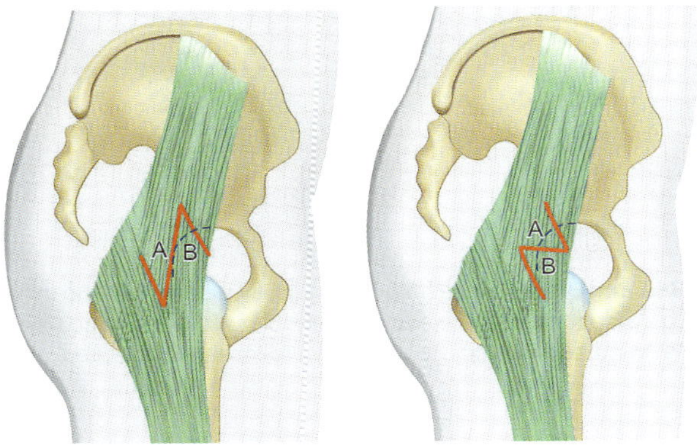

Fig. 36: Illustration of the incision and transposition Z-plasty technique originally described by Brignall and Stainsby.

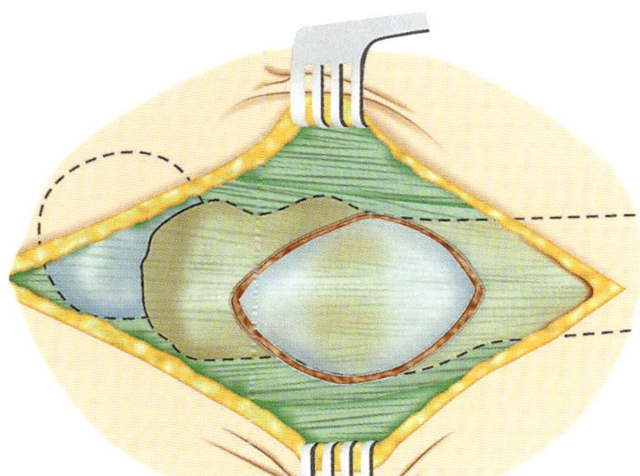

Fig. 37: Ellipsoid-shaped segment excision of the iliotibial band over the greater trochanter described by Zoltan et al.

Larger resection of the posterior half of the iliotibial tract can be also done at its insertion at the gluteus maximus. Brooker (1979) described a cruciate incision of the ITB over the greater trochanter that successfully relieved pain from severe trochanteric bursitis **(Figs. 38A and B)**. Endoscopic procedures are being tried in the form of bursoscopy that may be extended to endoscopic ITB release also.

For patients with internal snapping surgery consists of partial or complete release of tendinous portion of the iliopsoas to eliminate snapping. Commonly, the posteromedial tendinous portion of the iliopsoas is released in partial releases leaving the anterior muscular portion intact effectively producing a lengthening of the musculotendinous unit **(Figs. 39A and B)**. Fractional lengthening of the iliopsoas tendon at pelvic brim has been proposed by Gruen et al. through an ilioinguinal approach **(Fig. 40)**. To reduce postoperative loss of hip flexion strength modification of fractional lengthening of the tendon through modified iliofemoral approach over the iliopectineal eminence has been proposed. This can also be done through a more cosmetic medial approach. Endoscopic release of the tendon has also been described done at the lesser trochanter **(Fig. 41)**. Also due to significant association of the internal snapping with intra-articular pathology, arthroscopy provides the advantage of simultaneous exploration of the hip joint and debridement if needed. After arthroscopic resection of the tendon, the tendon retracts exposing its muscular remnants which are preserved. This endoscopic release of the iliopsoas tendon is now preferred by many surgeons for treating even recalcitrant cases also and is an effective alternative to conventional open techniques. It can be done in outpatient setup and offers excellent cosmesis.

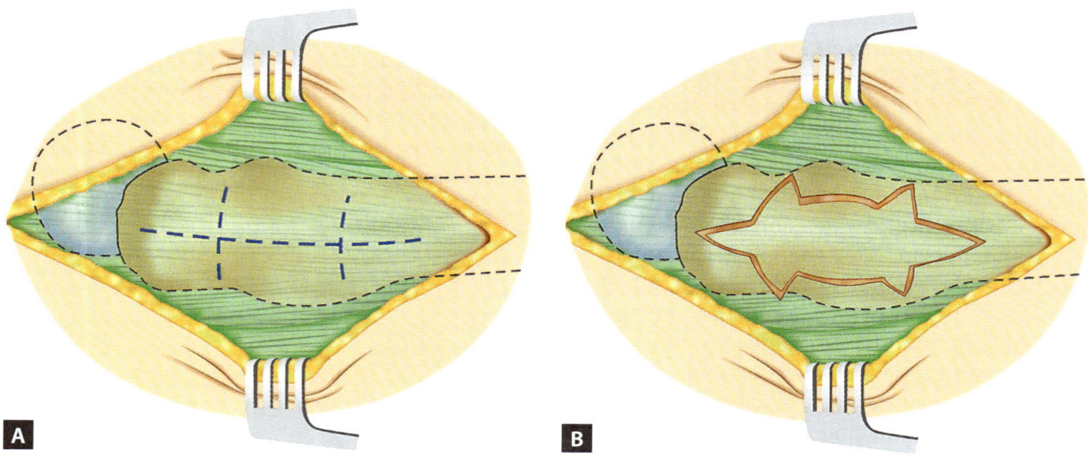

Figs. 38A and B: Brooker technique is basically placing relaxing incisions over the ITB. An 8- to 10-cm longitudinal incision, posterior to the midpoint of the greater trochanter is made centrally followed by two transverse incisions at the thirds division of the initial longitudinal incision. This relaxes the iliotibial band, eliminating the snapping. No repair is attempted.

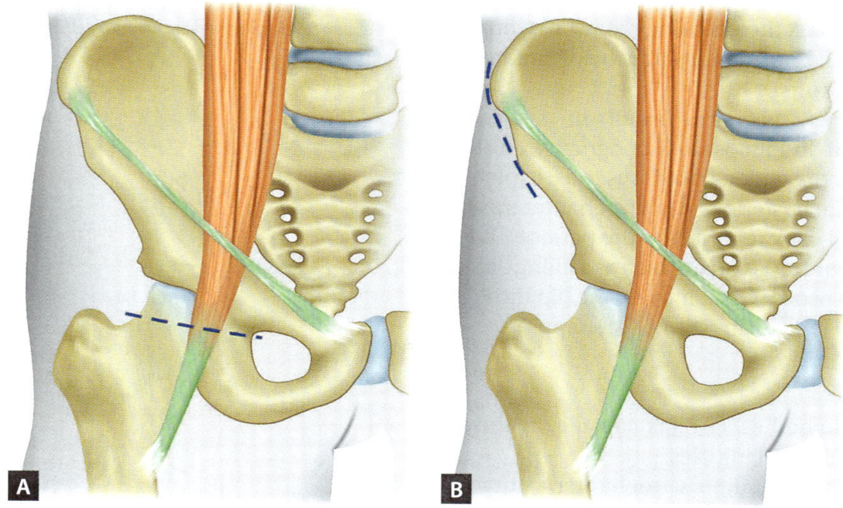

Figs. 39A and B: Releasing the posteromedial tendon of iliopsoas. (A) Anterior approach of Allen and Cope using a cosmetic transverse incision; (B) Modified iliofemoral approach described by Dobbs et al.

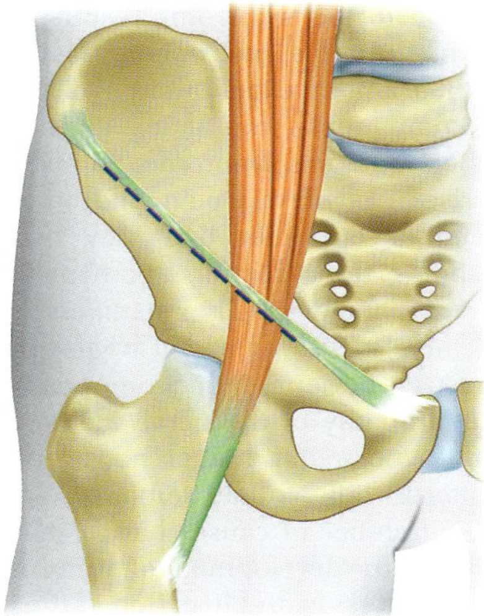

Fig. 40: Illustration of Ilioinguinal approach for release of the iliopsoas over the pelvic brim described by Gruen et al.

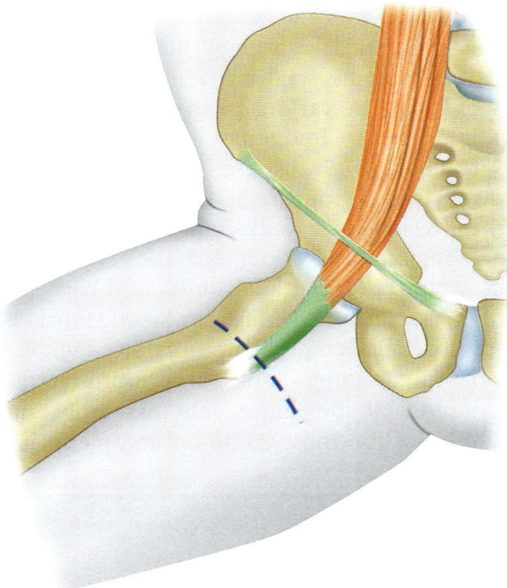

Fig. 41: Medial approach for release of the iliopsoas from its insertion on the lesser trochanter described by Taylor and Clarke.

PIRIFORMIS SYNDROME (DEEP GLUTEAL SYNDROME, PELVIC OUTLET SYNDROME, INFRAPIRIFORM FORAMEN SYNDROME)

The piriformis syndrome represents an entrapment neuropathy of sciatic nerve almost always accompanied by an anatomical abnormality of the piriformis muscle that may be intrinsic to the muscle or extrinsic to it. These cases represent nearly 6% of cases in clinical practice causing lower back pain and/or sciatica. Piriformis syndrome has been a controversial diagnosis debated hotly in the past. Due to elusive literature and nonagreement, there is high possibility of underdiagnosis or overdiagnosis by nonbelievers and proponents respectively. Yeoman in 1928 first linked the piriformis muscle to sciatica but attributed sacroiliitis as the primary cause of pain. SI joint as cause of piriformis syndrome-related pain has been rejected, and piriformis syndrome currently is recognized as having primary and secondary causes.

Robinson in the 1947 is credited with naming the syndrome and identified six diagnostic features:
1. Traumatic insult—injury to sacroiliac and gluteal region (now refuted)
2. Radiation from and spread of sacroiliac joint pain (now refuted) or other pain causing pathologies from greater sciatic notch or the piriformis muscle itself, extending down the leg and causing difficulty walking
3. Exacerbations of pain brought by stooping forward or lifting weight. The pain is relieved by traction on the affected leg
4. Palpable tender, sausage-shaped mass over piriformis
5. Positive Lasegue sign
6. Atrophy of gluteal muscles

Anatomical Considerations

The anatomy, functions, and relationship of the muscle to sciatic nerve are essential in understanding the etiopathogenesis of the syndrome.

Piriformis muscle originates from anterior surface of the sacral 2nd–4th vertebrae, sacrotuberous ligament, and the roof (superior margin) of sciatic notch. Muscle then passes through the greater sciatic foramen and inserts on to the posteromedial region of greater trochanter near the piriformis fossa **(Fig. 42)**. The functions of the piriformis vary with the position and attitude of hip.
- In extension, the piriformis serves as external rotator of the hip.
- In flexion, it becomes an abductor.
- When the person is standing, its trochanteric attachment becomes its origin and the muscle works to pull pelvis forward, elevating the opposite side (Trendelenburg sign).

Piriformis is the only muscle that crosses greater sciatic notch transversely. It is innervated by the first and second sacral nerves. Sciatic nerve normally passes beneath the piriformis muscle but variants are noted **(Figs. 43A to F)**. The anatomical association has classically been thought to potentiate irritation of the sciatic nerve by dysfunction of the piriformis but all anomalies have not been documented to potentiate the piriformis syndrome.

The sciatic nerve forms from the lumbosacral plexus and receives components from L4-S1 nerve roots. It divides to form the tibial and peroneal nerves distally at a variable course. Once the sciatic nerve exits the sciatic notch, it normally lies below the piriformis muscle belly though variations are seen. Throughout its course from lumbar spine to proximal posterior thigh sciatic nerve is susceptible to compression and entrapment. For theoretical purpose, one must understand structures that pass from the greater sciatic notch apart from sciatic nerve which are as follows:
- The superior gluteal nerve and artery (above the piriformis)
- The inferior gluteal nerve and artery (below the piriformis)
- Pudendal nerve
- The internal pudendal vessels
- Posterior femoral cutaneous nerve.

Etiology

The primary pathophysiology is compression of the nerve by piriformis muscle. This can be primary or secondary as related to the piriformis muscle:

- Primary piriformis syndrome includes all pathology intrinsic to the muscle, such as myofascial pain, pyomyositis and myositis ossificans.

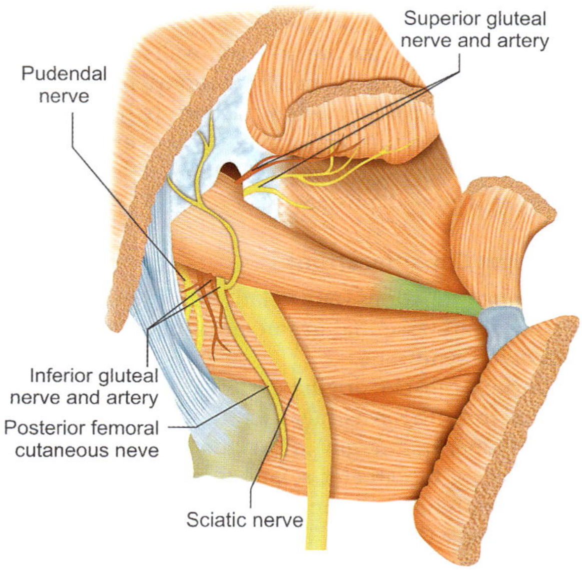

Fig. 42: Illustration of the piriformis muscle and various structures in relation to the muscle.

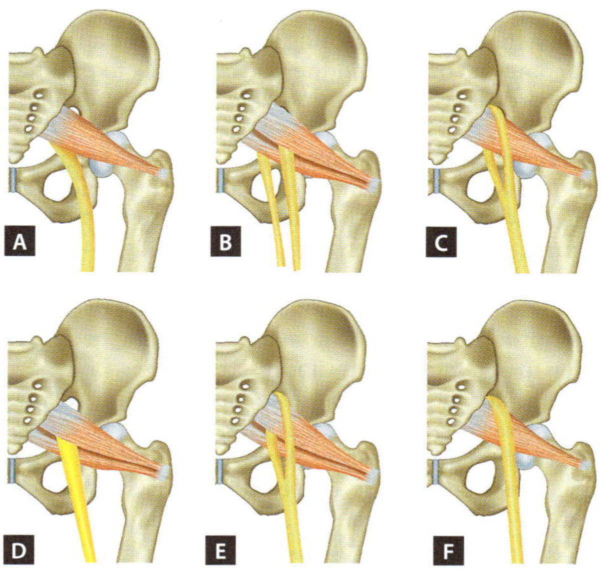

Figs. 43A to F: The anatomic variations of relationship between sciatic nerve and piriformis muscle. (A) This is the most common variant where the undivided nerve passes below the piriformis muscle (seen in ≈ 80% individuals); (B) This is seen in about 12% individuals where the tibial and peroneal divisions of sciatic nerve pass through the bifid piriformis (12%); (C) Uncommon variant where the nerve divisions encircle around the undivided muscle (3%); (D) Uncommon variant where undivided nerve passes through the bifid muscle bellies of the piriformis (1–2%). Rare variants (E and F) include passage of divisions around the upper part of bifid muscle seen in <1% or passage of the whole nerve superficial to the muscle <1%.

- Secondary piriformis syndrome results from external influences on the nerve, such as compression, etc.

This is not just a point event but it involves somatic and neuropathic components, the latter developing usually later but predominate the syndrome. Somatic component usually comprises of myofascial pain syndrome and intrinsic pathology mentioned earlier that may be additionally modified by short external rotators and hamstring muscles. The somatic component usually emanates from a gluteal trauma that causes development of trigger points in and around the muscle. The neuropathic component is the typical entrapment neuropathy of the nerve in the infrapiriform foramen. It does not really matter however with respect to the treatment to differentiate somatic and neuropathic components. A number of causes have been reported by various authors for the development of piriformis syndrome that result in compression and irritation of the nerve in and around the piriformis muscle **(Box 2)**.

Clinical Features

The syndrome is six times more common in females presenting commonly as a deep, boring, ill-defined buttock pain or posterolateral thigh pain that may be referred along the course of the sciatic nerve also. Radiated pain resembles sciatica. The variously reported pains according to descending order of frequency in piriformis syndrome include gluteal pain (97.9% of cases), pain (and paresthesia) in the lower back, groin region, perineum (including sometimes the testicles), buttocks, hip, posterior region of the thigh (saddle region, 81.9%), calf (59%), foot (outer border), even in the rectum (during defecation), and coccygodynia. Low back pain is seen in 18.1% of cases, so one must evaluate cases of low backache. The symptoms are aggravated by sitting, walking, climbing stairs, or performing squats or repetitive rotations on the planted foot (assembly line work, dancing, etc.), but the most common complaint is sitting

BOX 2: Etiology of piriformis syndrome.

- *Idiopathic:*
  - Trauma
  - Gluteal region
  - Sacroiliac joint
  - Anatomical variants
  - Double piriformis
  - Split nerve
  - Anomalies of posterior cutaneous femoral nerve
  - Inferior gluteal nerve
  - Superior gluteal nerve
  - Myofascial trigger points
- *Hypertrophy and spasm of piriformis muscle:*
  - Abscess, hematoma, myositis, piriformis bursitis, neoplasms in the infrapiriform foramen, colorectal carcinoma, myositis ossificans of piriformis
- *Sciatic nerve pathology:*
  - Neuroma of sciatic nerve (idiopathic or after injury)
  - Miscellaneous
  - Intragluteal injections
  - Episacroiliac lipoma
  - Femoral nailing
  - Klippel-Trenaunay syndrome
  - Post-laminectomy
  - Gynecological conditions

intolerance, especially on hard surfaces (60–100% patients). This is frequently associated with joint dysfunction. Trauma or a fall involving the gluteal region is commonly reported. Pregnancy also has been associated as a possible risk factor. Symptoms can often be relieved initially by externally rotating the leg but soon become fixed and intolerant. Because of the proximity of the piriformis muscle to the lateral pelvic wall, patients may also complain of dyspareunia, sexual dysfunction (13–100%) or pain with bowel movements. Some people mix the sacroiliac dysfunction with piriformis syndrome. I feel sacroiliac joint dysfunction should be kept aside from the piriformis syndrome. The latter may though include not only the myofascial pain from trigger points of the muscle and structures adjacent to it but also the entrapment of nerve from adjacent structures as discussed earlier.

Examination findings: The patient may walk with antalgic gait, overpronation of the foot and has leg-length inequality; there may be foot flare on the involved side. There is often gluteal atrophy. The following should be further noted along with special tests:

- *Piriformis sign:* On gross inspection, the patient may hold the leg in an externally rotated position while lying supine.
- *Buttock tenderness* over the greater sciatic foramen is present in almost all patients. This is specifically elicited over the piriformis line—it overlies the superior border of piriformis that can be surface marked by a line that extends from immediately above the greater trochanter to the upper border (roof) of the greater sciatic foramen at the sacrum **(Fig. 44)**. The line can be divided into equal thirds, and trigger point is commonly present over junction of middle and medial thirds.
- Specific piriformis tests have been reported with most relying on either active contraction of the muscle in resistance or by passive stretching of the muscle.
  - The Pace test is an active contraction test. It elicits pain with resisted abduction and external rotation of a flexed thigh.
  - The Freiberg test is a passive stretch test and causes pain with internal rotation during thigh extension.
  - *Beatty maneuver:* Patient lies on the uninvolved side and abducts the involved thigh upward causing contraction of the ipsilateral piriformis muscle causing pain.
  - *The FADIR test (Lasegue's sign, piriformis test):* Eliciting pain with flexion, adduction and internal rotation (**Fig. 45**; passive stretch test).
  - *Huge's test:* External isometric rotation of the affected lower extremity following maximal internal rotation elicits pain.
- Reduced ROM (reduced active and passive hip rotation, reduced active and passive hip abduction)
- Neurological findings are minimal and mostly absent, specifically the sensory findings are absent in most patients.
- Per rectal (PR) or per vaginal (PV) examination to palpate medial end of piriformis elicits pain in the muscle and trigger point
- Tests that are positive but neither specific nor sensitive for piriformis syndrome:
  - Positive SLRT
  - Bonnet's sign
  - Positive Hibb's test

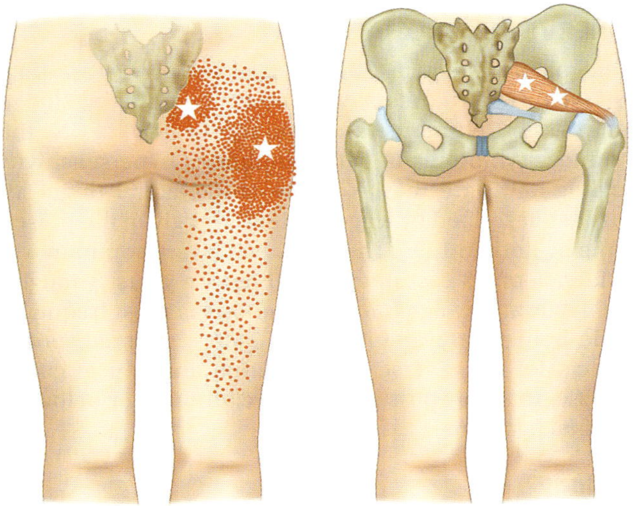

Fig. 44: The location of buttock pain (superficial marking) in patient of piriformis syndrome.

Investigations

- Radiographic and other imaging studies are usually not helpful with the diagnosis; they are useful to rule out pathology in pelvis, lumbar spine, sacrum and coccyx. A MRI can evaluate for a mass effect, anomalous sacral attachment of piriformis muscle (usually extending medially over S2 foramen).
- Neurophysiologic testing provides more consistent and reliable results. Results affect the peroneal division of the sciatic nerve that supplies the hamstrings, but the tibial nerve innervations are spared. Peroneal H-reflexes are elicited in the anatomic position while H reflexes are recorded in FADIR test. A prolongation of 1.86 msec in the FADIR test is acceptable as an electrophysiological criterion by many for diagnosing piriformis syndrome; also, delayed F-waves are seen in such cases. The Ehlers-Danlos syndrome (EDS) specifically helps in differentiating proximally located root or spinal involvement.
- Diagnostic and therapeutic injections with anesthetics and corticosteroids can be attempted.

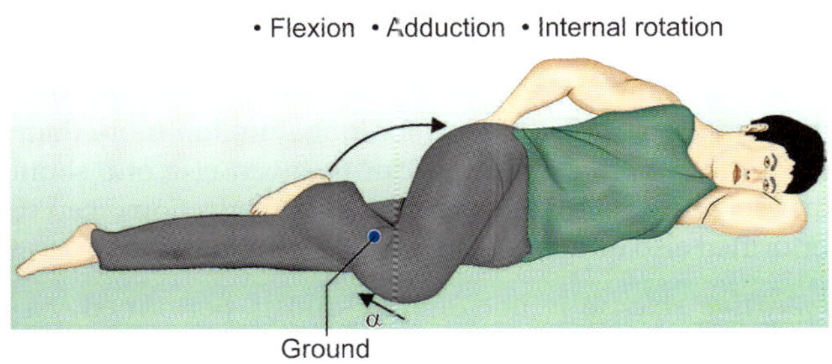

Fig. 45: The FADIR test for piriformis. Internal rotation is then produced by lifting foot above maintaining adduction. Improvement can be noted/monitored by measuring angle alpha.

Differential Diagnosis

Sacroiliac joint dysfunction, prolapsed intervertebral disk (PIVD) and spinal lesions, femoroacetabular impingement and acetabular labrum tears, iliac vein thrombosis, post-laminectomy syndrome, coccygodynia, pseudoaneurysm of inferior gluteal artery, gluteal varicosities, vascular compression of sciatic nerve, posterior facet syndrome of lower lumbar vertebrae, pseudo-S1 syndrome, pelvis fractures and pseudofractures, lumbar osteochondroses.

Diagnosis

The diagnosis of piriformis syndrome should be favored when the following are found:

- Buttock pain worse with sitting and with activity
- Variable component of radicular symptoms (usually not remarkable)
- Pain with active or passive provocation/stretch of the piriformis (See tests earlier)
- Reproduction of symptoms on intrapelvic palpation/pressure on piriformis as it exits from the sciatic notch
- Reasonable, reliable and conforming diagnosis is relief in pain from anesthetic injection in the area of the piriformis muscle; one should be sure to elicit the dye distribution in the region of muscle during injection for surety.

Management

Most patients with piriformis syndrome respond successfully to ***conservative treatment***. The strategies commonly used are combination of NSAIDs, muscle relaxants, local ultrasound treatment and physical therapy. The *physical therapy* comprises of stretching with hip internal rotation with adduction and flexion, myofascial therapy, massage, hip muscle strengthening, sacroiliac manipulation, ice and hydrotherapy, and possibly acupuncture. These modalities can be combined with neural mobilization to improve the yield of successful result. Lifestyle changes are an essential component comprising of reducing the sitting time; change sitting or standing position; remove wallet from hip pocket; and avoid pivoting on planted foot.

Trigger point injections may be used in those patients that fail conservative treatment for 1–2 months. Various injections have been used like the lidocaine hydrochloride, steroids (often combination), botulinum toxin type A, and prolotherapy. The injection is given at the maximum tender point usually medial to posterior hip joint margin toward the sciatic notch. When mixed with local anesthetic, the patient should experience numbness in the region of sciatic nerve or at least relief of his pain symptoms. If the relief is for long duration more than 6 weeks then another injection can be given else one should consider surgical decompression. The injections can be performed also under ultrasound or CT guidance.

Operative release is not difficult and is performed via a limited posterior approach. Only proximal portion of modified Moore's approach to hip is used. Piriformis is identified and tendon tagged **(Fig. 46)**. The tendon is released off the femur; a neurolysis is performed; and any obstructing lesions are also removed. Muscle is explored for its relationship to nerve. Distal 1–2 cm of tendon is excised to let the muscle retract and reduce compression or irritation of the nerve. If bifid muscle was found on exploration, then the two parts should be made complete to prevent undue tension on the nerve causing compression and palsy! Patients are made to ambulate with crutches and progress to full weight bearing by 5–10 days after surgery. The clinical success of the procedure is essentially dependent on careful patient selection. This comprises of following factors:

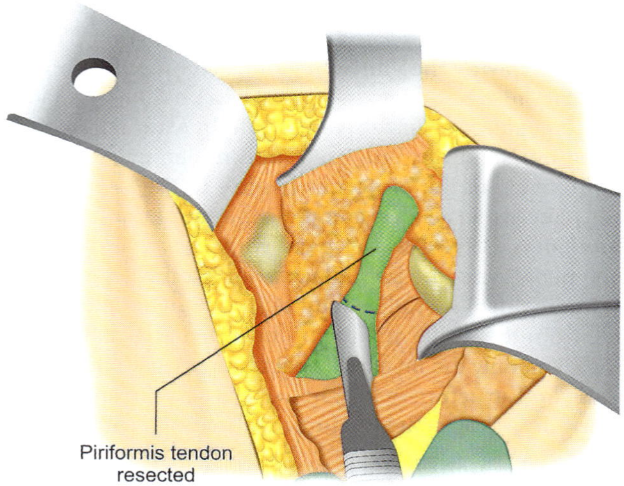

Fig. 46: Release and resection of piriformis tendon. The tendinous insertion of the piriformis is released, tagged and tension is maintained with a tag suture, and a portion is resected within the muscle fibers proximal to the tendon.

- Conclusive diagnosis of piriformis syndrome
- Good patient motivation and interest in recovery
- The patient must have reasonable expectations from the procedure.

MERALGIA PARESTHETICA (BERNHARDT-ROTH SYNDROME, LATERAL CUTANEOUS NERVE NEURALGIA)

Meralgia paresthetica (MP) (Greek words *meros*—thigh and *algos*—pain) refers to sensory neuropathy due to compression/entrapment or injury to the LFCN that produces symptoms of pain, numbness, hypersensitivity, tingling and paresthesias in the anterolateral thigh. MP was first described by Hager in 1885 and given the present name by Roth in 1895. The entity is not very common with incidence of 4.3 cases per 10,000 person years. Though it can occur at any age but the diagnosis is most frequently made between 30 and 40 years. Males are predisposed. The causes are diverse due to varied anatomical course of LFCN that may pass either above, through or below the inguinal ligament.

Etiology

- *Spontaneous:*
  - Idiopathic

- *Metabolic:* Lead poisoning, alcoholism, hypothyroidism, diabetes mellitus
- *Mechanical:* Pressure of belt, corsets or tight garments. Military armor, police uniforms, leg-length discrepancy (LLD), iliacus hematoma.

▪ *Iatrogenic injury:*
- Autogenous iliac crest bone grafting
- The ilioinguinal approach and neuroma formation for fracture acetabulum
- *Other causes:* Retroperitoneal dissection (traction injury), total hip arthroplasty, laparoscopic cholecystectomy and myomectomy, surgery for morbid obesity, transplantations for coronary bypass surgery.

▪ Local direct trauma say during pelvic injuries, road traffic accidents.

The various risk factors for development of meralgia paresthetica due to the inconsistent anatomy of the nerve or patient profile include:

▪ Pregnancy
▪ Morbid obesity (BMI ≥ 30)
▪ Surgery around anterior iliac crest and inguinal ligament
▪ Diabetes mellitus (incidence rises to 247 cases per 100,000 patient years)
▪ Too petite patient
▪ Sports, especially gymnastics, baseball, soccer, body building.

Anatomy and Related Considerations

The nerve originates from lumbar plexus receiving isolated or combination contribution from L1 to L3. The nerve then emerges at the lateral border of psoas major, crosses iliacus to reach near the ASIS where it can be medial **(Fig. 47)** or lateral to it. The nerve usually passes underneath the inguinal ligament over the Sartorius and enters the thigh dividing into anterior and posterior branches. Variations have been reported **(Figs. 48A to D)** in this classically accepted course of the nerve. The following is as reported by Azman et al.

▪ *Type A (4%):* LFCN runs posterior to the ASIS across the crista iliaca.
▪ *Type B (27%):* LFCN runs anterior to the ASIS superficial to the tendinous origin of sartorius but is embedded in the tissue of the inguinal ligament.
▪ *Type C (23%):* LFCN runs medial to the ASIS, embedded in the tendinous origin of the sartorius.
▪ *Type D (26%):* LFCN runs medial to the tendinous origin of the sartorius, between the tendon of sartorius and a thick fascia of the iliopsoas under the inguinal ligament.
▪ *Type E (20%):* LFCN runs further medially and is embedded in the connective tissue under the inguinal ligament and lies on the thin fascia of iliopsoas where it branches off toward the genitofemoral nerve contributing the femoral component to it.

Lateral femoral cutaneous nerve following the types A, B, and C course are most sensitive to trauma. Apart from above, branching pattern variations of the LFCN have also been described (1–3 branches with variable course), the nerve can even have one or two vertebral origins. Isolated compression of the branch of LFCN in the thigh has also been documented.

Clinical Features

Patients describe numbness, tingling, pain, hypersensitivity, burning or coldness, buzzing (such as cellphone vibration),

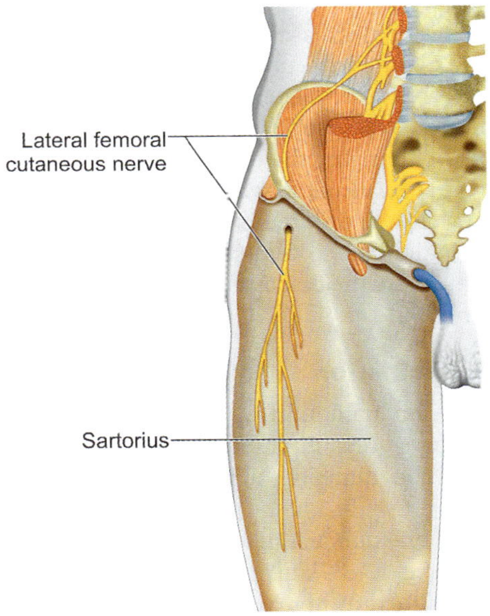

Fig. 47: The usual course of lateral femoral cutaneous nerve.

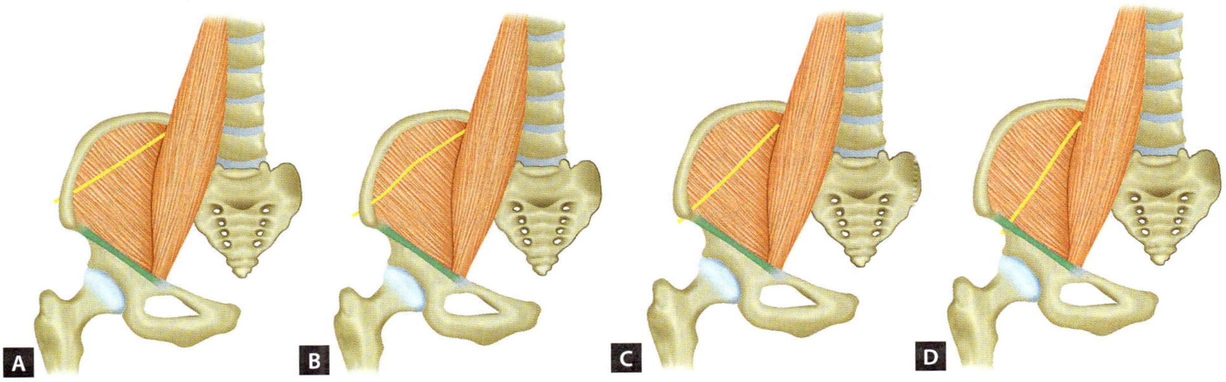

Figs. 48A to D: The anatomical variations of lateral femoral cutaneous nerve of thigh (see text for description).

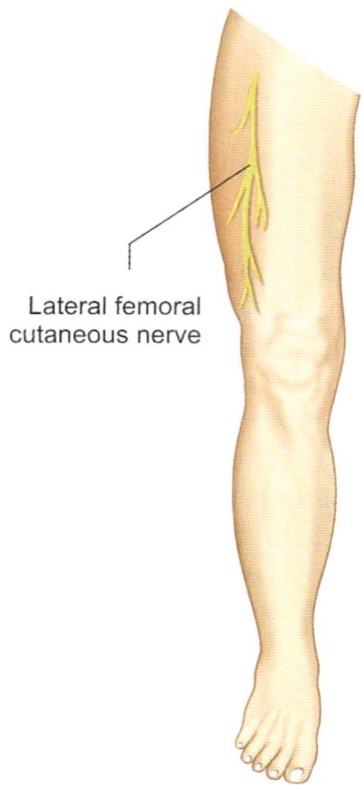

Fig. 49: The distribution of symptoms in meralgia paresthetica.

lighting pain and decreased sensitivity to pain, touch, and temperature in the distribution of the LFCN **(Fig. 49)**. Direct palpation often exacerbates symptoms. Prolonged standing and walking often worsen while sitting decreases (possibly by reducing or changing the tension in the LFCN or inguinal ligament) the severity of the symptoms. Hip extension during walking puts stretch on the nerve and hence aggravates the symptoms. Patients are often seen massaging the region to attempt to alleviate the discomfort. This may produce loss of hair in the region!

Physical Examination

There is pain on palpation of the lateral part of inguinal ligament. Sensory examination in the distribution of the nerve should be done. Other tests that may be helpful include:

- *Pelvic compression test of Nouraei et al. (sensitivity 95% and specificity 93.3%):* In lateral position with the affected side up, the examiner applies downward pressure on pelvis maintaining pressure for 45 seconds. Positive test is indicated by relief in symptoms due to relaxation of the inguinal ligament.
- *Tinel's sign*—performed over the inguinal ligament where the nerve exists. Ultrasonic Tinel's is also described (from the ultrasound probe) and is useful in interventional procedures (like injections) given under ultrasonic control.
- *Neurodynamic testing (Butler's test)*—the patient in lateral position with affected side up. The examiner passively bends the knee and adducts and extends the hip. Positive test indicates tension on the nerve in the region by reproduction of the patient's symptoms.

Motor examination for muscles innervated by L1-3 roots should be done. Also loss of cremasteric reflex would indicate damage to L1 nerve root. Any muscular weakness or abnormality of reflex would rule out the diagnosis of meralgia.

Patients should also be evaluated for neuropathy as a result of diabetes or deficiency of vitamin B_{12} and folate.

Investigations

Radiography can be performed to rule out bone tumors and other pathology. Ultrasonography and advanced imaging can be done to study the pathology further.

Electrodiagnostic testing using somatosensory-evoked potential and a nerve conduction test of the LFCN can be performed for difficult clinical presentations. These also help to evaluate the compression at other places (intrapelvic and spinal). For difficult clinical presentations diagnostic blockade with 8 mL local anesthetic, performed by locating the LFCN using a nerve stimulator, can usually confirm the diagnosis.

Differential Diagnosis

- Bone metastasis to the iliac crest
- Lumbar disk herniation with radiculopathy at L1–L3
- Avulsion fractures of the ASIS
- Uterine fibroids or pelvic mass that compress the nerve
- Chronic appendicitis

Management

Conservative treatment is usually effective for most patients with spontaneous onset disease. The inciting event should be properly controlled by making the patient aware of identified lifestyles changes (weight loss or the wearing of tight clothing and/or belts). Physical therapy like active release techniques, pelvic manipulation, myofascial stimulation therapy for the rectus femoris and iliopsoas, inguinal ligament transverse friction massage to relieve adhesions, hip and pelvic muscular stretching exercises, and pelvic stabilization exercises has been combined to improve the effectiveness of conservative therapy. Medications in the form of anti-inflammatories, pregabalin or other anticonvulsants or nortriptyline or other tricyclic antidepressants are administered. The latter drugs reduce the paresthesia and dysesthesias. For patients not responding to these measures, anesthetic injections with corticosteroids (bupivacaine 0.25%, 1:200,000 epinephrine and 40 mg methylprednisolone) may be beneficial to decrease inflammation. The injection should be performed 1 cm medial to the ASIS and may be performed under ultrasound control. For subsequent injections 20 mg methylprednisolone is effective given at a difference of 3 weeks. The results of the injections in literature have been but variable.

Pulsed radiofrequency (PRF) treatment has been sparingly reported. It is a minimally invasive and relatively nontraumatic procedure and when used properly (output below 0.6 V, using a 23-G RF needle with an active 5 mm tip, PRF current of 45 V lasting for 120 seconds with local temperature not exceeding 42°C) does not damage the nerve. Similarly, *cryolesioning* of the nerve has been described.

Spinal cord stimulation using a quadripolar lead implanted at T10 level could be effective for occasional refractory patient.

The literature for *kinesio-taping* is not available, but it has been also found effective in allaying the symptoms. The effectiveness could be due secondary to increase in lymphatic and vascular flow, reduction of pain, enhancement in normal muscular function, improved proprioception, and correction of possible articular malalignments/periarticular dyskinesias. *Acupuncture and acupressure* are regionally practiced methods with nondocumented efficacy.

Surgical intervention such as neurolysis/decompression of the constricting tissue, neurolysis and transposition (laterally by cutting a slot in iliac crest) of the LFCN, and transection with excision of a portion of the LFCN may be considered for severe symptoms at presentation or intractable symptoms. Decompression and neurolysis is "ethically" better than transection but the possibility of recurrence could be high; we use it as initial procedure anyways and resort to transection if it fails. If neurolysis is not feasible or not required then isolated decompression of the nerve can be done as by cutting the posterior slip of inguinal ligament. Decompression is but effective in nearly half of the patients. Transposition involves lateral shifting of the nerve by cutting a slot in the iliac wing or by medially transposing the nerve by cutting the posterior slip of inguinal ligament.

It is recommended that persons with moderate but uncontrolled symptoms on conservative management should be considered for decompression ± transposition. Patients with long-standing symptoms (>1 year) or those with severe symptoms should be considered for primary resection. Resection should also be considered in patients who fail by decompression alone.

Nerve transection leaves patients with permanent anterolateral thigh anesthesia, but other symptoms are alleviated. Resection should be done several centimeters posterior to the ASIS. Always the resected sample should be submitted for histopathology for documentation.

TROCHANTERIC BURSITIS (GREATER TROCHANTERIC PAIN SYNDROME)

Bursitis around hip is most commonly seen at the greater trochanter bursa (other less prominent regions include lesser trochanteric, or psoas bursa, and occasionally the bursa about the ischial tuberosity). Greater trochanteric pain syndrome is a common clinical complain and better describes the symptomatology rather than the term "trochanteric bursitis". The latter term may be better dropped in view of frequent findings of degenerative or overuse gluteus maximus and medius tendinopathy or tears without any documentable bursitis or collection.

Anatomical Considerations

The primary abductors of hip-gluteus medius, tensor fascia lata and gluteus minimus are involved in various pathologies around hip causing GTPS as they insert into the greater trochanter. The greater trochanteric bursa is a small fluid filled pouch that reduces friction between the tendons and bony structure **(Fig. 50)**. Deep to gluteal muscles there are various bursae of which two larger ones are most consistently found—the subgluteus maximus bursa and the subgluteus medius bursa **(Fig. 50)**. The former one is commonly implicated in trochanteric bursitis. Greater trochanteric pain syndrome has a prevalence of 10–25% with a female to male ratio of 4:1. The annual incidence is 1.8 out of 1,000. Bilateral cases are not very frequent, representing 5–8% of the cases.

Etiology

The inciting factors in bursitis appear to be related to overuse and/or excess friction between tissues. The common causes/risk factors are:

- Direct trauma
- Wider pelvis in women—mainly responsible for the prevalence difference between sexes
- *Mechanical disturbances:*
  - Gait disturbances
  - Limb-length inequality
- A prominent trochanter
- *Repetitive injuries:*
  - Runners who adduct beyond the midline or those who run on banked surfaces (this cause uneven pelvis and abnormal stress at the trochanter precipitating inflammation)
  - Snapping hip (external type)
  - *Iliotibial band friction syndrome:* Repetitive friction between the ITB and the greater trochanter causes chronic trochanteric bursitis presenting a characteristic symptomatology. It can be considered one step ahead of the external snapping hip syndrome.

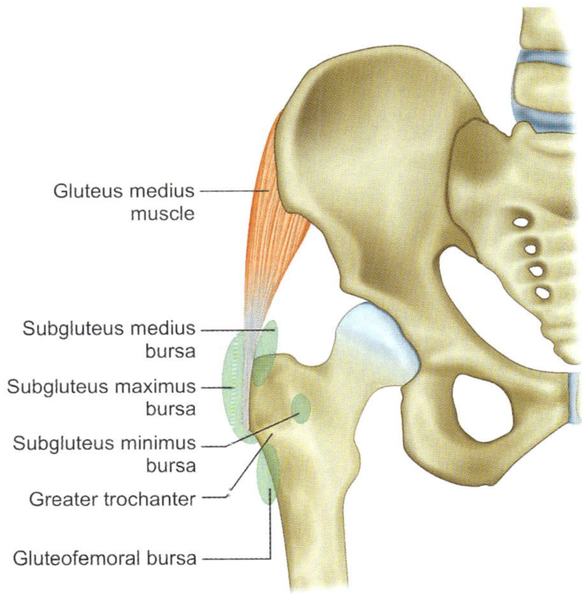

Fig. 50: The anatomy and location of trochanteric bursa and structures in vicinity producing lateral femoral pain syndrome.

ITB friction syndrome presents with pain typically over the lateral (outside) aspect of the knee. The onset of this pain usually occurs toward the middle or ends of running or bicycling and may persist for some time after completion of the exercise. Mostly in these cases, the ITB is tight due to weak tensor fascia latae (TFL) or glutei. The predisposing factors for ITB friction syndrome are:
- Genu varum
- Weak TFL or glutei
- Leg-length discrepancy
- Pronated foot and ankle
- Overuse with inappropriate training and stretching

- *Systemic disorders:*
  - Inflammatory arthritis
  - Gout
  - Paget's disease
  - Chondrocalcinosis
  - Diabetes mellitus

Associations: The GTPS has been found to be significantly associated with lumbar degenerative disease and arthritis of the lower limb joints.

Clinical Features and Diagnosis

The typical complaint is that of lateral thigh pain while these patients often also present with diffuse pain in the hip, thigh, and leg. Proximal or distal radiation is uncommon. The pain is increased by pressure on the region or when the patient lies on the affected side. Maneuvers such as pivoting, climbing or running also aggravate the pain. On examination, there is tenderness in the region of posterolateral aspect of greater trochanter **(Fig. 51)** that can be aggravated by flexion, abduction and external rotation. The tenderness in the region of the greater trochanter, buttock, or lateral thigh often mimics the symptoms of lumbar nerve root compression. The diagnosis of bursitis can be confirmed by response to anesthetic corticosteroid injection.

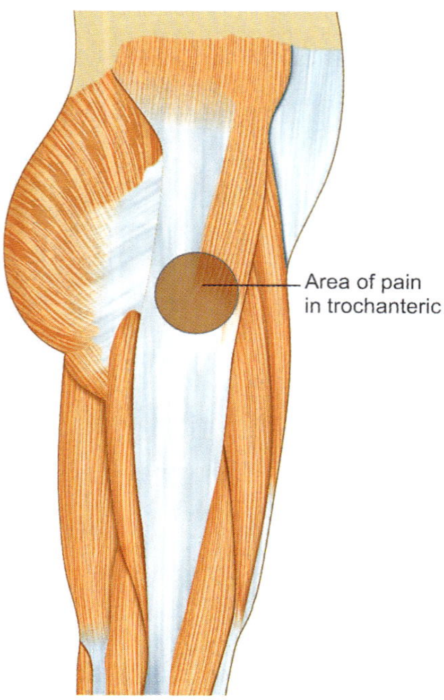

Fig. 51: Location of pain in trochanteric bursitis.

Investigations

Radiographs are needed in the setting of acute trauma to rule out fractures or trochanteric prominences or neoplasia [like germ cell tumor (GCT)]. The modalities like MRI may be useful for evaluating additional pathologies, viz. tendon degeneration or tear, thickening of gluteal tendons, edema, high signal intensity and discontinuation of tendon at insertion site, ITB friction and thickening, etc. Ultrasonography though handy is highly user dependent but remarkably has the advantage of possible dynamic imaging.

Management

The treatment includes rest, stretching of the involved tendons, and NSAIDs. Gait abnormalities, leg-length discrepancies should be corrected and activity modification like avoiding the aggravating factors should be practiced. In refractory cases, a corticosteroid injection provides good relief and is frequently prescribed. Local ultrasonics and shock wave therapy are seldom used due to limited benefits and inconsistent response. The steroid injections provide immediate relief but symptoms often recur for which injections can be repeated as early as 3 weeks and rarely more than three injections are prescribed. No relief with injections indicates either a wrong site or discrete pathology (like pain coming from spine). Injections have been shown to play significant role in preventing the bursitis from becoming chronic.

Patients who do not respond even after repeated injections are managed with surgical excision of the trochanteric bursa (less than 10%). Arthroscopic management of trochanteric bursitis has now become common place for the surgical management of the disease. Often with the surgical excision of bursa additional pathologies should be addressed like release or lengthening of ITB, gluteal tendon repair or osteotomy of the greater trochanter. ITB release or debridement of gluteal tendons can be done endoscopically also. Hip joint may also be examined along with the bursoscopy but is unnecessary.

Trochanteric Reduction Osteotomy (Fig. 52)

This has been used as a salvage procedure if the symptoms do not relieve even after bursa excision. Primary use of this modality for treatment of trochanteric bursitis is unconventional but may be done if there is trochanteric prominence to cause the symptoms. The treatment for ITB friction syndrome comprises of removal of trochanteric osteophytes with ITB release and excision of the bursa. Various options of release for ITB have been discussed previously in snapping hip. Trochanteric reduction osteotomy may be considered advancement over these procedures which can also be used to salvage the previous

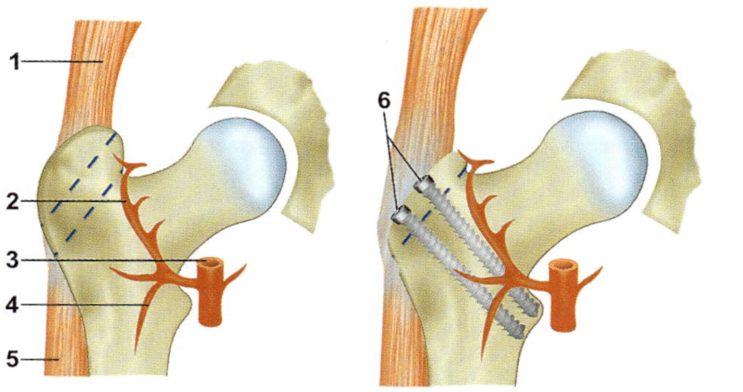

Fig. 52: Trochanteric reduction osteotomy: This is done to reduce the prominence of greater trochanter. A slice of 5–10 mm in thickness is removed from trochanter to reduce its prominence.

methods if they fail. The relief from trochanteric reduction osteotomy is possibly due to three factors:

1. Reduced prominence of trochanter produces less friction.
2. Distal transfer increases strength of the abductors by increasing resting length (the laxity is taken up and muscular weakness as one of the cause of ITB friction syndrome is hence addressed).
3. Postoperative hyperemia may resolve the tendinitis/tendinopathy due to enhanced repair.

OSTEITIS PUBIS

Osteitis pubis is the most common inflammatory affection of the pubic symphysis. It is classically aseptic as separate from the infected variety. The onset is insidious and radiologically characterized by erosion of one or both joint margins followed by sclerosis. The condition is self-limiting in majority with variable time duration to resolve. Some cases may even take few years to resolve. Osteitis pubis was first described in 1924 by Beer (urologist) following suprapubic surgery. Till late 1950s, osteitis pubis was considered to be a complication of urologic or gynecologic surgeries and child birth attributing it to subacute infection. It was considered a difficult to diagnose and hard to treat chronic condition. Spinelli first described the condition in athletes in 1932. In the athletic population, the incidence of osteitis pubis ranges from 0.5 to 7.0%. Now the pathophysiology is centered upon chronic stress syndrome and repetitive microtrauma. This mechanical theory has many proponents but a few cases might definitely arise out of infection.

Anatomy of Symphysis Pubis

The symphysis pubis is a secondary cartilaginous joint formed by articulating pubic bones covered by hyaline cartilage with an intervening fibrocartilage disk. The joint is rigid and provides relative stability to pelvis anteriorly except physiologically during pregnancy when it gains some laxity. It is covered superiorly by the suprapubic ligament and inferiorly strength is imparted by arcuate ligament; these are supported by the anterior (superficial and deep layers) and posterior pubic ligaments. Development of the symphysis is usually complete by 26 years of age whence it settles with a mean width of 3 mm. The disk is thickest in the superior and anterior regions and undergoes continued narrowing throughout adult life eventually osteoarthritic degeneration. The disk functions to absorb and dissipate axial and shear forces. The latter are typically greatest during mid-stance, when the unsupported pelvis begins to drop. It interdigitates between the apposed pubic bones.

The muscle attachments about the symphysis tend to maintain vertical balance. Superiorly, the rectus and abdominal musculature are attached while inferiorly the adductors and gracilis counter their pull. The blood supply to the symphysis comes from periosteal vascular plexus has its venous outflow through pudendal plexus and is valveless. Pubic symphysis is supplied by both sympathetic (L1, L2) and parasympathetic (S2-4) system. The former is stimulated by ischemia and causes pain that can induce muscle spasm, while the latter respond to mechanical stimuli and is responsible for causing referred pain to the groin, thigh and perineum.

Mobility as mentioned earlier, about the symphysis is limited (<2 mm); however, it is influenced by hormonal changes like in pregnancy to adjust the birth canal physiologically.

Pathophysiology and Pathoanatomy

The most probable cause of osteitis pubis is repetitive microtrauma. Abnormal and unequal muscle balance is also postulated in athletes that may result in osteitis. Following an initial muscle strain in an athlete, a progressive cycle of events develop that run a downhill course and ill-effects of poor muscular balance also get exacerbated by further activity. Excessive firing of the rectus abdominis or adductors, or imbalance between these muscles has been identified in activities like unilateral leg support. The imbalance is exacerbated in sports involving sudden acceleration-deceleration, and multidirectional cutting from sports such as soccer, rugby, ice hockey and football. The muscle imbalance between thigh adductors and the abdominal muscles produces anterior pelvic tilt as described in athletic pubalgia. This causes periosteal inflammation, osseous resorption, or osteolysis along the symphyseal margin of the inferior pubic ramus, and in chronic cases sclerosis. The possible biomechanical causes of osteitis pubis are:

- Instability of the sacroiliac joint leading to secondary stress reaction at the symphysis pubis
- Excessive frontal or up-and-down pelvic motion or horizontal side-to-side sway
- Limitation of hip movement with resultant shearing stress being applied to the hemipelvis on the opposite side
- Repetitive adductor muscle pull

Though uncommon infection of the symphysis has been reported in various locoregional surgeries from gynecologic and surgical faculty (herniorrhaphy) and also from hematogenous spread in intravenous drug users, the most common pathogen identified has been *Pseudomonas aeruginosa* (Staphylococci and *E. coli* are others). There often is destruction of the periosteum and hyaline cartilage with infection and is associated with protracted osteomyelitis of the pubic bones.

In mechanical osteitis pubis, histology shows moderate lymphocytes, plasma cells and an inflammatory reaction along with marrow fibrosis. The articular lining undergoes hyaline cartilage degeneration and subchondral bone resorption.

Etiology

Infective (now it is better called osteomyelitis of pubic symphysis):

- Direct inoculation—surgery near symphysis
- Seeding by nearby orgonal infection (via pelvic plexus)

Noninfective:

- Athletics and sports like soccer, sprinting, ice hockey, etc.
- Rheumatologic disorders
- Pregnancy and child birth
- Trauma (major single event or repetitive microtrauma)

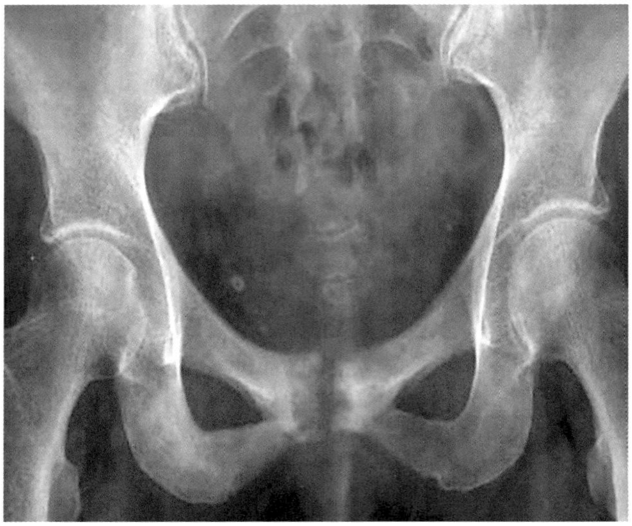

Fig. 53: Osteitis pubis. Note the lysis and widening of the joint with erosion of the joint surfaces and sclerosis of bones on either side.

Clinical Evaluation

History

The patient complains of insidious onset deep groin (adductor pain), anterior pubic pain or lower abdominal pain that is typically exacerbated by activity. Diagnostic delay is related to nonspecific nature of presenting complaints. An audible or palpable click over the symphysis might be detected during daily activities. Pain is exacerbated by activities such as running, pivoting on one leg, kicking, or pushing off to change direction, as well as by lying on the side. Exclusion of genitourinary and obstetric-related causes, and seronegative arthropathies should be done through meticulous history.

Physical Findings

The most consistent finding on physical examination is tenderness on palpation over pubic symphysis. Functionally, pain can be reproduced with resisted hip adduction and active contractions of anterior abdominal muscle. Pelvic compression test is also positive. Asking the patient to squeeze examiner fist placed between knees is painful. Pushing the pubic rami produces pain centrally over symphysis.

Imaging

Plain radiographs demonstrate articular surface irregularity, erosion **(Fig. 53)**, sclerosis and osteophyte formation. Subtle symphyseal joint laxity or disruption is better elicited on Flamingo views of the pelvis. Symphyseal laxity is defined by widening of greater than 7 mm or otherwise greater than 2 mm of malalignment of the upper margins of the superior pubic rami.

One must note that radiological severity of sclerosis does not correlate with clinical symptoms.

Scintigraphy with Tc-99 is more sensitive and quite useful to confirm the diagnosis, especially in radiographically equivocal cases. A positive bone scan demonstrates focal radionucleotide accumulation at or adjacent to the symphysis pubis.

Magnetic resonance imaging demonstrates abnormal marrow signal at the symphysis pubis and may additionally show displacement of symphyseal fibrocartilaginous disk or its extrusion. MRI is also helpful in identifying concomitant lesions of the sacroiliac joint or pubic rami, such as stress fractures. Even muscle tendon lesions like those of adductor magnus may be identified. The classic diagnostic findings are:

- Reciprocal bone marrow edema across the entire symphysis, anterior to posterior, with or without subchondral cysts, erosions, and posterior or superior osteophytes
- Characteristics of a true arthritis
- More severe cases can manifest as osseous or osteochondral erosion and resorption
- Often there is concomitant rectus abdominis/adductor aponeurosis injury.

Classification

As is clear from the discussion above, two types of osteitis pubis can be clinically identified—one infectious and the other due to mechanical causes (often microtraumatic). Osteitis pubis due to mechanical causes has been divided into four stages by Rodriguez et al. as follows:

1. Stage 1 includes unilateral symptoms that subside after warm-up but again return after training.
2. Stage 2 involves bilateral symptoms.
3. Stage 3 players are functionally limited by pain and are unable to continue playing.
4. Stage 4 players have severe pain and difficulty with even activities of daily living.

Osteitis pubis may exist isolated or in association with a larger syndrome such as athletic pubalgia or sports hernia.

Differential Diagnosis

- Stress fractures
- Injury or diseases of the hip
- Nerve entrapment
- Sports hernias

Treatment

Nonoperative

Nonoperative treatment for osteitis pubis is in itself usually effective. This includes rest, use of ice, ultrasound stimulation and NSAIDs. Oral corticosteroids for short duration may be added. Phonophoresis with topical ketoprofen has also been utilized with some benefit. When the acute pain subsides, stretching and strengthening is initiated to reduce the forces across the pelvis (especially the hip flexors and external rotator muscles). With good progress, the exercises (low-impact activities) that will not stress the pubic symphysis are introduced gradually followed by progression to biking, running, cutting, and ultimately high-level sporting activities.

Corticosteroid injection into the symphysis (4 mg dexamethasone or depot preparations of methyl prednisolone or triamcinolone with 1 mL 1% lidocaine, and 1 mL of 0.25% bupivacaine) in athletes that do not respond to simpler treatment modalities has been found quite impressively successful in cases refractory to conservative management.

Some unconventional treatment methods found to have success in discrete authors' experiences include intravenous pamidronate infusions (two injections per month for 3–6 months) for refractory osteitis pubis or botulinum therapy to relax nearby muscles. With the difficulty in availability of injectable palmidronate, zoledronate may be prescribed as 5 mg infusions 3 months apart keeping the precautions in mind.

Operative

This is obviously reserved for refractory cases and recurrences only (5–10% of patients fail to respond to nonoperative management). Absolute indications include:

- Acute symptomatic infection of the joint
- Excessive widening (the upper limit usually in >2 cm) of the symphysis with/without associated sacroiliac joint disruption
- Severe unrelenting symptoms that limit even activities of daily living.

Surgical options include:

- Arthrodesis **(Figs. 54 and 55)**
- Wedge resection
- Curettage of symphysis
- Open/mini-open curettage and bone grafting with rigid fixation
- Extraperitoneal retropubic synthetic mesh—possibly enhances support to conjoint tendon and posterior pubic symphysis
- Endoscopic pubic symphysiotomy.

Ideal operative treatment is still undecided. Wedge resection (cutting a wedge of bone 5 mm wide on each side of symphysis anteriorly to preserve arcuate ligament and 2 cm posteriorly) carries risk of progressive sacroiliac arthrosis and posterior pelvic instability. The complications may need a secondary procedure to fuse sacroiliac joint. Curettage only is met with suboptimal results. Rigid plate fixation has been advocated for athletes with refractory osteitis pubis; however, the data on long-term biomechanical/functional effects are unknown. Also there is risk of nonunion that may further lead to implant failure and complications. Also another concern is unknown effects of anterior arthrodesis biomechanically on the posterior pelvic ring and SI joint. These make arthrodesis an option only for those patients who radiologically demonstrate large osteophytes, gross instability, and complete loss of joint space and have refractory symptoms. Endoscopic methods are very new and need expertise, and the clinical outcomes need to be further documented.

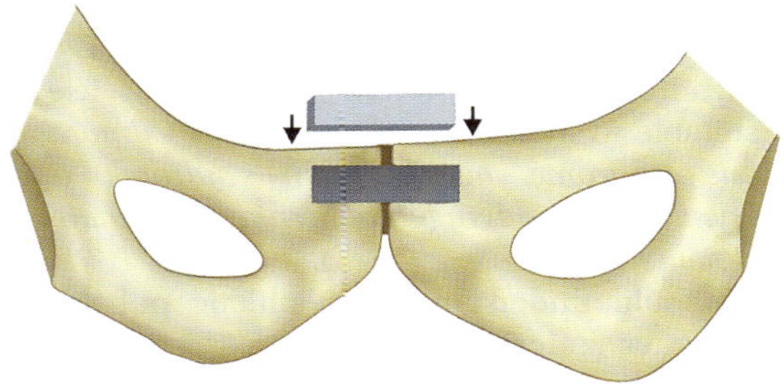

Fig. 54: Arthrodesis of symphysis pubis using phemister type graft alone.

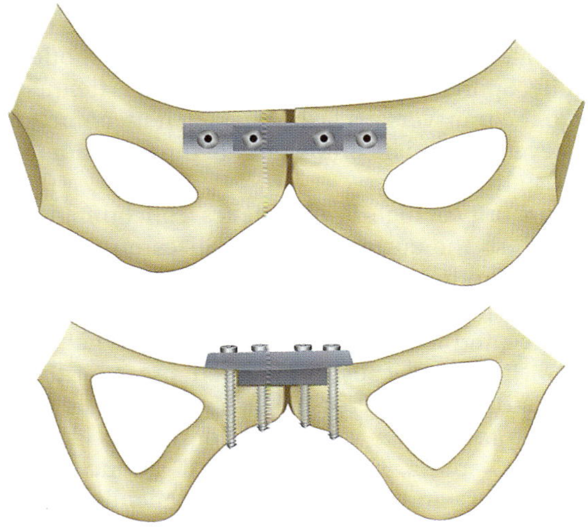

Fig. 55: Illustration of arthrodesis and plating (rigid fixation) for stabilizing symphysis pubis.

GROIN PAIN (ATHLETIC PUBALGIA AND SPORTS HERNIA)

These syndromes (along with osteitis pubis—discussed earlier) are debilitating exertional groin pain syndromes that have increasingly been recognized in high level athletics and have raised serious concerns. The concept was first described by Gilmore in 1980 as a "*groin disruption*". The irony remains that there is still no consensus on classification of the syndromes and eminent authors thus use varied terms suitable to their experience such as *Gilmore's groin, symphysis syndrome, hockey groin syndrome, adductor gracilis syndrome, occult inguinal hernia, sportsman's hernia and incipient hernia.*

One should understand that athletic pubalgia is by itself a biomechanical concept, whereas sports hernia is best considered from an anatomical perspective. Athletic pubalgia arises from muscle injury around pubic symphysis and is defined as an injury to the rectus abdominis insertion on the pubic symphysis. This is often accompanied by injury to conjoined tendon insertion forming the floor and strained adductor longus attachment to the pelvis. There may also be associated muscular dyskinesia to cause subtle pelvic instability. Sports hernia on the other hand is defined as an injury to the transversalis fascia making it incompetent and leading eventually to incompetency of the posterior inguinal wall and herniations.

In a majority of high-level athletics, concomitant FAI has been seen, so the current theory realizes on a continuum of disorder around the hip of which the patient has groin pain over majority of the time period. The FAI leads to ROM disturbance and limitations (flexion and internal rotation). The ROM limitation causes increased stress on the extra-articular structures. Increased stress on the neighboring structures produces a variety of conditions like athletic pubalgia or sports hernia, proximal adductor/gracilis/pectineus injury and/or osteitis pubis depending on which tissue gives way first and how the person tends to balance the increased stress. This may be followed or concomitantly associated with subtle pelvic instability.

Anatomical Considerations

Both athletic pubalgia and sports hernia have locus of injury around the medial extent of the inguinal canal in the region of transversalis fascia that lies posteriorly. Rectus abdominis and conjoined tendon lie anterior while the bony pubic symphysis is medial. The distal adductor tendons originating from inferior pubic rami and adjoining region define the distal extent of the injury zone. Quite often due to close proximity, the various nerves of the inguinal region are involved and hence cutaneous pain is typically distributed to the region around and including scrotum (ilioinguinal nerve), ipsilateral and contralateral inguinal area (genitofemoral nerve), and medial thigh (obturator nerve). The term sports hernia came from surgical literature: "nonpalpable, nonvisible inguinal hernia". "*Sportsman's hernia*" is an incipient hernia (no true hernia) possibly appearing as a posterior bulge found in 80–85% of the operations due to absence of striated muscle at the posterior inguinal wall (only thin transversalis fascia supports the structures here) and the passage of the spermatic cord. Literature however now even reports an actual tear typically 3–5 cm in length in the transversalis fascia in the posterior inguinal wall between the internal inguinal ring and the pubic tubercle. Most authors describe "sportsman's hernia" due to this tear that subsequently results in progressive weakness of the posterior inguinal wall. Under endoscopic visualization, a defect in the posterior wall in Hesselbach's triangle is seen with/without true herniation. The pain generators in groin pathology have been variedly reported as:

- Enthesopathies of adductor or rectus abdominis tendinous regions
- Internal oblique muscle avulsion injury near the pubic tubercle
- Osteitis pubis
- Inguinal canal disruption that consists of tearing of the superficial inguinal ring and thinning of the posterior wall
- Incompetency of external oblique muscle and aponeurosis
- Nerve entrapment involving ilioinguinal, genitofemoral and/or obturator nerve.

Due to inconsistency of reports causing groin pain and poor acceptance of the term groin hernia (as there is no true hernia!) universally, it is prudent to use the term "athletic pubalgia" an umbrella term, under which the variously reported causes of groin pain can be classified. "*Gilmore's groin*" is due to torn external oblique aponeurosis and falls under the category of athletic pubalgia. It is also associated with tearing of the conjoined tendon and avulsion from the pubic tubercle, and a dehiscence between the conjoined tendon and inguinal ligament. There is no reported hernia however. *Hockey player's syndrome*, hockey groin syndrome or slap shot gut represents a tear in the external oblique aponeurosis associated with inguinal nerve entrapment (entrapment neuropathy of ilioinguinal nerve). This indicates that the ilioinguinal nerve and the genital branch of the genitofemoral nerve play important roles in chronic pain associated with occult groin injuries that resolves with nerve decompression after "sports herniorrhaphies". The phrase "*symphysis syndrome*" describes the combination of abnormalities of the rectus abdominis at its small attachment area in the pubis, and chronic adductor pain from overuse and incorporates pelvic instability as one of the causes of athletic pubalgia. Number of adductor syndromes are described all causing groin pain (all classified under athletic pubalgia) and include:

- Adductor longus (AL) variant is due to tear or attenuation of AL tendon without tear of the rectus tendon. It is commonly observed in runners and kicking athletes, such as soccer players, rugby players and sprinters.
- Adductor avulsion (AA) variant is due to partial or complete avulsion of pubis origin of the common adductor tendon resulting in instability with anterior subluxation of the symphysis. Hockey players, skaters and swimmers are particularly susceptible to this injury.
- Adductor calcification (AC) variant is due to calcification at the common adductor/AL tendon insertion from repetitive microtrauma.
- The *hockey goalie/baseball pitcher syndrome* is a localized painful condition characterized by infolding of the adductor muscle fibers between the torn fibers of the epimysium.

As reiterated above also, most of these muscle injuries result in an imbalance of dynamic muscle stabilizers. In the anterior pelvic region, the strong adductors easily overpower torn rectus muscles causing subtle anterior pelvic tilt. This increased anterior tilt has an effect similar to high heel biomechanically but is more severe in the sense that triggered abnormalities in the biokinetic chain get amplified due to associated muscle injury ultimately causing more pain around the anterior groin. The athlete is usually crippled functionally and is unable to compete at a high level.

Biomechanics

The biomechanical concept is related to the instability of pelvis but is not completely understood. The initial insult occurs at the muscles as mentioned earlier that stabilize the pelvis. The mechanism seems to be an overuse syndrome due to repetitive hip hyperextension and truncal rotational movements. This causes initially a stress and tear and ultimately failure (acute or acute on chronic) of the musculotendinous attachments of rectus abdominis, both the obliques (external and internal), and transversus abdominis in the upper region and injury to adductor group of muscles, namely the adductor longus, pectineus and gracilis inferiorly. The ultimate failure can be precipitated in athletes by the tremendous moments generated at the level of the pelvis. These forces generated by contraction of many muscles, especially the rectus abdominis and adductor longus, are typically concentrated in the anterior compartment that takes the major brunt. Moment force imbalance is created when one on the muscle weakens in the cycle of injury causing unequal distribution of pelvic forces. This generates pelvic instability that is not clinically identified (termed microinstability). Once there is pelvic microinstability, the rectus attachment is rendered incompetent and allowing it to tilt anteriorly shifting the pressure in the adductor compartment generating the so called "adductor compartment syndrome" and adductor pain. Development of pathology and incompetent support mechanism on one side of the pubis (right or left) obviously creates an overly stressed region for the contralateral rectus and adductor group and the process is repeated causing pubalgia. If unchecked, it transforms into deteriorating cycle and later massive damage.

Clinical Evaluation

History

High performance pivoting athletes like the football players and hockey players are more likely to develop athletic pubalgia/sports hernia. Males are almost exclusively affected. Women though should also be evaluated carefully. The athletes present with a long-standing history of lower abdominal pain with exertion. In early course of disorder, commonly the athlete will report pain while getting out of bed in the morning. Initially, the pain is localized to the inguinal area in the region corresponding to insertion of the rectus abdominis on the pubic tubercle just medial to the external inguinal ring. It is usually unilateral but may be bilateral. Uncommon location of pain is along the insertion of adductor tendon. The pain may radiate to the scrotum, laterally in the upper thigh, or to the opposite groin though uncommonly. The pain is aggravated by rotational movements such as lateral cutting, kicking, shooting a slap shot, pushing off with ice skates, and sudden torso rotation and is relieved by rest.

Physical Findings

Examination of the unaffected side should be performed first for comparison. The first goal is to rule out a classic hernia. Observe for any injury tell-tale marks like mass, bruising, or other soft tissue lesions of the groin. Next examine the inguinal canal that is best done patient lying supine with the hips slightly flexed and externally rotated to relax the abdominal fascia. The tip of pinkie finger is inserted through the scrotum negotiating the external inguinal ring. Commonly in sports hernia, there is slight enlargement of the inguinal ring associated with tenderness of the posterior wall of the canal. In chronic cases, a subtle defect may be noticed in the transversalis fascia sometimes. A cough impulse may also be evident. These findings help differentiate athletic pubalgia where most are absent. Instead in athletic pubalgia, the most common finding is adductor tenderness. Maneuvers such as sit-ups, resisted hip adduction and Valsalva reproduce exacerbate the symptoms in athletic pubalgia and are more suggestive. Additionally diffuse tenderness over the pubic tubercle and the peripubic region is noted. Gait and clinical examination of the hip joint are usually normal.

Imaging

Radiographs are obtained to rule out avulsion fractures and osteitis pubis. They are otherwise normal in athletic pubalgia or sports hernia. "Secondary cleft sign" may be found in patients with osteitis pubis or in patients with adductor tendon injury.

Magnetic Resonance Imaging

Magnetic resonance imaging is possibly the best tool to help rule out serious diagnoses in the differential diagnosis but the identification rate is unfortunately low. STIR and T2-weighted sequences and gadolinium enhancement are recommended. The following are some of the findings:

- Bone marrow edema common but isolated to anterior cortex of pubis in tears of rectus or adductor muscles. Secondary or accessory cleft sign is common—tenoperiosteal disruption at the anterior, inferior pubis on sagittal views approximately 1 cm lateral to primary cleft or symphysis
- Attenuation of the abdominal wall musculofascial layers was seen most often.
- Lateral bundle of rectus abdominis is disrupted or atrophic on axial cuts.
  - Common adductor tendon is torn and retracted on coronal cuts
  - Increased signal within one or more of the groin muscles
  - Rectus abdominis insertion appears "lifted" from its normal pubic attachment.

Ultrasound

Dynamic ultrasound examination can demonstrate posterior wall insufficiency of inguinal canal in young males where no clinical signs of hernia are elicited but the greatest limitation is that the investigation is highly user-dependent. Experienced sonologists can demonstrate a weak, bulging posterior inguinal canal wall. There are high chances that ultrasound may become the future modality of choice in identifying inguinal region pathologies for athletes having unresolved chronic groin pain with increased dedicated usage.

Bone scan is of limited help in pathology identification but may be used to rule out other causes of the groin or inguinal pain, especially bone infections or metabolic disorders.

Herniography

Currently, the indications are ill-defined; however, it has the capability to demonstrate occult hernias. Herniography is performed by intraperitoneal injection of the contrast material followed by fluoroscopy to visualize spread of dye. Demonstration of any extraperitoneal extravasation of dye is diagnostic of an occult hernia. One should however balance the risk involved with the procedure. Complications such as bowel perforation and peritonitis are reported in 5–6% cases. The utility and indications are however not completely defined.

Differential Diagnosis

- *Bone pathology:*
  - Stress fractures
  - Osteoid osteoma
- *Intraperitoneal pathology:*
  - Endometriosis/fibroids
  - Inflammatory bowel disease
- Arthritides—sacroiliitis and primary synovial diseases
- Apophysitis of AIIS or ASIS
- True herniations
- Internal derangements of hip

Management

Adductor pain with minimal or no pubalgia only is treated conservatively. Most established pubalgias with above-mentioned physical findings fail conservative management as is also true of sports hernia. Persistent adductor pain despite conservative treatment needs adductor release along with an open pelvic floor repair. The latter is specifically needed as adductor symptoms are often secondary to pelvic microinstability that need to be addressed. The concept of adductor release is highly controversial.

Surgical Treatment

For pelvic instability, an open procedure should be performed; we prefer a modified Bassini herniorrhaphy pelvic floor repair that also takes care of most sport hernias should they coexist. Another method is open repair of the transversalis fascia with mesh augmentation. For patients with overt defects of external oblique aponeurosis, reinforcement of the external oblique aponeurosis with mesh is advocated. Ilioinguinal nerve entrapment is commonly seen in such cases and simultaneous ablation of the ilioinguinal nerve is recommended.

For patients with established diagnosis of sports hernia surgical repair should focus on reconstructing the posterior inguinal canal wall deficiency. Both laparoscopic [total extraperitoneal (TEP) and transabdominal preperitoneal (TAPP)] and open procedures are successful in this regard. Prophylactic repair of the unaffected side is debated.

Complications

The complications of surgical procedures for athletic pubalgia or sports hernia are minor and include:

- Wound infections
- Hematoma
- Peri-incisional numbness
- Failure of repair and recurrence of symptoms

HIP STRESS FRACTURES

Stress fractures are most common in the lower extremities in the athletes. These types of fractures are typically overused and overload injuries sustained during endurance running, jumping and dance. These fractures can occur in normal bone exposed to persistent abnormal stress, or in abnormal bone exposed to normal stress.

The **mechanism** involves microfractures sustained during repetitive and cyclical impact loading that overwhelm the body and bone's ability to remodel and heal. Once a certain threshold is crossed, the fractures become symptomatic. Influence of various factors that predispose patients to stress fractures:

- Structural alteration (gross/microscopic anatomy) of bone
- Altered load patterns or change in mechanical/anatomical axis—includes joint deformity
- Altered chemical structure of bone as by metabolic imbalances:
  - Medications
  - Nutritional deficiencies
  - Hormonal disturbances (females)

Stress fractures in hip can occur on either the femoral or pelvic aspect. The pelvic side fractures occur in the medial wall or roof of the acetabulum, and in the pubic rami. These occur due to metabolic or structural abnormalities as most occur due to bone insufficiency. These fractures can usually be treated symptomatically. Femoral side stress fractures occur in the femoral neck region and are typically stress-related **(Figs. 56A and B)**. Only rarely do they arise from metabolic abnormalities. Uncommon stress fractures of femoral head are also described (see later). The metabolic related fractures of femoral neck are better called spontaneous fractures of femoral neck as is seen in osteoporosis. Renal osteodystrophy, metastatic and neoplasia-related fractures are better called pathological fractures. Bilateral femoral neck fractures may arise due to various causes and may also be idiopathic. The mentioned causes for bilateral spontaneous fractures of femoral neck (pathological or otherwise) include:

- Repetitive trauma (stress fractures)
- Renal osteodystrophy
- Seizures
- Abnormal anatomy
- Osteoporosis

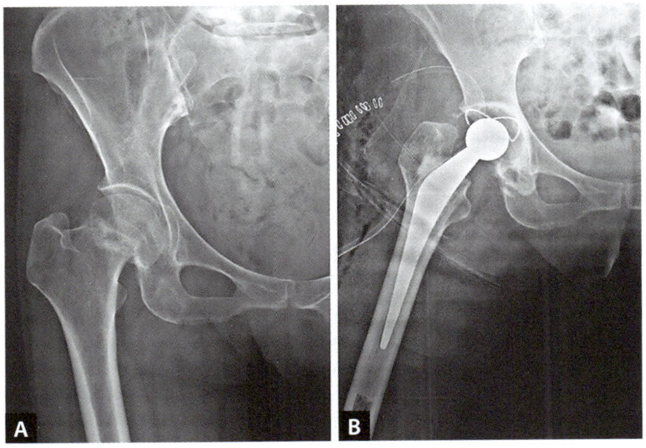

Figs. 56A and B: Stress fracture neck of femur. The patient had pain for 3.5 months and was taking Ayurvedic treatment for groin pain that used to increase with walking. One day however excruciating pain developed while patient was walking, and on radiographs, right subcapital femoral neck fracture was noted with sclerotic margins. The patient was treated with total hip arthroplasty.

Clinical Presentation

There is vague onset of groin and anterior thigh pain that initially bothers the patient and later becomes unremitting and activity limiting. Trauma as a history is usually not mentioned. There is usually a reported recent increase or change in activity or training program or episodes of extreme muscle fatigue. Examination findings are nonspecific and difficult to interpret. Pubic rami fractures are tender to palpation. Slight limitation of internal rotation in flexion may be observed in proximal femur stress fractures. Single leg hopping provocates pain but predisposes to possible completion of fracture.

Investigation and Management

Plain radiographs are likely to be normal in patients with stress fractures 2–4 weeks after the onset of symptoms. They help in evaluating other problems like unsuspected and metabolic abnormalities. With normal plain radiographs but high index of suspicion, there is controversy as to the best modality for evaluation—bone scintigraphy or MRI. Bone scans have been classically prescribed and were the investigation of choice previously but it should be remembered that they give radiation exposure to patient. The sensitivity of both tests approach 100% for stress fracture. Bone scan lacks specificity however and when positive is typically followed by an MRI for characterization of pathology. MRI has thus become investigation of choice as the scans are now readily available, identify stress fractures, and localize and quantify the lesions **(Figs. 57A to D)**. Additionally, it also defines the periarticular soft tissue and can identify other pathology.

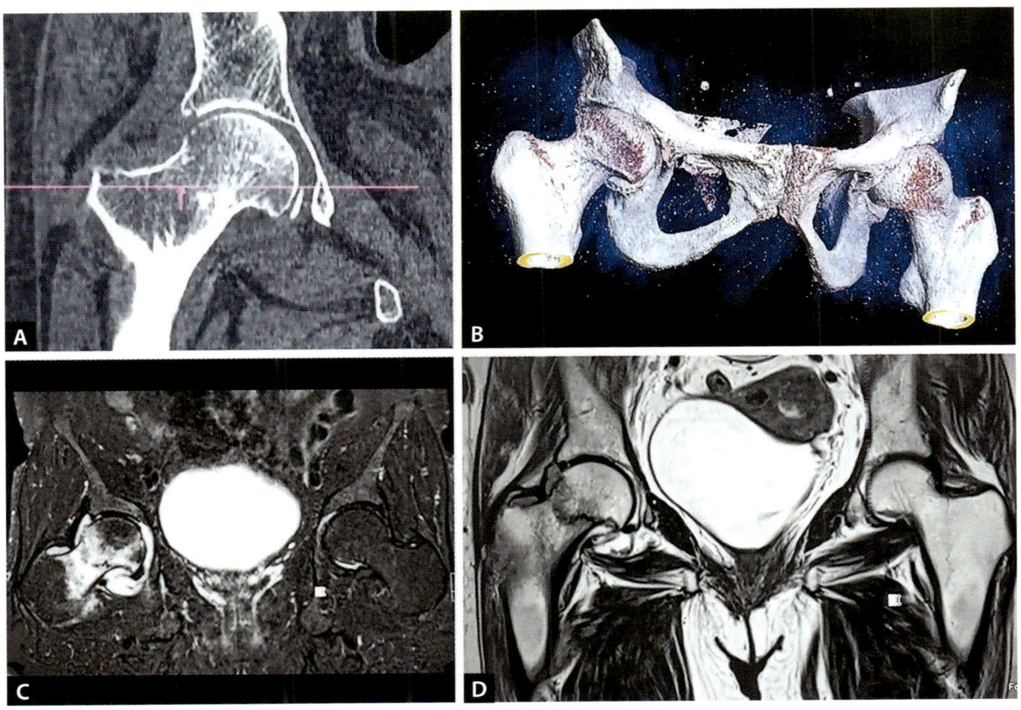

Figs. 57A to D: Tension type stress fracture of femoral neck. The patient presented with pain in right hip developing after intense 3 weeks defense services training. The radiographs (not shown) were normal. CT-scan of the hip was also unremarkable (A and B). MRI of right hip revealed classical tension type stress fracture of femoral neck (C and D). The fracture line appears complete but conventionally the fractures occurring in superior portion of femoral neck are called tension type while those in inferior portion are designated compression type stress fracture.

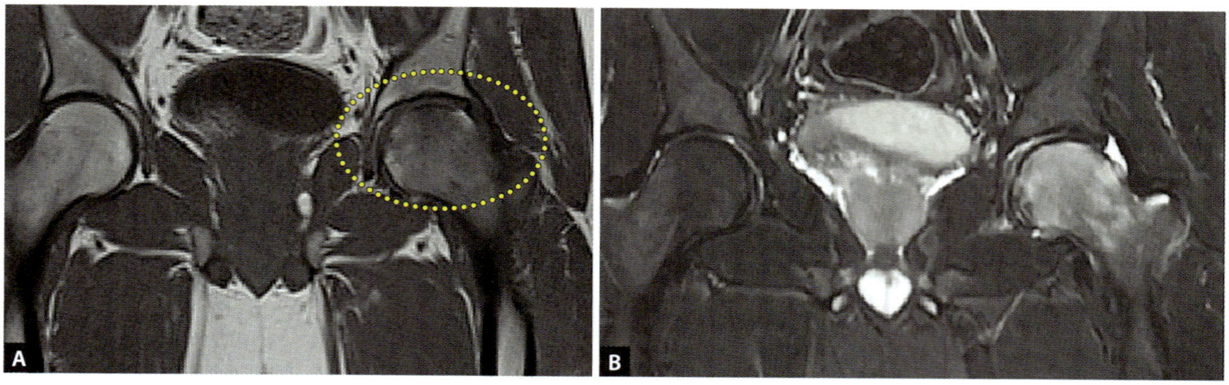

Figs. 58A and B: This 21-year-old male patient had pain for 6 months in shifting between left hip and groin region and knee making diagnosis difficult with local practitioner. He had aggravation of pain in groin and buttock region while attempting running in college level event. The radiographs (not shown) were unremarkable but MRI scans demonstrated characteristic subchondral fracture (yellow oval) of the head in weight bearing zone (A) and edema in the proximal femur (B), findings characteristic of fatigue fracture of femoral head.

Femoral neck stress fractures are classified into types based on location, cause and biomechanical stability:

- ***Lateral "tension-side":*** The tension-side fractures are inherently unstable and are best treated with operative fixation.
- ***Medial "compression-side":*** These fractures are biomechanically stable and have been treated successfully with rest, limited weight-bearing, and activity restriction in dependable patients. Unfortunately, these stable fractures can go on to nonunion, so further refinement of the classification specifically guiding treatment has been proposed. The modification suggests that compression-side fractures with a visible fatigue line greater than or equal to 50% of the width of the femoral neck should be treated operatively with screws. Those being treated nonoperatively should be followed with biweekly serial radiographs, and if delayed healing or fracture progression is noted, internal fixation is recommended.

Uncommon entity of *fatigue fractures of femoral heads* has also been reported. The radiographic presentation mimics osteonecrosis, so a brief detail is pertinent. Fatigue fractures of the subchondral femoral head are more likely to occur in individuals with poor bone quality. Even the advanced diagnostics may be confusing so in a healthy athlete with no risk factors for osteonecrosis radiologist evaluating hip MRI should be alerted to the possible diagnosis. In a hip with a subchondral fatigue fracture, the signal changes and bone marrow edema patterns differ **(Figs. 58 A and B)**. Treatment is conservative and protected weight-bearing for patients without collapse but those with collapse need bone grafting (light bulb procedure).

The clinician should have a high level of suspicion for these lesions (stress fractures of femoral neck or head) as displacement of fractures or collapse respectively has a dismal prognosis even after surgery. The reported complications of surgical fixation include infection, malalignment, LLD, nonunion and osteonecrosis.

CONCLUSION

- Arthroscopy of the hip is a new tool that is gaining popularity for management of various labral, capsular and chondral injuries in patients with this disorder. The technique is quite specialized and has steep learning curve for even experienced arthroscopist due to unique instrumentation and difficult access.
- Labral injuries are quite common that mostly arise out of hip impingement syndromes. The management involves prompt identification and refixation of the labral injuries (or debridement as the case demands) to preserve rest of the structures and prevent progression of disease. Osteoarthrosis of hip is a morbid condition that limits functionality in later life if the labral or chondral tears are not promptly addressed.
- Hip (femoroacetabular) impingement syndrome has been recognized over last two decades as important harbinger of hip osteoarthrosis that can be captured early in life and treated appropriately to prevent this complication from occurring. The two types have unique disposition in patient population and well-defined diagnostic and treatment protocols exist for their management.
- Snapping hips and lateral trochanteric pain syndromes should not be neglected as benign as some of them have pathological lesions that can be given specific surgical remedy.
- The piriformis syndrome is entrapment neuropathy of sciatic nerve with lot of controversy surrounding around its diagnosis. The existence is probably real and one should make a careful diagnosis of the disorder excluding most other causes though most of them are relieved by conservative management alone.
- Osteitis pubis is a disorder of significant concern to the sports athlete as it may even be the carrier of the person if recurrent. Accurate diagnosis and proper management should be introduced with graded rehabilitation to ensure successful outcome. It should be differentiated from athletic pubalgia, which is more a cluster of unrelated disorders in the region.
- Stress fractures are commonly missed as nonspecific groin pains or tendinitis, but have dramatic consequences if untreated. One must be vigilant in patient evaluation and have high index of suspicion in order not to miss them and institute immediate treatment.

CHAPTER 48

Sports Medicine: Elbow

Manish Kumar Varshney

INTRODUCTION

Elbow injuries are common in sports persons. Most are related to chronic overuse or friction syndrome but a few results from direct injury to susceptible ligaments of the restricted mobility. The joint has comparatively high bony congruity leading to mobility restriction in a single plane. The joint had been classically thought to be "touch me not" for frequent occurrence of stiffness following open surgical procedures. Arthroscopy has developed lately but the vision is not as well as for large joint arthroscopy, also the surrounding structures make the approach difficult. The various affections of elbow joint are discussed in separate Chapter on "Anomalies of Pediatric Upper Limb" but we will discuss elbow arthroscopy and terrible triad injury here.

ELBOW ARTHROSCOPY

The procedure was attempted early in 1931 but was considered unsafe and modern procedure was described only in 1985 (Andrews and Carson).

Indications

- Loose body removal
- Olecranon osteophyte debridement **(Fig. 1)**
- *Synovectomy:* Inflammatory arthritides, etc.
- Capsular releases for stiff elbow
- *Osteochondritis dissecans (OCD) of capitellum (Panner's disease):* Examine by radiocapitellar compression test (place the elbow in full extension and load with supination and pronation to produce mechanical symptoms)
- Lateral epicondylitis (chair test—standing behind the chair patient is asked to lift it with elbow extended, forearm pronated, and wrist dorsiflexed)
- Arthrofibrosis
- *Plica excision:* Identify plica by flexion-pronation test—place the forearm in maximum pronation and passively flex the elbow to 90–110° to cause snapping.
- Assisted fixation of fractures of coronoid (for exact repositioning) and capitellum (check intra-articular screw penetration)

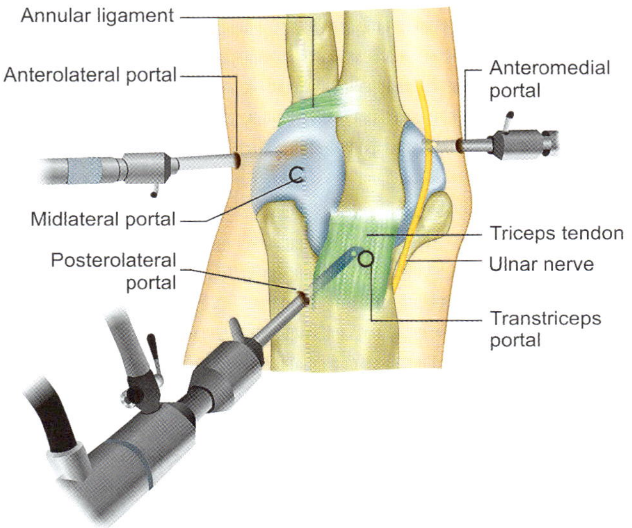

Fig. 1: The portals for elbow arthroscopy as viewed from posterior aspect.

Contraindications

- *Prior trauma:* Causing deformity and loss of prominent superficial bony markers for portal placement
- *Surgical scarring:* It may tether important structures near or into the site of portal placement.
- Previous ulnar nerve transposition
- Ankylosed joint
- Local soft tissue infection at the portal sites
- Ulnar nerve subluxation is not a contraindication, but it should be identified prior to surgery.

Patient Evaluation

Detailing the evaluation is out of the scope of current text, but the following points should be noted:

- The site of pain, i.e., from which part of the elbow is the complaint originating (lateral, medial, anterior, or posterior):
  - *Lateral:* Radial head fracture, radiocapitellar chondromalacia, osteochondritis dissecans, and osteochondral loose bodies.

- *Medial:* Medial epicondyle avulsion, ulnar collateral ligament (UCL) sprain, ulnar neuritis, ulnar nerve subluxation, and students elbow.
- *Anterior:* Distal biceps rupture, anterior capsular strain, and brachialis muscle strain.
- *Posterior:* Posterior impingement, valgus extension overload syndrome, triceps tendinitis, triceps tendon avulsion, osteochondral loose bodies, olecranon stress fracture, and olecranon bursitis.

- Examine for ulnar nerve symptoms and signs:
- Examine for UCL strain or insufficiency, elbow instability as outlined in section on upper extremity (*see* Chapter on "The Unstable Elbow")
- Evaluate the integrity of muscles in the region.

Radiological Help for Arthroscopy

Evaluate the radiographs for degenerative changes, osteophytes, previous fractures and malunion, and loose bodies. Obtain stress views and compare with the contralateral elbow for subtle changes. Magnetic resonance imaging (MRI) is a better investigation to evaluate the integrity of ligaments, articular surface, and joint capsule.

Procedure

Elbow arthroscopy may be performed in lateral, supine, or prone position. We prefer a regional anesthesia for its low morbidity but surgeons may prefer general anesthesia for muscle relaxation, immediate postoperative evaluation of nerve function and avoid positional discomfort to the patient in regional anesthesia. Either a 4-mm 30° or a 2.7-mm 30° scope is used.

Use a tourniquet. The elbow joint is first insufflated with 20–30 mL of normal saline. Portals should be placed only after proper marking of the important landmarks and on a distended joint capsule as the neurovascular structures are pushed away from the portal site with capsular distention. Use the "nick and spread" technique. Posteromedial portal may be avoided for its proximity to ulnar nerve and no additional details are provided by its use. The following are brief description of the various portals **(Figs. 2 to 4)** used in elbow arthroscopy:

- *Distal anterolateral:* This is the primary portal made during supine position. It is made 1 cm lateral and 1–3 cm distal to the lateral epicondyle. It gives excellent view of the radial head, medial side of the joint, coronoid, trochlea, brachialis insertion and coronoid fossa. The radial and lateral antebrachial cutaneous nerves should be protected.
- *Direct lateral (midlateral portal):* This is situated at the soft spot of elbow (triangle formed by olecranon, radial head, and lateral epicondyle). It is a relatively safe portal. It is used for viewing posterior compartment of elbow (capitellum, radial head, and radioulnar articulation).
- *Proximal anterolateral:* It is not a common portal to establish and does not have any specific utility. It is situated 2 cm proximal and 1 cm anterior to lateral epicondyle.

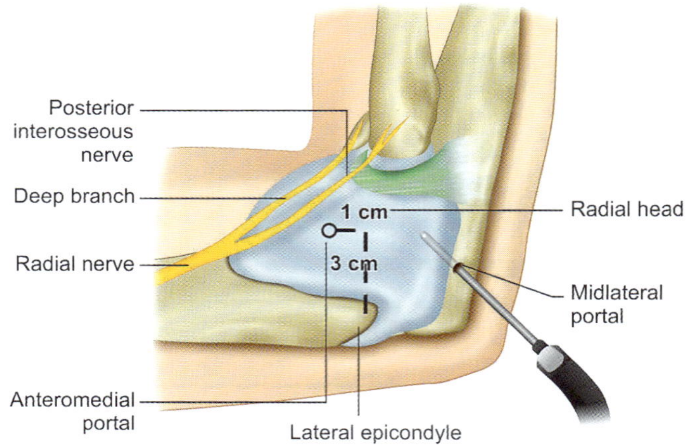

Fig. 2: The arthroscopy portals as viewed from lateral aspect.

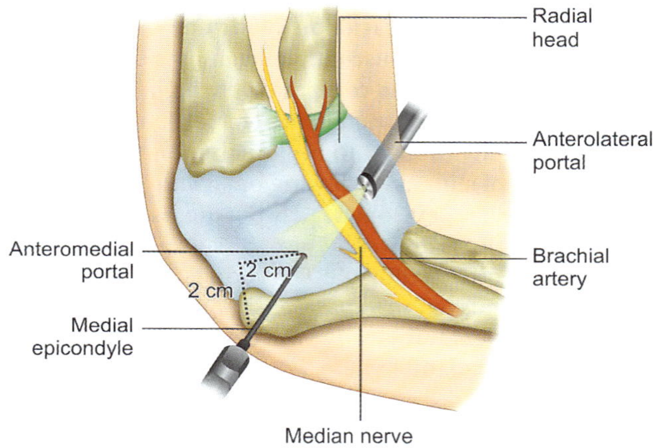

Fig. 3: The elbow arthroscopy portals as viewed from medial aspect.

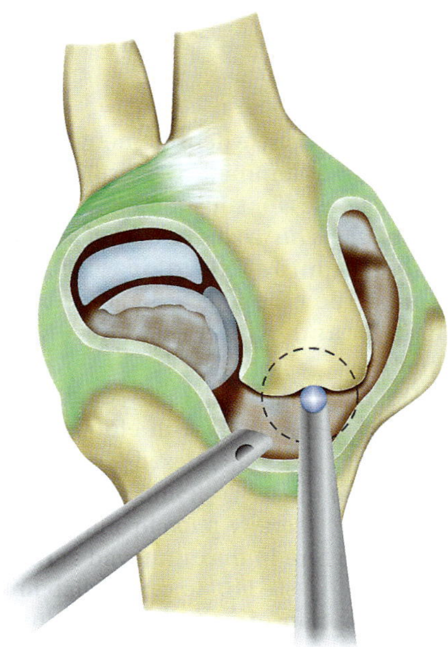

Fig. 4: Illustration of arthroscopic removal of olecranon osteophytes.

- *Anteromedial:* This portal is made 2 cm anterior and distal to medial epicondyle. Protect medial antebrachial cutaneous and median nerves.
- *Proximal medial (superomedial):* Situated 2 cm anterior and distal to the medial epicondyle, anterior to intermuscular septum. The portal is used to visualize entire anterior compartment, radial head, capitellum, coronoid, and trochlea. A good portal for survey. Ulnar and median nerves should be protected.
- *Posterior portal (transtriceps):* Made 3 cm proximal to olecranon through the triceps muscle in midline at musculotendinous junction. It is good for removing the olecranon osteophytes and loose bodies from the joint and posterolateral compartment. Protect the ulnar and posterior antebrachial cutaneous nerves.
- *Posterolateral portal:* This is the best portal to assess the posterior compartment and radiocapitellar joint for debriding OCD lesions. Protect the posterior antebrachial cutaneous nerve, medial brachial cutaneous nerve, and the ulnar nerve.

Commonly, the midlateral, posterolateral, transtriceps, and the proximal anterolateral portals are used.

Elbow arthroscopy is still not much popular though it has its own stern proponents. The joint is difficult to assess with limited mobility for instruments and has no definite indications.

Advantages of Elbow Arthroscopy

- Visualization of nearly all of the joint with this technique (open surgeries give limited exposure)
- Decreased postoperative pain
- Faster postoperative recovery.

Disadvantages of Elbow Arthroscopy

- Technically demanding
- Limited space for instrumentation
- Cumbersome compared to faster open arthrotomy
- High risk of damage to neurovascular structures due to their proximity to the joint

Complications of Elbow Arthroscopy

- *Nerve palsy (1-5%):* The nerves around elbow are at greatest risk with the procedure. The risk increases in patients with underlying rheumatoid arthritis, elbow contracture, stiff elbow or ankylosed joints and frequent use of transtriceps, and proximal lateral portal (inexperience). The nerves at particular risk have been mentioned with the specific portals but commonly injury is seen to:
  - Ulnar nerve palsy (the most common and commonly transient)
  - Radial nerve palsy (second most common)

  The mechanism of nerve injury is either a direct injury by trocars and instrumentation (failure to use blunt dissection causing neuroma formation) or indirect injury say due to compartment syndrome (aggressive distention and fluid extravasation) or stretching.
- Joint ankylosis or heterotopic ossification
- Articular cartilage injury
- Synovial fistula formation
- Instrument breakage
- Infection

TERRIBLE TRIAD INJURY OF ELBOW (HOTCHKISS TRIAD, 1996)

A terrible triad injury of elbow is, basically, a complex posterior dislocation of the elbow associated with radial head and coronoid process fractures. It is termed terrible due to poor outcomes of the injury complex even after best of reconstructions.

Anatomy

- The coronoid process provides an important anterior and varus buttress to the elbow joint. It consists of a tip, body, anterolateral facet and anteromedial facet. At the inferomedial aspect is the insertion of the anterior bundle of the medial collateral ligament (MCL). The coronoid process provides stability against axial, varus, posteromedial, and posterolateral rotatory forces.
- The lateral portion of radial head does not articulate with capitellum or proximal ulna (site for plate fixation).
- Radial head provides an important anterior and valgus buttress to the elbow.
- The anatomy of medial and lateral collateral ligaments has been detailed in Chapter on "The Unstable Elbow". The stabilizers of elbow can be categorized into primary and secondary:
  - Primary stabilizers (an elbow with intact joint surfaces only requires two ligaments for stability—(i) the ulnar lateral collateral ligament (LCL) and (ii) the anterior band of the medial collateral ligament):
    - *Medial collateral ligament:* Anterior bundle provides stability against valgus stress.
    - *Lateral collateral ligament:* Resists varus force
    - *Ulnohumeral articulation:* Beyond 30° of flexion, the coronoid provides stability against posterior dislocation.
  - Secondary stabilizers:
    - *Radial head:* Axial support to forearm and secondary stability against varus force
    - Joint capsule
    - Common flexor and extensor origin

Pathogenesis

- Dislocations or subluxations typically occur as a result of a fall on an outstretched hand (FOOSH) result in axial load and supination and valgus moments at elbow.
- Soft-tissue disruption proceeds sequentially in three stages from medial to lateral as displacement increases (Hori's circle described by O'Driscoll, see below). This typical pattern of soft tissue disruption is associated with fractures of the coronoid and radial head.
- The coronoid fracture commonly occurs at the tip including the anterior capsular insertion site. Less commonly, the coronoid fracture is large or may primarily involve the anteromedial facet.

Stages of soft tissue injury as described by O'Driscoll:

Stage 1:
- Lateral collateral ligament disruption
- Posterolateral rotatory subluxation that reduces spontaneously
- Positive lateral pivot shift

Stage 2:
- Additional anterior and posterior soft tissue disruption
- Elbow subluxes so that the coronoid is perched under the trochlea

Stage 3:
- *Stage 3A:* Anterior band of MCL is intact. Elbow is stable to valgus stress test after reduction.
- *Stage 3B:* Anterior band of MCL is ruptured and elbow is unstable to valgus stress after reduction.
- *Stage 3C:* All soft tissues stripped from distal humerus. Elbow grossly unstable from 0 to 90° but partially stability gained when flexed to >90°. If there is no associated fracture of the coronoid or radial head, the instability is due to extensive soft-tissue tearing. Typically, the common flexor and extensor tendons are torn as well. However, fractures of the radial head and coronoid (terrible triad injury), when present, absorb energy and there is secondary soft tissue tearing which is less severe.

Clinical Features

One should thoroughly look for and evaluate the stability of elbow; the various ligament disruptions and their tests have been detailed elsewhere (*see* Chapter on "The Unstable Elbow"). The most important aspect is immediate reduction of elbow that should not be delayed for understanding the mechanism of injury. After closed reduction, it is imperative to test and document stability in all planes with the forearm in pronation, neutral, and supination.

Imaging and Diagnostic Studies

Once reduction has been achieved, a computed tomography (CT) scan assessment should be systematically performed to investigate the associated bone lesions and plan the most adapted therapeutic management. Plain radiographs are obtained mainly for documentation purpose though the details they reveal are much inferior to a CT scan. MRI and magnetic resonance (MR) arthrograms are not actually needed unless one does not believe his clinical examination. In acute injury setting, overdiagnosis of injuries is common with MRI.

Regan Morrey classification of coronoid fractures:
- Type I fracture involved an "avulsion" of the tip of the coronoid process.
- Type II involved a single or comminuted fracture representing ≤50% of the coronoid process.
- Type III involved a single or comminuted fracture of >50% of the coronoid.

These are further classified into types A and B, which represent associated absence or presence of a dislocation, respectively.

Mason's classification of radial head fractures is preferable for operative decision-making:
- Type I, nondisplaced fracture
- Type II, displaced partial articular fracture with or without comminution
- Type III, comminuted radial head fracture involving the whole head.

Hotchkiss modification of Mason's classification includes:
- Type I fractures are those displaced <2 mm, with no mechanical block
- Type II fractures are those with >2 mm of displacement that are repairable and may have a mechanical block to motion.
- Type III fractures are comminuted fractures that are judged to be not repairable by radiographic or intraoperative findings and that require excision or replacement.

Treatment

All terrible triad injuries require surgical repair unless contraindicated in patients too morbid to undergo operation or those who are terminally ill due to other reasons.

Operative Treatment

The principle of surgical management is based on two main objectives:

1. Restoration of bony stabilizing structures (radial head and coronoid process):
   - It is now well admitted that type II radial head fractures and, as long as it is possible, type III fractures should be preserved and treated with osteosynthesis in case of terrible triad injuries of the elbow. If type III injuries cannot be reconstructed then arthroplasty should be envisaged for proper reconstruction of lateral column.
   - Coronoid fractures are importantly addressed to maintain posterior stability. Though some advocate nonoperative management of type I fractures, we prefer anterior capsular reinforcement using suture anchors **(Figs. 5A and B)**. Types II and III should be repaired or fixed with a screw or plate osteosynthesis.
2. *Radial (lateral) collateral ligament repair:* Reinsertion of the lateral ligament complex in the management of elbow joint instabilities was first described by Osborne and Cotterill. We recommend a transosseous suture of ligament at the isometric point carefully identified by O'Driscoll and Morrey.

Management of MCL is more contested in the contemporary literature. We feel that MCL should only be addressed in case of persistent instability after above repair. Since the common finding in repaired elbows is the injury to MCL when opened medially. One should aim for sagittal stability in 30–130° arc of motion.

There are a few cases where instability will persist despite all above measures. In such cases, external fixation should be applied to the reconstructed elbow. The hinged external fixator centered at elbow joint should be used that allows early mobilization while providing supplementary stability during range of motion (ROM).

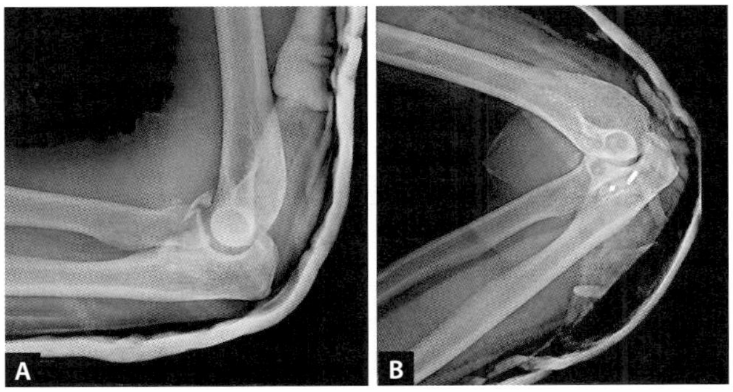

Figs. 5A and B: (A) The patient suffered from dislocation of elbow that was unstable anteroposteriorly; (B) Type 2 coronoid fracture was present with comminution so a hammock loop was taken from behind the fragment and capsule to fix to the ulna using suture anchors.

Some key aspects of the surgical technique:

- Use lateral Kocher's approach between anconeus and extensor carpi ulnaris (ECU) for lateral repair and reconstructions.
- Combine medial approach for MCL repair
- Direct anterior transbrachial approach is sometimes necessary for coronoid plate fixation.
- A standard surgical protocol should be followed with repair or reconstruction of radial head followed by LCL and then coronoid.
- Use safe zone for fixation of radial head (with the forearm in neutral rotation, bisect the anteroposterior diameter to the radial head and make a mark at this point. The safe zone extends 65° anterior and 45° posterior to this mark (total arc = 110°). Do not overstuff the joint during arthroplasty.
- Repair LCL by transosseous sutures at the isometric point
- Coronoid osteosynthesis can be eased from additional medial approach if lateral is insufficient.
- After treatment of the radial head fracture, coronoid process fixation and LCL repair/reconstruction test elbow stability under live fluoroscopy. The elbow should remain concentrically reduced from 30° to full flexion in one or more positions of forearm rotation. If this is the case, repair of the MCL is not necessary. If elbow is still unstable, repair the medial collateral ligament.
- If elbow is unstable after repairing the MCL, place the patient in a static or hinged external fixator (ulnohumeral transfixation is an option as well).
- Before leaving the operating room (OR) test and document the stable arc of motion for rehabilitation purposes.

Postoperative Immobilization or Rehabilitation

For a satisfactory result possibly this is as important as the surgical procedure itself. Most cases fail due to surgeon unawareness of a proper postoperative protocol. This should be carefully practiced and impressed upon the patient that the surgery was just the beginning of treatment and not the end of it (of course, surgeons should also be convinced with this approach).

Postoperative splinting position depends on the ligament reconstructions or repairs that have been done as they have differential lengths at varying positions. The aim is optimal healing of both the ligaments:

- *Medial collateral ligament intact, LCL repaired:* Splinted at 90° or full pronation
- *Medial collateral ligament and LCL repaired:* Splint in neutral
- *Lateral collateral ligament repaired and MCL unrepaired:* 90° flexion and full supination
  Range of motion is begun 2–5 days postoperatively within stable arc of motion determined intraoperatively. Include pronation or supination with elbow at 90°.
- Resting splint is used between exercises for 6 weeks.
- Static progressive extension night splint is begun at 6 weeks.
- Strengthening of muscles around elbow and forearm at 8 weeks or when fractures and ligamentous repairs are secure.

CONCLUSION

- Involvement of elbow is quite frequent in throwing athletes.
- Most of the disorders involve either tendinitis or impingement syndromes. The management has been marked by change from conservative approach to aggressive operative intervention of most of the disorders with gaining popularity of elbow arthroscopy and development of higher end diagnostic interventions including MRI and MR arthrography.
- Quite a complicated lesion around is the terrible triad of elbow as it is popularly called due to quite dismal prognosis despite meticulous reconstruction. One has to be perfect in dealing with all the aspects of injury in order to provide best possible outcome to the patient.

CHAPTER 49

Sports Medicine: Hand Injuries

Manish Kumar Varshney

INTRODUCTION

Injuries to hand and fingers are common in outdoor and competitive sports. Tendon disruptions and injuries to various finger bones are commonly encountered. Their appropriate management is imperative to restoration of competitive sport levels.

JERSEY FINGER

Jersey finger refers to avulsion of the tendon of flexor digitorum profundus (FDP) from the distal phalanx **(Fig. 1)**. This is a volar aspect injury to distal phalanx. The injury is caused by forcible extension of the digit while attempting to flex at the distal interphalangeal (DIP) joint, such as in football or rugby when the athlete grabs an opponent's jersey and the finger is involuntarily extended as the opponent attempts to elude tackle, thus gathering its name "jersey" finger. Three-fourths of FDP avulsion injuries involve the ring finger.

Presentation

There is loss of the normal cascade of the fingers with swelling and prominence of the digit and patients are unable to flex the DIP joint. The injury is commonly missed as there is no classic diagnostic deformity, and the pathognomonic sign of loss of active flexion at the DIP joint may be dismissed because of swelling and pain. The other reason of missing the injury is that radiographs are often negative, and pain, swelling, and ecchymosis are not always present. It is, hence, imperative to specifically test for active flexion of the DIP joint. One must also attempt to localize precisely the area of maximum tenderness to try to identify the distal end of the retracted tendon.

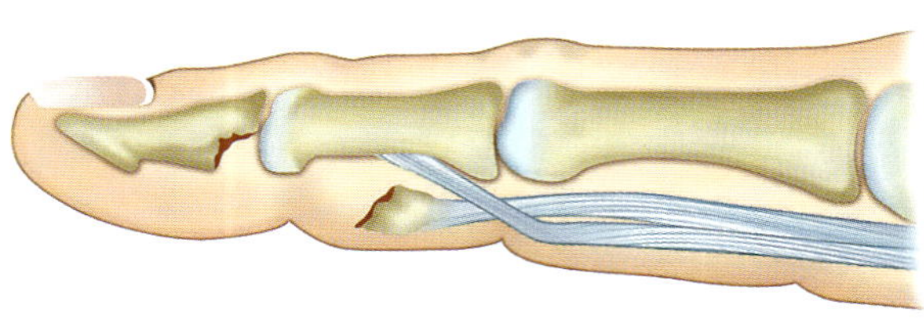

Fig. 1: Jersey finger—avulsion of the bony fragment from distal phalanx.

The Jersey finger is classified into four types:

1. Type I, retraction of the tendon to the palm with rupture of the vincula
2. Type II, retraction of the tendon to the proximal interphalangeal (PIP) joint with intact vinculum
3. Type III, avulsion with a large bony fragment which catches on A4 pulley at the middle phalanx
4. Type IV, a partial avulsion or bony avulsion and the tendon lies near to the phalanx.

Prognostic Factors

Various factors determine the success of treatment as follows:

- Time from injury to treatment
- The level to which the tendon retracts
- *The presence and size of bony avulsion:* Three-view radiographs are recommended to identify bony avulsions.
- The remaining blood supply of the tendon

Treatment

The goal is quick diagnosis of avulsion injuries and prompt anatomic repair. The tendon to bone repair is slow and during the first 6 weeks following repair significant increase in the repair site strength is not gained. Thus, deploying suture anchors to insert the tendon into cancellous bone troughs provides the best opportunity for rapid tendon repair. Delay in treatment can result in fibrosis and scarring of the tendon sheath. Pure tendinous injuries allow the FDP to retract to the palm, whereas injuries with bone fragments tend to limit retraction to the level of the middle phalanx (bony fragment gets stuck at the chiasm).

Management of types I to III injuries has been discussed in detail in Chapter on "Tendon Injuries of Hand and Management". Type IV injuries are conservatively managed with dynamic rehabilitation of the tendon involving passive flexion, dorsal block splint, and active extension exercises.

MALLET FINGER

Mallet finger deformity is also known as "Baseball Finger" and "Drop Finger" Zone I Injuries of Extensor Tendon. It is most commonly seen in softball, baseball, basketball, and football players, the extensor tendon attachment is disrupted from the dorsal aspect of distal phalanx. The extensor mechanism over the DIP joint gets disrupted. The resultant deformity results from unopposed flexion of the distal phalanx.

The common mechanism of mallet finger in sports injury is by a direct blow to the tip of extended finger. This acutely flexes the distal phalanx resulting in strained tendon at the insertion due to existing tenodesis effect. The other mechanism is a direct blow to the dorsum of the DIP joint. The mallet finger may lastly be also produced by hyperextension injuries that fracture the dorsal base of distal phalanx.

The patient or athlete presents with pain and swelling on the dorsum of the DIP joint with lack of active extension at this joint.

The mallet deformity may be purely soft tissue caused by tear of the terminal extensor mechanism through its substance or bony, associated with an avulsed bony fragment (the "bony mallet", **Fig. 2A**). The speed and degree of flexion present during disruption of the extensor tendon will determine whether there is an associated bony avulsion or not. The radiographs are normal in case of soft tissue mallet, except for a flexion deformity at the DIP joint. The injury may be complicated by concomitant skin lacerations. The open injuries have an impact on the tendinous gaps. There is 30° extension lag with a 1.5 mm gap. On flexion of the DIP, the gap increases by 0.5 mm per 10° of flexion. Flexing PIP has an opposite effect and the tendon gap at DIP closes.

Four types of mallet finger injuries have been described by Doyle **(Box 1)**.

The thumb can also uncommonly sustain a mallet injury. The injury at thumb usually consists of a tendinous avulsion with little or no bony component.

Treatment

The treatment for a mallet finger deformity is determined by the patient's age, mechanism of injury, associated fractures, and the chronicity of the injury.

- Closed acute stable mallet fingers are best treated by continuous splinting in extension for at least 6 weeks. Maintaining slight hyperextension is recommended while standard splinting. The patient is gradually weaned from splinting after 6–8 weeks. If deformity recurs during weaning then splinting is further continued for two more weeks. Weaning involves night-time splinting for nearly 6 more weeks. Regular follow-up should be maintained to identify complications of splinting such as skin necrosis, fungal infection, excoriation, etc. Active PIP joint motion should be done during splinting to avoid a swan neck deformity. Extension block wiring **(Figs. 2B and C)** is another option for displaced bony mallet finger deformity if the patient is noncompliant for splinting or adequate reduction is not obtained for the bony fragment with splinting. I prefer extension block wiring for the latter case or for patients that present late >3 weeks seeking treatment.
- Type II mallet finger deformity is treated with a simple figure-of-eight suture through the tendon. Tendon and skin may also be taken in the same suture (tenodermodesis/dermatotenodesis). I feel that because the tendon is so thin and small the most reliable method of repair is that of tenodermodesis that utilizes skin to increase the strength of repair. Capsulotenodermodesis sutures the capsule also along but may be associated with increased chances of DIP stiffness. The sutures should be removed at 3 weeks. Because the repair is fragile, one

BOX 1: The different types of mallet finger deformity.

- *Type I:* These are closed injuries, with or without avulsion fractures.
- *Type II:* These are open injuries where the laceration is located at or proximal to the DIP joint with loss of tendon continuity
- *Type III:* These are open injury associated with soft tissue loss—deep abrasion with loss of skin, subcutaneous soft tissue, and tendon substance
- *Type IVa:* These are bony injuries in pediatric patients—transepiphyseal plate fracture in children
- *Type IVb:* These are also bony injuries but stable—hyperextension injury with fracture of the articular surface ranging from 20 to 50%
- *Type IVc:* These are bony injuries but are unstable—fracture of the articular surface >50% with palmar subluxation of the distal phalanx

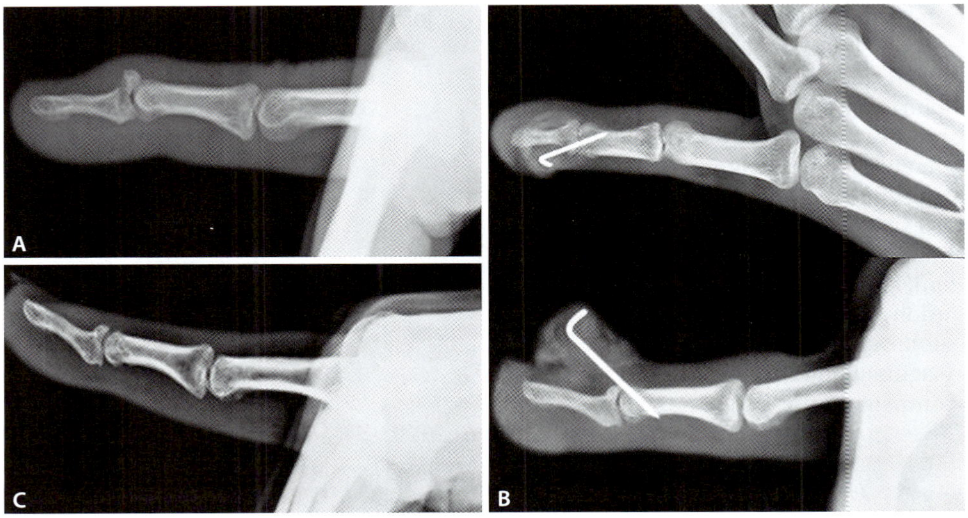

Figs. 2A to C: Bony mallet finger (A) treated with extension block wiring (B). Note the resolution of deformity (extensor lag) in final postoperative film (C).

should consider placing transarticular K-wire through DIP additionally (recommended for 6 weeks).
- Type III injuries usually require soft tissue coverage and primary grafting or other soft tissue reconstruction along with correction of mallet deformity. The tendon avulsion can be repaired using suture anchors or tying them through button on volar aspect using a pull through suture.
- Type IVa usually is a Salter-Harris type II injury and should be managed with closed reduction and splinting.
- Type IVb injuries heal well with closed treatment for articular surface remodeling. Late presenting injuries with displaced bony fragment (>2 mm) can be treated with extension block wiring.
- Type IVc injuries with palmar subluxation of the distal phalanx are usually treated with open reduction internal fixation (ORIF) with a K-wire and possibly using a pullout suture with a button.

Chronic mallet finger refers to injuries that are up to 12 weeks old and are still flexible may respond to conservative treatment with full-time splinting. Failure of response to splinting (around one-third of patients) is an indication for advancement of the terminal tendon to bone using suture anchors or pull-through sutures. The repair can be augmented with dermodesis and a transarticular K-wire. If the deformity is rigid to begin with, arthrodesis may be a better treatment choice.

A swan-neck deformity occurs with late and neglected chronic mallet finger deformity resulting in hyperextension of the PIP joint as the central extensor tendon retracts and the lateral bands subluxate dorsally. Treatment then includes ligament reconstruction using the spiral oblique retinacular ligament (SORL) or a superficialis tenodesis or conservative treatment with long-term splinting for an unwilling patient.

BOXER'S KNUCKLE (BOXER'S FRACTURE)

The term "boxer's fracture" was classically applied to fracture of fifth metacarpal neck but is a misnomer because boxers are more likely to fracture their index and middle metacarpals than their fifth metacarpal. The term has also been modified to boxer's knuckle rather than boxer's fracture so that the range of problems about the metacarpophalangeal (MCP) joint may be taken under this definition such as fractures, dislocations, tendon ruptures, and open injuries. The major impact for the trained boxer is on the flexed MCP joint. Rarely, the strike is with the flexed PIP joint on an extended MCP joint. The index finger and the long rays are the primary punching tools of the trained boxer, only amateur street fighters use ulnar border metacarpals fracturing them in a street scuffle.

The MCP joint is exposed to repeated trauma leading to an entire spectrum of disorders such as contusion, rupture, fracture or dislocation, extensor tendon or capsular fibrosis, collateral sprain, effusion or synovitis and sagittal band rupture **(Fig. 3)** leading to subluxation of the extensor tendon.

The last entity (sagittal band rupture) is most intriguing and challenging comprising the major part of so-called "boxers knuckle".

Anatomy

The extensor tendon is positioned centrally over an irregularly shaped metacarpal head (with slight ulnar inclination called the metacarpal descent) by the investments of the sagittal bands. These sagittal bands invest the extensor tendon crossing both volar and dorsal to it and interweaving with the fibers from the opposite side. Other restraints helping the stabilization of the tendon are the juncturae tendinum present proximally and the extensor mechanism insertions present distally **(Fig. 4)**. The extensor mechanism has no bony insertion at the MCP level as the sagittal bands originate from the volar plate and the deep transverse intermetacarpal ligaments.

Pathoanatomy

The subluxation of the extensor mechanism is caused by a post-traumatic longitudinal rent in the sagittal band **(Fig. 3)**. The most common finger injured is the middle finger but any finger can be involved. The longitudinal slit often develops more due to microtrauma than a single acute event. The extensor subluxates in an ulnarward direction because of a loss of dorsoradial support.

Clinical Features

There is an MCP extensor lag, which may be accompanied by a snapping of the extensor tendon over the MCP joint through an arc of flexion and extension. In advanced cases, the tendon can be seen or palpated as it subluxates from a central position to a more lateral or medial position.

Metacarpal neck fractures present with swelling, dorsal angulation deformity, tenderness, and crepitus. Often the fractures are impacted in flexion.

Treatment

Surgical repair is the best chance for an athlete to return to sports or improve the function of extensor mechanism from a sagittal band injury. The typical surgical procedure for repair of the extensor hood includes the following steps:
- A C-shaped incision to permit wider exposure of the ruptured sagittal band.
- The thickened capsule should be debrided only as much as needed, tight repair may cause inability to flex the MCP joint.

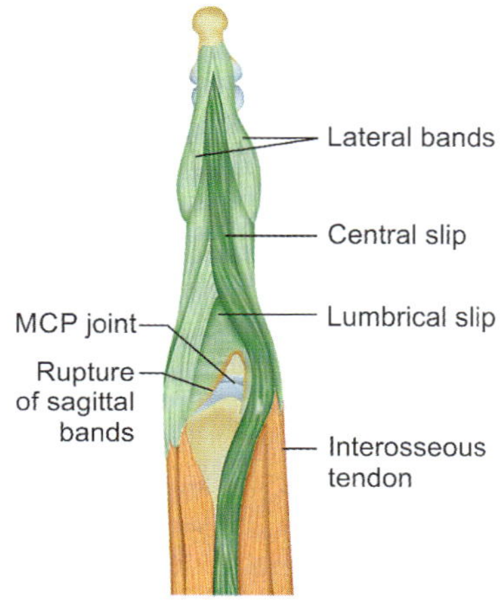

Fig. 3: Sagittal band rupture resulting in extensor tendon subluxation. (MCP: metacarpophalangeal)

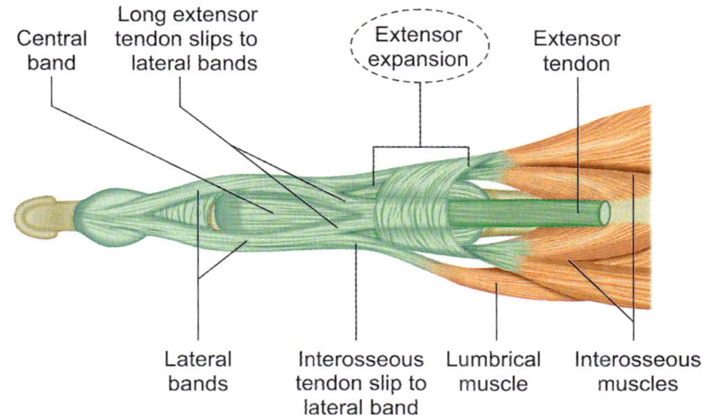

Fig. 4: The illustration of extensor mechanism of finger. The extensor expansion is also called dorsal expansion/the hood/juncturae tendinum.

- Extensor tenolysis and preparation of the hood
- Centralization of the hood and coaptation of the sagittal band in MCP flexion of about 60°. Metacarpophalangeal joint should be immobilized for 4–6 weeks. A systematic program for graduated movements is begun. Boxing is resumed when the tendon position throughout the range of motion of MCP is stable and painless.

Metacarpal neck fractures are mostly managed closed without surgery. Although the degree of acceptable angulation is variable and debated in the literature, it differs from finger to finger. Up to 30–50° of angulation can be accepted with little or no functional deficits, especially in the fourth and fifth digits. Fixation should be strongly considered in unstable patterns.

JAMMED FINGER

This incorporates a spectrum of potential injury, from minor sprain to severe fracture-dislocation of the PIP joint. It is also called *coach's finger* because it commonly occurs in almost all athletic pursuits and a coach often tends to attempt reduction on the sidelines.

Pathomechanics and Evaluation

The PIP joint is a gingivotrochlear joint. The stability against rotational forces, direct mediolateral translation, and lateral deviation is provided by the articular fit. The collateral ligaments (accessory and proper) and the volar plate provide stability against lateral deviation **(Fig. 5)**. Secondary restraints are the flexor tendon sheath, parts of the extensor apparatus coalescing about the PIP and the joint capsule.

Clinical Features

Assess the ligament injury in terms of direction and stability. Open injuries usually result with the phalanx protruding out from volar aspect resulting from an inside-out injury in hyperextension.

For closed injuries, swelling is global but tenderness can be localized to the volar, lateral, or dorsal areas.

Pathoanatomy and Treatment

Proximal interphalangeal dislocations or fracture-dislocations are of two types: (1) dorsal and (2) volar. A pure lateral dislocation is usually an element of one of the major types.

- *Dorsal PIP joint dislocations and fracture-dislocations (the middle phalanx dislocates dorsally):* It is the most common PIP dislocation or fracture-dislocation and is caused by axial loading and hyperextension. There can be isolated soft tissue or a combination of soft tissue and bone injuries. A small avulsion fragment from the volar lip of the middle phalanx can be seen attached to the volar plate. Classification is only important to group the injury patterns into stable versus unstable. A volar fracture percentage of <40% is considered stable whereas fractures with 50% articular involvement are unstable. The main concern is whether there is enough bony and soft tissue support to maintain concentric reduction through the normal range of motion. The steps that should be employed to assess whether a PIP dislocation or fracture-dislocation is *stable* or *unstable* should include reduction and arc of motion testing under metacarpal or wrist block anesthesia, provocative stress in lateral and anteroposterior planes, and lateral imaging at various points throughout the arc of motion.

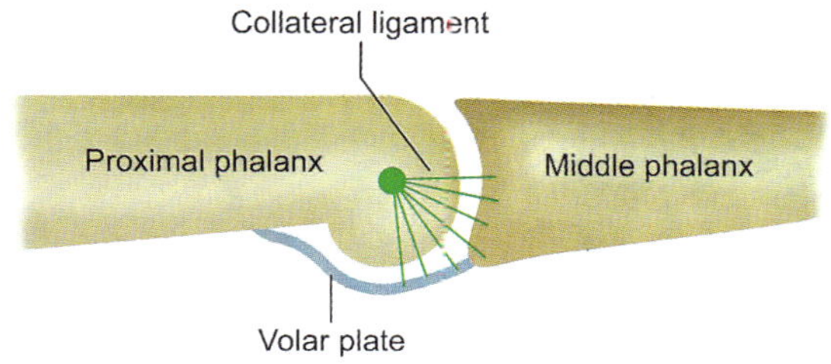

Fig. 5: The structures providing support to the proximal interphalangeal (PIP) joint that get frequently injured in a sprain.

Treatment

Most can be reduced closed. The behavior of fracture fragments and the joint itself can be appreciated and documented if this reduction is performed under fluoroscopic guidance. The closed treatment of these injuries must include a dorsal extension block splinting to block the PIP joint extension when the patient flexes the MCP joint.

Operative reduction is indicated in:

- Middle phalanx impaction fracture where the base splays
- Pilon fracture-dislocation
- The leading edge of the fracture hinges instead of coapts with the proximal phalanx condyles
- If mismatch at the joint is seen as a V sign at the dorsal articulation.

For pilon fracture-dislocation, either bone grafting and repair (early treatment) or volar plate arthroplasty (late cases) is good option.

CONCLUSION

- Competitive sports involve frequent injury to the hand and wrist. Jersey and Mallet finger involve avulsion injury to tendon insertions at distal phalanx. These need meticulous diagnosis and specific management.
- Fracture of metacarpal neck and development of stiff fingers by involvement of ligaments around small joints are common after accrual of trauma. Treating surgeon should have thorough knowledge of the anatomical structures of complex hand that should be managed meticulously else the outcomes are not acceptable often.

CHAPTER 50

Head Injuries in Sports

Manish Kumar Varshney

INTRODUCTION

Head injuries represent a wide range of trauma. In sports-related head injury, concussion is the most common injury. Other intracranial lesions such as intracranial hemorrhage and cerebral contusion that represent severe injuries however must always be considered with any head injury.

The injury pattern can be divided into two types depending upon sequence of events:

1. *Primary injuries* are those that are a direct result of the initial traumatic event. Like scalp and skull injuries diffuse axonal injury (DAI), cortical contusion, extraparenchymal hemorrhage, concussion, and DAI.
2. As highlighted by the concept of damage control orthopedic (DCO), head injury patients may suffer from *secondary injuries* which are devastating because of the inability of cerebral tissue to repair or to regenerate. These secondary injuries include herniation syndromes, diffuse cerebral edema, secondary infarcts and bleeds, hypoxic and ischemic injuries, and hydrocephalus.

So, the fundamental goals as a physician get prioritized to recognizing primary injuries and to prevent secondary lesions.

PATHOPHYSIOLOGY

The primary causes of head injuries are either a direct impact and/or deceleration-rotational events that produce the following patterns of injuries:

- *Coup injuries:* These injuries result in brain contusions from a forceful blow to a stationary head. The injury occurs directly beneath the point of impact.
- Countercoup injuries occur due to brain mobility and floating nature in cerebrospinal fluid (CSF). The energy of impact makes it to glide against the fixed, sharp surfaces of the dural reflection or skull base ridges, thus resulting in a contusion at a site opposite that of the initial external trauma. The effects of forces on the brain parenchyma are quite negated by the CSF. The CSF converts focal stresses to more uniformly distributed compressive stress acting as a shock absorber.
- When there is a skull fracture, the depressed fragment directly injures the adjacent parenchyma.

Three types of stresses are commonly imparted to brain tissue in any injury (often a combination is seen):

1. *Compression:* Compressive forces result in direct impact to the brain parenchyma, as in the case of depressed skull fractures.
2. *Tensile:* It is produced by the small filaments that tether the brain to its membranes pulling it as the brain floats under impact force. Tensile and compressive forces may occur with linear acceleration injuries, such as in the coup/countercoup injury patterns.
3. *Shear:* Shearing injuries are caused by rotational forces and are poorly tolerated by brain parenchyma. These are thought to be related to differences in the physical properties of gray matter and axonal fibers (density differences), typically occur at gray matter-white matter junctions. The differently dense tissues decelerate at different velocities resulting in shearing injuries.

SPECTRUM OF HEAD INJURIES

- Epidural hematomas **(Fig. 1)** often are arterial (middle meningeal arterial injuries) and associated with temporal bone fractures. These rapidly enlarge from blood that rapidly accumulates between the skull and dura and can be fatal in 30–60 minutes. The classically taught lucid interval after an initial loss of consciousness may occur only in one-third or less of patients. It is essential to diagnose and remove an expanding hematoma as an unrecognized bleed may be fatal.
- Subdural hematomas **(Fig. 1)** are venous bleeds caused by tear of bridging veins and occur between the dura and arachnoid. They are three times more common than epidural hematomas resulting in most deaths.
  Also subdural hematomas result from such injuries to brain tissue that are by themselves serious and make recovery guarded. Acute subdural hematomas can lead into herniation-induced brainstem dysfunction that is mostly fatal even with neurosurgical intervention.
  - Clinical features of acute subdural hematomas are rapid in onset and include focal neurologic signs such as hemiparesis, aphasia, and a "blown pupil".

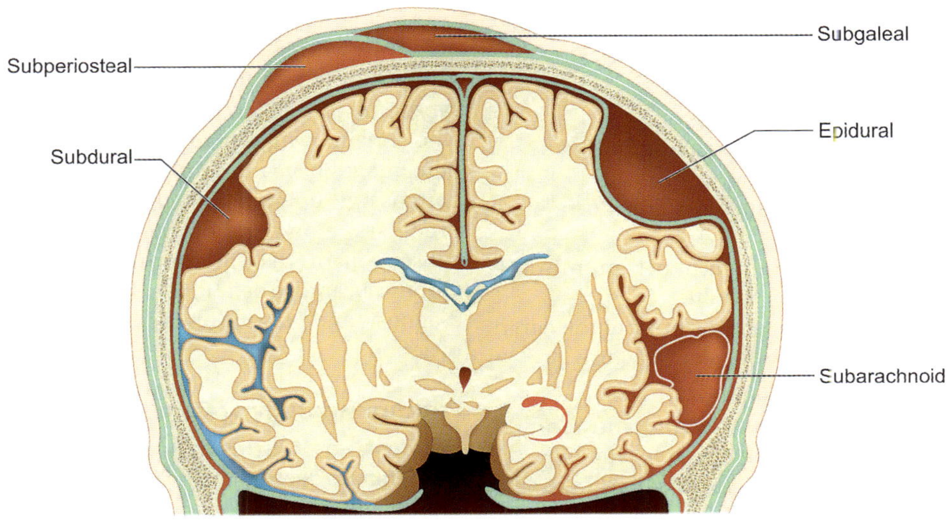

Fig. 1: Anatomic depiction of intracranial and extracranial hemorrhages.

- Clinical features of chronic subdural hematomas manifest in a delayed fashion with symptoms of headache and subtle changes in mental, motor or sensory function.

- Subarachnoid hematomas **(Fig. 1)** are bleeds that are restricted to the CSF space along the surface of the brain and are a result of rupture of the small, surface brain vessels. Meningeal irritation is produced due to nuchal rigidity and secondary vascular spasm may cause infarcts.
- Cerebral contusion or "bruise" of the brain parenchyma occurs due to depressed skull fracture or by countercoup mechanisms where acceleration-deceleration forces cause the brain to press against inner table of the skull. They are supratentorial and are associated with concussion. Close monitoring with repeated computed tomographic evaluation is required as they may progress to focal neurologic deficits.
- Diffuse axonal injuries are caused by high-velocity rotational forces causing multifocal microhemorrhages and edema at gray matter-white matter junctions, deep gray matter, upper brainstem, corpus callosum, and internal capsule. These are best detected with magnetic resonance imaging (MRI).

TABLE 1: Glasgow coma scale.

Eye opening:	
• Spontaneous	4
• To voice	3
• To pain	2
• None	1
Verbal response:	
• Oriented	5
• Confused	4
• Inappropriate words	3
• Incomprehensible sounds	2
• None	1
Motor response:	
• Obeys commands	6
• Purposeful movement	5
• Withdraw to pain	4
• Flexion to pain	3
• Extension to pain	2
• None	1
Eye opening + verbal response + motor response = 3–15	
• GCS ≥ 13 = Possible mild brain injury • GCS 9–12 = Moderate injury • GCS 8 = Severe brain injury • GCS ≤ 7 = Coma • 90% of those ≤8 are in coma • GCS ≥ 11 = Usually excellent prognosis	

Clinical Evaluation

The presentation may range from subtle headaches to loss of consciousness and neurologic deficits. Blood being an irritant to brain tissue may precipitate a seizure.

On-the-field Evaluation

- The levels of consciousness are ascertained.
- Injuries to cervical spine are always assumed until ruled out, especially in the unconscious patient, so stabilize the neck immediately.
- Assessment of the patient's airway, breathing, and circulation (i.e., ABCs).
- Quantitate level of consciousness by Glasgow coma scale **(Table 1)**. Also assess the orientation to person, place, and time and for the presence of retrograde amnesia.
- Visual changes, dizziness, and head or neck pain must be specifically looked before removing the athlete from the field.

On-the-bench Evaluation

Perform a specific survey—questioned for specific symptoms as dizziness, visual changes (e.g., photophobia, double vision or blurriness), headache, nausea, vertigo, and tinnitus. Absence does not ascertain normality as mostly symptoms are often delayed. Vomiting is suggestive of head injury with elevated intracranial pressure.

Inspect and palpate the head and neck:
- Evaluate crepitus of skull and facial bones.
- Malorientation with teeth clenching and grinding occur with mandibular fractures.
- Leakage of CSF from the nose suggests cribriform plate fracture.
- Spinal fluid adjacent to the tympanic membrane indicates fracture in the temporal bone.
- The Battle sign which ecchymosis posterior to the ear in the mastoid region shows posterior skull fracture.

Cranial nerve examination is imperative:
- Changes in pupil size shows elevated intracranial pressures or a unilateral sympathetic nerve response.
- Deficient oculomotor function is indicative injury to the third cranial nerve from a skull fracture or subdural hematoma.
- Asymmetric upward gaze is seen in infraorbital blow-out fractures causing impingement of the inferior rectus muscle and cranial nerve VII palsy from basilar skull fractures.
- Transient nystagmus is indicative of shearing or rotatory injury to the brainstem.

The neurologic examination is completed by performing tests for strength, sensation and coordination.

Higher mental functions are then assessed by neurocognitive assessment. These include concentration levels, recent memory, orientation to person, place, new learning, and delayed recall. Specific tools include the Mini-Mental Status Examination can be used.

CONCUSSION (COMMOTIO CEREBRI)

The terminology has been used interchangeably to mild traumatic brain injury (mTBI) especially in US; however, physicians elsewhere use the terms to refer to various injury constructs. Concussion may refer to milder low-velocity injures that cause brain "shaking" resulting in clinical symptoms and which may not be necessarily related to a pathological injury (in this sense concussion represents a subset of mTBI). We will continue to use the term concussion throughout the chapter to maintain distinction unless more clarity is dictated. Concussion is the most common athletic head injury, and is defined as a "clinical syndrome characterized by immediate and transient post-traumatic impairment of neural functions, such as alteration of consciousness, disturbance of vision, equilibrium, etc. due to brainstem involvement" (Committee on Head Injury Nomenclature of the Congress of Neurologic Surgeons) or "complex pathophysiological process affecting the brain, induced by biomechanical forces (4th International Conference on Concussion in Sport, Zurich, November 2012). The cardinal diagnostic features of concussion are:
- Altered mental status after head injury
- Glasgow coma scale ranging from 13 to 15
- Negative findings on neuroimaging
- Loss of consciousness (±).

Most athletes fully recover from a concussion (80–90%) only a few will have persistent sequelae that can be disabling. Always be aware of the possibility or dangers of second-impact syndrome (see below) that can be catastrophic in a patient who remains symptomatic from a previous concussion. A few percentages have more subtle chronic sequelae of repetitive concussive episodes, such as impairment of cognitive processes, mood and behavior as well as increased risk of subsequent mTBIs. There are no available methods to predict chronicity, and no definitive guidelines for return to play. Early diagnosis and prevention of sequel is the present best course of action.

Pathophysiology of Concussion and Etiology

Concussion injuries represent DAIs caused by rapid acceleration/deceleration of the head resulting from stretching of nerve fibers. There is a growing consensus that mTBI is a result of temporary neuronal dysfunction rather than cell death as the defects do not occur with significant anatomic disturbance and appear to resolve over time. Thus, the neural cells are not irreversibly destroyed by mTBI but remain in a vulnerable neurometabolic state before recovery, which explains the etiology of postconcussive symptomatology and vulnerability.

The metabolic dysfunction is the key physiological event after a concussive event. There is disorganized release of neurotransmitters which causes poorly regulated neuronal depolarizations and abnormal ionic shifts. This altered cellular physiology leads to hypermetabolism of glucose and a "cellular energy crisis" which is attenuated by a decrease in cerebral blow flow. This puts the brain to increased vulnerability for a second concussive event. For a balanced event after the hypermetabolic glucose consumption, the concussed brain enters a period of depressed metabolism impairing neural connectivity. This is responsible in part to lasting changes in cognitive potential.

The majority of concussions occur by impact with another player's helmet. Combination of rotation coupled with translation produces high likelihood of concussion and reduces tolerance as (in the face mask injuries) the impact twists the head in addition to accelerating it. The accelerating/decelerating force along with rotational component forces brain into a complex shear injury responsible for DAI (discussed above).

Epidemiology

Difficult to define in India (as is always the case for absence of central registries), data from the United States indicates that 3.9–7.7% of high school and college athletes sustain a concussion each year. Contact sports are the most common cause for head trauma (football has the highest risk; other sports include basketball, softball, soccer, baseball, rugby, and ice-hockey). There is increased predisposition to future concussive events after an initial mTBI. There is a threefold increase in concussive risk and an eightfold increased risk of experiencing loss of consciousness if a player had suffered three or more mTBIs over a period of 7 years. Recurrent concussive events also may also lead to slower recovery and more severe symptoms.

Diagnosis of Concussion

Any head trauma associated with a loss of consciousness is a concussion. The signs and symptoms vary **(Table 2)** with location, duration, and severity of impact. Change in an athlete's behavior is an indication of altered neurologic functioning. Features of concussion are dizziness, slow and uncoordinated motor function, disorientation, delayed verbal responses to questions, blurred vision, short-term memory deficits, blank stare, slurred speech, and emotional liability. On physical examination (see above also), the most common findings are information-processing problems, problems with immediate recall and retrograde amnesia.

Standardized Assessment of Concussion

Standardized concussion assessment forms are used for initial evaluation. They help to detect and quantify initial cognitive deficits and provide an objective and standardized mental status examination (they yield uniform data and allow longitudinal and multicenter studies to better define the significance of postconcussion symptomatology).

- *Neuropsychological testing:* These are functional cognitive instruments that quantify cognitive weakness by assessing changes in memory, attention, concentration, information-processing, motor speed and coordination. They act as tool for measuring both the initial and recovery stages of athletes after concussive events. Neuropsychological tests are most useful when baseline data on the athlete exist and can be longitudinally compared to serial tests after concussive episodes.

It has been demonstrated with these standardizations that high school athletes with the postconcussive symptom of headache had significantly worse performance on reaction time and memory neurocognitive scores compared to athletes without headache after concussion.

TABLE 2: Common signs and symptoms of concussion (any one or more should strongly arouse suspicion of concussion, combination is usually present). The Pittsburgh card is a quick reference guide.

- Symptoms—somatic (e.g., headache), cognitive (e.g., feeling like in a fog) and/or emotional symptoms (e.g., liability)
- Physical signs (e.g., loss of consciousness and amnesia)
- Behavioral changes (e.g., irritability)
- Cognitive impairment (e.g., slowed reaction times)
- Sleep disturbance (e.g., insomnia)

University of Pittsburgh Medical Center's sideline concussion card: signs and symptoms of concussion

Signs observed by staff	*Symptoms reported by athlete*
• Appears to be dazed or stunned • Is confused about assignment • Forgets plays • Is unsure of game, score or opponent • Moves clumsily • Answers questions slowly • Loses consciousness • Shows behavior or personality change • Forgets events prior to play (retrograde) • Forgets events after hit (post-traumatic)	• Headache • Nausea • Balance problems or dizziness • Double or fuzzy/blurry vision • Sensitivity to light or noise • Feeling sluggish or slowed down • Feeling "foggy" or groggy • Concentration or memory problems • Change in sleep pattern (appears later) • Feeling fatigued

Functional MRI

Structural neuroimaging modalities, such as MRI and computed tomographic, are normal in cases of concussion as there is no anatomically demonstrable neurological injury. Functional MRI examines the metabolic/physiological state of the brain so may assess and monitor concussion. Functional MRI provides task-specific information about neural function. It is also capable of detecting defects in neural function during cognitive load. This tool may allow mapping of neural injury patterns to quantify injury load and more accurately direct return-to-play guidelines in recent future.

Blood investigations: There are no definitive well-documented markers for cellular damage in brain injury, but some that have been proposed are myelin basic protein (MBP), S-100, neuron specific enolase (NSE), GFAP, tau, etc.

Electrophysiological tests: Different electrophysiological recording techniques, like evoked response potential (ERP), cortical magnetic stimulation and electroencephalography, show some abnormalities in the postconcussive state but complete characterization for diagnosis is lacking.

Postconcussion Syndrome

Approximately 20% (one-fifth) of patients suffer from post-concussive symptoms. Postconcussive symptoms are thought to represent the clinical manifestation of the neurometabolic derangements (see above). Many of these symptoms are short-lived, and resolve spontaneously however. Characteristic symptoms of postconcussion syndrome are persistent headache, fatigue, impaired memory and concentration, mood and sleep disturbances, dizziness, etc. Treatment includes nonsteroidal anti-inflammatory drugs (NSAIDs) and rest (no play strictly).

Second-impact Syndrome

This is a syndrome which occurs when an athlete without completely recovered from an initial concussive event sustains a second head trauma (second impact). This is a life-threatening consequence of premature return-to-play but fortunately rare, around just more than a dozen cases have been reported till now. It can occur up to 2 weeks postinjury and is seen most often in athletes younger than 21 years of age.

The second event need not be a high-energy force and even minor injuries cause a dangerous increase in intracranial pressure because by dysregulation of cerebral blood flow in a recuperating brain. The second impact results in vascular engorgement, cerebellar herniation and death. Clinically, the athlete appears to be stunned with the injury and often does not lose consciousness initially but within seconds to minutes, he/she collapses, becomes semi-comatose and develops dilated pupils as well as respiratory failure. The patient expires more quickly than those with intracranial hemorrhage syndromes even before one clearly understands the cause of sudden collapse. Even with fastest and best of care mortality rate are very high, approximately 50%, and the morbidity is nearly 100%.

Chronic Traumatic Brain Injury

It is the long-term sequelae of multiple concussive events (mostly in boxers, street fighters and uncommonly in college football players). As an example the dementia pugilistica or punch drunk syndrome in boxers typified by a pattern of ataxia, impaired memory, pyramidal tract dysfunction, tremor, dysarthria and behavioral changes. The general symptoms of chronic traumatic brain injury (CTBI) are a general feeling of fogginess, concentration deficit, decreased processing speed, short-term memory impairment, irritability or depression, fatigue, sleep disturbance, and academic difficulties.

Management of Concussion

There is no definite treatment for concussion and the cornerstone of concussion management is physical and cognitive rest until the acute symptoms resolve. The guidelines of management basically focus on four considerations:

1. Identify immediate neurologic emergencies—careful patient history and physical examination
2. Prevent the second-impact syndrome
3. Minimize the risk of recurrent concussive episodes
4. The cumulative effects of repeated concussion that lead to CTBI must be avoided.

For points 2, 3, and 4 above determining the time to return-to-play had been classically decided based on the presence and duration of loss of consciousness or amnesia. However, neither symptom is necessary for an injury to be classified as a concussion nor do they guide the treatment option/duration. More objective assessment tools help in grading the injury pattern and hence the course of further management. These include the Cantu guidelines, the Colorado guidelines **(Table 3)**. These criteria specifically dictate that any loss of consciousness is considered a grade 3 concussion and should be treated as a severe injury. The American Academy of Neurology (AAN) modified the Colorado guidelines in 1997 and these criteria seem to help in deciding the permission for return-to-play (e.g., following a grade 1 concussion if the athlete is asymptomatic he can return to play 15 minutes after the episode).

TABLE 3: Grading systems for concussion.

	Grade 1 (mild)	*Grade 2 (moderate)*	*Grade 3 (severe)*
Cantu	No LOC or post-traumatic amnesia <1 hour	LOC < 5 minutes or post-traumatic amnesia 1–24 hours	LOC > 5 minutes or post-traumatic amnesia >24 hours
Colorado Medical Society	No LOC, confusion without amnesia	No LOC, confusion with amnesia	LOC
American Academy of Neurology	No LOC, symptoms <15 minutes	No LOC, symptoms >15 minutes	LOC

(LOC: loss of consciousness)

Concussion by itself is difficult to categorize and reliable return-to-play decisions are difficult to make. Neuropsychological testing has shown that complete normalization takes 6 days after the concussion event, indicating that some current return-to-play recommendations, which allow athletes with grade 1 concussions to return to the game after the symptoms resolve, may be too liberal.

Return to Play

Being ill-defined currently two basic approaches are used to manage concussion and to make return-to-play decisions.

- First approach is to grade the concussion using one of the grading systems **(Table 3)** at the time of the event and within 15 minutes of the concussion to assess immediate estimation of the injury severity and progression if any. Using this approach the following have been recommended [American Orthopedic Society for Sports Medicine (AOSSM Concussion Workshop Group, 1999)]:
  Return to play the same day is permitted if signs and symptoms cleared within 15 minutes or less both at rest and with exertion, there is a normal neurologic evaluation and there is no documented loss of consciousness.
  Delayed return to play (not the same day) is recommended if signs and symptoms did not clear within 15 minutes at rest or with exertion and there is documented loss of consciousness.
  These guidelines also dictate few generalizations that are outside the grading system:
  - New symptoms arising after an asymptomatic period should preclude play.
  - Symptoms that last for 20–30 minutes should be considered as prolonged symptoms and disqualify the athlete from returning to competition on the same day.
  - Asymptomatic athletes should be subjected to provocative test before a return to play (to increase the intracranial pressure with physical stress and determine if symptoms occur). The common provocative tests recommended are a 40-yard dash, five sit-ups, five push-ups, five deep knee bends, or reclining in a supine position with the legs elevated for several seconds.

Return to play must always be accompanied by serial examination to assess for recurrence of symptoms.

1. As there is absence of evidence-based recommendations, a cautious approach involves a gradual return to school and social activities (prior to contact sports) so as not to result in a significant exacerbation of symptoms. This second approach shuns the grading system due to lack of ability to capture all events. It monitors the athlete's recovery based on symptoms, serial neurocognitive testing, and postural-stability testing. The athlete's symptoms are closely monitored; once the athlete is asymptomatic, a progression of activities is instituted that increases demands over several days in a stepwise

TABLE 4: Graduated return to play protocol (4th International Conference on Concussion in Sport Held in Zurich, November 2012).

Rehabilitation stage	*Functional exercise at each stage of rehabilitation*	*Objective of each stage*
No activity	Symptom limited physical and cognitive exercise	Recovery
Light aerobic exercise	Walking, swimming or stationary cycling keeping intensity < 70% maximum permitted heart rate. No resistance training	Increase HR
Sport specific exercise	Skating drills in ice-hockey, running drills in soccer. No head impact activity	Add movement
Noncontact training drills	Progression to more complex training drills, e.g., passing drills in football and ice-hockey	Exercise, coordination, and cognitive load
Full contact practice	Following medical clearance participate in normal training activities	Restore confidence and assess functional skills by coaching staff
Return to play	Normal game play	

(HR: heart rate)

fashion (endorsed in consensus statement from Conference on Concussion in Sport, 2012). Each step in this approach takes a minimum of 1 day, and a recurrence of symptomatology mandates that the athletes drop back to the previous asymptomatic level and then try to progress again after 24 hours **(Table 4)**.

2. The guidelines need a systemic research for adequacy and sufficiency, however, as both are more empirical than evidence based.

CONCLUSION

Head injuries in sports entail a serious event. Though concussion is the most common pattern of head injury seen one should be aware of other types of injuries also. Being a sports physician primary knowledge of on-field and out-of-field examination is necessary so as to provide early care to the patients. Management is done by specialists but the injury usually has a protracted course of recovery keeping the player out of sports for a prolonged period in moderate disruptions or may be forever in severe cases.

CHAPTER 51

Doping (Drugs and Legal Aspects)

Manish Kumar Varshney

INTRODUCTION

The word doping originally was used for a mixed remedy containing opium given to "dope" horses. "Dope" was also a concoction prepared from grape used by zulu warriors as a stimulant during war and religious activities ("doop"—Afrikaans or Dutch). Chinese physicians recommended the use of Ma Huang (ephedra extract) to increase performance. Indian physician Sushruta recommended consuming testicles around 300 BC to enforce virility. In any form, the term referred to any form of medication (blend/potion/concoction/mixture) used to improve performance and hence had been adopted to refer to illegal and illicit substance abuse in sports. Hallucinogenic mushrooms were used in Olympic competitions (between 776 BC and 393 AD) for the same purpose. "Doping" during those Olympic games were as prohibited as it is today but the penalties were much more severe, including death. It is believed that emperor Theodosius abolished the Olympics possibly on these premises only as he mentioned in his note that games had become "a hotbed of cheating, affronts to the human dignity and doping".

The use of doping still continues and substances such as caffeine, cocaine, heroin, strychnine, alcohol, etc. Continue to be used in not so well-regulated sporting events internationally. "Mariani wine" produced by Angelo Mariani was a popular doping drink that was later banned in Germany in 1920 under opium law. Not only doping to increase performance but its negative use has also come up. "Negative doping" or drugs that decrease performance had been given to the competitors to impede their performance. The international athletic foundation was the first to ban the use of these illicit substances but the full effect of ban was not perceived till biochemical testing abilities were installed.

Modern attempts to stop the doping and protect the athletes' fundamental right to participate in doping-free sport and promoting health, fair play, and equality for Athletes worldwide have led to development of world antidoping program and code. This also permits coherent, synchronized, and effective antidoping program at international and national level with regard to detection, penalization, and prevention of doping. The World Anti-Doping Agency (WADA) considers doping to be "fundamentally contrary to the spirit of sport".

DEFINITION

The definition has been expanded to capture even most remote violator that works against the spirit of sport. Doping according to WADA 2021 code is defined as occurrence of one or more of the following antidoping rule violations:

1. Presence of a prohibited substance or its metabolites or markers in an athlete's sample.
2. Use or attempted use by an athlete of a prohibited substance or a prohibited method.
3. Evading, refusing or failing to submit to sample collection.
4. Whereabouts failures—any combination of three missed tests and/or filing failures, as defined in the International Standard for Testing and Investigations, within a 12-month period by an athlete in a Registered Testing Pool.
5. Tampering or attempted tampering with any part of doping control.
6. Possession of a prohibited substance or a prohibited method.
7. Trafficking or attempted trafficking in any prohibited substance or prohibited method.
8. Administration or attempted administration to any athlete in-competition of any prohibited substance or prohibited method, or administration or attempted administration to any athlete out-of-competition of any prohibited substance or any prohibited method that is prohibited out-of-competition.
9. Complicity—assisting, encouraging, aiding, abetting, conspiring, covering up or any other type of intentional complicity involving an antidoping rule violation, attempted antidoping rule violation.
10. Prohibited association—this is a broad term and actually prohibits any athlete or athlete support person to have any association with a person who is ineligible or serving a period of ineligibility in context to doping or violation of antidoping rules.

11. Acts by an athlete or other person to discourage or retaliate against reporting to authorities. This also includes any act to intimidate or threaten any person who intends to or provides information/evidence pertaining to antidoping rule violation.

TESTING

The sample testing is carried out at WADA accredited laboratories and the burden of establishing violation of antidoping rule lies on antidoping organization. Any athlete may be required to provide a sample at any time and at any place by any antidoping organization with testing authority over him or her. Each major event organization, including the International Olympic Committee and the International Paralympic Committee, has in-competition testing authority. All testing is conducted in conformity with the international standard for testing and investigations.

The *list of prohibited substances* is very long and is available from the WADA website. Broadly these have been categorized into (only broad classes mentioned) the following:

- Substances prohibited at all times:
  1. Anabolic agents like steroid and its derivatives
  2. Erythropoietins, peptide hormones, and growth factors related substances and mimetics
  3. β-2 agonists
  4. Hormone and metabolic modulators
  5. Diuretics and masking agents
  6. *Nonapproved substances:* This is a new category added and refers to any pharmacological substance not listed in above categories but is not approved by any governmental regulatory authority for health or therapeutic use including drugs under trial or clinical development.
- Substances prohibited during competition (apart from above):
  1. Stimulants
  2. Narcotics
  3. Cannabinoids
  4. Glucocorticoids

One should realize that some of the drugs may come under therapeutic use exception (TUE) for which prior permission and intimation with proper documentation have to be provided to the authority in advance.

CONSEQUENCES OF ANTIDOPING RULE VIOLATIONS

- Disqualification of results in the event during which an antidoping rule violation occurs—disqualification of all of the athlete's individual results obtained in that event with all consequences, including forfeiture of all medals, points, and prizes.
- Ineligibility for presence, use or attempted use or possession of a prohibited substance or prohibited method:
  - A. The period of ineligibility shall be of 4 years for violation of rule 1, 2, and 6 (discussed earlier):
    - i. The antidoping rule violation does not involve a specified substance, unless the athlete or other person can establish that the antidoping rule violation was not intentional.
    - ii. The antidoping rule violation involves a specified substance and the antidoping organization can establish that the antidoping rule violation was intentional.
  - B. If the above does not apply, the period of ineligibility shall be of 2 years.
- For violation of rules 3 and 5, the period of ineligibility is of 4 years.
- For violations of rule 4, the ineligibility is for 2 years subject to reduction of 1 year depending the found degree of fault.
- For violations of rules 7 and 8, the ineligibility is a minimum of 4 years which may be extended to lifetime depending on seriousness.
- For violation of rule 9, the ineligibility is for 2 years for a maximum of 4 years.
- For violation of rule 10, the ineligibility is for 2 years that can be reduced to 1 year depending on degree of fault. The period of ineligibility in a normal course begins from the date of the final hearing decision. If an athlete or other person establishes in an individual case that he or she bears *No Fault* or *Negligence*, then the otherwise applicable period of ineligibility shall be eliminated. However, in cases of repeat violation of rules, the period of ineligibility varies and is usually extended to more than above mentioned periods. The financial costs are decided by the preceding antidoping organizations.

During the period of ineligibility:

- No athlete or other person who has been declared ineligible may, during the period of ineligibility, participate in any capacity in a competition or activity.
- Athlete may, however, return to train with a team or to use the facilities of a club or other member organization of a signatory's member organization during the shorter of:
  - The last 2 months of the athlete's period of ineligibility
  - The last one-quarter of the period of ineligibility imposed.

CONCLUSION

- Doping is an international crime that mars the basic sporting spirit.
- The most idealistic environment entails ethical competition in the basic essence of sports but lure for medals and name often forces athletes into malpractice.
- Regulations are quite stringent to avoid such practices and penalty is also quite severe if found guilty.

CHAPTER 52

Skeletal Muscle: Structure and Function

Manish Kumar Varshney

INTRODUCTION

There are over 400 skeletal muscles in human body that make up 40–50% of body weight (in ideal sittings). The skeletal muscle functions to produce:

- Force for locomotion and other vital functions such as breathing
- Force for postural support and maintaining stability
- Heat during cold stress (shivering).

Muscle is a conglomeration of muscle fibers that share the common properties of conductivity, distensibility, irritability, contractility, relaxation, and elasticity. Muscle fibers are multinucleated cells with a cylindrical shape. Muscle fibers range a few millimeters to several centimeters in length having diameters ranging between 10 and 100 µm, surrounded progressively by following connective tissue layers:

- Sarcolemma is the membrane of individual muscle cell.
- External lamina is situated just below the endomysium.
- Endomysium that surrounds individual muscle fibers.
- Perimysium fibers are arranged into larger units known as fascicles (visible to the naked eye). Fascicles are surrounded by perimysium.
- The whole muscle is surrounded by the epimysium that blends with the individual muscle investing fascial layer. The connective tissue surrounding muscle carries blood vessels and contains satellite cells that play a role in muscle growth and repair. These satellite cells play important role in strength training. The epimysium, perimysium, and endomysium extend to provide a broad attachment surface for muscles to join to bone at one end and form tendons at the other **(Fig. 1)**. The perimysium is continuous distally with the endotenon sheath at the myotendinous junction. This allows tendon to transmit the force generated by muscle without much losses. It is now considered that the force is transmitted by shear through the endomysium that also contributes to the final connection at myotendinous junction.

Fibers in muscle can be arranged either in a parallel fusiform arrangement (common) or at an angle to the longitudinal axis of muscle giving a pennate (pinnate) arrangement. Angular arrangement produces the unipennate, bipennate, and multipennate types. This orientation of muscle fibers not only affects the muscle's physiological cross-sectional area but also determines the contractile properties. The fiber length is smaller in pinnate arrangement while the fibers are longer in fusiform muscles. The force produced by a muscle is proportional to physiological cross-sectional area and the amount of shortening of muscle fibers which is dependent on muscle fiber length. Shorter fibers produce greater force due to less need of take up of slack compared to longer fibers **(Figs. 2A and B)**. This portends that a pennate muscle will generate more power due to greater force of contraction than a muscle of equal mass but fusiform arrangement of fibers. Pinnation provides more fibers per unit volume for contraction and also the angle of pinnation in relation to tendon fibril increases during contraction reducing the speed of contraction but increasing the force production. The amount of force generated is given by cosine of the angle of insertion, which; at rest, is usually 10°.

CYTOLOGY

Each muscle fiber is surrounded by sarcolemma. Fibers are further divided into smaller units as follows:

- Myofibers or myofibrils containing the contractile proteins and their subsidiaries (myosin, actin, tropomyosin, and troponin) are made of sarcomeres arranged in "series" alignment.
- Sarcomeres ("sarx"—flesh, "mere"—part) is the basic functional unit of muscle contraction and is divided into Z line, M line, H zone, A band, I band.
- Sarcoplasmic reticulum serves as cistern to store the calcium.
- Transverse tubules (T-tubules) (discussed later).

The amount and type of proteins being synthesized is determined by the nuclear DNA that can be quickly upregulated and downregulated for adaptation to various tasks. Cellular mitochondria are the most abundant organelle and accounting for up to 20% of cell volume. Mitochondria are abundant in highly oxidative slow-twitch fibers as they are responsible for production of adenosine triphosphate (ATP) through oxidative metabolism (essential for muscle contraction).

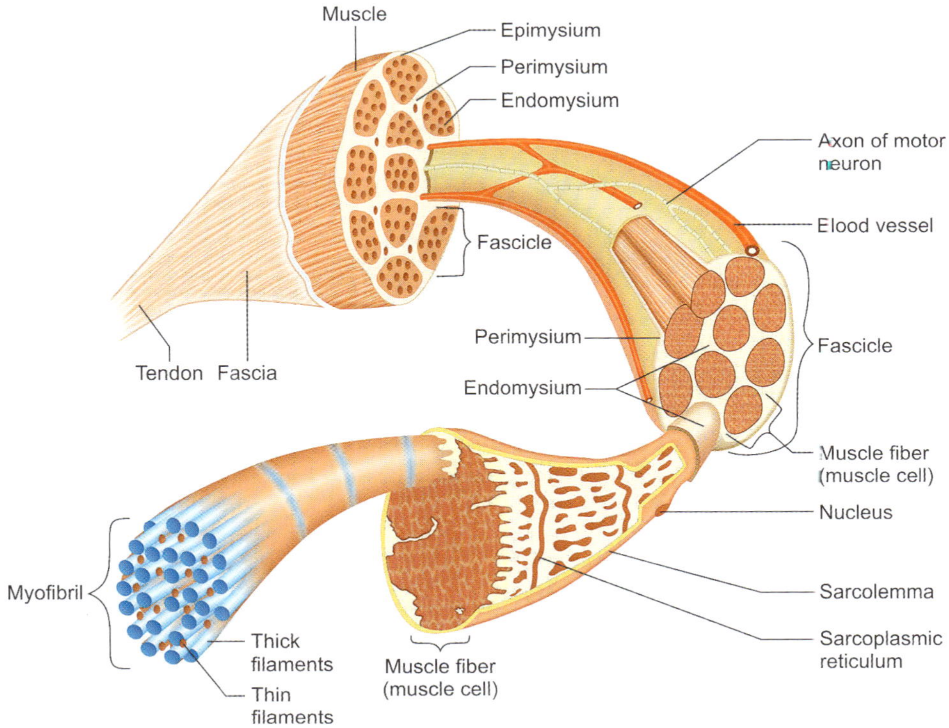

Fig. 1: The gross structure of muscle and muscle fibers.

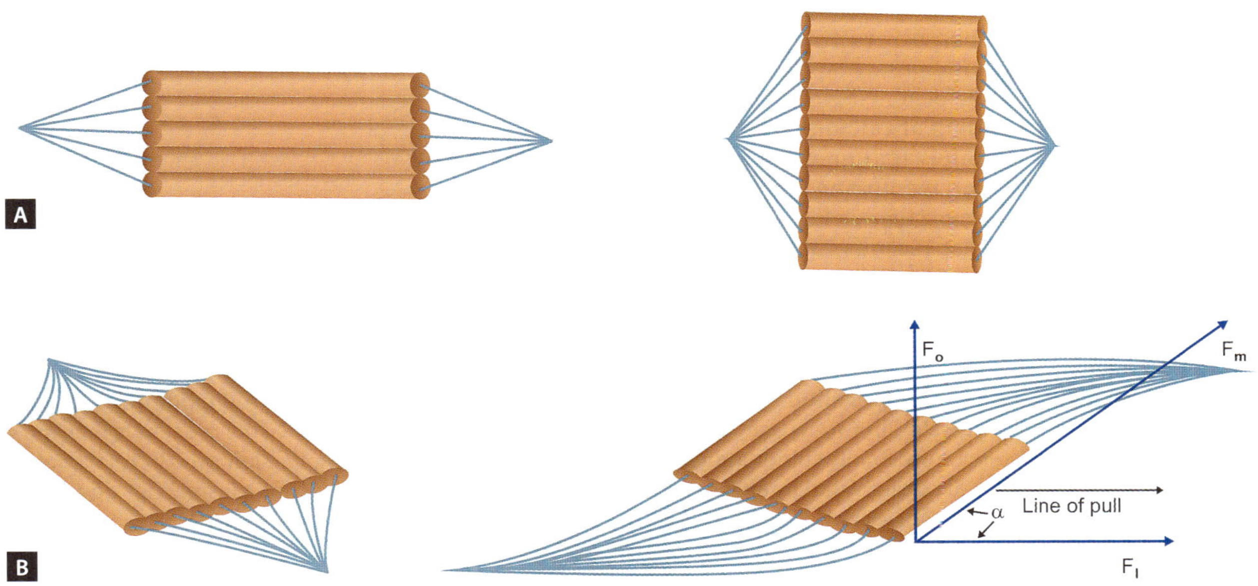

Figs. 2A and B: The role of muscle architecture in force production. Parallel arrangement: Tendon fibers project from the muscle fibers directly transmitting the force generated (A). Pennate arrangement: Tendon fibers extend obliquely forming two sides of the parallelogram, so the ultimate force generated is a resultant vector of the pennate angle (B).

MOTOR UNIT

The junction between motor neuron and muscle fiber is called motor unit or myoneural junction. The muscle fiber motor unit is composed of a single alpha motor neuron (somatic efferent) and the skeletal muscle fibers that are innervated by its axon terminal. Motor end plate is a pocket formed by sarcolemma around the axon terminal. There is no overlap in the innervation of muscle fibers, and single muscle fiber receives innervation from only one efferent motor neuron. The sizes of motor units differ and they are not all identical. A single motor neuron may innervate as few as 10 (ocular muscles needing fine motor control), or as many as several thousand muscle fibers (force-generating muscles such as the quadriceps). Each muscle fiber, whatever type may be, will be contacted by a single nerve ending at the motor end plate (usually at the myofibril midsection). There are three groups of motor units each having distinctive group of motor neuron and muscle fiber. Fibers belonging to the same motor unit share similar fiber type and contractile characteristics, i.e., fast glycolytic, fast oxidative, and slow oxidative. The smallest

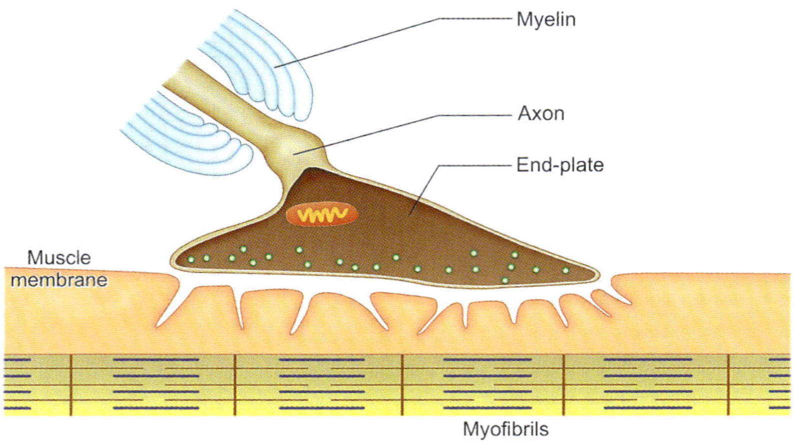

Fig. 3: Illustration of neuromuscular junction.

muscle fibers (viz., slow oxidative) are innervated by the smallest motor neurons and also have low myosin ATPase activity.

At the motor end plate, the axon expands into a Schwann cell—enveloped synaptic terminal. The action potential arising from the nerve cell when reaches the muscle at the motor end plate or neuromuscular junction **(Fig. 3)** causes release of the acetylcholine (Ach)-containing vesicles from nerve terminal of the presynaptic axon (active zones). These active zones are adjacent to the postsynaptic folds of the sarcolemma known as the sole plate. Progressing neuronal depolarization causes an influx of calcium ions through voltage-gated calcium channels that mediate fusion of synaptic vesicles with the axon membrane and hence the release of Ach into the neuromuscular cleft. The sole plate on muscle cell has numerous Ach receptors in the junctional folds along with chemically gated ion channels. Ach binds to these receptors in turn depolarizing the muscle sarcolemma, thereby initiating an action potential in the muscle. The resting end-plate potential is disturbed with the activation of these ion channels initiating muscle depolarization. This action potential spreads along the muscle fiber to trigger calcium release (from sarcoplasmic reticulum) finally culminating into muscle contraction. Ach is rapidly deactivated by enzymes in the synaptic cleft (acetylcholinesterase) and choline is then reabsorbed by the terminal axon to recirculate to form Ach for future transmitter release.

SARCOPLASMIC RETICULUM

With depolarization of muscle, calcium ions are released from system of membranous sacs (cisterns) known as the sarcoplasmic reticulum. The sarcoplasmic reticulum is organized into longitudinal and lateral sacs and T-tubules. The T-tubules carry action potential from fiber's surface to the inner fiber for homogeneous and complete contraction. The T-tubules penetrate the muscle fibers near the Z-line **(Fig. 4)**. Sarcoplasmic reticulum actively sequestrates calcium and maintains a low resting calcium concentration in the resting state. This low concentration is needed for continuing with the resting equilibrium of muscle fiber and is aided by calcium adenosine triphosphatase (ATPase) pumps that transport calcium ions even against concentration gradient. With muscle action potential, the sarcolemma and the sarcoplasmic reticulum become increasingly permeable to Ca^{2+} that egresses from the sarcoplasmic reticulum into myoplasm. They release free calcium then bind to troponin initiating contraction. This process is referred to as excitation—contraction coupling followed by relaxation of the muscle with restoration of low myoplasmic Ca^{2+} concentration via the Ca^{2+} ATPase pumps.

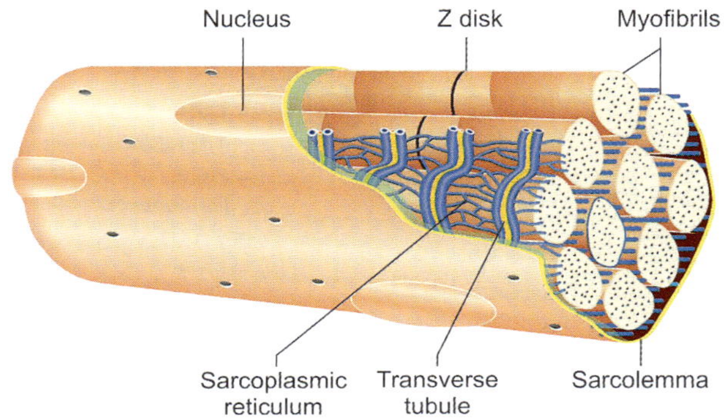

Fig. 4: The sarcoplasmic retinaculum. Longitudinal and transverse tubules.

STRUCTURAL PROTEINS OF MUSCLE

Actin, myosin, tropomyosin, and troponin are the main structural proteins of muscle with other minor proteins. These proteins form the foundation of sarcomere. Banding pattern of striated skeletal muscle visualized in polarized microscopy comes from the repeating arrangement of thick filaments and thin filaments.

- Thick filaments composed primarily of contractile myosin molecules arranged in staggered side by side complex (*cf*—thin filaments) accounting for 55% or so of the total percentage of main proteins. It has two heavy chains and four light chains. In addition to myosin, the thick filament also contains M protein, C protein, and titin having individual distinct functions in muscle contraction.

The C protein is involved in cross-bridging of the thick filament whereas the M protein contains the creatine phosphokinase enzyme involved in supplying phosphate to ATP. Titin (elastic protein) protects against overstretch of muscle fiber.

- Thin filaments are made up primarily of globular actin monomers that are weaved around with tropomyosin and troponin proteins (serving a regulatory function during contraction) like a cable to form an alpha double helical cylinder. Actin only is anchored to the Z-line at the end of sarcomere. The actin is composed of G-actin and F-actin (filamentous portion) that are weaved together. Troponin comprises troponin C, I, and T subunits with discrete functions of calcium binding, inhibition of ATPase and tropomyosin binding respectively. Thin filaments also contain nebulin that regulates the length of the thin filament during contraction and stretch.

The sarcomere extends from one Z band to another. The Z band or Z disk (from Zwischenscheibe, which is German for "interim disk") contains α-actinin forming an embedding matrix or anchor for thin filaments (actin) at either end. Similar to the Z-line, the A band in the center of the sarcomere is a protein dense band known as the H (Heller) zone that contains the M (middle) line **(Fig. 5)** serving as an attachment to myosin filaments (thick filaments). The I (isotropic) band represents zone of thin filaments and is composed of actin, troponin, and tropomyosin. This band is isotropic due to less dense packing of proteins and, therefore, appears lighter under a polarizing microscope. The A (anisotropic) band is composed of entire length of single thick filament myosin and the actin-tropomyosin complex that lies within the length of thick filaments.

SLIDING FILAMENT MODEL OF CONTRACTION

The sliding filament model was proposed by both Huxley and Simmons in 1971. According to this model, the shortening occurs due to the movement of actin filament over the myosin filament that intimately requires the ATP and muscle proteins noted above. The length of the myosin and actin remains constant during contraction, but the overall sarcomere length becomes shorter. This occurs by formation of cross-bridges between actin and myosin generating power stroke. Ca^{2+} binds to troponin C, which causes shift in tropomyosin to uncover active sites and facilitates cross-bridge formation. Deformation of the actin and sliding brings the two Z disks together. This is the most accepted hypothesis explaining the molecular basis of muscle contraction.

MUSCLE TWITCH AND TETANUS

Muscle twitch is the basic response of a motor unit to a single stimulus of adequate strength that causes a momentary rise in tension. There are three phases of muscle twitch:

1. Latent period is the delay (approximately 15 milliseconds), during which the muscle depolarization occurs and Ca^{2+} is released from the sarcoplasmic reticulum into myoplasm. The muscle maintains a constant length without force production. There is also cross-bridge formation before sarcomere shortening occurs.
2. Contraction period involves actual sarcomere shortening (*see* Sliding Filament Model).
3. Relaxation phase is defined by restoration of resting low myoplasmic Ca^{2+} concentrations and release of cross-bridges. The stage ends with relaxation of muscle to its original length.

If a second stimulus reaches the muscle fiber after adequate relaxation of first twitch → another twitch identical to previous one takes place. If the second stimulus reaches the fiber before completion of the relaxation phase, an increase in tension above that of the first twitch results which is called wave summation. The motor unit responds more forcefully to the stimulus that reaches a plateau after few twitches causing Treppe effect or an unfused tetanus. As the frequency of stimulation is increased, the individual twitches fuse and amount of tension then produced increases proportionally until reaching a maximum level known as a "fused tetanus" **(Fig. 6)**.

The rate of muscle shortening depends on the muscle fiber type and the load being lifted. Fibers can be Type I (red or slow twitch) or Type II (white or fast twitch) based on their biochemical properties (oxidative capacity, type of myosin ATPase) and contractile properties (maximal force production, speed of contraction, and efficiency). Type I fibers take longer time period before reaching peak tension, whereas

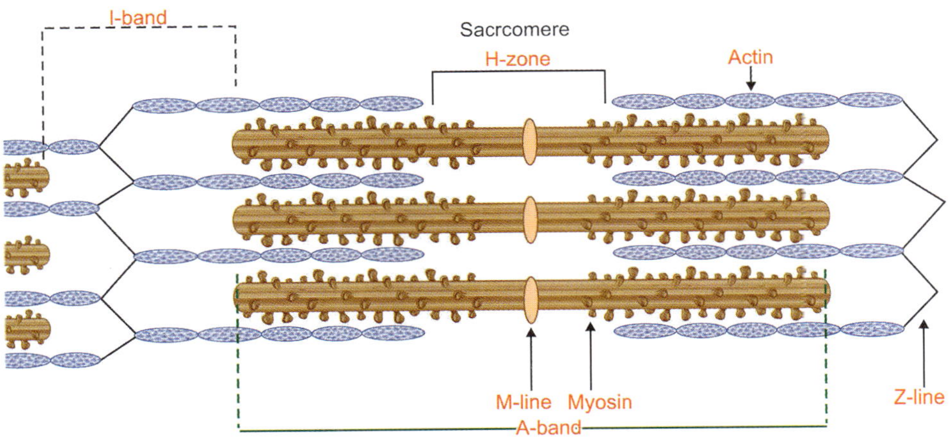

Fig. 5: The structure of sarcomere and various terminologies used (*see* text).

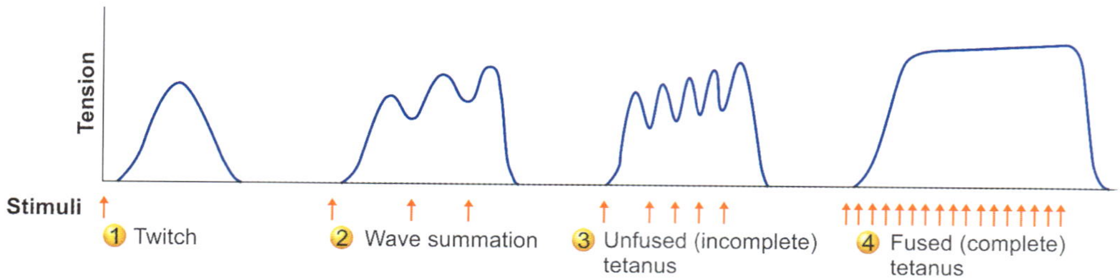

Fig. 6: Graphical illustration of twitch, wave summation (also called paired twitch), unfused tetanus, and fused tetanus. As the frequency of stimulation increases, the generation of muscle force rises until the point of fused tetanus.

Type II fibers reach peak tension in short time. They can be distinguished by staining for myosin ATPase.

- Concentric contraction also called shortening contraction occurs when the force generated by the contraction is greater than the resisting load and produces muscle shortening.
- Eccentric contraction occurs when the resisting load is greater than the amount of tension being produced. In this case, there will be a lengthening contraction.

The force generated by muscle contraction depends on the frequency of motor unit stimulation and the absolute number of motor units stimulated. Recruitment is a process for modulating the quantity of motor units being stimulated with each contraction. Optimal combination for force production and limb movement is fine-tuned by adjusting/synchronizing the frequency of motor unit stimulation and recruitment.

FIBER TYPES AND MUSCLE ADAPTABILITY

As detailed above, there are different types of muscle fibers based on biochemical, histological, and physiologic properties **(Table 1)**. Myosin ATPase (that determines contraction velocity) staining produces dark fibers corresponding to Type I fibers, while the Type IIa fibers stain lightest. Type IIx fibers stain in between. Large fibers expressing rapid myosin ATPase produce tension at a faster rate. Smaller fibers produce tension slowly. Immunohistochemical staining with selective antibody against unique myosin proteins identify fibers by color difference. Gel electrophoresis can also be used to this effect.

Type I Fibers (Slow-Twitch, Slow-Oxidative Fibers)

These fibers contract slowly and also relax slowly. They have high fatigue resistance as they are rich in mitochondrial and myoglobin concentration as required for marathon running.

Type IIA Fibers (Fast-Oxidative Glycolytic, Intermediate Fiber Type)

They contract faster than Type I fibers but are slower compared to Type IIB fibers. For fatigue resistance, they are intermediate between Types IIx and I fibers.

Type IIx Fibers (Fast Glycolytic Fibers with Predominant Anaerobic Mechanism)

They have least fatigue resistance but are highly responsive to stimuli with fastest contraction velocity as required for sprint running. These fibers also generate higher force per unit area (15–20% higher than Type I fibers).

TABLE 1: The types of different muscle fibers.

Characteristics	*Type I (Red, slow twitch slow oxidative)*	*Type IIA (White, fast twitch fastoxidative glycolytic)*	*Type IIx (Fast glycolytic)*
Contraction speed	Slow	Fast	Fast
Mitochondrial density	High	Moderate	Low
Metabolism (predominant)	Aerobic	Combination	Anaerobic
Capillary density	High	High	Low
Strength of contraction	Low	High	High
Specific tension	Moderate	High	High
Fatigue resistance	High	High/moderate	Low
Efficiency (aerobic capacity)	High	Intermediate	Low
ATPase activity	Low	High	Highest
Motor unit size	Small (coordination)	Larger	Largest (power generation)

The relative percentage of Type I or Type II fibers varies in general population and is believed to be genetically determined. Nonathletes have nearly equal percentages of fast and slow fibers. Their numbers do not change through training, but for sure development and maturation of specific types are influenced by endurance activities. Endurance athletes like marathon runners have higher percentages of fatigue resistant Type I fibers, whereas power athletes like sprinters or long jumpers have higher percentage of Type II fibers. Predominant fiber type does not determine success in athletic events so muscle biopsy for selecting sport specific athletes is not accepted, real ability is dependent more on training, reflex development and psychological factors rather than fiber type. Endurance training improves the oxidative capacity and increases the percentage of Type IIA fibers conditioning the muscle for fatigue resistance. Strength training, on the other hand, increases the percentage of Type IIB fibers. Strength training would increase the size of fibers (hypertrophy) and possibly also hyperplasia (increased number, uncertain in humans). Similarly, muscle atrophy results with prolonged bed rest, limb immobilization, and in space flights due to reduced protein synthesis. This can be reversed with resistance exercises. Apart from above, there is age-related loss of muscle fibers—10% between 25 and 50 years and added 40% between 50 and 80 years, this cannot be, however, eliminated by exercises.

LENGTH-TENSION RELATIONSHIP

Initial length of muscle (resting length, before stimulation) is an important determinant of force generation. Higher resting length (within physiological limits) is proportional to ultimate force generation. Two components determine the increased force generation with increased resting length—the elastic recoil of connective tissue and improved sliding distance between thick and thin fibers. The connective tissue and fascial components store the stretch force in the form of elastic tissue potential energy that gets released in the form of recoil improving the force of contraction. With passive stretch the actin and myosin filaments are optimally placed and can slide to a greater length generating greater force. If the passive stretch is too much, the filaments would uncouple or the myofibrils will rupture reducing force generated as might happen in eccentric contractions.

- Isometric contraction would generate maximal force at a length (L_0) where there are maximal numbers of mechanical couplings between thick and thin filaments **(Fig. 7)**. Isotonic contractions are produced in response to a fixed load with limb movement against resistance. They can be concentric (muscle shortening with contraction) or eccentric (muscle lengthening with contraction).
- Lengths greater than L_0 would produce proportional decrease in force generated as lesser number of actin-myosin cross-bridges are available for overlap of thick and thin filaments and would ultimately uncouple at the fiber rupture limit **(Fig. 7)**.
- Resting lengths shorter than L_0 would result in excessive overlap of thick and thin filaments reducing the sliding distance and causing disordered cytoskeletal geometry.

FORCE-VELOCITY RELATIONSHIP

Muscle shortening velocity during contraction is proportional to fiber length and the load placed on the muscle. Rate of myosin ATPase induced cross-bridge deformation cycle between myosin and actin helices is reduced as the load on the cross-bridges increases (higher weight). These heavier loads increase the time needed for flexion at the globular-filament actin fibril junction and hence prolong the cross-bridge cycling. This reduces the shortening velocity of muscle. At a finite load (endurance limit), the velocity of shortening would approach zero and then only isometric force will be generated. An unloaded muscle with same corollary would generate maximum shortening velocity. The peak power generation, however, is maximal for velocities up to 200–300 degrees/sec and beyond this the force decreases with increasing speeds.

MUSCULAR TRAINING, CONDITIONING, AND STRENGTHENING

Muscular conditioning and training play an important role in sports medicine. They are important not only for preparing athletes for competitive sports but also indispensable during recovery from injuries sustained in sporting events. Proper conditioning, training, and strengthening of muscles is needed for optimal outcome that is aimed to:

- Enhance musculoskeletal performance
- Mitigate risk of injury
- Minimize injury severity
- Accelerated rehabilitation and return to activity during recovery phase post injury
- Prevention of re-injury.

The musculoskeletal conditioning works on Davis law or the SAID (specific adaptation to imposed demands) principle. Davis law is a corollary of Wolff's law as applied to soft tissue. It states that soft tissues heal in accordance to the mechanical stress they are subjected to. Not only healing but tissue modeling is also guided by imposed demands. It is an extension of the Harold frost "stretch-hypertrophy" rule, which is applicable to all fibrous collagenous connective tissues such as ligaments, tendons, bones, and fascia that are capable of modeling and remodeling. The rule basically states that controlled intermittent stretch causes collagenous tissue to hypertrophy until resulting increase in strength reduces elongation in tension to some minimum level (Frost). The different physiotherapy training and exercise programs

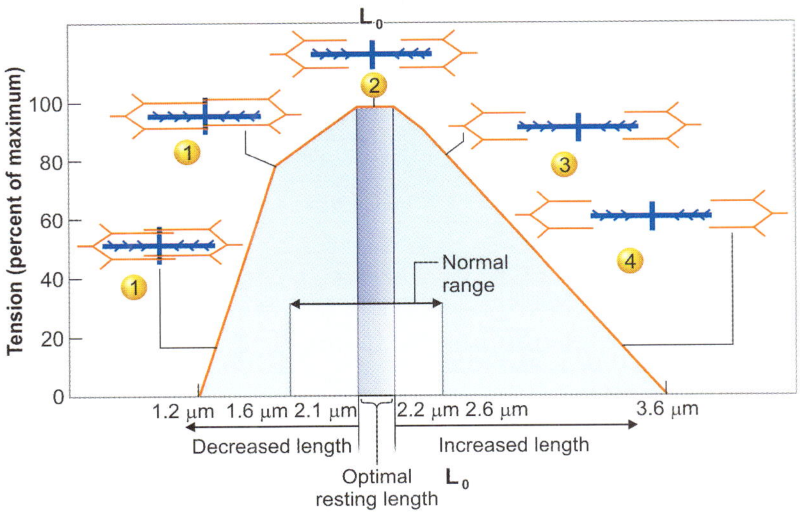

Fig. 7: The length tension relationship of muscle fibers.

exploit this rule to improve competitive musculoskeletal biomechanics. Based on the speed of movement and resistance applied, there are three types of exercises; used for conditioning muscles viz.:

1. *Isometric exercises:* These exercises do not produce any joint movement. The exercised muscle maintains fixed length (thus as per physics no work is done!) so it is called "isometric". The static tension developed is very high and causes rapid deoxygenation of muscles due to compression of capillaries, promoting anaerobic metabolism. The primary advantage of these exercises is that they can be initiated very early in rehabilitation even when joint mobilization is not begun. The strength increase is very fast with these exercises which also prevents wasting. The basic problem is the fact that dynamic balancing and muscle coordination needed for rhythmic movements is not gained. Also stopping these exercises leads to rapid loss of strength and atrophy. The other most important limitation is limited physiologic strength overflow, i.e., strength gain in a particular plane will not be reproduced at other angle of joint motion. At maximum, this strength will be appropriate for the angle at which strength development is done ±10°. At other angle of joint motion, the muscle will behave weak!
2. *Isotonic exercises:* These exercises inherently involve movement of joint across which the muscle acts. The tone developed in the muscle against resistance during contraction remains same so it is called isotonic. If the muscle shortens with joint movement and the joint moves then it is called "concentric" contraction while if the tense muscle lengthens while the joint moves then it is called "eccentric" contraction. Because displacement occurs in isokinetic exercises so there is definite dynamic muscular work done physically. The strength training involves alternating cyclic use of concentric and eccentric contractions. Compared to concentric movements, eccentric movements produce two to three times force helping gain muscle mass and strength. Multiple repetitions of the exercise cycles produce initial anaerobic metabolism but the replenishment of blood supply is so fast and massive (15–20 times normal) during relaxation that the metabolism is ultimately aerobic. Because the exercise involves agonist and antagonists across a joint so the neurophysiology of muscular dynamics is more reliably maintained. The resistance against which the muscle contracts can either remain static (like fixed weights) or may be made to vary (using commercial devices). The former usually simulates real-life conditions while the latter is used to smoothen muscle strength generation throughout range of motion in athletes if there is variability identified in muscle strength.
3. *Isokinetic exercises:* This is essentially opposite of isokinetic exercises. Here, the velocity of muscle contraction is same (so called as "isokinetic") but the dynamic loading of muscle varies so there is variable resistance throughout range of motion. In isotonic contractions against fixed resistance, the velocity of contraction gradually increases and peaks in the middle where power generation is highest and then reduces again so the period for which strength generation is high is comparatively small. In isokinetic exercises, this high-strength generation phase is prolonged markedly. This type of exercise, hence, can be tailored for specific sporting activity.

The differences between isometric, isotonic, and isokinetic exercises are detailed in **Table 2**.

Kinetic Chain Exercises

The different parts of limbs are connected to each other through mobile joints. It is logical that movement of one part alters how the other part will move in a predetermined manner so these parts are anatomically distinct but connected kinetically. This was first realised by Dr Arthur Steindler in

TABLE 2: The differences between isometric, isotonic, and isokinetic exercises.

Characteristics	*Isometric*	*Isotonic*	*Isokinetic*
Definition	Static muscle contraction without altering length against stationary resistance ("iso"-same; "metric"-length)	Dynamic muscular contraction altering its length maintaining muscle tone against resistance where speed is not constant ("iso"-same; "tone"-tension)	Dynamic muscular contraction against variable resistance at fixed speed of movement ("iso"-same; "kinetic"-speed)
Strength development	Focuses on maximal strength development in muscle contraction	Focuses on explosive strength, improving the instantaneous burst of muscle strength at peak of contraction	Improves both the explosive strength and strength endurance
Rehabilitation of immobilized joint	Possible	Not possible	Not possible
Coordination and skill training	Poor	Excellent	Good
Endurance and speed development	Poor	Good	Speed development better than isotonic
Durability of strength development	Short (depletes very fast on stopping exercise)	Persists longer	Prolonged development of strength
Utility	Rehabilitation of immobilized joints/limb, postsurgery beginning of rehabilitation and strength training. Some sporting activities like wrestling, weight-lifting, and gymnastics	Long-term rehabilitation of joint motion postsurgery. Almost all sporting activities need this training and conditioning	Sport specific development of muscle strength, endurance, and speed Controlled by a preset protocol for specific sport

TABLE 3: The differences between open and closed chain kinetic exercises.

Characteristics	*Open chain exercise*	*Closed chain exercise*
Joint stress	Rotatory and shear	Linear
Targeted joints	Single	Multiple simultaneous
Movements of segments	All segments distal to the moving joint remain stationary	Barring the distal fixed segmental other segments are moving
Number of moving joints	Single	Multiple
Planes of movement	Single plane movement	Multiple planes allowed
Muscular involvement	Isolated muscle/group is focused during contraction	Contraction of all related muscles
Clinical utility	Nonfunctional movement so clinically discrete usage for joint or muscle focused activity	Functional movement so clinically commonly used for rehabilitation in postoperative period, e.g., lower limb function following anterior cruciate ligament reconstruction
Posture and balance	Poor in improving dynamic balance but as good as closed chain for static balance	Good dynamic and static balance

1955 describing human movements as a kinetic chain. The chains are further connected to the torso. There can be two type of kinetic movements one where the distal extremis is fixed and does not move while the individual components are moving or it may remain free in space with the movements of individual parts, distinguishing **(Table 3)** two subtle but dynamically important concepts as follows:

1. *Closed kinetic chain movements and exercises:* Here, the most distal component of the successively arranged connected parts is fixed and does not move. The individual components move connected to one another, the common examples are push-ups and dead-lifts. Here, the body moves against a permanent fixture (usually ground). There exercises target multiple joints, movements, and muscle groups together. Because the load is shared between related muscles of the limb so stress on joints is minimized. This also logically derives into the fact that related muscle group strengthening will improve joint stability. Usually in activities of daily living, coordinated combined movements are needed as also in sporting activities so all units should be simultaneously strengthened. This also improves postural control because maintaining posture need simultaneous work of many groups of muscles. If a single element is "off" then posture cannot be maintained. Closed chain would focus on a limb in totality so it improves joint and limb stability and functional movement patterns. For example, following anterior cruciate ligament (ACL) reconstruction, the knee function is to be improved in coordination with hip and ankle movements so that the lower limb acts as a stable dynamically functional unit. In addition, the shear stress has to be minimized on the ACL graft so closed chain kinetic exercises are best.
2. *Open chain movements and exercises:* The most distal segment of the connected parts is free to move in space, e.g., leg extension exercises. Here, the movement is at knee and one can discretely focus on quadriceps muscle. So, open chain exercises are specifically used when focus is on a particular joint or muscle. In cases where there is specific muscle inhibition like biceps inhibition following humerus plating, one can use open chain exercises for activation of muscle. Mobilizing a stiff joint like elbow or knee also uses open chain exercises focusing on the specific joint. Third utility of open chain exercises is for improving muscle coordination. Correcting uncoordinated movements like in scapular dyskinesia need individual muscle training for coordinated firing and correct dyskinetic movements.

CONCLUSION

- Skeletal muscles provide the "motor" power to the locomotor system. Without them the body is merely equivalent to effigy.
- Competitive sports usually are a measure of the efficacy of locomotor system in specific fields. To provide the best outcome of sporting activity trainers need to focus on specific aspects of skeletal muscle function and development. This, hence, entails a good knowledge of the structure and biomechanics of the skeletal muscle.
- Understanding the physiology of different types of muscle training and kinetic exercises forms the basis of optimal postoperative rehabilitation. This also helps in individualizing the patient care which is often neglected and a general "completely inadequate" prescription like *"mobilization and strengthening exercises or isometric exercises"* should be avoided. Every patient has different needs and one should be aware of the functional aspects of dynamic muscular rehabilitation and concepts; to prescribe patient-specific scheme of functional rehabilitation protocol.

SECTION 7

Regional Orthopedics: Shoulder

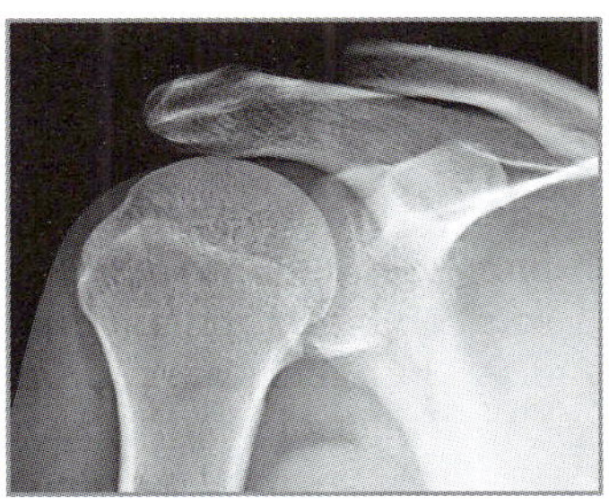
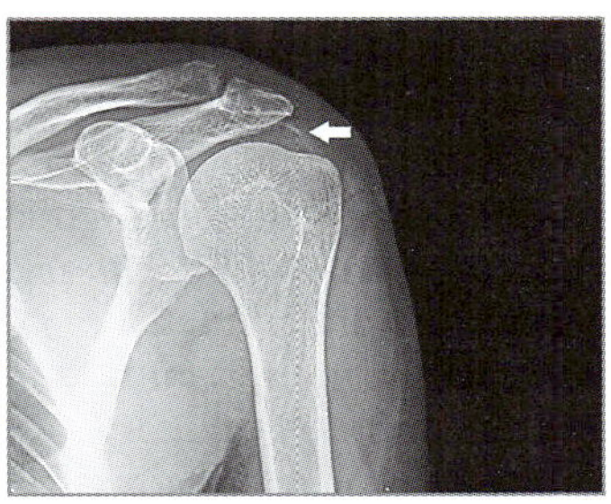
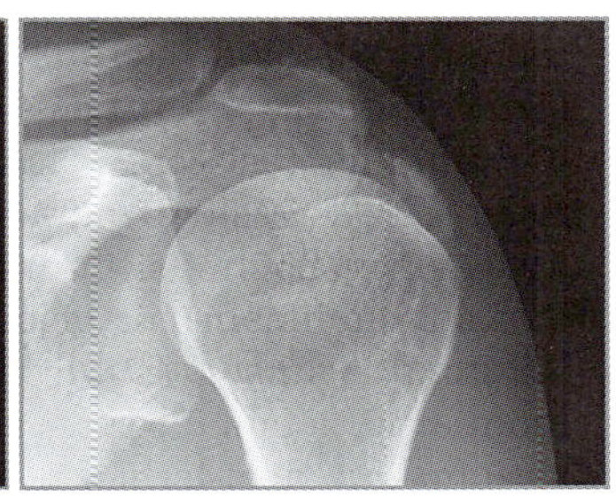

CHAPTER

53 Shoulder: Functional Anatomy

Manish Kumar Varshney

INTRODUCTION

Shoulder is an interesting ball and socket joint with large degrees of freedom due to unique disposition of osseous components. The small congruence of humeral head to glenoid surface (likened to "golf ball on tee") provides minimal restraint in space achieving large range of motion but compromises inherent stability. Soft tissue components hence play very important role in stabilizing the joint. This also makes the joint vulnerable to injuries because soft tissue bears the major brunt of forces. Understanding anatomy hence is paramount to restore the soft tissue balance and force couples which are very important in maintaining the rhythmic movements at shoulder.

SHOULDER JOINT

There are typically four articulations in the shoulder complex **(Figs. 1A to C)**:

1. Sternoclavicular

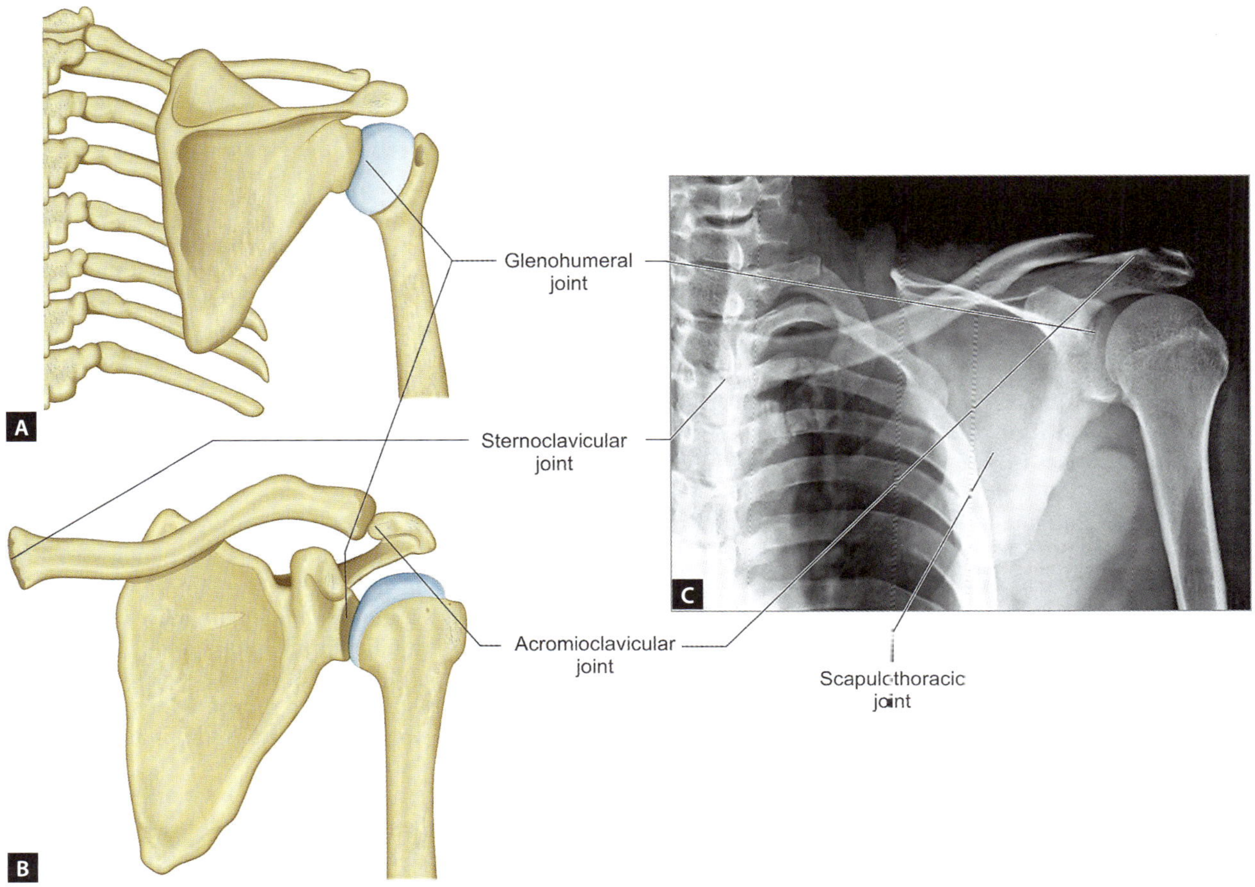

Figs. 1A to C: Articulations of shoulder complex. (A and B) Illustrate from the posterior and anterior aspect while (C) Demonstrates the same on a radiograph.

2. Acromioclavicular
3. Scapulothoracic
4. Glenohumeral joint

These are supplemented by a fifth "pseudojoint" between humeral head and the coracoacromial arch.

The fifth joint (scapulohumeral joint) was described as a concept by Matsen R. This joint is occupied mostly by the subacromial and subdeltoid bursa and gets mostly involved in "adhesive capsulitis".

The glenohumeral joint is commonly referred to as *the shoulder joint*. The shoulder joint has the largest range of motion among all the joints in the human body. Due to its flexibility it has its own unique share of problems. The *stability of shoulder* is outcome of complementary and in tandem working of various stabilizing structures. These structures have been typically classified into static and dynamic types **(Table 1)**.

- ***The static ones*** include the labrum, ligaments (discrete thickenings of capsule), capsule and to a certain extent the bones. The shoulder capsule has twice the surface area of humeral head and accepts 25–30 mL of fluid normally. The capsule fibers blend with ligamentous structures to provide static support.
- ***The dynamic stabilizers*** include the rotator cuff muscles, scapular muscles, scapulothoracic rhythm, and even the axial core muscles of the body.

Proprioception connects the dynamic stabilizers to each other and to the static ones. The most active **primary stabilizers** are the glenohumeral ligaments.

There are four ligaments: (1) superior glenohumeral ligament (SGHL), (2) middle glenohumeral ligament (MGHL), (3) inferior glenohumeral ligament (IGHL, its split anterior and posterior part), and (4) the posterior glenohumeral ligament (it is the posterior split part of IGHL) better visualized from inside than outside **(Figs. 2 and 3)**.

- Superior glenohumeral ligament (present in 90% individuals) arises from the glenoid rim from approximately 12 or 1 o'clock and runs inferiorly and laterally to insert on the anatomical neck near the medial ridge of the intertubercular groove. It limits the external rotation and inferior translation of the humeral head with arm at side.
- Middle glenohumeral ligament (present in 70% individuals) arises from 2 to 3 o'clock and runs inferiorly and laterally to insert on the anatomical neck, medial to the lesser tuberosity. It limits the external rotation and anterior translation of the humeral head with the arm in 0° and 45° of abduction.
- Inferior glenohumeral ligament is like a hammock and comprises different ligaments together forming a complex. The anterior band (arises from 2 to 4 o'clock position) restrains external rotation and inferior translation of the humeral head with the arm abducted to 90° while the posterior band of IGHL (arises from 7 to 9 o'clock position) restrains against internal rotation with the arm in all positions of abduction. Both counter the anterior and posterior translation in 90° of abduction.

The secondary stabilizers include the rotator cuff and the core muscles of the body. All work together to center the humeral head into glenoid (glenoid is too small and covers only one-third of the humeral head articular surface, so it is like stabilizing the golf ball on the "Tee").

TABLE 1: Stabilizers of shoulder joint.

Structures	***Pathoanatomy***
Static	
Osteochondral articular surface	• *Humeral articular surface:* Hill–Sachs lesion, post-traumatic defect, osteonecrosis, abnormal humeral version • *Glenoid articular surface:* Bony defect, erosion, or fracture (recurrent dislocations), dysplasia, and abnormal version
Capsulolabral complex • Glenoid labrum • Glenohumeral ligaments • Coracohumeral ligament	Recession of capsule from glenoid, tear of capsule and anterior ligamentous complex, labral tear or deficiency. The labrum is strongest posterosuperiorly and anteroinferiorly. Anterior ligaments tighten in extreme ER and abduction; IGHL forms a hammock sling inferiorly that supports head during abduction
Coracoacromial ligament (arch)	Anterosuperior support. Lost in advanced rotator cuff tear or trauma
Negative intra-articular pressure	Negative intra-articular pressure aids in centering the head; this is enhanced by "suction cup" effect of labrum
Cup (glenoid) and humeral head (ball) + Labral suction cup mechanism	Disturbed in various pathologies including joint degeneration
Synovial fluid adhesion-cohesion	Degenerative joint, rheumatoid arthritis, and crystal arthropathy
Rotator cuff	Tear (sport injury and degenerative)
Dynamic	
Long head of triceps (fifth rotator cuff muscle)	Fraying, subluxation, and attrition tears
Rotator cuff and scapular muscles	Weakness proportionately reduces joint stability. Infraspinatus and teres minor reduce strain on IGHL in abduction and ER. They are called the "hamstrings" of shoulder. Subscapularis provides anterior stability. The scapular muscles are key chain in Kibler kinetic chain mechanism that describes transfer of potential energy of trunk to kinetic energy at shoulder (Kinetic chain)
Scapulothoracic rhythm	Neurologic disorders, poor training during endurance
Concavity compression	Weakness of shoulder muscles, anatomical damage to bony surfaces
Proprioception	Spinal cord damage, degenerative joint disease, Charcot's and Milwaukee shoulder

The *muscles around shoulder* joint have been functionally classified (modified from Saha) into:

- *Scapular elevators:* Levator scapulae, trapezius, rhomboideus major, and rhomboideus minor
- *Scapular depressors:* Pectoralis minor and major, serratus anterior, and trapezius
- *Protractors of scapula:* Serratus anterior and pectoralis minor
- *Retractors of scapula:* Trapezius and rhomboideus
- *Rotators of scapula:* Trapezius and serratus anterior (upward rotator), rhomboideus, and levator scapulae (downward rotator)

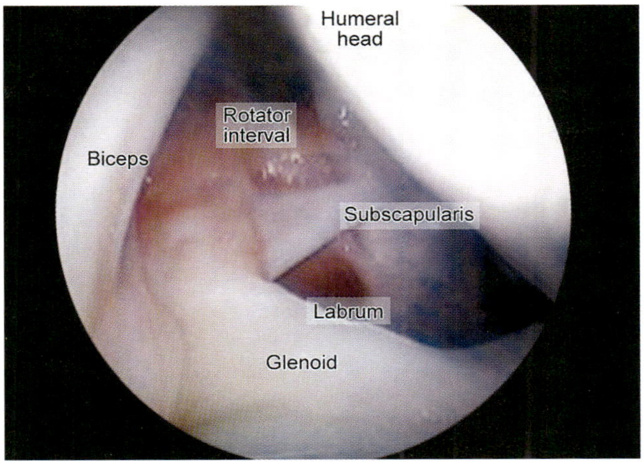

Fig. 2: The normal shoulder arthroscopic picture details as viewed from posterior portal. The prominent structures are biceps tendon (light house for shoulder arthroscopy), glenoid labrum, subscapularis tendon, humeral head, and rotator interval.

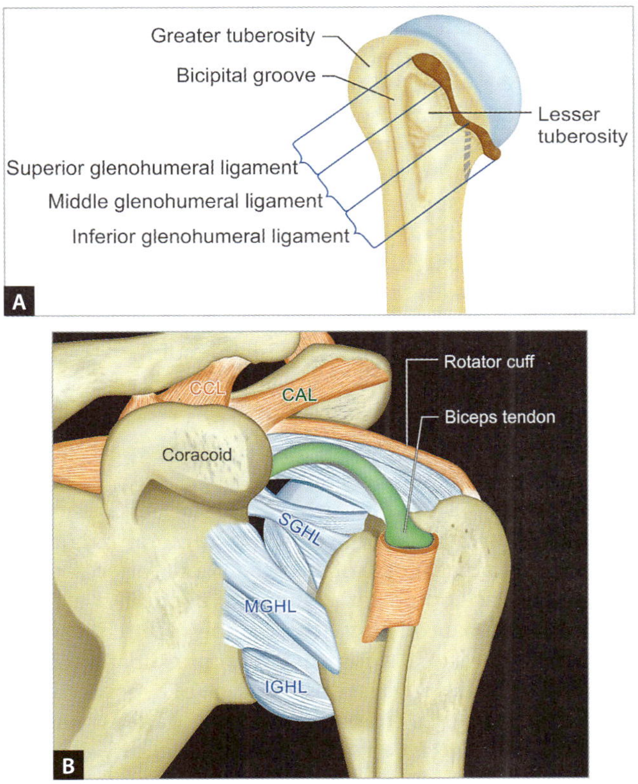

Figs. 3A and B: (A) The attachment of glenohumeral ligaments. The superior glenohumeral ligament (SGHL) attaches to the fovea capitis just above lesser tuberosity. Middle glenohumeral ligament (MGHL) attaches medial to lesser tuberosity. Inferior glenohumeral ligament (IGHL) attaches either as a collar or as a "V-shaped" scarf along the humeral neck (shown as serrated curve); (B) The static ligamentous shoulder stabilizers. Also shown are the rotator cuff and the biceps tendon. (CAL: coracoacromial ligament; CCL: coracoclavicular ligament)

- *Compressors of shoulder joint:* Subscapularis (anterior compressor), supraspinatous (superior compressor), infraspinatous (inferior compressor), deltoid (the posterior and middle portions are important than the anterior part in producing concavity compression). Kindly note that there are *no* "depressors" of shoulder joint as was once thought.
- *Internal rotators of humerus:* Deltoid (anterior), pectoralis major, subscapularis, teres major, and latissimus dorsi
- *External rotators of humerus:* Infraspinatous, teres minor, and deltoid (posterior)
- *Abductors:* Supra- and infraspinatous and deltoid
- *Adductors of humerus:* Coracobrachialis, pectoralis major, teres major, and latissimus dorsi

The *subacromial space*, as the name suggests is the space under the surface of the acromion and the under surface of the coracoid process of the scapula with the coracoacromial ligament (aka "roof of shoulder") stretched between them **(Figs. 4A and B)**.

- The roof of space is formed by the coracoacromial arch and the acromioclavicular joint.
- The floor of the space is formed by the greater tuberosity and upper portions of the humeral head.
- The space is occupied by the rotator cuff tendons, the tendon of the long head of biceps brachii, and the subacromial and subdeltoid bursae.

ROTATOR CUFF ANATOMY AND PATHOANATOMY

This is a conjoint tendon of the four muscles originating from scapula and inserting onto the humeral tuberosities (supra- and infraspinatus, teres minor attaching to greater tuberosity, and subscapularis to lesser tuberosity). The fused tendons act together and with significantly augmented strength to bear the forces across the shoulder keeping the humeral head centered in glenoid fossa and contributing to rotation in stability. *Rotator interval* is a triangular structure **(Fig. 5)** that lies between superior aspect of subscapularis tendon and anterior aspect of supraspinatus tendon. The base of triangle is located at coracoid. The interval contains coracohumeral ligament (protecting supraspinatus tendon and restraining inferior translation of humerus in adduction), SGHL, and transverse humeral ligament (protecting the biceps tendon and roofing the bicipital tunnel). The microstructure of rotator cuff has been detailed into five layers near the insertion of supraspinatus and infraspinatus **(Figs. 6A to C)**.

1. ***First layer:*** Composed of the superficial fibers of the coracohumeral ligament.
2. ***Second layer:*** The main portion of the cuff. The tendon fibers are closely packed parallel to each other and grouped in large bundles extending directly from the muscle bellies to the insertion on the humerus.
3. ***Third layer:*** Random orientation of collagen fibers with a weaved pattern. The fascicles are smaller than layer two and have less uniform orientation. The tendon is as thick as layer two here.
4. ***Fourth layer (transverse band, pericapsular band, and rotator cable):*** Loose connective tissues with thick band of collagen fibers running perpendicular to the primary fiber orientation as seen in layer two. This layer has deep extension of the coracohumeral ligament. The

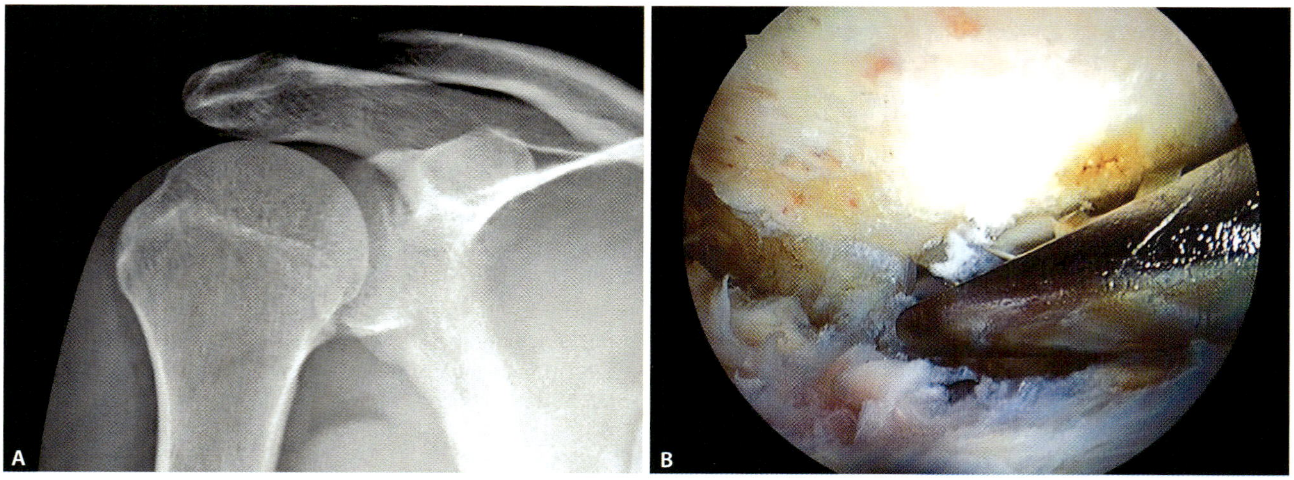

Figs. 4A and B: Subacromial space lies beneath the acromion. The patient has a hooked acromion with impingement symptoms, so he was treated with subacromial decompression and bursectomy. (A) Radiograph shows the subacromial space with hooked acromion (better delineated on Y-view—not shown); (B) The arthroscopic appearance of subacromial space as in this patient requiring decompression and acromioplasty.

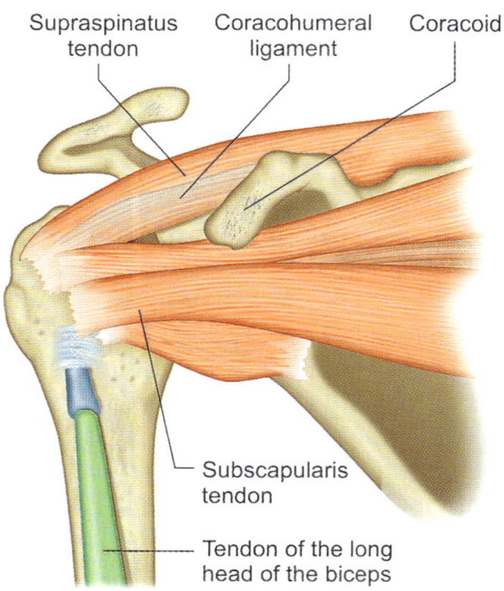

Fig. 5: Rotator interval. This is the triangular layer between subscapularis and supraspinatus with coracoid at its base.

layer is thought to distribute the forces across the different muscle tendons explaining why some rotator cuff tears are clinically asymptomatic. This layer is also the site of *intrasubstance cuff tears* possibly due to transmission of shear forces and concentration.

5. ***Fifth layer:*** This is the continuous capsule layer running from humerus to glenoid.

The collagen fiber orientation differs along the rotator cuff tendon. The fibers are regularly and uniformly arranged parallel to each other near the musculotendinous junction while near the insertion into bone they become flat ribbon-like crossing at about 45°. The tendon of supraspinatus contains type 2 collagen with abundance of aggrecan. The fibrocartilage portion of the insertion resembles the histopathology of tissues subjected to compressive stress with prominent proteoglycan content and may be responsible for frequent finding of degenerative tears due to constant tensile forces. There is another interesting concept of **"rotator cable"**. This is a ligament (ligamentum semicirculare humeri) demonstrable in anatomic specimens and on MRI. It has been divided into three segments—(1) anterior, (2) middle, and (3) posterior. The anterior segment of this cable lies in the lateral part of rotator interval. The middle part of the cable lies under supraspinatus tendon while the posterior part lies under infraspinatous tendon. The fibers of the ligamentum semicirculare humeri remain perpendicular to the longitudinal axes of the supraspinatus and infraspinatus tendons. The ligament may have a reinforcing function contributing to the strength of the rotator cuff.

Clinical Anatomy of Rotator Cuff

- With tendinopathy, there is an increase in type 3 collagen and glycosaminoglycan content.
- *Vascular supply and anomalies:* Rotator cuff is supplied by anterior branch of ascending humeral circumflex artery, acromial branch of thoracoacromial artery, and the subscapular and posterior humeral circumflex arteries. There is a debate on the vascular supply of the critical zone (8–10 mm proximal to insertion) of supraspinatus tendon. Cadaver studies suggest this as a zone of hypovascularity while the studies from symptomatic patients suggest that there is in fact a zone of hypervascularity. It seems that the neovascularization is in fact secondary to the impingement rather than being the cause of degeneration of tendon. More recent studies utilizing the polarization spectral imaging suggest this as a normovascular zone. The hypovascular theory (quite popular in past) is not well supported in literature and is not linked to development of pathology directly in my view.
- The pathology of impingement is more related to acromion anatomy **(Figs. 7A to C)** and biomechanical strain. Anteriorly hooked acromion (type 3 Bigliani) is associated with friction and degenerative tear due to extrinsic

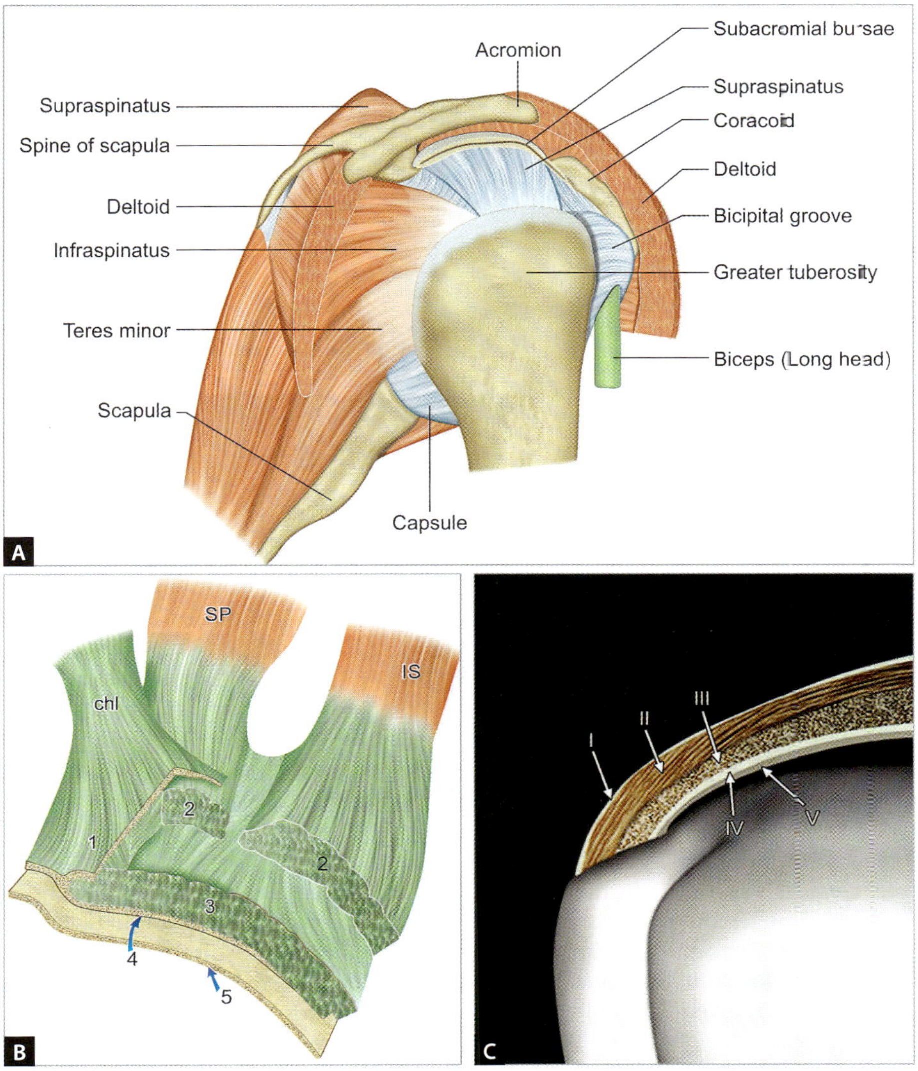

Figs. 6A to C: Rotator cuff anatomy. Rotator comprises four tendons (subscapularis, supraspinatus, infraspinatus, and teres minor) blending together into a cover-like structure to the capsule more so toward bony insertion (A). The cuff has five distinct layers appreciated near the insertion of supraspinatus (SP) and infraspinatus (IS) (B). The layers from the coracohumeral ligament to main tendon structure from above to below (C). This is supported by a randomly oriented collagen layer further supported below by the investing deep layer of coracohumeral (chl) ligament forming the fourth layer. The deepest layer is the capsule.

impingement on the tendon. Type 1 (straight) and type 2 (curved) do not cause supraspinatus impingement **(Figs. 7A to C)**. The different shapes of acromion are not congenital but develop in response to traction forces applied by the coracoacromial ligament on it.

- Biomechanical causes of impingement are discussed in the subsequent chapter that mainly lead to intrinsic impingement.

Long Head of Biceps Tendon and its Clinical Significance

The long head of biceps tendon (LHBT) originates from the superior aspect of glenoid labrum commonly referred to as 12 o'clock position. The labrum acts as a fibrous tether to the tendon but continuous traction by the tendon may produce superior labral tears [the superior labrum anterior and posterior (SLAP) lesions]. The LHBT and labrum were considered distinct entities but are now referred to as a continuum of structures with interdependent functions forming a biceps tendon-labral complex. This is further subdivided into three distinct zones:

1. *The inside* represents the tendon labrum anchor.
2. *The junctional* is the intra-articular portion of the tendon with bicipital pulley. The pulley is formed by the coalescence of fibers from coracoacromial and glenohumeral ligaments. This region can be evaluated by standard glenohumeral arthroscopy.

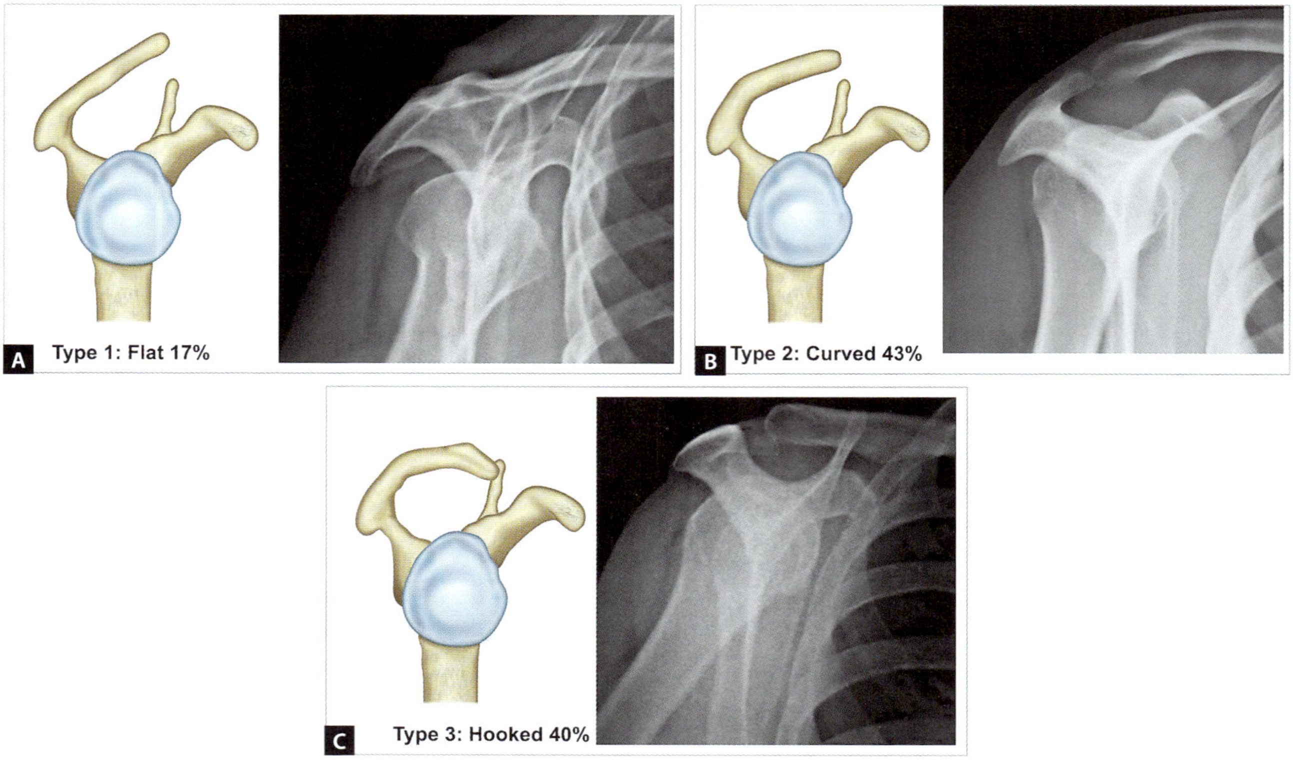

Figs. 7A to C: Types of acromion. The three types of acromion as described by Bigliani et al. The type 1 is a flat structure proving a spacious subacromial space while the majority of population has an arched acromion maintaining the concentric symmetricity with humeral head. Type 3 has anterior hook that may impinge and injure the rotator cuff.

3. *The bicipital tunnel zone:* The tunnel is further divided into three zones. Zone 1 is the region from intra-articular margin to the lower edge of subscapularis. Zone 2, also known as "no man's land" due to its inaccessibility by standard operative procedures, extends from lower edge of subscapularis to the upper edge of pectoralis tendon. Zone 3 is the infrapectoral region. Tunnel commonly harbors lesions that are inaccessible to the arthroscopic procedure and hence hidden.

CONCLUSION

- Shoulder joint is unique in two aspects as it is the largest suspended joint in the body and has the highest mobility in all directions enabling humans' access to majority of the surrounding environment with ease.
- The joint is most importantly stabilized by ligamentous structures that are also, hence, the most common source of pathology when injured.
- The capsuloligamentous structures primarily represented by rotator cuff act to locate the joint while maintaining mobility simultaneously.
- Thorough anatomy of the structures is imperative in comprehensive management of the patients so that optimal function can be restored. The different shapes of acromion are not congenital but develop in response to traction forces applied by the coracoacromial ligament on it.

CHAPTER 54

Biomechanics of Shoulder Joint

Manish Kumar Varshney

INTRODUCTION

It is important to understand the mechanism of shoulder joint to decipher shoulder instability and other disorders. Shoulder differs from hip in having a shallow socket (acetabulum is a deep socket) and from knee in that the knee ligaments remain isometric providing stability in most of movement range. Other differences from hip include retroversion of humerus vis-à-vis anteversion of femur and nearly two-thirds coverage of head of femur in acetabulum while shallow humeral head containment in shoulder. Maintenance of congruent bony articulation in shoulder is thus very important and a function of soft tissue biomechanics and disposition. The articular surfaces are already compromised (in the sense that glenoid only provides coverage to one-third equivalent of humeral head). Loss of >20% of anterior glenoid surface leads to shoulder instability. Humeral head depression fracture leading to Hill-Sachs lesion can produce recurrent instability with the eburnated glenoid falling into the position during external rotation.

GLENOID LABRUM

Labrum is the first anatomical and biomechanical restraint to instability that limits the gliding and sliding of humeral head on glenoid **(Figs. 1A and B)**. It is a fibrous structure

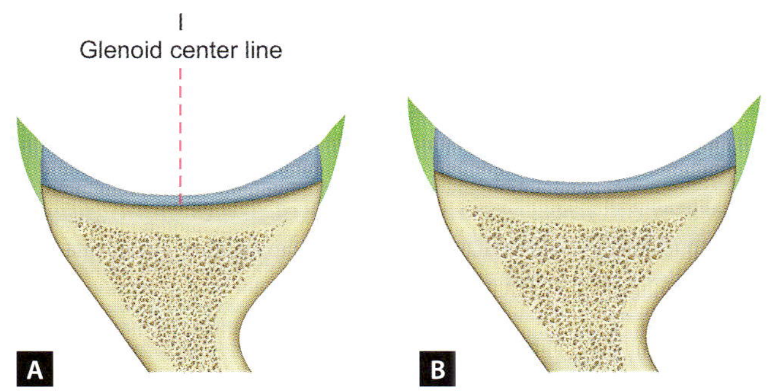

Figs. 1A and B: The glenoid is itself a shallow cavity that is quite prominently conformed to humeral head by the labrum. This also acts like the suction cup for holding the humeral head through motion.

that attaches to the rim of glenoid and improves stability by following mechanisms:

- Increase the glenoid depth by 50%
- Increase the surface contact area with the humeral head
- Act as a static stabilizer through a buttress effect
- Serve as an attachment site for the shoulder capsule, glenohumeral ligaments, and long head of the biceps tendon

The labrum may be normally deficient in anterosuperior quadrant. This when combined with cord-like middle glenohumeral ligament (MGHL) is termed "Buford complex".

The humeral head is stabilized within the glenoid by the combined action of shoulder muscles maintaining the position by a mechanism called "concavity compression". This mechanism operates due to supplementary action of shoulder compressors and glenoid concavity. Importantly, this mechanism is active in all positions of shoulder unlike the ligaments that come into play in specific positions only. The "glenohumeral ligaments" limit extremes of glenohumeral movements and need to slack and tighten in different positions. Most of the pathology that develops in the glenohumeral joint can be understood in terms of net force acting on the joint (humeral head) and the shape of glenoid fossa. The basic law of glenohumeral stability is that the glenohumeral joint will not dislocate as long as the net humeral joint reaction force is directed within the effective glenoid arc. Effective glenoid arc in a given direction is also known as the "balance stability angle (BSA)", the maximal angle that the net humeral joint reaction force can make with the glenoid center line in a given direction before dislocation **(Figs. 2 and 3)**. BSAs vary for different directions around the glenoid. The requisite for a stable glenohumeral joint is that the net humeral joint reaction force be maintained within the BSAs. Trauma, congenital deficiencies, excessive tissue compliance or wear of glenoid compromises the BSA that can be restored by Bankart lesion repair, rim augmentation, congruent glenoid bone grafting, and glenoid re-orientation osteotomy. Calculating the net joint reaction force is complicated as the forces acting are controlled by rotator cuff muscles, biceps long head, deltoid, gravity and externally applied force. The compressors of shoulder joint along

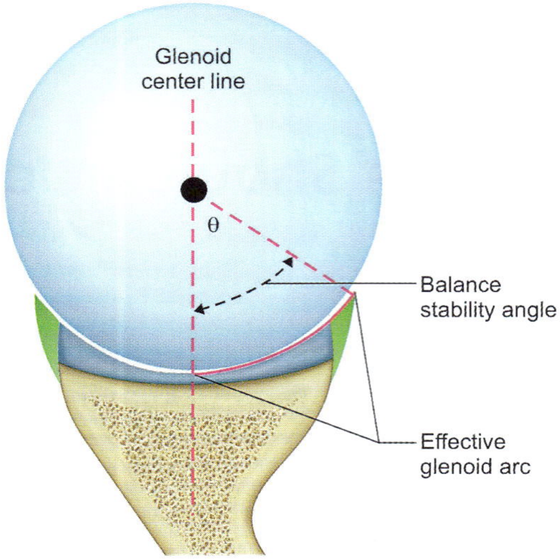

Fig. 2: The mechanism of stability of glenohumeral articulation as enhanced with labrum.

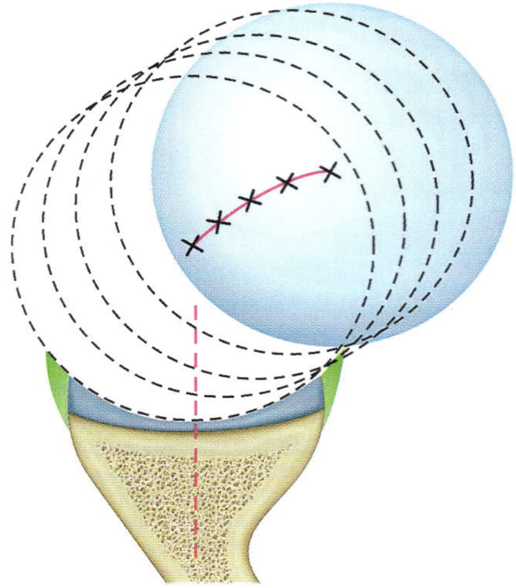

Fig. 4: Glenoidogram is a good way to explain the importance of depth of glenoid cavity. The more the depth the greater is the work required for displacing the humeral head out of the socket.

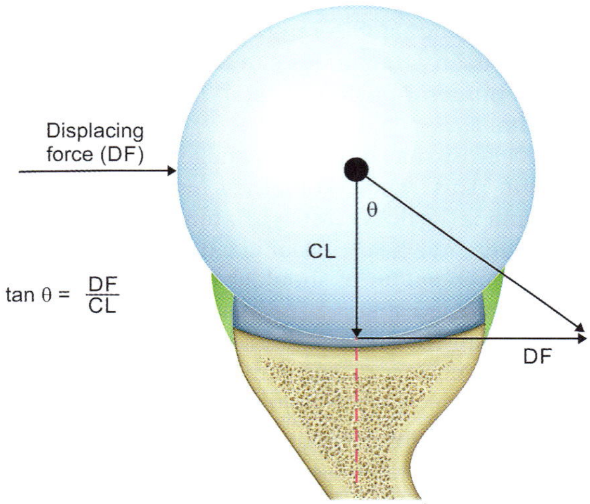

Fig. 3: Stability ratio is the maximal displacing force that can be stabilized by specified compressive load and is represented by tangent to balance stability angle. DF is magnitude of displacing force; and CL is the magnitude of compressive load.

with biceps are important in this regard to center the head in glenoid. The neuromuscular stabilization by capsular feedback and pattern generators coupled to muscular activity is very important. It is imperative to mention here that many muscle builders receive poor training producing a distorted scapulohumeral rhythm due to lack of muscle optimization and have shoulder problems and instability.

Stability Ratio

A tangent drawn to BSA vector is the ratio between its displacing component and its compressive component, which is known as the "stability ratio" **(Fig. 3)**. The displacing force vector operates perpendicular to glenoid center line while the compressive force biomechanically acts along the glenoid center line to position humeral head in centric stable congruence **(Fig. 3)**. The stability ratio, hence according to principles of physics, is the maximal displacing force in a given direction that can be stabilized by a specified compressive load, assuming frictional effects to be minimal. The stability ratio is preferred in the laboratory being relatively easy to measure—usually a fixed compressive load is applied, and the displacing force is progressively increased until dislocation occurs. Clinically, the stability ratio is judged by the load and shift test, wherein the examiner applies a compressive load pressing the humeral head into the glenoid while noting the amount of translating force necessary to move the humeral head from stable position. It gives a fair idea of the adequacy of the glenoid concavity and is one of the most practical ways to detect deficiencies of the glenoid rim.

Glenoidogram

It is a better idea to understand how glenoid "works" rather than to determine how it "looks". Glenoidogram is an ingenious tool to explain this. The glenoidogram is the path taken by the center of the humeral head as it translates across the face of the glenoid in a specified direction away from the glenoid center line **(Fig. 4)**. The height of the glenoidogram reflects the amount of work (and hence the stability) needed to dislocate the humeral head for a given compressive load **(Fig. 4)**. The shape of the glenoidogram indicates the extent of the effectiveness of glenoid arc in that direction. The glenoidogram is oriented with respect to the "glenoid center line", a reference line perpendicular to the center of the glenoid fossa. A good example of use of glenoidogram is from the poor glenoid version that can arise from loss of part of the glenoid rim **(Fig. 5)**.

Anterior Restrictors

The inferior glenohumeral ligament (IGHL) is stretched in "abduction and external rotation" ("ABER" position) becoming an important stabilizer. Failure of anterior

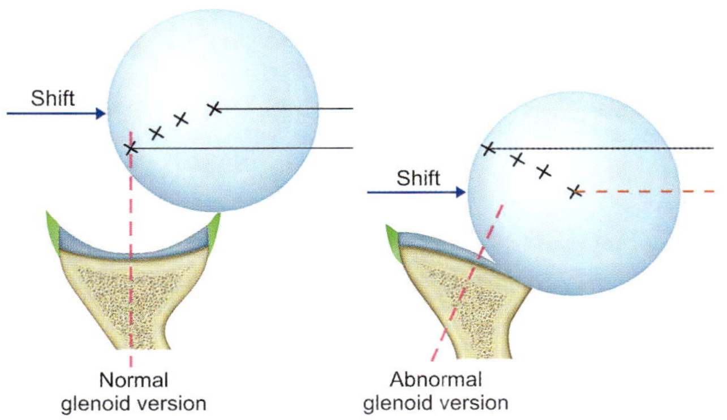

Fig. 5: A shallow glenoid or a damaged glenoid will have a reverse glenoidogram so that the humeral head will remain unstable even at rest when there are no movements occurring at the joint. This is a harbinger of recurrent shoulder instability in bony Bankart or glenoid dysplasia.

structures capsulolabral-periosteal sleeve in this position is imminent to anterior dislocation.

Posterior Restrictors

Adducted and forward flexion of shoulder places the joint prone to force transmitted along the humerus. Posterior glenoid, capsule, and labrum are stressed in this position, getting damaged in case of dislocation.

Repetitive submaximal stress on the structures leads to plastic deformation and laxity with increased joint range of motion. This produces the typical "*A*traumatic, *M*ultidirectional, *B*ilateral, *R*ehabilitation, and *I*nferior capsular shift (AMBRI)" form of instability in multiple directions and scapulohumeral rhythm dysfunction.

SCAPULOHUMERAL RHYTHM

The angle between the glenoid and the moving humeral head has to be maintained within a safe zone of 30° of angulation during activities to decrease shear and translatory forces. So for all the complementary movements of humerus, the scapula must be actively positioned muscularly. This also entails stabilizing the scapula to act as a stable base during movements. Losing scapular controls imbalances the length-tension relationships. The combined and synchronized movements between the scapula and the humerus during abduction is termed "scapulohumeral rhythm". The "rhythm" involves a scapular rotation during abduction, which decreases the shearing effect between the humeral head and the glenoid and allows the glenoid to stay centered under the humeral head. This counters the inferior dislocating tendency of the humerus. The rhythm ensures that at full abduction, the glenoid completely supports the humerus. There is a ratio of 3:1 for humeral rotation to scapular rotation that varies with the stage of abduction and also with loading of the arm. For every degree of rotation at scapula, the humeral head has rotated by 3°. The abduction has been described into five equal phases (each phase of 20% progressive abduction). With external loading, there is considerably increased movement at humeral head than the scapular rotation which increases with increasing phase of abduction. Scapular rotation occurs about an axis that passes through the base of the spine of the scapula during arm elevation in various phases. In the normal abduction mechanism, the scapula moves laterally in the first 20–50° of glenohumeral abduction. Also there is a total of 40–50° of clavicle rotation predominantly occurring at sternoclavicular joint and only 5–8° at the AC joint. The final 30–60° of upward rotation of the scapula is essentially the result of 30–45° of posterior rotation around the long axis of the clavicle and an elevation of the acromion. For each 10° of arm elevation, there are approximately 2° of clavicular elevation, with the maximum elevation occurring at approximately 130°.

The rotation of the scapula helps to maintain an effective length-tension relationship between the force couples that attach to the scapula. A force couple consists of two forces acting in opposite directions and are usually equal in magnitude to rotate a part about its axis of motion. This eliminates the translational force and linear motion while producing the torque and rotational movements. During the first 30° of upward rotation of the scapula, the serratus anterior muscle and the upper and lower divisions of the trapezius muscle are considered the principal upward rotators of the scapula. Together these muscles form two force couples; one formed by the upper trapezius and the upper serratus anterior muscles, the other formed by the lower trapezius and lower serratus anterior muscles. The trapezius appears to be more critical for abduction, whereas the serratus is more critical during flexion. Normal motion of the scapula on the thorax is believed to include consistent contact between the thoracic wall and the medial border and inferior angle of the scapula. Loss of this contact has been clinically implicated as evidence of abnormal scapular kinematics. The abnormal scapular kinematics may put additional stress on the anterior shoulder stabilizers.

FORCE COUPLE MECHANISM ON HUMERAL HEAD

Rotator cuff and long head of biceps (considered the fifth tendon of rotator cuff) generate force couples in coronal and transverse planes. It is essential to stabilize shoulder for varied and large rotational movements, thus force couples are the predominant stabilizing mechanism as mentioned above. There are two force couples coronal and transverse acting across the glenohumeral articulation. Deltoid and supraspinatus give abduction moment equally. So one would assume that the coronal abduction moment is unbalanced; however, the resultant of force vectors of these both muscles are so oriented that actually a compressive force is produced that improves the stability of joint. The supraspinatus force (coronal force couple) is directed medially and inferiorly that nullifies upward force of deltoid in a moment advantage **(Fig. 6)**. The supraspinatus is responsible for approximately 50% of the torque occurring with shoulder abduction and flexion, rest contributed by deltoid. As the weight of the arm pulls downward, the force of the supraspinatus pulls slightly above horizontal, helping to steer the humeral head and producing abduction of the arm. Initially, it was thought that the only function of the supraspinatus was to help in the initiation of abduction. Loss of coronal force balance (say supraspinatus weakness/inhibition or tendon tear)

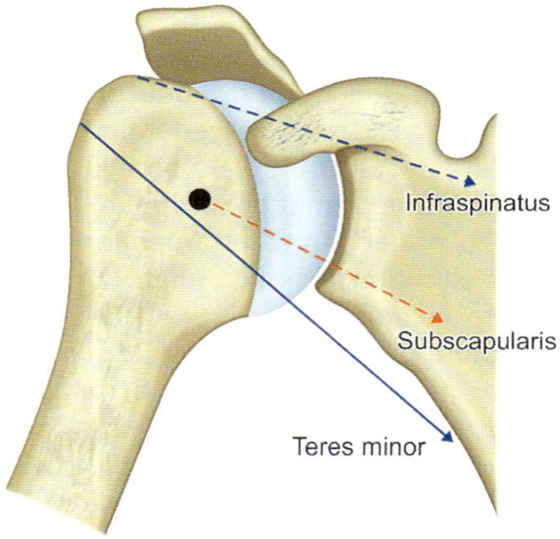

Fig. 6: The force couple in coronal plane prevents superior migration of humeral head during abduction by maintaining predominant vector of pull directed below the horizontal line. This pull is provided by the orientation of all four rotator cuff muscles while abduction force is tangentially placed away from humeral head center to act as rotatory force and not a translatory one.

results in superior migration of the head but may not restrict function (gradually, however, it does produce rotator lesions and impingement and pain). Loss of transverse couple (subscapularis anteriorly and teres minor and infraspinatus posteriorly, **Figs. 7A and B**) results in pain and loss of function and disrupts the concavity-compression mechanism. This leads to pathological translation and subluxation of humeral head toward deficiency. There is also a loss in active abduction.

Altered scapulohumeral rhythm is associated with impingement syndrome and later with rotator cuff tears. This occurs due to alteration in the force-couple mechanism and hence altered position of scapula at rest and with dynamic motion. Typical scapular dyskinesis is characterized by lost upward motion of acromion, excessive internal rotation of scapula, and excessive anterior tilt. These produce scapular protraction which actually reduces subacromial space and decreases rotator cuff strength. Clinically, this is seen as prominent medial scapular border. The altered scapular movement becomes evident when the patient is asked to raise and lower arm 3–5 times or asking him to hold a 2–3 kg weight. Further scapular assistance and scapular retraction test are dynamic maneuvers to evaluate the impingement. In the former, examiner applies gentle pressure to assist upward rotation and posterior tilt as the patient raises arm resulting in relief of the pain and improved arc of rotation. In the scapular retraction test, the examiner stabilizes scapula in a retracted position that results in an increase in the supraspinatus strength. These tests show that the dyskinesis is directly producing the symptoms of impingement than anything else (secondary impingement).

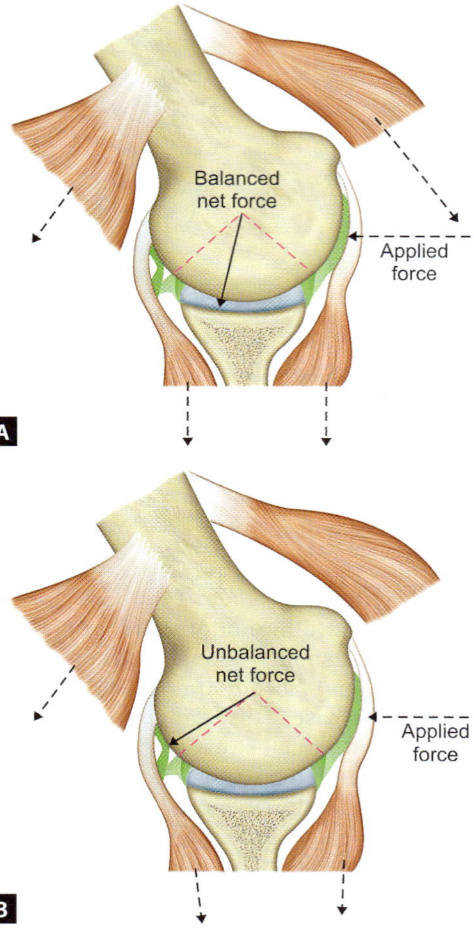

Figs. 7A and B: The transverse force couple maintains the anteroposterior stability of humeral head so that the balanced force vector remains within the curve of glenoid (A) else the humeral head may displace out of the glenoid cup (B).

CONCLUSION

- Understanding the bony articulation and forces across the joint is important to comprehensively manage the patients. This is important especially in those complex cases that have additional bony component of instability apart from the involvement of ligaments of capsular structures/rotator cuff. Performing only ligamentous reconstruction is bound to fail in such cases.
- Quite a lot of stress is being paid on the force couple mechanisms across the shoulder joint and problems of scapulohumeral rhythm that impairs the functional outcome even after adequate reconstructions. Alteration in scapulohumeral rhythm is also responsible for pathogenesis of disorders like impingement syndrome and cuff tears so conservative management of these disorders in early stages should include directed rehabilitation.

CHAPTER 55

History and Clinical Examination

Manish Kumar Varshney

INTRODUCTION

Like any other branch of medical science, a foolproof history and clinical examination will diagnose majority of the shoulder pathologies. The common primary information used to diagnose shoulder conditions is given in **Box 1**. The diagnostic tests should only act as an adjunct to a proper clinical examination and not be the substitute.

AGE

This has an important bearing on the diagnosis of shoulder pain. A young cricket player who is complaining of pain may have instability. A middle-aged lady who has shoulder pain which increases at night, with activity and with jerks may have adhesive capsulitis; a middle-aged executive who has pain on overhead activity without any major loss of motion probably has impingement syndrome; a 65-year-old lady complaining of pain and gradual loss of motion may be having early onset of glenohumeral osteoarthritis and lastly a 75-year-old man complaining of pain and inability to abduct may be suffering from rotator cuff arthropathy. Younger patients mainly have history of trauma and associated deformity like superior labrum anterior and posterior (SLAP) tears, labral tears or biceps tendinitis, mainly secondary to shoulder joint dislocation (glenohumeral dislocation). Recurrent dislocation may lead to shoulder instability in these patients. In older patients, these dislocations result in rotator cuff tear more often than labral tears. Having strong bones, clavicular fracture is less common in younger patients than in older ones, instead, *acromioclavicular* (AC) joint disruption occurs more commonly in them. Shoulder dislocation is common in all ages barring children.

BOX 1: Primary information that helps decipher shoulder conditions.

History-based diagnosis: Shoulder instability

Physical examination based diagnosis:
- Scapulothoracic crepitus
- Impingement syndrome
- Glenohumeral internal rotation deficit (GIRD)
- Scapular malposition, inferior medial border prominence, coracoid pain, dyskinesis (SICK) scapula—either winging or dysrhythmia

Mixed origin diagnosis:
- Adhesive capsulitis
- Biceps tendinitis

Anatomic diagnosis:
- Fracture
- Calcific tendinosis
- Rotator cuff tear
- SLAP lesion
- Biceps tendon rupture
- AC joint dislocation
- Osteoarthrosis
- Dislocated shoulder

Functional diagnosis:
- Dysfunctional Thrower's shoulder
- Scapular dyskinesis

(AC: acromioclavicular; SLAP: superior labrum anterior and posterior)

GENDER

Sex difference has a varied effect on prevalence of various conditions affecting shoulder. Some conditions occur with equal frequency in both sexes such as arthritis, infection, cuff tears, osteonecrosis, calcific tendinitis, idiopathic stiff and painful frozen shoulder, and gout (rheumatoid arthritis though has bit of female predominance). Some conditions have high prevalence in females, notably multidirectional shoulder instability (mainly seen in younger females), adhesive capsulitis (mainly in middle-aged and elderly females) and rotator cuff arthropathy (a sequelae to rotator cuff tear leading to painful collapse of humeral head with superior migration). Although it should be noted that massive rotator cuff tears are more common in males.

PAIN

The following points while pain evaluation should be inquired in detail.

- *Character of pain:* Pain resulting from acute fracture is severe and disabling that responds to nonsteroidal anti-inflammatory drugs (NSAIDs) or narcotic analgesics temporarily. The pain of external/internal shoulder impingement and rotator cuff pathology is commonly described as dull, boring, and toothache-like in quality. In advanced stages of rotator cuff pathology or frozen shoulder pain is typified as all or none, i.e., if present at the endpoint of available motion it is truly disabling, whereas within available shoulder arcs of motion, pain does not exist. Pain from osteoarthritis remains at a chronic lower level of pain during less-demanding activities but suddenly becomes sharp stabbing in intensity under high compressive joint loads. Destructive rheumatoid disease so conditions the chronic pain that their description is often inconsistent with the degree of joint destruction. The functional loss is more compared to the perceived pain. Acute calcific tendinitis is akin to the ureteric stone disease in terms of pain description for which it is also called "kidney stone of the shoulder". These patients seek a dark and quiet room with minimal competing stimulation and may visit emergency department. The clinical picture and the radiographs are contributory to diagnosis.

- *Onset of pain:* Pain of acute onset usually follows traumatic event. Impingement and rotator cuff disease are more insidious and if patient can date it weeks or months in the past without a clearly identifiable event then the physician should be highly suspicious for cuff-related pathology. For patients reporting recent onset of pain despite absence of trauma inquiry for past traumatic event should be made. Radicular pain of cervical origin is likely to have an insidious onset that may be aggravated by turning head. Often, sharp and stabbing pain occurring intermittently in the scapular muscles nearly always originates in the cervical spine.
- *Location of pain:* The site of perceived pain is rarely the origin of the pain. The rotator cuff disease and associated bursitis commonly presents as pain down the arm toward deltoid muscle insertion. The pain and inflammation of bicipital tendinitis radiates to anterior arm. Pain originating from acromioclavicular pathology usually radiates medially along the mid and medial clavicle. Intrinsic shoulder pathology has a pattern of pain that radiates down the arm to the level of the elbow and not below unlike the cervical radicular pain. Pain from adhesive capsulitis also does not follow a dermatomal pattern and often radiates along the trapezius muscle and periscapular muscles.
- *Aggravating and relieving factors:* Activities that need long lever arm with elbow extended result in shoulder pain in rotator cuff disease. Impingement results in pain during specific overhead activities that also involve internal rotation bringing greater tuberosity under acromion. Pulling bedcovers in night is also painful in impingement. Positional night pain is very frustrating and is commonly seen with cuff disease and is associated with loss of internal rotation. AC joint arthritis is also painful in night especially while sleeping on the same side. Adhesive capsulitis is typically painful in defined positions like shoulder external rotation or external rotation while abduction. Repetitive activities are typically painful in arthritic shoulders like wiping, mopping, cleaning floors, etc. Patients with adhesive capsulitis do not report any meaningful relief with NSAIDs. Patients with cuff disease report relief in symptoms with arm placed above the shoulder level and hand behind head (Saha position), enabling them also sleep in night.

BOX 2: Guide to examination points for instability.

- Onset (traumatic or atraumatic, voluntary or involuntary, details of trauma, and repeated trauma if present)
- Does the shoulder dislocate completely or it just perches (subluxates) and returns? Also, ask the direction of instability
- How easy is it to dislocate shoulder?
- Number of episodes and frequency (daily or intermittently)
- Associated symptoms (apprehension, pain, and paresthesias)
- Treatment of dislocation and duration of immobilization. Also ask if the reduction occurs spontaneously or requires external help

INSTABILITY

Instability usually has a preceding traumatic history often a fall on outstretched hand (FOOSH) though it may occur without having such history. In shoulder instability due to ligamentous laxity, pain is the main symptom, in contrast, patients with instability due to trauma have apprehension more often. These two groups can be described by acronyms as:

- *AMBRI:* Atraumatic, multidirectional, frequently bilateral, responds to rehabilitation and rarely requires an inferior capsular shift.
- *TUBS:* Traumatic unilateral lesion with Bankart lesion and usually requiring surgery.

Posterior shoulder instability is more frequently seen with electric shocks and epilepsy. A guide to broader evaluation of history on instability and its subsets are presented in **Box 2**.

Other things to consider: Thoracic pathology and even abdominal pathologies can be a cause of shoulder pain. It is important to know that various systemic diseases such as inflammatory arthritis, spondyloarthropathy, and hyperuricemia can be a cause of shoulder pain. Various tumors around the shoulder joint also can at times lead to diagnostic dilemmas.

PHYSICAL EXAMINATION

The three cardinal rules of any orthopedic examination are look, feel, and move. A short systemic examination is always helpful. Both the shoulders should be exposed properly. Look for bony prominences, muscle wasting over deltoid and scapular region, and local skin condition including axilla.

Feel for tenderness around the coracoids, AC joint, bicipital groove, just over greater tuberosity (GT), anterior and posterior joint lines.

Check for the range of motion (active and passive). Choose your standard reference point for describing shoulder motion considering in mind the existence of Codman's paradox **(Fig. 1)**. The special tests for the shoulder joint will help in diagnosing a specific disorder. The examination should include a neurological examination to evaluate the power of shoulder girdle muscles, mainly deltoid, supraspinatus, infraspinatus, teres minor, and subscapularis. The neurological examination should include the cervical nerve roots.

SPECIAL TESTS

Impingement Tests

Neer's Impingement Sign

In 1972, Charles Neer stated that rotator cuff impingement beneath the anteroinferior portion of acromion could be the

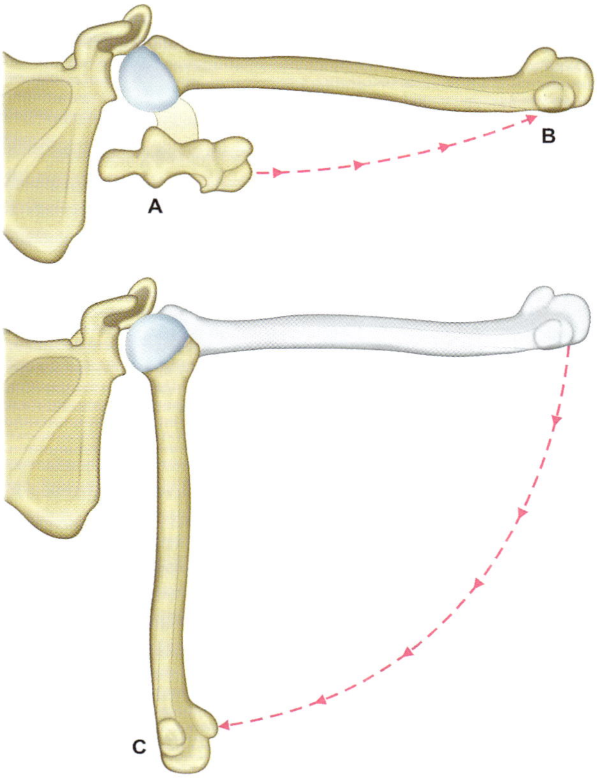

Fig. 1: *Codman's paradox:* With medial epicondyle facing medially the arm is abducted without rotation, when brought down by the side of the body the medial epicondyle faces to front. This externally rotates the arm by 90°. On repeating this maneuver the arm gets rotated by 90°, however, there is no rotational component incorporated in this maneuver! The phenomenon arises from the fact that serial translations or angular movements are not additive and may result in a different final position or rotation. So while describing multiple serial movements around shoulder, the sequence of such movements must be defined. These are termed "Eularian angles" (Yaw, Pitch, and Roll).

cause of pain in impingement syndrome, especially when shoulder is flexed forward and internally rotated. The pain mainly originated from inflamed bursa and/or the rotator cuff. The inflamed structures get stuck between the humeral head and the undersurface of acromion and coracoacromial arch. In the classic maneuver, the examiner stabilizes the scapula while standing behind the patient and passively internally rotates and forward flexes the patient's shoulder >90° **(Fig. 2)**. The pain is reproduced in the anterolateral part of the shoulder due to approximation of GT to acromion compressing the inflamed supraspinatus and bursa. In the modified version, the examiner stands at the head side of supine patient and elevates the shoulder fully then gives internal rotation torque to the flexed elbow. This eliminates the need of stabilizing the scapula. Both these are too nonspecific and can be positive in Bankart and SLAP lesions and AC joint arthritis. Also isolated bursitis and long head of biceps impingement can produce the pain.

Neer's Impingement Test

This is to improve the specificity of Neer's sign. It is performed after Neer's sign is positive. 5 mL of 1% lidocaine is injected

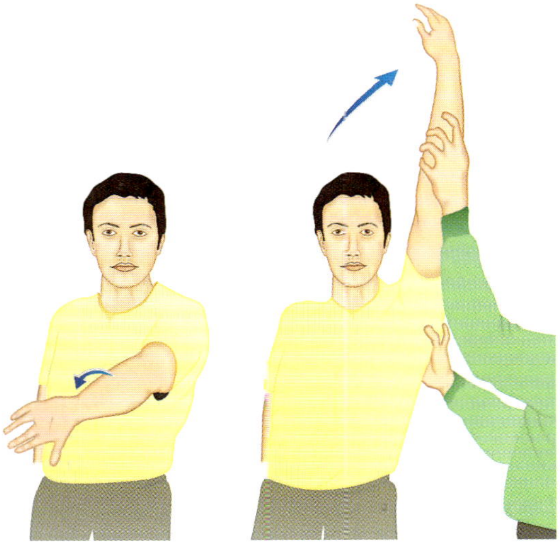

Fig. 2: Classic Neer's impingement sign and test. The examiner stabilizes the scapula and passively internally rotates and forward flexes the patient's shoulder >90°.

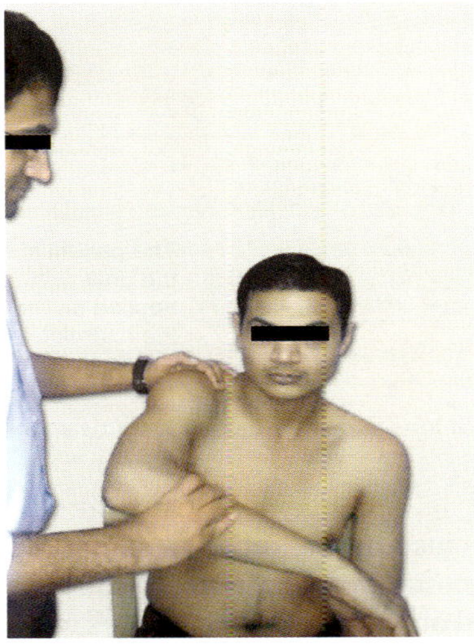

Fig. 3: Modified Neer's test (Hawkins-Kennedy).

into subacromial space and the maneuver repeated. Positive test is indicated by reduced or absent pain.

A modification of Neer's test is the *Hawkins-Kennedy test* (described in 1980). The examiner flexes the patient's shoulder to 90° and forcibly internally rotates the shoulder **(Fig. 3)**. The pain is reproduced in the anterolateral shoulder. Interpretation is similar to Neer's sign.

Internal rotation resistance stress test (of Zaslav) differentiates between intra-articular pathology (internal impingement) and subacromial impingement (SAI, external impingement) with a positive Neer's test. With the patient standing and the arm in 90° abduction and 80° externally rotated, the examiner tests the isometric external rotation and internal rotation strength by supporting the elbow (flexed at 90°) and applying counterforce at wrist **(Fig. 4)**. Relative weakness of internal rotation is a positive test and suggests internal impingement while external rotation weakness

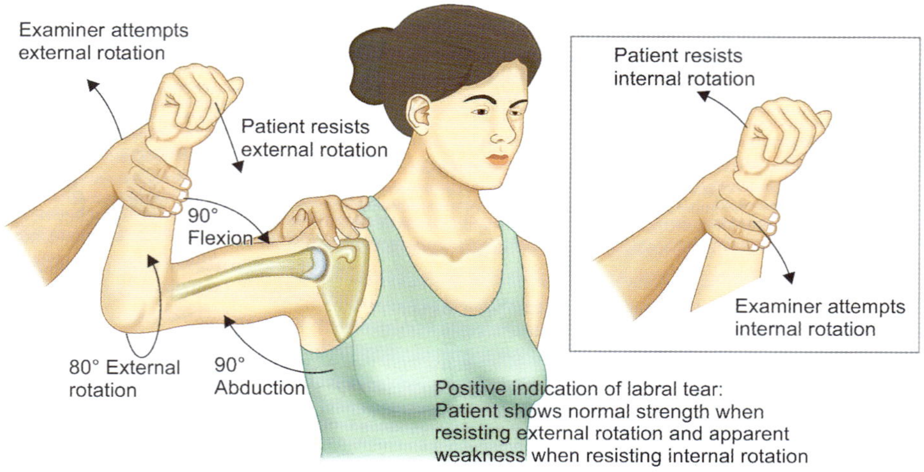

Fig. 4: Internal rotation resistance strength test of Zaslav.

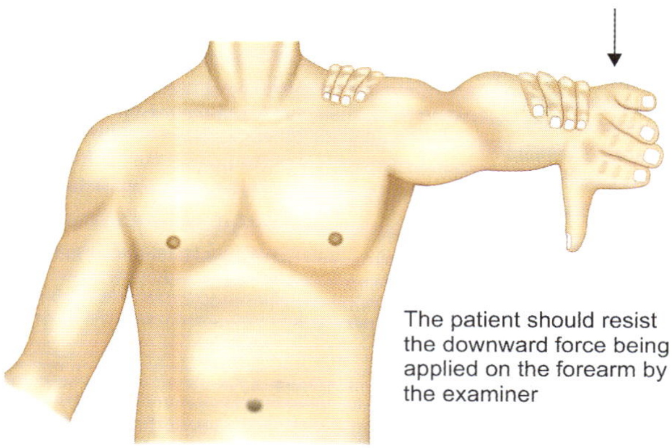

Fig. 5: Jobe-Yocum test (see text for description).

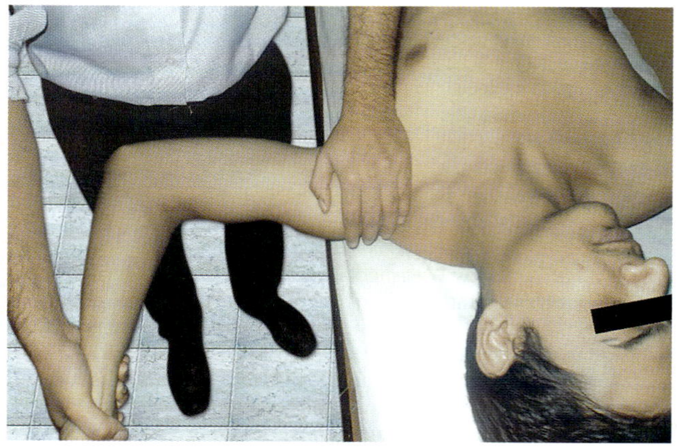

Fig. 6: Modified relocation test.

suggests external impingement. Only the relative strength of internal versus external rotation is important and tested and it is not compared to healthier shoulder. The test is recommended only with a positive Neer's test.

Jobe-Yocum test is used to detect any tear or tendinosis of the supraspinatus. The patient's arm is held at 90° of abduction and 30° of forward flexion with full internal rotation (with thumbs down). The patient maintains this position against downward resistance **(Fig. 5)**. A positive test is concurred when the patient is unable to keep the arm up against resistance secondary to pain or weakness. Once positive, the test should be repeated with limb in full external rotation that should have minimal or no pain.

Modified Relocation Test

Hammer's Modification of Jobe's Test: It is for testing the internal impingement. In supine position, arm hangs on side of the table with shoulder on outside of the edge of the table. The arm is positioned sequentially in 90°, 110°, and 120° of abduction and maximal external rotation. In each of three abduction angles, anterior (dislocating force) and posterior force (relocating force) is applied **(Fig. 6)**. Pain produced by anterior force that gets relieved by posterior force indicates impingement of the undersurface of rotator cuff and posterosuperior labrum.

Painful Arc Test

Ask patient to put arm in full elevation and slowly bring the arm down to his side. Note that the position of arm is neutral, else some patients try to externally rotate (to avoid pain) the arm. By this external rotation, impingement is prevented as GT stays away from undersurface of the acromion **(Fig. 7)**. If in between 60° and 100° of the abduction arc, patient feels pain, then the test is positive.

Combining the tests improves the yield of diagnosis **(Table 1)**. A positive drop-arm test, painful arc sign, and weakness in external rotation are best to diagnose rotator-cuff tear when combined together with accuracy of greater than 90%.

Tests for AC Joint

O'Brien active compression test is useful to indicate potential labral tears (like SLAP lesion) or AC lesions as cause for shoulder pain. In sitting or standing position, the patient's upper extremity is kept in position of 90° forward flexion of shoulder and 10–15° of horizontal adduction with fully extended elbow. Patient then completely internally rotates his arm and pronates the forearm so that thumb points downward **(Figs. 8A and B)**. The examiner applies a downward force with the patient trying to resist. The same maneuver is done with the arm in external rotation. A positive test means that the pain is elicited with the first maneuver and is reduced in the second maneuver. Pain at the top of the AC joint is suggestive of AC joint pathology. Pain or a painful click inside the shoulder joint points toward a SLAP lesion.

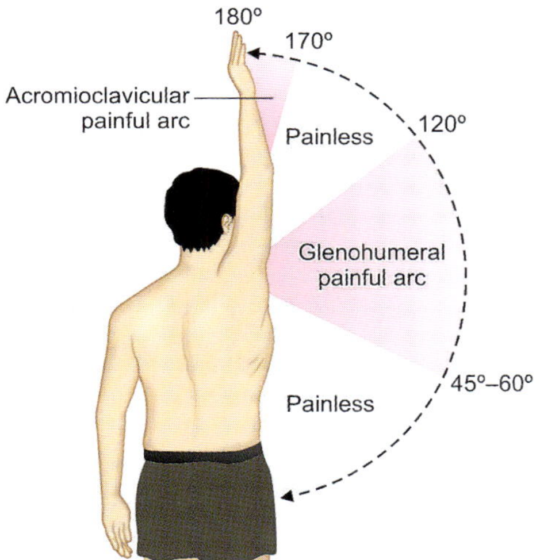

Fig. 7: *Painful arc test:* Here the patient's arm is fully elevated overhead and passively then the patient is asked to bring down the arm gently keeping the limb in neutral rotation. Patients with impingement will have pain in 60–100° of abduction arc.

TABLE 1: Utility of various tests for detecting shoulder impingement.

Test	*Sensitivity (%)*	*Specificity (%)*
Neer's sign	70	70
Hawkins–Kennedy test	70–75	65–70
Painful arc test	75	80
Jobe's test	45	90
Zaslav's test	>90	90

The SLAP Test (SLAP-prehension Test)

With arm in 45° of adduction, the same maneuver used in O'Brien's test is performed **(Fig. 9)**. Higher adduction causes entrapment of labrum and bicipital complex between the glenoid and humeral head and thus creating pain but it may elicit pain from AC joint abutment also.

Tests for Biceps Tendon and Superior Labrum (See Tests for Acromioclavicular Joint also)

Yergason's Test

It indicates pathology of long head of biceps in its sheath. Patient stands with the arm by his side with 90° flexion of elbow and pronated forearm. The patient supinates against resistance **(Fig. 10)**. If there is pain in the anterior shoulder or bicipital groove, the test is positive.

Speed's Test (Fig. 11)

Originally described to detect pathology in long head of biceps muscle, Speed's test also detects SLAP lesions. In sitting or standing position, patient flexes his arm in 60–90° of forward flexion, fully extends the elbow and supinates the forearm. Examiner applies downward force at wrist, which is resisted by the patient. In patients with inflamed or having lesion of long head of biceps (also in SLAP lesion), pain is felt in bicipital groove or in the anterior aspect of shoulder, and the test is considered to be positive.

Ludington's Test (Fig. 12)

This test is used to detect rupture of the tendon of the long head of biceps. In sitting position, patient puts his both hands on top of the head with fingers interlocked. While examiner

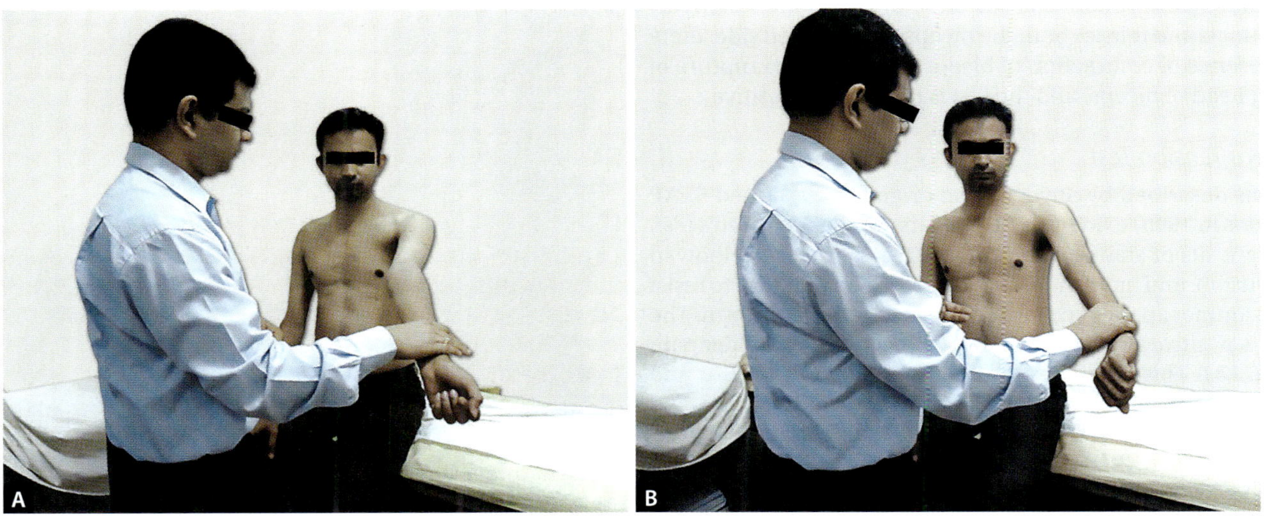

Figs. 8A and B: O'Brien's test.

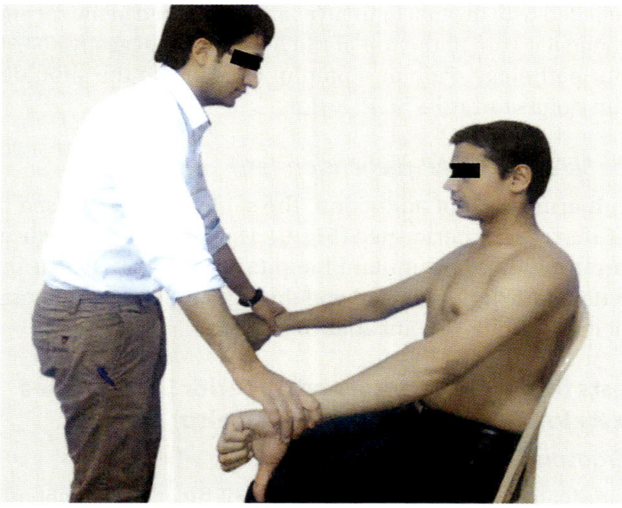

Fig. 9: SLAP-prehension test (The adduction is increased whence the patient reports pain). (SLAP: superior labrum anterior and posterior)

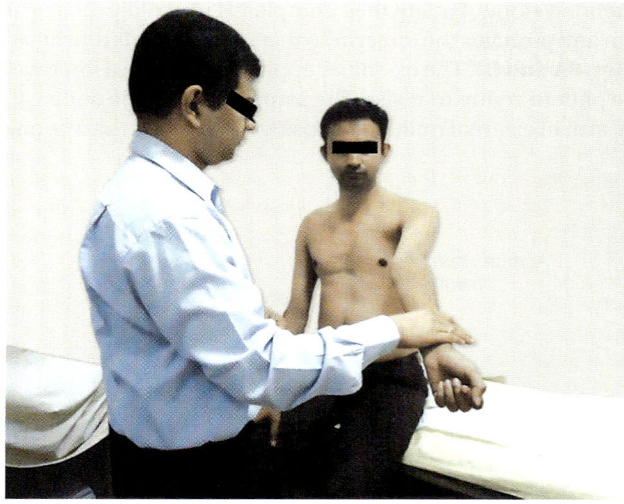

Fig. 11: Speed's test.

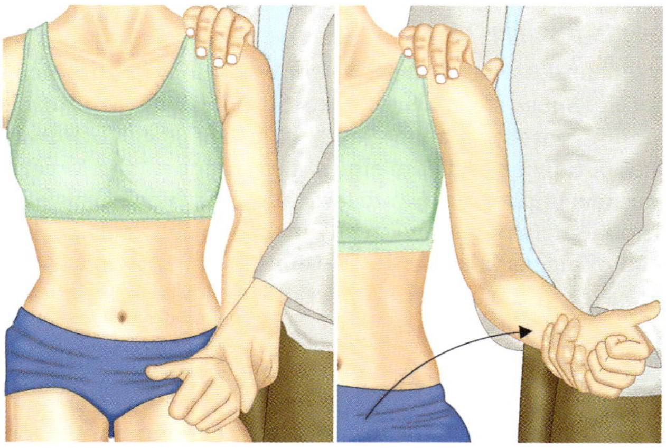

Fig. 10: Yergason test.

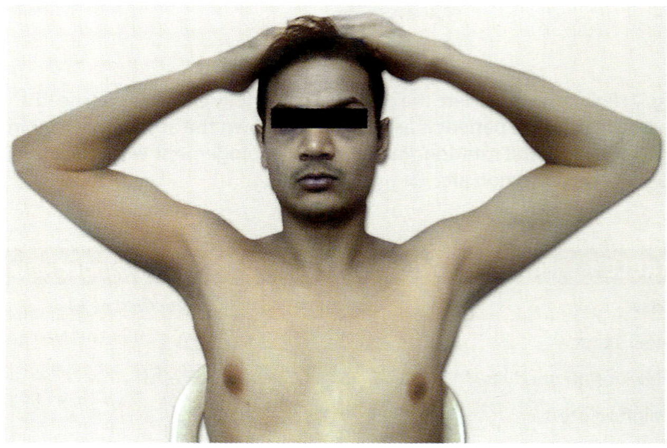

Fig. 12: Ludington's test.

palpates both the biceps simultaneously, patient actively contracts and relaxes both the biceps. On involved side, there is absence of contraction of biceps muscle due to rupture of long head of biceps, and the test is considered positive.

Biceps Tension Test

It was described by Snyder (who originally described SLAP lesions in 1990) to identify SLAP tears. Similar to Speed's test, patient sits or stands with arm in 90° of abduction, elbow in extension, and hand in supination. While patient tries to resist it, examiner applies eccentric adduction force to the arm. The test is positive when patient feels deep anterior shoulder pain **(Fig. 13)**. This generates tension on the biceps anchor and superior labrum.

Anterior Slide Test of Kibler

It is useful to evaluate the SLAP lesion. Patient stands or sits with both hands on hips with thumbs facing posteriorly. Standing

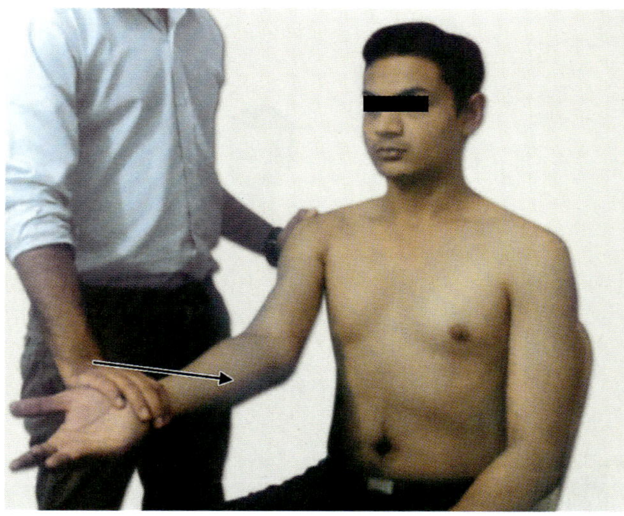

Fig. 13: Biceps tension test (arrow).

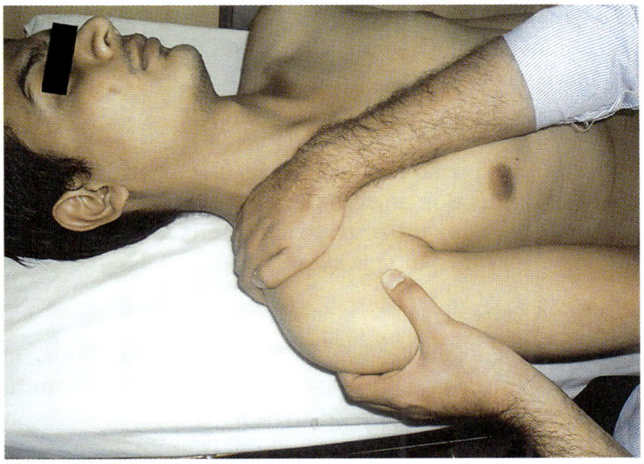

Fig. 14: Anterior slide test of Kibler.

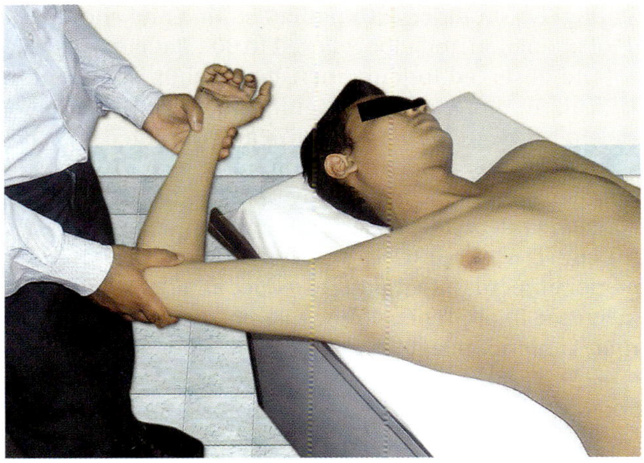

Fig. 15: Kim II.

behind the patient, the examiner places one hand over the acromion of the involved side with fingers extending over the anterior aspect of acromion. With other hand, he applies anterosuperior force over the patient's elbow and patient tries to resist it **(Fig. 14)**. Pain or a click over the anterior shoulder is considered as a positive sign indicating an SLAP lesion.

Biceps Load Test I of Kim

In 1999, Kim described this test to diagnose SLAP lesion in patients having history of recurrent anterior instability. In supine position, patient abducts his arm up to 90° and fully externally rotates it. The examiner further externally rotates it until the patient begins to feel apprehension. In this position, the patient flexes the elbow against resistance. The test is considered negative if the apprehension is relieved with active biceps contraction. The test is said to be positive if there is no change or increased apprehension with active biceps contraction and it indicates an SLAP lesion.

Biceps Load Test II of Kim

Kim described this test in 2001 to detect SLAP test for patients without anterior instability. In supine position, the patient abducts the arm up to 120° and fully externally rotates it with 90° flexion of the elbow and full supination of the forearm. The patient then flexes the elbow against resistance **(Fig. 15)**. If the pain is increased, it indicates the SLAP lesion and the test is said to be positive.

Crank Test

This test is useful in evaluation of superior labral pathology as well as different glenohumeral ligaments and for anterior shoulder instability. In standing or supine lying down position, examiner passively elevates the shoulder to 160° in the scapular plane. He then applies axial loading on humerus through proximal hand while with distal hand, he internally and externally rotates the humerus **(Fig. 16)**. Reproduction of symptoms of pain, catching, or a click indicates a positive test.

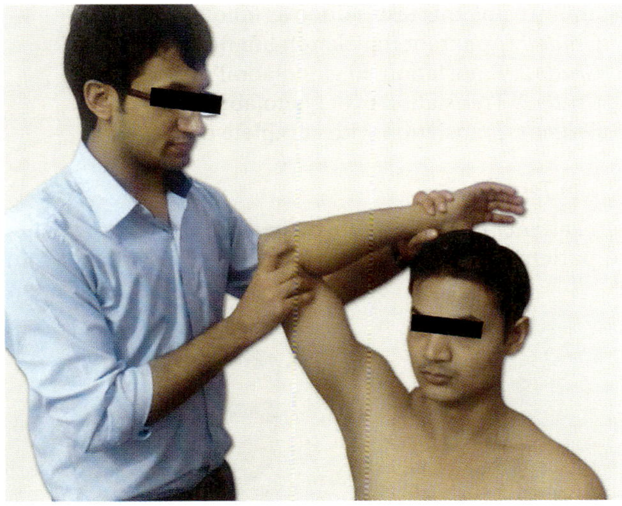

Fig. 16: Crank test.

Kim Test

It is used to diagnose posteroinferior labral pathology. In sitting position, the arm is in 90° of abduction and elbow in 90° of flexion, the examiner supports the patient's elbow with one hand and applies axial compression to the glenoid with the same hand. With the other hand, he applies downward and backward force on the humerus while patient tries to resist it. Pain in the posterior shoulder is a positive test.

Subcoracoid Impingement Test of Gerber (Fig. 17)

Gerber described two variations to reproduce subscapularis impingement between the humeral head and coracoid. In the first technique, patient elevates the arm to 90° in the scapular plane and internally rotates it. The test is said to be positive if this maneuver produces impingement symptoms and radiating pain toward upper arm and forearm. In second method, patient forward flexes the arm instead of elevation in the scapular plane and internally rotates it; this will reproduce impingement symptoms and radiation of pain into the arm.

Tests for Shoulder Instability

The *apprehension-relocation test* **(Fig. 18)** is performed to diagnose suspected anterior instability cases. Apprehension test as described by Rowe consists of maximally externally rotating the shoulder with patient supine and shoulder in 90° of abduction and elbow flexed to 90°. Patients are asked for (and observed for apprehension) feeling of impending dislocation, mere pain is insignificant. Then either elbow is taken backward or a posterior to anterior force is applied to the posterior aspect of the humeral head. Increase in apprehension and retraction by patient are positive signs. *Relocation test* of Jobe is performed in conjunction to above and consists of applying a posteriorly directed force on anterior humerus (attempting to reduce anterior subluxation); a decrease in apprehension with a posterior directed force implies anterior instability.

Load-shift Test

The humeral head is compressed into glenoid and then noting the amount of force needed to displace the humeral head "out" in anterior and posterior direction. The grading of instability using this test is done as follows:

- *Grade 1:* Apparent translation but not to rim
- *Grade 2:* Translation till glenolabral rim
- *Grade 3:* Translation over glenolabral rim
- *Grade 4:* Translation with complete dislocation.

Drawer Test

The examiner holds the humeral head while standing behind the patient and pushes forward (for anterior laxity) and pulls backward (for posterior laxity) in the glenoid to access translational stability **(Fig. 19)**. A clunk or snap on anterior subluxation can suggest Bankart lesion.

The Push-pull Test for Posterior Instability

Done in supine position with shoulder off the edge of bed and arm in 90° abduction and 30° flexion. Examiner pulls on the wrist while pushing the proximal humerus down. Normally, 50% posterior translation is allowed.

The Sulcus Sign

The sulcus sign signifies anteroinferior labral tear/inferior shoulder laxity/instability. The patient is seated or standing with the arm relaxed by the side. The patient's arm is grasped by the examiner and pulled inferiorly. Dimpling of the skin below the acromion suggests widening of the subacromial space between the acromion and the humeral head with inferior subluxation of humeral head **(Figs. 20A and B)**. The sulcus sign is graded as follows:

- *Grade 1+:* Acromiohumeral interval <1 cm
- *Grade 2+:* Acromiohumeral interval 1–2 cm
- *Grade 3+:* Acromiohumeral interval >2 cm.

Fulcrum Test

This tests the anterior shoulder laxity. The patient is made to lie supine on examination couch and arm is abducted to 90°.

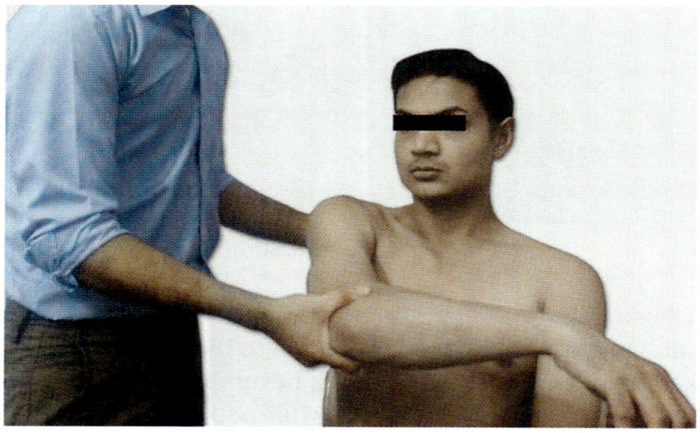

Fig. 17: Subcoracoid impingement test of Gerber.

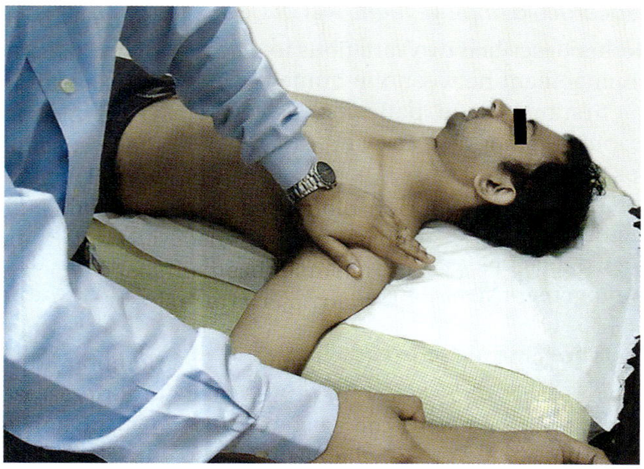

Fig. 18: Apprehension-relocation test.

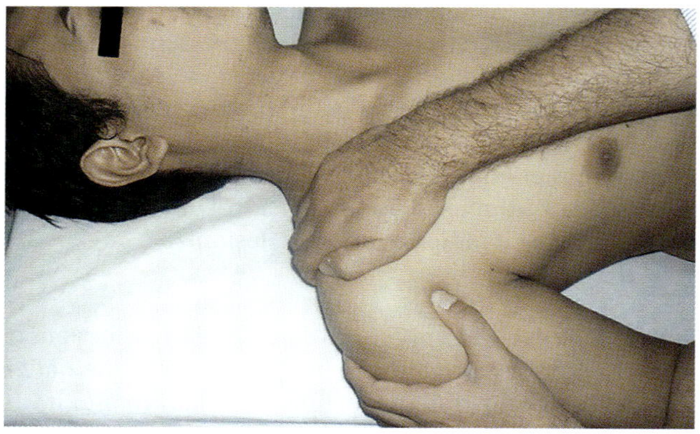

Fig. 19: Drawer test.

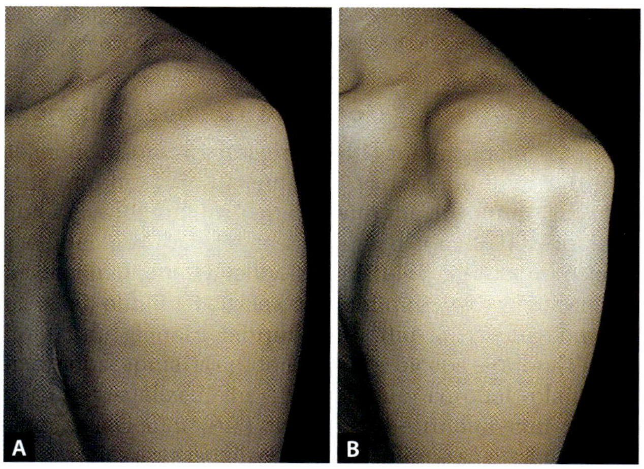

Figs. 20A and B: Sulcus sign.

The examiner places his fist on the table under the proximal humerus. The arm is then extended with the fist as fulcrum in external rotation to elicit apprehension **(Fig. 21)**. Apprehension of the patient may cause subscapularis contraction to mask instability which can be fatigued by maintaining external rotation for a minute and hence revealing the anterior instability.

Jerk Test

The patient's arm is internally rotated and flexed forward to 90°. Axial load is applied by examiner toward a plane tangent to glenoid while moving the arm across the body **(Fig. 22)**. Sliding of humeral head off the posterior border of glenoid in a jerk indicates positive test. Jerk of return can be felt when the arm is returned to original position.

Tests for Rotator Cuff Lesion (Table 2)

Drop arm test is helpful in diagnosing massive rotator cuff tear. The examiner abducts the patient's shoulder to >90° and then asks the patient to hold it in that position as the examiner withdraws support **(Fig. 23)**. The patient with a rotator cuff tear will not be able to hold it and the arm will drop down suddenly. The drop of the arm may be accompanied by severe pain.

Hornblower's sign will test the integrity of infraspinatus and teres minor tendons. The patient's elbow is flexed to 90° and then arm is elevated to 90° of abduction. Patient rotates the arm externally against examiner's resistance **(Fig. 24)**. Weakness indicates incompetency in one of the components while test is positive if there is pain and/or inability to maintain the externally rotated position. In complete rupture as in massive rotator cuff tears the arm drops back to neutral position.

The "lift-off test" assesses the integrity of the lower subscapularis muscle **(Fig. 25)**. Another test is the "belly press test" which requires less internal rotation and tests the upper portion of subscapularis. The patient presses against the belly with wrist extended and elbow in front of body. "Napoleon test" is a further modification of "belly press test". Here the patient puts his hand on belly with elbow resting by his side, then he is asked to bring the elbow forward/anteriorly while maintaining the position of hand. Positive test is when patient is unable to bring the elbow to front without moving the shoulder girdle. "Bear hug test" **(Fig. 26)** also assesses subscapularis muscle. In this test, the patient crosses his hand and keeps it over the other shoulder. He is asked to push against the shoulder down where a subscapularis muscle produces pain.

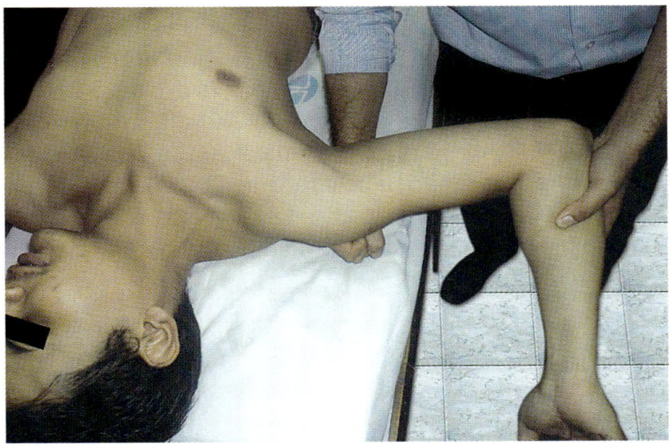

Fig. 21: Fulcrum test.

TABLE 2: Various signs for rotator cuff lesions and their utility in localizing the muscle concerned.

Test	*Finding*	*Muscle*
Drop arm test	Patient unable to maintain arm in 90° elevation	Supraspinatus
External rotation lag test	Patient unable to maintain arm in maximum external rotation in adduction	Infraspinatus
Hornblower sign	Patient unable to maintain arm in external rotation 90° abduction, 90° external rotation	Teres minor
Belly press test	Pain while pressing on abdomen with hand and elbows anterior to midsagittal plane of body	Upper subscapularis
Lift-off test	Patient unable to maintain hand off lumbosacral spine in full internal rotation	Lower subscapularis

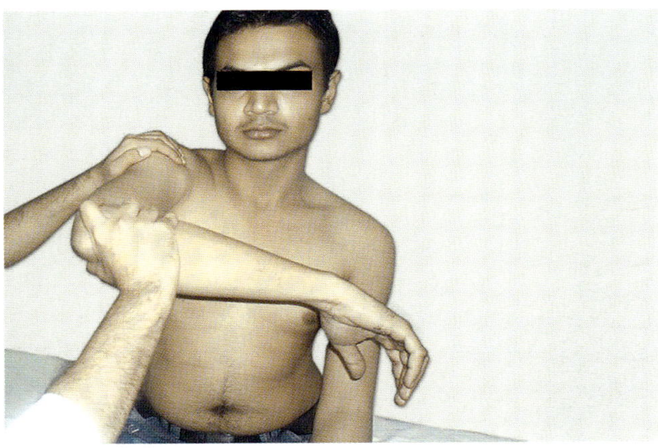

Fig. 22: Jerk test.

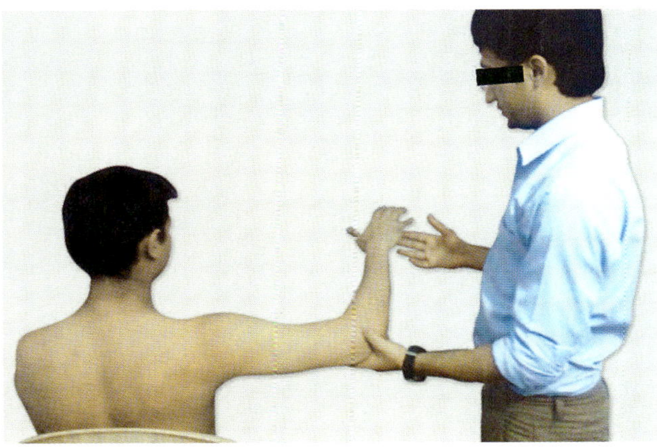

Fig. 23: Drop arm test.

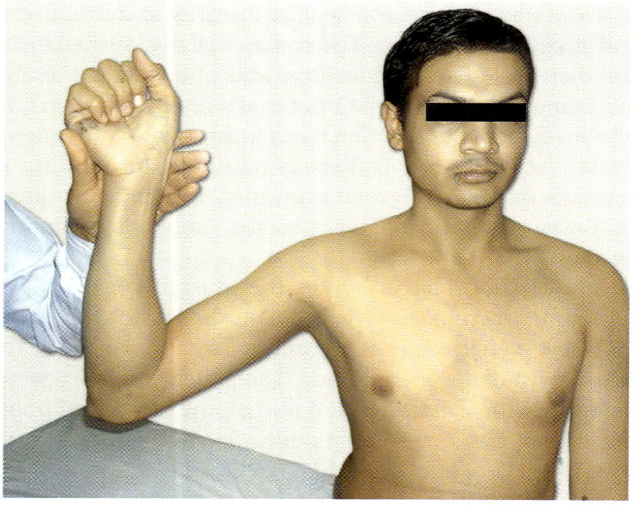

Fig. 24: Hornblower sign.

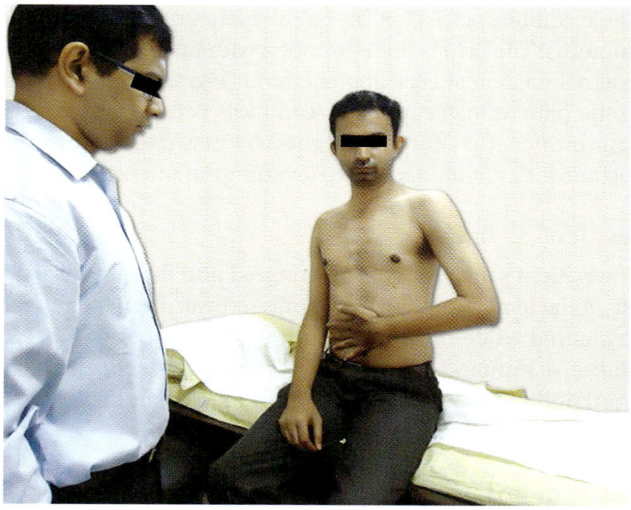

Fig. 26: Bear hug (Belly press).

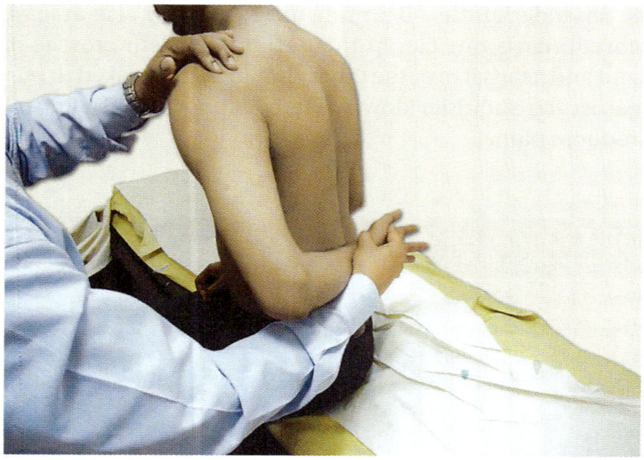

Fig. 25: Lift-off test.

CONCLUSION

- History and examination of shoulder joint is important in the evaluation of shoulder disorders and making a diagnosis, despite the preponderance of use of advanced diagnostic imaging for financial and otherwise purpose.
- Mere obtaining the MRI does not produce diagnosis as a lot depends on the observer and the evaluation of this spherical joint with complex orientation of ligaments is often incomplete.
- Despite >125 tests described for shoulder pathologies only a few are adequate to make a diagnosis to near certainty that can then be confirmed by imaging studies. The tests should be performed in a defined order so that the diagnosis is not missed and differentials can be safely excluded.

CHAPTER 56

Imaging of Shoulder Joint

Manish Kumar Varshney

INTRODUCTION

We need imaging to establish the diagnosis, plan surgery, and evaluate the change in patients' shoulder anatomy with time. The approach should be directed by history and defined individually taking into consideration the following points:

- The shoulder is a three-dimensional (3D) structure that is difficult to project on a single planar view just like mapping the earth.
- Critical relationships like the centering of the humeral head changes with the position of the arm.
- Pathology for current symptoms may be found in a large number of different bones and soft tissues that should have adequate representation in the ordered investigation.
- There is often difficulty in evaluating irregular bones like scapula placed obliquely as there is significant overlap and superimposition of structures. Placing metallic or nonmetallic implants may complicate imaging the structures of interest.

All these suggest a surgeon to use a judicious approach that yields the information necessary to treat the patient while avoiding the tendency to "over-image". The importance of radiography, computed tomography (CT) scan, and magnetic resonance imaging (MRI) cannot be overstated but use should be justified. Radiography is the usual first screening tool serving as quick peek into the joint. It demonstrates some instability patterns, developmental, and post-traumatic changes. CT scan is preferred for demonstration and quantification of bony changes. MRI is indispensable for identifying and characterizing soft tissue changes but recent techniques dedicated to bone window tend to replace CT scans for quantification of bone pathology. The imaging is generally prescribed for instability evaluation or otherwise for degenerative/arthritic conditions including cuff pathologies so the description below is also divided into two main sections for simplification and discrete understanding.

IMAGING FOR SHOULDER INSTABILITY

Radiography

Radiographs are helpful in diagnosing a variety of pathologies. The plain radiograph of the shoulder is the basic investigation to rule out a suspected/unsuspected serious shoulder pathology such as tumor, infection, or arthritis. At least three views (two of which should be orthogonal) should be obtained to diagnose subtle pathologies. For suspected acute shoulder dislocation, straight anteroposterior (AP) view (neutral or with internal/external arm rotation) is commonly coupled with Scapular Y-view **(Fig. 1)** due to humeral head overlap on glenoid in AP view. Grashey glenoid profile view **(Fig. 2)** also serves the same purpose. Glenoid bone loss can be seen in an axillary view **(Fig. 3)** that also helps to identify posterior shoulder instability that may be missed on AP radiographs. Humeral head bone loss (Hill–Sachs lesion) is better demonstrated in the Stryker notch view **(Fig. 4)**.

For recurrent shoulder instability—dislocation/subluxation/positive apprehension a complete radiographic study is needed. The glenoid profile view [West Point **(Fig. 5)** or Bernageau **(Fig. 6)** view] assesses the anteroinferior glenoid rim where large glenoid defect is seen as a "cliff sign" and blunting with rounding off of anterior glenoid is visualized as "blunted angle sign". West Point view has a good correlation with CT scan findings of bone loss while Bernageau view is quite accurate in detecting anteroinferior glenoid bone loss. In recurrent anterior shoulder instability blurring of anterior

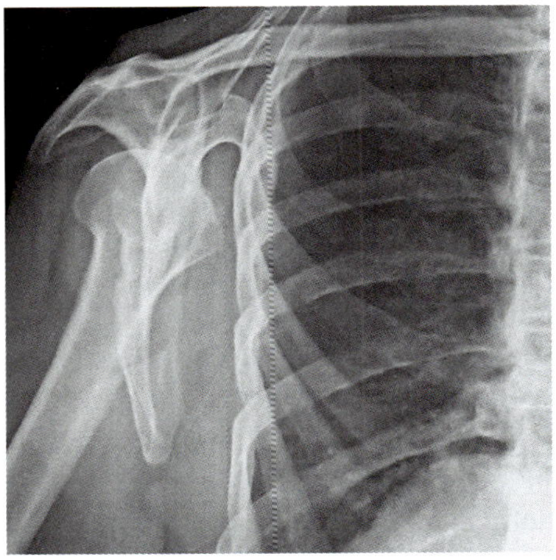

Fig. 1: ScapularY-view.

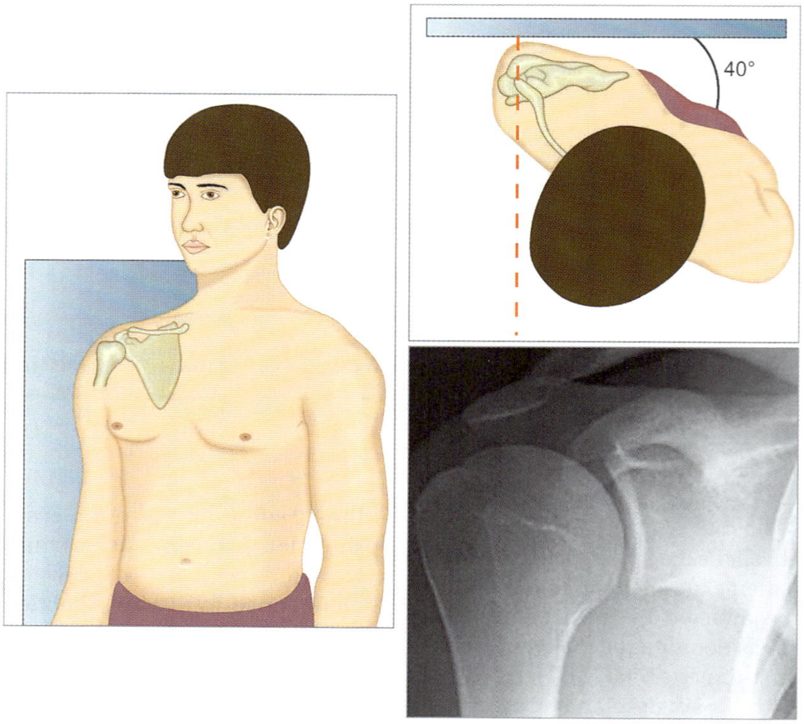

Fig. 2: Grashey glenoid profile view. The patient is rotated (usually 40–45°) until the cassette is parallel to the scapula so glenoid is perpendicular to the setup. Dotted red line indicates the direction of X-ray beam.

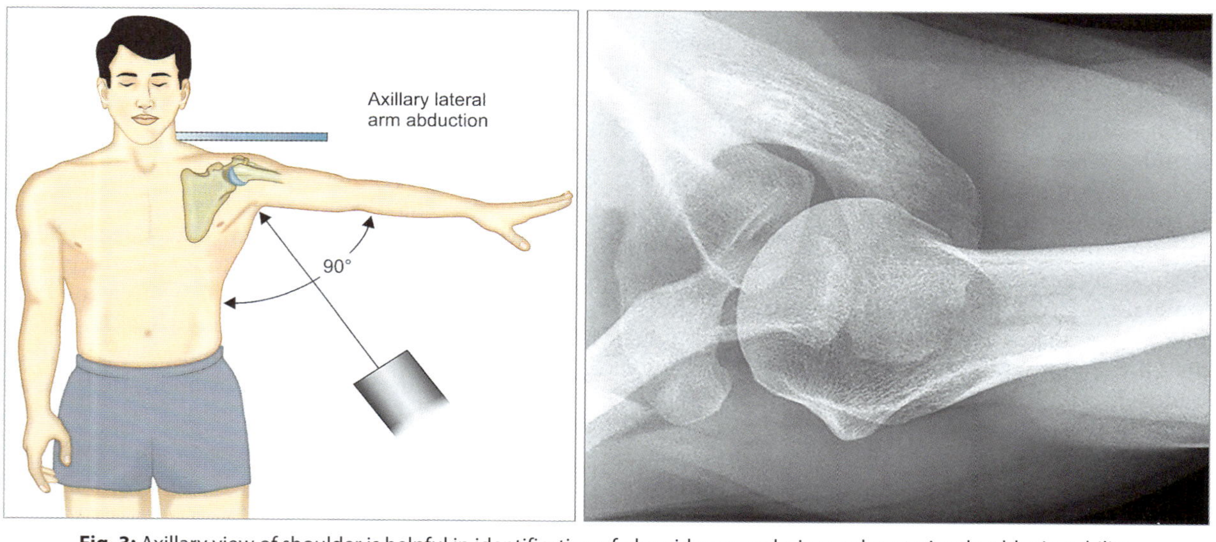

Fig. 3: Axillary view of shoulder is helpful in identification of glenoid osseous lesion and posterior shoulder instability.

glenoid is seen suggesting bony Bankart rather than actual bony fragments. For posterior instability, demonstration of reverse Hill–Sachs sign on a scapular Y and axillary views serves as a good clue.

Computed Tomography Scan

Multidetector CT scan better delineates the bony pathology and most commonly performed imaging in post-traumatic instabilities for quantification of injuries. Bony Bankart fragment (anteroinferior glenoid bone fragment) involving >25% of anteroinferior glenoid width **(Fig. 7)** that corresponds to fracture fragment ≈ 6–8 mm in width would need open repair ± bone grafting. The glenoid appears as "inverted pear" structure due to this bone loss as against its normal pear shape **(Figs. 8A and B)**. This percentage of bone loss is now most commonly calculated on 3D *en face* (pronounced "on fass") view of glenoid using one of the two "best-fit circle methods":

- *Glenoid width (index) method:* The best-fit circle is drawn over the inferior two-thirds of the glenoid and radius of circle is calculated **(Fig. 9)**. The deficient radius in

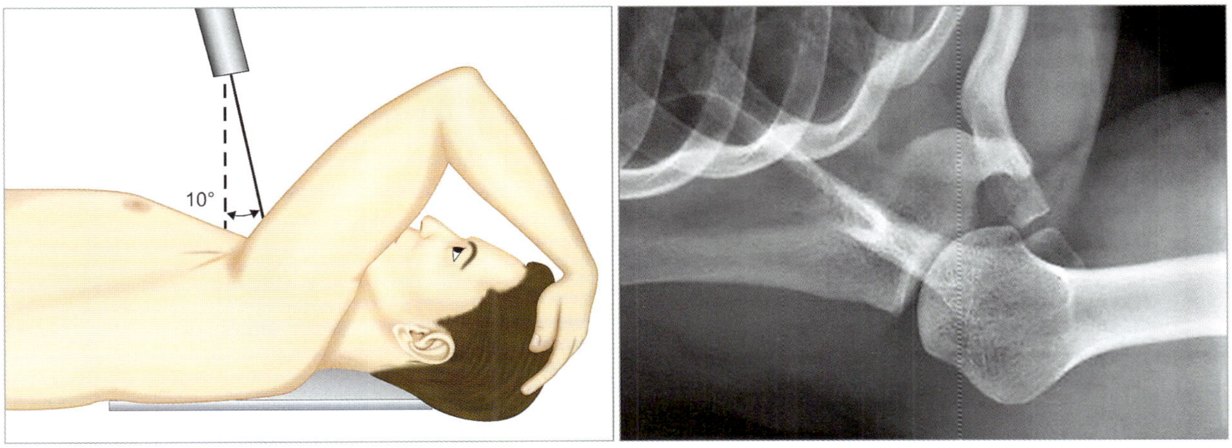

Fig. 4: Stryker notch view is commonly used for assessing humeral head bone loss.

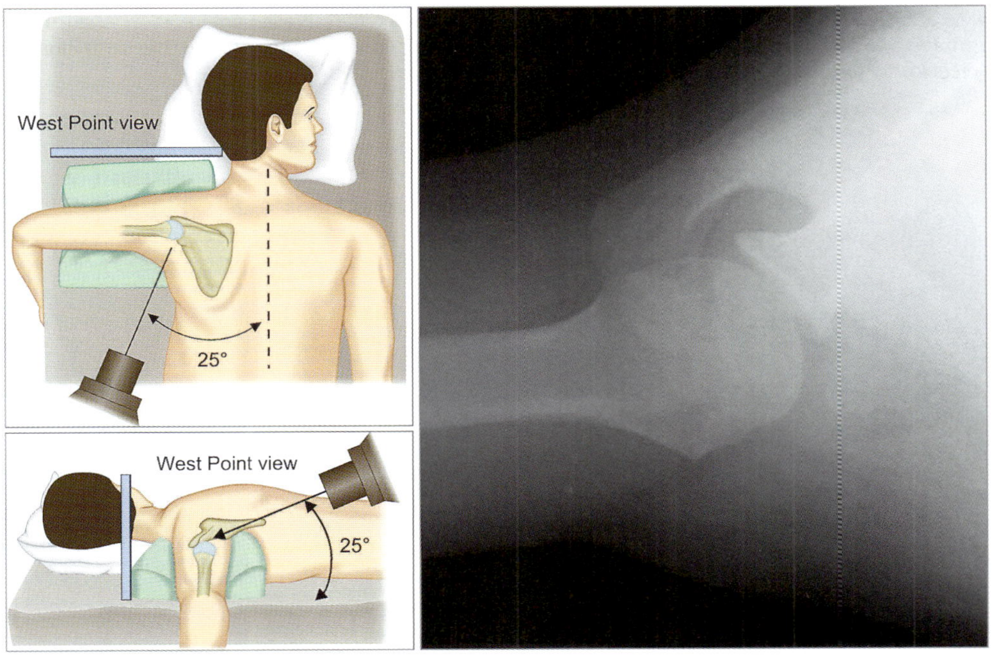

Fig. 5: West Point view better reveals the glenoid profile view demonstrating glenoid bone lesions.

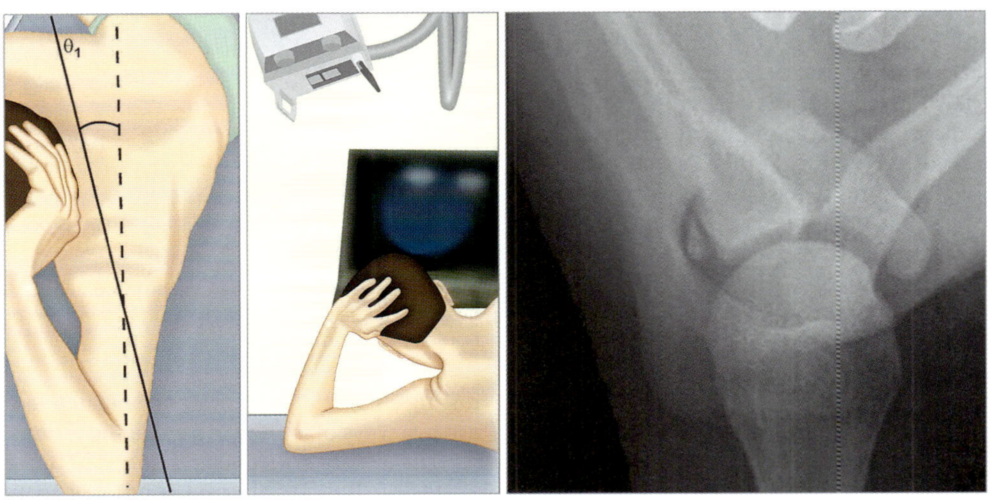

Fig. 6: Bernageau view is preferred by some surgeons for identification of glenoid bone profile and lesions.

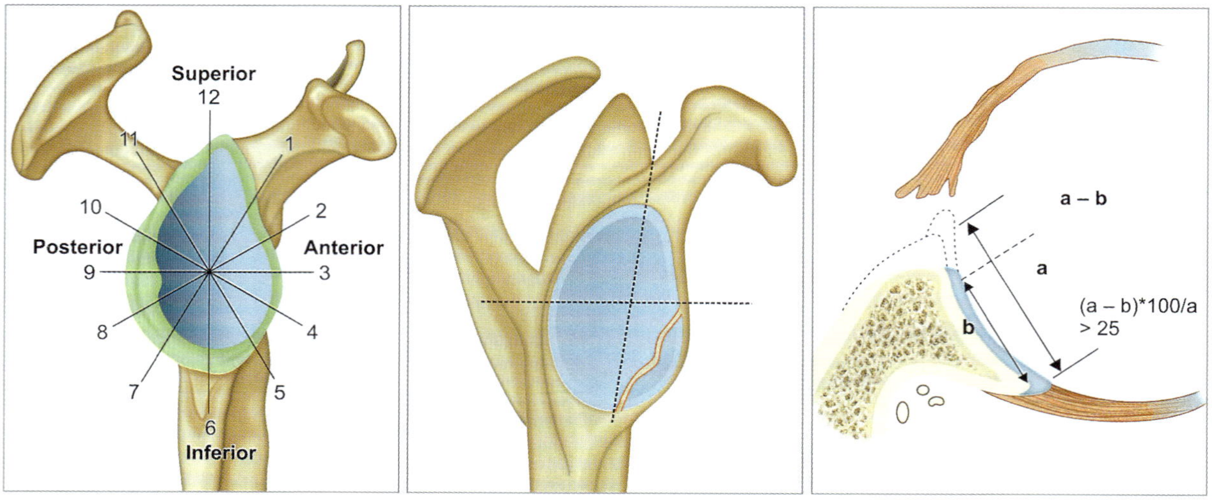

Fig. 7: The *en face* view of glenoid is divided according to face of clock for better interobserver communication as illustrated on left image. The central image demonstrates a common bony bankart lesion present in anteroinferior portion of the glenoid. The illustration on right demonstrates calculation of the percent loss of glenoid articular surface region using linear method.

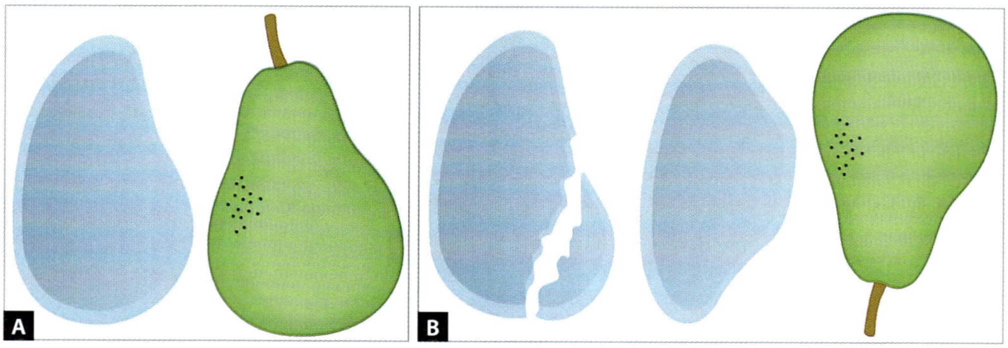

Figs. 8A and B: The normal bony glenoid appears pear-shaped while following fracture of the anteroinferior portion of the glenoid, the remaining intact portion appears as "inverted pear".

anteroinferior portion is calculated and percentage bone loss calculated by formula:

$$\% \text{ bone loss} = \frac{(R - r)}{2R} \times 100$$

where, R = radius of the circle and r = radius at the deficient portion of glenoid.

- *Pico method:* Here, the same best-fit circle is drawn and the deficient area is calculated as a percentage of the area of circle **(Fig. 10)**. It is better than glenoid width index in estimating the bone loss as deficient radius ("r") in above equation is subjective. Percentage of bone loss >20% using Pico method is associated with recurrent dislocations.

Other methods like Nofsinger technique and clock-face method need substantiation. Hill-Sachs lesions are a common association in patients with traumatic glenohumeral instability occurring in two-thirds of the patients. The combination of glenoid bone defect and humeral head lesion (Hill-Sachs lesion) is called "bipolar bone lesion". The importance of its identification and quantification is that an "engaging" Hill-Sachs lesion may cause engagement of the defect with the anterior labrum even after anterior glenoid reconstruction so it needs to be simultaneously addressed

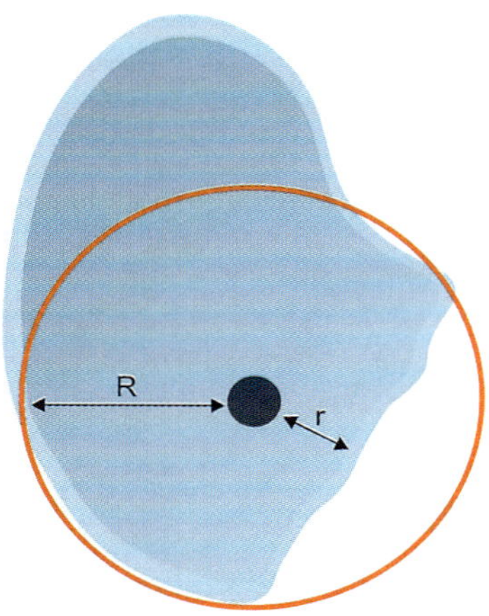

Fig. 9: Glenoid width index estimation on *en face* (2D or 3D) view of glenoid. The best-fit circle is drawn matching the posterior and inferior border of glenoid.

during surgery. The prevalence of such lesions is 7%. There are two ways of identifying engaging lesions:

1. *The axis of Hill-Sachs lesion:* The engaging Hill-Sachs lesion has an oblique long axis in neutral shoulder position. This becomes parallel to anterior glenoid edge

in abduction-external rotation position [(ABER) of 90° abduction and 30° external rotation] whence it engages easily. If the long axis of lesion is vertical in neutral shoulder position, then it does not engage as during ABER it becomes diagonal.

2. *"Off-track" glenoid lesion of Di Giacomo et al.:* We know that humeral head surface area is massively large compared to glenoid so tracking of humeral head on glenoid should maintain a delicate balance by maintaining contact and humeral head centered throughout motion. Yamamoto introduced the concept of "glenoid tracking". With the arm in variable abduction, external rotation, and maximal horizontal extension, the glenoid moves along the posterior articular margin of humeral head. This contact zone of glenoid with humeral head is called "glenoid track". The width of the glenoid track is approximately 83–85% of the maximum glenoid width **(Fig. 11)**. Small defects in glenoid and large Hill-Sachs lesion alter the contact area of the posterosuperior humeral head with the glenoid when the arm is raised in ABER position. If the Hill-Sachs lesion is large enough that its medial border is medial to lateral glenoid track, then the humeral surface would miss the glenoid support in ABER and will fall off the track producing anterior dislocation because now Hill-Sachs defect engages into glenoid. If the medial border of Hill-Sachs lesion remains lateral to glenoid track, then support is maintained, and the lesion is considered "on-track" maintaining shoulder stability. Bipolar lesions exacerbate the chances of engagement. From above it is clear that in bipolar lesions Hill-Sachs defect that is smaller than the track ("on-track") will maintain contact and not engage/cause instability. A Hill-Sachs defect larger than the track will engage on the contrary. Here, there are two determinants if the lesion is on-track or off-track:

a. *Anteroinferior glenoid bone loss:* This is calculated again by the best-fit circle method but some alteration in computation due to evolution in knowledge. On *en face* 3D view (better) draw a best-fit circle matching the posterior and inferior portion of glenoid. Calculate the diameter (D) of this circle.

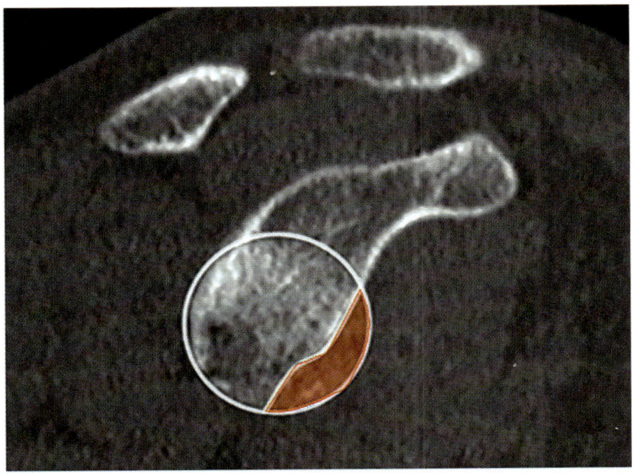

Fig. 10: Pico method: The area of deficient sector (shaded) is calculated by the software itself. I would reiterate that whether manual or automated method; the area of damaged sector would nearly always be a bit overestimated as the normal glenoid would never fill the damaged sector completely. Still, this is the most useful method as a guiding principle for management.

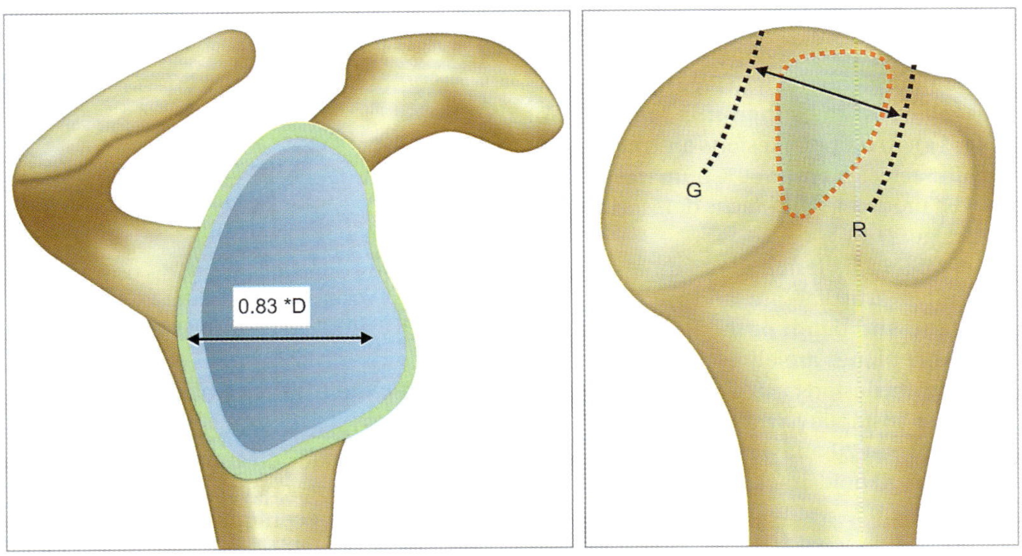

Fig. 11: The glenoid track occupies nearly 83% of the maximal anterior-to-posterior glenoid diameter (we can denote this by variable "D") so the glenoid track will be mathematically 0.83*D as illustrated on left side. This diameter can be easily obtained by drawing a best-fit circle in the lower two-thirds of glenoid tracking the posterior and inferior portions of glenoid as done in previous figures. The diameter of the circle is the maximal diameter of glenoid ("D"). The figure on right demonstrates the corresponding Hill–Sachs interval that includes bone surface from rotator-cuff attachment (R) + bare area or Hill–Sachs defect if present + humeral articular surface till the limit of glenoid track (G). The sum of all these should be < (0.83*D) for it to be "on-track". The track width is demonstrated by double-headed black arrow. Till the glenoid track (0.83*D) is greater than the pathology at Hill–Sachs interval (marked small Hill–Sachs lesion with red-dotted curved polygon) the humeral head would not engage and joint would remain stable.

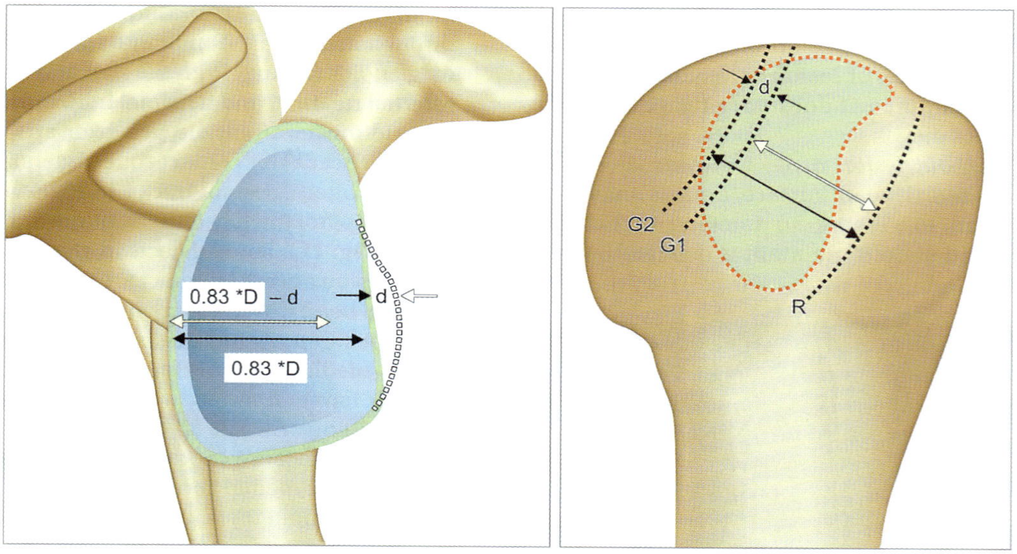

Fig. 12: When there is damage to the anteroinferior glenoid, the glenoid track is reduced by an amount [(0.83*D) – d], where "D" is the maximal width of glenoid as determined by the best-fit circle, "d" is the defect of glenoid in the anteroinferior region as measured from the anterior extent of the best-fit circle. The original glenoid track [= (0.83*D)] is shown on left by double-headed black arrow while the remaining glenoid track [= {(0.83*D) – d}] is represented by the white double-headed arrow. The corresponding markings of tracks on Hill–Sachs interval are illustrated on right side. It can be seen that with a large Hill–Sachs lesion (dotted red curved polygon) the humeral head may or may not engage; compatible with apprehension in the patient, while with the added glenoid defect (bipolar lesion) the humeral head is bound to engage in abduction and external rotation (ABER) position.

Then measure the width of anterior glenoid defect (d) by drawing horizontal line from anterior aspect of glenoid to the anterior circle. The glenoid track width is then calculated by formula [(0.83 × D) – d] **(Fig. 12)**.

b. *Hill–Sachs interval:* This is measured in axial plane as the Hill–Sachs defect + bone bridge between the rotator cuff attachment and lateral aspect of Hill-Sachs defect **(Fig. 11)**.

Bipolar lesion will be called engaging or off-track if Hill-Sachs interval > remaining glenoid track **(Fig. 12)**, else if the Hill–Sachs interval < glenoid track then it is "on-track" or "nonengaging" **(Fig. 11)**. In unipolar lesions off-tracking can occur from large Hill–Sachs lesions (>40% humeral arc) but in bipolar lesions even moderate Hill–Sachs defects (20–40% humeral arc) can engage.

Quantification of Hill-Sachs lesion is not quite standardized. Humeral residual articular arc and percentage of articular arc loss, width, and depth of the lesion **(Fig. 13)** on the axial and coronal planes are all used to assess Hill-Sachs lesion. Generally, the lesions >40% of humeral arc are clinically significant for instability while <20% are mostly benign (Flatow). In between 20 and 40%, it is better to use other measures such as glenoid tracking, etc. The critical values for Hill-Sachs lesions needing intervention are a depth > 16% of the head diameter, an area > 20–25% of the humeral articular surface, a volume > 250 mm^3 (calculated on 3D-CT).

In addition to demonstrating bony injuries, it also assesses humeral and glenoid version. Normal glenoid version in 0° or <10° retroversion. Higher retroversion is associated with posterior instability.

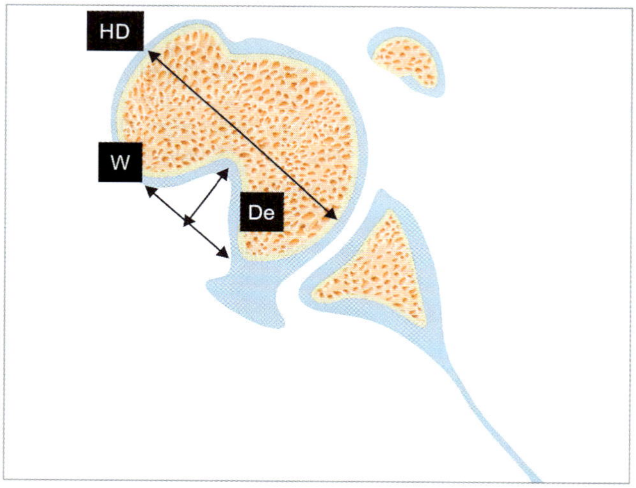

Fig. 13: The assessment of Hill–Sachs defect on proximal humerus on axial images. Volumetric calculations are commonly done on 3D images. (De: depth of the defect; HD: humeral head diameter; W: width of the defect)

Magnetic Resonance Imaging

Magnetic resonance imaging (MRI) and magnetic resonance arthrography can diagnose a variety of lesions of the shoulder with great accuracy. With the advent of latest MRI machines and techniques, the need for MR arthrography has declined considerably. The MRI is done in three planes, i.e., axial, oblique coronal, and oblique sagittal. In the axial plane, the glenoid labrum with the ligaments, humeral head, subscapularis tendon, and the biceps tendon **(Fig. 14)** can be visualized. In the oblique coronal plane, the acromioclavicular (AC) arch and the rotator cuff tendons and muscles are visualized. In the oblique sagittal plane, the supraspinatus tendon, the AC joint, the biceps anchor, and the subacromial bursa are seen. The MRI diagnosis should correlate with the clinical findings and symptoms. Many a times, it has been seen that when surgery is done solely based on MRI findings, the final outcomes are unsatisfactory. This is mostly because the soft tissue evaluation is rendered incomplete on a standard MRI.

MR arthrogram gives much detailed information with regard to capsular laxity and capsular insertion sites. It is the gold standard for diagnosis in patients younger than 40 years with shoulder instability. Intra-articular injection of gadolinium-DTPA (diethylenetriaminepentaacetate) at 2 mmol/L has been shown to safe and the contrast completely diffuses from the joint within 6–24 hours. MR arthrogram very well delineates anatomic variations of the labral signal intensity, form, and size along with caspular and ligamentous structures. The sensitivity to identify the pathology is greatly increased while minimizing the chances of missing them and is especially helpful in failed reconstructive surgeries. MR arthrogram has been considered better than plain MRI for evaluation of Bankart lesions [especially in ABER, Perthes lesions (difficult to otherwise diagnose in their chronic form), anterior labral periosteal sleeve avulsion (ALPSA) lesions (that usually become occult with resynovialization), and humeral avulsion of the glenohumeral ligament (HAGL) lesions].

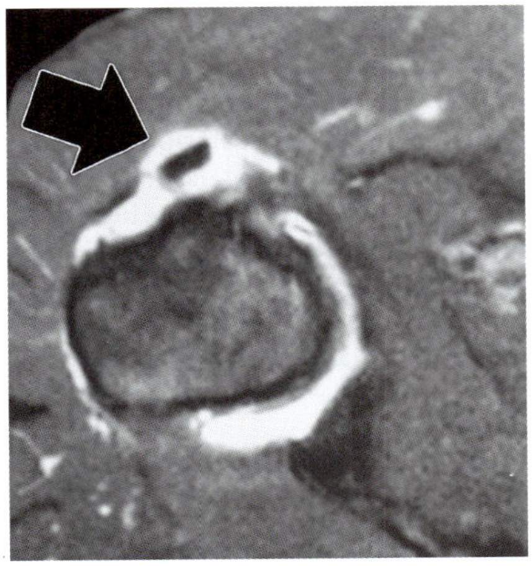

Fig. 14: The MRI shows displaced biceps tendon out of its groove anteriorly representing subluxation (arrow).

The MRI findings for instability are best grouped under traumatic (anterior/posterior), atraumatic, and minor shoulder instability.

Traumatic Anterior Instability

More than 80% shoulder instability patients have anterior instability. Anterior dislocation is mostly associated with Bankart lesion in 86% patients. Bankart lesion comprises avulsed inferior labral complex from glenoid rim + periosteal disruption **(Fig. 15)**. If there is avulsion of osseous glenoid rim, then it is called "bony Bankart" **(Fig. 15)**. Bony lesions >

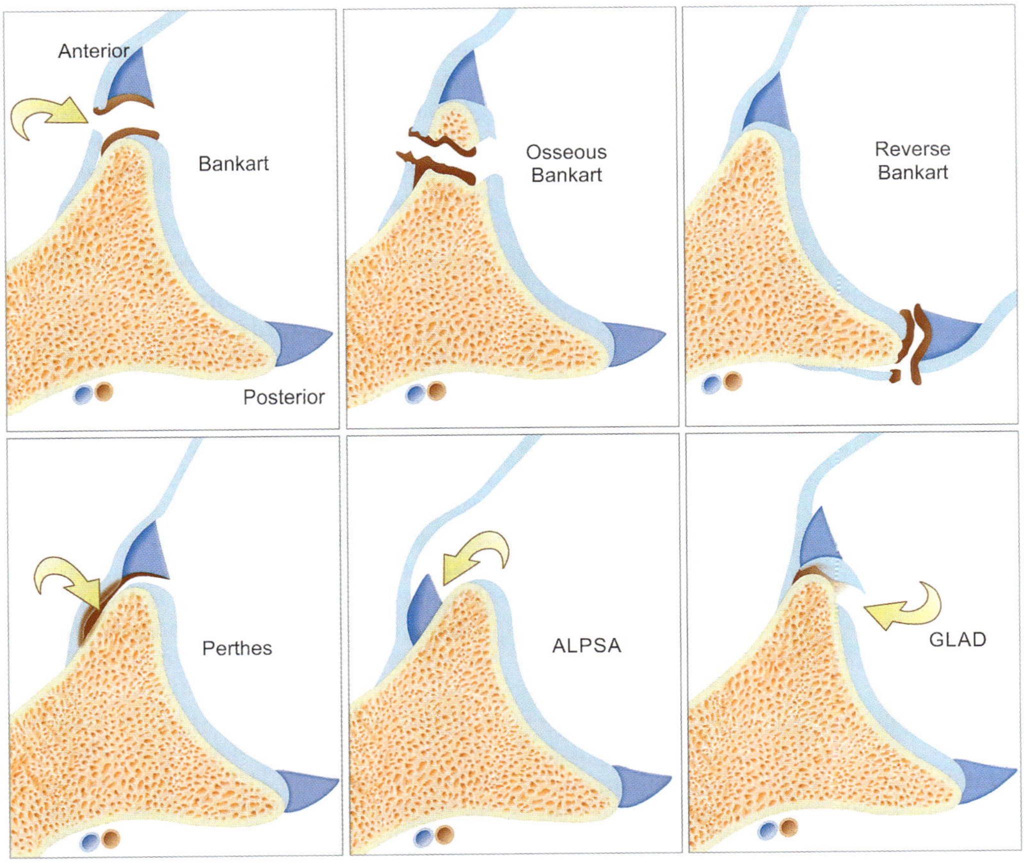

Fig. 15: The Bankart lesion and its variations. (ALPSA: anterior labral periosteal sleeve avulsion; GLAD: glenolabral articular disruption)

6–8 mm produce glenoid width defects of 20–25% and need open repair (acute) or reconstruction (Latarjet procedure). If the Bankart lesion is associated with intact periosteum that has stripped from the glenoid anterior surface, then it is called Perthes lesion **(Fig. 15)**. It is better detected in ABER position. Another variant of Bankart is anterior labral periosteal sleeve avulsion (ALPSA) which consists of complete disruption of the anteroinferior labrum with medial displacement and inferior rotation of the torn fragment **(Fig. 15)**. This is much more common (one-third of patients) in recurrent shoulder instabilities. Anterior ligamentous periosteal sleeve avulsion (ALIPSA) lesion has avulsion of anterior band of inferior glenohumeral ligament (IGHL) from glenoid origin but with intact labrum. Forced adduction of shoulder from ABER position produces another variant of Bankart called "glenolabral articular disruption" (GLAD) lesion which comprises superficial anterior inferior labral tear with an associated articular cartilage injury **(Fig. 15)**. The patient has pain, but GLAD is not associated with instability as the anterior fibers of the IGHL remain attached to glenoid and labrum.

Humeral avulsion of glenohumeral ligament (HAGL) lesions consist of ligament disruptions at glenoidlabral insertion in 40% of cases, intrasubstance in 35%, and at the humeral insertion in 25% of patients **(Fig. 16)**. In 20% cases, the humeral HAGL has bony component (BHAGL, **Fig. 16**) and is associated with Bankart lesion causing bifocal detachment and is termed as "floating IGHL" that appears as a J-shaped structure instead of "U" on oblique coronal images **(Fig. 16)**.

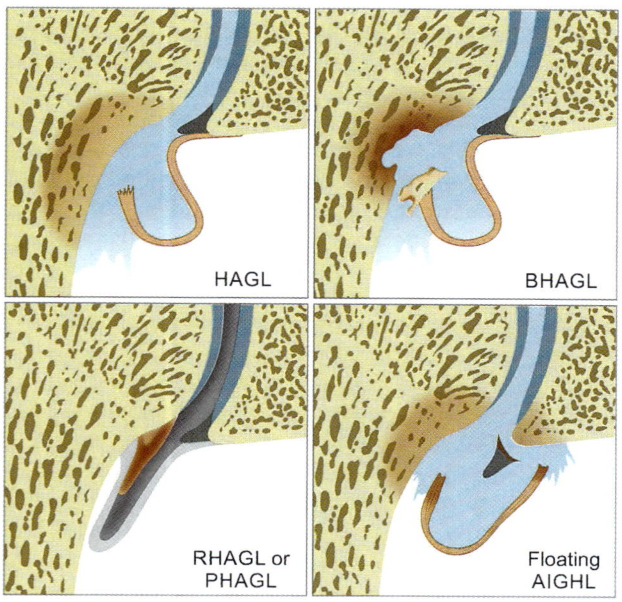

Fig. 16: Illustration of humeral avulsion of glenohumeral ligaments (HAGL) and its variations. (AIGHL: anterior inferior glenohumeral ligaments; BHAGL: bony humeral avulsion of glenohumeral ligaments; PHAGL: posterior humeral avulsion of glenohumeral ligaments; RHAGL: reversed humeral avulsion of glenohumeral ligaments)

Traumatic Posterior Instability

This is seen in a small percentage of patients (2%) presenting with posterior dislocation of shoulder and has a variety of labral lesions ranging from nondetached tear, crushed or frayed labrum, and detached tear. There is commonly a "reversed Bankart lesion" **(Fig. 16)** and "reversed Hill-Sachs lesion". When the posterior periosteum is partly avulsed, and labrum displaces medially posterior labroscapular sleeve avulsion (POLPSA) lesion develops. Kim lesion represents incomplete and concealed superficial tear in the posterior glenoid labrum causing reduction in glenoid labrum's height and abnormal contour. It produces posterior instability if untreated. Glenoid rim articular divot lesion (GARD) lesion results form posterior glenoid rim and/or cavity bone impaction but is not associated with instability like GLAD lesions. Bennet disease may be identified on MRI in chronic cases where calcification develops in posterior capsule at glenoid insertion due to chronic traction injury from instability. Posterior HAGL (PHAGL) injuries may be identified similar but reverse of HAGL **(Fig. 16)**.

Multidirectional Instability

The characteristic MRI findings in multidirectional instability are failure of rotator cuff interval and laxity of inferior capsular pouch. The rotator interval is occupied by capsule + superior glenohumeral ligament + coracohumeral ligament that limit inferior translation and external rotation. The disruption usually causes three patterns of instability (all have inferior instability with variable anterior/posterior component):

1. Anteroinferior dislocations and posterior subluxations
2. Posteroinferior dislocations and anterior subluxation
3. Dislocations in all three directions

These are usually associated with labral and cuff pathologies in athletes.

Minor Shoulder Instabilities

Matsen classical classification into TUBS (*T*raumatic, *U*nidirectional, *B*ankart lesion, and *S*urgery) and AMBRII (atraumatic, multidirectional, bilateral, responds to rehabilitation, inferior capsular shift, and interval closure) does not cover all instability patterns. Minor instability patterns such as acquired instability, overstressed shoulder (AIOS) and atraumatic minor shoulder instability (AMSI) in clinical practice. AIOS results from overuse overhead injuries causing injury to capsular structures mostly in dominant shoulder. The microinstability may produce labral injury like superior labral tear from anterior to posterior (SLAP), capsular fibrosis or calcification, and tears of the rotator cuff secondary to internal impingement. SLAP lesion may extend to adjacent structures producing numerous variants (at least 10 are described) where most have type II lesion with some variable extension of injury **(Figs. 17A to J)**. SLAP is commonly associated with thickened posterior capsule that results in glenoid internal rotation deficit (GIRD) lesion. GIRD lesion has thickened posterior-inferior capsule with

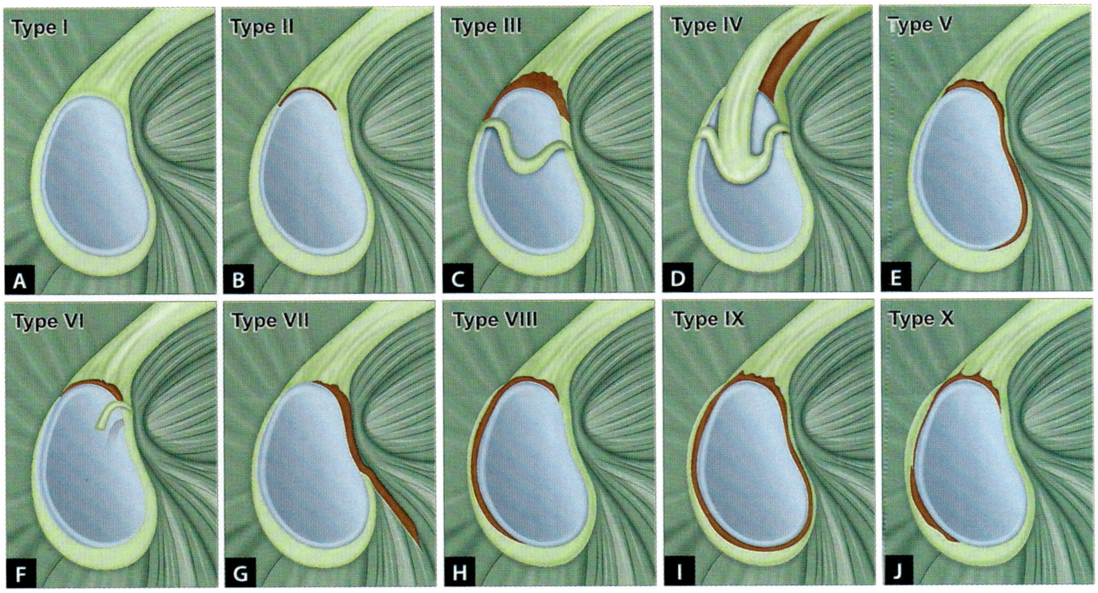

Figs. 17A to J: The different types of superior labral tear from anterior to posterior (SLAP) lesions recognized in clinical practice (more are being described). Type I—Fraying of superior labrum biceps anchor intact; Type II—Superior labrum detached with detachment of biceps anchor; Type III—Bucket handle type tear of the superior labrum (biceps anchor intact); Type IV—Bucket handle tear with extension into biceps tendon; Type V—SLAP lesion with anterio-inferior extension (Bankart + SLAP); Type VI—Anterior or posterior flap tear like type IV or III with bucket handle component; Type VII—Extension of SLAP lesion into glenohumeral ligament; Type VIII—Extension of SLAP lesion into posterior labrum; Type IX—Circumferential labrum detachment; Type X—Extension of SLAP to rotator interval and articular abnormalities.

tight IGHL and may have complete Bennet lesion (see above). There is commonly associated pathology of posterior labrum, infraspinatus, and teres minor tendons. AMSI is rare and is seen due to overload of congenital insufficient static stabilizers in patients with muscle atrophy (commonly after prolonged immobilization). Commonly, insufficient, stretched, or loose middle glenohumeral ligament (MGHL) is seen.

IMAGING FOR ROTATOR-CUFF PATHOLOGY

The imaging and diagnostic modalities in RC pathology are aimed to:

1. Determine presence, extent, and orientation of RC tear.
2. Quality of tendons and their healing capacity.
3. Assess associated pathology like biceps tendon pathology, AC joint abnormality, glenohumeralarthrosis, etc.

Radiographs

Rotator cuff (RC) is radiolucent so its pathology (barring dystrophic calcification) will not be revealed on plain radiographs **(Figs. 18A and B)**. They, however, serve as a good indirect pointer to RC pathology and do not too much cost burden. The biggest disadvantage is that the radiographic signs develop late in RC pathology so if they are demonstrated then the disease is already significantly advanced. Usually AP, axillary lateral, supraspinatus outlet is ordered but in some cases AP active-abduction view is also obtained. AP active-abduction image is obtained with the patient holding a 1 kg weight in 45° of abduction. This demonstrates humeral head migration especially anterosuperior escape and dynamic instability. Following are the common pathologies identified in RC tears:

- Acromio-humeral interval <7 mm is associated with RC pathology **(Fig. 19)** like supraspinatus tear (most common). It is also reduced in infraspinatus or subscapularis tear.
- Measuring critical angle of shoulder (normal = 31–35°). The critical angle is drawn as a line from glenoid inclination to the outer edge of acromion on true AP view **(Fig. 20)**. Increase in this angle is associated RC pathology (>38°) while a reduction (<28°) is seen in glenohumeral osteoarthrosis.
- Scapular Y-view helps to evaluate the shape of acromion. Bigliani et al. classified acromion into three types **(*see* Fig. 1)**:
  1. *Type I:* A flat acromion
  2. *Type II:* A curved acromion
  3. *Type III:* An anterior downward hook on the acromion—this is commonly associated with RC tear.
  4. *Type IV (added later):* Upward curved acromion.
- Rotator cuff arthropathy is seen as degeneration of the glenohumeral articulation with changes like femoralization of humeral head (prominence of the tuberosities) and acetabularization of acromion (deep spherical glenoid socket) **(Fig. 21)**.
- Finding *os acromiale* (unfused center of ossification of acromion) is associated with RC tear.
- Features of impingement such as greater tuberosity changes and sourcil sign (sclerosis of undersurface of

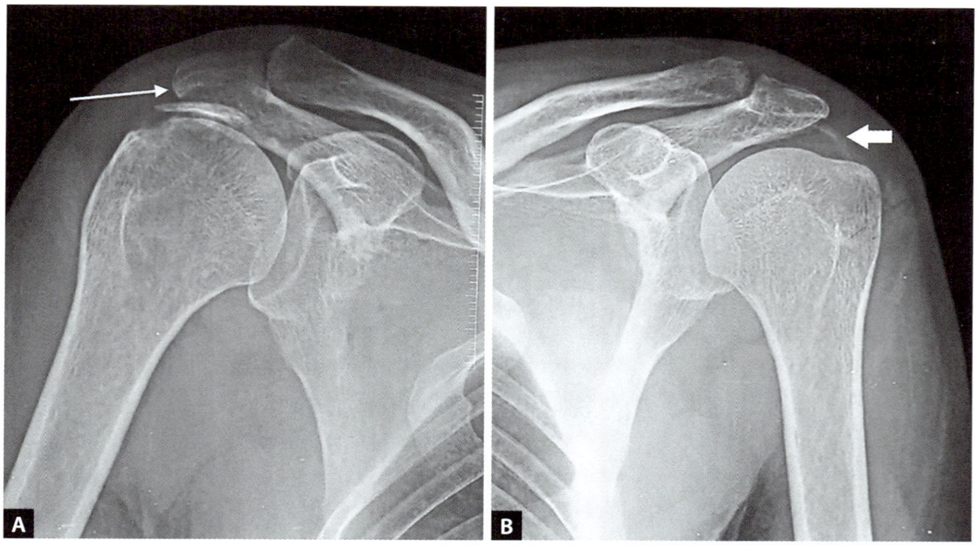

Figs. 18A and B: The radiographs of right and left shoulders of same patient. (A) The right shoulder demonstrates long-standing advanced pathology with well-developed dystrophic calcification in the region of rotator cuff above humeral head. The region had avulsed from humeral head a month ago from trauma causing pain and loss of function for which the patient presented. Also notable is the traction spur of coracoacromial ligament (thin arrow). (B) The left shoulder radiograph demonstrates developing pathology with emerging calcification in the rotator cuff (block arrow). The acromioclavicular joint is also arthritic.

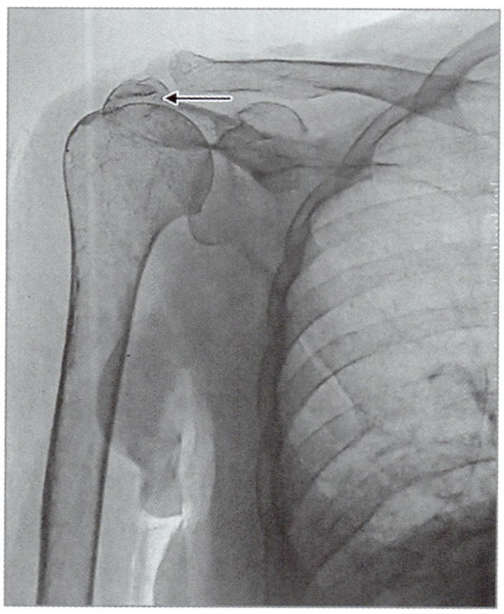

Fig. 19: The radiograph demonstrates reduced acromiohumeral space (arrow) suggestive of near total rotator-cuff tear here.

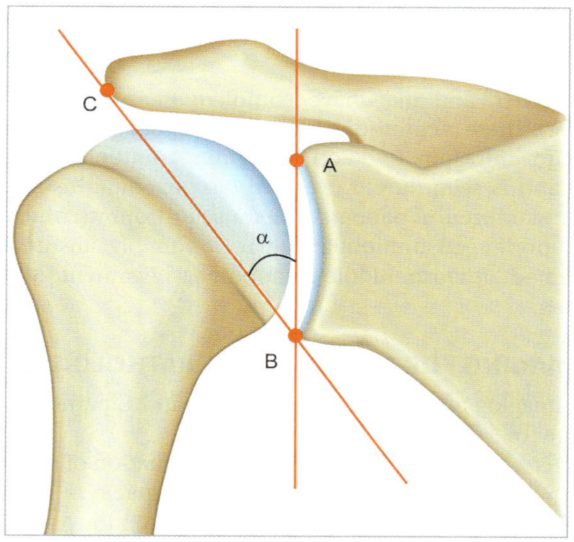

Fig. 20: The critical angle of shoulder can be used to indirectly evaluate the presence of rotator cuff pathology or shoulder joint arthrosis (see text for details).

acromion) in early cases **(Fig. 22)**, calcific tendonitis and traction spur in coracoacromial ligament in late cases **(Figs. 18A and B)** may be appreciated on radiographs.

Ultrasonography of Shoulder Joint

Ultrasonography of shoulder has evolved over a period and has replaced radiography at some centers as a screening and even definitive diagnostic tool. It can evaluate all the soft tissue pathologies in real time and can also provide dynamic evaluation of the musculoskeletal tissues around shoulder. Bone pathologies such as greater tuberosity cortical roughening can also be demonstrated. Postsurgical evaluation of surgical repair and follow-up is also relatively easy and cost-effective. The following structures are evaluated on a routine shoulder ultrasound examination:

- Long head of biceps for tendinosis, instability, synovitis, or synovial hypertrophy. Tendon enlargement, reduced echogenicity, and splitting are seen in tendinopathy. Proximal and chronic distal tear of tendon with loss of motion can be dynamically evaluated. Biceps subluxation (loss of at least two supporting structures) or dislocation (tendon resting on subscapularis or posterior to it in case of complete subscapularis tears).
- Rotator interval and structures within

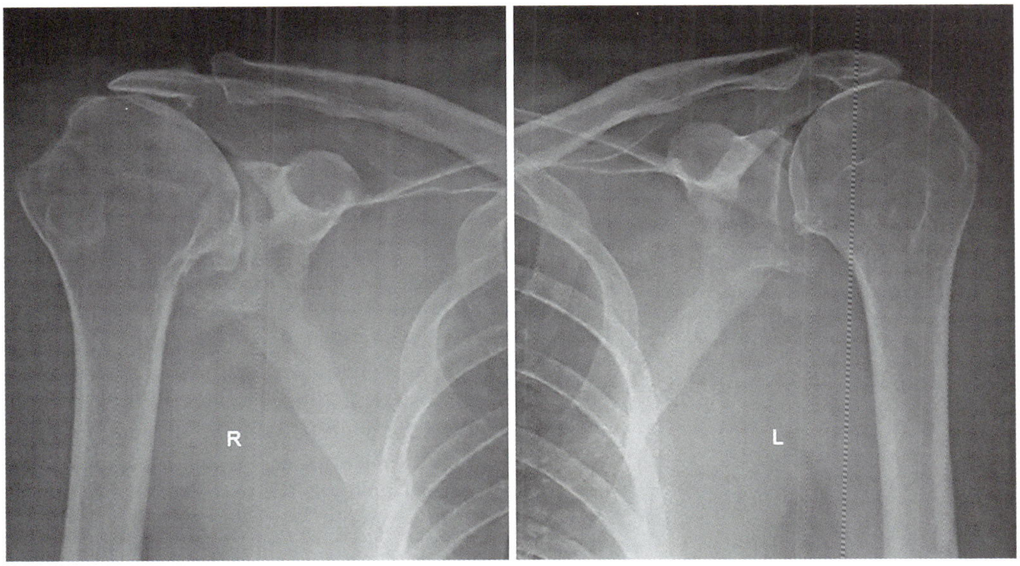

Fig. 21: The radiographs of right and left shoulders of a patient demonstrating advanced rotator cuff arthropathy. There are numerous humeral head and tuberosity osteophytes (femoralization) exhibited on right shoulder prominently. The acromion shows flattening due to attrition while glenoid is deepened (acetabularization) in a way that whole glenoacromial arch seems to have become an acetabulum. Loss of acromiohumeral space is obvious.

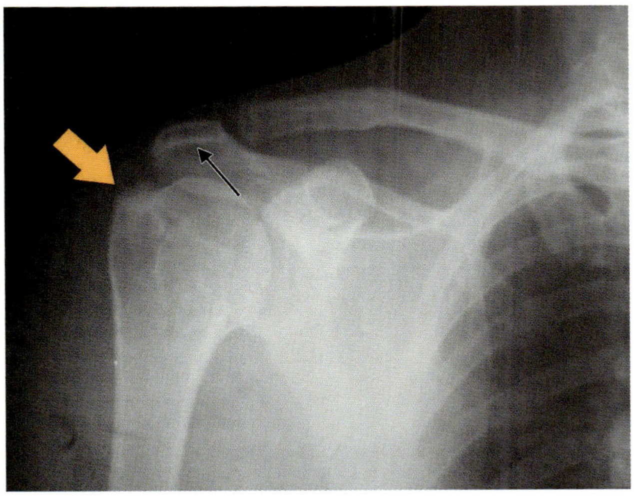

Fig. 22: The radiograph demonstrates signs of impingement and rotator cuff involvement in the form of "sourcil sign" of acromion undersurface (black arrow) and prominent greater tuberosity with fluffy osteophytic excrescence (orange block arrow).

- Evaluation of rotator cuff components:
    - Subscapularis (normal thickness 4.4 mm in males and 3.8 mm in females)
    - Supraspinatus tendon (normal thickness 5.6 mm in males and 4.9 mm in females)
    - Infraspinatus tendon (normal thickness of 4.9 mm in males and 4.4 mm in females)
    - Teres minor tendon
    - Rotator cable—thick deep bundle of fibers originating from coracohumeral ligament traveling deep to supraspinatus and infraspinatus from anterior to posterior.
    - Crescent—portion of tendon distal to the cable.

Rotator cuff tendinosis is visualized as an ill-defined hypoechoic region, focal tendon enlargement due to edema, and loss of normal fibrillary structure. Neovascularity can be demonstrated on Doppler evaluation. Supraspinatus tendinosis is commonly seen at coracoacromial ligament or acromioclavicular joint. Subscapularis tendinosis is seen at coracoid level. Partial RC tear can be articular or bursal sided and is visualized as cuff delamination, intrasubstance tearing, and cyst formation within the tendon. Bursal tears demonstrate focal tendon thinning and deltoid dipping into the defect. Articular side tears show naked cartilage sign due to more sound being transmitted to and reflected from cartilage. Ultrasonography has been reported to detect full-thickness tears in 92–95% cases. It is better than arthrography (now obsolete). The direct signs of RC tear on ultrasound are nonvisualization of the supraspinatus tendon and hypoechoic discontinuity in the tendon. Indirect signs are double cortex sign, sagging of peribursal fat, and compressibility of the cuff. Absence of cuff motion on real-time ultrasound is a reliable sign for full-thickness cuff tear. Deltoid is seen to lie directly on humeral head in chronic large tears. The grading of RC tears on ultrasonography is done as follows:

1. *Grade 1:* <3 mm deep
2. *Grade 2:* 3–6 mm deep (Up to 50% thickness of cuff involved)
3. *Grade 3:* 6 mm deep (>50% thickness of cuff enveloped)

- Extrinsic impingement at subacromial, coracoacromial, and subcoracoid space. This can also include dynamic evaluation.
- Suprascapular nerve especially at suprascapular notch and spinoglenoid notch
- Acromioclavicular joint

Magnetic Resonance Imaging for Cuff Pathology

MRI of shoulder is the current standard for imaging the pathologies and their identification and detailing. Useful information like type of tear (partial vs. full), shape and dimensions of full-thickness tear, tendon retraction, and assessment of tissue quality is all possible with this modality.

- *Partial-thickness RC tears:* Partial articular surface tears or tendon avulsions (PASTA, **Fig. 23**) are most common that appear as focal signal change along the articular aspect of the rotator cuff with fluid in the subacromial-subdeltoid bursa. Other partial RC tears are bursal side tears, intrasubstance (interstitial) tears and cysts **(Fig. 24)**. Normal RC is 10–12 mm thick and tears are graded into three types according to thickness of tendon involved as detailed in ultrasonography. Grade 3 tears are significant and need surgical interventions. Additionally, identification of tendon thinning guides toward surgery.
- *Shape and dimension of RC tear:* Full thickness of RC tears on MRI appears as a focal discontinuity in the tendon extending from the articular to the bursal surface typically viewed as fluid signal intensity on T2W images **(Fig. 25)**. Sometimes intermediate- to high-signal granulation tissue and/or synovial hypertrophy may fill the tear defect. Secondary signs such as superior humeral head translation and muscle atrophy are commonly present. RC tears nearly always involve supraspinatus tendon with variable involvement of other components. The sensitivity and specificity of MRI in identification of full-thickness RC tears vary from 85–100% to 93–99%, respectively. Arthroscopically, the tears are classified as crescent, U-shaped, and L-shaped. This has discrete bearing on surgical repair method. DeOrio and Cofield classified rotator cuff tears on the basis of greatest dimension into:
    - Small (<1 cm)
    - Medium (1–3 cm)
    - Large (3–5 cm)
    - Massive (<5 cm): Massive contracted tears on MRI are classified into massive crescentic tears (large anteroposterior dimensions) and massive longitudinal tears (spared anterior cuff tissue at rotator interval).

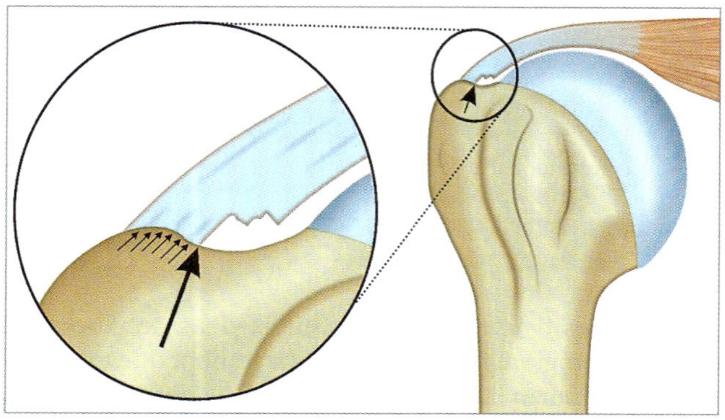

Fig. 23: The PASTA (partial articular surface tears or tendon avulsions) lesion is a partial articular side tendon avulsion of supraspinatus tendon as illustrated in the figure.

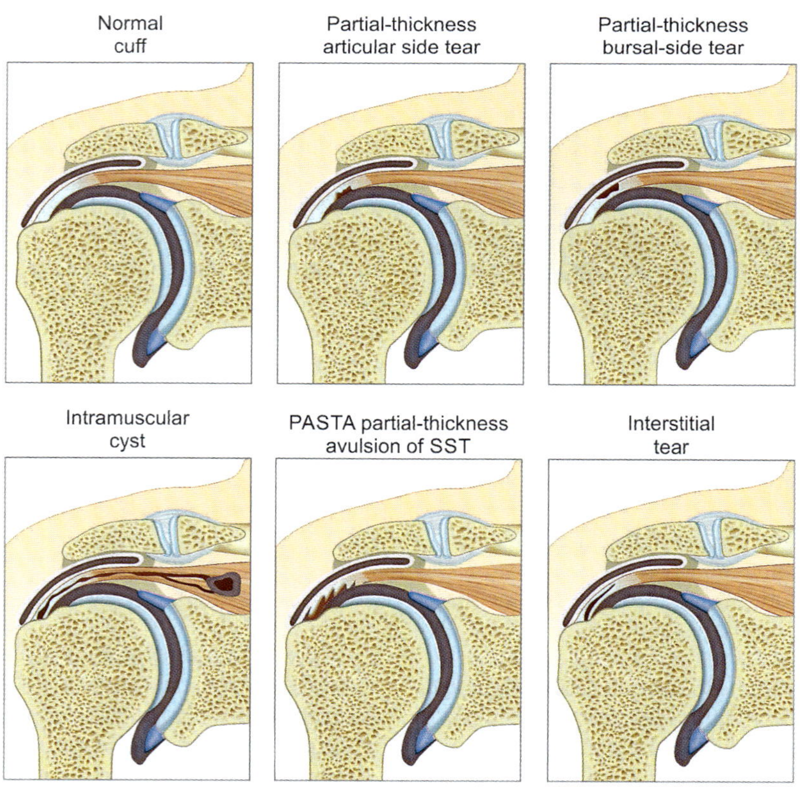

Fig. 24: The different types of partial rotator cuff tears. (PASTA: partial articular surface tears or tendon avulsions; SST: supraspinatus)

These have bearing on deciding if surgical repair is possible or not and the modality of repair. Tears with dimensions greater than 4 cm in both length and width are generally not reparable.

- *Retraction of tendon:* This is possibly the most important ancillary information revealed on MRI that guides surgical method. It is classified according to Patte classification **(Table 1 and Figs. 26A to C)**. Retraction of torn edge medial to glenoid fossa makes it unrepairable. This is not but always definite as the mobility of tear also has important bearing on reparability.
- *Tear extension:* Extension of the RC tear has important prognostic implications. Supraspinatus tear may extend anteriorly into RC interval to involve medial aspect of coracohumeral ligament and superior subscapularis fibers. This significantly reduces the chances of successful repair. Supraspinatus tendon tears may also extend posteriorly to involve infraspinatus tendon reducing the external rotation power.
- Associated biceps tendon pathology such as tendon fraying, disruption, subluxation **(*see* Fig. 14)** or dislocation should be appropriately identified because it has important prognostic implications.
- Muscle atrophy, cross-sectional area, and fatty degeneration—loss of muscle function can be identified by atrophy of fibers on MRI. Measurement of cross-sectional area correlates with muscle strength. Direct volume estimation is possible, but it is impractical, so two other measures are commonly deployed—the scapular ratio (occupation ratio) and the "tangent sign". Scapular ration is calculated at the level of the medial coracoid process in sagittal oblique plane images. Here, the fossa is largely encompassed by osseous boundaries. If the ratio of area occupied by supraspinatus muscle to area of supraspinatus fossa is <50% in sagittal oblique plane, then it indicates supraspinatus muscle atrophy. In the similar images supraspinatus muscle should cross the line joining superior borders of the scapular spine and the superior margin of the coracoid process (tangent sign, **Figs. 27A and B**). If the muscle fails to do so, then muscle atrophy is present. Fatty degeneration of muscle not always occurs with aging, it may also be seen with neurologic impairment, glenohumeral osteoarthritis, and rotator cuff tear. It is classified as per Goutallier D, et al. classification scheme. It occurs even in unrelated muscles in the presence of large chronic tears. Infraspinatus muscle degeneration may occur in

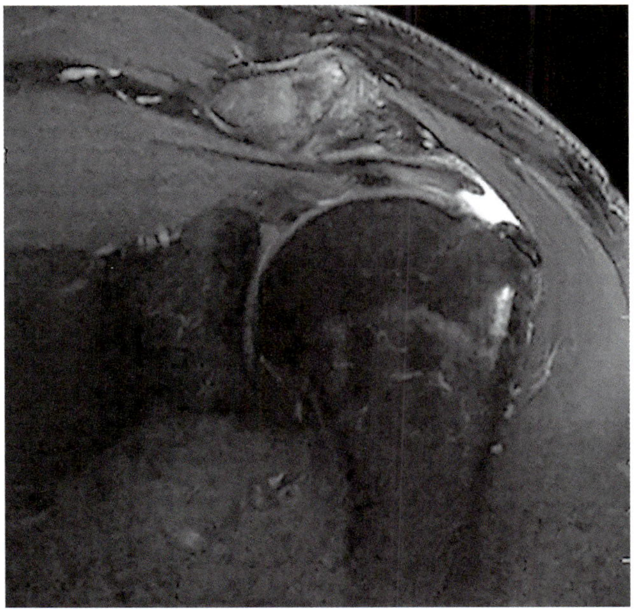

Fig. 25: The typical appearance of a complete rotator cuff tear on MRI, the void is usually fluid-filled in acute cases appearing intensely radiodense; however, in chronic cases it may be filled with granulation tissue reducing the signal intensity in the void.

TABLE 1: The Patte classification of rotator cuff (RC) tendon retraction as applied on sequence in frontal (coronal) plane.

Stage 1	Proximal stump near the bony insertion
Stage 2	Proximal stump is at the level of the humeral head.
Stage 3	Proximal stump at the level of glenoid or more proximal

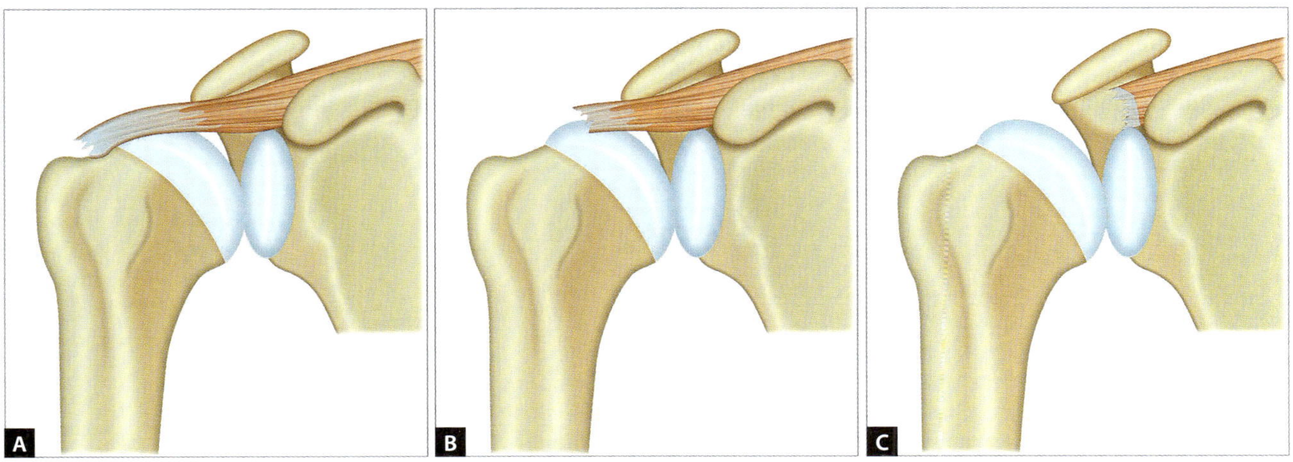

Figs. 26A to C: The Patte classification of rotator cuff retraction, in stage 1 the proximal stump is near the bony insertion (A), in stage 2 the proximal stump retracts till the level of humeral head (B) while in stage 3 the proximal stump retracts at the level of glenoid or more proximal (C).

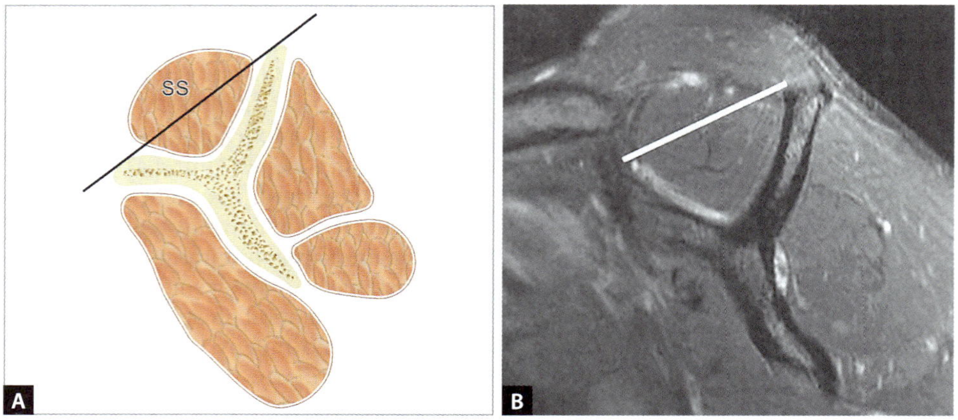

Figs. 27A and B: (A) The "tangent sign" as drawn on oblique sagittal MR image (see text for details) is illustrated; (B) The image demonstrates the muscle crossing the line comfortably indicating good muscle bulk. (SS: supraspinatus muscle)

large anterosuperior tears not involving infraspinatus tendon and with intact subscapularis tendon its muscle fibers may undergo fatty degeneration. It is not typically degeneration rather an infiltration of lipid tissue between atrophied muscle fibers. Occurrence of fatty degeneration is correlated to the extent of the supraspinatus tendon tear, retraction of tendon stump, and an increase in the number of torn tendons. Infraspinatus and subscapularis muscle fatty degeneration is correlated with recurrence of supraspinatus tendon tears.

- Muscle denervation can also be identified on MR as denervation edema of the involved muscle or muscle groups. Subacute muscle denervation mimics as massive rotator cuff tears and pseudoparalysis. The edema is homogenous within the muscle not involving adjacent soft tissue. Post-traumatic edema has a feathery appearance.
- *Coracoacromial arch and impingement:* Coracoacromial arch comprises anterior one-third of acromion + coracoacromial ligament + coracoid process. Supraspinatus tendon glides below this in the impingement interval (space between arch and humeral head) separated by subacromial and subdeltoid bursa. Type III (mostly) and II (to some extent) acromion compromise this tight space further causing tendinosis and tears. Thickening of coracoacromial ligament and presence of osacromiale also reduce the available space causing impingement. Similarly, variations in coracoid morphology may cause sib-coracoid impingement and lead to subscapularis muscle pathology.

Other Investigations

Sometimes nerve conduction studies and electromyography studies may have to be done in cases with suspected deltoid muscle paralysis, brachial plexus lesion (Parsonage-Turner syndrome), suprascapular nerve entrapment or in any symptoms which arouse the suspicion of a neurological pathology.

CONCLUSION

- Diagnostic imaging is indispensable in shoulder pathologies and is highly helpful in global assessment of the pathology along with clinical examination.
- The imaging modalities are not only focused on the primary pathology but also on the very pertinent and important associated structures that have direct bearing on the outcome of surgical procedure.
- Ultrasonography of the shoulder has fast emerged as an important diagnostic modality that has replaced MRI as screening and definitive modality of investigation for rotator cuff pathologies.
- Surgeon should control the tendency to over-image and present a concise clinical summary for guiding radiologist in providing directed useful reports.

CHAPTER 57

Rotator Cuff Disease

Manish Kumar Varshney

INTRODUCTION

This encompasses the full spectrum including impingement syndrome, subacromial bursitis, supraspinatus tendinitis and rotator cuff tear. The term "impingement syndrome" is considered outmoded by dedicated orthopedic surgeons as pathologies can be pinpointed to specific structures that produce the symptoms. Even International Classification of Diseases (ICD) classification has replaced the term impingement syndrome by "Disorders of bursae and tendons in shoulder region, unspecified". But, due to its vast usage and broad understanding of the "mechanism" the term is used for understanding at a basic level throughout the text here. We will discuss them in detail here.

SUBACROMIAL IMPINGEMENT SYNDROME

Impingement as a causality event is discussed for broader understanding here, otherwise the consensus now emerging is that most of the rotator cuff tears and related pathologies are degenerative in nature. Rotator cuff tendinosis, partial tears, and complete tears could be reliably differentiated and diagnosed by clinical examination and sonography, magnetic resonance imaging (MRI), and arthroscopy. These pathologies progress as a continuum of the degenerative spectrum (previously solely attributed to impingement instead of degeneration) but any one of them can also have traumatic origin. The prevalence varies widely in different populations due to population characteristics but one thing is common that increasing age is associated with increased prevalence of rotator cuff (RC) pathology. This is not to say that everything is degenerative but only to impress upon the fact that degeneration also has a defined role and impingement is not the only pathology bringing up nontraumatic rotator cuff disease.

Subacromial impingement syndrome (SIS) or simply impingement syndrome is closely related to rotator cuff tear and often precedes nontraumatic cuff tears. With normal rotator cuff function, the humeral head translates <3 mm superiorly during the midranges of active elevation, whereas at extreme movements, anteroposterior and superoinferior translations of 4–10 mm do occur **(Fig. 1A)**. An increase in superior translation with active abduction may result in encroachment of the coracoacromial arch. This encroachment produces a compression of the suprahumeral structures against the anteroinferior aspect of the acromion and coracoacromial ligament **(Fig. 1B)**. Repeated compression of these structures, when coupled with other predisposing factors, results in SIS. It was first recognized by Jarjavay in 1867, and the term *impingement syndrome* was popularized by Neer in the 1970s. Now with detailed study, various intrinsic and extrinsic factors have been implicated into the impingement process including the shape of acromion, cuff vascularization, functioning of dynamic stabilizers, acromioclavicular (AC) joint degeneration, position of arm during activities, capsular tightness, and repetitive activities **(Table 1)**. A number of impingement types and subtypes have thus evolved. Two of those broad types include the outlet (intrinsic) impingement and the nonoutlet (extrinsic) impingement.

Outlet Impingement

"Outlet impingement", classically described by Neer, is called so because it occurs at the supraspinatus outlet formed by the coracoid process, the anterior one-third acromion, the AC joint, and the coracoacromial ligament. Supraspinatus tendon glides freely in the space protected by subacromial and subdeltoid bursa. The space volume reduces considerably in abduction and can be pathologically reduced by type III or II acromion, thick tendon (tendinosis), thick coracoacromial ligament or presence of os acromiale, etc. pressing on the tendon during movement. The term "impingement syndrome" refers to this outlet impingement per se. This type of impingement classically presents as a painful arc. It is thought to be the cause of symptoms in 90–95% cases, however, with better understanding and evaluation of elderly, the role of degenerative changes is gathering importance. Neer divided the outlet impingement process into three stages, although the condition is a continuum of symptoms. These stages have specific findings and the intrinsic or extrinsic factors contributing to the problem.

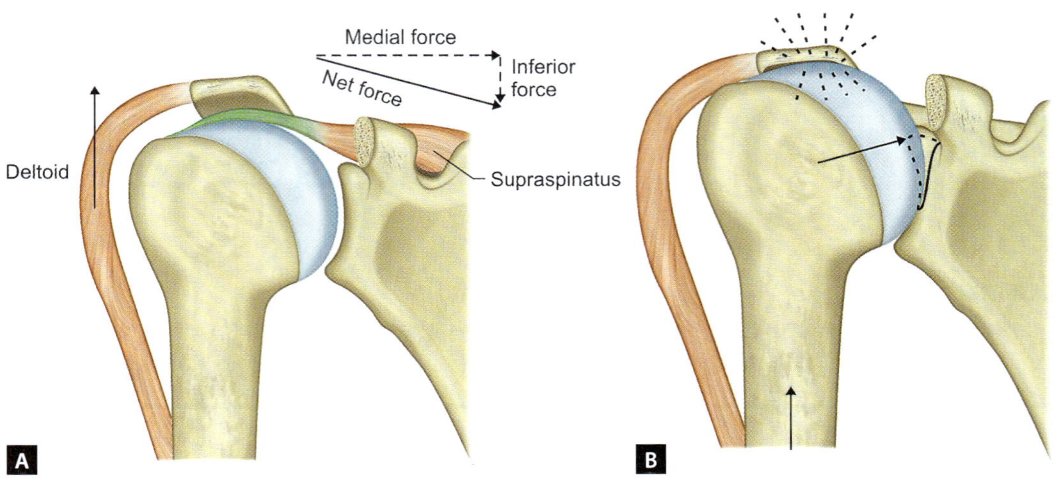

Figs. 1A and B: (A) The normal coronal force couple tends to maintain the humeral head by providing a resultant vector acting in inferior direction to the top of humeral head that allows rotational moment to act instead of superior translation by the deltoid pull. The inferior moment acts at a point medial and superior to the pull of deltoid so that deltoid force does not translate the humerus instead its pull is converted to rotational moment and maintains the humeral head in the glenoid socket; (B) The deficiency of coronal force couple leads to superior translation of the humeral head and impingement of the superior structures (biceps tendon, rotator cuff, etc.) and glenoid abrasion.

TABLE 1: Clinical diagnosis associated with impingement syndrome.

Diagnosis	*Type of factor*
Subacromial factor: • Bone spurs • Thickened coracoacromial ligament • Calcific enthesopathy • Synovitis/bursitis	Intrinsic
Acromioclavicular joint injury: • Arthrosis • Bone spurs • Instability	Intrinsic
Rotator cuff injury: • Tear • Tendinopathy	Extrinsic
Labral injury	Extrinsic
Shoulder instability	Extrinsic
Biceps tendinopathy	Extrinsic
GIRD	Extrinsic
Scapular dyskinesis	Extrinsic
Neurologic	Extrinsic

(GIRD: glenohumeral internal rotation deficit)

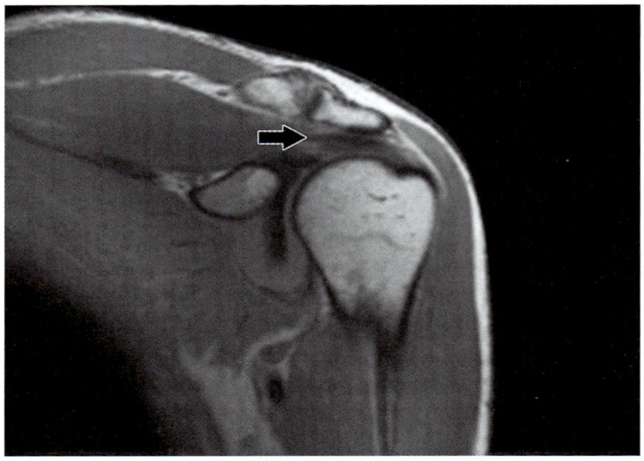

Fig. 2: Subacromial impingement seen on an MRI due to inferior acromioclavicular (AC) joint spur pressing the supraspinatus tendon (arrow).

Stage I

This stage consists of localized inflammation, and edema of the rotator cuff typically observed in younger (<25 years of age) patients, although it can also be seen in older patients as a result of overuse **(Fig. 2)**. The patient has painful shoulder and a history of associated trauma or microtrauma. There is tenderness at the supraspinatus insertion and anterior acromion, the range of motion (ROM) is painful, and weakness arises due to pain. Scapular stabilization is jeopardized due to painful inhibition of the serratus anterior and trapezius.

Stage II

This represents a progressive deterioration in the tissues of the rotator cuff typically seen in the 26- to 40-year-old age group. With continued irritation of the subacromial structures, secondary changes develop in the tissues **(Fig. 3)**. The subacromial bursa loses its ability to lubricate and tendonitis of the cuff develops. Especially the overhead activities are painful with pain commonly located on the top of the shoulder radiating to arm in the deltoid insertion region.

Stage III

This is the end stage with destruction of the soft tissue and tear of the rotator cuff. It is commonly seen in patients above 40 years age group. The wear of the anterior aspect of the acromion on the greater tuberosity and the supraspinatus tendon eventually results in a full-thickness tear of the rotator cuff. Degeneration of nearby AC joint is seen with osteophyte formation **(*see* Fig. 5A)**. Muscle atrophy is quite prominent especially of the infraspinatus and supraspinatus. There is progressive limitation in active and passive ROM. Rotator cuff tears hence develop.

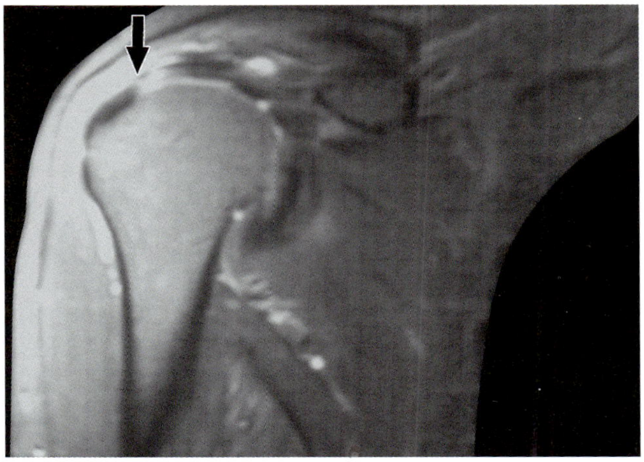

Fig. 3: In the next stage, the impingement leads to supraspinatus tendonitis visible on MRI as a bright signal in the supraspinatus area (arrow) which can be confused with a tear.

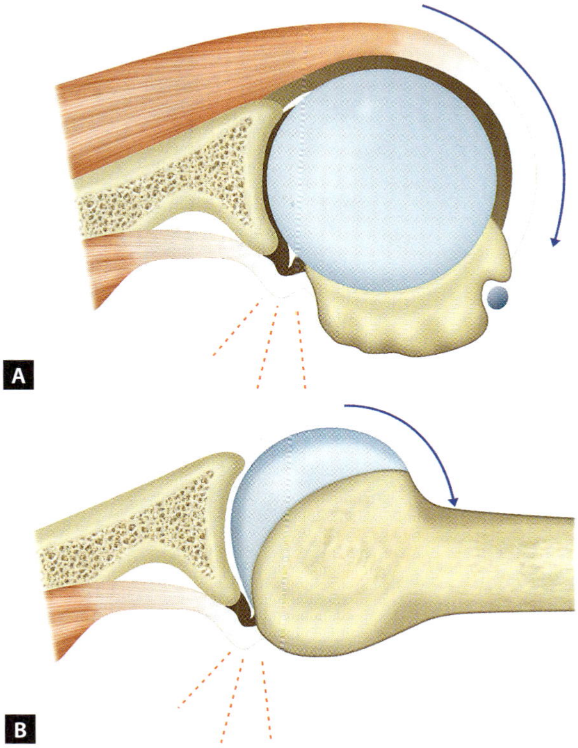

Figs. 4A and B: Posterosuperior impingement (external impingement) seen due to abnormal transverse force couple (arrow: A) and/or abnormal scapulohumeral rhythm (B) and/or increased anterior capsular laxity.

Nonoutlet Impingement or Posterior Superior Glenoid Impingement

This is a lately recognized source of rotator cuff pathology seen in athletes performing repetitive overhead motions and is associated with superior labrum anterior and posterior (SLAP) lesions (possibly they represent a spectrum of the disorder). It has been found that a triad of anterior capsular laxity, posterior contraction, and *internal impingement* occurs in overhead athletes. It results from impingement of the in-folded rotator cuff between the greater tuberosity and the posterior superior glenoid labrum during forced humeral elevation and internal rotation. During extreme overhead abduction, the articular surface of the cuff gets stuck between the posterosuperior labrum and humeral head **(Figs. 4A and B)**. Also stress concentration has been found to occur in the so-called critical zone of cuff in varying degrees of abduction. This leads to degenerative tears being initiated on the articular side, bursal side, and the intratendinous portion. This can eventually result in posterior superior tears in the glenoid labrum (reverse Bankart lesion), and lesions in the posterior humeral head. The pathoanatomy, pathophysiology, and treatment are discussed below with SLAP lesion.

Primary and Secondary Impingement

Jobe and Pink proposed two other types of impingement, which relate to chronic disorders of the rotator cuff.

1. Primary impingement same as outlet impingement of Neer occurs when the superior aspect of the rotator cuff is compressed and abraded by the surrounding bony and soft tissues due to a decreased subacromial space. In primary impingement, the impingement itself creates the clinical presentation so that treatment should be directed to the impingement itself.
2. Secondary impingement is a condition found in both older and younger individuals. This type results in tensile overload of the rotator cuff resulting in poor control of the humeral head during overhead activities and may be associated with instability. In secondary impingement, the signs and symptoms are those of impingement; however, they result from factors other than impingement of the tissues "directly", e.g., instability of shoulder might lead to secondary impingement of the tissues as in the posterosuperior corner or scapular dyskinesis. In this sense, the term "diagnosis" of secondary impingement is not apt in these cases as actual disease is something else that should be treated masterly.

Apart from SIS, another entity called "subcoracoid impingement" has also been described. The condition arises from a laterally placed coracoid process that impinges on proximal humerus with forward flexion and internal rotation.

ROTATOR CUFF TEARS

The understanding and treatment of rotator cuff tears **(Figs. 5A to C)** is still evolving since Codman published his comprehensive evaluation in 1934. He proposed a traumatic origin to cuff tears. Soon in 1937, the theory of outlet impingement was introduced envisaging the friction and attrition of cuff between greater tuberosity and the acromion due to repetitive movements. Still later three stages of outlet impingement describing the spectrum of disease severity and need of anterior acromioplasty to remove the offending structures gained popularity among shoulder surgeons. As we age the subacromial space narrows down and the supraspinatus tendon undergoes degenerative changes. Due to repetitive abduction movements, the supraspinatus

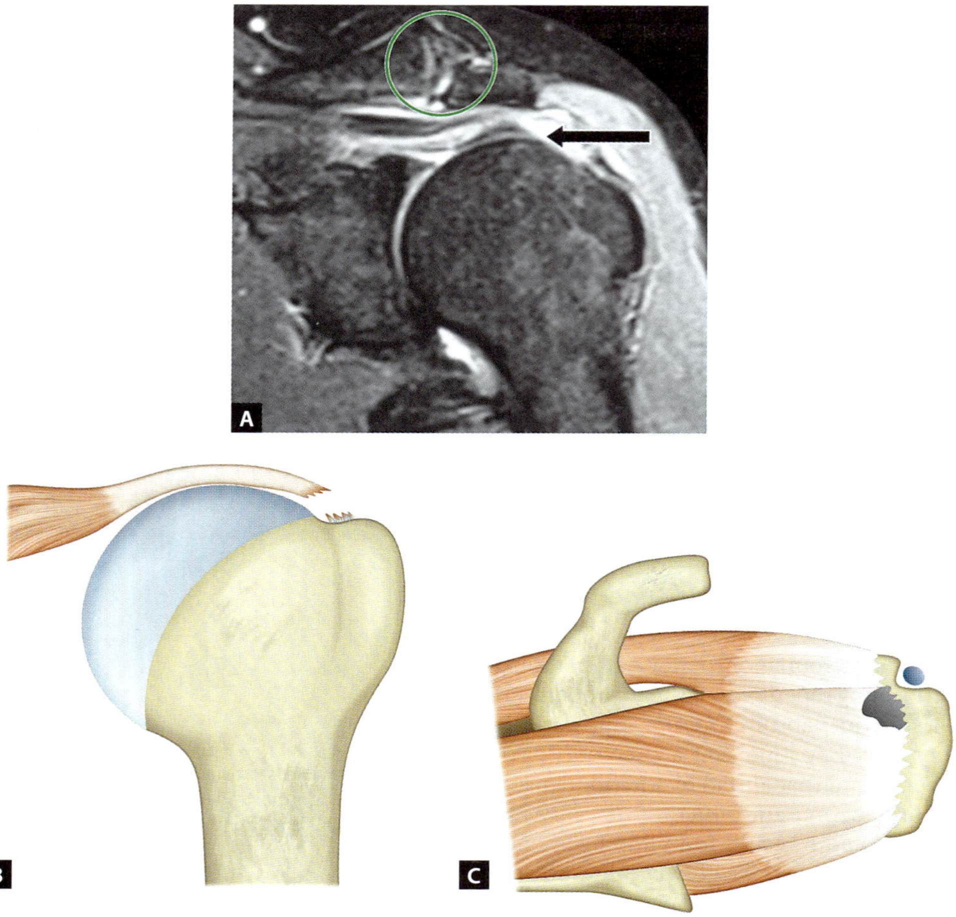

Figs. 5A to C: (A) The MRI shows a supraspinatus insertional complete tear (arrow), the green circle highlights the presence of acromioclavicular joint arthrosis which is not an uncommon finding; (B) Illustration showing the same; (C) The cuff tear as visible from superior aspect while doing open repair.

tendon glides against the undersurface of the acromion. Acute trauma also plays a significant role in etiopathogenesis. The current understanding of rotator cuff pathology can be summarized into four mechanisms:

1. *Tensile overload:* The rotator cuff is subject to stretching forces when it attempts to resist horizontal adduction, internal rotation, anterior translation, and distraction forces eventually damaging the collagen fibers.
2. *Compression:* Compression of the cuff can either be primarily due to a reduction in the size of the subacromial space, or secondary (dynamic) due to joint instability.
3. *Internal impingement:* Stretching and impingement of the rotator cuff tendons in internal impingement leads to articular side tear of supraspinatus and infraspinatus [partial articular surface tendon avulsion (PASTA)]. The PASTA lesion term was coined by Snyder et al. to describe the articular side lesions at junction of supra- and infraspinatus tendons **(Figs. 6A and B)**. Rotator cuff tears in throwers can extend into middle layers of infraspinatus tendon delineated by Conway et al. and termed partial articular-sided intrasubstance tears (PAINT) lesion.
4. *Acute trauma:* Tearing of the tendon results when forces generated by the trauma exceed the tensile strength of the tendon.

These mechanisms also entail possibility of existence of some associated lesions that should be looked for during the workup of pathology. These include commonly the AC joint arthritis and sometimes the involvement of glenohumeral articulation. The long head of biceps may be involved with fraying or detachment (in SLAP lesions). Some uncommon findings include the presence of os acromiale (8% of population) and suprascapular nerve compression pathology. The suprascapular nerve compression can cause shoulder pain and weakness mimicking full-thickness supraspinatus and/or infraspinatus tears. The compression can also come secondary to excessive retraction (>2 cm) following complete tear of tendon.

Classically, traumatic rotator cuff tears affect patients between 40 and 50 years of age. The symptoms are vague to begin with. Pain is classically along the deltoid region and upper arm. Pain increases on active abduction. Origin of pain is unclear but should definitely be not linked to tendon tear. The findings that suggest pathology other than tendon as cause of pain includes the fact that 12–40% population older than 60 years have cuff tears but most have no pain, moreover, more than one-third of the surgeries for cuff tears fail, still patients report improvement in pain. Degenerative tears are common in elderly. In these patients the cuff may

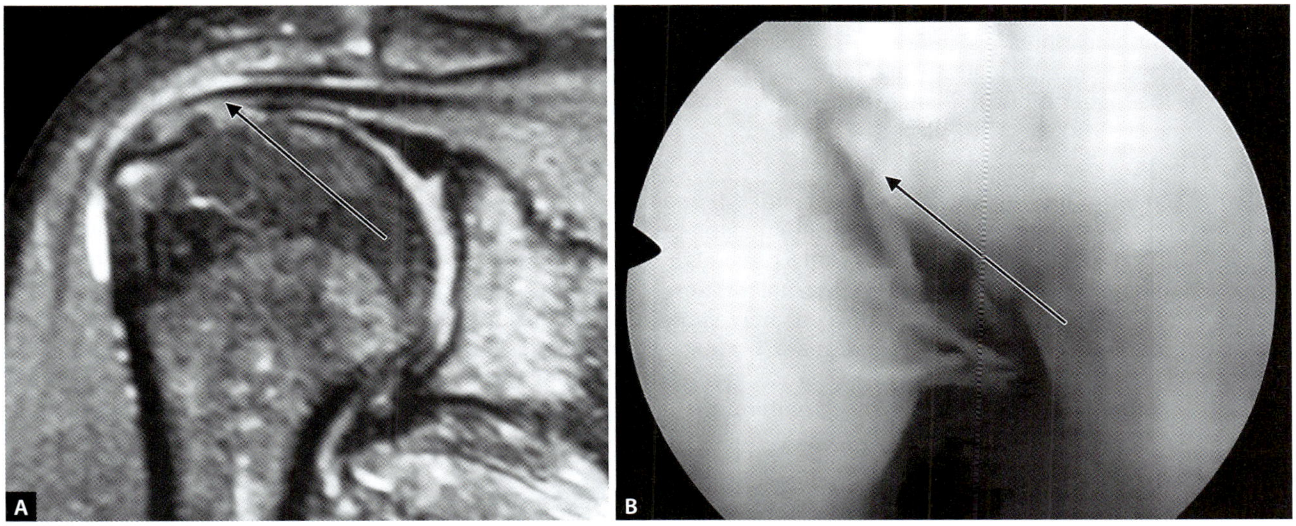

Figs. 6A and B: MRI showing the supraspinatus partial tear of articular surface (PASTA lesion) and arthroscopic view of the same (arrows).

be overpowered by deltoid muscle pulling and impinging the humeral head into coracoacromial arch. This results in development of coracoacromial ligament enthesiophyte (bony spur) which may be the reason for progression of Stage II to Stage III disease described above. Smoking has negative impact on cuff disease and its treatment as it impairs healing. Similarly, hyperlipidemia increases the risk of rotator cuff disease and recurrent tears. Genetic factors have been identified lately pointing to specific genetic loci in these patients but biological pathways are undefined. Age >60 years, full-thickness tears, fatty infiltration (and hyperlipidemia), smoking, and genetic factors have been linked to progression of the RC tear overall but precisely pointing specific individuals that will progress is difficult. The progression of tendinosis to full-thickness cuff tear is failure of biology, despite inflammation the tissue somehow fails to productively respond to the insult resulting in deposition of disorganized connective fatty and fibrous tissue at the pathological site. Clinical examination reveals generally preserved motion of shoulder especially external rotation (it is usually restricted in adhesive capsulitis). Empty-can test has high sensitivity and specificity for full-thickness supraspinatus tear. Lift-off and Belly-press test have high specificity but low sensitivity for full-thickness subscapularis tears. Patients with external rotation lag sign have a large posterosuperior tear involving infraspinatus (it is a powerful external rotator when limb is by side of body). Massive posterosuperior RC tear precluding positioning of limb in space is better detected by positive Hornblower sign.

BOX 1: Patte classification of rotator cuff tears.

Extent of tear:
- Group I: Partial tears or full-substance tears <1 cm in sagittal diameter at bony detachment
  - Deep, partial tears
  - Superficial tears
  - Small, full-substance tears
- Group II: Full-substance tears of entire supraspinatus
- Group III: Full-substance tears involving more than one tendon
- Group IV: Massive tears with secondary osteoarthritis

Topography of tear in sagittal plane:
- Segment 1: Subscapularis tear
- Segment 2: Coracohumeral ligament tear
- Segment 3: Isolated supraspinatus tear
- Segment 4: Tear of entire supraspinatus and one half of infraspinatus
- Segment 5: Tear of supraspinatus and infraspinatus
- Segment 6: Tear of subscapularis, supraspinatus, and infraspinatus

Topography of tear in frontal plane:
- Stage 1: Proximal stump close to bony insertion
- Stage 2: Proximal stump at level of humeral head
- Stage 3: Proximal stump at level of glenoid

Quality of muscle:
- Minimal fatty streaking
- Less fat than muscle
- Equal fat and muscle
- More fat than muscle

State of the biceps tendon:
- Intact
- Subluxated
- Dislocated

Classification of Rotator Cuff Tears

The origin of tears has always been elusive and classical thought was that the tears originate in anterior supraspinatus just behind the biceps tendon (watershed vascular zone) and then propagate posteriorly. Ultrasonography based findings have challenged the notion and suggest that the tears originate in the "rotator crescent of Burkhart" located nearly 15 mm behind the biceps tendon separate from rotator cable, and the tears then propagate anterior or posterior from this region.

Rotator cuff tears have been classified according to the depth (full- versus partial-thickness), etiology (traumatic vs. degenerative), age of the tear (fresh vs. chronic with secondary changes), size (partial to massive), and number of tendons involved (single, multiple to massive). The Patte classification **(Box 1)** is the most elaborated system and includes anatomic and pathologic considerations that are important for defining an individual treatment plan for each patient. Full-thickness tears are 1.5 and 4 times more likely to propagate compared to partial-tears and muscle degeneration is also much more common in them. It is also seen that tear propagation is a significant risk factor for pain development and as can be logically drawn the more severe the tear type the higher is the incidence of pain.

Investigations

Detailed discussion on investigations, their utility, and significance has been done in the Chapter on "Imaging of Shoulder Joint" previously, the following only provides a summary. Radiographs (AP in internal and external rotation, scapular Y-view) are usually unremarkable but may show subtle or prominent (depending on duration) greater tuberosity sclerosis, subacromial spurs or sclerosis (sourcil sign, **Figs. 7A and B**), and narrowing of the acromiohumeral distance. Glenohumeral arthritis should also be noted. Few patients may show a type 2 or type 3 acromion which has no bearing on the intensity of the symptoms. Cuff tear arthropathy **(Figs. 8A and B)** obviously tells long-standing disorder. Rotator cuff arthropathy is described in detail in Chapter on "Osteoarthritis of Shoulder Joint". CT scan is useful particularly for its ability to grade tears based on the Goutallier grading system **(Table 2)** which describes grades consequent to muscle fatty infiltration. A higher preoperative degree (≥grade 3) is associated with recurrent tears and lower constant scores. MRI is an excellent method to confirm the diagnosis and the extent of involvement for a rotator cuff tear images shows hyperintense signals of the supraspinatus tendon in T2-weighted images. MR arthrogram is beneficial

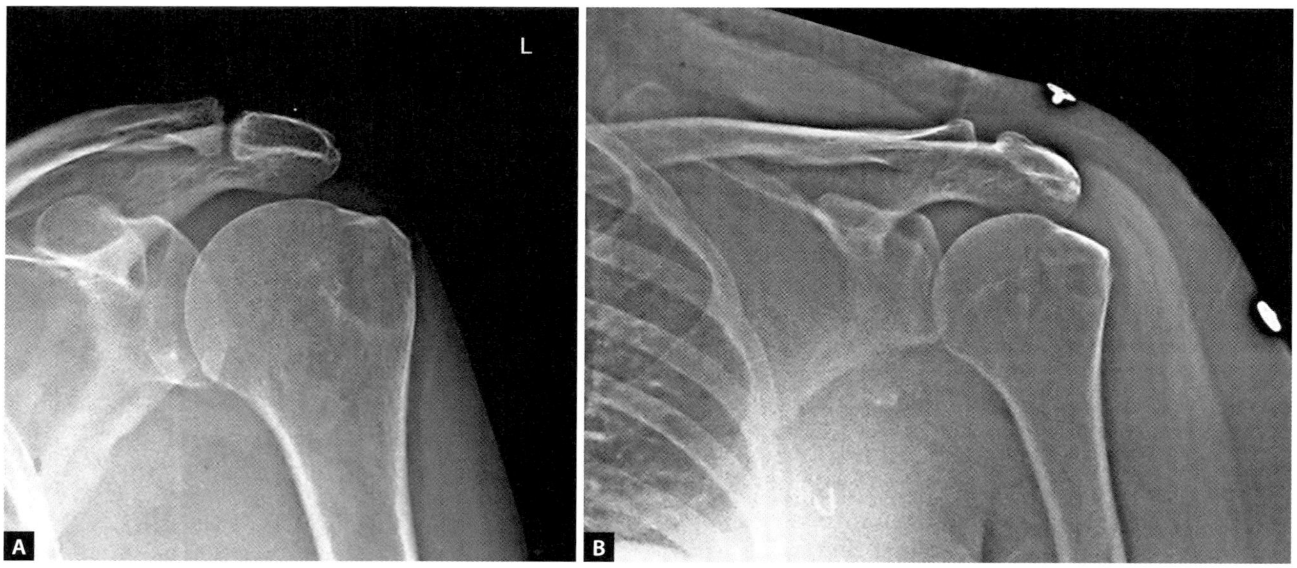

Figs. 7A and B: Radiograph showing the sourcil sign (A) visible as a sclerosis of the inferior aspect of the acromion, and reverse sourcil sign (B) visible as a sclerosis over the greater tuberosity near insertion of rotator cuff. With experience, it seems that reverse sourcil sign better predicts the rotator cuff lesions.

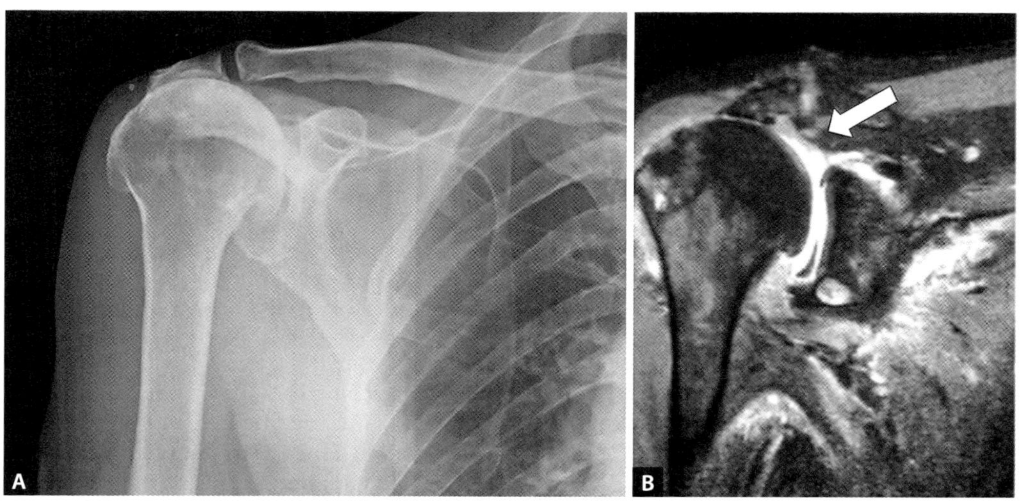

Figs. 8A and B: Rotator cuff arthropathy. Radiograph showing superior migration of the rotator cuff impinging directly on the acromion and eroding the same (A). MRI scan of the patient showing advanced rotator cuff arthropathy (B) with superior migration of humeral head and erosion of acromion. The rotator cuff is crumpled medially (arrow).

TABLE 2: Goutallier classification for fatty infiltration of muscle.

Grade	*Finding on CT scan*
0	No fat within muscle
1	Some fatty streaks
2	Fat < muscle
3	Fat = muscle
4	Fat > muscle

for detecting small, full-thickness tears, and depicting the extent of partial articular-sided tears. Ultrasound is an accurate, highly user-dependent, noninvasive, and less expensive method of detecting rotator cuff tears. It can be as useful as MRI but requires a highly experienced person.

TREATMENT OF SUBACROMIAL IMPINGEMENT SYNDROME AND ROTATOR CUFF LESIONS

Depending on the demands and activity level in relation to the self-perceived disability, conservative or operative treatment is offered to the patient. Operative treatment (especially arthroscopic) has been refined and significant progress has been made so that the conventional notion of preferable conservative treatment has mitigated. There are few circumstances where the conservative management suffices and, in fact, can also serve to prevent progress. In this respect, conservative therapy is best suited for patients having cuff symptoms with incomplete (partial thickness) tears. Partial-thickness RC tear progresses slowly compared to full-thickness RC tear providing adequate time for nonsurgical dedicated rehabilitative treatment to provide improvement without risk of terminal degeneration. This includes rest, activity modification, gentle passive and active motion exercises, anti-inflammatory medication, and biological therapy like platelet-rich plasma injection **(Box 2)**. Nonsteroidal anti-inflammatory drugs, physical therapy which includes the ultrasound massage and cryotherapy should be liberally used, especially in the Stage I of SIS. Scapular and rotator cuff exercises, neuromuscular training exercises, and plyometric exercises will build the muscles around the shoulder girdle and are appropriate in Stage II of SIS. This is usually effectively combined with passive joint mobilization and ROM. Conservative management should always include training for proper use and strengthening of core body and shoulder girdle musculature, and avoidance of aggravating activities that helps in preventing tear progression. Operative management is prescribed for patients whose symptoms are not relieved by above conservative measures for a minimum of 2–3 months, or for those who have a full-thickness symptomatic rotator cuff tear. Some partial-thickness tears are precarious for progression and may not be amenable to conservative treatment. The commonly relied "50% rule" as critical defect (this refers to footprint defect and not thickness of tear) is based on a classic 1999 article but may not be a suitable single measure to define the cut-off mark for deciding surgery. Instead surgical option may be preferred in a young and active patient with traumatic larger partial-thickness RC tear without any medical complications. For patients

BOX 2: Conservative management of rotator cuff tears/pathology.

One should consider a combination of modalities individually in the conservative management of rotator cuff pathology.
- *Obtaining pain relief:*
  - Avoid pain aggravating/producing movements
  - Nonsteroidal anti-inflammatory drugs or a combination of paracetamol and low dose narcotic analgesic
  - Physiotherapy including physical modalities
  - Subacromial platelet-rich plasma injection
  - Bupivacaine suprascapular nerve block—identify the patients properly, better to locate the notch ultrasonologically than a blind procedure
- *Improvement of joint motion and function:*
  - Stretching exercises
  - Restoring the scapulohumeral rhythm by physical therapy of parascapular and scapula-stabilizer muscles
  - Restoration of strength of the rotator cuff muscles
- *Improving proprioception:* Proprioceptive exercises must complement strengthening exercises especially in young individuals

of impingement syndrome and partial thickness of RC tear that failed with conservative management, surgical treatment gives good results.

Surgical Management of Partial-thickness Rotator Cuff Tears

For managing partial-thickness RC tear, there are three primary options discussed here.

Debridement and Acromioplasty

Subacromial decompression can be done by open or arthroscopic methods. The principles of surgery include removal of the subacromial bursa and removal of any bony spurs and, at times, the coracoacromial ligament. It should be considered in small articular side tears in elderly patients with low-risk of progression. The results are good in 90% patients at 1 year but failure is seen in bursal-sided large-sized tears. One must consider other modalities more strongly in younger patients because isolated debridement does little to prevent tear progression.

In Situ Repair

This is the most common addendum to acromioplasty as it has shown superior properties in cyclic loading and load to failure in biomechanical studies.

Completion of Tear and Proceeding with Repair as in Full-thickness of Rotator Cuff Tear

Repair with tear completion and transtendinous repair have produced good and excellent results, similar to in situ repairs. Completing a partial tear may sound unethical but it improves the geometry and margins can be better freshened to stimulate biology as proposed by proponents. There is no difference between this technique and in situ repair technique.

Surgical Treatment Options for Full-thickness of Rotator Cuff Tear

Surgical repair of rotator cuff tears can be performed through open, arthroscopically assisted mini-open, or all-arthroscopic techniques. Various anatomic types and

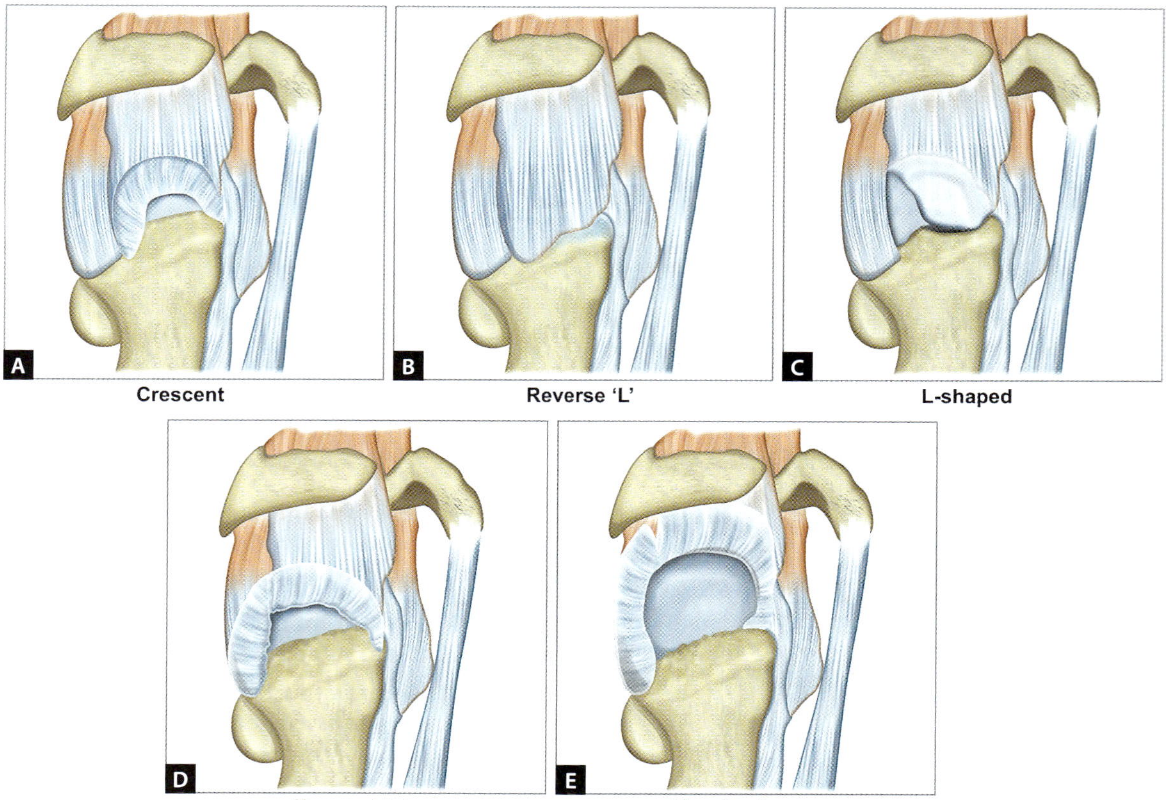

Figs. 9A to E: Rotator cuff tears (illustration). The shape of tears determines the tear type in Ellman classification for full-thickness rotator cuff tears.

configuration patterns of tears have been described **(Figs. 9A to E)** but they are not helpful in defining the treatment. Acromioplasty and subacromial decompression are usual accompaniments to relieve pressure on the cuff preserving deltoid function. Current evidence demonstrates no benefit of adding acromioplasty routinely with arthroscopic RC repairs and there is a trend of moving away from performing acromioplasties nowadays.

Open Rotator Cuff Repair

A diagnostic arthroscopy is recommended to be performed before open repair as restaging and visual examination often differs from the clinical and imaging picture.

Also concomitant pathologies can be simultaneously identified. In large and massive tears **(Fig. 10)**, the degree of glenohumeral arthritis may be more severe than suggested by preoperative evaluation precluding repair. Typically, the biceps tendon pathology (subluxation, fraying, tenosynovitis, and insertional detachment, or hypertrophy) is not appreciated well on imaging and needs proper addressal in the form of tenodesis or tenotomy as the case may be. Skin incisions are planned with respect to addressing all current pathologies (including massive tears) and keeping in mind the future requirements of revision surgery including arthroplasty. An oblique incision from the posterior edge of the AC joint to the anterolateral corner of the acromion that extends 2–3 cm distally between the anterior and middle deltoid provides excellent visualization for cuff repair

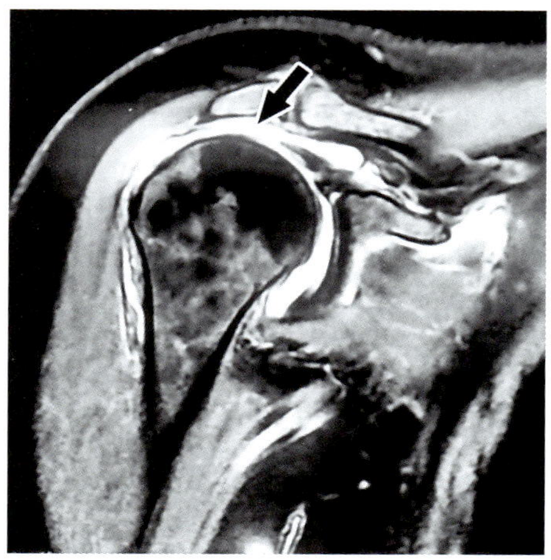

Fig. 10: MRI of a patient with massive tear of rotator cuff (block arrow in the tear region) and significant functional deficit needing repair.

(simultaneously also it allows for anterosuperior access for revision surgery including reverse shoulder arthroplasty). With open repair, the arthroscopic portals should be closed and the shoulder draped again to prevent infection. Often a distal clavicle resection and acromioplasty and subacromial bursectomy is added to improve access to the subacromial space without compromising deltoid anatomy. The coracohumeral ligament is palpated in external rotation, adduction, and released if it is tight. This gives excellent exposure to the rotator cuff pathology for evaluation, mobilization, and repair. The open repair technique has been summarized in **Figures 11 to 14**. Open RC repair with transosseous sutures provides the best stability for construct. Other techniques are compared to this transosseous repair. The deltoid should be meticulously repaired.

Arthroscopic Repair

Arthroscopic rotator cuff surgery as stated above has become increasingly popular and more standardized. Arthroscopy allows much better diagnostic evaluation of the intra-articular and extra-articular pathology that opens technique. It also allows easier management of associated pathologies. With improved techniques and training, the surgeons have been able to match the repair strength of open repairs with lesser complications. Beach chair and lateral positions are both equivalent for RC repair where the former allows for easier conversion to open procedure if needed but is associated with risk of reduced cerebral perfusion. The risk can be mitigated if mean arterial pressure of 60 mm Hg is maintained at the level of brain in normal individuals else in higher risk individuals 80 mm Hg is recommended.

There are many described techniques and configurations for fixation of torn cuff to bone **(Fig. 15)**. They have evolved over time to improve outcomes and reduce failure. The controversy of single-row versus double-row repair is unsettled by and large. Double-row fixation is costly, time-consuming, and technically more difficult when performed arthroscopically but, biomechanically, has higher initial fixation strength and stiffness, improved footprint restoration, and decreased gap formation. It is suggested that for larger tears (>3 cm), double-row fixation may be better as recent studies have reported higher American Shoulder and Elbow Surgeon Shoulder Score (ASES) and constant scores with double-row fixation in tears larger than 3 cm. Also better healing has been demonstrated with CT arthrography following double-row fixation but clinical superiority for

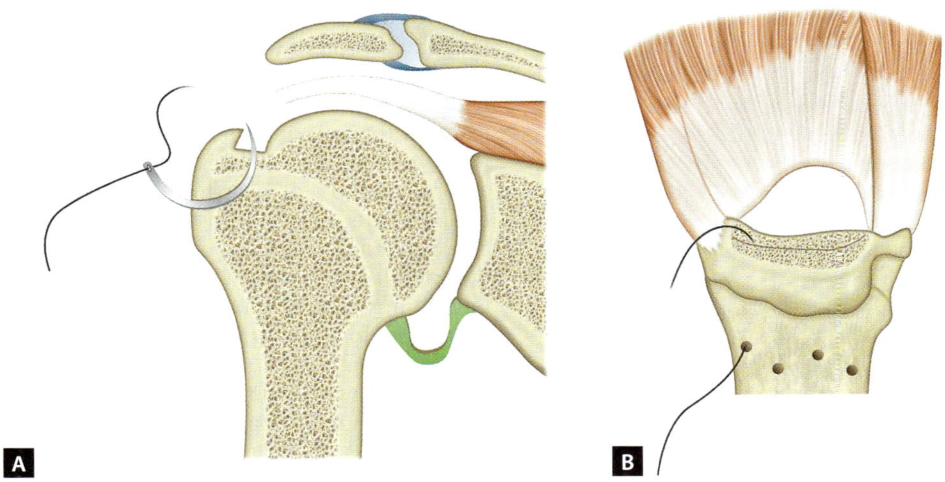

Figs. 11A and B: Mini-open rotator cuff repair. The cuff is mobilized and notch made into the greater tuberosity to position the cuff for attachment site. The drill holes are made onto the greater tuberosity and needle passed across and through the cuff.

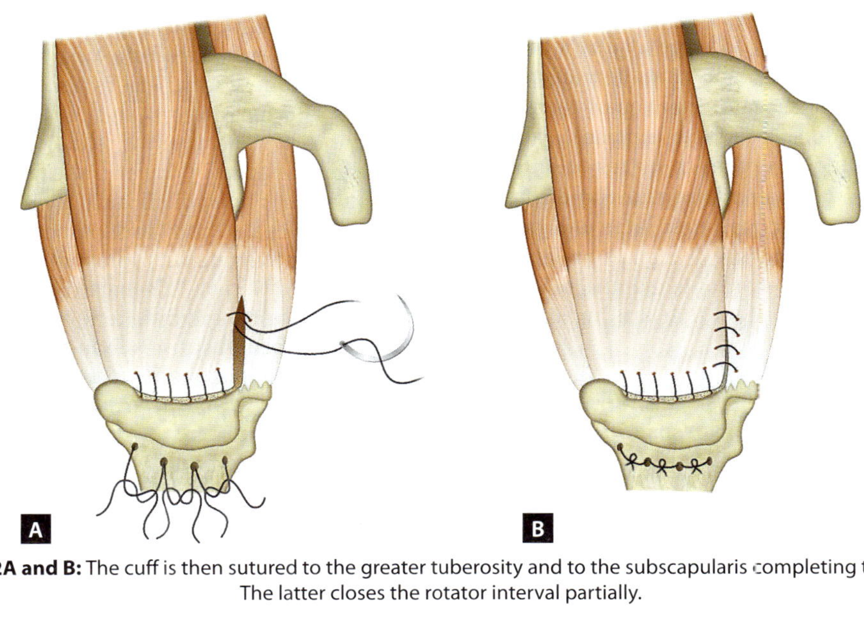

Figs. 12A and B: The cuff is then sutured to the greater tuberosity and to the subscapularis completing the repair. The latter closes the rotator interval partially.

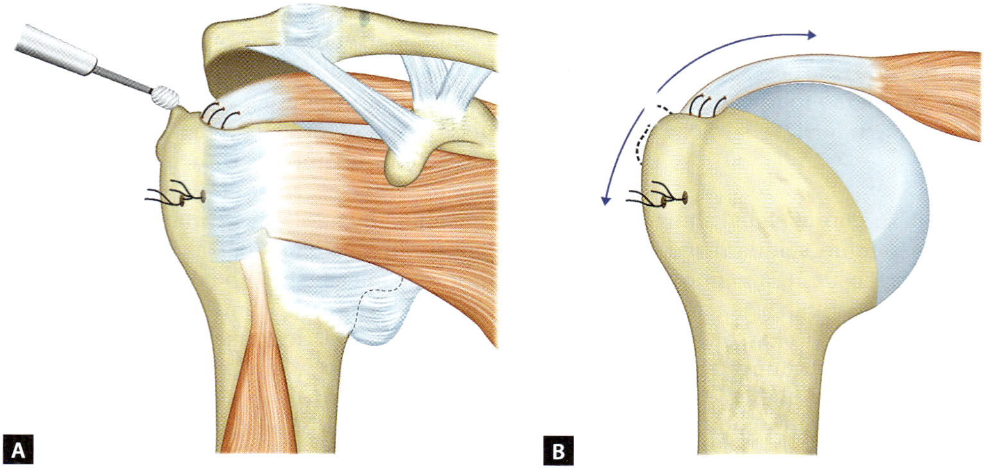

Figs. 13A and B: The greater tuberosity is shaved to smoothen the excrescences formed while notching the insertion site.

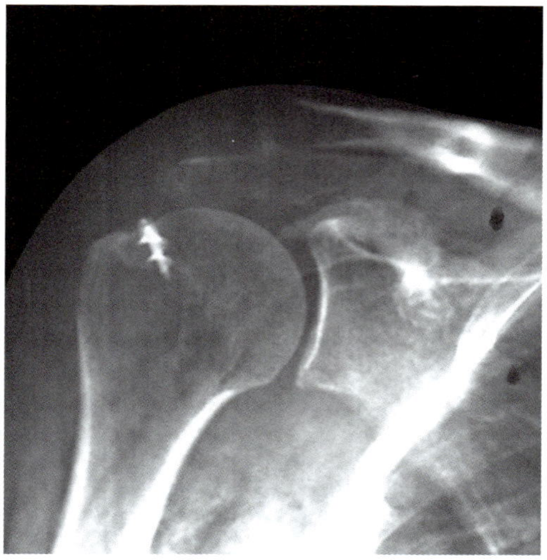

Fig. 14: A better way is to suture the rotator cuff back at footprint is by using titanium anchor. This allows repair to be done faster and with a smaller incision.

smaller tears is unsubstantiated for smaller tears between the two methods. Further, it is notable that the transosseous and transosseous equivalent rotator cuff repair techniques produce low bone-tendon interface motion, excellent footprint restoration, a high number of cycles to failure in biomechanical and clinical evaluations and could improve the current repair technique scenario for large and massive tears but are technically demanding. They are preferred for cuff tears that can be adequately mobilized and reattached to bone (through anchors) or tears that are juxtaposed to tuberosity.

Management of Massive Rotator Cuff Tears

There are yet instances where tears are so large and massive that repair is not possible with standard methods. For such cases, especially in young patients or active individuals with higher functional demands, *tendon transfers* are a viable option to reduce pain and restore function. Latissimus dorsi tendon transfer is recommended for patients with an intact subscapularis, an irreparable, painful posterosuperior rotator cuff tear with external rotation deficit. Though grade 2 or less fatty infiltration of the teres minor on preoperative imaging is ideal condition but satisfactory results are reported even with teres minor dysfunction. The tendon transfer improves external rotation and forward flexion. The pectoralis major tendon transfer is designed for treating symptomatic anterosuperior tears with an irreparable subscapularis tendon. The tendon transfer is commonly done over the conjoint tendon whereas underneath repairs have also been described. Interestingly like the confounding influence of teres minor on latissimus dorsi tendon transfer, an irreparable supraspinatous tear produces worse outcome with pectoralis major transfer so it should be concomitantly addressed. Pectoralis major transfer can be done for irreparable anterosuperior RC tear. One technique involves transfer of the pectoralis tendon over conjoint tendon while in other the sternal component is split and tendon passed under conjoint tendon. Both the techniques seem to be equally effective but the latter procedure is technically challenging. For chronic subscapularis tear, transfer of latissimus dorsi and teres major to lesser tuberosity is proposed. The technique is safer and the pull of transferred muscles provides better anterior to posterior moment arm. This is also a phasic transfer (all are shoulder internal rotators) and can be done arthroscopically. Irreparable posterosuperior tears (infraspinatus tears) may be better managed by lower trapezius tendon transfer. The disadvantage is need of allograft for reconstruction.

Partial repair and margin convergence is another approach for irreparable supraspinatus tears. The tendinous segments of "U"- or "L"-shaped tears are first sutured to converge margins and then tendon edge to tuberosity repair is done. The former sutures reduce strain on the latter repair. For massive supraspinatus tears if posterior force couple is restorable then at least partial repair of the supraspinatus tendon should be done.

The other approach is *"smooth and move"* of Matsen where the irregularities in the scapulohumeral space are smoothened by debridement and decompression and patient mobilized immediately to prevent adhesion formation. The procedure is well suited in a motivated

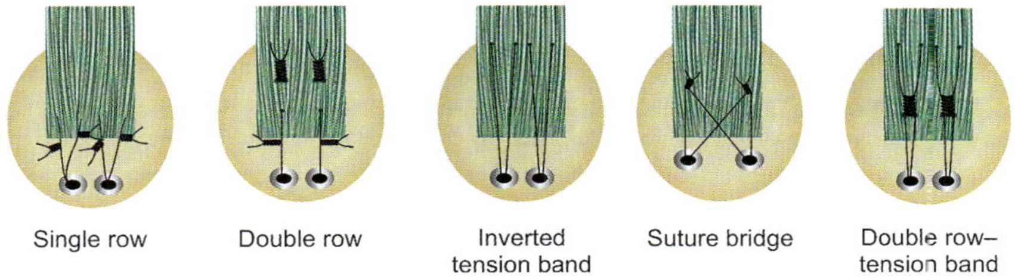

Fig. 15: The various methods for fixation and repair of rotator cuff to bone footprint. The double-row techniques are biomechanically superior but no distinctive advantage has been seen in small- to medium-sized tears.

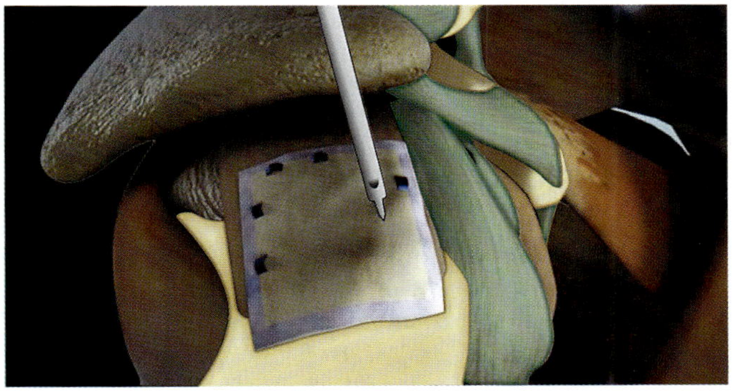

Fig. 16: Large massive rotator cuff tears frequently fail with standard techniques of repair, so augmentation of the repair site is done with collagen synthetic or allografts to improve repair strength.

patient with symptoms of pain, crepitus, and stiffness associated with an irreparable tear or a failed prior repair. The shoulder is approached as for mini-open repair and the hypertrophic bursa and adhesions between the cuff and acromion are removed and uneven surfaces under acromion and prominence of the greater tuberosity are smoothened. Additionally rough superior surface of the rotator cuff, frayed edges of torn tendons, residual suture anchors, etc. are cleaned. Fukuda-lite test with saline (injected into the joint to inflate the joint and assess the cuff integrity, methylene blue previously used may cause chondrolysis) can be performed to evaluate shoulders with suspicious cuff integrity. Coracohumeral ligament should be preserved to prevent anterosuperior escape. Patient should be encouraged to immediately undergo shoulder mobilization and strengthening program to prevent adhesion formation.

Reconstruction of superior shoulder capsule to provide stability to chronic massive irreparable cuff tears is also being explored. It is logical that large and massive tears have high failure rates (up to 94% at 1 year) with standard techniques so *augmentation techniques* are yet another tool to strengthen the repair techniques. The recurrent tears are currently managed with augmentation; however, it is recommended to augment large and massive tear primary repair with allograft or xenograft tissues to improve repair strength and provide a bioreplaceable collagen network in an effort to decrease failure rates **(Fig. 16)**. Human dermal allograft is possibly the best method (not available in India currently) as porcine dermis, and porcine smooth intestine submucosa has been found to induce adverse immunological graft reactions. Biodegradable spacers are being used in elderly patients with massive unrepairable RC tears to improve function. These spacers are placed in the subacromial space and inflated to reverse proximal humeral migration. This partially restores glenohumeral mechanics and improves glenohumeral abduction, external rotation, and elevation. Placement of the spacer is also simple and does not require extensive postoperative rehabilitation.

Postoperative Rehabilitation

Postoperative rehabilitation plays an important role and should be directed by the physician individually for the patients depending on the repair and requirement. In general, patients are maintained in a shoulder sling/immobilizer with an abduction pillow to keep arm in approximately 20–30° of abduction. This takes tension off the repair. Conventionally, passive-assisted forward elevation and external rotation are started immediately but internal rotation is delayed for 3–6 weeks (depending on size of initial tear, higher for larger tears). Active motion is started at around 6 weeks while resistive motion is added after assessing individual's progress, usually at 10 weeks. Recently, a decelerated protocol has been utilized to reduce the chances of recurrent tears in an effort to improve tendon healing. This, particularly, delays the initial passive elevation and external rotation for few days to couple of weeks.

Role of Biceps Tendon

Long head of biceps tendon often becomes painful in chronic RC pathology and inflammatory conditions (like rheumatoid arthritis). Isolated tears of long head biceps tendon are usually not operated if Popeye deformity is acceptable to patient. Only in patients not tolerating deformity or tear in a young laborer in dominant arm needing good strength for work, surgical tenodesis is done. In patients undergoing SLAP or RC repair suprapectoral tenodesis **(Figs. 17A to E)** may be done if full supination strength and endurance is needed. Otherwise in such patients with painful tendonitis arthroscopic tenotomy may suffice though there are 30% chances of formation of Popeye deformity. If the pathology lies in the biceps groove then it is better to do arthroscopic or open subpectoral tenodesis fixing the tendon with one of the methods, viz., bone sutures, anchors, screw, or button.

Complications of Rotator Cuff Repair

The following is a list of common complications of standard RC repair that should be borne in mind during counseling patients and performing surgical procedure so that they can best be avoided:

- *Recurrent RC tear:* This is the most common issue following RC repair. The most important factors

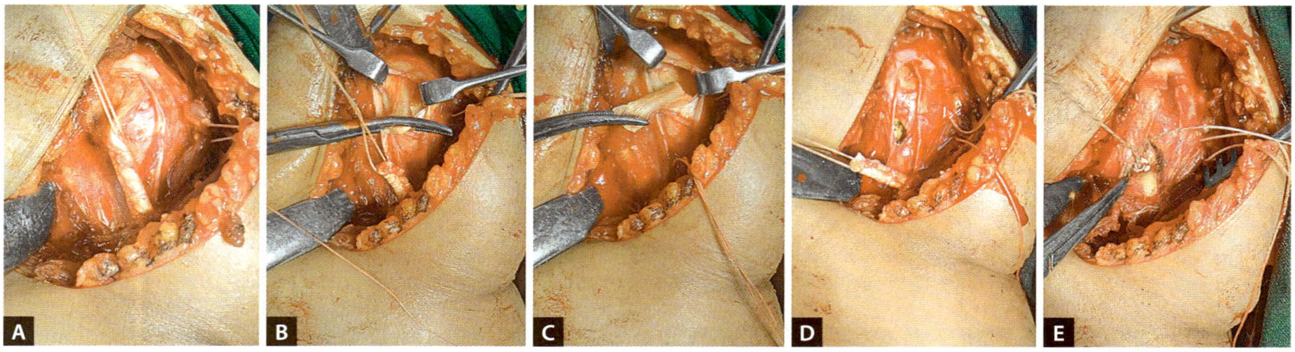

Figs. 17A to E: The biceps tendon is tenodesed if diseased and symptomatic. The tendon is exposed (A) and distal part prepared by braiding strong sutures. Cut at appropriate site is made (B) and proximal stump excised (C). The site for fixing biceps tendon is marked (D) and tendon fixed using tenodesis anchor (E).

associated with this is individual's age. Retear is rare in younger patients with increase in 5% per decade after 50 years and is very high (>35%) in patients >80 years of age.

- *Shoulder stiffness and arthrofibrosis:* Stiffness is seen in 10% patients after RC repair where 3% may need some surgical release for improving function.
- Slow return to function
- Implant loosening
- Neurovascular injury
- Thromboembolic events
- Deep infection
- Development of complex regional pain syndrome type 1

CONCLUSION

- Involvement of structures in subacromial space is a common source of morbidity and pain.
- Involvement of rotator cuff affects the function of shoulder joint and in later stages makes it nearly "pseudoparalyzed".
- Outlet impingement and posterior glenohumeral impingement are commonly missed or ignored conditions that should be carefully looked for and addressed.
- Mini-open repair of rotator cuff with transosseous repair was considered gold-standard but development of improved arthroscopic techniques have outsmart the open methods.

CHAPTER 58

Shoulder Instability

Manish Kumar Varshney

INTRODUCTION

The shoulder joint is precariously unstable due to its high mobility and low congruence. Excessive movements beyond permissible limits would compromise one or more static or dynamic stabilizers (*see* Chapter on "Shoulder: Functional Anatomy") resulting in instability of the joint in that direction. Over a period the shoulder instability becomes a broad and complex pathoanatomy generally classified by direction **(Table 1)**. The reader is encouraged to refresh the knowledge on anatomical restraints and shoulder biomechanics and a thorough understanding of imaging of shoulder instability discussed in previous chapters.

It has been a task to define instability of shoulder and different experts have given various descriptions, all of which incorporate excessive glenohumeral (GH) translation and inability to maintain the functional relationship with applied physiological loads.

TABLE 1: Common terminologies used in description of various types of shoulder instabilities.

Pathoanatomic term	***Comment***
Bankart lesion	Anteroinferior capsulolabral tear
Bony Bankart	Bankart + Glenoid rim fracture
Reverse Bankart	Posterior/posteroinferior capsulolabral tear
ALPSA (anterior labroligamentous periosteal sleeve avulsion) lesion	Anteroinferior Bankart lesion that heals on the glenoid neck medially
GLAD (Glenolabral articular disruption) lesion	Shear injury involving articular cartilage
HAGL (Humeral avulsion of glenohumeral ligament)	It is a failure of capsule at the humeral side where the capsuloligamentous structures tear near humerus
Kim lesion	Describes an incomplete posteroinferior labral tear or a posterior labral crack
Hill–Sachs lesion	Posterosuperior humeral head impaction defect
Reverse Hill–Sachs lesion	Anterior/anterosuperior humeral head impaction defect

The different types of shoulder instability:

	Anterior	***Posterior***	***Multidirectional***
History	Trauma to externally rotated abducted arm	Aches or clicks in shoulder on FADIR (flexion, adduction, and internal rotation). Microtrauma commonly. Acute trauma in flexed, adducted, and internally rotated arm. Following seizures or electrical shock	Vague activity related pain and dysfunction usually in overhead athletes
Clinical examination	Apprehension test, relocation test, load, and shift test	Posterior load and shift test, Jerk test, and apprehension test	Sulcus sign and ligamentous laxity
Imaging features	Bankart, Bony Bankart, Hill–Sachs lesion	Reverse Bankart and reverse bony Bankart, Kim lesion, and reverse Hill–Sachs lesion	Capsular laxity and increased intra-articular volume
Treatment and pitfalls	Physical therapy, arthroscopic capsulolabral repair, open repair, Remplissage, open augmentation, and glenoid bone reconstruction. Failure to recognize glenoid bone loss.	Conservative muscle strengthening program, arthroscopic capsulolabral repair and/or capsular plication, McLaughlin procedure, glenoid reconstruction. Missed diagnosis common	Muscle strengthening/stabilization program, Neer's capsular shift, arthroscopic capsular plication Failure to recognize connective tissue disorder, voluntary dislocation and unscrupulous advice to surgery

- Instability is defined as increased GH translation of the humeral head in relation to the glenoid and inability of the humeral head to remain centered in the glenoid fossa (Matsen).
- Instability is excessive symptomatic translation of the humeral head relative to glenoid articular surface during active motion (Allen).
- Instability is a pathologic condition that presents as pain or discomfort in association with excessive translation of humeral head on glenoid fossa during active shoulder motion (Cole and Warner).
- Instability is pain associated with shoulder dysfunction due to excessive translation of humeral head on glenoid fossa (Friedman).
- Instability is abnormal limit of motion associated with a functional deficit (dynamic instability) or subluxation/dislocation (static or dynamic instability). Dynamically unstable load configuration will be one in which an incremental load will cause pain and inability to continue the function (functional buckling). A statically unstable configuration and load state would be one in which an incremental increase in load leads to large displacements with subsequent subluxation or dislocation (Lew et al.).
- Instability is a condition of joint characterized by abnormal increased mobility secondary to ligaments, capsule or bone; when applied to shoulder, instability is typically used to describe a clinical condition characterized by physical signs and symptoms of increased or excessive displacement of the GH joint (Rodkey et al.).

All definitions involve some pathological displacement/translation of glenohumeral joint. The amount of translation can range from mild subluxation to complete dislocation.

- *Dislocation* of the GH joint is complete separation of the articular surfaces (spontaneous relocation usually does not occur).
- *Subluxation* is defined as symptomatic translation of the humeral head on the glenoid without complete separation of the articular surfaces; it is usually transient and the humeral head returns spontaneously to its normal position in the glenoid fossa.
- *Apprehension* refers to the fear that the shoulder will subluxate or dislocate but may not necessarily so.
- *Laxity* is the physiologic motion of the GH joint that allows a normal range of motion (ROM). It is normally asymptomatic and not synonymous with instability.

Shoulder instability is a spectrum of disorder that can be classified into categories with respect to the timing (acute vs. chronic or locked shoulder), etiology [congenital (Ehlers-Danlos syndrome, glenoid dysplasia) vs. traumatic vs. atraumatic colloquially called "born loose", "torn loose", or "worn loose"], conditioning (voluntary vs. involuntary), direction of instability, severity (mild, moderate, and severe), frequency (solitary, frequent, and recurrent), static versus dynamic, bilateralism, etc. Instability can be acute or insidious in onset, can occur after a single traumatic event (acute), or can be the result of repetitive microtrauma (chronic). Instability can occur in a single plane (unidirectional—anterior or posterior) or in multiple directions (multiplanar). Matsen's classification of instability into traumatic unidirectional Bankart surgery (TUBS) and atraumatic multidirectional bilateral rehabilitation inferior capsular shift (AMBRI) pattern is very useful, especially as it correlates the etiopathogenic events. But, these possibly represent the extreme ends of the spectrum of disorders and patients often seem to lie "in-between". Frequency, etiology, direction, and severity (FEDS) classification attempts to incorporate most of the above parameters to classify GH instability **(Box 1)**. The surgical management perspective has become so specific these days that often the surgeons talk of predominantly anterior and posterior instability that requires specific repair/reconstruction or multidirectional instability (MDI) requiring an altogether different approach to management. So, we will use and discuss the instability by dividing it under the two groups:

- *Unidirectional:* Anterior, posterior, inferior, or superior.
- *Multidirectional:*
  - With primary structural changes
  - Without structural changes but with muscular dyskinesia

BOX 1: FEDS (frequency, etiology, direction, and severity)—classification of shoulder instability.

Frequency:
- Solitary (1 episode)
- Frequent (2–5 episodes)
- Recurrent (>5 episodes)

Etiology:
- *Traumatic:* History of injury
- *Atraumatic:* No history of injury

Direction (determined by provocative testing):
- Anterior
- Inferior
- Posterior

Severity:
- *Subluxation:* Reduced without help
- *Dislocation:* Help needed to reduce

Recurrent instability can be initiated with or coexist with acute event. Recurrent inferior and superior events are uncommon but recurrent inferior instability has now been recognized as a hallmark of MDI.

ANTERIOR INSTABILITY

Traumatic anterior shoulder instability often results following shoulder dislocation; a brief introduction of shoulder dislocation, hence, is hereby presented. Anterior dislocation of the shoulder **(Fig. 1)** is most common so also is the anterior subluxation. Glenohumeral joint is most susceptible to dislocation in 90° abduction and 90° of external rotation as dynamic support and ligament stabilization is minimal in this position. Subcoracoid dislocation is the most common form resulting from humerus abduction, external rotation, and extension. With increased force of dislocation, the humeral head may lie (and is sometimes used for classifying dislocation) into subglenoid, subclavicular position and rarely intrathoracic, and even retroperitoneal dislocations have been described. Inferior dislocation results from hyperabduction force with the shaft

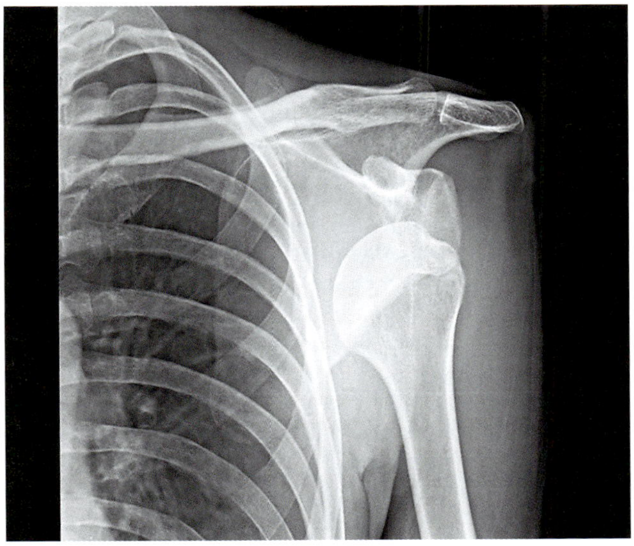

Fig. 1: Radiograph of anterior dislocation of humeral head (note how anterior glenoid rim abuts against humeral head to cause impression fracture).

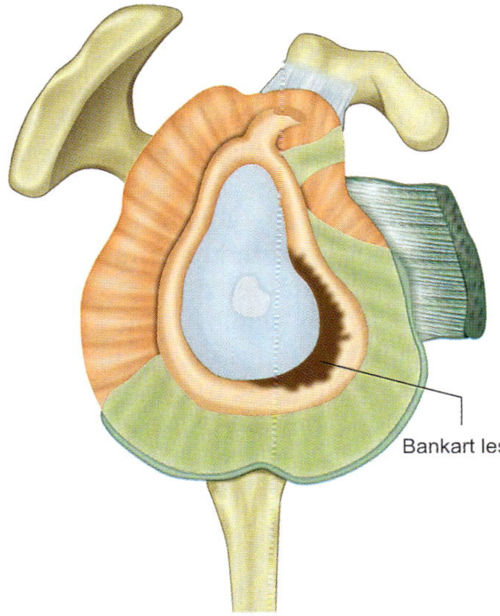

Fig. 3: The illustration for Bankart lesion as viewed end on, typically involving the anteroinferior portion of the glenoid labrum.

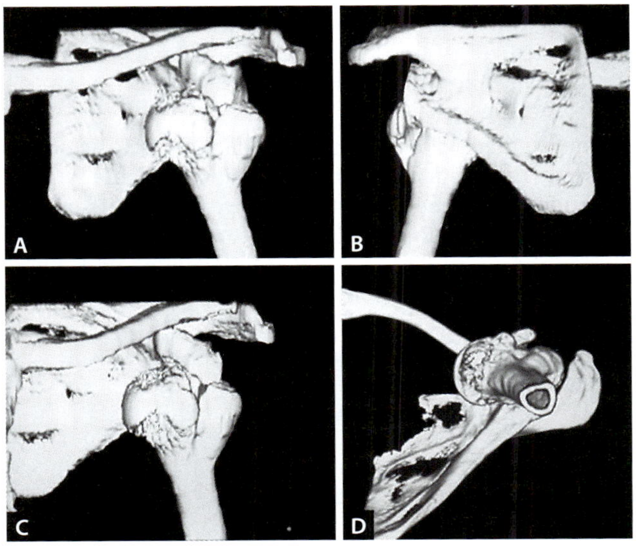

Figs. 2A to D: Noncontrast computed tomography (NCCT) of shoulder depicting the fracture dislocation of the shoulder joint in various views (A—Anterolateral, B—Posterior, C—Anterior, D—Inferior). Such cases have unfavorable prognosis if repaired, however, they do well if managed with arthroplasty particularly due to the fact that cuff tendons are relatively preserved due to absorption of major trauma force by the bone.

of humerus pointing overhead—a condition called "luxatio erecta". Severe high energy injuries with head pouting out of axilla due to skin breach and avulsion of pectoralis major, capsule and subscapularis may be seen. Superior dislocation occurs from severe forward and upward force on an adducted arm which is usually associated with fracture of acromion, acromioclavicular (AC) joint, clavicle or humeral tuberosities **(Figs. 2A to D)**. The earliest report of anterior dislocation is mentioned from the papyrus (3000-2500 BC) and nearly all the famous authors including Hippocrates and Perthes have described the lesion and various methods of treatment. Hippocrates described the lesion in lucid detail and criticized the then prevailing "burning" techniques of shoulder to reduce capsular volume by poking rods in various directions that caused complications. His surgical technique was to burn the inferior part of capsule using red hot oblong iron rod. Anatomical details of posterolateral humeral head defects (Hill-Sachs lesion described first by Flower) and capsular and labro-periosteal-ligamentous defects (Bankart lesion) then followed in detail.

Pathoanatomy and Development of Instability

The anterior band of the inferior glenohumeral ligament (IGHL) is the primary stabilizer that limits anterior translation in 90° of abduction. Perthes and Bankart described the detachment of this intra-articular ligament from the anterior glenoid rim as the typical lesion found in recurrent anterior dislocation **(Figs. 3 and 4)**. With anterior dislocation specific pathology develops in the anterior aspect of shoulder. All these lesions result into recurrent dislocation and instability in different patients.

- The detachment of labrum from anterior glenoid (Bankart lesion) is common to most if not all. The Bankart's lesion is seen in 87–100% of initial dislocation.
- The Bony Bankart lesion (a piece of glenoid fractures along with the ligamento-labrocapsular complex; **Figs. 5A and B**) called the glenolabral articular disruption lesion.
- *Anterior labroligamentous periosteal sleeve avulsion (ALPSA):* ALPSA results from healing of Bankart lesion to medial glenoid and is more often a feature of recurrent instability.
- *Bankart lesion associated with superior labrum anterior and posterior (SLAP) (Taylor and Arciero):* They result

from a more extreme trauma and can be seen both in acute and recurrent instability.

- *Superior labrum anterior cuff (SLAC) lesion:* This is superior labrum anterior cuff lesion in which the anterior supraspinatus exhibits a partial or complete tear resulting from instability.
- *Humeral avulsion of glenohumeral ligament (HAGL):* Capsuloligamentous stretching and detachment of capsule/ligament from humerus
- *Massive rotator-cuff tear* seen by Robinson et al. is cited by him as an important cause of recurrent dislocation of shoulder. Apart from acute trauma, chronic recurrent strain or *stretching of anterior structures* also results in anterior instability despite absence of recurrent trauma but is uncommon to find. Though it may only rarely produce acute shoulder dislocation but it is commonly responsible for failure of anatomical repairs done for anterior instability.
- *Bony pathology seen with anterior dislocation shoulder:* Greater tuberosity fracture, glenoid rim fracture, and Hill–Sachs lesion (posterosuperior impaction fracture of humeral head; **Figs. 6A and B**) are found frequently. Other associated injuries include lesser tuberosity fracture and rotator-cuff tears (seen in 30% patients >40 years of age; 80% patients above 80 years of age). Rotator-cuff injury is responsible for development of arthritis in long run. For this reason, dislocations in patients younger than 25 years of age are protective against arthritis as rotator cuff is commonly spared.

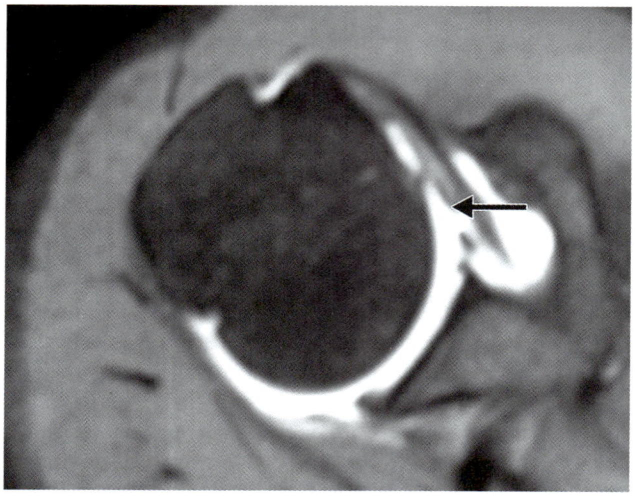

Fig. 4: The axial section of MRI of shoulder joint depicting the avulsion of the capsulolabral structures from the anterior aspect of glenoid rim and subluxed labrum fallen anteriorly (arrow).

Loss of 20–30% glenoid rim is associated with instability as is presence of large Hill–Sachs lesions in isolation. Glenoid bone loss is common in high-energy injury or if the arm is abducted >70° and/or extended >30° during dislocation. *Bipolar lesions*—combined anteroinferior bone loss and posterosuperior humeral head lesion are of interest in redislocations. Recurrent instability is responsible for attritional anteroinferior bone loss. It has been found that glenoid deficiency of as small as 2 mm may compromise labral repair if a moderate Hill–Sachs lesion is present due to "off-tracking".

The characteristics that increase chances of a dislocation becoming recurrent after acute dislocation include:

- Young age at first dislocation (<20 years); male sex
- Ease of dislocation with applied force (the less the force required to initially dislocate is associated with higher incidence of dislocation)

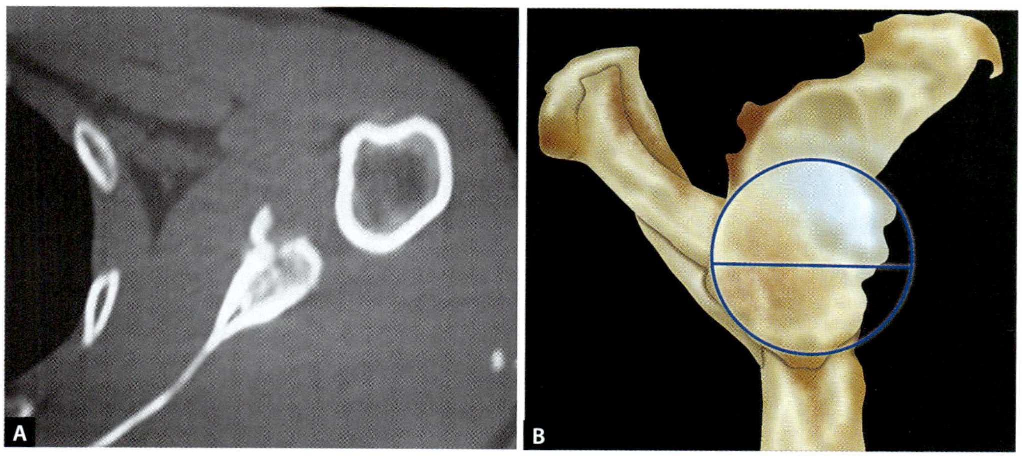

Figs. 5A and B: Bony Bankart lesion the noncontrast computed tomography (NCCT) showing anterior glenoid bone loss in recurrent dislocation of shoulder and measurement of bone loss can be better done in a three-dimensional (3D) reconstruction model (Illustration here). The commonly used technique uses the diameter of the "best-fit circle" circumscribed around the inferior glenoid. This circle is drawn around the inferior portion of the glenoid and defect can be measured either as percentage of anteroposterior glenoid width (diametric method) or as percentage of surface area. In the diametric method the linear bone defect is measured from anteriormost aspect of the circle to the anterior edge of the defective glenoid. This is then divided by the "diameter" of the circle to reveal the percentage width defect from the formula: Percent bone loss = (Defect width/Diameter of inferior glenoid circle) × 100%. Softwares also provide the surface area determination where the free-hand drawing is done for glenoid defect whose area is calculated by the software and it can be divided by the area of complete circle/ellipse to reveal area of glenoid bone loss. Arthroscopically Burkhart similarly determined the glenoid bone defect using the "bare spot" technique where the bare spot corresponded to the glenoid defect in an imaginary circle drawn circumscribing the inferior glenoid.

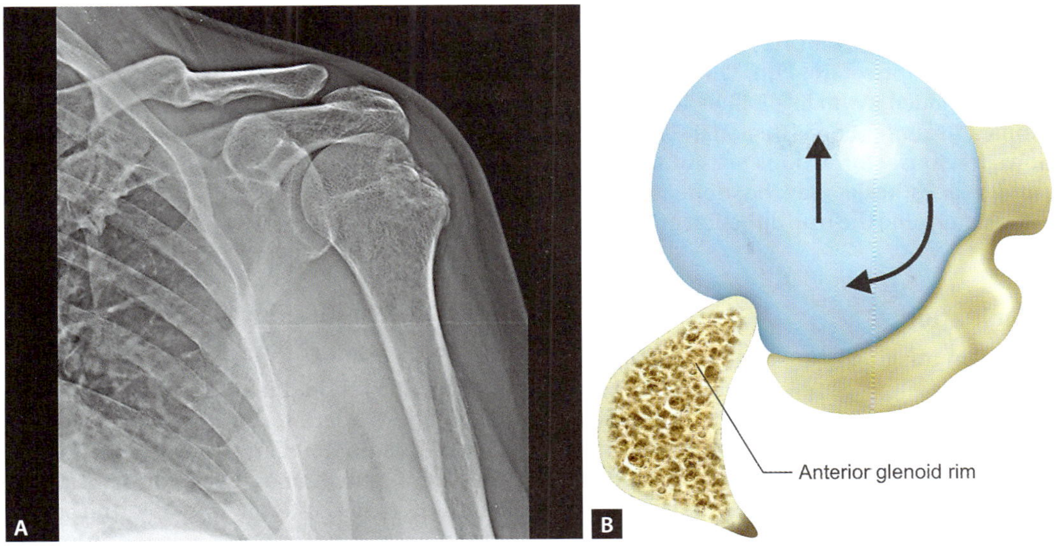

Figs. 6A and B: The radiograph demonstrating the Hill–Sachs lesion in a patient with reduced shoulder dislocation (A). Illustration of the Hill–Sachs lesion (B). The lesion is an impression fracture due to impaction of the anterior glenoid rim in the cancellous humeral head more prominent in delayed cases.

- Ligament hyperlaxity
- Possibly shorter time of immobilization (not proven)
- Presence of associated lesions as described above. Bipolar lesions should be especially considered in this setting.

Preoperative MRI scan of the shoulder is helpful in detailed assessment of intra-articular pathology. Sometimes, bone defects in the glenoid can only be detected and quantified better with a CT scan with three-dimensional (3D) reconstruction of the glenoid. If specific bone-sensitive sequences are used then 3D MRI quantification of glenoid bone is possibly as good as a CT-based measurement.

Examination and Findings (See also the Chapter on "History and Clinical Examination")

Acute Anterior Dislocation (see also Table 1)

The patient has intense pain with characteristic posture of asymmetric deltoid bulge, presence of sharper shoulder contour, loss of external rotation and inability to adduct the limb. The limb lies in internal rotation and an adducted attitude. There is loss of abduction and external rotation, loss of deltoid contour, and prominent acromion on the dislocated side. The humeral head is palpable anteriorly and all movements are painful (if attempted). There may be palpable fullness below coracoid. Looking at the axillary fold it is lower on the affected side (Bryant's sign). Girth of shoulder (vertical axillary circumference) may be compared on the two sides which is increased on dislocated side (Callaway sign). If patient is asked to place the hand of affected extremity on opposite shoulder while trying to simultaneously touch the chest with elbow, he will be unable to do so (Dugas test). Radiographs are not needed if one is pretty sure; however, for litigation purpose people obtain the standard views to document a dislocation and presence of any fracture (like greater tuberosity). Also, mainly for litigation purpose neurological examination is done to document axillary nerve injury (rupture), suprascapular nerve injury (traction injury) and long thoracic nerve injury else they can be comfortably performed postreduction. Examine for vascular insult if present. In severe injuries (and also fracture-dislocations, intrathoracic dislocation; retroperitoneal dislocations) vascular injury may be seen as may be the injury to brachial plexus.

Recurrent Shoulder Instability

Young age at first dislocation is the most important risk factor for recurrence. Average recurrence rate approaches 50% in patients suffering from first dislocation in 15–30 years of age group. The complaint of a recurrent dislocation is usually of the shoulder "slipping" or "popping out" during overhead activities, especially external rotation and extension. The patient with recurrent subluxation describes a sudden catch, followed by sudden inability to move the arm with a "numb" feeling the so-called "dead arm syndrome" (the feeling of dead arm syndrome can also arise in SLAP lesion). Most patients with instability are athletic adolescents or young adults with joint laxity. Such individuals may have pain with overhead movements due to an inability to control their laxity by means of their muscles. They may develop enough instability directed superiorly that they present with impingement-like symptoms (instability-impingement overlap), especially in positions of abduction and external rotation. These patients have usually normal asymptomatic shoulder function until some event precipitates symptoms which is usually relatively minor (compared with traumatic causes of unidirectional instability), or repetitive microtrauma as occurs in gymnasts. The most common presenting complaint is pain. Loss of internal rotation in young patients may be an important finding suggestive of posterior capsular contracture that is often associated with subtle instability. Chronic recurrent dislocations of the shoulder can also lead to degenerative arthritis. An older person who dislocates a shoulder is likely to have concurrently torn the rotator cuff. The apprehension test typically identifies patients with instability [*see* Chapter on "History and Clinical Examination" (Regional Orthopedics: Shoulder section) previously for various tests of instability]. Examination under anesthesia may be done to identify unusual cases and determine the true direction of functional instability.

Radiological Evaluation

Detailed discussion on imaging of unstable shoulder is provided in Chapter on "Imaging of Shoulder Joint". Radiographs may be obtained to evaluate the bony lesion of anterior glenoid deficiency or Hill–Sachs lesion. Patients with engaging Hill–Sachs lesion and inverted pear-shaped glenoid have recurrence rate of 67%. Engaging Hill–Sachs lesions are those that lock and catch the humeral head in functional abduction and external rotation **(Figs. 7A to C)**. The problem is exaggerated in bipolar and off-track lesions. Computed tomography may be obtained in the following situations:

- Instability at markedly low abduction
- Marked apprehension at low abduction and external rotation
- Instability at little provocation of the maneuver
- Multiple instability events
- Revision surgery
- Bone loss detected on radiographs

Despite the fact that bone loss (anteroinferior glenoid; posterosuperior humeral head or both) is associated with recurrent instability; very few surgeons obtain a CT scan. I feel it is the gold standard for identification and quantification of bone loss especially 3D reconstruction in plane of glenoid surface **(Fig. 5B)**. Even the instability severity index score (ISIS) incorporates glenoid bone loss as one of the parameters for predicting recurrent instability. The correlation is typically strong with glenoid bone loss than humeral head defect. Frank recurrent dislocation rate increases in likelihood if AP glenoid defect measures >20% of glenoid length (corresponding to absolute glenoid articular surface area loss of 20–30%). Once the glenoid AP width reduces by 25% or more its shape changes to "inverted pear" (I strongly recommend going through Chapter on "Imaging of Shoulder Joint" for conceptual understanding).

MRI is the modality of choice to evaluate the soft tissue injuries including capsulolabral lesions, ligamentous, and rotator-cuff injuries. Adding intra-articular contrast (MR arthrogram) hastens the sensitivity to detect lesions significantly.

Treatment of Anterior Instability

First Time Shoulder Dislocators

The shoulder should be reduced as early as possible using one of the standard techniques described. The Hippocrates (described six different techniques but most commonly used was levering the humeral head into position over examiner heel placed just inferior to axilla and not within it) and Kocher's maneuver (maneuver in the order-traction, external rotation, flexion, internal rotation, and adduction to opposite shoulder, actually a confusing description where humeral head is levered against glenoid and shaft of humerus is levered against the chest wall) are older methods for shoulder relocation that have been nowadays fallen into disfavor due to higher associated complications of additional soft tissue and neurological injury. Especially the Kocher's method is quite confusing in its original description and is prone to cause fractures of humeral head and spiral fracture of shaft and also predisposes to recurrent dislocations. Various other methods such as the Legg maneuver, Eskimo technique, Manes method, Cunningham's method, Hennepin method, Stimson's maneuver, traction-countertraction, strap method, scapular manipulation, external rotation and Spaso technique are used by identified people. We prefer Milch technique **(Fig. 8)** in which the arm is gently abducted and further taken into overhead position; this eliminates all the cross forces on humerus. The humeral head is then gradually pushed over the glenoid into the socket. This should not be done if humeral head is incarcerated into anterior glenoid due to large Hill–Sachs lesion. Failure of closed reduction is uncommon but if fails then surgical reduction is imperative.

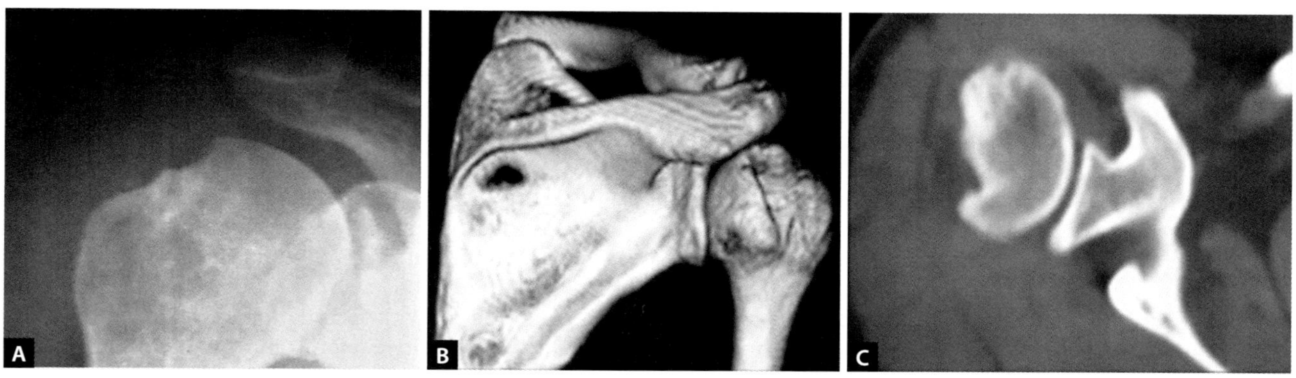

Figs. 7A to C: Engaging Hill–Sachs lesion involve usually >40% of the articular surface of humeral head as in this case. (A) Radiograph shows the abrupt end of humeral articular surface; (B) Three-dimensional (3D) reconstruction from noncontrast computed tomography (NCCT) shoulder; (C) Image showing the extent and plane of the lesion. These views are needed for planning reconstruction of the defect to ameliorate recurrent instability.

Patient's upper limb is immobilized for around 2–3 weeks (Itoi et al. found immobilization in neutral rotation or external rotation of 30° to be better and associated with much less incidence of recurrent dislocation as the Bankart lesion heals in well approximation; compliance is an issue however; **Fig. 9**). The finding of improved anatomical healing with external rotation has not however been reproduced in the literature elsewhere. The patient is allowed to return to activity if majority of the following criteria are met:

- Little or no pain
- Restoration of preinjury ROM
- Normal functional capacity
- If a sports person then sport specific skills

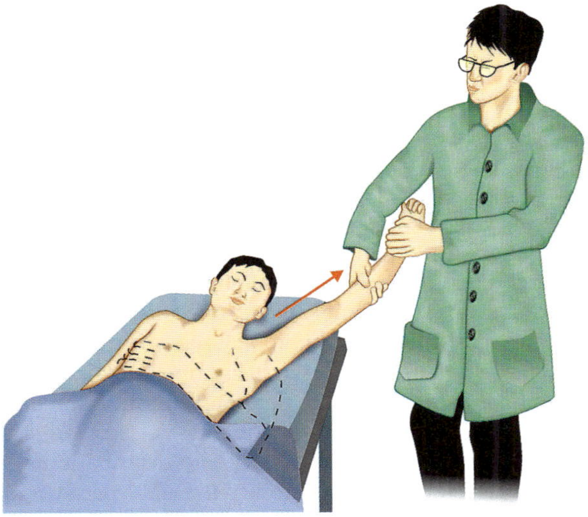

Fig. 8: Milch technique for reduction of the anterior glenohumeral dislocation (see text for description).

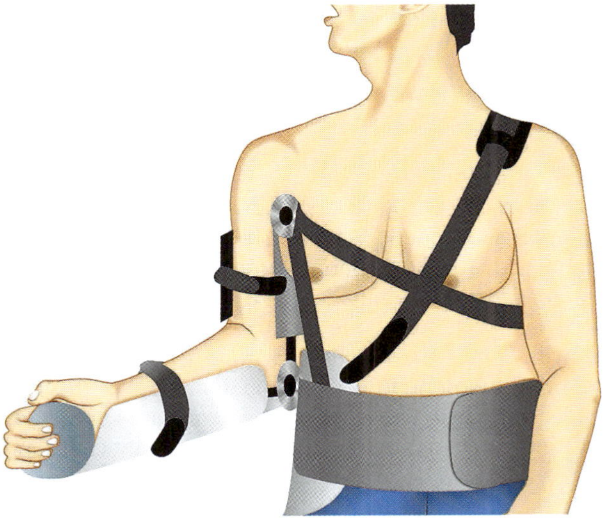

Fig. 9: The immobilization brace after reducing the shoulder dislocation. Note the external rotation at glenohumeral joint better approximates the avulsed capsulolabral structures back to glenoid encouraging better anatomical healing. As evident, this brace is cumbersome to wear and compliance hence is an issue.

The period of sling immobilization is being shortened to 7 days in most clinical practice followed by structured rehabilitation focusing on cryotherapy, restoration of full ROM, scapular muscle stabilization, and rotator-cuff strengthening exercises to culminate into sport-specific drills. The above-described closed reduction and nonsurgical regime is most suitable for preadolescents, patients aged >30 years of age and those with low demands. With increasing demonstration of development of recurrent instability in patients aged 22–30 years managed conservatively a consensus shift toward primary surgical management is getting build-up. This is particularly interesting because recurrent dislocations further complicate the future procedure due to increased attritional glenoid bone loss and humeral head defect needing bony procedures and grafting. These patients can be given a well-informed option for surgery after closed joint reduction.

Surgical treatment: The surgical treatment is required for acute anterior dislocation in the following instances:

- Many surgeons prefer arthroscopic repair of the capsulolabroligamentous avulsion during acute stage itself for the management in athletic injury as the incidence of chronic instability is high. The treatment is specifically pertinent in patients with no glenoid bone loss, minimal humeral bone loss, and good capsulolabral tissue quality. The standard treatment is anatomic repair and restoration of static capsulolabral restrains often accompanied by capsular plication. The difference from Bankart repair for recurrent instability is the limited capsular plication done in these cases to prevent stiffness. There are still high chances of recurrent instability (10–50%). It is largely accepted that not all patients are suitable to undergo arthroscopic only stabilization following anterior shoulder dislocation. Instability severity index score (ISIS) as suggested by Balg and Boileau **(Table 2)**

TABLE 2: The instability severity index score (ISIS). This is a 10-point simple scoring system to identify patients at risk of failure following arthroscopic Bankart repair. Patients with a score >6 points have unacceptable recurrence risk so may be considered for open procedure like Latarjet procedure.

Instability severity score		
Variable	***Parameter***	***Score (Total possible = 10)***
Age	<20 years	2
	>20 years	0
Degree of sports participation	Competitive	2
	Recreational/None	0
Type of sport participation	Contact/Forced overhead	1
	Other	0
Shoulder hyperlaxity	Hyperlaxity (anterior/inferior)	1
	Normal	0
Hill–Sachs on AP X-ray	Visible on external rotation	2
	Not visible on external rotation	0
Glenoid contour loss on AP X-ray	Loss of contour	2
	No lesion	0

(AP: anteroposterior)

is a measure to possibly determine future risk of development of recurrent instability (score >6 associated with high recurrence rates). There are problems as regard the ISIS validation by other studies and absolute value for triage to open surgical stabilization (Latarjet etc.) may not have been correctly determined as the risk of recurrent instability is unacceptably higher even if the score is as less as 4. The issue may be related to cut-off value for age, use of poorly sensitive external rotation AP view for Hill–Sachs lesion instead of a CT scan, etc.

- Open reduction is needed in failed closed cases. It should be accompanied with labral repair and pants-over-vest capsular shift providing some soft tissue stabilization. This is equivalent to open Bankart repair. Studies report lower redislocation rates after open surgery. It is demonstrated that recurrence tends to occur earlier after arthroscopic repair (2.5 years) than after open repair (3.7 years). Irrespective of the technique literature has demonstrated higher than previously reported failure for soft-tissue stabilization. Redislocation rates are high in athletes participating in contact sports and vary by as much as twice after open stabilization to thrice after arthroscopic stabilization compared to noncontact athletes. Some surgeons advocate Latarjet procedure for primary and recurrent instability because of its low recurrence rates. The issue between arthroscopic versus open versus Latarjet can be better answered by understanding and incorporating the concepts of glenoid bone loss, bipolar lesions, and on-track and off-track lesions as detailed below.

Recurrent Shoulder Instability

Conservative management: A subset of patients will be able to avoid surgery by doing rotator cuff and scapular rehabilitation exercise under the guidance of a physiotherapist and this is specifically true of AMBRI shoulders. The stabilizing mechanisms require muscle strength, coordination, and training. Many people with sedentary lifestyle learn to avoid provocative activities and never dislocate again. Optimizing neuromuscular control helps balance the humeral head in the glenoid and is preferred for children, for patients with voluntary instability, posterior GH instability, and for those requiring a supranormal ROM (such as baseball players and gymnasts). A strict routine is needed to be followed for patients starting with use of shoulder in the most stable position, followed by gradual introduction and conditioning of more unstable positions. Taping the shoulder to avoid unstable positions is a good method to remind patients. Conditioning is finalized to avoid all positions that lead to increased GH instability. However, for patients with troublesome recurrent instability nearing "TUBS type" and with failure of conservative treatment surgery is strongly considered as an option.

Operative management: As a basic rule, the preoperative clinical tests should suggest anterior or anteroinferior instability. The mechanism is often the lost support of the labrum **(Fig. 10)**. Bone defects that involve >25% of the glenoid surface area are a contraindication for arthroscopic treatment. The choice of surgery varies from arthroscopic or open Bankart repair (anatomical repairs) versus non-anatomical repairs (that usually aim to augment bone defect or capsular laxity). Primary determinants for chosing a surgery are capsulolabral quality, glenoid or humeral bone defect, and bipolar lesions. Arthroscopic repairs done in recurrent shoulder instability patients without bone defects and good capsulolabral tissue quality is associated with high rate of revision surgery (nearly one-third patients) and complaints of subjective instability in >60% patients. This procedure is hence mostly unsuccessful reasoned possibly on progressive tissue stretching and insufficiency, labral degeneration and attritional bone loss. These patients without critical glenoid or humeral bone loss or bipolar lesions are better suited for open repair as it inherently tends to stabilize soft tissue by pants-over-vest capsular shift.

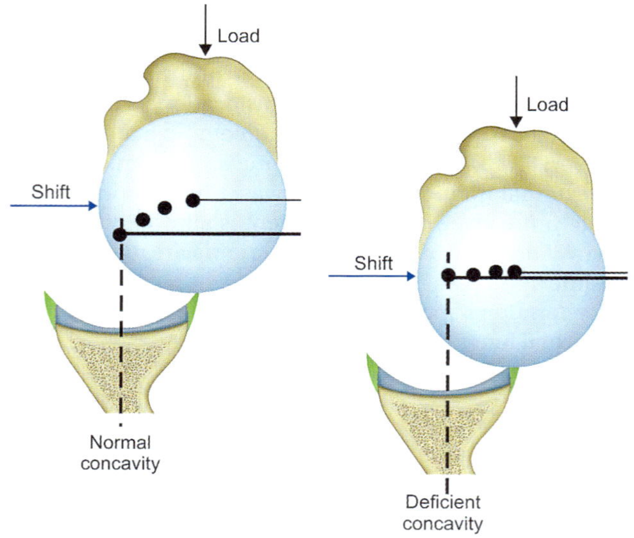

Fig. 10: Recurrent instability due to deficient labrum. Note with deficient labrum the glenoidogram is flattened and causes easy subluxation of the humeral head with minimal applied forces.

Glenoid bone defect: One must understand that if glenoid fragment is large enough for primary fixation then it is preferably fixed in acute dislocations. Nonfixable or chronic bone loss is considered here. Classically, 20–25% glenoid bone loss was considered critical above which bony augmentation is needed; however, it has been realized that patients with 13.5–20% glenoid bone loss also fare poorly in shoulder function if managed with arthroscopic repairs. So patients with glenoid bone loss up to 20% are better managed with open repairs. Patients with >20% glenoid bone loss need bony augmentation of glenoid definitively. The various popular options in the order of preference are Latarjet coracoid transfer (benchmark procedure), Bristow capsular tip transfer, autograft bone augmentation using distal clavicle or iliac crest, or osteoarticular distal tibial allograft augmentation. Latarjet procedure improves shoulder stability by three mechanisms, viz., creating dynamic sling of conjoint tendon across subscapularis in abduction and external rotation, bone augmentation of glenoid, and capsular reconstruction anteriorly using coracoacromial ligament. The augmentation bone grafts should be placed a bit medially (2–3 mm medial) to prevent late osteoarthrosis.

Humeral defect and bipolar lesions: Here, consider glenoid tracking. If there is glenoid bone loss of >25% with an off-tracking bipolar lesion then it is better to do a bone grafting procedure along with remplissage of the Hill-Sachs defect. If the glenoid defect is <25% with off-tracking humeral lesion then Bankart repair with remplissage is recommended. If the Hill-Sachs defect is >40% of the humeral articular surface then structural augmentation of humerus defect is needed. The text below describes some of the procedures with their pros and cons.

Anatomical Procedures

The *Bankart operation* or capsulolabral reconstruction is an essentially anatomical repair of the capsulolabral structures which has been avulsed from the anterior glenoid rim **(Figs. 11A and B)**. This is the gold standard treatment for shoulder instability. Today Bankart operation can be performed arthroscopically in most cases owing to development of specialized instruments, implants, and better surgical techniques. Arthroscopic classification of anterior labral Bankart lesions was proposed by Green and Christensen as follows:

- Type I is the normal intact labrum.
- Type II is a simple detachment of the labrum from the glenoid.
- Type III is an intrasubstance tear of the glenoid labrum.
- Type IV is a detachment of the labrum with significant fraying or degeneration.
- Type V is complete degeneration or absence of the glenoid labrum.

The principles of arthroscopic Bankart surgery involve identification of the pathology, proper elevation and mobilization of the capsulolabral complex, denuding the glenoid anterior surface of any soft tissues and repair of the capsulolabral complex onto the face of the glenoid using metal or bioabsorbable suture anchors. Arthroscopic repair provides 270° access to the labrum which can be extensively repaired. Arthroscopy can also be combined with remplissage (French—"to fill in") of infraspinatous tendon into the Hill-Sachs defect that is one of the reasons of recurrent instability after conventional arthroscopic Bankart repair in "off-track" bipolar lesions. Remplissage procedure is a capsulotenodesis of infraspinatous tendon into the humeral bone defect effectively rendering it extra-articular. This also provides posterior restraint to anterior translation of humeral head thus preventing its engagement. There is some compromise of shoulder rotation in overhead athletes after remplissage so one must discuss this possibility thoroughly preoperatively.

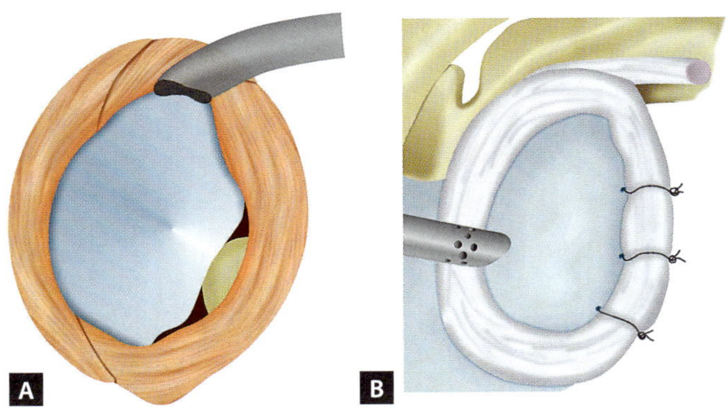

Figs. 11A and B: In the arthroscopic repair of Bankart lesion (A) the labrum is relocated using suture anchors. The inferiormost anchor is the most important and also helps pull the inferior glenohumeral ligament (IGHL) (B). So, it should be placed nicely and well.

Open repair was first performed by Perthes in 1906 popularized later by Bankart who did it in 1923 and detailed in 1939. The modified procedure (Modified Bankart procedure) is done these days that does not osteotomize coracoid or shave off bone from anterior glenoid and attach the labrum to glenoid lip rather than anterior surface as described by Bankart. The capsulolabral structures can be attached via suture anchors or by creating holes through the glenoid. The former has disadvantage of less strength of repair and difficulty in recreating the effective glenoid depth. Also, when placed in ideal position, there is a chance of anchor suture rubbing off of the humeral articular surface. Excessive tightening of the anterior capsule should be avoided as it may lead to limited function and comfort and capsulorrhaphy arthropathy. Some key points for a successful repair are as follows:

- It is imperative that inferior aspect of the capsule is tightened and secured by adequate number of suture anchors.
- Surgeon should re-establish the labral anatomy, IGHL tension and fix associated lesions.
- Capsular plication should be done using a pinch and tuck method 1 cm lateral to labrum taking care that the shoulder reaches neutral rotation after the surgery.
- Rotator interval closure should be performed in patients with positive sulcus sign of one or more with arm in external rotation.

Open Bankart repair with capsular shift: It has been observed that there occurs stretching of the anterior capsule and ligamentous structures at the time of injury. This led to advocacy of adding a capsular shift or capsulorrhaphy to the Bankart repair by many authors. The procedure helps ligament plication along with repair of the labrum. Capsular microtears have been reported in simian studies that caused pathological increase in anterior laxity when seen with a Bankart lesion. This type of combined surgery is especially favored in contact athletes as these athletes if treated with open Bankart repair only had a high redislocation rate that reduced to <3% with addition of capsulorrhaphy. There is one drawback however, excessive tightening of the anterior capsule and subscapularis can restrict external rotation and function and may be a harbinger of secondary degenerative joint disease known as *capsulorrhaphy arthropathy*. The degeneration occurs after nearly a gap of 15 years but is highly variable. There exists a correlation between loss of external rotation and development of degenerative arthropathy. Functional loss may be restricted by limiting immobilization to just 2–3 days and the motion and function of the extremity are gradually increased.

Nonanatomical Repairs

These are specifically needed for management of critical bone defects on humeral or glenoid side or both (bipolar lesions) or for associated soft tissue lesions.

- *Hill-Sachs lesion:* These impression fractures occur on the posterosuperior surface of humeral head (first identified by Malgaigne in 1832 and associated to anterior instability by Hill-Sachs in 1940) due to the impaction of rounded cancellous head in anterior dislocations onto the relatively sharp cortical glenoid rim. These fractures may also occur onto the anterior aspect of humeral head as a result of posterior shoulder dislocation (reverse Hill-Sachs lesion) but less frequently. Mere presence of the lesion does not entail instability but the size and direction/orientation of the defect describes unstable pattern (*see* Chapter on "Imaging of Shoulder Joint"). The unstable lesion was termed "engaging" Hill-Sachs lesion by Burkhart and De Beer as one which engages the glenoid within functional range of shoulder motion. Lesions < 20% of the humeral head articular surface are quite benign while lesions 20–40% in size cause moderate instability. Significant instability is imparted by lesions > 40% of humeral head articular surface. Also, the lesion should parallel the glenoid rim to engage successfully **(Figs. 7 and 12)**. There are various methods of addressing the Hill-Sachs lesion:
  - First-line treatment of humeral head defect is remplissage with tenodesis of infraspinatous tendon arthroscopically. The tendon is advanced over proximal lip of defect making the defect extraarticular.
  - Second is by way of tightening the shoulder to restrict external rotation as by double breasting subscapularis (Putti-Platt operation, **Fig. 13**). This is not at all popular due to its restrictive nature, future development of capsulorrhaphy arthropathy, and better available methods.).
  - Another approach is by filling the humeral head defect by matched or unmatched osteoarticular allograft. This is needed if the defect is >40% of the humeral articular surface.
  - Partial articular resurfacing is available in select centers that avoids the issue of disease transmission or the need of dedicated bone bank for osteoarticular grafts.
  - Glenoid augmentation also indirectly increases the arc of contact (glenoid tracking) preventing humeral head engagement.
  - Failed primary surgery with shoulder remaining unstable at <90° of abduction and <90° of external rotation with large Hill-Sachs lesion can be successfully managed by *tendon transfers*. The *Saha procedure* involves transfer of latissimus dorsi muscle at the infraspinatus insertion, thus pulling the humeral head backward during abduction. Infraspinatus tendon transfer acts as an anterior block to humeral defect engaging the glenoid. Reverse Hill-Sachs lesions can be managed with subscapularis transfer.
  - Older patients with large defects >45% of articular surface can be very well managed with arthroplasty (hemi or total). Arthroplasty can also be used for chronic unreduced dislocations. Total arthroplasty is preferred for associated glenoid side degenerative changes.
- *Humeral avulsion of glenohumeral ligament and posterior avulsions:* HAGL involves avulsion of the capsule from humeral neck which should be suspected in all cases of

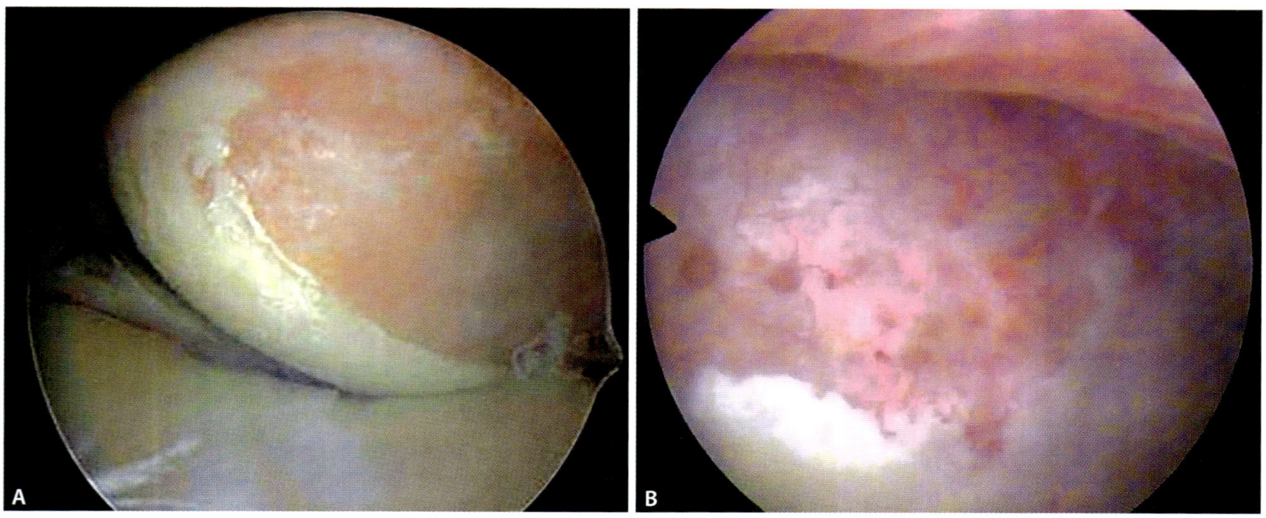

Figs. 12A and B: Arthroscopic picture of Hill–Sachs lesion in the same patient (A). This patient also had patulous capsule evident by easy anterior translation of the humeral head as shown here. To show the difference an arthroscopic picture of the bare area of humerus (B) has been put by the side that shows nutrient foramina, small vessels and irregular articular surface to help differentiate and mark the anatomically "bare" region of humerus frequently confused by young arthroscopic surgeons.

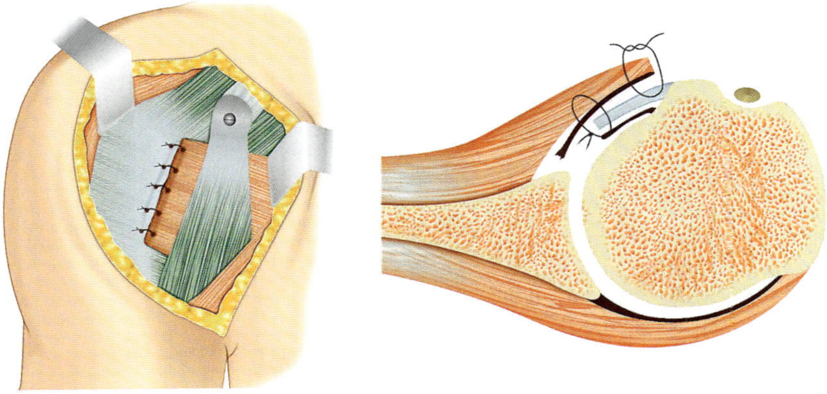

Fig. 13: Putti–Platt procedure: Double breasting and tightening of anterior capsule to restrict the external rotation of the humeral head.

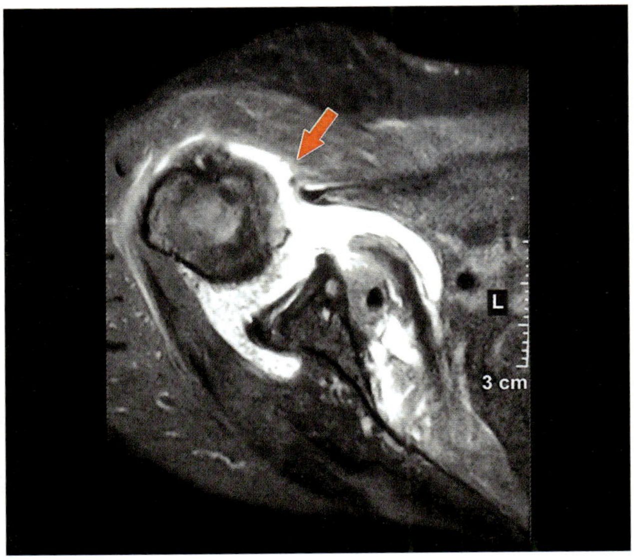

Fig. 14: Uncommon case of recurrent anterior glenohumeral instability. The MRI shows subscapularis tendon tear (arrow) and humeral avulsion of glenohumeral ligament (HAGL) lesion.

recurrent instability without a Bankart lesion, especially if the subscapularis muscle is seen exposed. There are arthroscopic methods described to treat HAGL lesion but most surgeons prefer open methods to treat them. There are descriptions of the posterior GH ligament avulsion from proximal humerus but it is very infrequently seen.

- *Subscapularis rupture* **(*Fig. 14*)***:* Subscapularis deficiency should be suspected in recurrent shoulder instability. The results of repair of subscapularis tendon are not very encouraging however. Pectoralis major tendon transfer may be done in which the superior 2.5–3 cm of the tendon is transferred lateral to bicipital groove lateral to greater tuberosity superficial to coracoid.
- *Glenoid bone defects:* Glenoid rim deficiency of 21% or more (Itoi et al.) is associated with instability, a deficit of >30% is associated with gross instability (Greis et al.). 30% loss of glenoid rim leads to 41% reduction in contact area and 100% increase in contact pressures **(*see* Fig. 5)**. Due to difficulty in defining the percentage loss of glenoid even radiologically, Burkhart and De Beer defined significant glenoid loss as one where the shape changes to inverted pear-shaped glenoid. The guiding principles for glenoid bone loss management are discussed above. The various procedures for augmentation are as follows:

The *Bristow–Helfet procedure* is usually done for glenoid bone loss anteriorly and as described first by Helfet consists of bone block of coracoid process resected just distal to the pectoralis minor insertion containing the conjoined tendons **(Fig. 15)**. The bone with tendons is then passed through a vertical slit in the subscapularis to anterior surface of glenoid neck and the conjoined tendons are sutured to subscapularis tendon. Various modifications are proposed and practices important being attaching the bone piece using a screw and passing the tendon-bone unit through horizontal slit. Though the bone block is suggested to be the primary restraint but it seems that the tenodesis effect on subscapularis primarily stabilizes the shoulder by prevention of superior migration of the lower half of muscle upward during abduction. This (or Eden-Hybbinette) is the preferred method for managing unstable shoulders with anterior glenoid defect.

Latarjet procedure is similar to Bristow but involves transfer of a larger portion of coracoid process and the bone-tendon unit transferred to anteroinferior aspect of glenoid rather than anterior surface. Placement of bone block should be rather precise with the bone placed 2–4 mm medial to the edge of glenoid. It is unknown as to the exact mechanism of providing stability to shoulder by this procedure. Some suggest "triple-block" providing stability postoperatively, viz.:

1. Increased bone surface area from coracoid transfer
2. Sling effect of the coracobrachialis muscle on subscapularis
3. Anterior capsular reconstruction-augmentation with coracoacromial ligament

It is conjured that at extremes of movements the sling effect of the conjoint tendon contributes to three-fourths of the stability while in mid-ranges only half to two-thirds is gained by this effect and bony reconstruction instead supplies remaining one-third to half of the stability. Complication rates (15–30%) for neurological injury, loss of motion, graft osteolysis, graft fracture, nonunion, and

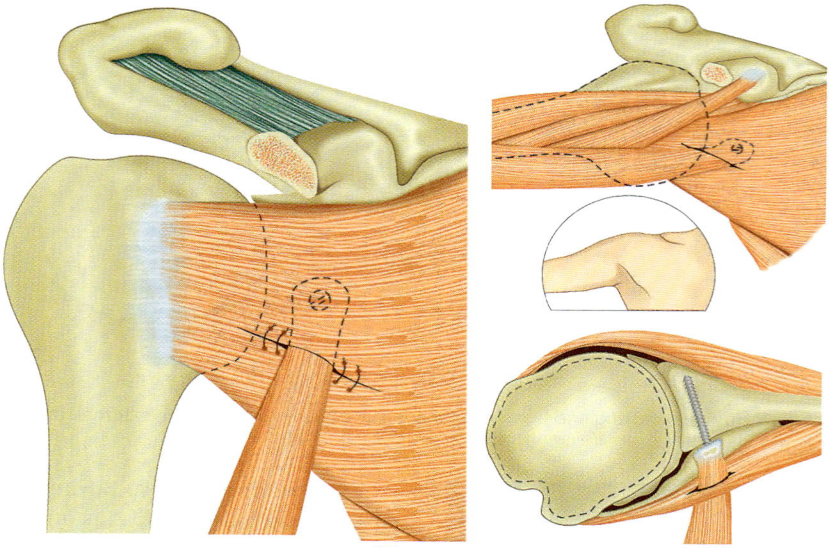

Fig. 15: Bristow–Helfet procedure for anterior glenoid deficiency. The coracoid process with attached muscles and ligament is attached to the anteroinferior glenoid rim. The soft tissue structures act as a check-reign to anterior dislocation of humeral head in shoulder abduction.

development of arthritis in longer term are quite higher, however, with this technique as intraoperative stretching and manipulation of structures is quite obvious. There is a high rate of injury to axillary nerve followed by suprascapular and musculocutaneous nerves.

Other less-used procedures are mentioned as follows. *Eden-Hybinette procedure* extends the bony glenoid anteriorly. Bone graft harvested from iliac crest is inserted into the substance of anterior glenoid rim. The *Oudard procedure* aims to create a bone block by elongating the coracoid process either by using a bone graft or by performing an oblique osteotomy and sliding the coracoid and refixing it. *Trillat* displaced the coracoid process downward and laterally after osteotomy at base to act as a bone block. The *Gallie procedure* reconstructs the ligament anteroinferiorly using fascia lata as a graft material. *Nicola procedure* uses long head of biceps tendon as a checkrein ligament. *Derotation osteotomy* is an interesting proposal based on finding by some authors that there is abnormal humeral torsion in a repeatedly dislocating shoulder. Weber described this procedure of increasing the humeral retroversion by transverse osteotomy of proximal humerus. This is combined with anterior capsulorrhaphy. There is effective alignment of the healthy anterior articular surface of humeral head abutting against glenoid surface and taking away the damaged posterior aspect of humeral head containing the Hill-Sachs lesion. Glenoid osteotomy has also been described to correct the alignment. These are rarely prescribed or used for their complexity and availability and practice of more anatomical repairs.

Complications of anterior stabilization procedures:

- Infection
- Recurrent/refractory instability
- Excessive tightening and capsulorrhaphy arthropathy—due to excessive anterior tightening, there is obligatory posterior nonanatomic translation of humeral head and resulting degeneration changes from altered biomechanics.
- Missed or wrong diagnosis
- *Nerve injuries:* Musculocutaneous nerve in Helfet or Bristow procedure, axillary nerve in Putti–Platt procedure
- *Implant loosening and failure:* Loose screw/staple
- *Reduced external rotation:* Magnuson–Stack and the Putti–Platt procedures
- *Subscapularis deficiency:* Usually occurs in multiply operated patients.

Revision Anterior Instability Surgery

This is a challenging endeavor for any surgeon and involves various patient specific innovations and some deviations from standard approach but ultimately aiming at stabilizing the shoulder joint. Attention should be paid to the original surgical procedure, reasons for failure, bone loss, demands, quality of bone, demands from activity level, hyperlaxity, etc. Revision arthroscopic soft tissue repair is fraught with high failure and recurrence rate. The only indication possibly is in patients with inadequate primary surgery (single suture anchor), no glenoid bone loss and good capsulolabral tissue quality. In patients with no glenoid bone loss, open repair with capsular shift is preferable. If >13.5% glenoid bone loss is present then Latarjet procedure is needed as is also in patients with "off-track" Hill–Sachs or bipolar lesions. This means that the threshold for bony augmentation is reduced for revision surgery. One must note that the results of remplissage in revision surgery is not at all encouraging and have high failure rates (nearly 35%).

POSTERIOR SHOULDER INSTABILITY

Posterior shoulder instability is a rare condition present in 2–10% of clinically unstable shoulders. Like the anterior instability it also encompasses a spectrum of laxity at one end to complete shoulder dislocation at the other. Posterior shoulder instability (PSI) may be defined as posterior glenohumeral translation that reproduces symptoms outside the normal physiologic translation in an individual. Asymptomatic translation is considered joint laxity. PSI is seen in active men usually within age group of 20–30 years that engage in contact sports.

Etiopathogenesis

Posterior shoulder instability is generally uncommon and rarely occurs alone. Common coexisting factors include scapulothoracic dysfunction or scapular dyskinesia, voluntary, trauma (micro/macro) due to previous shoulder dislocations producing soft-tissue and/or bony abnormalities. The last is the most common cause of PSI seen in competitive athletes but in most it is the pattern of recurrent posterior subluxation rather than frank posterior dislocation. Microtrauma due to the repetitive shearing forces and loads to the posterior shoulder in flexed, adducted, and internally rotated position is an important mechanism for development of PSI. Posterior capsule is the most important structure preventing posterior translation that may get degenerated in weight lifters doing bench-presses, overhead sport athletes, swimmers, and military personnel due to microtrauma. Macrotrauma from a blow to the anterior shoulder or axial load on flexed shoulder is seen in contact sports such as football. These mechanisms produce structural abnormalities in posterior band of the inferior glenohumeral ligament, glenoid, coracohumeral ligament, posterior capsule, the rotator-cuff muscles, and the biceps tendon **(Box 2)**. Scapulothoracic dysfunction in PSI is poorly understood. Winging of the scapula is seen during provocative testing but that may be compensatory also. Subscapularis majorly resists the posterior translation of humerus as is serratus anterior muscle, so a weakness or dysfunction in both or any one may contribute to instability. Voluntary posterior subluxation of shoulder can be psychogenic or may be associated with secondary gain for attention. These patients are poor surgical candidates.

BOX 2: The bony and soft tissue structural abnormalities seen in posterior shoulder instability.

Soft-Tissue structural abnormalities include:
- Posterior capsular redundancy from recurrent subluxation
- Soft-tissue and osseous reverse-Bankart lesion (posteroinferior tear of the capsulolabral complex)
- Kim lesion (avulsion of posteroinferior labrum)
- Posterior labral cyst—this is an MRI finding and may actually represent a covert Kim lesion.
- Chondrolabral erosion of the glenoid rim
- Rotator-cuff tear
- Avulsion of the glenohumeral ligaments especially the posterior band of the inferior glenohumeral ligament

Bony abnormalities comprise:
- Posterior glenoid fracture
- Glenoid retroversion
- Reverse Hills–Sachs lesion
- Glenoid erosion

Clinical Presentation and Classification

The common presentation is of poorly localized aching/pain and/or clicking in the posterior aspect of involved shoulder instead of frank instability symptoms. Overhead athletes usually feel symptoms during their follow through phase (bowlers) or pull-through phase (swimmer). Patients usually prefer carrying arm in an internally rotated position with a prominent humeral head posteriorly. The coracoid process is also more prominent. There patient may be tenderness on palpation of posterior glenohumeral joint line. Provocative testing elicits sensation of instability in the position of 90° forward flexion, adduction, and internal rotation. There usually is weakness of the rotator-cuff muscles and scapular stabilizers. The subluxation or the patient's symptoms of pain and instability may be reproduced during Jerk Test, Kim Test, Load-and-Shift, and Posterior Drawer Test.

Differential Diagnosis

Due to vague presentation of PSI, one needs to rule-out other conditions that may present in a similar way like superior labral anterior to posterior (SLAP) tear or rotator-cuff tear. Subacromial impingement tests may be positive in PSI and one needs to also differentiate internal impingement from PSI. Multidirectional instability closely resembles PSI so instability of the joint in other directions should also be tested.

Imaging

Plain radiographs are often normal in patients with PSI. Even posterior shoulder dislocations are missed on radiographs by an unquestioning observer. Magnetic resonance imaging, especially MR arthrography, is the radiological tool of choice and an important diagnostic tool to identify any possible soft tissue lesions that may be contributing to or associated with the instability. Computed tomography (CT) scans are recommended for determining bone quality and glenoid morphology.

Classification of Posterior Shoulder Instability

Degree of instability, direction, mechanism of injury, and volition are all used to classify PSI but I feel direction of instability is quite useful to understand the underlying pathology. Unidirectional (posterior), bidirectional (postero-inferior), and multidirectional (posterior, inferior, and anterior) instabilities have been described where the latter two are the most common. Atraumatic instability that is voluntary should be additionally identified due to its altogether different treatment.

Treatment of Posterior Shoulder Instability

Mild instability symptoms are better left alone. Fair trial of conservative management is given to patients who have functionally disabling symptoms. Activity modification and a conservative physical therapy protocol followed for 6 months is usually the first-line treatment except if there is evidence of bony pathology of the glenohumeral joint and traumatic instability as conservative treatment fails in them. *Conservative management* for acute dislocations usually consist of immobilization for 3 weeks followed by gradual return to movements over next 3 weeks. Younger patients are at higher risk for redislocation so should be followed under supervision more strictly. "Locked" posterior dislocations commonly occurring after violent trauma or seizure should be promptly recognized and reduced. Delay results in dismal posterior contracture and anterior laxity which is generally associated with large reverse Hill–Sachs lesion that would need surgical intervention. Rehabilitation consists of gradual incremental mobilization with strengthening of the rotator-cuff (supraspinatus, infraspinatus, teres minor, and subscapularis) muscles especially the infraspinatus muscle and subscapularis. Scapular stabilizers and posterior deltoid are also gradually build. *Operative stabilization* should be considered in patients who fail to return to activity or continue to experience pain or instability, are psychologically stable, and have failed a trial of physical therapy. One must understand the caution that surgical management is contraindicated for patients with voluntary instability due to psychological problems and in patients with seizures it should be controlled before attempting repair/reconstruction. Operative treatment may involve more than one procedure to address all the underlying factors contributing to the instability depending on structural abnormalities, and direction of instabilities.

The *soft tissue procedures* commonly performed include anchor-based posterior capsulolabral repair and/or retensioning of the redundant posteroinferior aspect of the capsule (open posterior-inferior capsular shift, arthroscopic capsular plication, or a reverse Putti–Platt procedure), Boyd–Sisk procedure, and biceps tendon transposition. Posterior capsular laxity is the most common lesion in PSI so posterior capsulorrhaphy not only adds to the success of soft tissue reconstruction but may be the sole needed procedure in many. Soft-tissue procedures are quite successful in managing posterior instability with low recurrence rates. Thermal capsulorrhaphy is not recommended due to variable results and redevelopment of capsular insufficiency. The *bony procedures* usually performed are posterior bone block, glenoplasty (in glenoid retroversion > 15°), posterior opening wedge osteotomy of the glenoid neck, or rotational osteotomy of the proximal humerus. They are indicated with posterior glenoid bone loss of >20% as in these isolated soft tissue repairs are inadequate. Large fragments can be acutely repaired/fixed. Additional procedures like correction of reverse Hill–Sachs lesion by McLaughlin's procedure (transfer of lesser tuberosity and subscapularis in humeral head defect) or its modification and allograft reconstruction of the humeral head (for severe defects) may be needed. Arthroscopy-only procedures have similar reported success to open procedures; however, I feel that the former is better suited to unidirectional instability while open procedures may better address instability in multiple directions.

Rehabilitation following surgery comprises in addition to gradual mobilization and isometric strengthening (see above) the neuromuscular re-education where scapular and glenohumeral muscles are activated during functional movements to produce full range and diagonal and spiral patterns. The posterior-deltoid specifically has been shown to respond to electromyography (EMG) training and this should be utilized as appropriate.

MULTIDIRECTIONAL INSTABILITY

This is a rare condition that is typified by Matsen concept of "AMBRI" unstable shoulder representing the extreme end of shoulder instability. The term multidirectional instability (MDI) was possibly first brought to literature by Neer who defined it as "abnormal amount of excursion of the humeral head on the glenoid in all (anterior, posterior, and inferior) directions". At the outset one should realize that instability is different from laxity so term like "global laxity" does not classify as MDI that may be also seen in asymptomatic hyperlax individuals. The laxity (clinical sign) should be able to cause instability (symptom) in the form of symptomatic subluxation or dislocation (that causes "dysfunction") in more than one direction to be labeled as MDI. Inability to understand the difference is the root cause of finding so-called MDI by amateurs often, though the real existence of MDI is in fact rare. Ability to sublux shoulder in multiple directions on examination in an otherwise asymptomatic patient or a patient having typical symptoms of unidirectional instability does not qualify labeling him as MDI.

Defining MDI as a discrete entity is difficult but the Neer's definition above is usually followed. This, however, needs finding instability in "all" planes and thus patients with lesser abnormalities may be left with no diagnosis! Finding inferior instability is quite universal in MDI so this leaves additional instability in anterior and posterior direction. Commonly followed definition for MDI is hence symptomatic instability in more than one direction to cover two-direction instability also. This definition would, however, overlap patients with posteroinferior instability and sure there is overlap in two-direction instability and MDI in current practice but this is possibly not of much concern as clinically the treatment remains same for two-direction or MDI. MDI classically affects young patients in 2nd–3rd decade and has no gender preference though females are a bit more clinically "lax" (but not unstable).

Pathoanatomy and Etiology

Pathoanatomically two hallmarks are common in most—redundant inferior capsule and patulous rotator interval that bulges on arthrograms (Neer). Other capsuloligamentous structures may be deficient (Bankart's, Kim's, HAGL, etc.) depending on additional instability. Recurrent instability left untreated exaggerates the deficiency of shoulder stabilizers. Patulous capsule diminishes the negative intra-articular pressure maintenance and over a time the scapulohumeral rhythm also alters in these patients due to deconditioning of dynamic stabilizers and development of trick movements to keep shoulder stable. If labral tear occurs, then concavity compression effect is also lost (see shoulder biomechanics for details). There is a subset of patients where the MDI is volitional, they can dislocate/subluxate the shoulder at will and may also have primary scapular dyskinesia. The changes most commonly result from accruing microtrauma during overhead activities in athletes and contact sports. Generalized ligamentous laxity may also predispose to development of MDI in high-level athletes but is not the direct cause of MDI per se.

Clinical Features and Classification

The patients usually have vague multiple complaints such as pain, instability, looseness, weakness, fatigue, paresthesias, popping, clicking, crepitus, traction paresthesias or "dead-arm syndrome" that lead clinician nowhere to make diagnosis at outset. Some complain of instability during sleep. Anterior instability is suggested with symptoms appearing in overhead activities, throwing and racquet sports; inferior instability is suggested with symptoms on carrying weight or traction paresthesia while posterior instability is associated with symptoms on bench press, pitching follow through or batting. It is the careful physical examination that ultimately deciphers MDI. Scapula is commonly protracted in these patients that also exacerbates multidirectional laxity. One should, hence, examine with scapula retracted. This is also a common finding in EUA when the impression of MDI actually reduced to unidirectional instability due to the effect of static muscle disposition. Specific tests like evaluation of laxity with Cofield's technique and Gagey test for inferior capsular laxity should be done. Perform apprehension test and anterior and posterior load-shift test in various positions. Also examine for muscle patterning and kinetic chain during active shoulder movements. In hyperlax, individuals do scoring as mentioned by Beighton.

Neer classification for MDI is usually followed that classifies it in three groups:

- *Group I:* Anterior-inferior + posterior subluxation
- *Group II:* Posteroinferior + anterior subluxation
- *Group III:* Global pattern of instability

Differential Diagnosis

Being vague in presentation some unrelated conditions might clinically resemble MDI including cervical spine disorder, periscapular myoclonus, scapular dyskinesis, suprascapular nerve entrapment, brachial plexopathy, thoracic outlet syndrome, and unidirectional instability.

Imaging

Radiographs are usually obtained to identify bony glenoid or humeral head abnormality. Standard series of AP (additional internal and external rotation views), axillary, scapular Y-views are obtained. CT scan may be used to determine retroversion. Magnetic resonance arthrography is the modality of choice for evaluation of soft tissues that usually reveals redundant inferior recess with patulous rotator interval. Additional Kim lesion, Bankart lesion, HAGL, SLAP tear, etc. might also be revealed. Electromyogram may be obtained in scapular dyskinesia and diagnostic arthroscopy would reveal patulous capsule and easy passage of scope to other side (*drive through sign*).

Treatment

As suggested by Neer, patients with MDI should be treated conservatively for at least 1 year before prescribing surgery; however, this is often not practical these days. The time duration might differ but a generous trial of physical therapy and other measures would help. Taping and brace for scapular retraction aid in stabilization of shoulder. One should work toward core stability by strengthening of muscles while simultaneously improving muscle patterning and proprioception and functional rehabilitation. For first 6–10 weeks, progressive resistance exercises are prescribed that are then gradually maintained with scapulothoracic and glenohumeral retraining. Overhead activities are added in the end. Failed conservative therapy for maybe 6 months in structural MDI without voluntary instability or secondary gain is the indication for surgical management. The goals of surgical management are to reduce capsular volume, close rotator interval, and possibly reinforce capsule so that it does not become lax again. Both arthroscopic and open techniques are utilized depending on surgeon training and comfort. Open inferior capsular shift has stood the test of time in providing lasting relief though recurrences are still seen. The most popular open procedure is the Neer's inferior capsular shift but in any case, the surgical procedures alone have limited ability to cure atraumatic instability. The patient should be carefully chosen with a major functional problem clearly related to atraumatic GH instability and clear understanding by the patient of the limitations of this static procedure and future requirement of strict discipline. In the Neer's inferior capsular shift (**Fig. 16**), the capsule in incised deep down inferiorly and medial capsule is

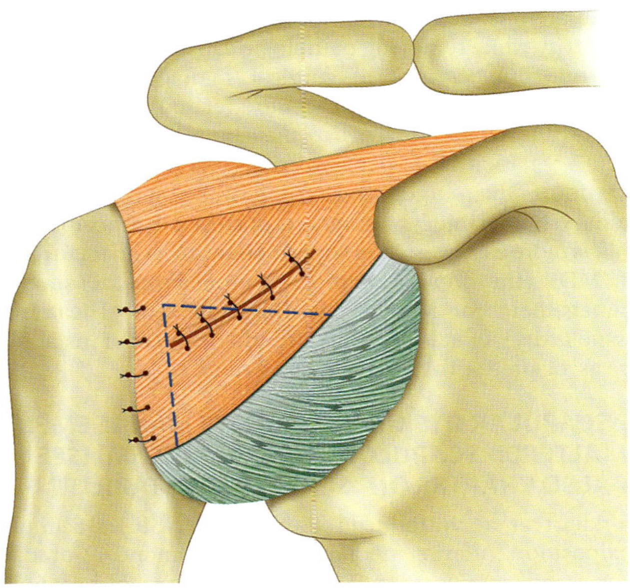

Fig. 16: The Neer's inferior capsular shift is done for a patulous and lax capsule causing recurring shoulder instability. Uncommon patients with atraumatic multidirectional bilateral rehabilitation inferior capsular shift (AMBRI) instability also benefit from it. One must be cautious, however, before prescribing or doing this procedure as voluntary dislocators frequently fail from even this procedure. It should never be considered a remedy for failed cases also.

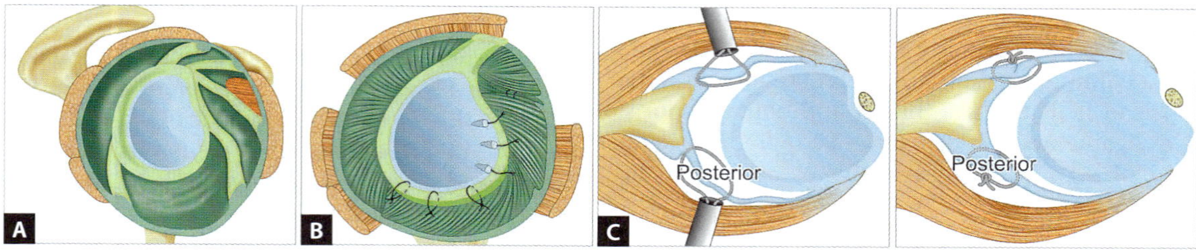

Figs. 17A to C: Capsular plication and rotator interval closure for multidirectional instability. (A) The lax inferior capsule and illustration of patulous rotator interval with defect; (B) The lower three stitches demonstrate capsulorrhaphy while anterior three stitch demonstrate additional labral repair. The rotator interval is closed separately; (C) Axial view illustration of the capsular plication showing tightening of the same.

taken *superiorly and laterally* under the lateral capsule. It is important that the capsule be pulled superiorly and not just an east-west shift. The sutures are placed and tied with arm in 20–30° of external rotation. Though named inferior capsular shift the procedure tightens the capsule inferiorly, anteriorly, and posteriorly all along. Bankart repair, if present, can also be simultaneously done with ease. Arthroscopic capsular plication is possibly as effective in a trained hand. Proponents of "key-hole" surgery say that arthroscopic tightening gives better visualization and control over the tissues. The arthroscopic treatment may be **(Figs. 17A to C)** simple capsulorrhaphy, "çombi-stitch" (where the capsule pleats are combined with labral imbrication) or "çombi-repair" (here the capsule is plicated along with labral repair). Plication of 5 mm reduces the capsule volume by 16.2% while 10 mm plication reduces it by 33.7%. Plication is usually done in inferiorly and progressively advanced superiorly. Thermal capsulorrhaphy should be avoided as this leads to further weakening of capsule hence contraindicated. In involuntary dislocators, the labral tears could be circumferential, that can be helped by arthroscopic stabilization with or without capsular plication. These procedures improve glenoid concavity while removing pathologic capsular redundancy.

The *complications* of surgical management include subscapularis deficiency (procedure related), loss of movements (due to tightening of capsule—but usually movements are all regained by 1 year), arthritis (this is a concern with overdoing the surgery restricting movements severely), axillary nerve injury, iatrogenic posterior subluxation (in shift is more east-west than superior inferior), and recurrence of MDI (the most common complication of surgical management for MDI). High Beighton score (ligament/tissue laxity), female sex, and atraumatic onset of instability are associated with high recurrence rates.

SCAPULAR DYSKINESIA AND ITS MANAGEMENT (ALTERED SCAPULOHUMERAL RHYTHM) (*SEE ALSO* CHAPTER ON "SCAPULAR INSTABILITY")

Burkhart et al. introduced the acronym SICK (*S*capular malposition, *I*nferior medial border prominence, *C*oracoid pain and malposition, and dys*K*ynesis of scapular motion) for scapular dyskinesis in overhead athletes. The pathophysiology of development of symptoms is quite complex and involves muscular (weakness), neurological (proprioceptive damage and neuropathy), and structural failure (usually a consequence of dyskinesia) as presented in **Flowchart 1**.

The disorder is not easy to recognize early and must be suspected in all patients with vague complaints of pain in the anterior and/or the posterosuperior aspect of the shoulder or upper arm below the acromion posteriorly. The pain may unusually radiate proximally into lateral aspect of the neck along the upper trapezius (UT) or may confusingly radiate along the upper extremity suggesting cervical radiculopathy. Two typical symptoms help to identify scapular dyskinesia—pain in the coracoid region (possibly due to tightening of the pectoralis minor resulting from downward tilt and lateral displacement of the coracoid) and posterosuperior scapular pain.

On examination, scapular dyskinesia is suggested by asymmetric positions of the scapula on movement and/or poor progression of muscle chain activity often resembling dancing jerks or fasciculations. Tests to identify dyskinesia include the scapular assistance test where examiner passively assists the scapula into upward rotation and posterior tilt during humeral elevation by pushing scapula upward and laterally on the inferior angle pulling the superior aspect of the scapula posteriorly. The assistance provides relief of symptoms and improves movements by increasing the acromiohumeral space. The other test is scapular retraction test where the examiner first performs Jobe's empty can test and then repeats it while stabilizing the medial scapular border. The second part of test improves supraspinatus strength and reduces pain.

Classification

Kibler et al. identified three dyskinetic patterns as follows:

- *Type I:* Here the inferomedial border of the scapula is prominent due to abnormal posterior tilt around a horizontal axis in the plane of the scapula. In unilateral cases the scapula may be lower than other side.
- *Type II:* Here the entire medial (vertebral) border is prominent due to excessive external rotation around a vertical axis through the plane of the scapula. There is a strong association of this type with simultaneous SLAP lesions (see below).
- *Type III:* In this type there is upward rotation of the superomedial border of the scapula around a horizontal axis perpendicular to scapular plane that results in superior migration of the scapula. This is the most symptomatic pattern and causes pain due to reduction in acromiohumeral space and development of rotator-cuff injuries.

Flowchart 1: Pathomechanism for development of scapular dyskinesia. There are usually multiple inhibitory loops that accentuate the inhibition and dyskinesia.

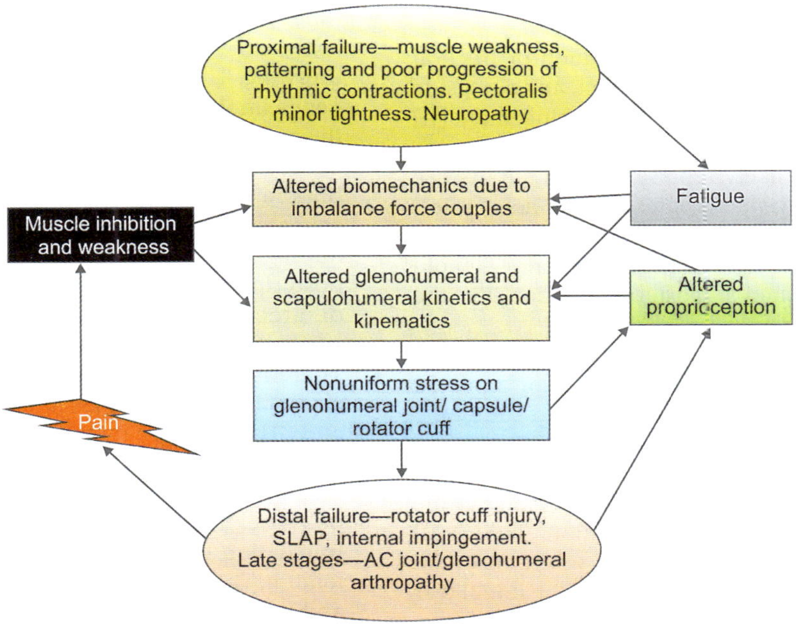

(AC: acromioclavicular; SLAP: superior labrum anterior and posterior)

Flowchart 2: General schema for multipronged approach to treatment of scapular dyskinesia.

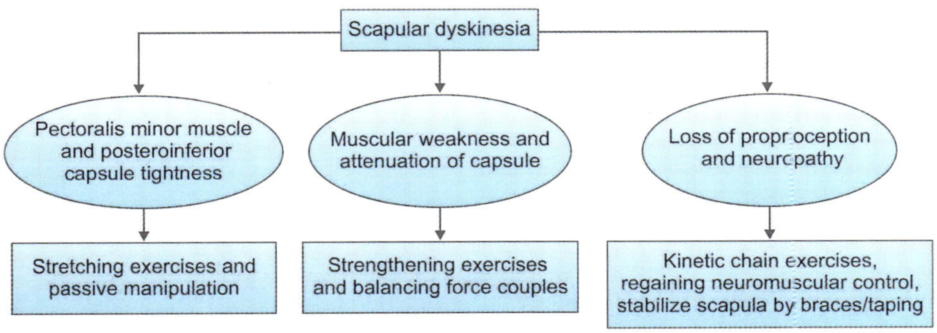

Imaging

Radiographs are mostly noncontributory and the investigation of choice is MRI to identify associated SLAP lesion or rotator-cuff injuries.

Treatment

It is best to prevent the development of dyskinesia by identifying a "shoulder at risk" in the throwing athletes. In its prodrome, the athletes have varying degree of glenohumeral internal rotation, scapular dyskinesis. Once identified, the treatment should be initiated by temporary cessation of activity and internal rotation stretching and strengthening of scapular stabilizers. This would also save the athlete from potential injuries to superior labrum and cuff tendons or a full-blown SICK syndrome. Once developed the scapular dyskinesis is predominantly managed by functional rehabilitation (vide **Flowchart 2** for a general schema of rehabilitative treatment). Commonly a set of four exercises (prone extension, side-lying external rotation, side-lying forward flexion, and prone horizontal abduction with external rotation) is deployed to induce activation of middle and lower trapezius and low contraction of UT. Additionally, focus should also be given to stretching of both the posteroinferior glenohumeral capsule and the pectoralis minor. Despite the effective treatment with muscular rehabilitation some patients develop muscular patterning which is difficult to reverse and produce permanent deficits. Little is known on the results of treatment as a whole and based on complex pathophysiology it is commonly recommended to include taping and bracing for scapula stabilization and proprioception improvement additionally.

Failed Primary Surgery for Glenohumeral Instability

The common causes of failure are choosing wrong patient (MDI), incomplete evaluation (bony defect missed), iatrogenic injury (capsular damage from cautery), or an unlucky patient with repeat injury. Failed surgeries are usually revised with Bristow–Latarjet procedure reinforcing both the defect and giving a tenodesis effect.

SUPERIOR LABRUM ANTERIOR AND POSTERIOR LESION AND INTERNAL IMPINGEMENT

Lesions of superior labrum develop with fall on an outstretched hand (FOOSH), sudden deceleration or traction forces such as catching a falling heavy object, and alongside anterior and posterior instability. Internal impingement (II) and superior labral tears are seen commonly in throwing athletes also. They most likely represent the same disease spectrum. *Internal impingement* represents the mechanical abutment of undersurface of the posterior supraspinatus and anterior infraspinatus against posterosuperior glenoid rim and labrum in abduction and external rotation (like the late cocking phase of a throw).

The *SLAP lesions* are defined as superior labral lesions that are both anterior and posterior. The superior aspect of labrum is in general more mobile and prone to additional injury due to close attachment of biceps tendon. So traction injury from biceps long head can peel the labrum. FOOSH directly impacts the vulnerable region by loading the superior labrum in flexed abducted position. The SLAP lesions are classified into at least 10 types where most are subtypes of type II with variable extension of the initial tear **(Figs. 18A to J)**.

Pathophysiology

The etiology remains controversial but the basic mechanism of production of internal impingement (II) and the anatomical lesions in II and SLAP lesions is increased external rotation at extremes of abduction. The following have been proposed as the possible mechanisms that rely on the basis of excess anterior or anteroinferior translation of humeral head causing impingement posteriorly or superiorly.

- Jobe proposed that the microinstability results from laxity of the anteroinferior capsulolabral complex during throwing. This causes anterior humeral translation and hence impingement of soft tissues (rotator cuff) against the posterosuperior labrum. The cuff gets "pinced" between glenoid rim and humeral head or tuberosities.
- Burkhart proposed posterior capsular contracture as cause of this anterior humeral head translation and impingement. This contracture produces increasingly posterior center of rotation and posterior translation of greater tuberosity relative to glenoid causing impingement.
- There is a high likelihood of II resulting from dyssynchrony between complex movements of scapulothoracic and GH joints.
- The anterior translation of humeral head and relative posterior translation of greater tuberosity increases peel-back forces at superior labrum. Also the anterior translation gives tractional forces through the biceps tendon. The magnitude of these forces equal body weight and can avulse the labrum from attachment of glenoid—the SLAP lesion.

Pathoanatomy

The areas at risk of injury and developing pathology from it are:

- Posterosuperior labrum
- Articular side of rotator cuff (PASTA and PAINT) lesions

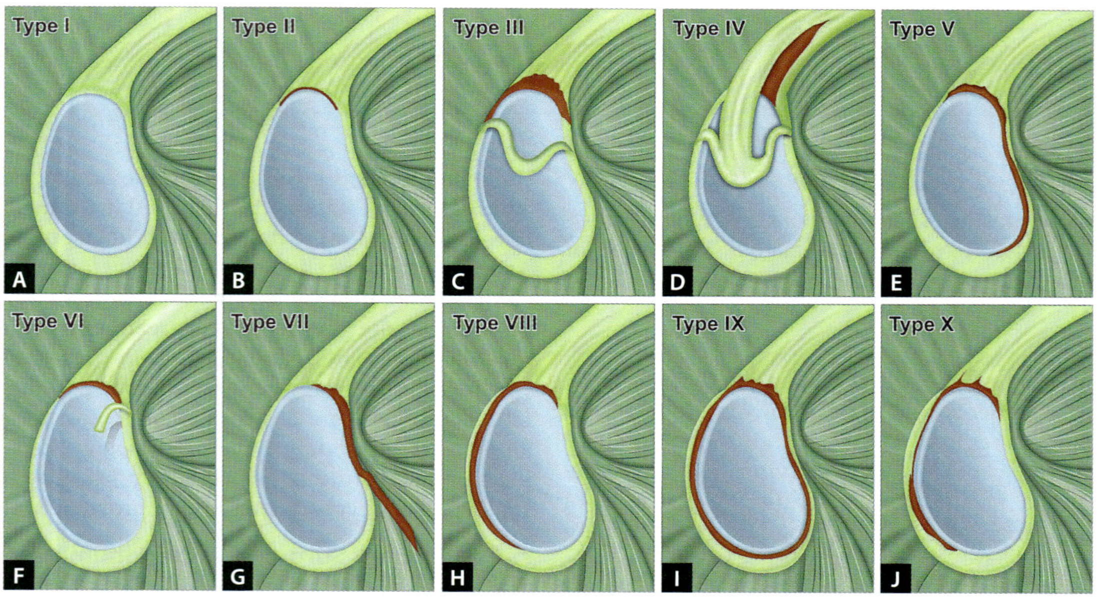

Figs. 18A to J: Superior labral anterior to posterior (SLAP lesions) classified according to location of the tear and its extent. The different types of SLAP lesions recognized in clinical practice (more are being described). Type I: Fraying of superior labrum biceps anchor intact; Type II: Superior labrum detached with detachment of biceps anchor; Type III: Bucket handle type tear of the superior labrum (biceps anchor intact); Type IV: Bucket handle tear with extension into biceps tendon; Type V: SLAP lesion with anterioinferior extension (Bankart + SLAP); Type VI: Anterior or posterior flap tear like type IV or III with bucket handle component; Type VII: Extension of SLAP lesion into glenohumeral ligament; Type VIII: Extension of SLAP lesion into posterior labrum; Type IX: Circumferential labrum detachment; Type X: Extension of SLAP to rotator interval and articular abnormalities.

- The greater tuberosity
- Anterior and anteroinferior capsulolabral complex
- Posterosuperior glenoid

Clinical Features

The patients report pain on overhead activity with gradual deterioration of faculty like slowing of the speed of throw or athletic activity and inability to reach preinjury levels often describing it as "dead arm syndrome". There is pain during particular phase of throwing motion. Throwers with II feel pain posteriorly and those with SLAP lesion feel it more anteriorly. Other symptoms with SLAP include "catching" or "locking" during overhead activity. Careful evaluation will point to SLAP lesion. There is atrophy and asymmetry of the musculature. Tenderness may be elicited over bicipital groove, greater and lesser tuberosities, posterior capsule, and sometimes even over AC joint. The throwers have been found to have GIRD and increased posterior shoulder tightness. A combination of positive O'Brien test, speed's test and apprehension with arm in 90° of abduction and maximal external rotation has been found to be 75% sensitive and 90% specific for diagnosis, though crank and Yergason tests are also positive. MRI will identify the lesion in doubtful cases though MR arthrogram is a more specific investigation it seems.

Treatment

Conservative treatment is the preferred modality in low-demand patients and even in high-grade athletes. This is called "thrower's paradox"—they need to have enough intrinsic laxity while also stability to prevent subluxation. Even minimal decreases in ROM are potentially dangerous to career. There should be stress on dynamic stabilization exercises and stabilizing the shoulder thus usually suffices. Focused core-strengthening, trunk stability, and pelvic stabilization exercises should be stressed. Labral and rotator-cuff pathologies are addressed by rotator-cuff stretching and strengthening and correcting the internal rotation deficits (GIRD).

Repair of the lesion is indicated in high-level athletes for restoring function if the conservative management fails after 6 months of faithful perusal. The order of repair is usually as follows:

- Rotator-cuff debridement
- Labrum debridement
- Posterior and superior labrum repair
- Articular-sided rotator-cuff repair (PASTA lesions)
- Anterior labrum repair
- Intratendinous rotator-cuff repair (PAINT lesions)

CONCLUSION

- Glenohumeral instability is a common cause of morbidity and loss of function in young individuals. This has been the most common indication for arthroscopy of the shoulder joint for restoring stability.
- Instability of shoulder joint should be carefully evaluated for identifying all the damaged structures so that comprehensive management is delivered.
- Most of the patients can be managed by arthroscopic reconstruction, however, some complex cases exist that need bony reconstruction or complex repairs (as in recurrent instability) by open methods additionally or completely.
- Atraumatic multidirectional bilateral rehabilitation inferior capsular shift type instability is a tricky problem that needs to be managed on individual basis else failures are common.

CHAPTER

59 Calcific Tendinopathy

Manish Kumar Varshney

INTRODUCTION

Also termed as "calcific tendonitis", it is characterized by a reactive deposition of calcium in the rotator cuff tendons almost always at the deeper layers where the collagen of cuff blends with capsule. Supraspinatus tendon is the most common site of calcific tendinopathy. Most often, the deposits are incidentally seen on radiographs but with significant growth, they are a common cause of shoulder pain **(Figs. 1A and B)**. Some 50% of patients with calcific deposits in rotator cuff tendons have shoulder pain and acute or chronic painful restrictions of the range of motion of the shoulders. The disease is uncommon in patients under 40 years of age and is seen in approximately 5% of population. Right shoulder is more commonly affected than left and females seem to be affected more commonly than males.

ETIOPATHOGENESIS

The etiopathogenesis of calcific deposits is unclear; however, it is definite that the calcification occurs in the metaplastic degeneration. Decreased vascularity, cuff degeneration, and increased levels of human leukocyte antigen class 1 (HLA1) are likely related. There seems to be no relation of tendon rupture and calcification. Various theories for this metaplastic degeneration have been forwarded including ischemia in the so-called hypovascular critical zone of the rotator cuff, degeneration of the tendons, and metabolic disturbances but none substantiated to complete the explanation. Somehow fibrocartilaginous transformation of the tendon tissue occurs that favors calcium deposition, however, the local factors that favor calcium deposition and nucleation still need detail. Intracellular accumulation of *microspheroliths or psammomas* has been identified in macrophages and other cells ultrastructurally; though the appearance of crystals is different from extracellular deposition. Interesting to the calcific deposition is that inflammatory reactive cells are conspicuously absent histopathologically. Inflammation is seen only during acute episodes but is still subdued. Granulation tissue and reparative fibrotic tissue is present during healing phase. Bilateral affection is seen in 20–30% patients suggesting a predisposition to disease rather than evolution from trauma or degeneration only. The course of the disease typically consists of intermittent increase in pain that is quite severe lasting for few days to weeks and

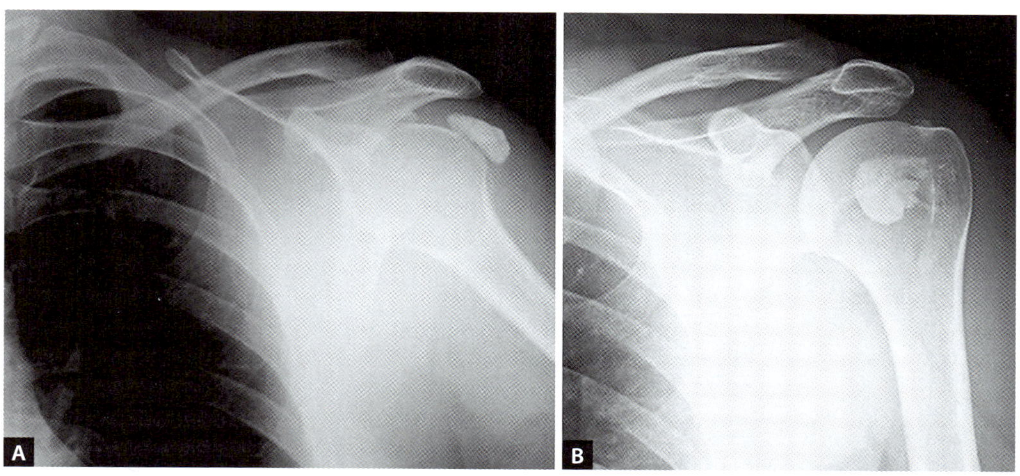

Figs. 1A and B: Calcific tendinopathy: The appearance of incidentally diagnosed lesion showing dense white deposit in the bursa or the tendon.

commonly subsiding with conservative means. The pain is so severe that the person often prefers somnolence in a dark area or may toss in bed. The patients often relate the severity to ureteric stone pain so colloquially calcific disease of shoulder is also called "kidney stone disease of shoulder". The pain often subsides with bursting of the calcific deposit out of the tendinous deposit commonly toward the bursal side (less commonly into the joint). This can be followed by spontaneous resorption of deposit and reconstitution of the tendon only for the disease to recur later. In some patients, the deposits are absorbed spontaneously with limited pain.

RADIOLOGIC APPEARANCE AND CLASSIFICATION

Usually two types are easily appreciable, one fluffy and amorphous type (representing the resorptive symptomatic phase) while other sharply defined and homogeneous (representing the formative/chronic phase) as described by DePalma. The calcific tendinosis is classified by French arthroscopic society into four types:

1. *Type A:* Dense, homogeneous, and sharply delineated appearance
2. *Type B:* Dense, fragmented, and sharply delineated
3. *Type C:* Fluffy heterogeneous appearance **(Fig. 2)**
4. *Type D:* Dystrophic spotted appearance occurring at the torn edges typically seen at the tendon insertion. This is associated with poor prognosis.

The calcific deposits appear hyperechoic on ultrasonography are hyperemic on Doppler scan. The deposits in less symptomatic individuals are arc-shaped, dense, and homogeneous while more painful ones appear fragmented, nodular and cystic but have higher chances of resorption.

CLINICAL COURSE OF DISEASE

The disease has a variable course and while the disease onset is acutely painful in some patients with progressively enlarging deposits disabling them to chronic mild symptomatic shoulders in others with intermittent increase in symptoms. In some patients, the disease fully subsides with complete remission of symptoms and resorption of calcific deposits. Chronic calcific tendonitis generally presents with impingement symptoms of pain with overhead motion. The deposits are commonly located 1–2 cm from the insertion of the supraspinatus tendon on the greater tuberosity. Uhthoff described four stages of calcific tendinopathy as follows:

1. *Precalcific phase:* This is asymptomatic and possibly entails the fibrocartilaginous metaplastic change.
2. *Formative phase:* The calcific nucleation and deposition begins but inflammation is minimal to cause pain. If at all the pain is usually mild and self-limited.
3. *Resorptive phase:* The solid calcium deposits change to "paste" like consistency and pain could be acutely severe developing abruptly. The movements are limited and patient is disabled for even the routine activities.
4. *Postcalcific phase:* This final phase sometimes called reconstitution phase is characterized by resolution of symptoms and possible recycling of events. Some tendon regeneration is seen with fibrotic changes in surrounding tissue.

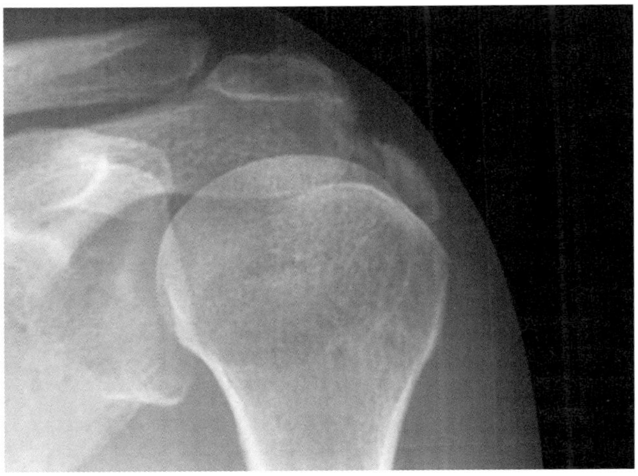

Fig. 2: Calcific tendinopathy. Note the fluffy deposit seen in the liquefactive stage of the disease.

TREATMENT

Initial management of calcific tendonitis is mainly conservative aimed at making the patient comfortable with typical ice application, analgesics, and symptomatic therapy. Passive mobilization and pendulum exercises are combined to prevent the development of adhesive capsulitis. The conservative treatment may fail in patients with bilateral disease, large calcifications, calcific tendonitis beneath anterior third of acromion and extension of calcific deposits medial to acromion. Alternative therapies are sought in these symptomatic patients. Variable benefits have been reported with shockwave therapy and locally applied ultrasonic therapy that are aimed to disintegrate the deposits and stimulate resorption. Lower-intensity ultrasound preferably stimulates inflammatory reaction to clear the debris by phagocytosis while higher-intensity ultrasonics directly shatter the calcium aggregates. The shockwave therapy is believed to produce dose-dependent changes in the calcific deposit that become more amenable to resorption but it has never been substantiated strongly. High-energy treatment is somewhat better than low-energy shock waves. It is contraindicated in patients with any type of infection, patients on pacemaker, presence of heterotopic ossification, osteonecrosis of osteomyelitis of humeral head and in patients <18 years (open growth plate). Open surgical removal of the deposits, needling and local anesthetic injection, closed lavage of the deposits with lidocaine and arthroscopic debridement are reserved for unresolved patients and offer the quickest relief from symptoms but may not be effective in all. Ultrasound-guided needling and aspiration involves needle insertion into the lesion and lavage with a solution of saline and anesthetic.

Some surgeons use two needles for safe egress of the lavage fluid. Multiple sites puncture may benefit by removing more deposits and stimulating healing. Arthroscopic evacuation and debridement of the calcific deposit is the most preferred mode of intervention. Associated rotator cuff tears are rare (<10%) but when found may be simultaneously repaired. The postoperative course in these repair patients is more protracted and marked by higher rate of shoulder stiffness and slow return to function. Radiation therapy has now no role, however, in France the concept of "anti-inflammatory radiation" is supported.

CONCLUSION

The calcific tendinopathy of shoulder represents possibly metaplastic deposition of calcium in degeneration tendons (most commonly supraspinatus) and/or soft tissues around shoulder. The etiopathogenesis is not completely clear; however, episodic pain is definitely a concern that needs prompt treatment. Surgical extirpation of the deposit gives the most consistent results but in patients with infrequent disturbance with the deposits one may consider other options such as ultrasound therapy or shock-wave therapy.

CHAPTER 60

Lesions of Biceps Tendon

Manish Kumar Varshney

INTRODUCTION

Long head of biceps tendon is an important structure (stepchild of shoulder joint) both for dynamic and static stability of shoulder and being an intra-articular structure it is vulnerable to various pathologies. Like the critical zone of rotator cuff the biceps tendon is subject to vascular compromise due to limited supply.

BICIPITAL TENDINOSIS

Primary inflammation (tendinitis) of biceps tendon is rare if at all. Commonly, there is tendinosis or tendinopathy. This can arise in following conditions:

- More often the condition is seen associated with subacromial impingement syndrome (SIS) as the tendon passes beneath the anterior edge of the acromion (anterior impingement of Neer) where it can get impinged in forward flexion and internal rotation. Otherwise, the tendon may get exposed to the stiff coracoacromial arch in complete rotator cuff tears (the type A impingement tendinitis of Slatis and Aalto). The type B bicipital tendinitis has been referred in context to subluxating tendon and type C represents attritional tendinitis. I feel type B is a separate disorder itself and would get rather less importance if grouped under tendinitis (rather tendinosis).
- Other cause is a narrow groove that tightens the tendon and under constant pressure that may even rupture following weakness from inflammation. This is the classic example of primary tendinitis still, however, the inflammation of intra-articular part is missing. One can see arthroscopically the inflammation of the extra-articular portion by pulling the tendon into the joint and also at the lips of bicipital groove (lipstick sign).
- The biceps tendon sheath is a direct extension of the glenohumeral (GH) joint whereby the involvement can be seen in periarthritis and other inflammatory conditions such as rheumatoid arthritis (referred to as secondary tendinitis).

The pain of bicipital tendinitis is typically felt along the anterior lateral aspect of the shoulder with radiation into arm. Often local tenderness can be elicited directly over the bicipital groove with arm in 10° of internal rotation. Pain can also be felt while resisting functional movements at shoulder joint like resisting forward flexion and even resisting the elbow flexion. Other tests have been mentioned in previous chapters (*see* also **Table 1** and **Figs. 1A to D**). The patients typically have full active and passive ROM with pain felt at the end range of flexion and abduction. Management is primarily aimed at controlling the inflammation of the tendon taking care not to exacerbate the acutely inflamed tissue. Once the inflammation and pain subsides, passive and active ROM exercises are begun within pain-free ranges. Intensive strengthening of muscles and program for it is initiated when full pain-free ROM is obtained. Prevention of rupture is the most important motive of therapy to retain function. Ruptured tendon is quite acceptable to elderly population, however, it has shown to reduce supination, pronation, and flexion strength by 20–30% that produces noticeable disability in young and active patients. Isolated tenodesis or tenotomy is not usually indicated. In patients with concomitant rotator cuff pathology (majority), the treatment should be primarily for cuff lesions. Detailed discussion is available in Chapter on "Rotator Cuff Disease".

SUBLUXATING BICEPS TENDON

The biceps tendon swings from one side to another in the bicipital groove with rotations at shoulder **(Fig. 2)**. Normally, this is a smooth process but if the groove is shallow or the movements are extreme the tendon may slide over one of the tuberosities tearing the transverse humeral ligament in the process. Repeated subluxation withers the tuberosity and tendon both with increase in the frequency of the subluxation. Mild pain with activity but an annoying click with rotation of arm is the primary complaint. The tendon subluxates out of tuberosity during abduction and external rotation motions and reduces back with adduction and internal rotation. Treatment is guided primarily by the activity level and participation of the individual. Conservative intervention involves the temporary avoidance of the pain and click-provoking movements, and the application of transverse friction massage. Subluxation of the biceps can be treated surgically by replacement of the tendon into the groove and reconstruction of the rotator cuff combined with subacromial decompression.

TABLE 1: Clinical tests for proximal biceps tendon pathology.

Test	*Method*	*Interpretation*
Ludington test for pathology of long head of biceps tendon	Ask the patient to flex I will go to 90° and keep forearm in full pronation while keeping his arm at their side. Grasp the patient's wrist and actively resist his effort to supination	The maneuvre produces pain in anterior shoulder or bicipital groove
Yergason test to check integrity of transverse ligament across the bicipital groove of humerus	The patient sits with arm by the side of body. The elbow is flex to 90°. The examiner resists supination movement of arm from fully pronated position	Localized pain is felt at the bicipital groove
Neer test for internal impingement syndrome (Neer demonstrated that long head of biceps tendon please closely involved in internal impingement)	Passively elevate the arm of patient maximally in full internal rotation while stabilising the scapula simultaneously	Patient reports pain/weakness in the subacromial space/edge of the acromion and in biceps region
Hawkins–Kennedy test (this tests impingement of greater tuberosity and coracoacromial ligament)	Forward flex the arm to 90° and quickly rotate internally	Pain is felt in the anterior shoulder
Speed test for pathology of biceps muscle or tendon	Ask the patient to flex his arm to 90° while keeping in full supination. Examiner provides resistance to this movement. Repeat the maneuvre in full pronation	Increased pain is felt in the bicipital groove especially during full supination

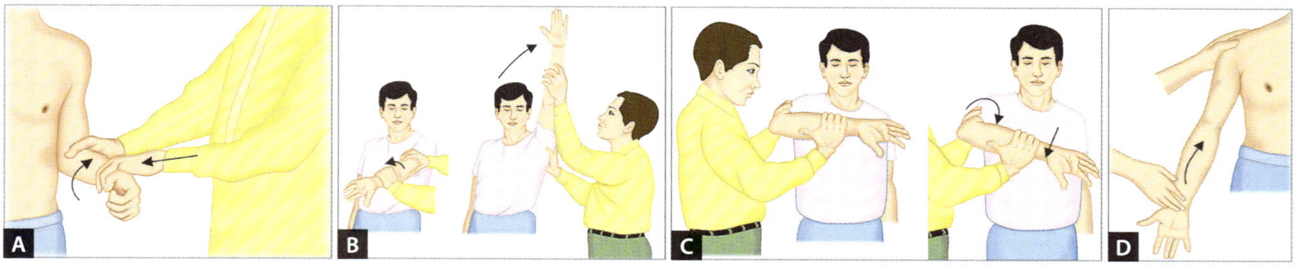

Figs. 1A to D: Tests for biceps tendon. (A) Yergason test; (B) Neer test; (C) Hawkins–Kennedy test; (D) Speed test (*see* **Table 1** for details).

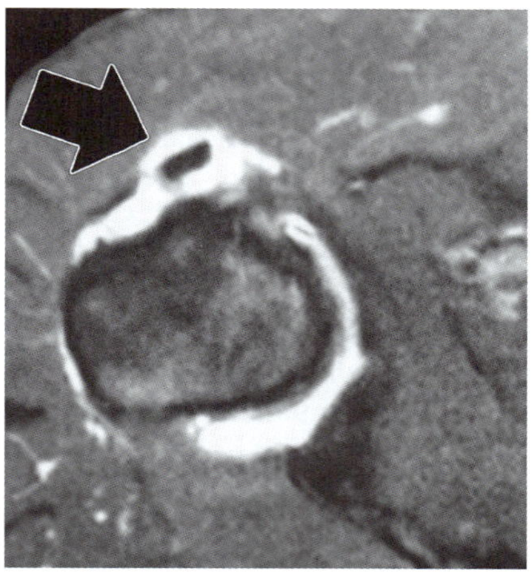

Fig. 2: Biceps subluxation: The biceps tendon is seen displaced anteriorly from its groove.

RUPTURE OF THE LONG HEAD OF BICEPS

Total rupture of the biceps muscle is usually seen in middle-aged patients, especially the parachutists. Rupture of proximal long tendon of biceps accounts for more than half of the tendon ruptures and is seen in patients aged 40–60 years. Younger patients with tendon ruptures are those commonly engaged in heavy weightlifting or other high-energy contact sports. Rupture is commonly located at the exit of tendon from joint into groove but may also be intra-articular or at the musculotendinous junction (less common). In the case of later site quite a significant ecchymosis may trickle down into the arm confusing with the muscle belly rupture. Ruptures at the glenoid origin are also seen and are commonly associated with SLAP (superior labrum from anterior to posterior) lesions. In elderly the rupture commonly occurs following impingement or attrition of tendon from friction of coracoacromial arch or anterior acromion inferior osteophyte. The condition can also get precipitated by weakening of collagen structure from repeated injections of steroid into the bicipital groove or in cases of chronic impingement.

Except in degenerative tears, the patients usually report feeling a "snap" at the time of the direct or indirect injury. Indirect injury often occurs via powerful contraction of the biceps against isometric position. Immediately following the feeling the patient has severe pain and swelling with feeling of loss of strength, especially in elbow flexion and shoulder external rotation. This is followed by a few weeks of mild-to-moderate pain, followed by resolution of the pain and restoration of normal function. The degenerative tears are usually painless and noted by the elderly patient for sudden change in the contour of the arm. When patient attempts to contract the biceps, the muscle belly rolls down the distal humerus, producing a characteristic swelling closer to the elbow instead of in the middle of the arm: the so-called *"Popeye" sign* (**Fig. 3**, based on the famous cartoon character). After a few months, there is usually no

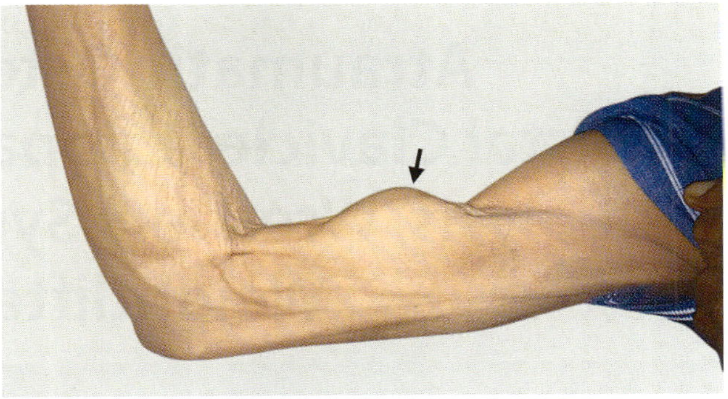

Fig. 3: Note the distal bulging of biceps muscle in the arm (arrow) due to rupture of long head of biceps resembling the biceps of cartoon character "pcpeye".

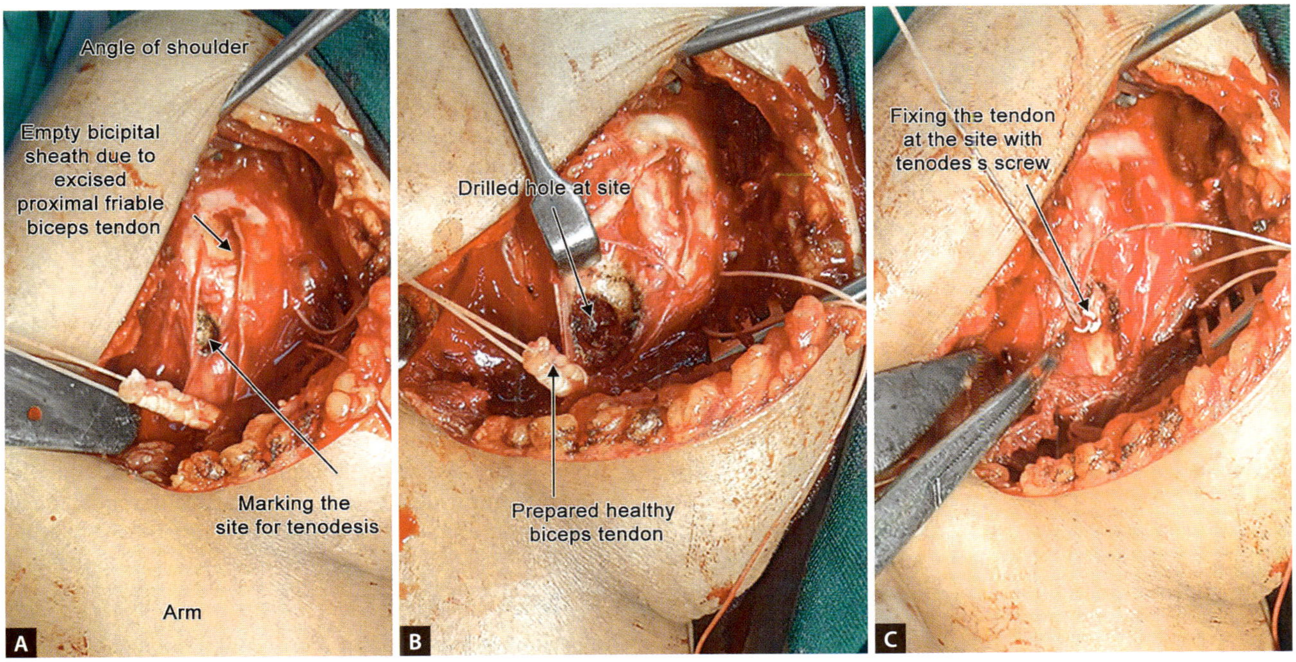

Figs. 4A to C: Open technique biceps tenodesis is performed in this patient with chronic rotator cuff tear and biceps tendon pathology troubling her. Open subscapularis repair is also performed in the patient.

demonstrable loss in strength and is especially common in elderly where they are not at all troubled by functional loss (as none remains). Careful clinical examination and evaluation of strength reveals loss of supination strength but powerful supination is hardly required in routine activities. The short head of the biceps remains intact and usually compensated for any significant functional deficits. Surgical repair is rarely indicated except in the younger, active population (<50 years), patients requiring powerful supination activities (carpenters) and in those chronic cases that are troubled due to cuff pathology (the biceps tendon is indirectly addressed). Tenodesis is preferred in young active patients that can be done either by an open **(Figs. 4A to C)** or arthroscopic approach. Tenotomy is reserved for elderly patients who are less troubled by weak supination. Rupture of the long head of the biceps increases the risk of developing a subacromial impingement syndrome resulting from the pull of short head of the biceps onto the humeral head, so acromioplasty and coracoacromial ligament excision should be combined.

CONCLUSION

Biceps tendon is an important dynamic structure of the shoulder joint, being quite mobile it is often subjected to frictional syndromes producing bicipital tendinosis. If it is let to continue, rupture of the tendon is inevitable outcome.

Subluxation of biceps tendon out of humeral groove can also produce bicipital tendinosis and ultimately attritional rupture of the tendon. If associated with rotator cuff injury it should be repaired in the groove if intervention is done for cuff tear.

Ruptured long head of biceps is commonly seen in elderly patients and is often not noticed by them for low functional demands. In young individuals that do not accept the functional loss, tenodesis of the tendon may be prescribed.

CHAPTER 61

Atraumatic Osteolysis of the Distal Clavicle (Idiopathic Clavicle Osteolysis, Wrestlers Syndrome, and Weightlifters Shoulder)

Manish Kumar Varshney

INTRODUCTION

The condition was first described by Dupas in 1936 as caused by trauma, while Ehricht in 1959 reported that osteolysis of clavicle can even occur in the absence of trauma. This leads to the division of the condition into two broad arms—traumatic and atraumatic. The atraumatic disease arises from repeated microtrauma where it is believed that the distal clavicle fails with propagation of repeated stress fractures, followed by cystic and erosive changes. The bone resorption occurs subsequently with continued stress. Haupt named the condition "weightlifter's shoulder" where he reported the radiological features in heavy-weightlifters who reported more severe pain after a weightlifting program. Inhibition of bone formation is poorly understood but seems to also result from continued stress on the joint. The condition is most common in athletes involved in prolonged weight training like weightlifters and the prevalence is reported to be increasing. Bilateral affection is seen in 20% patients. Atraumatic osteolysis of clavicle represents a subset of acromioclavicular (AC) arthritis so the following description is also appropriate for AC joint arthritis.

PATHOGENESIS

Like for most other conditions the pathogenesis is debated between traumatic and atraumatic. As noted above even the atraumatic pathology involves repeated microtrauma so in essence also incorporates trauma in pathogenesis. For atraumatic osteolysis, synovial invasion of subchondral bone has been suggested by Brunet that is partly supported by magnetic resonance imaging (MRI) findings of synovial proliferation in the AC joint, but the microscopic examination findings of Matthews and associates demonstrated increased osteoclastic activity representative of repeated microfractures. Cahill reported microfractures in >50% of cases and he reported in a case series suggesting also that repetitive microtrauma and development of microfractures followed by cystic changes is responsible for the osteolysis. The articular cartilage undergoes fissuring and degeneration secondarily due to lost support from subchondral bone.

PATHOANATOMY

Histopathologically, three characteristic findings are reported in osteolysis of lateral end of clavicle viz.:

1. Poorly mineralized trabecular bone (seen also radiologically) seen replaced by dense scar tissue in lateral end of clavicle. Also there is thin unorganized hyperplastic fibrocartilage.
2. The above findings are dominated by prominent metaplastic bone formation due to reactive osteoblastic activity in an environment of increased osteoclastic activity consistent with repetitive stress on the bone as proposed in pathogenesis.
3. Due to loss of hard bone the histological sections passing across the AC joint demonstrate articular cartilage degeneration, destruction, synovial proliferation, chronic inflammatory tissue, and fibrosis.

CLINICAL FEATURES

The patients report a painful and dull ache localized to the AC joint. Pain is worse at the beginning of exercise often radiating down into the deltoid and trapezius. Patients find bench presses, and push-ups particularly painful. Abduction of the arm beyond 90° and throwing causes pain with disease progression, but the movements at glenohumeral joint are usually full. On examination, localized point tenderness and pain at the AC joint can be elicited. Stability of AC joint should be assessed by stressing the joint in anteroposterior and superoinferior directions by grasping the clavicle between thumb and index finger. Forced arm adduction across the chest is painful **(Table 1)**.

DIFFERENTIAL DIAGNOSES

Differential diagnoses include cervical spondylosis, rotator cuff disease, hyperparathyroidism, gout, Gorham's disease, scleroderma, infection, rheumatoid arthritis, multiple myeloma, etc. Injecting lidocaine into subacromial bursa and relief from same distinguishes rotator cuff disease, alternatively AC joint could be injected in patients with clavicle osteolysis who get prompt relief.

TABLE 1: Tests for nontraumatic acromioclavicular (AC) joint pain.

Test	Comment
Cross-body adduction test	Passively abduct patient's arm to 90° then cross the arm horizontally across the patient's chest anteriorly—positive if pain at AC joint
O'Brien's active compression test	Place patient's arm in 90° forward flexion then completely internally rotate the arm (thumb pointing downward) and give 10–15° adduction. Push patient's arm down while he resists this push—pain at AC joint suggests pathology
Hawkins–Kennedy test	Patient's arm in 90° forward flexion with the elbow flexed to 90° and the scapula fixed. Examiner forces the glenohumeral joint into internal rotation—pain perceived as discomfort in AC joint region is positive
AC joint tenderness	Palpation of AC joint—pain on palpation localized to AC joint is suggestive

RADIOLOGICAL FINDINGS

Zanca view of clavicle (cephalad tilt of the beam by 15°) helps in visualizing the AC joint without overlapping of the scapular spine. Acromion is spared in the disease process while lesion is seen in the distal clavicle. Osteolysis could be seen on 5 mm–3 cm region of the distal clavicle. Early in the course of disease Tc-99 scintigraphy demonstrates marked uptake in the clavicle; however, the findings are not characteristic.

MRI demonstrates bone marrow edema in all the cases that may also be seen in the acromion but is never seen "only" in the acromion in the formed of increased signal intensity on T2-weighted images and fluid-sensitive (fat-suppressed) STIR images in the distal clavicle. Additional findings of AC joint osseous irregularity, fluid in the joint, and osseous fragments may be present but are not characteristic of the disease.

TREATMENT

Prohibiting the stressful exercises and weight-training give relief in majority of patients but the disease recurs with resumption of activities, so restriction is to be for life long. The provocative maneuvers are completely avoided, weight-training techniques may be modified to avoid putting stress on the AC joint, nonsteroidal anti-inflammatory drugs (NSAIDs) for control of symptoms are few of the measures. To reduce the stress on the AC joint during bench-press, narrowing the grip by placing the hands no farther than 1.5 times the bi-acromial width is recommended. Ancillaries to conservative management include local heat, NSAIDs, range of motion, and stretching and strengthening exercises. Intra-articular injection of steroid does not provide lasting relief but a lot of surgeons do use it for diagnostic purpose and temporary relief.

Surgical treatment is indicated in patients failed on conservative management and consists of resection of the distal clavicle (open or arthroscopically) distal to coracoclavicular ligament insertion to prevent instability. The indication for surgical treatment is finding point of tenderness at the AC joint with supportive evidence in the form of characteristic radiographs, abnormal uptake in scintigraphy, unwillingness of the patient to avoid/modify the training or manual labor. Amount of distal clavicle resection is debated; however, as proposed by Cahill, a resection of 1–2 cm (Mumford procedure, resection of distal clavicle with small amount of acromion) provides good relief, however, arthroscopic resection of as less as 4 mm of the bone has been found to give significant relief from symptoms. In any case, the idea is to prevent AC joint impingement when shoulder is taken through complete range of motion. All attempts should be made to preserve AC ligaments that can be closed later. Transferring the coracoacromial ligament to distal clavicle as suggested by Flatow may provide additional stability to the clavicle in weightlifters. Damage to the AC ligaments may result in abutment of distal clavicle on acromion causing failure of open procedure.

"Arthroscopic procedure" is advantageous in the sense that less tissue damage occurs at the site and patient has a shortened postoperative hospital stay and rehabilitation period. Pain relief is also fast and it is portended that lesser bone removal would relieve the symptoms than that needed in open procedure. Usually 5 mm–1 cm of bone is removed in arthroscopic procedure. The approach in arthroscopy can be made indirectly through the subacromial region (Ellman and Esch) that has the advantage of preserving stability at the AC joint better. Small portion of acromion can also be resected but it is now considered useless. In any case, the AC ligaments should be preserved else impingement is a likely possibility. If it is found that the ligaments have been disrupted then it is recommended to bevel the distal clavicle posteriorly to avoid impingement. The approach is a bit difficult in tight joints with medial inclination especially those that are osteoarthritic, here direct superior approach could be more useful. The other approach is the direct superior approach to AC joint described by Lanny Johnson. The direct approach is based on the notion that there is no reason to disrupt the bursa for isolated involvement of the AC joint. The distal clavicle can be resected under visualization. Using a 4.0-m or 2.7-mm scope in the joint, the bone is exposed subperiosteally through direct anterosuperior and posterosuperior portals. The intra-articular debridement is done and meniscus is resected along with shelling-out the distal clavicle to preserve soft tissues and AC ligaments. The burr is then used to remove 5–9 mm of the clavicle.

COMPLICATIONS OF SURGICAL PROCEDURES

The complications of surgical procedures are:

- Disruption of the AC ligaments and instability—this causes impingement of clavicle and persisting pain.
- Heterotopic bone formation
- Muscular injury
- Bleeding and hematoma formation

- Lateral clavicle fracture
- Infection

CONCLUSION

- Atraumatic osteolysis of distal clavicle is an uncommon and unique disease most likely linked to overuse syndrome resulting in continued stress at the distal clavicle producing microtrauma.
- Once developed life-time restrictions on the provocative maneuvers are necessary.
- If activity modification fails or patient is unwilling to continue the same, it is usual to go for surgical excision of the distal clavicle. This entails preserving the ligament attachment at the distal clavicle else operative procedure would fail.
- Open (Mumford procedure) is the gold standard but arthroscopic releases have recently become popular. Limited clavicle resection through arthroscopy (using indirect or direct approach) gives adequate pain relief in experienced hands.

CHAPTER 62

The Stiff Shoulder

Manish Kumar Varshney

INTRODUCTION

The stiff shoulder could arise primarily or could develop secondarily following trauma or surgery. The frozen shoulder syndrome was first described by Duplay in 1872 in France calling it "periarthritis scapulohumerale" while Putnam described similar condition in the United States. In 1934, Codman used the term "frozen shoulder" to describe a clinical pattern of muscle spasm and stiffness. In 1945, Neviaser coined the term "adhesive capsulitis" to describe a chronic inflammatory process with secondary thickening and adhesion of capsule to humeral head, at surgery and autopsy in patients treated for a painful and stiff shoulder. True shoulder stiffness can be a primary condition arising independent of any other abnormality or illness (so called "idiopathic stiffness") or it can be a primary condition arising in conjunction with another medical condition (such as diabetes mellitus) also it can develop secondary to another condition (such as prior surgery, arthritis, or trauma). The term "adhesive capsulitis" should be used only to classify idiopathic frozen shoulder and not the secondary forms of stiffness.

A lot of factors have now been associated with adhesive capsulitis and include female (70% cases) gender, age >40 years, trauma, diabetes (11% diabetics suffer from adhesive capsulitis and stiffness in other peripheral joints—"limited joint motion syndrome"), cervical disk disease, pulmonary tuberculosis, prolonged immobilization, chest wall tumors, thyroid disease, stroke or myocardial infarction, parkinsonism, cerebral tumors, certain psychiatric conditions, and the presence of autoimmune diseases. The disease occurs simultaneously or sequentially bilaterally in 20–30% cases. The underlying problem and details of the condition are unknown but the most common explanation favors underlying synovial inflammation with subsequent reactive capsular fibrosis and thickening. Thus, adhesive capsulitis is an inflammatory fibrosing condition but the initial trigger and subsequent development (progression into) fibrosis is unknown. Some cases occur seasonally so even viral etiology has been proposed.

ADHESIVE CAPSULITIS

It is characterized by an idiopathic, progressive, and painful loss of active and passive shoulder motion, particularly external rotation. It is aptly defined as "a condition of uncertain etiology characterized by significant restriction of both active and passive shoulder motion that occurs in the absence of a known intrinsic shoulder disorder" by the American Academy of Orthopedic Surgeons in 1993. There may be syndromic association of diabetes but is not primarily responsible for it. The individual gradually limits the use of the arm. Inflammation and pain can cause muscle guarding of the shoulder muscles without true fixed contracture of the joint capsule. Disuse of the arm results in a loss of shoulder mobility, whereas continued use of the arm through pain can result in development of subacromial impingement. Compensatory movements of the shoulder girdle develop in order to minimize pain. With time, there is resolution of pain and the individual is left with a stiff shoulder with severe limitation of function.

Clinical Course

Patients of adhesive capsulitis have in general pain as the primary complaint with restriction of movements (so called "frozen shoulder"). Typically, two presentations can be seen:

1. In a subset, the pain is predominant complaint while the movement restriction does not corroborate to quantity of pain. Often this gets confused with rotator cuff disorder or impingement syndrome with incarcerated tendon. This condition is self-limiting, and the patient spontaneously recovers within 6 months to a year—the so-called connotation of 1-year disease. The treatment here is majorly supportive with stretching exercise program aimed to restore function and pain control with analgesics.
2. In the other subset, the pain is as prominent as restricted movements at shoulder and a radiation component is commonly noticed with pain going laterally from arm to elbow. The patient complains of pain at rest and sleep disturbance due to pain noticeable in specific postures. Typical restriction of external rotation is noticed.

Because fibrotic component is predominant fibrolysis with manipulation, repetitive steroid injections, and distention therapy, and arthroscopic release is indicated individually or in combinations.

The natural history of adhesive capsulitis follows a pattern of escalating disability and then recovery moving through three phases—the "painful phase" lasting 9 months, the "adhesive phase" lasting 3–12 months, and the "resolution phase" lasting 3 months to 3 years. Four stages of adhesive capsulitis have been described by Neviaser based on pathologic changes in the synovium and subsynovium.

1. *Stage I (symptoms for <3 months):* The patients have mild-to-moderate dull aching pain even at rest similar to impingement syndrome and rotator cuff tendinosis. Immediately, however, the patients report progressive loss of motion. There is loss of external rotation and abduction with a mild decrease in internal rotation in adduction. In patients with concomitant type 1 diabetes mellitus, there is typically equal limitation of external rotation and internal rotation, which is greater than the limitation of abduction. Capsular contracture is absent and most symptoms arise from synovitis.
2. *Stage II (symptoms for 3–9 months):* This stage is a continuum of stage 1 with more scarring and similar synovitis. Physician injects local anesthetic into the joint and evaluates the patient. Patient in stage 1 will have significant improvement in pain and movements while in stage 2, the pain will relieve but movements will still be restricted due to capsular scarring. The loss of motion is present in all planes and full ROM is painful.
3. *Stage III (symptoms for 9–14 months):* The patients have initial history of painful stiffness of shoulder that burns into relatively painfree but stiff shoulder. Poor scapulohumeral rhythm with a dominance of the upper trapezius activity is demonstrable which is attributable to decreased inferior glide of glenohumeral joint.
4. *Stage IV (stage of thawing):* This stage is characterized by the slow and steady recovery of shoulder function. There is capsular remodeling with increased movements and shoulder usage. Pain is resolved but the functional residue persists and possibly patient accepts the disability so is much less complaining. Functional restriction is evident with use of function evaluation tools like disabilities of the arm shoulder and hand (DASH).

Arthroscopically, four stages can be differentiated based on the findings:

1. *Stage 1:* There is patchy fibrinous synovitis with localized capsular adhesions.
2. *Stage 2:* Capsular contraction with fibrinous adhesions is visible along with active synovitis.
3. *Stage 3:* There is increased capsular contraction with difficult fluid distention of shoulder. The synovitis undergoes resolving stage and is replaced by disorganized fibrous tissue.
4. *Stage 4:* Advanced capsular contraction and poor negotiation of arthroscope or joint visibility.

Epidemiology

The overall incidence of adhesive capsulitis has been reported to be between 2 and 5%. It is commonly observed in patients in their fifth and sixth decade of life and females are affected more than males. There is a correlation between incidence of adhesive capsulitis and certain chronic illnesses like Parkinson disease (13%), head injuries (25%), diabetes mellitus (10–35%), autonomic disorders of the upper extremity (such as post-stroke shoulder-hand syndrome with an incidence of approximately 25%), thyroid diseases, cardiopulmonary diseases, and lung carcinoma.

Pathogenesis

The recent understanding in gross and microscopic pathological changes in the capsule of shoulder joint shows active fibroblastic proliferation, accompanied by some transformation of fibroblasts to myofibroblasts by the activity of polypeptide growth factors and matrix metalloproteinases. Many of the histologic characters of Dupuytren's disease are shared by adhesive capsulitis. The changes, hence, produce gross restriction of movements that is often painful.

Diagnosis

The diagnosis is purely clinical with investigations required only to rule out the secondary causes of shoulder stiffness. The physical examination in a patient with adhesive capsulitis of shoulder reveals a global reduction of shoulder range of motion with marked decrease in glenohumeral translation (the average range of motion described in literature being 98° of abduction, 117° of flexion, 33° of external rotation, and 18° of internal rotation). Apart from the limited range of motion, an imbalance in the shoulder complex muscles leads to altered shoulder motion (shoulder dyskinesis). The upper trapezius has been found to be more active than the lower trapezius. Pain though reported to be present diffusely throughout the shoulder girdle by patients, the tenderness on examination is often greatest over the anterior subacromial bursa, the proximal biceps tendon, the rotator interval area, and the anterior capsule.

Differential Diagnosis

The following closely resemble a stiff shoulder clinically:

- Glenohumeral arthritis
- Rotator cuff tendinosis, and
- Calcific tendonitis.

Radiology

Radiographs are silent and demonstrate osteopenia in initial stages; they should be done to exclude other pathologies like arthritis. MRI demonstrates synovitis, obliteration of the infraglenoid capsular recess, fluid in the joint, fibrosis, and capsular thickening. Increased vascularity is also evident with active inflammation in initial stages. Rotator cuff tears are a common accompaniment of adhesive capsulitis.

Treatment

The advances in histopathological characterization or clinical judgment over time with recognition of various patterns have not contributed much to guide the treatment, which has been classically symptom based. Various modalities have been prescribed to basically improve movements and control pain without any logical reasoning as to how fast and how complete the relief of symptoms should be. Treatment options for adhesive capsulitis range from nonoperative to operative modalities. The various proposed methods by different authors for the treatment of frozen shoulder are education/watchful waiting; physical therapy (including physiotherapy, cryotherapy, and acupuncture), oral corticosteroids, nonsteroidal anti-inflammatory drugs (NSAIDs), injections (corticosteroid, local anesthetic, and sodium hyaluronate), articular or arthrographic distention, manipulation under anesthesia, arthroscopic and open surgery, or a combination of these.

Conservative management is aimed at symptomatic relief and gradual return of shoulder function by stretching exercises. Patients need to be informed and counseled for protracted course of physiotherapy so that compliance is better. Interventions like local ultrasonics and guided program for intensive stretching in movement restricted patients. The steroids should be used to control pain and ongoing fibrosis keeping also in mind the prohibiting effects on collagen. Despite aggressive maneuvers significant percentage of patients (30–50%) have long- term restriction of movements. Various interventional measures have been reported to dilate capsule. Capsular distention or *brisement* relies on rupturing the capsule by fluid injection. Closed manipulation under anesthesia is recommended as a measure to stretch capsule but may be associated with recurrence of disease due to subsequent pain, neurological damage, uncontrolled damage due to stretching of tissue and fractures in osteopenic patients. Sequential stretching of inferior, anteroinferior, anterior, posterior, and postero-inferior capsule should be done using force from only two fingers else arthroscopic release is recommended. Long-term diabetics are usually resistant to manipulation techniques. I have found good return of function by arthroscopic anterior release **(Fig. 1)** and synovectomy combined with steroid injection. Prior to arthroscopic release, we manipulate the shoulder to improve external rotation and abduction. This facilitates the arthroscopic visualization in an otherwise stiff, tight shoulder. Intra-articular steroid suppresses synovitis well compared to any oral therapy and controls the re-occurrence of fibrosis. Early intervention is the rule that we follow and the technique is effective even in long-term diabetics. In general, the more the patient is delayed for treatment, the more protracted course he undergoes and takes longer time to recovery. Open release is rarely needed but may be used for recalcitrant shoulder stiffness following arthroscopic release. Periarticular trigger point injection of subscapularis tendon and pericapsular muscles provide at best temporary relief and are not effective in long term. Suprascapular nerve blocks improve patient's tolerance to deep pressure and may have possible role in patients associated with reflex sympathetic dystrophy.

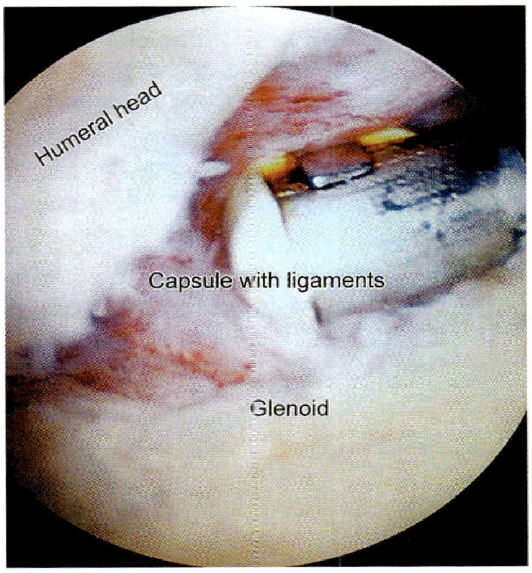

Fig. 1: Adhesive capsulitis: It is being released with a radiofrequency device anteriorly. Usually, the anterior release suffices to improve external rotation. Less frequently, if ever a posterior release is needed.

CONCLUSION

- Stiff shoulder is a disabling condition that significantly limits the activity of patients due to difficulty placing the hand around the body even for day-to-day activities.
- Adhesive capsulitis refers to idiopathic involvement of the shoulder joint without any demonstrable primary condition causing shoulder stiffness.
- Diagnosis is mainly clinical and is based on finding of gross restriction of movements at the affected shoulder joint.
- Manipulation under anesthesia and arthroscopy with or without intra-articular depot steroid injection are both good methods for management of the patients with adhesive capsulitis.
- Compared to manipulation under anesthesia (with local steroid injection) the arthroscopic capsular release (with steroid injection) significantly improves the overall outcome of patients with adhesive capsulitis (at least in our hands, unpublished report).

CHAPTER 63

Hemorrhagic Shoulder (Milwaukee Shoulder, L'épaule Sénile Hémorragique)

Manish Kumar Varshney

INTRODUCTION

The hemorrhagic shoulder of the elderly was first described in 1968 in a subtle form with not much details. It consists of recurrent blood-streaked effusions of the shoulder along with severely destroyed glenohumeral joint evident radiologically. The process is associated with chronic massive tears of rotator cuff and was labeled "cuff tear arthropathy" by Neer et al. now the disease is thought to be a destructive shoulder arthropathy due to deposition of hydroxyapatite crystals identification of which in synovial fluid is the mainstay of diagnosis. The destructive changes are attributed to unrelenting collagenase activity released in response to hydroxyapatite crystals released from pathologic cuff, capsule, synovium and possibly cartilage as described by McCarthy in 1981. McCarthy hailed from Milwaukee so possibly somehow this disorder now comes to be known in the name of "Milwaukee" shoulder. He is credited with the use of term "Milwaukee shoulder syndrome" where he described four elderly women from Milwaukee (Wisconsin, USA) with characteristic finding of recurrent bilateral shoulder effusions and radiologic description of advanced destructive changes in glenohumeral joint. The patients also had massive tears of the rotator cuff. Now it is known that though shoulder is most commonly involved, the disease can also be found in wrists, hands, elbows, neck, lumbar spine, hips, knees, and feet.

PATHOGENESIS

The cuff-tear theory of Neer and colleagues (1983) postulates that untreated chronic and massive tears would lead primarily to a degenerated joint. The destructive changes evolve from combined mechanical and nutritional alterations in the shoulder with a rotator cuff tear. It is now clear that cuff arthropathy is not the primary event rather the presence of aggregates of calcium hydroxyapatite crystals in the synovial fluid cause release of lysosomal enzymes (primarily collagenase and neutral proteases from synoviocytes) that eat away the periarticular tissues, including the rotator cuff. The anteroposterior instability resulting from a massive tear of the rotator cuff, and rupture of the long head of the biceps (producing proximal migration of the humeral head) sort of creates "global" impingement of humeral head in every direction and movement. This creates accelerated wear of glenohumeral articulation from repetitive trauma due to altered biomechanics associated with loss of primary and secondary stabilizers. Inadequate diffusion of nutrients and the diminished quantity of synovial fluid produce changes in the composition of the articular cartilage.

PATHOANATOMY

There are two characteristic findings:

1. First is the finding of numerous aggregates of calcium hydroxyapatite crystals in the synovial fluid along with a noninflammatory effusion.
2. The second is presence of massive rotator cuff tears and associated instability.

EPIDEMIOLOGY

Milwaukee shoulder syndrome occurs commonly in elderly patients aged between 60 and 90 years with a characteristic female preponderance in the ratio of 4:1. To this end higher life expectancy of females may be a contributory factor. Unilateral shoulder joint involvement is much more common than bilateral disease and is typically seen in the dominant side. When the disease is bilateral then also the shoulder on the dominant side almost always presents with more advanced involvement. Few risk factors for the development of the disease have been identified as follows:

- Female gender
- Calcium pyrophosphate crystal deposition (CPPD) disease
- Trauma
- Overuse syndrome
- Neuropathic joint
- Dialysis associated arthropathy
- Joint denervation
- Advanced age

CLINICAL FEATURES AND RADIOLOGY

The patients are typically elderly with long-standing history of shoulder pain. The shoulder somehow starts hurting

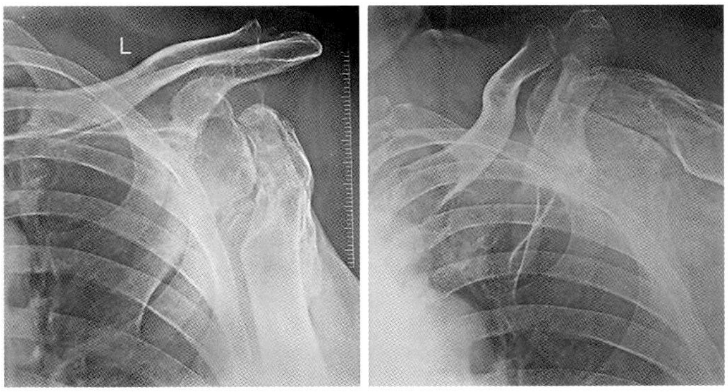

Fig. 1: Milwaukee shoulder. The radiographs of two different patients reveal deshapening of humeral head with large osteophyte formation, cystic sclerotic subchondral changes and extensive narrowing of joint space. The radiograph on right shows complete lysis and resorption of the humeral heads of both shoulders.

more and becomes swollen and unstable over a few months. There is marked crepitus in the joint and loss of active movements. A characteristic finding has been reported by some authors of multiple small dilated blood vessels around the shoulder that produce repeated subcutaneous hemorrhages and ecchymosis in untreated shoulder. The vascular ectasia seems to disappear after surgical intervention spontaneously. Radiographs demonstrate joint space narrowing, advanced degenerative changes and loss of architecture of humeral head with flattening, osteophyte formation **(Fig. 1)** and mixed subchondral sclerotic and cystic changes at the articular surface. Additionally, there may be calcification of the capsule and presence of multiple intra-articular loose bodies.

Ultrasonography demonstrates intra-articular synovial proliferation and large effusions associated with rotator cuff tears.

DIAGNOSIS

The diagnosis is made by clinic-radiological correlation of the above findings. Demonstration of the hydroxyapatite crystals in aspirate is not easy as they do not appear with characteristic findings on light or polarized microscopy. Aggregates of the crystals, however, appear as clumps of "shiny coins". These can be made conspicuous by the use of alizarin-red S stain that produce a characteristic "halo" of orange-red stain around the clumps of hydroxyapatite crystals. Synovial histopathology reveals noncharacteristic findings like synovial cell hyperplasia, giant cell formation, and deposition of fibrin along with calcium phosphate crystals.

DIFFERENTIAL DIAGNOSIS

The differential of this disorder includes:

- Septic arthritis
- Tuberculosis of the shoulder joint
- Rapidly destructive arthropathy of unknown cause
- Neuropathic arthropathy
- Osteonecrosis
- Other crystal-associated arthropathy
- Inflammatory arthritis like rheumatoid arthritis
- Vanishing bone disease
- Syphilitic arthropathy (late)

TREATMENT

Mostly the treatment is supportive and for a less troublesome shoulder initially a conservative approach serves to improve functionality. Mild anti-inflammatory medication and gentle stretching exercises to maintain or regain a functional range of motion (ROM) usually helps to gain patient confidence and reassess the situation. Colchicine has been found useful in management of Milwaukee shoulder syndrome. Physiotherapy is, however, the mainstay and a strengthening program should follow to improve the active use of the arm for activities of daily living.

If conservative management fails or is unacceptable then resurfacing procedure will help pain relief and provide functional improvement. The functional gain is, however, much better with a reverse shoulder arthroplasty that takes care of the poor superior coverage and stability of shoulder. It only depends on the deltoid function rather than conventional arthroplasty that require good cuff integrity for functionality. It should be emphasized that reverse shoulder has higher chances of failure and glenoid loosening in young patients due to inferior glenoid rim impingement (inferior notching).

CONCLUSION

- Milwaukee shoulder syndrome is an uncommon destructive arthropathy that is commonly seen in elderly females.
- The disease is characterized by hydroxyapatite induced destruction of the soft tissues around the shoulder with rapid progression of degeneration due to lack of tissue support (rotator cuff) and joint balance.
- Alizarin-red stain may help in establishing diagnosis by characteristic demonstration of the crystal aggregates.
- Treatment is mainly supportive based primarily on physiotherapy but patients who fail to respond to the same may be benefitted in a limited extent by shoulder arthroplasty.

CHAPTER 64

Osteoarthritis of Shoulder Joint

Manish Kumar Varshney

INTRODUCTION

The shoulder is the third most common joint affected by degenerative joint disease after knee and hip, but incidence is significantly less in India. Risk factors for development of glenohumeral arthrosis include genetic predisposition, female sex, age >70 years, heavy manual labor, and many secondary causes **(Table 1)**. The pathophysiology of development of glenohumeral arthrosis is possibly same with minor differences as at knee or hip. As femoroacetabular impingement is specific to causing arthrosis of hip joint, rotator cuff disorders in advanced stage produce arthropathy/arthrosis of the shoulder joint. The rotator cuff arthropathy (coined by Neer in 1983 for end-result of massive rotator cuff tears) is a specific disorder that results in a defined pattern of shoulder joint degeneration characterized by:

- Insufficiency of rotator cuff
- Glenohumeral joint destruction
- Proximal (superior) migration/subluxation of humeral head
- Osteoporosis of humeral and glenoid components and osteosclerosis under acromion
- Variable destruction and collapse of humeral head.

The deficiency in structure/function of rotator cuff results in abnormal glenohumeral wear pattern and loss of joint congruence. Loss of glenoid concavity compromises joint stability making it susceptible to recurrent dislocations unless soft tissue contractures stabilize the joint thus reducing the movements. The arthropathy is seen more commonly in dominant shoulder of females and superior migration of humeral head is a harbinger of the disorder. The rotator cuff arthropathy has been classified by Seebauer into two types with two subtypes each **(Table 2)**.

Inflammatory arthritis including crystal-induced, rheumatoid, and other seronegative arthropathies produces synovitis that leads to osteopenia erosion of articular cartilage, osteophytes, cystic changes, joint space narrowing, and glenoid erosion. The term "dislocation arthropathy" was coined by Neer and is linked to recurrent instability. It takes years to develop (>20 years) and is also seen after treatment of instability. Overtightening of anterior capsule produces contracture and abnormal mechanics causing capsulorrhaphy arthritis. The degenerative changes involve posterior glenoid

TABLE 1: The etiological associations of glenohumeral arthritis.

Primary glenohumeral arthritis	***Secondary glenohumeral arthritis***
Idiopathic: • Female sex • Age >70 years • Genetic predisposition	*Post-traumatic:* • Proximal humeral fracture • Recurrent instability • Heavy manual labor • Repetitive stress on shoulder *Inflammatory:* • Rheumatoid, systemic lupus erythematosus, seronegative arthropathy • Crystal-induced *Iatrogenic:* • Intra-articular hardware • Tight capsulorrhaphy *Osteonecrosis:* • Traumatic and nontraumatic causes similar to femoral head osteonecrosis *Septic arthritis* *Tuberculosis of shoulder joint* *Rotator cuff arthropathy* *Neuropathic arthropathy* *Hemophilic arthropathy* *Chondrolysis*

TABLE 2: Seebauer classification of rotator cuff arthropathy.

Type	***Description***
Type IA (Centered and stable)	Humeral head is centered and stable, minimal superior migration, coracoacromial arch acetabularization and femoral head acetabularization, anterior restraints are intact, and dynamic joint stabilization
Type IB (Centered and medialized)	Humeral head is centered but medialized, minimal superior migration, medial glenoid erosion, coracoacromial arch acetabularization, intact or compensated anterior restraints, and compromised joint stability
Type IIA (Decentered and limited stability)	Humeral head is decentered, superior translation, superior-medial erosion, significant coracoacromial arch acetabularization, compromised anterior restraints, and limited joint stability
Type IIB (Decentered and unstable)	Humeral head is decentered and unstable, anterior superior escape, coracoacromial arch and anterior structures deficient, nonexistent dynamic stabilization, and no coracoacromial arch stabilization

wear and posterior subluxation of humeral head. Rapid chondrolysis has been seen after arthroscopy and is called postarthroscopic glenohumeral chondrolysis.

Humeral head is the second most common site for developing osteonecrosis. The predisposing factors following proximal humeral fractures for causing ischemia include anatomic neck involvement, posteromedial metaphyseal extension of >8 mm and medial hinge disruption (Hertel et al.). Nontraumatic causes are similar to those discussed for femoral head osteonecrosis elsewhere. The treatment varies with stage and age of patient ranging from arthroscopic debridement, core decompression to arhroplasty that may be resurfacing or standard one.

Uncommon forms of shoulder arthritis include hemophilic arthropathy due to repetitive leak of blood into the joint causing synovial hyperplasia, fibrosis, and precipitation of iron complexes in the joint tissues. Charcot and neuropathic arthropathy (diabetes and syringomyelia) produces rapid destruction of the articulating surfaces due to loss of proprioceptive and protective sensations. The use of continuous pain pumps in shoulder joint has been abandoned due to cytotoxic effects of bupivacaine on chondrocytes.

CLINICAL FEATURES

Patients suffering from primary glenohumeral arthritis complain of activity related joint pain that can radiate posteriorly. The movements at the shoulder are not smooth and they report crepitus and catching sensations during ROM. As the disease progresses patients have morning pain and stiffness along with difficulty sleeping on the affected side. Advanced disease has even rest pain. The muscles around the shoulder are atrophic especially seen in the periscapular region as the shoulder itself is swollen and may mask deltoid atrophy.

The patients with cuff tear arthropathy are usually aged 50–70 years and may give past history of trauma. The early features are similar to impingement syndrome while with evolution of disease the patients have chronic and dull pain located at the joint initially at extremes of motion gradually restricting all movements. Slowly the pain starts occurring at rest becoming increasingly resistant to analgesics. On examination, patients have disuse atrophy potentiated by pain and restricted mobility of the shoulder joint in all planes particularly the external rotation. The patients with rotator cuff arthropathy also present with limited movements at shoulder and sometimes pseudoparalysis due to inability to abduct the shoulder joint. There is anterosuperior prominence of humeral head due to "escape" and coracohumeral ligaments wear in late stages. The movements (especially external rotation) are restricted and massive cuff tears are associated with positive external rotation lag sign (inability to maintain passive external rotation of the shoulder with elbow at 90°—infraspinatus tear) and positive Hornblower's sign (Teres minor dysfunction).

DIFFERENTIAL DIAGNOSIS

Differential diagnosis includes adhesive capsulitis, subacute infections, tuberculosis of the shoulder, cervical spondylosis, and locked posterior dislocation.

RADIOLOGY

Radiographs reveal typical osteophyte formation, wear of the joint, decreased joint space **(Figs. 1A and B)**. CT scan may be done to assess eccentric wear of the joint prior to planning arthroplasty. Levigne and Franceschi classified glenohumeral arthritis based on glenoid and humeral wear **(Table 3)**.

In rotator cuff arthropathy standard radiographic series reveal the following signs:

- Acetabularization of acromion
- Femoralization of the humeral head
- Superior glenoid wear
- "Sourcil sign"—subchondral sclerosis at the inferior aspect of acromion
- Variable osteopenia and osteosclerosis
- Absence of osteophytes (Milwaukee shoulder)
- Anterosuperior escape of humeral head

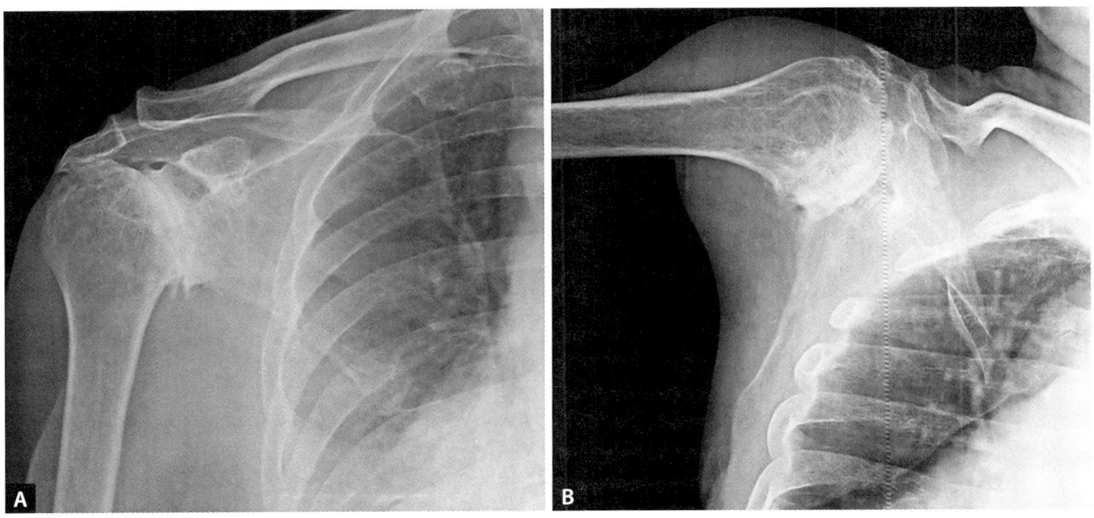

Figs. 1A and B: Degenerative arthritis (osteoarthritis) of shoulder joint. Note the loss of radiological joint space and presence of dense osteophytes some even in the rotator cuff tendon.

TABLE 3: Levigne and Franceschi classification of glenohumeral arthritis based on humeral and glenoid wear.

Stage	*Glenoid wear*	*Humeral head wear*
Stage 1	Subchondral bone intact or minimally deformed	Subchondral bone intact
Stage 2	Erosion reaching the base of coracoid	Anatomical neck deformed by notch > 10 mm
Stage 3	Erosion going beyond the base of coracoid	Loss of spherical form of the head
Radiological classification of shoulder in rheumatoid arthritis		
Ascending form	Most common form, there is upward migration of humeral head, head retains sphericity, head ascends, and then medializes	
Centered form	No upward migration, uniform glenoid wear, humeral head pushes into glenoid, progressive head medicalization, reduced acromio-humeral distance	
Destructive form	Destruction of humeral head, loss of sphericity, notching of humeral neck, and simultaneous glenoid destruction	

Magnetic resonance imaging (MRI) is indicated in rotator cuff arthropathy to evaluate the rotator cuff muscles and deemed function as excessive fatty infiltration is associated with poor function postoperatively.

Computed tomography (CT) scan is now a standard modality for evaluation of glenoid morphology, version, inclination, and bone loss. The images are obtained in scapular plane. Glenoid is classified morphologically into various types **(Table 4)** by Walch et al. that have been modified since proposal **(Fig. 2)**. Walch classification has been found useful for:

- Predicting natural history of glenohumeral osteoarthritis—A1 glenoids rarely develop posterior glenoid wear.
- Guiding surgical reconstruction—Glenoid with posterior wear is not an optimal candidate for anatomical total shoulder arthroplasty and needs augmentation.

CT scans have also proved very useful in assessing rotator muscle quality and function. Fatty infiltration (Goutallier classification) of the muscle significantly alters its strength and

TABLE 4: The Walch classification for glenoid wear.

Type		*Description*
Type A		Concentric wear, no humeral head subluxation, and centered head
	A1	No or minor central erosion
	A2	Deeper central erosion such that a line connecting anterior and posterior edge of glenoid transects humeral head
Type B		Biconcave glenoid due to asymmetric glenoid wear and humeral head subluxation
	B0	Preosteoarthritic and posterior subluxation of humeral head
	B1	Posterior joint narrowing (no posterior bone loss), osteophytes, subchondral sclerosis
	B2	Posterior rim erosion and retroverted glenoid
	B3	Monoconcave glenoid, posterior wear, humeral head subluxated >70% else glenoid retroversion >15°
Type C		
	C1	Glenoid retroversion >25°, regardless of erosion
	C2	Biconcave, posterior bone loss, posterior translation of humeral head
Type D		Glenoid anteversion or anterior humeral head subluxation <40%

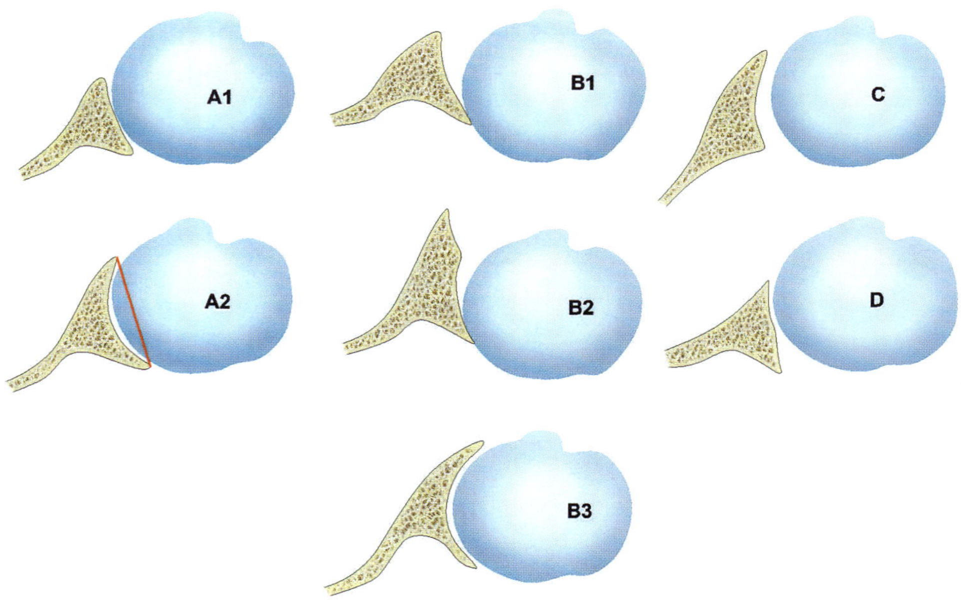

Fig. 2: The Walch classification for glenoid wear based on CT scan.

postoperative range of motion (ROM) and functional outcome following arthroplasty is compromised.

TREATMENT

Education, rest, and activity modification are essential part to improve the patient compliance. Pain can be controlled by titration with least effective dose of analgesics.

There are no disease modifying drugs or curing drugs so patient should be prepared for surgical treatment to provide lasting relief. Intra-articular steroids have not been successful in providing lasting relief while they may result in detrimental effects on bone and soft tissues. It may also increase the future incidence of periprosthetic infections. Viscosupplementation with hyaluronic acid may improve symptoms in moderate arthritis. Platelet-rich plasma injections into the joint for degenerative arthritis have equivocal effects only and stem cell has not been dedicatedly studied. As an interim measure, arthroscopic lavage and debridement can provide temporary but significant pain relief (unlike knee joint where it is equivalent to placebo). It is indicated in relatively young and active patient with mild-to-moderate glenohumeral arthritis and minimal glenoid deformity. Significant relief in symptoms is obtained in these patients provided symptoms were limited to pain and stiffness and humeral head is well-centered. Extensive chondroplasty, capsular release, subacromial decompression, excision of osteophytes, loose body removal, and microfractures have not shown any improvement and instead may result in poor outcome. Resection arthroplasty is a mutilating surgery and is only indicated in salvage of a failed arthroplasty where reconstruction is impossible by current methods or in infection associated arthropathy where control of the primary disease is not otherwise possible. Total shoulder arthroplasty (preferred, **Figs. 3A and B**) or hemiarthroplasty **(Fig. 3C)** are the preferred modalities to reconstruct the shoulder providing good pain relief but functional gains are often modest. Reverse shoulder arthroplasty has shown promise as far as functional gain and stability are concerned (see further). Arthrodesis of glenohumeral articulation is not a modern logical option for degenerative disease but may be prescribed for hard laborer, unaffording patient, or a failed shoulder arthroplasty.

Arthrodesis of Shoulder Joint

Shoulder joint arthrodesis involves obtaining bony fusion of the glenohumeral joint alleviating pain while permitting function through scapulothoracic motion. In the modern world, there are few if any indications of arthrodesis due to specific advances in the joint arthroplasty. In essence, it is prescribed when no other alternative reconstructive option will provide the desired functionality. The following are the indications for shoulder arthrodesis currently:

- Septic arthritis and concurrent damage to joint
- Failed shoulder arthroplasty
- Resection—reconstruction for shoulder neoplasms (proximal humerus)
- Reconstruction for paralytic disorders of shoulder (flail shoulder)
    - Brachial plexus palsy—especially when good elbow and hand function are obtainable or present
    - Poliomyelitis
- Complete rotator cuff tear with superior instability
- Nonreconstructible glenohumeral instability especially after failed reconstructive procedures
- Painful arthritic shoulder that is not suitable for arthroplasty (extremely rare).

Advantages

- Stable painless shoulder
- Lifelong once successfully done.

Disadvantages

- Limited function
- Disuse atrophy and cosmetic concern
- Extremely low potential for reversal to arthroplasty and poor results if done at all.

Prerequisites

- Sufficient strength of the axial and scapular musculature to maintain stability of the scapula
- Understanding patient.

Contraindications

- Flail scapula

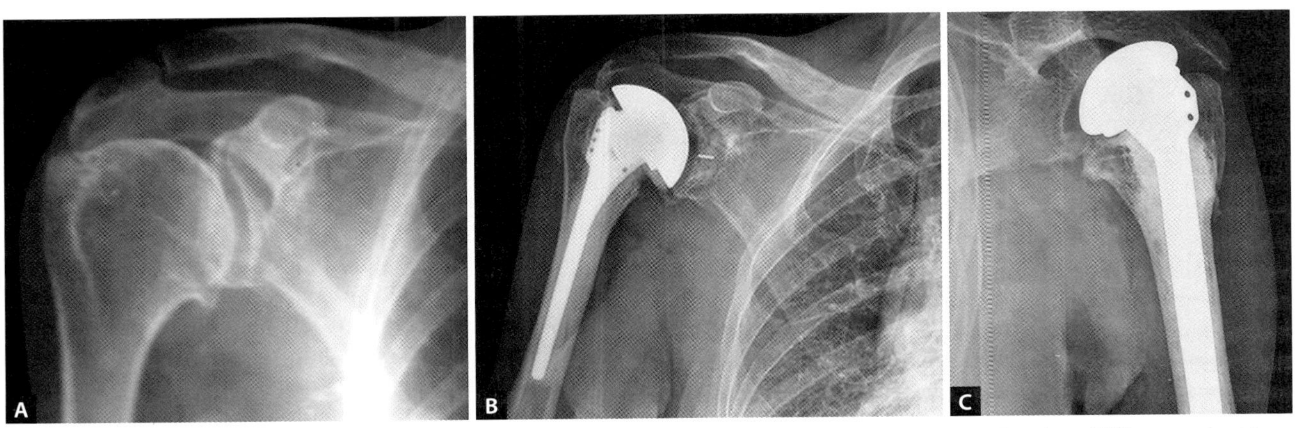

Figs. 3A to C: (A and B) Osteoarthritis of shoulder joint treated with total shoulder arthroplasty; (C) Hemiarthroplasty (different patients).

- Rotator cuff or deltoid or both intact—arthroplasty and other procedures can obtain reliable painless function and are worth trying
- Age >70 years as the procedure would be too morbid for them.

Position of Arthrodesis

- 20° of abduction, 15–30° of forward flexion, and 40° of internal rotation with side of body as reference point is the most commonly acceptable position to many surgeons.
- 45–50° of abduction, 15–25° of forward flexion, and 25–30° of internal rotation. This much abduction was advised by the American Academy of Orthopedic Surgeons to provide axillary hygiene. It is however found that this leads to uncomfortable scapular winging with arm at side.
- Richards et al. suggested that the acceptable position is one that allows hand to be raised in midline with elbow flexion to reach the mouth. He prescribed 30° of abduction, 30° of forward flexion, and 30° internal rotation as ideal position of arthrodesis.

Procedure Details

- Prefer beach chair position and using extensile deltopectoral approach from spine of scapula to deltoid insertion exposes the deep structures.
- Protect deltoid and incise the rotator cuff to repair later.
- Retract humerus and decorticate glenoid using reamer and humeral head using curettes.
- Place bone graft between humeral head and acromion to bridge the gap and fix humeral head to glenoid using screws in the position of arthrodesis as above. Use side of body as reference point. Richards advocated translating the humerus head upward to acromion and did not use bone graft. Additional screw can be placed from acromion to humeral head.
- Place a long reconstruction plate **(Fig. 4)** from spine of scapula to proximal humerus as in many patients there is osteopenia of the bones.

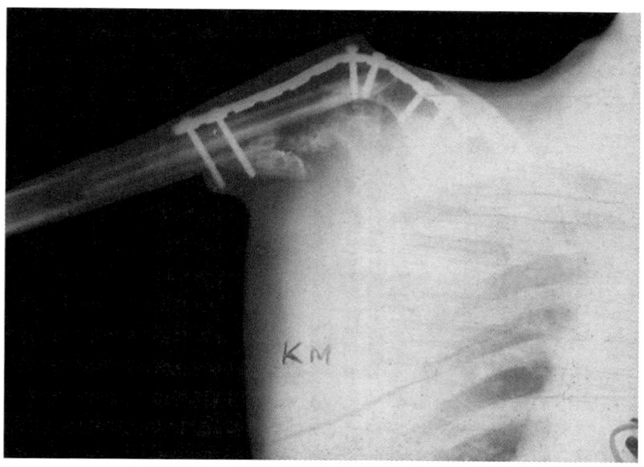

Fig. 4: Arbeitsgemeinschaft für Osteosynthesefragen (AO) type shoulder arthrodesis done using a reconstruction plate spanning across the glenohumeral joint on to the spine of glenoid.

Postoperatively place the upper limb in abduction pillow or a shoulder spica for 8–12 weeks. The former is preferred for better hygiene. Once fusion is demonstrated radiologically focus is shifted to periscapular muscle strengthening. The elbow and hand should be mobilized as early after the surgery as possible.

Arthroplasty of Shoulder Joint

Arthroplasty of shoulder is well-accepted, however, the choice between total shoulder arthroplasty and hemiarthroplasty is a bit arbitrary and is strongly biased by surgeons' preference. Classical indications for glenohumeral replacement are:

- Glenohumeral arthritis (osteoarthritis, rheumatoid, or post-traumatic)
- Osteonecrosis
- Three or four part of proximal humerus fractures
- Rotator cuff arthropathy
- Capsulorrhaphy arthritis
- Symptomatic anterosuperior shoulder deficiency.

This has been made possible by the availability of modern improved implants including the reverse total shoulder arthroplasty.

Total Shoulder Replacement (see Figs. 3A and B) versus Hemiarthroplasty

Hemiarthroplasty for proximal humeral reconstruction can be performed with resurfacing, short-stemmed or stemless implant options that may be combined with glenoid resurfacing. There is reported significant incidence of glenoid erosion that has been unsuccessfully improvised by augmentation with biological resurfacing by meniscus, fascia lata, anterior capsule, and acellular dermal allograft or Achilles tendon. The "ream and run" procedure aims at improving congruence of glenoid to humeral head by concentric reaming of the former and also fibrous tissue layer growth may serve as biological augmentation. The revision rates for ream and run are higher at 14–25% at 2 years of follow-up. While total shoulder arthroplasty (TSA) has shown consistently good results for treatment of primary shoulder arthritis compared to hemiarthroplasty **(*see* Fig. 3C)** the latter has the advantage of being less time consuming, cheaper, and technically easier and is preferred for other indications. Anatomical total shoulder replacement has demonstrated excellent results in patient with intact rotator cuff and ample glenoid bone stock. Lasting implant survival and relief in symptoms have made it the benchmark for surgical treatment of primary glenohumeral arthritis. Comparing the patient-reported outcomes, ROM, and symptom relief it has proven itself much better than hemiarthroplasty. Joint stuffing, impingement, and subscapularis rupture are primary concerns with TSA. Glenoid component loosening is the most common complication after TSA. The all-poly-pegged glenoid component seems to fare better than metal backed or keeled designs. The main factors related to glenoid loosening include patient-related [rotator cuff status (fatty infiltration), female sex, glenoid morphology (Walch B2), infection], surgery-related (cementing technique and implant seating),

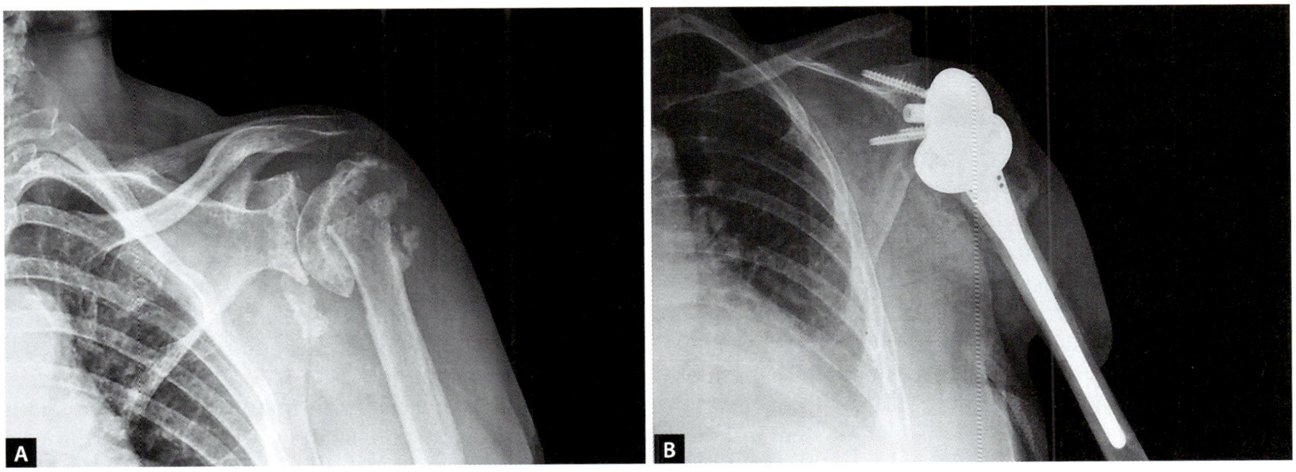

Figs. 5A and B: Reverse shoulder replacement for an ununited four parts proximal humerus fracture with cuff damage.

and implant design/conformity. Humeral side implant components have been shortened from standard stem to short stem, stemless and resurfacing components. Resurfacing components make placing of glenoid components difficult as they obscure a good glenoid view.

Cemented versus Uncemented Implants

Cemented components fare better than the cementless counterparts, however plasma-sprayed, hydroxyapatite coated, convex glenoid components, and recently introduced double radius glenoid components have improved results for cementless shoulder arthroplasty. Important measures to reduce the rate of failure of arthroplasty are proper size and version of stem, anatomic component sizing, anatomic glenoid version (eccentric reaming preferential to increasing humeral anteversion) and to avoid keeping the arm at end range of motion.

Reverse ball and socket design [*reverse total shoulder arthroplasty* (*RTSA*), **Figs. 5A and B**] had been in vogue since 1984 in European countries that was once abandoned due to catastrophic glenoid component failure. Due to improved design and component fixation, the prosthesis has been able to deliver very good results that even exceed that of total shoulder arthroplasty in peer comparisons for certain disorders. RTSA is now preferred for refractory rotator cuff arthropathy, multiple failed rotator cuff repairs with poor function and anterosuperior escape. TSA is bound to fail in these cases due to absent rotator cuff support necessary for its function. The concept of RTSA was reintroduced by Professor Paul Grammont in a rheumatology journal in 1987 that was based on specific principles **(Box 1)** and proposed to circumvent some of the problems of conventional shoulder arthroplasty by:

- Reversing the component design so that the weight-bearing part is convex and located at glenoid while the supporting moving part would acquire a concave shape attached to the humeral shaft. Initially, the glenoid component was two-thirds of a sphere centered at the center of rotation of native glenoid this was then changed (1991) to a hemisphere positioning the glenohumeral center of rotation at the interface of the glenoid component and scapula (neck, see further). Also the stemmed humeral component was introduced.
- Restricting glenoid translation by making the weight-bearing part at glenoid convex along with two essential modifications:
  1. Center of the sphere (glenosphere) should lie within the glenoid neck. This eliminated the neck totally and its associated complications. Neckless hemisphere was found to induce compressive forces at the implant bone interface rather than creating shear forces that were responsible for failure of initial designs.
  2. The center of rotation must be medialized and shifted a bit distally. Medialization of glenosphere by 10 mm increases deltoid moment by 20% at an abduction angle of 60°. Medializing the center of rotation in an almost horizontal humeral concave component however produces the so-called "inferior scapular notching" by impingement of humeral poly component and inferior glenoid bony rim. This necessitates distalizing the component so that ROM is impingement free. Also with distalization of the glenosphere by 10 mm the abductor moment is further increased by 30% (increased deltoid efficiency). Some authors prefer to lateralize the glenoid component by using a convex baseplate, however, increasing the tilting forces at the baseplate-bone interface. Medialization and distalization also impact the excursion of humerus tuberosities by increasing it, so for a given diameter of TSA humeral sphere the tuberosities have to travel a greater distance when instead RTSA is used, the implications are unclear but some authors did

BOX 1: The principles of reverse total shoulder arthroplasty as proposed by Grammont.

- Fixed fulcrum of rotation
- Inherent stability of constrained joint design
- Medialization of center of rotation
- Distalization of humerus

find tuberosity impingement at the spine of scapula levering out the humeral socket and the risk in fact increases the more the humerus is lateralized.

- Providing intrinsic stability (albeit with some loss of movements)—this biomechanically implies zero mismatch in the radii of curvature of convex and concave surfaces as is provided in RTSA components. In the conventional TSA, the spherical humeral component has shorter radius of curvature to that of the glenoid by a proportion of at least 5.5 mm to basically prevent rim loading, but in effect this is responsible for pseudoparesis of abduction (despite full ROM passively and absence of any neurological disease) in patients with inadequate rotator cuff. In a conventional TSA the joint reaction force should be within 30° of the glenoid center line so that effective abduction can happen. In the absence of rotator cuff the unopposed action of deltoid results in superior translation of the spherical head and the joint reaction force vector lies beyond the required <0° of glenoid center line. So most of the effort goes waste in translation of the head instead of producing rotation at the joint—causing pseudoparesis. In RTSA, the deeper concave component and smaller convex component with shorter radius of curvature is responsible for increasing the joint force vector to 45° and even more without the risk of dislocating, hence increasing the inherent stability. Also rotation is quite subtly induced in a concave stem component oriented at 155° (neck-shaft angle) that is pulled up by deltoid against a spherical component, rather than translating superiorly.
- Compensating for deltoid dysfunction partially—RTSA offers methods to increase tension in the deltoid by distally translating the humerus (increasing the size of poly insert) and also distalizing the glenosphere. The other benefit is that even if the anterior deltoid is damaged by previous surgeries the elevation in RTSA is effected by lateral deltoid which is commonly preserved.

The success of RTSA is also contributed by avoiding the problem of fixation of ultra-high molecular weight polyethylene (UHMWPE) on metal base plate and associated back side wear. The reverse prosthesis works by changing the direction of deltoid pull and hence intact deltoid with adequate glenoid bone stock is a prerequisite. Patients with glenoid deficiency (rheumatoid, traumatic, etc.) fare better with hemiarthroplasty. The current recommendations for use of a reverse total shoulder prosthesis are:

- Primarily, the prosthesis is considered when shoulder pain due to arthritis and functional loss say rotator cuff tear or deltoid dysfunction cannot be managed by conventional surgical reconstruction methods. Such patients usually have paresis of anterior and/or lateral elevation of the arm. Fixed upper displacement of humeral head (anterosuperior escape) relative to glenoid and massive rotator cuff tears managed with hemiarthroplasty had inconsistent results due to recurrent instability and glenoid arthrosis but results have been superior with reverse prosthesis. One should notice that patients with both advanced arthritis and massive rotator cuff tears are ideal candidates for RTSA and not patients with any one of them.
- Other indications for reverse total shoulder arthroplasty include a failed prosthetic reconstruction with superior, anterior, or posterior instability (i.e., revision surgery); chronic unreduced dislocations, three or four part fractures in elderly older than 70 years of age, revision shoulder arthroplasty, rheumatoid arthritis with adequate glenoid bone stock, tumors, revision of failed fracture fixation and revision of failed RTSA itself!

Though the indications of RTSA have expanded a lot but the results are best for rotator cuff tear arthropathy. One emerging indication for RTSA is for severe bone loss with intact rotator cuff but results are only limited to few case series. The primary advantage of RTSA over TSA or hemiarthroplasty for proximal humerus fracture is the minimal dependence of RTSA on tuberosity healing. Instead of medialization of glenosphere as originally proposed nowadays lateralization has been found to place the center of rotation in a more anatomic position and has become popular. This is even more desirable with the use of 135° humerosocket inclination instead of original 155° which avoids scapular (glenoid neck) notching. The improvement in internal rotation after RTSA is less as compared to TSA and overall complication rates are higher for RTSA that should be borne in mind while counseling patients.

Contraindications: These referring to the mentioned prerequisites for use of RTSA one can draw the contra-indications for use of RTSA as:

- Irreparable loss of deltoid function—complete axillary nerve palsy, scapulohumeral myopathy, etc.
- Severe loss of glenoid bone stock and poor glenoid bone quality—poor fixation of glenosphere is bound to loosen and ultimately fail.
- Infection.
- Neuropathy.
- Severe osteopenia as in long-standing rheumatoid on steroids—complication rates of RTSA are three times that of conventional TSA.
- Pain only or paralysis of external rotation only is also contraindication for sole use of RTSA. The RTSA cannot reconstruct the external rotation power and anterior translation of deltoid insertion as proposed by Grummont does not have universal acceptance. RTSA with latissimus dorsi transfer for external rotation pseudoparesis is a better option.

Technique of RTSA: Commonly the deltopectoral approach is used which is also the approach of choice for revision surgeries for shoulder. For concern of instability and experience of the surgeon a superolateral approach may be chosen. After resecting the humeral head, the biceps tendon is tenotomized. Exposure of glenoid is completed with resection of labrum and capsule circumferentially. The tendon of triceps is released but the axillary nerve should be protected. While reaming the glenoid avoid creating anteversion or retroversion or a superior tilt. Position the component slightly distally (inferiorly). Keeping the baseplate (also called "metaglene") flush with inferior border helps that actually causes the glenosphere to overhang the glenoid margins. Fixation is achieved by screws anchoring to lateral pillar and coracoid base. Whenever in doubt, chose a larger glenosphere for the patient. Humerus should be inserted into neutral torsion but the height of polyethylene component should be such that arm is lengthened by 2–3 cm. Test for stability in abduction and internal rotation. The issue of resuturing the subscapularis tendon is still uncertain and possibly the current assessment scores fail to capture positioning of the hand to back which is a significant disability if the tendon is left unrepaired. Close the wounds over drain as hematoma formation in subacromial space is quite frequent.

Complications of shoulder arthroplasty (including all types) surgery:

- *Infection:* Florid infections are less common than indolent smoldering infections. The common organisms are *Cutibacterium acnes* and coagulase negative staphylococci. The standard management is two-stage revision with intermediary spacer and long-term antibiotics followed by revision implantation. Indolent infections are being increasingly managed by single-stage revisions.
- Humeral fractures or perforations during surgery.
- Glenoid complications—intraoperative fractures, late (after 2 years usually) loosening (around 4%).
- Instability—usually anterior instability occurs especially with arm in adduction, internal rotation, and extension due mostly to inadequate soft tissue tension following implant malposition, deltoid dysfunction, proximal humeral bone loss, and mechanical impingement. Prevention can be afforded by avoiding humeral retrotorsion, using a superolateral approach and avoiding glenoid anteversion. Lengthening the arm also helps to prevent instability.
- Acromial fracture—avoid overtensioning of deltoid especially in osteoporotic bone. Conservative treatment with abduction pillow is better than operative fixation.
- Inferior scapular notching—distalize (preferred) the glenosphere or lateralize it. This complication is unique to RTSA especially with large humerosocket inclination (older designs had angle of 155°). It causes impingement of polyethylene humeral liner with scapular neck in adduction and external rotation.
- Hematoma formation.
- *Late humeral shaft fracture:* It is commonly associated with revision surgery, osteoporosis, rheumatoid arthritis, prolonged steroid use, and elderly patients with unstable gait.

Construing from the elucidation above it is apparent that a wide range of "technologically advanced options" are available that can tackle most of the surgical challenges, however, a wise choice between these is imperative as no single one is the total solution. Reverse shoulder is associated with quite frequent complications (nearly one-fourth of all patients would have some or other complication) and should be done only by surgeons versed extremely well with performing conventional shoulder arthroplasty regularly.

CONCLUSION

- Osteoarthrosis of shoulder is an uncommon disease in Indian subcontinent compared to the knee and hip joint.
- The radiology is quite characteristic with reduced joint space and formation of osteophytes. This may or may not be accompanied by deformation of the humeral head/glenoid.
- Treatment as for other joints is either providing painless mobile joint in the form of arthroplasty (preferred) or giving painless fixed joint relying on the compensation at other articulations (less preferred).
- Advent of reverse shoulder arthroplasty has improved the outcomes in difficult situations where conventional total shoulder designs or hemiarthroplasty would have been rendered less effective.

CHAPTER 65

Scapular Instability

Manish Kumar Varshney

INTRODUCTION

The scapula normally follows very rhythmic movement with the shoulder girdle. Movements of scapula, however, can become dyskinetic making the bone unstable for a number of reasons. A dysfunctional (as in arthritic joint) or nonfunctioning (as in distal clavicular resection) acromioclavicular joint or sternoclavicular joint (viz. post-traumatic) produces shoulder girdle abnormality causing an unstable scapula due to altered biomechanics. Seventeen muscles attach to the scapula; imbalance of muscular activity that primarily stabilizes the scapula can also, hence, cause an unstable scapula. Specifically, the muscles that stabilize scapula are the trapezius, the serratus anterior, the rhomboids, the levator scapulae, and the subscapularis. Abnormality in the stabilization of scapula produces broadly two groups of dysfunction—scapular dyskinesia which involves nonrhythmic scapular rotations seen associated with the glenohumeral movements and the other is winging of scapula which is the most recognizable form of scapular instability. The former is discussed in Chapter on "Shoulder Instability", following discussion will focus mainly on the latter, i.e., winging of scapula as it is the most characteristic and prominent clinically appreciated scapular dysfunction.

ETIOLOGY

Winging of scapula (also called "scapula alata") is a common dysfunction of shoulder. Conditions as benign as poor posture may produce scapular winging. Though some people classify scapular winging into neurological and musculoskeletal causes, I find it useful to put scapula alata into two major etiological groups that can be devised from clinical findings of scapular winging.

1. *True scapular instability resulting from unbalanced action of muscles acting on scapula:*
    - *Injury to long thoracic nerve:* There is serratus anterior weakness resulting in superior elevation with medial scapular translation and the inferior angle is rotated medially. This is called scapular winging of the "medial type". The damage to nerve can occur from direct damage during mastectomy or from brachial plexus injury from compression or pull as in young athletic patients. Medial winging is the most common type of scapular winging. Athletic activities that involve repetitive stretch of the nerve with head tilting away during overhead arm activity as in weightlifters and volleyball players cause traction damage to the nerve. Medial type winged scapula may also be seen in posterior capsular contracture of the glenohumeral joint and shortening of the latissimus dorsi muscle, but is quite less common this way.
    - *Injury to spinal accessory nerve:* There is trapezius weakness causing shoulder depression with lateral scapular translation and the inferior angle is also rotated laterally unopposed by serratus anterior pull. This is called scapular winging of the "lateral type". The condition can be seen in patients with history of neck surgery. Uncommonly, the condition may also be seen with shortened pectoralis minor muscle.
    - Myopathies involving shoulder girdle like facio-scapulohumeral muscular dystrophy.
    - Excessive shortening of pectoralis minor or scapulo-humeral muscles.
2. *Winging due to affection of nearby structures:*
    - Glenohumeral joint stiffness
    - Shoulder instability
    - Rotator cuff disease

CLINICAL FEATURES

The patients with medial winging of scapula often report discomfort while sitting against chair and are mostly painfree. Presence of shoulder or scapula pain is not frequent. Patients also report weakness when lifting objects away from body. On clinical examination there is peculiar "scapular winging syndrome" characterized by an inability to elevate and/or lower the arm without the scapula winging (vertebral border getting prominent) or its inferior angle tilting. To test for the muscle ask the patient to push against the wall with both arms apart at the shoulder width and elbows straight. This maneuver makes the vertebral border of the scapula prominent by lifting it. If there is no winging ask the patient to repeat the maneuver with head forward or while putting pressure on cervical spine from above. This accentuates the long thoracic nerve dysfunction revealing the serratus deficiency especially in cases with anterior C5 or C6. Atrophy and weakness of the involved group of muscles may be overtly evident. Else examine for "vicinity" causes (as mentioned in etiology above) of winging.

TREATMENT

The resulting disability is usually mild and treatment is mainly rehabilitative. Most of the programs are aimed to stretch the pectoralis minor and other scapulohumeral muscles. If the disability is astounding then scapula can be fixed to rib cage (scapulothoracic fusion) for providing a stable platform to good shoulder function. Dynamic stability can be given by attaching pectoralis major muscle via fascia lata graft to lower pole of scapula (Pectoralis transfer). For lateral winging apart from scapulothoracic fusion lateralization of levator scapulae and rhomboids (Eden-Lange transfer) may be done.

CONCLUSION

- Scapular instability is not an uncommon finding. There are two broad categories of scapular instability: (1) the scapular dyskinesia and (2) winging of scapula with the latter being much more prominent.
- The winging of scapula can arise from neurological or musculoskeletal causes but medial winging of scapula due to damage to long thoracic nerve or weakness of the serratus anterior muscle is most common.
- The problem is mostly managed conservatively, however, surgical management by pectoralis transfer or scapulothoracic fusion may be also done.

CHAPTER 66

Suprascapular Nerve Syndrome

Manish Kumar Varshney

INTRODUCTION

The suprascapular nerve has recently gained popularity in terms of managing intractable shoulder pain as well as a cause itself of some of pain syndromes associated with shoulder joint. It should be aptly remembered that shoulder pain that persists despite extensive conservative approaches could be of neural origin and one should have high index of suspicion for this syndrome if patient has scapular dyskinesia. Stretching of the nerve due to unstable scapula can secondarily produce shoulder dysfunction to cause impingement syndrome and rotator cuff tendon and muscle lesions. Apparently the syndrome was first mentioned in literature by Leaf in 1993 where he described applied kinesiology and demonstrating weakness in the infraspinatus muscle in a position of shoulder putting stretch on the suprascapular nerve for an otherwise normally testing muscle.

ANATOMY

The suprascapular nerve is a mixed nerve originating as a branch from upper trunk of brachial plexus receiving contributions from cervical fifth and sixth roots (± fourth cervical root). The nerve then passes under omohyoid and anterior border of trapezius in posterior triangle of neck to reach the scapular notch. It passes through the scapular notch beneath the superior transverse ligament to enter the supraspinous fossa supplying the supraspinatus muscle, coracohumeral, coracoacromial ligaments, the subacromial bursa, and acromioclavicular joint. The nerve then traverses around the spinoglenoid notch into infraspinous fossa to supply the infraspinatus muscle, shoulder joint, and scapula.

ETIOLOGY

The nerve may be injured by trauma (direct/indirect), traction, or compression neuropathy and the pathology is commonly unilateral. Bilateral nerve involvement is uncommonly reported in weightlifters.

- Traumatic injury to the nerve can occur from direct blow to Erb's point, scapular fracture and malunion or hematoma from fall on outstretched hand (FOOSH).
- Tractional damage occurs in pallbearers or repetitive strain in volleyball players. Stretch can also occur in scapular instability where the scapula moves to such a large extent so as to cause traction on suprascapular nerve. Commonly the dysfunction of rhomboids, anterior serratus, levator scapulae, and lower or middle fibers of the trapezius muscles are seen in scapular instability leading to suprascapular nerve syndrome.
- Entrapment (compression) neuropathy of the suprascapular nerve classically occurs in the scapular notch under the transverse scapular ligament or at the spinoglenoid notch. This compression can occur through extraneural inflammation (resulting from overuse injuries from overhead movements), lipoma or cyst (ganglion) development in the notch, space occupying lesions (like synovial sarcoma, Ewing's sarcoma, chondrosarcoma, metastatic renal cell carcinoma, etc.), following distal clavicle resection or from thickened ligament. The other site of compression is in the spinoglenoid notch where uncommon space occupying lesions like neoplasia or ganglion may compress the nerve.

CLINICAL PRESENTATION

Patients usually have low intensity vague pain at the posterior and lateral aspects of the shoulder. The pain usually radiates across scapula. This may have paresthesia of a burning quality. Pain is specifically induced with cross body adduction and full external rotation. Muscle atrophy of the supraspinatus and infraspinatus may be present. The scapulohumeral rhythm initiation is altered with initial elevation of scapula with start of abduction producing impingement like symptoms. Combined sensory-motor symptoms are seen in involvement of the suprascapular nerve trunk at the suprascapular notch region. Uncommonly, the sensory branch of the nerve may remain uninvolved producing painless paralysis or paresis, which is typically seen in professional volleyball players due to entrapment of nerve at spinoglenoid notch.

On examination of the patient, the findings that commonly suggest suprascapular nerve syndrome are excessive scapular motion on protraction and retraction, scapular dyskinesia (asymmetric movement of the two scapulae), weakness of the infraspinatus and supraspinatus when tested with arm flexed to 90° in anterior rotation of shoulder.

INVESTIGATIONS

Radiologically, the scapular notch view may reveal cause of bony impingement. Magnetic resonance imaging (MRI) may be obtained to identify soft tissue causes of nerve compression and inflammation of surrounding structures. Electromyography (EMG) of the supraspinatus and infraspinatus muscles usually confirms the diagnosis.

DIFFERENTIAL DIAGNOSIS

Rotator cuff tendonitis or tear, facioscapular muscular dystrophy, cervical disk disease, neuralgic amyotrophy, and disuse wasting of shoulder (as in adhesive capsulitis or elderly).

TREATMENT

Conservative

The management includes symptom control and local steroid injections to help reduce neural and local inflammation. Exercises to control and improve scapulohumeral rhythm and coordination should be initiated. Suprascapular nerve may be injected for control of inflammation and pain **(Fig. 1)**. Strenuous overhead activities should be restricted.

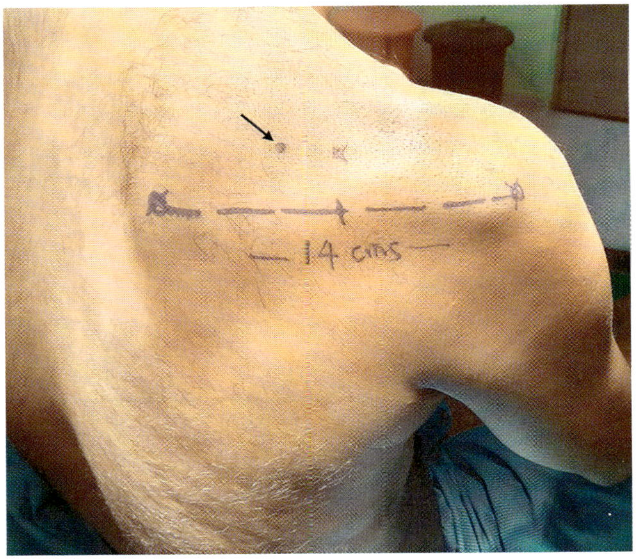

Fig. 1: The Meier technique for suprascapular nerve block. Mark the angle of acromion and the vertebral aspect of spine of scapula. Mark point 2 cm superior and medial to the midpoint of the above line (arrow). This is the needle insertion point. Pass the needle inferomedially from here under ultrasonological guidance to place it beneath supraspinatus fascia. Avoid injecting into vessels that accompany the nerve or too anteriorly into the pleural cavity.

Surgical Intervention

This is considered for failed conservative management and persistent symptoms or presence of muscle wasting. Typical intervention includes neurolysis and nerve decompression by removing the underlying pathology (cyst removal, etc.) and division of the transverse scapular ligament. Posterior (Swafford and Lichtman) approach is quite popular using oblique incision along the spine of scapula. Trapezius is elevated subperiosteally to expose the supraspinatus muscle that is carefully elevated superiorly and inferiorly to expose the suprascapular nerve and vessels. Identify the suprascapular notch and transverse scapular ligament to decompress the nerve and remove pathology like cyst or ganglion if present. The muscles are then reposed and sutured well to the bone. Postoperatively the patient is kept in a sling support for 2 weeks followed by gradual physiotherapy for shoulder mobilization and muscle strengthening program.

CONCLUSION

- Suprascapular nerve involvement can occur due to various causes that compress the nerve at suprascapular or spinoglenoid notch.
- The syndrome is often missed even on a systematic shoulder examination, one should have high index of suspicion for this pathology of there is scapular dyskinesia.
- Once diagnosis is made, treatment is quite effective with decompression of the nerve if patient fails to respond to conservative management.

CHAPTER 67

Tuberculosis of Shoulder Joint

Manish Kumar Varshney

INTRODUCTION

Tuberculosis of the shoulder joint is rare having an incidence of 1–3% of skeletal tuberculosis. There are few reports about it in the literature. There is preponderance of males affected with the disease and the left side is more often affected.

PATHOANATOMY AND CLINICAL FORMS

The head of the humerus is probably a prime target location as destructive changes are maximally seen in it. Tuberculosis of the shoulder is predominantly a disease of adults but may also be encountered in children. Specifically, the presentation of disease is distinct in the two age groups that have been colloquially called the sicca form (in adults) and the fulminant form (septic or wet form in children).

- *Type I (sicca form and dry form):* Caries sicca is well-documented and is seen in adults. Here, the disease more or less presents like osteoarthritis with degenerative changes in the shoulder and pain that is aggravated by movements. The presence of inflammatory symptoms for pain (aggravation in night and morning, cold intolerance, stiffness, etc.) should raise suspicion. The rapidity of joint space loss in tuberculosis is highly variable and is often a late finding, occurring after marginal and central erosions of large size have initially appeared. In others, loss of joint space can be seen early when only small marginal osseous defects are apparent.
- *Type II (Caries exudata, wet form, and fulminant form):* The florid form with swelling and cold abscess formation is seen more commonly in children. Such inflammatory changes in the synovial membrane are usually more marked if infection follows the penetration of a caseous bone focus into the joint space than if it starts in the membrane itself. There is joint effusion, inflammatory thickening of the periarticular connective tissue, and fat contributing to soft tissue swelling. The synovial membrane thickens and is covered by heavy layer of fibrin.
- *Destructive form* of caries shoulder has also been reported but not classified—this has combination of features of rheumatoid arthritis and Charcot's joint.

Pathologic abnormalities in tuberculosis arthritis involve synovial membrane and cartilaginous and osseous abnormalities. Accurate diagnosis mandates synovial fluid aspiration or synovial membrane biopsy.

CLINICAL FEATURES

In the sicca form, the patients present with pain of insidious onset that is often more at night. The consultation to a physician is delayed by 3–6 months due to indolent nature of the disease initially and even misdiagnosis in a primary care. On examination, the patient has atrophy of the shoulder girdle muscles and prominent bony landmarks. The movements are reduced in all directions and often painful. These are commonly misdiagnosed as adhesive capsulitis or frozen shoulder. The typical inflammatory components of the disease should be evaluated in history and examination. Tenderness is initially present on the posterior aspect of shoulder that quickly becomes generalized a finding uncommon in adhesive capsulitis. In the exudative form of disease, features are clearer with swelling effusions and cold abscess formation around the joint. The child often is malnourished and has cachectic look. Joint aspiration or biopsy readily helps in confirming the diagnosis by an alert physician.

RADIOLOGY

A triad of radiographic finding (Phemister's triad) is characteristic of tubercular arthritis. This includes severe periarticular osteoporosis, peripherally located osseous erosions and gradual narrowing of the interosseous space. In addition, there are subchondral erosions, reactive sclerosis, and periosteal reactions in the sicca form **(Fig. 1)**. Exudative form presents with soft tissue swelling and edema and periarticular osteopenia that is prominent. There are reports of misdiagnosis as a neoplasm so histological correlation should be promptly obtained.

DIFFERENTIAL DIAGNOSIS

Pigmented villonodular synovitis, synovial chondromatosis, gout, rheumatoid arthritis, Milwaukee shoulder, Charcot's joint, and osteoarthrosis.

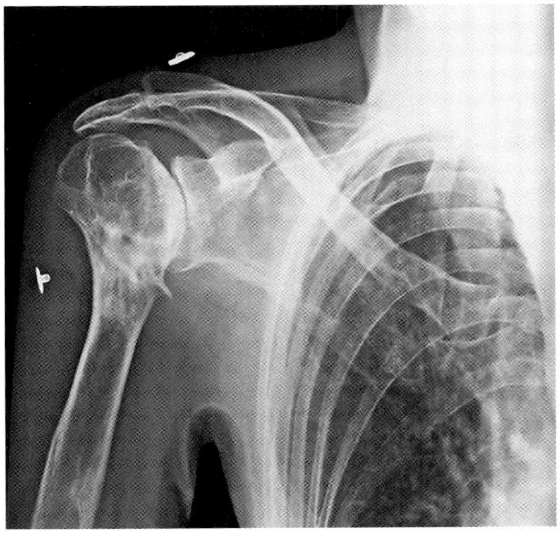

Fig. 1: Tubercular affection of shoulder joint in a 62-year-old lady presenting with caries sicca. The patient was managed elsewhere as an osteoarthritis of shoulder joint. Note the osteomyelitic changes and possible sequestrum at the surgical neck site.

TREATMENT

Antitubercular chemotherapy is the standard form of treatment. There had been recommendation of shoulder spica immobilization with chemotherapy but is possibly unnecessary in the present scenario. Instead of immobilization, the availability of successful and proven chemotherapy opens avenues for early gentle mobilization to improve and retain as much function as possible. Cases where shoulder arthrosis develop, arthrodesis is commonly preferred but with successful use of hip arthroplasty in treated cases of TB hip, a shoulder arthroplasty may have a definite place for patients who desire so and are good candidates (not doing hard labor). It should be, however, remembered that the periarticular soft tissues and muscles get weaker by the disease process and so reverse shoulder may have an appropriate role in these cases.

CONCLUSION

- Even in endemic regions, tuberculosis of the shoulder joint is a rare disease. It is mainly seen in adult population.
- Two clinical forms have been realized—one dry form (without any pus formation) which is more common and seen in adults. The other wet form (pus formation) is seen in children and is less common. An even uncommon destructive form has been seen.
- Not missing the disorder by meticulous clinical examination supplemented by radiological findings is essential for instituting correct treatment.
- Diagnosis has to be made by histopathological confirmation ideally or high suspicion of an experienced surgeon when no other possibility is seen despite noncharacteristic histopathology.
- Antitubercular treatment is the mainstay of treatment that should be instituted as early as possible. In late cases when shoulder arthrosis has developed—arthrodesis/arthroplasty is recommended.

SECTION 8

Regional Orthopedics: Hip

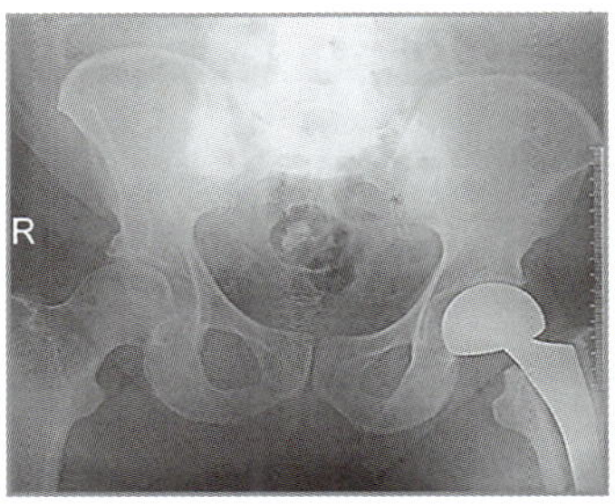

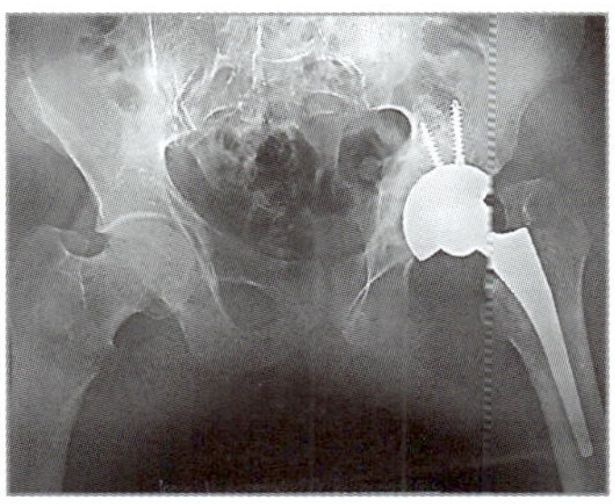

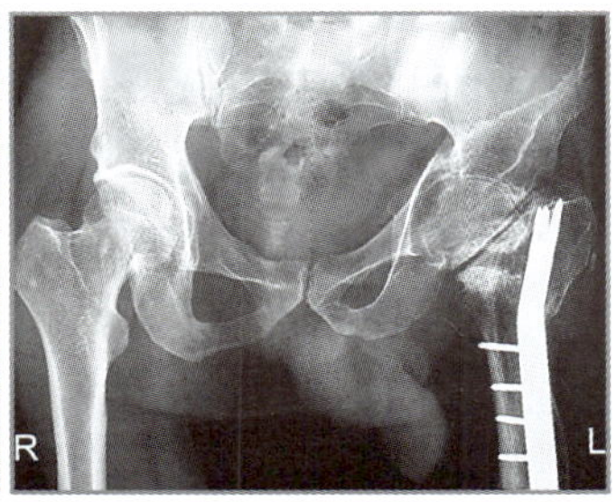

CHAPTER 68

Surgical and Functional Anatomy

Manish Kumar Varshney

ANATOMY OF THE HIP

The hip is a true ball-and-socket joint with high congruity. It meets all four characteristics of a synovial joint, viz., it has a joint cavity; joint surfaces are covered with articular cartilage; it has a synovial membrane producing synovial fluid; and it is surrounded by a ligamentous capsule. Embryologically, the acetabular fossa is discernible by 8–9 weeks of fetal development. By the 17th week of development, the joint cavity has cleaved with the formation of a synovial layer. Ossification of this physeal complex is completed by the age of 16–18 years. The hips not only transmit forces from the ground up but also carry forces from the trunk, head and neck, and upper extremities. The anatomy of the joint can be studied by dividing it into bony, ligamentous, muscular, and neurovascular structures.

Bony Anatomy

The cup-shaped acetabulum (os coxae) is formed from three separate primary ossification centers forming the ilium (40% contribution to formation of acetabulum), the ischium (40%), and the pubis (20%) **(Fig. 1)**. The secondary centers form the iliac crest, the anterior inferior spine, the ischial tuberosity, the pubic symphysis, and the triradiate cartilage at the center of the acetabulum. By 14 years of age, the ossified bones of the ilium, ischium, and pubis unite in the acetabulum, forming a Y-shaped triradiate cartilage that, in turn, fuses by 15–16 years of age. The other secondary centers unite and fuse between the ages of 20 and 22 years with the ischial tuberosity being the last one.

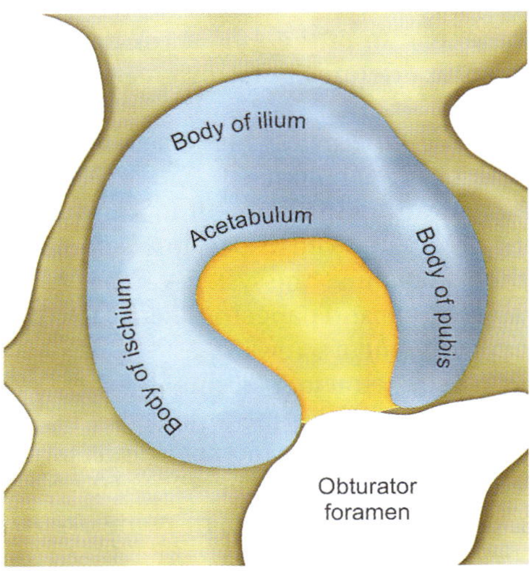

Fig. 1: The os coxae: Ilium and ischium contribute 40% each in the formation of acetabulum while pubis contributes 20%.

Acetabulum

The acetabular fossa is orientated inferiorly (45°) and anteriorly (15°) and laterally. The acetabular rim is circular but deficient in the lower one-fifth where it is completed by transverse acetabular ligament (TAL) **(Fig. 2)**. The depth of acetabulum provides coverage to 170° of the femoral head. This depth is augmented by the labrum, which runs circumferentially around its perimeter to the base of the fovea, where it becomes TAL. The labrum receives a vascular supply from the obturator and the superior and inferior gluteal arteries. Functions of labrum are:

- Increases depth of acetabulum by 20%
- Increases joint stability
- Increases acetabular contact area by 25%—reduces contact stress
- Forms a sealed cavity for lubrication

The acetabulum is reinforced by anterior and posterior column that encompass the cotyloid fossa as they pass across **(Figs. 3A and B)**. The thickness of columns varies but as a general rule they make up for thickness 30% greater than the acetabulum [to understand this, one can remember that expanding the acetabulum (say by reaming during total hip arthroplasty, THA) more than one-third beyond the acetabular diameter will cause pelvic discontinuity, up to one quarter is safe].

Applied anatomy of acetabulum and ilium: There are some important aspects of anatomy relevant to total hip arthroplasty (THA) and are discussed below:

- The anterior and posterior brim of the base of the fovea and the transverse acetabular ligament serve as important landmarks for THA. The anterior and posterior brim

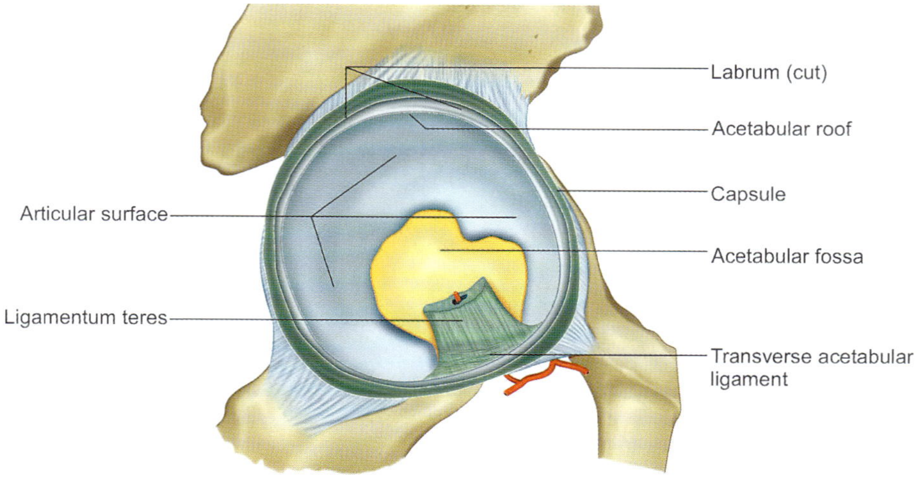

Fig. 2: The anatomy of acetabulum and surrounding structures.

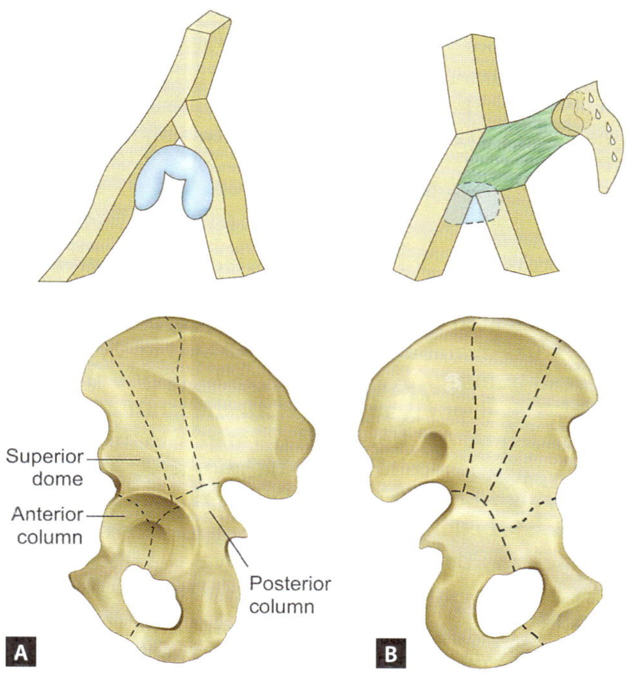

Figs. 3A and B: The columns of acetabulum: (A) End on view from outside; and (B) Viewed from inside of pelvis.

help to determine acetabular component anteversion and flexion. The base of the fovea guides the extent of possible medial reaming of acetabulum, this is especially important when a large medial osteophyte compromises view of acetabulum.

- Medialization of acetabulum in THA has advantages (*see* Chapter on "Biomechanics of Hip Joint") but it is contraindicated in patients with inflammatory arthropathy where protrusio may occur.
- Transverse acetabular ligament provides a landmark to identify the inferior-most aspect of the acetabulum especially in dysplastic hips. The landmark is quite often preserved in most pathologies and nearly always in dysplasia.
- Transverse acetabular ligament provides a restraint to inferior drifting of the acetabular reamer in cases where the superior acetabular bone is sclerotic. Even in ankylosing spondylitis, the ligament is fairly preserved.
- The anterior superior iliac spine (ASIS) should always be relied upon for identifying the location of competent bone to fix the acetabulum. It also guides the placement of transacetabular screws.
- Over-reaming the acetabulum during THA will remove the hard subchondral bone and prevent adequate circumferential hoop stresses for press-fit acetabular components.
- Excess reaming decreases the space for placing screws.
- With superior migration of acetabulum the safe zone for transacetabular screw placement reduces. The quadrant systems, as described by Wasielewski et al., are useful in avoiding injury to neural and vascular structures.

Acetabular quadrant systems **(Figs. 4A and B)** demonstrate the nerves and vessels that course around the acetabulum and proximal femur. The quadrants are formed by two perpendicular lines:

- A line drawn from the ASIS through the center of the acetabulum defines anterior and posterior quadrant locations.
- Second line is perpendicular bisector of the first line at midpoint in acetabulum.

The quadrant helps surgeon to know the location of intrapelvic structures with respect to fixed points of reference within the acetabulum. The system can be used to:

- Locate the safe and dangerous zones for the transacetabular placement of screws
- As a guide for retractor placement
- For drilling acetabular anchoring holes for graft fixation
- To estimate bone depth in a specific acetabular zone
- Anterior quadrants should be avoided for the placement of screws or anchoring hole. Sharp-pointed retractors should not be used here (injury to external iliac artery and vein and the obturator nerve, artery, and vein). The external iliac vessels lie opposite the anterior-superior quadrant,

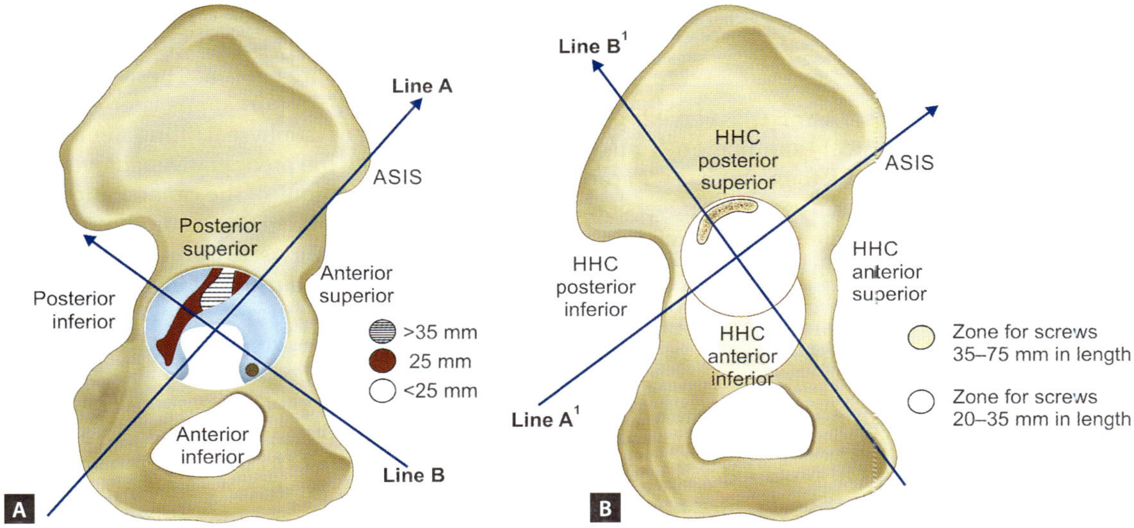

Figs. 4A and B: The quadrants of acetabulum. The quadrant system at the normal (anatomic) hip center (see text for details). The high hip center (HHC) quadrant system, superimposed on one-half of an acetabular diameter proximally over the original anatomic acetabular quadrant system (see text for details). The recommended and usual sizes of screws are also mentioned in the adjoining text. (ASIS: anterior superior iliac spine)

and the obturator neural and vascular structures lie opposite the anterior-inferior quadrant. The risk to these structures is increased during aging by the relatively small obturator internus muscle and the shallow acetabular bone depth opposite the structures. The anterior retractor should be placed with utmost care, one can err on the superior side in unsure.

Posterior quadrant—sciatic nerve and the superior gluteal nerve and vessels course opposite the posterior superior quadrant, and the inferior gluteal and internal pudendal structures are opposite the posteroinferior quadrant. The bone depth in the posterior quadrants is 25 mm or greater so screws and anchoring holes can be placed relatively safely in these zones. Sciatic nerve can be protected by gentle retraction. The superior gluteal nerve and vessels can be protected in the greater sciatic notch. The inferior gluteal and internal pudendal neural and vascular structures are relatively mobile and can be protected by retractors placed directly against the bone of the posterior column.

High hip center quadrants: The peripheral halves of the posterior superior and posterior inferior high hip center (HHC) quadrants contain the best available bone stock and are relatively safe for transacetabular screw placement. The entire anterior superior and anterior inferior HHC quadrants, as well as the central half of the posterior superior and posterior inferior quadrants, should be avoided because of the close proximity of intrapelvic structures and minimal protective musculature on the inner wall of the pelvis.

Femur

The femur is the longest and strongest bone in the human body. It is mostly cylindrical throughout its length, and it is anterolaterally bowed in its midportion. The extent of bowing is clinically relevant because, if excessive, it may not be possible to pass long straight implants (one of the reasons for failure of first generation Gamma nail). The head of the femur forms approximately two-thirds of a sphere and is covered by articular hyaline cartilage in approximately 60–70% of a sphere also the fovea centralis is devoid of cartilage **(Fig. 5)**. The hyaline cartilage is thickest in the superior, medial, and posterior surface that contacts with the acetabular surface. The neck of the femur is approximately 5 cm long **(Fig. 5)**. The proximal metaphysis and neck are anteverted by approximately 14°. The angle between the femoral shaft and the neck is approximately 125° **(Figs. 6A to C)**. In most hips, the center of the femoral head is at the level of the tip of the greater trochanter. As the neck-shaft angle increases, the center of the head comes to lie above the level of the trochanter (resulting in coxa valga). A decreased neck-shaft angle results in coxa vara. Also, the distance between the center of the

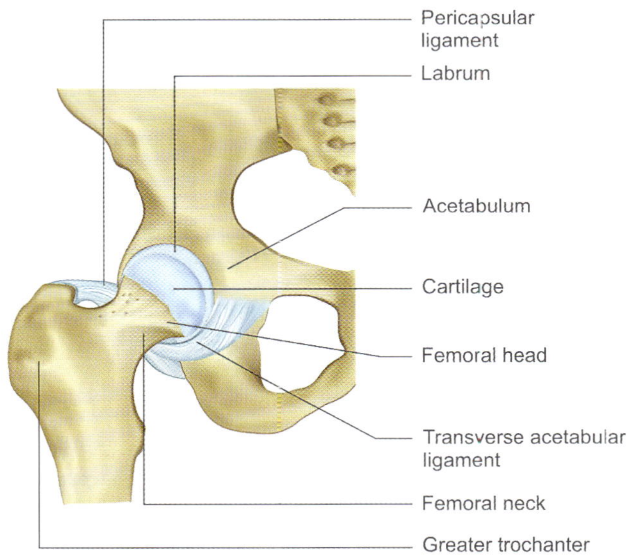

Fig. 5: The anatomy of proximal femur and its articulation with acetabulum.

femoral head and the lateral aspect of the trochanter can vary independent of the neck-shaft angle.

Applied anatomy of femur:

- The extent of anteversion **(Figs. 7A and B)** is variable and should be determined by clinical examination (Craig's test). If it comes grossly abnormal, then obtain a CT scan and arrange modular stems that can vary the anteversion. For a surgeon comfortable with different approaches in a patient with high anteversion [as in congenital dysplasia of the hip (CDH)] use an anterolateral surgical approach and for retroverted hip (the old slipped capital femoral epiphysis) use a posterolateral approach to dislocate femoral head.
- The proximal femoral metaphyseal orientation and shape have great variability that may create problems for a cementless stem with fixed proximal geometries. Cementless stems must fit the anterior, posterior, and medial-lateral dimensions of the canal that should be maintained for variable lengths down the canal for maximum contact. The length of contact of prosthesis depends on anatomy of canal and prosthesis design, so chose prosthesis based on specific needs of patient; usually for primary THA proximal contact stems with low-profile taper are chosen. These can be revised with calcar replacing/support stems later and still later they can be revised to diaphyseal fitting stems if needed. One should evaluate the preoperative radiographs for what is called "funnelization" of the canal. Endosteal expansion of the isthmus with age results in the stovepipe femoral configuration in contrast to the proximal femur of younger patients who have a trumpet like or champagne-fluted configuration. Dorr and Spotorno have developed indexes to characterize proximal femoral configuration **(Figs. 8A to C)**. The Dorr index is a ratio of the canal diameter at the level of the lesser trochanter to the canal diameter at a point 10 cm distal. As the canal calcar isthmus ratio (the Dorr index) approaches 1, prosthesis fill proximally and distally is compromised. Patients with stovepipe configurations should either be treated with thick fully porous-coated stem or better a cemented implant.
- Singh's index **(Fig. 9)** (*see* Chapter on "Metabolic Diseases of Bone") can be used to assess the osteopenia but osteopenia measurement is likely to be less important than the quality of bone for ingrowth. Presently, there are no available parameters for determining the quality of bone.

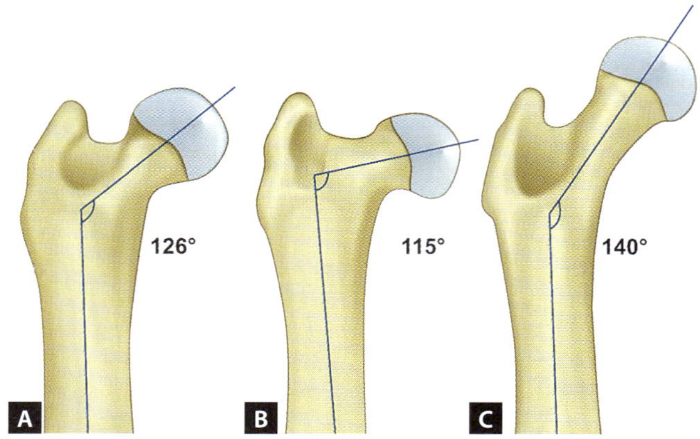

Figs. 6A to C: (A) Normal femoral neck angle; (B) A decreased femoral neck angle (coxa vara); (C) An increased femoral neck angle (coxa valga).

Capsular and Ligamentous Anatomy (Figs. 10A to C)

The capsule is attached along the anterior and posterior periphery of the acetabulum just outside the acetabular labrum. Inferiorly, the capsule is attached to the transverse acetabular ligament. The capsule is attached to the femur anteriorly along the intertrochanteric line, but posteriorly it attaches to middle of the neck so that the basicervical portion and intertrochanteric crest are extracapsular posteriorly. The iliofemoral and the pubofemoral ligaments, reinforce anterior portion of the capsule while ischiofemoral ligament reinforces the posterior capsule.

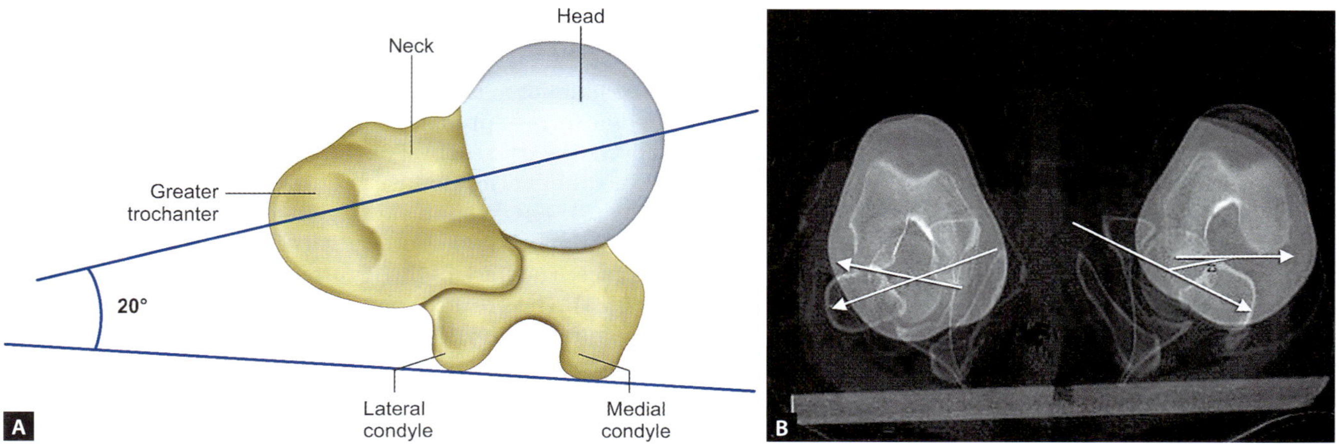

Figs. 7A and B: The anteversion of femoral neck is measured with reference to the transepicondylar axis. It has a mean value around 12–14° depending on sex of the person and race. (A) Illustration of method for determining the angle of anteversion, here the anteversion is increased; (B) Radiographic determination of the same.

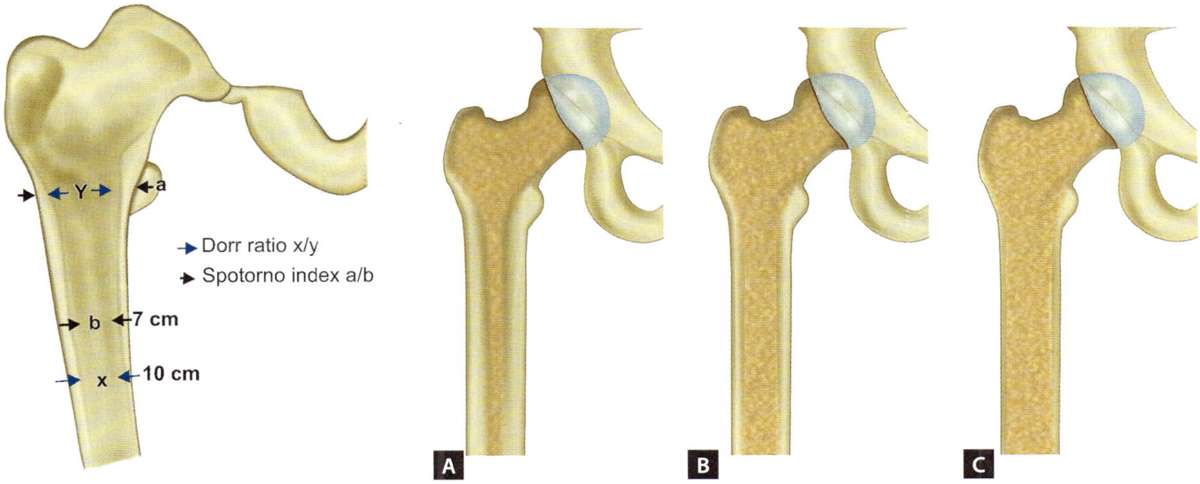

Figs. 8A to C: The Dorr and Spotorno indexes for evaluating proximal femoral bone configuration are depicted in the left figure. Dorr classification of femoral bone quality is depicted in the right figure—Dorr Type A has thick medial and lateral cortices giving a champagne-flute appearance (A). In Dorr type B (intermediate), the proximal femur shows bone loss at the medial and posterior cortices (B). Dorr Type C is seen in osteoporotic femora (also called "stovepipe appearance") and forms due to complete loss of both the medial and the posterior cortices. The intramedullary canal is very wide.

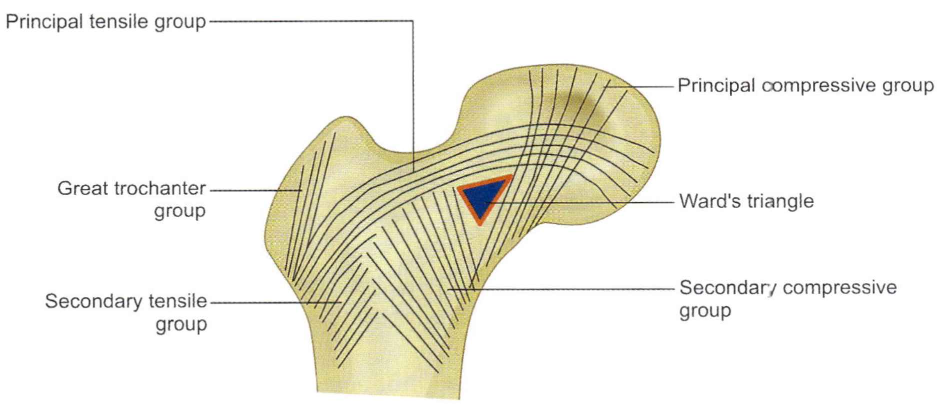

Fig. 9: Singh's description of proximal femoral bony trabeculae (the details of reading Singh's index are provided in Chapter describing Osteoporosis).

- ***The iliofemoral ligament*** **(Figs. 10A to C)**, the Y ligament, ligament of Bigelow—this is fan-shaped modified "λ" structure that resembles inverted letter Y. It is the strongest ligament in the body with a tensile strength >350 N. The apex of ligament is attached to the lower portion of the anterior inferior iliac spine and the diverging fibers of the Y fan out to attach along the intertrochanteric line. The ligament is taut in full extension, superior portion additionally resists excessive external rotation. Contracture of this ligament produces flexion/internal rotation deformity requiring release at THA. Anterolateral approach is preferred in this case as it will inescapably release this contracture.
- ***The pubofemoral ligament*** attaches to the inferomedial part of the anterior capsule. It arises from pubic portion of the acetabular rim and the obturator aspect of the superior pubic ramus and blends with the inferior-most fibers of the iliofemoral ligament. The ligament becomes taut in hip extension and abduction. Contracture of ligament may cause adduction deformity so in cases with adduction contracture mere release of the adductor tendons may not be enough and these fibers may need to be additionally released.
- ***The ischiofemoral ligament*** blends with the posterior surface of the capsule and zona orbicularis (the sparse circular capsular fibers in posteroinferior region, otherwise the capsule has predominantly longitudinal fibers, **Figs. 10A to C**). It arises from the ischial portion of the acetabular rim and spirals laterally and upward to blend in the capsule. The ligament tightens during extension and transverse fibers restrict excessive internal hip rotation.
- ***Zona orbicularis—"annular ligament"*** encircles the femoral neck like a button hole and again plays little role in stability. It is actually the horizontally oriented fibers of capsule separate from the longitudinal fibers that reinforce the hoop stresses encountered by the acetabular labrum.
- ***Ligamentum teres***—it is intra-articular but actually extrasynovial as it is surrounded by synovial membrane.

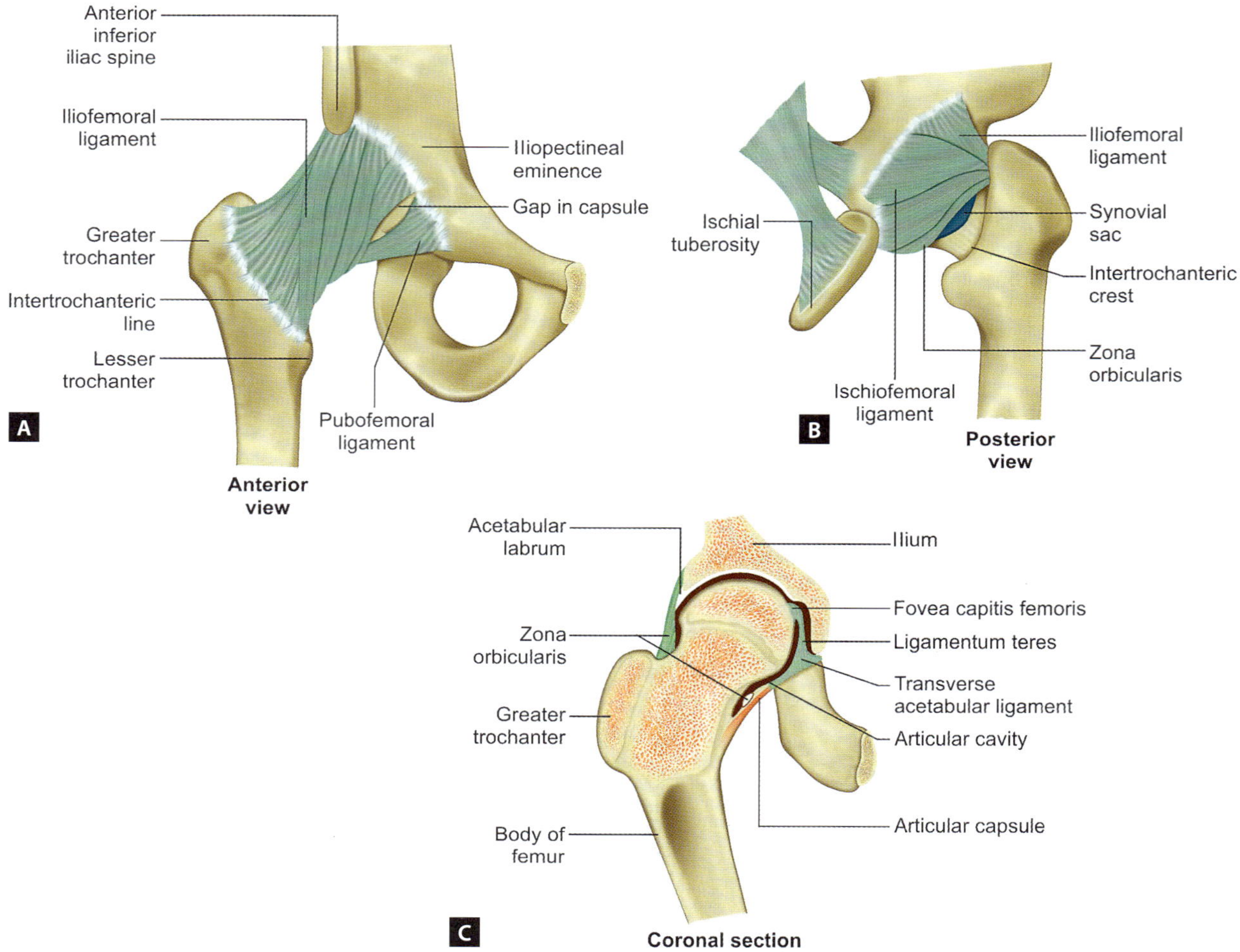

Figs. 10A to C: The capsular and ligamentous anatomy of the hip joint.

The ligamentum attaches to the fovea of the femoral head and acetabular central fovea. It contains a small vessel (80% population) that may contribute to the blood supply of femoral head in perifoveolar region but does not contribute to stability of the joint.

Screw Home Effect for Hip

As can be gathered from above, all ligaments around hip joint restrict extension and the special disposition of the ligaments make them fully taut in extension. The hip joint "screws-in" and locks in full extension gaining maximum stability by virtue of peculiar disposition of ligaments. This is needed also as the articular surfaces of the joint are not in optimal contact in extension. The position of maximum articular contact is hip flexion, abduction, and external rotation (FABER) and is loose-packed position where the ligaments are lax. In flexed and adducted position, the ligaments are not tight and also the articular surfaces are not congruent so hip is prone to dislocation.

Movements at Hip

- Flexion of 120°
- Extension of 30°
- Abduction of 45–50°
- Adduction of 20–30°
- Internal rotation of 35°
- External rotation of 45°

Functional range of motion (ROM) of hip needed for walk on level surface is 30° of flexion, 10° of hyperextension, 5° of both abduction and adduction and 5° of both internal and external rotation.

Muscular Anatomy

The muscles around hip region are the bulkiest and strongest muscles and operate as part of a closed kinematic chain-link system.

Flexors (Fig. 11)

The primary hip flexors are:

- The iliopsoas (N. supply—femoral nerve) has three separate muscles: the iliacus, the psoas major, and psoas minor, that converge to insert as a tendon on lesser trochanter. The origin of the muscle is possibly the most vast in human body taking origin from iliac crest and fossa, sacral ala, and iliolumbar and sacroiliac ligaments (the iliacus portion); and the sides of the bodies of the

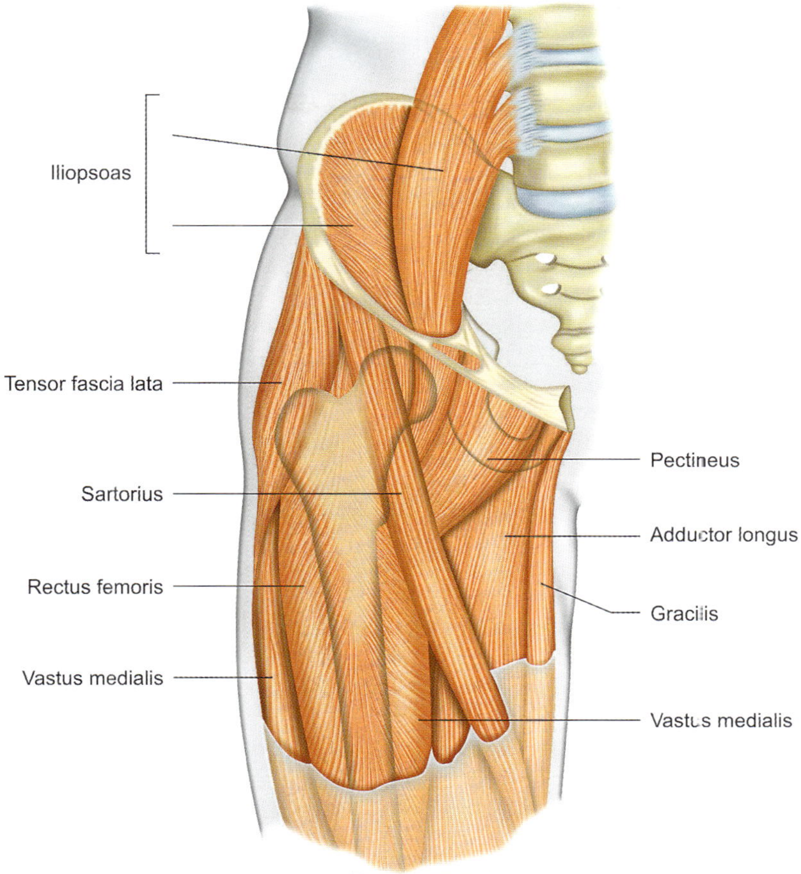

Fig. 11: Muscles around hip as seen from anterior aspect.

12th thoracic through fourth lumbar vertebrae, transverse processes of the first through the fifth lumbar vertebrae, and the intervertebral disks (the psoas portion). The inserting tendon crosses hip joint inferiorly [prevents relocation in developmental dysplasia of hip (DDH)]. If tight, it causes flexion deformity and tendon can be released (just distal to where it crosses pelvic brim protecting the muscular portion) if the flexion deformity is 20° or more after performing THA.

- Rectus femoris (N. supply—femoral nerve)—crosses both the hip joint and the knee joint, flexing the former while extending the latter. It has two heads of origin (straight and reflected) but single insertion into retinaculum-patella-patellar tendon and tuberosity. The flexion strength of muscle is highest with knee flexion. In flexion deformity of hip due to tight rectus, release of the reflected head and transverse release of the fascia along the undersurface of the rectus helps in regaining knee flexion and hip extension.
- Sartorius (N. supply—femoral nerve, tailor's muscle)—arises from the ASIS. It crosses the hip and knee joints to insert on the medial aspect of the proximal tibia in association with the other pes anserinus muscles. It flexes and abducts the hip, and it also flexes the knee.
- The tensor fascia lata (N. supply—superior gluteal nerve) originates more laterally than the sartorius. The muscle fibers blend together to form the iliotibial band. The tensor fascia flexes, abducts, and internally rotates the hip but its predominant role is maintaining tension in the iliotibial band to maintain the knee in extension during stance.
- Secondary flexors of hip are pectineus (N. supply—femoral nerve), adductor longus (N. supply—obturator nerve), brevis, magnus, the gracilis and the anterior portions of the gluteus minimus and medius muscles. Gracilis is a hip flexor only when the knee is extended but not when it is flexed.

Extensors (Fig. 12)

The gluteus maximus (N. supply—inferior gluteal nerve) and hamstring muscles (N. supply—sciatic nerve, tibial br.) are the primary hip extensors with secondary contribution from adductor magnus. Gluteus maximus originates from the sacrum, coccyx and the sacrotuberous ligament, and its uppermost fibers insert into the iliotibial band while the inferior fibers insert into the gluteal tuberosity and the lateral intermuscular septum. Gluteus maximus also externally rotates the femur and stabilizes the knee through its insertion in the iliotibial tract.

The hamstrings (N. supply—sciatic nerve, tibial br.) include the long head of the biceps femoris, the semitendinosus, and the semimembranosus all originating from the ischial tuberosity. The primary action of these is to extend the hip and

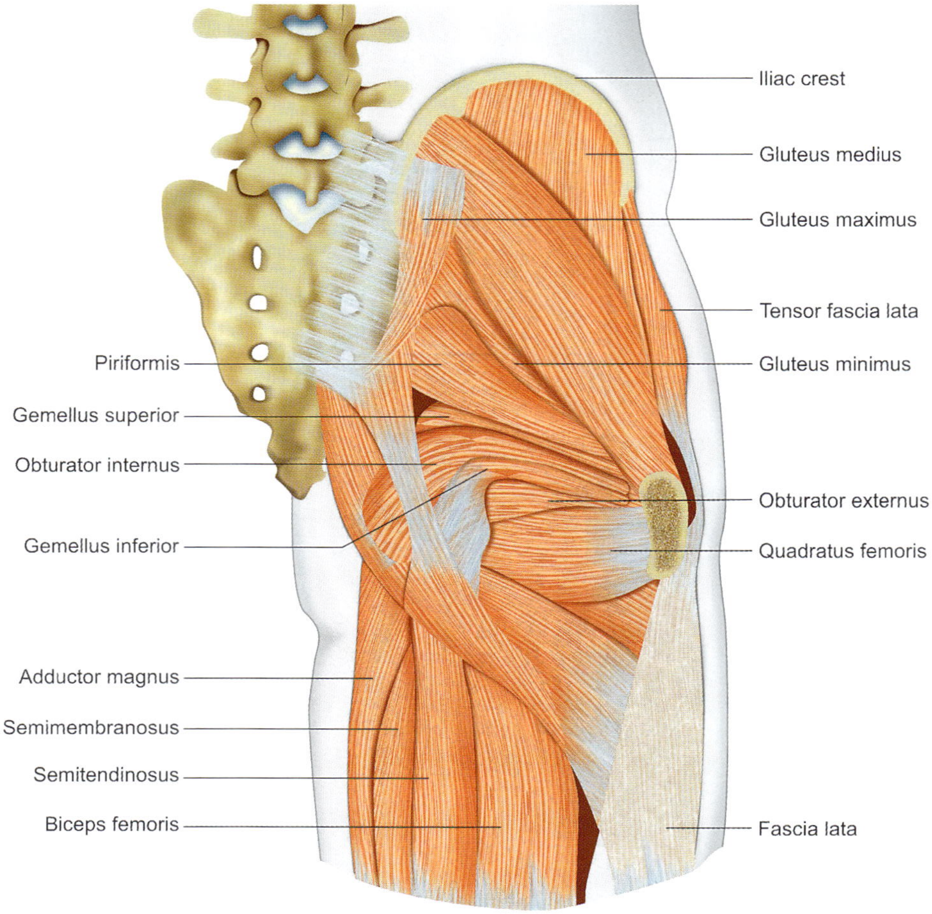

Fig. 12: Muscles around the hip as seen from posterior aspect. It is a see through gluteus maximus to appreciate the deeper structures.

flex the knee. Their power increases with hip flexion whereas decreases with as the hip flexes beyond neutral.

Abductors (Fig. 12)

- ***Gluteus medius (superior gluteal nerve):*** The muscle has anterior, middle, and posterior parts that function asynchronously:
  - Anterior fibers of the gluteus medius are active in hip flexion and medial rotation.
  - Posterior fibers function during extension and lateral rotation.
  - Middle are involved in abduction predominantly.

The gluteus minimus and medius muscles function together to abduct the hip during the stance phase of gait countering the effects of the adduction moment created by the patient's weight (*see* Chapter on "Biomechanics of Hip Joint"). The combined force is equal to 2.5 BW normally when the ratio b/a is 2.5 (*see* Chapter on "Biomechanics of Hip Joint"). After THA, patient has Trendelenburg gait until the abductor musculature can generate this force.

- ***Gluteus minimus (superior gluteal nerve):*** It lies deep to the gluteus medius, arising from the outer surface of the ilium, and inserting on the anterosuperior angle of the greater trochanter. The muscle needs to be released from bone surface to prevent internal rotation contracture in long-standing deformities when regaining length by THA else posterior dislocation is common.
- ***Tensor fascia lata (superior gluteal nerve):*** It may significantly contribute to abduction but only during concomitant hip flexion along with the gluteus minimus muscle.

Adductors (Fig. 12)

- Adductor brevis (obturator nerve)
- Adductor longus (obturator nerve)
- Adductor magnus (obturator nerve)
- Pectineus (femoral nerve)
- Gracilis (obturator nerve)—this is a part of pes anserinus and originates on the inferior pubic ramus and the edge of the symphysis pubis, to insert on the medial surface of the proximal tibia.

Adduction contractures are frequently found in pathologic conditions of the hip and as their strength is more than the abductors adductor tenotomy through a separate medial incision should be done to prevent recurrent dislocation (also consider release of the pubofemoral ligament and inferior capsule in these cases—discussed earlier).

External Rotators (Fig. 12)

The short external rotators include the obturator internus and externus (N. supply—nerve to obturator internus and obturator nerve, respectively), the superior and inferior gemellus (nerve to gemelli), the quadratus femoris (N. supply—nerve to quadratus femoris), and the piriformis muscles (N. supply—nerve to piriformis). The convexity of the neck and backward projection of the intertrochanteric crest gives these muscles excellent mechanical advantage in externally rotating the hip joint. Piriformis syndrome is described in detail in the Chapter on "Sports Medicine: Hip and Thigh".

Internal Rotators

There are no primary internal rotators of hip and the muscles that do so is a part of their secondary function.

These muscles include anterior fibers of the gluteus medius and minimus and the tensor fascia lata muscles. Other internal rotators include: Semimembranosus, semitendinosus, and pectineus.

Vessels around the Hip Joint

Common Femoral Vessels (Fig. 13)

The common femoral artery is an extension of the external iliac artery as it passes under the inguinal ligament. It lies directly anterior and medial to the hip capsule separated from it by only the iliopsoas tendon. The common femoral vein lies medial to the artery and becomes the external iliac vein as it passes under the inguinal ligament after receiving contributions from the profunda femoris and greater saphenous vessels. The causes of arterial injury in THA have been reported due to various mechanisms:

- Aberrant retractor placement during the surgical approach (placed too far medially over the anterior inferior acetabular margin during the anterior lateral approach)
- Bulk allograft placement for acetabular reconstruction
- Osteophyte resection and resection of scar tissue from the anterior inferior acetabulum
- Extrusion of excess cement anteromedially can cause—pseudoaneurysm formation, thrombus formation, peripheral femoral arterial embolization due to intimal damage from the heat of polymerization
- Prolonged cement spicule pressure has resulted in postoperative vessel erosion and pseudoaneurysm formation and the formation of an arteriovenous fistula.
- Complete restoration of length in severe shortening or correction of severe flexion contractures.
- Intraoperative plethysmographic monitoring is recommended in high-risk patients.

Profunda Femoris Vessels (Fig. 13)

- Arises from the lateral side of the femoral artery approximately 3.5 cm below the inguinal ligament.

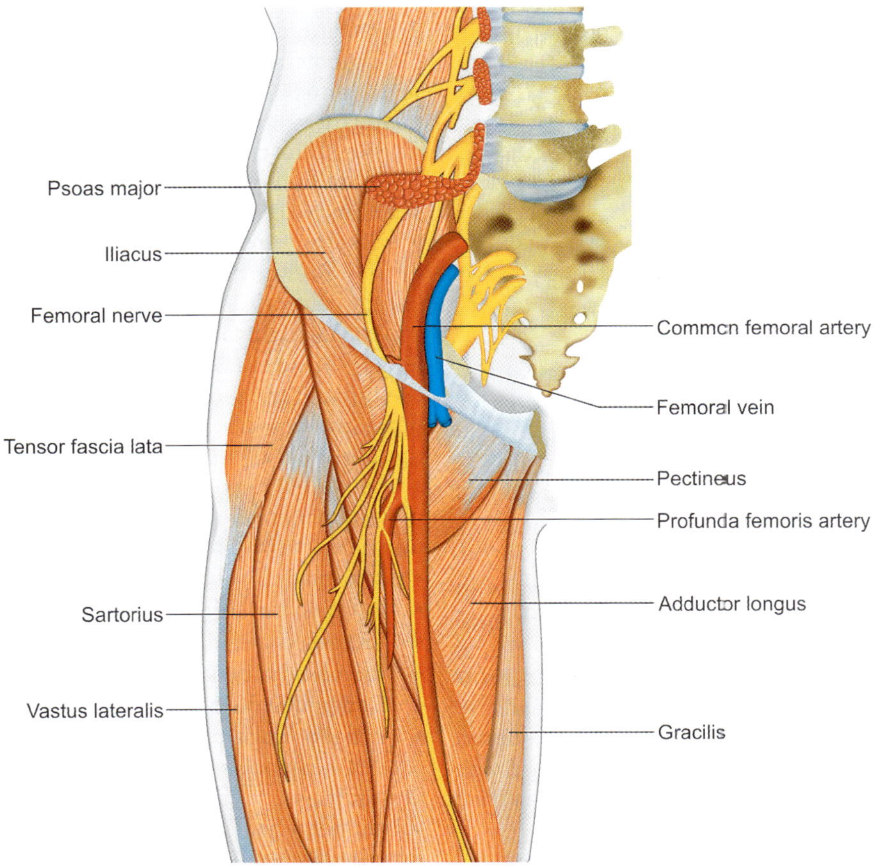

Fig. 13: The course and disposition of femoral neurovascular structures.

- The lateral circumflex artery arises from the lateral side of the proximal profundus femoris artery. It passes laterally beneath the sartorius and rectus femoris muscles and divides into ascending and descending branches.
- The medial circumflex artery usually arises from profunda but may also arise from the femoral artery. It winds medially around the femur between the pectineus and psoas muscles and posteriorly along the intertrochanteric line to appear at the upper border of the quadratus femoris.

The arteries may get injured by various mechanisms:

- Retractor placement too far medially over the anterior inferior quadrant can damage medial circumflex artery.
- Extruded cement may also injure the medial circumflex vessel.
- Hohmann retractor placed over the anterior hip capsule can cause severe arterial hemorrhage from profundus femoral and lateral circumflex artery laceration.
- Removal of scar and retracement of anteroinferior capsule during revision surgery can also damage the lateral circumflex artery.

Superior Gluteal Vessels

The superior gluteal vessels are branches of the posterior division of the internal iliac artery and exit from the greater sciatic notch along with the nerve and vein. They are relatively fixed at exit above the piriformis muscle. The artery can be injured by:

- Fixation screw in the area of the sciatic notch
- A pin retractor inserted in the direction of the notch.

Inferior Gluteal and Internal Pudendal Vessels

The inferior gluteal and internal pudendal vessels are the terminal branches of the anterior division of the internal iliac artery. These vessels exit the pelvis between the piriformis and coccygeus muscles to enter the gluteal region. The inferior gluteal vessel is commonly injured by excessively long transacetabular screw used for acetabular component fixation.

External Iliac Artery and Vein

The external iliac artery is the anterior division of the common iliac artery after its bifurcation at the level of the L5-S1 intervertebral disk. It runs down the medial border of the psoas muscle, anterior and lateral to the external iliac vein distally; the vein becomes lateral to artery. Injuries to these vessels have been commonly reported with the vein being injured more commonly.

- Atherosclerotic and arteriosclerotic diseases have both resulted in limb ischemia in these patients due to prolonged positioning and thrombus formation.
- Retractors placed too far medially over the anterior column cause direct laceration—risk is decreased by proximal retractor placement along the anterior column.
- Excessive medial reaming and cementing the cup through defect causing cement extrusion into the pelvis—a pelvic cement restrictor or bone graft is recommended.
- The use of transacetabular screws for uncemented acetabular component fixation.
- Delayed injury to the external iliac vessels occurs due to socket migration, cement spicules, and aneurysm formation.
- Revision surgery—removal of a cemented acetabular component, with cement extruded toward the iliac vessels, can tear the external iliac vessels. Arteriography or contrast-enhanced CT scanning is indicated in such cases.

Obturator Vessels

The obturator nerve, artery, and vein traverse the lateral wall (quadrilateral surface) of the pelvis with the nerve located most superior and the vein most inferior. The obturator internus muscle and fascia separate them from the quadrilateral surface. The obturator nerve, artery, and vein exit the true pelvis via the obturator canal where they are relatively fixed at by the obturator membrane and surrounding peritoneum. An aberrant (accessory) artery and a vein may also descend across the pelvic brim from the external iliac vessels to the obturator foramen forming anastomoses (corona mortis anomaly, *see* Chapter on "Surgical Approaches to Hip Joint" for detailed discussion). Injury could occur if the anterior inferior quadrant is violated or if a retractor is placed under the transverse acetabular ligament into the superolateral aspect of the obturator foramen.

Nerves Across the Hip Joint

Sciatic Nerve

The sciatic nerve is the continuation of the upper sacral plexus roots from the anterior and posterior divisions of L4, L5, S1, S2, and S3. The sciatic nerve has two divisions contained within the same connective tissue sheath: the tibial (anterior divisions) and common peroneal (posterior divisions) nerves. The common peroneal nerve is located more laterally. The sciatic nerve lies anterior and medial to the piriformis muscle. It exits from the greater sciatic notch below the piriformis muscle (infrapiriformis fossa), passing over the posterior lateral surface of the posterior acetabular column. It lies superficial to the obturator internus, gemelli, and quadratus femoris muscles **(Figs. 14 and 15)**. The tibial component has less funiculi and more connective tissue allowing it to sustain more stretch so it is a common finding that in stretch injuries the peroneal component is commonly damaged. Sciatic and peroneal nerve palsies are the most common forms of peripheral nerve injuries following THA, incidences ranging from 0.5 to 2.0%. The risk factors for sciatic nerve injury are:

- Minimally invasive hip surgeries
- Revision hip surgery
- Increased surgical time
- Increased blood loss
- Congenital dislocation
- Lengthening and/or lateral displacement of the extremity

Peroneal component palsies may be seen with lengthening as small as 2.7 cm (range, 1.9-3.7 cm) while complete sciatic nerve palsies have been associated with an average lengthening of 4.4 cm (range, 4.0-5.1 cm). Uncommon causes of injury include entrapment by trochanteric wiring,

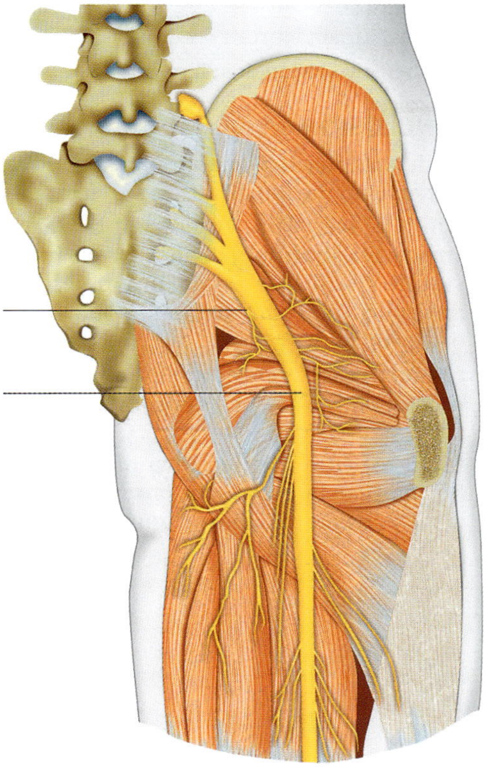

Fig. 14: Disposition of sciatic nerve.

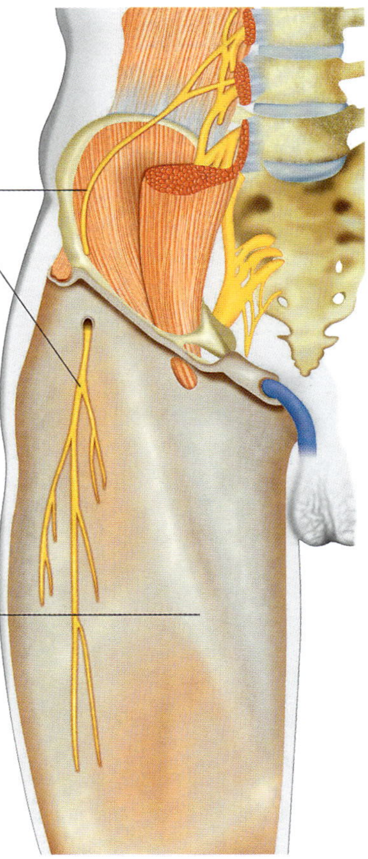

Fig. 15: The relations and anatomy of lateral femoral cutaneous nerve.

compression of the nerve over a spur of cement, migration of broken trochanteric wires, etc.

Damage to peroneal nerve fares much better than complete sciatic palsy. Stretch injuries do not fare as well as direct injury (retractor, electrocautery burn, suture, and intraoperative femur fracture). Patients who retain some motor function after surgery or who recover some function while in the hospital are more likely to have a good recovery.

Femoral Nerve (Fig. 13)

The femoral nerve is formed from the posterior branches of the second, third, and fourth lumbar nerve roots. It lies in the femoral triangle that is located directly anterior and medial to the hip joint. It supplies motor innervation to the iliacus, pectineus, sartorius, and quadriceps muscle groups. The causes of nerve injury include:

- Minimally invasive anterior approach
- Cement extravasation
- Lengthening or stretch
- Hematoma formation—the femoral triangle area is quite unyielding and nerve is prone to compression here.
- Retractor placement

Most femoral nerve palsies recover with conservative care. Complete entrapment of the femoral nerve by cement has a bad prognosis. Surgical decompression and neurolysis may be considered for impingement by spurs of polymethylmethacrylate (PMMA) or hematoma in the femoral triangle. Stretch-induced femoral neuropathy does not appear to do well.

Lateral Femoral Cutaneous Nerve (Fig. 15)

The anatomy is detailed in topic "meralgia paresthetica". The nerve is at increased risk of damage in the Smith Peterson incision for cup placement in the two-incision minimally invasive technique.

Obturator Nerve

The damage to this nerve is rare and manifests as persistent groin pain after THA. The common mechanism is cement extrusion inferomedially. Injury by drills is also reported. Damage to medial acetabular wall as well as defects in the pubic ramus have been noted to cause obturator nerve damage. Wire mesh is inadequate in preventing cement-induced damage and bone grafting is indicated. Anteroinferior screw (gross malpositioning of screw) may theoretically cause damage to the nerve.

Stability of Hip Joint

Stability of hip joint is provided by the combination following as individually discussed above and in Chapter on "Biomechanics of Hip Joint":

Osseous structures:

- Head/neck offset

- Acetabular coverage of femoral head
- Acetabular anteversion
- Femoral anteversion

Ligamentous structures:
- Capsular ligaments
- Iliofemoral (limits extension)
- Pubofemoral (limits abduction)
- Ischiofemoral (limits internal rotation)
- Ligamentum orbicularis
- Internal ligaments
- Ligamentum teres (secondary constraint to external rotation)
- Transverse ligament
- Torn/stretched/lax ligaments → greater excursion, marginal contact

Neuromuscular factors:
- Strength of muscles bridging hip joint
- Balanced strength of opposing muscles
- *Muscle tone*: Complex neural feedback

Cartilaginous structures:
- Normal, intact labrum
- Concentric seal against femoral head

CONCLUSION

- Understanding hip anatomy is imperative to functionally understand the hip disorders and treat them.
- Hip is a deep joint supported by various soft-tissue structures that play dynamic role in maintaining its stability and function. They need anatomical and physiological reconstruction to optimize reconstruction of the hip joint.
- Anatomical references are used while performing joint arthroplasty and their reproduction is the essence of success of THA.
- Injury to neurovascular structures during surgery around hip joint can be avoided by proper understanding of their disposition around the hip joint.

CHAPTER 69

Surgical Approaches to Hip Joint

Manish Kumar Varshney

INTRODUCTION

The hip joint has been subjected to varied pathology and has spherical shape so there is requirement of various exposures from all sides to address localized versus global pathologies. The anatomy involves various internervous and intervascular planes. The hip joint is hence amenable to many approaches depending on the authors and surgeons who described them. The choice of approach depends on:

- Type of surgery—trauma or elective, replacement versus conservative surgery
- What part of the hip needs to be exposed—acetabular or femoral or both
- Age of the patient—adult versus child
- Surgeon's preference and expertise

The characteristic of a good approach to be chosen for a particular procedure depends on features that it should:

- Provide adequate approach to both femoral head and acetabulum so that it can be universally applied
- Involve minimal dissection of soft tissues
- Reduce operative time and blood loss
- Be between intervascular and interneural plane to minimize morbidity
- Provide least postoperative pain and early mobilization
- Be associated with minimal chance of damage to neurovascular bundles and other vital structures and with minimal risk of infection or thrombosis
- Reliably restore the anatomy after procedure so that functional deterioration is minimal and stability of joint is maintained.

There is not any ideal approach, therefore, multiple approaches have been described, over the years, in search for better approaches. Not all described approaches are important or necessary to be learnt so limited number of commonly used exposures are described in the following section.

CLASSIFICATION OF APPROACHES TO HIP JOINT

Surgical approaches to the hip joint can be classified in multiple ways:

- ***Based on the direction (Fig. 1):***
  - *Anterior approach*: Smith-Petersen approach and modified mini-incision approach, Somerville "bikini" incision.

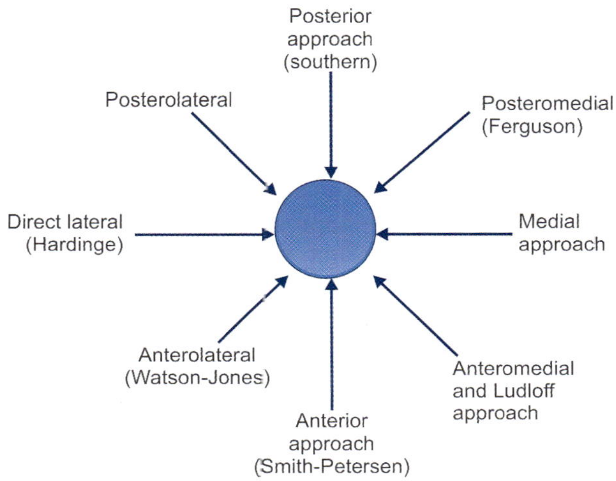

Fig. 1: The various described approaches to hip joint. As obvious from the figure, hip joint can be approached from all around except from inside the pelvis!

  - *Lateral*: Hardinge, Harris, McLauchlan approach, McFarland, and Osborne
  - *Anterolateral*: Watson Jones, Cave, and Gonder
  - *Posterior*: Moore/Southern, Osborne
  - *Posterolateral*: Kocher-Langenbeck, Gibson
  - *Medial*: Anteromedial, posteromedial (Ferguson approach), and Ludloff's
  - Combination of anterior and posterior approaches
- ***Based on incision size and level of invasiveness:***
  - Standard incision
  - Mini incision
  - Minimally invasive surgery (MIS)
- ***Based on type of surgery:***
  - Open surgical (surgical dislocation of hip)
  - Arthroscopic
- ***Combination approaches:***
  - Using Ganz trochanteric flip osteotomy
  - Modified anterolateral
  - Anterolateral MIS
  - Mini-incision or two-incision posterior approach

TECHNIQUES OF VARIOUS SURGICAL APPROACHES TO THE HIP JOINT

Principles

The basic principles are:

- Thorough knowledge of anatomy and variations.
- Basics of surgery should be always followed including hand scrub, part preparation, positioning the patient, draping and secondary preparation of the area, identification of landmarks and making the incision along skin creases, following surgical planes and standard descriptions.
- All incisions should be made best in the mid-half of classical incision line so that it can be extended. The concept of "Big surgeons make big incisions" does not hold true in current practice and actually we are moving toward mini-incisions and keyhole surgery to improve the cosmetic outcome.
- *Focused dissection:* Directly approach the operative area whether it is a bone or a joint, thus minimizing dissection and unnecessary damage to soft tissues such as nerves and vessels.
- As far as possible, follow "internervous plane" to avoid damage to and denervating the muscles. It is, however, not always possible to dissect along the internervous plane and muscle splitting approaches are needed often. These muscle splitting incisions should:
  - Split muscle longitudinally along the line of the fibers.
  - Splitting is done as far as possible from the neuromuscular junction to avoid denervation.
  - Bulk of the muscle should be retracted along with the nerve to retain the nerve supply.

Anterior Approach (Smith-Petersen Approach)

Indications

- Hip arthroplasty (increasingly approach for better early results)
- Hip resurfacing is done through this approach (now abandoned due to prosthesis complication, see tribology).
- Hip arthrodesis (anterior plating)
- Decompression of the joint and pus drainage in septic arthritis
- Developmental dysplasia of the hip (DDH)
- Sartorius-based muscle pedicle bone grafting
- Extended approach for exposing inner and outer tables of ilium, anterior hip, and acetabulum

Steps

1. ***Position:*** Supine with a sand bag under the hip on the same side.
2. ***Incision:*** Incision is carried along the iliac crest border about 2–3 cm lateral to the iliac crest beginning at the junction of the middle and anterior third of the crest leaving a small strip for later closure **(Fig. 2)**. At the anterior superior iliac spine (ASIS), the incision is carried distally toward the knee, slightly lateral along the anterior border of the tensor fascia lata (TFL) muscle sheath.
3. ***Soft-tissue dissection:*** The lateral femoral cutaneous nerve should be protected **(Fig. 3)**. Develop plane between sartorius and the TFL and deep between rectus femoris and gluteus medius **(Fig. 4)**.
   - The superficial dissection is internervous between the sartorius (femoral nerve) and the TFL (superior gluteal nerve) and the deep dissection proceeds between rectus femoris (femoral nerve) and gluteus medius/minimus (superior gluteal nerve) which is also internervous, so it is a true internervous approach.
4. ***Arthrotomy:*** Rectus femoris tendon is released near its origin to expose the medial capsule **(Fig. 5)**. Incise the capsule longitudinally T-shape **(Fig. 5-inset)**. Adduction and external rotation of the leg facilitates arthrotomy.
5. ***Dislocation:*** Externally rotate the leg and placed in a sterile pouch.

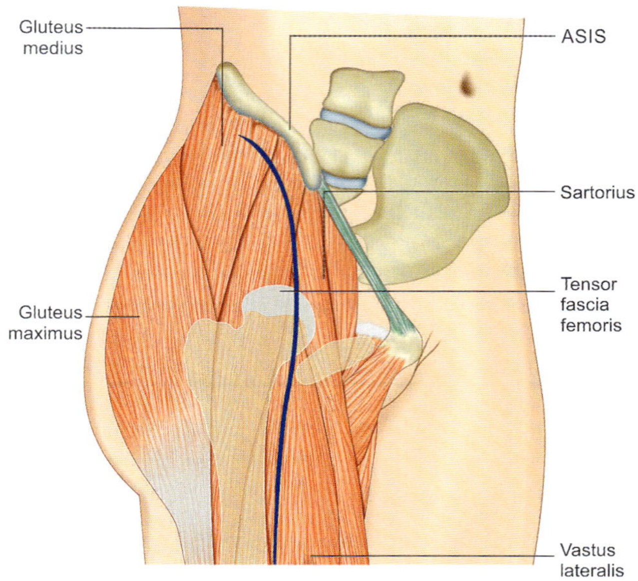

Fig. 2: Incision for Smith-Petersen approach. (ASIS: anterior superior iliac spine)

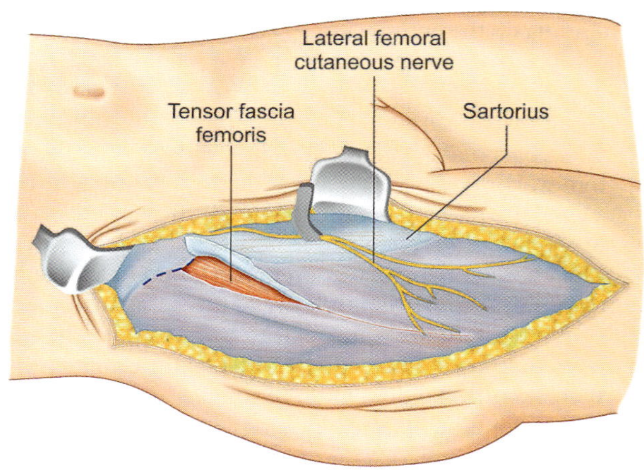

Fig. 3: Incision of the fascia of tensor fascia lata exposing the muscle, protecting the lateral femoral cutaneous nerve (LFCN).

Advantages

- Preservation of the vascularity—the medial circumflex femoral artery and its branches are preserved.

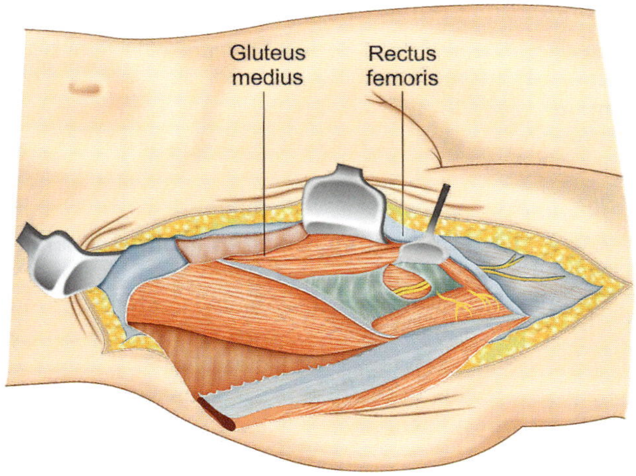

Fig. 4: Releasing tensor fascia lata (TFL) to expose gluteus medius and rectus femoris.

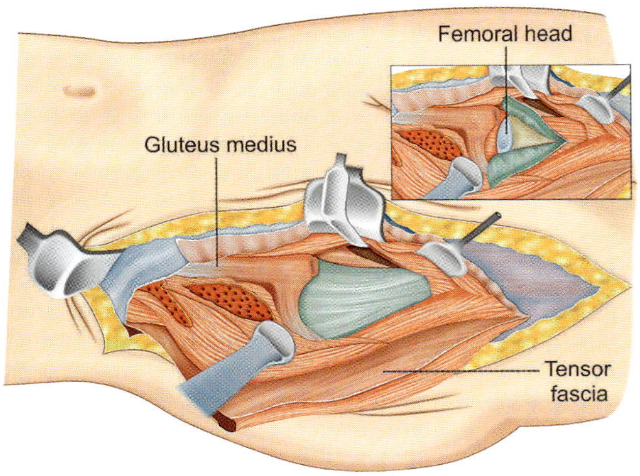

Fig. 5: The rectus femoris tendon has been released near its origin to allow further exposure of the medial hip capsule. Inset shows the capsulotomy.

- Better stability following the procedure with less chance of dislocation—key muscle groups such as the extensors and the abductors are intact.
- Less intraoperative bleeding
- Easier to take intraoperative radiographs as the patient is supine. Easier patient positioning especially in spinal and fixed pelvic deformity. Bilateral surgery is also facilitated.
- Less postoperative pain.
- Shorter length of hospital stay and faster postoperative recovery

Limitations and Complications

- Limited access makes it technically demanding to place components in arthroplasty as the femoral exposure is limited.
- Damage to lateral cutaneous nerve and the anterior cutaneous nerve.
- Complicated reconstructions pose a challenge through this approach and have reported higher occurrence of intraoperative fractures.
- Not a good approach to perform revision total hip arthroplasty (THA) as implant retrieval through extended trochanteric osteotomy is very practically possible. Also it is restricted in extensibility for complex acetabular reconstructions.
- Determining version of hip using combined anteversion technique is not possible (it is described for posterior approach).
- Wound complications are quite significant due to stretching of skin.

Modifications to the Approach

- Two incision direct anterior approach
- MIS direct anterior approaches

Anterolateral Approach (Watson-Jones Approach)

Indications

- Hip arthroplasty
- Surgical dislocation of hip
- Fracture of femoral head
- Open reduction of femoral neck fractures
- Surgical management of femoro-acetabular impingement (FAI)
- Muscle pedicle bone grafting (TFL based)

Steps

1. ***Position:*** Supine or lateral (preferred for hip arthroplasty) on the table.
2. ***Incision:*** Curvilinear incision centered over the greater trochanter running posteriorly along the shaft of the femur with hip in 30–40° of flexion starting 2–3 cm behind the ASIS **(Fig. 6)**.
3. ***Soft-tissue dissection:*** Plane is developed **(Fig. 7)** between the TFL and the gluteus medius (protects the inferior branch of the superior gluteal nerve). Original description described a partial release of the anterior fibers of the gluteus medius from the trochanteric insertion. TFL is retracted medial and anterior, and the gluteus medius retracted posterior and lateral exposing gluteus minimus posteriorly and rectus anteriorly. External rotation, abduction, and flexion help in exposure. Rectus is retracted anteriorly and gluteus minimus posteriorly (they can be released partially/completely to improve exposure) to expose the capsule **(Fig. 8)**. Along the capsule, do not go anteriorly—femoral vascular injury or inferiorly—circumflex injury.
   - *The dissection is not in the true internervous plane* as superior gluteal nerve supply both gluteus medius and TFL.
4. ***Arthrotomy:*** The capsule is divided with an L-fashion at the anterior superior femoral neck.
5. ***Dislocate*** the hip by external rotation, traction, and adduction.

Advantages

- Stability and reduced chances of posterior dislocation
- Less risk of sciatic nerve damage (unless too much stretch has been put on the nerve). Precautions should also be taken not to extend the knee producing sciatic nerve stretch.

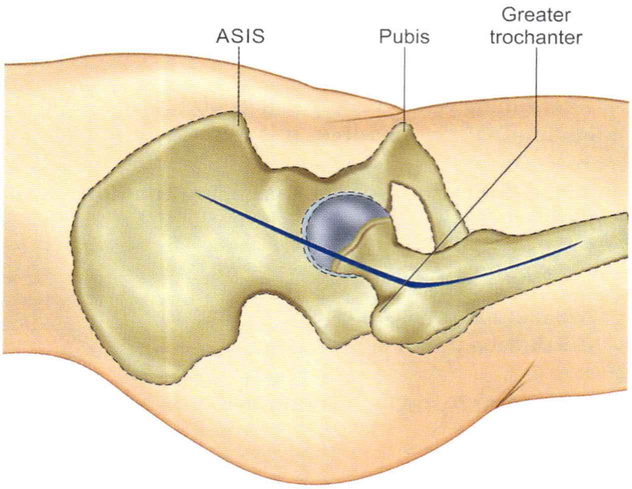

Fig. 6: The incision for Watson-Jones approach. (ASIS: anterior superior iliac spine)

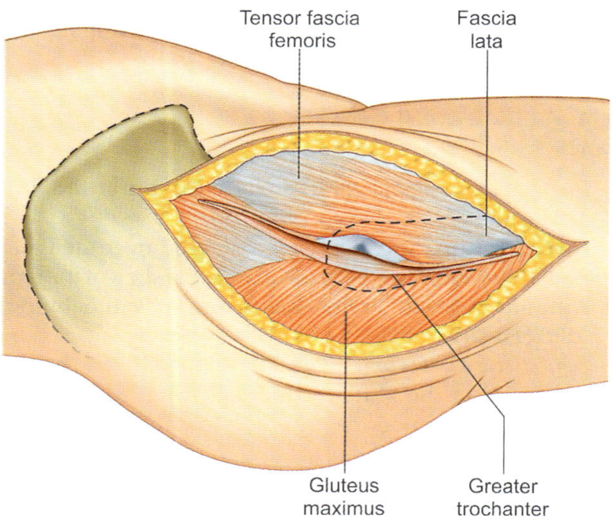

Fig. 7: Developing plane between the tensor fascia and gluteus medius.

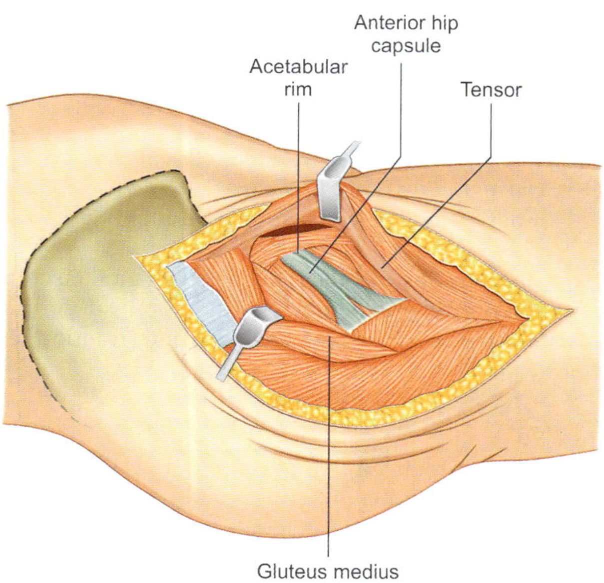

Fig. 8: Retracting the tensor and gluteus to expose hip capsule.

Limitations and Complications

- Weakening of abductors during dissection or by denervation
- Injury to the superior gluteal nerve
- Injury to lateral circumflex femoral artery
- Rarely injury to the femoral nerve and vessels

Modifications

- The Müller modified approach to avoid trochanteric osteotomy.
- Minimally invasive approach—Anterolateral MIS approach which has reduced hospital stay, surgical time, blood loss, morbidity, and encouraged early mobilizations and recovery. Higher complication rates have been reported with this approach.

Direct Lateral Approach (Bauer Approach as Modified by Hardinge)

Indications

- Total hip replacements, hip resurfacing
- Fracture of femoral neck
- Open reduction of femoral neck fractures
- Slipped upper femoral epiphysis (SUFE)
- Proximal femoral osteotomy

Key Steps

1. ***Position:*** Lateral or preferably the supine position.
2. ***Incision:*** It is centered over the midpoint of greater trochanter and extends distally longitudinally along the femoral shaft for about 8–10 cm with proximal extension in line of femoral shaft **(Fig. 9)**.
3. ***Soft-tissue dissection:*** Gluteal fascia and iliotibial band are cut and plane between TFL and gluteus maximus is developed. The fibers of the gluteus medius are divided a short distance proximally **(Fig. 10)**. The dissection is carried distally into the vastus lateralis, and the entire muscle and tendinous attachment is elevated off the trochanter sharply. Exposed gluteus minimus is dissected to expose the capsule.
   - Dissection is not in the true internervous plane as gluteus medius and vastus lateralis are split.
4. ***Dislocation:*** Leg is externally rotated and abducted for dislocation.

Advantages

- Good access to the hip with preservation of vascularity
- Minimal risk of damage to sciatic nerve

Limitations and Complications

- Damage to gluteal muscle mainly gluteus medius and loss of abductor function.
- Heterotopic ossification may be a problem.

Modifications

The modifications are:

- Trochanteric slide modification was added by Dall that removes a fragment of bone from trochanter along with the

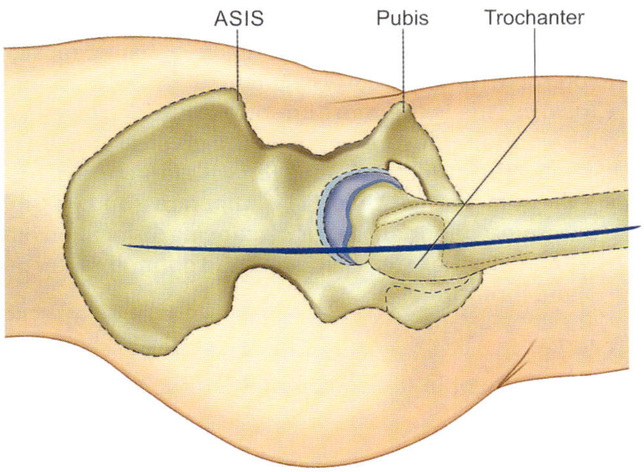

Fig. 9: Incision for the direct lateral approach.

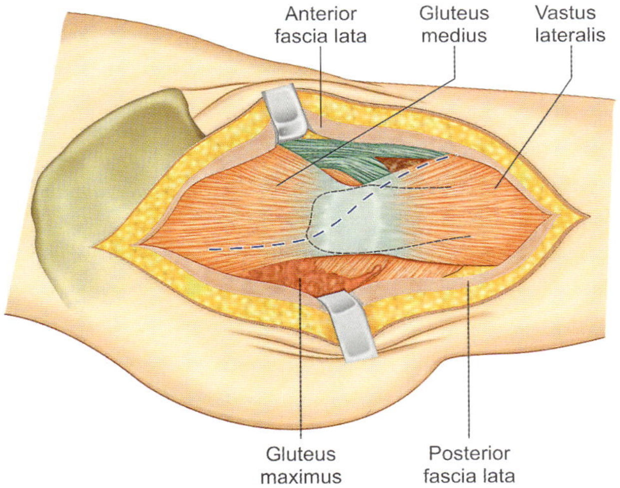

Fig. 10: The deep incision that releases the majority of the insertion of the gluteus medius and minimizes the release of the vastus lateralis.

attached muscles **(Fig. 11)**. The extent of slide is, however, limited and is not useful in revision surgery.

- Transgluteal approach originally described by Bauer the dissection of gluteus medius and vastus is altered.
- Lateral transtrochanteric approach first described in 1881 by Ollier and popularized by Sir John Charnley for revision arthroplasties. It also allows the lateralization of greater trochanter.
- Extensile modification for revision arthroplasty—here the gluteus medius and minimus are released from the anterior trochanter by performing osteotomy to allow exposure of the anterior hip capsule.

Posterior Approach

Moore's approach (or Southern approach) is one of the most common approaches used by the orthopedic surgeons at present for arthroplasty. It was originally described by Austen Moore in 1957. The original posterior approach was described by Langenbeck in 1874 and since then different people added modifications to it so by 1957 when Moore described his approach there were 13 different posterior approaches.

Indications

- Hip arthroplasty
- Acetabular reconstruction during revision
- Muscle pedicle bone grafting (quadratus femoris based)
- Acetabular fractures for fixation of posterior wall/column

Steps

- ***Position:*** Lateral position
- ***Incision:*** 10–15 cm long curvilinear extending from 10 cm distal to posterior superior iliac spine (PSIS) to greater trochanter and extends down along the shaft of the femur as required **(Fig. 12)**. Small incisions ≈ 10 cm are also enough however and can always be extended.

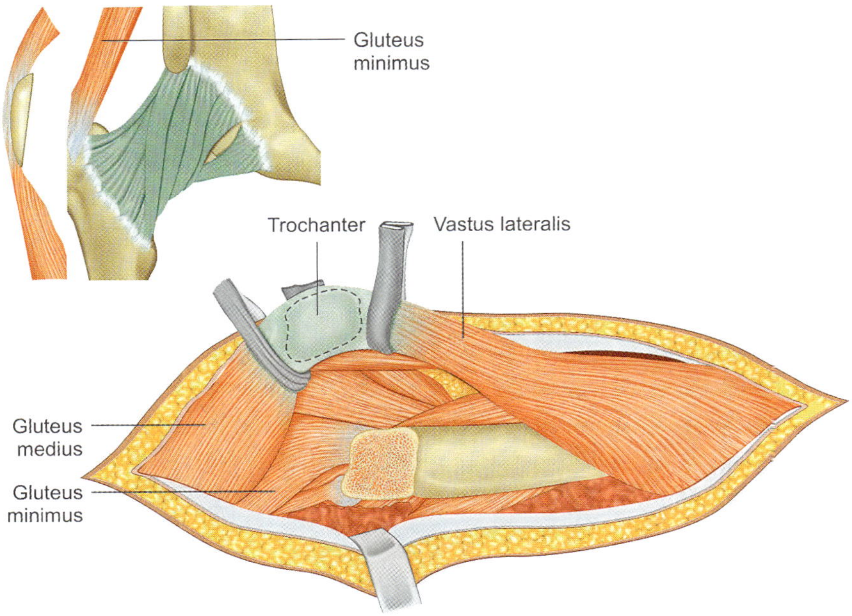

Fig. 11: Trochanteric slide modification by Dall for lateral approach.

- ***Soft-tissue dissection:*** The gluteus maximus fibers are split and upper part of fascia lata is split **(Fig. 13)**.
    - The hip is internally rotated and short external rotators are identified and held with stay sutures **(Fig. 14)**.
    - Obturator internus and externus, two gemelli and piriformis are detached and reflected backward to protect the sciatic nerve **(Fig. 15)**. I personally preserve the piriformis in most hemiarthroplasty procedures and some of the total hips. Quadratus femoris is commonly separated from femur shaft in proximal thirds or half to improve exposure of the joint. For THA, the muscle may be detached at its attachment but for hip-preserving procedures the muscle is cut at least 1 cm away from its femoral attachment to prevent injury to medial circumflex femoral artery.
    - Superior extension and reflection of gluteus minimus may be done for acetabular reconstruction as needed.
- ***Internervous plane:*** No internervous plane
- ***Arthrotomy:*** Capsule is incised with a classical T-/H-shaped incision **(Fig. 16)** or better an L-shaped incision to preserve the iliofemoral ligament.
- ***Closure:*** This is the most important after arthroplasty as meticulous closure only has the greatest impact on reducing the dislocation rate seen with this approach:
    - Capsular closure **(Fig. 17)** is imperative and possibly the most important factor in reducing dislocation rate.
    - Re-attach the external rotators and obturator inter nus and piriformis.

Advantage

Good exposure of both acetabulum and the femoral head and neck.

Disadvantages and Complications

- The blood supply to femoral head is likely to get damaged resulting in osteonecrosis restricting its use in conservative

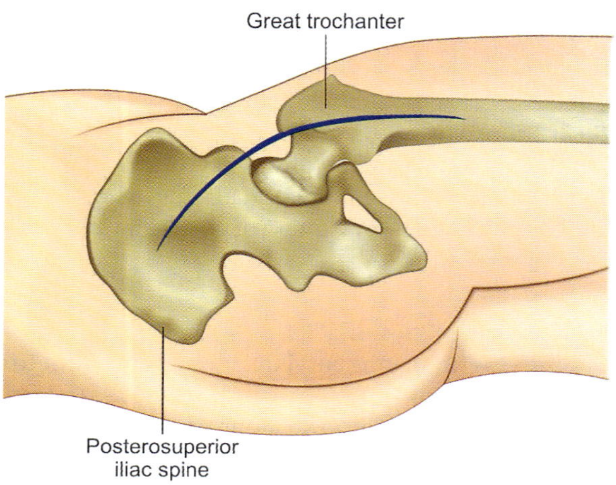

Fig. 12: Moore's (or Southern's) posterior approach.

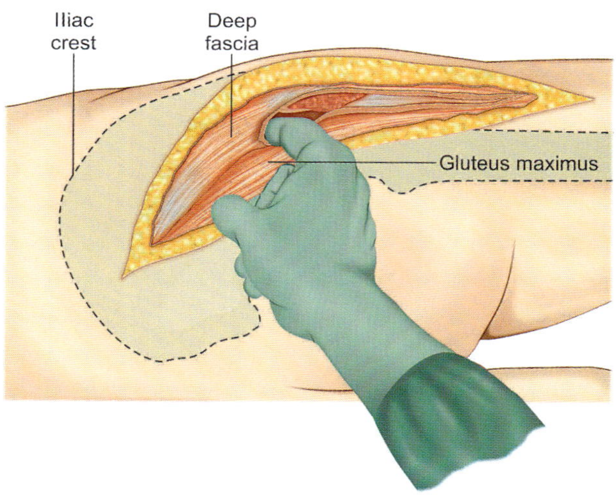

Fig. 13: Splitting the gluteus maximus.

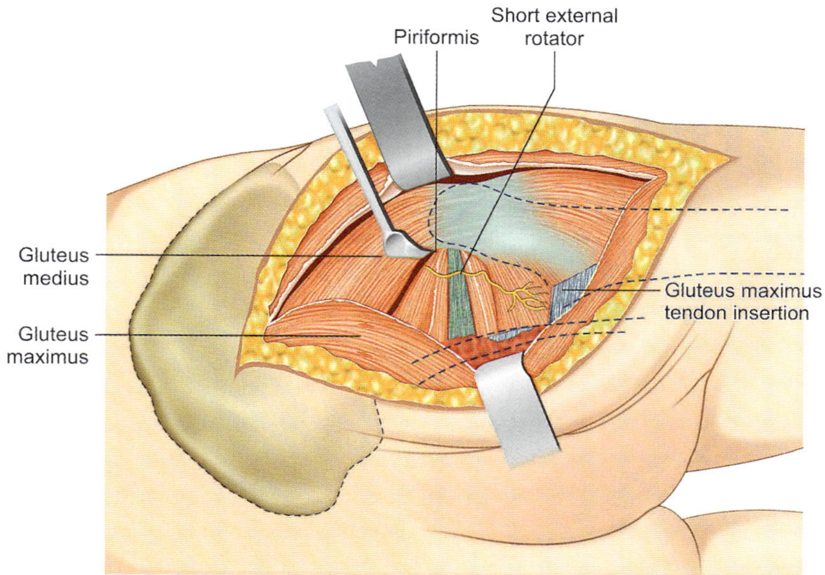

Fig. 14: Releasing gluteus maximus tendon insertion and identifying the short external rotators.

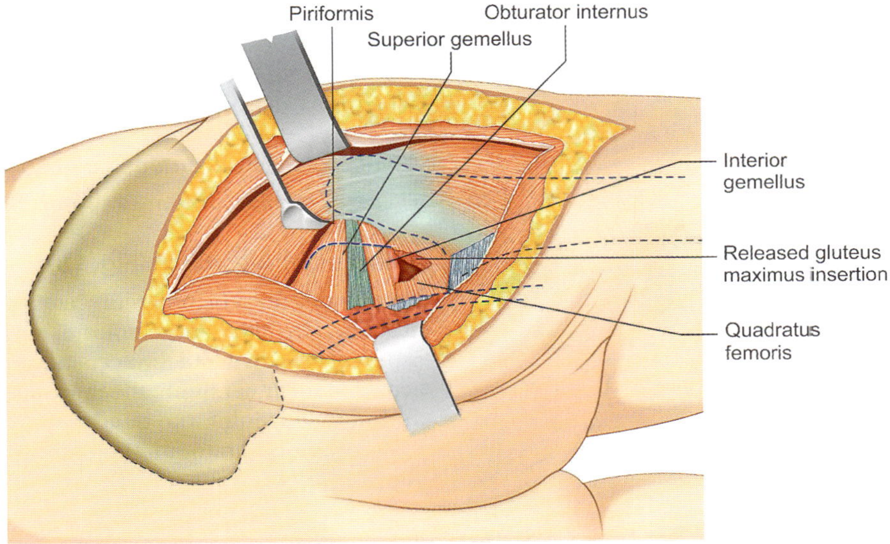

Fig. 15: Releasing the short external rotators and piriformis after tying them.

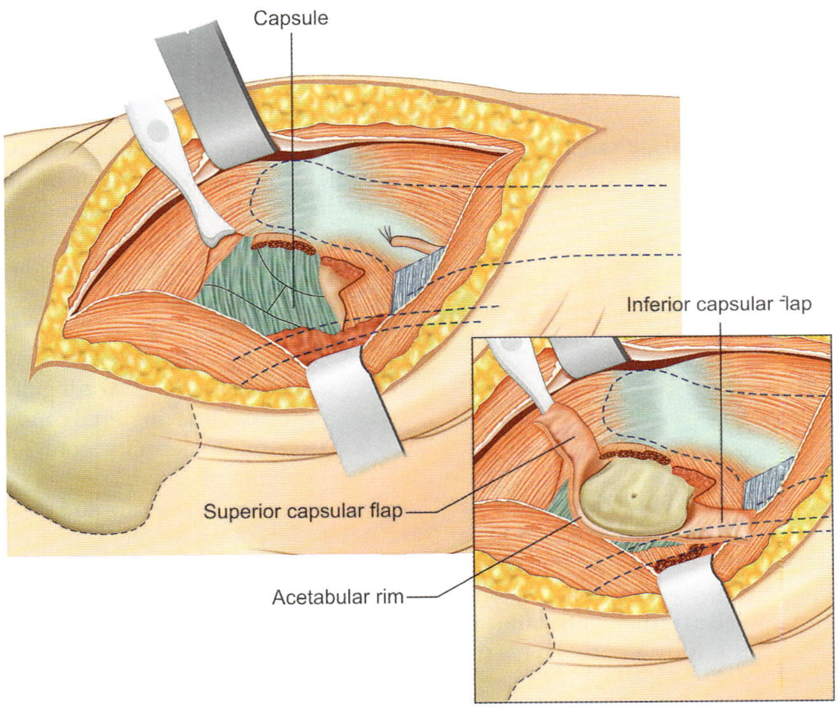

Fig. 16: Making the capsulotomy "H-shaped". The short external rotators have been reflected.

hip surgery such as open hip debridement, open surgery for hip impingement.

- Damage to sciatic nerve—palpate the nerve through fat pad to identify its lateralized variation. The nerve is retracted by the reflected cut short external rotators (not piriformis—it lies superficial to nerve). The knee should be kept flexed minimum 45° throughout to prevent traction on the nerve.
- Injury to inferior gluteal vessels, branches of profunda femoris vessels and rarely femoral vessels.
- Higher dislocation rate if soft-tissue reconstruction is inadequate.

Modifications

- Minimally invasive posterior approach—it has similar outcomes in the early postoperative period (such as surgical duration, blood loss and hospital stay) but long-term results such as Harris Hip Score are better in the MIS.
- Gibson approach

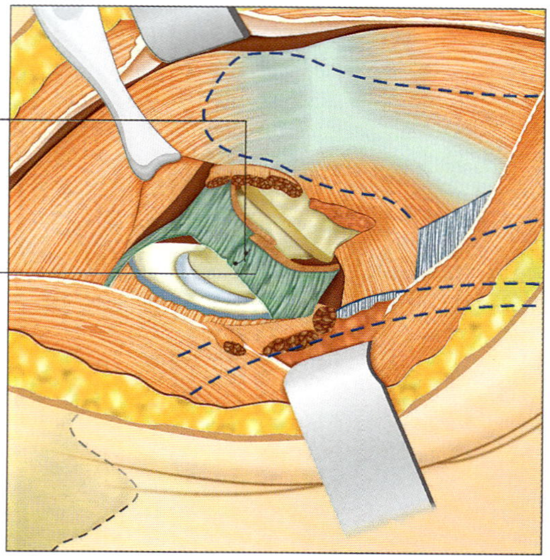

Fig. 17: The repair of capsule is an integral part of closure followed by tying of the short external rotators.

- Iyer modification—splits a portion of the gluteus medius, and a portion of the greater trochanter is osteotomized and re-attached (preserves the original soft-tissue attachments of the posterior hip).

Posterolateral Approach (Langenbeck in 1873 and Kocher 1887)

Indications

- Total hip arthroplasty
- Revision hip arthroplasty
- Fixation of fractures of acetabulum posterior wall and column
- Tumor surgery

Steps

1. ***Position:*** Lateral position
2. ***Incision:*** Langenbeck incision extended from the PSIS to the trochanter tip with the hip held at 45° of flexion (Kocher modified to place the incision at the anterior aspect of trochanter). Kocher also added distal extension in line with femur. Harros added a further limb at the distal aspect of incision curved posteriorly 45° (this is useful in bulky individuals).
3. ***Soft-tissue dissection:*** Gluteus maximus is split (blunt dissection) and fascia lata may be split proximally for 3–4 cm to release the attachment of gluteus maximus. Hip is internally rotated. Trochanteric bursa is excised followed by gentle teasing of the fat pad overlying gemelli and obturator internus. Branches of inferior gluteal artery are cauterized. Piriformis tendon is identified just beneath the gluteus medius. These are tagged and released. Quadratus can be released proximally to gain internal rotation. The capsule is hence exposed. For further acetabular exposure, gluteus medius and minimus can be reflected superiorly and retracted. Piriformis and obturator internus can be dissected free of tissues and bone deeply to expose the posterior wall. The soft-tissue dissection posteroinferiorly would expose the ischium.
4. ***Capsulotomy:*** H-shaped capsulotomy is made.
5. ***Dislocation:*** Hip is dislocated by internal rotation.

Advantages, Disadvantages, and Complications

These are similar to Moore's approach.

Ilioinguinal Approach (Fig. 18)

It is a modification of the Smith–Petersen iliofemoral approach described by Judet and Letournel for access to the anterior aspect of the pelvis and the acetabulum. The approach allows access to the inner ilium, the inner surface of the true pelvis and sacroiliac joint, the quadrilateral plate to the spinous process and obturator foramen, the anterior column to the superior pubic ramus, and the symphysis pubis.

Indications

- Fixation of anterior column and wall of acetabular fractures
- Reduction and fixation of T-type, tectal fractures, and fractures involving quadrilateral plate
- Tumor surgery
- Periacetabular osteotomies

Steps

I. ***Position:*** Supine with a bump underneath the hip. Insert Foley catheter to empty the bladder.

II. ***Incision:*** The incision extends from 2 to 3 cm above the symphysis pubis toward the ASIS and then posteriorly from the ASIS to beyond the gluteus medius tubercle of the iliac crest **(Fig. 19)**.

III. ***Soft-tissue dissection:***
   - The external oblique fascia is incised parallel **(Fig. 20)** and just proximal to the inguinal ligament as far medial as the external inguinal ring.
   - Isolate the spermatic cord/round ligament and open the inguinal canal.
   - The internal oblique and transverse abdominis fascia are incised adjacent to the conjoined tendon and beneath the spermatic cord from lateral to medial **(Fig. 21)**.
   - Protect and preserve the lateral femoral cutaneous nerve (LFCN) in lateral part of incision.

- Medially, the transversalis fascia can be dissected off the inguinal ligament and the rectus abdominis fascia.
- The exposed iliopsoas is retracted laterally with the femoral nerve using penrose drain.
- The iliopectineal fascia is identified as a vertical stout band. The fascia is an extension of the fascia iliaca presenting as an investing fascia extending from SI joint posteriorly along the pelvic brim to anteriorly. Release this carefully under full direct vision. Take care for the presence of Corona mortis anomaly that may produce profuse bleeding if cut carelessly.
- Dissection is then performed deep to the vessels bluntly using fingers and then the vessels are retracted using another penrose drain.

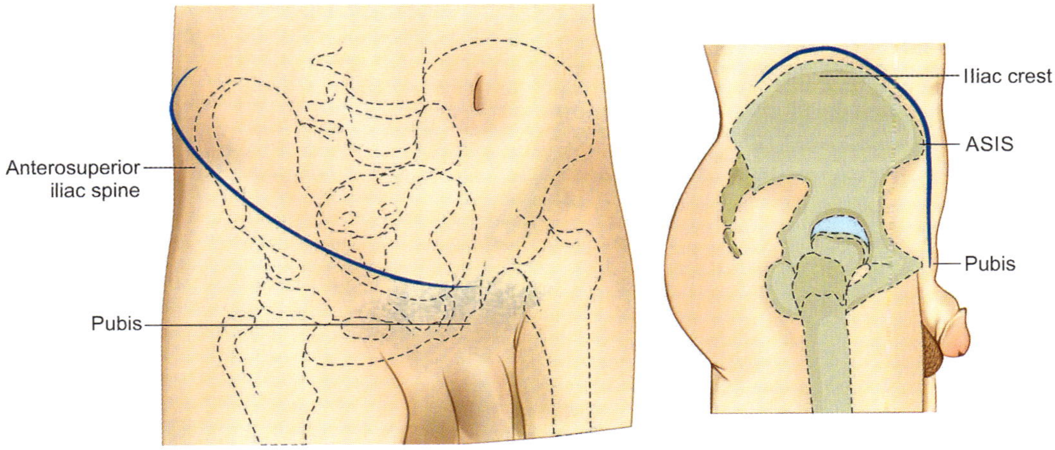

Fig. 18: Incision for ilioinguinal approach.

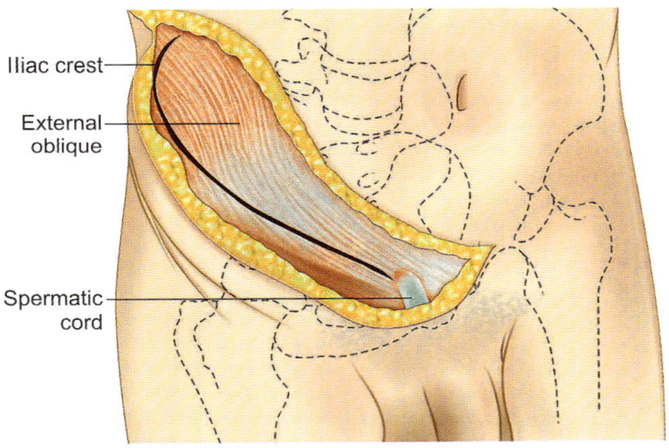

Fig. 19: Incising the external oblique aponeurosis.

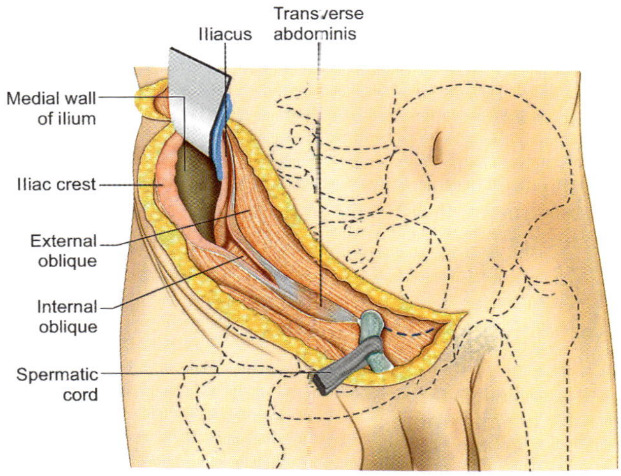

Fig. 20: The transverse abdominis and internal oblique are incised adjacent to the conjoined tendon which is also released to expose the vessels and iliopsoas muscle.

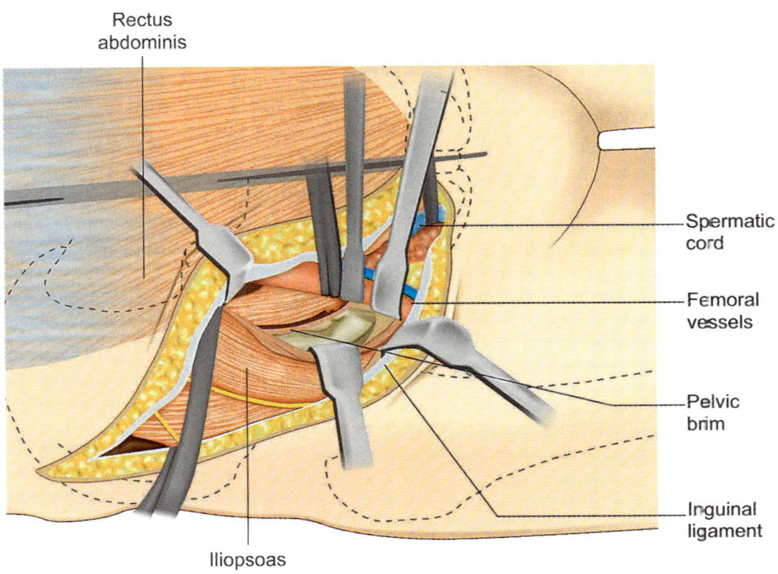

Fig. 21: Exposed iliopsoas with femoral nerve separated medially from the vessels showing the middle window, the lateral window lies lateral to the psoas muscle. The muscle and vascular bundle are retracted with penrose drain.

- The dissection hence exposes three windows **(Fig. 21)**:
  1. Lateral window is lateral to iliopsoas that exposes inner table of iliac wing and pelvic brim
  2. Middle window between the iliopsoas and the femoral vessels
  3. Medial window between the rectus and femoral vessels

Modification

Stoppa approach.

Complications

- Hernia—if closure is not perfect
- Vascular injury
- ***Injury to corona mortis (crown of death) anomaly:*** It is basically an anastomosis between the obturator and the external iliac or inferior epigastric arteries or veins **(Fig. 22)** that can be life-threatening, if neglected. It is found behind the superior pubic ramus at varying distance from the symphysis pubis (range 40–96 mm). Obturator artery (OA) is usually a branch of the anterior division of the internal iliac artery. This artery has significant and frequent (40% cases) variations. The most important and surgically relevant is accessory OA. "Aberrant" obturator artery means abnormal origin of OA from the external iliac artery or its branches that may be accessory or not. Accessory OA specifically refers to presence of an extra OA in addition to the normal counterpart. The "aberrant" vessel is actually the enlarged pubic branch of the inferior epigastric artery and may not be "accessory". When both the normal and accessory obturator arteries are present with rich anastomoses that pass over Cooper's pectineal ligament and posterior to the lacunar (Gimbernat's) ligament **(Fig. 23)**, it is known as "corona mortis" or "crown of death". It is an anastomosis between the pubic branch of the inferior epigastric (aberrant-accessory) and the obturator arteries so in fact connecting the two iliac arteries (*arteria ilica communis*). Venous corona mortis has also been described and has been considered to be present in higher number of patients than arterial anastomosis. The corona mortis has been characterized into three morphological patterns by Rusu et al. as follows:
  - *Arterial corona mortis:*
    - Obturator artery arising from the external iliac artery (EIA)
    - Obturator artery arising from the inferior epigastric artery (IEA)
    - Anastomosis between the OA and IEA
    - Pubic branches of the OA, without any anastomosis with the EIA system
  - *Venous corona mortis:*
    - Obturator vein (OV) which drains into the external iliac vein (EIV).
    - Obturator vein which drains into the inferior epigastric vein (IEV)
    - Venous anastomosis of the OV and IEV
  - Combined, arterial, and venous corona mortis

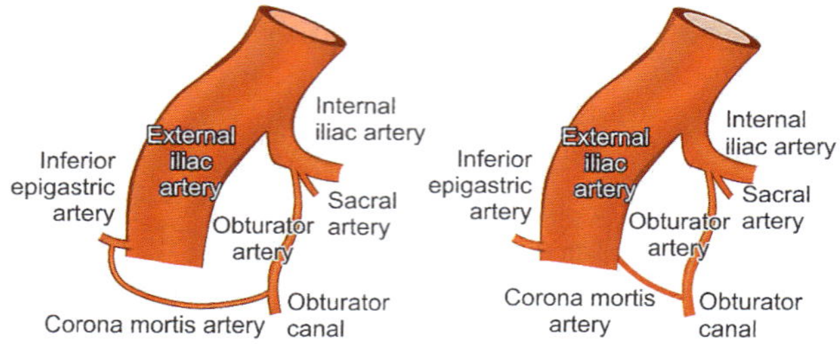

Fig. 22: Schematic drawing explaining the formation of corona mortis anomaly, the two most common ways of formation.

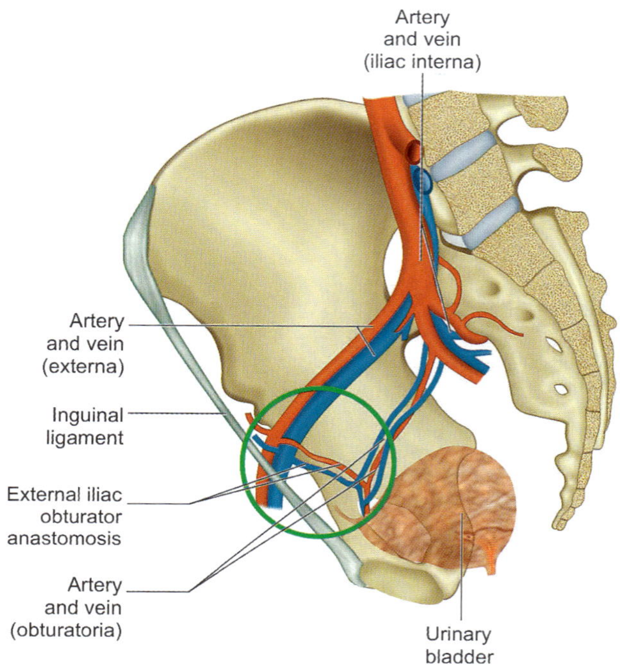

Fig. 23: Anatomical localization of the anomaly with respect to the lacunar ligament and true pelvis.

Clinical significance of corona mortis:

- In case of pelvic fracture, massive extraperitoneal hemorrhage may arise due to the presence of corona mortis.
- If it is medial to the femoral ring widening the neck of the hernial sac of femoral hernia during surgery by releasing the lacunar ligament may cause injury to the anomaly.
- In ilioinguinal approach, the vessel may be damaged if the iliopectineal ligament is cut blindly or the medial lacunar ligament is overenthusiastically released to improve exposure.

Medial Approaches

Mainly used for DDH; these can be further divided into:

- *Anteromedial approach:* Longitudinal incision is made 15–20 cm long, 2–3 cm medial to femoral artery and 2 cm distal to inguinal ligament. Pectineus and adductor longus are exposed. The external pudendal and medial circumflex femoral vessels are identified and retracted laterally. Muscles are then separated by sharp dissection and retracted to expose the lesser trochanter. Iliopsoas tendon is released and retracted to expose the capsule.

- Posteromedial approach (Ferguson's approach)
- *Ludloff approach (1908):* It was initially developed for surgery on a congenitally dislocated hip.
  - ***Position of patient***—hip placed in flexion, abduction, and external rotation.
  - ***Incision:*** Placed on medial aspect of thigh beginning 2.5 cm distal to pubic tubercle and over the interval between gracilis and adductor longus muscle **(Fig. 24)**.
  - ***Soft-tissue dissection:*** A plane is developed between sartorius and adductor longus superficially that changes to the interval between adductor brevis and pectineus in deep **(Fig. 25)**. Posterior branch of obturator nerve and neurovascular bundle to gracilis is exposed and protected while exposing the lesser trochanter.
  - ***Arthrotomy:*** Capsule is located in the floor of wound. Capsulotomy is done and the hip dislocated.
  - ***Complication:*** Injury to the nerve to gracilis and obturator nerves.

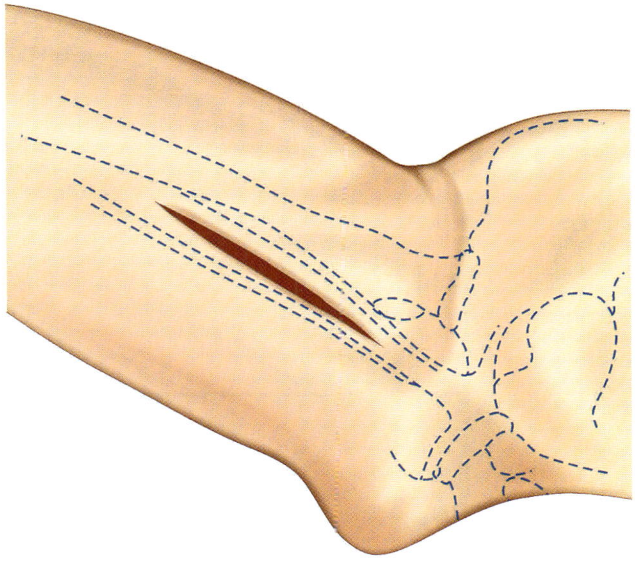

Fig. 24: Incision for Ludloff approach to hip. The incision is made directly over the adductor longus muscle.

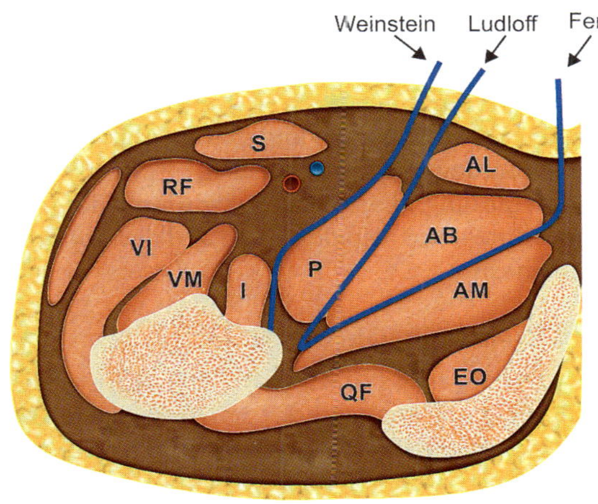

Fig. 25: The planes of various medial approaches to hip. (AB: adductor brevis; AL: adductor longus; AM: adductor magnus; EO: obturator externus; I: iliopsoas; P: pectineus; QF: quadratus femoris; RF: rectus femoris; S: sartorius; VI: vastus intermedius; VM: vastus medialis)

Minimally Invasive Approaches

They are to be less invasive with lower intraoperative complications such as blood loss, less tissue dissection and less operative time, with early recovery, early mobilization and early discharge from hospital with the availability of navigation, modern instrumentation and specific reamers, these approaches have been feasible. These are usually modifications of existing approaches. The most common MIS approaches are MIS anterolateral, MIS direct lateral, MIS posterior, and MIS anterior.

Initial results have shown increased soft tissue and wound healing complications due to excessive retraction, however, with improvement in the same comparable outcomes have been reported. Also there had been issues with optimal placement of the implant. The principles include shorter skin incision which may be single or multiple, minimal soft-tissue dissection, without compromising the access or the quality of the surgery.

Presently, there is debate over the long-term outcomes of the quality of surgery including implant positioning and need for long-learning curve to use them and the true benefit of being MIS. It is difficult to "quantitate" invasiveness in terms of real tissue damage. In a constricted space with limited visibility in a fat patient, excessive dissection may be done by the surgeon, in fact, that compromises the real goal of minimally "invasive" approach.

CONCLUSION

- The hip joint is buried in the soft tissues all around and it is impossible to approach the joint from perineal surface due to acetabular floor. The soft tissue envelop, however, provides various internervous and intervascular planes through which the joint can be exposed for elective and emergency procedures.
- The choice of approach depends on the type of surgery, selective exposure of femoral versus acetabular side and often surgeon's expertise and preference.
- Recently, the approaches have been modified to shorten the incision length in an attempt to shift to minimally invasive surgery.
- Commonly the anterolateral and posterior approaches are used for elective surgical procedures while surgeons should be also well versed with anterior approach especially for children to decompress the joint in septic arthritis. Anterior approach is also getting quite popular for primary uncomplicated THA.
- Trochanteric flip osteotomy is commonly added to lateral and anterolateral approaches to ease the hip exposure.
- Exposure of acetabulum entails learning special approaches that allows visualizing anterior and posterior columns through ilioinguinal and Kocher-Langenbeck approaches, respectively.

CHAPTER 70

Biomechanics of Hip Joint

Manish Kumar Varshney

INTRODUCTION

Biomechanics is a science that deals with the study of forces (internal or external) acting on the living body. Understanding biomechanics of hip is essential in keeping pace with the advances in sports medicines and joint reconstruction procedures. It constitutes an important background for diagnosis and treatment of various hip disorders. Evolving concepts of injuries to capsulolabral structures in development of femoroacetabular impingement (FAI) and etiopathogenesis of degenerative diseases can be understood in light of static and dynamic loading of hip joint. These ultimately help in proper understanding, diagnosis of disorders, planning of surgical procedures, and also designing and development of total hip prosthesis.

FUNCTIONAL ANATOMY (FIG. 1)

With the increasing recognition of the fact that soft-tissue disruption occurs more frequently for many hip joint disorders and they are essential early component of hip degeneration, a closer look at the functional and mechanical aspect of hip joint and geometry in imperative. The hip joint is a mobile but also highly stable joint supported by body's most powerful muscles and the strongest ligament. The innocuous looking hip joint capsule is critical to preventing hip dislocation. Strong anterior iliofemoral and arcuate ligaments are not sufficiently balanced in strength by posterior ischiofemoral ligament accounting for more frequent posterior dislocation of hip. Acetabular labrum hence occupies an efficient role in maintaining hip biomechanics:

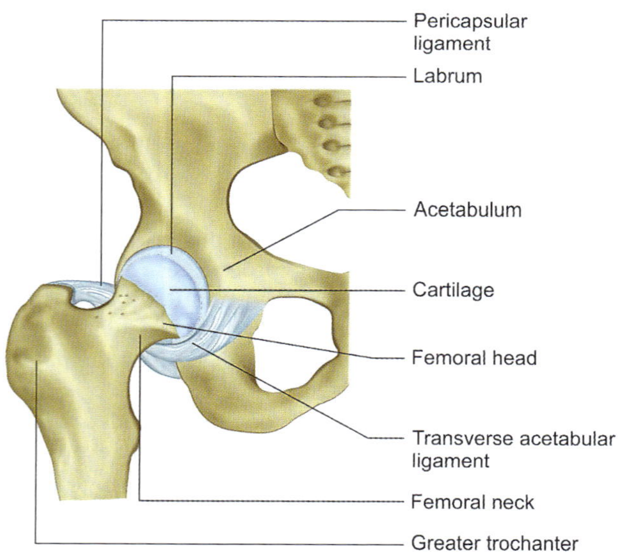

Fig. 1: Hip anatomy.

- The acetabular labrum increases the depth of the joint and acts as a seal.
- It increases the volume of joint by 33% and contributes 22% to articular surface.
- This increases stability of hip joint by dissipating large forces across the hip joint during outdoor activities.
- Function as a seal increases the effective hydrostatic pressure of the joint enhancing lubrication and reducing friction during weight-bearing also this resists joint distraction.

Labrum, thus, primarily acts to dissipate the high contact forces generated at various flexion angles and damage to labrum produces abnormal cartilage gliding during strenuous twisting and pivoting motions accelerating degenerative changes. Labral tears occur most often at junction of labrum and articular cartilage—the watershed region leading to abnormal sliding of articular surfaces under dynamic torsional sporting activities. Recent surgical techniques are aimed at preserving and repairing damage to acetabular labrum.

Inherent stability afforded by acetabular depth also defines the limits of motion of hip joint before anterior bony impingement occurs. These are 120° of flexion, 25° extension, 45° abduction, 25° adduction, and 40° internal and external rotation with interpersonal variability. However, for a normal gaitonly 35° flexion, 10° extension, and a rotational arc of 40° is required. Mobility is due to the long neck which is narrower than the diameter of the head.

Cartilage is mechanically designed to bear repetitive forces applied slowly. Rapid impulsive loading above threshold levels damage the cartilage and repetition leads to degeneration of the tissue with development of osteoarthrosis over time. This is probably the reason of joint degeneration in elite athletes;

however, contributions of subchondral sclerosis can also be substantial. Cartilage can possibly tolerate repetitive loads indefinitely if the pressures at articular surfaces are kept below 2 MPa. Normal activities such as walking produce peak pressures of up to 4 MPa while stumbling and generate pressures as high as 8 MPa, further rising from chair can triple pressures to 9–15 MPa so that degeneration frequently observed in the posterosuperior region of acetabulum is inevitable. Weight-bearing regions of hip vary according to the flexion angle and activity. Significantly, higher amount of forces is transmitted through anterior, superior, and posterior part of femoral head forming two columns of force transmitted within acetabular margin. The maximum thickness of articular cartilage, hence, is found in the ventral-cranial region of acetabulum and ventral-lateral surface of femoral head.

Joint geometry especially neck length, inclination, and neck-shaft angle has significant influence on joint forces and degeneration. For given neck length, the abductors gain mechanical advantage with reduced neck-shaft angle (varus hips). This also improves joint stability by increasing head coverage of acetabulum. However, increasing the neck length in a varus hip will lead to increased bending moment on the femoral stem (for hip arthroplasty); generating stresses in implant and its bony interfaces predisposing to loosening. On the contrary shorter valgus stem though will have lesser bending forces but mechanical disadvantage to the abductors will demand more work from them and higher forces. This produces muscle fatigue and higher joint reaction forces increasing the wear.

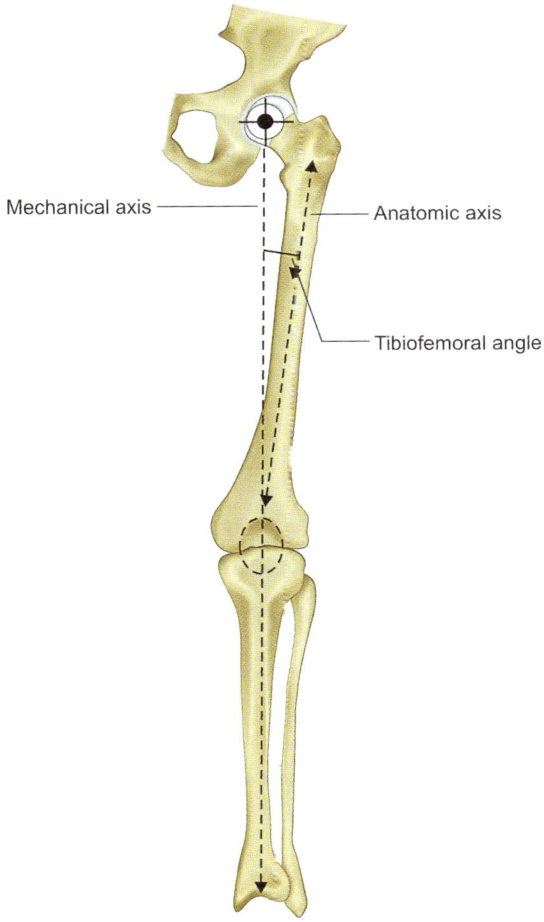

Fig. 2: Mechanical and anatomical axes of the femur.

Axes of Lower Limb and Center of Gravity (Figs. 2 and 3)

- Mechanical axis line passes between center of hip joint and center of ankle joint.
- Anatomic axis line is between the tip of greater trochanter and center of knee joint.
- Angle formed between these two is around 7°.
- Weights of any object act through center of gravity, in humans the center of gravity passes just anterior to second sacral vertebra.

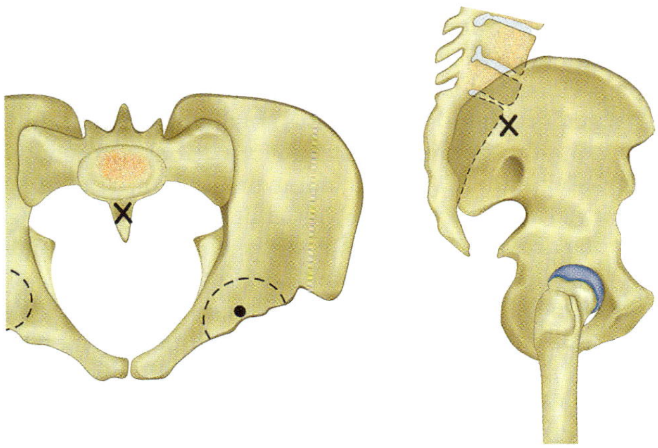

Fig. 3: The center of gravity of human body.

FORCES TRANSMITTED ACROSS HIP JOINT

The hip joint is never fully unloaded during daily activities and even though it may not be bearing weight (say during swing phase of gait); there is a residual compressive force across the joint from muscle action approximating the body weight (BW). Pauwels described the *"balancing moments"* across the hip joint. Moment is the effective force and is simply a product of force (F) times the distance (D) from which it acts (= F × D). For balancing the weight moment the hip acts like a class 1 lever **(Fig. 4)** where the fulcrum is the hip joint that lies in the center balancing the forces applied on either side of it **(Fig. 5)**. (Remember, hip joint does not always act as a class 1 lever. For supporting the weight of limb in lateral position with joint in abduction the hip acts as a class 2 lever where the abductor force is distal to the fulcrum and load of limb weight applied further distal at the foot). The abductors act to balance the force moments to maintain level pelvis **(Fig. 6)**. The joint reactive force (defined as force generated within a joint in response to forces acting on the joint) is primarily the compressive force at femoroacetabular articulation resulting from pull of abductors balancing the moment arms to maintain a level pelvis **(Figs. 5 and 6)**. Abductor force of contraction must balance the resultant forces on head of femur **(Fig. 6)** to balance the pelvis else it will drop (Trendelenburg sign). The joint reaction force is sum

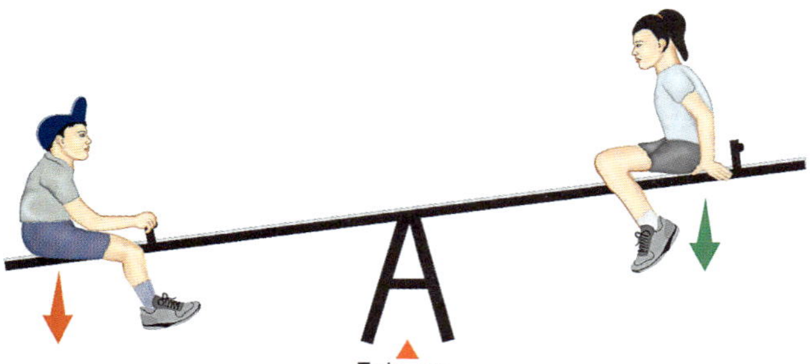

Fig. 4: Class 1 lever has fulcrum in the center and load and force acting on either side of it, i.e., the fulcrum is between load and effort.

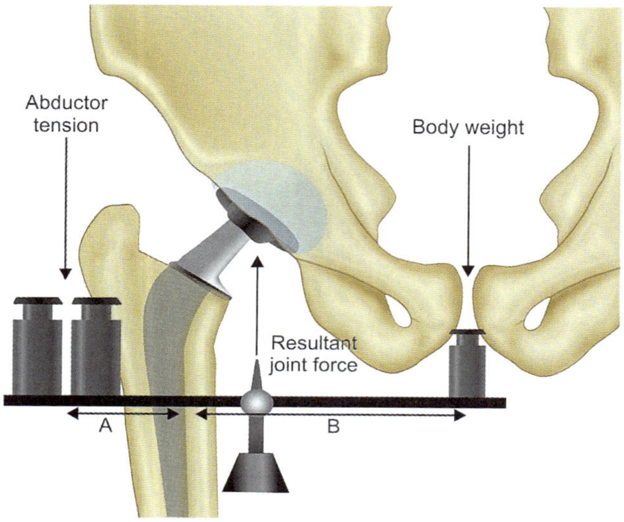

Fig. 5: The action of hip as a type 1 or class 1 lever.

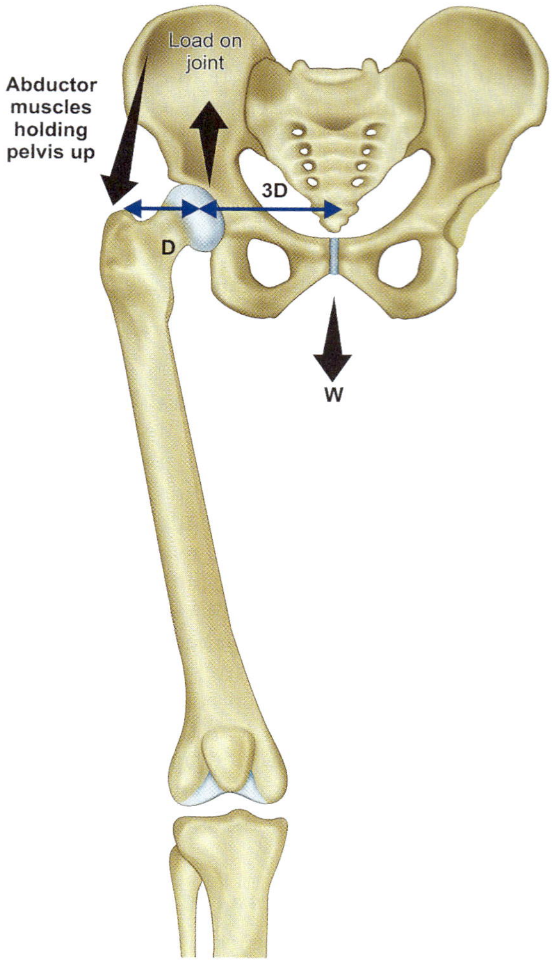

Fig. 6: The forces across hip joint. Abductors have to maintain the pelvis level. The force of body weight acts at larger distance than the abductor balancing force. So at the hip center (instant center) the torque or moment of body weight will be W multiplied by the distance from hip = [3 D × W]. To balance the force abductors act at a fixed distance of "D" from hip center.

of BW and the abductor contraction force **(Fig. 7)**. It is not a moment but a pure force depicted with the units of Newton (N). The equation is not but as simple and the moment will be W' × D. These forces must be equal to level the pelvis so, 3 D × W = W' × D, hence W' = 3 W this entails that abductors will have to produce a three times larger force to balance pelvis on a single-leg stance. This is an approximation the real ratio is around 2.5 muscle force is not just abductors but a combined muscular activity across the joint and the BW is also "effective BW". Also not all forces act parallel or perpendicular.

For analytical purpose, let us say that "effective BW (K)" exerts a turning moment on femoral head through its moment arm "b". The combined muscular activity "M" balances the moment K × b through the moment arm "a" **(Fig. 8)**. This arm acts approximately at 30° (θ) to the center of femoral head.

So, M × a = K × b

The lever arm ratio (a:b) typically decides the magnitude of forces. As b > a so, from above "M" > "K". This analytic estimate typically reveals joint forces range of 2.3–4.6 BW (for a short statured female to heavy muscular male) for one-legged stance.

Complexity of Measurements

Simple explanation given above is just for understanding; however, the determination of forces across hip is much more

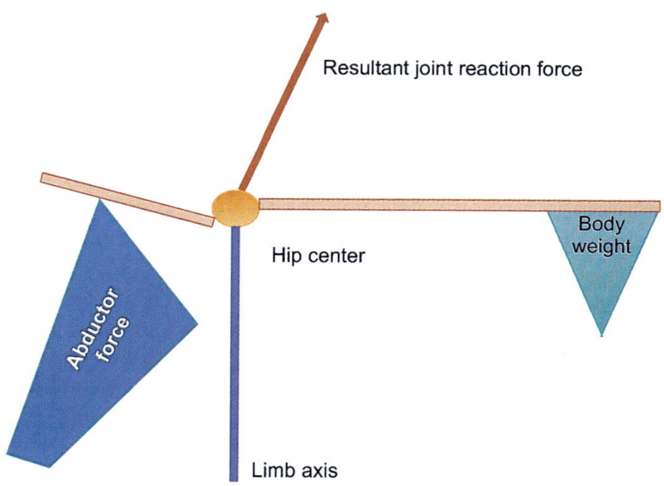

Fig. 7: Determinants of joint reaction force.

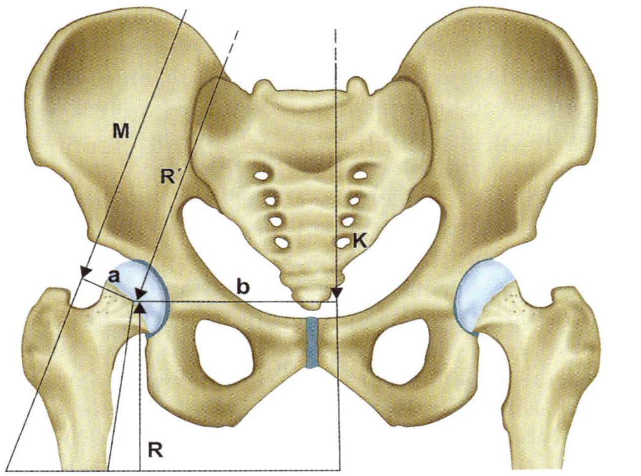

Fig. 8: The resulting balance of moments of effective forces and weight (load) across the hip joint and the calculation of the resultant forces.

complex. The hip joint supports the BW (minus weight of lower limbs during standing, minus weight of one limb during walk) presented to it with vectorial disposition generating resultant forces (vectorial summation of BW, joint reaction forces, and lever vectors). Simply stating the hip joint supports the BW and joint reaction forces that vary with activity (running, walking, getting up from chair, etc.), and as the BW passes through center of gravity (not at hip joint) so there is a variable vectorial component to it (described as moment). This makes the evaluation of forces directly at hip using static measures or simulation difficult. But in keeping with the ethical and practical problems of measuring joint forces in vivo the forces across hip joint can be measured (rather approximated) by theoretically balancing the moments. We know that lower limbs constitute 2/6 (1/6 + 1/6) of BW while the upper limb and trunk constitute 4/6 of the total BW. In a two-leg stance as there is no muscular contraction so no force is needed to maintain equilibrium. The BW is equally distributed across both hips. Each hip carries one-third of BW (6/6 – 1/6 – 1/6 = 4/6 ≡ 2/3 → 1/3 + 1/3).

In the free body diagram analysis for single-leg stance, hip is assumed to be in the resting position at one-legged stance and only abductors acting at 30° are active. It should be noted that it is impossible to determine instant center of rotation of hip joint **(Fig. 9)** as movements occur simultaneously in all three planes. Core assumptions here include position of center of gravity minus one leg [so, effective body weight = 5/6 BW **(Figs. 10 and 11)**; approximately 81% of BW], the muscles active in position of the test (abductors for single-leg stance), and lastly that the forces in a system of mechanical links of various lengths and areas in the test will correspond to the forces developed in the muscles of living body (difficult to approximate).

Now considering a = 5 cm and b = 12.5 cm (a:b will be 1:2.5) and the moments of forces to be balanced, the muscle forces acting at 30° to trochanter are around 2.5 BW. For hip to remain static, the sum of forces should be zero, so:

- R' – (M + K) = 0 (R' is joint reaction force acting at 30°)
- R' = 3.5 K (M = 2.5 × BW = 2.5 K)

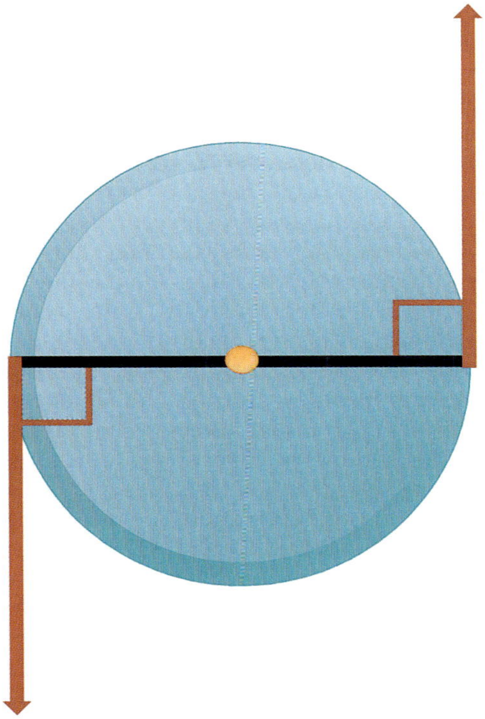

Fig. 9: Instant center of rotation. Point at which a joint rotates, normally lies on a line perpendicular to the tangent of the joint surface at all points of contact.

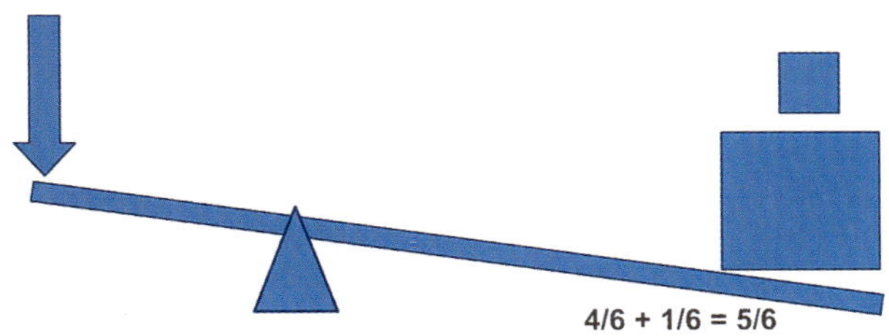

Fig. 10: The mechanics of single-leg stance. The weight supported in single-leg stance = 5/6 (Total body weight – Weight of one lower limb). Hip abductors must, hence, balance the forces equal to the moment produced (see text for details).

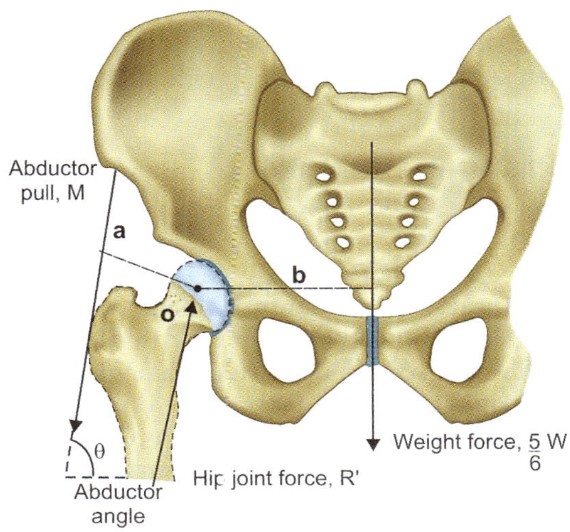

Fig. 11: Mechanics of single-leg stance (see text for details).

- $R = R'/\cos\theta = R'/\cos 30°$ (R is joint reaction force)
- $R = 4\,K \approx 4\,BW$

From above it can be seen that joint reaction force can be reduced by shifting BW over the hip (reducing "a") as in Trendelenburg gait, by tilting toward the affected hip. Holding cane in other hand reduces the "K" partially as the weight is supported also on the cane, here the "R" will be dependent on how much force passes through cane moment (usually 60%). People with shorter necks have higher hip forces, more so people with wider pelvis have higher forces due to far away distance of hip center from line of BW. Conceivably females (wider pelvis–higher "b" and smaller "a" due to shorter neck) are at mechanical disadvantage with respect to hip forces (and hence more hip fractures, arthritis, and athletic activities) though this does not translate always to clinical effects.

Direct measurements of resultant joint forces using endoprosthesis instrumented with transducers by various authors provided variable records. The peak forces varied 2.1–4.3 times BW during gait, 2.3–5.5 BW during stair-climbing to exceeding 8 BW during stumbling. The forces vary much more in sagittal plane than in frontal plane where they are directed medially and inferiorly. Direction and magnitude, in particular, are affected by type of activity (jogging, running, stair-climbing, squatting, etc.), stride length, and cadence. Out of plane loads like anterior and posterior components of joint reaction forces and torsional forces have significant bearing on the longevity and survival of implants. Torsional forces are higher by 23% during stair-climbing compared to normal walking. The magnitudes of forces experienced in hip during walking are biphasic, with a zenith reached at heel strike and terminal stance of the gait cycle. A slower unassisted gait produces higher peak forces compared to brisk walk; similar association has been found between being overweight and higher hip moments for obvious reasons predisposing to injury and joint dysfunction.

For a Moore type endoprosthesis, maximum forces (measured in MPa) transmitted across hip joint during gait were found to occur between heel strike and early midstance. Anterosuperior surface of femoral head bears the maximum pressures (Mean: 5.6 MPa) during gait corresponding to superior acetabular dome. These data are difficult to extrapolate to normal hip as they are from few subjects and often assistive devices were required after surgery for ambulation.

CLINICAL APPLICATIONS

1. *Femoroacetabular impingement* results in abnormal contact of bone of proximal femur and acetabulum due to altered osseous morphology. Repeated impingement of femoral head-neck junction to acetabular margin damages labrum and secondary changes of the acetabular cartilage. The clinical syndrome manifests into anterior hip pain and restriction of joint motion. Various deformations, such as wide femoral neck, reduced head-neck offset, reduced femoral anteversion, malunited femoral neck fracture, acetabular retroversion, coxa profunda, etc., can produce such symptoms, grouped under FAI. Two distinctive types have been recognized first one arising from reduced joint clearance and acetabular overcoverage (pincer type). This occurs due to repeated linear contact between acetabular rim and femoral head-neck junction damaging labrum and is seen more often in middle-aged women. There is further ossification at the rim deepening the acetabulum and impingement occurs at the "extended" rim. The rim "pinches" the femoral head-neck junction. Second type more common in young athletic males arises from femoral head abnormality (cam type) where the head has higher anterolateral diameter and/or decreased offset between femoral head and neck junction. The neck is most narrow midway down and most pathologies widening this region produce cam lesion. This contact generates outside-in abrasion/compression of acetabular labrum damaging the acetabular cartilage and labrum in anterosuperior region. FAI has been now considered to evolve into degenerative disease of the hip joint and is possibly the most common cause of development of idiopathic osteoarthrosis.
2. *Hip arthroplasty and its biomechanics:* Achievement of *proper soft-tissue tension* around reconstructed joint is paramount to success of hip arthroplasty. Longevity can also be achieved by reducing the wear by minimizing the joint reaction forces. Altering the hip geometry can help to achieve these goals. Medial, inferior, and anterior shifting of joint center minimizes joint reaction forces, maximizing the abductor moment and reducing the foot-floor reaction forces. Higher joint forces and wear have been associated with superior and lateral displacement of joint center (reduced medial offset) and neck lengthening. Valgus stem position has provided better clinical results than varus positions possibly due to increased bending moments and implant-bone interface micromotion in the latter.

The length and inclination of the femoral neck also influence the bending moments generated within the proximal femur. For a given neck length, joint contact forces decrease as the neck-shaft angle is reduced (varus disposition of hip). These lower angles also improve joint stability by increasing joint coverage. The mechanical advantage of the abductors may be increased by moving the greater trochanter laterally, and deepening the acetabulum **(Figs. 12A and B)**. This was also the rationale of developing varus osteotomies for proximal femur. But the effect of shortening the abductor length did not produce the desired advantages. The result of varus osteotomies was in fact much poor when they were made to improve hip mechanics (one should not confuse this from the use of varus osteotomy for repositioning the femoral head to bring healthier lateral area into weight-bearing zone for osteonecrosis of femoral head, which is reasonably successful). A varus hip and an increase in neck length will both increase the bending moment within the proximal femur by increasing the moment arm of the joint reaction force. Predisposing to tension type stress fracture and weakened abduction both.

The effect of placing the femoral stem in varus results in increased stress transmitted to the femur due to increased moments being transferred through higher bending moment of a varus neck **(Fig. 13)**. The increased stress

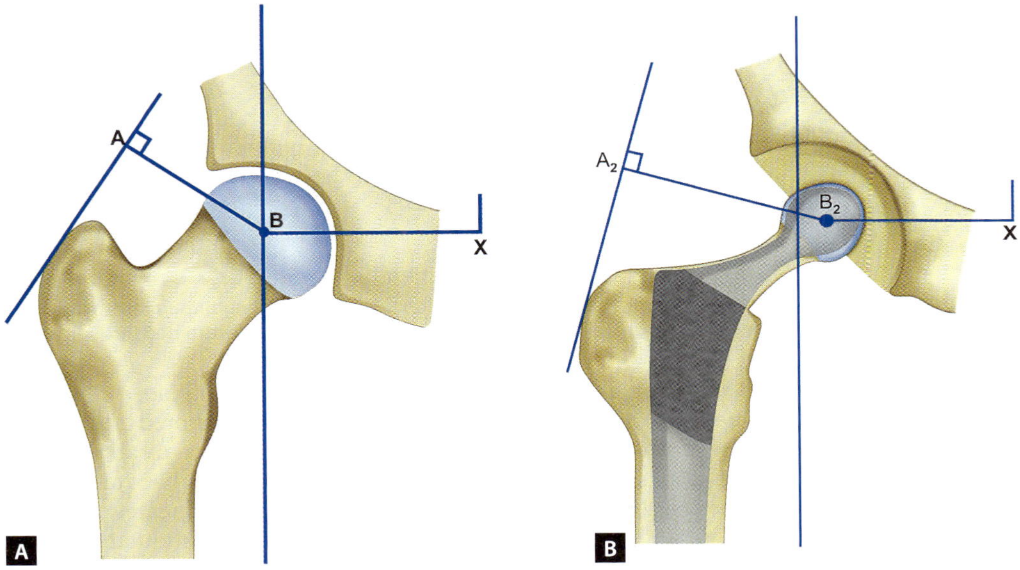

Figs. 12A and B: The joint reaction forces are reduced by deepening the acetabulum (A) and simultaneously optimally (not excessively) advancing the trochanter (B) distally.

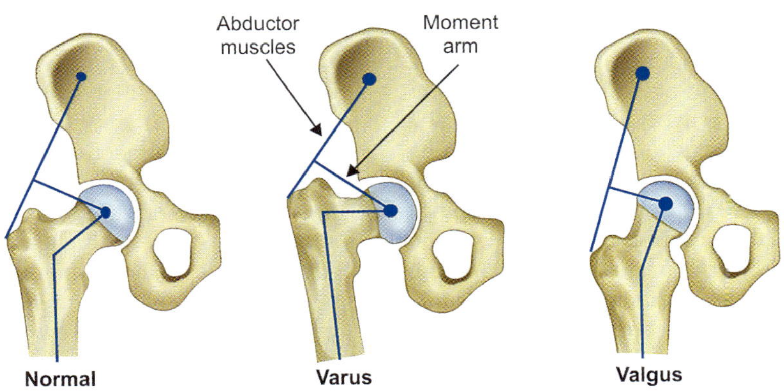

Fig. 13: A valgus neck angle decreases the moment arm, while a varus neck angle or an increased neck length increases the moment arm.

predisposes to failure of stem and/or loosening at various interfaces. Conversely, a shorter or more vertically inclined (valgus) femoral neck reduces the bending moment in the stem. However, the reduction in head offset requires larger abductor forces to balance the weight of the body, leading to an increase in the joint reaction force (increased product M*a) **(*see* Fig. 8)**. This produces a significant increase in the wear rate of the artificial joint and a greater incidence of implant failure secondary to wear and osteolysis. Thus, optimal horizontal and vertical offset of femoral stem is necessary for successful arthroplasty. The joint reaction forces are minimized when the joint center is moved medially, inferiorly, and anteriorly. This maximizes the working length of the abductors and brings the joint center closer to the line of action of the foot thus improving the moment generating capacity and reducing the floor reaction force, thereby reducing the external moment that must be balanced by the muscle forces acting at the hip. Increasing the neck length and advancing the trochanter partially compensates for these losses. So, in nutshell reduced offset—increases wear and reduces efficiency of muscles, unoptimally increased offset (especially horizontal)—femoral stem loosening. As the horizontal offset should not be increased (higher product M*a increased joint reaction forces) the alternative is medializing the cup that effectively increases "a" so improving the abductor moment **(Fig. 14)**. I personally recommend placing the hip as near to the anatomy as possible.

3. *Role of cane in painful hip:* For a painful hip, patients reduce the time of weight-bearing on the affected joint and tilting the trunk ipsilaterally (antalgic gait). This is but natural as this maneuver brings center of gravity closer to the joint and reduces bending moments and forces transmitted across painful hip. However, this is much less efficient means of ambulation and is energy consuming. Better and effective way is to use a "cane" in the other hand (*see* also Chapter on "Osteoarthritis of Hip Joint"). The cane-floor reaction forces on other side significantly nullifies (rather counters) the foot-floor joint reaction

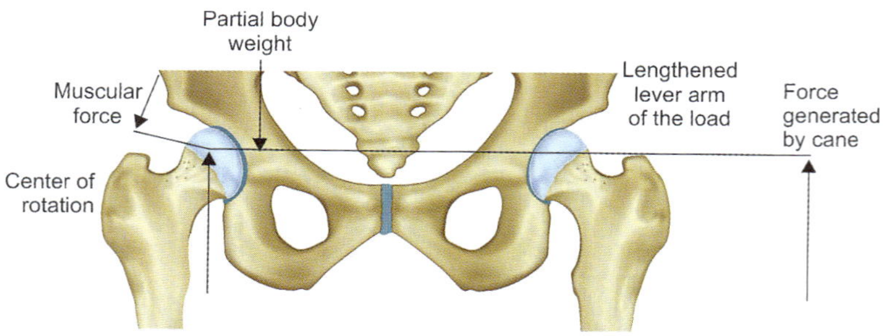

Fig. 14: The efficacy of force transmitted through cane. The cane has longer lever arm acting through the handle of cane this produces higher moment (product of distance to force) despite smaller force transmitted through it.

forces so that the work required for abductors reduces and hence the joint reaction forces. It creates an additional force that keeps the pelvis level in the face of gravity's tendency to adduct the hip during unilateral stance and decreases the moment arm between the center of gravity and the femoral head. Cane transmits part of the BW to the ground thereby decreasing the muscular force required for balancing by reducing the effective BW (effective K). One can also understand it this way normally in a single-leg stance, the unaffected leg is dangling conferring a weight = 3.5 K on the affected hip that has to be balanced (see above). Now with the use of cane, the cane acts as a "bipedal gait" transmitting part of BW through the upper extremity so reducing the effective K. We know that if cane transmitted full BW as in a bipedal gait, there would be no muscular contraction needed, but the fact that upper limb cannot transmit all of BW the effect is partial retrieval of BW. It is estimated that bearing just 15% BW to the cane reduces the joint reaction forces by half (50%). The higher efficacy of smaller cane force can be explained by the lengthened lever arm of the cane. Longer lever arm produces a higher moment even for less force transmitted through cane to counter the BW passing near center of gravity **(Fig. 14)**.

4. Osteotomies around hip should be properly planned balancing the abductor moments and centring the hip for correcting excessive varus and valgus.
5. Fixation of proximal hip fractures is of special concern for proper function. Extramedullary devices will have to bear higher moments compared to intramedullary devices while the proximal fixation screws are same for both. This translates that for preventing implant failure of extramedullary devices weightbearing has to be delayed to avoid them reaching break point. For intramedullary fixation as the device is placed closer to hip center and the fixation screw is anchored close enough, there will be some respite with respect to earlier mobilization.
6. *Coxa vara and coxa valga:* In coxa valga **(Fig. 13)**, the neck shaft angle is increased, greater trochanter is lower than normal. This increases abductor length and efficiency but reduces the lever arm "a" **(*see* Fig. 8)**. Thus, the joint reaction forces are increased in single-leg stance as more work has to be done by the abductor muscles (to keep the product of load to distance balanced). Muscles have to but apply less force due to better resting length. In coxa vara, trochanter is higher than normal reducing the resting length but increasing the lever arm due to higher horizontal offset. So, effectively "a" is increased, this reduces the joint reaction forces during single-leg stance as the product of muscle force to "a" will be higher. But, the muscles have to apply more force and will get fatigued easily due to poor resting length.
7. Hip arthrodesis should be done in 25–30° of flexion and 0° of abduction (and rotation) as excessive abduction will produce lurch and excessive truncal shift. Patient will have to bend on the affected extremity to lift the normal leg, this will produce degenerative changes in spine and low back pain.

CONCLUSION

The hip joint complex comprises complex interplay of osseous, ligamentous, and muscular structures providing weight-bearing stability and tremendous global movement capability. The evaluation of symptoms can be challenging provided multiplicity of causes that can produce similar symptoms. Detailed understanding of the complex anatomy and biomechanics of normal and pathologic hip can help in better understanding, diagnosis, and treatment of the complex pathologies of the joint.

CHAPTER 71

Osteoarthritis of Hip Joint

Manish Kumar Varshney

INTRODUCTION

"Osteoarthritis" (OA) is the most common cause of joint pain and stiffness in patients with heterogeneous conditions resulting in common clinical features and radiological changes [details in Chapter on "Joint Disorders Including Inflammatory and Noninflammatory Arthritis and Infective Arthritides (Including Mycobacterial Infection and Prosthetic Joint Infection)" in Section on Joint: Structure, Function, and Related Disorders]. In elderly, OA of hip joint is the most common cause of hip pain. In adults, hip OA has prevalence rate of 0.4–27%. In about 5% of the general population over the age of 65 years, radiographic evidence of hip OA is present, including osteophytes or spurs, subchondral bone sclerosis and cyst formation **(Figs. 1A and B)**. In Indian and Asian population, the OA hip is mostly secondary to some preceding cause unlike the western population where the incidence of primary idiopathic form is significantly common. From the current maintained registry, the incidence of primary OA hip in India appears to be 11% but is likely to get further updated. Though historically considered a disease of cartilage, OA hip involves the whole joint, affecting structure and function of the entire joint. Range of motion (ROM) of the hip joint becomes limited because of joint capsular changes and subsequent articular cartilage damage occurs. As the disease progresses, periarticular tissues undergo atrophy due to muscle weakness (mainly abductors of the hip joint). However, these symptoms are not seen in all the patients having radiographic changes of OA. There is wide spectrum of symptoms as well as radiographic changes and the inconsistent relationship between them results in discrepant findings in the prevalence studies.

RISK FACTORS

- *Age:* As the condition mainly affects middle-aged and elderly people; age is considered as the most common predisposing factor. Most of the patients are above the

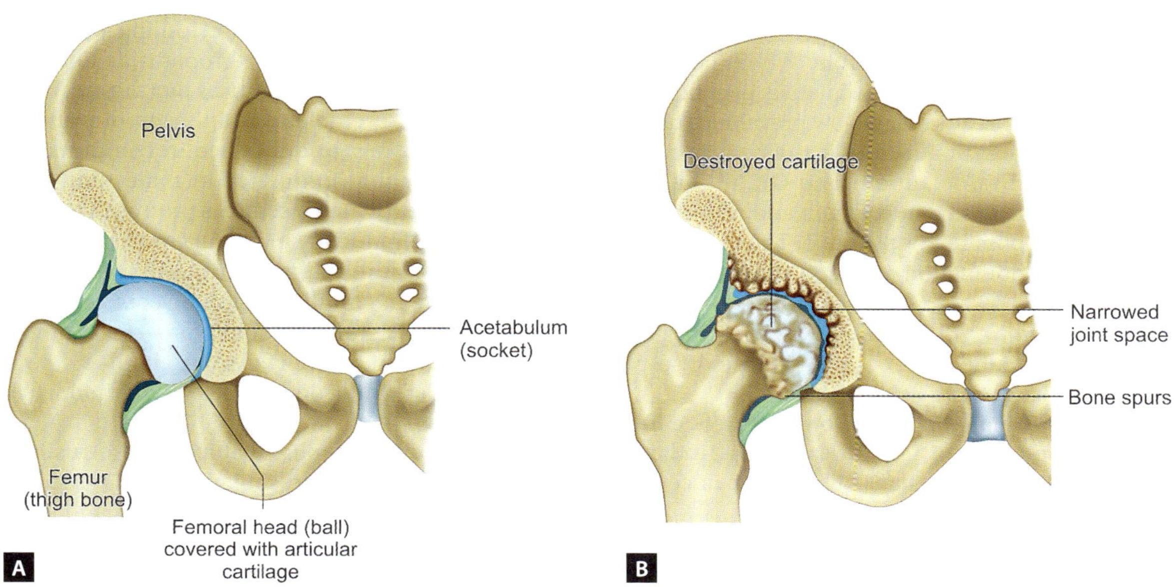

Figs. 1A and B: Osteoarthritis of hip. (A) Normal hip illustration; (B) Osteoarthritic hip—the hip joint space is reduced with destruction and wear of cartilage, formation of osteophytes and bony spurs.

TABLE 1: The differences between arthritic hip and aging of joint.

Characteristic	*Osteoarthritic joint*	*Aging joint*
Water content in synovial fluid and cartilage	Increased	Decreased
Collagen structure	Disorganized	Remains same
Proteoglycan synthesis	Increased (but is also degraded fast so actual content remains same)	Same or some reduction (degradation is also reduced so proteoglycan content remains constant)
Chondrocyte size	No alteration	Increased chondrocytes and rounding
Chondrocyte numbers in cartilage	Same	Reduced over time
Modulus of elasticity of cartilage	Decreased	Increased

age of 60 years. But aging and OA are not synchronous terms and cannot be used interchangeably, these are two distinct processes; the former being physiological while the latter is pathological. The changes in joint are also different in aging and arthritis **(Table 1)**.

- *Developmental disorders:* These are all incorporated in the secondary causes of OA hip. All these are responsible for premature OA of the hip as it occurs in patients in middle age itself due often to poor mechanics. The list includes:
  - Developmental dysplasia of hip (DDH)
  - Legg-Calve-Perthes disease
  - Slipped capital femoral epiphysis (SCFE)
  - Osteoarthritis is commonly seen in patients with femur and acetabular dysplasia. Dysplasia is defined as abnormal growth of the hip in which acetabulum and proximal femur are not in orientation with each other, resulting in change of femoral-acetabular articulation. Types of dysplasia include:
    - Femoral anteversion
    - Femoral retroversion
    - Acetabular anteversion
    - Acetabular retroversion
    - Coxa vara
    - Coxa valga
    - Coxa profunda
- *Genetics:* Siblings show a high association of hip OA, suggesting a possible genetic role. While the nature of the genetic influence is still speculative, genetics is often linked to hip OA because of the low prevalence of hip OA in Asian and African populations in their native countries and the familial association of hip OA in Caucasians. Genetic polymorphisms in collagen and minor proteins of cartilage are possibly responsible. The environmental influence and modulation of genetic factors all need to be determined.
- *Femoroacetabular impingement (FAI):* This is now considered to be the most common cause of so-called "idiopathic" osteoarthrosis of hip **(Fig. 2)**.
- *Race*: Primary hip OA has very low prevalence in non-Caucasian population of Asia, Africa and East India, while high prevalence in Caucasians of European ancestry.
- *Endemic forms of OA of hip:* Occasionally, OA is found in entire community, acting like an endemic disease. The cause is unknown, though dysplasias in genetically isolated community or some environmental factors are thought to be responsible for that.

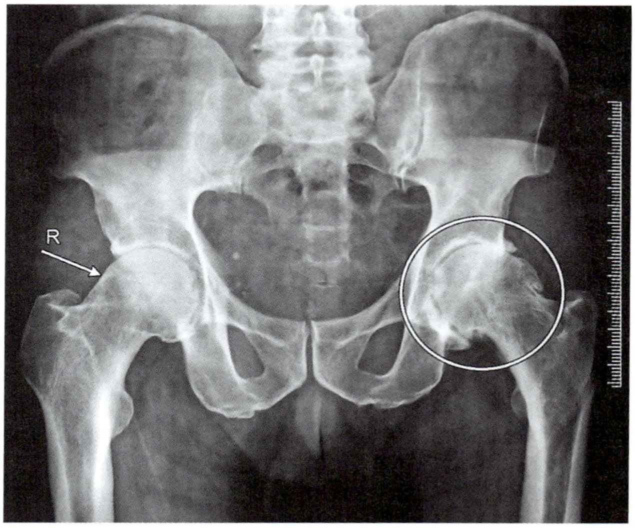

Fig. 2: Development of osteoarthrosis in femoroacetabular impingement (FAI). The radiograph demonstrates development of osteoarthrosis of left hip joint (encircled) while right hip demonstrates "cam" lesion of the femoral head-neck junction (arrow), there is also narrowing of right hip joint space.

- *Some of the endemic forms of hip OA found so far are:*
  - *Mseleni joint disease:* Mseleni is a district in Northern Zululand in South Africa, in which around 2,000 people suffer from a crippling joint disease with degenerative osteoarthropathy, mainly involving hip joint. It mainly comprises two distinct disorders: One which resembles multiple epiphyseal dysplasia has no sex or age difference in community, occurring with equal frequency in males and females. And another which resembles protrusion acetabuli occurs more frequently in young females and the frequency increases with age. In the first group, the disease starts in childhood with discomfort in major joints of lower limb, gradually progressing over time and results in severe OA with painful and swollen joints and crippling deformities in adulthood. In the second group, pain in the hip joint starts in teenage girls, with radiographic features of protrusion acetabuli, gradually progressing, resulting in secondary OA in adult life. Various environmental and genetic causes are proposed, but by far, no causal relationship is found for this disease.
  - *Handigodu joint disease:* First found in 1975 by a social worker named Chandrashekhar in a patient from

Handigodu village, it is a crippling disorder endemic in Shimoga and Chikmagalur districts of Karnataka, Southern India. The disease starts in childhood or early adulthood with painful swollen hip and knee joints, and stunting of growth. In extreme cases, crippled patients become prone to crawl because of pain. It is defined genetically as autosomal dominant inheritance, with a form of spondylo epi (meta) physeal dysplasia. No specific cure is available at present for this disease.

- *Gender:* Males have a slightly greater prevalence of hip OA compared to females (3.2% compared to 3.0%). Though the difference is minimal, men and women appear to have different patterns of hip OA. Women have a more superomedial femoral migration while men have a more superolateral migration. There is strong evidence that superolateral migration is an important prognostic factor in the progression of hip OA.
- *Occupation:* There is higher prevalence of hip OA in male workers involved in lifting very heavy loads over a prolonged period. Suspected risk factors include regular heavy lifting, framing—tractor driving (vibration), and walking on uneven ground. Even then the incidence of hip OA in Indians is small. The possibility could be frequent habit of squatting that maintains the movement of joint to extremes (higher force transmission to knee, however, produces OA knee commonly in these patients). The role of this environmental factor needs to be further evaluated.
- *Sports:* While running is found to decrease the risk of OA development and subsequent hip replacement, other strenuous sports activities increase the risk for OA. Sports like American football and hockey, which include direct-impact activities, increase the risk of hip OA.
- *Previous injury:* History of previous injury causing proximal hip fractures **(Fig. 3)** is found to have high association with development of hip OA, secondary to changes in articular surfaces creating abnormal joint load bearing. Acetabular fractures cause joint surface irregularities causing increased wear and osteoarthrosis as for any intra-articular fracture.

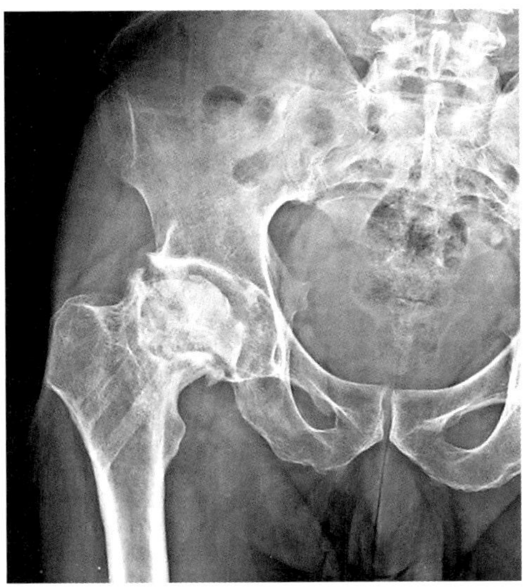

Fig. 3: Radiographic features of osteoarthrosis of hip joint (osteophyte formation, reduction of joint space, sclerosis of acetabular roof). This is a case of osteoarthritis of the hip joint secondary to osteonecrosis of femoral head following fracture intracapsular neck of femur.

- *Body mass index (BMI):* There is a controversy regarding role of BMI in development of hip OA. Some studies have shown positive relationship between them, while other studies have not. Logically, obesity seems to be associated with OA progression, rather than its onset, and weight loss is important controlling measure.
- *Leg length inequality:* Leg length disparity may be associated with increased risk for OA according to some studies, but more research is needed to confirm this probability.
- Rapidly destructive OA hip or rapidly progressive OA hip is a rare disease of unknown etiology that is marked by rapid chondrolysis often progressing to complete destruction of femoral head. It is mostly seen in middle aged to elderly females beginning as a hip pain present for 6 months to 3 years. This is associated with narrowing of joint space that suddenly undergoes chondrolysis (>2 mm/year or >50% joint space narrowing/year) to complete destruction of femoral head within a short period of time.

Pathophysiology and Natural History

Destruction of cartilage lies at the core of development of OA hip. This is primarily mediated by the action of various cytokines although accrual of microtrauma may also be a factor. So OA hip is a combination of biomechanical and biochemical process where the latter is mediated by cytokines and growth factors like interleukin-1 and tumor necrosis factor-α (catabolic) and insulin-like growth factor (anabolic). When the catabolism takes an upper hand OA develops. Collagenases are primarily responsible for breakdown of cartilage matrix that include collagenase-1 [matrix metalloproteinase (MMP)-1, a fibroblast collagenase], collagenase-2 (MMP-8, a neutrophil collagenase), and collagenase 3 (MMP-13). OA of hip is a progressive disorder with different rate of progression in different patients. The radiographic and clinical changes of the progressive arthritic hip are as follows:

- Asymmetric narrowing of the joint space between the femur and the acetabulum, e.g., narrowing occurs more commonly superolaterally than over medial side (superolateral portion is the weight-bearing portion of the joint).
- Shortening of the fibrous joint capsule
- Irregularity of femoral head, it becomes flat.
- Development of bridging osteophytes extending from ilium to sacrum, and around the margins of femoral head and acetabulum (it may be absent in some individuals)
- Migration of femoral head superolaterally or medially
- Cystic changes in femoral head and acetabulum (subchondral cyst, also known as "geode") along with sclerotic changes in subchondral region

TABLE 2: The classification of osteoarthritis (OA) hip joint.

Primary osteoarthritis of hip joint	*Secondary OA hip*
Due to genetic and racial predisposition the hip joint catches the disease state and cartilage and bone degeneration. Endemic forms of the disease are also included in this (see risk factors)	*Abnormal stress on hip joint:* • Joint subluxation (reduced center-edge angle)/dislocation • Anatomical abnormalities of bones – Coxa magna – Coxa vara – Coxa profunda (increased center-edge angle) • Protrusio hip with acetabular abnormality
	Defective cartilage: • Infection/septic hip/postseptic sequel • Rheumatoid arthritis • Urate/crystal arthropathy • Chondrocalcinosis • Hemophilia • Hemochromatosis
	Abnormality of bone: • Femoroacetabular impingement • Fracture (acetabular or femoral head fracture/impaction) • Osteonecrosis and collapse • Paget's disease of bone • Fluorosis • Dysplasia (developmental or multiple epiphyseal) • Slipped capital femoral epiphysis • Perthes disease

- Range of motion of hip joint decreases, mainly internal rotation followed by flexion become limited.

Progressive difficulty in ambulation due to muscle weakness, mainly in abductor musculature

CLASSIFICATION OF HIP OSTEOARTHRITIS

The two main categories in which hip OA can be classified are: (1) Primary (idiopathic), a more common type in western countries but much less common in Asian population, in which no identifiable cause can be defined, or (2) secondary (systemic or localized) in which degeneration occurs due to some pre-existing conditions **(Table 2)**.

CLINICAL FEATURES AND EVALUATION

Pain, stiffness, and altered function are the main symptoms of hip OA. Pain is activity related, increased with weight-bearing and ambulation, and decreased with rest, though not resolved completely. As the disease progresses, the duration of pain and morning stiffness increases (though not exceeding 1 hour) and night pain becomes evident. It should be noted that night pain may reflect inflammatory arthritis.

The main idea of clinical examination is not to diagnose OA which is quite obvious on primary look, but to assess the disability and document the level of functional performance that can be repeatedly evaluated over time and follow-up:

- *6-minute walk test:* Measures the distance a person can walk in 6 minutes.
- *Self-paced walk test:* Measures the speed of a person who walks for 4 meter and for 40 meters.
- *Stair measure:* Measures the efficiency of a person while ascending and descending the stairs.
- *Timed up-and-go tests:* Measures the efficiency of a person who gets up from a chair, walks for 3 meters, turns around, returns, and sits down again.
- *Movements at hip joint:* The first two motions that are diminished are usually hip internal rotation and hip flexion.
- Strength testing of muscles especially abductors
- Pain assessment visual analog scale (VAS score) including the flexion, abduction, and external rotation (FABER) and Scour test for determining the irritability of hip joint, etc.
- Antalgic gait
- Locking or sticking of the joint and a grinding noise during movement caused by loose fragments of cartilage and inflammation
- Deformities are examined as usual for hip examination (flexion deformity by Thomas test, adduction and abduction deformities by squaring pelvis, rotational deformity by foot progression angle and thigh foot angle, etc.)
- Examine for contracture of iliotibial band (ITB), rectus, and Hamstring contractures.

As clinical features precede the development of radiological changes, early diagnosis can be made by appropriate clinical findings as described by Bierma-Zeinstra et al. (joint space narrowing to <2.5 mm):

- Tenderness over inguinal ligament
- Age >60 years
- Decreased external rotation <21°
- Decreased internal rotation <21°
- Decreased adduction <10°
- Bony restriction in one direction during passive hip movement
- Muscle weakness—hip abductors

(Sensitivity 98% and specificity of 72% if five of above present, however, if more than five are present the specificity reduced to <50% despite 100% sensitivity).

Radiology

In patients with hip OA, joint space narrowing is found to be best and most important indicator of the severity of the disease (Normal hip joint space: 3–5 mm, moderate loss: <2.5 mm, severe loss: <1.5 mm). Other radiological findings include osteophytes spurs, subchondral sclerosis, and cysts. The hip joint OA can be graded radiographically using various criteria and newer MRI grading are also proposed **(Table 3)**. Detailed MRI-based scoring systems such as HOAMS and HIMRISS are also available but not very useful in clinical practice as they do not have direct bearing on treatment currently.

Diagnosis of Osteoarthritis Hip

The diagnosis of OA hip based only on clinical criteria is sensitive but not very specific. Additional objective criteria

TABLE 3: The radiological grading of osteoarthritis (OA) hip joint.

Kellgren–Lawrence radiographic grading	***Tonnis radiographic grading***
• *Grade 1:* No radiographic evidence of OA • *Grade 2:* Doubtful narrowing of joint space and possible (minute) osteophytes • *Grade 3:* Moderate multiple osteophytes, definite narrowing of joint space, some sclerosis and possible deformity of bone contour • *Grade 4:* Large osteophytes, severe joint space narrowing, subchondral sclerosis, and definite deformity of bone contour. A potential caveat when using the Kellgren/Lawrence scale is spurred or osteophytes are emphasized and not all patients with hip OA have osteophytes	• *Grade 1:* Minor joint space narrowing, subchondral sclerosis of the femoral head and/or acetabulum, small osteophytes • *Grade 2:* Moderate joint space narrowing, small subchondral cysts of the femoral head and/or acetabulum, moderate loss of sphericity of the femoral head • *Grade 3:* Severe joint space narrowing or obliteration, large subchondral cysts, and severe deformity of the femoral head. The original classification had three grades only. Grade "0" was latter added to denote no signs of osteoarthritis
Scoring hip osteoarthritis with MRI (SHOMRI grading system) *Grading of acetabular cartilage:* 1. SHOMRI 0—No damage to the cartilage surface 2. SHOMRI 1—Partial thickness defect of articular surface 3. SHOMRI 3—Full-thickness defect of articular surface *Grading of femoral head cartilage:* 1. SHOMRI 0—No damage to cartilage surface 2. SHOMRI 1—Partial-thickness defect of articular surface 3. SHOMRI 2—Full-thickness defect of articular cartilage	

BOX 1: The American College of Rheumatology (ACR) criteria for diagnosis of hip osteoarthritis (OA) (1991) using combined clinical and radiographic methods.

- Hip pain
  "and"
- At least two of the following three features:
  1. Erythrocyte sedimentation rate < 20 mm/1st hour
  2. Radiographic femoral and acetabular osteophytes
  3. Radiographic joint space narrowing (superior, axial, and/or medial)

need to be added to make the scoring-based diagnosis more specific and reproducible. There are various diagnostic scores available like the American College of Rheumatology (ACR) criteria for hip OA **(Box 1)**, and Lequesne criteria for OA hip joint. For the Lequesne criteria, the inclusion criteria includes:

- Reduced ROM in three of the seven spheres (flexion/extension/adduction/abduction/internal/external rotation and flexion with adduction)
- Radiographic joint space narrowing [anteroposterior (AP) or oblique standing radiographs]
- Osteophytes, subchondral sclerosis, and subchondral cyst formation.

Exclusion criteria: Secondary forms of OA including rheumatoid arthritis.

Differential Diagnosis

In patients presenting with hip pain and clinical findings suggestive of hip OA, other conditions to be considered are as follows:

- Bursitis or tendinitis
- Athletic pubalgia
- Chondral damage or loose bodies
- Femoral neck or pubic ramus stress fracture/pseudo fracture, osteomalacia
- Iliotibial band syndrome
- Labral tear
- Lumbar radiculopathy—(mainly L2-3 radiculopathy)
- Meralgia paresthetica
- Metastasis/neoplasm
- Muscle strain
- Hamstring syndrome
- Osteonecrosis of the femoral head
- Paget's disease
- Snapping hip syndrome
- Piriformis syndrome
- Inflammatory or infective arthritis
  - Psoriatic arthritis
  - Gout/pseudogout
  - Septic hip arthritis
  - Rheumatoid arthritis
- Sacroiliac joint dysfunction

Prognosis

Except in some rare cases of rapidly destructive OA of hip joint, OA of hip has slow progression in most of the cases, with total hip arthroplasty (THA) as the end result. As the patient diagnosed with radiographic OA may not have symptomatic OA, distinguishing between these two is important. Oxford hip score (OHS) appears to be the best guide for identifying patients that need active treatment. Score <20 needs aggressive/operative treatment, e.g., hip arthroplasty while patients with score >40 can be managed conservatively. Patients between 20 and 40 of OHS need individualized management and close observation for progression of OA. Among different radiographic parameters predictive of the disease such as osteophytosis, subchondral cysts and sclerosis, femoral head migration and severity (joint space narrowing in mm, Kellgren-Lawrence score), the prognostic predictors found to be most important are narrowing of the joint space and Kellgren-Lawrence score.

- In structural progression of OA of hip, narrowing of the joint space is found to be best prognostic indicator. Those having slowly progressive OA hip have rate of joint space narrowing of <0.2 mm/year, while rate of >0.2 mm/year is associated with rapid progression of OA hip.

- Kellgren-Lawrence score is another important predictor, with higher chances of progression of hip OA in grade II or higher, with strong chances of THA as the ultimate treatment option in grade III and IV.

According to Altman et al., to detect OA progression, more important than Kellgren/Lawrence score are the measurement of individual radiographic features **(Box 1)**. A change in joint space narrowing on AP radiograph along with cyst formation has high sensitivity for detecting progression of OA hip.

Management

Osteoarthritis of the hip is treated conservatively initially with total hip arthtoplasty/replacement (THA/THR) as the end result of failure of conservative measures. Criteria for optimum time regarding surgery are not specified yet. A rough guideline followed throughout the world is failure of conservative management, the criteria for defining the same are also not clear. Conservative intervention can be considered to have failed if a patient:

- Complains of pain despite continuation of conservative treatment with <20–25% reduction of pain on Western Ontario and McMaster Universities (WOMAC) index.
- Has rate of >0.2 mm/year for progressive joint space narrowing.

Interventions in conservative management [**(Table 4)** *see* also the Section on "Joint: Structure, Function, and Related Disorders", Chapter on "Joint Disorders Including Inflammatory and Noninflammatory Arthritis and Infective Arthritides (Including Mycobacterial Infection and Prosthetic Joint Infection)"]:

- *Anti-inflammatory agents:* Nonsteroidal anti-inflammatory drugs (NSAIDs), COX-2 inhibitors, steroid injections.
- *Complementary medication:* Diacerein, univestin, etc. are used variably [*see* details in Chapter on "Joint Disorders Including Inflammatory and Noninflammatory Arthritis and Infective Arthritides (Including Mycobacterial Infection and Prosthetic Joint Infection", Section on "Joint Structure, Function, and Related Disorders)"]
- *Patient education—"hip school":* This concept highlights the need for educating patients with hip OA, especially understanding the importance of preserving hip ROM and muscle function, understanding what therapy is effective. Other methods that should be incorporated include activity modification, exercise, weight reduction, and methods of unloading the arthritic joints.
- *Gait and balance training:* Due to pain in the joints, the patients of hip OA may develop abnormal gait patterns to unload the affected joint. To reduce the pain and improve activity level, assistive devices are helpful in these patients. An appropriately selected cane in the contralateral hand and carrying load in ipsilateral hand can reduce hip loading and abductor muscle activity by 20–30% (**Fig. 4**, *see* also the Chapter on "Biomechanics of Hip Joint"). When cane is used in contralateral hand, pain reduces in the affected hip, abduction moment of the affected hip decreases and of opposite hip increases by one-fourth, there by load on the operative hip decreases and so, soft tissues and bone can heal.
  - *Insoles:* They may reduce the forces across the joint, thereby may reduce pain in the affected joint and progression of the disease, but have not been found to be useful when studied on a large scale **(Table 4)**.
  - *Functional, gait, and balance training:* As these patients may develop balance, strength, and proprioception impairment, they have higher risk of fall, especially elderly individuals. Functional exercises which simulate activities of daily living (such as gait, rising from a chair, reaching, stepping, and squatting down) with different levels of speed and difficulties are highly recommended in these patients. They have shown to improve performance in elderly.
- *Manual therapy:* It may help in increasing hip joint ROM and reduce pain. It is applied by physical therapist (or medical doctors) with special training in manual therapy. Manual therapy mainly improves the elasticity of the joint capsule and the surrounding muscles. It includes:
  - Manipulation and stretching exercises
  - *Traction:* To expand the hip joint space
  - Traction manipulation (high-velocity thrust technique)
  - Traction is based on the premises that when attempting to mobilize the hip joint, the amount of movement produced at the hip is facilitated by distraction of joint surfaces overcoming impingement from various irregularities in joint surface.

TABLE 4: What works and what does not in conservative management of hip osteoarthritis (OA) [based on the American College of Rheumatology (ACR) 2019 recommendations].

Recommended modalities for symptomatic relief in OA hip	*There is no supportive evidence (~) for these modalities, or the evidence is against (#) their use for managing OA hip*
• Guided exercise program • Self-efficacy and self-management programs • Weight loss • Tai chi (Yoga has not been found beneficial!) • Use of cane • Heat or therapeutic cooling* • Cognitive behavioral therapy* • Acupuncture* • Balance training* • Oral NSAIDs • Intra-articular steroids • Acetaminophen and tramadol* • Duloxetine*	• Transcutaneous electrical nerve stimulation (TENS)# • Manual therapy~ • Massage therapy~ • Modified shoes~ • Wedged insoles~ • Bisphosphonates# • Glucosamine# • Hydroxychloroquine# • Methotrexate# • TNF inhibitors# • IL-1 receptor antagonists# • Platelet rich plasma# • Stem cell injection# • Chondroitin# • Intra-articular hyaluronic acid# • Intra-articular botulinum toxin~ • Prolotherapy~ • Colchicine~ • Nontramadol opioids~ • Fish oil~ • Vitamin D~
**Conditionally recommended*	*#Evidence is against their use#* *~No supportive evidence~*

(IL-1: interleukin-1; NSAIDs: nonsteroidal anti-inflammatory drugs; TNF: tumor necrosis factor)

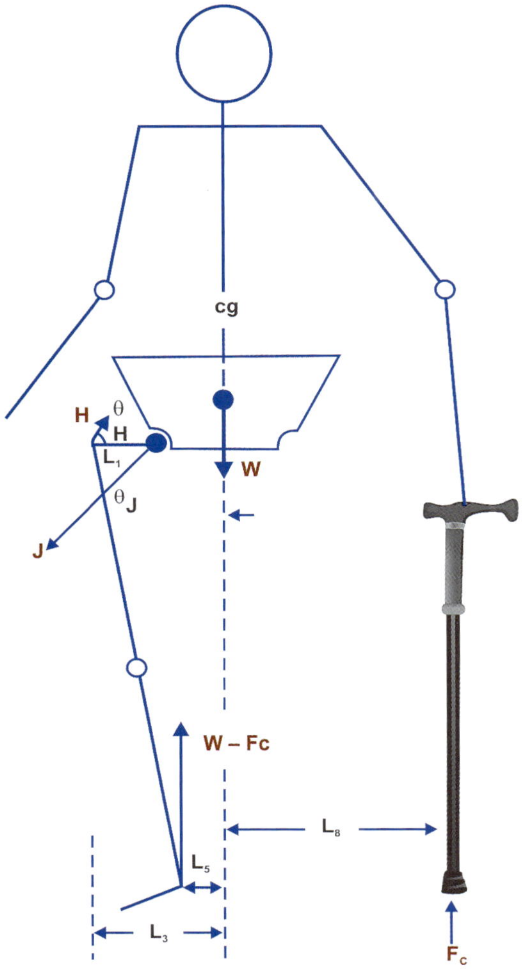

Fig. 4: Effect of cane on hip biomechanics: An assistive device like a cane creates an additional force that keeps the pelvis level in the face of gravity's tendency to adduct the hip during unilateral stance (W). The cane's force must substitute for the hip abductors (vector H). A force that levels the pelvis efficiently by virtue of its relatively long lever arm is directed upward from a point of application on the pelvis (vector C). The force originates on the side opposite the involved hip. The aim of cane is to reduce the Vector H by substituting vector C. Hence, to produce a force like vector C with a cane, one must push the cane firmly into the ground in a vertical direction. Doing so generates an upward reaction force (vector Fc) whose magnitude equals the downward force one exerts on the cane. The vector Fc is transferred to vector C by the muscles of the wrist, elbow, shoulder girdle, and trunk that connects vectors Fc and C. Thus, the work of abductors of involved hip will be reduced as C is now partly compensated by Fc, (hence, H = C – Fc) this reduces the joint reaction force J. Also the moment Fc*L8 is large so even small forces reduce the adduction moment of the involved hip and the patient need not adduct the involved hip allowing muscles and soft tissues to heal well. The adduction moment force is also reduced to W – Fc.

- *Strengthening and endurance exercises:* These exercises are aimed to improve and maintain motion and flexibility without increasing the pain. These exercises can be categorized into three types:
  1. *Range of motion/flexibility exercises:* To improve overall movement of the arthritic hip joint.

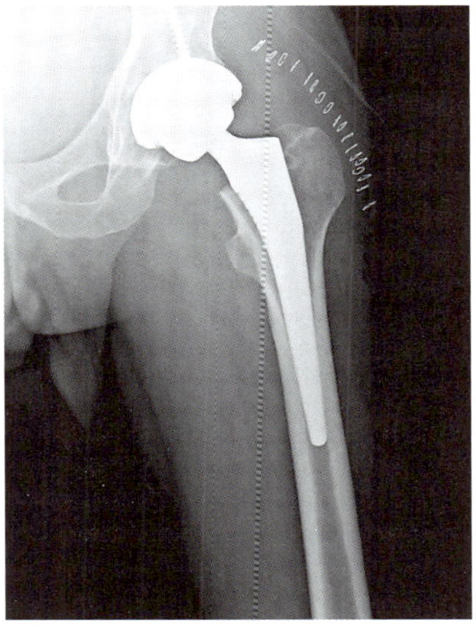

Fig. 5: Total hip arthroplasty.

  2. *Muscle-strengthening exercises:* To strengthen the muscles while limiting tissue injury.
  3. *Aerobic conditioning/endurance exercises:* By providing workload to cardiovascular and pulmonary system.

  Other measures such as hydrotherapy can be useful when deployed in specific patient groups.
- *Surgical treatment:* Artificial replacement of joint is the preferred method, however, osteotomy may be done in an occasional patient unwilling or inappropriate for THA **(Fig. 5)**. OHS is a useful guide to identify patients needing surgical treatment. Various functional outcome measures have been validated by researchers that can be used by clinicians for evaluation of treatment modalities. Some of these scores for patient evaluation include the lower extremity functional scale, the WOMAC osteoarthritis index, and the Harris hip score. These scores can be used before and after treatment/interventions that are intended to alleviate the impairments of body function (and form), limitations in activity, and functional restrictions associated with hip OA.

CONCLUSION

- Osteoarthritis of hip is a disabling disease causing significant functional limitations.
- In Indian subcontinent, the disease is mostly post-traumatic but some endemic forms are also encountered.
- The deforming nature of disease makes it imperative to replace the affected joint by arthroplasty ultimately, however, conservative means of providing symptomatic relief like analgesics and unloading the joint are tried in most patients in early course of the disease.

CHAPTER 72

Protrusio Acetabuli (Otto-Chrobak Pelvis, Otto Pelvis, Arthrokatadysis, Osteoarthritis Deformans, and Osteoarthritic Protrusion of the Acetabulum)

Manish Kumar Varshney

INTRODUCTION

Protrusio acetabuli is a radiological diagnosis on antero-posterior (AP) radiographs of the pelvis where the acetabular line projects medial to the ilioischial line. Arthrokatadysis is a Greek word meaning "subsidence of joint". The condition is often bilateral and has slight female predominance. Primary protrusio is a diagnosis of exclusion. Primary protrusio is now a less recognized entity as more and more underlying disease states associated with this condition are recognized and classified so diagnosis of protrusio becomes secondary only. The prevalence of the disease process is unknown, but the natural history of those with the condition appears to be one of relentless progression of the deformity, worsening of function, and increase in pain.

HISTORICAL CONSIDERATIONS

Intrapelvic protrusion of the acetabulum was first recognized by Otto in 1824 on a desiccated specimen from the Natural History Museum of Breslau in Poland **(Fig. 1)**, who attributed it to "abnormal gout". The pathology, however, gained little attention over the ensuing century due to unclear causes and pathophysiology. Initially, it was considered a primary growth abnormality of the pelvis or that the acetabulum in most cases is too deep to begin with (Rechtman) that is still deeply remodeled by the femoral head. Eppinger postulated chondrodystrophy. Alexander suggested that the protrusio is physiological in children while persistence in adults is due to failure to remodel this physiological disposition. Gilmour reported an abnormal "rhythm of adolescent development" in patients with protrusio where the girls showed accelerated epiphyseal growth and fusion. Now, however, a lot of causes have been identified that modulate the bone physiology and growth producing abnormal shape (see below).

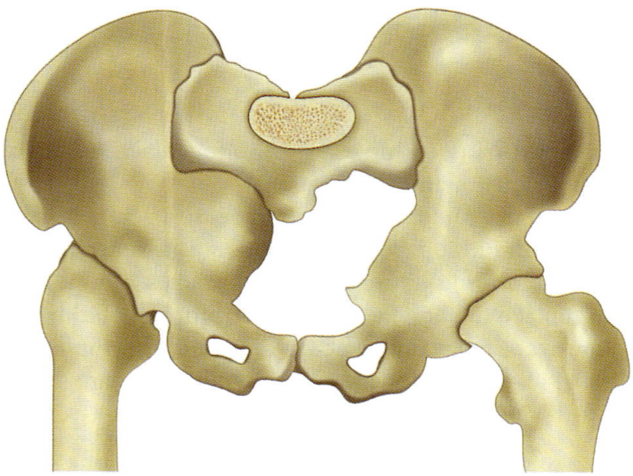

Fig. 1: Lithograph of pelvic specimen originally described by AW Otto.

CLASSIFICATION

Protrusio had been classified by Overgaard (1945) to mainly distinguish between primary (idiopathic and osteoasthenic protrusion) and secondary protrusio (osteoarthritic protrusion) that was simplified by Gilmour in 1939. By convention now only the primary bilateral idiopathic form is called "Otto pelvis" that may be familial, all other secondary varieties are bunched under "protrusio acetabuli". Gilmour classified primary protrusio as one where no other cause can be identified while "secondary" as any protrusio where underlying pathology can be demonstrated **(Table 1)**. The disorders can be actually classified into three main categories:

1. *Primary qualitative deficiency of the acetabular bone:* This encompasses the genetic causes. The bone matrix is weak to begin with and the joint reaction force acts at 69° from the horizontal. The femoral head migration occurs just medial to this at 65°.
2. *Secondary qualitative deficiency of the acetabular bone:* This acquired deficiency in bone quality encompasses the inflammatory, infectious **(Fig. 2)**, metabolic, traumatic, and neoplastic causes. It is easy to understand the weakening of the bone; however, it is difficult to explain the progressive nature of the disease in them.
3. *Developmental growth abnormality:* This also takes some of the genetic and metabolic conditions.

Apart from the detailed list presented above, it is practically useful to remember unilateral causes of protrusio acetabuli, viz., post-traumatic, postirradiation, failed hemiarthroplasty, tuberculosis, Paget's disease, and neoplastic.

TABLE 1: Classification and causes of protrusio.

Primary (idiopathic):	***Secondary (known pathology that causes protrusio):***
"Otto pelvis"	• *Genetic:* – Trichorhinophalangeal syndrome – Stickler syndrome – Trisomy 18 – Ehler–Danlos syndrome – Marfan syndrome – Sickle cell disease • *Inflammatory:* – Rheumatoid arthritis – Juvenile rheumatoid arthritis – Psoriatic arthritis – Ankylosing spondylitis – Reiter's syndrome – Acute idiopathic chondrolysis – Osteolysis following hip replacement • *Infectious:* – *Gonococcus* – Syphilis – *Echinococcus* – *Staphylococcus* – *Streptococcus* – *Mycobacterium tuberculosis* • *Metabolic:* – Paget's disease – Osteogenesis imperfecta – Osteomalacia – Hyperparathyroidism – Ochronosis – Acrodysostosis • *Neoplastic:* – Hemangioma – Metastatic carcinoma (breast, prostate) – Neurofibromatosis – Radiation-induced osteonecrosis • *Traumatic:* – Sequelae of acetabular fracture – Surgical error during hip replacement

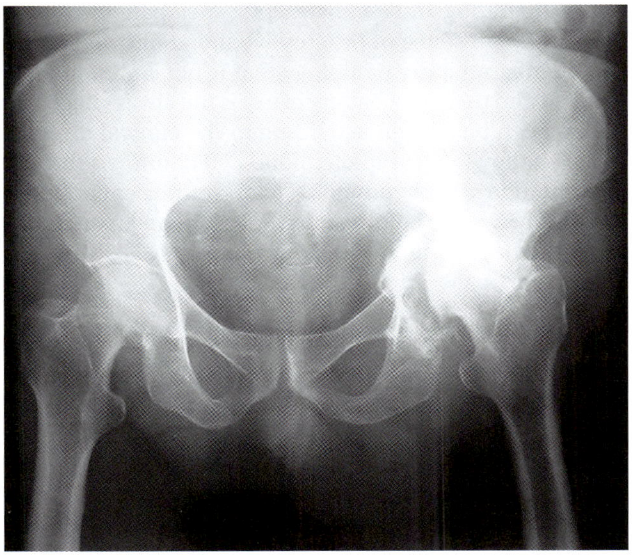

Fig. 2: Protrusio acetabulum post-tubercular infection of the left hip.

BIOMECHANICS OF PROTRUSIO

The consequence of acetabular protrusio is secondary osteoarthritis (OA) and has been characterized by a loss of medial joint space, while the craniolateral (superior) joint space initially remains largely unaltered. The mechanism has been explained by higher load transmission through the medial aspect of the joint.

CLINICAL FEATURES

- The condition is most prominently seen in the middle age group between 35 and 50 years of age; however, patients in their teens and those between 51 and 85 years of age also show higher prevalence than other age groups. The condition is female preponderant and also has racial distribution. The Bantu females in Natal have high prevalence of the Otto pelvis with as many as one-fourth of them affected.
- Typically, patients with primary protrusio acetabula present with activity-related increasing stiffness rather than pain. Often, stiffness has been noticed in adolescence as the OA is not prominent in this age group, so pain is less reported. The deepening effect of acetabulum relatively shortens the femoral neck and reduces offset. Arising from a seated position frequently exacerbates the symptoms. Pain is reported in the groin with some patients reporting radiating pain to the knee. There is impingement during hip movements of abduction and flexion. This causes labral tears and repetitive attacks of synovitis. The changes degrade the cartilage, and hence, progression to OA is very prominent. Secondary changes due to limitation of hip movements are seen in the form of increased lumbar lordosis
- Family history should be obtained as the genetic associations have been found and also metabolic defects may affect the siblings altogether. Past history of hip trauma and surgery should also be obtained
- On examination, there is often global limitation of active and passive movements with terminal pain. Impingement signs are often positive. Pain is also reproduced in active straight leg raise. Trendelenburg sign may be positive due to reduced offset, and hence abductor effectiveness. The gait is a combination of antalgic and Trendelenburg gait.

RADIOGRAPHS

The features are best appreciated on true AP radiographs of the pelvis with both hips [coccyx positioned in the midline, about 1 cm above the pubic symphysis (neutral tilt) and the obturator foramina and the greater trochanter symmetrical (neutral rotation)]. Various parameters are used to diagnose and grade the protrusio **(Fig. 3)** as follows:

- The center-edge angle (CE) of Wiberg of over 46° is diagnostic of protrusio acetabuli while <20° indicates developmental dysplasia of the hip **(Fig. 3)**. Normal range lies between 25° and 40° and the angle ranges 20–25° and 40–46° represent gray areas amenable to measurement errors also. The CE angle has, however, been a subject of debate to quantitate or diagnose protrusio with wide values reported in literature. The primary reason is formation of osteophytes, and difficulty in ascertaining the center of femoral head.
- Armbuster et al. considered protrusio to be present if the medial wall of the acetabulum protruded medial to the ilioischial line (Kohler's line) by 3 mm in males or 6 mm in

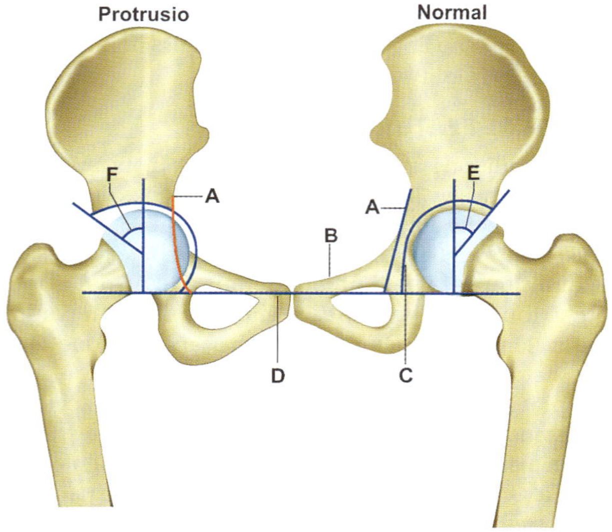

Fig. 3: Radiographic landmarks used in the diagnosis of protrusio acetabuli: A = ilioischial (Kohler) line; B = iliopectineal line; C = acetabular wall; D = interteardrop line; E = normal center-edge angle; F = abnormal center-edge angle indicative of protrusio acetabuli.

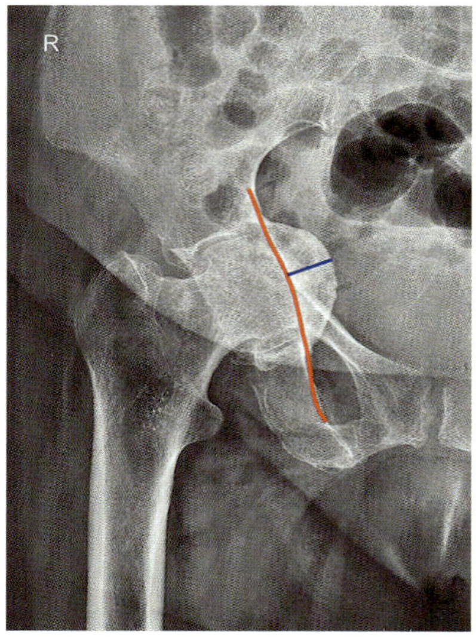

Fig. 4: Measurement of acetabular floor from Kohler's line. The Kohler's line is drawn on the radiograph (deep red line) and a perpendicular is dropped from it to the acetabular floor (blue line). The length of this line determines the grade of protrusion (Here, it is moderate—9 mm).

females **(Fig. 3)**. The line is, however, sensitive to rotation of pelvis as it is formed by the quadrilateral plate that lies posterior to the acetabulum.

- Sotelo-Garza and Charnley used the ilioischial line on an AP radiograph of the pelvis as a reference point from which to measure the location of the acetabular floor **(Fig. 4)**. The acetabular floor is normally lateral to Kohler's line on a true AP projection of pelvis. If the acetabular floor abuts the Kohler's line and the distinction is obscure then it is called "Coxa Profunda" (profunda = deep). If the acetabular floor crosses the Kohler's line then it is called "protrusio". The magnitude of this protrusion medially beyond the Kohler's line is used to grade protrusio as:
  - Mild (1–5 mm)
  - Moderate (6–15 mm)
  - Severe (>15 mm)
- Goodman et al. and Gates et al. suggested that the teardrop **(Figs. 5A to D)** is the most consistent landmark representing the medial and lateral walls of the floor of the acetabulum, varying little with minor degrees of pelvic obliquity. They recommended distance of the hip center in relation to teardrop (using Cartesian coordinates) as the most useful way to assess and track progression of protrusio. Crossing of teardrop is consistent with protrusio.
- *Tonnis angle*: This is negative in moderate-to-severe cases; it is a measure of the tilt of acetabular roof **(Figs. 6A to C)**.

These grading systems and quantification of protrusio do not help planning of management. The primary aim of radiology is identification of protrusio and if present then looking for arthritic changes, status of medial wall, and presence of proximal migration of femoral head in addition to medial protrusion. Dynamic gadolinium MRI of cartilage is useful to evaluate the degree of cartilage degeneration MR arthrography in the early stage of degeneration. MR arthrogram in early stages may reflect changes similar to pincer impingement. These studies are especially important if joint preservation surgeries are being planned to determine the status of cartilage.

LABORATORY WORKUP

This should be done to evaluate the inflammatory causes, metabolic causes, and infectious causes of protrusion as listed in **Table 1**. One needs to identify the primary cause because operating and reconstructing such patients is likely to fail in the presence of progressive metabolic disorder or ongoing inflammatory pathology that is not simultaneously identified and treated. A battery of test is not always necessary and tests can be chosen according to the clinical direction from the following: complete blood cell count, erythrocyte sedimentation rate, rheumatoid factor, antinuclear antibody, blood culture, urine culture, and serum chemistry including liver and renal function tests. Synovial biopsy is obtained, if inflammatory causes are suspected.

MANAGEMENT OF PROTRUSIO

Conservative management is mostly supportive and utilizes approaches such as strengthening exercises, maintaining mobility, and relieving pain by appropriate medications. Ultimately, surgery is needed and conservative management serves only as an interim measure. Primary pathology should always be looked for and treated, as this may prevent progression and reduce the amount/extent of surgical intervention later.

The surgical management broadly falls into two measures (**Flowchart 1** describes about choosing surgical option for protrusio):

1. ***Joint compromising methods:*** These disturb the normal anatomy and/or function of joint.

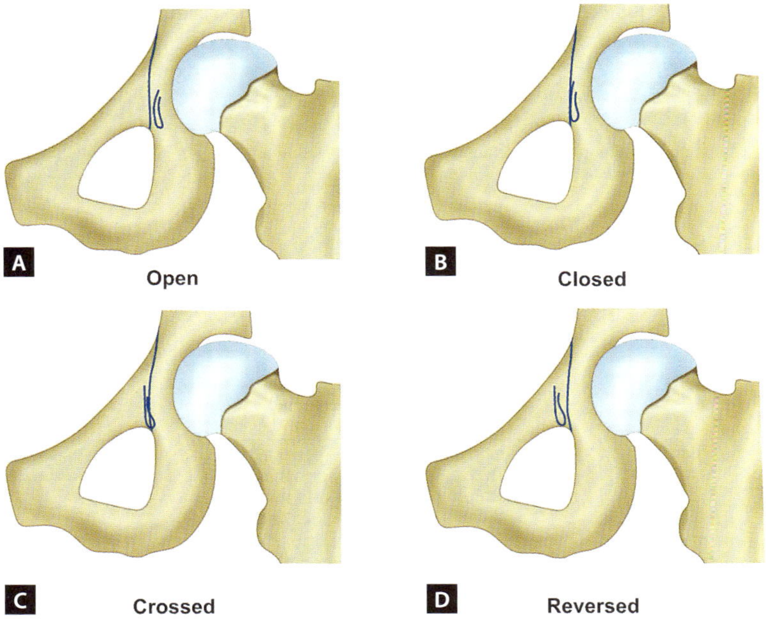

Figs. 5A to D: Role of teardrop and its varied morphology.

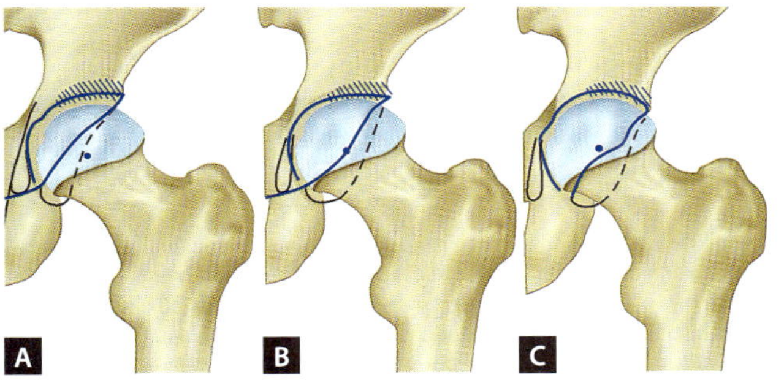

Figs. 6A to C: In a normal hip, (A) the acetabulum sufficiently covers the femoral head; (B) Coxa profunda, the head is more medial—the "acetabular fossa" is at or medial to the ilioischial line; (C) Protrusio, the "femoral head" is close, at or medial to the ilioischial line, the acetabular roof is negatively tilted (negative Tonnis angle). The center of the femoral head being medial to the anterior and posterior acetabular walls

- *Total joint arthroplasty:* Quite popular and the bias toward this procedure has reduced tremendously. The procedure is first choice in patients past their middle age and obvious arthritic changes in the hip joint. Most important concern is anatomical repositioning of the cup. Cemented cups placed 1 cm away from the anatomical position resulted in failure in all the three zones. Higher medial stresses are produced with medial placement of the cup. Methods to circumvent this are use of morselized bone graft, use of protrusio cage, lateralization of cup by using metal-backed implants or protrusio cup itself. Augmenting the medial wall by bone graft only has little benefit as the stresses are ultimately transmitted to it. Still successful results have been reported by the use of "concavoconvex" femoral head graft for filling medial acetabular defect and cementing the acetabular cup. The femoral head articular cartilage was denuded using reverse reamer, and the center of head was scooped of the bone resulting in typical concavoconvex graft that was impacted in the protrusio defect and augmented with the retrieved bone graft from center of femoral head. I prefer medial morcelized bone graft and using a porous-coated metal-backed cup. Rim augments (antiprotrusio rings) have also been used that transmit the stress on acetabular rim rather than the center. In general, as recommended by Ranawat and Zahn, protrusio up to 5 mm does not require any bone graft, protrusio >5 mm and intact medial wall need bone graft but augmentation devices may not be needed. Gross deficiency would need above described methods. Some technical keypoints in reconstruction of protrusio acetabulum with a total hip replacement are provided in **Box 1**.
- Hip arthrodesis (*see* Chapter on "Hip Arthrodesis" for details)
- Excision arthroplasty

2. ***Joint preservation methods:***
   - *Hanging hip of Voss (not used at all today):* This was based on premises that gravity will distract the joint and resultant forces will be reduced. I am unaware of any current indications for this procedure.
   - *Acetabuloplasty (rimectomy of Smith-Peterson):* This may be appropriate for mild-to-moderate protrusio in a middle-aged patient where the symptoms are more of pincer type impingement. Hip is exposed through surgical dislocation of hip, and the peripheral osteophytes are cleared followed by reattachment of labrum.
   - *Valgus intertrochanteric osteotomy (VITO) (Pauwel's):* This is known to reorient the resultant forces of the hip to a more cranial position, thus controlling the

Flowchart 1: Surgical management of protrusio acetabuli.

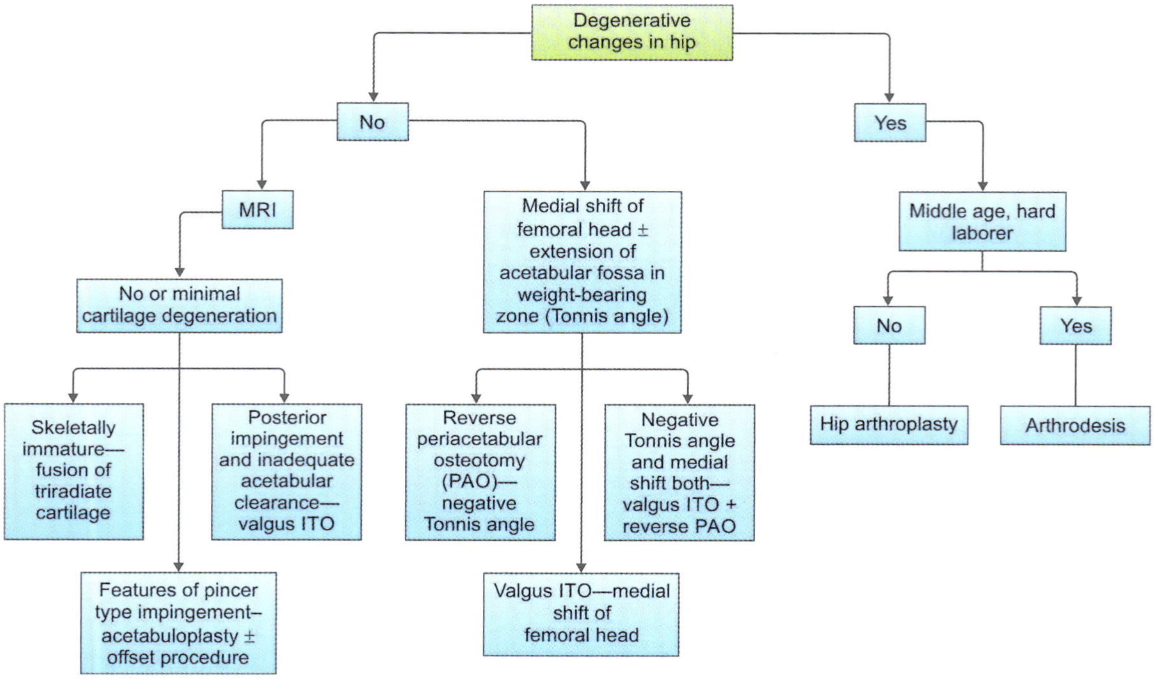

(ITO: intertrochanteric osteotomy)

BOX 1: Some keypoints while planning and performing total hip replacement in protrusio acetabuli.

Evaluate the patient on these parameters first as they have their own importance discussed later:
- Depth of medial migration
- Status of medial wall
- "Mouth" versus "cavity" of the defect—this essentially means whether the defect is convergent type ("mouth" > "cavity" inside) or divergent type ("mouth" < "cavity")
- Protrusio has only one component, i.e., medial migration or it is a complex variety having additional superior migration of the femoral head.

Where to place the cup? Do not place it too medially in situ or lateralize it too much. One simple rule of thumb is to place the cup in center within 1 cm of the native acetabular center. Now this may be difficult to determine in bilateral deformities so the other simple guide is to place the medial wall of cup at the Kohler's line (i.e., at the coxa profunda level) undercorrecting the deformity. Restoring anatomical offset in these patients make them uncomfortable because they are used to lower offset and the hip will become unusually tight for them. Anatomical restoration may be desirable only in unilateral causes of protrusio.

Depth of medial migration: Protrusion till "coxa profunda" is easier to dislocate and one should attempt dislocation in these cases instead of in situ osteotomy. Moderate-to-severe variety protrusion are difficult to dislocate and the neck is obscured by "curtain osteophytes" from acetabulum preventing any motion. Surgeons get easily tempted by the common recommendation of in situ neck osteotomy and proceed in such cases but one must realize that the tissues have not been mobilized so despite implanting the prosthesis the patient will not have any useful function. Decent attempt at releasing soft tissues should be done before proceeding with in situ osteotomy even if it is obvious at the first go.

Status of medial wall: Medial wall continuity is very important in proper reconstruction of the acetabulum. I would say X-rays are enough, but most recommend CT scans to judge the continuity of the medial wall. The wall is sclerotic **(Fig. 7A)** but thin even if it is complete so one must be careful in not penetrating or reaming it overzealously. Alongside one must also pay attention to the intactness of anterior and posterior columns. If both are intact and cup can get a good rim fit on these, adequately also supported superiorly then just impacting trabecular metal backed cup or antiprotrusio cup without filling medial defect would suffice (if medial defect is <5 mm). Filling medial defect >5 mm is commonly recommended **(Figs. 7A to C)**. Use bone graft harvested from the femoral head to fill the medial defect. The graft need not be "sludge-like" reamings as I find it difficult to impact and it also comes off during washing, instead particulate graft of size 5–7 mm prepared using rongeur interlocks much better during impaction **(Fig. 7B)**. Impact graft also anteriorly as the defect in protrusio is both medial and anterior. If there is a small to moderate medial wall defect (up to 1 cm) one can reinforce using a metal mesh and graft above it. Larger defects in isolation are rare [unless one is doing total hip arthroplasty (THA) in acute fracture of acetabulum!] but would need antiprotrusio cage (APC). One can then use an uncemented **(Fig. 7C)** or a cemented cup (surgeon preference). Sometimes the walls of the acetabulum may not be strong enough (e.g., in metabolic disorder) to hold uncemented cups wherein cemented cups do well.

Convergent versus divergent protrusio: The convergent is the easiest type of protrusion because as we go deep from the mouth the acetabulum tightens so one prepares acetabulum in the usual manner and ± graft as above and gets out. Problem is a divergent type protrusio where as soon as surgeon negotiates and reams the mouth; the inner cavity keeps enlarging like a cave and implanting a cup will be unstable. One needs to carefully bone graft the whole cavity medially and anteriorly (posterior wall is usually safe) using impaction bone grafting and provide strong floor for cup to stay there. The cups need additional screw support to prevent migration with initial graft resorption. Use of antiprotrusio multihole cups is recommended.

Complex protrusio: Sometimes the femoral head does not only migrate medially but also superiorly. If medial migration is larger than superior migration then reconstruction methods described as above suffice but if superior migration is more than medial migration then standard bone grafting + reconstruction will not work. This makes the situation complicated partly in the sense that anterosuperior bone grafting along the axis of weight-bearing is not very successful in restoring the bone and it resorbs very fast. Medial bone grafts are excellent. In these cases, a high hip center is acceptable option and partial compensation can be done for limb length on the femoral side. The other option is of trabecular metal (TM) spacers/offsets, if one intends to still center the cup anatomically. Here, one must remember than after obtaining bleeding subcortical/cancellous bone of the acetabular cavity place the acetabular trial supported on anterior and posterior columns as desired anatomically then trial superiorly for TM spacers. But during final implantation first fix the TM spacers and then implant the acetabular cup for good fit. The third possibility is use of APC cage + bone graft and then implanting the acetabular shell/cup. This is especially indicated if complex protrusio is present along with medial wall defect that cannot be grafted well.

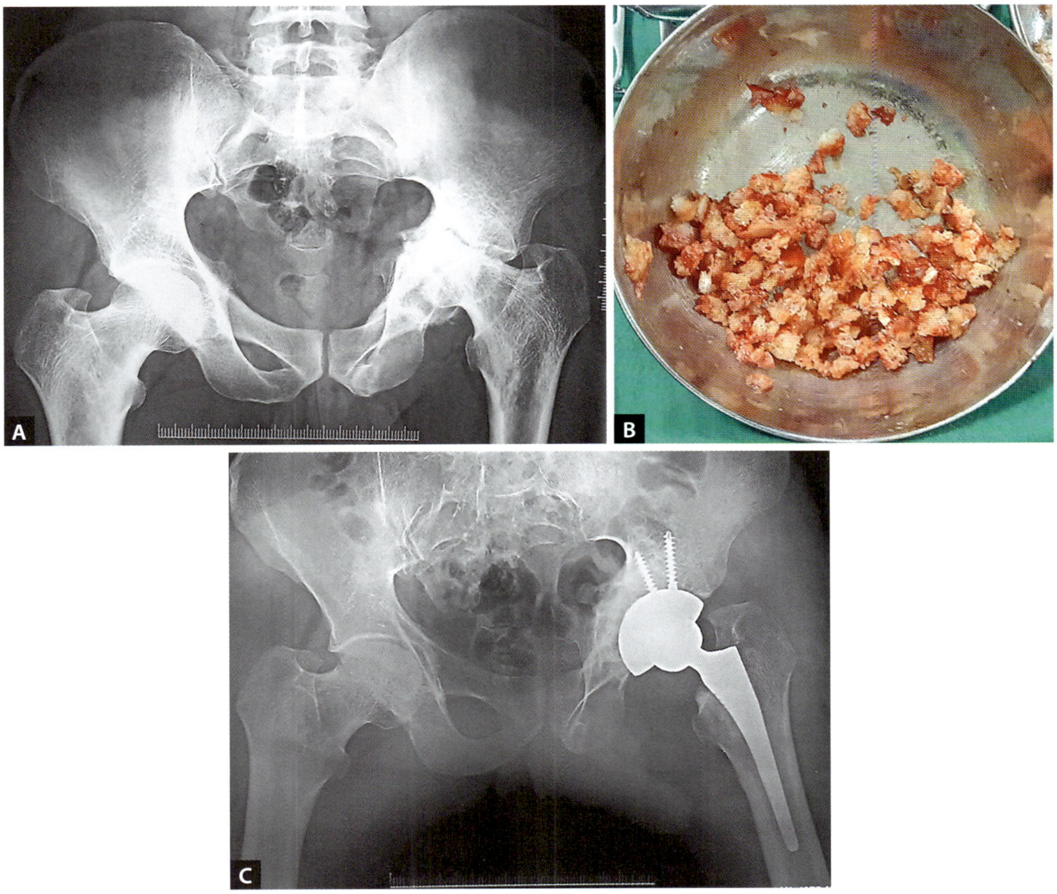

Figs. 7A to C: The left hip joint suffered from fracture acetabulum and femoral head 3 years ago and was neglected resulting in advanced degeneration of the joint and protrusion of the medial wall (A). The medial defect was quite significant (>5 mm) so medial and anterior grafting was done with graft harvested from retrieved femoral head (B). Implantation of the uncemented cup with proper seating was done (C) The malunion of rami and resulting deformity of acetabulum should be evaluated using CT scan before planning such cases (not shown) else there are high chances of intraoperative surprises in these cases. The malunion was left untouched and functional reconstruction was aimed in this case using standard principles **(*see* Box 1)**.

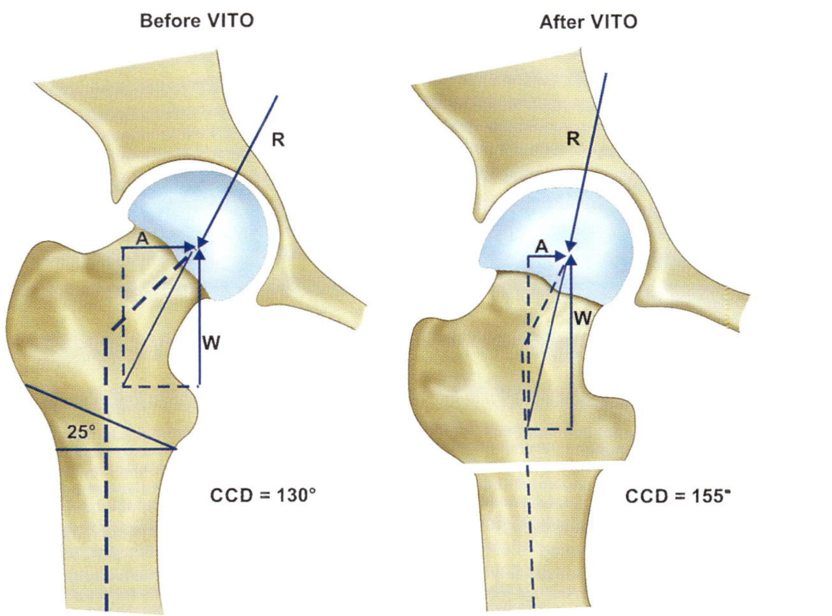

Fig. 8: Effects of valgus intertrochanteric osteotomy (VITO) on the medializing force (vector Q) in the hip. The angle of resultant force increases from 130° to 155°. (CCD: centrum-collum-diaphyseal)

superomedial migration of the femoral head **(Fig. 8)**. Correction of 20–30° is desirable; overcorrection causes abductor contracture. The added advantage of the procedure is reduced impingement at the superior acetabular margin. If correction is done >40° then abductor tension should be released by opening wedge osteotomy of trochanter, and limb-shortening may also need to be performed. This procedure should not be performed on patients over 40 years of age or in whom significant degenerative changes were evident on plain radiographs.

- *Surgical closure of triradiate cartilage:* This is indicated in skeletally immature patients with open triradiate cartilage and absence of inflammatory pathology. It is, however, difficult to determine which protrusio will progress as opposed to those where there is more likelihood of indolent course (not needing surgery). This procedure is, hence, recommended for Marfan syndrome and genetic causes of protrusio.

CONCLUSION

- Protrusio acetabuli involves inward migration of the acetabular floor beyond the ilioischial line. The diagnosis is radiological as the clinical features are not much characteristic until the protrusion is marked.
- There are various measures used to determine the medial migration of acetabular floor but importantly one should follow a particular technique to perform planning and treatment of individual cases.
- Joint preserving methods are appropriate for mild-to-moderate protrusion, however, in late stages and particularly with the onset of joint degeneration arthroplasty is a better choice.
- Arthroplasty should be done by experienced persons only as not just the reconstruction of acetabulum but even the exposure and dislocation of hip is also difficult in advanced cases. Often the head has to be removed piecemeal else one is liable to fracture the acetabulum if dislocation of hip is attempted by conventional method in a protrusio.

CHAPTER 73

Transient Synovitis of Hip (Transitory Coxitis, Acute Transient Epiphysitis, Coxitis Fugax, Coxitis Serosa, Seu Simplex, Phantom Hip Disease, Toxic Synovitis, and Observation Hip)

Manish Kumar Varshney

INTRODUCTION

Transient synovitis is a clinical diagnosis and is a common cause of limp in children aged 3–8 years. The first description of transient synovitis was published in 1892, where a short lived (transient) hip disease with classic symptoms was noted that spontaneously disappeared completely over a span of weeks to months. The pathology essentially involves synovitis of the joint lining and effusion. The etiology of transient synovitis remains elusive, while many have been proposed including trauma, hypersensitivity, and perhaps most notably infections of both viral and bacterial origin (none though substantiated). The biggest challenge for clinician is to distinguish this from septic disease of the hip that has long lasting and poor outcomes, if left untreated.

EPIDEMIOLOGY

Transient synovitis occurs mainly in children of age 3–8 years. Children have lifetime risk of around 3% for developing transient synovitis with annual incidence of about 0.2%. Although common between ages of 3 and 8 years, transient synovitis has been reported in infants of 3 months as well as in adults. Though males have a higher incidence (nearly double) of females in adult onset disease the incidence is nearly equal among the sexes. In about 4–17% of children, transient synovitis may recur, mostly with benign course, though in about 10%, it presents with features of chronic inflammatory condition. In patients who have recurrence have 20 times higher risk over general population for developing it again. Bilateral disease is uncommon (1–4%) of the cases.

ETIOLOGY

The exact etiology of transient synovitis is elusive, but transient viral infections or an immune reaction to it is the strongest contender. Parvovirus-19 and human herpes simplex virus-6 have been plausibly associated with it. The association is strengthened by the following findings:

- Children with transient synovitis have higher chances of having history of viral infections with symptoms such as malaise, mild pyrexia of common cold.
- Interferon concentration is found to be on higher level in them with more chances of them to be in antiviral state.
- High incidence in humid environment of October than in dry environment of February.

Though not strongly proved, allergic reactions and history of trauma are thought to be possible causative factors for transient synovitis.

DIAGNOSIS

Clinical Presentation

The typical presentation is acute onset of groin or thigh pain. The pain is often associated with flexion, abduction, and external rotation deformity at hip (position of rest—comfortable position due to raised intracapsular pressure). The patient walks with a limp (antalgic gait) and the pain increases on weight-bearing. On examination, there is limited passive range of motion and hip is irritable to examination. Bilateral involvement is seen in minority of patients. Ask for a history of upper respiratory, gastrointestinal, or urinary tract infection or minor trauma.

Imaging

Plain radiographs: These are mainly helpful to exclude bony lesions (like occult fracture) and other disorders such as slipped upper femoral epiphysis (SUFE) and Perthes disease (increase in teardrop distance). In transient synovitis, mostly the X-rays are normal with occasional finding of medial joint space widening comparison with asymptomatic contralateral hip helps on a pelvic radiograph.

Ultrasonography (USG): It is probably the most reliable investigation that noninvasively detects the presence of even small hip effusion though distinction with septic arthritis is not possible with it. Lack of fluid also does not exclude septic arthritis, so it needs to be repeated.

Magnetic resonance imaging (MRI): It has been shown to help distinguish transient synovitis from septic arthritis. In transient synovitis, the differentiating features are contralateral joint effusion and the absence of signal intensity abnormalities in the bone marrow. It may become the investigation of choice with improved characterization of the findings and population study. The following features have been suggested to distinguish transient synovitis from septic arthritis on MRI:

- In septic arthritis, there is decreased perfusion at the femoral epiphysis (mainly seen in coronal plane) on fat-suppressed gadolinium-enhanced T1-weighted MRI (Kwack et al.).
- On fat-suppressed contrast-enhanced T2-weighted MRI, high-signal intensity in bone marrow of the affected hip along with contrast enhancement of the soft tissues is found in septic arthritis (Yang et al.).
- Utilizing dynamic contrast-enhanced MRI, Kim et al. distinguished between septic arthritis and transient synovitis, reporting a negative predictive value of 88.9%. In lesions other than septic arthritis, invasive procedures like arthrocentesis can be prevented with the help of these MRI findings.
- Though cost and availability as well as possible requirement of general anesthesia are limiting factors for MRI, when clinical features and USG findings are nonconclusive, it helps to distinguish between transient synovitis and septic arthritis.

Bone scan: "Cold hip sign" is often seen on bone scans of patients referred with irritable hip due to fluid under pressure in the hip joint that impairs perfusion of the structures in the joint capsule. In the most initial stages, however, increased perfusion due to synovitis causes nonspecific increased periarticular perfusion. Bone scintigraphy may show mildly elevated uptake, though transient decrease of technetium-99 (Tc-99) uptake is not uncommon. Due to lack of enough sensitivity and specificity, it is not helpful to differentiate between transient synovitis and septic arthritis. It may identify other conditions like multifocal musculoskeletal infections.

Hip aspiration: This is the gold standard to diagnose septic arthritis. It should be performed in all patients with moderate-to-high suspicion of septic arthritis. It can be done either under USG or fluoroscopically guidance.

Aspiration can be done by spinal needle under fluoroscopic guidance. If there is doubt about the position of needle then 10 mL of either iothalamate meglumine contrast or nonbacteriostatic saline may be done followed by subsequent reaspiration. US-guided aspiration of hip synovial fluid is a preferred procedure. Hip aspiration can be done by anterior, medial, or lateral approach. In anterior approach, femoral artery is palpated in femoral triangle and a needle gauge of 18–21 is inserted 1 inch lateral to the artery and 1 inch below the inguinal ligament straight down in the lateral half of the joint cavity. In lateral approach, greater trochanter is palpated and needle is inserted from anterior side of its tip, parallel to femoral neck into the hip joint. In medial approach, needle is inserted between gracilis and adductor longus muscle, fluoroscopy is necessary for further procedure with this approach.

- Findings suggestive of septic arthritis are positive culture results, positive Gram stain or a white blood cell count (WBC) > $50 \times 10^9/mm^3$ in the synovial fluid with predominance of polymorphonuclear cells. Limitations are painful and invasiveness of the procedure and need of general anesthesia.

DIFFERENTIAL DIAGNOSIS

Transient synovitis is a diagnosis of exclusion, and all other known hip disorders and causes of pediatric hip pain ranging from benign conditions to surgical emergencies should be excluded before labeling the child as being suffering from transient synovitis. The list includes:

- Septic arthritis
- Tuberculosis of hip joint
- Legg-Calve-Perthes disease (LCPD)
- Slipped capital femoral epiphysis (SCFE)
- Osteomyelitis
- Juvenile rheumatoid arthritis
- Primary or metastatic lesions
- Iliopsoas bursitis
- Lyme arthritis
- Sacroiliitis
- Uncommon and rare misdiagnosis:
  - Osteitis pubis
  - Tibia torus and Toddler's fracture
  - Pelvic abscess
  - Labral tear
  - Psoas abscess

Difference between septic arthritis and transient synovitis: Differentiating septic arthritis is most important. **Table 1** summarizes the differences between the two conditions.

TABLE 1: Differentiating features of septic arthritis and transient synovitis.

Characteristic	*Septic arthritis*	*Transient synovitis*
Fever	+	–
Limitation of movements	+++	+
Failure to thrive	+	–
Local raised temperature	+++	+
Constancy of symptoms	Pain and fever increases, if no treatment done	Symptoms remain more or less constant
Preceding ailments	Usually none or pyogenic focus may be present	Viral diseases such as common cold or diarrhea
CRP levels	>20 mg/L	Raised but mild
MRI	Reduced perfusion of the femoral epiphysis	–
Radiographs	Osteopenia is marked	Mild osteopenia
Spontaneous resolution	Occasional	Often
Residual changes	Often if untreated (see squeal of septic arthritis)	Never (as of now, some authors consider this to be a prelude to Perthes, etc., but need substantiation)

(CRP: C-reactive protein)

In 1999, Kocher et al. found four clinical predictors to differentiate between septic arthritis and transient synovitis:

- Fever (temperature > 38.5°C)
- Nonweight-bearing on the affected limb
- Erythrocyte sedimentation rate (ESR) ≥ 40 mm/h
- Serum WBC > 12 × 10^9 cells/L

The predicted probabilities of septic arthritis on the basis of one, two, three, and four predictors were 3.0%, 40.0%, 93.1%, and 99.6%, respectively. Craid added the fifth predictor, namely C-reactive protein (CRP) > 20 mg/L and found the predicted probabilities of three, four, and five factors to be 83%, 93%, and 98%, respectively. Despite these attempts, the criteria have not been substantiated by other studies. Fever (temperature above 38°C) is the most significant predictor, followed by elevated CRP. A value of CRP of >20 mg/L is the strongest independent risk factor for septic arthritis.

TREATMENT

Transient synovitis is a self-limiting condition that resolves spontaneously and is managed conservatively through observation (so-called observation hip). The following modalities are employed:

- Rest and immobilization—intracapsular pressure is greatest when the joint is extended hence, immobilization of the hip in 45° of flexion is recommended that can be reduced with subsidence of symptoms.
- Nonsteroidal anti-inflammatory drugs (NSAIDs)
- Role of aspiration—though this can give immediate relief long-lasting benefit is unknown.
- In cases refractory to conservative management, search for other related problems like cartilage defects. Synovium debridement by arthroscopy may help sometimes.

NATURAL HISTORY AND PROGNOSIS

The natural history of transient synovitis is benign and it resolves over a period of 1–3 weeks.

- There is an increased possibility of developing a recurrence of the condition.
- The incidence of LCPD following an episode of transient synovitis has been estimated to be 3% as opposed to the incidence of LCPD in the general population of 0.9/100,000. The association is unclear, however, and large scale prospective studies are needed (difficult due to rarity of both diseases).

CONCLUSION

- Transient synovitis of the hip joint is a common condition in children presenting as a limp while walking.
- The condition is benign in itself but should be differentiated from more severe pathologies such as infection, slipped upper femoral epiphysis, and neoplastic lesions.
- Once it is ascertained that the child has transient synovitis only, reassurance and symptomatic treatment usually suffices. Long-term risk of Perthes disease is a bit elevated in these children but there is no conclusive evidence to this effect for initiating surveillance.

CHAPTER 74

Osteotomies Around Hip Joint

Manish Kumar Varshney, Shalinder Kumar Sharma

INTRODUCTION

Osteotomies around hip joint had been in fashion since long and various variants had been described for different hip joint pathologies. The use of osteotomies now is, however, commonly limited to management of deformities and hip pathologies in pediatric age group. The loss in popularity is mainly due to successful and acceptable outcomes of hip arthroplasty and quite extensive training of the new orthopedic surgeons in joint replacement surgery. Osteotomies but definitely have an important place in the orthopedic practice where native joint preservation is indicated and needed (described later in specific places). Trochanteric osteotomies are now in fashion for arising need of complex surgeries like revisions and complex primary arthroplasty, a detailed knowledge of the same is also important for the orthopedic surgeons.

DEFINITION AND RATIONALE

An osteotomy is the transaction of a bone to correct axial malalignment or to lengthen or shorten the bone or to relocate the joint in a way that distributes (rather than concentrating) the load-transmission across joint surfaces. There are three groups of osteotomies that can be done around the hip joint:

1. Periacetabular osteotomies [discussed with "developmental dysplasia of the hip (DDH)" in pediatric orthopedic section]
2. Proximal femoral osteotomies
3. Combined type

Proximal femoral osteotomies have been in vogue till last decade of last century whence they have been superseded by advancements in arthroplasty. First femoral osteotomy was performed by John Rhea Barton in 1826 to obtain movement in ankylosed hip. In 1835, Sourvier performed first subtrochanteric osteotomy for the treatment of congenital dislocation of hip (CDH). In 1918/19, von Baeyer and Lorenz described proximal femur bifurcation ("Y" osteotomy)/split osteotomy to secure stability in old CDH. In 1922, Schanz reported his famous low subtrochanteric abduction pelvic support osteotomy (PSO). In 1936, McMurry performed oblique displacement osteotomy for osteoarthritis of hip that is now also used for nonunion fracture neck of femur. In 1959, Pauwels described varus osteotomy (much less popular) at intertrochanteric level for severe osteoarthrosis of hip (Pauwels' I) followed by a valgus osteotomy in 1975 (highly popular and used for most osteotomies with modifications). Blount and Moore described excellent blade plate for fixation of high subtrochanteric osteotomy.

Despite the popularity of hip arthroplasty, there are specific situations that can be managed better with osteotomies and conserve the hip than replacing it. Typically, such a situation is clinically encountered for correction of deformity or achieving stability (compensatory) in a population that cannot be managed by replacement arthroplasty (say in pediatric group). The progression and severity of hip deformities are linked to the remaining growth potential. Osteotomies about the hip are most useful when there are morphological abnormalities present that can be corrected with an osteotomy in the presence of viable articular cartilage. Apart from deformity correction, the osteotomies have been utilized for various unrelated conditions such as nonunions, joint subluxations/instability, painful hip, etc. The primary goal of an osteotomy, hence, depends on the specific condition for which it is used and can be summarized as follows:

- To increase the joint contact area, thereby decreasing the load about the hip to a level that is compatible with normal articular function; or
- To relieve an impingement problem; or
- To improve joint mechanics to achieve a more functional range of motion by eliminating fixed deformities; or
- To redistribute stress in periarticular region fostering union (as in ununited fracture neck of femur).

It has been realized that femoroacetabular impingement is a common harbinger of painful hip conditions. The effects such as cam-effect or hinged abduction and femoroacetabular impingement results in progressive deterioration of the labrum and the articular cartilage instability, limits mobility, and is the source of pain, limping, and early arthritis. So, additional procedures such as osteochondroplasties, labrum procedures, osteotomies for acetabular realignment, or acetabuloplasties are commonly combined in current practice.

The proximal femoral osteotomies achieve the above goals by producing changes in the anatomy that have bearing on hip biomechanics and biology later.

A typical proximal femoral osteotomy permits following corrections:

- *Angulation:*
  - Valgus-varus
  - Anterior-posterior
- *Rotational deformity:* Internal and external rotation
- *Limb-length discrepancy:* Lengthening or shortening of limb (virtual by changing angulation or true by say lengthening femoral neck)
- *Translations:*
  - Medial or lateral
  - Anterior or posterior displacement

CLASSIFICATION AND TYPES OF PROXIMAL FEMORAL OSTEOTOMIES

Commonly, an anatomical or functional name is added to the type of osteotomy nowadays, as there are so many authors describing modifications of various classical procedures. Still some procedures that cannot be described by these descriptives are called by the name of their originator (such as McMurray's osteotomy, Lorenz osteotomy, Chiari osteotomy, etc.).

Depending on the functional correction that osteotomy achieves, it can be classified as:

- *Lineal:* When it is performed to correct shortening or lengthening.
- *Torsional:* When performed to correct internal or external rotation deformity.
- *Translational:* When the fragments are displaced medially or laterally, e.g., McMurray's osteotomy.
- *Angular:* When performed to correct the angular deformities, e.g., Blount osteotomy, Schanz osteotomy.

Depending on the type of bone cut, osteotomy can be grouped into following types:

- *Transverse osteotomy:* This is ideal for correction of rotation and is performed in metaphyseal or diaphyseal region. It is easy to perform but is unstable and not ideally suited for interfragmentary compression. Angular corrections are difficult to control by this osteotomy, so not indicated.
- *Oblique osteotomy:* Gives superior bending and rotational stability as it is easily compressed with interfragmentary lag-screw. Oblique osteotomy is especially useful in metaphyseal/diaphyseo-metaphyseal area.
- *Crescentic osteotomy (dome or reverse dome-shaped):* This osteotomy maintains good bony contact and preserves length while correcting angulations and rotational deformity. It is difficult to plan and is technically difficult to perform. It is a very good option (preferable) to correct varus/valgus deformity close to joint if one is experienced in performing crescentic osteotomies.

Depending on the relative position of two fragments after bone cuts:

- *Displacement or transpositional osteotomy:* Usually a transverse metaphyseal osteotomy and one of the fragments (usually distal) is shifted/rotated so that the corner of fragment is impacted into medullary canal of the other fragment. Longitudinal axis of distal fragment remains parallel to the longitudinal terminal axis of proximal fragment. This osteotomy relies on biological changes induced and preserves or improves the joint forces and physiology. By specific translation of fragments, the bending and loading forces are converted into compressive load. The osteotomy preserves length and joint alignment, e.g., McMurray's osteotomy, Dimon-Hughston osteotomy, etc.
- *Angulation osteotomy:* Most other osteotomies fall into this category where the longitudinal axis of distal fragment forms an angle with that of proximal fragment. This is done to reorient the joint and/or realign the limb to maintain proper mechanical axis or improve load transmission across the joint. Extra-articular deformities are commonly corrected by this method.

Today the majority of osteotomies include displacement and angulation both to achieve a multiplanar correction. In addition to alterations in the frontal plane, rotation and sagittal plane corrections are also combined together.

Depending on the location of proximal osteotomy, it can be referred to as:

- *Intertrochanteric osteotomy:* It is of various types and depending on the use it has been variedly described by authors:
  - Pauwels' osteotomy (this is a valgus or varus repositioning osteotomy)
  - McMurray's osteotomy (for osteoarthrosis and also used for nonunion neck femur; it is a pelvic support medial displacement intertrochanteric osteotomy)
  - Modified osteotomy of Muller
  - Ball and socket osteotomy
  - Dimon–Hughston osteotomy are for improving the stability of intertrochanteric fractures.
- *Trochanteric displacement osteotomy:* These are done to reposition the trochanter for either:
  - An abnormal pathologic position of the greater trochanter compromising abductor function; or
  - Short femoral neck and elevated greater trochanter
- *Subtrochanteric osteotomy:* These are mainly done either as a part of PSO or to correct rotational deformity:
  - *Milch-bachelor type*—improves stability of the hip; for nonunion of femoral neck fracture and unstable hip with positive telescopy test and Trendelenburg limp
  - Blount osteotomy
  - Schanz osteotomy similar to Milch osteotomy
- *Femoral neck osteotomy:* These are done for:
  - Slipped capital femoral epiphysis (SCFE)
  - Sugioka osteotomy (avascular necrosis of head of femur)

Depending on pathology (this is not a classification but instead a list of available options):

- *Osteonecrosis of femoral head:* The choice of osteotomy depends on the site of collapse and amount of collapse (arc) (*see* Section 1: Bone Anatomy, Physiology, Pathology

and Related Diseases, Chapter on "Osteonecrosis and Osteochondrosis"):
  - Varus/valgus/flexion/extension or a combination of osteotomies
  - Sugioka rotational transpositional osteotomy
  - Atsumi osteotomy
  - Merle d'Aubigné osteotomy
- *Osteoarthrosis of hip joint:*
  - McMurray's osteotomy
  - Pauwels' I and II osteotomy
- *Proximal femoral nonunions:*
  - Ununited proximal femoral neck fractures:
    - McMurray's osteotomy
    - Pauwels' II (valgus) osteotomy
    - Schanz angulation osteotomy (modified Pauwels' osteotomy)
    - Dickson's osteotomy
    - Putti osteotomy
  - Ununited intertrochanteric fractures or unstable (four part fracture, medial cortical comminution, reverse obliquity fractures, large separate posterior trochanteric fracture, subtrochanteric extension) intertrochanteric fractures:
    - Dimon-Hughston
    - Sarmiento
    - Valgus resection osteotomy
- *Neglected dislocation of hip joint:*
  - Schanz PSO
  - Lorenz bifurcation osteotomy
  - *Perthes disease:* Varus derotation osteotomy (VDRO)
- *Slipped capital femoral epiphysis:*
  - Closing wedge osteotomy of neck:
    - Fish osteotomy technique
    - Technique of Dunn (just distal to slip)
    - Base of neck technique osteotomy by Kramer et al.
    - Osteotomy technique of Abraham
  - Compensatory osteotomies:
    - Ball and socket osteotomy
    - Biplanar IT osteotomy (Southwick)
- *Coxa vara:*
  - Cuneiform osteotomy
  - Pauwels' "Y" osteotomy
  - Basilar osteotomy
- *Paralytic hip:*
  - Derotation osteotomy
  - Varus osteotomy (Pauwels' I)
  - Extension osteotomy

GENERAL WORKUP FOR OSTEOTOMY

A preoperative drawing is essential before carrying out a corrective osteotomy to determine the various components of the deformity. In general, the following are essential components for evaluation of patients:

- Full length X-rays of the limb in anteroposterior (AP) and lateral views (obtain special views to localize and define pathology, if needed)
- Assess the shortening and limb length inequalities, pelvic tilt associated bony abnormalities at acetabulum, degeneration, etc.
- Distant joints (knee and spine) should be also evaluated for compensatory changes.
- Mark the osteotomy site and perform paper osteotomy, clearly defining wedges to scale.
- Plan the fixation device in advance and obtain any special fixation material needed preoperatively.
- Plan the unexpected under guidance of experienced surgeon.

CLINICAL EXAMINATION

Following must be examined:

- Hip contractures
- Duchenne-Trendelenburg limp and sign
- Power of muscles around hip especially the abductors for varus/valgus osteotomies
- Knee deformities, spinal deformities, and flexibility for required postoperative compensation
- Examine the other limb always
- Passive range of movements of the hip
- Measure and note all deformities (abduction/adduction, flexion and rotational deformities, etc.)
- Measure true and apparent lengths of limbs

RADIOLOGICAL EVALUATION OF THE INVOLVED HIP

- An AP view is taken in internal rotation with the patient supine and beam centered on pubic symphysis (the patellae should be pointing toward roof).
- The cross table lateral view of the hip is taken with the normal leg crossed over the involved leg.
- *Contour projections:* These are performed to look for sphericity of the femoral head [to be frank noncontrast computed tomography (NCCT) scans are more reliable and three-dimensional (3D) reconstructions are easily obtainable nowadays and are recommended).
  - The lower limb is supported in 45° straight leg raising test (SLRT) position and standard AP projection is taken to evaluate the congruity of the cranioventral part of the femoral head under the weight-bearing zone of the acetabulum.
  - In the same position, the beam of the X-rays is directed 30° obliquely from cranial to caudal to evaluate craniodorsal head segment.
- *Functional radiographs:* These are obtained to assess the postosteotomy configuration of joint in advance. They check the anatomical advantage that can be obtained by repositioning the head and hence portended improvement in function.
  - *Abduction and adduction projections:* In supine position, the affected hip is abducted to its maximum and internally rotated and a standard AP radiograph is taken. Similar position is used for adduction views only the hip is placed in maximal adduction.
- In pediatric patients, magnetic resonance-arthrogram is a better investigation due to cartilaginous nature of femoral head that better evaluates the morphology of femoral head. Condition of articular cartilage and labrum.

Contraindications

Contraindications for performing osteotomy:

- *Absolute:*
  - Neuropathic arthropathy
  - Active infections
  - Advanced arthritis/ankylosis
- *Relative:*
  - Inflammatory arthropathy
  - Severe osteopenia
  - Advanced age
  - Smoking, obesity

INTERTROCHANTERIC OSTEOTOMY

Intertrochanteric osteotomy permits the corrections of various deformities (and in various planes) as mentioned above, also depending on the wedge cuts taken combined corrections can also be obtained depending on site and type of pathology (like varus flexion osteotomy or valgus extension osteotomy, etc.). There are two broad classes of proximal femoral intertrochanteric osteotomies, classified on the basis of procedure done for correction of deformity:

1. Varus, valgus, flexion, and extension intertrochanteric osteotomies
2. Simple or double osteotomies of the greater trochanter with lengthening of the femoral neck

Indications

- Typical indications:
  - Malunions of the fractures in the trochanteric region with preserved joint (cartilage) and normal feasibility of reconstructing anatomical relationship
  - Ununited femoral neck fracture with a viable head
  - Congenital coxa vara
  - Avascular necrosis involving a small well-circumscribed area
  - *Oval head with capital drop osteophyte:* Bombelli named the medial femoral head osteophyte in DDH as "capital drop osteophyte". A valgus producing osteotomy would load it and open the superior joint surface, helping acetabulum remodeling and improving coverage.
  - Spastic cerebral palsy
- *Uncommon indications:*
  - Deformity after healed acetabular fracture
  - Hip arthrodesis healed in malposition
  - Coxa valga
  - Chronic slipped capital epiphysis
  - Excessive anteversion in a child
  - Perthes disease—varus derotation in subtrochanteric region is preferred.
- *Doubtful indications in modern orthopedic practice:*
  - Young patients with advanced osteoarthrosis. It is difficult to find such patients in clinical practice and even then the advances in arthroplasty outweigh the need of osteotomy in such patients. The rationale portended behind the practice of osteotomy in such cases is mainly of theoretical concern and the author is personally unaware of any current practice of doing osteotomy for this indication. The intertrochanteric osteotomy helps by a combination of the following mechanisms in primarily relieving pain:
    - Results in local hyperemia
    - Improved venous drainage
    - Helps remodeling of the architecture
    - Increase in the joint contact area with a resultant decrease in stress
    - An increase in the length of the muscle effort arm
    - Relaxation of the periarticular musculature

Indications for osteotomy must account for subsequent future total hip arthroplasty considering its popularity. Implantation is difficult after an osteotomy which can cause important technical problems. The rate of failure of arthroplasty following osteotomy is also very high.

Rationale of Intertrochanteric Osteotomy

Intertrochanteric osteotomy has both a "mechanical and biological effect" producing relief in various pathologies as follows:

- Altering the mechanics by medially shifting the line of weight-bearing
- Correction of deformity
- Realignment of the limb during movement
- Relaxation of contracted joint capsule
- Improved stability
- Psoas relaxation (similar effect as "hanging hip of Voss")
- Improved congruity of joint surfaces
- Improved leverage
- Change of weight-bearing region reducing contact stress and degeneration
- Wider surface of contact
- Relief of pressure by release of muscles
- Redistribution of tensile forces at the fracture line to compression forces

Prerequisites for Performing Intertrochanteric Osteotomies

- The hip should be mobile in >90° of flexion (assessment of articular range of motion should be performed under general anesthesia with or without tenotomy)
- Abduction >15° is necessary for varus correction.
- Adduction >15° for valgus osteotomies

General Operative Technique

- An intertrochanteric osteotomy is performed principally proximal to the lesser trochanter with a transverse cut.
- A varus-producing osteotomy is usually performed with a transverse osteotomy at the superior aspect of the lesser trochanter and a 90° blade plate for reduction and fixation of the osteotomy fragments. If the blade is inserted at a 110° angle to the femoral shaft in the frontal plane, a 20° correction will be obtained when the 90° blade plate is inserted and the osteotomy is reduced **(Figs. 1A to D)**.

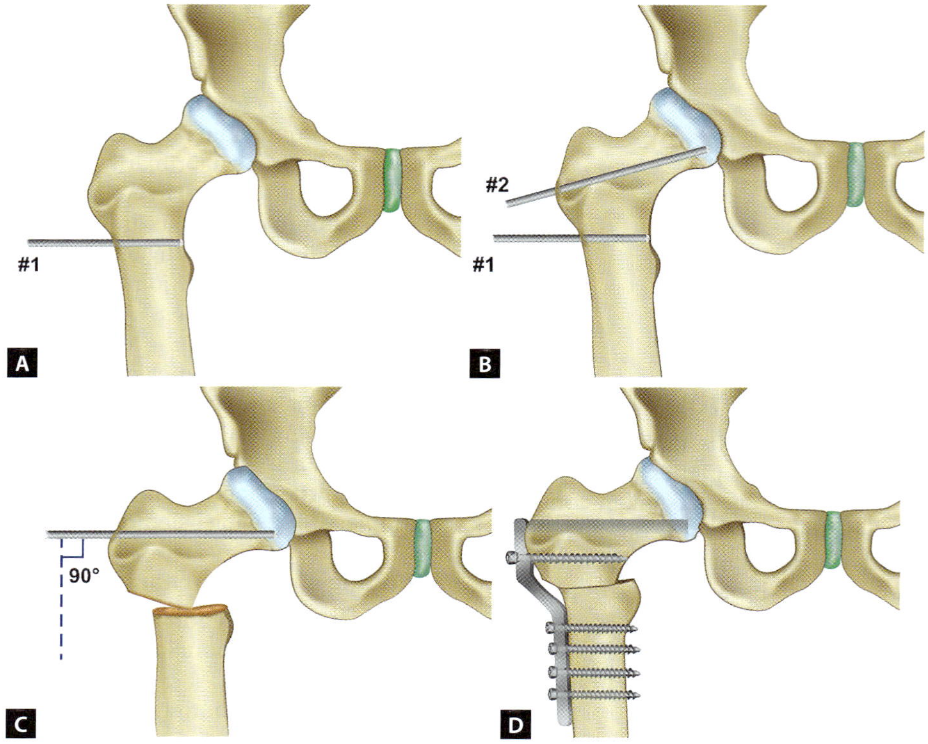

Figs. 1A to D: Varus intertrochanteric proximal femoral osteotomy. (A) Horizontal guidewire insertion at the site for anticipated transverse intertrochanteric osteotomy; (B) Second guidewire at predetermined site for blade plate chisel position to obtain varus correction; (C) Osteotomy reduction and fixation with a 90° blade plate; (D) Osteotomy and reduction with varus correction and medial displacement of the femoral shaft.

For valgus osteotomies the procedure is reversed. Here, an angled-blade plate (usually 120° or 130°) is utilized. The amount of valgus correction is determined by the angle of insertion and the blade-plate angle, a 40° correction is obtained by inserting a 130° blade plate at a 90° angle to the femoral shaft in the frontal plane. With reduction of the osteotomy and fixation of the plate, a 40° correction will be obtained **(Fig. 2)**, but this is not as simple always (see below). Sagittal plane correction say flexion is added to the osteotomy by inserting the blade plate with anterior angulation with respect to the sagittal plane of the femur. Upon reduction of the osteotomy, a relative apex posterior angulation is produced between the osteotomy fragments **(Fig. 3)**.

- The rotational malalignment is corrected before the displacement or angular corrections are made.
- Once the rotational corrections are achieved, appropriate wedges are removed in frontal or sagittal planes. Varus osteotomies cause shortening so transverse osteotomies are made to preserve as much bone as possible, while as valgus osteotomies lengthen, the limb wedge is removed to equalize limb lengths.
- Osteotomy is then fixed with one of the implants as follows:
  - Varus intertrochanteric osteotomy—90° double-angle-blade plate
  - Valgus osteotomy—120° or 130° double-angle-blade plate

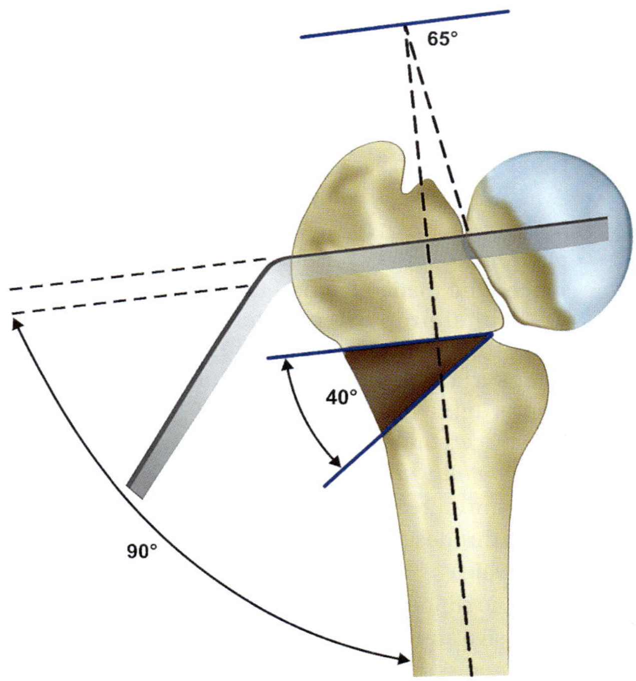

Fig. 2: Valgus intertrochanteric osteotomy. The 130° blade plate is inserted at 90° to the femoral shaft. When it is reduced for fixation 40° correction will be obtained (helped by wedge removal).

  - Locked compression plate is a new implant suitable for most of the osteotomies including weak bone of osteoporosis or dysfunctional/paralytic limbs.

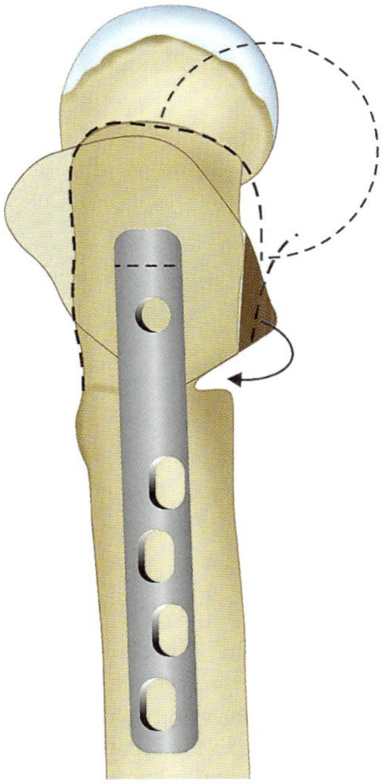

Fig. 3: Producing sagittal plane correction in addition to coronal correction. For an extension osteotomy, the blade is inserted with the "L" limb (to be fixed to shaft) pointing posteriorly (toward floor in operation theater) at an angle equal to the desired correction. When it is fixed to the shaft, the proximal fragment has to be rotated superiorly/anteriorly producing anterior angulation at the osteotomy site and thus an equivalent extension osteotomy. Same step is done for flexion osteotomy only the "L" limb is kept anterior (toward roof) to start with.

VARIOUS COMMONLY PERFORMED OSTEOTOMIES

Modified Muller Osteotomy for Pseudoarthrosis of Femoral Neck Fracture (Also *see* Chapter on "Nonunions and Malunions" for details on Its Rationale to Use in Nonunion Fracture Neck of Femur)

Pauwels' Type II Valgus Osteotomy as Modified by Muller (also called "Y"-shaped Pauwels' Osteotomy)

The aim of surgery is to achieve Pauwels' angle at fracture site from 25° to 30° to bring the fracture site under compression to achieve sound union of the fractures. The other option for nonunion fracture neck of femur is McMurray's type osteotomy.

Rationale of Pauwels' II Osteotomy as Modified by Muller for Ununited Fracture Neck of Femur

The mechanical axis passes through the center of the head of the femur, center of the knee, and then through the center of the ankle. It subtends an angle of 3° with the vertical and 5–7° with the anatomical axis of the femoral shaft. Thus, the vertical axis forms an angle of 9–10° ('3°'+ '5° to 7°') with the anatomical axis of the shaft of the femur. The resultant of the body weight forms an angle of 16° with the vertical. Therefore, the anatomical axis of the femoral shaft forms an angle of 25° (16° + 9°) with the resultant of the compressive forces **(Fig. 4A)**.

- *Compression effect:* Hence, a pseudoarthrosis of the femoral neck fracture will sustain compressive forces if it is kept inclined at 25° with the perpendicular to the femoral shaft axis.
- *Lengthening effect for a short limb:* Valgus intertrochanteric osteotomy results in rotation of the upper segment of the femur in a clockwise manner for the left hip and counterclockwise direction for the right hip. The osteotomy line is oblique running downward and laterally, hence, its lateral end gets displaced distally, resulting in lengthening which is desirable for shortened limb.

Prerequisite

The patient should have requisite adduction available at hip for good postoperative movements and compensation after the osteotomy. When kept in complementary adduction (say 25° adduction for 25° valgus producing osteotomy) the hip should be painless preoperatively.

The angle of osteotomy for the pseudoarthrosis is determined by subtracting 25° from the angle which the pseudoarthrosis makes with the perpendicular dropped to the femoral shaft axis. Say for a Pauwels' angle of 65° the osteotomy angle would be 40° **(Fig. 4B)**. Still, care should be taken not to extend the proximal fragment > 25–30° or future hip arthroplasty may be more difficult.

Advantages

- Limb length equality can be achieved.
- Lateralization can be achieved to prevent genu valgum.
- Osteotomy can be fixed and patient can be mobilized at the earliest.
- Subsequent total hip replacement (THR) can be performed.

Disadvantages

- Stresses per unit area of femoral head increased.
- Reduced abductor efficiency (reduced offset) though this is compensated by increased length of abductor muscles. Still limp may be persistent due to abductor weakness.

Steps of Surgery **(Figs. 5A to D)**

- Stabilize the femoral neck fracture with a 6.5-mm cancellous screw prior to insertion of the seating chisel.
- Entry point for chisel is made in the anterior half of the greater trochanter to locate the chisel/blade in the center of the femoral neck.
- The seating chisel is inserted into the femoral neck along the wire k3 (the chisel is not parallel to this k-wire) with its vertical flap "i" set at an angle of 100° (the angle is made with the hammering side of chisel). The chisel in this instance will hence be seated at an angle of 80° to the femoral shaft (= 120°—osteotomy angle). The flap is always kept parallel to the vertical axis (If one uses 130° blade plate then seating angle would be 90°).
- With the chisel in situ in the femoral head, the 35° intertrochanteric wedge of bone "k"-based laterally is excised. The distal osteotomy cut is made first followed by proximal complete cut to protect come calcar medially to

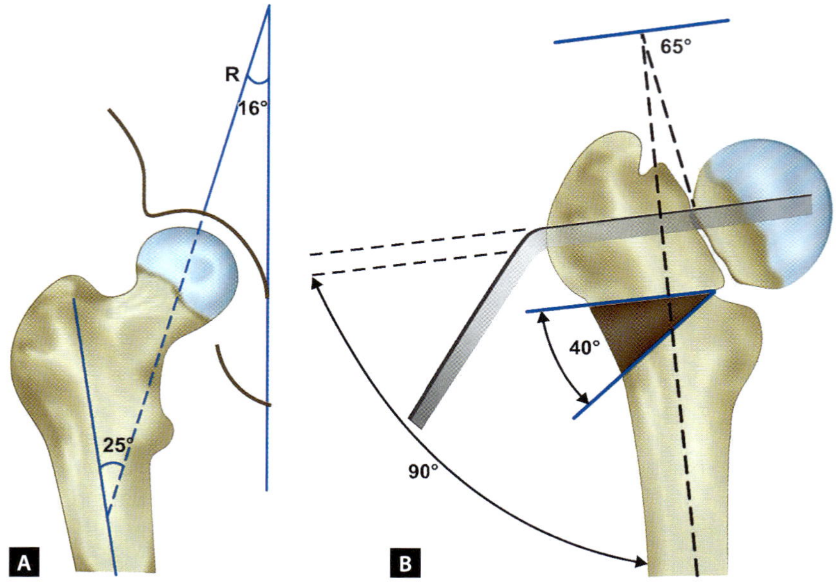

Figs. 4A and B: (A) The resultant of forces across hip form an angle of 25° to the anatomical axis of femoral shaft and 16° to the vertical; (B) For valgus intertrochanteric osteotomy, the osteotomy angle is calculated as the angle of fracture line –25°. This is due to the fact that if the fracture line/plane is oriented at 25° then the forces will pass perpendicular to the fracture producing maximal compression and minimal shear. In this example, the osteotomy angle hence is 65° – 25° = 40°.

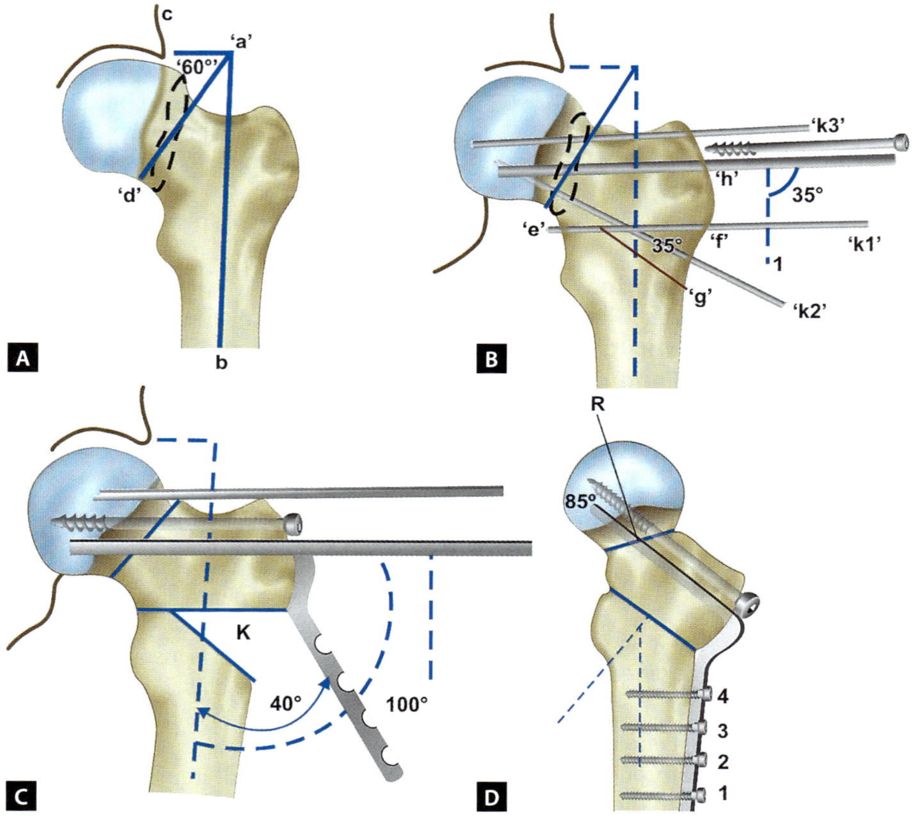

Figs. 5A to D: Steps of Muller modification of Pauwels' osteotomy. (A)"ab" femoral shaft axis, "ac" perpendicular to femoral axis, "ad" fracture line forming angle to the perpendicular ("ac") to femoral shaft axis ("ab"); (B) Draw a line "ef" at right angle to the femoral shaft a little above the superior margin of lesser trochanter. Draw a line "eg" making an angle equal to the osteotomy angle. Angle "feg" = osteotomy angle. "h" represents the entry point of chisel which is 2–2.5 cm from the line "ef" and accommodates the curve of osteotomy blade plate. Three k-wires (k1, k2, and k3) are passed along the lines "ef", "eg", and one perpendicular to vertical from point "h"; (C) The osteotomy blade plate's blade is inserted. The plate should subtend an angle equal to the osteotomy angle with the vertical axis. The blade/chisel will subtend an angle of 100° to the vertical axis; (D) The shaft is abducted and fixed to the osteotomy plate by screws.

act as a hinge. There are two ways of calculating the size of wedge:

1. *Approximation method:* It is generally considered that 1° of angle corresponds to 1 mm of wedge size (which is really crude but very easy). This means that for angle of correction of 40° we need a wedge of 40 mm. The approximation method is often incorrect but if one sees practically up to 3–4 mm error in the correct direction will not make much difference, if still performed meticulously.
2. *Geometric method:* This relies on the tangent to the angle of correction and diameter of the bone at osteotomy site. The size of wedge is given by the formula:

Wedge in mm = Tangent to angle of correction × Angle of correction × Diameter of bone

This is a bit difficult for general calculation purposes so a simpler version is as follows:

Wedge in mm = 0.02 × Angle of correction × Diameter of bone at the osteotomy

- Remove the chisel and insert the osteotomy blade plate into the slot.
- Abduct the limb to close the osteotomy by inserting screws from distal to proximal direction one by one.

Complications

- Avascular necrosis of femoral head
- Loss of position of the fragments
- Infection
- Technical failures

Pauwels' Type I (Varus Intertrochanteric Osteotomy)

This is a rarely performed osteotomy and has limited indications.

Indications

- Developmental dysplasia of the hip—only if little or no acetabular dysplasia to improve coverage. Center-edge (CE) angle should be >15–20°.
- Perthes—to improve coverage
- Osteoarthritis with severely deformed flattened hip enlarged by medial osteophyte (Pauwels' original indication)
- Osteonecrosis of femoral head—if medial head involved (unusual)
- Coxa valga > 135°:
  - Lateral subluxation of head
  - Signs of lateral overload, i.e., eccentric sourcil
  - Adduction contracture

Requirements

- Spherical head
- Increased congruity in maximal abduction
- Minimum 15° abduction

Contraindication

Head osteophyte

Valgus Intertrochanteric/Pauwels' Type II

Indications

- *Osteonecrosis:* To unload anterolateral head—usually valgus-flexion combined osteotomy
- Nonunion fracture neck of femur
- Severe osteoarthritis (OA) with medial osteophytes—the capital-drop osteophyte (inferomedial femoral head osteophyte):
  - Acts as fulcrum against acetabular osteophyte
  - Widens the superolateral joint surface
- Coxa vara:
  - Congenital/developmental
  - Fibrous dysplasia
- Protrusio in young patient
- Fixed abduction contracture

Requirement

Preserved ROM of hip joint—90° flexion and 15° adduction/abduction, normal contralateral hip.

Technique

The osteotomy is aimed for restoring the neck-shaft angle or increasing the same to reorient the forces across the neck. Mostly one aims for neck-shaft angle 145–150°.

CURVED VARUS OSTEOTOMY FOR OSTEONECROSIS (FIGS. 6A AND B)

Initially it was devised as a treatment for OA of the hip by Pauwels' and later adapted for osteonecrosis by Merle d'Aubigné et al. and Kerboul et al.

Technique

- The greater trochanter is exposed by detaching the posterior sections of the insertion of gluteus medius and minimus.
- A curved Kirschner wire (K-wire) is prepared by adjusting it according to the preoperative radiograph in the line from the greater to lesser trochanter.
- Under fluoroscopic guidance, this wire is introduced into the intertrochanteric region and multiple drill holes are made from the posterior to anterior cortex.
- An intertrochanteric curved osteotomy is then carried out from the greater to lesser trochanter using a 5-mm osteotome.
- The anterior periosteum is then dissected along the line of the osteotomy and the femoral head rotated into a varus position by displacing the femoral neck in a cranial direction.
- Fixation of osteotomy is done using compression hip screws.

Advantages

- Similar to dome type osteotomies
- Provide good stability
- Possibility to add flexion or adduction component

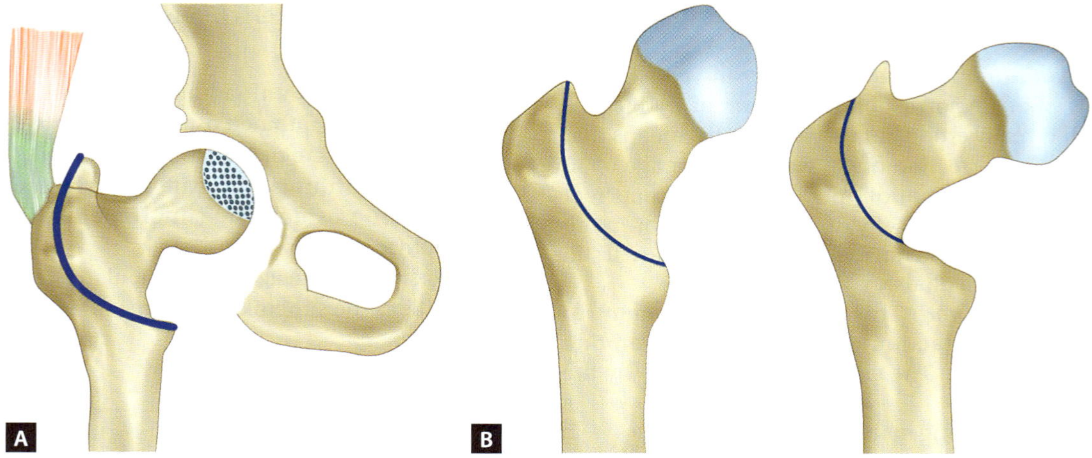

Figs. 6A and B: (A) Site for creating the curved varus producing osteotomy for superomedial osteonecrotic location; (B) The needed displacement for shifting the weight-bearing region.

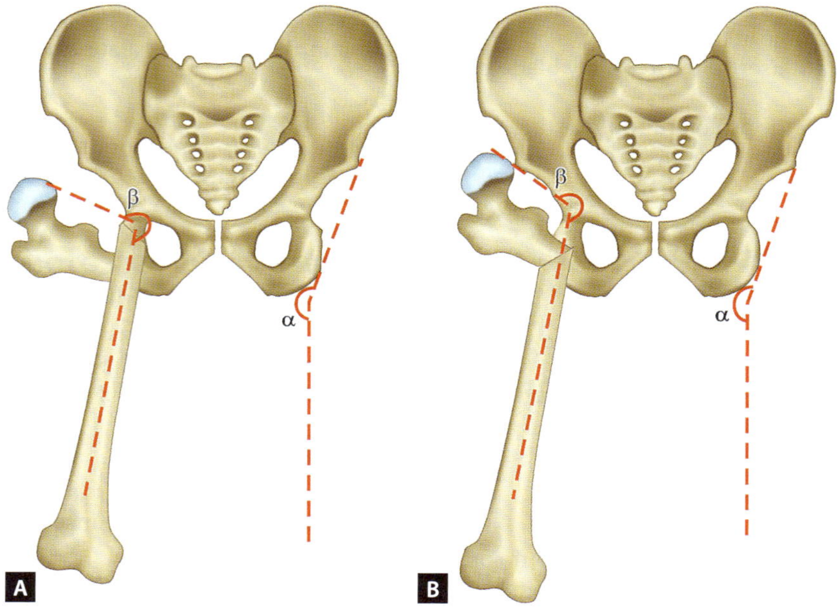

Figs. 7A and B: The pelvic support osteotomy of (A) Schanz; and (B) Lorenz. Milch described a postosteotomy angle (β) which predicted abutment against the lateral wall of the pelvis when it exceeded the angle of pelvic inclination (α).

Disadvantages

- Cumbersome when simpler alternatives are available.
- Fixation is tenuous.
- Nonunion, malunion
- Abductors are put at disadvantage causing weakness and possible lurch.

PELVIC SUPPORT OSTEOTOMY (PSO) ALSO KNOWN AS RESECTION ANGULATION OSTEOTOMY

The PSO is a double-level femoral osteotomy with the objective of eliminating a Trendelenburg and short-limb gait in young patients with unstable hips. It can also be done to stabilize hips after resection arthroplasty or infected prosthesis removal to stabilize hip. The surgery is performed at two levels in femur:

1. The proximal valgus-extension osteotomy is performed with the femur in maximum adduction and at a level where the femoral shaft is seen to abut the pelvis.
2. The second distal osteotomy restores the limb alignment by bringing the knee and ankle joint lines in the coronal plane.

Femoral lengthening at the distal osteotomy site is optional (propagated by Ilizarov).

The proximal osteotomy component (hip component) can be of various types and modifications described by Schanz, Lorenz **(Figs. 7A and B)**, Gruca, Milch, Bachelor, Carry, McMurray's osteotomy, etc. This osteotomy component is detailed below. The primary aims of proximal osteotomy are to:

- Lateralize greater trochanter
- Distally displace greater trochanter—improve abductor strength

- Eliminate adduction between femur and pelvis preventing pelvic drop
- Reduce limp by abolishing Trendelenburg lurch
- Equalize limb length by stabilizing the hemipelvis
- Produce energy efficient gait

Depending on the type of osteotomy and methodology used to obtain pelvic support to the femoral shaft the osteotomy can be of two types, as has been exploited by different authors:

1. Medial displacement osteotomy (McMurray)
2. Valgus angulation and alteration of mechanical axis (Schanz, Milch)

History

- The term "pelvic support" was first used by Lance in 1936, where he performed subtrochanteric osteotomy in DDH.
- Medial displacement osteotomies have been described even earlier.
- Lorenz designed a valgus osteotomy coupled to proximal and medial displacement of the shaft of femur but this resulted in prominence of the displaced femoral shaft until it gets remodeled or is surgically removed. Also it resulted in abutment of femur to pelvis that reduced movements.
- Schanz osteotomy is a valgus, extension osteotomy without proximally displacing the femoral shaft. It also resulted in abutment however.
- Milch studied the problem of abutment and described the pelvic inclination (α) and postosteotomy angle (β) and their mutual relationships to prevent it **(Figs. 7 and 8)**.
- Ilizarov circumvented the problem of excessive angle β by adding the distal femoral osteotomy to realign the parallelism and bring knee and ankle in coronal plane, so that no ankle eversion is needed and the opposite hip adduction contracture does not develop. Also, lengthening of the limb can be done in such circumstances.

Current Indications

The current indications for PSO include the following:

- Neglected DDH
- Sequel of septic arthritis with Hunka types 4 or 5
- Instability following girdlestone resection arthroplasty (now girdlestone arthroplasty is considered mutilating, so not performed; however, this is in reference to context where a prosthesis has been removed due to intractable infection literally producing a girdlestone hip)
- Neglected traumatic hip dislocation with instability
- Femoral neck nonunion

Contraindications

For pediatric uses of PSO:

- Age older than 12 years (reduced remodeling capability, shortening, and reduced movements)
- Total hip replacement could be an alternative later.
- Chronic paralytic hip dislocations in nonambulatory patients

For failed reconstructions in elderly:

- Too osteoporotic bone
- Unresolved/continuing infection

Clinical Assessment for Performing PSO

Measure the adduction/abduction/flexion/extension contracture. The amount of adduction contracture needs to be added to the maximum extent of hip adduction possible to determine the size valgus correction at the proximal osteotomy **(Fig. 8)**. One must, however, note that the femur is at 9° varus to vertical axis **(Fig. 9)**, so:

Size of valgus correction = (Adduction contracture + Amount of maximal adduction) – 9°

Overcorrection by 15–25° has been recommended by various authors in anticipation for remodeling and some atrophy of the soft tissue between proximal femur and pelvic wall **(Fig. 8)**. Radiologically, the angle α is better measured by double leg weight-bearing stance rather than the single stance drop-angle of pelvis. The angle for distal osteotomy (corrective) will be given by the difference between measured angle α and determined valgus angle with overcorrection **(Fig. 10)**.

Level of Osteotomies

The level of proximal osteotomy varies with the pathology for which it has been planned. The classical level at horizontal plane passing through ischial tuberosity holds true for many, but in cases with extreme proximal migration of femur (such as congenital dislocations, etc.), level at superior border of obturator foramen is chosen.

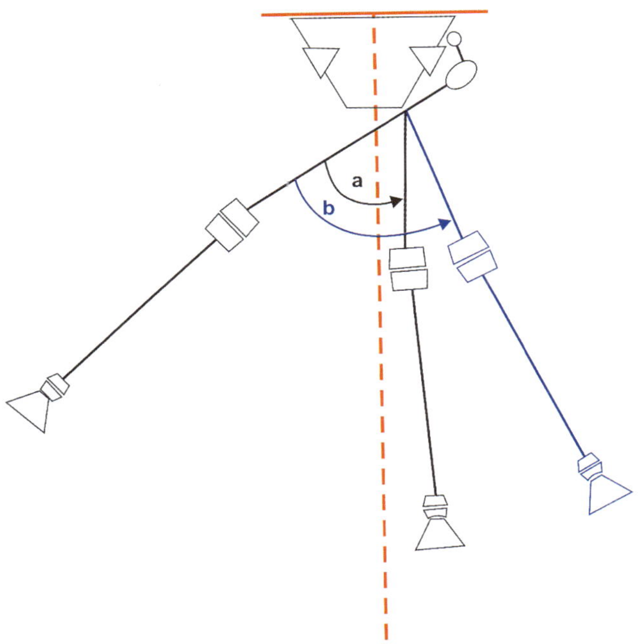

Fig. 8: Performing a valgus osteotomy equal in size to the maximum range of adduction (gray schematic representation of the limb) plus any adduction contracture will bring the femoral shaft to its normal inclination of 9° to the vertical. Bringing the shaft to vertical therefore overcorrects by 9° (black-colored limb schematic diagram). This does not lateralize the shaft or knee joint sufficiently. But, the limb is still positioned too close to the midline. Also, therefore, an overcorrection in the region of 25–30° is preferable to allow a shift of the limb from the midline (blue-colored lines) which is achieved by adding 15–25° to calculated osteotomy angle.

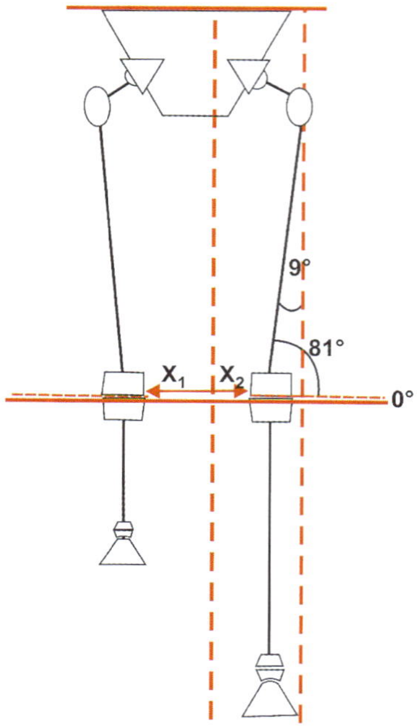

Fig. 9: In single stance, the knee and ankle joints of the weight-bearing limb are horizontal and parallel to the pelvic line. There is slight adduction at the hip. The femoral shaft subtends an angle of 9° to the midline vertical axis.

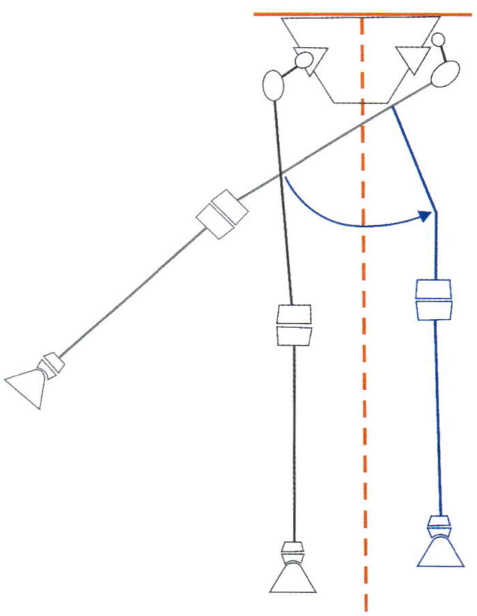

Fig. 10: The second osteotomy removes the excess abduction created by the subtrochanteric osteotomy. It allows both limbs to be parallel, with the knee, ankle, and the pelvis horizontal. Also lengthening at this osteotomy corrects limb length inequality.

The level and size of distal osteotomy is planned so as to bring the knee and ankle in coronal plane **(Fig. 11)**. The site of the distal osteotomy varies with the amount of valgus overcorrection introduced and also varies if the position of the proximal osteotomy is in line with the medial edge of the ischial tuberosity as compared with its lateral edge. The site should be appropriately chosen as proximal osteotomy location will medialize the whole limb. Size of correction and level may be determined trignometrically or by radiographic method.

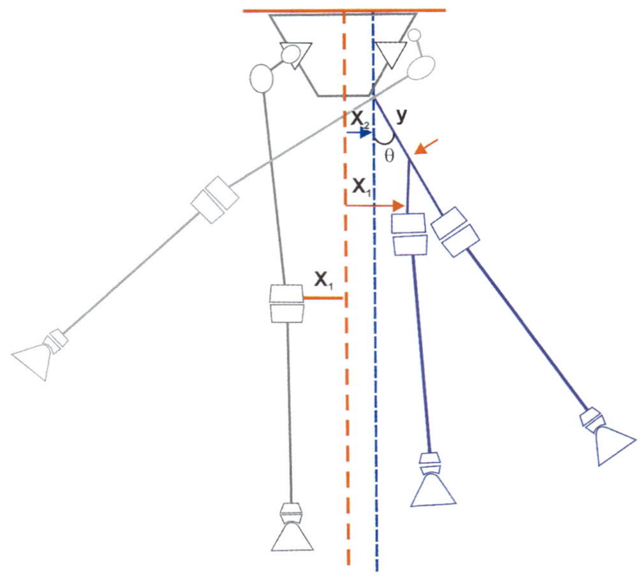

Fig. 11: The level of the second osteotomy can be determined by radiographic method.

- *Radiographic method* ***(Fig. 11):*** Measure distance of the center of the contralateral knee to the midline axis of the body. Also measure distance of the proposed proximal osteotomy site from the midline axis of the body. Leave 10–12° of valgus overcorrection at knee. 9° of overcorrection is needed for aligning femur parallel to vertical axis. So total overcorrection is usually in the range of 20–25°.
- *Trigonometric method:* The following equation gives the level of distal femoral osteotomy:

$$\text{Sin } \theta = (x_1 - x_2)/y$$

Where, *y* is the distance along the shaft of femur to second osteotomy. θ is angle of overcorrection = 9°; x_1 and x_2 are the distances from the midline **(Fig. 11)**.

Amount of Valgus

One thing important is that even with overcorrection of 15–25° the Milch recommendation of 240° is not reached for which 30–40° overcorrection is needed. One should not be wary of overcorrection which will improve stability as this will be compensated by second osteotomy being done at distal femur.

Amount of Extension and Derotation

Extension is added to compensate for flexion deformity/contracture. Normally, a correction of around 20° is added. Rotational correction is done based on foot-progression angle profile of the patient and the rotational malalignment of foot in full adduction.

MILCH-BACHELOR OSTEOTOMY

The two stage resection angulation osteotomy as described in 1943 by Henry Milch (New York) and Bachelor JS (London) separately comprises two stages:

1. Release of pelvis and restoration of femoral mobility (resection of femoral head and neck)
2. Re-establishment of stability by means of PSO (Schanz)

Problems

- Traction is needed after first stage to prevent upward migration of femur followed by immobilization for second stage for osteotomy. This causes stiffness and often restriction of movements.
- If osteotomy is done first then resection of femoral head and neck is difficult in second stage.
- Therefore, one stage resection angulation surgery was proposed by Milch and Gruca.

Indications of PSO (Milch Bachelor Type)

- Bilateral neglected DDH in underprivileged patients, too young for total hip arthroplasty (THA) or inability to bear the hip arthroplasty or its stringent precautions
- Failed hip arthroplasty
- Ankylosing spondylitis in younger patients

Postosteotomy Angle (β)

The postosteotomy angle (angle of osteotomy) should be congruent to the lateral pelvic wall tilt/inclination [α, the inclination of pelvic wall is a mean of 205–210° (males = 211° ± 5.8°, females = 206.4° ± 4.7°, in DDH it reduces to 190° approximately)] of acetabulum. The angle β should always be determined before performing any osteotomy and should be between 210° and 240°.

- If angle is more than the angle of pelvic wall α, it will produce increased stability but at the expense of:
  - Limited movements
  - Excessive downward ipsilateral tilting
  - Relative shortening of the contralateral limb
- If angle is less than the acetabular tilt α then:
  - Ipsilateral tilting is discouraged.
  - Impaired stability
  - Disparity in limb length remains uncorrected.

The principle of Milch type PSO is to compensate for the shortening produced by resection of femoral head and neck by inducing compensatory lengthening of the limb by pelvic tilt. The problem of increased β can now be successfully handled by a second distal femoral osteotomy to realign the limb and also do lengthening (ilizarov).

Procedure Details

The site of osteotomy is predetermined by radiological planning on radiographs. It is at the level of ischial tuberosity. There is a limit to which the pelvis can tilt for compensation. Usually the upper limit of pelvic tilt is 20–25° so the degree to which the postosteotomy angle can be permitted to exceed the determined angulation of lateral pelvic wall should not be >15–20°. His tilt permits correction of disparity up to 5 cm, for any more deformity it is better to use shoe-raise than increasing the angle, else problems mentioned above will come.

The osteotomy is performed through a lateral iliofemoral approach extending from anterior superior iliac spine (ASIS) to the base of trochanter and downward along the lateral aspect of femur. The nerve to tensor fascia lata is usually sacrificed. The plane between the gluteus medius and tensor fascia is developed and neck is resected at the intertrochanteric line. Subtrochanteric osteotomy is performed at the predetermined level and distal fragment is abducted and internally rotated to 20–25°. Internal rotation is done to compensate for the external rotation that is produced due to loss of pelvic support.

Complications

- Wound infection
- Excessive postosteotomy angle causes postoperative pain.
- Genu valgum (due to tendency of the limb to undergo external rotation)
- Limp is produced dueto shortening and flexion contracture.

McMURRAY'S OSTEOTOMY

The osteotomy is an intertrochanteric medial displacement of PSO **(Fig. 12)** wherein the body weight is transmitted to the distal fragment displaced under the head of the femur.

- The osteotomy begins just below the level of lesser trochanter at the lateral cortex of femur and proceeds in an oblique manner to exit proximal to the lesser trochanter medially. The obliquity of osteotomy permits:
  - Medial displacement of shaft
  - Psoas major pull at lesser trochanter maintains the displacement.
  - The distal fragment to come in direct contact with the fracture site and the femoral head permitting weight transmission directly
- The lower fragment is displaced medially (not >50% width of medullary canal) by manual pressure and abduction so that it is placed under the head of the femur.
- The fracture has been classically fixed using wainwright spline but osteotomy blade plate or other suitable implant (S-P nail with Tupman plate, etc.) may also be used.

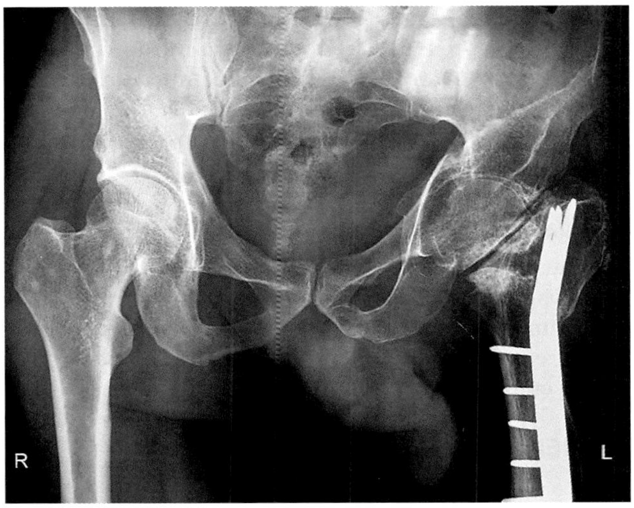

Fig. 12: McMurray's intertrochanteric medial displacement osteotomy—even if the fracture did not unite (as is often the case) the osteotomy serves to act as a good support to the pelvis.

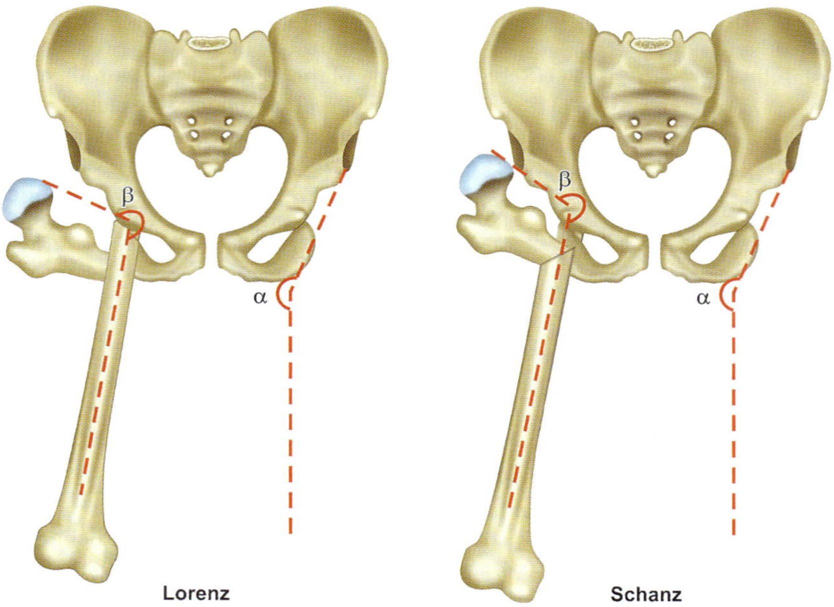

Fig. 13: The Lorenz and Schanz proximal femoral osteotomies.

- Abduction is maintained at the osteotomy site during implant fixation which is gradually reduced later after 3 weeks.

McMurray's displacement osteotomy is effective in treating nonunion of transcervical fracture neck femur in the following two ways:

1. *By making the fracture line more horizontal:* The osteotomy is fixed in abduction of distal fragment, when the abduction is reduced the fracture line becomes more and more horizontal (effect similar to Pauwels' valgus osteotomy). With weight-bearing the psoas pull also helps in adduction and valgus rotation of the head. This renewed horizontal orientation converts shearing forces to compressive forces and promotes union.
2. *"Arm chair effect":* This refers to bypassing of shear forces across the fracture site; actually, the forces across the fracture site are reduced so shear displacement of the fracture is prevented, encouraging union. The distal fragment bears weight partially transmitted directly from the head-capsule-ligament region to the distal fragment. Even if the fracture does not unite, painless weight-bearing is possible.

Disadvantages

- It causes shortening.
- Predisposes knee to genu valgum
- Proximal fixation of the osteotomy is difficult and prone to failure, so one must slowly produce abduction.
- Subsequent THR is difficult due to canal abnormality.

LORENZ BIFURCATION OSTEOTOMY

The idea of the Lorenz osteotomy is to convert the abnormal upper end of the dislocated femur into a fork at the top of the shaft or, more usually, into an inverted L. The angle rests in the true acetabulum, while the tip of the short limb remains in or near the false acetabulum in the region of the anterior inferior spine, and the long limb is represented by the femoral shaft. Commonly, a variant of osteotomy is used where the shaft is divided in the subtrochanteric region **(Fig. 13)**. The distal fragment is then pushed into the lower aspect of acetabulum creating significant shortening.

Lorenz principle is to make an intertrochanteric osteotomy in the coronal plane, the frontal plane of the body, so that when the upper end of the shaft is guided into the true acetabulum, its raw posterior surface continues in contact with the raw anterior surface of the upper fragment; this prevents it from slipping backward and makes hyperextension of the limb easy and also induces early bone union.

- Incision—curved incision convex downward
- Exposing acetabulum—done along the anterior aspect of the undivided shaft and neck of femur.
- Osteotomy cut—passes from the top of greater trochanter downward and inward, to the region of the small trochanter, with the blade of the osteotome held in the frontal (coronal) plane. The bone must be cut clean and not broken to allow smooth seating of the shaft into acetabulum.

SCHANZ OSTEOTOMY (LOW SUBTROCHANTERIC OSTEOTOMY)

The osteotomy is similar to Milch osteotomy **(Fig. 13)** but no angle β is calculated. The major emphasis is providing stability to the pelvis through malformed or absent hip joint. The corrections in flexion, adduction, and external rotation are made by making the osteotomy at ischial tuberosity level.

Advantages

- Lurching gait will be diminished.
- The depression of the trochanter also improves the leverage of the glutei.

Contraindication

Before 15 years of age, because loss of angulation occurs during growth period later.

TROCHANTERIC OSTEOTOMIES

The trochanteric osteotomies include surgical procedures that are concerned with repositioning of greater trochanter or displacement of the same to provide improved exposure of the hip joint. They can be divided into two types:

1. Repositioning osteotomies (these are dealt with in appropriate chapters in Section on "Pediatric Orthopedics"):
   a. Trochanteric advancement osteotomy
   b. Trochanteric arthroplasty
2. Trochanteric osteotomies for exposure of hip joint and arthroplasty **(Fig. 14)**:
   - For primary hip arthroplasty or management of fracture of head of femur (a part of surgical dislocation of hip). It is needed in patients with previous osteotomies of proximal femur that distort the anatomy precluding direct access to the femoral canal.
   - Revision arthroplasty for removal of stem often

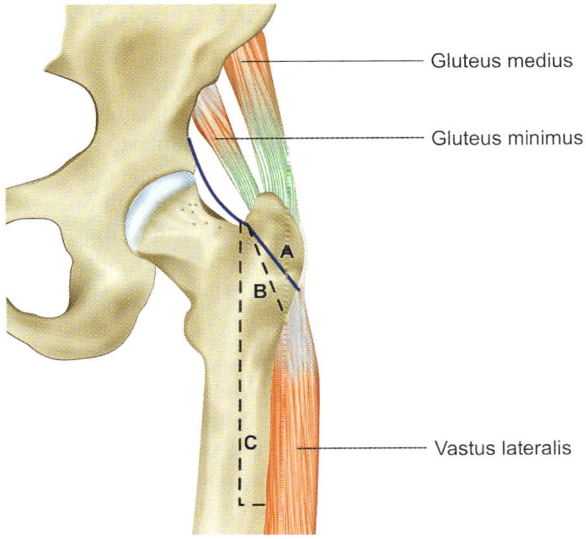

Fig. 14: The planes for the standard trochanteric osteotomy (A), the trochanteric slide (B), and the extended trochanteric osteotomy (C). The standard osteotomy spares vastus lateralis.

Standard Trochanteric Osteotomy

Indications

Wider than normal exposure of the hip needed:

- Complex primary THA, e.g., in patients with previous femoral osteotomy or in ankylosed hips fixed in external rotation where exposure is done with posterior approach.
- Protrusio acetabuli (trochanteric slide is better suited.)
- Complex acetabular reconstruction
- Total hip arthroplasty in a patient with unacceptable laxity of abductors that cannot be corrected otherwise as in DDH.
- Cases where femur needs to be shortened as in high hip center making the hip lax.

Contraindication

Total hip arthroplasty or revision done using Hardinge approach.

Steps

- Expose the hip joint.
- Protect capsule by placing Hohman retractor between it and gluteus minimus
- Release the origin of the vastus lateralis from the vastus tubercle.
- Make an osteotomy cut 1 cm distal to the vastus tubercle at the sulcus between the lateral portion of the origin of the vastus intermedius muscle and the insertions of the gluteus medius and minimus in a distal to proximal direction. When using a gigli saw proximal to distal direction, osteotomy progression is done **(Fig. 15)**
- The trochanter is released from short external rotators and flipped proximally.
- Reattachment—after completion of procedure the attachment is made by a four-wire technique **(Fig. 16)** In cases with poor bone quality (revision, osteoporotic, rheumatoid, etc.) it is recommended to use a wire mesh for reattachment.

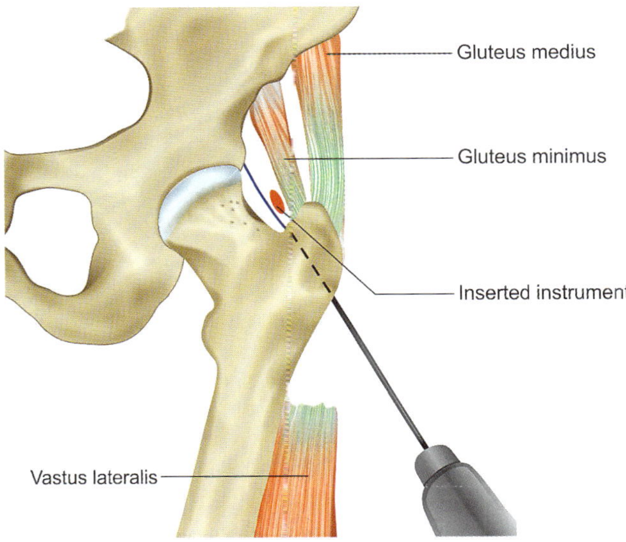

Fig. 15: Standard trochanteric osteotomy. The plane of cut spare abductors (by a retractor), capsule (under direct vision), and vastus lateralis. Osteotomy. It traverses from the sulcus between the origin of the vastus intermedius muscle and the insertions of the gluteus medius and maximus distal to the vastus tubercle and extending medially to the junction of the greater trochanter and the lateral portion of the femoral neck.

Complications

- Nonunion
- Migration
- Abductor insufficiency
- Instability
- Lateral hip pain, mainly due to hardware but removal does not guarantee alleviation
- Heterotopic ossification

Chevron (Biplane) Trochanteric Osteotomy (Figs. 17A and B)

The chevron osteotomy was developed to:

- *Improve intrinsic stability:* The geometry of the cut provides inherent stability with resistance to rotation and displacement.
- Reduce the incidence of trochanteric nonunion.

The chevron osteotomy can be done using either an osteotome or an oscillating saw to create a fragment with a concave, chevron-shaped medial surface.

Trochanteric Slide

Here, the distal attachment of vastus lateralis remains intact and is not removed as for standard osteotomy **(Figs. 18A and B)**. This preserves the blood supply and prevents proximal migration of the greater trochanter, but the thickness of trochanteric bone is significantly less than the standard osteotomy. Rest all the steps are more or less same. This technique was described in detail in 1987 by Glassman et al. The trochanteric slide can be converted to a conventional osteotomy by releasing the vastus lateralis muscle origin for additional exposure. The indications are similar to standard osteotomy, few more additions could be—impaction bone grafting and cemented revisions, protrusio acetabuli, and surgical dislocation of hip joint.

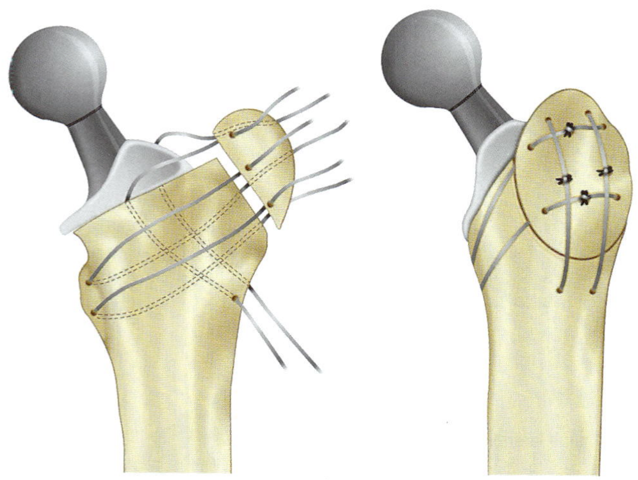

Fig. 16: The four-wire technique for fixation of the standard trochanteric osteotomy.

Contraindication

Absence of medial bone for wire or cable placement and insufficient trochanter thickness, resulting in an inadequate bed for repair and healing.

Steps

- Expose the hip using direct lateral incision.
- Elevate vastus lateralis subperiosteally from lateral and anterior aspect of femoral shaft region (till 15 cm below the vastus lateralis ridge) and retract anteriorly.
- Osteotomize trochanter and retract anteriorly with the muscular sleeve. The attachment of short external rotators and gluteus minimus are sharply incised.
- Dislocation is then done by external rotation and adduction.
- Reattachment—trochanteric reattachment is done with two wires (**Fig. 19**, arthroplasty) or cancellous fully threaded screws (fixation of Pipkin fractures).

Oblique Trochanteric Osteotomy

This was devised for increasing the somewhat limited exposure that is sometimes obtained with a direct lateral approach for primary total hip replacement while minimizing the risk of posterior dislocation. The advantage is preservation of the continuity of the gluteus medius and vastus lateralis muscles and the posterior half of the trochanter with attached posterior gluteus medius and short external rotators.

Indications

- Noncompliant patient (e.g., elderly or with Parkinson's disease) at risk for posterior dislocation
- Desire to leave posterior capsule and short external rotators intact

Steps

- The osteotomy begins anteriorly at the sharp ridge that is the limiting structure of the anterior aspect of the insertion

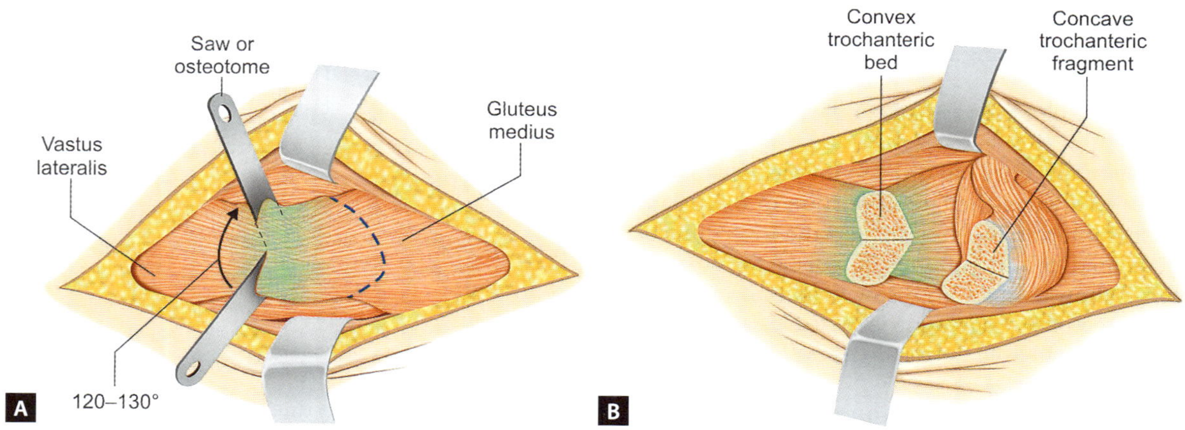

Figs. 17A and B: The chevron, or biplane, osteotomy. (A) The two limbs of the osteotomy directed at the center to converge at a 120–130° angle; (B) Released trochanteric fragment has a concave medial surface that has increased surface area and improved stability.

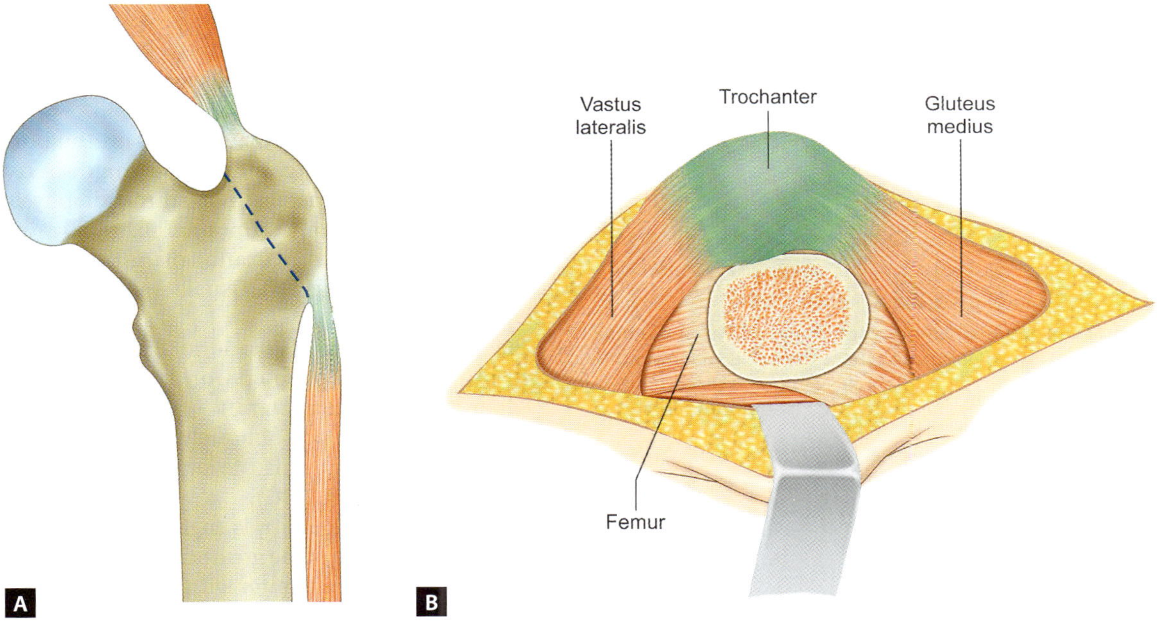

Figs. 18A and B: Trochanteric slide osteotomy. (A) Osteotomy cut begins just medial to the tendinous insertion of the gluteus medius into the greater trochanter and includes the origin of the vastus lateralis laterally; (B) The trochanteric fragment attached to the glutei and vastus lateralis maintaining continuity.

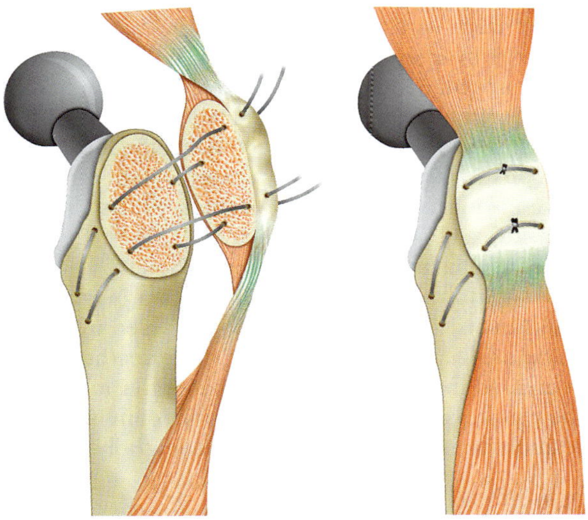

Fig. 19: Two trochanteric wires are used to fix the trochanteric slide osteotomy.

of the abductors, lying along the most cranial aspect of the sulcus between the abductor insertions and the lateral half of the cathedral roof-shaped origin of the vastus intermedius **(Figs. 20A and B)**

- Posterior aspect of osteotomy is conservative and remains superficial to the intertrochanteric ridge and the insertion of the short external rotators, which are left attached to the femur.
- These cuts make the fragment wider anteriorly than posteriorly (so called "oblique").
- Reattachment—performed with two horizontal and three vertical wires.

Horizontal Trochanteric Osteotomy

This is done in revision cases where there is not enough bone available at the standard osteotomy site due to implanted prosthesis/cement/lysis that reattachment would not be feasible. Horizontal bone cut is made as far proximal as possible without compromising abductor function **(Fig. 21)**. The remaining fragment should be large enough to be reattached. The attachment is done using two horizontal and two vertical wires.

Vertical Trochanteric Osteotomy

This is the only feasible option in cases where the trochanter has been already advanced over lateral femoral cortex. The vastus intermedius and lateralis are completely released distal to the trochanter **(Fig. 22)**. Osteotomy is made 3–5 mm lateral to lateral cortex of femoral canal for proper attachment. Reattachment is done using horizontal wires.

Extended Trochanteric Osteotomy

Extended osteotomy of the proximal femur has been successful in dealing with:

- Removal of well-fixed femoral stems
- Complex revision problems such as loose femoral implants but well-fixed cement mantle
- Varus remodeling of proximal femur—eccentric reaming and high likelihood of cortical perforation
- Retained bone cement
- Proximal femoral deformity

Contraindication

Need of impaction of bone grafting.

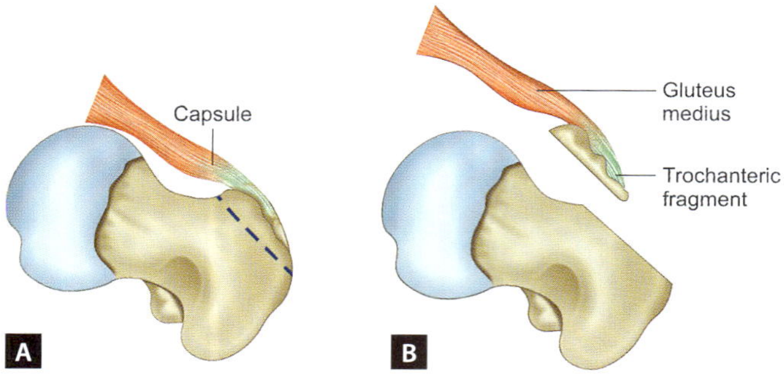

Figs. 20A and B: Oblique trochanteric osteotomy: (A) This is a modification of the direct lateral approach where the cut is made on the anterior aspect of trochanter; (B) A thin wafer of bone is osteotomized that contains both gluteus medius and vastus lateralis attachments, sparing the short external rotators.

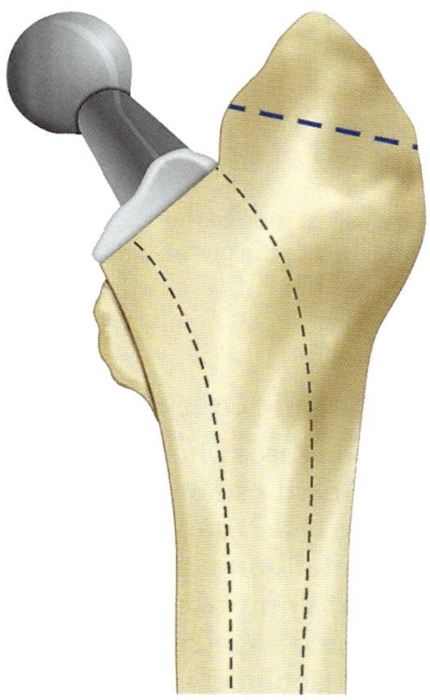

Fig. 21: Horizontal trochanteric osteotomy. The cut starts proximally on the lateral surface of the greater trochanter without dividing the fibers of the abductors inserting into the trochanter.

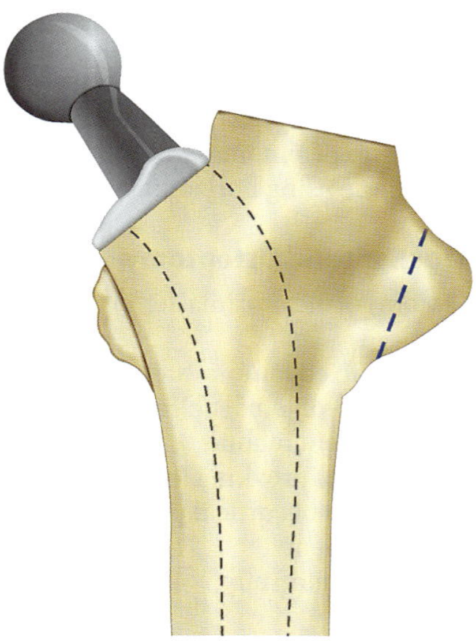

Fig. 22: Vertical osteotomy is only utilized on a femur in which the greater trochanter was advanced previously to the lateral femoral cortex.

Steps

- Wider exposure is needed.
- The vastus lateralis and vastus intermedius are detached anterior to the linea aspera and elevated.
- The proposed osteotomy is drawn on the bone with a sterile marking pen/cautery—the length of osteotomy should permit at least 5 cm of isthmic diaphyseal cortex available for revision component fixation (minimum 10 cm is needed for secure fixation of the fragment to medial cortex, **Figs. 23A and B**). Usual length is 12–15 cm from tip of trochanter.
- Place cerclage wire distal to the distal end of osteotomy to prevent crack propagation form osteotomy while separating the fragment.
- The distal cut is made obliquely, from proximal to distal encompassing one-third to one-fourth of the femoral circumference **(Fig. 23C)**.
- Proximally, the osteotomy is angled medially at the level of the vastus tubercle of the greater trochanter to incorporate all of the greater trochanter with the osteotomy fragment.
- Elevate the osteotomy using broad osteotomes **(Figs. 23C and D)**.
- Remove and clean the fragment.
- Insert the fully porous-coated revision prosthesis and replace the osteotomy fragment after modifying its shape to match the prosthesis. Tightening is done using cables and circlage wires **(Fig. 24)**. The cables are passed from posterior to anterior to protect the sciatic nerve. The distal cable is tightened the most followed by the middle cable and proximal the least tightened but none left loose. This is to prevent fracture of the fragment at the most tenuous part proximally. Trochanteric advancement can be done by removing a portion of the osteotomy fragment distally **(Fig. 25)**.
- For cemented revision, gelatin foam should be used along the osteotomy edges to act as a gasket **(Fig. 26)**. The fragment is repositioned and compressed into the site using cables and wires. The revision prosthesis is then cemented in standard fashion. It is better to bone graft the whole osteotomy site. The gelatin foam is eventually resorbed and does not interfere with new bone formation.

Complications

- Migration
- Nonunion
- Fracture propagation
- Shattering of the fragment
- Cement leakage
- Subsidence of stem

Other osteotomies that can serve as alternatives to extended trochanteric osteotomy include:

- Posterior longitudinal split osteotomy
- Femoral bone slot osteotomy
- Rail-road osteotomy

SUBTROCHANTERIC OSTEOTOMIES

Osteotomies at this region are usually used to correct the limb alignment or provide stability to the pelvis in case of

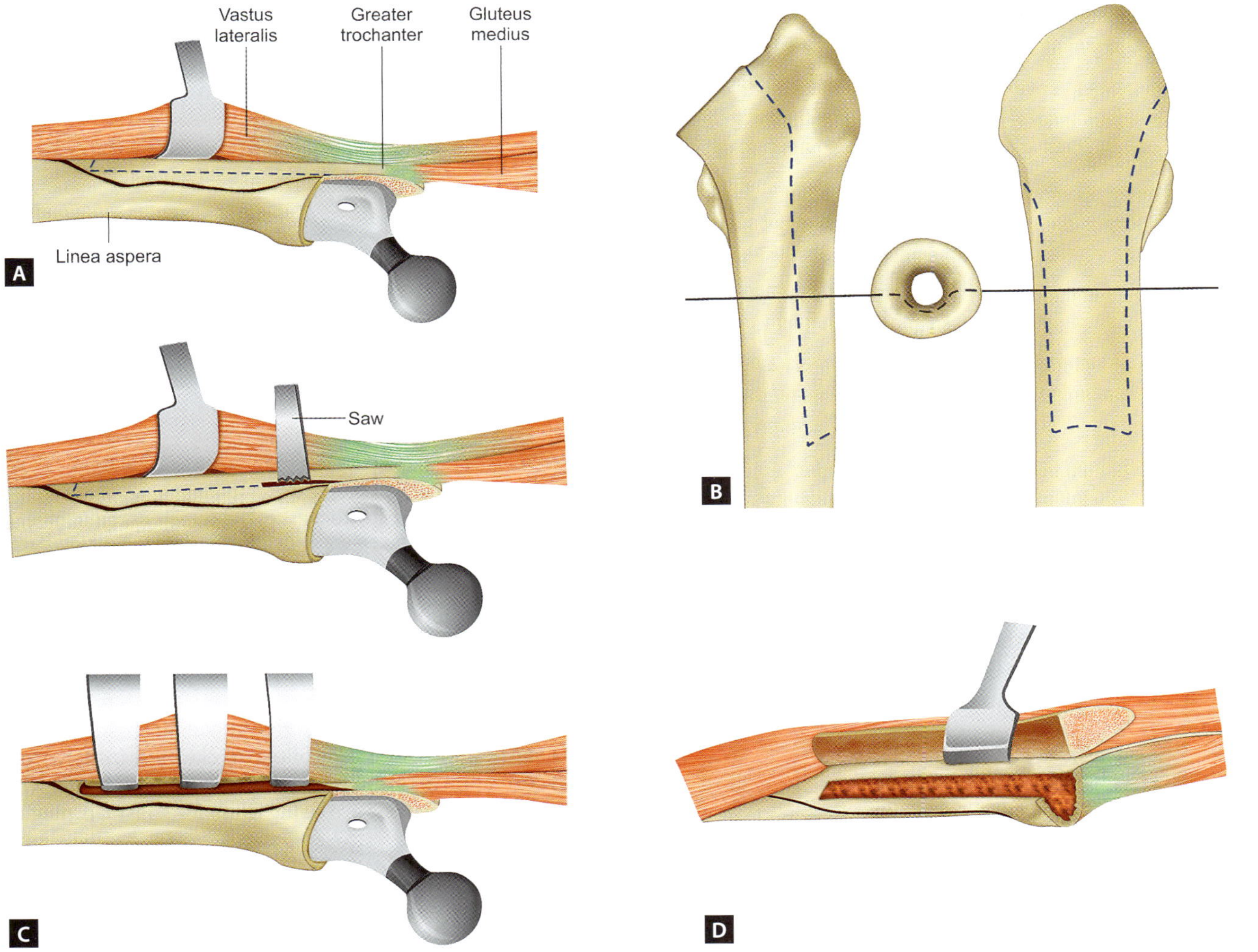

Figs. 23A to D: The extended trochanteric osteotomy is done by cutting posteriorly from the greater trochanter distally (dashed line, A); (B) The transverse portion is cut to incorporate one-third of the diaphyseal circumference obliquely so that the fragment can be dovetailed into the femur when it is replaced; This creates a tight fit and is stable enough upon reposition; (C) The osteotomy is scored and opened with a series of broad osteotomes. The fragment is elevated (D) by everting it in continuity with overlying muscle.

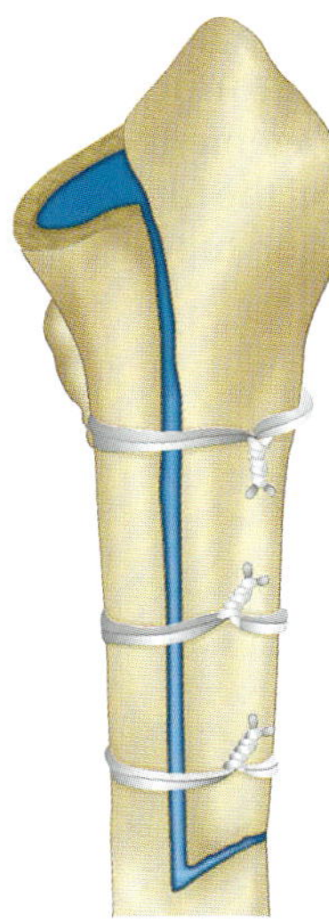

Fig. 24: The osteotomized fragment is repositioned and tightened with doubled monofilament circlage wires.

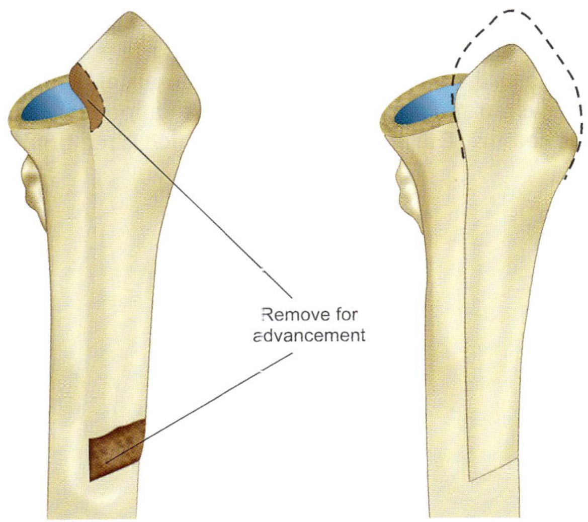

Fig. 25: To facilitate advancement of the trochanter, the distal portion of the fragment is excised by making a cut parallel to the oblique distal cut in the osteotomy.

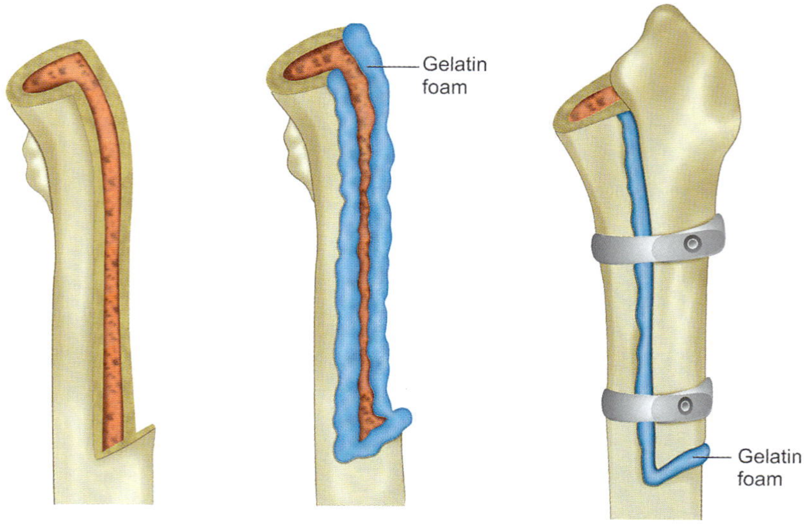

Fig. 26: Technique for cemented revision. Dry gelatin foam serves as a gasket throughout the osteotomy site. The osteotomized fragment is pretightened and cement pressurized into the canal in a standard fashion. The gelatin foam prevents cement from intruding into the cut interface of the osteotomy.

compromised hip joint. Valgus/varus correction is usually done distally along the shaft of femur but rotation correction of the limb in paralytic hips is usually done at the subtrochanteric region. Schanz osteotomy and other PSOs are also done at this region.

DEROTATIONAL OSTEOTOMY

Femoral derotation osteotomy (FDO) may be indicated in intoeing gait principally due to medial femoral torsion that interferes with gait and function. The other indication is in spastic hips that cause gradual subluxation and dislocation of the hip joint, in such cases a VDRO is done similar to Perthes disease. In the former cases with intoeing gait, the femur is derotated axially into external rotation distal to osteotomy. The site of osteotomy in such cases is a bit controversial with advantages specific to proximal and distal site for osteotomy:

- Proximal femoral osteotomy is obligatory when there is both intoeing and subluxation of the hip. The proximal osteotomy allows varus angulation of the femoral neck to ensure stability of the hip with internal rotation of the femur proximal to and external rotation distal to the osteotomy. The muscle dissection which is required for a proximal osteotomy is more extensive than that for a distal osteotomy and may interfere with abductor and extensor function of the hip. The delay in mobilization may lead to decompensation and prolonged loss of extension of the hip and an increase in anterior pelvic tilt.
- Distal femoral osteotomy offers quicker, less invasive form of correction for intoed gait. This is especially chosen when multilevel surgeries are being done for spastic diplegia.

CONCLUSION

- Osteotomies around the hip are a specialty surgery cherished by experienced practitioners in the field. Though the indications have diminished over time there are situations where osteotomy provides a much more viable alternative to arthroplasty.
- Many hip pathologies in children are amenable to osteotomy and correction of deformity so surgeons should be aware of the technique of performing the same.
- Trochanteric osteotomies are being increasingly performed for management of unusual cases requiring extended exposure of the hip joint as in complex primary arthroplasty or revision hip surgeries.

CHAPTER 75

Total Hip Replacement Arthroplasty (Rationale, Design, Complications, and Revision)

Manish Kumar Varshney

INTRODUCTION

Total hip arthroplasty (THA, total hip replacement arthroplasty, or total hip replacement) is a procedure where both articulating surfaces of hip joint are replaced by specific prosthetic components. This includes the resurfacing arthroplasty (trimming and covering by a metallic cap). THA has now become so successful that it has been referred to as "the operation of the century". It is the main surgical procedure in elective orthopedics. Despite its popularity and widespread use, the technique and technology are constantly under review for improvements on various fronts to make it perfect, the perfection is still not achieved.

PRINCIPLES OF TOTAL HIP ARTHROPLASTY

The defective hip joint is replaced by an artificial acetabular cup and femoral head, which replace the damaged painful/dysplastic/unstable natural articulating surfaces. Therefore, the materials must have low friction and withstand wear and oscillating mechanical load, provide stable articular surfaces, and improve the function of hip joint. For the arthroplasty to be suitable for masses with varying dimensions of the hip joint, the prosthesis has to be modular enough, so there are femoral stem, acetabular sizes, liners, and femoral heads of various sizes and combination. Over the years, the basic principle of hip arthroplasty had been *low-friction torque arthroplasty* as propounded by Sir John Charnley (Charnley low-friction torque arthroplasty, CLFTA, or simply CLFA). The specific principles of Charnley's low friction arthroplasty are discussed in the Chapter on "Tribology and Bearing Surface."

The other principles of arthroplasty that are considered essential for success include:

- *Prosthetic component alignment:* Based on the "safe zone" concept of Lewinnek, the anteversion for the cup should be 15–30°, and the coronal tilt (theta angle) should be 35–45°. For the femoral stem, an anteversion of 10–15° is generally acceptable. This principle is hotly challenged now with the identification of various other important variables such as spinopelvic alignment, soft tissue tensioning, composite measures such as combined anteversion and combined offset discussed later.
- Soft tissue tension as well as adequate repair of the abductor complex and function is very important to the stability of THAs and will help to minimize the risk of Trendelenburg gait.
- Equalizing limb lengths and femoral offset
- Placing the hip in normal center of rotation achieved by optimizing **(Fig. 1)**:
  - *Vertical height (vertical offset)*—determined primarily by the base length of the prosthetic neck plus the length gained by the modular head used.
  - *Medial offset (horizontal offset or, simply, offset)*—distance from the center of the femoral head to a line through the axis of the distal part of the stem.
  - *Version of the femoral neck (anterior offset)*—refers to the orientation of the neck in reference to the coronal plane. The normal femur has 10–15° of anteversion of the femoral neck.

Despite the surgery being performed for so long and extensively, the following design features or philosophies

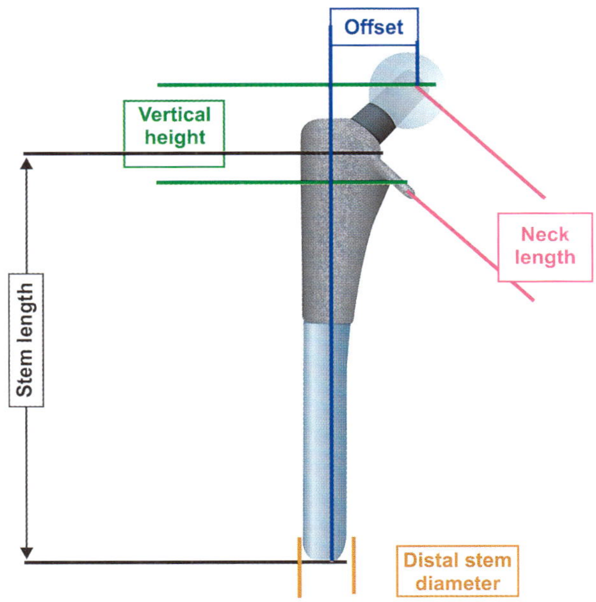

Fig. 1: Illustration of some terms in relation to hip arthroplasty. (offset = horizontal offset; vertical height = vertical offset)

are under constant evolution and a matter of debate (though it is "the operation of century", we always feel we are still beginning to perfect it but alas never!). We will address these issues individually in the text below.

- Femoral head size
- Linear geometry
- Bearing surfaces (*see* Chapter on "Tribology and Bearing Surface")
- Modularity
- Acetabular fixation—cemented versus cementless
- Screws versus no screws in cementless acetabular fixation
- Cemented femur—smooth versus rough, small versus large mantles (French paradox)
- Cementless femur—extensively coated versus proximally coated
- Acetabular cup alignment and version
- Surgical approach to perform THA

HISTORY OF TOTAL HIP ARTHROPLASTY

- THA is not a modern procedure and the earliest documented attempt to replace a femoral head dates back to 1891 (Glück ivory prosthesis fixed with nickel plated screws). But, it was an obvious failure. Glück was far ahead of his time, discussing and experimenting on uncemented versus cemented fixation, stress-shielding, and issues of biocompatibility. He was disheartened by the failures of his prosthesis (he even performed a total knee arthroplasty in 1890, that too though failed later) and published a repentance under peer pressure and force.
- Interpositional arthroplasty possibly started in France where Auguste Stanislas Verneuil (1823–1895), from Paris France, performed soft tissue hip interpositions in 1860, but the method was highlighted by Lèopold Ollier's (1830–1900) work in Lyon, France. In 1885, Ollier described the use of adipose tissue in uninfected hip joints, but this procedure failed because he did not fix the interposed fat to the bone (Ollier, 1885). A Czech surgeon, Vítězslav Chlumský (1867–1943), experimented with various interpositional materials that included muscles, celluloid, silver plates, rubber struts, magnesium, zinc, glass, pyres, decalcified bone, wax, etc. Pig bladder was later suggested as a good interpositional material by a French surgeon known as Foedre. Sir Robert Jones (1855–1933) used a strip of gold foil to cover the surface of the femoral head.
- Delbet used a rubber femoral prosthesis in 1919 to replace one-half of the hip joint.
- Smith-Petersen in 1923 performed a synthetic interpositional arthroplasty with a glass mold prosthesis (mold arthroplasty).
- Smith-Petersen in 1937 used Vitallium (an alloy of 60% cobalt, 20% chromium, 5% molybdenum, and other substances) on the advice of his dentist friend that became a good success.
- In 1938, stainless steel prosthesis was first introduced to replace the femoral head and the acetabular cup but was quickly modified to cobalt-chromium alloy (developed for dental applications) in 1940. This was reasonably accepted and led to development of Austin Moore prosthesis, introduced in 1952 (uncommonly used now).

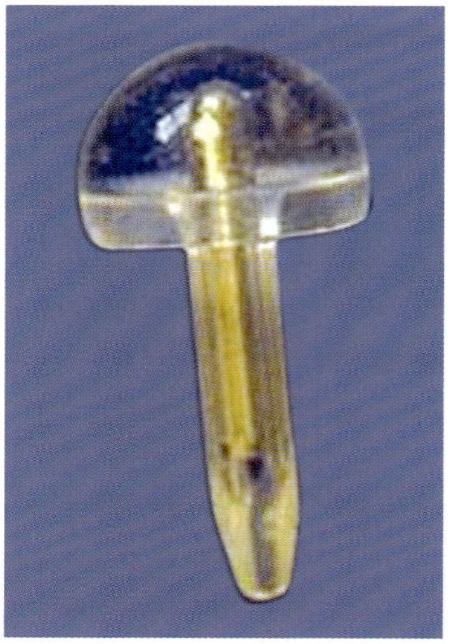

Fig. 2: The Judet acrylic femoral prosthesis.

- Robert Judet and Jean Judet (Paris, France) used an acrylic prosthesis in 1948 that was but highly susceptible to wear **(Fig. 2)**.
- Based on Judet experience, Thompson produced a refined prosthesis made of Vitallium with a distinctive collar and a curved stem that was placed in femur. The prosthesis was monoblock in design. The design encouraged the development of Moore's prosthesis, which was used first in a patient of giant cell tumor. This prosthesis had fenestrations to improve bone integration.
- Because of engineering predominance, metal-on-metal (MoM) hip arthroplasty was introduced in clinical practice in 1953 (concept rediscovered by McMinn) that failed quickly. The improved McKee-Farrar design, introduced in 1958, is regarded as the first generation of widely used MoM prostheses made of cobalt-chromium alloy. This design but also had the common problems of failure and were soon unpopular partially also due to success of Charnley's hip.
- Charnley hip **(Fig. 3)** marked the beginning of the era of a new specialty within orthopedics—total hip joint replacement surgery as stated by Wroblewski et al. The first hip replacement surgery was performed by Charnley in 1962 using a prosthesis design based on a stainless steel femoral component and a Teflon [polytetrafluoroethylene (PTFE)] acetabular cup both fixed with acrylic bone cement describing his so-called low-frictional torque arthroplasty (*see* Chapter on "Tribology and Bearing Surface"). The cup wore easily, so it was later replaced with high-molecular weight polyethylene. Its success superseded the failures of MoM arthroplasty.
- The success of Charnley's prosthesis was partially marred by aseptic loosening (osteolysis) due to polyethylene wear particles. This polyethylene disease taught orthopedics a lot about the prosthesis design and delved heavily in the world of tribology (*see* Chapter on "Tribology and Bearing Surface").

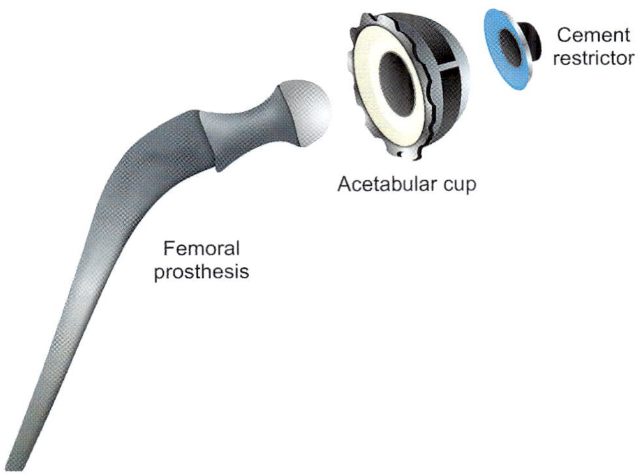

Fig. 3: The Charnley prosthesis.

- The research for a better material led to three advancements:
  1. The development of ultrahigh-molecular weight polyethylene (UHMWPE) and cross-linked UHMWPE.
  2. The resurgence of MoM devices because osteolysis was not reported as failure mechanism in earlier MoM hip prostheses.
  3. Development of alternate bearings such as ceramics, the search, however, still continues.
- A second generation of MoM prostheses was developed and introduced in clinical practice in the late 1980s. This also gave the chance to reintroduce the surface replacement arthroplasty. Resurfacing arthroplasty interested orthopedic surgeons, as it expanded the horizon of THA to younger patients. Revision is inevitable in younger patients, so a prosthesis that minimally damaged or utilized the bone would ease revision surgery where one may be more liberal at bone cuts and implant adjustments to provide better outcome. Additionally, larger diameter femoral heads are used that give the joint more stability. It was expected to achieve lower failure rates because femoral stem loosening would be less probable. The theoretical interest and advantages disguised the thinking ability (of complete understandings of historical failures), and there was a boom in the late 1990s and early decade of this century toward MoM implants. Slowly, however, the failures creeped up and initial warning tuned out finally into complete withdrawal of the system from world over. The MoM era has again eclipsed.
- Simultaneously, however, the need of hip prostheses to withstand higher load for extended time periods mobilized a lot of research into materials with improved wear resistance. Ceramic bearings were found to be satisfying for most of these characteristics. This has led, since the late 1970s, to the development of ceramic-on-ceramic (CoC) hip prostheses that exhibit excellent wear performance but factually also the risk of fragile fracture. Currently, their main disadvantage seems to be an audible squeaking that occurs in 1–20% of the patients.
- Finally though should have been included above in the evolution history, the ultimate salvage still remains conversion to Girdlestone—the Girdlestone-like excisional arthroplasty (advocated for infected hips as a drainage measure from Oxford, UK).

COMPONENTS OF A MODULAR HIP PROSTHESIS

Femoral Stem

The femoral stem firmly fixes the femoral side of the hip prosthesis to the femoral bone. Stem fixation can be achieved either by a surrounding layer of bone cement or by press-fitting the stem against the medullary canal walls. The primary function of stem is to ensure a uniform load transfer from the prosthesis to the lower limb. The fixation strategy influences the stem design, the choice of the material, and the surface finishing. The rationale for different designs available for stem is as follows:

- The stem is the component of the hip prosthesis subjected to the highest mechanical stresses so its material must have high mechanical strength and fatigue resistance. Metals are the only option for stem manufacturing to this effect.
- Stem length influences its stability. A longer stem would improve stability; however, more reaming of medullary canal would be required, cement would have to be injected more distally, and less bone would be available for revision surgery. In primary THA, a stem in the range of 130–140 mm presents a reasonable compromise. Some other terms used to define various parameters are mentioned in **Figure 1**.

Cemented Femoral Stems

In *cemented stems*, the force is transmitted to the cement while the stem should remain mechanically stable in long term. Charnley stem had been the prototype cemented femoral stem. Not many complications were encountered with the use of original 1962 stem until Charnley realized that cantilever mechanism is responsible for stem fractures in a significant number of cases. Charnley addressed this problem by changing the surface finish of the stem to a vaquasheened surface in 1969. This mainly was surface hardened design and was quickly improved by changing the material to 316 low-carbon vacuum-melted stainless steel in 1971 to improve corrosion resistance and fatigue properties. Charnley continued improving his stems and introduced his second generation femoral stem in 1973 that had a rounded cross sectional profile. But being unsatisfied, he introduced yet another stem (third generation) that was Cobra flanged vaquasheened stem intended to provide improved proximal loading. Also, the offset was reduced to 40 mm to reduce bending moment and head–neck ratio reduced by reducing neck length from 12.5 to 10 mm in 1984. Cobra flange addition actually changed the whole biomechanics of Charnley from taper-slip to shape-closed design (see below). There have been characteristically two design philosophies for a cemented stem:

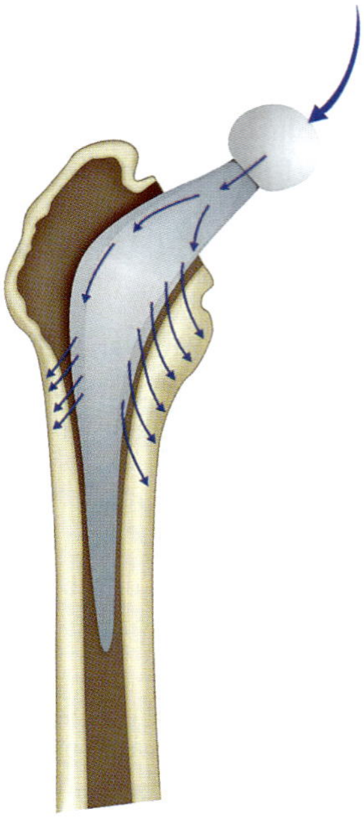

Fig. 4: Force transmission in a taper slip cemented stem reconstruction.

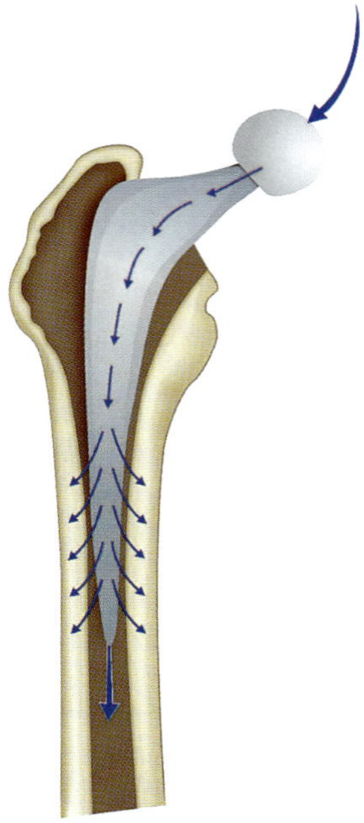

Fig. 5: Force transmission in a composite beam cemented stem reconstruction.

1. *"Loaded-taper" model ("taper-slip", "force-closed" fixation):* Exeter stem is the classical example. The stem is tapered in two (e.g., CPT stem of Zimmer) or three planes (C-stem of DePuy). The stem locks as a wedge in the cement transmitting the stress through mid-portion of fixation **(Fig. 4)** and reduces proximal and distal stress. These stems characteristically "creep" up to 1 mm over the 1st year and subsequently stabilize until radial compressive forces are transmitted to the mantle and bone as hoop stresses. To prevent stress on cement distally during this subsidence, air-filled centralizer is used to act as a cushion. The design rationale includes a polished, round, collarless, straight, tapered stem that facilitates creep while generating minimal particle debris.
2. *"Composite-beam" concept ("shape-closed" fixation):* These are nonsubsiding implants, i.e., their shape itself limits the subsidence required to achieve a stable position and hence the stem is to be bonded firmly to the cement mantle. These stems employ an interference fit with the bone and cement and have higher initial stability in the longitudinal direction; however, some stem migration is definitely seen (0.3–1.4 mm in 1st year). They are often rectangular, can be straight or anatomic, and occasionally have a collar. These stems are often roughened to improve bonding, and hence require a thick cement mantle well fixed to bone (very poorly tolerating the mantle defects). There is also a concern of loosening at the stem–cement interface due to micromotion and the loosening at cement–bone interface due to excessive stress transfer added by torsional stresses especially distally **(Fig. 5)**. If micromotion occurs then excess wear particles will get generated to cause osteolysis and implant failure.

- Surface finish of stem has been a topic of considerable debate. For loaded-taper design stems, the surface should be polished. Though initially, it was thought that integration would be better with a rough surface and the cement would interlock with femoral stem better. It was found, however, that rough surface finish has high lysis due to micromotion at the interface and increases transmission of shear and tensile stress. Three types of stress are transmitted by the stem–cement interface. The cement has good strength in compression but fares poorly with shear and tensile stress. If the cement–stem bond will be tight then all the stress will get concentrated on this interface and there will be high likelihood of failure. So, surface is polished to minimize this cement–stem bond. Poor bonding causes minimal accumulation of tensile stresses and shear forces, but compressive forces are transmitted due to subsidence. In composite beam designs, this shear force is high and leads to so-called second space wear (primary space is the articulation itself); this increased release of wear particles increased osteolysis and failure rate. The latter stems are also sensitive to the presence of incomplete and thin cement mantles with a poor cement–bone interface than polished stems. Precoating the stem has been attempted to reduce wear; however, it was found that when debonding finally occurs at the precoated or roughened cement–stem interface, there will be damage to the cement and large quantities of polymethyl methacrylate (PMMA) and/or metal particles will be generated causing increased wear and osteolysis. This problem with polished stems is minimal as micromovement at the cement–implant interface produces less debris. Preheating of the stem to 50°C reduces the porosity of cement and improves shear strength and fixation at the stem–cement interface.
- Material is also important for cemented stem. If titanium is chosen for a rough cemented stem, the wear is much

faster as the wear resistance of titanium is much low. Though polished titanium stems perform fairly well as the friction is low then.

- The stem cross-section is designed to ensure rotational stability and to reduce stress concentration around the device. Cross-sectional shape influences the distribution of cement within the femoral canal, the rotational stability of the implant, and the stress distribution within the cement mantle. Stems with a square cross-section have more rotational stability than oval stems but their sharp edges create peak stresses in the cement, which could lead to microfractures. Oval broaches fit well into the femoral stem and occupy more of the cavity. The canal is more uniformly broached in these circumstances so that the distribution of cement is more uniform (e.g., CMKII® of Smith and Nephew, and Centralign® of Zimmer). Rectangular broaches (as for Exeter® of Stryker, CPT® Zimmer) are limited in size by their contact against the inner cortex of the oval cross-section of the medullary canal. This leaves extracancellous bones in the intervening spaces while less cancellous bone at the edges. The weak cancellous bone, if not pressurized well, will lead to weak cement mantle. Use of cement gun is hence mandatory as this causes cement penetration of up to 3 mm in the cancellous bone. The cancellous bone can also be removed by the use of curette to increase the space for cement. The use of modern cementing technique (pressurization) entails the presence of around 3 mm of cancellous bone for proper interdigitation of the cement into bone.
- *Anatomical versus nonanatomical (straight) stems:* Anatomical stems have been designed to better fit the femoral canal and allow even distribution of cement mantle. These anatomical stems are shape-closed design and have limited subsidence. They also limit the area of anterior proximal contact and posterior distal point contact.
- *Addition of third taper:* Third proximal taper in the axial plane from lateral to medial has been found beneficial to load the proximal femur posteromedially and prevent the proximal osteolysis due to stress shielding. The design features have been incorporated in C-stem®.
- *Collared cemented stem:* The collar in a cemented stem has its own advantages and disadvantages as follows:
    - It promotes direct transfer of load from the implant to the medial cement mantle and the bone. This unloads the vulnerable proximal cement mantle. Medial part of the cement mantle proximally is most vulnerable to cracks and if these cracks propagate to the distal tip then implant failure is imminent.
    - Collar reduces the tensile stresses and reduces overall migration (helpful for shape-closed design)
    - Collar controls the insertional length of the stem. This is useful especially in the composite-beam stems that are undersized with respect to broach and may get inserted more than needed.
- In loaded-taper stem design, the collar is contraindicated as it will prevent the final subsidence of stem in the cement mantle to reach a stable position during cyclic loading.
- *Stem-broach mismatch* **(Fig. 6)**: This should allow enough cement present between the stem as bone as is required for the design. Normally, a mantle 2–5 mm in thickness is considered adequate. Thinner mantle crack easily. The controversy is, however, too much and it extends to the extent that there is a recommendation that taper-loaded stems may not be as theoretically sound as it seems. The better results have been found with stems that are more in contact with bone than with intervening cement mantle so the theory of subsidence is questioned, and it appears that composite beam design is what improves the long-term survival. Also undersizing the stem with respect to broach has been found to be of no relevance. "Line-to-line" cementing (same size broach and stem) has been found to be successful and may improve the long-term results (French paradox). I personally feel that cement is a graveyard for the mistakes one makes during various crucial surgical steps and does a beautiful cover-up. Instead of too much relying on a thick flawless cement mantle, one should be more concerned about the best intramedullary fit. Canal filling stems remove most of the weak cancellous bone offering direct points of contact with cortical bone through a thin cement layer and the stem alignment is better as the cortical bone guides the stem rotation during insertion. Finally, if few errors remain, they are "filled" by the cement.

Cementless Femoral Stems

These rely on osseointegration (the attachment of lamellar bone to implants without intervening fibrous tissue) described by Albrektsson et al. in 1981. This was based also partially on the findings of Lord (1979) that "living bone that undergoes remodeling provides for long-term anchor of the prosthesis". This implies firm fixation (press-fit) of the implant minimizing micromotion. Micromotion of >150 μm leads to fibrous tissue formation, between 40 and 150 μm leads to a combination of bone and fibrous tissue formation, and <20 μm results in predominantly bone formation. In contrast to the cemented stems that are either undersized or "line-to-line", the uncemented stems are oversized. Possibly, the composite beam design of cemented stems has encouraged the development of uncemented stem. The evolution of cementless stem is interesting for academic purpose and also for understanding the design rationale.

- *Tapered stem:* Classic tapered stem was the Zweymüller prosthesis (Allopro, Switzerland) now manufactured by Zimmer in the name of Alloclassic®. The stem was first used in 1979 and has a taper of 3° from proximal to distal portion on sagittal and coronal planes. The rectangular cross-section has four corners and surfaces. This achieves axial rotational stability. The similar stems developed later such as Taperlock® and Tri-lock® also have taper and a flat anteroposterior (AP) surface but the medial and lateral surfaces are rounded. All these tapered stems use diaphyseal fixation below lesser trochanter.

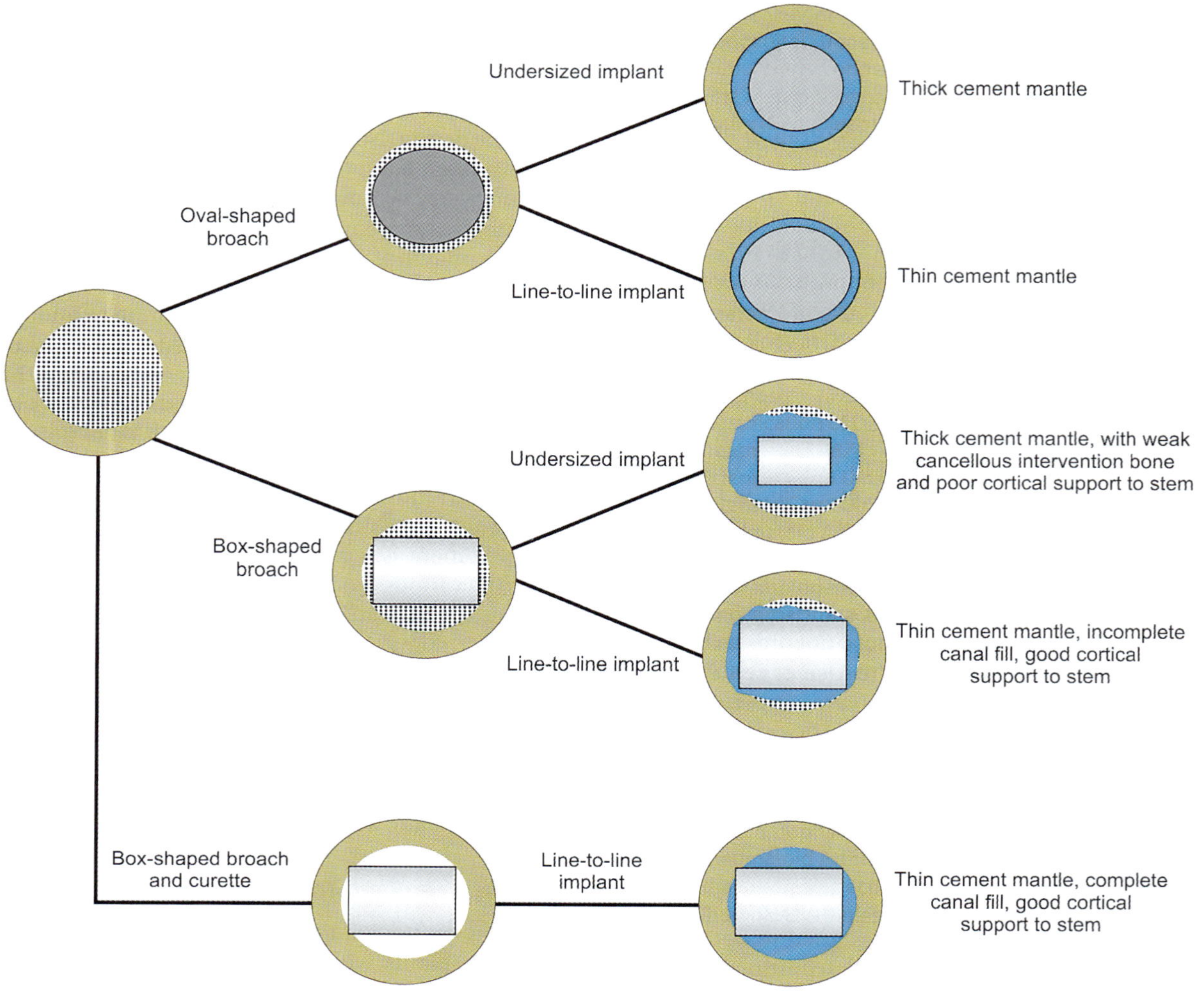

Fig. 6: The influence of the stem–broach matching and cross-sectional shape of the stem on the appearance of the cement mantle.

- *Anatomical stems:* Porous-coated anatomic (PCA®, Howmedica) and anatomic porous replacement (APR®, Zimmer) stems were introduced around the same time and had anatomic sagittal curve and proximal porous coating with a posterior bow to match the anatomical characteristics of femoral canal. These stems maximized the bone contact and worked on the philosophy of "fit and fill" to achieve highest possible three-point fixation and initial stability. The main concerns are the high variability of femoral canal anatomy in population so the stem may not fit in one of the other patient and the high reported incidence of proximal femoral fracture due to posterior bow. The stem had been highly successful with studies reporting even 100% survivorship. Due to close anatomical fit, this stem in particular suffers from high incidence of thigh pain.
- *Short cylindrical stem:* The anatomic medullary locking (AML) stem was the first cementless femoral implant approved for use in the United States having success serving benchmark for future stems too. Though termed anatomic, the stem was neither anatomic nor tapered. It relied on distal diaphyseal fixation at isthmus using "scratch fit" and was fully porous coated. The initial design though achieved high fixation rate had high rate of cortical atrophy, proximal stress-shielding, and bone loss. So, the stem was modified to include porous coating only in proximal thirds. This led to changed philosophy of metaphyseal fixation.
- *Composite stems:* These stems were introduced to mimic the natural flexibility of the human femur, and thereby in theory prevent bone resorption due to stress shielding—the concept of "isoelastic" stems. The concept failed rapidly, however, due to high proximal stem/bone interface stresses, causing interface debonding and nearly all of the implants had to be revised. "Epoch" stem is a modern version of isoelastic stem introduced by Zimmer but the long-term widespread results are awaited.
- *Distally fixing and revision stems:* With the diseased pathology in proximal femur, in revision cases, the proximal fitting are often unreliable. These stems have to be extensively coated long anatomically contoured designs that provide distal fit at and below the isthmus. Also, the stress are all loaded on the proximal portion

of stem where the bony calcar may be missing so some calcar replacing/substituting designs have to be incorporated. The concerns are obviously proximal bone loss due to stress shielding.

- With the introduction of these implants for younger population, the modern stems tend to incorporate double-taper metaphyseal filling designs (proximal fixation). Double-taper design allows for "fit and fill" of the proximal femur so that there is higher rotational stability, and less stress shielding.
- The cementless stems have been classified based on their shape (straight/curved), cross-sectional geometry (wedged, tapered, rounded, splined, rectangular, etc.) and surface coating. Simply stating the stems are either straight or curved and either engages proximally (metaphysis) or distally (diaphysis). With incorporation of various features, the surgeons now refer to stems as either proximally porous-coated tapered or fully coated cylindrical. The detailed classification of uncemented femoral stems divides them into following six types (modified Berry classification of Khanuja et al.). Here, with progress in number, the fixation area increases.
  - Type 1—straight, single wedged, tapered, proximally fitting. These fit in the metaphyseal region and are proximally coated (one-third). The stem is collarless, narrows mediolaterally, but is flat in the AP plane.
  - Type 2—straight, double-wedged, tapered, and proximally fitting. These are same as type 1 but are wider and narrows both mediolaterally and in AP plane. Thus, these stems obtain the cortical contact in two planes in contrast to type 1 stems. They may be fluted to reduce the modulus of elasticity and minimize stress-shielding to lessen thigh pain.
  - Type 3A—straight, round, tapered proximally fitting. They are conical stems that are coated in proximal two-thirds and fit in the metaphyseodiaphyseal region.
  - Type 3B—straight, splined. Tapered distally fixing stems. They have a conical shape but splined circumferentially and fix in the metaphyseodiaphyseal region and proximal diaphysis. They are usually fully coated.
  - Type 3C—straight, rectangular, and tapered distally fixing stems. Being rectangular, they get four-point rotational stability in the metaphyseodiaphyseal region and proximal diaphysis.
  - Type 4—cylindrical, straight stem, and fully coated. These are extensively porous coated with a proximal collar. Fixation is primarily diaphyseal along entire length of prosthesis.
  - Type 5—modular stems. The metaphyseal and diaphyseal components are separately chosen so that the contact is both metaphyseal and diaphyseal. Modularity, however, predisposes to fretting corrosion (*see* Chapter on "Tribology and Bearing Surface").
  - Type 6—curved anatomic stems. They fit anatomically in proximal and distal regions. The proximal portion is wide laterally and posteriorly so the primary fixation is metaphyseal.
- Some femoral stems have a collar **(Figs. 7A and B)**; this feature is mostly located for uncemented stems. Collar ensures transfer of loads to calcar bone and avoids prosthesis subsidence. It also prevents wear debris to enter the canal, if the contact to bone is intimate enough.
- The neck angle is an important parameter influencing the load transfer to the whole stem and its long-term resistance. Modular necks impart ability to adjust the anteversion and offset especially in revision surgeries. Though, this also increases chances of fretting corrosion.
- Neck design may impart a sleeve that improves the ability to bear stress; this structure is important in patients where the posteromedial buttress of calcar is missing. Such designs are popularly called calcar replacing designs.
- *Implant material:* Uncemented stems are either made of cobalt-chromium-molybdenum alloys or titanium-aluminum-vanadium (Ti-6Al-4V) alloys. The latter has modulus of elasticity closer to that of bone-mitigating thigh pain and stress shielding. Not much clinical difference has been, however, seen.

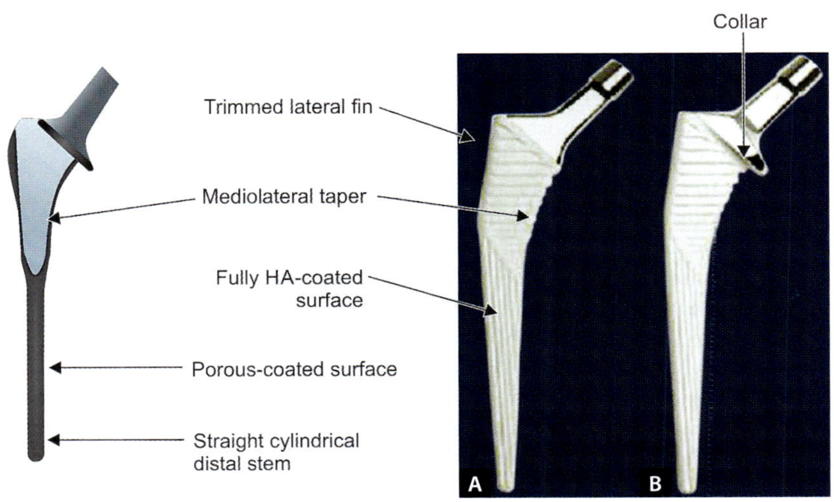

Figs. 7A and B: Some design features of stem and Collarless stem (A) versus Collared stem (B).

- *Surface coating of uncemented femoral stems:* This is an integral part of uncemented stems. The surface should be such that bone can ingrow and cause stem fixation (integration) to bone. If this does not occur then fibrous intervening surface will result, which is neither strong enough and also cause persistent pain. Ingrowth requires a pore size between 50 and 400 μm, and the percentage of voids within the coating should be between 30 and 40% to maintain mechanical strength. Various methods have been proposed for bone ingrowth and integration that either include direct surface modification of the implant stem (creating an ongrowth surface) or applying material from outside for bone to grow into the pores (ingrowing surface). Both basically serve the same purpose, but in the former technique, one has to take cognizance of retaining the implant fatigue strength.
  - *Ongrowth surfaces:* The most popular methods of creating an ongrowth surface is by:
    - Grit blasting involves high-pressure bombarding the implant with small abrasive particles such as corundum (aluminum oxide). The surface roughness ranges from 3 to 5 μm. The mechanical and fatigue strength of the implant reduces with this method, hence, it is mostly used as adjunct to ingrowth methods such as combining the fiber mesh or sintered beads to increase friction and retaining strength of them.
    - Plasma spraying involves high-temperature metal spray on the surface of implant to create a textured surface. The metal powder is mixed with an inert gas that is pressurized and ionized under very-high temperature usually generated from arc. The molten material is then sprayed onto the implant. This method retains most of the mechanical properties of the implant.
  - *Methods used for creating an ingrowth surface include:*
    - *Sintered beads:* These are microspheres of either titanium alloy (preferred) or cobalt chrome welded to implant surface under high temperature. They impart highly rough areas.
    - *Fiber mesh:* This process involves attaching metal pads by diffusion bonding to the implant.
    - *Porous metals:* These are the most porous constructs by virtue of their geometry (but costly too). Trabecular metal (tantalum) is most popular in use. They create the most uniform highly interconnected voids with high porosity (75–80%) compared to other methods that barely reach 50% mark.
    - *Hydroxyapatite-coated stems (HA coated):* This involves plasma spraying calcium phosphate on the porous-coated surface (often grit blasted surface). The surface is deemed to be more osteoconductive but as a matter of fact, not much difference has been achieved. There is a concern of interface degradation where the plane between HA coat and underlying porous coat may get delinked. For optimal mechanics and biological ingrowth, the coating should be minimum 50-μm thick, ideally between 50 and 75 μm and the calcium-to-phosphorus ratio is approximately 1.67. The benefits of the use of HA coating are not substantiated by studies that yield varying results.
- Whatever the method used, surface coating should be circumferential and continuous so that:
  - Maximal bone can grow and minimize shielding
  - Prevent wear particles from circulating around the stem
  - Reduce the incidence of thigh pain

Femoral Head

The material for metallic femoral heads is Co-Cr (titanium has poor resistance to wear). The diameter of the femoral head plays an important role in determining the achievable range of motion (ROM) of the artificial joint and its stability against dislocation. Charnley used the smallest heads in history of THA. Potential for a better contact area and greater motion **(Figs. 8A and B)** before impingement or dislocation led to the use of larger femoral heads **(Figs. 9A and B)**. The problem with larger heads has been of wear and increased wear is seen due to longer distances covered, so this has actually led to search for improvement in bearing surfaces to reduce wear.

The size of the femoral head, the ratio of head and neck diameters, and the shape of the neck of the femoral component influence the ROM of the hip, the degree of impingement between the neck and rim of the socket, and the stability of the articulation. Early impingement associated with smaller head diameter (28 mm and less) predisposes

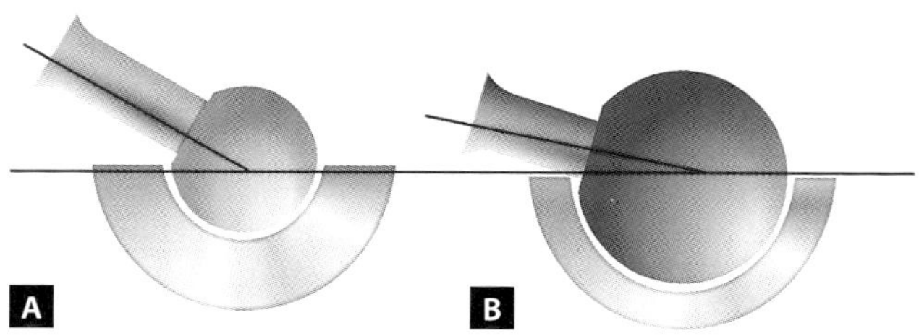

Figs. 8A and B: (A) Implant with smaller femoral head have lesser arc of motion than; (B) Larger one. This also increases the range of movement after which the impingement occurs.

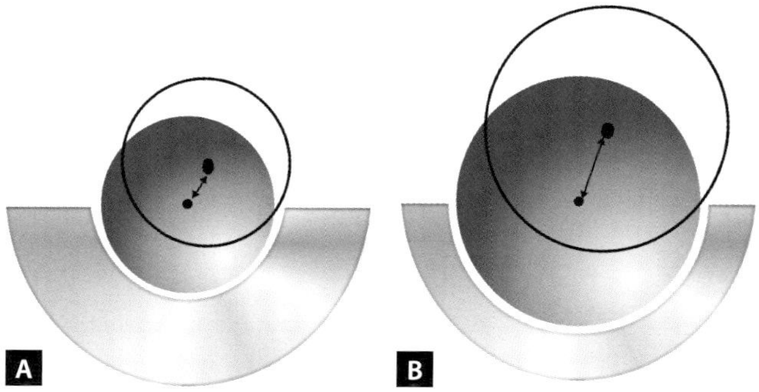

Figs. 9A and B: Jump distance. With subluxation, for example, with terminal impingement of (A) neck to bone/cup smaller head will have shorter distance to travel before escaping rim of acetabular component than (B) larger one.

to dislocation, accelerated polyethylene wear (due to edge impingement, recurrent subluxations, and relocations), acetabular component loosening, and liner dislodgment or fracture. A larger femoral head increases the head–neck ratio and increases the distance head moves before neck impinges on the rim of the socket **(*see* Figs. 8A and B)** and levered out. "Jump distance" is the distance head must travel to escape the rim of the socket and is generally approximated to be half the diameter of the head **(*see* Figs. 9A and B)**. Larger diameter head is theoretically more stable than a smaller one, and it is found that head size of 32 mm or more virtually eliminates impingement. Due to increased movement at the bearing surface, the frictional wear increases; however, hence there is a concern for wear and osteolysis especially at the modular head–neck junction—Trunnionosis. This was seen with MoM hips in particular. The other concern with large femoral heads is impingement against native soft tissues such as the anterior hip capsule and the iliopsoas muscle/tendon (especially iliopsoas), leading to anterior hip pain (or groin pain).

Other critical parameters for the manufacturing of the femoral heads are:

- *Minimum achievable surface roughness (influences friction and wear rate):* Ceramic heads feature the highest smoothness, resulting in the lowest friction coefficients, but their maximum diameter is limited by the manufacturing techniques to about 38–40 mm.
- Mechanical resistance of the material to the tensile stresses generated along the taper junction.

Acetabular Cup

The liner has been discussed in detail with the description and choices of bearing surfaces in the Chapter on "Tribology and Bearing Surface".

Cementless Acetabular Cup and Its Design Features

Here, the metallic acetabular shell provides the outer face of the acetabular cup, which is fixed into the pelvis. The fixation can be enhanced by use of screws. Uncemented components present porous surface finishing (e.g., sintered titanium beads) or hydroxyapatite coatings to foster improved bone integration. In a cementless acetabular component, the liner is locked in the shell. Here, the limiting factor for the choice of liner material is the minimum thickness of the shell, as it has to ensure the mechanical stability of the acetabular cup. For larger head diameters, the liners have either to be hard or for polysurfaces modular choice are needed. Maximum external diameter is limited by the space available in the iliac bone that has to host the acetabular cup. A minimum thickness of poly is needed to accommodate large heads, else it will break or wear fast. So, modularity has to be there in the same implant, a large head say 36 mm will fit only with the larger acetabular cup sizes (say >50 mm) while for smaller acetabular shells, smaller option head will be needed (32 mm) to maintain adequate poly thickness.

Three generations of acetabular cups have been described according to their evolution:

1. *First-generation cementless acetabular cups:* This was the first attempt to improve upon the concerns with loosening of cemented acetabular components. These were porous ingrowth acetabular components aimed to provide long-term biologic fixation to bone. Most designs offered cementless monoblock component, however, some were modular too, providing reasonably satisfactory fixation. The typical cause of failure was result of UHMWPE wear or dissociation between the liner and metal shell. Dissociation was associated with deformation or fracture of the UHMWPE at the linerlocking mechanism due to relatively poor congruity between the dome of the liner and metal shell and thin UHMWPE rim. The other problem was use of gamma-irradiated in-air UHMWPE, which has reduced fatigue strength.
2. *Second-generation cups with highly cross-linked UHMWPE:* This began with the use of highly cross-linked UHMWPEs in combination with the clinically successful second-generation modular acetabular components since early 2000s. The wear rates were improved but unique problem creeped up of edge impingement. Due to improved wear, surgeons started the use of larger femoral heads that have greater ROM. A larger head size resulted in a thinner acetabular liner compared with a smaller-diameter head in the same shell size. To use a large-diameter head in a relatively small acetabular shell and to maintain adequate thickness of UHMWPE at the weight-bearing region of the dome, thicker poly has to be used lateralizing the head **(Fig. 10)**. The poly is thicker at the dome than at the rim, in the region of the locking mechanism. This eccentric relation of head center to acetabular shell center causes peripheral impingement especially at the elevated liner margin. This further leads to liner fracture. A crescent-shaped fracture occurs

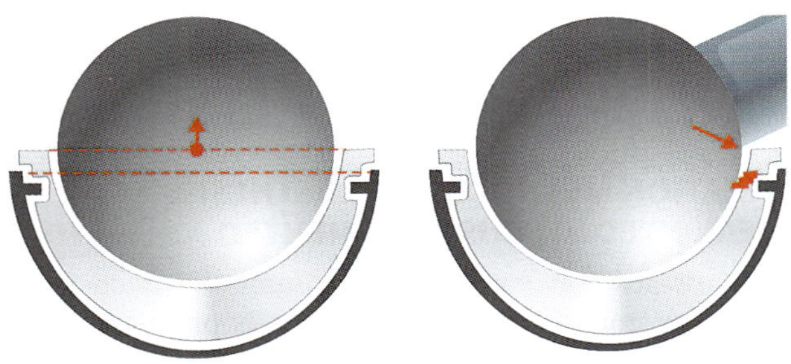

Fig. 10: A cross-sectional diagram to illustrate the effect of a thicker UHMWPE (ultrahigh molecular weight polyethylene) at the dome than at the rim on the use of a large femoral head in a relatively small shell. We know that there is a minimum thickness of poly needed for weight bearing or else it will fail (8 m for older and 6 mm for newer). If one uses a large head size (as has recently been in fashion) then the liner thickness will be compromised but to prevent failure of poly thickness needs to be maintained at the weight-bearing dome increasing the thickness there but simultaneously thinning the poly at periphery to accommodate larger heads. This increased thickness at dome pushes the head center laterally (arrow). Also the "relatively" thin UHMWPE at the rim near the liner-locking mechanism is prone to failure. The reduced coverage of head from pushing of head out has to be addressed by skirting the poly out to cover the protruding head. This makes liner prone to impingement from the femoral neck and rim. Contact forces are transmitted to the unsupported liner rim that hence cracks and a fracture along the outer part of the liner develops failing the locking mechanism resulting in liner-shell dissociation.

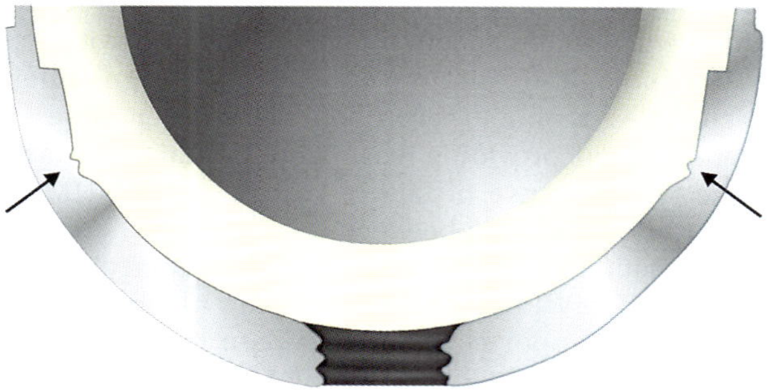

Fig. 11: A third-generation modular cup design where the ultrahigh molecular weight polyethylene (UHMWPE) liner is not elevated above the shell rim. The locking mechanism (arrows) is recessed into the interior of the shell to avoid fracture of the liner rim if impingement occurs.

along the liner rim, which also damages the liner-locking mechanism causes liner-shell dissociation.

3. *Third-generation cementless modular acetabular cups:* Third-generation modular acetabular cups have been developed to reduce the risk of fracture of the liner rim when large-diameter femoral head are used with highly cross-linked UHMWPE. The following design changes have been incorporated **(Fig. 11)**:
   - Eliminating UHMWPE protruding above the rim
   - Minimizing sharp corners at the liner-locking mechanism
   - Recessing the locking mechanism into the interior of the metal shell

The other method to improve the risk of liner fracture is to use the process of annealing just below melting temperature, retaining much of mechanical properties of UHMPE rather than cross-linked poly (it has reduced mechanical properties). Similar features are incorporated into modular ceramic liners to protect the relatively brittle ceramic material from impingement-related damage.

FIXATION METHODS OF PROSTHESIS: CEMENTED VERSUS UNCEMENTED

Two basic fixation methods are commonly practiced for placing the implants in the bone. One is press-fit method without the use of any intermediary method (cementless fixation). The other is fixation of the stem and acetabular cup component in THA by using acrylic bone cement (cemented prosthesis). Both schools are successful in providing reasonably good functional outcomes to the patient, but they are always at loggerheads for gaining superior position. Whatever one portends to be, the unique benefit of one system has been countered by an equally forceful argument by the other school. Till date, the issue is unsettled and I personally feel that the surgeon should be trained in both with an "open mind" without any bias to one system. Then he should apply the unique advantages for each patient to devise the best possible fixation or optimal system suitable. To this effect even the hybrid and reverse hybrid systems have evolved so that one has absolute liberty to use cemented or uncemented femoral stem or acetabular cup or any combination depending on the merits and needs of individual case.

Unlike building construction, the cement used for implantation of prosthesis does not bind the prosthesis to bone. It merely acts as a grout filling the canal space so that the load from prosthesis can be uniformly transferred to bone. A homogeneous, complete continuous layer of bone cement between implant and bone is hence required to achieve this and to prevent stress concentration. Mantle defects are liable to cause local crushing of the bone (leading to periprosthetic fractures) and implant loosening. The characteristics of prosthesis for cemented systems are:

- The prosthesis must have smooth surfaces in order to avoid stress concentrations.
- They must be sufficiently stiff to avoid mechanical loading of cement by elastic deformation of the metal. Co-Cr has the sufficient rigidity and other mechanical parameters for a suitable cemented component.

The disadvantages of acrylic bone cements, however, are:

- *Absence of osseointegration:* Due to dense polymerized structure of cement, it does not allow osseointegration for improved bone fixation.
  - Exothermal polymerization reaction causes bone necrosis
  - Monomer toxicity
- Shrinkage during polymerization of methyl methacrylate (MMA) may compromise the fixation of a component. Improvement in cementing techniques has improved most of the disadvantages [*see* generations of cementing in the Chapter on "Poly (Methyl Methacrylate) (PMMA; Plexiglass, Bone Cement, and Acrylic Bone Cement)"].

  Noncemented THA is characterized by a direct press-fit contact between implant components and surrounding bone close enough to facilitate bone integration. The shape of uncemented stems exhibits edges and grooves to mechanically enhance primary fixation. For long-term stability, osseointegration is an essential component that relies on the patient's health status, so factors reducing the capability of bone growth, such as age or pathological conditions, limit the use of uncemented THA.

  The utility of cemented system and the cause of gradual shift from cemented to cementless system:
  - *Pros for cement includes:*
    - In general for older patients with less vital bone tissue, cemented implants do better that aid to provide additional buttress for metallic fixation.
    - Patients with Dorr type C femurs are most benefited as cementless implants supporting such bone are not available or successful.
    - Cementing also compensates for some reaming errors in acetabular side and bone defects.
    - Moreover need of revision has low probability in these patients where implant life is deemed to outlast patient's life.
    - Cemented fixation has the highest survival rate in most registries when failure has been defined as a revision of the primary implant for aseptic loosening. The surgeons were, however, concerned

with the difficult acetabular side revisions, "cement disease"-related pelvic osteolysis, etc., so that the cementless fixation was sought for.

(*Note:* Pelvic osteolysis has now been shown to result from hydrostatic flow and not due to PMMA.)

- *Pros for uncemented fixations (as also cons for cemented fixation) includes:*
  - As younger patients have biologically more active bone tissue, uncemented THA is preferred in them for permanent bondage.
  - Moreover, this group will more likely undergo revision surgery, which will be complicated by the presence of cement and cement debris.
  - Cemented implants primarily remove larger amount of bone compared to the uncemented implants especially on the femoral side so bone loss is more of a concern in younger patients that are more likely to have revision; this is further compounded by bone necrosis due to exothermic cement curing reaction.
  - Cemented implants provide an immediate postoperative advantage (intimate contact between the prosthesis cement and the bone, which permits dramatic early relief of pain and more weight-bearing) and short-term outcome is very good; there were doubts raised over mid- and long-term results. Some thought that the cemented total hip replacement (THR) had a gradual but discernible diminution in quality over time.
  - Cementless implants provide a broader range of options especially for the acetabulum where liner exchange may be required for postoperative instability, which is the most common cause for early reoperation in all primary THR.
  - Uncemented implants offer more modularity and variety in terms of femoral head size and bearing surfaces.
  - Bone loss is not seen in uncemented stem despite loosening as against the osteolysis quite commonly seen with cemented systems. (There is strong argument to counter this, and the fact that osteolysis has been definitely seen with the use of cementless components now.)

Development of Hybrid Systems

Mainly concerning the above two arguments, there has been a worldwide trend toward uncemented fixation in THR especially by the increased prescription to relatively younger population by virtue of improved component designs. It was observed in mid-1990s that the cemented cups tend to fail much frequently than the stems, and loosening and bone lysis are much more prominent there. Also, revision of an enlarged destroyed acetabulum was cumbersome due to anatomical location and requirement of bone graft not easily available. The popularity of noncemented prostheses also, however, began to wither with cases of "noncement disease" with worse outcomes. This brought up the use of hybrid systems where the femoral stem was cemented; however, the acetabular fixation was primarily uncemented to utilize best of the two philosophies. This trade-off found better use in younger patient as this was also a bit cost-effective. There is no clear evidence till date that the cementless acetabular cup is superior to the cemented cup, however. Furthermore, in the initial findings, it was seen that once fixed, the femoral cementless stems become permanent and even if they get loose bone, loss is minimal as no osteolysis is seen (proven untrue now), so another philosophy of "reverse hybrid" system cropped up where the stem was cementless fixation but the acetabular cup was cemented due to proven record.

Settling Controversy of Cemented versus Cementless versus Hybrid Fixation

The picture is still more confusing when we find that the literature reports better osteolysis, migration properties, and aseptic loosening survival for uncemented acetabular components, but in terms of wear and overall survival, the cemented acetabular components excel. Cemented femoral component undoubtedly provides an immediate postoperative advantage in terms of better integration between bone, cement, and the prosthesis, which permits dramatic early relief of pain and early weight-bearing but the cementless fixation is favored for its deemed permanency.

The overall picture is, however, not so bleak. Some *conclusions* are defined. The cemented fixation is significantly cost-effective than the uncemented components. With respect to revision rates, both cemented and uncemented components are equivalent; however, uncemented components fare better in population <55 years. Moreover, the uncemented femoral stems fare better in this age group than the uncemented acetabular components. Cemented components have an overall higher survival rates when taken together for all revisions for all causes for all age groups in most registries, but on deeper analysis, it appears that the cemented acetabular component does not fare so well for young active population. Thus, cemented acetabulum and stem (cemented THA) may be a better choice for patients aged >60 years. Cementless acetabular cup and femoral stem (cementless THA) are better in younger population but because femoral cemented stem has equivalent results in both younger and elderly population, it can be used to reduce the cost in patients <55–60 years of age by providing a hybrid construct comprising cemented femoral stem and uncemented acetabular cup. This cemented femoral stem also takes into account the unusual proximal femoral anatomy in young like Dorr C type canal and the osteoporotic femora in elderly that do not hold uncemented stems well. Surgeon should, hence, be rationale, ultimately to the patient for the likelihood of the implant he receives! Combinations should be used that best allow the reconstruction of the proper physiological function of the hip joint considering the anatomic situation of the patient. Bone shall be conserved as much as possible and geometries should be preferred allowing for this.

ACETABULAR CUP POSITIONING AND VERSION

Placing acetabular cup in appropriate alignment and version is one of the most crucial aspects of THA. This has been the biggest deterrent for classical surgeons shifting from conventional surgeries to performing THA. It is surprising that even today <50% of the best and high-volume hip surgeons can achieve the ideal target for acetabular cup placement (both inclination and version taken together) for individual patients. The biggest reason for this is that acetabulum is not a static structure and hitting target on a moving component is not at all easy and always possible. There are other associated factors such as spinopelvic dynamics (some call it hip-spine syndrome) and population variance for which single figures cannot be standardized. The optimal cup positioning is important for the following reasons:

- Preventing impingement and resulting instability and liner/component complications
- Improving ROM of the prosthetic component
- Optimal abductor muscle function
- Gait dynamics improvement
- Equalizing limb lengths
- Reducing implant and bearing wear
- For hard-on-hard bearings, it reduces noise generation.

The acetabular cup is implanted in three dimensions, so its position is defined in three distinctive planes:

1. Mediolateral position defines the depth of cup implantation. The acetabular offset is dependent on the center of rotation of acetabulum. This influences the "combined" offset **(Fig. 12),** which is the sum of femoral and acetabular offset, and hence ultimately influences "global" offset (= vertical offset + "combined" offset). Nowadays, the horizontal offset is referred together as a "combined offset" like the "combined anteversion" instead of classical concept of femoral or acetabular offset. Deep cup implantation was classically suggested by Charnley in his low-friction torque arthroplasty. Here, the cup was medialized to reduce the joint reaction forces (shortens the body weight lever arm and increased abductor lever arm) where because of medialization of the cup, the forces were converted into rotatory torque (*see* Chapter on "Biomechanics of Hip Joint"). This is expected to improve bearing surface longevity but increases chances of impingement between cup and femoral components causing cup microseparation and shell/cup failure itself. Also, one must realize that the work of abductor muscles increases because center of rotation is shifted far away medially so more force is needed producing early fatigue, discomfort, and pain. Also, because of excessive medial reaming if the patient needs future arthroplasty, then acetabular bone is already compromised. On the contrary, excessive lateralization is still more harmful because it reduces superolateral support to the cup and brings the construct in line with joint reaction forces increasing bearing wear and abductor dysfunction (their lever arm is reduced). So, the present concept is restoring the anatomic center of rotation to reduce impingement and improve ROM. This also preserves medial bone stock.
2. *Height of cup:* Placing the cup superiorly in iliac bone (high center of rotation cups) as is done for some cases of dysplasia and superior protrusio shortens the abductor muscles increasing joint reaction forces, increased wear of bearing resulting in aseptic loosening and implant failure. This also produces gait disturbance and predisposes to hip instability. Lower center of rotation causes unacceptable lengthening of the limb.
3. *Angular acetabular cup alignment:* This has two components—one is the coronal plane alignment called the acetabular inclination and the other is sagittal plane alignment called cup "version" **(Fig. 13)**. These have important bearing on stability, impingement, ROM, and long-term survival of implant. Classical proposal and often reiterated "safe zone" placement of cup as suggested by Lewinnek (1978) is vehemently challenged now. He suggested that cups placed out of 15 ± 10° of anteversion and 40 ± 10° of inclination have high dislocation rate (6.1% vs. 1.5%). So, this was accepted as the "ideal" placement for acetabular angular position for years. It was also supported by other studies to follow. However, dislocations never ended despite placing the cup within these "ideal" limits and cups outside this safe zone also functioned well, raising scepticism to this as the "holy-grail" cup alignment. Studies comparing the alignment of components in dislocated versus uncomplicated hips found no difference strongly pointing to other factors that compromise stability. We know that factors such as proper surgical exposure respecting soft tissues, soft-tissue tensioning, restoring length, and proper surgical closure of wound are important for THA stability but prosthetic component alignment plays most important role affecting the THA stability. Anteversion of the acetabular cup and, to some extent, its inclination are specifically important in this regard. Because hip instability is a dynamic process, static radiographic measures such as offset, version, inclination do not correlate with a stable hip. It is being increasingly

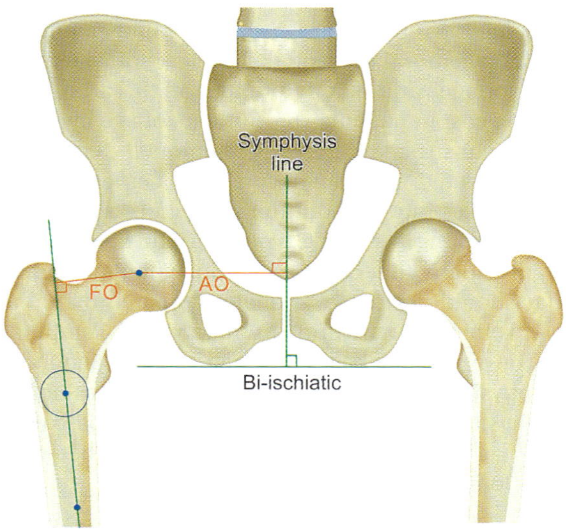

Fig. 12: The acetabular offset (AO) and femoral offset (FO) together determine the combined horizontal offset. FO is measured from anatomical longitudinal femoral canal center.

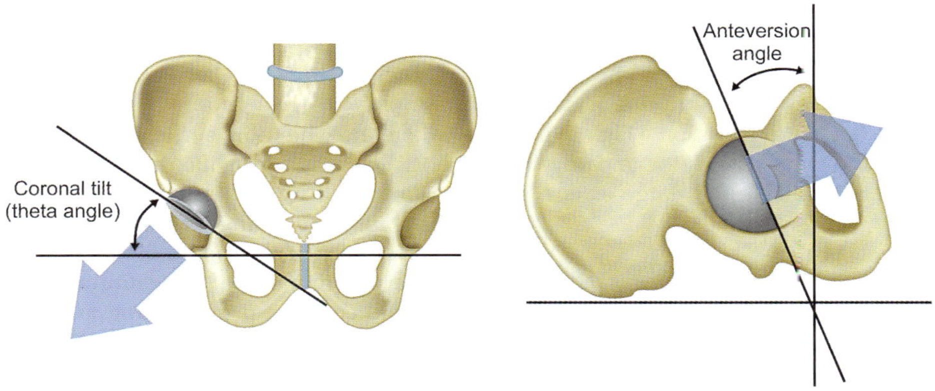

Fig. 13: Angular alignment of cup as assessed in coronal plane determines its inclination as shown on left. The tilt is also measured in transverse plane determining its version as illustrated on right.

recognized that every patient is different, and "NO" "safe zone" will universally work. The concept of functional personalized safe zone has emerged but is in a nascent stage because it can be defined but not determined! It is a range of acetabular anteversion/abduction angles that provides impingement-free ROM during basic activities such as standing, sitting, sitting-to-standing, bending, and laying down. This safe zone is unique for each patient. Femoral head diameter plays an important role in this safe zone as larger diameter heads will provide a wider safe zone. Femoral anteversion should also be considered strongly to acetabular alignment for stability. So, the present accepted methods to plan and execute patient specific variability in angular placement of cup include:

a. *Preoperative assessment of spinopelvic alignment:* This is a large topic now in itself that basically states that status of spine (alignment, deformity, and mobility) affects the dynamic position of acetabular cup. The proposal of acetabular alignment is getting shifted from conventional coronal alignment to sagittal plane functional alignment, which is still undefined and elusive. In a nutshell, the spine-pelvis-hip alignment categorizes patients into two types, viz., hypermobile (kyphosis) and stiff spinopelvic alignment. For hypermobile category, general recommendation is reducing acetabular version and inclination while for stiff category, it is reverse, i.e., increasing anteversion and coronal acetabular inclination (but not >45°). It is a topic in its own and is discussed separately but a very useful practical (but "crude") tip is that if a pelvis looks like "inlet" view on a standard radiograph then increased acetabular anteversion but if the radiograph looks like an outlet view then reduced acetabular anteversion.
b. *Intraoperative assessment of combined anteversion angle (see below):* This does not improve angular cup orientation but more so affects overall hip anteversion because cup version during implantation should not be changed.

The other component is improper coronal plane alignment of acetabular cup (acetabular inclination),

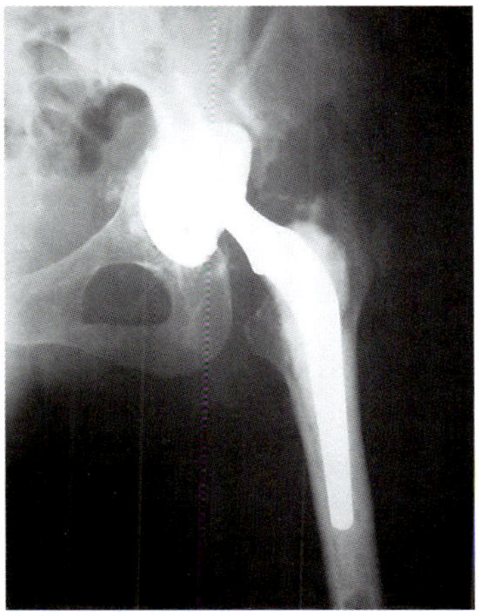

Fig. 14: The acetabular cup here is too vertical approaching inclination of 75–80°. This is likely to cause excessive stress and edge loading of liner, if the hip remains articulated. Such high cup angle causes hip instability and dislocations.

which leads to increased polyethylene wear. Cup implanted in abduction angle of >45° **(Fig. 14)** has high linear and asymmetric polyethylene wear rates resulting in lower implant survival rates. High abduction angles >65° result in catastrophic wear and bearing failure. Cups implanted at 45° of inclination improve ROM of hip particularly the internal and external rotations compared to those with angles >45–50°. Implantation of cup in retroversion leaving it uncovered anteriorly produces psoas impingement that may later need arthroscopic or open release **(Fig. 15)**.

Methods to Optimize Cup Positioning

Various techniques are proposed to optimize cup positioning and reduce ensuing complications **(Box 1)**. *Preoperative planning* is an important aspect of performing THA that is a dwindling art and often bypassed by young aggressive surgeons. It is 2D projection of the 3D acetabulum so does not exactly reproduces the anatomy but is still useful in understanding the center of rotation, implant size, depth/height/angular position of placement and offset. It is discussed in detail later. Very shortly, 3D printed or projected acetabulum from imaging with available templates will be available that will have tremendous impact on preoperative planning. *Patient positioning* is an important variable specially in the lateral decubitus position **(Fig. 16)**. The pelvis may tilt anteriorly 25° to posteriorly 20° and anywhere in-between which is uncontrollable to a large extent. This

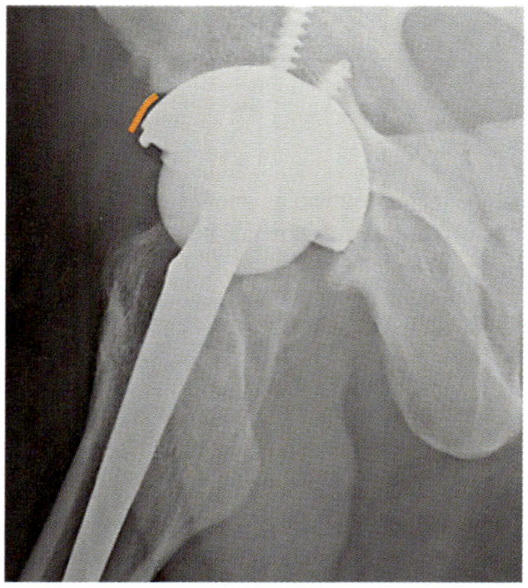

Fig. 15: The anterior uncoverage of acetabular cup (marked as orange line) predisposes to psoas impingement and anterior groin pain.

BOX 1: The techniques to optimize acetabular cup positioning.

Preoperative:
- Templating

Intraoperative:
- Patient positioning
- Assisted surgery—robotic/navigation
- External jigs for cup positioning
- Bone and soft tissue landmarks
- Combined angle of anteversion and coplanar test
- Intraoperative fluoroscopy

should be kept in mind while placing cup in anteversion using external jigs or eyeballing. The operated limb is also adducted tilting the pelvis down in coronal plane, thus if one plans to give cup a 45° inclination from horizontal it will actually be more vertical. Typically, the down tilt is –4° (±12°), so it is very difficult to perfectly position cup in 45° inclination. External jigs are highly inaccurate and have wide variability depending on patient positioning. They just give a false sense of security to the unaware surgeon and are no longer recommended. Navigation and robotic surgery reduce the outliers in cup positioning and improve cup position but are not widely available due to prohibiting costs. For implanting the cup at proper depth, one should identify true floor of the acetabulum by removing the medial osteophyte and reaching the fat pad in cotyloid fossa **(Box 2)**. Ream till the acetabular wall reaches this floor and it usually indicates proper depth of cup placement. Proper angular positioning of cup by various methods has been proposed and described in literature such as:

- *Combined anteversion angle:* Proposed by Ranawat as coplanar test and propounded by Dorr as combined anteversion angle, it is one of the most practical ways of positioning hip in proper angular alignment. The combined angle of anteversion as the name suggests is the sum of femoral stem anteversion and the anteversion of the acetabular cup. This is assessed by "coplanar test" of Ranawat. This is relevant in posterior approach to the hip particularly, as it cannot be done in other positions. Once the femoral stem + head has been implanted or femoral trial is in place (+ femoral head trial), the acetabular component trial is put in the prepared socket (femur first technique). Now, in 10° of adduction, the leg (tibia + fibula) is rotated to produce internal rotation at the implanted hip. The position at which the femoral head and acetabular cup become coplanar, the rotation is stopped and the angle between leg (tibia + fibula) and horizontal (floor) is noted **(Fig. 17)**. This

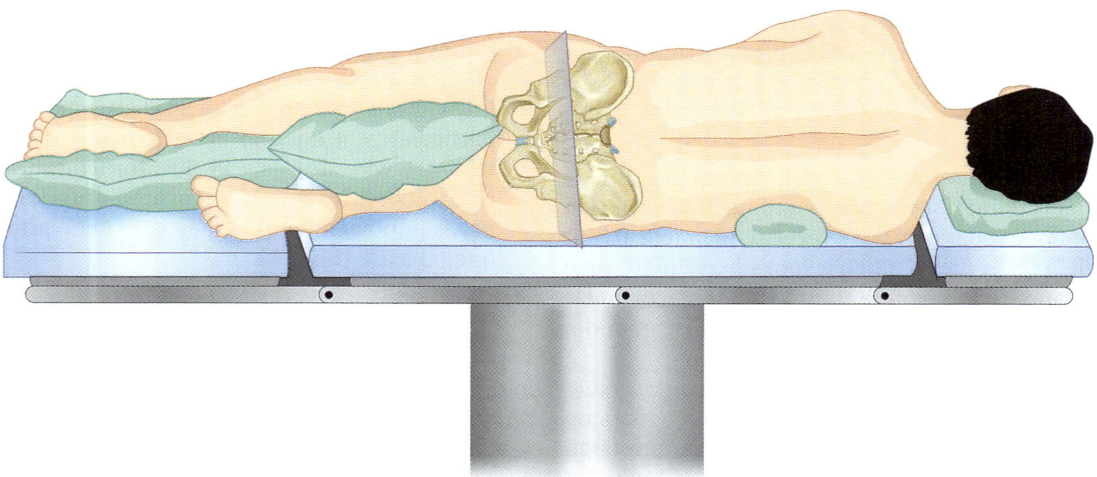

Fig. 16: The lateral position of patient causes pelvic tilt inadvertently. In such a position, the acetabulum faces down, but if horizontal line is used to put cup in 40–45° of inclination then always the cup will get placed in higher inclination and will be open. So, it is recommended to reduce inclination by 5–8° from the measured while implanting cup. Similarly, due to anterior roll of the patient, anteversion of acetabular cup should be increased.

BOX 2: The intraoperative assessment and execution of acetabular cup positioning and overall optimal hip placement.

It is not clear to any one as to what is the "true" acetabular/femoral/combined alignment that will be absolutely stable and will always work. The following is an attempt to provide surgeon reach closer to "functional patient alignment" of his hip (please remember, all this pertains to *posterior approach*). There are three aspects to acetabulum—native size, native version, and native inclination. Out of these three, native size is most important for primary hip replacement, and one should always try to reproduce it. Native version is second important component, which should be restored "in most cases" by placing the cup parallel to transverse acetabular ligament (TAL, there are four described types of TAL but for general discussion, this finer variable can be ignored). Why "in most cases" and not all? The acetabulum may be in excessive anteversion in developmental dysplasia or may be in pathologic retroversion in some patients (identified as crossover sign radiologically), here it may be a better idea to consider overall hip version (combined anteversion) instead of just looking at acetabular version. Version also changes with pathological spinopelvic alignment, but we do not have current methodology to place cup-free hand in this alignment (robotic systems may do this). The last component is inclination which by popular convention and literature support is maintained at 40–45° regardless of patient's native value.

Step 1: Anatomical placement of acetabular cup (template cup size in preoperative plan)—identify floor of acetabulum which is just beneath the cotyloid fossa fat pad and is preserved even in ankylosed hips. Reach this with initial reamers and then expand the cup by incremental reaming. Native size is mostly reached when the expansion of cup reaches floor medially and just starts taking off bone at the posterosuperior margin. Do not ream beyond floor. The reamer is always parallel to the TAL and braces it, do not push reamer far medially from TAL. This technique will prevent too deep a cup and too high a cup maintaining it in anatomical position **(Fig. 19)**.

Step 2: Implant the trial cup parallel to TAL (native version, we are discounting dysplastic and naturally retroverted hips here)—place the cup parallel to TAL and gently tap it for a "soft fit", stand perpendicular to the handle and look for cup inclination. Eyeballing is a bad idea and jigs are not very accurate. Better use a protractor to measure inclination of handle from horizontal. Maintain inclination of 40–45° and then push the cup deep into acetabulum.

- *Useful tip*: Always err on the side of *reducing inclination* by 5–8° from the chosen 40 or 45° because in lateral position, the hip is more adducted. Similarly, people have recommended *increasing anteversion* while cup implantation by 6–10° because of common forward roll of patient.
- Literature says that TAL is not good for assessment of inclination, but I disagree. If cup is not medialized and is not too high using above technique, then we lower the handle down so that the inferior sector of cup parallel to TAL is rotated inside medially (maintaining parallelism) then inclination will be reduced. This will also produce uncovering of superior region of the cup, which is desirable for reducing inclination to 40°. Lastly, inclination can also be checked by the amount of uncovering of the cup that was seen in preoperative templating but this is not very accurate and reproducible.

Step 3: Now, prepare and implant the femoral trial. Maintain limb length by appropriate technique such as coaxial stich technique. Once the limb length is restored that means vertical offset is restored. Now, we need to equalize horizontal offset only. This can be done by intraoperative projection of femoral offset (measured from center of femoral head/neck to tip of trochanter), it can be measured using ruler. Acetabular offset will be constant because cup size is determined already. Now, when vertical and combined horizontal offsets are restored then global offset will automatically fall in place. Perform coplanar test of Ranawat **(Fig. 17)** to obtain target "combined anteversion angle" (for Asian population is near 30–35°). Cemented stems offer leeway of changing anteversion much better. For uncemented stem, acetabular version will need adjustment! In this case, femur first technique is much better as follows. Prepare femur and obtain global offset as above (so this becomes step 2 here), now use combined anteversion technique to place acetabular cup in correct version.

Step 4: Check abductor tightness (palpation) or by the "shuck test". If the soft tissues are loose then offset needs to be altered usually. Recheck leg length, if leg is shortened then it is very easy—use a higher size head (not a larger diameter head, this size is implant "+" size heads). If leg length is equal, then only horizontal offset needs to be changed. To increase this offset, one can sink stem and choose a "+" size head. If hip is too tight then soft tissue tension without altering limb length can be achieved by keeping stem proud and choosing a "-" size head **(Fig. 20)**.

Step 5: Perform hip stability check for sitting position, sleeping position, and anterior/posterior/abduction impingement (as described by Ranawat). Instability is specific position and will need appropriate tweaking.

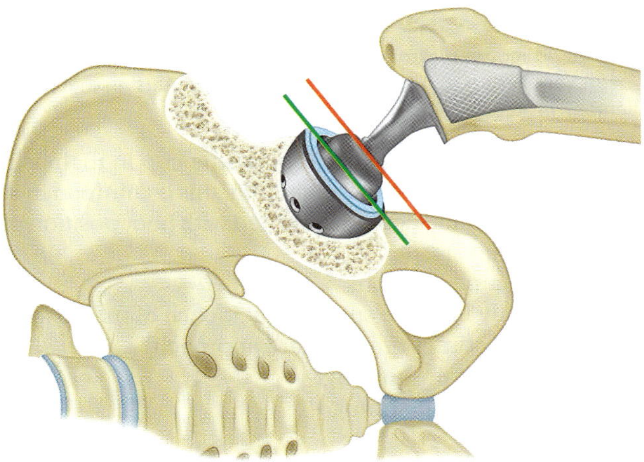

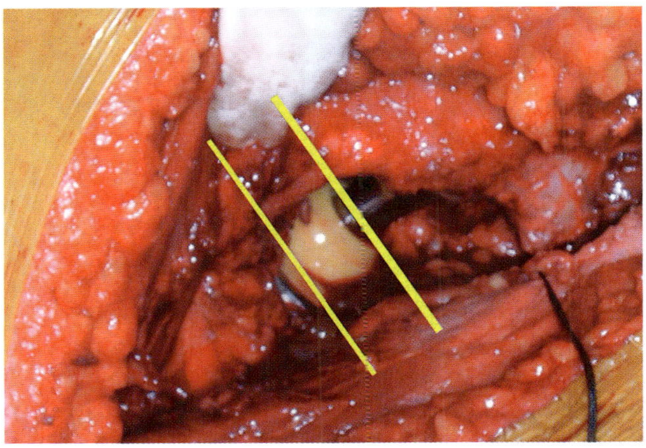

Fig. 17: The Ranawat's coplanar test to implant acetabular cup in correct version as done for femur first technique using a posterior approach. It is assessed in 10° of limb adduction. Notably, the acetabular liner should be nonlipped one, else it will be very difficult the coplanarity.

angle is the combined angle of anteversion (CAA). The recommended CAA is 30–50° but there is suggestion that in Indian (Asian) population, the lower value near 30° is more apt.

- Archbold-TAL technique **(Fig. 18)**
- Gray and McCollum
- Sotereanos
- Notch-acetabular angle of Maruyama

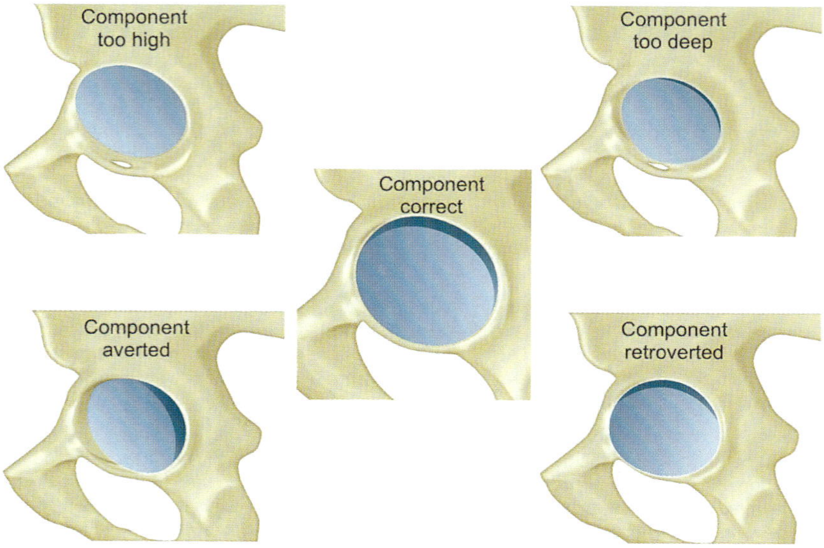

Fig. 18: As suggested by Archbold, the transverse acetabular ligament provides a good alignment guide in nondysplastic hips for placing the cup in correct anteversion.

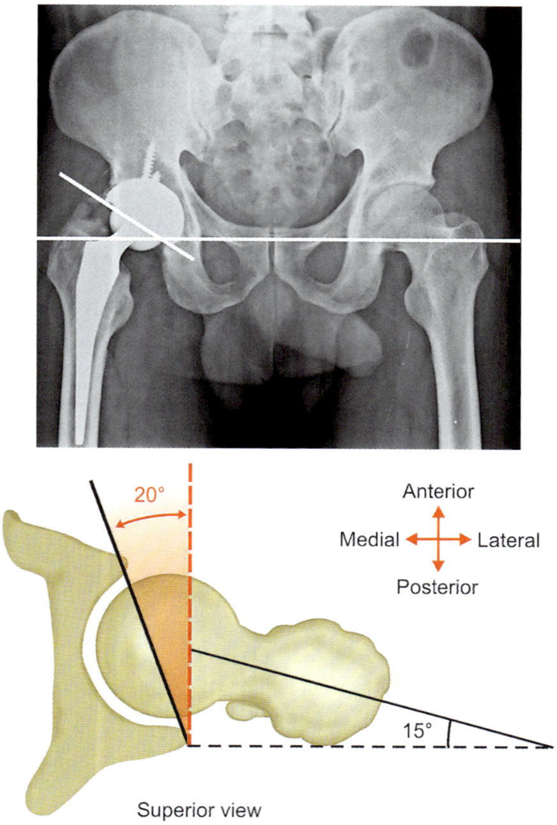

Fig. 19: The radiograph on left demonstrates acetabular cup implanted at correct depth and of correct size. The acetabular cup in correct height lies below teardrop—between tear drop and "cotyledon" (inferior posterior acetabulum). The cup should be just shy of Kohler's line and not touch or cross it, else it will be deeper than native acetabular floor. After correct size, depth and inclination look for correct version as illustrated on right.

Risk Factors for Cup Malposition

The chief factors that lead to malposition of cups are *inexperience* (young surgeons in first few cases fail to understand the dynamics fully so are liable to place the cup in malposition) and poor exposure of the acetabulum, this is common in *obese patients*. The other factors associated with poor position of the acetabular cup are:

- Low-volume surgeons
- Minimally invasive surgery (incidence of malposition as high as six times the standard approach)
- Poor patient positioning
- Inappropriate planning

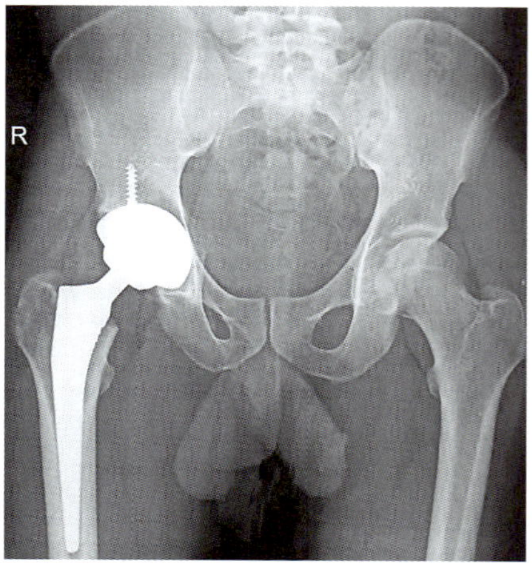

Fig. 20: To reduce horizontal offset in this patient, the femoral stem has been kept proud to maintain limb length while using a "minus"-size femoral head.

ROLE OF SURGICAL APPROACH

There is conventionally stated increased dislocation rate associated with posterior approach. This has considerably improved with better understanding of the approach and technique. There are >15 described variations of posterior approach and poor understanding of the same by young surgeons and not following basics such as capsular and posterior sleeve repair is associated with instability.

Anterior approach has been promoted as an approach that has less dislocation rate and faster postoperative recovery especially in the first 6 weeks but has various wound-related complications. I do not find any substantial advantage of one approach over another that would strongly one to shift the ground in the literature, there are proponents of each and presently it does not seem that approach has great variability in altering outcomes. It is recommended to continue using the approach, which one is familiar is and makes the surgeon comfortable in case some unusual scenarios arise intraoperatively. One should gain knowledge of alternative approaches to the hip so as to understand the scarring and tissue damage for revision cases and also in specific scenarios, one approach may be better than other (*see* Chapter on "Surgical Approaches to Hip Joint").

GOALS OF TOTAL HIP ARTHROPLASTY

There are only two specific goals for performing a THA:

1. Relieving pain emanating from hip joint
2. Improving function due to disease affecting the hip joint

The glamour of being called a replacement surgeon or revision surgeon comes nowhere near to these primary goals for performing THA.

INDICATIONS FOR TOTAL HIP ARTHROPLASTY

There are many absolute and extended indications. Basically, any hip joint pathology that terminally limits the hip function and/or causes pain that can be improved upon by performing THA is an indication for THA itself—the list includes among others:

- *Osteoarthritis:*
  - Primary
  - Secondary:
    - Osteonecrosis (most common), sickle cell disease
    - Post-trauma
    - Developmental dysplasia of the hip
    - Legg–Calvé–Perthes disease
    - Slipped capital femoral epiphysis
    - Sequel of septic arthritis
    - Crystalline disease
    - Paget's disease
    - Acromegaly
    - Hypothyroidism
    - Hyperparathyroidism
    - Multiple or spondyloepiphyseal dysplasia (SED)
    - Ehlers–Danlos syndrome (EDS)
    - Thalassemia
    - Hemophilia
    - Gaucher's disease
    - Ochronosis
    - Wilson's disease
    - Hemochromatosis
- Rheumatoid and other terminal inflammatory arthropathies:
  - Lupus
  - Psoriatic arthritis
  - *Spondyloarthropathies:*
    - Ankylosing spondylitis
    - Reiter disease
- Hip dysplasia that has evolved into degenerative joint disease
- Patient who desires movement at hip after arthrodesis
- Patient who wants a stable hip after Girdlestone type hip resection arthroplasty
- Failed reconstruction of hip (osteotomy, previous dynamic hip screw for fracture intertrochanteric, etc.).

CONTRAINDICATIONS FOR HIP ARTHROPLASTY

- *Absolute:*
  - Active sepsis
  - Severely damaged hip that cannot be restored by standard or even extravagant attempts
  - Medical comorbidities outweigh the gain from THA.
- *Relative:*
  - Renal failure (increased sepsis)
  - Intravenous drug abuser
  - *History of high-dose pelvic irradiation:*
    - Charcot arthropathy
    - Patients with dementia
    - Unstable patients suffering from psychiatric illness, excessive alcohol consumption and those who will be unable to understand that THA is merely start of treatment for them and not the end of it
    - Unrealistic expectations of patient

PREOPERATIVE PLANNING

Clinical examination is the most important preoperative assessment. Examine the hip and limbs as we do for all hip patients including flexion/adduction/abduction deformities, true lengths, apparent lengths, ROM, gait and most importantly spine examination. Also, perform peripheral neurological examination. Symptoms pertaining to spine problems should never be ignored as now it is very clear beyond doubt that spinepelvic-hip system functions as a unit and affection in one will have consequences in other component. The detailed discussion on spinopelvic alignment is presented below. Evaluate medication history from patients especially the inflammatory arthritis, as they may be on synthetic disease-modifying antirheumatic drug (sDMARD), biologic disease-modifying antirheumatic drug (bDMARD), or biosimilar disease-modifying antirheumatic drug (bsDMARD) [*see* Chapter on "Joint Disorders Including Inflammatory and Noninflammatory Arthritis and Infective Arthritides (Including Mycobacterial Infection and Prosthetic Joint Infection)"] and these drugs need to be stopped for a fare delay between surgery. Cardiorespiratory assessment is a must as most deaths after joint arthroplasty are due to compromised and nonoptimized cardiorespiratory status and it is important for planning alternative short surgery and prognostication or avoiding surgery altogether in some cases. Age, gender, obesity, and neurological diseases such as parkinsonism have their implications on outcome of specific implants and surgical technique. In the end, always look for skin, previous scars, and drug (opioid) abuse in these patients. Patients with low hemoglobin such as ankylosing and inflammatory arthropathies, and renal osteodystrophies need specific measures for blood conservation during and before surgery to avoid and minimize complications of blood component transfusions. For radiographic assessment, always obtain true standing AP radiographs of the pelvis and full-length femur with hip joint AP and lateral projections. If spine symptoms are present, always obtain sitting and standing lateral lumbosacral spine radiographs for spinopelvic assessment. Dysplasia or distorted anatomy will need additional assessment by dedicated CT scans.

Templating

Apart from the routine workup and evaluation of patient, templating is of paramount importance in obtaining reproducible results. It is the process of anticipating the size and position of implants prior to hip arthroplasty. It is not at all a guesswork, but a systematic procedure that helps the operating surgeon in many ways. The *goals* of templating are:

- Analyze hip anatomy and variations
- Determine anatomic hip center that needs to be restored also for correcting the leg length and femoral offset.
- *Determine implant size and position:* This reduces inventory by and large, and one is clear as to what is to be done in the operation theater.
- Rehearse surgery in mind as one is clear he can communicate to the staff and assistants better so the speed of surgery also increases.
- Identify problems in advance and correct them for smooth surgery.

Templating the hips should be a habit and unless developed one is bound to fail or struggle with frustration at least once while operating after which he will automatically switch to templating. It is a good habit to documented the templated size on the operating room board for comprehension of the whole operating team **(Fig. 21)**. Templating allows the surgeon to anticipate potential difficulties in advance that can be addressed intraoperatively, the hip biomechanics is more accurately reproduced as in fact, the surgery is double checked and also discrepancy in leg length is minimized **(Box 3)**. Templating is not but a straightforward process and bears a learning curve, experience over time teaches the accuracy of templating and overall templating is 52–98% accurate for sizing to near of ±1.

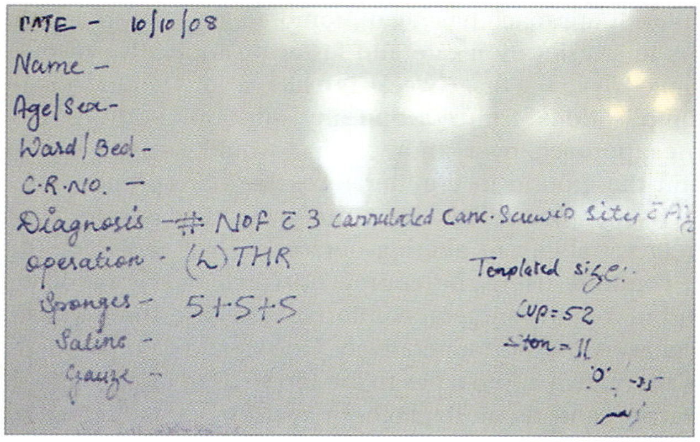

Fig. 21: The hip should be templated at least a day before surgery and the obtained sizes, etc. should be written clearly on the operating room patient information board for understanding of the whole operating team.

BOX 3: Role of templating in total hip arthroplasty (THA).

Templating is a must for all cases (even if one considers a case simple and obvious). It must be done at least 1 day prior to surgery and not in operating room. Implant inventory is never complete in our country always, so templating gives a very good approximation of what to ask from the particular company and what implant to choose. The five basic things to note down while templating that have direct bearing on surgical procedure and reproducing best possible THA are:

1. Acetabular cup size—measure it from just below the tear drop. Typically speaking the acetabular cup is best positioned at a point midway between teardrop and the cotyledon (this is the inferior posterior rim of acetabulum) visible on radiograph inferior and lateral to teardrop
2. Femoral stem size and type
3. Femoral offset
4. Neck cut line (must for cementless stems and collared prosthesis)
5. Limb length discrepancy (to be adjusted as part of vertical offset)

Digital templating is fully acceptable, it is of two broad types—manual templating on digital films (to know the magnification used place a known size marker on the radiograph so that it can correlate with sizes or ask the radiographer to give 1.2× magnification to the radiograph itself reproducing real size images for templating) and templating using commercial digital software.

Prerequisites for Proper Templating

Standard radiographs or given templates the radiographs should be standardized. The magnification should be known (use a marker) from the correlation of distance from bone to cassette. For a cassette into table slot ≈15–20% magnification while for a cassette under buttock ≈10% magnification is seen (for a beam placed 1 meter away and cassette placed 5 cm below the buttock the magnification is 20 ± 6%). Obtain AP radiographs of pelvis, hip, and lateral projection of the hip along with the contralateral hip. The styloid process radiograph of pelvis gives valuable information for leg-length discrepancy, determination of anatomic hip center, and assessment of contralateral hip pathology. The AP projection of hip should be obtained with hip in 15–20° of internal rotation to bring the hip into plane of acetabulum and allows accurate assessment of femoral neck-shaft angle, femoral offset, adduction/abduction contracture, and metaphyseal dimensions. It gives a more accurate assessment of proximal femoral dimensions that may be evaluated by the Dorr index; it often helps to decide between the uses of cemented versus cementless implants. Evaluate the radiographs for bone quality and other bone diseases likely to influence the implant placement (Paget's disease, previous osteotomies, or fibrous dysplasia). If the affected hip cannot be brought into internal rotation then it is better to evaluate the contralateral hip (if normal) or obtain the posteroanterior (PA) views. Lateral views are taken often in a table down position (Lowenstein). The bone is typically closer to the cassette, and this reduces magnification so one should be aware of this fact. These radiographs are important to determine anterior femoral bow, femoral neck version, and intramedullary canal dimension. Mark the following references on the radiographs:

- Ilioischial (Kohler's) line for protrusio assessment
- Interischial line for determining leg lengths
- *Interteardrop line:* Teardrop is the most accurate landmark from a conventional radiograph. The teardrop represents an actual anatomic landmark of the inferomedial acetabulum rather than a radiographic image. Make a line joining the base of the teardrops.
- *Vertical teardrop line:* These lines bisect the teardrop and are perpendicular to the interteardrop line.
- *Femoral head center:* Use circular templates to mark the center of femoral head.
- *Femoral offset:* The perpendicular distance from the neutral long axis of the femur and the center of rotation of the hip.
- *Femoral neck-shaft angle:* The angle between the central axis of the femur and the axis of the femoral neck
- Lesser trochanter
- *Saddle point:* The junction of superior aspect of femoral neck and the greater trochanter.

The next step is determining the following characteristics that need to be addressed during surgery and are to be corrected:

- *Leg-length estimation:* Vertical distance from interischial or interteardrop line to lesser trochanter. Use medial most aspect of lesser trochanter, as it is least affected by rotations of pelvis.
- *Acetabular dysplasia (Ranawat method):* Draw line connecting inferior teardrop to superolateral lip of acetabulum. Normal angle made from the interteardrop line is 45°. Any deviation indicates dysplasia.

Templating Procedure

First, template the acetabulum. Place acetabular template adjacent to lateral edge of teardrop at 40–45° angle relative to interteardrop line and adjust component size to maximize cup coverage and avoid excessive bone resection. At this angle, the medial border should approximate the ilioischial line and the cup has adequate lateral bone coverage, with minimal removal of the supportive subchondral bone. For a cemented cup, select size which allows a uniform 2–3 mm cement mantle. Mark acetabular component center of rotation from template. For a destroyed acetabulum with distorted anatomy, template the normal acetabulum and transpose it to the affected side. In case of protrusio, it is imperative to lateralize the template adjacent to the lateral edge of the teardrop to increase offset and reduce cup-neck impingement. On the other hand, for a lateralized acetabulum, medialize template to the teardrop. For dysplastic acetabulum with superolateral migration, it is better to restore the anatomic hip center and augment the defect; however in case of nonrestorable hip center, choose a high hip center.

Template the femur based on the chosen stem type (cemented versus noncemented) or proximal versus distal filling stem. The stem size is best determined on AP film. In case of a cementless chosen stem, for a proximally coated stem, it is better to emphasize on the proximal fit and fill of the canal; however, for an extensively coated film, one should be giving emphasis to the diaphyseal isthmic fill. For cemented stems, allow 2–3 mm of the clear space for cement. Place the femoral template along the longitudinal femoral axis and adjust it vertically to position the femoral head center at the same vertical height as the previously marked acetabular component center. There will be few situations that arise in this sitting:

- If head/cup centers overlap (best scenario), length/offset restored
- If head center medial, increased femoral offset
- If head center lateral, reduced femoral offset
- If head center higher, increased leg length and cause adduction deformity reducing head coverage
- If head center lower, reduced leg length and will cause abduction deformity increasing head coverage.

Adjust the femoral component size (modular necks) to obtain desired offset and length in above situations. Offset may further be adjusted by choosing a stem with different neck-shaft angle or choosing a stem with built-in higher or lesser offset.

Newer methods include the use of digital templating. These provide an improved measure of magnification but results are probably similar to manual templating.

Spinopelvic Alignment

The optimal component position is still undefined and has been a topic of intense investigation since the inception of THA. This is now being redefined considering hip–spine relation and femoral implant orientation.

Historical "Safe Zone"

Lewinnek et al. (1978) suggested an abduction angle of 40 ± 10° and an anteversion angle of 15 ± 10° in a paper that seems to be significantly flawed. Critically reading the paper, it is found that the acetabular implant was within this safe zone in 3 out of 9 dislocations (33%). Also, hip dislocation did not occur in 35 out of 113 patients (30.9%) in whom the acetabular implant was outside the safe zone. The femoral anteversion and offset was neglected in original assessment.

Functional Personalized Safe Zone

As stated previously, it is defined but not determined. From recumbent to standing position, the acetabular cup position does not change significantly (<5°) but from standing to sitting or vice-versa, there is a significant change in acetabular anteversion and inclination in a normal patient **(Figs. 22A and B)**. This is the reason Lazennec et al. discussed the sagittal "functional" cup position in THR as opposed to the coronal inclination and anteversion achieved at surgery. This spine–pelvis–hip relationship can be captured on a lateral radiograph of lumbar spine and pelvis. There are lots of sagittal angles and measurements explained for assessment of spinopelvic imbalance, a simplified description is presented here. Sagittal sacral slope

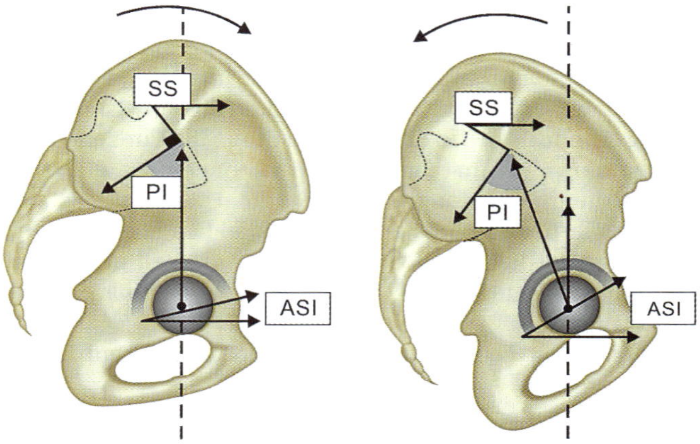

Figs. 22A and B: The sagittal sacral slope (SS) changes significantly in sitting (lower angle) to standing position (higher angle) and vice versa. This alters SS the acetabular sagittal inclination = version of the acetabular cup which if not optimal then may impinge in particular position. The pelvic incidence (PI) is constant for a patient and does not change with position of sitting or standing.

(SS) is a good measure and determines pelvis tilt. It is 40° in standing and 20° in sitting. In seated position, the pelvis tilts posteriorly (↓SS) producing increased anteversion and inclination of the acetabulum—biological tilt of acetabulum. The posterior pelvic tilt (PT) from standing to sitting is normally 20°, and the femur flexes only 55–70° to accomplish sitting. The patterns of spinopelvic mobility abnormalities are divided into two types:

- *Hypermobility:* It is defined as pelvic motion (change in SS) of ≥30° between standing and sitting. It may be normal also and is advantageous to the patients because it reduces required hip motion and minimize impingement. Hypermobility is considered to be unbalanced when it is a result of the lumbar spine tilting into kyphosis (≡ flexible and unbalanced type of Phan et al.) with sitting (seated sacral tilt of <10° and is considered severe when <5°). This is associated with three conditions:
  1. Stiff hips that have flexion ROM of ≤50°, which forces increased posterior tilt of the pelvis during sitting.
  2. Patients with a body mass index (BMI) of >40 kg/m^2, who have a large trunk mass that forces increased posterior tilt of the pelvis with sitting to balance their body.
  3. Patients with neuromuscular imbalance (Parkinson's disease).
- *Spinopelvic stiffness:* It is defined as ≤10° change in sacral tilt between standing and sitting positions (as may occur in lumbar degenerative disk disease, facet spondylosis of the lumbar spine, lumbar fusion, or ankylosing spondylitis). Stiffness can occur in three patterns (Stefl et al.):
  1. The pelvis tilts posteriorly from standing to sitting ≤10°, such that the sacral tilt crosses a value of 30°—decreased pelvic motion but is not fixed anteriorly or posteriorly.
  2. Stuck standing—loss of posterior tilt when sitting so that the pelvis is fixed in anterior tilt (sitting sacral tilt is >30°) ≡ Phan et al. rigid and balanced.
  3. Stuck sitting—the pelvis is fixed in posterior tilt and never tilts anteriorly with standing (standing sacral tilt is <30°) ≡ Phan et al. rigid and unbalanced **(Table 1)**.

TABLE 1: The recommendations on altering acetabular cup version based on spinopelvic imbalance as proposed by Phan et al.

Parameter	*Balanced*	*Unbalanced*
Flexible	Cup version from 5 to 25°	Spinal realignment followed by THA—component anteversion from 15 to 25° Or Primary THA with decreased component anteversion
Rigid	Cup version from 15 to 25°	Spinal realignment followed by THA—component anteversion from 15 to 25° Or Primary THA with decreased component anteversion

(THA: total hip arthroplasty)

Both 2 and 3 increases the risk of impingement and dislocation.

While sitting, the acetabulum anteverts more to contain the flexed and internally rotated femoral head. After THR, dislocation can occur because of the loss of functional anteversion, resulting in anterior impingement. Always remember that impingement is the harbinger of dislocation in most hip instabilities thus outlining the importance of implant positioning. Diagnosis of hip impingement is difficult following THR because no currently available imaging or computerized technique can reliably identify it. Dislocation is the most recognized consequence of impingement, which may be either between implant components, implant-bone or only osseous. The highest risk for impingement from spinal imbalance is pathologic stiffness (rigid and unbalanced hips, according to Phan et al.) like in spinal fusion. Such a pelvis does not achieve the anterior tilt that physiologically occurs in the transition from sitting to standing → acetabulum fails to retrovert → femur itself must hyperextend to compensate for the relative lack of anterior PT → high chance of posterior impingement and anterior hip dislocation.

Similarly, in "stuck standing" position, the pelvis is never able to reach SS <30° (lack of posterior tilt) while sitting → the acetabulum does not undergo normal physiologic transitional anteversion → the femur must hyperflex to facilitate sitting → this produces impingement anteriorly and hence predisposes to posterior hip dislocation.

It is possible that sagittal cup measurements can provide a more predictable "safe zone" for optimal cup position (the combination of anteversion and inclination) than coronal safe zones, but a way to measure and reproduce it is not available. For flexible and balanced spine, a component range of 10° appears optimal. For functional activities such as bending, low sitting, and squatting, a smaller safe zone than that described by Lewinnek et al. is required. Not complicating it any further, simple practical tricks are presented here:

- For patients with stiff spinopelvic motion (change in SS ≤10°)—the acetabular cup requires more coronal inclination (45–50°, 50° only in elderly patient else keep it near 45°) and anteversion (combined anteversion of 35–40°).

- For hypermobility types (change in SS ≥30°)—the cup needs less coronal inclination (35–40°) and anteversion (combined anteversion of 20–30°).
- If one is not comfortable with SS measurements, then further simplification could be (this is very crude however)—for a pelvis that looks more like inlet view on a standing AP pelvis radiograph—increase anteversion and inclination. If the look is more like an outlet view, then reduce acetabular version and inclination.

This discussion makes it clear the importance of examination of spine for a hip case and relevance of standing and sitting lateral spine-pelvis-hip radiographs in revision THR for acute or late dislocation, and primary THR in patients with spinal fusion or known spine disease. EOS imaging reveals coordinated motion of the spine-pelvis-hip joint during postural change such as from lying to standing and from standing to sitting. But, this is a static measure only. For those who are keener on finer detailing to understanding spinopelvic alignment, it is also described in relation to pelvic incidence (PI) and lumbar lordosis (LL). PI determines the position of the femoral heads in relation to the spine **(Figs. 22A and B)** and is fixed for an individual patient irrespective of standing/sitting position. This is, however, variable in population for unknown reasons. PI is the sum of SS and PT, if SS changes PT changes compulsorily **(Fig. 23)** keeping PI constant. Normally, PI is within 10° of LL measured using Cobb method **(Fig. 24)**, i.e., difference between PI and LL is <10°. The algorithm based on PI and LL is presented in **Figure 25**.

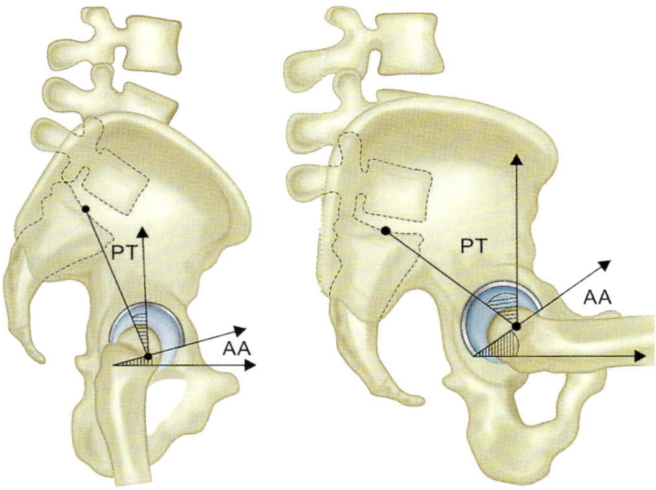

Fig. 23: The pelvic tilt (PT) changes in sitting and standing positions and reciprocates sacral slope. The PT is ess in standing when the sacral slope (SS) is higher (illustrated on left) and vice versa. This reciprocation makes the pelvic incidence (PI) remains constant irrespective of position. Lesser the PT lesser is the acetabular anteversion (AA), while increased PT as in sitting increases acetabular anteversion.

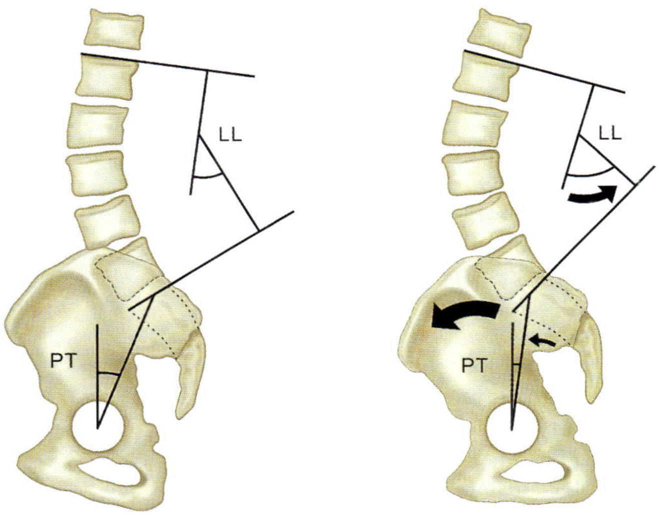

Fig. 24: The lumbar lordosis (LL) can be measured using Cobb's method and normally, it varies within 10° of pelvic incidence (PI). Pelvic tilt (PT) varies with sitting (higher angle, illustrated on left) and standing (lower) due to change in sacral slope, which varies inversely to PT. difference between PI and LL can be used to define spinopelvic imbalance and it helps in optimal acetabular cup version positioning.

CLINICAL RESULTS AND POSSIBLE COMPLICATIONS

To recover pain-free mobility and overcome restrictions in their private and professional activities are the main expectations of patients. Based on these grounds, >80% of the patients are satisfied with the result after THA. Durable solutions of THA can only be achieved, if the surgeon manages to reconstruct the hip joint in a way that it can fulfill its proper function. This requires a high degree of skill and practice. Deviations from the perfect biomechanical alignment will increase hip loads and result in failure.

COMPLICATIONS OF ARTHROPLASTY

Arthroplasty as a procedure by itself indicates a major undertaking. Most of the surgical procedures are encased under the term major if they have significant morbidity or mortality associated with them. The only other reason why some surgeries are called major is because of the surgical time. Various complications are associated with THA that can be summarized by dividing them into early and late as follows:

- *Early complications:*
  - *Cardiopulmonary:*
    - Chest pain
    - Palpitations
    - Dyspnea
    - Pulmonary embolism
    - Congestive heart failure
    - Atelectasis
    - Fat embolism
    - Blood loss
  - *Neuropsychiatric:*
    - Altered sensorium
    - Postsurgical psychosis

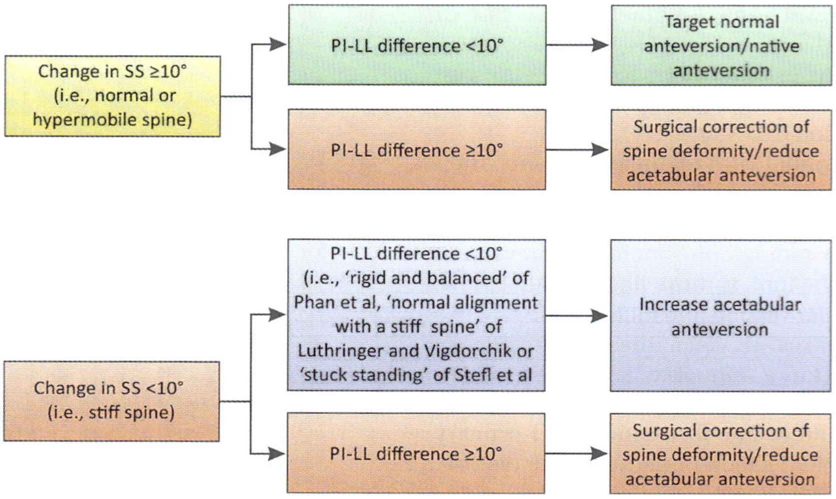

Fig. 25: The algorithm for adjusting acetabular cup anteversion based on pelvic incidence and lumbar lordosis.

    - Hyponatremia
    - Delirium
  - *Nonspecific:*
    - Fever
    - Nausea
    - Abdominal pain
  - *Renal:*
    - Oliguria
    - Chronic renal failure
    - Urinary retention
    - Urinary tract infection
  - *Wound complications:*
    - Superficial infection
    - Wound necrosis
    - Instability and dislocation
    - Neurovascular injury
- *Late complications:*
  - Aseptic loosening
  - Heterotopic ossification (HO)
  - Malignancy
  - Metal hypersensitivity
  - Late instability
  - Stress fractures
  - Periprosthetic fractures

Below are discussed some of the orthopedically relevant and common complications.

Deep Infection

Infection in THA or for any arthroplasty has great negative impact on patient satisfaction, causes morbidity and mortality, and places a large financial burden on the healthcare system. The incidence of infection after THA is 1–2% for primary THA and 3–5% for revision THA. The pathogenesis of periprosthetic infection is dealt elsewhere. *Staphylococcus aureus* and *Staphylococcus epidermidis* account for >50% of the pathogens, Gram-negative aerobic and facultative organisms for 11% of pathogens, and anaerobic bacteria 12% of pathogens. The most frequent source of infection includes the patient's skin (most frequent), blood, or the operating room environment. Risk factors for infection include:

- Advanced vascular disease
- A history of multiple operative procedures
- Extensive scarring
- A history of wound infection
- Rheumatoid or psoriatic arthritis
- Renal disease
- Immunosuppressive medication
- Diabetes mellitus
- Hemophilia
- Obesity
- Malnourishment

Classification

- Acute postoperative infections (type I, within first month) are usually caused by wound colonization, infected hematomas, or superficial infections spreading to the periprosthetic space. It is better treated by wound debridement while retaining the prosthesis.
- Late chronic infections (type II) are indolent infection presenting after 1st month. They originate at the time of surgery itself but owing to either a small inoculum or low virulence of the organisms; the presentation is often delayed to between 1 and 24 months. This mandates prosthesis removal.
- Acute hematogenous infections (type III) are the least common. They present with sudden deterioration in a previously well-functioning THA. These may be associated with a history of pyogenic infection elsewhere in body (usually skin) or recent dental work. The treatment includes prosthesis removal and debridement.
- Positive intraoperative cultures (type IV) are fourth type to include patients with two out of five positive intraoperative cultures without any other features of obvious infection. They may be treated by extended organism-specific antibiotics.

Prevention [*see* periprosthetic infection in Chapter on "Joint Disorders Including Inflammatory and Noninflammatory Arthritis and Infective Arthritides (Including Mycobacterial Infection and Prosthetic Joint Infection)"]:

- Proper identification of risk factors
- Surgical technique
- Operating room environment
- *Prophylactic antibiotic use:* Systemic antimicrobial prophylaxis be given 30–60 minutes before the skin incision is made. Prolonged procedures require an additional intraoperative dose of antibiotic.
- Use of body exhaust suits
- Laminar flow (vertical laminar airflow units)
- Ultraviolet lights (which destroy airborne bacteria)
- Proper sterilization of instruments
- Careful preparation of the operative site
- The use of double gloves
- Reduction of traffic flow in the operating room
- *Characteristics of prosthesis:* Cobalt–chromium surfaces have been found to be more conducive to infection than titanium surfaces (at least nine times); porous surfaces are more conducive to infection than polished surfaces.
- Dental procedure prophylaxis (associated with gingival hemorrhage) includes amoxicillin 2 g PO (or clindamycin 300 mg PO) administered 1 hour prior to procedure. The American Society of Colon and Rectal Surgeons and the American Society for Gastrointestinal Endoscopy do not recommend prophylactic antibiotics for colonoscopy, sigmoidoscopy, or endoscopy.

Aseptic Loosening

This is defined as implant loosening as a result of noninfective osteolysis resulting from various factors primarily the inflammatory reaction to wear particles. The main reason for aseptic loosening had been poly (UHMPE) wear. Polyethylene wear debris starts a subtle chronic granulomatous inflammatory response, which becomes more pronounced as osteolysis progresses. Polyethylene particles above a critical size of about 0.2–0.8 μm can be phagocytosed by macrophages and initiate a series of physiological reactions, which finally lead to osteolysis and aseptic loosening of the implant. This particle-induced periprosthetic osteolysis may affect both the acetabular and the femoral prostheses' components.

Polyethylene debris is created with a typical size of 0.2–5 μm, whereas metallic debris released from MoM prosthesis (no longer in use) exhibits typically a size of 50 nm. Debris particles can also be generated and released from surfaces not designed for tribological applications, such as conical taper junctions or in case of micromotion between stem and bone or stem and cement along the stem surface and analogously on interfaces on the acetabular side that should not be subjected to movements under normal conditions.

The dissemination of wear particles to liver, spleen, or abdominal lymph nodes after hip or knee replacement is a common feature. But usually size and concentration of such disseminated debris particles appear to be pathologically irrelevant. The disseminated particles are mostly generated by wear of metal against bone cement, metal against bone or in taper junctions between femoral head and stem, or by micromotion between shell and liner of the acetabular cup. Large femoral head diameters increase the mechanical stress at the taper junction between stem and head (trunnions); they had been in focus for release of the small metallic debris **(Box 4)**. This implies that even for CoC bearings, a certain amount of metallic debris particles can be disseminated in the body.

BOX 4: Trunnionosis.

Trunnion is the part of stem where femoral head fits (it is commonly in the form of taper either 11/13 taper or 12/14 taper). Wear of this head–neck interface is called trunnionosis. Mostly, it is the neck side that undergoes wear and generates metal debris but the electrochemical corrosion can also involve the head side. Interestingly hence in a nonmetal-on-metal hip also, metal debris and related adverse local tissue reaction may occur. This has been recognized as a cause of failure of total hip arthroplasty and revision in 3% of the cases independently.

Cause of trunnionosis:

Design concerns:

- The most popular hypothesis is that large head size bearings have higher frictional torque that gets transmitted on the femoral–head–neck junction. Thus, this is specific for modular implants where femoral head is a separate component, monoblock designs with fused femoral head to neck will not have this complication. Maximum stress is located on the medial aspect of the femoral neck and is proportional to the size of femoral head size (but this relationship is not all correct). The increased stress at this modular junction causes fretting of the components producing wear and corrosion.
- Length of trunnion has also a bearing where longer trunnions have higher chance of impingement during ROM. Thus, trunnion length was reduced in newer designs and also, they had lesser flexural rigidity. This led to stress concentration at the base of trunnion, as it completely engaged within the head taper and hence increased chances of corrosion.
- The older trunnions were 14/16 taper, so were thicker while newer popular designs have 12/14 thinner tapers reducing the surface area for contact length and fitting. This possibly increases the chance of fretting corrosion.

Implant material concern: The implant material is also important in the development of trunnionosis. Cobalt–chrome (Co-Cr) bearings have high incidence of this wear so electrochemical corrosion is considered an important component of the wear. Co-Cr on titanium will have less wear and titanium or ceramic will have still lesser wear.

Surgical technique: Poor position of implant components and component damage during insertion has also been implicated in generation of increased local stress on modular junction.

Clinical presentation:

The adverse reaction to metal ion debris produces specific reactions termed adverse reaction to metal debris (ARMD) or aseptic lymphocyte-dominated vasculitis-associated lesions (ALVAL) that have been described in Chapter on "Tribology and Bearing Surface". This produces tissue necrosis, lymphocytosis, vasculitis, and production of exudates, pseudotumors, or sinuses. Patient presents with pain and in late cases with swelling/mass. High index of suspicion is necessary in these cases, as radiographs may not be much helpful. Serum concentration of cobalt in excess of 1 ng/mL is suggestive, if it not a metal-on-metal hip. Metal artifact reduction sequence (MARS) MRI helps in diagnosis.

Treatment:

The treatment involves debridement and exchange of fresh components. If liner or shell damage is also present, then revision THA will be necessary. Complete synovectomy and removal of metal debris is essential. Change femoral head with that of ceramic head and if stem is changed then choose a titanium stem for revision.

(ROM: range of motion; THA: total hip arthroplasty)

Loosening of implant on radiographs is categorized into three types:

1. Definite loosening is defined as migration of the stem, new appearance of a continuous radiolucent line at the stem–cement junction, fracture of the stem, or fracture in the cement mantle.
2. Probable loosening is defined as a continuous radiolucent line at the cement–bone interface on either the AP view or the lateral view.
3. Possible loosening is defined as a radiolucent line extending between 50 and 100% of the cement–bone interface on either the AP view or the lateral view, or both.
4. Debonding between the metal and the cement seen at the proximal and the distal end of the prosthesis is often one of the earliest signs of loosening of a cemented femoral component.

Cancer Risk

See also Chapter on "Tribology and Bearing Surface". Total hip arthroplasty seems to affect the risk profile of cancer since the incidence of malignant melanoma, multiple myeloma, prostate, and bladder cancer appears to be slightly increased whereas the incidence of stomach cancer seems to be decreased compared with the general population. The reduced stomach cancer risk might be related to the use of antibiotics in THA patients that may eliminate *Helicobacter pylori*, which is considered as a major risk factor in stomach cancer. The increased incidence of melanoma in THA patients points toward an effect of metal release from implants. Though risk of leukemia has been reported to be higher by three times, the statistical significance could still not be reached. The most recent investigation did not distinguish between different cancer types, but concluded that the cancer mortality in MoM patients is higher during the first 20 years after surgery than in metal-on-polyethylene patients. The slight changes of the cancer risk profile that might so far be associated with THA will not change the medical indications for hip joint replacement since the benefits for the patients' quality of life outweigh the marginal increase of risk for a few specific cancers.

Neurovascular Injury

These are among the most uncomfortable complications of THA for both patient and surgeon.

- The prevalence of nerve palsy after THA is between 0.6 and 3%, which increases to around 5% for revision THA, or THA done for congenital dysplasia. The sciatic, femoral, obturator, and gluteal nerves can be injured.
- Vascular injury is extremely rare (0.2–0.3%). Injuries to the iliac, femoral, obturator, and gluteal arteries have been described.
- The causes of nerve or vascular injury include direct trauma, constriction by wire or suture, traction or pressure from retractors, extremity positioning, excessive tensioning (often from lengthening the extremity), ischemia, thermal injury from cement, or dislocation of the components. The placement of acetabular screws into major intra-abdominal vascular cavities has also been reported with catastrophic results (*see* Chapter on "Surgical and Functional Anatomy").

Prevention and Management

A thorough knowledge of the neurovascular structures about the pelvis helps the surgeon to avoid injury to these vital structures (see anatomy). Care must be undertaken during surgical dissection, retractor placement, insertion of acetabular screws, and the passing of cerclage wires. Preoperative angiography is indicated for high-risk situations, such as intrapelvic migration of a failed acetabular component or intrapelvic extravasation of cement in revision cases. Intraoperatively, help from vascular surgeon should be sought. A knee immobilizer should be worn in patients with a femoral nerve injury to prevent knee buckling. Patients with sciatic or peroneal nerve injury should have the foot splinted postoperatively to prevent equinus deformity.

Instability

Dislocation is one of the most common complications for a patient following THA. The incidence of dislocation varies widely (0.3–9%) with most large series averaging 2–3% for primary THA. The rate of early dislocation after THA has decreased from 4.2% in 1998 to 2.14% in 2007.

Risk factors for dislocation of THA include:

- *Disease conditions:*
  - Developmental dysplasia of the hip
  - Prior hip surgery
  - Nonhealed fracture
  - Rheumatoid arthritis
  - Prior sepsis.
- *Surgical factors:*
  - Posterior approach
  - Retroverted acetabular cup
  - Excessively anteverted components predispose to anterior dislocation
  - Vertical orientation of the acetabular component (>55°) **(Fig. 26)**
  - Small femoral head size and the re-enforcement at the base (skirted heads)
  - Large acetabular components (diameters >62 mm) have also been shown to have greater dislocation rates than when components <60 mm were used. Elevated rim and lipped liners have also been shown to improve stability, provided they are used to maximize restoration of femoral offset and avoid impingement.
  - Less experienced surgeons
  - Reduced femoral offset
  - Trochanteric fracture and avulsion

The greatest risk of dislocation occurs within the first 3 months after surgery. Dislocations that occur beyond 5 weeks have been shown to have a higher rate of recurrent dislocation than those in patients who had their initial dislocation within the first 5 weeks.

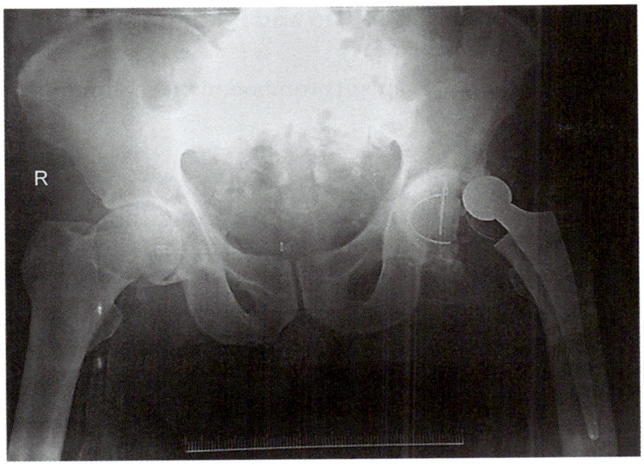

Fig. 26: Vertical orientation of cup approaching 90° is in no case going to articulate with femoral head and the result is instability of implanted hip and dislocation as in this poorly done total hip arthroplasty (THA).

- *Patient factors:*
  - Twice as frequently in females as in males
  - Elderly frail patients higher dislocation rates
  - Alcohol abuse
  - Neuromuscular disease
  - Obese
  - Emotionally unstable

Classification

Posterior dislocation is the most common and is followed by anterior. Dorr and associates have proposed a classification system based on increasing severity of the cause:

- *Type I dislocations:* These occur due to malposition of extremity
- Type II dislocations are caused by soft tissue imbalance
- Type III by component malposition

Prevention and Treatment

The best prevention is to recognize all of the contributing factors that can lead to dislocation and avoid them. There is no substitute to good surgical planning. The immediate treatment for a dislocated hip is closed reduction that may be better done in operation theater. Care must be taken not to dislodge or dissemble a well-seated, modular component. Postreduction immobilization is done with long knee brace, traction is not of much use and should be avoided for complications. For recurrent hip instability, the underlying cause of dislocation should be addressed. And if found correctable (like retroversion or offset problem, etc.) then resurgery should be done. In some cases, the cause is unknown and such cases need constrained cups or dual mobility cups with large head designs. Bipolar or a tripolar prosthesis is a good rescue in recurrent dislocation with unidentified pathology.

Heterotopic Ossification

Heterotopic ossification is a frequent complication of THA, with a reported incidence between 0.6% and 62%

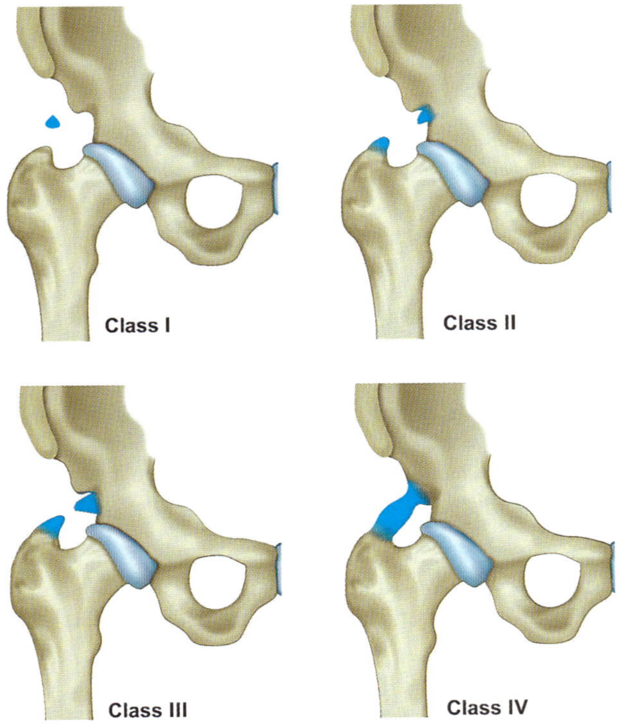

Fig. 27: Schematic diagram of the Brooker classification for heterotopic ossification.

[*see* Chapter on "Orthopedic Oncology (Bone Tumors and Metastasis) and Heterotopic Ossification"]. The HO may be complete or incomplete with still elusive pathogenesis. Anterior and anterolateral approaches have an increased possibility of HO.

Classification (Brooker, Fig. 27)

- Grade 0 has no ossification
- Grade I represents one or two isolated areas of ossification each <1 cm in diameter **(Fig. 28)**.
- Grade II represents more widespread isolated areas of ossification along the proximal femur or acetabular rim, the exostoses are separated by a distance >1 cm.
- Grade III ossification covers more than half of the distance between the femur and pelvis but does not bridge the entire distance; the exostosis are separated by a distance <1 cm.
- Grade IV ossification bridges the entire distance between the femur and pelvis (extra-articular ankylosis).

Della Valle proposed a modified classification and reduced the Brooker groups into three. Here, type A is either absence of HO or exostoses <1 cm in length. Grade B is the presence of one or more islands of bone at least 1 cm in length and separated by a distance >1 cm in-between. Grade C is the presence of exostosis from the pelvis or femur with <1 cm distance between and/ or complete fusion.

Risk Factors for Heterotopic Ossification

- *Patient factors:*
  - Previous HO (90% probability of occurrence)
  - Previous trauma to the hip

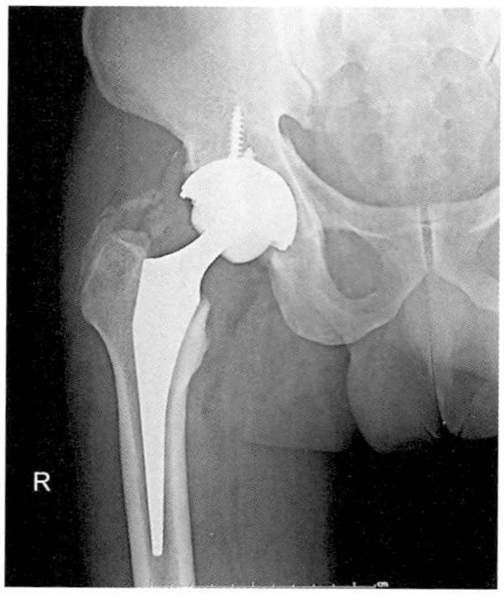

Fig. 28: Grade 1 mature heterotopic ossification in a patient with avascular necrosis (AVN) and renal transplantation treated with uncemented total hip arthroplasty (THA).

    - Hypertrophic osteoarthritis
    - Diffuse idiopathic skeletal hyperostosis (DISH)
    - Male gender
    - Ankylosing spondylitis
- *Surgical factors:*
    - Surgical approach—anterolateral and transtrochanteric
    - Type of implant fixation—cementless > cemented
    - Surgical trauma to the gluteus medius/minimus
    - Postoperative hematoma
    - Dislocation
    - Femoral fracture
    - Infection

Prevention

- Minimize tissue trauma
- Irradiation—single preoperative or postoperative (800 cGy) dose, shield the noncemented implants for preventing injury to bone and retain its regenerative capacity.
- Nonsteroidal anti-inflammatory drugs (NSAIDs)
- Bisphosphonates [*see* Chapter on "Orthopedic Oncology (Bone Tumors and Metastasis) and Heterotopic Ossification"].

Treatment of Heterotopic Ossification

Only when the HO is matured enough and the signs of active disease are absent, one should plan excision, if HO is symptomatic and restricting functions.

Leg–Length Discrepancy

Patient dissatisfaction from this complication is the most common cause of litigation against the orthopedic community. Preoperative templating is the best way to avoid this. Intraoperative references are not accurate but do help. Use a combination of various methods such as coaxial stitch method and Ranawat method. Knee ankle/foot position assessment is totally inaccurate for even gross assessment.

Venous Thromboembolism and Pulmonary Artery Embolism

(*see* Chapter on "Venous Thromboembolism Prophylaxis and Treatment")

Periprosthetic Fracture

Periprosthetic femur fractures are divided into intraoperative and postoperative fractures. Intraoperative fractures occur during the course of surgery, and postoperative fractures usually occur within days to several years after the procedure. Intraoperative femoral periprosthetic fracture occurs with rate of 1% in primary THA and 7.8% in revision THA. Postoperative periprosthetic fractures of the femur occur in from 0.1 to 2.1%. To be specific from Swedish registry data, the mean time to postoperative fracture is reported to be around 7 years for primary THA and 4 years for revision surgery. The incidence of intraoperative acetabular periprosthetic fracture has been reported to be <0.2% that results from impaction forces incurred while employing a press-fit technique into an acetabulum that has been under-reamed by 1 or 2 mm in relation to the acetabular component. Postoperative periprosthetic acetabular fractures usually occur as a result of bone loss from osteolysis but can also occur because of traumatic fracture. Revision THA with impaction grafting is associated with a higher incidence of intraoperative and postoperative fractures.

Etiology and Risk Factors

The most frequent mechanism for sustaining these fractures is a low-energy fall from sitting or standing. The main risk factor for sustaining a periprosthetic femur fracture is osteolysis associated with implant loosening. Any pathologic process, however, that weakens bone may contribute to these fractures, viz.:

- Osteoporosis
- Rheumatoid arthritis
- Paget's disease
- Polyneuropathies
- Tumors
- Cortical defects
- Trauma
- Revision surgery
- Extruded cement
- Stress risers
- Varus stem position

Classification

Callaghan classification of intraoperative periprosthetic acetabular fractures is based on anatomical region:

- Anterior wall
- Transverse
- Inferior lip
- Posterior wall fractures

Peterson and Lewallen classified postoperative periprosthetic acetabular fractures into two types:

1. Type I is a clinically and radiologically stable acetabular component.

TABLE 2: Vancouver classification of intraoperative and postoperative periprosthetic fractures.

Intraoperative fracture	*Subtypes*	*Postoperative fracture*	*Subtypes*
A. Proximal metaphyseal fractures not extending into the diaphysis	1. Simple cortical perforation 2. Undisplaced linear crack 3. Displaced or unstable fracture	A. Fractures around the trochanteric region	G. Around the greater trochanter LT. Around the lesser trochanter
B. Diaphyseal fractures not extending into the distal diaphysis	1. Simple cortical perforation 2. Undisplaced linear crack 3. Displaced or unstable fracture	B. Fractures around or just distal to the femoral stem	1. Femoral implant well-fixed 2. Femoral implant loose but good bone stock 3. Femoral implant loose and poor-bone stock
C. Distal fractures extending into the distal metaphysis	1. Simple cortical perforation 2. Undisplaced linear crack 3. Displaced or unstable fracture	C. Fractures distal to the femoral stem	

(LT: lesser trochanter)

2. Type II is an unstable acetabular component.
   The Vancouver classification proposed by Duncan and Masri is more appropriate and is most commonly used **(Table 2, Fig. 29)**. It was developed for THAs with cemented femoral components and considers three important factors:
   a. The site of the fracture
   b. The stability of the implant
   c. The quality of the surrounding bone stock

The advantages of the classification include:

- Simple and reproducible
- Useful for devising a treatment strategy based on easily identifiable characteristics
- Helps the surgeon to differentiate between a stable fracture (managed with osteosynthesis) and an unstable fracture (revision surgery).

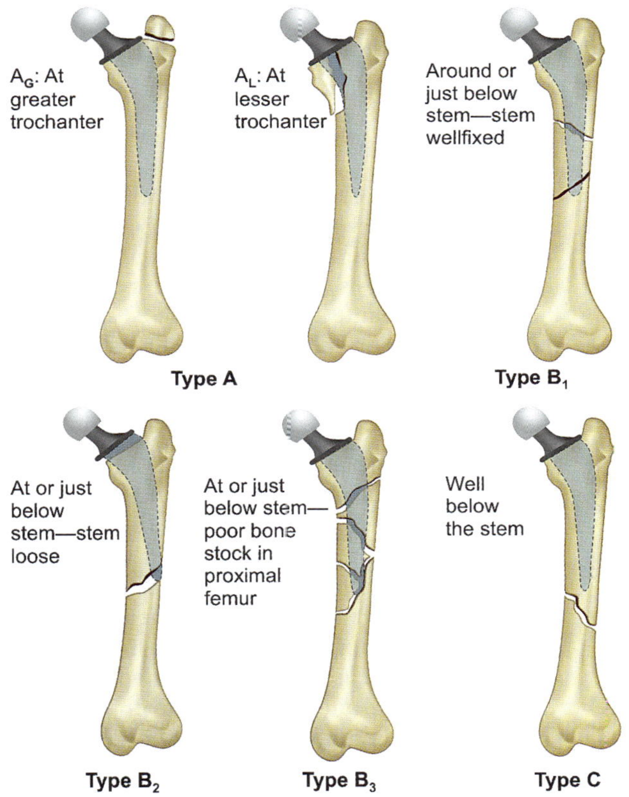

Fig. 29: The Vancouver classification of periprosthetic femur fractures around total hip arthroplasty.

Prevention and Management

Intraoperative fractures:

- Assess acetabular fractures for stability. Stable fractures can be treated conservatively whereas unstable fractures require fixation and weight-bearing restrictions. Early postoperative acetabular fractures are treated according to their pattern. Patients with stable, minimally displaced acetabular fractures can be treated conservatively with union expected in most cases. Late postoperative acetabular fractures are usually associated with significant osteolysis and often warrant operative intervention.
- *Intraoperative femoral fractures are managed as follows:*
  - Simple bone grafting (type A1)
  - Cerclage wiring (type A2)
  - Wires, cables, cortical strut grafts, trochanteric claw plates, and a diaphyseal-fitting stem (types A_3, B_1, B_2, and B_3).
  - Diaphyseal fractures should be bypassed by at least two cortical diameters with a diaphyseal-fitting stem.
  - If the fracture occurs distal to a well-impacted femoral stem (type C), the stem should be retained and the fracture should be treated with extramedullary strut and cable augmentation or formal open reduction and internal fixation.

Intraoperative fractures that are identified in the immediate postoperative period should be evaluated fully with radiographs to determine extent. Most of these fractures are stable, minimally displaced, do not compromise the fixation of the prosthesis and will unite successfully without complication.

- Postoperative periprosthetic femoral fractures are commonly treated as follows:
  - *Type A_{LT}:* Usually nonoperative treatment unless a large portion of calcar is compromised with loss of medial buttress. In the latter case, cerclage wiring is appropriate **(Fig. 30)**. Some authors recommend

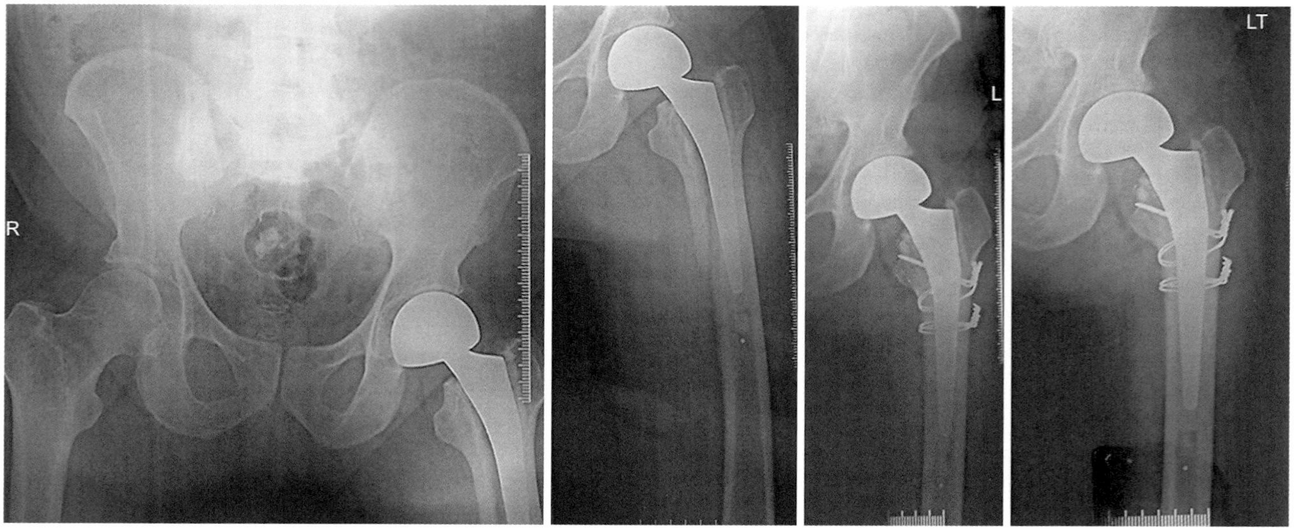

Fig. 30: Type A_{LT} periprosthetic fracture managed with cerclage wiring.

revision in such cases, this is true, if cement mantle is fractured along.

- *Type A_G:* Fractures, if stable and undisplaced, are managed conservatively with protected weight bearing and avoidance of abduction for 6–12 weeks if there is no osteolysis. Internal fixation is considered if the greater trochanter has displaced >2.5 cm or if the patient has pain, instability, and abductor weakness. In the presence of osteolysis, operative treatment includes bone grafting, the lytic lesion, trochanteric fixation as above, and acetabular liner revision to address the cause of osteolysis.
- The type B fractures are the most common accounting for 80% cases. Perforation of the femur led to a 44% reduction in the original strength of the femur and osteosynthesis with a plate that bridged the fracture area by two femur widths re-established the stability of the bone to 84% of its original strength (Larson).
    - Type B_1 fractures should be treated with open reduction and internal fixation with or without cortical strut bone grafts. Metallic bone side plates have the problem of implant failure, weak construct due to cerclage or unicortical screw, and fractures at plate tip. Also, the transcortical screws weaken the bone that can fracture there. Trochanteric plate with unicortical screws proximally and distal bicortical screws is a sufficiently strong construct. Cortical strut grafts is the preferred modality that can be used alone in B_1 fractures or combined with adjunct osteosynthesis. The grafts can be applied at 90° or 180° and have the advantage of being osteoconductive and biological. Also being isoelastic to bone, the stress-shielding effect is minimal. The host bone is strengthened after union and incorporation of graft. The disadvantages of strut grafts are their high cost, limited availability, increased danger of infection, and potential for transmitting disease.

    The other reliable implant available is the locked plates—these have the advantage of increased axial and angular stability, indirect fracture reduction, less soft tissue dissection, preservation of periosteal blood supply, strong fixation in bone of poor quality, and less damage to cement mantle or sable implant. They are stiffer than the Ogden construct (plates with just proximal cerclage and distal bicortical screws) but are not mechanically superior to conventional plates. The locked plates, however, offer few perks to fixation and improve the surgical horizon by preserving the blood supply and allowing minimally invasive fixation. In a nutshell, the author prefers a locked plate with proximal unicortical fixation combined to cables and distal bicortical screws with cortical strut grafts.

- B_2 fractures are best treated with revision to a longer femoral stem preferably cementless (bypassing the fracture by a minimal distance of two femoral diameters with at least 5 cm of diaphyseal fit) and fracture fixation with cerclage wires with or without cortical strut grafts. Fluted modular noncemented stem is preferred, if there are concerns of rotational stability and/ or soft tissue tensioning. Cemented stem is recommended only for patients with osteoporosis and capacious canals that cannot be filled by implant or those with irradiated bones. Cement-in-cement fixation is preferred for cement mantles that are reasonably fixed to bone and fractures have no to minimal comminution. It is a faster and technically less demanding technique. I especially prefer this for frail elderly patient with a cemented implant in situ. Another interesting approach is the use of extensively porous-coated stems with distal interlocking screws that have reported reasonable results. These stems have high initial axial and torsional stability.
    - Patients with B_3 fractures often require structural allograft replacement of the proximal femur with an allograft-prosthetic-composite revision, tumor prosthesis (I prefer), or a custom implant.

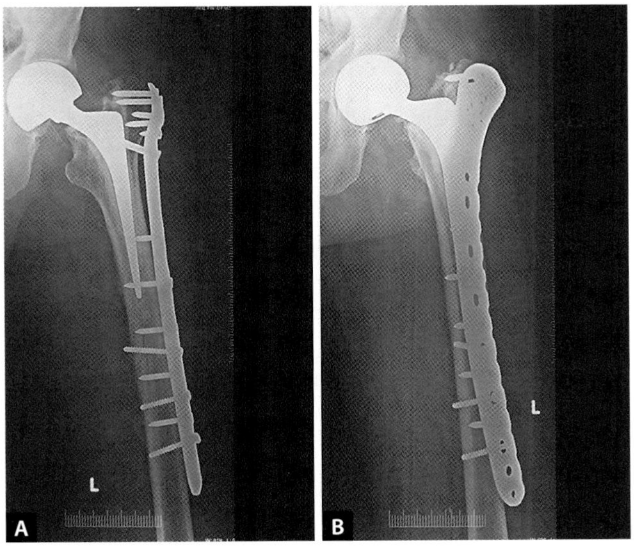

Figs. 31A and B: Treatment of periprosthetic fracture with locking plate. In this, type C periprosthetic fracture reversed distal femoral locking plate of contralateral side was used and unicortical screws were additionally used to improve purchase. One needs to have good cortical purchase and overlap the prosthesis adequately else the fixation device may avulse and fail.

- Patients with type C fractures are treated with standard open reduction and internal fixation **(Figs. 31A and B)**. I prefer a locking plate with unicortical and bicortical screw and cable hybrid construct with bypass "butterfly"/clamp, if available.

REVISION HIP ARTHROPLASTY

Even the good things come to an end! At present, the success rates of THA at 10 years or longer exceed 95% survivorship in patients >75 years. The number of revision procedures is expected to increase in the near future despite improvement in fixation systems and surgical approaches. The primary reason is that the surgery is being offered more liberally to even younger population, which is comparatively more active and for any given argument, the fact remains that the implanted joint is artificial one incapable of its own repair, so one day, it will succumb needing revision with a newer one. Now itself in the high-volume centers, revision surgeries account for one-fourth of the volume of arthroplasties. Potential reasons for hip revisions can be stratified into four groups: (1) patient-related factors, (2) implant-related factors, (3) failures related to inadequate surgical technique, and (4) the most common one is ungroupable and I call it miscellaneous causes.

- *Miscellaneous causes:*
  - Aseptic loosening and osteolysis (most common cause)
  - Infection
  - Metal allergy
- *Implant related:*
  - Implant (bearing) wear out
  - Periprosthetic fractures
  - Delamination of porous coating
  - Manufacturing problems
- *Patient-related factors:*
  - Poor-bone quality
  - Sickle cell anemia
  - Obesity
  - Smoking
- *Surgical technique related:*
  - Malpositioning of components
  - Recurrent dislocation

  The mean time to failure of implant varies with the age of patient, being earliest in the younger population while latest in the elderly population possibly related to the demand and activity level differences. As a matter of fact, nearly half of the hips are revised within <5 years of the primary index THA. The mode of failure of the implanted hips is dependent on the length of the time interval following the index surgery—more or less than 5 years. In the late group, the primary reason for revision is aseptic loosening and implant wear out followed by fractures, whereas for the early failures, instability and deep infection are the most important causes. A cemented stem may not just fail by the above mechanisms or factors. It may fail "primarily" by one of the four modes (Gruen) unique to it as follows:

  1. Pistoning
  2. Medial mid-stem pivot
  3. Calcar pivot
  4. Bending cantilever fatigue

During evaluation, the three most important factors that need attention are the physical condition of the patient and fitness, presence or absence of infection, and the quality of bone. The first part is aided by an anesthetic check-up while for the second concern, blood investigations and radiological parameters help evaluation, and in case of any doubt, aspiration of hip settles the issue most often. The evaluation and classification of bone defects are the third most critical part that needs to be addressed before embarking upon surgery and planning. Briefly, the following are some radiological evaluation points for patients with hip pain following arthroplasty due to procedure-related complications.

- Loosening of femoral stem (see above)
- *Migration of the implant:* Measured as the distance from the tip of the greater trochanter to the shoulder of the prosthesis
- *Bone pedestal* formed when there is a lack of initial firm fixation to provide vertical stability to implant
- *Atrophy of the calcar:* Due to stress shielding when there is distal load transfer either due to ingrowth in the distal part of the stem or due to wedging of a tapered implant at the level of the isthmus
- Cemented acetabular cup loosening is defined by observing the demarcation of >2 mm in the DeLee and Charnley zones (*see* **Fig. 8A**, Chapter on "Tribology and Bearing Surfaces").
  - Demarcation in all three zones indicates loose cups in >90% cases

- Demarcation in zones 1 and 2 indicates loosening in 70% cases
- Loosening in zone 1 only is much less predictive and <10% cups are loose

- Socket break-in is the medial migration of the cup and cement mantle, and socket break-out is the migration of the acetabular component relative to the cement mantle. Both of these are definite indicators of a loose acetabular component.
- Cementless cup loosening is less predicted by the radiolucent lines. Migration of the shell, breakage of a screw, fracture of the metal shell, and shedding of the porous surface are some of the indicators of loose cementless cups.
- Presence of infection radiologically is predicted by a lacy periosteal reaction, loss of the subchondral sclerosis superior to the acetabular component, and unusual osteolytic lesions.

In any case, radiographs usually underestimate the extent of osteolysis, but better methods to quantitate are either expensive or futile. Aspiration arthrograms are futile in indicating loosening. CT scans are good, if infection is to be ruled out. The positive signs are fluid collection in muscle planes (100% sensitivity to predict infection) and absence of distended joint space (96% negative predictive value). Dynamic CT scan can also predict loosening by measuring the version of stem in internal and external rotation with 92% sensitivity and 90% specificity.

Classification of Bone Deficiency

Once the decision to do a revision is made, the crucial step is defining the bone loss and deficiency in the femoral and acetabular components. The loss of bone around an existing arthroplasty directly affects the reconstruction options. Different methods are available to classify the bone defects as follows:

Acetabular bone defects: Here, the primary distinction is to be made between segmental and cavitary bone defects. Though various classification systems are available, the American Association of Orthopedic Surgeons (AAOS) system comes in handy **(Box 5)**.

- A segmental defect is a complete loss of bone in the supporting hemisphere or the medial wall.
- Cavitary defects involve a volumetric loss of bone in the acetabular cavity or the medial wall with an intact rim.
    - Both segmental and cavitary defects are further classified as superior, anterior, posterior, or medial.
- Combined defect incorporates both segmental and cavitary defects (e.g., failed, migrated endoprosthesis, or in developmental dysplasia).
- Pelvic discontinuity causes separation of the superior half of the acetabulum from the inferior half.
- Though in arthrodesis, there is no actual loss of bone but the "deficiency" is in terms of inability to locate the acetabulum itself.

BOX 5: The American Association of Orthopedic Surgeon (AAOS) classification of acetabular bone defects.

Type I: Segmental deficiency **(Fig. 32)**
- *Peripheral (rim defect)*:
    - Superior
    - Anterior
    - Posterior
- Central (medial-wall defect)

Type II: Cavitary deficiencies **(Fig. 33)**
- *Peripheral*:
    - Superior
    - Anterior
    - Posterior
- Central (medial-wall intact)

Type III: Combined deficiencies **(Fig. 34)**
Type IV: Pelvic discontinuity
Type V: Arthrodesis

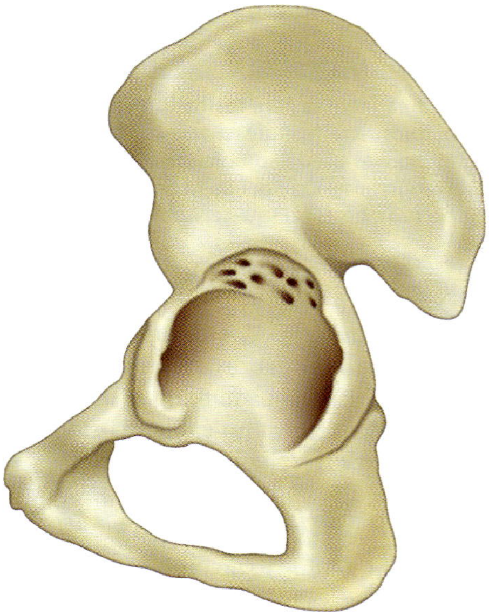

Fig. 32: Type I acetabular segmental defect.

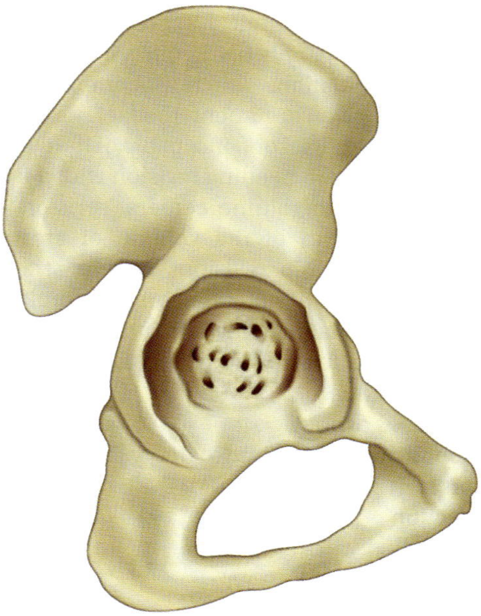

Fig. 33: Type II acetabular cavitary defect.

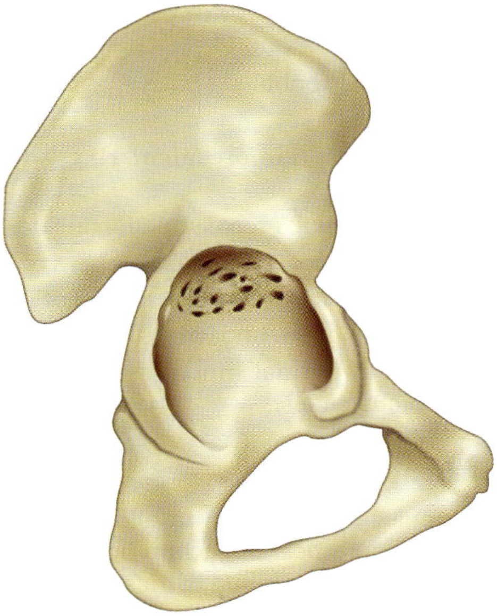

Fig. 34: Type III acetabular defect.

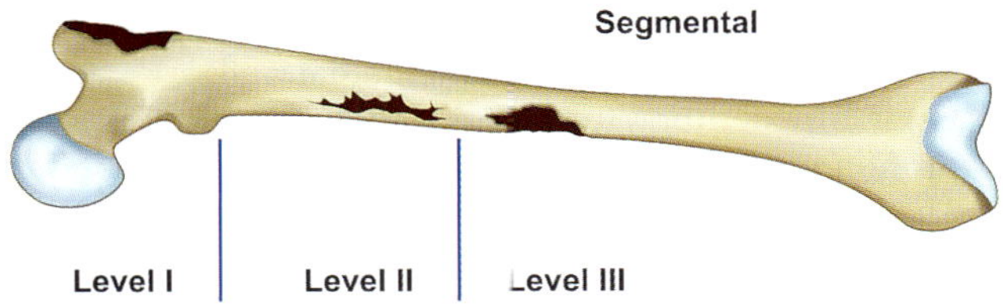

Fig. 35: Segmental defect.

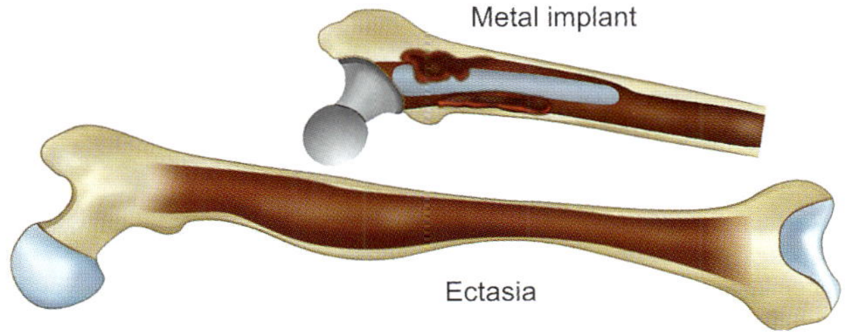

Fig. 36: Cavitary defect, also shown is a subtype—canal ectasia.

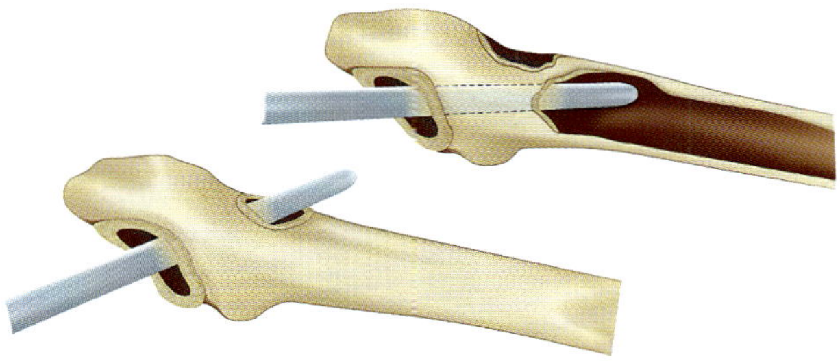

Fig. 37: Combined segmental and cavitary defect.

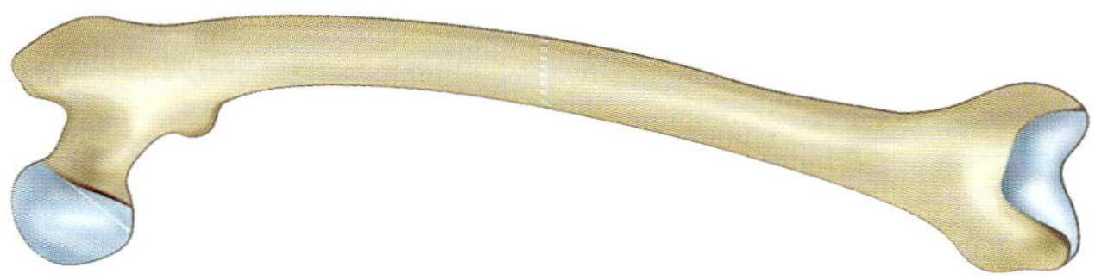

Fig. 38: Malalignment.

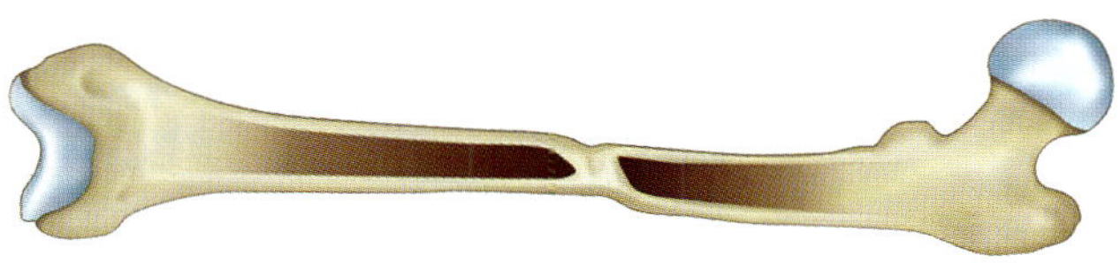

Fig. 39: Stenosis of femur.

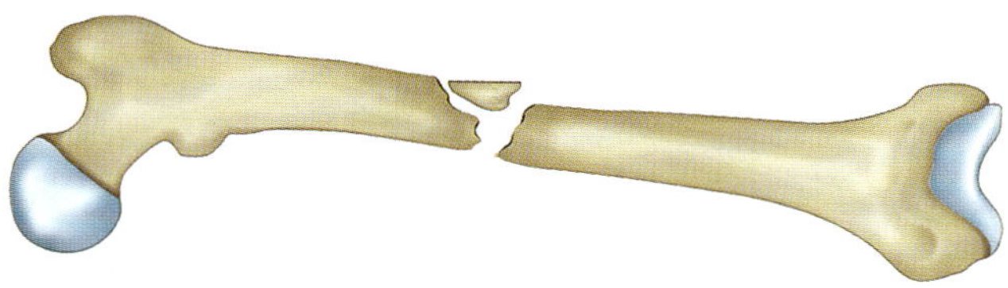

Fig. 40: Discontinuity.

BOX 6: The American Association of Orthopedic Surgeon (AAOS) classification of the femoral bone defects.

Type I: Segmental deficiency **(Fig. 35)**
- Proximal
- Partial
- Complete
- Intercalary
- Greater trochanter

Type II: Cavitary deficiencies **(Fig. 36)**
- Cancellous
- Cortical
- Ectasia

Type III: Combined deficiencies **(Fig. 37)**

Type IV: Malalignment **(Fig. 38)**
- Rotational
- Angular

Type V: Femoral stenosis **(Fig. 39)**

Type VI: Femoral discontinuity **(Fig. 40)**

Femoral deficiencies **(Box 6)** can also be segmental or cavitary. In addition, however, the medullary canal anatomy, malalignment, and loss of bony integrity affect the reconstruction. Cavitary defects are "contained" lesions with an intact outer cortex. Segmental defects can be partial (perforations) or intercalary (circumferential loss of bone). Remodeling of bone may produce rotational or angular malalignment. Femoral stenosis implies narrowing of the femoral canal while discontinuity is a fracture of the femur.

Overall, the AAOS classification is theoretically simple, but more complex in its application. Other classification systems such as the Engh classification, Chandler–Pennenberg classification **(Table 3)**, and the Paprosky system **(Table 4)** are used individually at dedicated centers.

Some *reconstruction options* for acetabular defects are as follows:

- Jumbo cup—minimum diameter of 60–70 mm, these were suggested as a more reliable alternative to structural allograft in treating cavernous acetabular deficiencies but have been also successfully applied for segmental loss of the anterior column and medial wall.

- High hip center—for bone deficiency that is most pronounced superiorly resulting in oblong acetabulum. The high hip center is defined at a minimum of 35 mm proximal to the interteardrop line. Because of nonanatomic location, cemented fixations have higher failure rates. Dislocation rates are not higher than conventional hips.
- Oblong cup/double bubble
- Impaction grafting
- Bulk allograft and reinforcement rings—for severe acetabular deficiency.

The principles of acetabular reconstruction include:

- Creation of a stable acetabular bed
- Secure prosthetic fixation with freedom of orientation
- Bony reconstitution (see impaction bone grafting)
- Restoration of a normal hip center of rotation with acceptable biomechanics

Impaction Bone Grafting

The aim of impaction grafting with allogeneic bone is to reconstruct the bone stock. Impaction bone grafting (IBG) of the acetabulum was described by Hastings and Parker in 1975 and subsequently popularized for revisions by Slooff et al. Slooff et al. also introduced the concept of using this procedure with cement in the proximal femur that became more frequently used common when Gie et al. developed specific instruments for the same. They demonstrated the incorporation-substitution of impacted cancellous allografts and repair of the surrounding cortical bone. Bone graft is impacted into a contained defect or a defect that can be made contained to create a stable bed into which the prosthesis can be placed. For acetabulum, most cavitary defects and combined defects, where a rim can be recreated, are amenable to impacted morselized bone grafting.

Both cemented and uncemented (extensively porous coated) implants can be used though initially cementing

TABLE 3: Chandler–Penenberg classification for femoral and acetabular defects.

Femoral bone defects	***Acetabular bone defects***
Calcar deficiency: • Intramedullary • Total *Trochanteric deficiency*: • Cortical thinning • Cortical perforation Femoral fractures about or below the stem of a femoral component • Fractures of the patient's femur • Fatigue fracture of an allograft Circumferential deficiency of the metaphysis and proximal diaphysis • Loss of the trochanter and metaphysis with a thin shell of the diaphysis remaining • Total loss of the proximal femur	• Rim defects • Intra-acetabular defect • Protrusio of the medial wall of the acetabulum • Perforation of the medial wall of the acetabulum • *Combined acetabular defects*: – Protrusio and perforation of the medial wall of the acetabulum – Superior rim and intra-acetabular defects – Superior rim and intra-acetabular defects with medial wall perforation – Superior acetabular defects and perforation of the medial wall – Global deficiency (complex anterior, superior, and intra-acetabular area deficient) – Column defects (anterior or posterior rim and intra-acetabular defect with medial wall perforation or pelvic discontinuity)

TABLE 4: Paprosky classification for acetabular and femoral defects.

Acetabular defects:

Defect	***Rim***	***Walls/dome***	***Columns***	***Migration***	***Teardrop lysis***
Type 1	Intact	Intact	Intact/supportive	None	
Type 2	Distorted	Distorted	Intact/supportive	<2 cm	
2-A	Distorted	Intact	Intact/supportive	Superomedial	Minimal
2-B	Missing	Distorted	Intact/supportive	Superolateral	Minimal
2-C	Distorted	Intact	Intact/supportive	Medial	Severe
Type 3	Missing	Compromised	Nonsupportive	>2 cm	
3-A	Missing	Compromised	Nonsupportive	Superolateral	Moderate
3-B	Missing	Compromised	Nonsupportive	Superomedial	Severe

Femoral defects:

Type	***Femoral defect***
1	Minimal metaphyseal and diaphyseal bone loss
2-A	Absent calcar extending just below the intertrochanteric level
2-B	Anterolateral metaphyseal bone loss
2-C	Absent calcar with posteromedial metaphyseal bone loss
3-A	2-A plus diaphyseal bone loss
3-B	2-B plus diaphyseal bone loss
3-C	2-C plus diaphyseal bone loss

techniques were popular where the implant was fixed using a cement interface onto the impaction bone grafted surface. Use of a porous-coated femoral stem was introduced by Retpen and Solgaard.

Goals of IBG:
- Restoration of the bone stock
- Contribute to the initial stability of the implant
- Restore hip center of rotation for acetabular components
- Creating/restoring intimate contact between the implant and host bone all over

Acetabular Impaction Bone Grafting

Role of uncemented acetabular cups: Though initially popular, the cemented acetabular cups for revision were not found suitable for the deficient mechanical support and the sclerotic or nontrabecular nature of revision acetabular defects. This led to the use of uncemented counterpart; however, the durability and reliability of the fixation depend on the contact between viable bone and the implant and also on mechanical stability.

Morselized autograft is considered the best but due to limited availability, allograft is used together [even bone graft substitutes (*see* Bone Grafting in Chapter on "Fracture Repair, Bone Grafting, and Bone Banking") can be combined]. The graft is packed using a combination of impaction (incremental sized impactors are commercially available) and reverse reaming to create a hemisphere. The reconstruction relies on the ability to gain biological fixation of the component to the underlying host bone. This requires intimate host bone contact and rigid implant stability.

In the presence of bone stock deficiency, bone grafting of contained defects and the use of an uncemented, porous, coated component (augmented by screw fixation) is now well-accepted. One must realize that it is important to minimize the interposition of bone graft between host bone and implant for bone biology to be able to incorporate the same effectively and provide better initial stability to the uncemented cup. Stuffing too much graft may not get incorporated and, in fact, may fail early. Currently, it is deemed important to achieve host bone contact in at least part of the dome and posterior column whenever possible. Also, when there is a good rim fit, it is not absolutely necessary to have contact with host bone over >50% of the surface. The minimum required host bone contact and the maximum amount of bone graft that may be tolerated without compromising stability and bone ingrowth, however, in uncemented cups are not known. Proximal migration of cups has been seen with IBG but neither the size of the acetabular defects nor the amount of morselized bone graft had any influence on migration, and when hydroxyapatite-coated acetabular implants were used in combination with more forceful impaction of morselized graft host bone contact of <50%, implant stability did not seem to be compromised. Some technical tips for successful IBG can be summarized as:

- Make a good exposure to define the complete defect.
- Clear the membrane and prepare the surface to make it more likely to allow bony ingrowth and incorporation of bone graft. A sclerotic surface can be reamed by hemispherical reamers and even drilled for bleeding to occur.
- As far as possible, try to achieve three-point (tripod) contact with the ilium, ischium, and the pubis bones. For pelvic discontinuity, it is imperative to restore the columns and continuity of pelvic ring by supplementary fixation else the procedure is bound to fail.
- Bone graft should be carefully prepared—the current recommendation is the use of a combined mixture of bone milling and bone chips of multiple sizes ranging from slurry to 1 cm bone chips. If the graft is insufficient then synthetic materials can also be used in a ration not exceeding 50:50. Insert pack (with impactors), reverse ream the graft into cavitary defects.
- Place the implant as previously planned using a cemented or uncemented component. When using an uncemented component, it is better to oversize the acetabular component by 2 mm and is important to achieve maximum peripheral press-fit to whatever limited portion of the acetabular circumference is available. It is recommended to augment the uncemented cups using screws nearly always.

Uncemented cups are specifically favored in severely osteopenic pelvis, pelvic osteonecrosis after irradiation, tumors, and metabolic bone disorders where there is high probability of a limited fit or poor regenerative capacity of bone.

Femoral impaction bone grafting: The goals here remain the same as above more or less. IBG is the best way to address the extensive femoral bone defects where the impacted bone graft creates a "neomedullary canal". In Retpen and Solgaard's technique, cancellous bone grafts are packed into the medulla corresponding to the upper half of the stem, which may be sufficient for uncemented stem, but we prefer as much distal packing as possible for a cemented stem. Both cemented and cementless techniques are used here too. Uncemented fixation is preferable, if a good proximal femoral stem contact fixation can be achieved along with three-point fixation of the stem as a whole. If the above cannot be sufficient then it is best to cement the femoral stem into the neomedullary canal. Both the techniques are well-accepted and successful.

There is a principle difference in IBG for femoral stem and that for pelviacetabular region. The bone is primarily cortical in femoral region and is liable to fracture with increased use of force, more than required. Also for the required amount of force, a weakened and thin femur may fracture undesirably. So, it is wise to provide temporary/permanent support (reinforcement) to the femur by way of plates, strut grafts, cables, wires or mesh, etc. Metal reinforcement mesh is preferred also for the segmental defects especially in the proximal femur. The perforated tip defects are most dangerous for postoperative fractures and should not only be bypassed sufficiently but also secondarily protected by strut grafts in my view. There is a high rate of subsidence of uncemented femoral stem, if the IBG is not done well enough or the three-point contact fixation is lost. The latter may arise due to defective cortex but the former is mainly due to poor incorporation of graft, so one must pay attention to detail the preparation of bone graft (see above). In the end, as it is a known fact that the radiographs underestimate the defect, so one must be prepared to completely bypass the defect (if not reconstructable) by the use of a long distal fitting stem without IBG.

Advancement to IBG and ancillary technique: Use of "vibration" has been recently advocated for better initial subsidence of the bone graft. Vibration is commonly used in civil engineering to improve compaction of aggregate particles and to increase the compressive and shear strengths of the aggregate. The prepared bone graft is impacted on the same principles using a vibration impaction device. It has been found that the addition of vibration at 60 Hz imparts more resistance to shearing force than graft impacted without vibration *in vitro*. Clinical experience is not available with this technique. Also, only theoretical but there is possibility of the use of bone morphogenetic proteins to increase the incorporation of bone graft. The reason why bone morphogenetic proteins are not used is that the IBG is by itself successful and not many failures with respect to poor incorporation have come up—most are technical errors to begin with.

CEMENT-IN-CEMENT REVISION

Traditionally, revision of a cemented femoral stem involved complete removal of the primary cement mantle followed by a cemented or an uncemented femoral stem insertion. Removal of cement mantle is a long, tedious, and complicated process. There is significantly high rate of femoral cortical perforation or fracture as well as blood loss while removing the cement. Complete removal of cement and insertion of an uncemented stem often require an extended trochanteric osteotomy and a distally fixing stem. These are quite aggressive procedures which have a substantial complication rate. The idea of cement-in-cement revision was developed by Greenwald, Narten, and Wilde. According to the principle, if the primary cement mantle is intact, rasping and drying the mantle followed by revision can increase the shear strength to 94% of that of a single cement block.

The technique involves removal of cement around the shoulder of the stem and then removal of the stem with punch. The collarless, tapered, and polished stems are usually amenable to such procedure, although the other types of stems can also be removed by removing extra cement from around the shoulder. After removal of the stem, the cement mantle is inspected for any break and loose fragments. After inspection, a trial stem of proper diameter, version, and offset is selected and trial reduction is done. The canal and mantle are then prepared by lavage and drying. New cement is then injected in the canal in a retrograde manner with a cement gun and the new stem is cemented. The new stem is usually slimmer in size to allow for proper thickness of the cement mantle around the stem. Current literature including both clinical and biomechanical studies advocates using this technique in selected patients with good to excellent short- to mid-term clinical results.

CONCLUSION

- Hip arthroplasty is a specialized and very popular surgical technique for ultimate reconstruction of hip joint especially when dealing with degenerative diseases that deform the anatomy of native hip joint.
- Understanding your implant is most important. Both cemented and uncemented implants have their pros and cons for usage and one must be thorough with the biomechanics of the implants before using them or prescribing to the patients rather than financial indulgences.
- Use of hybrid systems is ingenious, if the surgeon has experience of combining the cemented and uncemented arthroplasty systems to utilize the best of both while reducing the disadvantages to minimum.
- The current controversy revolves around bearing surfaces and the size of head diameter to be used for the arthroplasty to be more successful. In any case, one should understand the available systems well and plan the surgery well so as not to get caught with surprises intraoperatively.
- Revision surgery is a niche procedure that entails lot of experience and a knowhow of different systems that have in them incorporations for management of various defects and deficiencies of the bone stock. One must also be well versed with augmentation techniques for bone stock such as IBG. This entails need of bone banking facility.

CHAPTER 76

Intertrochanteric Resection Osteotomy/Arthroplasty of Girdlestone (and its Modifications)

Manish Kumar Varshney

INTRODUCTION

Excision arthroplasty of a damaged joint was a popular procedure done in 18th century. Henry Parker (1744–1831) was one of its early advocates who practiced this procedure in knee and elbow. Girdlestone arthroplasty in essence comprised of extensive debridement of septic hip joint and surrounding soft tissue with free drainage creating a "type" of excisional arthroplasty. Excisional arthroplasty of hip per se was first described by A White (1849). In extensive review of literature, various interesting facts are revealed and there is quite a great misconception for the procedure. Gathorne Girdlestone described his operation in 1923 (not the other oft quoted dates) as a modification of Robert Jones operation (1921) done for ankylosis of hip joint, whereby greater trochanter with its attached muscles used to be attached to resected end of neck to produce pseudarthrosis. Since then there are as many modifications as there are descriptions.

INDICATIONS

The decision to perform a Girdlestone operation is in fact a last resort. It is typically chosen for medically suboptimal and functionally compromised patients with high anesthetic and operative risk for revision surgeries in modern orthopedic practice **(Figs. 1A and B)**. Girdlestone resection arthroplasty should be considered only as a salvage procedure, primarily aimed at pain relief and infection control. Such patients must be warned to expect 2–3 inches of limb shortening and the need of a walking aid postoperatively.

- Periprosthetic infection—as a salvage procedure in patient whose infection is uncontrolled or not willing for surgery.
- Aseptic loosening—patient unwilling for surgery or medical condition does not permit revision.
- Recurrent dislocation—ultimate salvage when even jumbo implants or constraint cups fail or refused.
- Infected destroyed hips in underprivileged population.

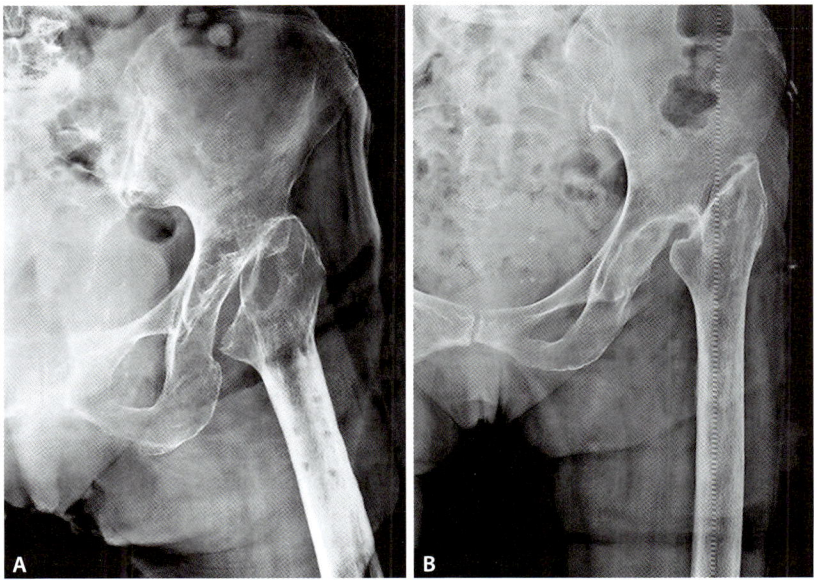

Figs. 1A and B: (A) Girdlestone resection arthroplasty performed for infected implant; (B) Following septic hip disease.

TECHNIQUE (CLASSICAL GIRDLESTONE)

The method and steps for performing intertrochanteric resection osteotomy in the original description of Girdlestone are briefly as follows:

- Transverse incision approximately 5 inches long, centered, 1 inch above trochanter is used to expose deep structures.
- Make two transverse cuts to remove all involved gluteal muscles, trochanter and 3–4 inches wide and 1 inch deep bone is removed from depths (this includes superolateral acetabulum) **(*see* Figs. 1A and B)**.
- Curette out all carious bone and decide whether to leave bone for ankylosis or remove further to create pseudarthrosis! [*Here it appears that this procedure was not to create pseudarthrosis only, rather a method to do joint debridement (saucerization for drainage) in long-standing infections of hip with outcome as either ankylosis or pseudarthrosis*].
- Suture the flaps to periosteum in depths to prevent proud granulation tissue to appear.
- Loosely pack the wound with Vaseline gauge.

MODIFICATIONS OF GIRDLESTONE ARTHROPLASTY

The most popular modifications are firstly that of Taylor (1950) using Smith-Petersen approach. Additionally, trimming of acetabular rim was done to provide opposing surfaces, pain relief, deformity correction, and movements. Nelson (1971) described soft-tissue interposition to achieve pseudarthrosis. The other is that of Grauer et al. (1989) who described four different levels of proximal femoral resections and one by Nagi (1997) who did a subcapital osteotomy and sutured anterior capsule. He reposed the neck back into acetabulum. Basically, now the concept is to retain adequate amount of bone and no acetabular surgery or extensive muscle debridement, using posterior approach.

POSTOPERATIVE COURSE

The basic aim is to develop a flexible but strong tissue in the region of pseudarthrosis that will allow painless mobility albeit with compromised stability. The tissue takes 6–12 weeks to form in the region and immobilization or splinting beyond this period is possibly not necessary. The limb is kept distracted for around 6 weeks in traction in order to provide enough space for the tissues to form.

COMPLICATIONS

- Severe lurch—there is often excessive proximal migration of the femur that is uncontrollable producing significant shortening. This is associated with abductor muscle dysfunction due to both abolished lever at the hip joint and proximal migration. The combination results in short-limb and Trendelenburg gait which is often associated with pain and antalgic gait
- Instability of hip
- Shortening
- Late onset pain due to erosion of bone
- Osteoarthrosis of knee
- Hyperextension deformity at knee
- Adduction deformity of other hip.

CONCLUSION

- Girdlestone arthroplasty is a mutilating and deforming surgery that finds no definitive primary indication in current orthopedic practice as a primary procedure.
- It is nowadays performed only as a salvage procedure in nonreconstructible hip arthroplasty when there is no option to save or redo hip arthroplasty or if the patient desires so or if the clinical scenario prohibits attempting another reconstruction.
- The only indication is probably a septic hip in an underprivileged female who has demands of housekeeping and squatting that would render arthroplasty or arthrodesis useless. The lurch will be a significant problem to her but shoe raise or performing pelvic-support osteotomy of Milch type or Lorenz type can reduce it.

CHAPTER 77

Hip Arthrodesis

Manish Kumar Varshney

INTRODUCTION

There are three general choices for restoring the functionality of hip joint following a pathology that restricts the hip movements/stability/function and which cannot be treated medically. They are:

1. Painless, stable, mobile hip with variable longevity of reconstruction—total hip arthroplasty (THA)
2. Painless stable hip with permanent loss of mobility with reconstruction—hip arthrodesis
3. Painless mobile hip but with shortening and loss of desired stability at the joint—resection arthroplasty.

All these methods aim at minimum one aspect, i.e., reduction of pain. The first is the most desirable as it restores also the stability and movements though the duration of restoration is variable and depending on the usage, age, fixation, etc. may have to be revised. The second option is less desirable as it leads to loss of movements at hip but they can be compensated a bit at nearby joints. The functional outcomes have been considered inferior to THA but strictly speaking if one considers the long-term results of arthroplasty, then we realize that revision rates are quite high for patients and they perceive it as a disappointment. Total hip arthroplasty has not been perfected to the point of adequately meeting the needs of the young active patient over a normal lifespan. Hip arthrodesis is a viable alternative for management of advanced hip pathologies in a select group of patients (summaritively, the best indication would be patient's age <30 years with a history of multiple hip surgeries, post-traumatic arthritis, and/or postinfectious hip disease without pre-existing lower back pain, ipsilateral knee or contralateral hip arthritis in a highly active individual). Currently, the procedure is practiced for two broad groups of patients:

1. ***Primary hip arthrodesis:***
   - Young active laborers with painful unilateral ankylosis after infection or trauma
   - Neuropathic arthropathy
   - Advanced unilateral osteoarthrosis [primary or secondary due to osteonecrosis, Perthes disease, slipped upper femoral epiphysis (SUFE), developmental dysplasia of hip (DDH), femoroacetabular impingement (FAI), etc.] of the hip in a patient (30–35 years) who is a laborer and needs to do hard manual labor, or those underprivileged that need to earn their daily living by laborious jobs
   - Tumor resection
   - Long-standing neglected pseudoarthrosis of fracture neck of femur.
2. ***Secondary/salvage procedure:***
   - For failed THA
   - Failed hip reconstructions in neoplastic conditions around hip.

HISTORY OF THE PROCEDURE

Till 1930s, the procedure was prominently practiced, whence the growing popularity of THA gradually reduced the indications and practice of the procedure.

- Hip arthrodesis was first attempted by Lagrane of France in 1886.
- Albee is the *Father of Hip Arthrodesis* in the United States who described two methods of doing the procedure:
  1. Intra-articular method in 1908 **(Fig. 1)**
  2. Extra-articular procedure in 1915 **(Fig. 2)**
- Brittain's procedure (1931) was an extra-articular hip arthrodesis developing the concepts from various previous authors (DeBeule, Maraglino, Trumble, etc.). The arthrodesis was accomplished with subtrochanteric osteotomy and medialization of the shaft to act as pelvic support and aid weight transmission in a linear rather than angular fashion **(Fig. 3)**. Subtrochanteric osteotomy is the first step followed by incising ischium just below the acetabulum through osteotomy. Then a massive tibial corticocancellous graft is pushed into the defect through osteotomy. Alternatively, in a healed case (ankylosed) with adduction and flexion deformity, a subtrochanteric McMurray's osteotomy can be done.
- Till this time, all above methods used bone grafts, the internal fixation era of hip arthrodesis was popularized by attempts and persistence from Van Nes (1922).
- Onji et al. (1965) described intramedullary arthrodesis **(Fig. 4)** but was cumbersome and frequently complicated.

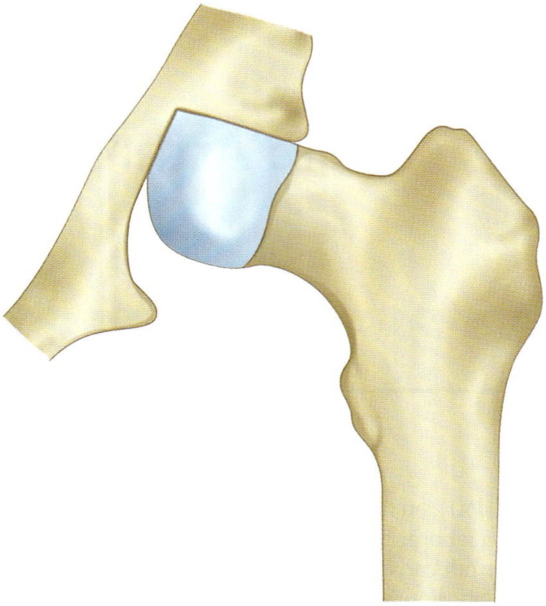

Fig. 1: The intra-articular arthrodesis described by Albee.

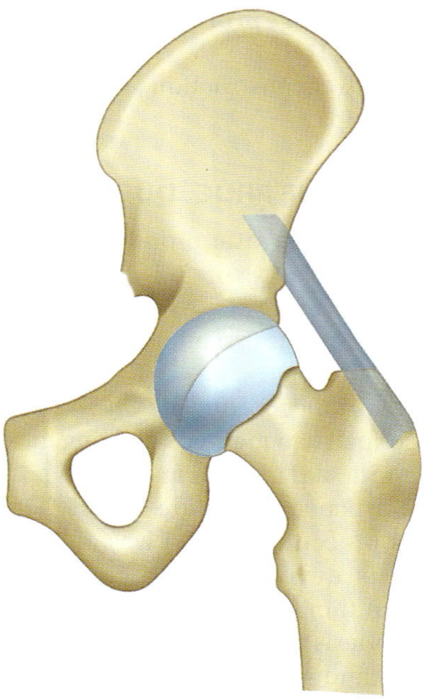

Fig. 2: The extra-articular arthrodesis described by Albee.

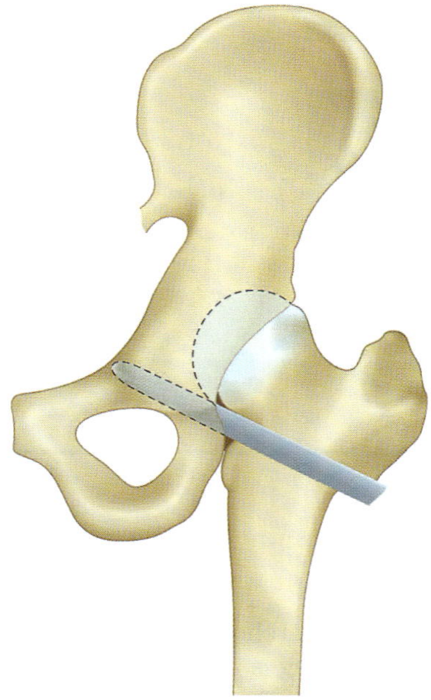

Fig. 3: The extra-articular arthrodesis with subtrochanteric osteotomy described by Brittain.

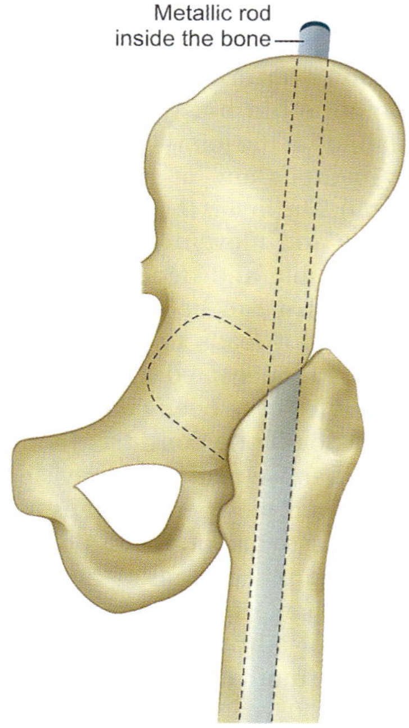

Fig. 4: The intramedullary arthrodesis described by Onji.

- Watson-Jones method **(Fig. 5)** was extremely popular using the transarticular triflange nail (to be replaced by Schneider procedure in future).
- Central dislocation and internal compression arthrodesis of Charnley **(Fig. 6)**.
- Due to often poor fixation in the iliac bone, the arthrodesis has high rate of nonunion despite opposing cancellous surfaces of the prepared bones. This was improved upon by two prominent methods:
  1. Davis (1954) muscle-pedicle iliac bone graft to augment hip fusion **(Fig. 7)**—this fell out of favor as it mutilated the hip pathology, and if in any case future THA would be planned the surgery will be unnecessarily complicated.
  2. The *cobra-head plate arthrodesis* described by Schneider in 1966 **(Fig. 8)**: This has been the most popular method for performing hip arthrodesis till recently but availability of the implant is limited nowadays so alternatives are emerging. Actually, Schneider took concepts from Charnley's medial displacement of hip for improving surface contact and rigid fixation. Medial displacement (as also

practiced by Brittain) was to lower the hip joint reaction forces by reducing offset and hence aligning the line of weight-bearing more centrally.

BIOMECHANICS AND NATURAL HISTORY OF THE PROCEDURE

The procedure is not very ergonomic to the body. There is a lot of increased energy consumption and expenditure by body.

The following are some of the changes brought upon by hip arthrodesis:

- Reduces efficiency of gait by approximately 50%.
- Increases pelvic rotation of contralateral hip.
- Increases stress at adjacent joints.
- Increases oxygen consumption.
- Requires 30% more energy expenditure for ambulation.

Optimal Position of Hip Arthrodesis

- 20–35° of flexion—minimum 20° else calculate as a general rule of 1° per year of age above 10 years till a maximum of 30° above 25 years of age (rationale is that ongoing compensation develops in children with flexible

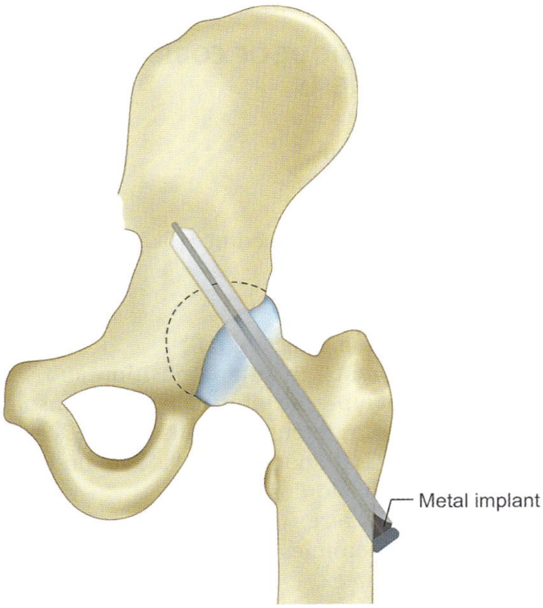

Fig. 5: The transarticular nail arthrodesis described by Watson-Jones.

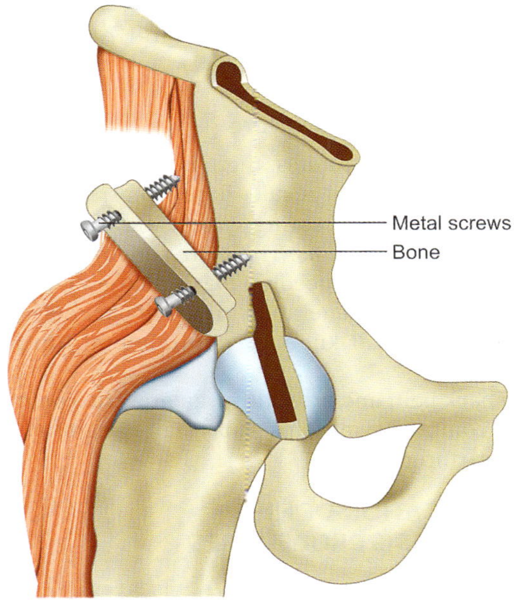

Fig. 7: The iliac bone graft augmentation described by Davis.

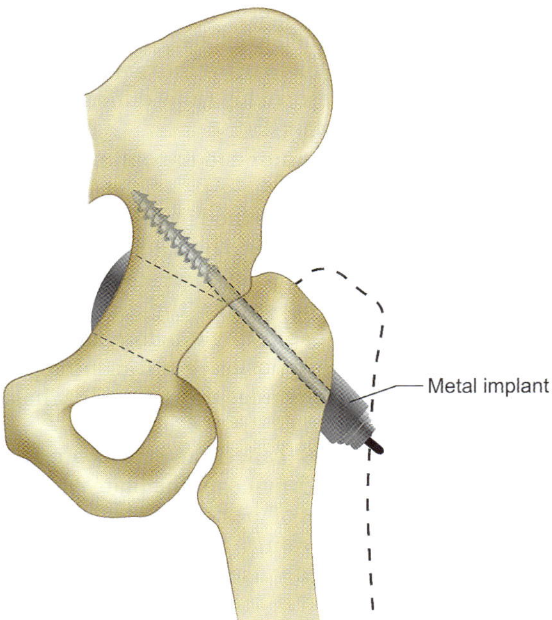

Fig. 6: The central dislocation and internal compression arthrodesis described by Charnley.

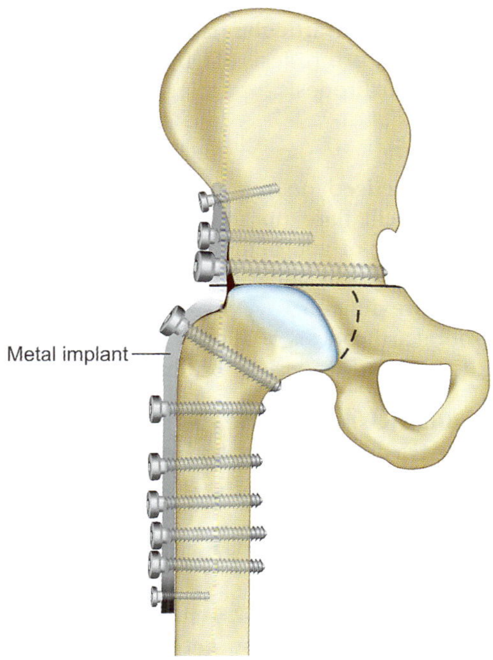

Fig. 8: Vancouver method—the cobra-head plate arthrodesis with pelvic osteotomy described by Schneider.

spine and in adults up to 30° of flexion can be hidden by lumbar lordosis). Flexion provides necessary ground clearance and lets one hide fixed joint while sitting. Inadequate flexion produces difficulty in sitting while excessive flexion puts stress on spine and increases limb length discrepancy.

- 0–5° adduction improves gait. Zero degree is preferred in children. An increase of 3° of adduction causes apparent leg shortening of approximately 1 cm.
- 5–10° external rotation prevents ipsilateral foot banging into the contralateral foot and aids in donning footwear when flexing the knee.
- Adduction is not favored as it creates pelvic obliquity, frontal plane knee deformity, and has chances of increased back pain.

Natural History of Procedure

Once the arthrodesis unites, there is prominent pain relief and reasonable clinical results have been reported by the authors (the objective scoring systems have not been used however) in most patients. There are still long-term sequel as expected from the procedure that limit the success:

- Adjacent joint degeneration in 60% of patients—Lumbar spine, ipsilateral knee, or contralateral hip may be affected.
- Low back pain and arthritic ipsilateral knee pain are the most common symptoms—may start as early as 25 years of hip arthrodesis.

CLASSIFICATION OF HIP ARTHRODESIS PROCEDURES

Intra-articular

- Central dislocation and internal compression arthrodesis of Charnley
- Watson-Jones transarticular nail arthrodesis
- Intramedullary arthrodesis of Onji
- Cobra-plate arthrodesis.

Extra-articular

These were practiced on the premises that opening up diseased joint will flare up the infection and there was lack of availability of good chemotherapy. However, these procedures destroy the anatomy of hip joint making any future procedure difficult.

- Iliofemoral arthrodesis of Albee
- Ischiofemoral arthrodesis of Brittain.

Para-articular (Usually Done to Augment Intra-articular Procedure)

Davis muscle-pedicle arthrodesis.

CONTRAINDICATIONS FOR HIP ARTHRODESIS

- Active infection
- Limb-length discrepancy >2.5 cm
- Bilateral hip arthritis or active pathology in the contralateral hip (like osteonecrosis of the other head of femur that would also need a surgery)
- Adjacent joint degenerative changes:
  - Lumbar spine
  - Contralateral hip
  - Ipsilateral knee
- Severe osteoporosis
- Degenerative changes in lumbar spine
- Contralateral THA—Increased failure rate (40%) in THA when there is a contralateral hip arthrodesis
- Psychologically unstable patient who fails to understand the merits and importantly demerits of procedure
- Tall patients (femur length > 72 inches) should be warned that sitting in crowded places (movie theaters, airplane seats) would be difficult.

SURGICAL TECHNIQUE OF COBRA-HEAD PLATE ARTHRODESIS

- Wide bony contact
- Rigid internal fixation
- Compression of surfaces
- Minimal shortening
- Minimally limit future procedures (like arthroplasty)
- Early mobilization.

Approach and Steps

(Vancouver Technique, Figs. 9A to E)

- Mid-lateral approach in supine position and a bump under ipsilateral hip—the interval between tensor fascia latae (TFL) and the gluteus maximus muscle is explored. The opposite leg is draped free and is kept under flexion to minimize lumbar lordosis.
- Standard trochanteric osteotomy is performed (*see* Chapter on " Osteotomies Around Hip Joint") to preserve the abductor complex.
- Surgical dislocation of the hip is done [*see* Chapter on "Surgical Dislocation of the Hip (Ganz Surgical Dislocation of Hip, Open Dislocation of Hip)"] and femoral head delivered anteriorly.
- The acetabulum is reamed to expose the cancellous bone and femoral head is reamed using the reamers for surface replacement arthroplasty of hip (now difficult to procure due to withdrawn implants!).
- Cobra-head plate is contoured to the optimal position of hip arthrodesis:
  - Adduction control is obtained by image intensifier.
  - Rotational control is judged by patella and foot.
  - Flexion is best assessed by long sterile goniometer or placing a bump under the posterior thigh preoperatively and adjusting it beforehand. It is also helpful to drape the opposite leg and an intraoperative Thomas test can help judge the flexion that has been obtained.
- Fix the plate with screws (cancellous screws proximally).
- Fix the trochanteric fragment over the plate with a screw through one of the holes of the plate and into femur.
- Close the wound over drain.
- Reamings can be tactfully used as bone graft to fill the irregularities.

Other easier methods have been described like debridement using Watson-Jones approach plus surgical dislocation

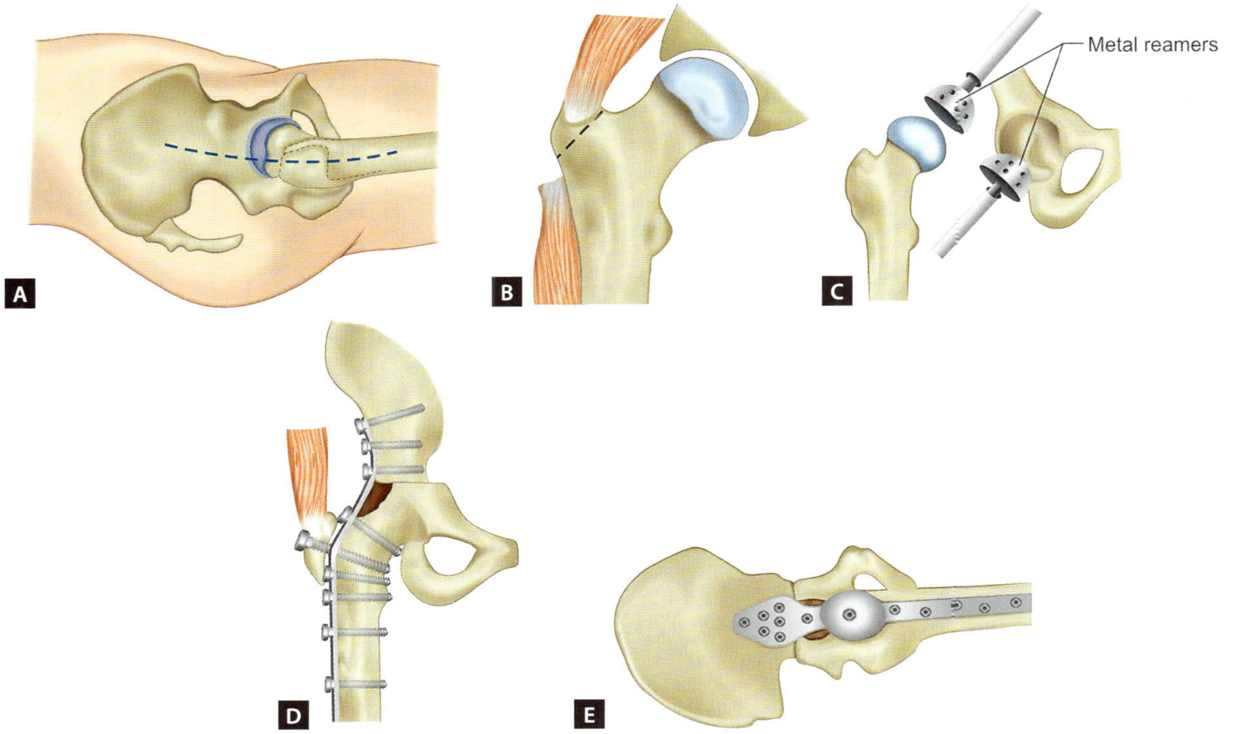

Figs. 9A to E: The steps of Vancouver method: (A) Exposure by direct midlateral approach; (B) Performing standard trochanteric osteotomy; (C) Reaming the acetabulum and femoral head; (D) Application of the cobra-plate; and (E) Fixation of trochanter fragment.

of head followed by fixation using 150°/160° dynamic hip screw (DHS) plate screw construct **(Fig. 10)** and are likely to become popular. This method has following advantages:

- Total hip arthroplasty is minimally compromised
- Less invasive
- Preservation of abductor mechanism fully
- Simple internal fixation device.

Hip arthrodesis by anterior plating method **(Fig. 11)**—due to lack of universal availability of cobra-head plate, alternative methods are designed for hip arthrodesis. In this method, hip is exposed through a modified Smith-Petersen approach.

- Exposure is deepened through the subcutaneous layer releasing the abdominal and abductor muscles from the iliac crest.
- Both sartorius and rectus femoris are detached from the tensor fascia muscular sheet. The vastus lateralis is elevated anteriorly.
- Surfaces are prepared and 6.5-mm lag screw fixation is done across.
- Broad dynamic compression holes (DCP) is contoured and placed along the inner table of ilium and across the joint surface to proximal femur.
- This approach preserves the vascularity of head, and uses the areas of good bone stock for fixation.

POSTOPERATIVE COURSE

Postoperative management includes hip spica cast immobilization until radiographic healing. Based upon

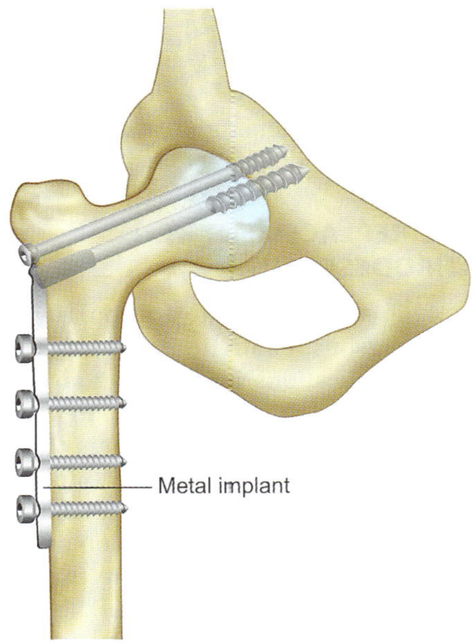

Fig. 10: Transarticular hip arthrodesis with a dynamic hip screw via the lateral approach.

clinical and radiographic findings, weight-bearing may be allowed after 12 weeks.

Complications

- *Immediate, early, and intermediate term:*
    - Blood loss
    - Infection

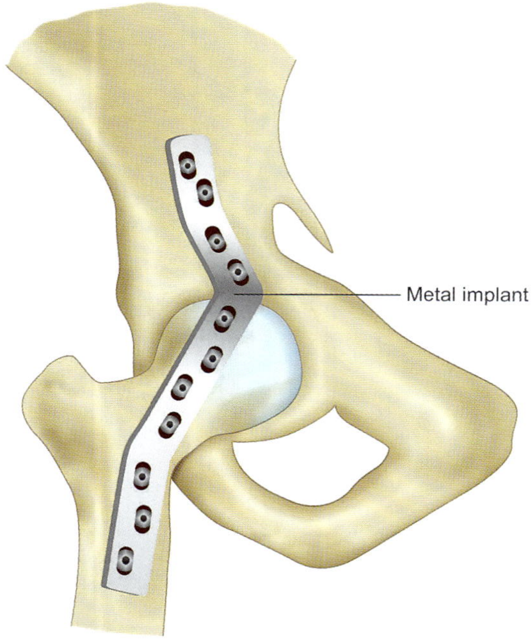

Fig. 11: Hip arthrodesis via anterior plating technique.

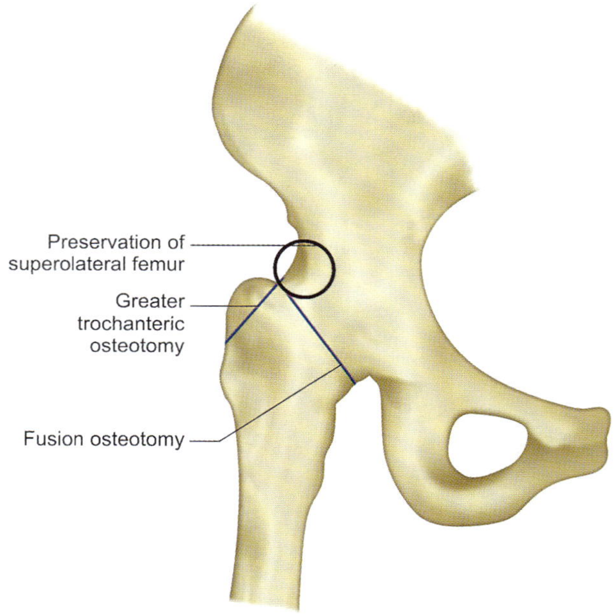

Fig. 12: The greater trochanter and fusion site osteotomy. Preserve the superolateral femoral neck and superolateral acetabulum to provide optimal acetabular component coverage.

- Implant failure
- Nonunion
- Malposition

- *Late and long-term:*
  - Low back pain
  - Ipsilateral knee degeneration and laxity
  - Contralateral hip degeneration.

TOTAL HIP REPLACEMENT IN AN ARTHRODESED HIP

Conversion of hip arthrodesis into arthroplasty is a difficult task and most surgeons refrain from this conversion due to intraoperative complications, inexperience and poor results. Indications for conversion of a fused hip to a THA include functional disability and continuous pain in the back, knee, and/or contralateral hip secondary to hip fusion. This operation should be performed only for disabling pain (and never on the patient's wish to have motion at the joint). In general, conversion of a fused hip to THA may relieve pain in adjacent joints and improve mobility of the hip (although not as good as with a primary THA). However, postoperative gait quality is strongly related to the preoperative abductor muscle function and it is likely that patients may require walking aids after conversion to THA. The following points summarize the intricacies of this conversion:

- If the arthrodesis was done for infection or there is even minimal suspicion of infection [raised erythrocyte sedimentation rate (ESR), C-reactive protein (CRP), counts, bone scan, etc.] a two-stage procedure is performed to ensure clearance of infection before any definitive total hip replacement (THR).
- A transtrochanteric approach is optimal. There should be a gap of 3 months between the placement of articulating spacer and THA with subsidence of laboratory parameters. Patient should also be informed that final outcome could be a Girdlestone hip.
- All dissection should proceed (whether the fusion was intra- or extra-articular) subperiosteally on bone when identifying the acetabulum and femur at the fusion site else vital structures may get damaged.
- Greater trochanter usually serves as a good landmark for osteotomy but in its absence pubofemoral arch is relied upon. Femur may need to be cut higher anteriorly or posteriorly, depending on the flexion at the fusion site.
- The lateral edge of the acetabulum and the superior lateral femoral neck should be preserved to allow optimal acetabular component coverage **(Fig. 12)**.
- Transverse acetabular ligament is usually preserved serving as guide to the lower limit of acetabulum. Place a retractor in the obturator foramen for orientation. To further gain orientation one should not hesitate in exposing the superior pubic ramus and ischial tuberosity.
- Reaming the acetabulum in fluoroscopy control is best.
- In patients with markedly deficient gluteus medius and minimus musculature, tenodesis of the iliotibial band into the greater trochanter may aid in obtaining hip stability.
- Constrained sockets or dual mobility cups may be a better choice, if too much instability is expected.
- Femur preparation is as routine.

CONCLUSION

- Arthrodesis of the hip joint is an uncommonly performed surgery—I should put actually it as a rarely performed surgery.
- It is difficult to find a patient fitting into all the requirements of arthrodesis of such a major joint who also accepts the disability and limitations that follow the procedure.
- There are various described classical methods of performing hip arthrodesis but the favored ones are cobraplate arthrodesis or newer methods of DHS plate arthrodesis.
- One should always consider the status of the other limb while prescribing hip arthrodesis and also patient should be given trial in the form of function limiting brace to understand exactly what the course of postoperative management would be like after the procedure.
- Arthrodesis can be converted to hip arthroplasty in experienced hands, however, the outcomes are inferior to that of procedure done on native hips with maintained muscular power.

CHAPTER 78

Surgical Dislocation of the Hip (Ganz Surgical Dislocation of Hip, Open Dislocation of Hip)

Manish Kumar Varshney

INTRODUCTION

By definition, it is a procedure that preserves blood supply to the femoral head maximally while also allowing repair of the hip joint pathology. It allows safe dislocation of the joint without jeopardizing blood supply and completing joint reconstruction or preservation procedures with minimal morbidity. Surgical dislocation of hip is considered powerful method or an essential technique in modern practice of joint preserving hip surgeries to allow correction of complex and intricate problems like femoroacetabular impingement. These problems mostly deal with elective surgeries, either cartilage damage or labral pathologies on acetabular side or correction of bony deformities that can be corrected while maintaining the overall integrity of hip joint. Some traumatic injuries like fractures of head of femur can also be managed by open surgical dislocation of hip. Traumatic fracture dislocations of hip have an osteonecrosis rate of around 10–15% that increases to 30% when surgical relocation is required. This may be due to rupture of external obturator muscle causing damage to the medial circumflex femoral artery (MCFA) which is the main blood supply to the femoral head via intermediary ascending retinacular vessels. Surgical dislocation of hip is indicated for the treatment of younger patients to treat specific disorders which will not permit violation of hip joint integrity using an open method. These patients have a relatively healthy hip and joint should not be sacrificed. Open surgical dislocation is apparently the most effective technique for major intra-articular hip pathologies that may not be adequately addressed with hip arthroscopy. Some surgeons consider this to the procedure of choice for intra-articular pathologies as arthroscopy may miss some critical areas and require specialized instruments. Hip pathologies that can be currently successfully managed with surgical dislocation include:

- Femoral head fractures (Pipkins fractures)
- Complex femoroacetabular impingement (FAI) deformities
  - Repairing of acetabular labrum
  - Reshaping the bony acetabular rim (acetabuloplasty)
  - Removing bony bumps (cam lesions) on femoral head (femoral osteoplasty)
- Correction of major structural abnormalities of the hip joint
  - Reduction osteotomy (intraosseous, head splitting) of femoral head in Perthes
  - A deformed femoral head as seen in Perthes disease (cheilectomy)
  - Slipped upper femoral epiphysis (SUFE)—intra-articular osteotomy of femoral neck
- *Articular cartilage defect reconstruction:* Autologous cartilage implantation (ACI), matrix autologous chondrocyte implantation (MACI)
- Loose body removal in fracture dislocation of hip
- Post-traumatic hip deformities
- Hip arthrodesis
- Other conditions:
  - Rheumatoid synovitis
  - Synovial chondromatosis
  - Pigmented villonodular synovitis.

PRINCIPLES

- Deep branch of the MCFA primarily supplies the femoral head that should be protected during most of the surgical procedures. The vessel crosses the intact obturator externus muscle from below and is violated during standard posterior approaches to hip. The main idea of surgical dislocation of the hip is to protect this vessel.
- The trochanteric flip allows hip joint to be exposed anteriorly. The femoral head can be dislocated in the same direction without violating the short external rotators and hence preserving the vascularity.
- Traction to femoral head can be given and the approach allows separating the femoral head from acetabulum by 11 cm. Visibility of head can be hence gained all around exposing it circumferentially and giving a simultaneous full 360° view of the acetabulum.

TECHNIQUE

Position and Approach

Patient is placed in lateral decubitus position and hip is exposed using posterior Kocher–Langenbeck approach.

The incision is made and fascia lata split. The leg is then internally rotated by assistant.

Superficial Dissection

- The posterior border of gluteus medius is only identified but neither mobilized nor retracted to view the piriformis.
- The trochanteric fine vascular plexus is cauterized superficially to minimize bleeding.
- Small length incision is made along the posterosuperior edge of greater trochanter that extends distally to the posterior border of the vastus ridge to expose the trochanter and identify landmarks for trochanteric osteotomy.

Deep Tissue Dissection

- Mark the tip of greater trochanter, region of piriformis fossa and vastus ridge.
- A trochanteric flip osteotomy is done (see osteotomies around the hip). One should try to maintain thickness of 1.5 cm at least for the osteotomized fragment **(Figs. 1A and B)**. One can also modify it into Z-osteotomy for improved stability.
- To make the cuts one must ensure that the osteotomy does not incorporate anterior portion of the femoral neck or hip joint capsule. The osteotomy exits proximally just anterior to the most posterior insertion of gluteus medius muscle. This protects the profundus branch of the MCFA at the soft spot where it becomes intracapsular to supply the ascending lateral retinacular vessels at the level of the superior gemellus muscle. To prevent the osteotomy becoming too oblique it is useful to ask the assistant rotate flexed leg internally by 15–20°. This makes head parallel to the floor and avoids inadvertent injury when saw is used to make osteotomy.
- The greater trochanteric fragment is translated anteriorly after releasing at posterior border of the tendon of gluteus maximus and inserting posterior fibers of gluteus medius. Usually, a part of the tendon of piriformis is attached to the fragment that has to be freed to accomplish this.
- To ease external rotation at hip the vastus lateralis and intermedius muscles are elevated from the lateral and anterior aspects of the proximal femur.
- Next the inferior border of gluteus minimus is separated from the relaxed piriformis; usually, there is a vascular anastomosis between underlying joint capsule and the muscle that needs to be preserved while freeing muscle. This anastomosis is formed by inferior gluteal artery and MCFA. The latter is seen running along the distal border of the piriformis.
- One should protect and retract the sciatic nerve from getting injured as the piriformis is mobilized and anomalous relationship of the nerve and muscle might cause nerve compression or traction damage.
- If the piriformis muscle is sandwiched between split branches of sciatic nerve then muscle should be released from greater trochanter to avoid stretching the nerve during dislocation/anterior flip of entire flap.
- After anterior flip of the fragment with attached medius and vastus lateralis, the gluteus minimus is retracted anteriorly and superiorly to expose the superior capsule. To further enhance exposure to anterior, superior, and posterosuperior capsule, the leg can be further flexed and externally rotated.
- Hip joint capsule is then incised in a straight line along the long axis of the femoral neck anterolaterally as this zone is relatively watershed/avascular and avoids the deep branch of the MCFA **(Fig. 2)**. The incision is extended distally in the anteroinferior capsular along the base of femoral neck **(Fig. 2)**.
- It is important that this vertical limb of osteotomy remains anterior to the lesser trochanter to avoid damaging the main branch of the MCFA. The artery lies here just superior and posterior to lesser trochanter.
- The anterior and inferior half of the labrum can be well visualized once the anteroinferior flap of capsule is reflected.
- To expose rest of the labrum and hip joint the first capsular incision (straight anterolateral) is extended along the superolateral acetabular rim using capsulotomy

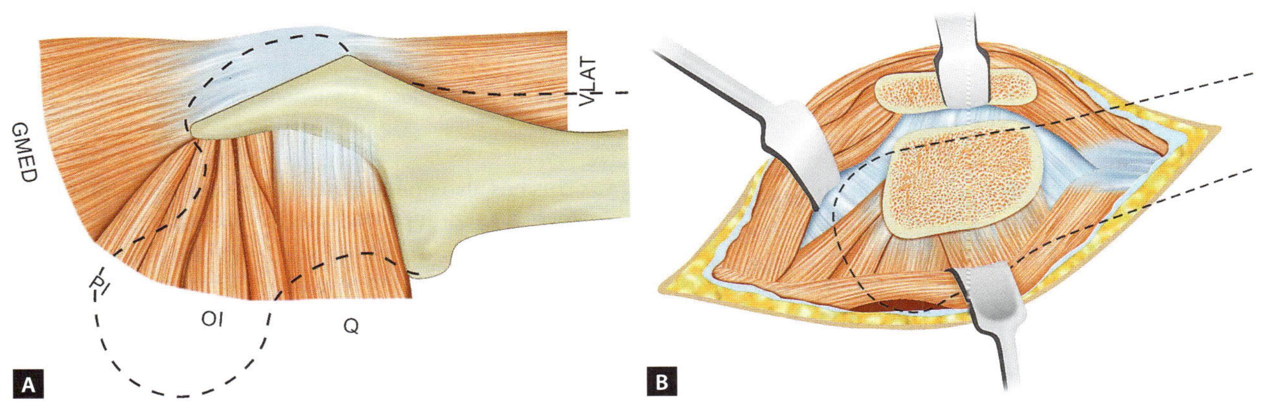

Figs. 1A and B: (A) The trochanteric flip osteotomy is made preserving significant thickness of greater trochanter; (B) The osteotomized fragment is retracted anteriorly to expose capsule. (GMED: gluteus medius; OI: obturator internus; PI: piriformis; Q: quadratus femoris; VLAT: vastus lateralis)

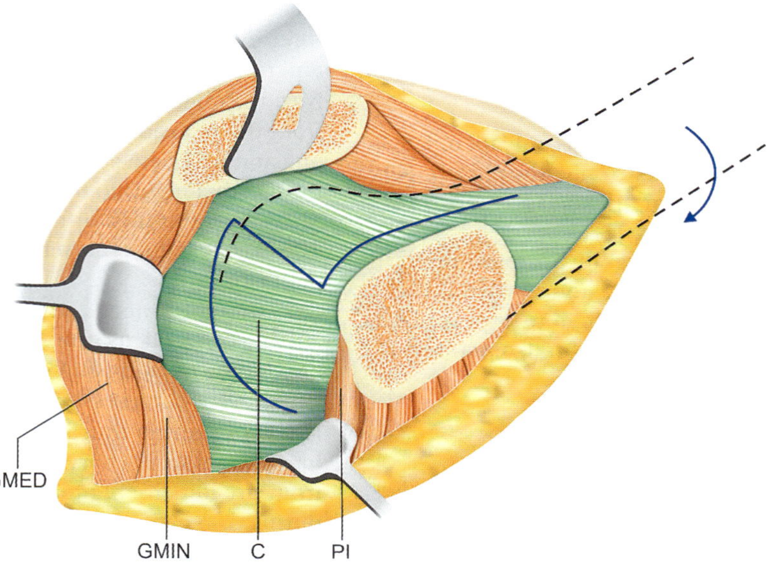

Fig. 2: Exposed capsule and making the incision. The anterolateral limb is marked on the capsule extending it vertically anteroinferiorly along the femoral neck base. The anterolateral limb is extended proximally along the acetabular side superiorly to complete the osteotomy. (C: capsule; GMED: gluteus medius; GMIN: gluteus minimus; PI: piriformis)

scissors or knife. The limb is extended till it sharply turns posteriorly. It may reach as far as the retracted tendon of piriformis protecting the labrum. This completes the capsulotomy **(Fig. 2)**.

- The hip joint is now dislocated by flexion, externally rotating the leg, and bringing it over the front of the operating table. The leg can be placed in a sterile bag allowing inspection of most of the acetabulum **(Fig. 3)**.
- After completion of the procedure, greater trochanter is reattached using two or three cancellous screws or better cerclage wire (*see* Chapter on "Osteotomies Around Hip Joint").

COMPLICATIONS

- Fracture of trochanter
- Damage to vascularity
- Injury to sciatic nerve
- Injury to intra-articular structures
- Nonunion of trochanteric osteotomy
- Migration of trochanteric osteotomy
- Lateral hip pain
- Heterotopic ossification
- Osteonecrosis.

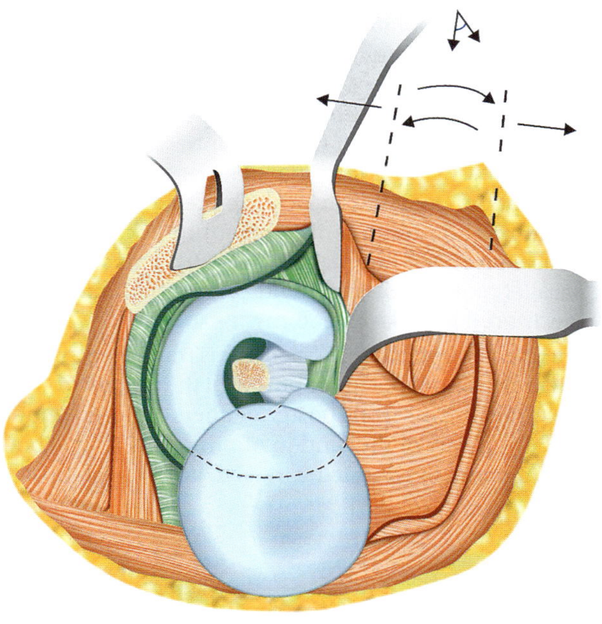

Fig. 3: The hip is dislocated anteriorly through the capsular incision.

CONCLUSION

- Surgical dislocation of hip is a special procedure for exposing the hip joint without damaging the vascular supply of the hip joint.
- With increasing realization of femoroacetabular impingement syndrome the safe surgical dislocation of the hip has been increasingly performed for osteochondroplasty and labral repairs.
- This has also opened the avenues for chondral repair and reconstruction procedures in sports persons.
- Attention to details of the procedure is essential else undesirable damage to the joint may occur or the exposure may not be adequate.
- This is a versatile procedure and substitutes to a large extent the need of hip arthroscopy.

SECTION 9

Disorders of Foot and Ankle

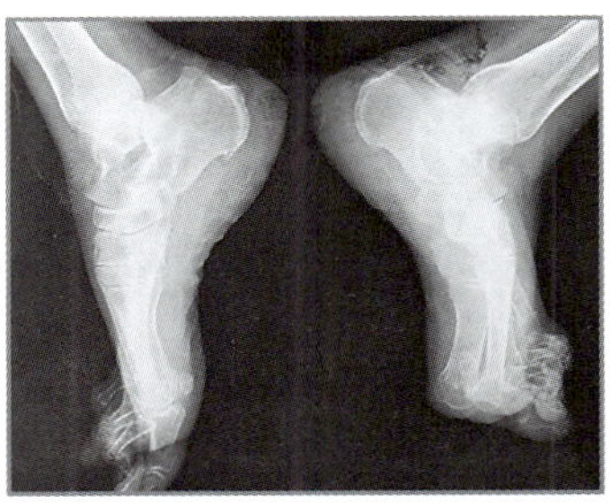
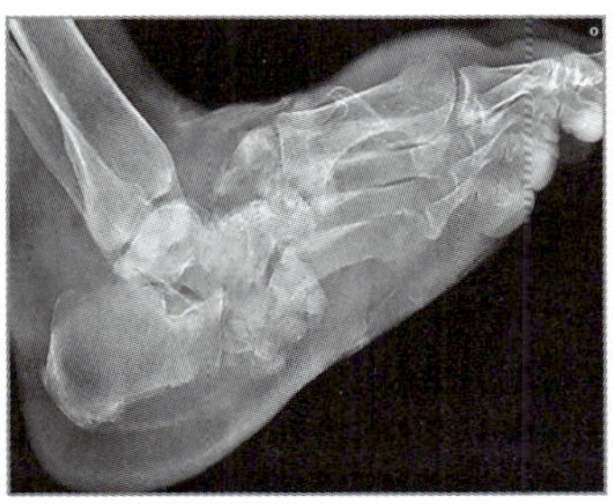
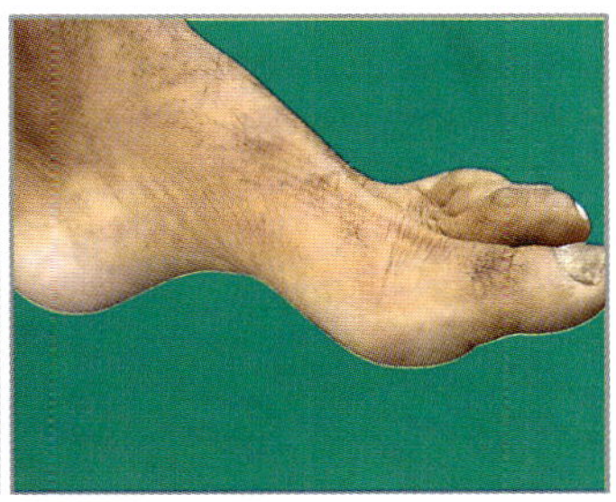

CHAPTER 79

Anatomy of Ankle and Foot

Manish Kumar Varshney

INTRODUCTION

Understanding anatomy of a region is paramount to discriminate abnormal from normal and hence make a correct diagnosis and also decipher the knowledge associated with them. This is especially important when the region is complex like foot that involves various articulations involved in bearing the weight of whole body. Here, even small deviations will produce amplified biomechanical consequences leading to rapid deterioration of the anatomy and function. The chapter focuses on the anatomical perspective of the ankle and foot region as clinically relevant and will be followed in other chapters by biomechanics and examination based on the same.

BONY ANKLE

The ankle joint (talocrural joint) is a compound synovial hinge joint **(Fig. 1)**. During walk the forces across the ankle exceed

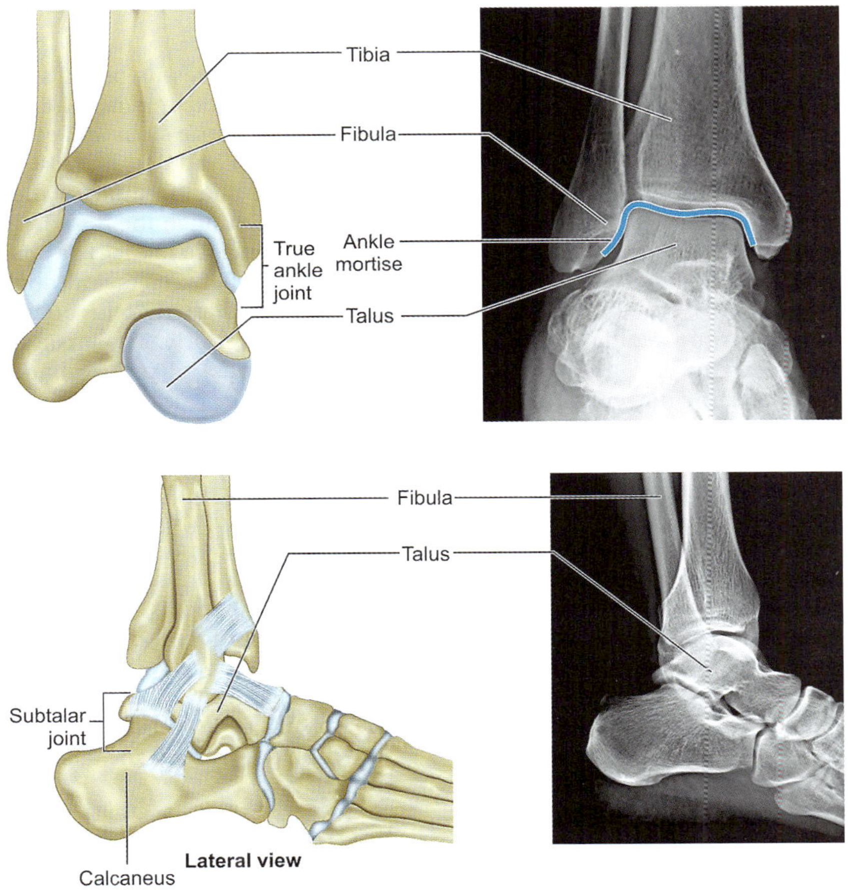

Fig. 1: Bony and radiographic anatomy of ankle joint.

five times the body weight and shear forces approach three times the body weight. It consists of:

- Talar dome
- The distal end of tibia, the tibial plafond—which includes medial malleolus and the posterior malleolus, articulating with the body of the talus
- The distal end of fibula, lateral malleolus

The ankle is a complex hinge joint considered saddle-shaped, with a talar dome covering a larger circumference more laterally than medially.

TIBIA

Five surfaces of the lower end of tibia forms the tibial plafond: (1) anterior, (2) posterior, (3) inferior, (4) medial, and (5) lateral. The inferior articular surface of tibia is transversely convex and concave anteroposteriorly, the width of the articular surface is more wide laterally and narrow medially and the distal extent of the posterior border is at a lower level as compared to the anterior border.

The distal medial extension of tibia is the medial malleolus. The lateral surface of which is covered with articular cartilage and articulates with the medial facet of talus. On the medial surface, a longitudinal groove divides it into anterior large and posterior small colliculus, the anterior one extends distally than the posterior. Both give attachment to the deltoid ligament. Also there is a groove at the posterior surface of the medial malleolus for the tibialis posterior tendon. The intercollicular groove gives attachment to the deep talotibial component of the deltoid ligament and the superficial fibers of the deltoid ligament take origin at the anterior border of the anterior colliculus.

The lateral distal border of the tibia is concave and has anterior and posterior tubercles. The anterior tubercle gives origin to the anterior tibiofibular ligament and the posterior tubercle gives attachment to the deep component of posterior tibiofibular ligament.

FIBULA

The distal end of the fibula gives rise to multiple ligaments and forms the lateral malleolus along with its articular surface. The lateral malleolus is a widened structure with three surfaces. The lower end of fibula twists on itself so that the lateral surface becomes the posterior border as traced distally, the interosseous ligament attaches to the fibula at the level of this twist. Strong ligaments attach anteriorly, posteriorly, inferiorly, and superiorly.

- *Anteriorly:* The anterior talofibular ligament (ATFL) and the main and secondary bands of the ATFL.
- *Posteriorly:* The posterior talofibular ligament and the superficial and deep components of the posterior tibiofibular ligament.
- *Superiorly:* The tibiofibular interosseous ligament.
- *Inferiorly:* The calcaneofibular ligament (CFL).

With the increased practice and gaining popularity of minimally invasive surgeries for ankle ligament reconstruction the fibular obscure tubercle plays an important role in surface marking of the lateral malleolus for incision placement. The fibular obscure tubercle (detected in 57% of patients) allows identification of origin of ATFLs and CFLs. As detailed by Kentaro Matsui et al., it is seen 1.3 mm proximal to the articular tip of the fibula, 2.7 mm to the intersection of the ATFL and CFL, 3.7 mm distal to the ATFL, and 4.9 mm proximal to the CFL origins.

TALUS

Talus, also known as astragalus, is the second largest tarsal bone. The talus is devoid of any muscular attachments and most of the surface of the talus is covered by articular cartilage (almost 60% of surface). The talus receives retrograde blood supply, which predisposes it to vascular insufficiency and trauma to talus associated with capsular and ligamentous disruption may result in osteonecrosis of the body of talus. The superior surface or the talar dome conforms the tibial articular surface. It is trapezoidal in shape with the anterior surface wider than the posterior providing much more ankle stability in dorsiflexion than planter flexion. The dome of the talus like the mortar is convex from back to back, the dome being much stronger than the plafond, so is protected in severe injuries. The superior articular surface is continuous with the medial and lateral articular surface. The ankle joint has variable axis of rotation probably because the lateral border is larger than medial and the anterior border is longer than the posterior, this configuration resembles a medial apex frustum of a cone. This architecture allows internal rotation during plantar flexion and external rotation during dorsiflexion.

Blood Supply

The talus receives its blood supply via its capsular and ligamentous attachments. The anastomosis of the vessels occurs in the tarsal sinus and canal, lying below the neck of talus **(Figs. 2A and B)**. The vessels from the canal and sinus perforate the inferior surface of the neck and supply the body of the talus through the intraosseous channels. The tarsal sinus is a cone of a funnel-like area lies on the lateral aspect of the surface between the calcaneus and talus, it is bounded by calcaneus inferiorly, talus body posteriorly, and talar head and neck anteriorly. The tarsal canal (not to be confused with tarsal sinus) is like the cylindrical part of the funnel that lies between the calcaneus and the talus just posteriorly and inferior to the medial malleolus.

Posterior tibial artery gives a branch the artery of tarsal canal, which further gives the deltoid branch and supplies the medial third of the body of talus. The talar body receives most of its blood supply from the anastomotic sling in the tarsal canal and sinus. Multiple branches from anterior tibial and the dorsalis pedis artery enter the dorsal aspect of neck. The posterior process of talus is supplied by branches from the peroneal artery.

The talar head receives majority of its vascularity from the dorsalis pedis, arising from the dorsal neck vessels and also from the artery of the tarsal sinus (perforating peroneal artery).

LIGAMENTS OF ANKLE JOINT

As in the elbow the stability is conferred by bony architecture and capsule-ligamentous structures. These ligaments primarily

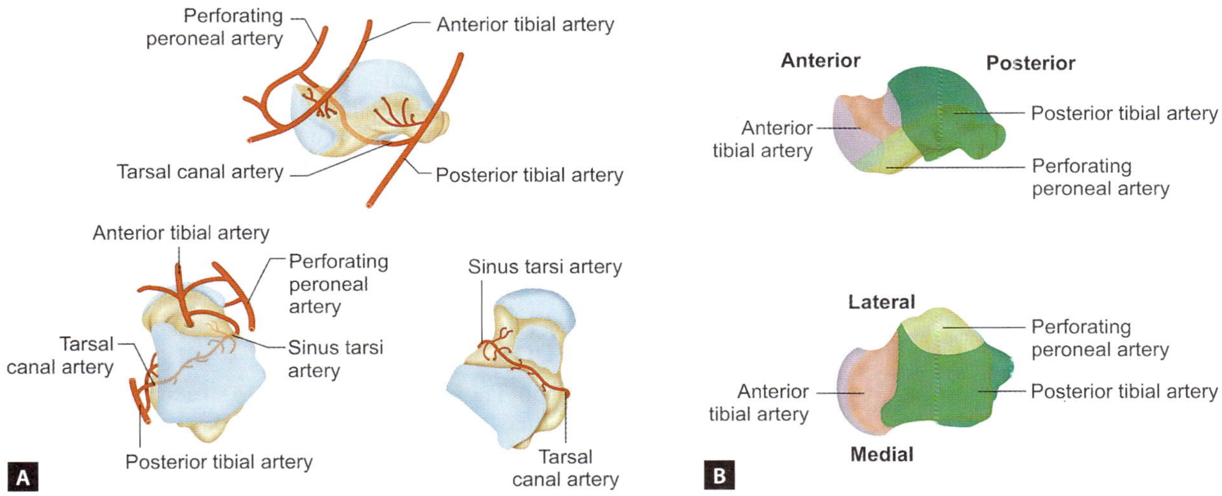

Figs. 2A and B: Blood supply of the talus. The talus receives blood supply from (A) anterior tibial artery, dorsalis pedis artery through anastomosis in tarsal sinus with the artery of tarsal sinus (branch of perforating peroneal artery), posterior tibial artery (through artery of tarsal canal), and the perforating peroneal artery itself. Sectoral blood supply of talus is illustrated (B) from top and side views.

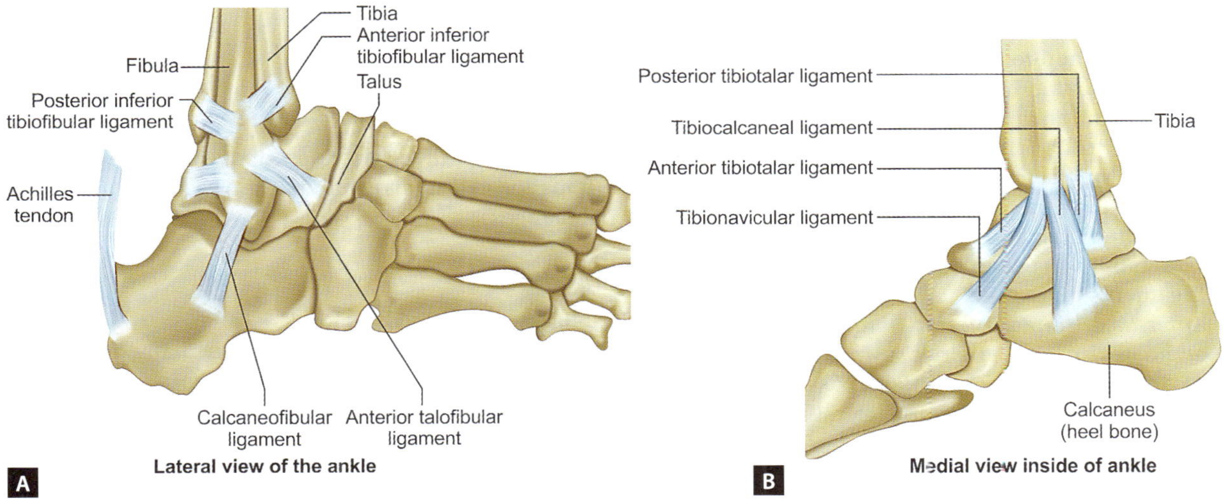

Figs. 3A and B: The ligaments of ankle joint articulation (see text for details). (A) Lateral view; (B) Medial structures.

perform three functions—providing proprioceptive information for joint function, providing static stability to the joint and prevent excessive motion, and guiding movements of the joint. There are three distinct groups of ligaments that include **(Figs. 3A and B)**:

1. The medial collateral ligament
2. The lateral collateral ligaments
3. The syndesmotic ligaments

The medial collateral ligament (Deltoid ligament complex): It provides anteroposterior stability to the medial side of ankle joint, and limits talar abduction at talocrural joint. It has five components.

- The "deep portion" of the deltoid ligament (most important structure) has two components, the anterior and posterior deep tibiotalar ligaments. It provides greatest restrain against lateral translation. The "anterior deep tibiotalar ligament" is a short ligament that originates from the most inferior and anterior areas of the medial malleolus. Its insertion is over the medial aspect of talus on its anterosuperior portions. The "other one is the posterior deep tibiotalar ligament" which is the largest, thickest, and strongest band among the superficial and deep layers. The deep posterior tibiotalar ligament originates near the distal center of the intercollicular groove and inserts on the posterosuperior aspect of the medial talar body. They are intra-articular but extrasynovial.
- The "superficial portion" of the deltoid ligament has three components:
  1. Anteriorly, tibionavicular component
  2. In middle, tibiocalcaneal component
  3. Posteriorly, posterior tibiotalar component

The valgus tilting of the talus is resisted by both, superficial and deep components equally. They secondarily resist anterior translation of the talus.

The lateral collateral ligaments: It is the most common ligament affected in ankle sprains. It is made up of three primary ligaments. Collectively, these ligaments stabilize the ankle joint.

- *The anterior talofibular ligament (2–2.5 mm thick, 15–20 mm long, and 6–8 mm wide):* In the lateral collateral group, this ligament is the weakest ligament and so it is most commonly injured ligament. Anteriorly, it is attached over the neck of the talus. It has posterior attachment on the anterior border of the lateral malleolus. Its main function is to resist the anterior translation of the talus and plantar flexion of the ankle.
- *The CFL (20–25 mm long, 6–8 mm thick):* It is stronger than anterior talofibular ligament. Contrary to the other lateral ligaments, this ligament is extracapsular. It originates from the tip of the lateral malleolus, runs obliquely downward and backward, passes deep to the peroneal tendons, and inserts over the lateral surface of the calcaneus. It bridges both the talocrural joint and subtalar joint.
- *The posterior talofibular ligament (30 mm long, 5 mm wide, and 5–8 mm thick):* Among the lateral ligament, this is the strongest one. It originates from the medial surface of the lateral malleolus, from malleolar fossa, passes horizontally toward talus to insert on its posterolateral aspect. It is taught in dorsiflexion and relaxed in plantarflexion and neutral position of the ankle. In posterior soft-tissue impingement syndrome of the ankle, this ligament may get involved.
- *The syndesmotic ligaments* ***(Figs. 4A and B)****:* Distal tibiofibular stability is maintained by these ligaments, which resist the axial, rotational and translational forces separating the tibia and the fibula. These ligaments also provide stability to the ankle joint. This group consists of four ligaments:
  1. *Anterior or anteroinferior tibiofibular ligament:* It originates from the anterior surface of the tibia, 5 mm proximal to the articular surface, passes inferiorly and laterally, and inserts over the lateral malleolus on its anterior margin. Occasionally, a thickened accessory slip of the anteroinferior tibiofibular ligament (Bassett's ligament) may insert too distally on the fibula, causing symptoms as it impinges against the anterolateral aspect of the talar dome.
  2. *Posterior or posteroinferior tibiofibular ligament:* The posteroinferior tibiofibular ligament is the strongest syndesmotic ligament in the ankle joint.

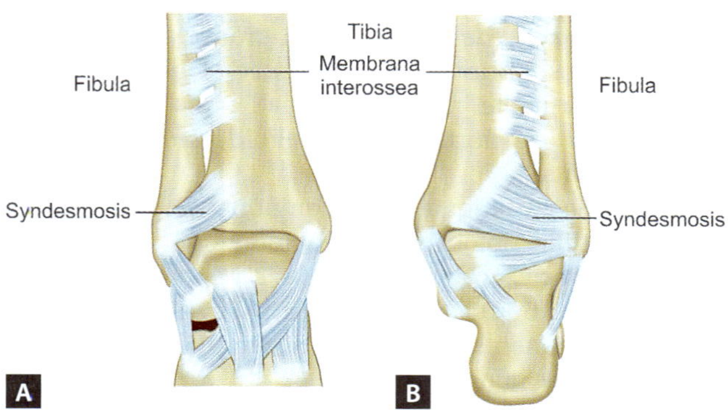

Figs. 4A and B: Syndesmotic ligaments of ankle. (A) Anterior view; (B) Posterior view.

  3. *Inferior transverse fibular ligament (also called transverse tibiofibular ligament):* This ligament originates on the posterior aspect of the fibula and extends to the posterior margin of the medial malleolus. In between, it forms the posterior labrum, which effectively deepens the tibiotalar joint.
  4. *Interosseous tibiofibular ligament:* The interosseous tibiofibular ligament continues as the interosseous membrane proximally and is attached to the contiguous rough surfaces of the tibia and fibula.

FOOT

The foot is a complex and flexible structure of 26 bones and 33 joints, layered with an intertwining web of >120 muscles, ligaments, and nerves. The foot supports body weight and helps in walking and running. It is organized in the form of arches that enable it to adapt to uneven surfaces. It also serves shock absorber in jumping.

Bones of the Foot (Fig. 5)

The bones of the foot are:

- The tarsal bones
- The metatarsals
- The phalanges

The foot is divided for descriptive purposes into hindfoot (talus and calcaneus), midfoot, and forefoot (metatarsals and phalanges).

Hindfoot

Talus as relevant to hindfoot:

- The neck of the talus deviates medially by about 15–20° and has multiple vascular foramina making it more susceptible to fracture than the body of the talus.
- The head of the talus articulate with the navicular anteriorly. The inferior side of the talus articulates with the posterior facet of the calcaneus. The lateral process of the talus is a large, broad-based, wedge-shaped prominence of the talar body that articulates:
  - Dorsolaterally with the fibula
  - Inferomedially with the anterior portion of the posterior facet of the calcaneus
- In the inferior surface of the talar head lies the spring ligament and the medial aspect of the talar body lies the deltoid ligament, the area of attachment of the deltoid ligament is wide extending from the body of talus to the medial aspect of the neck. The tip of the lateral process gives attachment to the talocalcaneal ligament.
- On the posterior surface of talus lie two tubercles medial and lateral, which are separated by a groove. The posterior process of talus is derived from these two tubercles. The medial tubercle is larger than the lateral. The tendon of flexor halluces longus passes through the groove. The posterior talofibular ligament is attached to the lateral tubercle. The posterior third of the deltoid ligament is attached to the medial tubercle.

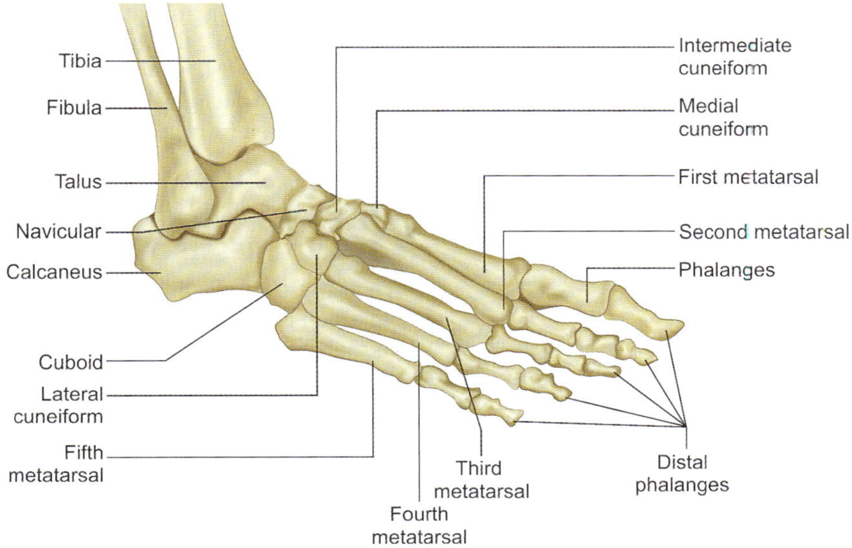

Fig. 5: Foot bony anatomy.

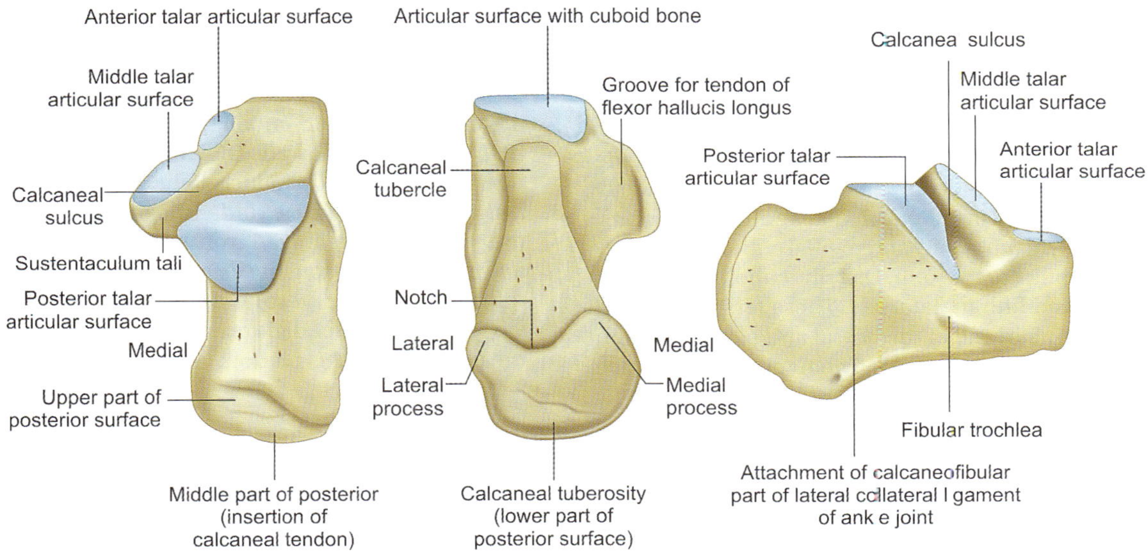

Fig. 6: The bony anatomy and landmarks of calcaneum as seen from above (left), lateral (right), and inferior aspect (center).

Calcaneus (Fig. 6)

- The superior surface has three articular facets (the anterior, middle, and posterior) that articulate with the talus. The posterior facet is the major weight-bearing surface and the largest facet.
- The middle facet is often contiguous with the anterior facet. The sustentaculum sits under the talar neck and is medial to the calcaneal body.
- It is attached to the talus by the interosseous talocalcaneal ligament and by the deltoid ligament medially. The flexor hallucis longus tendon runs below sustentaculum. Laterally, the peroneal tendons run obliquely along the lateral wall of the calcaneus and sit in two shallow groves, with a bony prominence between them known as the peroneal tubercle.
- The entire calcaneal surface behind the posterior facet is the posterior tuberosity. On its plantar surface, there are two processes: (1) the lateral and (2) the medial. The lateral process is the origin of the abductor digiti quinti (minimi) muscle. The medial process is weight bearing and is the origin for abductor alluces muscle and plantar fascia. The Achilles tendon inserts on the posterior surface of the tuberosity.

Midfoot

Five bones comprise the midfoot, the navicular, cuboid and medial, middle, and lateral cuneiforms. The stability imparted to the midfoot is due to the tight bonding of the midfoot structures by the strong and dense plantar ligaments, also a strong mechanical linkage is made between the hindfoot and the medial forefoot by these ligaments. The normal arch shape of the weight-bearing foot can be maintained without the need for muscle action. The tibialis posterior has multiple insertions on the plantar surface of the midfoot bones intertwined with the plantar ligamentous structures which provide dynamic support and mechanical overload protection. The medial arch provides a protective conduit. The midfoot is also responsible for the weight-bearing relationship of the hindfoot to the forefoot.

Navicular

It is the keystone of the medial longitudinal arch of the foot. It is wider dorsally and medially. The medial prominence, known as the "navicular tuberosity", provides the interim attachment point for the tibialis posterior on its medial inferior surface. The talonavicular joint is the point at which inversion and eversion of forefoot takes place. It also transmits the motion of the subtalar joint to the forefoot. Distally, navicular articulates with the three cuneiforms through the broad facets. There is little motion at naviculocuneiform joints as thick plantar and dorsal ligaments support this joint. Also a strong medial support is imparted by the spring and the superficial deltoid ligament to the talonavicular joint.

Cuboid

It is considered as a part of the lateral support column of the foot. Calcaneocuboid joint compensates for the imperfectly matched movements of the talonavicular and subtalar joints. The dorsal calcaneal tuberosity and medial cuboid tuberosity provide bony stability to the joint. Distally, cuboid articulates with the fourth and fifth metatarsals. These tarsometatarsal joints provide for nearly all of the dorsal and plantar motion of the lateral column of the foot. The overall importance of the cuboid in the function of the foot lies primarily in its structural position as a lateral column spacer, secondarily, in the function of the fourth and fifth tarsometatarsal joints and thirdly in calcaneocuboid joint motion.

Three Cuneiform Bones

The three cuneiforms make the medial longitudinal arch rigid. The apex of the transverse arch lies at the cuneiforms and also they provide a stable conduit for the plantar musculotendinous and neurovascular structures. Each cuneiform articulates with approximately one-third of the distal navicular and with its respective metatarsal distally. Numerous ligaments attachments between these three cuneiforms stabilize the joints and the arches. Between each of the two cuneiform pairs, there are three distinct connecting ligaments. There are no ligamentous connections between the first and second metatarsal to stabilize the first ray and dissipate any rotatory forces (causing lisfranc injuries). Stress across the first metatarsal is hence resisted only by the strength of the medial cuneiform attachments.

The foot has two important functions: (1) to support the body weight and (2) to serve as a lever to propel the body forward in walking and running. As the lever is segmented with multiple joints, the foot is pliable and can adapt itself to uneven surfaces. Moreover, the foot is organized in the form of arches that transmit the forces along columns so that the foot is protected from getting fatigued easily or losing its lever functions.

TENDONS AND NEUROVASCULAR STRUCTURES AROUND ANKLE

Five nerves (sural, tibial, nerve accompanying saphenous vein, deep peroneal nerve, and superficial peroneal nerve), two major arteries, and veins (anterior and posterior tibial) and 13 tendons cross the ankle joint. The tendons can be divided into four groups:

1. *The posterior group:* Achilles and plantaris tendons. The Achilles is the strongest tendon in the body and most powerful plantar flexor of the ankle. Plantaris is a weak plantar flexor of ankle and is a vestigial structure. It may or may not be present in all the subjects; it can be, however, used to supplement tendon or ligament repairs.
2. *The medial group* ***(Fig. 7)****:* The laciniate ligament attaches from medial malleolus to the calcaneus gives several septa and covers the flexor tendons. From anterior to posterior, the structures organized in the tarsal tunnel are the tibialis posterior tendon, the flexor digitorum longus (fDL) tendon, the posterior tibial artery and vein, the tibial nerve, and the flexor hallucis longus (fHL) tendon.
3. *Anterior group* ***(Fig. 8)****:* Under the extensor retinaculum, the structures organized from medial to lateral are the anterior tibial tendon, the extensor hallucis longus (EHL) tendon, the deep peroneal nerve and anterior tibial vessels, the extensor digitrorum longus (EDL) tendon, and the peroneus tertius tendon.

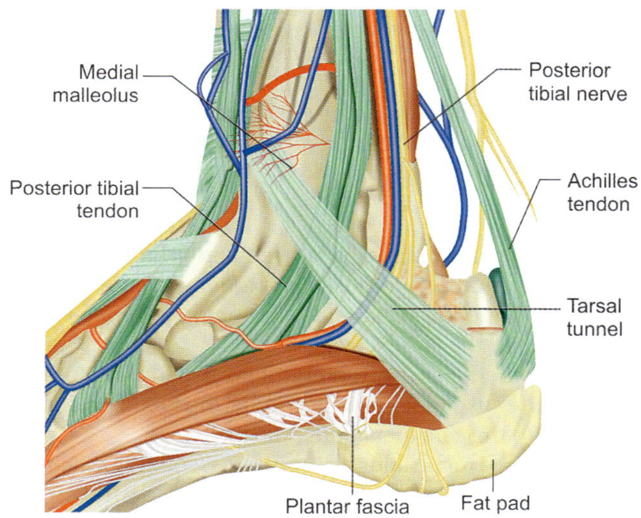

Fig. 7: The medial aspect of ankle demonstrating the disposition of tarsal tunnel and structures passing through it.

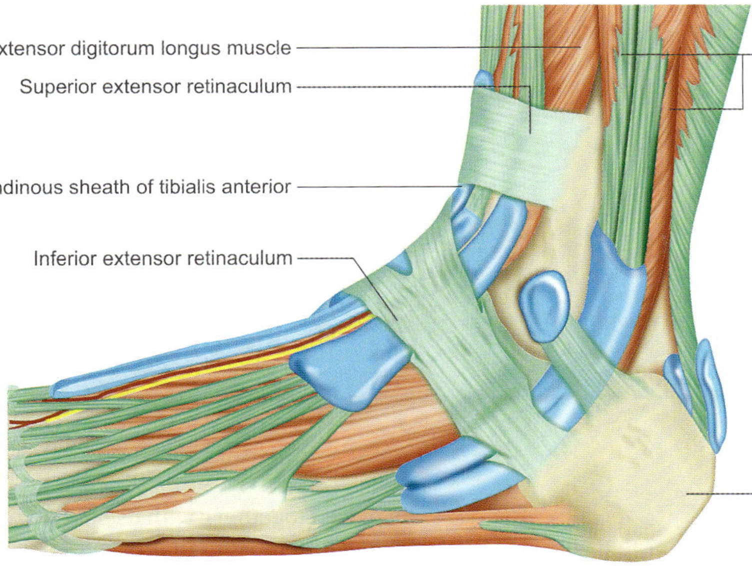

Fig. 8: The anterior aspect of ankle and structures passing under extensor retinaculum.

4. *Lateral group:* The tendons of peroneus longus tendon and peroneus brevis.

CONCLUSION

- The advances in arthroplasty and arthroscopy of foot and ankle region entail more detailed understanding of the anatomy.
- The proper understanding and preoperative assessment of the landmarks help in smooth execution of the surgical procedure.
- Specific disposition of the bones of foot makes possible the arrangement into arches and tripod action of the foot to provide stability in standing and walking.

CHAPTER 80

Arches of the Foot

Manish Kumar Varshney

INTRODUCTION

The foot as a segmented structure is capable of bearing weight, as it is in the form of arch. The foot has three arches maintained by the bony anatomy, muscular activity, and the ligaments. They are present at birth.

1. *Medial longitudinal arch* **(Fig. 1A)**: The medial margin of the foot, from the heel to the first metatarsal head, is arched above the ground because of the important medial longitudinal arch. This part is missing from the wet footprints as it is too tall and does not normally touches the floor.
2. *Lateral longitudinal arch* **(Fig. 1A)**: This is formed by the lateral margin of foot to the lateral two toes and bears most of the weight during ambulation. The pressure exerted on the ground by the lateral margin of the foot is greatest at the heel and the fifth metatarsal head and least between these areas.
3. *Transverse arch* **(Fig. 1B)**: The transverse arch involves the bases of the five metatarsals and the cuboid and cuneiform bones. This is, in fact, only half an arch (the other half being provided by the other foot; when both feet are placed together), with its base on the lateral border of the foot and its summit on the foot's medial border.

BONES OF THE ARCHES

Medial longitudinal arch: The medial half of calcaneum, whole talus, the navicular bone, the three cuneiform bones and the first three metatarsal bones.

Lateral longitudinal arch: This consists of the lateral half of calcaneum, the cuboid and the fourth and fifth metatarsal bones.

Transverse arch: This consists of the bases of the metatarsal bones, the cuboid, and the three cuneiform bones.

MECHANISMS OF THE ARCH SUPPORT (MASONRY CONCEPT)

- *The shape of the stones:* The stones are wedge-shaped, with the thin edge of the wedge lying inferiorly preventing it from slipping. This applies particularly to the important stone that occupies the center of the arch and is referred to as the "keystone" **(Fig. 2)**.

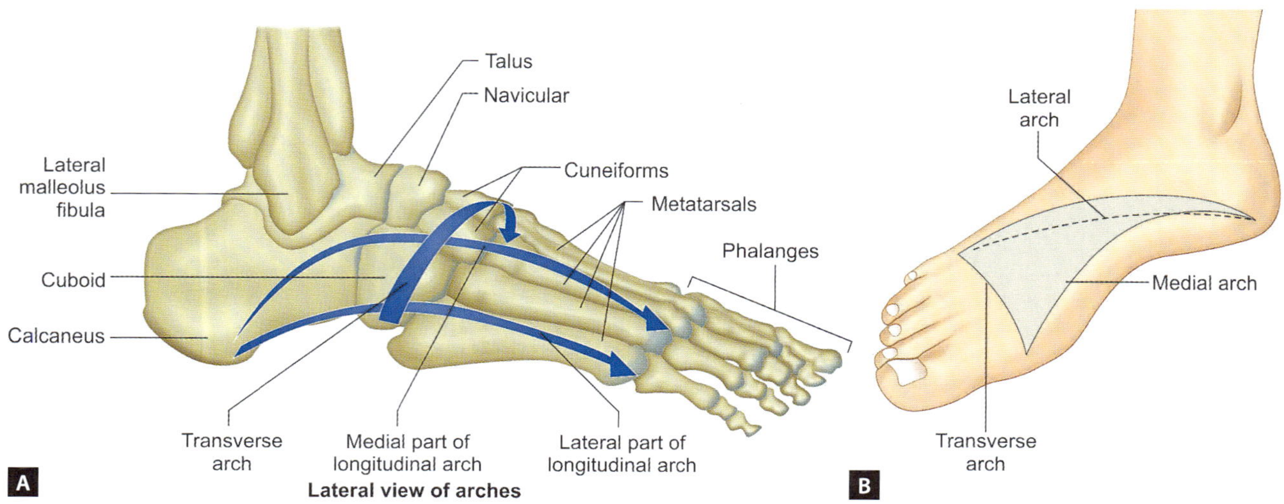

Figs. 1A and B: Arches of foot. (A) The disposition of arches in the foot; (B) Illustration showing how the arches support foot as a spring sheet.

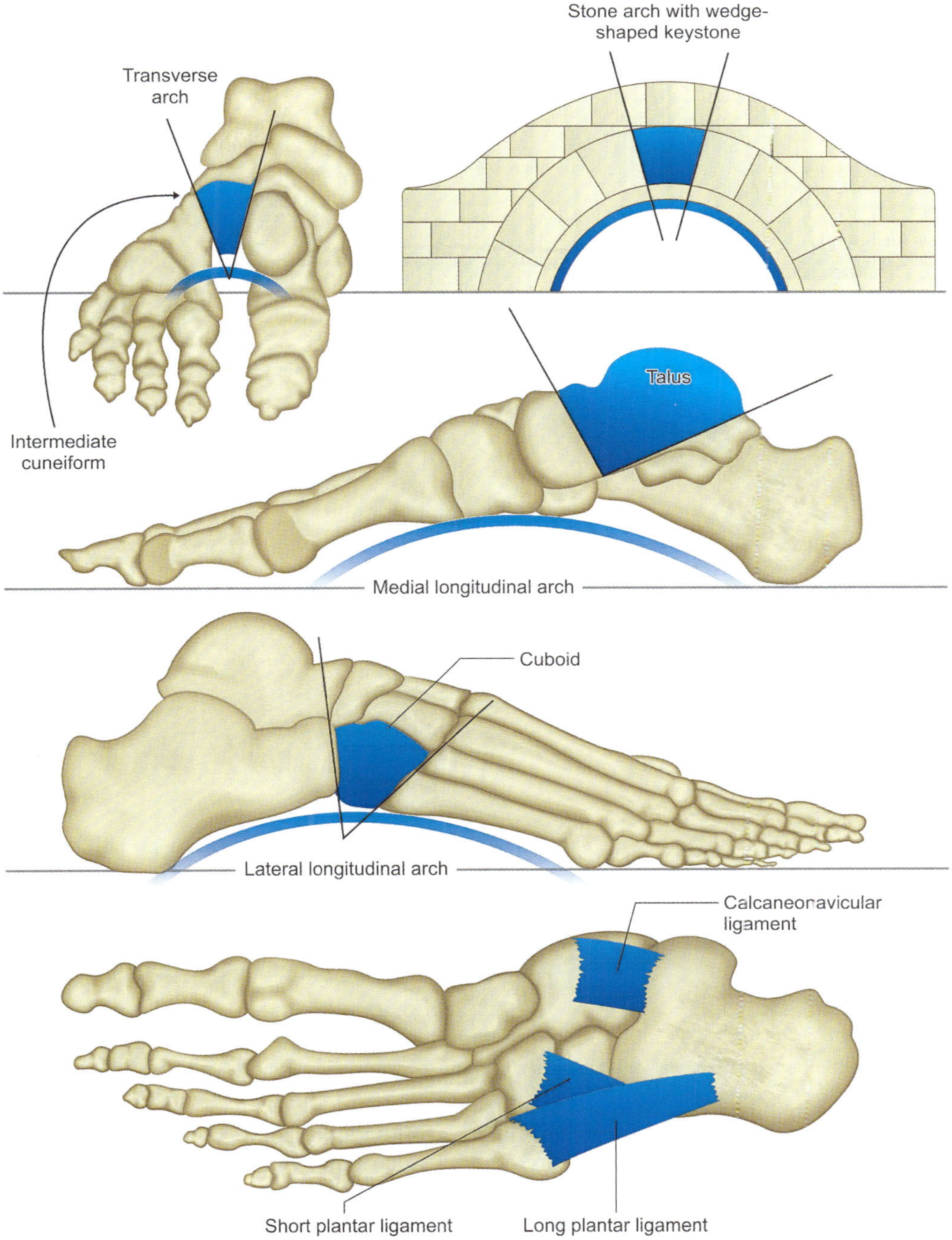

Fig. 2: Keystone bones of various arches and "cementing" of the stones by the ligaments.

- *Cementing the stones:* This is accomplished by interlocking the stones (bones) or binding their lower edges together with strong cords (ligaments). This method binds the lower edges of the stones together, when the arch is weight-bearing.
- *The use of the tie beams* ***(Fig. 3A)****:* These connect the distant pillars of long arches by preventing their separation. This is especially useful when the foundations at either end are shallow or base insecure, a tie beam effectively prevents sagging of the arch in such cases.
- *Suspension mechanism* ***(Fig. 3B)****:* The structure of the arch is maintained by suspension cables from above to prevent from sagging or collapsing.

MAINTENANCE OF THE MEDIAL LONGITUDINAL ARCH (FIGS. 4A AND B)

- *Shape of the bones:* The rounded head of the talus is the keystone in the center of the arch. The sustentaculum tali holds up the talus, the concave proximal surface of the navicular bone receives the rounded head of the

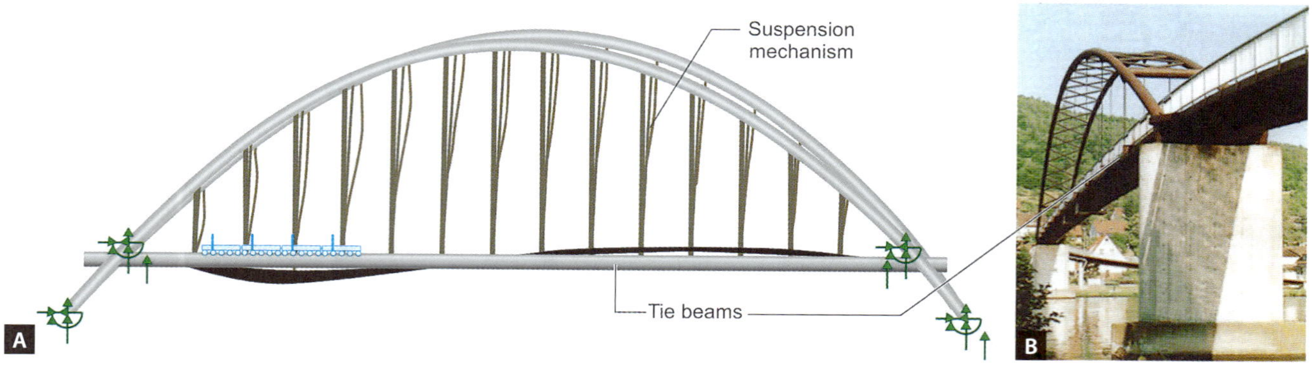

Figs. 3A and B: (A) Role of tie beams and suspension in maintaining the arches (B) as they suspend the bridges.

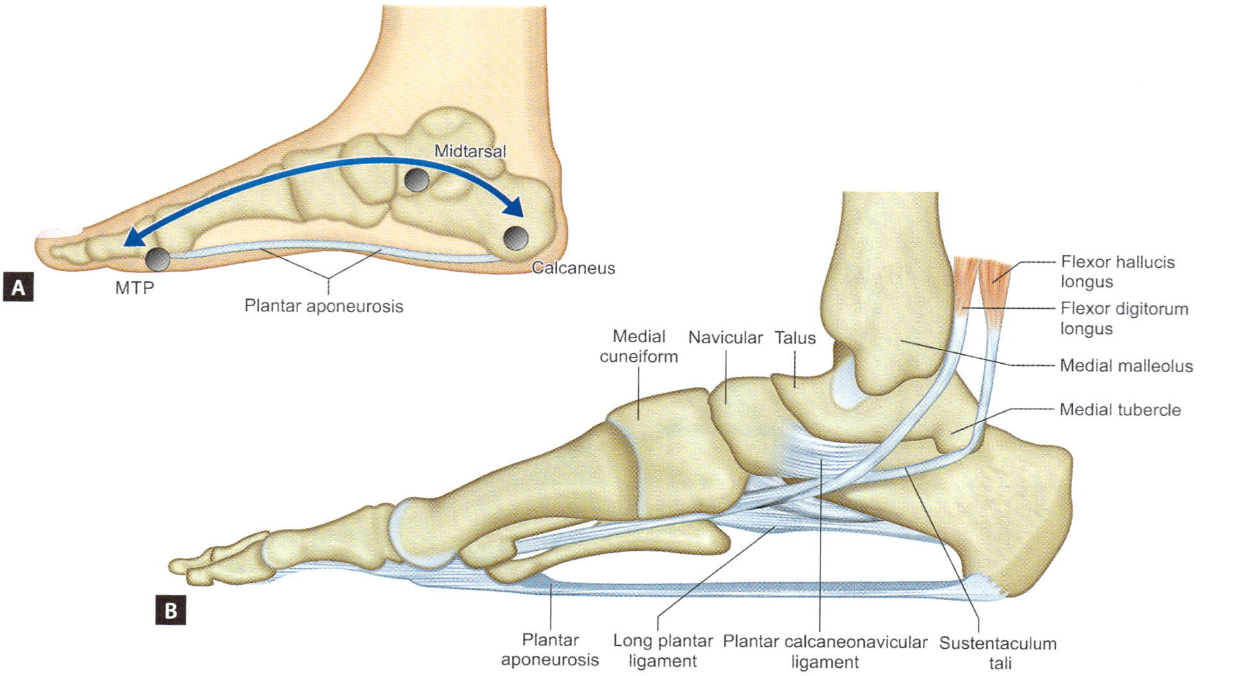

Figs. 4A and B: (A) The components of medial longitudinal arch; (B) The structures supporting it (see text). (MTP: metatarsophalangeal)

talus and it itself fits into the proximal surface of the medial cuneiform bone. The medial longitudinal arch is supported by the spring ligament, which shoulders the head of the talus.

- *Interosseous ties (cement and staples):* The inferior edges of the bones are tied together by the plantar ligaments, which are larger and stronger than the dorsal ligaments. The most important ligament is the plantar calcaneonavicular ligament. The tendinous extensions of the insertion of the tibialis posterior muscle also hold the small bones together.
- The tie beams for medial longitudinal arch are the plantar aponeurosis, the medial part of the flexor digitorum brevis, the abductor hallucis, the flexor hallucis longus, the medial part of the flexor digitorum longus, and the flexor hallucis brevis.
- *Arch suspension:* Suspending the arch from above are the tibialis anterior and posterior and the medial ligaments of the ankle joint. Though previously considered very important structure for static maintenance of the arches; the tibialis anterior, the peroneus longus, and the small muscles of the foot have been now found to play no important role in the normal static support of the arches. They provide support only while walking and running.

MAINTENANCE OF THE LATERAL LONGITUDINAL ARCH (FIG. 5)

- *Shape of the bones:* The cuboid is the keystone.
- The inferior edges of the bones are tied together by the long and short plantar ligaments and the origins of the short muscles from the forepart of the foot.
- *Tie beams:* The plantar aponeurosis, the abductor digiti minimi, and the lateral part of the flexor digitorum longus and brevis.
- *Arch suspension:* The peroneus longus and the brevis.

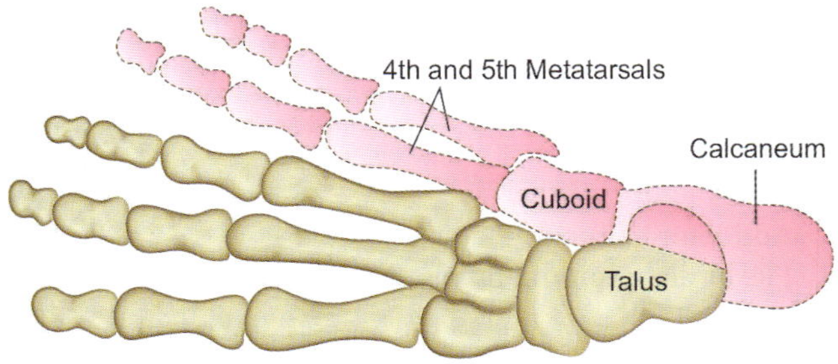

Fig. 5: The bony components of lateral longitudinal arch.

MAINTENANCE OF THE TRANSVERSE ARCH

- *Shape of the bones:* The marked wedge shaping of the cuneiform bones and the bases of the metatarsal bones.
- The inferior edges of the bones are tied together by the deep transverse ligaments, the strong plantar ligaments and the origins of the plantar muscles from the forepart of the foot, the dorsal interrossei and the transverse head of the adductor hallucis are particularly important in this respect.
- *Tie beam:* The peroneus longus tendon.
- *Arch suspension:* The peroneus longus tendon and the peroneus brevis.

PROPULSIVE ACTION OF THE FOOT

- The bodyweight in foot is distributed through the heel posteriorly and the heads of the metatarsal bones anteriorly (including the two sesamoid bones under the head of the first metatarsal).
- While walking, as the bodyweight is thrown forward, the weight is born successively on the lateral margin of the foot and the heads of the metatarsal bones—the Tripod concept (*see* Chapter on "Biomechanics of the Foot and Ankle Joint and Related Examination").
- As the heel rises, the toes are extended at the metatarsophalangeal joints and the plantar aponeurosis is pulled on thus shortening the tie beams and heightening the longitudinal arches (Windlass mechanism, **Fig. 6**). The energy is hence stored in the form of potential energy in arches (energy of deformation). The slack in the long flexor tendons is taken up, thereby increasing their efficiency.
- The body is then thrown forward by the actions of the gastrocnemius and soleus (and plantaris) on the ankle joint, using the foot as a lever and converting the energy of deformation stored in arches into kinetic energy. The toes are strongly flexed by the long and short flexors of the foot providing the final thrust forward (the push off).
- The lumbricals and interossei contract and keep the toes extended, so that they do not fold under because of the strong action of the flexor digitorum longus. In this action, the long flexor tendons also assist in plantar flexing the ankle joint.
- In running, the weight is borne on the forefoot and heel does not touch the ground. The forward thrust to the body is provided by the mechanisms described for walking (discussed above).

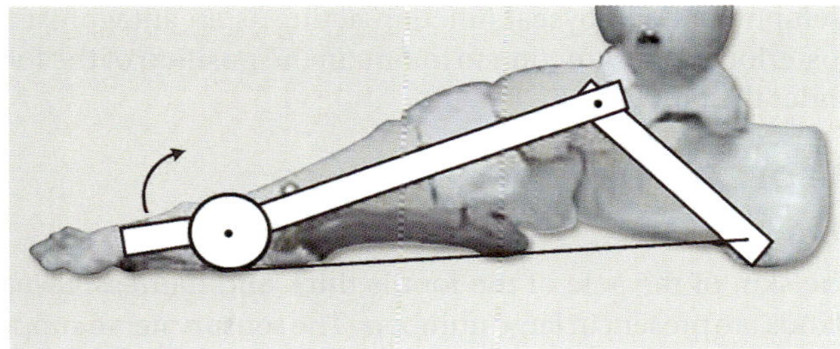

Fig. 6: Windlass mechanism—as the toes dorsiflex, the drum (metatarsophalangeal joints) rotates clockwise pulling the tie rod (plantar fascia) increasing tension in the same. This effectively supports the arch and raises its height.

FOREFOOT

It provides a broad plantar surface for load sharing. The two sesamoids and the four lesser metatarsal heads share an equal amount of the forefoot load in normal gait. Being mobile in sagittal plane also it has the ability to alter position and maintain a relatively even pressure distribution on the plantar skin, protecting it from local injury.

First Metatarsal

It is shorter and wider than that of the lesser four metatarsals. The lack of interconnecting ligaments between the first and second metatarsal bones allows independent motion, but makes it susceptible to dislocations. Strong and thick ligaments that make up the capsule of the first tarsometatarsal joint support its resting position. The anterior tibialis inserts on the plantar medial aspect of the first metatarsal base, it elevates the first metatarsal. The peroneus longus attaches onto the plantar lateral base of the first metatarsal, it plantarflexes the head. These two muscles exert significant influence on the position of the first metatarsal head. The first metatarsal head supports two sesamoid bones that provide two of the six contact points of the forefoot. By these mechanisms the first ray supports 33% of bodyweight at any time.

Central Metatarsals

Each of the four metatarsals provide one contact point on the plantar weight-bearing surface. The central three have only intrinsic muscular attachments; no extrinsic muscle gets attachment here. The main function of central metatarsals is in providing structural support to the arches. The dorsal and plantar interossei take origin from them. The distal plantar surface of these bones provides attachment to transverse metatarsal ligaments; these ligaments are thick and connect indirectly the metatarsals by linking the adjacent metatarsophalangeal joint plates. The middle metatarsals impart enhanced mobility in the sagittal plane which help in adapting the shape of the foot while moving on uneven terrain.

Fifth Metatarsal

The peroneus brevis attaches on the dorsal aspect of the tubercle of the fifth metatarsal counteracting the natural inversion tendency of the tibialis anterior. The peroneus tertius attaches on the dorsal aspect at the proximal metaphyseal diaphyseal junction acting as an antagonist to posterior tibialis function to maintain the position of the foot under the talus.

SOLE OF THE FOOT

Skin

The skin of the sole of the foot is thick and hairless. Sweat glands are present in large numbers. The sensory nerve supply to the skin of the sole of the foot is derived from the medial calcaneal branch of the tibial nerve, which innervates the medial side of the heel, branches from the medial plantar nerve, which innervate the medial two-thirds of the sole and branches from the lateral plantar nerve, which innervate the lateral third of the sole.

Plantar Aponeurosis

The plantar aponeurosis is a thickened and triangular connective tissue forming the deep fascia of the sole of the foot which supports the arches of the foot from the plantar side of the foot by acting as a tie rod. It serves to protect the underlying nerves, vessels, and muscles. It spans from the medial calcaneal tubercle to the proximal phalanges of the toes. Its apex is attached to the medial and lateral tubercles of the calcaneum; the distal base of the aponeurosis divides into five slips that pass into the toes. The collagen bundles are oriented longitudinally and the thickest and the strongest part is the central portion of the aponeurosis.

Muscles of the Sole of the Foot

The muscles of the sole are described in four layers. The sole muscles are chiefly concerned with supporting the arches of the foot.

First Layer

- Abductor hallucis
- Flexor digitorum brevis
- Abductor digiti minimi.

Second Layer

- Quadratus plantae
- Lumbricals
- Flexor digitorum longus tendon
- Flexor hallucis longus tendon.

Third Layer

- Flexor hallucis brevis
- Adductor hallucis
- Flexor digiti minimi brevis.

Fourth Layer

- Interossei
- Peroneus longus tendon
- Tibialis posterior tendon.

An aid to remember muscles is by understanding the mnemonic (though I am never fond of them) "three muscles in layer one and three and four muscles in layers two and four". For layer one it is "1Abs Flex 5Abs" (the numerical denote the digit on which the muscle acts), and for layer three it is "1Flex Add 5Flex".

The vascular supply of the sole of foot comes from medial and lateral plantar artery with accompanying veins and dorsalis pedis artery.

Compartments of the Foot (Table 1)

There are following separate compartments of the foot:

- The medial compartment of foot lies medial and plantar to the first metatarsal. It contains two muscles the abductor hallucis and flexor hallucis brevis.
- The lateral compartment lies inferolaterally to the fifth metatarsal and contains the abductor digiti minimi and flexor digiti minimi brevis muscles.
- The central compartment is divided into superficial and deep portions:
    - The superficial portion contains the flexor digitorum longus and brevis muscle.
    - The deep or calcaneal compartment contains the quadratus plantae muscle.
- Dorsally, between each of metatarsals lie the dorsal and plantar interosseous muscles, which appear to lie in a separate compartment defined by each intermetatarsal space.

TABLE 1: Compartments of the foot.

Compartment	*Location*	*Boundaries*	*Contents*
Medial	Entire length of foot	Fascia, abductor hallucis, medial and lateral intermuscular septum	Abductor hallucis, flexor halluces brevis
Superficial (central)	Entire length of foot	Plantar aponeurosis, medial, and lateral intermuscular septum	Flexor digitorum brevis, flexor digitorum longus tendon, 4 lumbricals
Adductor	Entire length of foot	Horizontal septum	Adductor hallucis
Interossei (4 in total)	Forefoot	Abductor compartment, metatarsals, fascia (plantarly)	Interossei
Lateral	Forefoot	Abductor digiti quinti, medial and lateral intermuscular septum	Abductor digit quinti, flexor digiti minimi brevis
Calcaneal	Rearfoot; communicates with deep posterior compartment of leg	Medial and lateral intermuscular septum, calcaneus, talus, fascial extensions	Quadratus plantae, posterior tibial and lateral plantar neurovascular bundles

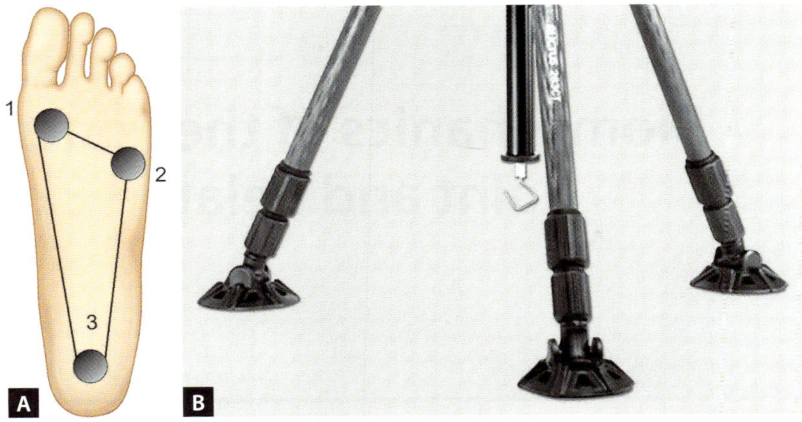

Figs. 7A and B: The tripod action of the foot. (A) Foot as a structure is itself stabilized by distributing pressure at the three points; (B) like a tripod.

- The oblique head of adductor hallucis lying on the plantar aspect of the forefoot distal and deep to the quadratus plantae has its own fascial compartment.

TRIPOD ACTION OF THE FOOT

To maintain perfect ground contact each foot acts as tripod, with legs of the tripod represented by the calcaneus and the heads of the first and fifth metatarsals **(Figs. 7A and B)**. The three points of contact during stance provide stability compared to a single point or two-point contact. The arches supplement this tripod contact acting as spring mechanisms to store and release energy during ambulation alternately. Reconstructions around the foot should aim at restoring this tripod structure for optimum outcome.

CONCLUSION

- The foot bears all the weight of human body. It should be strong enough to bear the weight on itself completely and effortlessly while also be resilient enough to allow locomotion.
- To serve both these purposes, the foot is divided into arches that bear the weight of body well allowing also spring like shock-absorption that stores and releases energy during locomotion making it more smooth.
- During reconstruction of the foot for various disorders, it is necessary to maintain this arched structure so that function of foot does not get lost and foot becomes painful.
- It is important to understand various structures and factors that maintain the unique foot structure to provide best clinical outcome.

CHAPTER 81

Biomechanics of the Foot and Ankle Joint and Related Examination

Manish Kumar Varshney

INTRODUCTION

The foot acts as a tripod that bears and distributes body weight collectively between the head of the first metatarsal, the heel, and the four lesser metatarsal heads during stance phase **(Fig. 1)**. Malalignment/malpositioning and alterations in biomechanics disrupt this crucial balance, resulting in various painful conditions. A cavus foot type (accentuated medial arch of foot), for example, would transmit excessive load under the first metatarsal head and lateral aspect of the foot. If there has dorsiflexion malunion of a metatarsal fracture then there develops increased risk for a painful callus under another metatarsal head. Similarly, distal foot deformity and malposition ultimately affect more proximal joints, as seen in patients with planovalgus foot deformities. The rotational forces created by the planovalgus foot may eventually result in attenuation of the deltoid ligament and valgus tilting of the talus. So, for any reconstruction or correction of deformity the tripod concept must be kept in mind.

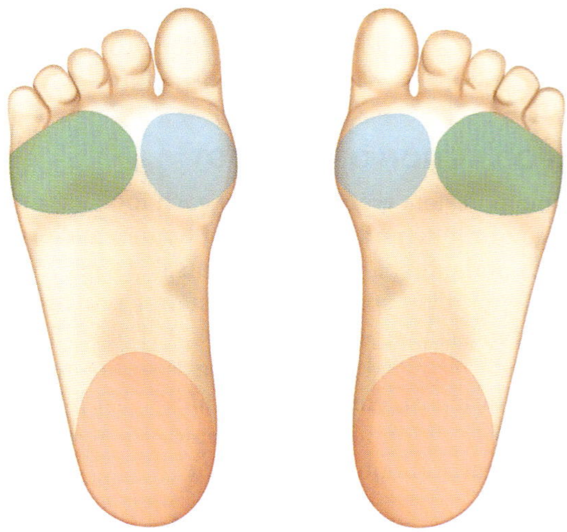

Fig. 1: The tripod concept of foot. There are three main areas of weight-bearing during stance phase (shown in different colors).

BIOMECHANICS OF ANKLE JOINT MOVEMENTS

- The ankle joint is a complex hinge. The main movements at the joint are plantar and dorsiflexion **(Figs. 2A to E)** and secondary movements are inversion/eversion and rotation.
- The ankle joint axis of rotation keeps on changing with ankle motion. Majority of the ankle motion takes place in the sagittal plane but there is subtle amount of motion taking place in the longitudinal and vertical axis. The plane of ankle plantar and dorsiflexion passes nearly 5 mm from the tip of medial malleolus distally and 3 mm distal and 8 mm anterior to the lateral malleolus **(Figs. 3A to C)**. The concept of a single axis may be helpful in understanding the basic biomechanics and simplifying the concepts. With dorsiflexion, the axis inclination is downward and laterally, whereas in plantar flexion the axis inclined downward and medially.
- The differential contouring of the talar head and trochlea may explain the changing axes of rotation; this is also responsible for mortise widening with dorsiflexion. There is approximately 1.5 mm increment in the intermalleolar distance during dorsiflexion of ankle because of external rotation of the fibula and lateral rotation of the talus as an attempt to match the wedge contour of the talus in the mortise.
- The deltoid ligament imparts rotational stability to talus in the ankle mortise and also maintains its closed pack configuration in the ankle mortise while dorsiflexion of ankle in the stance phase of gait cycle. Also the syndesmosis firmly binds the tibia to the fibula, preventing any additional movements.
- About five times the body weight is transmitted by the ankle joint while walking. Most of the stability of the joint is imparted by the articular congruity. The mortise view is taken with the patient's leg internally rotated approximately 15° so the beam of the X-ray is perpendicular to the transmalleolar axis **(Fig. 4A)**. The articular surface of the talus should be congruous with the distal tibia and the clear space between the talus and the medial malleolus, distal tibia, and lateral malleolus should be equal.
- The talocrural angle is the angle subtended by a line drawn parallel to the articular surfaces of the distal tibia and one connecting the tips of both malleoli. Normally, range of

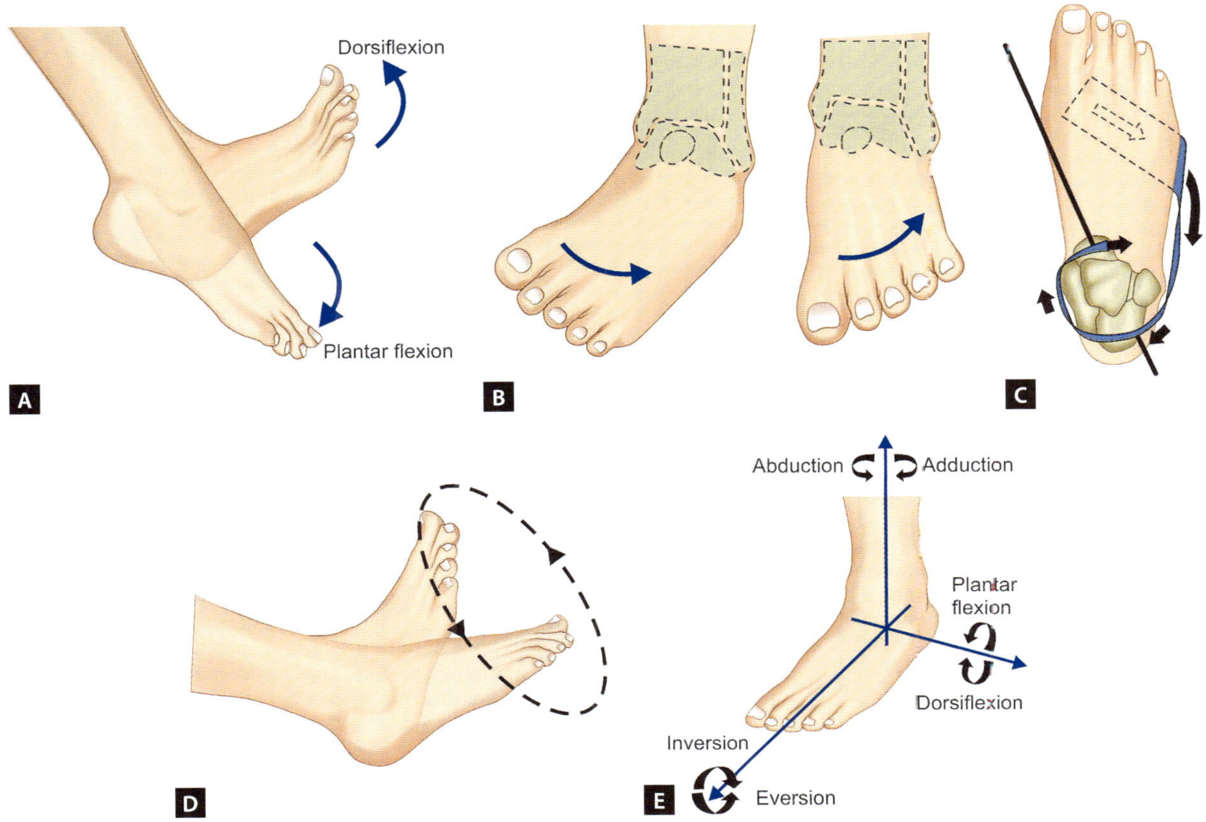

Figs. 2A to E: Various movements at the ankle joint. (A) Flexion-extension; (B) Inversion and eversion—predominantly at subtalar joint; (C) The combination supination and pronation involve ankle, external and internal rotation; (D) Circumduction; (E) Axes of various movements.

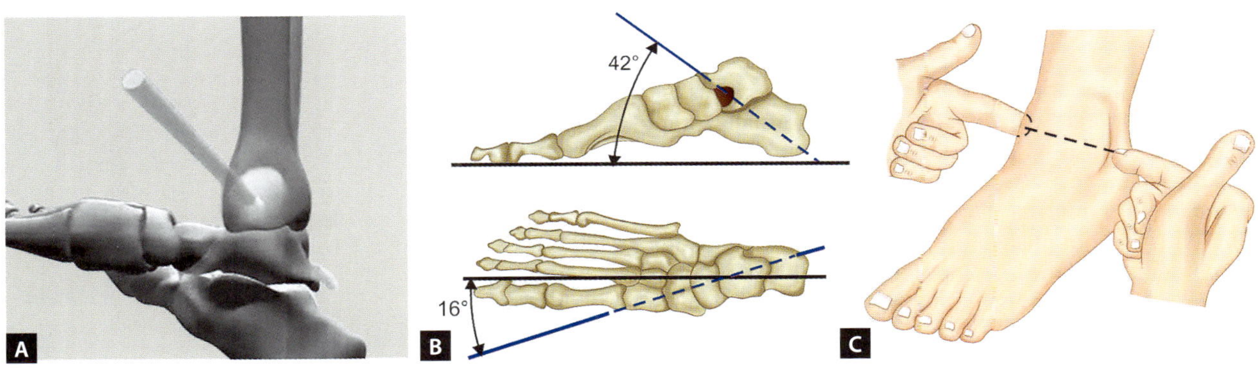

Figs. 3A to C: (A) Detail of axis for plantar and dorsiflexion at ankle joint; (B) Eversion-inversion at subtalar joint; (C) Method to locate the axis of ankle joint.

talocrural angle is from 83° ± 4°. It is used to judge the anatomical restoration of the ankle by comparing to other side. Fibular shortening is indicated by a difference >2–3°. Medial clear space is the distance between the lateral border of the medial malleolus and the medial border of the talus. It should be equal to the superior clear space between the talus and the distal tibia. A space >4 mm is considered abnormal and indicates a lateral shift of the talus.

- The radiological distance between the medial wall of the fibula and the incisural surface of the tibia, the tibiofibular clear space should be <6 mm **(Fig. 4B)**.

Ankle Joint Movements

Measure plantar flexion from zero position. This lies at right angles to the line of the leg. Normal range is 50–55°.

Dorsiflexion and plantar flexion: Normal range is 15–20°. If dorsiflexion is restricted, bend the knees. If this restores normal range, the Achilles tendon is tight due to gastrocnemius component. If it makes no difference, joint pathology (osteoarthritis, rheumatoid arthritis or infection) is the likely cause in an adult or both gastrocnemius and soleus are tight in children.

The axis of rotation of the tibiotalar joint comprises a series of instant centers of rotation. This results from translation of

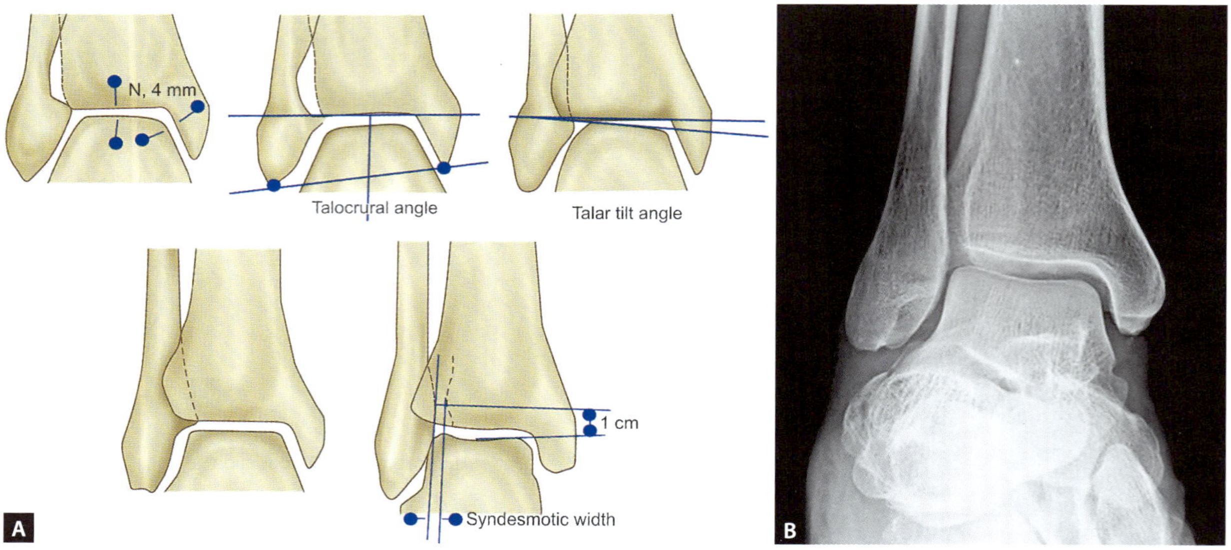

Figs. 4A and B: Various angle and measurements around ankle joint that help in deciding adequacy of reduction while doing open reduction internal fixation (ORIF) or other surgical bony/joint procedures (A). A good mortise view (B) showing symmetrical reduction of the ankle mortise is essential. Anatomical reduction of the fibular fracture and restoration of fibular length should be confirmed. The stability of the syndesmosis can be tested directly once the fibular fracture has been fixed. This can be done using a small bone hook or a Hohmann retractor which is inserted into the syndesmosis and rotated. Any instability is readily appreciated. The medial mortise width should be <4 mm. The talocrural angle, talar tilt angle and width of the syndesmosis 1 cm above the joint can be compared to that of the opposite limb. The posterior edge of the tibia (reverse Tillaux fragment) should overlap the fibula by 6 mm.

talus in the horizontal plane with dorsiflexion and plantar flexion. But for descriptive purposes, the axis is represented by a single line drawn horizontally through the distal aspects of both malleoli (see above). This axis lies in 20–30° of external rotation with respect to the coronal plane and is tilted down laterally (oblique laterally) at 82° instead of being perpendicular to axis of the tibia. With the foot free and the leg in a fixed position, the oblique ankle joint axis causes the foot to externally rotate with dorsiflexion and internally rotate with plantar flexion **(Fig. 5)**. But in more practical instance like walking when the foot is fixed to the floor, the oblique axis forces the leg into internal rotation as the body passes over the foot. With the foot push-off, ankle plantar flexion results in external rotation of the leg. Rotation of the tibia is coupled with the inversion and eversion motion of the subtalar joint.

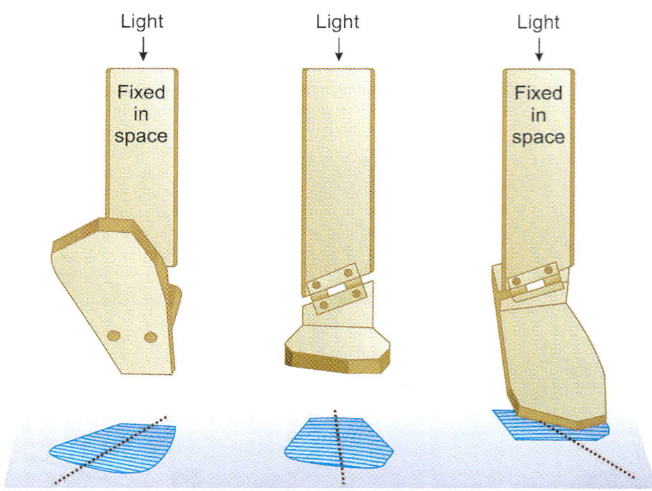

Fig. 5: The oblique ankle joint axis causes outward rotation of foot with dorsiflexion and inward rotation with plantar flexion, if not fixed to ground.

Movements of Foot (Figs. 6A to C)

- In the X-axis, nearly all movements occur in the ankle.
- In the Z-axis, supination and pronation occur mostly due to inversion and eversion at the subtalar joints.
- In the Y-axis, a very limited range of abduction and adduction occurs mostly at the midtarsal joints.

Subtalar Joints Movements

- The subtalar joint involves two pairs of highly complex articular surfaces. The axis of movement is relatively fixed passing through the center of the head of the talus in front and through the posterolateral tubercle of the calcaneus behind.
- The complex pattern of calcaneal movements that occurs in inversion is sometimes compared with three plane movements of ships or aircrafts: the calcaneus pitches and yaws (turns) under the talus.

Inversion and Eversion

Inversion of the heel occurs when the calcaneus tilts into varus at the subtalar joint. With the heel tilt, the foot is carried with it and forms a part of supination of foot. Eversion is the mirrored opposite movement (valgus tilting of the heel resulting in pronation of the foot).

Heel varus and valgus are a combination of two different movements. Heel varus is a combination of inversion and

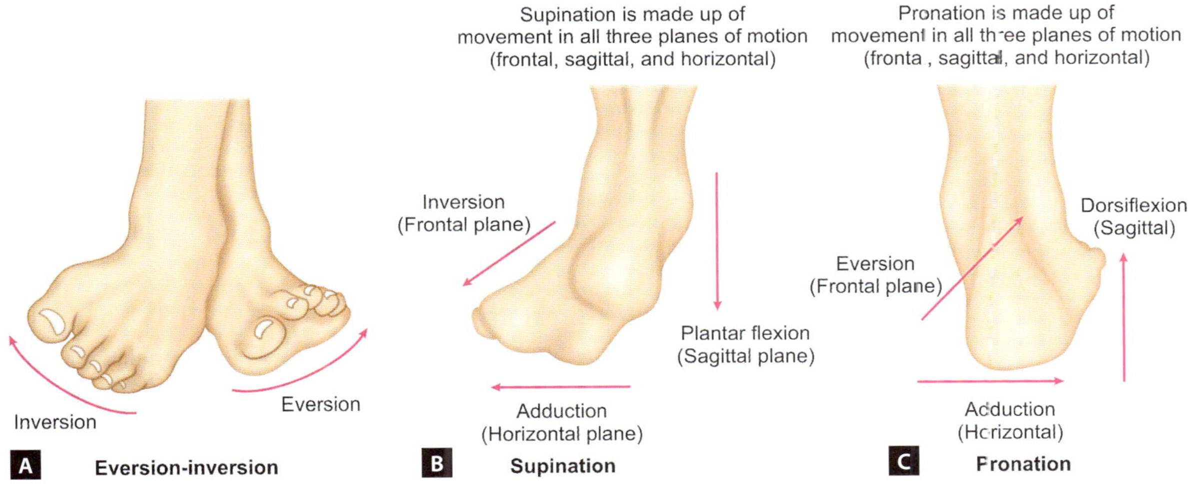

Figs. 6A to C: The movements of foot. (A) Illustration depicts the eversion-inversion movement of foot at subtalar joint; (B and C) Supination and pronation are compound movements occurring simultaneously at various joints combining different movements.

adduction of calcaneum while heel valgus is a combination of eversion and abduction movements of the calcaneum.

Midtarsal Joint

The joint has in effect two axes of movement. First, it acts as a hinge, allowing slight dorsiflexion and plantar flexion (like the ankle). The axis of this hinge passes the center of the head of the talus, so that this movement is coordinated with subtalar movement. The plane of this axis is tilted at 45° relative to the horizontal. The transverse, sagittal, and longitudinal planes of motion at midtarsal joint are explained better by understanding the "acetabulum pedis" concept **(Fig. 7)**. The midfoot is separated from the hindfoot by the talonavicular and calcaneocuboid joints (transverse tarsal joint or Chopart joint). The talonavicular joint is a ball-and-socket-type joint. The head of talus is larger than navicular and also articulates with calcaneum. The socket (acetabulum) for the talar head (similar to femoral head) is thus deepened by the anterior and middle facets of the calcaneus, the calcaneonavicular slip of the bifurcate ligament, and the superomedial and inferior calcaneal navicular ligaments (spring ligament). The superomedial component of the spring ligament serves to suspend the head of the talus, functioning like an anatomic hammock. Movements at talonavicular or subtalar joint thus also involves motion at the calcaneocuboid joint due to close linkage.

In addition, a limited amount of pronation and supination. The navicular slides and rotates around the head of talus and the cuboid slides on the calcaneus. This axis of rotation also passes through the center of the head of the talus.

Tarsometatarsal Movements

The tarsometatarsal junction is called the "Lisfranc joint" that separates forefoot from midfoot. Elevation and depression of the first metatarsal head and of the other (particularly the fourth and fifth) can contribute to overall supination of the foot.

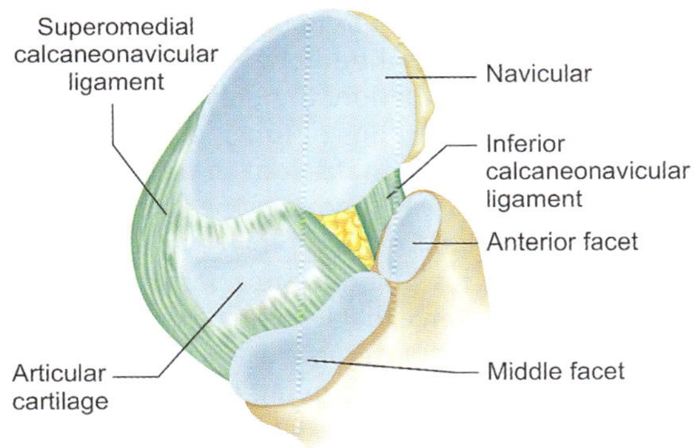

Fig. 7: The acetabulum pedis concept. The illustration depicts socket (acetabulum) for talar head (removed).

The examination of all these movements should be discretely performed as follows:

- *Supination:* Ask the patient to turn the soles of the feet toward one another. The patellae should be vertical. Normal range is approximately 35°.
- *Pronation:* Ask the patient to turn the feet outward. Normal range is approximately 20°. If supination and pronation are restricted, fix the heel with one hand and with the other, assist the patient to repeat the movements. No further reduction in the range indicates a stiff subtalar joint.
- *Eversion:* In prone position with the feet over the edge of the couch. Evert the heel and note the presence of movement in the subtalar joint by position of the heel. Normal range is approximately 10°.
- *Inversion:* Repeat the above procedure, forcing the heel into inversion. Normal range is approximately 20°. Loss of movement indicates a stiff subtalar joint (e.g., old calcaneal fracture, rheumatoid or osteoarthritis and spastic flat foot).
- Test for mobility in the first, fourth, and fifth metatarsal joints, by steadying the heel with one hand and attempting

to move the metatarsal heads individually in a dorsal and plantar direction.

Motion of the subtalar joint and transverse tarsal joint (also called the triple joint complex) are intricately linked. The talonavicular joint plays a key role in this compound movement. If talonavicular joint is fused (as in triple arthrodesis), movements through the remaining joints of the triple joint complex is virtually cease. The dynamic and static soft-tissue stabilizers act in concert to effect the smooth movements. At heel strike, the tibialis anterior eccentrically contracts to control foot descent, dissipating the acutely applied forces and prevent slapping of the foot against the ground. The tibialis posterior produces hindfoot inversion during push-off across the transverse tarsal joint. The tibialis posterior also adducts the navicular over the head of the talus, helping to invert the calcaneus, which follows the cuboid. This adduction-inversion enables an efficient heel rise. The triceps surae additionally helps by pulling the Achilles tendon making it the strongest hindfoot inverter at heel rise. This ensures the midfoot will remain locked for toe-off. The clinical scenario becomes evident during tibialis posterior tendon disruption where this transverse tarsal midfoot locking mechanism is compromised. In this situation, the only support to medial longitudinal arch (see arches of foot) is the plantar soft-tissue structures that are inefficient in bearing the body weight and slowly give way producing pes planus (flatfoot). Further, the Achilles tendon pulls on an everted hindfoot to ensure that midfoot locking does not occur and this then becomes a deforming force that leads to further accentuation of deformity now producing valgus—so the progressive planovalgus deformity. The coupling of movements within foot can be exploited to correct deformity because correction of one of them would alter and improve other associated movements/deformity components. This is especially useful in management of CTEV by corrective cast technique. The following are commonly used corrective maneuvers that utilize the coupling of movements at the ankle:

- Abduction of calcaneum corrects heel varus and calcaneal plantar flexion.
- Abducting the foot causes abduction of calcaneum.
- Abduction at calcaneum + eversion + dorsiflexion occur simultaneously.
- Adduction of calcaneum + inversion + plantar flexion occur simultaneously.

Great Toe

- Normal extension at the metatarsophalangeal joint is 65°.
- Normal flexion at the metatarsophalangeal joint is 40°. Metatarsophalangeal joint movements are severely restricted in hallux rigidus.
- Range of motion in the *interphalangeal* (IP) joint. Normal flexion is 60°. Normal extension is 0°. Restriction is common after fractures of the terminal phalanx, and is generally regarded as a contraindication to metacarpophalangeal joint fusion.

During late midstance and toe-off, the hallux and lesser toes dorsiflex tightening the plantar fascia. This adds to the stability of the midfoot during toe-off and push-off phase. Arthrodesis of great toe joints as in modified Jones procedure partially compromises this ability producing sudden break in the push-off phase where the foot has to be lifted and dragged by leg muscles resulting in abnormal gait.

CONCLUSION

- Ankle is surrounded by numerous tendons all over and it transmits all the weight of body through it to the foot.
- Alteration in the biomechanics of ankle due to altered force transmission is a common cause of pain in the joint.

CHAPTER 82

Examination of the Foot and Ankle

Manish Kumar Varshney

INTRODUCTION

The examination of foot and ankle involves not only the three common components or inspection, palpation, and movements but also the examination of the footwear as it reveals various disorders related to foot movements and deformities. The examination should be comprehensive so that proper understanding of the disease condition is made and that would also help in planning the treatment.

INSPECTION

- Note the general state of the skin and nails. If there is evidence of ischemia, a full cardiovascular system (CVS) examination is required. The dorsalis pedis pulse should be sought routinely.
- *Signs of ischemia:* Thinning of the skin, diminished hair growth, loss of subcutaneous fat, shininess and trophic changes in the nail, which becomes brittle and show transverse ridges, minor ulcerations in pressure areas such as heel, malleoli, ball of the foot, and tip of the toes.
- *Deformity* of shape (old fracture, sinus scars, macrodactyly), of posture (calcaneus deformity, talipes deformity and drop foot).
- Look for bruising swelling (with all its characteristics) or edema.
- Note whether the foot is normally proportioned. If not, look at the hands and assess the rest of the skeleton.
- Heel—for calcaneal prominence (calcaneal exostosis), with overlying callus or bursitis.
- Dorsum—for any prominence of the fifth metatarsal base or exostosis, for prominence of the fifth metatarsal head (Bunionette or Tailor's exostosis). Both can be a source of local pressure symptoms.
- *Great toe*—for any hallux valgus deformity, any bursa over the first metatarsophalangeal (MTP) joint (bunion) and whether active inflammatory changes are present. Discoloration of the joint with acute tenderness is suggestive of gout. Note for toe thickening at the MP joint, suggesting hallux rigidus (osteoarthritis) or hallux flexus (osteoarthritis). Note the presence of excess callus under the great toe. This is highly suggestive of hallux rigidus.
- *Great toenail*—note whether the great toenail is deformed (onychogryphosis), ingrowing (accompanied by inflammation), elevated (suggestive of subungual exostosis) or uneven in texture and growth (fungal infection or psoriasis).
- *Toes*—a second toe longer than the first may be associated with Freiberg's disease. Flex the toes to note the relative lengths of the metatarsals. Abnormally short first and fifth metatarsals are potential causes of forefoot imbalance and pain. The various deformities of toes are depicted in **Figure 1**.
    - *Curly toes:* Fixed flexion deformity develops in the interphalangeal (IP) joint and the MP joints. It is generally caused by interosseous muscle weakness.
        - *Grade A:* The toe is mildly flexed (with or without adduction).
        - *Grade B:* There is some degree of under or overriding.
        - *Grade C:* The nail is not visible from the dorsum.
    - *Claw toes:* Flexion at IP joint with hyperextension at metacarpophalangeal (MCP) joint. In pes cavus or some form of intrinsic muscle insufficiency, all toes are involved.
    - *Hammer toe deformity:* The toe is flexed at the proximal IP joint and extended at the MP joint and distal IP joint. The second toe is most commonly

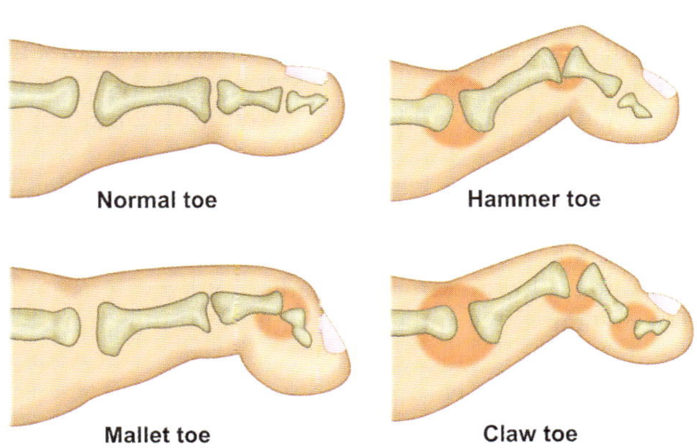

Fig. 1: Toe deformities.

affected, often due to an associated hallux valgus deformity. There is usually a callus formation at the proximal IP joint (as opposed to mallet toe where the callosity is under the tip of toe), as a result of pressure against the shoe.
  - An overlapping fifth toe or quinti varus is often congenital.
- *Note the presence of:*
  - Hard corns that represent the site of pressure from abnormal bony excrescence localizing the pathology often.
  - Hyperhidrosis causing fungal infection.
  - Athlete's foot and ulceration of sole suggesting pes cavus or neurological disturbance.
  - Callus indicating uneven or restricted area of weight-bearing.
  - Verruca (plantar wart)—classically occurs at the heel, under the great toe and in the forefoot in the region of the metatarsal heads.
  - Localized fibrous tissue mass typical of Dupuytren's contracture of the feet. Always inspect the hands, as both the upper limbs are often involved in this process.
  - *Tennis toe:* This painful condition arises from repetitive trauma to the big toe causing accumulation of small or large hematoma under the toe nail. It may arise from ill-fitting shoes or repetitive start-stop activities producing stress locally (as in tennis sport). Tennis toe is also known by skier's toe or runner's toe as it may arise in them also. Clinically, there is blackish discoloration of the nail plate and patient feels pressure building-up in the great toe associated with throbbing pain.

POSTURE

- *Examine the patient standing:* Are both the heel and the forefoot squarely on the ground? If the heel does not touch—equinus deformity (shortening of the tendocalcaneus).
- Intoeing and out-toeing deformity (causes discussed in section on pediatric conditions).
- *Genu valgum:* It is frequently associated with flatfoot.
- *Eversion:* A peroneal spastic foot or if less marked, pes planus.
- *Inversion:* Muscle imbalance from stroke or other neurological disorder, hallux flexus or rigidus, pes cavus, residual talipes deformity or painful condition of the forefoot.
- *Splaying:* Note whether there is any broadening of the forefoot. This is often the result of intrinsic muscle weakness and may be associated with pes cavus, callus under the metatarsal heads, hallux valgus, anterior metatarsalgia, and trouble with shoe fitting.

MEDIAL ARCH

- In weight-bearing position, assess the medial longitudinal arch. Slip the index finger under the navicular. In pes cavus, the finger may go to a distance of 2 cm or more. Look for clawing of toes, callus, or laceration under the metatarsal heads and alteration of footprints.
- In pes planus, the medial arch is obliterated. The navicular is often prominent and the fingers cannot be inserted under it. Ask the patient to stand on toes of foot. In mobile pes planus, the arch can often be restored. Examine the Achilles tendon, shortening of which can cause flatfoot.
- In pes planus examine for an increase in the area of the sole involved in weight-bearing. The footprint will be abnormal in these cases. Examine knees for genu valgum.

HEELS

- Look from behind to observe the heel varus or valgus. Ask the patient to stand on his toes observing the heel. If the heel posture corrects, it indicates a mobile subtalar joint. Persisting deformity suggests loss of movement due arthritic changes, tarsal coalition, loss of spring ligament or posterior tibialis function or shortening of the tendocalcaneus.
- *Gait:* Examine patient walking barefooted and then with shoes on.
- *Skin temperature:* A warm foot is indicative of inflammatory arthritis or gout.

SHOES

Shoe examination is a major part of the foot examination. Different parts of shoe **(Fig. 2)** need to be inspected for defining the wear patterns in different deformities **(Figs. 3A to C)**.

- Examine for wear patterns in shoe. In the normal, sole wear is fairly even, being maximal across the tread and the tip at the back of the heel. Maximum wear is also to the lateral side.
- In too short shoe, excessive wear occurs at the toe and heel. The toe cap bulges and the inside of the shoe are marked by the toes. The heel may give-way at the seam. There may be blistering of the heel and excessive wear. A gap may appear between the quarter and the ankle.
- *Pes planus:* Wear on the medial side of the sole extending to the tip, increased wear on outer heel and in severe cases wear on the diagonal corner of the heel. The shoe may be twisted when viewed from behind (the heel and the sole are on different planes) with scuff marks on the medial side. The upper will bulge over the sole on the medial side while the quarter bulges away from the foot.
- *Splay foot:* Excess wear in region of the first and second metatarsal. There is an upper bulge over the sole anteriorly.
- *Pes cavus:* Excessive wear under the metatarsal head region, excessive wear at the back of the heel, raising of toes, creases, and giving way of lacings.
- *Hallux valgus:* There is often excessive wear of the first and second metatarsal heads and bulging of the upper to accommodate the prominent first metatarsal head.

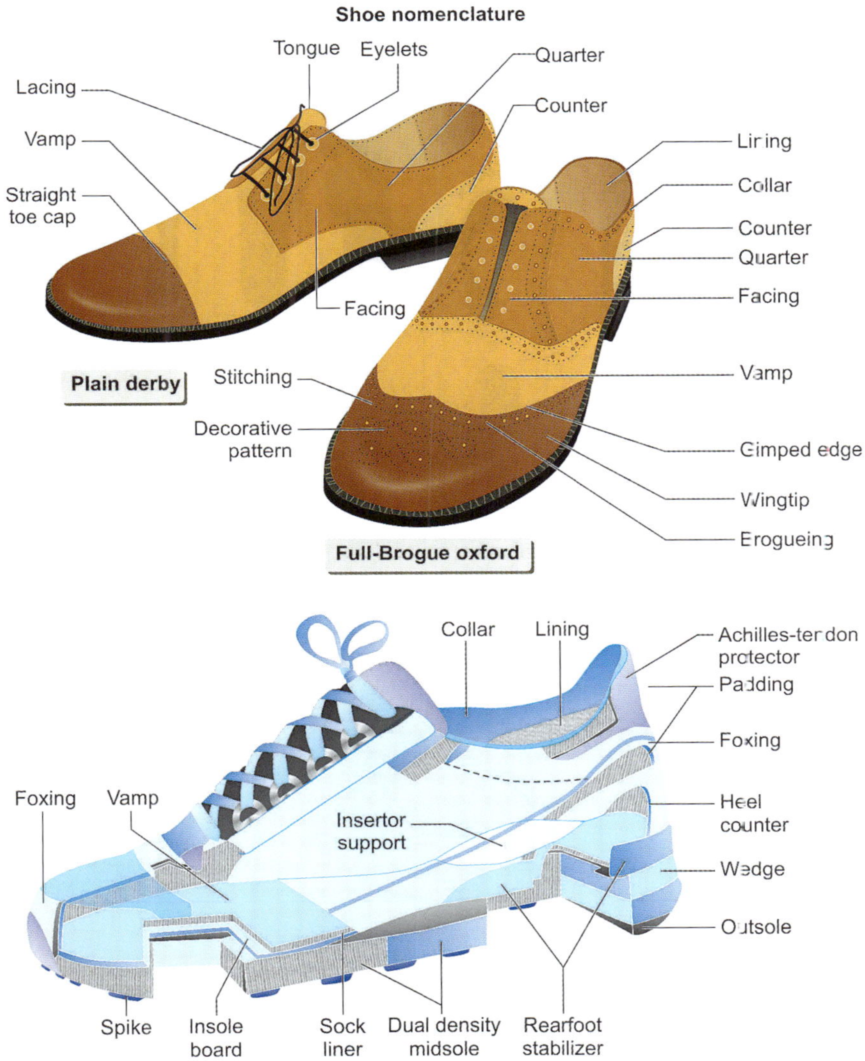

Fig. 2: Shoe and its various components.

- *Hallux rigidus:* Excessive wear under the first metatarsal head and at the tip of the sole, excessive wear on the lateral side (walking on the side of the foot) and lateral overhang. The toe of the shoe may be upturned.

PALPATION

Soft-tissue palpation of the foot points to probable diagnosis in many instances **(Box 1)**. The forefoot pain is a common complaint and the issue of differential diagnosis may be settled to some extent by algorithm presented in the **Flowchart 1**.

Bony Palpation

Medial Aspect

- With the feet dangling free, stabilize the foot and lower leg with one hand holding the foot around the calcaneus and support the head of first metatarsal bone and metatarsophalangeal (MTP) joint. MTP joint is most frequently involved in gout and bunions.
- *Navicular tubercle:* Along the medial border of the foot palpate the navicular tubercle.
- *Head of the talus:* It is present immediately proximal to the navicular and can be easily palpated during eversion and inversion of the foot. Eversion causes the head of the talus to become more prominent.
- *Medial malleolus:* From the head of the talus proximally the bony medial malleolus can be palpated.

Lateral Aspect

- The fifth metatarsal bone and fifth MTP joint
- Calcaneus
- *Peroneal tubercle:* It separates the peroneus brevis and the longus tendons.
- Lateral malleolus
- Dome of the talus
- *Inferior tibiofibular joint:* It lies immediately proximal to the talus. Since the anteroinferior tibiofibular ligament overlies this joint, clear palpation is impossible and the bones of the joint may be separated following ankle injury (diastasis).

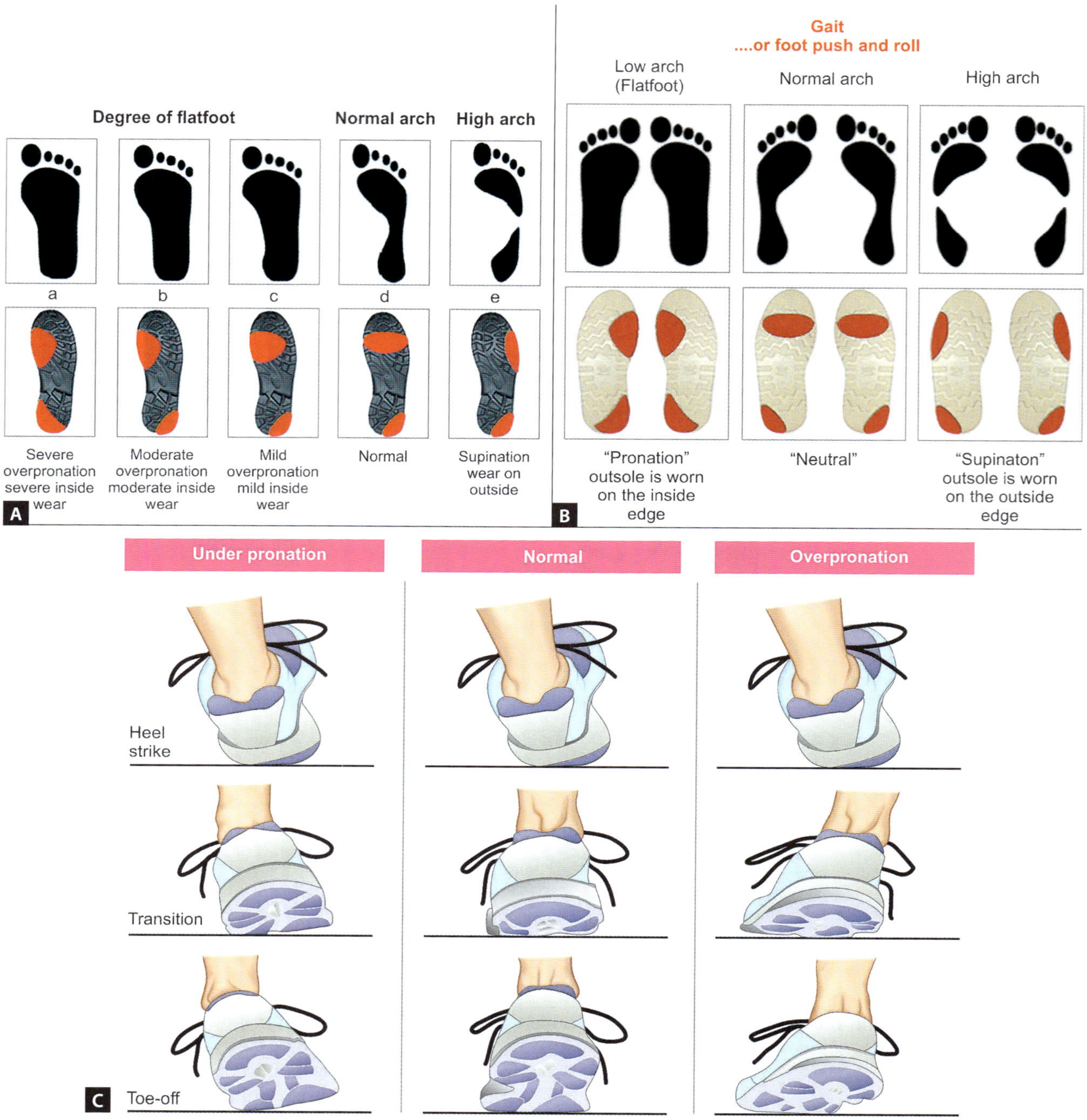

Figs. 3A to C: (A) Wear pattern of shoe in various foot deformities and (B and C) gait patterns that may indirectly help to identify foot problems.

- *Sinus tarsi area:* It is palpated as a soft-tissue depression just anterior to the lateral malleolus. This depression lies directly over the sinus tarsi. It is partly masked by the extensor digitorum brevis muscle and overlying pad of fat. It is the area for performing subtalar arthrodesis.

Hindfoot

- Palpate the Achilles-tendon attachment (common site of inflammatory pain).
- Palpate the fat pad anterior to tendo-Achilles that gets frequently inflamed.
- Palpate the tendo-Achilles itself for discontinuity (complete tear) or nodule formation (partial tear that is healing).

Plantar Surface

- Sesamoid bone within the flexor hallucis brevis tendon.
- *Metatarsal heads:* Move laterally and palpate each metatarsal head placing the thumb over the plantar surface and the index finger over the dorsal aspect. Tenderness under the metatarsal heads is common in anterior metatarsalgia, pes cavus and pes planus, gout,

and rheumatoid arthritis. Puffy localized swelling on the dorsum of the foot, palpable thickening on the second MTP joint, pain on plantar flexion of the toe and joint tenderness are diagnostic of Freiberg's disease.

- Tenderness on both plantar and dorsal surface of the second or third metatarsal necks or shafts occurs in March fracture.
- Tenderness around the heel is present in Sever's disease, superior calcaneal exostosis and tendocalcaneus bursitis, plantar fasciitis and inferior calcaneal exostosis and pes cavus.

Soft-tissue Palpation

Lateral

- *Complete tear of lateral ligament complex:* Swelling is rapid and is egg-shaped and placed over the lateral malleolus (McKenzie's sign).
- *Stress testing (use local anesthetic):*
    - Under forced inversion, note any opening up of the lateral side of the ankle between the tibia and the talus
    - Perform a stress X-ray.
    - Anterior drawer test—for testing the anterior talo-fibular component, with the patient prone, press downward on the heel, looking for anterior displacement of the talus, which is often accompanied by dimpling of the skin on either side.
- Perform stress test by forcing the foot into plantar flexion and inversion. This will give rise to pain and increase tenderness along the line of the peroneal tendons, if tenosynovitis is present.
- Lightly scratch the side of the foot. In the normal foot, the child will respond by dorsiflexion of the foot, eversion, and fanning of the toes. This reaction does not take place in fixed clubfoot deformity.
- Look and feel for displacement of the tendons, as the patient everts the foot against light resistance. Displacements occur in a condition known as snapping peroneal tendons.

BOX 1: The disorders associated with common points of tenderness at the foot.

- On the undersurface of metatarsal heads—Metatarsalgia
- At insertion of Achilles-tendon—Insertional tendinitis
- At tendon of Achilles—Achilles tendinits
- Anterolateral aspect of ankle joint line—Lateral gutter impingement in post-traumatic cases
- Fifth metatarsal base—Fracture, tendinitis of peronei
- Posterior or lateral to lateral malleolus—Peroneal tenosynovitis
- Tip of lateral malleoli—? Fracture as per ankle Ottawa rules
- Anterior joint line of ankle—Impinging osteophyte in osteoarthritis
- On the dorsal aspect of first MTP—Hallux rigidus, gout (usually involves all over the joint)
- Third interspace—Morton neuroma
- Retrocalcaneal bursa to tendo-Achilles—Bursitis
- Posterior aspect of medial malleoli—Tendinitis of tibialis posterior
- At the plantar fascia—Plantar fasciitis
- On the undersurface of first MTP—Sesamoditis
- On the medial aspect of first MTP—Bunion

(MTP: metatarsophalangeal)

Inferior Tibiofibular Ligament

Grasp the heel and try to move the talus directly laterally in the ankle mortise. Lateral displacement indicates a tear in the ligament.

Deltoid Ligament

It is palpable just beneath the medial malleolus (eversion ankle sprain). Feel for tenderness, discontinuity, etc.

Tendocalcaneus (Achilles Tendon)

- Examine the patient prone with the feet over the edge of couch. Note for local or diffuse swelling, redness of the skin or Hagelund deformity (a bony excrescence affecting the posterosuperior aspect of calcaneum). Look for tenderness, normally situated 3–5 cm proximal to the tendon insertion. Gently squeeze the tendon. Marked pain is a feature of tendinosis and if it changes with dorsiflexion and plantar flexion then it indicates tendinitis, in paratendinitis the site of maximum pain will remain fixed.

Flowchart 1: The algorithm for evaluation of forefoot pain.

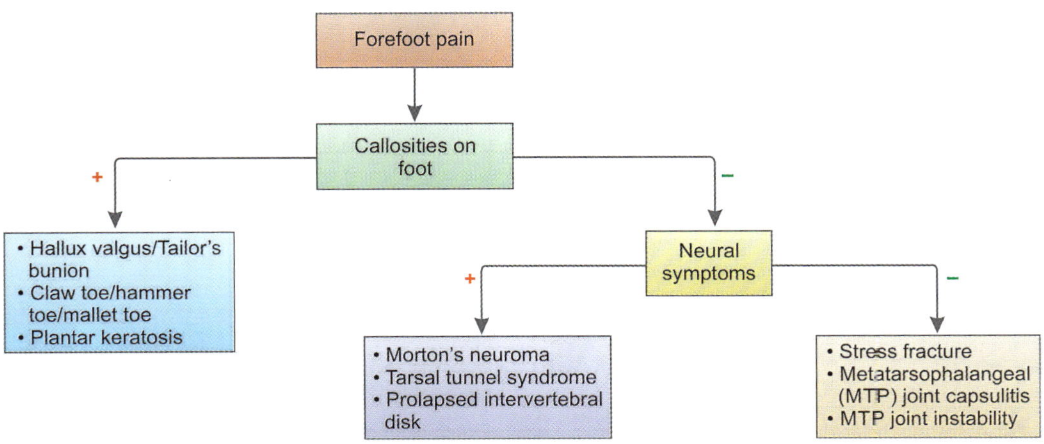

- Test the power of plantar flexion, by asking the patient to press the foot against your hand, compare one side with the other and note the shape of each contracting calf and the shape of the tendon. Note for any gap in the tendon.
- Perform the Thompson and O'Brien's test, if gap was found.

Medial

- Look for synovitis (tenderness along the course) in relation to the flexor tendons.
- Demonstrate the presence of any excess fluid, by milking the sheaths in a proximal direction.
- Plantar flex and evert the foot for involvement of tibialis posterior tendon.
- Also look for tenderness or gaps in the line of the tibialis posterior tendon. Spontaneous rupture is seen most frequently in flatfoot and rheumatoid arthritis.

Crepitus

- Palpate for crepitus at MTP and the IP joint of great toe. Crepitus, indicating osteoarthritis change is constant in the MP joint in hallux rigidus. IP joint crepitus is considered as a contraindication for MP joint fusion.
- Palpate for crepitus of peroneal tendons posteriorly—may indicate impingement or tendinitis.
- Place a hand across the front of the ankle and passively dorsiflex and plantarflex the foot. Crepitus suggests articular surface damage.

The examination of foot and ankle movements has been discussed in Chapter on "Biomechanics of the Foot and Ankle Joint and Related Examination".

BLOOD CIRCULATION

- Note the skin temperature gradient along the limb. Observe any trophic changes or discoloration of the skin suggestive of ischemia.
- *Palpate for the pulsations of:*
    - Posterior tibial artery
    - Dorsal pedis artery
    - Anterior tibial artery

NEUROLOGICAL EXAMINATION

Muscle Testing

Dorsiflexors: Majority lie in the anterior tibial compartment. They share a common innervation and paralysis results in foot drop.

- *Tibialis anterior (deep peroneal nerve L4):* Ask the patient to walk on his heels with the foot inverted. Paralysis produces characteristic drop foot or steppage gait. Manual testing is done by asking the patient to reach your finger by dorsiflexion and inversion of foot while sitting on the edge of the bed. Power is tested by asking the patient to plantarflex and everts the foot against resistance applied against the head and shaft of first metatarsal **(Fig. 4)**.
- *Extensor hallucis longus (EHL) (deep personal nerve, L5):* The patient is asked to walk on his heels, by doing so the tendon of the EHL becomes prominent on its way to its insertion on the proximal end of the distal phalynx of great toe. For the manual test, support the foot as above and place your thumb in such a way that he must dorsiflex his toe to reach it. Oppose his dorsiflexion by placing your thumb on the nail bed of the great toe or by pinkie finger of hand **(Fig. 5)**. If the thumb is placed across the IP joint, the extensor hallucis brevis is also being tested.
- *Extensor digitorum longus (deep peroneal nerve L5):* The tendon fans out on the dorsum of the foot to insert on the dorsal surface of the middle and distal phalanges of the four lateral toes. For the manual test, secure patient's calcaneus and place the thumb of your free hand in such a position that he must extend his toes to reach it. Then oppose this motion by attempting to bend them plantarward **(Fig. 6)**.

Plantar Flexors

- *Peroneus longus and brevis (superficial peroneal nerve, S1):* They become prominent when the patient walks along medial border of foot. For manual testing, secure the

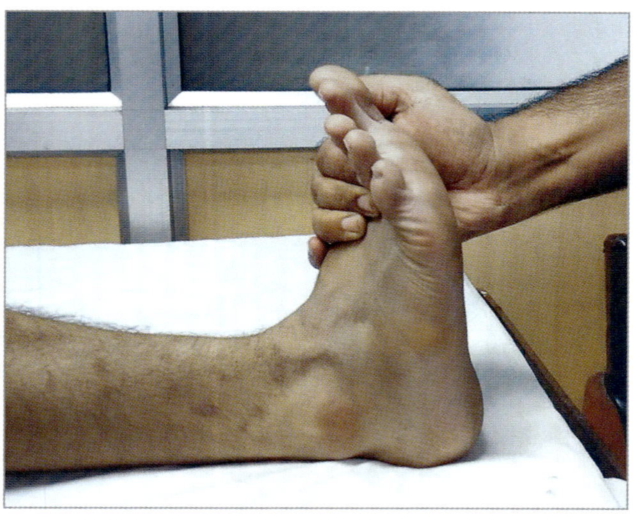

Fig. 4: Testing the ankle dorsiflexors.

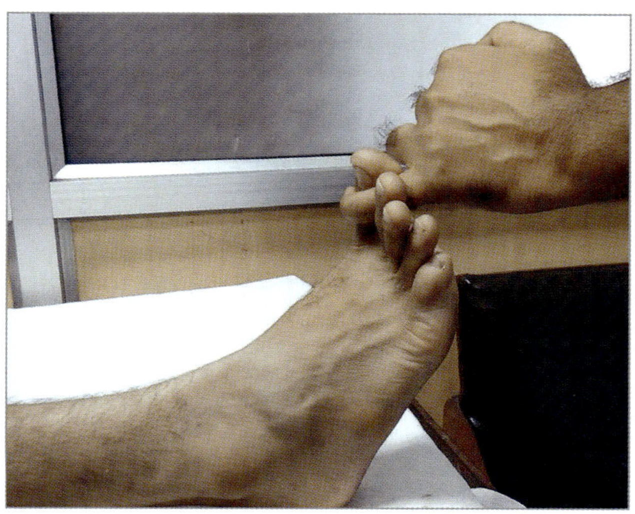

Fig. 5: Testing the extensor hallucis longus (EHL)/great toe extensors.

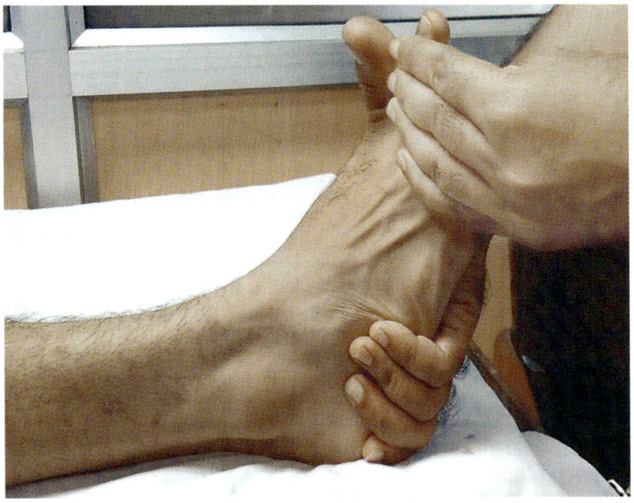

Fig. 6: Testing the evertors of foot.

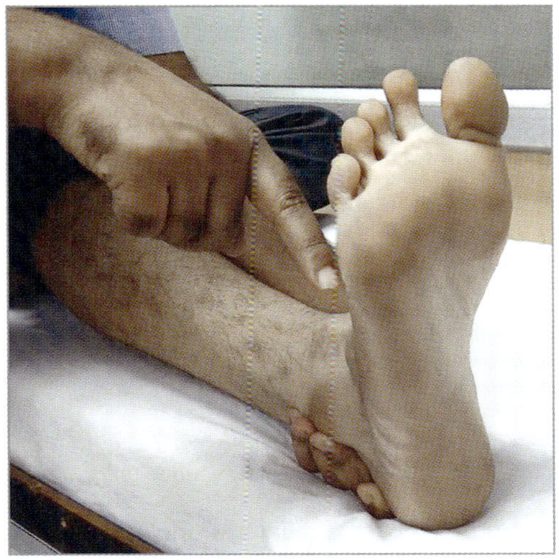

Fig. 7: Testing the toe extensors.

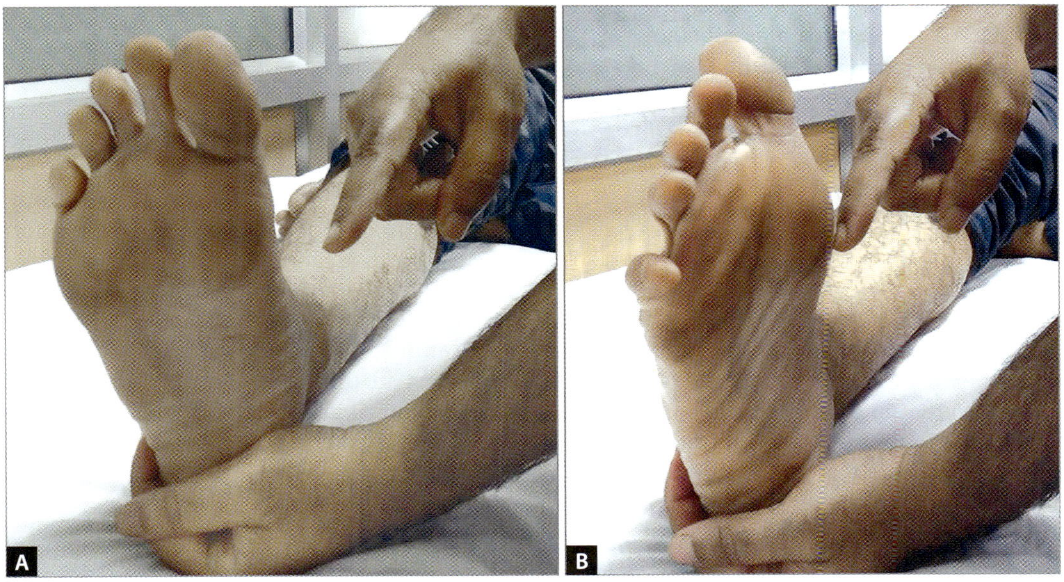

Figs. 8A and B: Testing invertor of foot (tibialis posterior).

patients ankle by stabilizing the calcaneus ask him to plantar flex and evert his foot to reach your finger **(Fig. 7)** with little toe and assess power by pushing against the fifth metatarsal head and shaft with the palm of your hand.

- *Gastrocnemius and soleus (tibial nerve S1, S2):* As it is difficult to detect any existing weakness of gastrocnemius by manual testing because it is stronger than all upper limb muscles therefore, observing these muscles in function is better to reveal weakness. First the patient is instructed to walk on his toes, and then he is asked to jump up and down on the balls of his feet, one at a time to force the calf muscles to support almost two and a half times the body weight, inability to do the above task reveals the weakness.
- *Flexor hallucis longus (tibial nerve, L5):* The muscle action is integral to the smooth toe-off phases of gait. For the manual test, make the patient sit on the edge of the bed and support his foot by stabilizing the calcaneus. Instruct him to curl his great toe and oppose this plantar flexion. Compare on both sides.
- *Flexor digitorum longus (tibial nerve L5):* Manually tested by having the patient bend or curl his toes and opposing the movement.
- *Tibialis posterior (tibial nerve L5):* With the calcaneus stabilized and patient sitting on the edge of table ask him to invert and plantar flex the foot so that his great toe touches your finger aptly placed **(Figs. 8A and B)**. Oppose the movement by pressing up the ball of great toe to assess power.

Sensation Testing

- L4 dermatome crosses the knee joint and over the medial side of the leg (medial to the crest, the medial malleolus and the medial side of the foot).

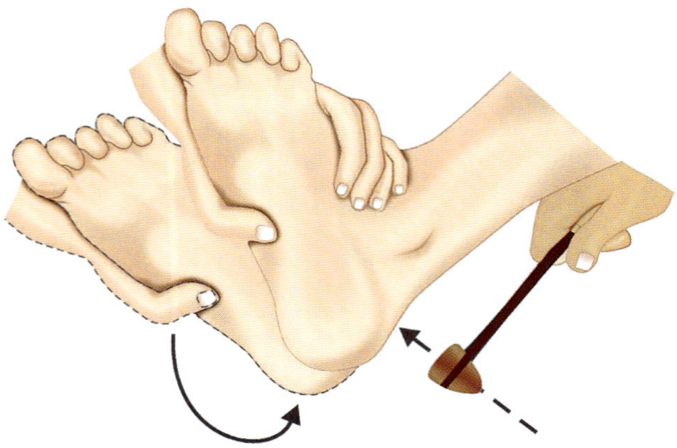
Fig. 9: Testing for Achilles-tendon reflex.

- L5 dermatome covers the lateral side of the leg (lateral to the crest of the tibia) and the dorsum of the foot.
- S1 dermatome covers the lateral side of the foot.
- The saphenous nerve supplies the medial side of the foot.
- The peroneal nerve supplies the dorsum of foot.
- The lateral side of foot is supplied by the sural nerve.

Deep Tendon Reflexes

Elicit the:
- Achilles-tendon reflex (S1, S2, **Fig. 9**)
- Tibialis posterior reflex (L5)

MEASUREMENTS

Foot

1. *Length measurements:* It is measured along lateral and medial aspect one from the most prominent point on the back of the heel to the tip of the great toe and another (medial) from the first point to the tip of the fifth toe. Compare these to the other foot for quantification.
2. *Lever arms of the foot:* The relationships between the long lever arm (tip of the medial malleolus to the tip of the great toe and tip of the lateral malleolus to the tip of the fifth toe on the outer side) and short level arm (tip of the medial malleolus to the most prominent heel point on the medial side and tip of the lateral malleolus to the tip of the most prominent heel point on the lateral side) of the foot should be symmetrical on both sides.

SPECIAL TESTS

- Anterior Drawer sign (Kindly see above)
- Test for rigid or supple flat feet [Kindly *see* flexible flatfoot in Chapter on "Anomalies of Pediatric Lower Limb" and Chapter on "Acquired Flatfoot (Pes Planus) and Posterior Tibial Tendon Dysfunction"]
- Tibial torsion test (Kindly *see* rotational and angular alignment of lower limb in Chapter on "Anomalies of Pediatric Lower Limb" of Pediatric Orthopedics section)
- Homan's sign (Kindly *see* Chapter on "Tendo-Achilles Rupture")

CONCLUSION

- It is important to evaluate all the structures in foot and ankle to make a comprehensive and correct diagnosis.
- The foot and ankle have complex anatomy with various structures intricately related and supported by tough structures to maintain the architecture. All of them need to be examined individually and in totality so that treatment can be well planned.
- Examination of footwear also comprises an important aspect in the evaluation of foot as most of the bio-mechanical alterations and deformities have characteristic wear patterns on the footwear that also indicate the abnormality well.

CHAPTER 83

Ligament Injuries Around Ankle

Manish Kumar Varshney

INTRODUCTION

It is the most common acute sports injury (occurring often in basketball and jumping sports) and even otherwise injury to human body. The mechanism of injury is inversion and plantar flexion of the foot (85%) injuring the anterior talofibular ligament most commonly and sometimes the calcaneofibular ligament (especially in the complete tears). Remaining 15% consist of eversion mechanisms, which are often the result of an outside force. Acute ankle sprain is commonly seen in individuals aged 10–19 years. Boys outnumber girls in the 15–24 years age group; while in patients aged >30 years, females are frequently affected. The lateral ligament complex is variably injured and proper initial management is needed to prevent long-term morbidity including instability of chronic injury.

Diagnosis

History and clinical examination are the most important aspects for making diagnosis. Palpate the commonly injured structures around the ankle and foot as follows:

- *Ligaments:* Anterior tibiofibular and calcaneofibular ligaments **(Figs. 1A and B)** are commonly injured while other ligaments that should be examined for severe injury include the bifurcate, syndesmotic, and deltoid ligaments—in case the injury extends medially.
- *Bones:* Both malleoli (medial and lateral), fifth metatarsal base and insertion of the peroneus tertius, anterior and lateral process of calcaneus, and lateral process of the talus.
- *Tendons:* Peroneal tendons, posterior tibial tendons, flexor hallucis longus, flexor digitorum longus, and the tendo-Achilles.

Findings

- Swelling **(Fig. 1C)**
- Ecchymosis
- Tenderness
- Decreased range of motion

Provocative tests (Inject local anesthetic into the peroneal sheath and lateral gutter of the ankle to reduce pain and muscle guarding).

- Anterior drawer test **(Fig. 2)**
- *Eversion stress test:* Knee is bent 90° to relax gastrocnemius. The heel is held from below by one hand, while the other hand stabilizes the lower leg. The hand on the heel is used to push the calcaneus and talus into eversion (eversion stress). It is to test deltoid ligament while the talus often shifts laterally with eversion stress.

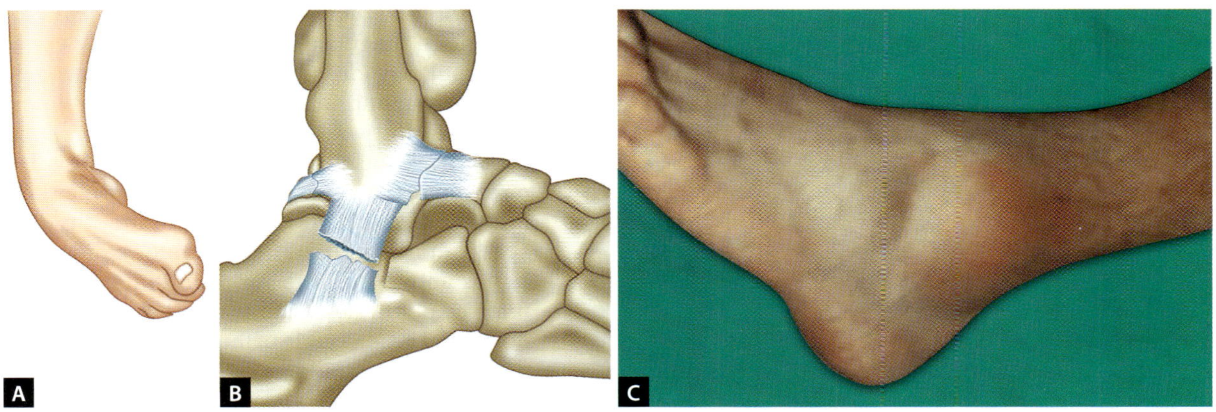

Figs. 1A to C: Ankle sprain. (A) Mechanism; (B) Pathoanatomy; (C) Clinical presentation.

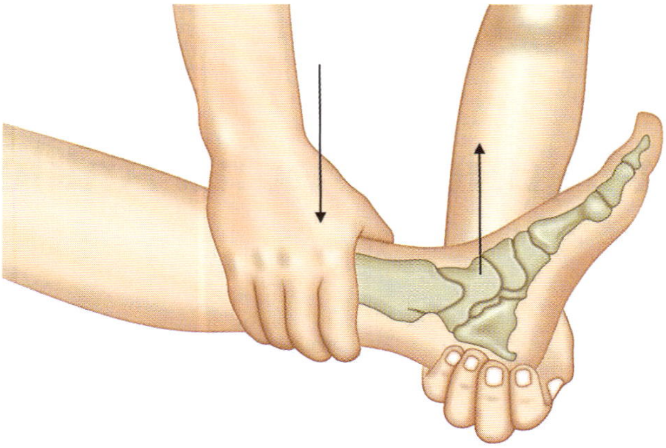

Fig. 2: Anterior drawer test.

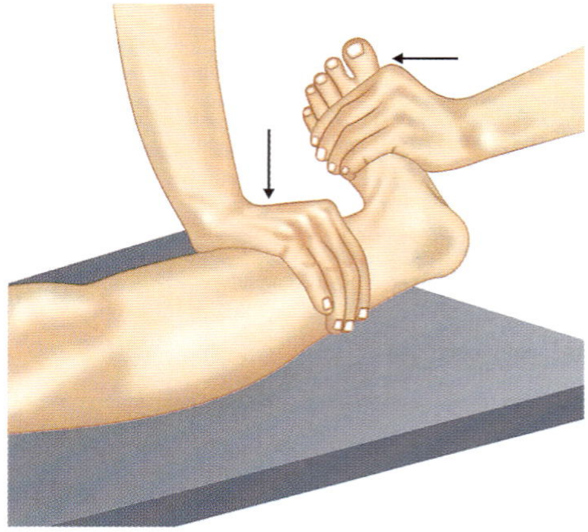

Fig. 4: Kleiger's test (please see text for details).

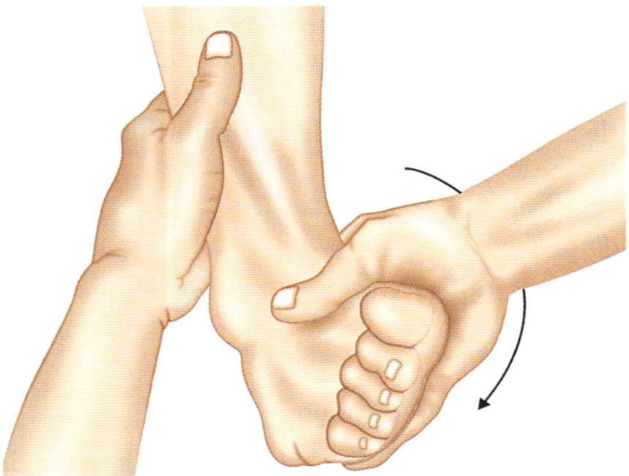

Fig. 3: Inversion stress test.

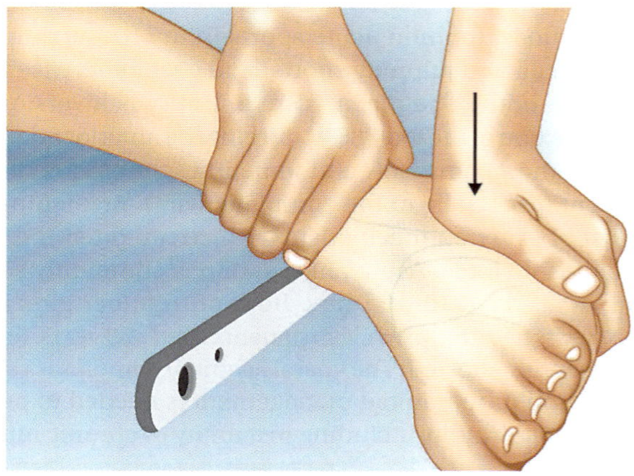

Fig. 5: Medial subtalar glide test.

- *Inversion stress test* ***(Fig. 3)****:* In the similar position as above, the inversion stress is applied. Note for a definite endpoint (if absent indicates complete tear). It is to test calcaneofibular ligament, posterior talofibular ligament and anterior talofibular ligament. The amount of talar tilt gives a rough indication of the component rupture:
  - Tilting of the talus >15° indicates rupture of the anterior talofibular ligament alone.
  - Tilting 15–30° indicates rupture of the anterior talofibular and calcaneofibular ligaments.
  - Tilting >30° indicates rupture of all three of the lateral ligaments.
- *Talar tilt test:* It is performed to determine extent of inversion or eversion injuries. The calcaneus is alternately inverted and everted, excessive motion in inversion indicates injury to calcaneofibular ligament and possibly the anterior and posterior talofibular ligaments. In eversion, the deltoid ligament is tested.
- *Kleiger's test* ***(Fig. 4)****:* With lower leg stabilized as above foot is rotated laterally to stress the deltoid. It tests primarily the deltoid ligament and may also be used to evaluate distal ankle syndesmosis, anterior/posterior tibiofibular ligaments and the interosseous membrane.
- *Medial subtalar glide test:* It is performed to determine stability of the subtalar joint by assessing the medial translation of the calcaneus on the talus. Talus is stabilized while other hand glides the calcaneus medially **(Fig. 5)**. A positive test is indicated by excessive movement, indicating injury to the lateral ligaments.
- *External rotation test (similar to Kleiger's test):* This test is done to diagnose high ankle sprain, i.e., to identify tibiofibular syndesmotic injury. It is performed with the lower leg stabilized and the foot in neutral position the examiner slowly externally rotates the foot, a positive test occurs if pain occurs at the site of syndesmosis. Depending on severity, the interosseous membrane may be involved.
- *Squeeze test:* This test is done to identify tibiofibular syndesmotic injury. The examiner squeezes both the bones above the anterior tibiofibular ligament at the midway up to the calf firmly and slowly, hold and then quickly release; a sprain of the ligament is highly suspected if the patient complains of pain at anterior tibiofibular ligament.

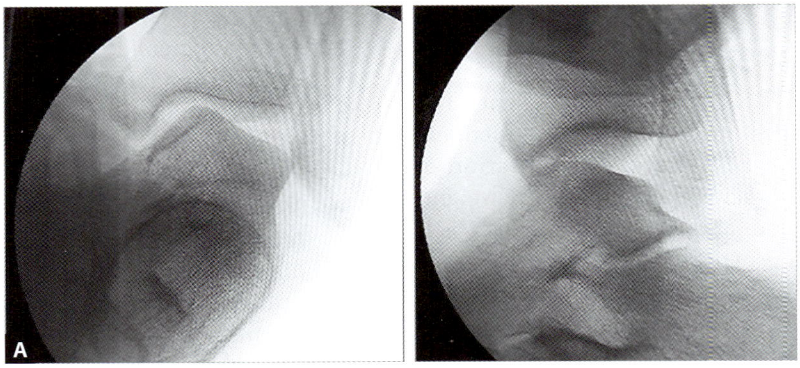

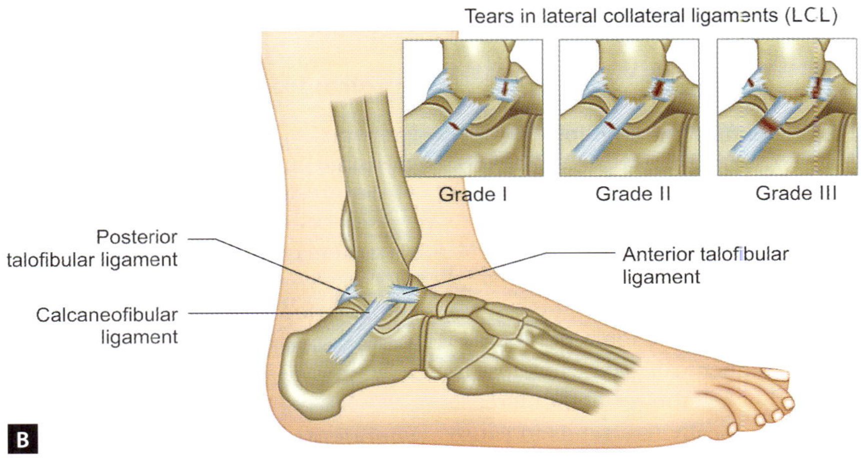

Figs. 6A and B: (A) Lateral joint space opening on stress views and demonstration of positive anterior drawer's test radiologically in awake patient under fluoroscopy; (B) Classification of ankle ligament sprain.

Functional Tests

While weight-bearing the following should be performed:

- Walk on toes (plantar flexion)
- Walk on heels (dorsiflexion)
- Walk on lateral border of feet (inversion)
- Walk on medial border of feet (eversion)
- Hopping on injured ankle

Imaging

- *X-rays*—obtain stress radiographs to document joint opening and assess the extent of opening. AP projection reveals a navicular fracture or Lisfranc injury, and the oblique foot view reveals an anterior process of the calcaneus fracture or a fifth metatarsal fracture. Lateral view may demonstrate talar chip avulsion fracture, etc.
- *Magnetic resonance imaging (MRI)*—done to determine the associated soft tissue injury. There is no definite role in the acute ligament injuries except if there is a high suspicion of associated osteochondral injury or peroneal tendon dislocation or to confirm a subtle syndesmotic injury. MRI has a specific role in chronic ligament injuries to identify the extent of injury and associated injuries.
- *Ultrasonography (USG)*—can be a good substitute for MRI in experienced hands.

CLASSIFICATION (FIGS. 6A AND B)

- *Grade 1 sprain:* The ligaments of the ankle are stretched with some damage to fibers but maintain their integrity.
- *Grade 2 sprain:* The ligaments are partially torn and on examination there may be laxity of the joint.
- *Grade 3 sprain:* There is complete tear of the ligament and on gross examination, gross instability is documented.

Classification of Ankle Ligament Injury and Treatment Recommendations (Clanton)

On the Basis of Stability

- Type I—stable ankle to clinical testing
- Type II—unstable ankle with positive anterior drawer test or positive talar tilt test or both.

On the Basis of the Type of Patient

- Grade 1, nonathlete or older patient—functional treatment
- Grade 2, athlete or high-demand patient—often needs reconstruction.

On the Basis of the Radiographic Stress Testing

- Type A, negative radiograph stress test—functional treatment
- Type B, positive tibiotalar stress test—surgical repair
- Type C, subtalar instability—functional treatment

TREATMENT

Conservative Management

This is the initial choice of treatment for most patients. The commonly followed protocol includes selective functional treatment, which consists of a short "select" period of protection with taping or bracing that allows early weight-bearing, followed by functional range-of-motion exercises and neuromuscular training of the ankle.

Protection, Rest, Ice, Compression, and Elevation (PRICE)—helps in limiting swelling, reducing pain, and early return to activity **(Flowchart 1)**.

- *Rest:* Immobilize in plaster of Paris (POP) slab or cast or aircast.
- *Ice:* Apply for 15 minutes four to five times a day
- *Compression:* This helps to control the swelling.
- *Elevation:* Keep ankle above heart level when possible, allows gravity to drain out swelling.

The modalities often used (these are used almost exclusively in sport injury center for high-demand athletes) are enumerated below:

- *Cold whirlpool:* It causes vasoconstriction around ankle and slows cell metabolism reducing the acute increase in demand due to injury and hence the resultant increase in metabolite concentration locally that tends to cause vasodilation.
- *Ultrasound:* Enhances edema subsidence. It assists in bringing digestive enzymes to clean debris cells or the injured ankle.
- *Rehabilitation exercises:* They improve range-of-motion and maintain mobility of the ankle. These comprise of:
  - Range-of-motion exercises
  - One leg stands
  - Toe pick-ups
  - Toe rises
  - Biomechanical ankle platform system (BAPS) board
  - Towel curls and Theraband
- *Taping and wrapping:* They help in psychological support to the athlete and preventing injury further.
- *Ankle braces:* They support the ankle and also restrict undue mobility. Many variants are available including lace up, hinged, aircasts, etc.

Surgical Treatment

Indications

- Large bony avulsions
- Severe ligamentous damage on the medial and the lateral sides of the ankle
- Severe recurrent injuries

Goal of the Surgical Treatment

- Prevent chronic instability
- Control and avoid the recurrent episodes

Various Methods for Surgical Management of the Ankle Ligament Injuries

- *Repair of acute rupture of the deltoid ligament:* Suture the ligament with nonabsorbable sutures or better using the suture anchors. Fix the bony fragments if associated.

Flowchart 1: PRICEMM [Protection, rest and immobilization, ice, compression, elevation, methods (physical therapy), and medication].

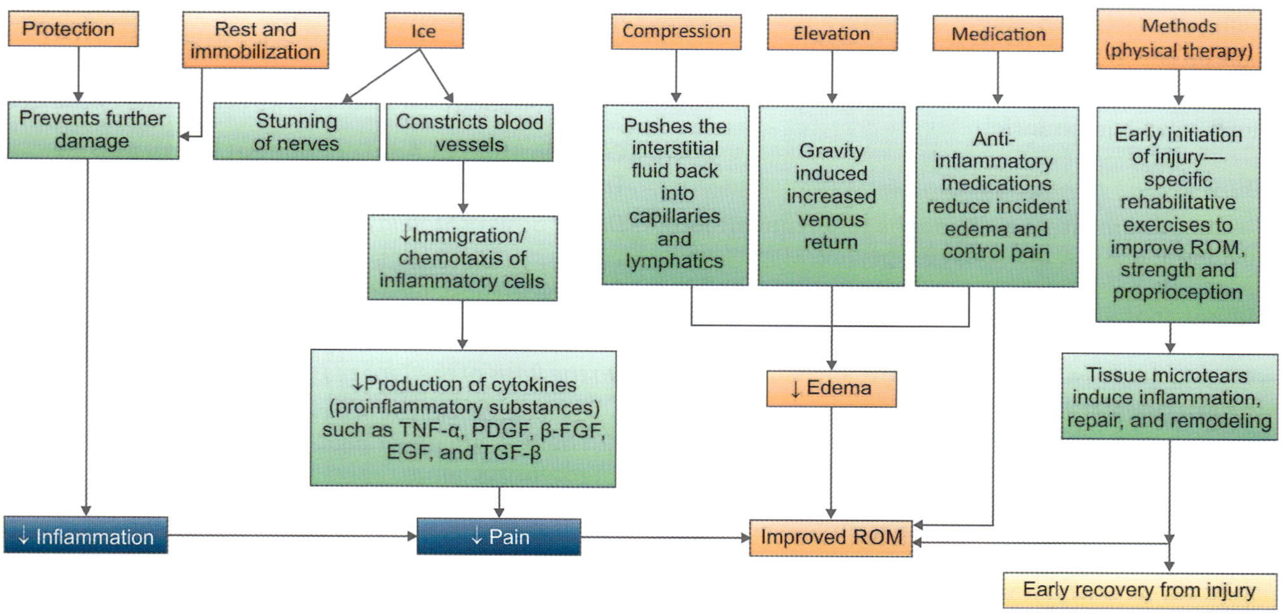

(EGF: epidermal growth factor; FGF: fibroblast growth factor; PDGF: platelet-derived growth factor; ROM: range of motion; TGF: transforming growth factor; TNF: tumor necrosis factor)

- *Repair of acute rupture of the ligaments of the distal tibiofibular joint:* Suturing or reattaching the ligaments here is unnecessary. Syndesmotic stabilization suffices for this injury. With the ankle dorsiflexed 30°, insert a screw transversely through the fibula into the tibia approximately 1–1.5 cm proximal to the ankle joint. If the foot is held in equinus during screw fixation, the narrowest part of the talus is engaged in the ankle mortise that limits the ankle dorsiflexion after healing. Check the position of the screw and the reduction of the talus by radiographs in the operating room, to ensure that the talus has been replaced precisely against the medial malleolus.
- *Repair of acute rupture of the lateral ligaments* ***(Figs. 7A and B):*** The technique described for Brostrom repair is commonly followed and is appropriate. Through a curved incision beginning 5 cm proximal to the distal tip of the fibula and 1.5 cm anterior to its margin to end distal to the fibula, the superficial peroneal nerve and its branches anteriorly and the sural nerve posteriorly and distally are identified and protected. The immediate structure below the incision is the ankle joint and tibiofibular joint capsule with their aponeurotic covering, the aponeurotic covering is incised and with blunt dissection the tear is exposed. To expose the calcaneofibular and the anterior portion of posterior tibiofibular ligament the peroneal sheath is incised and the tendons are retracted. The lateral ligaments are stressed for stability of the ankle and the subtalar joint. The torn ends of the ligaments are approximated and if there is any bony avulsion, suture anchors are used **(Figs. 8A to C)**. For talocalcaneal ligament tear with subtalar instability, the subtalar joint is stabilized by suturing the calcaneofibular ligament. Wound is then closed in layers over drain and joint protected in a cast. Commonly the ligament ends are friable so it is recommended to augment the repair by pulling up and suturing the transverse portion of extensor retinaculum (Gould technique) onto the Brostrom repair.
    - *Karlsson technique:* Expose the calcaneofibular ligament. Open the peroneal tendon sheath, and identify the talofibular and calcaneofibular ligaments. The joint is opened and using a 2-mm drill bit 5–6 holes are drilled in the fibula. Using mattress sutures and the foot in dorsiflexion and pronation the capsule and ligaments retightened and the periosteal flaps are duplicated.

After Treatment

The initial cast should be changed after 2 weeks and the sutures should be removed. After 2 more weeks, weight-bearing with crutches is allowed. At 6 weeks, range-of-motion exercises and manual resistive exercises are begun to gain inversion and eversion. For distal tibiofibular ligaments, the cast is removed at 3 weeks and a walking boot cast is applied and worn for 4 weeks. The syndesmotic screw is removed at 8 weeks and movements (dorsiflexion and plantar flexion) begun. If screw is not removed, it either becomes loose and painful or breaks.

CHRONIC INSTABILITY AFTER INJURY

It is a common complication of acute ligament injury. Around one-third patients with grade 3 injury continue to have lingering symptoms for up to 3 years. The patient has persistent disability and disabling pain and stress radiographs show talar tilt.

Patient should first be treated conservatively if symptomatic by stirrup brace, ankle tape, and muscle-strengthening program.

Surgical reconstruction is indicated for failed conservative program for 3–6 months and patient suffering from recurrent instability. The predominant surgical procedure is ligament reconstruction for which various methods are available as described later. Usually the ligament reconstructions are performed in isolation but it is recommended that if the injury is <6 months old, the Brostrom-Gould repair may be combined additionally. The other indication of using the anatomical ligament reconstructions is for augmentation of acute lateral ankle repairs done especially if it is felt that the repairs may not fair well.

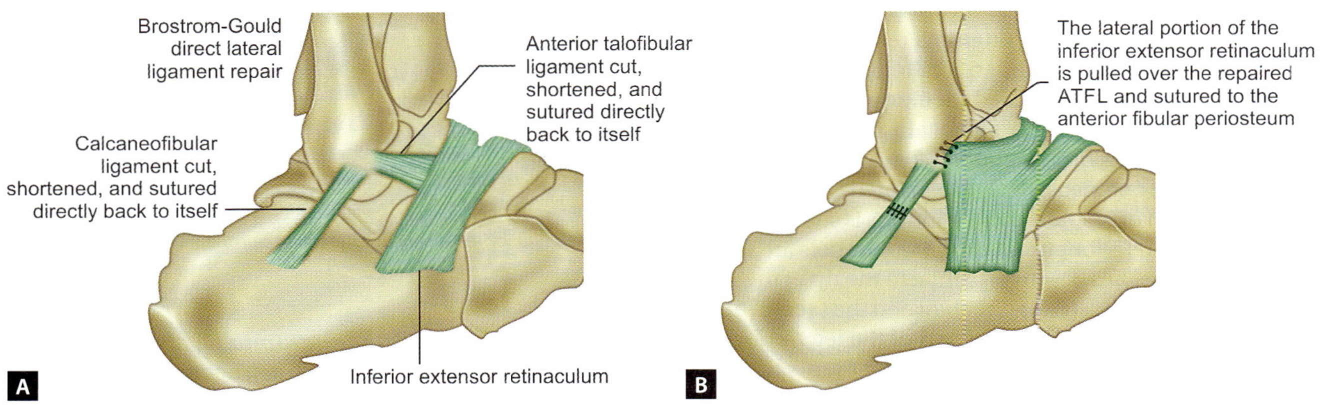

Figs. 7A and B: Direct lateral ligament repair of Brostrom-Gould. (A) The cut ends of anterior talofibular ligament (ATFL) and calcaneofibular ligament (CFL) are refreshed and sutured directly; (B) The lateral portion of the inferior extensor retinaculum sutured over the repaired ATFL and anterior fibular periosteum.

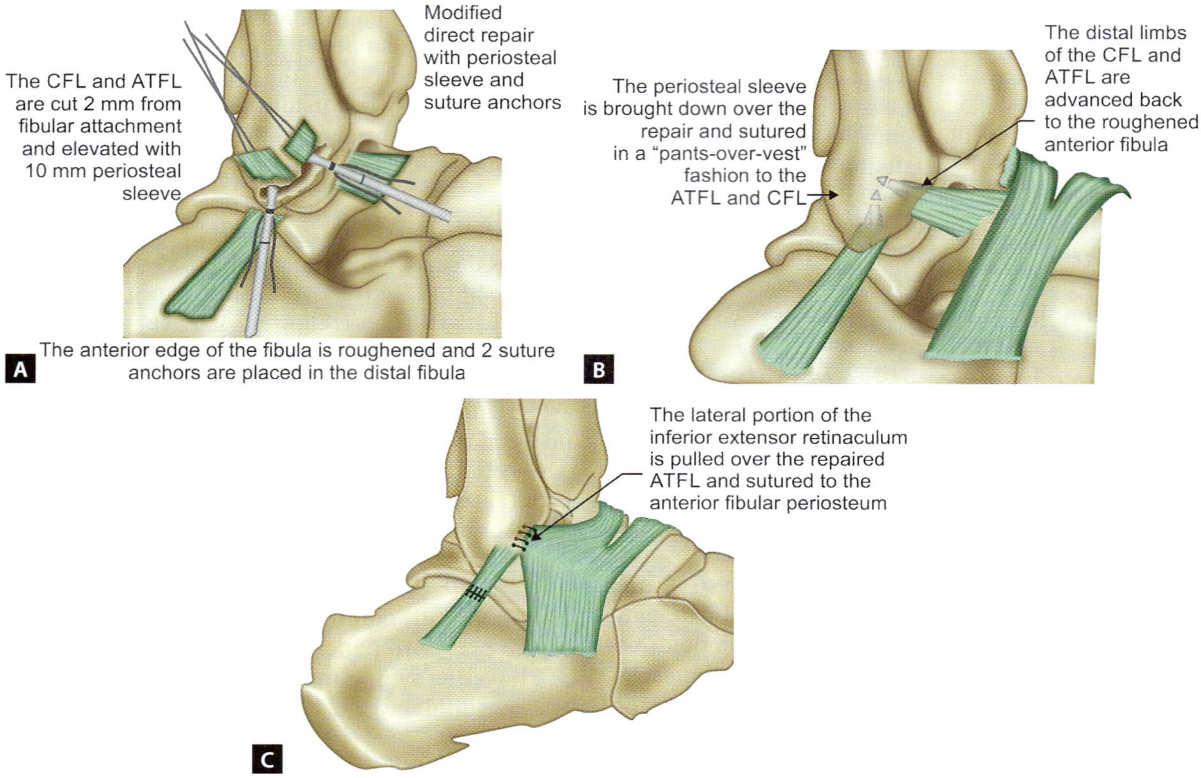

Figs. 8A to C: Modified repair using suture anchors. (ATFL: anterior talofibular ligament; CFL: calcaneofibular ligament)

Techniques for Reconstruction of Lateral Ankle Ligament(s)

There are various procedures that reconstruct the anterior talofibular and the calcaneofibular ligaments using either peroneus brevis tendon or hamstring tendons. The reconstruction could be done in a fashion that anatomical constraints are restored or may involve functional restoration by nonanatomical reconstruction. The following are the commonly used methods:

- *Watson-Jones procedure (nonanatomic):* It is one of the standard procedures for tenodesis for lateral instability of ankle joint using peroneus brevis tendon. The Watson-Jones technique **(Fig. 9)** attempts reconstruction of the calcaneofibular and the anterior talofibular ligaments but has following two technical difficulties:
  1. The tunnel in the neck of the talus is difficult to drill.
  2. The peroneus brevis tendon often falls too short. The tendon of peroneus brevis is separated from the muscle by a clean dissection and the muscle is sutured back to the peroneus longus tendon. Two tunnels are drilled, first tunnel lies 2.5 cm proximal to the tip of the fibula in the anteroposterior direction and the second tunnel lies along the longitudinal axis of the leg through the lateral part of the neck of talus just anterior to the talofibular joint. The peroneus brevis tendon is passed from the first tunnel in posterior to anterior direction and in inferior to superior direction from the second tunnel.

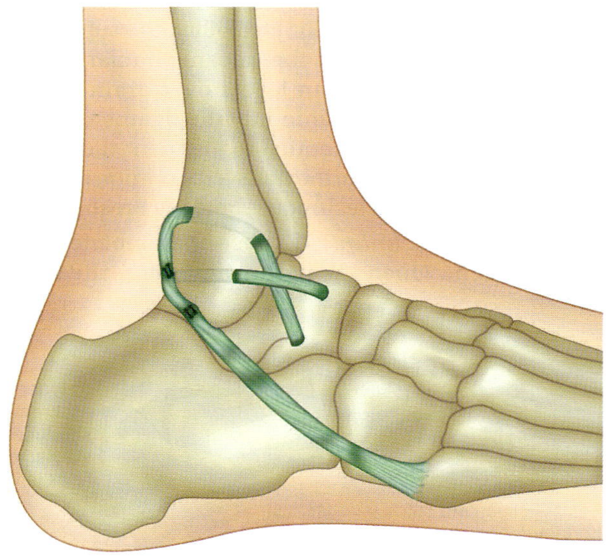

Fig. 9: Watson-Jones technique using peroneal tendon (see text).

- *Evans technique (nonanatomic):* This procedure is used only if anatomical reconstruction of lateral ankle ligaments is not possible. The Evans technique **(Fig. 10)** was designed to overcome difficulties of Watson-Jones procedure, but it reconstructs only the calcaneofibular ligament. Proximally, the peroneus brevis tendon is

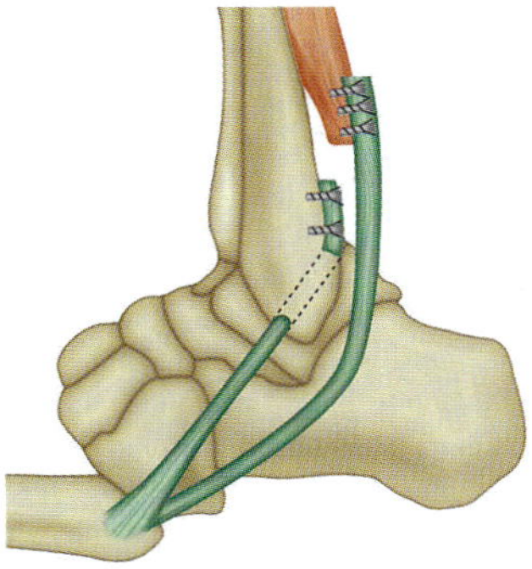

Fig. 10: Evans technique of reconstruction of lateral talofibular ligament.

divided from its muscle belly. A tunnel is drilled in the lateral malleolus in an anteroposterior direction starting from the tip of malleolus anteriorly and progresses in superior and posterior direction to come out from the posterior cortex about 2.5–3 cm from the tip. The foot is maintained in eversion and the tendon of peroneus brevis is passed through the tunnel in inferior to superior direction and is sutured under tension to the adjacent soft tissue.

- *Larsen's technique (nonanatomic):* Depending on the type of instability, the direction of peroneus brevis tendon can be changed. The tendon of peroneus brevis is fixed in a hole in the calcaneus through a tunnel made in the lateral malleolus.
- *Split peroneus brevis tendon graft (nonanatomic):* The procedure was described by Sammarco in which the routed tendon of peroneus brevis is sutured to the reconstructed anterior talofibular and calcaneofibular ligaments. The tendon is passed through tunnels made in the talus, fibula, and the calcaneus.
- *Chrisman-Snook (nonanatomic):* Here, the peroneus brevis tendon is first split into two. One half is mobilized and it is threaded through anterior talocalcaneal ligament which is held by sutures. The tendon is then passed through hole in fibula **(Fig. 11)**. The free end of tendon is wrapped and sutured to its anterior portion near fibular tunnel.
- *Modified Coughlin technique (anatomic, **Figs. 12A and B**, and **Figs. 13A to I**):* Using the free hamstring tendon graft (Semitendinosus). I prefer this technique for simplicity and being anatomic. The hamstring tendon reconstructions are as such being increasingly preferred.

Cavovarus malalignment correction should be included in the surgical plan, if it is believed to contribute to the patient's instability or pain. Such procedures include plantar fascia release, dorsiflexion first metatarsal base closing-wedge osteotomy, lateralizing calcaneal tuberosity osteotomy, and peroneus longus to peroneus brevis transfer. Also, intrinsic ankle abnormalities are quite common in chronic instability. Soft-tissue impingement lesions, distal tibial osteophytes, loose bodies, synovitis, and osteochondral lesions of the talus are commonly dealt with arthroscopy. It is a common practice nowadays among foot and ankle surgeons to perform arthroscopy with ligament reconstruction procedure.

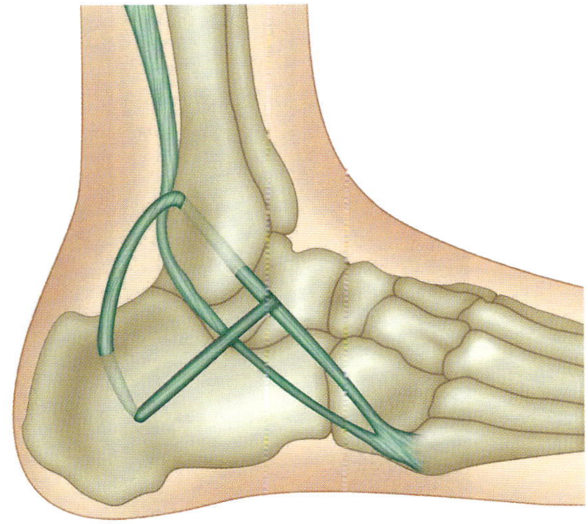

Fig. 11: Chrisman–Snook procedure.

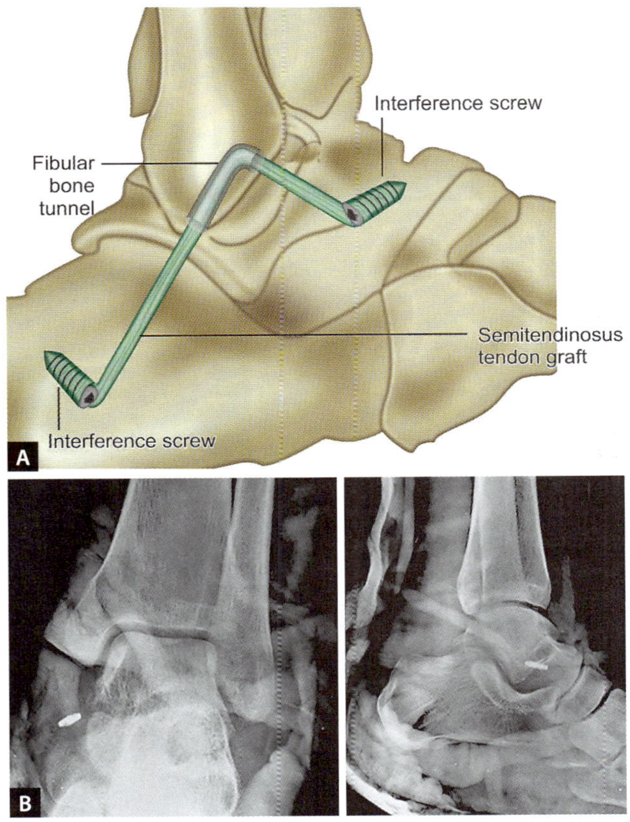

Figs. 12A and B: Modified Coughlin technique—illustration (A); I use endobutton instead of screws as there are chances of fracture with them, (B) Note the reduced joint space same patient as shown in stress radiographs previously. Endobutton was used to hold the tendon in the neck of talus and bioscrew to fix it to the calcaneum.

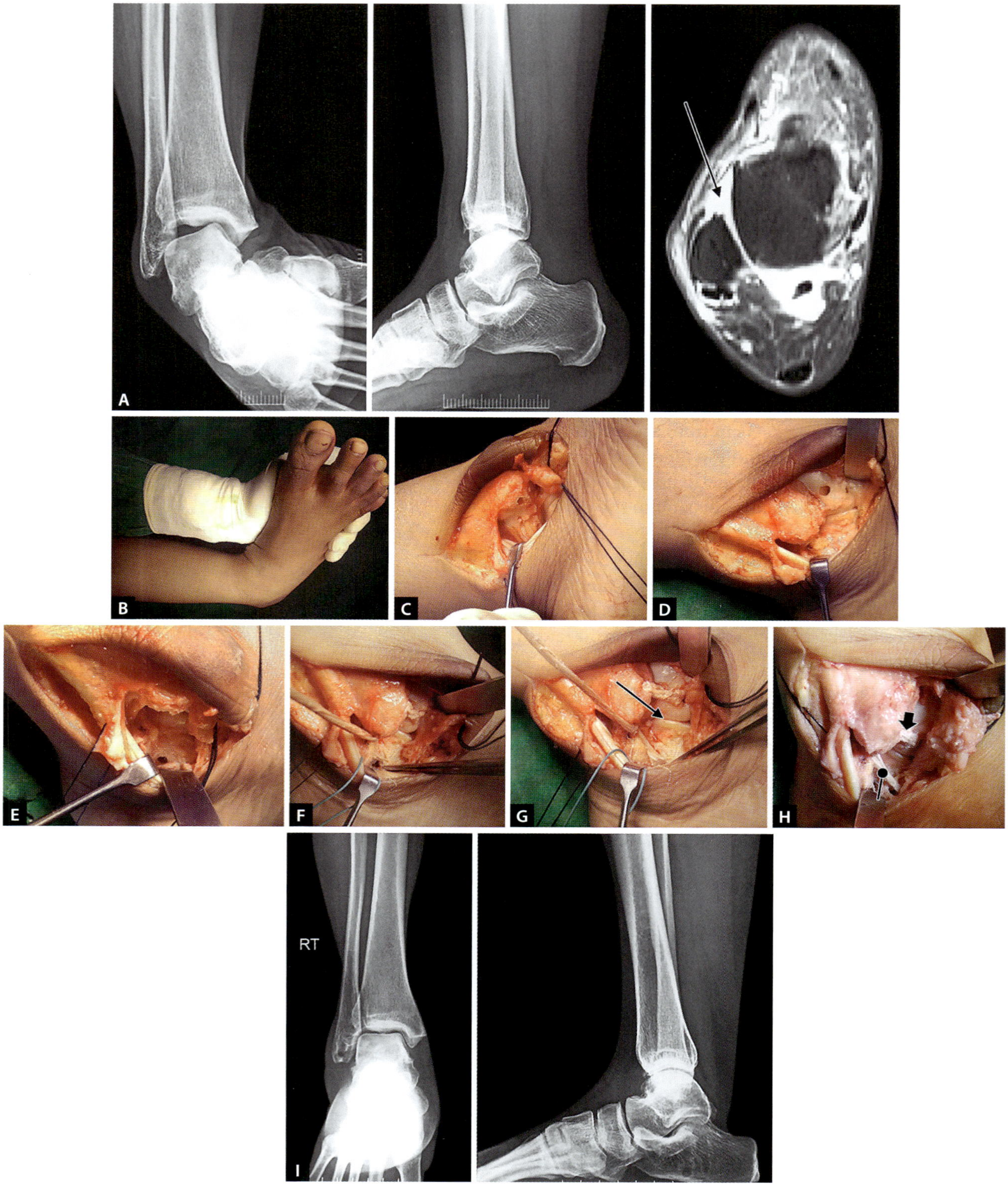

Figs. 13A to I: (A) Stress radiographs of patient with chronic (8-month-old) injury to right ankle producing complete tear of the calcaneofibular and talofibular ligaments as also demonstrated on axial MR image (arrow). Clinical demonstration of the lateral ankle laxity (B); The reconstruction of torn ligaments was done using ipsilateral semitendinosis hamstring graft. Tunnels were made in fibula (C) and talus (D) after retraction of retinaculum as a flap and identifying the footprints of torn ligament. Similarly, drill hole for anchoring the ligament into calcaneum (E) was done. The graft was passed from talus → fibula → calcaneal anchorage (F) and reversed to improve strength (G). Anchorage in talus and calcaneum was done using bioabsorbable 6 mm and 7 mm screws, respectively. The subtalar joint and ankle joint were reduced (arrow, G) and ligament sutured back in appropriate tensioning without compromising the ankle or subtalar movements. Final construct showing the talofibular (block arrow) and calcaneofibular (pointer) limbs of the reconstructed ligament (H); (I) Postoperative radiographs demonstrating well-reduced ankle joint and tunnel position in fibula, talus, and calcaneum.

Medial Repair of Chronic Instability

This is seldom symptomatic and more importantly the repair of short fibers of deltoid ligament is nearly impossible. The short span of deltoid ligament also lends it less amenable to reconstruct. The technique of DuVries has been commonly followed in dedicated sports injury center.

DuVries technique: Expose the deltoid ligament and make two incisions, one transverse and the other longitudinal, through the full thickness of the ligament, forming a cross with equal arms. Free the resulting four flaps of ligament from the underlying bone. Suture the margins of the flaps together in an imbricated manner to tighten the structure.

CONCLUSION

- Ankle sprain and ligamentous injuries to ankle are probably the most common conditions encountered in emergency room for orthopedic care.
- Conservative management in acute setting usually suffices, there are distinctive indications for operative repair of the injured ligaments.
- Some ligament injuries become chronic and need operative reconstruction later if instability and/or pain persists in a patient kept on conservative trial.
- Anatomical ligament reconstructions for managing chronic instability are gaining popularity and are possibly better, as in our experience.

CHAPTER 84

Tendo-Achilles Rupture

Manish Kumar Varshney

INTRODUCTION

Tendo-Achilles is the largest and strongest tendon forming a very important component of rhythmic ambulation apparatus. Rupture of Achilles tendon **(Figs. 1A and B)** is commonly encountered in young athletes and those engaged in recreational sports. The incidence has been increasing due to increased popularity and engagement in recreational sports and currently 10 persons in a lakh may be seen to have Achilles tendon tear. Peak age for tear is between 30 and 40 years, whence the strength has relatively declined vis-a-vis activity level of the persons. Achilles tendon ruptures are less common in developing countries where physical work and exercise are part of daily living. Not only recurrent strain but various anatomical and biomechanical factors are also responsible for tendo-Achilles tear **(Box 1)**.

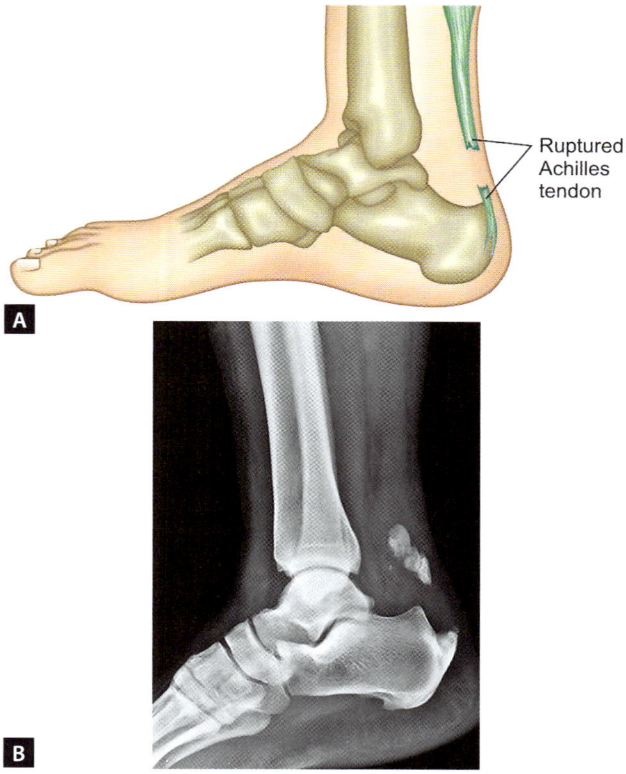

Figs. 1A and B: (A) Tendo-Achilles rupture; (B) Avulsion from bony attachment.

SITE AND MECHANISM OF TEAR

The site of rupture has been reported to occur in the myotendinous junction in 12.1%, the insertion of tendon in 4.6%, and 3.5 cm proximal to the insertion in 83%. Most of the tears occur while trying to push-off or balance with the weight-bearing forefoot on extended knee. This causes excessive strain on the tendon to push the foot down in a situation where there is already dorsiflexion of the ankle. Failure to do so results in violent dorsiflexion of the plantar flexed foot exceeding the limit of forces that tendon can bear, especially in unexpected positions and uneven surfaces. Other cause includes blow with a sharp or angulated surface directly over the tendon.

Various factors lead also to development of weakness of this tendon that would ultimately fail under less than "excessive" load. The pathological changes that have been proposed to cause weakness, and hence rupture of tendon are tendinosis, paratendinitis, and paratendinitis with tendinosis. The term tendinosis describes various degenerative changes within tendon (hyaline, mucoid, myxoid, fatty, fibrofatty, etc.) that may arise out of various above-listed

BOX 1: Predisposing and etiological factors in Achilles tendon tear.

Collagen disorders (genetic):
- Inflammatory and autoimmune mechanisms (vasculitis causing ischemia)
- Anatomical and biomechanical (eccentric loading/sudden loading with incomplete synergism of agonist muscles/inefficient plantaris which is not able to maintain tension in tendo-Achilles) predisposing factors:
  - High body mass index
  - Aging
  - Subtalar hyperpronation with hindfoot valgus
  - Equinus deformity due to tendo-Achilles contracture
  - Increased femoral anteversion
  - Short limb
  - Muscle weakness/imbalance

Environmental factors:
- Unusual endurance training in duration and intensity
- Drugs—corticosteroids especially those injected locally, fluoroquinolones
- Previous tendinopathy, tendinitis, peritendinitis with unrelenting activity (as in professional runners and jumpers)

BOX 2: The Achilles tendinopathy.

Achilles tendinopathy presents as pain and dysfunction of Achilles tendon. The term tendinitis is a misnomer as inflammatory features are missing from the tendon. It is most usefully classified into insertional (at calcaneal tuberosity) and noninsertional Achilles tendinopathy (2–6 cm proximal to insertion; watershed vascular zone). The most common cause of tendinopathy is degeneration related to overuse/increased activity. Insertional tendinopathy presents as pain and swelling at the insertion while noninsertional tendinopathy typically presents with pain and fusiform swelling/thickening/nodularity 4–6 cm proximal to insertion. There is commonly associated contracture of gastrocnemius-soleus complex. One may find intratendinous calcification on plain radiographs in noninsertional tendinopathy, while insertional pathology commonly shows Haglund deformity/insertional osteophyte.

Treatment: Nonsurgical treatment consists of rest, activity modification, heel lifts/shoe lift and shoe modification of a boot. Eccentric strengthening exercises are effective in healing phase of tendinopathy. Extracorporeal shock wave therapy is effective in tendon healing. Patients may be temporarily immobilized in ankle-foot orthosis to neutralize Achilles's tendon. Surgical treatment of insertional tendinopathy is indicated for failed conservative treatment of 4–6 weeks. The usual procedure is resection of Haglund deformity and insertional osteophytes, debridement of degenerative tendon and tendon repair to calcaneal tuberosity [±flexor hallucis longus (FHL) transfer]. If tendon degeneration is minimal, then lateral exposure + exostectomy is sufficient. For more severe degeneration midline tendon splitting approach is mostly needed for debridement and Haglund exostosis excision. More than 50% tendon detachment or complete detachment needs repair by multiple suture anchors (better in a double row fashion) which is commonly combined with FHL transfer. FHL transfer can also be considered for elderly and obese patients even with preservation of >50% of tendon.

For noninsertional tendinitis, several minimally invasive procedures have been proposed like ultrasonography guided percutaneous tenotomy, endoscopic debridement using tendinoscopy, isolated gastrocnemius recession or mini-open scraping/debridement of peritendinous hypervascular tissue. Usually, a posteromedial approach is utilized, and if paratenon is severely thickened and inflamed, then partial excision can be done. Debride the tendon to healthy tissue, if <50% of the tendon is involved the rest of tendon may be tubularized while for >50% involvement augment repair with FHL tendon transfer.

causes **(Box 2)**. Often tendinosis is not symptomatic and is realized only on rupture of tendon. Repetitive trauma or inflammatory conditions produce paratendinitis which may be later accompanied with tendinosis and is often painful before rupture. This when combined with eccentric loading/sudden loading with incomplete synergism of agonist muscles leads to rupture of tendon in an "unexpected" manner. Steroid injection(s) at the site of insertion have also been suggested to induce degenerative changes in the tendon by halting collagen remodeling and weakening fibers making it susceptible to rupture. Rupture of gastrocnemius musculotendinous junction is specifically called *tennis leg*.

PATHOANATOMY AND PATHOPHYSIOLOGY

The Achilles tendon is formed by the aponeurosis of the soleus muscle and gastrocnemius muscle at the distal end of their muscle bellies inserting terminally into posterosuperior aspect of calcaneum. The tendon derives its name from the famous legend Achilles who was the warrior of Homer's Iliad and was made invincible by his mother by immersing him in the river Styx holding his heel which remained untouched by water, and hence vulnerable. It is also interesting to note that the unit for measuring length "foot" used by Greeks originated

BOX 3: The risk factors for tendo-Achilles rupture.

- Intermittent athletics (so-called weekend warriors)
- Advancing age
- Extreme change in training level
- Tight gastrocnemius
- Poor vascularity
- Over pronation
- Cavus foot
- Recent steroids or fluoroquinolone therapy
- Infectious diseases
- Neurologic conditions
- Arteriosclerosis
- Genetic collagen abnormalities
- High serum lipid concentration

from the length of Achilles foot that was used as a standard unit to measuring length. The Achilles-tendon is the strongest ("invincible" like the Achilles) in human body called so as it bears 4–5 times the body weight during walking and up to 20 times the body weight during landing after jump. Even with these requirements the blood supply to tendon and its intrinsic repair mechanisms are not adequate. The major blood supply of the tendon is through its mesotendon, with the richest supply through the anterior mesentery which gets reduced with age-related vascular changes and atherosclerosis accounting for age-related degeneration of the tendon fibers. Thus, repetitive microtrauma may not heal well. This is the reason for increasing incidence of tendinopathy and nodular tendinitis in athletes with increasing age.

There are three major sources of blood supply coming from both posterior tibial and lateral peroneal artery:

1. Musculotendinous junction
2. Surrounding connective tissue
3. Bone-tendon junction

The vascular supply is disputably precarious in midportion or 2–6 cm from insertion of tendon, and skin directly posterior to the tendon is relatively sparsely supplied as demonstrated by the dedicated perfusion studies. This is also the site for rupture of the tendon commonly. Traumatic ruptures can, however, occur in any part of the tendon. Tenocytes from a degenerative or fatigue rupture of tendon produces more type III collagen. This collagen is less resistant and elastic to tensile forces than type I collagen predisposing to re ruptures of the tendon if similarly loaded as before. The risk factors for rupture of tendo-Achilles are given in **Box 3**. Based on the compiled etiopathogenesis various theories are forwarded for tear of the tendon as follows:

Degenerative Theory

Chronic degenerative changes and reduction of vascularity (hypoxia and impaired metabolism) with increasing age leads to rupture even in absence of excessive loads being applied. Chronic overloading, microtrauma, and physiologic alterations in the tendon structure were the factors associated with degeneration.

Biomechanical Theory

Sports play an important role in the development of tendon rupture, especially when training sessions are poorly performed. Repetitive microtrauma to the tendon without

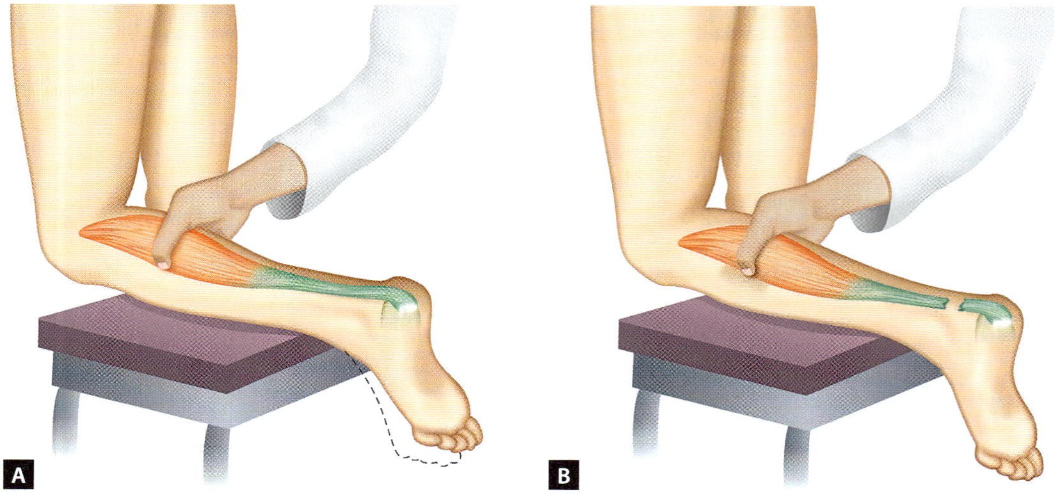

Figs. 2A and B: Thompson test. (A) Squeezing the calf muscle produces plantar flexion in normal anatomy; (B) While it is absent with a ruptured tendon.

enough time for interim repair leads to rupture even in healthy tendons without prior degenerative changes. Uncoordinated muscle contraction also may cause rupture of the tendon that is seen in athletes who return to sports too early after a long period of inactivity. Also functional over pronation, gastrocnemius-soleus insufficiency, overtraining, and repeated microtrauma from an eccentric loading of a fatigued muscle are possible causes of rupture.

Drug-associated Tendon Rupture

Steroids and quinolones are responsible for the rupture of Achilles-tendon as they decrease the tensile strength and increase the risk of rupture due to dysplasia of the collagen fibrils. Steroids instilled locally or used systemically over a long time lead to depletion of collagen reducing its strength and healing capacity. Steroids also mask the onset of symptoms of a damaging tendon due to its analgesic effect, making the patient continue their physical activity. Giving local steroid injection directly into the tendon (accidently or using wrong technique) also weakens the tendon. Fluoroquinolone causes disruption of the extracellular matrix of the cartilage, depletion of collagen, and necrosis of chondrocytes.

CLINICAL FEATURES

One must understand the difference between tendinitis and tendinosis. The former is an inflammatory condition presenting as pain and swelling that demonstrates inflammation in histopathological specimens. Tendinosis on the contrary is a degenerative condition of the tendon that may arise from disuse atrophy, aging, drugs or loss of vascularity. This predisposes to tendon rupture by virtue of weakening the same. There is no sign of active inflammation on biopsy. The most common patient profile for human Achilles tendon rupture is a male in his third or fourth decade of life that plays sport occasionally. Ratio of men to women rupture rate has been reported from 2:1 to 12:1. The mean age has been estimated between the 30s and 40s with the left Achilles being ruptured more commonly than the right, probably reflecting right side dominance with left leg pushing off. In females, the incidence increases as one reaches 60 years and more so the etiology seems to be more toward degenerative tears. One must divide the tears into acute versus chronic. The distinction is made on the basis of delay in presentation such that tears presenting after 4–6 weeks are labeled chronic. These need separate reconstruction methods from acute tears. The chronic tears arise primarily from missed initial diagnosis in up to 25% of cases.

The patient reports:

- Sudden onset of pain over back of ankle associated with snap and inability to walk (common)—the common reporting by young population is of a sudden shot or being kicked at the back of ankle without any actual contact occurring.
- Sudden feeling of jerk or snap without pain and slowness of walk (less common)
- Acute onset swelling, formation of hematoma
- Previous history of minor trauma

On examination, there is:

- Palpable gap/irregularity (old cases) on posterior aspect of lower leg in the region of tendo-Achilles
- Inability to toe-walk
- Weakness of gastrosoleus and painful plantar flexion
- *Positive test(s) for tendo-Achilles discontinuity:*
    - *Thompson-Simmonds-Doherty test* **(Figs. 2A and B)**—patient prone—squeeze the calf muscle of patient—passive plantar flexion of foot demonstrates continuous tendon [after 7 days (neglected cases) due to intervening scar formation the test may be falsely negative].
    - *Needle test of O'Brien:* Insert a hypodermic needle 10 cm above the insertion of tendo-Achilles so that its tip is just inside the tendon. Alternately, plantar and dorsiflex foot. If the outer portion of needle points cranially on dorsiflexion the tendon is supposed to be intact.
    - *Sphygmomanometer test:* Wrap the cuff around calf region and inflate it to 100 mm Hg, if then on

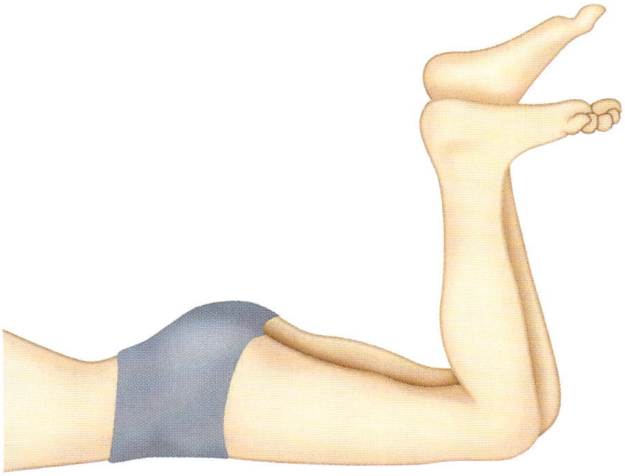

Fig. 3: Knee flexion test (Matles test) demonstrating ruptured tendon on the left side.

dorsiflexion of foot pressure rises to 140 mm Hg, then it indicates intact tendon.

- *Knee-flexion test, Matles test* ***(Fig. 3)****:* With patient prone, ask the patient to flex knee to 90°, neutral position or dorsiflexion of ankle suggests torn tendon.
- *Reverse Silfverskiöld test (not very popular):* With knee in full extension (ankle dorsiflexion here is solely restricted by tendo-Achilles) measure the range of dorsiflexion at ankle (more on injured side compared to the normal side).
    - *Single leg heel raise test:* Ask the patient to stand on injured leg with heel raised (not possible with torn Achilles tendon).

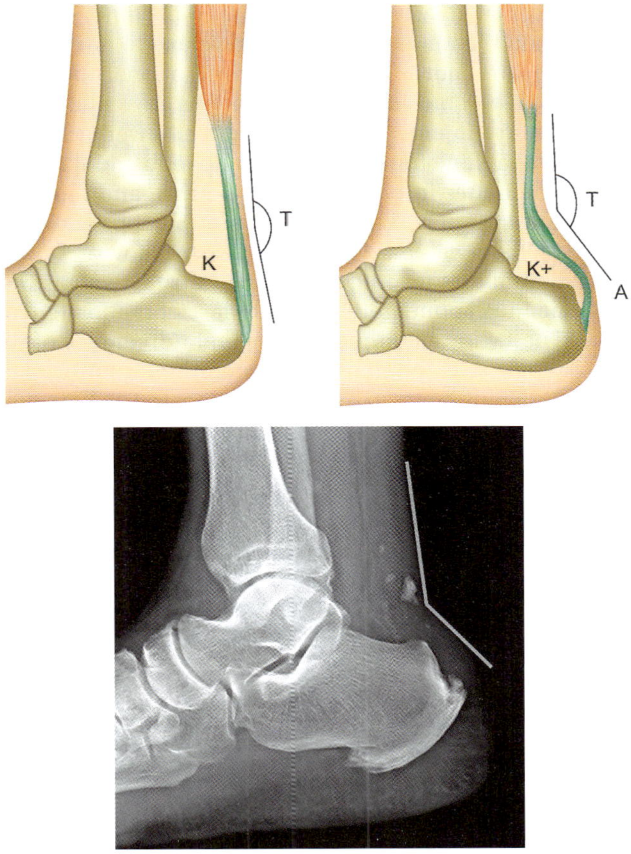

Fig. 4: *Toygar's sign*. The reduced T-angle is demonstrated in radiograph of a patient with tendo-Achilles rupture.

INVESTIGATIONS

Radiology

- Loss of posterior border of Kager's triangle (fat-filled triangular space in front of tendo-Achilles) or complete disappearance is suggestive of torn tendon
- *Toygar's sign* ***(Fig. 4)****:* It involves measurement of angle of posterior skin-surface seen on lateral projection. With disappearance of triangle and tendon rupture the angle reduces to 130–150°.

Ultrasonography

Ultrasonography is the investigation of choice provided it is done by an experienced radiologist. It reasonably demonstrates the tear, edema at the ruptured ends, fibrosis, hematoma, tenosynovitis, etc.

Magnetic Resonance Imaging

It is done, if infective pathology is suspected or good ultrasonography is unavailable as often a "short-cut" to good clinical examination.

MANAGEMENT

Primarily for high complication rates of surgery ***conservative treatment*** had been classically followed comprising mainly of immobilizing ankle in below-knee cast in plantar flexion for 4 weeks followed by plantar flexion orthotics for another 4 weeks and then gradual mobilization. They are aimed to preserve the mesentry and paratenon that helps regenerate the tendon. The results had been equivalent to surgical repair but possibly the re-rupture rates could be higher as often the surgeons now do a repair with augmentation that should be superior to the repaired fibrous tissue. John Hunter suffered from Achilles-tendon tear himself that was managed conservatively by calf bandaging and raising the shoe heel. Conservative management is preferable, if there is less than 5 mm gap in ultrasonography, <10 mm on neutral position and "reasonable apposition" of the tendon (say 75% minimum) on 20° of plantar flexion. Eccentric strengthening exercises are essential part of rehabilitation.

The *surgical management* of Achilles-tendon tear depends on the chronicity and defect size. The contraindications for surgical treatment include arterial insufficiency, poor skin and soft-tissue quality, poorly controlled medical comorbidities (diabetes, immunocompromised states, Cushing's, smokers, BMI >30, vascular disease), inability to follow the prolonged rehabilitative protocol.

- For an acute tear, if the tendon ends can be approximated then an end-to-end suturing with modified Kessler method (**Fig. 5**, other like Bunnell and Krackow are equally effective) and plantaris augmentation is preferable. Percutaneous method of Ma and Griffith is acceptable in experienced hands. The tendon is approximated by passing sutures multiple times through skin and the tendon using tiny incisions to bury knots. The repair is not as strong as the conventional open end-to-end repair but wound complications are reduced. The sural nerve injury is reportedly higher. Newer technique using a midline transverse incision (Webb and Banister) may be better in preserving sural nerve and reducing re-rupture rates. If the ends cannot be approximated, then reinforcements will be required as follows:

- Lindholm's technique **(Fig. 6)**—turn down gastrocnemius aponeurotic flap with fascial reinforcement. The Lynn technique involves reinforcement of the repair with plantaris augmentation. Teuffer used peroneus brevis to reinforce the repair. The last one is uncommonly used.
- Other reinforcements uncommonly practiced (if ever)—artificial tendon implants, marlex, and collagen prostheses.
- Use of fibrin glue—not favored clinically but may be used as supplement to suture repair.

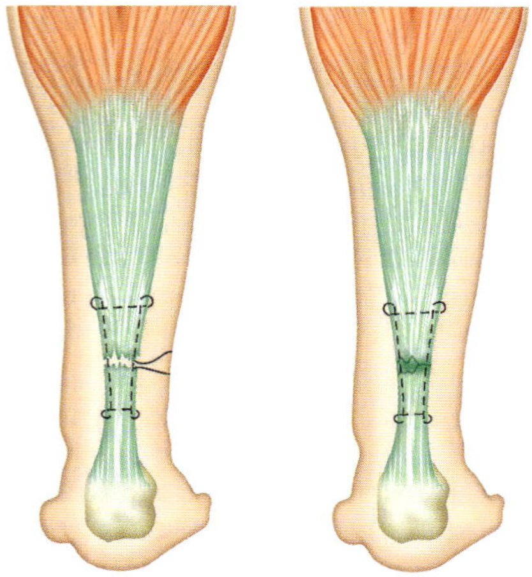

Fig. 5: Kessler technique of repairing ruptured Achilles tendon.

- Use of PPRP—this may bring the platelet derived growth factors that improve repair speed and quality, literature support for routine use and advantage is lacking.
- *Mini-Open Indirect Repair using Achillon System (Newdeal, Lyon, France):* Wound complications are the greatest worry after conventional open repair of Achilles-tendon. This has led improvement in techniques to minimize soft tissue trauma logically. This system reduces wound complications and scarring but the repair is less powerful than the Krackow technique especially if there is a previous history of severe tendinosis. In latter case with double Krackow technique is required.

▪ For old tears (>2 days to 8 weeks old), the management is better guided by classification system as follows:
  - *Myerson's classification:*
    - *Type-1 defect:* 1–2 cm long → End-to-end repair and posterior compartment fasciotomy
    - *Type-2 defect:* 2–5 cm → V-Y lengthening with or without tendon transfer
    - *Type-3 defect:* >5 cm → Tendon transfer alone or combined with V-Y advancement and augmentation.
  - *Kuwada's classification:*
    - *Type I:* Partial tear → Conservative management
    - *Type II:* Complete tear <3 cm defect → end-to-end repair
    - *Type III:* 3–6 cm defect → debride + tendon transfer ± augmentation
    - *Type IV:* >6 cm defect → debride + tendon graft ± augmentation.

I prefer flexor hallucis longus (FHL) tendon augmentation **(Figs. 7A to D)** for defects up to 5 cm. Usually after debridement and freshening; the ends can be approximated with 30° of plantar flexion, and then they are sutured with number 5, ethibond. The repair is then augmented with FHL tendon located from the same wound and tunneled through

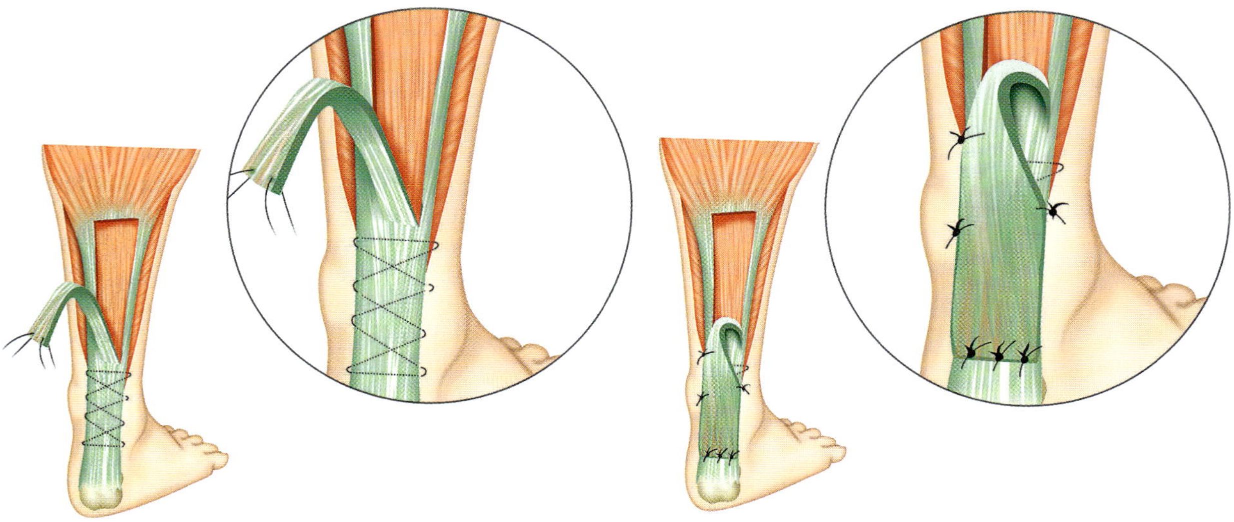

Fig. 6: Lindholm's technique of augmenting repair using tendon sheath turndown.

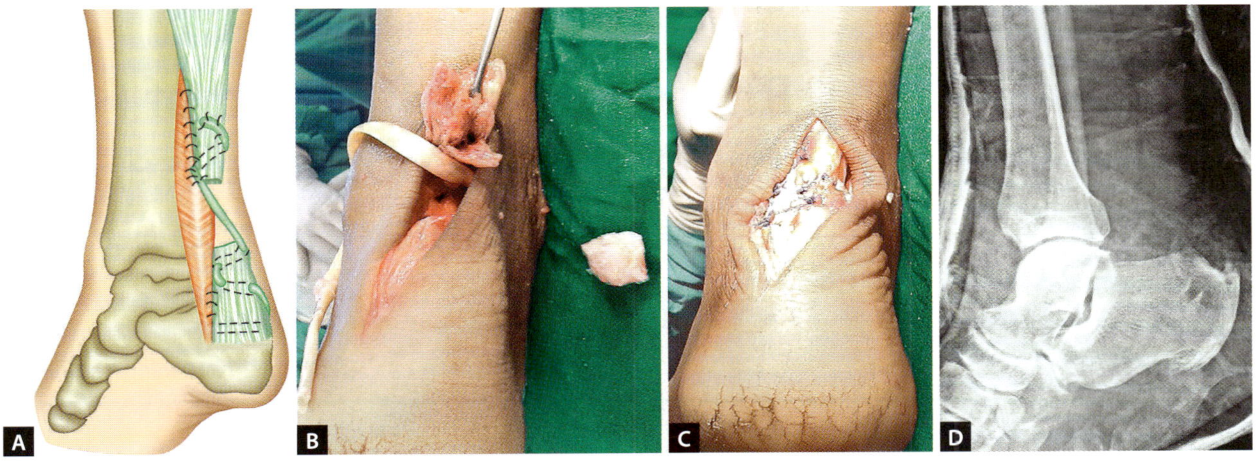

Figs. 7A to D: Flexor hallucis longus (FHL), augmentation for reconstruction of chronic rupture of tendo-Achilles (my preference). (A) Illustration of the technique; (B) Harvesting the FHL and cleaning dystrophic calcification from the tendon rupture site; (C) suturing and reconstruction; (D) Postoperative radiograph.

calcaneum distally. The tendon is long enough to be wrapped around the repair one and half times. Also I suture the FHL tendon loop to the Achilles-tendon using 1-0 vicryl suture, the strength of FHL tendon is 13 times less than the native Achilles-tendon strength, while the flexor digitorum longus (FDL) is 27 times as weak. The chief advantages of using FHL are that it is in phase to the tendo-Achilles in the gait cycle, and provides a strong tendon for repair. Some surgeons used to prefer peroneus brevis + plantaris combination previously (White and Kraynick and Teuffer), but it is 18 times weaker and there are concerns of sural nerve damage and loss of eversion strength. Also the tendon is located in a separate compartment that is slightly distant from the operative site.

For defects >5 cm approximation is not possible so additional V-Y technique of Abraham and Pankovich is done proximally followed by FHL tendon augmentation. The Bosworth technique of using the median raphe of tendon and turn down into the repair site is another described method, I find it is weaker than the FHL tendon augmented repair and also the technique requires a large incision.

Free Tendon Transfer

Tobin described using fascia lata for chronic tendo-Achilles rupture. Though the results were satisfactory but delayed wound healing was the complication in some patients. Free gracilis tendon grafts can also be used and patients returned to work by 2 years. Achilles-tendon allograft has also been used which can act as a scaffold for migrating host cells.

Complications of Surgical Management

- Skin necrosis
- Inability to close the skin
- Infection
- Hematoma formation
- Wound dehiscence
- *Formation of chronic ulcer/sinus:*
    - Re-rupture
    - Secondary deformities such as equinus and valgus, if the repair was too tight with augmentation
    - Dorsiflexion lag for lax repair
    - Functional deficit and chronic pain is seen in half of the patients irrespective of the method chosen
    - Deep vein thrombosis (DVT), pulmonary embolism may be seen as in all orthopedic lower limb surgeries.

Postoperative Management Protocol

- Immobilize in cast or slab in plantar flexion (20°) for 2 weeks
- Apply posterior splint in plantar flexion after 2 weeks till 4 weeks maintaining plantar flexion
- Remove sutures at 14–18 days
- Allow passive plantar flexion and active dorsiflexion between 2 weeks and 4 weeks. Provide a boot with heel raise.
- 4–6 weeks—allow partial weight bearing and physiotherapy as above.
- 6–8 weeks—remove heel from boot and start passive dorsiflexion stretching.
- 8–12 weeks—allow full weight bearing on crutch support. Continue muscle strengthening exercises and gradually wean crutches by 12th week.

CONCLUSION

- Although tendo-Achilles is the strongest tendon of the body, it is prone to rupture following trauma or attrition of the fibers in elderly.
- Most of the tendon ruptures occur in the high stress pure tendinous region 3–4 cm proximal to insertion.
- The diagnosis is quite obvious clinically by palpating the discontinuity of the tendon fibers and inability to perform a powerful push-off or toe-walk. Various tests are described additionally to confirm the findings. Ultrasonography is a good aid in determining the gap at the rupture site, as mostly the treatment guidance can be obtained by this investigation.
- For small gaps <5 mm conservative treatment by immobilizing in plantar flexion would suffice. However, for larger gaps repair of the tendon (for acute tears) or reconstruction of the tendon by using variously described augmentation techniques is better.

CHAPTER 85

Rheumatoid Affection of Foot, Diabetic Foot Disease, and Neuropathic (Charcot) Foot

Manish Kumar Varshney

INTRODUCTION

The ankle joint and small joints of the foot commonly get involved in various inflammatory disorders. The stress at the joints and incurring microtrauma possibly are responsible for their frequent involvement. Also, being peripheral; the joint temperature changes make the environment a bit challenging to maintain homeostasis. The common inflammatory disorders affecting the foot include:

- Autoimmune diseases
- Rheumatoid arthritis (RA)
- *Seronegative inflammatory arthritis:*
  - Ankylosing spondylitis
  - Psoriatic arthritis
  - Inflammatory bowel disease
  - Reactive arthritis (Reiter's syndrome)
  - Crystalline arthropathies (metabolic)—gout, pseudogout, and calcium hydroxyapatite crystal arthritis
- Infective (septic, tubercular, and fungal)

RHEUMATOID AFFECTION OF FOOT

Rheumatoid arthritis commonly affects the foot. 17% of patients with RA present with symptoms affecting the joints of the feet initially. With progress, 89% of patients have arthritis of foot and ankle. The foot degeneration progresses in various stages in rheumatoid affection **(Box 1)**. To improve the understanding, feet can be divided into three regions as they have characteristic involvement that is treated specifically.

Rheumatoid Affection of Forefoot (Figs. 1A and B)

Forefoot involvement is seen often within 1 year of diagnosis.

- The earliest manifestation of RA of the forefoot is synovitis of the metatarsophalangeal (MTP) joints. There is articular cartilage disruption and weakening of the ligament-bone structures.
- Due to fluid distention of the joint capsule the toes sublux dorsally at the MTP joint.
- The balance between flexor and extensor mechanisms and joint capsules maintains the normal alignment of MTP joints. In RA, imbalance occurs with progressive dorsal subluxation of MTP joints due to overpowering antigravity muscles.

BOX 1: Stages of progression of deformities in rheumatoid foot.

- *Stage 1:* Discomfort, synovitis without significant joint space narrowing; no bony deformity
- *Stage 2:* Minimal erosive articular changes; early involvement without fixed deformity
- *Stage 3:* No significant joint erosion; soft-tissue deformity present
- *Stage 4:* Severe hallux valgus, lesser MTP-joint dislocation with fixed hammer-toe or claw-toe deformities, articular destruction, pes planovalgus, and hindfoot arthritis

(MTP: metatarsophalangeal)

- With disease advancement, there is pressure atrophy of fat pad over protruding metatarsal heads formation of callosities and ulceration.
- Flexion contracture of the middle and distal digital joints of the lesser toes and interphalangeal joint of the great toe **(Figs. 1A and B)**.
- Finally, dislocation of MTP joint occurs and the proximal phalanx is ankylosed to dorsal aspect of metatarsal head.

Management

Nonoperative treatment is aimed to:

- Maintaining a good gait pattern
- Independent ambulation or restoring adequate gait by minimizing inflammation, reducing pain, and supporting inflamed joints

Patients are advised extra deep shoes with a wide, high toe box, and a molded insert that allows for bony prominences. Orthotic devices help to redistribute plantar weight-bearing forces. Semirigid orthosis is more effective than a soft orthosis. Rocker soles and steel shanks may help to relieve midfoot pain and counteract stiffness. Toe sleeves and spacers, corn pads and debridement of plantar callosities may also help.

Surgery

Surgery usually is required in advanced disease due to pain and increasing deformity and disability.

Synovectomy

Synovectomy of the MTP joints is indicated for the treatment of painful joints early in the disease process, before significant

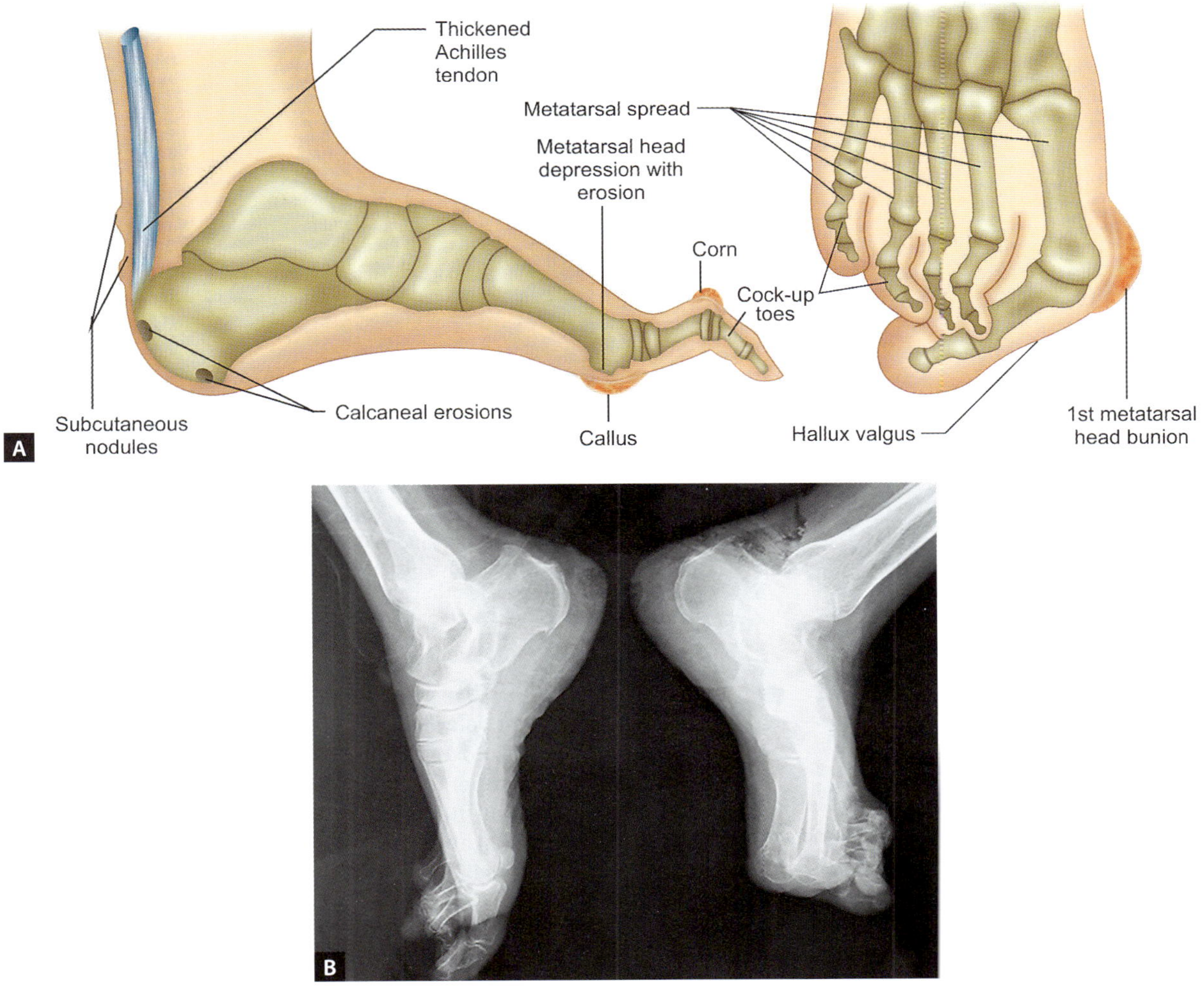

Figs. 1A and B: Rheumatoid foot. (A) Pathoanatomy and deformities; (B) Radiograph.

deformity has occurred. This procedure is contraindicated in the presence of MTP joint subluxation or dislocation or with the formation of intractable plantar keratoses. Synovectomy decreases distention of MTP joints and reduces the soft-tissue deformation. For multiple joint synovectomies, use a second and/or fourth interspace incision to expose adjacent joints. Resect proliferative synovial tissue on the medial and dorsolateral aspects especially any synovium beneath the collateral ligaments. Carry the resection as far in the plantar direction as possible.

Forefoot arthroplasty is done primarily for the MTP joint deformity. Joint resection is done to realign phalanges loosely with the metatarsals. Forefoot arthroplasty relieves pain, corrects deformity, and potentially improves ambulatory function. Importantly, it allows to wear footwear.

Techniques of Forefoot Arthroplasty

- *Fowler's procedure* ***(Figs. 2A and B)****:* Through a dorsal transverse incision, removal of the base or up to one-half of the proximal phalanges, shortening and contouring of the metatarsal heads to provide a uniform weight-bearing surface. Also an ellipse of plantar skin is removed to provide a good fat pad.
- *Hoffmann's procedure:* Removal of metatarsal heads through transverse plantar incision.
- *Thompson and Mann technique* ***(Fig. 3)****:* Metatarsophalangeal joint is exposed through dorsal approach (through incisions in second and fourth webspaces). Metatarsal head and base of proximal phalanx are removed and joint realigned.

Commonly the Kirschner wires for stabilization of the arthrodesis are used but interfragmentary screw can be used if bone stock is strong.

Rheumatoid Affection of Midfoot

Involvement of the first metatarsocuneiform joint is most common and may lead to instability with collapse of the medial longitudinal arch, with or without hallux valgus **(Fig. 4)**. This is partly managed by arthrodesis of the first metatarsocuneiform joint and also possibly fusing the medial cuneiform navicular articulation. A percutaneous lengthening of the Achilles tendon should be added, if the tendon is tight and dorsiflexion of the ankle to at least 10° is not possible.

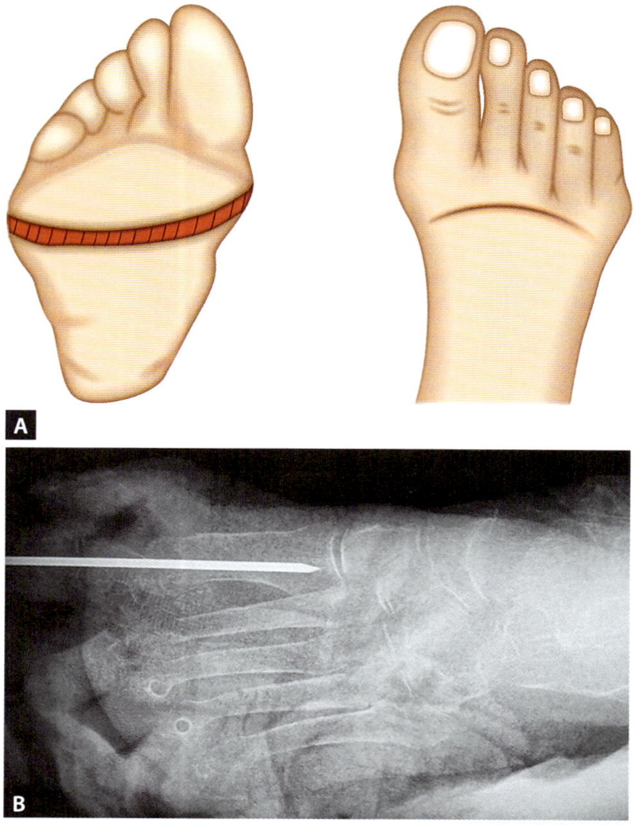

Figs. 2A and B: Fowler's procedure. (A) Incisions; (B) Radiographs after reconstruction.

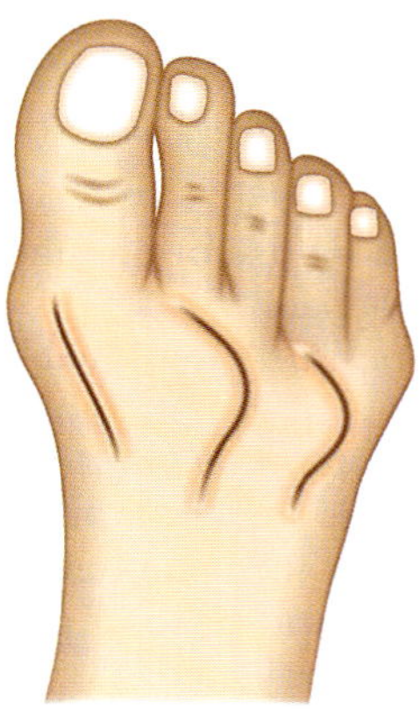

Fig. 3: Thompson and Mann procedure incisions.

Rheumatoid Affection of Hindfoot

Involvement of the hindfoot is not uncommon in chronic RA. More than half to three-fourths of the patients (females more common) with chronic RA have involvement of the subtalar and midtarsal joints. Isolated talonavicular arthritis may be one of the earliest findings with rheumatoid arthritis.

The typical findings with chronic RA are midfoot and hindfoot pain, swelling, flattening of the longitudinal arch, and progressive valgus of the hindfoot.

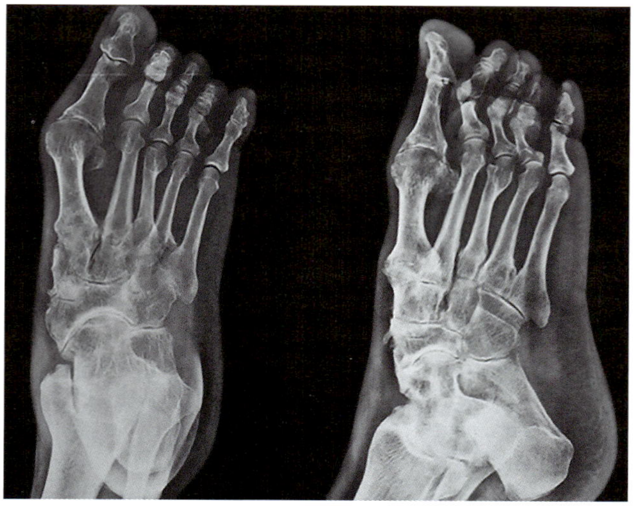

Fig. 4: The involvement of midfoot in rheumatoid arthritis especially the first metatarsophalangeal joint with associated hallux valgus. There is prominent talonavicular arthrosis. In the forefoot, there is claw toe and hammer toe deformity of the toes. The hind foot is also involved but less than midfoot and forefoot.

Management

Conservative approach should always be tried due to poor results of mostly joint mutilating surgeries. The measures include proper footwear, rest to relieve swollen and inflamed joints from the stresses of weight-bearing, padding, and longitudinal arch supports.

Surgery is only indicated in progressive deformity with unrelenting pain refractory to conservative treatment. The following methods or a combination of these can be used.

- *Synovectomy:* May give good pain relief if significant articular damage has not occurred.
- *Subtalar arthrodesis* ***(Figs. 5A and B)****:* A subtalar joint arthrodesis is indicated to correct heel valgus, if the midtarsal joint and tibiotalar joint have been spared by the rheumatoid destructive process. Instead a triple arthrodesis is indicated if the latter structures are also involved. The goal of surgical treatment is to restore hindfoot stability in the appropriate-position 5–10° of hindfoot valgus. Subtalar arthrodesis results in less rigid foot but still it limits talonavicular motion to about 26%, and limits calcaneocuboid motion to about 56%. Flexor digitorum longus (FDL) tendon transfer to navicular or first cuneiform has been suggested to improve function and stabilize talonavicular joint. Subtalar arthrodesis can be performed both by an open or arthroscopic technique. The open procedure is associated with higher rate of sural nerve damage and a painful scar while the arthroscopic procedure is associated with hardware related complications. One of the common complications is nonunion following arthrodesis and that has minimally improved over time. The risk factors for nonunion are obesity, smoking, and previous infection.
  - Standard approach to the subtalar joint involves two incisions, one medial and one lateral. Lateral incision provides exposure to the entire subtalar joint complex.

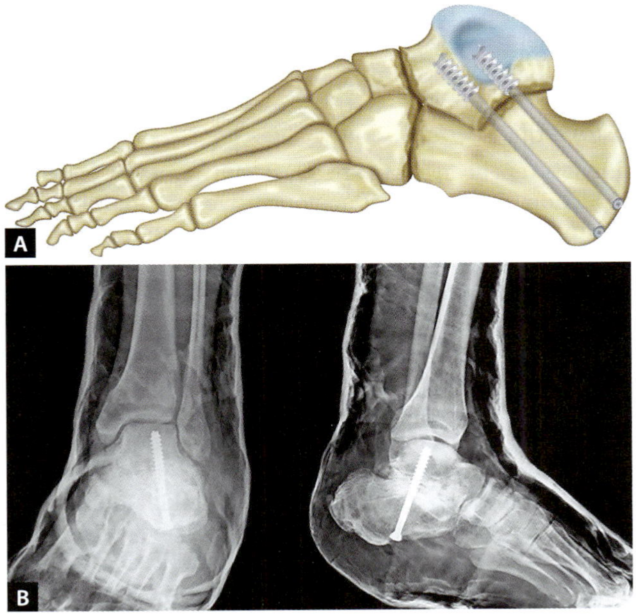

Figs. 5A and B: Subtalar arthrodesis. (A) Illustration of the procedure; (B) Radiographs after subtalar arthrodesis procedure.

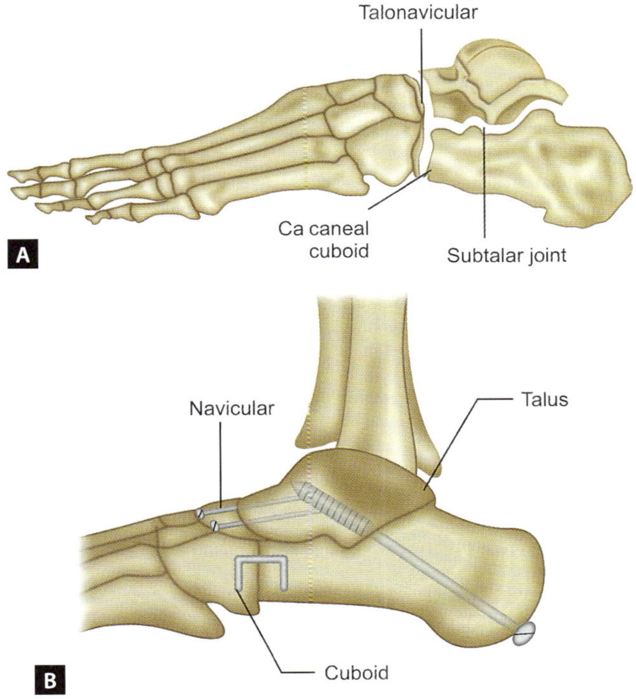

Figs. 7A and B: Triple arthrodesis. (A) The joints that are fused; (B) Illustration of various hardwares that can be used for obtaining fusion.

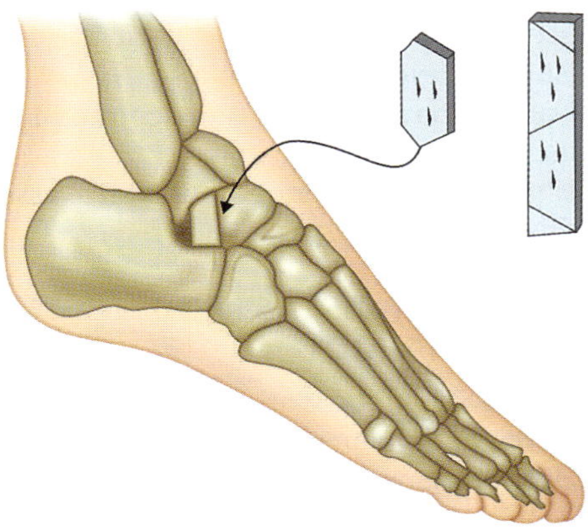

Fig. 6: Grice subtalar arthrodesis.

Resection of the joint surfaces is readily achieved through this approach after removal of the fibro-fatty contents of the sinus tarsi. Identify the calcaneocuboid joint which is found just distal to the anterior beak of the calcaneus. The talonavicular joint lies superior and medial to calcaneocuboid joint. The cartilage of the posterior facet of the calcaneus is "scraped" to its subchondral bone plate. The cartilages of both joint surfaces are removed by this "scrapping" or "chipping" technique. Small power burr and needle-nose rongeur are helpful to do this. The medial incision provides exposure to the head and neck of the talus to allow insertion of the fixation screw (AO/ASIF 6.5 mm cancellous screw) from neck of talus to calcaneus to give rigid fixation.

- Extra-articular method of subtalar arthrodesis has been advocated by Grice **(Fig. 6)** in patients with no gross skeletal deformities but having instability of hindfoot. This technique is typically favored in children as it does not affect further bone growth. It involves placing a bone graft (typically obtained from tibia) laterally in the sinus tarsi to prevent valgus malalignment of the foot. Grice advocated this for the management of pes valgus due to flaccid paralysis muscle imbalance due to poliomyelitis, but it has also been popularly used for patients with cerebral palsy (spastic valgus deformity). This procedure has also been used by the favorites for management of calcaneocavus, calcaneovalgus, talocalcaneal coalition, congenital vertical talus, and isolated post-traumatic arthritis of the subtalar joint. In patients with prior calcaneal fracture there is already a loss of heel height and a relatively horizontal talus which limits ankle dorsiflexion. Subtalar bone block wedge restores native talus alignment. Varus deformity is not well corrected by the procedure so Grice procedure should not be used for the same; also the procedure is contraindicated for rigid deformed hindfoot. After Grice arthrodesis if triple arthrodesis is ever needed then it is easier as the method minimally affects the alignment of the joint. Prerequisite for performing the Grice arthrodesis is that the foot should be flexible and correctable passively to a plantigrade position.

- *Triple arthrodesis* ***(Figs. 7A and B)****:* This is a preferred method as RA is a progressive disorder and gradually involves nearby joints other than subtalar joint even if subtalar arthrodesis is done. Typically, it is done for advanced disease with involvement of the subtalar joint

BOX. 2: The indications and contraindications of triple arthrodesis.

Definition statement—triple arthrodesis is the fusion of three joints around calcaneum that include talonavicular, calcaneocuboid, and talocalcaneal joint. The method was described primarily from the increased risk of talonavicular arthritis emanating from the subtalar fusion and continued pain.

Indications:
- Rheumatoid arthritis
- Valgus foot deformity that fails conservative management
- Collapsing pes valgus deformity
- Ruptured tibialis posterior tendon with advanced collapse of the foot
- Tarsal coalition
- Tarsal arthritis—post-traumatic
- Varus foot deformity as it is not addressed by subtalar arthritis well
- Cavus foot
- Cavo adductovarus
- Talipes equinovarus late stages and neglected cases in adolescence or later
- Lateral ankle instability
- Ankle equinus
- Neuromuscular disease—cerebral palsy, polio, Charcot-Marie-tooth disease

Contraindications:
- Feet that can be otherwise managed with bracing or soft-tissue procedures
- Smoking as it is associated with nonunion or painful fibrous union especially of the talonavicular joint

with more severe and irreducible valgus of the hindfoot. The triple arthrodesis not only stabilizes the hindfoot but also corrects the deformity. The objective is to obtain a plantigrade foot. Therefore, a triple arthrodesis **(Box. 2)** is usually necessary. Ryerson, in 1923, originally described the procedure that underwent various modifications primarily related to the fixation methods. Ryerson originally used cast treatment for fixation of the surfaces.

Technique

Classically, the Ollier incision was used for performing the procedure that ran from the tip of the fibular malleolus across the sinus tarsi to the dorsal region of the talonavicular joint. Ollier incision poses obvious potential hazards to specific vital structures including sensory nerve/extensor tendons, and deeper neurovascular structures. To avoid the same, many surgeons prefer two-incision approach. The lateral one is a straight incision, 1 cm inferior to the tip of the fibular malleolus. Extend it distally over the anterolateral border of the calcaneus and cuboid to expose the subtalar and calcaneocuboid joints. The medial incision extends from the region of the medial malleolus distal to the level of the naviculocuneiform joint and provides exposure of the talonavicular joint, as well as access for fixation of the subtalar joint. Traditionally, the triple arthrodesis procedure involved resecting wedges of bone from the joint surfaces of the tarsal area and applying plaster cast to compress the surfaces against each other. The modern approach involves anatomic dissection with minimal bone resection and rigid internal fixation. Midtarsal joint surface preparation followed by subtalar joint surface resection is done. The forefoot is then positioned by derotating it, correcting the plantar or dorsiflexion as required and abduction of the hindfoot is done finally. If there is bone defect or otherwise for larger deformity correction bone grafting may be necessary if the cut surfaces do not appose well. After temporary fixation, the joints are fixed by rigid internal fixation using 6.5 mm cancellous screws or staples.

Postoperative Period

Patient is kept in an above knee cast with a window for wound inspection. During initial postoperative period, the patient is managed for wound by dressing and managing drain that is quite significant due to cut cancellous surfaces. From 5th day to weeks, the patient is kept in cast and bone surfaces are allowed to heel. Patient is encouraged to move knee and is allowed nonweight-bearing walk. Sutures are removed at 14 days and the cast can be bivalved for wound inspection regularly initially. After 4 weeks, the cast is generally removed and movements at ankle, toes, and foot are encouraged though the patient is still kept nonweight bearing. It is preferable to keep the patient in ankle brace [knee-ankle-foot orthosis (KAFO)] that helps to reduce edema associated with ongoing physiotherapy. Physical therapy and weight-bearing is allowed from 8th week in the form of toe-touch for 3–4 weeks then partial weight-bearing on foot for 3–4 weeks followed by full weight bearing at 4.5–5 months if radiological union is seen.

Complications

- Wound complications—Eschar formation, necrosis and dehiscence, and infection
- Persistent or reversed deformity
- Bony nonunion typically is more common at the talonavicular joint.
- Persistent pain due to poor preoperative assessment and arthritis at other joints

DIABETIC FOOT DISEASE AND NEUROPATHIC FOOT

Approximately, 7% of the world's population is estimated to have diabetes, and the percentage is expected to reach 8.3% by 2030. Its prevalence in developing countries especially is rising at an alarming rate and added to it are the undetected cases comprise vast majority due to lack of awareness. Diabetes mellitus (DM) was considered a dismal disease before the discovery of insulin in 1922, as the morbidity was unrelenting resulting in quick mortality. Diabetes affects nearly all the vital systems over a period of time resulting in reduced function, limiting the repair process, and hence a progressive downhill course. Due to chronicity of course of the disease, it is responsible for substantial consumption of healthcare resources. To an orthopedic surgeon diabetic foot disease, surgical complications, and osteoporosis are the relevant changes associated with DM. Complications associated with diabetic foot disease are the most common reason and patients with DM are admitted under orthopedic care. Diabetic foot disease presents over a spectrum of neuroarthropathy and foot deformity, infection (subtle infections to wet gangrene), and ulceration. The lifetime risk of diabetic foot ulcer is nearly 15%. Patients who previously had foot ulcer or infection, or have undergone a partial or whole foot amputation are at the greatest risk of developing a foot ulcer or infection. The optimal care in these situations depends not only on the vascularity of the limb but also on the good glycemic control, patient cooperation, and preventive foot care. Because DM is multiorgan dysfunction, care should be provided by a team that includes an orthopedic surgeon, an endocrinologist, an infectious disease specialist, a vascular surgeon, a plastic surgeon, a physical therapist, and an orthotist (pedorthist).

Etiology

The primary factor responsible for the development of diabetic foot disease is diabetic neuropathy and the severity of foot disease is proportional to neuropathy. Neuropathy is the result of both metabolic and vascular factors. Neuropathy also limits patient's functional ability, balance, and coordination; and sensations and autonomic function are disturbed. Sensory neuropathy affects 75% of patients suffering from DM. It begins distally and progresses proximally in a stocking glove pattern. Somatic sensory neuropathy is length dependent; involving the longest nerves, so a taller person with longer nerves is at greatest risk. There is a decreased awareness of light touch and diminished proprioception (large-fiber neuropathy) that is quickly followed by loss of pain and temperature perception (small-fiber function). Loss of proprioception is estimated by using Semmes-Weinstein 5.07 (10 g) monofilament. Significant population report neuropathic pain that is worse in the evening that is commonly bilateral and symmetric. The pain may be reported as paresthesia (burning, tingling, allodynia, electric shock, deep-shooting pain, cramping, or aching). Vibratory sensation and deep tendon reflexes are last to disappear.

Motor neuropathy causes intrinsic muscle dysfunction producing claw and hammer toes secondary. The fixed toe deformities increase pressure under the toe tips and metatarsal head. This is accentuated by progressive Achilles-tendon contracture. These changes with loss of sensation predisposes to pressure ulcerations. Autonomic neuropathy presents as resting tachycardia, exercise intolerance, loss of thermoregulation, orthostatic hypotension, constipation, gastroparesis, erectile dysfunction, sudomotor dysfunction, impaired neurovascular function (loss of blood vessel tone), "brittle diabetes", and hypoglycemic autonomic failure. The normal hyperemic response following injury is lost, so ability to fight infection is reduced. Dry and scaly skin predisposes to cracks and fissures allowing easy access to bacteria causing infection. Vascular disease is extremely common in patients with DM and typical atherosclerotic findings in patients with diabetes include diffuse and circumferential plaque formation in the middle layer of blood vessels (as opposed to intimal layer in general population). The advanced glycation end-products accumulate in the walls of blood vessels impacting local perfusion and triggering cytokine release. Secondary degenerative calcification thins the lumen and gives vessels a rigid pipe-like consistency. Typically, disease begins at or just distal to the popliteal trifurcation involving all the three arteries; and in later stages, the femoroiliac vessels are also involved. This further compromises the blood flow.

Loss of sensation, increased pressure due to deformity, poor blood flow, and cracked skin make the person vulnerable to progressive infected ulcers that are difficult to control unless above factor(s) are mitigated. Sores are fast to develop, as tissue dies within 1 hour in such conditions, even walking that intermittently puts pressure causes development of preulcerative conditions that progress to complete ulceration. The triad of neuropathy, foot deformity, and repetitive trauma creates a high risk of ulcer formation. All attempts must be made to identify peripheral neuropathy and vascular disease to limit risk of ulceration/infection by appropriate intervention(s).

Examination

Examination should include evaluation of the patient's gait, posture, sensations, motor examination, range of motion (ROM) of various joints, and skin coverage. Fixed deformities increase chances of pressures ulcerations. Corns and calluses should be recorded in detail. Thin, shiny, atrophic, and hairless skin with thick toe-nails indicate vascular insufficiency. Preulcerative conditions include areas with intradermal hemorrhage or blistering. Record foot deformities and their suppleness. Sensation should be charted and acceptable limit is the ability to perceive a Semmes-Weinstein size 5.07 nylon monofilament wire applied perpendicular to the skin. Vibration sensation may carry a greater sensitivity for detecting impaired sensation. Record all peripheral pulses and capillary refill. Examination of the sole should include identifying any sharp irregularities in the inside or presence of foreign body, deformity of foot produces specific abnormal wear patterns.

Imaging

Plain radiographs provide information on joint alignment, soft-tissue gas (infection and wet gangrene), vascular calcifications, foreign bodies, and osteomyelitis. Focal demineralization is the earliest radiographic change related to osteomyelitis. The classical findings of osteomyelitis—periosteal reaction, osteolysis, and bone destruction are not commonly seen due to altered physiology. Ultrasonography may help in identifying associated abscess that can be simultaneously aspirated. Doppler studies are valuable in evaluating the vascularity status. The results of arterial Doppler are reported in terms of toe pressures and the ratio of ankle pressure to arm Doppler arterial pressure. An acceptable level for healing is toe pressures > 40 mm Hg or an ankle-brachial index > 45 mm Hg. Absolute toe pressure is a better predictor of healing than the ankle-brachial index. MRI is considered the best modality for evaluating the soft-tissue and bone marrow changes associated with osteomyelitis. There is confluent hypointensity on T1-weighted images that is further elaborated on gadolinium-contrast injection and also differentiates abscess and necrotic tissue. The problem is differentiating midfoot neuroarthropathy (Charcot joint) from infection changes. Usually, changes that extend beyond subchondral bone proximally indicate infection. Triple-phase bone scanning using technetium Tc-99m (99Tc) phosphonates has 94% sensitivity and 95% specificity for the diagnosis of osteomyelitis of the bone with a high-negative predictive value, but the advantage is lost in the presence of neuroarthropathy, trauma, recent surgery, or tumor. Complementary Tc-99m sulfur colloid bone marrow imaging helps to distinguish bone marrow changes from that caused by infection. Indium-111 white blood cell (WBC) scintigraphy in general is more accurate than 99Tc bone scanning for diagnosing osteomyelitis, but has limited availability. Other emerging WBC labeling modalities include radiolabeled granulocytes, antigranulocyte monoclonal antibody fragment, radiolabeled polyclonal immunoglobulin, and Tc-99m hexamethylpropylene amine oxime (HMPAO) labeled WBCs. Positron emission tomography (PET)-CT/MRI is highly accurate and specific for the differentiation of osteomyelitis from neuroarthropathy, if the issue needs to be finally settled.

Laboratory Studies and Vital Signs

White blood cell count may be normal even if an infection is present in diabetics due to impaired immune response. Leukocytosis > 11×10^9/L is associated with a 2.6-fold increase in the risk of amputation, and fever >100.5°F (38°C) has been associated with a 1.3-fold increased risk of amputation. Albumin levels > 30 g/L are necessary for satisfactory healing. Erythrocyte sedimentation rate (ESR) of <40 is more common with cellulitis or local soft-tissue infection, while >60 suggests osteomyelitis. C-reactive protein (CRP) level is highly sensitive but not specific for inflammation, so is a better marker for follow-up and monitoring of patients with diabetic foot infection. Worsening blood sugar level is one of the earliest signs of uncontrolled or spreading diabetic foot infection.

Diabetic Ulcer

It is a serious complication accounting for a quarter of all hospital stays for diabetic patients. The pathogenesis of foot pressure ulceration is described above. A lot of factors are responsible to their causation including:

- Loss of skin integrity
- Neuropathy
- Decreased vascularity
- Foot deformity
- Increased body weight
- Poor vision
- Malnutrition
- Poor glucose regulation
- Need for insulin
- Impaired leukocyte function
- Use of immunosuppressive drugs
- Tobacco use

The ulcerations are troublesome to heal primarily due to poor vascular supply, deep infection, and difficulty in unloading the affected area **(Figs. 8A and B)**. Initial wound size, duration, and grade are directly linked to likelihood of wound healing by the 20th week of care. The Scottish Foot Ulcer Risk Score classifies an ulcer as mild, moderate, or high-risk based on palpable pulses, sensory neuropathy, foot deformity, and a history of ulcer or amputation. It can be used to predict ulcer development and ulcer healing. The Brodsky classification system, which is based on ulcer depth and ischemia, helps to determine the need for hospitalization and possible surgery **(Figs. 9A and B)**. Some people use the Wagner-Meggitt system to grade ulcers. Both systems do well in clinical assessment and management.

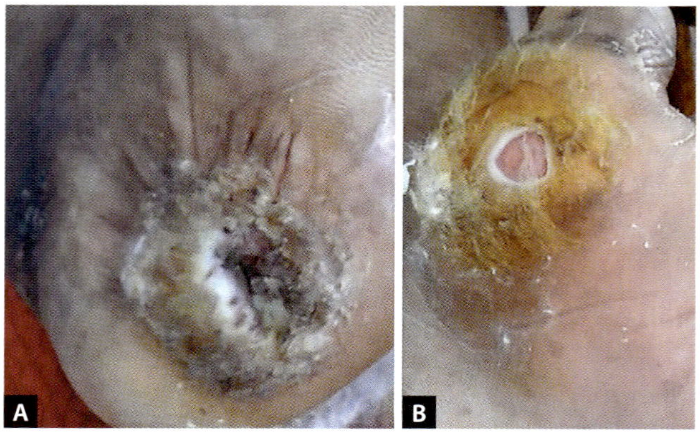

Figs. 8A and B: The close-up views of diabetic foot ulcers. The heel ulcer (A) is deep (Grade 2) but has not reached bone while the one on ball of great toe (B) is developing lately and is still grade 1, these two are the most common pressure regions on the foot of a patient predisposing for ulceration.

Management of Diabetic Foot Ulcers

- The first step in ulcer management is to remove all necrotic tissue and unhealthy repair tissue. Also perform bone debridement. Ultrasonic clearing may help in removing the necrotic tissue. This induces acute injury with reducing the necrotic load to encourage healing. Elliptical wounds heal better than circular wounds. Wound debridement needs to be repeated quite frequently.
- Offload pressure on the area by distributing it elsewhere over a larger surface area. One must be opportunistic to lengthening of the Achilles-tendon as soon as possible, as it decreases plantar pressure and enhances healing of forefoot ulcers. Plantar fascia release has also been found to result in healing of forefoot ulcers. Best nonoperative method is to obviously avoid bearing weight on the limb; however, compliance is an issue. Total contact casting remains the gold standard to hasten healing of ulcer in the shortest time than other contemporary methods. One must, however, be vigilant of complications such as stiffness, other pressure ulcers, etc. The time taken for ulcer to heal increases with its location progressing from toe to midfoot. Alternatives to total contact cast are healing shoe, custom orthotic device, or a pressure-dissipating insole.
- Hyperbaric oxygen therapy has been promoted highly as adjunct therapy but is costly, not readily available and of unproved effectiveness. Though transcutaneous oxygen tension at the affected extremity level is improved, but it is just one aspect of addressing the pathology. If screening arterial Doppler reveals occlusion then arteriography and stenting of the vessel can be done for improvement in blood supply and oxygenation. Vascular consult should be obtained to determine possibility of improving circulation.

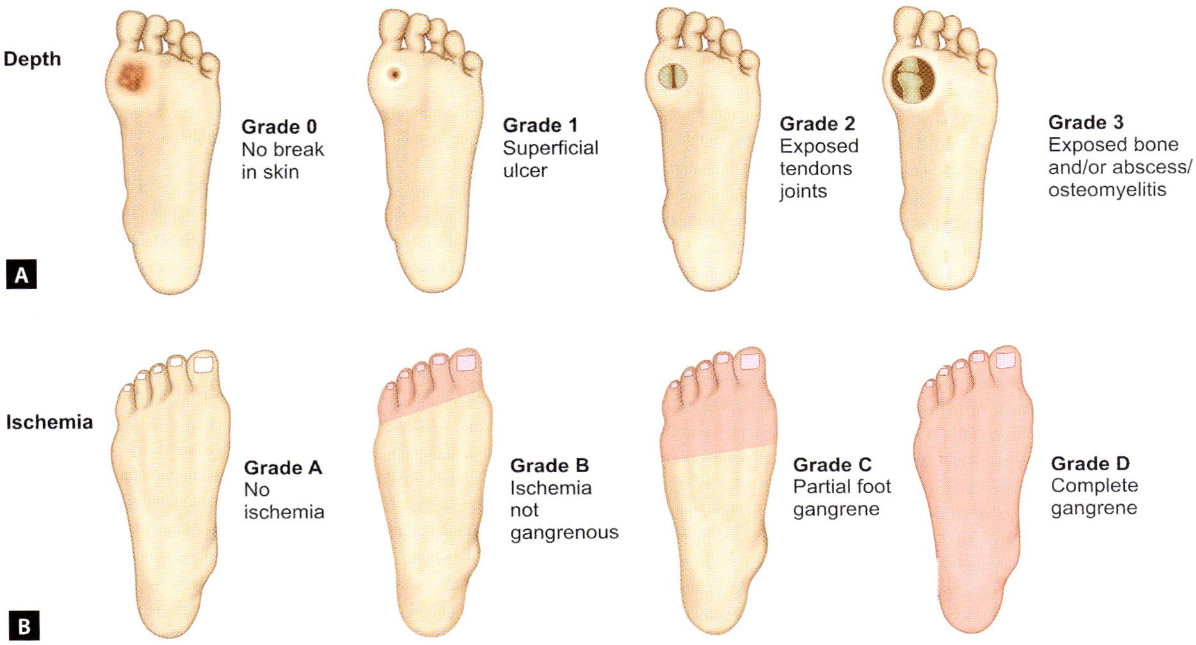

Figs. 9A and B: Illustration depicting the classification of diabetic foot ulcer based on the depth of ulcer (A) and ischemia (B).

Inpatient Management of Diabetic Foot Ulcer

Patients with exposed tendon and necrotic tissue with abscess formation, osteitis, osteomyelitis, or gangrene would need thorough surgical debridement or amputation and parenteral antibiotics for which inpatient care is mandatory. These patients usually have signs of sepsis at presentation. The most commonly used test to determine deep infection and the need for surgical intervention is "probe-to-bone test". The ulcer or wound is probed using a sterile applicator stick and if it contacts bone then it certifies deep infection necessitating surgical management. Negative test, however, does not rule out deep infection. The surgical management consists of repeated debridement reducing the necrotic load, management of osteitis (shaving the bone), osteomyelitis (removal of necrotic bone and stabilization if needed), amputation, etc.

After the ulcer is healed, maintenance takes priority by customizing the footwear to offload the pressure site, improving the gait by training, improving nutrition, and tight glycemic control.

Diabetic Foot Infection and Its Management

Patients with DM are at an 80% greater risk for cellulitis, a fourfold increased risk for osteomyelitis, a twofold higher risk for sepsis and death (septicemia), and a 10-time greater risk of amputation. Antibiotics are the mainstay of controlling infection where oral antibiotics are effective for infection that does not threaten the limb while intravenous antibiotics are prescribed otherwise. Suppressive therapy with long-term oral antibiotics to remit osteomyelitis has not been uniformly successful. One must be balancing the risks of such therapy with complications of progression threatening limb or life in the long run. So, surgical management should be the primary focus of therapy with intravenous antibiotic therapy serving as adjunct. Topical antibiotic alone has no recommendation for treating an infected ulcer barring the use of topical metronidazole to control odor for necrotic ulcers. Topical silver-containing dressings or pexiganan acetate cream [a synthetic analog of the antimicrobial cationic peptide magainin 2 (a host-defense peptide isolated from frog skin)] may be used for managing mildly infected ulcers. Bacterial biofilm precludes ulcer healing, and its surgical removal is extremely important. Swab culture is futile, as it confuses by growing commensals and instead culture should be obtained from deeper specimens (bone or granulation tissue). With increasing ulcer depth, anaerobic bacteria become more abundant than gram-positive cocci. The most commonly isolated pathogens in osteomyelitis are gram-positive organisms; especially *Staphylococcus aureus*, however, it has been determined that deeper infections usually contain gram-negative pathogens alone or in combination with a gram-positive organism. Infections with gram-negative pathogens more often are associated with a fetid odor, necrotic tissue, and clinical signs of severe infection than those with gram-positive pathogens alone. The risk of ulcer-associated infection is increased with hyperglycemia, as it defunctions neutrophil degranulation. Poor glycemic control is also associated with ulcer cluster, and very poor glycemic control is associated with an increase in the concentration of *Staphylococcus*-rich and *Streptococcus*-rich ulcer clusters. Multidrug-resistant bacteria increases with deep and recurrent ulcers, history of previous hospitalization, elevated HbA1c level, and nephropathy. A 2004 consensus report of the Infectious Diseases Society of America (IDSA) described four grades of severity in diabetic foot infection that has been reworked by the International Working Group on the Diabetic Foot (IWGDF) in 2012. IDSA and IWGDF agree that a severe diabetic foot infection is accompanied by two or more of the signs of a systemic inflammatory response, viz., a body temperature > 39°C or <36°C, a heart rate > 90 beats/min, a respiratory rate >20 breaths/min or an arterial partial pressure of carbon dioxide ($PaCO_2$) < 32 mm Hg, and a WBC count > 12 × 10^9/L or <4 × 10^9/L **(Table 1)**. Hyperglycemia, azotemia, and acidosis that were a part of earlier system have been dropped from the IDSA-IWGDF consensus. Wet gangrene or soft-tissue emphysema represents severe infection.

Weight-bearing on an infected foot should be discouraged because it encourages infection spread from an area of high pressure to areas of lower pressure. Most commonly infection spreads from the plantar foot to the dorsal foot. The infections spread usually along the tendons within their sheaths or along intermuscular fascial planes that get damaged by liquefaction and loss of vascularity. With progressive involvement of compartments within the foot, pressures within the compartment increase and can cause extensive tissue damage due to strangulation of blood supply, accrual of necrotic tissue, and increased bacterial growth. Antibiotics also do not reach target site, as the vascularity is compromised. Surgical intervention, hence, becomes imperative. Simple surgical intervention may include abscess drainage, aggressive debridement of ulcers, and application of negative pressure wound therapy. Negative pressure wound therapy is more effective than topical moist wound dressings. The involved compartment must be opened and all necrotic tissue is removed performing effective debridement. More aggressive surgical measures include exostectomy, deformity correction, muscle or microvascular free flaps, or amputation. Repetitive debridements are more a rule than chance need. Staged reconstructive surgical procedures sometimes are necessary until healthy tissue is obtained.

TABLE 1: Classification of diabetic foot wound infections (International consensus).

Grade	Characteristics
I	No symptoms/signs of infection. Lesion of 0.5–2.0 cm limited to the skin (no subcutaneous tissue lesion or systemic disorder) with local warmth and erythema
II	Tenderness+, pain+, local swelling+, induration+, pus discharge+
	Erythema >2 cm along with at least one of:
	• Local tenderness or pain • Local swelling or induration • Purulent discharge • Absence of other causes of inflammation (trauma, gout, acute Charcot arthropathy, fracture, thrombosis, and venous stasis)
III	• Local infection involving deeper structures beneath the skin and subcutaneous tissue—deep abscess, lymphangitis, osteomyelitis, septic arthritis, or fasciitis • No systemic inflammatory response • Regardless of local infection, the presence of systemic signs corresponding to body temperature >39°C or <36°C and pulse >90 beats/min
IV	• Respiratory rate >20 breaths/min • $PaCO_2$ <32 mm Hg • Leukocytes >12 or <4 × 10^9/L • Proportion of immature leukocytes >10%

Amputation

Nonhealing and resistant foot wounds often need lower extremity amputations. Similarly, extensive abscess formation, wet gangrene, and proximal extension of lesion into legs or knee region will be difficult to control by simpler methods. The rate of major amputation is three times higher in patients with severe diabetic foot infection. More than half of the patients with severe infection would need amputation compared to 40% in patients with moderate infection [moderate vs. severe defined by IDSA consensus **(Table 1)**]. There is a strong correlation between morbid obesity and diabetes-associated morbidity. The risk of amputation is highest in socially deprived patients, older than 50 years, males, or those who smoke tobacco.

Thirty percent of patients with a unilateral amputation undergo amputation of the contralateral limb within 3 years. Two-thirds of patients die within 5 years of the amputation. Level of amputation has to be meticulously decided by considering both the optimal level for healing (the vascular supply) and optimal residual limb function. The factors contributing to the decision making include the quality of the tissue, the extent of the infection, the vascularity of the limb, and the patient's nutritional (serum albumin > 3.0 g/dL), immune, and ambulatory status. The various levels of amputation needed include partial digital, digital, ray resection transmetatarsal, Chopart, Syme, transtibial, and transfemoral. For hallux amputation, it is recommended to retain insertion of flexor hallucis brevis at the level of proximal metaphysis for maintaining medial column stability. Long plantar flap provides optimal soft-tissue cover. If ray amputation is needed then amputation of first ray should be avoided as much as possible in young individuals as it causes apropulsive gait. For a fifth-ray amputation, late varus deformity can be avoided by retaining the base of metatarsal with the attachment of peroneus brevis tendon. For a midtarsal or tarsometatarsal amputation, a plantar-based flap provides the best soft-tissue envelop. Late varus or equinus can be avoided by performing a percutaneous tendon Achilles or gastrocnemius muscle lengthening and application of short leg walking cast while the ankle is positioned at 90° for 1 month. Hindfoot amputations are better avoided as they lead to development of equinus deformity and these patients are better treated by Syme's ankle disarticulation. Osteomyelitis of the heel is more likely to require transtibial amputation. Midfoot amputation may require tendon lengthening or releases and possibly tendon transfers to balance the foot. After metatarsal head resection, the greatest risk of reulceration is at the first metatarsal head, and the lowest risk is at the fifth metatarsal head. The risk of major reamputation after minor foot amputation in patients with diabetes is strongly associated with the presence of peripheral vascular disease. Transmetatarsal and Chopart amputations result in better ambulatory ability and longer durability than other partial foot amputations.

CHARCOT NEUROARTHROPATHY

Charcot neuroarthropathy involves progressive destruction of the joints, most commonly in the feet and ankles. The condition is named after Jean Martin Charcot who noted the occurrence of mutilated feet in syphilis (1868), and the disorder was later related to diabetes in 1936. It is characterized by pathologic fractures, joint dislocation, and overt loss of normal pedal architecture. DM is the most common cause while others being syphilis, alcoholism, leprosy, and idiopathic neuropathy. It is seen in <1% of the general population of patients with DM but in high-risk patients with diabetes the incidence may go to as high as 13%. The distribution in men and women is equal and one-third of the patients have bilateral involvement. The common findings in Charcot foot include a combination of vascular, neuropathic, and infective features:

- Erythema
- Warmth
- Cellulitis
- Ulcer
- Swelling
- Varied deformity mostly destruction of the natural features of foot
- Joint dislocation
- Loss of/reduced sensation

Pathogenesis

Two theories are proposed to explain the development of Charcot neuroarthropathy.

1. *The theory of neurotraumatic destruction:* This explains that the joint destruction is the result of accrual of repetitive trauma unrecognized by an insensate foot.
2. *The theory of neurovascular destruction:* This states that bone resorption and ligament laxity are secondary to a neurally controlled vascular reflex.

It is highly possible that both the mechanisms are at interplay with dominance of one of them in some patients. There is a role of osteopenia in diabetic neuroarthropathy where weak bones fracture easily and then deform and resorb under continued stress. Excessive osteoclastic activity is found in Charcot-reactive bone mediated by cytokines.

Increased expression of nuclear transcription factor NF-κβ (nuclear factor kappa-light-chain-enhancer of activated beta cells) results in increased osteoclastogenesis, inhibition of which may control osseous destruction. It is interesting to note here that the patients with Charcot dislocation often have normal bone density while those with Charcot fracture often have decreased bone density. The severity of diabetes is not correlated with the risk of Charcot neuroarthropathy.

Charcot neuroarthropathy is seen to progress in three classic stages (*Eichenholtz classification*):

1. *Stage I,* the fragmentation phase, is clinically characterized by hyperemia, edema, increased warmth, and erythema around the affected joint. Radiographically, this stage is characterized by fragmentation of bone associated with fracture and joint subluxation.
2. *Stage II* (the subacute or coalescence phase)—here, the acute inflammatory findings decrease. Radiographs show evidence of bone debris and new bone formation.
3. *Stage III* is the chronic or consolidation phase. Swelling and warmth surrounding the joint resolves, but there may be considerable residual deformity. On radiographs, the fragmentation is seen to have consolidated, but residual joint deformity and bone loss are evident **(Figs. 10A and B)**.

Charcot neuroarthropathy of foot and ankle is classified in anatomical terms (*Brodsky classification*, **Figs. 11A and B**). In general, the more proximal the Charcot joint involvement, the higher the risk of subsequent joint instability.

- *Type I (60% of patients)* affects the midfoot, tarsometatarsal, and naviculocuneiform joints. Collapse of these joints results in a residual deformity involving a plantar medial bony exostosis that places the foot at risk of pressure ulceration.
- Type II (30–35% of patients) involves the hindfoot with subsequent instability resulting in foot subluxation and ulcer formation.
- Type IIIA (5% of patients) involves the ankle joint and is the most unstable pattern.

Type IIIB involves fracture of the calcaneal tuberosity and results in weak push-off, pes planus, and risk of ulceration associated with the avulsed bony prominence.

Another *classification by Schon et al.* divides Charcot foot into four types **(Figs. 12A and B)**. Type I is destruction of the

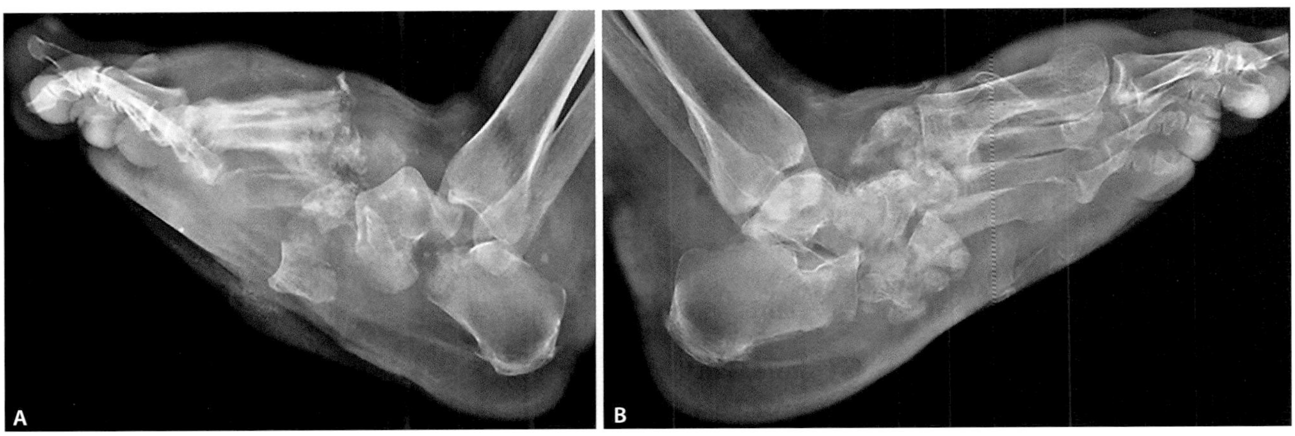

Figs. 10A and B: The radiographs of Charcot neuropathic disease. There is gross disruption of intertarsal and tarsometatarsal joints with bones showing massive destruction, fragmentation, and lying dislocated free. In the right foot even, the ankle joint is dislocated. The complete architecture of foot is lost. Forefoot is relatively preserved especially in left foot.

MTP joint with medial plantar prominence and abduction deformity. Type II is involvement of naviculocuneiform joint with residual plantar lateral prominence under the fourth and fifth metatarsocuboid joints. Type III affects the navicular and the medial column with collapse resulting in an adducted-supinated deformity and a plantar lateral prominence under the cuboid. Type IV involves the transverse tarsal joints with associated prominence under the calcaneocuboid and talonavicular joints. Further detailed substages A, B, or C are assigned based on the severity of the rocker-bottom sole **(Fig. 13)**.

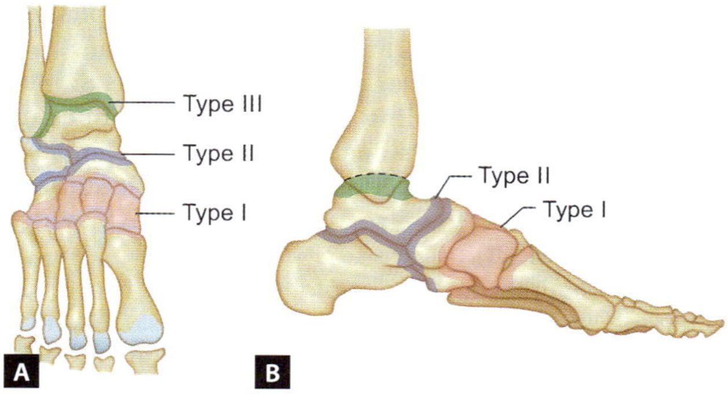

Figs. 11A and B: The schematic drawings depict the anatomical regions in (A) frontal and lateral (B) projections for classification of Charcot neuroarthropathy according to anatomical region(s). Type I—midfoot (tarsometatarsal and naviculocuneiform joints), Type II—hindfoot (subtalar, talonavicular, and calcaneocuboid joints), Type IIIA—involvement of tibiotalar (ankle) joint, and Type IIIB—involvement of calcaneum–calcaneal tuberosity.

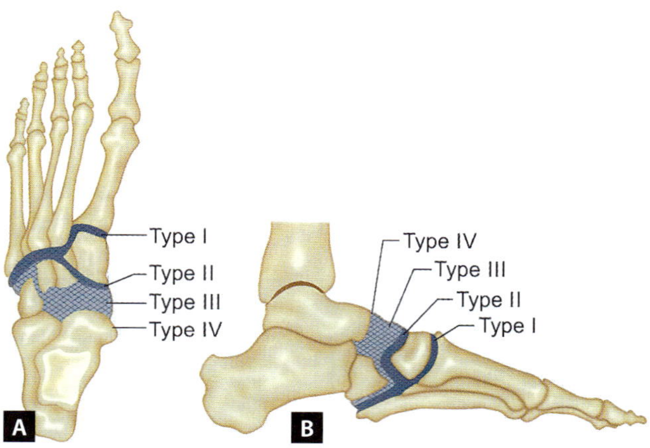

Figs. 12A and B: Schematic illustration of four types of chronic Charcot rocker-bottom foot in frontal (A) and lateral (B).

Management of Charcot Foot Disease

The goal of treatment after stage III (Eichenholtz classification, the consolidation phase) is to stabilize foot making it plantigrade, and amenable to bracing and customized shoes. This entails correction of residual deformity also; for achieving these goals and keeps the foot free of ulceration and infection. The following are common recommendations for management according to the stages:

- The nonsurgical treatment is the mainstay at stage I that includes rest, elevation, and protection. A total contact cast with weekly cast changes is prescribed. Patellar weight-bearing molded ankle–foot orthosis (AFO) is frequently used. Weight-bearing is restricted until the acute process resolves. Immobilization seems to turn off the destructive process. With improvement, the cast change is prolonged to every 2 weeks. Limb elevation and elastic bandaging of the foot and limb is another option.
- At stage II, the swelling and temperature in the foot begin to stabilize. Immobilization is changed to removable boot walker or AFO, but pressure distribution is improved by customized modifications. Ancillary therapy in the form of early introduction of pharmacotherapy, bone stimulation, and physiotherapy is gaining popularity.
- In stage III due to difficulty in achieving stability, accommodative shoes with a custom-molded protective orthotic device is used. Extradepth custom-molded orthosis shares weight and prevents ulceration. Exostectomy is done for nonhealing ulceration.

Residual deformity can result in chronic pressure and subsequent ulceration. These patients with nonplantigrade foot are candidates for surgical correction of deformity. Another new indication for surgery is the presence of pain at the site of unstable Charcot arthropathy deformity. The first step is usually lengthening of Achilles tendon or gastrocnemius muscle lengthening to achieve muscle balance. Next step is to perform a wedge resection at the apex of deformity. Internal fixation, external fixation, or a combination can be used to stabilize foot and ankle and also correct deformity. Amputation may be needed for unmanageable feet with severe deformities precluding footwear and multiple/recurrent nonhealing ulcerations. In morbidly obese diabetic patients with renal failure, knee disarticulation should be considered because fitting a prosthetic joint is difficult in them due to volume fluctuation of the extremity.

Complications of Surgery in Charcot Foot and General Rehabilitation

Patients are at risk of various complications including failure

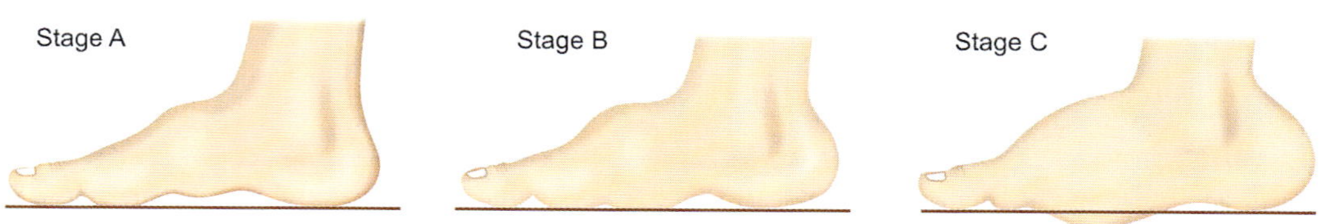

Fig. 13: Illustration depicting the three substages of development of Charcot rocket-bottom deformity.

BOX 3: General foot care instructions counseled to patients for prevention and maintenance.

- *Washing your feet:* Wash feet daily. Wipe carefully especially between the toes. Do not soak or immerse your feet
- If your feet are dry, apply a thin coat of oil or cream after bathing and drying them avoiding region between your toes
- *Inspecting your feet:* Keep a check on changes and note them. Use mirror to aid inspection of sole. Note for scratches, cuts, or blisters. Always check between your toes
- *Cutting your toenails:* Cut your toenails by following the contour of the nail. Keep corners smooth. Do not trim into the corners or cut ingrown toenails. Contact physician immediately, if redness appears around your toenails
- *Treating corns and calluses:* Do not cut corns or calluses. Do not use corn plasters or chemicals. Do not use adhesive tape on your feet
- *Avoid extreme temperatures:* Do not walk on hot surfaces like beach-side sand. In winter, wear wool socks, do not use heat
- *Use shoes:* Do not walk barefoot. Do not wear sandals with thongs between your toes. Wear shoes with stockings or cotton socks. Check shoes for sharp object or irregularities, foreign objects, nail points, torn linings, and rough areas
- Avoiding harm to your legs
- Avoid tobacco and alcohol

of wound healing, infection, malunion, delayed union, and nonunion.

To prevent these complications, optimal glycemic control, maximization of limb vascularity, meticulous soft-tissue care, and prolonged avoidance of weight-bearing after the surgery should be practiced.

Patients are encouraged to participate in a comprehensive foot-care program that includes risk assessment, foot-care education, and preventive therapy. All patients with diabetes should undergo an annual foot examination.

These patients should be taught the importance of blood glucose monitoring and self-examination of the feet **(Box 3)**. The risk factors for development of a diabetic ulcer include insensate foot, diminished pulses, foot deformity, abnormal reflexes, increased age, past history of a foot ulcer, and an abnormal neuropathy disability score. The risk of foot complications is scored from 0 to 3 **(Table 2)**. A normal-appearing foot with intact sensations and minimal deformity is assigned risk category 0. For risk category 3, the patient requires interventions such as foot-risk education, foot self-examination three to four times daily, etc. Foot protection by customized gear should be done during walking and other activities. These high-risk patients should undergo a foot examination by a podiatrician every 2 months. In addition, any new skin or nail issue should immediately be clinically evaluated.

TABLE 2: Risk category for developing foot complications.

Category	*Recommendation*	*Risk factors*
0	(Yearly foot examination and regular footwear)	• No history of ulcer/deformity/ sensory loss/amputation • Pedal pulses present
1	(Daily foot self-examination and 6-monthly visit to physician, total-contact orthotic device)	• No history of ulcer/deformity/ previous amputation • Sensory loss present, pedal pulses present
2	(Daily foot self-examination and every 4-monthly physician visit, custom-molded orthotic devices)	• No history of ulceration • Moderate deformity (prominent metatarsal head, hallux rigidus, claw/ hammer toes, etc.) • Single lesser ray amputation done, sensory loss present, pedal pulses intact
3	(Daily foot self-examination, 2-monthly physician visit, custom pressure-dissipating orthosis, inlay depth, soft-leather, adjustable lacing shoes, patellar tendon-bearing brace, and podiatric evaluation of any new lesion)	History of ulceration present, deformity present, previous amputation present (>1 at different sites), sensory loss present, pedal pulses±

CONCLUSION

- Involvement of small joints of foot and ankle is common in inflammatory disorders. Infection in foot is also common due to frequent wear and tear, this holds true particularly for diabetic patients who develop neuropathy and insensate foot.
- Rheumatoid affection of foot produces deformity at the joints resulting in significant disability due to altered biomechanics.
- As most of the inflammatory affections produce deformation of the joints and degeneration of articular cartilage, salvage is not usually possible if symptomatic treatment fails. The stabilization of foot and reconstruction hence mostly relies on arthrodesis of various joints or excision arthroplasty of small toe joints to make it functional and painfree.
- Diabetic foot disease is a morbid condition that cripples the patient. Incidence is increasing with the rising incidence of diabetics. Proper foot care and preventive measures are the most important aspects of management of diabetic foot disease.

CHAPTER 86

Deformities of the Hallux and the Lesser Toe

Manish Kumar Varshney

INTRODUCTION

The great toe is the most important phalanx of the foot and is subject to major pressure bearing. It also provides stability and ball of great toe forms one spot of the tripod for pressure transmission to floor. The following are some of the commonly encountered great toe deformities while some uncommon forms are also discussed below:

- Bunion (Hallux valgus)
- Hallux rigidus
- Hallux flexus

BUNION OR HALLUX VALGUS

Bunion is a bump on the side of the big toe. The deformity is often seen and referred to as hallux valgus. The hallux valgus deformity is characterized by lateral (fibular) deviation (away from midline of body or toward midline of foot) of the proximal phalanx on the metatarsal head **(Figs. 1A to D)**. This is often associated with disorders of lesser toes. In describing hallux valgus, it is still uncertain as to which is the primary deformity metatarsus primus varus or lateral deviation of the great toe, though considering the pathogenesis (see below), it appears that the latter is primary.

Etiology

The following is a comprehensive list of disorders that are associated with the hallux valgus deformity:

- *Metatarsophalangeal (MTP) joint arthritis (inflammatory, metabolic conditions, and connective tissue disorders):*
  - Rheumatoid arthritis
  - Psoriatic arthritis
  - Gouty arthritis
  - Ehlers–Danlos syndrome, Marfan syndrome, Down syndrome, and ligamentous laxity
- *Traumatic:*
  - Dislocations
  - Malunions
  - Intra-articular damage
  - Soft-tissue sprains
- *Neuromuscular disease:*
  - Charcot–Marie–Tooth disease (CMTD)
  - Cerebral palsy
  - Multiple sclerosis
- *Primary structural deformity:*
  - Metatarsus primus elevatus
  - External tibial torsion
  - Malalignment of articular surface or metatarsal shaft
  - Abnormal metatarsal length
  - Genu varum or valgum
  - Femoral retroversion

Pathogenesis

Biomechanical instability: This involves a complex interplay of disorders of bones, articular surfaces, and the capsuloligamentous structures. The angle between the first and second metatarsals is normally up to 10°, more than this is pathological. The valgus angle of the first metatarsophalangeal joint (MTP angle) measured up to 20° is normal. Following are some of the pathogenic mechanisms explaining development of this progressive deformity:

- Great toe pronates if this MTP angle exceeds 35° → this produces plantar shift of the abductor hallucis longus compared to the metatarsal axis and precludes its power to adduct the great toe **(Figs. 2A and B)**.
- Excess lateral pull results from the unopposed pull of the adductor hallucis that is only countered by medial capsular ligament along with the capsule-sesamoid portion (tight slightly thickened structure inserting into the sesamoid, **Figs. 2A and B**) and capsulophalangeal portion (part of capsule inserting onto base of the proximal phalanx).
- Constant pull produces a creep effect and hence gradually the capsule attenuates, elongates, and the metatarsal head becomes prominent medially.
- The first ray is pulled laterally by the flexor hallucis brevis, flexor hallucis longus, adductor hallucis, and extensor hallucis longus all of which have a medially directed moment along with their primary action, increasing the valgus deformity.
- Attenuation of the sesamoid ridge under the first metatarsal head. This causes displacement of the fibular sesamoid partially (subluxation) or completely (displacement) into the first intermetatarsal space **(Figs. 3A and B)**.

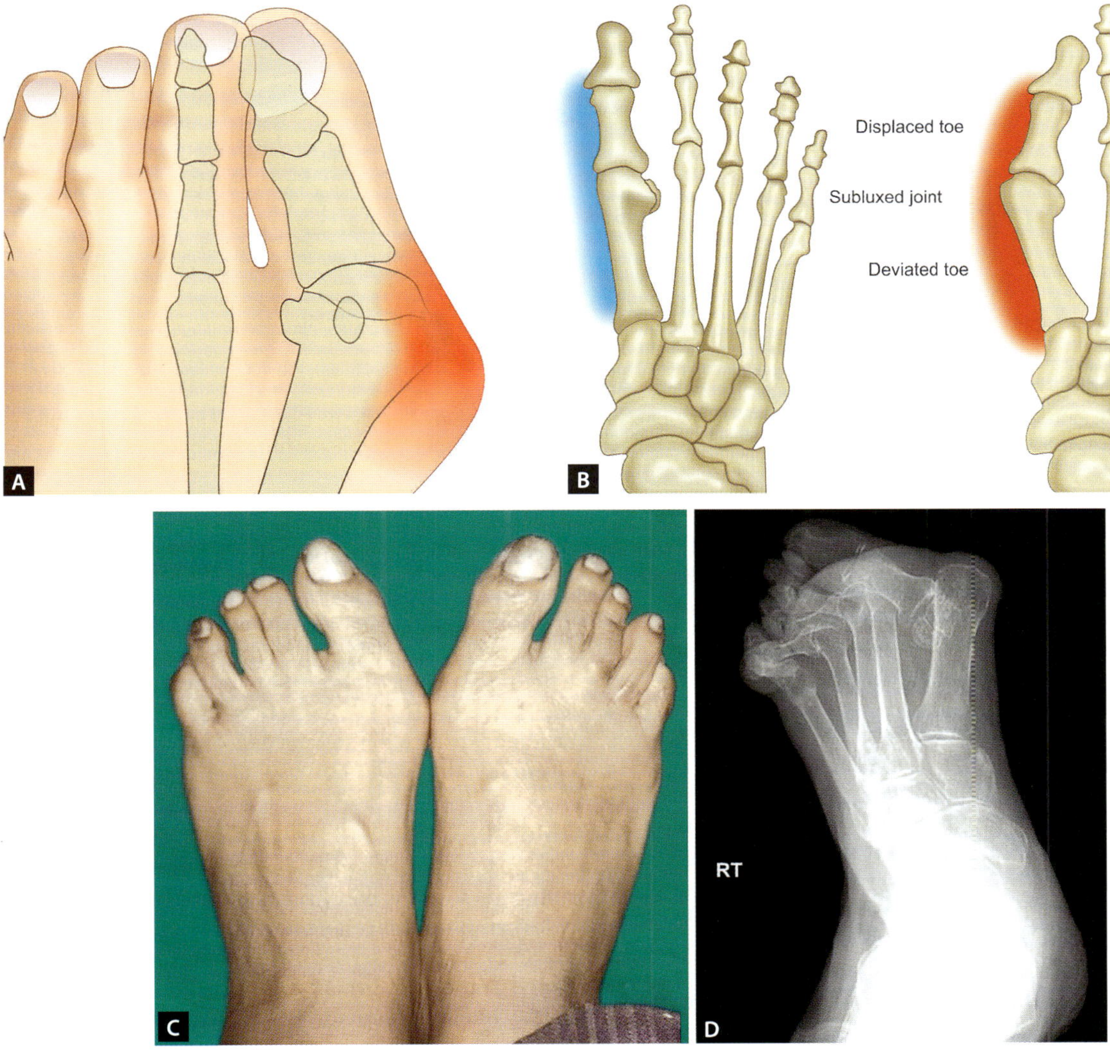

Figs. 1A to D: Bunion: (A) Pathoanatomy; (B) On the left is shown a well-oriented metatarsophalangeal (MTP) joint while on the right is shown an illustration of bunion for comparison; (C) Clinical photograph; (D) Radiograph.

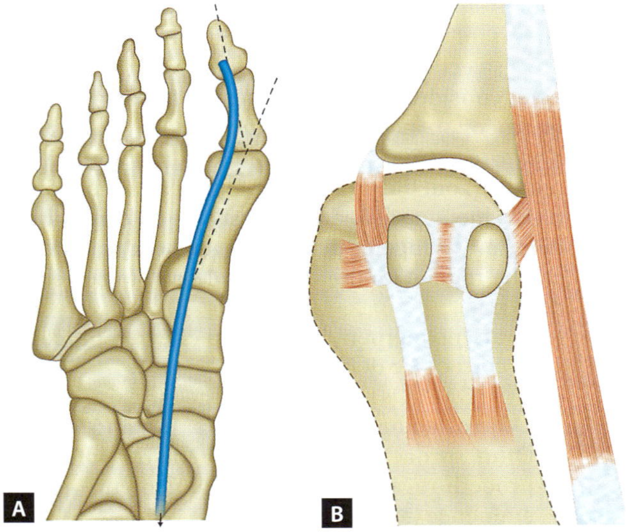

Figs. 2A and B: Pathogenesis of bunion formation (see text). (A) Subluxation; (B) Abnormal pull moment from the tendon.

- Apart from above, the articular offset between the phalanx and the metatarsal head is also responsible for producing the deformity. The distal metatarsal articular angle (DMAA) is offset (the articular surface of the metatarsal head appears like an ice-cream scoop placed at an angle on cone, **Fig. 4**) and the phalangeal articular angle is offset (measured as the articular angle of the base of the proximal phalanx in relation to its longitudinal axis). The former is considered as an important factor in recurrence of deformities if it is not adequately addressed.

Some associated factors contribute to progression of the deformity and if present they may exacerbate it. These include:

- Equinus due to gastrocnemius or gastrosoleus complex involvement (dynamic)
- Flatfoot (pes planovalgus, flexible, or rigid)
- Rigid or flexible forefoot varus
- Dorsiflexion of first ray
- Hypermobility or short first metatarsal

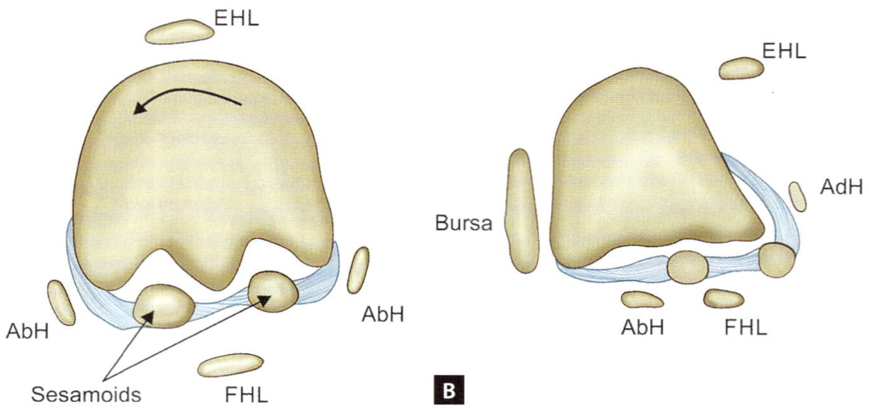

Figs. 3A and B: Pathogenesis of bunion (contd.). (A) There is subluxation of the sesamoids laterally; (B) Development of bursa medially. (AbH: abductor halluces; AdH: adductor halluces; EHL: extensor hallucis longus; FHL: flexor hallucis longus)

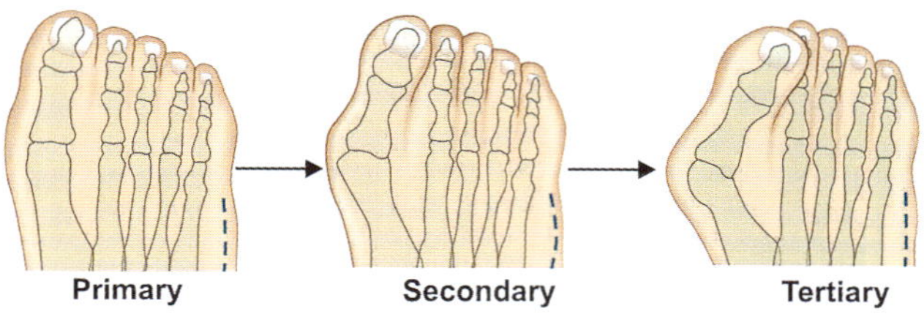

Fig. 4: The three stages of bunion development.

Pathoanatomy: The following deformations are commonly seen in a hallux valgus deformity (so it is called a complex deformity). As a result of this lateral subluxation of the proximal phalanx (which is now considered as a primary deformity) on the metatarsal head, several secondary changes occur, **Figs. 5A and B**).

- Medial deviation of the first metatarsal, giving rise to an increase in the intermetatarsal angle (first metatarsal varus), great toe valgus, and bunion formation.
- Hammer toe-like deformity of the second toe due to overlapping of the second toe on valgus great toe underneath.
- Contracture of the lateral joint capsule
- Attenuation of the medial joint capsule
- First MTP joint degenerative arthritis
- Corns, calluses, and metatarsalgia
- Pronation of the hallux, as the deformity becomes more severe
- Formation of the medial eminence (may actually represent hypertrophic component or from the medial deviation of the metatarsal head itself)

As the deformity increases, the weight-bearing capacity of the hallux and first metatarsal is diminished, resulting in increased weight-bearing by the second metatarsal head, which results in metatarsalgia.

Clinical and Radiological Features

Note the typical features mentioned above in "pathoanatomy". Note any pain about the MTP joint, synovial thickening or crepitation. The foot should be examined for mentioned etiological conditions.

Radiographic Examination (Figs. 6A and B)

- Measure the first MTP joint angle, which should be <15°.
- The intermetatarsal angle should be <8°.
- Look for arthrosis in the first MTP joint and assess whether the joint is congruent or incongruent.
- Measure the DMAA, which is the relationship of the articular surface to the long axis of the metatarsal.
- Normally, this should be <10° of lateral deviation.

Treatment

Conservative management: For initial deformities and patients unwilling for surgery, conservative management is tried that provides symptomatic relief often and retards the progression of deformity. In any case, deformity being progressive; surgery is needed at the end. Broad and soft-soled shoes, preferably with a low heel, that provide adequate room for the great toe and the medial eminence are prescribed. Silicon spacer for abducting the great toe is also worn the whole day and can be taken off at night or better worn even then.

*Principles of surgical correction **(Flowchart 1)**:* One of the most important factors in the outcome of bunion surgery is the correct selection of the operative procedure.

- The first consideration is whether the deformity is in a congruent or an incongruent joint.
  - *Scenario 1 **(Fig. 7)**:* The joint is congruent (DMAA reduced) but the proximal phalanx cannot be rotated on the metatarsal head to correct the deformity or the deformity is incongruent, however, proximal phalanx can be rotated on the metatarsal head to correct the deformity.
    - In an incongruent joint, use a chevron procedure to correct the deformity.
    - If the DMAA is reduced, use a medial closing wedge (Akin osteotomy) (see later **Figs. 15A and B**).
    - Other procedures include a distal soft-tissue procedure along with excision of the medial eminence (exostectomy).
    - *Scenario 2:* The hallux valgus deformity in an incongruent joint with noncorrectible proximal phalanx.

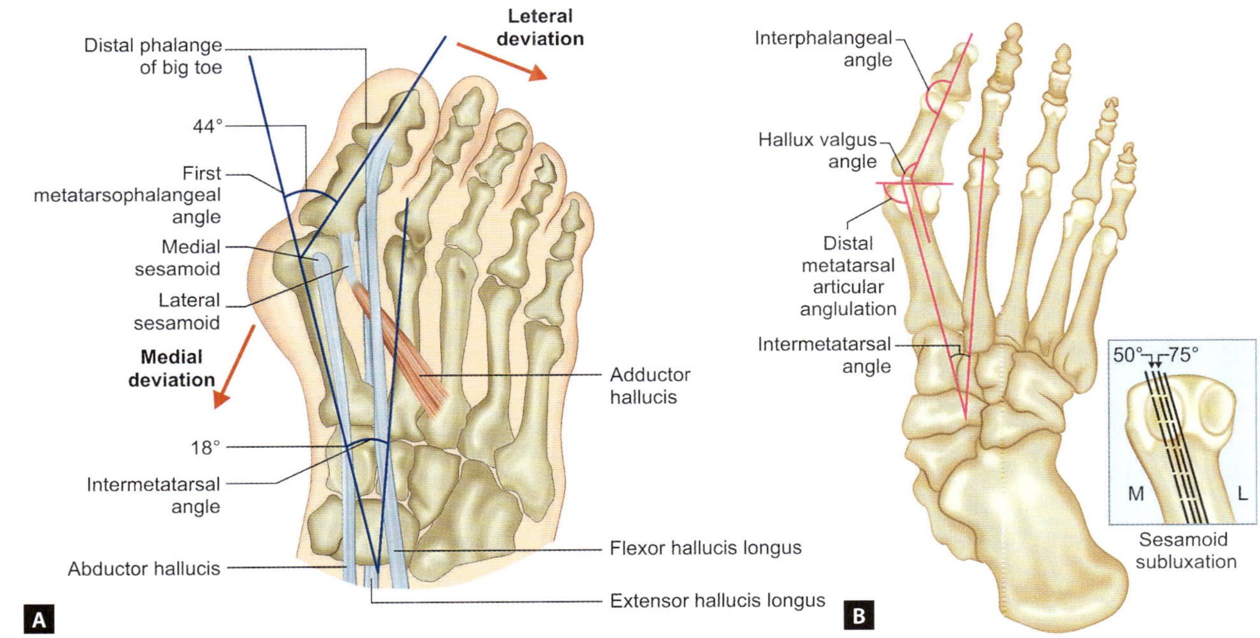

Figs. 5A and B: Illustration summarizing: (A) The pathoanatomy and pathogenesis of hallux valgus; (B) Determining various measurements for grading deformity and choosing procedure for deformity correction. Inset shows method to determine tibial sesamoid subluxation—the sesamoid is considered medial if 75% of its width is medial to the central line, lateral if 75% is lateral to the central line. Otherwise, the sesamoid is considered to be centrally located.

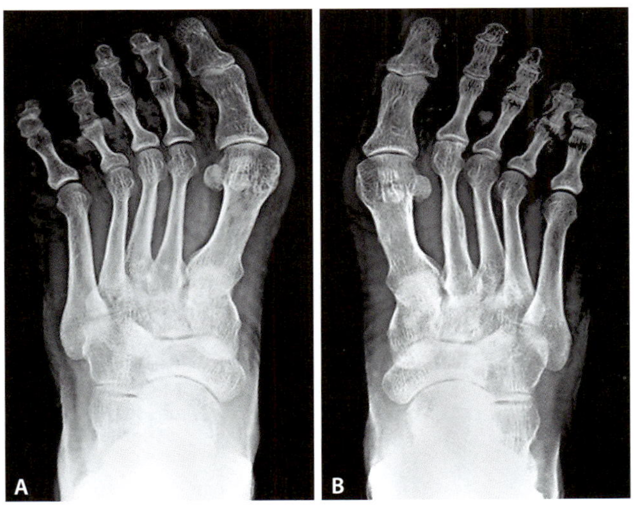

Figs. 6A and B: Radiograph of a moderate hallux valgus deformity.

Here, the operative procedure depends on the severity of the deformity.

- Mild hallux valgus deformity (hallux valgus angle of <20° and the intermetatarsal angle <11°)—use a chevron osteotomy or distal soft-tissue procedure to correct the deformity.
- If the deformity is moderate (hallux valgus of 20–40° and the intermetatarsal angle is 11–16°)—use a distal soft-tissue procedure and a proximal metatarsal osteotomy (Scarf or alike) to correct the deformity. Note that a chevron osteotomy cannot correct a deformity of this magnitude.
- If the deformity is severe (hallux valgus angle of >40° and the intermetatarsal is >16°) use a distal soft-tissue procedure with proximal osteotomy (arthrosis should be minimal). These severe deformities usually quickly develop arthrosis so threshold for arthrodesis should be low.

- The second consideration is of arthrosis which if present or the deformity is too severe and then consider an arthrodesis. If there is significant arthrosis of the MTP joint, an arthrodesis is probably the procedure of choice.

  Place the hallux at about 15° of valgus and 10–15° of dorsiflexion in relation to the ground.

In general, any chosen surgical procedure must correct the following structural components of deformity for optimal outcome:

- *Hallux valgus deformity per se:* Valgus deviation of the great toe
- First metatarsal varus
- Pronation deformity of hallux, first metatarsal or both
- The medial eminence (bunion)
- First MTP arthritis and stiffness
- Maintaining length of short first metatarsal
- The displacement of the sesamoid apparatus
- Pathology (excessive mobility or obliquity) at first metatarsomedial cuneiform joint
- Muscle-tendon imbalance at the MTP joint and hallux
- A variety of procedures are available to the foot and ankle surgeon to choose from for correction of the hallux valgus deformity **(Flowchart 2)**. Most commonly the hallux valgus deformity correction is divided into four chronological steps described below:

  1. *Lateral release of the metatarso-sesamoidal phalangeal complex (MSPC)* ***(Figs. 8A to C)****:* This is the common

Flowchart 1: Simplified algorithm for management hallux valgus.

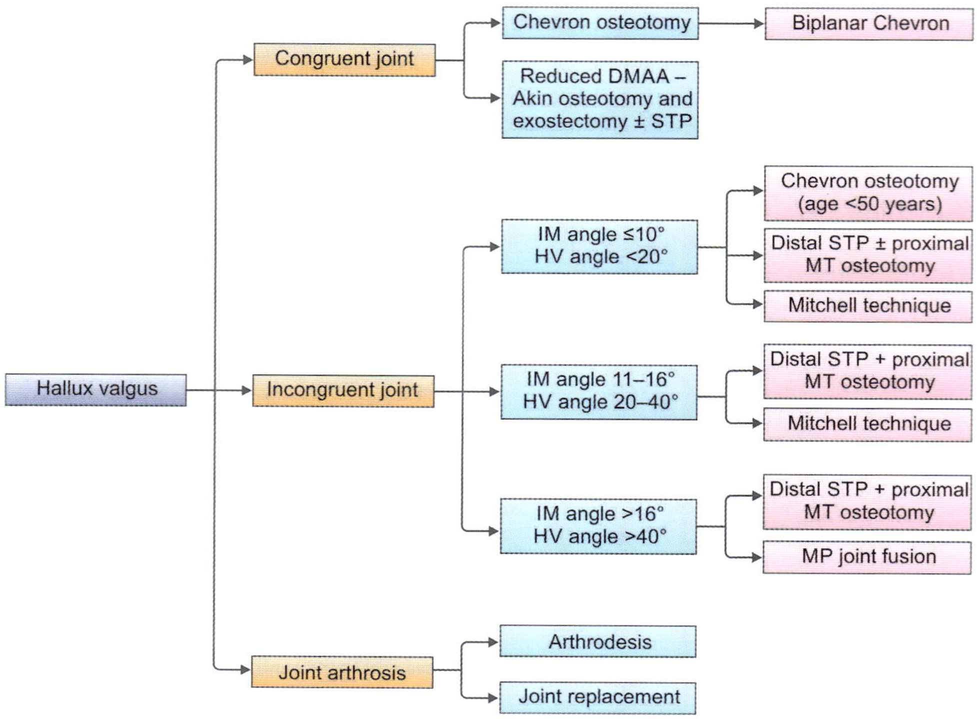

(DMAA: distal metatarsal articular angle; HV: hallux valgus; IM: intermetatarsal; MC: metatarsocuneiform; MP: metatarsophalangeal; MT: metatarsal; STP: soft-tissue procedure)

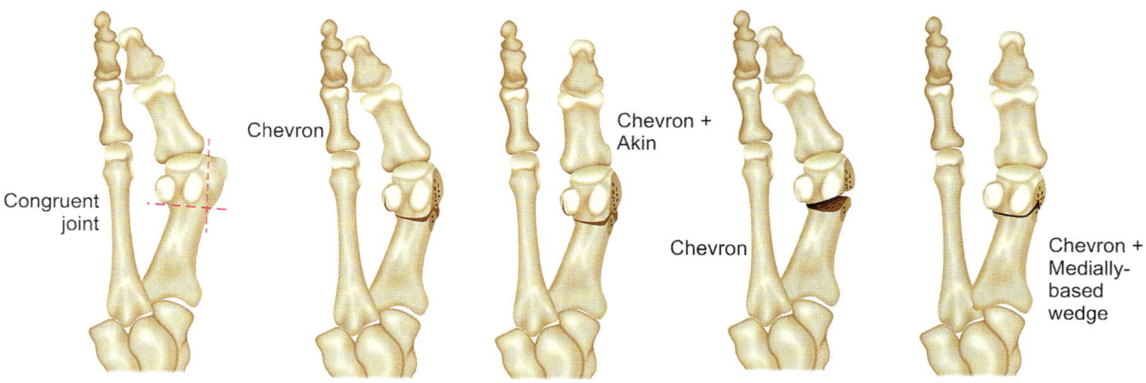

Fig. 7: Surgical management of congruent hallux valgus deformity.

step and should be done even in mild deformities. The release achieves two main goals:

i. Releasing sesamoids from the head of the metatarsal places them correctly after deformity correction.
ii. It marks the first step by releasing the phalangeal insertional band. MTP joint collateral ligament should be preserved in every case to avoid overcorrection. The phalangeal insertional band can be preserved in mildest of the deformities.

2. The first metatarsal osteotomy
3. *The medial soft-tissue tightening* ***(Fig. 9)****:* Medial capsulorrhaphy is done by tightening the medial capsular cut (dorsal medial sensory nerve is isolated and positioned more laterally to protect). The rotation point suggested by A Lahm should be understood and followed which is the center of metatarsal head where the suture is placed. The suture should be placed with great toe in plantar flexion so that the great toe makes ground contact after procedure. The long extensor tendon should lie straight and not "bent" to reduce plantar flexion and decrease risk of overcorrection.

Flowchart 2: Various procedures at disposal of surgeon for correction of hallux valgus deformity.

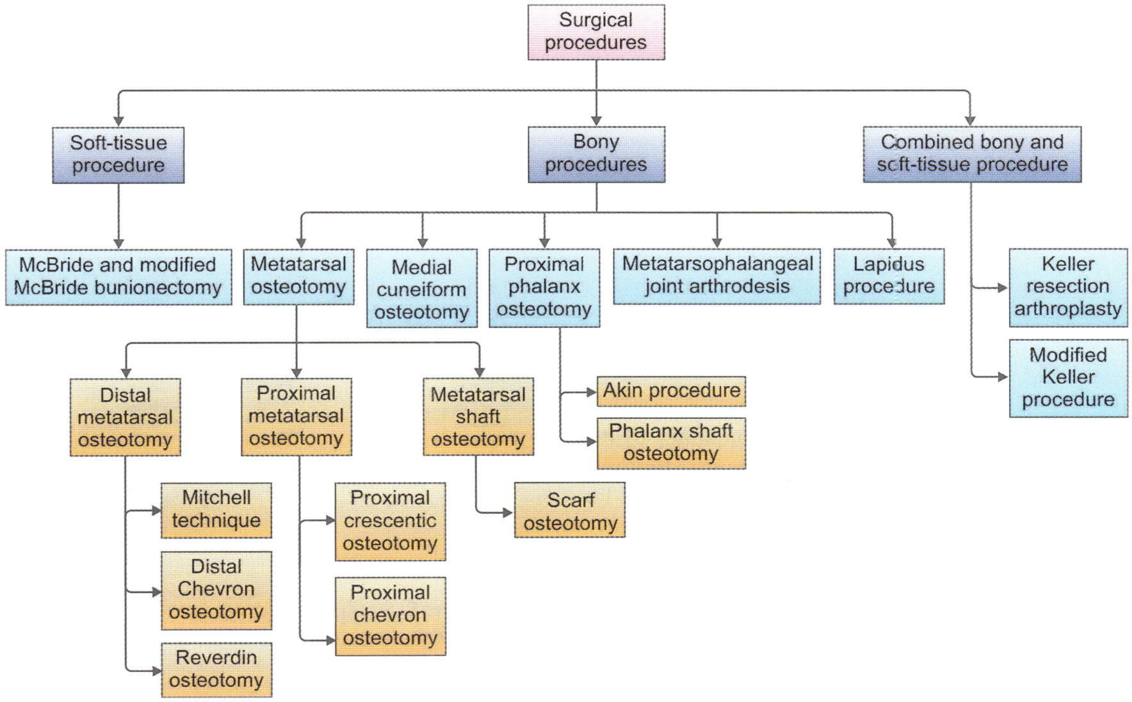

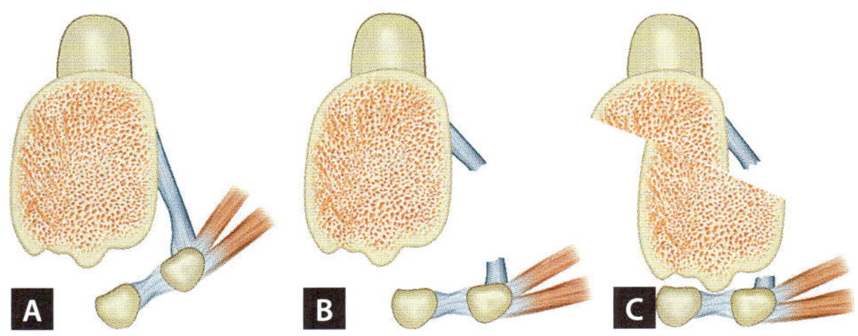

Figs. 8A to C: Bunion correction steps—the steps common to nearly all reconstructive procedures are: (A) release of the metatarsosesamoidal phalangeal complex and (B) first metatarsal osteotomy (C) that replaces the seramoids underneath and in horizontal plane.

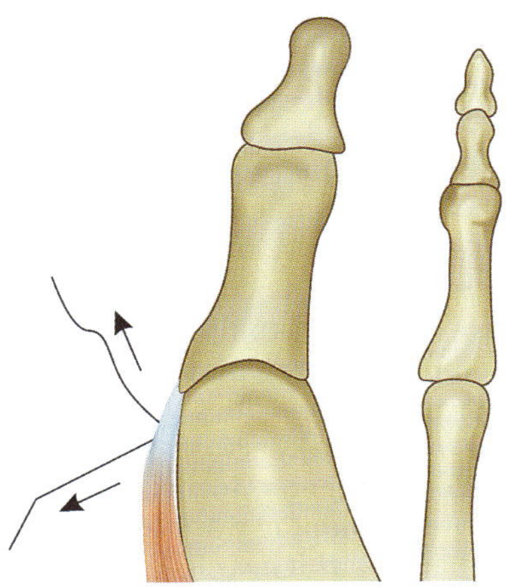

Fig. 9: Medial soft-tissue tightening by capsulorrhaphy is also an essential step.

4. The first phalanx great toe osteotomy (performed in most cases, see **Fig. 10**). The osteotomy can be done at two locations—"basal" or at "shaft".
   i. Basal osteotomy is typically indicated for a short toe when enough length cannot be obtained for osteotomy. Healing of osteotomy is good as it is performed in the proximal cancellous bone. To improve stability, a lateral hinge should be preserved at the lateral cortex. The varusization (varus producing) osteotomy allows large medial displacement despite smaller wedge. It can also be combined with rotation. It is easily fixed with a staple.
   ii. Shaft osteotomy is performed in toes of enough length. A cut perpendicular to the shaft is made to allow maximal correction (the range of correction possible with this osteotomy is much larger). As it is performed in midshaft, the stability is a bit compromised compared to basal osteotomy so stronger fixation is needed. Three different kinds of shaft osteotomy have been described, viz. shortening, derotation, and shaft varusization.

In mild deformities (intermetatarsal angle <9°) usually no osteotomy is needed. Medial eminence excision and reefing of soft tissues with a modified McBride procedure (see below) suffices. For moderate deformities (intermetatarsal angle between 10 and 14°) a Chevron osteotomy is done. In severe deformities (intermetatarsal angle >14°) a proximal metatarsal osteotomy is required. A variation of the hallux valgus is hallux valgus interphalangeus in which the

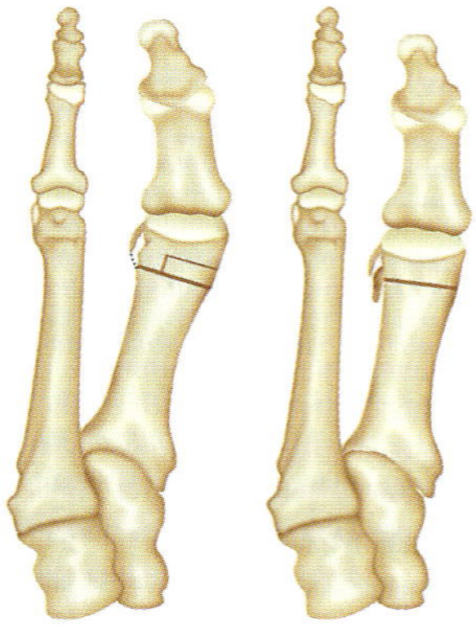

Fig. 10: Mitchell technique.

deformity is between proximal and distal phalanges of the hallux. Here, proximal phalanx medial closing osteotomy of Akin is needed. The various popular techniques used for correcting the hallux valgus are described below.

Modified McBride Operation

This soft-tissue surgery attempts to correct the abnormal biomechanics around the MTP joint. In this surgery, the lateral deforming forces of the conjoined tendons of adductor halluces and the lateral head of flexor halluces brevis are transferred from the lateral sesamoid/proximal phalanx to the lateral side of head of first metatarsal. The tendon is passed through a hole in the metatarsal and this releases the deforming force on the proximal phalanx. In addition, a lateral capsular release and medial imbrication are done. The structures released in order are second metatarsal to lateral sesamoid "intermetatarsal" ligament, adductor hallucis muscle inserting into lateral base of the proximal phalanx, lateral sesamoid suspensory ligament, and lateral MTP joint capsule. Inadequate reduction of the sesamoids back to their anatomic position under the first metatarsal is the greatest predictor of procedure failure and recurrent deformity. In the original McBride procedure lateral sesamoidectomy was done.

Metatarsal Osteotomy

Metatarsal osteotomy is a common procedure done for correction of moderate-to-severe deformities. It is almost always combined with medial reefing or a formal complete distal soft-tissue procedure. MTP arthritis should not be present as it only addresses the medial deviation of metatarsal. It corrects deformity by shifting the axis of the metatarsal laterally toward the second metatarsal and is supplemented by soft-tissue procedures, which involve tightening of the medial capsule of MTP joint to realign the toe in correct position.

- *Mitchell technique:* Metatarsophalangeal joint is exposed by dorsal incision and the small exostosis is removed from medial aspect of metatarsal head. This is a distal *"Step Cut"* metatarsal displacement osteotomy with the primary gain of displacing the metatarsal head fibular wards (laterally) achieving correction of hallux valgus deformity, **Fig. 10**). Transverse cut is made through metatarsal neck preserving lateral 3 mm of metatarsal cortex, just proximal to the level of sesamoids. To create the step, lateral cortex is then cut proximal to the first cut. The head is then pushed laterally and also slight degree of plantar flexion is incorporated to accommodate shortening produced as a result of removing the section of bone. Fixation is done with a suture or screw.
- *Other types:*
  - *Scarf procedure:* Scarf originates from carpentry term "a joint made by bevelling two beams to correspond" **(Figs. 11A and B)**. The cut traditionally described for scarf osteotomy resembles "flash of lightening" on a thunder sky. This is why this osteotomy has a unique name in France: "trait de Jupiter (Jupiter = Zeus in France, the god of thunder)" (in Spain "rayo de Jupiter"). The metatarsal is exposed through proximal plantar exposure through which the cuts and fixation can be done best. The osteotomy is designed to create two fragments—one proximally based dorsal fragment that should be handled carefully on the lateral side, and a second plantar fragment that incorporates the metatarsal head. The cuts are so made to maximally preserve the blood supply to metatarsal **(Fig. 12)**. The longitudinal cut is first performed from medial aspect through given specificities. Then the longitudinal cut is made transversally across the metatarsal. One must be a skilled "carpenter" to make this cut as it is oblique laterally and plantar-ward also cutting the lateral cortex of metatarsal near its plantar border **(Fig. 13)**. Obliquity of cut permits lowering of the plantar head fragment (plantar flexion slightly) when it is laterally displaced. Short cut is commonly done for milder

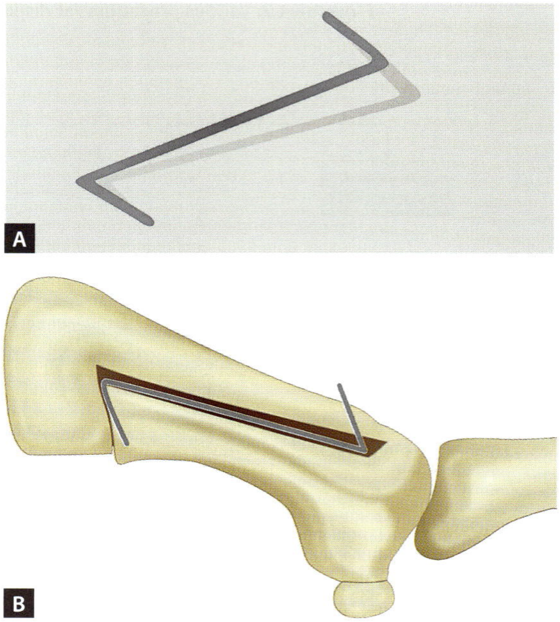

Figs. 11A and B: Scarf osteotomy. (A) As in "carpentry" a "joint" is created by doing oblique cuts; (B) Similarly, the metatarsal in scarf osteotomy is cut in a "Z" fashion.

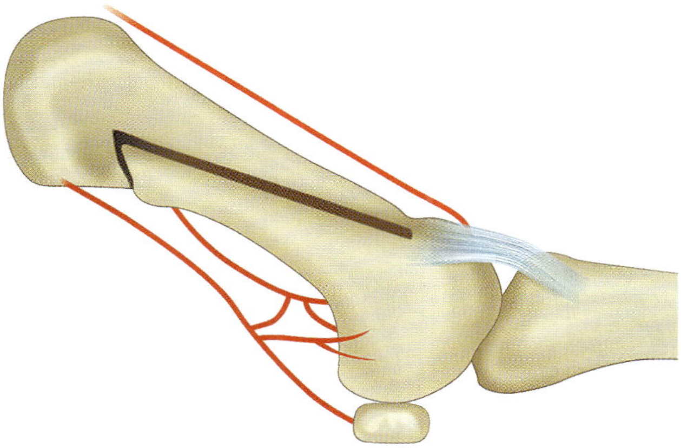

Fig. 12: Blood supply preservation of metatarsal is essential performing the osteotomy so cuts should be appropriately made.

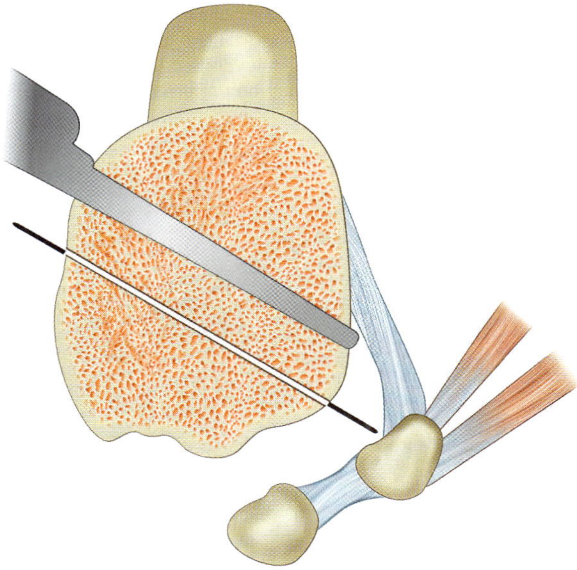

Fig. 13: Oblique longitudinal cut of scarf osteotomy.

deformities while longer cuts are done for moderate-to-severe deformities. The longer the cuts are in general, the more stable are the two solid fragments contacting each other in distal and the proximal cancellous bones of the first metatarsal and this also prevents “channel effect” in osteoporotic bones. The transverse cuts are meticulously placed at 60° to the primary longitudinal cut. First make the proximal cut in order not to jeopardize the distal fragment. The “distal cut” is then performed to complete osteotomy. The fragments are then rotated and translated for deformity correction **(Figs. 14A and B)**. If >20° of angle correction is needed then possibly short scarf is appropriate. If the hallux valgus is associated with cavus, then elevation of head fragment is indicated. In mild-to-moderate deformities, lateral push of head fragment is sufficient while additional medial tightening is needed in severe deformities. Intraoperative check should be performed by “load simulation test”.

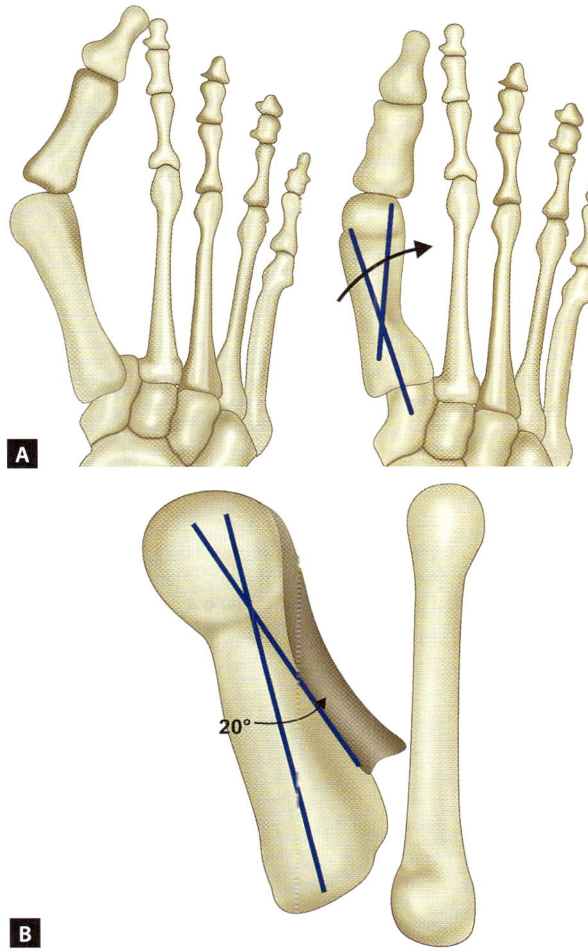

Figs. 14A and B: After making osteotomy, the fragments are rotated and translated to obtain desired correction.

Distal metatarsal articular angle is also important—if DMAA is not decreased, then mere lateral shift will correct deformity. If DMAA is decreased (as in juvenile hallux valgus, iatrogenic hallux valgus or arthritic hallux valgus) the joint is already congruent. Here, the main role is of medial soft-tissue tightening **(Figs. 15A and B)**.

- Metatarsal neck wedge osteotomy (Reverdin, **Fig. 16**)
- *Chevron osteotomy (**Fig. 17**):* This procedure is done for mild to low-moderate hallux valgus deformity. Involves a V-shaped cut in the metatarsal head that allows it to be displaced up to 5 mm laterally. Avascular necrosis of the metatarsal head is an unusual complication.
- Hohmann neck osteotomy
- Oblique neck osteotomy

Keller's Operation

This is indicated when osteoarthritis is established in an old patient. It involves the removal of bunion and excision of the proximal half of the proximal phalanx of great toe and shortening of the toe. Stabilization is achieved by transarticular K-wire.

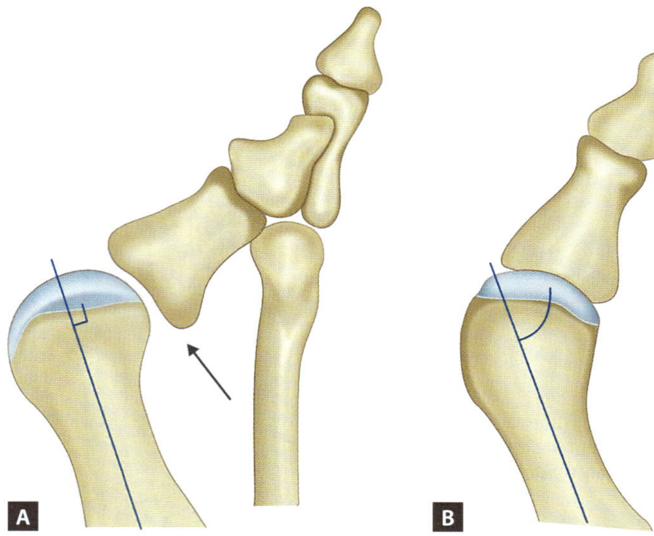

Figs. 15A and B: Significance of distal metatarsal articular angle (DMAA). If the DMAA is normal or nearly normal (A), metatarsal osteotomy and lateral shift is a good procedure but avoid Akin procedure in increased DMAA. If the DMAA reduces as in juvenile patients (B), soft-tissue procedure is indicated and one should bank less on correction from osteotomy, Reverdin-type osteotomy may be preferred in reduced DMAA.

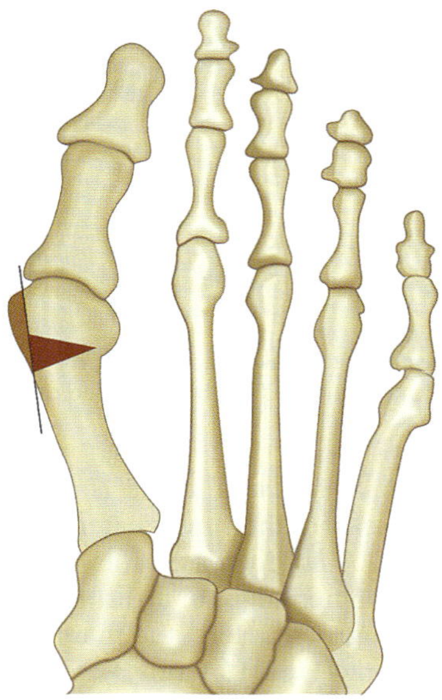

Fig. 16: Reverdin medially base wedge osteotomy of metatarsal neck with bunionectomy.

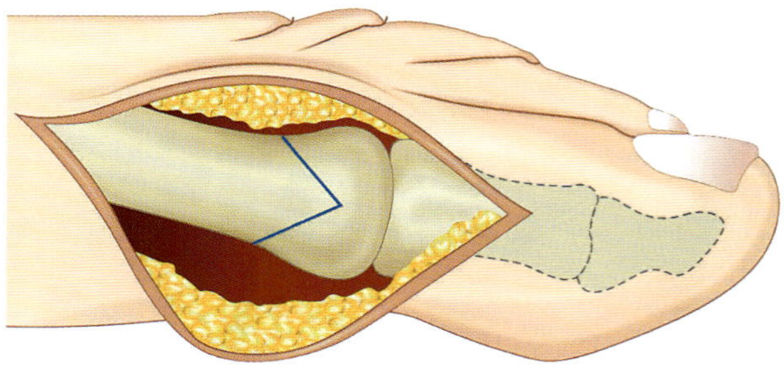

Fig. 17: Chevron osteotomy—V-shaped osteotomy at metatarsal neck.

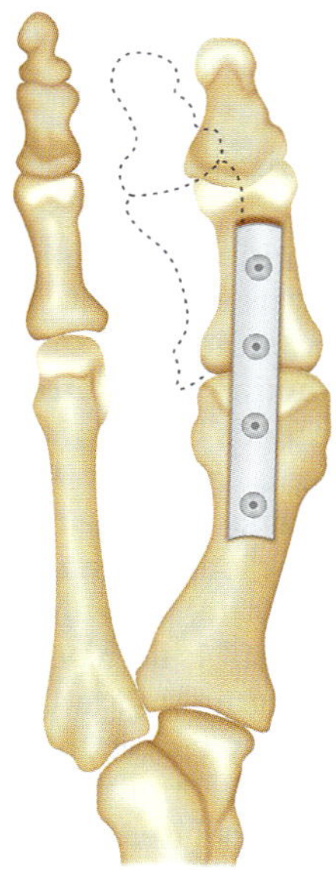

Fig. 18: First metatarsophalangeal joint arthrodesis.

Arthrodesis of First Metatarsophalangeal Joint

The base of the phalanx and the head of the metatarsal are denuded of the articular cartilage and the osteophytes are trimmed. Alignment should be 15° of valgus, 25° of dorsiflexion in relation to the metatarsal shaft, and 15° with respect to the plantar aspect of the foot **(Fig. 18)**.

Bunionectomy

Bunionectomy consists of removing the exostosis with a careful reefing and repair of medial joint capsule. It is indicated in elderly patient with slight valgus deformity. It is mostly combined with other procedures like metatarsal osteotomy.

Akin Procedure (Fig. 19)

This is a medial closing-wedge osteotomy of proximal phalanx. It can be utilized as an isolated procedure or in conjunction with excision of the medial eminence. Do not perform this procedure if the MTP joint is incongruent (DMAA increased). It is a useful salvage procedure for a mild recurrent hallux valgus deformity with a stable MTP joint. Through a medial incision, "make a dorsomedial capsular incision to expose the medial eminence", "expose the medial eminence by sharp dissection and excise it with a sharp thin osteotome".

Lapidus procedure

Lapidus procedure **(Fig. 20)** may be done in patients with hypermobile great toe or even large, severe bunions, and recurrent cases. The philosophy of hallux valgus developing as a result of unstable tarsometatarsal joint was propounded by Dr Paul W Lapidus who proposed arthrodesis of the first cuneiform-metatarsal joint. It comprises arthrodesis of metatarsal cuneiform joint and this fusion also reduces the angle between first and second metatarsal. It is imperative to avoid shortening. The bunion is corrected medially and tightening of soft-tissue structures (distally) is performed.

Distal Soft-tissue Procedure

The distal soft-tissue procedure with and without a proximal metatarsal osteotomy is indicated for a wide range of deformity from mild to severe. It involves proximal transfer of the adductor to the metatarsal neck, lateral sesamoid and intermetatarsal (IM) ligament recession (lateral MPSC as described above), and medial capsular reefing. The procedure is more or less similar to McBride's procedure detailed above.

CROSSOVER SECOND TOE

The deformity occurs secondary to a significant hallux valgus deformity that can cause pressure on the second toe and lead to dorsal subluxation or dislocation of the second toe. There is attenuation of the second metatarsophalangeal (MP) joint's fibular collateral ligament and later even the formation of a rent in it. The tibial collateral ligament often contracts secondarily. As the deformity progresses, dorsal subluxation

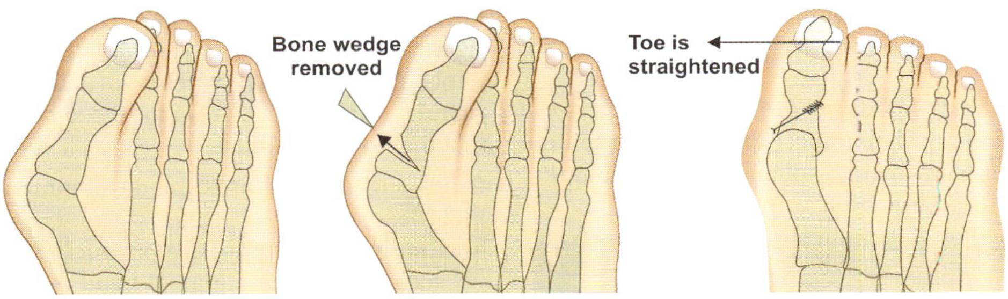

Fig. 19: Akin procedure (see text).

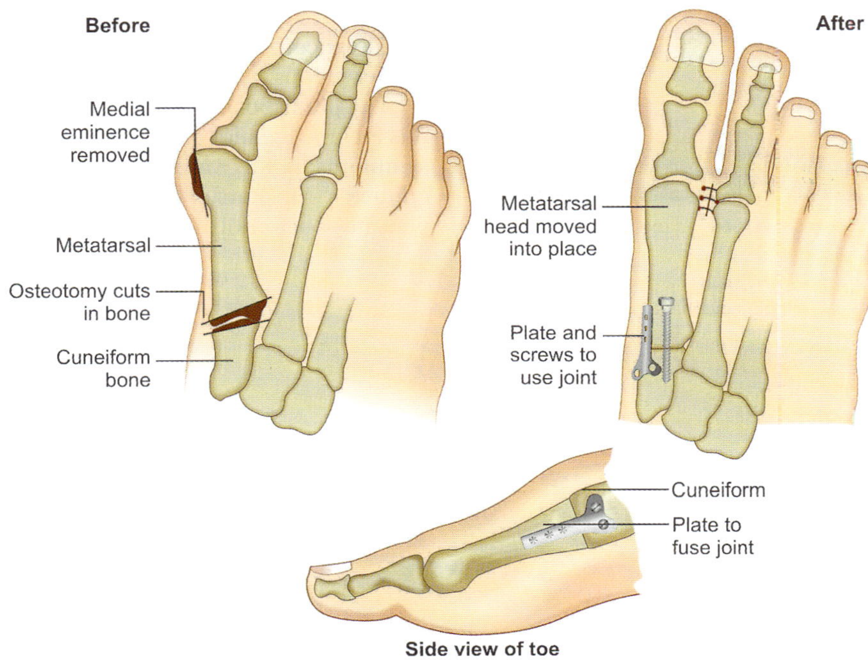

Fig. 20: Lapidus procedure (please see text).

and dislocation of the second MP joint can occur. The uncommon cause is varus deformity of second toe **(Fig. 21)**.

Clinical Features

Apart from the characteristic deformity, evaluate instability of the joint by anterior drawer sign. This anterior drawer sign (Thompson and Hamilton's) consists of grasping the proximal phalanx of the lesser toe between the thumb and index finger (while stabilizing the metatarsal with the other hand) and manipulating the toe in a vertical fashion. If instability exists, there is subluxation at the MP joint and pain may occur.

Treatment

- Nonsurgical treatment includes taping the second toe in a reduced position or using open-toed or extra-depth shoes.
- Surgical repair includes extensor tenotomy, dorsal capsulotomy of MTP joint, and tibial collateral ligament release, with intramedullary K-wire fixation of the toe. Reefing of the lateral capsule may also be used to strengthen the reconstruction; this also helps to reduce the recurrence of deformity.
- For severe deformity, MP joint arthroplasty to both decompress the joint and allow reduction of the proximal phalanx is done.

It is necessary with all these procedures to perform correction of the hallux valgus deformity at the same time to prevent the hallux from again displacing the second toe.

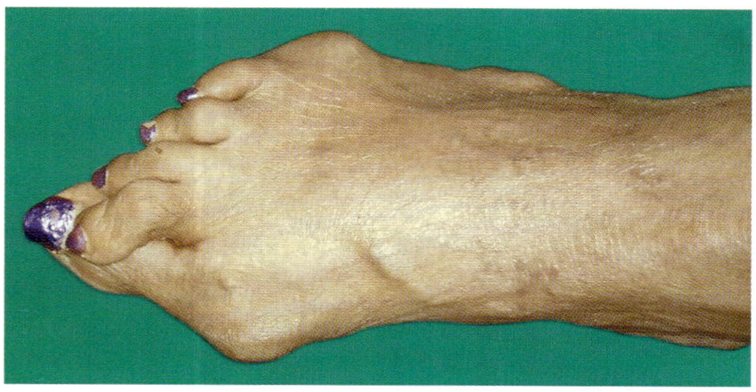

Fig. 21: Crossed-over second toe.

Complications

- Swelling
- Recurrence
- Loss of motion at the MP joint, from postsurgical scarring and fibrous arthrodesis is a common complication.

HALLUX RIGIDUS

Hallux rigidus is painful limitation of movements of the MTP joint of the great toe. Its pathogenesis is still elusive but it closely resembles osteoarthritis or a degenerative pathology. As for degenerative joint disorders, cartilage damage appears to be the primary event that initiates synovitis. Pannus formation from relentless synovitis further causes cartilage destruction, osteophyte formation and proliferation and in advanced cases subchondral bone destruction **(Figs. 22A and B)**. Although mostly considered idiopathic, the process may begin in adolescence, when an unrecognized traumatic event at the MTP joint causes damage to dorsal articular surface of metatarsal head. This may slowly progress to degenerative joint disease being in constant use, weight-bearing and motion under an altered biomechanical environment due to inciting event. Repeated microtrauma has also been suggested to cause articular cartilage damage further progressing to degenerative joint disease. Adult hallux rigidus is usually due to degenerative arthritis of first MTP joint **(Figs. 23A and B)** whereas in adolescent, patient's hallux rigidus usually results from localized cartilage damage of the first metatarsal head.

Other suggested causes for development of hallux rigidus include:

- Osteochondral fracture producing osteochondritis dissecans of first metatarsal head over dorsal convexity of the joint surface.
- First metatarsal hyperextension injury
- Abnormally long first metatarsal
- Advanced pronation deformity of the foot as in severe pes planus

The predisposing factors for development of hallux rigidus include female sex, positive family history with bilateral symptoms, hallux valgus interphalangeus, and metatarsus adductus. Metatarsus primus elevatus seems to be a compensatory deformity instead of being a risk factor for devel-

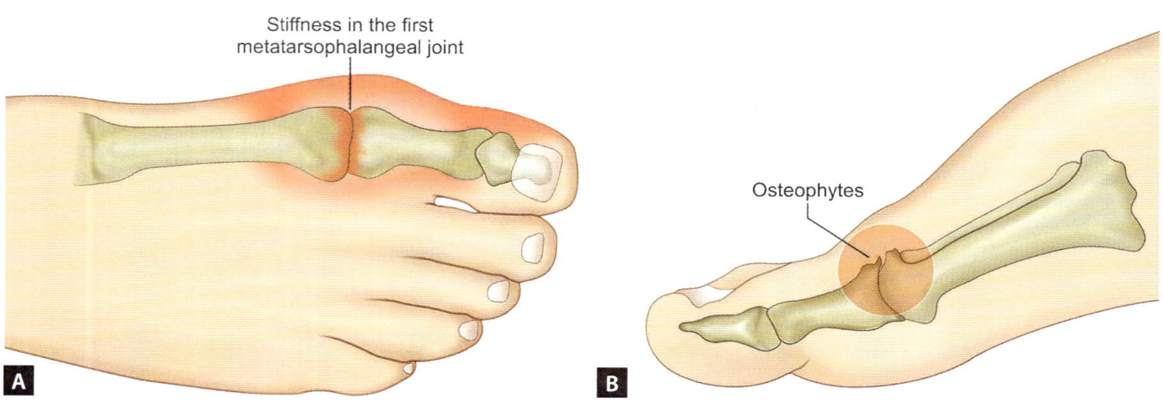

Figs. 22A and B: Hallux rigidus—degeneration and stiffness of the first metatarsophalangeal joint.

opment. Hindfoot contracture, abnormal foot posture, first ray hypermobility, and metatarsal length, or the patient's occupation or shoe wear do not seem to have any documented association with development of hallux rigidus.

Pathoanatomy and Classification

- *Cleavage lesion:* This is the most common microscopic finding in patients with hallux rigidus which is always between the apex of the dome and the dorsal margin of the articular surface. The underlying subchondral bone is not detached.
- Abutment of the proximal phalanx against the cleavage lesion in the articular cartilage on hallux extension causes pain, also causing an indistinct flexion deformity as an avoidance mechanism.
- Later there is osteophyte formation at this site which mechanically blocks joint extension. This is when the patient usually presents to clinician. The earliest radiological finding in hallux rigidus is a small depression in the dome of the metatarsal head.

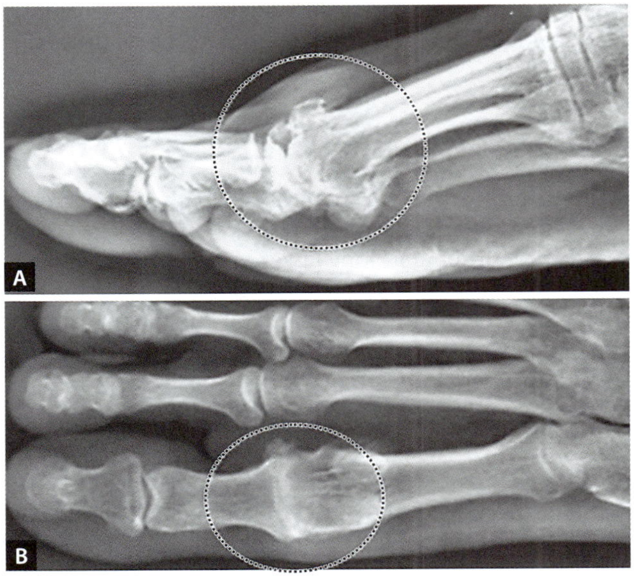

Figs. 23A and B: The hallux rigidus deformity in adult commonly results from degenerative joint disease. There is reduced joint space (B) with osteophyte formation seen prominently on the lateral projection (A).

Clinical Features

The patient reports painful limitation of movements of great toe initially appearing in load-bearing activities such as running and jumping and later limiting a casual walk also. The symptoms are intermittent initially that subside easily with simple analgesics but become functionally limiting over a period of time with development of synovitis and dorsal osteophytes. There is dorsal impingement with foot-wear and a careless patient may present with dorsal skin ulceration. Palpation of the joint may reveal tenderness due to tendinitis, bursitis, capsulitis, synovitis, and painful dorsal spur.

Radiographic Evaluation

Standard radiological examination involves obtaining AP, lateral and oblique views of the involved foot. Joint space narrowing and arthritic changes are better seen in AP projection while dorsal osteophytes are best seen on a lateral projection. Coughlin and Shurnas proposed grading of Hallux rigidus **(Table 1)** that partly correlates with clinical findings.

Differential Diagnosis

The following must be borne in mind while evaluating painful first MTP joint:

Gout and pseudogout, rheumatoid arthritis, septic arthritis, sesamoiditis, sesamoid fracture, turf toe injury, acute isolated osteochondral injury to the hallux MTP joint, hallux varus, and hallux valgus.

Treatment

Commonly for a surgically unwilling patient, use of a shoe with an ample toe box is advised. However, in most patients, operative correction is required to give symptomatic relief and improve function.

The various operative options exercised for management of Hallux rigidus are:

- *Cheilectomy:* Chiselling away bony irregularities at osteochondral margin is especially useful in older patients with degenerative joint disease.
- *Dorsal wedge osteotomy:* Done at the base of the proximal phalanx or distal first metatarsal. This option is commonly prescribed for adolescent patients.
- Arthrodesis of first MTP joint is done only if loss of joint space is evident not only on standard anterior-posterior

TABLE 1: Grading of severity of hallux rigidus (Coughlin and Shurnas).

Radiological grade and description		*Reported pain*	*Movements at MTP joint*
0	Normal	None	Stiffness or slight loss
1	Narrowing (early) of MTP joint space	Intermittent	Mild movement restriction at MTP
2	Moderate narrowing of joint space + osteophyte formation	Intermittent	Restricted joint extension with pain
3	Severe joint space narrowing + extensive osteophyte formation around the metatarsal and phalanx base	Constant (no pain at midrange of MTP joint motion)	Severe joint movement restriction (<20° total motion)
4	Same as grade 3	Pain at midrange of passive MTP joint motion	Same as grade 3

(MTP: metatarsophalangeal)

(AP) and lateral views but also on the oblique views of the joint as is common in grade 4 or 3 hallux rigidus. There had been cases of painful nonunion and formation of short fibrous nonunion at the site using cross pins and K-wires but with newer fixation techniques, locked plate osteosynthesis, and use of interfragmentary compression screws or dorsal plates fusion rates are high.
- *Resection arthroplasty (Keller procedure):* Here, the pathological joint is resected below the subchondral bone removing all osteophytes, synovium, etc. and the created space is filled with extensor halluces brevis tendon and capsular tissue for interposition.
- Hemiarthroplasty of the proximal phalanx is new introduction but not very popular among surgeons as the results of other procedures described above are quite satisfactory for improving function.

HALLUX FLEXUS

This is a static deformity which occurs initially during walking but may become fixed and rigid later. There is dorsal bunion formation due to marked plantar flexion of the proximal phalanx of the big toe, with some degree of dorsiflexion of the first metatarsal **(Fig. 24)**. Normal medial longitudinal arch is lost and the talonavicular break is often present with abnormality of the cuneiform which is tilted upward. Soft-tissue contractures occur particularly of the first MTP joint capsule, flexor hallucis longus, and brevis tendons so that there is loss of mobility of the first MTP joint.

Etiology

Unbalanced flexion pull at the great toe that causes plantar-flexion of the phalanges results in flexion deformity; this mechanism can be produced by various conditions:
- Paralysis of all the foot muscles (as in poliomyelitis) but preserved gastrocnemius-soleus group posteriorly and normal flexors of the toes, as well as flexor hallucis brevis.
- Certain tendon transfer operations in which there is failure to achieve balance between the peroneus longus with its insertion into the lateral side of medial cuneiform and first metatarsal base and the tibialis anterior which is inserted into the medial surface of these bones.
- Arthritic hallux rigidus with soft-tissue contractures involving the plantar capsular structures
- Rocker bottom deformity of vertical talus or congenital flat foot

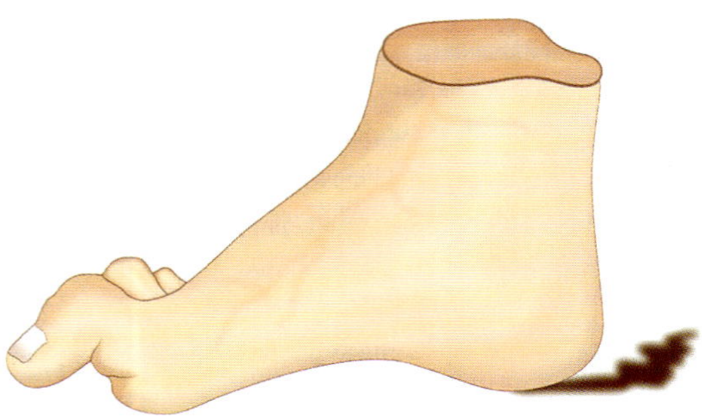

Fig. 24: Hallux flexus deformity.

Treatment

- Lapidus procedure along with transfer of the insertion of tibialis anterior backward to be attached at the site of insertion of tibialis posterior at the navicular tubercle.
- A plantar-based wedge osteotomy is carried out at naviculocuneiform-metatarsal joints.
- The flexor hallucis longus tendon is divided at its insertion and transferred proximally to be inserted through an oblique hole drilled in the neck of first metatarsal.
- Plantar capsulotomies may be necessary.

DEFORMITIES OF THE LESSER TOE

The following two deformities are commonly observed in lesser toes:
1. Rigid hammer toe
2. Flexible hammer toe

Hammer toe deformities involve flexion deformity of the proximal interphalangeal (PIP) joint with extension (not hyperextension) at the MTP joint.

Rigid Hammer Toe

A rigid hammer toe is defined as a fixed flexion deformity of the PIP joint that cannot be passively corrected to the neutral position.

Etiology

- Flexible hammer toe often results from a tight flexor digitorum longus (FDL) tendon which if uncorrected develops into rigid deformity.
- A disproportionately long lesser toe or a shoe with a tight toe box can also cause a fixed hammer toe deformity.
- Hammer toe deformity can also be due to the formation of a hallux valgus deformity which can push the second toe into a hammered or overlapped position.

Symptoms

- Pain over dorsum of the PIP joint where toe rubs against the top of the shoe box or at the tip of toe where the toe hits the sole of the shoe. Later there is development of callus or callosities at the pressure regions.
- If there is sufficient distal migration of the plantar fatty cushion, pain under the metatarsal head can result.

Treatment

Shoe modifications are primarily used:
- Extra depth shoes
- Soft insoles and metatarsal pads

Surgical correction is often necessary for rigid hammer toe deformity:
- Evaluate for related deformities, such as tight FDL tendon or a hallux valgus deformity.
- A hallux valgus deformity can reduce the space lateral to the hallux, which prevents reduction of a second toe into a reduced position. If this condition exists, a hallux valgus repair should be strongly considered.

- A PIP joint arthroplasty (some alternatively perform bony arthrodesis of the PIP joint), such as described by DuVries consists of the resection of the distal condyle of the proximal phalanx. It results in a fibrous ankylosis that allows approximately 15° or 20° of motion. If the method is not fully successful then additional procedures can be done like:
    - Extensor tenotomy [Releasing both the extensor digitorum longus (EDL) and extensor digitorum brevis]
    - Releasing dorsal aspect of MTP joint capsule
    - If still the deformity is not fully corrected then perform an MTP arthroplasty (arthrotomy → expose metatarsal head and remove a 2-mm wafer of bone with microsaw → fix with K-wire).
- Weil osteotomy is an alternative to MTP arthroplasty—here the metatarsal is shortened by an osteotomy done along the metatarsal shaft in the axial plane. The osteotomy starts at the junction of the articular cartilage and dorsal shaft of the metatarsal and continues along a plane parallel to floor (weight-bearing position of the foot). The osteotomy is fixed after translation of the metatarsal with screw and redundant cortex removed. For unstable MTP joint additionally plantar plate reconstruction can be done. Remove the plate from proximal phalanx → pass suture transversely through it, advance it and pull sutures through the holes drilled in proximal phalanx while maintaining the MTP joint in extension or slight flexion.

Complications of Surgery

- Swelling, infection, and wound dehiscence
- Recurrence of deformity
- Floppy toe, if too much of the shaft of the proximal phalanx is removed along with the distal condyle in excision arthroplasty.

Flexible Hammer Toe

A flexible toe deformity can be passively corrected. They are completely eliminated with the plantar flexion of the MP joint or of the ankle indicating tightness of the FDL tendon.

Treatment

- Strapping of the toe is helpful for a flexible deformity. Tape is placed dorsally over the proximal phalanx, the MTP joint is plantarflexed. The strapping reduces the deformity by exerting a plantarflexion force at the MTP joint with compensatory extension at the PIP joint.
- Surgical therapy involves releasing the FDL tendon and reducing the flexion force.
- Girdlestone-Taylor flexor to extensor tendon transfer often combined with the release of deforming forces at the MP joint is usually satisfactory. An arthroplasty of the PIP joint is, sometimes, combined with the tendon transfer if there is some element of a fixed component.

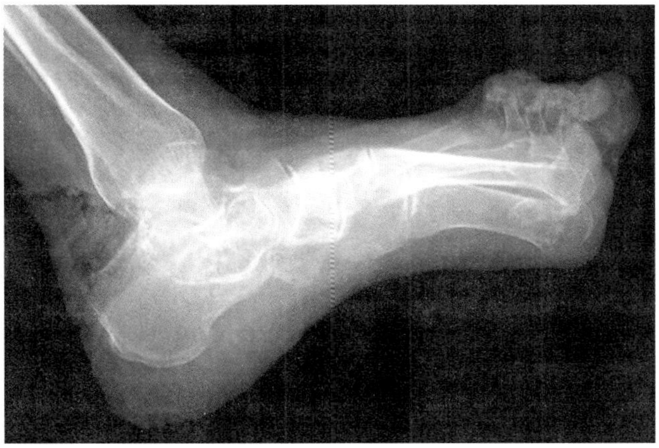

Fig. 25: Clawing of toes (radiographic appearance).

Technique

The FDL tendon is released from the base of phalanx percutaneously and split into half. They are delivered dorsally near the base of proximal phalanx and sutured to the soft tissues. While suturing, the toe is maintained in a flexed position at the metacarpophalangeal (MCP) joint and extension at the interphalangeal (IP) joint, a K-wire can be used to maintain this position. Close all wounds and hold the toe in neutral position with a postoperative dressing. Fix the toe with a K-wire, if a fixed PIP joint deformity was treated.

Complications

The most significant complication is possible neurovascular injury from pressure or swelling around the area of the tendon transfer, producing vascular or neurologic compromise.

CLAW TOE

A claw toe is a hyperextension deformity of the MP joint along with a flexion deformity of either the proximal or distal interphalangeal joints (clawing, **Fig. 25**). The word is derived from the appearance of claws of animals. Evaluate both the MTP and the involved IP joint for flexibility at each joint.

Treatment

- Resection arthroplasty as described for hammer toe. This may be supplemented with extensor tenotomy and capsulotomy with release of the medial and lateral collateral ligaments as necessary.
- For deformities that recur or are not fully addressed with above, a flexor tendon transfer, as described in the treatment of flexible hammer toe may be required.
- If severe subluxation or dislocation at MP joint is present then a resection arthroplasty of the MP joint might be necessary.

Complications

- *Redislocation of the MP joint:*
    - It can result from inadequate shortening of the MP head or stiffness from inadequate rehabilitation after pin removal.

- Incomplete soft-tissue release may also be a factor contributing to recurrence.
- Compromise of the vascular supply at the toe can occur from tension or spasm of the interdigital vessels.

MALLET TOE

Mallet toe is a flexion deformity of the distal interphalangeal (DIP) joint. It is painful due to rubbing of the tip of the toe on the inner sole of the shoe. Mallet toe is usually a fixed deformity and is less common than hammer toe.

Treatment

Being commonly fixed, the deformity needs surgical correction often:
- If there is some flexibility at the DIP joint and passive correction can be done forcefully then treatment with percutaneous tenotomy of the FDL tendon may restore the alignment.
- When the deformity is rigidly fixed then it is necessary to decompress the DIP joint and perform a resection arthroplasty. Excise an ellipse of skin from the dorsal aspect of the DIP joint and after release of the extensor apparatus and the collateral ligaments, excise the distal condyle of the middle phalanx with a bone cutter to create a resection arthroplasty. Capsular tissue is commonly interposed into the space.

Complications

- Possible neurovascular injury
- Swelling
- Recurrence of deformity

TAILOR'S BUNION OR BUNIONETTE

Tailor's bunion or bunionette is a term used for an enlargement of the lateral aspect of the fifth metatarsal head. This is associated with pain, swelling, and tenderness. Pathological enlargement of the lateral aspect of fifth metatarsal head can occur due to (or a combination of):
- Hypertrophy of soft tissue overlying the fifth metatarsal
- A congenitally enlarged or dumbbell-shaped fifth metatarsal head
- An abnormal lateral angulation of the fifth metatarsal shaft

Etiology

Structural Causes

- Supernumerary bone growing from or attaching to the lateral aspect of the fourth metatarsal head pushing the fifth metatarsal head outward.
- Congenital splaying of the fifth metatarsal due to incomplete or imperfect development of the transverse intermetatarsal ligament
- Wide intermetatarsal angle resulting from spreading of the metatarsals
- *Professional:* Persons used to sitting crosslegged or forced to sit in this position (like tailors) suffer from persistent pressure on the lateral side of the fifth metatarsal head.

The Functional Causes

Tailor's bunion may result from abnormal biomechanics resulting from:
- Excessive subtalar joint pronation
- Uncompensated varus position of the forefoot
- A congenitally plantar-flexed fifth metatarsal
- Idiopathically, an enlarged fifth metatarsal head

Clinical Features

- *Bursa formation and bursitis:* With continuous pressure over this bony prominence there is development of skin thickening, corn formation, and an adventitious bursa develops because of chronic irritation.
- *Corn formation on lateral aspect:* Due to prominent bunionette that may get exacerbated with shoe wear.
- Ulceration due to chronic pressure and ensuing infection. This complication occurs in neuropathic foot due to diabetes mellitus, CMTD or spinal dysraphism with compromised sensibility. Infection locally may result in loss of the entire fifth ray or, sometimes, even the foot.
- *Corn formation on the plantar aspect:* Localized intractable keratosis may develop beneath the fifth metatarsal head.

Treatment

Support and protection is primarily tried. Metatarsal pads or bars (usually made of silicone), wide toe box shoes, and semirigid shoe insert beneath the plantar aspect of the condyle usually help. In some cases, one-eighth to one-fourth inch foam rubber between the prominence and the shoe may be useful. It is recommended to perform pressure point study before designing the sole for these patients as some compensatory or trick movements to avoid pain may have developed that causes symptoms elsewhere.

Surgical treatment may be required for intractable symptoms and one of the following or a combination can be used:
- Resection of the lateral third of the fifth metatarsal head
- Osteotomy of the fifth metatarsal
- Resection of the fifth metatarsal head

INGROWING TOENAIL (ONYCHOCRYPTOSIS)

This is a common complaint caused by pressing of the shoe against the toenail that causes nail to get driven into the soft part of the toe and result in pain **(Figs. 26A to C)**. Importantly, such patients should be asked to cut the nails square at right angles to its long axis and not in a lunar shape.

Treatment

Conservative Treatment

Correctly cutting the nail as above and wearing of easy fitting stockings and shoes to avoid pressure. It can also be controlled

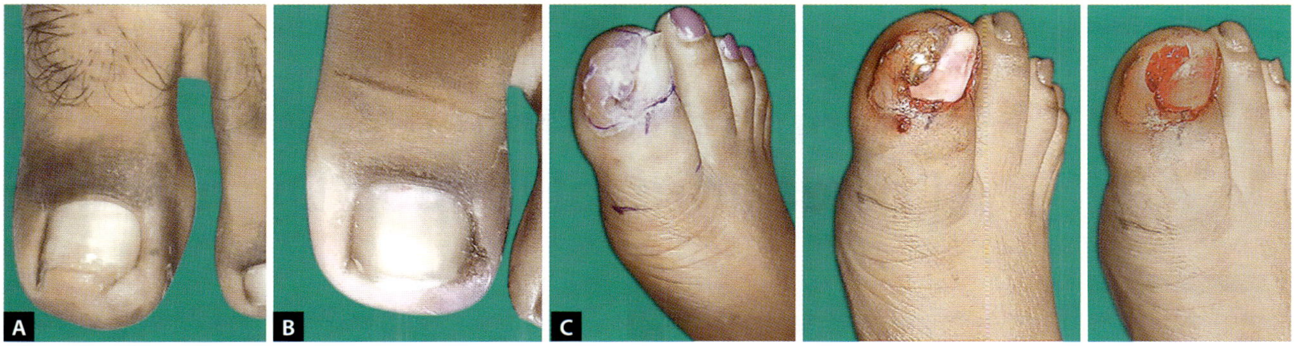

Figs. 26A to C: Ingrowing toenail is a common deformity of the great toe nail (A) that often leads to sepsis due to poor hygiene (B, different patient). This requires nail removal and proper toileting (C, different patient).

by separating the anterior tip and lateral edges of an ingrowing toenail (IGTN) from adjacent soft tissues by cotton.

Surgery is needed for painful nail ingrowth, infection, recurrent infection and abscess formation, paronychia, and recurrent IGTN despite initial nail removal.

Operative Treatment

If nail is infected, remove it under general anesthesia and allow regrowth. If further ingrowing occurs, ablation of nail bed is required.

Zadik's procedure (marginal nail avulsion and phenolization)—excision of all of the nail bed especially on the sides of the distal phalanx. I prefer to use trichloroacetic acid instead of phenol for better safety reasons and ease of handling to ablate the germinal layer.

CONCLUSION

- Deformities of hallux are functionally disabling to the patients as they alter the gait (push-off). These are also many a times not cosmetically acceptable for the patients.
- Most of the deformities are due to inflammatory affection of the foot (rheumatoid arthritis) that is also accentuated by pointed footwear. Trauma comprises a small subset of these patients.
- Understanding the pathogenesis is essential for providing comprehensive correction of deformity. Patient should also be counseled for the need to maintain correction afterward else recurrence is also common.
- Various osteotomies are described (>100) for correction of hallux valgus deformity but only a few are practiced. Even in such case the bony procedures are to be adequately supplemented by soft-tissue procedures otherwise failures are bound to happen. Choice of osteotomy is usually guided by surgeon's practice, however, type and extent of the deformity, patient's age, and joint congruity also make an important bearing.
- Other problems of great toe such as hallux rigidus, hallux flexus, mallet toe, and claw toes must be promptly recognized and correction often entails bony procedures.

CHAPTER 87

Acquired Flatfoot (Pes Planus) and Posterior Tibial Tendon Dysfunction

Manish Kumar Varshney

INTRODUCTION

The human foot is a well-arched structure both in longitudinal and transverse disposition (as discussed in Chapter on "Arches of the Foot"). The loss of arches produces altered mechanics and clinically presents with pain, instability, and difficult ambulation. The posterior tibial tendon (PTT) dysfunction is closely related as a cause of the flat foot and at other times as a consequence of it. Both these conditions are discussed in detail in the chapter here.

ACQUIRED FLATFOOT (PES PLANUS)

Flatfoot is a frequently-encountered pathology in the adult population affecting females more than males peaking at 55 years of age. It refers to partial or complete loss of the normal medial longitudinal arch that develops after skeletal maturity **(Figs. 1A to C)**. Pes planus may arise out of various osseous, ligamentous, muscular-paralytic, spastic or postural causes **(Flowchart 1)** resulting from mostly a benign process reflecting continuation of a congenital problem, trauma, or a condition associated with systemic pathology:

- Osseous—trauma (run-over fracture, fracture of navicular or calcaneus) or from osseous diseases
- Ligamentous variety develops from rupture or avulsion of plantar ligaments.
- Paralytic and spastic muscular types—the flattening of the arch is secondary to altered muscle balance.

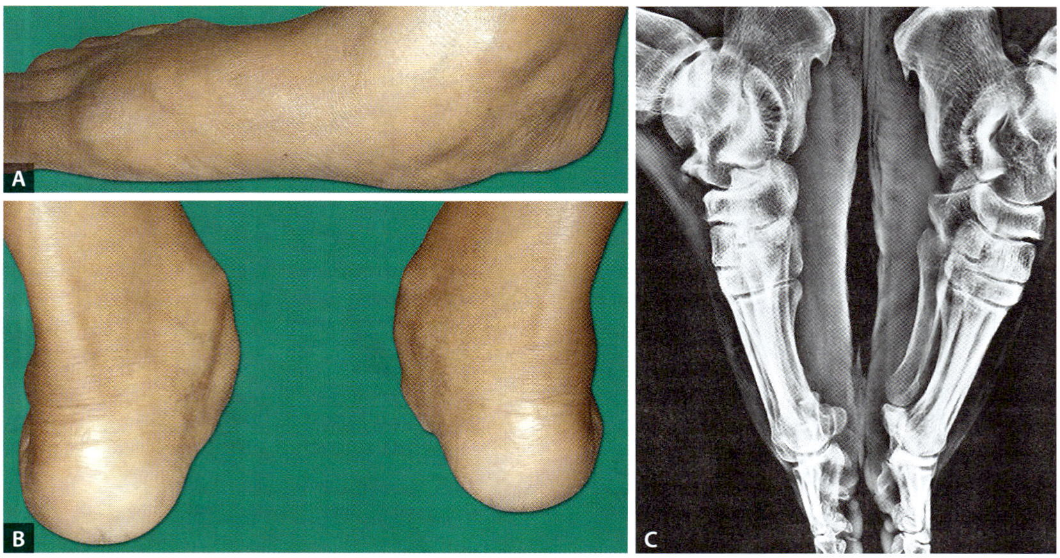

Figs. 1A to C: (A) Flatfoot deformity as visible from side; (B) Posterior aspect; (C) Radiographic appearance.

Flowchart 1: Types of (cause-wise) adult flatfoot.

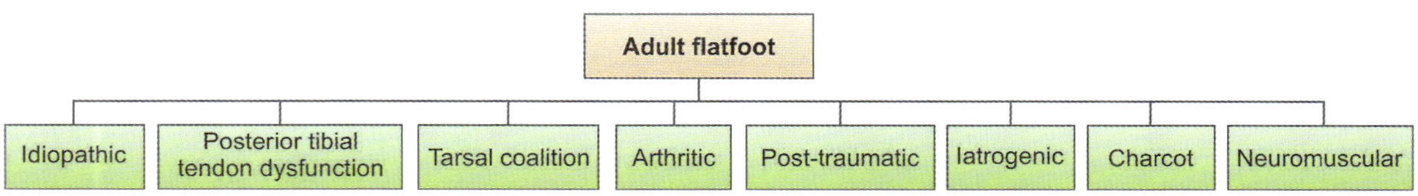

PTT dysfunction/insufficiency is the most common cause of adult acquired flatfoot.

Note: See also chapter on "Anomalies of Pediatric Lower Limb"

PATHOMECHANISM

- There are two main pathological mechanisms for development of pes planus or loss of longitudinal arch:
  1. Calcaneus may be at fault and heel gets drawn up resulting in equinus deformity.
  2. The medial anterior pillar may be pulled up keeping the big toe off the ground as a result of the varus deformity.
- The common causes of flatfoot resulting from muscular causes are excessive fatigue of normal muscles as in:
  - Occupations which require standing or working for long hours
  - Rapid gain in weight (e.g., menopause)
  - Shoe wear
  - Severe trauma

These may get exaggerated by some predisposing factors like general muscle hypotonia after illness or during rapid growth. The risk factors for development of adult flatfoot otherwise are obesity, diabetes, hypertension, trauma, and steroid injections.

PATHOANATOMY

Posterior tibial tendon insufficiency is central to development of adult flatfoot in most of the cases. PTT inverts the hindfoot normally that locks the transverse tarsal joints to provide a platform for push-off. With PTT degeneration, the hindfoot goes into valgus stressing and stretching the medial ligaments. This PTT dysfunction is associated with failure of both capsular and ligamentous structures at midfoot region for complete expression of the deformity. Peritalar subluxation defines the pathologic malalignment of the talus about the subtalar and midtarsal joints resulting from the combined ligamentous, capsular, and tendon insufficiency.

- As the calcaneonavicular ligament yields, the head of the talus is pressed forward, downward, and medially. The navicular translates laterally.
- The calcaneum may deviate medially and its anterior end is depressed, resulting in sustentaculum tali and head of the talus and tuberosity of navicular forming prominences on the medial side of foot.
- The long and short plantar ligaments yield, followed by yielding of deltoid ligament. Dysfunction of the deltoid ligament results in medial ankle instability with development of ankle and foot deformity occurring in the most advanced cases of flatfoot deformity.
- With lateral shift in axis of pull the gastrocnemius contracture develops further exacerbating valgus alignment.

SYMPTOMS

- Feet feel tired after activity. With progression, the feet feel stiff even after sitting or resting. The discomfort is most prominent in the morning. Patient has pain that is more severe on standing than on walking. Muscles in the leg and foot tend to fatigue and cramp because of overuse.
- Tendency to walk with feet everted
- Tenderness is felt over navicular, inferior calcaneonavicular ligament, sole of the foot, and below the first metatarsal head. Lateral ankle pain arises from subfibular impingement.
- Gait is inelastic and clumsy, rising of the heel is avoided, to prevent strain on tarsal and metatarsal ligaments. Patient carefully lifts ball and heel of the foot together. The toes are turned outward.
- Medial parts of shoe wear out more quickly.
- Skin, along the medial border of the heel and foot, is thickened and painful. Callosities may form in weight-bearing areas, and over little toe.

PHYSICAL EXAMINATION

- Depression of the medial longitudinal arch
- Everted or valgus heel in relaxed stance
- Abduction of the forefoot relative to the rearfoot
- Localized tenderness at PTT, plantar fascia, and lateral rearfoot
- *Assess:*
  - Range of motion at various components
  - Flexibility and reducibility of deformity by the Hubscher's maneuver (Jack's test)
  - Single heel rise and double heel rise test (reducibility of rearfoot valgus, **Figs. 2A and B**). If on single heel rise, the hindfoot inverts then it indicates patent and functional PTT and that the deformity is flexible. If hindfoot does not invert then it indicates rigid deformity.
  - Gastrocnemius contracture is assessed by the Silfverskiöld test.

RADIOLOGY OF FLATFOOT

The following findings are often seen in the radiographs taken from a flatfooted patient **(Figs. 3A and B)**:

- Calcaneal pitch is decreased in a flatfoot deformity and becomes negative in the presence of a rocker-bottom deformity.
- The "cyma line" **(Figs. 4A and B)** is the radiographic visualization of the talonavicular and calcaneocuboid joints on the lateral radiograph. The joints should be visualized as a continuum, whereas in a pronated foot type, the talonavicular joint space is positioned anterior to calcaneocuboid joint space.
- Talocalcaneal angle is formed by the long axis of the rearfoot and the midtalar line. This angle is increased in pronated feet on both the anteroposterior and lateral views.
- Increased talar-first metatarsal angle.

ANCILLARY STUDIES

- Magnetic resonance imaging (MRI)
- Computed tomography (CT) scan
- Bone scan

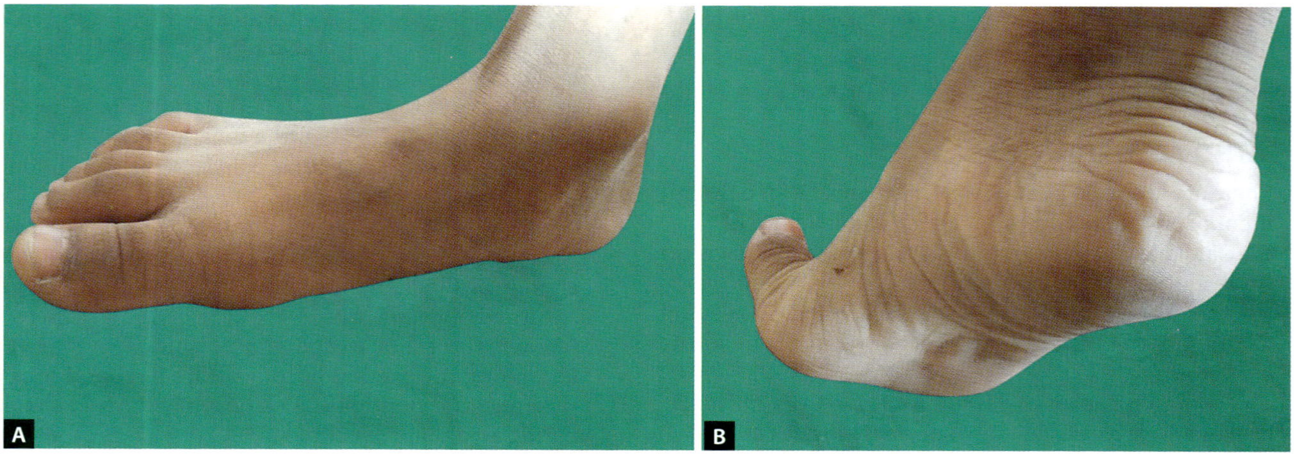

Figs. 2A and B: (A) Single heel rise; (B) Restores the arch in flexible flatfoot.

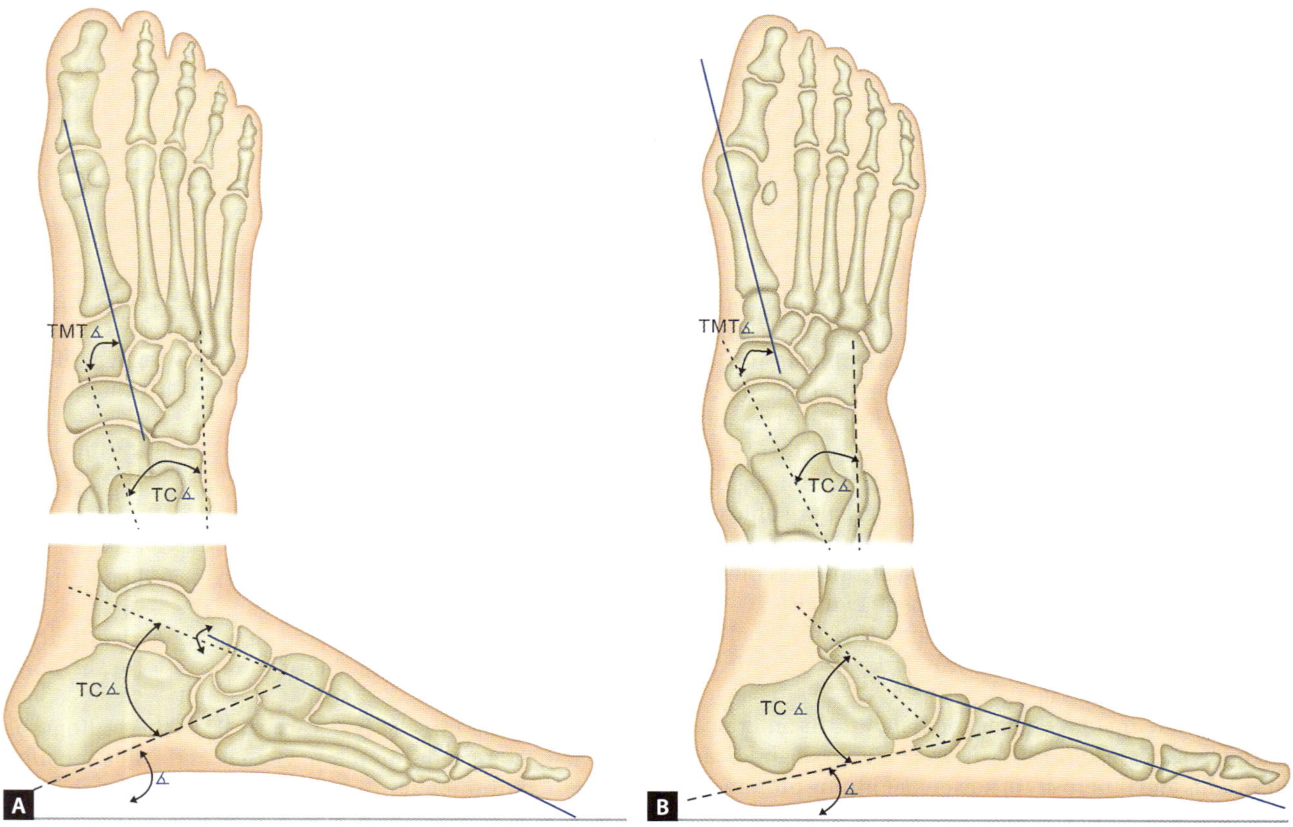

Figs. 3A and B: Radiography in flatfoot. (A) The TC angle in normal foot on anteroposterior (AP) and lateral views; (B) This angle is increased in flat feet. (TMT: tarsometatarsal; TC: talocalcaneal)

- Gait analysis
- Nerve conduction studies (NCs) electromyogram/nerve conduction velocity (EMG/NCV)
- Diagnostic anesthetic injections

STAGES OF DEVELOPMENT OF FLATFOOT

- Foot strain or incipient flatfoot. It is the earliest stage and corresponds to the period, when foot is undergoing deformation and bearing pressure. The ligaments absorb the pressure and undergo stretching and lengthening changes. There is no evident deformity.
- Mobile or flexible flatfoot
- Rigid flatfoot

FLEXIBLE PES PLANUS

The arch may not develop fully until the child is 7–10 years old. Even then once the child is made to stand on toes, the arch appears (*See* Chapter on "Anomalies of Pediatric

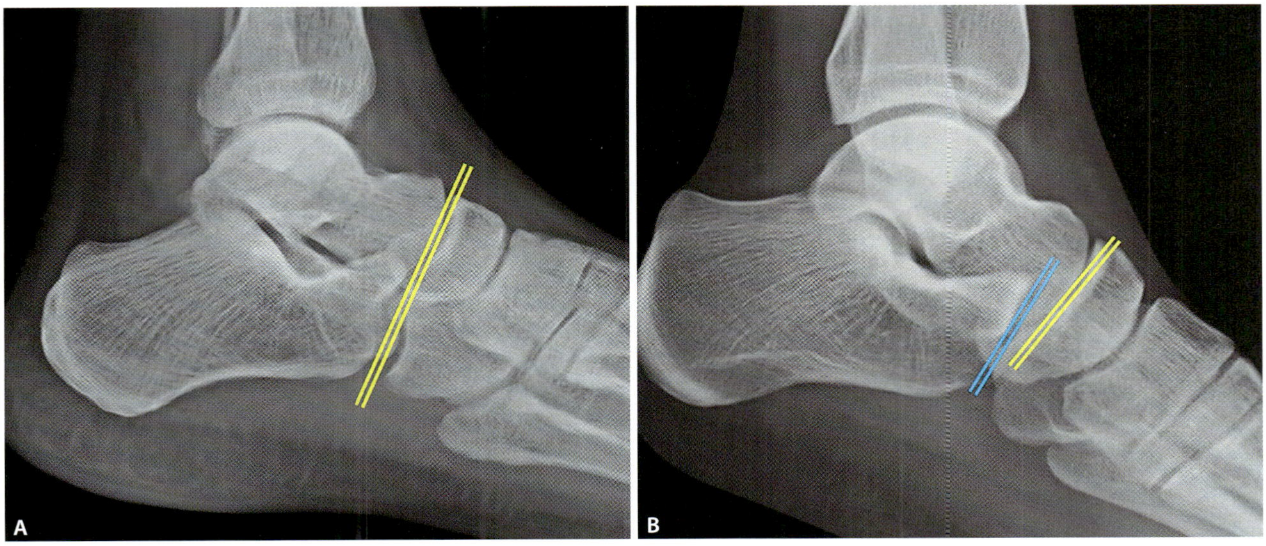

Figs. 4A and B: Cyma line—both talonavicular and calcaneocuboid are in same line in a normal foot (A), while in a pronated foot (B) the former (yellow) is in front of the latter (blue).

Lower Limb"). Generally, adult flexible pes planus is a progression of a pediatric condition in unilateral or, more commonly, as bilateral frequently associated with a short or contracted TA. In its late stages of progression, degenerative arthritis may occur, leading to loss of flexibility or ankylosis ± peroneal spasm due to arthritis produces pronation of rearfoot causing long arch collapse. The talus adducts and plantarflexes on the calcaneus, which simultaneously everts and plantarflexes. Subtalar joint pronation unlocks the midtarsal joint, making it unstable and leading to various degrees of transverse plane abduction.

Etiology

The following conditions are commonly implicated in the development of flexible pes planus:

- Faulty postural activity of the muscles
- Short tendo-Achilles
- Varus deformity of forefoot (skewfoot)
- Spinal dysraphism (e.g., spina bifida, diastematomyelia, lumbosacral lipomata)

Causes of pronation of foot include:

- Compensated forefoot varus
- Compensated flexible forefoot valgus equinus
- Congenital talipes calcaneovalgus
- Torsional abnormalities of adduction or abduction
- Muscle imbalance
- Ligamentous laxity
- Neurotrophic feet
- Anything that contributes to a medial shift in weight bearing (e.g., genu valgum, obesity, and wide base of gait).

Anatomically, the following changes are appreciated:

- Valgus posture of the heel
- Mild subluxation of the subtalar joint, in which the head of the talus tilts medially and plantarward, appearing foreshortened on the standing dorsoplantar radiograph
- Eversion of the calcaneus at the subtalar joint
- Medial angulation (abduction) at the midtarsal joint (talonavicular and calcaneocuboid joints)
- Pronation of the forefoot relative to the hindfoot, which places the first ray plantigrade
- Achilles tendon shortening

Clinical Examination

- When the child stands, there is a flattening of the longitudinal arches, which disappears on standing on toes.
- Short tendo-Achilles is apparent when the foot is correctly aligned and equinus is revealed.
- Valgus deformities of the knees
- Tender areas may be seen at:
  - Sinus tarsi—suggestive of lateral subtalar impingement
  - Talonavicular joint
  - Plantar arch and heel
  - Posterior tibial tendon
  - Anterior tibial tendon
  - Anterior or posterior tibia
  - Subfibular impingement pain

Radiograph

- Talocalcaneal divergence is apparent on the dorsoplantar view and plantar flexion of the talus on the lateral view.
- The "C" sign on lateral radiographs of the ankle originally proposed to indicate talocalcaneal subtalar coalition is found to be more specific for pes planus.
- "Sag" at the talonavicular and naviculocuneiform joint or tarsometatarsal (TMT) joint or both can be assessed.

TREATMENT

Conservative

- *Shoe modification:* An arch support is placed in shoe with a firm heel counter, an extended medial counter, a steel shank, a Thomas heel, and a medial heel wedge. Continuous use of a molded orthosis over an extended

period can result in an improved arch radiographically and clinically.
- Analgesics
- Orthotic management [ankle-foot orthosis (AFO)] and activity modification

Surgical Management

Surgical management is done for controlling disabling pain (and disability) after exhausting every means of conservative management (symptomatic nonresponder). It should not be performed for cosmetic reasons only. The surgeon should explain the loss of inversion and eversion of the foot resulting from surgical correction for the relief of pain and disability. The commonly used techniques are as follows.

Osteotomy

- Evans—lateral column lengthening. The Evans procedure involves lengthening the lateral column, by placing a bone graft from the tibia into the anterior process of the calcaneus. Medial and lateral columns are equalized in length. This procedure preserves the calcaneocuboid joint and pushes the navicular bone medially in relation to the talus. This procedure reduces forefoot abduction and realigns midtarsal joints. The first metatarsal is plantarflexed and also talocalcaneal subluxation is reduced.
- Posterior calcaneal displacement osteotomy (Koutsogiannis)—restores the inverter capability of gastrosoleus and decreases medial arch load. In a symptomatic patient with flexible pes planus and excessive heel valgus, this calcaneal osteotomy is intended to displace the posterior part of the calcaneus medially to restore normal weight-bearing alignment.
- Double calcaneal osteotomy (Evans + posterior calcaneal displacement osteotomy)
- Plantar flexion osteotomy of medial cuneiform (Hirose and Johnson)
- Cotton's medial cuneiform opening wedge osteotomy
- Anterior calcaneal lengthening-distraction wedge osteotomy (Mosca)

Arthrodesis

- Medial column—naviculocuneiform joint(s) and/or metatarsocuneiform joint when medial column collapse is noted. Durham pes planus plasty (Caldwell Coleman) combines advancement of the PTT and osteoperiosteal flap with arthrodesis of the navicular-first cuneiform joint.
- Talonavicular—corrects talar head subluxation
- Calcaneocuboid distraction—similar to evans procedure
- Double (midtarsal joint)—talonavicular and calcaneocuboid joints. These produce lesser subtalar joint arthrosis than isolated talonavicular arthrodesis.
- Subtalar—better done for flatfoot with a reducible deformity without midtarsal joint arthrosis or fixed forefoot varus
- Triple—more suitable for rigid flatfoot. The patient's bone age should be 12 years or older. Arthrodesis for relieving painful pes planus has been most successful when subtalar joint is included, although midtarsal arthrodesis without inclusion of the subtalar joint has gained popularity.
- Pantalar—long-standing deformities with rearfoot and ankle degenerative changes
- Ankle—for ankle joint arthrosis
- Tibiotalocalcaneal (retrograde intramedullary nail)—if midtarsal joints are spared of arthrosis.

Arthroereisis

Blocking the talocalcaneal movement.

Soft Tissue Procedures

- Kidner PTT advancement
- Flexor digitorum longus (FDL) transfer
- Young tenosuspension
- Spring ligament reconstruction + medial arch reconstruction
- Achilles tendon lengthening
- Gastrosoleus recession

RIGID PES PLANUS

The rigid pes planus deformity results from bony abnormality such as tarsal coalition or congenital vertical talus or arthritis (subtalar or midtarsal). PTT dysfunction is the most common cause of adult acquired flatfoot. Other causes such as charcots/post-traumatic are less common.

Clinical Examination

In rigid flatfoot deformity in adults: There may be medial pain from posterior tibial tendonitis, lateral pain from talocalcaneal impingement, or fibulocalcaneal impingement. Patients examined from behind revealing medial flatness of arch and heel valgus. In advanced deformities "too many toes" are visible laterally but is not pathognomonic. Ankle range of motion should be evaluated that may be limited due to tendo-Achilles tightness. Tender areas may be seen at:
- Sinus tarsi
- Talonavicular joint
- Plantar arch and heel
- Posterior tibial tendon
- Anterior tibial tendon
- Anterior or posterior tibia
- Subfibular impingement pain

Harris Mat score has shown correlation with lateral talometatarsal angle and first metatarsocuneiform height. This can be utilized to quantify the extent of acquired flatfoot deformity.

Radiographic Examination

One should obtain weight-bearing AP, lateral foot, and ankle AP radiographs. Measure the Meary's angle (Kindly *see* Chapter on "Pes Cavus and Accompanying Deformities" for radiographic parameters), forefoot abduction, talar head uncoverage, and talar tilt. Talar head uncoverage may be calculated as percentage or may be alternatively assessed by lateral talonavicular incongruency angle that indirectly indicates 30% or more talar head uncoverage. Look also for naviculocuneiform and first TMT joint collapse. Radiographs also help in identifying arthritic changes that develop in advanced deformities. MRI is as such not indicated but in large deformities assessment of spring ligament is only possible by MRI as this would then decide surgical planning and need for reconstruction.

POSTERIOR TIBIALIS TENDON DYSFUNCTION

The PTT is the primary dynamic stabilizer of the medial longitudinal arch. The tendon inserts mainly on the navicular, but has minor additional attachments to the cuneiforms and metatarsal bases. Insufficiency of tendon is caused by an elongated or degenerative tendon over the course of its watershed area from the tip of the medial malleolus to 2 cm distal. Over a course of evolution other structures also get involved like the spring ligament, talonavicular capsule, and deltoid ligament exacerbating the pathology. The superior medial portion of spring ligament combines with the deltoid ligament and is frequently initially involved. In rare instances, isolated spring ligament rupture may initiate the pathology of adult acquired flatfoot deformity (AAFD). With the progressing insufficiency of PTT unopposed peroneus brevis causes further attenuation of the spring ligament. This causes plantar flexion and downward tilt of the talar head and the Achilles or gastrocnemius-soleus complex develops a contracture. The forefoot then abducts, creating talonavicular uncoverage. With advanced disease, flexible deformities can become rigid, limiting treatment options. The following are the common features of PTT dysfunction:

- Typically unilateral
- Usually progressive and result in flexible to rigid flatfoot depending on stage
- Common in women 45–65 years of age
- Family history common

CLASSIFICATION—MODIFIED JOHNSON STROM

The "modified Johnson strom" classification was originally published in 1989 and since then various modifications detailing subgroups have been published by different researchers most recent being in 2015. The simplistic version is presented in **Table 1**. The classification basically represents the stages of progression of adult flatfoot deformity over time if uninterrupted. A patient may present with any of the stage depending on the severity at seeking consultation. Following are the clinical features of different stages that can be identified at presentation.

- *Stage 1:*
    - Pain and edema along the medial aspect of the rearfoot indicating tenosynovitis or early tendinosis
    - Increased warmth, edema, and tenderness along the course of the tendon. Spondyloarthropathy has also been associated with stage I AAFD in a subgroup of patients.
    - The patient is able to complete single heel rise with ease.

TABLE 1: The clinical staging of posterior tibial tendon dysfunction.

Stage	*Description*
I	Pain over tibialis posterior without deformity
II	Flexible deformity—variable degree of midfoot abduction measured as percentage uncoverage of talonavicular articulation
IIA	Medial pain only (<30% talonavicular uncoverage)
IIB	Lateral pain (>30% talonavicular uncoverage)
III	Deformity no more flexible—no hindfoot inversion with single heel rise test
IV	Deformity is not flexible with significant arthritis at ankle joint (IVB) or flexible with mild arthritis (IVA)

- *Stage 2A:*
    - Medial rearfoot pain, edema, and tenderness along the course of the PTT, and mild valgus of the heel, with or without lowering of the medial longitudinal arch
    - Abduction of the forefoot on the rearfoot (too many toes sign)
    - Complete single heel rise with difficulty
    - Increased talo-first metatarsal angle, peritalar subluxation on radiographs. There is <30% talonavicular uncoverage on a standing AP radiograph of the foot.
- *Stage 2B*—stage 2A + lateral pain (sinus tarsi, subfibular, cuboid), more severe valgus, medial arch collapse. There is >30% talonavicular uncoverage on AP radiographs representing higher grade failure of spring ligament and other midfoot restraints. Lateral subtalar joint impingement will also come under stage IIb.
- *Stage 3:*
    - More severe and fixed deformities. The rigidity classically arises at the triple joint complex (talonavicular, subtalar, and calcaneocuboid joints) leading to fixed hindfoot valgus and abduction through the midfoot
    - Loss of subtalar joint motion
    - Posterior muscle group contracture
    - Unable to perform single heel raise test
    - Rearfoot remains everted with double heel eversion
    - Degenerative changes in rearfoot, increased angular deformities
- *Stage 4:*
    - Medial soft tissue restraints become weak. The deformity at foot is basically aggravated by valgus deformity at ankle joint. There is valgus tilt of talus in anteroposterior view on radiographs.
    - Degenerative changes in ankle joint also. The deformity is further divided into two stages—4A is characterized by hindfoot valgus, flexible ankle valgus without significant ankle arthritis. Stage 4B refers to hindfoot valgus with rigid or flexible ankle valgus with significant arthritis.

TREATMENT

Nonsurgical Treatment

- *Stage 1:*
    - Cast [Cam type cast or removable boot **(Fig. 5)**] or brace for 4 weeks → physiotherapy [strengthening

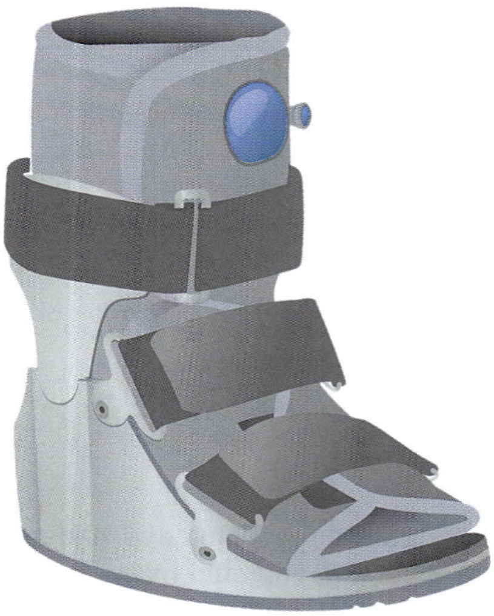

Fig. 5: Cam type removable boot.

exercises for the posterior tibial, peroneals, anterior tibial, and gastrocnemius and soleus muscles. Also incorporate isokinetic exercises, exercise band, heel rises (double and single support), and toe walking].
- Nonsteroidal anti-inflammatory drugs (NSAIDs)

- *Stage 2:*
  - Orthosis with deep heel cup
  - Extended medial counter and medial heel wedge
  - Immobilization for painful foot
- *Stage 3:* Short-articulated AFO or custom brace (viz., Arizone brace)
- *Stage 4:* Nonarticulated AFO

Surgical Treatment

Brace wear is quite cumbersome and so the compliance rate is low. Obesity is also a contributory factor for failure of conservative treatment. This entails frequent need for operative management.

- *Stage 1:* Synovectomy if noninvasive method ineffective. Conservative management is attempted for 3 months initially. Some recommend additional medializing calcaneal osteotomy to correct heel valgus with the PTT procedures as heel valgus if uncorrected will predispose to recurrence.
- *Stage 2A:* Synovectomy or tendon debridement is done. Posterior calcaneal displacement osteotomy or Evans procedure may be required in some cases as above. This is often combined with FDL transfer to navicular with/without tendo-Achilles/gastrocnemius lengthening. For elevated medial column precluding the tripod function of foot, one can do open dorsal medial cuneiform osteotomy (cotton osteotomy) to bring down first metatarsal if TMT joint is stable. For arthritis/unstable joint arthrodesis of the joint is better. Subtalar arthroereisis is an interesting option as suggested for the treatment of flexible pes planus. Blocking the movement at subtalar joint (hindfoot valgus) and reorienting the calcaneus vertically using implant (usually screw-like spacer) at sinus tarsi often ameliorates the symptoms but pain may not subside until screw removal. Arthroereisis also dorsiflexes the talus and corrects talonavicular subluxation. Though this procedure saves patient from arthrodesis and other morbid surgeries, it opens door to different set of complications such as persistent pain, implant dislocation, implant fracture, talar cysts or osteonecrosis, and foreign body reaction.
- *Stage 2B:* Synovectomy or tendon repair and tendon transfer. Realignment procedures as osteotomy for stage 2A may be required. Medial column arthrodesis or calcaneocuboid interpositional bone block as isolated procedure has also been recommended. Lateral column lengthening such as Evans-like procedure or calcaneocuboid distraction is commonly performed to improve foot arch by correcting talonavicular joint abduction. The complications of lateral column lengthening procedures, however, are lateral discomfort, nonunion, fifth metatarsal stress fracture, and stiffness. Arthroereisis is not a favorable option here.
- *Stage 3* requires one of the arthrodesis procedures. Triple arthrodesis for whole foot involvement® is commonly prescribed but attempt should be made to preserve calcaneocuboid joint as far as possible. Fusing all three joints produces a stiff foot that is unable to adapt to uneven surfaces. Heel valgus should be corrected to <5° and if this is not possible during arthrodesis then calcaneal osteotomy is an option. The forefoot should be neither in pronation or supination. Elevated first ray is corrected as detailed for stage 2A.
- *Stage 4* deformity (valgus deformity without arthrosis) correction needs triple arthrodesis in combination with deltoid ligament repair and a medializing calcaneal osteotomy. Pantalar arthrodesis/ankle replacement is needed for involvement of foot and ankle joint arthrosis.

PERONEAL SPASTIC PES PLANUS

It is an acutely painful condition commonly seen in young adolescents. The common presentation is with pain, tightness or spasm of the peroneal muscles, and an eversion deformity of the foot. Predisposing factor usually seen is starting work or changing to an occupation involving much standing.

Etiology

- *Congenital:* Tarsal coalition or synchondroses of calcaneo-navicular, talocalcaneal bars, calcaneocuboid bars
- *Acquired:*
  - Inflammatory—tuberculous lesions, rheumatoid arthritis, and nonspecific tarsal joint synovitis
  - Degenerative—osteoarthritis
  - Trauma
  - Occupational strains

Pathology

The pathology of the peroneal spasm is probably that of a reflex muscle reaction, but there is no established relationship between the sensory innervation to talonavicular joint and that supplying peroneal muscles.

"Tarsal coalition" is the most common cause and can present as peroneal spastic flatfoot. Other causes include secondary degenerative changes in subtalar and midtarsal joints due to clubfoot, old trauma rheumatoid arthritis, or osteoarthritis. They complain of difficulty with sports activities or even with standing and walking.

Clinical Features

Physical examination shows a rigid hindfoot. Loss of the medial longitudinal arch and fixed forefoot abduction due to spasm of the peroneal tendons can be appreciated by placing the foot into inversion. This results from contraction of the peroneus brevis or longus or both.

Radiology (Figs. 6 and 7)

Radiographs (Harris-Beath views) may show a naviculo-calcaneal coalition on the oblique view of the foot. The Harris view (posterior axial) can show a talocalcaneal coalition, but CT scans are more helpful in demonstrating this.

Management (*See* also Chapter on "Anomalies of Pediatric Lower Limb")

Nonoperative Treatment

Rest, nonsteroidal anti-inflammatory medication, and cast immobilization are prescribed initially. Cast immobilization for at least 3 weeks and usually 6–8 weeks is required for relief of symptoms. Immobilization in a knee-ankle-foot orthosis (KAFO) or below knee slab usually controls the symptoms well. Later, a shoe modification, such as a heel cup, a medial arch support or a medial heel wedge, may allow patients to return to weight-bearing activities.

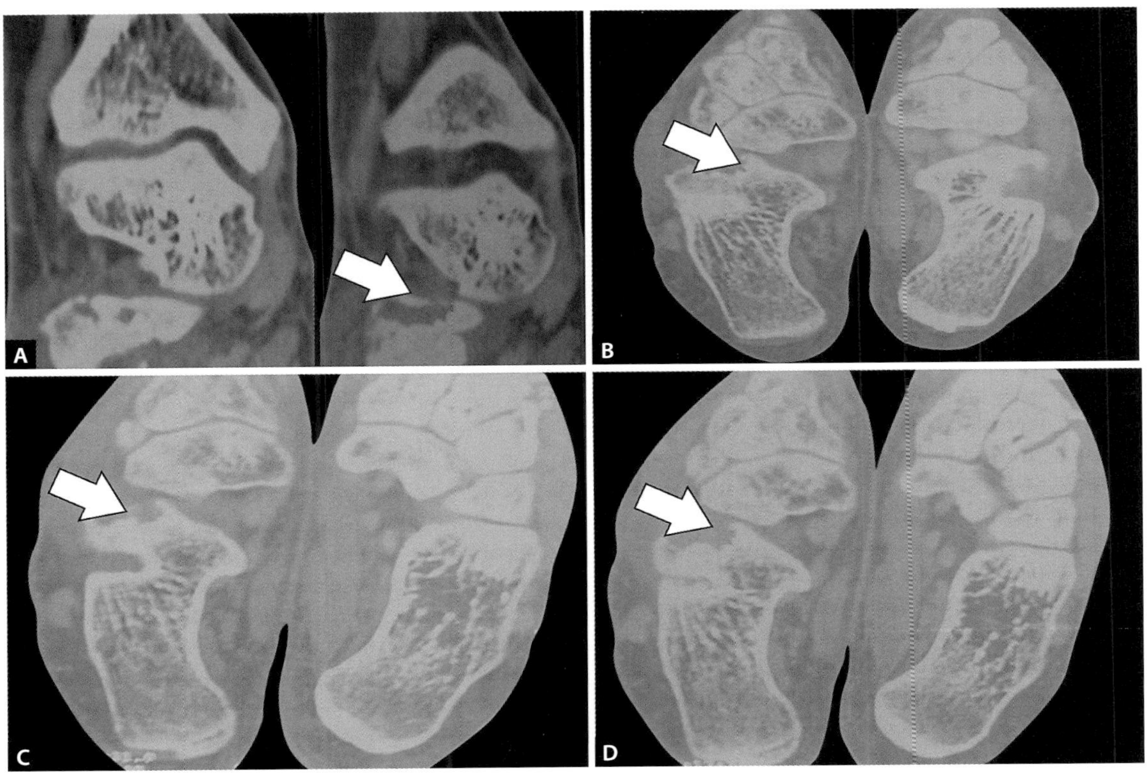

Figs. 6A to D: Talocalcaneal incomplete (fibrous) coalition (block arrows in various cuts of CT scan).

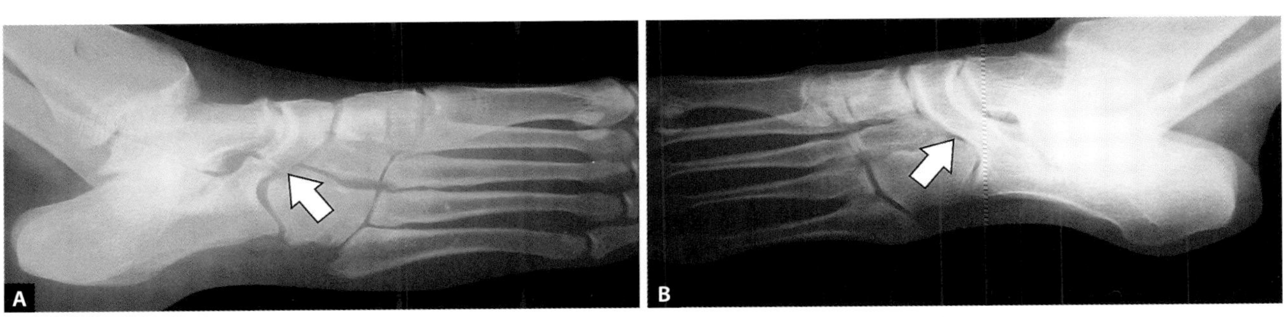

Figs. 7A and B: (A) Incomplete and (B) complete calcaneonavicular coalition.

Surgical Treatment

Resection of tarsal coalition is the treatment of choice with middle or posterior facet coalition that comprises <25% of the joint surface and that is symptomatic and unresponsive to nonoperative treatment. Contraindications to coalition resection include degenerative arthritis, associated deformity, and involvement of >50% of the posterior facet. In such cases, arthrodesis is preferred.

CONCLUSION

- Flatfoot is a common foot disorder that produces flattening of the arches of foot to variable extent.
- Loss of arched structure produces increased stress on the joints and ligaments of the foot producing pain and reducing the efficacy of the foot for ambulation by altering biomechanics.
- Flatfoot is also common in the children aged <8 years but it is more due to incomplete development and should not raise much concern. Asking the child to stand on toes brings in the arch in flexible flatfoot.
- Symptomatic rigid flatfoot due to tarsal coalition (rigid pes planus) needs excision of the coalition bar to treat the patient. Midtarsal realignment procedures are needed for managing nonrigid flatfoot that fail to respond to conservative management. Various arthrodeses and fusion procedures are also available that should be decided individually.
- Flatfoot due to neuropathic arthropathy should be managed by protection and stabilization with the use of orthosis unless one is forced to perform surgery due to severely unstable foot. The surgery is usually arthrodesis but is associated with high rates of nonunion and failure so patient should be explained the need of amputation if the reconstruction surgery fails.

CHAPTER 88

Pes Cavus and Accompanying Deformities

Manish Kumar Varshney

INTRODUCTION

Cavus foot is a deformity of the foot characterized by an excessively high longitudinal plantar arch (sagittal plane deformity, **Figs. 1A and B**) with either a plantarflexion of the forefoot on the rearfoot, or dorsiflexion of the rearfoot on the forefoot. Cavus deformity *per se* is commonly present in general population with the prevalence of around 10%. There are commonly associated secondary multiplanar forefoot and rearfoot deformities [like hindfoot varus **(Figs. 2A to C)** forefoot adduction and complex torsional changes in other areas of foot]. The forefoot deformity predominates and is commonly flexible. Rearfoot involvement occurs with evolution to rigid deformity.

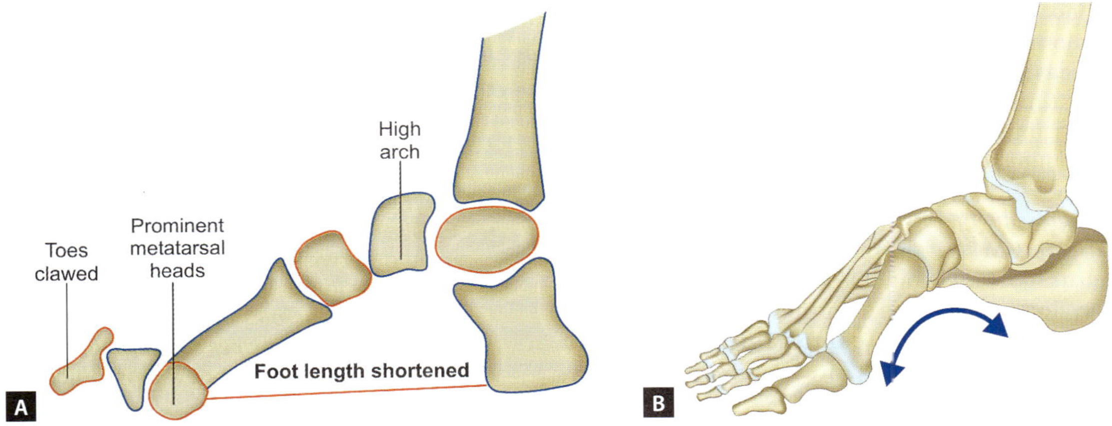

Figs. 1A and B: Pes cavus. (A) Illustration of various structural components; (B) Appearance in an articulated foot.

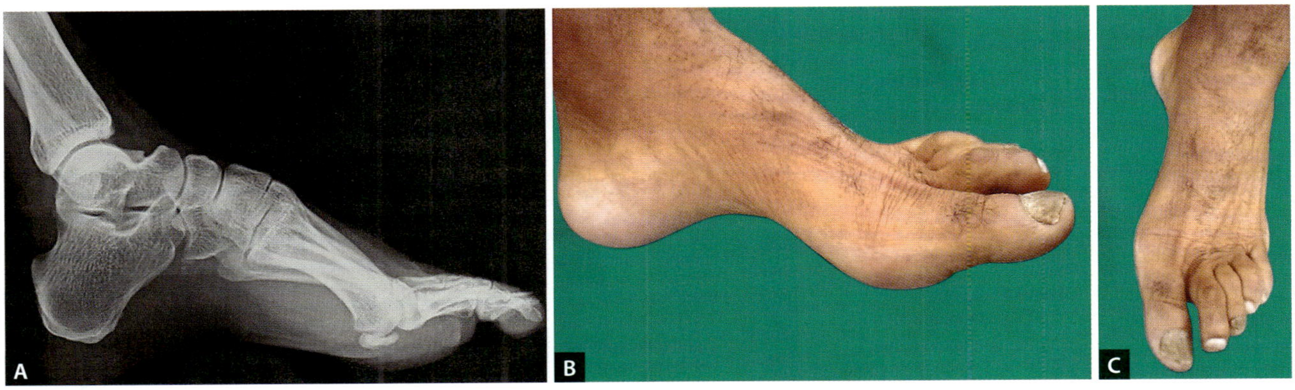

Figs. 2A to C: The radiological (A) and clinical appearance of cavus foot, the clawing has started to appear in the lateral four toes (B). Heel varus is a common accompaniment of the developing cavus deformity, in fact heel varus (C) is mostly detectable in as "peek-a-boo" sign when the foot is examined from front (see later in text).

ETIOLOGY

Three main patient groups have been identified to develop cavus deformity:

1. Idiopathic or postural deformity
2. *Paralytic foot:*
    - Contracture during acute stage, e.g., poliomyelitis
    - Charcot-Marie-Tooth disease (CMTD)
    - Muscle imbalance during growth period
3. In association with certain neurological diseases or developmental deformity of spine

Classification

There are various classification schemes of cavus foot depending on severity of the deformity (mild, moderate, and severe/rigid), severity of cavus itself, etiological, etc. We will follow a simple format based on pathogenesis of the deformity.

- *Idiopathic:*
    - Most common
    - Develops after 3 years of age
    - Males and females are equally affected.
    - Often associated with spina bifida occulta
- *Secondary:*
    - *Neurologic disease:*
        - Spinocerebellar hereditary degeneration of Mollaret, multiple sclerosis
        - Friedreich's ataxia
        - Poliomyelitis
        - Diseases of conus medullaris or cauda equina—diastematomyelia, cauda equina tumor, and syringomyelia
        - Pyramidal or extrapyramidal syndromes, cerebral palsy
        - *Progressive peroneal palsy, Charcot-Marie-Tooth disease:* CMTD is the most common cause of cavovarus foot and should be suspected in all cases of developmental cavus deformity.
    - Direct trauma to foot (compartment syndrome, malunions, and talus fracture nonunion can cause cavus foot)
    - Myopathies, e.g., muscular dystrophy
    - Plantar fibromatosis
    - Congenital talipes equinovarus

PATHOGENESIS OF DEFORMITY

It is imperative to understand the balance of muscular forces that maintain the function of foot (**Table 1**). The tibialis anterior acts as primary dorsiflexor and secondary inverter of the ankle. It is antagonized by peroneus longus that acts as a plantar flexor and weak evertor. The tibialis posterior has a wide insertion along the medial and plantar medial aspect of the medial column. It acts to invert the foot and plantarflex it secondarily. The action of tibialis posterior is opposed by the peroneus brevis that is a strong evertor and inserts at the base of the fifth metatarsal. The intrinsic muscles flex the metatarsophalangeal (MTP) joints and extend the proximal interphalangeal (PIP), and distal interphalangeal (DIP) joints. The extrinsic extensor muscles [extensor hallucis longus, extensor digitorum longus, extensor digitorum brevis, and extensor hallucis brevis (EHL, EDL, EDB, and EHB)] extend the toes through the MTP, PIP, and DIP joints. The extrinsic long flexors [flexor digitorum longus and flexor hallucis longus (FDL and FHL)] and the short flexors [flexor digitorum brevis and flexor hallucis brevis (FDB and FHB)] flex the toes at the PIP and DIP joints. The various theories principally relate to muscle imbalance that are responsible for development of deformity:

1. *Intrinsic weakness theory of Duchenne:*
    - The intrinsics fail to flex the MTP joints and extend the interphalangeal (IP) joints.
    - Theory is questionable because paralysis of intrinsics produces a planovalgus foot.
2. *Overactivity of intrinsics:*
    - Persistent function of short toe flexors and intrinsics in an otherwise flatfoot results in the development of cavovarus foot.
    - *Sharrard principles of development of deformity for paralytic secondary pes cavus (poliomyelitis):*
        - Acute contracture—develops rapidly in acute stage of paralytic disease.

TABLE 1: The understanding of normal anatomy and action of various muscles involved in the pathogenesis of cavus deformity.

Muscle	*Insertion in foot*	*Action*	*Antagonist*
Peroneus longus	First metatarsal base and medial cuneiform	1°: plantar flexion, 1st metatarsal 2nd: weak eversion	Tibialis anterior
Peroneus brevis	5th metatarsal base	Everter of foot	Tibialis posterior
Tibialis anterior	Navicular and medial cuneiform	1°: foot dorsiflexion 2nd: inversion	Peroneus longus
Tibialis posterior	Medial and plantar midfoot andforefoot	1°: inversion 2nd: plantar flexion	Peroneus brevis
Lumbricals and interossei (the intrinsic muscles of foot)	Extensor expansion near proximal phalanges	MTP flexion, PIP, and DIP extension	Long flexors and extensors
Long and short extrinsic extensors (EHL, EDL, EDB, and EHB)	Extensor hood at MTP joint, distal phalanges	MTP, PIP, and DIP extension	Intrinsic and extrinsic long flexors
Extrinsic long flexors (FDL, FHL, FDB, and FHB)	Flexor sheath and plantar aspect of distal phalanges	PIP and DIP flexion	Extrinsic long extensors

(DIP: distal interphalangeal; EDB: extensor digitorum brevis; EDL: extensor digitorum longus; EHB: extensor hallucis brevis; EHL: extensor hallucis longus; FDB: flexor digitorum brevis; FDL: flexor digitorum longus; FHB: flexor hallucis brevis; FHL: flexor hallucis longus; MTP: metatarsophalangeal; PIP: proximal interphalangeal)

- Postural contracture—immobility and edema encourage deposition of collagen.
- Muscle imbalance—in the growing child with muscle imbalance the deformity progresses in spite of stretching and splinting.

3. *Muscle imbalance:*
   - *Weakness in the peroneus brevis and tibialis anterior:* This causes unchecked peroneus longus and tibialis posterior function. Dorsiflexion and eversion are hence compromised. The overpull of the tibialis posterior causes medialization of the talonavicular and calcaneocuboid joints locking the subtalar joint in supination. The peroneus longus pulls the first ray into plantar-flexion producing cavus. To compensate for tibialis anterior the long toe extensors become overactive and they hyperextend the toes at the MTP joints. Additional weakness of the intrinsic muscles produces clawing of the toes and distal migration of the plantar fat pad. The first metatarsal drop and forefoot equinus produce forefoot pronation. As the forefoot deformity becomes fixed slowly, the hindfoot becomes fixed in varus to keep the foot plantigrade.
   - In poliomyelitis, triceps surae weakness causes the long toe flexors to compensate, leading to forefoot plantar flexion and the development of cavus.

Subsequent tibialis posterior muscle contracture can additionally produce equinus and cavovarus.

Pathoanatomy

Anatomy of cavus foot varies massively particularly with respect to the associated components. Cavus foot per se represents an abnormal elevation of the medial arch that persists with weight-bearing. Biomechanically, cavus deformity of foot may include high calcaneal pitch, varus hindfoot, high-pitched midfoot (defined by the navicular height), and plantar-flexed and adducted forefoot. Idiopathic or primary pes cavus is seen to have the following deformities:

- *Dropping of forefoot:*
  - Initially develops in first ray
  - The naviculocuneiform and cuneiform metatarsal joints become rigid.
  - The first metatarsal gradually loses its passive range of dorsiflexion, while other metatarsals remain mobile until late.
  - Entire foot becomes pronated which becomes rigid and resists passive correction.
- Lengthened lateral border of the foot
- Shortened medial border of foot
- *Contracture of plantar fascia:* Increases the height of longitudinal arch
- Pronation of the forefoot and inversion of heel increase the cavus deformity.
- *Varus of heel:*
  - As the forefoot becomes pronated, there is compensatory inversion at subtalar and midtarsal joints in order to place all metatarsals evenly on the floor.
  - The inversion produces heel varus that becomes fixed and pronounced.
- Clawing of toes
- A "bony" dorsum of the midfoot with wrinkled skin folds on the medial plantar aspect.
- Calluses beneath the metatarsal heads

The clinical implications of altered pathomechanics are presented in **Box 1**.

Examination

Examine the parents and siblings because of high incidence in idiopathic pes cavus, degenerative disease of spinocerebellar tracts and spina bifida. Include examination of feet, a neurologic evaluation including examination of muscles and X-ray studies of feet and entire spine. Clinically, the "peek-a-boo" sign and Coleman block test form the most important components for assessing pes cavus deformity. The "peek-a-boo" heel sign was described by Manoli et al. in 1993. Ask the patient to stand with feet straight ahead and examine the medial border of foot from front. The heel "peeks out" medially around the ankle in cases of subtle pes cavus deformity (in normal feet due to slight valgus; the heel is not visible). It may be false positive in patients with large heel pad or those with metatarsus adductus.

Coleman block test ***(Figs. 3A to C)*** *(also known as Coleman lateral block test):* This test is used to determine the flexibility

BOX 1: The clinical implications of the altered mechanics due to cavus foot.

- Varus of the hindfoot leads to recurrent sprains and abnormal ankle loading.
- The lateral rays are overloaded due to hindfoot varus and altered pitch of the midfoot. These patients have, otherwise, uncommon stress fracture of the navicular and metatarsals for this reason.
- Uneven forefoot loads due to variable metatarsal alignment have varied effects on metatarsals and stability during heel rise.
- Hyperplantar flexion of first metatarsal and medial foot produces pain under the first metatarsal (MT) and lateral overload. This plantar flexion deformity of first metatarsal is responsible for the dynamic heel varus and adduction thrust seen in heel rise. Other causes of foot pain include pain under the sesamoid region, development of painful callosities, ankle arthritis and Achilles tendinitis.

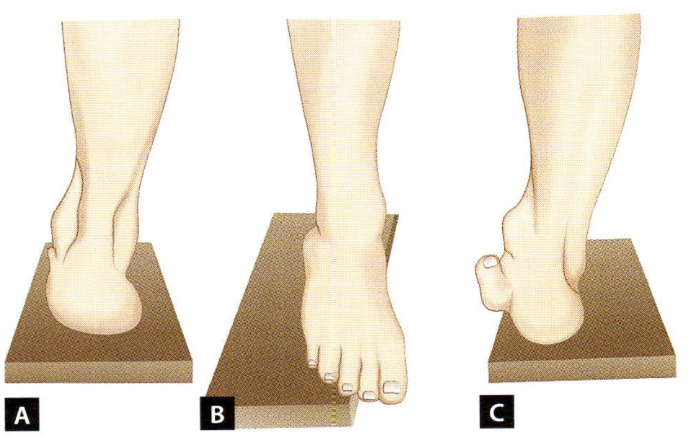

Figs. 3A to C: A Coleman block test. A foot rests fully on the block with the hindfoot in mild varus (A). The foot is on the block to test for flexible cavus, with the first metatarsal off the block to allow it to plantarflex (B). The foot from behind, after the deforming force of the first ray is eliminated by the block; the hindfoot is now in valgus (C).

of hindfoot in a patient with pes cavus and heel varus and ultimately guide treatment. Principle of test is that in some cases the hindfoot varus is produced by excessive plantarflexion of the first metatarsal (metatarsal drop), and if that is eliminated, then the varus corrects. The test is performed by asking the patient to stand on a wooden block in such a way that the heel and lateral edge of forefoot (fifth metatarsal) rests on the block but the first metatarsal is off the block. Usually, the block is 1 inch in height. The examiner observes from rear side of patient. Standing in such a way allows the first metatarsal to drop to the floor (plantarflex) without driving the rest of the foot. If the heel varus corrects and returns to neutral position (or even valgus), it indicates that the deformity is due to first metatarsal plantarflexion and the foot would be correctable by reducing the plantar flexion of the first ray and/or balancing the dynamic cause (peroneus longus overdrive).

- If the hindfoot remains in varus, then it indicates rigid hindfoot deformity and pes cavus is due to tripod effect of fixed varus. This deformity will not correct with correction of first metatarsal flexion. This may also arise from tibialis posterior spasticity.
- *Reverse Coleman test:* This is mentioned here only for completing the discussion on Coleman test and has nothing to do with a cavus foot. Instead the reverse Coleman test is done in an acquired flatfoot deformity (reverse test for reverse deformity!) to identify medial column insufficiency. In this test, the patient is made to stand on medial aspect of forefoot (first metatarsal head) that corrects the mobile valgus heel to neutral position. The foot is radiologically studied for any instability with this position of neutral heel and forefoot in relative supination. Medial column instability in an otherwise acquired planovalgus foot is commonly missed. The reverse Coleman test helps to identify it and also quantification is aided by magnifying the level of deformity already present that needs correction.

TYPES OF DEFORMITY

- *Simple pes cavus:*
  - Forefoot equinus evenly distributed.
  - All metatarsals bear weight equally.
  - Heel in neutral position or slight valgus.
- *Pes cavovarus:*
  - Medial column alone in rigid plantar flexion. Other metatarsal easily dorsiflexed.
  - Forefoot pronated 20–30°.
  - Hindfoot inversion is flexible and reducible initially that later becomes fixed and requires separate correction.
- *Calcaneocavus:*
  - Results from paralysis of triceps surae
  - Heel assumes vertical position (calcaneus deformity).
  - Forefoot in equinus in relation to hindfoot
- *Equino cavovarus:* Typical deformity of uncorrected clubfoot. This also develops in poliomyelitis.

ROENTGENOGRAPHIC FINDINGS

They are not useful for making diagnosis as it is clinical and descriptive from deformity itself, however, some radiographic features may help to evaluate the severity of deformity and judge the deformity correction.

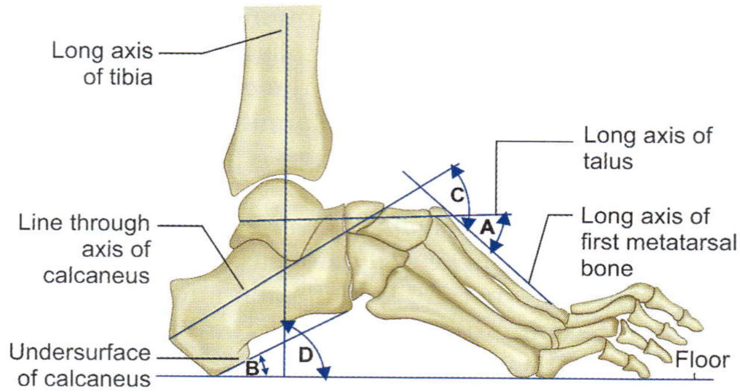

Fig. 4: A: Meary's angle; B: Calcaneal inclination angle (calcaneal pitch angle); C: Hibb's angle; and D: Tibioplantar angle.

- Normally the proximal and distal articular surfaces of the inner cuneiform are parallel. In pes cavus, forefoot downward inclination is maximal at inner cuneiform and proximal and distal articular surfaces of the cuneiform converge outward to the plantar aspect of foot.
- In anteroposterior standing view the talocalcaneal angle is decreased when heel inversion is fixed.
- In lateral weight-bearing view, the angle of the cavus can be demonstrated by the intersection of two lines corresponding to the axis of first metatarsal and the other through the axis of either talus or calcaneus.
  - Characteristic of cavus foot is the plantar flexion of the first metatarsal relative to the axis of the talus, a relationship described as Meary's angle **(Fig. 4)**. It is the angle between line drawn from the centers of longitudinal axes of the talus and the first metatarsal. Normally Meary's angle is 0° (angle with convexity up >4° → pes cavus). It can also be used to assess severity of the deformity:
    - Angle <15°—mild deformity
    - Angle 15–30°—moderate deformity
    - Angle >30°—severe deformity
  - Increase in the calcaneal inclination angle **(Fig. 4)**
- A standing lateral view of ankle joint allows radiological assessment of calcaneal pitch and midfoot and forefoot position. An estimate of the degree of first ray plantar flexion can also be made.
- The standing lateral radiograph is useful to assess the individual contribution of the hindfoot (talus and calcaneus), midfoot (navicular and cuboid-cuneiform), and forefoot (Lisfranc) to the cavus deformity.
- Hibb's angle < 150° (Hibb's angle is formed by the lines running along the axes of the calcaneus and the first metatarsal. The intersection of the lines represents apex of the deformity) **(Fig. 4)**. Normally Hibb's angle is >150°. Hibb's angle <150° is pathological and indicates pes cavus.

Other radiographic findings that may be helpful in deciding the treatment include:

- Degenerative changes in the ankle, subtalar, midtarsal, and Lisfranc joints.

- *Talar rotation in ankle mortise:* This is caused by dorsiflexion of talus and inversion at the subtalar joint.
- Oblique views help in identifying soft-tissue dystrophic ossification that suggests soft-tissue (tendon/ligament) injury.

NATURAL HISTORY OF DEVELOPMENT OF PES CAVUS IN PARALYTIC FOOT

Development of deformity may be divided into a series of stages.

First Grade

- Only physical sign positive at this stage is slight extensor weakness, which can be demonstrated by difference in circumference of two calves.
- Child is clumsy with history of repeated falls and the child catches his toes against low objects such as edge of the carpet.

Second Grade

- Flexion of forefoot and flexible clawing of great toe. Clawing can be made to disappear by upward pressure on the ball of great toe.
- Plantar fascia is tense and contracted.

Third Grade

- *Involvement of other metatarsals:* The arch of the foot is markedly raised, while all the toes are clawed.
- Hind foot inversion
- Tendocalcaneus starts contracting.
- Painful corns appear.
- Foot tires easily.

Fourth Grade

- In addition to cavus and hammer toes there is adduction at tarsometatarsal joints resulting in varus deformity.
- Rigid and painful foot to walking

Fifth Grade

- Seen in advanced paralytic conditions such as polio.
- Whole foot is contracted into rigid equinovarus with high arch.
- Tender callosities
- Foot is highly painful to walk.

Weak plantarflexors (gastrocnemius-soleus) against a strong tibialis anterior produces calcaneus deformity of the hindfoot, hindfoot varus or valgus may or may not be present. The post-poliomyelitis cavus foot has both the anterior (forefoot component) and posterior (hindfoot component) deformed regions unlike CMTD. Postpoliomyelitis cavus feet respond better or have a predictable outcome to treatment as they have intact sensation and deformity is usually nonprogressive as compared to patients with CMTD who would have Charcot's component to deformity and it may progress further.

PRINCIPLES OF TREATMENT

- *Correct primary deformity:* Equinus and pronation of forefoot.
- When the deformity is recognized early, it should be treated conservatively.
  - Forefoot is forced into inversion and dorsiflexion.
  - Heel is manipulated into eversion.
  - Toes are plantarflexed at MTP joint.
- Correction that is limited to secondary deformities, such as contracted plantar fascia, clawed toes, and varus heel affects partial improvement so forefoot pronation should always be addressed in the manipulative/surgical correction.
- Progressive and increasingly resistant cavus deformity requires surgical correction, but before surgical intervention, the neurologic disturbance should be clearly defined and muscle imbalance analyzed.
- In immature foot, the operative procedure is mainly directed to soft tissues to avoid compromising growth of foot and future movements and flexibility.
  - Manipulative stretching takes precedence.
  - Surgery is limited to soft tissues.
  - If at all done, surgical trauma to bone structures should avoid growth areas and midtarsal joints.
- When late structural changes have occurred, the forefoot is fixed in marked equinus and bony procedures are necessary. These should always be preceded by plantar release (Steindler release). The type of surgical procedure is determined by:
  - Nature of hindfoot deformity
  - Stability of heel
  - Apex of cavus deformity
  - Type of pes cavus
  - Toe deformities
  - Degree of muscle weakness

Treatment

First Grade

- Passive manipulations to flatten arch by supinating forefoot and everting heel
- Anterior arch bar in shoe
- Night splint-dorsiflexion pressure applied behind metatarsal heads
- Re-educating the small muscle function by intrinsic exercises
- *Soft-tissue procedure:* Girdlestone flexor to extensor transfer is performed.

Second Grade

- Shoe fitted with metatarsal bar for interim relief.
- The plantar fascia is divided percutaneously for milder cases.
- If the contracture is greater, the aponeurosis and the underlying muscles are stripped from the calcaneus-Steindler stripping.
- *Modified Jones procedure gives good results:* The tendon of extensor halluces longus is divided at its insertion

and passed through the neck of first metatarsal (Jones tenosuspension). Arthrodesis of IP joint is done with tenodesis of extensor halluces brevis to improve take off.

Third Grade

In immature foot, dynamic correction is accomplished by transferring the long extensors to metatarsals to effectively reinforce weak anterior tibialis.

Calcaneal muscle slide: All the structures on the sole of the foot that arise from undersurface of calcaneum are separated from bone. Structures are erased right forward to the calcaneocuboid joint laterally and talonavicular medially.

- *Extensor shift procedure:* To remove the deforming force that hyperextends the MTP joint and uses it to elevate the metatarsals. The EHL overcompensates to aid in ankle dorsiflexion due to weak tibialis anterior. However, this produces hyperdorsiflexion of the first MTP joint and clawing of the big toe. The peroneus longus pulls first ray into plantar flexion causing first metarsal drop and cavus. Transferring the extensor by the modified Jones procedure **(Figs. 5A to D)** would correct this deformity. In this procedure, the IP joint is fused first. Using a small dorsal incision, the IP joint is prepared, compressed, and fixed with crossing screws or a single 4.0 screw across the joint. The EHL is released from its insertion. Distal part of first metatarsal is exposed, and a transverse drill hole is made across the neck level. The EHL is passed through the hole and sewn back onto itself while the ankle is held in 10° of dorsiflexion.
- *Dwyer procedure:* Osteotomy of the posterior portion of calcaneus restores the valgus position of the heel. This operation is effective only in growing foot.

Fourth and Fifth Grades

The deformity becomes pronounced and resists passive correction. Wedge tarsectomy helps to achieve correction by dividing the bones at the level of midtarsal joint like tarsal osteotomy of Japas (anterior tarsal wedge osteotomy and fusion of first metatarsocuneiform navicular joints).

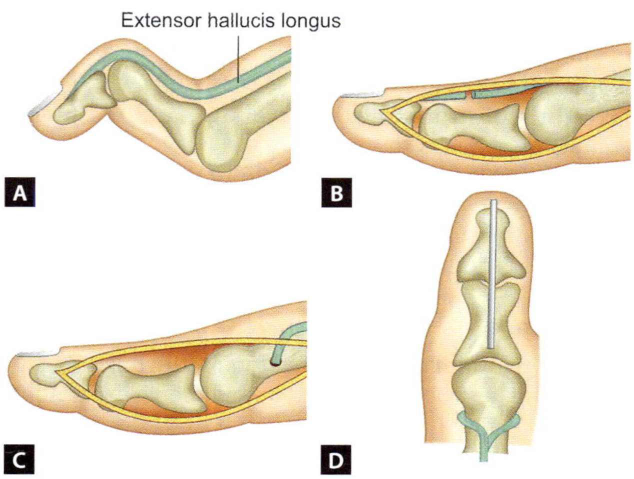

Figs. 5A to D: For correction of claw toe deformity of big/great toe (A); The modified Jones procedure involves release of extensor deforming force (B); From the tendon of extensor hallucis longus (EHL) and performing distal interphalangeal joint arthrodesis (C); The EHL is used to suspend the metacarpal neck instead to correct clawing (D).

Surgical Correction of Pes Cavus

"Various Surgical Techniques" that are recommended for correction of individual components of the cavus deformity are briefed below:

- *Claw toes:* Traumatic pes cavus may have only surgically correctible claw toe deformities with additional tight plantar fascia. The bony midfoot deformity can be corrected with appropriate shoe and orthotic management. Fixed contractures at the MTP and IP joints are corrected by:
  - Lengthening of long extensors of toe (the extensor halluces longus and extensor digitorum longus) along with tenotomy of the short extensors (the extensor digitorum brevis and the extensor halluces brevis). The other procedure involves flexor-to-extensor transfer (Taylor's procedure). Here, the FDL is released and brought laterally or split into two and sutured medially and laterally to the extensor expansion.
  - Opening the MTP joint dorsally by dorsal capsulotomy
  - *For great toe:* The IP joint is arthrodesed along with releasing the plantar plate. The collateral ligaments are sectioned for the IP joint of the hallux and temporary stabilization is done by inserting Kirschner wire.
  - For severe and fixed deformity excision arthroplasty by resection of the head and neck of the proximal phalanges is performed.
  - Plantar fascia release
- *Forefoot equinus:* Occasionally, in an adolescent foot, soft-tissue procedures alone correct the forefoot equinus sufficiently to avoid osteotomy or arthrodesis. Other commonly done procedures for forefoot equinus are:
  - *Gould technique:* Plantar fasciotomy, closing wedge greenstick dorsal proximal metatarsal osteotomies.
  - *Modified Jones technique:* Tenosuspension (see above) of the first metatarsal and IP joint arthrodesis.
  - The Hibbs procedure involves transfer of the extensor digitorum longus to the middle cuneiform.
  - Jahss procedure involves dorsal bone wedge resection at the tarsometatarsal joints and arthrodesis of all tarsometatarsal joints without plantar fascial release.
- *Midfoot cavus:* Midfoot cavus occurs at the midtarsal joints—most commonly at the talonavicular—calcaneo-cuboid and, sometimes, at naviculocuneiform joints. Most of the surgical procedures include release of the plantar fascia along with osteotomy of calcaneus or metatarsal bone depending on the rigidity of deformity. In patients with mild-to-moderate fixed deformity the following osteotomies have been described:
  - Tarsal wedge osteotomy by Cole **(Figs. 6A to C)**.
  - Jahss technique for tarsometatarsal truncated wedge arthrodesis.
  - *Japas V-osteotomy* ***(Figs. 7A and B):***
    - A V-osteotomy is formatted in the midtarsal region with the apex of the V proximally located at the highest point of the cavus (commonly at navicular bone).
    - The lateral limb of the V extends to cuboid and medial through the first cuneiform at its medial border.

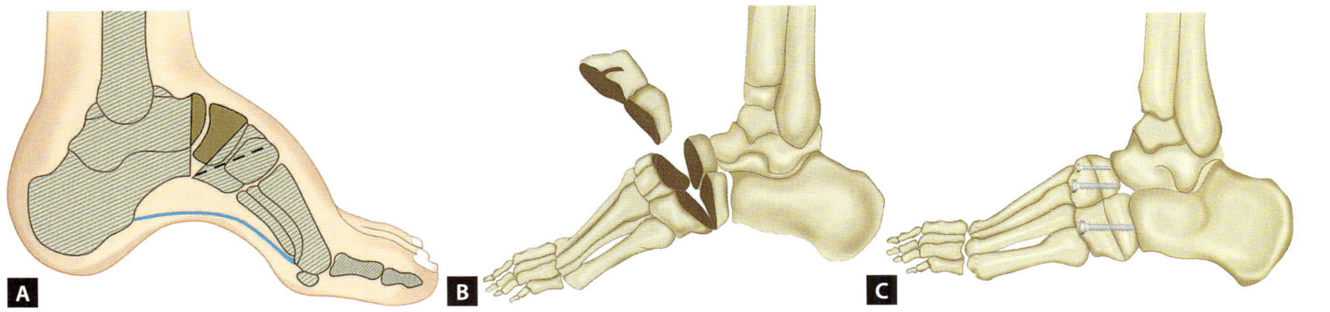

Figs. 6A to C: Tarsal wedge osteotomy. (A) Marking of wedge in planning; (B) Removal of the wedge; (C) Osteosynthesis correcting the deformity.

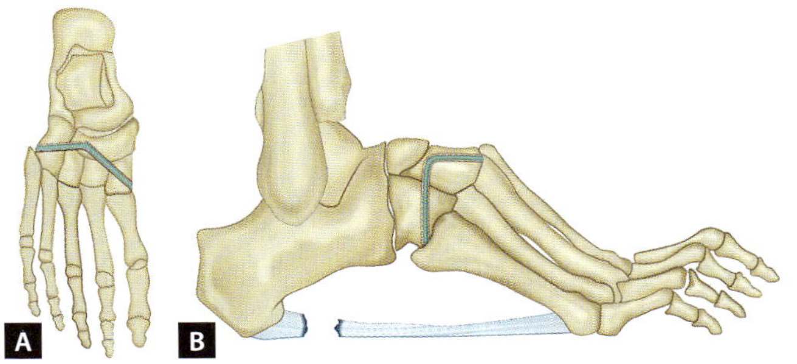

Figs. 7A and B: Japas "V"'osteotomy at midtarsal region. Marking and planning in anteroposterior (A) and lateral (B) views. The plantar fascia has to be simultaneously released to effect correction.

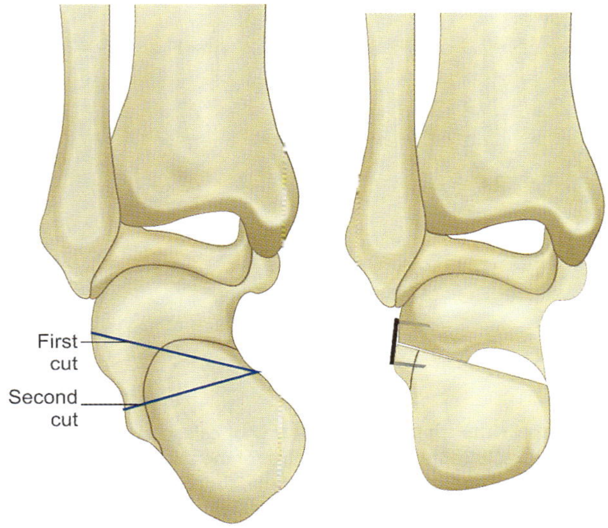

Fig. 8: Calcaneal osteotomy [Dwyer's type (modified)].

- The proximal border of the distal fragment of the osteotomy is depressed plantarward, while the metatarsal heads are elevated to correct the deformity. This also lengthens the plantar surface of the foot.
- Japas osteotomy is recommended for moderate midfoot cavus deformity in children 6 years or older. It does not address the deformities of the hindfoot or midtarsal joint.

- *Combined-cavus (calcaneocavus deformity):* The deformity is better treated by hindfoot crescentic calcaneal osteotomy (with or without midtarsal osteotomy). The Dwyer procedure can correct the varus and calcaneus posture of the hindfoot if appropriate wedges are removed. A triple arthrodesis usually is a better choice for severe and fixed equinocavovarus deformity.
  - *Dwyer-calcaneus osteotomy:* This is used to correct fixed hindfoot varus deformity (as determined by Coleman block test). The osteotomy moves the heel into a physiologically neutral or slightly valgus position. Achilles tendon lengthening is often combined through either gastrocnemius recession or direct tendon lengthening. Dwyer osteotomy not only corrects hindfoot varus but also shifts the center of force laterally at the ankle joint. It can be performed as a wedge resection osteotomy or a lateral slide osteotomy. The calcaneus bone is exposed laterally through a straight incision and laterally based wedge of bone is marked depending on the needed correction **(Fig. 8)**.

Remove a wedge of bone (8–12 mm wide) from the calcaneus just inferior and posterior to the peroneus longus tendon and parallel with it. It is useful to leave the medial cortex intact for stability that can be manually broken to close the gap maintaining the strength from interdigitation of spikes. Wedge osteotomy shortens the bone and often weakens the tendo-Achilles strength so it is considered better to use lateral sliding osteotomy in mild-to-moderate varus deformity. The osteotomy cut is made perpendicular to the long-axis of the calcaneus and the heel is slid 1 cm laterally. The posterior fragment can also be moved superiorly to reduce the calcaneal pitch. The osteotomy is fixed using two screws. Overhanging lateral bone is trimmed or resected for bone graft. For severe varus, Z-osteotomy (triplanar osteotomy, **Figs. 9A to C**) is a better method that also allows multiplanar correction of the deformity.

- *Crescentic calcaneal osteotomy of Samilson:* The calcaneus must be relatively vertical on a lateral radiograph and the apex of the cavus must be posterior to the midtarsal joints. The operation does not correct midtarsal or forefoot cavus.
  - *Calcaneocavovarus and cavovarus deformity:* These deformities are commonly seen in patients with CMTD, but occasionally may also occur after poliomyelitis or malunion of displaced fractures of the talus.
  - Post-traumatic cavovarus feet (as after talus malunion) with forefoot adduction and supination in which talonavicular and calcaneocuboid joints are

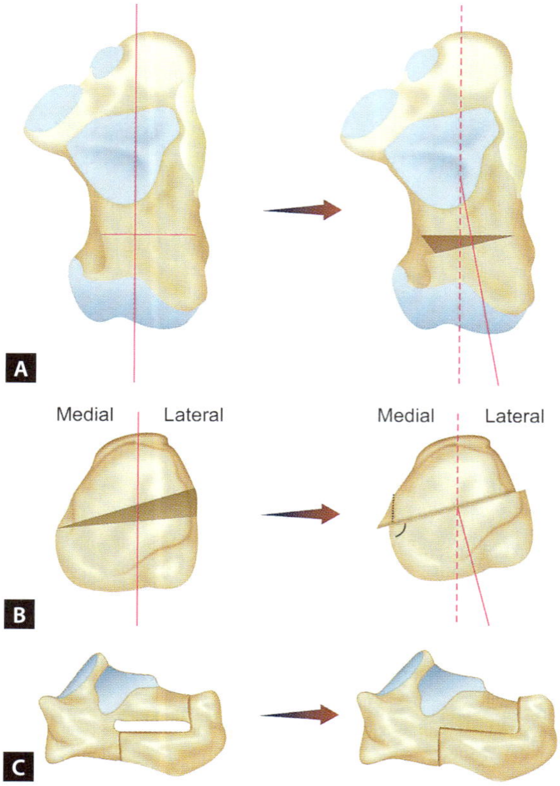

Figs. 9A to C: The triplanar z-osteotomy of calcaneum. The solid and dashed vertical lines show the central axis of the calcaneus in each plane. (A) Top view of the calcaneal osteotomy, that is corrected by lateral rotation of the osteotomy producing medial gap (right); (B) Posterior view shows the removal of laterally based wedge cut that is closed by tilting and lateral rotation correcting varus (right); (B) Lateral view also demonstrates the lateral wedge removed and closed down creating valgus (right).

radiographically preserved are best treated by subtalar arthrodesis. This can be combined with lateral closing wedge osteotomy of the anterior aspect of the calcaneus 1 cm proximal to the calcaneocuboid joint (to shorten lateral column) is a good option. In case these joints show arthritic changes on radiographs, triple arthrodesis is recommended else the patient will have continued pain.

- *Triplanar osteotomy and lateral ligament reconstruction by Saxby and Mayerson:* The triplanar calcaneal osteotomy corrects all three planes of the cavovarus deformity. It is a difficult procedure but all deformities are corrected by a single plan in which lateral translation of the tuberosity fragment and closing wedge osteotomy laterally corrects the varus component while a proximal slide of the tuberosity fragment corrects the calcaneal component of the hindfoot deformity. If the ankle joint is unstable and degenerative changes are not present, then it can be combined with lateral ligament reconstruction. In the presence of degenerative changes, however, a triple arthrodesis with lateral ligament reconstruction is preferred.
- Triple arthrodesis—the Siffert "beak" triple arthrodesis combines osteotomy and triple arthrodesis to correct varus and cavus in severe and rigid deformity. Lateral approach is used to prepare and fuse subtalar and calcaneocuboid joints while talonavisular joint is exposed and prepared through a medial approach. Smaller cuts are made in the plantar aspect of the talar head leaving a "beak" dorsally **(Figs. 10A to C)** and larger wedges are made in dorsal navicular correcting cavus when the navicular is closed into the talus. Compensatory shortening of lateral side is done through the calcaneocuboid joint.

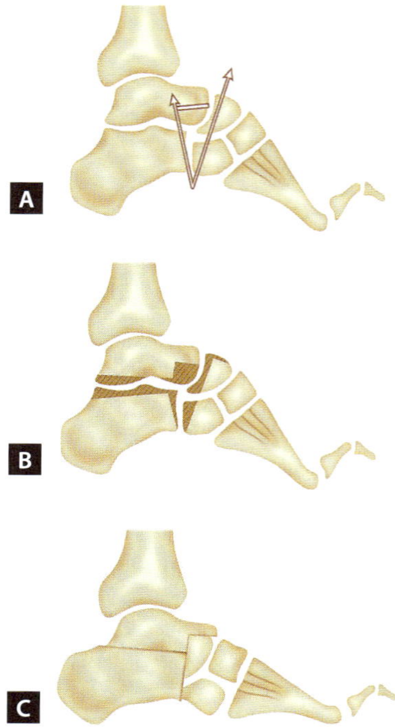

Figs. 10A to C: The Siffert "beak" arthrodesis for midfoot cavus correction. (A) Determining the apex of deformity and planning the cuts; (B) Making the respective–preserving the beak of talus to preserve vascularity of talus and prevent AVN; (C) Final correction.

- Lambrinudi technique (Kindly *see* the Chapter on "Poliomyelitis").

CONCLUSION

- Pes cavus involves accentuation of the longitudinal foot arch. This also reduces the foot length so alters the biomechanics by altering the lever arm.
- The deformity is seen in various disorders and most likely results from intrinsic overactivity.
- The deformity is also commonly associated with varus of the heel and/or calcaneus deformity.
- If uncorrected, the deformity develops into painful foot due to altered weight transmission and biomechanics.
- Treatment involves principally preventing any further progression of the deformity and correcting the deformity by manipulation and stretching in initial stages but failure of them or in late stages surgical correction is necessary. Surgical procedures mostly involve bony procedures and one can follow a rough guideline by dividing the deformity into various grades.

CHAPTER 89

Hindfoot Deformities and Plantar Heel Pain

Manish Kumar Varshney

INTRODUCTION

The deformity of hindfoot is commonly seen with various midfoot deformities as discussed in previous chapters. Malunited fracture of calcaneum produces primary hindfoot deformity that is better dealt in dedicated text for trauma. We will discuss here the commonly seen hindfoot varus and valgus deformities. We will also discuss the very commonly encountered plantar heel pain that is commonly attributed to plantar fasciitis but in reality has various differentials.

HINDFOOT VALGUS DEFORMITY

Spastic pes valgus foot is a flexible deformity until adolescence as detailed in pes planus and peroneal spastic flatfoot discussed elsewhere. The talus becomes vertically oriented, as calcaneum is abducted in this deformity. The forefoot and the plantar ligaments are pulled laterally by spastic plantar ligaments. Talus remains on its position with plantar flexion, but all the other structures including forefoot and calcaneum along with their supportive ligaments are abducted and pulled laterally. The midfoot sags down and if the condition is left untreated, complete breakdown in the midfoot may occur.

Pathoanatomy

- Plantar flexed talus with abduction of calcaneum
- Widening of talocalcaneal angle with dorsiflexed calcaneum in relation to talus
- With plantarflexed talus, navicular displaced dorsally and laterally
- Supination of forefoot in relationship to the hindfoot

Examination

- Note how much deformity can be corrected in hindfoot with manipulation.
- If the hindfoot can be placed in varus, look for equinus contracture.

Treatment Methods

- Grice arthrodesis (*See* Chapter on "Poliomyelitis")
- Subtalar arthrodesis (*See* Chapter on "Poliomyelitis")
- Triple arthrodesis (*See* Chapters on "Poliomyelitis" and "Pes Cavus and Accompanying Deformities")
- *Calcaneal lengthening:* Modified Evans calcaneal lengthening technique.

HINDFOOT VARUS DEFORMITY

Presents as an inverted and small heel, a tight tendocalcaneus forefoot abduction and inversion rotation at the mid-tarsal joints. There may also be some cavus deformity as well as clawing of the toes and lateral rotation of tibia. It is usually accompanied by equinus deformity and isolated deformity is rare.

Etiology

It is often an accompaniment of other deformities or residue of partial correction of a bigger or complicated deformity:

- An uncorrected or relapsed club foot
- As part of arthrogryposis multiplex congenita
- As part of pes cavus deformity
- As a result of neurological disorders, such as spina bifida or cerebral palsy or poliomyelitis

Treatment

- *Dillwyn Evans operation:* Extensive medial soft-tissue release with lengthening of tight tendons together with calcaneo-cuboid arthrodesis.
- *Dwyer operation* (discussed multiply elsewhere, viz., pes cavus, clubfoot, poliomyelitis, etc.): Aimed at correcting varus by increasing the medial height of calcaneus and placing it directly under the line of weight-bearing.

PLANTAR HEEL PAIN

Plantar heel pain is quite common and has multiple etiologies. This is different from posterior heel pain as occurs in retrocalcaneal space at the Achilles tendon insertion or in the Krager fat pad. *Plantar fasciitis* is the most common condition, but following etiologies should be distinguished before finalizing the diagnosis:

- Plantar fasciitis
- Tarsal tunnel syndrome

- *Nerve entrapment syndromes:*
  - Lateral plantar nerve entrapment
  - First branch of the lateral plantar nerve involvement (central heel pad syndrome) also known as Baxter's neuropathy
  - Medial plantar nerve entrapment
  - Entrapment of calcaneal nerve, and sural nerve
- Neuroma formation
- Calcaneus osteomyelitis
- Stress fracture of the calcaneus
- Ruptured plantar fascia
- Foreign body of the heel pad
- Neoplasia

A careful history and physical examination are essential to differentiate pathologies. The history helps in differentiating mechanical, neurogenic, neoplastic, infectious, or traumatic etiologies. Traumatic event (recent/ past) may involve the skin, fat pad, fascia, nerve, vascular system, or bone. There may be an impaled foreign body due to trauma that may also be associated with infection. The trauma may also be just an incidental finding. History of intense program of walking, running, or weight-bearing activity (as in practicing for defense entrance) may strain the plantar tissues and produce insidious or acute spontaneous pain. Nerve pain may be aggravated with changes in foot position or activity level. Some characteristics of foot pain should be recorded as pain appearing with first step in the morning, disappears with further walking (plantar fasciitis), and reappears when arising after sitting (plantar fasciitis); or is the pain made worse by standing or walking (nerve entrapment). Does the pain occur at night (infectious/nerve entrapment) and wake the patient from sleep? Note the location of pain—medial, central, or lateral heel and any radiation. In examination, locate the precise area of tenderness. Nerve entrapments like the central heel pad syndrome or others occurring at the medial soft spot where the neurovascular bundle enters the foot can be often localized this way. Plantar fasciitis presents as tenderness over the medial tubercle of the calcaneus at the origin of the plantar fascia. Subcutaneous foreign body or a lack of prominence of the medial border of the plantar fascia may also be diagnosed by careful examination. Ruptured plantar fascia may also be diagnosed by dorsiflexion of the ankle and the great toe.

Plain radiographs may demonstrate bony lesion or foreign body. Soft-tissue lesions of the heel, neoplasia, tendinopathy, neural entrapments, foreign bodies, and plantar fascia defects may be demonstrated by MRI but it is quite nonspecific in the absence of clinical correlation. Ultrasonography is a less expensive and dynamic investigation but area that can be examined is limited and interpretation of the test results is much more difficult than with MRI. Infectious cause may be also substantiated by blood tests for infection markers such as raised white blood cell count and differential, erythrocyte sedimentation rate, C-reactive protein level, and if possible a labeled white blood cell scan.

Plantar Fasciitis

This is enthesopathy and inflammation involving the origin of the plantar fascia on the medial tubercle of the calcaneus. The usual cause is repeated minor trauma to the fascial origin that lies plantar and superficial to the origin of the flexor digitorum brevis. A broad shelf of bone may form into this muscle origin, it is more of an incidental finding and is not the cause of heel pain despite being prominent on a lateral radiograph as a heel spur **(Fig. 1)**.

Plantar fasciitis typically develops with an increase in activity related to weight bearing or a change in running shoes or other types of shoes. The risk factors for development of plantar heel pain are tightness of tendo-Achilles, limb length discrepancy, sedentary lifestyle, overpronation, obese person with high BMI, pes cavus and frequent long distance running. Sometimes the symptoms arise spontaneously, however. Patient classically reports pain in the heel during the first step in the morning that disappears after a few steps but may reoccur with prolonged sitting. The pain does not occur at night, does not disturb sleep or develop before arising in the morning. It also does not become worse with activity. Windlass mechanism explains the etiological development of plantar fasciitis. On examination, there is a specific tenderness limited to the origin of the plantar fascia. The plantar fascia is intact otherwise (differential from ruptured plantar fascia). The plain radiograph may demonstrate a spur. MRI may show reaction in the plantar fascial origin and the adjacent bone.

Treatment

Various nonspecific treatments are prescribed usually in combination with plantar fascia stretching exercises which is the real effective treatment. Spontaneous remissions are common but the symptoms usually recur after a gap of 2–3 months or sometimes a year. Maintenance after remission is

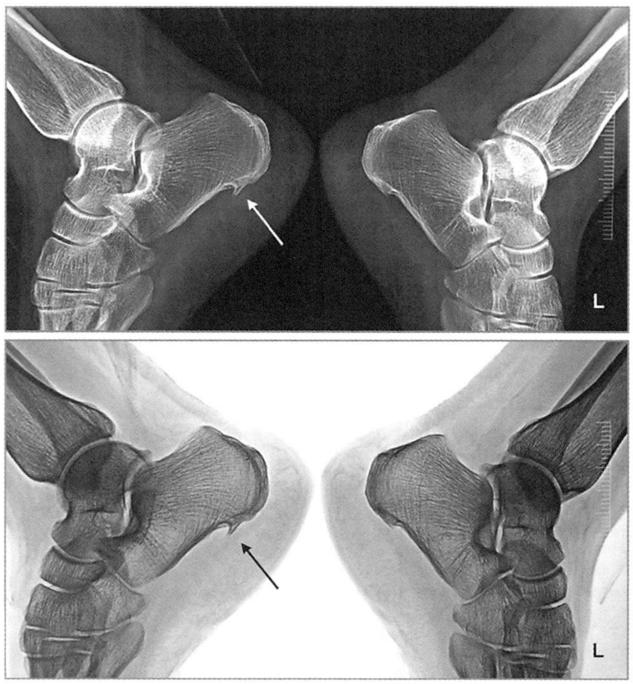

Fig. 1: The calcaneal spur (arrow) is commonly seen as an incidental finding and is not the common cause of heel pain. This patient had both heel pain but only the right calcaneus had the typical spur.

hence important and may be achieved by simple measures like using a simple heel cup or soft sole shoes. Orthotic devices that splint the plantar fascia and gather heel pad fat reduce the contact of the irritated plantar fascia with the weight-bearing surface. Walking on hard surfaces and repetitive microtrauma should be avoided or prevented. Oral nonsteroidal anti-inflammatory drugs (NSAIDs) also are helpful for symptomatic relief as is local use of ice or heat for inflammation control. Phonophoresis or iontophoresis has been found to be helpful in selective studies. Local injection of depot or nonparticulate steroids has been found to be variably helpful and often gives drastic but temporary relief. This may be used as interim measure to relieve pain and begin physiotherapy that may later take effect for long-term pain control. Open surgical release of the plantar fascia historically has been used to treat persistent symptoms, with or without removal of the so-called heel spur. The outcome had been extremely variable and may, in fact, sometimes lead to persistent and worsening pain, pain on the lateral border and dorsum of the foot, and classic neurogenic symptoms.

Denervation of the heel by division of the calcaneal nerves has also been attempted by some with variable results. Release of only the medial plantar fascia has had variable outcomes though it can be done endoscopically. One should take care of laceration of the tibial nerve or nearby vascular structures. The addition of acupuncture was found to add some benefit to a standard protocol using ice, NSAIDs, and stretching. It has been found that most of the patients with chronic pain from plantar fasciitis have a contracted gastrocnemius and can get relief by gastrocnemius recession. This is also the basis for proximal medial gastrocnemius release in patients with resistant or recalcitrant plantar fasciitis. The use of ESWL, local PPRP injection, and prolotherapy are investigational only. I would recommend tissue-specific stretching, NSAIDs, and a simple full-length orthotic device/soft sole support for initial cases that can be tried for 3–5 months and may be supplemented with local steroid injections (conservatively though). In recalcitrant cases, medial endoscopic plantar fascia release and/or gastrocnemius recession are possible options.

Ruptured Plantar Fascia

The plantar fascia may tear during an acute dorsiflexion stretch regardless of associated condition. There is usually a history of local steroid injections. A sensation of popping or suddenly giving way is classic. The patient presents with acute pain in the heel and medial foot arch, pain/ache on the lateral border of the foot, and in the dorsal region. There may be associated neurogenic symptoms in the tibial nerve distribution.

On examination, one can elicit tenderness in the proximal fascia, midfoot ecchymosis, and a fascial defect. Tear can also be confirmed using ultrasonography or MRI in chubby feet or in noncooperative patients or for documentation.

Treatment generally is immobilization in a cast or walking boot for 1–2 weeks supplemented by analgesics. A custom-molded orthotic device with posting of the longitudinal arch can be placed after cast immobilization for 4–6 weeks. At the healing site, irregular hypertrophic scar usually forms that can be superficially palpated also. Pain may not relieve in a number of patients even for prolonged duration. Spontaneous rupture commonly involves the medial border of the plantar fascia sparing the central and lateral portions that may cause mechanical symptoms and hence prolonged pain. Complete release of the remaining fascia may be tried in these cases to relieve the mechanical symptoms. Some patients may have neurogenic pain due to neural impingement/involvement that can be relieved by complete release of the remaining plantar fascia along with tarsal tunnel release.

Heel Pad Bursitis

Bursa present at the heel pad acts as a cushion between tendons and bone. Prolonged pressure over the bursa leads to bursitis at the heel pad. Trauma is another etiological factor. Patient presents with pain and swelling over the heel. They give history of prolonged standing or walking that accentuates pain. On palpation, the tender point is posterior to the insertion of plantar fascia. USG evaluation helps in diagnosing bursitis although clinical suspicion is all that is required. Other imaging modalities are usually not required. Conservative treatment is given with avoidance of nearing weight and RICE (Rest, Ice, Compression, and Elevation) therapy. NSAIDs help to alleviate pain. Silicon heel cups are highly useful in this condition.

Heel Fat Pad Atrophy

This disease occurs in middle age usually after 40 years as there occurs reduction in size of fat pad in the heel. As the age advances, there is decrease in water and collagen content as in degenerative disorders. The elastic nature of the tissue that acts as shock absorber is reduced gradually. The pain usually is bilateral, aggravates by bearing weight, and also occurs at night-time. Conservative treatment is all that is required as in plantar fasciitis. Silicon cups are recommended as they give relief when the patient starts bearing weight.

Nerve Entrapments

Lateral Plantar Nerve Involvement

The lateral and medial plantar nerves branch from tibial nerve proximal to the abductor hallucis. The lateral plantar nerve then enters foot crossing the soft spot obliquely while medial plantar nerve runs under the muscle of the abductor accompanied by medial plantar artery and vein. The medial plantar nerve is free from the usual constricted region formed by the distal edge of the abductor hallucis fascia and proximal edge of the plantar fascia. The lateral plantar nerve, however, due to its disposition gets entrapped in distal tarsal tunnel syndrome. Once involved, it is managed with the total-contact orthotic shoe insert, and surgical release as is also commonly performed during surgical release performed also for chronic plantar fasciitis. It is important to note here that partial release of the plantar fascia and the tarsal tunnel is not reliably successful.

First Branch of the Lateral Plantar Nerve Involvement (Central Heel Pad Syndrome)

This is also called Baxter's neuropathy. The first branch of the lateral plantar nerve (the inferior calcaneal nerve or Baxter's nerve, **Fig. 2**) occasionally may emerge from the tibial nerve itself. The branch sends a sensory branch to the central heel pad while running posteriorly under the abductor halluces and over quadratus plantae to innervate it. It also supplies the flexor digitorum brevis and the abductor digiti quinti. The first branch of the lateral plantar nerve may get entrapped between the deep fascia of the abductor hallucis and the medial third of the plantar fascia causing pain over central heel pad in runners. Central heel pad syndrome may also be produced by contusion of the central heel with a neuroma of the nerve causing persistent pain that aggravates with running or brisk walking. Flat-soled shoes also may aggravate the pain.

Treatment may be initially tried with use of total-contact orthotic shoe insert, with widening of the nerve relief channel posteriorly on the medial and plantar surfaces, and modifying the patient's running regimen. If this fails, then surgical release of the above-mentioned structures may be attempted. Neuroma of the nerve needs to be surgically excised through tarsal tunnel incision, with excision of the branch, insertion into a conduit, and placement of the conduit into the retrocalcaneal space.

During surgery one must differentiate the first branch of the lateral plantar nerve from the calcaneal branches of the tibial nerve. The latter usually emerges more proximally and ends in the subcutaneous tissue and skin of the medial and posteromedial heel.

Medial Plantar Nerve Involvement

The medial plantar nerve can be involved in tarsal tunnel or it also can be involved over the course of the lateral plantar nerve as it passes under the abductor hallucis muscle with the medial plantar artery and veins. It may also be affected by tenosynovitis of flexor hallucis longus (FHL) or flexor digitorum longus (FDL) tendons.

Involvement/entrapment produces pain typically in the arch and occurs with active or passive movement of the nearby structures/involved tendons. When the nerve is affected posteromedially under the abductor hallucis there is referred pain into the tarsal tunnel and the heel. For conservative management, total-contact orthotic shoe insert is modified by extending the nerve relief channel anteriorly.

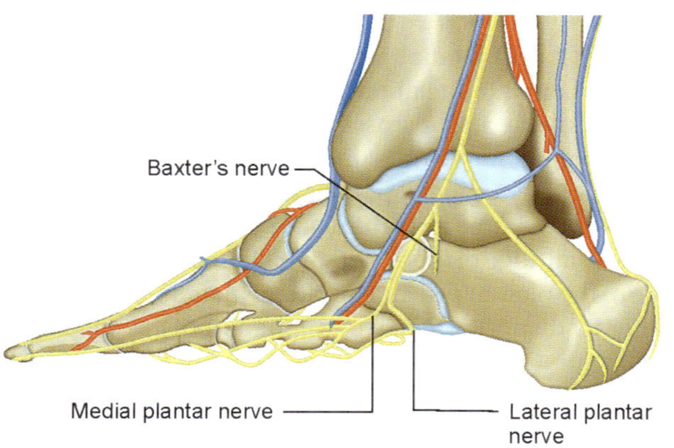

Fig. 2: The anatomy of Baxter's nerve. The nerve emerges from the tibial nerve itself higher up instead of emerging from lateral plantar nerve thus gets predisposed to entrapment over its course.

A shoe with a stiff rocker sole is used, or the insert is stiffened with an extended steel shank or a Morton extension and is used with rocker sole. Medicines are prescribed for symptomatic relief.

For intractable symptoms, combined tarsal tunnel and plantar fascia release are done. The medial plantar nerve should be completely exposed by incising the abductor hallucis. If the patient has had both heel pain and tenderness along the nerve then release is carried beyond the bifurcation under the muscle longitudinally. If the patient has tenosynovitis of the FDL and/or FHL without significant tarsal tunnel or heel pain; then nerve release is done along the longitudinal arch and simultaneous synovectomy is performed without opening tarsal tunnel.

Calcaneal Branch Involvement

Calcaneal branch(es) of tibial nerve innervate medial plantar heel that can cause medial plantar heel pain if contused or entrapped or suffer from neuroma formation. Palpation of the nerve localizes the site of the lesion. Conservative treatment with cushioning and manual desensitization is usually unsuccessful but the use of a backless shoe is recommended. The calcaneal nerves can be excised and placed in a vein or collagen conduit directing the conduit into the retrocalcaneal space.

Sural Nerve Involvement

Sural nerve and its branches innervate lateral plantar heel, lateral border of the foot, the fifth toe (plantar surface), and fourth and fifth toes (dorsal surface). Involvement of first branch of the lateral plantar nerve can cause pain in central and lateral heel pad. Traumatic injury to sural nerve or a surgery may result in pain over the lateral heel region. There may be associated loss of sensibility in the area and localized tenderness or a positive Tinel sign. One may resort to sural nerve block as an adjunctive tool for diagnosis. Backless shoe and manual desensitization are recommended along with symptomatic treatment. If intractable neurolysis of nerve can be performed but excision of the nerve is curative.

Stress Fractures of the Calcaneus

This is seen in runners. Young amenorrheic women and osteoporotic patients are particularly prone to develop stress fractures. The patient notices pain at the moment of injury or shortly after. The pain is initially constant but gradually gets worsened with activity. Over a course of time the pain appears with activity but is relieved by rest. Examination reveals point tenderness with palpation. On radiographs, the fracture may not be apparent until 10–14 days after the injury. MRI shows localized signal changes.

CT can be used to confirm the diagnosis. The typical fracture in a patient with pain in the plantar heel is a break in the plantar cortex without displacement. The treatment is rest and immobilization for minimum 6 weeks in a cast.

Osteomyelitis of the Calcaneus

Infection and osteomyelitis of calcaneus usually develops following direct inoculation of the bone from a penetrating foreign body but it may also develop following hematogenous or contiguous spread. Diagnosis is easy to make with radiographic confirmation. Pain usually increases at night and is unaffected by activity or rest. Definitive diagnosis requires Gram staining and culture of organism from material obtained through sterile aspiration guided by ultrasonography (the preferred method) or fluoroscopy. The treatment is debridement with immobilization and use of intravenous antibiotics.

CONCLUSION

- Deformities of hindfoot commonly are an accompaniment to other midfoot deformities. Only in post-traumatic cases (fracture of the calcaneus bone) do they occur isolated.
- The deformity can produce either heel varus or valgus. Correction of deformity is often bony osteotomy that is usually associated with the correction of primary deformity at midfoot. Correction also, however, commonly requires some alteration of the tendo-Achilles as commonly its contracture is seen.

CHAPTER 90

Tarsal Tunnel Syndrome

Manish Kumar Varshney

INTRODUCTION

The term "tarsal tunnel syndrome" embraces entrapment neuropathy of posterior tibial nerve or its associated branches as it passes through the porta pedis (tarsal tunnel) deep to flexor retinaculum (laciniate ligament). "Posterior tibial neuralgia" is another name for it. It is easier to understand the syndrome when we consider the analogy with a common disorder the carpal tunnel syndrome (CTS) where median nerve is compressed beneath the transverse carpal ligament, similarly in tarsal tunnel syndrome, the tibial nerve gets constricted. Compromise of the space at porta pedis causes compression of the tibial nerve causing symptoms. The condition was first described in 1960 but Keck and Lam in 1962 dubbed the entity as tarsal tunnel syndrome detailing its treatment and pathology.

ANATOMY (FIGS. 1 AND 2)

Tarsal Tunnel

Akin to carpal tunnel the tarsal tunnel (also known as "porta pedis") is a fibro-osseous structure formed from the bones of foot on one side and covered by overlying fibrous tissue on the other. The tarsal tunnel anatomical landmarks are as follows:

- *Roof:* The unyielding fibrous roof is an extension of the deep fascia of the leg that blends with the deep transverse fascia (flexor retinaculum also known as "Laciniate ligament") of ankle joint at its posteromedial aspect. Hence, the proximal extent of roof is contiguous with the investing deep fascia of calf posteriorly while distally it merges with deep fascia and aponeurosis on medial aspect of sole. It is about 2.5–3 cm wide and extends from medial calcaneal tuberosity and proximal border of abductor halluces with indistinct borders to the medial malleolus. From this fibrous roof, septa extend toward the calcaneum that form compartments through which tendons of tibialis posterior, flexor digitorum longus (FDL), and long flexor of great toe pass separately encased in their synovial sheath. The neurovascular bundle passes through its independent compartment where the vessels lie superficial to the nerve.
- *Floor:* It is formed by superomedial aspect of the calcaneum, medial part of talus, and the terminal portion of medial malleolus.
- *Contents:* Tibialis posterior, flexor hallucis longus (FHL), FDL and the tibial nerve, and posterior tibial artery and accompanying veins. The neurovascular structures pass between the FHL and FDL. In the proximal region, the

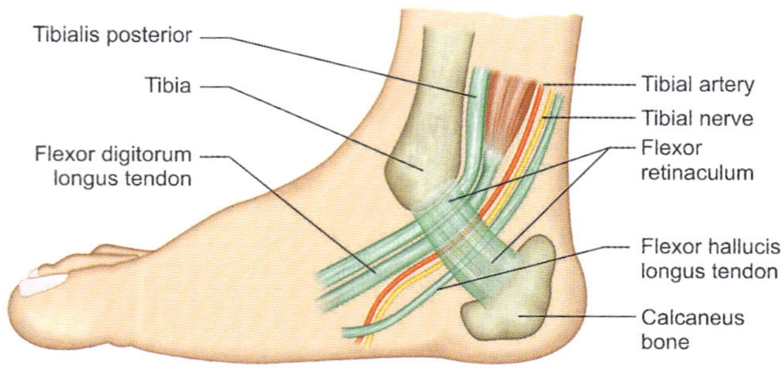

Fig. 1: Tarsal tunnel anatomy.

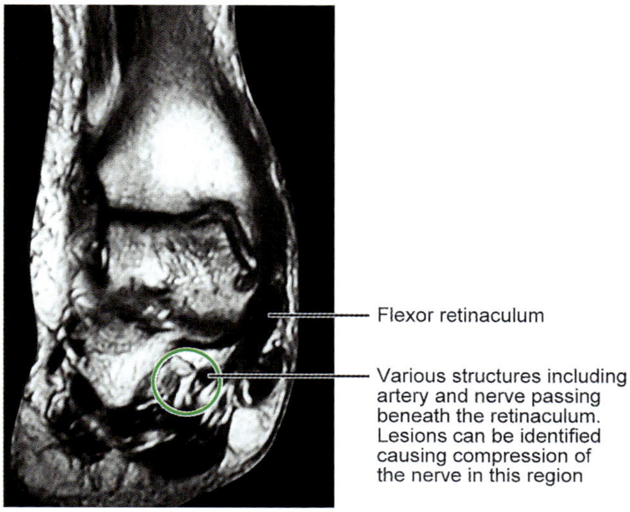

Fig. 2: Tarsal tunnel anatomy MRI. The region of tarsal tunnel is encircled.

tibial nerve passes between the tibialis posterior and FDL tendons and distally between the FDL and FHL tendons. The nerve then courses behind the medial malleolus and anterior to the Achilles tendon dividing into three prominent and often consistent branches: (1) the medial calcaneal, (2) medial plantar, and (3) lateral plantar. The nerve always bifurcates before the posterior tibial artery ramifies into its branches. The division is also intratunnel in 93–96% cases while in the rest division may occur even proximally. The calcaneal branch travels to the heel, the lateral plantar nerve traverses through the belly of the abductor hallucis muscle supplying the sole of foot. The medial plantar nerve is the thickest branch that crosses superior to the abductor hallucis and FHL tendon and terminally gives three medial common digital nerves of the foot and the medial plantar cutaneous nerve of the hallux. The individual components may also get compressed so their distribution should be known—

1. Calcaneal branch—supplies the sensations to heel in medial and posterior distribution.
2. Medial plantar branch—lies at a distance averaging 20 mm (range 11-30 mm) from medial malleolus and provides sensation to the medial aspect of sole of foot including the hallux and three toes and gives motor branches to the abductor hallucis (while traversing through it) and flexor digitorum brevis muscles.
3. Lateral plantar branch—lies at a distance of 21–40 mm from medial calcaneal tubercle and gives cutaneous sensation to the fifth digit and gives motor supply to the abductor digiti quinti and quadratus plantae muscles.

ETIOLOGY

Any condition that compromises the volume of tarsal tunnel by virtue of altering the spatial configuration of elements will produce the syndrome, so tibial nerve may get constricted by either external pressure or lesions constricting space within the tunnel. The common causes producing tarsal tunnel syndrome hence include:

- *Fractures and malunion:* Bone fragments from displaced calcaneal fracture fragments (commonly), medial malleolus or talus.
- *Inflammatory conditions:* Tenosynovitis, rheumatoid arthritis.
- *Space occupying lesions:* Lipoma, ganglia, amyloidosis, schwannoma, or exostosis.
- *Doublecrushsyndrome:* Thisisnotasyndromebutageneral phenomenon that is common to various compression neuropathies such as radial nerve compression at elbow and cervical spondylosis, sciatic nerve compression near piriformis muscle and lumbar spondylosis, etc. A double-crush phenomenon occurs when a proximal nerve root pathology diminishes axoplasmic flow, making it more susceptible to injury (*see* Chapter on "Foot Drop" also). Double-crush phenomenon is based on the work of Upton and McComas (1973) who summarized their findings that "local damage to a nerve at one site along its course may sufficiently impair the overall functioning of the nerve cells (axonal flow), such that the nerve cells become more susceptible to compression trauma at distal sites than would normally be the case". So in case of lumbar spondylosis or prolapsed intervertebral disk at S1 the tibial nerve may be more susceptible to compression at the flexor retinaculum. Double-crush phenomenon may be seen in up to three-fourths of the patients with compression neuropathy.
- Varicosities.
- *Intrinsic:* Neural tumor (neurilemmoma) and perineural fibrosis, other space occupying lesions like enlarged veins, hypertrophic retinaculum. Trauma leading to hematoma formation may cause adhesion formation later.
- Valgus deformity of hindfoot may stretch the tibial nerve and cause perineural fibrosis by increasing tensile load on the nerve.
- Tarsal coalition.
- Inflammatory—fibrous enlargement.
- Congenital deformity.
- Systemic disorders such as diabetes, vascular disease.
- Extensive vascular supply to the posterior tibial nerve in the tarsal tunnel may cause vascular congestion predisposing the nerve to symptomatic compression.

CLINICAL FEATURES AND EXAMINATION

- Patients report a nonspecific vague pain in the foot and sole often confusing with plantar fasciitis.
- Pain, paresthesia, and numbness are not uncommon **(Figs. 3A and B)**. The paresthesia most commonly presents as nocturnal burning type of pain. The paresthesia and pain are normally referred distal to the site of compression but in one-third of patients, the pain may also radiate proximally into the midcalf (Valleix phenomenon). It is defined as pain that radiates proximal to the tarsal tunnel instead of distal radiation and is sometimes seen in double crush syndrome. One needs to palpate along the course of the nerve to identify pain points to confirm the diagnosis and not be misled by proximal radiation of pain to lumbar disk herniation. Pain of tarsal tunnel syndrome gets aggravated by walking/standing and is relieved by rest.
- Tenderness may occur over the posterior tibial nerve in this syndrome, where the presenting symptoms are usually of local pain and paresthesia in the foot.
- In patients with leprosy and amyloid neuropathy perineural thickening may be palpable.
- Tapping over the posterior tibial nerve (Tinel's test) may give rise to paresthesias in the sole of the foot, medial heel, the instep of the sole and the toes in the area corresponding to supply of the medial calcaneal, the medial and lateral plantar nerves. It is always imperative to compare both sides.
- Sensory loss in the plantar foot area of medial (base of great toe and its ball) and lateral plantar nerves is a characteristic finding which extends dorsally till over distal phalanges of toes only. This can be examined by diminished two-point discrimination and hypoesthesia to prick.

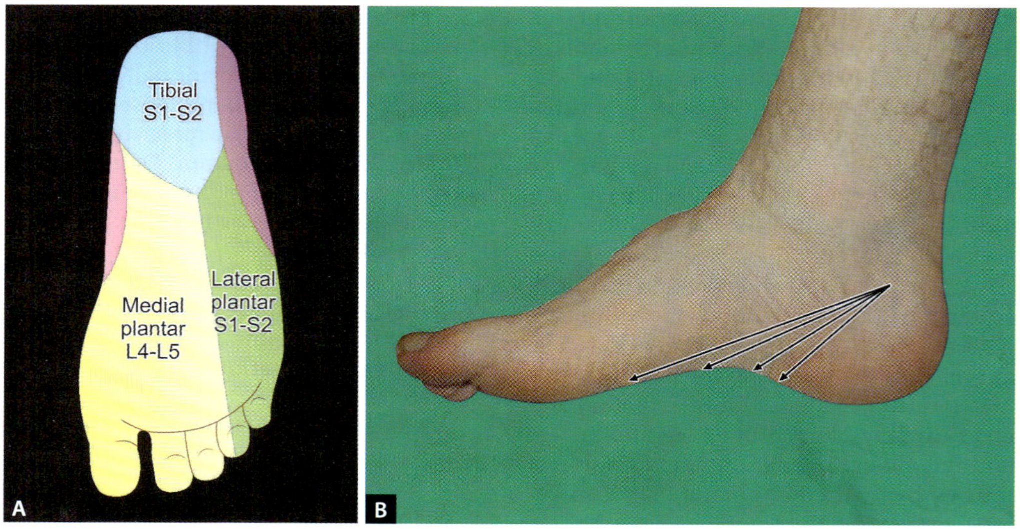

Figs. 3A and B: Symptoms tarsal tunnel syndrome are commonly distributed in (A) the region of medial plantar nerve; (B) Often radiating from the nerve compression site in the tunnel.

- Only in late cases, one may note atrophy of the intrinsic foot muscles, but it is clinically difficult to appreciate.
- In long-standing cases, neuropathic changes may be noted including deformity like pes cavus, and atrophic changes such as loss of hair and skin ulceration. Also, note the heel valgus that may predispose to neuritis and development of pain.
- *The dorsiflexion-eversion test (Kinoshita et al.):* Maximally dorsiflex the ankle and the metatarsophalangeal (MP) joints of all three toes, firmly evert the foot and hold this position **(Fig. 4)**. In a positive case, the patient's symptoms will be reproduced. Look also for increased local tenderness, accompanying the maneuver.
- *The tourniquet test:* In doubtful cases, apply a tourniquet to the calf and inflate to just above the systolic blood pressure if this brings on the symptoms the diagnosis is confirmed.

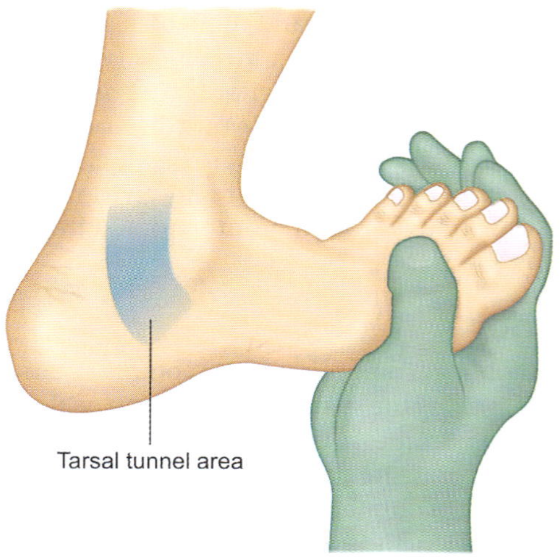

Fig. 4: Dorsiflexion-eversion test.

INVESTIGATIONS

Standard radiographs of the ankle and foot may demonstrate the fracture fragment protruding into the canal, exostosis, and bony deformities. MRI may demonstrate the soft tissue causes of compression neuropathy. Nerve conduction studies (NCS) are the best and reliable diagnostic modalities to demonstrate the site of compression, type (sensory, motor, both), pathophysiology (axonal versus demyelinating), and changes in the muscles if performed by experienced person. Hematological investigations include evaluation for diabetes mellitus and long-term glycemic control (HbA1c), erythrocyte sedimentation rate (ESR), blood urea nitrogen (BUN), creatinine, and vitamin B_{12} levels.

DIFFERENTIAL DIAGNOSIS

Plantar fasciitis, Morton's metatarsalgia, tendinitis and tendinopathy, inflammatory arthropathy, and urate arthropathy.

TREATMENT

Medical Treatment

This is indicated in the absence of demonstrable nerve compression.

- Initially, the nonsteroidal anti-inflammatory drugs (NSAIDs), oral steroids, neurotropic vitamins are commonly tried for mild-to-moderate symptoms.
- For nonresponsive patients, local injection of steroids into the tarsal canal may give temporary to permanent relief in some.
- Correction of planovalgus deformity with physiotherapy or orthosis may also relieve symptoms in specific patients.
- Use of night splints to maintain plantar flexion and inversion may also be tried for symptomatic relief (similar to carpal tunnel extension splint).

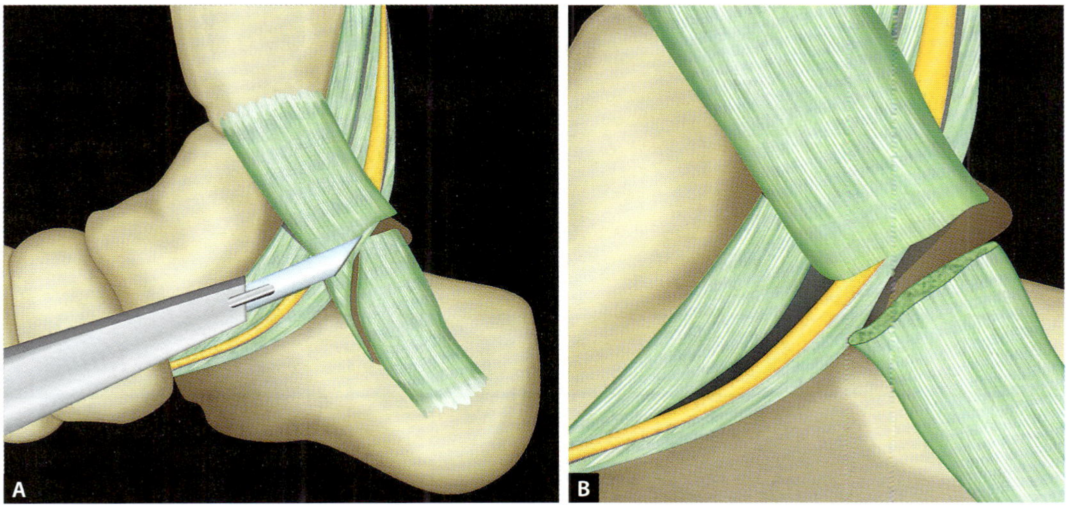

Figs. 5A and B: Surgical tarsal tunnel release.

Surgical Treatment

Surgical treatment is done in patients unresponsive to conservative therapy or if there is identified pathology on MRI or clinically or a deformity is present. Also, surgical release of the nerve is required in electrodiagnostic study (like NCV)-demonstrable nerve compression. Predictors of failed nonsurgical treatment included longer motor nerve conduction latency (7.4 ms or greater) and greater predominance of foot comorbidities. Tarsal tunnel release **(Figs. 5A and B)** is the commonly performed surgery. Clinically, it is seen that pronation and plantar flexion significantly increase pressures in the medial and lateral plantar tunnels causing nerve compression. The greater effect on the lateral plantar tunnel could be the result of greater angularity of the passage from the medial ankle to beneath the foot. It has been seen that intraoperatively measured pressures were similar to cadaver pressures except for higher lateral plantar tunnel pressures in particular positions. Tunnel release and septum excision greatly reduce those pressures. Additionally, one or more of the following may be required.

- External neurolysis is an acceptable procedure especially if, on surgical exploration, there are adhesions or scar tissue formation causing the nerve impingement.
- Space-occupying masses require specific removal. Also, correction of deformity of feet as needed for planovalgus correction, calcaneal malunion, bone spurs, etc. should be done.
- Decompression of the nerve should be attempted by those versed with anatomy. Expose the nerve through incision made posterior to the tibia. Release the retinaculum in entirety and identify the tibial nerve. Leave it undisturbed unless there is fibrosis for which neurolysis is required. Neuroma or compressing lesions should be identified and removed. Identify the medial plantar branch of posterior tibial nerve along the margin of flexor sheath of flexor hallucis longus. Any fibrous band constricting the branches of nerve should be released.

CONCLUSION

- Entrapment neuropathy of posterior tibial nerve is not an uncommon disorder and a commonly missed condition of foot pain.
- The disorder has various similarities to carpal tunnel syndrome but is not necessarily present in the patients suffering from it.
- Making a diagnosis by careful examination makes the treatment easy as decompression of the nerve is often curative.

CHAPTER 91

Foot Drop

Manish Kumar Varshney

INTRODUCTION

Foot drop is a crippling and complex problem that can be defined as a significant weakness of ankle and toe dorsiflexion so that the foot takes up a plantarflexed position. It is not a disease in itself but an inability to lift the forefoot resulting from various disorders. There are so many conditions that can lead to foot drop. Some of the associated conditions are stoke, trauma to foot or lower limb, nerve damage, diabetes, adverse drug reaction, alcoholic neuropathy, Parkinson's, multiple sclerosis, etc.

Generally, foot drop can be categorized into three groups:

1. *Neurologic [peripheral (commonly) or central]:*
   - Injury or neuropathy of deep peroneal, common peroneal or sciatic nerve. Leprosy was the most common nontraumatic cause of foot drop but with reduced infection and improved management, its incidence has fallen.
   - Prolapsed intervertebral disk (PIVD) (mainly L4–L5), injury to lumbar or sacral segments of spinal cord. Spina bifida and neoplasia of the spine or cord are other causes.
   - Cerebral lesions involving motor area of foot (parasagittal region) or motor neuron disease
   - Compression of common peroneal or deep peroneal nerve at the fibular head **(Fig. 1)** is the most common compressive neuropathy in the lower extremity seen as a result of varied pathology. Peroneal nerve injury may arise iatrogenically due to ischemia, mechanical irritation, and traction (poor technique of insertion of Steinman pin for skeletal traction itself may injure the nerve), crush injury, laceration intraoperatively during total knee or hip arthroplasty, proximal tibial osteotomy, correction of a severe valgus or flexion deformity at knee or postoperatively by hematoma or constrictive dressings.
   - *Sciatic nerve injury:* Posterior hip dislocation, hip, and acetabular fractures are commonly associated with sciatic nerve injury where involvement of the common peroneal component is much more common that tibial component injury. Intramuscular injections in gluteal region due to poor technique (nerve palsy occurs due to drug injected directly into the nerve tissue and not due to needle injury to nerve) is another cause.
   - In patients having rapid weight loss after operation (e.g., bariatric surgery), neuropathy leading to foot drop may occur. Vitamin B_{12} deficiency may be an involved factor.
   - Central causes include stroke, multiple sclerosis, Charcot-Marie-Tooth disease.
2. *Muscular:*
   - Direct injury to the dorsiflexors, subcutaneous tendon (tibialis anterior) rupture
   - Muscular dystrophy, polio, amyotropic lateral sclerosis (Lou Gehrig's disease)
3. *Anatomic:*
   - Compartment syndromes (anterior leg compartment syndrome resulting in weakness of the dorsiflexors), deep posterior compartment Volkman ischemic contracture causing tethering of the foot in plantar

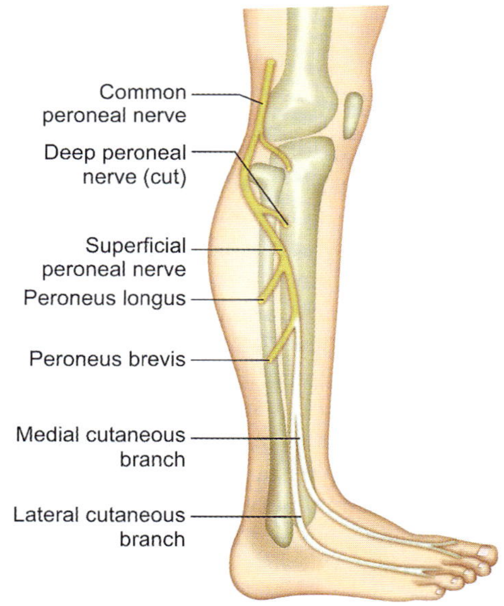

Fig. 1: Site of compression near fibular head for peroneal nerve.

flexion, chronic compartment syndrome slowly causing the symptoms especially in the soldiers—march gangrene (see compartment syndromes)
- Habitual crossed leg sitting
- Charcot joints

PATHOPHYSIOLOGY

Axoplasmic flow is necessary for functional integrity of an axon (basic unit to transmit the electric impulse in a nerve) and its target. A laceration interrupts the anatomical axon unit. Axoplasmic flow may also be compromised by crush injury. It may also be diminished by an injury proximally in nerve root, rendering it more susceptible to subsequent injury (double-crush phenomenon). Foot drop occurs when distal lesion occurs resulting in clinical palsy. Double-crush phenomenon may be the cause for increased prevalence of foot drop in spinal stenosis patients undergoing total hip joint replacement. The proximal insult occurs by spinal stenosis and the distal insult may result from sciatic nerve stretch during the surgery.

CLINICAL PRESENTATION

There can be either equniovarus or equinovalgus deformity in foot drop. Equinovarus type is more common and occurs due to central nervous system (CNS) insult as in stroke, trauma whereas equinovalgus type occurs in peripheral nerve injury, polio, direct trauma to tibialis anterior and posterior (rare). Cerebral palsy may lead to either equinovarus or equinovalgus.

In equinovarus type, spasticity of plantarflexors and tibialis posterior leads to equines and varus, respectively with weakness of dorsiflexors and peronei. The patient stands with foot everted and has loss of dorsiflexion when attempting to heel walk. Hindfoot varus is further evaluated for whether it is rigid or flexible as rigid deformity needs bony procedure (osteotomy or fusion).

Gait

Patients have a step-page gait or a high stepping gait like that of soldiers in paretic foot drop. Foot-lift is an important part of swing phase of the gait. To clear the foot off ground the patient bends hip and knee more than usual producing an uncomfortable sluggish high step. In paralytic foot drop, the foot slaps on the ground after heel makes the initial contact as the dorsiflexors are unable to hold the foot during heel strike. This produces "slapping foot gait".

DIAGNOSIS

Laboratory Studies

Workup of foot drop proceeds according to the suspected cause. Investigation of metabolic cause includes:
- Fasting blood sugar
- Hemoglobin A1c
- Liver function test (alcoholic)
- Erythrocyte sedimentation rate
- C-reactive protein
- Serum protein electrophoresis
- Renal function test
- Vitamin B_{12} levels

Imaging Studies

- *Plain films:* To look for exostosis or Charcot joint.
- *Ultrasonography:* If bleeding is suspected in a patient with a hip or knee prosthesis.
- *Nerve conduction studies (NCS):* To assess the regeneration of nerve fibers, site of lesion and document the damage to nerve. Electromyogram additionally helps to identify peripheral neuropathy, myopathy, nerve radiculopathy, motor neuron disease, peripheral nerve compression (peroneal of common peroneal nerve), etc.

TREATMENT

Conservative and Medical Therapy

The condition is commonly managed conservatively at detection for establishing diagnosis and preventing contracture. Also in cases of incomplete neural injury this may be the definitive management till the nerve function recovers. An ankle-foot orthosis (AFO) is used to control the position of ankle and toes during swing and stance phase, to compensate for ankle dorsiflexors, to minimize abnormal gait pattern and to increase the efficiency of walking **(Figs. 2A and B)**. Foot stretch and isometric dorsiflexion

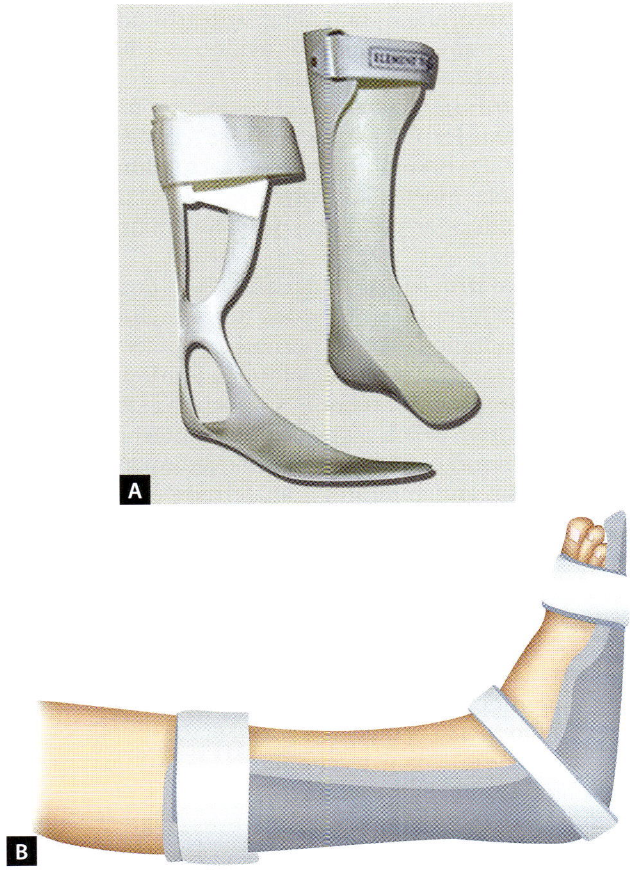

Figs. 2A and B: An ankle-foot orthosis (AFO) splint for foot drop. (A) The splint and (B) its method of application.

are encouraged continuously. Sympathetic blocks help to control painful paresthesia. Managing metabolic etiologies such as diabetes, alcohol liver damage, and neuropathies with supplements of B_1, B_6, or B_{12} can also be useful. Peroneal nerve stimulation can help faster recovery of neuropathy (especially successful for stroke and multiple sclerosis patients). Electrical stimulation should be refrained in patients with pacemaker installed, uncontrolled epilepsy, and those with poor skin condition.

Surgical Repair

Depending on the cause of foot drop that is finally identified, the surgical intervention is planned.

- Foot drop secondary to lumbar disk herniation needs diskectomy.
- Decompression of sciatic nerve may be necessary after foot drop following hip arthroplasty, especially following hematoma collection compressing the nerve is suspected and the nerve has not been surgically damaged.
- Direct damage to the peroneal nerve needs neural repair.
- In acute foot drop due to deep peroneal nerve injuries (<1 year duration); tibial or superficial peroneal nerve fascicle transfer can be done.
- For chronic foot drop, contracture needs to be corrected by Achilles tendon lengthening.
- Foot drop due to polio or Charcot joint cannot be corrected by above-mentioned modalities and these patients require arthrodesis of ankle joint. Along with arthrodesis, if there is severe contracture, Achilles tendon lengthening needs to be done to correct equinus.
- *Tendon transfers:* In surgical correction for foot drop, tendon transfer procedures involve a transfer of a tendon that is still working in place of the tendon that is not functioning. Mostly, it involves transfer of the posterior tibial tendon for providing dorsiflexion and reducing inversion.
  - *Bridle procedure:* It is called so because in this procedure, three tendons are attached in bridle configuration, namely posterior tibial tendon, tibialis anterior, and peroneus longus tendon. Normally, tibialis posterior tendon is inserted on the navicular bone from which it is taken off and attached to second cuneiform bone, and it is attached to anterior tibial tendon and anteriorly transferred peroneus longus tendon in bridle configuration. Now, the posterior tibial muscle will pull the foot up when it contracts, and thus balance the foot in dorsiflexion.
  - In neurotendinous transposition, the lateral head of the gastrocnemius is transposed along with the proximal end of the deep peroneal nerve to the tendons of the anterior muscle group. The nerve is neurotized to the motor nerve of the lateral head of the gastrocnemius. This restores active voluntary dorsiflexion of the foot and automatic walking.
- *Bone-block procedures for foot drop* ***(Fig. 3)****:* Gill and Campbell, or Inclan posterior bone block were preferred methods of management of paralytic foot drops that resulted from polio in children who specifically had a limited involvement. Limited involvement in the sense that they do not require large callipers for walking and the predominant disability in them was flail foot or severe foot drop. The posterior bone block serves as an interim measure till a pantalar arthrodesis or Lambrinudi triple fusion could be undertaken on a skeletally mature foot. For the sheer reasons of uncommon post-polio feet in children and creation of nonanatomical deformity, the procedure is less commonly followed if at all.

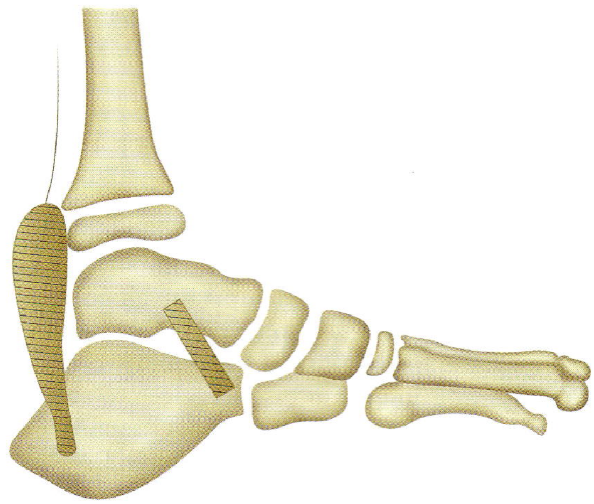

Fig. 3: Posterior bone block to prevent foot drop.

- *Arthrodesis:* For patients with unacceptable power in peroneals and a flail foot that cannot be managed by reconstruction of adequate dorsiflexion power, ankle or pantalar arthrodesis is a good option. The former is preferred for limited damage done to bone unless there are arthritic changes in the tarsal bones where latter is preferable.
- In equinovalgus type, plantarflexors pull foot in equinus and pull of peroneus brevis causes valgus. First equinus is evaluated whether it is flexible or rigid and treated accordingly. Then valgus is evaluated upon whether it is fixed requiring calcaneal osteotomy/subtalar fusion. For flexible deformity, both peronei are transferred to lateral cuneiform.

COMPLICATIONS

The complications are procedure-specific but some common complications that may arise are:

- Wound infection
- Nerve graft failure
- Recurrent deformity
- Pseudoarthrosis, delayed union or nonunion

CONCLUSION

- Foot drop occurs due to loss of dorsiflexion power of the foot that may be neurological, or muscular in origin.
- The patient is disabled as the gait changes to toe-first rather than heel first stance.
- Management consists of keeping the foot supple by stretching and maintaining passive dorsiflexion by splints. Reconstruction of motor power needs active and preserved muscles.

CHAPTER 92

Avascular Necrosis of the Metatarsal Head (Freiberg's Disease)

Manish Kumar Varshney

INTRODUCTION

Also known as Freiberg's infraction or Kohler's second disease, avascular necrosis of the metatarsal (MT) head was first described by Freiberg in 1914. Mostly, it affects the second MT (68%); third MT (27%), and fourth MTs are occasionally involved. It is also referred to as anterior metatarsalgia **(Figs. 1A and B)**. It mainly occurs in puberty during growth spurts, females are mostly involved with female to male ratio of 4:1, this is in contrast to the Kohler's disease (osteochondrosis of navicular tarsal bone) where boys are commonly affected and is unrelated to level of activity. Bilateral disease or involvement of multiple sites simultaneously has been rarely reported.

ETIOLOGY

Traumatic Insult or Repetitive Stress with Microfractures

The microcirculation is compromised. Many theories are there to explain the loss of microcirculation which include chronic repetitive microtrauma, impaired vascularity, systemic diseases, mechanical factors, and endocrine disorders. During walking, the highest stress is borne by second metatarsal head. As the cuneiform metatarsal base has a stable configuration, stress is transferred distally to the metatarsal head. The disease is more commonly seen in patients having shorter first metatarsal, with more transfer of weight and stress on the comparatively long second metatarsal head. Lesser metatarsal excess load transfer can also occur in conditions such as gastrocnemius contracture, an unstable first ray, and relatively long lesser metatarsals.

CLINICAL FEATURES

- Diffuse pain, generally along the plantar and dorsal aspect of second metatarsal. Symptoms also may be present for transfer metatarsalgia—pain in multiple lesser metatarsals due to longer metatarsal lengths or gastrocnemius contracture. The causes for transfer metatarsalgia should also be thoroughly evaluated hence.
- Periarticular edema and pain during range of motion of second metatarsophalangeal (MTP) joint. The range of motion gradually becomes limited, with progressive articular collapse and osteophyte formation. Absolute dorsiflexion varies and movements need to be compared to the contralateral foot. Palpation of dorsal osteophyte of second metatarsal is quite highly suggestive of Freiberg's infraction.

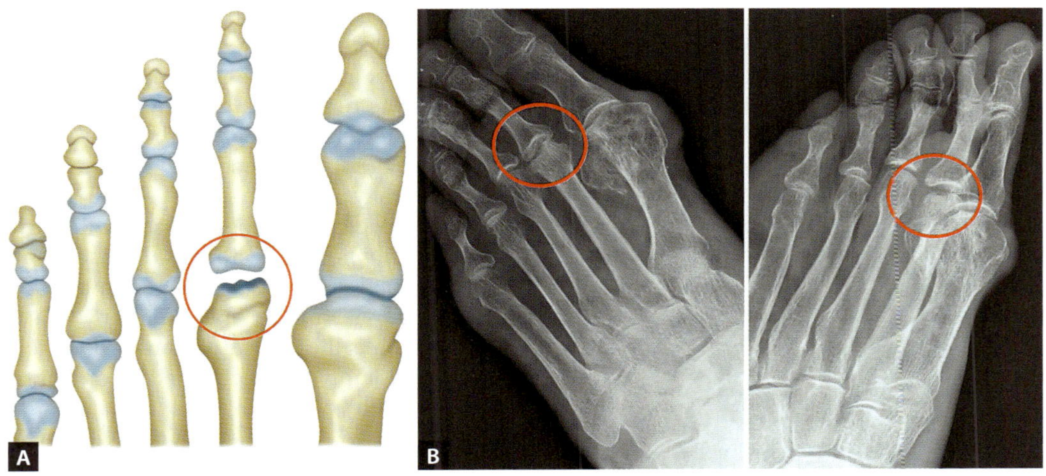

Figs. 1A and B: Freiberg's disease. (A) The head of second metatarsal undergoes osteonecrosis (encircled); (B) Radiographs depicting the healed Freiberg's disease with osseous deformity in anteroposterior (AP) and oblique projections (encircled).

INVESTIGATIONS

Radiography: The radiological changes with progressive pathology are as follows:
- Initially, metatarsal head may show hyperemic response, it may have osteoporotic appearance. There may be sclerotic epiphysis with initial widening followed by narrowing of joint space.
- With progression of the disease, there is flattening of metatarsal head and appearance of loose bodies in the joint.
  - There may also be flattening of the base of the proximal phalanx.
  - In a classic radiographic picture, there is fragmentation of epiphysis followed by osteolysis and reconstitution of bony architecture.
  - If the patient is misdiagnosed in these initial progresses, arthritic changes develop subsequently with formation of a dorsal or dorsotibial osteophyte.

Bone scan: Demonstrate photopenia due to reduced uptake initially followed by increased uptake in late stages when the metatarsal head is reconstituted.

Magnetic resonance imaging (MRI): Better depicts the full extent of the lesion **(Fig. 2)**.

DIFFERENTIAL DIAGNOSIS

- Osteomyelitis (particularly tubercular)
- Stress fracture
- Osteosarcoma
- Inflammatory arthritis
- Degenerative arthritis

STAGING BY SMILLIE

- *Stage I:* The earliest sign is subtle fracture line through the epiphysis, visible only on MRI and usually missed on plain X-rays.

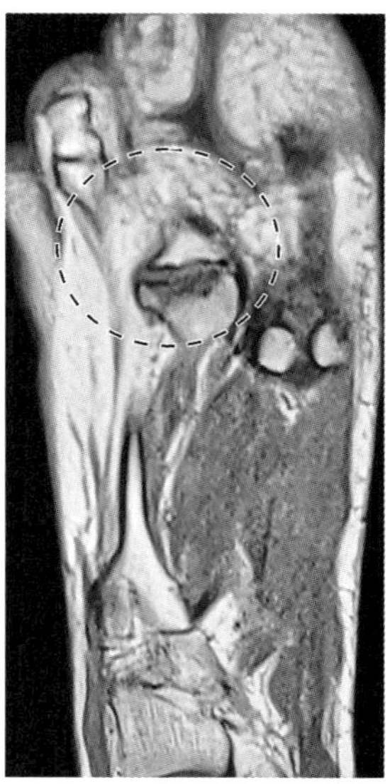

Fig. 2: MRI of Freiberg's disease reveals the involvement of bone better. It also demonstrates presence of synovitis or other associated soft-tissue abnormalities.

- *Stage II:* Central depression of the articular surface from resorption of subchondral cancellous bone.
- *Stage III:* Further collapse of the head with residual medial and lateral projections at the margins but the plantar hinge remains intact.
- *Stage IV:* The central portion of the head becomes free from intact plantar hinge and becomes a loose body, along with fractures of the medial and lateral projections.
- *Stage V:* Shows arthritic changes along with deformity and flattening of the metatarsal head, and joint space obliteration. At this stage, there may be resorption of the central loose body.

TREATMENT

The treatment plan depends on the severity of the disease and duration of the disease. Conservative measures may be helpful for stages I, II, and III disease which may occasionally resolve spontaneously. Surgical treatment is necessary in stages IV and V disease and when conservative measures fail.

Conservative Treatment

If patient presents with severe acute pain, nonweight-bearing cast and immobilization for 4–6 weeks are advised. If the pain is present since a long time, modifications in shoe-like metatarsal bar or pad-placed beneath the involved bone may help. Immobilization is necessary for 4–6 weeks to allow healing process to proceed. If the symptoms are severe, immobilizing foot in short leg walking cast or hard sole are the other options. Adjuvant therapies such as nonsteroidal anti-inflammatory drugs (NSAIDs), cortisone injections, ultrasound, and physical therapy may help.

Surgical Treatment

Several surgical options have been advocated aimed to diminishing pain and restoring joint function. They are described below:
- *Simple debridement:* Described by Freiberg, if there is limited damage with presence of loose bodies, removal of the loose bodies by simple debridement is performed. This can be metatarsal head resection, but it has disadvantage of increasing load on neighboring metatarsal heads.
- *Bone grafting procedure of Smillie:* This is done in an attempt to restore joint congruity. Drilling of metatarsal head is first done, the depressed articular surface is elevated and cancellous bone graft is inserted. Intact cartilage flap is necessary for this procedure, which is generally present in stages I, II, and III disease. If cartilage is damaged, it can be replaced with cartilage allograft.
- *Osteotomies:* In Freiberg's disease, generally the dorsal articular surface is damaged and plantar surface may remain healthy. So, the osteotomy procedures are aimed to redirect the healthy plantar cartilage toward more dorsal side. Mainly it is performed by one of the following two procedures:
  1. *Dorsal closing wedge osteotomy* ***(Fig. 3)****:* Modified Weil's osteotomy (dorsal closing wedge osteotomy) is performed by rotating plantar cartilage dorsally

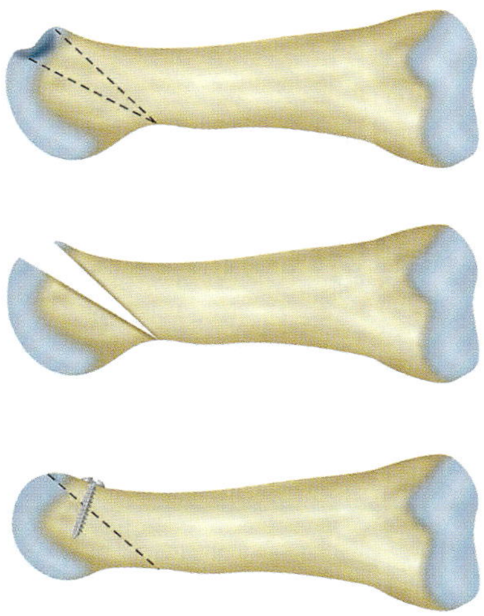

Fig. 3: Dorsal closing wedge osteotomy for Freiberg's disease.

by dorsal based "V" osteotomy. This is done in conjunction with thorough debridement of synovitis, abnormal cartilage, osteophytes, and necrotic bone. Some surgeons have suggested additional joint distraction with miniexternal fixator for 6–8 weeks to allow cartilage to heal itself and prevent joint contracture to form. The utility of joint distraction is not fully established.

2. *Shortening extra-articular osteotomies:* Based on the observation that the second metatarsal usually is the longest of the metatarsals in Freiberg's disease, it is assumed to bear excess loads. With shortening overloading of the metatarsal is believed to get reduced, and thus giving relief.

- *Resection arthroplasty:* Not favored now. The metatarsal head or base of the proximal phalanx is resected with or without soft tissue interposition. After resection of metatarsal head, it becomes short and may become incompetent causing joint instability, transfer lesions may develop and progressive hallux valgus may complicate the process.
- *Total small joint arthroplasty:* Usually performed utilizing silicone prosthesis, and is preferred over resection arthroplasty. The metallic/ceramic or carbon implants are now favored over silicone prosthesis that has become obsolete. As it replaces articular surface without resection of metatarsal head, it is more advantageous than the resection arthroplasty. Some of the proposed advantages are:
  - Avoidance of shortening and subsequent increased stress to adjacent metatarsals
  - Preserved or increased joint motion
  - If condyles are not resected, better weight distribution

Complications include the following surgical treatment:

- Synovitis
- Infection
- Dislocation

Other Uncommon Miscellaneous Procedures

- *Core decompression:* For early stage lesions by multiple drilling of metatarsal head with K-wire (0.45 inch) has been suggested by some on principles similar to core decompression of femoral head.
- *Osteochondral plug transplantation:* Done for late stage lesions. The osteochondral plug is harvested from a nonweight-bearing site of the upper lateral femoral condyle of the ipsilateral knee.

Surgical Algorithm

Helal and Gibb algorithm is logical and comprehensive that is favored at dedicated institutions:

- For early-stage disease, collapsed articular surface is elevated and bone grafting is done.
- For advanced lesions, i.e., stages III to V treatment depend on the patient's symptoms.
  - If patient has only pressure metatarsalgia, an osteotomy is performed.
  - With advanced lesions having arthritic joint and pain while joint motion, replacement arthroplasty is performed.

CONCLUSION

- Freiberg's disease is the osteochondrosis of the second metatarsal heads, third and fourth metatarsals are also uncommonly involved.
- Once diagnosed, the treatment is guided by symptomatology. Early cases respond to conservative measures while late cases and those that fail on conservative management may be managed by osteotomy or bone grafting to control symptoms.
- In general, the treatment of Freiberg's disease requires dedicated doctor–patient relationship. The patient should be informed that it is a progressive disease and more than one procedure may require in the future. First conservative treatment should be tried in early disease, failure of which may require less invasive surgical processes first followed by more invasive joint altering procedures for only advanced or resistant cases.

CHAPTER 93

Morton's Metatarsalgia (Morton's Toe, Interdigital Neuroma)

Manish Kumar Varshney

INTRODUCTION

This was first described by Durlacher in 1845 as interdigital plantar neuralgia and detailed by Morton in 1876 to bear his eponym with the condition. He treated the painful condition of the fourth metatarsophalangeal (MTP) joint with resection of the joint and additional removal of soft tissue surrounding the joint including digital branches of the third and fourth webspace nerves. He described removing the swollen portion of the tissue wrongly interpreting as a neuroma. The disease refers to sharply defined tenderness between the metatarsal heads resulting most probably from entrapment neuropathy of common digital nerve and its irritation (wrongly termed a "neuroma") beneath the transverse intermetatarsal ligament. Women are more commonly affected than men (8:1), and the condition is usually unilateral.

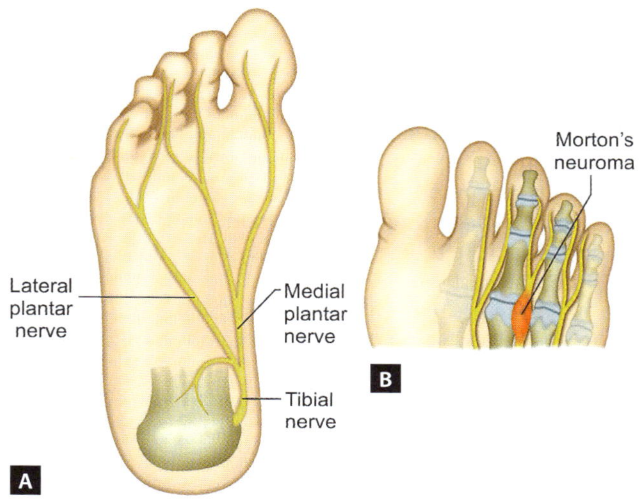

Figs. 1A and B: Morton's metatarsalgia. (A) The third webspace receives nerve supply from both medial and lateral plantar nerves; (B) The thickening arises in this interspace most commonly.

PATHOGENESIS

The nerve supply to plantar aspect of the foot comes from the medial plantar nerve (MPN). The MPN divides into the first, second, and third digital nerves and the lateral plantar nerve (LPN). The LPN then provides the common digital nerve to the fourth interspace and a proper digital branch to the lateral side of the fifth toe. One study observed that the second and third intermetatarsal spaces are narrower than the first or fourth and theorized that this could be the reason for the more common entrapment of the nerves in these interspaces. Morton's metatarsalgia is the most common in the third interspace as due to dual supply to digital nerve from medial and LPNs that causes tethering and traction. After third interspace, second interspace is the second most common site of nerve entrapment. The following are some of the proposed theories of development of interdigital plantar neuralgia:

- Morton—the neuroma resulted from pinching of the common digital branch of the LPN to the fourth webspace between the mobile fourth and fifth metatarsal heads. The view is largely abandoned.
- Betts—puts reasoning on the anatomy of fourth digital branch of the MPN itself. The common digital nerve to the third web is thicker to communicating branch it receives from LPN **(Figs. 1A and B)**, so it is more likely to be compressed against the unyielding deep transverse intermetatarsal ligament dorsal to it. This is also not clinically supported.

Flattening of transverse metatarsal arch and instability of the fifth MTP joint—plantar displacement of the central metatarsal heads puts pressure on the adjacent digital nerve. This produces "pressure neuralgia" from pressure on the nerve during weight-bearing.

Direct compression by the intermetarsal ligament is the most possible mechanism. The area of pathology has been found always distal to the deep transverse metatarsal ligament supporting the pressure theory especially as may result during push-off phase. Fat pad atrophy with advancing age may additionally make the nerve more vulnerable. Other causes of interdigital plantar neuralgia include direct injuries to the interdigitial nerve such as stepping on sharp objects, and crushing or traction injuries. Repetitive activities and walking on hard surfaces with uncushioned shoes might also result in interdigital neuralgia by provoking perineural ischemia.

In runners, dancers, or athletes, high forefoot forces result in overuse injury of the interdigital nerve. Quite unusual but another mechanism relates to modern footwear that allows excessive dorsiflexion of the MTP joint, causing forced plantarflexion of the metatarsals and hence injury to the interdigital nerves. Space occupying lesions like metatarsophalangeal synovitis, ganglion cyst, and trauma leading to hematoma and swelling in the region may also cause the pain syndrome. A communicating branch between the third and fourth common digital nerves is present in up to 28% of feet and an injury to one of these communicating branches could result in pain, which might be responsible for recurrent pain after neuroma resection.

PATHOANATOMY

The findings observed on histopathology of the excised specimens show sclerohyalinosis consisting of perineural fibrosis, increased number of intrafascicular arterioles with thickened and hyalinized walls. There is demyelinization and non-Wallerian degeneration of nerve fibers with a decrease in the number of axis cylinders and increased elastic trauma. Interestingly, there are no inflammatory changes. These findings differ from neuroma where a haphazard proliferation of axons is seen. The deposition of hyaline and collagenous material accounts for the enlargement in Morton's metatarsalgia. The perineural fibrosis, ischemia from vasa nervorum occlusion, and endoneural edema are possibly the reason for development of the symptoms of interdigital neuroma. Hence, it should be better called interdigital neuritis.

CLINICAL FEATURES

The patient presents with pain in the region of the metatarsal heads, usually the third and fourth **(Fig. 2)**. This is associated with paresthesias (burning and cold sensations) and sometimes aching or cramping. Symptoms are perceived more with activity and wearing tight shoe. Some patients may also feel a lump or mass while rolling up their socks. Tenderness is commonly located in the third webspace which is a useful sign for pain originating from neuroma, especially if there is no pain on the plantar aspect of proximal phalanx or dorsally near the MTP capsule. Sometimes, the neural thickening is felt popping back and forth on compressing the metatarsals.

- On compressing the metatarsal heads, the patient's symptoms of pain are reproduced with paresthesia and click of slipping of neuroma into the sole of foot that can be felt with examiner's thumb placed at the site (Mulder's sign, **Fig. 3**). Repeat, while simultaneously pressing in a coordinated fashion from the sole toward the dorsal surface and back with the other hand. This painful click is associated with a mobile neuroma.
- Sometimes the patient complains of paresthesia in the toes and sensory impairment.

INVESTIGATIONS

The diagnosis is clinical and radiology is of limited help if any. MRI and ultrasonography have not been found to be of much help as are the neurodiagnostic studies. Ultrasonography is quite inaccurate for lesions <5 mm and for larger lesions the modality is highly user dependent. It reveals an ovoid, hypoechoic mass in the intermetatarsal space proximal to metatarsal head but the sensitivity and specificity are both low. MRI has been used to settle the issue (higher sensitivity) but a negative scan does not rule out the disease (high false negative). For confirming the diagnosis, small amount of local anesthetic can be injected and the positive findings should be repeated that should have subsided.

TREATMENT

Initially, a supportive trial consisting of a variable combination of metatarsal bars or pads, local injection of a steroid preparation into the affected webspace, and wide toe box shoes should be tried that often relieves symptoms albeit temporarily. Most patients develop symptom with other

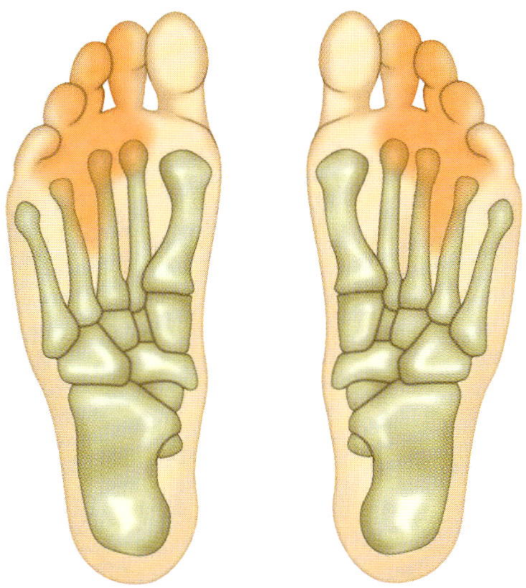

Fig. 2: The distribution of pain in foot in Morton's neuroma.

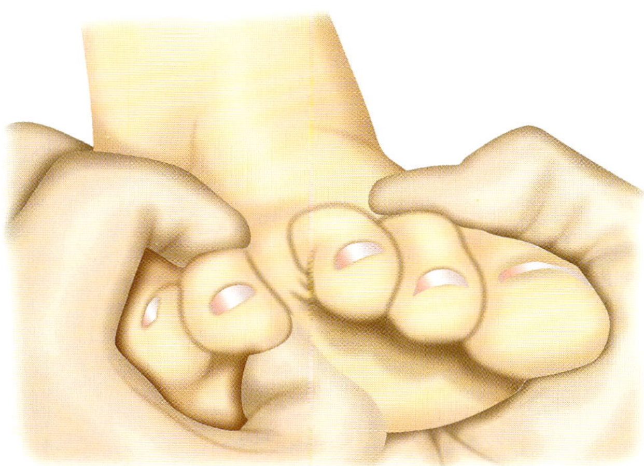

Fig. 3: Mulder's test.

casual or formal footwear. Surgery is, hence, indicated in many for reasonable and durable relief.

Excision of the interdigital neural thickening (neuroma) gives, as far as possible, a long lasting relief to the patients. There are, however, many conflicting reports that indicate unpredictable results and persistence of symptoms. Though excision of the neuroma can be done through both dorsal and plantar approach in a fresh case, the latter is better for a recurrent interdigital neuroma for better localizastion to the stump of origin. Scission of the transverse metatarsal ligament is often combined to prevent recurrence. Keratosis is a concern with the plantar approach, while dorsal approach is associated with excision of artery rather than nerve and a bit higher incidence of postexcision neuralgia. This may be related to the fact that nerve is very plantar and easily identified by plantar approach. Better technique for excision improving the success rate and lesser wound complication make it more popular for excision in a primary case. Endoscopic approach for resection of transverse metatarsal ligament is gaining popularity and is quite safe also. Postexcision neuralgia may result from bulb neuralgia formation at the end of excised nerve and may be prevented by burying the nerve in surrounding tissue or laying it in a vein conduit.

COMPLICATIONS

- Dorsal approach—incomplete excision or missed nerve, keloid formation
- Plantar approach—keratosis and scar pain
- Injury to other digital nerves and surrounding anesthesia
- Infection
- Wound gaping and dehiscence
- Recurrent neuroma—the surgery for recurrent neuroma and symptoms is highly unpredictable and is often associated with unsatisfactory results.

CONCLUSION

- It is the entrapment neuropathy of common digital nerve of the foot seen commonly in females.
- The symptoms of entrapment neuropathy are all present such as pain, aching, cramps, and paresthesia.
- Diagnosis is commonly evident on clinical examination with typical findings of pain on compressing the metatarsals together and positive Mudler's test.
- In most patients, a conservative trial is instituted to reduce irritation of the common digital nerves, failing of which needs surgical excision.

SECTION

10 Regional Orthopedics: Spine

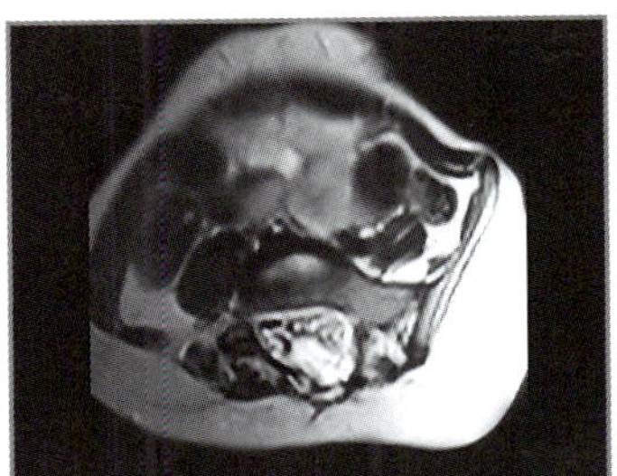

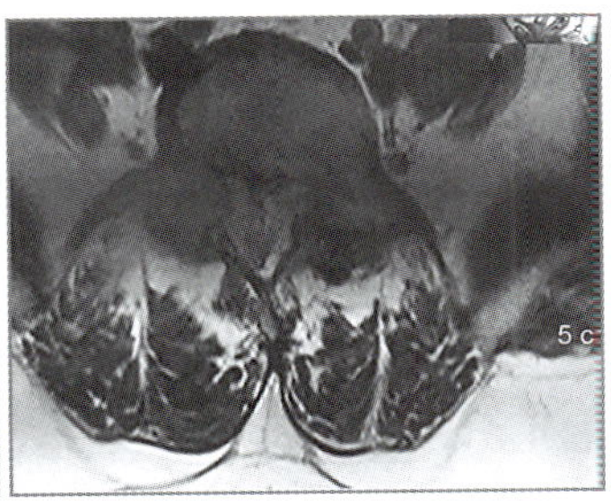

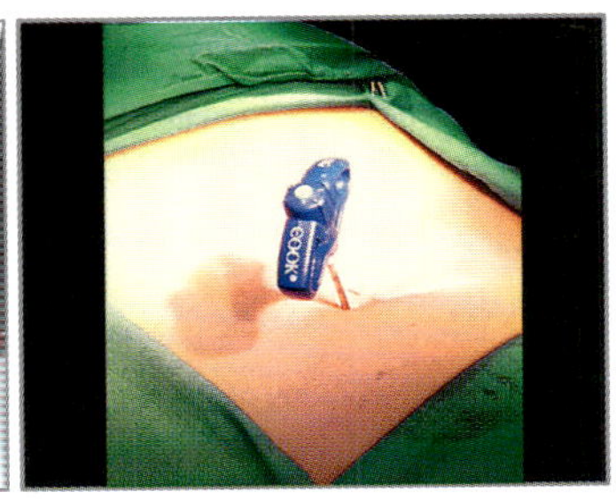

CHAPTER 94

Anatomy of the Spine and Spinal Cord

Manish Kumar Varshney

INTRODUCTION

Spinal column represents a complex mix of osseous and nonosseous structures. The latter provides the dynamic stability to the curvilinear arrangement of vertebral column. To understand the degenerative disorders, approaches to the spinal column and injury mechanisms a thorough understanding of the anatomy is necessary. The chapter basically reviews the concept of spinal anatomy keeping the relevance to a spinal orthopedic surgeon in mind instead of providing theoretical details.

VERTEBRAL COLUMN

The vertebral column (backbone or the spine) is a wavy pillar composed of approximately 33 small bones (that fuse to form 26 bones in adult) called vertebrae **(Fig. 1)**. The vertebral column runs from the cranium to the tip of coccyx on the posterior aspect of the trunk. It serves the following purpose:

- *Houses and protects spinal cord:* Shielding it from damage while providing safe exit for spinal nerves.
- *Support and weight transmission:* It transmits the weight of the body to the lower limbs through pelvis.
- *Axial disposition:* The vertebral column forms the central axis of the body around which the organs are dispositioned.
- *Provides attachment of the muscles:* Muscles of back, head, upper extremity, and thorax.
- *Movement:* It has roles in both posture and movement.

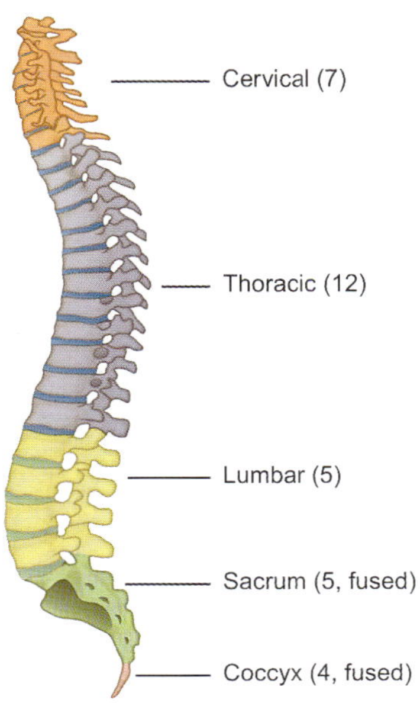

Fig. 1: The vertebral column.

The vertebral anatomy differs from region to region. A typical vertebra contains following elements **(Fig. 2)**:

- *Body:* Anterior solid part that transmits weight.
- *Vertebral arch:* This is the part of vertebra posterior to vertebral body and it surrounds the vertebral canal and contained spinal cord. It comprises of:
  - *Pedicles:* Project from body
  - *Laminae:* Unite to form arch posteriorly
  - *Transverse and spinous processes:* Projections from arch for muscle, ligament attachments
  - Articular process

Embryologically, each vertebra is formed from caudal portion of one sclerotome and rostral portion of the lower adjacent sclerotome while the space between them converts

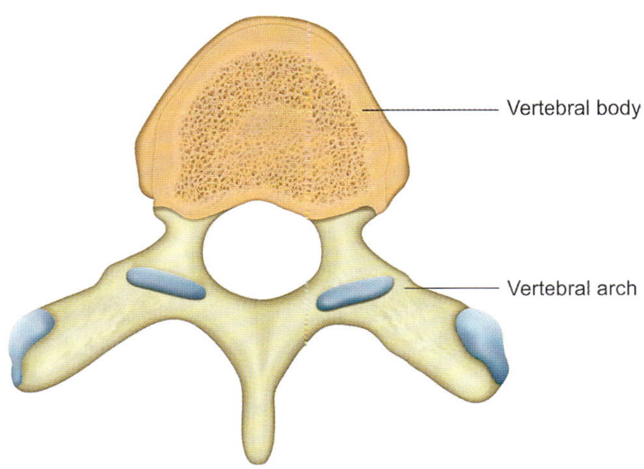

Fig. 2: The parts of a typical vertebra.

into intervertebral disk. Additional features according to the region involved are mentioned below:

Cervical vertebra (Fig. 3)—body is small with a large triangular spinal canal. Foramen transversarium in transverse process (C1–C7) for vertebral arteries and veins (C7 transmits only vein and not artery). The spinous process is bifid (divided) for ligamentum nuchae (except for C7 vertebra). The articular facets are angled superiorly and medially but are oriented in a more horizontal direction facilitating greater freedom in flexion, extension, axial rotation, and lateral bending. The pedicles are directed from dorsolateral to ventromedial direction obliquely. The occipito-cervical and atlantoaxial articulations provide the 50% movements to cervical spine. Atlas supports the weight of cranium over its two saddle-shaped superior articular processes and is a ring-like vertebra lacking anterior vertebral body. The second cervical vertebra (axis) articulates at the atlantoaxial articulations and atlantodens articulations. The latter is present between the superiorly projecting odontoid process from axis anteriorly and atlas ring. It is heavily stabilized by ligaments. The subaxial cervical spine (C3–C7) comprises vertebrae that more closely resemble the general vertebral body structure. Superior endplate of the vertebral body is concave and it curves upward laterally into uncinate process that articulates with the vertebral body above forming uncovertebral joints (joints of Luschka). Hypertrophy of the posterior part of uncinate process may compress the passing nerve root causing radiculopathy.

Thoracic vertebra (Figs. 4A and B): Their body is heart-shaped; larger than cervical vertebrae (bodies of vertebrae increase in size in rostral-caudal sequence). Costal facets for ribs on vertebral body (demi-facets) and transverse process are prominent. The demi-facet (because it is a partial articulation) for same level rib head is present on the superolateral aspect of vertebral body. 1st, 11th, and 12th vertebral bodies have single articulation. The transverse process ventrally articulates with the rib (of same number) at costotransverse joint. The transverse process projects superolaterally to reach rib. T11 and T12 vertebrae have no costotransverse articulation. Spinous process is slanted inferiorly and posteriorly. The vertebral foramen (spinal canal) is circular and smallest in this region (not much space for cord manipulation). The pedicles arise more superiorly than in cervical vertebra and project more obliquely. T1 and T2 pedicles have generous cross-sectional area but project more medially, while the medial projection and diameter reduces till T6 vertebra. The cross-sectional diameter starts increasing again thereafter. The superior articular facets originate from junction of lamina and pedicle articulating with the inferior articular facets that are essentially contiguous with ventral aspect of the lamina. The orientation of facets permits minimal movements.

Lumbar vertebra (Figs. 5A and B): Largest vertebrae with heavy kidney-shaped bodies with stout pedicles, the lamina are thick with broad spinous process. Pedicles project more horizontally than thoracic vertebrae and medial orientation increases from L1 to L5 significantly. The pedicles arise from superior aspect of vertebral bodies. The articular processes are in sagittal plane where superior facet faces dorsomedially. This orientation allows flexion/extension movement but restricts axial rotation and translation. The vertebral foramen is triangular-shaped and capacious.

Sacrum and coccyx (Figs. 6A and B): The sacrum is a large-expanded bone formed from the fusion of five vertebral bodies that transfer weight from spine to iliac wings. The upper three-fused vertebrae take part in formation of sacro-iliac joint. Sacral ala represents fused anterior costal and

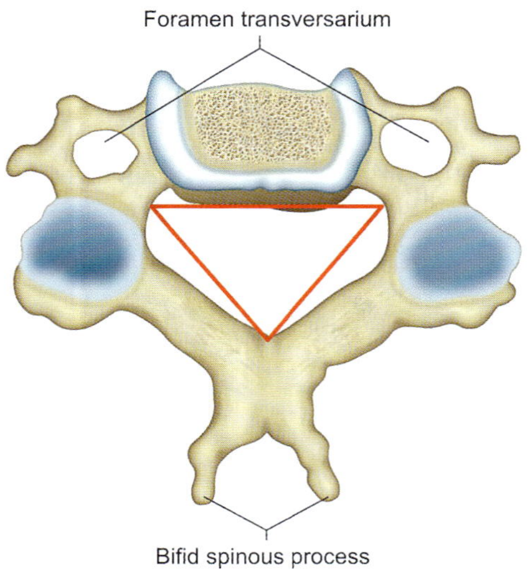

Fig. 3: A typical cervical vertebra (C3–C6).

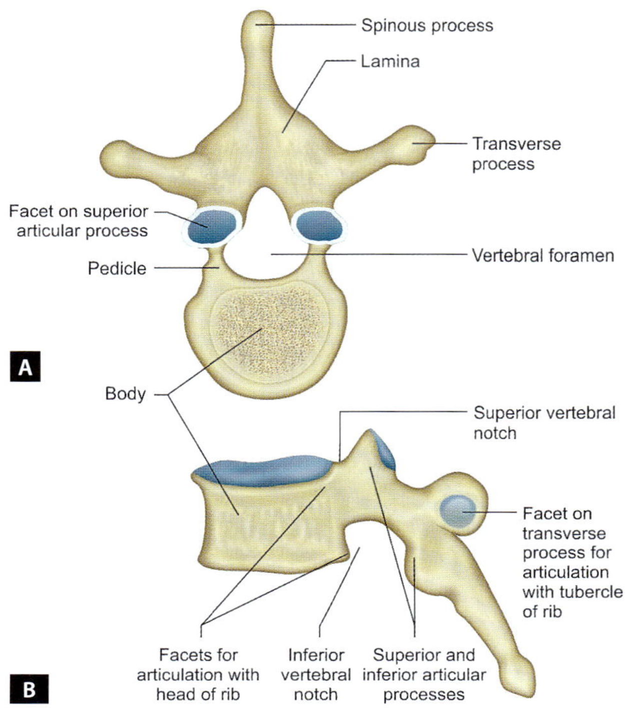

Figs. 4A and B: A typical thoracic vertebra. (A) Axial view; (B) Lateral view.

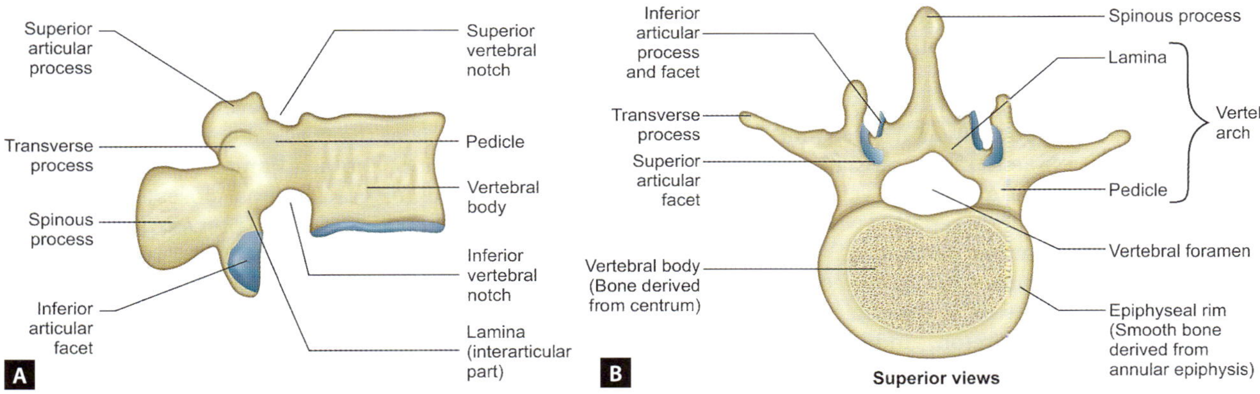

Figs. 5A and B: A typical lumbar vertebra. (A) Lateral view; (B) Superior view.

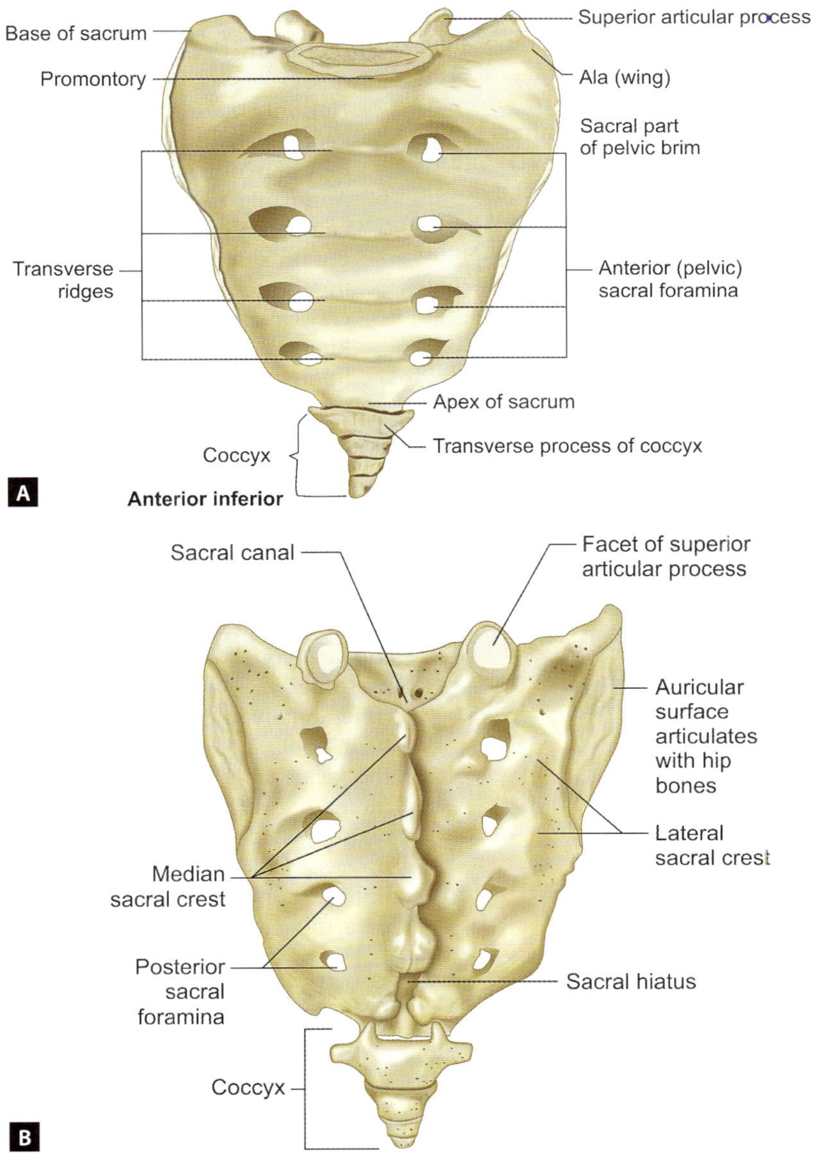

Figs. 6A and B: The anterior (A) and posterior (B) views of the bony sacrum and coccyx along with their prominent features (see text for details).

posterior transverse processes. The fused spinous process forms middle sacral crest, on both sides of it, is medial sacral crest or articular crest (formed from fused articular processes) that runs just medial to dorsal foramina. The medial crest projects superiorly as a facet that articulates with fifth lumbar vertebrae to resist translation. The coccyx is formed from four or five rudimentary vertebrae where the first coccygeal segment is often separate with the remaining fused to serve attachment for pelvic muscles and gluteus maximus. They do not have any dorsal elements.

In between there are atypical vertebrae (atlas, axis, C7, T11, and T12), their description, and characteristics are better referenced from dedicated anatomy texts.

CURVATURES OF VERTEBRAL COLUMN

In a newborn, the spine has a single dorsal-facing convex curve in the sagittal plane. This curvature straightens out in the first few years of life and by third year it is reversed to form the cervical and lumbar lordosis. The adult spinal curvatures are attained after the 10th year converting spine from a "C-shape" to an irregular S-shaped structure. The sagittal plane lordosis of cervical and lumbar regions and thoracic (and sacrococcygeal) kyphosis is determined by the differential morphology of intervertebral disk (IVD) and to a lesser extent the vertebral bodies in the ventral and dorsal aspects **(Fig. 7)**. The cervical spine is in 15° of lordosis while thoracic spine has a kyphosis of 20–40°. The lumbar spine has a sharper lordosis of 40–50°. Apart from these general values, the variability is large depending on posture, stature, and race of individual. The vertebral bodies and IVD are wedge-shaped having higher height on the ventral side in

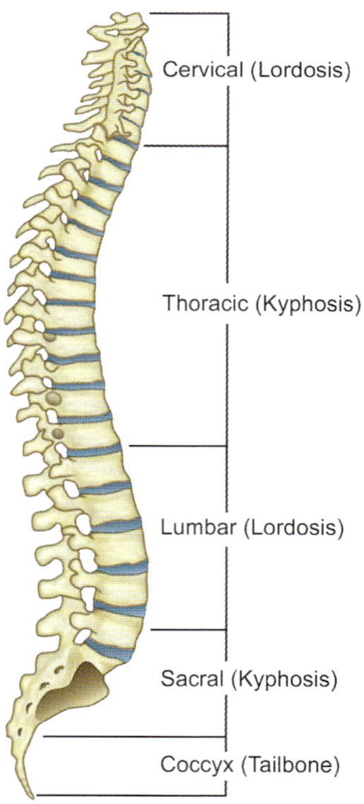

Fig. 7: Curvatures of vertebral column.

lordotic regions than on their dorsal aspect and vice versa in the thoracic region. The thoracic and sacral kyphosis are called "primary curves" because they are present since birth while the lordotic curves develop "secondarily" later in life. The lordosis of the cervical and lumbar spine helps to bear the weight of the head and the torso. Despite the curves, the center of gravity runs close to the vertebral column running from the odontoid process proximally to the sacral promontory caudally. The presence of a curved spine instead of straight spine was explained by Kapandji (1974), who proposed that higher number of curves improves the load-bearing capacity. He gave formula:

$$R = N^2 + 1$$

Where, R is load-bearing capacity, and N is number of curves. So, it indicates that the load/weight-bearing capacity is directly related to square of number of curves. But, this has been shown to be incorrect as a straighter column is always more stable under compressive loads than a curved column.

The curvature in vertebral column has additional functional advantages:

- Not only the individual vertebrae move with respect to each other, but also the segmental division of movement between individual curves also occur.
- Abnormal movements in the lumbopelvic region get compensated by equivalent, but opposite movements in the proximal regions. Also, for most normal movements the segments have summative movements, i.e., for deemed cervical spine movement some movement will also occur at lumbosacral and thoracic spine. If not for the compensation in movements a small range of caudal movement would need a significantly greater range of cervical movement.
- S-shaped curvature of spine can absorb great amount of energy because of its resistance to deformation and multiplanar movements.

Functional Spine Unit

The motion segment of spine consists of "functional spine unit" comprising two vertebrae, the disk between them and the facet joints. The functional spine unit limits the motion of spine while protecting the contained neural elements differentially in different portions of spine. Vertebral bodies bear 70–90% of the axial load, the rest being taken up by the facet joints. Postural changes alter load on facet joints increasing with extension to 30% while in flexion they may be subjected to 50% of anterior shear load. The spinous processes and transverse processes act as lever arms providing mechanical advantage for the muscles to counter the deforming forces on spine.

VERTEBRAL JOINTS

The vertebrae are connected to each other by following articulations **(Fig. 8)**:

- Intervertebral disk (discussed below)
- Intervertebral joint (zygapophyseal, facet joints)—synovial joints at facets with the articulating surfaces covered with hyaline cartilage.

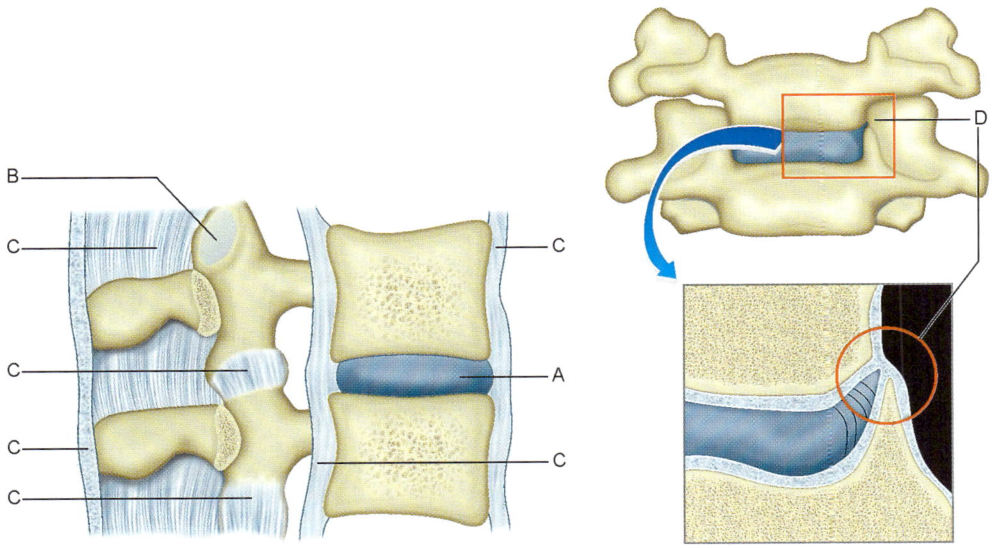

Fig. 8: The joints between vertebrae: A–intervertebral disk; B–facet joints; C–ligaments; D–uncovertebral joint in cervical spine.

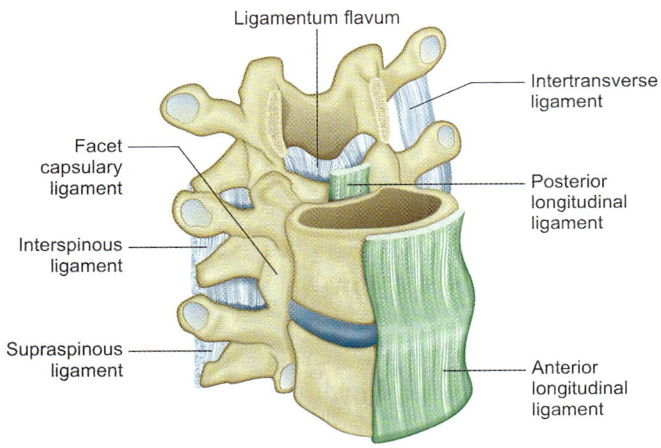

Fig. 9: Various ligaments joining the vertebral bodies.

- Ligaments and the joint capsule **[Figs. 8(C) and 9]**—These are the intertransverse ligaments, interspinous ligaments, anterior longitudinal (ALL), posterior longitudinal (PLL) ligaments, and ligamentum flavum (thickens caudally—it is also highly elastic its length increases by 40% during flexion). ALL runs along ventral aspect of vertebral bodies and at the most cranial end it forms anterior atlanto-occipital membrane. It prevents hyperextension of spine. PLL lies within spinal canal beginning cranially as tectorial membrane, moving down covering the dorsal aspect of vertebral bodies and intervertebral disks intermingling with their fibers. It limits hyperflexion of spine. The interspinous ligaments are present between spinous processes and are separate for every level. The supraspinous ligaments run as a continuous structure from sacrum to C6–C7 level, joining the spinous processes at the tips. It becomes ligamentum nuchae cranially. The ligamentum flavum originates at the leading upper edge of lamina of the lower vertebra both ventrally and dorsally and runs upward to insert along the ventral surface of the lamina above it. The insertion point is half-way up the ventral surface of lamina. There are two ligamenta flava (right and left) at each level that meet in midline but do not fuse and can be separated to lift it up from dura during surgical exposure.
- Uncovertebral cervical joint (Luschka's joints)—seen in cervical vertebrae where the bony ridges articulate with each other and provide lateral stability. It is at these joints where decompensation caused by excessive strain will show up in radiographs (uncarthrosis).
- Intrinsic lower back musculature.
- *Craniocervical junction* ***(Figs. 10A and B):*** This is a complicated arrangement so it is discussed separately. It provides stability to the most mobile portion of spine. The apical ligament runs from tip of dens to the basion. The alar ligaments run horizontally to the anteromedial aspect of occipital condyles laterally from the dens. The cruciate ligament has both a transverse and craniocaudal component. The transverse ligament spans from the lateral masses of C1 supporting and restricting dens to subluxate posteriorly. The vertical component of cruciate ligament runs in midline from transverse ligament cranially to the basion and caudally to the C2 vertebral body. The posterior atlanto-occipital membrane runs from opisthion (posterior foramen magnum) to the posterior arch of C1. It has a gap laterally for vertebral arteries.

THE INTERVERTEBRAL DISK

The total number of disks in humans is 23:6 cervical, 12 thoracic, and 5 lumbar. The structure of the disk is referred to as that of "jelly-filled candy" having three components:

1. ***The nucleus pulposus:*** This represents the remnant of notochord constituting the central portion of disk. It is made up of chorda reticulum (mixture of bladder-shaped notochord cells and notochord strands). This extensively

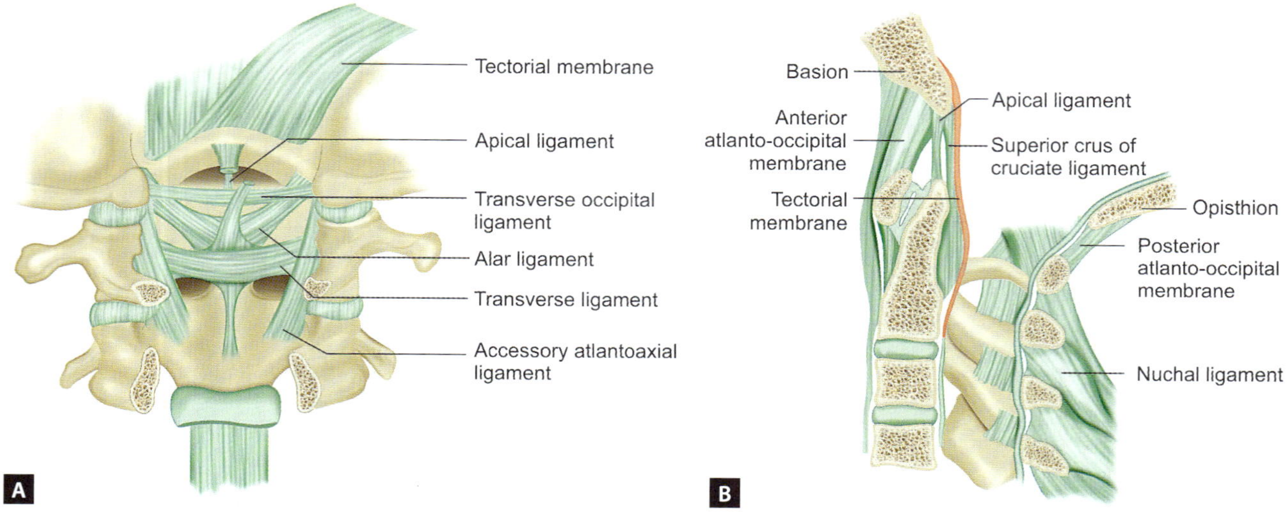

Figs. 10A and B: The craniocervical junction as viewed in coronal (A) and sagittal (B) planes. The disposition of various ligaments and their attachments are illustrated.

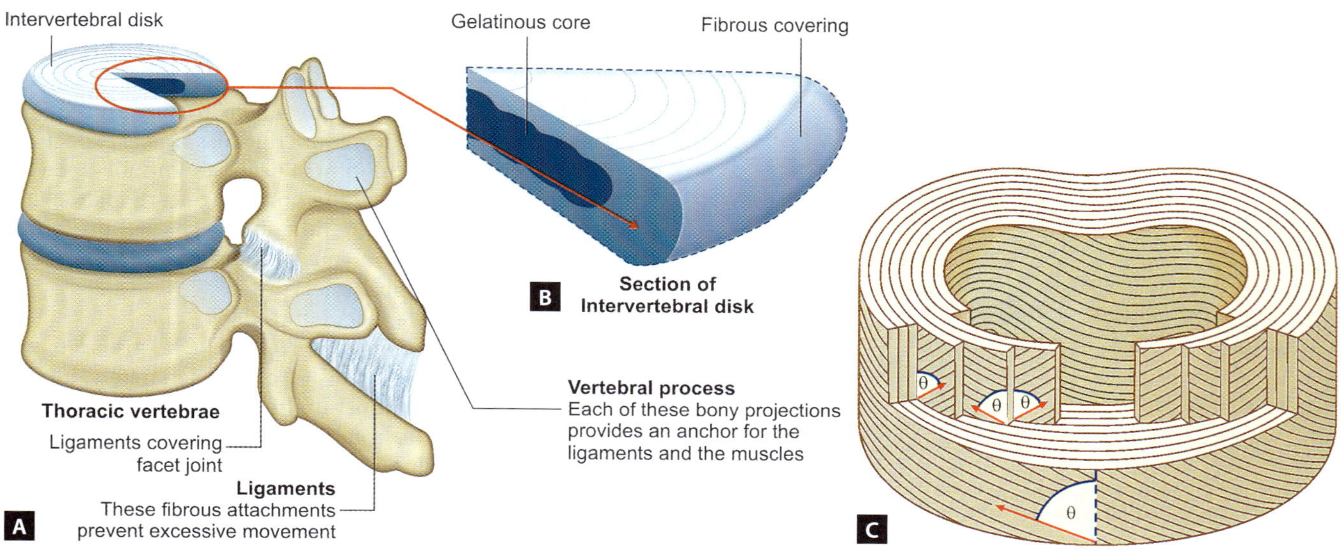

Figs. 11A to C: The intervertebral disk. (A) The disks are situated between the vertebral bodies; (B) Laminated annulus surrounds the nucleus pulposus like a "jelly-filled candy"; (C) The laminations have collagen layers oriented at an angle to each other in each successive layer (θ = 30°) that confers flexibility and increased strength to the disk.

branched hollow mesh is filled with synovial fluid initially and later replaced by Gallert tissue (jelly-like substance produced by connective tissues, **Figs. 11A to C**). With aging this Gallert tissue becomes less homogeneous and loses its elasticity. The nucleus pulposus bears 75% of the weight transmitted across. This is the only uninnervated structure in the disk. The cervical and lumbar regions have well-developed nucleus pulposus. It has 88% water and acts like a shock absorber during various movements of the spine. With age, this water content decreases.

2. ***The annulus fibrosus:*** The annulus is primarily composed of interwoven fibers that are likened to thread on a screw. The annulus has a thin outer collagenous layer while a thick inner fibrocartilaginous layer. The Sharpey's fibers (outermost boundary of the annulus) radiate outward anchoring to the bony outer wall of vertebral body. The concentric lamellae of collagenous fibers lie obliquely from one vertebra to other; allowing rotational movement. The collagen bundles crisscross to form a cross woven structure which ensures that in any direction of movement the fibers are always tight. These fibers are strongest at the ventral and lateral aspect and weakest dorsally. This imparts flexibility and also stability to the disk and is similar to arrangement of collagen in "shark skin" imparting the needed flexibility to it. The outer annulus bears 25% of the weight.

3. ***The vertebral endplates (cartilaginous endplates):*** These form the upper and lower margins of the disk and form principle junction between the disk and vertebral body, so on one side they are connected to vertebral bodies and the peripheral part (circumferentially) is fused to the vertebral ring apophysis. They are made of hyaline cartilage. The vertebral endplate has a terminal layer of calcium toward the vertebral side that has pores that forms a transition zone connecting with the vertebral body side lamina cribrosa (sieve-like surface toward bone). The pores and sieve allow diffusion of metabolic substances across (**Figs. 12A and B**).

Molecular Composition of the Intervertebral Disk

The three major constituents of the disk are water, fibrillar collagens, and aggrecan **(Fig. 13)**. The annulus has 50–70% water content and collagen forms 40–50% of weight of annulus. The nucleus has 70–85% water. The aggrecan in nucleus pulposus contains highly sulfated glycosaminoglycan (GAG) chains which are highly negatively charged conferring the same to matrix. This negative charge attracts various positively charged solutes (cations, like sodium) increasing their concentration in the tissue through the Gibbs-Donnan equilibrium. This develops a high concentration (three times) than negatively charged chloride ions which are maintained by the local GAG concentration (small and large balloons, discussed below). High solute concentration attracts water to maintain equilibrium and the osmotic pressure, thus resulting in adequate swelling pressure inside the disk nucleus. The nucleus has the highest concentration of aggrecan that is hydrated by the above mechanism and relatively low collagen content than seen in other regions. The nucleus due to limited space available to accommodate collagen contains only type II collagen in contrast to annulus that contains both types I and type II collagen. With aging the amount of aggrecan and hence also the water in the nucleus reduces, while the concentration of collagen rises. Similar changes are seen in degenerated disks (remember, however, that

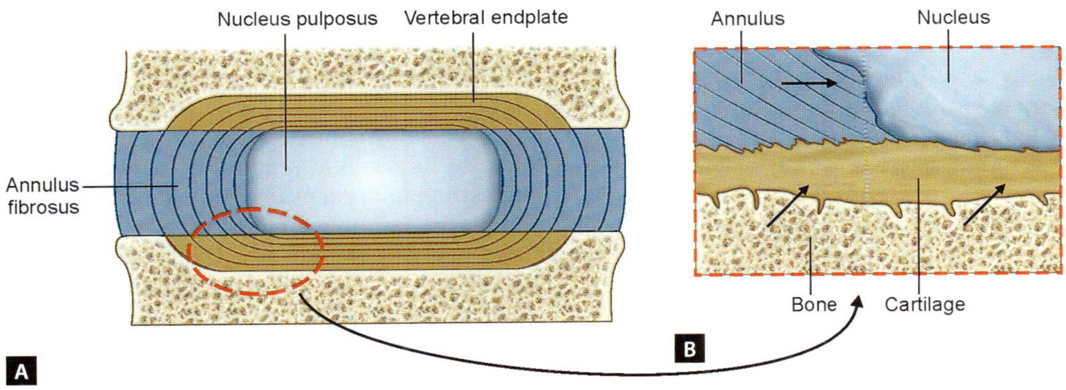

Figs. 12A and B: (A) Vertebral endplates. The hyaline cartilage is bonded to the perforated cortical bone of the vertebral body and collagen fibers of the annulus and the nucleus; (B) Arrows indicate routes for nutrient transport from blood vessels into the central portion of the disk.

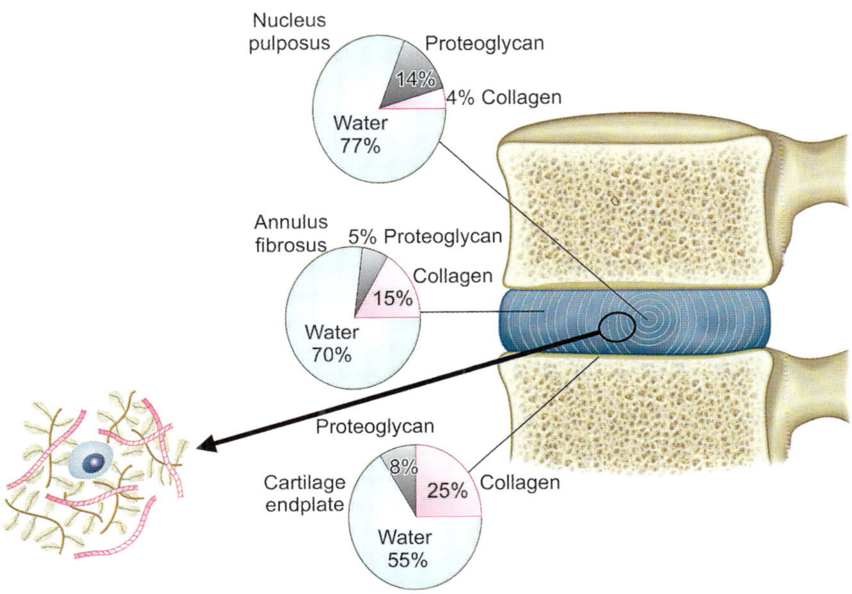

Fig. 13: The differential composition of the disk in different regions. Aggrecan in the nucleus pulposus retains water by virtue of highly negatively charged branches (inset).

degeneration is not equivalent to aging). The primary change is overall reduction of aggrecan gradually rather than an increase in the amount of collagen which is actually secondary to reduced aggrecan. In specific locations around the cells few minor collagens such as type IX, VI, and III are found that possibly have a functional role. Small leucine-rich proteoglycans (SLRPs), such as decorin, biglycan, lumican, and fibromodulin also exist in the nucleus in minor percentages that serve to repair the matrix and in homeostasis by aiding fibril formation and preventing mineralization along collagen fibers. The disk also contains proteases (collagenase, gelatinase, and stromelysin) that cleave molecules, such as collagen and aggrecan at specific sites. To understand the progression of disk degenerative disease and for research purpose of understanding disk turnover (gathering information on natural history of disease) antibodies against these “neoepitopes” serve as markers.

Functions of Intervertebral Disk

- Physiological—separation of vertebral bodies
- Providing a strong and flexible structure for movements between vertebrae
- Responsible for 25% of spinal column height
- Shock absorber for axial loads and water bed effect for flexion and twisting movements
- Counter the compressive loads from weight of body and muscle contraction
- It anchors vertebral bodies to each other.

CHANGES IN THE INTERVERTEBRAL DISK WITH AGE (FIGS. 14A AND B)

- Due to reduced proteoglycans the nucleus becomes more rigid and less hydrated or resilient and more collagenous.
- There is decrease in absolute number of viable cells.
- Discoloration of nucleus pulposus to yellow-brown instead of white.
- Loss of distinction in the boundary between nucleus and annulus—there is thickening of annular rings that also becomes more disorganized.
- Annulus tears at multiple places.
- There is increase in keratin sulfate to chondroitin sulfate ratio and lactate content.
- Increasing concentration in type X collagen in the matrix of elderly patients, the same effect is also seen in scoliotic disks. This may be related to abnormal calcification in these stressed disks or calcification of degenerated disks.
- At about 9 years of age in the cervical spine a process known as pseudo-degeneration occurs in which there is tearing of fibers in the outer annulus which is complete in the middle. This tearing of the cervical annular fibers causes the disk to split into two parts: (1) caudal and (2) cranial. This possibly accounts for higher rotational capability of cervical disks. Normally with rotation, one component of the fibers becomes taut and restricts further rotation for stability due to oblique angulated arrangement of fibers, which over time gets torn forming brush border surfaces (only in posterior part and anterior annulus remains intact).

The loss in disk height produces various secondary changes **(Figs. 15A and B)** in the nearby structures (facet joints, ligaments, etc.).

BIOMECHANICS OF INTERVERTEBRAL DISK

The IVD demonstrates creep which allows for deformity over time and hysteresis which allows for energy absorption with repetitive axial compression. The compressive resistance and shock absorber function can be explained by the balloon on string model.

The **“balloons on string”** model—cartilaginous tissues form the string network filled with balloons (aggrecan filled by water, drawn into the tissue by the high swelling pressure due to its osmotic properties). The inflated balloons put the string under tension while the string hold the balloons in place. Both the components need to act in conjunction and neither component is individually capable of bearing loads. If left alone, the string would break and the balloons would fly apart. When the conjugate is well-established they successfully bear tensile and compressive loads together. It is obvious that a network containing a few small and few large balloons of which the smaller ones are floppy, will deform more than one stuffed full of highly inflated ones, so the aggrecan molecules are of different molecular weights and charge density **(Figs. 13 and 16)**. Pressure in the disk depends more on muscular activity than on body weight solely. The intradiskal pressure, hence, varies with body posture and activity. The disk pressure is lowest when lying prone (at around 0.1–0.2 MPa) that increases five to eight times when person stands or sits. The equilibrium is here reached by ingress and egress of water from the nucleus primarily. Throughout the day nearly 20–25% of the disk’s water is expressed out under compressive loads transmitted through body weight and muscular activity; this water is regained under rest at night increasing the height in morning

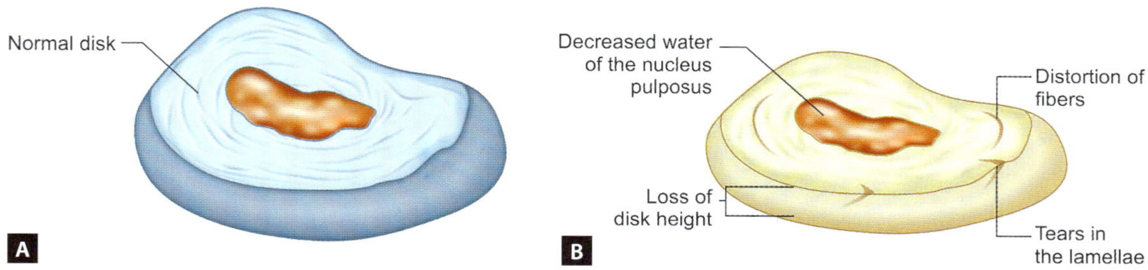

Figs. 14A and B: The changes in intervertebral disk (IVD) with aging. (A) Normal disk; (B) Aged disk.

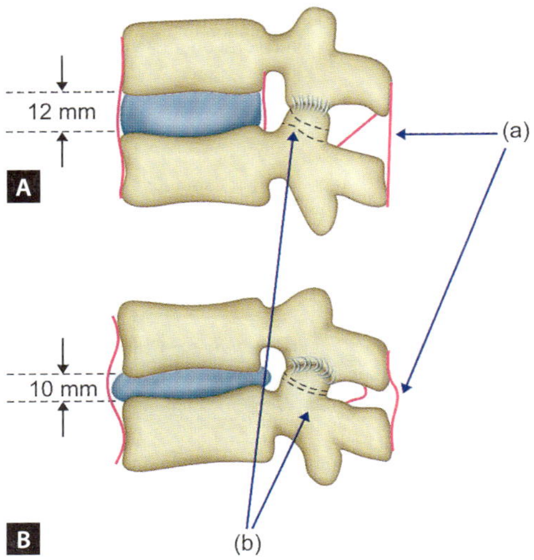

Figs. 15A and B: The effect of loss in height with load on other spinal structures. The degenerate disk bulges due to weakened annulus and nonresilient nucleus. The loss in height results in (A) buckling of ligaments and (B) loss of apophyseal joint space and secondary degeneration.

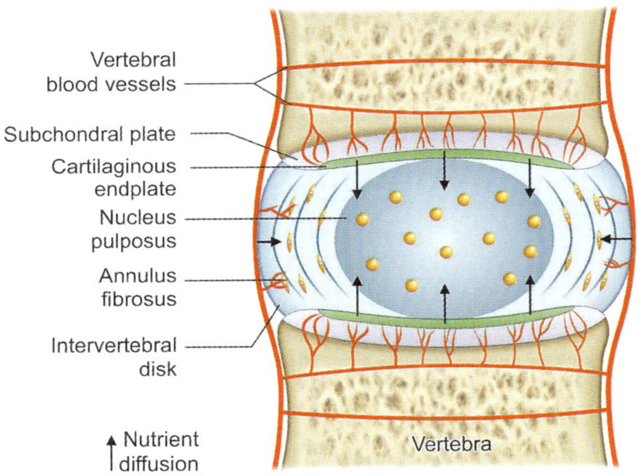

Fig. 16: The water is carried in the nucleus pulposus and retained due to the aggrecan molecules. The disk has limited vascularity and hence the water diffusion in the nucleus pulposus is restricted. The egress of water is also similarly restricted. Most substance diffuses into nucleus pulposus through the vertebral endplates only, and is a slow process. These are responsible for creep and elastic behavior of the disk.

by 1–2.5 cm. This alteration in height, however, puts stress on the adjoining joints.

BLOOD SUPPLY AND INNERVATION OF INTERVERTEBRAL DISK

Disk is avascular and is the biggest such avascular structure in humans. Its capillaries terminate at the level of endplates so that in an adult the cells at the center in the lumbar disk are about 8 mm from the blood supply. Nutrition reaches nucleus pulposus by diffusion through pores in the endplates that in turn reaches them via a complicated route originating from the vertebral body blood vessels to form a separate capillary network. Diffusion of nutrients from these capillaries across the cartilaginous endplate supplies the cells located within the matrix and is really a slow process. The outer annulus has some penetration of capillaries but gets most of its nutrients from soft-tissue blood vessels at its periphery.

The annulus and endplates are innervated with free nerve endings that act as pain receptors and reach the dorsal root ganglion through sinuvertebral nerve. The action potential generated here continues to the axon of the small C-fibers or A-delta fibers and goes into the dorsal horn of spinal cord. After synapse there the second neuron ascends into the spinal cord through the spinothalamic tract which reaches the thalamus and second synapse occurs there. The third neuron reaches the somatosensory cortex.

BLOOD SUPPLY OF SPINE (FIGS. 17A AND B)

Arterial Circulation

The arterial blood supply to the vertebral segment (bony vertebrae, intervertebral joints, and nearby area) varies according to the region (cervical, thoracic, lumbar, etc.). Throughout the entire spine there is copious intercommunication between the intervertebral joints, arterial network of dorsal rami at similar networks above and below, and contralateral plexus. The lumbar and posterior intercostal arteries which are the segmental arteries in the lumbar and thoracic region give rise to the articular branches. There are 62 segmental arteries as 31 paired structures branches arising from:

- Aorta
- Subclavian
- Vertebral
- Internal iliac arteries

The lumbosacral region of spine is supplied by a branch originating in the iliolumbar arteries; sacral vertebrae have additional contribution from lateral sacral and middle sacral artery. In the cervical spine arterial supply is derived from branches of the vertebral artery and the cervical ascending pharyngeal artery. The vertebral arteries enter the sixth cervical vertebra and run proximally to C1 where they exit and course posteriorly over C1 ring before turning proximally again and enter foramen magnum to unite and form basilar artery. Typically, one side is more dominant and has larger caliber. There are significant variations to above anatomy and need to be well evaluated before instrumentation. The lower cervical spine additionally receives contribution from the deep cervical artery and the supreme intercostal artery. The transitional area of cervicothoracic region receives blood supply from the inferior thyroid artery. The arterial branches to intervertebral joint also supply adjacent periosteum of the vertebral body and hence the surrounding attached muscles also.

Venous Circulation

As described by Batson (1957) and Clemens (1961) two dense venous plexuses are found adjacent to the spinal column:

1. *Posterior external vertebral venous plexus:* This plexus is formed near the vertebral arch and is close to the bases of the spinous process, transverse process, and posterior aspect of the intervertebral joints.
2. The second lies longitudinally inside the spinal canal and has connecting transverse veins. It is called the posterior

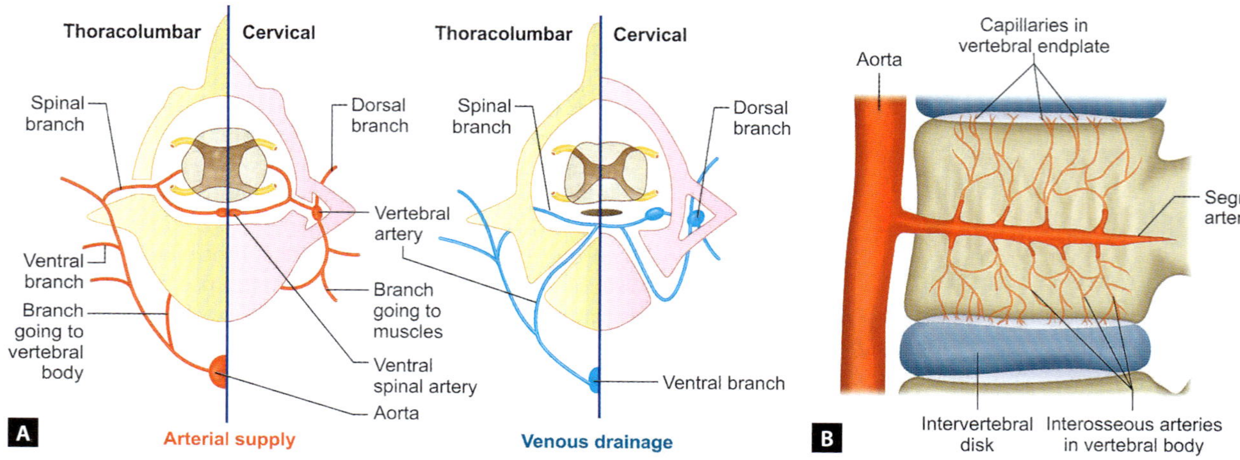

Figs. 17A and B: (A) Blood supply of spine; (B) The blood vessels branch from the segmental artery and enter the vertebral body and end as capillaries in the endplate.

internal vertebral venous plexus. Veins from bones of the vertebral arches and the articular processes flow into the adjacent plexus.

There are no valves in the vertebral plexus. Hence, the flow of blood varies as per the local pressure into either the dorsal or ventral plexus.

The vertebral venous system forms a chain of anastomoses which extends from the base of the skull to the sacrum. Spinal plexus veins are connected by small veins to the vertebral, intercostal, and lumbar veins as described by Putz (1981). The lumbar epidural veins respond to central venous pressure and their filling is dependent on it. Thus, posture [Ghazvinian and Kramer (1974)] plays an important role in blood flow in this venous system. A crawling position reduces pressure while coughing, sneezing, or pushing increases it and promotes retrograde flow. This mechanism would be responsible for metastasis to vertebral column from abdominal neoplasms and even from thoracic region.

SPINAL CORD

The spinal cord serves the most important anatomical and functional link between the whole body and the brain. It provides a vital link between the brain and the body carrying information from and to the systems. Individually, the spinal cord plays a major role in the reflex activity that is also under the control of neural pathways linking higher nervous centers. The spinal cord extends from the level of foramen magnum to the level of the intervertebral disk between first and second lumbar vertebra. The spinal cord is 40–50 cm long and 1–1.5 cm in diameter. By weight the spinal cord contributes only 2% of the central nervous system. All the three meninges namely the pia, arachnoid, and dura mater cover the spinal cord **(Fig. 18)**. It is attached to the dura mater by a series of lateral denticulate ligaments emanating from the pial folds.

The spinal cord is a continuous cylindrical structure lying within the vertebral column and has two enlargements:

1. The "cervical enlargement" extends between C3 and T1.
2. The "lumbar enlargement" extends between L1 and S2.

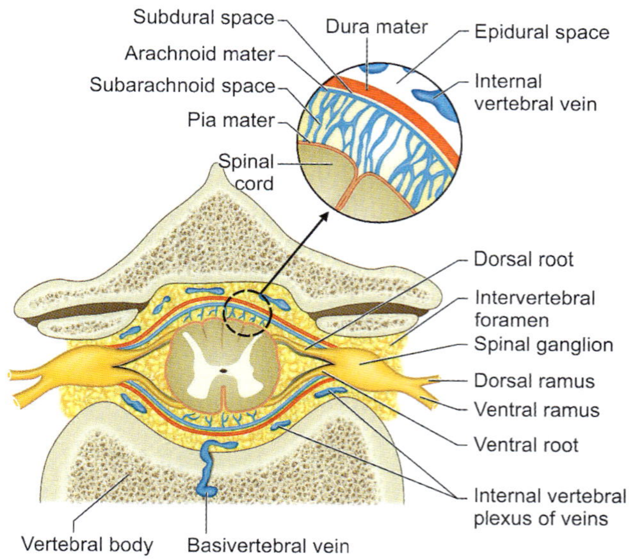

Fig. 18: The spinal cord contained in the three membranes.

Spinal Nerves

Spinal nerve is formed by joining of nerve roots that emerge as two consecutive rows on each side of the cord and then join distally. There are in all 31 pairs of spinal nerves **(Fig. 19)** in human body. Each spinal nerve, hence, contains motor (from ventral root) and sensory (from dorsal root) nerve fibers carried to and from all parts of the body respectively. As for regional distribution there are 8 cervical, 12 thoracic, 5 lumbar, 5 sacral, and 1 coccygeal spinal nerve. Intervertebral foramen at respective vertebral segments serves as passage for entrance or exit of the spinal nerve containing the dorsal and ventral roots. During the embryonic period the foramen corresponds to the respective spinal nerve, however, with differential growth of the cord and vertebral column over years, the lower parts of the spinal cord segments differ from the anatomical location of the vertebral segment. In anatomical terms, the part of the spine that gives rise to one spinal nerve is considered a spinal segment. It is defined by dorsal roots and ventral roots. Some spinal segments also contain autonomic fibers to and from smooth muscle, the cardiac muscle and/or exocrine or endocrine glands. In a nutshell, all spinal nerves, except the cervical, exit below their corresponding vertebrae **(Fig. 20)**. Spinal nerves from C1 to C7 exit above their corresponding vertebrae, whereas the eighth cervical nerve exits below the C7 vertebra. This particular spinal nerve leaves between the C7 vertebra and the first thoracic vertebra. Hence, each subsequent spinal nerve leaves below the corresponding vertebral level, but the location of the spinal segment in cord and the anatomic vertebral level do not correspond. In the upper thoracic (T1–T3), the difference between the vertebrae and cord level is one segment, while the difference between T4 and T6 is two segments which increase to three behind T7 and T8. The T12 spinal segment lies behind T8–T9 disk. Lumbar segments lie behind T9–T11 vertebrae and sacral segments lie behind T12–L1 or L2. At these levels, the roots of the segments have to travel longer to exit from the intervertebral foramen. At the level of the lumbar enlargement, they form a structure that looks like a horse's tail and hence called the "cauda equina".

Inside the intervertebral foramen dorsal (sensory) and ventral roots (motor) combine to form the *spinal nerve roots* **(Fig. 21)**, which is a mixed nerve root. The spinal nerve, thus, has fibers that are motor and supply a particular group of the muscles and sensory to skin region developing from one

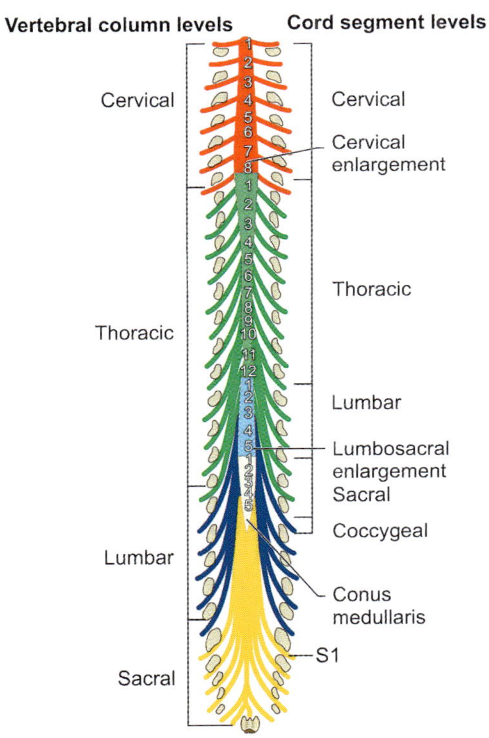

Fig. 19: The 31 pairs of spinal nerves.

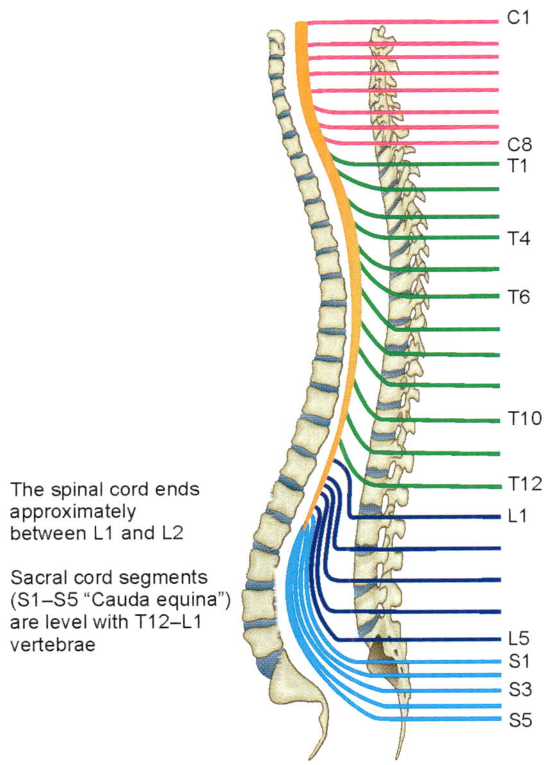

Fig. 20: The differential disposition of spinal segments to vertebral levels.

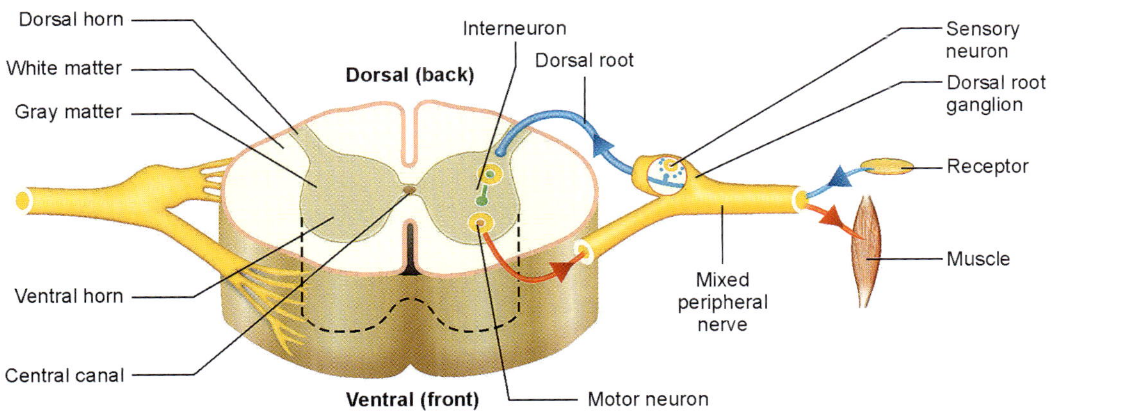

Fig. 21: The formation of spinal nerve. Ventral and dorsal roots combine to form the spinal that exits through intervertebral foramen.

body *somite* (segment). A *dermatome* represents an area of skin supplied by peripheral nerve fibers originating from a single dorsal root ganglion and can be mapped.

- *The dorsal root:* Sensory stimuli from the skin, voluntary muscle and joints are conveyed to the spinal cord by sensory cells located in the dorsal root ganglia. Sensory dorsal root ganglion cells give rise to the axons of dorsal root fibers. These axons serve as primary sensory afferents and the dorsal root neurons are the first order (1°) sensory neuron in the sensory pathway. The dorsal root fibers are divided into lateral and medial divisions. The lateral division terminates in the "Rexed laminae I, II, and IV of the gray matter (discussed below)", it carries pain and temperature sensation through unmyelinated and small myelinated axons. The medial division, on the contrary, comprises predominantly of myelinated axons that conduct sensory information through dorsal or posterior column and terminate finally in the ipsilateral nucleus gracilis or nucleus cuneatus in the medulla oblongata.
- *The ventral root:* This comprises the axons that arise from motor neurons in ventral horn of spinal cord. These are predominantly motor to voluntary (skeletal) muscle. Some fibers arise from the lateral horn in the region of thoracic, lumbar, and sacral enlargements to synapse on autonomic ganglia and then supply internal thoracic and abdominal visceral organs. Ventral root fibers arise as ventral rootlets from ventrolateral sulcus that join to form the ventral root and contain motor nerve axons to skeletal muscle and visceral motor neurons. The alpha (α) motor nerve axons innervate the extrafusal muscle fibers, while the small gamma (γ) motor neuron axons innervate the intrafusal muscle fibers. The visceral motor neuron sends preganglionic fibers to supply the visceral organs.

STRUCTURE OF THE SPINAL CORD

The adult spinal cord being an extension from the brain contains white matter and the gray matter. However, while the former is in periphery and the latter is inside (opposite to that of brain). There is a tiny central canal at its center. The canal is surrounded by a single layer of ependymal cells similar to the lining of ventricles of brain. The gray region containing cell bodies surrounds the ependymal layer which is shaped like the capital letter "H" or a "butterfly" **(Figs. 22A and B)**. The two vertical arms of the H-shaped gray matter are connected centrally across the midline by the dorsal gray commissure and below it is the white commissure. Because the nerve fibers keep exiting the tracts and fibers in descending tracts keep reducing, white matter keeps thinning till the end of cord so at the lower levels the ratio between gray matter and white matter is higher than in higher levels.

The gray matter containing the cell bodies of neurons and glia is visibly grossly divided into four main columns:

1. *The dorsal horn (sensory column):* This contains cell bodies of somatic and visceral sensory neurons.

2 and 3. The intermediate column and the lateral horn column comprise autonomic neurons innervating visceral and pelvic organs and the ganglia, so this is the thickest in the spinal cord enlargements.

4. The ventral horn—contains α and γ motor neurons that innervate extrafusal skeletal muscle.

Only for comprehensive mention, the nerve cells in the gray substance are multipolar and have been classified into Golgi type I and type II nerve cells according to microscopic appearance. Functionally, these can be grouped into root cells, column or tract cells, and propriospinal cells depending on their predominant characterization.

- The *root cells* present in ventral and lateral gray horns have no fixed size. These provide axons to form ventral root of the spinal nerves and are divided into two functional separations:
  1. Those supplying the skeletal musculature form the somatic efferent root neurons.
  2. Preganglionic autonomic axons supply various autonomic ganglia and form visceral efferent root neurons.

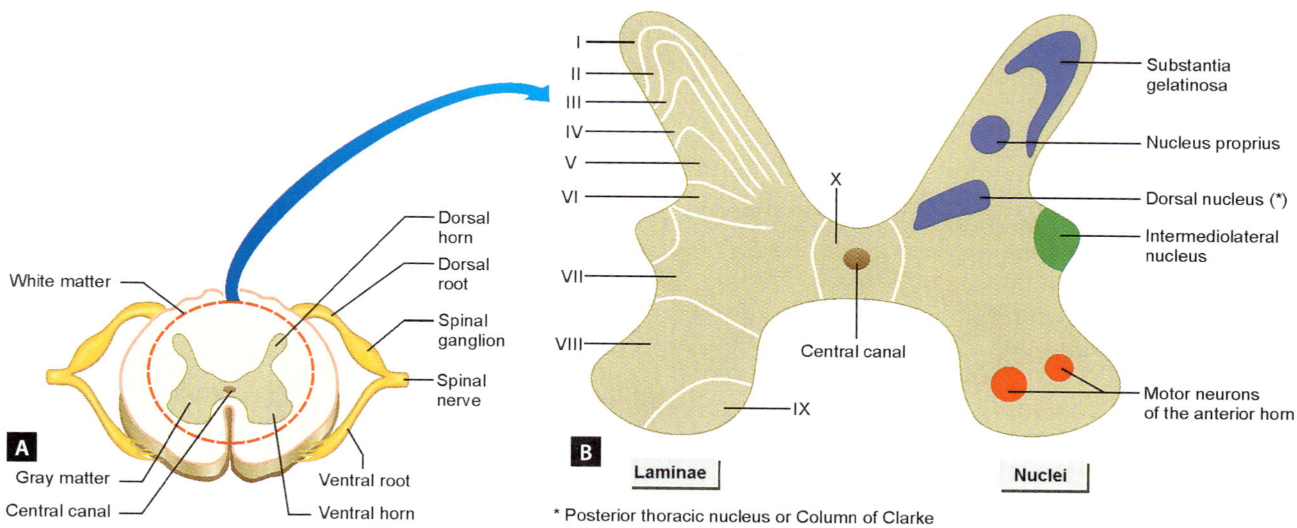

Figs. 22A and B: (A) The gray matter is distributed in a pattern of "H" or butterfly in the spinal cord; (B) The disposition of various nuclei and later described Rexed laminae.

- The dorsal gray horn contains the *column or tract cells* and their processes. Their axons form the ascending tracts that ascend in the white columns and terminate in the brainstem, cerebellum, or diencephalon.
- The *propriospinal cells* form nearly 90% of intraspinal neurons that do not leave spinal cord. Some of these fibers can be located around the margin of gray matter of the cord that aggregate to form the fasciculus proprius or the propriospinal tract (also called "archispinothalamic tract").

Spinal Neurons are Organized into Nuclei and Laminae

Nuclei (Figs. 22A and B)

Describing from dorsal to ventral aspect the prominent nuclear groups of cell columns that can be located within the spinal cord are:

- ***Marginal zone***—Appears as a cap over the tip of the dorsal horn. Its neurons partially form the lateral spinothalamic tract involved in relaying pain and temperature sensation.
- ***Substantia gelatinosa*** is present at the head of the dorsal horn and forms a cap-like structure. Anatomically, it is made up of intersegmental column cells which form synapse with cells in "Rexed layers IV–VII" and then form the anterior and lateral spinal thalamic tracts. Functionally, it is responsible for transmission of pain, temperature, and light touch.
- ***Nucleus proprius*** (also known as "chief sensory nucleus")—located below the substantia gelatinosa, it is associated with mechanical and temperature sensations. Its neurons contribute to the formation of the ventral and lateral spinothalamic tracts and also to ventral spinocerebellar tracts.
- ***Dorsal nucleus of Clarke*** (found only in segments C8–L3) is located in the dorsal horn and its fibers contribute to the formation of the dorsal (posterior) spinocerebellar tract (DSCT). This tract is involved in transmitting unconscious proprioception from muscle spindles and Golgi tendon organs to the cerebellum.
- ***The intermediolateral nucleus*** as the name implies is present in the area between dorsal and ventral horns of the H. At the C8–L3 levels, there is a sensory input to these nuclei from visceral organs. They also contain the preganglionic sympathetic neurons in the lateral horn which send preganglionic fibers via the ventral spinal roots and white rami to the sympathetic tract. At the S2–S4 level, these nuclei contain the preganglionic parasympathetic neurons.
- ***Lower motor neuron nuclei:*** They contain motor nuclei of α, β, and γ motor neurons (root cells) and are located in ventral horn of spinal cord. The α motor neurons as mentioned above innervate the involuntary and voluntary muscles.

Rexed Laminae (Figs. 22A and B)

It is interesting to note that the cells and fibers within the gray matter of the spinal cord are distributed in laminated pattern **(Figs. 22A and B)**. The cellular pattern (cytoarchitecture) of each lamina is distinctive that can be divided into 10 layers (laminae was proposed by Rexed). This classification into laminations is more accurately correlated to function than the previous classification scheme (based on major nuclear groups, discussed above). In short, the laminae I–IV are concerned with peripheral sensation and form part of dorsal horn, the laminae V and VI are primarily involved with proprioceptive sensations (dorsal column), whereas lamina VII can be considered equivalent to intermediolateral zone and functionally acts as a relay between muscle spindle to midbrain and cerebellum. The laminae VIII and IX are motor to skeletal muscles and are formed by ventral horn. Lamina X contains neuroglia and surrounds the central canal of the spinal cord.

- ***Rexed lamina I:*** This is similar to the marginal zone (nucleus posteromarginal). The layer is thin and forms cap at the tip of the dorsal horn. The cells in this lamina contain small dendrites and unmyelinated axons. As mentioned above, the primary function is transmission of pain and temperature and joins the contralateral spinothalamic tract.
- ***Rexed lamina II:*** These are tightly packed interneurons and correspond to the substantia gelatinosa. The cells here respond to noxious stimuli and majority of neurons receive information from sensory dorsal root ganglion cells and descending dorsolateral fasciculus fibers. It acts as a relay to send axons to "Rexed laminae III and IV (fasciculus proprius)". The lamina is rich in substance P and cells contain high concentration of opiate receptors. Due to the presence of these, it is considered that the main function of this lamina is pain modulation by altering the sensory input. This may act as a "mini-brain" to possibly differentiate which pattern of incoming information would produce "painful" sensation in higher nervous system.
- ***Rexed lamina III:*** This is more of a plexus of axons emanating from cell of variable size that divides several times to form a dense network. Cells within this layer function as propriospinal or interneuron cells for receiving axodendritic synapses from Aβ fibers entering dorsal root fibers. This layer contains dendrites of cells from laminae IV, V, and VI to which the axons of cells synapse.
- ***Rexed lamina IV:*** It is distinctively thicker than previously described laminae. The cells in this layer receive Aβ axons through lamina III and carry predominantly non-noxious inputs. These also respond to light touch via connections with dendrites of neurons in lamina IV. Nucleus proprius is located in this lamina.
- ***Rexed lamina V:*** Formed by neurons that have dendrites in lamina II. These neurons receive monosynaptic information from Aβ, Aδ, and C axons which also carry nociceptive information from visceral organs, possibly after modulation of sensory input from lamina II. These neurons ultimately project to the brainstem and the thalamus traveling in contralateral and ipsilateral spinothalamic tract and they are also modulated by descending corticospinal and rubrospinal fibers.

- ***Rexed lamina VI:*** This broad layer is best developed in the cervical and lumbar enlargements. It receives group Ia afferent axons from muscle spindles finally giving rise to ipsilateral spinocerebellar pathways.
- ***Rexed lamina VII:*** The region occupied by this lamina is called the "zona intermedia (or intermediolateral nucleus)". This lamina contains all the visceral motor neurons which innervate neurons in autonomic ganglia. The neurons in this lamina get input from Rexed laminae II–VI and visceral afferent fibers. An oval-cell column is formed from C8 to L3 by the dorsal nucleus of Clarke from which arise the uncrossed nerve fibers of the DSCT. Similar uncrossed fibers arise from the cells in laminae V–VII to form the ventral spinocerebellar tract. The preganglionic sympathetic fibers that innervate postganglionic cells in the sympathetic ganglia arise in the lateral horn of the cord in segments T1 and L3. The preganglionic sacral parasympathetic fibers that innervate postganglionic cells arise from the lateral horn neurons at level S2–S4.
- ***Rexed lamina VIII:*** This is the terminating area of the descending vestibulospinal and reticulospinal fibers. The function of the neurons of lamina VIII is to act as modulator of motor activity. They probably act through the γ motor neurons innervating the intrafusal muscle fibers.
- ***Rexed lamina IX:*** This lamina is made up of large α, and the smaller γ and β motor neurons which together form large groups. At the level of cord enlargement, there are higher number of α motor neurons. Extrafusal skeletal muscle fibers get supply from α motor neurons supply and the intrafusal muscle fibers get supply from the small γ motor neurons.
- ***Rexed lamina X:*** The neurons in this lamina are present commissural lateral area of the gray commissure and they surround the central canal. They also contain the decussating axons.

WHITE MATTER AND SPINAL CORD TRACTS (FIG. 23)

White matter surrounds the gray matter and contains myelinated and unmyelinated nerve fibers arranged in cords that transmit information upward (ascending) or downward (descending). These nerve fibers are arranged in the white matter in form of columns which are the dorsal (or posterior) column (or funiculus), lateral column, and ventral (or anterior) column. Crossing nerve fibers from the spinothalamic tracts, spinocerebellar tracts and anterior corticospinal tracts constitute the anterior white commissure. The nerve fibers in the spinal cord white matter are of the following types:

- *Long ascending nerve fibers:* These fibers arise from the column cell and connect to various brainstem nuclei, centers in cerebellum, and dorsal thalamus.
- *Long descending nerve fibers:* These fibers arise from cerebral cortex and various brainstem nuclei and synapse in various Rexed layers in the spinal cord gray matter.
- The fibers that interconnect various spinal cord levels and coordinate flexor reflexes are the short nerve fibers.
- All columns contain ascending tracts, but descending tracts are located only in the lateral and the anterior columns. The axon groups found in the white matter can be described as: funiculus, fasciculus, tract, and pathway.

The term "funiculus" denotes a conglomeration of large group of nerve fibers present in a given area (e.g., anterior or posterior funiculus).

- *Fasciculus:* This represents distinct groups of fibers within a funiculus having common features, but from different origins. They are arranged in smaller bundles (e.g., fasciculus proprius). This is primarily a morphological definition.
- Tract is a group of nerve fibers having similar origin, destination, and course along with similar function. They derive their names from their origin and their termination:

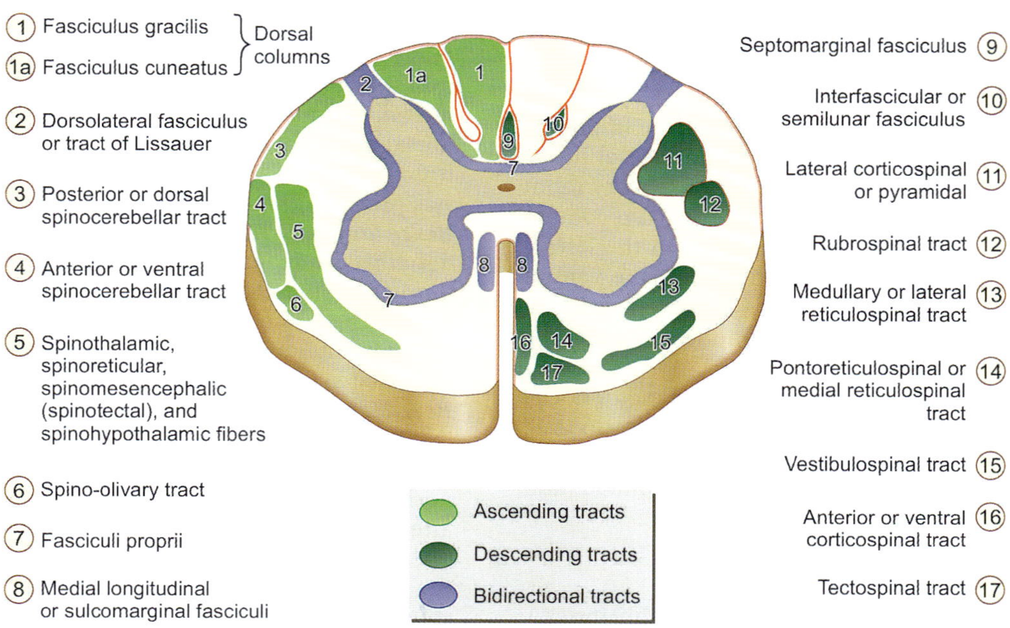

Fig. 23: The various tracts as disposed in white matter of spinal cord.

- *Corticospinal tract:* This descending tract originates in the cerebral cortex and ends in the spinal cord (Rexed laminae).
- *Lateral spinothalamic tract:* This ascending tract originates in the lateral part of spinal cord and terminates in the thalamus.

- The entire neuronal circuit including all nuclei and tracts that together carries out a specific function is called a pathway. The spinothalamic pathway, for example, has one function but originates in the dorsal root ganglia and synapses in the spinal cord via the dorsal roots. The second and third order neurons of this tract cross at white commissure and end in the thalamus.

Ascending Tracts (Fig. 23)

The primary function of ascending tracts is to transmit sensory information from sensory receptors located in skin, visceral organs, etc., to the central nervous system. The nerve fibers emerge from the first order neuron located in the dorsal root sensory ganglion.

- The dorsal funiculus is formed by ascending gracile and cuneate fasciculi. These tracts carry following informations:
  - Fine touch
  - Two-point discrimination
  - Vibration and position sense
  - Conscious proprioception and joint movement sensation
- Pain, temperature, and crude touch (somatic and visceral) are carried by the neospinothalamic tract (or lateral spinothalamic tract).
- The proprioception signals from muscles and joints of the lower limbs are carried to the cerebellum via dorsal and ventral spinocerebellar tracts.
- Signals for pain, temperature and touch are carried to the brainstem nuclei and to the diencephalon by the paleospinothalamic tract (or anterior spinothalamic tract).
- Signal from the Golgi tendon organs is carried to the cerebellum by the spino-olivary tract.
- The spinoreticular tract and the spinotectal tract
- Pain signals to the brainstem and diencephalon are carried by intersegmental nerve fibers which travel for several segments (2–4) and are located around the gray matter. These are known as fasciculus proprius, spinospinal, or archispinothalamic tracts.

Descending Tracts (Fig. 23)

These tracts arise from different areas of the cortex and brainstem nuclei. They carry signals for motor activities such as muscle tone, posture, balance, and visceral and somatic reflex activity. These include:

- The lateral corticospinal and rubrospinal tracts are located in the lateral column (funiculus)—these carry signals for voluntary movement.
- Mediation of balance and posture is function of the reticulospinal, vestibulospinal, and the anterior corticospinal tract.
- Regulation of incoming pain sensation at the spinal level is by Lissauer's tract carries the descending fibers of the dorsolateral funiculus.

BLOOD SUPPLY OF THE SPINAL CORD

The spinal cord receives its arterial supply from various sources that include:

- Vertebral artery
- Ascending cervical arteries
- Deep cervical artery
- Intercostal arteries
- Lumbar arterial system
- Lateral sacral arteries

Anatomically, these basically constitute three longitudinal arteries on the surface of spinal cord that supply specific geographical regions of the cord **(Figs. 24A to C)**:

1. Anterior two-thirds by an anterior spinal artery
2. Posterior one-third by a pair of posterior spinal arteries
3. The lateral columns are supplied by an anastomoses between the spinal arteries known as "arterial vasocorona".

The anterior and posterior spinal arteries are formed from vertebral arteries in the apical region (cervical) at or near the cervicooccipital junction and then they travel down longitudinally along the spinal cord **(Figs. 24A to C)**. These arteries are small in caliber may even be discontinuous along their path. The little blood flow and small caliber limits capacity of the anterior and posterior spinal arteries in sustaining the supply to the spinal cord on their own and hence in reality, independently they can supply only to the superior portion of the spinal cord (till cervical cord levels), it is only the reinforcement received from segmental medullary and radicular arteries that vascular supply is maintained till the most caudal aspect. The medullary segmental arteries receive contributions from the ascending cervical, deep cervical, posterior intercostal, lumbar, and sacral arteries (discussed above) that reach the primary anterior and posterior spinal arteries through the intervertebral foramen to augment and maintain flow throughout. This segmental reinforcement is especially provided at the cervical and lumbar enlargement. The anterior and posterior radicular arteries that travel along with the anterior and posterior nerve roots arise from the segmental spinal arteries when they enter the vertebral canal. The most important segmental artery is called the artery of Adamkiewicz (arteria medullaris magna, the great anterior segmental medullary artery), which arises directly from the aorta mostly in the lower thoracic or upper lumbar vertebral levels (anywhere between T8 and L1). This vessel reinforces circulation to lower two-thirds of the spinal cord and chiefly to the lumbosacral enlargement. The artery is mostly unilateral entering the spinal cord from left side. Any injury to this vessel can cause spinal cord infarction and paraplegia.

The anterior and posterior spinal arteries have numerous interconnecting vessels sort of forming a plexus on the surface of the spinal cord over its entire length to provide continuous and uninterrupted blood supply. This anastomotic connection is called the "arteria vasocorona" present on the surface of the cord. The segmental reinforcement of vascularity is also important in the sense that even if blood supply from

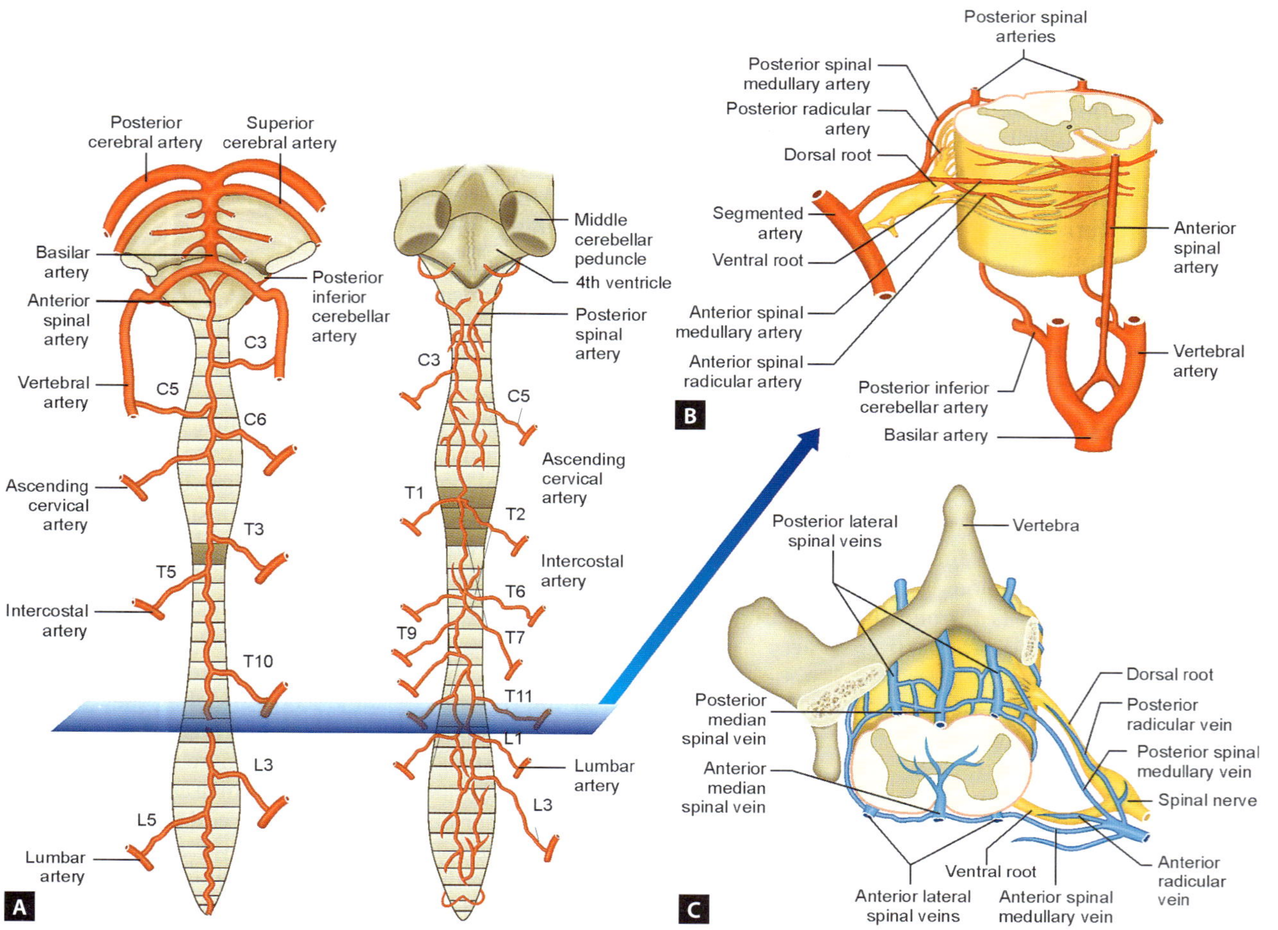

Figs. 24A to C: (A) The blood supply of spinal cord. The posterior spinal arteries are quite inconsistence and discontinuous at places; (B) The formation of segmental artery and radicular arteries; (C) Venous drainage is through six main channels that have extensive anastomosis.

the aorta gets interrupted say by surgery or trauma then collateral arterial flow from reinforcements through internal thoracic and lateral thoracic arteries that form a network with the posterior intercostal arteries will keep the cord surviving.

The dorsal and ventral roots of the spinal nerves along with their coverings are supplied by radicular arteries derived from spinal segmental arteries; there is distinct dorsal and ventral radicular artery for respective roots.

Venous Drainage

Venous drainage of spinal cord follows the arterial supply. Anatomically, disposed parallel to the arteries are the anterior and posterior spinal veins, and anterior and posterior radicular veins that form six tortuous longitudinal channels that freely connect to network within the internal vertebral plexus present in the epidural space **(Fig. 24C)**. The epidural plexus drains into the cerebral dural venous sinuses and cerebral veins as well as the external vertebral plexus. These veins are all valveless.

CONCLUSION

- The bony anatomy in various spinal regions is adapted to the discrete functions performed and specific requirements. This introduces significant anatomical variability that needs to be carefully acknowledged during surgical management.
- The ligamentous stability is particularly important at the craniocervical junction and is conferred by a mix of structures.
- Nucleus pulposus functions to maintain disk height and resist compressive loads providing adequate cushion between bony segments and flexibility to the column.
- Within the spinal cord, nerve fibers destined those for upper extremities are located deeper while those for thoracic and lumbar regions are sequentially located in periphery.
- Augmentation of vascular supply to spinal cord by artery of Adamkiewicz is important in supplying the lumbosacral segments and its damage may incur serious vascular damage and infarction.

CHAPTER 95

Low Back Pain, Intervertebral Disk Degeneration, Lumbar Spondylosis, and Degenerative Conditions of Cervical Spine

Manish Kumar Varshney

INTRODUCTION

This is the most common problem seen in orthopedic outpatient clinic and is the most common cause of activity limitation in adults younger than 45 years. Low back pain (LBP) could be acute or chronic. Acute attacks of back pain (pain duration is <3 months) are usually self-limited. Chronic LBP is defined as persistent or fluctuating pain that lasts longer than 3 months. There are many factors such as mechanical, genetic, chemical, social, nutritional, and psychological factors which can influence the onset of LBP. On the basis of clinical history and physical examination, LBP can be categorized into one of the following categories:

- Back pain associated with symptoms and signs of radiculopathy or spinal stenosis
- Back pain related to a nonspinal source
- Back pain associated with a specific spinal cause
- Back pain without a specific or definitive cause

Each of these has their differential diagnosis and etiology **(Table 1)**. One should evaluate further by special tests, investigations, imaging to identify the exact etiology of chronic LBP. The pathogenesis is still unclear and genetics, smoking, specific occupations and comorbidities such as coronary artery disease, psychiatric disorders, and body mass index have all been correlated with LBP. Contrary to the common notion of association of degenerative disk disease (DDD) with LBP, it has not been found to be the cause of LBP in significant number of cases. Thus, lot still needs to be defined and studied for LBP.

TABLE 1: The differential diagnosis of low back pain.

Nonspecific or idiopathic (70%)	***Mechanical (27%)***
Lumbar sprain or strain	• Degenerative of disks disease (DDD) process and facets • Internal disk disruption (IDD) or diskogenic pain • Herniated disk • Spinal stenosis • Spondylosis and spinal instability • Transitional vertebrae • Spinal deformity—kyphosis/scoliosis • Fracture—osteoporotic/traumatic
Nonmechanical (1%)	*Referred pain (2%)*
• *Neoplasia*: – Multiple myeloma – Metastatic carcinoma – Primary bone tumors – Spinal cord tumors – Retroperitoneal tumors • *Inflammatory:* – Seronegative spondyloarthropathy – Rheumatoid arthritis • *Infection:* – Osteomyelitis – Septic diskitis – Epidural abscess • *Miscellaneous:* – Scheuermann's disease (osteochondrosis) – Paget disease of bone – Arachnoiditis – Sickle cell disease	• *Visceral origin:* – Urinary system—kidney stones and pyelonephritis – Reproductive system (endometriosis, retroverted uterus, and ectopic pregnancy) – Gastrointestinal tract (duodenal ulcers, pancreatitis, and biliary colic) – Abdominal aortic aneurysm – Retroperitoneal tumors • *Musculoskeletal origin:* – Myofascial pain – Hip arthrosis – Sacroiliac joint pathology • *Miscellaneous causes:* – Psychogenic – Central pain syndromes

Source: Modified from Deyo RA and Weinstein JN.

INVESTIGATIONS

History gives a good idea of the pain origin by its characteristics. History and investigations are discussed together here as they are highly complementary and substantiation of LBP history needs assistance of investigations essentially. The further evaluation basically is designed to identify the pain generator (see below).

Laboratory assessment is as follows:

When red flag signs **(Table 2)** indicate the possibility of a presence of serious underlying condition, the following tests should be obtained:

- Erythrocyte sedimentation rate (ESR)
- Complete blood count
- C-reactive protein (CRP) level

Consider the possibility of multiple myeloma in elderly, prostrate screening is recommended for elderly males.

If urinary tract infections are suspected urinalysis may be useful. Alkaline phosphatase and calcium levels can help identify conditions, such as Paget disease of bone, that affect bone metabolism. However, all these tests are only done in

TABLE 2: Red flag signs for evaluation of chronic low back pain.

Clinical feature	*Comment ("and" denotes simultaneous use, "followed by" denotes second line investigation)*
Age older than 50 years	Laboratory investigations (include PSA for males) followed by MRI
Fever; chills; recent urinary tract or skin infection; penetrating wound near spine	Laboratory investigations and MRI
Significant trauma	Radiology followed by MRI
Unrelenting night pain or pain at rest	Laboratory investigations (include PSA for males) and radiology followed by MRI
Progressive motor or sensory deficit	Emergent MRI
Saddle anesthesia; bilateral sciatica or leg weakness; difficulty urinating; fecal incontinence	Emergent MRI
Unexplained weight loss	Radiology and laboratory investigations (include PSA for males) followed by MRI
History of cancer or strong suspicion for current cancer	Radiology and laboratory investigations (include PSA for males) followed by MRI
History of osteoporosis	Radiology followed by MRI
Immunosuppression	Radiology and laboratory investigations followed by MRI
Chronic oral steroid use	Radiology and laboratory investigations followed by MRI
Intravenous drug use	Radiology and laboratory investigations followed by MRI
Substance abuse	Radiology and laboratory investigations followed by MRI
Failure to improve after 6 weeks of conservative therapy	Radiology and laboratory investigations (include PSA for males) followed by MRI

(PSA: prostate-specific antigen)

patients with high level of suspicion and every patient with chronic LBP do not require these tests. Most patients with chronic LBP have nonspecific findings on imaging studies, therefore, imaging have limited utility. Even highly sensitive investigations like magnetic resonance imaging (MRI) will reveal anomalies that are more nonspecific than true the cause. However, red flags do mandate initial imaging with MRI (or CT), which is the preferred study. Also, patients with radicular symptoms that do not subside after 6 weeks need MRI evaluation. The primary reason for delaying imaging for 1–2 months in patients with chronic LBP is the fact that there is no evidence of improved outcomes with basic (radiographs) or advanced (MRI) studies in patients without red flags for serious disease.

How to identify:
- Keep high index of suspicion
- Give full attention to history (majority of information in history)
- Inspection of back during movement
- Neurological examination
- Observe during heel/toe walk and squat

When and how to investigate red flags:
- Urgent when red flags present
- To include: Myeloma screen, ESR, CRP, serum electrophoresis, free light chain assay, full blood count (FBC), U+E, Ca^{2+}
- Plain X-ray, particularly when osteoporosis/infection suspected
- Consider MRI

The recommended approach as follows:
- All patients with "red flags" should be investigated further and referred to a specialist if clinical findings and test results suggest some serious concerns.
- Cauda equina syndrome is a medical emergency and requires urgent hospital referral. All patients with symptoms or signs of cauda equina syndrome should be referred immediately to hospital for neurosurgical assessment. Features of cauda equina syndrome are urinary retention, fecal incontinence, neurological symptoms and signs in the lower limbs, gait abnormality, saddle area numbness, and a lax anal sphincter YY. Investigations in the first 4–6 weeks of an acute LBP episode do not provide clinical benefit. However, if red flags are present, investigations should be done early for proper diagnosis.
- A FBC and ESR must be performed and other tests may be indicated depending on the clinical situation.
- Radiological investigations (X-rays and CT scans) may be avoided if not required for diagnosis or management at least in early part of management.
- Keep high level of suspicion to observe red flags as "red flag" pathology may lie outside the lumbar region and may not be detected by radiology.
- Nonspecific acute LBP is not an indication for MRI scan. MRI findings at times are misleading because many people without symptoms show abnormalities on MRI. However, MRI is justified if "red flags" are present for early and proper diagnosis.
- Red flags algorithm **(Fig. 1)** helps in decision-making and further management plan of patients with "red flags". In patients with "red flags", the history and clinical assessment should be reviewed weekly until the symptoms have resolved and the patient has returned to their usual activities.

The aim of the review of clinical assessment is to:
- Exclude "red flags"
- Identify any neurological deficit and if require urgent referral for specialist management
- Assessment of functional limitations due to pain
- Determine and suggest options for clinical management

An important aspect in clinical evaluation is the presence of psychological issues. They play an important role in guiding the treatment of patients with chronic LBP. Patients with chronic LBP who have a reduced sense of life control, disturbed mood, negative self-efficacy, high

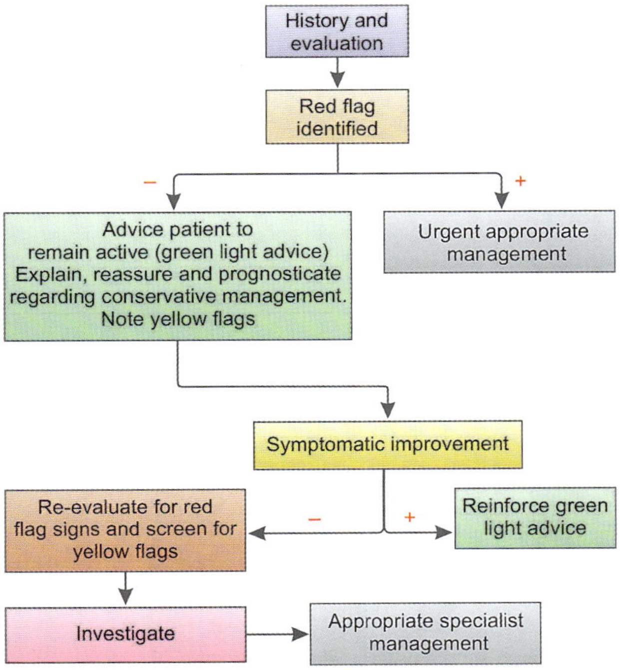

Fig. 1: Evaluation and management in accordance with red flag and yellow flag signs.

TABLE 3: Yellow flag signs predicting poor outcome of management of chronic low back pain.

Affect	Feeling of uselessness; anxiety; depression; and irritability
Behavior	Impaired sleep because of pain; passive attitude about treatment; adverse coping strategies; withdrawal from activities
Beliefs	Thinks that pain is harmful or uncontrollable, or that it needs to be eliminated (before returning to activities or work)
Social	History of physical abuse, sexual abuse, or substance abuse; lack of support or overprotective family; and older age
Work	Expectation that pain will increase with work and activity; problems with compensation or claims; poor job satisfaction; pending litigation; and unsupportive work environment

anxiety levels, and mental health disorders, and who engage in catastrophizing respond poorly to treatments. "Yellow flags" are psychosocial risk factors for long-term disability **(Table 3)**. Evaluation of psychosocial problems and "yellow flags" are useful in identifying patients with a poor prognosis. Psychosocial barriers to recovery may increase the risk of long-term disability and work loss. Yellow flags do not contraindicate the interventional procedure; however, early identification of "yellow flags" may help in management to prevent unnecessary delay in improvement.

THE CONCEPT OF PAIN GENERATOR AND COMMON RECOGNIZED PAIN GENERATORS IN LUMBAR SPINE

Low back pain can arise from a variety of different anatomical sites in concert with complex mechanical and neurophysiological processes that arise in response to trauma and disease.

Definition

Pain generator is a pathoanatomic site or a pathological structure (deranged structure that develops de novo or has discretely gone beyond the physiological limits to be identified as separate) from which the primary cause of patient's LBP is thought to originate and implies certain premises that make the term clinically meaningful. A pain generator is considered the primary or sole cause of patient's illness.

It is difficult to however believe that a single structure can be always pin-pointed and it has been repeatedly proven directly or indirectly that other associations work together in modulating the pain symptomatology. Adjacent tissue injury and collateral damage are two most important associations. For any pathological structure adjacent tissue is also frequently damaged that has been shown to ensue "hyperalgesic effect", this hyperalgesia can also be produced by a distant structure as in double crush phenomenon. Collateral damage refers to pain generators in complexes, e.g., the intervertebral joints comprise intervertebral disk (IVD) and facet joints (zygapophyseal joints or z-joints or ZAJs), it is highly unlikely that pathology of disk would spare z-joints and they would be normal. This association of collateral damage has been shown in the frequent persistence of pain after total disk replacement (TDR).

The above discussion hence entails a thorough examination for evaluation of pain generation in totality (multifactorial school of LBP) and not prefixed ideas for an isolated cause (single disabling pathology school). The following is a list of common pain generators that have been implicated in LBP:

- *The lumbar IVD (see also diskogenic pain below):* Afflictions of the cartilaginous endplate (CEP), annulus fibrosis, and nucleus pulposus.
    - For CEP, development of Schmorl's nodes due to herniation of nuclear material into the vertebral body **(Fig. 2)** indicate breech in the integrity and communication of blood into the nucleus and a subsequent initiation of a clinically-relevant chemical cascade. The CEP injury is prominent in younger population and produces central pain.
    - In the nucleus, autoimmune activities induce release of bradykinin, serotonin, and collagenase; the aggregation of T-lymphocytes; and the production of phospholipase A2 (PLA2). These chemical agents aggressively irritate nerve roots and sensitize **(Fig. 3)** previously silent nociceptors. Interleukin-1 from inflammatory cells stimulate vascular endothelial growth factor (VEGF), nerve growth factor (NGF), and brain-derived neurotrophic factor (BDNF) producing a combination of neurovasculature promoted inflammatory state in the disk.
    - The outer third of annulus is innervated by fibers of the sinuvertebral nerve **(Fig. 4)**. The nerve endings can get activated by the chemicals mentioned above or directly by annular tear.

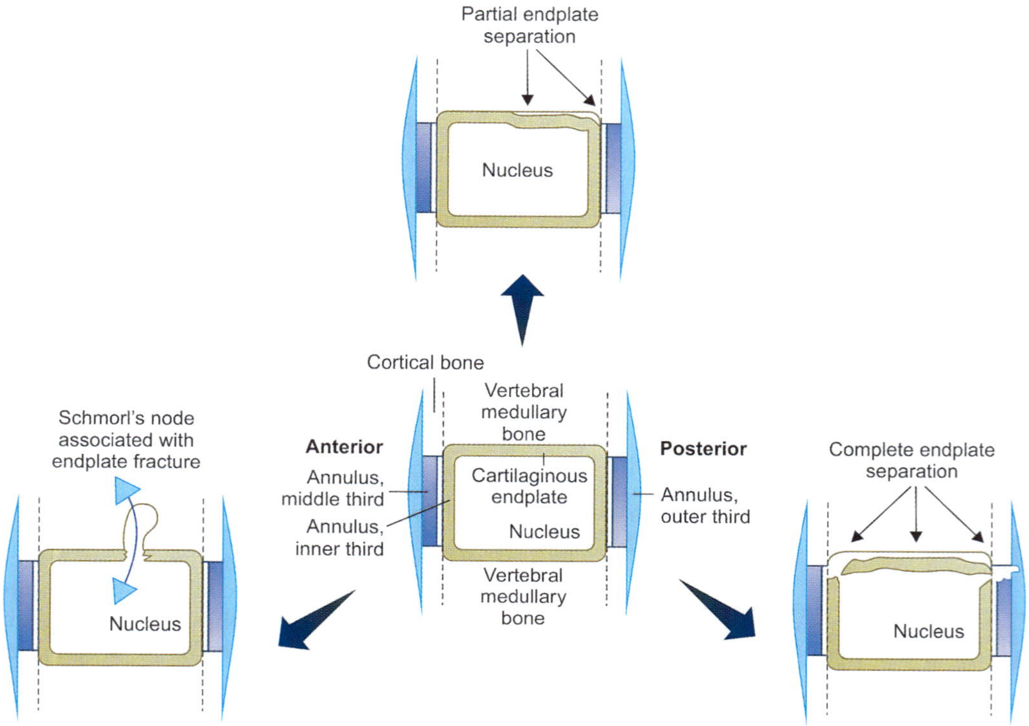

Fig. 2: Endplate damage as pain generator.

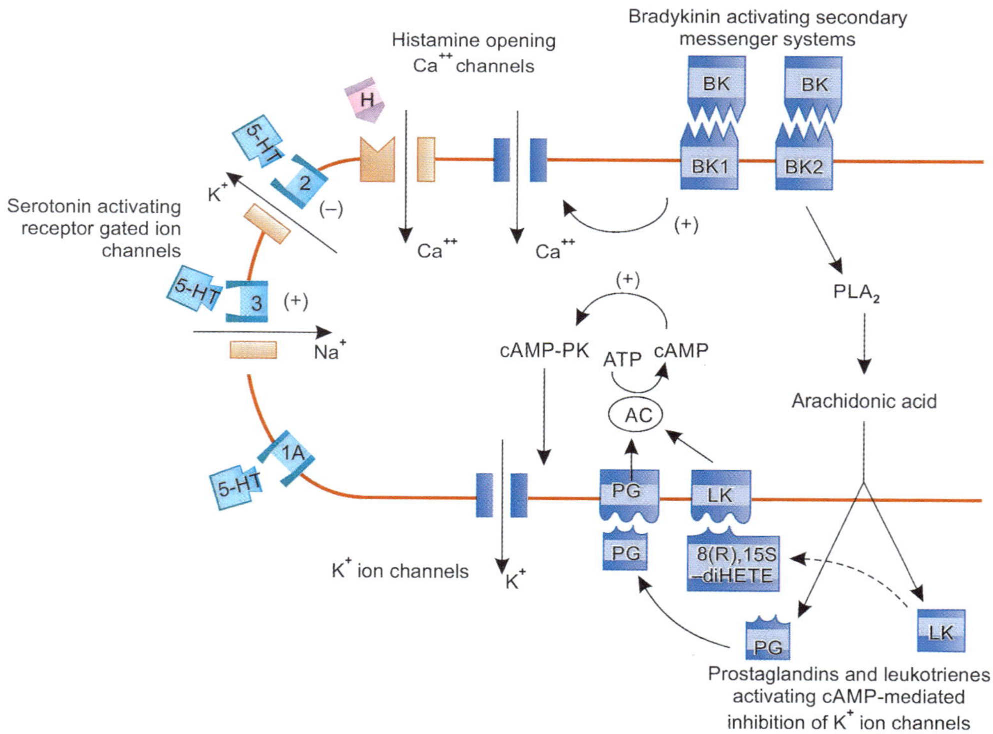

Fig. 3: Chemical sensitization of nociceptive nerve endings.

- *Vertebral body—usually a traumatic event or neoplasia produces pain from vertebral body:*
  - Osteoporosis
  - Infection
  - Multiple myeloma
  - Paget's disease
  - Metastatic tumor
  - Primary neoplasia

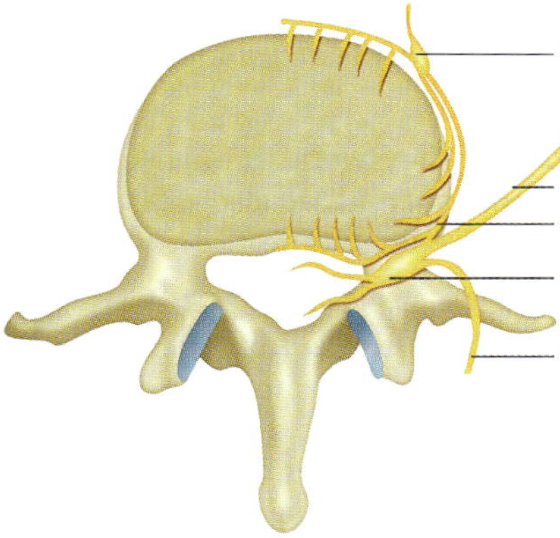

Fig. 4: Illustration showing the origin, course, and structures innervated by the sinuvertebral nerve [annulus, vertebral endplate, posterior longitudinal ligament (PLL)].

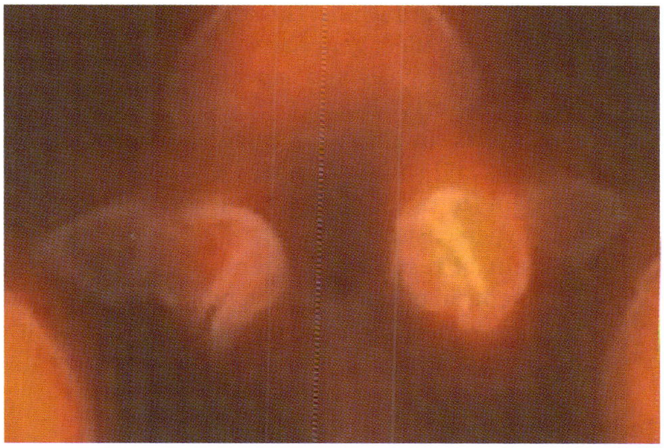

Fig. 5: Firescan showing left L5-S1 facet joint arthrosis.

- Nerve roots—primarily they are pain insensitive but in the presence of inflammatory mediators, they have been demonstrated to develop pain:
  - Lateral recess stenosis
  - Radiculitis
- Facet joints—they contain high-threshold mechanosensitive afferent nerve fibers that serve as nociceptors. They are innervated by the medial branch of the dorsal rami of vertebral nerve at the same level.
  - Degeneration is the most common cause
  - Fracture of facet joints has been also observed to cause pain
  - Pain is produced with extension of the spine
- *Spinal musculature:*
  - Myofascial pain produced from trigger points
  - Accumulation of potentially toxic metabolites during anaerobic metabolism
  - Noncongruent firing of irritated nerve—muscle spasm and dysfunction
- *Sacroiliac joint—the joint is involved in 5-10% of cases of LBP. Various pathologies can involve the joint causing pain:*
  - Spondyloarthropathy
  - Crystal arthritis
  - Infection (tuberculosis of sacroiliac joint)
  - Sacral and pelvis fracture
  - Ligament laxity and joint dysfunction during pregnancy
- Spinal ligaments—the ligaments are commonly secondarily involved with primary damage to the surrounding structures such as IVD and facet joints.
  - Primarily the posterior longitudinal ligament (PLL), anterior longitudinal ligament (ALL), and supraspinous and interspinous ligaments may be involved in chronic lifting stress and twisting forces/maneuvers
  - Posterior longitudinal ligament and ligamentum flavum are supplied by the sinuvertebral nerve (*see* **Fig. 10**)
  - Ligamentum flavum is buckled in DDD and gets hypertrophied
  - Anterior longitudinal ligament in innervated by gray rami communicantes and ventral rami

Identification of Pain Generator

This is a difficult aspect but history and physical examination do indicate the primary site of involvement. For confirmation various investigations can be done as guided by clinical examination. In case of doubt locally injecting the structure by local anesthetic (e.g., facet joints) or provocation of pain in diskography (detailed below) would help localization. For facet joints intra-articular injection or medial branch block is considered diagnostic. The diagnostic power of injections is limited by false positives (40%) and technically challenging facet joint anatomy.

Use of "Firescan"

This is a newly reported technology that digitally fuses bone scan with single photon emission computed tomography (SPECT) to a CT scan. "Firescan" word denotes the appearance of pathological structure that lights up in images **(Fig. 5)**. This scan combines sensitivity of bone scan to the anatomic details and specificity of CT scan. The studies are ongoing for demonstration of specificity and sensitivity to diagnose pain generator and its ability to predict response to facet injections and radiofrequency neurotomy.

MANAGEMENT

It is difficult to lay down a simple plan encompassing all presentations and patients. The general goals of management for LBP include:

- Pain relief
- Rehabilitation
- Improving quality of life

One must understand that there is a large gap between physicians' role and patient expectations. Most patients consider treatment of back equivalent to treating fever that will go away with pills and ultimately settle completely over a short span of time leaving minimal or no residue. This thinking needs to be modified aggressively else the result will be complete patient dissatisfaction and even litigations. They should be made to realistically understand the problem and minimum percentage of improvement that would make a treatment worthwhile. The integral components of management to this effect hence are:

- Documenting the goals and expectations and revisiting them on follow-up visits.
- All the patients should be informed about effective self-care options and should be advised to remain active to reduce pain (muscles that do not move can eventually become hypersensitive to pain).
- Assessment of response to therapy should focus on improvements in pain, mood, and function.

A general flow-diagram highlighting the components of managing patients with LBP is presented in **Flowchart 1**.

Medications

Analgesics and anti-inflammatory: It is worthwhile to begin patients on nonsteroidal anti-inflammatory drugs (NSAIDs) initially to give symptomatic relief even in those that are being still evaluated for possible red flags or yellow flags. They work by inhibiting prostaglandin synthesis [specifically prostaglandin E2 (PGE2)]. Choice is quite empirical but one should balance the needs (anti-inflammatory versus analgesic component) and the adverse effect profile. For patient with past history of gastritis cyclooxygenase-2 (COX-2) could be better or NSAIDs may be altogether avoided instead a combination of paracetamol and narcotics may be prescribed. COX-2 inhibitors are avoided in patients with past history of cardiovascular events as they have been shown to cause deterioration. Some herbal medications have been found to be as effective as NSAIDs in management of LBP. Though not popular but may be tried in selected group of patients, these include *Harpagophytum procumbens* (Devil's claw), Univestin (bioflavonoids derived from *Scutellaria baicalensis* and *Acacia catechu*). There is no specific recommendation and dedicated studies are needed before use.

Narcotics and tramadol: They work through μ-receptor binding (substantia gelatinosa) and are also weak reuptake inhibitors of serotonin and epinephrine. They also inhibit release of substance-P.

Membrane stabilizers (anticonvulsants): They are useful for radiating pains (radiculopathy) and specifically for the control of lancinating or burning pains (neuropathy). Carbamazepine, topiramate, gabapentin, or pregabalin falls into this group that are commonly used specifically pregabalin. One should withdraw or taper them slowly lest seizures may be precipitated. Pregabalin causes pedal edema and potentiates congestive heart failure (CHF) so should be used with caution.

Antidepressants: Tricyclic antidepressants are most effective for pain modulation, amitriptyline and nortriptyline are commonly used drugs. They block the uptake of norepinephrine and serotonin into presynaptic nerve terminals.

Muscle relaxants: This is a nonhomogenous group commonly combined to NSAIDs in fixed dose combination and possibly most irrationally prescribed. They are supposed to ease the muscle spasm associated with neural irritation. Cyclobenzaprine, tizanidine, thiocolchicoside, diazepam, and metaxalone are some of the examples. There is no recommendation to their use as first line agents.

Topical medications: These act as counter irritants and act in relation to gate theory of pain.

Flowchart 1: Management algorithm for low back pain.

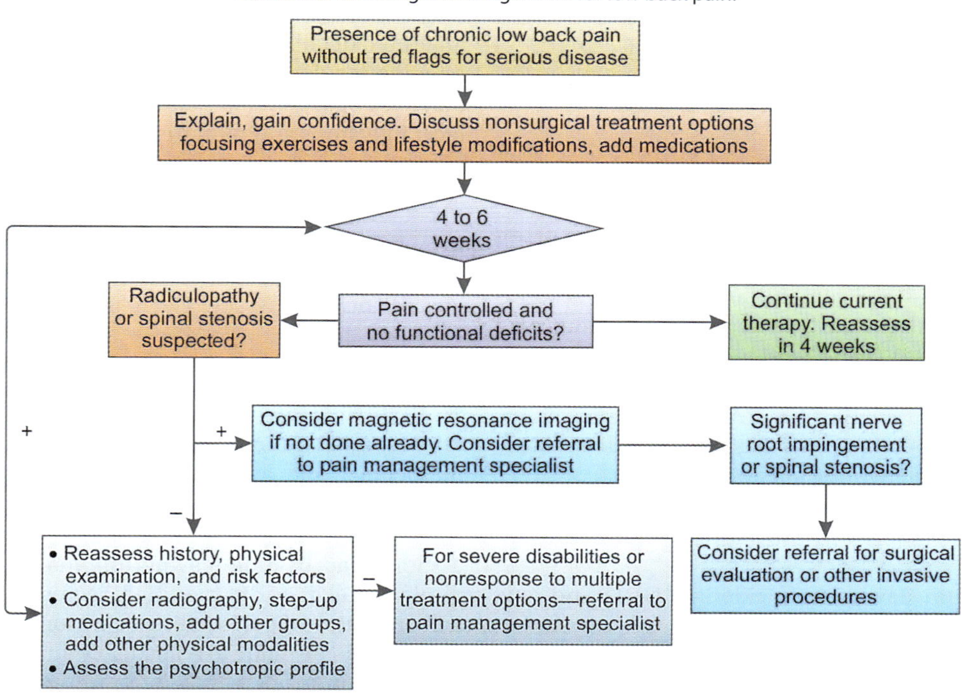

Lifestyle Modifications

Cessation of smoking: LBP has been related to 50 packs per year of smoking. Causes are not fully understood but possibly acceleration of degeneration is one of the mechanisms.

Limiting alcohol use: Alcohol use should be ideally curtailed as it hampers the basic muscle tone. Immediate cessation may not always be feasible so the least such patients can do is to reduce the usage quickly culminating to completely cessation.

Weight management: Overweight persons put strain on back muscles and IVD.

Exercises: These are cornerstone of chronic LBP management. The goals of exercise are:
- Strengthen lumbar extensors and abdominal flexors
- Centralize the pain in setting of radiculopathy
- Strengthen weak muscles
- *Stretch tight* muscles
- Provide an aerobic program
- Improve mechanics of patient
- Prevent development of myofascial trigger points

Pilates: This was developed by Joseph Pilates and incorporates Zen meditation and yoga. This utilizes open and closed chain exercises, in a home-based program, to strengthen and stretch muscles. It aims to improve joint proprioception and flexibility. The muscle soreness is minimal compared to other forms of exercise therapy.

Other Supportive Therapies

Transcutaneous electric nerve stimulation (TENS): TENS uses pulsed electric current through the skin to stimulate underlying muscle. Conventionally 10–30 mA of current is used at 50–100 Hz. They provide pain control by:
- *Gate control theory:* Stimulation of large Aβ fibers activates the dorsal horn and action potentials from small diameter afferent nociceptors (Aδ and C fibers) are selectively suppressed.
- May involve release of endorphins.

Acupuncture: This works on the principle of reorganization of hypothetical Qi energy, disruption of which is the cause of pain. Specific points are identified that serve as nodes for control of energy flow and are activated/suppressed by placement of solid metal needles. Acupuncture provides short-term relief of chronic LBP, improves functioning, and works as an adjunct to other therapeutic options.

Osteopathic manipulation: Nonthrusting manipulation techniques are used by trained physical therapists to relieve pain. The mechanism is unclear but release of restrictions, malfunction of joints, and improved flexibility may improve pain characteristics. Various contact-relax, controlled pressure, and high-velocity low-amplitude techniques are used. Person should be experienced else fractures and secondary muscle damage may ensue.

Magnets: Static and electromagnetic therapy had been used in orthopedics, while the latter is sometimes used for delayed or nonunions of fractures. Static magnets generating 300–5,000 gauss of field are placed strategically to relieve symptoms. Possibly they act by generating local electric currents that stimulate muscles and reduce spasm or work through gate theory of pain. Magnets are also supposed to reduce the sensitivity of nociceptive fibers.

Yoga therapy: One therapeutically directed style of *Yoga* (*Viniyoga*) may provide some relief of chronic back pain. 6 weeks of treatment can has shown moderate improvement in pain relief and gain in self-esteem.

Back schools, low-level laser therapy, lumbar supports, prolotherapy and short-wave diathermy, and traction: All have conflicting evidence to recommend any use. The same however also applies for transcutaneous electrical nerve stimulation TENS, magnets, manipulation, and acupuncture.

The current evidence is not complete to recommend any of the above therapy in isolation and a combination is often prescribed. There is a very high possibility that these ancillary therapies keep the patient psychologically occupied while the disease improves over course.

Injections

For those with severe functional disabilities, radicular symptoms, or refractory pain, referral for epidural steroid (or root block) injection or surgical evaluation may be reasonable. They have been found useful in controlling pain and providing relief significantly. There is no evidence to support the use of epidural steroid injections in patients without radicular symptoms also injections are less effective in patients with severe spinal stenosis and those with stenotic lesions encompassing more than three lumbar levels. The details have been discussed separately in management of DDD.

Surgical Management

This is specifically discussed in detail with the individual pathologies. In general, conservative management is the mainstay of managing diskogenic back pain. NSAIDs and omega-3 fatty acids provide good symptom relief. Biological therapies aimed at inhibiting inflammatory cytokines have not shown much benefit. Similarly, cell-based therapies and platelet-rich plasma has limited success. Surgical intervention for control of diskogenic back pain is very limited. Fusions have mixed results. TDR is appearing to provide promising results in various studies and the long-term results are better compared to fusion or multidisciplinary rehabilitation.

INTERVERTEBRAL DISK DEGENERATION

INTRODUCTION

Back pain is a major public health problem and is strongly associated with degeneration of the IVD. Degeneration is not a diagnosis but an expression of the state of the disk, which is the result of several factors acting individually or collectively. This is the reason why there is no universally accepted definition of DDD. DDD is viewed differently by persons, to surgeons and radiologists DDD usually means the presence of osteophytes, loss of disk height, and reduced signal intensity on MRI. To a biochemist degeneration means changes in the content of proteoglycans or water whilst a pathologist sees degenerated disk as dry with cracks and fissures. This entails that there are different views for degenerated disk.

Disk degeneration in symptomatic patients is also associated with sciatica and disk herniation or prolapse. So, it is instead useful to focus on the term "diskogenic pain" for making a differentiation. Diskogenic back pain refers to a pain syndrome that theoretically originates from a lumbar disk, creating LBP without concomitant radicular symptoms. Diskogenic pain syndromes have been divided into two separate categories—internal disk disruption (IDD) (radiology normal but MRI/diskography reveals pathology) and DDD (DDD, radiological degenerative changes in spine visible). The alteration in disk height from IDD alters the mechanics of the rest of the spinal column, possibly adversely affecting the behavior of other spinal structures such as muscles and ligaments. In the long-term, it can lead to spinal stenosis and DDD, a major cause of pain and disability in the elderly. Over the decades research has revealed that spinal degenerative cascade involves interplay of both biologic and biomechanical factors. Biochemical events are important in the pathogenesis of the degenerative process as well as in the pain-signaling pathways responsible for the clinical features of the condition. As the biologic aspects of spinal degeneration are better understood, less invasive, nonablative treatments designed to reverse these biologic processes and restore the disk and facet functioning may become a reality.

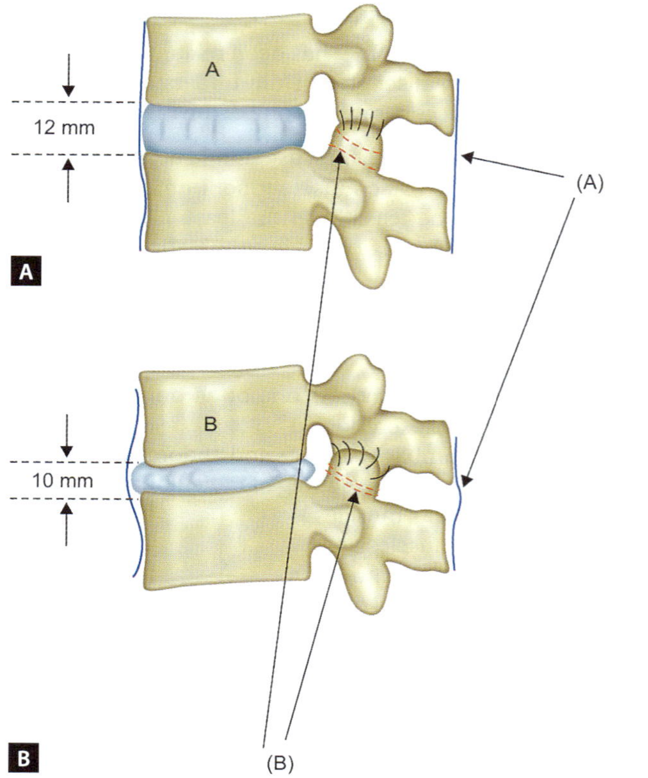

Figs. 6A and B: The effect of loss in height with load on other spinal structures. The degenerate disk bulges due to weakened annulus and nonresilient nucleus. The loss in height results in (A) Buckling of ligaments and (B) Loss of apophyseal joint space and secondary degeneration.

PATHOANATOMY

"Morphologic alterations"—seen with IVD degeneration.

- *Reduced disk height:* A posterior disk height <4 mm or a foraminal height <15 mm correlates with symptomatic nerve root compression. The decrease in disk height results in loss of tension in the ligamentum flavum causing its buckling into the canal **(Figs. 6A and B)**. A decrease in tension within the posterior annulus fibrosus also contributes to bulging of the disk within the canal.
- Degeneration of the disk can lead to annular fissures and tears. Decreased osmotic pressure by itself may actually enhance the opening of small cracks and fissures in the annulus. The propagation of these fissures into the periphery has been implicated in the etiology of disk herniations and diskogenic back pain. Three types of annular tears have been described:
  1. The radial tear is most commonly located in the posterior annulus fibrosus. It has been reported that radial tears are most commonly associated with disk degeneration.
  2. Circumferential tears may be secondary to interlaminar shear stresses and are more likely to be observed in older disks.
  3. Peripheral rim tears are more commonly located anteriorly and may be associated with trauma.
- *Facet joint degeneration:* Facet cartilage degeneration, especially thinning of the cartilage, causes capsular ligament laxity. Capsular laxity may allow abnormal motion or hypermobility of the facet joint. The facet joint complex protects the IVD from rotational stresses. As disk disease progresses, increased stress is applied posteriorly, accelerating facet osteoarthrosis. The resultant facet joint osteoarthritis is likely to change the segmental spinal motion, altering the mechanical forces experienced by the IVD.

PATHOBIOMECHANICS

Spinal Motion Segment and the Tripod Vertebral Joint

The motion segment (lumbar spine) consists of an anterior IVD and two posterior facets. This three-joint complex allows for motion and simultaneously resists the compressive forces across the vertebral column. IVD provides the most resistance to compression, whereas the facets allow for rotation, lateral bending, and extension.

Degree of disk degeneration decides the stress distribution across the IVD and vertebral end-plate. The healthy lumbar IVD demonstrates a uniform stress distribution across the entire end-plate area under pure compressive and eccentric compressive loading **(Fig. 7)**. In degenerated disks, the asymmetry of the stress distribution is increased with both angle of inclination and degree of degeneration **(Fig. 8)**. Relatively solid nature of the degenerated disk and its inability to conform to the eccentric loads is presumed reason for asymmetric stress distribution. With advancing degeneration, the proportion of load transmission shifts to the posterior elements. Degenerated disks cause significant increase in facet load for that segment **(Figs. 6 and 8)**. Due to eccentricity of the applied compressive load this increased load is more prominent posteriorly. What we observed clinically in disk degeneration is this biomechanical sequence of disk degeneration leading to posterior element load bearing which typically precedes facet arthrosis **(Fig. 8)**. The motion segment ultimately becomes less mobile and more painful with advancing degeneration. Degenerative changes in facet joints are similar to those of osteoarthritis seen in other synovial joints as the facet joints are also true synovial articulations. With progressive spinal degeneration, the load-bearing patterns of the facet joints get altered. Progresses of the degenerative cascade leads to loss of anterior column support the facet joints bear more weight and the fulcrum moves dorsally to balance the motion segment **(Fig. 8)**.

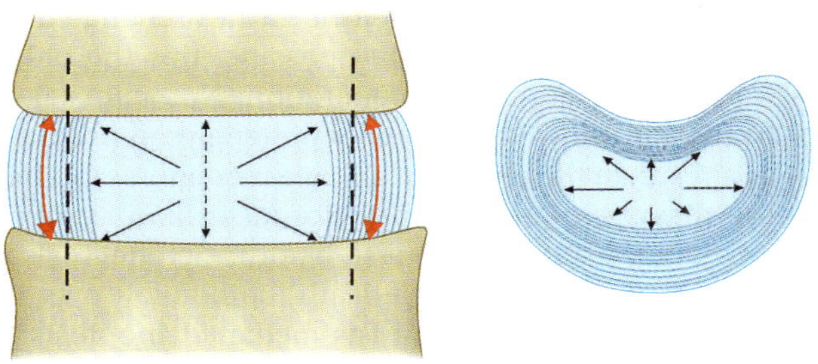

Fig. 7: Under compressive forces, the pressure in the disk is uniformly transmitted to the annulus fibrosus.

More recently, a term so-called internal disk derangement has received considerable attention. It is a disk dysfunction giving rise to axial back pain. The high-intensity zone (HIZ) has been described as a focally increased T2-weighted MRI signal believed to be representative of an annular tear extending to the periphery of the disk. The HIZ can be seen on T2-weighted MRI scans as a high-intensity signal located in the substance of the posterior annulus fibrosus. The HIZ has been suggested as, but by no means confirmed to be, associated with diskogenic axial back pain.

Disk Loading

Unlike most other mammals, humans walk upright and place large compressive loads on their IVDs. The normal nucleus pulposus is relatively noncompressible. Compressive loading causes slight deformation of the cartilaginous end-plate and vertebral body as well as bulging of the annulus fibrosus **(Fig. 7)**. Lateral bending and rotation of the spine places significant tensile stresses on the fibers of the annulus fibrosus and result in fiber failure if the stresses exceed the tensile strength of the tissue.

In disk degeneration, the integrity of the annulus fibrosus becomes compromised by the development of fissures. When the intact facet complex is lost because of vertebral spondylolysis, pathologic stress applied to the tissues can lead to early degeneration of the IVD. To dissipate compressive loads in the spine, the normal disk converts the load into tensile hoop stress in the outer annulus fibrosus while allowing controlled motion of the intervertebral segment. The vertebral end-plates transmit the compressive load to the nucleus pulposus, leading to elevated pressure on the hydrated gel of the nucleus pulposus. In a young, healthy disk, the load is transmitted evenly outward in all directions to the surrounding tissues of the disk. The result is a viscoelastic deformation of the circumferential fibers of the outer annulus fibrosus, which dissipates some of the stress.

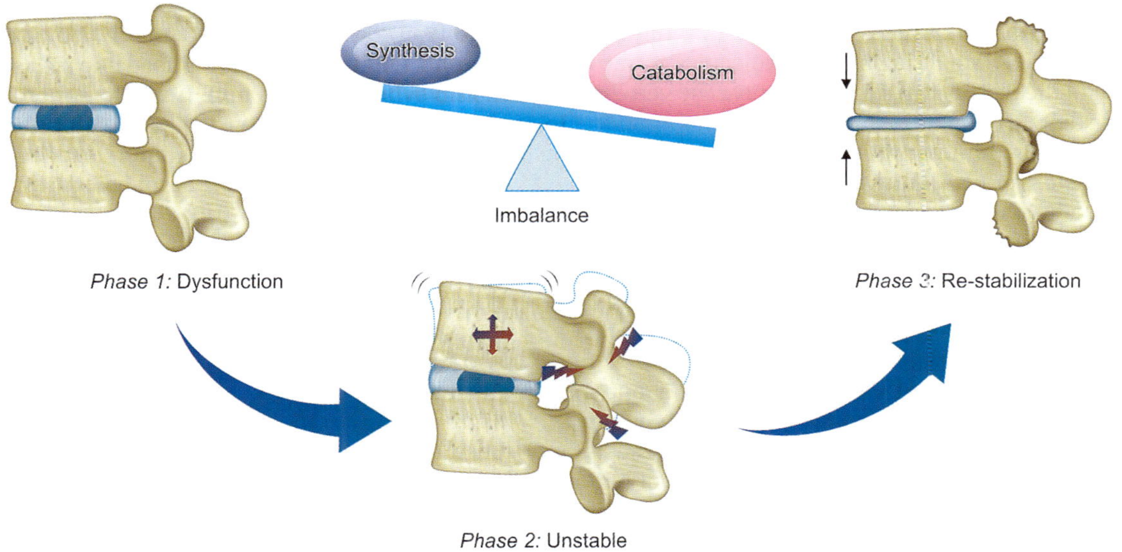

Fig. 8: Eccentric loading and imbalance of compressive loads on the disk causes degeneration and facet arthrosis.

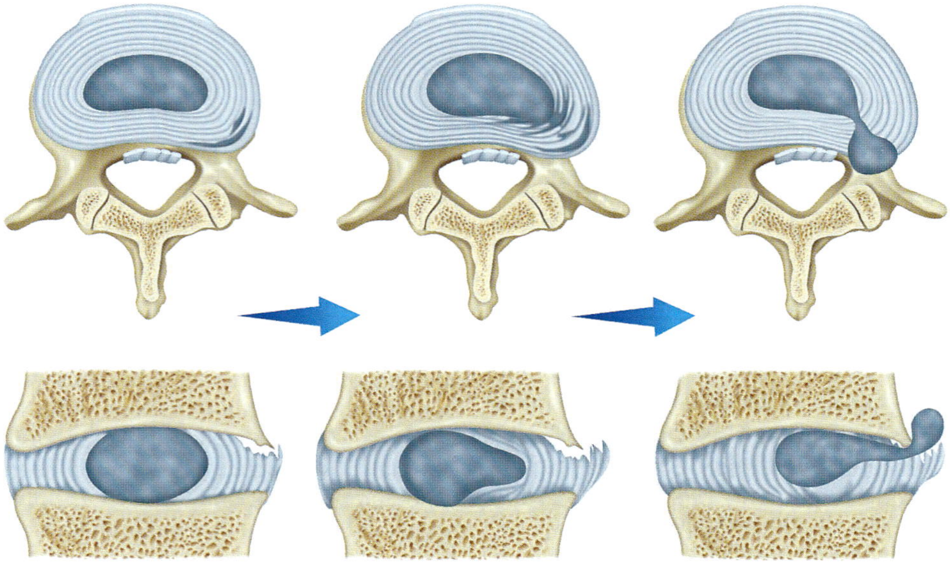

Fig. 9: The progressive tearing of the annular fibers with increased compressive forces that put increased pressure on the circumferential annular fibers.

But in degenerative disks, the annular tear weakens the structure causing increased bulging and fiber tear that may ultimately give way and cause herniation of nucleus **(Fig. 9)**.

The loss of the normal biomechanical function of the nucleus pulposus and annulus fibrosus leads to overloading of the bony end-plates, which become sclerotic and form peripheral osteophytes, as is seen in vertebral spondylosis.

DEGENERATIVE PROCESSES

Changes in nucleus pulposus and vertebral end-plates harbinger the molecular degenerative process. Notochordal cells (nucleus pulposus) are believed to stimulate and maintain regenerative process. Large notochordal cells remain active until the second decade of life, after which they are rarely seen. The bony vertebral end-plates are covered with a hyaline cartilage layer acts as a diffusion barrier allowing only small uncharged molecules to move into and out of the disk in significant quantity. The vertebral end-plates calcify as they age, and the calcification affects disk metabolism by limiting the delivery of nutrients and removal of waste products. Thus, the cells inside the disk live in a nutritionally challenged environment that worsens with age.

In all tissues, the balance between synthesis and degradation of matrix macromolecules is crucial to tissue homeostasis. Degenerative processes predominate when synthesis of new macromolecules is decreased or the rate of product breakdown increases. Disk degeneration is one of the earliest forms of tissue degeneration seen in the human body; early signs are often present by the second decade of life. About 20% of people in their teens have disks with mild signs of degeneration; degeneration increases steeply with age, particularly in males, so that around 10% of 50-year-old disks and 60% of 70-year-old disks are severely degenerated.

- The loss of notochordal cells is earliest change in disk (physiological process) that possibly tips the balance from regeneration to degeneration. Notochordal cells have been shown to stimulate proteoglycan production as a result of the release of soluble mediators, and hence the disappearance of notochordal cells may remove a necessary stimulus to disk health. Cell necrosis and apoptosis (programed cell death) both follow over time. Two primary pathways for Fas-mediated apoptosis have been identified: type I cells carry the Fas receptor on their cell membrane and type II cells carry the Fas receptor intracellularly at the mitochondrial level. A recent study suggested that type II cells predominate in human disk fragments.
- The supply of nutrients has been shown to control the density of disk cells. Because the supply of oxygen to the disk is limited, cell metabolism is largely anaerobic, and it produces lactate as a by-product. Lactate increases the acidity of the disk to a pH level between 6.9 and 7.2, although a pH level as low as 6.1 can be observed when the disk is under stress.
- Disk enzymes including cathepsin, lysozyme, aggrecanase, and several matrix metalloproteinases (MMPs) have been found to participate in the disk degeneration process. Disk metabolism is regulated by a host of cytokines, including interleukins, prostaglandins, and tumor necrosis factor. Interleukin-1, for example, decreases proteoglycan synthesis and upregulates the expression of stromolysin-1 and PGE2. Interleukin-8 has been found in patients with sciatic pain. Interleukin-6, tumor necrosis factor-α, and PGE2 are believed to play a role in producing diskogenic pain. These cytokine molecules may be used in the future as targets of therapies to diminish disk-related pain.

PRODUCTION OF PAIN AND RADICULAR SYMPTOMS IN DEGENERATIVE DISK DISEASE

Diskogenic Pain

An ingrowth of blood vessels and free nerve endings occurs in full-thickness annular fissures. In a normal disk, only the outer 1–2 mm of the annular surface is innervated, and the inner region of the disk has no nerve supply **(Fig. 10)**. In some degenerative disks, nerve fibers with a receptor for nociceptive substances such as substance P and calcitonin gene-related peptide have been found in annular disruptions. These nerve structures may play a role in the production of diskogenic symptoms. Diskography, which is widely used to establish a particular disk as a source of pain, has well-documented limitations. Better diagnostic tests are needed to guide both the assessment of patients with symptomatic disk degeneration and the development of new forms of treatment. Other mechanisms of development of pain proposed variously are as follows:

- Production of inflammatory cytokines (see above)
- Brodsky and Binder in 1979 characterized the mechanisms for provocation of pain with diskography and suggested the following:
  - Stretching of the fibers of an abnormal annulus
  - Extravasation of extradurally irritating substances such as glycosaminoglycans, lactic acid, and acidic media
  - Pressure on nerves posteriorly caused by bulging of the annulus
  - Hyperflexion of posterior joints on disk injection
  - Presence of vascular granulation tissue, with pain caused by scar distension
  - Pain generators in the end-plate (speculative still)

Pain pathways of diskogenic pain—though still elusive some insight has been provided by the investigators.

- It had been proposed that the irritation of nerve adjacent to the disk transmits pain signal from that root into the dorsal root ganglion and into spinal cord.
- Newer findings suggest that pain signals from lower disk levels (L4-5) would get detoured up the sympathetic nerves (gray ramus communicans) and upper lumbar dorsal root ganglion especially the L2 level producing in effect a referred pain to the L1-2 region for pain originating in L4-5 region.

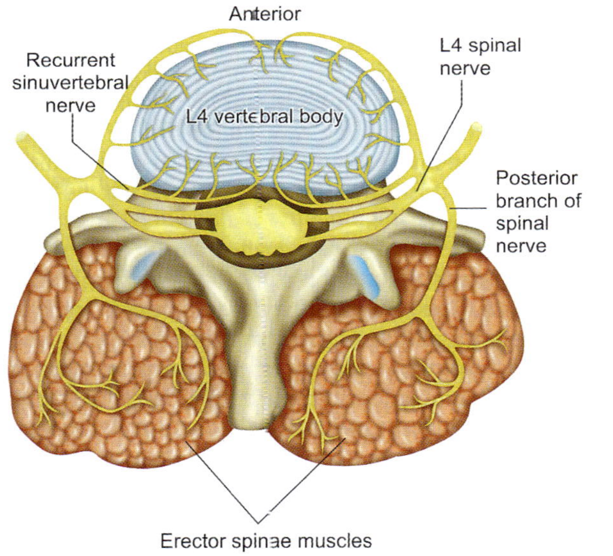

Fig. 10: Sinuvertebral nerve, which innervates the posterolateral region of the disk. The nerve exits from the dorsal root ganglion and enters the vertebral foramen, where it divides into a major ascending and a lesser descending branch. The posterior longitudinal ligament is richly innervated by nociceptive fibers from the ascending branch of the sinuvertebral nerve.

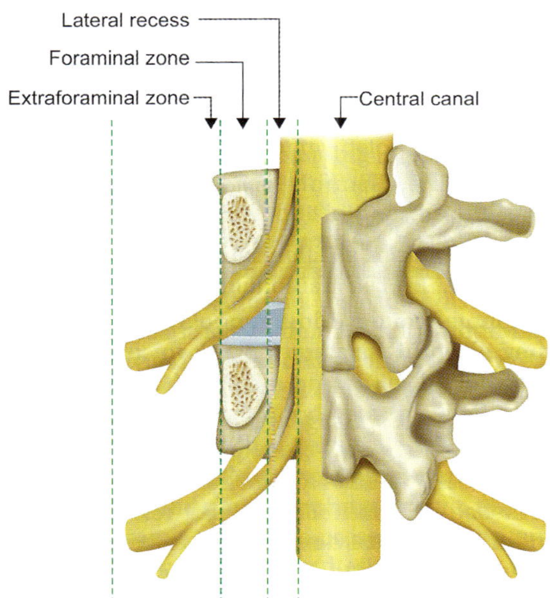

Fig. 11: The divisions of the lumbar spinal canal.

Radicular Symptoms

To understand the development of radicular symptoms, we need to study the sagittal subdivisions of the spinal canal:

- The lumbar spinal canal is divided into three regions from midline to lateral **(Fig. 11)**
  1. The central zone is defined as the region between the lateral margins of the dura
  2. Lateral recess lies between the lateral margin of dura and the medial border of the pedicle
  3. The foraminal zone lies between the medial and lateral margins of the pedicle and contains the intervertebral foramen. The lateral recess and foraminal zones have been further defined.
     - The entrance zone is bordered anteriorly by the posterior surface of the disk and posterolaterally by the facet joint
     - The midzone is bordered anteriorly by the posterior vertebral wall and posteriorly by the pars interarticularis
     - The exit zone is the area of the intervertebral foramen bordered posteriorly by the lateral margin of the facet below, and anteriorly by the intervertebral disk of the level below.

The presence of osteophytes on the superior medial articular process can result in nerve compression in the entrance zone. Hypertrophy of fibrocartilage from a pars interarticularis defect results in nerve compression in the midzone. Causes for nerve root compression in exit zone include a far lateral disk herniation and osteophytic facets.

Facetogenic Pain

Facet joints are amply supplied by nerve fibers. Facet joint degeneration is an integral part of disk degeneration as detailed in morphology and biomechanics above. This degenerative process not only limits the mobility of spine but also produces pain similar to osteoarthritis anywhere else **(Fig. 12)**.

ETIOLOGY OF DISK DEGENERATION

The rate and degree of disk degeneration are affected by several factors.

Aging

This is possibly the most consistent physiological reason explaining the disk degeneration. Undoubtedly changes occur as the disk ages. Individually and collectively these changes reflect impaired synthesis of the matrix. In a nutshell, the following changes occur:

- The concentration of cells in the disk declines with age (especially in annulus).
- The rate of synthesis and concentration of proteoglycans decreases.
- The quality of proteoglycans produced is poorer (smaller and less aggregated).
- The concentration of chondroitin sulfate falls (causing increased ratio of keratan sulfate to chondroitin sulfate).
- The collagen content of the nucleus increases and quality changes (type II replaced by type I which is vulnerable to calcification).
- Noncollagenous proteins in the nucleus increase. There is less proteoglycan available to bond to water.
- The nucleus becomes progressively more solid, dry, and granular.
- The collagen lamellae of the annulus increase in thickness and cracks and cavities develop within it.

Although this is deleterious, why body takes this path is not known. The possible causes could be declining nutrition, cell senescence, accumulation of degraded matrix products, and fatigue failure of the nucleus.

One should bear in mind that not all features/changes in disk are age related:

- Narrowing of the IVDs has previously been considered one of the signs of aging of the lumbar spine but this is untrue as substantiated by postmortem studies that have shown that lumbar disks do not narrow with age.
- Similarly, radial tears (considered a harbinger of degeneration) do not correlate with age.
- It is also interesting to consider the fact that despite all disks being of same age in an individual, those at lower lumbar levels exhibit degenerative changes far more often than in the upper levels (possibly better related to mechanical loading than aging).

Genetic Factors

The most intriguing and highly supported by studies in twins, there seems to be a strong genetic predisposition to disk degeneration. Genetic predisposition has emerged as perhaps the strongest factor leading to symptomatic DDD. Siblings of patients with disk degeneration were found to have a higher prevalence of both disk degeneration and osteoarthritis than the general population. Though difficult to understand or remember for a surgeon the following changes have been described that assert a genetic cause rather than environmental/mechanical factors related to disk degeneration **(Fig. 13)**.

- Taq I and Fok I of the vitamin D receptor gene have been implicated in disk degeneration in several studies.

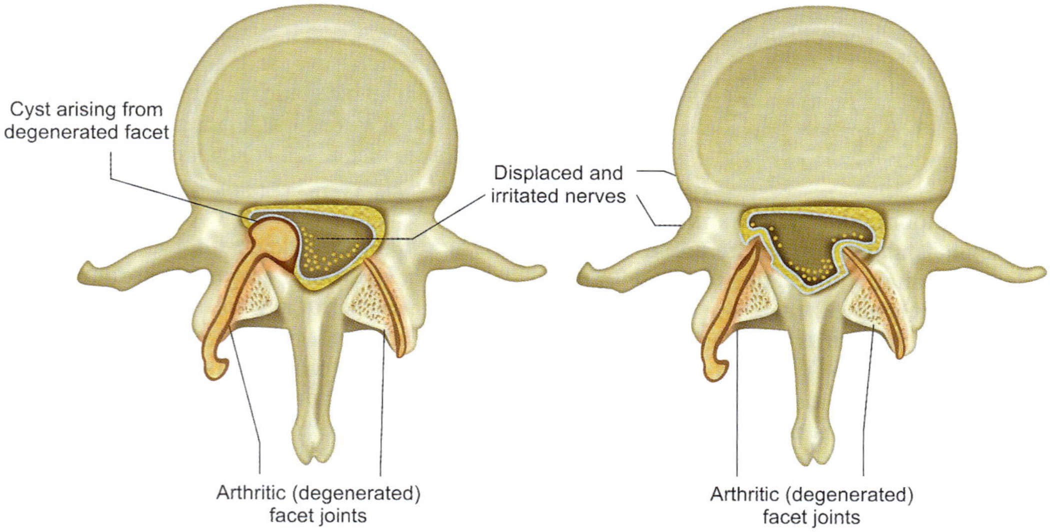

Fig. 12: The degeneration of facet joints of spine with osteophyte and cyst formation and consequent irritation of the nerves.

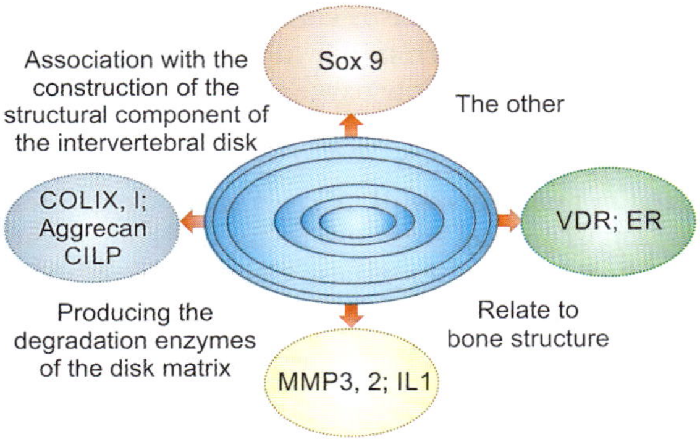

Fig. 13: Genetic factors involved in disk degeneration.

Taq I increases the decay of the messenger ribonucleic acid (RNA) by 30% which impairs the sulfation of glycosaminoglycans by vitamin D. The prevalence of the t-allele of Taq I, and hence the risk for disk degeneration, differs among races. It is present in 43% of Caucasians and 31% of Africans, but in only 8% of Asians.

- Polymorphism (5A and 6A alleles) commonly occurs in the promoter region of the gene that regulates MMP-3 production (elderly Japanese patients). The 5A allele is a possible risk factor for accelerated degenerative changes of lumbar disks in the elderly.
- Trp2 and Trp3 alleles result in the substitution by tryptophan of the amino acids in type IX collagen (producing an unstable triple helix) encoded by *COL9A2* (type IX collagen α-2 gene) and *COL9A3* genes. Patients with these variants of type IX collagen have an increased risk for lumbar disk disease and chronic sciatica due to susceptibility to mechanical stress. Those having Trp3 allele (α-3 chain of type IX collagen) are at an increased risk of developing disk degeneration if they are obese (implicating the role of environmental factors also).
- In the human *AGCI* gene, the region coding for the CS1 [Chondroitin sulfate (CS)] domain exhibits specific polymorphism which is associated with disk degeneration.
- A single nucleotide polymorphism (1184C allele) results in an amino acid substitution in the *CLIP* gene that encodes cartilage intermediate layer protein. The presence of an 1184C allele increases inhibition of growth factors, such as transforming growth factor-beta (TGF-β), reducing the growth factor mediated induction of matrix formation genes.
- The alleles (IL-1αT889 and IL-1βT3954 that code for interleukin-1) are associated with disk bulging (correlated with diskogenic pain and sciatica), suggesting a genetic predisposition to disk degeneration through alterations in the function of proinflammatory mediators.

Mechanical Factors

Apart from genetics and age the mechanical factors are most commonly purported in the etiology of disk degeneration as supported by the fact that for same age degeneration is more common and more severe at lower lumbar levels.

- *Vibration:* Vibration can adversely affect the nutrition and metabolism of the disk, especially if the vibration matches the resonant frequency of the lumbar spine (4–6 Hz). Helicopter pilots and drivers of trucks, buses, and tractors have a high rate of back pain. Driving has been proposed to adversely affect the IVDs with a higher rate of herniation in occupational drivers (not supported by epidemiological studies however).
- *Torsion:* Due to criss-cross arrangement of fibers in the annulus, torsional movements generate tension in half of the collagen fibers in the annulus, whereas the other fibers tend to become slack. For the fibers to incur damage, they must be elongated by >4% of their resting length that requires an axial rotation of >3° at each individual segment. This is possible only if ZAJs are damaged as they resist rotation beyond 1.5–3°. When the spine is flexed, however, the facet joints offer less constraint to rotation leading to annular tear without damage to the facets. Such torsional injury results in tears at the peripheral posterolateral region of the annulus, which slowly extends radially toward the center. Such tears are seen in professional bowlers in cricket often associated with stress fracture of pars interarticularis.
- *Compression:* Compression is the physiological stimulus for matrix turnover to disk. Physiologically, it induces MMPs and nitric oxide to clear the matrix in preparation for new synthesis, and induces matrix synthesis. Excessive loading can have negative effects in the disk by reducing gene expression of all anabolic proteins including formation of aggrecan. When compression is excessive, the endplate fails by fracturing that leads to degeneration by a variety of mechanisms. Callus formation may cause occlusion of blood vessels in the endplate, thereby interfering with cell nutrition and maintenance of the extracellular matrix (ECM). Endplate damage causes depressurization of the nucleus and increase in stress in the posterior annulus. Due to reduced pressure the inner lamellae of the annulus buckle inward and the outer lamellae buckle outward, particularly posteriorly producing interlaminar shear and concentric tears. The term "Schmorl's nodes" was given by German pathologist Christian George Schmorl (1861–1932) who was first to describe diskal protrusions into adjacent vertebral bodies in patients with adolescent kyphosis. Schmorl's nodes **(Fig. 14)** have shown a strong association between degeneration and defects in the endplate and fractures with an increased incidence of disk prolapse, particularly at the lower lumbar levels. Other than "Schmorl's nodes" a number of endplate abnormalities have been described including:
  - *Vascular channel defects:* These are radiographically referred to as "limbus" vertebre. This residual vascular channel is often misdiagnosed as post-traumatic when trauma has not occurred. The vertebra is, however, weak here and avulsion fracture can result from trauma.
  - *Centrum abnormalities:* These occur between centrum and ring apophysis. The defect is congenital

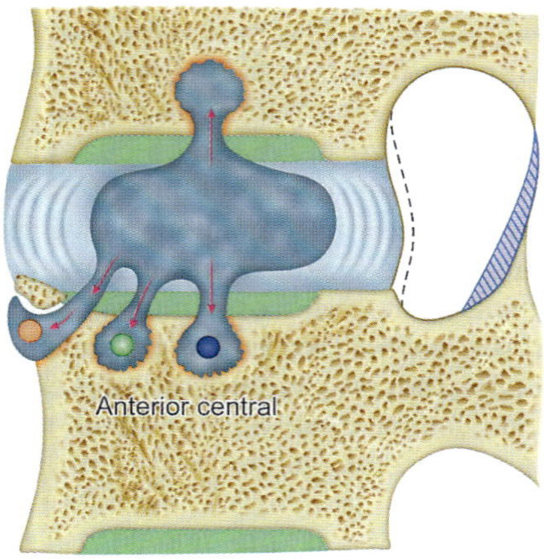

Fig. 14: Development of Schmorl's nodes as a result of endplate fracture and migration of nucleus in various directions.

but can be expanded by trauma and increased axial pressure that causes nucleus migration. This is the most common type of Schmorl's node.

- *Notochord endplate defects:* Residual notochord endplate deformities can be prominent and are often the result of poor development in embryonic period. These are quite commonly seen in the genomic spine disorder "juvenile diskogenic disease". The deficiencies also compromise the IVD nutrient diffusion and convection to and from the disk across the endplate. The defects are often in the anterior half of the endplates.

Nutrition

The disk relies on diffusion for its nutrition, and pivotal to this is movement, which pumps water and nutrients into the disk.

- Calcification of the endplate occludes the vascular openings within it, acting as a barrier to transport of nutrients because of lowering of endplate permeability.
- Smoking is associated with an increased incidence of disk herniation and degeneration implying a systemic effect by constriction of arterioles or anoxia to cells in the disk induced by carboxyhemoglobin (not verified in humans).
- First signs of disk degeneration become evident after the first decade of life with the diminishing capillary network at the bone-cartilage endplate junction.
- Atheromatous lesions in the abdominal aorta or congenital hypoplasia of the lumbar arteries may lead to insufficient blood supply to the lumbar spine.
- Reduced supply of nutrients leads to an increase in oxidative stress markers in the nucleus of young disks. A distinct cellular reaction to increased oxidative stress and possibly impaired function may reflect deposition of carboxylmethylolysine.
- A low level of oxygen and an acidic pH from the anaerobic metabolism lead to a fall in protein and synthesis of proteoglycan.
- The activity of disk cells is very sensitive to extracellular oxygen and pH, with matrix synthesis rates falling steeply at acidic pH and at low oxygen concentrations and the cells do not survive prolonged exposure to low pH or glucose concentrations.
- A fall in nutrient supply → lowering of oxygen tension and/or pH (arising from raised lactic acid concentrations) → reduced ability to synthesize and maintain the disk's ECM → disk degeneration.

Toxic Factors

Smoking and ill effects of nicotine have been reported in animals, but need to be substantiated in humans.

Metabolic Disorders

Metabolic disorders can cause disk degeneration either by interfering with the normal biochemistry of matrix synthesis or by deposition of foreign materials in the disk, but these are one-off events and do not explain the widespread prevalence of DDD.

- In diabetes mellitus, nucleus pulposus demonstrates a significant decrease in hexosamine content, an increase in hydroxyproline and deficiencies of 35S-sulfate during proteoglycan synthesis. This indicates a reduced rate of glycosylation and a decrease in the number of sugar side chains per core protein.
- In patients with alkaptonuria, disk degeneration is induced by intradiskal deposits of a black pigment which is characterized by calcification appearing as elliptical opaque wafers.

Low-grade Infection

Disk degeneration may be caused by low-grade infection (sporadic and inconsistent data). Up to one-third of the disks harvested after microdiskectomy tested positive for low-virulence gram-positive bacteria, and 84% of these were infected with *Propionibacterium acnes* in one study.

Neurogenic Inflammation

Antidromic release of substance P into the disk innervated by the dorsal root ganglion neurons might produce degeneration by stimulating the synthesis of inflammatory agents and degradative enzymes in the disk. This argument appears farfetched as it requires a cause of irritation of the ganglion before the disk degenerates or herniates and this effect is not the cause but rather other way around.

Autoimmune Theory

The nucleus is thought of, as a concealed antigen and trauma after compression injury exposes the antigenic components of the nucleus pulposus to the circulation triggering an immune response. This may be responsible for a chronic inflammatory reaction leading to resorption of the affected disk and activation of Fas ligand guided apoptosis (*see* Chapter on "Spinal Cord Injury").

PATHOPHYSIOLOGY OF DISK DEGENERATION

A lot of factors take part in degeneration of the disk. The predisposing factors are etiological factors on which molecular and immunologic interactions are superimposed to produce disk degeneration **(Fig. 15)**. Initiation of inflammatory pathway with interleukin-1 (increase innervation and vascularization) and tumor necrosis factors-alpha increase cellular distress and death altering the ECM remodeling.

Loss of Proteoglycan

This is the most significant biochemical change to occur in disk degeneration. The aggrecan molecules become smaller and get leached from the tissue more readily than larger portions. This reduces glycosaminoglycans and water holding capacity and thus there is fall in the osmotic pressure of the disk matrix. The amount of decorin and biglycan is elevated in degenerated human disks to fill the space as compared with normal ones.

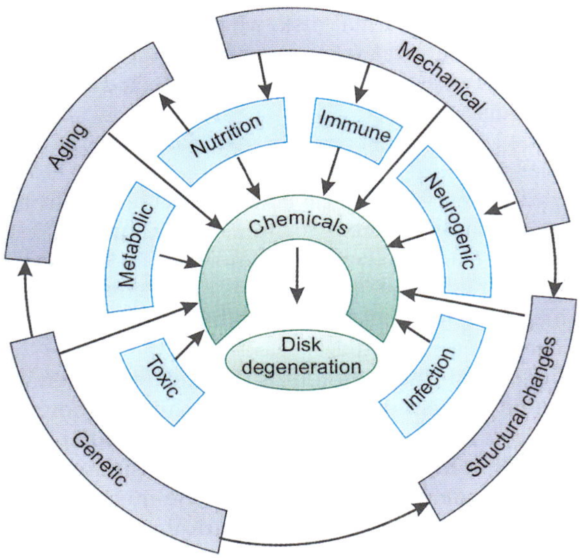

Fig. 15: The pathophysiology of disk degeneration.

Loss of Collagen Fibers

The absolute quantity of collagen does not change much but the types and distribution of collagens get altered. The fibrillar collagens such as type II collagen become more denatured and get replaced by type 1 collagen.

Increase in Fibronectin

Fibronectin content increases with increasing degeneration and it becomes more fragmented. They downregulate aggrecan synthesis and also simultaneously upregulate the production of some MMPs in in vitro systems.

Enzymatic Activity

Increased fragmentation of the collagen, proteoglycan, and fibronectin is mediated by increased enzymatic activity including cathepsins, MMPs, and aggrecanases. Cathepsins have maximal activity in acid conditions (seen in degenerative disks).

FUNCTIONAL CHANGES OF THE DISK DUE TO DEGENERATION

The normal mechanics of the disk **(Fig. 16)** in response to axial compression and shear forces is disrupted due to the molecular disorganization mentioned above, chief among which is the loss of proteoglycans in nucleus pulpous.

Reduced proteoglycan in degenerated disks alters the disk's load-bearing behavior.

- The osmotic pressure of the disk falls → the disk is less able to maintain hydration under load → when loaded they lose height and fluid more rapidly → the disks tend to bulge.
- Loss of hydration → degenerated disks develop nonhydrostatic loads and inappropriate stress concentrations

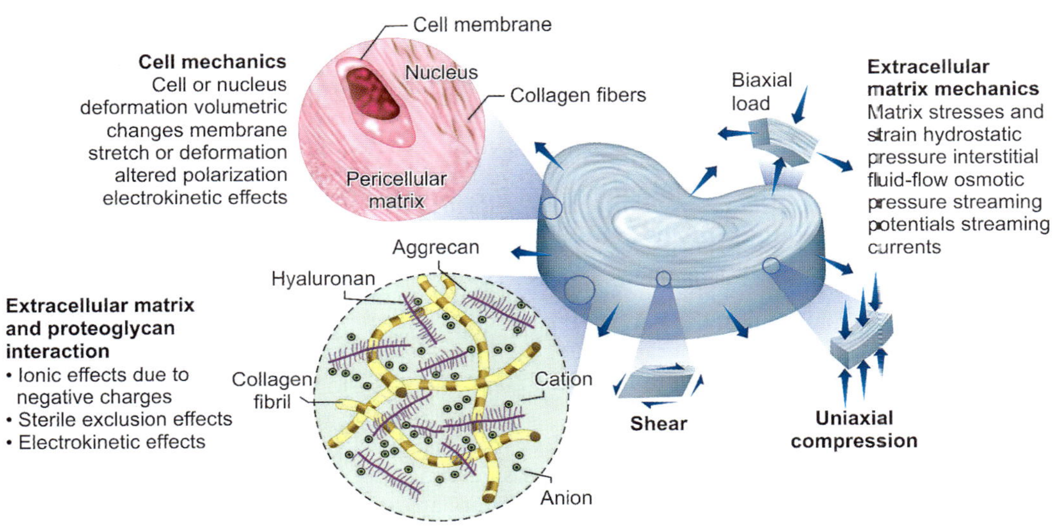

Fig. 16: The normal mechanics of disk under axial compressive loading that induces shearing and tensile stresses on annulus and radial expansion generating hoop stresses. Loading of the intervertebral disk provide mechanical stimuli to the cells. The cell-matrix interactions ultimately determine the biologic response of intervertebral disk to local mechanical events.

along the endplate or in the annulus → annular tear → diskogenic pain produced during diskography

- Rapid loss of disk height under load in degenerate disks → Z-joint osteoarthritis, reduced tensional forces on the ligamentum flavum causing remodeling and thickening → the ligament tends to bulge into the spinal canal → all three leading to spinal stenosis
- Fall in concentration of aggrecan in degeneration → allow increased penetration of large molecules such as growth factor complexes and cytokines into the disk → progression of degeneration
- Aggrecan is an inhibitor of neural growth, its loss hence allows pathological neural ingrowth seen in degenerate disks and hence causing chronic back pain
- Pressure from a disk bulge is asymptomatic in normal individuals but in those with degenerated disks the increased migration of cytokines like PGE2, thromboxane, PLA2, tumor necrosis factor-α, the interleukins (see above), and increased neural density (see above) would predispose to development of pain by sensitizing these new dense nerves in close vicinity. Thus, even slight pressure would be painful in them.

CLASSIFICATION OF PATHOLOGY OF DISK DEGENERATION

The disk lesions can be classified as contained or herniated (*see* Chapter on "Pes Cavus and Accompanying Deformities").

The annular tear is the harbinger of disk degeneration process producing characteristic symptoms. Progression of disk degeneration can be classified as follows:

- *Grade 0:* Normal nonleaking nucleus.
- *Grade 1:* Annular tears confined to the inner region of the annulus fibrosis. In grade 1, a tear or fissure becomes visible extending radially into the inner one-third of the annulus fibrosus—grade 1 radial annular tear, or grade 1 IDD.
- *Grade 2:* The annular tears have completely disrupted the full disk width but do not affect the outer contour of annulus (Sharpey's fibers PLL intact and competent). The entire width of annulus is disrupted but there is no leakage of injected dye on diskography from neither the disk, nor bulging nor protrusion of the disk. This is classified as grade 2 IDD or a grade 2 radial annular tear. The exiting nerve root is not compressed but these patients have lower back pain, which may travel into the lower limb and even past the knee into the lower leg and foot (thermometer pain).
- *Grade 3 (grade 3 IDD or grade 3 radial annular tear):* Tears have completely disrupted the annulus and PLL and there is deformation of the contour of the posterior portion of the disk due to disruption of Sharpey's fibers and PLL. Contrast material leaks out of the back of the disk into the epidural space during diskography. The presence of a disk bulge and/or disk herniation is also included in this category.

Computed Tomography Classification of Annular Tears

The computed tomography (CT) classification of annular tears on axial CT image (modified Dallas classification, **Fig. 17**) is considered gold standard. Bogduk et al. in 1992 modified this classification which has been further modified by Schellhas et al. in 1996.

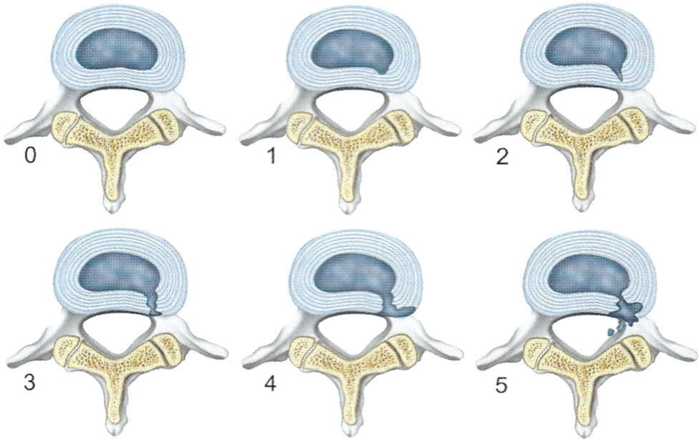

Fig. 17: Modified Dallas classification of annular tears on CT image.

- Grade 0—is a normal disk, where disk has no leak for contrast material from the confines of the nucleus pulposus when, contrast material is injected in the center of the disk.
- Grade 1 tear—when contrast material leaks only into the inner one-third of the annulus.
- Grade 2 tear—when the contrast has leaked from the nucleus into the outer two-thirds of the annulus.
- Grade 3 tear—the contrast completely leaks through all three zones of the annulus. This represents painful tear since the outer one-third of the disk has many tiny nerve fibers that are irritated.
- Grade 4 tear—now the contrast spreads circumferentially around the disk, often resembling a ship's anchor but not into epidural space (PLL intact). The spread of contrast must encompass >30° of the disk circumference to be called grade 4 tear. It represents the merging of a full thickness radial tear with concentric annular tear.
- Grade 5 tear—includes either a grade 3 or grade 4 radial tear + completely ruptured the outer layers of disk. The contrast material leaks from the disk into the epidural space. This tear can induce an inflammatory reaction in the nerve root despite no objective compression and produce radicular pain.

DIAGNOSIS OF INTERNAL DISK DISRUPTION

Provocative Diskography

This has been considered the gold standard in confirming the diagnosis of diskogenic pain (it is considered that spinal instability may be a better marker; *see* also Chapter on "Nonsurgical Interventional Techniques for Management of Back Pain"). "Provocation diskography" (painful invasive test) should be followed up with CT diskogram. Diskography should only be used as a confirmatory test to evaluate a vertebral level in question and should not be used as a screening tool because of high false-negative test results. There are two components of provocation diskography and both are important to make a definitive diagnosis.

- Provoke the concordant pain (awake patient) by pressurizing the disk with a contrast material

- The second is a painless diskogram in the adjacent disks—it is as important to demonstrating pain in the pathological disk else if pain is present even in the normal disks, then there are high chances of a false positive test

Results are interpreted according to the disk injection pressure, volume of fluid accepted by the disk, the pattern of contrast distribution in the injected disk **(Fig. 18)** and the subjective pain response to the injection compared with the patient's typical symptoms. Criteria for diagnosing IDD (The International Society for the Study of Pain):

- No visible disk herniations seen on MRI or CT
- During provocation diskography injection of the suspected disk, recreation of the patients' exact back, and/or leg pain must occur
- Injection of the disk above or below the suspect disk must be nonpainful, and this acts as a control disk or normal disk
- A grade 3 or 4 radial annular fissure must be demonstrated on CT diskography

Cons of diskography—it is invasive and painful but the biggest concern is a possible spread of the tear and further damage to the disk.

Confounding factors in interpretation of results of diskography:

- Asymptomatic patients who have had a prior diskectomy have the same risk of diskography-induced pain at the diskectomy site as are patients with LBP who undergo diskography at a previous diskectomy site
- High injection pressure has been implicated in false-positive diskography results. However, even in asymptomatic patients receiving low-pressure (22 psi) diskography, a 25% incidence of painful injection has been reported.

Discogram type		Stage of disc degeneration
1. Cottonball	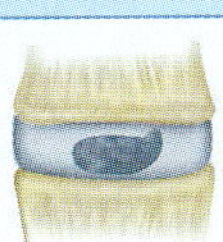	No signs of degeneration. Soft white amorphous nucleus
2. Lobular	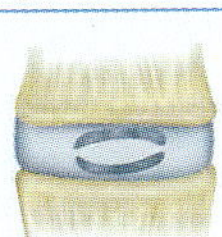	Mature disc with nucleus starting to coalesce into fibrous lumps
3. Irregular	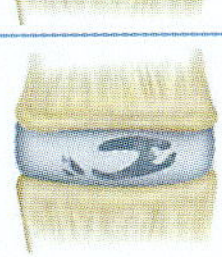	Degenerated disc with fissures and clefts in the nucleus and inner annulus
4. Fissured	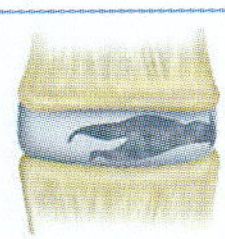	Degenerated disc with radial fissure leading to the outer edge of the annulus
5. Ruptured	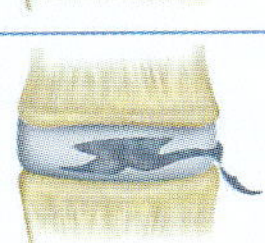	Disc has a complete radial fissure that allows injected fluid to escape. Can be in any state of degeneration

Fig. 18: Classification of disk degeneration produced by diskography.

- The correlation of future development of LBP in positive diskography test as was previously thought is poor as even after 4 years of positive diskography in asymptomatic volunteers there was no significant complain of back pain over general population.

Gadolinium-DTPA-enhanced MRI

The gadolinium (gadolinium dimethoxypropane, contrast) increases visibility of the granulation tissue that forms within a healing/healed full thickness annular disk tear.

Hyperintensity Zone

A hyperintensity zone is a focal high-intensity signal in the posterior annulus fibrosis distinct from the nucleus without disk protrusion (referred to represent annular tear). This phenomenon also gives another clue that IDD might be involved in the patient's pain syndrome although considered important by many, but some do not pay much importance to this finding and merely treat it more corroborative than diagnostic.

TREATMENT OF DISKOGENIC PAIN

Conservative management is the basis of management of patients and is effective in 90% of patients. One should be tolerant enough for the modalities to take effect and trial up to 3–6 months may be given (unless symptoms keep increasing or are too severe to start with). For nonresponsive patients or those with too severe symptoms that fail to subside by conservative means following strategies are described:

- Total disk excision and arthrodesis—preferred by orthopedic surgeons (*see below* Lumbar Disk Degeneration)
- Total disk replacement (*see below* Lumbar Disk Degeneration)
- Dynamic stabilization systems (*see below* Lumbar Disk Degeneration)
- More conservative measures—preferred by pain physicians. This group includes following methods:
  - *Annuloplasty:*
    - Intradiskal electrothermal therapy IDET (*see* Chapter on "Failed Back Surgery Syndrome")
    - Radiofrequency posterior annuloplasty
    - Biacuplasty
  - Percutaneous disk decompression
  - Laser diskectomy
  - Radiofrequency coblation (plasma diskectomy)
  - Mechanical disk decompression
  - Manual percutaneous lumbar diskectomy
- Endoscopic percutaneous diskectomy
- *Chemonucleosis:*
  - Enzyme-based
  - Ozone-based

CHEMONUCLEOLYSIS

Chymopapain was derived from the papaya by Jansen and Balls. Thomas demonstrated the softening of the cartilaginous material in the ear (rabbit) due to the chymopapain.

Smith et al. tried to find the use of the enzyme to treat chondroblastic tumors, but failed. His experiments, however, did show that when injected into the intradiskal space of rabbits the nucleus pulposus disappeared (annulus remained intact) so in 1963, Smith injected the first human patient with chymopapain to treat sciatica. Chymopapain primarily depolymerizes the proteoglycan and glycoprotein molecules in the nucleus pulposus reducing the water content within the disk and disk shrinkage follows. The bulging disk, therefore, shrinks. Chymopapain has been in use for >30 years. After approval by the United States Food and Drug Administration (US FDA), in 1982, early complications were reported but overall the procedure had been reasonably safe. Indications for chymopapain include patients unwilling for surgery:

- Who present with radicular pain as the chief complaint
- Confirmation of the contained disk herniation via MRI, CT, or myelogram
- Patients having failed conservative treatment

Procedure

- The patient is placed in either a lateral or a prone position and under fluoroscopy, a 6-inch, 18-gauge needle is inserted posterolaterally and placed centrally within the disk **(Fig. 19)**.
- Diskography (pain provocation) is performed for evaluation of the affected disk.
- Chymopapain is then injected into the nucleus pulposus (1,000–4,000 U). The number of units injected decreases if more than one disk is to be treated (to maintain the maximum total dose).

Complications

- Anaphylaxis, reported in 1% of cases, proved to be the most severe complication. This can be avoided by good patient selection, proper surgical training and technique, preoperative hypersensitivity testing and antihistamine administration.

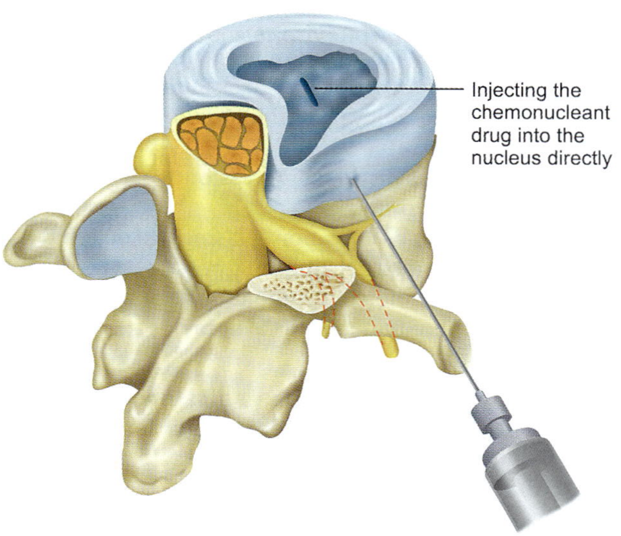

Fig. 19: Chemonucleolysis procedure.

- Chemical neuritis
- Infection
- Chemical diskitis

Determinants of good outcome with chemonucleolysis:

- Patients with moderate-to-severe positive straight leg raise had a significantly higher success rate as compared to those with no or mild straight leg raising pain.
- The younger the patient, the better the outcome.
- Those patients in whom the pain provocation test was positive had a 91.7% success rate compared to those who did not experience pain provocation (73.1% success rate).

Ozone Chemonucleolysis

It gained popularity in Europe for the treatment of herniated IVDs. This therapy was developed by C Verga in 1983. Verga stated that the relapse of pain occurred in <2% of cases (over 15 years of experience). The method involves the administration of 40/60 mL of ozone gas (O_2-O_3 mixture) at a concentration of 20/30 micrograms per mL, repeated 8–14 times. The injection is generally made into the paravertebral musculature, and in the hernia zone and is generally painless and well-tolerated. The results of Verga have not been decisively reproduced and controversy remains over its real efficacy.

RADIOFREQUENCY ANNULOPLASTY

This is a minimally invasive method of delivering radiofrequency thermal energy to the disk to treat diskogenic lower back pain. Ideal candidates for this procedure are patients with IDD grade 3/4/5 as per CT classification (see above) with chronic LBP. The procedure is typically performed on an outpatient basis in a clinical setting under mild sedation and local anesthesia. Under fluoroscopy guidance the diskTRODE™ (Valleylab, Boulder, CO, USA) cannula is inserted into an IVD. The radiofrequency catheter electrode is passed into the outer disk tissue **(Fig. 20)** and tissue adjacent to electrode is heated to a specific treatment temperature. Complications of this procedure include catheter breakage, nerve root injuries, diskitis, disk herniation, cauda equina syndrome, infection, epidural abscess, and spinal cord damage.

Biacuplasty

The intradiskal biacuplasty utilizes a bipolar system that includes two cooled radiofrequency electrodes placed on

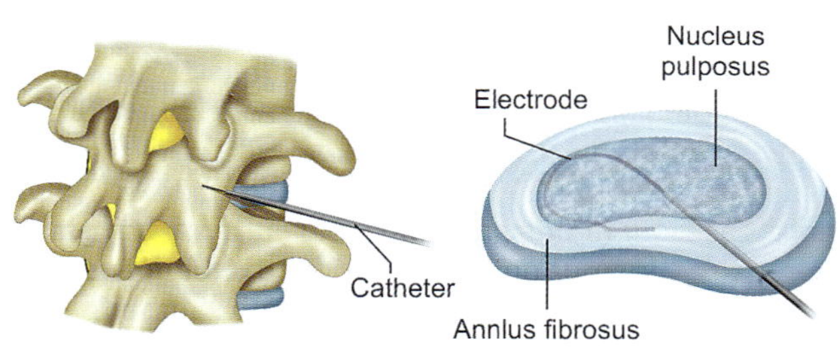

Fig. 20: The technique of radiofrequency annuloplasty. The electrode is inserted posterolaterally in the posterior annulus.

the posterolateral sides of the intervertebral annulus fibrosus. The radiofrequency probes are positioned through two introducers bilaterally to create a bipolar configuration and temperature is gradually increased to 55°C for over 11 minutes. Further studies are needed to determine the efficacy, complication rates, and possible comparative advantages of this procedure with other minimally invasive procedures for disk lesions.

PERCUTANEOUS DISK DECOMPRESSION

Laser Diskectomy

Ascher, Choy et al. published the use of a neodymium:yttrium-aluminum-garnet (Nd:YAG) laser on the lumbar spine for nucleolysis. Holmium:yttrium- aluminum-garnet (Ho:YAG) laser is most commonly used (potassium-titanyl-phosphate laser is also used but not as popular) as it can be paired with the endoscope for disk ablation and removal capabilities. Combining with endoscope allows two advantages:

- *Ablation:* As the affected tissues absorb the laser, light is converted to heat. At 100°C, tissue vaporizes and ablation takes place. As a small amount of nucleus pulposus is vaporized, intradiskal pressure decreases, allowing the disk to return to its normal state.
- *Disk removal:* If any disk material needs to be removed, endoscopic tools can be used to do so.

Best candidates for laser diskectomy include those with back and leg pain with a confirmed disk herniation.

Procedure

With the patient prone or in lateral position under conscious sedation a guiding needle is introduced through "triangular safe zone" (just anterior to the superior articular process and superior to the transverse process) under fluoroscopy guidance **(Fig. 21)**. The needle is placed 1 cm beyond the annulus into the nucleus pulposus just parallel to the disk axis half-way between the superior and inferior endplates. The Ho:YAG laser is pulse-fired. Side-firing capabilities provide more control of laser placement and reduce the risk of injury to several areas, especially those anterior to the spinal column. Smaller fragments can be removed through endoscope while larger fragments are laser ablated.

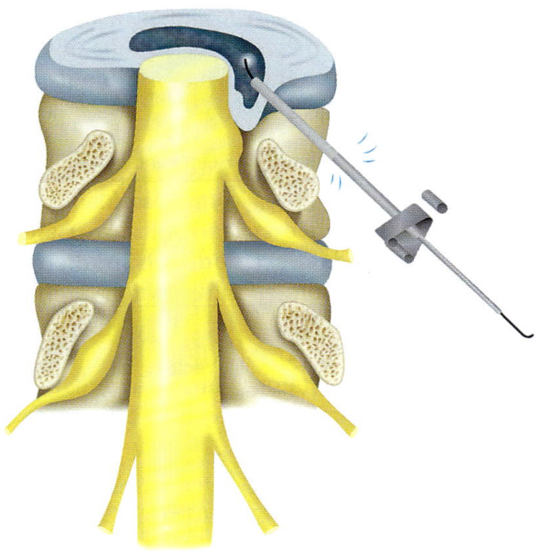

Fig. 21: Illustration of laser percutaneous disk decompression (see text for details).

Newer transforaminal procedures can treat those patients with fragments in the epidural space. There is a scarcity of clinical trials regarding percutaneous lasers.

Cons of Laser Diskectomy

- Steep learning curve
- Difficult technique especially the concurrent use of endoscope
- No long-term, large-scale support to the technique

Radiofrequency Coblation (Plasma Diskectomy)

Radiofrequency coblation (plasma diskectomy) was first was performed in 2000. It combines disk removal and thermal coagulation to decompress a contained herniated disk. After diskogram confirmation the nucleus pulposus is first ablated with radiofrequency waves as the wand is advanced. The tissue gets converted into gas, which is removed through the needle. As the wand is withdrawn, coagulation takes place thermally closing and denaturing collagen along the channel ablating the nerve fibers along in the process. This process is repeated up to six times within an individual disk. Patients with spinal stenosis and those with a loss of disk height of 50%, severe disk degeneration, spinal fracture, or tumor should be excluded.

Mechanical Disk Decompression

Dekompressor is a disposable, self-contained, battery operated handpiece connected to a helical probe which was introduced in 2002. It has one outer cannula (measures 1.5 mm), an inner rotating probe and a suction chamber at the base of the handheld unit. The inner probe during rotation creates suction which pulls milled nucleus pulposus from the disk up to the suction chamber at the base of the handheld unit. It can remove approximately 0.5–2 cc of nucleus pulposus. Total procedure time takes approximately 30 minutes where actual time of the probe being used is about 10 minutes. This procedure is usually performed under fluoroscopic guidance. Percutaneous diskectomy has a reported success rate of 60–87% but needs to be studied on a larger basis.

Manual Percutaneous Lumbar Diskectomies

Percutaneous lumbar diskectomies have always remained contentious for >30 years with results ranging from disappointing to good. The procedure includes use of 3–5 mm cannulas from the posterolateral approach, curettes, and time-consuming manual removal of the nucleus pulposus with pituitary forceps. It is primarily a decompressive surgery aimed to reduce irritation of the nerve root and the nociceptive nerve receptors in the annulus. Development of a new and smaller type of aspiration probe by Onik et al. in 1985 reduced risk of injury to the peripheral nerves and the annulus, facilitated easier removal of the nucleus pulposus and decreased surgical time.

Percutaneous Endoscopic Diskectomy

Pool introduced the concept of intrathecal endoscopy and reported the outcomes of >400 myeloscopic procedures but complication rates were high. Percutaneous nucleotomy by means of arthroscopy instruments for disk removal for the treatment of posterior or posterolateral lumbar disk herniation under local anesthesia was demonstrated by Hijikata et al. in 1975. Kambin described the safe triangular working zone (Kambin's triangle) of arthroscopic microdiskectomy. This technique is based on arthroscopic visualization of the herniation via the posterolateral approach for diskectomy of contained herniations. Onik et al. reported the use of a 2-mm blunt-tipped automated percutaneous suction cutting probe for transforaminal endoscopic microdiskectomy **(Fig. 22)**.

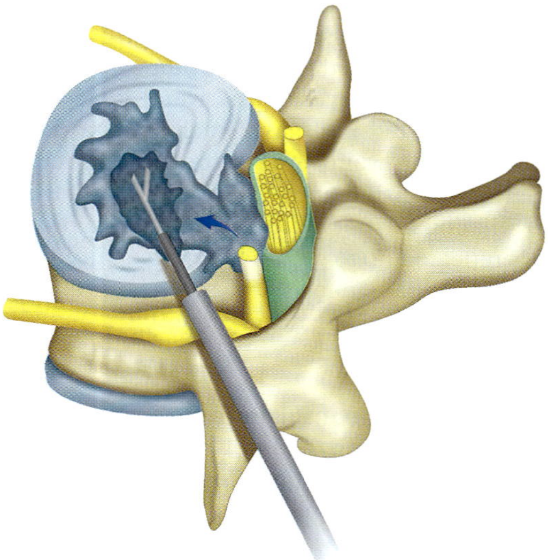

Fig. 22: Transforaminal endoscopic diskectomy.

It is performed through epidural endoscopy (*see* Chapter on "Failed Back Surgery Syndrome"). There is direct visualization of the epidural space, the pathology, and neuroanatomic structures. Closed decompression of spinal roots with lasers, epidural biopsies, percutaneous interbody fusion, and lysis of epidural adhesions are now possible. Ideal patient for this procedure is one who has paramedian, foraminal, or extraforaminal contained herniation, or one that is noncontained at <50% of the canal diameter.

GENE THERAPY/CELL-BASED THERAPIES

These are therapies to achieve repair of the degenerated disk matrix. The following approaches are under consideration:

- One approach has been to stimulate the disk cells to produce more matrices. Growth factors can increase rates of matrix synthesis by up to fivefold. These proteins have thus provided targets for genetic engineering. Direct injection of growth factors (TGF-β and BMP-7) or cytokine inhibitors (TIMM) has but proved unsuccessful because their effectiveness in the disk is short-lived.
- To obtain sustained improvement in matrix regeneration gene therapy is now under investigation. In this in vivo method, the gene-vector complex is directly injected into the target tissue producing the requisite growth factor **(Fig. 23A)**. The ex vivo strategy **(Fig. 23B)** differs significantly as the targeted cells are isolated and removed from the living host. These cells are then cultured with transduction of the therapeutic gene occurring in vitro. The final step includes the reimplantation of the genetically altered cells back into the host. Due to harsh conditions of the nucleus pulposus (low pH, low oxygen tension, etc.) the cells in ex vivo therapy get altered when cultured in vitro for transduction and when transplanted may not function well. The in vivo method is thus more popular. It has the potential to maintain high levels of the relevant growth factor or inhibitor in the tissue. The details of therapy are dealt with in Chapter on "Gene Therapy in Orthopedics". The gene transfer techniques

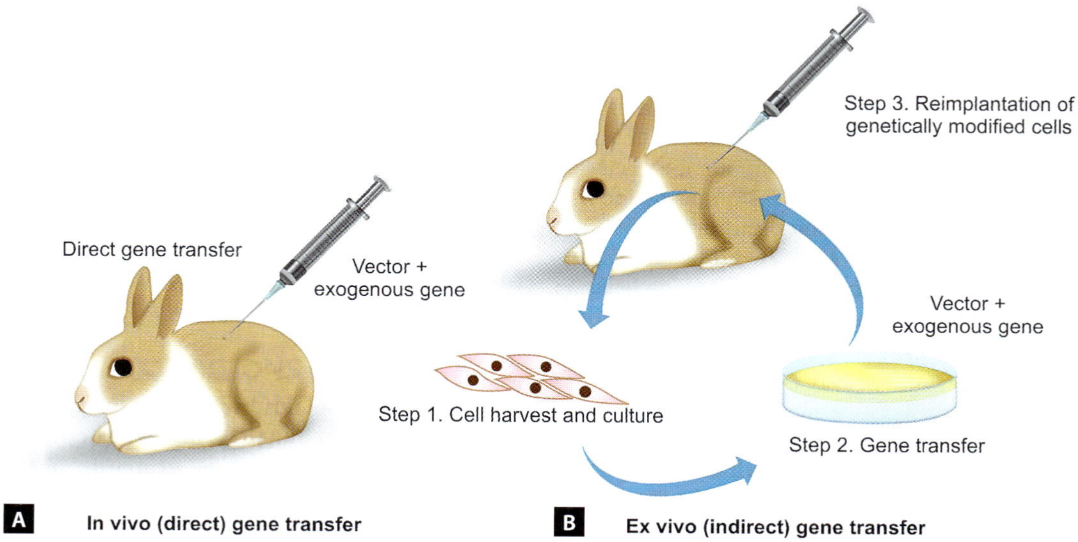

Figs. 23A and B: In vivo and ex vivo gene therapy.

using adenovirus have been employed to increasing TGF-β1 production by disk cells in animals to improve proteoglycan production. Other target genes have been identified for increasing local production of IGF-1, BMP-2, and TIMP-1 that have been successfully utilized following the use of TGF-β gene therapy. Two other potentially disease altering genes being investigated include LIM mineralization protein (LMP-1) and Sox-9. LMP-1 is a regulatory protein that upregulates the anabolic activity of bone morphogenic proteins (BMP) in the disk. Sox-9 is a transcription factor which has many responsibilities including type II collagen expression, an essential component of the nucleus pulposus ECM. Human IVD cells treated with adenoviral vector Sox-9 complex in vitro showed increase type II collagen production compared with controls. However, at present this therapy has limited clinical use because correct choice of therapeutic genes further requires improved understanding of the pathogenesis of degeneration. One more limiting factor is the cell density of normal human disks which is low, and many of the cells in degenerate disks are dead.

- Cell implantation alone or in conjunction with gene therapy is an approach that may overcome above difficulty. In this approach, the cells of the degenerated disk are supplemented by adding new cells [mesenchymal stem cells (MSCs) either on their own or together with an appropriate scaffold (as used for articular cartilage)]. There are two problems to this approach:
    - There is no obvious source of clinically useful cells for the human disk, particularly for the nucleus, the region of most interest.
    - There is obvious nutrient compromise in the disk and milieu change that is hostile for cell growth.
- Culturing MSCs with nucleus pulposus cells in a coculture system, allowing for cell-to-cell contact is another approach. Cell-to-cell contact stimulates MSCs to differentiate toward a chondrocytic lineage, ameliorating the need for predifferentiation in vitro. There is increased mRNA expression of type-II collagen and aggrecan in co-cultured cells. Cells also aggregate to form three-dimensional micromasses expressing collagen-2, aggrecan, and Sox-9 at RNA and protein levels. Adipose-derived stem cells (ADSCs) are also able to differentiate into nucleus pulposus cells.

    Embryonic stem cells (ESC)-based regeneration for use in human IDD/DDD is in progress. ESCs may be useful for repairing IDD as evidenced by their ability to differentiate into a chondrocytic lineage and yield notochordal-type cells in IDD models, but clinical use is undefined.
- *Regulation of pathologic gene expression:* This method alters the genetic information flow in the cells. Ribonucleic acid interference (RNAi) reduces the overall production of a targeted gene product by the use of small interfering RNA (siRNA) which binds to the targeted mRNA in a sequence specific manner leading to either suppressed translation or enhanced degradation of the message. Thus, catabolic genes within the disk tissue can be targeted and silenced through siRNA-mediated destruction preventing translation of those genes. Expression of firefly luciferase has been inhibited 93.7% in human nucleus pulposus cells cultured in vitro that was treated with siRNA targeting this gene. However, this inhibitory effect was gone 3 weeks after initial treatment.

AUGMENTATION OF NUCLEUS PULPOSUS/ NUCLEUS REPLACEMENT

Nucleus replacement therapy aims to replace the IVD nucleus while preserving the annulus and vertebral endplates. This would prevent disk height loss and the associated biomechanical and biochemical changes. Additionally, this can be done in minimally invasive manner. Two indications for nucleus replacement have been considered.

- Replacement of the nucleus following microdiskectomy surgery
- For the treatment of DDD

The greatest concern is that in an IDD annulus is additionally disrupted that will not be addressed by nucleus replacement.

Historically, various materials have been tried to replace the nucleus of the IVD like polymethylmethacrylate (PMMA), polyvinyl alcohol/polyvinylpyrrolidone copolymer, polycarbonate urethane, albumin, silicon, and stainless steel. The mechanical devices have fallen out of favor. Newer elastomeric devices made of hydrogel or a nonhydrogel substance, and are available in "injectable" (free-flowing, **Fig. 24A**) or "preformed" shapes. Prosthetic disk nucleus (PDN) developed by Ray consists of a predefined geometry core enclosed in a polyethylene cover. This has been used as an adjunct to disk surgery following removal of the nucleus in cases of disk herniation. The free-flowing materials may be injected via a small incision, allowing minimally invasive access to the disk space **(Figs. 24A and B)**. Fluids can further interdigitate with the irregular surgical defects and may even physically bind to the adjacent tissue. Injectable biomaterials (copolymer consisting of amino acid sequence blocks) allow for incorporation and uniform dispersion of cells and/or therapeutic agents (recombinant protein). NuCore™ injectable nucleus developed by Spine Wave (Shelton, CT, USA) consists of a solution of the protein polymer and a polyfunctional cross-linking agent. This nucleus material closely mimics the protein content, water content, pH, mechanical properties, and complex modulus of the natural nucleus pulposus. It is a nontoxic and biocompatible material which is able to restore the biomechanics of the disk following microdiskectomy. Clinical evaluation trial on human is under way in a multicenter clinical study.

REGENERATION OF THE CARTILAGE ENDPLATE

This is a new focus area due to stress on nutritional factors for IDD/DDD. Methods for repair and regeneration of the cartilage endplate are being explored to restore the endplates as closely as possible to their natural state prior to disease or degeneration. Endplate therapy is a potential means of

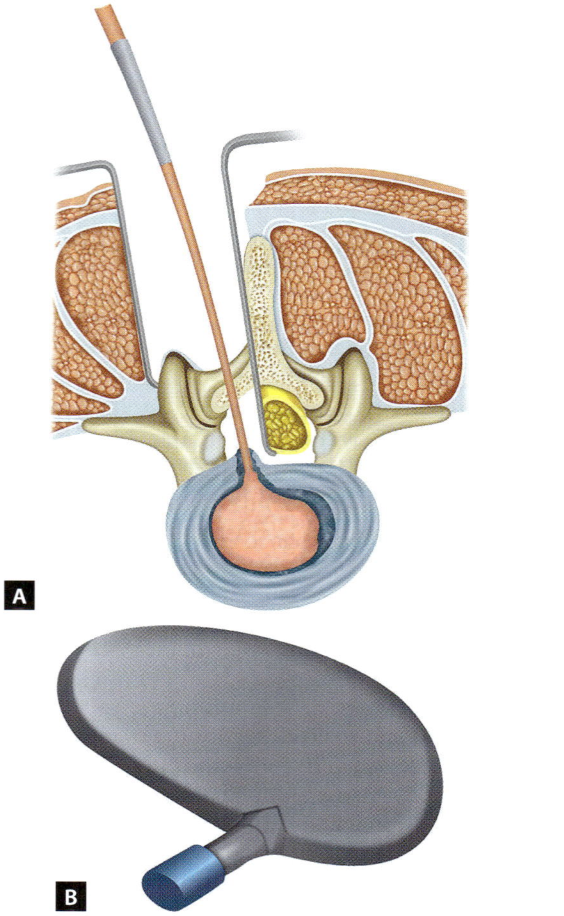

Figs. 24A and B: Nucleus pulposus replacement. (A) The injectable free flowing form; (B) Preformed shapes for replacement.

enhancing biomaterial integration and cell survival but is a far-fetched concept currently.

LUMBAR SPONDYLOSIS AND LUMBAR DEGENERATIVE DISK DISEASE

INTRODUCTION

The pathoanatomy, pathomechanics, and pathophysiology of disk degeneration have been already covered previously in detail. Here we will review the clinical and surgical management aspects.

EPIDEMIOLOGY

Degenerative changes in the lumbar spine occur in most of the population. It is also estimated that 80% of the United States population will experience LBP. However, only 7% of individuals with LBP have symptoms that last longer than 2 weeks; of these individuals, only 1% will require long-term treatment.

CLINICAL FEATURES

As already discussed, diskogenic back pain refers to a pain syndrome that originates from a lumbar disk, presenting as LBP without concomitant radicular symptoms. Diskogenic pain syndromes have been divided into two separate categories:

- *Internal disk disruption:* The plain radiographs are normal but disk space changes are seen. The pathology promulgates as annular tears and "dark disk disease" that are detectable on MRI scans. Symptoms associated with IDD include deep, midline, low lumbar, and aching pain. The pain is exacerbated by bending and rising from sitting and does not resolve with rest. Nonradicular leg pain is another presentation that can present similarly.
- *Degenerative disk disease:* This encompasses lumbar spondylosis and isolated disk resorption. The degenerative changes are detectable on plain radiographs and typically include **(Fig. 25)**:
  - Disk space narrowing
  - End-plate sclerosis
  - Osteophyte formation

Degenerative disk disease presents with midline back pain and referred pain over the sacroiliac joints and posterior thighs. Buttock and posterior thigh aching with ambulation is common, but this pain does not radiate below the knee and should be differentiated from neurogenic claudication.

Lumbar range of motion is consistently painful for patients with diskogenic back pain. Nonorganic causes of back pain should be specifically evaluated (Waddell signs). The association of LBP has been found significantly with:

- Disk space narrowing
- Radial disk fissures
- Disk prolapse
- Disk signal intensity change on MRI has minimal relationship to pain, if any

DIAGNOSTIC IMAGING

Plain radiographs may be normal in IDD (except some reduction in disk space). In DDD, the radiographs show:

- Variable degrees of spondylosis
- Including disk space collapse
- End-plate sclerosis
- Marginal osteophytes
- Facet hypertrophy

Segmental instability **(Box 1)** should be evaluated on lateral projection flexion-extension films.

Magnetic resonance imaging: This has emerged as important modality to evaluate degenerative changes in disk, though the findings have still not reached a prominent diagnostic value vis-à-vis patient symptoms. The sensitivity of investigation is high but specificity is low. The significance of MRI findings has not been fully elucidated.

- High-intensity zones detected in the annulus fibrosus on T2-weighted MRI scans are thought to (but highly controversial for diagnosis, see below also) represent annular tears consistent with IDD (see above also).
- Loss of normal disk signal and the presence of dark disks represent loss of disk hydration and early degeneration (poor correlation with symptoms), similar changes have been shown to be present in up to 57% of asymptomatic volunteers.

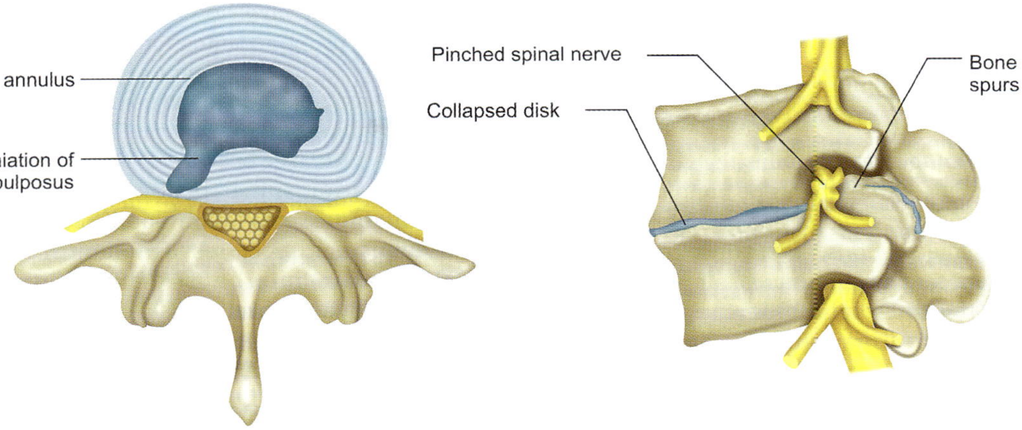

Fig. 25: Illustration of changes in the spinal segment in patients with degenerative disk disease and consequent neural irritation.

BOX 1: Radiographic criteria for spine instability.

Resting radiographs:
- Sagittal displacement >4.5 mm or 15%
- Relative sagittal plane angulation >22°

or

Flexion-extension radiographs:
- Sagittal displacement >4.5 mm or 15%
- Relative sagittal plane rotation

>15° at L1–2, L2–3, L3–4
>20° at L4–5
>25° at L5/S1

TABLE 4: Modic classification of degenerative end-plate and vertebral body MRI changes.

Stage	*Endplate*	*Vertebral body*
Type I	T1 = Decreased signal	T1 = Decreased signal
	T2 = Increased signal	T2 = Increased signal
Type II	T1 = Increased signal	T1 = Increased signal
	T2 = Isointense to mild hyperintense	T2 = Isointense to mild hyperintense
Type III	T1 = Decreased signal	T1 = Decreased signal
	T2 = Decreased signal	T2 = Decreased signal

- Degenerative progression of the vertebral body and end-plate as seen on MRI scans are now referred to as Modic changes **(Table 4)**.
  - Type I Modic changes reflect acute vertebral body and end-plate inflammation.
  - Type II Modic changes represent chronic changes (including end-plate disruption and fatty degeneration of the adjacent vertebral body).
  - Type III changes correlate with end-plate sclerosis and loss of vertebral cancellous bone.

Provocative diskography is often used to evaluate diskogenic LBP (see above). Positive test (i.e., high likelihood of diskogenic back pain) is considered if it demonstrates annular disruption, reproduces the patient's symptoms (concordant pain), and the control levels are negative.

DIAGNOSIS

There are a lot of controversies in labeling the disk as prime pain generator:

- As mentioned previously also; the clinical implications of Modic changes and HIZ lesions have not been fully elucidated.
  - One study reported no difference in the prevalence of HIZ lesion in patients with LBP and asymptomatic controls.
  - Another study found that patients with LBP had a higher incidence of HIZ lesions compared with asymptomatic control subjects.
- Disk segments with HIZ lesions were more consistently positive on provocative diskography in patients with LBP but the same is also true of asymptomatic control group.
  - 50% of disks with an HIZ lesion were positive on diskography among patients with normal psychometric testing, whereas 100% of disks with an HIZ lesion were diskography-positive in patients with abnormal psychometric testing or chronic pain.
  - The high prevalence of HIZ lesions in asymptomatic individuals (25%) and the similar percentage of asymptomatic and symptomatic patients with a diskography-positive segment with an HIZ lesion suggest that HIZ lesion does not reliably indicate the presence of symptomatic IDD.
- The validity of provocative diskography remains unproven because there is no current gold standard to which diskography can be compared. The only method is to compare the clinical results following spinal fusion of diskography positive levels. Interestingly multiple studies have demonstrated low clinical success of spinal fusion to relieve LBP.
- The psychometric profiles strongly and independently predicted the development of LBP.
- Segmental instability as demonstrated by radiographs **(Box 1)** possibly better guides the intervention in symptomatic patients.

So, in a nutshell annular fissures and HIZ lesions were weakly predictive of LBP and routine use of diskography for diagnosis heralding intervention is uncertain. Consequently, diskography remains controversial and should be used only as an adjunct in the assessment of patients with LBP.

TREATMENT

Nonsurgical management remains the cornerstone for the treatment of LBP as >90% patients respond to it. It comprises of a multidisciplinary approach including education, rehabilitation, medications, and injections. The "back school" program may help in increasing awareness but has not been shown to prevent LBP. Exercise therapy appears to be effective for decreasing pain and improving function in adults with chronic LBP but may not be effective for acute LBP. TENS and topical magnets are no better than placebo. Traction has no definite indication or demonstrable benefit in treating LBP while it may be associated with increased morbidity. NSAIDs are effective in treating acute LBP; however, chronic NSAID use is associated with hepatic dysfunction, gastric ulceration, and hemorrhage. Selective COX-2 inhibitors limit most of these adverse effects, but have been found to provoke cardiovascular complications. Narcotics and muscle relaxants should be rationalized for use in acute LBP because of associated addictive and central nervous system (CNS) adverse effects.

- Facet joint injections and medial branch nerve blocks have also demonstrated short-term relief for chronic LBP.
- Facet denervation by radiofrequency dorsal neurotomy has demonstrated variable results.
- Intradiskal electrothermal therapy (IDET) utility is limited as the benefits recently demonstrated are no better than placebo when treating symptomatic disk degeneration confirmed by CT diskography.
- Other measures are discussed in detail above.

The "**surgical measures**" (typically fusion) are indicated if there is:

- Failure of aggressive conservative treatment
- Prolonged chronic pain, disability for >1 year
- Advanced disk degeneration as identified on MRI limited to one or two disk levels

The surgical methods commonly used for management of diskogenic LBP include:

- *Fusion (arthrodesis):* Spinal fusion has been practiced since the beginning of the 20th century and was mainly used for spinal deformities and infections in particular in spinal tuberculosis cases (Pott's disease) with vertebral collapse and kyphosis. Fusion is the most commonly performed spinal operation. As of date given the debatable efficacy of spinal fusion and its possible implication in the degeneration of the adjacent segments, various nonfusion techniques are being developed.
- Artificial TDR
- Dynamic stabilization

Lumbar Fusion Techniques

The rationale of fusion is to stabilize the motion segment and eliminate the progression of disk degeneration and relative pathological motion between vertebrae to relieve pain. Spinal fusion involves the use of bone tissue, classically achieved using an autograft (e.g., iliac crest or lamina), to bridge two or more vertebrae. Alternatives to autologous bone grafts have been developed consisting of the use of allografts, demineralized bone matrix (DBM), ceramics, and more recently BMP (see below).

- Posterior spinal fusion *aka* posterolateral fusion/intertransverse fusion—applying bone graft between the transverse processes of the lumbar vertebrae.
- Lumbar interbody fusion—advocated for more effective removal of diskogenic pain generators, greater elimination of painful disk space motion, and greater fusion rates compared with posterior spinal fusion alone.
  - *Anterior lumbar interbody fusion (ALIF):* This is the oldest method used since thirties of last century. The spine is approached anteriorly for removal of pathological disk and fusion **(Fig. 26)**. It involves minimal or no posterior muscle dissection when performed in isolation. ALIF removes large portion of the annulus and ALL and there is better restoration of the disk height compared to posterior lumbar interbody fusion (PLIF). It also has reduced surgical time and favors load transmission due to graft location. The problem is that when used in isolation (standalone procedure) the complication rates are high including high nonunion rate up to 30%, revision rate and overall complication rate. Additional concerns are with relation to surgical procedure—vessel damage (2–5% incidence), retrograde ejaculation (0.5–1% incidence), and difficulty of a repeat anterior approach if revision is necessary. Newer ALIF techniques using cylindrical cages and BMP have shown good results.
  - *Posterior lumbar interbody fusion:* It was popularized by Cloward, this is the most popular technique. Obviates the need for an anterior approach. Consists of inserting a cage filled with bone graft or bone substitutes, within the allowable disk space clearance

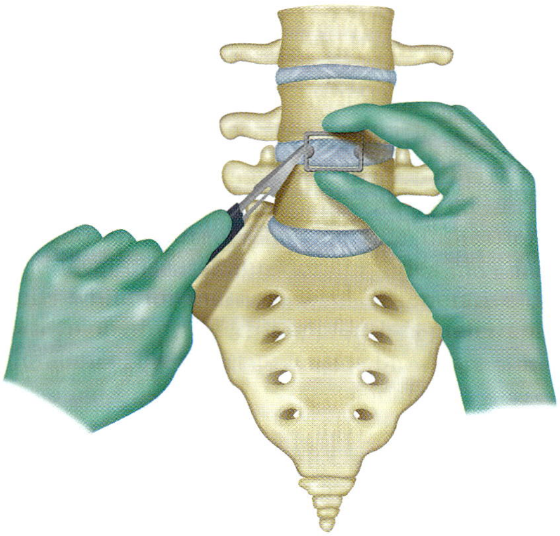

Fig. 26: Anterior lumbar interbody fusion. The graft is placed in the involved segment anteriorly through a retroperitoneal approach.

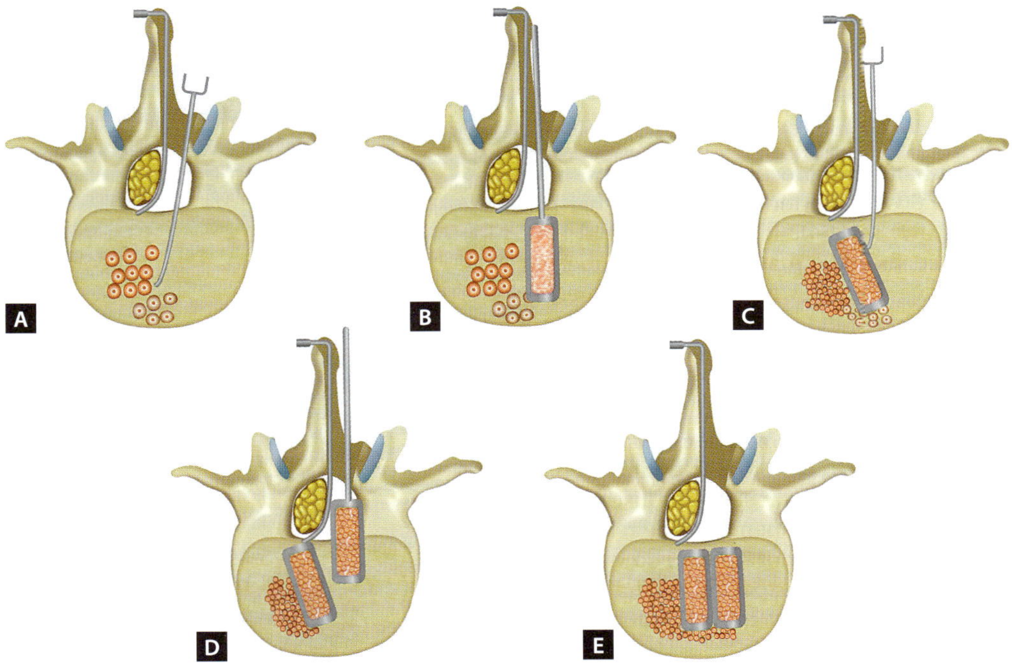

Figs. 27A to E: Posterior lumbar interbody fusion using unilateral approach.

with the addition of pedicle instrumentation **(Figs. 27A to E)**. Early experience with PLIF indicated good results but flip side includes increased need for neural element manipulation, high rates of cage subsidence, cage migration and retropulsion, bleeding, subsequent scar formation within the spinal canal. There is an increased pseudoarthrosis rate when PLIF is not supplemented with posterior instrumentation.

- *Transforaminal lumbar interbody fusion (TLIF):* This popularized by Harms and Rolinger, obviates the need for an anterior approach, like PLIF. Additionally, it has the advantage of avoiding exposure of the spinal canal since the cage is introduced unilaterally through the intervertebral foramen **(Fig. 28)**. TLIF thus includes the advantages of a posterior approach, but less neural retraction is required than for PLIF. There is increased stability when TLIF is combined with posterior instrumentation.
- Extreme lateral approaches
- Circumferential fusion

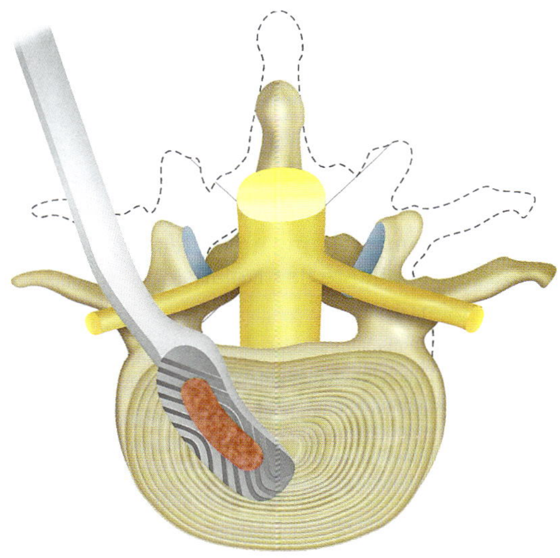

Fig. 28: Transforaminal lumbar interbody fusion. The graft or cage is pushed through intervertebral foramen of each side.

Combined Techniques

Role of Bone Morphogenic Protein

In an effort to improve lumbar fusion rates and reduce donor morbidity recombinant human BMP (rhBMP) as a substitute for autogenous iliac rest bone graft has been popularized. The two current US FDA approved applications for rhBMP in the spine include:

1. rhBMP-2 carried on a type I collagen sponge in conjunction with a tapered, threaded ALIF cage for the treatment of degenerative lumbar disk disease
2. rhBMP-7 as a humanitarian device exemption in the posterolateral lumbar spine for established nonunions or for patients at high risk for nonunion

Clinical outcome following lumbar fusion for diskogenic LBP has been variable. While the Swedish Lumbar Spine Study Group reported superior outcomes for pain, disability, depressive symptoms, and return to work among patients treated with lumbar fusion other studies have demonstrated 40–70% satisfactory clinical outcomes, despite 60–90% radiographically demonstrated solid arthrodesis.

Artificial Total Disk Replacement

In this procedure, the biological injured or degenerated disk material is removed and an artificial disk is implanted in the spine. Total disk replacement (TDR) technology is not totally new and first attempts were made in the1950s using the Fernstrom steel-ball endoprosthesis. Attempts have been made since the 50s to produce an implant that can mimic (at least partially) the function of the normal IVD. The technology has been used for many years in Europe, but is still mostly in trial stages in the United States of America, >100 designs were developed but only few are in use. More widespread application of TDR followed after the mid-80s developments of a TDR designed at the Charité Hospital in Berlin, Germany. The principle of replacing almost the entire IVD is based on the success of hip and knee replacements. Proponents of TDR view it as a technology to treat back pain while attempting to decrease adjacent segment disease. The initial excitement with TDR got tampered by the realization that specific cause of LBP is still not known, so complete relief in all patients is far-fetched expectation and the fact that mechanical failure of devices was quickly reported.

Aims of Total Disk Replacement

The typical objectives are to:
- Restore the physiological kinematics of the IVD
- Relieve pain
- Improve stability and resist wear
- Protecting the adjacent disks and facet joints from undue degeneration.

Indication

The classic indication for TDR includes failure of aggressive conservative treatment with disabling LBP attributed to the lower lumbar spine affecting no more than two disks. Other indications are similar to those of fusion.

Prerequisite

- Demonstrable disk degeneration as the cause of pain
- Intact facet joints posteriorly and no other pain generators demonstrated

Contraindications

- Lumbar spinal stenosis
- Facet disease
- Old fractures
- Previous laminectomy
- Instability as seen in spondylolisthesis
- Osteoporosis
- Pars fracture
- Infection
- Relative contraindication—patients with a steep lumbosacral angle at the intended TDR level. It is difficult to implant disk in such situation.

Total Disk Repair Designs

The materials that have been used for TDR are similar to those that have been employed in other major joint arthroplasties

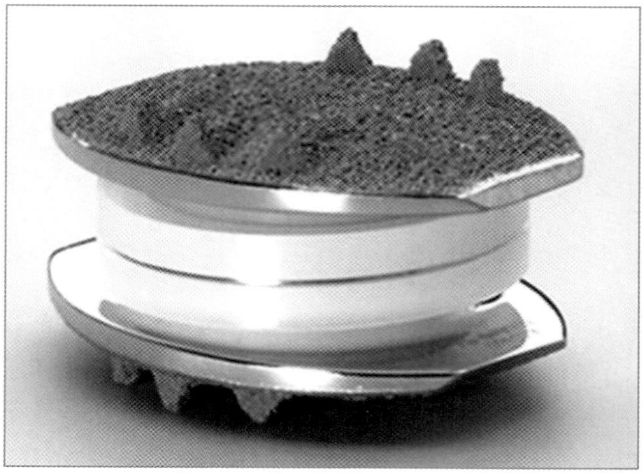

Fig. 29: Charité lumbar total disk replacement.
Source: DePuySpine, Raynham, MA.

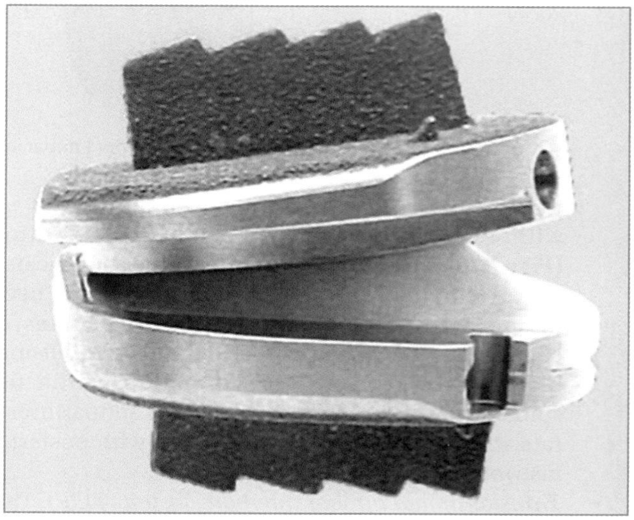

Fig. 30: ProDisc lumbar total disk replacement.

(e.g., polyethylene, chrome cobalt, and titanium). And to this effect the replacement designs are also available in varying conformities:
- *Unconstrained [Charite™* ***(Fig. 29)****]:* Two concave metal end-plates and an unconstrained biconvex polyethylene core
- *Semiconstrained [Maverick, ProDisc™, Synthes, Paoli, PA* ***(Fig. 30)****]:* Two metal end-plates, one of which has an attached concave polyethylene inlay and the other has a metal convex articulating surface
- Constrained (FlexiCore™).

The surgical approach is similar to the one used to obtain an ALIF and carries similar rates of vascular complications.

Outcome of Implantation

The reports have been encouraging and in most cases have not been found to be inferior to fusion surgery.
- A randomized controlled trial (RCT) comparing lumbar TDR using the Charité with spinal fusion demonstrated TDR clinical outcomes to be equivalent to those with ALIF (Blumenthal et al.)

- In another RCT, the authors conclude that TDR is safe and efficacious, and that ProDisc-L is superior to circumferential fusion by multiple clinical criteria (Zigler et al.)
- Total disk repair as compared to spinal fusion is superior to the latter technique 6 months following surgery (Zigler), but at 12 months the difference appeared to be less pronounced (Delamarter et al.).

A retrospective study on the Charité disk, including some earlier designs of the implant, showed that at 17 years the majority of operated levels lost mobility and resulted in ankylosis (Putzier et al.). This finding is very prominently highlighted in systematic reviews. Also, there is evidence that the range of motion at the segment is similar to preoperative segment and normal spine mobility is not restored.

The long-term complications and benefits of TDR are yet to be realized, especially in terms of preventing adjacent level disk degeneration (Freeman and Davenport; Resnick and Watters). The current evidence with respect to adjacent segment disease is not encouraging.

Complications

- Osteolysis
- Implant fracture or wear
- Vertebral body fracture
- Failure of ingrowth
- Instability with dislocation

The revision surgery is technically difficult as there is prominent anterior fibrosis after the procedure increasing the chances of vascular injury and other complications.

Dynamic Stabilization

With a view to address some of the shortfalls of spinal fusion, alternative options for the last decade have included the use of semirigid or dynamic stabilization implants. The theory is that dynamic stabilization could potentially stiffen the symptomatic level while preserving some motion, which in theory decreases the risk of adjacent segment disease.

- Semirigid stabilization aims to achieve fusion without stress shielding at the bone graft that may disrupt or delay bridging
- Dynamic stabilization aims to stabilize while restricting painful motion without the need for diskectomy and fusion. The devices most studied are:
  - *The Graf®:* It consists a non-elastic band (like a prosthetic ligament) attached between pedicles screws maintaining the motion segment in lordosis. The idea was to prevent flat back and limit flexion to within the normal range while distressing the adjacent vertebral segments. It was associated with worse clinical outcomes at one year and higher revisions with poor outcome after 2 years so fallen out of favor.
  - *The Dynesys®:* The design of the Dynesys® is similar to the Graf® with the exception that it has an additional polycarbonate-urethane spacer around the polyethylene terephthalate band between the pedicle screws. This added spacer also limits extension while providing flexion constraint as for the Graf®. In simpler terms, it consists of pedicle screws that are attached by a rope and a plastic cylinder **(Fig. 31)**. The rope is threaded through the cylinder and tensioned to 300 N. The Dynesys® system aims to restore the biomechanics of the posterior annulus and facet joints.

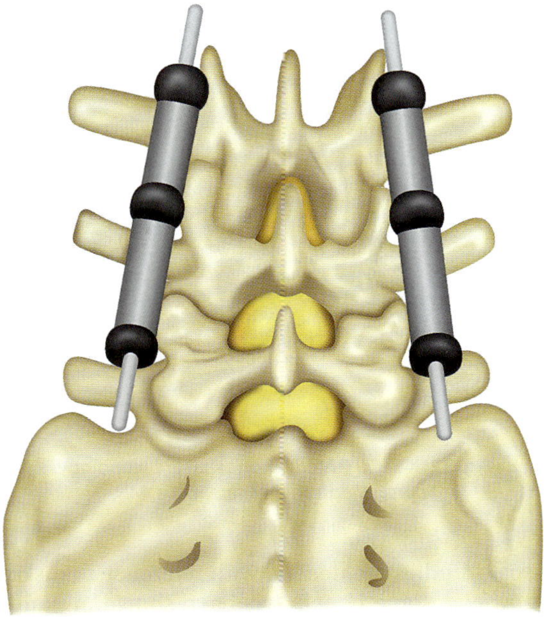

Fig. 31: Dynesys™ dynamic stabilization system.

Indications for Dynamic Stabilization

- Low back pain due to early disk degeneration
- To stabilize degenerative spondylolisthesis or scoliosis following decompression laminectomy (The Dynesys® system)
- Protect a degenerated disk above a fusion to prevent the progression of adjacent segment disease
- After diskectomy to protect the disk against further degeneration

Results from the literature are mixed while even this is unclear that the system provides any mobility or not. As it has been showed by studies that there is no effect between the Dynesys® and fusion with regard to increased motion at the adjacent segments. The systems have still to prove their superiority over fusion in RCT, but one thing is clear that reoperation rates due to loosening/implant failure are quite high with the use of this system.

Another concept is using 'interspinous implants" which are floating devices **(Fig. 32)** not attached to vertebral bodies and have the advantage of limiting the possibility of loosening during motion. These are also classified as dynamic stabilization devices and aims to avoid excessive extension while also unloading the posterior annulus, which is regarded as the primary pain source. Different designs are available (compressible or noncompressible implants) some limiting flexion and/or extension. They have the added advantage of being introduced in minimally invasive manner.

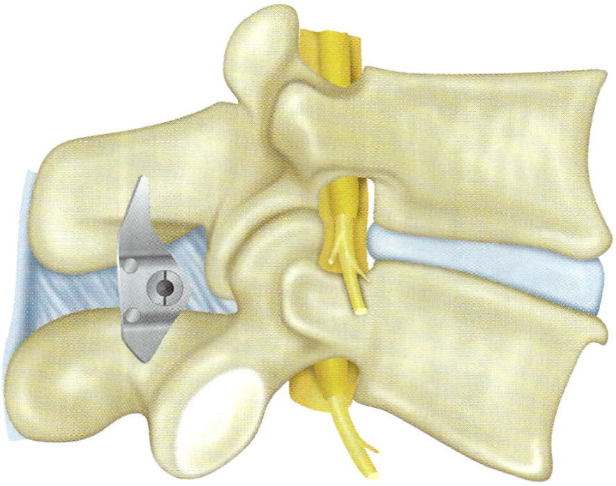

Fig. 32: X STOP® interspinous spacer technology.
Source: Medtronic, Minneapolis, MN.

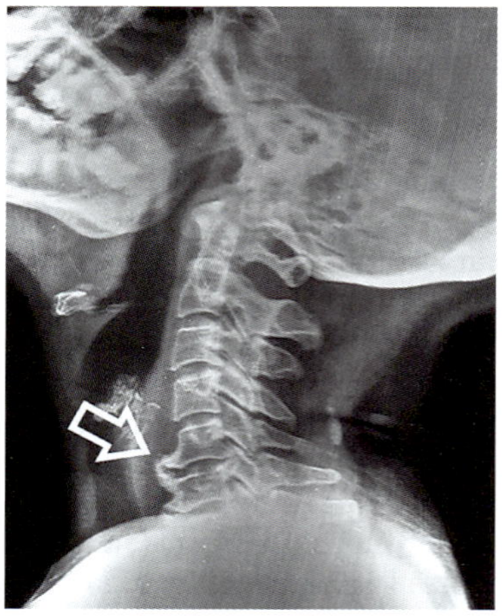

Fig. 33: The cervical spondylosis presents with osteophyte formation (arrow) and reduced disk spaces. There is often subtle or overt facet joint and uncovertebral joint arthrosis.

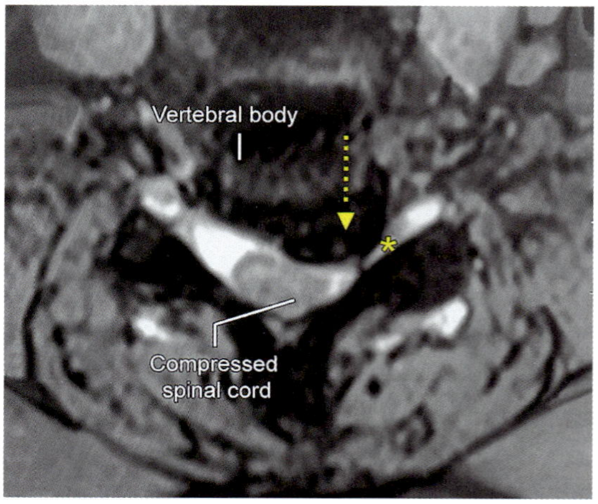

Fig. 34: The herniated nucleus pulposus compresses (arrow) exiting nerve root producing radicular symptoms. The left side foramen is reduced in dimensions (asterisk) by the left paracentral herniated nucleus pulposus in this patient producing symptoms along fifth cervical nerve root.

Large scale studies are needed with reference to diskogenic pain; however, some benefit has been shown in patients of spinal stenosis.

FACET REPLACEMENT

This is the newest arthroplasty technology developed in criticism of disk replacement. TDR substitutes for only one articulation leaving behind the posterior pain generators. Facet replacement replaces both facet joints, and in conjunction with TDR, all three pain generators would then be eliminated. Indications are similar to those of dynamic stabilization.

Two types of designs are available:

1. The first is a relatively unconstrained anatomic design in which two unlinked components articulate with each other and rely on its anatomic design for its motion and stability.
2. The second design is a linked system that attempts to reproduce the stability and motion properties but is anatomically different from normal facets.

Both methods aim to achieve stabilization without fusion while allowing decompression of the neural elements.

Complications

It is not known fully as studies are underway but expected complications from experience of other arthroplasty techniques include:

- Implant loosening or failure—more prevalent in the presence of osteoporosis
- Subluxation may occur in unconstrained models.

DEGENERATIVE CONDITIONS OF CERVICAL SPINE (CERVICAL SPONDYLOSIS, RADICULOPATHY, AND MYELOPATHY)

The cervical degenerative disorders represent a clinical spectrum where the mildest presentation is intermittent nonbothering neck pain and stiffness to severe presentations of cervical myelopathy and cervical spine deformity (kyphosis/scoliosis). In between are the symptoms emanating from cervical spondylosis (localized symptoms), root compression from osteophytes (radicular symptoms/cervical radiculopathy), herniated nucleus pulposus, disk-osteophyte complexes, canal compromise, and stenosis from ossified posterior longitudinal ligament (OPLL). Cervical spondylosis represents a noninflammatory condition of cervical spine resulting from DDD **(Fig. 33)**. There is often associated facet joint and uncovertebral joint arthrosis and in folding of ligamentum flavum compromises canal space. Cervical radiculopathy results from root compression from bony (osteophyte) or soft tissue (herniated nucleus pulposus **(Fig. 34)**, hypertrophied ligament) or both. Cervical myelopathy results from cervical cord compression and is characterized by demyelination **(Fig. 35)**. The myelopathy in cervical degeneration is due to a combination of mechanical compression and ischemia resulting in oligodendrocyte death.

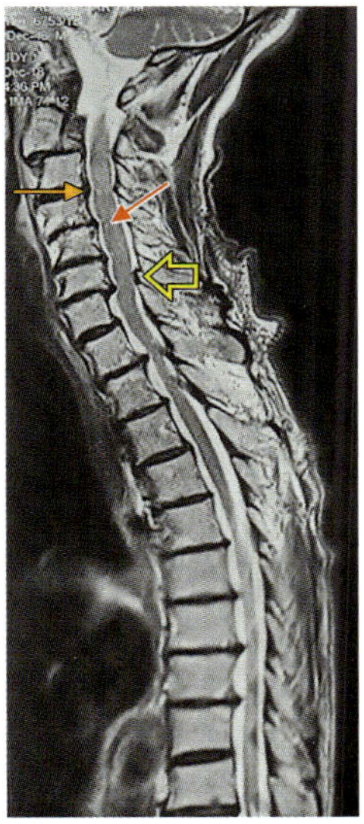

Fig. 35: The cervical cord gets "pinched" between anterior and posterior pathological structures ultimately leading to demyelination. The osteophytes and ossification of posterior longitudinal ligament (orange arrow) reduces canal diameter, while posteriorly the buckling ligamentum flavum (yellow block arrow) digs into the cord compressing it. There is relative ischemia due to vascular compression and it leads to death of oligodendrocytes. The MRI demonstrates hyperintensity changes within the cord suggestive of myelopathy (red arrow) with edema, demyelination, cystic changes, and Wallerian degeneration.

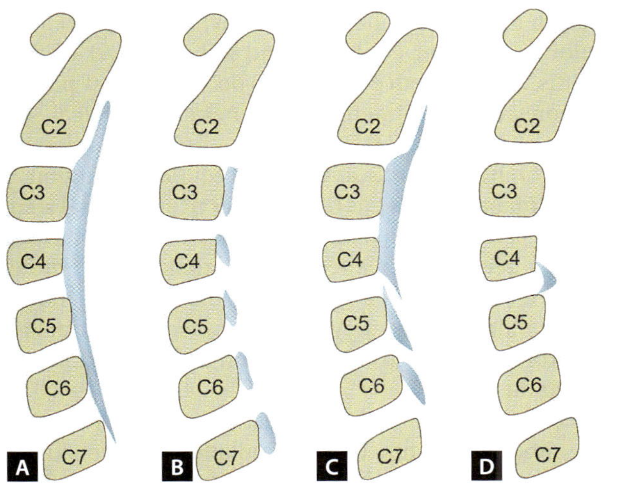

Figs. 36A to D: The different variants of ossified posterior longitudinal ligament. (A) Continuous type; (B) Segmental type; (C) Mixed type; (D) Localized type.

The causes of myelopathy can be spinal (degenerative spondylosis, OPLL, tumor, infection, syringomyelia, Chiari malformation, epidural abscess and trauma) or nonspinal (multiple sclerosis, vitamin B_{12} deficiency, tabes dorsalis, and hereditary spastic paraplegia). OPLL and its variants **(Figs. 36A to D)** may have genetic interplay and its incidence is nearly 25% in Caucasians further increased by diabetes and obesity. The compression of cord by buckling of ligamentum flavum and pincer mechanism with anteroposterior (AP) combined compression exacerbated by cervical spine movements has been postulated as prime mechanical factor in cord compression. The cord compression results in cystic cavitation, gliosis, and Wallerian degeneration. Vertebrobasilar insufficiency arises from compromise of vertebral arteries resulting in insufficiency of the basilar arterial system to brain. This occurs in severe advanced cervical spine degeneration in elderly associated with deformity.

BOX 2: The common upper motor neuron (UMN) signs that are assessed for evaluation of spinal cord compression.

- *Hoffman sign:* Flexion of both thumb and index finger as the middle fingernail is snapped
- *Inverted radial reflex:* There is flexion of fingers without flexion of forearm as the distal end of radius is tapped in patients with root and/or cord compression at C5 level
- *Pathological clonus:* Abnormal reflex movement of the foot in plantar flexion induced by sudden dorsiflexion caused by alternate contraction and relaxation of triceps surae. The number of ties foot plantar flexes should be noted and if it does not stop then it is sustained clonus which is highly significant
- *Babinski reflex:* The big toe moves upward and toward the top surface of the foot while other toes fan out when the outer border of foot is firmly stroked
- *Finger escape test:* The patient is asked to forcefully keep his fingers adducted and extended. The small finger spontaneously abducts escaping the voluntary effort
- *Grip and release test:* The patient is unable to make a grip and release 20 times in 10 seconds
- *Romberg test:* Due to dorsal column dysfunction the patient is unable to maintain balance while standing with arms forward and closed eyes
- *Lhermitte sign:* Demyelination of nerves in dorsal column causes hyper-excitability resulting in an electric shock like sensation traveling down the vertebral column and into extremities on flexion of the neck

CLINICAL PRESENTATION

Pain in neck, loss of sensation in upper limbs, and weakness of discrete muscle groups are the common clinical presentations. The pain is commonly localized axially to neck and paraspinal region that may involve trapezius muscle variably in spondylosis. It is chronic and insidious in nature. Sudden, acute, intense, and radicular pain is seen with disk herniation that radiates to specific cervical nerves down the upper limb and may be associated with weakness and/or loss of sensation in long-standing cases. Myelopathy may additionally present with loss of manual dexterity in hands, weakness, difficulty with gait and balance, urinary symptoms, and spasticity. The patient walks with wide-based gait with frequent loss of balance and falls. The sensory findings include loss of proprioception and patient may have difficulty in buttoning clothes, changed handwriting, and dropping objects. Motor weakness is usually subtle and may not be successfully identified in many patients with root or cord compression; only in long-standing cases, it is more overt. More crude expression of motor power like grip strength is a more sensitive measure to identify weakness. Fine and crude touch, pain, temperature, pressure sensation should be evaluated. Hyperreflexia suggests spinal cord compression with upper motor neuron (UMN) signs. The common UMN signs seen are Hoffman's sign, inverted radial reflex, pathological clonus, and Babinski reflex **(Box 2)**. These signs may be masked in conditions that produce peripheral neuropathy like diabetes mellitus. Combination of myelopathy and radiculopathy is called myeloradiculopathy (spinal stenosis + concurrent compression of neuroforaminal contents) where there are lower motor neuron signs at the level of cervical cord lesion while UMN signs appear caudal to the lesion. One must remember that vertigo is not a usual complaint of cervical degenerative disease contrary to the common belief.

DIFFERENTIAL DIAGNOSIS

Cervical spine lesions mimic many other related lesions that emanate from cervical spine of CNS. The following are common differentials for cervical spine degenerative pathology:

- Multiple sclerosis (it produces progressive loss of sensation and weakness)
- Normal pressure hydrocephalus (gait and bladder dysfunction is seen, presence of cognitive dysfunction helps distinguish from cervical spine lesions)
- Transverse myelitis
- Cerebrovascular disorder
- CNS trauma
- CNS tumor (hyperactive jaw reflex suggest brainstem or intracranial tumor)
- Meningitis/encephalitis
- Peripheral nerve compression disorders (carpal tunnel, cubital tunnel syndrome; they may coexist with cervical spinal lesions producing double crush syndrome)
- Myelopathy due to vitamin B_{12} deficiency
- Shoulder pathologies such as extrinsic impingement, bursitis, adhesive capsulitis, and rotator cuff tears
- Amyotrophic lateral sclerosis [electromyography (EMG) studies are diagnostic for diagnosing it]
- Guillain-Barré syndrome (it produces subacute onset of progressive weakness)

IMAGING

Plain radiographs, especially the lateral projection, help in localizing the degenerative lesion and its severity. Performing AP and flexion-extension views in addition also help in identifying deformity and instability. Cord pathologies and compression are best evaluated with MRI scans. Signal changes within cord are suggestive of spinal cord compression and injury. T2 weak signal hyperintensity [less than cerebrospinal fluid (CSF)] that appears diffuse without clear bordering is associated with potentially reversible changes such as edema, Wallerian degeneration, demyelination, and ischemia. Higher intensity levels on T2 images with sharp bordering and T1 hypointensity represent suggest irreversible changes such as cavitation, neural tissue loss, myelomalacia, necrosis, and spongiform changes in the gray matter **(Fig. 35)**. CT myelography is good in patients who cannot undergo MRI for specific reasons (cardiac pacemakers, aneurysm clips, claustrophobia, metal implant/scar tissue).

TREATMENT

The management of cervical spondylosis aims at symptomatic relief and improvement in function. Rest, lifestyle modifications, and short period of immobilization (soft cervical collar) are commonly tried first to control the symptoms. Rest prevents reinjury to the muscles and tendons giving good pain relief, especially in acute period. Muscular strain and inflammation to the disks and facet joints are controlled with NSAIDs. Short course of steroids may be beneficial. Gabapentin or its derivative may be beneficial in radicular pains that may be combined with amitriptyline or nortriptyline. Narcotics may be given under supervision for severe pain. Patients using computers should be counseled for good ergonomics (adjusting screen height, sitting posture, use of special whale mouse, and split keyboards). Rest and immobilization should not be prolonged as it causes atrophy of muscles. Strengthening exercises of neck and shoulder muscles help reducing muscle-related spasms and fatigue. Physical therapy often worsens the symptoms in acute setting and may result in prolonging duration of pain. They should be only started after resolution of acute symptoms. Gentle cervical traction and massage may be added to maximize benefit of therapy. The role of cervical traction is however equivocal and has low-level evidence that it is more effective than placebo. Myofascial pain is a common accompaniment to degenerative cervical spine disease. Trigger point injections, epidural injections, medial branch blocks, and radiofrequency ablation are used for managing pain as needed. Cervical epidural steroid injections are less much less frequently that lumbar region primarily because it has been conventionally very difficult to determine in which patient would the injection be effective. Additionally, they have their own substantial risks of neurological deficit, epidural hematoma, and possible vascular infarct.

The treatment of cervical radiculopathy aims to resolve pain, improving functional limitations, reversing, or improving neurological deficits and preventing further neurological deterioration. It has been observed that progression of radiculopathy to myelopathy is quite rare so unless there is severe motor deficit [motor power of Medical Research Council (MRC) grade <3], prolonged course of nonoperative treatment is usually provided. Surgery is indicated in patients with cervical spine disease with specific clinical presentations **(Box 3)**.

BOX 3: The indications for surgery in patients with cervical spine degenerative disorder.

- Progression of neurological symptoms
- Presence of myelopathy for >6 months
- Compression ratio (ratio of smallest sagittal cord diameter to the largest transverse cord diameter) approaching 0.4
- Transverse area of the cord <40 mm^2

Surgical Treatment

Duration and degree of symptoms and cord dysfunction, general health of patient, and degree of functional deterioration guide surgical procedure. The choice is also frequently influenced by radiographic findings and predominant anterior versus posterior disease.

Anterior versus Posterior Surgery

The details of anterior and posterior approaches to spine can be read from dedicated texts. The anterior approach is useful in:

- Direct decompression of pathologies in anterior cervical spine
- Reducing postoperative pain by virtue of sparing muscles in dissection
- Ability to correct cervical kyphosis simultaneously with decompression
- Better postoperative infection rates

Generally, anterior approach is preferred for small segment pathologies (1–2 levels) because complications increase with long segment disease using it. Posterior approach is preferred for posterior spinal pathologies and longer segment disease (3 or more). Kyphotic patients are better managed by anterior or combined approach. The combined approach is especially better for posterior compressive pathologies associated with kyphosis. Lordotic patients have comparable benefits with both approaches. Cobb's method has been conventionally used to determine lordosis or loss of it from C2–C7 measurements (other measures such as Jackson physiological stress lines, Harrison's posterior tangent method, and Ishihara index are not commonly used). Sagittal vertical axis from C2–C7 (the distance between the C2 plumb line and the posterior superior end plate of C7 vertebra, **Fig. 37)** has been shown to correlate with postoperative disability scores. Increase in the distance of >40 mm is associated with significant pain and disability. The T1 slope, neck tilt angle, and thoracic inlet angle are discretely used.

Anterior Cervical Spine Surgery

The three most common anterior techniques for managing cervical spine pathologies are:

1. Anterior cervical diskectomy and fusion (ACDF)

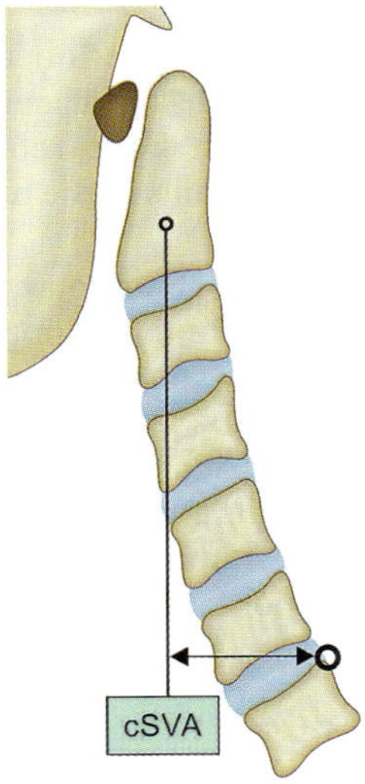

Fig. 37: The C2–C7 sagittal vertical axis deviation is measured from 2nd cervical vertebra to the posterosuperior corner of the superior end-plate of C7 vertebra. (cSVA-cervical sagittal vertebral axis)

2. Anterior cervical corpectomy and fusion (ACCF)
3. Cervical diskectomy + arthroplasty

Hybrid procedures using a combination of 1 and 2 are also common. The success (decompression) and fusion rates after single level ACDF **(Fig. 38)** are high and commonly it is done in younger patients. For multilevel fusions and decompression also the success rates are good but rate of nonunion increases with increase in the number of levels. Anterior plating mitigates this risk somewhat, but it is better to do a corpectomy that also allows wider decompression **(Fig. 39)**. It is considered prudent to perform posterior segmental fusion to increase fusion rate and decrease implant/graft-related problems in multilevel surgery.

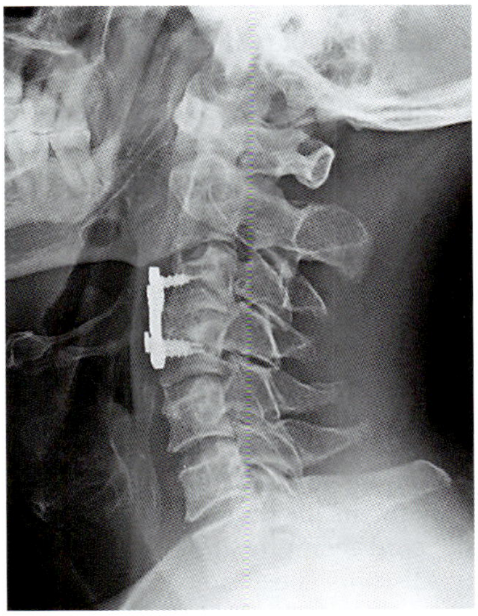

Fig. 38: Anterior cervical diskectomy and fusion (ACDF). The fusion rates get improved by adding anterior plate but one must bear in mind the implant-related complications in such situation.

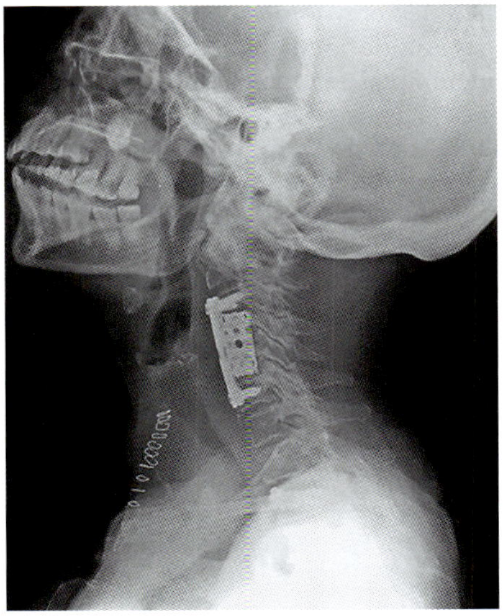

Fig. 39: The anterior cervical corpectomy and fusion involves removing the vertebral body for wider area of decompression and maintaining lordosis with cage and fusion.

Arthroplasty may be associated with lower incidence of degenerative changes in adjacent levels compared to fusion. It preserves motion at the segment maintaining normal biomechanics and has shown better functional outcomes compared to ACDF for single level disease. The results were more pronounced for disease at two levels as arthroplasty resulted in reduced rates of subsequent surgery. However, it should not be used in patients with associated facet joint degeneration (causing persistent pain), kyphotic deformity, acute or chronic infection at the level, ankylosing spondylosis or severe ankylosis at the level, and poor bone quality. There is high potential for future osteophyte regrowth at the level in younger patients due to continued motion so thorough foraminal decompression is a must. Complications of anterior surgery are as follows:

- Postoperative dysphagia
- Hoarseness in voice (commonly temporary but may be permanent in 0.33% patients)
- Vertebral artery injury
- Implant-related problems (screw-plate disengagement, cage displacement, breakage of implant, and failure)
- Graft-related problem (graft resorption/subsidence, expulsion, nonunion, migration, etc.)

Posterior Surgery

Posterior approach to cervical spine is preferred in patients with short neck, obesity, barrel chest, or those with previous anterior cervical surgery. Commonly laminectomy or laminoplasty is used for spinal cord decompression that can be combined with fusion. Laminectomy has been regarded as standard treatment for multilevel cervical degenerative disease with cord compression. Performing multilevel laminectomy disrupts posterior cervical tension band resulting in delayed kyphosis and segmental instability. This has necessitated adding posterior instrumentation and fusion. Instrumentation and stabilization have its own set of complications related to implant so some surgeons resort to skip-level laminectomy to preserve posterior tension band. Laminoplasty is performed in stable cervical spine with good lordosis and minimal neck pain. It preserves natural cervical biomechanics to a greater extent. It may be done using open door or double door or various muscle-sparing laminoplasty alterations. In open door method, hinge is created on one side while the other end is complete osteotomy that can be opened on the hinge on other side. Later the complete osteotomy site may be reconstructed with small plate osteosynthesis. In double-door laminoplasty ("French-door" procedure), central decompression is achieved by splitting the spinous process in midline and it is hinged open on both sides. Muscle-sparing techniques (preserving semispinalis cervicis, multifidus, and musculoligamentous attachments) limits postoperative axial neck pain, kyphosis, and segmental instability. Complications of posterior surgery:

- Loss of range of motion
- New-onset kyphosis
- Neck pain
- Delayed C5 nerve palsy (this was classically linked to laminoplasty but has been found with various forms of cervical decompression and also laminectomy)

CONCLUSION

- Low back pain is the most common orthopedic problem encountered in general practice. Despite being common most cases are symptomatically treated without much of a complete diagnosis as the pathophysiology is evolving and not fully clear.
- One should primarily differentiate between pain developing locally and a pain emanating from a faraway site. This should be followed by identifying the exact pathology as far as possible. Specific signs that dictate seriousness of the problem should not be missed.
- Investigating the cause of pain that fails to respond to preliminary treatment usually involves radiography and supplementation with advance imaging modalities such as MRI and bone scan, the rationale of which should, however, be always balanced on their specific need in individual patients.
- Intervertebral disk degeneration is a common cause of pain in the middle aged and the elderly. The cause is not limited only to increasing age and many factors play their role. Diskography is a useful investigation to identify the pathological disk.
- Lot of interventional techniques (nonsurgical) are available that claim to relieve pain from a degenerated disk disease, but variably. Specific consensus for using them has never emerged. Even gene therapy has found its way in modifying the course of degeneration of disk in degenerative process.
- For symptomatic disk degeneration with otherwise unrelieved pain, fusion or disk replacement are viable surgical options but must be carefully chosen in experienced hands only. Results in the hands of learners are usually unsatisfactory.
- Cervical spine degenerative condition ranges from mild neck pain to gait imbalance and myelopathy. Most of the spondylotic and radicular pains can be conservatively managed and surgery has specific indications. For single level disease, anterior surgeries have fantastic results while for multiple level degenerative disease and myelopathy posterior approach is preferrable with restoration of the posterior tension band.

CHAPTER 96

Lumbar Disk Herniation and Spinal Stenosis

Manish Kumar Varshney

LUMBAR DISK HERNIATION

DEFINITION

Lumbar disk herniation (LDH) has been defined as a focal displacement of nucleus, annulus or end plate material beyond the normal margins of intervertebral disk space (**Fig. 1**), resulting in displacement of epidural fat, nerve root and/or the thecal sac causing pain, weakness or numbness in a sclerotomal or dermatomal distribution. Herniation is separate from disk bulge, which is a diffuse symmetrical outpouching of annulus fibrosus beyond the confines of the normal disk space associated with varying disk degeneration, with no evidence of neural impingement.

TERMINOLOGY OF DISK PATHOLOGY (FIGS. 2A TO E)

- ***Disk bulge (as known as prolapse):*** Diffuse symmetrical outpouching of annulus fibrosus beyond the confines of the normal disk space associated with varying disk degeneration, with no evidence of neural impingement. Disk extending < 3 mm beyond the end plates, can be a normal variant.
- ***Disk protrusion:*** Focal or asymmetric extension of disk beyond the vertebral border. Disk origin is broader than the extent of protrusion. Annulus involvement is generalized or broad based versus localized or focal based.
- ***Disk extrusion (ruptured disk):*** More extreme extension of disk beyond the vertebral border. Base of disk extrusion at the site of disk origin is narrower than the diameter of the extruding material. Connection exists between the extruded material and disk.
- ***Sequestration:*** No connection between the fragment and parent disk. Intermediate signal on T1 and increased signal on T2.
- ***Migration:*** Displacement of disk material from the site of origin. It is difficult to find connection between disk and fragment in such cases. It may or may not be sequestrated.
- ***Intermittent disk herniation of "falconer" or "concealed disk" of dandy:*** This is not obvious in position of flexion on table, but can be reproduced by hyperextension of spine.

Contained herniations: Displaced disk is still covered by annulus, "subligamentous" refers to disk being covered by posterior longitudinal ligament (PLL) (annulus ruptured).

Uncontained herniations: There is no annulus covering over the displaced disk. It may also be subligamentous (beneath PLL).

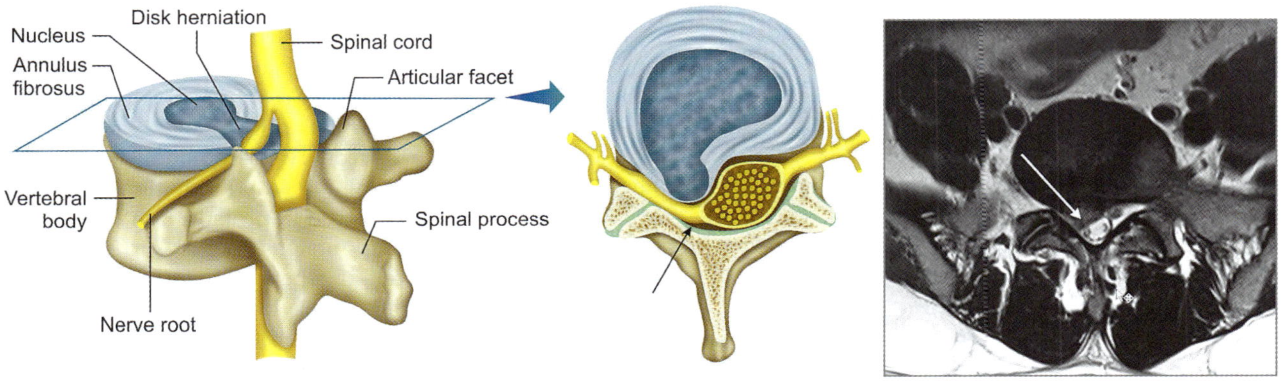

Fig. 1: Herniation of nucleus pulposus. Herniated nucleus pulposus still contained in the thinned annulus compressing exiting nerve root. Also shown is the MRI of lumbar spine demonstrating disk extrusion (arrow) displacing and compressing the right traversing nerve root.

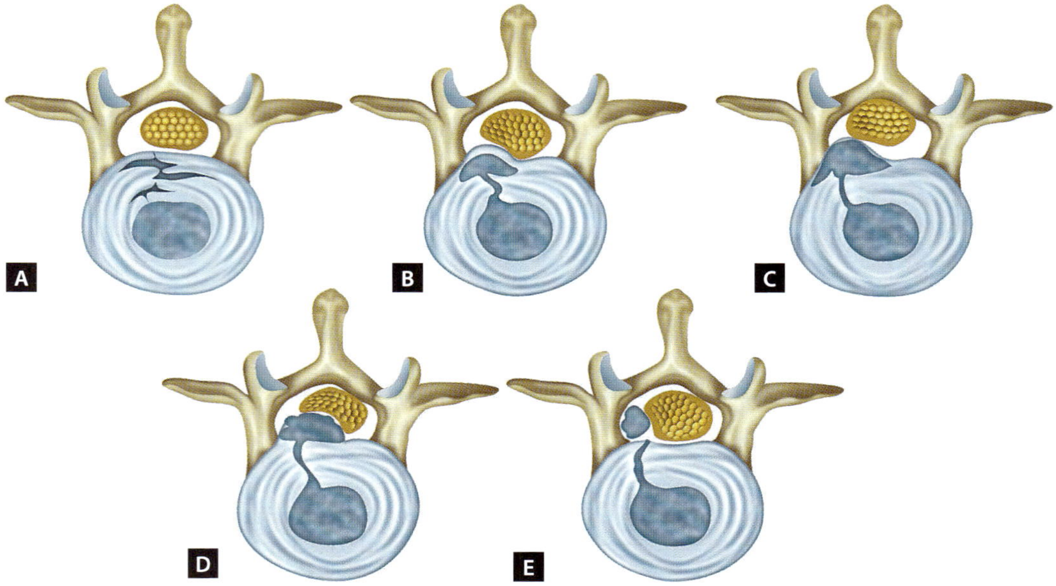

Figs. 2A to E: Illustration of morphologic types of disk pathology. (A) Disk bulge due to annular weakness; (B) Contained disk protrusion; (C) Noncontained subligamentous disk extrusion; (D) Noncontained transligamentous disk extrusion; (E) Noncontained disk sequestration.

PATHOPHYSIOLOGY

The radicular symptoms are likely generated by a combination of mechanical and chemical irritation.

- Nerve root compression alone has been demonstrated to generate only mild local discomfort and is not painful.
- However, when the same patients sustained neural compression following nerve root exposure to nucleus pulposus extract, they reported symptoms consistent with radicular pain.
- Exposure to nucleus pulposus increases nerve tissue edema, fibrosis, demyelination, and Schwann cell hypertrophy.
- Tumor necrosis factor-alpha (TNF-α) is produced by the chondrocyte—like cells of the nucleus pulposus, and has been implicated as the key chemical mediator that sensitizes the nerve root to stimulation. The local effects of TNF-α include sodium channel upregulation (predisposing the nerve root to depolarization) and chemotaxis (causing local inflammation), which may then lead to further nerve root irritation.
- TNF-α may also mediate dorsal root ganglion apoptosis. Inflammatory cytokines, such as interleukin-1β, interleukin-6, prostaglandin-E2, and phospholipase A2 are found in significant concentrations in the nerve root and dorsal root ganglion, suggesting they play a role in the inflammatory process.

The localized back pain may develop due to one of the following:

- Stretching and friction of sinuvertebral nerve or irritation by torn annulus fibers/local inflammation
- Occlusion of vasa nervorum
- Pain from facet joint arthropathy may get amplified due to sensitized nerves
- Engorgement of extradural veins
- End plate changes

EPIDEMIOLOGY

- Symptomatic LDH is seen in lifetime of 2% population.
- 90–95% of LDH is seen at L4–L5 (most common) and L5-S1 levels and most patients are between the ages of 20 and 50 years.
- The risk factors for sustaining an LDH are:
  - Male gender
  - Age 30–40 years
  - Heavy weight lifting and twisting motion
  - Poor job satisfaction and low income
  - Cigarette smoking
  - Exposure to vibration

PATHOANATOMY

The disk material may present as a central disk or a peripheral herniation. The weakest portion of annulus is posterolateral region that causes common posterolateral herniations. Posterocentral and central herniations are next in frequency.

For peripheral herniations, the disk material may present beneath the nerve root displacing it laterally (axillary presentation) or the disk material may compress the nerve root laterally displacing it medially (shoulder presentation). This produces characteristic posture of the trunk as the patient tries to reduce nerve root irritation by taking the root away from the disk. This is done by "tilting" trunk toward the affected side in axillary presentation and away from the affected side in shoulder presentation. This presents as the typical list observed in prolapsed intervertebral disk (PIVD). The herniated nucleus pulposus irritates the nerve roots physically and biochemically producing pain. The former causes local increase in nociceptive chemicals, viz., substance P and somatostatin that disrupt diffusion across involved nerve roots. Biochemical mediators like TNF-α activate a proinflammatory environment in the dorsal root ganglia.

NATURAL HISTORY

Majority of patients will improve independent of treatment. Disk herniations will often shrink/regress over time. Many studies have demonstrated a clinical improvement with decreased size of disk herniations.

CLINICAL FEATURES

Lumbar disk herniation causing radicular symptoms will produce features of lower motor neuron pathology.

Symptoms include:

- Mannequin's posture
- Pain and/or paresthesias in dermatomal distribution
- Numbness in a dermatomal distribution [for L5 nerve root the positive predictive value (PPV) is 76% while for S1 it is 50%]
- Coughing/sneezing increases pain
- Weakness in myotomal distribution [lateral four toe weakness has PPV of 76% for L4-L5 disk herniations, additional extensor hallucis longus (EHL) weakness increases PPV to 86%].
- Sclerotomal (referred) pain (not to be confused with radicular pain) originates from mesodermal tissue (muscle, ligaments, and periosteum). Sclerotomal pain is confined to the low back, buttock, and posterior thigh and does not radiate below the knee.

Physical Examination

- Sciatic list (depending on disk presentation to the root—axillary or shoulder) **(Figs. 3A and B)**.
- Dermatomal sensory loss—most important localizing sign.
- Atrophy and hyporeflexia—patellar tendon reflex has no diagnostic value for lower disks. Loss of Achilles reflex with S1 sensory abnormalities—80% PPV.
- Cough impulse test has been found to increase pain in patients with LDH.
- *Special tests:*
  - ***The passive straight leg raise test (Lasegue's test)*** defined as production of ipsilateral, concordant leg pain at 35–70° of leg elevation **(Fig. 4)** in supine or sitting positions, has demonstrated a high sensitivity, but low specificity for L4-5 and L5-S1 disk herniations. The test is sensitive (true positive in 72–97% of patients), but not specific (false positive in 11–66% of patients). The straight leg raise will not produce pain, if nerve root pathology is cephalad to the L5 nerve root because the straight leg raise test maneuver tensions lower nerve roots (L5-S1).
  - ***The contralateral or crossed straight leg raise test*** or crossed Lasegue or well-leg raise test (production of concordant leg pain with contralateral leg elevation) has a lower sensitivity (false positive in 85–100% of patients) of patients, but higher specificity (true positive in 23–42%) This test signifies that the disk is central or that there is a large lateral recess herniation and it is more specific for a "free" disk fragment.
  - ***Sciatic tension accentuation test (Figs. 5A to D):***
    - Bowstring test
    - Bragard sign
    - Dorsiflexion of foot
  - Upper lumbar root irritation (L1-4) is reproduced by the ***femoral stretch test*** **(Fig. 6)**, defined as anterior thigh pain generated by hip extension and knee flexion with the patient in the lateral or prone position.

The clinical findings in various lumbar and 1st sacral nerve root involvement are compiled in **Table 1**.

Cauda equina syndrome (CES) is caused by severe compression of lumbar and sacral nerve roots and occurs

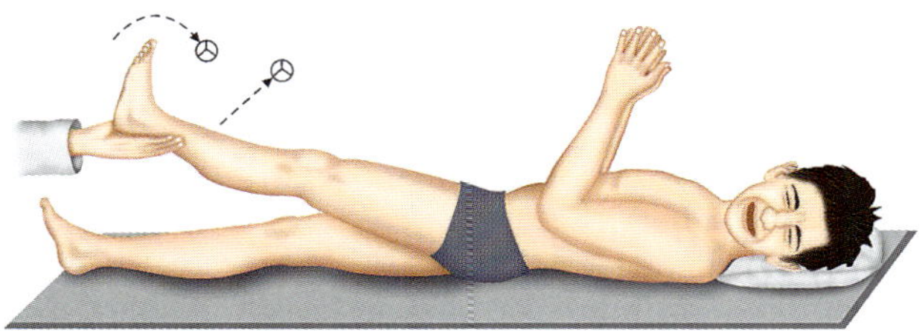

Fig. 4: The passive straight leg raise test.

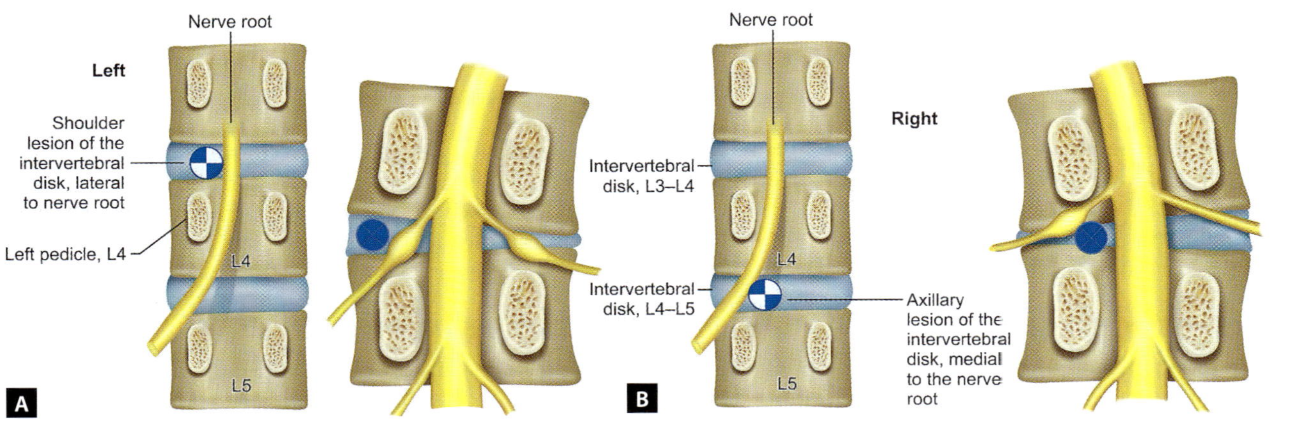

Figs. 3A and B: The presentation of pathological disk material in relation to the nerve root. (A) In shoulder presentation of the extruded posterolateral disk, the patient will bend to opposite side (sciatic list) to relieve neural irritation; (B) In axillary presentation of the disk, the patient will have sciatic list to the same side to relieve nerve irritation.

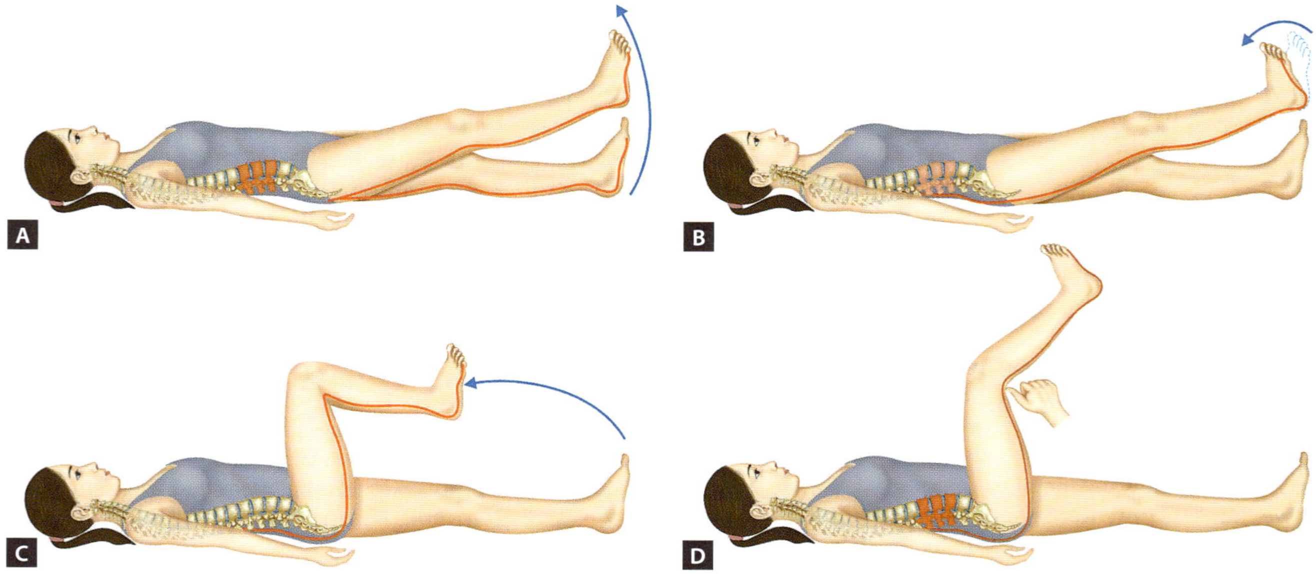

Figs. 5A to D: (A) The sciatic tension is produced by passive straight leg raise (SLR) and (B) is accentuated by foot dorsiflexion, (C) the knee is then flexed to 90° to relieve tension in nerve and hip is also brought to 90° flexion. (D) The knee is then extended with passively tensing the nerve at knee biceps tendon.

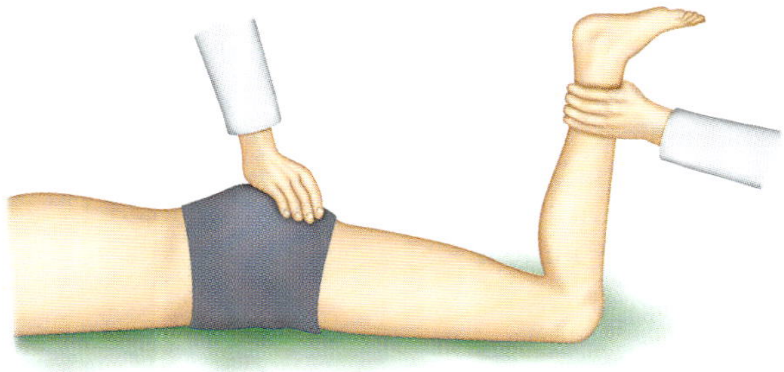

Fig. 6: Femoral nerve stretch test.

in approximately 2% of all patients with LDH. Symptoms include **(Flowchart 1)**:

- Severe bilateral leg pain
- Numbness in buttocks, back of legs, and sole (Saddle anesthesia)
- Perineal sensory deficit decreased rectal tone
- Paralysis in L5 and S1 supplied muscles of foot and tensor fascia lata (TFL) and gluteus medius
- Loss of tibialis posterior, medial hamstring, and ankle (gastrocsoleus) reflex
- Trendelenburg sign and gait
- Bowel/bladder symptoms (urinary retention early, then urine and bowel incontinence as the condition progresses)
- Impotence
- Babinski's reflex would be mute.

DIAGNOSTIC IMAGING

Plain radiographs of the lumbosacral spine in standing position—anteroposterior, lateral, and flexion/extension views.

- No help in diagnosis, but they provide a global overview of the lumbar spine alignment.
- Help to rule out other potential sources of low back pain and nerve root dysfunction including trauma, tumor, infection, and spondylolisthesis, and aid in surgical planning by defining the regional anatomy.
- Magnetic resonance imaging (MRI) is the diagnostic imaging modality of choice for LDH:
  - Allows localization and classification of the herniated material
  - T2-weighted images are most commonly used to identify and assess primary LDH. The disk fragments appear hypointense on T2 imaging with or without focal intensity with annular rupture.
  - Contrast enhancement is recommended to the T1-weighted images to differentiate between scar tissue and herniated disk material in patients who have had prior lumbar spine surgery. Herniated disk material has low signal intensity on postcontrast T1-weighted images because it is not vascularized, whereas scar tissue has high-signal intensity.
- Computed tomography (CT) may be used to visualize bony anatomy in regions of prior surgery or local pathology (e.g., in patients with spondylolysis or spina bifida).
- Myelography and CT myelograms are often poorly tolerated and have no place currently in the diagnosis of LDH, when MRI is available. Only in absolute contraindication to MRI (cardiac valves or pacemakers) one may resort to them.

DIFFERENTIAL DIAGNOSIS

The low back pain **(Table 2)** and radicular pain have long list of differentials that need to be ruled out before labeling the pathology emanating purely from disk herniation. The radiating pain from lumbar or sacral segments should be differentiated from the following:

TABLE 1: Clinical symptoms and signs from compression/impingement of various lumbosacral nerve roots.

Lumbar 2nd-3rd spinal segment involvement/disk herniation compresses L3 traversing nerve root (very rarely L2 exiting nerve root in far lateral or foraminal herniations)	*Compression of lumbar 2nd nerve root (uncommon):* • Pain radiating over anterior mid-thigh and anterolateral aspect • Hip flexors are weak • Femoral nerve stretch test is positive • Screening test—pulling thighs up during sitting position (flexing hip) *Compression of lumbar 3rd nerve root*: • Pain radiating over distal anterior thigh • Hip flexors and knee extensors (quadratus femoris) are weak • Absent patellar reflex, in some cases it may be diminished • Femoral nerve stretch test is positive • Screening test—getting up from squatting position
Lumbar 3rd-4th disk herniation compresses L4 nerve root commonly and only uncommonly L3 will be involved in far lateral large disk herniations	*Compression of 4th nerve root:* • Pain radiating to leg and foot • Paresthesia and sensory blunting in medial lower leg/foot • Weakness of tibialis anterior and/or knee extension (quadriceps muscle) • Patellar tendon reflex may be diminished (nonsensitive and nonspecific) • Straight leg raising test (SLRT) is positive • Screening test—patient is unable to walk over heel (or in weakness with power more than three-fifths there would be fanning of toes with loss of arch)
Lumbar 4th-5th disk herniation compresses L5 traversing nerve root. Exiting L4 nerve root rarely involved with far lateral pathology	*Compression of 5th lumbar root*: • Pain radiating to leg and foot till toes • Sensory loss over lateral and anterolateral leg and dorsum of foot (typically in the first web space—deep peroneal nerve territory) • Weakness of EHL, extensor digitorum longus (EDL), knee flexion (hamstrings), tensor fascia lata (TFL), gluteus medius (hip abduction) • Weakness or mute posterior tibialis reflex and medial hamstring reflex • Screening test—positive Trendelenburg sign (variable) and inability to walk on heels • Trendelenburg gait is variably observed
Lumbar 5th and sacral 1st spinal segment involvement/disk herniation commonly involves 1st sacral nerve root	*Compression of 1st sacral nerve root:* • Radiating pain over leg and foot • Paresthesia over lateral aspect of foot • Ankle plantar flexors (gastrocsoleus complex) and evertors (peronei) are weak • Hip extension is also weak with variable weakness of knee flexion (hamstring) • The ankle reflex is diminished or absent • Screening test—walking on toes is difficult or not possible

Flowchart 1: Cauda equina syndrome.

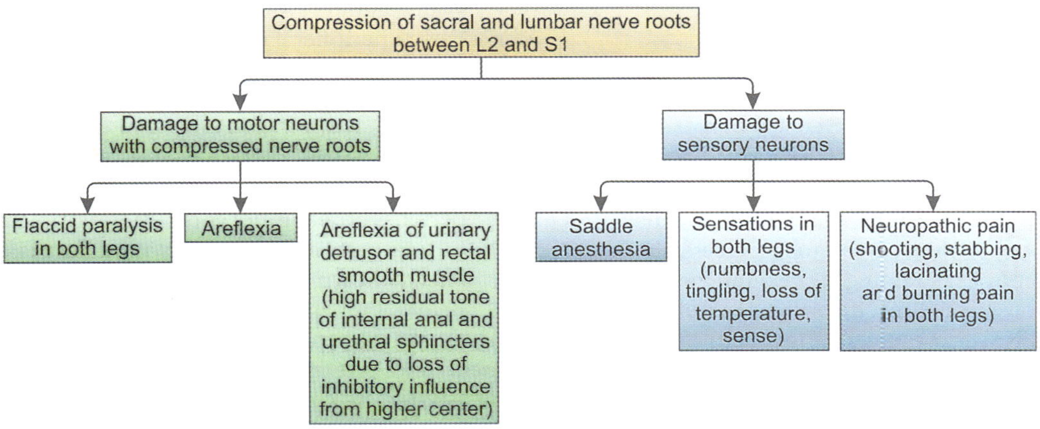

- Low back pain **(Table 2)**
- Thoracic disk herniation
- Pseudoradicular syndrome
- Inflammatory/metabolic abnormalities:
  - Diabetes mellitus
  - Osteoporotic compression fractures and nerve root compression
  - Ankylosing spondylosis
  - Arachnoiditis
  - Sarcoidosis
  - Paget's disease
- Pyriformis syndrome
- Polymyalgia rheumatica
- Eosinophilic granuloma
- Cauda equina
- Intraspinal synovial cysts

TABLE 2: Differential diagnosis of low back pain that should be kept in mind while evaluating a patient. Basically, this is again a comprehensive list of causes of low back pain presented in a different manner.

• *Myofascial:* – Myalgias and myositis – Fibromyalgia • Vertebral joint pathologies: – Facet joint pain – Sacroiliac joint pain - Infection - Sacroiliitis – Spondylolysis (pars interarticularis defect) • *Discogenic pain:* – Internal disk derangement – Annular tears – Herniated nucleus pulposus – Diskitis – Spondylolisthesis • *Osseous pathology:* – Osteoporosis – Osteomyelitis – Malignancies – Spinal stenosis – Scoliosis	• *Epidural (intraspinal extradural pathologies):* – Epidural adhesions – Epidural abscess – Epidural hematoma – Epidural lipomatosis • *Visceral pathology presenting as low back pain:* – Abdominal aortic aneurysm – Urinary tract pathology – Prostatitis – Endometriosis – Gastrointestinal tract pathology – Chronic pancreatitis – Duodenal ulcers – Colonic pain – Rectal pain • *Uncommon pain syndromes:* – Bertolotti's syndrome (lumbosacral transitional vertebra) – Baastrup's disease (kissing spine syndrome or spinous process impingement syndrome) – Maigne's syndrome (thoracolumbar junction syndrome) – Forestier's disease (DISH—diffuse idiopathic skeletal hyperostosis) – Cluneal nerve impingement syndrome • *Inflammatory disorders:* – Rheumatoid arthritis, ankylosing spondylosis – Psychosocial issues (yellow flags)

- Intraspinal metastasis
- Lumbosacral plexopathy
- Iliopsoas or retroperitoneal hematoma irritating lumbosacral plexus

TREATMENT

Nonsurgical Management

Approximately 90% of patients with LDH report improvement of symptoms in concordance with the natural history of disease. This implicates that nonsurgical modalities used to treat LDH [rest, lifestyle changes, tobacco cessation, limited alcohol intake, physical training, ultrasound massage, microwave or shortwave diathermy, transcutaneous electrical nerve stimulation (TENS)—acupuncture, osteopathic manipulation, magnets] may only reflect the ability to make the patient comfortable and passing time, while the natural history of LDH takes its course and symptoms dissipate. There has been no thorough documentation that nonoperative modalities truly alter the course of the disease.

Nonsteroidal anti-inflammatory drugs (NSAIDs) have definite role in pain control, but they should be rationally used:

- Avoid continuous use for >2–3 weeks.
- Provide adequate protection and stratify risk.
- Choice of NSAIDs should be tailored to meet cost, patient tolerance, and efficacy objectives.
- COX-2 inhibitors have doubtful cardiovascular safety.
- Muscle relaxants may be added as they have efficacy better than placebo in treating acute low back pain associated with LDH.
- Restrict the use of narcotic to no more than SOS basis.

The use of systemic [oral or intravenous (IV)] glucocorticoids for acute radiculopathy has demonstrated inconsistent results, but some short-term benefit is seen. They have no effect on functional recovery, clinical findings, or long-term relief.

Use of TNF-α inhibitors (infliximab or etanercept) for sciatica associated with LDH showed no difference in outcomes at 3 months or 1 year.

Epidural steroid injection (ESI) and selective nerve root injections (SNRIs)—this modality is under limelight for treatment of LDH.

- It has been found that though surgical management demonstrates better results than ESI [Injection therapy with corticosteroid (betamethasone) combined with local anesthetic (bupivacaine)]; approximately half of the patients treated with ESI could be spared of surgery over long term. Also, any delay in surgical treatment because of failed ESI does not affect surgical outcome.
- Selective nerve root injection also has a diagnostic and prognostic utility—91% of patients with symptom relief following SNRI had good surgical outcomes, whereas 60% of patients who had no symptom relief had good surgical outcomes.

Surgical Management

Various techniques are available for surgical removal of the disk fragment. The indications of operative treatment for LDH are:

- Progressing neurological deficit
- Cauda equina syndrome
- Severe peripheral neurological deficit, viz., foot drop
- Failure of conservative treatment to relieve pain and neurological signs and symptoms after aggressive compliance for 6 weeks to 3 months.
- Severe persistent pain and disability for more 3 months. Previous recommendation of 1 year or 6 months waiting period is probably not good. There is indication that delay in treatment of >6 months may decrease therapeutic affect and symptomatic improvement of surgery.

Before embarking on surgical treatment, one should ensure that patient is motivated enough for surgical management and one has exhausted most of the conservative measures. The compressive pathology must be concordant to the patient's signs and symptoms and that there are no secondary gains involved (psychometric testing is a good method). The following are some of the surgical methods for removing the offending disk:

- *Open diskectomy* **(Fig. 7)**: Usually the standard care. It offers better visualization. Due to increased muscle dissection, the hospital stay is prolonged. This can be done through laminectomy, laminotomy, or fenestration techniques depending on surgeon preference and training.

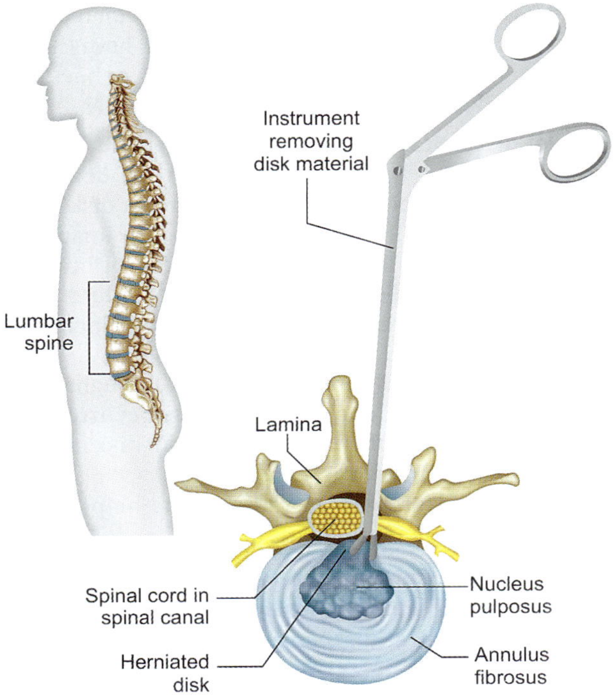

Fig. 7: Open diskectomy.

- *Open microdiskectomy* has recently gained popularity above open diskectomy (and is now accepted as gold standard by many). It is becoming more standard. The muscle damage is more limited so there is significantly reduced postoperative pain and hospital stay. The procedure is performed through either laminotomy or fenestration. The problem is limited visualization of nerve and there is potential for nerve injury because of smaller incision. Headlamps, loupes should be used for improved visualization. Unilateral, limited, open diskectomy (unilateral laminotomy or interlaminar fenestration and removal of free fragments without curetting the disk space and end plates) have demonstrated reduction in postoperative back pain compared with radical or subtotal diskectomy, and reduce the risk of neurologic and vascular injury without significantly increasing the risk of reherniation.
- Microscope-assisted diskectomy—limited muscle dissection, better lighting and magnification are so good delineation of structures. The hospital stay is very less and some centers do this on a day care basis. The operative time is increased for set-up and cost of surgery goes up.
- Endoscopic and percutaneous diskectomy—*see* Chapter on "Low Back Pain, Intervertebral Disk Degeneration, Lumbar Spondylosis, and Degenerative Conditions of Cervical Spine".

Long-term success rates vary between 76 and 93% for open, interlaminar diskectomy. The likelihood of recovery of neurologic deficit is independent of surgical intervention. The predictive factors for improved outcome of surgery for LDH include:

- No workman's compensation claim
- Large, anteroposterior herniations
- More severe symptoms preoperatively
- Married status
- Absence of diabetes
- No joint problems
- Sciatica present for <6 months (true radicular pain—pain that extends to the foot)
- Extruded or sequestered fragments with intact or minimal annulus fissure
- Nonsmoker
- Absence of back pain
- Positive straight leg raise

Comparing Nonoperative and Operative Management

This issue is most commonly referred by quoting the report on long-term outcomes for surgical versus nonsurgical treatment of LDH published in 1983.

- This study indicated that surgery improved short-term outcomes (1-year); however, there was no difference in long-term (4–10 years) outcomes between the surgical and nonsurgical groups. The study has met with the following criticisms (but still this is the most quoted study).
  - High crossover rate of patients initially randomized not to undergo surgery and then proceeding to surgery (25%)
  - Lack of intent-to-treat analysis
  - Small sample size
  - Insensitive outcome measures
- The Spine Patient Outcomes Research Trial (SPORT)—The SPORT randomized trial for patients with LDH better relief of pain, function, decreased disability, and better satisfaction in surgically treated patients at 8-year follow-up compared to nonsurgical cohort.
- The Maine Lumbar Spine Study reported results similar to the 1983 study. Ten-year patient follow-up for surgical and nonsurgical LDH treatment demonstrated that 69% of surgically treated patients reported improvement of their predominant symptom, compared with 61% in the nonsurgical group. Both groups had similar work and disability status at 10-year follow-up; however, patients treated surgically reported better functional status, greater satisfaction with treatment, and greater magnitude of improvement than those treated nonsurgically, despite having worse preoperative symptoms and functional status.

As the differences in clinical outcome between surgical and nonsurgical management for LDH are still vague, the current rationale for surgical management is fostered by the finding that surgical treatment of LDH that was unresponsive to nonsurgical therapy was more cost-effective and provided an increase in quality-adjusted life in comparison with continued nonsurgical treatment. The cost-effectiveness of diskectomy has been reported superior to medical treatment of moderate hypertension or to coronary artery bypass grafting for single-vessel coronary artery disease, but it is inferior to total hip replacement and cervical cancer screening.

FAILURE OF DISKECTOMY (FAILED BACK)

The following are the causes of failure of diskectomy procedure resulting in poor outcome (Kindly also *see* Chapter on "Failed Back Surgery Syndrome").

- Removal of lamina > 25% or facet > 50% predisposes to facet fracture and/or instability.
- Recurrent/persistent disk herniation - SPORT had a 15% revision surgery rate overall and 85% of those patients were treated for recurrent LDH. Outcomes of revision surgery are poor.
- Epidural fibrosis
- Arachnoiditis
- Lumbar canal stenosis
- Wrong level and wrong side
- Emotionally unstable patient/patient requiring workman's compensation

Indications for Fusion after Diskectomy

Posterior fusion can be done after laminectomy or facetectomy during disk removal. The indications are as follows:

- Associated listhesis
- Congenital malformation
- Advanced intervertebral arthrosis
- Instability due to bone removal
- Need to return for heavy manual work

McNab's indications for fusion:

- Less than 50-year-old with normal disk height and root entrapment associated with changes in posterior facet joint necessitating joint excision.
- Progressive history of backache-associated severe sciatic pain and nerve root irritation where mechanical instability is deemed to be the most important cause.
- Recurrent episodes of low back pain in otherwise emotionally stable patients.

Use of dynamic stabilization after diskectomy instead of fusion (*see* Chapter on "Low Back Pain, Intervertebral Disk Degeneration, Lumbar Spondylosis, and Degenerative Conditions of Cervical Spine").

Management of Cauda Equina Syndrome

Emergent decompression is traditionally advocated to prevent permanent weakness and loss of bowel/bladder and sexual function.

- The practice was questioned by a meta-analysis which indicated statistically equivalent postoperative outcomes when comparing patients who underwent decompression within 24 hours of symptom onset with those treated 24–48 hours after symptom onset. A subsequent analysis of this study showed poor methodology and conclusion of the meta-analysis and in repeat evaluation it was found to suffer from too many drawbacks (inconsistent definitions of symptom onset when calculating time to surgery, variable follow-up periods used to report outcomes, lack of inclusion of patients with partial recovery, and too small a sample size for meaningful statistical analysis).
- Repeat analysis demonstrated an increased risk for poor outcome for surgery at 24–48 hours compared with surgery within 24 hours.

There is no concrete evidence till date to reject the increased risks for surgery performed at 24–48 hours or later.

RECURRENT HERNIATION AND REVISION

Recurrent herniation occurs in 5–11% of patients following open diskectomy. Recurrent herniation is defined as recurrent radicular pain onset following lumbar diskectomy, with evidence of neural impingement by disk material at the concurrent level. There should be a gap of minimum 6 weeks with pain relief after the index procedure (else it would qualify for persistent herniation and/or incomplete removal).

- Fat-saturated, gadolinium-enhanced T1-weighted MRI is the modality of choice to evaluate recurrent disk herniation and differentiate between disk material (nonenhancing) and scar (enhancing).
- CT scans and/or oblique radiographs help rule out iatrogenic pars interarticularis fracture.

Surgical treatment options for recurrent disk herniation include repeat diskectomy or fusion.

- Outcome of repeat diskectomy is good (sometimes as good as primary surgery).
- The problem is that these patients are at increased risk for further spine surgery.
- Fusion is often recommended to treat symptomatic recurrent herniations at the involved level though it is difficult to justify completely.

DISK HERNIATION IN PEDIATRIC PATIENTS

Pediatric disk herniations constitute 1–3% of all instances of LDH. Common causes are previous trauma and vertebral column abnormalities such as congenital stenosis or transitional vertebrae. The clinical presentation is similar to that for adults but neurologic deficits in these patients are typically uncommon. The herniation is frequently an avulsed fragment of the ring apophysis of the vertebral body. Surgery usually results in good relief of symptoms though conservative measures are always tried. A unilateral hemilaminectomy/laminotomy (with partial diskectomy) is the procedure of choice, but bilateral laminectomy is occasionally necessary when the avulsed apophysis fragment is large.

LUMBAR SPINAL STENOSIS

INTRODUCTION

Lumbar spinal stenosis (LSS) is a reduction in the dimensions of the central or lateral lumbar spinal canal that occurs most frequently as a result of chronic degenerative changes at the lumbar motion segment. There are various causes of LSS that can be grouped into congenital or developmental and acquired **(Box 1)**.

PATHOANATOMY

The normal cross-sectional area of the lumbar canal is 150–200 mm^2. Absolute central canal stenosis is defined as a decrease in the midsagittal lumbar canal diameter of <10 mm, whereas

10–13 mm represents relative stenosis. Decrease in cross-sectional area to <100 mm^2 is a more reliable indicator of the combined central and lateral lumbar stenosis. Central canal stenosis commonly results from combination of disk bulging anteriorly combined with ligamentum flavum hypertrophy and superior articular process hypertrophy. This compresses several nerves within the dura. The lateral portion of the lumbar canal is divided into three zones: (1) the lateral recess, (2) foraminal zone, and (3) extraforaminal zone **(Fig. 8)**.

- The most common pathology in the lateral recess is bony overgrowth of the superior articular process caused by degenerative facet joint arthrosis. This space is further compromised by bulging disk compressing the traversing nerve root.
- Foraminal height normally ranges from 20 to 23 mm, and anteroposterior depth ranges from 8 to 10 mm in the upper foramen.
    - A foraminal height of <15 mm and a posterior disk height of <4 mm are associated with nerve root compression in 80% of patients.

The lumbar nerve roots lie in the upper foramen and occupy approximately 30% of the available foraminal area. Stenosis in foraminal zone is commonly the result of cartilaginous overgrowth or facet osteophytes, callus/fibrosis from pars defect, foraminal disk and loss of disk height **(Fig. 9)**. Other causes of foramen narrowing are congenital stenosis, achondroplasia (short and narrow pedicles), osteopetrosis, neoplasms, infection, and postsurgical changes.

During extension of the lumbar spine, there is reduced interlaminar space and buckling of the ligamentum flavum causing spinal stenosis. Also foraminal height and width decrease by 14–18% and area decreases by 20% during extension. CT studies show that the cross-sectional area of the foramen increases by 12% in flexion, and that nerve root compression is least in flexion and highest in extension.

Central canal stenosis results from congenitally short pedicles diffuse posterior protrusion of the degenerative disk, and unfolding of the ligamentum flavum **(Fig. 10)**.

BOX 1: Etiological classification of lumbar spinal stenosis.

Congenital/Developmental:
- Degenerative—age related
- Achondroplasia
- Congenital small spinal canal
- Congenital meningeal cysts
- Osteoporosis

Acquired:
- Degenerative—age related
- Degenerative spondylolytic/spondylolisthesis
- Degenerative scoliosis
- Ankylosing spondylitis
- Rheumatoid arthritis
- Pseudogout
- Acromegaly
- Diffuse idiopathic skeletal hyperostosis (DISH)
- Iatrogenic—postdiskectomy/laminectomy/fusion, scarring/fibrosis postchemonucleolysis
- Malunited vertebral fractures
- Spinal infections with abscess bone collapse
- Paget's disease
- Fluorosis
- Pseudogout

Combined - here both congenital and acquired components (above) may co-exist together in variable combination

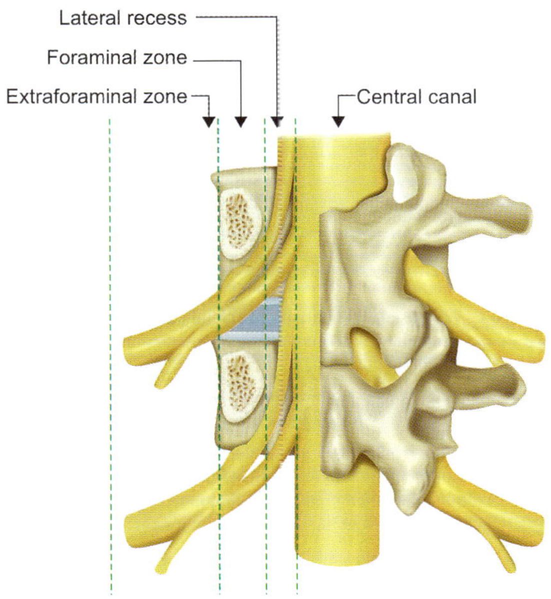

Fig. 8: The central canal, lateral recess, foraminal zone, and extraforaminal zone.

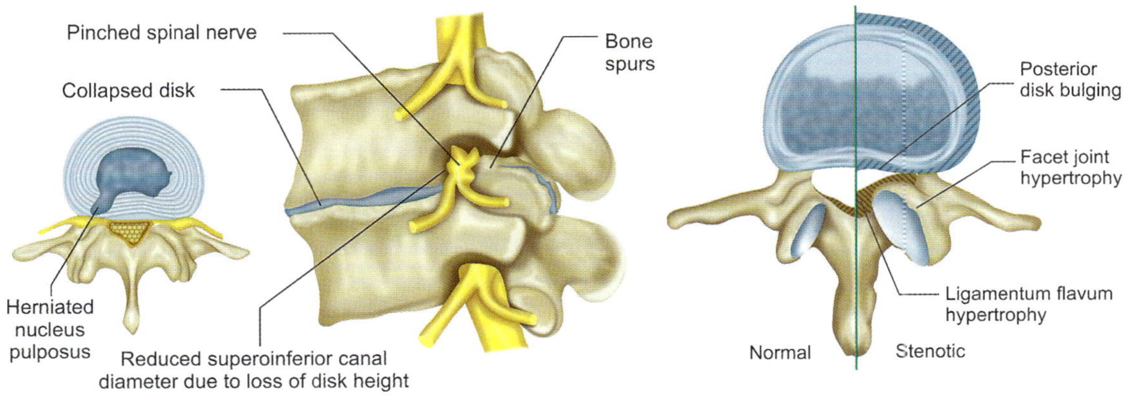

Fig. 9: Illustration of some causes of lateral recess and foraminal stenosis.

PATHOPHYSIOLOGY

Similar to LDH, the symptoms of LSS likely result from a combination of mechanical compression and local inflammation.

- The rate of onset of compression determines symptom atology, as rapid onset results in more severe symptoms.
- Multilevel compression may also have a greater impact than single-level compression.
- Mechanical compression may lead to decreased nutrition, reduced neural activity, and ischemic neuritis. At least 50% of spinal nerve root, nutritional support is dependent on cerebrospinal fluid diffusion.

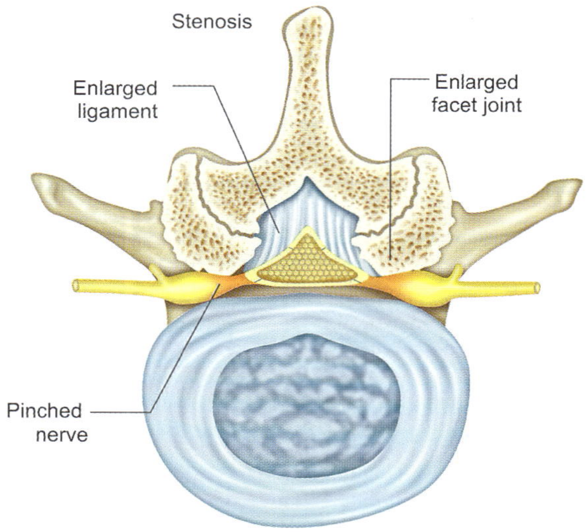

Fig. 10: The causes of spinal stenosis.

The cause of pain in LSS is due to a combination of increased neural tension, local irritation from mechanical compression, and local ischemia.

CLINICAL FEATURES

Patients are usually older than 50 years of age. Low back pain and stiffness are commonly reported as a baseline pain along with neurogenic claudication—refers to buttock and leg pain that worsens with lumbar extension and ambulation and is relieved by lumbar flexion and/or rest **(Table 3)**. The lumbar flexion as in case of walking with the help of walker or walking uphill provides good pain relief but walking downhill produces spinal extension and reduces foraminal diameter exacerbating pain and symptoms. Lying down is more comfortable than sitting and standing. The neurogenic claudication must be differentiated from vascular claudication and degenerative disk disease. Over the years the patients develop lower extremity weakness, persistent radiculopathy and symptoms compounded by concomitant cervical stenosis causing cervical myelopathy. The prevalence of combined cervical and lumbar, or tandem spinal stenosis (TSS) is reportedly 5–25%.

Physical Examination

Physical examination is mostly normal in patients with LSS. In SPORT study, only 50% patients had concurrent physical examination findings such as depressed reflexes, sensory-motor deficits, or positive nerve tension signs.

- Reduced lumbar extension
- Muscle atrophy
- Difficulty in toe/heel walking

TABLE 3: Differentiating features of neurogenic and vascular claudication and segregation from degenerative disk disease (spondylosis).

Findings	*Neurogenic claudication*	*Vascular claudication*	*Lumbar spondylosis*
Pain type and location	• Lower extremity vague, cramping acheslocated to back/buttocks/legs • Sharp burning and paresthesias in legs	Calf tightness and cramping	Dull low back aching
Radiation	Commonly seen, proximal to distal	Often localized in legs, distal to proximal radiation if at all	Low back and hips maximum to thighs
Exacerbation	Lumbar extension, standing, walking upright no change with cycling (unless trunk extended)	All lower extremity exercise	General activity including twisting, bending, standing, and lifting
Walking distance	Variable and reducing	Constant	Variable
Relief	Sitting, lumbar flexion, squatting and rest.Only standing does not relieve pain, spine needs to be flexed	Standing, cessation of lower extremity exercise	Decreased activity, rest
Back pain	Common	Uncommon	Common
Bicycle/treadmill test	Bicycle generates minimal symptoms; treadmill generates symptoms	Bicycle and treadmill generate symptoms	Variable
Time to relief of pain	Slow	Rapid	Slow
Walking uphill	Walking uphill generates minimal symptoms due to postural spine flexion; walking downhill generates symptoms dueto extended spine	Walking uphill or downhill generate symptoms	Variable
Lower extremity appearance	Normal	Vascular changes including hair loss, toenail atrophy, edema	Normal
Pulses lower extremity	Normal	Diminished	Normal
Lumbar range of motion	Diminished, painful	Normal	Diminished, painful

- Absent long tract signs
- Sensations and motor examination are usually normal except in advanced cases.
- Patients walk with lumbar flexion and avoid lying flat or standing straight.

The manifestations of central and lateral canal stenosis are not easily distinguished.

- Unilateral radicular pain from foraminal stenosis is worsened by extension to the painful side (Kemp sign)
- Presence of paresthesia indicates dorsal root compression in foramen.

DIAGNOSTIC IMAGING

Plain radiographs: Upright anteroposterior, lateral and flexion/extension radiographs.

- Delineate the amount of lumbar degeneration:
  - Disk space narrowing and degenerative disk disease
  - Endplate osteophytes and sclerosis
  - Facet enlargement and osteophyte formation
  - Narrowed neuroforaminal canal
  - Loss of lumbar lordosis
- Evaluate for congenital stenosis
- Evaluate associated scoliosis and spondylolisthesis; and rule out trauma, infection, or malignancy as a potential source of symptoms.

Magnetic resonance imaging is currently the recommended advanced imaging modality to evaluate LSS. MRI is as accurate as CT myelography and is noninvasive. Contrast is needed only in postoperative cases. Obtain both axial and sagittal—coronal cuts **(Figs. 11A to C)**. Evaluate the following on MRI scan:

- Spinal and lateral recess stenosis
- Disk bulge and herniations
- Facet changes (degeneration, osteophyte, hypertrophy, cyst formation)
- Evidence of obliteration of perineural fat on images is an early indicator of foraminal stenosis.
- Ligamentum flavum hypertrophy
- Tumors, lysis, infection, etc.

Electrodiagnostic testing using electromyography has high specificity for diagnosing LSS (and in differentiating LSS from other neuromuscular disorders including peripheral or diabetic neuropathy, myopathy, and inflammatory neuropathies). In combination with MRI, it reduces the high false-positive rate associated with the former.

TREATMENT

The natural history of LSS is variable and most patients will not experience severe neurologic deficits or impairment. Paralysis as is often used by surgeon to bewilder patient for accepting surgery is uncommon. Three-fourths of the patients who are not operated or who refuse surgery remain unchanged or improve at long-term follow-up. Studies have also shown inconsistent correlation between the severity of clinical symptoms and/or treatment response and the severity of stenosis, the location of the stenosis (central or lateral), and the number of stenotic levels. So, a fair extended and aggressive nonsurgical treatment trial is warranted. Options include activity modification, NSAIDs, narcotics, antidepressants, physical therapy, and ESI/SNRI as discussed for LDH. There have been concerns raised that these symptomatic treatments might be less effective for LSS compared to LDH; however, good outcomes with physical therapy for patients with LSS have been reported and benefits increase with increasing duration in responsive patients.

Surgical treatment is needed in patients who fail and do not progress on conservative measures. These patients should be however willing for possible limited benefit of surgical intervention. The indications are patients having

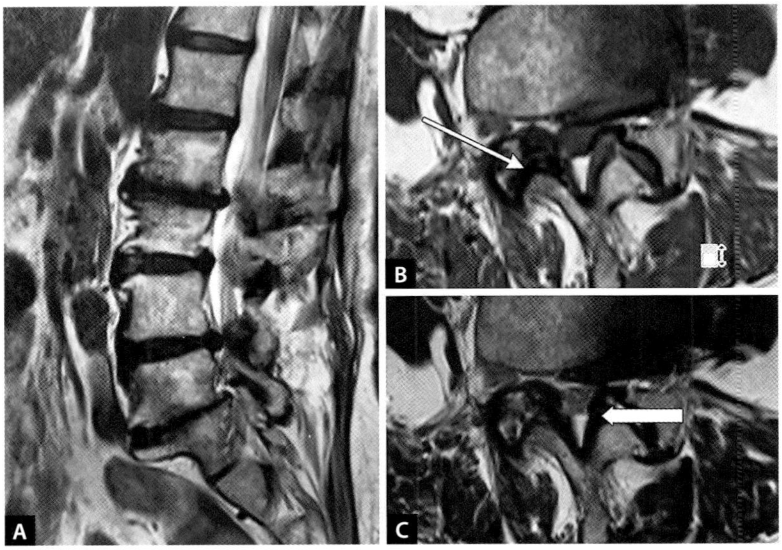

Figs. 11A to C: Sagittal (A) and axial T1 (B) and axial T2 (C) MRI scans of a 67-year-old female demonstrating multilevel degenerative disk disease from L2 to S1 (A) in sagittal images. The axial images show lumbar canal stenosis secondary to facetal arthrosis prominent on right side with osteophyte formation and joint space destruction (arrow, B). The subarticular bone shows cystic degeneration. Ligamentum hypertrophy is marked on axial T2 image (C) as thickened black structure compromising the canal space (block arrow) dorsally.

radicular pain or those with neurogenic claudication with small walking distance say < 100 m sort of making them home bound. The goals of surgery should be communicated to the patient clearly and include:

- Pain relief (that may not be complete)
- Increased mobility
- Prevention of further neurological damage
- Improvement in quality of life

The cornerstone of surgical treatment of LSS is decompression of the compressed neural elements in particular the nerve roots. Treatment is dictated by the severity of myelopathy, radiculopathy, and canal stenosis. The choice of surgery depends on:

- Level of stenosis (one or many)
- Number of involved segments
- Location of stenosis (central/foraminal)
- Associated deformities (listhesis, degenerative scoliosis)
- Presence of instability

Canal stenosis: Resection of approximately 50% of the cephalad and caudad lamina and the intervening ligamentum flavum often provides adequate central decompression. Decompression should then extend laterally into the lateral recess to the medial wall of the pedicle and into the foramen. Care must be taken to preserve > 50% of the bilateral facets because resection of > 50% of the bilateral facets or complete unilateral facetectomy may result in iatrogenic instability.

Lateral recess and foraminal stenosis: Decompression can be achieved using one or multiple level laminotomies decompressing individual roots.

Decompression with fusion: The role of spinal fusion following decompression depends on the presence of associated coronal or sagittal instability. Fusion is associated with longer hospital stay, increased bleeding, longer surgical time, and increased cost. Fusion is recommended when one or more of the following are present:

- Unstable degenerative kyphosis or scoliosis
- Degenerative spondylolisthesis
- Iatrogenic instability following decompression
- Recurrent same level or adjacent level stenosis

In cases of tandem canal stenosis (combined cervical and lumbar stenosis), it is better to treat patients with a cervical spinal canal of 10 mm or less by an initial cervical surgery. Whereas patients with predominant lower extremity radiculopathy and a cervical canal of 11–13 mm or more may be initially managed with lumbar surgery. Cervical decompression usually improves myelopathic symptoms; however, neurogenic claudication may worsen and would need subsequent lumbar decompression.

Dynamic stabilization, nonfusion technologies, including interspinous implants and motion-sparing rods (discussed in Chapter on "Low Back Pain, Intervertebral Disk Degeneration, Lumbar Spondylosis, and Degenerative Conditions of Cervical Spine") may be used instead of fusion.

Outcome of surgical treatment:

- The Maine Lumbar Spine Study for surgical and nonsurgical treatment of LSS demonstrated greater relief of predominant symptoms, demonstrated greater functional improvement, and reported greater satisfaction with functional status at short-term and intermediate-term follow-up, despite having worse preoperative symptoms.
- Instrumentation and fusion were associated with superior clinical outcomes compared with patients with a pseudarthrosis at long-term follow-up.

CONCLUSION

- Herniation of nucleus pulposus causes typical symptomatology that should be quickly recognized and treated appropriately.
- Most cases respond well to conservative treatment but in some the regression of the herniated material and symptoms both are incomplete. These patients especially if having progressive, neurological symptoms should be managed by surgical removal of the disk material after appropriate imaging confirmation.
- Not all patients should be given a conservative trial and surgery is indicated on an emergency basis in patients with CES or those with advanced neurological damage at presentation.
- Lumbar canal stenosis is a common finding in degenerated spine with typical development of neurological claudication. As patients frequently respond favorably to the conservative treatment, an aggressive and prolonged conservative trial is warranted for patients with canal stenosis. Surgery is reserved for those not improving or worsening on conservative treatment and principally comprises of decompression of the neural elements at the identified level(s).

CHAPTER 97

Lumbar Spondylolysis and Spondylolisthesis

Manish Kumar Varshney

INTRODUCTION

Spondylolysis is a disruption or insufficiency in the pars interarticularis (bony connection between the superior and the inferior articular process) of the posterior spinal arch **(Figs. 1A and B)**.

Spondylolisthesis (Greek *spondylos—vertebra, olisthesis—slippage*)—is an anterior vertebral translation, or slippage, in relation to the caudal vertebra **(Figs. 2A and B)**. The common sites for this are the fourth lumbar vertebra (L4) on the fifth (L5), and the L5 on S1 (most common). Spondylolisthesis can occur with or without spondylolysis.

[The inferior articular process of each lumbar vertebra articulates with the superior articular process of the subjacent vertebra in an overlapping or shingle fashion. The pars interarticularis is the bony connection between the superior and the inferior processes **(Figs. 3A and B)**].

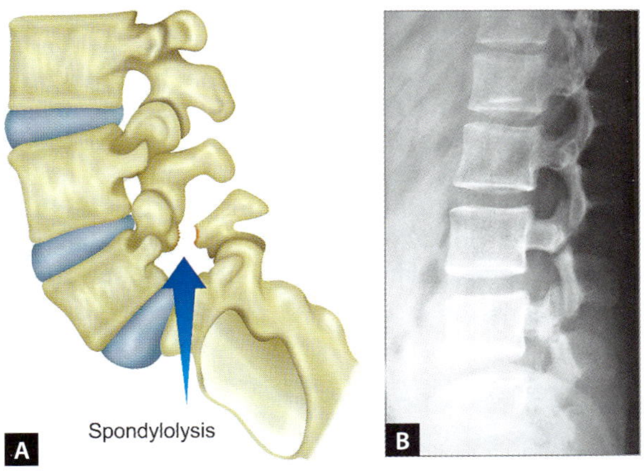

Figs. 1A and B: Spondylolysis: Pars defect, radiograph depicting the clear pars defect in lumbar 4th vertebra (note the subtle defect in lumbar 5th vertebra—one should not be too engrossed by seeing a clear finding as to miss a subtle one).

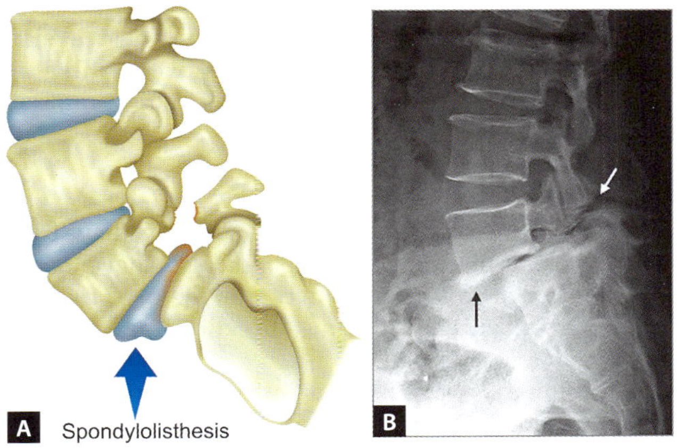

Figs. 2A and B: Spondylolisthesis: (A) Anteroinferior slip of 5th lumbar vertebra over 1st sacral vertebra; (B) Radiograph depicting the same—grade II slip of L5 over S1.

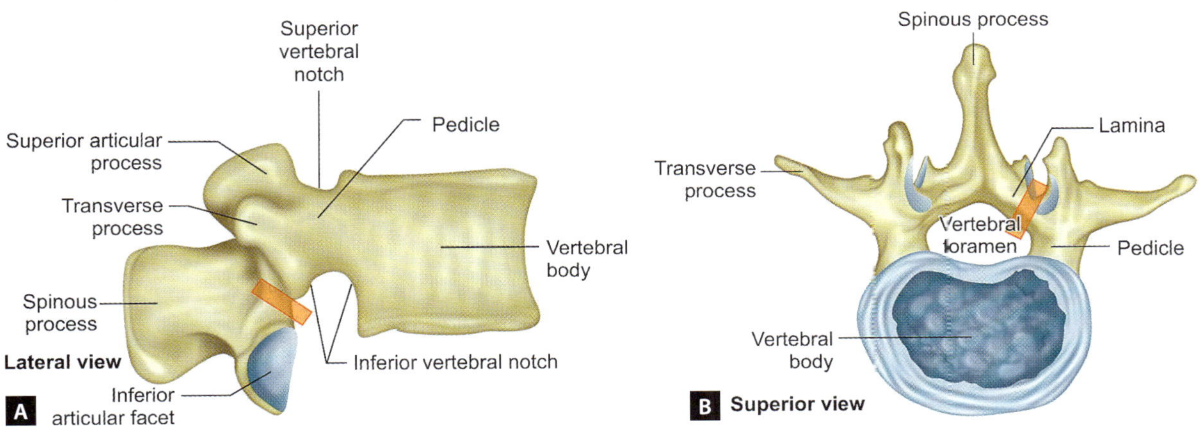

Figs. 3A and B: Pars interarticularis: (A) The pars region as depicted in the side; and (B) Axial view.

SPONDYLOLYSIS

Robert and Lambl revealed a neural arch defect at the pars interarticularis, termed spondylolysis in their anatomical studies. The term spondylolysis, in addition to above simplistic definition, has now been expanded to include a spectrum of other pathologies such as:

- Stress reaction—there is no cortical or trabecular disruption but just an intraosseous edema with associated sclerosis of the pars interarticularis, lamina, or pedicle.
- Stress fracture—a stress fracture is a disruption of pars trabecular or cortical bone but without separation of the fracture fragments.
- Pars fracture—a pars fracture is a separation of the pars interarticularis fragments with associated displacement.
- Pars nonunion—the most common spondylolytic defect is chronic nonunion of the pars interarticularis, with associated bony sclerosis and fibrous tissue.

Causes: Exact etiology is elusive but certain risk factors have been identified:

- Repetitive trauma—sports that require frequent or persistent hyperextension of the lumbar spine, viz., gymnastics, diving, wrestling, weight lifting, etc.
- Genetics—developmental defect of the pars and spondylolisthesis (Inuit Eskimos have a much greater overall incidence). About 15–70% of first-degree relatives affected with the disorder. Lysis is two to three times common in boys but slippage is two to three times most common in females.

PATHOPHYSIOLOGY

- Repetitive impacts can produce a stress or fatigue fracture of the pars interarticularis. Spondylolysis never has been reported in individuals who cannot walk.
- "Nutcracker" mechanism—direct compression of the region under stress.
- Tension mechanism—pars interarticularis is subjected to traction in various sports and athletic activities.

SYMPTOMS

- Midline low back pain is most prominent.
- Radicular symptoms are much less common than back pain. The pain and numbness are caused by nerve root compression due either to fibrous tissue hypertrophy within the pars defect or foraminal stenosis resulting from an associated spondylolisthesis.
- The symptoms are exacerbated by extension-based activities.

NATURAL HISTORY

- Spondylolysis is present in 5% of the general population.
- 15% of individuals with a pars interarticularis lesion had progression to a spondylolisthesis.
- Slip is most susceptible to occur during growth spurt.
- Progression to a slip is not a cause of pain.
- Nearly half of the patients with lysis do not have a slip.

CLINICAL FEATURES

There is no detectable deformity. Most patients with spondylolysis are asymptomatic. When symptoms occur, they are due to muscle contraction and spasm, as the body tries to limit movement around a painful pseudarthrosis of the pars interarticularis, a tear in the annulus fibrosus, or compressed spinal nerve roots.

IMAGING

Anteroposterior (AP) radiographs are given much less importance as in classic texts the defect is prominently always shown in lateral projections. When unilateral the defect is often missed on conventional lateral radiographs. Unilateral defects in the pars interarticularis can usually be seen on AP radiographs, and, if the spondylolysis is bilateral, it can be seen on lateral radiographs. Additional features should also be evaluated on radiographs including a coexisting degenerative disk disease or spondylolisthesis. Differential diagnosis of back pain like the presence of fracture, tumor, or infection is also commonly revealed on a radiograph. Oblique views **(Fig. 4)** show defects or sclerosis of the pars interarticularis that are not visible on AP or lateral images. Standing long films should be used to assess global sagittal balance, thoracic kyphosis, lumbar lordosis, pelvic incidence, sacral slope, and pelvic tilt.

Computed tomography (CT) scan is useful in detecting subtle pars defects that are difficult to see on routine radiographs, but having high suspicion. It should be understood that even on a CT scan the spondylolytic defects may be missed as they lay in the plane of axial cuts so sagittal and coronal reconstructions should be obtained. A technetium bone scan or single-photon emission CT (SPECT) can demonstrate spondylolysis by showing abnormal uptake in the pars interarticularis despite normal plain radiographs.

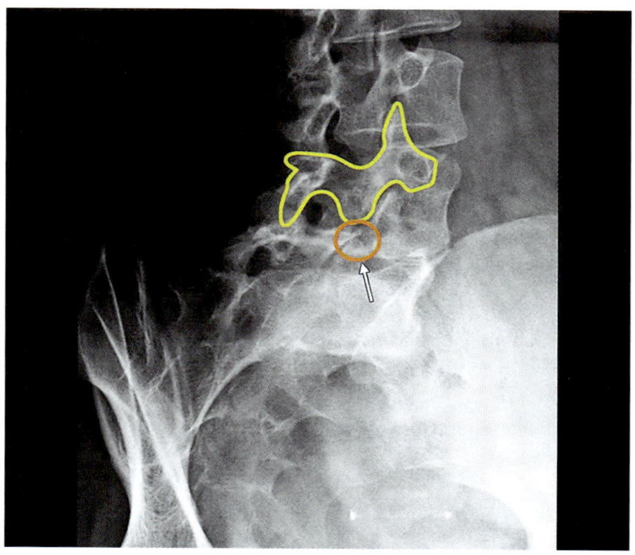

Fig. 4: X-ray spondylolysis (oblique view)—one can appreciate the normal looking scotty dog in the 4th lumbar vertebra (outlined) while the neck in the 5th lumbar vertebra is broken (encircled and arrow).

Magnetic resonance imaging (MRI) is possibly most useful investigation to:

- Identify any coexistent pathology
- Identify stress patterns
- Differentiate union [(high signal changes) from nonunion absence of signal] in the ipsilateral pedicle

DIFFERENTIAL DIAGNOSIS

- Patient ≤ 18 years—primary spinal neoplasms, infection
- Older patients—degenerative disk disease, facet arthrosis, infection, and malignancy

SPONDYLOLISTHESIS

INTRODUCTION

First written description of spondylolisthesis is attributed to Herbiniaux, a Belgian obstetrician (1978) who described narrowing of birth canal by bony prominence anterior to sacrum (for definition see earlier). The term spondylolisthesis was coined approximately one century later, in 1854, by Kilian. The severity of the spondylolisthesis is commonly accessed and communicated by the magnitude of the slip and the slip angle using plain lateral radiographs, despite availability of various classification systems.

CLASSIFICATION SYSTEM

Several classification systems exist for spondylolisthesis following are the most commonly used:

Meyerding system describes slippage as a percentage of uncovering of the caudal vertebral superior end plate based on Taillard method *radiologically* **(Figs. 5A and B)**. Taillard method (Wiltse et al., 1983)—the degree of the slip is expressed as a percentage of the anterior displacement of the inferior vertebral end plate of the cephalad body over the superior end plate of the caudal vertebra:

- Grade I (0–25% slip)—low grade
- Grade II (26–50% slip)—low grade
- Grade III (51–75% slip)—high grade
- Grade IV (76–99% slip)—high grade
- Grade V (Spondyloptosis or 100% slip)—high grade

Marchetti and Bartolozzi classification system classifies spondylolisthesis by *anatomic etiology and prognosis* **(Table 1)** and is considered more rational. The two primary categories distinguish between developmental slips, which are at high risk of progression, and acquired slips, which are relatively stable. Some confusion in organization might arise as pars defects developing later in congenitally abnormal

TABLE 1: Marchetti and Bartolozzi classification system for spondylolisthesis.

Developmental	*Acquired*
• High dysplastic • Low dysplastic	• *Traumatic*—includes acute injuries and stress fractures • *Degenerative*—could be primary (intact bony arch with degeneration in the disk and the facet joints) and secondary (adjacent to nonsurgically fused segments) • *Pathologic*—may arise out of local pathology (e.g., malignant) or systemic pathology (e.g., metabolic bone disease, Marfan syndrome or osteogenesis imperfecta) • *Postsurgical*—this is again divided into direct (from excessive removal of both facet joints) and indirect (usually immediately above a spinal fusion) types

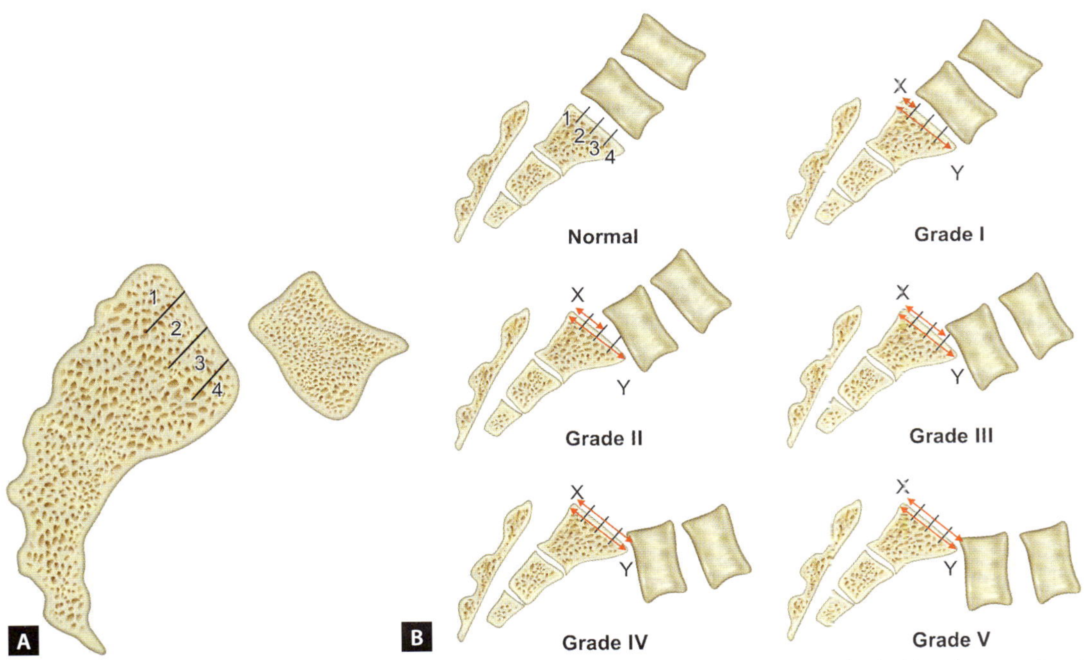

Figs. 5A and B: Meyerding classification of spondylolisthesis: (A) The superior sacral plateau is divided into four equal parts; (B) Relative subluxation of 5th lumbar vertebra is measured with this reference diving into progressive grades.

TABLE 2: Modified Wiltse, Newman, and Macnab classification of spondylolisthesis.

Type	*Name*	*Comments*	*Commonly involved vertebral level*
I	Congenital/ dysplastic	Forward displacement due to dysplasia of sacrum or fifth lumbar arch, facets, etc. (see text for various dysplasias in Marchetti and Bartolozzi system)	L5-S1
II	Isthmic or spondylolytic	Defect in pars inter-articularis	L5-S1
III	Degenerative	Forward displacement due to segmental instability and disk degeneration, facetal arthropathy	L4-L5 (90%), L5-S1 or L3-L4 (10%)
IV	Traumatic	Fracture of neural arch other than spondylolysis	L5-S1
V	Pathologic	Secondary forward displacement due to pathological lesion in pars interarticularis, pedicle or facet or generalized metabolic disturbance	Any level
VI	Postsurgical	Iatrogenic displacement of facet, ligament, disk or bone	Any level

vertebra are strictly speaking acquired but may be labeled developmental. Developmental spondylolisthesis is further divided into high-dysplastic or low-dysplastic categories (depending on which set of facets is involved). Dysplastic abnormalities like incompetence of the posterior arch (the pedicle, lamina, and pars interarticularis), an abnormal structure or orientation of the facets, a trapezoidal L5 body, and a rounded S1 superior end plate can lead to instability and slip progression.

Wiltse system classifies spondylolisthesis based on their *etiology* **(Table 2)**. The three of the Wiltse categories (degenerative, traumatic, and pathologic) can be considered subcategories of acquired spondylolisthesis in *Marchetti* and *Bartolozzi system*, because they are similar in prognosis (specifically, slip progression) and treatment.

NATURAL HISTORY

- Slip progression appears to slow with each decade.
- Patients with higher grades of spondylolisthesis and higher slip angles, a measure of lumbosacral kyphosis, have a higher risk of progression.
- Patients with low-dysplastic spondylolisthesis have a lower prevalence of progression than those with high-dysplastic spondylolisthesis.
- The risk factors for slippage are:
  - Preoperative slip angle > 40°
  - Slip of >50%
  - Kyphotic slip angle
  - Female patient
  - Dysplastic spondylolisthesis
  - Presence and increasing back pain
  - Abnormal gait with protuberant abdomen

CONGENITAL OR DYSPLASTIC SPONDYLOLISTHESIS

This type almost always occurs at the lower end of the lumbar spine, primarily between L5 and the sacrum. Displacement occurs early, usually during the adolescent growth spurt. By the age of 5 years, the prevalence is approximately 5%, rising to approximately 7% in adult life. There is a 2:1 female-to-male ratio. Most Grades IV and V subluxations occur during the adolescent growth spurt (more in females) or during pregnancy. Congenital spondylolisthesis represents 14–21% of all spondylolisthesis cases.

Etiology and Pathogenesis

- There is a congenital or dysplastic abnormality of the L5-S1 facet joint that prevents proper articulation. This allows the superior vertebra to slide forward over the inferior vertebra. Displacement is early but limited due to intact neural arch. The pars interarticularis is intact but poorly developed, elongated or lysed.
- Hook and catch mechanism—the hook is made up of the pedicle, pars interarticularis and the inferior articular process of the higher vertebra, and the catch is the superior articular process of the one below. Slippage occurs due to imperfect organization, either anomaly in the hook or the catch which may also be supplanted by deformation or stretching of abnormal ligaments. The hook and catch no longer function properly.
- An intact neural arch increases the chance that even low-grade slips (25–35%) will have associated compression of the cauda equina or exiting nerve roots.

Subtypes

- Dysplastic articular process in horizontal direction. Patient has severe hamstring spasm. Often associated with spina bifida (occulta).
- Dysplastic facet with asymmetric sagittal orientation and intact neural arch. Patient has leg pain and radicular symptoms. There is high chance of developing cauda equina syndrome and nerve root compression.
- Failed vertebral body formation. Angular kyphosis of the involved region (congenital kyphosis).

Clinical Presentation

- Radicular symptoms due to nerve of root compression—pain radiates into lower extremities (rarely below the knee) with little or no back pain. Fatigue or weakness in lower extremities.
- Cauda equina compression:
  - Incontinence of bowel or bladder
  - Saddle anesthesia

Radiological Evaluation

Plain radiographs in standard projections and oblique X-ray films with lateral flexion and extension views should be considered and repeated every 4–6 months until skeletal maturity to follow slips considered stable.

Treatment

Most congenital spondylolisthesis patients with progression of the slip require decompression and arthrodesis of the involved motion segment.

ISTHMIC SPONDYLOLISTHESIS

Isthmus refers to pars interarticularis—the portion of the neural arch that connects the lamina with the pedicle, facet joints and transverse process. Defect in the isthmus may cause vertebral body subluxation producing the isthmic spondylolisthesis. This is the most common spondylolytic disorder among children and young adults. About 50% patients have spondylolysis alone. Males predominate in a 2:1 ratio. Males are as twice as likely to have a pars interarticularis defect, but females are more likely to have a high-grade slip as mentioned earlier. The disorder is unique to upright posture and is absent in quadrupeds. It occurs only after walking begins, most commonly from 7 to 8 years and is not seen in nonambulators or bedridden patients. The incidence increases with age as in dysplastic form.

Etiology and Subtypes

There are three described subtypes **(Fig. 6)**:

1. Early fatigue fracture that persists because of the constant motion of a poor mechanical environment. This is the classic lytic lesion of the pars indicative of a stress fracture. Fibrous tissue exists between fracture edges.
2. Elongated but intact isthmus; this is thought to represent healed repetitive microfractures.
3. Acute fracture of the pars interarticularis is the rarest of the subtypes. Slippage is rare, often heals with immobilization.

There are various theories to explain the defect in pars:

- Hereditary dysplasia of the pars interarticularis causing isthmic defect.
- Nutcracker mechanism—an erect posture, combined with the normal 40–60° of lumbar lordosis, produces a constant downward axial force or thrust on pars interarticularis. This repetitive trauma causes microfractures, which heal incompletely forming fibrous tissue and nonunion. Also repetitive extension activities cause increased loading of posterior elements of the spine.
- Fatigue fracture of the pars interarticular is due to tensile forces—risk factors include vigorous exercise, participation in competitive sports involving repetitive lumbar extension and flexion, and Scheuermann's disease.
- A strong genetic component is involved:
  - Inuit race—Persistent stooped posture during common employment in harvesting seal blubber; high incidence (26–50%) continues to increase in this population until individuals are 34 years old.
  - A known relative will have 25–70% chance of having the disease.

Four histopathologic patterns have been observed: (1) thin fibrous bands, (2) thick fibrous columns, (3) a bony bridge, or (4) a false joint but significance is unknown. The abnormal pars interarticularis tissue is richly innervated and may be a source of pain during movement.

Signs and Symptoms

Though the onset occurs in early childhood the symptoms appear late with patients presenting in late adolescence for evaluation. There is a dull aching pain in the back, buttocks, or thighs beginning during the adolescent growth spurt and exacerbated by activity. There is no relation of pain to the degree of slip or development of lysis. So, most patients with spondylolysis or even low-grade slips are asymptomatic. This makes it imperative to search for other causes of the pain (infection, neoplasm, fracture, or disk herniation) before attributing symptoms to the spondylolisthesis. Of symptomatic children, 92% complain of recurrence during adulthood; 55% complain of sciatica at the affected nerve root or roots. True radicular symptoms are rare but if present are often restricted to L5 root distribution (irritation, compression, or tension due to L5-S1 listhesis). The symptoms develop due to:

- Compression of the root by the hypertrophic callus at the pars interarticularis defect (L5)
- Degenerated, herniated disk at the level causing compression (S1)
- Higher-grade slips may cause stretching of the nerve root (L5). Even the distal root say S1 may also get stretched (S1).

Pain appearing after patients are 40 years old is unlikely to be related to a pars interarticularis defect. Disk degeneration in spondylolytic spine is the main cause.

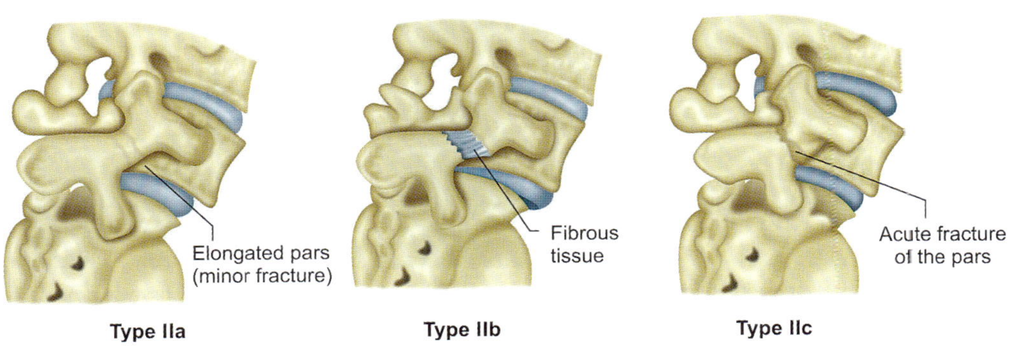

Fig. 6: Types of isthmic spondylolisthesis.

Physical Findings

- In L5 pars lesion, the neural arch remains with S1 but the rest slides forward with the L4, so during palpation the defect will be palpated at L4-L5 region as the neural arch of L5 remains at place! A posterior step-off along the spinous processes can be seen in patients with a grade II or higher slip.
- Angular displacement may cause lumbosacral kyphosis.
- Lumbosacral kyphosis and trunk shortening is apparent with an absence of a waistline, abdominal, and flank skin folds with higher-grade slips. To maintain the sagittal balance patient compensates by:
  - Hyperextension of the lumbar spine and rotation of the pelvis such that the sacrum is vertical.
  - Flexion of the knees and hips (Phalen–Dickson sign).
- Deep palpation over the affected area may reproduce local pain.
- 80% have spasm and foreshortening of the paraspinal and hamstring muscles.
- Limited forward flexion and decreased straight leg raise correspond to hamstring tightness.
- A flexible scoliosis occurs in 5–7% of all patients with spondylolisthesis (which usually corrects spontaneously following surgery for the slip).

Natural History

- About 68% patients with lysis have slip. Lysis destined to develop slip will have so by adolescence.
- Of adults with a slip:
  - 40% will not progress.
  - 40% will progress < 5 mm.
  - Only 15% will progress > 1 cm.
- Female patients with a documented slip often experience progression more than males.
- Disk degeneration adds to the potential for slip progression.
- High slip angle has higher likelihood of progression.

Diagnostic Evaluation

- Plain radiographs in the standing position in standard projections.
- Oblique views increase the sensitivity of plain radiography by a small amount but at significantly increased gonadal radiation. Thirty-degree oblique cranial tilt X-ray films may be more sensitive than traditional oblique X-ray films for demonstrating spondylolysis. Instability can be assessed by dynamic lateral flexion and extension plain radiographs.
- Classically, the defect in the pars interarticularis is seen as the "Scottie dog's neck with collar" on oblique views **(Figs. 7A and B)**.
- In high-grade slips especially the spondyloptosis, the posterior body of L5 rests on the sacral promontory. This results in a trapezoidal or wedge-shaped L5 body and a rounded sacral dome, which can be seen on AP radiograph as the "Napoleon's hat" sign **(Figs. 8A and B)**. The slip is classified and graded based on the following systems:
  - Meyerding classification (discussed earlier) measured by defining percentage slip **(Fig. 9)**.
  - Slip angle or angle of kyphosis or sagittal rotation **(Fig. 10)** is measured as the angle between the superior endplate of L5 and a line perpendicular to the posterior border of the sacrum. It is the most sensitive indicator of potential instability and clinical symptoms. Risk factor for slippage includes preoperative angle > 35–40° or a kyphotic slip angle.
  - Lumbar index **(Fig. 11)** is a measure of the wedging of the anterior L5 vertebral body, expressed as the quotient between anterior and posterior height of the slipped vertebra.

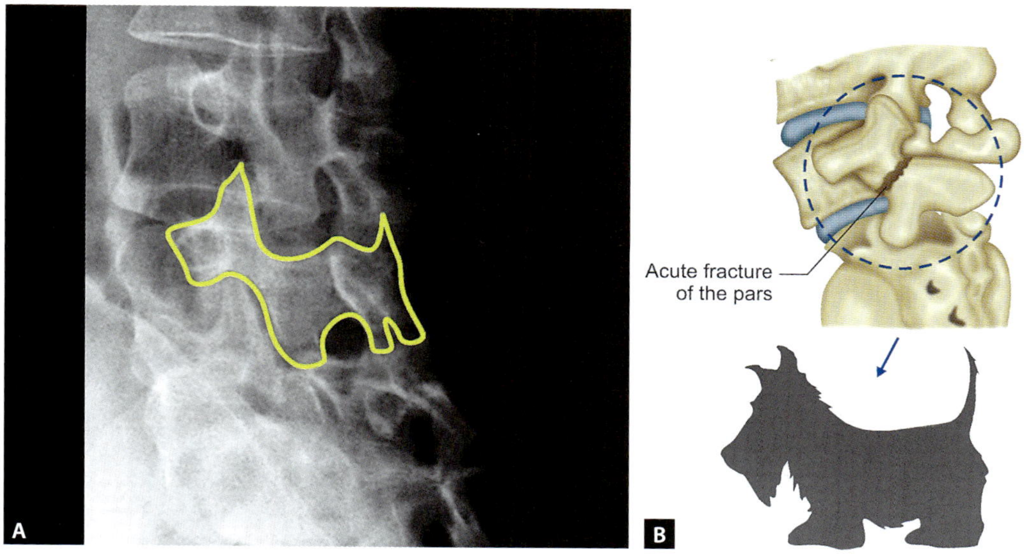

Figs. 7A and B: (A) Scottie dog appearance on oblique radiograph; (B) The mouth and nose are formed by transverse process, ears are formed by the superior articular process, neck region is formed by pars interarticularis, trunk and abdomen are formed by the lamina and spinous process, front legs are formed by the ipsilateral articular process while rear legs are formed by the opposite side inferior articular process as detailed in this illustration. When the pars interarticularis is broken and gets elongated showing a fracture it resembles a "Scotty dog wearing collar".

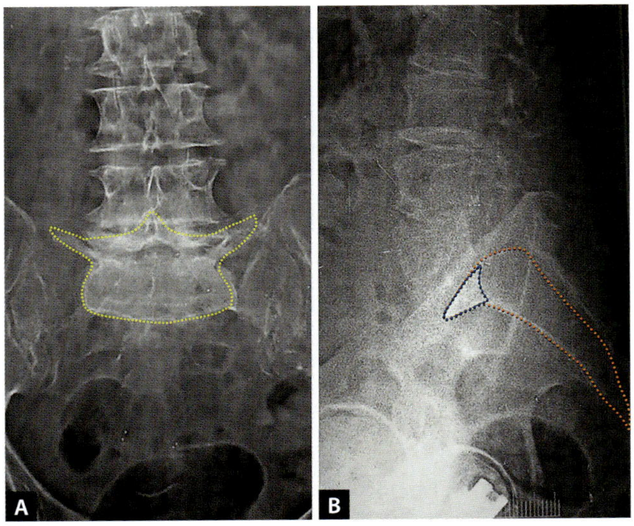

Figs. 8A and B: The "Napoleon's hat sign" in severe grade spondylolisthesis (A). The silhouette of Napoleon hat is marked over the subluxed vertebral body (yellow dotted closed polygon). The lateral projection demonstrates rounded sacral dome with anterior shelf formation to extend support for falling 5th lumbar vertebral body (B). The whole sacrum is outlined in orange dotted closed polygon while the shelf is outlined in blue polygon.

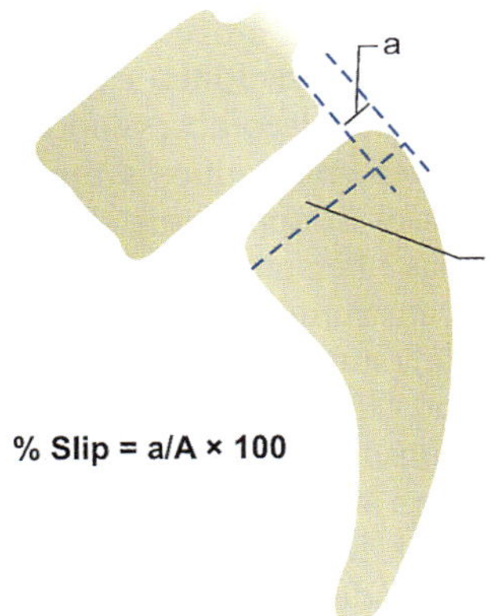

Fig. 9: Measuring percentage slip: Slip is measured by dividing amount of displacement of cephalad vertebra by diameter of caudal vertebral body, expressed as percentage.

- Sacral inclination **(Fig. 12)**
- Percentage of rounding of the sacral dome
- The degree of lumbar lordosis
- The degree of sagittal rotation
- Measure pelvic incidence, pelvic tilt, sacral slope (see adult-onset scoliosis)

▪ 36-inch AP and lateral radiographs obtained to evaluate coronal and sagittal balance and the presence of scoliosis.
▪ Normal radiographs and high suspicion can be evaluated by SPECT that illustrates the metabolic activity at the region of a suspected pars interarticularis defect.
▪ CT scan can be used to define the bony anatomy more clearly (discussed earlier in spondylolysis).
▪ MRI is the study of choice for spinal stenosis and defining the neural elements. It is also invaluable for demonstrating the presence of disk degeneration.

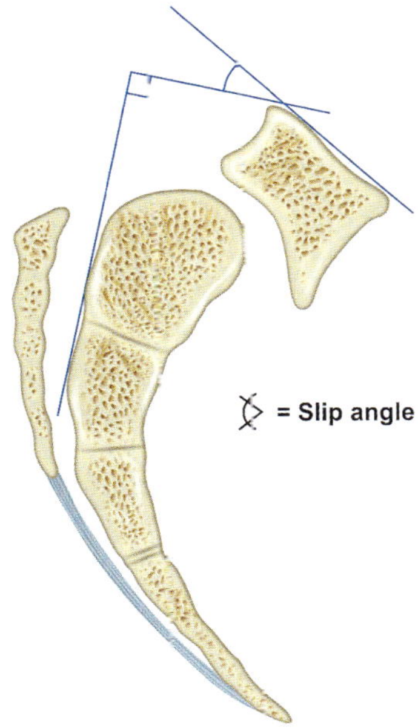

Fig. 10: Slip angle or angle of kyphosis. The progressive slip of rostral vertebra produces a sagittal rotation and is measured as an angle (see text).

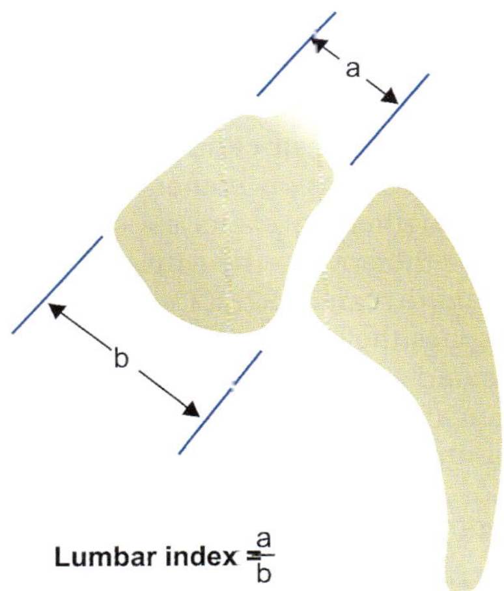

Fig. 11: Lumbar index (see text).

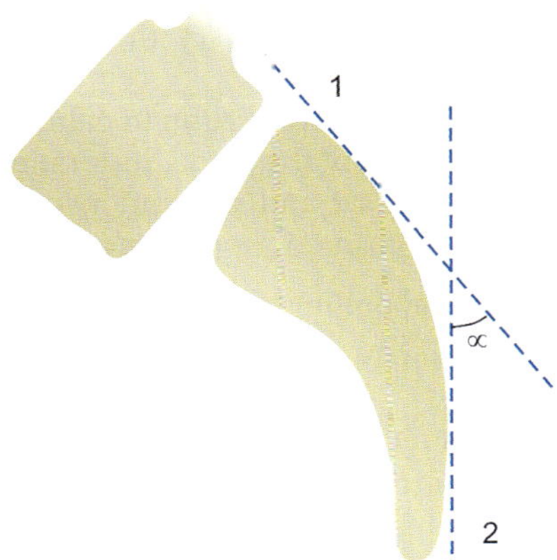

Fig. 12: Sacral inclination.

- The "wide canal sign" or ratio, measured as the AP diameter of the canal at the slip level divided by the AP diameter at the L1 level, has been offered as a means of detecting the presence of bilateral pars interarticularis defects with spondylolisthesis when the ratio is >1.25.

- Provocative discography is a useful study to assess the presence of coexisting symptomatic disk disease. If concordant pain is reproduced at the level of the spondylolysis or olisthesis, this contraindicates direct repair of the pars interarticularis defect in favor of arthrodesis in patients considering surgical intervention.
- Correction of the kyphotic deformity, as measured by the slip angle, is the most important goal of surgical reduction.

Treatment

Most patients are asymptomatic with an incidental finding of a pars interarticularis defect without a slip. They can be followed on an as-needed basis if symptoms develop. With a listhesis serial radiographs on a 3- to 6-month basis may be done to determine the stability of the slip until skeletal maturity. In the pediatric and adolescent population, spondylolisthesis is the predominant cause of low back pain and sciatica. In them also conservative management is quite successful.

Nonoperative Treatment

Activity modification—restriction of high-risk athletics, avoiding repetitive extension maneuvers, physical therapy and graded strengthening exercises, selective nerve/pars injections, brace therapy are the conservative management tools. Positive bone scan or SPECT scan in a young child or adolescent implies the potential for possible healing at the pars interarticularis defect with external immobilization and may be an indication for brace therapy. Also traumatic lysis heals well so immobilization should be considered.

Operative Treatment

The accepted criteria for surgical intervention include:

- Persistence of pain or neurological symptoms despite an adequate course of nonoperative treatment
- Progression of slippage > 30%
- Presentation with greater than grade II subluxation
- Cosmetic deformity secondary to postural and gait difficulties

Goals of surgery include reduction in pain, prevention of further slip, stabilization of the spine, restoration of normal posture and gait, reversal and prevention of neurological deficit, and improved cosmetic appearance.

The following surgical options are available:

Decompression: Suitable in adults with only radicular symptoms.

- Gill's procedure **(Fig. 13)**—removal of loose posterior elements and cartilaginous tissue. The disadvantage is potential for increasing the subluxation postoperatively. The procedure is controversial as slip progression rates have been found to be as high as 27%. Nerve root symptoms quite

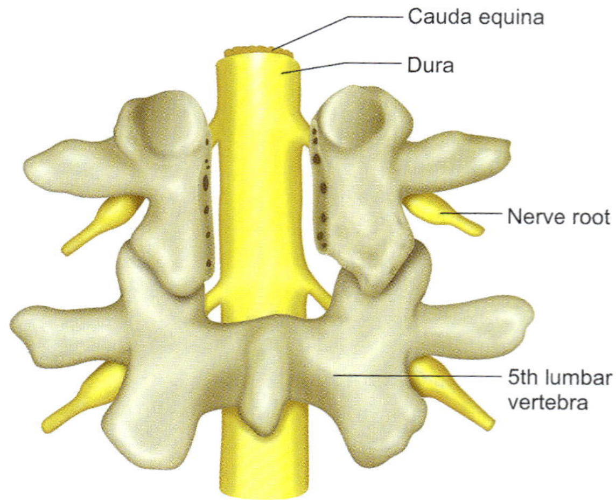

Fig. 13: Gill's laminectomy.

successfully resolve with fusion without decompression so the procedure might be futile indeed. Also in adults decompression increases pseudoarthrosis rates.

In situ bone fusion: Patients with axial low back pain are benefitted with noninstrumented fusion of the lumbar spine. Fusion can be achieved in various ways including anterior interbody, posterior interbody, transforaminal interbody or intertransverse. The last two are mechanically most apt to treat isthmic lysis and listhesis (often called posterolateral in situ fusion). Simultaneous decompression can also be done. Stabilization of the elements reduce symptoms in children. Pseudarthrosis develops in approximately a third of patients with spondylolisthesis after attempted posterolateral in situ arthrodesis without instrumentation because of the altered anatomy of the slip, low surface area for fusion, increased stress across the fusion, and difficulty in exposing the L5 transverse process without exposing the L4 transverse process. Slip progression (translation and angulation) occurs in 33% of cases despite presence of "solid fusion" (noninstrumented), especially in patients with high-grade slips, after a Gill's laminectomy, or when no postoperative immobilization is used.

Instrumented bony fusion (instrument-assisted bone fusion): Instrumented assistance is used to improve fusion rates, to repair a pars defect directly, or to reduce the dislocation in high-grade spondylolisthesis. Pedicle screw devices are the universal choice. In pediatric patients, instrumentation is used only for direct repair of the defect or to reduce listhesis. The repair is done by passing a wire around the transverse and spinous processes of the affected level or by placing a screw through the lamina and pars defect into the pedicle. In any case, direct repair should be done only for low-grade subluxation. For high-grade listhesis greater than grade II, it is always better to correct deformity and spinal alignment by simultaneous anterior interbody release and fusion. The indications for reduction (and anterior column fusion) in the adult patient with isthmic spondylolisthesis include:

- Vertebral slippage > 60%
- Slip angle > 50°
- Age between 12 and 30 years
- Symptoms uncontrollable by nonoperative means

DEGENERATIVE SPONDYLOLISTHESIS (FIG. 14)

By definition this is an acquired anterior displacement of one vertebra over the subjacent vertebra associated with degenerative changes without an associated disruption or defect in the vertebral ring (no spondylolysis). This most often occurs at the L4-L5 level. Normal lumbar lordosis of 40–60° create anterior force vector across L3 level. The L5-S1 articulation is inherently stable forming foundation to the spine by virtue of coronally oriented facets, strong iliolumbar ligaments and often sacralization of L5 vertebra. These factors concentrate stresses most frequently across the L4-L5 and sometimes the L3-L4 motion segment. The facets at these levels are more sagittally oriented and with disk degeneration these joints are further stressed due to shift of stress posteriorly. The facet joints thus give way under increased stress and unfavorable orientation; this is also supplanted by ligamentous laxity in susceptible population causing anterior slip of the vertebral body. Lateral subluxation and rotatory instability occurs with hypertrophy and osteophyte formation in facet joints that in addition cause nerve root compression and symptoms.

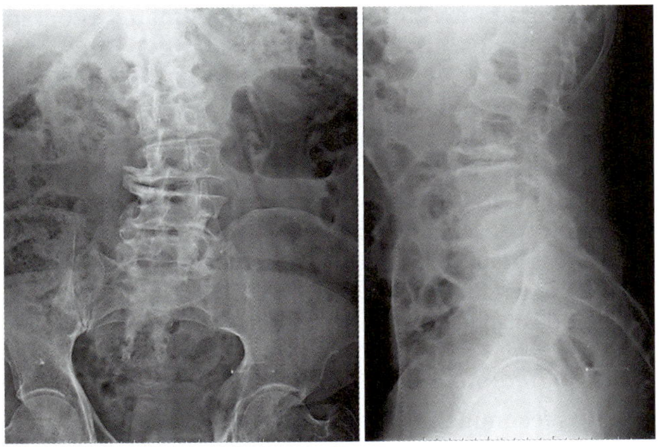

Fig. 14: Degenerative spondylolisthesis. Note there is also degenerative adult-onset scoliosis in this patient.

It is 15–16 times more frequent in women than men. Approximately, 10% of women older than 60 years have a degenerative slip. Black women are three times more likely to develop degenerative slips than the average population (they have high incidence of L5 sacralization). Presenting symptoms usually appear after the patient is 40 years old.

Etiology

- Multiple factors contribute to the development of a degenerative spondylolisthesis, including disk degeneration, degenerative arthritis of the facet joints, and anatomic factors specific to the affected motion segment.
- The slip rarely exceeds 33% and progression occurs in only 30% of patients.

Signs and Symptoms

- Patients typically complain of low back pain radiating into the buttocks or lateral thighs. Stiffness is not a common finding.
- Hyperflexibility may be a feature in many (suggesting generalized ligamentous laxity).
- Hamstring spasm is not a feature generally.
- Radicular symptoms are much frequent than in other types seen in more than half of the patients and are often referable to the L5 nerve root. Tingling and numbness can occur down the lateral calf into the lateral toes. Mild weakness exists in 15–20% of patients in extensor hallucis longus (EHL) (L5), and sometimes the tibialis anterior (L4), or gastrocsoleus complex (S1).
- The following symptoms of spinal stenosis are extremely common and are usually the reason these patients seek medical attention.
  - Proximal muscle weakness
  - Intolerance to walking or even standing, relieved by leaning over or sitting
  - Intermittent neurogenic claudication **(Table 3)**

TABLE 3: Differentiation between neurogenic and vascular claudication.

Characteristic	*Neurogenic*	*Vascular*
Pain location	Lower back, thigh, calves, buttocks	Calves and leg muscles mainly, buttocks uncommon
Pain quality	Burning, vague cramping aches	Cramping
Radiation	Commonly seen proximal to distal	Localized in legs may climb up
Aggravating factors	Erect posture, extension of spine, continued walking. Not seen with cycling (provided back is not straight)	Leg exercise that increases metabolic stress. Will come-up with cycling also
Relieving factors	Squatting or even just bending forward, sitting	Rest only, no change with alteration of posture
Walking through pain	Possible if patient just flexes his trunk forward	Not possible
Walking uphill	Walking distance might improve due to flexed trunk	Walking distance will reduce due to increased effort
Time to relief	Slow improvement	Rapid relief with rest
Leg pulses	Normal	• Reduced pulses (?absent) • Reduced blood pressure • Bruits and murmurs may be present
Skin	No trophic changes	Trophic changes present (reduced/absent hair, pallor, nail dystrophy, thin shiny skin)
Autonomic changes	Bladder incontinence (uncommon)	Impotence may coexist

Investigations

Plain radiographs—the standing lateral radiograph is the most appropriate, noninvasive test for detecting degenerative lumbar spondylolisthesis. AP film is used to detect degenerative scoliosis, lateral olisthesis, or sacralization of L5.

- Flexion and extension lateral X-ray films **(Fig. 15)** can reveal the unusual translational or angular dynamic instability.
- Excessive translational motion is generally defined as >4 mm of motion with flexion. Angular instability is considered to be present when there is >10° difference between flexion and extension radiographs.

Plain myelography and/or CT myelography are useful studies to assess spinal stenosis in patients with degenerative lumbar spondylolisthesis especially in those who have contraindications to MRI. CT also gives valuable information about the amount of osteoporosis and a detailed view of the facet joint hypertrophy. Myelography had historically been the test of choice to evaluate spinal stenosis. The classic findings are traversing nerve root cutoff due to facet hypertrophy and spondylolisthesis. Complications of myelography like headache and nausea and wide availability of MRI has diminished its usage.

MRI is the most appropriate, noninvasive test for imaging stenosis and has become the standard in evaluating these patients because it provides information about the nerve roots and about the soft-tissue component of stenosis, such as hypertrophied ligamentum flavum or synovial cysts in the facet joint.

- Facet joint effusion > 1.5 mm on supine MRI may be suggestive of the presence of degenerative lumbar spondylolisthesis.

Changes at the posterior elements including the joints **(Figs. 16A to D)** can be a source of compression of the nerves and an indicator of instability at the motion segment.

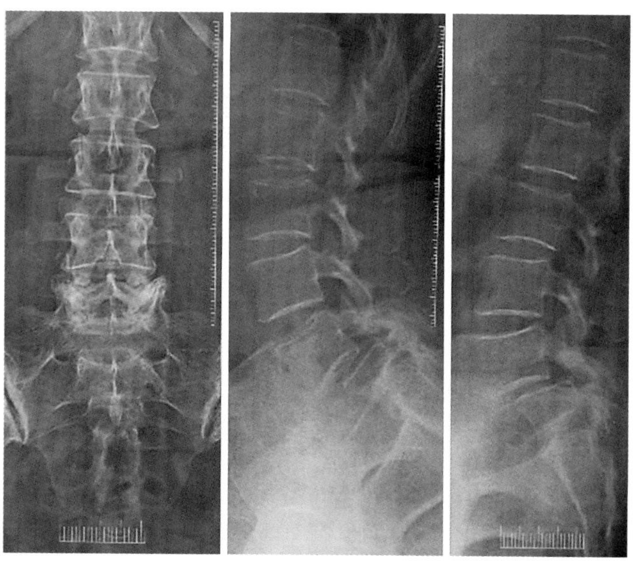

Fig. 15: Lateral projection of lumbosacral spine in neutral, forward flexion and extension. The grade II listhesis is stable and does not change with spinal movements.

Electromyography and nerve conduction studies differentiate neuropathy from neurogenic claudication in diabetics.

Treatment

Nonoperative treatment guidelines have not been universalized for degenerative spondylolisthesis but in general a nonoperative management is tried for stable symptoms (nonprogressive symptoms) initially. The treatment is logically similar to treatment for symptomatic degenerative lumbar spinal stenosis. Nonoperative measures succeed in most patients because a progressive neurologic deficit is rare.

- Basic intervention—short-term bed rest (1–2 days) followed by activity modification, combined with anti-inflammatory medication.
  - Nonsteroidal anti-inflammatory drugs (NSAIDs), aspirin or acetaminophen are conventionally used. Opioids may be added for severe pain.
  - Steroids are best reserved for acute exacerbations of leg pain in the older patient.
  - Additional treatment in the form of physical therapy is commonly introduced in a graduated program. Isometrics are first prescribed till reduction of symptoms whence active flexion exercises and strengthening exercises for lower back paraspinal muscles and abdominal muscles are taught. Aerobic conditioning is introduced in the end. Weight reduction is stressed throughout the course of treatment.
  - Epidural steroids and selective nerve root injections are valuable adjuvants (*see* Chapter on "Low Back Pain, Intervertebral Disk Degeneration, Lumbar Spondylosis, and Degenerative Conditions of Cervical Spine").

Operative Treatment

Surgery is recommended for treatment of:

- Patients with symptomatic spinal stenosis associated with low-grade degenerative spondylolisthesis whose symptoms have been refractory to a trial of medical/interventional treatment.
- It is also recommended in the presence of symptomatic spinal stenosis and cauda equina syndrome.

Goals of operative treatment include:

- Pain relief
- Improvement or prevention of neurological deficit
- Increased tolerance to walking and standing
- Improvement in quality of life

Decompression alone: Considered for the treatment of patients with symptomatic spinal stenosis associated with low-grade degenerative lumbar spondylolisthesis whose symptoms have been recalcitrant to a trial of medical/interventional treatment. It involves removal of lamina and part of medial facet joints. The following are notable for "decompression only" as treatment:

- Indirect surgical decompression is often recommended for treatment of patients with degenerative spondylolisthesis. It is the least invasive surgery and provides rapid, substantial relief of pain. Avoids morbidity of fusion.

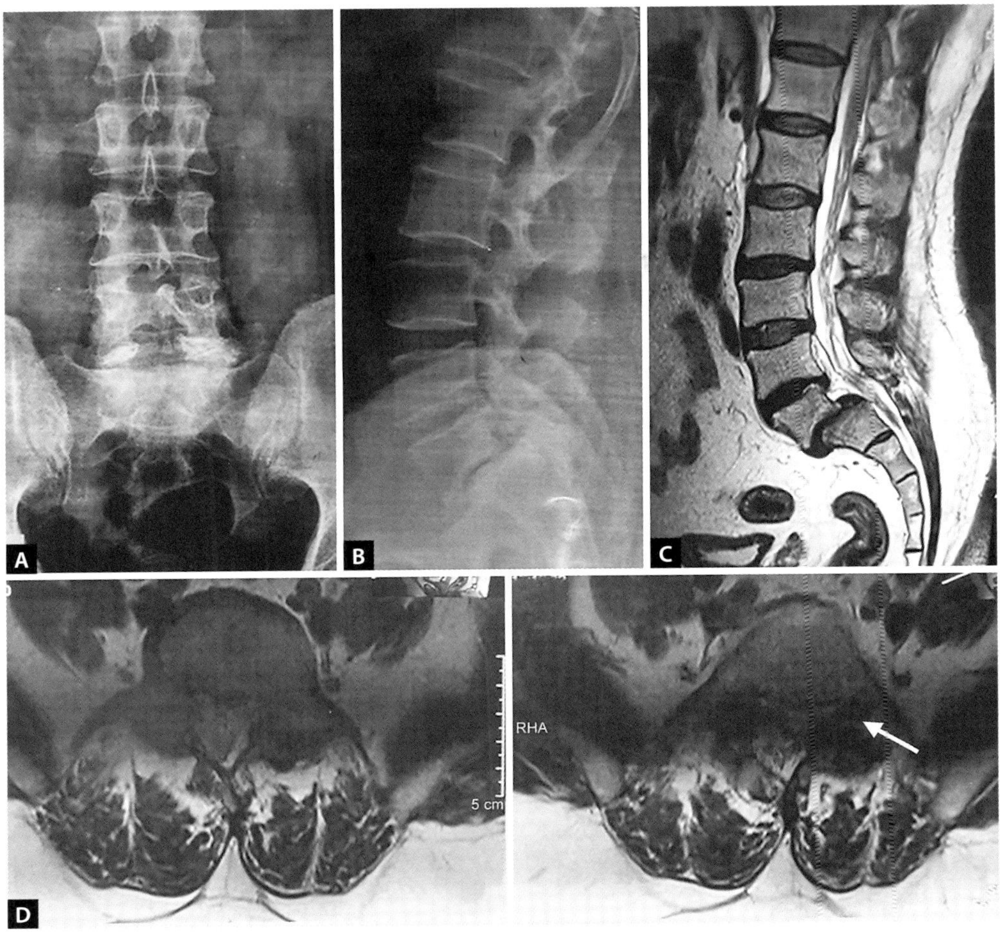

Figs. 16A to D: (A and B) The radiographs and MRI of patient with grade II spondylolisthesis; (C) Sagittal section demonstrates minimal compression if any by intervertebral disk; (D) Axial views demonstrate root compression by osteophytes at facet joint and the fibrous tissue at the pars defect prominent on left side (arrow).

- Does not address instability. May cause iatrogenic instability.
- Slip progression occurs in 25–50% of patients and may correlate with a poor clinical outcome.

Surgical decompression with posterolateral fusion: It is suggested for the treatment of patients with symptomatic spinal stenosis and degenerative lumbar spondylolisthesis to improve clinical outcomes compared with decompression alone. It involves full laminectomy and partial facetectomy with exposure and fusion of the transverse processes. It may decrease slip progression if fusion is solid which often fails in many.

Surgical decompression with fusion, with or without instrumentation, is suggested to improve the functional outcomes of single-level degenerative spondylolisthesis compared to medical/interventional treatment alone. It also provides satisfactory long-term results for the treatment of patients with symptomatic spinal stenosis and degenerative lumbar spondylolisthesis. Segmental instrumentation is commonly added for the following:

- Addition of instrumentation is suggested to improve fusion rates in patients with symptomatic spinal stenosis and degenerative lumbar spondylolisthesis.
- Instrumentation also lends space for more aggressive fusion and deformity correction. Problem is occurrence of flat back deformity in a significant population and longer operative time.
- The added complications of instrumentation include—implant failure, infection, etc., that should be borne in mind as for any implant-related surgery in orthopedics.

Some studies suggest that for symptomatic single-level degenerative spondylolisthesis that is low-grade (<20%) and without lateral foraminal stenosis, decompression alone with preservation of midline structures provides equivalent outcomes when compared to surgical decompression with fusion.

TRAUMATIC SPONDYLOLISTHESIS

Trauma results in acute fracture if the posterior neural arch especially the facet or lamina that creates instability. These are extremely rare injuries in isolation. Treatment should follow the guidelines for isthmic spondylolisthesis, with a bias toward conservative treatment and immobilization. One must keep in mind, however that the posterior fracture may be part of a much larger injury, including a fracture or dislocation of the spine that has spontaneously reduced so the evaluation must be comprehensive.

PATHOLOGIC SPONDYLOLISTHESIS

Osteoporosis and osteomalacia are the most common causes of instability resulting from continuous fatiguing stresses applied to the weakened structures by the disease process. The structures undergo microfractures that heal in an elongated position leading to segmental instability. Other causes include Paget's disease, osteogenesis imperfecta (high-grade slips related to elongation of the pedicle), and tumors (that disrupt bony architecture leading to instability).

IATROGENIC SPONDYLOLISTHESIS

This results from surgical disruption of ligaments, bone, or the intervertebral disk. The most common cause is wide decompression without fusion. Diskectomy further destabilizes the motion segment. Resection of >50% of each facet joint or an entire facet joint unilaterally predisposes the spine to increased instability. Treatment is by instrumented posterolateral fusion with or without an interbody fusion depending on the degree of instability.

CONCLUSION

- Break in the pars region of vertebrae results from various factors and is commonly seen in the middle age or later.
- Isthmic and degenerative types are the most common ones commonly managed conservatively for nonprogressive disability but need specific management for an unstable symptomatic spine not responding to conservative management.

CHAPTER 98

Failed Back Surgery Syndrome

Manish Kumar Varshney

INTRODUCTION

Failed back surgery syndrome (FBSS or post-laminectomy syndrome or simply FBS) is defined as persistent or recurrent chronic pain with or without sciatica after one or more surgical procedures on the lumbosacral spine. The other very general definition for FBSS could be when the outcome of lumbar/lumbosacral spine surgery does not meet the presurgical expectations of the patient and the surgeon. This definition does not only rest on pain in defining failed back but also includes a constellation of symptoms. FBSS is not uncommon and constitutes a heterogeneous group of patients which have either their original cause of pain amenable to treatment or their original causes of pain nonamenable to surgery due to induced anatomical changes.

Failed back surgery syndrome can arise from several causes either related to the initial surgery like poor patient selection (most common), mismatch of the procedure with patient pathology, failure of the procedure to achieve its goals, recurrent disk herniation, scar tissue, muscular deconditioning or due to patient predisposition on account of systemic diseases such as diabetes, autoimmune disease, psychiatric disease or vascular disease. FBSS may also arise from new sources of pain that may or may not be related to the initial surgery. So, FBSS may present as unresolved symptoms or new onset of symptoms following index procedure.

INCIDENCE

The correct incidence is not reported but it may be as high as 15%. The incidence would increase with the complexity of surgery, reduced vigilance due to time pressure of finishing procedure, and revision surgeries. The complication rates are already more than double for complex surgeries (5.6%) compared to simple surgeries (2.3%). Success rates of spine surgery reduce with revision procedure and hence FBSS would rise with more and more revisions. It is generally accepted that the success rate of index primary surgery is >50% which reduces to 30% for first revision. Third surgery will have satisfaction rate of around 15% and fourth surgery will be nearly nonsatisfactory mostly (success—5%). Highest success rates are seen for purely decompressive surgeries (75–85%).

ETIOLOGY

The several common identifiable causes of failure of back surgery include:

- *Poor patient selection (most common cause):* Chronic pain behavior, unreachable expectations, psychological problems (depression, anxiety, poor coping, somatization, and hypochondriasis)—evaluate the yellow flags.
- *Incorrect/incomplete diagnosis:* Degenerative or age-related changes, such as disk herniation, spondylolysis, or spondylolisthesis attributed for pain that may actually arise from quadratus lumborum, iliopsoas or gluteal syndrome, and mimic disk pathology. Missing a conjoint nerve root or far lateral disk would result in continued symptoms.
- *Wrong procedure:* Wrong surgery, wrong level operated, wrong side, missed additional component of pain generator (e.g., associated spinal stenosis)
- *Revision surgery*
- *Poor technique:* Inadequate or overaggressive surgery, battered root syndrome, residual deformity, and creation of iatrogenic instability.
- *Failure to achieve surgical goals:* Nonunion, incomplete decompression (inability to remove far lateral disk), incomplete deformity correction, and creation of flat back (inability to restore physiological curves).
- *Progressive disease:* Recurrent disk herniation (5–15% of patients, mostly at a new level or on the contralateral side), recurrent spinal stenosis like formation of disk osteophyte complex **(Figs. 1A to C)**, epidural fibrosis and tethering of nerve roots and new instability/altered biomechanics.
- *Systemic disorders:* Diabetes, neuropathy, vascular disorders, myofascial pain syndrome, and autoimmune disease.

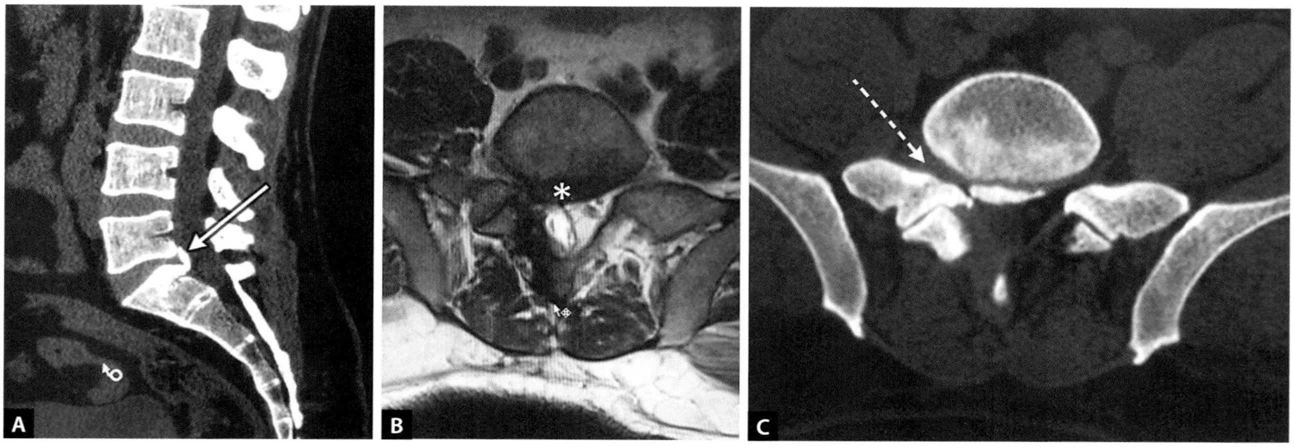

Figs. 1A to C: Failed back syndrome and recurrence of symptoms in a patient with intervertebral disk herniation at L5–S1. The patient was treated previously by endoscopic diskectomy 3 years ago and developed disk-osteophyte complex (pointing arrow in A and asterisk in B) causing foraminal stenosis (dotted arrow) on right side (C)

- *Postoperative complications:* Infection, hematoma, dural tear or pseudomeningocele, and arachnoiditis
- *Unclassifiable:*
  - *Transition syndrome:* Stability of a fused segment will increase load onto the adjacent segments and accelerate disk degeneration in a process called "transition syndrome". This syndrome occurs within 10 years in up to 25% if patients who undergo anterior cervical fusion with similar or higher rates for lower spine possibly.
  - Personal injury
  - Workman compensation

Overall both biological and psychological issues play a significant role in the outcome of lumbar spine surgery.

CLASSIFICATION OF PATIENTS WITH FAILED BACK SURGERY SYNDROME

There is no accepted classification for FBS. There are three ways of classifying the patients:

1. ***Time duration of appearance of pain (temporal factors):***
   - *Early (no improvement):* Pain or symptoms either present immediately following surgery or recur within 2–3 weeks. Usually, the pathology is not addressed and either wrong-level surgery (most common surgical cause) or the wrong procedure is the cause like inadequate removal of an extruded disk fragment and incomplete decompression. Inadequate work-up also contributes like missing the L4–5 adjacent disk in L5–S1 spondylolisthesis. Partial relief with varying degrees of persistent pain may be seen in patients with chronic intrinsic neuropathy.
   - *Intermediate (1–6 months):* It may be related to recurrent disk herniation, or hardware or graft failure or displacement. Symptoms from iatrogenic instability such as progressive scoliosis, rotatory subluxation, or spondylolisthesis that may develop after wide decompression may also develop during this postoperative phase.
   - *Late (>6 months):* Recurrent pathology (like recurrent stenosis) at the same or adjacent segments is the common cause here. Altered biomechanics, transition syndrome, and nonunion are other causes. A difficult problem to address is fibrosis (whether perineurial, epidural, or arachnoiditis) that may develop at variable period after index surgery.
2. ***Etiological:***
   - Patients in whom the surgery was never indicated, or the surgery performed carried a low likelihood of achieving the desired result (95% cases).
   - Patients in whom the surgery was indicated but the surgical procedure was inadequately or incompletely performed, failing to achieve the intended result (5% cases).
3. ***Pain distribution (not a good method of classifying as there is a lot of overlap and pain is not always the only reason for FBSS):***
   - *Spine (lower back):* Apart from recurrent or missed disk herniations [pelvic inflammatory disease (PID) in females]; inflammation/infection of abdominal organs such as cholelithiasis/cholecystitis, psoas abscess, renal system, and pancreatitis should be evaluated. Other conditions that are known to produce lower back pain include seronegative spondyloarthropathies such as ankylosing spondylitis, regional enteritis, diffuse idiopathic skeletal hyperostosis (DISH), and Reiter's syndrome and rheumatoid arthritis. Degenerative and inflammatory conditions of the sacroiliac joint are known to cause back pain in association with radiation often to groin and thigh. Tumors and infections of thoracic and abdominal structures also can cause flank and back pain, as can rare instances of aortic aneurysms in thoracic or abdominal region.
   - *Lower extremity:* The radicular pain from recurrent disk herniation or stenosis should be differentiated from entrapment syndromes of the locoregional

nerves such as the sciatic, common peroneal, femoral and lateral femoral cutaneous nerves that may cause pseudoradicular pain. Patients with associated diabetes may have diabetic neuropathy to confuse the clinical diagnosis. Compression of lumbosacral plexus due to pelvic tumors, infections, inflammatory processes, and aneurysms. Patients that report leg pain immediately after surgery that has different nature or is more severe than the original should raise suspicion of inappropriate placement of pedicle screws or cage.

- *Widespread:* More often indicate a psychogenic and/or neuropathic component (label it after extensive exclusion of other causes such as malpositioned implants, neural compression, infection, or tumor). Complex regional pain syndrome or reflex sympathetic dystrophy is an important cause of widespread pain syndrome.

PATIENT EVALUATION

History

- Obtain details of postoperative symptoms and their relation to preoperative clinical symptoms.
- Careful review of medical records to identify events such as wrong-level surgery or incorrect initial diagnosis.
- The current degree of nociceptive back pain and neuropathic leg pain (planning treatment)
- Assessment for possibility of somatization or addiction disorders (depression, sleep disturbance, loss of appetite, weight change, feelings of despair, loss of sexual desire, irritability, and inability to make decisions) Constitutional symptoms (e.g., night sweats, fever, chills, and weight loss) may indicate occult infection.

Physical Examination

- *Nonorganic physical findings (Waddell's signs):* This is a group of physical signs to aid in diagnosing nonorganic low back pain. Waddell signs are grouped into five types or categories:
  1. *Tenderness:* Superficial (skin is tender to light touch over the lumbar spine) and nonanatomic (deep tenderness over a wide area in the lumbar spine not confined to an anatomic structure).
  2. *Stimulation tests:* Axial loading (axial load on the standing patient's skull causes low back pain) and rotation (rotating the patient through the lower extremities while keeping the spine straight causes low back pain).
  3. *Distraction tests:* Indirect observation (patient can move without pain when not being examined) and the straight-leg raise test (which produces symptoms when the patient is lying supine but not when distracted while sitting).
  4. *Regional disturbances:* Weakness ("cogwheeling" or multiple muscle group weakness that cannot be explained neuroanatomically) and sensory ("stocking," nonanatomic sensory changes).
  5. *Overreaction:* Inappropriate or disproportionate verbalization, facial expression, muscle tension and tremor, collapsing, and sweating.

  The presence of three or more Waddell's signs has been considered clinically significant and has been used to detect malingering and/or nonorganic low back pain. The prognostic value of Waddell signs has demonstrated variable results in studies. Some reports indicate that the Waddell signs might interfere with optimal response to treatment, whereas other studies have indicated that Waddell's signs are not predictive for outcomes following intensive, nonsurgical programs such as functional restoration.
- Standard tests are performed for gait examination, tenderness, movements of nearby joints (hips and spine), radiculopathy evaluation (nerve root tension signs) and standard neurologic examination.
- *Flat back syndrome:* The human spine has natural curvatures. The instrumentation of a sagittal transition area or the majority of the lumbar spine may cause loss of this natural back curve to become flat. The shape and rigidity of the rods along with poor contouring to straighten the deformity would produce this condition. Patients may have difficulty in standing straight. Most of them compensate this loss of curvature by bending at the hips and/or knees, resulting in even poorer posture.

Investigations

Investigations are primarily focused at confirming the pain generator or in rare circumstances to find an unidentified pain generator.

- Biplanar standing radiographs (changes in alignment and progressive degenerative changes)
- Flexion-extension radiographs are indicated in the patient who has had fusion or has any possibility of instability. Pseudarthrosis is likely when motion is present on flexion-extension. The iliac crest bone graft site also should be evaluated clinically and radiographically to evaluate the possibility of a pelvic fracture or sacroiliac joint dysfunction.
- Assess overall sagittal balance. A good estimate is that the weight-bearing line passes from C7 to the sacrum if a straight line is drawn on standing lateral 36-inch radiographs. If this line is displaced anteriorly it indicates flat back syndrome.
- Magnetic resonance imaging (MRI) (nonenhanced) or gadolinium-diethylenetriamine penta-acetic acid (Gd-DTPA) enhanced MRI is the most sensitive test for evaluation of these patients and is now considered standard investigation. It is particularly useful for evaluation of recurrent disk prolapse, arachnoiditis, epidural fibrosis, and infective diskitis.
- Computed tomography (CT) myelography is not a common investigation prescribed but is indicated in patients where MRI is contraindicated (stainless steel hardware, pace maker, etc.), in the evaluation of patients

with dynamic problems (e.g., instability and facet impingement) or grotesque spinal deformities that are not well-visualized by MRI (e.g., severe scoliosis).

- Electrodiagnostic studies may evaluate extraspinal neural compression, assess the severity and location of nerve injury and discriminate from other causes of neuropathic pain.
- *Laboratory tests:* Assess for occult infection (diskitis). Erythrocyte sedimentation rate (ESR) and C-reactive protein levels are usually elevated, C-reactive protein returns to a normal level sooner than ESR (usually 14 days) and may be useful in determining response to treatment.
- *Psychological assessment:* The most popular is the Minnesota multiphasic personality inventory (MMPI). High scores on the scales of hysteria, depression, and hypochondria predict the probability of a poor outcome.
- Diagnostic block of selective nerve root is helpful to confirm exact localizations of neural abnormalities (their abilities to predict outcome in the patient group with FBSS are lacking).
- Diskography can identify painful disk segments after posterior fusion and indicate good clinical outcomes following interbody fusion. Diskography also can be used to identify painful transitional motion segments. The latter can also be identified by diagnostic facet blocks.
- *Chronic pain evaluation:* This indicates possible poor outcome. Plasticity occurs in the pain modulation system, creating increased pain sensitization to noxious stimulation.

PREVENTION AND MANAGEMENT

It is best to prevent FBS. Accurate diagnosis is fundamental to prevention of all surgical complications including the failed back syndrome. The presurgical patient assessment includes the following parameters:

- Symptoms of sufficient severity to justify further surgery.
- There should be sufficient correlation between symptoms and abnormalities found on clinical examination and imaging studies. Assess findings of pain behavior (i.e., Waddell's signs).
- Other differential diagnoses discussed above in etiologies such as hip arthrosis, vascular disease, and peripheral neuropathy that would explain the pain symptoms should be excluded.
- Intraoperatively during time-out, the correct level to be operated on should be confirmed by the responsible person that could be a circulating nurse, anesthesiologist, and/or surgeon. The Joint Accreditation Commission on Healthcare Organizations mandates all institutions to develop a program for preventing wrong-site surgery which has been accepted by North American Spine Society that further includes using intraoperative radiology in all cases.
- Postspinal decompression the check nerve root for adequate mobility and sufficient opening in the neuroforamina should be ensured. The instrumentation that has been placed, the spinal cord and neuroforamina all should be inspected for misplaced metal.
- Postoperatively complications should be promptly identified and aggressively treated. One should not shy away even if revision is required in the good interest of patient. The acceptance level for human error should be high instead of fighting with emotions otherwise delays are bound to cause further neural injury. Often the first indications for failed surgery are reporting of severe leg pain or finding differences in extremity temperature immediately after the surgery. Vascular occlusion or injury or from compartment syndrome should be appropriately excluded. With absent pulses a Doppler examination of the extremities should be performed. If all of the above are normal then nerve root injury should be considered. Position of pedicle screws or fusion cages should be assessed. CT myelography is helpful in identifying compression of the thecal sac or nerve roots as MRI would be compounded by metal artifacts. Fusion cages or interbody bone graft placed through anterior approach may displace the disk tissue posteriorly into the canal and cause severe radicular pain. These cases require early reintervention to address the offending implant or disk tissue.

CONSERVATIVE MANAGEMENT

Conservative management should be tried first. It is common for patients to report some new pain due to active postoperative rehabilitation program. It can be usually addressed with standard nonsteroidal anti-inflammatory drugs (NSAIDs) and/or reduced activity, followed by reintroduction of rehabilitation program slowly and gradually advancing it. Only a few clinical circumstances would ask for immediate surgical management shunning the conservative approach like:

- Severe spinal instability
- Infection
- Impending neurologic

Spinal Cord Stimulation

Spinal cord stimulation (SCS) has been in use for over 30 years and widely utilized with good outcomes in FBS especially in those suffer from intractable sciatic pain. The first spinal cord stimulator was placed in 1967 by Shealy by a D2–D3 laminectomy and the first indication was cancer pain.

Spinal cord stimulation involves placing percutaneous leads in the epidural or intrathecal space and providing electrical stimulation over a specified portion of the spinal cord based on the patient's pain pattern. Thorough evaluation is necessary before final implantation. It is clear that not all pains are sensitive to treatment with SCS.

Spinal cord stimulation is based on the theory that electrical stimulation of large fibers would close the gate to input from the smaller diameter and unmyelinated A-delta and C fibers mediating pain (exploiting the "gate control theory" of pain). The principle is to stimulate the dorsal column and interfere with the sensory information coming from the painful area. The analgesic mechanisms of SCS are, however, not fully clear. Endorphins and opioids are not involved in the mechanism; however, GABA and adenosine have been suggested from animal studies. Dorsolateral funiculus (DLF) is one such preferred stimulation target that contains descending pain controlling pathways.

There are three components of SCS system: (1) The epidural electrode; (2) the connection between the epidural electrode and the battery; and (3) the implantable-pulse generator (IPG). Out of the wide range of electrodes available, percutaneous and surgical leads are commonly used, the later (surgical leads) requiring laminotomy for implantation. For FBSS, a trial period implantation of electrode is performed for 1–4 weeks. IPG is then implanted under general anesthesia (GA) if there is minimum 50% pain reduction with test-lead, paresthesia covers the area of pain and is well-tolerated and there is mood, sleep, and activity improvement with trial electrodes.

Spinal cord stimulation is done by a voltage-controlled pulse generator that creates a potential difference between two electrodes. The transmitted current gets distributed in a three-dimensional (3D) space that can be characterized by potential distribution and current density distribution presented as isopotential line and isocurrent lines, respectively. The stimulation induces mainly a depolarization of the nerve large myelinated fibers; both orthodromically and antidromically inducing paresthesia and confusing brain. This, in turn, reduces painful sensory perception.

Complications:

- Electrode migration (most common)—use multichannel devices and paddle electrodes
- Infection, meningitis (sometimes life-threatening)
- Lead breakage
- Cerebrospinal fluid (CSF) leak
- Weakness

Success rates are on the order of 50% improvement in 50% of patients at specialized centers. The concerns raised over this technique had been:

- Decreased effect over time
- High incidence of adverse reactions

In a Canadian study, SCS has been found to be cost-effective compared to conventional medical management in patients with various intractable and refractory disorders such as FBSS, peripheral arterial disease, complex regional pain syndrome (CRPS), and refractory angina pectoris. In FBSS particularly, leg pain responds better than local back pain to SCS and neuropathic pain is better improved compared to the nociceptive or mechanical pain. In particular, the latter is almost nonresponsive to SCS. The same authors also reported that probability of SCS being cost-effective is 75–95% for different pathologies when projected over long-term (20 years).

Intrathecal Analgesia

Spinal narcotics such as diamorphine, bupivacaine, clonidine, and baclofen may be administered epidurally or intrathecally for pain relief in the form of a permanent delivery system such as pain pump. Intrathecal drug infusion is now well-accepted as a treatment option when all conservative and etiologic treatment has failed. In addition to the SCS, intrathecal medication also covers the nociceptive aspects of pain. Morphine is the most common analgesic agent used (other medications have been used in patients who have inadequate pain relief or adverse effects from morphine). To reduce the side-effect of morphine and prevent "escape" mixtures have been used like morphine + bupivacaine (maximum 30 mg/day), morphine + clonidine, and morphine + bupivacaine + clonidine. Combining drugs maximize effect and reduce adverse effects but there is no definite strategy that is universally followed. Other newer agents being used or under development for intrathecal delivery include midazolam, ketamine, neostigmine, gabapentin, and ziconotide.

Failed back surgery syndrome is the most common indication for pain pump insertion and anywhere from 60 to 80% of patients achieve good pain relief from intrathecal drug administration. The technique is but cumbersome and most importantly constant refills have to be made unlike in SCS patients, so in dedicated centers this technique is used after SCS has been ineffective or failed. For mixed pain patterns, however, intrathecal drug infusion is probably the first choice.

Complications

- Pump malfunction causing overdose or withdrawal symptoms
- Infection and meningitis
- Catheter granuloma
- Respiratory failure
- *Drug adverse effects:* Urinary retention, constipation, nausea, and pruritus.

Overall significantly improved quality of life measures and pain have been reported with the technique especially the improvement in chronic back pain. Work interruption and effect of pain on sex did not improve.

Intradiskal Electrotherapy

Intradiskal electrotherapy (IDET) was developed by Saal and Saal in 2000 as an alternative for selected patients with chronic diskogenic pain who have failed all conservative treatments and to whom the next step offered was arthrodesis. Arthrodesis has known complications and significant failure rate and no specific treatment were available. IDET is based on modification of collagen making it thicker and causing it to contract decreasing its ability to revascularize. This, in turn, also prohibits the reinnervation and inflammation which may be causing root irritation. The indication for IDET is demonstrated long-term diskogenic pain (positive provocative diskography), normal neurologic examination, negative straight leg raising (SLR) test, no neural compression demonstrated and positive diskography. Contraindications include inflammatory arthritis, nonspinal conditions that mimic lumbar pain, and any medical or metabolic condition that would preclude proper follow-up.

Procedure: With patient lying prone under conscious sedation provocative diskography is performed after the skin is infiltrated with local anesthetic, a 17-G introducer needle is inserted into the disk posterolaterally, guided by oblique fluoroscopic imaging. One intradiskal catheter 30 cm long with a temperature-controlled thermal resistive coil is then deployed and inserted under guidance as far as possible adjacent to the inner posterior annulus. After ascertaining the optimal position, the catheter tip (5–6 cm long) temperature is gradually raised according to a uniform protocol to 90°C over a period of 13 minutes and maintained for 4 minutes. The 90° intradiskal catheter temperature creates annular temperatures of 60–65°C. This high temperature possibly seals the radial fissures and destroys the nerve endings in the annulus.

Complications: Catheter breakage, nerve root injuries, post-IDET disk herniation, cauda equina syndrome, infection, epidural abscess, and spinal cord damage.

Medial Branch Radiofrequency Lesioning

The treatment evolved when no/minimal improvement was seen from intra-articular steroid injection in the z-joint (zygapophyseal joint). z-joint denervation was, hence, supposed to provide a lasting relief. The zygapophyseal joint is innervated by the medial branch of the dorsal rami which is ablated by the radiofrequency waves transmitted through coated needle. The radiofrequency generator produced waves are propagated into a small oval area around the noncoated tip of the needle causing thermal lesion. The temperature is usually preset to 90°C and is given over a defined time. However, this small oval area must capture the medial branch so for perfect lesioning, the needle must be placed parallel to the nerve.

SURGICAL MANAGEMENT

Surgery for FBS is controversial and good indications for elective surgical procedure for FBS are few. The indications for initial surgery must be thoroughly reviewed to demonstrate reasonable pathology for which appropriateness of the given treatment and completeness of it must be adjudged. It is imperative that prior to undergoing another procedure the reasonable chance of correcting the identified pathology must be determined. The general rules for prognostication of patient and judging the outcome of surgery include:

- Patients with root compression syndromes or instability usually respond very well. The second surgery is expected to have outcomes that would match for primary surgery.
- Similarly surgery aimed at correcting anatomical abnormalities or restoring sagittal alignment and balance by reversing flat back syndrome are likely to be successful.
- Simple revision of previous surgery is likely to fail.

Percutaneous Adhesiolysis [Percutaneous Epidural Neuroplasty (Racz Procedure)]

The epidural space is accessed through a caudal or transforaminal approach. "Epidurogram" is performed by injecting nonionic contrast material to detect "filling defects" (representing adhesions) in the epidural space. A metal reinforced catheter is then gently manipulated in order to release adhesions (visualized as "filling in of the defects"). Steroid is injected at the end of procedure. Other medications used are hypertonic saline, or hyaluronidase injection. Epidural neuroplasty provides effective treatment for FBSS. It is best reserved for patients with FBSS who have failed other treatment for radicular symptoms. The potential complications of this technique are:

- Nerve root irritation/damage
- Catheter shearing
- Spinal cord compression
- Blindness secondary to high epidural hydrostatic pressure causes excessive subarachnoid pressure with reduced retinal perfusion or macular bleed.
- Dural tear
- Infection

Spinal Endoscopy (Epiduroscopy)

Percutaneous adhesiolysis is performed under fluoroscopy control and hence gives two-dimensional (2D) control which can be obviously misleading. For real-time, 3D coverage along with color view of the anatomy spinal endoscopy was developed that accesses the epidural space with a fiberoptic flexible catheter passed from sacral hiatus. Procedure is performed under local anesthesia continuously monitoring the intraepidural pressures and patient response. Normal nerve roots when touched cause paresthesia while diseased ones cause pain. Targeted medication/injection hence can be given at the identified pathology additionally adhesiolysis and retrieval of foreign bodies can be also done, if needed (e.g., broken implanted SCS electrode).

By the pioneers, it had been seen that fibrosis resulting into chronic radiculitis will be aggravated by repeat surgery so is contraindicated. Adhesions compromise the blood supply especially the venous drainage and cause engorgement further promoting adhesion formation by propagating intraneural edema. Spinal endoscopy and adhesiolysis will be the best modality in this circumstance that also helps by dilution of cytokines and wash-out of the phospholipase A2. The technique may even be extended to treatment of spinal stenosis causing radicular symptoms, the concern being raised intraepidural pressures in a "restricted" space.

As per the discussion we would know that the indications often overlap between the choice of procedures and it is really difficult to define the treatment guide for an individual patient. Not all patients should go through such diagnostic processes and treatments. Nonreversible procedures should take place only when a valid diagnostic strategy has been undertaken; a restrictive algorithm is presented in **Flowcharts 1 and 2** to serve as a common guide in deciding the combination of patient to procedure.

Flowchart 1: Algorithm for patient with predominant low back pain.

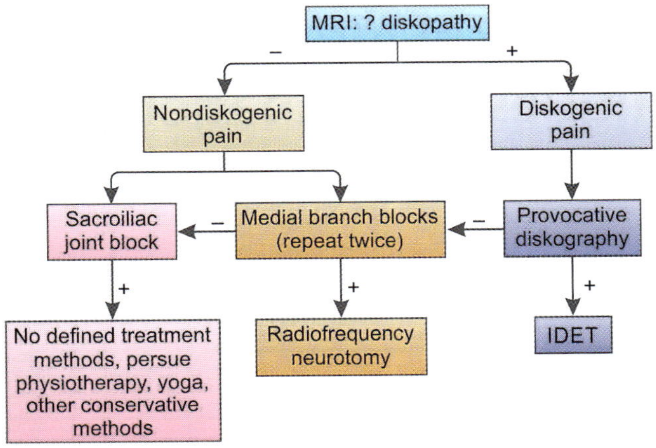

(IDET: intradiskal electrotherapy; MRI: magnetic resonance imaging)

Flowchart 2: Algorithm for patient with predominant radicular pain.

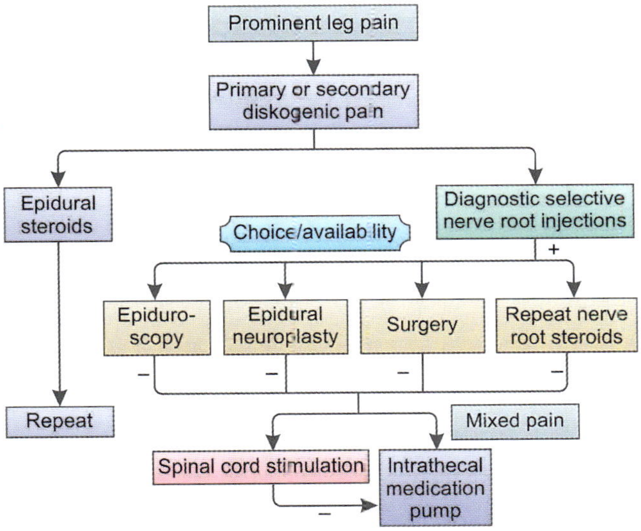

CONCLUSION

- Failed back surgery syndrome is the most common cause of dissuasion among patients as regard surgery for back. Failure of previous surgical intervention causes loss of trust and a strong negative psychological reaction.
- There are various causes of FBSS, most of which are either modifiable or avoidable but some factors are beyond the domain of current medical practice to avert. Prevention is the best cure for patients.
- It is important to identify the current cause of pain and evaluate it carefully to provide effective care by careful clinical evaluation supplemented with requisite investigations. Interventional measures have been developed to treat the patients by various methods. SCS has been quite successfully used for long and spinal epiduroscopy appears to be a promising upcoming method but has several limitations currently.

CHAPTER 99

Nonsurgical Interventional Techniques for Management of Back Pain

Manish Kumar Varshney

INTRODUCTION

Back pain is a very common problem which brings a patient to orthopedic clinic or pain clinic. It is estimated that it affects about 40–80% of general population in the whole life and at any point of time, it affects 14–20% of adult population. Back pain is associated with significant economic, social, and health implications. Patients usually present with activity intolerance due to lower back or back and leg symptoms. Symptoms may be acute in onset or chronic; however, it is important to carefully differentiate between the presentations of acute (symptoms lasting < 3 months), recurrent (symptoms reappearing after at least 6 weeks of total relief), and chronic low back pain (symptoms persisting for >3 months) because the risk factors for developing long-term problems may differ among different type of back pain.

Diagnostic interventional pain management (IPM) procedures have revolutionized the diagnosis of low back pain. Conventional evaluation of low back pain has many pitfalls **(Box 1)**. Through IPM (diagnostic block), diagnosis can be ascertained in most of the situations **(Box 2)**.

Another fallacy in making diagnosis is that, we look for abnormal anatomy when we look for the cause of pain from a particular structure; however, an important aspect that must be considered in diagnosis of back pain is pathologic process that converts a normal anatomical structure into a pain generator. Additional investigations are needed to confirm the disease or pathologic process **(Box 3)**. To make a successful management plan, we must identify both nociceptive source and pathologic process.

Interventional pain management is aimed to the diagnosis and treatment of pain and related disorders by the application of interventional techniques in managing subacute, chronic, persistent, and intractable pain. There are many interventional procedures to help in the diagnosis as well as therapeutic needs of the patient in back pain due to various etiologies and source of pain **(Box 4)**. The following discussion consolidates the various modalities that have been discussed in relevant chapters.

BOX 1: Pitfalls with conventional evaluation of low back in.

- Specific anatomic etiology is clearly and objectively identified in only 10–20%, because radiographic "abnormalities" are frequently clinically irrelevant.
- No universal criteria are established for scoring the presence, absence, or importance of particular signs.
- Quantification of the degree of disability and the association to treatment outcomes is difficult.
- Interpretation of findings relies on "clinical judgments," "physician's experience" and "diagnostic criteria".
- Routine clinical assessment/physical examination is frequently subjective and unreliable.
- Reliance on general "clinical impression" to detect gross psychological disturbances is "hopelessly inaccurate".
- It is usually not possible to make a precise diagnosis or identify anatomic origin of the pain by routine clinical assessment.

FACET JOINT INJECTION AND MEDIAL BRANCH BLOCK

Facet joints have been implicated for symptoms in 15–45% of patients with low back pain and it mostly remains undiagnosed even with CT/MRI. The capsule of facet joint is

BOX 2: Common nociceptive source and their contribution in etiology of back pain.

- Facet joint (most common source of back pain in elderly) 24–40%
- Annulus fibroses of disk (internal disk disruption is the most common cause of back pain in young and middle-aged population) 7–26%
- Sacroiliac joint (3rd common source of back pain in all age group) 4–30%
- Vertebral body (tumor or osteoporotic fracture are not uncommon)
- Nerve root (nerve root compression or inflammation is common cause of leg pain, but uncommon cause of back pain) 13–20%
- Myofascial pain which can be independent or more commonly secondary to other nociceptive source 20–85%
- Endplate of disk (with trauma up to 30%)

BOX 3: Pathologic process in back pain diagnosis.

- Degenerative (most common)
- Inflammatory
- Congenital abnormality
- Osteoporotic fracture
- Malignancy
- Trauma
- Infection
- Metabolic diseases
- Autoimmune process

richly innervated by sensory nerves and the medial sensory branch of spinal nerves is in close association with the facet joint capsule especially its lower half laterally **(Fig. 1)**. The inflammation of the facet joint irritates and stimulates the nerve causing pain. Facet joint pain usually has following characteristics:

- Pain on paramedian aspect of spine. Pain from cervical facet involvement is commonly felt in head, neck, shoulder and rarely arm, thoracic facet involvement produces pain in upper back and chest. Lumbar facet joint emanating pain is felt in lower back, hip, or buttock.
- Pain is predominantly on one side of back.
- Patients are comfortable on sitting and bending forward as facet joints are less loaded when spine is flexed forward.

BOX 4: The various interventional techniques in pain management of spine and back.

Facet joint interventions:
- Intra-articular injections
- Medial branch blocks
- Radiofrequency ablation of medial nerve and capsular denervation

Epidural steroid injections:
- Transforaminal
- Caudal
- Interlaminar

Epidurolysis/epidural adhesiolysis/neuroplasty:
- Percutaneous
- Endoscopic

Interventions for intervertebral disk:
- Percutaneous disk decompression/diskectomy
- Intradiskal electrothermal therapy (IDET), radiofrequency annuloplasty, intradiskal biacuplasty
- Nucleoplasty
- Ozone nucleolysis

Miscellaneous:
- Trigger point injection
- Sacroiliac (SI) joint steroid injection/radiofrequency neurotomy
- Vertebroplasty/kyphoplasty
- Gray ramus block
- Spinal cord stimulation
- Lumbar sympathetic block

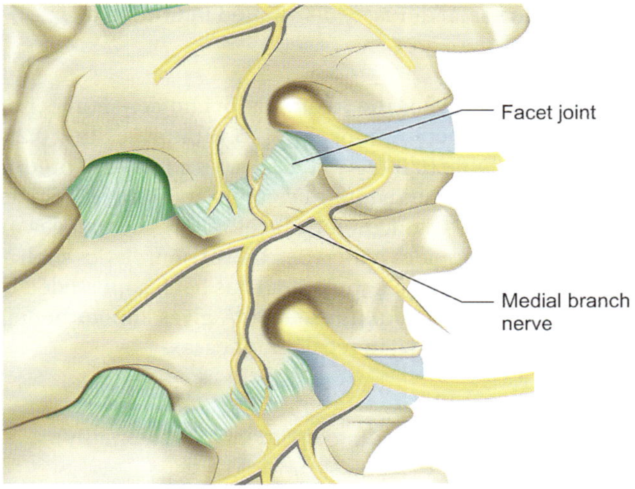

Fig. 1: The medial nerve branch emanates from dorsal ramus of spinal nerve supplying the facet joint and remains in close contact with the lower part of joint capsule.

- Sitting to standing, turning side on bed is painful.
- Extension, lateral bending, and rotation provoke pain as facet joints are maximally overloaded by these movements.
- Pain might be referred to leg, but that will be nondermatomal in distribution.
- There will be no neurological deficits.

The facet joint injections have both diagnostic and therapeutic utility. Intra-articular local anesthetic injection or medial branch block (*see* also Chapter on "Failed Back Surgery Syndrome") with 0.5–1.5 mL local anesthetic confirms diagnosis of facet joint as source of pain **(Figs. 2A and B)**. The medial branch nerve emerge from dorsal rami of spinal nerves and possess mostly sensory fibers (in cervical spine they also contain motor to small muscles). Once it is diagnosed, radiofrequency (RF) ablation procedure of medial branch gives good and sustained pain relief **(Figs. 2C and D)**. Intra-articular injection of local anesthetic with depot preparations of steroids can also be used though it is less effective than RF. Therapeutic facet joint injection with steroid/RF ablation of medial branch of dorsal rami gives long-term relief. The injection treatment or RF is done under fluoroscopy or ultrasound guidance. The effect may be permanent but mostly repeat sittings are needed because some fibers may get spared or pain may shift position to other facets (nerve may innervate other facets also, usually the lower one). Sometimes, chronic pain creates de novo pain circuit in the brain and despite successful nerve blockade the pain "feeling" persists, so not everyone gets pain relief. Recovery from procedure is fast and can be done as a day-care procedure, the relief is also immediate.

Contraindications

Contraindications for intra-articular facet injection and medial branch blocks are similar to contraindications of other neuraxial blocks.

Absolute contraindications: Patient refusal, systemic infection, skin infection at injection site, coagulopathies and low platelet count which can cause internal bleeding.

Relative contraindications: Needle phobias, physical conditions which restrict prone position, pregnancy and allergy to contrast and local anesthetics, psychiatric disorder, and preexisting neurological dysfunction.

Complications

- Postprocedure pain (in 1% of patients)
- Capsular rupture (if large volumes of drug is injected)
- Infection (use strict aseptic measures and sterile instruments)
- Dural puncture with or without spinal anesthesia/total spinal (avoid too deep penetration of needle; in lateral view, confirm the needle position that it should not be in intervertebral foramen or near the spinal nerves)
- Allergic reaction to contrast or local anesthetics (proper history of allergy should be taken and appropriate measures for prophylaxis and treatment should be taken.)

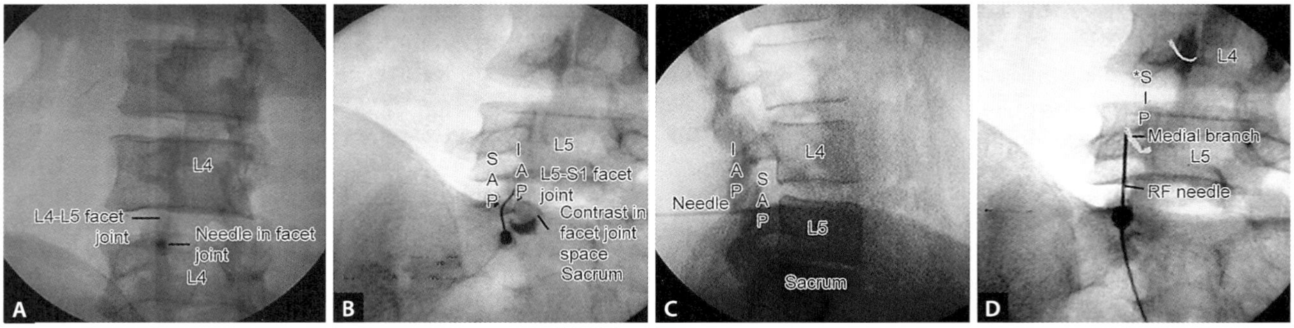

Figs. 2A to D: (A) Needle in L4-L5 facet joint inserted in parallel to X-rays (Gun barrel); (B) Contrast in facet joint confirms intra-articular position of needle; (C) In lateral view RF needle at junction of transverse process and SAP; (D) RF needle in close proximity to medial branch of L4. (IAP: inferior articular process; SAP: superior articular process)

Source: Dr Ashok Jadon, Chief Consultant and Head, Department of Anesthesia; Incharge, Pain Relief Services, Tata Motors Hospital, Jamshedpur, Jharkhand, India.

- Paraspinal abscess, septic, and chemical meningitis (these are rare complications and can be avoided by proper aseptic preparation and sterile techniques.)
- Inadvertent vascular injection and bleeding (Also rare complication, proper study of contrast flow before final injection and meticulous unhurried approach with adequate anatomical knowledge are prerequisites for any interventional procedure.)
- Radiofrequency treatment may result in changes similar to seen with infection.

MYOFASCIAL PAIN AND TRIGGER POINT INJECTION

Myofascial pain is a common dysfunction of skeletal muscles causing back pain with a lifetime prevalence affecting up to 85% of the general population. Presence of sensitized myofascial band called trigger point (TP) is the hallmark of the condition. They are mostly fibrotic bands with neurovascular core sensitive to touch, deformation and inflammation. These trigger points are commonly located in the trapezius and paraspinal muscles. The iliopsoas and quadratus lumborum are two muscles commonly involved in the origin of low back pain in the lumbar region. Pain patterns involving these muscles are referred to as superficial (lateral) or deep (medial), depending on the location of the TP. One should differentiate between myofascial pain syndrome that contains few localized trigger points; from fibromyalgia where the distribution is diffuse and mostly the trigger points are latent causing pains.

Characteristics of myofascial trigger points: Trigger points possess specific motor and sensory characteristics. Diagnosis of TP can be made if only a few of those characteristics are present:

- Trigger points are small (25 mm in diameter) palpable nodules of hypersensitivity located in taut, "rope-like" bands of skeletal muscle.
- Palpation of myofascial TPs will produce radiating or referred pain. This pain may be referred to distal or proximal area (zone of reference) and the intensity may vary from a dull ache to severe incapacitating.
- Palpation or needling of a myofascial TP may provoke an involuntary twitch in the muscle and/or skin.
- Patient will quickly flinch away from the palpation area in reaction which is known as the "jump sign".
- Verbalization may accompany the jump sign.
- TP activation may evoke an autonomic phenomenon, including dermal flushing, lacrimation, sweating, vasoconstriction (blanching) and temperature changes.

Types

Myofascial TPs can be classified as either *active* or *latent.*

Active

Trigger points remain symptomatic and painful even at rest. Palpation of active TPs produces a predictable local or referred pain of spreading or radiating nature. Jump sign and local twitch response will also be present.

Latent

Trigger points are not associated with spontaneous pain but are tender to palpation. They can be inactive for years. Muscle shortening and weakness, stiffness, and restricted range of motion may be present. Unlike active TPs, latent TPs usually do not require treatment unless activated. Large number of latent TPs are seen diffusely distributed in fibromyalgia.

Treatment

Neutralization of TP is the treatment of choice. TP injection with local anesthetic, [lidocaine (1%), bupivacaine (0.25–0.5%), ropivacaine (0.2–0.75%)] deposteroid (methylprednisolone acetate, methylprednisolone sodium succinate, dexamethasone, triamcinolone acetonide), ozone gas or even dry needling gives pain relief. Use of neurolytics such as sarapin, phenol (3%), alcohol (50%) has been superseded by above medications. Botulinum toxin A gives similar benefit and may be considered in recalcitrant cases.

Contraindications

Local infection and bleeding disorders (coagulopathy).

Complications

Increased pain in the area of the injection, infection, or hematoma in the muscles.

EPIDURAL STEROID INJECTION

Epidural deposition of anti-inflammatory medication **(Fig. 3)** is a popular technique of pain relief in low back pain and radicular pain. Epidural corticosteroids are indicated for acute pain, chronic benign pain, cancer-related pain, perineal and rectal pain and in the treatment of acute herpes zoster **(Box 5)**. The success rate is also remarkable but it is temporary mostly. Patients with degenerative disorders have to often take repeat injections.

History

First time in 1952, Robecchi and Capra utilized epidural steroid injections in the treatment of radicular pain syndromes via the first sacral nerve root. The first case series of interlaminar epidurals performed using loss of resistance technique was reported in 1966 by Harley et al.

Fluoroscopic-guided versus Blind Approach

Initial studies used the loss of resistance technique only (blind or without fluoroscopic guidance) for interlaminar epidural injection. This technique results in high failures to deposit drugs at intended place. Even in experienced hands, the blind technique has improper localization in 13–30% of injections. The use of fluoroscopy allows proper localization within the epidural space and assures placement of corticosteroid and anesthetic to the target areas. Fluoroscopy also helps to manage the significant anatomical anomalies in the epidural space like midline septum and spinal deformities such as scoliosis or postlaminectomy/fusion. Fluoroscopy is now considered "the standard of care" for epidural injections since 2007.

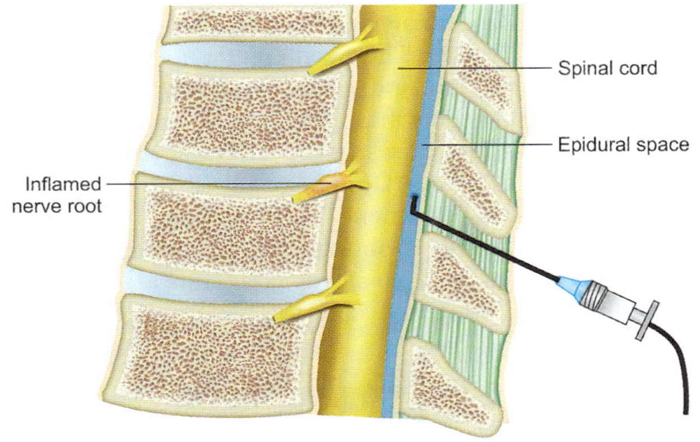

Fig. 3: The epidural injection delivers the drug into epidural space (above the duramater) that distributes in the space locally and downwards providing relief from inflammation associated pains.

BOX 5: Indications of epidural injections.

- Herniated nucleus pulposus
- Degenerative disk disease
- Nonspecific radiculitis
- Spinal stenosis ± facet arthropathy
  - Osteophytes impinging spinal nerves
  - Thickened ligamentum flavum
- Failed back syndrome
- Postherpetic neuralgia
- Intercostal neuralgia
- Spondylolysis and spondylolisthesis associated with nerve root irritation
- Spinal deformity causing nerve root irritation
- Diabetic polyneuropathy
- Complex regional pain syndrome of lower extremity
- Chemotherapy-related neuropathy

Contraindications

Absolute

- Patient's refusal
- Pregnancy (under fluoroscopy, particularly early pregnancy, weigh advantages against the risk after second trimester)
- Known true anaphylactic reaction and/or allergy to any constituents of the epidural injection (steroid, anesthetic, or contrast agent)
- Cauda equina syndrome
- Anticoagulation therapy and coagulopathy
- Suspected local or systemic infection

Relative

- Hypovolemia
- Diabetes mellitus
- Glaucoma

Rationale to Use Epidural Steroid

The epidural steroid in treatment of back pain is used with the premise that the pain source lies in intervertebral disks, nerve root, dura, facet joints, ligaments, fascia or muscles. The pain is generated by pressure on the annulus fibroses, posterior longitudinal ligament, and swollen, stretched or compressed nerve roots. This pressure or dysfunction may occur due to vascular compromise, inflammation or change in biochemical environment of the tissue. There is another proposed mechanism that vascular compromise (venous stasis) causes defect in nutrition to the nervous tissue and makes them susceptible for pain generators. The placement of corticosteroids as close as possible to an inflamed nerve root (other inflamed tissues) should help to lead to relief of pain in patients with sciatic symptoms related to inflammation from disk herniation, spinal stenosis, postsurgical fibrosis failed back surgery syndrome (FBSS) or chemically sensitive disk [internal disk disruption (IDD)].

Mechanism of Action of Steroids

The pathophysiologic mechanisms by which corticosteroids relieve back pain remain controversial. There have been several proposed mechanisms of action, which include anti-inflammatory, direct neuromembrane stabilization effects, and modulation of peripheral nociceptors input. Corticosteroid blocks C-fiber conduction, inhibits prostaglandin synthesis, reduces nerve root edema which improves microcirculation, reduces ischemia and decreases sensitivity of dorsal horn neurons. Steroids also interact with norepinephrine and 5-hydroxytryptamine neurons within the dorsal horn of spinal cord which are involved in the transmission of pain. Steroids modulate nociceptive inputs of peripheral nociceptors, reduce inflammatory reactions, and inhibit inflammatory mediators.

Approaches for Epidural Steroid Injection in Back Pain

There are three commonly used approaches to inject epidural steroid in treatment of back pain: lumbar interlaminar, caudal, and transforaminal approach **(Fig. 4)**. Each one has distinct advantages, limitations, and complications.

Lumbar Interlaminar Approach

Technique

Needles: There are numerous needles of different gauges and lengths that are appropriate for lumbar interlaminar epidural injections. The Tuohy needle is specifically designed needle for epidural injections. It gives a distinct loss of resistance feel and allows easier passage of a catheter through the needle into the epidural space if required. Some physicians may choose standard spinal needle (Quincke-Babcock needle). However, this needle may result in higher risk of dural puncture. 17–20G is appropriate for epidural injection because thin needles result in poor localization of epidural space, inadvertent dural puncture and resultant postdural puncture headache (PDPH).

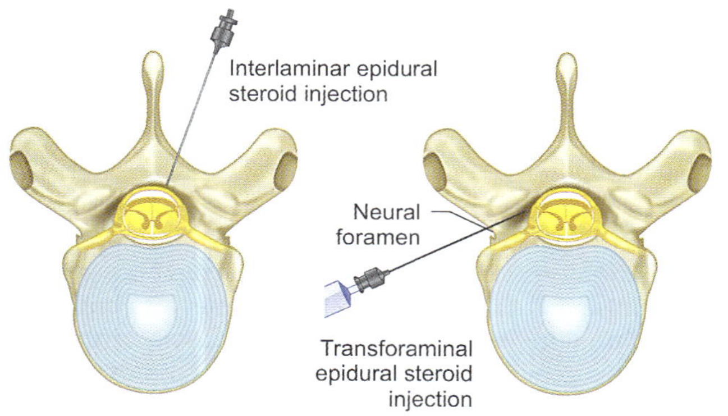

Fig. 4: The two of the most common methods of giving epidural injection are interlaminar and transforaminal techniques. While the former deposits the drug in epidural space the latter specifically targets one nerve root. They have unique indications, rationale, and complications (see text for details).

Identification of the epidural space: A syringe filled with either air or saline (some have stated saline is better than air) is used to locate epidural space by loss of resistance (resistance is offered by ligamentum flavum).

Injection procedure and positioning: A lumbar epidural injection can be performed with the patient in a seated, lateral, or prone position **(Figs. 5A to C)**. When fluoroscopic guidance is used, patient is usually placed in the prone position and desired interlaminar space is identified. The injection can be performed with either a midline or a paramedian technique. Skin at the needle entry site is anesthetized with 1% lidocaine. The Tuohy needle (18 G) is placed in the direct midline position. Continuous pressure is applied on the syringe plunger with the other hand, and the needle is advanced. Intermittent use of fluoroscope is useful in proper placement and advancement of the needle in the anteroposterior (AP) position **(Fig. 5A)**. As the needle is advanced through the interspinous ligament, the fluoroscope is positioned in a lateral view in order to ascertain the needle depth **(Fig. 5B)**. The needle is then advanced into the ligamentum flavum, and subsequently into the epidural space. Once the needle has reached the epidural space with appropriate loss of resistance to either air or saline, nonionic contrast 1–3 mL (Omnipaque or Isovue) is injected to confirm epidural placement. A lateral fluoroscopic image as well as an AP image is obtained. The contrast spread in epidural space has an areolar appearance **(Fig. 5C)**. If no intravascular or soft-tissue contrast pattern is seen with

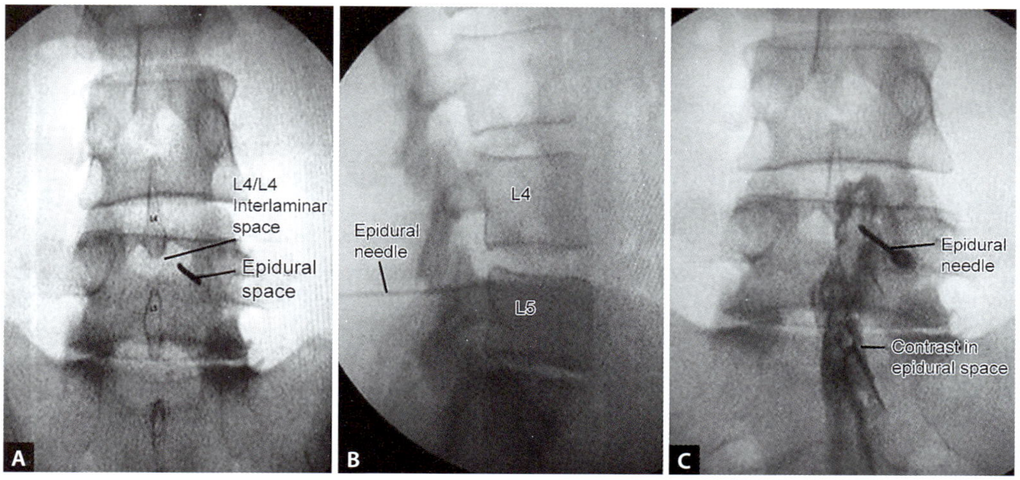

Figs. 5A to C: Interlaminar epidural injection. (A) AP view epidural needle in interlaminar space; (B) Lateral view showing needle in epidural space; (C) Epidural contrast spread and areolar appearance of contrast in AP view.
Source: Dr Ashok Jadon, Chief Consultant and Head, Department of Anesthesia; Incharge, Pain Relief Services, Tata Motors Hospital, Jamshedpur, Jharkhand, India.

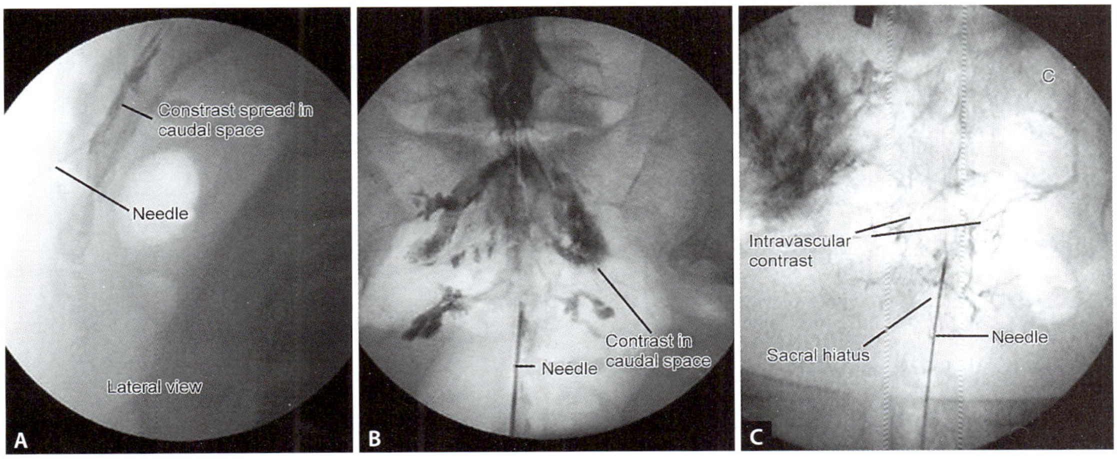

Figs. 6A to C: Contrast spread in caudal space. (A) Lateral view; (B) AP view (Inverted X-mass tree appearance); (C) Vascular injection of contrast.
Source: Dr Ashok Jadon, Chief Consultant and Head, Department of Anesthesia; Incharge, Pain Relief Services, Tata Motors Hospital, Jamshedpur, Jharkhand, India.

1-3 mL of contrast, mixture of local anesthetic and steroid can then be injected into the epidural space. Commonly 3-5 mL of 1% lidocaine without preservative and 1.0-2.0 mL of corticosteroid [Depomedrol (methylprednisolone acetate) 40-80 mg] or [40-80 mg Kenalog (triamcinolone acetonide)] is injected. The lumbar paramedian technique is identical to the midline approach except for the specific site of injection.

Caudal Epidural

Caudal epidural injections should also be performed with fluoroscopy because failure to enter the epidural space with needle placement is common (8-38%). Use of fluoroscopy improves the accuracy of needle placement and decreases the risk of subarachnoid puncture, reducing chances of intrathecal or intravascular injection (3.7-14% with blind approach) **(Figs. 6A to C)**. Use of fluoroscopy facilitates accurate delivery of medications and improves outcomes.

Injection Procedure and Patient Position

The procedure is performed with the patient in the prone position and fluoroscope in lateral view. Patient is placed on two pillows, one under the head and one under the hips to make sacral hiatus more prominent **(Fig. 7)**. Legs are abducted to relax the gluteus muscles for easy identification of the sacral hiatus. After palpation of sacral cornua and anesthetizing overlying skin, a 20-22 G needle (preferably with stylet) is introduced in the sacral hiatus. A distinct "pop" is felt while sacrococcygeal membrane is pierced. Needle position is checked by fluoroscope and proper placement is confirmed by injection of 2-3 mL contrast (Omnipaque). Contrast is seen like inverted X-mass tree in AP view and linear spread in lateral view **(Figs. 6A and B)**. If intravascular placement is ruled out (tortuous web formation if the contrast is in veins or quick run-off in arterial injection; **Fig. 6C**), 10 mL 0.5-1% xylocaine mixed with 40-80 mg depomedrol can be injected slowly. On pain on injection, needle position should be rechecked. Due to large volumes of local anesthetics used, patients are observed in recovery for potential side effects of local anesthesia.

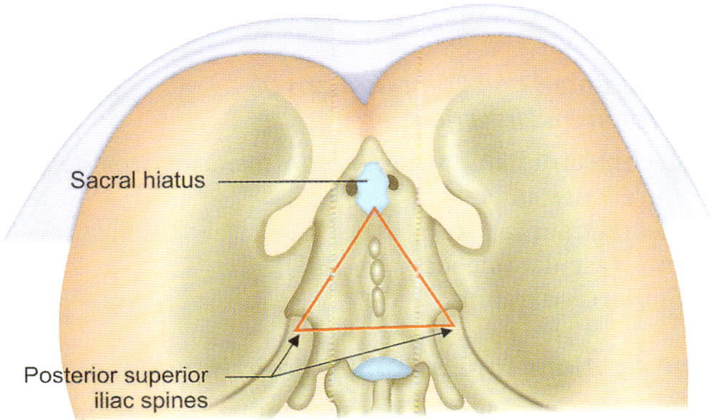

Fig. 7: The surface anatomy of sacral hiatus as used for caudal epidural steroid.

Transforaminal epidural Injection (Selective Nerve Root Block or Nerve Root Sleeve Injection)

Transforaminal epidural injection (TFEI) or a selective nerve root injection consists of injection of contrast, local anesthetic or other substances like deposteroid around spinal nerve root under fluoroscopy **(Fig. 8A)**. TFEIs are used for diagnostic as well as therapeutic purpose. Therapeutically, TFEI is more effective than simple lumbar interlaminar or caudal epidural steroid injection as drug is deposited more anteriorly right close to the target. The amount of drug dose is also much less in TFEI (e.g., 10-20 mg vs. 40-80 mg in lumbar/caudal epidural). In cases of failed back surgery syndrome (FBSS) and presence of scar, transforaminal becomes the choice of approach to the epidural space. The efficacy of TFEI is good in disk herniation and spinal canal stenosis and limited in FBSS.

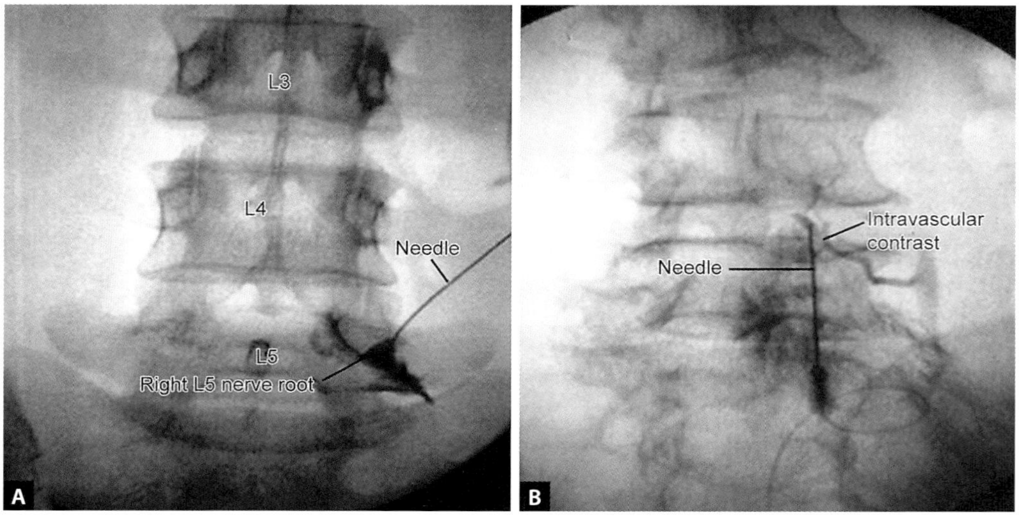

Figs. 8A and B: (A) Transforaminal injection at right L5 nerve root; (B) Accidental intravascular contrast injection during right L4 transforaminal injection.
Source: Dr Ashok Jadon, Chief Consultant and Head, Department of Anesthesia; Incharge, Pain Relief Services, Tata Motors Hospital, Jamshedpur, Jharkhand, India.

Disadvantages and Complications of Transforaminal Injection

- Technical difficulty in presence of fusion and/or hardware
- Intraneural injection
- Neural trauma
- Intravascular injection **(Fig. 8B)**
- Spinal cord trauma

Complications for Epidural Steroid Injections

- *Infections:* Epidural abscess, meningitis, osteomyelitis/diskitis
- *Neurologic:* Nerve injury, paresthesias, paralysis, seizures, increased sciatic pain, and headache
- *Ophthalmologic:* Retinal hemorrhage and acute retinal necrosis.
- *Others:* Dural puncture, epidural hematoma, pain at injection site, anaphylaxis, dysphonia, adverse effects of contrast media, and local anesthetics

Adverse Effects

Used cautiously at recommended therapeutic dosages the epidural steroids are safe and rarely produce complications. Prolonged and excessive use of corticosteroid administration (especially indiscriminate additional oral and other forms combined) may lead to suppression of pituitary adrenal axis, Cushing's syndrome, osteoporosis, osteonecrosis of the bone, steroid myopathy, epidural lipomatosis, weight gain, fluid retention, and hyperglycemia.

Outcome of Epidural Steroid Injections

The short-term relief is good with all three modalities of steroid instillation, however, long-term relief is better with transforaminal and caudal compared to interlaminar approach. Immediate relief occurs in >85% patients but long-term relief reduces to nearly 50%. If epidural injection is given at early stage of pain, success of pain relief is more with longer duration of pain relief. Best results are obtained in disk herniation and poor outcome is observed in nonspecific back pain.

EPIDUROGRAPHY AND EPIDUROSCOPY

Epidurography is a procedure of injecting nonionic water-soluble radio-opaque dye in the epidural space under C-arm guidance. Normal epidurogram looks like an inverted Christmas tree where dye enters into the dural extension of each nerve root. Epidurography has been used to increase success of interlaminar epidural injection. In cases of nerve root edema/inflammation or epidural fibrosis (postsurgical scar or failed back surgery), the dye may not enter into the neural foramen and around the nerve root. Epiduroscopy (a fiber-optic scope to visualize epidural space) helps in establishing the diagnosis of such adhesions and also site of these adhesions (*see* also Chapter on "Failed Back Surgery Syndrome"). These adhesions can be managed by adhesiolysis during epiduroscopy under vision. Epidural fibrosis is better diagnosed with epidurography or epiduroscopy than CT/MRI. Epidural fibrosis may account for as much as 20–36% of all cases of FBSS.

Epidurolysis/Epidural Adhesiolysis/Neuroplasty

Epidural fibrosis is seen in FBSS or in postinflammatory adhesion following extrusion/sequestration of nucleus pulposus. Breaking the adhesions around the nerves in epidural space is known as "epidurolysis/epidural adhesiolysis or neuroplasty". It is done with normal saline, hypertonic saline with or without hyaluronidase. It may be done with Racz catheter after performing an "epidurogram", procedure called Racz adhesiolysis.

PROVOCATIVE DISKOGRAPHY

Diskogenic pain may contribute up to 26% of spinal pain. Provocative diskography is a very useful test to diagnose diskogenic back pain due to internal disk disruption. Diskography literally means the opacification of the nucleus pulposus of an intervertebral disk to render it visible under radiographs. Sterile needle is placed into the center of the intervertebral disk (nucleus pulposus); radio-opaque contrast is injected to provoke pain. Radiological assessment of disk morphology, clinical assessment of the intensity and concordance of evoked pain in relation to baseline pain and the measurement of intradiskal pressure at which the pain is provoked are measured. It is not a very reliable imaging technique with high false positive rate but provides both anatomical and functional information about a diseased disk (details in Chapter on "Low Back Pain, Intervertebral Disk Degeneration, Lumbar Spondylosis, and Degenerative Conditions of Cervical Spine").

PERCUTANEOUS DISK DECOMPRESSION/ DISKECTOMY

If surgical intervention is not possible where disk protrusion is the causative factor for back pain, part of the disk can be removed percutaneous with the help of specialized instruments. Usually, a 17 G needle is introduced into the diseased disk under C-arm guidance then a special motorized probe or similar instrument is introduced through this needle. Nucleus pulposus is broken into fine particles and removed out. Percutaneous nucleotomy and hydrodissection are other similar procedures done for contained disk herniation with varied success.

OZONE NUCLEOLYSIS

Introduction

Ozone is naturally present in atmosphere and near sea shores. In nature, it is formed by superoxidation of oxygen mostly by lightening. In laboratory also, it is produced by passing oxygen over electrically charged electrodes. The concentration of ozone is controlled through dial setting which regulates the mixture of O_2/O_3. Oxygen-ozone mixture (70:30 ratio) is commonly used for intradiskal injections.

Mechanism of Action

Primary mechanism of action of the oxygen-ozone mixture injected into the herniated disk is volume reduction (disk decompression). Disk contains aggrecan (major. proteoglycan of the disk) responsible for maintaining tissue hydration through the osmotic pressure provided by its constituent chondroitin and keratan sulfate chains. Ozone reacts with the glycosaminoglycan (GAG) in the nucleolus pulposus (NP) which ultimately results in dehydration of the disk.

Secondary mechanism of action is related to analgesic and anti-inflammatory factors. It is well-known that ozone can react with organic compounds like prostaglandins (PG). Ozone inhibits synthesis of prostaglandins; liberation of bradykinin and other pain-inducing products; secretion of proteinases from macrophages, polymorph, and neutrophils. Ozone treatment is done for both contained and non-contained disk prolapse causing diskogenic pain. 2–3 mL of oxygen-ozone mixture (30–40% O_3) is injected intradiskally and about 10–20 mL injected in paravertebral space of affected disk subsequently.

Technique

In prone position, under fluoroscopic guide intended level of disk is identified and marked. In 30° ipsilateral tilt of C-arm 21 G long spinal needle (120–150 mm) is inserted in the disk (very strict aseptic measures are must for this procedure and it is always better to use needle through needle approach to prevent possible diskitis). Position of needle is confirmed in AP view and depth is confirmed with lateral view. 1 mL water soluble contrast is injected which further confirms the safe needle position. 2–3 mL of 30:70 (O_3–O_2) mixture is injected **(Figs. 9A to D)**. Subsequently, peripedicular injections of same mixtures are used weekly for 3–4 weeks.

Contraindications

Thyrotoxicosis and pregnancy are only known contraindications.

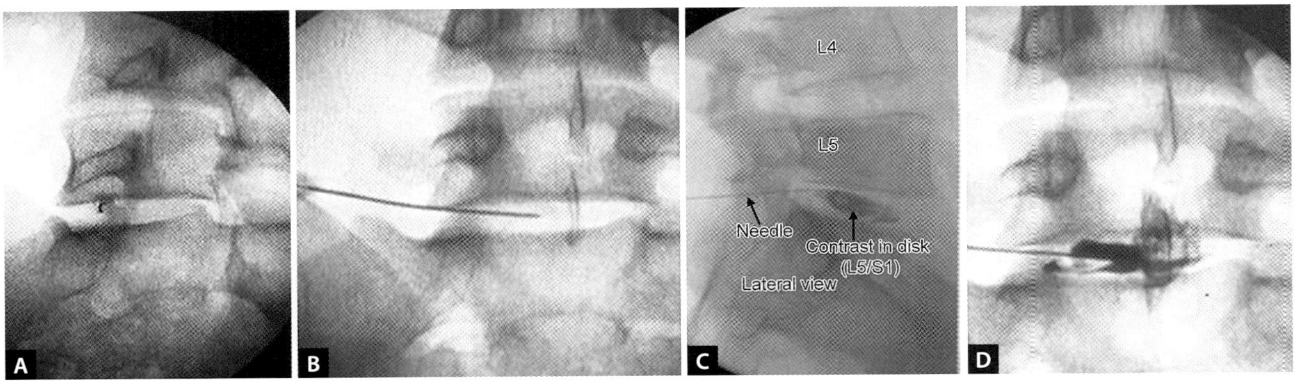

Figs. 9A to D: Steps of ozone nucleolysis. (A) Needle inserted in the intervertebral disk left oblique view; (B) Needle position is checked in AP view; (C) Contrast injected to confirm the needle position in lateral view; (D) Ozone-Oxygen mixture injected.
Source: Dr Ashok Jadon, Chief Consultant and Head, Department of Anesthesia; Incharge, Pain Relief Serv ces, Tata Motors Hospital, Jamshedpur, Jharkhand, India.

Complications

It is very safe agent to use; however, potential complications related to technique, e.g., nerve injury, intravascular injection, gas embolism can still occur. There are few reports of diskitis, however, it is difficult to prove that whether it is because of poor aseptic precautions or ozone.

The current status of ozone nucleolysis is discussed in Chapter on "Low Back Pain, Intervertebral Disk Degeneration, Lumbar Spondylosis, and Degenerative Conditions of Cervical Spine".

Methylene Blue Nucleolysis

Recently, methylene blue injection in intervertebral disk for diskogenic pain has been tried. The postulated mechanism of methylene blue is denervation of small nociceptive fibers that grow into the annulus fibrosis, which are implicated in diskogenic pain. The results are mixed; till more controlled studies are done, there is no clear-cut recommendation for this technique.

SACROILIAC JOINT PAIN AND ITS MANAGEMENT

The sacroiliac joint (SIJ) has been implicated as the primary source of pain in 16–30% cases. Pain from the SI joint is generally localized in the gluteal region. Referred pain may be perceived in lower limb lumbar region, groin or abdomen. There are many provocative tests to diagnose SI joint pain clinically and they are positive when they reproduce a patient's typical pain. Seven most important clinical tests to identify SIJ as a pain source are listed below:

1. *Compression test (approximation test):* The patient lies in lateral position with the affected side up. Patient's hips are flexed 45°, and the knees are flexed 90°. The examiner stands behind the patient then exerts downward medial pressure with both hands on the front side of the iliac crest.
2. *Distraction test (gapping test):* The patient rests in supine position and the examiner stands on the affected side. Then pressure in the dorsolateral direction is applied by examiner keeping hands on anterior superior iliac spine of the affected side.
3. *Patrick's sign (flexion abduction external rotation test):* The patient is in supine position and examiner stands on affected side. The foot of affected side is positioned under the opposite knee and then downward pressure is applied to the knee of the affected side.
4. *Gaenslen's test (pelvic torsion test):* Affected side is kept on the edge of the examination table while patient lies in a supine position. The unaffected leg flexed until the knee is pushed against the chest. The affected side is brought into hyperextension by applying light pressure to that knee.
5. *Thigh thrust test (posterior shear test):* The patient lies in the supine position with unaffected leg in extension and examiner stands on affected side. Examiner flexes the extremity on the affected side at the hip approximately 90° with slight adduction while applying light pressure to the bent knee.
6. *Fortin's finger test:* Consistently, patient indicates the location of the pain with one finger just inferior and medial to the posterior superior iliac spine.
7. *Gillet's test:* The patient stands on one leg and pulls the knee of other leg up to his or her chest.

Radiological imaging is important to exclude "red flags"; however, it does not contribute much in the diagnosis. Diagnostic blocks are the gold standard for diagnosis. Multidisciplinary approach is required to treat pain of SIJ. Intra-articular SIJ infiltrations with local anesthetic and corticosteroids are effective to treat SIJ pain and have highest evidence of success. If steroid injection provides only short-term relief then cooled RF treatment of the lateral branches of S1–S3 (S4) is recommended. Pulsed RF procedures targeted at L5 dorsal ramus and lateral branches of S1–S3 may be considered if cooled RF is not available. Percutaneous RF neurotomy of SIJ provides long-term relief; however, cooled RF neurotomy of lateral branch has better evidence over conventional RF.

Technique of Sacroiliac Joint Injection

The patient is positioned prone and under fluoroscopy lower end of posterior SI joint is identified and marker is placed **(Fig. 10A)**. A 25 or 22 G, 3.5-inch spinal needle is directed into the SIJ using a posterior approach. Once the needle has entered the joint space **(Fig. 10B)**, intra-articular placement

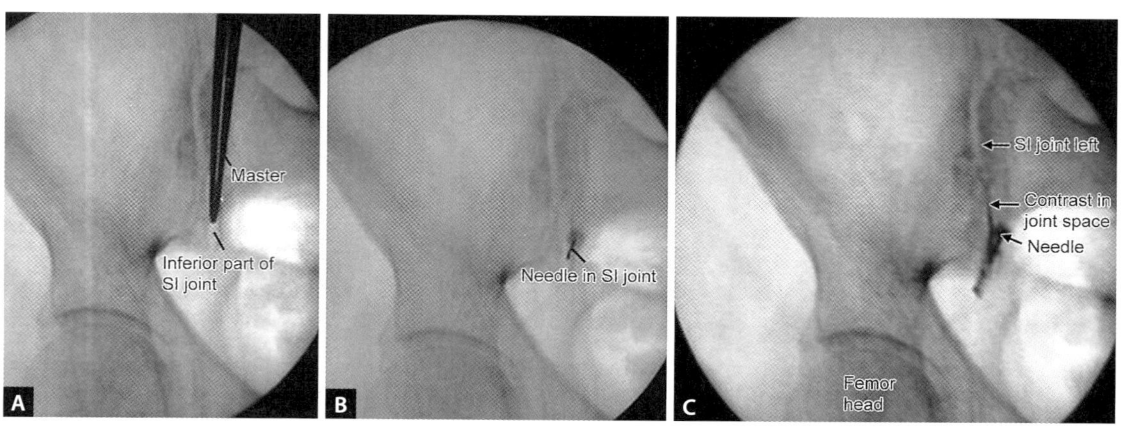

Figs. 10A to C: (A) Marker on SI joint; (B) Needle in SI joint; (C) Contrast filling the joint space.

is confirmed with an injection of contrast medium. If the needle has been correctly placed, injection of the contrast medium will outline the joint space **(Fig. 10C)**. Only a minimum volume of contrast medium (0.3–0.5 mL) is required to establish intra-articular injection.

Common Contraindications for Sacroiliac Joint Interventions

- Needle phobia
- Psychogenic pain
- Inability of the patient to understand consent
- Allergies to contrast, local anesthetic, steroids, Sarapin or other drugs
- Proven diskogenic pain, disk herniation or facet joint pain
- Infection
- Anticoagulant therapy/antiplatelet therapy or bleeding diathesis
- Pregnancy

PERCUTANEOUS VERTEBROPLASTY AND KYPHOPLASTY

Vertebroplasty is a minimally invasive procedure that is effective in the treatment of pain resulting from pathologic compression fractures, osteolytic bone lesions, myelomas, hemangioma, and osteoporosis. Vertebroplasty stabilizes the spine and gives immediate pain relief possibly due to thermal effect on small nerve endings responsible for pain. Balloon kyphoplasty is an advancement over vertebroplasty and attempts to restore vertebral height also. The techniques are discussed in detail elsewhere.

NEW TECHNIQUES

In view of persistent problem of back pain and nonavailability of ideal treatment, research is still on to find newer treatment. Few recently added treatments in the existing armamentarium to manage back pain are given below.

Nucleoplasty (Coblation)

This technique is used for disk herniation (contained disk) with premise that if volume of disk is reduced, it will shrink and back pain will be reduced. Nucleoplasty utilizes coblation technology in which ablation and coagulation of nucleus pulposus reduces the size of contained herniated disk. In this technique, through an introducer needle special RF catheter is inserted up to the disk and very high RF energy is delivered through tip of catheter which generates high-energy plasma and evaporates the nucleus. Thereby, it reduces the size and intradiskal pressure. Few short-term complications such as numbness and transient soreness in back have been observed. No long-term or serious complications are reported.

Annuloplasty

It is a group of minimally invasive procedures done on the disk. The concept is to denervate the outer annulus fibrosus which became painful because of ingrowing new nerve ending due to degenerative changes, resulting annular fissures and

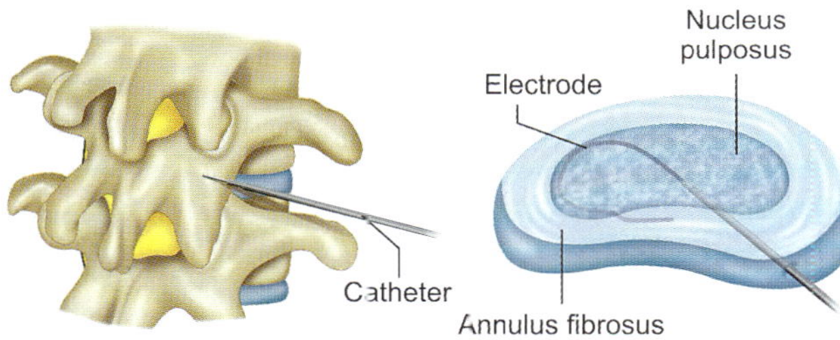

Fig. 11: The technique of intradiskal electrothermal therapy annuloplasty.

inflammatory reaction with nucleus pulposus. The common annuloplasty techniques are intradiskal electrothermal therapy (IDET), RF annuloplasty, and intradiskal biacuplasty (cooled RF).

Intradiskal Electrothermal Therapy

In this technique, thermal energy is gradually delivered to the posterior annulus through intradiskally placed resistive coil. Under fluoroscopic guidance, a 17 G introducer needle is inserted in the anterolateral part of the disk **(Fig. 11)** through which a special catheter is inserted which has metallic end to transmit the heat to target area (outer annulus fibrosus). The catheter rests on the posterolateral part of the disk and seals annular defects thermally (*see* also Chapter on "Failed Back Surgery Syndrome"). This technique is quite safe; however, complications such as paresthesias, occurrence of new radicular pain, foot drop, kinking and fracture of heating element have been reported. Other rare complications are cauda equina syndrome and disk herniation. The risk of complication can be reduced if procedure is done under light sedation as patient can communicate any undue discomfort due to probable harm.

Radiofrequency Annuloplasty

In this technique, a flexible RF probe disk-TRODE® (Covidien, Mansfield, MA) is inserted up to the painful annulus under fluoroscopic and electric impedance guide. The results are not promising. No complication has been reported; however, considerations will remain same as other intradiskal techniques.

Intradiskal Biacuplasty

It is new novel approach to treat diskogenic pain. Two RF probes are placed one from each side into the posterior annulus. RF current is then passed between these two probes which denervates annulus fibrosus. The hollow lumen of internally water-cooled probes allows delivery of high energy to target area without increasing temperature of the probes and preventing heat injury to surrounding tissue. The cooled RF probe produces larger therapeutic lesions than conventional RF.

GRAY RAMUS BLOCK

Gray ramus block (GRB) is effective to relieve low back pain caused by diskogenic pain. This procedure is used when surgery is not an option to relieve pain from disk. To

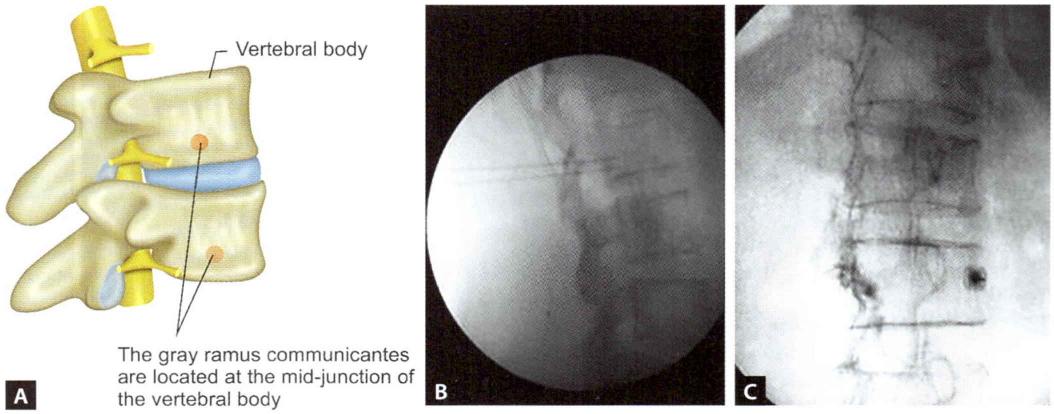

Figs. 12A to C: (A) Location of gray ramus on vertebral body; (B) Lateral view; contrast injection and safe localization; (C) AP view after contrast injection.

know that which disk(s) are causing pain, a diskography is performed before the procedure of GRB. After affected levels are identified, diagnostic block of gray ramus is done to predict the efficacy of subsequent GRB. Under fluoroscopy, 2–3 mL of local anesthetic with or without steroid is injected after contrast confirmation of safe needle placement **(Figs. 12A to C)** at three levels. One level which is affected and one level each upper and lower side. It is necessary to repeat the diagnostic block procedure two times to confirm the appropriate course of treatment. If the patient gets significant relief from both injections, the patient is a candidate for RF neurotomy of the gray ramus communicans nerve.

If back pain is due to internal disk disruption (IDD) or fracture of vertebral body, GRB with local anesthetic with or without steroid can be used as diagnostic tool as well as therapeutic intervention to provide temporary pain relief; longer duration of pain relief can be achieved by RF ablation. In cases of failed back surgery (FBS), if conservative measures fail in the treatment and if there is no indication for further surgery, interruption of nerve pathways conducting noxious stimuli by local anesthetic or by RF may be attempted. Treatment with RF lesions is well tolerated and it has few adverse effects in patients who are very difficult to manage otherwise. Osteoporotic vertebral compression fracture (OVCF) is a common complication of osteoporosis in the aging population, which leads to refractory chronic pain. Gray ramus communicans nerve block is a novel treatment approach for painful osteoporotic vertebral compression fracture.

SPINAL CORD STIMULATOR

The role of spinal cord stimulator (SCS) in back pain is mainly to manage FBS patients (*see* Chapter on "Failed Back Surgery Syndrome" for details) when other therapies have failed. The therapy masks pain signals before they reach CNS. So it has also been used to treat intractable pain not responding to other therapies and chronic low back pain **(Box 6)**. Stimulating electrodes (leads) are placed in epidural space either percutaneously or by surgery **(Fig. 13)**. These leads are connected to a pulse generator which acts as a source of stimulation. The action of spinal cord stimulation (neurophysiologic mechanisms) is not completely understood; however, effects at local and supraspinal levels through dorsal horn interneuron and neurochemical mechanisms have been suggested. The success of treatment depends upon successful trial and proper patient selection. Appropriate patients for neurostimulation implant must meet the following criteria: other conservative therapies have failed; the patient should have a diagnosis of neuropathic

BOX 6: Indications for spinal cord stimulation therapy.

- Failed back surgery syndrome
- Complex regional pain syndrome
- Angina pectoris
- Ischemic limb pain
- Chronic painful peripheral neuropathy or plexopathy
- Multiple sclerosis
- Postherpetic neuralgia
- Phantom limb pain following amputations
- Post-thoracotomy pain
- Intercostal neuralgia
- *Off-label indications:*
  - Improving locomotion in Parkinson's disease
  - Gastrointestinal motility disorders
  - Genitourinary and sexual dysfunction
  - Occipital nerve stimulation for chronic migraine/headache

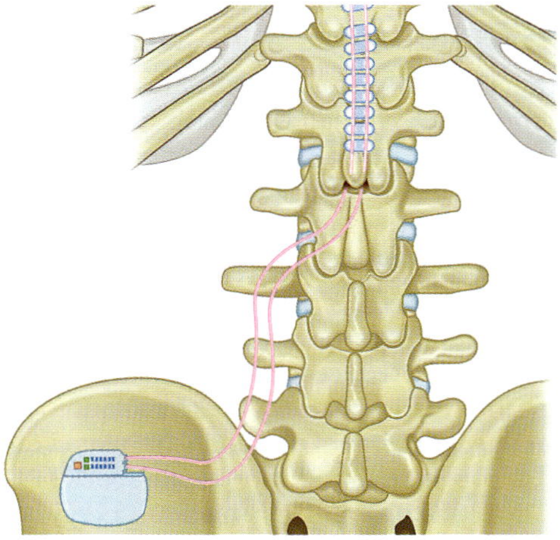

Fig. 13: Spinal cord stimulator electrodes are placed over the cord and the device is placed in a superficial pocket elsewhere.

pain syndromes; a trial has demonstrated pain relief; significant psychological issues have been ruled out. Careful trial period is advocated to avoid the failed implant. Trials of different lengths have been advocated. The risk of infection is more with long trials of 5–7 days where use of antibiotics is recommended. SCS is effective to improve quality of life in resistant FBS patients; however, it is an invasive and cost-intensive procedure, therefore its use is restricted for refractory cases.

Intradiskal Steroid Injection

In the past, intradiskal steroid injections were used for diskogenic pain in premise that it will reduce the inflammation within the disk; however, results remain inconclusive. The most serious complication of intradiskal steroid was epidural calcification which was symptomatic in 14–68% patients. There are reported cases of diskitis also with this technique. Although in patients with inflammatory endplate disease, it has shown some beneficial effects, it is rarely used now due to significant risks.

CONCLUSION

Back pain is a complex clinical situation with multiple pain sources. IPM procedures have revolutionized the management of spinal pain by providing definitive diagnosis and treatments. The "target specific" interventional pain management techniques are now integrated into the treatment plan of patients suffering from back pain. There are different choices of IPM procedures for similar type of problem. Before choosing a particular procedure, diagnostic intervention is advisable to assess the outcome of therapeutic procedure.

CHAPTER 100

Spinal Dysraphism (Spina Bifida, Myelocele, Meningomyelocele, Diastematomyelia, and Tethered Cord Syndrome)

Manish Kumar Varshney

INTRODUCTION

Spinal dysraphism encompasses a spectrum of congenital conditions resulting in a defective neural arch through which meninges or neural elements may herniate. The spinal dysraphic states are either overt (aperta form)—obvious at birth the overlying skin is not intact, pending leakage of cerebrospinal fluid (CSF) or occult (occulta) the defect is well-covered with full-thickness skin with only vague external marks that indicate an underlying pathology. The various conditions include:

- Spina bifida aperta—general term (see below)
- Spina bifida occulta **(Fig. 1)**—general term (see below)

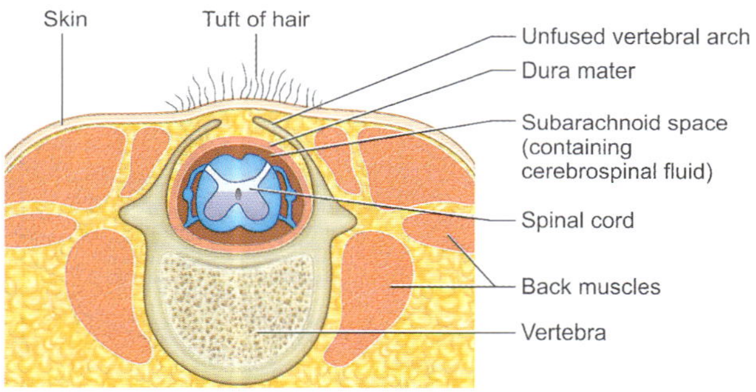

Fig. 1: Spina bifida occulta.

- Meningocele **(Figs. 2A and B)**
- Myelomeningocele **(Figs. 3A and B)**
- Lipomyelomeningocele **(Fig. 4)**—(lipo, fat; myelo, spinal cord; meningocoele, thin ballooning out of the coverings of the spinal cord) are malformations in which a fatty tumor (lipoma) under the skin is fused to the back of the lower spinal cord. The fat may engulf nerve roots or extend deep within the cord making complete removal extremely difficult or impossible. They are usually slow growing but growth rates can vary
- Myeloschisis [myelocele, **(Fig. 5)**]—most severe type of spina bifida resulting into open spinal cord presenting at the surface defect (bare—no coverings) exposed to surroundings as a flattened mass of nervous tissue.
- Rachischisis (complete spina bifida, rachi meaning *spine* and schisis meaning *split*)—There is a severe or complete defect involving the entire spine from the cervical region through to the sacrum.
- Tethered cord syndrome (**Fig. 6**, see below)
- Diastematomyelia (see below)
- *Dermal sinus*—dermal sinus is a tract, lined by skin cells that leads from the skin to anywhere along the back of the spine. The tract may end anywhere to just below the

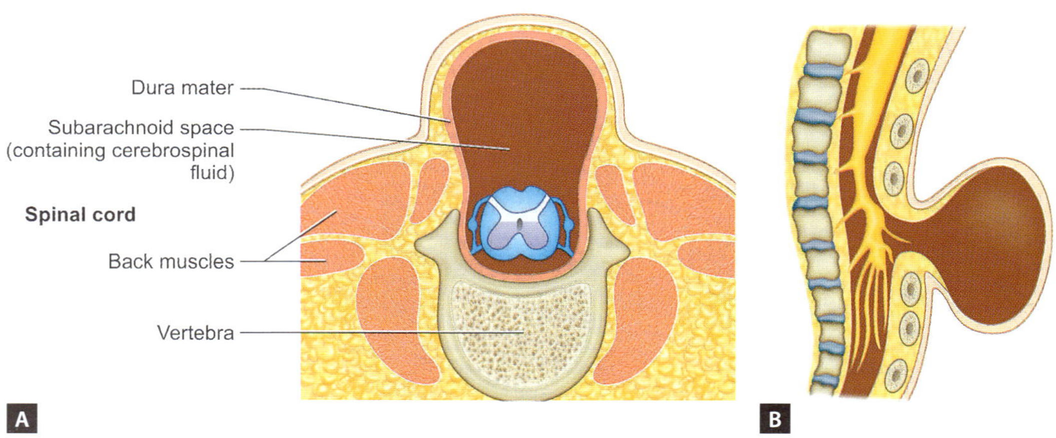

Figs. 2A and B: Meningocele: (A) Axial view; (B) Sagittal view.

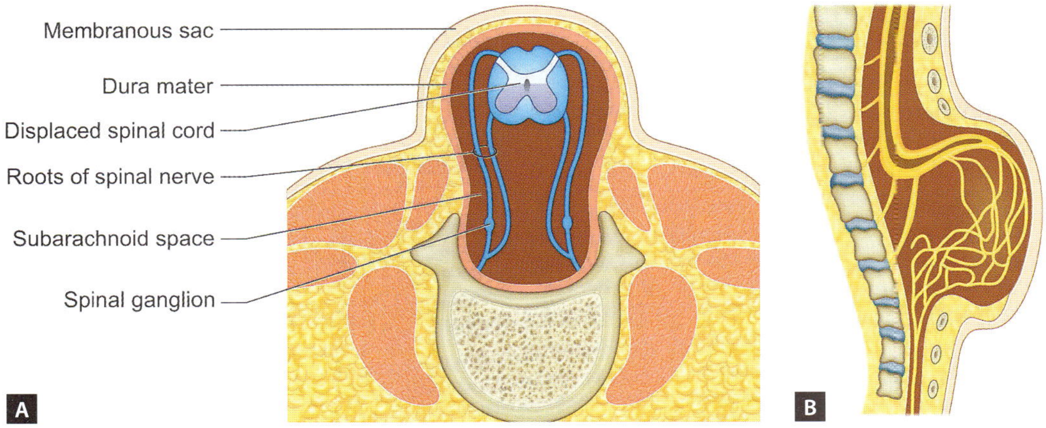

Figs. 3A and B: Meningomyelocele: (A) Axial view; (B) Sagittal view.

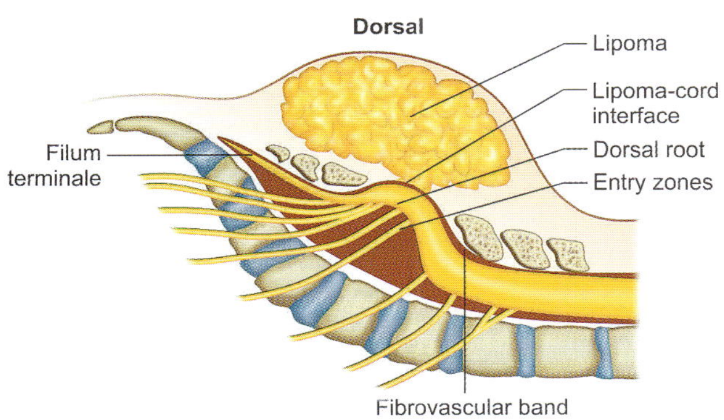

Fig. 4: Lipomyelomeningocele.

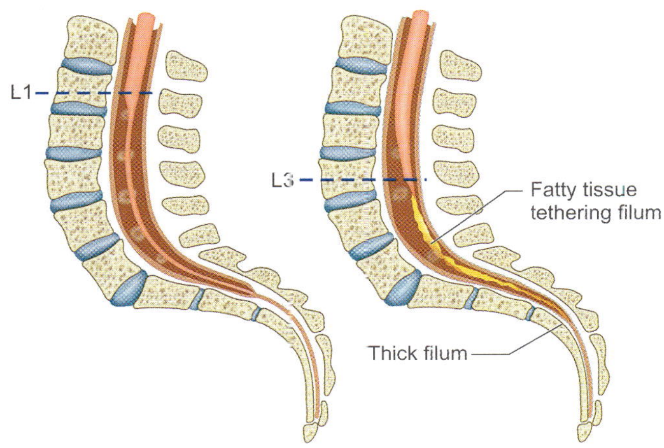

Fig. 6: Tethered cord syndrome.

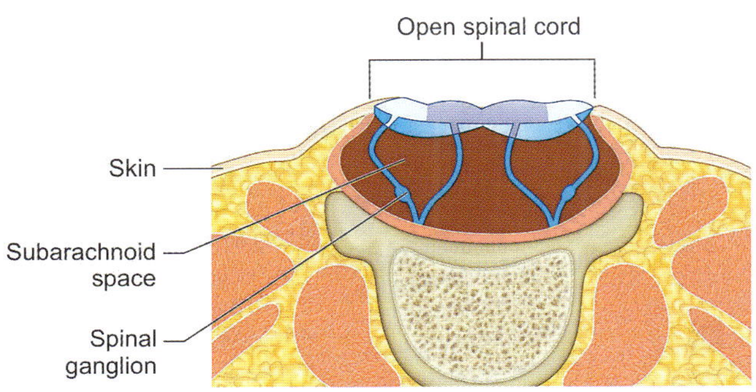

Fig. 5: Myelocele.

skin to the spinal cord. In the latter situation tethering can occur. This connection can be well-developed and lined by skin posing a risk of infection of the nervous system.

- Myelocystocele is a complex malformation of the distal tethered spinal cord in which the end of the spinal cord is ballooned into a cystic and associated with syringomyelia. It is often associated with malformations of the bladder and anus.
- Lipoma of filum terminale

Both overt and occult forms may produce signs and symptoms either at birth or in early childhood. The early signs are usually due to developmental defects of the embryonal spinal cord, whereas the late presentations of dysrhaphic states are due to tethering of the cord, either to the skin or to deeper structures, such as bone, fascia, and dura. Meningomyelocele (MMC), the most frequently encountered form of overt dysraphism, is almost always accompanied by various degrees of limb and sphincters paralysis. The occult forms, however, such as dermal sinus, lipoma of the filum terminale, diastematomyelia, and primary tethered filum, may stay unnoticed for several years before signs evolve.

EPIDEMIOLOGY

Fortunately, the prevalence of spinal dysraphism has been on a decline over the past 2 decades contributed by:

- Better nutrition of women
- Timely folate replacement
- Better antenatal care with high resolution ultrasound resulting in an available option for medical termination of pregnancy (MTP) for defective fetuses
- Liberal assay of maternal serum alpha-fetoprotein (AFP) are all contributing factors.

CLINICAL FEATURES (IN GENERAL FOR SPINAL DYSRAPHISM)

Interestingly, almost all occult forms of dysraphism have dermal signs at birth, such as dimples or sinuses, patches of hair **(Fig. 7)**, pigmentation or angiomata and nevi, almost always along the midline of the back. The signs and symptoms produced by spinal dysraphism have been grouped into orthopedic and neurological manifestations. The common orthopedic manifestations include—scoliosis, kyphosis, club feet or asymmetric feet, atrophy of muscles, increasing back and leg pain and progressive limb and sphincter paralysis.

EMBRYOLOGICAL AND DEVELOPMENTAL ASPECTS

Normal development of cord and meninges: In the earliest stage the embryonic disk is two layers thick formed by:

- The ectoderm on the dorsal aspect **(Figs. 8A to E)**
- The ventral endoderm, these two layers are separated by intervening mesoderm (develops immediately) containing the notochord **(Figs. 8A to E)**.

In a nutshell, the embryological development is as follows—the ectodermal thickening in the mid-dorsal region gives rise to the *neural plate* **(Fig. 8A)**. The margins of neural tube rise above the surface due to differential growth forming *neural folds* ***(Fig. 8B)***. These neural folds fuse **(Fig. 8D)** at the level of future cervical region, proceeding cranially and caudally and start the formation of *neural tube* **(Figs. 8D and E)**. Meanwhile notochord appears between ectoderm and endoderm. This is a midline rod of cells which extends to the level of the future hypophysis.

Mesodermal somites **(Fig. 9)** form on both sides of the tube during the 2nd week of gestation that give rise to sclerotomes (developing from paraxial mesoderm). These sclerotomes later form the centrum of the vertebra. Paired mesenchymal concentrations then start extending dorsally and laterally to later form the vertebral arches. The next stage involves conversion to cartilage, until a cartilage

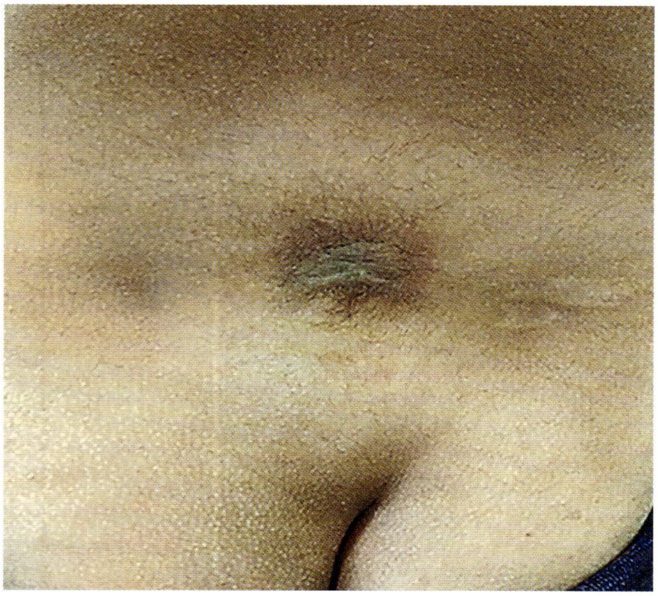

Fig. 7: Hairy patch over lower lumbar spinal region in a child suffering from spina bifida (occulta).

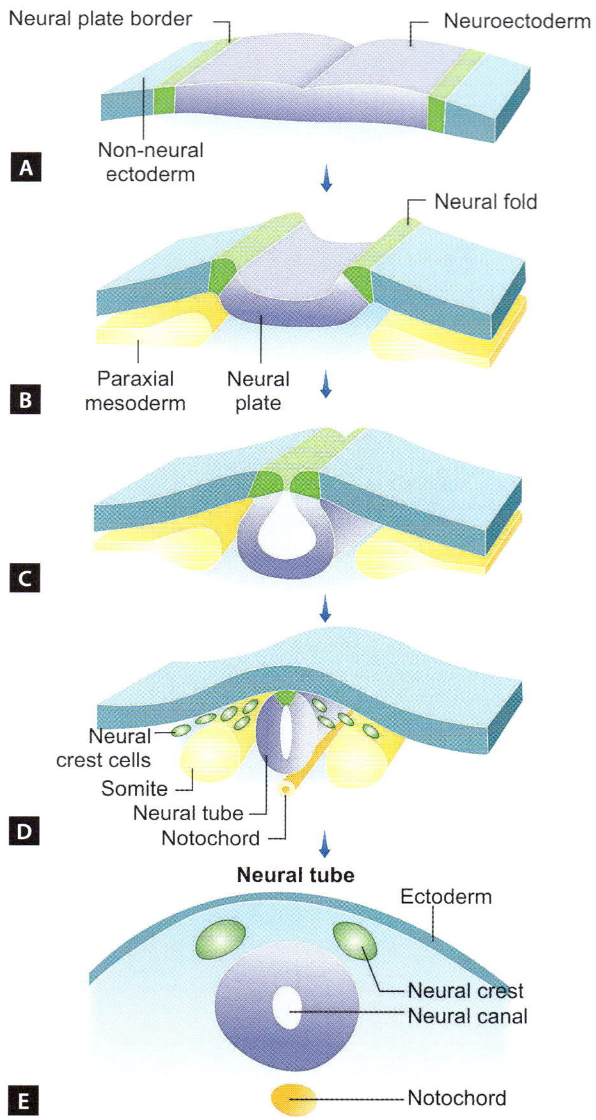

Figs. 8A to E: (A) The embryonic disk and neural plate; (B) The development of neural folds; (C) The formation of neural groove and fusion of folds forming neural crest; (D and E) Formation of neural tube.

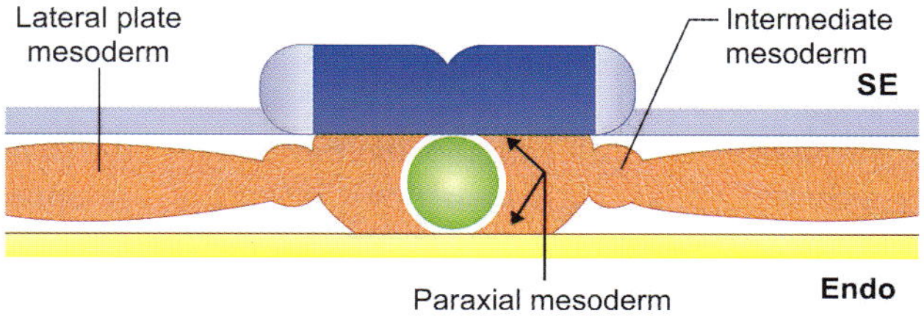

Fig. 9: The formation of mesodermal somites and segregation into paraxial, intermediate, and lateral plate. The paraxial mesoderm begins to migrate around the notochord near the surface ectoderm (SE) and the endoderm (Endo).

miniature of the vertebra is thus formed. This ends at about 60 days of gestation. The cells within the somites also give rise to myotomes and dermatomes forming muscles, bones, cartilage, fat, connective tissue, blood vessels, and the meninges later.

Neuropore **(Figs. 10A and B)** closure is completed by stage 12 around day 28. When caudal neuropore fails to close, open dysraphism occurs (see details below). On the contrary, defective secondary neurulation results in occult dysraphism in which the caudal part of the spinal cord remains connected with the epidermis causing tethering later in life.

The Development of Spinal Cord Proper

It is convenient to divide the development of the cord into three stages:

1. *Neurulation (**Figs. 8 to 10**, neural tube closure and differentiation)*—this is further divided into subphases. During phase I, the neuroectoderm is in contact with the amniotic cavity. Phases II and III refer to complete covering of the neural tube by ectoderm which separates it from the amniotic space. Further growth occurs rapidly and the neural plate (now 1–1.5 mm length) becomes evident during stage VIII at 10 days of gestation, formed by the induction of the notochord. The notochord gives rise to a ventral canal, the neurenteric canal, which connects it to the primitive gut. Stage VIII ends with formation of neural folds when stage IX begins. The tubulation of the plate now beings. Stage X (now 2–3.5 mm length at 22–25 gestational days) is marked by beginning of fusion of the neural folds that start first from the level of the third and fourth somites. The fusion first proceeds caudally down to the 12th somite and simultaneously, it also progresses rostrally toward the developing forebrain. *Once fusion is* initiated, the open ends of the neural tube form the cranial and caudal neuropores that still communicate with the overlying amniotic cavity. At the end of stage XI (now 4.5 mm length at 25–28 days of gestation) the tube is rostrally completely closed (18–20 somite stage, *closure of the cranial neuropore—a bit complex process)* at a region later known as the lamina terminalis. The newly formed central canal is now in continuity with the amniotic cavity only through the caudal neuropore, which finally closes during stage XII (4.5 mm length, 28–30 days), 2 days after cranial neuropore closure. The closure level is about L1–L2 segments. This completes the neurulation and there is no longer a connection between central canal and amniotic fluid. The wall of a recently closed neural tube consists of only one cell type, the "neuroepithelial cells", which extend over the entire thickness of the wall and form a thick pseudostratified epithelium. Once the tube is closed, the neuroepithelial cells give rise to the "primitive nerve cells or neuroblasts". The neuroblasts form a zone that surrounds the neuroepithelial layer, called the mantle layer (the future gray matter of the spinal cord). The outermost layer of the cord contains the nerve fibers emerging from the neuroblasts in the mantle layer—the "marginal layer". As a result of myelination of the nerve fibers, the marginal layer takes on a "white" appearance and is called the white matter of the cord.
2. *Canalization:* Now that the tube is completely covered with ectoderm it lacks the lower lumbar (L2 and beyond), sacral and coccygeal segments. These segments are formed by aggregation of vacuoles, which enlarge and contact the central canal at the lowest portion of the closed tube finally fusing with latter **(Fig. 11)**. This is the process of canalization. This begins at stage XIII and finishes by stage XX (4.5–20 mm, 29–50 days) whence accessory lumens are sometime seen in a dorsoventral or lateral plane, surrounded by neural cells during the canalization. Most of these disappear during the last phase of cord development (retrogressive differentiation). Simultaneously, filum terminale is formed at stage XIII (30 mm length, 52 days) as a result of caudal neural tube atrophy. Ependymal rests are found within it and the filum is divided into a rostral intradural part and a caudal part fused with the anterior leaf of the dura.
3. *Retrogressive differentiation:* This starts at stage XX and continues until sometime after birth. The central

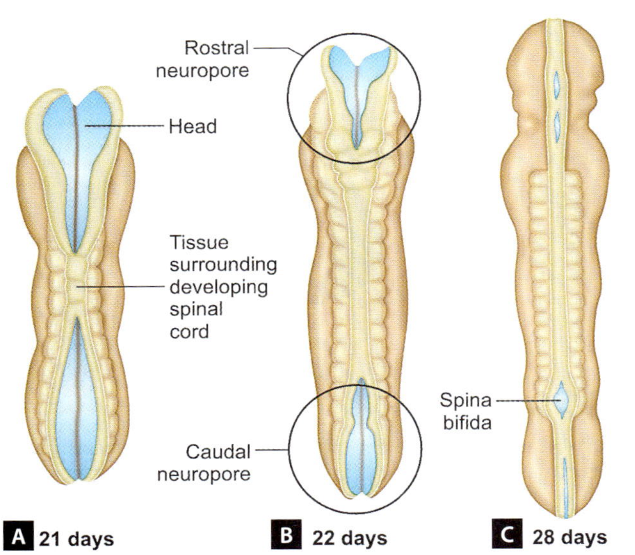

Figs. 10A to C: (A) The formation of neuropores at each end of the neural tube that starts fusing in center and (B) progresses rostrally and caudally. In the end pores are left at the rostral and caudal end. The pores ultimately close and any failure leads to spinal dysraphism and spina bifida (C).

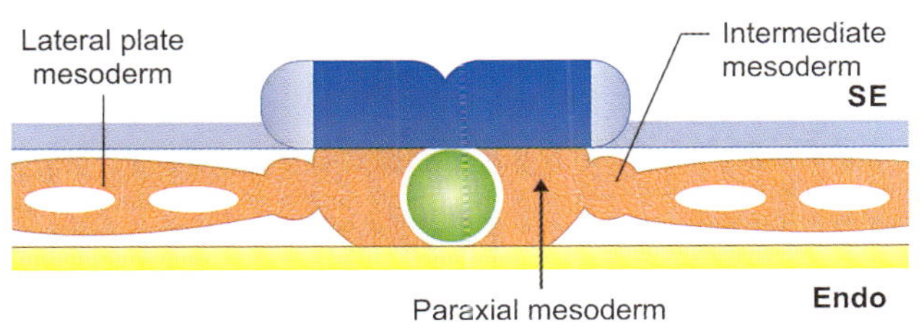

Fig. 11: Vesicles form within lateral plate mesoderm and then coalesce. (SE: surface ectoderm; Endo: endoderm)

canal progressively narrows in size (except for a small dilatation at the conus level—the ventriculus terminalis). The stage is marked by migration of the lower part of the tube rostrally/cranially. The specific landmarks of tube migration are as follows:
- Reaches level of the second coccygeal vertebra by stage XXIII (30 mm length, 52 days)
- Reaches second sacral vertebra at 67 mm length (73 days)
- Reaches fifth lumbar vertebra at 111 mm length (100 days)
- Reaches second lumbar vertebra at 221 mm (4th month of gestation)

The Meninges

The dura (pachymeninges) and leptomeninges (pia and arachnoid) are derived from the primitive mesoderm—from the meninx primitiva (it is a matter of controversy though). In the thoracic and caudal regions, these are derived from paraxial mesoderm while in the skull anterior to diencephalon they are derived from neural crest cells.

- The piamater is visible by day 24 of embryonic development while the duramater is evident by day 41. The ventricular fluid first escapes through the roof of the fourth ventricle at 29 days of gestation, and dissects the mesenchymal layer surrounding the neural tube forming the subarachnoid space, first of the cisterna magna, then progressively around the brainstem to the base of the cerebrum and into the spinal canal. The final separation of arachnoid from dura occurs at about 6 month of gestation.

The Vertebrae and Vertebral Column

- The vertebrae and annulus fibrosus of the intervertebral disks are derived from sclerotomal somitic mesoderm a derivative of paraxial mesoderm **(Figs. 12 to 14)**. The nucleus pulposus of the intervertebral disk is derived from the notochord.
- With the condensation of the myotomes and the sclerotomes, bone, cartilage, fat, connective tissue, blood vessels, and meninges form and surround the neural tube. The vertebral laminae are developed and fused by the 11th week of gestation **(Figs. 15 to 17)**.
- During the 2nd and 3rd months of embryonic life, the spinal cord and spinal canal are of equal length. As development continues, there is an upward shift of the cord due to unequal growth rate of bone and spinal cord. The conus at birth lies next to L2–L3 and by 6th month of age it lies at the final level of T12–L1.
- The filum terminale is 20 cm long and <2 mm thick. Its proximal 5 mm contain the central canal and neural

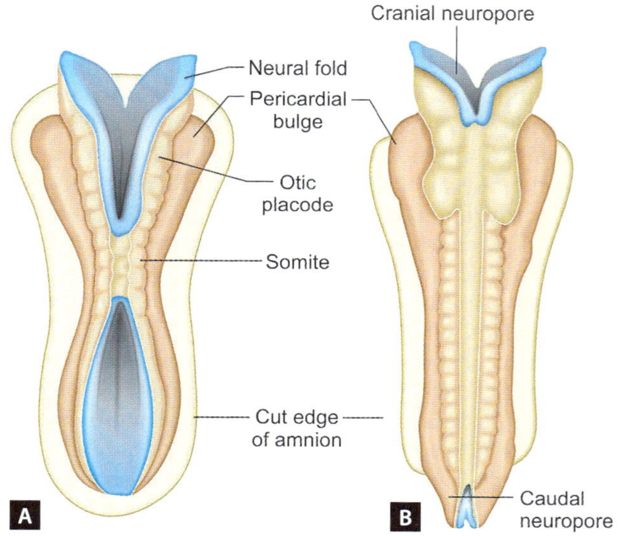

Figs. 13A and B: The paraxial mesoderm separates into blocks of tissue, called somites. There are 44 pairs of somites adjacent to the notochord.

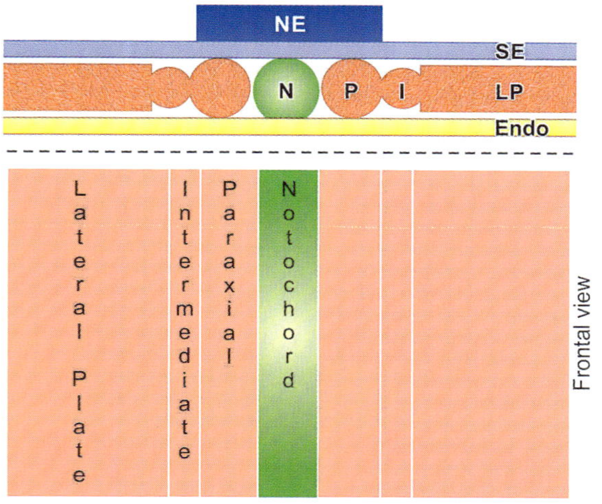

Fig. 12: The mesoderm segregates into three solid rods of cells paralleling the notochord. (Endo: endoderm; I: intermediate mesoderm; LP: lateral plate mesoderm; N: notochord; NE: neural ectoderm; SE: surface ectoderm; P: paraxial mesoderm)

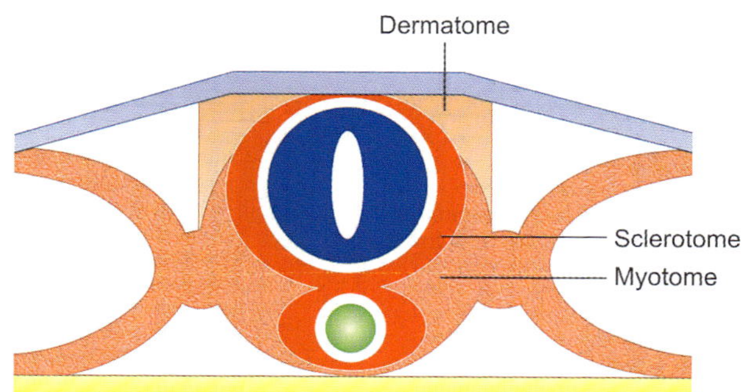

Fig. 14: Each somite divides into three regions: (1) Dermatome; (2) Sclerotome; and (3) Myotome. Sclerotomal somitic mesoderm will form the bone (vertebrae), cartilage, tendons, ligaments, annulus fibrosus of the intervertebral disk, fibrous connective tissues, and meninges of the axial skeleton. The dermatomal somitic mesoderm will form the dermis portion of the skin overlying the vertebral column (from tip of transverse process to tip of transverse process). The myotomal somitic mesoderm will form the deep back and neck muscles associated with the vertebral column. These particular skeletal muscles are innervated by the dorsal rami portion of a mixed spinal nerve.

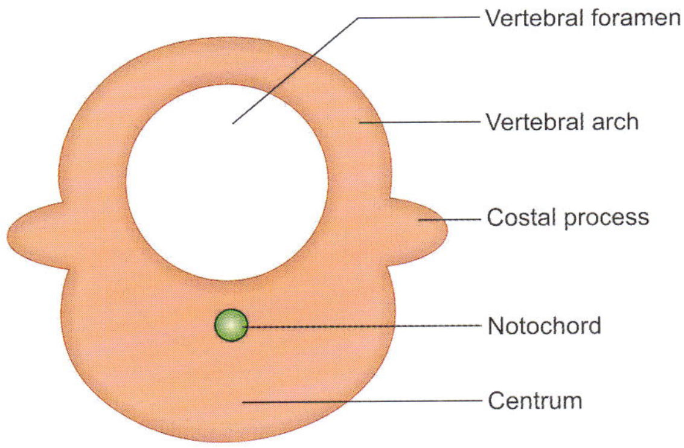

Fig. 15: The sclerotomal somitic mesoderm of the vertebrae surrounding the neural tube forms the vertebral (neural) arch that is eventually composed of the pedicles, lamina, transverse process, and spinous process.

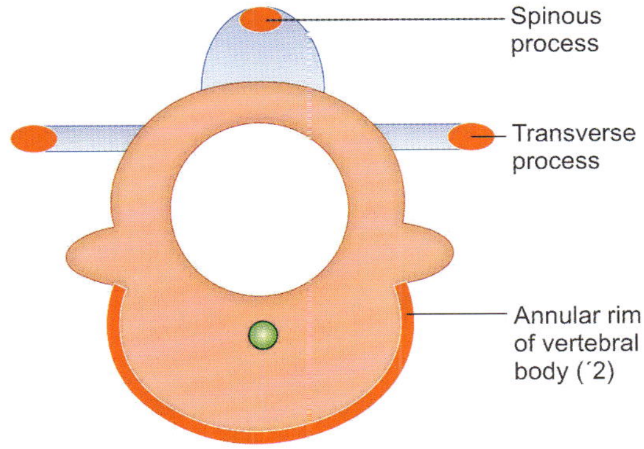

Fig. 17: Five secondary centers of ossification appear in the vertebrae after puberty: one at the tip of the spinous process, one at each tip of the transverse process, and two annular epiphyses, one on the superior and one on the inferior rim of the vertebral body.

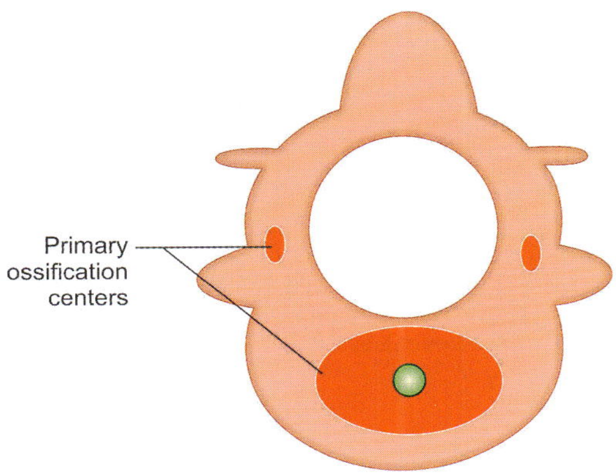

Fig. 16: Three primary ossification centers are present by the end of the embryonic period: one in the centrum and one in each half of the vertebral arch.

tissue. The rest consists of connective tissue. The upper 15 cm is within the dural sac, the rest is outside and is attached to the dorsal aspect of the first coccygeal segment. This fibrous band elongates by interstitial growth to adapt itself to the lengthening spinal column.

ANOMALIES OF DEVELOPMENT

Spina bifida is a "general term" for neural tube defects (NTD) affecting the spinal region. It consists of a splitting of the vertebral arches and may or may not involve underlying neural tissue. Two different types of spina bifida **(Figs. 18A to E)** are commonly described:

1. Spina bifida occulta (Virchow, 1875) is a defect in the vertebral arches that is covered by skin and usually does not involve underlying neural tissue. This defect in the vertebral arch is the result of the failure of the embryonic halves of the neural arch to grow together and fuse in the midline. It occurs in the lumbosacral region (L4–S1) and is usually marked by a patch of hair overlying the affected region. The L5–S1 spina bifida may also occur in 10% of otherwise normal persons.
2. Spina bifida cystica (aperta) is a severe NTD in which neural tissue and/or meninges protrude through a defect in the vertebral arches and skin to form a "cyst-like sac". The term "cystica" denotes the cyst-like sac that is associated with these anomalies. It includes meningocele, MMC, myeloschisis (myelocele), etc.

As mentioned that spina bifida is a general term, it is difficult to discuss individual pathologies by using this as a base term. We will instead describe the NTDs based on embryological pathogenesis. The difference can be appreciated from the fact that meningocele is included in spina bifida cystica but embryologically, it comes under defects of canalization and not defects of neurulation which encompasses MMC.

MALFORMATIONS OF NEURULATION

Meningomyelocele (Fig. 3)

Definition: Hernial protrusion of the spinal cord and its meninges through a defect in the vertebral arch as a cyst **(Fig. 3)**.

Development of MMC: In general, if there is a defect in embryological cord development during the first phase (neurulation, stage VIII–XII) then the nervous tissue will be found externally. MMC develops no later than stage XII (3–5 mm length, 25–29 days of gestation). MMC can appear.

- As a flat open lesion (myelocele, **Fig. 5**) with leaking CSF, or
- As a bulging membranous sac, MMC, in which there is an enlarged subarachnoid space ventral and dorsal to the plate, filled with CSF. The center of the lesion is called zona medullovasculosa, and the remainder periphery is referred to as zona epithelioisa. This thin layer, if allowed, will gradually cover the skin defect and will cause tethering of the cord to the skin.

Theories of Faulty Neurulation

There are three possible theories postulated for development of MMC:

- Nonclosure of the developing neural tube—dysraphia can arise from a neural tube that never closed properly or that had apparently not even begun the folding process;

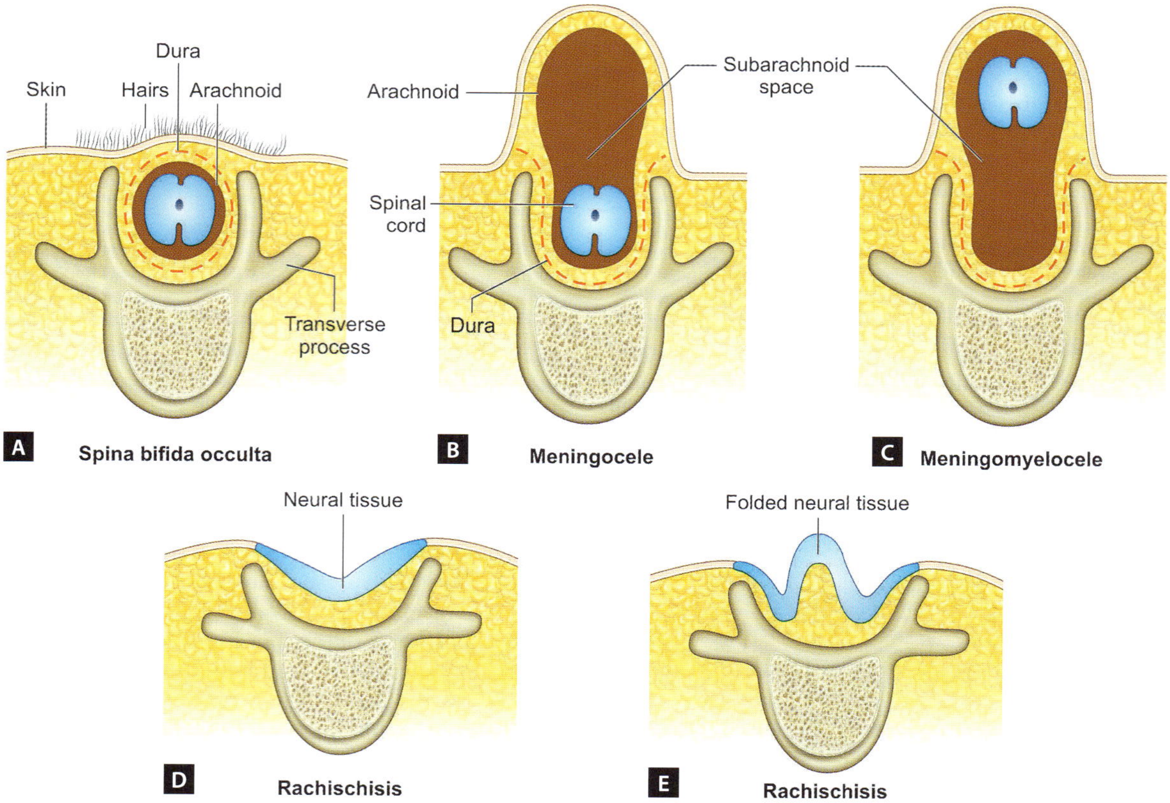

Figs. 18A to E: Various types of spina bifida.

in early stage embryos, this will result in unfused neural tubes that still contain portions of primitive neural plate. The first to suggest this etiology was Von Recklinghausen in 1886. The proposed mechanism for his theory was a sudden arrest of development in a normal neural tube, due to some external "noxious influence". Later, Patten (1953) suggested that the abnormal closure is not just the cessation of neural development, but the result of abnormal proliferation in the neural plate at the site of the lesion (Overgrowth Theory).

- Rupture of a previously closed well-developed neural tube (normal closure followed by reopening). This theory was popularized by Gardner (1960) and by Padget (1970). The basis to this theory is that an abnormality in the roof of the fourth ventricle prevents normal rupture of the roof causing distention of the primitive central canal (hydromyelia). Four stages of hydromyelia may develop:
  1. Transient overdistention resulting in normal central canal but enlarged bony canal and possible spina bifida. Syringomyelia may appear in adult life.
  2. Dorsoventral splitting the cord producing two hemicords (diastematomyelia)
  3. Internal hydromyelia becomes external and the expanding subarachnoid space bulges beneath the cutaneous ectoderm—meningocele.
  4. Forcible rupture of the tube and of the cutaneous ectoderm producing MMC. CSF escapes through the spinal opening.
- ***Induction theory:*** It is still not clear whether the primary defect is in the ectoderm or in the mesoderm but as is evident that all forms of dysraphic state involve not only the cord (ectoderm) but also the surrounding dura bone, muscle, fat, and connective tissue (mesoderm) as well as the skin, so it is postulated that pathogenesis could embrace the mutually inductive influence of the three germ layers on each other. This theory was first suggested by Lichtenstein (1940) and induced experimentally in chicken embryos by a dorsal midline incision of the caudal spine. However, this fails to explain conditions in which the neural tube is intact and the dura, bone, and dermal tissues have not developed.

Whatever the pathogenesis, the defect of closing or rupture of the tube most commonly occurs at either end of the tube and gives rise to the anencephaly (rostral region) or MMC (caudal region). In both conditions, nervous tissue is directly exposed to the outside of the body. All cases with MMC also have the Arnold–Chiari malformation (ACM), and about 85% will also develop hydrocephalus, usually within 1 week following closure of the spinal defect. Hydrocephaly is common in MMC (and also myelocele-spina bifida cystica) because the spinal cord is tethered to the vertebral column. As the vertebral column lengthens, tethering pulls the cerebellum into the foramen magnum, cutting off the flow of CSF. The MMC may be associated with various disorders/ syndromes **(Box 1)**.

Suggested etiological factors for development of MMC:

- *Drugs:*
    - Teratogenic agents
    - Hyperthermia
    - Valproic acid
    - Trypan blue (animals)
    - Cytochalasin B (animals)
    - Vitamin A
    - Salicylates
- Potato consumption! Renwich (1972) suggested a connection between potato consumption and neural tube defects due to teratogenic effect of a fungus affecting the potatoes (not got popular as the null hypothesis got easily rejected—many MMC babies were born to mothers who never ate any potatoes!)
- Environmental etiological factor—suspected due to variation of MMC with time, place, social class, parity, maternal age, and ethnic group.
- Genetic factors though intriguing but have been highly questioned by the finding of twins born in which only one was affected.

Investigations

Early detection is possible by maternal blood or amniotic fluid AFP levels. Three-dimensional (3D) ultrasound can identify spinal cord anomalies well. The diagnosis is clear at birth and MRI may be done to reveal or study other malformations/associations **(Figs. 19A to C)**.

BOX 1: The associations of meningomyelocele (MMC).

The myelomeningocele is associated with various syndromes/conditions like:
- Trisomy 18
- Trisomy 13
- Arnold–Chiari malformation
- Diastematomyelia
- Syringomyelia
- Arachnoid cysts
- Tethered cord syndrome

Treatment

The treatment of MMC has historically passed through interesting phases:

- John Holter, the engineer father to his son born with spina bifida, developed the first effective differential pressure valve to control hydrocephalus. This was perceived as the ultimate answer to the problems of the child with spina bifida.
- In the 1960s, surgeons around the world treated the birth of an infant with spina bifida as an emergency. Open neural tissue was immediately surgically covered and ventriculoatrial shunts were installed to control hydrocephalus. The early mortality rate decreased rapidly, almost reversing the previous 90% mortality to a survival rate of 80% but soon a number of problems previously not anticipated such as incontinence, paraplegia, and scoliosis, shunt malfunction, infection, and mental retardation overwhelmed the medical team.
- To prevent deaths from renal failure, the technique of clean intermittent catheterization (CIC) almost eliminated renal loss.
- Reigel's technique for repair of the open myelomeningocele offers an anatomically correct repair with the hope that it may also reduce the possibility of retethering of the spinal cord, still if retethering does occur the untethering procedure is made much easier after this repair.

Prevention

It has been proved beyond doubt that folic acid supplementation reduces the risk of MMC by 50–70% when instituted early (within around 4th week or so) of gestation.

Arnold–Chiari Malformation

It is the result of abnormal development of the cerebellum and brainstem but affects the spinal cord also. The main feature of ACM is elongation of the cerebellar vermis into

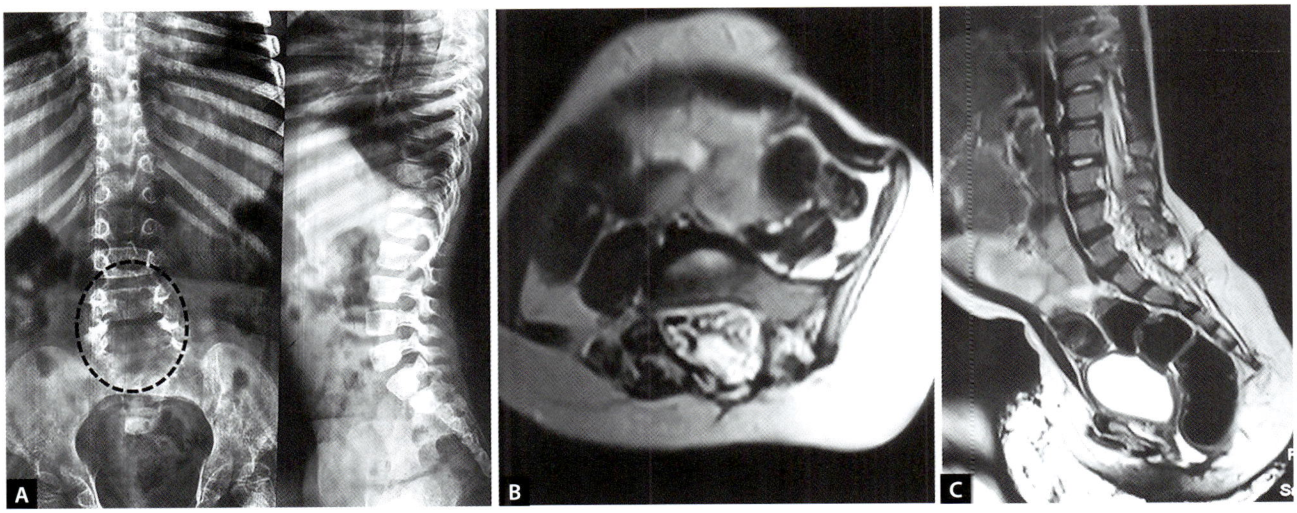

Figs. 19A to C: The radiographs (AP and lateral projections, A) of a patient with myelomeningocele showing spina bifida as unfused spinous processes peculiarly prominent in lower lumbar region (encircled). The MRI scan reveals lipomeningocele with fibrous components (B) in lumbosacral region with spina bifida with low lying cord (C) and vertebral anomalies.

the spinal canal via the foramen magnum. The tonsils may reach as low as even thoracic spine. The medulla is dorsally kinked, and there may exist other malformations such as aqueductal stenosis, subependymal heterotopias, beaked collicular plate, and syringobulbia and syringomyelia.

Pathogenesis

- ***Traction theory:*** The spinal cord is tethered to the skin and dura at the MMC site and cannot ascend by the process of retrogressive differentiation. With development, additional traction is put on the cord pulling the cerebellum and medulla into the spinal canal. This theory is supported by the finding of cervical spinal roots that run an upward oblique course.
- Other hypotheses attribute ACM to maldevelopment of the cerebellum and medulla as a primary fault in the developing tube, and not as the result of tethering.
- The relatively omnipresent association of ACM with MMC has been also explained by Cameron, 1957 who proposed that the CSF that escapes through the open distal neuropore into the amniotic sac produces amniotic fluid pressure that is greater than the intracranial pressure thus squeezing its contents caudally.

The malformation is indeed a multifocal abnormality involving the telencephalon (subependymal heterotopias), the diencephalon (enlarged massa intermedia), the mesencephalon (aqueduct stenosis and forking), the rhombencephalon (elogated herniated brainstem), spinal cord (MMC), and even the mesoderm (digital impression of skull, hypoplastic tentorium, and small posterior fossa).

MALFORMATION DURING THE SECOND PHASE (CANALIZATION, STAGES XIII-XX) AND THE THIRD PHASE (RETROGRESSIVE DIFFERENTIATION, STAGES XX THEREAFTER)

These malformations are covered by intact skin (occult dysraphism). They differ from defects of neurulation in that none is associated with the ACM and that the distal neuropore is closed and the neural tube is formed.

Spinal Lipomas

Spinal cord lipoma is the most common entity of occult dysraphism. The caudal cell mass seems to have multipotent characteristics (primitive cells). The developing lipoma interferes with normal development of the bony structures of the canal at that area permitting abnormal connections between subcutaneous and intradural fat.

Spinal lipomas may be classified into three groups:

1. *Dorsal:* Lipomas associated with abnormal development of the spine (lipomyelomeningocele, lipomas of cauda, and conus).
2. *Terminal:* Lipomas of the fIlum terminale.
3. *Transitional:* Intraspinal (intramedullary) lipomas.

Only the first two forms are accompanied by vertebral and dural as well as cutaneous abnormalities. Cutaneous manifestation of intradural lipoma with an obvious fatty lump is noted in more than 70% of cases. Other cutaneous stigmata include capillary hemangioma, dermal dimple, bifurcating or eccentric intergluteal cleft, skin tags, and hairy patch on the midline at the lumbosacral level **(Fig. 20)**.

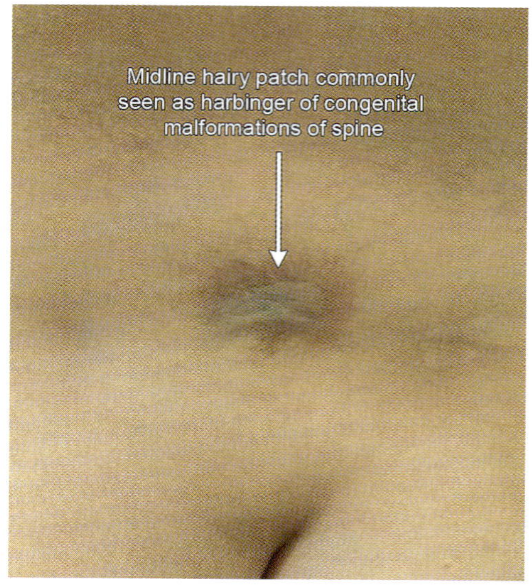

Fig. 20: The cutaneous manifestation as midline hairy patch in spinal malformations.

The third type of lipomas (transitional) is not considered dysraphic states (considered more to be hamartoma). Unfortunately because of the extensive involvement, motor deficit is more common in these patients. Loss of motor neurons results in smaller calves and/or buttocks. If passed unnoticed, abnormal gait as the child starts to walk and run would alert parents of the problem.

Meningocele

The development of the dura begins ventral and lateral to the neural tube in stage XIX. The caudal part of the tube remains very close to the skin until the vertebral lamina fuses in the early fetal period (stage XXIII and on, 30 mm length, 53 days of gestation). Meningocele occurs at that stage.

Myelocystocele

This is a cystic dilatation of the central canal associated with meningocele and covered by skin. It is often associated with malformations of the bladder and intestinal tract. It may be explained by Gardner's theory, which is based on an abnormal rhombic roof preventing the CSF from escaping from the central canal into the forming subarachnoid space. The fluid thus vents into the terminal ventricle after cannalization occurs. The terminal ventricle dilates, bulges into, and then disrupts the dorsal mesenchyme, but not the superficial ectoderm. The large cyst tethers the cord.

Diastematomyelia

[(Diastema = cleft; myelos = cord), diastomyelia, split spinal cord]

Diastematomyelia is a form of spinal dysraphism characterized by partial or complete clefting of one or more

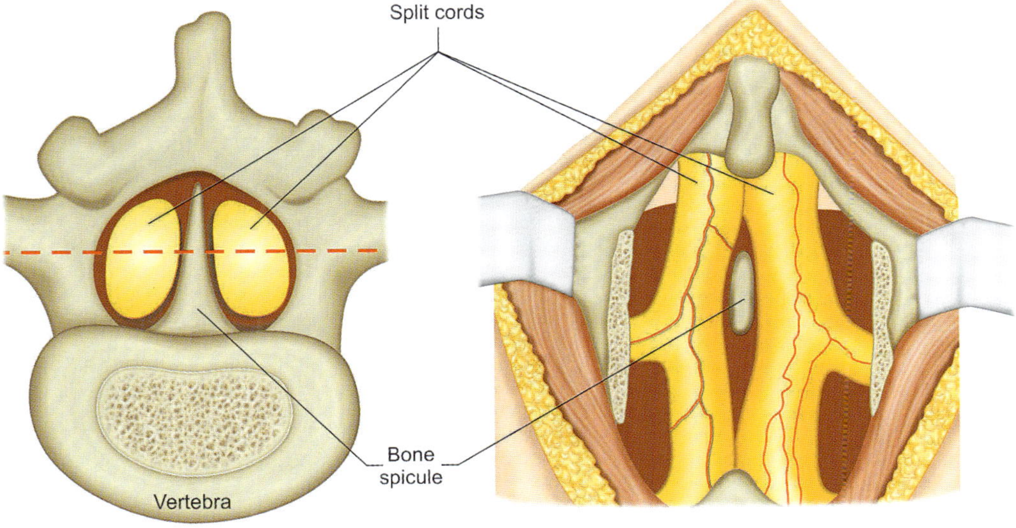

Fig. 21: Illustration of diastematomyelia.

segments of the spinal cord, conus medullaris and/or filum terminale. The abnormality most commonly occurs between the T9 and S1 vertebral bodies (85% cases) and is rare within the cervical region. Thoracic lesions account for one-fifth of the cases while thiracolumbar clefts occur in around 15% cases, the majority are in the lumbar region (approximately 62%). It is more common in women than men (1.6:1). It is believed to be the result of a failure of midline integration of the newly formed notocordal cells leading to the formation of two hemicords. The bifid cord is not by itself necessarily the cause of symptoms; they are produced by the septum or other associated lesion.

Pathoanatomy

In diastematomyelia, there may or may not be a septum passing dorsoventrally between the two halves of the spinal cord. If present, the midline ecto-endomesenchymal tract goes on to develop into fibrous, cartilaginous or osseous septum that tethers the cord **(Fig. 21)**. The sagittal cleft produces two variably asymmetric/symmetric cords each of which contains one central canal, one dorsal horn that gives rise to ipsilateral segmental dorsal root and one ventral root that gives rise to ipsilateral segmental ventral root. Very rarely one hemicord may give rise to three roots while the other to only one. Mostly the cleft is complete and only is it partial dorsal or ventral one—partial dorsal diastematomyelia or partial ventral diastematomyelia, respectively. The cleft is usually only focal (91%) in the sense that the cord reunites below the cleft of variable length. If the cord extends too far distally then bifid filum or bifid conus may be observed that may also be associated with bifid filum terminale. The split cords are nearly equal in size in 70% cases. The nerve roots that should have decussated in the region of the cleft may persist as commissural bands that bridge the intermedullary space. The hemicord usually have their own anterior spinal arteries supplying them.

Pathogenesis

- ***Persistence of the neurenteric canal:*** It connects the embryonic gut or yolk sac with dorsal surface of the embryo and the amniotic cavity (Bremer, 1952). The persisting canal contains endodermal, ectodermal, and mesodermal cell rests which are capable of giving rise to a variety of vertebral anomalies, including a split cord by a bony spur or a cartilaginous one.
- ***Mechanical pathogenesis [Gardner (1960)]:*** Hydrocephalomyelia causes increase in intracanal pressure and separates roof plate. As the roof plate is thinner than the floor plate it separates more readily. Dilatation of the neural tube then displaces the developing somites producing spina bifida, hemivertebrae, widening of the canal or fused vertebrae.
- ***Tsou et al. (1980) suggested two possibilities:***
  1. *Enterogenous fistula* which leads to neuroectoderm adhesions without a bony spur.
  2. *Sequestration of notochordal cells in the neural plate.* These cell nests remain loosely connected by a pedicle to the rest of the notochord somehow (supported by finding that the spur is always attached anteriorly to the centrum disk unit).

Classification

Initial classification systems were based on the arrangement of pia and dural tubes along the hemicords dividing it into two types:

1. In type 1 diastematomyelia there is duplication of arachnoid and dural tubes that individually surround each hemicord. While there is no bony spur, these patients can have fibrous septa associated with the split cord (50%). The dural and arachnoid sacs merge proximally and distally below the cleft. Patients with this type of abnormality are usually asymptomatic.
2. The type 2 deformity is characterized by an extradural bony spur that produces two separate dural sacs with two

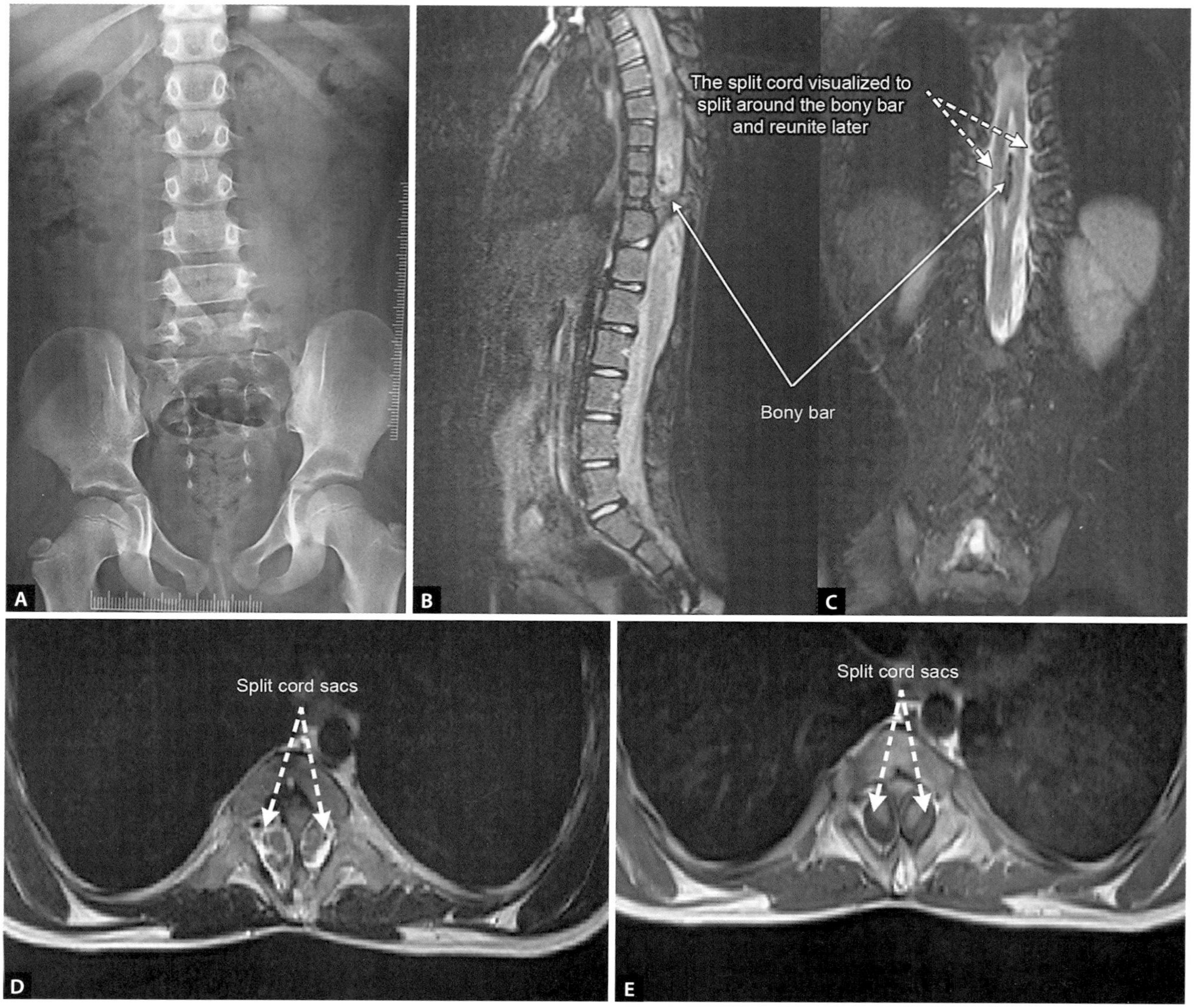

Figs. 22A to E: The radiographs of a patient who presented with recent onset lower limb weakness (<3 months) and gait disturbance. The radiographs (A) revealed spina bifida, while MRI obtained for high suspicion of tethered cord revealed bony bar (arrows) splitting the cord at dorsal 10–11 levels (B and C). The cord can be seen split into two sacs completely separated by the bony spur (dotted arrows). The two sacs (dotted arrows) can be seen on the T2-weighted (D) and T1-weighted (E) axial MR images separated by the central bony bar.

arachnoid sacs for each separate hemicord **(Figs. 22A to E)**. Both the hemicords are surrounded coaxially by single arachnoid and single dural tubes but they individually have their independent piamater. These patients nearly always have a fibrous or osteocartilaginous partition. The partition extends sagittally between vertebral body and lamina as a synchrondrosis. This is the type that usually produces symptoms.

Improvised classification has been proposed based on embryological development. Currently, the conditions with split cords are classified into one of two split spinal cord malformations (SSCM).

1. *Type 1 SSCM* consists of abnormalities that occur when two hemicords are separated by an extradural bony spur, resulting in two spinal canals and two dural sacs. The condition arises due to persistence of precursor mesangial cells in the accessory neurenteric canal (ANC). The mesangial cells make the medial parts of the hemicords and dural sac while the lateral sac develops and the ANC forms the bony spurs.
2. *Type 2 SSCM* arises when ANC is devoid of mesangial cells. On this condition it regresses but sometimes leaves behind a fibrous spur in the dura. Previously, this was termed diplomyelia. Now, diplomyelia is defined as a type 2 SSCM. Here anatomically, there is one dural sac with two hemicords and one spinal canal. There may be a fibrous band in-between the cords or sometimes just a fatty tissue.

Associations

Diastematomyelia has been associated significantly with other NTDs and malformation of spine, important of which are:

- Scoliosis
- Visceral malformations
- Myelomeningoceles

- Lipomas
- Chiari malformations
- Tethered spinal cords
- Hypertrichosis
- Syringomyelia

Investigations

- Spine radiographs are the initial modality of investigations. It must be remembered that diastematomyelia is more of a clinical suspicion that needs radiological confirmation rather than other way around. Radiographs are too insensitive to diagnose this serious condition. They may show widening of the spinal canal, a bony ridge at midline, scoliosis, and other vertebral anomalies.
- CT or MRI is frequently used to confirm or rule out the diagnosis. CT scans can show a bony septum and separation of the cord. MRI shows the cord separation and dural sacs in greater detail but may not be as beneficial as CT for the bony abnormalities.
- Prenatal or neonatal diagnosis can be made by ultrasound that demonstrates split cord as well as the echogenic formation of a bony spur.

Treatment

Asymptomatic patients with diastematomyelia do not require treatment. However, if the patient has symptoms related to the abnormality, they can be treated surgically. Treatment in these patients includes surgery to remove bony spur and reconstruct the dura around the two separated cords.

TETHERED CORD SYNDROME

"Tethered spinal cord" (thick filum terminale, primary tethered cord) was first coined by Hoffman in 1976 to refer a low-lying conus medullaris with a thickened (>2 mm diameter) filum. It may also include fibrolipomatous infiltration **(Fig. 6)** and, rarely, abnormal extension of the central canal. The cord reaches up to lower lumbar and the sacral vertebrae. Though generally associated with a low-lying conus (the "classic" type), tethered cord syndrome (TCS) is also seen in a normally positioned conus (dorsal or ventral tethering of the cord).

Pathogenesis

The mechanism of development of TCS is obscure.

Tethering of cord is theoretically possible at two points—one at the site where an extrinsic lesion such as a dermal sinus tract traverses through the dura and another at the caudal attachment of the conus to a taut or fatty filum. Either or both tethers **(Fig. 23)** may be present in any given case and they need to be individually addressed. Filum terminale normally anchors the conus to the sacral bony vertebral canal and suspends the entire lower cord in the buoyant CSF. A taut (short fibrous) or a thick (fat infiltrated) filum is inelastic and results in tension on the conus.

Not only the filum abnormalities but the cord movement may also be limited by anomalous fixity to a dorsal [e.g., lumbosacral lipoma, dermal sinus tracts **(Fig. 23)**, congenital inclusion tumors like dermoids and epidermoids] or ventral structure (e.g., bony diastem and neurenteric cyst).

There is a high likelihood of reduced blood supply to stretched cord due to diminished microcirculation producing ischemia, hypoxia, and impaired oxidative metabolism at cellular level. Traction injury probably results due to an altered growth rate between the spinal cord and column, combined with traction forces implied by contraction of the tissue within the abnormal filum. The process of tethering is more dynamic than this. Mechanisms additionally suggested that may finally culminate into tethering include:

- Hemorrhage and inflammation in the developing caudal cord in early fetal life
- Non-neoplastic growth of fat in the fatty filum
- Lumbosacral cord lipomata
- Progressive accumulation of putty material in congenital inclusion tumors and ensuing chemical meningitis
- Exogenous infection tracking along a dermal sinus tract

These or mostly a combination of these results in evolution of fibrous intradural bands which tether the cord. This is not the Holy Grail of pathogenesis, however, as none explains the ectatic dural sac, the bifid vertebrae and the associated cutaneous and subcutaneous lesions. TCS is associated with various disorders enlisted in **Box 2**.

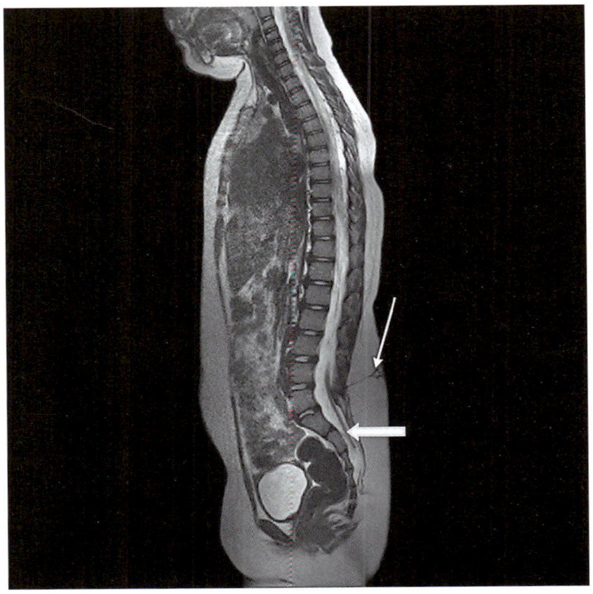

Fig. 23: The tethered cord syndrome. In this patient, the spinal cord was low-lying and ended behind S2 due to dural tethering from dorsal sinus tract (arrow) and thick filum (block arrow). Unfortunately, the same patient also had diastematomyelia at a higher level (not visualized here).

BOX 2: The various disorders associated with tethered cord syndrome.

- Spina bifida occulta/aperta
- Vertebral abnormalities like scoliosis
- Limb deformities
- Caudal regression
- Tail-fold anomalies
- Anorectal malformations
- Split cord malformations and diastematomyelia
- Dermal sinus tracts
- Congenital inclusion tumors complex

Clinical Features

The functional deficits in TCS may result from traction, compression or a combination of these. The lower motor neuron (LMN) symptoms are considered to be an effect of mechanical compression while the upper motor neuron (UMN) symptoms apparently result from ischemia and traction injury. The large fibers of the tracts cranial to the site of tethering are the most susceptible to injury.

Neurological Deficits

Often a patchy, asymmetric combination of UMN (spasticity and hyperreflexia) and LMN (atrophy, hyporeflexia) symptoms referable to the conus and the lumbosacral nerves occurs. Motor deficits are more evident than sensory aberrations.

Orthopedic Manifestations

Trophic ulcers (painless) and deformities (foot deformities most commonly pes cavus, limb length discrepancies, scoliosis, gluteal asymmetry, and gait disturbances).

Urological Abnormalities

Frequency, urgency, incontinence, and urinary infections.

Cutaneous stigmata are often multiple and they occur in 50–70% of all. These neurocutaneous markers can be classified into:

- *High-risk category*—atypical midline lumbosacral dimples (larger than 5 mm, located >25 mm cranial to the anal verge, directed cranially), hemangiomas, protruding lesions (masses, hairy patch, and tails) and multiple cutaneous stigmata. These require further investigations to evaluate underlying TCS or occult spinal dysraphism.
- *Low-risk category* markers include coccygeal pits, simple dimples, discolorations, and deviated gluteal fold.

Investigations

Plain radiographs—these are too insensitive to detect spinal cord malformations to merit any use. Occasional L5-S1 bifid spine or scoliosis may even be a normal finding Ultrasonography is a useful investigation but quite operator dependent:

- Pulsations are reduced in tethered cord.
- Level of conus can be easily documented.
- Detailed images of meninges and cord can be documented along within the filum terminale till 4–5 months of gestation after which the acoustic window is dampened and details not very prominent.

MRI—modality of choice for anatomical detailing.

- Sagittal T1- and T2-weighted images demonstrate the level of the conus.
- T1-weighted axial images illustrate the fat in the terminal filum and facilitate measuring its diameter.
- Voiding cystourethrogram and urodynamic studies—the earliest features of subclinical neurovesical dysfunction are detrusor hyperreflexia and detrusor sphincter dyssynergia resulting in vesicoureteral reflux.

Treatment

Operative treatment is preferred in many and is essential in symptomatic patients. Only in asymptomatic patients the views of surgeons regarding surgical release of tether is controversial. The aim of surgical management is restoring the normal mobility of spinal cord by eliminating the tethering structures and resuspending the freed conus and spinal nerves in the CSF. The following are some of the commonly performed surgical procedures:

- Sectioning of the filum reverses clinical and urodynamic deficits in a subset of the symptomatic tight or fatty filum terminale.
- Laminectomy and detethering of the cord
- Excision/debulking of cord lipoma/dermoid or epidermoid
- Excision of the bony/fibrous diastem

CONCLUSION

- Spinal dysraphism is an unfortunate complication of developmental anomaly of the spinal cord and central structures, often producing significant morbidity.
- Developmental arrest at various levels would produce discrete anomalies and need specific management. The severe forms that involve developmental arrest in initial stages have poor prognosis.
- Treatment often needs specialized and dedicated care to commission independency in patient.

CHAPTER 101

Spinal Cord Injury

Manish Kumar Varshney

INTRODUCTION

The term "spinal cord injury" (SCI) denotes any lesions to the spinal cord, conus medullaris, or cauda equina. The injury has predominantly two components where primary injury is the direct result of inciting event while secondary injury occurs by vascular perfusion abnormalities, edema, free radical generation, lipid peroxidation, excitotoxicity, inflammation, and cell death. In SCI, there is deranged motor, sensory, or autonomic function in the cord. This could be temporary or permanent, complete, or incomplete. Management should encompass all these lesions and deficits to optimize outcome.

ETIOLOGY

The injury may result from traumatic or nontraumatic causes:

The following are the chief causes of traumatic SCI:

- Trauma due to fall
- Trauma due to road traffic accidents (this is overall the most common cause of SCI)
- Occupational injuries (construction and agriculture and mining)
- Sports injuries
- Violence

The following are the chief causes of nontraumatic SCI:

- Infection (tuberculosis in India is the most common cause)
- Tumor
- Musculoskeletal disease such as osteoarthritis (compressive myelopathy)
- Vertebral subluxations in rheumatoid arthritis
- Congenital problems such as spina bifida, diastematomyelia
- Nutritional deficiencies—vitamin B_{12} deficiency and thiamine deficiency
- Iatrogenic—complication of medical care
- Multiple sclerosis (MS)
- Amyotrophic lateral sclerosis
- Vascular insults/diseases
- Transverse myelitis

EPIDEMIOLOGY

The global estimate of the incidence of SCI is approximately 40–80 new cases per million population per year covering all causes. This gives a rough figure of approximately 250,000–500,000 population that suffer from SCI from all causes.

Anatomical considerations: The vertebral column encloses the spinal cord **(Fig. 1)**; it extends from the foramen magnum as a continuation of the medulla to the level of the first or second lumbar vertebrae. Its end part is the "conus medullaris". The spinal cord is a vital link between the brain and the body. The cord is 40–50 cm long and the diameter varies from 1 to 1.5 cm, being more at the cervical and lumbar levels. The spinal cord terminates into the "cauda equina" (or "horse's tail"). Spinal cord is divided into neurological segments corresponding to the nerve roots exiting the spinal column. These spinal roots are numbered 8 cervical, 12 thoracic, 5 lumbar, 5 sacral, and 1 coccygeal, totaling 31. The neurological level of the cord is not the same as the vertebral segment as the length of the cord and the vertebral column differs.

MECHANISMS OF INJURY

Various mechanisms, often in combination, produce SCI. Most frequently, the injury results from indirect forces produced by movement of the head and trunk. Some areas of the spine are more vulnerable to injury due to mobility and lack of stability.

Pathophysiology of Spinal Cord Injury

There are both primary and secondary mechanisms of injury that may affect the final outcome of SCI. The best prognostic indicator is the patient's neurologic grade at presentation (primary injury, **Flowchart 1**), there are a further majority of patients that deteriorate or fail to respond to optimal treatment given due to secondary injury mechanisms. Both will, hence, be discussed below:

Primary Injury

The central gray matter sustains most damage by the initial trauma and the white matter is relatively spared possibly due

ASIA — INTERNATIONAL STANDARDS FOR NEUROLOGICAL CLASSIFICATION OF SPINAL CORD INJURY (ISNCSCI) — ISCOS

Patient Name ______ Date/Time of Exam ______

Examiner Name ______ Signature ______

RIGHT

MOTOR — KEY MUSCLES | SENSORY — KEY SENSORY POINTS: Light Touch (LTR), Pin Prick (PPR)

C2
C3
C4

UER (Upper Extremity Right)

Elbow flexors C5
Wrist extensors C6
Elbow extensors C7
Finger flexors C8
Finger abductors (little finger) T1

Comments *(Non-key Muscle? Reason for NT? Pain?)*:

T2
T3
T4
T5
T6
T7
T8
T9
T10
T11
T12
L1

LER (Lower Extremity Right)

Hip flexors L2
Knee extensors L3
Ankle dorsiflexors L4
Long toe extensors L5
Ankle plantar flexors S1

S2
S3
S4-5

(VAC) Voluntary anal contraction *(Yes/No)*

RIGHT TOTALS (MAXIMUM) (50) (56) (56)

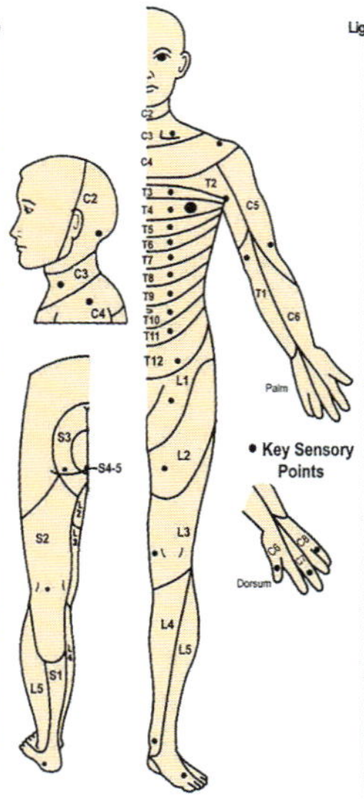

LEFT

SENSORY — KEY SENSORY POINTS: Light Touch (LTL), Pin Prick (PPL) | MOTOR — KEY MUSCLES

C2
C3
C4

C5 *Elbow flexors*
C6 *Wrist extensors*
C7 *Elbow extensors*
C8 *Finger flexors*
T1 *Finger abductors (little finger)*

UEL (Upper Extremity Left)

T2
T3
T4
T5
T6
T7
T8
T9
T10
T11
T12
L1

MOTOR *(SCORING ON REVERSE SIDE)*

0 = total paralysis
1 = palpable or visible contraction
2 = active movement, gravity eliminated
3 = active movement, against gravity
4 = active movement, against some resistance
5 = active movement, against full resistance
5 = normal corrected for pain/disuse*
NT = not testable

SENSORY *(SCORING ON REVERSE SIDE)*

0 = absent *2 = normal*
1= altered *NT = not testable*

L2 *Hip flexors*
L3 *Knee extensors*
L4 *Ankle dorsiflexors*
L5 *Long toe extensors*
S1 *Ankle plantar flexors*

LEL (Lower Extremity Left)

S2
S3
S4-5

(DAP) Deep anal pressure *(Yes/No)*

LEFT TOTALS (MAXIMUM) (56) (56) (50)

MOTOR SUBSCORES

UER ___ + UEL ___ = *UEMS TOTAL* ___ ; *MAX (25)* (25) (50)

LER ___ + LEL ___ = *LEMS TOTAL* ___ ; *MAX (25)* (25) (50)

SENSORY SUBSCORES

LTR ___ + LTL ___ = *LT TOTAL* ___ ; *MAX (56)* (56) (112)

PPR ___ + PPL ___ = *PP TOTAL* ___ ; *MAX (56)* (56) (112)

NEUROLOGICAL LEVELS — *Steps 1-5 for classification as on reverse*

1. SENSORY R ___ L ___
2. MOTOR R ___ L ___

3. NEUROLOGICAL LEVEL OF INJURY (NLI) ___

4. COMPLETE OR INCOMPLETE? ___ — *Incomplete = Any sensory or motor function in S4-5*

5. ASIA IMPAIRMENT SCALE (AIS) ___

(In complete injuries only) *ZONE OF PARTIAL PRESERVATION* — *Most caudal level with any innervation*: SENSORY R ___ L ___; MOTOR R ___ L ___

 REV 02/13

Muscle Function Grading

0 = total paralysis

1 = palpable or visible contraction

2 = active movement, full range of motion (ROM) with gravity eliminated

3 = active movement, full ROM against gravity

4 = active movement, full ROM against gravity and moderate resistance in a muscle specific position

5 = (normal) active movement, full ROM against gravity and full resistance in a functional muscle position expected from an otherwise unimpaired person

5* = (normal) active movement, full ROM against gravity and sufficient resistance to be considered normal if identified inhibiting factors (i.e. pain, disuse) were not present

NT = not testable (i.e. due to immobilization, severe pain such that the patient cannot be graded, amputation of limb, or contracture of > 50% of the normal range of motion)

Sensory Grading

0 = Absent

1 = Altered, either decreased/impaired sensation or hypersensitivity

2 = Normal

NT = Not testable

Non Key Muscle Functions (optional)

May be used to assign a motor level to differentiate AIS B vs. C

Movement	Root level
Shoulder: Flexion, extension, abduction, adduction, internal and external rotation **Elbow:** Supination	C5
Elbow: Pronation **Wrist:** Flexion	C6
Finger: Flexion at proximal joint, extension. **Thumb:** Flexion, extension and abduction in plane of thumb	C7
Finger: Flexion at MCP joint **Thumb:** Opposition, adduction and abduction perpendicular to palm	C8
Finger: Abduction of the index finger	T1
Hip: Adduction	L2
Hip: External rotation	L3
Hip: Extension, abduction, internal rotation **Knee:** Flexion **Ankle:** Inversion and eversion **Toe:** MP and IP extension	L4
Hallux and Toe: DIP and PIP flexion and abduction	L5
Hallux: Adduction	S1

ASIA Impairment Scale (AIS)

A = Complete. No sensory or motor function is preserved in the sacral segments S4-5.

B = Sensory Incomplete. Sensory but not motor function is preserved below the neurological level and includes the sacral segments S4-5 (light touch or pin prick at S4-5 or deep anal pressure) AND no motor function is preserved more than three levels below the motor level on either side of the body.

C = Motor Incomplete. Motor function is preserved below the neurological level**, and more than half of key muscle functions below the neurological level of injury (NLI) have a muscle grade less than 3 (Grades 0-2).

D = Motor Incomplete. Motor function is preserved below the neurological level**, and at least half (half or more) of key muscle functions below the NLI have a muscle grade ≥ 3.

E = Normal. If sensation and motor function as tested with the ISNCSCI are graded as normal in all segments, and the patient had prior deficits, then the AIS grade is E. Someone without an initial SCI does not receive an AIS grade.

** For an individual to receive a grade of C or D, i.e. motor incomplete status, they must have either (1) voluntary anal sphincter contraction or (2) sacral sensory sparing with sparing of motor function more than three levels below the motor level for that side of the body. The International Standards at this time allows even non-key muscle function more than 3 levels below the motor level to be used in determining motor incomplete status (AIS B versus C).

NOTE: When assessing the extent of motor sparing below the level for distinguishing between AIS B and C, the ***motor level*** on each side is used; whereas to differentiate between AIS C and D (based on proportion of key muscle functions with strength grade 3 or greater) the ***neurological level of injury*** is used.

ASIA — AMERICAN SPINAL INJURY ASSOCIATION

INTERNATIONAL STANDARDS FOR NEUROLOGICAL CLASSIFICATION OF SPINAL CORD INJURY

ISCOS — INTERNATIONAL SPINAL CORD SOCIETY

Steps in Classification

The following order is recommended for determining the classification of individuals with SCI.

1. Determine sensory levels for right and left sides.
The sensory level is the most caudal, intact dermatome for both pin prick and light touch sensation.

2. Determine motor levels for right and left sides.
Defined by the lowest key muscle function that has a grade of at least 3 (on supine testing), providing the key muscle functions represented by segments above that level are judged to be intact (graded as a 5).
Note: in regions where there is no myotome to test, the motor level is presumed to be the same as the sensory level, if testable motor function above that level is also normal.

3. Determine the neurological level of injury (NLI)
This refers to the most caudal segment of the cord with intact sensation and antigravity (3 or more) muscle function strength, provided that there is normal (intact) sensory and motor function rostrally respectively.
The NLI is the most cephalad of the sensory and motor levels determined in steps 1 and 2.

4. Determine whether the injury is Complete or Incomplete.
(i.e. absence or presence of sacral sparing)
*If voluntary anal contraction = **No** AND all S4-5 sensory scores = **0** AND deep anal pressure = **No**, then injury is **Complete**.*
*Otherwise, injury is **Incomplete**.*

5. Determine ASIA Impairment Scale (AIS) Grade:

Is injury Complete? **If YES, AIS=A** and can record ZPP (lowest dermatome or myotome on each side with some preservation)

NO ↓

Is injury Motor Complete? **If YES, AIS=B**

NO ↓ (No=voluntary anal contraction OR motor function more than three levels below the motor level on a given side, if the patient has sensory incomplete classification)

Are at least half (half or more) of the key muscles below the neurological level of injury graded 3 or better?

NO ↓ **AIS=C** | YES ↓ **AIS=D**

If sensation and motor function is normal in all segments, AIS=E
Note: AIS E is used in follow-up testing when an individual with a documented SCI has recovered normal function. If at initial testing no deficits are found, the individual is neurologically intact; the ASIA Impairment Scale does not apply.

Fig. 1: ASIA worksheet.

Flowchart 1: The mechanisms underlying spinal cord injury.

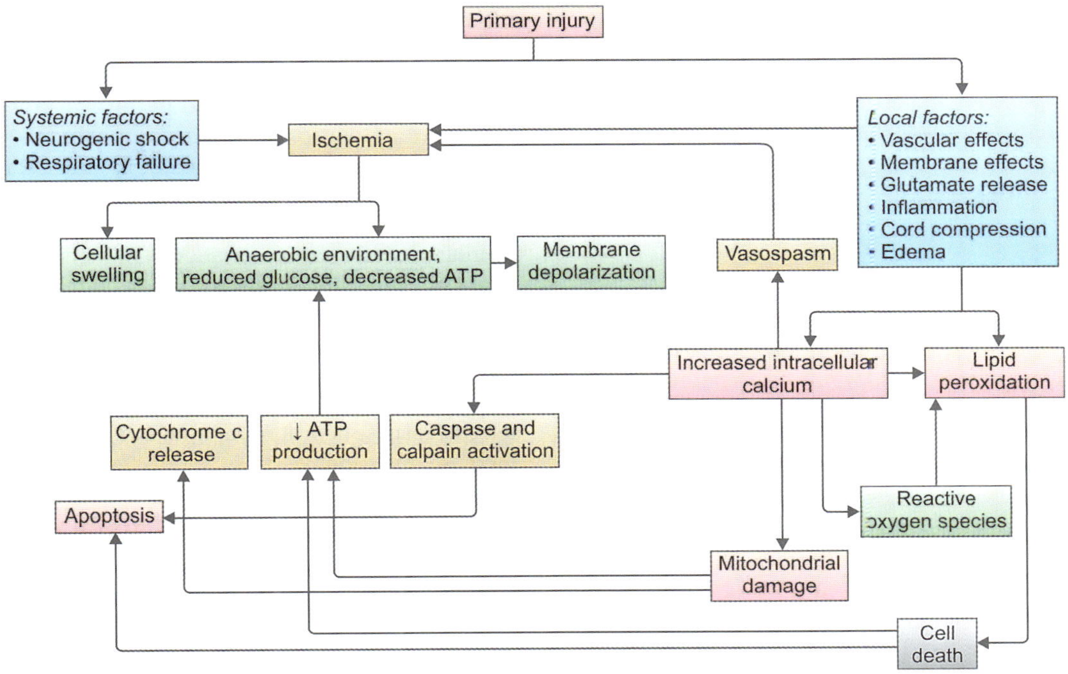

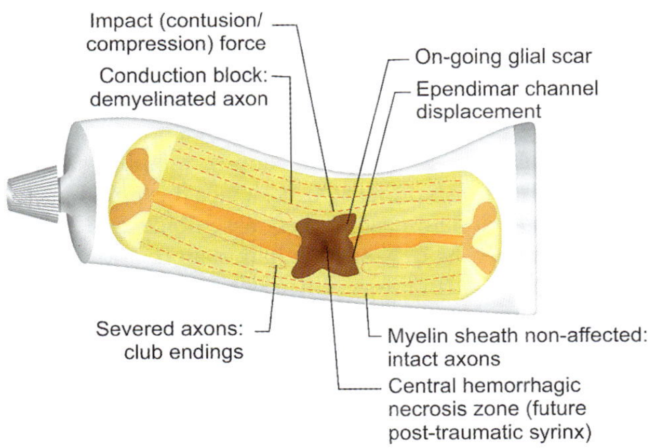

Fig. 2: The toothpaste theory to explain the mechanical morphometric early damages in spinal cord (primary injury).

to the softness of former. These primary mechanisms cause blood flow disruption and hemorrhages within the cord. This leads to hypoxia and ischemia. A central hemorrhagic area of necrosis marks the "epicenter" injury. This is surrounded by surviving axons in a centrifugal distribution. This centrifugal pattern of loss occurs due to longitudinal displacement of the cord's central content. The toothpaste theory **(Fig. 2)** explains these events that are similar to those occurring in a compressed toothpaste tube.

The main five features of the primary injury are:

1. *Pinching or contact pressure:* The former is due to pressure on the cord from opposite side (hematoma, neoplasia, etc.) while latter is the pressure transmitted from same side (prolapsed disk, infolded ligaments, and osteophytes). In cervical spinal injuries, there may be persistent pinching, such as from bilateral facet interlocking or temporary pinching such as from hyperextension sprains.
2. Impact plus persistent compression (e.g., burst fractures with retropulsed bone fragment)
3. Impact alone with transient compression (hyperextension injury in patients with degenerative spine)
4. *Distraction:* The shearing and forcible stretching of spinal cord is a component of various SCI mechanisms. Possibly this is the common mode of injury in SCI without radiographic abnormalities (SCIWORA) in adults with degenerative spine and in children with cartilaginous vertebrae.
5. *Laceration/transection:* This results often from missile injury, sharp bone fragment dislocation, or severe distraction. The injury may be complete or incomplete as described above.

Axonal tear is caused in the cord when tissue velocity exceeds 0.5–1 ms^{-1}. As the central part of the cord is the place where stretch velocities are maximum, it becomes the most common site for tears due to stretch and shearing forces. Most of the neural stretch injuries are seen at nodes of Ranvier.

Secondary Mechanisms of Injury

These build upon the primary mechanisms at the primary injury sites as a focus of injury. The secondary mechanisms are either the continuations of primary injury (continued compression) or more or less the reactions of body to primary injury and in time though meant for recovery, prove to be deleterious. The disturbances ultimately lead to neuronal necrosis, apoptosis, scarring and cyst formation, demyelination, and disruption of the morphofunctional nerve pathways (see below in rehabilitation). The most common secondary mechanism is persistence of compression from primary injury. The other causes of secondary injury are neurogenic shock, reperfusion injury after hemorrhage and ischemia, secondary injury mediated by intracellular calcium release, fluid electrolyte imbalance, immunologic injury, and injury due to apoptosis and disturbed mitochondrial function and excitotoxicity. These will be discussed below one by one.

Neurogenic Shock

This comprise of a triad of:

- Hypotension
- Bradycardia
- *Hypothermia:*
  - More commonly seen in injuries above T6.
  - Primarily there is disruption of sympathetic outflow from T_1–L_2 that causes loss of vasomotor tone, and hence pooling of blood.
  - Loss of cardiac sympathetic tone causes bradycardia, increased vagal tone also contributes.
  - Vasopressors are indicated for management along with atropine used to treat bradycardia.
  - Blood pressure (BP) will not be restored by fluid infusion alone and massive fluid administration may lead to overload and pulmonary edema.

Vascular Insult and Oxidative Overload (Flowcharts 1 and 2)

These produce both hemorrhagic and ischemic damage. Microcirculation and small venules and capillaries are an increased risk while the large vessels like anterior spinal artery are relatively preserved. There is a progressive post-traumatic ischemia in the locus of injury that also gradually spreads peripherally. The mechanism includes:

- Vasospasm
- Intravascular thrombosis
- Autoregulatory homeostatic mechanisms that actually cause more injury than repair
- Systemic hypoperfusion—causing ischemia
- Gross increase in BP—hemorrhages

There is an interlude of reactive hyperemia with increased perfusion resulting from reduced perivascular pH caused by excess of acidic metabolites (lactate). This is thought to be made even more deleterious by generation of free radicals and superoxide, hydroxyl, nitric oxide, and peroxynitrite (high-efficiency oxidant) molecules. These free radicals are produced by multiple mechanisms and pathways such as calcium-mediated activation of phospholipases, the Fenton and Haber–Weiss reactions, nitric oxide synthases, inflammatory cells, and xanthine oxidase. The highly reactive oxygen and nitrogen species cause oxidative stress and damage the critical cellular processes by inactivation of mitochondrial respiratory chain enzymes, inactivation of glyceraldehyde-3-phosphate dehydrogenase, inhibition of Na^+-K^+ adenosine triphosphatase (ATPase), inactivation of sodium membrane channels, and further advance the damage by activation of lipid peroxidation pathway. Calcium overload, mitochondrial cytochrome-c release, caspase activation, apoptosis, and excitotoxicity further increase the oxidative stress.

Spinal Cord Injury (*see* Flowchart 1)

Tumor necrosis factor-alpha (TNF-α) and interleukin-6 (IL-6) are strongly upregulated after SCI, the former potentiates glutamate mediate neuronal cell death while the latter is responsible for astrocyte proliferation and scar formation. IL-1α and IL-18 mediate inflammation and amplify a wide variety of effects associated with innate immunity. NALP1 inflammasome, part of nod-like receptor (NLR) superfamily consisting of NALP1, adipose-derived stem cell (ASC), caspase-1, and caspase-11, has also been implicated in the pathogenesis of secondary SCI. They form a protein assembly with the inhibitor of apoptosis family member, X-linked inhibitor of apoptosis protein (XIAP). Once this protein (XIAP) is cleaved, the inflammasome gets assembled and leads to rapid secondary SCI. Neuron-inflammation and transient paralysis are caused by the myelin basic protein (MBP)-reactive T-cells. In SCI, their levels reach similar to those seen in MS.

Excitotoxicity

Olney introduced the term "excitotoxicity" to describe processes which result from excessive activation of glutamate receptors [N-methyl-D-aspartate (NMDA) and α-amino-3-

Flowchart 2: The influence of local factors on cell death

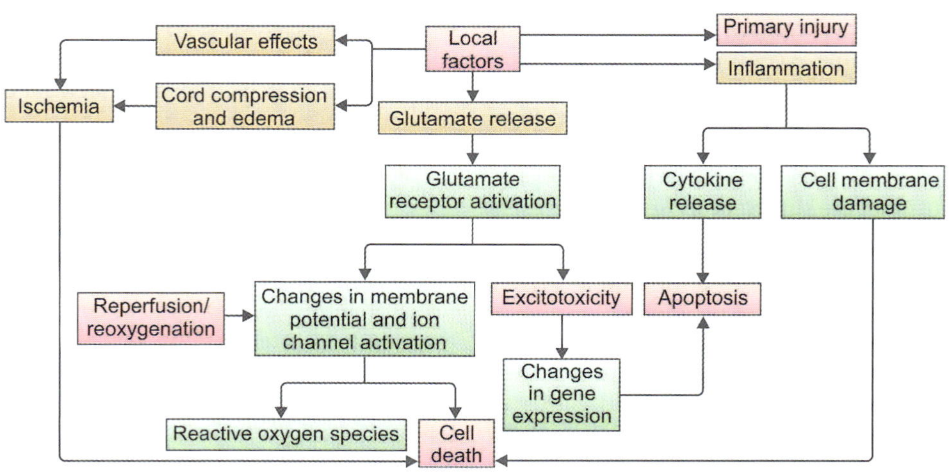

hydroxy-5-methylisoxazole-4-propionate-kainate (AMPA-kainate] leading to neuronal injury **(Flowchart 2)**. There are two mechanisms that get activated from the release and activation of excitatory neurotransmitters (especially glutamate) and produce further cytotoxicity.

- *Increased intracellular concentration of sodium ions:* Glutamate receptor activation causes increased sodium ion accumulation → cytotoxic edema and intracellular acidosis → inactivation of Na^+-K^+ ATPase → reduces sodium efflux → further edema → cell death.
- *Increased intracellular concentration of calcium ions:* Increased intracellular sodium → increases intracellular calcium by activation of Na^+-Ca^{2+} exchanger → increased intracellular calcium.

Increased intracellular calcium is the final common pathway for cell death. NMDA further induces cytotoxicity by inactivation of membrane sodium channels and glyceraldehyde-3-phosphate dehydrogenase, by causing inhibition of Na^+-K^+ ATPase activity and mitochondrial respiratory chain enzymes and by initiation of lipid peroxidation. Magnesium blocks the NMDA receptors, and has a protective role on neuronal cells. Magnesium depletion causes accumulation of intracellular calcium which contributes to the pathophysiologic changes. The third protective mechanism of magnesium is possibly by the modulation of binding of endogenous opioids that may cause alteration in the resulting aberrations.

Calcium-mediated Cytotoxicity

As mentioned increased intracellular calcium heralds cell death. The final blow comes from activation of various calcium-dependent mechanisms that kill cell ultimately as follows:

- *Interference with mitochondrial function:* "The cell stops breathing".
- *Stimulates calcium-dependent proteases and lipases:*
  - Calpains get activated in the glial and inflammatory cells present in the penumbra of SCI lesions. They cause damage by degrading the structural proteins of the axon-myelin unit.
  - *Phospholipase A2, lipoxygenase, and cyclooxygenase:* Increased generation of arachidonic acid metabolites such as thromboxanes, prostaglandins, and leukotrienes that reduce blood flow by causing platelet aggregation and vasoconstriction.
  - Calcium-dependent proteases and kinases get activated by the increased intercellular calcium and they destroy cell membranes and critical components of the cell ultrastructure such as neurofilament, this destruction leads to more lipid peroxidation **(Flowchart 3)** and free radical formation and then more cell death and dissolution. This self-feeding vicious cycle continues and can be stopped only by endogenous antioxidants such as α-tocopherol and superoxide dismutase.

Immunological Mechanisms

Immunologic activation inhibits neural regeneration and promotes progressive tissue injury after injury to the central

Flowchart 3: Lipid peroxidation and the inhibitory effects of steroids and lazaroids on it.

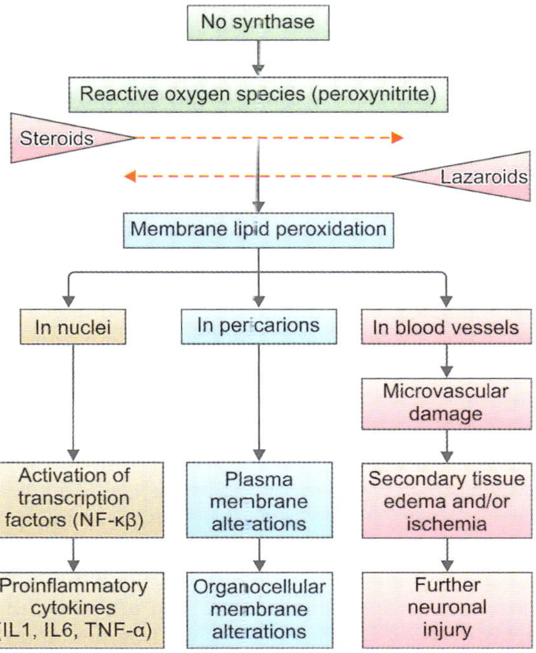

nervous system (CNS). Microglia, the primary CNS immune cells, is similar to peripheral macrophages. They phagocytose dead cells and play an important role in neural regeneration. They also have important function in demyelination, neuronal death and contribute to oligodendrocyte lysis using a process that involves TNF-α and nitric oxide production. The demyelination process of axons begins within 24 hours of injury and leaves a discernible area of cavitation visible in the gray and white matter. After trauma, process of Wallerian degeneration starts and scarring takes place. This scarring is a function of fibroblasts, astrocytes, and other glial cells. Various messengers and processes involved in this complex system serve as potential therapeutic targets:

- The immune response is further promoted by intercellular adhesion molecule 1 (ICAM-1) that causes infiltration of neutrophils into tissues. Antagonism or gene knock-out reduces neutrophil infiltration.
- The immune response is suppressed by IL-10 via reduced production of TNF and reduced activation of monocytes and other immune cells.

Apoptosis (Flowcharts 1 and 2)

This process starts at about 4 hours after injury and lasts for up to 3 weeks. Apoptotic cascade in SCI is activated in neurons, oligodendrocytes, and microglia mediated by a sequence of caspases. The apoptosis occurring in the microglia leads to inflammatory changes and secondary injury to the cord. The same apoptosis when it occurs in the neurons and oligodendrocytes could aggravate the neuronal injury. There are two mechanisms that start the apoptosis:

1. The first is the extrinsic pathway, which is receptor dependent. This pathway is mediated by *Fas* ligand and *Fas* receptor and also by macrophages producing

inducible nitric oxide synthase. In this pathway, there is an inducible TNF that activates a sequence of caspase in which caspase 8 is the inducer caspase, and caspase 3 and -6 are the effector caspases. This alternative pathway for caspase activation involves the nitric oxide synthase.

2. *Intrinsic pathway (receptor independent pathway):* Involves direct activation of caspase-3 proenzyme along with mitochondrial damage. There is release of cytochrome c along with activation of the inducer caspase-9 via apoptotic protease activation factor 1 (Apaf-1) (alternative programmed sequence of caspase activation). This pathway is activated by the high intracellular concentration of calcium and/or H_2O_2 and is receptor independent. The other potent nonreceptor-mediated pathway for apoptosis comes from glutathione/glutathione disulfide (GSH/GSSG) redox system. The change in cellular GSH-to-GSSG ratio specifically mediates cell apoptosis and that this imbalance in redox induces apoptosis is preceded by caspase-3 activation.

Caspase-3 is involved in the expression of an apoptotic phenotype by cleaving several essential substrates involved in its expression in vitro, including fodrin, gelsolin, nuclear lamins, p21-activated kinase 2, (PAK2) and the inhibitory subunit of deoxyribonucleic acid (DNA) fragmentation factor.

Role of Mitochondria (Flowcharts 1 and 2)

Mitochondrion is the central spot for cellular respiration and providing the energy to maintain homeostasis especially the intracellular calcium levels. It is like a nuclear reactor with unending supply of energy if properly maintained but if leakage or damage happens, then reactive and oxidative substrates get leaked in the cytosol causing damage to the cellular elements and activation of various mechanisms detailed above. Mitochondria has been found to actively sequestrate calcium and this increased intramitochondrial calcium is now considered key to induction of apoptosis (leakage and release of substances in the cytosol), and production of excitotoxicity. The calcium-induced mitochondrial permeability changes are most prominent and subject of therapy. If targeted well the medications that protect the mitochondria can be neuroprotective (like cyclosporine A).

Miscellaneous Mediators Implicated in Secondary Spinal Cord Injury

Certain neuropeptides and neurotransmitters have been implicated as a possible cause of secondary SCI. Prominent of them includes—the effect of reduced blood flow is attenuated by activation of μ- and δ-opioid receptors (prolongs excitotoxic process), κ-receptors, serotonin (5- HT) as they cause vasoconstriction and promote platelet activation.

CLASSIFICATION

The SCI is evaluated in systematic manner **(Fig. 3)** to classify the injury and determine level.

Mostly, the SCI are classified in terms of lesion level for which they can be categorized according to:

- Level of lesion is defined as the most distal uninvolved nerve root segment with normal function. Whereby normal function describes that the muscles innervated by the most distal nerve root must have at least a 3+/5 manual muscle test (MMT) grade indicating sufficient strength for functional use.
- *Complete or incomplete:*
  - *Complete lesions:* No sensory or motor function below the level of the lesion. It is caused by a complete transection (or severing), severe compression, or extensive vascular impairment to the spinal cord. Practically, complete lesions can be identified by absence of voluntary anal contraction, absence of anal sensation and absence of S4/S5 sensations.

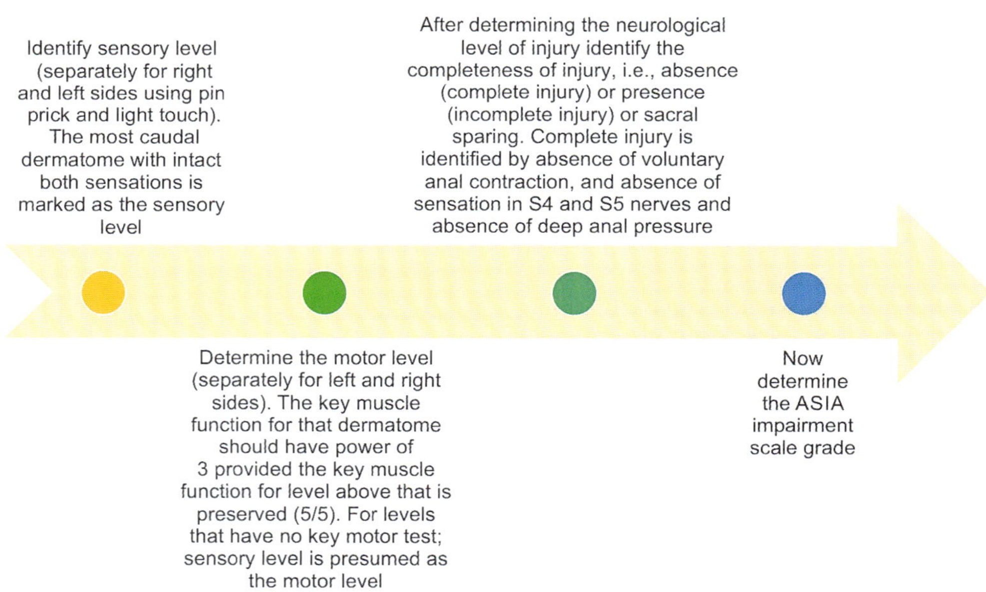

Fig. 3: The step-wise evaluation and assessment of spinal cord injury.

- *Incomplete lesions:* In this, some sensory or motor function below the level of injury is intact. Often result from contusions produced by pressure on the cord or swelling within the spinal canal. Clinical picture is unpredictable. For all practical purposes, check for sacral sparing—if present then incomplete lesion.
- *Extent of involvement:*
  - *Tetraplegia (aka—quadriplegia):* It arises from lesion of cervical cord. There is loss of sensory and motor function in the arms, body, and legs, usually also includes respiratory muscles.
  - *Paraplegia:* Loss of sensory and/or motor function in the trunk and both legs. It results from lesions of the thoracic or lumbar spinal cord or sacral roots.

A comprehensive grading scale as recognized by International Standards for Neurological Classification of SCI is the American Spinal Injury Association (ASIA) impairment scale **(Fig. 1)**. This scale provides a detailed and concise information about spinal cord and peripheral nerve function. It provides common nomenclature to document and communicate the neurological status.

- 28 dermatomes are checked for sensation on both sides by pin tip (nociceptive) and graded as in **Table 1**.
- Motor function is also graded as mentioned in **Table 1**.
- 10 bilateral myotomes representing key spinal motor segments are identified and manually tested. For a normal healthy adult the score will be 100. General reference can be taken as below:
  - C5: Deltoid
  - C6: Wrist extensors
  - C7: Elbow extensor
  - C8: Finger flexors
  - T1: Little finger abduction
  - L2: Hip flexion
  - L3: Knee extension
  - L4: Ankle dorsiflexion
  - L5: Toe extension
  - S1: Plantar flexion

TABLE 1: Muscle power and sensory grading for American Spinal Injury Association (ASIA) neurological examination.

Muscle grading		Sensation grading	
Grade	**Definition**	**Grade**	**Definition**
0	Absent	0	None
1	Palpable contraction	1	Impaired
2	Full ROM with gravity eliminated	2	Normal
3	Full ROM with gravity present	NT	Not tested
4	Active movement with resistance		
5	Normal strength		
NT	Not tested, patient unable to reliably exert effort or muscle unavailable for testing due to factors such as immobilization, pain on effort or contracture		

(ROM: range of motion)

- **Table 2** shows a further grading using ASIA modification of Frankel neurological classification system.

The incomplete forms have a distinctive presentation depending on the region of involvement within the cord. As has been detailed in the anatomy of spine and spinal cord there is a unique disposition of various tracts and nuclei in the cord that subserve specific function, so involvement of a particular region would result in a stereotypic distribution of motor and sensory abnormality. Though intriguing it is not always the case and mixed lesions are more often encountered in clinical practice. Specific incomplete lesions are described below for academic understanding.

- ***Anterior cord syndrome (Fig. 4):*** It is usually caused by cervical flexion ± rotation, which compresses and damages the anterior part of the spinal cord or anterior spinal artery. It usually occurs in an elderly patient with stenotic cervical spine due to osteophytes and ligament hypertrophy. It may also be produced by anterior dislocation/compression fracture of a vertebral body encroaching the ventral canal. Uncommonly, it may be seen in vascular lesions with thrombosis of the anterior spinal artery and resultant spinal infarction.
  - Corticospinal and spinothalamic tracts are damaged either by direct trauma or ischemia of blood supply (anterior spinal arteries)
  - Motor function below the lesion is lost bilaterally.
  - Pain and temperature sensation are lost bilaterally below the lesion.
  - Dorsal columns (vibration and proprioception) remain intact.
- ***Brown-Séquard syndrome (Fig. 5):*** Result of hemisection of spinal cord caused by gunshot or stab wound. It is usually associated with fractures of lateral mass of vertebrae. The nontraumatic causes include neoplasms, MS, disk herniation, cervical spondylosis, direct herniation of the spinal cord through a defect in the dura, pressure due to an epidural hematoma, dissection in the vertebral artery, transverse myelitis, radiation, intravenously drug abuse, TB, decompression sickness, etc. A slowly progressive Brown-Séquard syndrome suggests spinal cord compression on one side, such as by a prolapsed intervertebral disk.
  - Ipsilateral upper motor neuron (UMN) paralysis (corticospinal) one-two spinal segments below, Babinski sign ipsilateral to the lesion
  - Ipsilateral lower motor neuron (LMN) paralysis or weakness at and/or just below the level of injury

TABLE 2: American Spinal Injury Association (ASIA) impairment scale.

Scale	Injury subtype	Motor
A	Complete	No preservation
B	Incomplete	No preservation
C	Incomplete	More than one-half of key muscles caudal to injury have strength graded less than 3
D	Incomplete	More than one half of key muscles caudal to injury have strength greater than 3
E	Normal	Normal or radicular loss

- There is same sided derangement of fine touch, proprioception, and vibration (dorsal column).
- There is same-sided derangement of pain and temperature sense but only at the level of lesion.

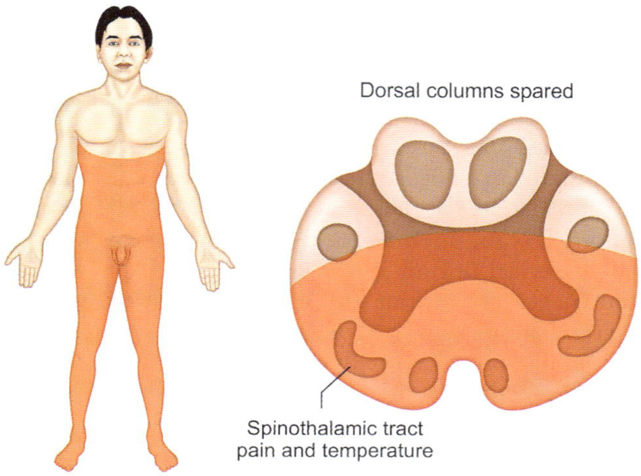

Fig. 4: Anterior cord syndrome.

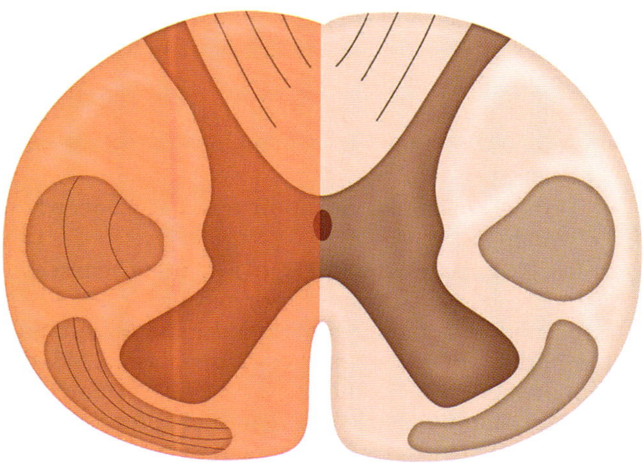

Fig. 5: Brown-Séquard syndrome—half of the cord is involved at the affected level.

- There is derangement of crude touch, pain, and temperature sense (spinothalamic) on the opposite side at one-two levels below the lesion.
- Horner syndrome could be present on same side due to deranged autonomic function.
- *Brown-Séquard-plus syndrome:* Pure syndrome is extremely rare in clinical practice whereas often there are partial signs of the syndrome along with that of the hemisection syndrome plus additional symptoms and signs referred to as Brown-Séquard-plus syndrome.
- If there is no traumatic hemisection, the motor recovery in this syndrome is good. The sequence of recovery is as follows:
  - The ipsilateral proximal extensor muscles recover before the ipsilateral distal flexors.
  - The extremity with sensory loss recovers first as compared to the opposite extremity.
  - It takes about 1–6 months for voluntary motor strength and a functional gait to recover.

- ***Cauda equina injuries:*** These are produced by injuries below the L1 vertebral level in the region of cauda equina that gets compressed by a large central disk or a bony fragment from trauma. It results in a lower motor neuron lesion (LMNL) and is usually incomplete but can be complete.
  - Bowel and bladder difficulties
  - Variable lower extremity motor and sensory deficits
  - Saddle anesthesia
  - Diminished rectal tone
  - Flaccidity and areflexia of the lower limb in severe affections.
- ***Central cord syndrome (Figs. 6A and B):*** Typically in older patients seen due to hyperextension injury. There is compression of the cord anteriorly by osteophytes and posteriorly by ligamentum flavum. The syndrome is also associated with fracture dislocation and compression fractures.
  - More centrally situated cervical tracts tend to be more involved—possible explanation is relatively

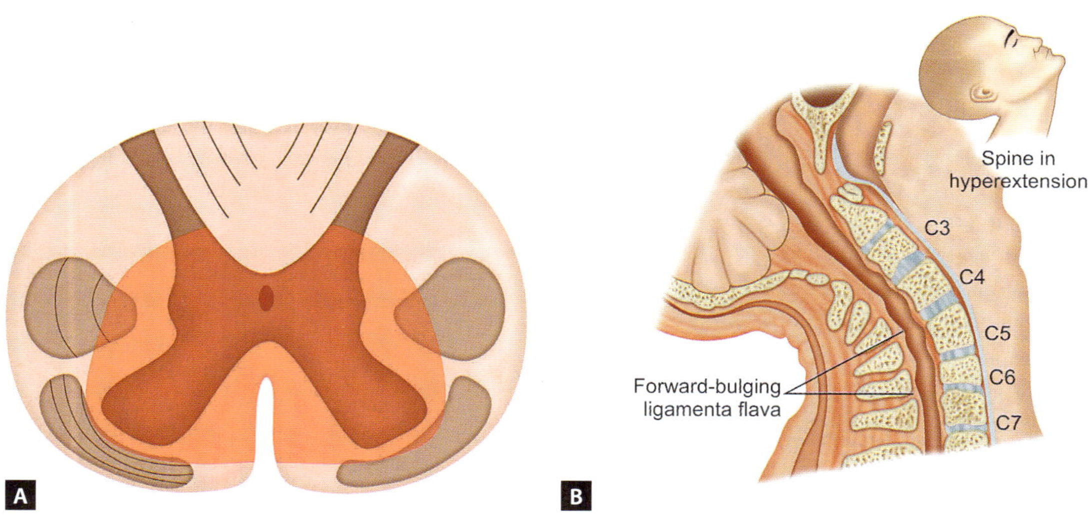

Figs. 6A and B: Central cord syndrome: (A) The involvement of region of cord; (B) The mechanism of injury.

loose texture and rich vascularization of the central cord region which allows the extension of edema and hemorrhage along the central canal in a longitudinal direction. The other possibility is relative vascular insufficiency in the terminal area of the anterior spinal artery.
- Disproportionally greater motor impairment of the upper than of the lower extremities
- Perianal sensation and some lower extremity movement and sensation may be preserved, hands are more severely involved than legs.
- In milder lesions, only the pain and temperature sensation are lost that are carried by the spinothalamic tracts and cross midline.
- High percentage of patients will attain ambulatory function, bladder and bowel control, and hand function.

- ***Posterior cord syndrome (Fig. 7):*** It is a very rare syndrome caused by compression from tumor or infarction of the posterior spinal artery.
  - Proprioception, stereognosis, two-point discrimination, and graphesthesia are lost below the lesion—these produce ataxia and a faltering gait.
  - Motor function is preserved.
- ***Dissociated sensory loss:*** This is caused by intramedullary lesions like neoplasms or syringomyelia.
  - There is a band of sensory loss with normal sensation below the area.
  - Decussating fibers located along the central canal (pain and temperature) are impaired, resulting in a decrease or a loss of pain or temperature sensation.
  - Position, touch, and vibration sense are not affected.
- ***Foix-Alajouanine syndrome:*** There is rapid loss of spinal cord function caused by venous engorgement and ischemic infarction of the spinal cord. The results are caused by obstructed venous flow, typically an arteriovenous malformation. There is presence of enlarged, tortuous, and thick-walled subarachnoid veins on the surface of the cord predominant on the posterior aspect. These enlarged veins are due to a dural arteriovenous shunt which causes reflux of arterial blood into the veins. The trauma to the cord is due to ischemic injury caused by the increased venous pressure. Usually, the lower thoracic level or the lumbosacral level or both are affected.
  - Gray matter structures are more severely affected compared to white matter structures.
  - There is gradually progressive weakness in one or both lower limbs along with sensory features of numbness or tingling that may be symmetric.
  - The initial symptoms are those of heavy feeling in legs with exercise that improves with rest.
  - Over a period of months, the symptoms worsen and patient may have even difficulty in standing over prolonged periods.
  - With progression, the bowel and bladder symptoms appear.
  - The lower back pain is nonradiating; weakness may progress to upper extremities later.
- ***Contusio cervicalis posterior:*** It is a reversible traumatic syndrome of the cord, characterized by pain, tingling, and hyperesthesia in a multisegmental area of the neck, arms, and hands, but sometimes also in the trunk. It is a common, mild, and reversible syndrome.

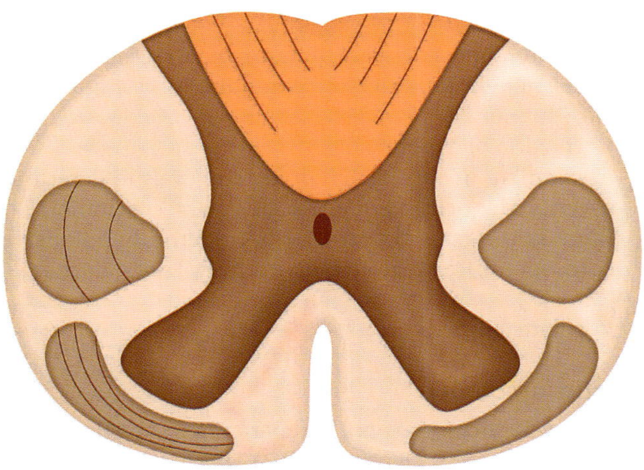

Fig. 7: Posterior cord syndrome.

CLINICAL MANIFESTATIONS

Spinal shock: The term spinal shock was introduced by Marshall Hall in 1841 to indicate the state of transient inexcitability or hypoexcitability of the isolated spinal cord below the level of a transection of the cord. Spinal shock may be due to the loss of facilitation from descending tracts, to persisting inhibition from below the transection acting upon extensor reflexes, or to the axonal degeneration of interneurons. The following are common features of spinal shock:
- There is a transient reflex reduction in cord function below the level of injury.
- Initially, hypertension due to release of catecholamines → Followed by hypotension
- *Flaccid paralysis:* The initial paralysis is always flaccid even if the injury is of UMN type.
- All cutaneous and tendon reflexes are depressed though bulbocavernosus and anal reflexes may persist.
- Bowel and bladder involved
- Sometimes priapism develops.
- Symptoms last several hours to days

The intensity and duration of shock vary on the level of involvement, the higher the cranial level the greater is the shock.

Reversal of shock: When the shock subsides the reflexes return back. In humans, the duration of the areflexia varies, with reflex activity sometimes appearing within a period of 3 days or 4 days in children or after 3–6 weeks in adults. The first reflexes to return are the anal and bulbocavernosus reflexes and as a rule further reflex return is in the cranial direction (the exception is probably the early return of knee reflex than ankle reflex).
- *Motor paralysis or paresis:* There is either complete or partial loss of muscle function below the level of the lesion.

- *Sensory loss:* Impaired or absent sensation below the level of the lesion due to disruption of the ascending sensory fibers.
- *Respiratory dysfunction:* Depends on level of injury, premorbid status of respiratory system, additional injury. Cervical injury commonly is associated with respiratory dysfunction. The impairments include decreased chest expansion and lowered inspiratory volume.
- *Impaired temperature control:* The connection with hypothalamus is lost so there is no temperature regulation through control of cutaneous blood flow or sweating. The person loses ability to shiver and there is absence of thermoregulatory sweating below the level of lesion. This lack of sweating is associated with compensatory diaphoresis above the lesion.
- *Spasticity:* Characterized by hypertonicity, hyperactive stretch reflexes, and clonus. It typically occurs below the level of the lesion after spinal shock subsides. The spasticity gradually increases during first 6 months and plateaus by 1 year. Spasticity is increased by internal and external stimuli [position changes, cutaneous stimuli, environmental temperature, tight clothing, bladder or kidney stones, fecal impaction, catheter blockage, urinary tract infection (UTI), decubitus ulcers, and emotional stress).
- *Bowel and bladder dysfunction:* Neurogenic bladder (*see* Chapter on "Neurogenic Bladder")
- *Sexual dysfunction:* Sexual function is a vital part of the rehabilitation process as is providing other information to enable the patient to better understand and adapt to his medical condition. Male erection and ejaculation are possible depending on the level of the lesion and complete/incomplete injury.

THERAPEUTIC INTERVENTION

The continuum of SCI care can be grouped into: initial and postinitial care, initial and ongoing medical rehabilitation, and life-long sustaining care.

Acute Presentation

The immediate treatments that need to be instilled (according to the flow, a clinician must practice) are:

- Triage
- Stabilization/immobilization
- Resuscitation and trauma care
- *Neuroprotection:* Administration of methylprednisolone (MP) (controversial, see National Acute Spinal Cord Injury Study (NASCIS) trials below) or GM-1
- Stabilizing the patient medically (associated injuries assessment and management)
- Definitive care (assessment and surgical decision) including pain management and anesthetic concerns
- Secondary prevention

Triage for SCI patients: This is especially important for mass casualties and remote areas. The most important period is the first 24 hours after trauma as it is the deadliest. Most of the death due to primary and secondary injuries to the CNS takes place during this period. Correct triage in this period leads to early evaluation by adequately equipped and trained providers in the correct healthcare setting, while maximizing the use of available resources.

Prehospital triage: Develop guidelines for transport of patients and identify regional centers for referral. Transfer the patient to level 1 trauma centers directly rather than passing through level 2 or 3 trauma centers (reduces mortality). It is best if patients are referred to specialized SCI centers after stabilization (reduces complications of SCI and rehabilitation period).

Early Immobilization and Stabilization of the Spine

- All trauma patients with suspected spine injury should have their spine immobilized while transporting.
- Patients with altered mental status, intoxication, fracture of extremity, distracting injury, neurological deficit, pain, or tenderness over spine are high-risk patients for cervical spine injury.
- The devices used for spine stabilization are rigid cervical collar, hard backboard, lateral support devices, tape, or straps. In cases where spinal or SCI is confirmed, the spine immobilization should be maintained till definitive treatment is provided.
- The best combination is a rigid cervical collar with supportive blocks on a backboard with straps. This secures the entire spine of patient.

During the process of immobilization, the following care should be taken:

- The patient should be cared for in the position of greatest comfort (especially at extremes of age)
- Logroll the patient
- Specialized bed for the patient (for prolonged immobilization)—water mattress or air ripple beds
- *Care of back to prevent sores:* Keep skin dry and avoid temperature elevation, mild massage, crease-free beddings, provide pressure relief every 30 minutes if patient will remain on board for >2 hours, regular turning (2 hourly) taking care to protect the spine, and apply astringent on skin to harden the epithelium for high-risk patients.

Resuscitation (only relevant points are mentioned):

- Cases of high tetraplegia will require airway and ventilator support.
- Correction of hypotension
- Assessment of base deficit or lactate levels to determine severity of shock and appropriate fluid resuscitation.
- Identify the cause of shock (neurogenic/hypotensive/cardiogenic) and treat accordingly (*see* Chapter on "Shock").
- Regulate temperature.

Neuroprotection

Inhibitory factors for axonal regeneration in myelin include myelin-associated glycoprotein (MAG) and Nogo-A. Downstream effects of these inhibitory pathways utilize Rho,

BOX 1: The various futuristic and research strategies deployed for limiting damage and improving outcome after SCI.

Improving axonal regeneration:
- Use of trophic factors, antibodies, or receptor blockers against inhibitory factors
- Agents that block inhibitory pathways like cethrin which is a Rho antagonist
- Enzymes that reduce glial scars like chondroitinase ABC
- Guidance molecules or physical scaffolds to steer axons for establishing proper connections
- Nerve tissue or material to bridge axonal gaps
- Gene therapy

Improving axonal conduction despite demyelination:
- Modulating ion channels by drugs to improve conduction in nerves

a guanosine triphosphatase (GTPase). The glial scar that forms in the recovery process can also inhibit regeneration by posing both a physical and chemical barrier. Proteoglycans have same effect. Research strategies for axonal repair and regeneration are presented in **Box 1**.

- One should note that no standard or definitive recommendation for use of any neuroprotective agent exists, this includes steroids.
- Methylprednisolone therapy if initiated is stopped as early as possible in neurologically normal patients and where prior neurologic symptoms have resolved.

Role of pharmacotherapy in immediate management: Based on the pathophysiology discussed above, there are a lot of experimental and evolutive strategies under development; some do have potential to become the future standard of care (none currently definitively recommended):

Anti-inflammatory Strategies

- ***Corticosteroids:*** Typically, MP has been evaluated in various studies over past few decades and has found favors, but more importantly criticisms to its use. Professional organizations have increasingly recommended against its use, citing lack of consistent compelling clinical evidence of effectiveness and demonstrated evidence of significant harmful side-effects. The applicability of MP was derived from animal studies and its theoretical ability to suppress or ameliorate many of the pathophysiological processes causing secondary SCI (vide above). The neuroprotective effects of MP have been proposed to be due to various mechanisms like:
  - Inhibition of lipid peroxidation **(Flowchart 3)**
  - Attenuation of anti-inflammatory cytokines
  - Suppression of proinflammatory cytokine expression
  - Prevention of calcium influx into cells
  - Improved microvascular perfusion
  - Inhibition of nitric oxide production
  - Inhibition of apoptosis

  The reason why MP was chosen was its higher efficiency to inhibit lipid peroxidation (compared to other peers). The use of MP has undergone three multicenter clinical trials collectively referred to as NASCIS; (Bracken, et al., 1984, 1990, and 1997). These trials promoted the role of clinical use of higher doses of MP to patients with acute SCI. The impact of trials was so high and lasting that the practice still continues despite criticism and lack of definite evidence. The following is a summary of the three NASCIS trials:

1. *First trial:* Two relatively low doses of MP after traumatic SCI (Bracken et al., 1984) given within 48 hours of SCI. 330 patients randomized and treated in two groups (MP 100 mg bolus, then 25 mg every 6 hours for 10 days and MP 1,000 mg bolus then 250 mg every 6 hours for 10 days). The results showed no significant difference in the neurological recovery in the two groups noted at 6 and 12 months.
2. Second trial much higher dose of MP (still currently practiced dose of 30 mg/kg bolus with 5.4 mg/kg/h infusion) compared to naloxone (opioid antagonist) and a placebo (Bracken et al., 1990). 487 patients randomized into the three arms and treated within 12 hours of SCI (*MP:* 30 mg/kg bolus followed by 5.4 mg/kg/h infusion for 23 hours, naloxone 5.4 mg/kg bolus then 4.5 mg/kg/h for 23 hours and Placebo). The results showed no significant difference in neurological recovery in the three groups at 6 or 12 months. Patients receiving MP within 8 hours of injury showed significant motor and sensory improvement at 6 months (Bracken, et al., 1990) and at 12 months (Bracken et al., 1992). Naloxone was not shown to be effective. In patients with incomplete lesions, naloxone was subsequently shown to promote significant neurological recovery (Bracken et al., 1993).
3. Third trial evaluated the timing of initiation and duration of MP treatment (Bracken et al., 1997). NASCIS-3 compared the 24- and 48-hour infusions of NASCIS-2 doses of MP against tirilazad mesylate (antioxidant that inhibits lipid peroxidation in steroid-independent pathway). The treatments were given within 8 hours of SCI. 499 patients randomized into three arms and all were treated within 8 hours of SCI (MP—30 mg/kg bolus, then 5.4 mg/kg/h for 23 hours, MP—30 mg/kg bolus, then 5.4 mg/kg/h for 47 hours, tirilazad mesylate—2.5 mg/kg every 6 hours for 48 hours).

   The results of third trial showed no significant difference in neurological recovery in the three groups after 6 months or 12 months of SCI. There was no benefit of prolonged administration of MP infusion in patients which were treated within 3 hours of SCI, but patients treated between 3 and 8 hours of SCI with 48-hour regime showed significant recovery over those who received MP for 24 hours ($p = 0.01$ at 6 months) (Bracken et al., 1997); $p = 0.53$ at 12 months after injury. Neurological recovery with tirilazad was equivalent to that observed with 24-hour MP.

Criticisms of NASCIS trials: There are detailed publications outlining the criticisms on the conduct of the NASCIS trials (especially, NASCIS-2), statistical analysis interpretations and conclusion drawn from them. A few are outlined below:

- Actually in none of the trials, any definitive benefit of the therapeutic interventions was ever revealed. In NASCIS-2, where there was a control group also, there were no differences in the groups while evaluating the primary outcome variables of motor and sensory recovery.

Only in posthoc analysis did a small significance was found for patients receiving steroids within 8 hours of the SCI.

- NASCIS-3 also revealed indifferent result with respect to the treatment duration and only posthoc analysis showed some benefit for earliest interventions. The trial failed to show improvement in primary outcome measures like motor scores, pinprick scores and light-touch scores which could mean that improved recovery with MP may be random events, thus weakening the overall study findings. The significant difference was only revealed after subgrouping the patients.
- None of the studies addressed the confounding variables. NASCIS-2 trial did not include information about other interventions such as radiology, surgical manipulations, or the extent of rehabilitative therapies, which could contribute to improvements.
- Methylprednisolone has been associated with serious complications such as higher infection and sepsis rates, respiratory complications, and gastrointestinal hemorrhage which are documented in both the NASCIS-2 and -3 studies. These were prominent with prolonged administration (48-hour regime) although statistical significance of this finding could not be substantiated. There is a high chance that the studies were not powered enough to capture this statistical significance as they were primarily directed at other end-point evaluation.
- One should clearly understand that the trials did not include pediatric spinal cord injuries, penetrating spinal cord injuries and cauda equine injuries so there is no rationale to use of MP in these patients (as is still blindly followed at some centers).

Conclusions that can be drawn from the above discussion are that:

- Methylprednisolone therapy should be avoided 8 hours after the SCI.
- In pediatric spinal cord injuries, penetrating injuries and possibly cauda equina injuries also, MP should not be used until specifically studied.
- Expecting benefit in neurological recovery in patients after SCI from MP administrations is more theoretically guided than experimentally substantiated so false hope to self or relatives of patient should not be given over the use of this drug.
- If used, one should adequately cover the patients with appropriate management for complications of MP, which can even be fatal in due course.

The other anti-inflammatory strategies that have been variably tried (but none clinically strongly recommended) include following:

- Lazaroids (21-aminosteroids)
- Nonsteroidal anti-inflammatory agents (NSAIDs)
- *Interleukin (IL) 10:*
    - *Rapamycin:* Neuroprotective effect in neurodegenerative diseases, brain injury, SCI through its anti-inflammatory effects. It belongs to the macrolide antibiotic group and also has anti-fungal, anti-tumor effects and inhibits the immune system.
    - Glatiramer acetate

Glutamate Receptor Antagonists (Antiexcitotoxic Agents)

As glutamate and NMDA receptors are intimately involved in excitotoxicity, it is an intriguing idea to incorporate NMDA receptor antagonists for preventing damage to cord after SCI (secondary injury).

- **Gacyclidine** was evaluated in a large trial in France for human SCI based upon its observed neuroprotective effect seen in animal models. In the trial, 200 patients were randomized into two groups (treatment with gacyclidine or a placebo within 3 hours of injury). All subjects had surgical decompression and stabilization, if they needed it. Subjects were examined for a 1 year period via blinded assessments. Till date no statistically significant improved neurologic outcomes have been shown in those patients who received gacyclidine over placebo.

Other strategies for antiexcitotoxic agents include:

- *α-amino-3-hydroxyl-5-methyl-4-isoxazole-propionate (AMPA) blockers:* The KDI tripeptide domain of γ1-chain of laminin is a synthetic tripeptide (Lys–Asp–Ile) which is a universal and potent inhibitor of NMDA, AMPA and of kainate subclasses of glutamate receptors. It facilitates axon guidance, modulated electrical activity and has been found to promote the survival of rat hippocampal neurons. Recently, it has been found that KDI neutralizes the glial- and myelin-derived inhibitory signals that limit the regeneration processes in CNS. KDI has not undergone any clinical trials yet.
- Metabotropic receptor-kainate-blockers.

Antiapoptotic Strategies

Block the apoptotic trigger: Drugs that scavenge free radicals, approaches target early premitochondrial alterations.

Activation of antiapoptotic pathways: This strategy works by inhibiting caspase-3 activity and protects neurons from ischemic injury. Caspase-3 activity is directly inhibited by proteins that are X-linked inhibitor of apoptosis and the neuronal inhibitor of apoptosis. These inhibitor of apoptosis proteins (IAP) such as XIAP, cellular inhibitor of apoptosis 1(cIAP-1), cIAP-2, neuronal apoptosis inhibitor protein (NAIP), Bruce, Survivin, and pIAP inhibit cell death by directly binding to and inhibiting certain caspases like caspases-3, -7, and -9. In the process of TNF family member Fas-induced apoptosis, XIAP is cleaved, separating the baculoviral inhibitory repeat 2 (BIR1-2) domains from the BIR3-Ring domain. This BIR1-2 fragment inhibits active caspases-3 and -7, but is not very active as it is turned over rapidly in cells. Increasing cleavage of XIAP would lower the threshold of caspase activity necessary for inducing apoptosis. A virus-mediated overexpression of NAIP or XIAP can in theory thus prevent apoptosis.

An NMDA receptor antagonist: MK-801 (dizocilpine) could reduce apoptosis and reverse impairment following SCI.

Protease inhibitors or caspase and calpain inhibitors: Direct caspase inhibitors (caspase-9 inhibitor Z-LEHD-FMK) decrease the morphological changes following SCI and improve outcome. Both upstream activators and downstream executioners converge on caspase-9 inhibition of which is hence more effective. Synthetic calpain inhibitors (4-quinolinone 2-carboxamides) administration reduces apoptotic cell death, reduces gliosis, and improves neurological outcome in preclinical trials.

- Poly (ADP-ribose) polymerase (PARP) inhibitors such as 3-amino benzamide may have role in SCI.

Stem Cell and Gene Therapy

- Silencing of gene can be achieved by micro-RNA (miRNA) and small interfering RNA (siRNA) mediated RNA interference (RNAi). This can be used to stop CC chemokine receptor 1 (CCR1) gene expression in MCCLM3 cells, and thus inhibit cell invasion. This process can act as an effective anti-inflammatory mediator but not yet used in SCI.
- Increasing local levels of cAMP enhances the efficacy of Schwann cell transplants and also reduces the production of inflammatory cytokine TNF-α. Stem cell therapy is being tried to increase the local cAMP levels.

Physical Therapy

Certain nonconventional modalities that have been tried are low-level light amplification by stimulated emission of radiation (LASER) therapy. Oscillating field stimulator—applying an oscillating, low-voltage, direct current generates an electrical field which is similar to the polarity guidance in the developmental stages of CNS. A battery powered device attached to the bone applies this field to the area above and below an SCI and stimulates the surrounding neural fibers to grow across the lesion. Repetitive transcranial magnetic stimulation (rTMS)—is a tool used in brain mapping and has shown positive results in Parkinson's disease, stroke, depression, and hallucinations. A changing magnetic field induces electric fields in the brain cord and improves motor and sensory function in patients with SCI.

Other modalities tried are local hypothermia, hyperbaric oxygen therapy, and functional electrical stimulation (FES).

Antagonists of Growth Inhibitory Signals in Central Nervous System

Some of the compounds that have been tried to suppress the growth inhibitory signals in the CNS are monoclonal antibodies to Nogo (11C7 and 7B12 compounds) which may stimulate axonal regeneration sialidase (derived from *Clostridium perfringens*) sialidase shows 2.6-fold increase in the amount of nerve regeneration compared to controls. MAG normally binds to sialoglycoconjugates on axons and gangliosides. Antibodies that suppress MAG show improved growth characteristics. Phosphodiesterase inhibitors (rolipram)—myelin-associated inhibitory proteins like phosphodiesterase 4 reduce the levels of cAMP which results in secondary tissue damage. Rolipram works by inhibiting this phosphodiesterase 4 and raising the level of cAMP. Dibutyryl cyclic AMP (db cAMP) is a synthetic analogue of cAMP which crosses cellular membranes and has same effect as rolipram. The effects of axonal growth inhibitors are mediated through Rho GTPase signaling. Cethrin (BA-210, biochemical analog of a bacterial toxin) is a recombinant protein-based inhibitor of Rho signaling. It has been used for cervical and thoracic acute SCI with encouraging results.

Neurotrophins: Glial-derived neurotrophic factor (GDNF), nerve growth factor (NGF), peptide mixtures with neurotrophic actions (Cerebrolysin and Actovegin), neurotrophin-3 (NT-3), brain-derived neurotrophic factor (BDNF), and ciliary neurotrophic factor (CNTF) may have role in regeneration of neural tissue that needs proper exploration.

Antioxidants: Included in this group are vitamins and nutrients such as B vitamins, thioctic acid, selenium, zinc, and magnesium. Free radical scavengers such as ascorbate, vitamin E, beta-carotene, alpha-tocopherol, penicillamine, superoxide dismutase, Q10 coenzyme, and L-cysteine.

Currently, there are five neuroprotective agents that are aggressively studied and appear to be of current clinical interest, these include:

- *Glyburide:* The use of this compound has been based on the fact that reduction of parenchymal hemorrhage promotes neuronal recovery. The drug primarily blocks sulfonylurea receptor 1 (SUR1)-regulated, Ca^{2+}-activated, adenosine triphosphate (ATP) i-sensitive nonspecific cation (NCCa-ATP) channels. This reduces secondary hemorrhages and also progressive hemorrhagic necrosis (frequently seen after SCI). The drug is already under clinical use for management of type 2 diabetes mellitus (DM). In SCI models, glyburide reduces hemorrhage and improves functional improvement over time.
- *Minocycline:* This drug is the current favorite for evaluation of neuroprotection after SCI. The drug targets various processes involved in secondary injury in SCI. It produces both anti-inflammatory and antiapoptotic actions by inhibition of caspase-1 and caspase-3 (which are involved in IL-1 generation, and cell apoptosis), by reducing microglial and macrophage activation and antibody blockade of the CD95 (FAS) ligand, by inhibiting production of glycosphingolipid-induced inducible nitric oxide synthase (iNOS) and mitigating the effects of matrix metalloproteinases. The reduction in production of nitric oxide reduces neuronal and glial apoptosis with concomitant improvement in neurological function, and enhances the efficacy of cell transplantation strategies. The attenuation effect on excitotoxicity provides neuroprotection in models of Parkinson's disease, autoimmune encephalomyelitis, amyotrophic lateral sclerosis (ALS), and adult and neonatal brain ischemia. Lot of preclinical trials have been done with reported varied effects most positive and some indifferent. Human trials on a large scale will probably bring an insight into the beneficial effects, if at all. The drug has been for the treatment of bacterial infections including acne at a maintenance dose of 50–100 mg taken orally once a day and also to treat rheumatoid arthritis. In SCI

models, treatment with minocycline reduces lesion size, improved white matter sparing, significant protection of oligodendrocytes. Clinical outcomes were variable but mostly positive.

- *Magnesium sulfate [±polyethylene glycol (PEG)]:* This has risen lot of interest recently and various preclinical animal trials have been done or are underway to evaluate the effect of $MgSO_4$ on SCI. The proposed mechanisms of action of $MgSO_4$ are reducing the levels of intracellular calcium by inhibiting of NMDA receptors and of voltage-gated calcium channels, and thus reducing controlling excitotoxicity, lowering free radical generation, lowering glutamate release, inhibiting the expression of p53-related proteins, and controlling lipid peroxidation and lactate accumulation.

  Magnesium sulfate is presently used for control of convulsions (preeclampsia and eclampsia) of pregnancy, in acute nephritis in children, in $MgSO_4$ deficiency with signs of tetany, to reduce premature contractions in pregnancy and to treat heart attack and asthma.

  Polyethylene glycol is a surfactant that has been shown to anatomically and physiologically fuse spinal cord axons in injury models. Additionally, PEG may facilitate physiologic repair of compressed spinal cord parenchyma. The results have been encouraging from phase 1 and 2 trials on dogs but the results were not reproduced in rodents. Currently, phase 3 trial is underway. PEG can be combined with $MgSO_4$ to improve the outcome of either compound.

  In SCI models, the drug reduces lesion volumes (effect enhanced with concomitant PEG), significantly improved white matter sparing, reduced caspase-3 activity, lower lactate and MDA (malondialdehyde) levels, improved vascularity, and clinical improvements in neuropathic pain and somatosensory evoked potentials (SSEP).
- *Calcium channel blockers:* Though expected to reduce intracellular calcium levels these agents work primarily by altering the tone of smooth muscles in the blood vessels. The reduction of calcium ions is minimal. Nimodipine functions as a calcium antagonist in CNS, it is a slow-acting channel blocker which causes elective vasodilation and improves spinal cord blood flow in SCI. Presently, it is approved for oral use in ruptured intracranial aneurysms and subarachnoid hemorrhage in a dose of 60 mg every 4 hours. This is because the effect of nimodipine on necrosis and hemorrhage of the spinal cord was found to be negligible by a number of studies.
- *Riluzole:* It is an inhibitor of voltage-activated sodium and calcium ion channels. It acts by inhibiting presynaptic glutamate release, and activating potassium ion channels. As detailed above that unchecked influx of sodium ions leads to downstream activation of various deleterious processes in the cell, so blocking the same may have positive effect on the survival. Also potassium stabilizes the resting membrane potential and reduces cell excitability in the central and peripheral nervous system. Presently, it has been used for treatment of ALS at a dose of 50 mg every 12 hours. In preclinical trials, it improved lesion size, significantly normalized residual tissue area and white and gray matter volumes, retained greater numbers of neurons and improved neuron counts, improved lipid peroxidation levels, glucose uptake, and mitochondrial function. Clinical improvements are, however, delayed and could take more than 1 month to manifest.

Miscellaneous neuroprotectors that cannot be classified into any one category definitely:

- *Gangliosides:* Gangliosides (sialic acid containing glycosphingolipids) especially GM-1 (monosialotetrahexosylganglioside, Sygen) is abundant in mammalian nervous system where they are abundantly expressed in the outer membranes of the neural cells. Animal studies have shown improved neurologic recovery after SCI following the administration of GM-1 (Sygen, Fidia Pharmaceutical Corporation, Washington, DC). They have been evaluated in human SCI based on various proposed mechanisms as follows:
  - Prevent apoptosis
  - Induce neuronal sprouting
  - Inhibits lipid peroxidation
  - Mimics or potentiates the effects of neurotropic factors
  - Attenuates excitotoxicity

  Basic science investigational data showed some benefits especially improved neuronal plasticity, regeneration, and a neuroprotective effect. The preclinical experimental data for SCI is equivocal not supporting its indiscriminate use.
- *Opioid antagonists:* Naloxone is a nonspecific opioid receptor antagonist. It was evaluated for its efficacy to reverse spinal shock in 1980s by improving spinal cord blood flow and enhance recovery by unknown mechanisms. It was also thought to antagonize the effects of endogenous opioids observed to increase after SCI. In human SCI clinical trials, it has not been demonstrated to be any more beneficial than a placebo (NASCIS-2), though a later posthoc analysis did show some benefit in incompletely injured patients.
- *Development of protective autoimmunity to control lipid peroxidation:* Immunization with neural-derived antigens has shown to modulate the autoreactive mechanisms that promote neuroprotective response and to render protective and restorative effects after SCI.
- Phospholipase A2 inhibition
- *Scar-preventing substances (chondroitinase ABC, cordaneurin, and EphA4 antagonists):* Chondroitinase acts by removing inhibitory signals of chondroitin sulfate proteoglycans and also removes partially the physical barrier; they form by digesting the chondroitin sulfate. Cordaneurin is developed in Germany for use with neurosurgical interventions done in first 3 hours.
- *Potassium channel inhibitors [4-aminopyridine (Fampridine)]:* It is under trial for treatment of spasticity in incomplete or partial SCI. It has been proposed to improve walking ability in MS but results in SCI are indefinite.

BOX 2: The uncommonly reported unconventional therapeutic agents used in spinal cord injury.

- Blockade of CD95
- Cell adhesion molecules (L1-CAM)
- Iron chelators (deferoxamine, 2,20-bipyridine, and quercetin)
- Squalenoyl adenosine nanoparticles
- *Lithium:* Studies are underway with administration of intrathecal lithium above and below the lesion with neonatal umbilical cord blood mononuclear cells. The results so far have not been impressive.
- *Erythropoietin:* In high doses, it acts by inhibiting lipid peroxidation and neuronal apoptosis. However, it also carries risk of polycythemia, hyperviscosity syndrome and hypertension. An isoform called "carbamylated erythropoietin" has been developed having no hematopoietic properties but having neuroprotective effects in animal models.
- Nitric oxide release inhibitors
- *Hormones:*
  - Thyrotropin-releasing hormone (TRH) and analogues
  - 17-estradiol/progesterone
  - Statins (simvastatin)
- Melatonin
- Inosine (Axosine)
- Dexmedetomidine a highly selective, potent adrenergic agonist effective in various regional and neuraxial anesthesia. It has not been shown to change somatosensory or motor-evoked potential responses during complex spine surgery by any clinically significant amount.

There are lots of other sporadically studied agents either in isolation or in combination to conventional drugs that have undefined role. These are presented in **Box 2**.

ASSESSMENT AND EVALUATION

The assessment starts with a baseline neurological charting of all the patients with suspected spinal injury or SCI. The neurological level and the completeness of injury are assessed. This is followed by serial examinations to determine neurological deterioration or improvement.

Radiographic evaluation: Imaging of entire spine is mandatory. Magnetic resonance frequency is done only of the known or suspected area(s) of SCI. There should be a high degree of suspicion of a fracture if there is stiff spine and midline tenderness. Magnetic resonance imaging (MRI), bone scan, and/or computed tomography (CT) may be done, if the plain X-ray is negative for fracture. This is especially important in cases of spondylosis, ankylosing spondylitis (AS), or diffuse interstitial skeletal hyperostosis (DISH). Awareness should be there for SCI without radiological abnormality or "SCIWORA".

Medical stabilization of patient *(Assessment of associated injuries and management) (tertiary trauma survey):*

- *Traumatic brain injury (TBI):* It should be assessed and document early in the form of loss of consciousness, post-traumatic amnesia, ear or nose bleed, vomiting, raccoon eyes, developing dizziness, or drowsiness (not otherwise explained).
- *Limb injuries:* Fractures elsewhere in the body should be stabilized.
- Chest and abdominal injuries should be checked for and a nasogastric tube may be placed for abdominal decompression.
- *Arterial injuries:* The possibility of an aortic injury should be considered in high energy injuries. CT or MR angiography may be done for cerebrovascular injury.
- *Penetrating injuries:* While maintaining inline stabilization, evaluate the wounds for vascular or internal organ injury. Life-saving procedures should also be performed taking care to minimize SCI.

DEFINITIVE MANAGEMENT

- In case of bilateral cervical facet dislocation with an incomplete SCI, a closed or open reduction is done as soon as permissible. This is done as a proactive measure to improve neurological recovery, in a setting of progressive neurological deterioration, although there is no compelling evidence that it will. In case of an unstable spine, early spinal stabilization should be done with the use of intraoperative spinal cord monitoring where spinal cord function has been spared.
- *Autologous nerve bypass grafts:* This is an experimental surgical procedure which is used to bypass the lesion site in cases of complete paraplegia. The corticospinal tract is connected with the main standing/walking muscles of the legs, using the sciatic nerve as a graft. One case was done in Germany on a young female patient with a complete T9 lesion. At about 17 months, the first voluntary movements were noticed and mobilization with the help of a walker became possible after 27 months. In any case, this is a very promising approach but as expected the technical expertise needed is immense.
- *Schwann cell transplantation:* This is a new basically experimental technique with no definite outcome. Usually, the Schwann or olfactory ensheathing glia cell is grafted into the injured site in combination with other neuroprotective factors. One of the approaches uses a three-step process. In the first step, Rolipram is administered subcutaneously at the time of injury. One week later, Schwann cells are injected into site of SCI. This is then supplemented by db cAMP injection above and below the graft.

  The results in treated animals had been impressive with reasonable functional recovery after SCI mobilization. Human trials are pending.
- Minimization of the pain through thoughtful patient handling. Adequate analgesia should be provided.

Some anesthetic points to remember are postoperative ventilator support, mean arterial pressure (MAP) maintenance using a balance of infusion and inotropes. Expect and correct bradycardia and hypotension during intubation especially in case of tetraplegia. Do not use succinylcholine after the first 48 hours postcord injury.

Secondary Care

Take in-bed care of patient, prevent, and manage deep vein thrombosis (DVT) (*see* Chapter on "Venous Thromboembolism Prophylaxis and Treatment") using pharmacotherapy for prophylaxis. A vena cava filter is used only in patients with active bleeding which is anticipated to persist for 72 hours or more.

Respiratory management: Patients with tetraplegia usually need ventilation. A baseline assessment of vital capacity, forced expiratory volume 1 (FEV1), and arterial blood gases should be obtained. Monitor patients for respiratory failure in first few days.

- Perform tracheostomy for patients who will need prolonged ventilation. Use expiratory aids to avoid retention of secretions [manually assisted coughing (quad coughing), pulmonary hygiene, and mechanical insufflation-exsufflation]. Use defined protocol to prevent ventilator-associated pneumonia (VAP).
- *Genitourinary tract:* An indwelling urinary catheter or suprapubic catheter, if required is part of initial management. In SCI, priapism does not need treatment as is usually self-limiting.
- *Gastrointestinal care:* Initiate stress ulcer prophylaxis. Prevent aspiration by careful assessment of swallowing function.
- *Nutrition:* Enteral nutrition in recumbent position to prevent aspiration using a polymeric enteral formula is started within 24–48 hours of SCI. The caloric requirement is assessed by a 30-minute energy expenditure measurement using indirect calorimetry.

REHABILITATION SUPPORT

These basically begin after stabilization and recuperative period of SCI, when definitive management has been administered and one is waiting for recovery (48–72 hours onward). The emphasis lies on maintaining range of motion (ROM), facilitating active movement in available musculature, and limited strengthening activities pending orthopedic clearance.

- Psychosocial rehabilitation is an important aspect often neglected in medical care. Healthcare professionals should pay attention to following during the hospital stay (and appropriately treat) and afterward:
  - Major depression, acute stress disorder/post-traumatic stress disorder (PTSD), or substance intoxication and withdrawal, cognitive functioning and learning style, concomitant health problems, medical conditions, medications, and history of TBI
- Concurrent life stressors
- Detect suicidal ideation

Low-level LASER therapy: It is done using an 810 nm-wavelength LASER. It works by stimulating axonal regeneration and reducing inflammatory reaction. It has been shown to improve the neurological outcome in animals with SCI. Human trials are pending.

Functional electrical stimulation (FES): FES helps in SCI by preventing atrophy, compensating muscle dysfunction, maintaining mobility and improving the quality of life ultimately.

It can be applied externally by means of simple electrodes or as a component of hybrid orthotic systems. Work is being done on implanted systems to improve gait.

Pharmacological and Psychiatric Stimulation of the Spinal Central Pattern Generator

Central pattern generator (CPG) consists of a neural network located in the spinal cord at the level of L1 and L2. This network can endogenously or quasi-independently generate rhythmic nervous outputs for locomotion. This can be modulated in a normal individual by treadmill training.

Pharmacological modulation of CPG: At the molecular level, it is seen that 5-hydroxytryptamine (HT) receptors are responsible for massive synaptic amplification in the CPG. Rhythmic but uncoordinated and asynchronous stepping movements can be elicited by administering 5-HT alone, with other monoamines, such as dopamine. Another pathway associated with locomotion induction in mammalian cord has been identified close to the CPG. This is a descending serotonergic pathway present in the Rexed's lamina 7 of the distal dorsal spinal cord. It has an abundance of serotonin receptors. Thus, the CPG can be stimulated for a short time by the following:

- Alpha-1 and alpha-2 adrenergic agonists (methoxamine and clonidine)
- Serotonergic agonists (quipazine)
- Glycine receptor antagonists (strychnine)

Psychiatric stimulation of spinal CPG: Progressive verticalization that is to make a person slowly stand utilizes the residual motor function in the lower limbs. This is done in a passive manner using a tilt table stimulating the lumbar CPG and encouraging ambulation. It has a positive influence on proprioception/sensory-motor feedback, postural reflexes, bone trophicity, urine drainage, intestinal transit, and psychiatric influence of enhancing self-esteem and quality of life.

In later rehabilitation process, a standing frame is used. Postural loads stimulate CPG activity via stimulation of the *Hox* genes which are essential in the organization/reorganization processes in the CNS.

Epidural electrical stimulation uses a combination of neurosurgery and physical therapy. Implanted epidural electrodes deliver low frequency electrical stimulation (2.2–50 Hz). This elicits stepping-like movements but a functional gait is not achieved. This technique has some complications such as infections, local hemorrhages, etc.

COMPLICATIONS OF SPINAL CORD INJURY

- *Pressure ulcers:* Frequent complication of recumbency.
  Autonomic dysreflexia: This is a worrisome complication occurring in patients with lesions above T6. A painful or noxious stimulus below the level of the lesion causes sudden fall in BP by triggering the autonomic nervous system. This if untreated can lead to convulsions, hemorrhage, and death. These patients can be identified **(Box 3)** by a cluster of symptoms of high BP, severe headache (HA), blurring of vision, presence of a stuffy nose, sweating, presence of goose bumps below, and vasodilation (flushing) above the level of the injury. Some conditions that can precipitate these catastrophic

BOX 3: Identifying autonomic dysreflexia.

The following are the common presentations and signs in autonomic dysreflexia:
- Sudden fluctuation in blood pressure
- Pounding headache
- Flushing of skin above the level of SCI or below
- Blurred vision
- Nasal congestion
- Profuse sweating above the level of SCI
- Bradycardia
- Cardiac arrhythmias
- Feeling of apprehension or anxiety
- Minimal or no symptoms
- Symptoms or signs of underlying noxious stimulus may or may not be present.

BOX 4: The common management of autonomic dysreflexia.

- Blood pressure—if elevated immediately prop-up the patient to sitting position this reduces blood pressure.
  - Loosen constructive clothing or devices (like DVT pump)
- Survey for instigating symptoms beginning from urinary system. Catheterize the patient if not done already.
- Check indwelling catheter for kinks, constrictions, or obstructions and correct placement—if blocked then flush the catheter with normal saline at body temperature.
- Remove a blocked catheter and replace it.
- If urinary system is clear but autonomic dysreflexia, persists then look for fecal impaction.
  - Per rectal examination using lidocaine jelly
- *Pharmacological management of raised blood pressure:*
  - Nitroglycerin patches (immediate release 10 mg) or titrated intravenous dose—contraindicated in patients who have taken sildenafil within 24–48 hours before.
  - Nifedipine (10 mg crush and swallow tablet)—exercise caution in elderly.
  - Captopril (25 mg sublingual)
- Admit the patient if further evaluation is needed for uncontrolled blood pressure in case above measures fail.

events are a distended or full bladder caused by blockage in the catheter, any bladder infection, pressure ulcers or in grown toenail, sudden and extreme temperature change, or tight clothing. The treatment is resuscitation and identification and treatment of the noxious stimulus. Sitting position is recommended as lying will further elevate the BP **(Box 4)**.

- Orthostatic hypotension
- *Contractures:* Most common contractures develop in hip as flexion, IR, adduction flexion-adduction-internal rotation (FADIR); shoulder—flexion/extension, internal rotation, and adduction.
- Deep vein thrombosis
- *Osteoporosis and renal calculi:* These develop as a result of changes in calcium metabolism following SCI. There is calcium leaching from bones producing osteoporosis and renal calculi. The patients are predisposed for fractures due to weak bones. Urinary calcium levels are elevated due to hyperactivity of osteoclasts caused by immobility (absence of Wolf's law), lack of weight bearing and possibly dietary deficiencies. The effects are similar to space disease (seen in astronauts, zero gravity situations).

PROGNOSIS OF SPINAL CORD INJURY

The potential for recovery from SCI is directly related to the extent of damage to the spinal cord and/or nerve roots. Formulation of a prognosis is initiated only after spinal shock has subsided, once it is known if the injury is complete or incomplete.

- *C8 and higher:* Functional ambulation is not feasible.
- *T1-9:* It may walk but not functionally, need of crutches or walker and knee-ankle-foot orthoses (KAFOs) imperative.
- *T10-L2:* Household ambulation only with support of crutches or walker and KAFOs
- *L3-4:* Community ambulator with crutches or walker and ankle-foot orthotics (AFOs)/KAFOs
- *L5 and below:* Community ambulator with or without cane and AFOs

Hysterical Paralysis

In patients with marked inconsistencies in their neurological findings, hysterical paralysis may be the diagnosis.

- Reassess the patient with neurological examination
- Consult independent evaluation by another expert/specialist before making this diagnosis
- The patient is encouraged to resume normal function.
- Magnetic resonance imaging or motor-evoked potential testing is done if the patient fails to improve in 2–3 days.

CONCLUSION

- Spinal cord injury causes motor, sensory, and autonomic dysfunction. There are various patterns of SCI producing specific pattern of deficits.
- Various medications have been proposed to reduce the damage to spinal cord but none has been approved with certainty. Antiapoptotic and stem cell strategies do hold promise for future.
- Currently, the care for a spinal cord injured patient is mainly supportive and involves rehabilitation support and symptomatic improvement.

CHAPTER 102

Deformities of Spine

Manish Kumar Varshney

INTRODUCTION

The spine is straight in coronal/frontal plane while there are physiological curves in sagittal plane. The vertebral column may deviate from this common disposition and develop coronal plane curves producing unacceptable mechanics, and deformity. Also the sagittal plane curves may get exaggerated surpassing its physiological range or may lose the normal curvature, both altering the biomechanics. These abnormalities may arise congenitally or developmentally during childhood or in adults. They have their own set of problems and consequences that need discrete discussion. The management is mostly extensive and need specialty care more or less leading to development of separate faculty at dedicated centers. The following description is a primer for understanding of the deformities of spine while also dealing with the advancements in management.

SCOLIOSIS

Scoliosis is typically defined as a lateral curvature of the spine **(Fig. 1)** on a radiograph of the spine taken in standing position (defined this way for the first time by Galen). Truly speaking, however, scoliosis is a three-dimensional deformity (some hence call it "rotoscoliosis", **Fig. 2**) of the spine that involves a curvature in the sagittal, frontal and transverse plane **(Fig. 3)** without the loss of osteoligamentous continuity, which develops over a segment or over the entire length of the spine. To take the argument further, there is assertion that the coronal plane deformity (used to define scoliosis) is actually secondary, the primary deformity is vertebral rotation (*see* biomechanical pathogenesis later). The understanding of scoliosis entails recognizing not only the local deformity but also the regional, spinal and global deformity as a whole **(Figs. 4A to D)**. The term "kyphoscoliosis" is wrong and should be dropped as the characteristic finding of rib hump from which the term "kyphosis" has been added actually represents a "hypokyphotic state" of thoracic spine (Robert Winter). Frontal plane curves of up to 10° are accepted as normal in human population (though ideally the spine does not have any frontal plane curve). Curves more than 10° are considered scoliotic.

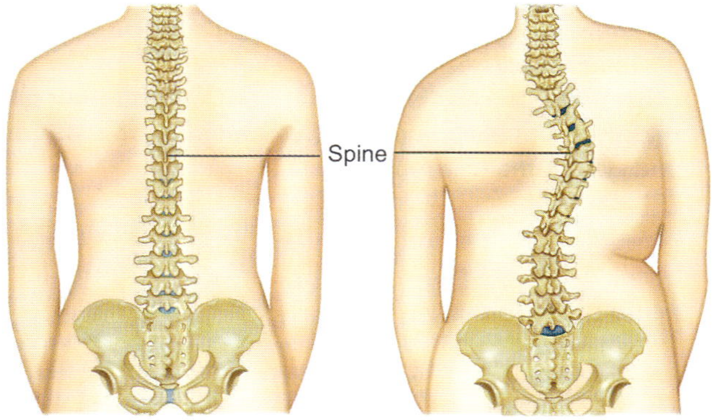

Fig. 1: Scoliosis—typically identified by lateral curvature of spine instead of normally straight spine in coronal plane.

Scoliosis can be structural due to spinal pathologies or nonstructural as a result of other skeletal abnormalities, for example, leg-length discrepancy, and pelvic obliquity. Scoliosis with Cobb's angle more than 10°, associated with vertebral rotational deformity, is regarded as structural scoliosis. The sidedness of curve (right or left sided) is defined by the side at which the apex of convexity points. Scoliotic curvature can arise out of many disorders and conditions **(Table 1)**.

Idiopathic scoliosis is a diagnosis of exclusion that can only be made after other causes of scoliosis deformity have been excluded. It is the most common type of spinal deformity and accounts for about 75% of patients with scoliosis.

It is handy to define terms related to scoliosis before describing individual conditions:

- *Nonstructural curve/scoliosis (functional scoliosis):* It has no structural component, it corrects on supine side-bending films **(Fig. 5)**. The curves correct passively and possibly arise from without the loss of osteoligamentous continuity, which develops over a segment or over the entire length of the spine. The most common causes of functional scoliosis are—lower limb length differences, unilateral paravertebral muscle contracture, torticollis, etc.

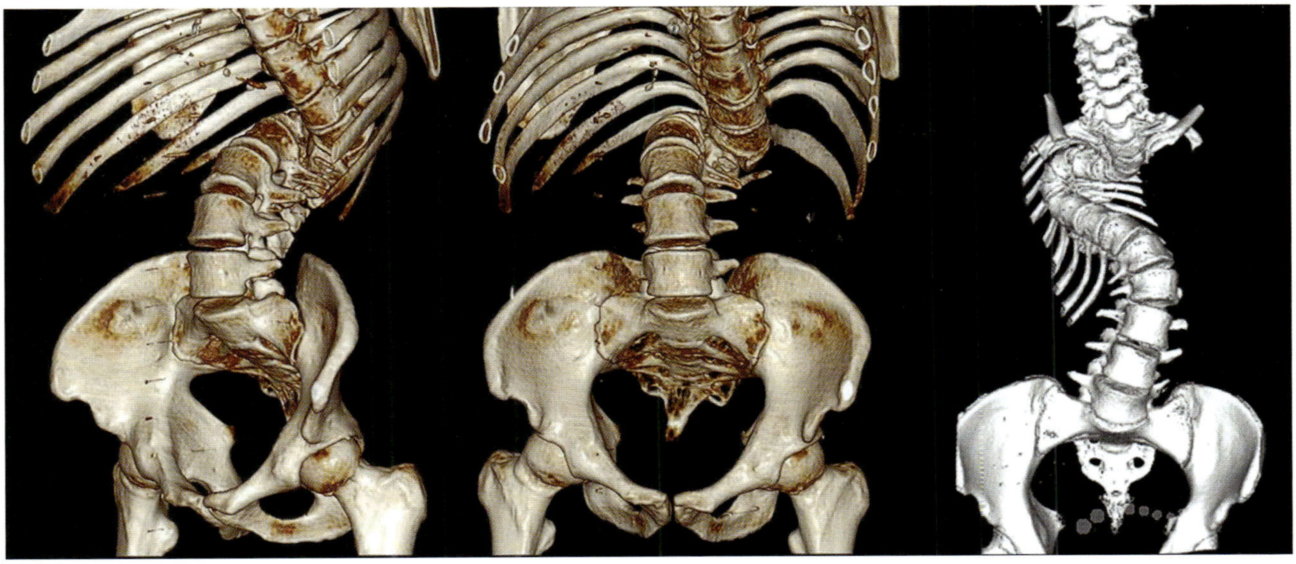

Fig. 2: Rotoscoliosis (invert and black and white) net images. Actually the scoliotic deformity is a rotational 3D deformity of spine in all planes so called "rotational scoliosis" or rotoscoliosis.

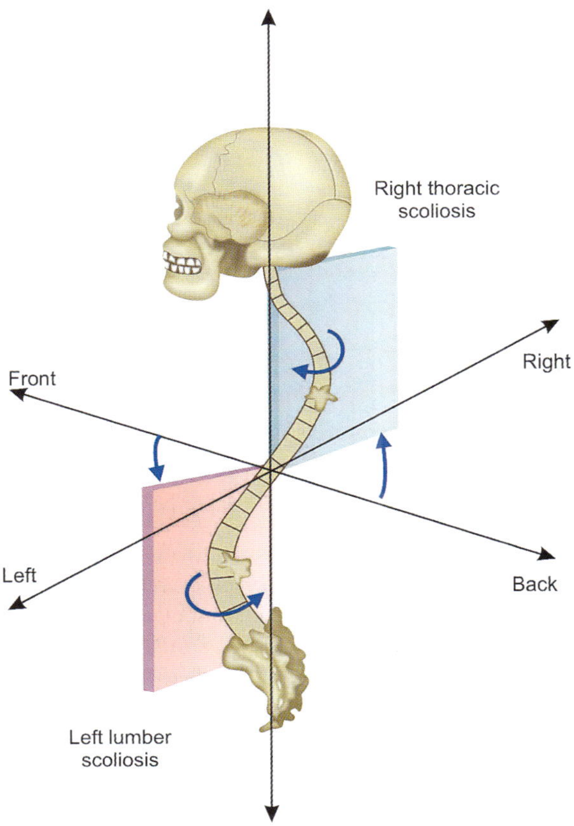

Fig. 3: 3D deformity exists in all three planes and now stress is being put to define the deformity in all the three planes for comprehensive management.

This type of scoliosis is classified into three types by Stagnara:

1. *Reducible scoliotic curvatures:* Reversible lateral curvature without rotation that usually arise out of painful spasms of muscles caused by vertebral and juxtavertebral abnormalities.
2. Compensatory curvatures develop due to defects located at a distance from the vertebral column, lower limb length differences, hip adduction or abduction fixed deformities, irreducible muscle retraction.
3. Postural defects are scoliotic postures without an obvious cause (often seen during childhood):
    - They can be intermittent or permanent
    - Not accompanied by vertebral rotation
    - Do not evolve into structural scoliosis
    - Disappear during the pubertal growth spurt.

- *Structural curve:* Lacks normal flexibility.
- *Structural scoliosis:* Irreversible lateral curvature of the spine with rotation of the vertebral bodies in the area of the major curve. It develops in all three spatial planes due to lateral inclination, curving and rotation movement.
- *Major curve:* The largest structural curve in magnitude that is least reducible and clinically most important **(Fig. 6)**.
- *Compensatory curve:* A curve that is above or below a major curve that serves to maintain normal body alignment. They can be nonstructural or become structural later **(Fig. 7)**.
- *Stable vertebra:* Most proximal vertebra that is most closely bisected by the central sacral vertical line (CSVL) **(Fig. 7)**.
- *Inflection vertebra:* It is the place where a curve changes direction from convex to concave or vice versa **(Fig. 6)**.
- *Stable zone:* The area (vertical strip) between lines drawn vertically from lumbosacral facet joints.
- A *superior end vertebra* is the vertebra at the upper limit of the curve, whose upper endplate has the greatest inclination towards the concavity of the curve **(Fig. 6)**.
- An *inferior end vertebra* is the vertebra at the lower limit of the curve, whose lower endplate has the greatest inclination toward the concavity of the curve.

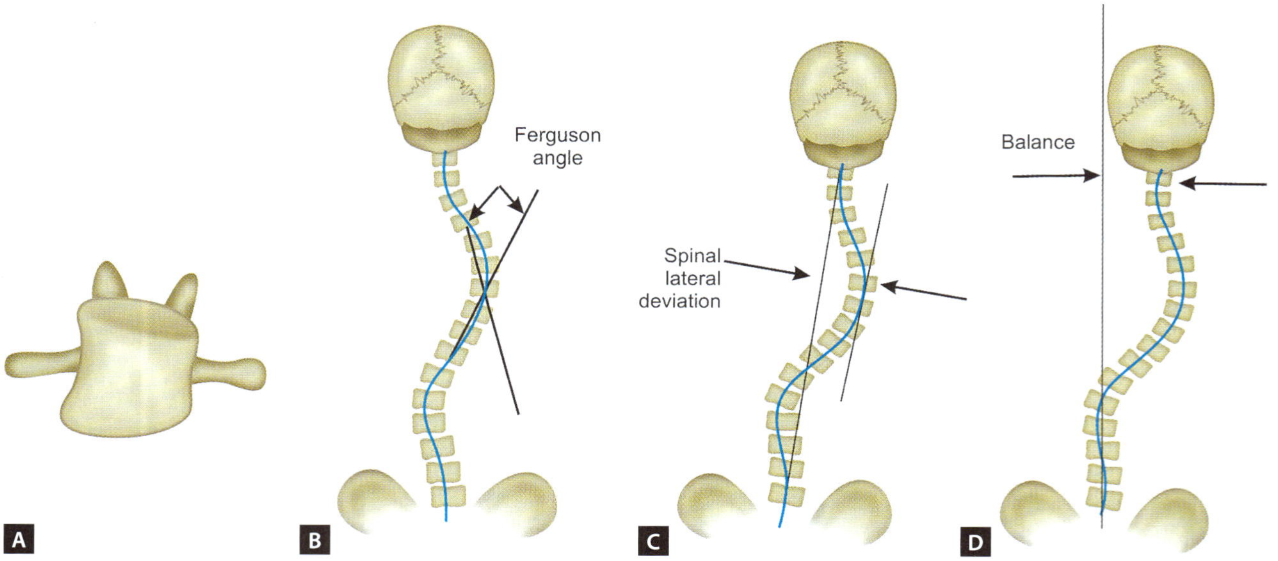

Figs. 4A to D: Splitting the deformity components of scoliosis into local, regional and global components helps in getting a better understanding: (A) Local deformity (Vertebra); (B) Regional deformity (Curve); (C) Spinal deformity (Spine); (D) Global deformity (Body).

TABLE 1: Causes of scoliotic deformity of spine.

- *Congenital:*
  - Failure of formation
  - Failure of segmentation
  - Mixed
  - Idiopathic
  - Infantile (0–3 years)
  - Juvenile (3–10 years)
  - Adolescent (10+ years)
- *Neuromuscular:*
  - *Myopathic:*
    - Arthrogryposis
    - Muscular dystrophy
    - Cerebral palsy
  - *Neuropathic:*
    - Upper motor neuron
    - Lower motor neuron
    - Dysautonomia (Riley-Day syndrome)
- *Others:*
  - Neurofibromatosis
  - Mesenchymal (Marfan's, Ehlers-Danlos)
  - Extraspinal contracture (after empyema)
  - Traumatic
  - Osteochondrodystrophies (Morquio's, diastrophic dwarfism)
  - Infection
  - Metabolic (osteoporosis, rickets)
  - Tumor
  - Associated with spondylolisthesis

- A *neutral vertebra* is the vertebra at the upper or lower limit of the curve, which is not rotated (pedicles are equidistant from the spinous process on PA radiograph). It can sometimes be a superior or inferior end vertebra. It is not same as stable vertebra **(Fig. 8)**.

HISTORICAL PERSPECTIVE

It is the scoliosis, its understanding and management that gave faculty "orthopedics" its name. The name is derived from the short book "*L'Orthopedie*" (*Orthopædia: or the Art of Correcting and Preventing Deformities in Children)* written by Nicolas Andry **(Fig. 9)** a French pediatrician in 1741. The name is derived from "orthos" (*Greek* straight) and "paidion" (*Greek* child). He believed the scoliosis arise from abnormal muscular tightness (convulsive muscular forces) in some places causing abnormal forces transmitted to spine.

Within the text he depicted the "crooked tree" that has been adopted by many orthopedic organizations around the world as a part of their symbol/emblem, now popularly known as Andry's tree **(Fig. 9)**. Not remembered for it but he was also the Father of Parasitology!

In ancient Indian literature (3500–1800 BC) reference to scoliosis correction is mentioned in "Bhagavata Purana" and "Sur Sagar" by Surdas. Lord Krishna is described to correct the scoliotic deformity of "Kubja" (mentioned as a low class maid servant for her deformities and ugliness) who had three curves ("trivakra"—triple deformity) in the spine **(Fig. 10)**.

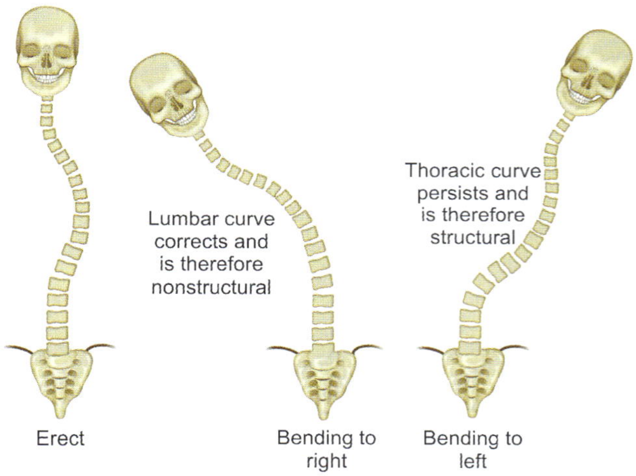

Fig. 5: Nonstructural curves correct on bending films.

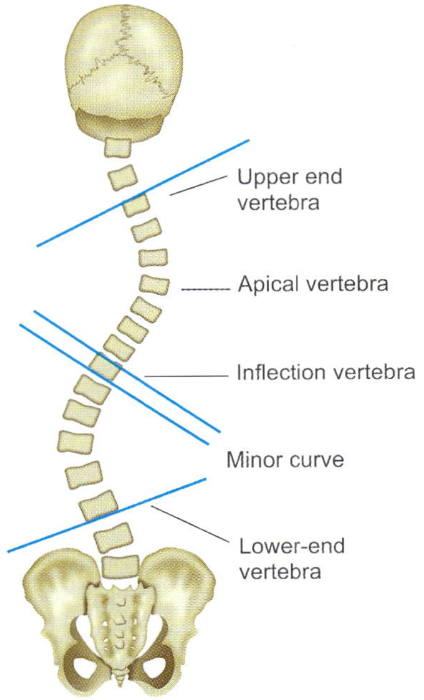

Fig. 6: In a structural curve, the spine may have major and minor curves defined by end vertebrae (see text for detail).

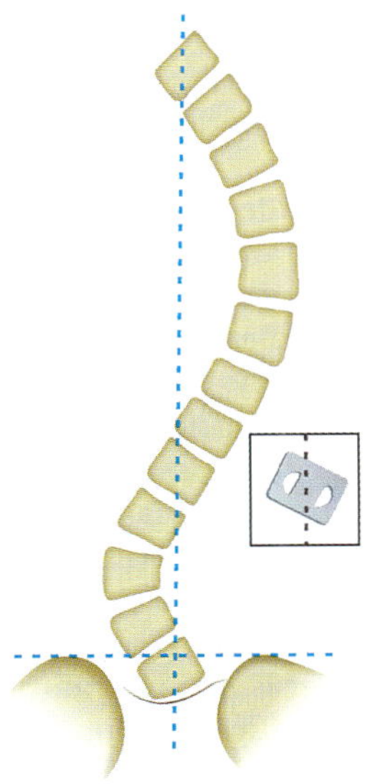

Fig. 7: For rigid major curves, body tries to compensate for balancing the head over pelvis by developing compensatory curves opposite to the major curve. This balance can be assessed by line drawn from the center of sacrum (central sacral vertical line). The vertebra most closely bisected by this line is called stable vertebra.

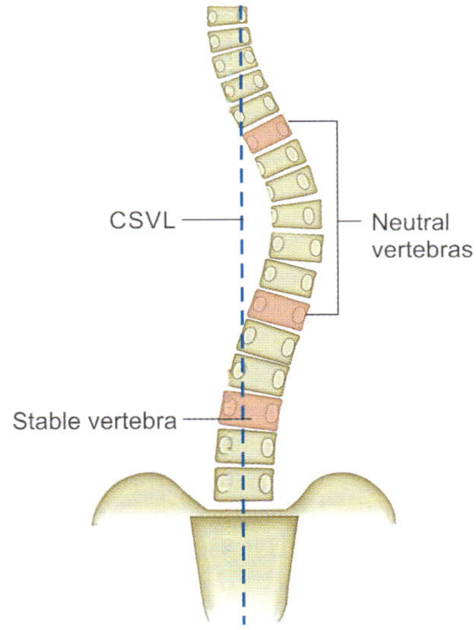

Fig. 8: A stable vertebra is defined by central sacral vertical line (CSVL) while neutral vertebra is defined by rotation.

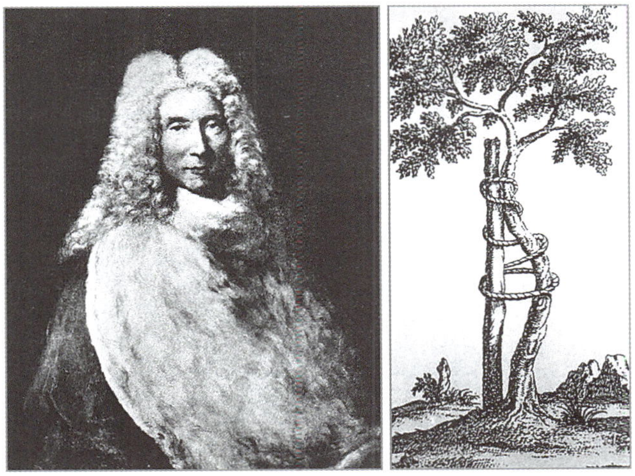

Fig. 9: Nicolas Andry and Andry's tree (see text).

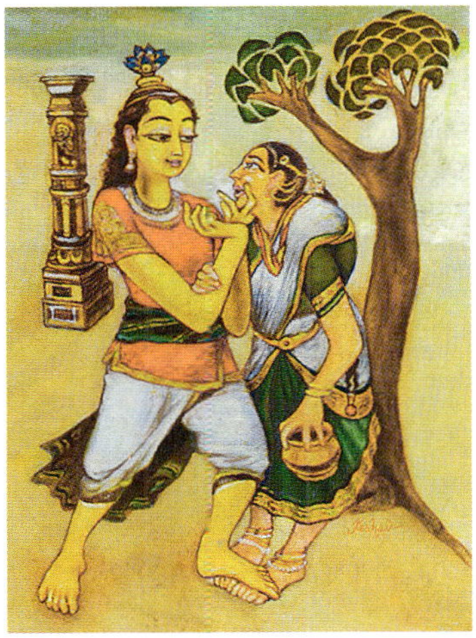

Fig. 10: Correction of scoliosis of Kubja by Lord Krishna as depicted in Hindu mythology. He used axial traction according to the descriptions (that may be incomplete though!).

Lord Krishna presses his toes on her feet and placed a finger of both his hands under her chin and raises the fingers, which straightened her body, finally turning her into a beautiful woman. "Kubja" (having crooked spine) is also mentioned as the reincarnation of "Surpanakha" (having "crooked nose" from Ramayana) possibly continuing the "genetic" element of deformity! Even "Manthara" the maid to "Kaikai" is said to have a crooked back just like her thinking.

Hippocrates (400 BC) postulated postural and muscular theories of scoliosis and used primarily spinal manipulation for the correction of deformity. He used a traction table called "scamnum" **(Fig. 11)** that was used with various modifications by medical practitioners later. Hippocrates also mentioned lesser used method of succussion **(Fig. 12)** for correction of deformity where the patient was tied upside down to a ladder and then dropped from height.

Ambroise Paré was the first person to treat scoliosis with braces and also noted that they are useless once the patient reaches skeletal maturity. He postulated the postural theory for scoliosis.

Jacques Mathieu Delpech devised graded exercises for strengthening muscles of the trunk to correct deformity considering it to develop due to muscular weakness.

Scoliosis is also credited with introduction of the "open criticism to scientific literature" in the form of famous Guerin versus Malgaigne trial. Guerin published his results of subcutaneous tenotomy and myotomy for correction of scoliosis in 1839 that was described by Malgaigne as "some orthopedic illusion". A defamation trial ensued that ended in Malgaigne's favor setting the precedence to criticize scientific literature if it is controversial or untrue!

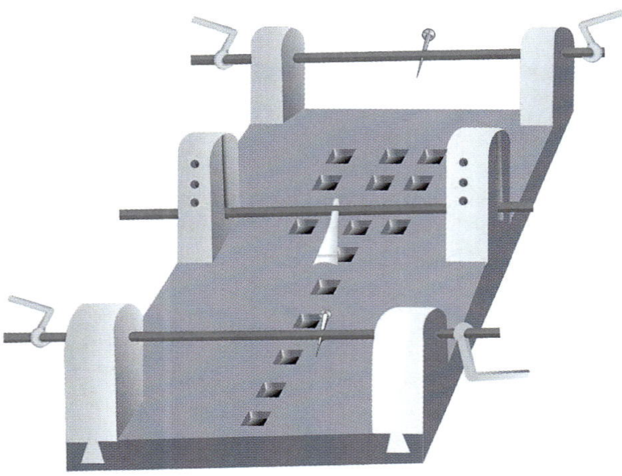

Fig. 11: Hippocrates scamnum: Traction machine to correct scoliotic curves. He also seemed to have used lateral corrective forces.

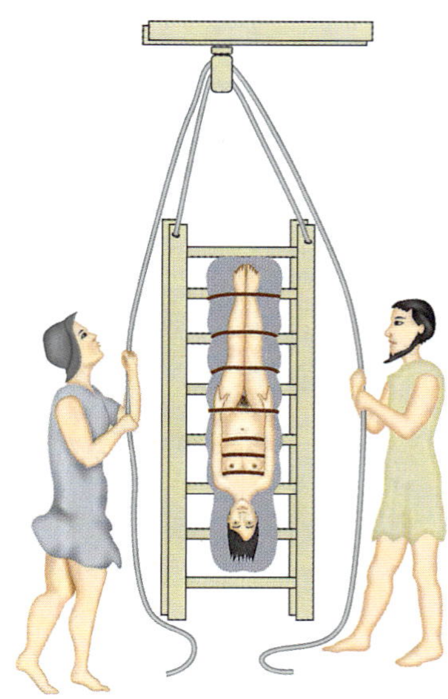

Fig. 12: Succussion method: Tying the patient on a straight board upside down.

Sayre popularized the cast treatment for scoliosis in the form of jackets.

Russell Hibbs is credited with the first surgical procedure done for treatment of scoliosis in the form of posterior fusion.

Harrington began the era of instrumentation for scoliosis that is still evolving.

IDIOPATHIC SCOLIOSIS

The term idiopathic was introduced by Bower in mid-1900s. Idiopathic scoliosis is unique as it occurs exclusively in humans. In other vertebrates, it is either congenital, cicatricial, neuromuscular or experimentally induced. As mentioned earlier because the cause of idiopathic scoliosis is not known, its diagnosis is not made until all other causes of scoliosis have been excluded. Idiopathic scoliosis has a familial tendency (pointing to genetic association still to be elucidated fully) and has a bimodal frequency distribution. The majority of the cases are seen during the adolescence while there is also an early small peak. The idiopathic is hence classified by Scoliosis Research Society into three varieties (initially used by JIP James) based on age of onset:

1. *Infantile scoliosis:* 0–3 years
2. *Juvenile scoliosis:* 3–9 years
3. *Adolescent scoliosis (most common):* Older than 9 years of age.

Infantile and juvenile are possibly not true idiopathic as in majority some or other congenital anomaly has been identified. Only a few cases do represent true idiopathic infantile or juvenile variety so few authors discard the use of these terms and only consider adolescent idiopathic scoliosis (AIS) as the true idiopathic variety. Early-onset variety in which a curvature develops before the age of 8–9 years is uncommon compared to adolescent scoliosis but has a poorer prognosis primarily because curvature progression is related to growth potential (rule of thumb for all types of scoliosis). Thus, the younger the age of onset of spinal curve the larger is the deformity at maturity. Taking this basic rule deformities developing in children before the age of 5 years have the potential of even exceeding 100° in magnitude. These curves compromise the developing cardiopulmonary system and also negatively influence the psychological development of the child. Early intervention is hence recommended.

ADOLESCENT IDIOPATHIC SCOLIOSIS

This is the most common variety and typically affects girls. Boys are affected 10 times less commonly than girls (for small curves the sex distribution is similar but larger curves are 8–10 times more common in females). The prevalence of AIS varies depending on the magnitude of the curvature used for the diagnostic criterion. For a minimum curve value of 10° it has been found that 2–3% of the adolescent population (10–16 years of age) has scoliosis. The prevalence for curves in excess of 20° is 0.3–0.5%, whereas that of curves in excess of 40° is fortunately only 0.1%. A typical curve of AIS is a right-sided thoracic curve with an accompanying functional left-sided lumbar curve. The etiology of AIS has not been elucidated; however, several theories have been studied and developed. At present, the general consensus is that the etiology of idiopathic scoliosis is multifactorial.

- ***Genetics:*** This is the most widely accepted factor presently is genetic association for which most frantic search is on and recently a DNA test has also been launched.
  - Autosomal dominant or multiple gene inheritance pattern is being pointed but not reaffirmed due to variable penetrance and genetic heterogeneity.
  - A definite familial predisposition.
  - Concordance rate in monozygous twins of 73%.
  - Using linkage analysis the possible chromosomes have been identified at 10 and 6 (primarily) and possibly at also 9, 16, and 17.
  - Using genome wide association study the Japanese investigators have found the locus at 6q24.1 in Japanese. The association is primarily located to *GPR126* (encoding G protein-coupled receptor 126). *GPR126* plays a role in human height and trunk length and is highly expressed in cartilage. Its suppression leads to delayed growth and bone tissue formation in the developing spine.
  - Other genes found to be associated with AIS include:
    - *SNTG1* (gamma-1-syntrophin) in 8q11.22
    - *ESR1* (estrogen receptor-1) in 6q25.1
    - *CHD7* (chromodin helicase DNA binding protein 7) in 8q12.1
    - *MTNR1B* in 11q21-q22—single nucleotide polymorphism at the Matrilin receptor level caused idiopathic scoliosis
- ***Effect of connective tissue:***
  - An abnormal collagen/proteoglycan ratio of the intervertebral disks has been found.
  - Elastic fiber abnormalities have been demonstrated in patients with AIS.
- ***Biomechanical spinal growth modulation:*** As mentioned earlier that idiopathic scoliosis is unique to humans and the fact that only we regularly have an erect posture, there is a prominent logic to support biomechanical mechanism (that may be facilitated by genetics or vice versa). Spine should be understood in three-dimension (3D). In the median plane, there are two symmetrical curves—the cervical and lumbar lordosis and sacral and thoracic kyphosis. ***L***ateral curvature in the coronal plane considered pathognomonic of scoliosis *is* actually a product of lordosis plus rotation (Adams). The rule of thumb is that the vertebral rotation occurs in scoliosis and kyphosis both but the bodies always rotate toward the same side in scoliosis (spinous processes rotated toward the concavity) while in kyphosis the bodies rotate toward the opposite side (spinous processes toward convexity). These changes cannot occur of its own as rotation takes a great deal of abnormal forces than bending. Growth modulation (genetic) or importantly by environmental and mechanical pull of muscles, etc., most likely influence the curve progression.
  - Typical thoracic vertebrae only extend from T3 to T9. Rest either resemble the cervical or the lumbar vertebrae.
  - Cervical and lumbar rotational instability is countered largely by the shape of vertebral bodies (increased lateral to anteroposterior width), while in thoracic region the poor heart like shape is vulnerable to rotational forces so additional stability is conferred by a kyphotic curve and rib cage. Still only a mild lordosis or lordotic deformity is enough to cause the spine to rotate to side.
  - The spine has to be symmetric also in transverse plane and not just median plane to balance rotational forces. This concept of *"biplanar symmetry"* explains the development of scoliosis **(Figs. 13A and B)**. Because the lateral profile in not disturbed in nonstructural scoliosis (no rotation) so the lateral curves do not increase with flexion with accommodation of the vertebral bodies anteriorly. While in structural scoliosis due to lateral rotation and reduction in the anterior length with flexion the vertebral bodies rotate still more laterally increasing the "lateral" or apical deformity.
- ***Muscular pathology and mechanisms:*** The changes in muscle fibers that have been identified may reflect secondary changes rather than primary pathology.
  - A decrease has been seen in type II (fast twitch) fibers in the paraspinous muscles, while some found normal fibers on the convexity but low frequency of type I (slow twitch) fibers on the concavity.
  - A decrease has been also found in the muscle spindles of the paraspinous muscles.
  - *Muscle contractile mechanisms:* The contractile systems (actin and myosin) of platelets and muscle

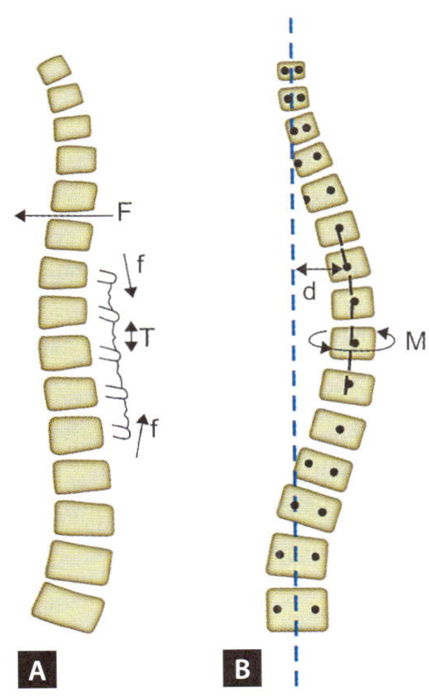

Figs. 13A and B: Simplified theoretical model of biplanar spinal asymmetry (see text). Lateral profile with lower thoracic lordosis (A): anteroposterior view of coronal plane asymmetry (B). (F = force of forward flexion; T = tightening of posterior structures, f = reactive force; d = distance of coronal plane asymmetry from midline; M = spinning moment)

are similar and are partially regulated by calmodulin. Calmodulin is the secondary indicator for melatonin and has an impact on muscle contraction.

- *Systemic melatonin-signaling pathway dysfunction:* Platelet calmodulin levels are higher in progressive curves. This is due primarily to low response to circulating melatonins. Higher calmodulin levels have been observed in progressive curves.
- *Systemic melatonin deficiency:* Melatonin (the antagonist of calmodulin) is lower in progressive curves.
- Higher levels of calmodulin are detected in the muscles on the convex side compared to the concave side in AIS
- Systemic platelet calmodulin dysfunction
- Osteopontin and soluble CD44 receptor dysfunction
- Contractile mechanisms have been studied in pinealectomized rats (produces decreased melatonin levels).

▪ ***Neurological abnormalities:***

- There is inconsistent data on presence of neurological abnormalities such as abnormalities of visual, vestibular, proprioceptive and postural control involving the brain stem, cerebral hemispheres and corpus callosum (Impaired peripheral, visual and spatial proprioception) producing pathological spinal curvature.
- Primary pathology in the hind brain causing a defect of central control, or processing in the central nervous system (CNS) that affects a normal growing spine has also been proposed as a causative mechanism. The four primary concepts for neurological abnormalities explaining development of AIS are:
  1. Visuospatial perceptual impairment producing a motor control problem
  2. Body-spatial orientation concept
  3. Neurodevelopmental concept
  4. Sensory integration disorder.

▪ ***Relative anterior spinal overgrowth (RASO theory):*** Hypokyphosis has been seen in AIS. It may be a result of imbalance of anterior and posterior growth. The theory explains the development of right-sided AIS but not the left-sided one.

- The overgrowth of vertebral bodies compared to posterior elements is partially explained by the enhancing effect of sympathetic nervous system on vertebral bodies producing RASO. This leads to cascading increasing defect and curve progression by virtue of "Hueter-Volkmann principle".

▪ ***The escalator concept (double neuro-osseous theory):*** This delves in the interaction between the growing skeleton and postural mechanisms of the maturing somatic nervous system. According to this concept AIS progression is dependent on the rapid skeletal enlargement that produces skeletal sizes for age beyond the capacity of postural mechanisms of the somatic nervous system to control the initiating deformity **(Figs. 14A and B)**.

- *Osseous escalator:* Increasing skeletal size and shape through posture and motion create ever-changing proprioceptive and visiospatial inputs.
- *Neural escalator and posture:* Central nervous system continuously calibrates itself with the osseous escalator specifically the posterior parietal cortex (area 7). This is modulated by Leptin that enhances N-methyl-D-aspartate (NMDA) receptors, increased leptin may explain the reduced gray matter in certain brain areas in obese subjects.

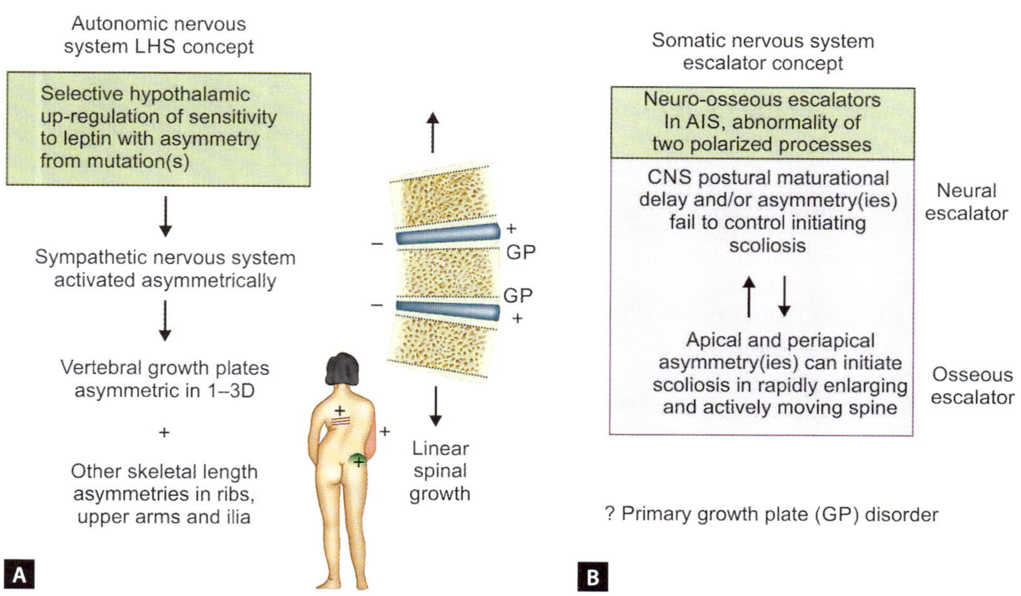

Figs. 14A and B: Double neuro-osseous theory for the pathogenesis of AIS in girls. (A) Autonomic [leptin-hypothalamic-sympathetic nervous system (LHS concept)]; (B) Somatic (escalator concept)

Thus the spine continues to grow rapidly with asymmetry while there is CNS postural maturation delay.

- ***Role of growth and development:*** Patients with scoliosis are taller with less kyphosis (especially right-sided curves).
    - Accelerated spinal growth starts earlier when compared with controls.

Clinical Features

Pain

It occurs in 30% of patients with AIS but is never bothering or prominent (virtually AIS has been described as a painless condition). Pain often arises due to associated muscular weakness, spasm due to imbalance or stretching of ligaments due to rapid change in curve. Uncharacteristic pain (awakens from sleep, continuous, radiating, or severe) should raise suspicion of other pathology that should be investigated. Nonstructural causes of scoliosis—tumor, infection and herniated disk are often painful.

Age at Onset

Patients may present symptoms in the adolescent period; however, they may have had earlier onset. It is important to determine the etiology—it may be juvenile or infantile onset. The presence of an important thoracic deformity before the age of 5 years increases the risk of altered pulmonary function and secondarily, cardiac function (cor pulmonale). Dickson opines that early onset scoliosis be considered between 0 and 5 years while late onset scoliosis is in patients older than 5 years of age. Shufflebarger for therapeutic reasons considers early onset scoliosis and late onset scoliosis be differentiated at 10 years as cut-point. Age of parents should be noted for Down's syndrome.

Growth Potential

Important to understand and plan for curve progression during growth spurts. Girls' peak growth occurs from 11 to 12 years; boys peak from 13 to 14 years. In girls, the menarcheal status is also important as the premenarcheal girls are the greater risk for progression and may crankshaft following posterior—only surgery.

Symptoms of spinal pathology (possible neuromuscular cause):

- Gait
- Coordination
- Bowel and bladder function and specifically late-onset bed-wetting.

Family history: Charcot-Marie-Tooth disease, Friedrich's ataxia, Marfan's syndrome, neurofibromatosis.

Physical Examination and Diagnosis

Assessment of Deformity

The extent of spinal curvature generally guides the treatment. The extent of spinal curvature and angle of trunk rotation (ATR) determine the severity of scoliosis. Spinal curvature and the ATR are generally correlated—a person with a spinal curve of 20° usually has an ATR of 5°.

Standing examination

- *Coronal imbalance assessment:* Plumb line to judge balance of curve
- *Coronal curve assessment:* Thoracic/thoracolumbar/lumbar curve with convexity to right/left side
- *Shoulder height or asymmetry:*
    - Raised shoulder on the convex side in thoracic curves (affected side), on concave side in lumbar curves.
    - Scapula rotated outward and forward with elevation on convex side:
        - Forward protrusion of chest wall on affected
        - Increased flank creases on opposite (concave side)
        - Higher anterior superior iliac spines (ASIS) and posterior superior iliac spines (PSIS) on concave side.

Adams forward bend test: This offers reasonable rotational deformity assessment of the upper thoracic, thoracic and thoracolumbar or lumbar curves. The patient bends at the waist with knees straight and the feet together until the trunk is at 90° and the arms dangling forward **(Figs. 15A to C)**.

- Assessment for symmetry of movement with flexion (absence of list to one side may denote nonidiopathic scoliosis)
- More prominence of structural curve on convex side with hump (rib hump in thoracic and thoracolumbar curves), partial/complete correction of compensatory curves or nonstructural scoliosis
- The spurious appearance of a kyphosis when the patient is viewed from the side is the scoliosis seen in a plane which is more an anteroposterior projection of the apex of the curve than an AP projection of the patient or specimen, compounded to a lesser extent by the deceptive rib hump.
- The test is not sensitive for lower curves occurring in lumbar region and hence misses 15% of scoliosis.

Flexibility testing (flexible/rigid curve)

- Forward bending
- Pushing the curve from convex side and noting the correction
- Lifting the patient up from head

Measurements

- Distance of plumb line from center (midline)
- Iliocostal distance reduced on concave side
- Ilio-occipital distance reduced on the side of decompensation (under correction)—often to the side of convexity
- Wasting in limbs
- Limb length inequality.

Neurologic Examination

- *Motor and sensory examination:* Usually intact even with intracanal pathology.
- *Deep tendon reflexes:* Knees and ankles.

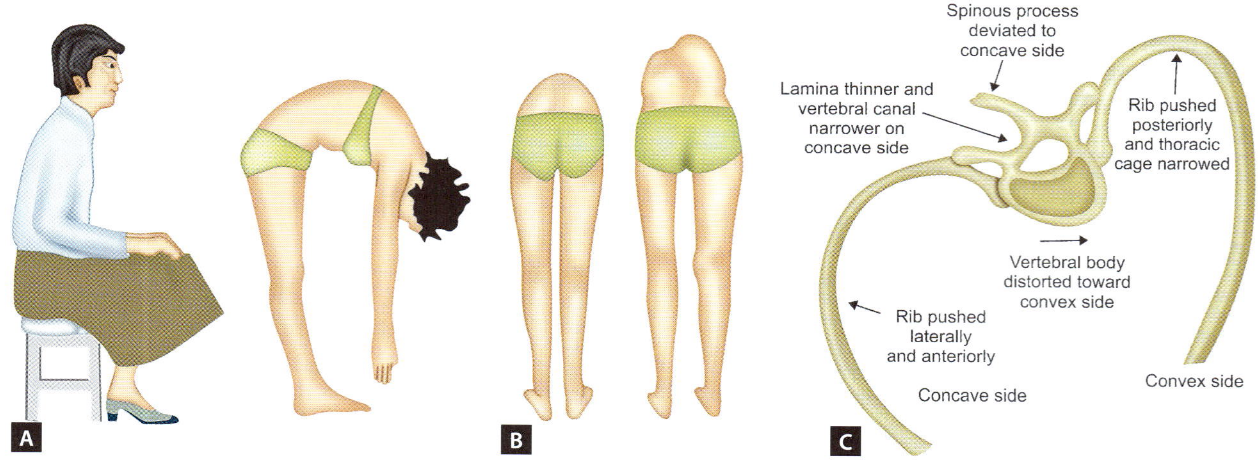

Figs. 15A to C: Adams forward bend test. (A and B) The examiner should be sitting so that his eyeline (A) is at the level of deformity for not missing subtle deformities (B); (C) The pathoanatomy of development of rib hump, this appears as "razor back" in advanced cases when a number of ribs are sharply angulated.

- Romberg's test for balance or proprioception
- *Abdominal reflexes:*
  - A lateral-to-medial gentle stroke of the abdomen, which elicits movement of the umbilicus
  - Should be symmetric (absent or present)
  - If asymmetric, then high correlation with neural axis pathology (syringomyelia, tethered cord) and is an indication to obtain magnetic resonance imaging (MRI).

Other Examination

- *Lower extremities:* Hip examination for fixed deformities and a quick look at knee and foot/ankle deformities, ensure no asymmetry in leg circumference, size, or length, (limb length discrepancy). Look for asymmetric foot deformities (intracanal pathology)
- Ober's test
- Gait pattern
- *Midline defects [possible neuromuscular scoliosis (NMS)]:*
  - Hairy patch
  - Swelling/mass
  - Port wine patch (Nevi)/Café-au-lait spots
  - Skin dimples
- *Congenital malformations (possible congenital scoliosis):*
  - Skull deformities
  - Cleft lip/palate
  - Mandibular hypoplasia/small chin
  - Tapering/small ears
  - Malformations of limbs
  - Transverse/longitudinal defects
- Tanner staging to estimate remaining growth.

Screening of scoliotic deformity: Screening for spinal curvature is quite strictly followed abroad but not so prominent in India. The screening programs started somewhere in 1940s and girls are screened twice, at ages 10 years and 12 years, and that boys be screened once at 13 years or 14 years. This schedule has been found to miss 40% of cases! So modified schedule to screen at ages 10, 12, 14 and 16 years is recommended by American Academy of Pediatrics (AAP). Adams forward-bending test (in conjunction with the use of a scoliometer/inclinometer) has been found to be an effective screening tool **(Fig. 16)**. Patients often referred from school screening where a 7° curve on scoliometer (measures ATR) during Adams forward bending test is considered abnormal. 7° correlates with around 30° coronal plane curve. There is an error of 10° in Cobb's angle measurement and an error of 2° in scoliometer so though a scoliometer reading of 7° ATR actually correlates with 30° of coronal curve it may be 5° and too many patients with benign curves may be referred if a cut-off of 5° is chosen. Curves 30° and more are taken as an end-point to intervene (brace or operate). So to prevent underreporting and miss cases, 7° is taken as cut-off for scoliometer reading.

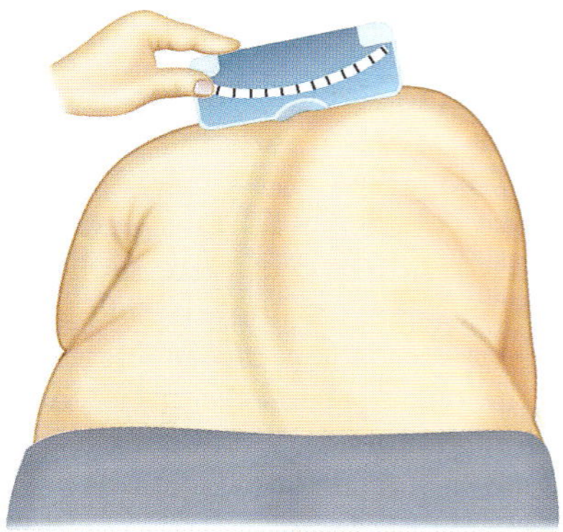

Fig. 16: Scoliometer use for screening scoliosis.

Cons of screening

- Tests are inaccurate and depend on examiner
- Over-referrals are very common burdening the health care system
- Early treatment may not have improved outcome (this statement is dicey and possibly curves intervened at 30°

do respond better). Experts state that as all curves are not destined to progress so too much overtreatment results.

Pros of screening

- Screening may provide data on knowledge of its cause and ways to prevent it.
- Bracing has been proven to be effective now for management of early cases.
- Without screening children are often missed as they do not have painful curves. Physicians do not even look at the back of children.
- Screening would be cost-effective if reasonable guidelines are setup so that over referral is prevented.
  - Scoliometer reading of 5° corresponding to 20° of coronal curve may be screened yearly as 80% do not progress
  - Curves between 20° and 30° will need screening every 6 months
  - Curves at 30° will be referred.

Radiographic Examination

This is important for the following purposes:

- Document severity—curvature and rotation
- Determine skeletal maturity—Risser's sign and Greulich and Pyle atlas
- Structural versus nonstructural (supine bending films)
- Evaluate for associated spondylolysis, listhesis, etc.
- Monitor progression
- Evaluate nonidiopathic causes of scoliosis (systemic pathology, spinal lesions, etc.)
- Ensure adequacy of bracing.

Posteroanterior-Anterior Standing (AP was previously used)

Contoured filter is used to balance higher density of abdomen and pelvis to lower density of thorax. High-speed films (to reduce exposure time) and rare earth screens (intensifying screens) are better. Shield breast and gonads and use collimation. For standardization all upright films are taken at a distance of 6 feet.

Remember: In contrast to reading other radiographs, spinal films for assessing deformity are conventionally viewed as if looking the patient from back so that the patient's right side is on viewer's right side! Measure upper thoracic, thoracic, and thoracolumbar or lumbar curves [Cobb's method (preferable, **Fig. 17**) or Ferguson method, **Fig. 18**]—universal standard for measuring the degree of curvature:

- *Cobb's method* ***(Figs. 17 and 19)****:* Identify end vertebrae (pedicle levels with greatest tilt from the horizontal plane)—construct lines along the superior endplate of highest vertebrae and inferior endplate of lowest vertebrae. Draw perpendicular lines to them. Determine angles.
- Determine the deviation **(Figs. 20A and B)** of C7 plumb line from the CSVL.
- *The apical rib vertebra relationship and the rib-vertebral angle difference (RVAD):* This is a useful parameter for evaluation of infantile scoliosis. It was first described by

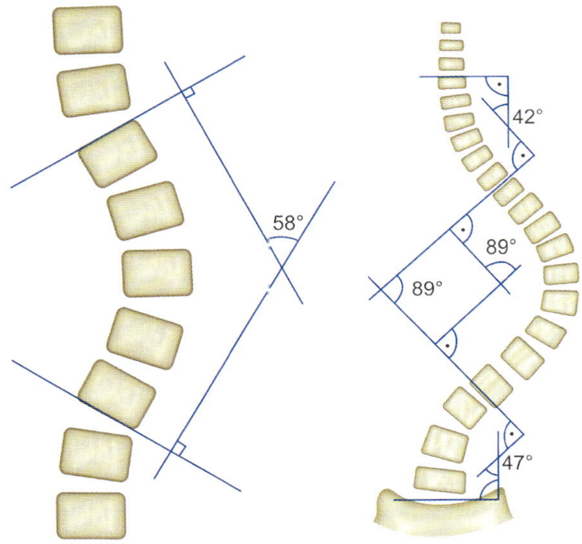

Fig. 17: Cobb's method of measuring curve(s).

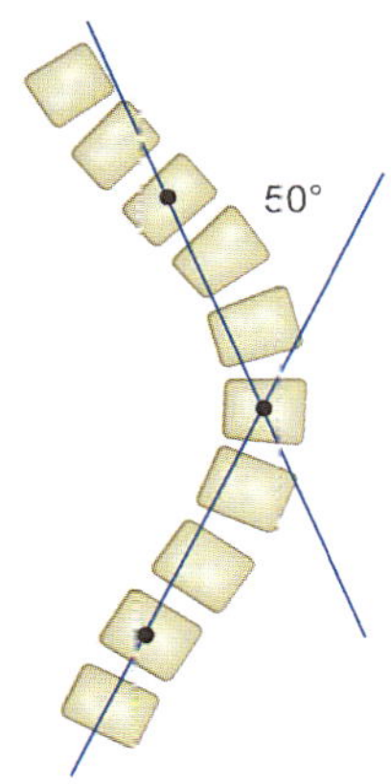

Fig. 18: Risser Ferguson method for measuring spinal curvature in coronal plane.

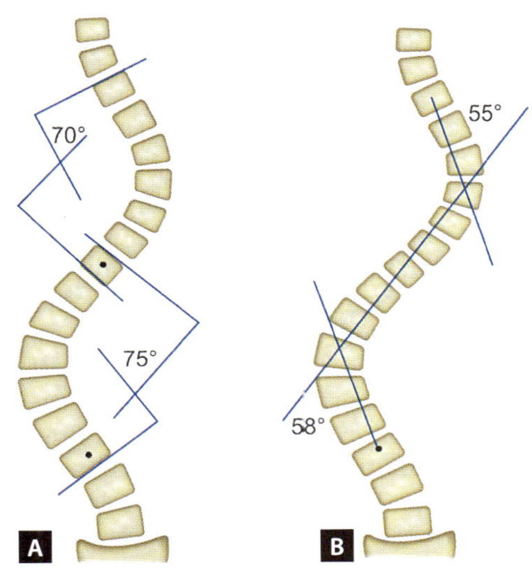

Figs. 19A and B: Comparative Cobb's (A) and Ferguson's method (B). Both the methods are good independently but the magnitude of curve varies by measurements. One should stick to their method once chosen (in the chapter, we have followed Cobb's method and recommendations are based on Cobb's measurement throughout where not mentioned).

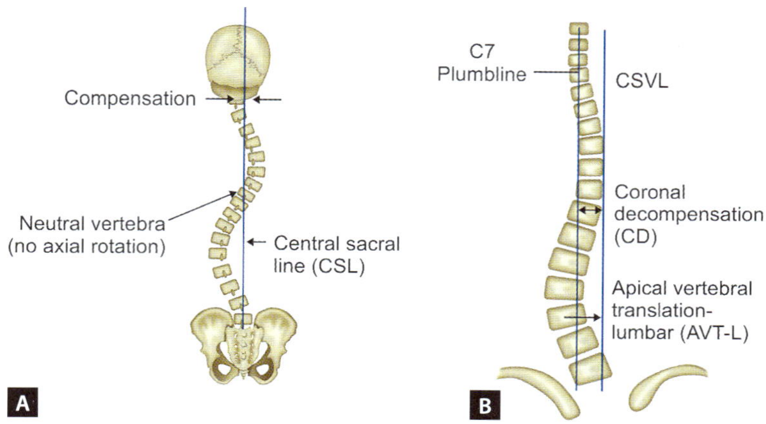

Figs. 20A and B: Coronal decompensation is assessed by drawing central sacral vertebral line (CSVL). The CSVL is perpendicular to a horizontal line across the iliac crest, passing vertically through the sacral spinous processes. Vertebrae bisected by the center sacral line are designated as the stable vertebrae. There is no stable vertebra in the Figure (A), had there been a compensatory thoracic curve, there would have developed a stable vertebra at the transition of the two curves that would also be most likely neutral vertebra (B).

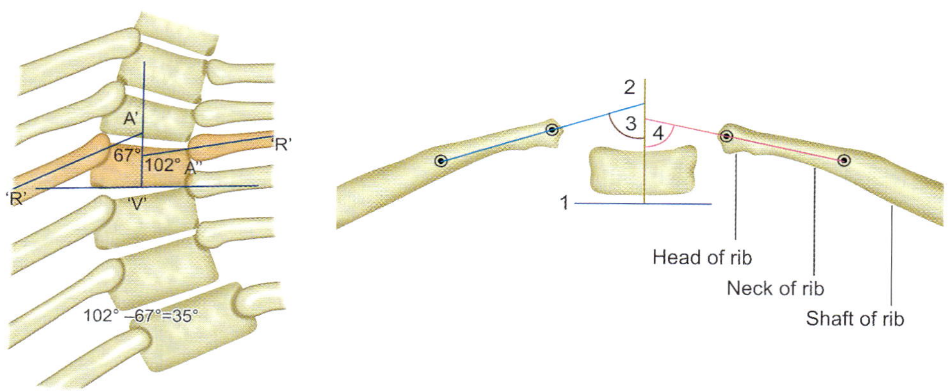

Fig. 21: Rib-vertebral angle difference.

Dr Min H Mehta who identified two primary radiographic findings that were useful for distinguishing resolving from progressive idiopathic infantile scoliosis curves on serial radiographs: the apical rib-vertebra relationship and the RVAD. These characteristics are measured on supine AP radiographs of the curve. In resolving or early progressive scoliosis, the rib head does not overlap the vertebral body, whereas in progressive curve the rib head on the convex side of the spine overlaps the apical vertebral body. Rib-vertebral angle is formed by the intersection of a line perpendicular to apical vertebral endplate and another line through middle of the corresponding rib. RVAD is the difference in values of angles on the convex from concave sides of the curve.

- Dr Mehta indicated that in 83% of the resolving curves the RVAD was less than 20°. If initial RVAD is greater than 20° then it indicates progressive curve until proven otherwise. These findings are supported by other investigators also.
- How to draw RVAD **(Fig. 21)**:
  1. Draw a line parallel to the bottom of apical vertebra
  2. Draw a line perpendicular to above line at its mid-point
  3. Join the midpoints of head and neck of the adjacent ribs to make central line of ribs on the concave side
  4. The angle formed by the intersection of the rib central line (step 3) and the perpendicular to apical vertebral line (step 2) is the RVA'
  5. Repeat the steps 2–4 for other side rib and find the RVA" for other side
  6. RVAD = RVA' – RVA".

- *Trunk shift:* Deviation of the mid-distance of the rib margins to CSVL.
- *Vertebral rotation* ***(Table 2)****:* As a curve increases the vertebrae rotate **(Fig. 22)**.
  - Spinous process deviates toward the concave side
  - Vertebral body rotates toward the convex side
  - Ribs become closer together on the concave side and separated on the convex side
  - Nash and Moe system **(Fig. 23)**.
- *Risser staging:* This is based on the ossification of the iliac apophysis that begins laterally (at the anterior superior iliac spine) and progresses posteromedially (towards the posterior superior iliac spine) to eventually cap the entire iliac crest **(Fig. 24)**.

TABLE 2: Vertebral rotation: The Nash and Moe method (*see* **Fig. 23**).

0 (Neutral)	Pedicle shadows are equal distance from the sides of the vertebral body
Grade 1+	"Pedicle shadow on the convexity has moved from the edge of the vertebral body". The convex pedicle migrates within first segment while the one on concave side may start disappearing
Grade 2+	Intermediate between grade 1 and 3. The convex pedicle migrates to second segment. The concave pedicle gradually disappears
Grade 3+	Pedicle shadow is in the middle of vertebral body. Convex pedicle migrates to middle segment. Concave pedicle is not visible
Grade 4+	Convex pedicle shadow is past middle of the vertebral body. Concave pedicle is not visible

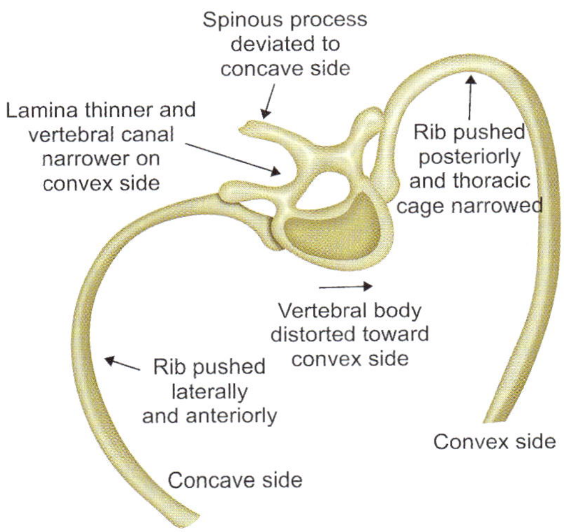

Fig. 22: Pathoanatomy of adolescent idiopathic scoliosis (AIS).

- Risser 1–5 used as measure of skeletal maturity and therefore to predict progressive of scoliosis.
- Incidence of curve progression is higher with Risser 0–1 compared to Risser 2 or more.
- Status of triradiate cartilage (acetabular physis)—open or closed.

Lateral Radiograph

- Measure thoracic kyphosis and lumbar lordosis (Cobb's method)
- Helps to locate Junctional kyphosis
  - Between the structural upper thoracic and middle thoracic curves
  - Between the structural middle thoracic and the thoracolumbar or lumbar curves
- Sagittal balance can be assessed only on lateral radiographs

  C7 plumb normally falls at the posterior edge of L5-S1

The stereoradiographic measurements of the spinal curves (3D assessment) are used for analysis the Cobb's angle, the apical vertebra, the axial rotation of the apical vertebra and the orientation of the apical vertebra in relation to the sagittal plane.

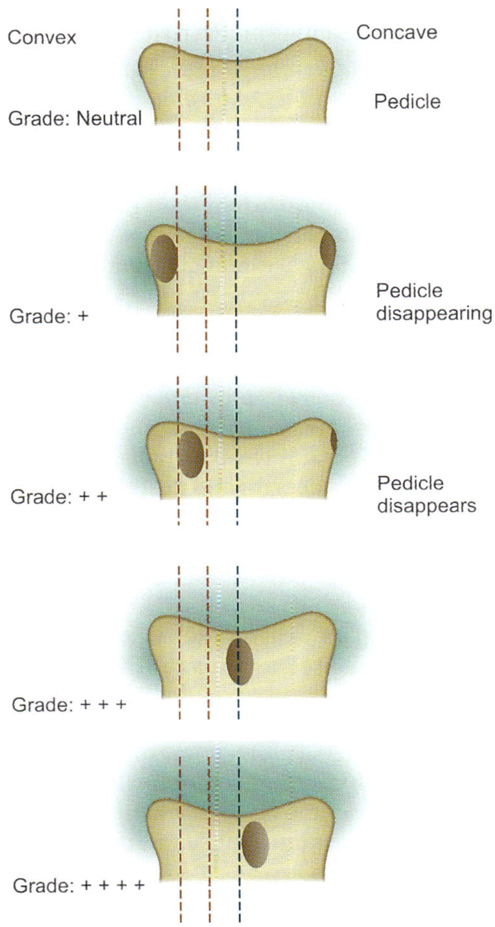

Fig. 23: Rotation of vertebra (Nash and Moe)—each half of vertebral body is divided into three segments and relative location of convex side pedicle noted with respect to it.

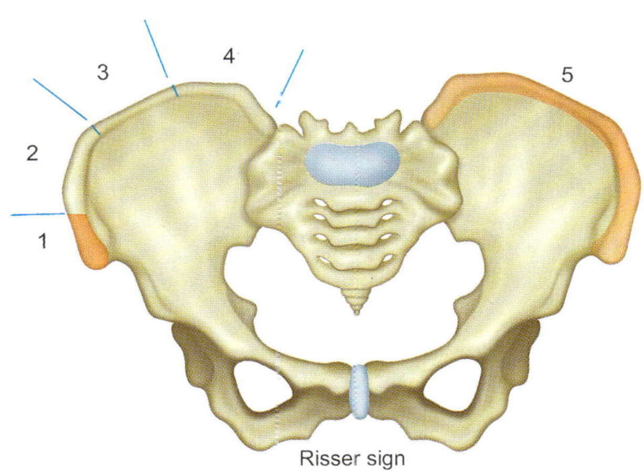

Fig. 24: The Risser stage of iliac ossification can be used to estimate remaining maturity and growth. Risser 1–4 takes around 2 years.

Bend Films

Supine bending films are important to understanding of purpose while evaluating the scoliotic spine.

- They help to determine the curve type—more than 25° is structural as described in Lenke system
- Determine the flexibility index (fI) for each curve:

$$Fl = \frac{(\text{PA radiograph Cobb's angle} - \text{Bend film Cobb's angle})}{\text{PA radiograph Cobb's angle}} \times 100$$

- *Determine fusion levels in the lumbar spine:*
    - Bend films help ascertain the flexibility of the disk below the distal fusion vertebra with which one can determine the distal extent of fusion
    - With bending films one can plan the distal fusion level to center over the sacrum.

Types of bend films:

- *Supine anteroposterior best-effort bend* **(Fig. 25A)**: This is the most commonly used method being easy to incorporate and obtain. The patient here lies supine on a table and bends to the right and the left.
- *Push-prone test:* Patient lies prone and the examiner pushes medially and anteriorly on the rotational prominence to judge passive correction.
- *Fulcrum bend film* **(Fig. 25B)**:
    - Patient lies in a lateral position with the apex of curve on a large roll used as a fulcrum to bend straighten the curve
- *Traction films:* The patient lies supine and manual traction is applied (more commonly) to judge the correction of curves (and rotation with traction). In a way, it also assesses the flexibility of the curves. Standing patient can have traction applied through halter traction.

Magnetic Resonance Imaging

Routine use of MRI is done in evaluating the children below 11 years of age to rule-out spinal pathology. The imaging is done from brainstem to sacrum. As a standard T1-weighted images ± Gadolinium (use especially for cord neoplasms or infection) is used. MRI is the investigation of choice for assessment of spinal canal contents and evaluation of soft tissue in the paraspinal area. Pathologies such as tumor, syrinx, neurofibromatosis, cord compression, atrophy, Chiari malformations, cord tethering, syringomyelia, diastematomyelia, spinal dysraphism, etc., are best evaluated with MRI.

Absolute indications for MRI:

- Presence of neurologic abnormalities
- Juvenile and infantile onset scoliosis
- Congenital vertebral abnormalities identified on radiographs
- Cutaneous manifestations of dysraphism (see above in examination)

Relative indications:

- Unusual curve pattern, i.e., left thoracic curve or thoracic kyphosis
- Very rapidly progressing curve
- Painful scoliosis
- Neck stiffness and headache.

Bone Scan

This is a useful investigation for identification of benign tumors (osteoid osteoma, osteoblastoma), metastasis to spine, osteomyelitis and stress fractures. It is indicated in painful scoliosis without known etiology. Technetium-99 labeled polyphosphonates are used to demonstrate areas of increased local blood flow and metabolic activity indicating the lesion as a "hot spot".

Noncontrast Computed Tomography Spine

This is used for preoperative evaluation of vertebral deformities that are associated with:

- Congenital scoliosis
- Dysraphism
- Diastematomyelia
- Meningomyelocele.

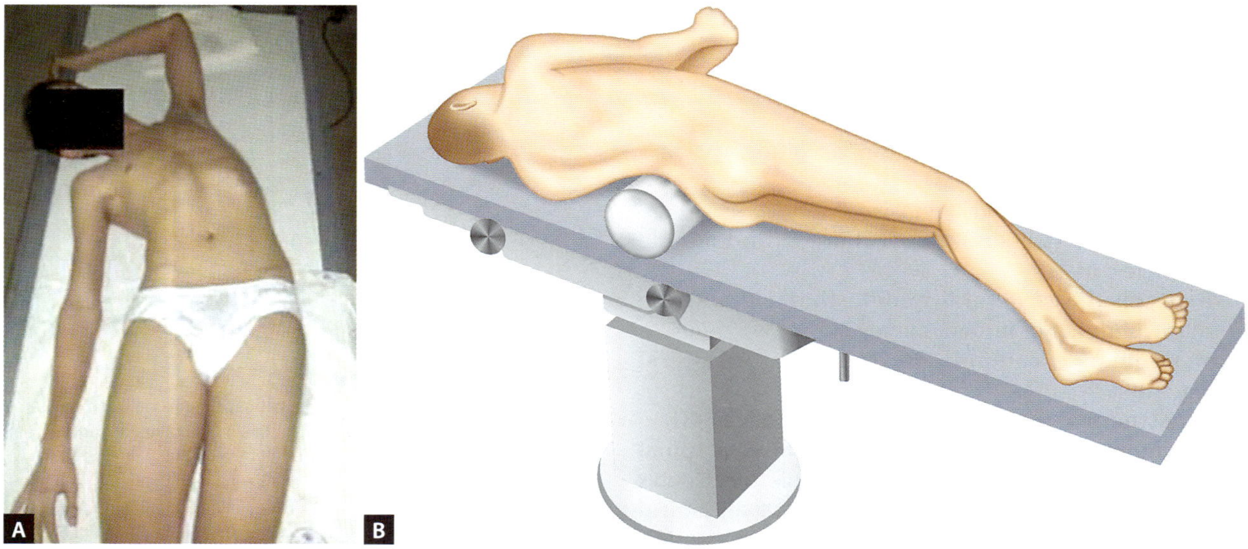

Figs. 25A and B: Bend film: (A) Supine bend film; (B) Fulcrum bend film.

It is indicated in known or suspected vertebral pathology. It is indicated in bone tumor cases to localize lesion and for planning surgery.

Natural History

Curves greater than 10° have prevalence of 2–3% in the adolescent population, of which 5% will demonstrate progression greater than 30°. There must be 5–10° (there is a measurement error of 4–8° using the Cobb's method, so 10° is a reasonable value) increase in the curves to *define progression*. Before planning treatment curve magnitude and remaining growth potential should be adjudged. The following points suffice the concept:

- Maturation can be assessed by the Risser's sign and the shape of the distal phalanx epiphysis—70% of the patients with Risser's sign 0, and curves of 20–30° progress 5° or more (Bunnell and Lonstein).
- Peak height velocity in girls should particularly be taken into account (period 6 months before menarche in girls). Progression in scoliosis is the fastest during this time. The peak growth velocity terminates with the menarche and growth decelerates gradually following this period.
- Large curves (30–40°) progress more than the minor curves (20–29°).
    - Curves greater than 25° before skeletal maturity will continue to progress
    - Curves greater than 50° thoracic curve will progress 1–2°/year
    - Curves greater than 40° lumbar curve will progress 1–2 /year
- Double curves progress more than single curves. Thoracic curves are more likely to progress that lumbar curves that are least progression is in the curves in the lumbar region.
- Curves greater than 80–90° are associated with cardiopulmonary dysfunction, early death, pain and decreased self-image
- The curve progression rate in girls is higher than that in the boys.

Risk factors for progression: During adolescence, curves typically progress a mean of 1°/month, and curves in excess of 50° are associated with a high risk of progression even after skeletal maturity.

- *Sex:* Girls have higher chances of curve progression.
- *Age:* Skeletal immaturity (open triradiate cartilage, Risser's sign 0–1, and premenarcheal)—younger patients have higher rate of progression
- *Curve location:* Thoracic curves progress less often than lumbar curves.
- *Curve magnitude:*
    - Larger curves progress more often than smaller ones
    - At maturity, thoracic curves greater than 50° progress into adulthood
    - Thoracolumbar/lumbar curves greater than 40° progress into adulthood (especially with coronal decompensation).

Curve Classification

Aims of Classification

- Categorize the disease into different patterns
- Improve communication by providing succinct information
- Should guide us in managing the disease
- Should help us to prognosticate the outcome

Following are some of the classifications used to describe the curve types in scoliosis aiming also to provide some treatment guideline.

Ponseti Classification (Ponseti and Friedman in 1950)

- Single-curve
- Double-curve
- Triple-curve patterns

Curve types were named after the location of the curve apex. Thoracolumbar curves had the apexes at T12 to L1, thoracic curves had the apexes above and lumbar curves have the apexes below these levels. The double curves had a higher chance to progress than single curves, and thoracolumbar and lumbar curves had a higher chance to progress than thoracic curves.

King's Classification (Howard King 1983, Table 3)

It is easier and useful for communication and prognostication **(Fig. 26)**. Some surgical guidance is provided by the classification particularly if one is using Harrington system. The problem is that it does not include the double major and triple curves so the system is not comprehensive enough and had a poor to fair interobserver variability. Originally for King's type II curves it was recommended by Harrington to selectively fuse the thoracic curves only but with newer systems high incidence of lumbar decompensation was seen and so not recommended now.

Lenke et al. (2001) Classification (Fig. 27)

To complete the King's classification and improve upon the drawbacks Lenke et al. proposed this classification. This system has three components:

TABLE 3: King's classification of the scoliosis into five subgroups based on primary and secondary curves.

Type	*Primary curve*	*Secondary curve*	*Lateral bending*
I	Lumbar, crossing midline	Thoracic, crossing the midline	Lumbar curve is larger
II	Thoracic, crossing the midline	Lumbar, crossing the midline	Thoracic curve is larger
III	Thoracic	Lumbar, not crossing midline	
IV	Long thoracic	Where L5 is centered over the sacrum	
V	Double thoracic, T1 is tilted to the upper thoracic curve		

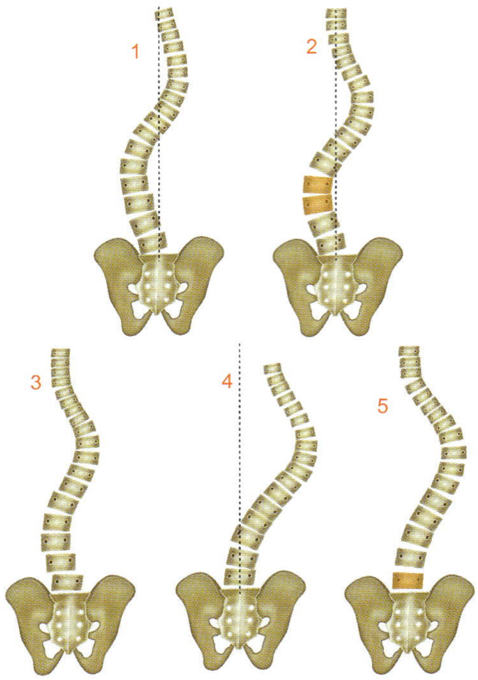

Fig. 26: King's classification of curve types (see text).

1. *Curve types (1 to 6):* Defined on both AP and lateral radiographs
   - The larger curve is always considered structural; smaller curves are structural if the patient fails to bend to less than 25°.
   - 1—Single thoracic
   - 2—Double thoracic
   - 3—Double major
   - 4—Triple major—proximal thoracic, main thoracic and thoracolumbar/lumbar curve
   - 5—Lumbar curve without thoracic curve
   - 6—Lumbar curve with compensatory thoracic curve
2. *Lumbar modifier:* Based on the relationship of CSVL to the apex of the curve
   - Based on where the CSVL falls in relation to the apical lumbar vertebra
   - A-CSVL falls between the pedicles
   - B-CSVL falls on the pedicle or lateral to the pedicle within the vertebral body
   - C-CSVL falls outside of the vertebral body.
3. *Sagittal thoracic kyphosis modifier:* Based on sagittal curve measurement from fifth to twelfth thoracic level.
   - Measured from T5 to T12
   - "–"-Kyphosis less than 10

Curve type

Type	Proximal thoracic	Main thoracic	Thoracolumbar/Lumbar	Description
1	Nonstructural	Structural (Major)*	Nonstructural	Main thoracic (MT)
2	Structural	Structural (Major)*	Nonstructural	Double thoracic (DT)
3	Nonstructural	Structural (Major)*	Structural	Double major (DM)
4	Structural	Structural (Major)*	Structural (Major)*	Triple major (TM)[5]
5	Nonstructural	Nonstructural	Structural (Major)*	Thoracolumbar/Lumbar (TL/L)
6	Nonstructural	Structural	Structural (Major)*	Thoracolumbar/Lumbar-Main thoracic (TL/L-MT)

Structural criteria
(Minor curves)

Proximal thoracic: - Side bending Cobb ≥ 25°
- T2-T5 kyphosis ≥+20°

Main thoracic: - Side bending Cobb ≥25°
- T10-L2 kyphosis ≥+20°

Thoracolumbar/lumbar: - Side bending Cobb ≥25°
- T10-L2 kyphosis ≥+20°

*Major = Largest Cobb measurement, always structural
Minor = All other curves with structural criteria applied
[5]Type 4 - MT or TL/L can be major curve

Location of apex
(SRS definition)

Curve	Apex
Thoracic	T2-T11/12 Disc
Thoracolumbar	T12-L1
Thoracolumbar/lumbar	L1/2 Disc-L4

Modifiers

Lumbar spine modifier	CSVL to lumbar apex
A	CSVL between pedicles
B	CSVL touches apical body(ies)
C	CSVL completely medial

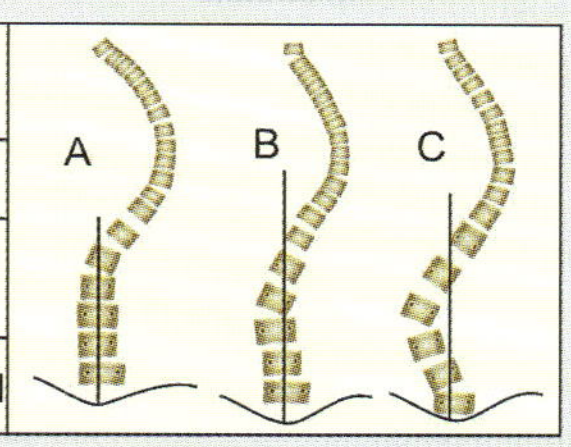

Thoracic sagittal profile T5–T12	
- (Hypo)	<10°
N (Normal)	10°–40°
+ (Hyper)	>40°

Curve type (1–6) + Lumbar spine modifier (A, B, C) + Thoracic sagittal modifier (–, N, +)
Classification (e.g. 1B+): ________

Fig. 27: Lenke system.

- "N"-Kyphosis between 10 and 40
- "+"-Kyphosis greater than 40.

Lenke system has high interobserver reliability and good results have been observed following the surgical strategy proposed by Lenke's classification.

Advantages over King's classification

- Lenke's classification is more comprehensive
- It separates the King's type 2 curves to Lenke's type 1 and type 3 curves and selective thoracic fusion is only indicated in type 1 curves.
- It addresses the sagittal alignment which was not mentioned in the King's classification.

Disadvantages

- It does not take into consideration the rotational deformity which is an important element of the 3D deformity of scoliosis.
- An important problem with this classification is that a "structural curve" is defined as a curve which is greater than 25° on side bending. Conventionally (and by SRS) a "structural curve" is defined by the presence of rotational component and not coronal plane deformity. This distinguishes it from the absence of rotation in a "nonstructural curve" (postural scoliosis). Side bending and curve change due to it actually represents the "flexibility" of the curve, possibly Lenke system confuses it with the structural character of the curve.

TABLE 4: Qiu Peking Union Medical College (PUMC) classification of idiopathic scoliosis.

Type 1: Single curve	
Subtype Ia	Thoracic curve
Subtype Ib	Thoracolumbar curve
Subtype Ic	Lumbar curve
Type II: Double curve	
Subtype IIa	Double thoracic curves
Subtype IIb	Thoracic curve plus thoracolumbar/lumbar curve, curve magnitude is >10°
Subtype IIb1	Meets criteria of no kyphosis; Cobb's angle <45°; rotation of curve <2°; flexibility of curve >70%
Subtype IIb2	Does not meet criteria
Subtype IIc	Thoracic curve plus thoracolumbar/lumbar curve, curve magnitude is <10°
Subtype IIc1	Thoracic curve is greater than thoracolumbar/lumbar curve; Cobb's angle of thoracic curve is <25°
Subtype IIc2	Thoracic curve is greater than thoracolumbar/lumbar curve; Cobb's angle of thoracic curve is >25°
Subtype IId1	Cobb's angle of the thoracic curve on convex bending X-ray is <25°
Subtype IId2	Cobb's angle of the thoracic curve on convex bending X-ray is >25°
Type III: Triple curve	
Subtype IIIa	Distal curve meets the criteria of the lumbar curve of IIb1
Subtype IIIb	Distal lumbar curve is larger and more rigid

Peking Union Medical College, Qiu et al. Classification (2005)

As it is now prominently established that scoliosis also has rotational deformity in the axial plane. A grading system for such rotational deformity was first described by Nash and Moe in 1969 **(Table 4, Fig. 28)**. The rotational deformity of scoliosis is focused by the PUMC classification (developed by surgeons at the Peking Union Medical College, China). This classification is based on:

- Location of the apexes
- Magnitude and flexibility of the scoliosis deformity
- Amount of apical vertebral rotation (AVR)
- Presence of a thoracolumbar kyphosis.

There are three main categories as type I (single curve), type II (double curve) and type III (triple curve) with a total of 13 subtypes **(Table 4)**, important ones being—

- *Single high thoracic (cervicothoracic):* It is usually a left thoracic curve that has a compensatory thoracic or thoracolumbar curve below, which can become structuralized during evolution.
  - Apex at T3 or T4
  - The superior end vertebra is usually T1 or T2, rarely C7
  - The inferior end vertebra is T7.
- *Single thoracic (most important and most frequent curve):* 95% of scoliosis cases in adolescents are right thoracic characterizing the AIS. It is frequently accompanied by a compensatory curve below that may be large enough to confuse with double major thoracic or even lumbar scoliosis. The right shoulder is elevated and the trunk is deviated to the right. It is most frequently located at T5–T12.
  - The apex is usually situated at T8 or T9
  - The superior end vertebra is between T4 and T6
  - The inferior end vertebra is between T11 and L2.
- *Single thoracolumbar:*
  - Apex at T12 or L1, or the disk between them
  - The superior end vertebra is between T8 and T10
  - The inferior end vertebra is usually L3.
- *Single lumbar*—the majority of the cases being left curves.
  - Apex at L2
  - The end vertebrae between T11–L1 and L4–L5.
- *Double major thoracic and lumbar*—has two curves of similar size and rigidity.
  - The thoracic curve is usually a right curve with the apex in T7 or T8 and the end vertebrae between T4–T6 and T10–T12
  - The lumbar curve, usually a left curve, has the apex in L2 and extends inferiorly up to L4–L5.
- *Double major thoracic:* High left thoracic curve and a right thoracic curve. The upper curve is short, extending to T5 or T6, while the lower curve extends inferiorly between T11 and L2.
- *Double major thoracic and thoracolumbar—usually:*
  - Right thoracic curve, with the apex at T6 or T7, extending between T4 and T9–T10, and
  - Left thoracolumbar curve, with the apex at the level of the disk between the vertebrae T12 and L1, extending inferiorly to L3
- Multiple curves.

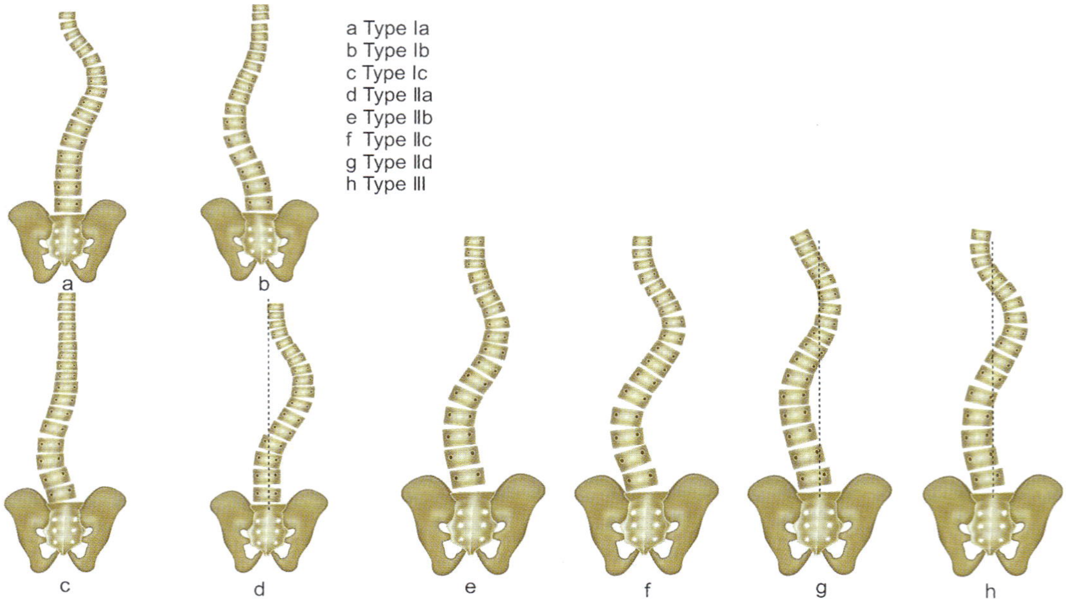

Fig. 28: PUMC classification.

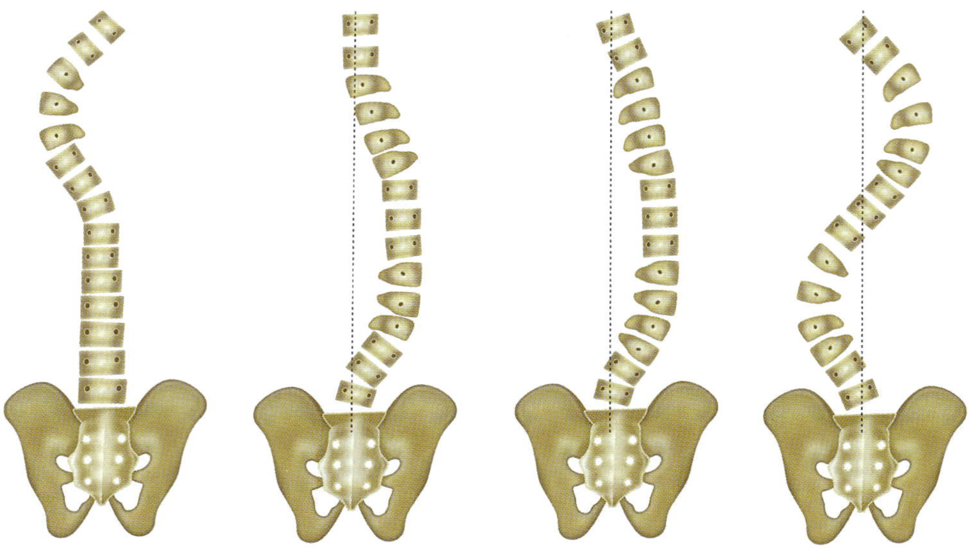

Fig. 29: Poncet's 3D classification (see text).

Selective thoracic fusion is advised only for patients with double curve pattern with thoracolumbar or lumbar curves less than 45°, flexibility greater than 70% and AVR less than Nash and Moe Grade 2.

Three-dimensional Classification (Fig. 29)

This incorporates again the rotational component of scoliosis comprehensively. Poncet et al. described four types of rotational malalignment in idiopathic scoliosis:

1. In type A curves, the maximum torsion is located in the upper-end vertebrae (UEV) region
2. In type B curves, torsional malalignment occurs in both the UEV and lower-end vertebrae (LEV) regions with geometric torsion in opposite direction, virtually neutralizing the torsion.
3. In type C curves torsional malalignment occurs again in both the UEV and LEV(LEV) regions, but the geometric torsion is in same direction, virtually increasing the torsion.
4. For **"double major"** scoliotic curves, the geometric torsion pattern is described by a combination of two types, one for each curve.

Nonoperative Treatment of AIS

This is based on the observation that most patients who have AIS do not progress to the point of treatment. However, it is not just observation rather a program aimed to prevent any progression if it is going to occur, that will really help the patient. Observation alone is not recommended. Scoliosis intensive rehabilitation program or scoliosis specific exercises help to reduce the lateral deviation and surface rotation. Radiographs should be performed every 4–6 months depending on the risk of progression.

Bracing for AIS

This is effective for curves less than 45° until skeletal maturity. The most ideal patient would be one whose curve progresses to 25–30° (30° correspond to ATR of 7°) and has still potential for growth (Risser's sign less than 4). It has been found that curves will worsen when they are 50° and more at maturity. Thoracic curves more than 80° are associated with shortness of breath and risks of cor pulmonale and death. Patients with curves less than 45° have lives with quality and length equal to those of control subjects. So the aim of bracing is to keep the curves below 50°. The indications of bracing according to maturity of patient as advised by SRS are as follows:

- *Risser 0–1:*
  - Curve 0–20° → observe
  - Curve 20–40° → brace
- *Risser 2–3:*
  - Curve 0–30° → observe
  - Curve 30–40° → brace
- *Risser 0–3:*
  - Curve 40–50° → ??
  - Curve 50° and more (Risser 0–4) → operate.

Goal of bracing is to maintain the present curve magnitude and prevent it from progressing to a level that would need surgical correction (patient reaching their full maturity and with curve greater than 45°). Milwaukee, SpineCor (dynamic bracing using elastic straps anchored to pelvic corset (no plastic or metal components), also called St Justine Brace), Wilmington, and Boston braces appear to be superior to the other types of braces.

History of bracing: Modern bracing is said to have started with Blount and Schmidt in 1946 with the use of Milwaukee brace (MB). The brace was intended to stimulate the patient to pull away from the contact points thus using muscle power to correct the curve. It was found that the brace was ineffective if the curve was more than 45°. There were lots of compliance issues with this rigid conspicuous brace. Hall and Miller developed a more total contact brace that works as a sleeve while applying lateral pressure over the apices of curves. This low profile "Boston brace" brace offered less conspicuous brace wear under clothing and had outcomes similar to MB. Then later braces were developed for night-time wear (Charleston bending brace, Providence brace, regulated force effect brace, etc.). The newest addition is the Chêneau style computer-aided design/computer-aided manufacturing (CAD/CAM) braces which is an example of asymmetrical bracing. Symmetrical bracing like the MB use pad inlays that push the most prominent areas on trunk while asymmetrical braces are constructed to overcorrect the deformity with foam pads to augment the pressure areas and having spaces on the opposing sides of pressure areas.

Effectiveness and Schedule of Bracing

- Still questioned with surgeons having individual views despite many studies (the confusion is primarily due to difficulty in judging/measuring compliance).
- Braces should be used for 18–23 hours a day on average.
- Preliminary results demonstrate that there is "dose response to bracing"; more than 12 hours in a brace was more effective in the skeletally immature patients. Part-time bracing was defined as 13–16 hours per day.
- Braces were reported to be effective for patients with curves less than 35° when used part-time or at night. That means for curves less than 35° part-time bracing may be effective (full-time wear is definitely effective).
- Braces should be used full-time by patients with curves equal to or greater than 35°. There is a big concern with full-time bracing as the patients are very sensitive to peers and comments in this growing stage where actually psychological development takes precedence. These patients with full-time bracing when enquired develop low self-esteem and prominent psychological stress. One should always consider this factor while prescribing braces.
- Bracing should be continued for 18–24 months by the end of 6th month following the end of growth (up to Risser's sign 4 in girls, Risser type 5 in boys, and following the menarche in girls).
- Bracing of curves over 40° is not likely to effectively change the natural history.
- The effects of bracing remain over a lifetime.
  - Curves that are kept under 50° at maturity are unlikely to progress over time to curves of 80° or more, preventing pulmonary effects or shortened life expectancy.

Milwaukee brace (Fig. 30): The Milwaukee brace (MB) is a cervicothoracic-lumbar-sacral-orthosis (CTLSO) originally

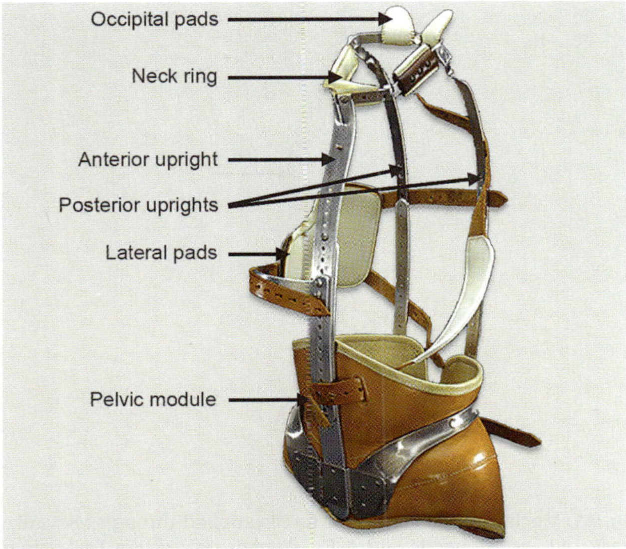

Fig. 30: The Milwaukee brace and its components (see text for details).

developed by Dr Walter Blount in Wisconsin in the 1940s. The brace was developed for postoperative management of polio patients following spinal fusion surgery in Milwaukee city (Milwaukee children hospital) from where it derives its name. The brace was first introduced publicly at the American Academy of Orthopedics meeting in 1946 by Dr Walter Blount and Dr AC Schmitt. Initially, it was used only for scoliosis correction by Dr Blount (1940s) and Dr Moe (1950s); later, Dr Blount also used it for correction of kyphosis (1958).

Designing principles: The basic concept was that the lumbar lordosis needs correction for correction of scoliosis. This designed the "foundation" of brace which remains in contact with the iliac crest and lumbar spine. From this base foundation three uprights are erected one anterior and two posterior connecting to the neck ring above the shoulders (chin rest was removed from brace due to production of malocclusion). The brace has an occipital pad or rest posteriorly to care for the occipital portion of the skull.

Biomechanics of brace: Following are the general biomechanical principles as applied for various braces:

1. Prevention of asymmetric compressive forces related to passive posture
2. Reduction of secondary muscle imbalance
3. Prevention of lordosing reactive forces
4. Prevention of asymmetric torsional forces from gait
5. Production of dynamic detorsional forces involving breathing mechanics.

The brace applies external corrective forces to the trunk with the aim to halt the curve progression or to correct it during growth or to avoid further progression of an already established pathological curve in adulthood. Specifically for MB, there are two forces that come to play in correction of deformity:

1. *Biomechanical effect* ***(Fig. 31)****:* The pelvic module in conjunction with the neck ring with or without a chin rest and the occipital pad did provide a longitudinal *traction force* to the spine. The second are the *corrective transverse forces* applied by placement of pads (ideally should be applied perpendicular to the curve). Pads placed laterally provide corrective forces to the apex of the convexity of scoliosis in the transverse plane. Alternatively, when placed posteriorly over the apex of the kyphosis, pads generate a corrective anteriorly directed force over the posterior prominence. The longitudinal and transverse forces applied by the brace are effective in correcting the sagittal and coronal plane deformities.

   By correcting the deformity partially the mechanical loading of spine is redistributed in a plane that allows more symmetrical and natural loading and will make possible proper spinal growth. This particular reinforcement has been termed "virtuous cycle" and as a result could lead to gradual reduction of the asymmetry present in scoliosis.
2. *Biological effect:* The other proposed mechanism of deformity reduction (or at least control) is the neuromotor reorganization (as opposed to mechanical discussed above) caused by changes in external and proprioceptive inputs and movement resulting from the constraint of bracing. Here the braces are considered to be the drivers while they increase external and internal bodily sensations. This changes the motor behavior and produces long-term effect on bone formation even after removal of brace.

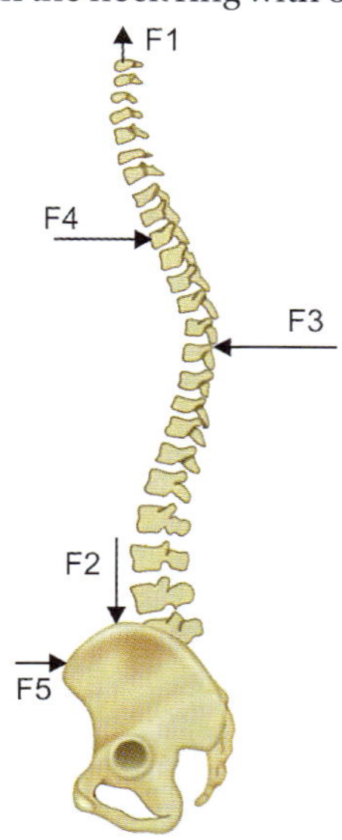

Fig. 31: Mechanism of corrective forces applied through Milwaukee brace—F1 and F2, traction force, F3—kyphosis correction, F4—anterior counterforce and substituted with lateral forces, F5—counter to pelvic tilt.

Components of Milwaukee brace:

The orthosis consists of three basic components: (1) Pelvic section; (2) the superstructure; and (3) the pads.

1. *The pelvic section:* It is carved from patient cast and is made of thermoplastics lined with foam interface (now prefabricated modules are commercially available). Custom molding of the pelvic component is needed especially with pelvic obliquity or atypical spinal deformity. It should be a snug fit to provide stable foundation from which pads gain a mechanical advantage.
2. *Superstructure:* It is composed of neck-ring and three metal bars that attach the pelvic structure to neck ring. The anterior bar is made of aluminum to give adequate radiolucency and posterior bars are made of steel to provide strength and rigidity. The chin attachment has been removed from the neck ring which was originally used due to concerns of malocclusion. The superstructure provides traction force and means of pad suspension to permit force application to body. The other function is to provide superior end point of control. In the high profile design the neck ring is placed with the throat mold just inferior to mandible. In the low-profile design the neck ring is placed at the level of sternal notch that makes it inconspicuous and more acceptable.
3. *Pads:* These are the most important parts of brace as they provide the corrective forces to the deformity. They need to be carefully and tactfully placed to provide benefit to the patient. The pads are made of rigid material like aluminum back with foam back and covered with

vinyl. The pads must be stiff enough to impart forces onto bone but prevent skin breakdown. Lumbar pads are incorporated in the "foundation" (pelvic section). Axilla slings and rings provide counterforce against the thoracic pads and permit maximal force to be applied. The force of thoracic pads can be altered by adjusting the axilla strap. Pads are "floating" when they are suspended from superstructure by straps. Gradually increasing pad forces applied produce decent correction provided brace is worn as scheduled.

Assessing the fit of brace:

- In the pelvic component after wear, even finger should not pass inside (say to palpate ASIS) to maintain a snug fit. If snug fit is not obtained then it will not serve as a strong foundation and control of forces will not be achieved. This entails use of custom-made component (plaster mold cast) rather than commercial or measurement derived build.
- The width of the posterior opening should be of magnitude equal to or slightly larger than that of the largest lumbar vertebral body. This ensures lateral counter rotation force exerted by the lumbar pad instead of central force.
- Superstructure should contour to the body walls.
- Thoracic pads are positioned posterolaterally so as to provide both a derotating force as well as a laterally directed force which can act in the coronal plane for correction of thoracic scoliosis.
- Lumbar pad should be positioned at the level of the apex of the lumbar curve "Null point".
- Axillary pad should be placed as superior as possible without patient experiencing pain or paresthesias.

Indications of Milwaukee brace:

- Scoliosis (see earlier)
- *Kyphosis:* MB is used in patient with Scheuermann's kyphosis with open vertebral ring apophyses and a kyphotic deformity of 45–50° or greater with vertebral wedging. Bracing is recommended for 20–23 hours/day until maturity including apophyseal closure on X-rays.

Other braces that have been used or are popular:

- Chêneau brace derivatives:
  - Rigo Chêneau system
  - ScoliOlogiC® Chêneau light
  - Gensingen brace
- Lyonnaise brace
- Dynamic derotation brace
- Progressive action short brace

Operative Treatment

Surgery is aimed most importantly to halt curve progression with fusion (primary goal) and also to reduce deformity using instrumentation (secondary goal). Increasing deformity has deleterious effects on cardiopulmonary system and future lifestyle of the patient. The other concern is to identify patients that may have continued rapid anterior growth producing a rotation of spine even after posterior procedures (Crankshaft effect), it is possible to partially identify these patients by low Risser grade and premenarcheal status but no definite indicators exist.

In general, curves greater than 45–50° should be treated by surgery. One should refrain from waiting and letting curves to progress as this increases complications of surgery including blood loss. The specific indications for operative treatment are as follows:

- *Thoracic curves:*
  - *Skeletally immature patients:* Curve magnitude greater than 40–50°
  - *Mature patients:* Curve magnitude greater than 50° (as they have high chances of progression even after maturity)
- *Thoracolumbar/lumbar curves:* Curve magnitude greater than 40° with significant coronal decompensation.

The surgical techniques can be divided mainly into fusion and nonfusion techniques. The former can be again classified into posterior or anterior or combined instrumentation methods.

Fusion Techniques

For all fusion techniques complete facetectomies at all instrumented levels is done as a mandatory procedure. The fusion is achieved using bone grafts (accessory procedures like implanting rhBMP-2 is individual preference and possibly overdone; it may have a role in failed fusion or revision cases). The concept of fusion emanated from the Russell Hibbs technique (first used for tuberculous spine in 1911, adapted for scoliosis in 1914), he corrected the deformity using plaster jackets however. Simple bone grafting is adequate and has stood the test of time. The bone graft can be obtained from:

- *Iliac crest:* Most common and easy but adds to pain after procedure.
- Rib is easily locally available but quantity is a bit limited.
- Allograft good quantitative supply but has problems of disease transmission, unknown quality. The results of allograft have been similar to autologous grafting. It requires additional logistic investment in the institute and often not very seriously maintained, standardization should be done and ensured.
- Local only from spinous processes, facets, etc. is a limited supply but may add to rib graft.

Posterior Instrumentation

All curves can be treated by posterior instrumentation and it is definitely indicated for double and triple curves.

- First used by Paul Harrington, he corrected the curves by distraction from the concave side using the rods.
- Second generation instrumentation system was developed by Cotrel and Dubousset. They attempted correction by rod rotation maneuvers. Rod contouring and placement on the concavity are followed by a counterclockwise rotation (for a right thoracic curve). Although conceptually correct the "derotation" of the

vertebrae has been found to be limited. Although some rotation may occur, most of the thoracic correction is achieved by distraction and apical translation.

- Modern systems and hybrid systems (third generation) allow various combinations where spine can be tightly attached to the rods by pedicle screws/wires/hooks. Suk used pedicle screws for surgical correction of deformity. Cheng found that transpedicular screws and hooks are similar in terms of correction.
  - All modern systems achieve correction by maneuvers that attempt to translate the spine posteriorly and laterally and to derotate the spine **(Figs. 32A and B)** in the axial plane. Modern segmental spinal instrumentation uses multiple fixation points and dual rods posteriorly and single or dual rods anteriorly.
    - Rod rotation as by Dubousset method **(Figs. 33A to C)**
    - *Translation or cantilever:* Distal attachment of a contoured rod and then translation of the spine to the rod
    - *In situ contouring:* The rod is attached to the contour of the spine and then shaped to improve spinal deformity.

The common tools used posteriorly:

Hooks:

- *Pedicle hooks:* Upgoing hooks are placed under the lamina or inferior facet engaging the pedicle. They can be placed in thoracic spine to T10.
- *Sublaminar hooks:* Can be up-going or downgoing.
- Transverse process hooks (not preferred as they are weakest construct and prone to failure): Can be placed as up-going or down-going.

Wires:

- *Sublaminar wires:* These have been long preferred (since Harrington instrumentation) and are excellent for translation (laterally and posteriorly).
- *Through the spinous process:* Wisconsin (Drummond) wires.

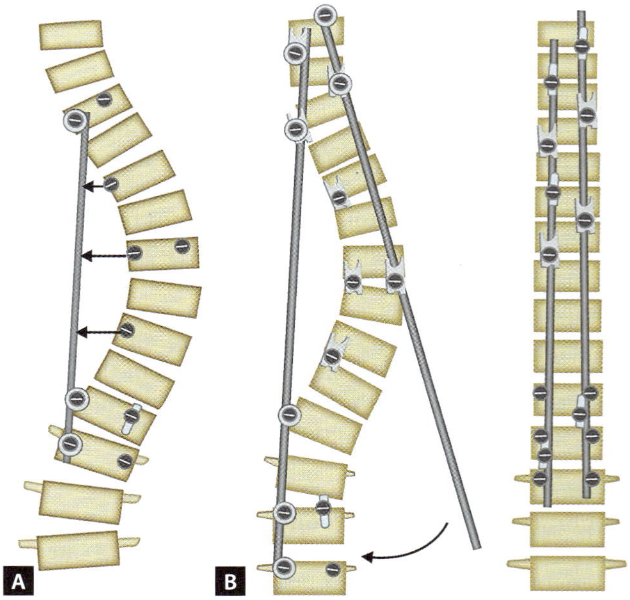

Figs. 32A and B: Correction of scoliosis curves: (A) Distraction across the concavity corrects scoliosis and produces kyphosis; similarly, (B) Compression across the convexity reduces scoliosis and produces lordosis. Hooks and pedicle screws can be used for sagittal or coronal tilting of the vertebrae as the axial force (distraction or compression) is applied; in addition, rotational forces can be exerted using pedicle and vertebral body screws.

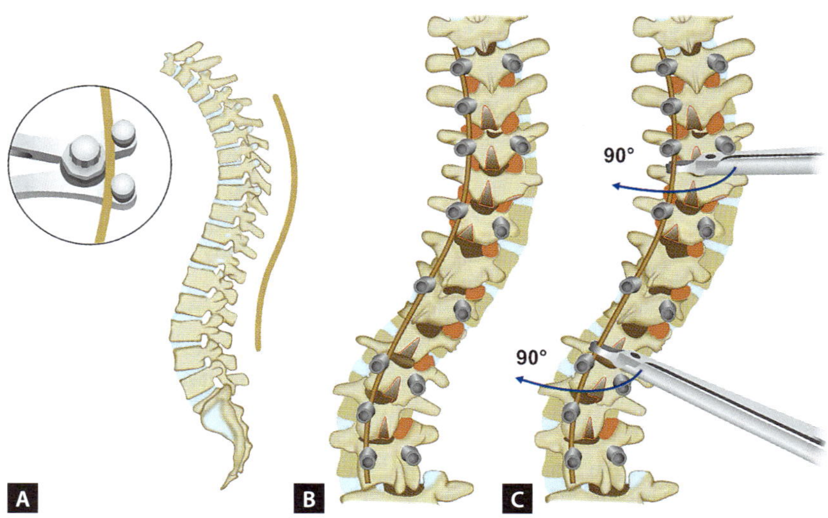

Figs. 33A to C: Rod rotation method of Cotrel and Dubousset (modified): (A) Rod is prebent according to the desired kyphosis and lordosis; (B) It is then inserted sequentially into the screws; (C) Using rod holders, the rod is bent to place into desired kyphosis and lordosis with simultaneous correction of scoliosis.

Pedicle screws:

- Provide optimal fixation of all three columns:
    1. Pedicle screws can produce sagittal-plane tilting, rotation, axial compression or distraction, and translation of instrumented vertebrae.
    2. Generally used in the lower thoracic and the lumbar spine. Various modifications have also permitted their use in upper thoracic spine too.
    3. They are not absolutely benign and have unique set of complications—screw breakage, pullout and attendant neurological injury.

Anterior Instrumentation

Dwyer in Australia developed the first anterior system. He envisaged better correction could be achieved by instrumenting the VBs after performing an anterior release procedure and discectomy. His prototype system (screw, staple and cable) has been replaced by newer vertebral body screws and rods. This is preferred by some as it needs shorter fusion levels to achieve correction especially in thoracolumbar or lumbar curves (it must be remembered that possibly due to limitation in exposure and accessibility of "unfriendly" region the magnitude of overall correction is lower than posterior approach.

- *Rod rotation:* The rod is contoured to the convexity of the spine, and rod rotation is performed to improve the coronal plane and restore or maintain lumbar lordosis.
- *Compression is done usually for thoracic curves:* The rod is seated completely or more often distally initially or proximally initially followed by compression.
    - A cantilever maneuver can be used (for the partially seated rod) followed by compression at each level.

Anterior structural support: Mesh cages or ring allografts are commonly used for disk space fusion after release and maintenance of lumbar lordosis.

- Provides improved structural stiffness when performing anterior instrumentation and fusion.

Video-assisted thoracoscopic surgery (VATS): Introduction of VATS has decreased postoperative pain and scar formation. This minimally invasive surgical technique is used for single thoracic curves and is aimed at decreasing operative morbidity. VATS is possibly similar to open procedure in experienced hands. The advantages of VATS include smaller incisions, less postoperative pain, less postoperative pulmonary problems and improved cosmesis. Disadvantages include technically demanding procedure (often converted to open due to lack of experience) and are more costly because of the use of disposable items.

Determining Fusion Levels

We will use Lenke system to define the fusion levels for curve types.

- *Lenke type 1:* Major curve in the main thoracic region proximal and distal curves are minor and nonstructural.
    - Fusion level proximally extends to between T3 and T5 stable vertebrae (as the case may be), while distally it is guided by lumbar spine modifier.
        - Lower instrumented vertebrae (LIV) in a patient with the lumbar spine modifier "A" should be the one that the CSVL intersects in the TL/l region (often one level below the LEV of main curve).
        - For 1B modifier similar technique is used with preserving some residual tilt due to lumbar apical deviation of curves.
        - For 1C modifier one should go down to the end vertebrae (usually the T11 or T12). One should attempt to incorporate junctional kyphosis in the fusion. Selective thoracic fusion would preserve the lumbar motion segments in patients with 1C modifier.
- *Lenke type 2:* These double thoracic curves often have left proximal thoracic and right main thoracic curves.
    - The most important rule while correcting the proximal curve is to maintain the shoulder balance (left shoulder higher).
        - This is achieved by compressing the convex and distracting the concave side of proximal curve.
        - For high right shoulder (right proximal and left main thoracic curve), the shoulder balance is achieved while correcting the main curve.
    - Upper instrumented vertebrae (UIV) should be T2 or T3 (for classical right thoracic cases), while the lower one is defined as for type 1 curves discussed above. Selected left main curve patients have UIV chosen at T4 or T5 (should be done only by experienced surgeons), leaving the proximal curve out of fusion.
- *Lenke type 3:* Double major curves (major curve in the thoracic region with structural thoracolumbar curve). The UIV is at T3–T5 as for type 1 while the lower level extends to L3 or L4.
    - *L4 is chosen if:*
        - Thoracolumbar curve is on or lower than l2
        - L3–L4 disk is convex or open on the convex side
        - L4 has rotation of 1° or more on Nash-Moe classification.
    - *L3 is chosen if:*
        - Thoracolumbar curve is on or higher than L1–L2
        - L3–L4 disk is neutral or closed on the convex side
        - L4 has a rotation of 1.5° and lower according to Nash-Moe.

    Distal fixation is best performed with pedicle screws for improved correction and maintenance of curve correction.
- *Lenke type 4 (triple major curves):* All three structural curves should be contained in the fusion. UIV is chosen as for type 2 curves while LIV is chosen as for type 3 curves. The fusion often extends from T2/3 to L3/4. Segmental fusion as proposed by Suk (2000) may be helpful. He showed good correction by fusing the spine in a segmental fashion (pedicle screw and rods) instead of long fusion segments.
- *Lenke type 5:* Main curve is in the thoracolumbar region. Upper curve if present is usually nonstructural. UIV is one or two level above the upper stable vertebra whereas LIV is one or two level below the lower end vertebra.

- *Lenke type 6:* The main and larger curve is the structural thoracolumbar/lumbar and is greater than the main thoracic structural curve. Proximal thoracic curve is nonstructural. Main thoracic and the thoracolumbar are contained in fusion. Fusion levels are determined as for type 3 curves.

Combined Anterior Release/Fusion and Posterior Instrumentation/Fusion

This is preferred for conditions where anterior release is needed. Stiff curves more than 75° that fail to bend to less than 50° will need some anterior release at least for reasonable correction (correction to below 50–40°). The release can be performed either open or thoracoscopically in the thoracic spine. The typical indications are:

- Large (>75°) stiff curves
- Skeletally immature
- Open triradiate cartilage or Risser 0–1, girls less than 11 years, boys less than 13 years
- Prevent crankshaft.

Nonfusion Surgery

This used either instrumented or noninstrumented epiphysiodesis on the convex side. This method is useful for AIS but not for the infantile scoliosis. The problem with this approach is that the body remains shorter than limbs and mars the pulmonary development. Instrumentation to correct the curves without compromising body growth has been developed in the form of Isula double rod system. The upper and lower parts of the curves are connected to the rods and the rods are interconnected by another rod. The rods are extended every 6 months.

Vertical expandable prosthetic titanium ribs (VEPTR) has been developed to treat the thoracic insufficiency syndrome caused by combination of rib fusion and curves. The deformity is acutely corrected by wedge thoracostomy and VEPTR device application which is expanded every 4–6 months.

Intraoperative Monitoring During Spine Surgery

Intraoperative neurophysiologic monitoring (IONM) is a technique for assessing the nervous system during spine surgery. For an awake patient spinal cord and central function can be evaluated using various tests while for a patient under anesthesia indirect assessment is needed using specialized techniques. These techniques help in assessment of neuromuscular junction, peripheral nerve, spinal cord, brainstem and cortex during surgery. Their relative utility has been compared in **Table 5**. The following are some of the commonly employed techniques:

- ***Transcranial motor evoked potentials (Tc-MEPs, Figs. 34A to C):*** The Tc-MEP involves applying a train of high-voltage stimuli to electrodes on the surface of the head to activate motor pathways. In a normal awake person these produce first a D-wave (direct wave) that is the orthodromic nerve action potential resulting from stimulation. D-wave is followed by I-wave (indirect wave) representing the volleys produced by the cortical

TABLE 5: Comparative characteristics of some IONM

Method	*Response speed*	*Anatomic region assessment*	*Criteria used to define injury*
Tc-MEP	Very fast	Corticospinal tract and anterior horn cell	• Disappearance of response • 100V increase in threshold • Reduction in amplitude of MEP
D-wave	Fast	Corticospinal tract	• Warning by reduction in amplitude by 50% • Absence indicates significant injury
SSEP	Slow	Dorsal column sensory pathway	• Decline of more than half of the amplitude • Increased latency by 10%
sEMG	Very fast	Large motor fibers	Short high frequency bursts
Triggered EMG	Very fast	Large motor fibers	• Reduction in amplitude by half or more • Increase in latency by 10% or more
H-reflex	Fast	Various (see text)	Variable and still undefined fully

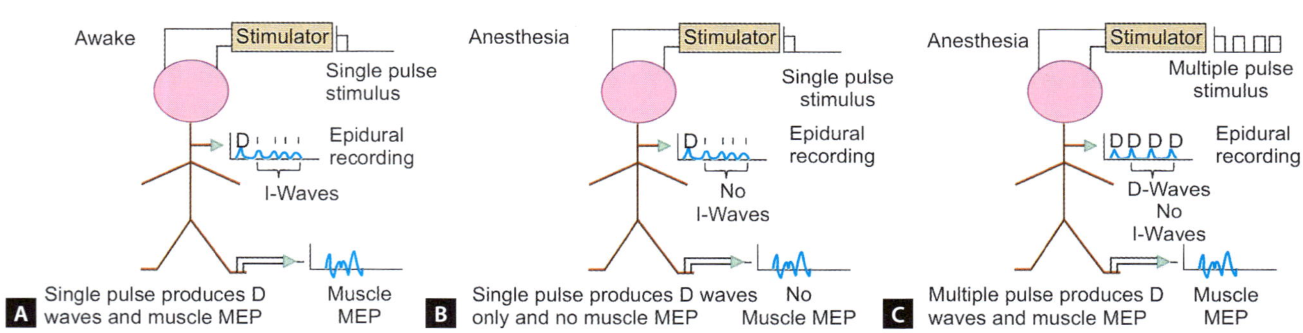

Figs. 34A to C: MEP and D-wave (see text).

neurons that were excited by the same stimulus. I-waves need synaptic activity and are hence suppressed by the anesthetic agents. So in an anesthetized patient to produce optimal response from anterior horn cell (final pathway for any motor response) a train of stimulus is used because anterior horn cells respond better to a train of stimuli and not a single stimulus (that may get easily suppressed by the anesthetic agent). Train of stimulus (3–12 pulses with the frequency of 150–500 Hz) typically placed over the C1 and C2 locations near the motor cortex produces.

- *Motor contraction (muscle MEP):* Transcranial motor evoked potential using muscle responses (muscle MEP) provides an effective means of monitoring motor pathways in the spinal cord. Changes in the muscle MEP during scoliosis surgery bear a strong correlation with cord injury (corticospinal tract and the anterior horn cell). Optimal criteria for diagnosis of cord injury have not been elucidated; however disappearance of the response serves as a good guide to cord injury. Other criteria to judge injury include:
  - Increases of more than 100 V in the threshold for obtaining a muscle MEP
  - Reduction in MEP amplitude of 50% or more
- *"or" Nerve action potential (D-wave):* D-wave monitoring is limited to cervical and upper thoracic cord (corticospinal tract) and requires an epidural recording electrode. It may be individually used or in association with MEP. The advantages of D-wave monitoring are that it is not anesthesia or neuromuscular blockade dependent and has simple criteria for interpretation.
  - 50% decline in amplitude indicates "alert" for possible cord injury
  - Disappearance of the D-wave is generally associated with a significant neurologic deficit

Complications of Tc-MEP: These include:

- Risk of tissue injury or shock to OR personnel (voltages as high as 900 V and current up to 0.9 A are used)
- Spread of current can cause direct stimulation of the trigeminal nerve and causing jaw contractions (the most common complication is hence tongue bite).
- The patient may move during the elicitation of the Tc-MEP
- Precipitate seizures in susceptible patients
- Patients with implanted defibrillator should not be subjected to Tc-MEP.

If evoked potentials remain abnormal after correction of physiological parameters, distraction should be relieved and implants should be removed to restore spinal cord function. Often with acute change in the evoked potential the immediately previous step reversal will restore potentials.

- ***Upper and lower somatosensory evoked potentials (upper and lower SSEP) (Figs. 35A and B):*** This was actually the first effective means for monitoring the function of the spinal cord during surgery. In contrast to Tc-MEP where the orthodromic conduction is evaluated, in SSEP the periphery is stimulated and response is recorded to evaluate the dorsal column (and possible dorsal spinocerebellar) sensory pathways during spine surgery. Commonly the median or ulnar nerve at wrist is stimulated or else radial nerve between the thumb and first finger on the dorsal surface of the hand is used. In lower limb posterior tibial nerve at the foot or peroneal nerve near fibular head is used.

From upper extremity the impulse is conducted to → brachial plexus (Erb's point) → dorsal column nuclei (N13 potential is evoked) → medial lemniscus in brainstem → thalamus (N20 potential) → sensory cortex, N20 and P22 potential are recorded

From lower extremity the impulse travels to cauda equina (N21 lumbar potential) → dorsal column nucleus → spinocerebellar pathway → P37/P40 potential.

These are slow potentials so interpretation requires continuous averaging and may even take 3–5 minutes. The impulses are also sensitive to anesthesia so subjected to interpretation error:

  - Injury to large fiber dorsal column pathways is suspected if there is a more than 50% decrease in amplitude or 10% increase in latency of any of the above potentials.

- ***Spontaneous electromyography (EMG):*** Muscles have a basal motor activity and modified activity with

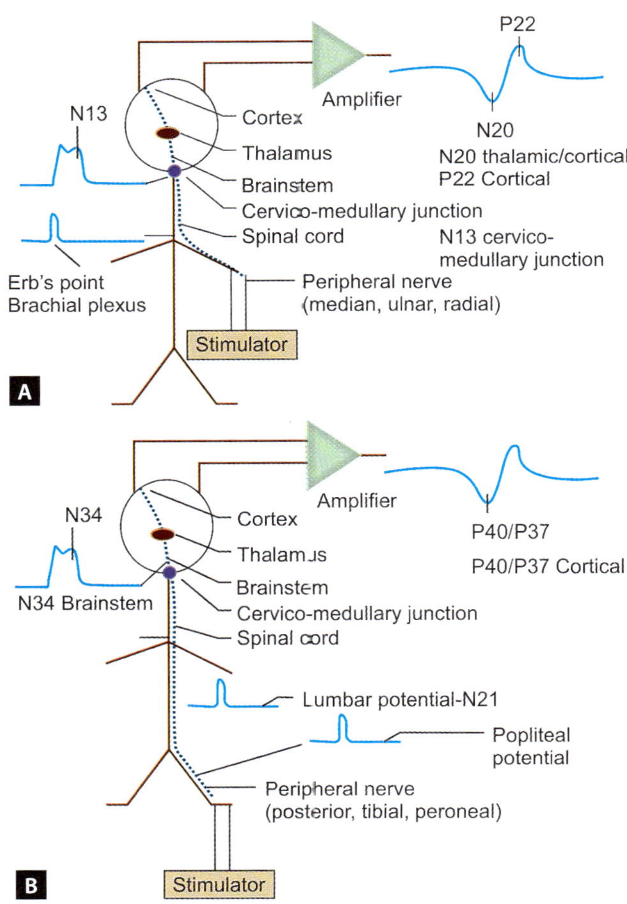

Figs. 35A and B: Somatosensory evoked potential.

nerve stimulation. Monitoring these changes in muscle will indicate the state of the innervating nerves. Nerve compression, stretch, hypothermia and ischemia all produce depolarization of nerve generating action potentials that can then be recorded. Determining the correct pattern of action potentials associated with nerve injury has been a task. Romstock classified three (A, B and C) different patterns:

- "A" trains—characterized by high frequency activity are the most likely to be associated with significant injury.

The most useful characteristic of sEMG is the instantaneous nature but the biggest disadvantage is high dependency on neuromuscular blockade (due to anesthetic drugs) faltering the evaluation of response.

- ***Triggered EMG (Pedicle screw simulation):*** Spinal instrumentation offers advantage to know if the screw is in vicinity of the nerve or injuring it. If the screw is electrically close (either in contact or presence of low-resistance pathway that can conduct electricity) to one of the nerve roots, then electrically stimulating the screw will activate the nearby nerve root at a lower current level. The cut-off point is taken as 10 mA or less with a stimulus duration of 0.2 msec for lumbar pedicle screws (stimulating potentials less than 5 mA nearly always indicated misplaced screws, greater than 10 mA often were safe). The problem is with nerve roots that have been already damaged, in that case higher stimulating potentials will be recorded. One should note that the values change with location of pedicle screw placement and given value is not true for thoracic spine.
- ***Direct spinal cord stimulation (Owen):*** This was a highly talked about method of recording nerve injury. The spinal cord is directly stimulated and the recordings were made from peripheral nerves. It was envisaged that motor function can be evaluated even in paralyzed patients as in them the muscle action potential will not be generated and only the nerve action potential will be recorded. However, it was later found that the responses evoked are no different from SSEP and MEP discussed above so offer no further advantage.
- ***Reflex monitoring:*** F-waves and H-reflex monitoring **(Figs. 36A and B)**. When a peripheral nerve is stimulated two waves are generated one that goes distally (orthodromic conduction) that terminates into M-wave or motor action potential. The other wave travels proximally (antidromic conduction) that goes toward the spinal cord reaching the anterior horn cell. The cell discharges and produces another impulse that travels peripherally as F-wave. Also this wave traveling through the sensory pathway will activate the monosynaptic reflex arc through activation of the dorsal horn of spinal cord and generate H-reflex. Both these F-wave and H-reflex help evaluate the proximal nervous system (propriospinal motor, corticospinal tract, spinal gray matter and anterior horn cell).
- ***Stagnara wake-up test:*** This is considered often the gold standard for monitoring spinal cord injury. The test consists of waking the patient up during the surgery and asking to move their feet. The test does not require any sophisticated apparatus or method but needs a skilled anesthetist who can quickly reverse the effect of anesthesia with return of enough cognitive function for patient to understand. Often short acting and fast reversing drugs are used like the desflurane and remifentanil. The method is however crude and does not tell the level of injury or mode of injury like direct nerve injury or cord injury due to ischemia/distraction, etc. So the basic purpose of removing or reversing the offending factor is not fulfilled and only the surgeon gets tense from cord injury! Contraindications to test include:
  - Mental retardation
  - Psychological problems
  - Preexisting neurological damage
  - Language problem

If a neurological complication is suspected based on an abnormal wake-up test result, immediate correction of hypotension and release of distraction should be undertaken. If the wake-up test continues to indicate abnormality, removal of the instrumentation is recommended.

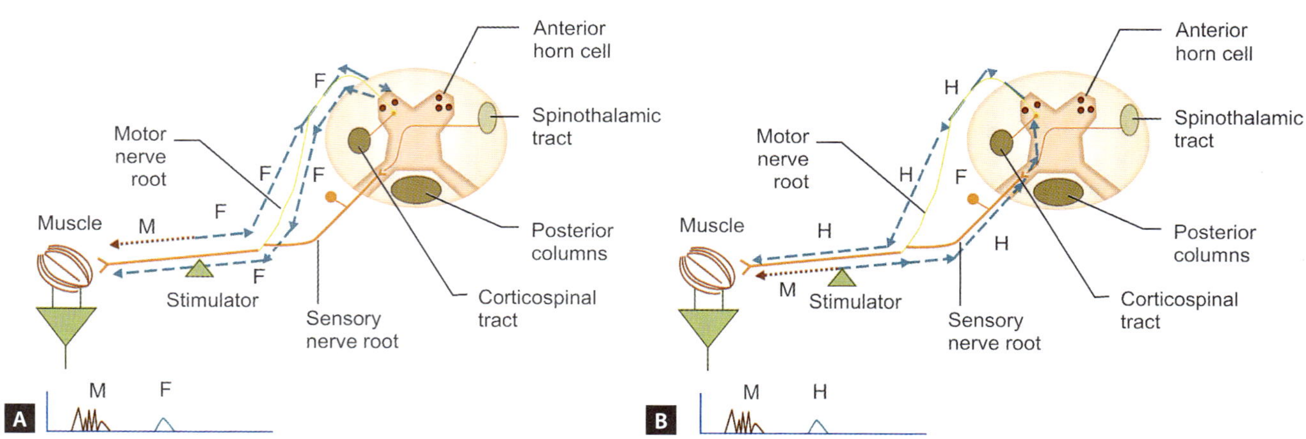

Figs. 36A and B: (A) F-wave; (B) H-reflex.

Postoperative Course

- Patients often need an intensive care for a couple of days
- Use of postoperative brace or casts has reduced dramatically with the modern instrumentation. It may be used with weak bones and anterior thoracic or thoracolumbar instrumentation. The brace is worn for 6 weeks continuously.
- Activities are slowly advanced until patients are performing full activities between 6 and 12 months
- Vigorous sports are restricted for at least a year (in some cases possibly forever!)
- Patients should be warned that some 20% cases of painless scoliosis become painful straight spine (usually interscapular pain).
- Fusion below L3 often produces a low back pain.

Complications of Surgical Management

- The reoperation rate for posterior spinal instrumentation is 5–19% for all causes
- Neurological injury (paraplegia occurs in 1:1,000). Risk factors being kyphosis, excessive correction, and use of sublaminar wires
- Delayed infection (often caused by low-virulence organisms like *Propionibacterium species is seen in* 1–7%. The treatment comprises of hardware removal and short-term antibiotics
- Disseminated intravascular coagulopathy (DIC) due to contamination of salvaged blood with the intraoperatively used gelfoam and thrombin
- Low back pain and interscapular pain are seen in 5% of patients after surgery and come under the category of late onset surgical pain. Unfortunately the treatment is removal of hardware that relieves pain still partially in most.
- Chylothorax and tension pneumothorax following VATS
- Superior mesentery artery syndrome
- Pseudarthrosis—late pain deformity progression and hardware failure is seen in 3% of patients. This needs to be managed by compression instrumentation and bone grafting to fuse the offending segment.
- Implant failure
- Flatback syndrome
- **Crankshaft phenomenon**—rotational deformity of the spine created by continued anterior spinal growth producing a progressive rotational and angular deformity in the setting of a posterior only spinal fusion done in younger patients. The term "crankshaft phenomenon" was coined by Dubousset. The posterior fused mass acts like a tethering bar producing continued lordosis and bending of the fusion mass as the unfused anterior vertebral bodies continue to grow. Radiologically the crankshaft phenomenon is diagnosed by:
  - Greater than or equal to 10° progression of Cobb's angle
  - Greater than or equal to 10° progression of RVAD—most useful.
  - Apical vertebral rotation by Perdriolle's method to be greater than or equal to 5°.

  Predicting factors for possible development of "crank" (as some call it) are still elusive but for sure just evaluating the Risser's stage and status of the triradiate cartilage at the time of surgery do not help (but with a closed triradiate cartilage the risk of crankshaft phenomenon is less than 5%).
  - "Peak height velocity" (6 months before menarche and continued through menarche) and a "multivariate method using chronologic/skeletal ages" and RVAD are effective but not entirely still. Potential of developing the crankshaft phenomenon is highest in (these are not the sole risk factors):
    - Girls less than 11 years
    - Boys less than 13 years
    - Risser grade 0–1
    - Juvenile scoliosis (normal growth potential of anterior vertebral body growth plates)
    - Open triradiate cartilage

  The most important risk factor is immature spine in a patient with difficult to objectively identify potential for rapid growth especially anteriorly (this is the reason why it is not common in congenital scoliosis as the anterior growth plates are defective often). In any case the standard of care for patients less than 10 years (females) and/or Risser 0–1 is combined anterior and posterior fusions that take care of more than 95% patients in whom crankshaft deformity might develop.

EARLY ONSET SCOLIOSIS (AGE <8 YEARS)

This includes the infantile and juvenile onset types. Some consider scoliosis diagnosed at age equal to or less than 5 years to be early onset scoliosis. It is a rather uncommon type and may represent congenital spine and thoracic malformations (congenital scoliosis) or may have normal vertebrae (idiopathic early onset scoliosis). These children need extra-care and aggressive management however.

- These children are at risk for rapid deformity progression, cosmetic disfigurement and pulmonary insufficiency.
- Pulmonary compromise is a concern in the rare cases of scoliosis developing before 5 years of age
- According to Nilsonne and Lundgren the severe curves (more than 100°) often result in death due to pulmonary (or cardiac) causes in 60% of cases. Children may die as young as 16 years and postmortem findings show reduced number of alveoli and markedly small lungs.

Evaluation

Because of rarity a detailed neurological, physical and radiological examination is mandatory to exclude congenital or neurological causes of the scoliosis. Routine brainstem and spinal cord MRI should be done to exclude CNS and spinal cord abnormalities such as a syrinx in patients with a spinal deformity of greater than 20°. In contrast to AIS and juvenile idiopathic scoliosis, the curves in infantile scoliosis are commonly (in 50–75% of patients) left thoracic curves, and boys are more commonly affected than are girls.

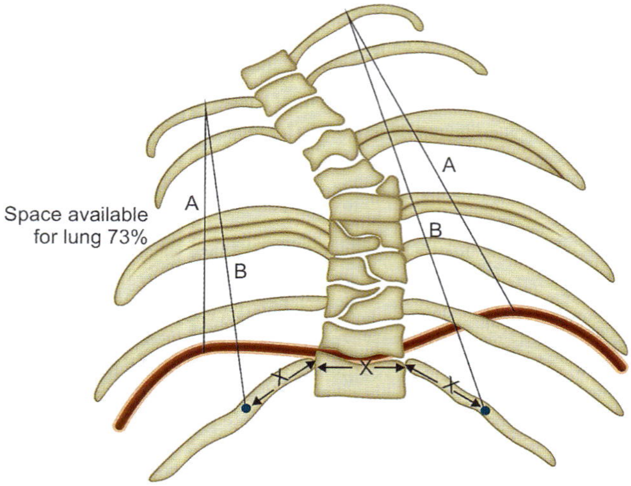

Fig. 37: Space available for lungs (after Campbell)—(SAL). The height of hemithorax is the distance from the middle of most cephalad rib down to the center of hemidiaphragm "A" lines. The ratio expressed as percentage obtained by dividing the height of concave hemithorax by convex hemithorax is defined as space available for lung. Alternatively, the inferior border is defined by points placed on each side of the vertebra of width "X" at distance equal to 'X' from the vertebra along the rib lines "B". The SAL is calculated as the ratio mentioned above.

- Rib-vertebral angle difference is a better indicator of curve progression for infantile scoliosis. This angle is formed by a line along the rib head and a perpendicular to the base of the apical vertebra. If the difference between the angles on the concave/convex side exceeds 20°, progression will likely occur.
- *Space available for lung (SAL)* ***(Fig. 37)****:* This measure has been introduced by Campbell only recently as a radiographic measure in the infantile idiopathic scoliosis population and congenital scoliosis to identify thoracic insufficiency syndrome. Declining SAl value indicates progressive thoracic deformity.
  - Space available for lung is calculated as the height of hemithorax. This height is defined by measuring the height of the most cephalad rib either from the hemi-diaphragm or from the most caudad rib.
  - In the first method the line is made and length calculated from the midpoint of the most cephalad rib to the center of the hemidiaphragm on the same side. Similar line is drawn on the other side. Ratio is calculated by dividing the height of concave hemithorax by convex hemithorax and expressed as percentage—defining SAL.
  - In the other method instead of measuring from hemidiaphragm the lower limit is measured at the most caudad rib at a distance equal to the vertebral width from the vertebral margin (distance "x").

Management

Until recently observation was considered reasonable course of action till the curve reaches 30–40° because brace therapy and application of a cast are difficult in small children. But it is believed that due to rapid progression of the curves in these children early bracing will possibly a better line of management.

Bracing

This is effective for progressive noncongenital deformities. Congenital and neuromuscular types of scoliosis do not respond to bracing. Curves less than 35° with RVAD of less than 20° have reportedly responded well to brace therapy, whereas those more than 45° with RVAD greater than 20° were associated with a poor prognosis. So the typical indication of brace management is:

- For minor curves in the range of 20–30°.
- Bracing requires prolonged usage and preferably worn full-time. MB is needed for proximal thoracic curves (but has poor compliance).
- If the early-onset curve fails to be halted by dedicated attempts at brace therapy, surgery should be considered once the curve exceeds 55–60°.

Fusion Surgery

The indications for fusion surgery in early-onset scoliosis are:

- Children with severe curves
- Deteriorating congenital spinal deformities
- Progression despite bracing.

The fusion requires combined anterior and posterior approaches to prevent crankshaft phenomenon (see above). Still however the growth continues and the rate of revision surgery is quite high needing circumferential fusion in young children. Due to suboptimal results of fusion and need of revision surgeries there is trend shift to nonfusion surgeries. The following are the arguments/facts identified to shun fusion surgery in early-onset scoliosis:

- Failure of the fusion to control the deformity fully and need of revision surgeries.
- Fused spine causes unacceptable physiological changes:
  - The most rapid period of spinal growth occurred in the first 5 years of life, when the spine increased 50% of its length. The spine still continues to grow albeit slowly till growth spurts. Fusion at 5 years will result in 12.5 cm loss of spinal growth.
  - *Thoracic insufficiency syndrome:* It is the inability of the thorax to support normal respiration or lung growth. Small thoracic height due to fusion and multiple congenital rib malformations interfered with normal respiration (Campbell). The greatest increase in number of alveoli occurs in first 2 years of life and alveolar growth completes by 8 years. Operating during these ages causes damage to the pulmonary system. Patients receiving fusion surgery at ages less than 10 years have forced vital capacity (fVC) of 41% of normal compared to those receiving fusion older than 10 years who have fVC of 68% of normal.

Nonfusion Surgery

The placement of spinal instrumentation without fusion is the preferred procedure in patients older than 9 years of age. These methods control growth, delay definitive fusion, increase thoracic volume. Various methods include epiphysiodesis on convex side with or without instrumentation, hemiepiphysiodesis, hemivertebral resection and short segment fusions. Usually biocompatible shape memory metal alloy staples are used. Once adolescence is reached, anterior instrumentation-assisted fusion may be performed. There are, however, still a lot of concerns with these techniques and inconsistencies observed. Complications related to this technique are common and include hook dislodgment, rod breakage, skin breakdown, and early fusion without bone graft.

Growing Rods

These systems were designed to overcome the disadvantages of braces and fusion surgery. The various distractible spine instruments are Harrington, Cotrel-Dubousset, Luque rods, isola dual rods and Shilla system. These are based on the premises that the spinal growth could itself provide the driving force for deformity correction and also if the apophyses are turned horizontal from vertical they will also contribute to vertical growth of spine and deformity correction. In all systems curve apex is fused as the apex of deformity is the culprit and the ends are normal growing centers.

The "isola dual rod" instrumentation devised by Akbarnia et al. is a recent addition that consists of two growing segments placed on each side and preformed to correct the sagittal balance. Foundation at ends are created using hooks and rods are interconnected by cross-links. Distraction is performed every 6-months by an open surgery under anesthesia. The rods control the deformity and also correct it.

Shilla Procedure (Shilla Growth Guidance Technique)

It is a growth enhancing pedicle screw system used for the treatment of spinal deformities in an immature spine (McCarthy). Limited fusion is done at the apex while spinal growth is guided at the ends of dual rods gliding through the extraperiosteally placed pedicle screws. The rods need not be elongated (*cf*- isola dual rod system) repeatedly as they can glide along the screws.

The **disadvantages of growing rods** and instrumentation include:

- Need for repeated surgeries (except Shilla system) under general anesthesia
- Proximal migration of devices with rib fractures
- Rod fracture or anchor failure
- Junctional kyphosis and curve decompensation
- These are not effective to control or correct kyphosis
- Progressive stiffness or autofusion of the spine causing decreased spinal length gain from repeated lengthening of the growing rods—the law of mechanical engineering "law of diminishing returns" applied to orthopedics.

Magnetically Controlled Growing Rods

This system (phoenix rod) was developed to avoid repeated surgeries and associated wound and cosmetic morbidity. The distraction can be done in outpatient clinic by a remotely distractible, magnetically-controlled (PEMf) growing rod system. The distractions can be done frequently (say monthly) that also avoids "law of diminishing returns".

Vertical Expandable Prosthetic Titanium Rib (Campbell et al.)

Another unique device is the VEPTR that also corrects the thoracic insufficiency syndrome to some extent **(Fig. 38)**. Opening wedge thoracostomy is created with acute correction and the device applied. The device is placed from the cephalad rib to caudal rib or lumbar spine or iliac crest. The devices are distracted at scheduled intervals of 5–6 months. There is an increase in the vital capacity and correction in deformity over time.

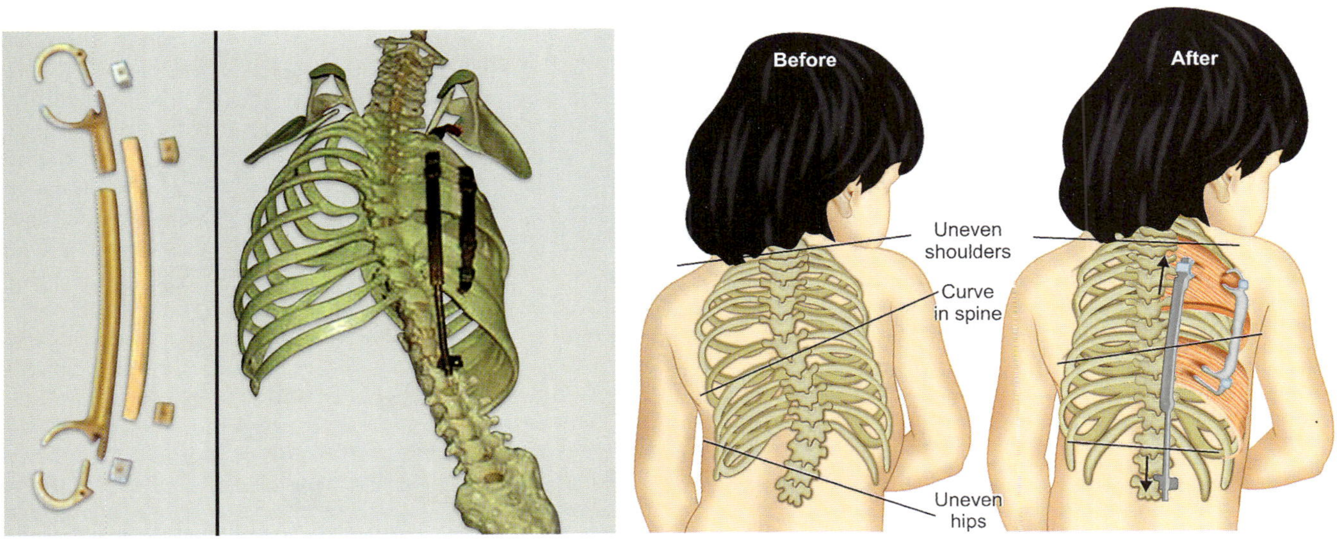

Fig. 38: VEPTR device.

Nitinol Staples (Spinal Growth Manipulation)

These memory staples limit the spinal growth asymmetrically while maintaining motion and disk physiology. They also prevent the need for spinal fusion for scoliosis. The current indications for their use include primary thoracic scoliosis 35–60° with 2–3 years of remaining growth, hypokyphosis and compensatory lumbar or upper thoracic curves less than 30–40°. The procedure can be done thoracoscopically/assisted in a minimally invasive manner.

CONGENITAL SCOLIOSIS

Congenital scoliosis (CS) is defined as a lateral curvature greater than 10° due to a developmental abnormality of the spine (curvature more than 10° without developmental abnormality is called infantile scoliosis). In congenital scoliosis the curve may not be present at birth or even may not develop until a significant time later but the vertebral anomalies are always present.

Epidemiology

- The incidence of congenital spinal anomalies approximately ranges from 0.5 to 1 per 1,000 births
- The deformities usually arise as sporadic cases with a 1% chance of transmission.
- When the anomaly is in isolated single vertebra the chance of a first-degree relative having a similar anomaly is approximately 1 out of 100
- For multiple vertebral anomalies the risk of similar anomalies in either siblings or children of the patient is between 10 and 15%
- When the spinal anomaly is one component of a multisystem anomaly, however, the risk of transmission rises to 5–10%.

Some definitions of terms used in congenital scoliosis are as follows:

- *Failure of segmentation* (***Figs. 39A to C***)*:* It means that one or more vertebrae are abnormally connected together on one side (the abnormal vertebrae did not separate properly). Bar formation due to fusion mass tethers the vertebral column restricting the growth on that side while it continues to grow on the opposite side producing progressive curvature.
- *Failure of formation* (***Figs. 40A to E****, most common type of congenital problem):* The normal shape of the vertebra is disrupted. Abnormally shaped vertebra may cause a wedge in the front back, or either side, or a combination, tilting the spine at that level.
- *Fully segmented:* It means that there is a growth plate and a disk on both the top and bottom of the abnormal vertebra.
- Semisegmented hemivertebrae—have disk and growth plate either above or below
- Nonsegmented hemivertebrae—are fused to the vertebra above and below. As these do not have any growth plate so curves due to lack of segmentation are least likely to grow.
- *Block vertebra:* It means that there is a missing disk space. They do not have a growth plate so unlikely to ever cause a progressive deformity.

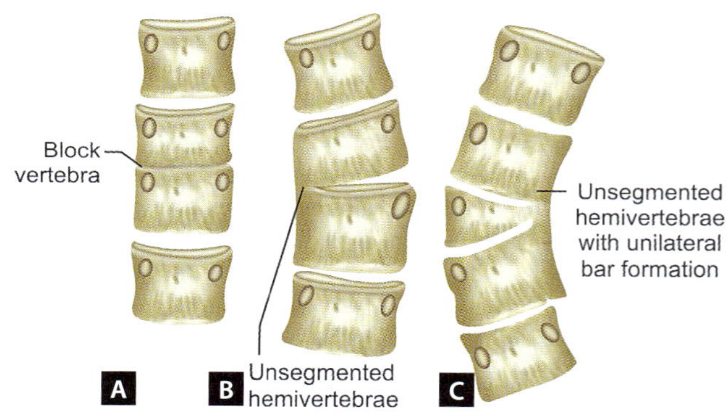

Figs. 39A to C: Failure of segmentation.

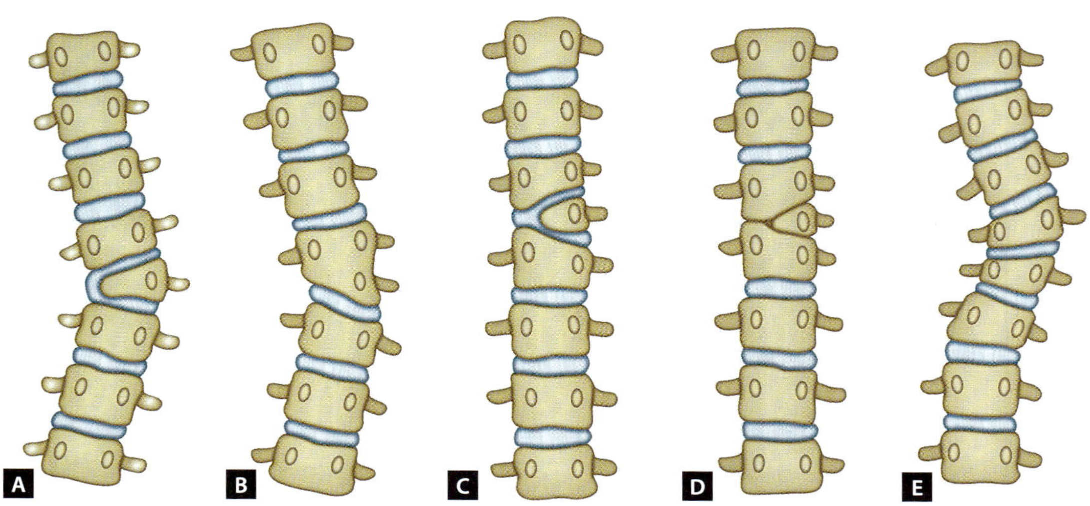

Figs. 40A to E: Failure of formation: (A) Fully segmented unbalanced hemivertebra; (B) Fused hemivertebra; (C) Fully segmented counterbalanced hemivertebra by wedge vertebrae; (D) Incarcerated unsegmented hemivertebra; (E) Wedge vertebra.

Etiopathogenesis, Associated System Anomalies and Natural History

Though epidemiology suggests strong genetic association, but the pattern of inheritance or the gene associated is still elusive. The following are some of the common associations reported (but not proven):

- Maternal exposure to toxins, such as carbon monoxide
- Associations with maternal diabetes
- Association with ingestion of antiepileptic drugs, alcohol, valproic acid, hyperthermia during pregnancy
- A wide variety of associated anomalies—genitourinary (25%, renal agenesis, horse-shoe kidney, duplicated ureters, etc.), cardiac (10%, tetralogy of Fallot, transposition of great vessels), and intraspinal—can accompany congenital spinal deformities.
- Intraspinal anomalies, such as stenosis, Chiari malformation, intradural lipomas, diastematomyelia (split cord seen in 20% patients) and spinal cord tethering occur in 5–35% of congenital spinal deformities. Diastematomyelia should be resected before corrective surgery as stretching of cord may cause permanent damage and paralysis.
- Understanding of multisystem can be understood on the basis of field concept by Opitz. The various associated syndromes that can occur with congenital scoliosis are:
  - VACTREL syndrome (see Radial club hand)
  - Joubert syndrome
  - Oculo-Auriculo-Vertebral syndrome (Goldenhar syndrome)—hemifacial microsomia and epibulbar dermoids)
  - Spondylocostal dysostosis (Jarcho-levin syndrome)—autosomal recessive, short trunk dwarfism, vertebral and rib defects, prominent thoracic insufficiency syndrome.
  - Klippel-Feil syndrome
  - Alagille syndrome—cholestasis, facial dysmorphism, pulmonary stenosis.
  - Basal cell nevus
  - Trisomy 18
  - Diabetic embryopathy.
- Rate of deterioration and the severity of final deformity are predictable according to the type of anomaly and curve location (see classification below).
- Upper thoracic curves tend to be less severe than thoracolumbar curves (these are most severe)
- Curve progression (caused by unbalanced growth of one side of the spine relative to the other) occurs more rapidly during the first 5 years of life and during puberty.
- Presence of either a bar or fused ribs indicates high chances of curve progression. The at-risk vertebral anomalies liable to cause curve progression (in order of severity) are:
  - Unilateral unsegmented bar combined with single or multiple contralateral convex hemivertebrae—fastest progression up to 10°/year.
  - Unilateral unsegmented bar
  - Double convex hemivertebrae
  - Single convex hemivertebra
  - Unsegmented hemivertebrae (incarcerated > unincarcerated)
  - Block vertebra—most benign producing curves less than 20°.

Development of Vertebral Column (Figs. 41A to C)

- To understand the anatomical development of various defects of congenital scoliosis we need to understand the development of vertebral column and potential for developing abnormalities.

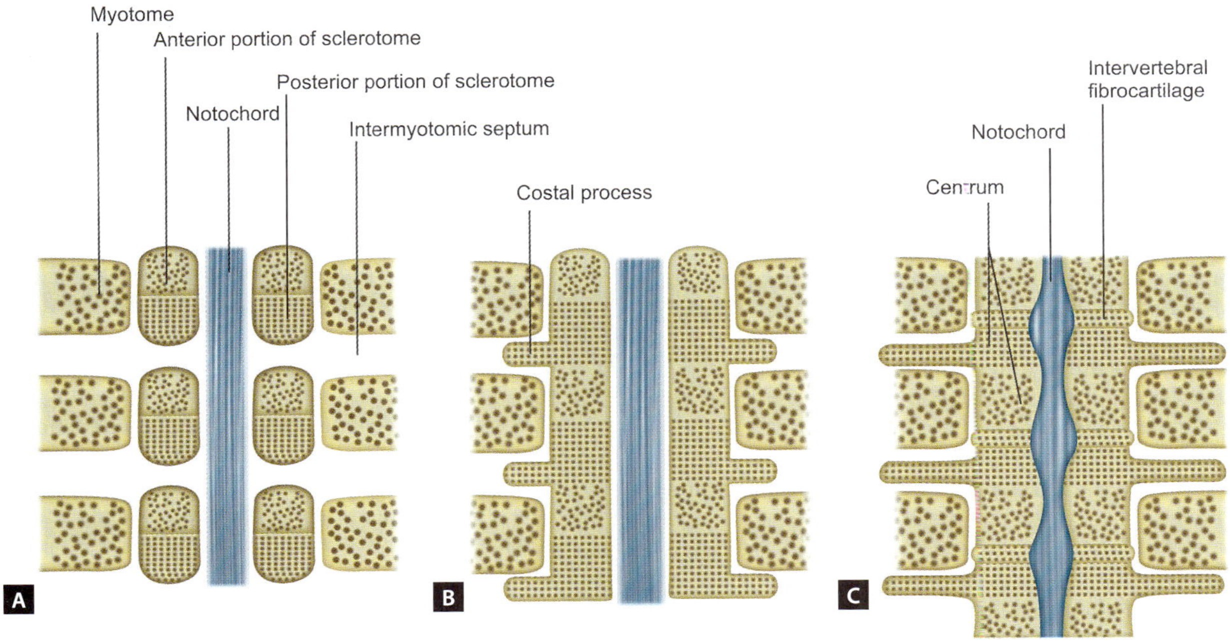

Figs. 41A to C: Vertebral column development (see text for details).

- Vertebral column develops from pairs of somites (mesenchymal segment on both sides of the neural tube), which begin to appear at 3 weeks gestation.
- Cells from the sclerotomes (anteromedial wall of the somite) spread out centrally to form an unsegmented, cellular perichordal sheath—form the centrum of the vertebral column.
- A zone of loose cells in the sclerotome forms superiorly where the intersegmental and spinal nerve pass through the plate
- A zone of dense cells forms inferiorly that later becomes the posterior neural arch of the vertebra and the rib
- Thus, in all one sclerotome pair forms one level of ribs and posterior elements of the spine
- In the notochord alternating zones of loose and dense zones appear
  - The superior zone of loose cells goes on to form the centrum of the vertebra
  - The inferior dense zone goes on to form the intervertebral disk.

Various theories have been proposed to explain congenital vertebral malformations (that occur by 4–6 weeks itself!) based on the understanding of development.

- Failure of ossification → defects of vertebra formation
- Osseous metaplasia of the annulus fibrosus → defects of vertebral segmentation
- Arrested vertebral development → due to persistent notochord.

Clinical Features and Evaluation of Patients

Prenatal history from mother—previous pregnancies, medications, health record and alcohol consumption. Details of length of gestation, type of delivery, birth weight and complications are recorded.

Examine for developmental milestones as cognitive development has been linked to curve progression.

There is variable presence of features that indicate presence of congenital anomalies. The following should be looked for as they serve signaling markers:

- *Spinal dysraphism:*
  - Posterior midline skin lesions (such as hairy patches or deep dimples)
  - Asymmetrical foot deformities (cavus or flat feet)
  - Muscle tone and power—weakness, or spasticity
- Sight and hearing can also be congenitally impaired
- Look for café-au-lait spots, axillary freckles (neurofibromatosis)
- Rib cage deformities and asymmetry
- Chest excursion (limitation indicates thoracic insufficiency syndrome)
- Rib hump—Adams forward bending test
  - In young children make them lay prone on examiners knee
- Curve flexibility
- *Spinal balance:*
  - Truncal balance
  - Shoulder inequality
  - Pelvic balance
- Detailed motor and sensory examination including superficial and deep reflexes—ABSENCE of abdominal reflexes may point to Chiari malformation.

Renal ultrasonography, cardiac consultation (and echocardiogram), and MRI of the entire brainstem and spinal cord are essential for complete evaluation. Systemic deficiencies are evaluated for anesthesia and general well-being of the patient to bear surgery.

The predominant congenital deformity usually exists as a scoliosis, kyphosis, or lordosis in a multiplanar distribution.

Radiographic description of deformity should include the involved area of the spine, type of vertebral anomaly and configuration of the deformity. CT scan should be judiciously used to detail the deformity and for classification.

The specific indications for MRI include:

- The presence of neurological defects such as weakness, sensory loss, bowel or bladder dysfunction
- Associated skin abnormality over the spine such as a dimple, hairy patches, or nevi
- Complaints of back or leg pain
- Patients with lumbosacral kyphosis
- Radiographic evidence of interpedicular widening
- Diastematomyelia
- Presence of a unilateral congenital bar with a contralateral hemivertebra
- Any patient who is to undergo spinal stabilization surgery (r/o tethered cord, syringomyelia intradural lipoma, etc.)

Pulmonary evaluation includes obtaining vital capacity and if it is less than 60% of normal then a full spirometry workup.

Classification of Congenital Scoliosis

A congenital scoliotic curve can be:

- Upper thoracic (33% of curves)
- Lower thoracic (31%)
- Thoracolumbar (20%)
- Lumbar (11%)
- Lumbosacral (5%)

In general, thoracolumbar curves tend to have the worst prognosis and the greatest progression, followed by lower thoracic curves and then upper thoracic curves. Anomalies tend to occur at the apex of a curve. A classification system for congenital spinal deformities based on the embryological development of the spine as visible on the plain AP and lateral radiographs was proposed and refined by Winter et al. Spinal anomalies are classified as failures of segmentation, failures of formation and mixed anomalies **(*see* Figs. 39 and 40)**.

- In this system 80% of deformities are classified; however, classification of the remaining 20% is obscured by the multiplicity of defects (better explained by the 3D CT-based classification of Kawakami et al. 2009, see below).
- This classification provides a prognostic guide for treatment.
- In general, 75% of congenital scoliotic deformities progress and the rate varies depending on the type.

- Defects of segmentation can be uni- or bilateral. Early in the course, a segmentation defect can appear as a narrow disk space that progressively narrows with growth until fusion occurs.
    - A block vertebra is a bilateral segmentation defect that causes the spine to shorten, but it has little propensity for scoliosis progression.
    - Unilateral unsegmented bars, however, have a high frequency of progressing because growth potential exists on only one side of the spine. This when combined with opposite hemivertebra (ae) is associated with most rapid curve progression due to growth on convex side (hemivertebra) and arrest on concave side by bar tethering, and should be surgically treated at an early stage to prevent severe deformity.
- Defects of formation are those in which absence or maldevelopment of a part of the spine produces deformity.
    - Bifid or absent dorsal elements
    - *Hemivertebra (complete):* There is absence of one pedicle and a region of the vertebral body. They are usually associated with extra rib. Hemivertebra are the result of abnormal cleavage of the primary chondrification center. These hemivertebra may involve mild wedging to complete absence of one side of the vertebra:
        - *Fully segmented hemivertebra:* There is normal disk space above and below.
        - *Semisegmented hemivertebra:* Hemivertebra fused to adjacent vertebra on one side, other side separated by disk space from vertebra.
        - Unsegmented hemivertebrae are fused to both proximal and distal adjacent vertebrae without any intervening disk space
            - Incarcerated unsegmented hemivertebra—found within lateral margins of vertebra above and below
            - Unincarcerated unsegmented hemivertebra—extends outside one of the lateral margins of adjacent vertebra
        - Wedge vertebrae (partial)—present with a height asymmetry with one side being hypoplastic. There are two pedicles. There is no extra rib and hence may involve a unilateral failure of development of the chondrification center.

          The prognosis varies and is based on the type, location and number of hemivertebrae. In general, 25% of hemivertebrae progress rapidly, 25% do not progress and 50% progress slowly.
    - Open vertebral growth plates dictate the tendency of curve to progress so a fully segmented hemivertebra, with a functional plate proximally and caudally will have the greatest propensity to progress.
    - Incarcerated and unsegmented hemivertebrae are infrequently associated with progression. Treatment is recommended only in cases of severe deformity or when curve documented progression is 10° or more.
- Mixed type—comprises of complex anomalies that include both segmentation and formation errors. They are difficult to identify as spine is only 30% ossified at birth.
- Congenital lordosis is due to posterior segmentation defects in contrast to kyphotic deformities that can result from both segmentation defects and failure of formation. Kyphosis that results from failure of formation results in a sharper more angulated deformity and may even cause paraplegia. This is more likely in thoracic spine and it progresses a mean of 7° per year if associated with failure of formation (hemivertebra). Kyphosis resulting from segmentation failure is more rounded but progression can occur. 95% of congenital kyphoses progress.

Three-dimensional classification of vertebral anomalies *(Kawakami et al.):* Plain radiograph cannot demonstrate the spatial relationship of each structure of the vertebrae. The relationship between anterior and posterior components cannot be fully evaluated on plain radiographs only. 3D CT images detail the various anomalies and define treatment algorithms better. It allows clearer observation of morphology and fusion compared to plain radiographs. Due to identification of various aspects of congenital anomalies the classification is quite complicated. Various identified morphologies, patterns of segmentation, solitary or multiple, and unison or discordant and descriptions of their combinations are out of the scope of current text and can be referred to by an interested reader. The system is not in practical use but may become important with further studies and for specific utility, if identified. In broader terms the system identifies three main types of congenital spinal deformity:

1. *Type 1:* Solitary simple
2. *Type 2:* Multiple simple
3. *Type 3:* Complex
4. *Type 4:* Segmentation failure.

Treatment

Observation and bracing has no known definitive role in management of congenital scoliosis. Either the curve will progress or need surgical treatment or it will not and will never require deformity correction. Observation (till skeletal maturity) is strictly done only for:

- Incarcerated hemivertebrae
- Nonsegmental hemivertebrae
- Some partially segmented hemivertebrae

Bracing has no role in management of congenital scoliosis either for prevention of curve progression or correction as it universally fails for these inflexible curves. The only known role of bracing is to control the supple compensatory curves if they develop [Milwaukee for upper curves, TLSO (thoracic/lumbar/sacral orthosis) brace for lumbar curves].

Surgical Management

Congenital spinal deformities are rigid and correction is generally achieved through the mobile segments above and below the anomaly. Instrumentation is the preferred modality these days compared to the cast management done previously. Instrumentation maintains or improves correction but the postoperative risk of neurological impairment is highest in this group due to the following reasons:

- Small spinal canal size
- Severe deformities
- Frequent presence of intraspinal anomalies such as diastematomyelia or tethering.

Ideally for early deformities surgical fusion is performed to prevent deformity progression and for patients presenting late with severe deformity correction of deformity becomes the goal. The goals of surgical management include in general:

- Achieve a straight spine
- Maintain a physiological sagittal profile while maintaining flexibility
- To arrest progression of the curve
- Short fusion segment preserving as much normal spinal growth as possible.

The principles of surgery include:

- Early and aggressive treatment of deformities
- In surgical planning the superior/inferior endpoints of instrumentation are so chosen that the head is centered over the pelvis in both the frontal and sagittal planes.
    - The compensatory curve need not be included in the fusion, unless it is anticipated that the structural component of the compensatory curve is the main cause of trunk decompensation. These compensatory curves must be however closely monitored.
- Posterior instrumentation is reserved for the thoracic and lumbar deformities in adolescents or in cases where spinal instability or unacceptable truncal shortening will result from combined anterior-posterior procedures/ osteotomies
- Preventing lengthening the spinal cord intraoperatively
- Routine use of MRI evaluation
- Tethered cords and diastematomyelia must be corrected before deformity correction
- Instrumentation appropriate to the patient's size must be chosen
- Monitored use of controlled hypotension
- Monitoring intraoperative neurology and postoperative neurological status.

As mentioned the surgery is done either to prevent deformity from occurring or correcting the deformity so two broad forms of surgical procedures are described. Out of the various surgical options posterior fusion (including in situ fusion), anterior fusion, combined anterior-posterior fusion, hemivertebra excision, and spinal osteotomy and fusion are used for preventing deformity while others for correction of deformity.

Procedures Preventing Deformity in Future

- *In situ fusion:* Posterior spinal fusion is the gold standard for both congenital scoliosis and kyphosis. To be successful, the posterior fusion must include the entire curve, from last stable vertebra to first stable vertebra. It is ideally suited for short curves like those with unilateral failure of segmentation (unilateral bar) with a curve less than 40°. Also deformities at the lumbosacral and cervicothoracic junction should be fused very early as they are cosmetically most disfiguring. The crankshaft phenomenon or bending of the posterior fusion mass may occur in some very young patients (<5 years of age) with congenital scoliosis and hence the major controversy is whether combined anterior and posterior fusion should be done routinely. It has been argued that there is less potential for anterior growth in a spine with congenital scoliosis because the growth plates may not be properly formed. So currently it is deemed that when thoracic lordosis is part of the deformity, anterior discectomy and fusion is preferable to prevent any crankshaft phenomenon and also to avoid progressive thoracic encroachment. Some recommend that for unilateral bars and contralateral hemivertebra the curve progression potential is high and should be managed by combined anterior and posterior procedures.

  In mild cases of congenital kyphosis, spontaneous correction after posterior fusion alone can occur in young patients (<5 years of age) with kyphotic deformity less than 50°.
- *Convex hemiepiphysiodesis (Roaf, 1955):* The common indication is a unilateral formation failure (hemivertebra). There should be potential for growth on the concave side so definite exclusion of contralateral bar should be made before the procedure. In convex hemiepiphysiodesis, the convex lateral half of disks adjacent to the hemivertebra are removed without touching the concave side and thus potentiate correction by preferential concave growth. This procedure should be reserved (Winter et al.) for patients younger than 5 years of age, with a progressive curve of less than 70° (ideally <40°) involving five segments or less (ideally <3) without any kyphosis or lordosis modifier. Hemivertebra excision or wedge resection is more predictable procedures than hemiepiphysiodesis.
- *Hemivertebra excision:* Here the culprit vertebra is removed by wedge resection where in situ fusion (or convex hemiepiphysiodesis) will not work as in kyphotic deformities and truncal imbalance. Ideally this procedure is reserved for an L-5 lumbosacral junction hemivertebra causing trunk decompensation. Excision of hemivertebrae at other levels is typically reserved for cases of severe kyphotic deformities, which may or may not be associated with neurological defects. Excision of hemivertebra decompresses the spinal cord tented over the apex of kyphosis. It is best done at and before 2 years of age as cast is less easily tolerated by patients older than this age. After excision compression instrumentation is mandatory. The procedure can be accomplished by posterior only or a combined anterior and posterior approach, having their individual pros and cons:
    - Posterior only approach—using pedicle screw instrumentation to correct deformity has been preferred for less operative time and morbidity and lesser risk to anterior vascular and visceral structures.

- Combined approach—is advocated by some for its capability to achieve higher correction including sagittal plane deformity correction. The growth plates can be removed and reduce the chances of development of crankshaft phenomenon.

Procedures Done to Correct the Deformity

- ***Gradual correction techniques:*** These include
  - *Hemiepiphysiodesis and hemiarthrodesis:* Used for failure of formation (there is no growth potential left in segmentation failure). Curves with limited growth potential on the concave side like the convex hemivertebra will not be benefitted by the procedure. The procedure is aimed to arrest growth on the convex side and relies on continued growth on the concave side for curve correction.
  - *Growing rods (see also in the management of early onset scoliosis):* For management of cases in early years of life (2–3 years of age), it is imperative to understand that sitting height reaches the adult height by the age of 5 years. So, long fusions will result in stunted growth. Also the thoracic volumes reach 30% of adult volumes by 5 years of age and similarly the fusion surgeries will produce a loss in the thoracic volume and thoracic insufficiency. Growing rods (Akbarnia and McCarthy system) permit growth of the spine and curve correction and apical fusion to correct the congenital anomaly (especially failure of segmentation) may be needed.
- ***Acute correction techniques:*** These include
  - *Correction and fusion with instrumentation:* The aim is to obtain a balanced spine in the safest way possible. High thoracic and lumbar spine needs particular care as they cause maximum imbalance. The best curves for these procedures are those with relatively preserved segmentation, partially flexible and less severe truncal deformity. If the disk spaces are well preserved then anterior fusion is combined. One should ensure, by preoperative MRI that there is no cord tethering or diastematomyelia.
  - Hemivertebra excision (see earlier)
  - *Reconstructive osteotomy:* Fixed curves are not amenable to manipulative correction either acute or gradual. The nonflexible curves with truncal decompensation need to be repositioned by corrective osteotomies. Other indications are pelvic obliquity and developing neurological deficit. The corrective osteotomies can be combined with hemivertebra resection or "fusion with instrumentation" procedures described above.
- ***VEPTR and expansion thoracoplasty:*** Thoracic insufficiency (introduced by Campbell et al.) refers to poor thoracic and lung parenchymal development that produces poor lung function resulting from restricted growth of the thoracic cavity. Tethering of the ribs is also responsible for curve progression that in turn reduces thoracic cavity exacerbating the insufficiency in pulmonary function with growth (contrary to the expectation of improving lung function with growth). The poor lung function primarily results from reduced height and volume of the thoracic cavity that precludes lung expansion and alveolar development that get arrested to infancy maturity. Both the numbers and size of alveoli are diminished. The growth of the lung and alveoli multiplication is greatest in the first 8 years of life reaching 50% of the adult thoracic volume. Early fusions will hence restrict not only the development of spine but also the thoracic height and volume (see radiographic evaluation for estimating the height of thoracic cavity). Children who have borderline lung function at maturity are at high risk for developing respiratory insufficiency in late adulthood due to the following reasons:
  - Approximately 400 cc of vital capacity is lost in aging process
  - Development of COPD will reduce the available lung volume
  - Acute respiratory infections and pneumonia will reduce the lung function to critical survival levels.

Thoracic insufficiency is a lately recognized complication of total growth inhibition of thoracic spine by combined anterior and posterior spinal fusion, convex anterior epiphysiodesis or arthrodesis performed with the ideology of having a "short straight spine instead of long crooked one". VEPTR technique (see above in early onset scoliosis) challenged the above concept by showing an increase in length of the unilateral unsegmented bars and equal increases in length of the concave and convex sides in congenital scoliosis. VEPTR expands thorax by rib distraction on the concave side of the curve achieving indirect correction.

When the focal kyphosis exceeds 50°, correction requires anterior release followed by posterior fusion. If the anterior release is not performed, the pseudarthrosis rate may be as high as 54% compared with 13% when combining anterior and posterior fusion. Winter et al. recommended routine re-exploration of the posterior bone graft 6 months after a posterior surgery if anterior fusion was not performed. In their series, however, instrumentation was not used.

ADULT SCOLIOSIS AND DEFORMITY

Adult scoliosis is defined as a coronal plane Cobb's angle greater than 10° in a patient older than 20 years. The scoliotic curves in adults could be due to persistent AIS curves (referred to as only "adult scoliosis" *cf-* "adult-onset scoliosis", **Table 6**) or may develop de novo. The persistent curves from AIS may have degeneration component (usually only after 40 years of age) or may not have any degenerative signs (benign persistence). The *de novo* curves are the real "adult-onset scoliosis" and are commonly secondary to degenerative changes of lumbar spine **(Figs. 42A and B)**. Adult-onset deformity progresses slowly and occurs in the elderly population with distinctive radiological and clinical features. Spinal canal stenosis, spondylolisthesis, rotational subluxation, lumbar hyperlordosis and rigid deformities often are seen with adult-onset deformities. This entails different forming mechanism and surgical management needed for adult deformity than that used for idiopathic scoliosis.

Theories of Pathogenesis

- Asymmetrical degeneration of disk → asymmetric loading of spine → asymmetric degeneration of facet joints → curve propagation
- Osteoporosis-induced asymmetrical loss of vertebral height → asymmetrical loading of spine → asymmetrical degeneration of spine → curve propagation. Anterior wedging causes sagittal imbalance.

  The natural history and clinical presentation: In both types of scoliosis females predominate.
- For adult scoliosis, the curves do not progress if less than 40°.
  - Curve progression averages 1° per year if more than 50°
  - Risk factors for the progression of lumbar curves include large apical rotation and/or lateral and rotatory listhesis
  - For double curves, the lumbar curve tends to progress more rapidly than the thoracic curve
  - There is no impact on pulmonary function
  - Incidence of back pain is not higher but those who have it are worse and have recurrent episodes compared to age-matched population
  - The reasons for presenting symptoms to the physician are either pain at the location of the curve or progression of the curve.
- De novo curves (adult-onset scoliosis) of the lumbar spine may progress rapidly and the rate of curve progression is not constant. Its prevalence is approximately 6%. The deformity develops quite insidiously. The degeneration is slow to start with and leads to loss in the intervertebral disk height. This progresses also slowly and finally most of the disk spaces are gone. Pain and disabilities are the main problems for progressive deformities. Foraminal stenosis causes sciatica and patients get bed-ridden in the end.
  - The average age at presentation is 6th–7th decade
  - The average curve progression is approximately 3.3° per year
  - A greater number of males are affected compared to those in adult scoliosis
  - *The common presenting symptoms are (often a combination):*
    - Neurogenic claudication—spinal stenosis is seen in 90% patients with de novo scoliosis. Foraminal stenosis is common than central stenosis. Stenosis is more common on the concave side. Facet joint hypertrophy and lateral subluxation is associated with foraminal stenosis.
    - Radicular symptoms—pedicular kinking and of the nerve beneath it commonly causes radicular symptoms present on the concave side. Symptoms on convex side of curve (uncommon) are due to

TABLE 6: Comparative features of adult scoliosis and adult-onset scoliosis.

Adult scoliosis, adult idiopathic scoliosis or persistent idiopathic scoliosis	*Adult-onset scoliosis or adult degenerative scoliosis (ADS), de novo scoliosis*
Persistence of previous curves	Curve develops due to degeneration of spinal motion segments
Younger patients mean around 50–55 years	Older patients mean age around 70 years
Cobb's angle usually less than 40°	Cobb's angle usually higher than 50°
The compensatory curve (usually lumbar or thoracic) is usually equal to the main/primary curve (usually thoracic)	ADS develops in lumbar region with no thoracic compensatory curves
Rotatory deformity present along the whole of major curve	Rotation limited at the apex of curve
No lateral subluxation	Lateral subluxation common at apex of deformity
Sagittal imbalance is limited	Sagittal imbalance prominent
Spinal stenosis and disk degeneration less common or develop only in late stages	Degenerative changes are consistently present and prominent. Spinal stenosis is seen in >90% of the patients

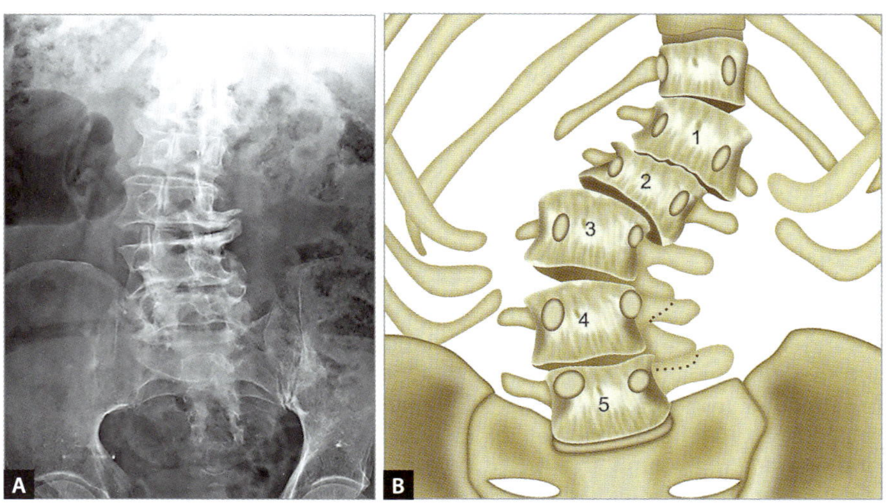

Figs. 42A and B: Adult-onset scoliosis in degenerative spine.

PIVD compression at L4/5 or L5S1. Nerve root compression and radiculopathy is seen on the concave side while nerve stretching is seen on the convex side.
    - *Back pain (in combined symptoms this is not the main complaint):* This is the most common (60–80% patients) but not the most prominent symptom. Back pain is usually present on the convex side of curve. The pain is mainly due to degenerated disk, facet joints or muscle fatigue. Rotational subluxation and sagittal imbalance increases back pain.
- Lumbar curves progress more rapidly than thoracic curves (contrast—AIS).

Risk Factors for Curve Progression

- Curve size over 30°
- Asymmetric disk above and below the apical vertebra
- Apical rotation greater than Grade 2
- Lateral subluxation (lateral listhesis) of the apical vertebra over 6 mm
- L5 vertebra being located above rather than below the intercrestal line

Classification of Adult Deformities

- Aebi made a deformity classification based on the etiology. It gives good insight in understanding the adult deformity.
    - *Type 1 scoliosis:* Primary degenerative scoliosis (de novo scoliosis) is usually seen at the thoracic and lower region in childhood. This is the most common. In this group patients start their lives with a healthy spine but the spine starts to curve at older ages. Degeneration begins from the intervertebral disk. As for any other joint the degenerations are often asymmetric creating asymmetric loadings. This initiates the curves slowly at the initiation site. Lysis of spine, instability, syndesmophyte formation, and foraminal narrowing due to lysis compress the roots causing symptoms.
    - *Type 2 scoliosis:* This is progression of adolescent thoracic, thoracolumbar and/or lower scoliosis (adult scoliosis).
    - *Type 3 scoliosis:* Secondary degenerative scoliosis
        - The idiopathic or other type of scoliosis progress and form this type. Also asymmetry of leg length, pelvic pathology or lumbosacral transitional anomaly causes this type of scoliosis which is usually at thoracolumbar, lumbar or lumbosacral regions.
        - Metabolic bone disease (osteoporosis) with asymmetric arthritis or/and vertebra fracture. In developed countries, osteoporosis is serious problem especially for women who live longer. Osteoporosis is also one of the main problems of older ages. Degenerations reduce vertebral resistance and thus excessive loading occurs and can cause acute vertebral fracture or progressive loss of vertebra height. The spine starts to curve.
- *King-Moe classification (**see Table 3**):* This classification is good for thoracic deformity. The classification provides for appropriate fusion levels and placement of distraction instrumentation. The principle problem with the classification system is that it is older for newer instrumented systems and does not fit. Other variously described limitations include:
    - The system does not include lumbar deformities
    - There is no inclusion of sagittal plane deformities which is fundamental to the adult deformities
    - Isolated triple major curves and thoracolumbar curves not described
    - Poor interobserver and intraobserver reproducibility.
- *Lenke system (seeearlier):* This system was more comprehensive and provides two dimensional analyses with emphasis on evaluation of sagittal plane deformities, providing appropriate treatment guidelines. However pain, degeneration and hence the formation of adult deformities required more than this classification, especially the complete definition of the sagittal deformity component.
- *Schwab clinical impact classification:* Based on the greater understanding of the pain and disability component of the adult deformity Schwab proposed a clinical impact classification by correlating the radiological parameters with poor health-related quality of life parameters. The initial classification underwent two important modifications to produce the final classification **(Table 7)**.
    - Lumbar lordosis, oliolisthesis and endplate obliquity are important radiological parameters that also correlate with poor HRQOL scores.
    - Global sagittal alignment measured by sagittal vertical axis (SVA; distance from the C7 plumb line to the posterior, superior corner of S1) also predicts poor HRQOL scores.
- *SRS-Schwab hybrid classification (**Table 8**, the SRS classification is not discussed here as it has been incorporated in this hybrid classification):* Schwab

TABLE 7: Schwab clinical impact classification for adult scoliosis.

Type: Location of the deformity (apical level of the major curve or sagittal plane only) • *Type I:* Thoracic-only scoliosis (no thoracolumbar or lumbar component) • *Type II:* Upper thoracic major, apex T4 to T8 (with thoracolumbar or lumbar curve) • *Type III:* Lower thoracic major, apex T9 to T10 (with thoracolumbar/lumbar curve) • *Type IV:* Thoracolumbar major curve, apex T11 to L1 (with any other minor curve) • *Type V:* Lumbar major curve, apex L2 to L4 (with any other minor curve) • *Type K:* Deformity in the sagittal plane only	*Lordosis modifier:* Sagittal Cobb's angle from T12 to S1 A: Marked lordosis greater than 40° B: Moderate lordosis 0–40° C: No lordosis present Cobb's angle less than 0° *Subluxation modifier:* Frontal or sagittal plane (anterior or posterior), maximum value 0: No subluxation +: Subluxation 1–6 mm ++: Subluxation greater than 7 mm *Global balance modifier:* Sagittal plane C7 Offset from posterior superior corner S1 N: Normal (0–4 cm) P: Positive (4–9.5 cm) VP: Very positive (>9.5 cm)

classification **(Fig. 43)** meets a high clinical relevance but does not include pelvic parameters. Lafage et al. have reported the fundamental role of pelvis as the main regulator of a chain of correlation between spine and lower limbs, and sagittal evaluation therefore addition of spinopelvic alignment gives a more complete description of mechanisms for upright standing posture and explains the pain and disability better. Pelvic tilt (PT), sacral slope (SS) and pelvic incidence (PI) are used to measure pelvic alignment (**Fig. 44**, also see the description on sagittal balance below).

TABLE 8: SRS-Schwab hybrid classification for adult scoliosis.

Curve type	Sagittal modifiers are pelvic incidence-lumbar lordosis (PI-LL), pelvic tilt (PT) and sagittal vertical axis (SVA)
Curve type T: Thoracic major curve is more than 30°, the apical vertebra is T9 and higher *Curve type L*: Lumbar and thoracic major curves are more than 30°, the apical vertebra is T10 or lower *Curve type D*: There is a double major curve and each curve much more than 30° *Curve type N*: Coroner curve or curves are not more than 30°. There is no major coronal deformity	*PI-LL modifier*: It shows the proportional relation between PI and LL. The PI is measured as the angle between the line drawn perpendicular to the sacral endplate at its midpoint and the line drawn from the midpoint of the sacral endplate to the midpoint of the bicoxofemoral axis **(Fig. 44).** The LL is the sagittal Cobb's angle measured between the superior endplate of L1 and the superior endplate of S1 • 0: Within 10° • +: Moderate 10–20° • ++: Marked greater than 20°
	Global alignment modifier is assessed by SVA. The SVA is defined as the offset between the sagittal C7 plumb line and the posterior, superior corner of the sacrum • 0: SVA <4 cm • +: SVA 4–9.5 cm • ++: SVA >9.5 cm
	Pelvic tilt is a compensatory mechanism that can affect and reduce the apparent extent of global sagittal malalignment. This is highly correlated with pain and disability. PT modifier assesses the degree of pelvic retroversion, with PT measured as the angle between the line connecting the midpoint of the sacral endplate to the midpoint of the bicoxofemoral axis and the vertical **(Fig. 44)**: • 0: PT < 20° • +: PT 20–30° • ++: PT > 30°

Evaluation and Investigations

Plain Radiographs

- Obtain initial PA and lateral long-cassette radiographs that should include the cervical spine down to the pelvis. Evaluate the following parameters:
  - *On PA films:*
    - Cobb's measurement of all curves
    - Coronal imbalance—measured as a trunk shift from the CSVL or a deviation of a C7 plumb from the CSVL (most important in adult deformity)
    - Rotatory listhesis or subluxation
    - Disk height and wedging
    - Osteophyte formation and degeneration
  - *On lateral films:*
    - Cobb's measurement—thoracic kyphosis (T5 to T12) and lumbar lordosis (L1 to L5)—Loss of lumbar lordosis is usually seen
    - Sagittal balance—the C7 plumb line should fall on the posterior aspect of the L5–S1 disk level
    - Disk space height and degeneration of facet joints
    - Osteopenia.
- Supine bend films should be used to assess flexibility (especially to evaluate the need for anterior surgery). They also are helpful when choosing fusion levels
- Traction films are also useful in assessing flexibility and choosing fusion levels
- Ferguson view—An X-ray beam directed 30° cephalad and focused on the lumbosacral junction" (to evaluate lumbosacral junction).

Computed tomography and myelography: Not an ultimate investigation to evaluate spine due to the much more decisive and versatile MRI, radiation risk is also high with CT. The current indications for obtaining CT scan are as follows:

- Inability to get MRI (pacemaker or claustrophobia)
- Primary presentation as canal stenosis—stenosis especially the central and lateral recess stenosis are well evaluated by CT scan. Also in setting of previous surgery, it is better to obtain CT scan for evaluating stenosis as MR often over-diagnosis and the picture is confusing. Patients with large curves are better evaluated by CT scan for stenosis

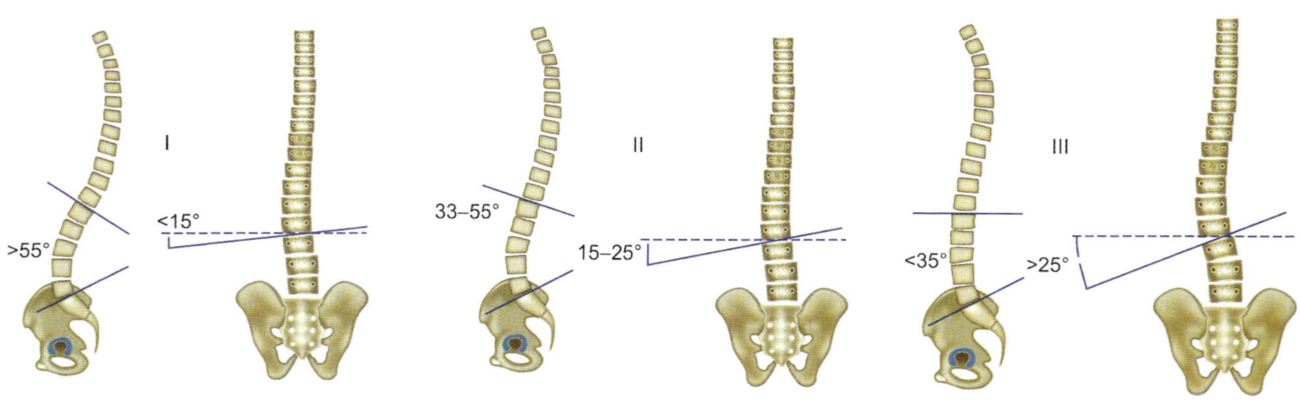

Fig. 43: Schwab adult lumbar classification of scoliosis.

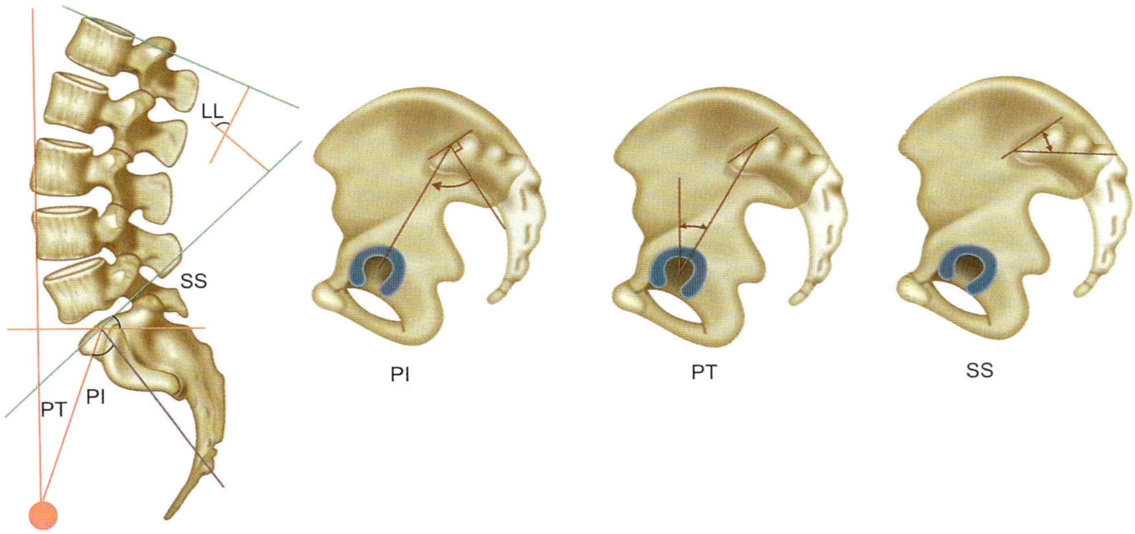

Fig. 44: Sagittal modifiers: PI-LL, PT and SVA (see text, Table 7). (PI: the angle between the line perpendicular to the sacral plate at its midpoint and the line connecting this point to the axis of rotation of the femoral head. PT: the angle between the line connecting the midpoint of the superior sacral endplate to the femoral rotational axis and the line extending vertically from the femoral rotational axis. SS: the angle between the superior endplate of S1 and a horizontal line extending from the anterior-inferior corner of the S1 endplate)

- Assessment of spinal fusion—no other investigation would surpass CT scan if one wants to evaluate spinal fusion and assessment of bony continuity
- Simultaneous assessment of bone quality—quantitative CT scan is best to evaluate the BMD and hence would guide the future quality of fixation and hence implant choice.

Magnetic Resonance Imaging

This is the investigation of choice to assess the pathologies associated with scoliosis that may represent the pain generators.

It is used to assess the:

- Spinal canal stenosis due to fibrosis/disk pathology, etc., that is not better represented on a CT scan
- Presence of disk herniation
- Morphology and degree of degeneration of the intervertebral disks—it helps to plan the fusion levels as usually all degenerated levels should be fused else the symptoms and disease recurs at the terminal fusion levels
- Patients who had been previously operated should also be additionally evaluated by gadolinium contrast study to study arachnoiditis/scar tissue or other inflammatory causes of pain.

Treatment

The treatment is related to the degeneration stage. Also the management depends on various other unique factors of adult deformity like:

- *Stiff curves:* It is difficult to achieve optimal correction with surgery. Due to reduced flexibility even the compensatory curves do not correct prominently.
- *Poor bone quality and implant purchase due to osteoporosis:* This leads to reduced fixation strength, loss of correction and pseudarthrosis. Segmental fixation improves fixation strength. Cement around the pedicle screw also improves fixation strength.
- Degeneration at spinal levels
- Medical comorbidities
- Need for simultaneous decompression prolonging the surgical time
- *Fixed sagittal imbalance:* This takes precedence over correction of scoliosis as poor results are seen with inadequate sagittal balance restoration.
- Multiple pain generators that contribute to postoperative failure if not addressed. It is difficult to identify all of them simultaneously.
- Requirement of longer fusions (blood loss, increased surgical time in a compromised patient!), also there is frequent need of combined anterior or posterior procedures.

Nonoperative Treatment

With degeneration at initial stage one can use a combination of physiotherapy and medications to provide relief to the patient. The common modalities include:

- Aerobic conditioning
- Strengthening and stretching exercises, "muscular re-education"
- Orthosis like a lumbar corset may help in improving back pain
- Radicular pain and/or neurogenic claudication often respond to nerve blocks or epidural steroid injections (*see* Chapter on " Preoperative Evaluation, Patient Optimization, and Pain Management in Orthopedic Patient").

BOX 1: The indications of operative management of adult spine deformity.

- Leg pain and radiculopathy not responding to conservative management and documented nerve
- Compression
- Curve progression or high potential for progression
- Coronal or sagittal imbalance or both
- Unresponsive to nonoperative treatment
- *Relative indications:*
  - Back pain not responding to conservative management
  - Pulmonary symptoms (uncommon indication)

Operative Treatment

The common "indications" for operative treatment of adult deformity are presented in **Box 1**.

The approaches commonly used based on curve types are as follows:

- *Curve type T:*
  - Posterior approach commonly used
  - Only the thoracic curve is fused lumbar motion is preserved
- *Curve type l:*
  - Anterior approach is the most common sometimes posterior approach is also combined
- *Curve type D:*
  - Posterior approach that includes both curves.

Anterior surgery has specific advantages and indications:

- It improves correction and fusion rates
- It recreates lumbar lordosis
- Anterior structural grafting in addition to improving fusion also creates a ligamentotaxis effect
- Anterior surgery has to be definitely added to posterior surgery at lumbosacral fusion to:
  - Improve fusion rate
  - Improve sagittal alignment.

Combined (anterior and posterior) fusion is a rigorous undertaking and should be used in:

- Large stiff curves
- Kyphosis and junctional kyphosis
- Rotatory subluxation or listhesis
- Lumbosacral fusion.

Fusion levels: Some principles are as follows:

- Manage adult scoliosis (Type 1, Aebi) according to principles for AIS
- End-instrumented vertebra should be neutral (horizontal, no rotation) and stable (bisected by the center sacral line)
- Fusion should not be stopped at the apex of the curve.
- For assessment of the distal lumbar disk levels below L3 an MRI is recommended to ensure that fusion of these levels is done due to presence of advanced degeneration. In any case if the fusion extends to L5 then sacrum should be included.
- For proximal level in ADS it is not known if the fusion should be carried to T10 levels or stopped at L1 but likely limiting fusion to L1 would produce degeneration at the T-L junction. Fusion till T11 or T12 is enough if the UIV is above the upper end vertebra.
- The junctional kyphosis is included in the fusion
- Levels of decompression for spinal stenosis should be included in the fusion levels
- The spondylolisthesis and retrolisthesis are included in the fusion.

Symptoms without Significant Deformity

Decompression alone is not usually recommended in adult degenerative scoliosis to treat the radicular symptoms. Nerve root compression on the concave side due to disk space narrowing causes radicular symptoms, but this is often associated with the lateral subluxation of the inferior vertebral body producing stretching of the nerve also. Instability may worsen with laminectomy and facet joint resection. Decompression may be done in an elderly frail patient with small curve and ideally without lateral subluxation.

- Decompression with limited short fusion—good choice in moderate scoliosis curve and mild subluxation of the apical vertebra. Problem is later development of disease in adjacent segments. Fusion should cross the apex of deformity else the degeneration progresses rapidly in out of fusion segments.

Deformity without Symptoms

Patient should be counseled that for large asymptomatic curves there are always significant chances of curve progression that may become symptomatic later.

- Manage the deformity with more minimally invasive surgery at the beginning period while sagittal modifier and sagittal balance are normal. This is done to prevent progression. Dynamic stabilization usually suffices.

Advanced Deformity

Scoliosis >30°, sagittal imbalance, coronal imbalance or both, lateral listhesis/rotatory subluxation with symptoms are the usual findings of advanced deformity:

- Hybrid system is recommended with segmental internal fixation. Segmental fixation is well done using pedicle screws. Pedicle screws are to be always used in lumbar spine and they provide good three-dimensional correction.
- Junctional kyphosis should be fused
- Fixation of lumbosacral region is another challenge. Combined procedure (anterior and posterior) should be done at L5-S1 region.
- Adding iliac screw or iliac instrumentation helps to add rigidity to the system. Various implants like Luque-galveston (developed by Allen and Ferguson it consists of contoured Luque rods placed between the cortical tables of the ilium and is used for scoliosis in which there is pelvic obliquity (frontal plane)), iliac screws, intrasacral rods and S2 screws provide fixation to "backup" S1 screws. In Dunn technique, contoured rods are passed through the S-1 foramen, coming to rest on the anterior sacrum between the internal iliac vessels.

Management of Fixed Sagittal Imbalance

Sagittal deformity has a more deformed appearance cosmetically and a higher degree of functional handicap of daily activity than a coronal deformity.

Indications for treatment: Risk to benefit should be aptly calculated before embarking on surgical management as the surgical complications and morbidity is significant. Aims of an osteotomy are to restore sagittal balance, so that the patient can stand erect without the need to flex the hips or knees, and to reduce the pain. Gross improvement in cosmesis and production of horizontal gaze are other advantages. The chief indications for osteotomy are:

- Painful fixed kyphosis
- SVA +/++ or C7 plumb line falling anterior to the L5-S1 disk.

Smith-Petersen osteotomy (1945, SPO): Smith-Petersen osteotomy was first described by Smith-Petersen as a one- or two-level osteotomy for ankylosing spondylitis. Opening of the anterior part (anterior column lengthening) and closing of the posterior part are performed after removing some of the posterior structures, such as lamina, spinous process, ligamentum flavum, lateral fusion mass, part of the inferior and superior articular process **(Figs. 45A and B)** in order to prevent neural impingement. The posterior part of the annulus acts as a pivot and pedicle is not resected. So

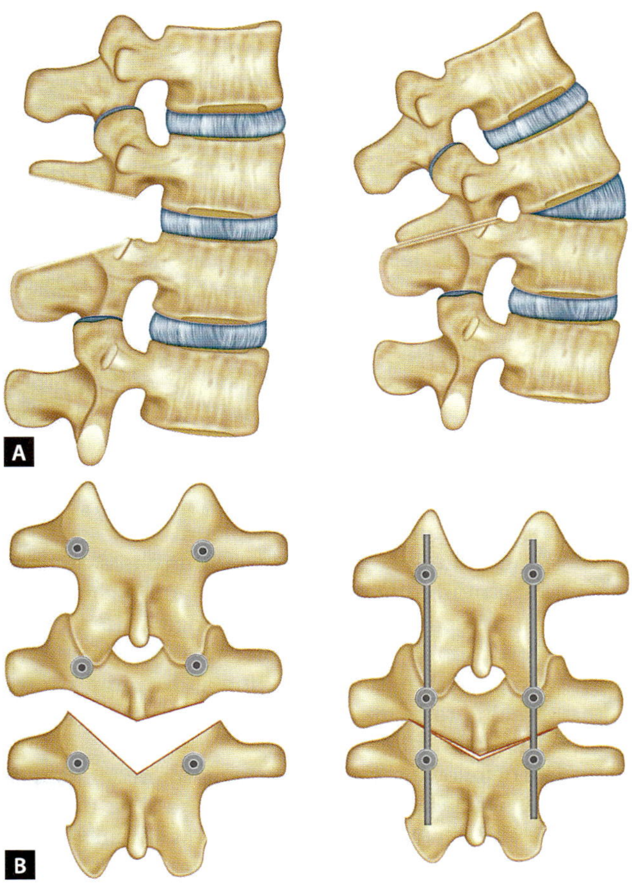

Figs. 45A and B: Smith-Petersen osteotomy. (A) The side; (B) Posterior views.

SPO can be only performed if there is mobile disk segment or anterior fusion mass is osteotomized. This osteotomy is indicated in cases requiring relatively small amount of correction (up to 30°, multilevel procedure has to be done as single level correction is averaged at 10°). SPO (thoracic spine) can be combined with PSO at lumbar spine (see below) for correction of long segment deformities from thoracic to lumbar spine. SPO can also be used to correct the kyphosis resulting from Andersson's lesion in ankylosing spondylosis. Due to lengthening of anterior column there is high chance of aortic or IVC rupture especially in cases with degenerative calcification. There have been various modifications to use of classical SPO:

- One-stage procedure at a single level is the classic SPO that achieves correction of 5–15°. 1 mm or resection achieves 1° of correction.
- Multiple osteotomies can be done posteriorly (polysegmental osteotomy—"Ponte procedure"): this achieves harmonious correction at various levels.
    - *Pushel and Zielke:* Multiple osteotomies at 4–6 levels and fixation with pedicle screws.
- *La Chapelle's procedure (1946) is a combined anterior and posterior procedure:* The ossified anterior ligaments of the spine are divided and correction is achieved by manual osteoclasis as in the Smith-Petersen technique. This combined procedure is indicated in:
    - Narrow disks that may not compensate for a significant correction of sagittal imbalance in a patient requiring greater than 30° of correction
    - Posterior only surgery is adequate in young patient but requires anterior procedure in multilevel osteotomies especially those patients having combined sagittal and coronal plane deformities.
- For the patient requiring 6–8 cm of correction of the C7 plumb line, it is more appropriate to perform a limited number of SPOs than one pedicle subtraction osteotomy (see below) unless the fixed deformity is fused anteriorly. The advantages of SPO are:
    - Technically easier and safer
    - Reduced operative time and blood loss intraoperatively.

Pedicle subtraction osteotomy (PSO): It is the posterior closing wedge osteotomy of spine. The patient best suited to undergo a pedicle subtraction osteotomy has a sagittal deformity and a solid anterior column, either from previous fusion or ankylosing spondylitis. Closing of the posterior part is performed after removing all of the posterior part, both the pedicle and half of the body. The anterior margin of the body acts as a pivot **(Fig. 46)**. There is no lengthening of anterior column and the correction of deformity is achieved through all three columns. Although it can be performed in a patient with open disk spaces (instead of a solid anterior fused column) the proximal and distal aspects of the wedged vertebral body will be left unattached to the hardware and hence difficult to control and bit unstable. Correction of up to 40° (some say 60°) can be achieved at a single segment. High amount of blood loss is a concern. The procedure is preferred in patients who require 30° or more correction

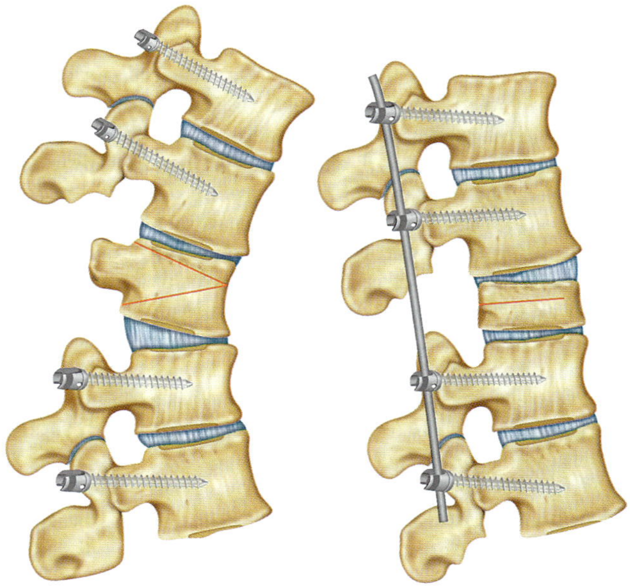

Fig. 46: Pedicle subtraction osteotomy.

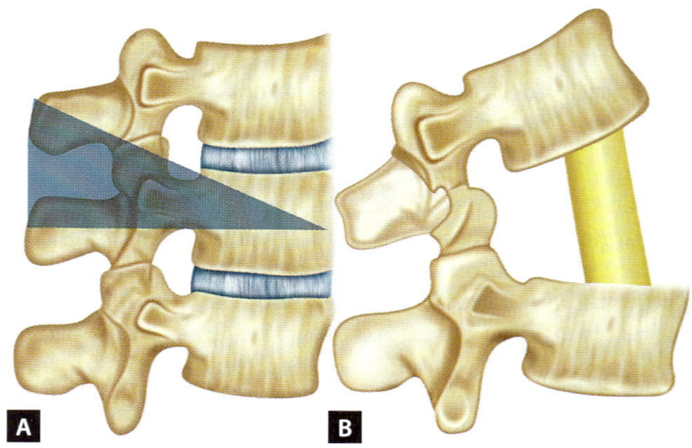

Figs. 47A and B: Vertebral column resection osteotomy.

at lumbar region, those with SVA (global modifier) "++" or more, those with sharp angular kyphosis and those having circumferential fusion between segments. It should be remembered that although subtle coronal imbalance may be manageable a prominent one may be made worse by the PSO. So if a concomitant coronal imbalance of more than 6 cm exists then better plan a vertebral resection (see later). The technical aspects of PSO are as follows:

- Three levels of fixation above and below the osteotomy should be planned and obtained before spine is destabilized by osteotomy
- The osteotomy resection begins with a wide laminectomy extending proximal and distal to the planned wedge resection
- This allows neural buckling and prevents neural compression upon closure of the osteotomy. The pedicles and lateral mass are resected and wedge is closed posteriorly
- The PSO closes the posterior and middle columns (hinges on the anterior column)
- Eggshell decancellation (Heinig and Chewning) may be combined with PSO for circumferential fusions
- Technically more challenging and associated with morbidity and complications
- To avoid cord injury it should be done at L1 or distal (below the conus medullaris)
- Advantages:
  - Posterior approach alone
  - Greater correction at a single segment—no need for multiple procedures
  - No lengthening of the anterior column
  - Better possibility for healing
  - Minimal concern of stretch on aorta or viscera.

Vertebral column resection osteotomy (1922, MacLenan, VCRO): Here combined opening of anterior structure and closing of posterior structure are performed. The procedure was popularized by Bradford and Tribus for correcting severe coronal deformity and combined coronal and sagittal deformity. Of the three osteotomies described above VCRO provides the greatest amount of correction.

- The three columns are completely removed at the apex of deformity and space replaced by a metal cage that is used as a pivot **(Figs. 47A and B)**. This minimizes shortening of the spinal canal and highest degree of correction is thus obtained.
- Vertebral column resection osteotomy is the only option in patients with rigid deformity and decompensation. The indications of VCRO are fixed trunk translation, severe scoliosis (congenital scoliosis or NMS) or congenital kyphosis. Other indications include spinal tumor, rigid sharp multiplanar deformities and spondyloptosis. In such cases translation of the spinal column is essential for restoring the truncal balance, correcting the deformity and rigid spinal deformities more than 80° in the coronal plane. More than one vertebral segment is completely removed.
- Usually both anterior and posterior approaches are needed. Suk et al. described posterior only approach (PVCRO) to reduce the operation time and complications. PVCRO is a single procedure compared to combined anterior and posterior VCR reducing the total operating time and the amount of blood loss and also avoiding opening of the thoracic cage and pleura.
- Vertebral column resection osteotomy is associated with high morbidity in the form of neurological injury that can arise out of direct neurologic injury during bone resection or deformity correction, subluxation of the spinal column, dural buckling and compression of the spinal cord by residual bone or soft tissues in the canal after correction.

Instead of following the above schema another treatment guideline is available in the form of Lenke-Silva treatment levels I–VI. The schema is mentioned below succinctly:

- I—Decompression alone—"limited utility". Strictly the curve should be less than 30° and patient should have neurogenic claudication but no low back pain (difficult to find such patient), radiological changes of degeneration but minimal subluxation (<3 mm).

- II—Decompression and limited instrumented posterior spinal fusion—the indications are:
  - Curves less than 30°, more than 2 mm subluxation but not grossly unstable/spinal imbalance
  - No anterior osteophyte in the area of decompression.
  - Spine should be well balanced and no thoracic hyperkyphosis should be present
  - Ideally back pain should be absent.
- III—Decompression and lumbar curve instrumented fusion (TLIF)—patients with complaint of back pain and curves 45° or more, greater than 2 mm subluxation.
- IV—Decompression with anterior and posterior spinal instrumented fusion—combined anterior and posterior fusion of lumbar spine. Imbalance in spinal curve is primary indication especially correcting the lumbar hypokyphosis. There should be no anterior osteophytes, or thoracic hyperkyphosis and greater than 2 mm subluxation.
- V—Thoracic instrumentation and fusion extension—the fusion is extended to thoracic region (due to thoracic hyperkyphosis) in addition to criteria for level IV above.
- VI—Inclusion of osteotomies for specific deformities—as detailed above in management of sagittal imbalance.

Complications of Surgical Management of Adult Spine Deformity

- Persistent and new development of pain
- Pseudarthrosis is the most common complication with an incidence of 5–25%. It is associated with revision surgery, use of allograft bone, and use of nonsegmental hardware
- Infection has an incidence of 0.5–8%. The risk factors are inadequate perioperative antibiotics, poor nutrition (use total parenteral nutrition in staged surgery), poor soft tissue handling and posterior surgery more common than anterior surgery
- Cerebrospinal fluid leaks
- Neurologic compromise is seen in less than 1–5% patients. The risk factors include combined anterior and posterior surgery, revision surgery, or osteotomy surgery
- Junctional kyphosis
- Adjacent segment degeneration
- Pulmonary embolism
- DIC and coagulopathy
- Myocardial infarction, ileus, pneumonia, DVT, superior mesentery artery syndrome, blindness, UTI, etc.

NEUROMUSCULAR SCOLIOSIS

Introduction

A neuromuscular disorder is defined as a defective function of the peripheral nerve system, the neuromuscular junction, or muscles, causing muscle weakness in the patient. Cerebral palsy (CP) is not included in this definition but for descriptive purpose and especially for describing spinal deformity not arising from growth abnormalities, the orthopedic literature groups CP also with neuromuscular disorders. Scoliosis is common in patients with neuromuscular diseases. NMS is a heterogeneous group with multiple and sometimes unknown underlying causes (see classification later). The common feature is weak musculature in all that fails to maintain axial balance and hence the spine bends into curvature. The clinical picture is also heterogeneous that varies from patients with mild curves and good function to severely debilitated patients with gross scoliosis. Typically the neuromuscular curves are long C-shaped thoracolumbar curves but some may have short-segment sharp angular focal scoliosis (as in neurofibromatosis) with compensatory curves or kyphotic deformities. Larger curves cause difficulties with sitting or ambulation. The curves in NMS are peculiar in few characteristics:

- The curves develop early
- Progress rapidly with growth
- Most importantly they deteriorate even after skeletal maturity in contrast to other types of scoliosis
- They are associated with pulmonary complications
- Pelvic obliquity is prominent in most of the patients

Neuromuscular scoliosis is in general associated with high morbidity; the children undergoing treatment have longer hospital stay, increased number of procedures and more hence complications. There are significantly higher chances of skin ulceration and bed sores, dislocation of the hip, ambulatory problems due to pelvic obliquity, etc. The total cost of treatment is also high. Management requires a multidisciplinary approach requiring teamwork of parents, physiotherapists and occupational therapists, pediatricians and intensive care physicians. Braces are poorly tolerated if at all and do not affect the natural history of scoliosis in these patients. Progressive severe curves require operative treatment. Surgery is indicated to correct sitting imbalance and lift the chest off the abdominal contents. Surgery may improve the deteriorating respiratory system and can be life-saving. Longer fusions up to pelvis are needed and have high complication rates. Impingement of the rib cage on the iliac spine due to trunk collapse is disabling and is relieved by deformity-correcting surgery.

Pathophysiology of development of NMS: There is neither any primary spine abnormality in scoliosis producing to or leading to deformity nor any growth abnormality that produces imbalanced growth in the spine. The primary reasons for development of curve in NMS are:

- *Muscular:* Spine and upper body muscles that are too weak or too tight (as in spasticity). They place abnormal forces on the spine pulling it in one direction (muscular imbalance that may have neurological origin—so NMS). This imbalance produces a curved spine (scoliosis) that can progress even after skeletal maturity as skeletal maturity has nothing to do with muscular balance.
- *Truncal shift:* Due to weak truncal muscles the head is no longer kept centered over the buttocks/pelvis causing gross malalignment in coronal and sagittal planes.

Classification

Neuromuscular scoliosis in orthopedic literature refers to patients with any neurologic disease, including CP. Neurologists, however, reserve the term neuromuscular to describe disorders associated with the peripheral nervous system causing flaccid weakness (rather than spasticity associated with CP). Despite this distinction we would stick to the classical orthopedic literature and classification. The NMS has been broadly grouped into neuropathic and myopathic forms with subdivisions in the former as follows:

- *Neuropathic:*
  - *Upper motor neuron:*
    1. Cerebral palsy
    2. *Spinocerebellar degeneration:*
       - Friedreich's ataxia
       - Charcot-Marie-Tooth disease
    3. Syringomyelia
    4. Spinal cord tumor
    5. Spinal cord trauma
  - *Lower motor neuron:*
    6. Poliomyelitis and other viral myelitis
    7. Traumatic
    8. *Spinal muscular atrophy (SMA):*
       - Werdnig-Hoffmann disease
       - Kugelberg-Welander disease
       - Letterer-Siwe
    9. Myelomeningocele
  - Dysautonomia (Riley-Day syndrome)
- *Myopathic:*
  - Arthrogryposis
  - *Muscular dystrophy:*
    - Duchenne's
    - Limb-girdle
    - Facioscapulohumeral
  - Fiber-type disproportion
  - Congenital hypotonia
  - Myotonia dystrophica

Cerebral palsy: See the Chapter on "Cerebral Palsy and Inherited Neuromuscular Disorders" for pathophysiology and genesis.

- Prevalence of scoliosis is around 25% in CP. Scoliosis is linked to motor involvement the severe the higher
- Spine is affected by spasticity and imbalance of the paraspinal muscles
- Spinal deformity is much more common in nonambulatory, quadriplegic, and spastic patients
  - Brace treatment is minimally effective if at all (somewhere 15% curves would be controlled by brace treatment). When used, a Boston-type underarm brace until puberty 0–12 years of age) is used with wheel chair modification.
  - Surgical treatment has to be individualized based on the overall patient condition and ambulatory status. In general progressive curves larger than 40–45° will be better managed by surgical fusion that will result in a well-balanced spine with level pelvis if the child is ambulatory with minimal assistance. The larger the curves are the faster they progress is a dictum for all forms of scoliosis and applies aptly here. The other indication is worsening pelvic obliquity with sitting imbalance (some call it type 2 curves, while those without pelvic obliquity as type 1 curves albeit not universally). Surgical fusion and instrumentation typically from T2 to pelvis is needed in nonambulatory patients, with a typical note to take care of osteoporotic bones. For ambulatory patients, fusion levels from proximal to distal stable vertebra may suffice. The instrumentation options include, Luque-Galveston (smooth rods in iliac wings, good initial fixation but loosening over time, needs dexterity to bend rods), Dunn McCarthy (S-contoured smooth rods over sacral ala, technically easy but has small moment arm to correct pelvic obliquity so less effective), Iliosacral screws (single implant engaging ilium and sacrum) and sacral screws (versatile and good purchase, can be connected to any system, see adult scoliosis for details), "MW" configuration of Arlet et al. (combining iliosacral screws with iliac screws for very strong fixation and posterior spinal fusion). Anterior surgery is advisable for immature curves and severe stiff curves. It is better to do both anterior and posterior fixation on the same day rather than staggering. The following are some of the commonly mentioned reasons to operate:
    - Improved sitting balance
    - Easier to nurse
    - Improved social and personal outlook, self- esteem and appearance
    - Improved pulmonary function
- Considerations for surgery and global assessment of child with CP includes—neurological (seizures, medications including baclofen pumps, previous treatments like rhizotomies), respiratory (pneumonia, aspiration), gastrointestinal (constipation, fecal impaction, reflux, fundoplication, etc.), nutritional status (serum albumin >3.5 g/dL, total lymphocyte count >1,500 cells/mm^3), genitourinary (bladder dysfunction, incontinence, UTI), infection (UTI, decubitus ulcer, aspiration, pneumonia, etc.).

Myelomeningocele

It is a birth defect characterized by exposure of the meninges and dysplasia of the underlying neural elements, resulting in bowel, bladder, motor and sensory paralysis distal to the malformation. Spinal deformities are seen in 50% of patients that may be congenital or acquired. The cause of disorder has been committed to dietary folate deficiency in majority. There is posterior element deficiency that is the hallmark. The clinical presentation is varied and depending on the level of the lesion the patient has been grouped functionally as:

- Thoracic level—sitter
- Upper lumbar—ambulatory with assistive devices
- Lower lumbar—ambulatory with ankle foot orthoses (AfOs)

- Sacral—Ambulatory with or without AfOs
- Beware of the 15% incidence of latex allergy, which leads to anaphylaxis and subsequent death.

The spinal deformity is associated with muscle imbalance and hydrocephalus. The incidence of tethered cord is also high, so evaluation by MRI is imperative. The spinal deformities are often complex and multiple. The reasons to operate include:

- Hygiene and skin care (prevent pressure sores)
- Improve pulmonary compliance
- Improve seating balance
- If the curve is more than 45–50° then surgery is needed to prevent progression and avoid imbalance.

Curve fusion from T2 to sacrum in often needed. Combined approach is often needed as the posterior elements are missing.

The kyphosis is a major problem and is of three types:

1. Collapsing—C-shaped, flexible, apex of deformity is lower thoracic
2. Congenital—most common, rigid S-shaped, centered at L2
3. With partial aplasia—quite rare

Management is with kyphectomies. Indications of kyphectomy include:

- Significant soft tissue breakdown over the gibbus
- Difficulty with sitting
- Levels—T2 to the sacrum
- Approach—all posterior with kyphus resection and ± spinal cord resection.

Duchenne's Muscular Dystrophy

This is an X-linked (xp21) recessive inherited disorder. Sporadic mutations are also found (where the disease is not inherited of course). The gene encoding for dystrophin protein is abnormal, leading to complete absence (Becker muscular dystrophy has a reduced dystrophin). Histology shows muscle necrosis and fibrofatty muscle infiltration. The affected individual has delayed milestones and rapidly progressive muscle weakness with muscle wasting. The dystrophy is characterized by progressive weakness in boys who begin walking late (18 months) and eventually lose ambulatory ability by 12 years making them wheelchair bound. Major changes during puberty are the progressive muscle weakness in hands, arms, and torso, the latter is associated with the development of scoliosis. Scoliosis typically develops only after the child is nonambulatory and is seen in nearly all children. Curves are relentless and associated with kyphosis. Respiratory system symptoms then also appear and may be exacerbated by associated cardiomyopathy. The life span is shortened to less than 25 years primarily because of pulmonary compromise. The disease is diagnosed by repeated determination of extremely elevated creatine kinase (CPK-MM) levels in the bloodstream or by the absence of dystrophin in a muscle biopsy. Genetic analysis will show loss of dystrophin gene.

There is loss of sitting balance (due also to pelvic obliquity), shortening of the trunk, and compression of the heart and lungs. The mobility of the ribs is reduced by rotation and deformation of the trunk, causing loss of vital capacity (VC). The development of curves and ensuing disability can be partially postponed by Deflazacort (corticosteroid, a prednisolone derivative), that may act in a minority of patients. Orthoses are not recommended to prevent the development or progression of scoliosis in DMD patients. Only for patients who refuse surgery or minimally benefit from it, a sitting orthosis to improve sitting comfort may be given. Total contact orthosis improve comfort and distribute pressure more evenly. The orthosis should be layered for flexibility and soft edges.

The typical indications for surgery are curves >30° in patients with >2 years of lifespan remaining and reasonable pulmonary function (>40% of normal, patients with VC <30% of normal have major complications postoperative). Trend toward earlier intervention when the curve is 20° is arising and is due to the fact that the surgery is less complicated (less complications hence), shorter and safer. Early surgery may also spare pelvic fusion. Posterior spinal fusion should be performed from high thoracic (Th2–3) at least to L4 or L5. Pelvic fixation is needed in larger curves and improves balance.

The children are at risk of development of malignant hyperthermia with anesthesia. Also before any intervention is planned the children should be evaluated for cardiac myopathy and pulmonary function. As a prerequisite the elbow power should be greater than 3/5 (serves as indirect measure to assess functional optimum).

Spinal Muscular Atrophy

Spinal muscular atrophy includes a number of genetic disorders all having weakness due to loss of anterior horn cells of the spinal cord and brainstem. The most common form of SMA is caused by a mutation of the survival motor neuron (SMN) gene, located on chromosome 5q13. It is an autosomal recessive disorder that affects individuals from infancy through adulthood. The spectrum of disease has been classified into four types:

1. *SMA type 1 (Werdnig-Hoffmann disease, severe infantile SMA):* Severe weakness in the neonatal period and death by 2 years from respiratory failure. The child never ever sits independently in his life.
2. *SMA type 2 (Intermediate SMA):* Normal development until 5–6 months then failure to stand or walk and are wheel-chair bound early in life. They have severe dystrophy associated with scoliosis by age 4 years universally that can be rapidly progressive. Respiratory assistance is often needed in the form of tracheostomy and may be required round the clock. It is difficult to distinguish it from type 1 till 3 years of age.
3. *SMA type 3 (Juvenile SMA):* Onset before 3 years and progressive loss of ambulatory ability by 15 years. Spinal deformity is common.
   - Type IIIb (Kugelberg-Welander syndrome)—Onset after 3 years and weakness is often mild (foot drop) with limited endurance. These patients retain

ambulation till 2nd–3rd decade and develop less scoliosis or respiratory problems.

4. *SMA type 4 (adult SMA):* Weakness begins in 3rd decade; disease is much slower with little impact on life expectancy.

The diagnosis is by clinical presentation (as above), hypotonia, areflexia, motor dysfunction, normal sensations and *SMA* gene test.

The curves are progressive in type 2 (others either do not need treatment or are never available). The curves grow to more than 50° by 10 years of age. Majority curves are low thoracic single curve types. Orthoses are not recommended to prevent the development or progression of scoliosis in SMA type 2 patients. A non-rigid spinal brace or sitting orthosis can be considered for the improvement of comfort and sitting balance. Surgery is to be considered in all patients at some point of time. In SMA type 2 posterior spinal fusion should be performed. Instrumentation should be segmental. Early scoliosis surgery is recommended in order to obtain a good and lasting improvement of the sitting balance but no beneficial effect on cardiac or pulmonary systems has been observed.

Friedreich's Ataxia

It is an autosomal recessive hereditary spinocerebellar ataxia with typical onset between 7 and 15 years of life. The clinical triad consists of:

- Ataxia
- Areflexia
- Babinski positive

The curves are progressive seen commonly in teens in nearly all patients. Bracing may be advisable in ambulatory patients with curves up to 30°. Surgery is indicated in curves more than 40°. Long posterior fusions are needed but often the pelvis is spared.

Complications of surgery: The incidence of complications is high following surgery for NMS. The major ones are:

- *Excessive intraoperative blood loss:*
  - Aggressive blood transfusion intraoperatively is necessary.
- Infection—often dependent on the nutritional status of the patient. It may be prevented by:
  - Good nutritional status prior to surgery (see CP earlier)
  - Preoperative and postoperative antibiotics
  - Intermittent irrigation of the soft tissues during surgery
  - Meticulous handling of the soft tissues
- Pulmonary compromise
- Implant failure
- *Gastrointestinal complications:*
  - Gastric distension
  - Obstruction
  - Gastroesophageal reflux disease (GERD)
  - Pancreatitis
- Neurological complications
- Wound dehiscence.

SAGITTAL PLANE DEFORMITY OF SPINE

The sagittal plane deformities of spine include the kyphotic deformity (of a previously flat/lordotic region) or a hyperkyphosis of kyphotic region or lordotic deformity (of a previously flat/kyphotic region) or hyperlordosis of an already lordotic region.

Kyphosis comes from the Greek word "kyphos"—"a hump, arched back" (vertebral deviations with posterior convexity), it is also called "roundback". Lordosis means "curved" and is applied to vertebral deviations with anterior convexity; it is also commonly referred to as sway back, hollow back or saddle back.

In the sagittal plane, a physiological thoracic kyphosis and a physiological lumbar lordosis can be specified with the morphotypology study **(Figs. 48A and B)**. During fetal life, there is global kyphosis of spine that is maintained in the early infancy. When the child begins to crawl the spine changes its conformation to a global lordosis between 6th and 9th month. This gradually assumes the adult curvatures while the child starts to learn walking. There is normal thoracic kyphosis (primary curve) and cervical and lumbar lordosis (secondary curves) in the human spine (sacrum is also in kyphosis, but the articulation is fused forming a kyphotic bony mass rather than an articulated curvature). Normal sagittal spinal balance is a result of mutual articulation of the pelvis and the spine in the sagittal plane. Kyphosis is the angle formed by the top plate of T4 and the lower plate of the vertebra, which is most inclined (usually T12) to the horizontal at the thoracolumbar junction. The average angulation is 37° ± 9° (range 10–40°) kyphosis and 40–60° of lordosis.

We will restrict the following description with respect to development, types, evaluation and management of kyphotic deformities. Kyphosis is defined as angle more than 40°. Most of the causes of kyphosis mentioned below either produce a shortening of anterior column, weakening or lengthening of posterior column or both.

Pathological (Morphological) Forms of Kyphotic Deformities

- *Angular kyphosis:* Focal sharply angulated kyphosis is referred to as gibbus deformity.
  - Congenital kyphosis with bone defect is mostly seen at birth. Congenital kyphotic malformations are less frequent but more severe than scoliosis, the risk of progressive paraplegia is important. Major forms found before the age of 3 years need surgery (epiphysiodesis performed as early as 6 months of age). There are two different types:
    - *Type I:* Hypoplasia of the vertebral body, the posterior arch is preserved and leads to kyphosis with growth. A night MB with crossbar centered on the defect can prevent the aggravation
    - *Type II:* Aplasia of the vertebral body. It is a congenital defect of the anterior segment of the vertebral body called "bars" or "block".

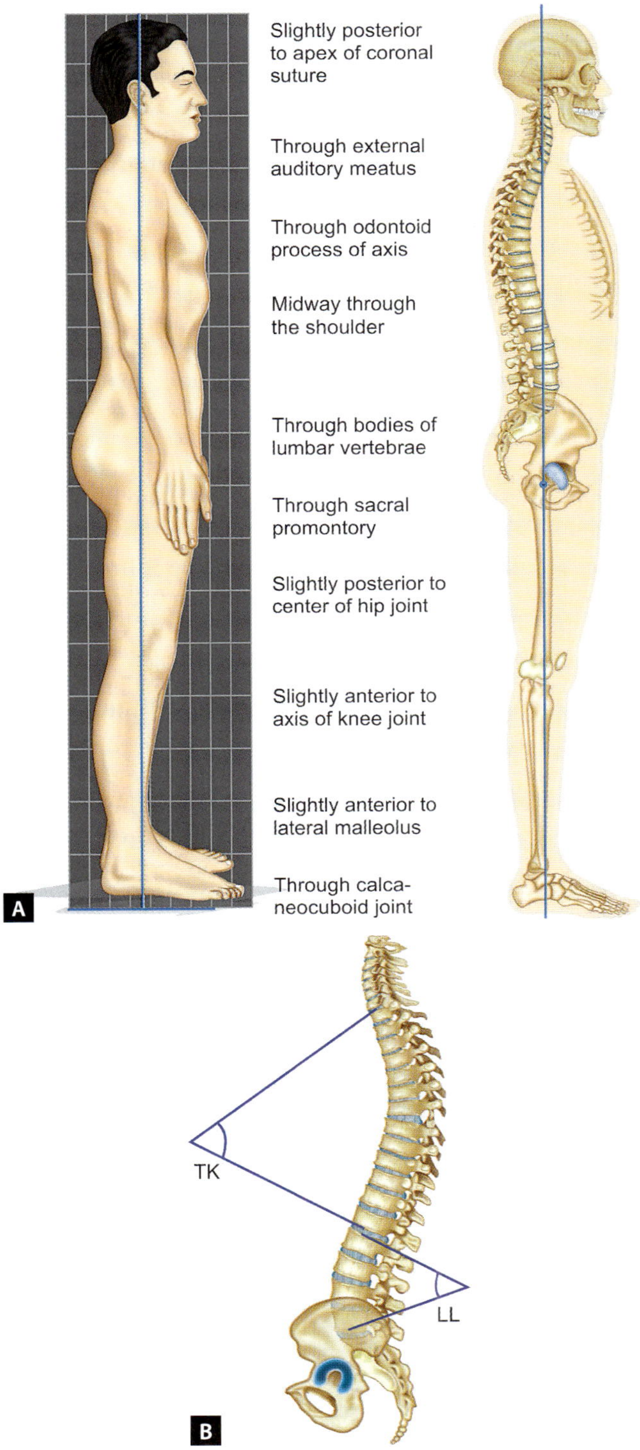

Figs. 48A and B: Sagittal plane alignment: (A) The various landmarks to assess sagittal balance; (B) The normal thoracic kyphosis (10– 40°) and lumbar lordosis (40–60°) in human spine.

- *Traumatic:* The compaction of the vertebral body fractures due to compression fractures (anterior wedging). These are usually seen at the thoracolumbar junction.
- *Achondroplasia:* Kyphosis is located at the thoracolumbar junction. In most severe cases, anterior surgery performed with a distractor needs to be performed.
- *Morquio disease:* Thoracolumbar kyphosis with platyspondyly. In these patients, there is also hypoplasia of the odontoid with unstable atlas/axis justifying caution in rehabilitation with neck mobilization.

- *Round or regular kyphosis*: The deformity is distributed over more than three vertebrae and can be seen in following situations:
  - *Idiopathic (Stagnara and de Mauroy):* Akin to AIS this progressive kyphosis is distinct from Scheuermann's/Calves disease. It is commonly seen during puberty.
  - Scheuermann's disease is a defect of the growth plate of the vertebral body that causes wedging. The vertebral rim or secondary nucleus of ossification is inhibited by hyperpressure related to kyphosis. The disease stops at the end of growth, when the growth of cartilage is no longer active.
  - *Neurological:* The paralysis of abdominal and spinal muscles is compensated by a lumbar kyphosis. The remaining muscles are utilized to maintain a position that can be effective. Global kyphosis develops in children who are on wheel chair, or lordosis, which are sometimes very unstable with athetosis.
  - *Postlaminectomy:* If the laminectomy extends and removes facet joints and posterior ligaments then kyphosis results in 80% cases that are very severe. Anterior fusion should be considered.
  - Radiotherapy in neuroblastoma and Wilms' tumor damages the growth cartilage of vertebral body and can cause kyphosis.
  - Ankylosing spondylitis results in disharmonious global kyphosis with loss of lordosis and forward projection of the trunk.
  - *Osteoporosis in adults:* Often results in painful high thoracic kyphosis.
  - *Adult camptocormia (forward flexion of the spine):* The camptocormia kyphosis is seen in aging population. It is due to weakness of the paraspinal posterior muscles as in Parkinson's disease. The deformity is flexible and disappears in supine position.

Clinical forms: Clinically, the following different types of kyphosis can be identified. They have their own compensatory mechanisms as mentioned:

- *Cervical kyphosis:* Kyphosis in the spine between the occiput (C0) and the first thoracic vertebra (T1). It is compensated by lumbar hyperlordosis or thoracic lordosis. There is forward projection of the neck and the shoulder in internal rotation.
- The thoracic kyphosis which is most common. Kyphosis between the first thoracic vertebra (T1) and the 12th thoracic vertebra (T12). It can be harmonious when compensated by lumbar hyperlordosis ± pelvic retroversion which is seen in rounded deformities however the angular deformities are often disharmonious with decreased lordosis.

- The thoracolumbar junctional kyphosis is the most common form of noncongenital angular kyphosis. Kyphosis between the 11th thoracic vertebra (T11) and the second lumbar vertebra (L2).
- *Lumbar kyphosis:* Kyphosis between the first lumbar vertebra (L1) and the sacrum (S1). It is compensated by thoracic lordosis ± pelvic retroversion (knee flexion).
- *Lower lumbar kyphosis:* Kyphosis between the fourth lumbar vertebra (L4) and the sacrum (S1). The compensatory mechanism is the upper lumbar hyperlordosis and/or pelvic retroversion.
- *Global kyphosis:* Lumbar kyphosis with normal or increased thoracic kyphosis. It can be only compensated by PT and/or flexed knees.
- *Pelvic kyphosis:* There is increased SVA with normal spine or minor regional kyphosis. It cannot be compensated.

Some uncommon forms that are mostly secondary and cannot be grouped into above forms are as follows:

- Kyphotic or lordotic attitudes seen in ligamentous laxity or muscular hypotonia.
- The paramorphism can be the result of a sport activity encouraging the kyphosis, such as, swimming (dolphin, butterfly).
- Constitutional kyphosis or lordosis, corresponding to a family morphotype is usually stable.
- *Kyphosis adaptation:* Seen with myopia and in children with infantile encephalopathy.

Clinical Evaluation

The age-related thoracic hyperkyphosis is seen in 20–40% of older adults and is more common in women.

Assessing Dynamic Balance

- Clinically, the C7 plumb line (a vertical line drawn from the center of the C7 vertebral body) should pass within a few millimeters of the posterior-superior corner of S1. Positive sagittal balance occurs when the C7 plumb line falls anterior to the posterior-superior corner of the S1 endplate. Negative sagittal balance occurs when the C7 plumb line falls posterior to this point.
- Other methods of evaluation of spinal sagittal curves are:
    - Flexible ruler
    - Occiput to wall distance
    - Block method (patient lying supine and distance of head from floor/table measured by measured blocks)
- In the sagittal plane, the axis of motion is a horizontal line across the two femoral heads. A virtual line joining the acromion to the trochanter is drawn; the position of this line from the vertical to maximal extension and flexion is recorded. The finger-floor distance corresponds to the stiffness in the spine and pelvis.
- In the frontal plane, a virtual line joins the top of the median gluteal fold (S2) to the C7 spinous process. The extreme positions of the virtual line during the left and right bending are noted.
- In the horizontal plane, the left to right rotation of the shoulder girdle (virtual line joining the two humeral heads) is measured in relation to the fixed pelvic girdle (line joining two femoral heads).
- The movements described above form together a cone of economy described by Dubousset **(Fig. 49)**. Within the cone the body may remain in an ergonomically favorable erect position. Beyond this cone the effort required to maintain the head over pelvis is high and may need external support to balance.

Assessing Direct Rigidity

In the prone position, the upper limbs are positioned laterally along the body and the patient is asked to move with hyperextension of the spine. The distance, manubrium-table, is measured appreciating the reducibility of kyphosis in this position.

Assessing Indirect Rigidity (The Stiffness of the Pelvic and Scapular Girdles)

- *Pelvic girdle stiffness:* Measure the popliteal angle (indicating hamstring retraction)—if the thigh is vertical, the popliteal angle is the angle between the vertical and the leg when trying to extend the entire leg.
    - If there is iliopsoas retraction then the patient is asked to hold his knee; starting from the vertical the leg is lowered in extension asking the patient to relax the trunk. The opposite limb is bent. At the end of the movement, a PT is seen and the distance heel-table is measured corresponding to the start of the PT.
- At the shoulder level, the upper limbs are lowered in extension and anterior retraction is assessed by the distance, table-elbow, ensuring that there is no hyperlordosis of spine.

Sagittal imbalance: Sagittal imbalance is different from sagittal deformity. Sagittal deformity refers to locoregional

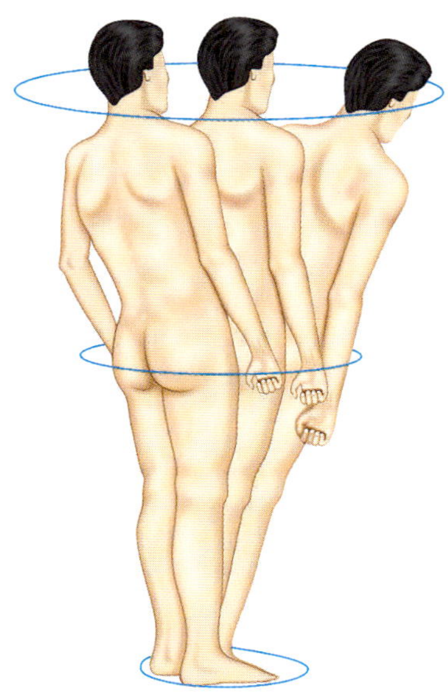

Fig. 49: Cone of economy: The body tends to remain in energy-efficient alignment within the "cone of economy" described by Dubousset. Deviations outside the cone require external support to body and increase the energy expenditure.

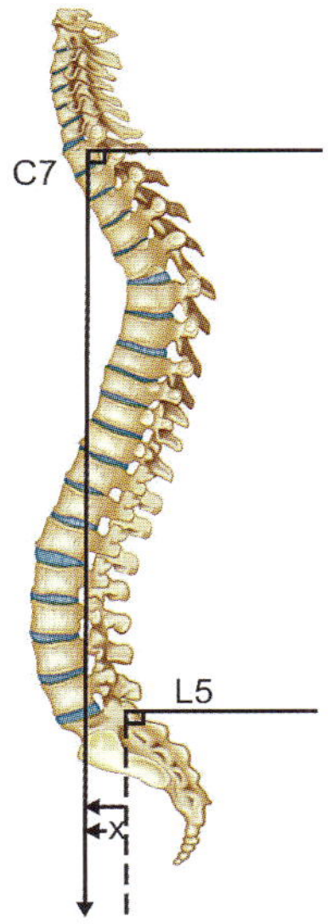

Fig. 50: Sagittal balance is determined by C7 plumb line drawn from the center of C7 vertebral body vertically down perpendicular to the floor. Normally this passes a few millimeters of the posterosuperior corner of S1. Positive sagittal balance occurs when C7 plumb line falls anterior and negative sagittal balance occurs when the plumb line falls posterior to the posterosuperior corner of S1.

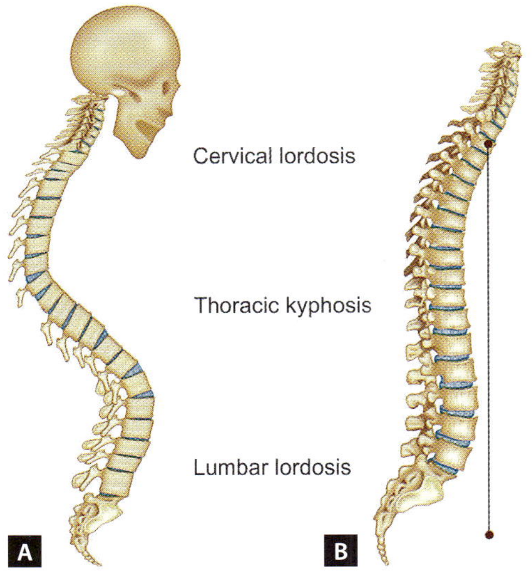

Figs. 51A and B: (A) Compensation of sagittal imbalance—the hyperlordosis is well compensated by the hyperkyphosis; (B) The lumbar kyphosis is not balanced by compensatory curves.

deformity of spine outside the physiological range (say >40° for thoracic region). Sagittal balance refers on the other hand to global positioning of spine with respect to the sacrum **(Fig. 50)**. Sagittal imbalance arises out of uncompensated sagittal deformities. Compensatory deformities "within" the spine produce congruent deformities **(Fig. 51A)**, while uncompensated deformities causing sagittal imbalance will produce positional changes outside the spine **(Fig. 51B)**.

Sagittal imbalance due to abovementioned various reasons produces various extraspinal compensatory mechanisms such as the pelvic retroversion, hip extension and knee flexion. Once a spinal deformity surpasses these compensatory mechanisms surgical intervention is necessary. The imbalance is evaluated radiologically on a full length AP and lateral radiograph obtained in "clavicle position" (hips and knees fully extended, the elbows fully flexed, the wrists flexed with the hands in a relaxed fist placed into the supraclavicular fossa) on 36-inch cassette.

- The mean C7 plumb line offset from the posterior-superior corner of S1 has been found to be 0.5 cm **(Fig. 50)**.
- An offset greater than 2.5 cm anteriorly or posteriorly is considered to be abnormal
- Thoracic kyphosis measurement described in starting of the chapter. Angle greater than 40° is defined as kyphosis.
- *Lumbar lordosis:* Measured from the superior endplate of L1 to the endplate of S1
- *Pelvic incidence, pelvic tilt, and sacral slope angles:* Pelvic incidence is a nonpositional anatomical parameter defined as the angle between the line perpendicular to the sacral plate at its midpoint and the line connecting this point to the axis of rotation of the femoral head. The PI angle is unique to each individual and becomes set at the end of growth. Low PI indicates a short pelvis ring while a high PI suggests a large AP axis of pelvis. SS is a positional parameter defined as the angle between the superior endplate of S1 and a horizontal line extending from the anterior-inferior corner of the S1 endplate. SS determines the position of lumbar spine in sagittal plane. PT is a positional parameter defined as the angle between the line connecting the midpoint of the superior sacral end plate to the femoral rotational axis and the line extending vertically from the femoral rotational axis. PT dictates the pelvic anteversion or retroversion thus defining the spatial orientation of pelvis. PI is usually equal to SS + PT and often determines these parameters.

Progression of Sagittal Imbalance (The Vicious Circle)

With initiation of the sagittal imbalance → pelvis moves into retroversion (the C7 plumb line goes backwards and the femoral heads are placed relatively forward) → the hips extend. Now considering the fact that PI = PT + SS (where SS cannot be negative), a higher PT would mean a high PI implying that PT can increase only in cases having a high PI (larger pelvis), so patients with a smaller pelvis will decompensate early. Increased kyphosis will produce a lordosis or hyperextended spine in a balanced curve. The hyperextension of spine produces retrolisthesis, facet joints overstress and even sometimes isthmic lysis. Further a forward tilting C7 plumb line due to kyphosis if not balanced by increased PT and hyperextension will produce knee bending to maintain the plumb line behind the femoral heads. This entails good quadriceps muscle power that usually gives way sooner than later and external support in the form of crutch or walker is needed. This produces classical late posture of a kyphotic deformity of a trunk tilted forward with pelvis retroverted, hips extended and knee bent.

Stages of sagittal imbalance: These include:

1. *Sagittally balanced:* The spine is able to align the gravity line and keeps horizontal gaze with little muscle effort. C7 plumbline is near posterior corner of S1 endplate (± 25–50 mm) *and* no compensatory mechanisms are present.
2. *Hidden sagittal imbalance:* The spine is able to align the gravity line and keeps horizontal gaze with increased muscle effort. C7 plumbline is near posterior corner of S1 endplate (± 25–50 mm) *but* compensatory mechanisms are present.
3. *Uncompensated sagittal imbalance:* The spine is unable to align the gravity line or keeps the horizontal gaze. C7 plumbline is beyond the accepted distance from posterior corner of S1 endplate (>50 mm). Compensatory mechanisms are lacking or insufficient.

Management of sagittal imbalance is based on the concerned regional deformities. To make it easy one can follow the Bridwell classification. The spinal sagittal deformities can be totally flexible, partially through mobile segments, and fixed deformity with no correction in the recumbent position based on curve flexibility. Flexible deformities can be addressed with anterior-posterior or posterior only surgery not requiring any osteotomy (discussed below in detail with individual regional deformity discussion). Commonly the sagittal balance is improved by lengthening the anterior column, either through an anterior or a posterior approach, using cages, structural allograft or structural autograft. The posterior column is then addressed with laminectomies when there is evidence of stenosis, facetectomies and fusion with instrumentation.

Fixed deformities can be managed by anterior-only, anterior and posterior combined and posterior-only approaches often needing osteotomies. The principles are discussed in management of adult-onset scoliosis as above with surgical correction by PSO, SPO and VCRO.

CERVICAL KYPHOSIS

Cervical kyphotic deformity is a debilitating condition. There is a lordosis from C2 to C7 of 30–40°, but there is no unequivocal definition of cervical lordosis. The cervical curve is a secondary curve developmentally, so the vertebral bodies have equal height anteriorly and posteriorly with anteriorly opened disk spaces. Vertebral bodies bear 36% while posterior elements bear 64% of axial load. The balance between both elements is needed to maintain the normal cervical curvature and the head in an upright position. Reduction of lordosis and development of kyphotic deformity **(Fig. 52)** leads to progression of kyphosis through a moment arm-induced bending moment "kyphosis begets kyphosis". The various causes of cervical kyphosis are presented in **Box 2**.

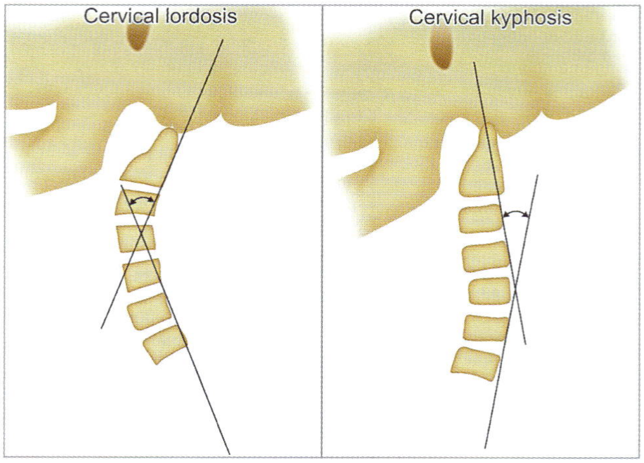

Fig. 52: Cervical kyphosis.

Clinical Presentation of Cervical Kyphosis

Patients often present with:

- *Neck pain:* Cervical musculature is placed at a significant biomechanical disadvantage causing neck pain. Also the degeneration of cervical intervertebral disks may add to symptom.
- *Neurological deficits:* Myelopathy, radiculopathy, quadriparesis, quadriplegia and Brown-Séquard syndrome—these occur due to:
  - Stenosis of the central canal and/or neuroforamina.
  - "Bowstring effect" occurs on spinal cord as it is stretched over the apex of kyphosis. This results in microvascular compression and ischemia causing myelopathy and cord atrophy.
  - The cord also gets tethered to the dentate ligaments anteriorly whereby micromovements during flexion extension result in repetitive trauma.
- Severe kyphosis may adversely affect forward vision, swallowing and respiration because of the settling of the chin onto the chest
- Low back pain due to lumbar compensatory hyperlordosis and subsequent lumbar degeneration.
- Functional evaluation is done based on the mJOA score to quantify motor, sensory and urinary function.

Radiological Evaluation

- Measure the local sagittal angle—kyphosis angle at the diseased segment
- Regional sagittal angle—C2–C7 kyphosis angle
- Dynamic flexion and extension radiographs to assess the flexibility, occult instability. Classify the kyphosis as fixed or flexible. Reduction of deformity of less than 50% classifies as fixed kyphosis. for fixed kyphosis perform CT scan.
- CT scan—obtain thin cut CT scan to identify anterior ankylosis or fact joint involvement.
- *MRI helps in management of patient:*
  - Intermediate vertebral bodies are identified by cerebrospinal fluid signal present dorsal to them on a T2-weighted sagittal MRI. These are retained to provide intermediate points of implant fixation during the anterior reconstruction procedure.
  - Iwasaki ratio—the ratio of the anteroposterior diameter between the spinal cord at the apex and the medullopontine junction on MRI—ratio below 0.3 indicates risk of myelopathy.

BOX 2: The various causes of cervical spine kyphotic deformity (the last two are the most common). Also briefed are the conventional/ standard pathways of management.

1. *Advanced degenerative disease:* Due to high mobility of the cervical spine, the region is prone to spondylosis.
   a. Degeneration produces arthrosis, altered mechanics and loss of physiological curvatures
   b. Treatment is usually conservative. Decompression is indicated if aggressive conservative treatment fails, or myelopathy develops. Restoration of alignment is simultaneously done
   c. Anterior approach is preferred while additional posterior stabilization is added for decompression of more than three levels
2. *Trauma:* Flexion-distraction and flexion-compression injuries are prone to development of post-traumatic kyphosis resulting from injury to posterior ligamentous structures, particularly in lower cervical spine
3. *Neoplastic disease:* Neoplasia may cause muscle denervation and weakness by the involvement of the anterior horn cells. The other possibility is a flexed posture that opens the spinal canal to relieve the symptoms
4. *Infection:* Tuberculosis of spine causes loss of disc space (diskitis), intervertebral fusion, loss of vertebral body (vertebral osteomyelitis) and loss of lordosis
5. *Dysplasias and congenital kyphosis:*
   a. Diastrophic dysplasia in cervical spine often causes anterior wedging of the apical vertebra. Surgery is performed only if there is no response to bracing or neurological symptoms appear
   b. Congenital cervical kyphosis is uncommon but may be seen in Klippel-Feil syndrome
6. *Systemic arthritides:* Ankylosing spondylitis or rheumatoid arthritis (*see* Chapter on "Rheumatoid Affection of Spine")
   a. In ankylosing spondylitis, there is a loss of flexibility of spine eventually developing a "chin on chest deformity"
   b. The patients become unable to perform activities of daily living
   c. Extension osteotomies may be considered to improve the deformity
7. *Iatrogenic processes:*
   a. Iatrogenically, there could be pseudarthrosis or any failure to restore the normal cervical lordosis during surgery ventrally or dorsally. There is disruption of cervical stabilizing structures like the interspinous ligaments, ligamenta flava, laminae and facet joint complexes
   b. Postlaminectomy kyphosis is the most common cause of cervical kyphosis (21%). It is commonly done for management of myelopathy. The kyphosis development depends on preoperative loss of lordosis, preoperative spinal stability, involvement of facet joints and age of patient
   c. Pediatric patients and young adults are more prone. This predisposition is due to ongoing spinal growth, the laxity of spinal ligaments, more horizontal orientation of the facet complex and poor resistance of incompletely ossified vertebral bodies to compression in pediatric patients
   d. Symptomatically there is recurrence of radicular and axial neck pain symptoms. The latter is caused by muscle fatigue and loss of horizontal gaze
   e. Usually combined anterior and posterior approaches are recommended for its management
   f. The risk of kyphosis is prevented at the time of initial index procedure by:
      i. Performing fusion at the time of laminectomy
      ii. Doing cervical laminoplasty that expands the area for neural elements but does not remove lamina

Management

Conservative Management

This is mainly used to address the symptoms and consequences of pain. This includes physiotherapy, intermittent cervical traction, proprioceptive exercises and retraining, bracing, and medications.

Surgical Management

The optimal indications are not defined but include:

- Neurological compromise
- Severe mechanical pain
- Dysphagia or difficulty with forward gaze due to progressive kyphotic deformity.

To address these problems the surgery aims to decompress, correct deformity and stabilize the spine with fusion. Attempting to correct the deformity by preoperative traction is a must that tells the further management as if the deformity corrects then a dorsal strategy that includes fixation and fusion is used to maintain correction. Patient is carried to OT with traction.

Anterior only surgery: This is performed for fixed deformity without posterior ankylosis of facet joints. The familiar approach permits ventral decompression, correction of deformity and spinal reconstruction. The previously practiced methods of anterior corpectomies and arthrodesis using rounded bone grafts without instrumentation met with unacceptable complications, especially if they attempted to correct the postlaminectomy kyphosis. This was mainly due to creation of additional instability anteriorly with poor support after surgery despite immobilization in a halo-vest. Modern day surgical approach uses hybrid decompression combined with multilevel instrumented fusions. Corpectomy is only used at levels with retrovertebral compression and discectomy is used at other levels combined with segmental fixation including plate and multilevel screws. This "hybrid" approach avoids consecutive corpectomies while simultaneously allowing multilevel strong fixation (through intermediate vertebral bodies). After distracting the spine and correcting the deformity the plate is fixed to the most caudal and rostral vertebral body and the intermediate vertebral body is pulled to the plate by tightening screws placed into it further decompressing and correcting the deformity. Most of the cases do not need a dorsal surgery whence managed hence.

With the availability of modern implant systems, this is the preferred approach by many to treat a fixed deformity. Rigid and dynamic implants are both available. The dynamic implants permit controlled subsidence and allow the graft to bear most of the axial load to promote bone fusion. These are preferred only cases with pseudarthrosis related to prior fusion however.

Combined anterior and posterior surgery: Dorsal spinal cord compression or the facet joint ankylosis cannot be corrected using anterior only approach. Other indication for posterior approach is to stabilize the spine circumferentially in postlaminectomy kyphosis correction or if the instability results due to three level corpectomy associated with laminectomy.

The advantage to this approach is that:

- Circumferential decompression can be achieved
- Deformity can be corrected effectively by lengthening anterior column while shortening posterior column.
- It also allows for ventrodorsal osteotomies to correct fixed deformities.

- Circumferential procedures minimize the translation and torsion of spine reducing graft and implant-related complications.

  Sequence of surgery (which one first anterior or posterior)
- *Anterior-posterior sequence:* The most common sequence of correction is the anterior–posterior sequence, where anterior discectomies and osteotomies are performed followed by interbody grafting. This is followed subsequently by posterior instrumentation placement, osteotomies and correction.
- *Anterior-posterior-anterior sequence:* for theoretical concerns of graft loosening in anterior–posterior sequence an anterior-posterior-anterior sequence has been proposed to place the grafts after posterior procedure, but this is associated with higher swallowing and airway complications.
- *The posterior–anterior-posterior sequence:* It is used when the kyphosis is too severe to perform the anterior approach in the first stage. Here posterior release of the ankylosis is performed, followed by anterior decompression correction and reconstruction. Finally, posterior instrumentation and fusion is performed.
- *The posterior–anterior sequence* is used in circumstances where there is no ankylosis of the anterior column of the cervical spine. The anterior procedure here aims to reconstruct the load-bearing capability of the spine.

Posterior only procedure:
- The typical indication is performing "cervical extension osteotomy". This osteotomy includes complete laminectomy of C7, partial laminectomies of C6 and T1, and the removal of the spinous process of C6, the ankylosed C7–T1 facet joints, and a portion of the C6 and T1 pedicles. The head is then extended and fixed using internal fixation. The procedure is but associated with complications and high morbidity.
- Now the consensus is emerging that patients with flexible deformity should be treated with the posterior—alone procedure (anterior ankylosis in a fixed deformity is better managed with either an anterior only procedure as above or a combined procedure in expert hands).

Improvement in posterior implants permits the stable fixation and newer screw rod systems also allow fixation at the cervicothoracic transition.

THORACIC KYPHOSIS

Thoracic kyphosis is defined earlier. Developmentally, the thoracic kyphosis is a primary curve. The vertebral heights are therefore increased posteriorly while reduced anteriorly to give a smooth shape to the thoracic curve. The thoracic spine is additionally stabilized by the rib cage. **Table 9** presents the common causes of thoracic kyphosis.

TABLE 9: The usual causes of thoracic kyphosis with brief description.

Postural kyphosis	Adolescents and young adults are commonly affected. The curves are smooth, and deformity is flexible measuring <60°. The curves are nonprogressive, so stress is on postural training and exercises for treatment.
Neoplastic diseases	Metastasis usually destroys anterior vertebral bodies causing kyphosis. The primary management is by anterior resection and posterior stabilization for neurologic involvement or instability. Primary malignant tumors need wide excision while benign lesions only need marginal excision.
Postinfection kyphosis	Tuberculosis is the most common cause of thoracic kyphosis **(Fig. 53)** in India. It causes diskitis and vertebral body destruction (discussed in detail in Chapter on "Vertebral Diskitis and Osteomyelitis and Other Spinal Infections"). Often the lower thoracic spine is involved but involvement anywhere in the spine has been reported. Bacterial diskitis and involvement of vertebral bodies by pyogenic organisms also causes destruction and kyphotic deformity. Antibiotic and brace treatment usually suffice initially, however resistant and advanced disease often needs debridement (excision of focus) and stabilization.
Osteoporosis	This is the second most common cause of kyphotic deformity in India, but slowly increasing in incidence with increasing "graying" population and would quickly surpass tuberculosis as the leading cause of kyphosis. Osteoporotic compression fractures occurring most commonly around the junctional region (thoracolumbar) result in anterior wedging and kyphosis **(Figs. 54A and B)**. They lead not only to deformity but also back pain and progressive disability by involving nearby and even distant vertebrae (kyphosis begets kyphosis). The person loses chest height and trunk sways forward making it difficult to retain a horizontal gaze. Noninvasive treatment is initially considered with bracing but for advanced deformity kyphoplasty or vertebroplasty should be aggressively considered.
Skeletal dysplasias	Achondroplasia is associated with thoracolumbar kyphosis. The deformity can be rigid or flexible. Brace treatment can be appropriate for the latter however surgery is indicated for specific instances: • Triangular apical vertebrae • Thoracolumbar kyphosis more than 30° • Thoracic kyphosis more than 50°
Scheuermann's disease	Described in detail separately

Scheuermann's Disease (Apprentice Spine, Juvenile Discogenic Disease)

This is the most common cause of adolescent kyphosis (incidence as low as 0.4% to as high as 10%, varying with region). It is a rigid juvenile kyphosis associated with a growth disturbance of the vertebral end plates. In 1920, Holger Scheuermann identified the radiographic characteristics of a fixed angular kyphosis with anterior wedging of the vertebral bodies and irregularities of the vertebral apophyses that he described a "juvenile round back" **(Fig. 55)**. The condition arises in prepubertal growth spurt becoming apparent by 10–12 years of age. The deformity is most commonly located in the thoracic spine (called type 1 with apex between T7 and T9) but could well be found in thoracolumbar (called type 2, apex between T10 and T12) and lumbar (L1 and below) region. The type 2 deformity is uncommon and was specifically referred to by Sorenson as "apprentice's spine". The etiopathogenesis has not been fully understood (the universal histological finding has been abnormal vertebral endplate cartilage, irregular mineralization and disorders in vertebral ossification) but the following causes of the disease have been proposed:

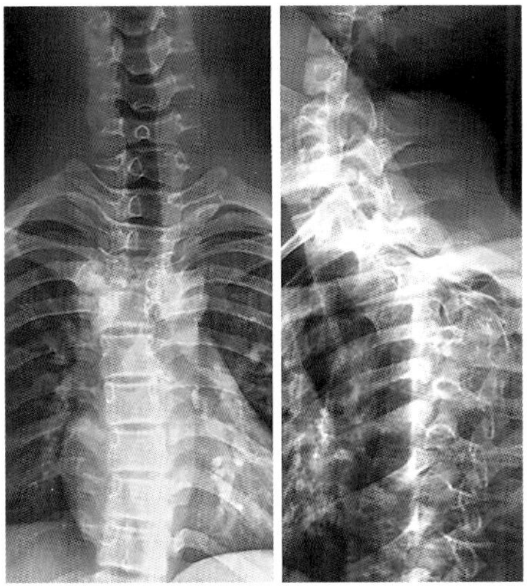

Fig. 53: Postinfection kyphosis. TB of upper thoracic spine involving dorsal third and fourth vertebra. There is kyphotic deformity of the spine at this level (seen in swimmer's view).

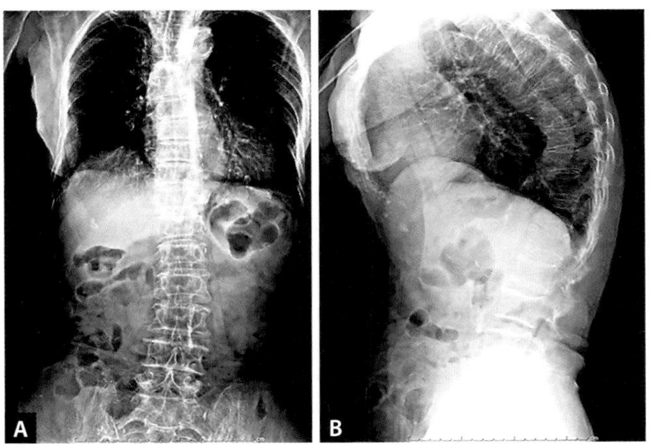

Figs. 54A and B: Thoracic osteoporotic kyphosis. The radiographic depiction in (A) Anteroposterior (AP); (B) Lateral projections.

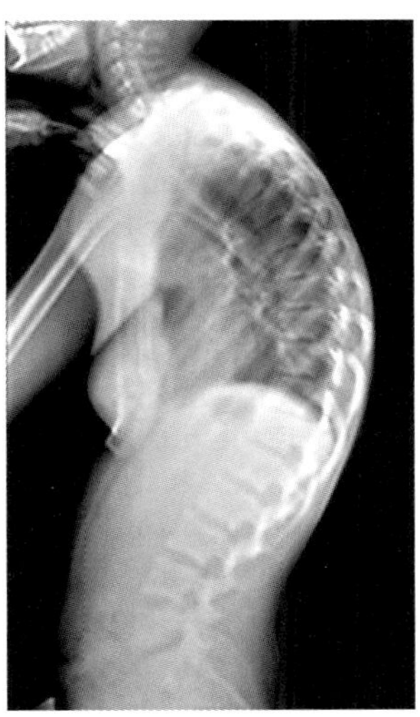

Fig. 55: Scheuermann's kyphosis.

- Osteonecrosis of the ring apophysis of vertebral body (Scheuermann, 1921)
- Herniation of the disk material into vertebral body (Schmorl nodes) causing disturbance of endochondral bone formation with subsequent wedging (Schmorl, 1930)
- Osteochondroses
- Persistence of anterior vascular grooves in vertebral bodies creating a point of structural weakness (Ferguson, 1956)
- Transient osteoporosis (Bradford, 1976)—refuted
- Hereditary (pattern still not established)
- Mechanical stress causing tightness of the anterior longitudinal ligament (Lambrinudi, 1934)
- Malabsorption, infection or endocrine disorders (growth hormone hypersecretion)
- Abnormal collagen and matrix of vertebral endplate cartilage, including decreased ratio between collagen and proteoglycan (Auf Der Maur, 1981)
- Biomechanical theory—vertebral body wedging is secondary to the increased anterior forces due to the first occurring kyphosis. Bilateral hamstring tension is a common finding resulting in focused bending stresses on the thoracic spine causing kyphosis consequent to Heuter-Volkmann law.

Natural history of disease: Ponte et al. demonstrated that all curves greater than 45° progressed during the adolescent growth spurt and continued to increase after the age of 30 years. Bradford et al. reported a higher incidence of disabling thoracic and lumbar back pain in untreated adults. There is often unremitting and incapacitating pain that is seen in 50% of patients during the adolescent growth spurt. These patients were more likely to have thoracic pain, had higher pain intensity readings, were more likely to work in sedentary jobs, and were more likely to be unmarried. There is usually no significant interference with the ADL.

Clinical presentation: Patients consult for their cosmetic deformity and back pain. The low back pain is due to lumbar hyperkyphosis compensation and consequent facet joint involvement. The pain may radiate to buttocks and lower extremities. It may awaken them from sleep in night.

Physical Examination

- Thoracic kyphosis with sloping shoulders
- Forward posturing of the head and neck due to cervical hyperlordosis
- *Adam's forward bend test:*
  - Slight truncal asymmetry associated with mild scoliosis
  - When viewed from side it shows posterior angulation of the thoracic spine
- The deformity is not correctible by manipulation or postural changes
- Protuberant abdomen due to hyperlordosis in lumbar region.
- Loss of lumbar lordosis (in lumbar kyphosis)—flattened lumbar region.

Radiology: Obtain large 36-inch films.

- AP films may show scoliosis not exceeding 25°. It also helps in assessing skeletal maturity—Risser's sign.

- Lateral projection demonstrates kyphosis greater than 40°. There are various ways Scheuermann's kyphosis is defined on a lateral projection.
  - Sorenson's criteria (1964)—more than 5° of anterior wedging of minimum of three consecutive adjacent vertebral bodies at the apex of the kyphosis
  - Drummond's criteria are minimum of two vertebral body wedging more than 5°.
  - *Bradford criteria for diagnosis of Scheuermann's disease on lateral radiographs:*
    - The presence of a hyperkyphosis greater than 40°
    - Irregular upper and lower vertebral endplates
    - Wedging of more than 10° in one or more vertebrae
    - The apparent loss of disk space height
  - Irregular, flattened and wedged vertebral apophyseal lines
  - Narrowing of the intervertebral disk spaces
  - Variable presence of Schmorl's nodes.
- Lumbar Scheuermann's will show—decreased lumbar lordosis or even a kyphotic deformity, the involved vertebrae have increased anteroposterior dimension than the uninvolved vertebrae. The lumbar vertebrae are scalloped with lucent defects at the anterosuperior corners.

Magnetic resonance imaging is needed in rapidly progressive cases of Scheuermann's disease as there may be thoracic spine stenosis. Also any neurological symptom mandates an evaluation of the spine by MRI. Preoperative evaluation by MRI is necessary for missing the neurology.

Differential Diagnosis

Postural kyphosis, osteochondral dystrophies, spondyloepiphyseal dysplasias.

Management

Conservative management is aimed to control deformity progression and improve vertebral height by applying hyperextension force (Heuter-Volkman law). It has been envisaged that any amount of deformity can be corrected by conservative management in skeletally immature patients (Risser stage 2 or less), but this seems to be an overstatement. There is finding that deformities large to begin with bracing (>70°) loose correction quickly after removal of brace, so there is little ultimate correction in the end. Thus ideally bracing will be indicated for immature spine with enough growth potential (Risser 2 or less) with curves around 60°.

Bracing the spine: Milwaukee brace is recommended for thoracic apex at T8 or above. There is also secondary impact on the lumbar curve and sagittal imbalance with the use of this brace. For curve apex below T9 a TLSO (thoracolumbosacral orthosis) is used with anterior sternal and infraclavicular outriggers to avoid extension moment superior to apex. Bracing should be done full time initially removing only for hygiene maintenance and exercises. There are two distinct radiological types of patients: one is the Sorenson type with multiple small wedging of vertebra distributed over few segments. These patients respond well to bracing and achieve faster correction so bracing is given full-time to them for 9–18 months (depending on individual correction). The other type is the Bradford type with single apical edging that is quite remarkable. These patients respond late and it is recommended to continue bracing in them full-time till apical remodeling is done (5° remaining wedge only). Programmed reduction in wearing time (2–4 hours intervals) can be advocated with deformity correction gradually; however, the bracing is continued till skeletal maturity in part-time (say night-time) application.

Risser casts: If passive correction on lateral bolster radiograph is less than 40%, brace treatment is not likely to be effective. Risser casts can be applied in a serial fashion to produce more correction of the kyphosis. Two or three casts (changed every 2–3 months) are applied to progressively correct the deformity. They provide better long-term angular correction, with lower loss of correction and lesser deterioration despite less initial correction. The cast correction is then maintained by brace application.

Surgical Treatment

Considering the limited functional loss and if there is no self-image distortion with the rounded back, surgical treatment was fraught with caution in these patients, particularly due to high complication rates. Now with newer implant systems and segmental fixation techniques interest has risen in improving the deformity and function of these patients. The typical indications for a Scheuermann's kyphosis are:

- Patients with pain
- Rigid deformity
- *Curve more than 70–75° or progressive deformity:* In immature patients the lower value is the indication (despite brace treatment) while in adults curves higher than larger value need surgery.
- Unacceptable cosmetic appearance.

The management principles for deformity correction in Scheuermann's kyphosis have been anterior column lengthening and posterior column shortening so a standard two-stage corrective procedure comprising of anterior release and fusion is commonly performed. Further there was observed a frequent loss of initial correction with previously practiced posterior only techniques and increased rigidity of large curves in adults often mandates anterior release. There is a concern that attempt to correct deformity more than 50% of the preoperative deformity may lead to development of junctional kyphosis, so commonly up to 50% of the deformity magnitude is corrected.

Fusion should include the proximal most tilted vertebral body into the kyphosis while distally the caudal extent of fusion should include the first lordotic disk space. Stable vertebra (till where the fusion should usually extend) can be defined for fusion. It is the lumbar vertebra most closely bisected by the posterior sacral line. The vertebra just proximal to the stable vertebra can be used for distal fusion level if the proximal disk is lordotic. In case the disk above the stable vertebra is kyphotic, then fusion has to be extended to one level below.

Anterior Release and Fusion

This is most advisable for skeletally immature patients having rigid large magnitude curves. The apex of deformity is fused in a partially corrected position after release that makes the posterior instrumentation more effective in controlling the deformity and correcting it better. If such large curves are managed only by posterior approach then there are high chances of pseudarthrosis because the "fused mass" will be in tension rather than compression. Anterior release should always be done prior to posterior surgery hence which can be done either open by right-sided thoracotomy or in experienced hands even thoracoscopically. In VATS, the apical 5–6 disks are removed with or without segmental vessel ligation. This can be followed by posterior instrumentation and then placing morselized graft in the spaces created and distracted. Prone VATS has the advantages of not needing to reposition the patient and improved lung ventilation (rather than single lung ventilation in lateral position).

Posterior Instrumentation and Correction

This involves correction of deformity by first creating space between adjacent laminae that are then closed during a cantilever compression maneuver **(Fig. 56)**. The inferior portion of the lamina is removed along with facet joint and the compression of space produces sort of closing wedge osteotomy. This closure is done by compression rod technique. The typical posterior construct involves using minimum eight anchors above and below the apex of kyphosis. Some authors have been able to achieve good correction by the use of posterior only technique without the need of anterior release and prefer this for most cases. We still think that for large rigid curves (thoracic kyphosis more than 50° on hyperextension radiographs or thoracolumbar kyphosis more than 20° on bending films) some anterior release is needed to make the curves a bit supple making posterior fiddling less and also reducing postoperative loss of correction.

Complications

Posterior only procedure (limited indications but has its proponents):

- Pseudarthrosis
- Hardware failure
- Hook pull-out
- Loss of correction

Combined Procedure

- Junctional kyphosis
- Wound infections
- Neurologic deficits
- Painful bursitis
- Deep vein thrombosis and pulmonary embolism
- Cardiopulmonary problems
- Pulmonary complications such as pneumothorax or hemothorax
- Gastrointestinal disorders
- Postoperative back pain or sciatica

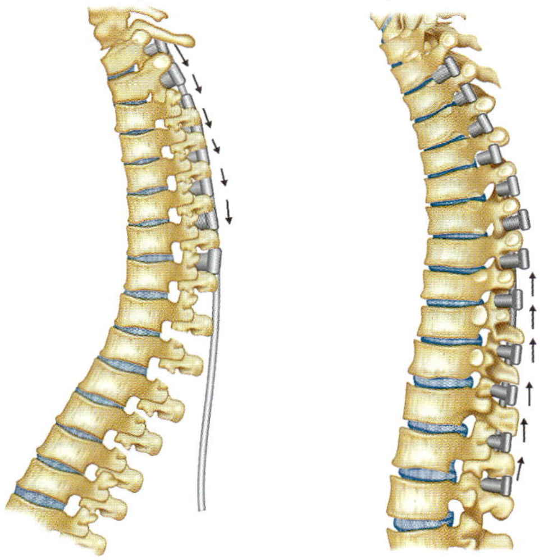

Fig. 56: Surgical correction of Scheuermann kyphosis.

- Dural lacerations
- Infected dural fistulas and postoperative meningitis and encephalitis

CONCLUSION

- Spinal deformities comprise possibly the third most common cause of referral to a spine surgeon after back pain and infections of spine.
- The spinal deformities can occur in coronal and sagittal plane (as is commonly perceived) but most deformities are three dimensional having an added rotational component often.
- Thorough evaluation of the cause of deformities and their description is important as both have bearing on the treatment prescription and planning.
- Surgical management must be undertaken only at the specialized centers and by experienced personnel, complications rates are very high and may even risk the neurology of patients in hands of young surgeons that have not undergone proper training. Intraoperative monitoring of the neurology is a versatile tool in order to minimize the neurological complications.
- Adult-onset scoliosis is an often neglected problem that needs proper and in-depth evaluation for comprehensive management. Evaluation principles are a bit different that childhood coronal plane deformities and surgical management is also discrete requiring advanced surgical skills, that needs to be conveyed to the patient and well understood by the surgeon.
- Neuromuscular scoliosis are a unique problem as they are rapidly progressive and need exacting treatment else the treatment also has high failure rates. The surgeon must be vigilant as regards treatment planning so that optimal treatment can be delivered.
- The sagittal plane deformities have been cumbersome to treat surgically and the apparent lesser degree of functional limitation improving acceptably with bracing, surgery was often considered late. Newer systems have, however, improved the outcome of surgery in management of deformity.

CHAPTER 103

Diffuse Idiopathic Skeletal Hyperostosis (DISH, Forestier Disease, Ankylosing Hyperostosis, Generalized Juxta-articular Ossification of Vertebral Ligaments, and Spondylosis Hyperostotica)

Manish Kumar Varshney

INTRODUCTION

In 1950, Forestier and Rotes-Querol described a disorder what they named "senile ankylosing hyperostosis" that was characterized by spinal stiffness, coalescing osteophytes, and "flowing" new-bone formation in the thoracic spine. Diffuse idiopathic skeletal hyperostosis (DISH) is characterized by exuberant bone formation in the spinal column and although men are affected most often, the condition occurs in women as well. The condition is however not limited to spine, and over the years, Forestier and various other authors have described numerous extraspinal findings such as type 2 diabetes mellitus, obesity, and dyslipidemia. The condition can be defined simply as a systemic bone-forming diathesis with primary spinal and various extraspinal clinical and radiographic findings. The term "diffuse idiopathic skeletal hyperostosis" was introduced by Resnick who also laid down the diagnostic criteria in 1970s (modified from Forestier, **Table 1**) that have been also largely used to define the disease.

ETIOLOGY

The etiology is unknown but the association with some syndromes have envisaged search for basic molecular defect that is though still elusive. Some strong contenders for diagnosis are:

- *Combined metabolic disturbances:* Diabetes mellitus, glucose intolerance, hyperuricemia, and dyslipidemia **(Flowchart 1)**
- The role of matrix Gla protein (MGP)
- *Abnormal levels of insulin-like growth factor-1 (IGF-1) and growth hormone:* IGF-1 stimulates alkaline phosphatase activity and type II collagen in osteoblasts. Growth hormone can induce the local production of IGF-1 and IGF-binding proteins in chondrocytes and osteoblasts.
- Endocrine and metabolic syndromes, such as acromegaly and hypervitaminosis A (exposure to low doses of the synthetic retinoids isotretinoin and etretinate in modern context)

TABLE 1: Diagnostic criteria for diffuse idiopathic skeletal hyperostosis (DISH).

Criteria (of Forestier as modified by Resnick and Niwayama)	*Comments*
Flowing ossification along the anterolateral aspect of at least four contiguous vertebrae	The first criterion, flowing ossification along the anterolateral borders of at least four contiguous spinal segments, is the essence of DISH. The number "4" has been specifically chosen to differentiate from spondylosis deformans. Although this requirement increases the overall specificity of the definition, it decreases the overall sensitivity and could also impede early detection of the condition, assuming that DISH progresses steadily over time.
Preservation of disk height in the involved vertebral segment; the relative absence of significant degenerative changes, such as marginal sclerosis in vertebral bodies or vacuum phenomenon	This criterion specifically eliminates the degenerative spine disease. Some patients with DISH do, however, have degenerative disk disease. So, it requires a more accurate definition.
Absence of facet-joint ankylosis; absence of sacroiliac erosion, sclerosis, or intra-articular osseous fusion	This criterion is to exclude the diagnosis of ankylosing spondylitis. It has been shown by some investigators that the two conditions can coexist.

Utsinger classification:

- Definite DISH—continuous ossification along the anterolateral aspect of at least four contiguous vertebral bodies, primarily in the thoracolumbar spine.
- *Probable DISH:*
  - (a) Continuous ossification along the anterolateral aspect of at least two contiguous vertebral bodies, and
  - (b) Symmetrical and peripheral enthesopathy (inflammation at the insertion of the tendons) involving the posterior heel, superior patella, or olecranon, with the entheseal new bone having a well-defined cortical margin.
- Possible DISH presence of either of the two criteria for probable DISH, especially if calcaneal spurs occur together with olecranon or patellar spurs.

Flowchart 1: Pathogenesis of diffuse idiopathic skeletal hyperostosis (DISH).

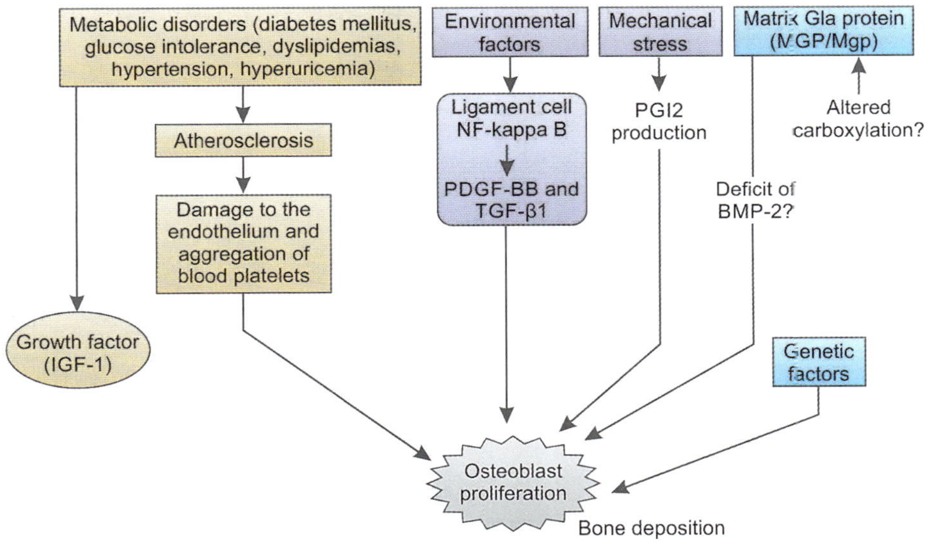

(BMP-2: bone morphogenetic protein 2; IGF-1: insulin-like growth factor 1; NF: nuclear factor; PDGF: platelet-derived growth factor; PGI2: prostaglandin I2; TGF: transforming growth factor)

- HLA-B8 is common among patients with both DISH and type 2 diabetes mellitus.
- HLA-B27 (unclear at best, probably no relation)
- Hypervascularity of ALL (anterior longitudinal ligament)
- *Speculative associations:* Neuroarthropathies, fluorosis, rheumatoid arthritis, and ankylosing spondylitis—historical importance assigned due to similar bony features. No established relationship.

PREVALENCE

Diffuse idiopathic skeletal hyperostosis is a common disease diagnosed predominantly in older male patients. So, age is possibly the most common but nonspecific association. Another factor is male sex, being at least twice as common in them, and also they have a more severe affliction. The average age is around 66 years. Racial differences are noted by some authors but most find the distribution—egalitarian and possibly is a nonfactor.

CLINICAL PRESENTATION

The presentation varies and is unequally distributed in patients between axial and extraspinal symptoms. One set of patients have predominant spinal manifestations while other have extraspinal symptoms that are more common. We will discuss these two groups separately although the axial manifestations of DISH are the most frequent and form the basis of the diagnosis. Overall, clinical findings are mild in comparison to the conspicuous radiographic findings. The minimal pain experienced by some patients may be a consequence of the relative stabilization of spinal segments through ankylosis. In fact, many patients are discovered incidentally.

SPINAL MANIFESTATIONS

The usual presentation is a middle-aged or older patient with mild, chronic back pain in the middle to lower spine, and stiffness. For extraspinal manifestations, bilateral involvement is characteristic.

- *Thoracic spine:*
  - The thoracic spine is the most commonly involved segment.
  - Thoracic myelopathy has been reported but is rare.
- *Cervical spine:*
  - Pain and stiffness of the neck may be prominent symptoms but are rarely, if ever, the presenting complaints. Involvement of the cervical spine is less reported than involvement of the lumbar or thoracic spine.
  - Dysphagia may result from large cervical syndesmophytes, which are present in as many as 28% of patients with DISH.
  - Hoarseness, sleep apnea, stridor, aspiration pneumonia, thoracic outlet syndrome, and difficulty with intubation have all been reported due to syndesmophytes.
  - Ossification of the posterior longitudinal ligament (PLL) not uncommon in DISH and cervical cord compression from osteophytes can cause cervical myelopathy, as well as C1–C2 atlantoaxial pseudarthrosis and subluxation.
- *Lumbar spine:*
  - Patients often complain of low back pain or stiffness but without the presence of changes on lumbar radiographs, so association of back pain with DISH is not established.
  - Significant compression of the inferior vena cava due to large anterior osteophytic excrescences has been reported.
- *Traumatic changes:*
  - Patients with DISH are vulnerable for fracture from even minor trauma (hyperextension injury) to the fused spine that may result in pseudarthrosis **(Fig. 1)**.

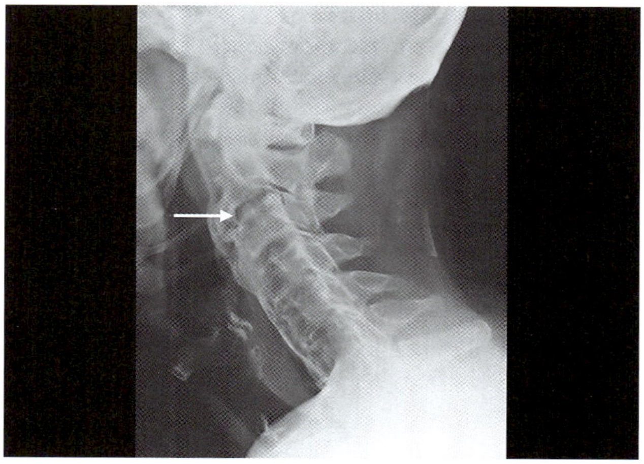

Fig. 1: Trauma resulting in pseudarthrosis (arrow).

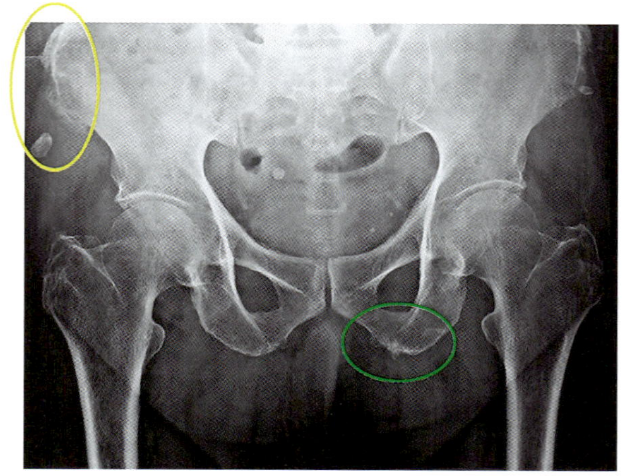

Fig. 2: Diffuse idiopathic skeletal hyperostosis of the pelvic region. Note the whiskering of the iliac crest (encircled in yellow). Ischium shows enthesopathy (encircled in green).

The increased incidence of fracture instability in these patients is due to long lever arm of fused vertebral segments proximal and distal to the fracture even in low-energy injuries. Concerns with these injuries include:
- Delay in diagnosis and a high rate of immediate and delayed neurologic consequences.
- They occur in the middle or at the ends of ankylosed segments so difficult to visualize and fix.
- Must be carefully evaluated for occult fracture with computed tomography or magnetic resonance imaging.

EXTRASPINAL MANIFESTATIONS

Tendinitis and enthesophytes (osseous outgrowths at the sites of attachment of tendon, ligament or capsule to bone) are the most common findings but their association with symptoms is unclear. Subtle periostitis at the site of ligament or tendon insertion is also common. The characteristic findings associated with DISH are usually bilateral and symmetrical.

Pelvis

- Enthesophytes are seen in the iliac wing and ischial tuberosity **(Fig. 2)** along with calcification of the sacrotuberous and iliolumbar ligaments.
- Periarticular osteophytes about the hip, sacroiliac joints, and symphysis pubis can often be found.
- Bone proliferation (whiskering) can be seen at sites of ligament and tendon attachment **(Fig. 2)**.
- To differentiate from ankylosing spondylitis, bone erosions in the sacroiliac joints and at the sites of ligament attachment are generally absent in DISH, but bridging or nonbridging osteophytes about the sacroiliac joint have been seen.

Hip

- Hip involvement is variable with some patients having few or no pathologic changes.
- Those with signs and symptoms may have periarticular bone proliferation with an intact joint space, hyperostosis with a narrowed joint space, or osteonecrosis, none of these findings are solely attributed to DISH and can be seen at any stage as due to age-related changes.

Knee

- Patients with DISH have a much higher prevalence (nearly 30%) of knee changes, compared to normal population.
- Tendinous ossification is seen in quadriceps mechanism associated with patellar hyperostosis and large osseous excrescences on the poles.
- A prominent tibial spine is the most common finding but incidence of symptomatic osteoarthritis of the knee is not higher than other population.

Foot and Ankle

- Most of the DISH patients (more than three-fourths) have manifestations involving the foot and ankle.
- Any bone in the foot may exhibit hyperostosis due to numerous sites of ligament and tendon attachment that make spur formation frequent.
- Achilles tendinitis is common.
- Calcaneal spurs are frequent (seen in three-fourths of DISH patient population compared to around one-fifth of normal population).
- The cortex of the calcaneus may be thickened.
- Calcification of the Achilles tendon or plantar fascia may be seen but have no definite relation with symptoms.
- The presence of large calcaneal spurs in the setting of Achilles tendinitis or plantar fasciitis should lead one to consider DISH as an underlying diagnosis.
- Talar beaking due to enthesophytes may be seen, other sites for spur formation include medial navicular, lateral and plantar cuboid, and the base of the fifth metatarsal.

Shoulder

Irregular osseous excrescences can occur at the deltoid tubercle, the greater and lesser tuberosities, inferior glenoid, distal clavicle, as well as at the sites of attachment of the coracoclavicular ligaments. These changes are variably associated with pain, stiffness, and loss of motion.

Elbow

- Enthesophytes around elbow contrary to other places are frequently symptomatic.
- Spurs on the olecranon are frequently seen in DISH.
- Hyperostosis can occur along the distal medial humerus.

Hand and Wrist

- Similar to feet, cortical thickening may be seen in the tubular bones, along with hyperostosis and spur formation in periarticular sites.
- The distal phalangeal tufts may appear pointed ("arrow-heading"). Soft-tissue and cartilage hypertrophy are present in acromegaly but not in DISH.

Ribs

Hyperostosis of the ribs also has been noted in patients with DISH. Typically, it affects the posteromedial aspect of the rib (no definite clinical significance).

RADIOLOGY

Diffuse idiopathic skeletal hyperostosis radiological changes in axial skeleton are thoracic spine centric, so much so that changes are most prominent in this region, and with cervical spine affection, the lower vertebrae, and for lumbar spine, the upper lumbar vertebrae are commonly affected. The characteristic features seen in axial skeleton are:

- *Thoracic spine:* Large syndesmophytes and flowing, laminated new-bone formation along the anterolateral margins of vertebral bodies.
- The syndesmophytes project horizontally from the vertebral bodies with the classic appearance of flowing candle wax, becoming confluent to form an extra-articular ankylosis (*cf.* vertically oriented "bamboo spine" outgrowths in ankylosing spondylitis).
- The syndesmophytes are more prominent on the right side (they are reduced to left side due to effect of pulsatile aorta), whereas they are commonly symmetrical in the cervical and lumbar spine **(Figs. 3A to C)**.
- Hyperostosis of posterior elements is rare, although hyperostosis of costovertebral joints may be present. Osteopenia (commonly seen in ankylosing spondylitis) is not a feature of DISH. Patients with DISH are quite protected against osteoporosis also.
- Facet articulations and disk spaces are generally preserved and their involvement goes in favor of age-related spine changes rather DISH.
- In *cervical spine* radiographic findings are most common in the lower segments and less prevalent at the more cephalad levels **(Fig. 4)**. Ossification and loss of elasticity occur along the anterior paravertebral tissues, such as the anterior longitudinal ligament.
- In the cervical spine, the changes in canal diameter, alignment, and mobility of motion segments not only cause neck pain and stiffness but put patients with DISH at risk for severe neurologic injury.
- Ligamentum flavum hypertrophy, dystrophic calcification of spinal ligaments (including ossification of the PLL), and mild cervical kyphosis can occur, occasionally resulting in cervical spinal stenosis and myelopathy.
- *Lumbar spine:* Radiographic evidence of DISH in the lumbar spine is most frequently seen in the upper levels and is less common caudally (thoracic centric disease); the syndesmophytes are more confluent and may take appearance of "parrot beak" **(Figs. 5A and B)**.
- Degenerative changes are common between the fourth lumbar and first sacral vertebrae due to the exacerbated stress imposed on the lumbosacral area by a stiff spine superiorly.
- Technetium bone scanning can show increased uptake in areas of involvement, which may be confused with evidence of periarticular metastatic disease.

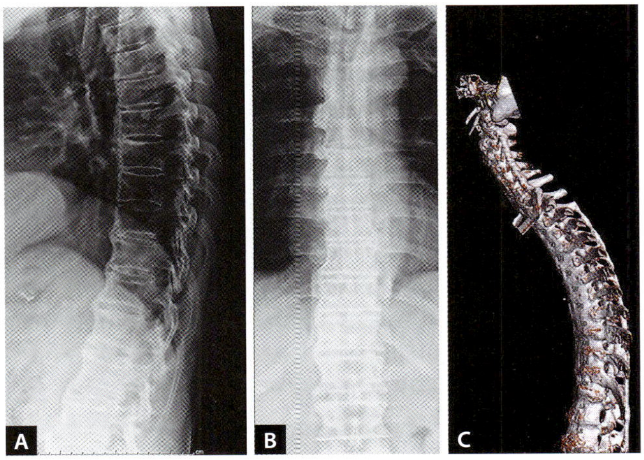

Figs. 3A to C: Diffuse idiopathic skeletal hyperostosis of the thoracic spine (A and B). Note the predominant lesions on the right side of lower thoracic vertebrae (C) (protection by aortic pulsations on the left side).

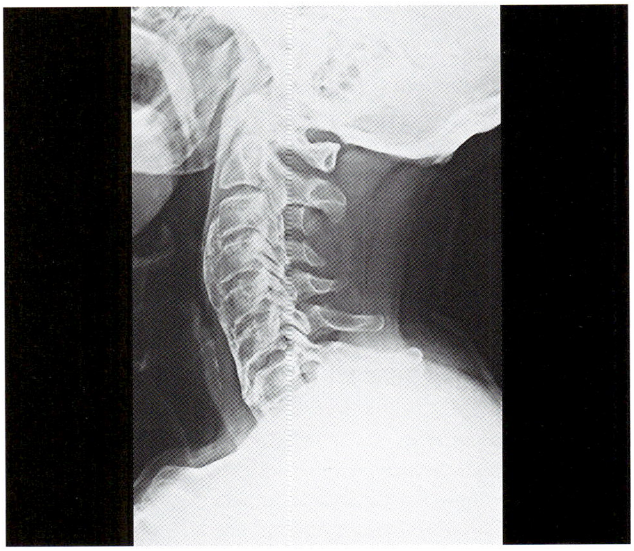

Fig. 4: Diffuse idiopathic skeletal hyperostosis of cervical spine. Note the flowing candle appearance of bone in the lower cervical vertebrae in the anterior aspect.

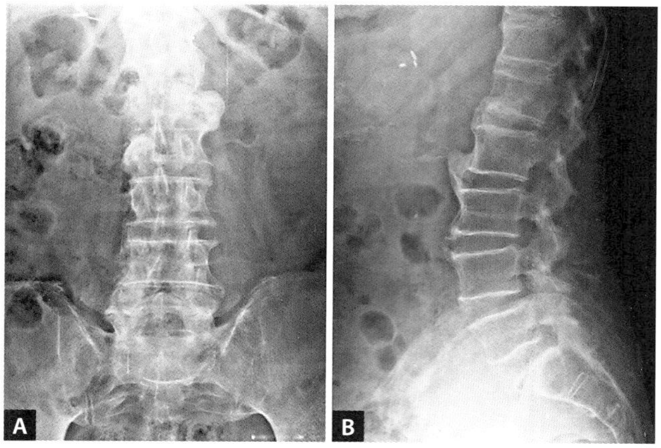

Figs. 5A and B: Diffuse idiopathic skeletal hyperostosis of the lumbar spine. Note that the osteophytes are predominantly seen in the upper lumbar spine (thoracic centric disease).

DIFFERENTIAL DIAGNOSIS

There are no diagnostic laboratory findings, but evaluation may exclude other potential diagnoses. The erythrocyte sedimentation rate and C-reactive protein, rheumatoid factor, and antinuclear antibody levels are typically normal. If DISH is suspected in an adult, the thoracic spine should be evaluated radiographically to establish the diagnosis. The condition should be separated from various related conditions as follows:

- Spondylosis deformans (age-related deformation, degenerative joint disease)
- Intervertebral osteochondrosis (degenerative disk disease)
- Ankylosing spondylitis
- Fluorosis
- Ochronosis
- Acromegaly
- Hypoparathyroidism
- Pseudogout
- Charcot spine
- Sternocostoclavicular hyperostosis
- Spondyloarthroses variants (psoriasis, Reiter's syndrome, inflammatory bowel disease, and Whipple's disease)
- Pachydermoperiostosis
- X-linked hypophosphatemic rickets

TREATMENT

The treatment of DISH predominantly involves nonoperative measures with occasional surgical intervention for specific sequelae.

Conservative Management

Activity modification, physical therapy, chiropractic manipulation and drop-table adjustments, corset or brace wear, nonsteroidal anti-inflammatory medications, and bisphosphonate therapy are the mainstays of treatment, but all are mainly symptomatic and may have a placebo effect. They are mainly directed to improve flexibility and daily living activities. Cervical traction may result in excessive distraction due to the lack of ligamentous structures and should be used cautiously.

Surgery

Surgery is indicated for DISH only for specific complications or conditions such as fracture/pseudarthrosis formation, stenosis, tumor, infection, or painful deformity.

- For hip joint involvement, the joint reconstruction surgeon should take proper precaution for possible increased chances of heterotopic ossification.
- If syndesmophytes are impinging on anterior structures say causing dysphagia, surgical resection can be palliative.
- Early stabilization of the fractured spine is needed to preclude nonunion, osteolysis, late instability, neurologic deficit and to prevent progression. Operative stabilization is usually required for significantly displaced or unstable fractures.
- In cases of multilevel cervical stenosis and myelopathy with preserved lordosis, laminoplasty or laminectomy may be indicated. In other cases, anterior decompression and stabilization may be necessary.
- The use of open reduction and internal fixation is recommended and delayed neurologic compromise.
- Most pelvic findings do not require surgical intervention.
- Symptomatic degenerative hip may require total hip arthroplasty. These patients may be at increased risk for heterotopic ossification. The clinical significance of heterotopic ossification in patients with DISH after total hip arthroplasty is debated.

CONCLUSION

- Diffuse idiopathic skeletal hyperostosis is a disabling condition of spine characterized by widespread ossification of the ligaments especially the anterior longitudinal ligament. Other axial bones like the pelvic bones are also commonly involved.
- Involvement of peripheral bones is not uncommon, but the radiology is most typical for axial skeleton.
- Management is usually symptomatic but surgical decompression may be needed in patients not responding to conservative management.

CHAPTER

104 Rheumatoid Affection of Spine

Manish Kumar Varshney

INTRODUCTION

Rheumatoid arthritis (RA) is a chronic inflammatory disease with inflammation of synovial joints. The end result is proliferative and erosive synovitis that causes destruction of articular cartilage. Cervical spine is the most commonly and significantly affected in RA compared to other regions, up to 86% of all RA patients may have cervical spine involvement. Cervical spine involvement is so common that it is only second to metacarpophalangeal joint involvement. Garrod, in 1890, reported involvement of the cervical spine while Davis and Markley were the first to describe medullary compression from atlantoaxial subluxation (AAS). The course is variable and that while some patients have benign process others develop instability. Within 7 years of serologic diagnosis, 30–50% develops subluxation. Prolonged persistence of RA for >14 years is responsible for development of AAS with myelopathy in 2.5% patients. Kornblum and colleagues documented the relationship of RA and cervical spine instability in 1952 that improved our perspective. Common presenting symptoms are neck pain and neurologic deficit and the patients are at risk for sudden death.

- Neck pain is seen in majority (40–80%) and though nonspecific, is a warning sign if present in any rheumatoid patient requiring further evaluation.
- Radiological instability is seen in 43–86% and needs further evaluation especially with respect to involvement of peripheral joint disease severity.
- Neurological deficit is not seen in many but 7–34% develop them over complete span of disease at some point (varies with risk factors, see below).
- Sudden death is seen in 10% and is the ultimate endpoint of untreated uncontrolled progressive disease.

The disease due to increased awareness often is now recognized in the form of asymptomatic radiological instability. Orthopedician's role is to identify those who are at risk and to stabilize them to prevent neurological damage.

PATHOPHYSIOLOGY OF DISEASE DEVELOPMENT AND JOINT DESTRUCTION

Rheumatoid arthritis at the best of our understanding is a multifactorial disorder triggered by some sort of antigenic exposure (arthritogenic) in an immunogenetically susceptible host. Disease has systemic manifestations both articular and extra-articular; joints are commonly involved in a symmetrical distribution and axial involvement predominantly is of the upper cervical spine.

- The inflammatory synovitis of RA is triggered by the antigenic expression of synovial cells that produce immunoglobulin M (IgM) against IgG (rheumatoid factor). Inflammation is initiated by the activated CD4+ helper T-cells, stimulating the release of monocytes, macrophages and synovial fibroblasts that secrete interleukin (IL)-1, IL-6, and tumor necrosis factor-alpha (TNF-α). Simultaneously, matrix metalloproteinase (MMP) is secreted via CD69 and CD11 mediated pathway through release from IFN-γ and IL-17 [*see* Chapter on "Joint Disorders Including Inflammatory and Noninflammatory Arthritis and Infective Arthritides (Including Mycobacterial Infection and Prosthetic Joint Infection)"].
- The above factors and proteases further cause proliferation of synoviocytes and destroy the articular structures with progressive proliferating fibrous tissue and fibrin within the basal layer of synovial membrane (pannus formation).
- The synovitis and pannus then destroys the ligaments and bone, leading to subluxation, pain, and neurological damage.

Pathoanatomy and Biomechanics of Forces on Cervical Spine

It is important to understand the various forces acting on cervical spine that are responsible for development of the various pathological forms seen as the peculiar anatomy and dynamic distribution of forces across makes cervical spine particularly vulnerable to effects of RA. The salient features important to context are mentioned below (detailed anatomy can be referred from dedicated textbooks):

- Compared to the relative size of vertebra in cervical spine, the synovial joints are quite big (percentage-wise) specifically when compared with lumbar or dorsal spine. The synovial joints are atlanto-occipital, atlantoaxial, and facet (apophyseal) joints. We know RA primarily affects the synovial joints.

- The cartilaginous intervertebral joints (intervertebral disks) are absent in atlanto (C1)-occipital joint and atlantoaxial joints both making them more vulnerable as they rely only on the synovial joints for stability as the cartilaginous joints that are spared in RA are absent.
- The transverse ligament articulates with dens through synovial joint.
- The C1 lacks a body and consists of lateral articulations that are highly mobile providing most of the flexion of cervical spine.
- The odontoid process (dens) of C2 articulation with transverse ligament and atlas accounts for >50% of rotation of cervical spine.
- Cervical spine is followed below by stiffer thoracic spine so that most movements are to occur through neck.
  - Weight of head from above followed below by stiff thoracic spine exacerbates the force transmission that can rupture weak ligaments or fracture eroded dens.
- The stability of C1–C2 articulation relies primarily on the integrity of transverse ligament **(Figs. 1A to C)**. The alar ligaments (between odontoid and occiput) are secondary stabilizers, and apical ligaments are tertiary stabilizers **(Figs. 1A to C)**. The facets of C1–C2 articulation are horizontally oriented providing no restraint via interlocking mechanism for stability.
  - Transverse ligament being primary stabilizer prevents anterior subluxation.
  - Complete insufficiency of the ligament produces, however, only 4–5 mm subluxations if the secondary restraints are patent.
  - 10–12 mm subluxation suggests complete loss of ligament restraints.
- In contrast to osteoarthritis, where the formation of osteophytes provides secondary stability by compensation, there is no osteophyte formation in RA so this mechanism also does not exist.
- The SAC (space available for cord, **Fig. 2**) is an important parameter referred below in the text. It is handy to know the referable values at various places:
  - 14 mm at the foramen magnum
  - 14 mm at C2
  - 12–14.5 mm in the subaxial spine

Pathophysiology and Development of Subluxations and Deformity

In the cervical spine, there are subtle differences in the involvement in upper and lower regions and a combination of these is not uncommon:

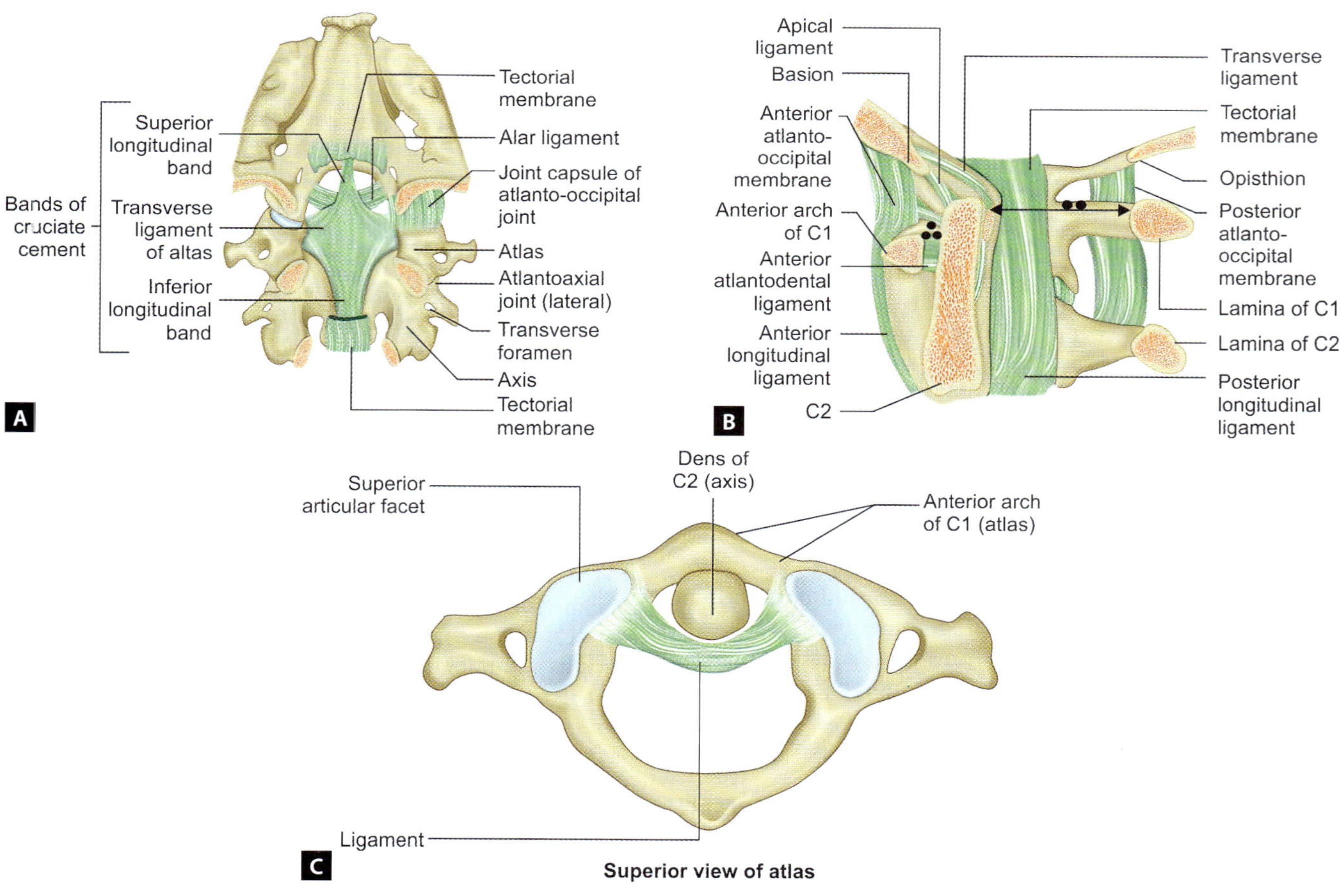

Figs. 1A to C: The atlantoaxial joint anatomy in: (A) Coronal section; (B) Sagittal section; (C) Axial section.

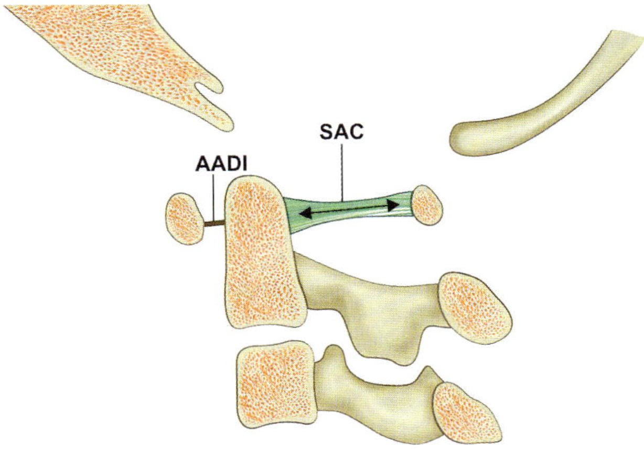

Fig. 2: The illustration depicting the space available for cord (SAC). (AADI: anterior atlantodental interval)

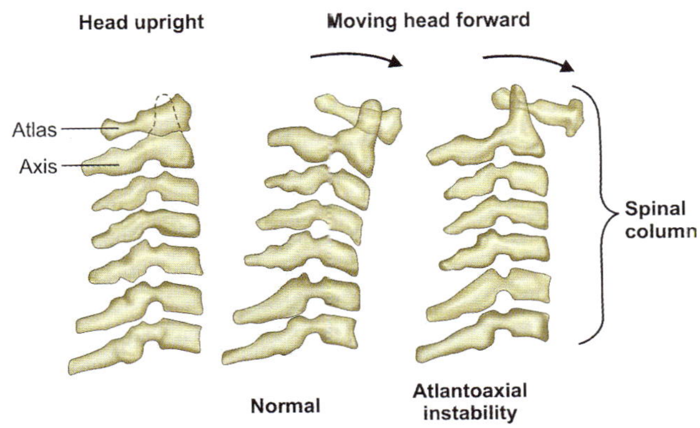

Fig. 3: Atlantoaxial instability in anterior direction.

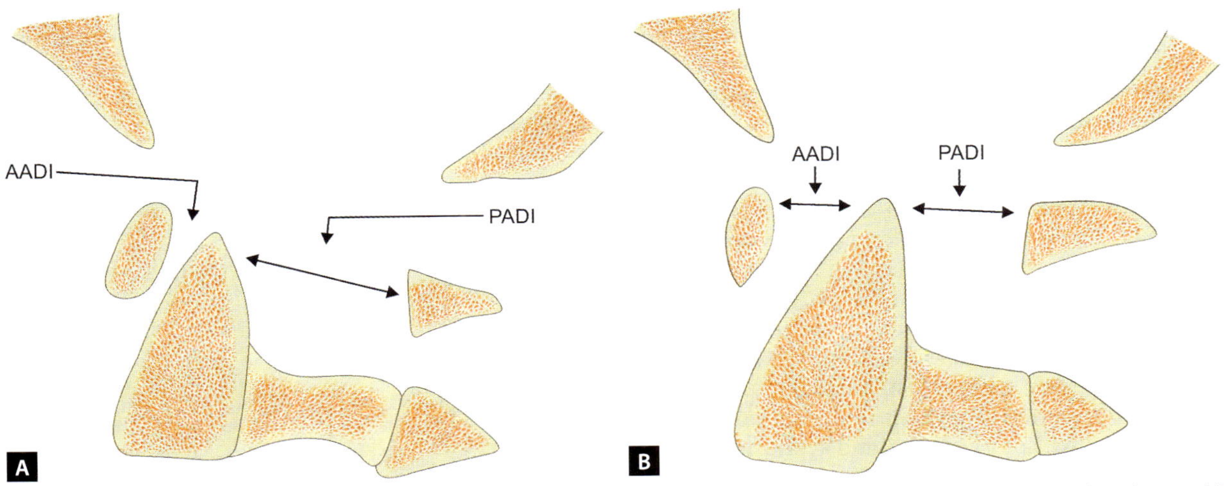

Figs. 4A and B: (A) The measurements at craniocervical junction anterior atlantodental interval (AADI) and posterior atlantodental interval (PADI); (B) Atlantoaxial subluxation is normally indicated by increased AADI and reduced PADI.

- *Upper cervical spine (two forms of subluxation):*
  - Primarily ligamentous destruction leads to *atlanto-axial subluxation* (AAS) which is seen in 65% of cases. This is the most common deformity resulting from involvement of primary and secondary restraints (see below). The AAS develops quite early in the disease process and usually develops in anterior direction **(Fig. 3)**, but may also be in lateral direction or even posterior (rare). The SAC decreases with anterior subluxation as there is reduced posterior atlantodental interval **(PADI, Figs. 4A and B)** and increased anterior atlantodental interval (AADI). PADI is further reduced by pannus formation in the region causing cord destruction and myelopathy. Lateral subluxation **(Fig. 5)** usually occurs in 20% of the cases and is associated with rotational deformity. Posterior subluxation is usually due to erosion or fracture of dens seen in 7% of cases but is prone to higher incidence of neurological complications.

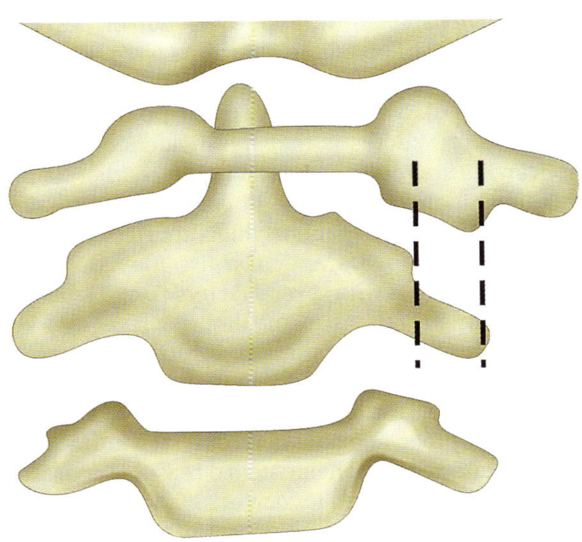

Fig. 5: Lateral atlantoaxial subluxation.

- Primarily bony destruction, later in the disease process, leads to *cranial settling,* also known as *superior migration of the odontoid* (SMO) or *basilar invagination/impression* (some prefer to call it translocation of the dens, atlantoaxial impaction, and vertical settling). SMO or basilar invagination (basilar invagination/impression is specifically used for osteogenesis imperfecta so better avoided here) is the second most common rheumatoid subluxation (20%). It is a late complication (always associated with AAS) but often fraught with neurological complications. SMO results form occipito-atlanto-axial erosion following AAS. Symmetrical rheumatoid destruction of the occipito-atlanto and atlantoaxial joints causes cranium to settle over cervical spine whereby dens enters foramen magnum. Due to bony destruction, therefore, SMO is rarely reducible and often associated with neurological damage (brain stem compression); prognosis is guarded. If there is only one lateral mass involvement, the erosion is eccentric and fixed rotational tilt of head may result. With SMO, there is relative reduction in the atlantoaxial space which residents may consider improvement in anatomic radiology and is called "pseudostabilization" **(Fig. 6)**.

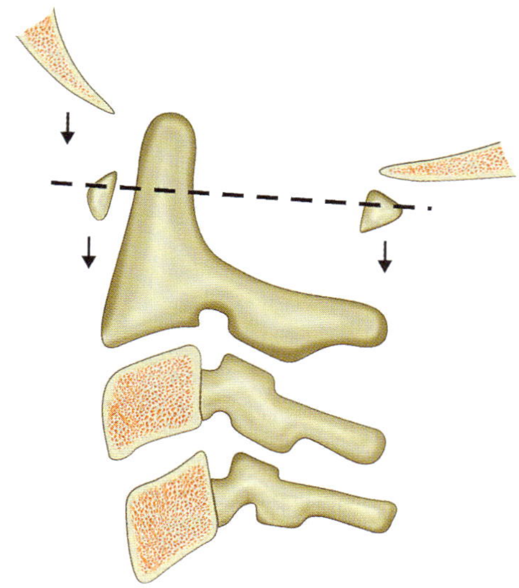

Fig. 6: "Pseudostabilization" occurs due to atlantoaxial impaction causing false or apparent reduction/normalization of anterior atlantodental interval (AADI).

- *Lower cervical spine:* Subaxial subluxation (SAS) is the result of combined destruction of diskovertebral and facet joints. The subluxation can appear as an isolated deformity or can affect multiple spinal levels resulting in "staircase/stepladder" deformity **(Fig. 7)**. SAS is found in approximately 15% of rheumatoid patients. There is appearance of anterior soft-tissue masses, posterior ligamentous thickening, and bony subluxation that produce osteophyte formation, ankylosis (subaxial postinflammatory ankylosis), bone collapse, and kyphosis.
- Patients may have a combination of any two or all three types of subluxation.

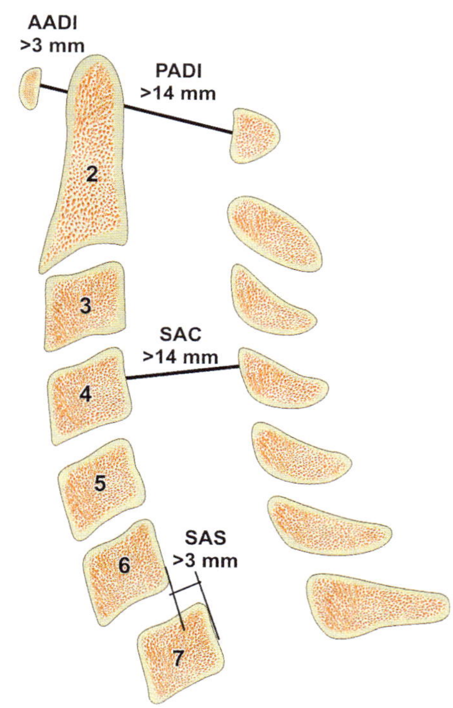

Fig. 7: Predictors of paralysis in rheumatoid affection of cervical spine. (AADI: anterior atlantodental interval; PADI: posterior atlantodental interval; SAC: space available for cord; SAS: subaxial subluxation)

EPIDEMIOLOGY AND NATURAL HISTORY

It is difficult to estimate the prevalence of cervical spine involvement in patients due to wide variation in presentation and therapeutic interventions. Reports vary widely with respect to prevalence (17–88%) and neurological complications (11–70%). The most important point from all the epidemiological studies is that the incidence of AAS and complications are much higher and much earlier than generally thought, and the disease in cervical spine is seen in much higher number of patients than reported.

- Subluxation appears after the first decade of active disease but varies with several factors **(Box 1)**. Instability depends on the severity of the disease process.
- Radiographic progression of subluxation has been observed in 35–80% of patients. The radiographic risk factors for progression of disease are detailed below.
- Neurologic progression has been observed in 15–36% of all patients affected with rheumatoid disease of cervical spine.
- There is a 5-year mortality rate of 17%.
- After the onset of myelopathy, 50% of patients die within 1 year.
- Peripheral disease coincides closely with the severity and progression of cervical subluxation.
  - Cervical subluxation is more likely to occur in patients with erosions of the hands and feet.
  - These subluxations have propensity to deteriorate progressively over time.
  - Both the timing and severity of cervical subluxation coincides with the progression of peripheral erosive disease.

BOX 1: Factors correlated with the severity/progression of cervical spine involvement in studies (some call them Lipson's factors).

- Severity and extent of peripheral joint involvement
- Rheumatoid nodules
- High seropositivity
- Vasculitis
- High-dose of steroid therapy
- Male gender

- Untreated AAS—there is high chance of myelopathy and death ultimately.
    - With the best of available methods and detailing (see below), it is still not possible to accurately predict as to which patients will have disease progression or neurological deficit.
    - Most patients succumb to paralysis and related complications following AAS within 4 years, if untreated.
    - Neurological deficits are irreversible and surgery only can prevent further deterioration.
    - Results of surgical stabilization are best in patients treated before development of myelopathy.

CLINICAL PRESENTATION

- Most cases are asymptomatic due to silent nature of disease and nearly a delay of 31 weeks has been reported from the first signs of myelopathy to diagnosis. Others have minimal pain. Most cases are nowadays often recognized at a preanesthesia checkup (PAC) for other joint surgery.
- Common presenting symptoms are the following:
    - Neck pain is seen in 40–80% and is often localized to craniovertebral junction, associated with occipital headaches. The latter may arise due to irritation of lesser occipital nerve (C1). Occipital pain with radiation to the vertex is one of the most common symptoms in patients with cranial settling. Neck pain may be a consequence of primary inflammatory disorder or potentially related to subaxial instability. The former may be identified by simultaneous involvement of peripheral joints and parallel waxing and waning of symptoms due to RA, while the latter is often disjunct to peripheral joint involvement or actual RA.
    - C2 (greater occipital nerve) nerve compression can present as occipital neuralgia. Similarly facial pain can arise from trigeminal nerve tract/nucleus involvement and earache develops with compression of greater auricular nerve.
    - Crepitus in the cervical spine and a palpable "clunk" on movement of the unstable joints of the cervical spine and patients may report feeling of head falling forward with flexion and clunk-like sensation.
    - Myelopathic symptoms (cord and medullary compression) include:
        - Weakness
        - Loss of endurance
        - Loss of dexterity
        - Gait disturbance
        - Paresthesias
    - *Lhermitte's phenomenon:* Electric shock sensation traveling through the torso and extremities with neck movement (flexion).
    - Vertebrobasilar insufficiency (with basilar invagination) due to compression of cervicomedullary junction presents as tinnitus, vertigo, loss of equilibrium, visual disturbances, nystagmus, diplopia, and dysphagia.
    - In patients with cranial settling, brainstem dysfunctions are frequently reported along with involvement of 5th, 9th, and 12th cranial nerves.
    - Urinary dysfunction is seen with severe disease.
    - Stiff shoulder, if seen, is often secondary to myelopathy instead of adhesive capsulitis.
    - *Warning clinical signs that necessitate further workup:*
        - Increased pain or weakness
        - Spasticity of the extremities
        - Changed ambulatory status, e.g., patient who has been using crutches or a walker for ambulation and progresses to the use of a wheelchair.
        - Bowel and/or bladder disturbance
        - Babinski sign
        - Lost proprioception
        - Hyperreflexia
- Neurological assessment is difficult and unreliable in cervical rheumatoid due to:
    - *Motor assessment problem:* Multifocal involvement is associated with muscle wasting, reduced range of motion of joints, arthritis and pain, and neuropathy.
    - *Sensory inaccuracies* due to entrapment neuropathies.
- Neurological deficit has been classified by Ranawat **(Table 1)**. It might be better to classify the functional capacity instead **(Table 2)** according to the American Rheumatological Association classification—a functional equivalent of Steinbrocker system.

TABLE 1: Ranawat classification.

Type	*Characteristic*
Class I	No deficit
Class II	Subjective weakness with hyperreflexia and dysesthesia
Class IIIA	Ambulatory
Class IIIB	Nonambulatory

TABLE 2: Functional capacity classification according to the American Rheumatological Association.

Class 1	Complete ability to carry on all usual duties without handicaps
Class 2	Adequate for normal activities, despite handicap of discomfort or limited motion at one or more joints
Class 3	Limited to little or none of the duties of usual occupation or self-care
Class 4	Incapacitated, largely or wholly bedridden, or confined to wheel-chair, little or no self-care

DIAGNOSTIC EVALUATION

Plain radiographs form the basis of the screening test. Standard evaluation includes obtaining the lateral, anteroposterior, open-mouth odontoid views, and lateral flexion-extension dynamic views. The flexion cervical spine radiographs are mandatory that are compared with neutral position radiographs. Recognize few critical landmarks to define the radiological changes like the opisthion (the dorsal border of the foramen magnum), basion (ventral border of foramen magnum), clivus, hard palate, atlas, pedicle of axis, and tip of odontoid. Earliest changes suggesting cervical spine involvement in RA are odontoid erosion, disk narrowing, and atlantoaxial and SAS. Cervical instability as detailed above has four main patterns:

1. Isolated AAS
2. Cranial settling associated with AAS
3. Subaxial subluxation
4. Combination of AAS, cranial settling and SAS

Atlantoaxial Subluxation

- Atlantoaxial subluxation is accentuated in flexion dynamic lateral films.
- The anterior atlantodens interval is the distance from the posterior aspect of the ring of atlas to the anterior aspect of the odontoid process, as measured along the transverse axis of the ring of the atlas and normally measures 3 mm in adults and 4 mm in children. AAS is defined as AADI >3 mm and not fixed in dynamic flexion and extension views **(Fig. 7)**. Lateral and rotatory AAS is identified by displacement of the lateral masses of the atlas >2 mm in relation to that of the axis and asymmetry of the lateral masses relative to the dens, respectively. This requires open-mouth anteroposterior view.
- The anterior atlantodens interval had been used clinically to define and follow RA cervical instability.
    - The critical limit of AADI that predicts an impending paralysis and need for surgery has been set to 8 mm, 9 mm, or 10 mm by different authors.
- The anterior atlantodens interval is now considered an unreliable predictor of paralysis because of poor correlation with the degree of cord compression shown by MRI. With increasing migration of the odontoid superiorly, the AADI reduces and also may become fixed on dynamic views (pseudostabilization).
- Posterior atlantodens interval has been found to be a more reliable predictor. PADI is measured from the posterior aspect of the odontoid process to the anterior edge of the posterior ring of the atlas. The critical lower limit for PADI is 14 mm (or less) and has 97% sensitivity and 52% specificity to predict paralysis.
- The negative predictive value of PADI at 14 mm is high, that is, when PADI measures >14 mm, the chance that the patient will *not* have paralysis is nearly absolute.
- Posterior atlantodental interval (radiological parameter) and SAC (anatomical parameter) are not the same—in RA patients, retro-odontoid synovial pannus may occupy as much as 3 mm of space.

Cranial Settling/Superior Migration of the Odontoid

Superior migration of the odontoid carries a higher risk of myelopathy and worse prognosis. Several radiological reference lines have been mentioned in literature to diagnose SMO **(Fig. 8)**, but possibly the Ranawat index and Redlund-Johnell values **(Fig. 9)** are the best. The hard palate and the atlas are the best recognizable landmarks while the tip of odontoid is least reliable reference due to attrition and being obscured by mastoid air cells.

- *Clark station* **(Fig. 10)** is the simplest method and importantly the relationship does not alter with flexion, extension or neutral views. Here, the odontoid process is divided into three equal parts from superior to inferior in the midsagittal plane. If the anterior arch of the atlas is level with the middle third (station 2) or the caudal third (station 3) of the odontoid process, basilar invagination is diagnosed. Station is mild while station three is severe variety. Station 1 where anterior arch/ring of atlas is level with superior third of odontoid is normal.
- *McRae's line* **(Fig. 8)** connects the anterior and the posterior margins of the foramen magnum (from the basion to the opisthion)—protrusion of the tip of the odontoid above this line indicates cranial settling.
- *Fischgold-Metzger line* ***(Fig. 11)****:* Drawn between the tips of mastoid processes on the anteroposterior open-mouth odontoid view. Protrusion of the tip of the dens above this line indicates cranial settling.
- *Chamberlain's line* **(Fig. 8)** is drawn from the posterior margin of the hard palate (easier to recognize on a lateral radiograph) to the posterior margin of the foramen magnum (opisthion). The odontoid tip should not project beyond 3 mm above this line.
- *McGregor's line* **(Fig. 8)** connects the posterior margin of the hard palate to the most caudal point (lowest point) of the occiput—the odontoid should not project beyond 4.5 mm above this line.
- *Wackenheim line* ***(Fig. 8)****:* Drawn along the superior surface of the clivus. Protrusion of the dens posterior to the projection of this line indicates settling.

The odontoid tip is often difficult to identify due to osteopenia or destruction. This makes Ranawat index and Redlund-Johnell values attractive and useful to many physicians.

- *Redlund-Johnell value* **(Fig. 9)** is the perpendicular distance from the middle of the lower endplate of the axis to McGregor's line. The normal limit is ≥34 mm in men and 29 mm in women. The value reduces as C1–C2 vertical subluxation occurs.
- *Ranawat index:* This is the distance between the center of the pedicle of axis and the transverse axis of the atlas. Normal range is 17 ± 2 mm in males and <15 ± 2 mm in females. The value reduces with C1–C2 subluxation.

When one combines the Clark station, the Redlund-Johnell value, and the Ranawat index the sensitivity of combined measure increases to 94% with a negative predictive value of 91% to diagnose cranial settling.

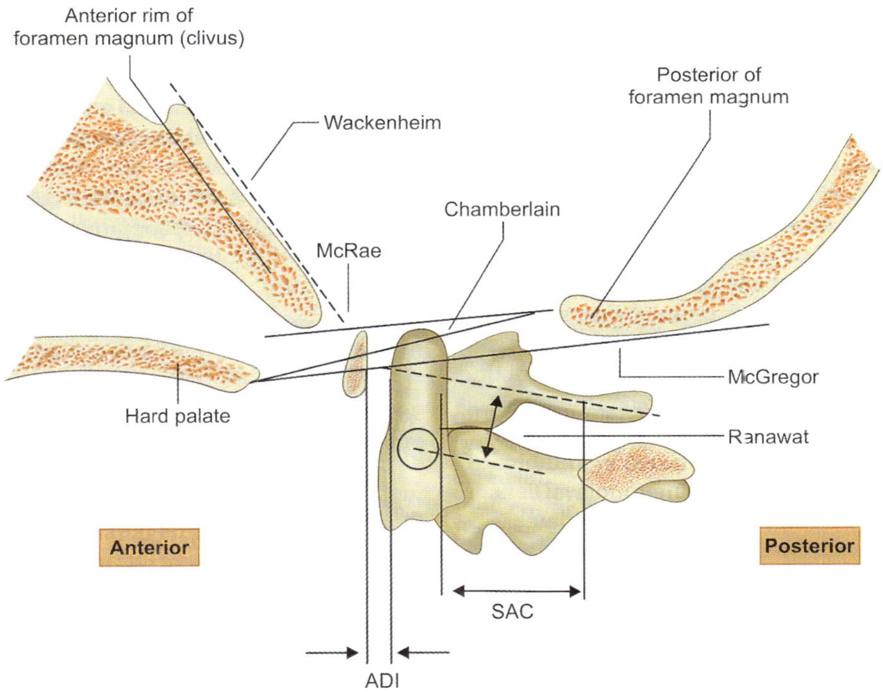

Fig. 8: Various lines for identification of superior migration of odontoid. (ADI: atlantodental interval; SAC: space available for cord)

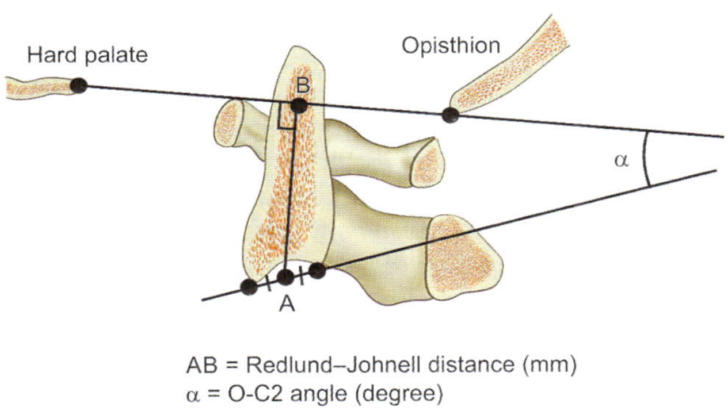

Fig. 9: Redlund–Johnell distance.

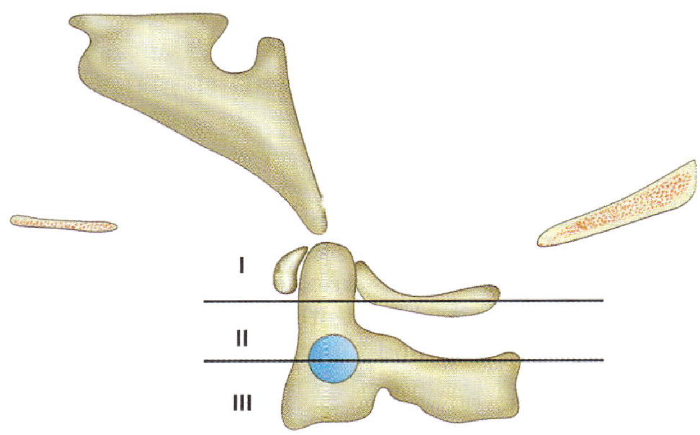

Fig. 10: Clark stations (see text).

Subaxial Subluxation

Subaxial subluxation tends to occur at multiple levels and should be differentiated from degenerative instability by a lack of osteophytes. It typically involves C2–C3 and C3–C4 levels unlike degenerative instability, which tends to occur around the C5–C6 level **(Fig. 7)**. *SAS* involves apophyseal joints, the joints of Luschka, interspinous ligaments and intervertebral disks, however, diskovertebral destruction and narrowing may not always accompany SAS. Endplate erosions are evident in 12–15% of patients.

- Relative translation of the vertebral bodies (>4 mm) is commonly expressed as percentage of the anteroposterior diameter of the inferior vertebral body. A flexion-extension view may indicate a dynamic instability.
- Alternatively SAC is measured behind the slipped vertebra which appears to be more reliable predictor. SAC of 14 mm or less gives a good measurement of

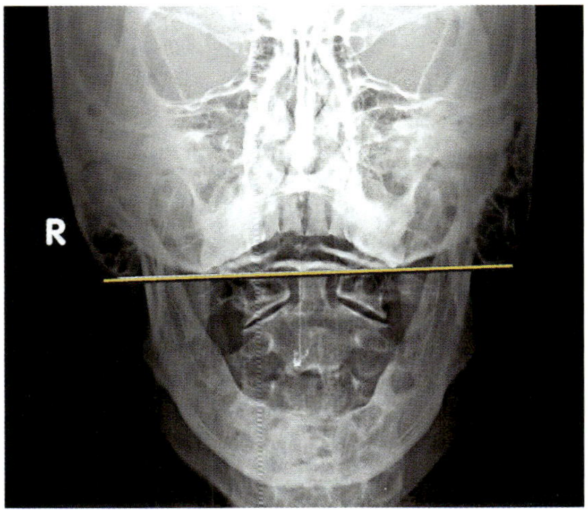

Fig. 11: Fischgold-Metzger line.

cord involvement and neurological dysfunction. Other measures that indicate progression of myelopathy are correlated with:

- Anterior subluxation (>2 mm)
- Axial shortening + progressive disk collapse, apophyseal joint erosion, and spinous process destruction

Cervical myelography and polytomography have become outdated while CT scan has been superseded by MRI scanning that is probably the most reliable investigation to evaluate RA of cervical spine. A CT scan, when used with a myelogram, may be particularly helpful in demonstrating cord compression. Measurement from a sagittal reconstruction CT scan may help to more accurately quantify the AAS and basilar invagination.

MRI scan shows "the exact space available for the cord". It should be obtained in all patients with neurological deficits.

- Although a PADI >14 mm is generally considered safe but depending on the amount of pannus, the patient may have as little as 8 mm or 9 mm of SAC. SAC may be further reduced in flexion. A flexion-extension MRI scan may show the actual space available for the cord in the presence of dynamic instability.
- It has been seen that spinal cord diameter of 6 mm or less in flexion predicts paralysis much better.
- *The cervicomedullary angle:* The angle between a line drawn along the anterior aspects of the cervical cord and another line along the medulla is normally 135–175°. It can only be measured from an MRI scan. It is reduced in the presence of cranial settling. When the cervicomedullary angle is <135°, there is definite cranial settling, and signs of C2 root pain, neural compression or myelopathy appear.
- *Dynamic flexion MRI:* This is useful in evaluating the subarachnoid space narrowing at the atlantoaxial level and below C2. Subarachnoid space encroachment is associated with a 12-fold increased risk of neurologic dysfunction.

Radiographic Predictors of Paralysis

- Posterior atlantodens interval of <14 mm
- Any combination of AAS with cranial settling
- Subaxial canal diameter of <14 mm
- *MRI findings:*
  - Cervicomedullary angle of <135°
  - A cord diameter in flexion of <6 mm
  - Subaxial canal measure of <13 mm
  - Subarachnoid narrowing
- Subaxial anterior subluxation (>2 mm)
- Axial shortening, accompanied by progressive disk collapse, apophyseal joint erosion, spinous process destruction.

Clinical and radiographic predictors of poor neurological recovery after operative stabilization with or without decompression:

- *Ranawat classification:* More severe preoperative neurologic deficit. Stage IIIB compared to stage IIIA and stage III compared to stage II has worse prognosis. The operative mortality of Ranawat IIIB (nonambulatory) patients is 12.5%, and the survivors have a 61% mortality rate in the first year. This raises the question of justification of surgical intervention in the presence of an advanced (IIIB) neurological deficit.
- *Location of disease:* Cranial settling with AAS has a much worse prognosis than isolated AAS or SAS.
- Isolated AAS or preoperative PADI of 14 mm or greater predicts a better chance of motor recovery after appropriate surgery. PADI of <10 mm indicates a poor prognosis for neurologic recovery.
- A postoperative subaxial canal diameter < 14 mm indicates poor prognosis for neurologic recovery.

DIAGNOSTIC STRATEGY

- Radiography is done in all RA patients with disease duration >2 years.
- Monitor patients with manifest peripheral erosions accompanied by rheumatoid factor (RF), and anti-CCP (antibodies to cyclic citrullinated peptide) positivity every second year and patients with few peripheral erosions and RF negativity at 5-year intervals.
- MRI is indicated in patients with neurological deficit, radiographic instability, vertical subluxation, and subaxial stenosis.

MANAGEMENT OF RHEUMATOID SPINE

One should aim to recognize the problem early (before an irreversible neurologic deficit) by reliable screening method for serial evaluation. On one hand, one needs to avoid sudden death because of unrecognized spinal cord compression, but on the other hand, one also needs to avoid unnecessary surgery because 50% of AAS patients may never develop neurologic symptoms.

Surgical Management

The various clinical and radiological factors predicting future paralysis are mentioned in the text above. More aggressive surgical approach is necessary for cranial settling as it is associated with morbidity and complications.

Indications

- *Relative:*
  - To prevent any myelopathy
  - To prevent further neurological deterioration in patients with a progressive cervical myelopathy.
- *Definitive:*
  - To treat intractable C2 root pain
  - Neurological deficit
  - To treat deformity, viz., chin-on-chest

General Considerations

- Preoperative cervical traction (halo for >2 days) should be used to relieve pain, reduce subluxation, arrest or reverse neurologic deterioration and correct deformity. This often scales down the surgical procedure needed.

- Halo traction **(Fig. 12)** is preferred over recumbent (risk of pressure sores and pneumonia) as it puts patient in functional position. It also facilitates intraoperative transfers.
- Posterior surgery (Atlantoaxial fusion or craniocervical fusion) is the preferred over anterior surgery (transoral decompression, subaxial corpectomy, and stabilization).
- Fiberoptic intubation is needed.
- Bone grafting is controversial but may be preferable in young fit patients.
- Assess oral hygiene and mouth opening for planned transoral approach.

Types of Surgical Stabilization

Atlantoaxial Subluxation

- Atlantoaxial subluxation usually fixed by a posterior atlantoaxial fusion. For small subluxations, C1–C2 fusion may be performed by the Gallie or Brooks wiring and autologous bone graft. C1–C2 transarticular screw fixation achieves better stabilization but requires reduction of subluxation before fixation.
  - The *Gallie wiring technique* (1939) consists of autologous bone graft fixed with a wire loop to the posterior arch of the atlas **(Fig. 13A)** and the spinous process of C2. Although simple, this provides poor stability against anteroposterior translation of C1 on C2. It is not indicated unless the AAS is reduced/reducible. Postoperative supplementation with additional external support is definitely needed.
  - The *Brooks wiring technique* (1978) involves two paramedial, wedge-shaped autologous bone grafts placed posteriorly between the arch of atlas and the lamina of the axis and secured by two wire loops **(Fig. 13B)**. The rotational stability is better than Gallie technique, but the wires need to be passed through spinal canal (risky).
  - *Transarticular fixation of C1–C2 (Magerl, 1979)* is done by one posterior screw crossing the atlantoaxial joints one on each side **(Fig. 14)**. Although it is superior to wiring and can be performed even after laminectomy of the C1 arch (better stability), the fixation requires good reduction of the atlantoaxial joint. Surgeons usually supplement this with wiring that further enhances stability and may ameliorate any need of external support postoperatively. To be on safer side additional external support is a better side to err however.
- For irreducible subluxations C1–C2 lateral mass and pedicle screw fixation is done.

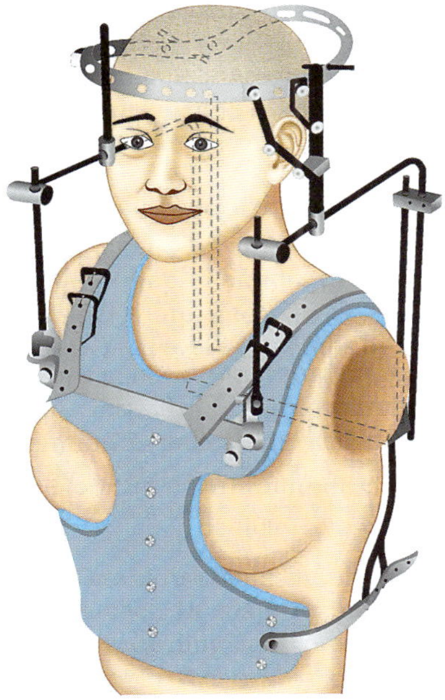

Fig. 12: Halo-vest traction assembly.

Cranial Settling

- Posterior occipitocervical fusion to C2 is the basic surgery.
- If cord decompression is not achieved by preoperative traction then decompression by C1 laminectomy in addition to occipitocervical fusion should be considered.
- Anterior decompression by transoral resection of the odontoid is indicated when there is:
  - Anteriorly placed pathologies such as odontoid pannus (>5 mm)
  - Subluxation of the odontoid

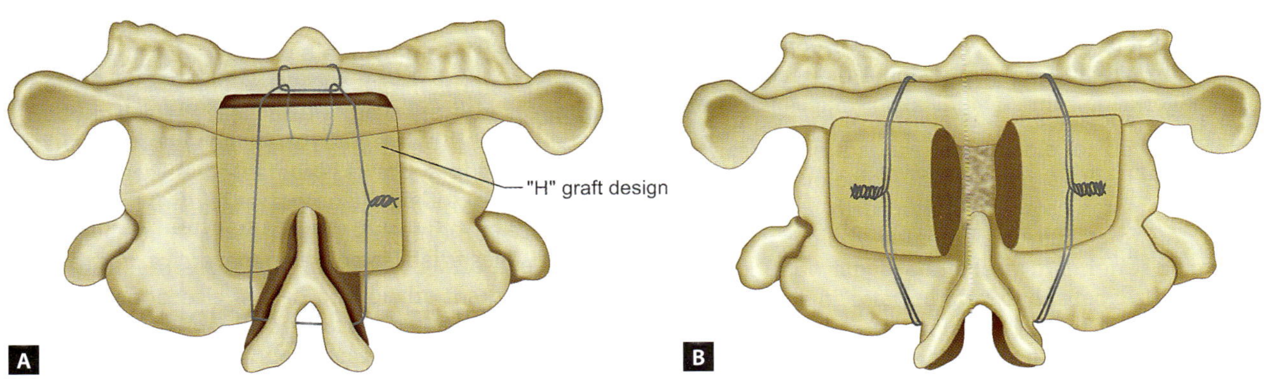

Figs. 13A and B: (A) Gallie-type fusion using wires tied in a loop to secure the onlay graft; (B) In a variant, a horizontal loop is added to form two loops for securing the onlay graft—Brooks-type fusion.

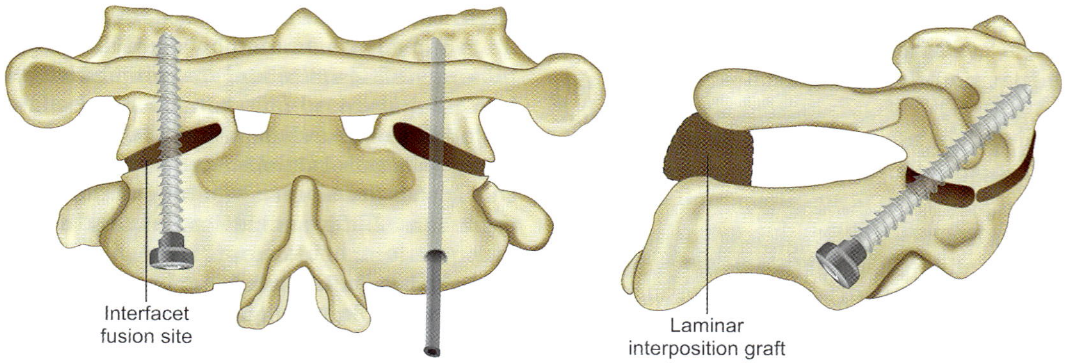

Fig. 14: Illustration of transarticular screw fixation of Magerl.

- Subaxial disk/osteophyte disease
- Kyphotic deformity

Transoral odontoidectomy is a well-recognized and safe procedure. One must, however, note the rotatory deformity at C1/C2, this brings the vertebral artery into midline and inadvertent injury if not recognized. *Transoral odontoidectomy* (Crockard, 1998) has an essential requirement: the ability to open the patient's mouth >25 mm. Temporomandibular joint ankylosis or flexion deformity of the neck may prevent adequate opening of the mouth. The alternative approach is then a midline mandibular split retracting the tongue downward. Poor dental hygiene, excessive damage to the pharyngeal mucosa, or dural tear may increase the risk of sepsis and meningitis. Postoperative intraoral swelling may be avoided by application of topical steroid in the oral cavity. A midline 4-cm incision is preferred identifying the anterior tubercle of atlas. The vertebral artery lies 20 mm away from the midline. On either side, 10 mm of the anterior arch may safely be exposed. The arch of atlas and odontoid are removed by a high-speed air drill to decompress the dura mater. Division of palate is not usually required and may be retracted by a suture. The segment is stabilized by posterior occipitocervical fixation and anterior fixation is not necessary.

Subaxial Subluxation

- Posterior cervical fusion with lateral mass instrumentation is most often needed.
    - C1–C2 *lateral mass and pedicle screw and rod fixation* provides very good stability. This is technically demanding and carries a significant risk of injury to the vertebral artery. An extensive preoperative evaluation using three-dimensional CT reconstruction image using thin-slice CT axial images is essential. Although it may be performed even in the presence of an unreduced subluxation, the chances of arterial injury increase manifold.
    - Decompression laminectomy is needed in cases of cord compression with fusion.
    - Subluxation that cannot be reduced needs anterior decompression with corpectomy and reconstruction with strut bone grafting. Graft resorption and progressive collapse is not uncommon so additional posterior stabilization is imperative.

Combined Subluxation

Here the occipitocervical fusion is performed extending to all the anatomically involved segments in the subaxial cervical spine.

Outcome and Complications

Complications are common and include death, infection, wound dehiscence, the loosening of hardware, or implant failure because of osteopenic bone and nonunion.

- The clinical success rate for cervical fusions ranges from 60 to 90%.
- Complications include death (5–10%), infection, wound dehiscence, implant breakage or pullout, loss of reduction, nonunion (5–20%), and late subluxation below the fused segment.

CONCLUSION

- Rheumatoid affection of spine is a common involvement in patients suffering from the disease. Of concern is the instability resulting at the atlantoaxial joint which could be life-threatening.
- Neck pain in any patient with rheumatoid arthritis should never be neglected as the consequences could be disastrous.
- A know-how of the various measures for determining changes in cervical spine is essential to identify the pathology and specifically manage the patients urgently having radiographic predictors of paralysis.
- Atlantoaxial instability, subaxial subluxation, and cranial settling are the three most important pathologies that need surgical management.

CHAPTER 105

Vertebral Diskitis and Osteomyelitis and Other Spinal Infections

Manish Kumar Varshney

INTRODUCTION

Spinal infection is an ancient entity being reported in Egyptian mummies and lots of reports from the Iron Age. Axial skeleton accounts for 2–7% of all cases of osteomyelitis, 1–2% of osteomyelitis cases in children. In 1779, Pott made the first detailed description of tuberculosis (TB) infection in the spine, Lanneloung, in France, used for first time the term pyogenic osteomyelitis of the spine. Spinal infections are of concern as due to the low specificity of signs and symptoms significant delay usually occurs until the establishment of diagnosis and treatment. There is often a delay of 2–6 months between first symptoms and diagnosis in most cases. The chapter focuses on TB of spine which is endemic to India and some other developing nations, also detail has been put on pyogenic affection of the spine.

TUBERCULOSIS OF SPINE (POTT'S SPINE, POTT'S DISEASE)

Tuberculosis of spine is the most common extrapulmonary form of disease. Approximately 10% of patients with extra-pulmonary TB have skeletal involvement. Spinal TB accounts for some 50% cases of skeletal TB.

Tuberculosis of spine is an ancient disease. First documented case of spinal TB cases dates back to 5,000-year-old Egyptian mummies **(Figs. 1A and B)**. In the modern literature, Percivall Pott **(Fig. 2)** described the first documented case of spinal TB in 1779. Spinal TB (Pott's disease) is the most dangerous form of skeletal TB and though thoracolumbar junction is the most common site of the spinal column involvement in spinal TB, any part of the spine can be affected. Pott's paraplegia (neurological complication of spinal TB) is estimated to occur in 10–43% cases. The exact prevalence and incidence in endemic nations appears to be underreported and is not well calculated that can also be partially attributed to increasing prevalence of multidrug-resistant (MDR) and extensively drug-resistant (XDR) cases and increasing prevalence of human immunodeficiency virus (HIV) infection in the population.

The risk of developing active TB is estimated to be 20–37 times greater in people coinfected with HIV than among those without HIV infection. One-third increase in incidence

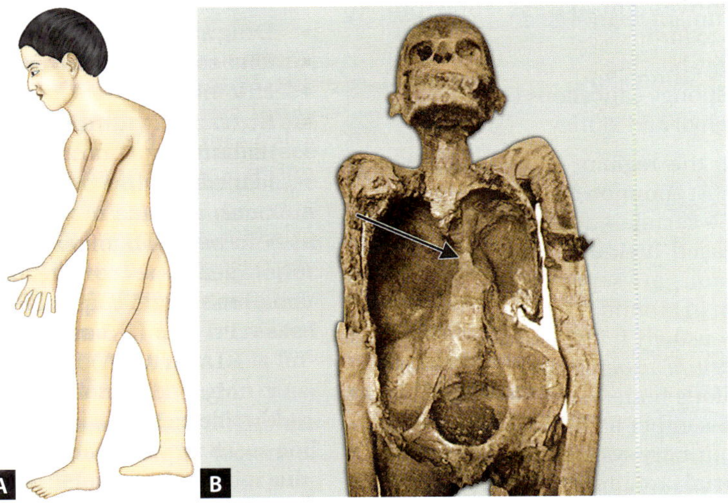

Figs. 1A and B: (A) This sculpture was produced in the 5th Egyptian dynasty that shows a male figure with upper spinal deformity quite representative for Pott's disease; (B) Image of Nespaheran (Egyptian mummy) that belongs to era of 21st dynasty with spinal tuberculosis (arrow).
Source: Wellcome Library, London.

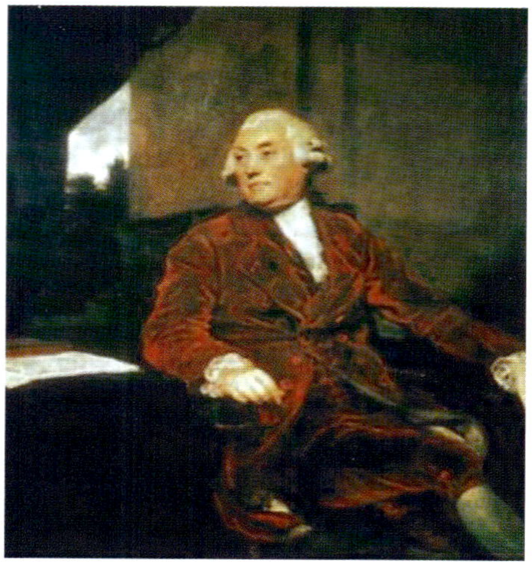

Fig. 2: Percivall Pott.

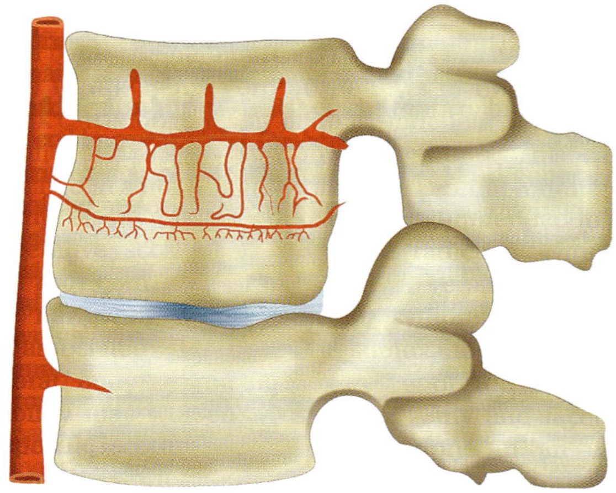

Fig. 3: Arterial supply of vertebral column.

of TB has been attributed to HIV infection. TB is the most common opportunistic infection, both pulmonary and extrapulmonary (62.2%) in India. The risk of having spinal TB is increased 12–20 times in HIV-positive patients compared to negative ones but vertebral destruction and resultant kyphosis is much less in this population due to disruption of type 4 hypersensitivity reaction causing granulomatous inflammation. There is greater epidural pus formation in the HIV-positive group, however.

Relative indication from pulmonary TB will give a rough idea of skeletal TB disease burden. About 35% of the incident cases world overcome from Southeast Asian countries contributing to the largest identified TB affected population (sub-Saharan African region has twice the incidence of Asian population but overall contributes less). Spinal TB accounts for 2% of all cases of TB, 15% of the cases of extrapulmonary TB, and 50% of the cases of skeletal TB.

Anatomy and Pathogenesis

Majority of the cases are reported in dorsolumbar region (lower thoracic and upper lumbar) due to:

- Greater extent of movement—stress zone due to transition of kyphosis to lordosis
- Higher degree of weight-bearing
- Large surface area of spongy cancellous bone
- Proximity to cisterna chyli and kidney

In order of involvement, the regions of spine affected in descending order from most common to least are: lumbar → upper dorsal → cervical → sacral → atlantoaxial

- Children have increased incidence of cervical spine involvement. Skip lesions are separated by 2–3 normal vertebrae and are seen in around 5% cases.
- Spinal involvement is usually a result of hematogenous spread of *Mycobacterium tuberculosis* into the dense vasculature of cancellous bone of the vertebral bodies. Primary infection site is either a pulmonary lesion or an infection of the genitourinary system.
    - *Arterial:* An arterial arcade, in the subchondral region of each vertebra, is derived from anterior and posterior spinal arteries; this arcade forms a rich vascular plexus **(Fig. 3)**. This vascular plexus facilitates hematogenous spread of the infection in the paradiskal regions.
    - *Venous:* Batson's paravertebral venous plexus **(Figs. 4A and B)** in the vertebra is a valveless system that allows free flow of blood in both directions depending upon the pressure generated by the intra-abdominal and intrathoracic cavities following strenuous activities like coughing. Spread of the infection via the intraosseous venous system may be responsible for central vertebral body lesions. Spread by venous system could be discontiguous and involve vertebrae at a distance explaining noncontiguous vertebral TB.

Predisposing Factors

Predisposing factors for TB include:

- Poverty
- Overcrowding
- Immunosuppressive treatment
- Alcoholism
- Illiteracy
- Malnutrition
- Drug abuse
- Diabetes mellitus
- HIV infection
- In Iran, older age, male gender, chronic peritoneal dialysis, imprisonment, and previous TB infection were identified.
- *Genetic predisposition:*
    - *FokI* polymorphism in *VDR* gene (especially the "ff" genotype) may be associated with the susceptibility to spinal TB in Chinese Han population.
    - Few reports suggest VDR TaqI polymorphism and risk of spinal TB but not substantiated in meta-analysis.
    - MCP-1-2518 GG genotype and presence of the G allele may be associated with susceptibility to spinal TB in the Chinese Han population.

Types of Vertebral Involvement (Fig. 5)

- *Anterior inferior portion of the vertebral body:* These are more common in thoracic spine region. Infection spreads

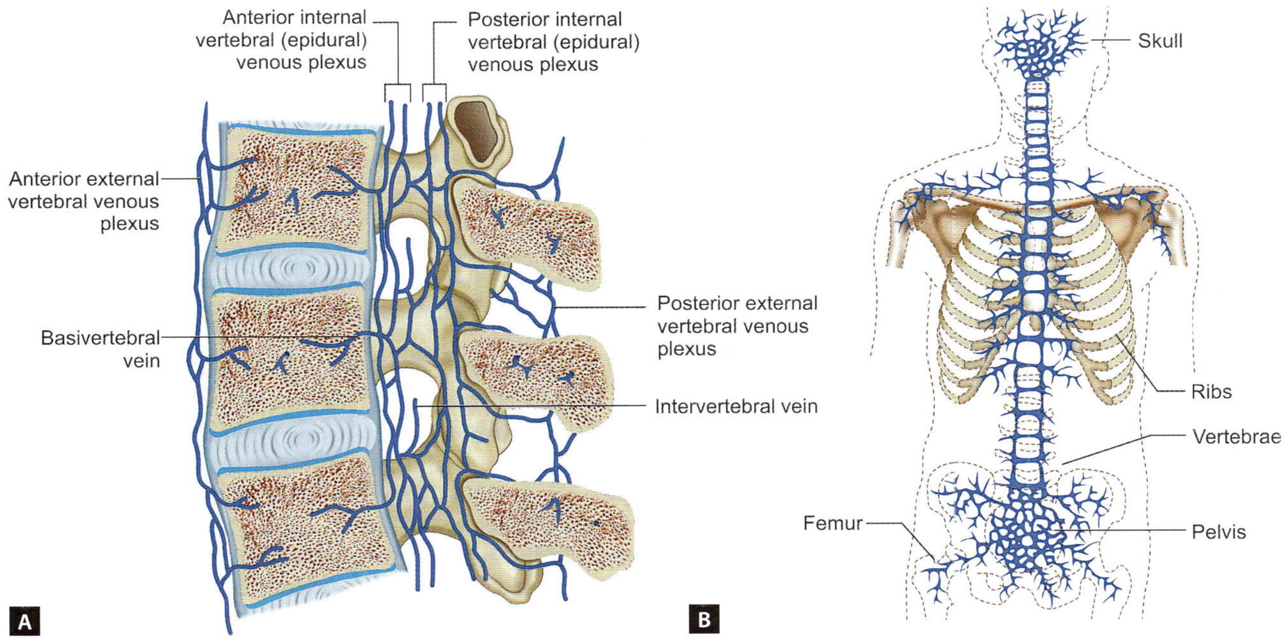

Figs. 4A and B: Vertebral venous plexus. (A) Detailed architecture of the vertebral veins illustrated; (B) The Batson's venous plexus and its connections with various body venous drainages.

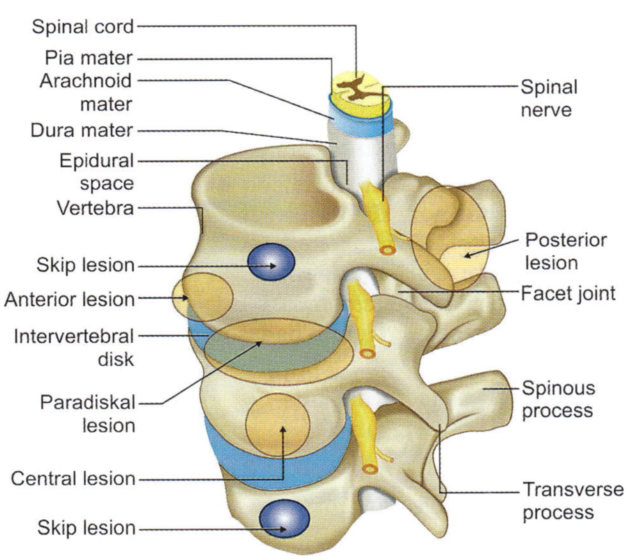

Fig. 5: Types of vertebral involvement.

under anterior longitudinal ligament. Shallow erosion of anterior surface of vertebral bodies occurs. Collapse and decreased disk space are uncommon and late if at all.

- *Paradiskal:* The infection spreads through epiphyseal arteries. Disk destruction occurs through loss of nutrition. The infection begins from the anterior vertebral body adjacent to the anterior endplate. With continued destruction anterior wedging of vertebra occurs, causing kyphosis. Intraosseous and extraosseous abscess formation are often found in this type of lesions which is major risk of cord damage due to pressure effect by the abscess, displaced bone, or ischemia from spinal artery thrombosis.
- *Complete lesion:* Destruction of one or two vertebrae. This type is seen in children <10 years of age, possibly associated with poor nutrition and lack of immunity. There is severe anterior column defect. They are prone to late-onset paraplegia.
- *Central lesions:* These are again common in children. The infection spreads through Batson's venous plexus and posterior vertebral artery. Radiograph shows patchy destruction and loss of bony trabeculae. Initially, there is expansion of the vertebral body and later in advanced lesions there is vertebra plana due to concentric type of collapse.
- *Posterior lesions (appendiceal lesions/apophyseal TB):* This is characterized by partial or complete involvement of pedicle, lamina, transverse process, and/or spinous process. Spread via the posterior external venous plexus of vertebral veins or direct spread. The lamina is most commonly involved followed by pedicles, articular processes, spinous processes, and transverse processes. The radiographs show destruction of one (winking owl) or both pedicles, loss of spinous process (beakless owl) or other processes. There is lateral translation and/or rotational deformities. There is increased chance of neurological deficit due to proximity to spinal canal and often a delay in diagnosis.
- *Skip lesion:* Poor general health in children with compromised immunological status is the predominant cause for this type of presentation. MDR TB also presents in this manner.
- *Spinal tumor syndrome:* The lesion starts at the posterior margin of vertebral body with proliferation of the granulation tissue in canal causing cord compression.
- *True tubercular arthritis:* This is seen in occipito-atlantoaxial type involvement.

Natural History of Disease

- In younger patients, the disk is involved due to higher vascularity but due to gradual age-related loss of vascularity the diskal lesions become less common.
- Average vertebral loss in children is twice that of adults.
- Spinal TB more often heals by bony ankylosis (**Figs. 6A and B**, as opposed to fibrous ankylosis in hip and knee joints). This is due to compression arthrodesis of large cancellous surfaces by paraspinal muscle spasm, gravity, and weight-bearing. Absence of bony fusion and fibrous pseudarthrosis are high-risk factors for late recurrence of disease. The two characteristic complications of spinal TB include collapse of segments and production of deformity and neurological involvement.
- Collapse before healing is more severe due to flexibility of spine (**Figs. 7A to C**). The collapse is of two types:
  1. Telescopic collapse—occurs along the long axis, more common in lumbar spine.
  2. Flexion collapse—occurs in sagittal plane of one spinal segment over another, more common in thoracic spine.
- Children show continuous change in deformity even after healing due to growth. The deformity at 5 years can be predicted from present deformity by the formula (Rajasekaran and Shanmugasundaram):

$$[Y = a + bx]$$

(where "Y" is the final deformity at 5 years, "x" is the initial loss of vertebral bodies (height in cm) at presentation, "a" and "b" are constants with value of 5.5 and 30.5, respectively.)

It is deemed that kyphosis >30° (approximates loss of one vertebral height) is likely to progress even after healing by many, but the author feels, it is the location of lesion that determines poor outcome with respect to progression of deformity (thoracolumbar lesions faring worst). The formula is limited by various parameters, it cannot determine deformity at 10 years, also cross-validation of the formula have found that the correct angle was predicted in only 34% cases with a margin of error of 10°.

- Another method has been proposed by Jutte et al. to measure the "indexed total bone height loss" (**Fig. 8**). This bone loss in individual vertebra is calculated by first measuring the anterior and posterior vertebral height (in mm) of the first normal vertebra cranially

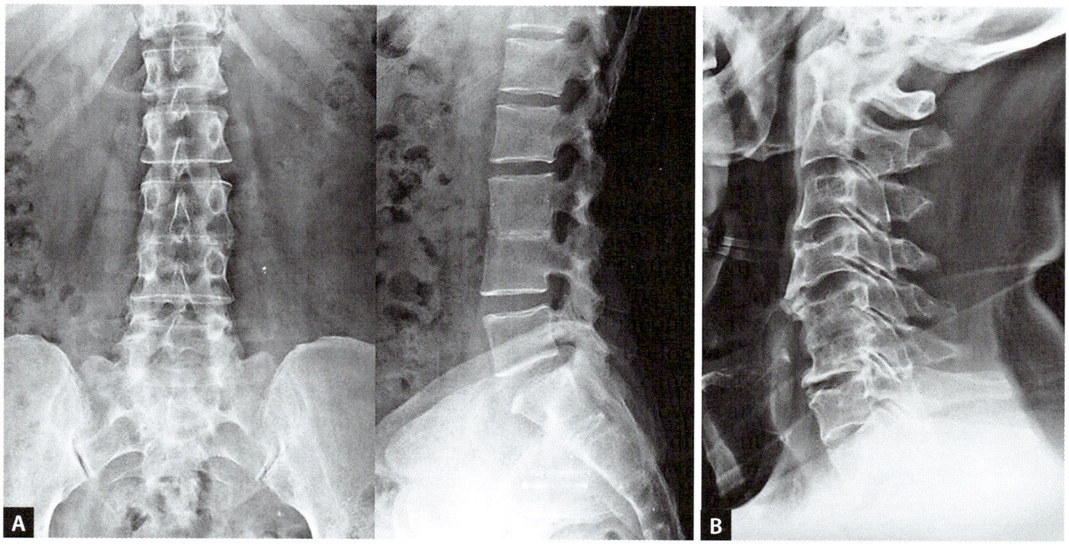

Figs. 6A and B: Healed spinal TB radiographs. (A) Note the completely fused lumbar 3rd or 4th vertebrae; (B) Cervical 5th and 6th vertebrae.

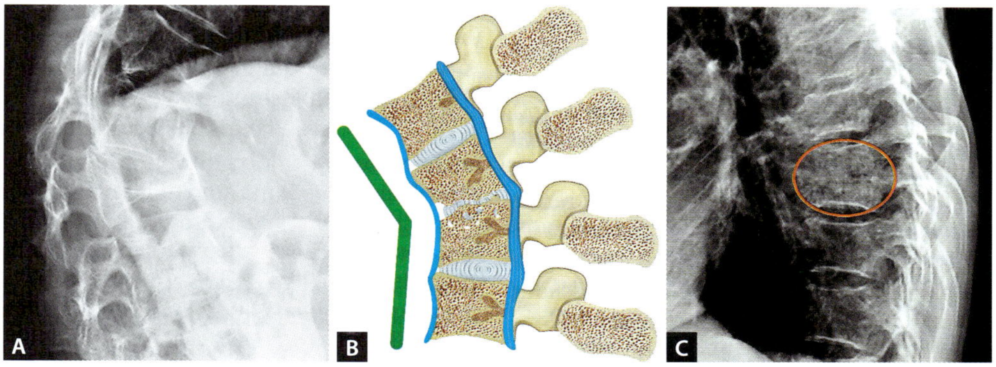

Figs. 7A to C: Types of collapse in spinal tuberculosis: (A) Collapse of central type TB producing vertebra plana; (B) Paradiskal type TB producing kyphosis (kyphos)—illustration; (C) Radiograph of paradiskal type TB.

and caudally from the affected lesion, divided by four. The mean height of each affected vertebra is calculated by adding the anterior and the posterior height of the affected vertebra and dividing by two. The bone height loss then is given by the formula:

1 – (Mean height affected vertebra/
mean height normal vertebrae)

The bone height loss is added up for each vertebra to give total loss of height. Value of 1 is equivalent to loss of entire vertebral body (this approximated to nearly 30–35° of kyphosis).

- *Natural history of kyphosis:* There are two phases of progression:
  1. Active phase—diagnosis is made in first 18 months
  2. Healed phase—diagnosis of deformity after the disease has been cured.
- *Risk factors for increase in deformity:*
  - Patients <10 years of age at onset
  - Initial kyphosis >30°
  - Vertebral body loss >1.5
  - Involvement >3 vertebral bodies
  - Evidence of instability in X-ray
  - Involvement of both anterior and posterior structures on radiology
  - Children who had partial or no fusion during adolescent growth spurt
- After cure during growth spurt, the children usually have five types of deformity (kyphosis) progression (Rajasekaran):
  - Type 1 (**Fig. 9**, 39%)—continued deformity throughout entire growth period
    - Type 1a—increase continuously after active period
    - Type 1b—lag period of 3–6 years
  - Type 2 (**Fig. 10**, 44%)—shows beneficial effects during growth with a decrease in deformity. This is characteristically seen only in post-tubercular kyphosis (in other deformities deterioration is the rule).
    - Type 2a—immediately after active period (good prognosis)
    - Type 2b—after lag period of 3–6 years
  - Type 3 (**Fig. 11**, 17%)—no major change in deformity

$$\text{Bone loss A} = 1 - \left(\frac{\frac{0+5}{2}}{\frac{10+10+10+10}{4}}\right)$$

$$\text{Bone loss B} = 1 - \left(\frac{\frac{5+5}{2}}{\frac{10+10+10+10}{4}}\right)$$

$$\text{Total} = 0.75(\text{A}) + 0.50(\text{B}) = 1.25$$

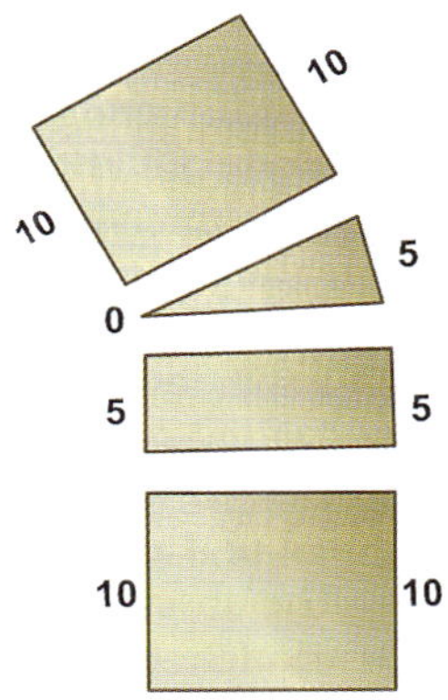

Fig. 8: Indexed total bone height loss.

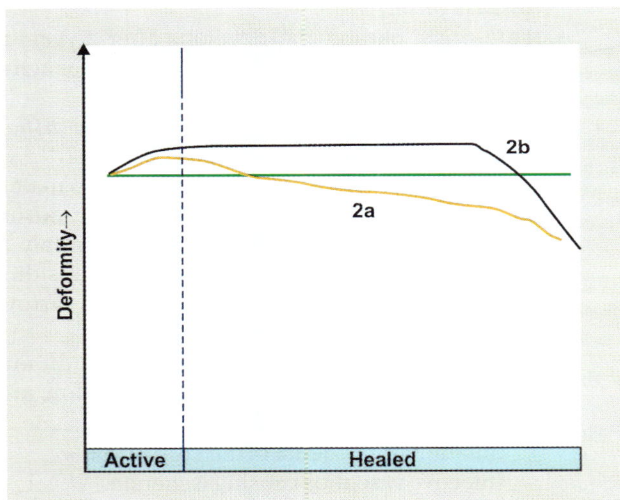

Fig. 10: Deformity progression during growth spurt (Type 2).

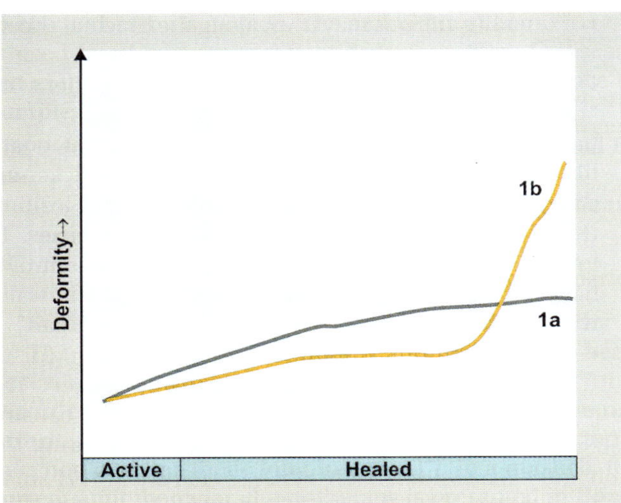

Fig. 9: Deformity progression during growth spurt (Type 1).

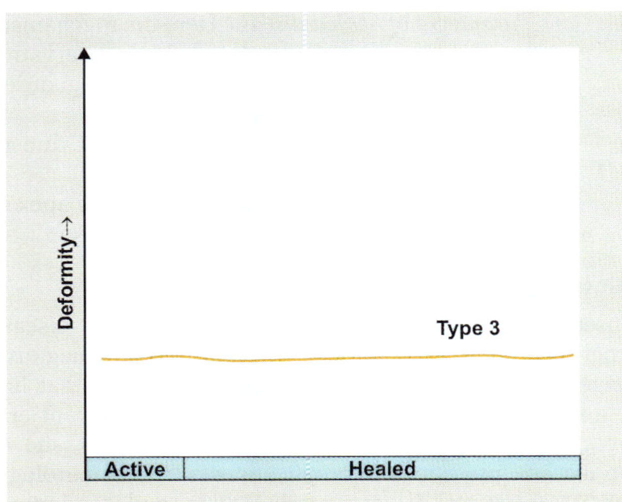

Fig. 11: Deformity progression during growth spurt (Type 3).

- *Influence of level on progression of deformity:*
  - Dorsal level—higher average deformity at presentation
  - Dorsolumbar has worst prognosis at this is the transitional zone and chances of higher instability. There is loss of protection of rib cage.
  - Lumbar spine has the best prognosis as it allows telescopic type of collapse.
- Paraplegia is the most unfortunate complication of spinal disease. The tubercular abscess or granulation tissue can directly compress the neuraxis leading to symptoms of cranial nerve involvement or spinal nerve root compression. The inflammatory exudates in cerebrospinal fluid can cause clumping of the nerve root leading to arachnoiditis. Children are more prone to late-onset paraplegia. The neurological complications can arise early in the disease or develop later as has been classified by Girdlestone or Hodgson.
  - *Girdlestone classification of onset of paraplegia:*
    - Early-onset paraplegia (develops within 2 years of disease onset)
    - Late-onset paraplegia (develops after 2 years of disease may even develop 2–3 decades after active infection)
  - *Hodgson's classification is more detailed differentiating the causes and types of paraplegia:*
    - *Paraplegia of active disease:* These develop mainly in response to the ongoing inflammation during active phase of disease, so respond favorably to conservative management and often subsiding with successful chemotherapy. The various proposed mechanisms are:
      - Compressive pathology like granulation and caseous tissue with abscess formation and sequestrated material. The other cause is inflammatory edema of the cord or roots.
      - Infective vasculitis causing ischemia
      - Spinal tumor syndrome
      - Pathological dislocation of spine
      - Direct infiltration of tubercular bacilli into cord
    - *Paraplegia of healed disease:* Here the mechanism is mechanical so chemotherapy or conservative management is likely to fail producing a guarded prognosis. The mechanisms are:
      - Progressive constriction of the cord due to extradural fibrosis
      - Cord stretching over bony ridge at the apex of deformity (internal gibbus)

Clinical Features

Onset of symptoms is usually insidious and disease progression is slow. Duration of symptoms prior to diagnosis ranges from few weeks to few years on average that has decreased to between 3 and 6 months in the recent era. Presentation depends upon stage of the disease, site of the disease, presence of complications such as neurologic deficit, abscesses or sinus tracts. Pain and tenderness localize the active disease. Back pain is the earliest and most common symptom. Paravertebral muscles remain in constant spasm to limit/abolish movement at the infected segment. Loss of spasm at the site in night causes relative translatory movements and causes night pains. Referred pain is often present along the costal nerves and involved roots. Tapping over spinous process can produce referred pain. Constitutional symptoms such as weakness, loss of appetite, loss of weight, evening rise of temperature, and night sweats may occur but are not very prominent or common. Careful evaluation is necessary to characterize the disease and guide treatment.

- Cold abscess develops around the lesion of variable sizes. Cold abscess is a collection of tubercular debris, disintegrated bone lamellae, serum, caseous material, granulation tissue, bone marrow, and tubercular bacilli. Due to continued development of cold abscess and migration of the pus, the abscess may track into different planes. The spread occurs beneath the anterior longitudinal ligament to variable distance then it takes one of the following course:
  1. *Tracking posteriorly into vertebral canal:* This is a dreadful complication as it causes compression and development of neurological complications.
  2. Tracking to skin through line of least resistance.
- *Cervical spine TB:* Patient has cautious and protected gait associated with torticollis. If there is >1 vertebral body, destruction the spine is unstable and patient then supports the chin or trunk with both hands. This is, however uncommon as mostly the deformity is limited and weight transmitted through posterior articular processes which is uncommonly involved. Same is true of lumbar lesions.
  - Cold abscess collects behind the prevertebral fascia forming retropharyngeal abscess that might be large enough to interfere with deglutition.
  - The abscess may track posterolaterally to posterior triangle of neck and present behind the posterior border or sternocleidomastoid muscle.
  - Abscess may track down into mediastinum and may even cause mediastinal syndrome.
  - Laterally, the pus may track along the brachial sheath into axilla or even cubital fossa.
- Dorsal spine—in upper thoracic spine, the patient has "military attitude"—raised shoulders, arm thrown backward and head shrunken. The patient has board like back rigidly straight and paravertebral thickening due to muscular spasm. In the midthoracic lesions, the anteroposterior diameter of chest increases. In lower thoracic disease, the thorax and head are thrown backward with a prominent abdomen, the patient walks with legs wide apart and waddling—"Alderman's gait".
  - Cold abscess of thoracic disease often forms paravertebral abscess in extrapleural space. The abscess may burst into intrapleural space causing pseudoempyema thoracis or may track along the intercostal nerves and vessels to point anteriorly.
  - The cold abscess may track along the rectus sheath or lower abdominal wall.

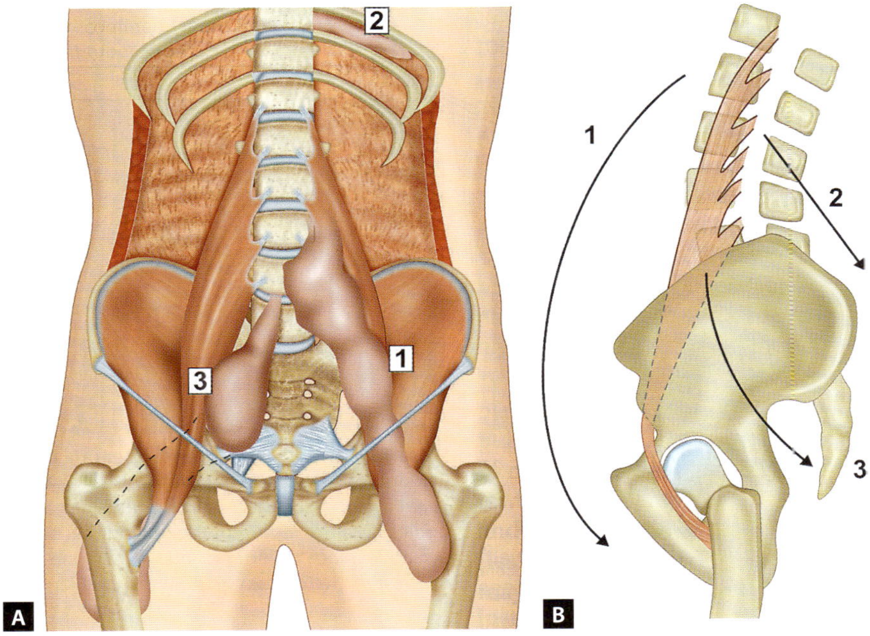

Figs. 12A and B: Psoas abscess and routes of spread. (A) Psoas abscess originating from spinal caries of the dorsolumbar vertebra and following the psoas muscle to the groin; (B) The different routes of spread of the abscess: (1) Spread to groin and thigh; (2) Spread to lumbar region and Petit's triangle; (3) Spread to gluteal region.

- *Spinal deformity is quite prominent in the thoracic lesions due to variable number of vertebral body destruction:*
    - "Knuckle" forms due to collapse of single vertebral body.
    - "Gibbus" forms when 2–3 vertebral bodies are involved forming the angular kyphosis.
    - "Short kyphus" is a gentle angular deformity spread over >3 vertebral bodies with a definite posteriorly palpable angle.
    - "Tubercular kyphosis" is an exaggeration of the normal kyphotic deformity with a gentle curve throughout and no angular deformity palpable.
- Lumbar TB—the presentation is similar to lower thoracic lesions.
    - Cold abscess in lumbar lesions (typically the psoas abscess) may track to form paravertebral abscess palpable posteriorly on one side of spine or may travel along the intercostal, ilioinguinal, and iliohypogastric nerves **(Figs. 12A and B)**.
    - It may go to Petit's triangle along the flat muscles of abdominal wall or in the ischiorectal fossa along the internal pudendal nerve.
    - Posteriorly, it may track to buttock along the gluteal nerve.
    - Anteriorly, it may form typical psoas abscess that may point anywhere from abdomen to groin to thigh to even popliteal region.
    - If it develops a connection in the inferior abdominal wall, it may form an inverted horseshoe abscess also (uncommon presentation).
- *Neurological complications:* Incoordination and clumsiness in walking is the earliest symptom (accompanied with spontaneous twitching of muscles) and clonus is the earliest sign. The physical examination usually reveals an extensor plantar response or ankle clonus. This evolves into incoordination during walking but patient is ambulatory with support. The paraparesis then becomes severe enough to confine patient to bed. The patient then develops paraplegia in extension with variable sensory blunting. This transforms into "paraplegia in flexion" with sphincteric involvement. In the end, complete cord involvement produces flaccid paraplegia.
- *Factors leading to poor recovery of cord:*
    - Inactive disease with poor mechanical compression
    - Complete paralysis
    - Paralysis for >1 year
    - Presence of severe kyphosis
    - Older age and poor nutrition
    - Presence of myelomalacia and syringomyelia on magnetic resonance imaging (MRI).
- *Good prognosis for neurological recovery is associated with:*
    - Inflammatory cause of cord involvement rather than mechanical compression
    - Incomplete involvement
    - Short duration of deficit
    - Minimal kyphotic deformity
    - Younger age
    - Good nutritional status

Radiology

Plain radiographs are the first to be obtained. The characteristic features of a typical lesion are osteoporosis (there must be 30% of bone mineral loss), reduced disk space **(Fig. 13)**, loss of paradiskal margins, and endplate changes **(Fig. 14,**

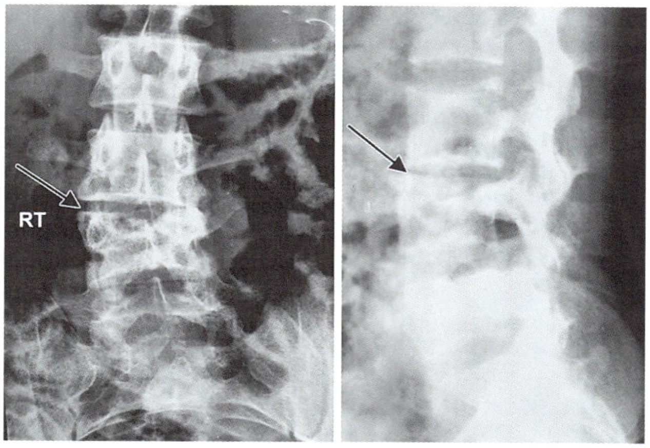

Fig. 13: Radiographs demonstrating typical disk space reduction in paradiskal type of involvement at L3–L4 region.

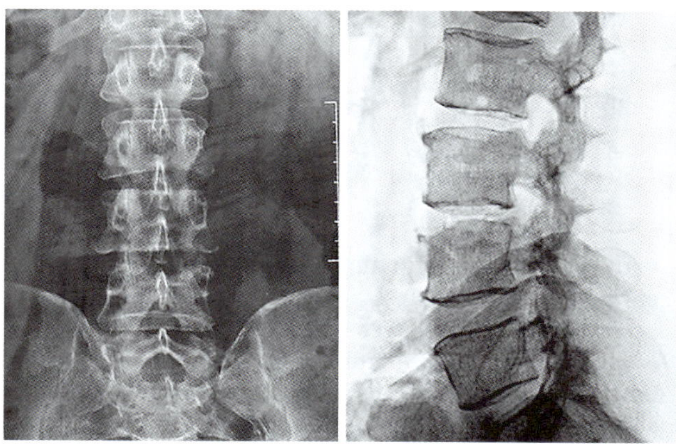

Fig. 14: Radiographs showing the involvement of L3–L4 disk space with endplate changes (erosion and irregularity) seen in the superior endplate of 4th lumbar vertebra. The reduction in disk space is not that conspicuous due to endplate destruction else there is definite reduction in disk space.

earliest finding). On an average, the reported number of vertebrae involved in spinal TB identifiable on radiographs at presentation classically vary to around 3 (3.4—Hodgson and Stock, 3.8—Mukhopadhyaya and Mishra, 3.4—Martin, it is more for children and lesser for adults). Now, with increased availability and frequent use of MRI, most of the lesions are diagnosed before such gross destruction.

- Increase in the prevertebral soft-tissue shadow on radiograph is useful to diagnose TB of cervical spine. The anterior convexity and forward displacement of tracheal shadow of >8 mm from the vertebral bodies in a lateral view of plain X-ray and widening of superior mediastinum in an anteroposterior X-ray are useful indicators of tuberculous involvement at cervicodorsal region.
- In thoracic spine, the destruction may appear like "bird's nest" on anteroposterior projection, due to crowding of ribs **(Fig. 15A)**. The eggs are represented by disintegrated vertebral bodies. Predominant involvement of posterior element may result in characteristic appearance of "winking owl" if one pedicle is involved **(Fig. 15B)** or a "beakless owl" if the spinous process is involved and disappears (Note the owl on anteroposterior projection is formed by two pedicles forming the eyes and the beak is formed by the spinous process).

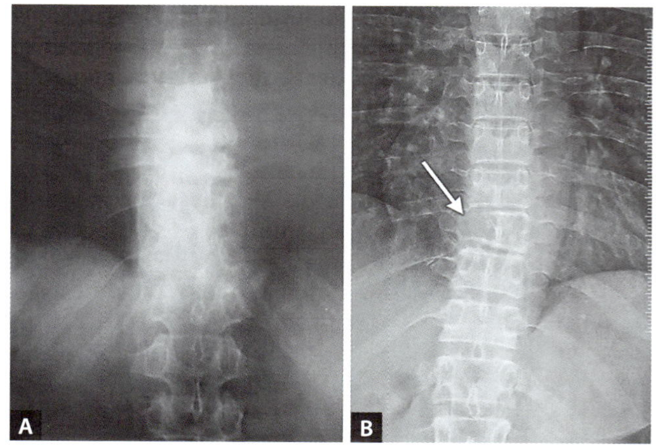

Figs. 15A and B: Bird's nest appearance of TB thoracic spine. (A) Radiograph shows the involvement of D7–D9 level that has produced crowding of associated ribs on both sides and disintegrated vertebral bodies in center represent the eggs in the "nest"; (B) The typical winking owl appearance of vertebral body when one of the pedicles is destroyed by the infective process [right in this case (arrow)].

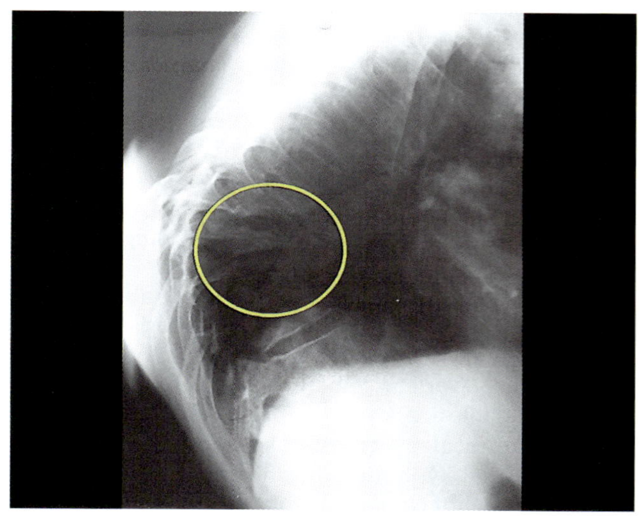

Fig. 16: Anterior wedging of vertebral bodies. This type of collapse is more common in children producing the typical kyphotic deformity as in this case. There is anterior wedging of the D8, D9 vertebral bodies (encircled).

- "Aneurysm phenomenon"—anterior vertebral body erosion producing a scalloped appearance in anterior spinal disease appears like aneurysmal erosion of anterior vertebral bodies. The disk spaces are spared.
- Anterior wedging **(Fig. 16)** is seen in thoracic spine and anterior type of TB seen commonly in children.
- Central collapse and production of vertebra plana is seen in lumbar spine and central lesion.
- Soft-tissue shadow—cervical region—well-defined globular

- Upper thoracic—there is squaring of upper mediastinal radiodense shadow if the lesion is above D4 vertebra.
- "Fusiform shadow"—is seen below D4 lesion **(Fig. 17)**.

Computed Tomography Scan

It provides greater bony detail of irregular lytic lesions, sclerosis, disk collapse, and disruption of bone circumference than plain radiographs. The presence of calcification within the abscess is virtually diagnostic of spinal TB. Contrast-enhanced scan demonstrates rim enhancement of the lesion. The details on epidural extent of disease are limited. It is the ideal investigation for guiding a percutaneous diagnostic needle aspiration biopsy in potentially hazardous or relatively inaccessible sites.

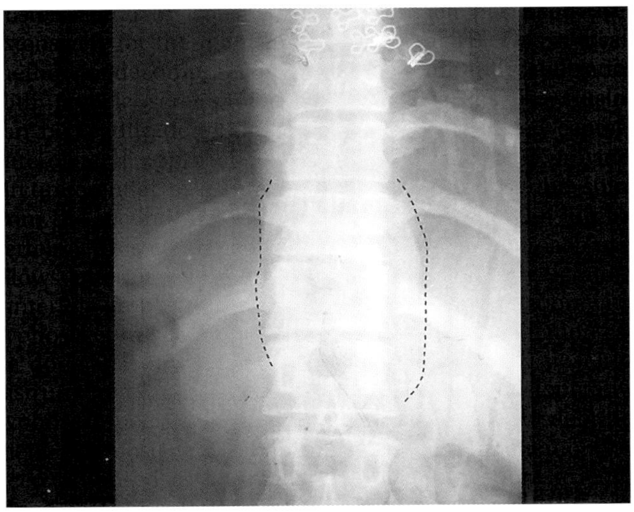

Fig. 17: Radiograph showing affection of dorsolumbar junction with reduction of D11–D12 and D12–L1 disk space with typical fusiform abscess shadow (outlined).

Magnetic Resonance Imaging

The usual sequences taken for spinal TB are noncontrast T1-weighted (T1W), T2-weighted (T2W), and short tau inversion recovery (STIR) sequences (to differentiate fluid from fatty component) in axial, sagittal, and coronal planes followed by contrast-enhanced T1W sequences. Abnormal signal intensities appear hypointense on T1W and hyperintense on T2W sequences with heterogeneous enhancement of the vertebral body. The characteristic findings are destruction of two adjacent vertebral bodies and opposing endplates; destruction of intervening disk; vertebral body edema; and occurrence of prevertebral, paravertebral, and epidural abscesses **(Figs. 18A to C)**. MRI has greatest sensitivity and specificity.

- Abscess formation and collection and expansion of granulation tissue adjacent to the vertebral body are highly suggestive of spinal TB. The details of epidural extension are quite productive in multiple planes.
- MRI is extremely useful in diagnosing the difficult and rare sites of disease like the craniovertebral junction. For sacroiliac TB, a coronal STIR T2W sequence is added to routine MRI of lumbar spine.
- MRI is also useful in detecting intramedullary or extramedullary tuberculoma, spinal cord cavitation, spinal cord edema, and possibly unsuspected noncontiguous lesions of the spine.
- Contrast helps in distinguishing granulation tissue from cold abscess. Administration of gadolinium with diethylenetriamine pentaacetic acid (Gd-DTPA) is useful to assess the extent of soft tissue mass and to differentiate postoperative spondylitis from a normal postoperative

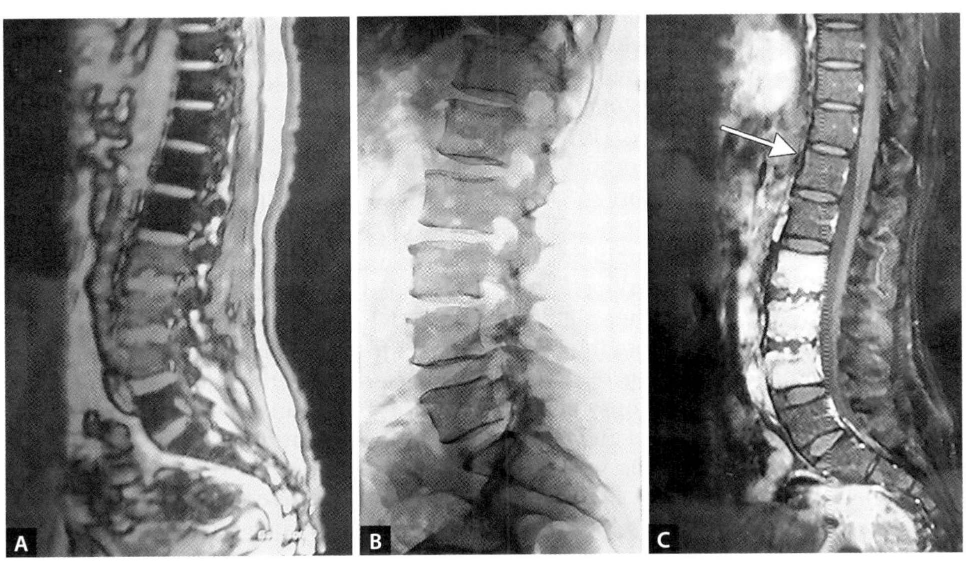

Figs. 18A to C: MRI of tubercular spine. The T1 (left, A) and T2 (right, C) images depict the characteristic changes of tubercular affection of spine. The lumbar 2–4 vertebrae show gross hyperintense shadow on T2-weighted images (right, C), while T1 is hypointense (left, A). The disk spaces are reduced with opposing endplate irregularities. The prevertebral abscess extends well-beyond the cephalad involvement up to D11 level (arrow). It is important to appreciate that comparative radiographs (B) demonstrate the involvement of L3–L4 levels only while involvement at multiple levels is readily evident on MRI making it the radiological investigation of choice for evaluation.

course, by showing disk enhancement (in tubercular spondylitis).

- MRI can also be used to assess radiological response to treatment in the early follow-up period around 6–8 weeks but the findings are variable.
- Diffusion-weighted MRI (DW-MRI) and apparent diffusion coefficient (ADC) values are recently introduced to differentiate tuberculous vertebral body involvement from metastatic lesions. DW-MRI provides information about the composition of tissues, physical properties, and the microstructure of the tissues. ADC values are a measure of the diffusion ability of molecules which provides the composition of the given tissue. High ADC value means increased diffusion of molecules suggesting less compact microstructure.

Diagnosis

[*See* also the diagnosis of TB in mycobacterial arthritis discussed in Chapter "Joint Disorders Including Inflammatory and Noninflammatory Arthritis and Infective Arthritides (Including Mycobacterial Infection and Prosthetic Joint Infection)"].

Diagnosis of spinal TB is mainly made on the basis of typical clinical presentation along with systemic constitutional manifestation. Substance to diagnosis is added by evidence of past exposure to TB or concomitant visceral TB, and neuroimaging modalities. Skin test should be a routine and other hematological investigations such as complete blood count (CBC) and erythrocyte sedimentation rate (ESR) are recommended to help differentiating the disease. Enzyme-linked immunosorbent assay (ELISA) is not well recommended. Modified interferon-γ release assays (IGRAs) may have a role that is being still studied but previous tests like QuantiFERON-Gold are not recommended at all for endemic regions and routine Bacillus Calmette–Guérin (BCG) vaccination settings. Obtain a chest radiograph to get circumstantial evidence.

Demonstration of the organism by microscopy, culture of the organism from samples or characteristic histopathology are the most definitive methods of diagnosing TB, in the absence of which the diagnosis always remains probable.

- *Sampling:* Bone tissue or abscess samples are obtained to stain for acid-fast bacilli (AFB) and isolate organisms for culture, antibiotic sensitivity, and histopathology. The yield of organisms can be improved by centrifugation of the sample and examining the residue. Other methods to improve the yield are taking curetting from the cavity lining and curetting from sinus. Sampling is best done using CT-guided or USG-guided needle biopsy and/or aspiration or surgical biopsy. In 88.5–96.4% of the cases, a CT/fluoroscopic-guided fine-needle aspiration cytology biopsy is helpful and yields a diagnosis.
- Smear positivity is seen with bacterial load of >10^4 bacilli/mm^3
- Culture remains the gold standard for diagnosis. *M. tuberculosis* is a slow-growing aerobic organism with a growth-doubling time of about 20 hours in conditions favorable to the bacillus. The load of *Mycobacterium* in the pulmonary lesions is 107–109, whereas in osteoarticular disease the load is <105, so the chances of isolating and growing the organism diminish manifold. Incidence for positive cultures for AFB in osteoarticular tuberculous lesion has been reported by various workers to be between 40% and 88%. Egg-based plate media such as Lowenstein–Jensen are used, but agar media such as Selective 7H11 and liquid-based media (Becton-Dickinson and Co., BACTEC™) now are the standard. Growth can be detected within 2 weeks.
- The characteristic pathology of tubercle [French physician, Laennec (1781–1826), discovered the "tubercle"] demonstrates epithelioid cells characteristic of the tuberculous reaction. These are large, pale cells with a large vesicular nucleus, abundant cytoplasm, indistinct margins and process that form an epithelioid reticulum. Langerhans giant cells are probably formed by the fusion of a number of epithelioid cells. These are formed only if caseation necrosis has occurred in the lesion, and they contain tubercle bacilli. These are then surrounded by a rim of lymphocytes forming the tubercle mass. Presence of caseation necrosis is almost diagnostic of tuberculous pathology (other being tuberculoid leprosy).
- Polymerase chain reaction (PCR) or nucleic acid amplification (NAA) assay could serve as a fast method in diagnosing spinal TB and is recommended as a diagnostic method for rapid diagnosis. PCR can provide both rapid results and an improved diagnostic accuracy by characterizing the microorganism (differentiating from atypical and nontuberculous forms). The specificity of PCR-based assays for *M. tuberculosis* is excellent at 98%, and sensitivity is at least 80%. *Mycobacterium* spp. probes for the rapid identification of mycobacteria are used to identify acid-fast organisms. The limitation of these NAA is that they detect nucleic acids from both living and dead organisms (thus may be false-positive even in inactive disease). Assays that detect mRNA remain positive only while viable mycobacteria persist, so they are sensitive indicators of treatment response and drug susceptibility. In culture negative cases with characteristic clinicoradiological findings, a positive PCR-mRNA can be considered diagnostic.
- Xpert® MTB/RIF should be done as recommended under EXPAND-TB initiative [*see* "Joint Disorders Including Inflammatory and Noninflammatory Arthritis and Infective Arthritides (Including Mycobacterial Infection and Prosthetic Joint Infection)"].
- Arthritis and Infective Arthritides (Including Mycobacterial infection and Prosthetic Joint Infection)'. It can also provide simultaneous result for drug-resistant disease.
- Drug susceptibility testing for both first- and second-line drugs (usually performed at the state laboratory or national referral center level) should be performed especially in areas with high incidence of MDR TB.

Classification of Spinal Tuberculosis

Classification of Tuberculous Paraplegia (Tuli)

- Stage 1 (negligible)—patient unaware of neurological deficit, physician detects plantar extensor response

- Stage 2 (mild)—patient aware of deficit but manages to walk with support
- Stage 3 (moderate)—nonambulatory due to paralysis (in extension), sensory deficit <50%—there is differential involvement of fibers in cord (predominantly related to the types of fibers) whereby, the inhibitory pathways to local reflexes are lost but motor power and intrinsic tone of muscles is still there, so this produces a "spastic" state and the antigravity muscles predominate producing paraplegia in extension and brisk reflexes with clonus.
- Stage 4 (severe)—stage 3 plus flexor spasm/paralysis in flexion/flaccid/sensory deficit >50%/sphincters involved. It is the end-stage in evolution of disease whereby all motor control and muscle tone is lost due to severe compression and possibly arachnoiditis.

Clinicoradiological Classification (Kumar; Table 1)

This system was based on site of involvement and stages of the disease. The main limitation of the classification is that it focuses on angular deformity only which does not give comprehensive picture.

Mehta and Bhojraj Classification

Mehta and Bhojraj classification system utilizing MRI (2001)—classifies patients to four groups **(Figs. 19A to D)**:

1. Group A consists of patients with stable anterior lesions and no kyphotic deformity—managed with anterior debridement and strut grafting.
2. Group B consists of patients with global lesions, who were treated with posterior instrumentation using a closed-loop rectangle with subluxation and strut graft.
3. Group C patients have anterior or global lesions along with a high operative risk for transthoracic surgery—managed with posterior global decompression. The anterior aspect of the cord is approached through a transpedicular route and posterior instrumentation performed using a closed-loop rectangle held by sublaminar wire.
4. Group D patients had isolated posterior lesions—managed with posterior decompression alone.

The classification is limited by description of only thoracic lesions.

GATA Classification (Oguz et al.)

Spinal TB is classified into three main types with few subtypes **(Figs. 20A to D)**:

1. Type I—one-level disk involvement and soft-tissue infiltration without abscess, collapse, and neurologic deficit
   a. Type I-A, lesions only limited to vertebra and therefore, manageable with fine needle biopsy and medical therapy.

TABLE 1: Clinicoradiological classification of Kumar (1988), K = K-angle (Konstam's angle as measured by Dickson's method).

Stages	*Features*	*Duration*
Stage 1 (predestructive)	Straightening of curvatures, spasm of perivertebral muscles, scintiscan would show hyperemia	Usually <3 months
Stage 2 (early destructive)	Diminished disk space plus paradiskal erosion (knuckle <10°), MRI shows marrow edema and break of osseous margins, CT scan shows marginal erosions or cavitations	2–4 months
Stage 3 (mild angular kyphosis)	2–3 vertebra involved (K: 10–30)	3–9 months
Stage 4 (moderate angular kyphosis)	>3 vertebrae involved (K: 30–60)	6–24 months
Stage 5 (severe kyphosis, Humpback)	>3 vertebrae involved (K: 60)	>2 years

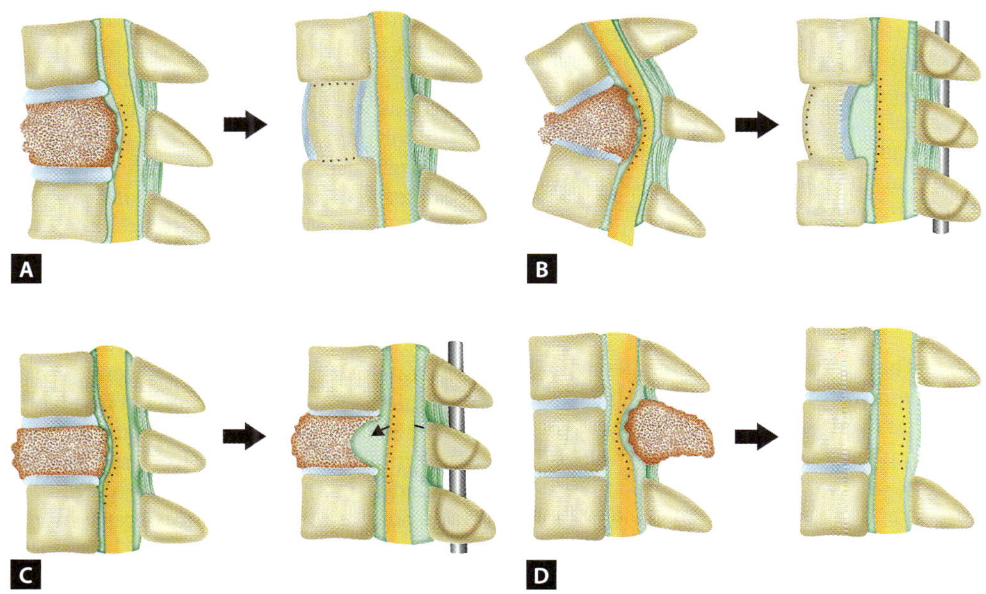

Figs. 19A to D: Illustration of Mehta and Bhojraj classification of tuberculosis of spine based on surgical protocol used in management.

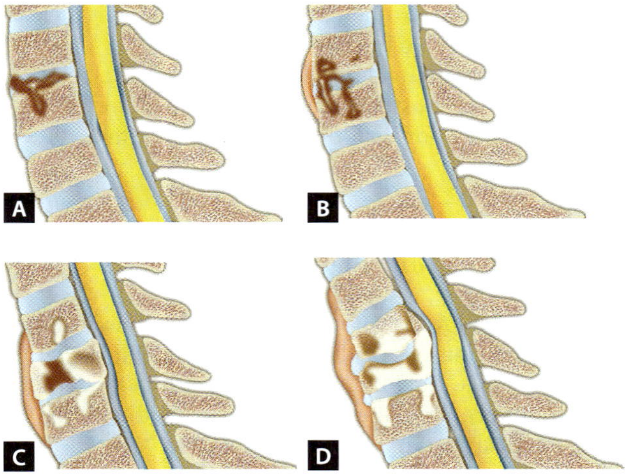

Figs. 20A to D: GATA classification.

b. Type I-B, abscess formation exceeds the vertebra and the treatment is debridement using an anterior, posterior or endoscopic approach.

2. Type II—one- or two-level disk degeneration, abscess formation and mild kyphosis correctable with anterior surgery. The spine may not be unstable but there is neurological deficit. Treatment involves debridement by anterior approach and fusion with tricortical graft.
3. Type III—one- or two-level disk degeneration, abscess formation, instability and deformity that cannot be corrected without instrumentation. Decompression and stabilization via anterolateral, posterior or combined approach.

Differential Diagnosis

Early thoracic disease in children—rickets, osteochondroses, Scheuermann's, Schmorl's nodes. Paradiskal type disease—pyogenic diskitis of tuberculosis should be differentiated especially from the one caused by *Brucella* (Lumbar spine is frequently involved but gibbus formation never seen), *Salmonella typhi*, and cholera. In bacterial pyogenic diskitis, bone destruction and homogeneous enhancement is more frequently observed compared to TB where there is heterogeneous enhancement. Central lesions have lymphoma and eosinophilic granuloma (EG) as important differentials latter especially with concentric collapse. Adults—metastasis (posterior elements most commonly involved and intervertebral disk heights normal), multiple myeloma, and lymphoma. In elderly patients, the important differential diagnosis is osteoporotic vertebral collapse and metastasis.

Management

The treatment of TB has basically drastically changed with the availability of chemotherapy from 1948 to 1951. This divides the management into pre- and postantitubercular era.

In the preantitubercular era, Hippocrates (450 BC) and Galen (131-201 AD) tried to correct kyphotic deformity by manual pressure, traction, and mechanical appliances (body cast, plaster beds, and braces) but failed. Bed rest was strongly advised and practiced by the two most popular personalities of the time namely, Sir John Hilton and Sir Hugh Owen Thomas along with domiciliary treatment. The results of conservative treatments were largely disappointing so some primitive attempts were made by the then practicing surgeons (most of them futile) to control the disease, as follows:

- Chipault Laminectomy (1896) and Fraser Laminotomy—abandoned the operation altogether due to disappointing results.
- Costotransversectomy of Menard (1894) fell into general disrepute because of the high incidence of sinus formation and of secondary infection.
- Posterior mediastinotomy of Obalinski was a bit more aggressive procedure for the evacuation of tuberculous paravertebral abscess.
- Calve's operation (1917) was primarily aimed to aspirate the contents of an abscess without sinus formation.
- *Lateral rachiotomy of Capener:* Norman Capener in 1933 devised lateral rachiotomy where decompression was obtained anterior to theca. He excised a part of the lamina and pedicle from one side to enter the spinal canal anteriorly.
- *Anterolateral decompression (ALD) of Dott and Alexander:* they modified Capener's operation and approached the spine a little more anterior by removal of a part of the body of the vertebra to gain access to the spinal canal. Lamina remains untouched.
- *Posterior decompression with posterior spinal arthrodesis:* Albee (1911, 1930) and Hibbs (1912, 1918). They were meant strictly to shorten the period of immobilization in the bed and to provide a permanent internal stability to the tuberculous spine to avoid recurrence of the disease and development of paraplegia. Just producing spinal fusion posteriorly did nothing to the diseased area and the organisms remain alive that may flare up at any chance or provocation.

With the evolution of chemotherapy and antitubercular drugs, the conservative school became powerful again. Not only that but aggressive surgical measures (the other school) were developed which evolved from primitive methods. The two basic methods of treatment hence persisted (depending on the followers and training), flourished and were practiced variably in different regions over time:

1. Conservative management with dedicated chemotherapy, bracing or cast immobilization to control deformity, etc.
2. Surgical management with complete excision of the disease focus and stabilization using instruments.

To evaluate the two diagrammatically opposite treatment methods and their rationale use MRC (Medical Research Council) trials were conducted independently in Africa, Korea, and India utilizing different pathways to manage the TB, and results assessed by achievement of "favorable status". The conclusions of these trials were:

- Patients without neurological involvement or risk factors for severe progress in deformity can be safely treated with ambulatory short course chemotherapy (Korean study, 1993). The patients were evaluated for ambulatory 6, 9, 18 months chemotherapy by dividing them into 6 or 9 months HR and 9 or 18 months HE/PH groups. It was concluded that 6 or 9 months HR was equivalent to 18 months HE/PH therapy. Nine months HE/PH was definitely inferior.

- Debridement has no advantage over short course chemotherapy (Chennai previously Madras, India 1999). The patients were divided into chemotherapy 6 or 9 months HR and 6 months HR plus surgical resection. It was found that the results after surgery were no better than ambulatory chemotherapy alone.
- There is no benefit of complete rest or domiciliary treatment for 6 months. Also plaster jacket treatment is not always necessary.
- Radical surgery may achieve favorable status quickly with earlier fusion or reduced tendency for progress in deformity (Hong Kong, 1986). In Hong Kong, the patients were randomized to HR for 6–9 months combined with bone grafting and streptomycin for 6 months for all patients. The reported fusion rates of surgery were but not reproduced consistently elsewhere.
- Daily addition of streptomycin is not necessary.
- Radical surgery has no advantage over ambulatory chemotherapy in preservation of life and health.
- It also came to realization that just two-drug chemotherapy has been used in the trials is inadequate due to rapid development of resistance and for faster initial clearance the four-drug regimen has to be opted.

The trials suffered from important lacunae that none included the severity of deformity in initial assessment for deciding favorable status. Considering this, a middle path regimen was developed by Tuli to rationalize the two diagrammatically opposite approaches. The following realizations from MRC trials helped devise the middle path regimen:

- Chemotherapy cures the disease but 15% have unacceptable kyphosis.
- "Hong Kong procedure" involving early radical debridement and fusion was successful in achieving good early fusion and less deformity but results were not reproduced everywhere. The expertise and infrastructure is not available everywhere and even in best hands the mortality and morbidity was 4%.

These disadvantages of surgery and possibly overtreatment and disadvantages of chemotherapy with possibly under treatment in some lead to development of *middle path regimen* by identifying the cases where some addition to chemotherapy is needed. The ambulatory chemotherapy is used in all and surgery is added when there is disease recurrence, threat of progressive deformity or presence of paraplegic (neurological) complications.

The indications of medical therapy in patients with spinal TB are:

- Single disk space involvement without significant vertebral body destruction
- Minimal or no instability
- Minimal or no neurologic deficit
- Medical comorbidities such as sepsis or coagulopathy

The ambulatory chemotherapy and regimen has been described elsewhere in the text [*see* Chapter on "Joint Disorders Including Inflammatory and Noninflammatory Arthritis and Infective Arthritides (Including Mycobacterial Infection and Prosthetic Joint Infection)"]. In a nutshell, the current antitubercular chemotherapy is presented in **Box 1** and associated **Tables 2 to 4**. Institutionalized aggressive or

BOX 1: General guidelines for management of tuberculous infection.

- The WHO now categorizes tubercular disease into only two types: (1) Drug-susceptible and (2) drug-resistant. Previous use of pulmonary/extrapulmonary/osteoarticular, and regimens based on them is dropped.
- Standard regimen for drug-susceptible tuberculosis (TB) is 6-month chemotherapy. This comprises 2 months intensive phase of HRZE (isoniazid, rifampicin, pyrazinamide, and ethambutol, respectively) followed sequentially by 4 months of HR. Four-drug intensive phase is routinely preferred especially because drug-susceptibility testing is not routinely done and isoniazid resistance is prevalent. In case susceptibility testing is done and the organism is susceptible to both isoniazid and rifampicin then use of ethambutol in intensive phase is futile.
- Daily dosing regimens are anytime preferable over intermittent dosing especially in intensive phase. Use of alternative regimens **(Table 2)** is not preferred for osteoarticular TB except in rarest of circumstances.
- Shortened regimens based on fluoroquinolones are not recommended.
- Directly observed therapy (DOT) is preferred in all situations over self-administered therapy (SAT), however, due to the disability associated with osteoarticular therapy; SAT is allowed with more frequent hospital visits for evaluation of compliance. If possible, healthcare workers may visit the patient daily at home to administer DOT (at least in intensive phase).
- DOT is especially recommended for patients with treatment failure, relapse, drug resistance, homelessness, current or prior substance abuse, HIV infection, previous nonadherence to therapy, children and adolescents, mental, emotional or physical disability (i.e., cognitive deficits such as dementia; neurological deficits; medically fragile patients; or patients with blindness or severe loss of vision) and previous treatment of active or latent TB.
- For patients with coinfection with HIV, the duration of antitubercular chemotherapy does not change (6 months as above with 2 months intensive and 4 months of continuation phase). In addition, initiate antiretroviral therapy within the first 2 weeks of TB treatment with CD4 cell counts <50/mm^3 and by 8–12 weeks of TB treatment for patients with CD4 cell counts >50/mm^3.
- Treatment interruptions are not uncommon and they should be managed appropriately **(Table 3)**.
- Drug-resistant TB (DR-TB) is very common in current day practice and clinician should be vigilant in determining and evaluating the same. The following are some of the variously used terms for drug-resistance:
  - *Monodrug-resistant TB:* TB caused by organisms that show resistance to a single anti-TB drug (e.g., isoniazid, rifampicin, ethambutol, or pyrazinamide).
  - *Isoniazid-resistant TB:* TB caused by organisms that show resistance to isoniazid (rifampicin susceptible).
  - *Rifampicin-resistant TB (RR-TB):* TB caused by organisms that show resistance to rifampicin, but may be susceptible to isoniazid, or resistant to isoniazid (i.e., MDR TB), or resistant to other first-line TB medicines (polydrug-resistant) or second-line TB medicines [e.g., extensively drug-resistant TB (XDR TB)].
  - *Polydrug-resistant TB (PDR-TB):* TB caused by organisms that show resistance to more than one anti-TB drug, but not including both isoniazid and rifampicin.
  - *MDR-TB:* TB caused by organisms that show resistance to at least isoniazid and rifampicin.
  - *Pre-extensively drug-resistant TB (pre-XDR TB):* TB caused by organisms that show multidrug resistance, and resistance to any fluoroquinolone or a second-line injectable (SLI) agent (i.e., amikacin, kanamycin, or capreomycin).
  - *XDR TB:* TB caused by organisms that show multidrug resistance, and resistance to any fluoroquinolone and at least one of the SLI agents
  - *Primary or newly diagnosed DR-TB:* DR-TB in a person who has previously received no or <1 month of anti-TB treatment.
  - *Acquired or previously treated DR-TB:* TB in a person who has previously received at least 1 month of anti-TB treatment.
- Drug-resistant TB should be managed primarily by infection care specialist in association with orthopedic surgeon in institutional care because new regimens are continuously evolving and the drugs have various complications that may not be manageable by orthopedic surgeon alone. The key recommendations are presented in **Table 4**, but the reader is highly encouraged to refer WHO or other appropriate agency dealing with standardized management of TB infection.

TABLE 2: The standard and alternative regimens of chemotherapy for drug-susceptible tuberculosis (TB). These are taken from treatment of pulmonary disease but due to unusual circumstances of osteoarticular TB the regimens other than "1" below are possibly not suitable for treatment of osteoarticular TB.

Regimen	Intensive phase Drug	Interval and dose	Continuation phase Drugs	Interval and doses	Range of total doses	Comments
1	HRZE	7 days/week for 56 doses (8 weeks) or 5 days/week for 40 doses (8 weeks)—if DOT is enforced	HR	7 days/week for 126 doses (18 weeks) or 5 days/week for 90 doses (18 weeks)	182–130	This is the preferred regimen for patients with newly diagnosed pulmonary TB
2	HRZE	7 days/week for 56 doses (8 weeks) or 5 days/week for 40 doses (8 weeks)	HR	3 times weekly for 54 doses (18 weeks)	110–94	Preferred alternative regimen in situations in which more frequent DOT during continuation phase is difficult to achieve
3	HRZE	3 times weekly for 24 doses (8 weeks)	HR	3 times weekly for 54 doses (18 weeks)	78	Use regimen with caution in patients with HIV and/or cavitary disease. Missed doses can lead to treatment failure, relapse, and acquired drug resistance
4	HRZE	7 days/week for 14 doses, then twice weekly for 12 doses	HR	Twice weekly for 36 doses (18 weeks)	62	Do not use twice-weekly regimens in HIV-infected patients or patients with smear-positive and/or cavitary disease. If doses are missed, then therapy is equivalent to once weekly, which is inferior

TABLE 3: The management of treatment interruptions.

Phase of interruption	Cumulative lapse or duration of lapse	Approach
Intensive phase treatment interruption	Lapse is <14 days in duration	Continue treatment to complete planned total number of doses (as long as all doses are completed within 3 months)
	Lapse is ≥14 days in duration	Restart treatment from the beginning
Interruption during continuation phase	Received ≥ 80% of doses	Continue therapy until all doses are completed
	Received <80% of doses and accumulative lapse is <3 months in duration	Continue therapy until all doses are completed (full course), unless consecutive lapse is >2 months
		If treatment cannot be completed within recommended time frame for regimen, restart therapy from the beginning (i.e., restart intensive phase, to be followed by continuation phase)
	Received <80% of doses and lapse is ≥3 months in duration	Restart therapy from the beginning, new intensive and continuation phases (i.e., restart intensive phase, to be followed by continuation phase)

prolonged regimens are not recommended for maintaining uniformity. Ultrashort-course chemotherapy (i.e., treatment with antitubercular drugs for <6 months) was reported to be as effective as short-course and standard anti-TB treatment especially when combined with partial excision of focus, but its utility is not completely documented. After 4–6 weeks of chemotherapy, TB symptoms and vertebral pain improve in almost all patients, and the ESR and C-reactive protein (CRP) also decrease. ESR and CRP are commonly used parameters for evaluating the response to treatment but their definitive role has not been comprehensively evaluated. Monitoring treatment response and guiding when to stop chemotherapy had been the biggest questions in minds of every clinician primarily because there are no definitive recommendations or known end-points to stop chemotherapy except following a fixed-course chemotherapy. Physicians follow all sorts of regimens from 6 to 18 months according to training and experience but this practice should be discouraged following the current recommendations.

Medical treatment alone even improves the neurological deficit in certain patient population. The following are the components of medical therapy generally practiced:

- Percutaneous biopsy
- Chemotherapy regimen
- Brace therapy with regular follow-up until stability
- Analgesic and nutrition build-up
- Controversial hyperbaric oxygen therapy

Thus, surgery as a primary indication for management of patients with spinal TB is not indicated.

Surgical Management in Spinal Tuberculosis

The most common indications are with regards to involvement of neurology with the disease; however, surgery may also be indicated in patients without neurological deficit **(Box 2)**. The typical indications for surgical management in patients on middle path regimen are:

- No neurological recovery even after 4 weeks of chemotherapy
- Development of neurological complications during chemotherapy

TABLE 4: Medicines and key recommendations from the WHO for management of drug-resistant tuberculosis.

Group and steps	***Medicine***
Group A: Include all three medicines	• Levofloxacin or moxifloxacin • Bedaquiline • Linezolid
Group B: Add one or both medicines	• Clofazimine • Cycloserine or terizidone
Group C: Add to complete the regimen and when medicines from groups A and B cannot be used	• Ethambutol • Delamanid • Pyrazinamide • Imipenem-cilastatin • Meropenem • Amikacin • Streptomycin • Ethionamide • Prothionamide • Para-aminosalicylic acid

Relative indications of different approaches:
- Fluoroquinolones (levofloxacin and moxifloxacin), bedaquiline, and linezolid (group A) were considered highly effective and are strongly recommended to be included in an MDR TB regimen unless contraindicated.
- Clofazimine and either cycloserine or terizidone (group B) are conditionally recommended as second-choice drugs.
- Drugs are in group C ranked by the balance of benefit to harm and can be considered when group A or B drugs are not available to build an adequate multidrug regimen.
- Injectable agents, amikacin and streptomycin, have been downgraded to group C and are not included if an adequate regimen can be built without them. Kanamycin and capreomycin are no longer recommended for use.
- Gatifloxacin and thioacetazone are either not available or not being used, and therefore are not included in the recommendations.
- High-dose isoniazid may have a role when there is confirmed isoniazid susceptibility or when only an inhA mutation is detected in longer MDR regimens and is a standard drug in the shorter MDR regimen.
- Clavulanic acid [only available in the combination amoxicillin-clavulanic acid form (Augmentin)] should only be given with a carbapenem (e.g., meropenem) and should not be individually counted as an anti-TB drug.
- There is no recommendation for the use of 4-thioureidoiminomethyl pyridinium perchlorate interferon-gamma, or sutezolid and no evidence that they increase likelihood of cure.
- Bedaquiline can be given to children ≥6 years of age.
- Delamanid can be given to children ≥3 years of age.
- There is no recommendation for giving bedaquiline and delamanid together.
- Bedaquiline and delamanid should be given for 6 months and, if extended, would be considered off-label use.
- Pyrazinamide should only be counted in the regimen if susceptibility is shown.
- Amikacin and streptomycin should only be used if susceptibility is confirmed (phenotypic conformation for streptomycin) and if high-quality audiology monitoring is available.

- Recurrence of neurological deficit after initial improvement
- Worsening of neurological complications during chemotherapy
- Advanced cases of neurological involvement (sphincter disturbances, flaccid paralysis, severe flexor spasms)
- Rapidly advancing paresis which is advancing daily

The surgical procedures commonly used for management in individual cases are:
- Abscess drainage around spine or pelvis (actually decompression surgery)

BOX 2: Surgical indications in patients without neurological deficit.
- Failure of clinical improvement after 6–10 weeks of treatment
- Recurrence of disease
- Primary drug resistance or history of irregular chemotherapy
- *To prevent deformity:*
  - *Adults:* vertebral body loss of >1 in dorsal and dorsolumbar regions and >1.5 in lumbar region
  - *Children:*
    - "Spine at-risk signs"score of >2
    - Vertebral body loss of >0.75 in dorsal and dorsolumbar regions and loss of >1 in lumbar region
    - Children who present with a kyphus >30° before start of chemotherapy
- *Uncommon indications:*
  - To establish diagnosis (only when CT-guided biopsy is inconclusive)
  - In patients with persistent sinuses and abscess
  - Tuberculosis of cervical spine with paravertebral abscess causing difficulty in deglutition and breathing

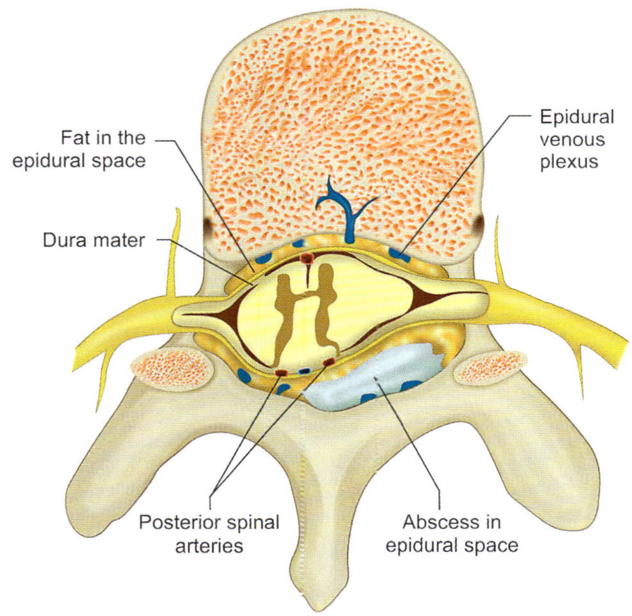

Fig. 21: Spinal epidural abscess.

- Posterior decompression plus fusion with bone grafts
- Anterior debridement/decompression plus fusion with bone grafts
- Anterior debridement/decompression plus fusion plus sequential posterior fusion with instrumentation
- Posterior fusion with instrumentation followed by simultaneous or sequential anterior debridement/decompression and fusion

Laminectomy per se has no place in TB of spine except for extradural granuloma/tuberculoma presenting as "spinal tumor syndrome" or a case of old healed disease presenting with secondary "vertebral canal stenosis" or posterior spinal disease.

Management of Abscess (Fig. 21)

Cervical spine (Fig. 22): Unless there is an emergency to drain the abscess an extraoral route through neck should be used. Direct posterior wall incision and drainage into pharynx is done only in emergencies but has potential of getting infected due to oral flora. The standard anterior approach between carotid sheath and esophagus (anterior

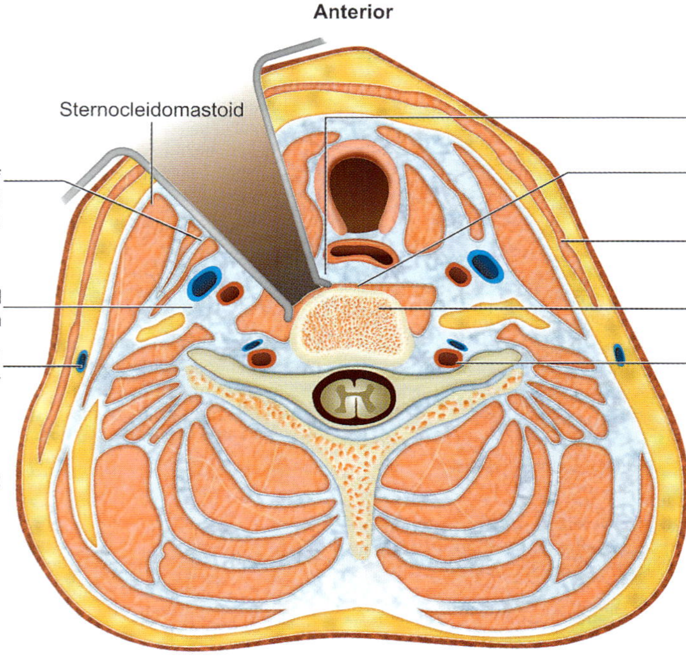

Fig. 22: Anterior drainage of cervical spine abscess.

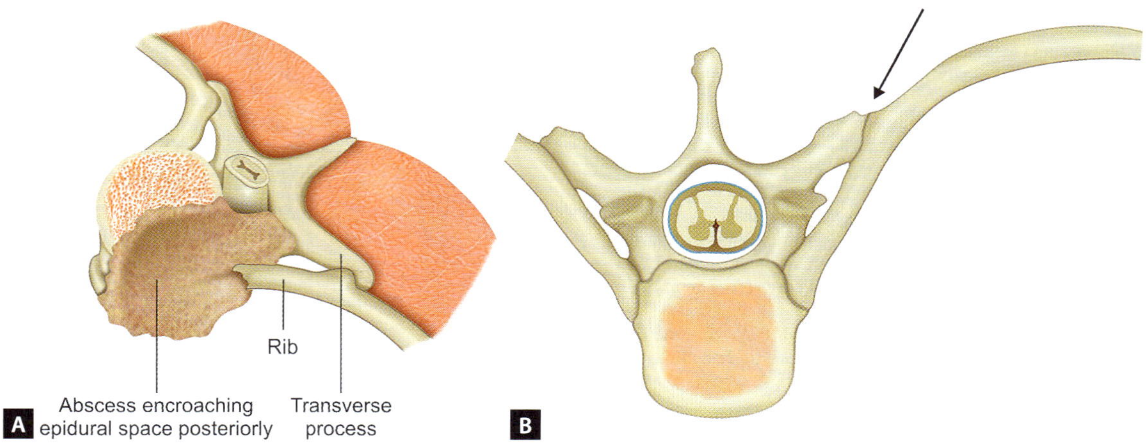

Figs. 23A and B: Costotransversectomy. (A) The relation of ribs and transverse process to the epidural abscess; (B) The approach in costotransversectomy.

triangle), or through posterior triangle is used. For C1 or C2, transoral approach is used often with supplementary fixation (occiput to C2 fusion).

***Thoracic spine*:** Abscess drainage is indicated, if there is dyspnea of spasmodic nature. The common procedure done in children is costotransversectomy **(Figs. 23A and B)**. The typical advantages of costotransversectomy include:

- Directly addresses the main cause of paraplegia (abscess itself).
- The drainage is done away from cord.
- Spine is not opened so chances of instability are minimal if at all.
- Simple procedure with minimal risk involved
- Produces greater area of drainage in the form of a big canal that can not only drain abscess, granulation tissue, caseous material, etc.
- For cervicothoracic region, it is better to use and anterior sternum-splitting approach.

***Lumbar region abscess*:** Direct drainage along lateral border of sacrospinous between last ribs and crest of ilium is the most appropriate method. Psoas abscess can be drained along the pointing regions or along the anterolateral region of iliac crest.

Factors affecting surgical outcome:

- *Good:*
  - Minimal destruction and short graft
  - Good intraoperative correction
  - Involvement of lower lumbar segments
- *Poor:*
  - Poor nutrition
  - No perioperative treatment

- Vertebral body loss >2
- Junctional lesions (cervicodorsal, dorsolumbar)
- Marked preoperative kyphosis
- Frank instability
- Postdebridement defects requiring grafts spanning more than two disk spaces. The grafts usually fail in such cases. The graft failure is of four types:
  1. Displacement
  2. Fracture
  3. Absorption
  4. Subsidence

Debridement Plus Decompression and Fusion

Posterolateral or transpedicular approach has been used extensively for the management of spinal TB. This is a safe method for decompression of thoracic spine and stabilization with pedicle screws **(Figs. 24A to D)**. Posterior fusion can be readily done altogether. In less privileged centers, anterolateral approach is feasible and safe, and provides circumferential exposure for lesions located in the spine from the second thoracic vertebra down to the 5th lumbar vertebra. This can be considered a universal approach as it allows anterior debridement, decompression, bone grafting (anterior or posteriorly), posterior implant fixation, and kyphosis correction all in one. Anterior instrumentation can be done that can be very well supplemented by posterior instrumentation as necessary to prevent postoperative kyphosis especially in children. Performing anterior debridement and posterior stabilization with instrumentation has been proposed as a "smaller" simpler procedure to combined instrumentation and is largely practiced. The only problem seems to be poor sagittal control and correction of the deformity with this approach. Biomechanically the combined anterior and posterior instrumentation and stabilization is better than either method alone in any case, so it is recommended for TB where there is ongoing bony destruction with a potential of increasing instability. The combined procedure can be done in two ways:

1. Anterior-posterior, anterior debridement/decompression and fusion is performed first
2. Posterior-anterior, posterior fusion with instrumentation is the first stage

Both approaches have been shown optimal and feasible equally. Video-assisted thoracoscopic surgery (VATS) can be combined for minimally invasive approach and reduction of morbidity.

Management of Complications of Spinal Tuberculosis

Kyphotic Deformity

Kyphosis is the predominant deformity. There is foreshortening of trunk, short stature, cosmetic problem and reduced pulmonary function. There are secondary cardiac and respiratory problems. The progression of kyphosis occurs in two separate phases either during the active phase of the disease (phase I) or after healing of the lesion (phase II), the latter is more serious as neurologic deficit and paraplegia after healing of the spinal TB lesion is associated with a worse prognosis. The angle of kyphosis increases by 10–30° in around 10% patients while some 3% patients have >30° increase in kyphosis. In the remaining 85%, the kyphosis either remains static or decreases or increases <10°. Progression of kyphosis is more common in children than adults, possibly due to the cartilaginous nature of bone (*see* the progression of kyphosis, five types in natural history of disease). Multiple vertebral involvement, active growth and location of the lesion in the thoracic spine are responsible for the excessive increase in kyphosis. Worsening of kyphosis is seen in 67% of the thoracolumbar region, 55% of the thoracic, and 33% of the lumbar lesions.

Prevention of Kyphotic Deformity

Children younger than 7 years of age, with three or more affected vertebral bodies in the thoracic or thoracolumbar spine and two or more "at-risk signs", are likely to have progression of the kyphosis. Patients having involvement of three or more vertebrae are benefitted by:

- Recumbency in the prone position in the early active stage
- Operative debridement and bone grafting posteriorly for panvertebral stabilization—radical excision and bone grafting as performed in Hong Kong by pioneers of the radical operation themselves during MRC trials. The Hong Kong procedure comprises of anterior approach for anterior pathology performing radical debridement (i.e., corpectomy) and removal of all necrotic tissue which is then filled with strut grafting or fusion using autograft or allograft. This restores the anterior column

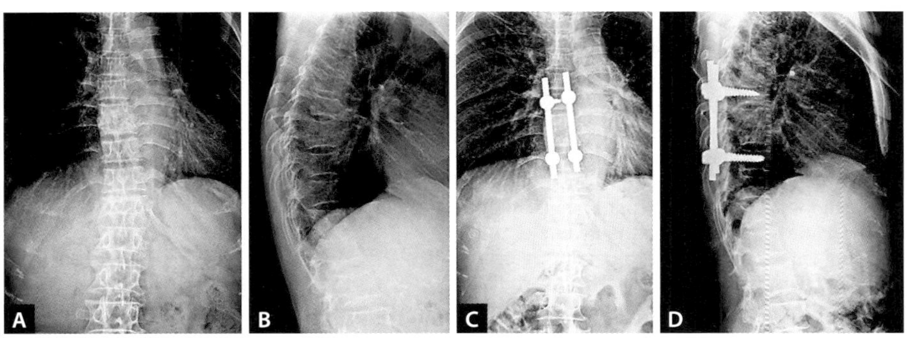

Figs. 24A to D: Debridement, decompression and posterior fusion for spinal tuberculosis. (A and B) Preoperative anteroposterior (AP) and lateral films showing tubercular involvement at dorsal 8th and 9th spinal segments; (C and D) Postoperative films following spinal decompression, debridement and posterior fusion giving complete relief in this patient who presented with paraplegia in extension.

and maintains sagittal balance. The fusion rates have been found to be >95%. The results are better when the infection is active (vs. "burnt out"). This single-stage decompression with fusion and kyphosis correction is very demanding surgery that should be performed by experts only. This surgery also prevents progression of neurological deficit and recurrence of late-onset paraplegia.

Indications for Surgery: Spine at Risk (Figs. 25A to D, Rajasekaran)

- *Facet dislocation* (separation of the facet joints): Facet joint at the apex of the curve gets subluxed followed by frank dislocation. There may be involvement of more than one level.
- *Retropulsion sign* (retropulsion of the diseased vertebral segments): This is assessed by drawing two lines along the posterior surface of the normal vertebra above and below the level of the lesion.
- *Lateral translation sign:* Translation is present when the line drawn from the center of a pedicle of the lower vertebra did not intersect the pedicle of the upper vertebra in anteroposterior radiographs.
- *Toppling sign*: The superior vertebra tends to tilt or topple, so that the anterior surface of the vertebra came into contact with the superior surface of the vertebra below the level of the lesion.

One score is assigned to each risk factor; these give a maximum score of 4 and minimum of 0. Score of >2 associated with higher increase in final deformity. Surgical correction of deformity is difficult.

Spinal "at risk" score (see above) higher than 2 seem to reliably predict patients who will have an increase of >30° kyphosis and a final deformity >60°. This often entails greater

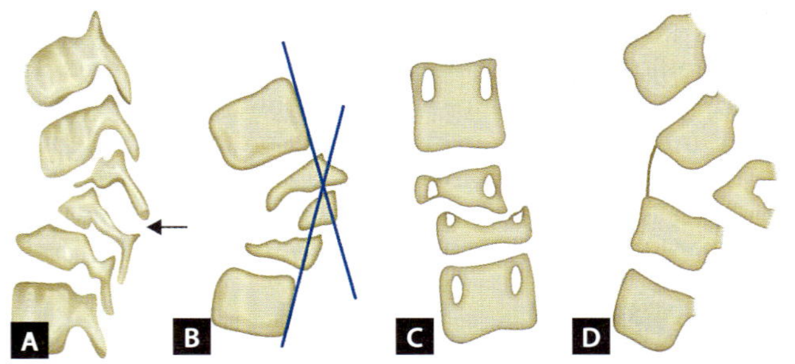

Figs. 25A to D: Spine at risk signs: (A) Separation of the facet joint. The facet joint dislocates at the level of the apex of the curve, causing instability and loss of alignment; (B) Posterior retropulsion. This is identified by drawing two lines along the posterior surface of the first upper and lower normal vertebrae. The diseased segments are found to project posterior to the intersection of the lines; (C) Lateral translation. This is confirmed when a vertical line drawn through the middle of the pedicle of the first lower normal vertebra does not touch the pedicle of the first upper normal vertebra; (D) Toppling sign. Often in the initial stages, a line drawn along the anterior surface of immediate lower normal vertebra intersects the inferior surface of the first upper normal vertebra usually. "Tilt" or "toppling" occurs when this line intersects higher than the middle of the anterior surface of the first normal upper vertebra.

need of surgical intervention. Early posterior stabilization and fusion with anterior debridement and reconstruction using graft/spacer and instrumented fusion is possibly good method. The methods described to correct kyphosis in cases deemed to progress later are:

- Single-stage transpedicular approach: This is the preferred method to prevent postsurgical progression of kyphosis. The pedicle of apex vertebra is used to decompress the spinal canal anteriorly through posterior approach. Kyphosis correction is achieved by removing the bone and tissues taking care to prevent cord stretch. Stabilization is done by fixing two vertebrae above and below, in dorsal spine while one on each side in lumbar spine. Anterior defect is then grafted.
- Anterior decompression (plus bone grafting and fusion) followed by correction of kyphosis and posterior instrumentation done in single or staged manner (preferable). The first stage is usually a transthoracic transpleural (dorsal spine) or retroperitoneal approach (lumbar spine) where after debridement and corpectomy the defect is filled with a graft (preferably using cage). Posterior surgery is then performed for instrumented fusion after 3–4 weeks.
- Correction by extrapleural anterolateral approach (single stage): Here the extrapleural exposure of deformity is done in a lateral position followed by anterior corpectomy and decompression. Sequentially posterior shortening and instrumented kyphosis correction is performed followed by bone grafting of the anterior gap.

Severe Kyphosis

Kyphotic deformity is unstable and progressive, particularly in childhood, and it is believed that a severe deformity in the presence of active disease should be an absolute indication for decompression, correction, and stabilization. Late reconstruction of tuberculous kyphosis is difficult. Correction of severe fixed kyphotic deformity involves anterior procedure at the site of disease, osteotomy at the posterior elements at the deformity, and halopelvic or halofemoral traction posteriorly. A single-stage posterior Smith–Peterson osteotomy or pedicle subtraction osteotomy (PSO) may not be useful for Konstam's angle >90° (see details of osteotomy in the adult onset scoliosis). Vertebral column resection osteotomy (VCRO, **Figs. 26A to D**) is associated with lot of intraoperative and postoperative complications. Newer approaches hence include multilevel VCRO through a single posterior approach. The other approach is to perform combined posterior closing anterior opening osteotomy (Rajasekaran). The anterior column reconstruction is done using cages. Paraplegia due to severe kyphosis is treated by anterior transposition of the cord through laminectomy and anterior kyphectomy. Laminectomy is performed first, and then enough spinal nerve roots are divided on both sides to permit retraction of the theca. Bone from the front of the vertebral canal is then removed to correct internal kyphosis. This can also be done through anterolateral approach to

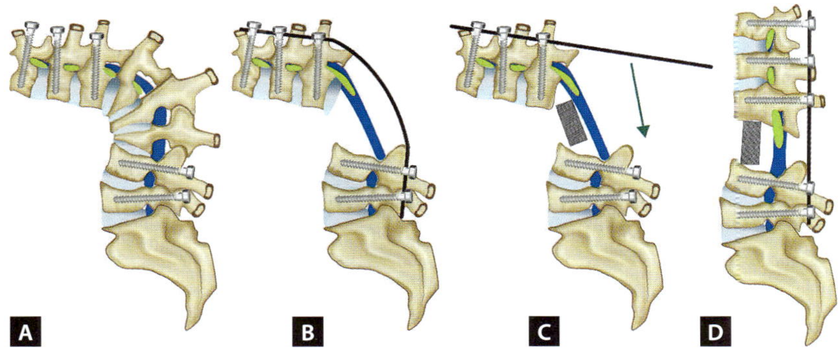

Figs. 26A to D: Vertebral column resection osteotomy (VCRO) for correction of kyphotic deformity. (A) Resection of three disease segments at the apex of kyphosis; (B) Temporary stabilization; (C) Anterior cage placement and revision of posterior stabilization; (D) Deformity correction and final fixation.

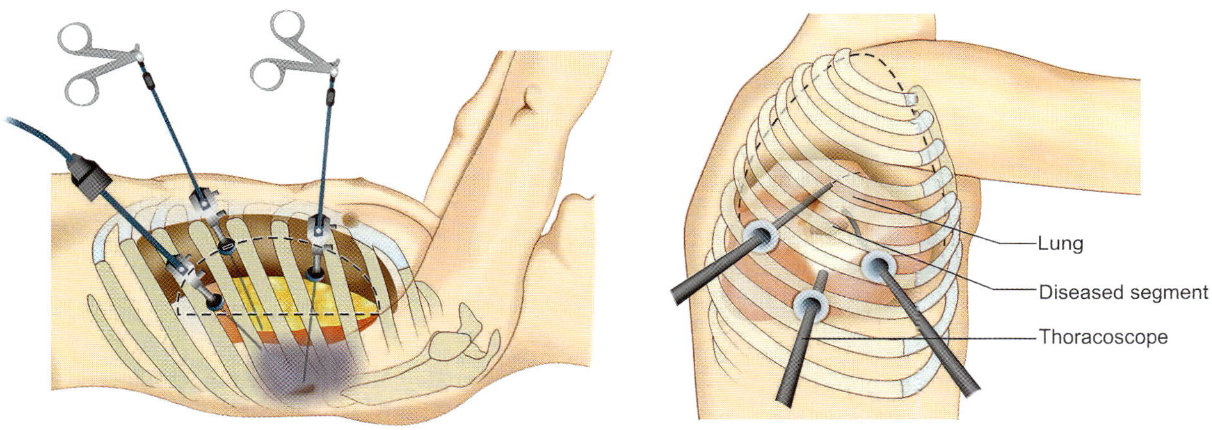

Fig. 27: Portals and basic schema for video-assisted thoracoscopic surgery.

permit cord to lie in a relaxed anterior position. Spine is then stabilized posteriorly.

Role of Endoscopy

Video-assisted thoracoscopic surgery procedure is a minimally invasive technique that allows adequate specimens to be obtained **(Fig. 27)**. It provides a significant advantage with minimum blood loss, less tissue damage, less pain in the postoperative period, and short hospital stay. The typical indications would be:

- For draining tubercle abscesses and biopsy
- Corpectomy and bone grafting for anterior fusion
- Obtaining samples in patients not responding to chemotherapy for 3 months

The main difficulty in performing VATS is poor distinction of tissues, adhesions, and bleeding granulation tissue.

Role of Implants

Anterior surgery alone is ineffective in management of Pott's spine, additional posterior instrumentation is often required. Adjuvant posterior stabilization hastens early mobilization and rehabilitation. Radical anterior debridement clears the diseased focus while simultaneously restoring the anterior column by cage. Healing of the disease and fusion of the graft across the affected vertebrae is improved. The incidence of graft-related problems and the progression of the kyphosis are significantly less by the combined approach when compared with anterior surgery alone. The postoperative loss of correction is insignificant for combined anterior and posterior surgery. Biomaterial centered infections are related to preferential bacterial colonization of inert surfaces and production of biofilm (glycocalyx) protecting them from host defenses and chemotherapy. As mycobacterial adhesiveness is less and there is decreased tendency to biofilm production so risk of persistence of infection is minimal.

Some Special Concerns

***Atypical forms of spinal TB*:** Atypical spinal TB is defined as compressive myelopathy with no detectable spinal deformity and the absence of radiological appearance of a typical vertebral lesion. It is seen in 2.1% of the cases. The "atypical" presentation could be in relation to atypical clinical presentation or atypical radiology (Pandey and Bhabhulkar). The three basic categories of atypical presentations include:

1. Type 1—posterior element (neural arch, appendiceal) TB
2. Type 2—single vertebral invasion and destruction with compressive myelopathy
3. Type 3—extradural extraosseous spinal TB (tuberculoma formation)

The Pandey classification of atypical spinal TB is as follows:

- *Atypical radiographic presentation:*
  - *Single vertebral disease:*
    - Concertina collapse of vertebra (concentric collapse)
    - Ivory vertebra
    - Neural arch (posterior elements) TB
    - Circumferential vertebral involvement
  - *Multiple vertebral disease:*
    - In continuity
    - Not in continuity (skip lesions)
- *Atypical clinical presentations:*
  - Presentation as prolapse of intervertebral disk (PIVD) or failed back syndrome
  - Cold abscess without bony lesion (primary cold abscess)
  - *Tubercular granuloma:*
    - Spinal tumor syndrome
    - Extradural granuloma
    - Subdural granuloma
    - Intramedullary granuloma

The various atypical clinical presentations of disease reported are astonishing and so unrelated to tubercular symptoms that the disease might be totally missed. Abdominal lymphadenopathy causing reversible renovascular hypertension, encephalopathy, etc., are some of the weird presentations. Early diagnosis is mandatory and management in lines of typical disease will yield good results if the condition is diagnosed early. The differential diagnosis for these atypical lesions includes pyogenic and fungal osteomyelitis, trauma, multiple myeloma, lymphoma, eosinophilic granuloma, and metastatic deposits. Though MRI has been the investigation commonly relied upon for differentiating the conditions, recently PET/CT imaging has been found useful for diagnosing the disease even in clinically unsuspected cases, though such scenarios are unlikely to present in routine practice. I feel that unless no diagnosis is possible PET/CT does not have a routine role in diagnosing even atypical TB cases.

***Multiple vertebral diseases*:** It is seen in 7% of spinal TB (possibly underreporting due to latent disease). Multiple level spinal TB may occur as continuous vertebral involvement or may affect different levels in different parts of the spine (skip disease). The lesion in continuity typically is seen in immunodeficient patients and in patients with hemoglobinopathies. In such patients before undertaking surgery accurate compression level should be preoperatively determined else surgical decompression may fail. Often there is concern of recurrence of compression at other levels so radical debridement followed by anterior spinal stabilization with a structural bone graft is used for interbody fusion and correction of the spinal deformity, in multilevel spinal TB.

VERTEBRAL PYOGENIC OSTEOMYELITIS

Vertebral pyogenic osteomyelitis (VPO) accounts for 2–7% of all cases of musculoskeletal infections. Its incidence varies between 1:100,000 and 1:250,000 in developed countries and its estimated mortality rate ranges between 2% and 4%. It can occur at any age, but literature supports a bimodal distribution with a peak below 20 years and another between 50 and 70 years of age (50% of cases in patients older than 50 years). A 2:1–5:1 male/female ratio has been reported. When infection affects the intervertebral disk only, the term to describe this condition is usually diskitis. If it invades the endplates or the vertebral body, the infection is more correctly designated as vertebral osteomyelitis or spondylitis (*see* Classification, **Table 5**). However, at the time of diagnosis in many cases, the infection has already compromised these two structures; therefore, spondylodiskitis is frequently used. So in general, it is considered that concomitant involvement of both bone and disk (i.e., spondylodiskitis) is the "rule". Isolated bone or joint involvement (each represents around 1% of adult cases)—isolated diskitis is more common in younger children but is still rare. Mortality rate is below 5%.

TABLE 5: Classification of spinal infection.

Descriptive factor	*Details*
Anatomic location	• Spondylitis—confined to bony elements (common with TB) • Diskitis—confined to disk space • Spondylodiskitis—involving bone and disk • Septic arthritis—confined to synovial joint (e.g., rare facet joint arthropathy) • Epidural abscess • Paraspinal abscess—outside the vertebral column
Regional classification	• Cervical • Thoracic • Thoracolumbar • Lumbar • Sacral • Occipitocervical
Organism	• Pyogenic (bacterial)—gram-positive/negative/ mixed/anaerobic, etc. • Tubercular • Fungal • Parasitic
Duration	• Acute (<6 weeks) • Subacute (up to 3 months, this duration is controversial as also organism type sometimes defines subacute—for example: less-virulent and indolent organisms often produce subacute infections) • Chronic (>3 months)
Route	• Hematogenous • Direct inoculation • Contiguous spread

The risk factors for development of pyogenic spondylodiskitis include:

- Previous spine surgery
- A distant infectious focus
- Diabetes mellitus
- Advanced age
- Intravenous (IV) drug use
- HIV infection
- Immunosuppression
- Oncologic history
- Renal failure
- Rheumatological diseases
- Liver cirrhosis

Increased incidence of pyogenic spondylodiskitis is due to a combined effect of an increase in susceptible populations (particularly history of previous spine surgery, IV drug abusers, HIV infection) and an improved accuracy in diagnosis.

Etiology

The majority of spinal infections are bacterial monomicrobial. *Staphylococcus aureus* is the most common isolate with an incidence between 30% and 80%. Recent increase in methicillin-resistant *S. aureus* (MRSA) is a growing concern. *Streptococcus* is the second most common followed by coagulase-negative *Staphylococcus* (20% and 15% of isolates in one series, respectively). Gram-negative bacteria such as *Escherichia coli* are responsible, in some series, for up to 25% of spinal infections, especially if there is isolated epidural abscess (no contiguous bony involvement seen). Gram-negative organisms responsible for urinary tract infections are the most common such as *E. coli, Pseudomonas aeruginosa* (also frequent in IV drug abusers), and *Proteus* species.

- Gastrointestinal tract organisms such as *Salmonella* is rare, but the following points should be noted for them:
  - Characteristically associated with hemoglobinopathies like sickle cell disease
  - Have been reported following acute gastroenteritis or cholecystitis
  - Has a tendency to localize in pre-existing diseased tissue
- Anaerobic bacteria are rare (e.g., foreign bodies, open fractures, wound infections, diabetes, or human bites).
- Low-virulence organisms such as coagulase-negative staphylococci and diphtheroids require prolonged incubation times. Infection is characterized by the following:
  - Indolent chronic presentations with delayed diagnosis
  - Frequently seen in elderly patients and those with immunocompromised
- The following must be realized regarding the identification of organisms in bacterial spondylodiskitis:
  - 25% of cultures show no growth.
  - 51% of cultures have one bacterium isolated.
  - 18% of cultures have two bacteria isolated.
  - 8% of cultures show more than two organisms and mixed growth.

Pathophysiology

Classically, there are three routes of pathogen spread:

1. *Hematogenous:* Urinary tract infections and transient bacteremia from genitourinary procedures are the most common sources, followed by soft tissue infections, oral infections, and respiratory tract infections. Pyogenic spondylodiskitis caused by hematogenous spread affects mainly the lumbar spine (58%), followed by thoracic (30%) and cervical (11%). Frequency increases in association with IV drug abuse. Batson's valveless venous plexus (a presumed mechanism of metastatic spine disease) that results in retrograde blood flow from pelvic venous plexus into perivertebral plexus is not considered to play significant role in bacterial hematogenous seeding. In the cervical spine, extensive prevertebral retropharyngeal venous plexus may however act as conduit for spread of infection.
   - Initial hematogenous spread into an adult disk is unlikely because of relative avascularity while a pediatric disk has a much richer vascular supply provided by numerous cartilage canals that end in "cul-de-sacs" without an associated venous outflow (physiological outflow obstruction).
   - Once seeded, the vertebral body metaphysis provides bacteria with a low-flow environment that facilitates direct spread into and across the disk into the adjacent vertebral body.
   - Like the physiological outflow obstruction seen in pediatric patients pathological outflow obstruction can be seen in osteoporotic fractures causing osteomyelitis.
2. *Direct external inoculation:* Direct inoculation is frequently iatrogenic as in discography, postsurgical lumbar procedures, after lumbar puncture or epidural procedures.
3. *Spread from contiguous tissues:* It is rare and may occur in the context of adjacent infection, including esophageal ruptures, retropharyngeal abscesses, or infections of aortic implants.

In children, the intraosseous and diskal arteries have extensive anastomosis. Any septic embolus from hematogenous spread hence will not cause bone infarction, and the infection is located essentially within the disk. The adult intervertebral disk is avascular and undergoes involution around third decade. The septic emboli hence cause formation of extensive infarcts and the infection spreads to adjacent structures producing the classic findings of:

- Erosion of vertebral endplates
- Osteolytic lesions
- *Compression fractures:*
  - Bacterial enzymes digest disk tissue (not ingested by the bacteria themselves)
  - Bone resorption by osteoclasts is activated by various inflammatory mediators (not bacteria specific).

Neurological Involvement

The neurological involvement can occur through a variety of means.

- The above pathological changes lead to spinal instability, deformity, and risk of spinal cord compression.
- The infection can cause paravertebral and psoas abscesses. If the pus spreads into the spinal canal, it can cause epidural abscesses, subdural abscesses, and meningitis causing neurological compromise.
- Neural tissue ischemia secondary to inflammation or septic emboli (rare)
- Spreading to the posterior structures is very rare and occurs more frequently in fungal and TB spondylodiskitis. Superior levels are more prone to developing secondary epidural abscesses and thus more likely to develop neurologic deficits.

Clinical Findings

The diagnosis is often delayed and requires high degree of suspicion. The delay is sometimes responsible for catastrophic outcome.

- Nonspecific back or neck pain are generally the first clinical features. The pain is present in >3 months before presentation in 50% of cases with a mean of 2 months. Pain is, however absent in up to 15% of patients. The pain worsens at night and is often associated with radicular pain.
- Dysphagia and torticollis are symptoms that may be caused by cervical location.
- Fever at presentation (>100°F) is seen in about 60–70% of cases with or without chills, often associated with limited range of motion, positive straight leg raise test or both. Fever of long duration and ill appearance are more common in VPO.
- Cachexia with generalized lymphadenopathy suggests HIV infection.
- The neurologic deficit on examination is seen in 17% of cases. Atypical, nonspecific complaints such as chronic chest pain, abdominal pain, and leg pain are present in 15% of cases.
- In children, a limp and a refusal to walk are characteristically present. Fever is usually absent and the most frequent sign in loss of lumbar lordosis.
- Neurological symptoms such as leg weakness, numbness, and incontinence are present in about one-third of patients.
- Pyogenic vertebral osteomyelitis and infectious endocarditis coexist in a significant number of patients especially if there is gram-positive infection. One should evaluate for symptoms such as new heart murmur, peripheral stigmata, or other metastatic foci and echocardiogram is recommended.

Laboratory Findings

- Erythrocyte sedimentation rate: It is a sensitive marker and elevated at presentation in >80% of cases, the specificity is however low. A 25% reduction of its initial value after 1 month of treatment is a good prognosis marker. In treated patients, ESR drops to at least two-thirds of the original value by the completion of antibiotic therapy.
- C-reactive protein: It is sensitive (elevated in >90% cases) and more specific than ESR for monitoring postoperative spine infections. It is also the best marker for monitoring treatment response.
- White blood cell (WBC) count: WBC count is the least useful of all inflammatory markers due to low sensitivity. The count is elevated *(>10,000/mm3)* in >50% of cases. A mean value of *8,000/mm3* has been reported in one series.
- Erythrocyte sedimentation rate and WBC are higher in the presence of a concomitant epidural abscess.
- Blood cultures: They are highly reliable but positive in only 24–59% of cases. They point the organism and are logical as more than half of the infections are monomicrobial. They are most useful in children. Anaerobic cultures should be obtained along with aerobic cultures as the incidence has risen. Urine cultures are not reliable.
- For definitive diagnosis, microscopic or bacteriological examination of infected tissue is a must. Craig needle is preferable unless there is an abscess. Needle biopsy can be obtained under fluoroscopic guidance or CT-guided biopsy. The latter is more reliable and useful and considered the mainstay in diagnosis with accuracy reported up to 70%. The following points must be noted:
  - Open biopsy is the gold standard for definitive tissue diagnosis. It has higher morbidity than closed biopsy but higher yield rate.
  - Nondiagnostic biopsy is the biggest frustration that may result from insufficient tissue or insufficient experience of pathologist.
  - False-negative examinations can occur when the patient is on antibiotics. It is recommended to specifically obtain prolonged cultures, preferably on liquid culture media.
  - Specimens should be submitted to microbiological analysis, such as Gram smear, aerobic and anaerobic cultures, and fungal and mycobacterial culture.
    - For mycobacterial infections, send the specimen for AFB microscopy and culture, PCR, Xpert® MTB/RIF [*see* Chapter on "Joint Disorders Including Inflammatory and Noninflammatory Arthritis and Infective Arthritides (Including Mycobacterial Infection and Prosthetic Joint Infection)"], and histopathology.
  - Histopathology is ancillary to diagnosis, if mycobacterial infection or tumor lesions are suspected.

Imaging

Imaging is an important ancillary for substantiating clinical diagnosis. A simplified diagnostic algorithm is suggested in **Flowchart 1**.

Plain Radiographs

- X-rays have low specificity in diagnosis. They have poor ability to differentiate pyogenic from nonpyogenic spine infections. The sensitivity is also low as there is a lag behind clinical presentation (at least 2 weeks from the onset of infection).
- Findings in spondylodiskitis include characteristically:
  - Reduction of disk space height with erosive changes (irregularity) in vertebral endplates (74% of cases). There is eventual fragmentation of the endplates.
  - Lytic changes, diffuse osteopenia, or focal defect (50% trabecular bone destruction before radiographic evidence is noted). In contrast, bony sclerosis may be seen in around 10% cases with slow-growing infections. The picture is more often of a lytic-sclerotic change in the vertebral body. This type of infection must raise suspicion of actinomycotic, mycobacterial, brucellar or fungal infection.
  - Involvement of appendiceal processes and posterior elements such as transverse, spinous, or both types of processes (7.5%) and articular processes.
  - Spontaneous bony fusion occurs in about 50% of cases in long-term follow-up.
- One should evaluate the coronal or sagittal balance of spine potential instability and deformity:

Flowchart 1: Management algorithm for vertebral pyogenic osteomyelitis.

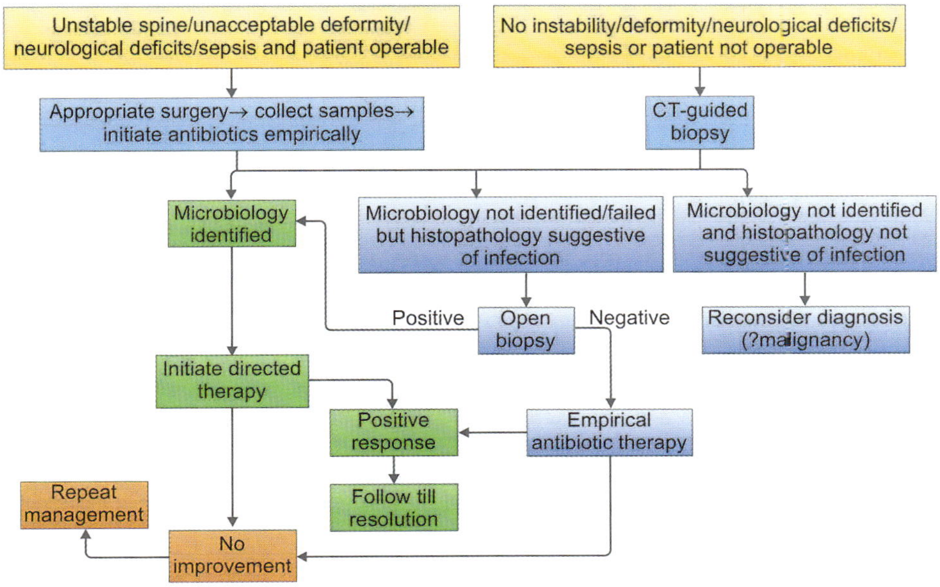

- Loss of height, kyphosis (acute gibbus at infected segment) or "scoliosis" (i.e., lateral angulation)
- Translational instability or lateral listhesis
- In children with VPO, plain films are diagnostic in only half of the cases compared with three-fourth of the cases of isolated diskitis.
- In infants, findings are at the extreme end and exaggerated:
  - Almost complete dissolution of vertebral body
  - Nearly normal adjacent endplates
  - Late findings mimic congenital kyphosis.

Nuclear Scintigraphy

- Good initial screening method to detect and localize the infection earlier than plain films.
- The combination of gallium (inflammatory) and technetium (bone) scans improves accuracy in diagnosis to 94%. The longer the duration of infection the higher are the chances for detection.
- Gallium scans normalize before technetium scans and serve as more useful parameter to monitor treatment response (like CRP vs. ESR) but their use has been demised and only few centers perform the study.
- Indium^{111}-labeled leukocyte (WBC) scans are not sensitive due to relative leukopenia.

Computed Tomography

- Best method for evaluating and quantifying bony changes including defining the early changes, bone necrosis and fragmentation and pathological calcification in abscess that is so pathognomonic of TB.
- It clearly depicts spinal canal compromise and its quantification.
- CT-guided biopsies are mainstay of collecting samples nowadays in this sort of "glamorous" practice of orthopedics.

Magnetic Resonance Imaging

- MRI is the gold standard modality of investigation for spondylodiskitis having high sensitivity (96%), specificity (94%), and greater capacity to provide detailed anatomical information about surrounding soft tissues.
- In children, 90–100% is diagnostic for both VPO and isolated diskitis. The characteristic changes include a hypointense signal of the disk and vertebral body on T1W images and a hyperintense signal of the same structures (due to edema) on T2W images. There is loss of definition of endplate-disk interface with irregular disk margins. There is absence of intranuclear cleft in the involved disk.
- Magnetic resonance imaging can detect and differentiate epidural and paravertebral abscesses.
- It is best to differentiate infection from malignancy, benign tumors, degenerative disk disease, and osteoporotic compression fractures. Contrast enhancement of the intervertebral disk, vertebral body, and surrounding soft tissues increases the accuracy of MRI. The tumor lesions (T1 hypointense relatively to normal bone marrow) are well differentiated from infection-related endplate changes (T2 hypointensity favoring Modic endplate changes)
- MRI plays an important role in the distinction between TB spondylitis and pyogenic spondylodiskitis **(Table 6)**. It should be remembered that due to constantly evolving nature of the disease pathology, there is no single pathognomonic finding that can differentiate infection from neoplastic disease or even between different infection etiologies, so ancillary investigations must be supplemented for strengthening diagnosis and initiating comfortable treatment.
- Follow-up utilization of MRI is futile till recent knowledge goes and use is not recommended to define treatment response as the resolution of MRI changes take much longer (loss of gadolinium uptake or restoration of bone) than "actual" extirpation of disease. The investigation

TABLE 6: MRI findings localizing the different etiological conditions and differentiation from tumors.

Feature	*Pyogenic*	*Tuberculosis*	*Fungal*	*Tumor/metastasis*
Spine segment	Lumbar	Thoracolumbar	Lumbar	Lumbar >thoracic for metastasis but primary thoracic >lumbar
Vertebral body	• Early stage—T1 hypointense and endplate T2 hyperintense • Late stage—vertebral body destruction—T2 hyperintense and homogeneous enhancement, adjacent vertebral body involvement	Early stage—paradiskal (disk involvement and contiguous spread), T1 hypointensity and T2 heterogeneous-hyperintensity. Anterior scalloping of vertebral body Late stage—T1 variable intensity with bone healing	Serrated margins of vertebral endplates without severe vertebral body destruction	• Osteoblastic—iso/hypo on T1 well-defined area of infiltrative edema, hyperintense on T2-weighted images • Osteolytic—hyperintense on T2-weighted images but no contrast enhancement • Lymphoma is not enhanced either in T1 or T2-weighted images • No endplate involvement • Pathological compression fractures—diffuse and complete often
Disk space involvement	Present early especially in children	Variable—from complete and early involvement to preservation till end	Typically spared, no change on T2 images	
Paraspinal and epidural space	Inflammation and small abscess with thick and irregular rim enhancement	Usually large paraspinal abscesses, thin and smooth rim enhancement	Small paraspinal abscesses with thick and loculated pus	Soft tissue masses are eccentric, large well defined and do not have pus pockets
Posterior elements	Typically spared	Can be involved but usually uncommon	Can be involved with rib heads	Pedicle commonly involved and quite characteristically differentiates
Anterior subligamentous spread	Uncommon	Present and common	Common	Not seen
Adjacent vertebral involvement	Present with endplate destruction	Common and conspicuous either in paradiskal form or anterior subligamentous spread	Uncommon	Infrequent
Multilevel involvement	Uncommon	Common—skip lesions	Skip lesions seen	Quite characteristic and most commonly seen

recommended for defining resolution of disease is possibly ^{18}F-FDG-PET in the absence of instrumentation, but cost and availability are limiting factors. In any case, the author has the opinion that a clinician should bank on investigations only if his clinical judgment is clouded else obtaining help form other experienced clinician is the best "modality". Patient should be subjected to radionuclide imaging only if the diagnosis is still uncertain or MRI remains inconclusive.

Differential Diagnosis

Benign: Infection, Scheuermann's disease, trauma, degenerative disease, osteoporotic compression fracture, neuropathic spinal arthropathy, Sarcoidosis, Paget's disease, hyperparathyroidism, benign tumor.

Malignant: Metastatic carcinoma, lymphoproliferative disease, lymphoma, myeloma, primary mesenchymal sarcoma, radiation-induced sarcoma, chondrosarcoma, malignant fibrous histiocytoma.

Treatment Goals

- Establish tissue diagnosis and identity the organism
- Prevent bacteremia and sepsis
- Provide long-term pain relief
- Prevent or relieve neurologic deficits
- Restore spinal stability and near-anatomic alignment

Treatment Principles

There are some principles that need to be followed for all infections and some related to the specific disease being encountered. Infection is a potentially life-threatening condition which if managed well will yield glorifying results; as most people the author believes, in this world take them for granted often complicating the condition by following a nonorganized approach. A simplified algorithm is presented in **Flowchart 1**.

The general treatment principles are:

- Optimization of patient (i.e., improve nutrition and immune response).
- Treat the identified source of infection (e.g., urinary tract, respiratory tract, and gastrointestinal tract).
- Spinal infections are usually not emergencies, so do not start antimicrobial chemotherapy prior to the identification of an organism, few exceptions to the rule are noted here:
  - If biopsy is not possible, nondiagnostic, or negative (but clinical suspicion is high), a full course of broad-spectrum antimicrobial treatment may be initiated.
  - In septic patients, broad-spectrum antimicrobial coverage should be administered immediately following biopsy and until a definitive diagnosis is made, which is then modified according to cultures.
  - Emergencies like rapidly evolving neurological deterioration will mandate antimicrobial administration immediately following promptly performed biopsy.

- IV antibiotics are recommended for 6 weeks followed by oral antibiotics (usually for 6 weeks to 3 months) until resolution (clinically and investigations).
- ESR and CRP levels are not substantiated but often found useful indicators of response to treatment in pyogenic infections (for tuberculous infection, their utility is still very much doubtful to monitor response).
- Immobilization is done for at least 3 months in absence of surgical stabilization.
- Nonoperative management can generally control infection, but surgery may be more effective in preventing neurologic deficit, instability, kyphosis, and chronic pain (26% vs. 64% with residual back pain for operative and nonoperative treatment, respectively).

The specific treatment principles are:

- Eradication of the underlying infection
- Early debridement and decompression of the spinal canal in the presence of neurological complications
- Stabilization of the affected segment to preserve or restore the spinal structure and stability

Conservative Management

This consists of antibiotic treatment as above and brace immobilization. The indications are patients at high risk for surgery, patients with no neurological deficits or those completely paralyzed for >72 hours. The more caudal lesions like thoracolumbar and lumbar respond better to conservative management unless operative indications exist (see here). Strict monitoring should be done however, and any worsening neurology or symptoms should be promptly responded.

Surgical Management

Indications

- Open biopsy—sample harvesting for microbiological and histological analysis when closed biopsy is nondiagnostic or negative (but there is high clinical suspicion)
- Neurological deficit attributable to the infection
- Decompression of a clinically significant abscess or granuloma
- Cases that have failed on conservative management
- Septic complications and failure to thrive
- Extensive bone destruction, progressive deformity or instability
- *Relative indications:*
    - Intractable pain not responsive to conservative measures
    - Presence of epidural abscess especially in cervical or thoracic region

Operative Principles

The surgical strategy is controversial and as such any standard surgical approach is sufficient. There is however a definite modifier in the form of neurological deficit that modifies the surgical exposure. The relative indications of different approaches are given in **Box 3**.

BOX 3: The various approaches used for surgical exposure of spine in tubercular disease.

Anterior approach is the most useful for:
- Vertebral body debridement (corpectomy) and reconstruction of anterior column support
- Decompression of the spinal canal, if offending elements are anterior (most cases)
- Cervical spine infections are mostly managed by anterior approach
- Thoracic spine—anterior approach (transthoracic, posterolateral, or thoracoscopic) is reserved for monosegmental lesions without involvement of posterior elements. Also in advanced bone destruction, it is recommended that anterior decompression and stabilization is done along with posterior stabilization
- To reconstruct the anterior column, either autogenous bone grafting (e.g., iliac crest, rib, or fibula) is used or even implanting metal (Cage) ± auto/allograft can be used. There are concerns of using metal in the presence of infection, but the results have not demonstrated any ill-effect of metal or persistence of infection in these cases provided adequate debridement and excision of focus is done. Fusion rates have been improved with the advent of bone morphogenetic proteins-2 (BMP-2).

Posterior fusion and instrumentation following anterior surgery (staged, 1–2 weeks) is indicated in:
- Thoracic spine with extensive bony destruction and kyphotic deformity
- Cases with multilevel disease requiring debridement or corpectomy
- Thoracolumbar lesions

Posterior approach only:
- In cervical spine, if the involvement is only epidural without body involvement
- Thoracic spine with preserved vertebral body and disk spaces when the involvement is mainly epidural
- Thoracolumbar region—posterior lumbar interbody fusion (PLIF) is recommended if there is moderate anterior bone involvement and minimal kyphosis deformity

- Thoracic and lumbar VPO are quite often successfully treated by combined debridement and internal fixation using only a posterior approach (either staged or as a single procedure).
- Laminectomy only as a procedure is generally contraindicated because it further destabilizes the spine.

Prognosis and Outcomes

Poor outcomes after pyogenic spinal infection have been reported with the following factors:

- *Elderly population or infection in infancy. In the infant, pyogenic spinal infection:*
    - There is poor prognosis and high recurrence rate.
    - Late radiographic appearance similar to congenital kyphosis
- Cervical or thoracic involvement, i.e., higher level of involvement. Somehow, the lower spinal levels respond favorably for unknown reasons.
- Medical comorbidities such as diabetes mellitus, rheumatoid arthritis or chronic heart disease
- Presence of paralysis or bowel/bladder involvement at presentation
- Delayed diagnosis—this is the most detrimental reason for neurological complication and their recovery.
- MRSA infection or other virulent infections. The author has found infection with gram-negative bacilli particularly difficult to treat somehow.
- Surgical time of >36 hours
- Immunocompromised patients. Surprisingly, vertebral osteomyelitis in IV drug abusers has an excellent prognosis.

- Neurologic recovery rates are higher with anterior than with posterior decompression.
- Residual deformity or instability is more common in the thoracic spine, in the thoracolumbar junction, and in cases with >50% destruction of the vertebral body.

PYOGENIC EPIDURAL ABSCESS

Epidemiology

These are most common in adults and adolescents. Incidence is 0.2–1.2 per 10,000 hospital admissions. Postoperative epidural abscesses represent 16% of all epidural abscesses. Nearly two-thirds have an identifiable source. Skin and soft tissue infections are the source in 21% cases. Thoracic involvement is seen in 51%, lumbar in 35%, and cervical in 14% (posterior 79%, and anterior 21%). Neurologic deficits are most common in the thoracic region.

Etiology

The most common association is with pyogenic spinal infections. The abscess may develop from:

- Hematogenous
- Contiguous spread, or
- Direct inoculation (usually iatrogenic)

Staphylococcus aureus is the organism responsible in about 60% of cases, gram-negative bacilli in 18% of cases. IV drug abusers may have infection with atypical and fungal organisms.

Clinical Presentation

The abscess develops from local spinal pain to radicular pain to weakness and finally paralysis. The clinical features are highly variable causing misdiagnosis and delayed treatment. Complaints depend on acuity of presentation.

The typical progression path of symptoms in terms of increasing severity and disease progression are:

- Fever
- Malaise
- Back pain
- Radiculopathy/paresis
- Bladder/bowel involvement
- Paralysis/plegia
- Sepsis/mental status change

Localized spine-tenderness often presents along with localized pain. Nuchal rigidity and other meningeal-type signs are also possible, depending on location of disease and its stage. Neurological deficit is usually late to come but may present suddenly.

Laboratory Evaluation

- Erythrocyte sedimentation rate—elevated in 100% of cases along with CRP, WBC counts are nonreliable.
- Drainage of abscess percutaneously (may be ultrasound guidance) reveals material in majority of cases that can be used to make bacteriological diagnosis.
- Blood cultures are positive and diagnostic in 60% of cases.
- Cerebrospinal fluid analysis may be done if there are meningeal signs.

Imaging

Without bony involvement, X-rays and even nuclear medicine studies are negative. MRI is the imaging modality of choice. MRI findings include a homogeneous-hyperintense signal on T2 representing the region involved which pathologically represents the granulomatous thickened tissue with embedded microabscesses without a significant pus collection (phlegmon). In other cases, there is a liquid abscess surrounded by inflammatory tissue which shows peripheral enhancement with gadolinium.

Treatment

Epidural abscess is a surgical urgency particularly of the cervical and thoracic spine. Also an epidural abscess in the presence of a worsening neurologic deficit is a surgical emergency. Bony involvement if present should be managed on lines of pyogenic spinal infection as above. Conservative management is practiced if:

- Comorbidities endanger the patient's life.
- There is absence of any neurologic deficits or signs when an epidural abscess is present in the lumbar spine.

Antibiotic Therapy

It is a must and patient is immediately put on broad-spectrum IV antibiotic therapy immediately after the culture specimen is obtained. In completely paralyzed patients for >72 hours or those unfit for surgical management, broad-spectrum antibiotic is started without culture. Gram-negative coverage should be added routinely but more so importantly for those with IV drug abuse. Antibiotics are usually given for 2–4 weeks after drainage or 6 weeks with concomitant pyogenic vertebral infection or diskitis followed by 6 weeks to 3 months of oral antibiotics.

Prognosis

If managed urgently, 78% of patients with either acute or chronic epidural abscesses have full or near full recovery. Poor prognosis is seen in patients with:

- Advanced age >60 years
- Complete paralysis for >72 hours
- Complete paraplegia within the first 12 hours
- Thecal sac compression >50%
- Complete sensory loss
- Comorbid conditions such as diabetes, renal or hepatic disease
- Immunocompromised patients
- Associated vertebral infection

CONCLUSION

- Infections of spine are a worrisome disease as they threaten the neural axis of the body.
- Tuberculosis of spine is the most common infection encountered in Indian subcontinent causing great morbidity if not treated early and even mortality in some cases.
- The treatment is mainly based on chemotherapy but for complications surgical treatment is often added.
- The nontubercular vertebral osteomyelitis or diskitis has varied etiology as is the flora for epidural abscess. The pathologies are fast to develop and produce rapid changes unless managed early so treatment comprises mainly eradicating the infection and debridement of the lesion.

CHAPTER 106

Miscellaneous Disorders (Vertebra Plana, CT-guided Biopsy, and Intervertebral Disk Calcification)

Manish Kumar Varshney

VERTEBRA PLANA

INTRODUCTION

"*Vertebra plana*" (platyspondyly, pancake vertebra, and Calves disease) is a radiological descriptive term for a vertebral body that has lost almost its entire height anteriorly and posteriorly so much, so that the two endplates approximate closely forming a plane rather than a rectangular disposition. Vertebra plana first became known as an entity in 1924 when Calve described it at the meeting of the British Orthopedic Association. Not many causes of this radiological finding were known then, hence, it was attributed to osteochondroses of vertebral body. Now the radiological feature of flattened vertebral body can be found in a variety of diseases including:

- Severe trauma that is an equivalent burst fracture and the body collapses altogether venting the cancellous bone anteriorly or causing its compaction.
- Osteoporosis—flattened architecture in this setting could be found at multiple levels.
- Eosinophilic granuloma—this is the classical diagnosis attached and the most common differential for nontraumatic platyspondyly.
- Osteogenesis imperfecta—the cause is similar to osteoporosis due to poor quality of bone that crumbles under axial body pressure.
- Vertebral metastases—lytic metastasis eats away the bony architecture that gets replaced by pathological neoplastic tissue and gets crushed under body weight or minor trauma. This can be seen at multiple levels.
- Hyperparathyroidism
- Injury in tetanus (very rare, now almost nonexistent)
- Osteonecrosis (vascular necrosis, pseudarthrosis, Kummell's spondylitis)—histologically there is necrotic granulation and fatty degeneration of the bone tissue, with a fibrocartilaginous membrane surrounding the fluid and absence of any new endochondral bone. The disease may be a harbinger of infection, liver cirrhosis, prolonged steroid treatment, sickle cell anemia, and Caisson's disease. It may also develop after trauma where the anterior vessels get injured. Magnetic resonance imaging (MRI) shows a dark zone on T1-weighted and a bright area on T2-weighted or short-tau inversion recovery images.
- *Bone infections:*
  - Osteomyelitis—infection weakens the bone primarily and also causes osteopenia.
  - Spinal tuberculosis—in advanced stage of spinal tuberculosis the vertebral body crumbles into a flattened structure and even may get completely absorbed if the infection is unchecked.
- *Primary neoplastic affections of bone:*
  - Multiple myeloma
  - Lymphoma (Hodgkin's)/leukemia
  - Vertebral hemangioma
  - Aneurysmal bone cyst (rare case described in literature)

FEATURES AND DIAGNOSIS

In about a third of the cases, there has been history of sudden onset; in the remainder the onset has been gradual. The speed of development of flat architecture probably directly related to the nature of underlying disease. There is no "idiopathic" cause and all cases have a primary diagnosis for this radiological aberration. Biopsy of the lesion is the most accurate way to diagnose the underlying disease.

RADIOLOGICAL FEATURES

Plain radiographs: The vertebral body characteristically has a flat structure on lateral films **(Figs. 1 and 2)**. The plain structure is often radiodense due to compaction of the cancellous bone. On an anteroposterior projection, there is approximation of the pedicles of the vertebra above and below the involved segment. Quite often a fusiform swelling is seen around the diseased vertebra possibly representing the disease component (pus in infection and soft-tissue extension in metastasis or primary neoplasms) and subtle increase in density can be due to nesting of soft tissues around the deformity. In Kummell's spondylitis, the radiographs (or better CT scan) show intervertebral cleft or "gas sign".

Magnetic resonance imaging: This is the investigation of choice particularly helpful in ruling out marrow abnormalities

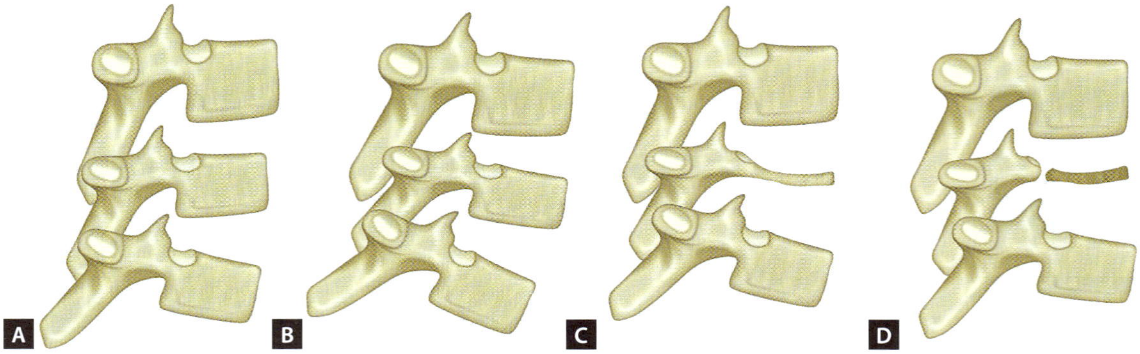

Figs. 1A to D: Illustration of appearance of vertebra plana on a lateral projection of spine. (A) Normal vertebral height; (B) Concentric compaction of bone with reduced height; (C) Concentric vertebra plana; (D) Vertebra plana with body and posterior elements disjunction.

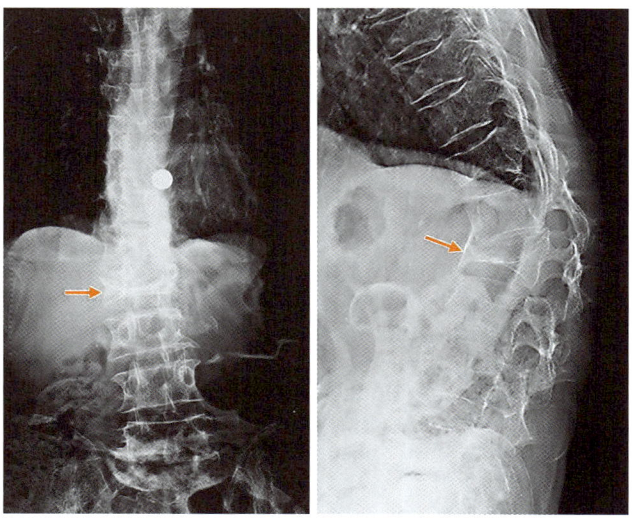

Fig. 2: Osteoporotic vertebra plana (arrow).

(lymphoma), finding multiple associated lesions (metastasis and tuberculosis), and defining the adjacent soft-tissue swelling (neoplasms, metastasis, and infection), by typical T1, T2, and STIR image findings. So, it quite plausibly hints at the probable diagnosis for which additional investigations can be done, e.g., PET scan for metastasis, hematological and other evaluation for finding the primary, substantiating tuberculosis by ancillary investigations, etc. The findings on MRI that suggest tubercular affection in a case of vertebra plana include:

- Signal intensity of the epidural soft-tissue mass on axial images, which is different from the vertebral body
- Presence of a thin, T2-weighted hypointense capsule of the paravertebral soft tissue
- Posterior element involvement characterized by intact hypointense cortical outline without expansion
- Involvement of the costovertebral joint

MANAGEMENT

The management is as per the primary disease. Once the primary disease is controlled and the patient has residual symptoms or deformity that he wishes to correct, reformation procedures like balloon kyphoplasty may be undertaken. It had been quite a concern as to difficult localization of the space for insertion of balloon, but a few authors have described the procedure in patients. The procedure is particularly amenable for metabolic causes of vertebra plana such as osteoporosis, trauma, and metastasis. The typical indications and timing of balloon kyphoplasty in osteoporosis is presented in **Flowchart 1**. It readily corrects the deformity and gives good pain relief. Balloon kyphoplasty applies the principles of balloon angioplasty to vertebroplasty. It was primarily devised for the treatment of osteoporotic vertebral compression fractures, and subsequently used in the treatment of metastatic osteolytic tumors.

Flowchart 1: Management of osteoporotic vertebral fracture with respect to kyphoplasty.

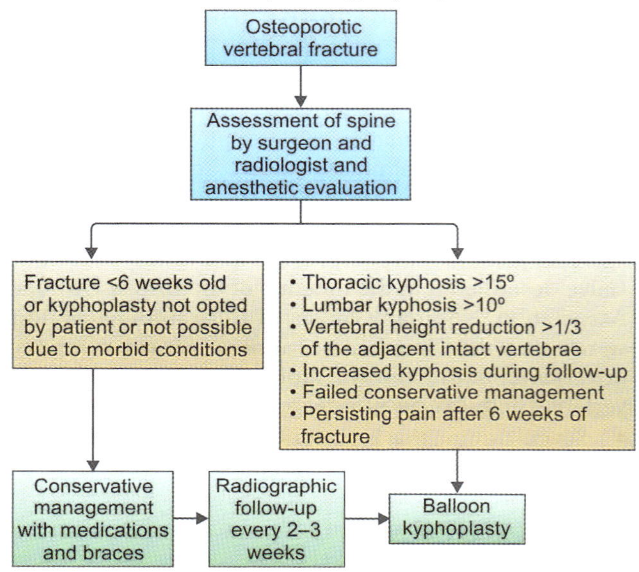

When osteonecrosis or pseudarthrosis is evident with vertebra plana, vertebroplasty is considered a more suitable option. Percutaneous vertebroplasty (**Figs. 3A to I**) was designed and introduced for the management of osteolytic tumors and later was successfully applied to osteoporotic vertebral compression fractures. It had been observed in a meta-analysis (Jason et al., 2008) that the vertebroplasty offered greater pain relief but also had higher incidence of

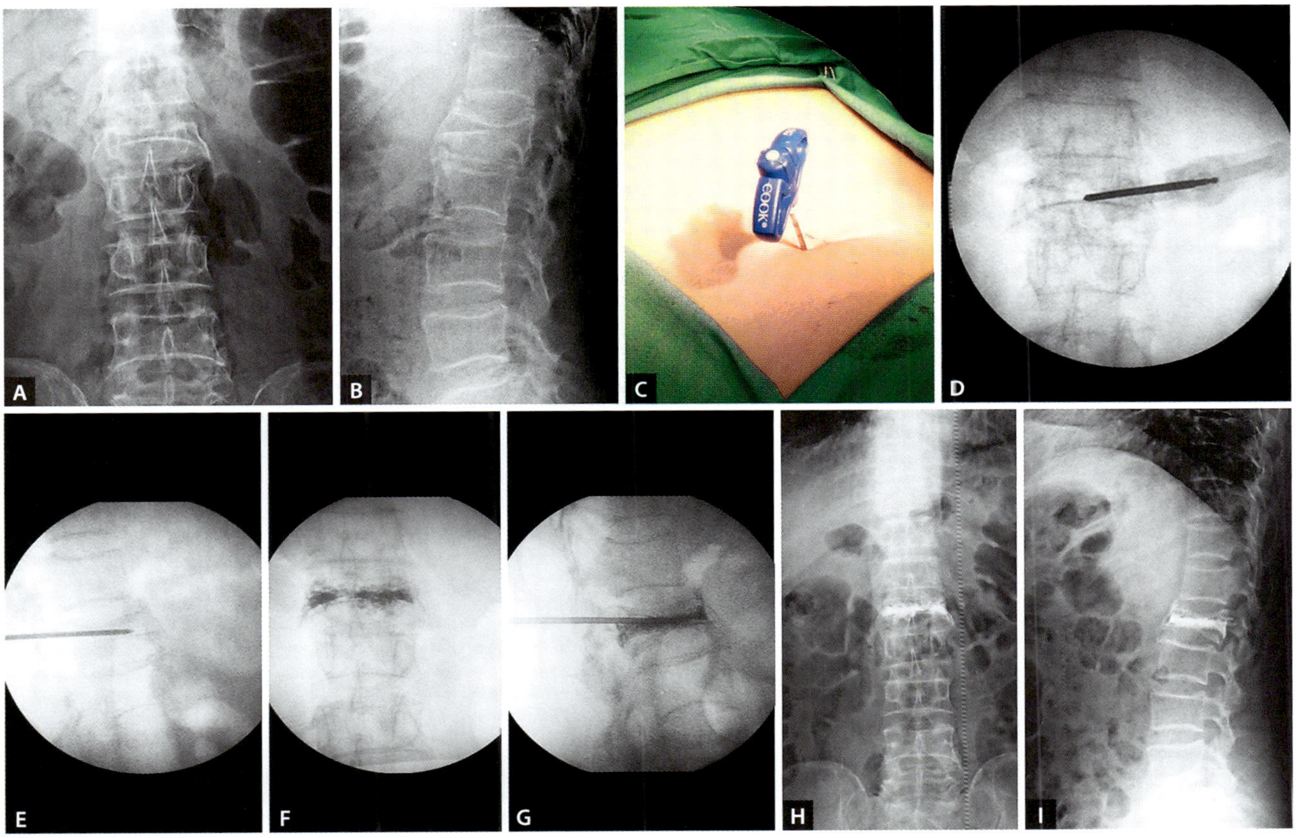

Figs. 3A to I: Vertebroplasty. (A and B) The patient with collapsed first lumbar vertebral body; (B) Placing the trephine biopsy needle; (C) Checking the ideal position in AP; (D and E) Lateral fluoroscopies (just across the midline and just ventral to the sagittal plane of vertebral body); (F and G) Injecting the cement; (H and I) Final radiographic pictures.

complications particularly with respect to cement leakage and new fractures. Possibly kyphoplasty may be safer in this regard and also restores the vertebral height much better.

Procedure of Balloon Kyphoplasty (Figs. 4A to N)

The aim is to restore the vertebral height as close to normal as possible and ameliorate deformity and related symptoms/ complications. The steps of the procedure are as follows:

- In a prone position, mark the vertebral level under fluoroscope.
- Using a 13-gauge needle (or other requisite instrument provided) puncture the pedicle region of the vertebra under C-arm control. Two C-arms in perpendicular planes are needed or better use an O-arm.
- Push the awl/provided introducer to make tract for balloon in the posterior part of vertebral body, through each pedicle
- Introduce the balloons of appropriate length into the created tract (usually 15 mm for upper thoracic region and 20 mm for lower thoracic and lumbar vertebra).
- In the lumbar region, lateral pedicular approach is preferred instead of transpedicular approach as used for thoracic region.
- Inflate the balloons according to the instructions for specific manufacturers (maximum 400 psi usually) using contrast medium.
- Once satisfactory "inflation" of the vertebral body is obtained, remove the balloons and inject liquid cement under low pressure through the same tract.
- To prevent collapse after balloon removal, it is recommended to keep one balloon inflated while injecting the other space (the technique of "maximum fracture reduction").

Advantages of Balloon Kyphoplasty

- Percutaneous (minimally invasive)
- Restores the vertebral height to a greater extent than vertebroplasty
- Much less chances of cement leakage compared to vertebroplasty
- Quicker recovery compared to open procedures and improved quality of life
- Reduced hospital stay

Complications of Balloon Kyphoplasty

- Cement leakage
- Pulmonary embolism and stroke
- Rib and sternal fractures
- Recollapse and loss of vertebral height after balloon deflation
- Late displacement of the cement mass

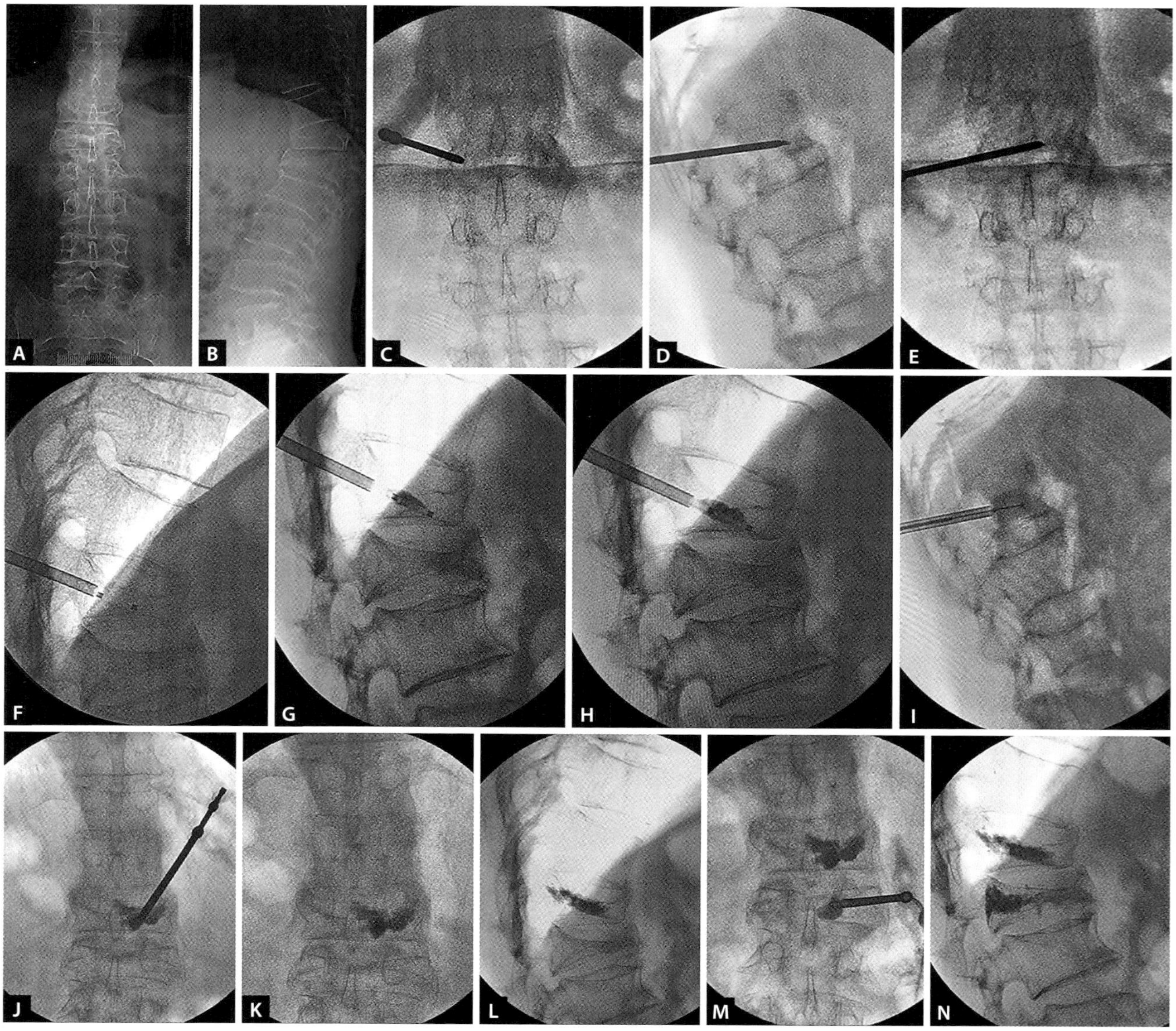

Figs. 4A to N: The procedural steps of kyphoplasty. The patient is having osteoporotic compression fracture of dorsal 12th and 1st lumbar vertebral body with painful gibbus deformity (A and B). The site for cannula entry at pedicle is marked in posteroanterior (C) and lateral (D) projections and the Jamshidi-type needle is progressed in the vertebral body targeting its center (E). After removal of trocar the balloon is passed so that its markers are well beyond the tip of cannula (F). Gradual inflation of the balloon is begun (G and H) to elevate the endplate of vertebral body (I) and create space for cement by compacting the bone. The pressure is monitored in the pressure gauge and should not exceed the inflation limit of system. Usually during gradual inflation one needs to stop intermittently so that the bone gets compacted and the pressure drops rather than single continuous inflation process. The cement is prepared and injected into the cannula using provided cement pusher (J) to fill the created void and confirmed in perpendicular views (K and L). The process is repeated for the 1st lumbar vertebra (M and N).

- Endplate fracture from balloon inflation
- Balloon rupture
- Spinal cord damage (faulty procedure or cement leakage into canal)
- Transient hyperalgesia
- *General complications:*
  - Infection
  - Scar tenderness
  - Bleeding and abandoning the procedure
  - Deep vein thrombosis (DVT)

COMPUTED TOMOGRAPHY-GUIDED BIOPSY

CT-guided biopsy is one form of image-guided biopsy. It is an interventional procedure which involves the insertion of a biopsy needle into the body under CT control in order to collect a tissue sample from the area of interest. It is overall less commonly used than ultrasound-guided biopsy, however, in some anatomical areas it has greater precedence especially lung and bone biopsies (others are kidney, liver mesenteric lymph nodes, etc.). It requires good teamwork with radiographic staff as it is not truly dynamic like ultrasound-guided biopsies. CT permits visualization of the inner structures of the human body. CT biopsies are usually performed using a coaxial needle technique to gain a stable position through which the biopsy may be performed. Most biopsies are performed to confirm that a mass is malignant and determine the specific type of tumor, so that appropriate therapy can be started. The other common indication is to evaluate the presence of infection and its type (viz., tubercular versus pyogenic). We will restrict the description below in orthopedic context of spine biopsy.

HISTORICAL PERSPECTIVE

Open biopsies had been the gold standard for two reasons—it permits biopsy under direct vision and multiple larger samples can be taken and secondly, it permits additional surgical procedures such as decompression and stabilization. The first percutaneous spine biopsy was performed by Robertson and Ball in 1935. This was performed without image guidance. The first image-guided (radiography-guided) procedure was possibly done by Siffert and Arkin using posterolateral approach. This was followed by fluoroscopy-guided spine biopsy in 1969 (Ottolenghi CE) and then CT-guided procedure (Adapton et al.) in 1981.

ADVANTAGES OF PERCUTANEOUS SPINE BIOPSY

- Faster
- More cost-effective
- Less morbidity
- Minimal hospital stay
- Overall less complications (bleeding, infection), etc.

INDICATIONS OF SPINE BIOPSY

Spine biopsy is often performed to evaluate destructive or space occupying lesions within the spinal axis. The common indications are:

- Suspected secondary spine tumor (i.e., metastasis) with either a known or an unknown primary tumor
- Suspected secondary spine tumor with a history of two or more pre-existing primary tumors
- Suspected primary spine or paraspinal tumor
- Pathological compression fracture
- Suspected infectious spondylitis
- Suspected inflammatory condition that involves the spine.

PROCEDURE DETAILS

Patient Preparation

- Nothing by mouth (NPO) for 8–10 hours
- Obtain hematocrit, hemoglobin, platelet count, prothrombin time (PT), partial thromboplastin time (PTT), International Normalized Ratio (INR), blood urea nitrogen (BUN), and creatinine. Give proper correction preoperative for any deficiency like platelet-rich plasma/single donor platelets (PRP/SDP), vitamin-K, etc., renal function-guided postoperative pain management by avoiding nonsteroidal anti-inflammatory drugs (NSAIDs) and giving renal sparing antibiotics.
- Platelet function antagonist drugs, such as clopidogrel, should be stopped minimum 7 days before the procedure. Aspirin® (Acetylsalicylic acid) should be stopped for 48 hours before the procedure.

Steps of CT-guided Spinal Biopsy

- The procedure is performed in prone position for thoracic/lumbosacral spine or supine for cervical spine in either a combination of local anesthesia and conscious sedation (benzodiazepines) or general anesthesia. If the patient cannot lie completely prone than a lateral decubitus position is chosen.
- Secure an intravenous line.
- Monitor patient for pulse rate, BP, O_2 saturation and electrocardiogram (ECG) (a digital monitor is the best).
- A CT-guided spine biopsy can be performed without or with the use of a stereotactic apparatus to guide the insertion of the biopsy needle. The CT scan gives approximate dimensions to entry point also that can be marked. It is better to however use standard radiopaque markers instead for making exact entry point.
    - Aspiration biopsy is performed with a 22- or 20-gauge stylet-bearing needle.
    - Core biopsy is performed with a trephine or beveled tip (usually 11-, 12-, or 14-gauge) bone biopsy needle or a soft-tissue-cutting needle (usually 18-gauge).
- There are two basic ways of doing CT-guided biopsy:
    - ***Tandem needle technique***: The biopsy needle is used along with the anesthesia needle. In a simultaneous tandem system, the biopsy needle is placed parallel alongside the anesthesia needle that was previously placed to anesthetize the biopsy tract. In a sequential tandem method, the biopsy needle is advanced along a tract previously created by the smaller anesthetizing needle.
    - ***Coaxial needle systems (more popular):*** The biopsy needle is advanced over the anesthetizing and localizing needle (long spinal needle usually, 22-gauge) that serves as a mechanical guide for the biopsy needle. A guiding cannula is left in place through which biopsy is taken. This method is particularly important for difficult to access places like cervical spine. They decrease procedure time, improve accuracy, and reduce procedure complications. A single biopsy tract avoids the risk of additional soft-tissue structure injury with a second pass. Fine-needle aspiration cytology (FNAC) can be done prior to trucut biopsy through the cannula. It is preferable to use an 18-gauge spring-loaded biopsy needle to obtain soft-tissue cores. Bone biopsy can be obtained by Craig, Ackerman, Jamshidi or similar needles commercially available.
    - Two or preferably three core specimens are obtained and placed in 10% formalin. Bone biopsy cores are kept for decalcification in 7% formic acid for a period (approximately 48 hours). The specimen is then embedded and embedded in paraffin for subsequent histological sectioning and staining. The reported diagnostic accuracy of core biopsy ranges from 77 to 97%.

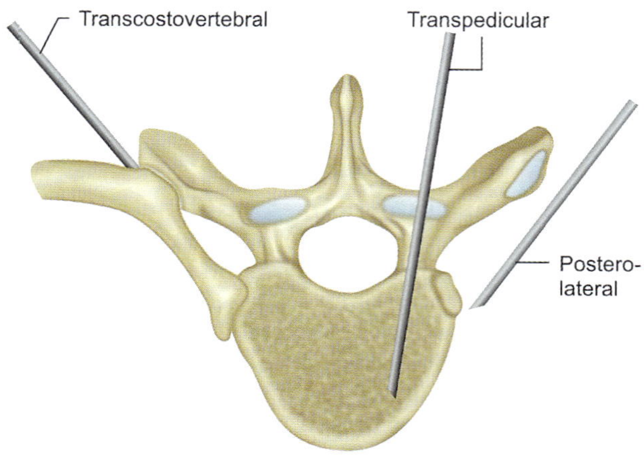

Fig. 5: The biopsy routes for the posterolateral, transpedicular, and transcostovertebral approaches.

Choice of Approach

The choice is guided by the location of lesion and its size.

- For bone biopsy paraspinal oblique approach is the best. Transpedicular and transcostovertebral approaches (**Fig. 5**) are preferred for thoracic spine. Lumbar spine is approached commonly through posterolateral approach (**Fig. 5**) as the pedicles are more straight and do not allow ready access to the vertebral body easily without risking the medial wall. Cervical spine is best approached anterolaterally in supine position. There is a higher possibility of false negative reports in transpedicular biopsies especially if the trocar has been removed too early. The best way here is to remove the trocar once deep enough tissue that represents the pathology has been reached, and take multiple samples. Slightly rock the biopsy needle to dismantle the core and let it carry with the needle. For cervical lesions, the neck is divided into supra and infrahyoid regions and the entry point is decided based on the relative position of the lesion with respect to the carotid vascular bundle.
    - ***Intervertebral disk***—the usual approach is the paraspinal oblique posterolateral for thoracic or lumbar spine. Cervical disks are best as usual approached through the anterolateral approach.
    - Soft tissues around bone—use posterolateral approach for thoracic or lumbar region while anterolateral approach for cervical spine.

Postoperative Care

Close the wound with a single 3-0 nylon stitch. Apply sterile dressing. Observe the site of bleeding. Keep the patient in recovery for type of anesthesia given.

CAUSES OF FALSE NEGATIVE BIOPSIES

- Biopsied core left in situ and does not withdraw with the needle—it is advised to rock the needle to break the core from parent bone, so that it becomes loose enough to carry with the needle. Most modern needles have a truncated tip that is slightly smaller than the needle. This traps the core and helps its extraction. The other method is to use a syringe (20 mL) and apply suction at the hub while extracting the sample core.
- Small lesion—it is better to increase the number of needle passes.
- Hypervascular lesion—increased bleeding and too fragile tissue that can be carried with the needle. Here, prefer FNAC. Submit the intraosseous blood always for histopathological examination as malignancy can be still diagnosed from the trapped cells within.
- Lesion identified on MRI and biopsied using CT scan assistance—in this case—the lesion may not be that prominent and might get missed. It would be better to perform MR-guided biopsy (too cumbersome) or open biopsy.
- In cases of infection—often the patient is already put on empirical therapy and the tissue would be sterile resulting in a negative biopsy.
- Calcified intervertebral disk—for biopsies from intervertebral disk the pathologist or the surgeon might be unable to negotiate through the disk.

COMPLICATIONS OF SPINAL BIOPSY

- Active hemorrhage—coagulopathy, renal, or thyroid metastasis
- Deep hematoma formation (viz., retroperitoneal hematoma)
- Vascular injury
- Neural injury (spinal cord or nerve) resulting in transient or permanent paralysis
- Pneumothorax, hemothorax, and hemoperitoneum
- Infection, including meningitis
- Tumor implantation/seeding, infection spread along the needle tract

INTERVERTEBRAL DISK CALCIFICATION

Intervertebral disk is normally a noncalcified structure composed of annulosus fibrosus on the outside and nucleus pulposus inside. Though an interesting finding on radiology, it is not usually associated with clinically significant findings. Still, however, it is a harbinger of many diseases that can be characterized on this finding of intervertebral disk calcification (IVDC). The first description of intervertebral disk calcification in adults has been attributed to von Luschka (Sandstrom 1951). Pediatric IVDC was first described by Baron in 1924. Calcification is thought to be related to developmental changes in the nucleus pulposus. Most patients are asymptomatic while a few would develop pain, stiffness, torticollis, reduced movements of the spine and hemogram abnormalities such as raised erythrocyte sedimentation rate (ESR) and total leukocyte count (TLC). The symptoms in children are caused only in patients with herniation of the calcified material anteriorly into the prevertebral soft tissue or posteriorly into the spinal canal. Containment of the calcified material is usually clinically benign and nonsignificant. Incidence of disk herniation is >30% in patients with symptomatic IVDC while asymptomatic patients have almost

BOX 1: The variously reported causes of intervertebral disk calcification [the common occurrence in pediatric (P) or adult (A) age group is indicated simultaneously].

- *Degenerative (A):* Relatively common and may occur in up to 6% in routine abdominal radiographs in adults.
- *Ochronosis (P, A):* Very dense central (nucleus pulposus) calcification associated with osteopenia. First appears in lumbar spine and ascends to thoracic spine.
- Transient intervertebral disk calcification (P) is seen in children, typically in the cervical spine and often spontaneously regresses.
- *Ankylosing spondylitis (A):* Associated findings should be visible.
- *Pseudogout [calcium pyrophosphate deposition disease (CPPD), A]:* Annulus fibrosis calcification
- Postoperative/traumatic (A)
- *Hemochromatosis (A):* Annulus fibrosis calcification
- *Hypervitaminosis D (P, A):* Annulus fibrosis calcification (uncommon manifestation)
- Juvenile chronic arthritis (JCA) (P)
- Amyloidosis (P, A)
- Poliomyelitis (P, A)
- Acromegaly (A)
- Hyperparathyroidism (P, A)

always no herniation. In any case neurological deficits are rarely if ever reported, instead anterior herniation may lead to dysphagia and posterior herniation can lead to neurological deficits or radicular pain. Contained IVDC in adults can be symptomatic especially pain with activity (see below).

The various causes of IVDC are presented in **Box 1**.

Imaging

In children, plain radiographs in pediatric IVDC show calcified round or ovoid masses within the disk space. CT better demonstrates the extent of calcification. The height of disk space is usually maintained. MRI is particularly useful to evaluate the extent of herniation and the effect on spinal cord. It shows pathological areas as hypointense lesions on T1- and T2-weighted images.

Natural History

In children, intervertebral disk calcification is seen mostly in boys between the ages of 6 and 10 years. More than 50% patients are symptom free within 3 weeks and 95% within 6 months. Radiological resorption of pediatric intervertebral calcification is usually seen within 3 months and no later than 6 months. Surgical management is needed only in cases which fail on conservative management or have severe sensorimotor symptoms to begin with.

In adults, the upper lumbar and lower thoracic spine are the most common sites of IVDC as against cervical disks in children. The deposits in adults are permanent which is also in contrast to IVDC in children. The cause of pain in adults is possibly related not to herniation of the material rather possibly the hydrophilic properties of the calcified material produce a rise in the pressure within the disks and cause pain. This pain, however, quickly resolves without radiological resolution.

Treatment

In children: Conservative and surgical in only selected cases (rare).

In adults: Conservative management is successful in most comprising analgesics, rest, cervical collar or thoracolumbosacral orthosis (TLSO) brace. Cervical traction may help in a few. Sports should be restricted till resolution of pain. Prognosis is very good, however, the patient should be counseled and explained for the possibility of degenerative spine disease later that may need surgical management (like fusion).

CONCLUSION

- Collapse of vertebral body commonly occurs in osteoporosis and also in some other pathologies.
- Vertebroplasty and kyphoplasty are commonly performed procedures to prevent further collapse and restore the vertebral height.
- Vertebrae are a common site for metastatic bony disease and obtaining specimen from them is a good method for making diagnosis.
- Intervertebral disk calcification is usually a benign pathology that is commonly a manifestation of disorder elsewhere and rarely if ever needs medical or surgical treatment.

SECTION

11

Regional Orthopedics: Hand and Upper Extremity (Except Shoulder)

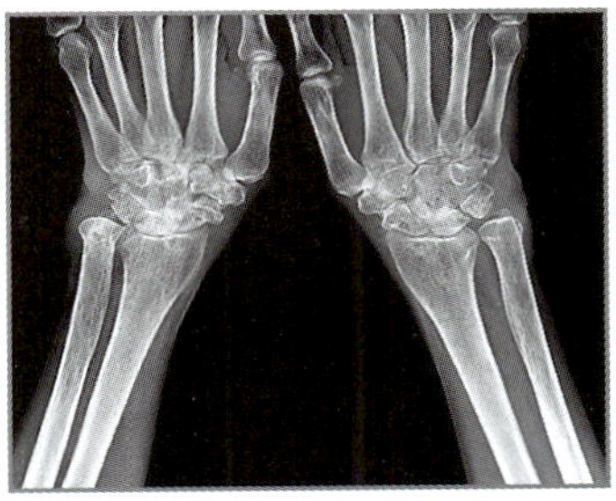

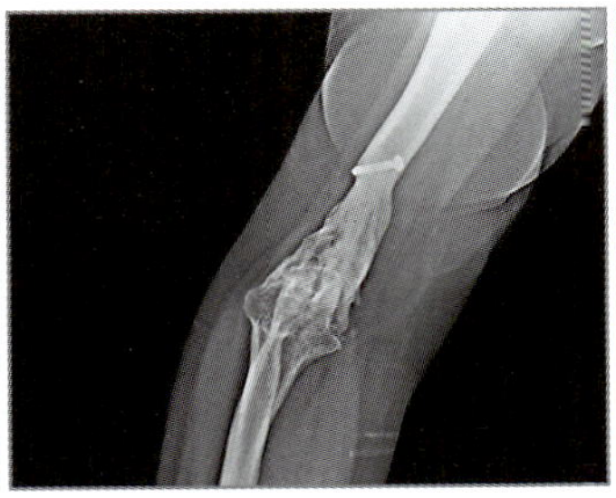

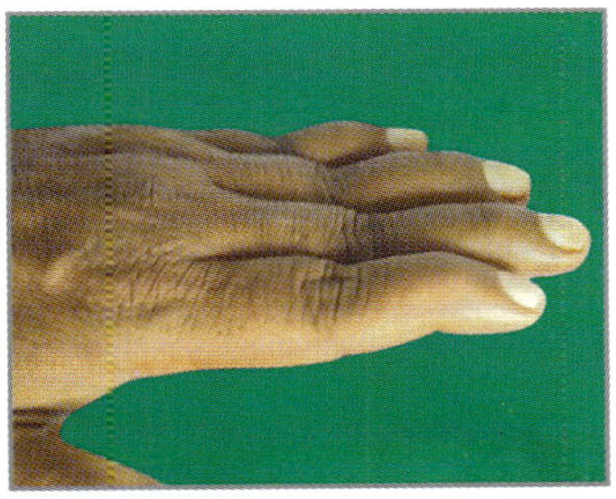

CHAPTER 107

Elbow Anatomy and Biomechanics

Manish Kumar Varshney

INTRODUCTION

Elbow is a unique complex articulation that is vulnerable to injuries being superficial in location and subjected to large lever arm forces on each side. It is a compound synovial joint formed by articulation of humerus, ulna, and radius. While the humeroulnar joint has some degree of congruence and bony constraint, the humeroradial articulation is primarily supported by ligamentous structures. The ligaments and musculotendinous structures are frequently subjected to repetitive strain and injuries producing various enthesopathies and overload syndromes especially in sports persons. It is pivotal to understand the anatomy of ligaments and their correct disposition with respect to underlying bones that helps to recreate the isometricity so important in reconstructions else stiffness and loss of movements is bound to happen. The bones around elbow has various ossification centers that also make the joint vulnerable to growth disorders in pediatric age group.

BONY ANATOMY

The elbow is a compound hinge joint **(Fig. 1)** better called as trochoginglymoid joint specifically having following articulations:

- Humeroulnar articulation is a hinge (ginglymus) joint and is the chief determinant of osseous stability.
- Humeroradial articulation is a gliding articulation that is more stable in extreme flexion and extension. It provides support to valgus strain.
- Radioulnar articulation is a pivot (trochoid) joint that plays a major role in supination and pronation of forearm rather than contributing any motion at elbow.

Bony anatomy largely contributes to the stability of elbow joint by virtue of its close congruity. The anatomy is highly congruent through 180° of articular contact, deficient only in strip-like bare area of greater sigmoid notch of ulna. The distal humerus is triangular in shape and has two condyles covered with hyaline cartilage supporting the joint surfaces of the spool-shaped trochlea which articulates with the saddle-shaped trochlear notch of the proximal ulna and the rounded capitellum articulating with concave proximal surface of head of radius. In a frontal plane, there is about 6° of valgus tilt of the condyles with respect to the longitudinal axis of the humerus. There is 5–7° of internal rotation with respect to the interepicondylar axis. The medial epicondyle provides the attachment for the flexor-pronator group of forearm muscles and the medial collateral ligament **(Fig. 2A)**. The lateral epicondyle serves as the site for forearm extensor and supinator muscles attachment **(Fig. 2B)**. Proximal ulna is composed of two processes, the olecranon and the coronoid with the trochlear notch between them. The radial head articulates with capitellum. The capitellum of the distal humerus is spherical and covered with a thick articular cartilage. The posteromedial capitellum is marked by a prominent tubercle separating it from the lateral lip of the trochlea, where the radial head articulates through the entire range of flexion. The orientation of the articular surface of the distal humerus is rotated anteriorly about 30° with respect to the longitudinal axis of the humerus **(Fig. 3A)**. The anterior humeral line passes through the center of axis of rotation which should be reproduced in all reconstructions so that flexion and extension movements are not lost. The axis of rotation is 6–8° angulated in the coronal plane projecting distally on the medial side contributing to the valgus in extension. This is lost in flexion so that axis of arm and forearm coincide. Proximal radius has radial tuberosity that

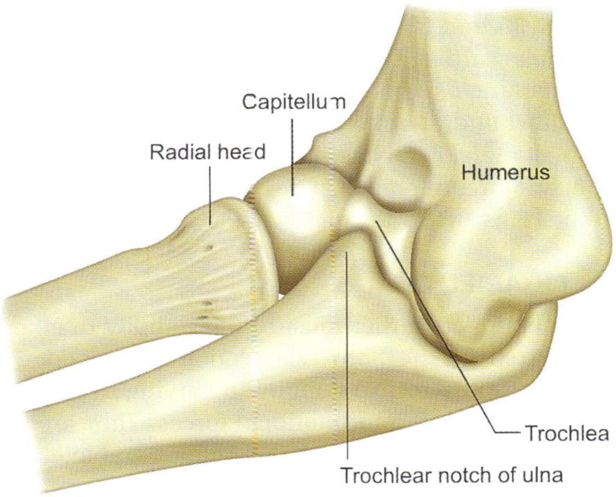

Fig. 1: The bony anatomy of the elbow.

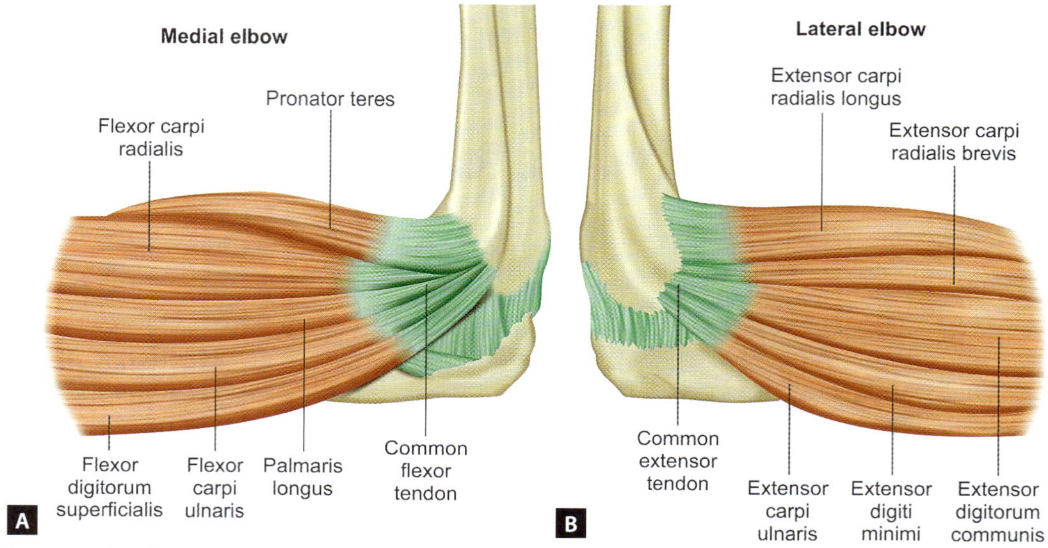

Figs. 2A and B: The medial (A) and lateral (B) aspects of elbow joint showing the various attachments (origins) of muscles and their relative disposition.

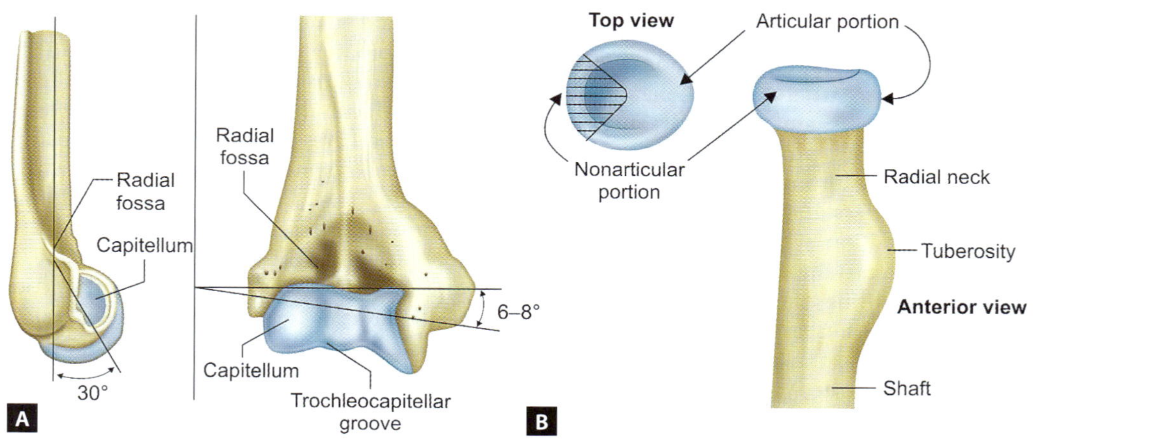

Figs. 3A and B: (A) The bony disposition of distal humerus and proximal radius demonstrating anterior rotation of the distal humeral articular surface by 30° and distal projection medially contributing to valgus in elbow extension; (B) Figure demonstrates the head of radius where a 120° sector does not articulate with the ulna. The tuberosity of proximal radius is a distinct projection that provides attachment to the biceps tendon.

provides attachment to the rounded tendon of biceps brachii **(Figs. 3A and B)**. The head of radius is largely covered with articular cartilage with the exception of the anterolateral one-third of the circumference of the head which is also devoid of subchondral bone and is hence weak. The concavity on roof of radial head has an arc of about 40°. About 240° of the outside circumference of the radial head articulates with the ulna **(Figs. 3B)**.

LIGAMENTS

As mentioned earlier most of the stability to elbow joint is conferred by the bony articulations. Ligaments, however, do contribute to the stability in varying degrees of flexion to varus, valgus, and rotational forces. They are mainly the thickenings in capsule. Medial (ulnar) and lateral collateral ligament complexes are the two primary ligament complex of elbow joint with discrete peculiarities.

Ulnar Collateral Ligament

Ulnar collateral ligament **(Fig. 4)** comprises various subparts that can be identified in anatomical specimens **(Table 1)**. These are primarily composed of the anterior oblique, posterior oblique, and transverse ligaments. The anterior oblique bundle has separate anterior (primary restraint to valgus stresses at 30°, 60°, and 90° of flexion) and posterior (secondary restraint to valgus stress with the elbow held at 120° of flexion) bands that tighten in reciprocal fashion as flexion (posterior band) and extension (anterior band) of the elbow occurs. This is the primary stabilizer of the elbow to valgus stress. Ulnar collateral ligament originates from the anteroinferior surface of the medial epicondyle not from axis of rotation except "Guiding bundle" isometric deep fibers of medial collateral ligament. This is the reason why different parts of the ligament are taught in different positions of elbow.

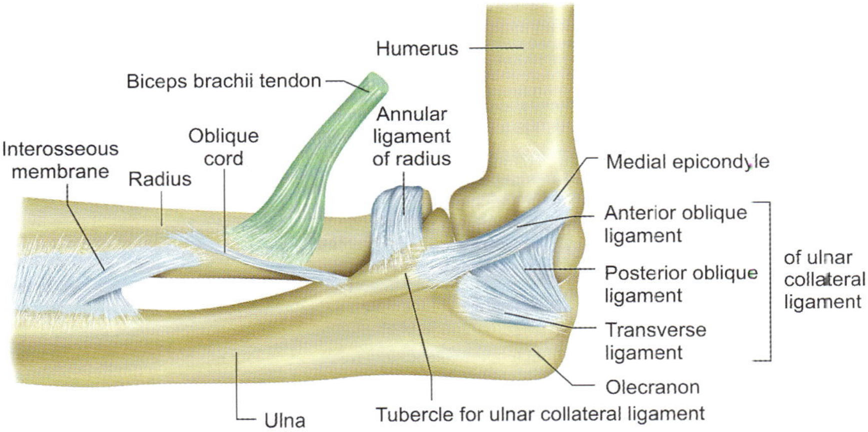

Fig. 4: The ulnar collateral ligament of elbow and its components. Also shown its relation to various bony and ligamentous structures in vicinity.

TABLE 1: The parts of ulnar collateral ligament.

Part	Origin	Insertion
Anterior	Medial epicondyle antero-inferior aspect	Sublime tubercle
Posterior	Medial epicondyle antero-inferior aspect	Greater sigmoid notch
Transverse band (ligament of cooper)	Traverses the medial border of greater sigmoid notch	

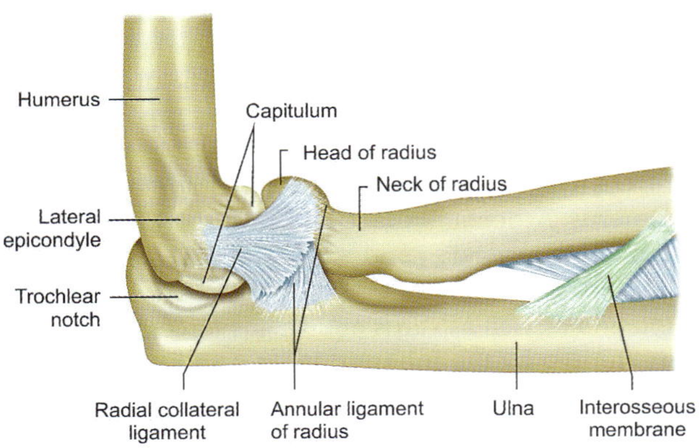

Fig. 5: The structural components and relation of lateral collateral ligament of elbow.

Lateral Collateral Ligament

Lateral collateral ligament **(Fig. 5)** has lateral collateral, lateral ulnar collateral, and annular ligaments components **(Table 2)**, but parts are not easily separable during dissection. The lateral collateral ligament origin is from the entire inferior surface of the lateral epicondyle as a blend of poorly demarcated fan-shaped ligamentous fibers. It provides external rotation and varus stability as the elbow flexes toward 110°. It remains taut throughout flexion and extension as lateral collateral ligament originates from axis of rotation on lateral epicondyle **(Figs. 6A and B)**.

Annular Ligament

The annular ligament attaches to the anterior and posterior margins of the lesser sigmoid notch. It becomes taut during supination at its anterior insertion and at its posterior insertion during extremes of pronation. This ligament is funnel-shaped and assists in stabilizing the proximal radius throughout the range of pronation and supination.

TABLE 2: The parts of lateral collateral ligament.

Part	Origin	Insertion
Radial collateral ligament	Lateral epicondyle	Lateral aspect of annular ligament
Annular ligament	Anterior margin of sigmoid notch	Posterior margin of sigmoid notch
Lateral ulnar collateral ligament	Lateral epicondyle	Supinator crest of ulna
Accessory radial collateral ligament	Distal margin of annular ligament	• Type I = bilobed • Type II = broad • Distal to lateral ulnar collateral ligament

The "stabilizers of elbow joint" hence comprise **(Fig. 7)**:

- ***Static:***
  - Bony articulation confer stability at <20° and >120° of elbow position.
  - Capsule
  - Medial collateral ligament
  - Lateral collateral ligament
- ***Dynamic:***
  - *Muscles:* Flexor carpi ulnaris is the predominant dynamic stabilizer of elbow, others include biceps anteriorly, triceps posteriorly, and anconeus provides restraint against posterolateral rotatory instability.

FUNCTIONS OF ELBOW

- Works primarily in conjunction with the shoulder to position the hand in space.
- Serves as a fulcrum for the forearm lever.
- Transmits load between the forearm and the upper arm.

MOVEMENTS AT ELBOW JOINT

It is a hinge joint in 5° axial rotation. It is a highly conformed joint with very small locus of rotation.

- *Range of motion (normal joint):*
  - Flexion = 0–140°

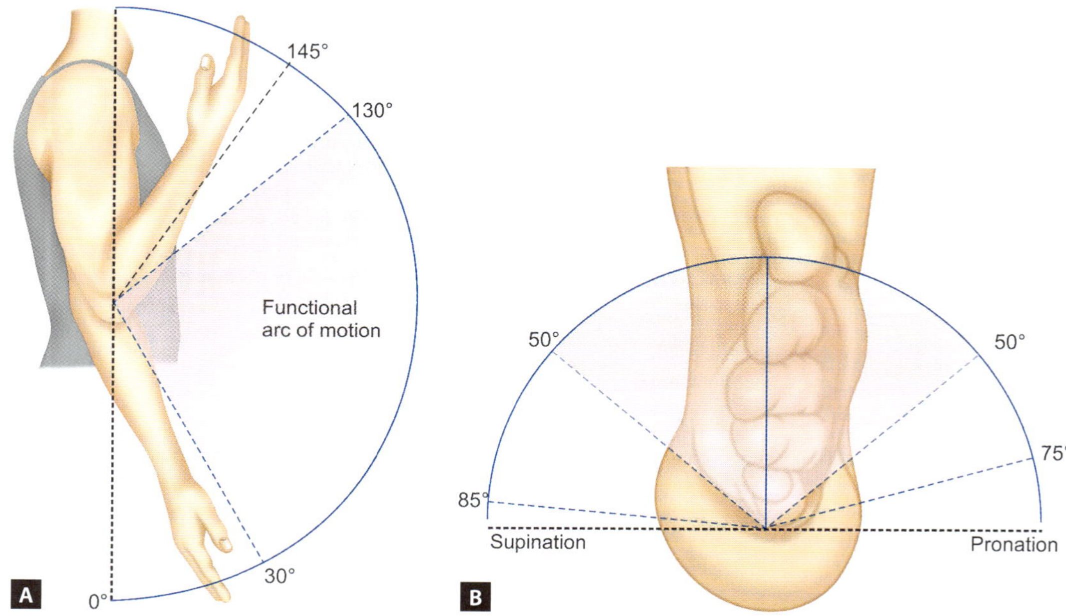

Figs. 6A and B: (A) Illustration of flexion-extension range of movements of elbow and (B) the supination-pronation movements at forearm [involves proximal radioulnar joint (PRUJ) of elbow also]. Also shown is the functional range of motion (ROM) needed to perform most of the activities of daily living independently.

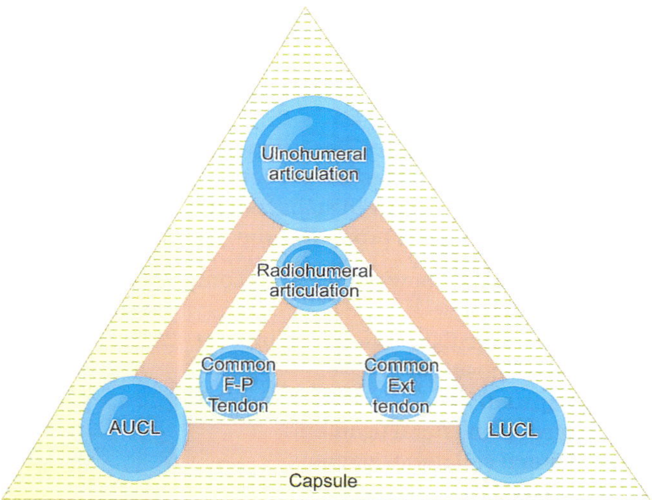

Fig. 7: Illustration of the "fortress" concept of constraints of elbow. (AUCL: anterior part of ulnar collateral ligament; Ext: extensor; F-P: flexor-pronator; LUCL: lateral ulnar collateral ligament)
Source: Modified from Mayo.

- Pronation = 75°
- Supination = 80°

- *Range of motion needed for activities of daily living:*
  - Flexion range = 100° (30–130°)
  - Rotation range = 100° (50° pronation and 50° supination)
- The elbow is a slightly loose hinge with small amounts of varus, valgus, and rotational laxity throughout its range of motion.
- The locus of center of rotation of the elbow is a circular area of the diameter 2–3 mm in the center of trochlea. This was first determined by Fischer in 1911.
- The center of the arc formed by the trochlea and capitellum form the axis of rotation of elbow lying on a straight line that is coplanar to the anterior distal cortex. Therefore, 5–7° of internal rotation is observed at the distal humeral articular surface with respect to midline.
- In a frontal plane, there is about 6° of the valgus tilt of the condyles with respect to the longitudinal axis of the humerus. Articular surface accounts for >50% of elbow stability in extension and >70% of elbow stability when the elbow is flexed 90°.
- Rotation as well as varus and valgus forces of the elbow are limited by the inherent bony stability as well as a significant restraint to varus and valgus forces from the collateral ligaments.
- The radioulnar joint plays an important role in pronation and supination. The axis of rotation runs through the center of the radial head and styloid process of the ulna. The ulna remains fixed in this movement and only radius rotates around.

CONSTRAINTS OF ELBOW JOINT

Role of various structures and primary constraints to different stress:

- ***Valgus stress:***
  - *Primary constraint:*
    - Medial collateral ligament:
      - *Anterior bundle:* Principle-stabilizer in 30–120° flexion
      - *Posterior bundle:* Co-restraint
  - *Secondary constraint:* Radial head
  - *Tertiary constraint:* Flexor-pronator muscle groups (flex carpi radialis, and flex digitorum superficialis)

- ***Varus stress:***
  - *Primary constraint:* Lateral collateral ligament and annular ligament complex
  - *Secondary constraint:*
    - Extensor muscles with fascial bands
    - Intermuscular septa

Salient Points

- Humeroulnar joint stabilizes elbow in <20° and >120° flexion.
- Radiohumeral joint provides secondary restraint in valgus stress.
- Division of nerve to anconeus—May predispose to posterolateral rotatory instability.
- If there is a fracture of coronoid process, do not remove the radial head.

BIOMECHANICS OF THROW

Competitive throw or pitching involves coordinated movement of upper limb, the torso and legs for rotational speed and stability. The movement of arm in arc motion is fast. The peak angular velocity during throwing is around 6,180° per second for shoulder internal rotation and 4,595° per second for elbow extension. Peak elbow acceleration has ranged from 225,000° to 500,000° per second. Stresses at the elbow occur during acceleration and follow-through phases for approximately 15 milliseconds. The throwing phase is divided into six phases **(Fig. 8)**: windup, stride, cocking (with subdivisions), acceleration (with subdivisions), deceleration, and follow-through.

Windup

It is like winding a spring. The thrower moves his leg to gain angular inertia and balance and the phase ends when the pitcher's forward knee has reached its maximum height. Elbow is kept flexed and hardly any forces are transmitted across.

Stride

This phase ends when the forward foot contacts the ground. In the beginning and middle periods of this phase, the elbow is extended. From the middle to the end of this phase, the elbow becomes flexed.

Cocking

This phase ends with the throwing shoulder reaches maximum external rotation—just before the ball starts in forward motion. A low-to-moderate flexion torque of 0–32 Nm is produced at the elbow throughout this phase. In the last 25% of the cocking phase (late cocking phase), upper trunk and pelvis rotate forward as the throwing shoulder externally rotates producing a large valgus torque onto the upper arm at the elbow. This force can be as large as 64 ± 12 Nm in baseball players and 60 Nm in tennis players. The flexor-pronator mass helps dynamically to stabilize the medial elbow from these distraction forces as the ulnar collateral ligament has only 32 Nm tensile strength, and it can break with every throw.

Acceleration

This is the shortest phase of a throw but with massive forces across the shoulder and elbow. This phase begins at maximal shoulder external rotation (the initiation of forward ball motion) and ends at ball release. In contrast to the cocking phase the "early" acceleration phase is the first 25% where greatest forces are generated. The elbow extends as the trunk continues to rotate. The maximum elbow extension velocity has been recorded at 1,800–2,700° per second (depending on the game) at approximately halfway through the acceleration phase.

Deceleration

Deceleration begins at ball release and ends when the shoulder reaches maximum internal rotation. There is

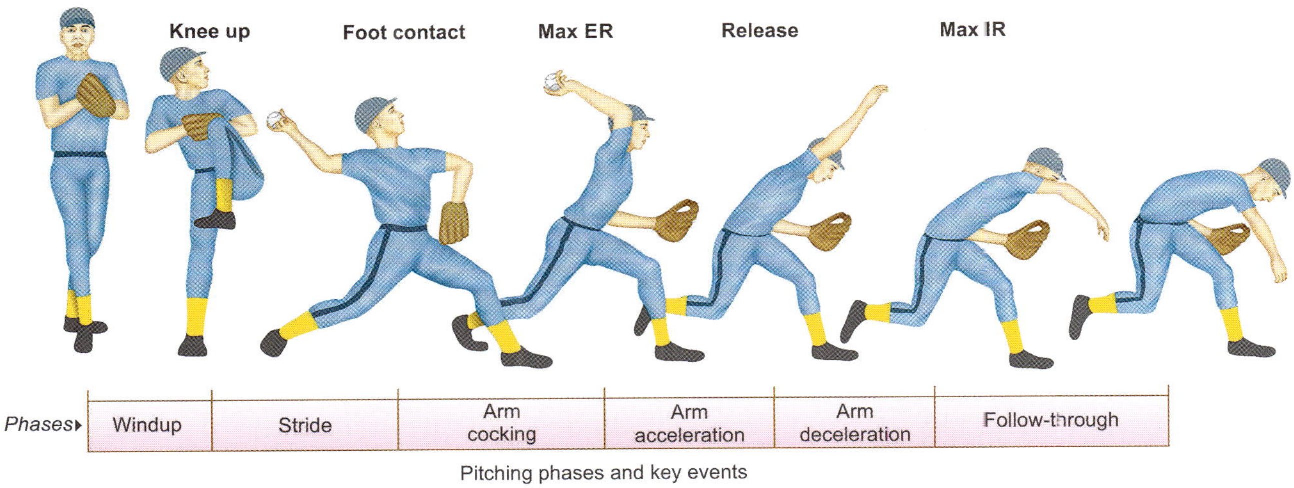

Fig. 8: Phases of a high-speed competitive throw. (ER: external rotation; IR: internal rotation, Max: maximum)

an elbow flexion torque produced by the elbow flexors of approximately 10–35 Nm to decelerate elbow extension. To prevent elbow distraction after ball release, the large proximal compression-contraction forces are also generated that increase with increasing skill of the thrower.

Follow-through

Follow-through begins when the shoulder reaches maximum internal rotation and ends when the pitcher reaches a balanced fielding position. The elbow flexes into a comfortable position as the trunk rotates forward and the arm moves across the body.

CONCLUSION

- The understanding of anatomy of elbow plays an important role in effectively diagnosing and managing the traumatic and nontraumatic disorders.
- The joint is like a fortress where disruption of any of its important structure has important bearing with respect to stability and mobility of the elbow. This is the reason why reconstruction and surgery around the joint was previously dreaded to be marred by stiffness.
- Improved techniques of surgery coupled with precise understanding of the osseoligamentous anatomy and biomechanics is paramount in functional reconstruction of the elbow joint.

CHAPTER 108

Tendon Disorders of Elbow

Manish Kumar Varshney

LATERAL EPICONDYLITIS (EXTENSOR ANGIOFIBROBLASTIC TENDINOSIS)

INTRODUCTION

Tennis elbow is a misnomer because most people that get this disease do not play tennis and lateral epicondylitis is a misnomer because of its pathophysiology different from an inflammatory condition, it is a tendinosis (i.e., chronic symptomatic degeneration of the tendon) that affects the common attachment of the tendons of the extensor muscles of the forearm [extensor carpi radialis brevis (ECRB), extensor digitorum, extensor digiti minimi, and extensor carpi ulnaris] to the lateral epicondyle of the humerus. The disease is idiopathic, benign, and self-limiting. Despite its relatively high prevalence, the development of a single effective and consistent management of lateral epicondylitis is still elusive.

HISTORY

- Lateral epicondylitis was first described in the medical literature by Runge in 1873.
- The term "tennis elbow" was attributed to description of the disorder as "lawn-tennis elbow" first in 1883 by Major.
- In 1936, Cyriax postulated that microscopic or macroscopic tears of the common extensor origin (ECRB) were involved in the disease process.
- Goldie described granulation tissue found at the origin of the ECRB.
- Coonrad and Hooper were the first to describe macroscopic tearing in association with the histologic findings. Nirschl termed these histologic findings angiofibroblastic hyperplasia. The term has since been modified to angiofibroblastic tendinosis.

ETIOLOGY

In most cases of lateral epicondylitis, no obvious underlying cause can be identified. However, the most common incriminated activities include any activity that involves overuse of the wrist extensor or supinator muscles. Individuals, who place high demands on the upper extremities, are prone to developing epicondylopathy.

Goldie attributed the onset of symptoms to overexertion of the extremity with repetitive wrist extension and alternating forearm pronation or supination. Repetitive tasks, especially involving heavy tools, are a significant risk factor. It has been suggested by some authors that work-related lateral epicondylitis in laborers may be related to handling tools >1 kg, lifting loads >20 kg more than 10 times/day with such repetitive activities continuing for >2 hours.

The popular association with tennis only signifies that lateral epicondylitis may result from activities involving repetitive use of the forearm extensors. These activities include but are not restricted to typing, household work in females like rinsing cloth and various types of industrial manual work in laborers. Biomechanically, it is shown that any movement that eccentrically stretches wrist extensors may cause pain, as it increases the load on inflamed and diseased common extensor tendon. For its classical association with tennis, Smidt and van der Windt identified several contributory factors that can be systematically avoided to relieve symptoms. They emphasized that racquet sports may be causative to it as a result of combination of following factors:

- Incorrect technique resulting in primary power generation from the wrist extensors rather than localizing to the rotator cuff. These now form an important part of sort training.
    - Back hand play causing wrist snapping
    - Poor feet positioning while countering a power shot
    - Hitting the ball late or with a bent elbow
- Overtraining and prolonged duration of play that give inadequate time to heal
- Frequency of play:
    - Frequent involvement in high-level competitive sport
- Choose optimal size of the racquet handle so as to completely grip it. Poorly fitting grip (too large or too small) would affect the lever arm of the force applied through the forearm.
- Racquet weight should not be unnecessarily high, as it will result in early fatigue.

ASSOCIATIONS

The disease has been found to be associated with the susceptibility to generalized tendinopathy. These patients were described as having a "mesenchymal syndrome" by Nirschl suggesting a genetic linkage to development of the disease. The patients have multiple problems including rotator cuff pathology, epicondylopathy, carpal tunnel syndrome, trigger finger, and DeQuervain's disease. It has been identified that patients with tennis elbow tend to have a higher incidence of rheumatoid factor positivity and human leukocyte antigen-B27 (HLA-B27) positivity—the significance of this finding is unknown but may be suggesting some form of autoimmune disorder of low severity. This may somehow justify the term "epicondylitis" as inflammation is a common final pathology here.

The historically suggested etiopathogenic mechanisms for tennis elbow include (none proved):

- Synovial fringe inflammation (Trethwan, 1927)
- ECRB (extensor carpi radialis brevis) tear (Cyriax, 1939)
- Hyaline degeneration of the annular ligament (Bosworth, 1954)
- Neuritis of the radial nerve (Kaplan, 1968)
- Radial nerve entrapment (Roles and Maudsley, 1972)
- Radial head fibrillation (Newman and Goodfellow, 1975)
- Inflammation in the anconeus muscle (Coe et al., 1993)

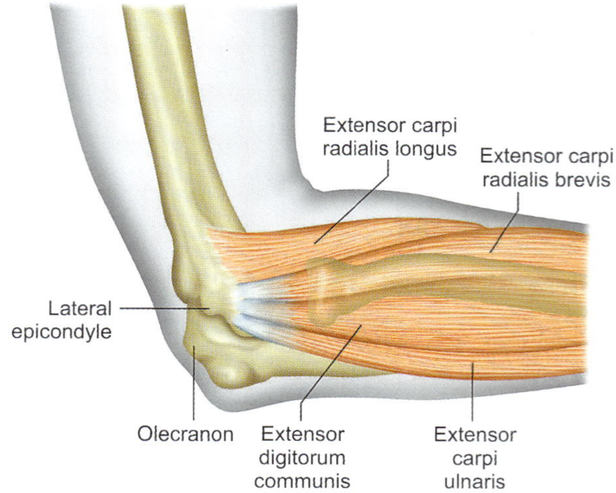

Fig. 1: The pathoanatomy of lateral epicondylitis. The marked oval is the area frequently involved in injury/degeneration/inflammation/angiofibroblastic dysplasia.

PATHOGENESIS

Lateral epicondylitis was previously considered to be a tendinitis, arising as inflammation of the tendon (that may in fact be partially true for above-mentioned newer theory and findings and also I personally feel that local steroid injections are highly effective possibly suggesting inflammatory mediator at least partially in the pathogenesis). However, it has been shown histopathologically to have a paucity of inflammatory cells such as macrophages and neutrophils, and the features more commonly resemble a tendinopathy. The condition is, therefore, now considered to be a tendinosis, which is defined as a degenerative process. Lateral epicondylitis pathology occurs in the more superior and slightly deeper fibers of the ECRB **(Fig. 1)**. Grossly, the abnormal region of the tendon looks gray and is slightly edematous and friable. It may contain small flecks of calcification. Histologically, under a microscope there is disordered healing superimposed on a degenerative process lacking inflammatory changes. At microanatomic and molecular level, the application of stress to a tendon normally leads to increased cross-linkage and collagen deposition. With increased stretching microtear results and the adaptation or repair of the tendon to multiple microtears leads to tendinosis. There are several well-defined histological stages that result from such repetitive microtrauma.

- ***Stage 1*:** An acute inflammatory response, which commonly resolves in initial episodes completely while with recurrence it persists and patients are inclined to seek medical help.
- ***Stage 2*:** Sustained stage 1 or recurrent cases cause histological appearance of "angiofibroblastic hyperplasia" with pathological tissue comprising of high concentration of fibroblasts, vascular hyperplasia, and disorganized collagen bundles in the region. The hypercellularity is seen both in the form of an organized and disorganized fashion in surrounding region. The combination of these factors results in tendinosis. Patients commonly present at this stage for treatment.
- ***Stage 3*:** Partial or complete tendon rupture—the pathological changes keep accumulating and lead ultimately to structural failure of the tendon.
- ***Stage 4*:** Along with features of stage 2 or 3 injury, there are also other associated changes such as fibrosis, soft-tissue calcification. The collagen is grossly disorganized and loose in hard osseous calcification.

Though degeneration had been considered to explain the pathoanatomy and cause of tendinosis, recent studies have also pointed to other causes.

- ***Altered mechanics:*** Cinematographic and electromyography (EMG) evaluation indicates that tennis players with epicondylitis demonstrate altered mechanics and increased ECRB activity as against the normal subjects.
- ***"Under-use" or stress shielding:*** This explains the occurrence of disease even in "not-so-laborious" patients. It envisages that certain sections of the tendon experience lower than usual amount of load during routine activities. This reduces their intrinsic strength and causes structural weakening of the tendon predisposing it to injury from even minor stress. Histopathological studies of the ECRB in patients with long-standing lateral epicondylitis demonstrate tendon defects and areas of necrosis manifesting as angiofibroblastic hyperplasia within fibers along with signs of disorganized muscle fiber regeneration. These defects are proposed to result from underuse and consequent weakness of the muscle. Pain-related inhibition or fear of pain could be one such cause of underuse or may result from disease. The shearing forces on the pathological tissue cause tissue metaplasia

to a progressively fibrocartilaginous composition of the ECRB enthesis. The tendon insertion into bone, hence weakens and initiates development of tendinosis.

- ***Compromised blood supply:*** Vascular supply and its loss has been proposed to be the culprit in most of the elusive pathologies where failure to heal to original tissue is the basic pathology. Tendons have an intrinsically limited blood supply compared to muscular tissue. Prolonged activities produce periods of ischemia by stretching the tendon and compressing the already precarious blood supply effectively rendering the tendon avascular. The damage is not just limited to reduced blood supply but on reperfusion there is generation of destructive free radicals causing additional destruction.
- ***Thermal injury:*** Tendons undergoing repetitive use develop increased internal temperature by virtue of friction in the collagen bundles that constantly stretch and regain elastic energy. The temperature may rise by 10% inducing hyperthermic injuries.
- ***Apoptosis:*** Injury to the tendon activates protein kinases, which lead to apoptosis.
- ***Altered local metabolic milieu in the tendon:*** Altered gene expression and an imbalance of matrix metalloproteinases and growth factors produce or predispose for the observed changes.
- ***Genetic:*** (*See* above in etiology)

There remain a lot to be explained despite the intensive research and mechanisms proposed as detailed above. Especially, there is a paucity of correlation between the histopathological findings and clinical features.

Histopathologico-clinical dissociation: Although it is known that the structure of the affected tendon in lateral epicondylitis is degenerate with multiple microtears, in itself that is not sufficient to explain the variability in patients' symptoms. The cause of pain in lateral epicondylitis is thought to originate both from intra-articular pathology and extra-articular structures:

- An increased concentration of excitatory neurotransmitters such as glutamate, which sensitizes the pain response and increased levels of neurokinin-1 (substance P) receptors.
- Direct irritation from chemicals, such as lactate, which have been found to be increased in tendinopathy.
- Both of above can lead to a cascade of changes in neurons in the peripheral nervous system that ultimately leads to sensitization of the central nervous system.
- Intra-articular pathologies have been reported by many investigators that may contribute to origin of pain and include plical fold, synovitis, and cartilage lesions in capitellum. For this reason, it is also recommended that the steroid be injected into the joint also.

This may be the explanation for why these patients get relief from local steroid injections and also that a significant number have pain in neurological regions distant from the site of injury. It has been reported that 56% of patients with lateral epicondylitis have associated pain in the neck (double crush syndrome). However, neck and shoulder pain could be due to the overuse of or change in biomechanics as a result of the elbow pain.

CLINICAL FEATURES

It affects approximately 1–2% of the population.

Signs and Symptoms

The disease is seen affecting the males and females equally in 4th to 5th decade but more prominently in their dominant arm.

- Usually affects patients between 35 and 55 years of age
- Pain on the outer part of the elbow (lateral epicondyle) region localized in stage one while diffusely located in later stages
- Gripping movements at wrist, especially those associated with wrist extension and lifting of heavy objects are painful.
- Pain in activities requiring wrist extension like emptying can, lifting jar from rim (palm down), sweeping floor using broom or mop
- Point tenderness just anterior and distal to lateral epicondyle and proximal region of the ECRB and EDC muscles
- Inability to extend the elbow completely after long sleep or rest (morning stiffness)
- Nonspecific symptoms that may be associated with tennis elbow include:
  - Radiating pain to the forearm and wrist
  - Pain during uncountered extension of wrist
  - Forearm weakness
  - Pain on shaking hands or opening a doorknob
- Tenderness can be elicited in the anterolateral aspect of lateral epicondyle.

Provocative Tests

Cozen's or Thompson's Test (Fig. 2)

Resisted wrist extension with radial deviation and full pronation causes pain in anterolateral elbow.

Mill's Test (Fig. 3)

Technique: The patient is seated, the clinician palpates patient's lateral epicondyle with one hand, while pronating the patient's forearm and fully flexing the wrist, the elbow is extended to stretch the tendon. A reproduction of pain in

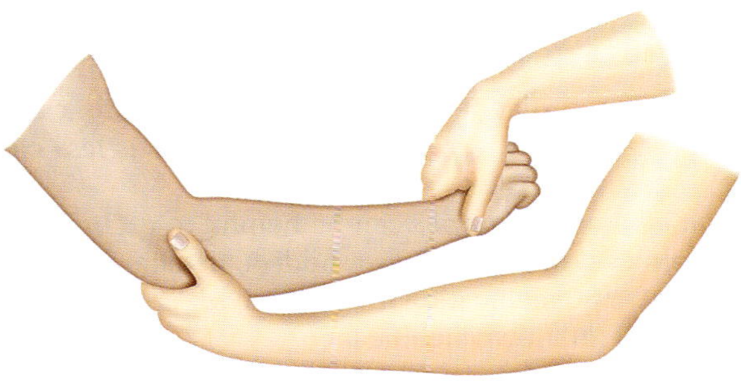

The image above demonstrates the most common location of tennis elbow and the examination technique that makes the pain worse with resisted wrist extension

Fig. 2: Cozen's test—pain at the lateral epicondylitis region is reproduced with resisted wrist extension.

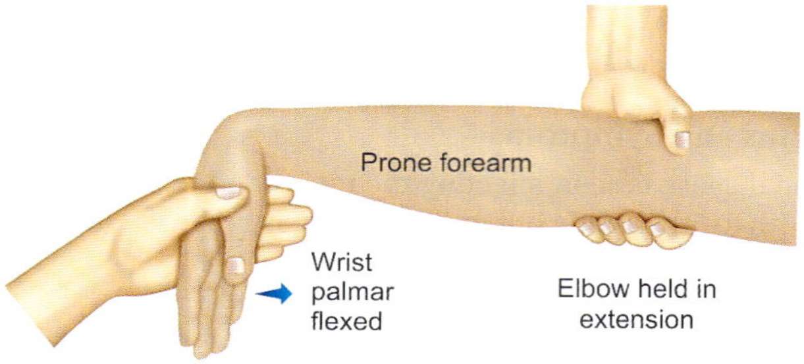

Fig. 3: Clinical method of performing Mill's test (see text).

the area of the insertion at the lateral epicondyle indicates a positive test.

Other techniques to diagnose lateral epicondylitis:
- ***Maudsley's test:*** Resisted third digit extension elicits pain at the pathology.
- ***Chair lift test:*** Lifting the back of a chair with a three finger pinch (thumb, index long fingers) and the elbow fully extended
- Injecting local anesthetic in the pathological region partially or completely abolishes the pain.

DIFFERENTIAL DIAGNOSIS

- Stenosis of the annular ligament
- Cervical spondylosis and/or C6 or C7 cervical nerve root compression
- Inflammation of the synovium adjacent to the radial head
- ***Posterior interosseous nerve (PIN) syndrome:*** Entrapment at arcade of Frohse is recognized in approximately 5% of patients.
- Radiocapitellar overload syndrome, early osteoarthritis (OA) of radial head or capitellum
- Bursitis
- Radial nerve entrapment
- Elbow overuse as a compensatory mechanism for ipsilateral frozen shoulder. The elbow is likely to continue to be painful despite local treatment until the shoulder pathology is addressed.
- Osteochondritis dissecans (OCD) of capitellum
- Lateral collateral ligament (LCL) laxity
- Inflammation and edema of the anconeus

INVESTIGATIONS

In most cases, a diagnosis of lateral epicondylitis can be made clinically. However, where the diagnosis is less clear, further investigations may be required.
- *Plain elbow radiographs* can be helpful to exclude bony pathologies, including loose bodies, osteoarthritis and OCD. Patchy calcification in the overlying soft-tissue may be seen of unknown significance.
- *Doppler ultrasound* is able to detect neovascularization. Gray-scale changes have been shown to rule out lateral epicondylitis.
- *Thermography* though not available for common use it has been found to correlate with clinical severity of the disease.
- *Magnetic resonance imaging (MRI)* is a more reproducible form of imaging than ultrasound (highly observer dependent) and can demonstrate other intra-articular pathology. Magnetic resonance (MR) scan can confirm the presence of degenerative tissue and tears within the tendon and underlying capsule. Positive MRI findings have been shown to correlate poorly with patients' symptoms. The length of separation within the ECRB tendon and extent of lesion are not related to the severity of symptoms. Computed tomographic (CT) arthrography identifies capsular tears better on the deep surface of ECRB (85% CT arthrograms correct compared with 64.5% for MRI using arthroscopy as defining measure).
- *Nerve conduction studies and EMG* can be used to help exclude PIN entrapment.
- *High-resolution real-time ultrasound* imaging can be useful by identifying structural changes in the affected tendons, including thickening or thinning, hypoechogenic foci indicating intrasubstance degenerative areas, tendon tears, and calcification.

TREATMENT

Principles of treatment: The aims of treatment for lateral epicondylitis include:
- Pain control
- Preservation of/restoration of movement
- Regaining grip strength and endurance
- Normalization of function
- Preventing recurrence and further clinical deterioration

Nonoperative

Approximately, 80–95% of patients have success with nonsurgical treatment though recurrence is common.
- ***Rest:*** Give proper rest by stopping participation in sports or heavy work activities for several weeks and activity modification.
- ***Nonsteroidal anti-inflammatory medicines:*** To reduce pain and swelling.
- ***Stretching exercise:*** Stretching exercise for wrist with elbow extended.
- ***Physical therapy:*** For strengthening the muscles of the forearm (eccentric exercise of forearm extensor muscles). Local application of low-intensity ultrasonic, ice massage to improve muscle healing and healthy scar formation.
- ***Brace (counterforce brace, Fig. 4):*** Using a brace centered over the back of your forearm may also help to relieve symptoms of tennis elbow. This can reduce symptoms by resting the muscles and tendons. A counterforce brace helps in many ways **(Box 1)**.
- ***Steroid injections (Fig. 5):*** These are very effective anti-inflammatory agents (I find them consistently helpful, if injected properly). Usually, depot preparations of triamcinolone (I prefer) or methylprednisolone are used. Caution the patient for development of swelling and increased pain for first few days and advice ice fomentation along with strong analgesics for couple of days. There is always a debate on the type, dose and number of injections that can be safely given. I tend to use

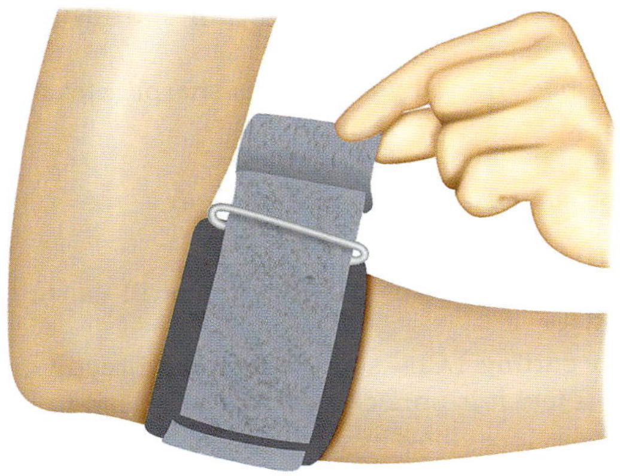

Fig. 4: Use of counterforce brace and correct place of applying the same.

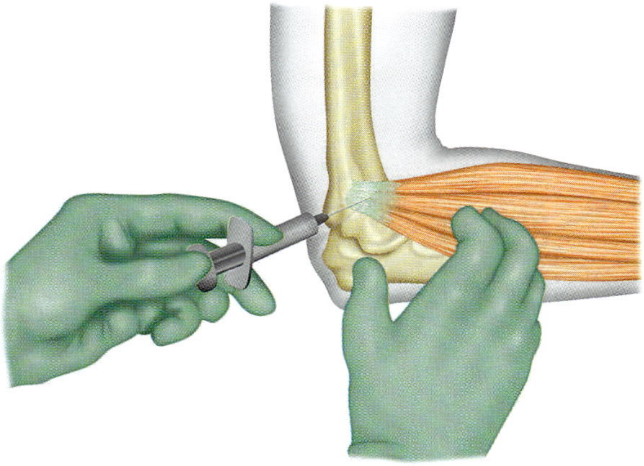

Fig. 5: The common method of injecting depot preparations of steroid in extensor carpi radialis brevis (ECRB) tendon in a case with diagnosed tennis elbow. Often small amount of the drug is also injected into the joint, around the annular ligament and intra-articularly.

BOX 1: Mechanisms of action of counterforce brace.

- Inhibit maximal contraction of wrist and finger flexor and extensors
- Restrict full muscle expansion, reducing intrinsic muscle force to vulnerable areas
- Reduce activity of forearm muscles decreasing overload
- Partially fix the muscle to the underlying forearm bone and soft-tissue, creating a new muscle origin that shortens the length of the muscle pull, slightly changing the direction of force and bypassing the inflamed and injured portion of the muscle that is proximal to the strap
- Reduce stress across the joint by passivating the proximal muscle.

a maximum of three triamcinolone acetonide injections 20–40 mg diluted in 3 mL 2% xylocaine at an interval of 4–6 weeks. Skin and fat atrophy and degeneration of tendon are some of the common side effects that should be borne in mind and the patient counseled thoroughly.

- ***Extracorporeal shock wave therapy:*** These waves cause "microtrauma" that promotes body's natural healing processes. Efficacy is not uniformly established and also availability is an issue, I feel this is more empirical and has no definite indication for standalone use.
- ***Autologous blood injection:*** This has been proposed to be effective. Blood collected from intravenous route is immediately injected to the affected area. Blood is by itself inflammatory outside the vessels and may "shell-out" the painful lesion causing relief. Again, the efficacy is not uniform and technique is also user dependent.
- ***Local injection of autologous concentrated platelets (Fig. 5):*** Platelet-derived growth factor (PDGF) is supposed to promote healing of the tissues particularly the damaged ones in inflammatory phase. Also, various epidermal growth factor (EGF) and vascular endothelial growth factor (VEGF) might help in the process by altering the local milieu. This has been a quite popular technique recently but is cumbersome for routine practice.
- Other methods of doubtful reliability that are used in some centers include:
    - Cryotherapy
    - Prolotherapy (with 25% dextrose)
    - Radiotherapy
    - Manipulation under anesthesia
    - Acupuncture
    - Local injection of botulinum toxin

Some patients inevitably fail on conservative manage ment. The poor prognostic factors include:

- Manual labor
- Dominant arm involvement
- Long duration of symptoms with high baseline pain levels
- Poor coping mechanisms

Such patients are better managed by operative treatment, if they accept it. Also, one should understand the compliance level of the patient and should exhaust all nonsurgical measures for 8 months to 1 year before embarking on surgery.

Operative Management

Various surgical methods have been described for management that can be done by open, percutaneous, and arthroscopic approaches. Historically, a number of methods have been tried by different surgeons but most are now abandoned for newer scientific methods. These include:

- Epicondylar osteotomy of Franke
- Incision of the ECRB of Hohmann
- Partial lateral denervation of Tavernier
- Partial resection of the annular ligament of Bosworth
- Distal lengthening of the ECRB of Garden
- Complete denervation and radial nerve decompression of Wilhelm
- Decompression of the PIN of Capener and of radial nerve of roles
- Extensor fasciotomy of Posch
- Proximal lengthening of ECRB and decompression of PIN by Narakas
- Modified Wilhelm procedure of denervation and decompression of PIN

Open Surgery

Despite the variously described procedures, "extensor slide" is the most common procedure done that partially releases the extensor origin. I personally favor excising the small pathological focus **(Figs. 6A to E)** if identified on MRI along with the extensor slide but keeping the dissection to minimum. In long-standing cases, I also perform decortication of the lateral epicondyle to improve vascularity of the region and healing. The steps for open release are:

- Making a 3–4 cm longitudinal incision just anterior to lateral epicondyle.
- Incising the fascia overlying the posterior edge of the extensor carpi radialis longus (ECRL) and expose the ECRB, which lies underneath the ECRL.
- Identify the abnormal anterior edge of extensor aponeurosis that lies just posterior to ECRL.
- Extensor carpi radialis brevis is inferior to the origin of the ECRL and deep to the extensor digitorum communis (EDC) (border between the ECRB and EDC is often poorly defined).
- Extensor carpi radialis brevis is sharply elevated and released.
- Degenerated tissue is excised.
- Decortication is performed with a burr.

Care must be taken to:

- Avoid the release of ECRL as that will cause elbow weakness.
- Avoid cutting LCL—some surgeons directly cut the LCL—I feel it is unnecessary and may lead to chronic instability (*See* elbow instability).
- Defect between the ECRL and the extensor aponeurosis should be firmly repaired.

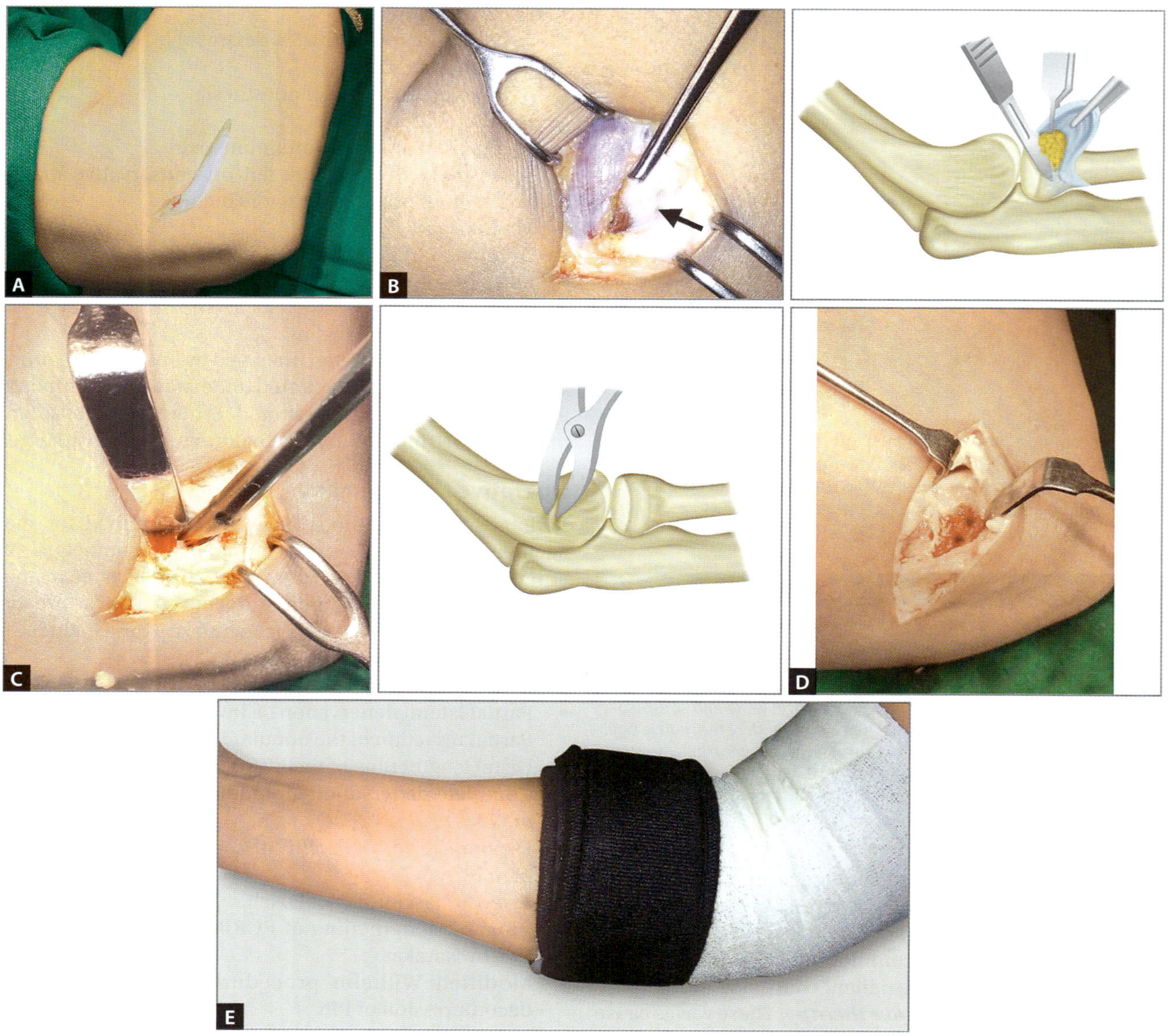

Figs. 6A to E: (A) Surgical release and decortication for Tennis elbow—incision; (B) Removal of the fibroelastic degenerative pathological tissue (arrow); (C) Decortication can be done using a rongeur or I prefer a high-speed burr; (D) Making drill holes help in healing and possibly also bringing stem cells into the region; (E) Postoperatively the patient is kept in a mild compression bandage and counterforce band may be applied to assist healing by removing stress.

- Bosworth procedure may be employed if one finds that intra-articular pathology is also the cause of pain.

Arthroscopic Management

First described by Grifka, Boenke, and Kramer in 1995. Three portals are needed—two working portals the "soft spot" posterior lateral portal, and anterolateral portal while an anteromedial viewing portal. The advantages of arthroscopic approach are:

- It can diagnose and treat concomitant intra-articular pathology.
- It also potentially minimizes damage to healthy tissue.
- It allows visualization of the undersurface of the ECRB tendon.

The disadvantage is that an arthroscopic procedure takes longer than an open operation, and is associated with the potential risk of damage to the radial nerve.

Percutaneous Release

"Extensor slide" or Hohmann's epicondylar stripping procedure can be performed as a day care or at an outpatient facility. For Hohmann's epicondylar stripping, the area around the lateral epicondyle is anesthetized with a local anesthetic. The common extensor tendon is incised just distal to the lateral epicondyle with a surgical blade. The displaced extensor tendon can be palpated through the skin approximately 1 cm distal from the epicondyle at the end of the procedure. The tourniquet is released, hemostasis is obtained and the wound is closed.

Postoperative common regime: After surgery, patients are advised to avoid the offending activity for a minimum of 3 months. For manual laborers, return to work is allowed by 4–12 weeks. Desk workers can go to work almost immediately but will still require modified activities, normally a period of rest followed by a period of gentle passive and active exercises.

Complications of Operative Management

The most serious complication is complete tendon rupture. Such an injury often causes a palpable defect in the extensors, which results in weakness on attempted wrist extension. Frequently, the treatment of this complication is surgical repair. The other most common complication is treatment failure.

CHRONIC REFRACTORY TENNIS ELBOW AND SALVAGE SURGERY FOR LATERAL TENNIS ELBOW

Some patients fail even surgical management (rare though) but then failures are the rule and can arise from wrong diagnosis or those with associated other symptoms that have not been addressed or true refractory tennis elbow. The treatment failures have been divided into two types by Morrey:

1. *Type 1:* Those whose symptoms are identical to their preoperative symptoms (improper patient selection and incomplete diagnosis or incorrect procedure)
2. *Type 2:* Those patients who have different symptoms following surgery resulting from possibly overzealous surgery resulting in elbow instability, capsular pathology, synovial herniation, bursitis or capsular fistula.

The treatment for refractory lateral epicondylitis is not consistent or rewarding being very vague and ineffective. The best possibility to treat is in fact those patients that had a wrong diagnosis. The opportunity now lies in treating the identified pathology provided patients trust is still maintained. I find PIN compression to be the most commonly missed associated pathology or confused pathology to tennis elbow, so one should always keep this in consideration while diagnosing a tennis elbow purely (one can easily differentiate by injecting local anesthetic distally into supinator and if it is due to PIN syndrome the symptoms will subside). To identify overtreatment (type 2), one should perform arthrography to identify capsular pathology and ligamentous injuries. The treatment is then directed to the same. As a matter of fact, only 15–20% of the refractory tennis elbow can be diagnosed and rest are more or less managed conservatively and majority improve surprisingly.

MEDIAL EPICONDYLITIS

HISTORY

Medial epicondylitis of the elbow, commonly referred to as "golfer's elbow," (wrongly called medial tennis elbow) is characterized by pathologic changes to the musculotendinous origin at the medial epicondyle. It is an inflammatory condition of the medial epicondyle of the elbow. It is in some ways similar to tennis elbow but not limited to golfers only. The golf swing is, however, a common cause of medial epicondylitis. Many other repetitive activities that result into overuse of the forearm wrist and finger flexor muscles [pronator teres (PT) and flexor carpi radialis (FCR)] can also lead to golfer's elbow like throwing, chopping wood with an axe, running a chain saw, etc. Other groups of patients that develop golfer's elbow belong to the "mesenchymal syndrome".

BIOMECHANICS

The biomechanics of the medial elbow and the flexor-pronator musculature are best described in terms of the baseball pitching mechanism that extall the forces across elbow in repetitive works. The acceleration phase of pitching (*See* biomechanics of elbow)—from the point at which the ball has virtually no forward velocity to the point of release—produces peak angular velocity and extreme valgus forces greater than the tensile strength of the medial ligamentous and musculotendinous structures. The forces are initially borne by flexor-pronator muscle group (the dynamic stabilizer of elbow) and then are transmitted to the deeper medial collateral ligament (MCL). Repeated microtrauma and its accrual progresses to the degenerative changes that cause epicondylitis. Similar to poor technique causing lateral epicondylitis in tennis (see above); medial epicondylitis in golf is also attributed to incorrect technique. When the club is "thrown" from the zenith of backswing toward the ball—termed "hitting from the top," it creates high-grade valgus forces upon the MCL and the medial epicondyle resulting in the overload pattern.

ANATOMY AND PATHOMECHANICS

- Musculotendinous structures of the medial elbow comprise flexor-pronator group. While looking from radial to the ulnar aspects, the muscles comprise pronator teres (PT), flexor carpi radialis (FCR), palmaris longus (PL), flexor digitorum superficialis (FDS) and flexor carpi ulnaris (FCU). The PT and FCR both attach anterior to medial epicondyle. The tendons of these muscles get stretched in the acceleration phase of throwing and swinging. Thus, the PT and FCR are most encountered culprit in golfer's elbow or the student's elbow.
- Professional throwing athletes develop hypertrophy of distal humerus and also of the flexor-pronator forearm muscles. This produces a subtle flexion deformity in nearly half of them, and a third has a cubitus valgus in comparison with the nondominant arm. Although these changes have never been directly implicated with the occurrence of medial epicondylitis, they may definitely contribute to occurrence of ulnar neuropathy due to frictional and stretching neuritis and medial elbow pain.
- The other possible cause for medial elbow pain is medial elbow instability that may result from repetitive stretching of the medial structures. Primary stability of the elbow is affected by the congruous bony articulation between the olecranon and trochlea. Static soft-tissue stability is provided primarily by the MCL and to some extent by anterior capsule, LCL. The flexor and extensor muscle masses provide dynamic stability. Cadaveric studies by Morrey and others have established that the MCL is composed of three bands: (i) anterior, (ii) posterior, and (iii) transverse. It is the anterior band of this ligament that stabilizes the elbow during valgus stress. Muscle strain can be caused by poor mechanics, improper conditioning, lack of flexibility or fatigue—all of which may lead to increased transmission of forces to the medial collateral ligament. Repetitive and excessive stress upon the MCL can lead to microscopic damage and ultimately to ligamentous insufficiency and elbow instability.

PATHOPHYSIOLOGY

Since Morris' first description of epicondylitis in 1882, a vast amount of literature has been dedicated to the pathophysiology of this disorder. Early descriptions postulated:

- Radial humeral bursitis or periostitis
- Synovitis
- Annular ligament degeneration/stricture/impingement

These theories are proven incorrect by the histologic analysis of Nirschl and others. From these studies, it has come out that the normal collagen architecture is disrupted by a fibroblastic and immature vascular response, an incomplete reparative process but minimal inflammatory response similar to one in tennis elbow. Initially like tennis elbow, there is inflammatory change in or near epicondylitis while later there is evidence of microtearing, characterized by tendon degeneration with or without calcification. The histologic alterations have been similar to "angiofibroblastic hyperplasia" seen in tennis elbow. Nirschl proposed four descriptive stages of epicondylar tendonosis:

1. *Stage 1:* Inflammatory stage often self-limited
2. *Stage 2:* Pathologically characterized by angiofibroblastic degeneration
3. *Stage 3:* Structural failure of tissues
4. *Stage 4:* Along with stages 2 or 3, there is also fibrosis or calcification.

In a nutshell, the accepted present theory for medial epicondylitis is that the insult results into microtearing of the tendon origin at the epicondyle that progresses to a failed reparative response and subsequent tendon degeneration, these pathological changes additionally alter the typical musculotendinous biomechanics of the elbow.

CLINICAL FEATURES

- The main symptom of golfer's elbow is pain at the medial epicondyle of the elbow. Pain usually starts at the medial epicondyle and may spread down the forearm.
- Bending of wrist, twisting the forearm down or grasping objects make the pain worse.
- There may be a feeling of weakness or less strength while grasping items or squeezing the hand into a fist.
- Ulnar nerve symptoms are associated in up to 50% of athletes with medial epicondylitis.
- Provocative test—resisted forearm pronation and resisting wrist flexion increases pain.

On Physical Examination

- There is palpable tenderness over the medial epicondyle.
- Increased point tenderness while extending the elbow with the forearm supinated
- Pain increases with resisted wrist flexion
- Pain increases with resisted forearm pronation
- In more chronic cases of medial epicondylitis, there may be pain with resisted elbow flexion
- The Tinel's sign should be checked over the ulnar nerve to rule out ulnar neuropathy.
- Palpate the ulnar nerve over its course, especially where it goes between the two heads of FCU. Examine for the weakness of muscles supplied in the hand.
- Always examine the ulnar collateral ligament (UCL). Chronic UCL deficiency is more common than medial epicondylitis in throwing athletes.

DIFFERENTIAL DIAGNOSIS

- Cervical radiculopathy
- Elbow and forearm overuse injuries
- Little league elbow syndrome
- Ulnar collateral ligament injury

INVESTIGATIONS

Investigations are hardly of any use as the diagnosis is often clinical. Still some do advise tests that also serve to exclude differentials.

- *Plain radiographs* may show calcification adjacent to the medial epicondyle in 20–30% of patients with medial epicondylitis, but radiography is not usually needed in the initial workup of this condition. Order radiographs, if:
  - There is a history of a traumatic injury.
  - The physical examination is suspicious for a fracture.
  - Recalcitrant cases
  - Suspicion of tumors and apophyseal injury
- *Bone scanning* is useful for evaluating stress fractures, infection and tumors.
- *CT scans* are useful for evaluating OCD and stress fractures.
- *MRI* helps in defining the OCD, fractures and soft-tissue injury and importantly excluding other pathologies. MR arthrography is useful for evaluating the UCL.
- *Ultrasonography* is user dependent as mentioned previously also and also contraindicated in children with open physes.

TREATMENT

Nonoperative

Most patients (above 90%) gain benefit from conservative means, and hence is the mainstay of treatment. Pain control is the initial treatment goal for patients with medial epicondylitis. The following modalities are used in combination:

- ***Nonsteroidal anti-inflammatory drugs (NSAIDs):*** Though deemed controversial, they are the first-line management as at least in some stage the disease has inflammatory component. They reduce swelling control pain and help in early recovery. If there are concerns of increased swelling (via platelet inhibition—I do not know how much of this is true but is debated in literature) then prescribe acetaminophen alone or a combination with tramadol.
- ***Rest:*** Protection, rest, ice, compression, and elevation (PRICE) method (mentioned before) is the mainstay for treating soft-tissue injuries. Ice should be applied after completing exercise, stretching, and strengthening ideally. The use should be limited to protect ulnar nerve. Ice packs are usually placed over the area for 15–20 minutes. Ice bath serves the same purpose.
- ***Modification of activities:*** Decreasing the amount, frequency or intensity of activity. Athletes are often more compliant with a decreased level of activity if they are allowed to increase other nonaggravating activities.
- ***Elbow braces:*** Counterforce bracing and cock-up wrist splints can be useful adjuncts for treating medial epicondylitis. The mechanisms of counterforce bracing are mentioned in **Box 1**, most prominent of which for medial epicondylitis is decrease in the contraction forces of the flexor-pronator muscles. Cock-up wrist splints are particularly useful for patients with morning pain and soreness. Elbow taping may also be useful.
- ***Local corticosteroids, platelet rich plasma (PRP, delivering PDGF) injection:*** Care should be taken not to inject the steroid into the ulnar nerve.

Operative

If conservative treatment fails (usually 6–12 months), surgical treatment should be considered for medial epicondylitis for persistent or recalcitrant symptoms. Surgical intervention is preponed often if the ulnar nerve symptoms are more prominent and persistent. Various techniques have been described, most of which consist of release/slide of the flexor origin or medial epicondylectomy and excision of the pathologic tissue. The standard surgical treatment I follow comprises:

- Flexor pronator release
- Excision of the pathologic portion
- Enhancement of local vascularity be decortication or a couple of low intensity drill holes into the epicondyle
- Repair of the resultant defect
- Management of concurrent ulnar nerve or UCL pathology

Flexor origin debridement, and repair and reattachment, is performed through a longitudinal incision over the medial epicondyle. Branches of the medial antebrachial cutaneous nerve are carefully protected. Depending upon the location and nature of the pathologic tissue, an incision of the PT-FCR interval is developed either longitudinally or transversely. If the pathology is focal, a longitudinal split; while for diffuse pathology, a transverse incision is performed and the abnormal tissue is completely excised. MCL lying deep should be protected as is the ulnar nerve. If there is ulnar neuritis or entrapment, then it should be relieved. It is a good idea to perform epineurolysis if fibrosis is seen in the nerve. Debridement alone without tendon release may be associated with frequent recurrence. Ulnar nerve transposition is a bit too much, I feel.

Potential Complications of Operative Treatment

- Persistent ulnar nerve symptoms
- Medial collateral ligament injury
- Recurrence of symptoms

Postoperative Management

An above elbow plaster of Paris (POP) plaster splint is applied posteriorly with the elbow at 90° of flexion and the forearm in neutral rotation. This splint and skin sutures are removed at 7–10 days postoperatively and isometric exercises are begun at 3–4 weeks postoperatively. This is followed by resistive exercises for wrist flexion and forearm pronation at 6 weeks. Full return to sporting activity usually takes 4–6 months as with most other ligament reconstruction procedures.

BICEPS TENDON RUPTURE

INTRODUCTION

The biceps brachii commonly known as the biceps is a two-headed muscle that lies in the upper arm between the shoulder and the elbow. Biceps have a short head and a long head that arise on the scapula and join to form a single muscle belly in anterior arm that inserts by a tendon and aponeurosis to radius (bicipital tuberosity) and upper forearm, respectively. The proximal insertional tears are often innocuous and partial (involving one head) and seen

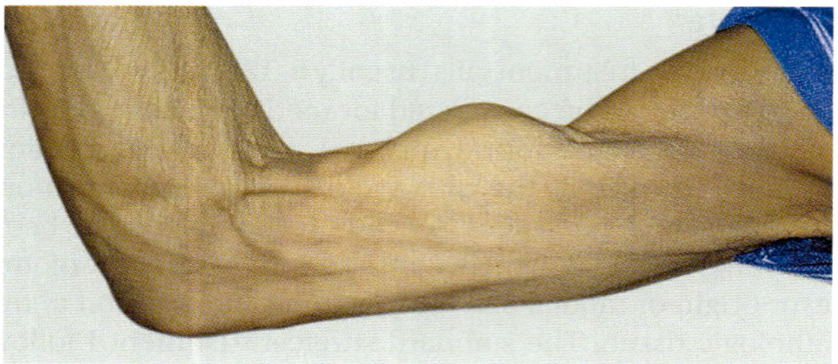

Fig. 7: Proximal biceps tendon rupture (Popeye biceps).

in elderly, especially the long head of biceps that produces mild-to-moderate elbow flexion weakness and a cosmetic deformity in the arm on flexing the elbow **(Fig. 7)**. Distal tears are quite disabling and vast majority are complete. Incomplete distal tears become complete in due course. The major impairment resulting from proximal biceps rupture involves limitations due to pain during the acute phase, but impairment ultimately relates to a decrease in strength during shoulder flexion, elbow flexion, and forearm supination.

ANATOMY

The biceps brachii muscle is involved in most of the functional activities of upper limb. The two distinct muscle bellies unite near the mid-shaft of the humerus and attach distally on the radial tuberosity. The distal tendon also blends with the bicipital aponeurosis (lacertus fibrosus) that fans medially over the flexor-pronator mass and affords protection to structures of the cubital fossa by forming its roof **(Fig. 7)**. This additional insertion allows distribution of forces across the elbow to lessen the pull on the radial tuberosity and improve the supination strength.

Nerve Supply

The biceps brachii is supplied by musculocutaneous nerve (C5, C6), a branch from the lateral cord of the brachial plexus.

PATHOPHYSIOLOGY

- The biceps muscle and its tendon lie most superficially in the arm and elbow.
- Distal intramural biceps tendon ruptures are relatively uncommon and account only for 3–10% of all biceps tendon injuries as most occur at the long head of biceps tendon proximally. The remaining ruptures occur distally at the insertion on the radial tuberosity or, even less commonly, at the short-head insertion on the acromion.
- As such the most common site for injury to the distal tendon is at its point of insertion into the radial tuberosity and not in the intramural portion of tendon **(Fig. 8)**.
- Most distal biceps rupture on a preexisting degenerative change within the tendon as for long-head rupture. The source of this preexisting asymptomatic degenerative change is considered to be the result of:
  - Friction and erosion of the tendon from repetitive rubbing against the bicipital tuberosity
  - Hypovascularity within areas of the distal portion of the tendon

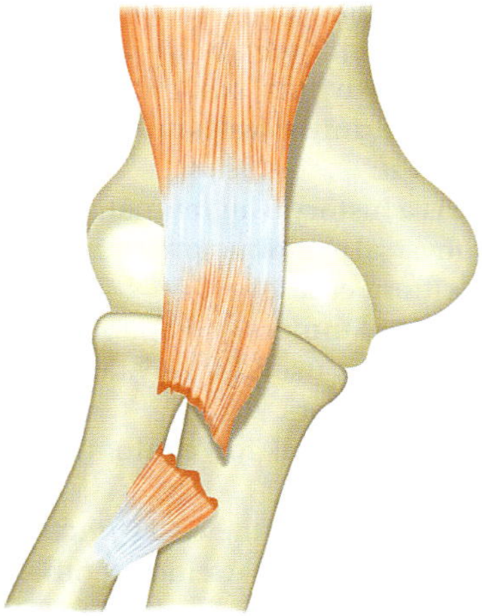

Fig. 8: Distal biceps tendon rupture.

Natural History

An untreated rupture of the distal biceps tendon leads to a 40% loss of strength in supination and a 30% loss of flexion strength of the elbow. In particular, sustained supination power is reduced by at least 50%. The tendon fails to heal naturally and will lead to chronic accrual of disability if left untreated.

EPIDEMIOLOGY

The injury is experienced most commonly in the individuals with history of shoulder problems aged 40–60 years, secondary to chronic wear of the tendon. In younger individuals, the tendon may rupture following a vigorous fall, heavy weightlifting or during sporting activities. Biceps tendon rupture is more common in males than females (related to activity levels probably). The dominant arm is involved more commonly, probably because it is used more often than is the nondominant arm.

CLINICAL PRESENTATION

Patient reports a sudden "pop" or "snap" when the flexed elbow is unacceptably loaded. Immediate severe pain follows with considerable swelling and bruising over the next few hours. On examination, there is localized pain and tenderness at the bicipital tuberosity. Proximal displacement of the distal biceps tendon with a bulge in the distal arm, inability to palpate the taut tendon within the antecubital fossa and marked weakness of forearm supination and elbow flexion (often associated with increased pain) are common findings. Various clinical tests have been described. There is discomfort in the antecubital fossa and loss of the normal biceps contour causing significant dissatisfaction in the patient. The special tests can be done to ascertain the pathology though most of the diagnosis is clear with presentation.

- ***Biceps squeeze test (similar to Thompson's test for tendo-Achilles):*** The patient is seated and elbow flexed 60–80° (to isolate supination action of biceps). The forearm is slightly pronated to take up the slack in muscle fibers and put tension on the biceps brachii tendon. The muscle belly is squeezed firmly in the midarm with both hands. One hand is placed at the distal myotendinous junction and the other hand around the muscle belly. Absence of forearm supination with this maneuver is considered positive test, suggesting rupture of the tendon or its muscle belly.

- ***The flexion initiation test:*** The patient is asked to attempt flexion of elbow with a 10-pound weight held in the hand starting with elbow extended. In an acute rupture of the tendon, this is not possible.
- ***The biceps hook test:*** Patient is asked to actively supinate with the elbow flexed to 90°. The biceps tendon fails to stand out at elbow.
- ***The biceps crease interval:*** The distance between antecubital crease and retracted distal edge of the tendon is measured using ruler. A value of >6 cm suggests poor prognosis but has good diagnostic accuracy to suggest a tendon rupture. The problem is that in acute cases ruptured tendon is not prominently palpable due to hematoma and associated swelling.

INVESTIGATIONS

- *Plain radiographs* may reveal hypertrophic spurring of radial tuberosity or bony irregularities suggesting frictional wear linked to rupture of biceps.
- *Arthrography* is not routinely used and has several drawbacks, including:
  - Invasiveness
  - Need for experienced interpreters of rarely seen images
  - Ionizing radiation
- *Ultrasonography* is useful for quick real-time examination of the biceps tendons. The problem lies with detection of intra-articular or partial thickness tears that are difficult to visualize, which interestingly is the most common site of rupture. Also, degenerative tears are often most difficult to detect ultrasonographically due to low echogenicity of whole tendon. Ultrasonography for musculoskeletal system as I always say is highly operator dependent and needs a dedicated sonologist. Advantages of ultrasonography include in general:
  - Absence of ionizing radiation
  - Dynamic "motion segment" evaluation is possible.
  - Painless
  - Easy and rapid interpretations
- *MRI* is the preferred modality to confirm a clinical rupture. It provides the greatest anatomic detail for the region. The only deterrent is the higher cost of MRI and ready availability as compared to costs of other imaging modalities.

TREATMENT

Conservative management is dismal and associated with poor prognosis. Surgical intervention undertaken within 2 weeks of rupture is the best method. There is little controversy that immediate reattachment of the distal biceps tendon is the procedure of choice.

Acute Injury

Two methods of reattachment have been described:

- The anterior Henry approach to the elbow and forearm **(Figs. 9A and B)**: This is more direct and a single incision is placed. It is technically more demanding than the two incision approach; also there is higher risk of damage to PIN if done by an inexperienced surgeon. One way to make the approach and fixation of the tendon easy is by using suture anchors that make it safer also. This is the reason now it is the preferred approach again.
- Boyd and Anderson described the dual-incision technique **(Figs. 10A and B)** due to the initial difficulty and complications of former. The tendon is retrieved anteriorly and passed through the forearm bones to be reattached through a posterior approach to the radial tuberosity, exposed by pronation of the forearm. The radial side of ulna should not be exposed, as there are high chances of synostosis formation and losing forearm rotations.

Delayed Presentation (2–3 Weeks after Injury)

Usually a straightforward reattachment of the tendon directly to the radial tuberosity is impossible (due to retraction). Nonanatomical replacement has been attempted by suturing the biceps tendon to the brachialis muscle tendon as closely as possible. Recovery of supination power gets substantially reduced by 50% though good flexion can be obtained by this method. The development of more sophisticated tendon-

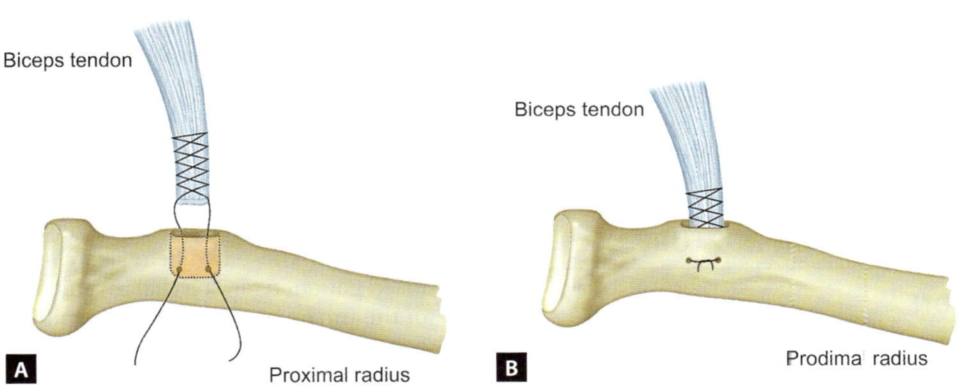

Figs. 9A and B: Biceps tendon repair—single incision technique (see text).

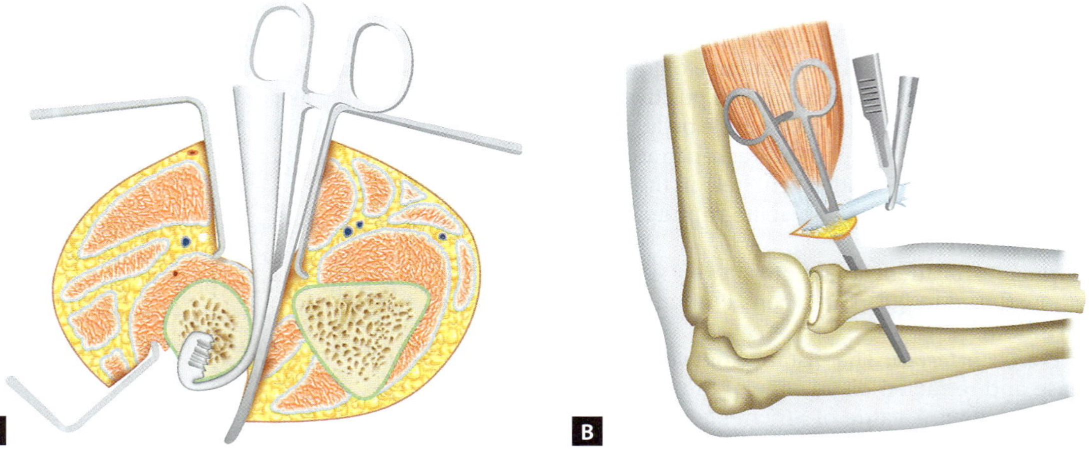

A B

Figs. 10A and B: Biceps tendon repair—two incision technique. The planes of anterior and posterior incisions (A) and final fixation with a soft tissue screw. Posterior incision can be located by passing a straight artery forceps from anterior incision (B).

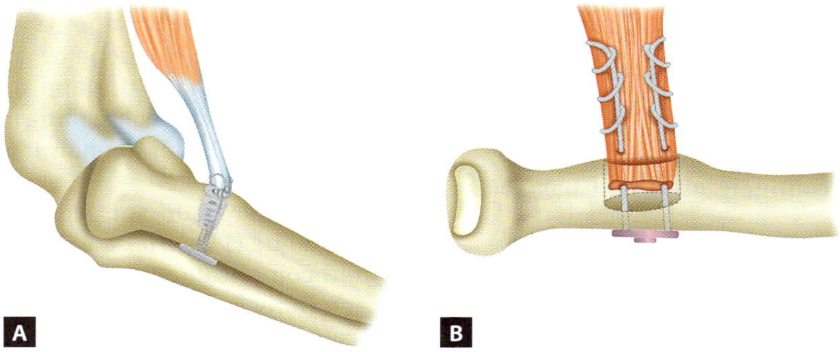

A B

Figs. 11A and B: Biceps tendon reconstruction: (A) the EndoButton technique; (B) Schematic illustration of passing the tendon through bone and placement of EndoButton.

to-bone fixation methods has enabled even long-standing ruptures to be repaired anatomically. To produce more anatomical repairs methods like applying sustained traction and/or epimysial relaxing incisions can be employed.

The EndoButton technique **(Figs. 11A and B)** can also be employed in these cases with reported good success.

Partial Ruptures

It is not clear whether true partial ruptures of the biceps tendon exist but surgeons have recommended repair in tears involving greater than 50% of the tendon width. Conversion of a partial to a complete tear with reattachment is the standard treatment in these cases.

Postoperatively, the patient's elbow is splinted at 90° of flexion. For next 3–4 weeks, patients are permitted to actively extend the elbow while passively flexing the joint followed by active flexion at elbow and active rotation of the forearm. Full activity is permitted after 6 months from surgery.

TRICEPS TENDON RUPTURE

INTRODUCTION

Triceps tendon ruptures are extremely rare and account for <1% of all tendon injuries. Partridge was the first to report this injury in the medical literature in 1868.

ANATOMY

Triceps has three heads: (i) The long head, (ii) The medial head, and (iii) The lateral head with three points of origin.

1. The long head of the triceps muscle arises from the infraglenoid tubercle.
2. The medial head originates from the inferomedial aspect of the radial groove of the humerus, medial to the origin of the lateral head at its proximal end. Medial head is more muscular and its origin widens to include the entire posterior surface of the humerus together with each intermuscular septum. It runs in arm deep to the long and lateral heads. For insertion, it gives rise to a separate tendon that inserts in part to the olecranon, in part to the flattened fused tendon of the long and lateral heads and in part to the posterior aspect of the elbow joint capsule, preventing impingement of the capsule on extension of the elbow.
3. The lateral head arises from the posterior surface of the humerus from a linear origin extending from the surgical neck to the deltoid origin and lies lateral to the long head. These two heads converge distally to form a fused flattened tendon that inserts into the posterior part of the proximal end of the olecranon. Superficial fibers continue as the triceps expansion and insert into the posterior crest of the ulna medially and the fascia of the extensor carpi ulnaris laterally.

PATHOPHYSIOLOGY

The cause of distal triceps tendon ruptures **(Fig. 12)** can be categorized into three groups:

1. The *traumatic group* includes healthy individuals (typically athletes) in whom the cause is violent trauma in which an extending elbow has been suddenly decelerated (eccentric contraction), say to break a fall on outstretched arm. The triceps tendon avulses from the olecranon sometimes with a small piece of bone. In the *pathological group*, the tendon is either weakened by chronic tendinosis, corticosteroids, infection, inflammation or the bone is weakened (such as renal osteodystrophy, osteogenesis imperfecta, osteoporosis, secondary hyperparathyroidism, and osteogenesis imperfecta tarda). Tendon injury occurs with normal physiological forces.
2. The *iatrogenic group* patients are those where the tendon ruptures following surgical mobilization or elbow arthroplasty (2%).

The most common site of triceps tears is at the insertion of the tendon with or without a bony avulsion.

CLINICAL PRESENTATION

History

For acute traumatic injuries, the typical history often is a fall onto an outstretched hand. The patient complains of pain and swelling at the insertion site of the triceps. Direct trauma to the extensor surface of the arm has also been reported as a method of rupture. Patients in pathological group usually have prodromal symptoms of elbow pain and give a history of low-energy trauma to the elbow. The iatrogenic group has history of a surgical procedure that required mobilization of the extensor mechanism of the elbow. Trauma is usually absent and extensor weakness is uncommonly reported because the elbow can be easily extended by relaxing the elbow flexors. It is often an examination finding.

Examination

Swelling and tenderness over the triceps insertion:

- There is a palpable defect.
- The patient has weakness of elbow extension that is most reliably demonstrated by fully elevating the arm with the elbow at 90° and asking the patient to extend the elbow against gravity.
- In chronic cases, an extensor lag of up to 30° may be identified at presentation.
- Triceps squeeze test can be performed similar to the gastrosoleus squeeze test. The arm is held in approximately 90° of abduction in scapular plane and the triceps muscle belly is squeezed. Extension of the elbow indicates a partial rupture of the triceps mechanism.

INVESTIGATIONS

- ***Imaging:*** Plain radiographs identify acute fracture of the olecranon or a bony avulsion.
- ***Ultrasound:*** It has been used to investigate distal triceps tendon ruptures.
- ***MRI:*** It is the preferred investigation. It can distinguish between partial and full thickness tears and also shows significant retraction of the tendon.

TREATMENT

Partial tears of the distal triceps tendon may be treated nonoperatively when up to 75% of the triceps tendon. Surgery is the preferred method of managing complete tears unless the patient is frail enough to be unfit for surgical repair or reconstruction. The extensor mechanism of the elbow is usually intact laterally, where the lateral border of the triceps muscle may retain its continuity with the medial border of anconeus. Patients with iatrogenic ruptures are best treated with a reconstructive procedure. This is because primary repairs often fail due to the pullout of sutures from an olecranon with poor bone quality.

A posterior approach is used and the triceps muscle, tendon, and olecranon are identified. A heavy nonabsorbable suture, such as Ethibond or FiberWire, is passed through the proximal portion of the tendon which is brought down and sutured to the transverse holes drilled in the olecranon **(Fig. 13)**. If there is a sizable piece of bone attached to the proximal portion of the tendon that has avulsed from the

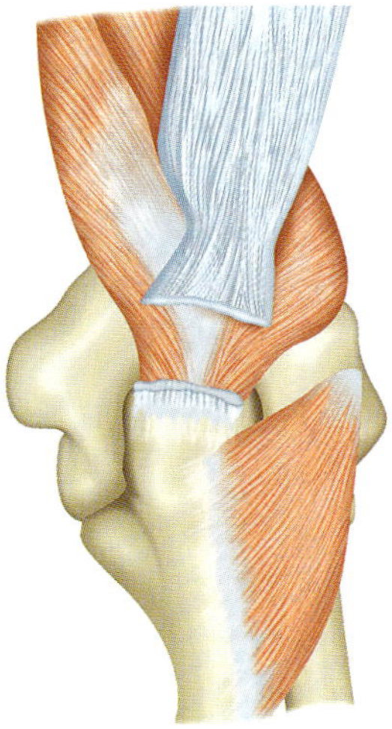

Fig. 12: Pathoanatomy of triceps tendon rupture.

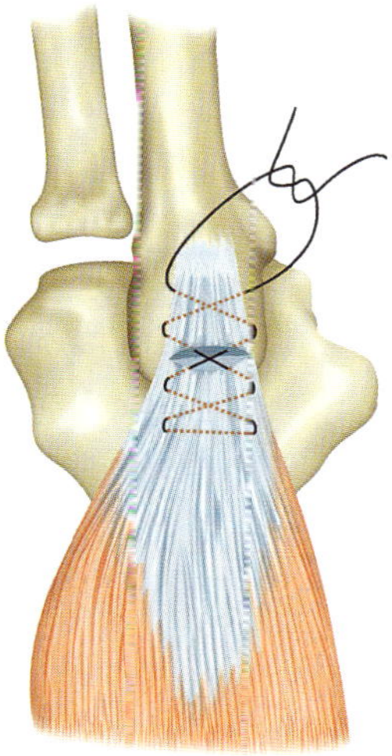

Fig. 13: Triceps tendon repair.

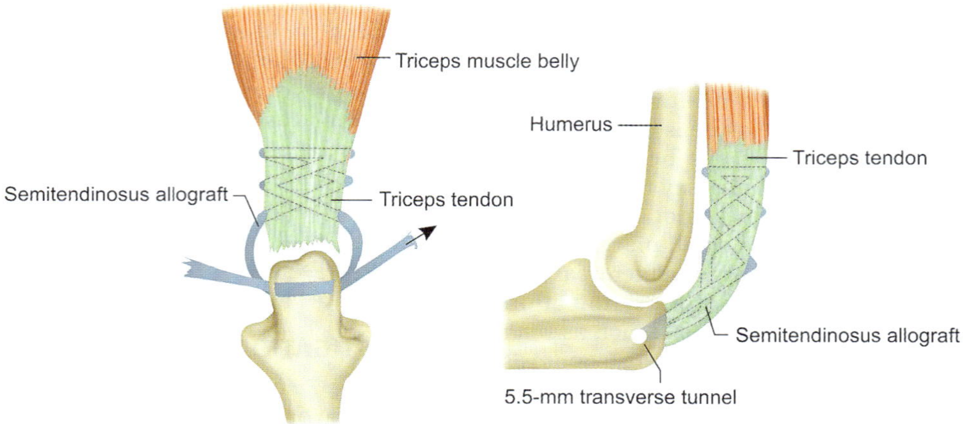

Fig. 14: Triceps tendon reconstruction.

olecranon, the repair is easier with internal fixation of the avulsion fracture. Tendon repair is effective if the injury is treated early (within 3 weeks) and there is no significant retraction of the tendon.

For chronic and iatrogenic full thickness, triceps tendon ruptures with retraction of the tendon into the muscle belly and subsequent scarring; reconstruction is a better option. Anconeus slide is performed for severe retractions. The distal portion of the anconeus is detached and reattached to the olecranon. The retracted triceps tendon is sutured to the medial border of the proximal portion of anconeus that augments and compensates for the deficiency in length of the triceps.

Reconstruction with ligament augmentation is done **(Fig. 14)** for even more severe retractions. Alternatively, Achilles tendon allograft with a small piece of calcaneus can be used.

COMPLICATIONS

The major complication of triceps tendon repair or reconstruction is rerupture.

CONCLUSION

- Tendon disorders are the most common cause of pain around elbow. Careful evaluation is needed to find the pain generator and differentiate it from some neurological and related causes so that correct treatment can be instituted.
- Tendinosis is usually treated conservatively to begin with that controls the disease process and symptoms in majority of patients, however, those who fail to respond to symptomatic treatment and activity modification or continue to progress symptomatically are managed by local injections (commonly as an intermediate measure) or operatively.
- Ruptures of chief flexor or extensor tendons need repair or reconstruction depending on acute or chronic presentation in younger patients, however, in older patients due to limited functional deficit they may be managed conservatively, providing strengthening exercises and activity modification.

CHAPTER

109 The Unstable Elbow

Manish Kumar Varshney

INTRODUCTION

Despite common finding of elbow dislocations (second most common joint to dislocate in adults and most common in children), chronic elbow instability remains uncommon in general population. Whenever present, however, it is debilitating particularly in an athlete or an active professional. The incidence of elbow dislocation is six patients in 100,000 but only 30 cases of recurrent dislocation reported in literature by 1966 and 40 cases by 1971. Of all the cases reported for chronic instability, half of the chronic instability occurred in conjunction with intra-articular fractures (treated/untreated). One-third of the cases have generalized joint laxity while one-sixth had simple dislocation. So even following quite complete and ominous looking elbow dislocation, instability occurs in only 15–35%.

CLASSIFICATION OF ELBOW INSTABILITY

Five criteria have been used to classify elbow instabilities **(Table 1)**. The various described patterns of elbow instability are as follows:

- Valgus instability:
  - Athletic chronic overuse injuries
  - Repetitive overload
    - Intrinsic (muscular)
    - Extrinsic (external tensile overload)
- Varus instability:
  - Posterolateral rotatory instability (PLRI)
  - Recurrent isolated radial head instability
- Anterior instability
- Posterior instability

TABLE 1: Classification criteria for elbow instability.

Articulation involved	Proximal radioulnar joint (radial head)	Ulnohumeral and radiohumeral (elbow)	Both (divergent)
Direction of displacement	• Anterior • Posterior	• Varus/valgus • Anteroposterior • Mediolateral • Posterolateral rotatory instability	Posterior
Degree of displacement	Subluxation	Perched	Complete
Timing	• Acute • Chronic	• Acute/chronic • Recurrent	Acute
Associated fractures	None	• Radial head • Olecranon • Coronoid	None

ETIOLOGY

- *Acquired/traumatic causes:*
  - Simple dislocation **(Figs. 1A and B)**
  - Fracture dislocation **(Fig. 2)**—there are increased chances of instability. In the decreasing order of contribution, the fractures responsible for producing instability include:
    - Coronoid (58%)
    - Radial head (17%)
    - Posterior capitellum
    - Medial and lateral epicondyle
  - Fractures in association with ligament injuries—"terrible triad injuries (see below)"
  - *Pure ligament injuries:*
    - "Valgus-extension overload syndrome":
    - Medial collateral ligament (MCL) attenuation, radiocapitellar joint compression, posteromedial ulnohumeral compression
    - Overuse injuries—cricketers and pitchers
    - Fall on outstretched hand
    - Apophysitis in children → functional lengthening of MCL
  - *Hyperextension injury:*
    - Anterior capsular tear
    - L-shaped rupture of flexor-pronator group
    - Elongation of lateral collateral ligament (LCL)
    - Incomplete rupture of LCL
- Congenital
- *Arthropathies:*
  - Joint erosion—loss of bony congruity
  - Periarticular ligament attenuation
  - Direction of nonspecific instability

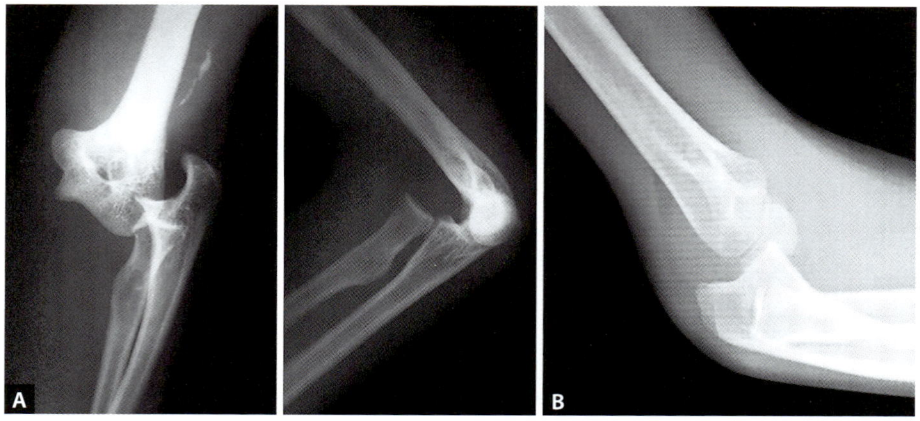

Figs. 1A and B: (A) Dislocation of elbow joint in an adult; (B) Pediatric age group.

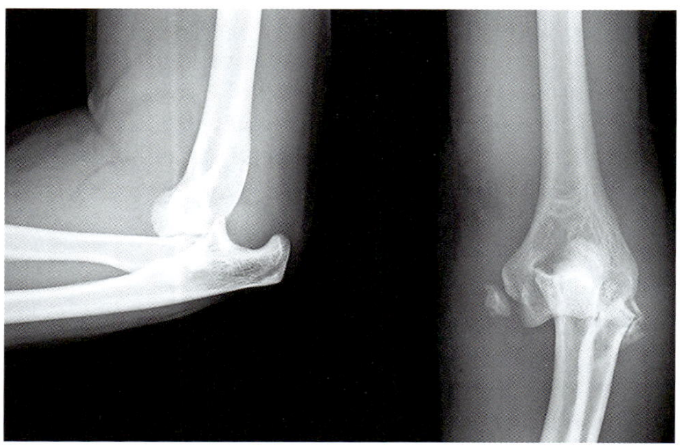

Fig. 2: Fracture dislocation of right elbow.

- *Iatrogenic:*
    - Overenthusiastic dissection of tissue in surgery for lateral epicondylitis
    - Kocher approach—if plain between anconeus and extensor carpi ulnaris not maintained then you divide LCL.
    - Radial head excision—functional lengthening of lateral ulnar collateral ligament (LUCL)
    - Excessive medial epicondylectomy for cubital tunnel syndrome
- *Repetitive valgus stress:* This produces chondromalacia, loose bodies, injury to LCL, injury to flexor group, osteochondritis dissecans, and ulnar neuritis.

PATHOMECHANICS

The inconsistent finding of chronic instability following trauma has led various thinkers and researchers for exploring and explaining the different possibilities as regard the sequence of events and specific events that produce instability.

Older Concepts

- 1966—"instability due to persistent defect"
    - Fall → axial compression and valgus strain → MCL stretched and avulsion of lateral epicondyle with fracture posterior ½ of capitellum.

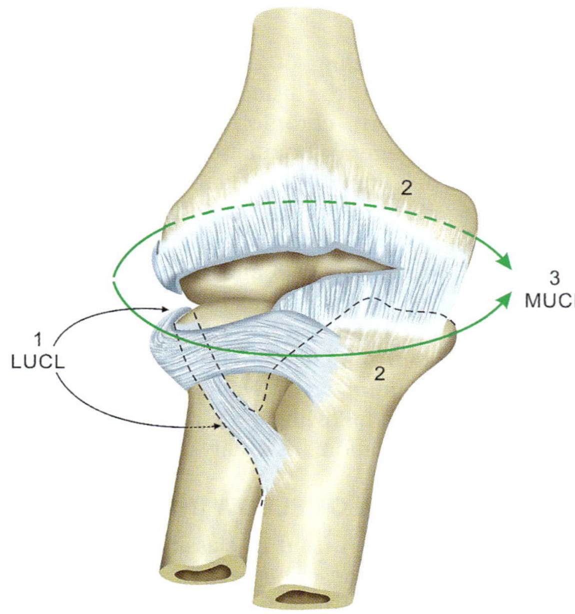

Fig. 3: Horii circle—this concept envisages progressive disruption of structures from lateral to medial across the periphery in the form of a circle. (LUCL: lateral ulnar collateral ligament; MUCL: medial ulnar collateral ligament)

- 1980 (Schwab et al.)—"hyperextension mechanism"
    - Olecranon levers against fossa → rupture MCL
- 1987 (Josefson)—"rupture of dynamic constraints" along with Schwab's concept
- 1989 (Söjberg)—"forced valgus and supination" as essential lesions
- 1991 (O'Driscoll)—combined Sjöberg and Osbourne's concept with classification as follows.

Unified Concept of Clinical Spectrum of Acute and Recurrent Elbow Instability—"Circle Concept" (Fig. 3)

- Three sequential stages of elbow instability
- The Horii circle **(Fig. 3)** progresses from lateral to medial side.
- It may pass through soft tissue or bone or both.

Stages:

- *Stage I:* LCL disruption → posterolateral rotatory subluxation → spontaneous reduction.
- *Stage II:* Additional anterior and posterior disruption → coronoid perched over trochlea → reduced with minimum force.
- *Stage III:* Subdivided into three parts:
  i. IIIA: Anterior MCL intact → stable in pronation
  ii. IIIB: Entire MCL disrupted → varus, valgus, and rotatory instability following reduction.
  iii. IIIC: Entire distal humerus devoid of soft-tissue attachment → unstable even in 90° flexion in cast.

Salient features of the Horii concept:

- As disruption can pass through bone/soft tissues or both → capsule may get spared if coronoid is fractured, energy gets dissipated.
- Supports the concept of immobilizing the limb in hyperflexion and pronation.

The support to unified concept comes from patients with recurrent elbow dislocation who do well with LCL reconstruction alone. Also reconstruction of anterior MCL has been shown to be no different than nonoperative treatment.

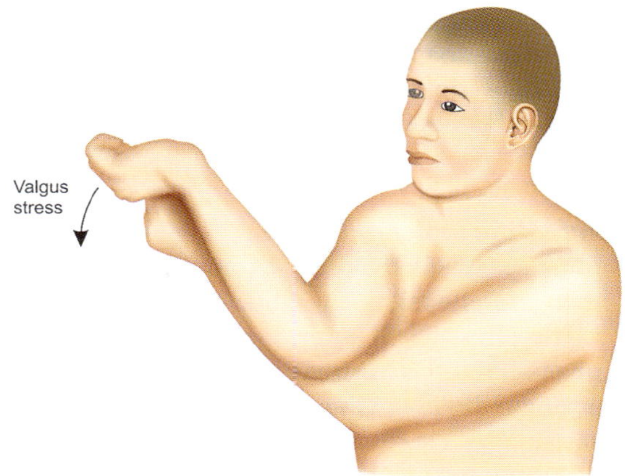

Fig. 4: Milking maneuver (see text).

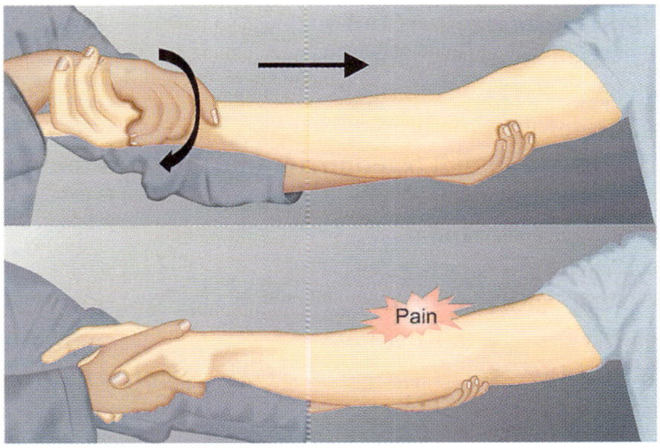

Fig. 5: The radiocapitellar compression test is elicited by forceful pronation of supinated elbow while applying axial load in the direction of proximal radius.

EVALUATION OF THE PATIENT WITH CHRONIC INSTABILITY

The following points should be evaluated for a patient to determine the cause of instability, extent of instability, and guiding the treatment.

History

- Antecedent trauma
- Overuse sports injury
- Congenital anomalies
- Surgery to elbow
- Erosive arthropathy
- Generalized ligament laxity
- Locking/clicking with clunk when elbow supinated in extension half way through range-of-motion (ROM)
- Assess patients' needs and demands.

Examination

Examine the patient for generalized joint laxity and features of arthropathy. Specific local examination of the elbow is done to look for:

- External signs of injury/surgery
- Tenderness over collateral ligaments.
- ***Stress tests:***
  - Valgus—patient's elbow is flexed beyond 25° to unlock the olecranon from its fossa and minimize the bony contribution to joint stability. While applying valgus stress, ulnar collateral ligament (UCL) is palpated while simultaneously applying a valgus stress. Local pain, tenderness, and end-point laxity are characterized with this maneuver.
  - Varus—in similar position as above, varus stress is applied to the elbow joint to assess the integrity of lateral collateral ligament. The assessment is done by palpating along the lateral humeroradial joint line to assess laxity of ligament and tenderness along the joint line for injury.
- ***Milking maneuver (Fig. 4)*** is a sensitive test for damage to the UCL and is performed with the elbow at 70–90° of flexion. Traction is placed on the thumb in a radial direction imparting a valgus force on the elbow. Local pain and tenderness indicate injury to the medial ulnar collateral ligament (MUCL).
- ***Radiocapitellar compression test:*** The forearm is placed in extension while pain is elicited over lateral side of elbow (radio-capitellar joint) on prono-supination of the forearm with axial force applied proximally in longitudinal direction **(Fig. 5)**. Alternatively, the elbow is moved in mid-flexion range while axial load is applied to the radius compressing the radiocapitellar joint that elicits pain over lateral elbow.
- ***Lateral pivot-shift test:*** Kindly see posterolateral rotatory instability later in the chapter.
- ***Valgus laxity in pronation:*** Increase in elbow valgus laxity in forearm pronation indicates subtle UCL deficiency and suggests predisposition to its injury on chronic repetitive valgus stress at elbow.

- Valgus-extension overload test—please see valgus extension overload syndrome later in the chapter.
- ***Ulnar nerve:*** Tinel's test and examine for subluxation of nerve and incident neuritis.

Investigations

- ***Examination under anesthesia:***
    - *Indication:* Positive history; no physical signs other than apprehension. The elbow is often stable to varus/valgus stress test if anterior band of MCL intact; only pivot-shift test is positive in such cases. So, to globally evaluate the following, tests should be done in these cases:
        - Varus stress test
        - Valgus stress test
        - Lateral pivot-shift test
        - Posterolateral rotatory drawer test
- ***Plain radiographs:*** Look for:
    - Associated bony injuries
    - Degenerative changes
    - Heterotrophic bone formation
    - Posteromedial osteophytes and calcification medial to medial epicondyle
- ***Stress radiographs:***
    - Varus stress
    - Valgus stress
    - Posterolateral stress
- ***MRI (57% sensitive and 100% specific) and MR arthrography:***
    - Rupture of collateral ligaments
    - Rupture of muscle groups
- ***CT arthrography (86% sensitive and 97% specific):***
    - Undersurface tear in MCL → T-sign **(Fig. 6)**.
- ***Arthroscopy:*** Unlikely to provide any further information.
    - Able to diagnose MCL strain/partial tear by observing opening of medial joint space on valgus stress (1994, Timmerman and Andrews)
    - Concept countered by Field and Altchek (1996).

DIFFERENTIAL DIAGNOSIS

Various disorders can mimic elbow instability with respect to the symptoms or examination findings or both. These can be divided based on different regions of the elbow.

Anterior

Brachialis tendonitis, biceps tendonitis, anterior capsular tear, distal biceps rupture, ectopic bone, pronator teres syndrome, annular ligament disruption, and loose bodies.

Posterior

Traction apophysitis, triceps tendonitis, triceps rupture, valgus-extension overload syndrome (VEOS), stress fracture olecranon, olecranon fracture, and olecranon bursitis.

Medial

Medial epicondylar physeal fracture, medial epicondylitis, flexor-pronator rupture, snapping elbow syndrome, medial elbow instability, ulnar neuritis, and loose bodies.

Lateral

Osteochondritis dissecans, Panner's disease, radial neck physeal fracture, radial head fracture, radiocapitellar overload syndrome (RCOS), lateral epicondylitis, extensor-supinator muscle rupture, radial nerve entrapment, and PLRI.

MANAGEMENT OF ELBOW INSTABILITY

The discussion will include both the management of acute and chronic cases:

For acute dislocation of elbow, the management guidelines depend on various examination findings as detailed in the Flowchart **(Fig. 7)**. Once surgical management is conceptualized based on the algorithm further planning can be done as detailed in the Flowchart **(Fig. 8)**. Repair and reattachment of ligament injury is quite straightforward using anchor sutures. Associated capsular tears, however, are best treated by immobilization for 10 days to 2 weeks and mobilizing gradually.

Management of chronic or recurrent instability depends upon following parameters:

- Frequency
- Severity
- Requirement
- Expectations of patient

The management can be conservative or operative, that has specific indications. **Conservative management** involves variable use of the following modalities.

- Activity modification:
    - Avoid aggravating movements
    - Attention to technique in athletes

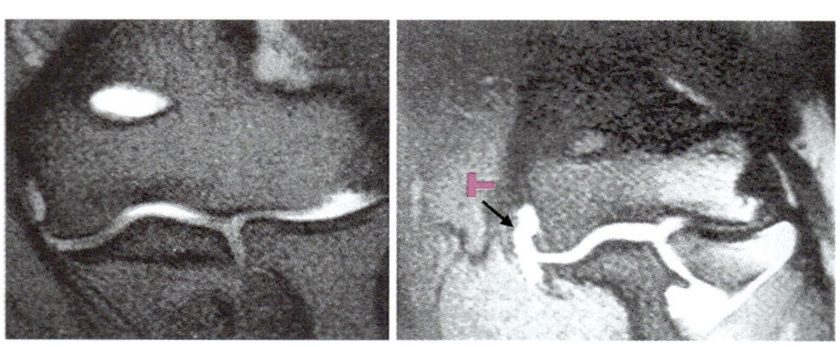

Fig. 6: The "T" Sign—in medial collateral ligament ruptures the contrast exudes out and forms a 90° rotated "T"-shaped image (right). On left is shown the plain MR image.

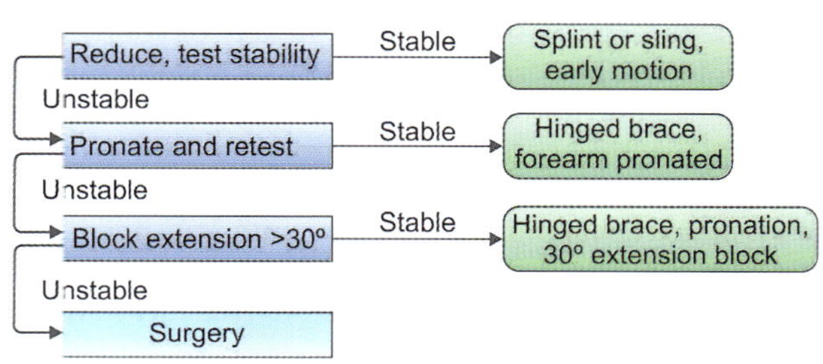

Fig. 7: Management of acute dislocation: Decision-making algorithm.

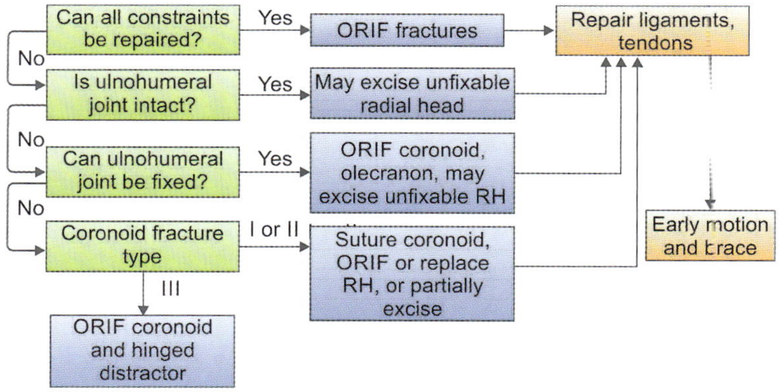

Fig. 8: Management of dislocated elbow: Surgical treatment algorithm. (ORIF: open reduction and internal fixation)

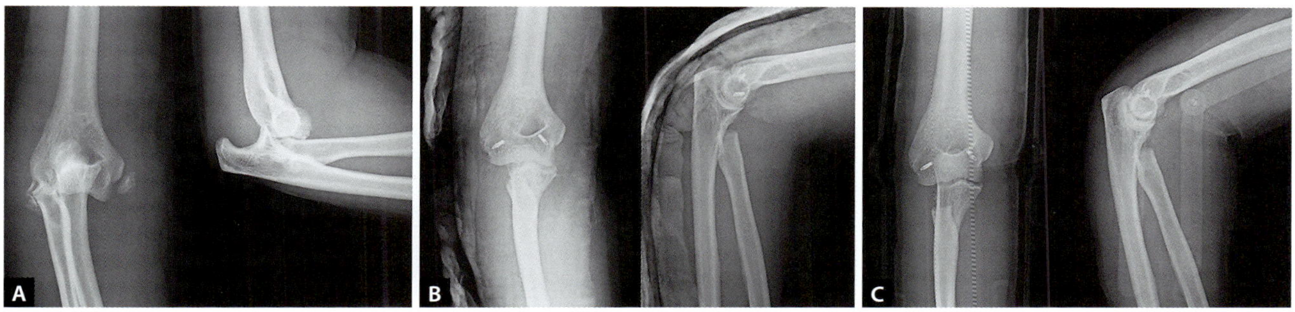

Figs. 9A to C: (A) Fracture dislocation of elbow; (B) Refixation of avulsed collateral ligaments using suture anchors; (C) Mobilization in hinge-brace.

- ***Functional bracing:*** Prevents excessive valgus strain
- ***Steroid injections and anesthetic*:** Do not address the pathology and are not useful.
- For overuse injuries:
  - P—protection
  - R—rest
  - I—ice
  - C—compression
  - E—elevation
  - M—medications
  - M—modalities: galvanic current, iontophoresis

Operative management of chronic instability is primarily cause-based and involves:

- Fracture fixation/refixation
- Reattach avulsed ligament (better for early fresh cases only, **Figs. 9A to C**)
- Reattach common flexor-extensor origins
- Ligament reconstruction with tendon fixation with synthetic ligament
- Hinge external fixator is indicated in patients with:
  - Persistent instability
  - Gross acute instability in a candidate not fit for surgery
  - Delayed treatment (≥4 weeks) of a dislocated/stiff elbow
  - Patients who have polytrauma.
- ***Distraction arthroplasty (Fig. 10):*** It is based upon the fact that there is a very small locus of center of rotation.
  - *Goal:*
    - Separate joint surface
    - Reorient joint surface
    - Protect ligament healing
    - Allow motion
  - *Indications:*
    - Ligament reconstruction/repair
    - Acute/subacute instability
    - Coronoid fractures
    - Humeral articular surface fractures
    - Interposition arthroplasty
    - Stiff elbow
- ***Total elbow arthroplasty/replacement arthroplasty of elbow:*** *Semi-constrained/linked prosthesis*—this is predominantly used in reconstruction of post-traumatic elbow instability. Coonrad–Morrey design **(Fig. 11)** is the prototype of linked prosthesis.
  - *Specific indications for use of total elbow arthroplasty (TEA) in unstable elbow include:*
    - Elderly patient with post-traumatic/arthritic joint destruction with deficit bone stock
    - Unstable capsuloligamentous support
    - Deformity at elbow that requires correction along with the management of capsuloligamentous structures.
  - *Contraindications:*
    - An active or a subacute infection
    - Neuromuscular deficiency of the elbow joint flexors
    - Soft-tissue scarring and poor tissue coverage
  - Posterior/Bryan–Morrey approach is best approach for performing this procedure in lateral position or supine position with support under ipsilateral scapula. The details of procedure can be obtained from dedicated texts.

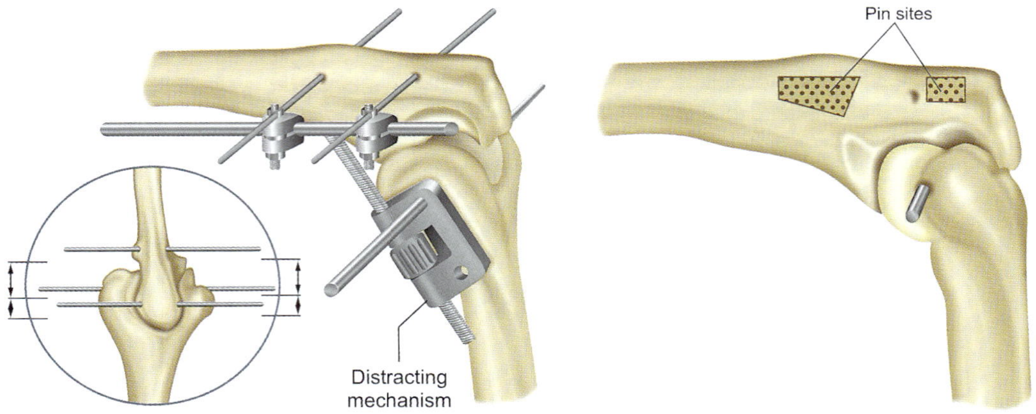

Fig. 10: Illustration depicting distraction arthroplasty apparatus and application for management of elbow ligament insufficiency and use while healing is awaited.

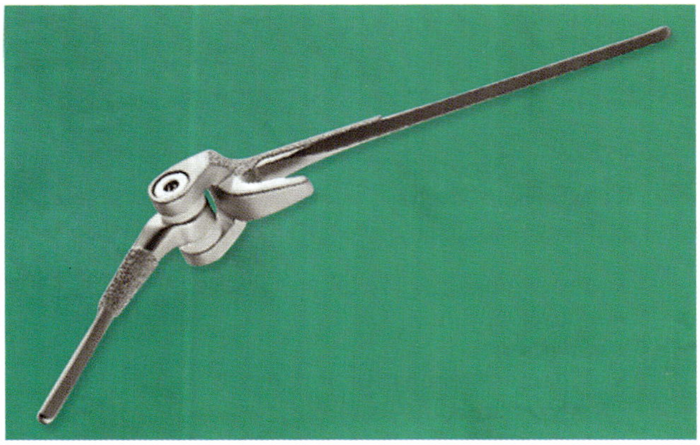

Fig. 11: Total elbow replacement: The Coonrad–Morrey design.

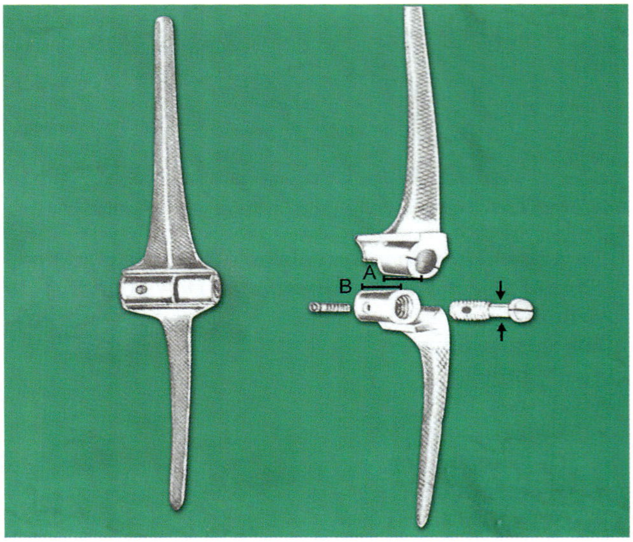

Fig. 12: Elbow arthroplasty: Bakshi's sloppy hinge prosthesis.

- *Postoperative management:*
    - Postoperative splintage in full extension
    - Assisted flexion and forearm rotation started 2nd day with gravity assisted extension
    - Daytime resting splint in 90o flexion for 6 weeks
    - Night-time extension splint for 12 weeks
- *Lifetime restrictions*
    - Lifting weight not >5 kg
    - Avoid upper limb impact sports.

Bakshi's sloppy hinge prosthesis (Figs. 12 and 13): This is another linked prosthesis. "Sloppy" design offers 5–10° of out-of-plane laxity (rotation) of the ulnar component → unloading stress at this point. Slowly the use of this design (indigenous to India) is decreasing.

Some specific conditions under the term elbow instability are discussed below due to their distinctive nature, presentation and treatment that is difficult to generalize.

CHRONIC VALGUS ELBOW INSTABILITY

This arises due to chronic MUCL instability or deficiency. The condition is quite prominent in overhead motion athletes. Injury to the UCL may be acute, chronically disrupted, or chronically attenuated. Anterior bundle of the UCL is the primary structure resisting valgus stress at the elbow (see elbow anatomy and biomechanics). Waris was the first to recognize and describe UCL tears, particularly isolated anterior oblique ligament disruption, in javelin throwers. Trauma (acute) to this ligament rarely leads to symptomatic instability in the majority of those injured but repetitive overuse interestingly produces instability. Overuse is the common cause of UCL insufficiency especially in throwing athlete that have been reporting inner elbow pain and discomfort with throwing for long. In a competitive sport throw, nearly 64 Nm of force is generated with around 60% forces transmitted through UCL. UCL can withstand forces up to 34.6 Nm. Plastic changes are seen in UCL at 22.7–34 Nm moment and above that the ligament fails. Chronic UCL insufficiency also induces formation of posterior medial gutter osteophytes, radiocapitellar degeneration due to overload and ulnar neuritis in advanced untreated cases.

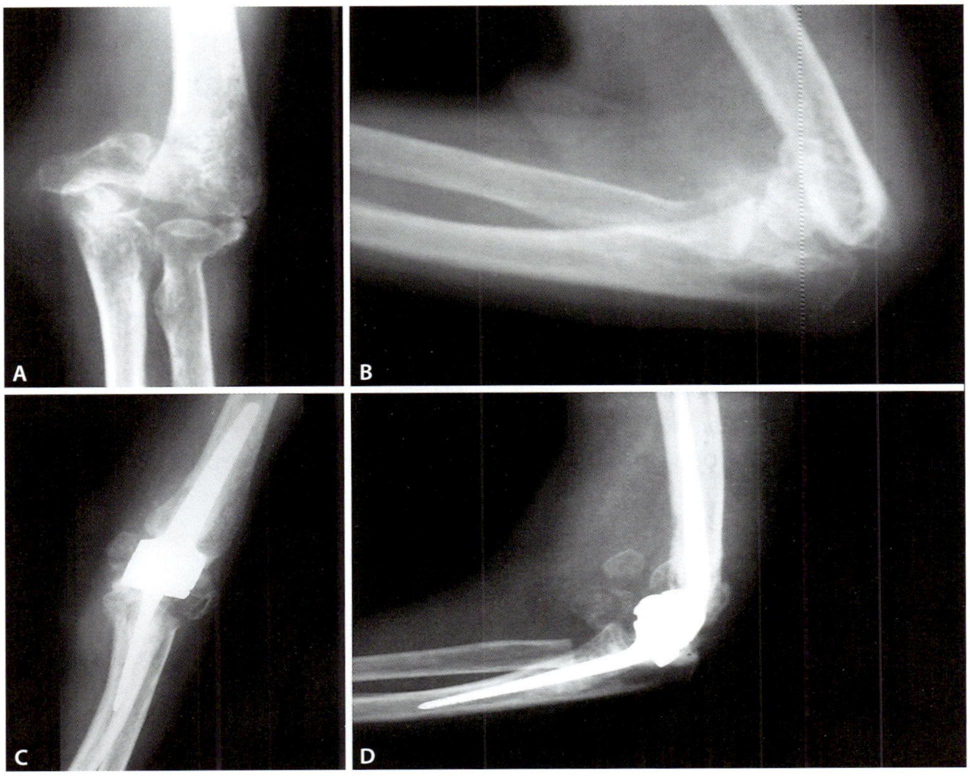

Figs. 13A to D: Bakshi's sloppy hinge prosthesis done for chronic unstable elbow.

Clinical Features

Patients report a pop or acute onset of pain but no true inciting event. Medial side elbow pain during throwing activity is reported. Pain is reported at two specific events of a throw predominantly first at the acceleration phase of throwing and second with ball release or point of impact in hitting the ball. There is point tenderness over the ligament 2 cm distal to medial epicondyle and pain on valgus stress testing. The tenderness is often located to the insertion at the sublime tubercle of ulna. Features of medial epicondylitis may be present causing pain on resisted wrist flexion. In chronic advanced cases, additional findings may be found:

- ***Ulnar nerve irritation due to neuritis and associated symptoms:*** The medial joint instability under valgus loading and the cubitus valgus deformity lead to nerve traction injury, whereas friction injuries result from recurrent subluxation of the nerve or abrasion by posteromedial osteophytes producing ulnar nerve lesions. Tinel's sign may also be positive.
- Locking due to loose body formation
- Lateral joint line tenderness due to radiocapitellar arthritis
- Swelling due to synovitis and collection and associated stiffness

Examination

Clinical findings include localized tenderness over the ulnar insertion of the ligament **(Fig. 14)**, posterior olecranon fossa tenderness due to impingement, swelling or fullness in soft spot. Ulnar nerve should be examined for neuritis (local tenderness and thickening) and weakness in the innervated muscles. Specific tests to evaluate the integrity of the ligament include:

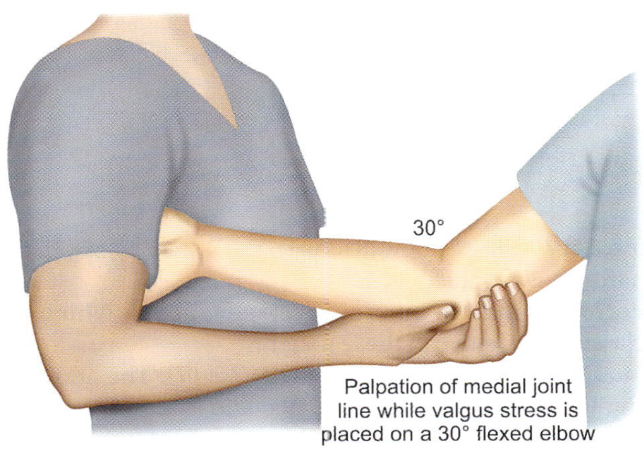

Fig. 14: Palpation for medial ulnar collateral ligament (UCL)] tenderness in valgus instability.

- Valgus-extension overload test is used to determine UCL incompetence: The examiner tries to bring the arm in extension while applying a valgus stress to the elbow.
- Valgus stressing the elbow **(Figs. 15A and B)** with the elbow flexed 30°. This test is less useful for two reasons, one that the humeral rotation is poorly controlled and second that UCL is most autonomous in resisting valgus

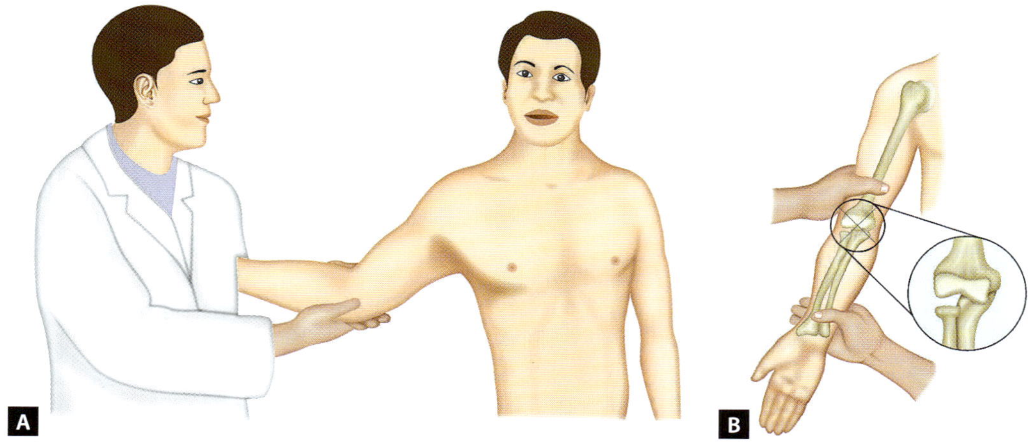

Figs. 15A and B: Valgus stress test. (A) Demonstrates the clinical technique of doing same; (B) Demonstrates the forces applied to ligaments with the test.

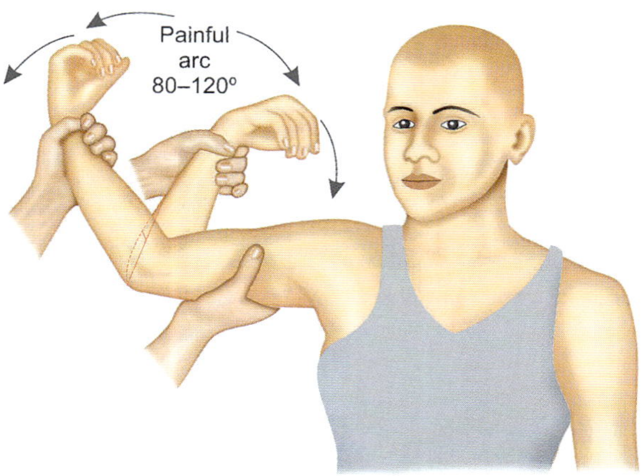

Fig. 16: Eliciting painful arc in elbow movements.

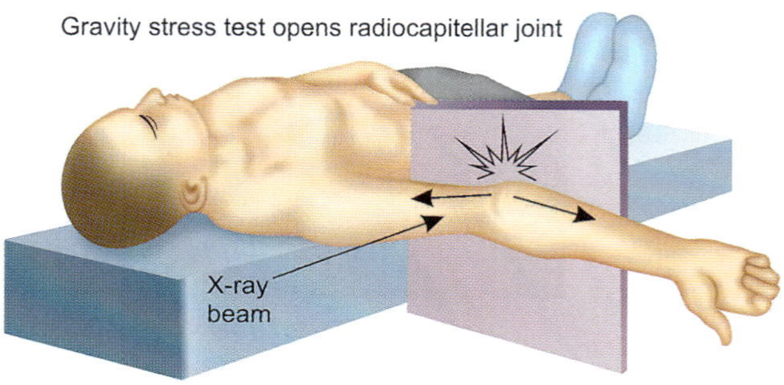

Fig. 17: Gravity assisted radiological evaluation of elbow joint for medial collateral ligament (MCL) insufficiency.

force at 70–90° of elbow flexion so the test in 30° of flexion hardly does evaluate it.

- Perform milking maneuver (see above) which is classically positive in these patients.
- ***Moving valgus stress test (of O'Driscoll):*** The athlete's shoulder is placed in an abducted and externally rotated position. The elbow is then flexed and extended while imparting a valgus force to the elbow. For those athletes with UCL insufficiency, pain is felt at a specific and reproducible point within the arc of 80–120° of elbow flexion **(Fig. 16)**.
- ***Gravity stress test (Fig. 17):*** Performed with the patient supine and the shoulder brought into maximal external rotation with the sagittal plane of the elbow parallel to the floor. In this position, the valgus stress is applied by the weight of forearm and resisted solely by the flexor-pronator mass and MUCL. Radiograph can be taken in this position to demonstrate the joint opening.
- ***Timmerman arthroscopic valgus stress test:*** Apparently the most sensitive and specific way to diagnose UCL disruptions, but need an experienced arthroscopist. Valgus stability of the elbow is best assessed in 60–75° of elbow flexion. Rupture of the anterior bundle results in only 1–2 mm of medial joint gapping when viewed arthroscopically, whereas complete release of the UCL results in 4–10 mm of medial joint opening.

Radiology

Radiographs in addition to opening of joint under stress may show ossification within the UCL (2 mm of relative increased laxity and 3 mm of absolute medial joint gapping are consistent with an incompetent UCL). Other findings include lateral compression symptoms like loose bodies in the posterior compartment, marginal osteophytes about the radiocapitellar or the ulnohumeral articulations or osteochondrotic lesions of the capitellum. Contrast MRI is a useful investigation supporting the ligament injury as primary pathology, its definition and localization. Dynamic ultrasonography provides a rapid means for evaluating the UCL; it also demonstrates increased medial elbow laxity with valgus stress but is highly user dependent.

Management

In early cases, return to function is most important. This can be partly achieved by nonsteroidal anti-inflammatory medications, alternating ice and heat and physical therapy modalities. These modalities provide good pain relief and encourage functional rehabilitation.

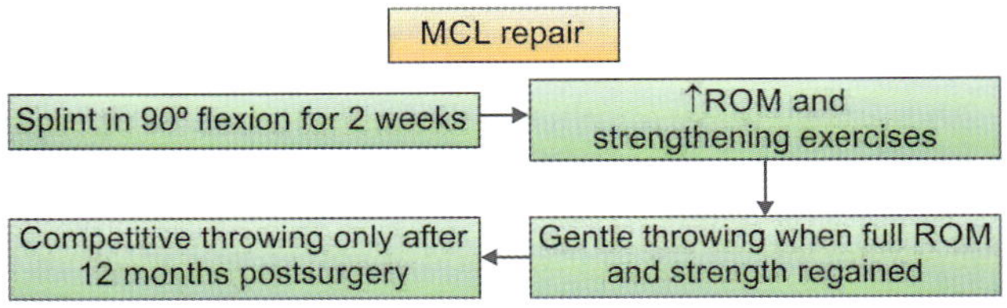

Fig. 18: Postoperative regime following repair of medial collateral ligament (MCL) injury.

Indications for surgical management:

- Return to overhead competitive sporting activity is difficult with conservative approach and needs definite surgical intervention.
- Ulnar neuritis or ulnar nerve symptoms may be present in up to 40% patients and need surgical remedial measures.
- Flexion deformity of elbow >30° if present needs surgical debridement and stabilization of elbow.
- Valgus instability that leads to degenerative arthritis (osteophytes and loose body formation) is also an indication for surgery.

Surgical management is primarily of two types:

1. *Repair of the ligament:* This is used less commonly as it is suitable only for proximal avulsion of the ligament and is uncommonly seen in chronic instabilities.
2. *Reconstruction using tendon graft:* This is the treatment of choice and is done with free autologous tendon graft often harvested from plantaris or palmaris longus. There are various described methods of MUCL reconstruction like Jobe's method (classic standard), docking technique, attachment with interference screws, zip-loop technique, etc.

Following surgery **(Fig. 18)**, the immobilization is done for 7–10 days followed by active elbow and shoulder and wrist ROM exercises. Muscle-strengthening exercises of the wrist and forearm are initiated at 1½ months postsurgery and valgus strain causing activities are restricted for 4 months.

Complications of surgical treatment:

- Injury to antebrachial cutaneous nerves
- Ulnar nerve compression
- Arthrofibrosis
- Heterotopic ossification
- Common complications otherwise include wound healing related complications of infection, dehiscence, etc.
- Graft loosening/unanchoring from the tunnel (tunnel fracture) and plastic elongation are uncommon if meticulous reconstruction is done.

EROSIVE ARTHROPATHIES

Elbow instability commonly occurs following damage by the arthritic conditions of the elbow. This involvement commonly affects the ligaments and capsule from inside and secondarily also damages the cartilage and subchondral bone. Frank instability occurs only in the advanced stages where variable but definite damage and loss of ligaments or bone stalk occurs. The following are the common erosive arthropathies that cause elbow instability:

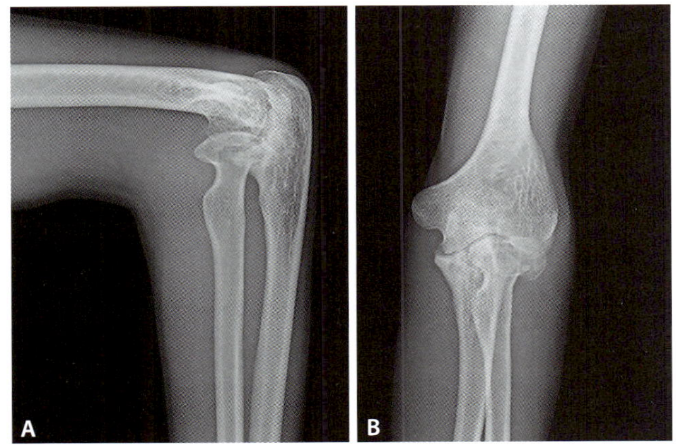

Figs. 19A and B: Sequelae of septic arthritis. Note the destroyed articular surfaces and deformed bones due to long-term non-use of elbow.

- Rheumatoid arthritis
- Psoriatic arthritis
- Gout
- Following septic arthritis in childhood **(Figs. 19A and B)**.

As with the involvement of soft tissue and simultaneous bony destruction only limited soft-tissue reconstructive options are left. The available surgical options in such cases include:

- Synovectomy and radial head excision
- Interposition arthroplasty (see stiff elbow for details)
- Resection/debridement arthroplasty (see stiff elbow for details)
- Total elbow arthroplasty/replacement arthroplasty (see above and stiff elbow).

TERRIBLE TRIAD INJURIES

This refers to combination of elbow dislocation and fractures of radial head and coronoid process. The nomenclature "terrible" refers to major disability resulting from this injury if untreated. The basis to understanding the management of this injury is converting this complex injury is to simple dislocation. If untreated, the injury complex is liable to produce persistent instability, nonunion, malunion, and osseous proximal radioulnar synostosis.

RECURRENT DISLOCATION OF ELBOW

This is an exceedingly rare condition seen in agenesis or dysplasia of trochlear notch of ulna, poor or insufficient collateral ligaments of elbow and only in untreated complex elbow dislocations. The elbow tends to dislocate posteriorly. Management is to treat the underlying condition. Congenital cases respond poorly and may need elbow arthrodesis. For insufficiency of collateral ligaments reconstruction may be attempted, however, stiff elbow is a common complication that should be explained to patient and borne in surgeon's mind. Arthroplasty may be attempted in neglected traumatic cases if patient is above 50 years of age or for a manual laborer elbow arthrodesis is an acceptable option.

VALGUS-EXTENSION OVERLOAD SYNDROME (VEOS)

This is a complex involvement of posterior elbow resulting from valgus strain **(Fig. 20)** *along with the hyperextension forces*. It may be considered similar to the valgus instability discussed above with two distinctions:

1. The primary pathology is located in the posterior elbow compartment **(Fig. 21)** and not medially in the UCL ligament
2. Intra-articular pathologies predominate rather than primarily ligamentous involvement seen in valgus instability. There is an exception that the lateral compartment symptoms are less prominent in VEOS, and they in fact make another pathology—the radiocapitellar overload syndrome (RCOS) discussed below.

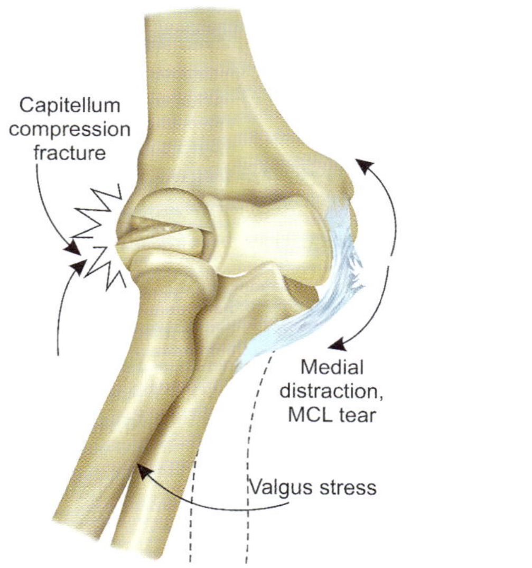

Fig. 20: Valgus extension overload syndrome—note the continuous stress on capitellum put by the radial head causing fragmentation and cartilage injury over time.

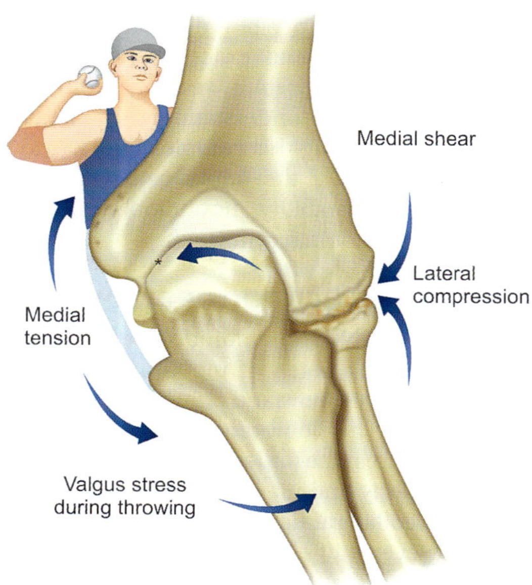

Fig. 21: Pathogenic progression of valgus extension overload syndrome where the posterior aspect of elbow is also predominantly involved and not just the lateral compartment.

Valgus-extension overload syndrome is an important component of sports injuries and involvement in athletes especially those participating in racquet sports, baseball, or javelin throw.

Pathogenesis

Repetitive impingement of olecranon in the fossa particularly the medial wall causes shear and friction between the translating bones producing pathology similar to osteoarthritis. The condition is made worse when there is concomitant laxity of the UCL. The consistent friction produces following pathologies in the joint:

- Local inflammation and chondromalacia and osteophyte formation
- Osteophytes can break off from the olecranon and become loose bodies within the elbow causing locking similar to that seen in knee joint.
- Stress fractures of olecranon
- Extension block and fixed flexion deformity
- Hypertrophy of distal humerus and narrowing of olecranon fossa

Clinical Features

The patients complain of:

- Posterior elbow pain
- Clicking or grating sensation especially while extension of elbow
- Intermittent locking of the joint

Examination of the Joint

Pain and tenderness is reproduced by hyperextension of the elbow specially on applying a valgus stress in hyperextension. Tenderness is felt in the olecranon fossa especially the ulnar margin more prominent with slight flexion and deep palpation. The extension impingement test and arm-bar test are commonly performed to examine the VEOS. In extension impingement test, continuous extension forces are applied to the elbow. If the pain occurs at the posterior aspect of elbow reproducing the pain or symptoms of the patient then it is positive indicating impingement by olecranon tip osteophytes. The Arm bar test is more sensitive; here, the patient's elbow extended, shoulder internally rotated, and hand is placed on the examiner's shoulder **(Fig. 22)**. The examiner then pulls down on the olecranon forcing elbow into extension that reproduces the pain associated with VEOS.

Radiology

- Calcification of the olecranon tip is seen along with thickening and irregularity due to osteophyte formation revealed better on a modified cubital tunnel view.
- Small olecranon fossa of humerus can be appreciated when compared to the opposite side.

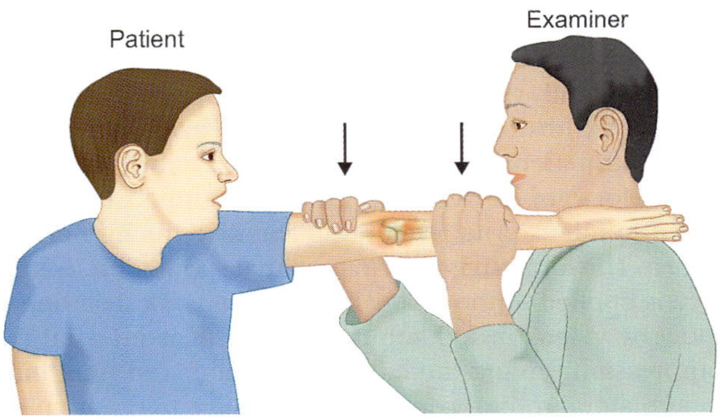

Fig. 22: The arm-bar test for assessment of valgus extension overload syndrome.

- Loose bodies are difficult to appreciate in standard radiographs but are better seen on arthrograms.
- CT arthrogram and plain CT scan are highly sensitive and diagnostic with typical clinical features.

Treatment

Conservative treatment with nonsteroidal anti-inflammatory drugs (NSAIDs) and strengthening of the flexor-pronator muscle group to reduce inflammation and symptoms and to protect the joint is done in early cases. Conservative treatment is ineffective in the presence of osteophytes when joint debridement (posterior) is the standard method. This can be done arthroscopically that also helps in removal of the loose bodies. The method is in general effective but in the presence of MUCL laxity or attenuation the recurrence rates are high as it does not address the pathology. Also there is a definite concern biomechanically that shaving the olecranon increases the stress on MUCL and hence leads to further attenuation. Open procedure with olecranon debridement and addressing the MUCL simultaneously could be a better option for long-term success.

RADIOCAPITELLAR OVERLOAD SYNDROME (RCOS)

This is the lateral counterpart of VEOS (and a subpart of valgus elbow instability) mentioned above but seen in a different subset of patients. It is more common in athletes involved in contact sports than in throwing athletes. One can safely commit this to be a late stage of the valgus elbow instability or the VEOS. About 500 N of compressive force is generated over the radiocapitellar joint during throwing activities. The increased load transmission (say by virtue of repetitive activity or lax/injured MUCL, etc.) across the radiocapitellar joint leads to chondromalacia **(Fig. 23)**. Chondromalacia has a tendency to progress to osteochondritis dissecans and degenerative arthritis. I feel that isolated RCOS should be predisposed in patients with some MUCL insufficiency or those with hyperlaxity but the findings have not been consistent.

Pathoanatomy

Pathologically finds variable stages of radiocapitellar chondromalacia, degeneration, osteochondral fracture fragmentation, and loose bodies in the radiocapitellar compartment are seen.

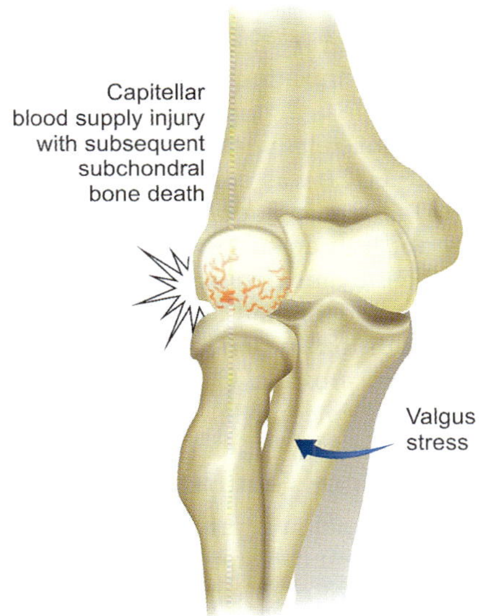

Fig. 23: Development of capitellar chondromalacia early in the course of valgus extension overload syndrome due to radial head impingement.

Clinical Findings

Patients present with predominant lateral elbow pain and joint line tenderness. This is frequently accompanied by the fullness in lateral soft spot and features of inflammation. The pain is more severe after rest and in morning gradually relieving with activity. There may be increased valgus angle at elbow (compared to the normal limb).

Treatment

Conservative treatment is adequate for skeletally immature patient. Rest NSAIDs and elbow support usually suffice. Low-dose corticosteroid injections may also be used. In skeletally mature patients, the symptoms have to be surgically managed especially with arthroscopic debridement. The treatment is most effective before development of loose bodies. Development of osteochondritis dissecans usually needs chondroplasty/microfracture followed by aggressive ROM exercise of elbow. Flexion contractures usually develop late and need release that can be successfully done by arthroscopy.

POSTEROLATERAL ROTATORY INSTABILITY

O'Driscoll is credited with the description and detailing of PLRI. Osborne and Cotterill were the first to appreciate fully the importance of the lateral ligamentous complex in recurrent instability and describe the findings of PLRI. The rotatory instability develops due to injury to lateral UCL that happens with a combination of axial compression, valgus stress and supination (or external rotation). The peculiar mechanism **(Fig. 24)** imparts a rotational force to the elbow resulting in a spectrum of soft-tissue injury. Contemplating the HORI circle concept, the initial injury is to the ulnar portion of the LCL that progresses to capsular disruption (anterior and posterior capsule) and eventually may involve the UCL complex if the injury is severe.

Pathomechanics (Fig. 25)

- Posterolateral rotatory instability of the elbow results from a rotatory subluxation of the radius and ulna (which move together in a "coupled" motion due to intact annular ligament) relative to the distal humerus.
- Although the LUCL was considered to be the primary stabilizer to PLRI recent literature suggests that the injury pattern is not limited to LUCL alone. The secondary restraints like the radial collateral ligament and capsule need to get injured for manifestations of PLRI.
- The only condition in which LUCL injury alone can produce PLRI is a proximal injury to the "Y" configuration of LUCL near the epicondyle.

Diagnosis and Clinical Features

A high degree of suspicion is primarily needed to diagnose PLRI as the findings and history are often subtle enough to miss the vigilance of even experts. Most patients have a vague elbow discomfort. Others often report nonspecific symptoms like painful clicking, snapping, clunking, locking or giving way.

For examination, the best method is to place the patient's upper limb in the position of reported discomfort and then apply rotatory stress. Otherwise the provocative test of instability described by O'Driscoll et al. (the lateral pivot-shift test of the elbow) is quite helpful **(Fig. 26)**. In this test, the elbow is converted into a position of knee and the hypermobility of shoulder is eliminated so that the stresses are more readily concentrated to elbow. The *pivot-shift test* is performed with the patient supine and the examiner standing above the patient's head. The upper extremity is brought into full forward elevation over the head and the shoulder is placed in full external rotation to stabilize the humerus for the test. The forearm is held in maximal supination. A valgus force is applied to the elbow holding the wrist. Loading the elbow by valgus in full supination produces an axial joint compression forcing the combined radius and ulna into a posterolateral rotatory subluxation relative to the humerus. Sensation of instability and apprehension or guarding is reported a positive test. The subluxation is maximal with elbow in 40° flexion and further flexion results in a sudden clunk (felt only in anesthetized patient) as a result of joint reduction. Other finding is dimpling of the skin proximal to radial head (posterolateral elbow) that is seen with PLRI in degrees of extension before the reduction.

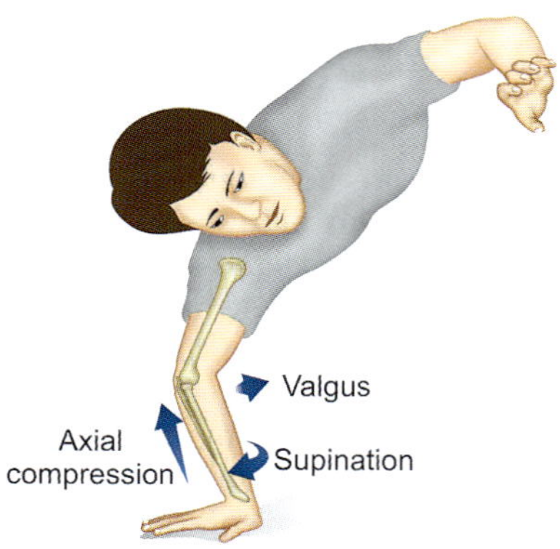

Fig. 24: Illustration depicting the mechanism of development of posterolateral rotatory instability.

Radiology

- Plain radiographs are usually unremarkable and uncommonly reveal a bony avulsion off the lateral epicondyle.
- Lateral stress radiographic studies or fluoroscopy during the pivot maneuver demonstrates posterolateral radial head dislocation and widening of the ulnohumeral joint (due to the subluxation of the ulna out of the trochlear groove). The ulna is rotated off the distal humerus (slight gapping of the ulnohumeral joint with otherwise maintained relationship) while the radial head is rotated with the ulna (differentiating from radial head subluxation) so that the radial head rests posterior to the capitellum.
- MRI allows good visualization of the LCLC and can be helpful in confirming the diagnosis in some cases. Most cases of PLRI still will be missed as it is more of a dynamic problem and the ligament may be stretched but intact.

Management

Posterolateral rotatory instability that markedly interferes with the patient's daily function only needs to be treated. For early cases, one can consider activity modification and

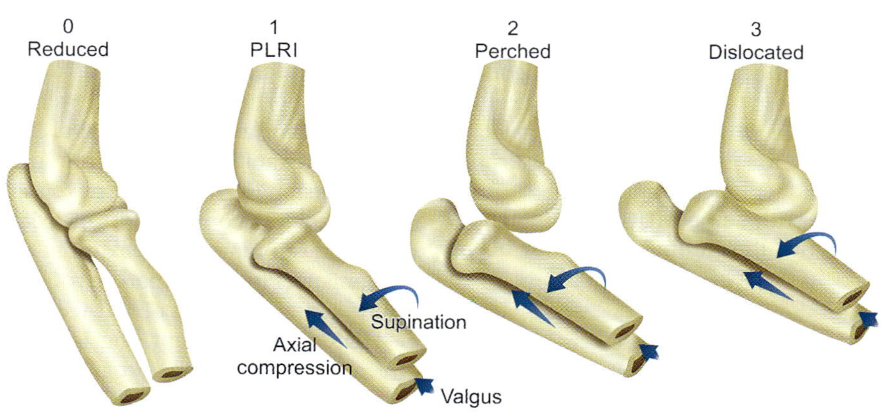

Fig. 25: Pathomechanics of the posterolateral rotatory instability (PLRI).

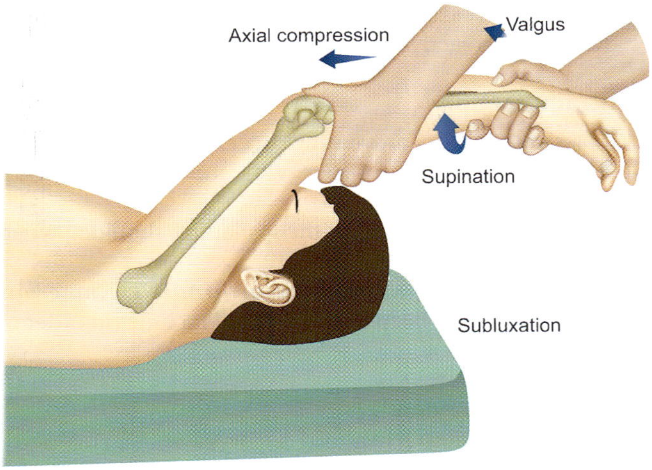

Fig. 26: Clinical examination for lateral pivot shift test (see text).

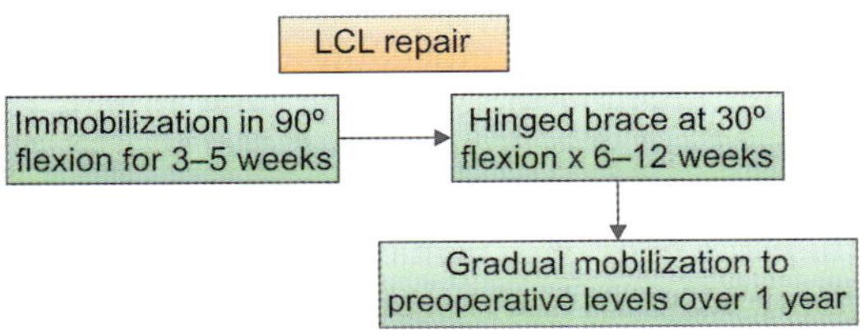

Fig. 27: Postoperative regime following repair of the lateral collateral ligament (LCL).

a hinged brace support that puts forearm in pronation and gives an extension block. The measures help in less than one-third of the patients but are the best method in a surgically unwilling patient.

Surgical treatment of PLRI is the treatment of choice. The primary aim is to restore the lateral ligamentous structures by reattaching the avulsed LCLC or reconstructing the LUCL with a free tendon graft to the lateral epicondyle. If the condition is diagnosed acutely, primary repair of the lateral UCL may be performed back to the bone. Various methods of surgical reconstruction are described in addition to the technique originally described by O'Driscoll and include making the distal connecting tunnels perpendicular to the isometric point to the lateral epicondyle, using interference screw, etc. Results for surgical reconstruction of the LUCL have been excellent in general. The general follow-up schedule is presented in **Figure 27**.

RECURRENT ISOLATED RADIAL HEAD INSTABILITY

This is an uncommon condition resulting from disruption of annular ligament and anterior dislocation/subluxation of radial head. There is instability of the proximal radioulnar joint associated with forearm rotations. The interosseous membrane is also very important in stabilizing the proximal radioulnar joint so the condition highlights anatomical and biomechanical importance of annular ligament, quadrate ligament and proximal half of interosseous membrane in stabilizing the proximal radioulnar joint in both transverse and longitudinal directions. The most common mechanism of injury is hyperpronation of already pronated forearm.

- ***Diagnosis and clinical features include:***
  - Locking/popping of elbow especially associated with forearm rotations
  - Decreased forearm rotations while maintained elbow flexion-extension
  - Crepitation over radial head
  - Apprehension with hyperpronation
- ***Differential diagnosis:***
  - Posterolateral rotatory instability
  - Monteggia fracture-dislocation
  - Congenital dislocation
  - Dislocation in association with cerebral palsy
- ***Treatment:***
  - Joint preserving procedures—annular ligament reconstruction (anatomical or nonanatomical like Bell-Tawse), proximal ulnar osteotomy, and interosseous membrane reconstruction. The nonanatomical procedure like Bell-Tawse is good in reducing anterior radial head dislocation but less effective in controlling lateral and posterior radial head instability.
  - Salvage procedures—Radial head excision, single bone forearm, and interpositional arthroplasty.
- ***Complications:***
  - Posterior interosseous nerve injury
  - Elbow stiffness
  - Recurrent instability
  - Heterotopic ossification

ELBOW ARTHRODESIS

Elbow arthrodesis is a rarely performed orthopedic procedure these days. Historically, it was performed for a tuberculous infection of the elbow. Now it is mainly a salvage procedure indicated to relieve pain and restore stability that cannot be otherwise restored. The elbow is one of the most difficult joints to fuse because of the long lever arm and strong bending forces across the fusion site. Early fusion rates were about 50%. With improved techniques, fusion rates approach 70–100%. The loss of motion significantly impairs the patient's functional abilities so it is least favorable option in modern orthopedic practice. It is mainly performed for severe nonreconstructible joint destruction. Following are the indications for consideration of elbow arthrodesis:

- Post-traumatic arthritis
- Chronic osteomyelitis especially tuberculous involvement
- Sequel of septic arthritis **(Fig. 28)**
- Young healthy laborers with posttraumatic arthritis who are too young for total elbow arthroplasty
- Juxta-articular pseudarthrosis
- Complex injuries (with large bone and soft-tissue defects precluding fixation and coverage)
- Severely comminuted intra-articular fractures of the distal humerus with joint destruction beyond reconstruction
- Failed elbow arthroplasty
- Failed internal fixation for nonunions

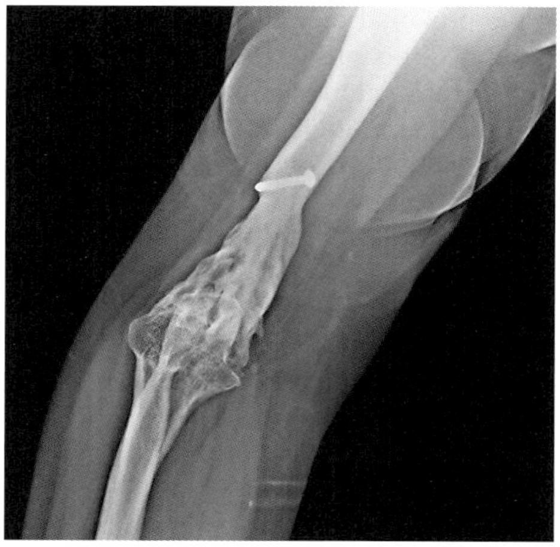

Fig. 28: Elbow arthrodesis performed in a patient with complex open fracture and septic arthritis. The screw used in primary fixation could not be removed due to complete incarceration.

Prerequisites

- Satisfactory shoulder function
- A functional hand is also desirable.
- ***Optimal position of arthrodesis*:** No optimal position for arthrodesis exists, though historically it was 90°. An arthrodesis at approximately 45° of flexion provides the best appearance and function for activities such as writing and bimanual tasks (but precludes self-care) while arthrodesis at 90° or 110° position allows the use of the arm for eating, but prevents many extra-personal activities and care of the perineum. The position of fusion is dictated by the needs of the patient, and for this, it is best to provide patient a brace that immobilizes the limb in different positions and let him decide the best position for himself. Other factors for fusion angle include:
    - *Gender:* Male—dominant arm at 90°, females seem to prefer lower angles of 40–70°.
    - Occupation
    - Hand dominance
    - Functional requirements
    - Associated joint involvement
    - *Unilateral versus bilateral arthrodesis:* Bilateral elbow arthrodesis—dominant arm at 110°, nondominant arm at 65°.
- Adequate skin and soft tissue for coverage
- Quiescent infection

Preoperative Evaluation

- Evaluate the need for bone graft or soft tissue coverage.
- Evaluate shoulder, wrist, and spinal column.
- Neurologic and motor deficits are documented.
- Blood flow to the hand is determined and in complicated injuries angiogram is helpful to evaluate the vascularity.
- The quality and quantity of bone available for fusion are assessed by standard radiographs and/or CT scans.
- For infected cases, complete blood count, sedimentation rate, and C-reactive protein.

Contraindications

- Massive bone loss preventing successful arthrodesis
- Massive soft-tissue loss not amenable to flap reconstruction
- Compromised function of the ipsilateral shoulder, wrist, and spinal column
- ***Methods of performing elbow arthrodesis: Numerous*** techniques have been described and include (in order of preference):
    - Plate fixation
    - External fixation
    - Limited internal fixation
    - Combined internal and external fixation

General Principles for Performing Arthrodesis (Procedural)

This is an intra-articular procedure unless off-course one refrains from opening the joint and does it with external fixator only.

- Use triceps-sparing posterior approach
- Fashion the bone ends to maximize bone apposition
- Prefer using graft for surface coaptation
- Perform staged procedure if active infection is found with repeated debridements—prefer external fixation for stabilization
- Transpose the ulnar nerve

Complications

- Nonunion in up to 50% cases
- Infection (aggravation or persistence)
- Implant failure

CONCLUSION

- The most common cause of elbow instability is repetitive ligament strain and plastic changes. Acute dislocations of elbow are uncommon cause of recurrent elbow instability unless managed badly.
- Terrible triad injuries are frequent cause of such chronic instabilities. Chronic instabilities are best managed by ligament reconstructions and bony stabilization (if needed).
- Chronic valgus instability needs ligament reconstruction by using a tendon graft for MUCL reconstruction. Chronic valgus overload syndrome on the other hand is mostly conservatively managed and only in failed cases open olecranon debridement and MUCL reconstruction is needed.
- Total elbow replacement is an uncommon procedure for management of nonreparable and chronic elbow instability unless degenerative changes have set in, performing elbow arthrodesis is even rarer.

CHAPTER 110

Stiff Elbow

Manish Kumar Varshney

INTRODUCTION

Elbow is affected more frequently than any other joint by post-traumatic loss of motion. Possible causes of peculiar affection of the elbow joint include (also see elbow anatomy and biomechanics for details):

- The presence of the three most congruous joints in a single capsule and a synovial space
- Delayed mobilization (inability to achieve rigid fixation)
- The lateral collateral ligament (LCL) and the medial collateral ligament (MCL) often remain taut through the whole range of motion (ROM)
- A very close relationship with tendons, muscles, and skin
- Brachialis muscle covers anteriorly (ectopic ossification)
- Requirement of high degree of articular congruity

ETIOLOGY

Involvement of structures within and around elbow joint by various disorders produces stiff elbow. A comprehensive (though not complete) list of such causes is presented below:

- *Soft-tissue contracture:*
    - Skin burns
    - Wound contractures (posttraumatic) due to retractile fibrosis of the capsule, ligaments, and muscular tissue. Retracted MCL posterior band can cause a flexion contracture beyond 60°, while a tauter anterior produces an extension contracture beyond 80°.
    - Hypertrophic scars
    - Spastic paresis (head injury) → contractures
    - Prolonged immobilization. Period of immobilization is directly proportional to elbow stiffness.
- Heterotopic ossification (HO) **(Fig. 1A)**
- *Osteoarticular incongruity:* Due to high congruity of the articular surfaces, any incongruity in the surfaces produces altered motion and stresses the ligaments in different positions; this cause reduced movements at the joint. Malunions of following fractures produce stiff elbow:
    - Intercondylar fractures **(Fig. 1B)**
    - Capitellum fractures **(Fig. 1C)**
    - Olecranon fractures
    - Radial head fractures (displaced fragments)
    - Malunited supracondylar fracture with overriding of the fragments **(Fig. 1D)**
- Triceps/biceps adhesions (posttraumatic/postsurgical)
- *Arthritis:* Coronoid/olecranon/radial osteophytes **(Fig. 1E)**

CLASSIFICATION

As proposed by Morrey, the post-traumatic stiffness of elbow can be grouped into three groups: extrinsic, intrinsic, and mixed contractures.

1. *Extrinsic contractures* **(Figs. 2A and B)** involve the contracture of the soft-tissue (posterior and anterior capsule and ligaments and muscles surrounding the joint).
    - Bony bridge also contributes to extrinsic contractures **(Fig. 3)**
2. *Intrinsic contractures* (usually associated with intra-articular fractures):
    - Intra-articular adhesions
    - Loss of articular cartilage (***see* Fig. 1E**)
    - Gross distortion due to inadequate or failed reduction **(Fig. 1F)**
3. *Mixed contractures* (most common): When both extrinsic and intrinsic factors are present. Extrinsic contracture could lead to intra-articular adhesion or to a secondary osteoarthritis. Intrinsic contracture is always associated with extrinsic contracture.

Just classification, however, does not guide the management perspective. There are definite treatment modifiers that should be specifically looked for in order to correctly judge, treat, and define planning. These treatment modifiers are presence of ectopic ossification and state of osseous articular anatomy. Following grades of clinical presentation can be identified when one combines the classification and treatment modifiers:

- ***Grade 1*:** A contracture of the capsular ligaments and periarticular muscle-tendons is present; the osteoarticular anatomy is preserved and HO is not present.
- ***Grade 2:*** A contracture of the soft-tissues is associated with HO without osteoarticular damage. In this type, "the HO excision is a greater surgical demand than soft-tissue contracture release".
- ***Grade 3:*** A contracture of soft-tissue with or without HO is in association with the osteoarticular damage. Here, the

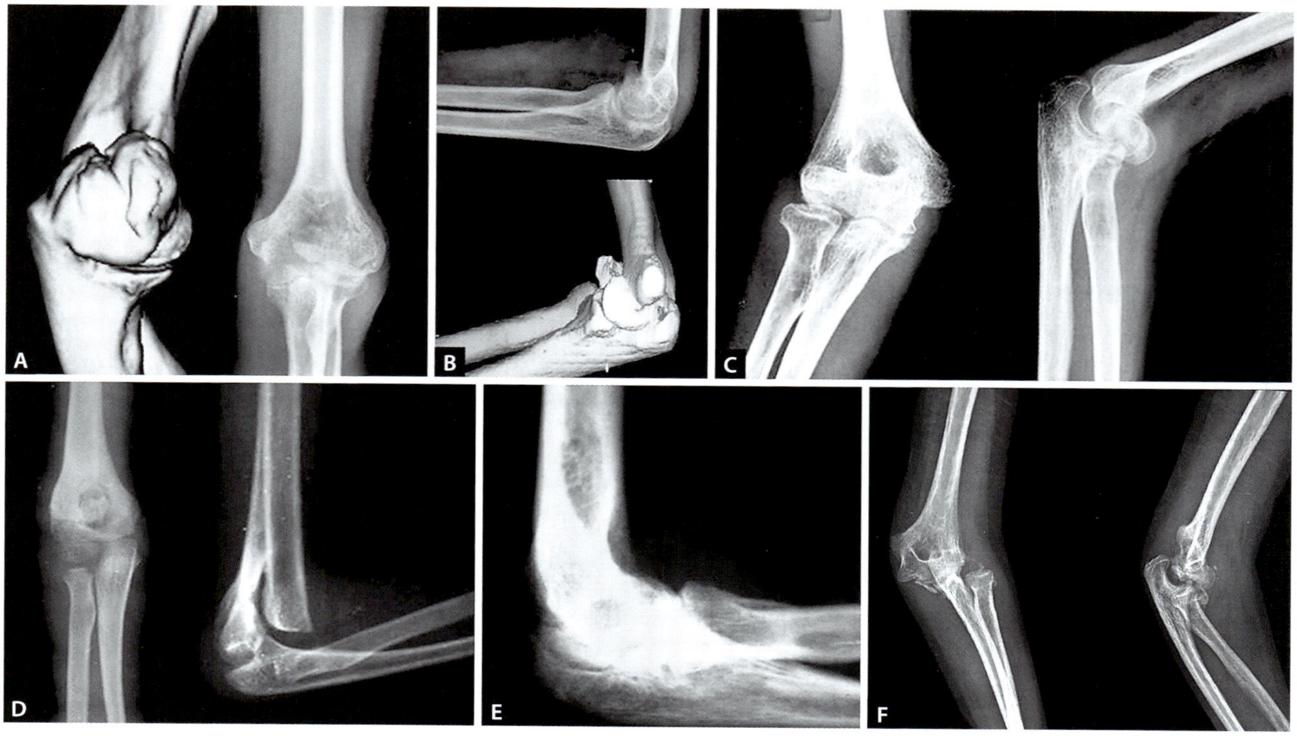

Figs. 1A to F: Various osseous causes of stiff elbow. (A) Heterotopic ossification causing bony fusion across the elbow joint and loss of all movements; (B) Intra-articular fracture; displaced fracture precluding joint motion; (C) A capitellum fracture left untreated causing flexion block; (D) Malunited supracondylar fracture again causing flexion block; (E) Arthritic elbow—look at the bony fullness in olecranon fossa and loss of joint space; and (F) Five-month-old neglected dislocation of left elbow with fracture capitellum treated by quack.

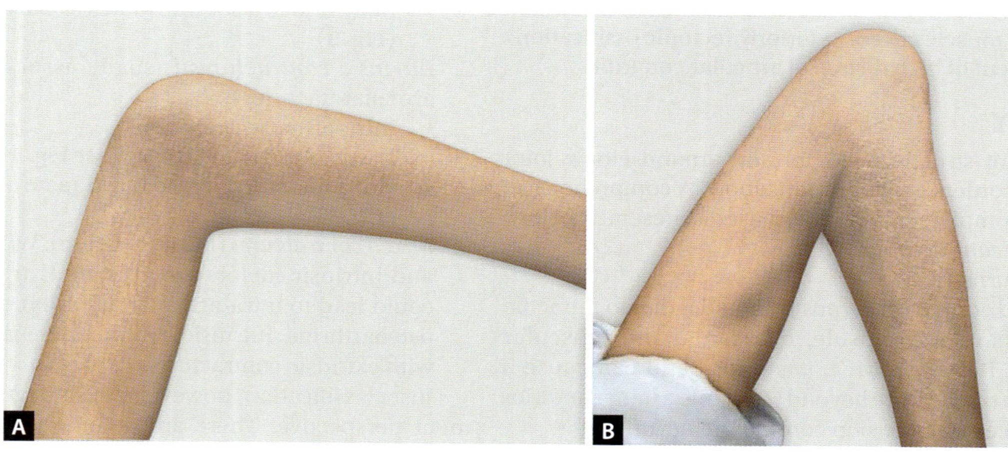

Figs. 2A and B: (A) Anterior elbow contracture causing loss of elbow extension but the flexion is unrestricted (B).

articular surface incongruity and surgical correction of the bone articular distortion are greater surgical demand than HO excision and soft-tissue contracture release. The joint loss, the articular surface congruity, and the bone are distorted such as:
- Malunions or nonunions of intra-articular fractures
- Chronic unreduced subluxation

CLINICAL FEATURES

History

Examine for the clinical symptoms and their progression, previous treatment, including duration of prolonged immobilization. Evaluate the internal fixation device, infection, reflex sympathetic dystrophy (RSD), etc. (if ever reported), and status of union.

Physical Examination

The movements are limited differently in patients with some having flexion block while others having extension block **(Table 1)**, all of which need evaluation as to ascertain the bony and soft-tissue causes of stiffness. Examine the skin of the involved limb around the elbow, the neurological state, patient's capacity to have normal motor strength and voluntary control of muscles, wasting, and soft-tissue

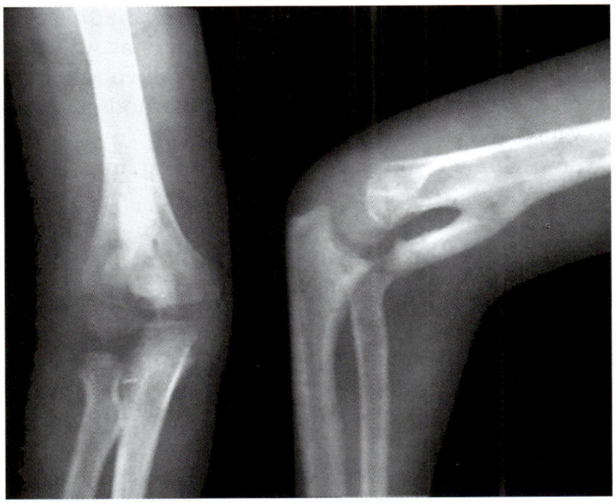

Fig. 3: Extrinsic bony bridge formation causing loss of all motion across the elbow joint. This is a type of extrinsic stiff elbow.

TABLE 1: The various causes for extension and flexion limitation in a post-traumatic stiff elbow.

Limited flexion	*Limited extension*
• Posterior capsular contracture more prominent on the lateral side • Posteromedial and transverse band MCL scarring • Triceps tendon scarring or impingement by posterior bony fragment • Coronoid tip osteophytes • Coronoid fossa bone or soft-tissue overgrowth • Radial head anterior osteophytes or malunited neck fracture • Articular adhesions, incongruity, or malunion • Anterior impinging heterotopic ossification	• Anterior capsular contracture • Anterior oblique band MCL scarring • Brachialis scarring • Olecranon tip osteophytes (common) • Olecranon fossa bone or soft-tissue overgrowth (common after surgical reconstruction of intercondylar fracture) • Radial head posterior osteophytes or malunited fracture • Articular adhesions, incongruity or malunion • Posterior impinging heterotopic ossification

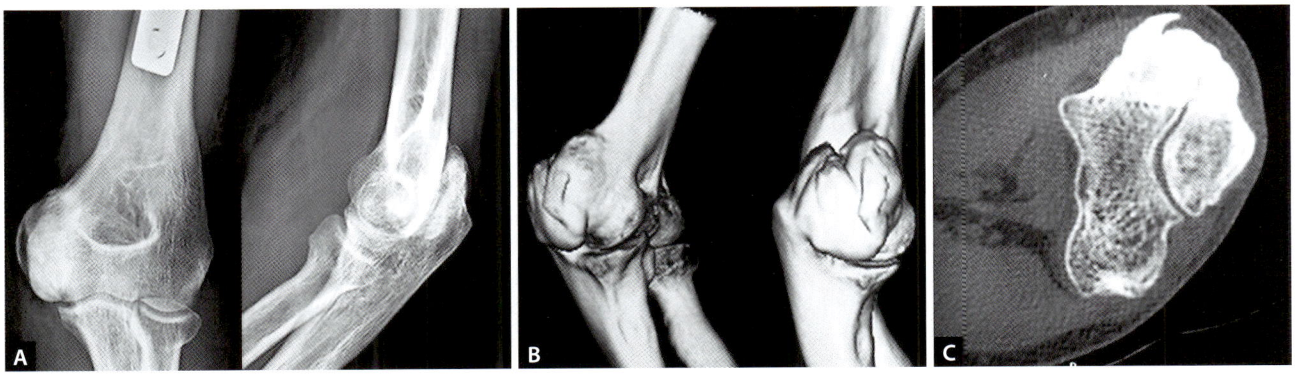

Figs. 4A to C: (A) It is difficult to understand the extent and location of ectopic ossification mass on two-dimensional projection of standard radiographs as in this elbow; (B and C) Computed tomographic SSD and axial images clearly demonstrate that the mass is attached both to the olecranon and medial condyle of humerus.

contractures. Evaluate for bony ankylosis, bony bar, ectopic ossification, etc., often one finds prominent bony landmarks in long-standing nonunion due to atrophy of the muscles and soft-tissues. Malunion and ectopic ossification make evaluation of the same a bit difficult. It is difficult to exactly pinpoint the intrinsic versus extrinsic category based on the clinical examination. The endpoint of ROM is springy in soft-tissue contractures rather than a firm block as in bone impingement. Ancillary investigations are commonly needed to make reasonably correct differentiation—in long-standing cases both intra-articular and extra-articular causes of stiffness usually develop irrespective of the initial location. However, type of previous injury like intra-articular fractures (intrinsic category) or prolonged immobilization (extrinsic category) can be evaluated from history.

INVESTIGATIONS

Routine lateral, oblique, and anteroposterior radiographs provide most of the information regarding the osteoarticular causes of elbow contracture.

Computed tomography (CT) scan can be employed to evaluate the articular congruity and precise location of ectopic/HO **(Figs. 4A to C)**. CT scan is also helpful as radiographs are difficult to obtain in fixed contractures where one or the other projection is compromised. MRI is not usually needed except to define any loose bodies if they are suspected (rare). Some often advise technetium bone scan to evaluate the maturity of ectopic ossification; however, it has been shown to be a poor investigation predicting the biological activity of the mass and is no better than radiographs.

MANAGEMENT

As for most orthopedic complications, the choices land on conservative and operative platforms:

Conservative approach is done if:

- The articular bone anatomy is preserved.
- The contracture is mild and has not been present for >6 months.
- The absence of the HO bridge (class II or class III in Hastings and Graham radiographic classification).

The various strategies for nonsurgical management include:

- ***Splints:*** These are used to preserve the gained arc of motion by other methods. They are most helpful in the

inflammatory and fibroplasia phase after the forced motion that stretches the periarticular soft-tissue.
  - Static
  - Dynamic
- ***ROM exercises:*** Short-term active or passive exercises, however, do not help and continuous passive motion (CPM) is often needed.
- ***Manipulation under anesthesia:*** This is not a common modality used to restore or gain elbow movements as the risks are far too many including:
  - Periarticular fractures
  - Ulnar nerve injury
  - Elbow instability
  - Increased risk of nonunion and secondary bone deformity
  - Ectopic ossification
  - Development of RSD or its aggravation
  - Failure of fixation

OPERATIVE MANAGEMENT

The logical considerations for surgery especially the type of intervention required is presented in **Flowchart 1**. However, this simplified version does not hold true always as most of the presentations of stiff elbow are mixed types (intra-articular + extra-articular).

Following considerations must be undertaken before planning surgery:
- Patient's expectations
- Functional needs
- Etiology of stiffness and clinical assessment
- Likelihood that procedure will satisfy these needs.

The surgical techniques are not to be ever considered as the end procedure or the most successful procedure as more often than not they produce poor results if not done well or planned well. The *common risks associated with surgery include:*
- Instability due to over release
- Weakness
- Recurrence of contracture
- Complete ankylosis
- Reflex sympathetic dystrophy

There are various surgical techniques described for treating elbow stiffness and the multiplicity of these lends support to the fact that none is uniformly successful. This is bound to be also partially true due the varied nature of etiology and presentation of elbow stiffness as well as the multiplicity of intra- and extra-articular involvement. In general, the principles of all surgical methods discussed below are as follows:
- Remove all the contracted structures and intra-articular deformities to obtain elbow motion.
- Maintain elbow stability by preserving the anterior band of ulnar collateral ligament (UCL) and the posterior band of the LCL.
- Avoid any damage to neurovascular structures.

Following are the commonly used approaches for surgical release of contractures:
- ***The posterior midline approach*** (global approach) is indicated for extensive elbow involvement as in multi-location joint involvement and ankylosis or extensive ectopic ossification that needs complete elbow exposure. I prefer this approach for most of the long-standing cases as they have combined intra- and extra-articular presentations.
- ***The lateral approach:*** This is the general approach used for treatment in most cases with limited disease.
  - *Limited "lateral column procedure* ***(Figs. 5A to C)****":* Proximal half of Kocher skin incision is utilized. The LCL complex is identified and preserved especially while identifying the annular ligament. This is best done before elevating the extensor carpi ulnaris. The LCL-sparing technique is useful to perform anterior and posterior capsulectomy without disturbing the extensor tendon insertion and LCL insertion. The advantage of this approach is to avoid instability after release. The disadvantage is, however, possible damage to posterior interosseous nerve and that there is greater difficulty in excising the medial half of the anterior capsule without disturbing the anterior bundle of the UCL. If full flexion is not achieved then the most common cause is scarred posterior oblique bundle of the UCL that should be excised through a separate posteromedial skin incision.
  - *Extensive Kocher approach:* This is rarely needed to additionally expose and clear the radiocapitellar joint space and adhesions, for example, after radial head excision.

Flowchart 1: Common surgical algorithm for management of stiff elbow.

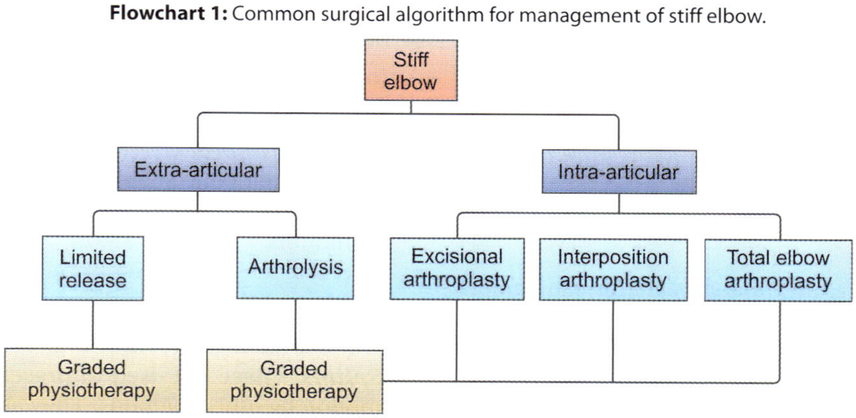

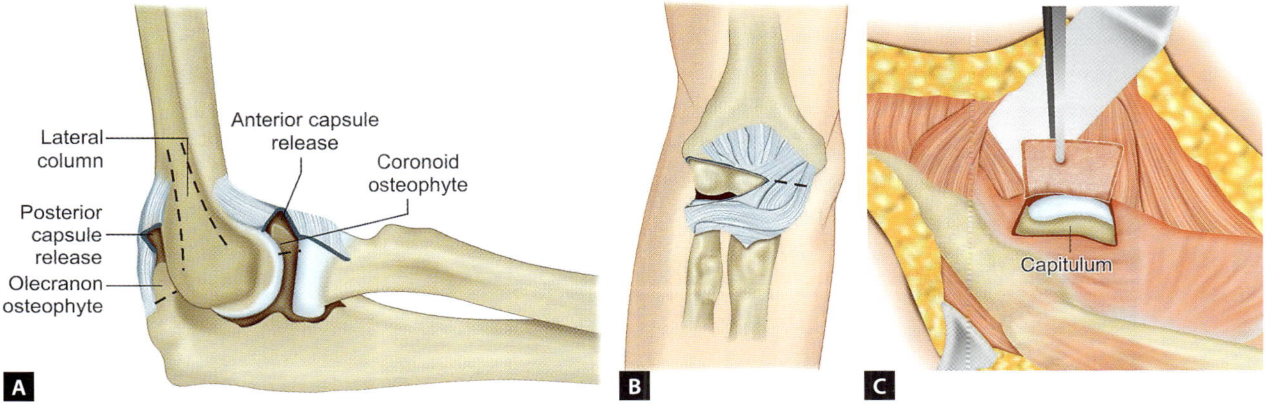

Figs. 5A to C: The column procedure: (A) Here, the elbow joint is exposed through one column removing the pathology anteriorly and posteriorly through single column. The initial step is identification of the supracondylar ridge (B and C) followed by sequential release of pathological structures followed by bony debridement.

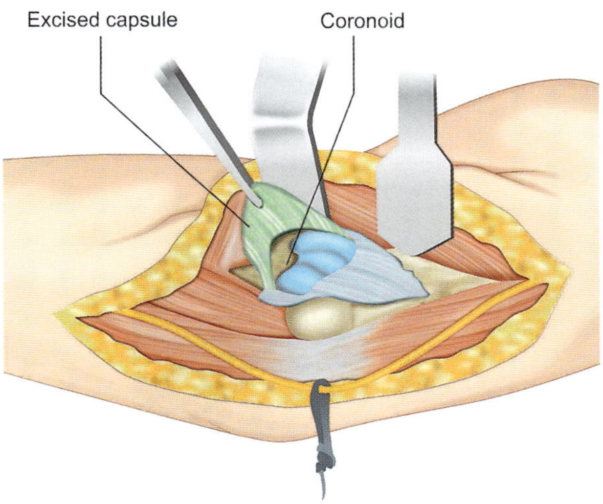

Fig. 6: The over-the-top approach.

- ***The medial approach:***
  - Limited "medial column procedure" useful for limited posteromedial bony bars or ectopic ossification.
  - Extensile "over-the-top approach" of Hotchkiss **(Fig. 6)** is indicated for treatment of post-traumatic elbow contractures with ulnar neuropathy or posteromedial ectopic ossification mass located over the posteromedial aspect of the elbow. This approach is also needed for severe capsule contracture is associated with posteromedial or anteromedial HO bone bars (class IIA, IIB, or III of Hastings and Graham classification). The ulnar nerve is commonly engulfed in the bony mass and should be carefully protected while release. After release, the ulnar nerve is transposed anteriorly.
- ***Anterior contracture release*** is indicated for loss of extension >45° and/or minimal articular surface changes.
  - *Contraindications:*
    - Altered articular contour
    - Loss of joint cartilage >50%
    - Pathology requiring release of collateral ligaments
- ***Arthroscopic approach*** is done in stiff elbows with intact articular surfaces with preserved congruity. Advantages of an arthroscopic procedure are that intra-articular debridement can be done with minimal soft-tissue trauma, and there are much less chances of recurrent adhesions, if they are limited to intra-articular region (uncommon to find such cases in practice as most are also associated with extra-articular contractures). This is a technically demanding procedure requiring experience. Ulnar and the deep motor branch of the radial nerve are at most risk as the capsular volume is reduced from 25 to 6 mL or so. The procedure in general involves:
  - Capsular detachment from the humerus or capsulotomy
  - Capsulectomy is only for most experienced arthroscopist as it is the most risky procedure.
  - Synovectomy
  - Debridement of the olecranon and coronoid osteophytes
  - Outerbridge-Kashiwagi procedure (fenestration of the olecranon fossa, see below)
- *Arthrolysis (Bhattacharya procedure):*
  - Removal of capsular contracture
  - Mobilizing Brachialis and Triceps from lower humerus
  - Minimal removal of bone block
  - After closure 25 mg *hydrocortisone acetate* is injected in joint with 2–5 cc of hylase.

Postoperative regime (in general for all approaches):

- Place drains anteriorly and posteriorly.
- Keep elbow in full extension for 24–36 hours.
- It is always useful to have intraoperative brachial plexus continuous block to examine elbow and start CPM through full arc of motion **(Figs. 7A to D)**. This is especially useful in early 2–3 days when the movement is reduced by fluid accumulation in periarticular soft-tissues.
- Remove catheter at 3 days and continue CPM.
- Use additional static splints **(Fig. 8A and B)** to maintain extremes of movements at home.

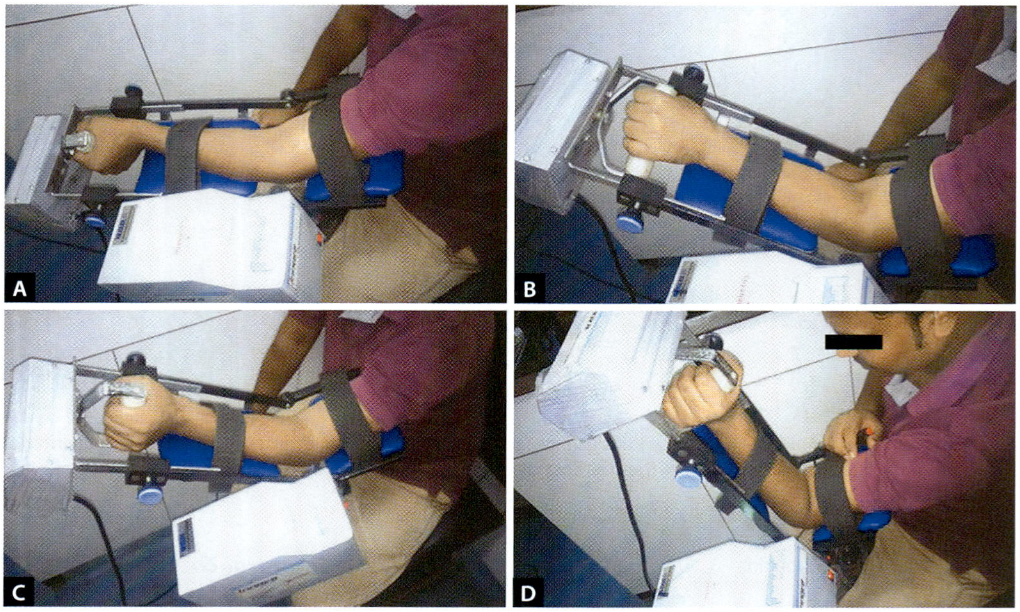

Figs. 7A to D: Continuous passive motion for elbow—this allows elbow movements during healing phase maintaining the same minimizing the chances of stiffness later. The machine also contains an emergency stop button in case the patient has too much pain or is uncomfortable.

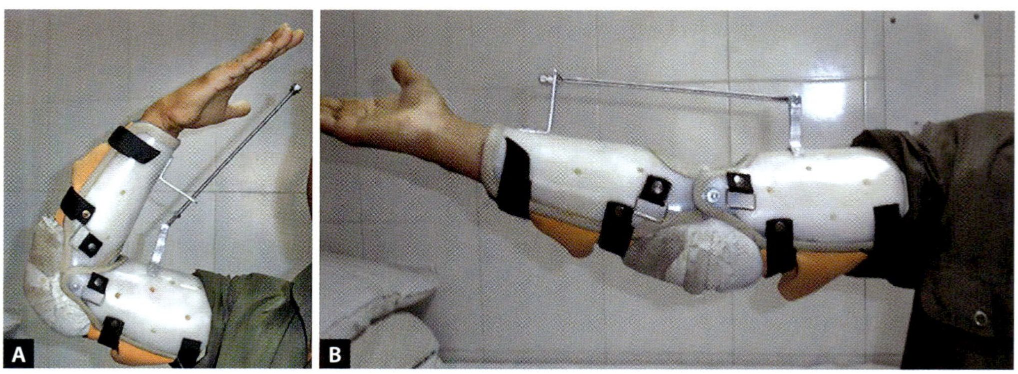

Figs. 8A and B: Improvised splint that the patient can use in home for continued mobilization of elbow.

- Indomethacin prophylaxis can be given to patients 25 mg three times a day or 75 mg sustained released for 6 weeks postoperatively.

Complications of contracture release:

- Ulnar nerve injury
- Median nerve injury, if contracture is >90°.

ECTOPIC OSSIFICATION AROUND ELBOW

Ectopic para-articular bone formation is a sequel of either a traumatic event or post-traumatic massage in which highly organized bone is formed and substitutes the surrounding injured soft tissues. The etiology is unclear and misunderstood (especially the role of massage that has been so consistently associated). Probably after trauma, the mesenchymal cells or fibroblasts in presence of a bone morphogenetic protein differentiate and proliferate into cartilage and osteoblasts [*see* Chapter on "Orthopedic Oncology (Bone Tumors and Metastasis) and Heterotopic Ossification"]. Ectopic ossification around elbow originates from direct trauma which is the minimum requirement; massage itself has also been seen to produce ectopic ossification while a combination of the two is more powerful factor in the development. This is further increased if head injury is associated; the mechanism is still more difficult to explain here. Simple dislocation and complex injuries to benign procedures like radial head excision all have been reported to produce ectopic ossification around elbow. Ectopic ossification typically localizes to swollen and hyperemic tissue. There is then progressive loss of motion followed by residual loss of mobility at the joint which may get impetus by the frequent practice of joint immobilization. On the contrary, practicing aggressive manipulation to avoid the progressive joint loss of motion has also been seen to hasten the process by increasing the already rampant local inflammation.

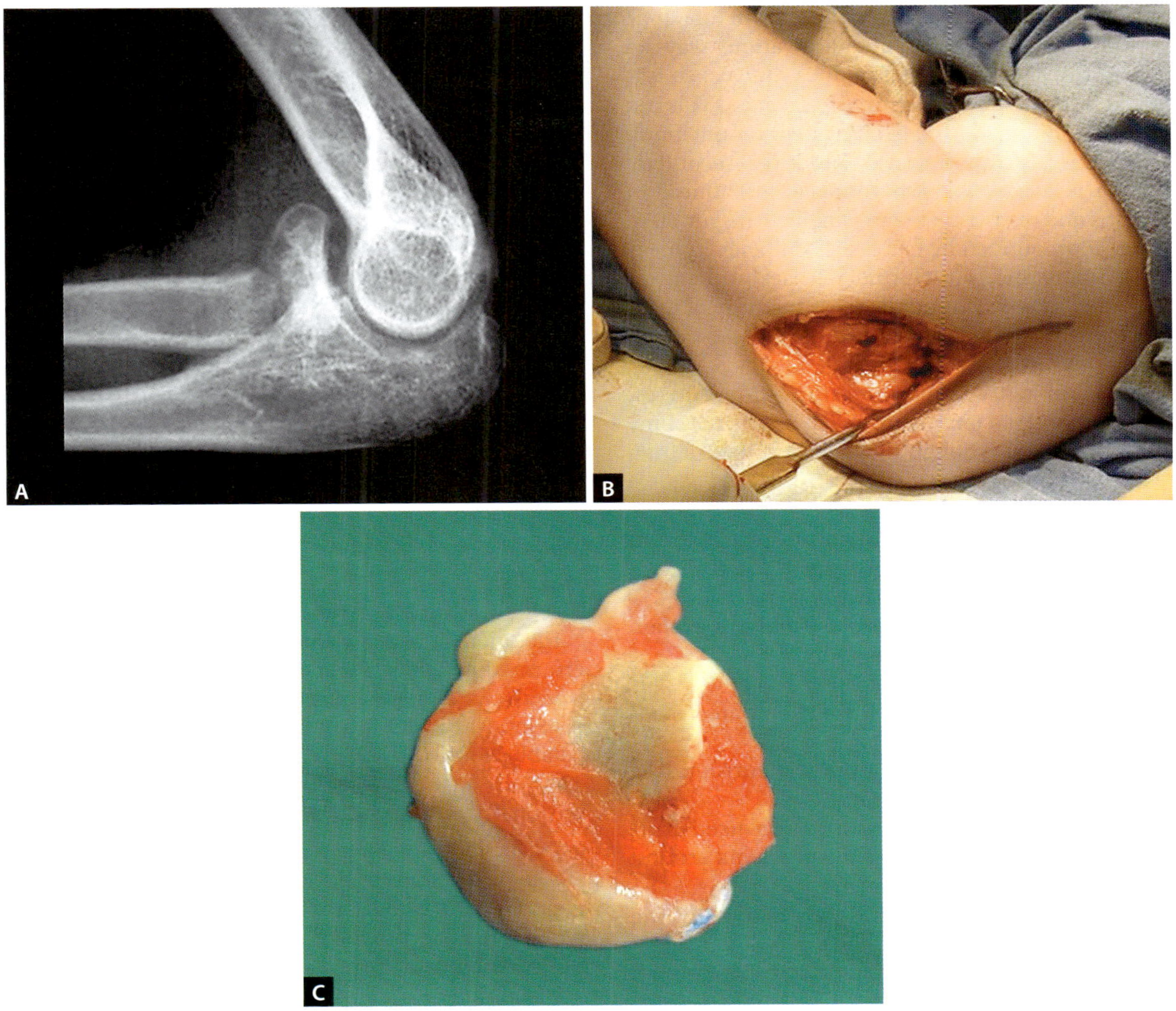

Figs. 9A to C: Excision of malunited radial head causing obstruction to elbow movements. (A) Lateral radiog-aph of the elbow causing obstruction to elbow complete flexion; (B) Excision of the malunited radial head; (C) The excised radial head.

Hastings and Graham proposed a useful radiographic and clinical classification distinguishing three classes of elbow HO:

1. *Class I:* HO with no functional limitation
2. *Class II:* HO further classified according to limitation in specific movement:
   - IIA—limited flexoextension
   - IIB—limited pronosupination
   - IIC—limited flexoextension and pronosupination
3. *Class III:* Ankylosis

Ectopic ossification is not limited to the anterior or posterior sites in elbow only (as identified by Garland). It can be found in any of the sites and any of the structures can be involved in it.

In anterior site:

- Coronoid
- Humeroulnar
- Humeroradial
- Periarticular soft tissue such as capsule or brachial muscle

In the posterior site:

- Olecranon
- Humeroulnar **(Figs. 9A to C)**
- Olecranon fossa

In the lateral site:

- Ulnar collateral ligament
- Lateral collateral ligament

MANAGEMENT

The obvious option is to excise the ectopic mass, but the procedure is not as benign to instigate.

- Indications/criteria for excision of the mass are as follows:
  - Functionally limiting elbow stiffness
  - Radiographic union of fracture
  - Intact ulnohumeral articular surface
  - Stage of maturation

The method is compounded by the ill-defined time when it should be done and the fact that the ectopic mass replaces the normal tissue and is not a separate mass, so excision will mean loss of normal tissue producing deficiency in function/structure specific to that tissue. There are various ways to assess the maturity of the mass but none is specific, so it is difficult to define when one should excise the mass. This has led to arbitrary definition of 1 year waiting period from injury to excise the mass. Delay, however, produces secondary changes in the periarticular tissue and cause stiffness in different regions and restriction in movements. This problem will be further compounded by increased tendency in these patients for ectopic ossification if further releases are planned! The common methods employed to assess maturity of mass are as follows (often a combination is used):

- ***Clinical:***
  - No signs of active inflammation—no redness, swelling, increased temperature. The skin is not shiny and has wrinkles (though they are always less than the normal limb).
  - No/minimal pain and tenderness
  - Reasonable movements at the joint—restriction of movements due to pain often indicates presence of inflammation (though not always)
  - There is sufficient delay from injury that can explain subsidence of signs of inflammation.
- ***Radiological:***
  - *Plain roentgenograms* show a well separated mass with trabecular bone pattern.
  - The mass is well separated from the surrounding tissue by smooth cortical outline.
  - MRI—presently a hyped investigation used irrationally for the purpose. Presence of edema around the mass indicates active lesion.
  - CT scan—this is not used to define activity of the lesion but is helpful in defining the three-dimensional extent of the irregular masses and their connection with the parent bone.
- ***Bone scans*** often prescribed but have no definite role as they have not been able to delineate the activity of the lesion in a timely fashion and consistently.

Postoperative management of HO is similar to that for other surgical procedures early mobilization and controlling inflammation is the goal. Postoperative indomethacin (75 mg sustained release) is necessarily given. Radiotherapy may also be used in dedicated centers. Other methods for prevention of HO are detailed in the section on bone tumors [*see* Chapter on "Orthopedic Oncology (Bone Tumors and Metastasis) and Heterotopic Ossification", Fibrodysplasia Ossificans].

Radial Head Excision (Figs. 10A and B)

This can be done especially if there is bony block due to malunited radial head that commonly blocks the flexion and/or supination-pronation movements. Disadvantages such as distal radioulnar joint instability pain is seen in acute injuries involving the interosseous membrane else for stable cases (after 6 months of injury) this is uncommon.

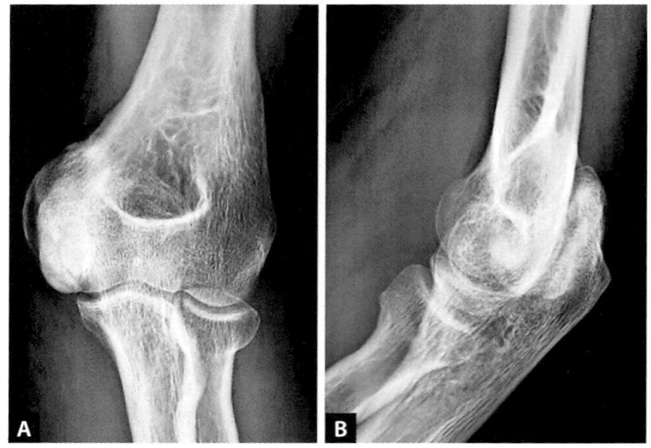

Figs. 10A and B: Ectopic ossification across the medial aspect of elbow visible as a calcified mass in AP (A) and lateral projections (B).

Elbow Arthroplasty Procedures

The term "total elbow arthroplasty" should be only reserved for elbow arthroplasty where elbow prosthesis is used to replace the existing joint surfaces. Interposition/debridement/distraction, resurfacing, remodeling arthroplasty are also elbow arthroplasty procedures.

Historically, extra-articular resection of elbow was performed by Ollier, Park, and Barton in Europe and USA, respectively. This was quickly abandoned to enter into the era of intra-articular resection due to invariable incidence of unstable elbow.

Excision Arthroplasty/Debridement Arthroplasty

First described by Tsuge, this involves removal of all the pathological tissue that distorts the articular anatomy provided >50% of the articular surface is preserved **(Figs. 11A to D).** The articular surfaces that undergo specific changes should be excised and include:

- Olecranon tip and fossa osteophytes
- Coronoid tip and fossa osteophytes
- Heterotopic bone between the ulna-olecranon and radiocapitellum joints
- Deformity and narrowing of the ulnohumeral joint space
- The intra-articular soft-tissue adhesion and triceps retraction

The olecranon fossa fenestration (Kashiwagi's procedure) should be performed only if the elbow loses the anterior rotation of the articular condyles (supracondylar malunion) with consequent ulnohumeral impingement in extension, but as a matter of fact, most surgeons prefer doing it. Morrey called this technique "ulnohumeral arthroplasty" and was also described by Kashiwagi for the treatment of osteoarthritis of elbow joint. Debridement arthroplasty is often performed with patient supine and utilizing posterolateral or longitudinal posterior skin incision (global approach). Laterally, the LCL-sparing approach is used with the dissection running between the extensor radialis longus and brevis. After performing the capsulectomies, an anterior trochlear recontouring osteotomy is often needed to instigate full flexion. All the pathological tissues as described above are then debrided, and postoperatively, the patient is placed in an extension slab for 24 hours.

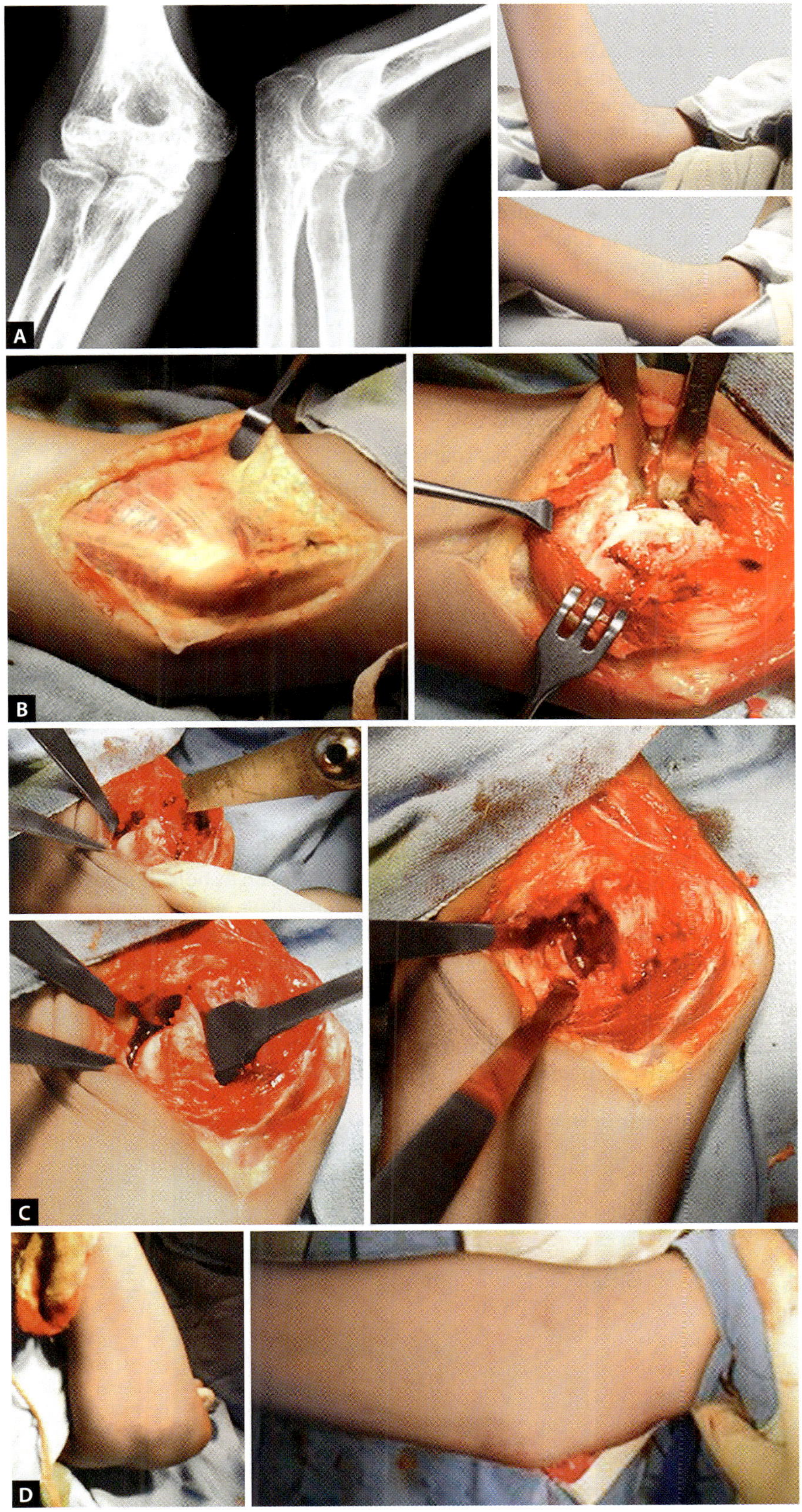

Figs. 11A to D: Excision of intra-articular malunited fragment from trochlear region causing limited arc of mction (90–125°). (A) Radiographs and the clinical movements under anesthesia; (B) Exposure of the pathological mass; (C) Excision of the mass; (D) Postoperative on-table movement at elbow.

Interposition Arthroplasty (Figs. 12A to C)

It is interesting to note that this was such a popular procedure that a number of materials have been tried as interposition materials by different authors. The primary aim is to reduce the initial pain associated with debridement arthroplasty in postoperative period during mobilization. So, the procedure is chiefly indicated in patients who seek pain relief but want to avoid restrictions associated with elbow arthroplasty. For an interested reader, a comprehensive list of materials used for interposition arthroplasty and techniques is presented below:

- Murphy introduced interposition arthroplasty in the USA using "fat" that he himself later changed to using "muscle" as the interposition material.
- Autologous fat and fascia were used by Lexer and Albee.
- Baer used animal membrane (pig's bladder).
- Putti used fascia lata fixed with catgut suture.
- Campbell method was using transtricipital approach where he carved the aponeurotic tricipital flap to be used as interposition material. He fixed this flap to the anterior portion of capsule.
- Froimson used abdominal skin.
- Kita used J-K membrane in 1977.
- Smith used a spongy gel and also utilized silicon membrane.
- Froimson and Morrey described the use of Achilles' tendon allograft in order to cover the humerus and to reconstruct the lateral and MCL.

Successful outcome following interposition arthroplasty is seen in patients with preserved elbow stability, relatively well preserved bony anatomy, good arthrolysis and stable resurfacing. Today the procedure is commonly done as distraction interposition arthroplasty though only interposition arthroplasty is also practiced by many. Patients should be thoroughly counseled about high revision rates and complications following this procedure.

- ***Indications:*** Typically where articular anatomy cannot be restored as in:
  - Post-traumatic ankylosis of elbow
  - Stage I and II rheumatoid arthritis (intact bone) in young
  - Loss of more than 50% articular cartilage.
- ***Contraindications:***
  - Active infection
  - Grossly unstable elbow
  - Congenital ankylosis (lacks soft-tissue support)

The procedure is performed as debridement arthroplasty followed by placing the interposition membrane on the carved surfaces. The membranes commonly used these days are fascia lata graft 8 cm by 20 cm, cutis graft from abdomen (Froimson's technique) or epidermis strips from groin or Bikini. This is followed by distraction apparatus application with considerable detail paid to pin placement.

Adjuvant procedures are often required with debridement and interposition arthroplasty and include:

- Lengthening of triceps aponeurosis
- Debridement and synovectomy
- Manipulation under anesthesia

Replacement Arthroplasty or Total Elbow Arthroplasty

(For description of prosthesis and types, *see* Chapter on "The Unstable Elbow")

This is advised to patients where no salvage is possible and particularly to aged, low-physical demand patients with osteoporotic bones. Patients with more advanced disease or distal humeral fractures not amenable to treatment by other procedures above may be offered distal humeral hemiarthroplasty. It is indicated in patients with preserved humerus and ulna bone stock where the patient wants to remain active continue to endorse high demand sports. This is an unlinked prosthesis with replacement of distal humerus only so later pain may arise from erosion of ulna or the radial head or both along with instability. If the collateral ligaments have doubtful integrity or the bone stock is not adequate then linked prosthesis is necessary. This procedure is especially considered in elderly lower demand patients who have failed (or refuse) conservative and other surgical alternatives and wish to maintain mobility at elbow. They should be able to comply with lifetime restrictions following the elbow arthroplasty. Patients with rheumatoid arthritis

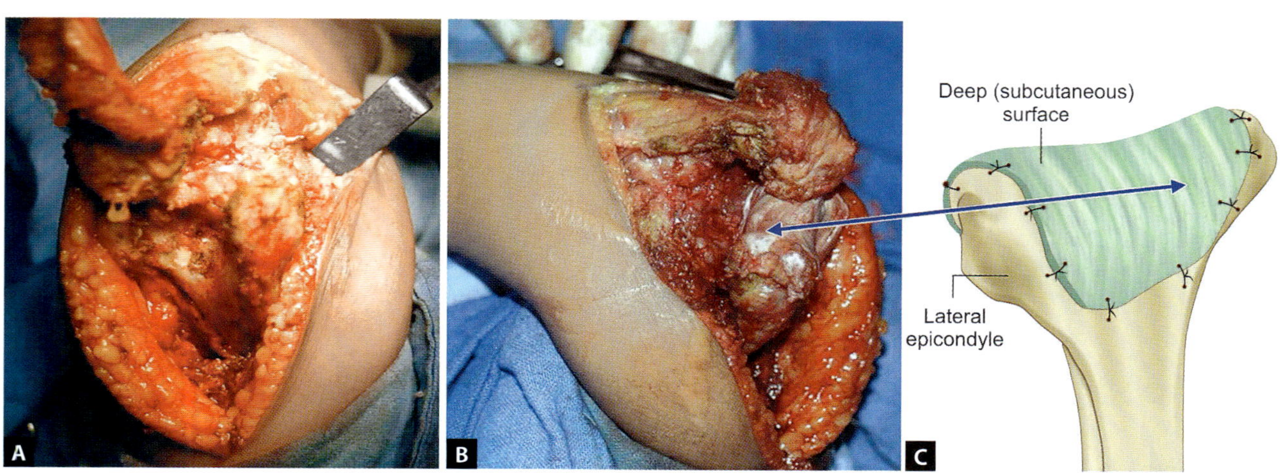

Figs. 12A to C: Interposition arthroplasty using cutis graft. (A) Exposure and debridement of the pathological structures; (B and C) Covering the distal humerus with the cutis graft.

Flowchart 2: Management algorithm for stiff elbow in a typical case.

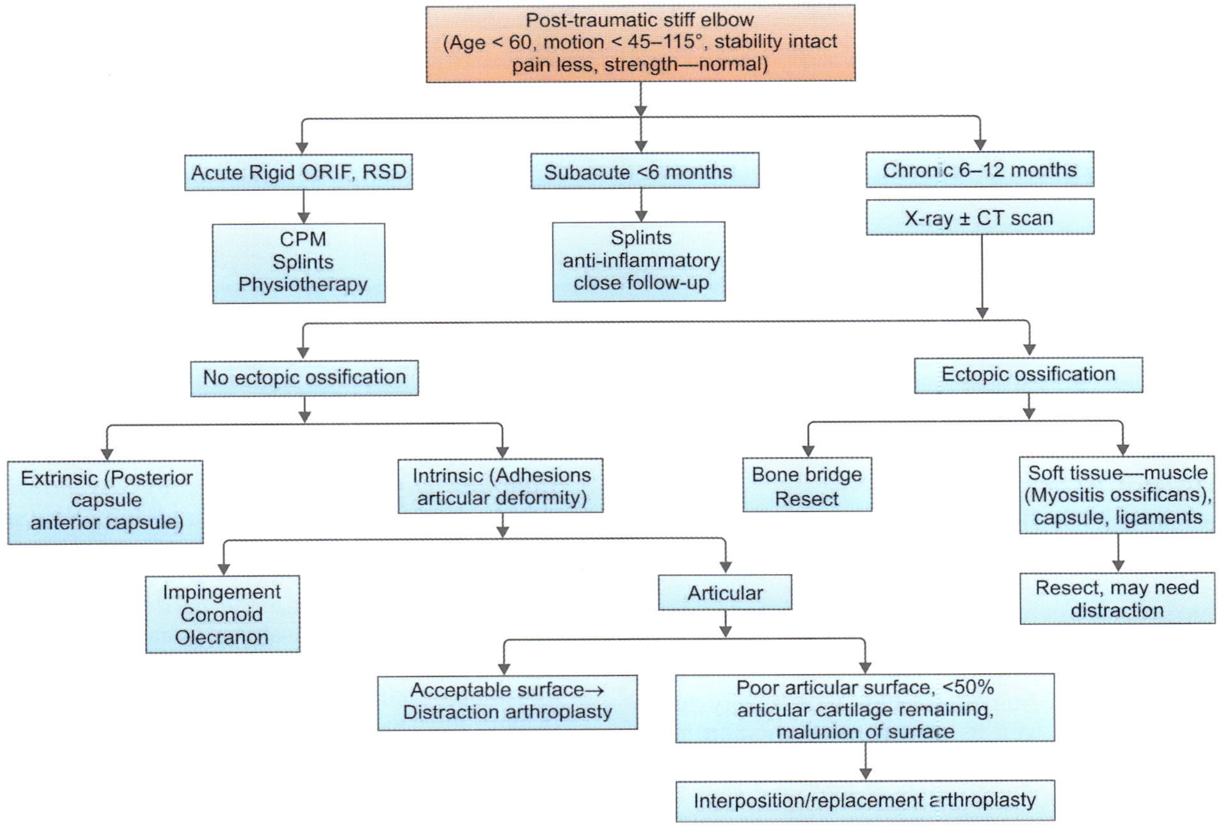

(CPM: continuous passive motion; ORIF: open reduction and internal fixation; RSD: reflex sympathetic dystrophy)

and secondary damage/degeneration of the joint are good candidates for total elbow arthroplasty. Implant failure is the biggest concern in younger patients so other methods described above should be preferred. Generally, a Coonrad-Morrey type prosthesis is preferred in post-traumatic elbow stiffness like those with old unreduced subluxation/dislocations in aged patients, else distal humeral arthroplasty can be done in younger patients that need reconstruction for malunion or osteonecrosis. The contraindications to total elbow arthroplasty include persistent infection, deficient motor function at elbow and patients noncooperative with stringent postoperative protocol (maximal allowable weight that can be lifted with treated limb is 5 Kg). Younger patients have high rates of complications including mechanical failure and need for revision. Recently radiocapitellar arthroplasty has been introduced for treatment of radiocapitellar compartment arthritis following trauma, degenerative arthritis, osteonecrosis or osteochondral lesions. The complications include loosening of radial head component, HO formation, and development of ulnohumeral arthritis. Elbow arthrodesis as a management option for disorders of elbow is discussed elsewhere.

Management algorithm differs from institute and teachings but commonly practiced ones are presented in **Flowchart 2**. For simplicity, considering the grades of elbow stiffness as detailed earlier, the broad principles of treatment in patients with HO can be stated as follows:

- *First grade,* the greater surgical priority is the soft-tissue release.
- *Second grade,* the most important surgical priority is excision of HO.
- *Third grade,* surgical treatment of the articular surface incongruity is the greater priority than HO excision and soft-tissue release.

CONCLUSION

- Stiffness in elbow joint is quite common to develop and often follows immobilization after trauma or reconstructive procedures. It is also a common site for formation of ectopic bone causing loss in range of motion.
- The functional range of motion for elbow to manage activities of daily living is quiet less. This logically explains the division of etiological factors causing loss of either extension or flexion. The division helps surgeon to recreate the movements around elbow by releasing or excising the affected structures selectively rather than performing extensive procedures.
- Elbow arthroplasty (replacement or interposition) is employed only if reconstruction of elbow movements is otherwise not possible.

CHAPTER 111

Hand Anatomy and Function

Manish Kumar Varshney

INTRODUCTION

It is well said that hand is the eye of blind and is tongue of the dumb. The hand should be regarded not only as an intricate mechanical device but as a sophisticated input device having precision sensory area and an accessory output device almost as important as the face that helps in communication.

The hand directed by the mind is responsible for the prominent status of human species. It is a very highly developed structure, with its area of representation in the cerebral cortex being disproportionately large. The hand is specialized to an infinite variety of tools and capable of complicated tasks of exploration, gripping and manipulation, requiring a great precision, power, and accuracy.

The intact hand provides four main functions:

1. ***Subjective sensory perception of the surrounding environment***—the tactile function is specialized for object identification, calibration, and distinction. Apart from the visual, auditory, taste, and smell such intricacy is not provided by any other part of body. Hand excels one step further that these functions can be done anywhere in space by virtue of mobility of upper limb and ability to place the hand anywhere (within limits) and does not require the object to be introduced to body.
2. ***Objective sensory contact***
3. ***Communication with others by direction and demonstration***—gestures are a very important part of communication, most of the sentences can be completed or emphasized by particular gestures that are common to community. It is amazing to see that dumb/mute persons are able to communicate almost as easily like others just by way of gestures.
4. ***Mechanical grips:*** Gripping is a very important function of hand and used most often in day-to-day activities. The following are the common grips of hand. The grips may be used for power function or the advanced precision function. Thumb is an essential component for both types of grips.
   - *Power grip* ***(Figs. 1A and B)****:* Most powerful grip (the fingers flex in one direction to hold the object while the thumb goes around in the opposite direction to provide the counterforce). This keeps the object supported in the palm and fingers. The strength of power grip is proportional to the range of flexion in the interphalangeal (IP) and metacarpophalangeal (MCP) joints, so that any cause of IP joint stiffness weakens the power grip. The final torque in; grasping objects comes from hand intrinsics and the loss of this transverse arch movement is noted in ulnar nerve palsy. The little finger is mechanically very important

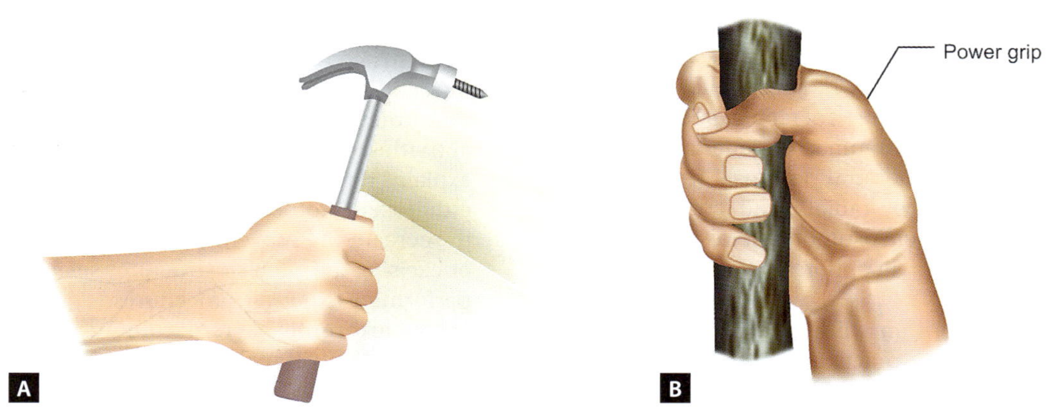

Figs. 1A and B: Power grip is used for holding objects with force and hence mostly uses all the fingers encircling the object tightly.

in power grip as it adds to the breadth of the palm and increases strength of power grip. Hence, amputation of little finger should not be lightly advised. The power grip is also aided by the typical distribution of fat and creases in the palm. The power grip is of three types:

1. *Cylindrical grip* **(Fig. 2)**: All fingers are flexed around the object which is usually at a right angle to forearm. The thumb overlaps the fingers wrapping the object around.
2. *Spherical grip:* All of the fingers and the thumb are adducted around an object, and unlike the cylindrical grip, the fingers are more spread apart. The palm of the hand is often not involved. This is further classified into **(Fig. 3)**:
   - Spherical
   - Box
   - Lateral
   - Cylindrical
   - Flipped cylindrical types
3. *Hook grip (briefcase grip,* **Fig. 4***):* Involves the second through fifth fingers flexed around an object in a hook-like manner. The MCP joints are extended, and the proximal interphalangeal (PIP) and distal interphalangeal (DIP) joints are in some degree of flexion. The thumb is usually not involved.

- *Precision grips:* Tend to hold the object between the tips of the fingers and thumb especially when the objects are small or fragile where no palm support is needed or proximal joints are not moving. They involve actions of both extrinsics and intrinsics. Thumb remains abducted in all. The grip is responsible for most of the fine movements and accuracy of hand. These are of four types:
  1. *Pinch grip (pad-to-pad,* **Figs. 5A and B***):* MCP and PIP of the fingers are flexed, thumb is abducted and the distal joints of both are extended bringing the pad of the finger and thumb together. If both the index and middle fingers are used then it is called "chuck pinch" (three jaw chuck). The pinch grip depends on the intrinsic muscles for posturing, stability, and strength. Weak or lost function of first dorsal interosseous weakens the radial abduction of the index against the thumb while the loss of action of adductor pollicis breaks the longitudinal arch of the thumb that collapses under pinch grip stresses.
  2. *Lateral prehension (pad to side,* **Fig. 6***):* Pad of the extended thumb presses an object against the radial side of the index finger as in holding the car key—"key grip" or in holding straps of objects. Most importantly, pen is held in this fashion!
  3. *Side-to-side grip ("smoking grip",* **Fig. 7***):* Requires adduction of two fingers, usually the index and middle fingers. It is a weak grip and does not permit much precision.

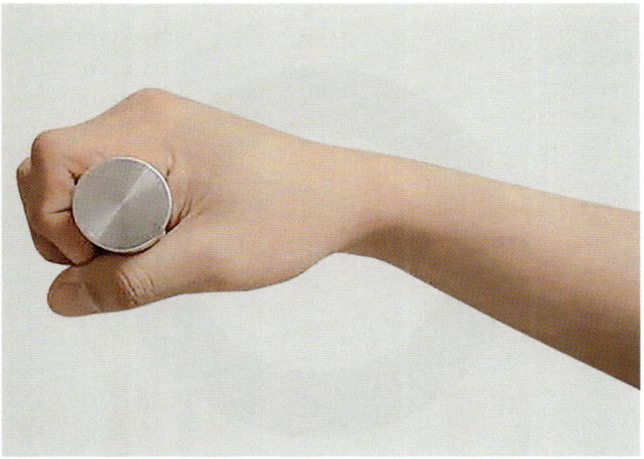

Fig. 2: Cylindrical grip (see text).

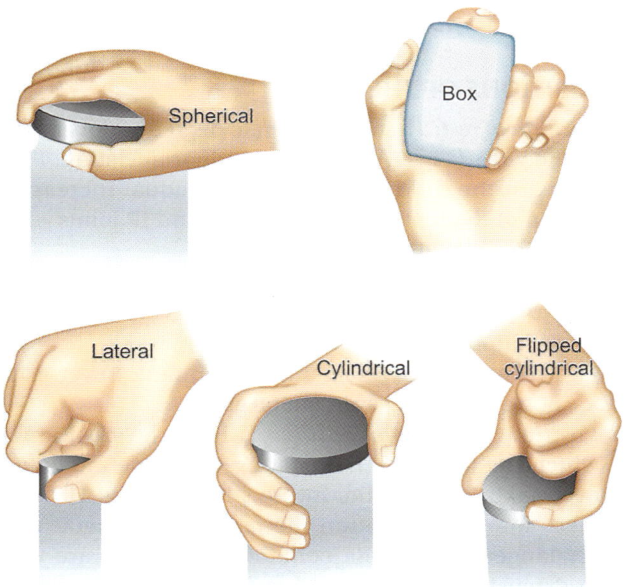

Fig. 3: Various types of power grip. As exception to use of all fingers there are other types of power grips where less number of fingers are used.

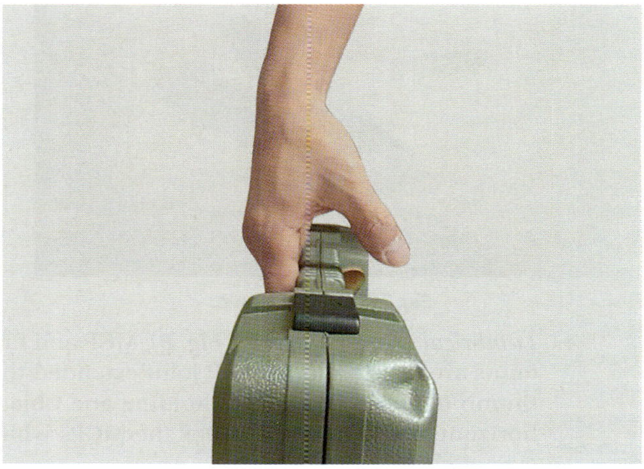

Fig. 4: Hook grip.

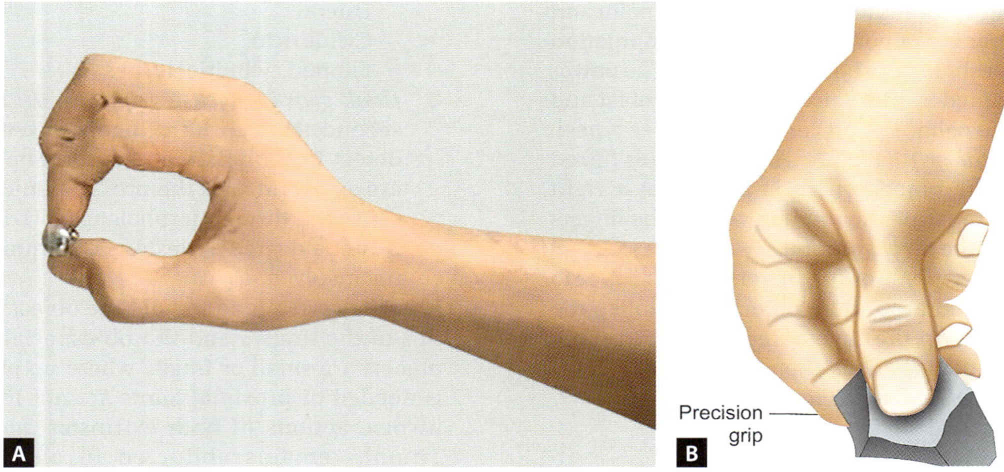

Figs. 5A and B: Precision grip (pad to pad).

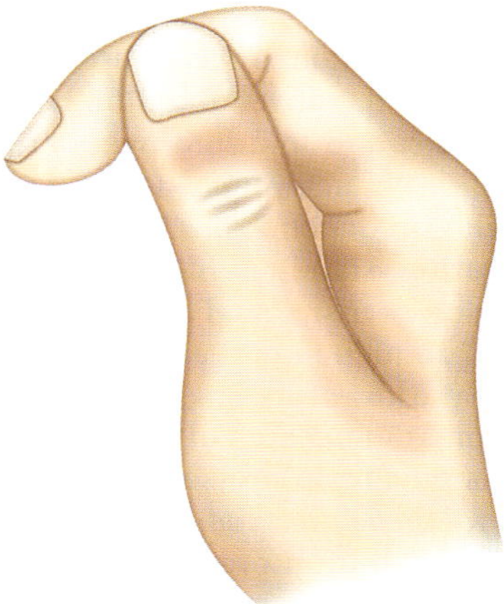

Fig. 6: Pad to side—lateral prehension grip.

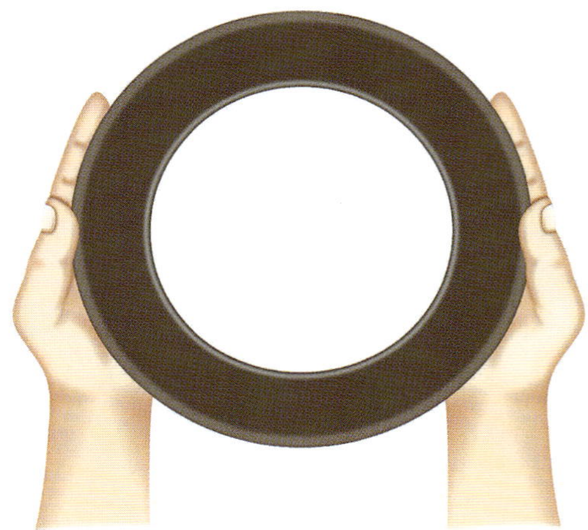

Fig. 8: Lumbrical grip—the plate holding grip.

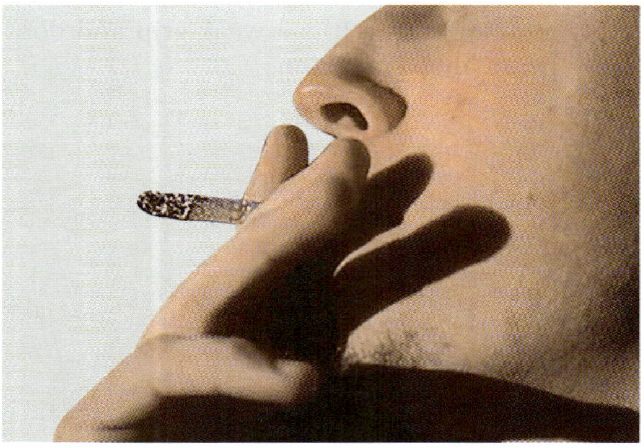

Fig. 7: Side-to-side grip.

4. *Lumbrical grip ("plate grip", **Fig. 8**):* MCP and PIP joints are flexed and the DIP joint extended the thumb opposed the fingers holding and object horizontal. The lumbricals flex the MCPs while extending the IP joints.

POSITIONS OF THE HAND

- *Position of rest:* There is moderate degree of dorsiflexion of the wrist **(Fig. 9A)** with slight ulnar deviation. From index to the little finger, there is gradual increase in flexion of the metacarpophalangeal and IP joints—"the cascade" **(Fig. 9B)**.
- *Position of function:* Various functions include:
  - *Nonprehensile:* Locomotion, in climbing, and swimming.
  - *Prehensile movements:* Precision and power grips, hook, ring, and key or lateral grips.
- *Position of immobilization:* This is the position in which the hand will be most useful to the individual, even taking care of the future stiffness **(Fig. 10)**. This takes into consideration the fact that, in metacarpophalangeal joints, the collateral ligaments are slack in extension and stretched in flexion, while collateral ligaments of proximal IP joints remain stretched for most of the range of flexion.

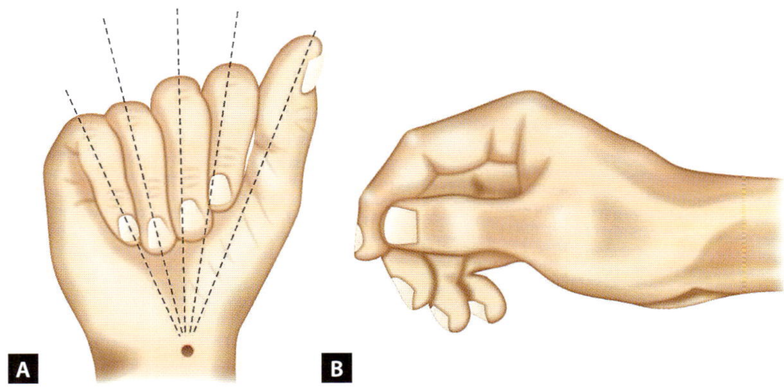

Figs. 9A and B: Position of rest (see text).

ANATOMY

Skin

The palmar skin is thick and well-fixed to the underlying tissues. The keratin layer is thick, compact, and laminated. The central area of the palm is thickest. Despite thickness, the skin has high resolution sensory receptors for tactile discrimination (a special function) acting as third eye. In dorsal skin, the keratin layer is thin and forms a loose covering, it is better for perception of temperature changes (so we use the palmar aspect of hand and finger for object identification while fever, etc., is judged from the dorsum of hand!). It is elastic and mobile. The dorsal skin is quite abundant over the back of IP joints. Tactile discrimination is also aided by the proprioceptive receptors located in the various joints (19 joints of hands) that give a three-dimensional (3D) detail of the object we touch by positioning effect, and the brain forms an image in mind. There is no fat in the superficial fascia and the dermis is directly continuous with the deep fascia. The skin folds onto flexor creases when movements take place at the articulations of hand.

Superficial Fascia

The superficial fascia in the dorsum is thin and stretches easily. On the palmar aspect, it consists of fatty tissues enmeshed in a network of fibers fixed at one end to the skin and at the other to the deep fascia. At the flexor creases, it is absent. Fat is more prominent in the medial and distal part of the thenar region, over the metacarpophalangeal joints, in the webs and in the hypothenar areas. These gripping pads surround triangular central area of palm, which is almost free of fat. This allows the palm to be molded to the object being held during the power grip.

Deep Fascia

On the dorsum of the hand, the deep fascia is arranged in two layers:

1. *Superficial layer:* It covers the extensor tendons and is continuous with the extensor retinaculum.
2. *Deep layer:* It covers the intraosseous muscles. The deep fascia on the palmar aspect of hand helps in preventing the bowstringing of the tendons by forming various large pulleys as follows:

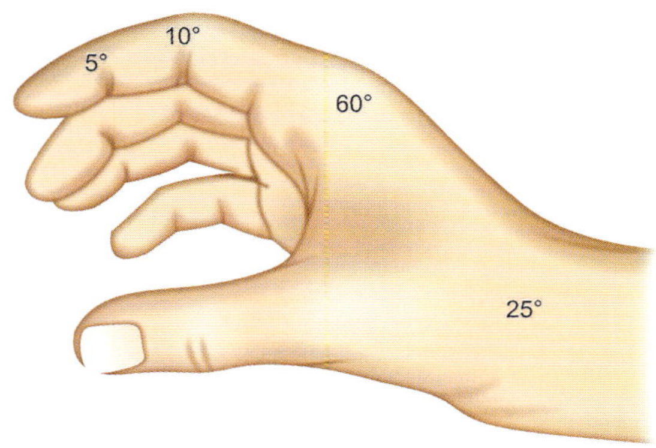

Fig. 10: Position of immobilization.

- The flexor retinaculum; also known as transverse carpal ligament
- Palmar aponeurosis
- Fibrous flexor sheaths of the fingers
- Guyon's canal

Carpal Bones (Figs. 11A and B)

They are divided into two rows, proximal (scaphoid, lunate, triquetrum, and pisiform) and distal (trapezium, trapezoid, capitate, and hamate). These eight bones have complex interlocking shapes and are stabilized by interosseous ligaments. Articulations and the interosseous ligaments link the carpal bones to each other. The blood supply reaches the bones along the ligaments. Volar ligaments are stronger than dorsal ligaments. They have a double "V" shape with a weak area in between (space of Poirier). The scapholunate and the lunotriquetral ligaments are the most important ligaments (*see* Chapter on "Carpal Instability"). Insufficiency of these ligaments leads to dorsal intercalated segment instability and volar intercalated segment instability (VISI), respectively **(Fig. 11B)**. Dorsal ligaments tend to converge on triquetrum. Wrist joint is formed by the distal radial articular surface along with scaphoid and lunate bones (in extreme flexion, the triquetrum also articulates with the radius partially).

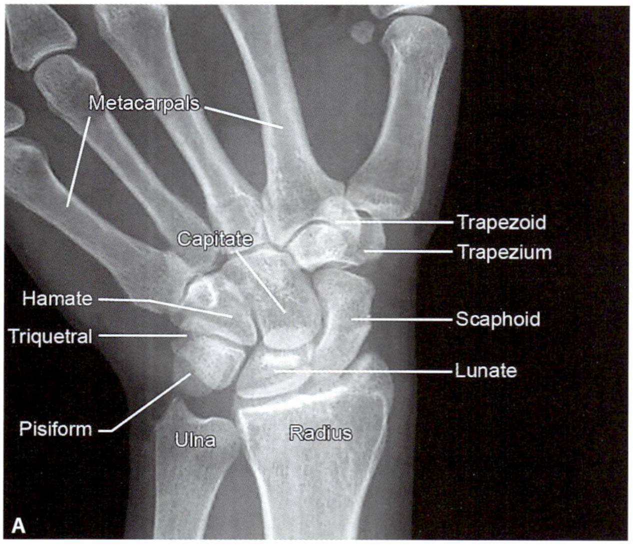

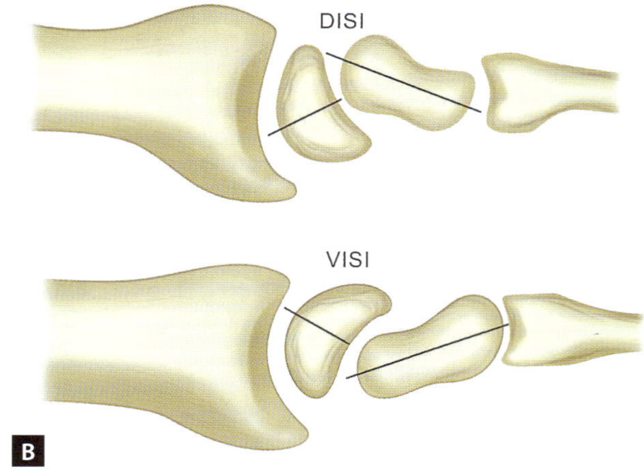

Figs. 11A and B: (A) Carpal bones of wrist; (B) Presentation of dorsal intercalated segment instability (DISI) and volar intercalated segment instability (VISI).

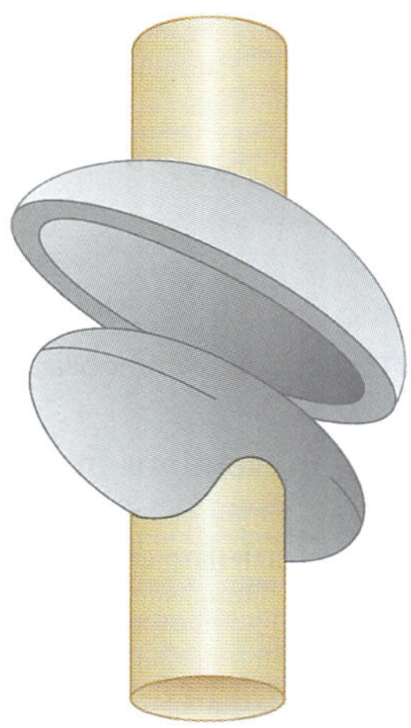

Fig. 12: Ellipsoid joint.

Kinematics of Wrist Joint

Radiocarpal joint is an *ellipsoid joint* (**Fig. 12,** oriented obliquely at a mean angle of 26.6° ± 4.4° to the sagittal plane of motion) with transverse and anteroposterior convexity. The articular complex has two degrees of freedom basically but when combined with pronosupination hand can be positioned virtually in any place in hemisphere. Movements have been classically described as that occurring in antero-posterior axis (frontal plane—radial and ulnar deviation) or transverse axis (sagittal plane—flexion and extension). These have been combined to a more complex "dart-throwers" axis now (see below). This is the most commonly used axis for wrist motion bringing it from radial-deviation extension position to ulnar-deviation flexion. The range of motion at wrist joint is as follows **(Figs. 13A to C)**:

- Flexion (volar flexion) = 80–90° (10° functional)
- Extension (dorsiflexion) = 65–80°
    - Flexion split between radiocarpal (40–50%) and midcarpal (50–60%) while extension is mainly radiocarpal (92%).
- Radial deviation = 20°
- Ulnar deviation = 25–35°
- Pronation (combined movement at various joints—*see* Chapter on "Distal Radioulnar Joint Disorders and Ulnar Wrist Pain") = 90°
- Supination (combined movement at various joints—*see* Chapter on "Distal Radioulnar Joint Disorders and Ulnar Wrist Pain") = 85–90°

Due to umpteen possibilities of wrist movement by addition of pronosupination, a concept of "coupled" wrist movements (amount of wrist flexion-extension per degree of radioulnar deviation) is being used to describe wrist movements.

Bryce, in 1896, described the carpal bone movements based on his own wrists radiographs. Since then a lot of mechanisms and theories have been propounded for weight transmission and its effect on carpal bone disposition. The distribution of carpal bones for explaining the kinematics has been varied according to the theory propounded for explaining the complex mechanism. Following are the common concepts propounded:

- *Rows (traditional concept,* ***Fig. 14****):* This is more described on the basis of anatomical disposition of the carpal bones. Proximal and distal rows are linked by scaphoid. The motion occurs between the rows and within the rows.
- Columns (Navarro, 1921; modified by Taleisnik 1976, **Fig. 14**):
    - Central (flexion/extension) lunate, capitate, and hamate
    - Lateral (mobile) scaphoid, trapezoid, and trapezium
    - Medial (rotation) triquetrum and pisiform. Taleisnik modified the columns by including trapezium and trapezoid in the central column and eliminated pisiform altogether.
- Oval ring concept of Lichtman and Lichfield **(Fig. 14)** signifies the reciprocal motion between distal and proximal row of the carpus during motion in opposite direction.

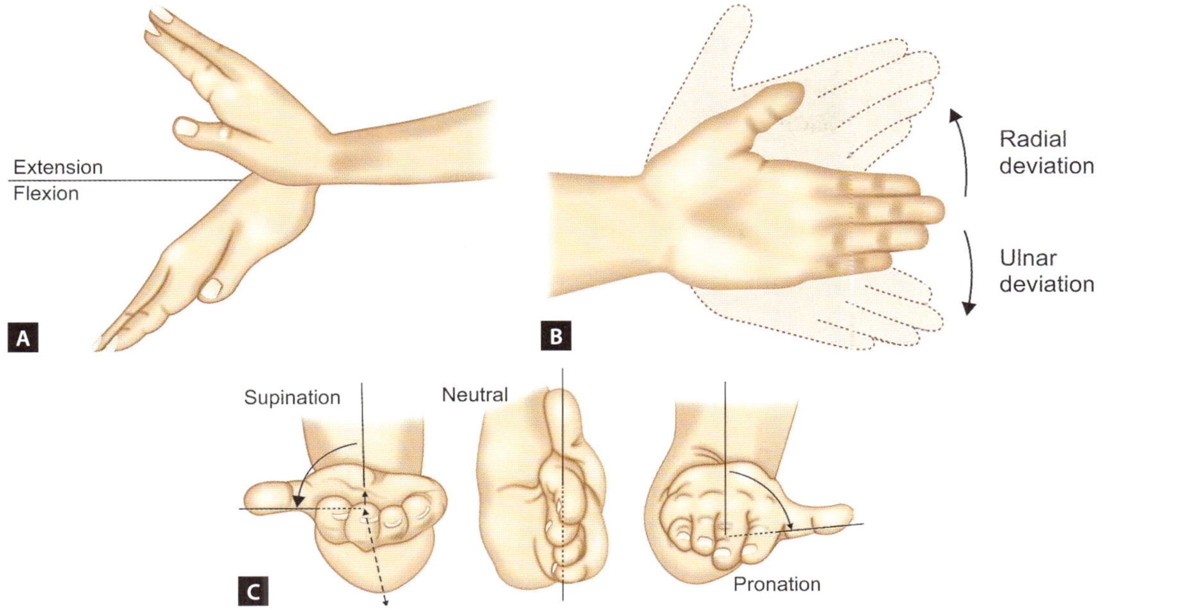

Figs. 13A to C: Various movements at the wrist joint: (A) Flexion-extension; (B) Radial and ulnar deviation; (C) Supination and pronation.

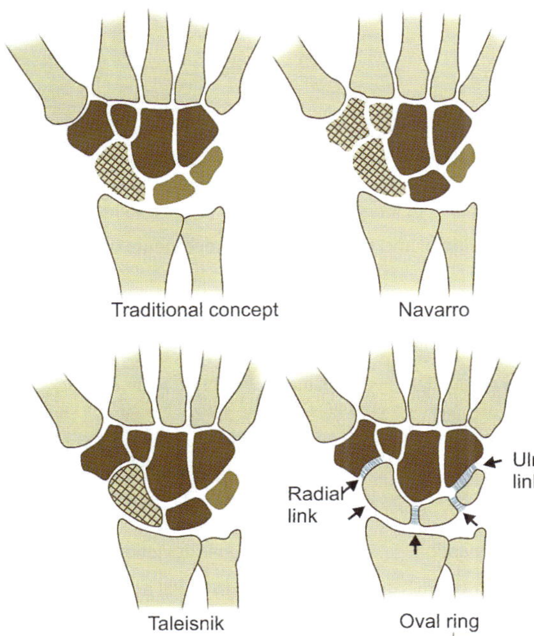

Fig. 14: Various concepts as prevalent to explain the carpal kinematics.

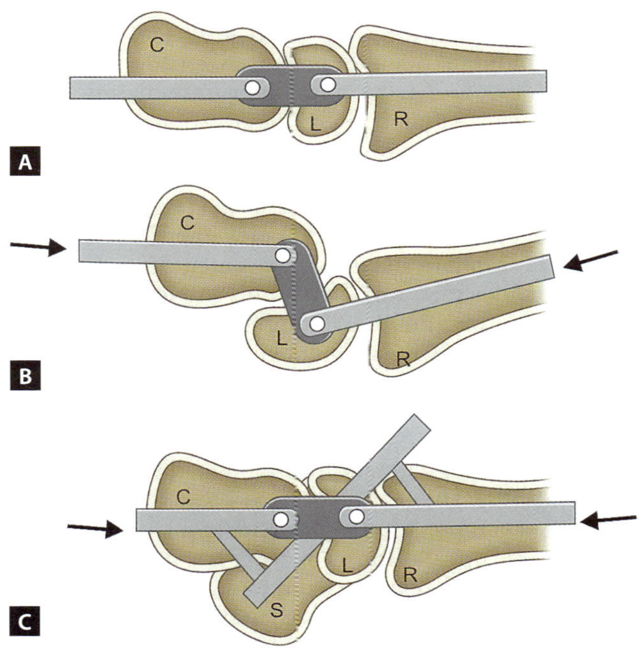

Figs. 15A to C: Link concept of Gilford. (A) The proximal represents an intercalated segment; (B) That rotates dorsally under compressive loads; (C) Scaphoid tends to maintain a fixed relation to this link axis (C: capitate; L: lunate; R: radius; S: scaphoid).

- *Link Joint (Gilford 1943,* ***Figs. 15A to C****):* This is a simplified concept explaining the movements as occurring in chains of three bones represented by radius, lunate, and capitate. The disadvantage of link concept is that scaphoid is out of main focus when describing dependent motions while this is considered by many as the bridge between two rows. However, the concept does include the fact that scaphoid links the radius to distal carpus and provides stability against compression forces in flexion and extension **(Figs. 16A to C)**.
  - Proximal row acts as a unit and is represented as "intercalated segment" (between radius and distal row) with no direct tendon attachments. The segment is represented by lunate bone. Intercarpal movement is significant between scaphoid, lunate, and triquetrum.
  - Distal row functions as unit and is represented by the capitate bone. It is motorized by tendons and by virtue of ligamentous attachments moves the proximal row. There is little intercarpal movement if at all.
  - Head of capitate acts as a center of rotation.

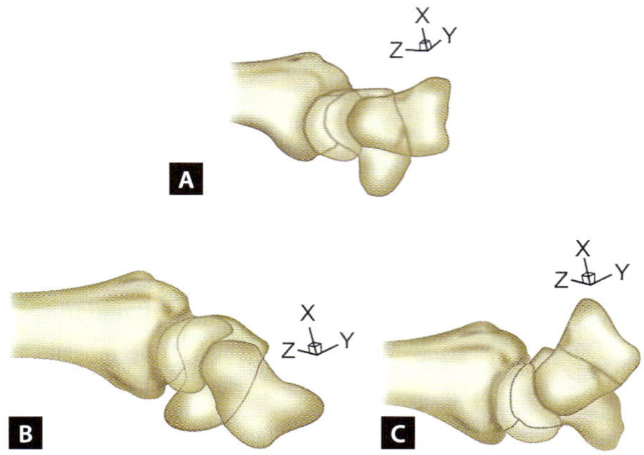

Figs. 16A to C: The flexion and extension of carpal bones in the link concept. (A) Normal relation; (B) Wrist flexion; (C) Compressive loading.

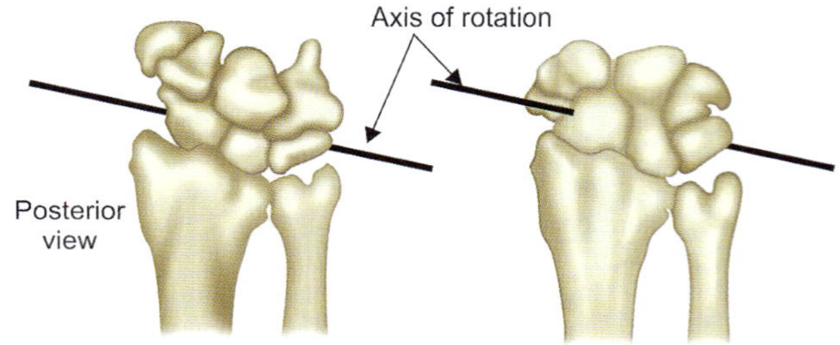

Fig. 17: Dart throwers axis (see text).

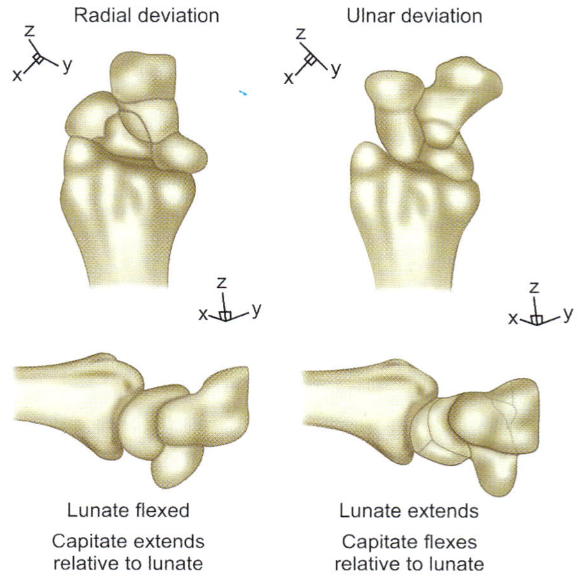

Fig. 18: Radial and ulnar deviation movements of scaphoid.

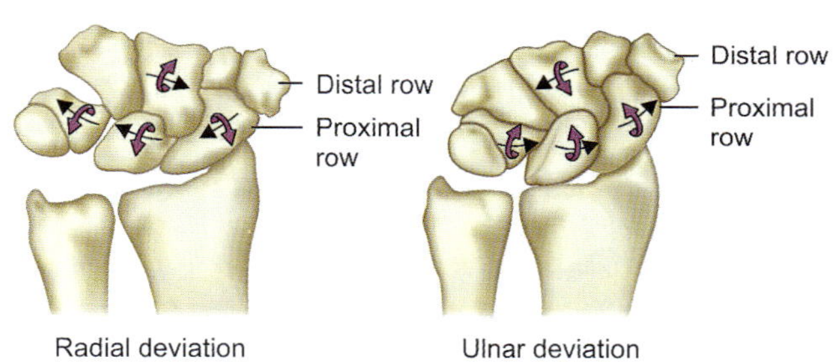

Fig. 19: The movements of carpal bones in radial and ulnar deviations, according to the triquetrohamate helicoid concept.

The following are the most important derivations from the various biomechanical theories of the wrist joint (should be always remembered while understanding carpal instability):

- Principal force transmission is through capitate lunate and proximal pole of scaphoid—75% through radius and 25% through ulna. Carpal bone movements are in conjunction to nearby bones and not at all isolated.
- The traditional plane of flexion-extension and radial-ulnar deviation have now been unified into "Dart-thrower's plane" of motion: This is an obliquely oriented plane of wrist motion that ranges from a position of combined radial deviation and extension to positions of combined ulnar deviation and flexion **(Fig. 17)**.
    - In a pure dart-throw (DT) movement, there is near zero scaphoid and lunate movement.
    - Activities requiring higher grip strength move along planes parallel to DT plane and have significant scaphoid and lunate motion.
- Wrist flexion is shared between the two carpal rows while the extension is primarily radiocarpal.
- *Radial deviation:* Scaphoid flexes; proximal pole goes dorsal "pulling" lunate into palmar flexion, capitate extends **(Fig. 18)**.
- *Ulnar deviation:* Scaphoid extends; proximal pole pulls lunate into dorsiflexion, capitate flexes.
- The triquetrohamate helicoid joint concept is another (albeit complex) way of understanding the lunate motion **(Fig. 19)**:
    - *Ulnar deviation:* "Low" position; the scaphoid is distal and dorsiflexed pulling lunate into dorsiflexion.
    - *Radial deviation:* "High" position; the scaphoid is proximal and palmar flexed pulling lunate into palmar flexion.
- The normal scapholunate angle (on lateral view) is 30–60° **(Figs. 20A and B)**, it is questionably abnormal between 60° and 80°, >80° is abnormal indicating instability.
- The capitolunate angle (on lateral view, **Fig. 21**) is ideally a single line (0°): angle >30° is abnormal indicating stability.

Radiological anatomy of wrist:

- The joint spaces of the wrist have a width of 2 mm or less. Radiocarpal joint is slightly wider while the carpometacarpal (CMC) joints are slightly narrower than the midcarpal joints **(Fig. 22)**.
- The capitolunate joint is considered the baseline joint width to which other joint spaces can be compared. Carpal joints should be symmetrical. Loss of symmetricity and variable overlap of carpal bones indicate carpal dislocation (commonly lunate and perilunate, **Figs. 23A and B**).
- The three carpal arcs (Gilula's arcs, **Fig. 24**): These are smooth curves joining the surfaces of the carpal bones.
    - The first arc is a smooth curve outlining the proximal convexities of the scaphoid, lunate, and triquetrum.
    - The second arc traces the distal concave surfaces of the same bones, and

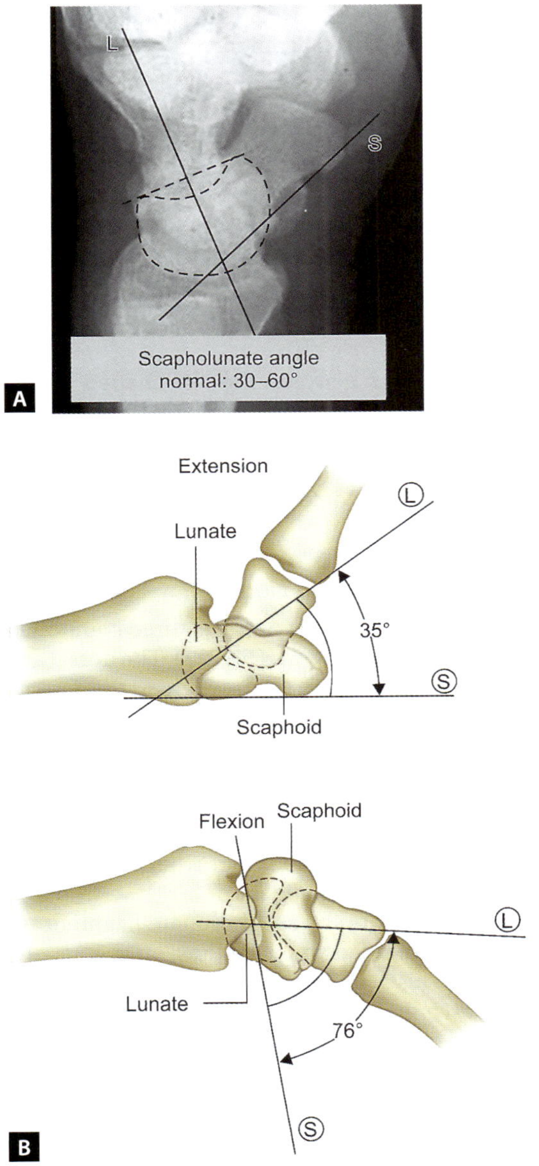

Figs. 20A and B: Scapholunate angle: (A) Normal; (B) Its relation during wrist extension and flexion (S—axis of scaphoid bone, L—axis of lunate bone).

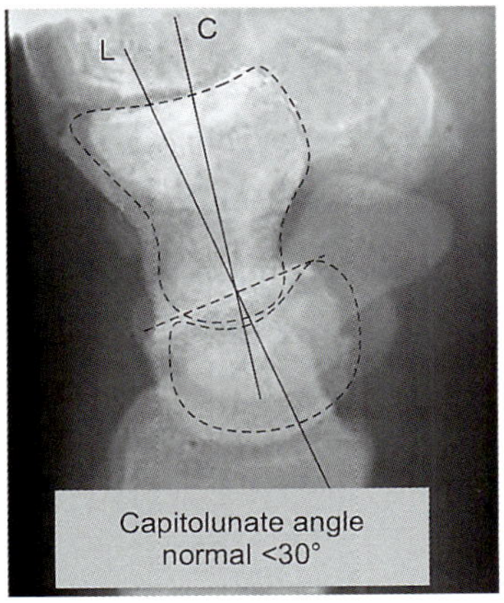

Fig. 21: Capitolunate axis derived from intersection of median capitate and lunate axes (C: capitate axis; L: lunate axis).

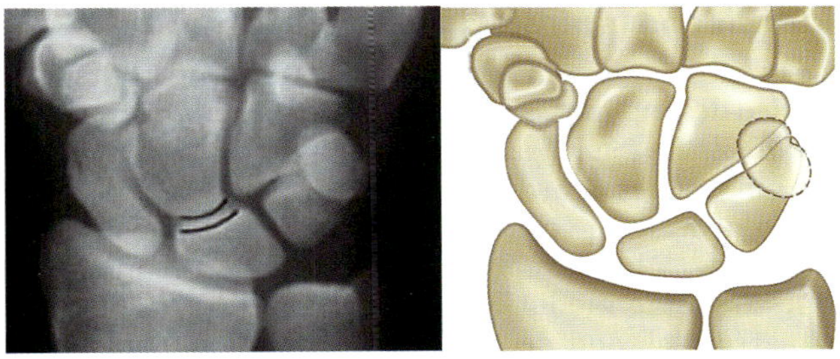

Fig. 22: The normal joint space between carpal bones.

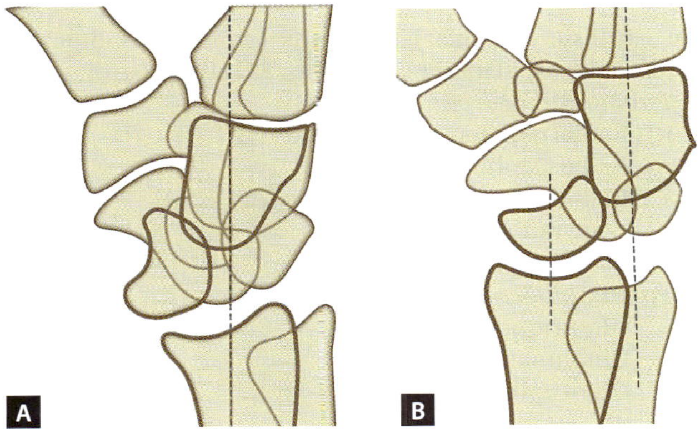

Figs. 23A and B: Lunate (A) versus perilunate (B) dislocations.

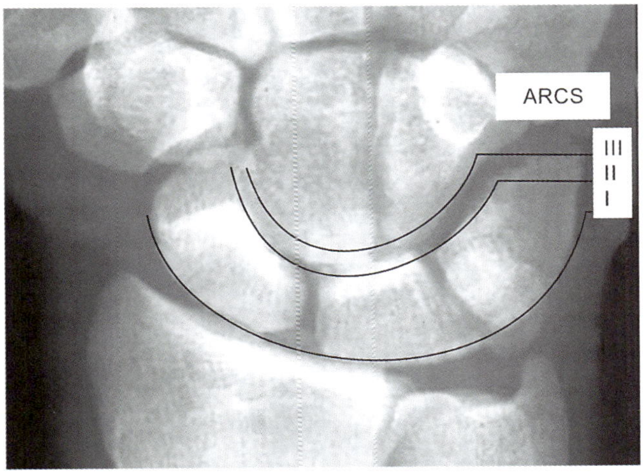

Fig. 24: Carpal arcs—these Gilula's arcs are smooth curves along the proximal carpal row and proximal aspect of distal carpal row.

- The third arc follows the main proximal curvatures of the capitate and hamate.
  Break in one of the arcs indicates a fracture or the disruption of a ligament leading to a subluxation or dislocation.

- The lunate and perilunate dislocations are differentiated based on capitate centering. If the capitate is centered over the radius and the lunate is tilted out, it is a lunate dislocation. If, however, the lunate centers over the distal radius and the capitate is dorsal, it is a perilunate dislocation.

Extrinsic and Intrinsic Ligaments of Wrist

The ligaments are so many with their attachments that their detailed description is of use to only dedicated wrist surgeon. We will list the main ligaments and discuss the scapholunate and lunotriquetral anatomy in detail. In general, as far as the nomenclature goes few terms help understanding the complexity, a bit. If more than two ligaments connect two bones then the modifying term is added, e.g., long, short, palmar/dorsal, and deep. The dorsal ligaments appear as distinct structures after elevating the retinaculum while palmar ligaments are better viewed from within the joint (dorsal arthroscopy portal).

The extrinsic (capsular) ligaments (cross the radiocarpal joint or midcarpal joint or both, **Fig. 25**) comprise of:

- *Palmar radiocarpal:*
  - Radial collateral
  - Radioscaphocapitate
  - Radioscapholunate (ligament of Testut)
  - Long radiolunate
  - Short radiolunate
- *Palmar ulnocarpal ligaments:*
  - Ulnotriquetral
  - Ulnolunate
  - Ulnocapitate
- *Dorsal ligaments:*
  - Radiotriquetral
  - Dorsal intercarpal
  - Radiolunate
  - Radioscaphoid

The intrinsic (interosseous) ligaments (between the bones of proximal or distal carpal rows) comprise of:

- *Proximal row:*
  - Scapholunate
  - Lunotriquetral
- *Distal row:*
  - Trapeziotrapezoid ligament
  - Trapeziocapitate ligament
  - Capitohamate ligament
- *Palmar midcarpal* (it is interesting to note that there is no ligament connecting *lunate and capitate*):
  - Scaphotrapeziotrapezoid
  - Scaphocapitate
  - Triquetral-capitate
  - Triquetral-hamate

Space of Poirier

Space of Poirier lies between the "V"-shaped volar radiocapitate and long radiolunate ligaments **(Fig. 26)**. The area expands when wrist is dorsiflexed and disappears in palmar flexion. Rent develops in this space in dorsal dislocations, and it is through this defect that lunate displaces into the carpal canal.

Scapholunate Interosseous Ligament

This is a U-shaped ligament and has three components the volar, dorsal, and interosseous **(Fig. 27)**. The dorsal and volar components are true ligaments, whereas the interosseous component is fibrocartilage.

- The dorsal component is 2–3 mm thick with transversely oriented bundles of collagen. This is the most important component and provides the most stability to diastasis. The ligament avulses from the scaphoid attachment and rarely at the lunate attachment whenever a diastasis is seen in symptomatic patients.
- The volar aspect of the scapholunate ligament typically is obliquely oriented and measures, on average, 1 mm in thickness. This is the weakest component. It lies volar to the radioscapholunate ligament attachment.

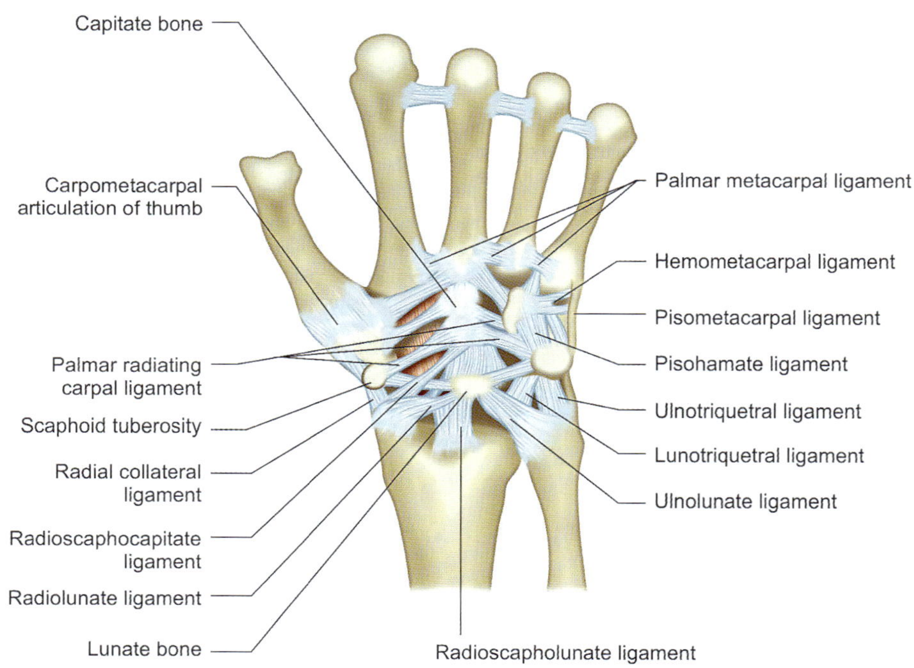

Fig. 25: The extrinsic wrist ligaments.

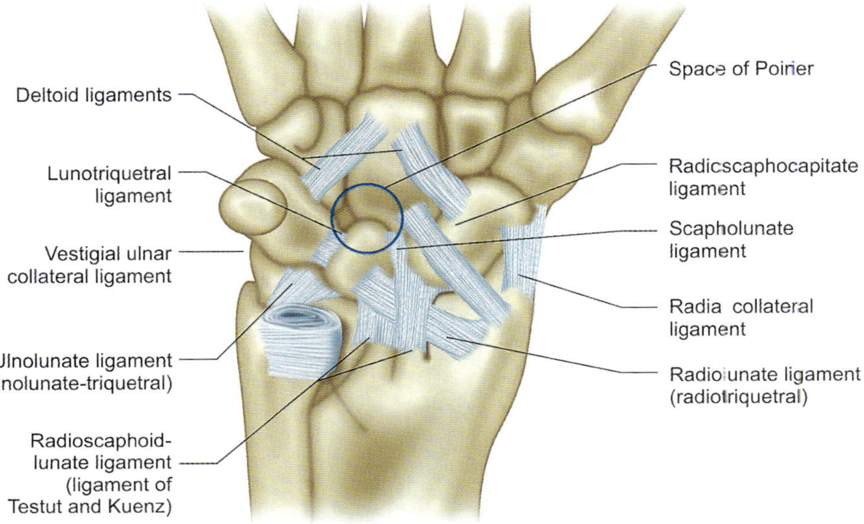

Fig. 26: Space of Poirier (see text).

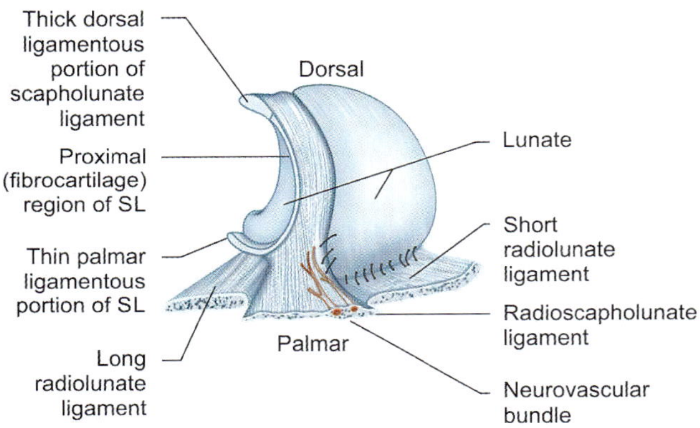

Fig. 27: Scapholunate interosseous ligament.

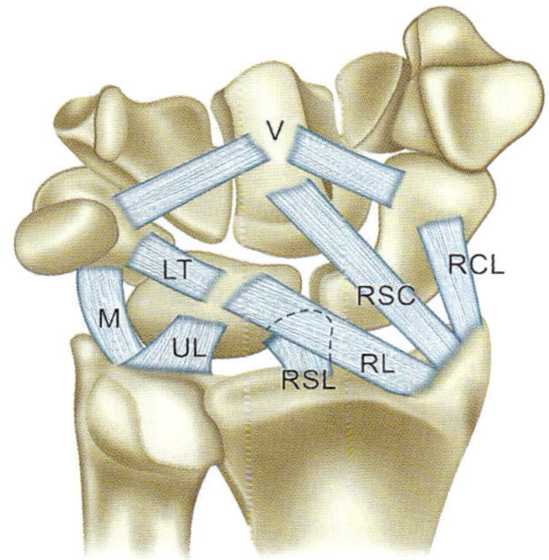

Fig. 28: Illustration depicting the intrinsic ligaments binding the carpal bones, also depicting the lunotriquetral ligament (LT) (RCL: radial collateral ligament; RSC: radioscaphocapitate ligament; RL: radiolunate/radiolunotriquetral ligament; RSL: radioscapholunate ligament [Ligament of Testut and Kuenz]; V: deltoid ligaments forming inverted "v"; LT: lunotroquetral ligaments; M: vestigial ulnar collateral ligament; UL: ulnolunate/ulnolunotriquetral ligament).

- Interosseous component is thin and fibrocartilaginous. It blends into the radioscapholunate ligament (Testut) and receives supply hence from branch of anterior interosseous nerve and artery and radial artery. The interosseous portion often ruptures in asymptomatic patients.

Lunotriquetral Interosseous Ligament (Fig. 28)

This is a C-shaped intrinsic ligament spanning the dorsal, proximal, and palmar edges of the joint lunotriquetral joint.

It is comprised of thick dorsal and volar regions and weak membranous portion.

- Dorsal lunotriquetral ligament has a triangular appearance and is most important as a rotational constraint. Its tears produce VISI.
- *Volar lunotriquetral ligament (linear appearance):* This is the thickest and strongest portion of the lunotriquetral ligament and transmits extension moment of the triquetrum.

Innervation of Hand

The nerve supply of the hand is obtained through the brachial plexus from the lower four cervical and first thoracic nerves (C5, C6, C7, C8, and T1). The pattern of distribution of median, ulnar, and radial branches in hand is shown in **Figure 29**. The motor innervation of the intrinsic muscles of hand is shared between the ulnar and median nerves while the radial nerve supplies the long-finger extensors along with wrist extensors.

Blood Supply of Hand

Blood supply of hand is derived chiefly from the distal parts of the radial and ulnar artery forming the palmar arches **(Fig. 30)**.

The *superficial palmar arch* is the main branch of the ulnar artery in the hand. The main branches of the arch are palmar digital artery to the little finger; three common digital arteries dividing into proper digital branches for the medial four fingers **(Fig. 31A)**.

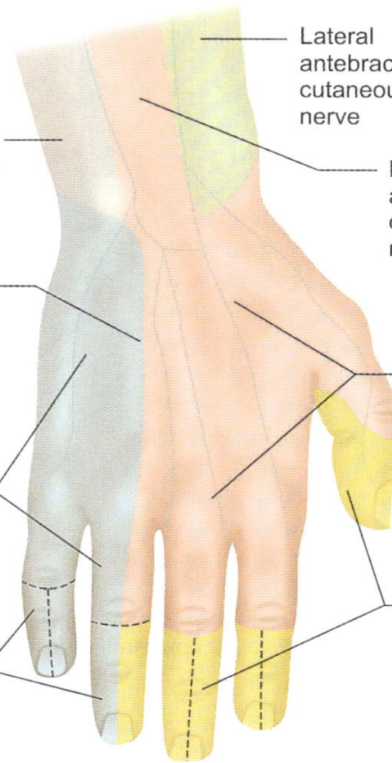

Fig. 29: Cutaneous innervation of hand.

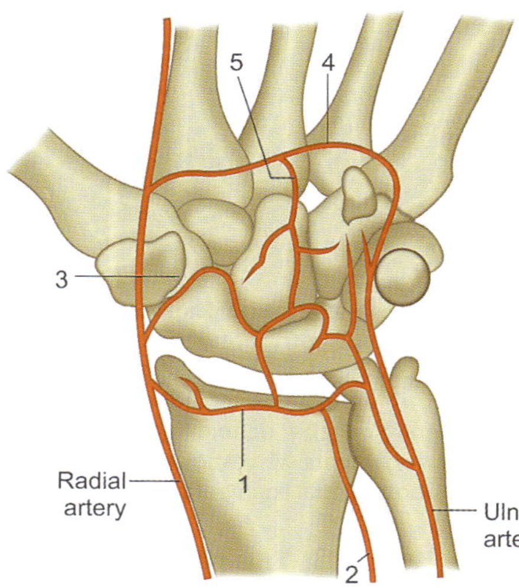

Fig. 30: Blood supply of wrist and carpals: Circulation of the wrist is obtained through the radial, ulnar, and anterior interosseous arteries and the deep palmar arch: 1—palmar radiocarpal arch; 2—palmar branch of anterior interosseous artery; 3—palmar intercarpal arch; 4—deep palmar arch; and 5—recurrent artery.

Deep palmar arch is the continuation of the radial artery into the palm, where it joins with the deep branch of the ulnar artery. It gives branches to the thumb, and also to the three palmar metacarpal arteries which pass distally to join the common palmar digital arteries **(Fig. 31B)**.

Functional position of hand:

- *Wrist:*
  - Extended 20°
  - Ulnar deviated 10°
- *Digits 2 through 5:*
  - MCP joints flexed 45°
  - PIP joints flexed 30–45°
  - DIP joints flexed 10–20°
- *Thumb:*
  - First CMC joint partially abducted and opposed
  - MCP joint flexed 10°
  - IP joint flexed 5°.

ANATOMY OF TENDONS

Hand movements are powered by 22 extrinsic reins called tendons that originate in forearm, the intrinsic tendons and muscles of hand guide their movement. Thus, hand possesses uniquely combined movements of strength and dexterity. Each tendon passes through osteofibrotic canal reinforced by number of pulleys **(Fig. 32)**. This is needed to prevent bowstringing and loss of power by getting mechanical advantage being as close to bone as possible.

Any disruption of the canal or main pulley system causes bowstringing increasing force needed to move the joint (distance from joint increases) and also the amount of torque placed on the articulation is increased tremendously. This also needs more tendon length (amplitude of gliding) to complete the same movement.

Flexor Tendons

The flexor carpi radialis and flexor carpi ulnaris are located at both sides of the carpal tunnel. The eight finger flexors and the flexor pollicis longus (FPL) pass through the carpal canal dorsal to the median nerve. The flexor digitorum superficialis and profundus tendons pass through a narrow

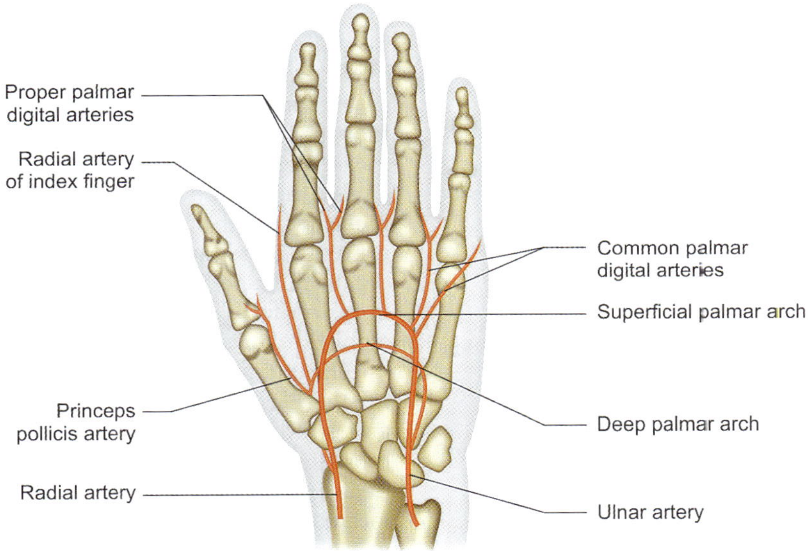

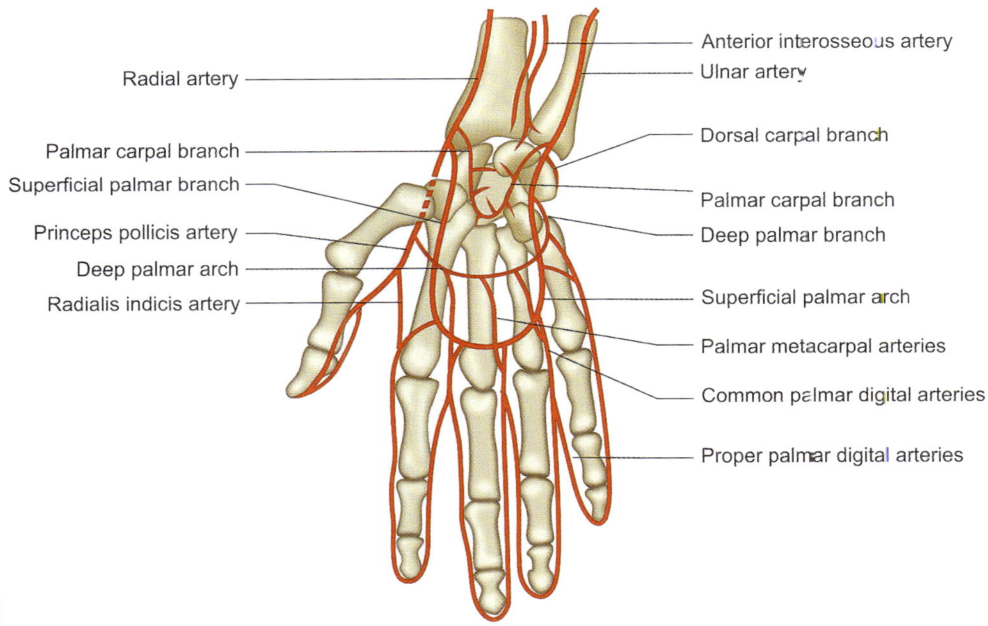

Figs. 31A and B: Blood supply of hand (see text).

osteofibrotic canal supported volar aspect by a pulley system to prevent bowstringing. The floor is formed by a sulcus that has been indented by the metacarpal's volar neck and the roof of the annular ligament. The tendinous sheath, at the finger level, is formed by a double layer of connective tissue; one is visceral and is in contact with the tendon, and other one is external parietal; separated by a virtual space, which creates a liquid circulating system.

Pulley system supports the tendon function throughout their length. This system spans from the transverse carpal ligament and the palmar aponeurosis pulley to the distant A5 pulley. There are *five annular and four crossed pulleys* supporting the tendon **(Figs. 33A and B)**. The annular pulleys are often thick and rigid.

- The pulley mechanism sacrifices force for efficiency. By keeping moment arms smaller, the pulleys decrease some of the available force for joint movement but precision of movement is increased.
- The palmar aponeurosis pulley (Manske and Lesker in 1983) is proximal to A1 pulley and lies 1 cm proximal to MCP joint. It is formed by the transverse fascicular fibers and paratendinous bands of the palmar aponeurosis.
- The A1, A3, and A5 pulleys are located over the MP, PIP, and DIP joints, respectively. The A2 and A4 pulley are located over the proximal and middle phalanges.
- The second annular (A2) pulley, which inserts itself on the proximal phalanx, and the fourth annular pulley are functionally the most important. The first annular (A1) pulley is released in trigger finger release.
- Major function of the A3 pulley is to reduce tendon pulley gliding resistance by decreasing the angle of attack of the flexor tendons during flexion.

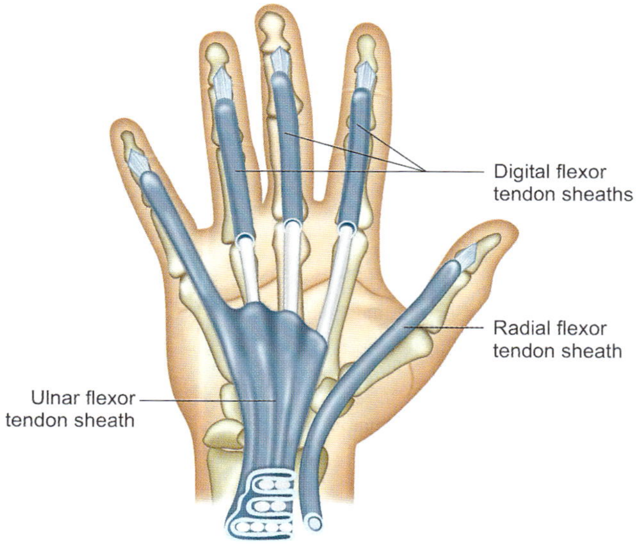

Fig. 32: Synovial sheath of the flexor tendons.

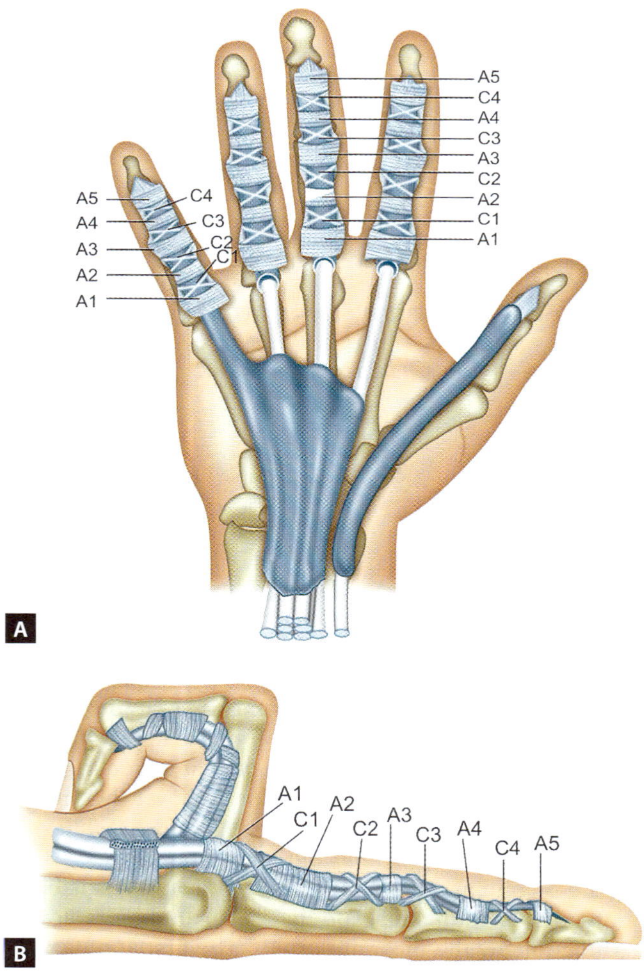

Figs. 33A and B: Flexor tendon anatomy: Flexor tendon pulley system of the fingers (A). Illustration shows that the flexor tendon pulleys maintain the tendon in close contact with the articulation throughout range of motion (A—annular; C—cruciate pulleys).

- Cruciate pulleys (each located distal to A2, A3, and A4 pulleys) modulate force transmission during finger flexion.

Flexor digitorum profundus tendon is responsible for most of the finger flexion. The tendon passes through the flexor digitorum superficialis split tendon at Camper's chiasm near base of middle phalanx **(Fig. 34)**. Along the metacarpals, the tendon gives origin to lumbricals that prevent its retraction during distal cut injuries. Flexor digitorum superficialis tendon is necessary to balance the finger as during flexion flexor digitorum profundus tendon alone is unable to balance the finger at all three joints.

The thumb—FPL tendon is also wrapped in a double sheath **(Fig. 35)**. The A1 pulley is approximately 7–9 mm wide and is situated on the palmar side of the MCP. The zone that more frequently constricts the thumb tendons from gliding freely is found at the level of the sesamoid bones, which are located on the sides of the articulation's capsule and at the point at which the two flexor pollicis brevis heads insert.

The most distally located oblique pulley has a width of approximately 9–11 mm, is oriented ulnoradially in a proximal-to-distal direction, and houses the distal fibers of the adductor pollicis.

Extensor Tendons

Extensor tendons pass through six different compartments, each one with its own synovial membrane, under the dorsal carpal transverse ligament **(Fig. 36)**.

- *Compartment one:* In classic description, this compartment houses the abductor pollicis longus (APL) and the extensor pollicis brevis (EPB). They are covered by a rigid structure formed by the extensor retinaculum's transverse fibers. The EPB is a phylogenetic structure that is specific to our species and is smaller and less bulky than the APL. Rather than a single compartment of classical descriptions, in 24–34% of population the compartment has been seen to be pluricompartmental with one ulnar canal housing the EPB, and one radial containing the APL. A third canal has also been reported containing anomalous tendon. So compartments should be specifically sought and released meticulously in De Quervain's disease else persistence of symptoms is common. Insertion of APL is also variable into on the base of the first metacarpal, the trapezium, the volar carpal ligament, the opponens pollicis, or the abductor pollicis.
- *Compartment two* contains the two extensor carpi radialis tendons—the extensor carpi radialis longus and extensor carpi radialis brevis.
- *Compartment three* has the extensor pollicis longus tendon. This tendon acutely rotates around Lister's tubercle to the base of the thumb's distal phalanx.
- *Compartment four* contains multiple tendons and is the largest. The extensor digitorum communis tendons of the four fingers and the second finger's extensor indicis proprius pass through the fourth canal.
- *Compartment five* houses the fifth finger's extensor digiti minimi.

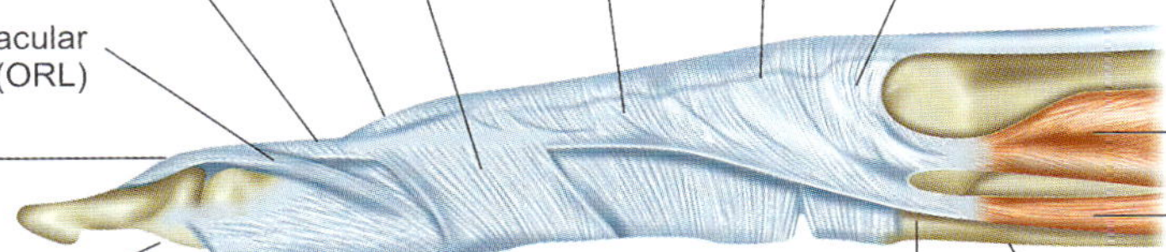

Fig. 34: The relationship of flexor tendon pulleys with the surrounding structures.

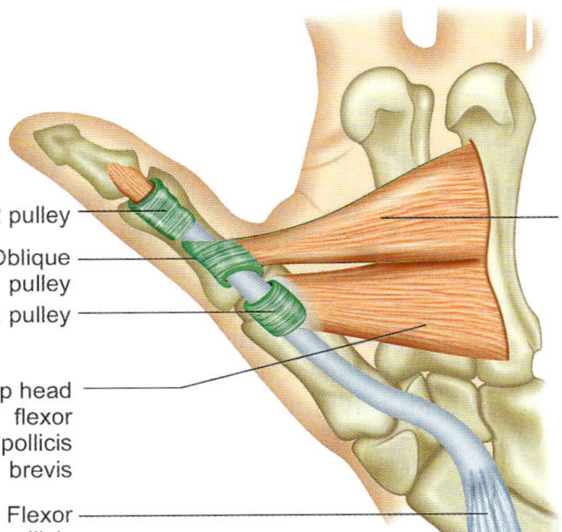

Fig. 35: Flexor tendon pulley system of the thumb (A: annular).

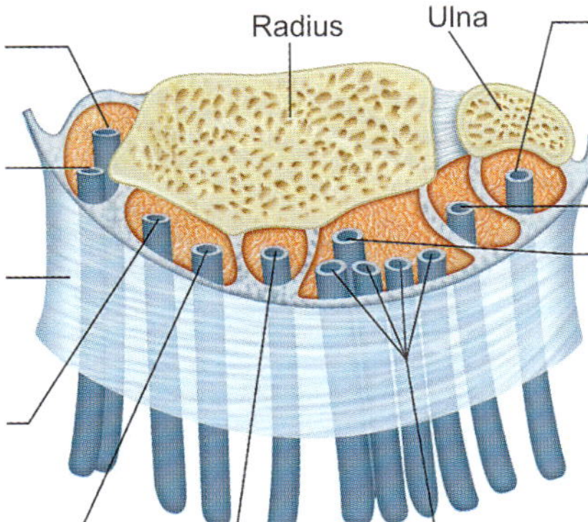

Fig. 36: Extensor tendon compartments.

- *Compartment six:* The extensor carpi ulnaris (ECU) to pinkie finger. The ECU's tendon sheath floor is partly formed by the triangular fibrocartilage complex.

Stenosing tenovaginitis most commonly involves the first and the sixth compartments.

Extensor Mechanism of Fingers (Figs. 37A and B)

This is an interesting apparatus and probably the most intricate mechanism to be reproduced mechanically (that is why any robotic hand is not a match to it!). We can actively extend the PIP and DIP joints without extending the MCP joints, but we cannot extend the PIP joint without extending the DIP joint at the same time. Also flexing only the DIP joint without flexing the PIP joint is difficult (actively). Full (active or passive) flexion of the PIP joint prevents active extension of the DIP joint. All these phenomenon are made possible by intricate disposition of various components of the extensor apparatus.

Structures that comprise the extensor mechanism ***(Figs. 37A and B)****:*

- The extensor digitorum communis *tendon* attaches by a tendinous slip to the proximal phalanx, through which it extends the MCP joint.
- The *central tendon* (or "slip") proceeds dorsally to attach to base of middle phalanx, where tension can extend the PIP joint.
- The *lateral bands* proceed on either side of dorsal midline and rejoin before attaching to the distal phalanx. Tension in the lateral bands extends the DIP joint.
- The *extensor hood* surrounds the MCP joint laterally, medially, and dorsally, and receives tendinous fibers from the lumbricals and interossei.

All the tendinous attachments transmit forces imparted to them by respective muscles.

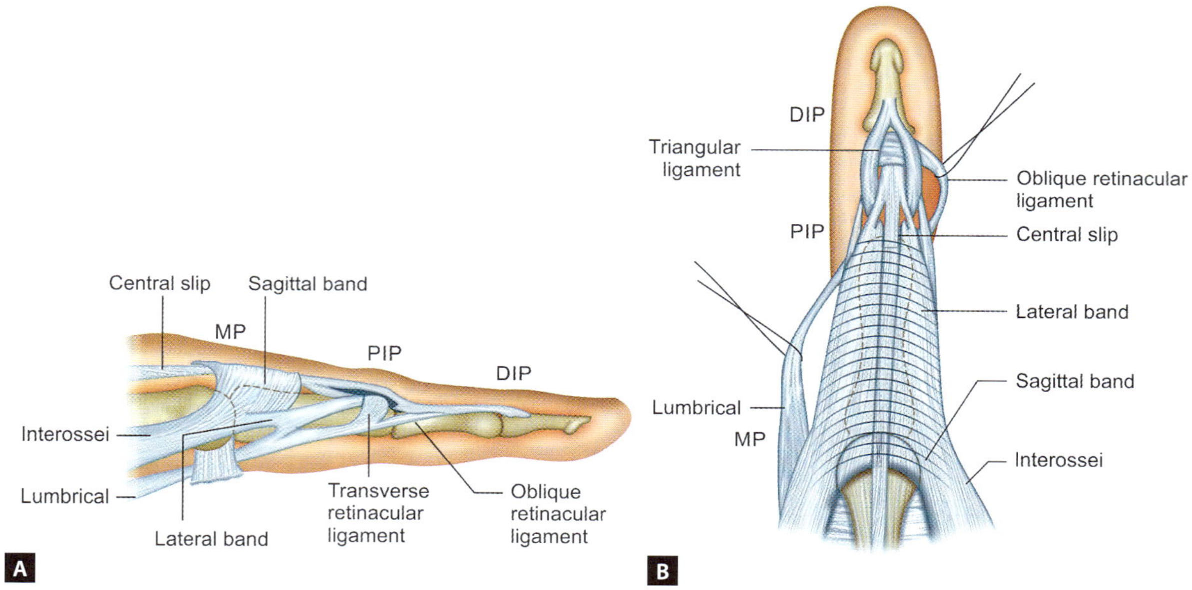

Figs. 37A and B: Illustration detailing the extensor mechanism/apparatus of fingers (see text for details).

Force develops in the extensor mechanism mainly in two ways:

1. *Active tension*—produced and transmitted by muscular contractions (hand intrinsics).
2. *Passive tension*—the extensor mechanism develops *passive tension* whenever it is elongated. This is generated by the reciprocal movements.
   The extensor mechanism's fibers have lines of application that are always dorsal to the lateral axes of the PIP and DIP joints. Therefore,
   - Activity in the intrinsic muscles that attach to the extensor mechanism always produces DIP and PIP extension.
   - Passive flexion of the MCP joint elongates the extensor mechanism and extends the PIP and DIP joints.

CONCLUSION

- The hand is a very complex anatomy, so complex that even the best of hand surgeons get baffled by the intricacies.
- The complexity is so combined into perfection that even minute disruption causes minor or major functional deficit.
- The small carpal bones and their articulation along with individually distinct fingers and thumb function need to be studied both individually and in totality so that optimal reconstruction is possible.

CHAPTER 112

Carpal Instability

Manish Kumar Varshney

INTRODUCTION

Carpal bones are arranged in an intricate manner within a small space that accommodates eight small bones bound together by intrinsic and extrinsic ligaments, articulating with each other and linking the five metacarpals distally with two forearm bones proximally. The requirement of movements and stability is immense, so the frequency of injury is also high. Even subtle changes in alignment of the small carpal bones or their stabilizing mechanism derails the finely balanced functional unit causing pain, loss of power, degeneration and limitation of movements ultimately disabling the person from using his hand fruitfully (disability). Because the demands are massive on the carpal bones, injury is also common in younger active population while degeneration is seen in elderly. Because of numerous articulations, involvement in inflammatory diseases is also frequent. The carpal bones hence get involved in a myriad of disorders such as trauma (fractures of carpal bones, dislocations and combined fracture dislocations), inflammatory and crystal deposition diseases (like rheumatoid arthritis, urate arthropathy, calcium pyrophosphate dihydrate deposition), and developmental abnormalities (like negative ulnar variance, Madelung's deformity). The carpal instability can be classified in different ways, but a simpler clinically useful classification and description of injuries is presented in the following text.

DEFINITION

It has been really difficult to give a precise definition of carpal instability that encompasses all observed forms. Quite often the term instability was adjudged similar to "malalignment" seen on radiographs so that in past the definition of carpal instability was restricted to *an alteration of the sagittal and/or anteroposterior alignment of the carpal bones beyond what was judged to be normal.* This limited definition identified four major types of carpal malalignment (mainly radiological):

- *Dorsal intercalated segment instability (DISI,* ***Figs. 1 and 2****):* The lunate, regarded as an intercalated segment between the distal row and the forearm bones, is abnormally extended relative to its proximal and distal links.
- *Volar intercalated segment instability (VISI,* ***Figs. 1 and 2****):* In the sagittal plane, the lunate appears abnormally flexed.
- *Ulnar translocation:* The proximal row is abnormally displaced (rotated or translocated) relative to the radius in an ulnar direction **(Fig. 3)**.
- *Dorsal translocation:* Due to a malunited fracture of the radius, the carpus is subluxed in a dorsal direction **(Fig. 4)**.

The concept received criticism due to two factors: one that not every alteration of radiological carpal alignment is pathological and second that dynamic instabilities did not show on static radiographs. Also wrists showing congenital hyperlaxity and radiologically malaligned are frequently asymptomatic.

Carpal instability was hence *redefined as the inability to bear physiological loads with an associated loss of the normal carpal alignment* taking into consideration the "dynamic aspect" and clinical findings. There is again a flaw, however, that it excludes patients who are asymptomatic for most of time due to consideration of only dynamic loading. This led

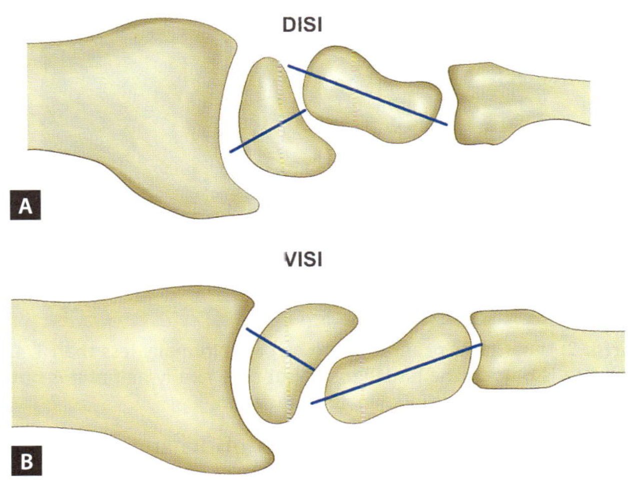

Figs. 1A and B: Simplified illustration of dorsal intercalated carpal instability (DISI) and volar intercalated carpal instability (VISI). Both are associated with malaligned carpal bones but in a DISI (A) the lunate faces dorsally while in VISI lunate faces volarly (3).

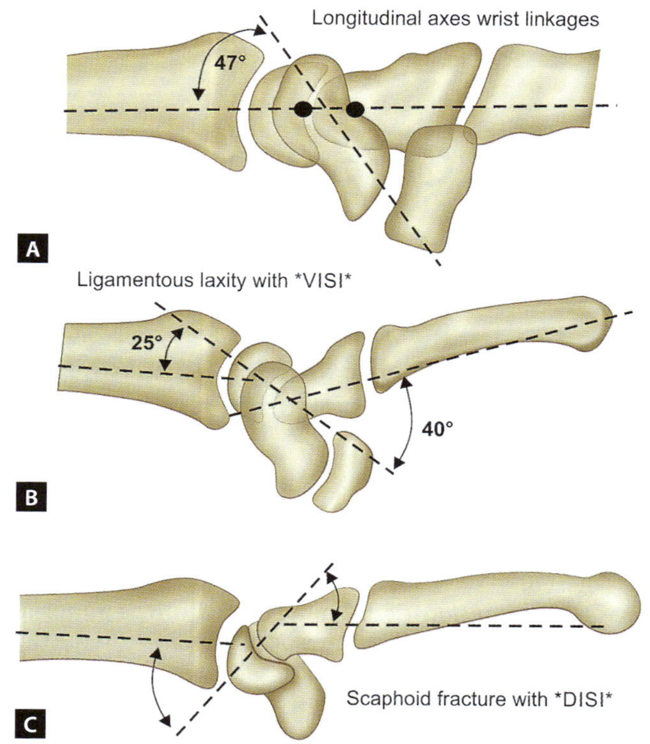

Figs. 2A to C: Detailed illustration of VISI and DISI. (A) Normal radiological longitudinal alignment of the carpal bones, the scaphoid axis is angulated at 47° to the long axes of the capitate, lunate, and radius. In volar intercalated segmental instability (VISI) deformity; (B) The lunate faces volarly and is usually associated with disruption of the lunatotriquetral ligament. In dorsal intercalated segmental instability (DISI) deformity the lunate is dispositioned facing dorsally (C) and it is associated with scapholunate disruption or a displaced scaphoid fracture.

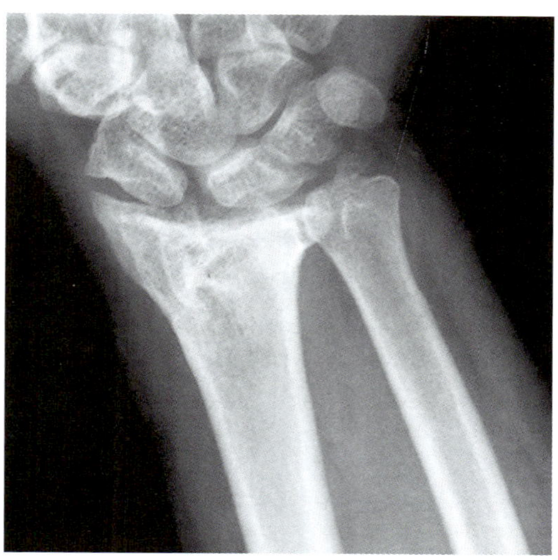

Fig. 3: Ulnar translocation of the carpals. Normally less than 1/4th of lunate is outside the lunate fossa, but here nearly half of it is outside, there is associated scapholunate dissociation.

to development of the concepts of dynamic versus static instability (taking into account the severity of injury) and kinetic versus kinematic instability (considering the ability to bear load).

- *Dynamic instability:* Carpal malalignment appears only under certain loading conditions.

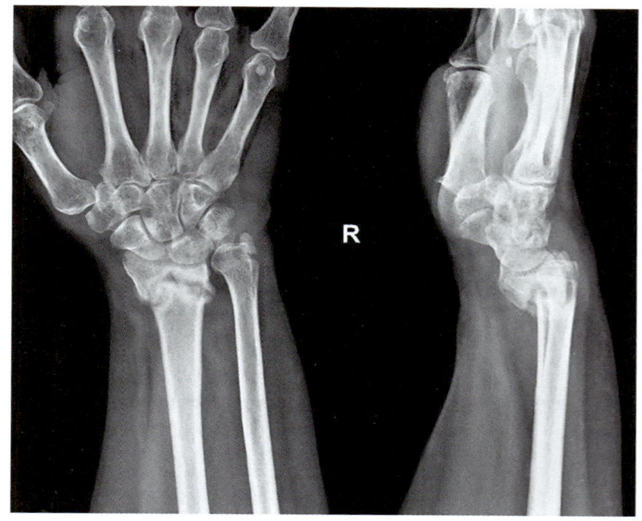

Fig. 4: Malunited fracture distal radius with dorsal angulation.

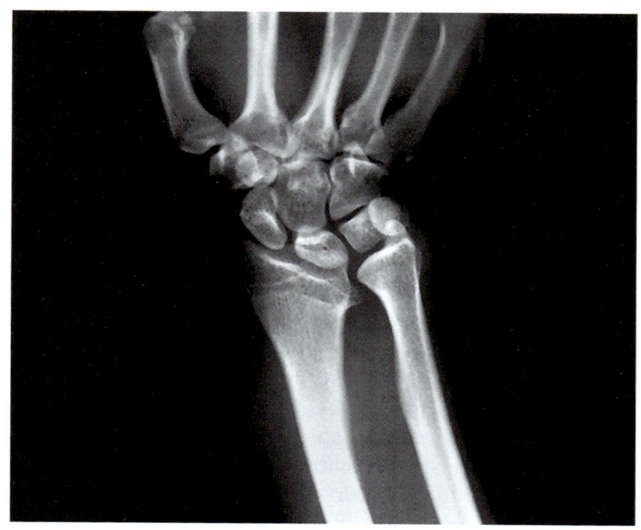

Fig. 5: Madelung deformity.

- *Static instability:* Carpal malalignment is permanent regardless of the amount of load being applied.
- *Kinetic carpal dysfunction:* There is problem of load transfer among the carpal bones.
- *Kinetic and kinematic dysfunction:* This occurs when there is problem of both load transfer *and* carpal bone movement. The latter arises due to alterations of intercarpal alignment.

Hence, clinicians often use a clinical definition for referring to the carpal instability. Instability is said to exist if there is symptomatic malalignment, i.e., person is not able to bear loads (with radiologically demonstrable malalignment) and does not have normal kinematics during any portion of its arc of motion. Carpal instability is not uncommon but most of the surgeons remain ignorant to observe it or are unaware at all of its existence. Nearly 10% of carpal injuries result in instability. There are various other causes of carpal instability:

- Congenital [Madelung deformity **(Fig. 5)**, transverse deficiency]

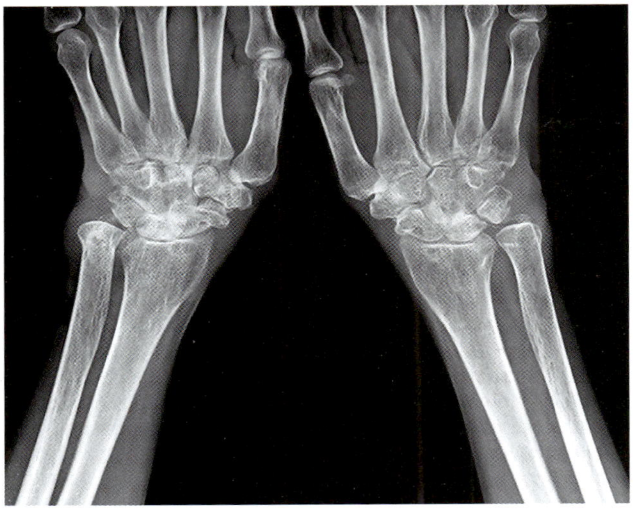

Fig. 6: Rheumatoid hand having grossly destroyed carpal bones and complex instability pattern.

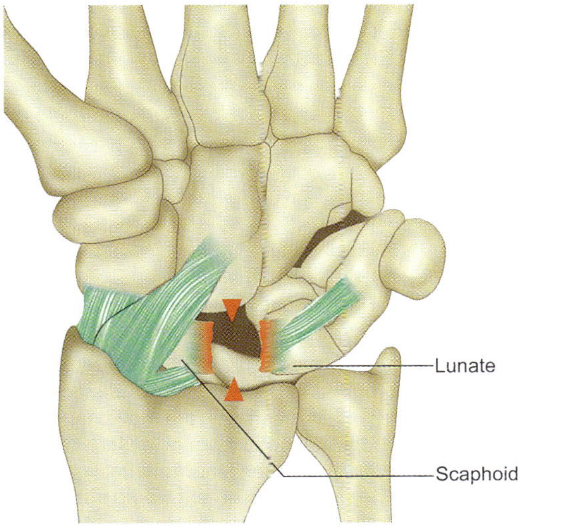

Fig. 8: Scapholunate dissociation, the red triangles depict the disruption of the interosseous scapholunate ligament.

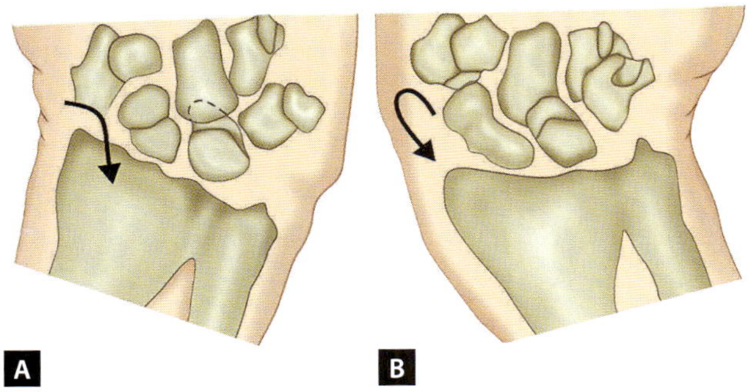

Figs. 7A and B: (A) Scaphoid movement with wrist radial; (B) Ulnar deviations.

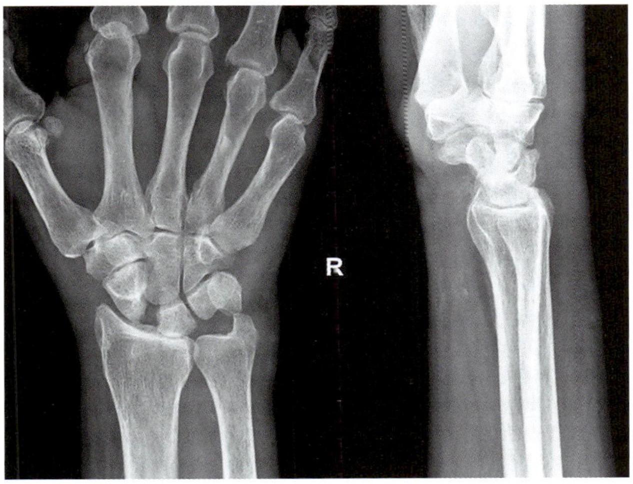

Fig. 9: Radiology of scapholunate dissociation.

- Trauma
  - Wrist "sprain"
  - Fracture ± dislocation
  - End stage of malunion or nonunion
- Rheumatoid arthritis **(Fig. 6)**
- Neoplastic

PATHOMECHANICS

To simplify the understanding of the carpal instability, we can understand the basic established carpal movement patterns during load transmission as follows:

- Lunate is in state of dynamic balance during wrist range-of-motion. It has a twisted and counterforce distribution across transverse axis so it can only flex or extend along the prominent force.
- Scaphoid flexes under compressive load (and radial deviation) and induces flexion force on lunate **(Figs. 7A and B)**.
- Triquetral extends and induces extension force on lunate during load bearing.

When this dynamic balance is interrupted, the lunate follows unbalanced force.

CLASSIFICATION

The classification system is still evolving with reports of uncommon patterns and understanding of the carpal biomechanics (especially the ulnar side carpals). In the current practice, the carpal instabilities are classified in the following four broad patterns (considering the kinetic versus kinetic and kinematic concept broadly) with some subgroups (Mayo).

1. *Dissociative carpal instability (CID)*: Major dysfunction between bones of the same carpal row (fracture/ligament disruption). There is loss of linkage *between individual carpal bones*. It usually affects the *smaller ligaments* such as scapholunate and lunotriquetral that are difficult to repair. It can be subclassified into:
   a. Proximal (scapholunate and lunotriquetral dissociations): It encompasses the terms DISI (scapholunate dissociation, **Figs. 8 and 9**) and VISI (lunotriquetral dissociation, **Figs. 10A and B**).
   b. Distal (capitate-hamate axial disruptions)

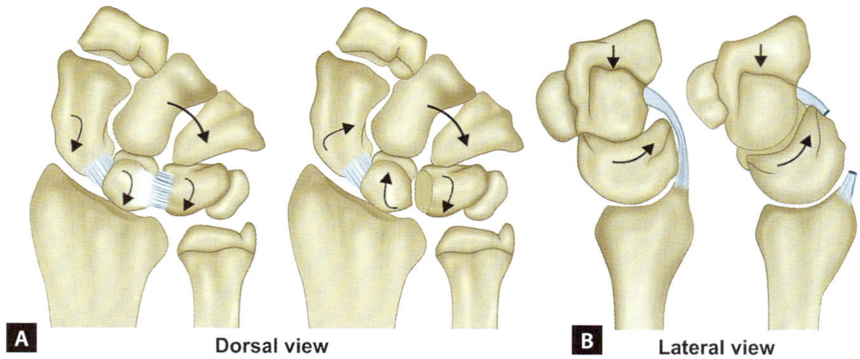

Figs. 10A and B: Lunotriquetral (LT) instability: LT dissociation in essence represents a separation of the bones that results in a lack of coordinated proximal carpal motion so that the triquetrum moves independently. In radial wrist deviation, the flexing scaphoid would pull the proximal row into flexion with the triquetrum staying extended. In ulnar deviation, as shown here [left side images of dorsal (A) and lateral views (B)], the triquetrum would move into extension. When the lunotriquetral ligament is intact the extending triquetrum brings the lunate in extension. If the ligament gets deficient or torn, then the extension moment would not be communicated to the scaphoid and lunate, and hence they would stay in flexion, creating the so-called VISI deformity.

2. *Nondissociative carpal instability (CIND):* Between carpal "rows", bones and intercarpal relation and function is maintained. It usually affects the longer ligament such as triquetral capitate, radiolunate, and radiocapitate. It is also subclassified into:
   a. Radiocarpal with rupture of several radiocarpal ligaments resulting in an ulnar translation of the carpus (often DISI).
   b. Midcarpal with rupture of the triquetral-hamate-capitate ligament complex (VISI).
   c. Ulnar translocation
3. *Complex carpal instability (CIC):* When CID and CIND are found together. Perilunate dislocations are a good example that involves radiocarpal (radiolunate and radiocapitate ligaments) and intercarpal levels (scapholunate and lunotriquetral) that later evolve into chronic scapholunate and lunotriquetral dissociation (CID patterns) and also an ulnar translation of the lunate (CIND pattern). Progressive perilunate instability **(Fig. 11)** passes through the following stages:
   a. Stage I: Scapholunate instability
   b. Stage II: Capitate dislocation
   c. Stage III: Triquetral dislocation
   d. Stage IV: Lunate dislocation
4. *Adaptive carpal instability (CIA):* When carpal instability originates proximal or distal to the wrist and is not located within the wrist (carpal bones individually or between rows). This instability arises secondary to adaptation of extrinsic pathology (like a malunited distal radius fracture, **Fig. 4**).

Amadio system (1995) was used previously but was very wide and bit imprecise to group the common patterns. It classified the instability on the basis of:

- Severity
  - Dynamic
  - Static with partial dislocation
  - Static with dislocation
- Direction
  - Volar versus dorsal

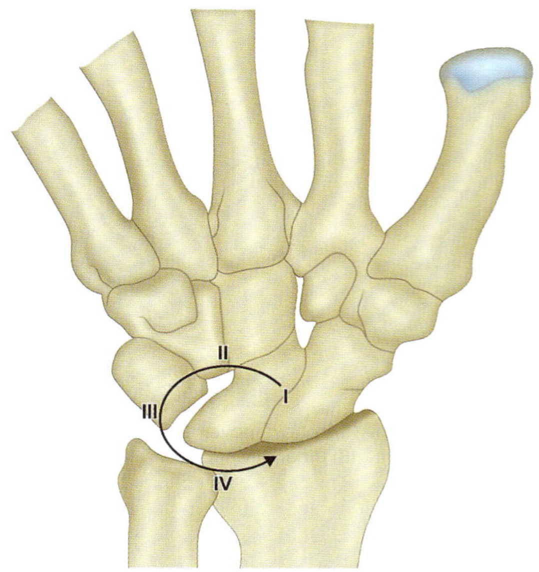

Fig. 11: Progressive perilunate instability.

- Site of injury
- Type of injury

MANAGEMENT

Management is guided by the primary pattern of injury as identified in the classification and radiological osseous/articular injury. Classification here comes in handy; the specifics are detailed as below:

Guiding principles (Larsen, 1995): The following factors must be considered while understanding the various instability patterns specifically to treat them.

- Chronicity (healing potential of the ligaments involved)
- Constancy (dynamic or static)
- Etiology (traumatic, congenital, inflammatory); location (site of the major dysfunction)
- Direction of the abnormal rotation and/or translocation of the carpal bones
- Pattern of instability (CID, CIND, CIC, or CIA)

DISSOCIATIVE CARPAL INSTABILITY

Proximal Dissociative Carpal Instability (Proximal CID)

The common conditions that are included in this pattern include:

- Unstable scaphoid nonunion **(Figs. 12A to J)**
- Scapholunate dissociation **(Figs. 8 and 9)**
- Lunotriquetral dissociation

Other less frequent disorders which produce proximal CID are Kienböck's disease and proximal fractures of the triquetrum.

Unstable Scaphoid Nonunion

The scaphoid is an important link between the proximal and distal rows and stabilizes the wrist when axially loaded.

Thus, proper function of scaphoid produces synchronous movement of the carpus. With unstable nonunion the "linking" function is lost due to independent proximal and distal fragments.

- The proximal portion of fractured scaphoid follows the unconstrained lunate and triquetrum. This results in extension of lunate relative to both the radius and the capitate (visible on a lateral radiograph as DISI).
- With dorsally rotated lunate, the forces cannot be transferred adequately and wrist movements are not normal. This instability is DISI pattern of carpal malalignment.

Treatment: Correction requires stabilization of fragments and restoration of the anatomical relationship between the scaphoid and the rest of the carpus.

Usually, there is a flexion deformity of the scaphoid with "humpback" on dorsolateral surface. There is also atrophy of its palmar cortex. This is corrected by a wedge-shaped graft inserted on the volar aspect to correct flexion malalignment and shortening. The correct length can be measured from the opposite wrist radiograph or better tomography. Some degree of rotational malalignment needs also to be corrected which is better observed and corrected from dorsal aspect. The reference for rotational correction is articular surface of capitate to maintain the scaphocapitate congruity. Using

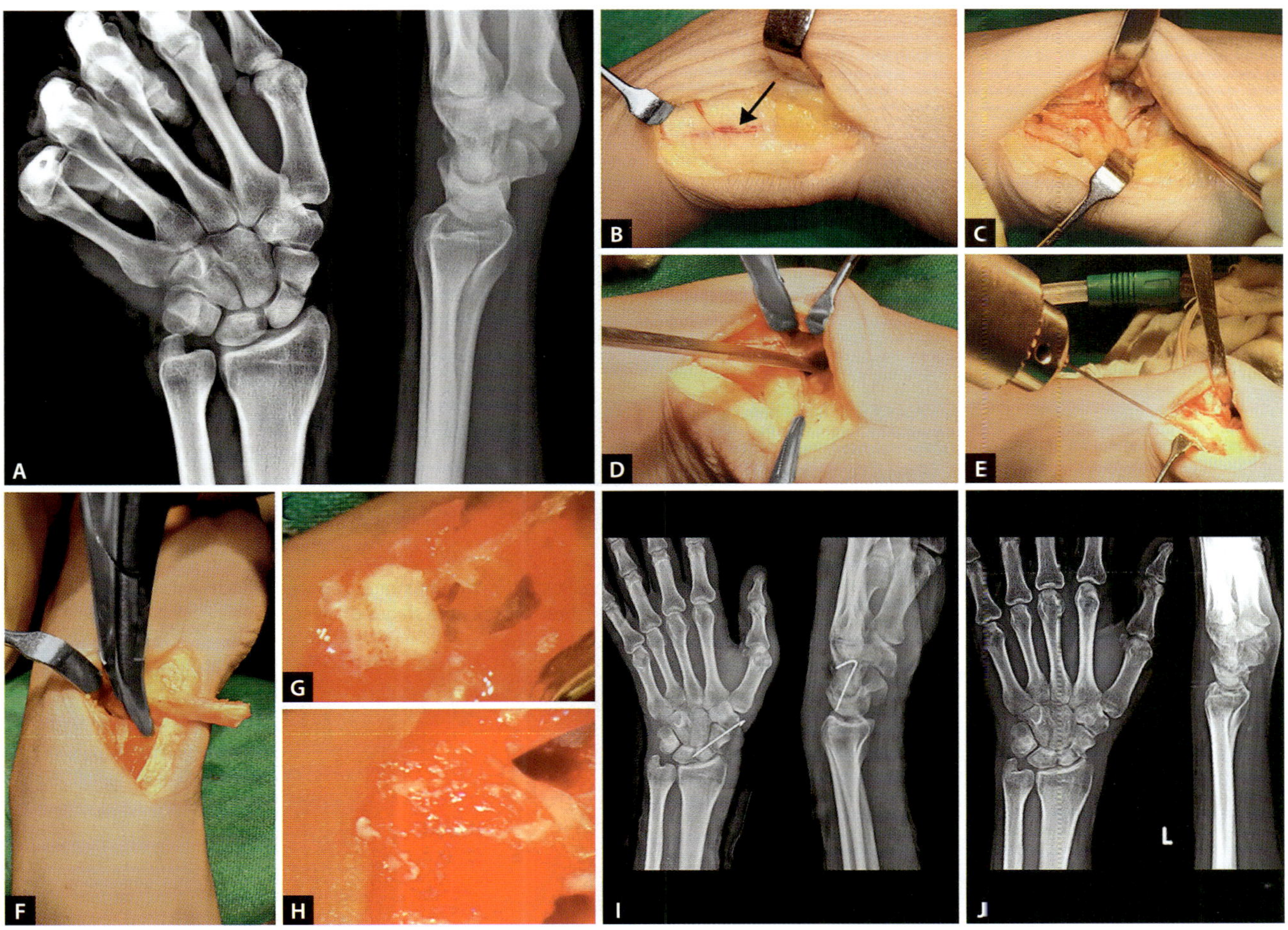

Figs. 12A to J: (A) Nonunion of fracture of scaphoid. This patient though does not have any overt carpal instability as he was diagnosed early. Long-standing nonunions become unstable and often present with DISI. The patient was managed by Zaidemberg vascularized graft technique for correction of nonunion and deformity. That went into uneventful union; (B) Exposure of the intercompartmental vessels (arrow); (C) Exposure of the nonunion site; (D) Preparation of the nonunion site and measuring the required graft size; (E) Marking the bone graft size by drill holes using K-wire; (F) Elevating the graft and performing partial radial styloidectomy; (G and H) Ensuring the vascularity of graft by deflating tourniquet; (I) Placement of the graft and fixing with smooth pin; (J) Radiograph of patient at 3 months showing well-placed graft and ensuing start of union, also note the partial radial styloidectomy.

the vascularized grafts for obtaining union is preferred as the chances of union possibly improve with the use of these vascularized grafts. I personally prefer the Zaidemberg technique for such reconstructions **(Figs. 12A to J)**.

Scaphoid Nonunion Advanced Collapse

The *scaphoid nonunion advanced collapse (SNAC, **Figs. 13A and B**) wrist* characterized by advanced carpal collapse and progressive arthritis of the wrist. Constant unrestricted instability producing aberrant movements are responsible for the production of arthritis at radioscaphoid articulation (early), followed by wrist joint (radioscapholunate) and then midcarpal joint (advanced). This is followed by carpal collapse due to loss of joint space and diffuse carpal arthritis. The following radiological classification has been followed (stage 13B):

- *Stage 1:* Arthrosis localized to the radial side of the scaphoid and radial styloid.
- *Stage 2:* Arthrosis of the entire radioscaphoid joint with sparing of the radiolunate joint.
- *Stage 3:* Arthrosis progressing to the capitolunate joint and midcarpal joints **(Fig. 14)**. Proximal migration of capitate (carpal collapse).

Clinically, the SNAC wrist is tender to palpation at the radioscaphoid region with swelling in the snuff box. The movements at the wrist are reduced with variable pain during movements. The patients experience stiffness during wrist movements and there is reduced grip and pinch strength.

Treatment for SNAC wrist:

- For stage 1, radial styloidectomy **(Fig. 15)** along with scaphoid reduction and fixation can be performed, bone graft should be used to correct the length of scaphoid, and open reduction is better to correct rotational malalignment.
- Stage 2 and above need salvage procedures. For stage 2, scaphoid needs to be excised. It can be done

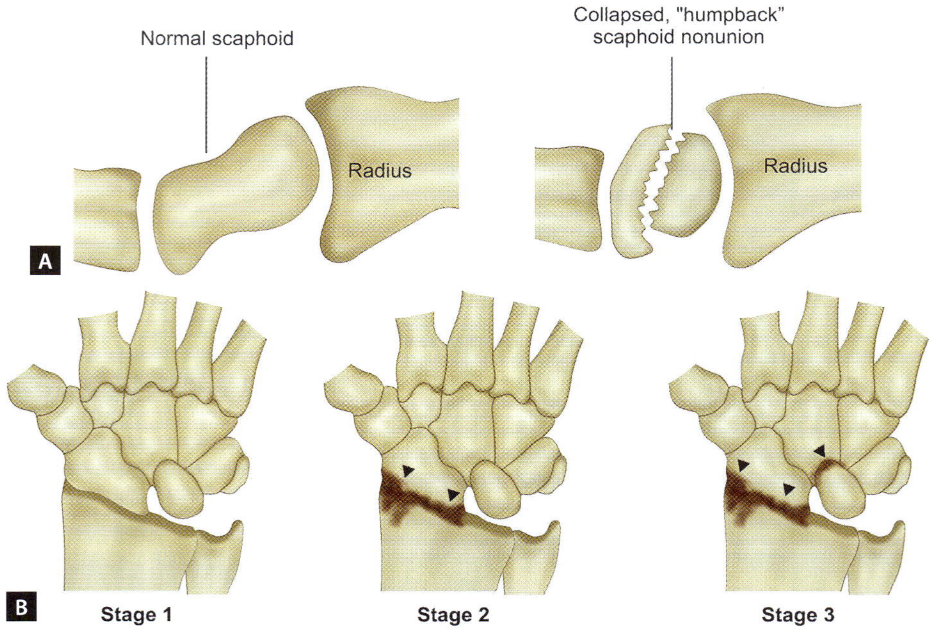

Figs. 13A and B: Scaphoid nonunion advanced collapse (SNAC). (A) The illustration demonstrates reduced length of the bone and hence altered kinematics; (B) Illustration of the three progressive stages of SNAC.

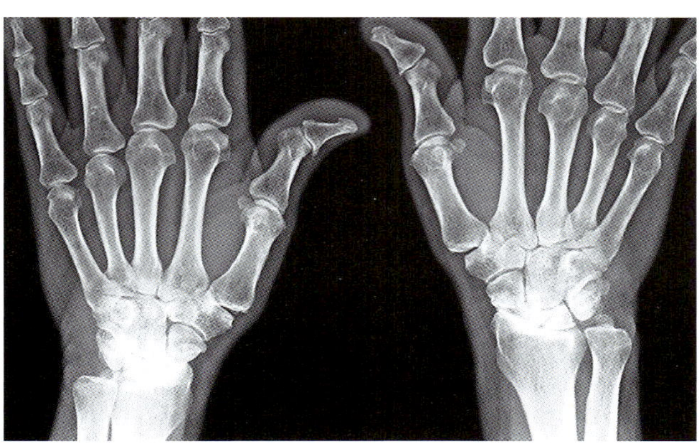

Fig. 14: Radiograph demonstrating stage 3 scaphoid nonunion advanced collapse (SNAC) wrist.

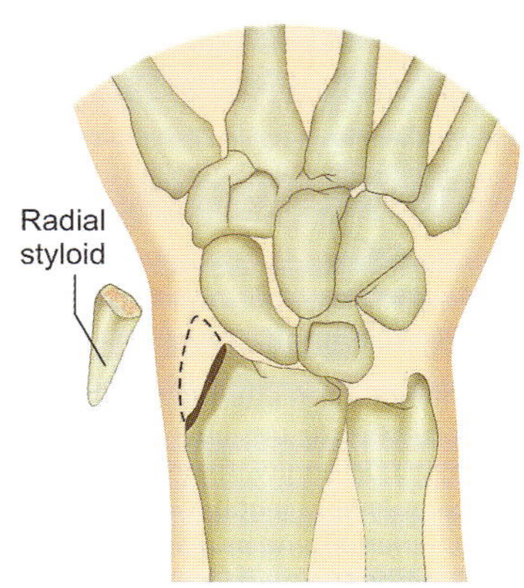

Fig. 15: Radial styloidectomy.

with excision of the entire proximal carpal row (as in *proximal row carpectomy, **Fig. 16***) or otherwise *four-corner fusion* can be done (scaphoid excision + fusion of lunate, triquetrum, capitate and hamate, **Fig. 17A**). The latter can be achieved with screws, K-wire, spider plate **(Fig. 17B)** or better a cervical H-plate.

- Proximal row carpectomy is contraindicated with incompetent radioscaphocapitate ligament and if there is advanced capitolunate arthritis leading to erosion of the proximal capitate (capitate head degeneration), as this will articulate with the lunate fossa.
- Following four-corner fusion, the wrist movements occur at the radiolunate joint and transmitted distally by the fused mass.

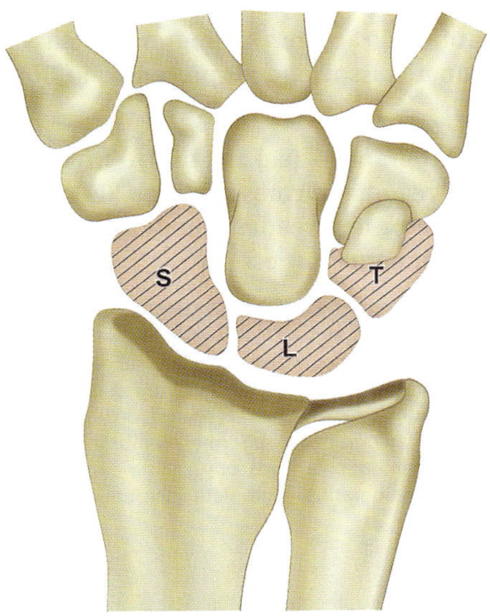

Fig. 16: Proximal row carpectomy: The three bones namely scaphoid (S), lunate (L), and the triquetrum (T) are removed.

- Proximal row carpectomy and four-corner fusion can be combined with *wrist denervation* procedure where the posterior interosseous nerve (PIN) and anterior interosseous nerve (AIN) are denervated to provide additional pain relief. Wrist denervation procedure is not recommended as an isolated procedure as without stabilization rapid joint destruction may occur.
- For advanced collapse of the carpal bones, it is better to fuse the wrist **(Fig. 18)** as the pain generators develop even in the carpometacarpal region that can only be controlled by obliterating any wrist movement.

Scapholunate Dissociation (Scapholunate Instability, Rotatory Subluxation of the Scaphoid, and Dorsal Intercalated Segmental Instability)

Mechanism of injury:

- Dorsiflexion-ulnar-deviation injury with an element of axial compression. Load causes injury to the scapholunate interosseous ligament (SLIL) and volar wrist ligaments (radioscaphocapitate and radiolunate ligaments).
- It may also be a component of the perilunate dislocation pattern or the reverse perilunate dislocation (discussed below).

Clinical features:

- Swelling and tenderness over the scapholunate joint
- Positive Watson's maneuver (palpable clunk when the wrist is brought from ulnar deviation into radial deviation while pressure is applied to the palmar aspect of the scaphoid tubercle).

Radiological features obtain five views for comprehensive evaluation (posteroanterior, lateral, scaphoid, 45° oblique and posteroanterior—clenched fist).

- *Posteroanterior view:*
  - Terry Thomas sign (named after the smile of British comedian Terry Thomas, **Fig. 19**)—increased gap between the scaphoid and lunate bones (accentuated

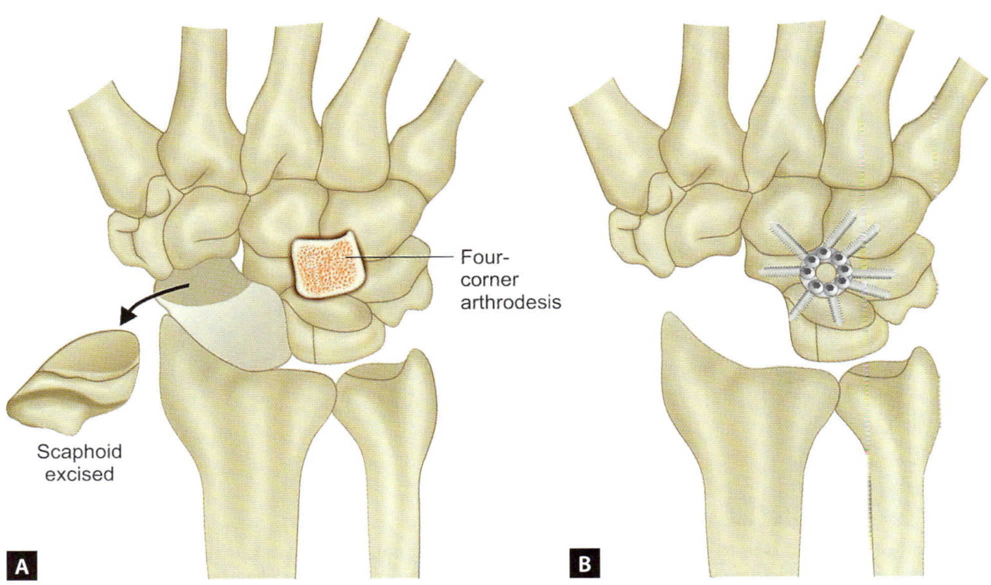

Figs. 17A and B: (A) Four corner fusion using a bone graft (B) or a spider plate.

on clenched fist view). Scapholunate gap should be measured from the proximal ulnar-most corner of the scaphoid to the proximal radial-most corner of the lunate. Scapholunate gap up to 5 cm (Cautillie and Wehbe) is normal in the absence of cortical ring sign (gap of 3 mm or more with cortical ring sign is positive

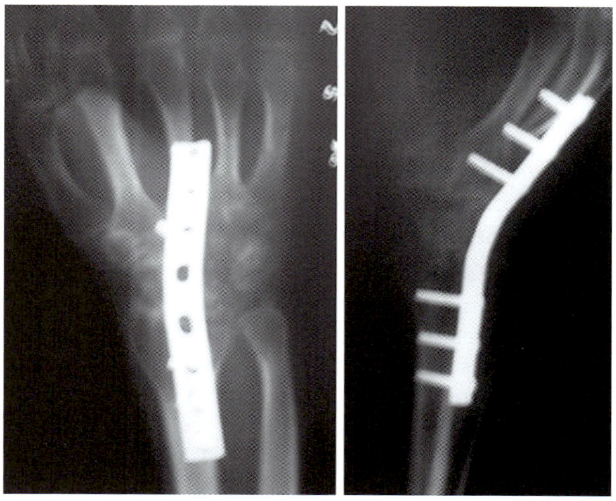

Fig. 18: Arthrodesis of the wrist joint—anteroposterior and lateral views.

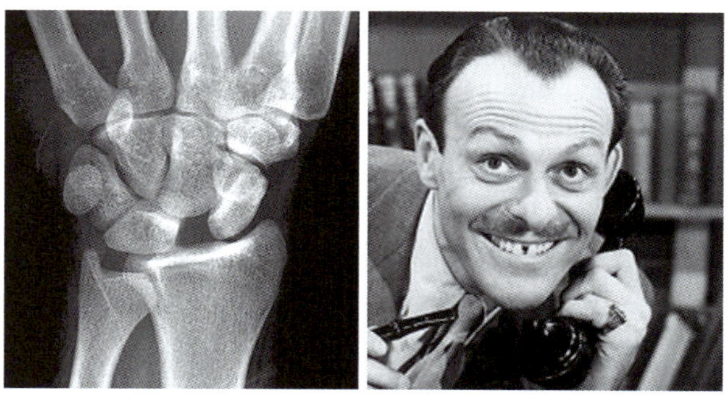

Fig. 19: Scapholunate disruption—the resultant gap between the scaphoid and lunate bones from torn interosseous ligament is likened to the gap between incisor teeth of famous comedian "Terry Thomas".

for dissociation). Increased gap with a triangular capitate is suggestive of congenital anomaly.
- Cortical ring sign (Signet ring sign) due to flexed scaphoid **(Figs. 20A and B)**. The distal tubercle of the scaphoid is seen end-on on a posteroanterior projection of the wrist.
- Reduced carpal height measured by carpal height ratio (carpal height divided by the length of the third metacarpal)
- Ulnar translocation
- Disruption of Gilula's lines
- Triangular lunate due to rotation

- *Lateral radiographs*
  - Scapholunate angle >60°
  - Lunate dorsiflexion >10° past neutral
  - Radiolunate angle >15°
- Oblique views help in identifying greater arc injuries and scaphoid fracture. Radiographic classification of scapholunate dissociation is presented in **Box 1**.

Other investigations:
- Wrist arthrography—leakage of dye from wrist joint to midcarpal region indicates ruptured SLIL.
- MRI—operator and reader dependent but can identify multiple ligament injuries.

BOX 1: The classification of scapholunate dissociation.
- Radiographs normal; conservative treatment successful.
- Radiographs normal but nonoperative treatment unsuccessful—ligament discontinuity (membranous portion disrupted).
- Abnormal stress radiographs—abnormal membranous and distal portion of the ligament on arthroscopy.
- Abnormal plain radiographs—complete ligament diastasis on arthroscopy
  - Reducible scaphoid
    - Repairable SLIL
    - Nonrepairable but reconstructible SLIL
  - Irreducible scaphoid
- Arthritis—mild (limited to radioscaphoid region) or advanced [associated with midcarpal arthritis and collapse, scapholunate advanced collapse (SLAC)].

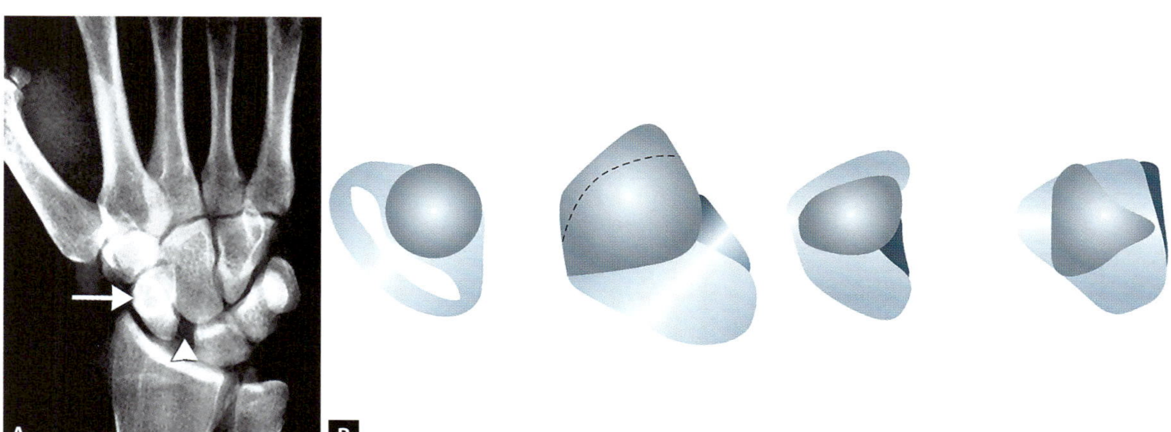

Figs. 20A and B: (A) Flexion of scaphoid due to deficient scapholunate ligament causes overlap of the proximal fragment on the "fallen" distal fragment appearing as a—Signet ring (bold arrow); (B) The characteristic is made prominent on radial deviation view. The radiological images with progressive flexion of scaphoid.

- Arthroscopy has high diagnostic accuracy and can also be utilized to treat the injuries simultaneously by judging the accuracy of reduction.

Pathomechanics and pathoanatomy: With complete disruption of the scapholunate ligament— the scaphoid, devoid of proximal constraints rotates with capitate (*cf.* above where the lunate guides scaphoid fragment) leading to dorsal subluxation of its proximal pole. The lunate has natural tendency toward extension again producing a DISI pattern of carpal instability. The primary restraint to scapholunate dissociation is the scapholunate interosseous ligament (especially the dorsal portion) while the secondary (minor) constraint is the distal scaphotrapezial ligament complex.

Treatment: Logically deriving from the understanding of pathomechanics, the treatment relies primarily on the repair/reconstruction of the ruptured ligaments and temporary stabilization of the scaphoid by Kirschner (K) wires. The remains of scapholunate ligament are usually found attached to lunate and is avulsed from the scaphoid. The ligament is repaired back to the scaphoid by nonabsorbable, transosseous sutures/suture anchors and immobilized in a cast for at least 2 months.

- For long-standing disruptions without intercarpal or radiocarpal arthritis reconstruction of the ligament is done using flexor carpi radialis or palmaris tendon. Surgical fusion of either the scaphoid-trapezium-trapezoid or the scaphocapitate joints has also been successful. It is but important to perfectly plan and execute the procedure else nonunion and/or secondary radioscaphoid osteoarthritis produces much poorer results and patient dissatisfaction. Another option is to fuse the midcarpal joint especially when there is extensive cartilage wear at the scaphoid-lunate-capitate joints.
- The management of chronic scapholunate instability with extensive degenerative changes at the radioscaphoid and lunocapitate joints is best done by midcarpal fusion with resection of the scaphoid (SLAC procedure).

Several methods of scapholunate and scaphotrapezial joint stabilization using adjacent wrist motor tendons have been reported. The tenodesis procedure of Brunelli and Brunelli, which is a double (distal and proximal) scaphoid stabilization using a portion of flexor carpi radialis, has shown good midterm results.

Scapholunate Advanced Collapse Wrist (Fig. 21A)

This is a specific condition that arises due to persistent dissociation between the scaphoid and lunate leading to advanced arthritis at the radiocarpal and midcarpal joints. The arthritis and degeneration arises due to abnormal distribution of the forces across the carpal bones while load bearing and movements. Arthritis progresses from the high-stress region of radioscaphoid joint to gradually involve the entre carpus, and finally a collapse of the carpal bones radiologically characterized by proximal migration of capitate (reduced carpal height ratio). The arthritis is classified by Watson as follows **(Fig. 21B)**:

- *Stage 1:* Radioscaphoid arthritis (arthritis limited to radial styloid), radiologically seen as beaking of the radial styloid, sclerosis and joint space narrowing of the scaphoid—radial styloid region.
- *Stage 2:* Advanced radioscaphoid arthritis (entire scaphoid fossa of radius involved), radiologically seen as reduced joint space between scaphoid and the entire scaphoid fossa.
- *Stage 3:* Capitolunate joint arthritis, radiologically the capitolunate joint space reduces with proximal migration of the capitate into the space created by scapholunate dissociation.
- *Stage 4 (modification):* Pancarpal arthritis (late cases or cases with additional pathology like inflammatory or crystal arthritis). The radiolunate joint is also affected.

Clinical features are similar to those described for a SNAC wrist. Additionally, Watson shift test is positive in early stages that later becomes negative due to arthritic changes.

Treatment of SLAC wrist involves conservative measures (rest, NSAID, steroid injections initially) followed by the operative procedures if conservative measures fail to control the symptoms. The operative measures are similar to the SNAC wrist (detailed above). Stage 1 is commonly treated with radial styloidectomy that can also be performed

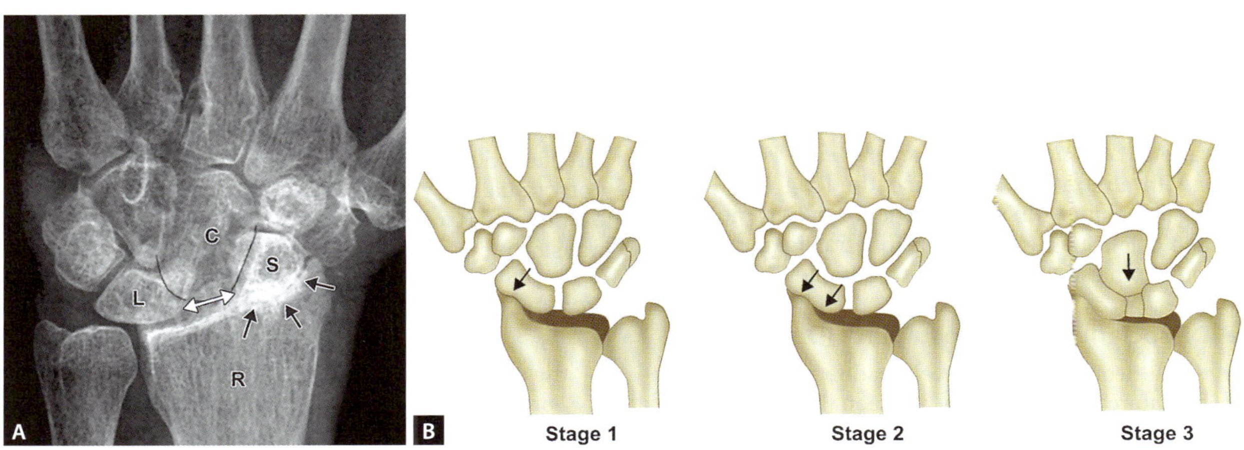

Figs. 21A and B: (A) Scapholunate advanced collapse (SLAC) wrist; and (B) The Watson's stages of SLAC wrist. (C: capitate; L: lunate; R: radius; S: scaphoid)

arthroscopically. Wrist denervation (AIN and PIN) is a symptomatic operative procedure that helps to reduce pain without any bearing on the disease. Stages 2 and 3 can be managed by four-corner fusion or proximal row carpectomy while for pancarpal arthritis wrist arthrodesis is needed.

Lunotriquetral Dissociation

Disruption of the lunotriquetral ligaments results in a dissociative VISI pattern of carpal instability. The instability is more prominent if it is associated with insufficiency of the dorsal radiotriquetral ligament (the dorsoradiocarpal ligament). To produce the complete VISI pattern additionally volar radiolunate ligament injury is also needed. It is caused by wrist hyperextension and radial deviation. Pathomechanically, due to inefficient constraints the scaphoid forces lunate into palmar flexion, while the triquetrum extends and translocates proximally producing the VISI pattern on lateral radiographs.

Clinical features: Patients have pain on ulnar aspect with pronation and ulnar deviation. The lunotriquetral ballottement test (Shuck test) is positive—grasp the lunate between the thumb and index finger of one hand while applying alternative dorsal and palmar loads across the triquetrum with the thumb and index of the other hand eliciting pain, crepitus or laxity at lunotriquetral joint. Pain is also produced with shear forces across the lunotriquetral joint as in Kleinman's shear test (stabilize the radiolunate joint with the forearm in neutral rotation, now with the contralateral hand load the triquetrum in the anteroposterior plane—producing shear across the lunotriquetral joint). On lunotriquetral joint compression as in ulnar deviation of the wrist, the triquetrum is ulnarly displaced producing pain.

Radiologically, there is volar flexion of the lunate on lateral views reducing the scapholunate angle to <30°. The capitolunate articulation is normally collinear while in VISI pattern the capitolunate angle increases to >15° producing a zigzag deformity. On anteroposterior views, there is disruption of the Gilula's arcs while there may or may not be widening of the lunotriquetral joint or proximal migration of the triquetrum.

For acute disruptions, anatomical reduction (usually open) and repair of both the intrinsic and extrinsic ligaments are done. Closed reduction and percutaneous pinning is acceptable for select cases. For delayed cases when there is cartilage degeneration and/or triangular fibrocartilage deterioration, a lunotriquetral arthrodesis is preferred. In cases with ulna positive variance, the long ulna may be impacting the triquetrum (ulna impaction syndrome) where arthroscopic debridement of lunotriquetral ligament can be combined to ulna shortening with acceptable results.

Distal Dissociative Carpal Instability (Distal CID)

This is very uncommon and develops due to rupture of the transverse intercarpal ligaments between the bones of distal row. The condition often arises in complex injury patterns like a blast injury. The intercarpal injury causes widening of the gap, and there occurs subsequent flattening of the palmar concavity. This pattern is characteristically identified as axial fracture dislocation. "Axial dislocation" refers to the fact that one column displaces while other remains aligned with one of the forearm bones (usually radius), and depending on the direction of displacement, this injury has been classified into three subgroups:

1. Axial-radial
2. Axial-ulnar
3. Axial-radial-ulnar

The treatment is basically open reduction of the displaced segment and ligament repair (acute cases) or surgical fusion.

NONDISSOCIATIVE CARPAL INSTABILITY

Radiocarpal Nondissociative Instability (Radiocarpal CIND)

Nondissociative primarily means intact (undissociated) carpal bones that remain as a unit together. Radiocarpal CIND develops in the following settings.

- The most common condition leading to a radiocarpal instability (nondissociative) is malunion of the distal radius. The dorsally angulated distal radius precludes axial transmission of the load across. The forces produce dorsal tilt of the lunate causing a DISI pattern. But this is included in CIA (see below).
- Distal radius developmental malposition (as in Madelung deformity) produces a volar tilt producing VISI pattern.
- Other less frequent cause is insufficiency of the extrinsic radiocarpal ligaments (traumatic or congenitally lax).

Distal Radial Malunion

If the radiocarpal ligaments are intact, the proximal carpal row remains aligned with the distal radius; thus the force transmission produces a DISI pattern at the midcarpal joint. In true sense of the term carpal instability, this pattern seems a misnomer as there is no carpal or intercarpal pathology rather a radiocarpal malalignment, but it is included with carpal instability as the consequential malalignment is at midcarpal region. The adaptation to malalignment causes DISI pattern (adaptive carpal instability, type 4). This is the classical CIA pattern according to the classification scheme already described and is not a part of CIND. On the other hand, radiocarpal CIND true develops if the radiocarpal ligaments are torn or become nonfunctional due to excessive stretch; as usually seen in association with distal radius malunion. The carpal bones (as a unit) sublux or occasionally dislocate in a dorsal, dorsoradial or palmar direction depending on the type of the malunion (dorsal, dorsoradial or volar angulation, respectively). This is an example of a radiocarpal CIND and is associated with ulnar translocation.

Treatment

- For adaptive instability, only a corrective osteotomy of the radius is necessary **(Figs. 22A to E)**.
- For CIND true type (associated with ligament disruption), correction of malunion + ligament reconstruction or a partial arthrodesis (radiolunate or radioscapholunate) is to be done.

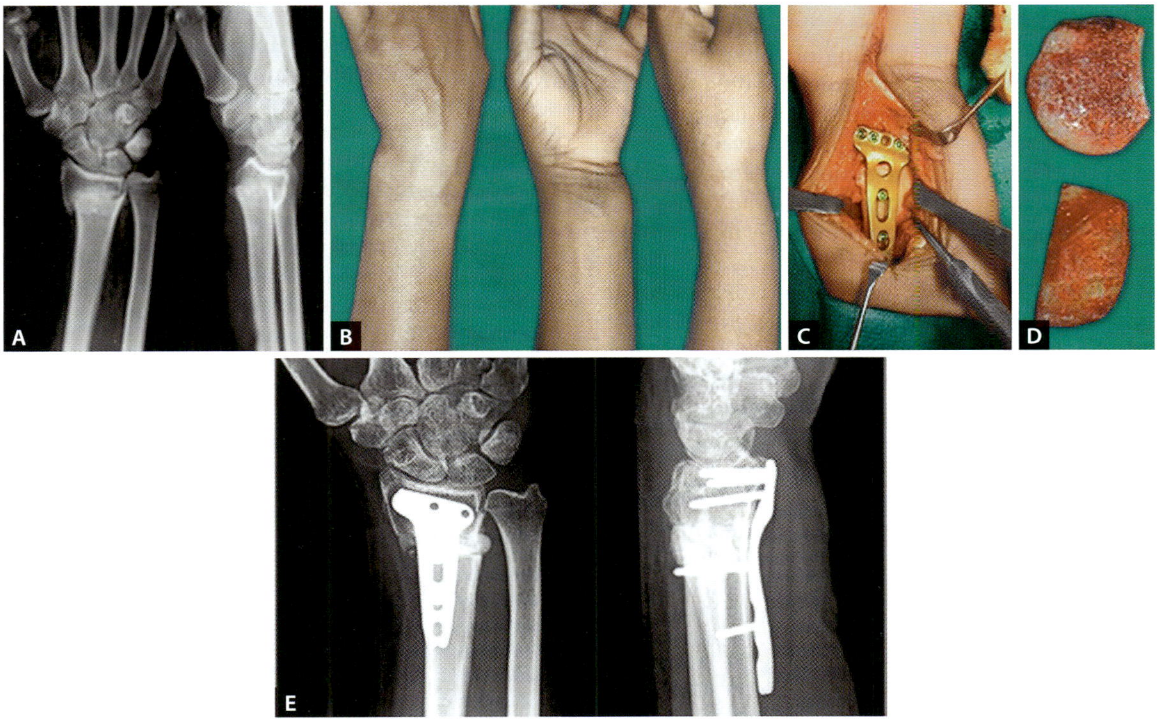

Figs. 22A to E: Radiocarpal nondissociative instability (CIND): This patient had symptomatic malunion of distal radius fracture (A) Radiographic appearance; (B) With DISI type instability, clinical appearance; (C) Intraoperative correction of deformity; (D) Using iliac crest bone graft; and (E) Final radiograph after deformity correction—note the restored radial length and inclinations and correction of DISI instability.

Midcarpal Nondissociative Instability (Midcarpal CIND)

We know from wrist biomechanics that under loaded conditions of the wrist:

- The triquetrum is pulled into extension by the palmar triquetrum-hamate ligaments.
- There is opposing movement of scaphoid to counter this which goes into flexion. This results in a twisted force transmitted across the lunate (scaphoid flexion and triquetrum extension) that remains neutral.

With torn palmar triquetrum-hamate ligaments (or its laxity), the lunate is forced by the scaphoid into palmar flexion that drags triquetrum along, resulting in a nondissociative VISI deformity of the proximal carpal row. This VISI relationship is maintained throughout the movements of the wrist. In full ulnar deviation, the scaphoid extends and the triquetrum-hamate joint is also fully engaged that throws the proximal carpal row to suddenly extend producing a quite typical snap (that can be tested clinically—positive ballottement test). This is the most commonly referred to "VISI pattern" in loose terms when unspecified.

Treatment

Soft-tissue reconstructions can correct this problem. Procedures described are palmar capsulorrhaphy or tenodesis but most have significant complications. So, commonly partial or total *fusion of the midcarpal joint* is done when causing symptoms are poorly controlled by conservative measures. For advanced cases with pancarpal arthritis, wrist fusion is best.

Combined Radiocarpal (Proximal) and Midcarpal Nondissociative Instability

It is an uncommon condition presenting as repetitive clicks while lifting the heavy objects. The common pattern described is a CLIP condition (capitate lunate instability pattern) that produces pain and click on lifting heavy weights. With traction produced by the lifted weight, dorsal subluxation of both the midcarpal and radiocarpal joints is produced along with dorsal translocation of the distal carpal row. In early phases, patients report snapping especially when lifting objects that progresses to painful clicks. In this type of instability, there is both a radiocarpal and midcarpal ligament insufficiency, commonly resulting from congenital laxity.

Most patients settle with conservative measures and activity modification with strengthening of the forearm muscles so surgery is seldom necessary. In selected nonresponsive patients, augmentation of the dorsal scaphotriquetral ligament (using extensor carpi radialis) may help.

COMPLEX CARPAL INSTABILITY

This injury pattern emanates from damage to both the intrinsic (smaller ligament, scapholunate and lunotriquetral that cause CID) and extrinsic (longer ligaments that cause CIND) radiocarpal ligaments. The typical example is a perilunate dislocation. It also includes the carpal instabilities that are otherwise unclassifiable. The perilunate injury pattern is detailed below to understand the development of carpal instability complex (CIC) followed by treatment of CIC.

Perilunate Injury Patterns

It is handy to have an understanding of Gilula's lines and greater and lesser arcs **(Fig. 23)** for understanding the injury pattern. The perilunar or perilunate is the most common of all wrist dislocations. There is progressive disruption **(Figs. 24A to D)** of most capsuloligamentous connections of the lunate to the adjacent carpal bones and radius. There may or may not be associated fracture (commonly the scaphoid, the classic transscaphoperilunate dislocation). The lunate commonly dislocates palmar wards in isolated lunate dislocations (the lesser arc injury). In transscaphoperilunate dislocation, the distal row (including the fractures scaphoid and triquetrum) dislocates in dorsal or dorsoradial direction, commonly (the greater arc injury, **Fig. 25**). Depending on the intensity and duration of the deforming force and position of the wrist during impact, several patterns are possible, and as it is a progressive event, where the ligaments are disrupted in a sequential manner, the progressive perilunar instability (of Mayfield) has been staged into four progressive stages (*see* **Fig. 11**):

1. *Stage I:* Scapholunate fracture or diastasis or both. With extension and supination force, the scaphoid bone is thrown into extension which is also transmitted to the lunate. The latter is, however, constrained by the long and short radiolunate ligaments so ultimately the scapholunate ligament is strained resulting in a tear.
2. *Stage II:* Lunocapitate dislocation—with persistent extension supination force, the capitate is next to dislocate dorsally relative to lunate.
3. *Stage III:* Lunotriquetral tear (perilunate dislocation)—following the capitate dislocation, the continuum of the force stress the triquetrum causing the triquetrum-hamate-capitate disruption (rarely) or lunotriquetral dissociation (common). The end stage is dislocation of the lunotriquetral dislocation.
4. *Stage IV:* Dorsal radiolunate tear (lunate dislocation). In the end the dorsal radiolunate capsule and the palmar radiolunate and ulnolunate ligaments remain keeping the lunate in position. Proximal pull on the capitate bone pushes the lunate volarly and commonly into the carpal tunnel due to the intact palmar ligaments.

Reverse perilunate instability with the above stage I–IV occurring in exactly reversed pattern (beginning from lunotriquetral dissociation and ending at scapholunate

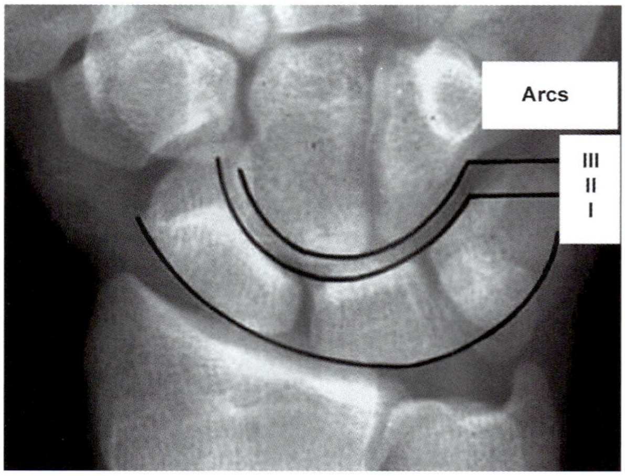

Fig. 23: Carpal arcs: These Gilula's arcs are smooth curves along the proximal carpal row and proximal aspect of distal carpal row.

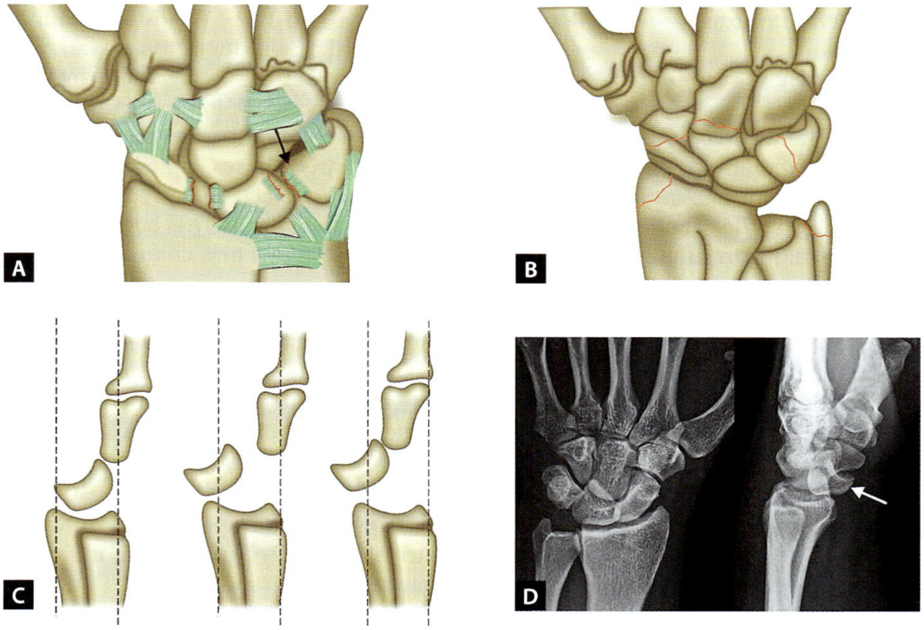

Figs. 24A to D: The preilunate injury patterns. (A) Illustrated are the commonly injured ligamentous structures; (B) They may or may not be associated with fractures of various bones, the various degrees of perilunate injuries; (C) (left to right) perilunate subluxation, perilunate dislocation and lunate dislocation at the right most figure; (D) The radiographic demonstration of isolated lunate dislocated displaced volarly (arrow) from the carpal alignment prominent in lateral projection, the AP projection is more subtle resulting in missing of injury by casual observer elsewhere though it shows carpal overlapping and lost Gilula's arc.

disruption) has been described in wrist positions of forced extension and radial deviation with pronation. These injuries are rare, however.

In general, the lesser arc perilunar injuries only produce ligament injury while greater arc perilunar dislocations have associated carpal fractures. The injury patterns are highly variable with intermediate forms between the greater and lesser arc injuries occurring. The proximal fractured scaphoid, triquetrum or the capitate may remain attached to lunate or may displace independently. The lunate may be partially or completely dislocated or even at times remain aligned to the radius.

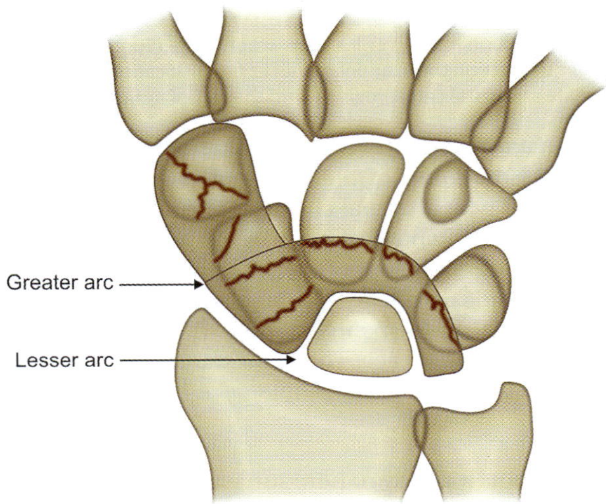

Fig. 25: Greater and lesser arc injuries: A lesser arc injury follows a curved path through the radial styloid, midcarpal joint, and the lunatotriquetral space. A greater arc injury passes through the scaphoid, capitate, and triquetrum.

To establish a common nomenclature to communicate uniformly, the system has met with some additions. Prefix *"trans"* indicates a carpal fracture, like trans-scaphoid means fracture through scaphoid, trans-capitate means fracture through scaphoid and capitate. The grade of lunate dislocation is also quantified into groups by Witvoet and Allieu as follows:

- *Grade 1:* The lunate appears normally aligned.
- *Grade 2:* Lunate is rotated palmarly <90°.
- *Grade 3:* Lunate is rotated >90° but still attached to the radius by its palmar capsular connections.
- *Grade 4:* Lunate is totally enucleated without any connection to the radius.

So, a trans-scaphoid perilunate dislocation grade 3 will mean dorsally displaced distal fragment of scaphoid with other carpal bones and lunate rotated 90° volarly.

Trans-scaphoid perilunate dislocation is the most common reported variety **(Figs. 26A to C)**. The dislocations are most commonly seen in young individuals, as in children the radial physis undergoes separation while in older people the forces are dissipated by the distal radius fractures. Lesser arc injuries are one-third as common than the "trans" injuries.

On examination, the patients have a dinner-fork deformity (as characteristic of distal radius extra-articular Colle's fracture). Swelling and radial deviation is also common. Patient will obviously have pain! Radiographs show undue overlap of carpals with loss of clear lines between them. The Gilula's arcs are discontinuous (like the disrupted Shenton's line in fracture neck of femur). The lunate appears more triangular shape and is proportional to the palmar dislocation. On a lateral radiograph, the lunate is "empty" of capitate and is volarly tilted or displaced or dislocated. With complete lunate dislocation, the lunate is volarly tilted and concavity facing palmar ("spilled tea-pot sign").

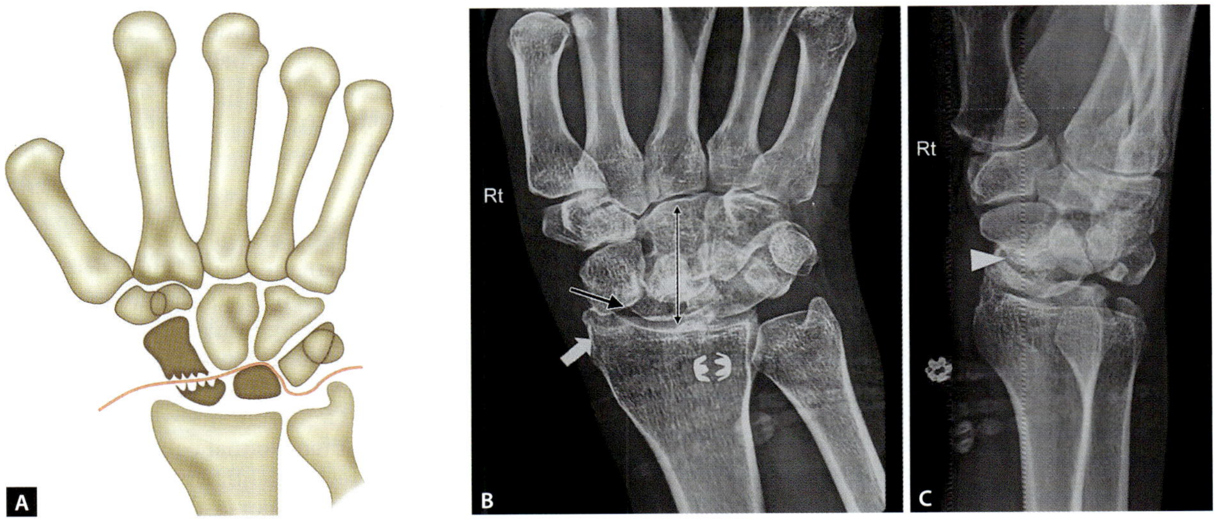

Figs. 26A to C: Trans-scaphoid perilunate dislocation means a perilunate dislocation associated with fracture of scaphoid where the force of injury passes through scaphoid taking proximal fragment with lunate; (A) The radiological appearance of neglected trans-scaphoperilunate dislocation, AP projection; (B) Demonstrates proximal migration of carpus (distal carpal row especially capitate) causing reduced carpal height (spanning arrow), non-union of scaphoid (arrow) and arthritic changes prominent at the radial styloid (block arrow); (C) The lateral projection demonstrates volarly dislocated lunate (pointer) disposed in a VISI pattern tilted volarly "spilled tea-pot sign".

Treatment

The injuries have always enticed the surgeon since the beginning of 20th century. The following methods have been commonly used:

- Closed reduction and casts
- Closed reduction and pinning
- Open reduction and internal fixation + ligament reconstruction

Closed reduction: Based on Gunn's law (by positioning the dislocated joint in the position it was in at the time of injury, and then reversing the force, any dislocation should be easily reduced). But, failures were common despite prolonged traction to overcome muscle spasm. It was expected that the lunate reduces back by the force of flexor tendons. Method as proposed by Watson-Jones and developed by Tavernier is the most popular one for reduction. It begins with axial traction (commonly given for over 10 minutes) and flexing the wrist to relocate the capitate onto lunate fossa and then reducing the capitolunate unit into the distal radius. Postreduction radiographs should show:

- Restored Gilula's arcs
- Symmetric scapholunate gap
- Scapholunate angle <80°
- Normal intercarpal relationship
- Reduced and aligned fracture

Plaster should be applied for 8–12 weeks followed by aggressive physiotherapy. The cast needs to be carefully molded on the dorsum of the capitate, the palmar scaphoid tuberosity, and the dorsum of the radius to counter the rotational instability of scapholunate region especially with scaphoid fractures. To reduce the period of external immobilization by cast (causing plaster disease) and maintaining a stable reduction, percutaneous pinning has been advised. The wire is obliquely inserted from radius to lunate. Other pins stabilize the lunotriquetral joint and scapholunate joint.

Optimal reduction in cases of perilunate dislocations is consistently achievable only through meticulous *open reduction*, so it is a preferred method especially and obviously if the closed one is ineffective **(Fig. 27)**. The classical combined palmar and dorsal approach described by Swanson is used. Here, the volar approach allows repair of the palmar capsular rent while from the dorsal approach the carpal reduction, and reconstruction/repair of the dorsal scapholunate and lunotriquetral ligaments is affected. In cases of scaphoid fractures, the volar approach is shifted radially like the Henry's volar approach to scaphoid for bone grafting and fixation, while in lunate dislocations the carpal tunnel approach is preferred to meticulously reduce lunate and repair the capsular rent. In patients with scaphocapitate syndrome, the capitate fracture is reduced and fixed through the dorsal incision. The repair can be protected by external fixator.

Chronic Instability

It is clear from above that the perilunate dislocations produce injury to both the intrinsic and extrinsic ligaments of the wrist joint so a combined CID and CIND pattern of instability

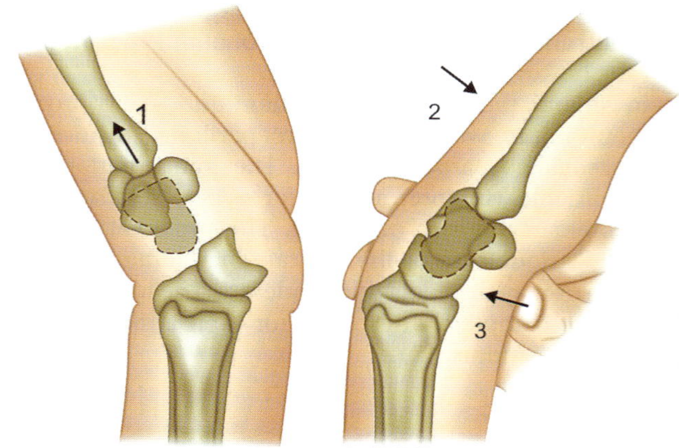

Fig. 27: Reduction maneuver for trans-scaphoid perilunate dislocations. After gentle traction the examiner reduces the dislocation by pushing on the lunate and distal carpal rows toward the axis of radius.

results in untreated cases (the CIC pattern). Failure to obtain stability of the joints of the proximal row may result in a chronic CID type of carpal collapse. The damaged extrinsic radiocarpal ligaments if do not heal or remain inefficient may lead to development of CIND (with ulnar translocation of the ulnar side of the carpus). On plain radiographs in CIC, the scaphoid is seen palmar flexed with widening of the scapholunate joint space. The ulnar translocation of carpus is prominent with dorsiflexed lunate.

Treatment

These patients logically require surgical stabilization of both CID and CIND to obtain a reasonably good outcome. Late ligament reconstructions are cumbersome and associated with poorer outcomes as the reduction of chronically dislocated joints and dissociated patterns make reduction difficult and incomplete. Distraction with fixators can be attempted in perilunate dislocations that were missed for up to 3 months followed by the open management as above. Still wrist stiffness and development of reflex sympathetic dystrophy is a concern. Midcarpal fusion with a tightening of the dorsal and volar radiocarpal ligaments is more appropriate. For even late cases and those with significant cartilage wear, a formal wrist fusion is probably the best.

CONCLUSION

- Carpal instability denotes malfunction of the bearing and linkage function of the carpal bones that presents in varied forms and is difficult to group into specific entities.
- Dorsal intercalated segment instability and volar intercalated segment instability are the commonly taught forms of carpal instability but various other important forms are also encountered, the surgeon should have information about them so that cause of wrist pain and dysfunction is correctly identified and proper treatment can be instituted rather than just hiving it off as another nonspecific wrist pain.
- Every carpal instability has a known cause to it and correction of it would cure the patient, missing them leads to progression of the pathology and wrist degeneration that is then managed by limited wrist fusions or wrist arthrodesis.

CHAPTER 113

Common Miscellaneous Conditions of Hand

Manish Kumar Varshney

INTRODUCTION

As is clear from the complex anatomy of hand, the myriad of intricate structures making up the mobile unit of hand are subjected to attrition or frictional injuries. Also overuse of the components in specific situations is bound to cause some disorders. Most involved structures are the long or short tendons of hand or the small joints subjected to degenerative changes. Some developmental conditions like Dupuytren's disease may also have in part associated traumatic component.

DE QUERVAIN'S STENOSING TENOSYNOVITIS (DE QUERVAIN'S TENOVAGINITIS, DE QUERVAIN'S DISEASE, WASHERWOMAN'S SPRAIN, STENOSING PERITENDINITIS)

Stenosing tenovaginitis is seen at locations where osteofibrotic canal houses the finger and wrist tendons, especially where the tendons brusquely deviate their gliding direction. De Quervain's disease is chronic inflammation of tendons of abductor pollicis longus (APL) and the extensor pollicis brevis (EPB) as they lie over the styloid process of the radius **(Fig. 1)**.

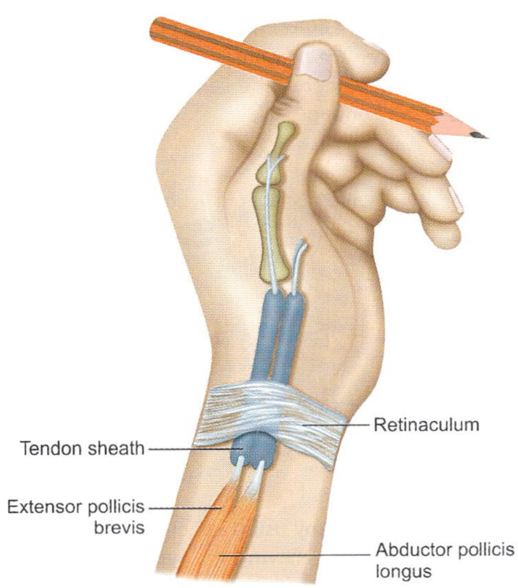

Fig. 1: Anatomical disposition of the tendons involved in De Quervain's tenovaginitis.

Pathophysiology

This condition has been related to friction syndromes. The repetitive passage of tendon (as in activities that require frequent thumb abduction associated with wrist ulnar deviation or repetitive hand pronosupination) through a narrow canal causes swelling or the formation of a fibrotic tendon nodule, which leads to poor tendon glide. Inflammatory changes cause edema within the surrounding area and incarceration of the tendon blocking its gliding in both directions. With disease progression the retinaculum thickens prominently and there is fibrocartilaginous metaplasia. Synovial hypertrophy is consistently seen during surgical exploration when disease has advanced to nodule formation. With further advancement of the disease there are signs of tendinous erosion, and an overall increase in the sheath's thickness. Findings in patients with De Quervain's disease or even a related condition the tenovaginitis of the flexor carpi radialis (FCR) are different from a typical friction syndrome in that they have more of endothelial proliferation with development of perisynovial fibrotic tissue latter with minimal inflammatory tissue. This presence of fibrosis without production of inflammatory tissue and associated increase in retinacular ligament thickness suggests intrinsic tendon pathology rather than an overuse/ friction syndrome. These findings have led to the use of term stenosing peritendinitis (Gartsen in 1951).

Etiology

Usually the disease is idiopathic but various causes have been suggested:

- Rheumatoid arthritis
- Pregnancy
- Recent trauma
- Occupational
- Malunited radius fracture
- Bony exostosis

Associated Conditions

Most of the conditions suggest an association with the systemic rheumatic syndrome.

- Carpal tunnel syndrome (CTS)

- Trigger finger
- Epicondylitis
- Subacromial bursitis

Clinical Features

Middle aged patients between 40 and 60 years are commonly affected and the disease is much more common in females than males. Classic triad consists of tenderness over the radial styloid, swelling over the first extensor compartment, and a positive Finkelstein's test. Persistent pain 1–2 cm proximal to radial styloid process occurs during certain movements. The pain is present often for few weeks to months and at times there is loss of function. Crepitus or squeaking with movements of involved tendons (wet leather sign) may be palpable. Swelling is found in 85% of cases. Finkelstein's sign is pathognomonic **(Fig. 2)**. It consists of ulnar deviating the partially flexed wrist, with thumb in opposition eliciting severe pain. Locking or triggering is uncommon but when present is a definitive indication of surgical release.

Differential Diagnosis

- *Intersection syndrome:* Pain, swelling, and, in more serious cases, a palpable crepitus that can be located at approximately 4 cm proximal to the wrist
- Carpometacarpal (CMC) joint arthritis
- Scaphoid fracture
- Intercarpal (scaphotrapeziotrapezoid) arthritis
- *Lindberg syndrome:* This involves an anomalous connection between flexor pollicis longus (FPL) and the index flexor digitorum profundus (FDP) causing simultaneous flexion of the index finger with active flexion of the thumb interphalangeal (IP) joint. Pathological form of this anomalous connection has been termed thumb-index flexor tenosynovitis. It is not associated with CTS as was previously thought. The patients have several months history of vague, poorly localized, and activity-related pain on the distal aspect of the volar forearm and wrist. There is often loss of independent flexion of the thumb and index finger preceding the symptoms. Pain is reproduced by actively flexing the thumb IP joint with passively extended index finger. Treatment is simple and consists of release of the intertendinous connection between the FPL and the index FDP.
- Flexor carpi radialis tendinopathy.

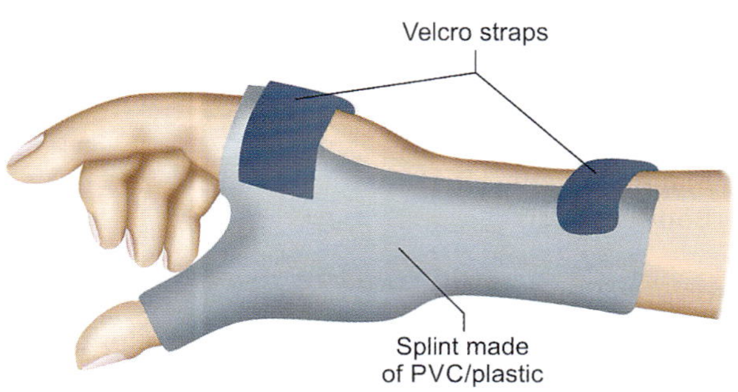

Fig. 2: Finkelstein test. (PVC: polyvinyl chloride)

Imaging

- Most of the bony differentials should be ruled out by plain radiographs of the wrist and hand.
- *Ultrasonography:* It is important for diagnosis if clinically dubious. It can verify that there is a reduction in tendon gliding and an increase in the APL or the EPB tendon sheath's thickness. Now this is considered a reliable test for diagnosis.

Treatment

Medical Treatment

Local ointments, plaster splint **(Fig. 3)**, physiotherapy, and heat and hydrotherapy are the mainstay of treatment along with the most useful drug—nonsteroidal anti-inflammatory drugs (NSAIDs). Injection of local steroids may give satisfactory results if the noninterventional management is not effective **(Fig. 4)**. It should be realized that most of the patients have anatomical variation with respect to first dorsal extensor compartment (see hand and wrist anatomy) so injecting all the stenotic canals is imperative else the relief will be partial or incomplete **(Fig. 5)**. Although commonly insoluble preparations of the steroid are used however local complications such as depigmentation, subcutaneous atrophy, and adipose necrosis are much more common.

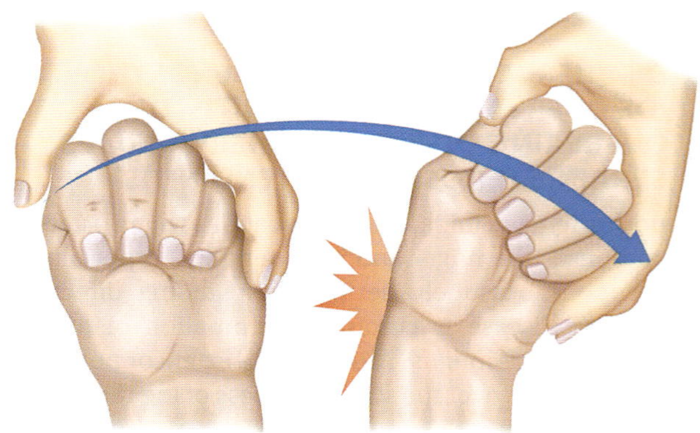

Fig. 3: Splinting for De Quervain's disease: Polyvinyl chloride (PVC)-based soft lined braces are commercially also available or they can be countered to patient's needs. The same can also be effected form a plaster of Paris (POP) bandage.

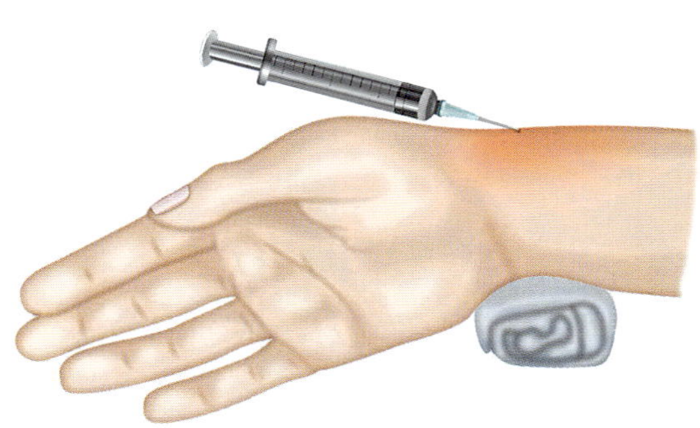

Fig. 4: Local injection therapy using various steroid preparations in the synovial sheath do help in relieving the symptoms quite promptly and for long-term. I prefer noncrystalline preparations like dexamethasone for acute flare-ups while depot preparations for long-standing chronic problem, if conservative therapy is otherwise ineffective.

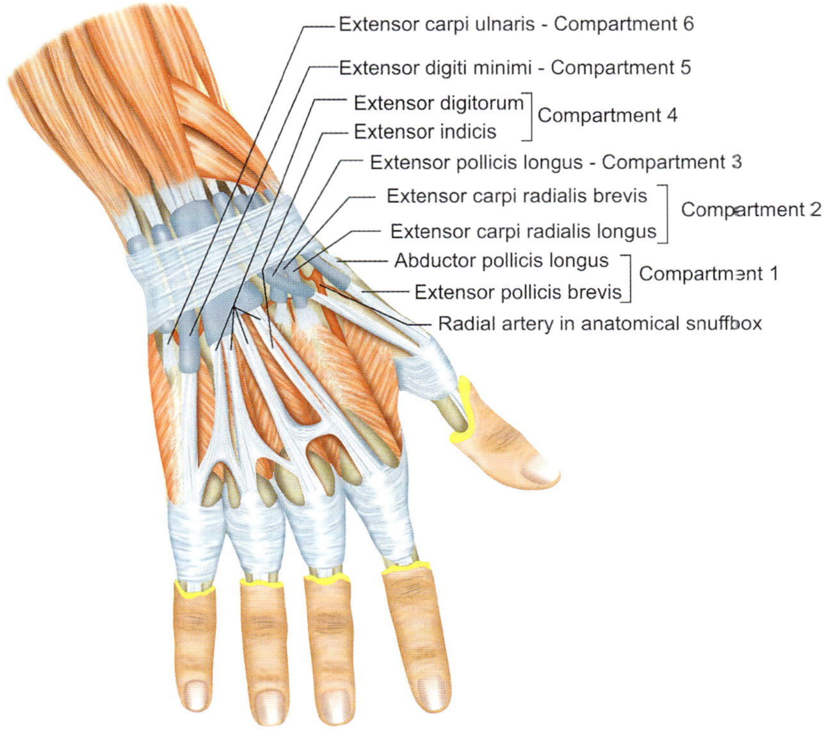

Fig. 5: Intersection syndrome occurs as a friction syndrome between first and second extensor compartment of wrist.

Preparations of dexamethasone are possibly more sober. Also only the tendon sheath should be infiltrated rather than injecting the steroid preparation within the tendon.

Surgical Treatment

This is indicated for recurrent disease or resistant one that does not respond to conservative management. Other definitive indication is extensor tendon triggering. Surgical release through a radial longitudinal or transverse incision aims at decompression of the twin tendons by the excision of the thickened sheath. Again the highly varying anatomy should be properly recognized and the multiple cutaneous branches of the radial nerve lying at the spot should be all protected.

Complications of surgical treatment:

- Radial superficial nerve laceration and neuroma formation
- Volar tendon subluxation
- Hypertrophic scarring
- Tendinous adhesions
- Persistence of symptoms (missed compartments)

INTERSECTION SYNDROME (ABDUCTOR POLLICIS LONGUS BURSITIS, CROSSOVER TENDINITIS, OARSMAN WRIST, SQUEAKER'S WRIST, AND PERITENDINITIS CREPITANS)

This consists of pain and swelling in dorsum of the distal forearm, approximately 4–6 cm proximal to the radial styloid where the APL and EPB (extensor compartment 1) intersect the extensor carpi radialis brevis (ECRB) and longus (ECRL) of extensor compartment 2. It represents classic example of friction syndrome occurring at the intersection point between the muscle bellies and tendons causing tendinopathy and bursitis. Forearm pain at the junction of these two compartments was first described by Velpeau in 1841 but the name "intersection syndrome" was given by Dobyn's in 1978.

Clinical Features

Symptoms (pain and swelling) occur after prolonged repetitive activity (flexion-extension of the wrist) with eccentric loading of the extensor compartment. Crepitus is palpable with flexion and extension of wrist. Weak pinch and diminished grasp may be seen. Finkelstein test produces pain proximal to the location of De Quervain's site. "**Bugaboo syndrome**" occurs in deep power helicopter skiers resulting from excessive radial deviation and repetitive extension while pulling out the implanted pole from deep snow while skiing. The pathognomonic finding is pain produced by direct pressure at the point of intersection producing pain and crepitus with wrist flexion/extension.

Differential Diagnosis

De Quervain's disease

Diagnostic Test

Ultrasound examination is very helpful in examining the pathological tendons and differentiating from De Quervain's disease. It shows a tendon gliding deficiency of the involved abductor pollicis brevis (APB), EPB, ECRL, and ECRB tendons.

Treatment

Medical Treatment

This consists of NSAIDs, alternate cold and hot fomentation, local ointments, and rest to the forearm. Activity modification consisting of avoiding the exacerbating movement is useful but needs to be done forever as recurrence is frequent. Local corticosteroids are useful as described for De Quervain's disease.

Surgical Management

Direct intervention: This attacks the primary pathological area and is considered standard operative decompression. Here, a longitudinal incision over the site of maximum swelling and tenderness is given at the point of intersection in line with the APB and EPB muscle bellies. The fascia and sheath around the APB and EPB are released (deroofed).

Indirect intervention: There is a school of thought that the basic pathology involves tenosynovitis of the second extensor compartment (ECRB and ECRL) causing referral of pain and swelling more proximally. This is similar to finding that in CTS if there is flexor tenosynovitis then pain is referred proximally to distal forearm. So, decompression only of the second extensor compartment will cause relief of the symptoms. This has been propounded by Grundberg and Reagan and has also shown relief in all patients.

I prefer opening the second extensor compartment through direct approach to APB and EPB at the swollen area and releasing the fascia of EPB to expose the compartment. ECRB and ECRL tenosynovitis is then addressed.

Complications

Radial nerve injury, scar tenderness, neuroma formation, and tendon subluxation.

TRIGGER FINGER (STENOSING FLEXOR TENOSYNOVITIS)

Trigger digits occur due to stenosing tenosynovitis resulting from various pathologies [including congenital **(Figs. 6A and B)**] causing hypertrophy of A1 pulley (commonly) or tendon thickening or both, however, in congenital form the tendon thickening is the primary pathology and not the pulley thickening. The flexor tendon becomes irritated as it slides through the tendon sheath tunnel causing tenosynovitis and thickening of the sheath causing the opening of the tunnel to become smaller **(Fig. 7)**. With continued irritation the tendon may thicken and nodules form, making its passage through the tunnel more difficult **(Fig. 7)**. The patient develops painful hand grasp or the finger/thumb triggers during finger flexion or extension movements (opening of the finger with sudden jerk).

Etiology

Triggering develops due to discrepancy between the flexor's circumference and that of its pulley system at the metacarpophalangeal (MCP) level (the region of A1 pulley). The pulley thickens especially at its distal margin where the tendon abruptly angulates causing "a white ring scar thickening" as described by Bunnell. The thickening is due to metaplastic fibrocartilage formation in the region.

The etiological factor directly responsible for trigger finger is usually unknown. There are some risk factors that put patients at increased risk for developing the acquired trigger finger as follows:
- Diabetes
- Rheumatoid arthritis
- Amyloidosis
- Workers doing repetitive hand job

Though mostly inflammatory condition of idiopathic pathogenesis, the trigger finger can also occur due to various uncommon pathologies as follows:
- Tendon or tendon sheath tumor
- Tight Camper's chiasm that causes FDP entrapment and trigger
- Sesamoid bone abnormalities
- Floating bodies in the MCP area
- Intrinsic tendon involvement due to metacarpal head abnormalities
- FDP thickening that causes trigger at the A3 pulley.

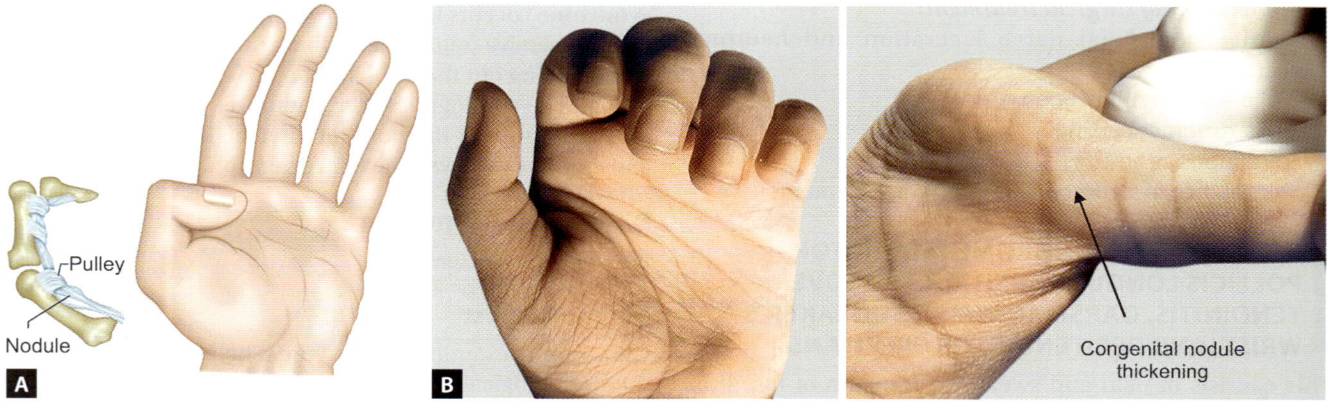

Figs. 6A and B: Congenital trigger thumb—involves formation of Notta nodule within the tendon and not a thickened pulley. The child presents with a flexed thumb that seldom opens bringing into notice the parents of some pathology to seek physician attention. Illustration of the tendon thickening (A) in a case with congenital trigger thumb (B).

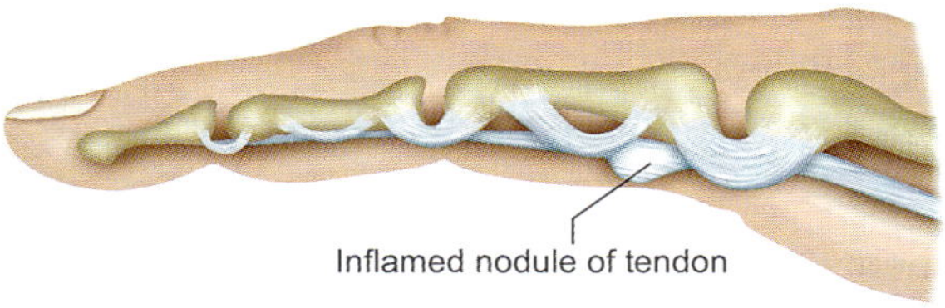

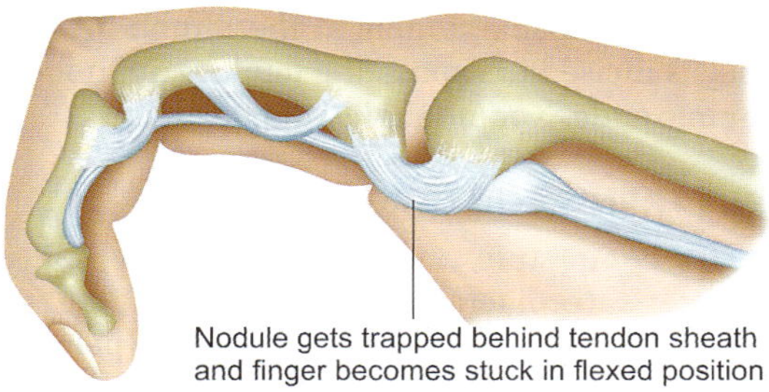

Fig. 7: Trigger finger: Illustration of thickening in A1 pulley causing trigger finger. Often in most cases the tendon also thickens due to collagen remodeling just proximal to the stenosed annular pulley accentuating the trigger.

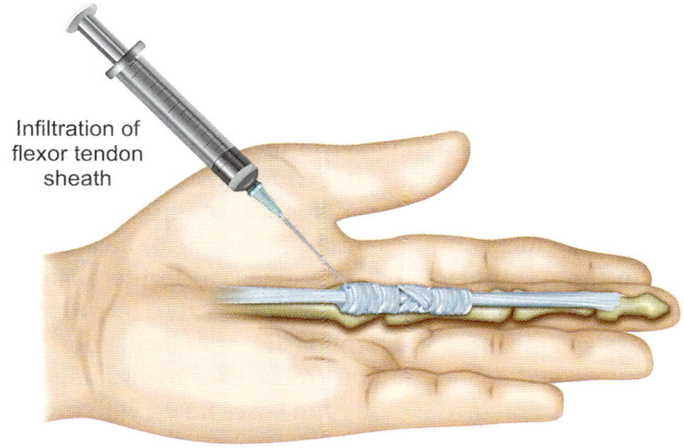

Fig. 8: Steroid infiltration: An ancillary to conservative management especially in cases where the symptomatic relief is inadequate. The steroid possibly acts by reducing the inflammatory edema and loosens the collagen.

Clinical Features

Trigger fingers are more common in women than men. They occur most frequently in people who are between the ages of 40 and 60 years of age. Thumb is the most commonly involved digit followed by fourth (ring), third (middle) and fifth (pinkie) finger, respectively. Symptoms of trigger finger are not associated with trauma although they may follow a period of heavy hand use. The symptoms commonly include:

- Pain on finger movements
- A tender nodule on volar aspect of the palm near the A1 pulley region often proximal to it
- Swelling
- Catching or popping sensation in finger or thumb, especially on extension stiffness and catching tend to be worse after inactivity, such as when you wake in the morning. Your fingers will often loosen up as you move them.
- Pain in proximal interphalangeal (PIP) region: The exact mechanism is unknown but may be related to excess stress put on the joint due to forceful pulling of the finger of snapping injury to the collateral ligaments. The other reason might be synovitis extending to the region and lastly may be related to referred pain.
- Without treatment the tendon meets one of the two fates:
    - Incarceration of the tendon and adhesions in the region: This prevents finger straightening and commonly the finger is fixed in mid-flexion.
    - The tendon breaks free and the finger fails to flex. There is a sensation of "dislocating" finger and complete weakness.

Diagnosis

Clinical evidence is enough and hardly any other investigation is needed to make the diagnosis. Radiographs help in identifying exostosis or malunited fractures. Ultrasonography may additionally reveal the thickening or swollen tendon.

Staging

This is based on the various clinical preoperative stages and has variable acceptance in orthopedic community due mainly to lack of treatment guidance:

- *Stage 1 (pretrigger):* Pain only; positive sign of trigger finger not demonstrated during the objective evaluation; A1 pulley is tender to palpation.
- *Stage 2 (active):* Positive trigger sign on objective evaluation; though with a snap the patient is able to extend finger actively.
- *Stage 3 (passive):* Positive trigger demonstrable:
    - *A:* Finger extension is possible only passively by applying external force
    - *B:* Active finger flexion also not possible
- *Stage 4 (rigidity):* Incarcerated trigger finger; the proximal interphalanx is stuck in a flexed posture.

Treatment

Rest, Medications, and Steroid Injections

If symptoms are mild in earliest stages resting the finger in neutral position may be enough to resolve the problem. NSAIDs or acetaminophen can be used to relieve the pain. Steroid injections resolve the inflammation quite quickly and insoluble preparations give a lasting relief **(Fig. 8)**. Some surgeons prefer soluble potent preparations in view of complications associated with the insoluble preparations. Injections may be repeated for one to two times but never more as there are tendon weakening and high chances of breakage of tendons. Late stages and long-lasting symptoms are less likely to resolve with this treatment. Steroid injections also often fail for thumb trigger.

Surgical Treatment

The definite indications of surgical treatment are incarcerated tendon and failed multiple injections. Broken tendon is also a definitive indication for surgical treatment, but management is done on the lines of tendon reconstruction rather than typically for the trigger finger. Long-standing cases with active disease are a relative indication for surgical release as conservative treatment often gives incomplete relief.

The goal of surgery is to widen the opening of the tunnel so that the tendon can slide through it more easily. A transverse incision is preferred for surgical release of the tendon the A1 pulley is partially released in the distal half else bowstringing of the tendon would occur. The procedure can be also done on outpatient basis under local anesthesia. We prefer needle percutaneous release for most stage 1 and 2 cases except recurrent cases and cases failed with multiple injections. Various authors have described the percutaneous procedure using custom-designed tenotome, a scalpel and a hook, or an extra-thin scalpel and a hypodermic needle. We prefer using a blood transfusion set needle as adequate force can be transmitted to cut the thickening in the pulley. Open release is also done for long-standing cases (>4–6 months of symptoms) and later stages. No attempt is made to repair the released sheath as the new sheath should be loose enough for tendon to glide easily. Local anesthesia is advantageous as adequacy of the release can be judged simultaneously by making the patient move finger through full flexion and extension. In children, the A2 pulley or one of the limbs of flexor digitorum superficialis (FDS) tendon may need to be simultaneously released.

Complications

- Incomplete extension following release of the pulley may occur due to tightness of the tendon sheath that may result from persistent flexed posture in a long-standing neglected stage 4 trigger finger.
- Persistent triggering more often represents a surgical failure and commonly occurs due to incomplete release of A1 pulley and sheath bowstringing of tendon is again a surgical failure caused by excessive release of the tendon sheath.
- Infection is a general surgical complication but is uncommon.

Postoperative recovery is fast and usually complete within a couple of weeks. In some patients swelling and stiffness may take up to 6 months to subside completely. Splint is provided for a few days to 1 week and patient is encouraged to move the finger actively.

CONGENITAL TRIGGER THUMB

Congenital trigger thumb is the most common cause for thumb rigidity in infants where the thumb is found in flexion or extension at IP joint. There is hypertrophy and tendon sheath proliferation, rather than an alteration in the pulley system (cf-adult trigger thumb). A nodule referred to as "Notta nodule" (named after Notta) described it in 1850 **(Fig. 6)**. The condition is rarely diagnosed at birth or within the first 6 months after birth but is characterized by the newborn assuming a thumb flexion posture. It is congenital found exclusively in the thumb often occurring bilaterally in monozygotic twins or in a hereditary fashion.

Differential Diagnosis

- Clasped thumb
- Absent or aberrant tendons
- Spasticity

Treatment

Surgical treatment is the method of choice. It consists of freeing up the FPL through a small transverse incision at the location of the palpable nodule at the thumb flexion fold. The pulley is incised to expose the tendon and nodule and check for free glide. Nodule should not be excised.

DUPUYTREN'S CONTRACTURE

Dupuytren's contracture (DC) is a thickening and hypertrophic fibrosis (proliferative fibroplasia) of the palmar aponeurosis and its extensions into the digits (palmodigital extensions, **Fig. 9**). It is the most common inheritable disorder of connective tissue of upper limbs in humans named after Baron Guillaume Dupuytren, who described an operation to correct the affliction in the Lancet in 1831, but he was not the one to describe it. Felix Plater described the palmar contracture in a master Mason (so "Mason hand" is some who call it) but he ascribed it to flexor tendon contracture which was corrected by Henry Cline Senior (1777, when Dupuytren was born!), one of John Hunter's (1728–1793) pupil by performing extensive dissections in affected hands and attributed it correctly to palmar aponeurosis. He kept the relation of disease to heavy manual labor as observed by Plater. Alexis Boyer (1826), personal surgeon to Napoleon Bonaparte and first patron and teacher of Dupuytren attributed the disease to a drying, hardening and stiffening of the flexor tendons and the overlying skin. These were corrected fully by Dupuytren who described it in a coachman and dismissed any association previously

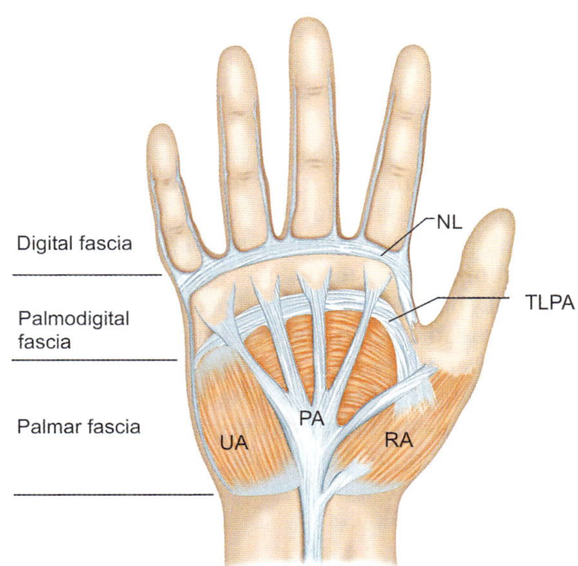

Fig. 9: Dupuytren's contracture. The fascial fibrotic bands extend longitudinally and contract gradually to cause fixed flexion deformity of fingers.

attributed to inflammatory conditions or rheumatic disorders propounded by contemporaries. He also vehemently dissuaded the notion of the disease resulting from trauma of the ligaments, joints, or bones. He firmly associated the condition with repetitive/chronic local trauma and demonstrated that the skin is tethered to underlying palmar aponeurosis by dense fibrous tissue without any adipose tissue. He advocated correction of retraction by dividing the aponeurotic bundles that insert on proximal phalanges and deep transverse metacarpal ligament without any intervention done to the tendons, essentially eliminating any role of tendinous origin to disease.

Contractures of the palmar aponeurotic fascia develop giving rise to flexion deformities of the distal palm and fingers. The fascia contains strands of fibers, like cords, that run from the palm upward into the fingers. In DC, these cords tighten, or contract, causing the fingers to curl forward. In severe cases, it can lead to crippling hand deformities.

Pathogenesis/Etiology

Dupuytren's contracture is the most common inherited connective tissue disease of humans and is hypothesized to be associated with aberrant wound healing of the palmar fascia. Both inherited and sporadic forms have been identified.

- Incidence among affected families has been reported to approach 70%. Autosomal dominant form of the disease has been mapped to the long arm of chromosome 16.
- Although, the genetic predisposition in Dupuytren's disease has been well established, the condition is seen more commonly in patients with epilepsy, patients who use alcohol and tobacco, and patients with diabetes, cirrhosis, and human immunodeficiency virus (HIV) infection. Diabetes could be a pathological cause as the combination of CTS, trigger finger, and DC has been increasingly found in the diabetic population.
- The disease is characterized by the appearance of small nodules of hyperproliferative cells within the palmar fascia that, over time, give rise to large bands of contracted, collagen-rich fibrotic tissue (diseased cords), a hallmark of the disease. The factors causing fibrosis and progressive contracture are poorly understood. Fibroblasts somehow transform to myofibroblasts with contractile elements (smooth muscle actin) and attach to the cells of the palmar aponeurosis. As the disease progresses, the affected tissues shorten as a unit, ultimately resulting in digital contractures. Along with the digital contractures, skin dimpling commonly occurs.
- Trauma may be a possible cause and explain a male gender bias.
- Dysregulation of multiple structural proteins in DC, including type I and type III collagens; the extracellular matrix (ECM) proteins fibronectin, tenascin C and laminin; as well as matrix metalloproteinases in the diseased fascial cords have been described.
- Unconfirmed dysregulation of various signaling proteins have been described like the transforming growth factor-β (TGF-β), epidermal growth factor (EGF), and platelet-derived growth factor (PDGF).
- The various other putative pathogenic pathways and proteins possibly involved in the pathogenesis are listed below:
    - Oxidative stress molecules, including superoxide radical (O_2^-), hydrogen peroxide (H_2O_2), and the hydroxyl radical (OH^-)
    - Serum/glucocorticoid regulated kinase (SGK) message is downregulated in DC
    - Downregulation of Chitinase-3-like 2 (CHI3L2)
    - Proteoglycan 4 (PRG4) and fibulin-1 (FBLN1) dysregulation. PRG4 has been implicated in camptodactyly-arthropathy-coxa vara-pericarditis (CACP) syndrome (where one or more fingers are curved inwards on the palm (flexed) and cannot be straightened); osteoarthritis; etc. *FBLN1* gene has been implicated in synpolydactyly, a congenital condition characterized by a union of fingers or toes and/or increase in the number of toes or fingers.

Pathology

The condition belongs to larger group of superficial fibromatosis (that may involve hand or foot) begins as fibrous nodules in the palmar fascia. The earliest change is the thickening of Grapow fibers (these connect the fascia to dermis). Initially, this tissue is hypercellular and vascular. Local proliferation continues to form a nodule or if skin retraction occurs then a pit. The palmar aponeurosis and the various ligamentous bands when involved in the disease process, form the classical nodules and cords giving rise to the characteristic flexion contractures of Dupuytren's disease. The pathoanatomy in fingers is much complex **(Figs. 10A and B)**. The two fibrotic structures that are clearly identifiable in Dupuytren's disease are the nodule and the cord **(Box 1)**.

Dupuytren's diathesis implies a more advanced form of the disease with multiple afflictions, presence of anyone should indicate a need to search for the other two:

1. "Knuckle pads" (Garrod nodes, thickening over the extensor surfaces of the PIP joints)
2. Plantar fibromatosis (Ledderhose disease)
3. Fasciitis of the penis (Peyronie's disease)

Clinical Features

The condition is commonly seen in Caucasians occurs more commonly in men between 50 and 70 years of age. It has a familial tendency (autosomal dominant with variable penetrance).

- The most commonly affected digit is the ring finger **(Fig. 12A)** followed by pinkie finger (then middle and index, uncommonly thumb), but any finger can be affected.
- Pain is never a characteristic feature. It is the deformity that concerns patient. Patient generally presents with a nodule in the palm **(Figs. 12A and B)** proximal to the base of the ring finger that has over the course of months or years become a thickened fibrous cord running along the palm to the fingers. Nodules typically are painless, unless nerve compression or tenosynovitis is present.

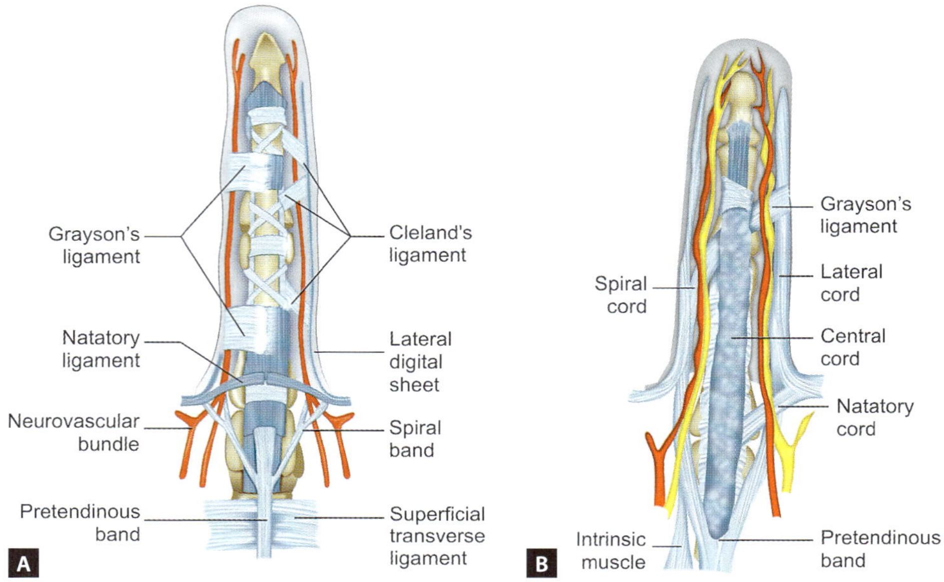

Figs. 10A and B: Pathology of Dupuytren's involvement in fingers. (A) Normal anatomy of ligaments and (B) structures on finger, pathological alterations in a Dupuytren's finger.

BOX 1: The nodule and cord of Dupuytren's disease.

- Nodule is a relatively vascular tissue containing a dense population of fibroblasts, with a high proportion being myofibroblasts. As the nodule hardens, it gets adhered to subcutaneous tissue and skin causing the cord formation leading to flexion contracture of the metacarpophalangeal joint (MCP) and proximal interphalangeal (PIP) joints **(Fig. 11)**.
  - In the palm they are located adjacent to distal palmar crease while in fingers the nodules are commonly found at PIP joint or at the base of fingers.
- The cord is a collagen-rich structure that is relatively avascular and acellular and with a lesser (but still significant) abundance of myofibroblasts.
  - The cords involve the palmar, palmodigital, and digital regions.

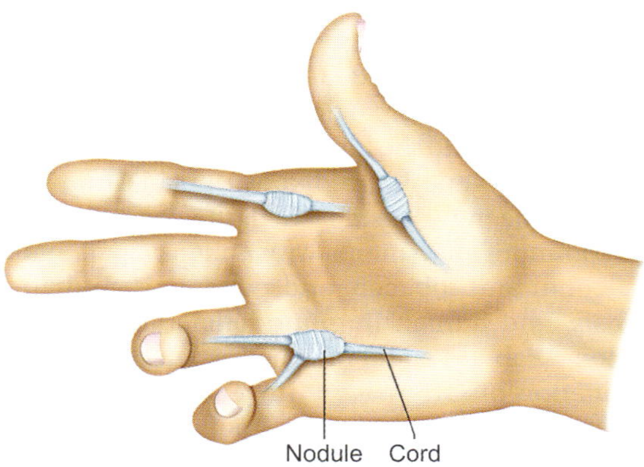

Fig. 11: Development of contractures in fingers in late presentation.

- Over time, as the contracture develops **(Fig. 12B)**, the fingers become clawed as they are pulled towards the palm.
- This leads to the flexion of the digit. The skin is adherent to this fibrous cord. Subsequently, other digits are involved and the patient has painful nodules in the pretendinous bands of palmar fascia of the ring and little fingers **(Fig. 13)**. Flexion contracture of the MCP joint occurs first **(Fig. 12B)**, followed by finger contractures. The hand bows and the fingers are completely pulled against the palm gradually. This produces difficulty in maintaining hygiene due to inability to open up the hand.
- Often, the skin of the palm is dimpled and puckered **(Fig. 12A)**.
- Associated conditions:
  - Plantar nodules
  - Peyronie's disease
  - Diabetes
  - Epilepsy
  - Chronic alcoholism
  - Smoking
  - Pulmonary tuberculosis (TB)
  - Vascular insufficiency

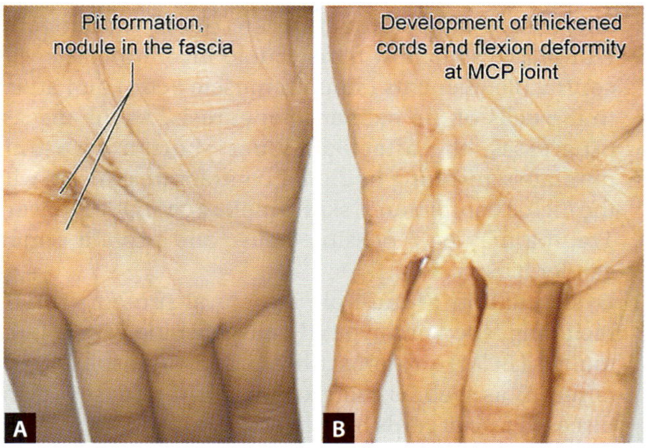

Figs. 12A and B: The earliest features are formation of a pit and nodule (A) along the ring finger long flexor tendons. Later cords and flexion deformity develops (B), the cord was stretched to make prominent for demonstration. (MCP: metacarpophalangeal)

Physical Examination

- Firm nodules (that may be tender to palpation) are closely adherent to the skin and their movement with finger motion suggests an association with the tendon and not DC.
- Thinning of subcutaneous fat.
- Painless cords proximal to the nodules causing finger flexion contracture.
- Active finger extension causes skin blanching.
- Pits or grooves represent skin adherence to the underlying fascia by vertical bands through the fibrous tissue.
- Garrod nodes are tender knuckle pads over the back of (dorsal aspect) the PIPs in a more aggressive disease. These occur in 40–50% of patients.
- Ledderhose disease is concomitant involvement of plantar fascia seen in 5–30% patients and should be always examined as this is associated with poorer prognosis.
- Presence of MCP and PIP joint contractures. True contracture is difficult to assess but objectively measure and record the degree of flexion deformity and also assess compensatory distal interphalangeal (DIP) joint hyperextension.
- *Hueston "table top test"* **(Fig. 14)**: If the patient is unable to lay the palm flat on a table top, the findings are considered positive. We do not consider this to be additionally of any help. It used to be a good guideline to decide need of surgical release. Positive table top test indicates flexion contracture of 30–40° at MCP joint, but is also affected by finger joint contractures. It has been found that the surgical release of PIP contractures yields better functional outcome while decisions based on MCP joint contracture either yield no improvement or produce worsening of contracture. So, now it seems that table top test that basically is an indirect indicator of MCP contracture may be useless.

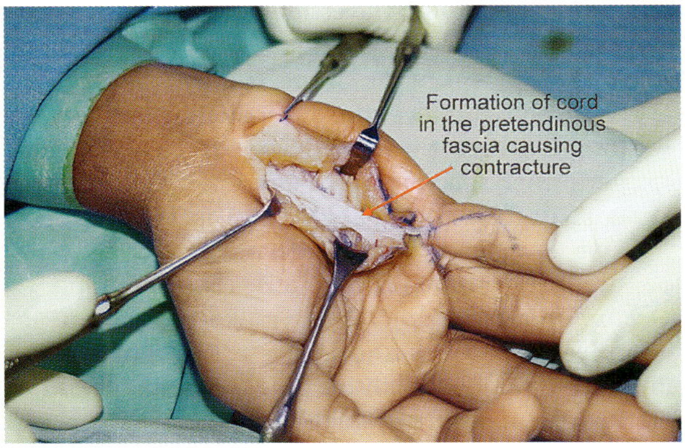

Fig. 13: Gross pathological location of fibrotic thickened cord in the pretendinous region.
Source: Professor PP Kotwal, Chairman, Institute of Orthopedics and Joint Replacement, Pushpawati Singhania Research Institute, New Delhi, India.

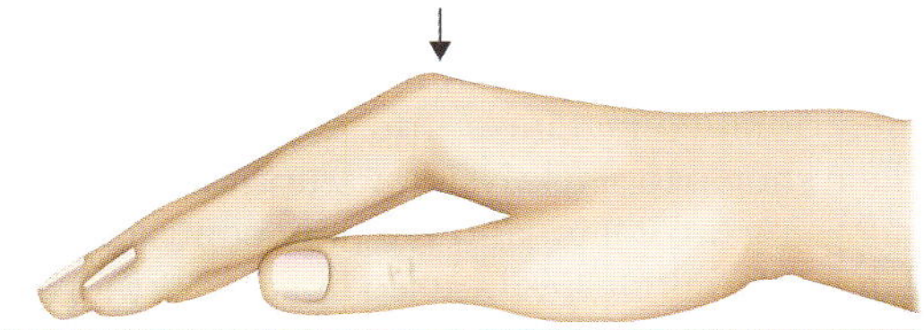

Fig. 14: Table top test.

Stages of Dupuytren's Disease

Pathologically, the Dupuytren's disease is seen to follow the following three progressive stages:

1. *Proliferative phase (nodular phase):* In this early phase, there is proliferation of myofibroblasts and formation of nodule. Some patients report tenderness and pain associated with the nodules initially that may be due to nerve fibers embedded in the fibrous tissue or local compression of sensitive nerves. Skin blanching of palmar skin is seen with finger extension.
2. *Involutional phase (cord phase):* In this phase, the disease/contracture spreads along the palmar fascia and its bands into the fingers resulting in the formation of continuous unyielding cord. Myofibroblasts are mainly responsible for the development of cord as they align themselves longitudinally along the tension lines within the nodule and cord. Skin pitting is evident.
3. *Residual phase:* The myofibroblasts contract causing characteristic flexion deformity of the fingers by tightening of the cord. The contraction of myofibroblasts end in suicide as the nodular tissue disappears and an acellular tissue with thick bands of collagen in the form of cords remain. The contractures are usually progressive to cause incremental deformity in the hand. It usually follows a pattern, e.g., a disease that begins in the ring finger following pattern usually applies:
   - Ring finger MCP joint contracture
   - (Ring finger MCP + PIP joint contracture) + little finger MCP
   - Above + (little finger PIP joint and MCP joint of middle finger)
   - Above + (DIP joint hyperextension of ring or little fingers or both)

Staging system of Tubiana **(Table 1)** is much more useful clinically in defining the severity with respect to further treatment and future comparison **(Fig. 15)**.

Grades of Severity

The grading system for Dupuytren's disease severity **(Fig. 16)** is as follows:

- *Grade 1:* Thickened nodule and band in the palmar aponeurosis; may have associated skin pitting
- *Grade 2:* Development of pretendinous and digital cords **(Figs. 11 and 13)** with limitation of finger extension
- *Grade 3:* Presence of flexion contracture

TABLE 1: Tubiana staging system for Dupuytren's contractures.

Stage	*Deformity*
0	No lesion
N	Palmar nodule with presence of contracture
1	Total flexion deformity (TFD) between 0° and 45°
2	TFD between 45° and 90°
3	TFD between 90° and 135°
4	TFD >135°

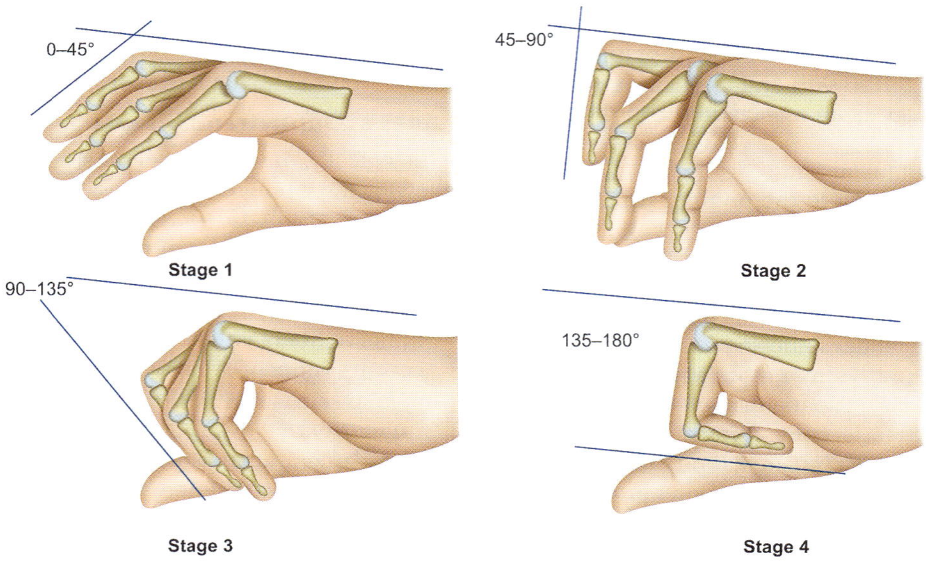

Fig. 15: Tubiana staging system.

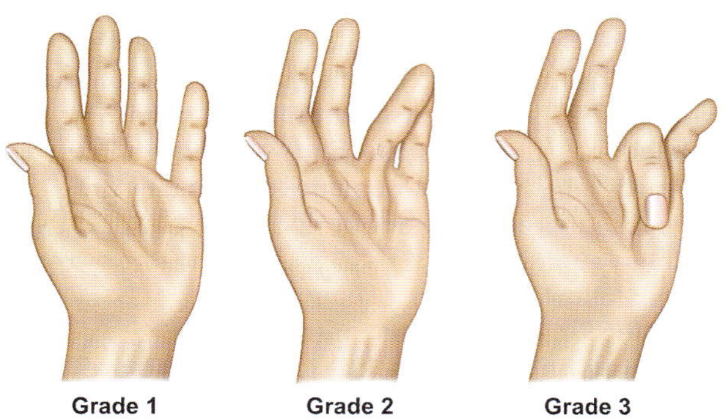

Fig. 16: Grades of Dupuytren's contracture (see text).

Differential Diagnosis

- *Nodular stage:*
  - Neurofibroma
  - Retinacular ganglion of the A-1 pulley
  - Epithelioid sarcoma
  - Ganglion cyst
  - Fibroma
  - Tophi
  - Giant cell tumor
  - Tendon nodule of stenosing tenosynovitis
  - Lipoma
  - Callus
- *Cord stage:*
  - Palmar fibromatosis
  - Palmar tendinitis
  - Traumatic scars
  - Intrinsic joint disease
  - Prolapsed flexor tendon
  - Ulnar nerve palsy
  - Camptodactyly
  - Changes secondary to rheumatoid arthritis
  - Hyperkeratosis

Treatment

Spontaneous resolution does not occur so nonoperative and operative regimes are followed depending on stage of disease, physician experience, and availability of resources.

Nonoperative Treatment

Lot of attempts to improve nonoperative management has occurred due to dismal overall findings of operative management.

- *Physical therapy:* Stretching with the application of heat and ultrasonographic waves may be helpful in the early stages of DC.
  - A custom splint or brace to stretch the fingers passively, worn over the day may slow progression.
  - Range of motion (ROM) exercises should be performed several times a day.
  - Postsurgical physical therapy is very important and comprises of wound care, massage, passive stretching, active ROM exercises, and splinting.
- *Occupational therapy:* These make the patient learn adaptive techniques and to use assistive devices that enhance functional abilities (like to open jars and wear clothes despite contractures).
- *Local injections* ***(Fig. 17)****:*
  - *Corticosteroid injection:* It may be effective for inflammatory tender nodules. The injection softens nodule and reduces inflammatory symptoms.
  - γ-interferon injections
  - Use of creams based on vitamin E, dimethyl sulfoxide
  - *Clostridial collagenase injection:* Direct injection of clostridial collagenase into nodules and cords has been shown to cause lysis and rupture of digital cords, releasing MCP joint and PIP joint contractures.
- Oral dugs like allopurinol—used by some orthopedicians and physicians but their efficiency is doubtful in controlling the disease.

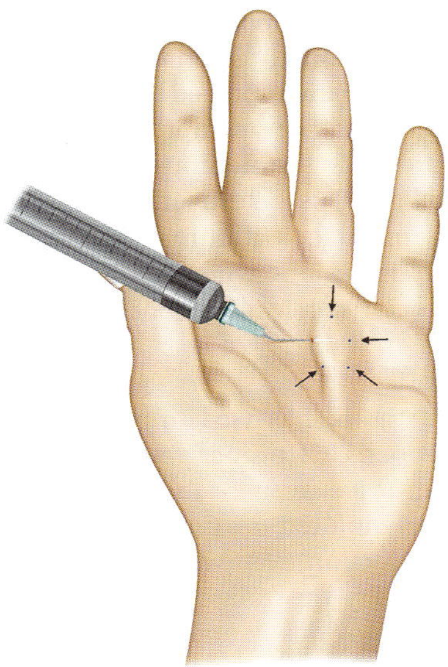

Fig. 17: Intralesional and perilesional depot steroid infiltration (or other drugs) for Dupuytren's nodules.

Operative Treatment

The best-known treatment is surgical. The surgical treatment is a partial or total excision of the palmar fascia depending on the extent of involvement. The contractures at the MCP joint are always correctable whereas the contracture at the PIP joint is more difficult to correct completely.

The surgical procedures used in treatment of DC are:

- *Subcutaneous fasciotomy [aka percutaneous needle fasciotomy (PNF)]:* This is the simplest of the procedures that has been popularized to relieve contracture in frail elderly who may be unable to bear anesthetic insult. It may also be done as a temporizing measure to improve skin hygiene before any definitive surgery or in those not willing for limited fasciectomy. It is usually performed as an outpatient procedure under local anesthesia. A large 16 gauge needle is used (as is available in some blood transfusion sets) to create multiple puncture sites and sectioning of the cord using the needle bevel. PNF is contraindicated in infiltrating disorders that would cause progressive and extensive contractures; rapid recurrence in a young patient, difficult to access multiple cords, long-standing digital disease that would cause contractures additionally in other structures and postsurgical recurrence.
- *Regional fasciectomy (open fasciectomy):* It is used to manage severe cases of DC. It is an outpatient procedure performed under local anesthesia. An incision is made over the diseased cord and direct visualization of the cord and neurovascular structures is possible. The offending cord is divided at a point immediately underlying the skin incision. Fasciotomy is usually most successful for MCP flexion contracture. The recovery is rapid, but the recurrence rate is high. Open fasciotomy is usually reserved for patients who cannot tolerate a more extensive procedure.
- *Limited fasciectomy* ***(Figs. 18A and B)****:* Popularized by Hueston (Hueston 1961), in this procedure, only the involved fascia is removed, preserving the overlying skin. This is the most widely used technique. Skin incisions may be transverse, longitudinal, or diagonal/zigzag with Z-plasty, Y-V-plasty and Bruner-type zigzag incision.
- *Extensive radical fasciectomy:* This involves extensive resection of the palmar and digital fascia. This technique though portended to be more successful due to extensive release of the pathological tissue but the recurrence rates have been similar to limited fasciectomy but with significantly higher complication rates. Patients are also prone to prolonged postoperative edema and stiffness.
- *Dermofasciectomy:* Now is known as the open palm technique (McCash 1964) **(Fig. 19)**. Here excision of the fascia and overlying skin is done. The wounds may be closed using skin grafts or left open. Skin grafts may reduce disease recurrence. Because of the radical nature of this procedure, it is usually reserved for patients with recurrent or severe disease.
    - The technique involves making two incisions, one from the DIP joint of the affected digit to the distal palmar flexion crease joined to a transverse palmar incision forming an "L" shape.
    - A selective fasciectomy is done with partial closure of the incision site to maintain some flexibility. The open portion is then covered with a full-thickness skin graft harvested from the hypothenar eminence. Padded dressing is applied with support to the skin graft and an extension splint is maintained to prevent any recurrence of contracture.

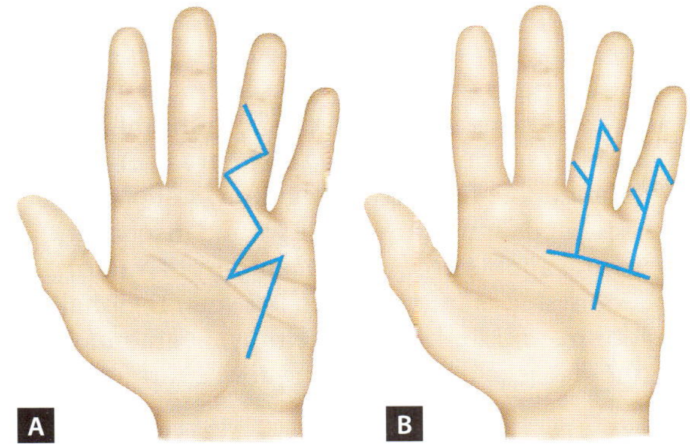

Figs. 18A and B: Limited fasciectomy approaches: (A) Hueston's and (B) Skoog's approaches.

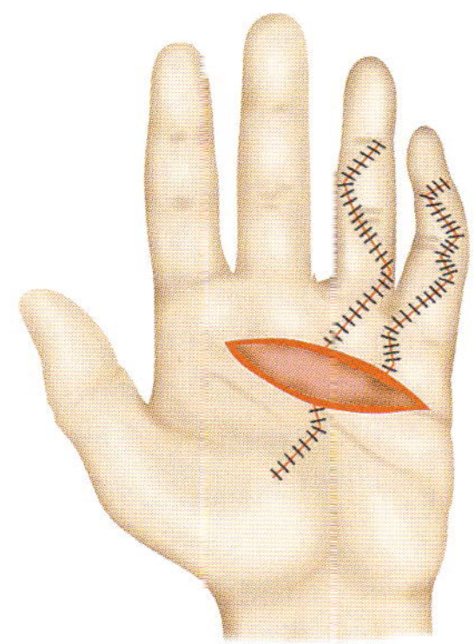

Fig. 19: Dermofasciectomy (McCash technique): The wound is kept open and covered with split thickness skin graft for secondary healing.

- In another technique, the harvested graft is applied after 4 days in another setting whence some vascularity and granulation tissue develops at the open raw surface. This also gives advantage of performing the first wound inspection simultaneously and then closing the wound for adequate time to allow graft to settle. The palm is resplinted for next 1 week till wound inspection.

- Segmental aponeurectomy/fasciotomy of Moermans is a procedure that is intermediate between regional (open) fasciotomy and limited fasciectomy. Segments (1 cm in length) of fascia are excised to relieve contractures albeit partially.
- *Amputation:* Sometimes, the contracture is so severe as to form an unyielding stricture of rolled up finger into palm that precludes any other function from the hand including activities of daily living. In such severe and neglected cases that often present late or else in multiple recurrences after surgery amputation may be indicated. The threshold is particularly low for little finger. Amputation is by no means any benign surgery and acceptance may be low particularly due to complications such as neuroma formation, neurogenic pain, increased stump sensitivity, development of reflex sympathetic dystrophy, reduced grip strength, and even proximal recurrence (1%) of disease. The cosmetic or psychological issues always exist with amputation.
- *Joint fusion:* This is considered a more cosmetic and ethical procedure to amputation. PIP fusion is a useful alternative to amputation. This is however achieved by shortening bone ends to account for the tight volar structures and then fused in a functional position.

Postoperative management: Early postoperative physiotherapy is required to prevent a stiff hand in these elderly patients. A static dorsal forearm splint with fingers strapped in extension is beneficial. A minimum of 3 months of splintage, followed by night splints for another 3 months is required.

FIRST METACARPOPHALANGEAL JOINT ULNAR COLLATERAL LIGAMENT INJURY (GAMEKEEPER'S THUMB AND SKIER'S THUMB)

Bertil Stener described a distinct instability of the first MCP joint caused by an insufficiency of the ulnar collateral ligament (UCL) in the MCP of the thumb.

Gamekeeper thumb and Skier's thumb: The term was first used by Campbell in Scottish gamekeepers who used to kill wounded rabbits by a special method. They used to lever the neck of rabbit by extending it against their thumb. Over a period of time the UCL would give way due to repetitive attrition and elongation. This UCL injury is chronic and results from repetitive actions. The ligament gets elongated, degenerated, and finally gives way. The entity is different from "Skier's thumb" that represents acute rupture of UCL of the thumb MCP joint. The term was first coined in Europe where forced thumb abduction occurred from falling on the outstretched hand while holding a ski pole.

Stener observed and detailed on the specific lesion where rupture of the distal UCL of thumb MCP joint is associated with simultaneous interposition of the adductor aponeurosis. The aponeurosis interposes between the site of distal attachment of the ruptured ligament and the detached ligament. The separation of ruptured ends of the ligament from bone prevents ligamentous healing and restoration of joint stability. This interposition is common in both gamekeeper and Skier's thumb specifically prominent in the later. Only in lesions where the adductor aponeurosis interposition occurs are called Stener lesion.

Pathoanatomy

The UCL of the thumb has two components: (1) the accessory and (2) the proper. UCL proper gets taut in flexion and loose in extension and vice versa for the accessory UCL. Both have to be completely injured for prominent instability but volar plate resists abduction even with complete UCL injury. For complete instability the volar plate also has to be injured. UCL inherently provides lateral support and prevents volar subluxation of the MCP joint also. This stability is vital for key pinch, tip pinch, and thumb opposition. In Skier's thumb and most of the gamekeeper's thumb, the distal attachment of the UCL is usually avulsed from the proximal phalanx of the thumb **(Fig. 20)**. Severed distal end gets caught under the adductor aponeurosis and gets separated from bone precluding healing (the classical Stener lesion). The severed ligament then folds on itself and loses its anatomical relationship and hence function (stability). Adductor aponeurosis serves as an active restraint to thumb abduction but has no passive role in MCP stability, so the MCP becomes unstable and symptomatic.

It should be understood that not every UCL injury will have a Stener lesion. Creation of Stener lesion requires significant radial deviation of phalanx (60° and more) along with tears of both proper and accessory collateral ligaments and volar plate in order for the ligament to be displaced above the adductor aponeurosis. This is the reason why gamekeeper's thumb will have less chances of having Stener lesion **(Fig. 21)**.

Clinical Presentation

Acute injury: Though disabling and painful this is a better counterpart to chronic instability as far as treatment is concerned. The patient presents with:

- Painful, swollen, and ecchymotic thumb MCP joint
- Palpation of a lump (the distal end of the ruptured UCL) on the ulnar aspect of the thumb MCP is highly suggestive of a Stener lesion.

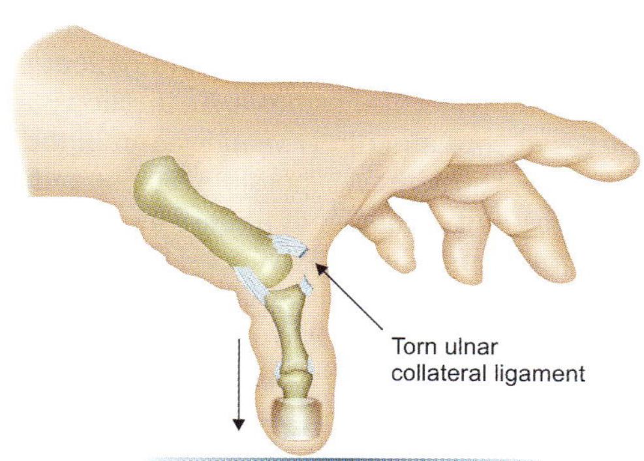

Fig. 20: Gamekeeper's thumb.

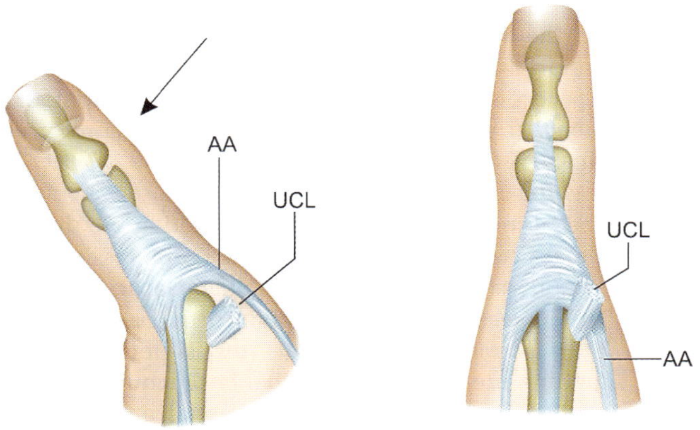

Fig. 21: Creation of the Stener lesion. (AA: adductor aponeurosis; UCL: ulnar collateral ligament)

Chronic insufficiency: This is a difficult part to treat as the ligamentous attachments are elongated and attenuated so that even with reconstruction there are chances of persistent laxity and instability. Recurrent injuries are also bound to happen. The clinical features and associated abnormalities of the chronic insufficiency are as follows:

- *Instability of MCP:* Proximal phalanx tends to volarly subluxate and rotate
- Medial joint line opening with thumb abduction
- Pain on the inner aspect of thumb (ulnar side)
- Dorsal expansion may attenuate and allow extensor pollicis longus (EPL) to shift ulnarly, compromising its extension effect on the joint.

Radiology

Plain anteroposterior (AP) and lateral radiographs may demonstrate bony chip avulsion (better prognosis). Valgus stress testing though intriguing is contraindicated as it may theoretically turn a nondisplaced disruption into a displaced Stener-type lesion. On a radiograph instability is indicated with radial deviation >40° in extension and deviation >20° in flexion. More than 3 mm of volar subluxation of the proximal phalanx also indicates gross instability.

Magnetic Resonance Imaging

For a strong suspicion of Stener lesion one can get an MRI from a dedicated center as most radiologist might still miss the lesion.

Classification (Louis and Colleagues)

- *Type I:* Nondisplaced avulsion injury.
- *Type II:* Displaced fracture of the ulnar aspect of the base of the proximal phalanx.
- *Type III:* Ligament strain. If resistance is felt as the thumb is radially deviated <35°, the patient most likely has a type III ligament injury.
- *Type IV:* Complete UCL tear. The thumb deviates radially >35° as it is stressed (never go beyond 40–50°). A type IV injury should be treated surgically, as it may reflect the presence of a Stener-type lesion.

BOX 2: The surgical steps for ligament repair/reconstruction of Stener lesion.

- S-shaped incision made over the dorsum of the thumb metacarpophalangeal (MCP) joint.
- Preserve any superficial radial nerve branches.
- The displaced ulnar collateral ligament (UCL) is identified at the proximal edge of the adductor aponeurosis. The ligament is held in a displaced position by the proximal edge of the adductor aponeurosis.
- The adductor aponeurosis is incised longitudinally parallel and just ulnar to the extensor pollicis longus (EPL) tendon, and elevated from the underlying capsule.
- A longitudinal capsulotomy is performed.
- A midsubstance tear may be repaired with a 3-0 nonabsorbable suture (uncommon). The results are also poor as the sutures usually do not hold well and there is bunching and shortening of the ligament.
- If avulsed from the distal insertion site the proximal phalanx is roughened and prepared for reattachment of the ligament using a suture anchor (preferable) or a pullout suture.
- The MCP joint then is held in position using K-wire in 20° of flexion and slight ulnar deviation prior to suture tying.
- The volar plate is repaired to the reinserted UCL to restore accessory UCL function.
- For a type 2 injury, tension band fixation without shattering the fragment is done.
- For chronic injuries, if there is significant arthritis of the joint then an arthrodesis is a prudent option.
- For a chronic ligament lesion without arthritis it is imperative to maintain the tension by imbricating the ligament or if the tissue is frail then better to reconstruct the ligament using pa maris longus/EPL/plantaris/flexor carpi radialis (FCR) tendon graft. This may be combined with adductor tendon advancement. An adductor advancement consists of relocating the adductor insertion distally to increase stability.

- *Type V:* Represents avulsion of the volar plate but no UCL injury. This injury is stable in flexion and is treated with a thumb spica splint or cast for 4 weeks.

Management

In the presence of Stener lesion, only operative intervention will allow apposition and healing of the traumatically displaced ligament in an anatomic position. In the absence of Stener lesion splinting of the thumb such that the torn ligament ends are reduced may produce healing and restoration of joint stability in selected patients—one should be fully sure that there is no Stener lesion and it is only a type 1 or type 3 injury.

The indications of surgical intervention (one should be a bit more biased to it):

- Gross radiographic instability
- Presence of palpable torn ligament ends (Stener lesion)
- Type 4 injury
- Type 2 injury (relative) as better and secure fixation would help early mobilization.

The surgical steps for ligament repair or reconstruction are presented in **Box 2**.

Postoperative regime: Wound inspection is done as a routine. K-wire is removed at 5 weeks and the thumb spica cast is removed. Active motion is begun by 6 weeks with joint mobilization. Abduction stress is avoided for approximately 3 months.

Complications of surgery include:

- Radial sensory nerve neurapraxia
- Stiffness of the thumb IP and MCP joints
- Recurrent instability

THUMB CARPOMETACARPAL JOINT ARTHRITIS (BASAL JOINT ARTHRITIS)

The CMC or trapeziometacarpal joint of the thumb is a saddle-shaped joint and allows a wide range of movement in three planes. Thus, it is also known as nature's universal joint. This increase in mobility, however, makes it prone to degeneration **(Fig. 22)**. The prevalence of basal thumb arthritis increases with age as for other degenerative diseases of joints and is seen predominantly in postmenopausal women. The female:male ratio is 6:1 (33% of postmenopausal women affected). The etiology is unclear but increased incidence is seen in patients with osteoarthritic diathesis. Other identified aggravating factors are presented in **Box 3**.

Clinical Features

- Pain localized to the base of the thumb: It may radiate to the thenar eminence and the MCP joint.
- Pain is increased by activity particularly after excessive use involving forceful pinch.
- Dorsoradial prominence of the thumb metacarpal base.
- Crepitus evident on examination implies erosion of the articular cartilage.
- Weakness or loss of motion is commonly reported in advanced disease.

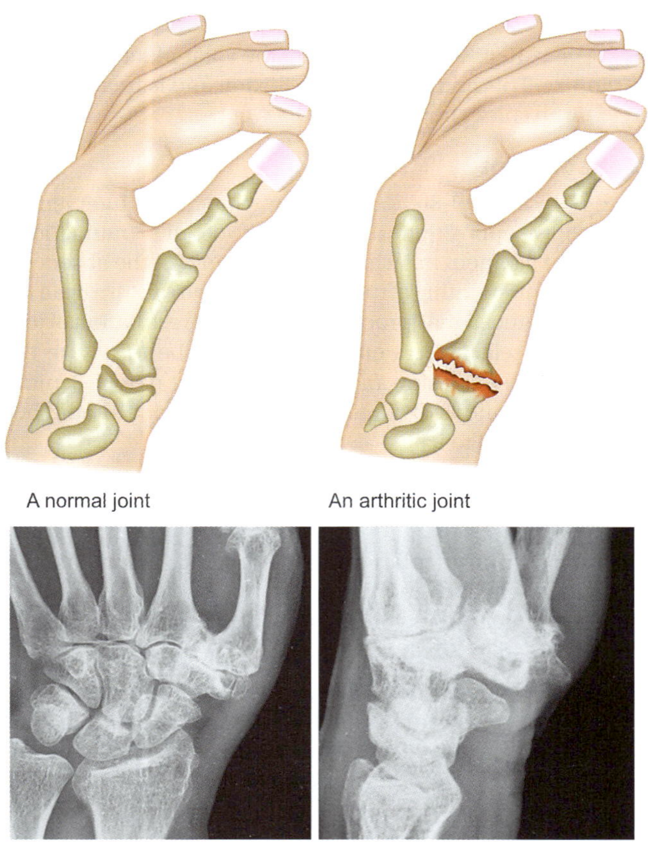

Fig. 22: Basal joint arthritis. The first carpometacarpal (CMC) joint space is reduced with development of osteophytes and subluxation of the joint. Illustrations depicting the normal CMC joint (left image) and the arthritic joint (right image).

- With increasing instability of metacarpal inability to abduct the thumb and a deterioration of hand function are important disabilities.
- With progressive adduction of the first metacarpal and compensatory hyperextension of the MCP joint produces a swan-neck deformity.
- *Aggravating maneuvers:*
  - The "grind" test is performed by rotating the thumb metacarpal base while applying axial compression (i.e., compression along the plane of the metacarpal bone): This increases pain due to rubbing of the bare surfaces.
  - The "distraction" or "torque" test is performed by rotating the thumb metacarpal base while applying gentle axial traction. A positive test indicates synovitis associated with milder disease as a result of traction on an inflamed joint capsule. It is much less specific.

Associated Conditions

- Carpal tunnel syndrome
- Scaphotrapezial arthrosis
- Trigger digits
- MCP hyperextension
- Tenosynovitis of the wrist

Radiology

Standard views rule out other osseous abnormalities and localize the areas of arthritis. Finding arthritis in associated joints has important implications. Basal joint stress views (Robert's view) can also be useful in assessing the laxity of the basal joint. There is however poor correlation between radiological and clinical features. Classification (radiology based) of basal joint arthritis of thumb is presented in **Table 2**.

There is currently no indication of ultrasonography or MRI for this condition.

Differential Diagnosis

Scaphotrapeziotrapezoidal (STT) arthritis.

BOX 3: The etiological/aggravating factors for thumb carpometacarpal joint arthritis.

- *Excessive basal joint laxity:* Ligamentous laxity is common in young women.
- *Previous trauma to the thumb:* Rolando or Bennett fractures of metacarpal if left malunited renders the joint more prone to arthritis.
- *Inflammatory arthritis, such as rheumatoid arthritis:* One-third of the patients have carpometacarpal (CMC) joint involvement.
- *Idiopathic:* It is most common and the disease development spontaneously points to some genetic predisposition.

TABLE 2: Radiological classification of basal joint arthritis.

Stage	*Description*
1	Normal trapeziometacarpal joint contour with <1/3rd joint subluxation
2	Trapeziometacarpal joint narrowing visible on plain radiographs and degenerative osteophytes or loose bodies <2 mm. Instability of joint is evident on stress views as ≥1/3rd joint subluxation
3	Trapeziometacarpal joint narrowing associated with findings of advanced degeneration like subchondral sclerosis, osteophytes or loose bodies >2 mm, ≥1/3rd joint subluxation
4	Advanced disease of trapeziometacarpal and also scaphotrapezial joint

Treatment

Initial treatment of basal thumb arthritis of any stage is:

- Activity modifications
- Rest: Specifically designed well-fitting splints should be given
- Nonsteroidal anti-inflammatory drugs to reduce pain from inflammation
- Thenar intrinsic and extrinsic muscle strengthening exercises.

Corticosteroid injections of the trapeziometacarpal joint can be useful when conservative measures have not worked. Pain relief is quite prominent but duration is variable. Repetitive injections should be avoided as there is evidence of collagen quality deterioration with repeated steroid injections.

Cartilage forming drugs such as glucosamine and hyaluronan have no defined benefit but an occasional patient unwilling for surgery may be given a trial till he accepts the surgery. Hyaluronidase injection has been tried but the relief duration, efficacy, etc., has not been completely determined.

Hyaluronic acid viscosupplementation is also an option but the complete efficacy of this treatment is unknown. This therapy may be associated with allergic reactions and synovial granulomatous inflammation.

If there is no improvement of symptoms after 2 months, surgical options can be given to patient.

Indications for Surgery

Persistent pain and functional disability after failed conservative treatment in the compliant patient is the most important general indication for surgery but none should be pressed up on the patient.

The various surgical options include joint preservation surgery and joint sacrificing surgery including joint replacement surgery or joint excision.

Joint preservation surgery: This is the first line of surgical approach that is tried in patients who fail conservative trial. The options include:

- *Ligament reconstruction:* This is based on stabilizing the painful, hypermobile trapeziometacarpal joint by reconstructing the palmar beak ligament with a portion of the FCR tendon. This is however suitable only for early disease and may slow the progression of disease. The surgery may be complicated with stiffness.
- *Osteotomy:* This is based on shifting the load bearing region reducing the symptoms with activities. Extension- or extension-abduction osteotomy of metacarpal improves thumb stability against dorsal translation. 20–30° wedge from dorsal cortex is removed and metacarpal refixed.
    - *Cheema osteotomy:* Osteotomy of the trapezium is an alternative.
- *Arthroscopy:* This is a specialized technique where various pathologies are addressed intra-articularly. Arthroscopic synovectomy, capsular shrinkage, and hemitrapeziectomy with or without tendon interposition may be done to improve the joint stability and remove disease.
- *Distraction arthroplasty:* Not commonly practiced.

Joint sacrificing surgery: These have been the standards for management of advanced arthritis. They basically work by removing the disease and relieving symptoms.

- *Trapeziectomy:* This may be done alone or combined with interposition of a spacer (autogenous or artificial) with suspension using tendon (LRTI—ligament reconstruction and tendon interposition). Interposition or ligament suspension has provided no concrete benefit in large trials over simple trapeziectomy (excision arthroplasty) but is associated with increased complications **(Fig. 23A)**. Moreover if at all interposition is preferred by surgeon then autogenous materials are better than artificial implants that increase complications and increase the cost. The most definite indication for ligament reconstruction is a patient with advanced arthritis with fixed adduction of the metacarpal and hyperextension of the MCP joint. Correction of the adducted metacarpal base with a tendon reconstruction readily corrects the adduction once the trapezium is removed. The various methods for stabilizing the metacarpal include:
    - Temporary K-wire fixation
    - Suspension of metacarpal using FCR tendon weaves **(Figs. 23B and 24)**
    - Suspension using APL

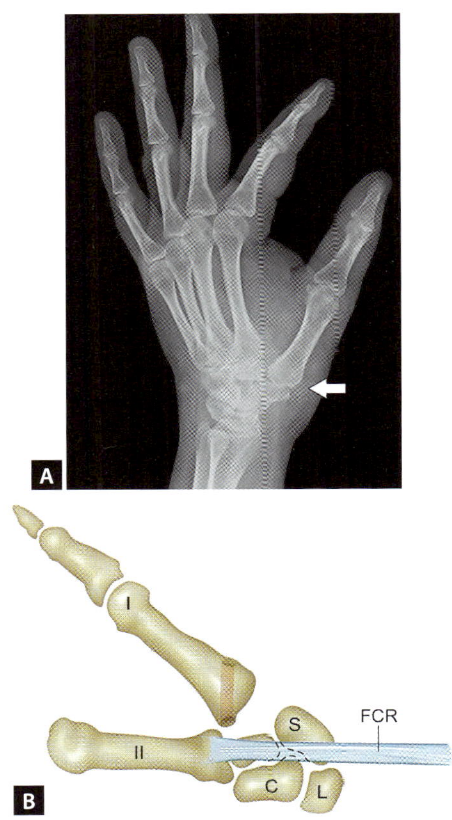

Figs. 23A and B: Simple excision arthroplasty often leads to proximal migration of the first metacarpal (A) into the void (white arrow) despite putting tendon spacers or so. Hence some sort of suspension arthroplasty mechanism is needed to maintain length adequately like the flexor carpi radialis (FCR) weave technique (B).

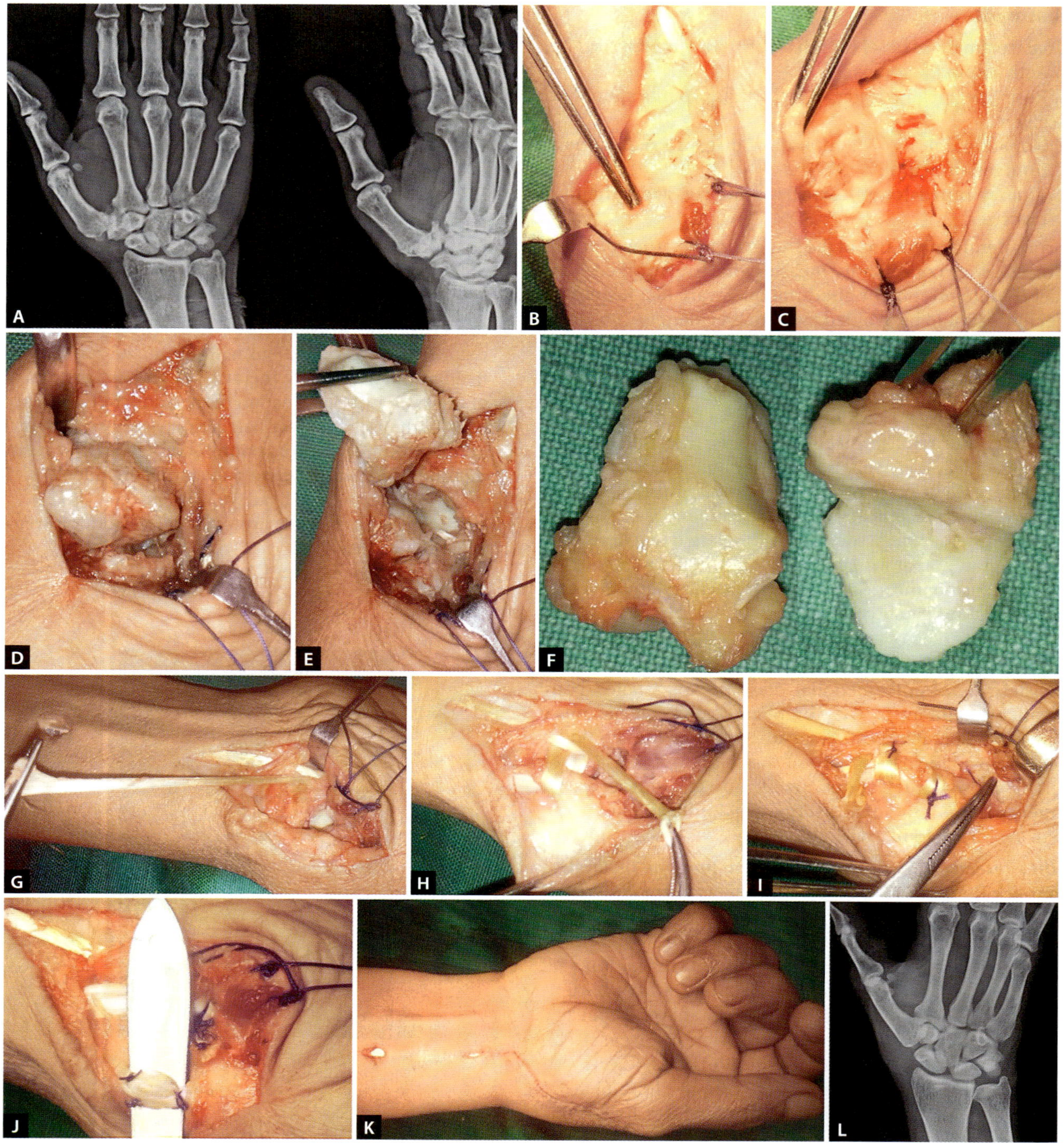

Figs. 24A to L: Flexor carpi radialis (FCR) weave suspension arthroplasty for management of basal joint arthritis (Burton and Pellegrini technique). (A) The preoperative radiographs for this symptomatic patient; (B) Localization of the arthritic joint; (C) Exposure of diseased joint; (D) Exposing the diseased trapezium; (E) Excising it completely in toto; (F) The excised diseased trapezium bone; (G) Harvesting partially (radial half) of the FCR tendon percutaneously; (H) Weaving the tendon in double figure-of-eight fashion across the abductor pollicis longus (APL) and remaining FCR tendon; (I) Distal advancement of the APL tendon; (J) Shortening by double breasting the extensor pollicis longus (EPL) tendon; (K) Closure of the capsule and wound; (L) Postoperative radiograph after 4 months.

- Suture-button suspensionplasty **(Fig. 25)**—"mini tight-rope" method. Here two metallic buttons joined together with several strands of fiber-wire sutures are introduced via drill holes in the thumb and index metacarpals and oppose the ulnar surface of the index metacarpal and the radial surface of the thumb metacarpal tethering the two metacarpals together (similar to cross-pinning metacarpals to prevent collapse in comminuted fractures).

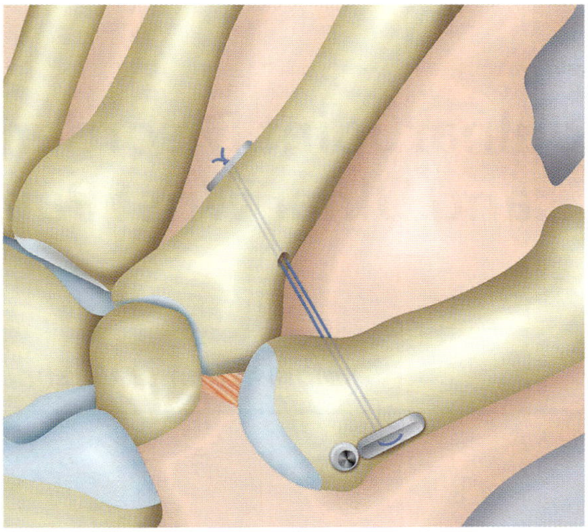

Fig. 25: The suture-button technique for preventing proximal migration of the metacarpal.

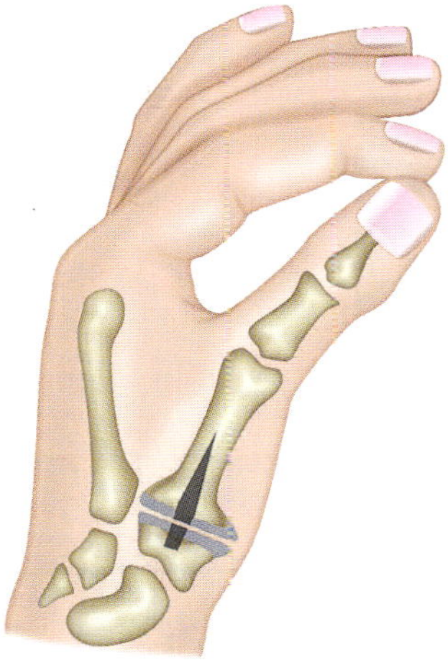

Fig. 26: Joint arthroplasty for management of carpometacarpal (CMC) arthritis, usually surface replacement options are chosen but at only selected centers.

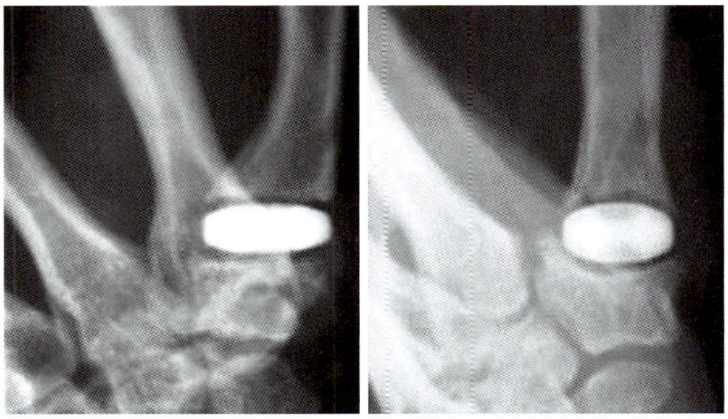

Fig. 27: Spacer arthroplasty for basal joint arthritis.

- *Trapeziometacarpal arthrodesis:* This is not a favorable option as thumb fixed in abduction, loss of opposition and an inability to place the hand flat on the table is of concern to many patients. Also there is potential to provoke arthritis in the adjacent STT or MCP joints so basal joint arthritis associated with other joint arthrosis is an absolute contraindication to arthrodesis.
- *Joint replacement:* This is aimed to provide a pain free, mobile stable joint. Total joint replacement gives faster pain relief and early function compared to any other procedure. The biggest challenge is reproducing the anatomy of "universal saddle joint" with that of ball in socket or other joints. Uncemented prosthesis has been in favor. Newer nonmetallic implants have been recently available for management of CMC **(Fig. 26)** arthritis like:
  - *Pyrolytic carbons:* This has been introduced as a hemiarthroplasty where the trapezium is replaced. These have low wear rates and devices are available also for MCP and IP joints. They have added advantage of phospholipids adhering to the surface improving the lubrication.
  - *Artelon spacer:* These are T-shaped biodegradable insert composed of polycaprolactone-based polyurethane urea. They are more of resurfacing arthroplasty (resecting 2 mm of bone on either side) that maintain the soft tissues around the joint. The joint capsule is augmented by their spacer action **(Fig. 27)**.

The difficulty with arthroplasty is the technical requirement, cost, and inevitable later loosening.

CONCLUSION

- Various attrition related, overuse related, and friction syndromes around the hand and wrist deserve special mention and description. Most of the tendinosis are managed conservatively for 6 weeks to 2 months whence with good relief the treatment is continued. Some definitely improve with steroid injections while only uncommon nonresponders need surgical release.
- Dupuytren's contracture is an unresolved issue for which adequate management is still not possible. The contractures are mostly progressive and cannot be halted medically. Surgical release is the most common method of correction of contractures provided arthritic changes or joint subluxations have not developed.
- Basal joint arthritis is a common disability seen in old age, more so in post-traumatic cases. Symptomatic patients are initially managed by rehabilitation but for progressive disability and unrelieved symptoms, surgical management by various methods gives adequate relief. Suspension arthroplasty provides reasonable relief from pain albeit with some loss of power.

CHAPTER

114 Distal Radioulnar Joint Disorders and Ulnar Wrist Pain

Manish Kumar Varshney

INTRODUCTION

The understanding of distal radioulnar joint (DRUJ) is very limited as this had been long considered a minor joint with limited contribution to wrist function. The development of sports and unusual sporting activity has led to increased focus on the chronic problems in this class and a review of anatomy and functional relation. Still due to late introduction into orthopedic community the association with pathogenesis has largely remained elusive till the beginning of the century whence it was termed "low back pain of the wrist".

Evolutionary, the DRUJ is a recent addition. Primitive wrist appeared in primitive fish crossopterygia 400 million years ago. This metamorphosed to multiple carpal bone—wrist in amphibian *Eryops* but was nonfunctional. Even in the reptiles, the wrist remained nonfunctional as ulna was the main weight-bearing bone. With the bipedal gait of hominids mobile wrist evolved with proximal retraction of ulna, development of triangular fibrocartilaginous complex and ulnocarpal meniscus and development of synovial DRUJ.

ANATOMY

The DRUJ per se comprises of following structures **(Fig. 1)**:

- Bony articulation of the joint (sigmoid notch of ulna and articulating ulna head "articular seat")—a synovial joint. Radial sigmoid notch is shallow and ulna head is asymmetric. Sigmoid notch is triangular with a dorsal, palmar and distal (carpal margin). Articular cartilage on ulna head covers 90–135° arc. The radius of curvature of ulnar head is 10 mm while for sigmoid notch is 15 mm so they are concentric. This nonconcentric location causes rotational and significant sliding movement at DRUJ (translation of 2 mm volar and 5 mm dorsal in pronosupination). This volar position of ulnar head during supination and dorsal position during pronation produces a "centrode of rotation" rather than a single center of rotation. One must remember that it is the radius that rotates around the ulna, and hence it is the radius that dislocates/subluxates and not the ulna! The bony articulation is unstable as the sigmoid notch has inclination of 7.7° from longitudinal axis while head of ulna has inclination of 21° **(Fig. 2)**. The articulation is primarily stabilized by the palmar and dorsal radioulnar ligaments.

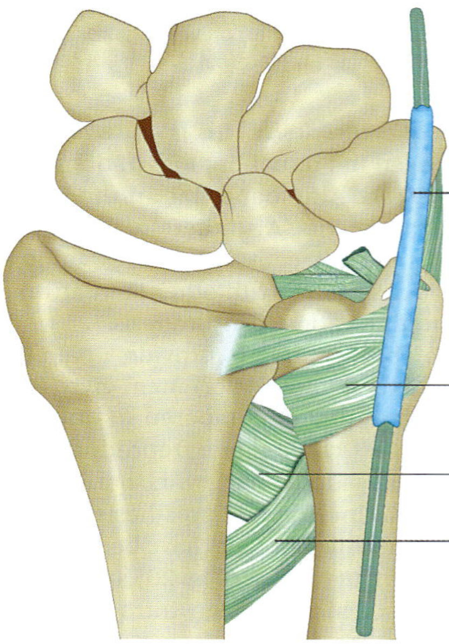

Fig. 1: The bony and ligamentous anatomy of distal radioulnar joint (DRUJ), volar view of the DRUJ.

- Interosseous membrane (IOM) of the forearm distally (syndesmosis).
- Soft tissue support system of DRUJ: These comprise of dynamic and static supports:
  - *Static supports of DRUJ:*
    - Triangular fibrocartilage complex (TFCC, **Figs. 3A and B**): This is an extensive, complicated, and recently studied in detail system comprising of structures originating from dorsal lip of sigmoid notch and attach to the ulnar base of 5th metacarpal and ulnar styloid (complex 3D structure). It comprises of five predominant structures:
      - Triangular fibrocartilage (TFC)—the disk having three components (see below)

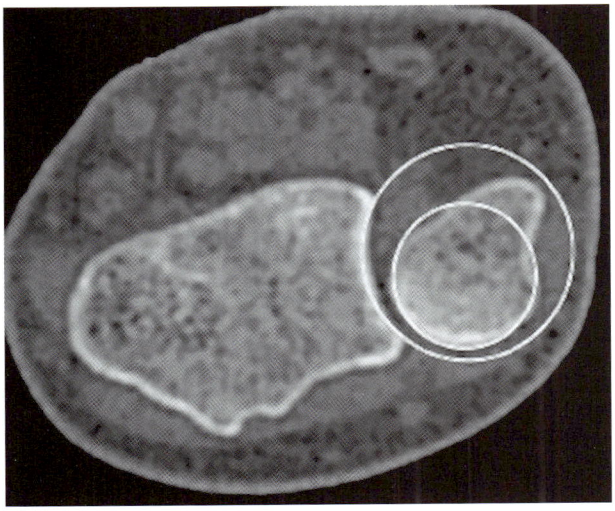

Fig. 2: Sigmoid notch ulna: The ulnar seat has a smaller radius (small circle) compared to the sigmoid notch.

- Ulnocarpal ligaments (two)—these comprise of ulnolunate and ulnotriquetral ligaments. The ligaments form a "V" configuration originating from the base of ulnar styloid (apex of "V") and attaching to lunate or triquetrum distally.
- ♦ IOM—transmits force between radius and ulna.
- • *Dynamic stabilizers:*
  - ♦ Extensor carpi ulnaris (ECU)—tension in supination provides stability
  - ♦ Infratendinous extensor retinaculum
  - ♦ Pronator quadratus—acts in conjunction with the distal oblique fibers of IOM to provide stability in supination.

Detailed anatomy of TFC (do not confuse with broader term TFCC): It has both a central and a peripheral component **(Fig. 4)**. It is bound dorsally and palmarly by the thickened collagenous bands called the radioulnar ligaments respectively **(Fig. 5)**. These dorsal and volar

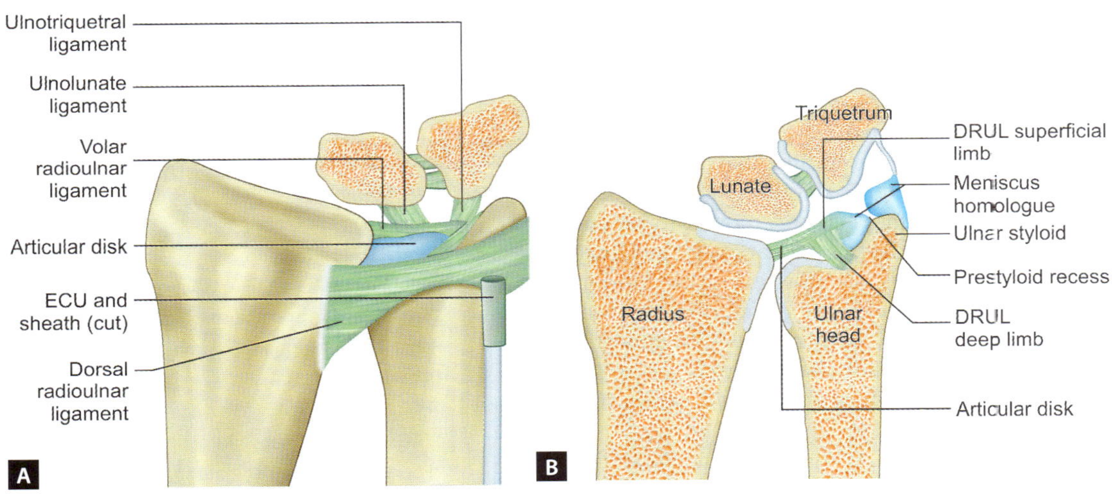

Figs. 3A and B: TFCC anatomy: (A) Gross anatomy in 3D illustration; (B) Illustration in cross-section. (DRUL: distal radioulnar ligament; ECU: extensor carpi ulnaris; TFCC: triangular fibrocartilage complex)

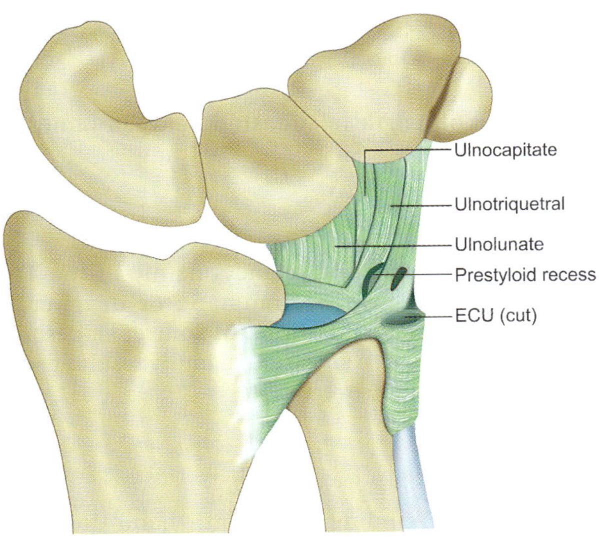

Fig. 4: The anatomy of TFC. (ECU: extensor carpi ulnaris; TFC: triangular fibrocartilage)

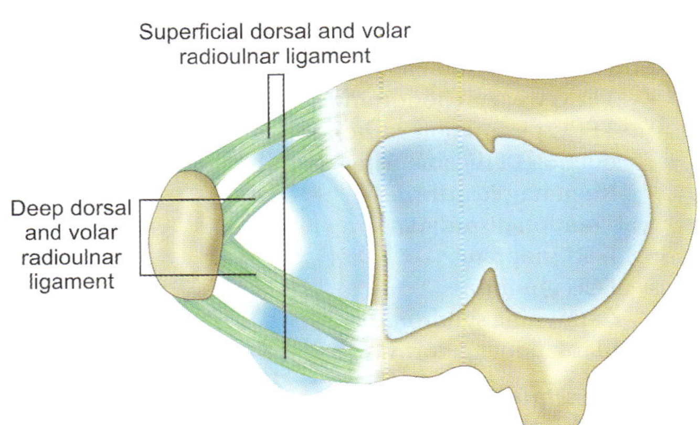

Fig. 5: The anatomical disposition of dorsal and palmar radioulnar ligaments.

radioulnar ligaments have superficial and deep (ligamentum subcruentum) components. These ligaments converge ulnarly toward the ulnar styloid encompassing the peripheral margins of TFC to form a triangle with base at the sigmoid notch (incisura ulnaris radii) and apex at the ulnar styloid (basistyloid fovea). The central portion is the fibrocartilage disk that transmits the compressive loads across. The dorsal ligaments provide stability in pronation and vice versa.

Functions of Distal Radioulnar Joint

- This joint is responsible for contribution to rotation of the forearm (supination and pronation) that occurs in conjunction with radiocapitellar joint, proximal radioulnar joint, and IOM. The combined rotation is 170–180°.
- Force transmission—20% of force across wrist is transmitted through ulnocarpal joint.

PATHOLOGY AT DISTAL RADIOULNAR JOINT AND PATHOGENESIS

The DRUJ may give rise to pain or instability in conditions such as arthritis and sports injuries. Hard manual laborers may additionally develop chronic instability. These problems arise either from injury (fractures), repetitive minor injury, or from degenerative arthritis. Symptoms may additionally arise from involvement of dynamic stabilizers and extensor tenosynovitis. The distal ulna becomes more prominent on the dorsum of the wrist during pronation (translatory movement; see above). This creates extensor tendon irritation and may lead to weakening or tendon rupture. **DRUJ disorders** have been succinctly classified by Bowers; a modified version is presented below as follows:

- Acute fracture—dislocation/subluxation [Galeazzi fracture dislocation **(Fig. 6)**]
- Acute joint injury mainly TFCC injury (*see* the classifications of TFCC tears in **Table 1**):
  - Central perforation
  - Distal avulsion
  - Radial or ulnar avulsion with or without fracture
- Chronic or late-appearing joint disruption mostly following malunited distal radius fractures:
  - Ulnocarpal abutment (and impingement) syndrome
  - Sigmoid notch or ulnar head deformity
- Chronic joint instability:
  - TFCC wear ± chondromalacia
  - TFCC perforation ± chondromalacia and/or lunotriquetral (LT) ligament injury and/or ulnocarpal arthritis
  - Rheumatoid arthritis
- ECU tendon disorders:
  - ECU snapping
  - ECU tendinitis
  - Caput ulna syndrome
- Fixed rotational deformity

Chronic instability of DRUJ can arise from three main aspects: These include

1. Fractures and their malunions (distal radius) and nonunions (ulna styloid)

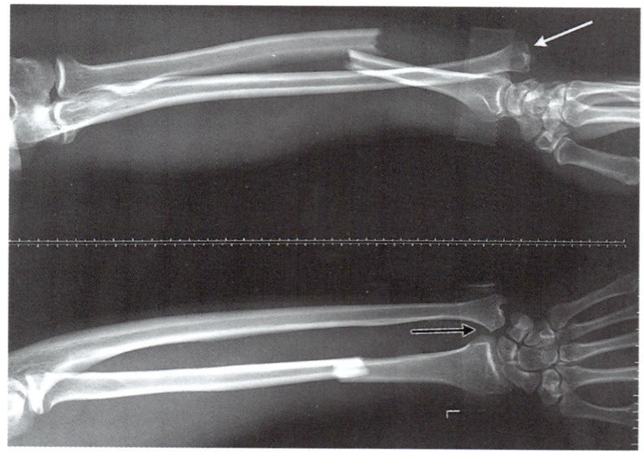

Fig. 6: The Galeazzi fracture dislocation by definition involves fracture of distal third radius typically with distal radioulnar joint (DRUJ) disruption. The triangular fibrocartilage complex (TFCC) is acutely disrupted causing dorsal ulnar head subluxation/dislocation. In this left forearm injury, there is radius shaft fracture with dorsal dislocation of the ulnar head (prominent on lateral projection; white arrow), note that the radiograph should also evaluate the elbow joint either in the same film or a separate film. The anteroposterior (AP) view shows acute distal ulna migration and widening at the distal radioulnar joint (black arrow).

TABLE 1: The classification of TFCC disorders (adapted from Palmer AK).

Type	*Description*
I	Acute traumatic tears
IA	Central TFC perforation
IB	Peripheral ulnar side TFCC tear (± ulna styloid fracture)
IC	Distal TFCC disruption (disruption from distal UC ligaments)
ID	Radial TFCC disruption (± sigmoid notch fracture)
II	Degenerative
IIA	TFCC wear
IIB	TFCC wear with lunate and/or ulnar chondromalacia
IIC	TFCC perforation with lunate and/or ulnar chondromalacia
IID	TFCC perforation with lunate and/or ulnar chondromalacia with LT perforation
IIE	Type IID + ulnocarpal arthritis

(LT: lunotriquetral; TFC: triangular fibrocartilage; TFCC: triangular fibrocartilage complex; UC: ulnocapitate)

2. Alteration of length relationship between radius and ulna:
   - Congenital
   - Traumatic
   - Iatrogenic
3. Chronic ligament insufficiency mainly of the TFCC complex—these can be traumatic or degenerative including rheumatoid arthritis. Melone et al. described TFCC disruption as a spectrum of injury resulting in five stages of increasing severity.

DIAGNOSIS

History

- Patient's age (guiding treatment), hand dominance (indicating pathology and guiding treatment), and occupation (telling pathology).

- Previous injury/problems/surgery, position reproducing pain, history of rheumatoid or osteoarthritis and detailed symptom characteristics.
- Ulnar-sided wrist pain and weakness in grip strength are classically reported in chronic and degenerative disorders.
- "Giving way" or a "clunk" in the wrist is often seen with chronic instabilities. There may be dorsal ulna head subluxation.

Physical Examination

Dorsal swelling indicates:

- Subluxing/dislocated ulnar head
- Caput ulnae syndrome
- Tendinitis
- Synovitis.

Limitation in the range of motion (due to pain or altered biomechanics) is a common finding. Ask the patient to reproduce the pain by positioning wrist. Observe clunk during movements (produced by chronic radial or ulnar-sided detachment of the TFCC) and in position of pain.

Check for grip and pinch strength. Perform special tests to localize TFCC tear and DRUJ pathology.

- The "piano key test"—"balloting" the dorsal ulna head is positive when there is very little resistance to ballottement and volar movement of the ulna head. This indicates DRUJ laxity.
- DRUJ grinding test—the examiner moves the ulnarly deviated wrist in a volar-to-dorsal direction while applying an axial load across the ulnar side of the wrist to transmit load across TFCC which may cause grinding and reproduce pain.
- Radius pull test of Essex-Lopresti—pull the radius proximally in longitudinal direction. Increase in ulnar variance (fluoroscopy) indicates IOM injury. The test was designed to find if there is IOM injury while performing radial head resection. More than 3 mm migration of cut radial neck toward capitellum is significant.
- DRUJ "shuck test" by holding the radius in one hand and the ulna with the other and moving the distal radius in a volar/dorsal direction, feel for crepitus and pain.
- Clunk test—press the radius and ulna together during pronosupination, palpating a clunk during the maneuver is significant and indicates injury to IOM.
- Test for ECU—with hand in ulnar deviation, the wrist is pronosupinated; abnormal motion suggests ECU tendon abnormalities.
- Press test—observe the patient pushing himself up from seated position with the help of affected wrist. This produces ulnar side wrist pain indicates TFCC pathology.

The ECU tendon/sixth extensor compartment should be palpated and evaluated during resisted pronation to identify any subluxation.

Perform a sensory, motor, and vascular assessment of the entire upper extremity.

Clinical Staging of Distal Radioulnar Joint Instability

The DRUJ instability progresses from dynamic to static in four stages:

1. *Stage 1 (dynamic):* The patient complains of a "giving away" sensation with no obvious clinical or radiographic signs.
2. *Stage 2 (secondary dynamic):* In addition to stage 1, clinically one can demonstrate joint subluxation and dislocation.
3. *Stage 3 (static):* Limited motion and pain are the important features. The joint is unstable but can be reduced and plain radiographs demonstrate subluxation and malalignment.
4. *Stage 4 (advanced static):* Limited motion is prominent with fixed deformity. There is increased risk for osteoarthritis development.

Imaging Studies

Plain Radiographs

Posteroanterior, lateral, ulnar deviation, radial deviation views at zero rotation, and posteroanterior and lateral views in full pronation and supination are taken. The following points are observed:

- Forearm rotation (assessed by comparison of the ulnar styloid to the shaft of the ulna and radius).
- Carpal deviation by comparing the position of the lunate with the position of the radius.
- Radioulnar widening
- Ulnar variance—compare with the other side always. The force distributed across the TFCC changes dramatically from 5 to 40% when the ulnar variance changes from –2 to +2.5 mm. Ulnar variance has been possibly linked to wrist arthrosis, Kienböck's disease and ulnar impaction syndrome.
- Ulnar dislocation (measured on true lateral radiographs, true lateral radiographs are judged by projection of pisiform bone over the scaphoid without overlap)—radioulnar distance of 6 mm or more between the most dorsal cortices indicates DRUJ instability. Indirect signs include:
  - 15° dorsal tilt of radius
  - Ulnar styloid fracture
  - Radial shortening of >4 mm
  - Radial inclination <0°
- Carpal height and features of carpal instability
- Wrist arthrosis
- Malunited fractures
- Ulnar styloid fracture and position

Computed Tomography Scan

This is the modality of choice to document DRUJ subluxation/dislocation. Congruity of sigmoid notch can be better evaluated.

Magnetic Resonance Imaging

Magnetic resonance imaging is the modality of choice to evaluate TFCC pathology (early reported rates being 100% sensitive, 90% specific, and accuracy of 97% for detecting TFCC tears). With increasing usage, it has been realized that tear

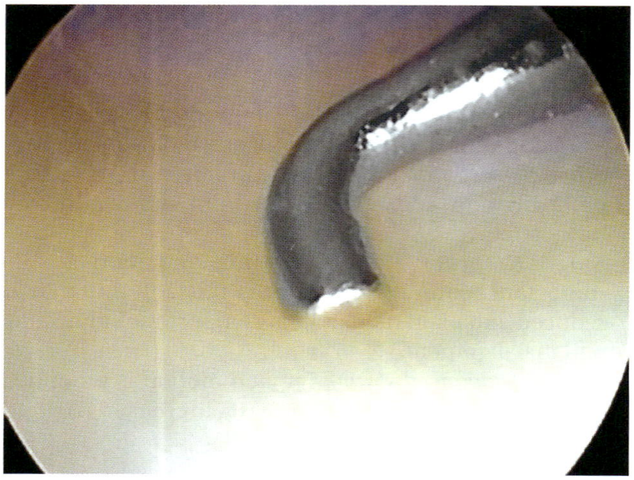

Fig. 7: Trampoline test.

localization and delineation is not as accurate and requires high resolution. Tears of the LT ligament are often missed.

Wrist Arthrography (Arthrogram)

The three compartment ("triple injection") technique has been shown to be the most sensitive wrist arthrogram technique in identifying ligament pathology (considered "gold standard" for TFCC tears); it also sensitively identifies pathology of the radioulnar, midcarpal and radiocarpal joints. The arthrogram is often the next step if plain films show no abnormalities. With the increasing use of wrist arthroscopy, it has been lately realized that arthrograms have a high false-negative rate.

Wrist arthroscopy allows the surgeon to directly visualize the TFCC and other wrist ligaments (I personally consider this to be the gold standard modality). An avulsion of the foveal TFCC insertion can be determined by a loss of the normal trampoline effect (trampoline test; **Fig. 7**), and a displacement of the TFCC radially by pulling on the TFCC using a probe (hook test; **Fig. 8**). The articular surface can be well evaluated and most importantly if central tears are found arthroscopic debridement of TFCC tears can be done simultaneously that relieves symptoms in three-fourths of patients. Peripheral tears are repaired and all this is done through a small hole; reducing fears of wrist stiffness (reflex sympathetic dystrophy excluded), infection and other complications of open surgery. The patients often have a faster return to normal range of motion and strength as compared to patients with an open excision. Slowly the arthroscopy is emerging as the modality of choice for diagnosis of DRUJ disorders.

CLASSIFICATION OF DISTAL RADIOULNAR JOINT INSTABILITY

From the above clinicoradiological correlation, Bowers and others have given a classification of DRUJ instability **(Table 2)**. Bowers has identified four types of instability based on abnormalities within the different structures that make up the DRUJ, while Scheker et al. have classified based on progressive severity.

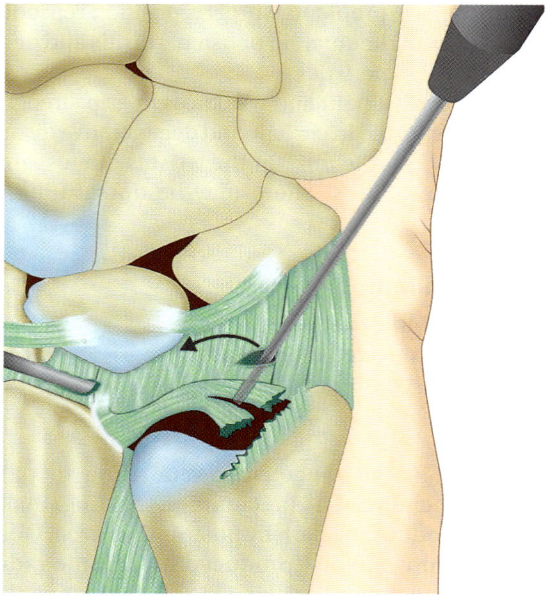

Fig. 8: Arthroscopy: Radial displacement of the triangular fibrocartilage complex (TFCC) by pulling on it using a probe indicates avulsion of the foveal TFCC insertion (hook test).

TABLE 2: Classification of DRUJ instability.

Bowers	***Scheker, Ozer, and Babb***
• *Group 1* has ligamentous defects only. • *Group 2* has loss of ligamentous tension due to loss of intra-articularjoint conformation. • *Group 3* is a combination of ligamentous and articular surface problems. • *Group 4* demonstrates ligamentous deficiency with extra-articular problems, such as distal radius metaphyseal malunion.	• *Stage 1:* TFCC attenuation. • *Stage 2:* TFCC disruption (no DRUJ dislocation or distal radius fracture). • *Stage 3:* TFCC disruption, DRUJ dislocation (no distal radius fracture). • *Stage 4:* TFCC disruption, DRUJ dislocation, fracture (distal radius fracture,malunion). • *Stage 5:* Radial instability following ulnar head resection.

(DRUJ: distal radioulnar joint; TFCC: triangular fibrocartilage complex)

TREATMENT

The management of chronic TFCC injuries is often surgical. Acute injuries that can be reduced congruously should be maintained in supination in an above elbow cast for 6 weeks. Many surgeons prefer arthroscopic TFCC repair intra-articularly when diagnosed early. The typical operative indications are:

- Noncongruous reduction due to soft tissue interposition
- Locked DRUJ
- Persisting DRUJ instability due to fractured volar lip of sigmoid notch

Central tears (TFC tear) are debrided while peripheral tears are repaired often arthroscopically intra-articularly or by open technique **(Figs. 9A and B)**. If successful, this anatomic intra-articular reconstruction may restore stability with minimal loss of motion. The intra-articular repair occasionally fails evidenced by continued instability and painful range of motion. These are managed by various

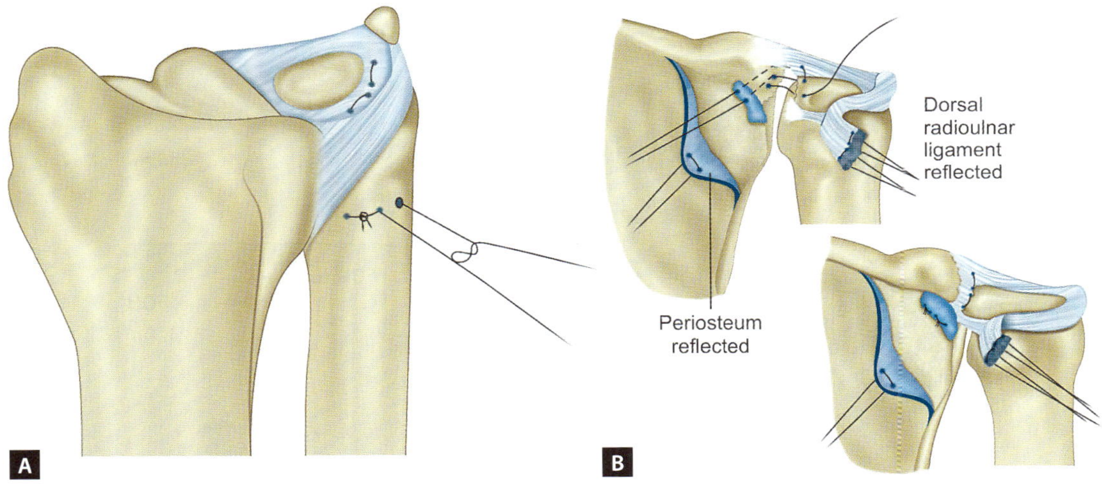

Figs. 9A and B: Open intra-articular triangular fibrocartilage complex (TFCC) repair. (A) Repair of peripheral tears; (B) Repair of radial base avulsion of triangular fibrocartilage (TFC) along with volar radioulnar ligament.

extra-articular soft tissue reconstruction methods. In addition to this reconstruction, the bony abnormalities (malunions and length discrepancies) should be addressed as they may be one of the reasons of recurrent instability. In general the methods of reconstruction involve reconstructing some elements of TFCC by creating ulnocarpal or radioulnar tether (all these are nonanatomic reconstructions).

Following are the Management Options for Acute Injury

- DRUJ instability following acute, isolated dorsal, or volar dislocation—6 weeks of forearm cast in forearm supination. Perform open reduction for irreducible joint and fix provisionally with K-wire that can be removed at 3 weeks.
- Acute distal radius fractures—assess for DRUJ instability using towel clip (perform lateral pull and dorsovolar translation to assess)—fix if unstable with K-wire.
- Ulnar styloid fractures—fix using K-wire of tension band technique.

Following are Some of the Commonly Used Methods for Reconstruction of the Chronic/Recurrent DRUJ Instability without Arthritis

- For **congruent ulnocarpal and radiocarpal joint,** the DRUJ can be successfully stabilized using the following procedures:
  - Anatomical palmaris tendon stabilization procedure of Scheker (1994) for reconstructing the radioulnar ligaments. Technique of Adams and Berger can be used alternatively.
  - Brachioradialis transfer (Gupta)
  - *Herbert plasty* for pure dorsal radioulnar ligament defects—reconstructed by ulnar based flap of extensor retinaculum.

  If the joints are not congruous, then the ligament reconstruction procedures are destined to fail. In such cases, the following techniques are used that either resect the incongruous joint or reconstruct them together.
- Breen and Jupiter **(Fig. 10)** involve both a dorsal and palmar approach. ECU tendon is mobilized dorsally while flexor carpi ulnaris (FCU) tendon is mobilized volarly.
  - Longitudinal and perpendicular tunnels are created in the bone for passing tendons.
  - Tenodesis is created by passing the ECU and FCU tendon.
  - ECU tendon is stabilized dorsally in the retinacular tunnel.
- Bunnell-Boyes reconstruction **(Fig. 11)**: This recreates the ulnocarpal ligament by harvesting FCU and inserting it into distal ulna near to the styloid process. The repair is completed with imbrication of dorsal capsule.
  - The technique can be used in addition to Darrach's procedure to stabilize distal ulna (see below)
  - To reduce dorsal translation of ulna advancement of pronator quadratus (in posterolateral direction) can be done **(Fig. 12)**.
- Osteotomy of bones to correct malposition and/or length discrepancies:
  - Distal radius osteotomy to correct the length and inclination (there is often radial shortening after the malunited radius fractures, **Figs. 13A to E**).
  - Osteotomy of the sigmoid notch where the radial articular surface of DRUJ is abnormally flat.
  - Ulnar osteotomies: For positive ulnar variance ulnar shortening is done, either in the diaphysis or within DRUJ; the former always needs rigid stabilization.
    - Milch procedure—resect a portion of ulnar diaphysis (we use coupled saw blades to create a uniform parallel gap) without causing bone necrosis. Fix them using rigid fixation.
    - Scheker transverse, diagonal or step-cut osteotomy.

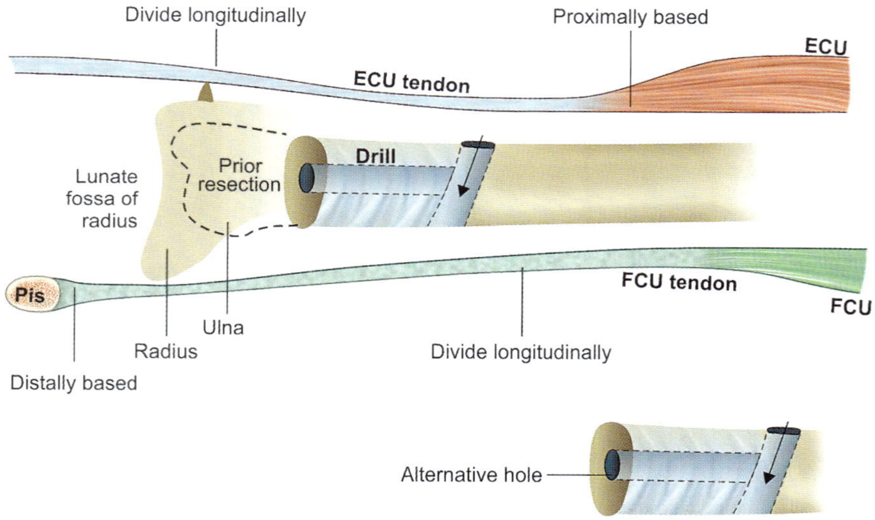

Fig. 10: ECU/FCU stabilization—Breen and Jupiter. Make the ECU slip and pass it through the drill hole made in distal ulna. Similarly make FCU slip and pass it across the transverse tunnel. (ECU: extensor carpi ulnaris; FCU: flexor carpi ulnaris)

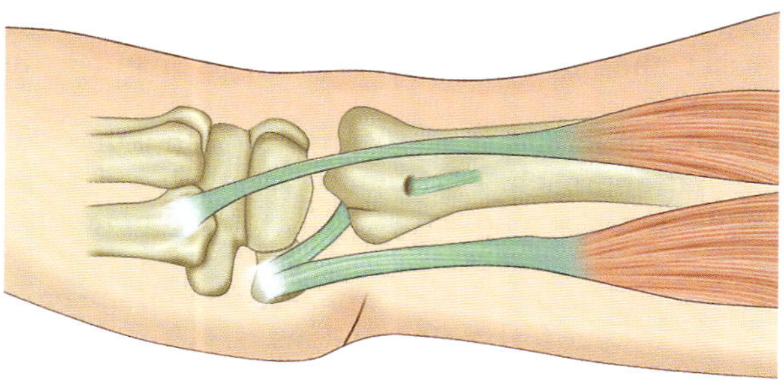

Fig. 11: Illustration depicting the Bunnell-Boyes reconstruction.

- Wafer procedure **(Fig. 14)**—involves excision of a 2–4 mm wafer of cartilage and bone from the ulnar articular bone just below the TFC. There is minimal disturbance of DRUJ, and there is no need of internal fixation. The procedure has gone into disrepute along with the so called arthroscopic wafer procedure. These procedure lead to cartilage ablation and hence should be discouraged. They have presently no role in the DRUJ reconstructive surgery, unless off course the articular cartilage is saved in the open procedure by doing subarticular resection.

Surgical Treatment in the Presence of Arthritis

These procedures mostly involve salvage procedures in the form of resection or replacement arthroplasty or arthrodesis including:

- *Darrach's resection arthroplasty (William Darrach in 1912):* This was the most popular procedure and today poses the benchmark against which all other procedures are compared **(Fig. 15)**.
  - 1 inch of distal ulna is exposed through and incision between ECU and FCU.
  - Distal 1 inch of ulna is removed keeping the ulnar styloid in position.

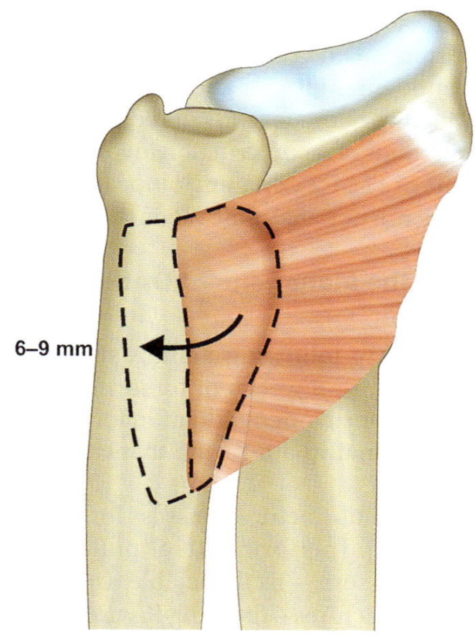

Fig. 12: Johnson's pronator advancement.

  - Periosteal sleeve is carefully repaired that is believed to act as a firm soft tissue tether for distal ulna keeping it in place.
  - It has been found that there is destabilization of the DRUJ and that the ulna has tendency to dorsally subluxate with pronation. The TFCC and ECU uncoupled from the remaining proximal ulna. Many patients are troubled by dorsal ulnar prominence and weakness of grip strength.
- *Hemiresection interposition technique (HIT) arthroplasty of Bowers (1984):* This is an unusual and nonanatomical procedure that reconstructs an incongruent DRUJ with autogenous tissue **(Figs. 16A to C)**. TFCC is maintained in this procedure.
  - Ulnar articular head is resected at the sigmoid notch saving a portion below TFCC to provide support. So

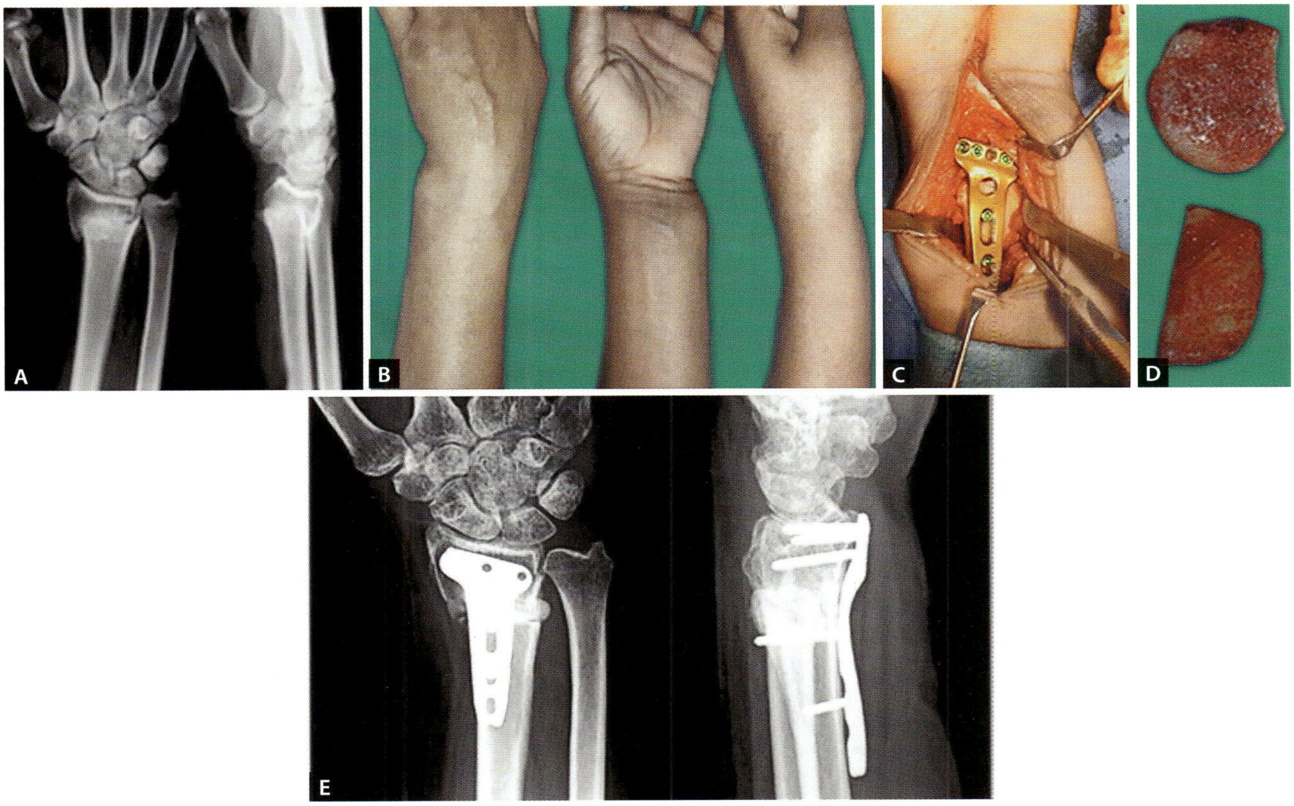

Figs. 13A to E: Malunited distal radius fracture correction—preoperative radiographic appearance (A), clinical appearance of deformity (B), intraoperative correction of deformity (C) using iliac crest bone graft (D), and final radiograph after deformity correction—note the restored radial length and inclinations (E).

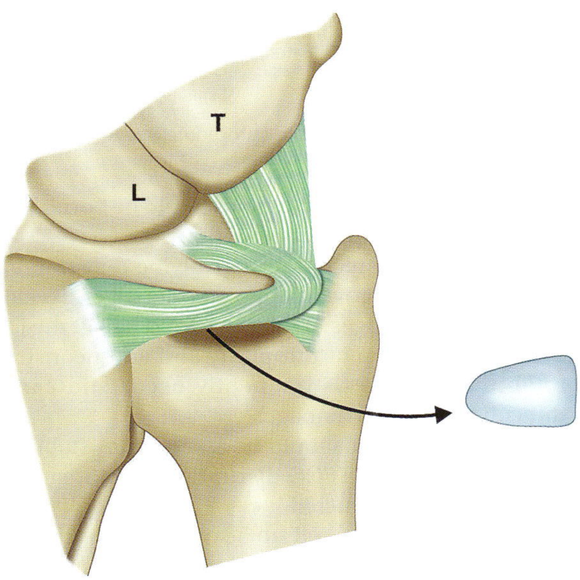

Fig. 14: *Wafer procedure:* Slice of distal ulnar articular surface is removed.

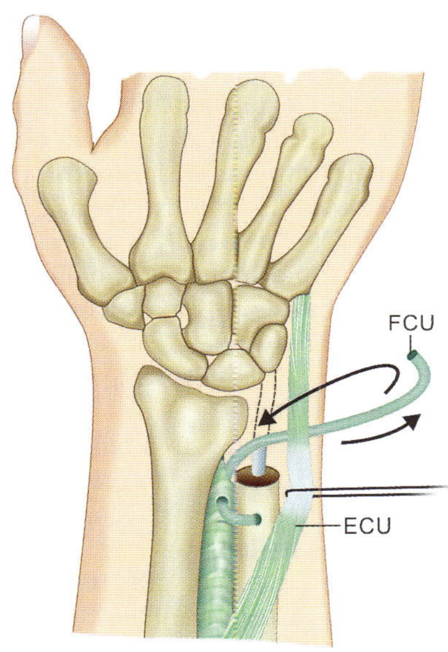

Fig. 15: Darrach's procedure: A modified Darrach's procedure using the flexor carpi ulnaris to stabilize the ulnar stump.

the resection is oblique maintaining the shaft styloid relationship.

- Soft tissue (muscle, tendon, or capsule) is placed between radius and ulna to act as interposition arthroplasty. This helps prevent impingement (ulnar impingement to radius—see ulnar impingement syndrome).

- *Matched distal ulnar resection of Watson (1986):* This can be simply described as a procedure of "penciling" the distal ulna **(Fig. 17)**. The distal 6 cm of distal ulna is exposed and shaped in a fashion using rongeurs that matches with the radial sigmoid notch, while maintaining the cuff of periosteum and ligamentous

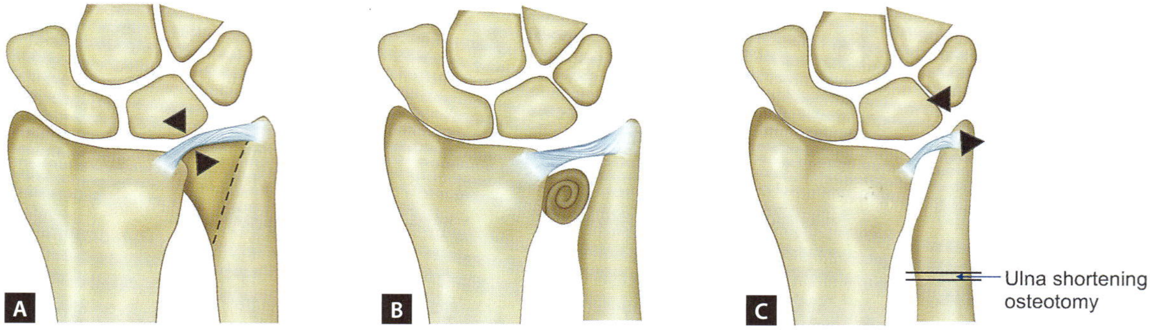

Figs. 16A to C: Hemiresection interposition technique (HIT) arthroplasty of Bower: (A) Resection of the distal ulna on radial aspect; (B) Interposition of autogenous tissue between the radius and ulna; (C) To avoid ulna impaction, it is better to shorten ulna simultaneously.

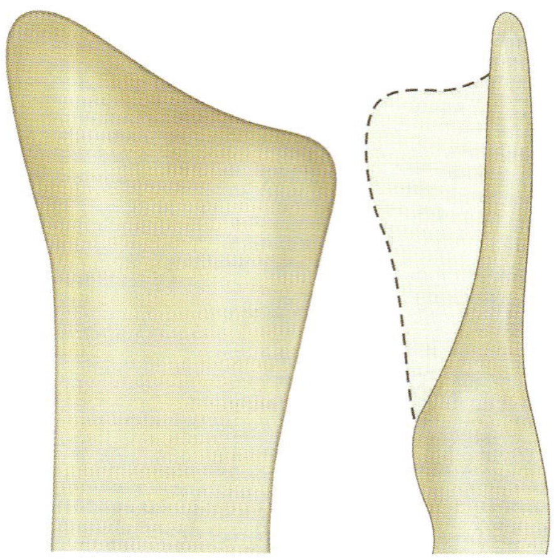

Fig. 17: Matched distal ulnar resection.

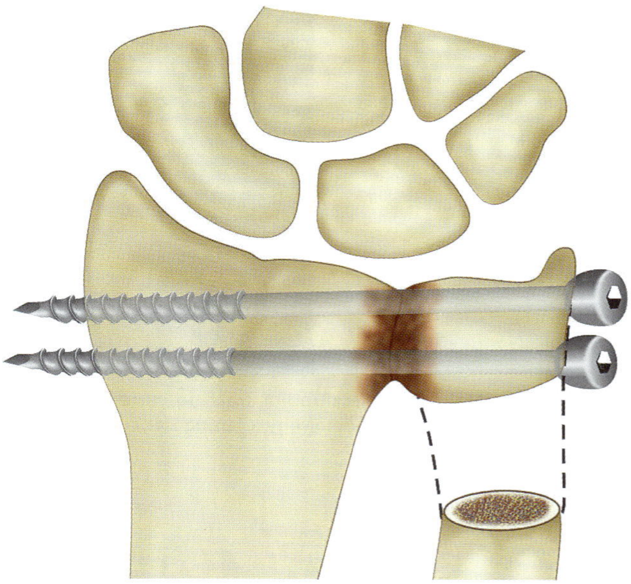

Fig. 18: Sauvè–Kapandji procedure (see text).

structures attached to the distal ulna. Watson proposed that adherence of ECU to rawed distal ulna increases stability. It is a cumbersome procedure and suffers from the same dorsal instability of ulna (albeit less).

- *Sauvé–Kapandji (1936):* The DRUJ arthrosis is primarily addressed by fusing the joint while mobility is restored by creating a pseudarthrosis proximal to this fusion **(Fig. 18)**.
  - To create pseudoarthrosis 1.5–2 cm of ulnar neck is resected with periosteum leaving the head and small portion of neck distally.
  - Fusion is achieved by freshening the articular surfaces (sigmoid notch and the ulnar head) and rigid compressed fixation achieved using screw (preferred) or K-wire in proper ulnar variance.
  - Pronator quadratus fascia is placed in the pseudarthrosis gap to prevent bony union and further development of stiffness.
  - The advantage of this procedure is that it recreates radioulnar surface and maintains physiological stress transmission across the ulnar aspect also.

Arthroplasty for Management of Distal Radioulnar Joint Disorder

Using silastic, metallic, or ceramic replacement for part or all of the ulna as well as total DRUJ replacement! The following are the current understandings that should be borne in mind before embarking on specific procedures:

- Hemiarthroplasty techniques involving only one-half of a load-bearing synovial joint run the risk of developing degenerative changes in the conserved half of the joint.
- Instability of a hemiarthroplasty and an unconstrained total joint prosthesis frequently occur and can be a difficult problem to manage.
- Before surgery joint should be assessed for stability and if unstable due to TFCC disruption then it should be repaired or reconstructed.
- Unipolar prosthesis needs to be correctly positioned, the soft tissue balanced and stabilized and the sigmoid notch needs to provide a volar and dorsal buttress.
- As for posterior exposure of hip requiring eminent closure—the hemiarthroplasty and an unconstrained prosthesis require a good quality dorsal closure.

Ulnar resurfacing technique: This is suited for involvement of the ulnar head only while relative preservation of the sigmoid notch **(Fig. 19)**. The ulnar head is partially replaced/resurfaced in radial half preserving the ulnar

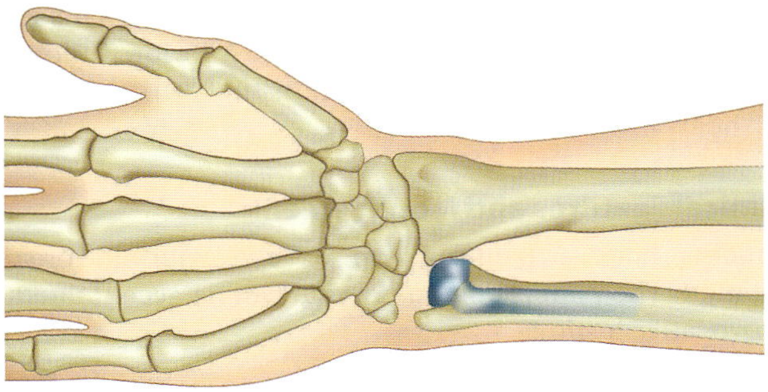

Fig. 19: Ulnar surface replacement illustration.

neck, ulnar styloid, ECU groove, ulnocarpal ligament attachments, ECU sheath, and the TFCC attachments to the ulnar styloid. Pyrocarbon prosthesis with bipolar components to reduce wear of the sigmoid notch and the surrounding soft tissues are available (EclypseTM). Exact sizing or undersizing the component is preferred else joint overstuffing occurs.

Total ulnar head replacement: Total ulnar head replacement has been suggested as often the involvement is global than partial. They replace the articular portion and remainder of ulnar head. Soft tissue balancing is an essential component as is the TFCC attachment to the eyelet that may break failing the reconstruction. Herbert sling can be used simultaneously to stabilize the ulnar prosthesis. The uHeadTM and E-CentrixTM are examples of available prosthesis.

Total distal radioulnar joint replacement: This is a suitable option for patients with advanced degeneration involving the distal ulna and sigmoid notch of radius.

- *Unconstrained prosthesis:* This is a suitable option for relatively stable DRUJ, good soft tissue envelop, and good bone stalk. The articulating surfaces are so designed that they tend to mimic the normal anatomic joint surfaces and hence the stability provided is around 20% while rest is provided by the soft tissue envelop. The sigmoid notch component comprises of a metal base plate and poly insert so depends on a good bone stalk. Often a Herbert sling (see above) is combined to improve stability.
- *Semiconstrained prosthesis:* If the joint is unstable (as is commonly the case) then semiconstrained prosthesis is a good option **(Fig. 20)**. It resists motion in planes other than the native plane/axis of the joint, so prevents the symptoms of instability and provides "created stability". Being semiconstrained, some out-of-plane movements do occur and are advantageous to prevent prosthesis loosening. The example is Scheker arthroplasty, that comprises an uncemented ulnar stem acting as a pivot around which is mounted a polyethylene ball. This ball is then encased in a cage attached to plate fixed to radius. The anteroposterior motion in this is completely restrained while rotations are fully free while allowing minor axial motion between the cage and poly ball and the ulnar stem and ball.

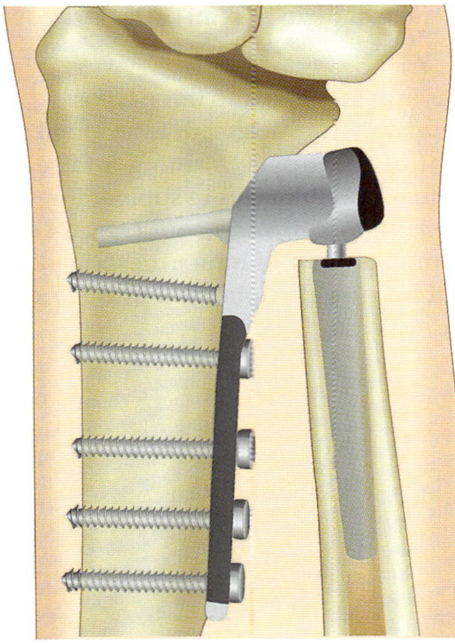

Fig. 20: Total distal radioulnar joint (DRUJ) replacement using a semiconstrained prosthesis.

EXTENSOR CARPI ULNARIS TENDON PROBLEMS AND EXTENSOR CARPI ULNARIS TENDINITIS

Anatomical considerations:

- The ECU tendon lies in a groove at the distal part of the ulna; that has variable depth **(Fig. 21)**.
- It is maintained within this groove during forearm rotation by the extensor retinaculum and a subsheath. These form the fibro-osseous tunnel.
- The *linea jugata* connects the subsheath to the epimysium and prevents subluxation of the ECU in a palmar direction during full supination **(Fig. 22)**.
- In pronation the course of tendon is straight while in supination the tendon forms an ulnar-sided obtuse angle that further increases in wrist flexion and ulnar deviation. There is maximal force on subsheath in this position.

Extensor carpi ulnaris subluxation/snapping syndrome: This occurs with injury (commonly) or with inflammatory degenerative disorders like rheumatoid arthritis. ECU tendon is no longer maintained within its fibro-osseous groove **(Figs. 23A and B)**. It is a chronic disorder and does not relieve by itself. The common pathology includes:

- If the sulcus is shallow then the ECU may displace volarly during supination moving out of the sulcus resulting in a painful snapping sensation and inflammation.
- Traumatic dorsal subluxation or dislocation of the ulnar head causes the ECU tendon to forcibly displace volarly along with disruption of the TFCC. The important restrains for ECU tendon may also rupture causing recurrent tendon instability later **(Fig. 24)**. Subsheath rupture without extensor retinaculum tear occurs with forceful radial deviation and flexion of the wrist (baseball and rodeo, **Fig. 23B**).
- In patients with rheumatoid arthritis attritional wear of the supporting structures often causes subluxation of the

ECU and extensor digiti minimi (EDM) without a specific traumatic event.

Injury patterns are classified into three types:

1. *Stripping injury:* The subsheath is stripped at the ulnar attachment of the groove forming a false pouch into which the tendon subluxates in supination.
2. *Ulnar-sided rupture of subsheath* ***(Fig. 24)****:* This is the most common pattern of injury (described above). The tendon subluxates in supination and relocates during pronation.
3. *Radial sided rupture of subsheath* ***(Fig. 24)****:* This is an interesting situation because the tendon following relocation lies above the sheath that will then never heal.

Clinical Features and Management

Patients have a painful snap or click during forearm rotation. The pain is dorsoulnar and can be accentuated by provocative testing:

- Active supination

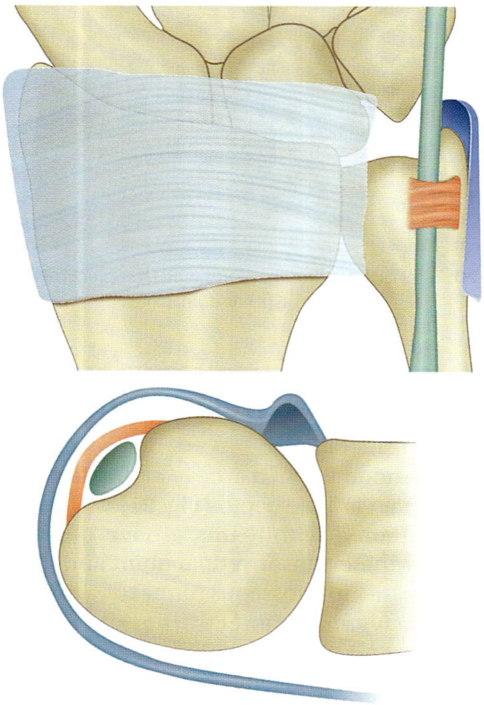

Fig. 21: The extensor carpi ulnaris tendon anatomy.

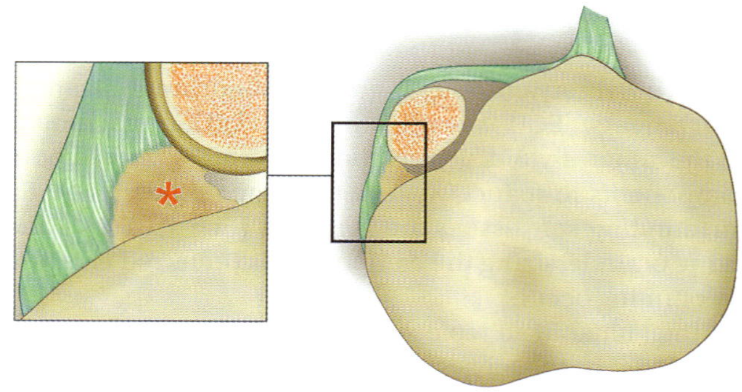

Fig. 22: The anatomy and disposition of linea jugata (marked by asterisk).

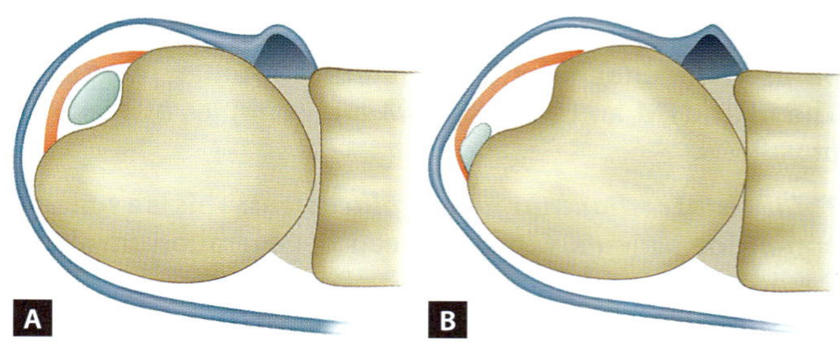

Figs. 23A and B: Extensor carpi ulnaris (ECU) tendon subluxation. (A) Normal location and maintained tendon in ulnar sulcus; (B) ECU subluxation due to subsheath rupture while still intact retinaculum.

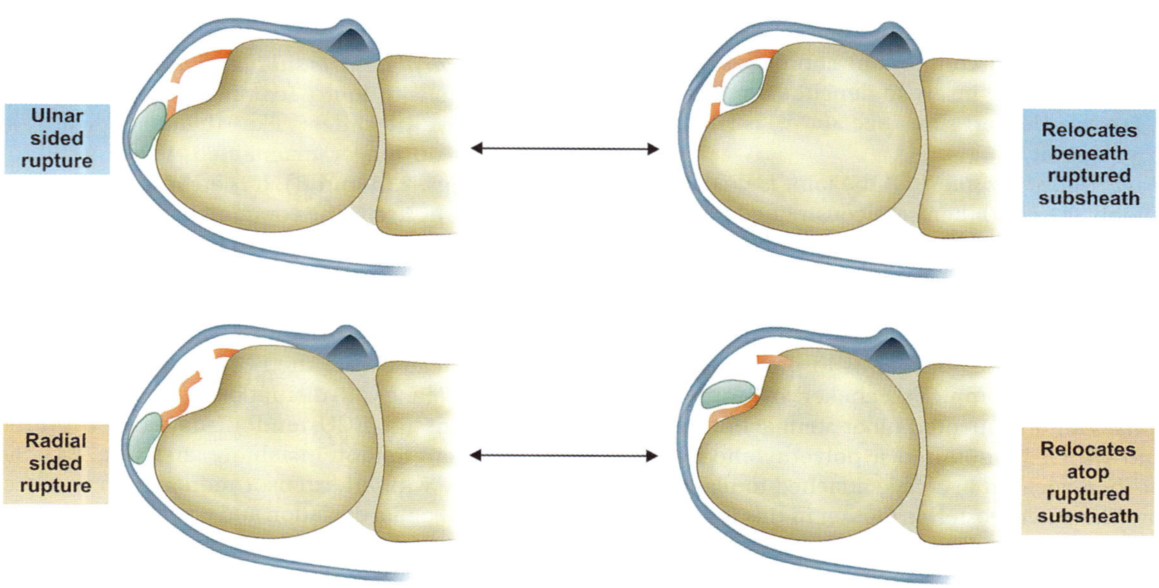

Fig. 24: Pathomechanism of extensor carpi ulnaris ECU subluxation due to various post-traumatic injury patterns.

- Passive supination
- Active supination, flexion, and ulnar deviation
- *ECU synergy test:* With the elbow flexed and forearm in full supination, wrist neutral, fingers fully extended, the examiner grasps patients thumb and middle finger. The patient is asked to abduct the thumb against resistance. The examiner simultaneously palpates the ECU tendon and confirms the contraction of ECU and FCU. This maneuver produces pain on dorsoulnar aspect suggesting ECU tendinitis.

  The subluxation of tendon can be confirmed on dynamic ultrasound. MRI is a bit too much of an investigation for this, but may also reveal tendinosis shallow groove, etc.

Acute treatment of a traumatic injury involving the ECU tendon is as follows:

- Reduce the DRUJ dislocation ± stabilization of the DRUJ ± repair of the TFCC.
- Immobilization of the wrist and forearm, rest, application of ice, and use of nonsteroidal anti-inflammatory medications followed by activity modification.
- We prefer neutral position of the forearm for immobilization (if associated with DRUJ injury); supinated forearm puts unnecessary stress and causes subluxation of the tendon. Pronation of forearm + extension at wrist is preferred for isolated ECU injury.
- Activity modification includes the use of "whale mouse" and "split keyboards" that promote a relaxed position of the hand and neutral deviation at the wrist **(Figs. 25A and B)**.
- The ECU tendon is stabilized by reconstruction of the ECU subsheath using a radially based flap of extensor retinaculum passed around the tendon as described by Spinner and Kaplan. The other methods of repair are:
  - Direct repair
  - Free retinacular graft
  - Tendon graft from palmaris longus

  Additional sulcus deepening may be needed or added to reconstruction. Immobilization following reconstruction is done in pronation and extension of the forearm-wrist.

RHEUMATOID AFFECTION OF EXTENSOR TENDONS

Subluxation

The patient must be managed by additionally stabilizing the dorsal subluxation of ulnar head in addition to reconstruction of the ECU subsheath.

Extensor Carpi Ulnaris Tendinitis/ Tenosynovitis/Tendinosis

This is a common accompaniment of tendon subluxation or otherwise. In recurrent subluxation, pathology stress is placed on the tendon causing inflammation of the synovial lining. Over time the tendon degenerates with/ without partial tears. There is tenderness at the distal part of the ulna, over the fifth (EDM) or sixth (ECU) extensor compartment. Inflammation at the insertion of the ECU presents with pain and inflammation at the dorsal base of the fifth metacarpal.

Treatment is mainly as for the ECU tendon subluxation. For nontraumatic tendinitis of ECU, the treatment mainly involves rest, brief periods of immobilization, nonsteroidal anti-inflammatory drugs, and judicious use of corticosteroid injections. Surgery is rare and is reserved for chronic, recalcitrant cases. Insertional tendinitis of the ECU is treated with dorsal transfer of the ECU to the hamate. Tendovaginitis within the extensor sheath is treated with release of the ECU subsheath and reconstruction of Spinner and Kaplan.

The "***caput ulnae syndrome***" **(Fig. 26)** as reported by Backdahl in 1963 consists of:

- Weakness of the hand and wrist
- Pain on rotation of the forearm
- Reduced range of motion of the DRUJ
- Unstable DRUJ—dorsal prominence of the ulnar head, reducible with painful crepitations, also called the piano key sign
- Bulging of the synovial bursae of the ECU and other extensor compartments—ECU tenosynovitis
- Rupture of extensor tendons—Vaughan-Jackson syndrome **(Figs. 27A and B)**

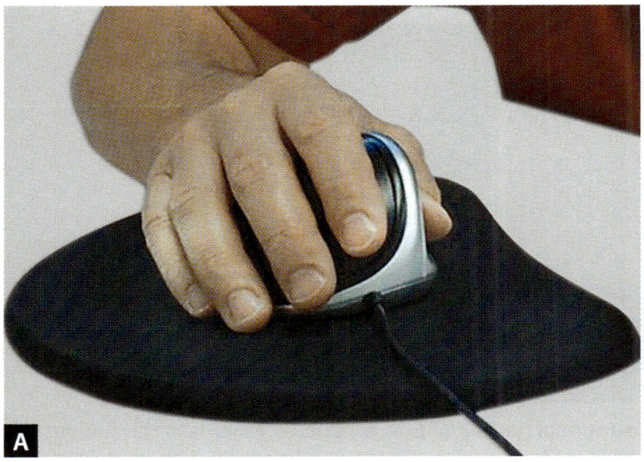

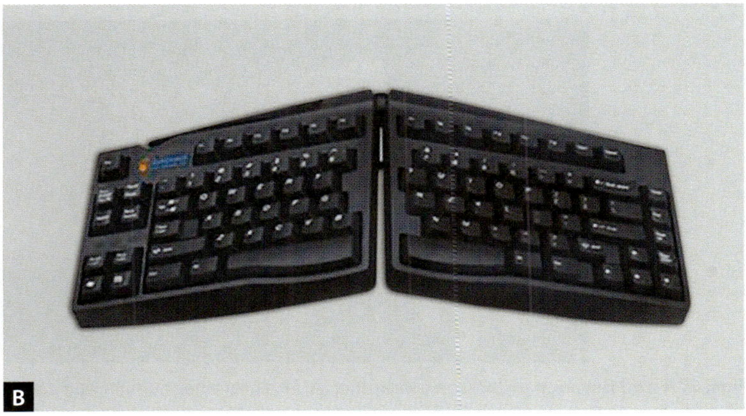

Figs. 25A and B: (A) Use of whale mouse; (B) Split keyboards is recommended in patients with subluxating symptomatic extensor carpi ulnaris (ECU) tendon.

The components of caput ulnae syndrome have been described above already with management. The last component is discussed below.

Vaughan-Jackson Syndrome

In 1948, Vaughan-Jackson reported on extensor tendon rupture due to the dorsally displaced ulnar head. A decade earlier he reported the rupture due to bony projections from ulna in two cases of DRUJ arthritis. The rupture begin on the ulnar side of the hand and wrist with the EDM and extensor digitorum communis (EDC) tendon of the small finger that if untreated (as in rheumatoid arthritis) leads to sequential rupture of the ring, long, and index finger EDC tendons **(Figs. 27A and B)**; and finally that of the extensor indicis proprius (EIP). The risk factors for rupture of extensor tendons include:

- Malunited fractures
- Ulnar head subluxation
- DRUJ arthritis
- Crystal arthropathy

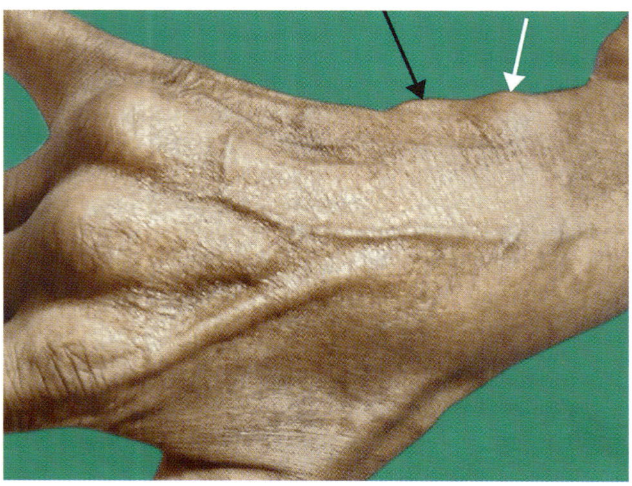

Fig. 26: The caput ulnae syndrome—note the swollen extensor carpi ulnaris (ECU) synovial bursa (white arrow) and prominent ulnar head (black arrow).

- Iatrogenic (DRUJ surgery like Darrach's procedure)
- ECU tendinitis.

Pathophysiology of tendon rupture:

1. *Biological cause:* The tendons rupture due to development of tendinosis from synovitis and inflammation (that is prominent in rheumatoid arthritis).
2. *Mechanical component:* The frictional component is predominant (serving like the attrition of rope on well) cause of rupture occurring due to rubbing of tendons against the dislocated/subluxated ulnar head. Mechanical component is important as similar ruptures are seen with DRUJ arthritis, extensor pollicis longus rupture following malunited distal radius and extensor tendon ruptures following Darrach's procedure.

Clinical Presentation

Symptoms develop suddenly and patients are unable to lift the pinky finger at the metacarpophalangeal (MCP) joint. Patient's report a swelling in past that would have been associated with pain. On examination, there is loss of active extension. Impending tendon rupture is indicated if there is:

- MCP joint extensor weakness
- Extension lag
- Active tenosynovitis on the dorsum of the hand and wrist
- Pain on the dorsum of the wrist associated with digital extension

Examine the joints for fixed deformity and DRUJ (for need of concomitant reconstruction/stabilization). Examine the peripheral nerves that may be involved, e.g., posterior interosseous nerve (PIN) palsy due to synovitis (causing symptoms similar to extensor tendon rupture—loss of extension at MCP).

Radiology

Radiographs show the classical signs of degenerative wrist with osteophyte formation at the DRUJ or findings of rheumatoid wrist such as carpal coalition, scallop sign (the sigmoid notch of the distal radius has an erosive scalloping concavity), articular erosions, severe osteopenia, and later

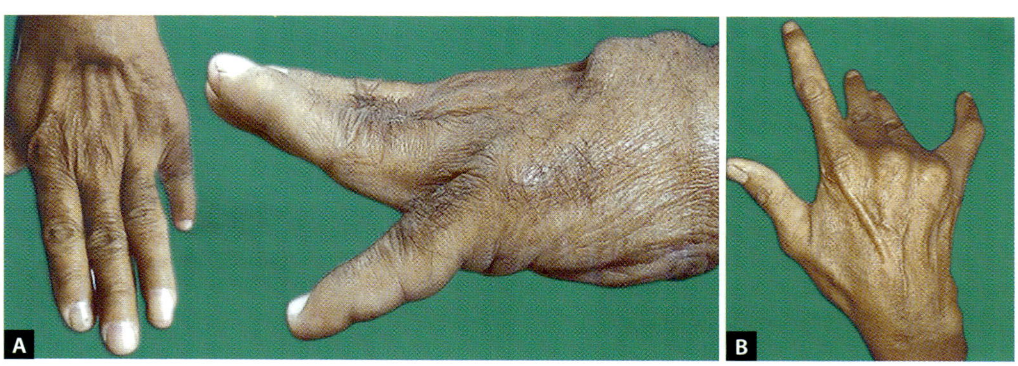

Figs. 27A and B: Vaughan-Jackson syndrome: (A) The prominent ulnar head causes attritional rupture of EDN tendon commonly in this patient also note the extensor carpi ulnaris (ECU) synovitis that indicates possible future rupture of ECU tendons also. (B) In the other patient, there is rupture of extensor digiti minimi (EDM) and extensor slips to ring finger (RF) and middle finger (MF) causing their drop, however the extensor index proprius maintains the extension of index finger (IF) and intact ADM causes abduction of the pinkie finger.

DRUJ destruction. Dynamic ultrasonography or MRI can be used to confirm tendon rupture if doubt remains.

Differential Diagnosis

- PIN palsy—the symptoms here begin from the middle and index finger rather than from the ulnar digits.
- Joint stiffness—traumatic precluding extension.

Treatment

Prophylaxis from tendon rupture (say if the patient has been seen in the impending rupture stage) involves active identification and supportive measures viz.:

- DRUJ stabilization
- Synovectomy
- Splinting to restrict pronation
- DRUJ fusion/replacement (degenerative disease)

Surgical restoration of the tendons: These procedures should be combined with correction of DRUJ problems, ulna head stabilization, debridement of the DRUJ, synovectomy, and retinaculum transposition.

- Direct repair—attritional rupture is not amenable to direct repair due to poor tendon strength and long zone of injury.
- Repair using tendon graft—this is a cumbersome procedure and amenable to fail due to adhesion formation. The procedure is long and needs another surgery to harvest tendons so not very popular.
- Tendon transfer—this is considered the most useful procedure to restore function. The following are some of the measures used to obtain functional extension:
  - For little finger—tenodesis of the distal stump (of EDC or EDM) to adjacent healthy EDC.
    - EIP transfer to EDM
  - For long, ring and small fingers—EIP transfer to EDM + EDC of ring finger + tenodesis of the long finger EDC to index finger EDC.
  - Loss of extension of all the fingers—use flexor digitorum superficialis (FDS) of ring finger to motorize the extensors of ring and pinky finger and long finger FDS to index and long finger EDC. Use subcutaneous route for transfer to prevent adhesion formation.

ULNOCARPAL IMPACTION/ ABUTMENT SYNDROME AND ULNAR IMPINGEMENT SYNDROME

Ulnar impaction syndrome (ulnocarpal impaction syndrome, ulnar abutment, or ulnocarpal loading) is a degenerative condition characterized by ulnar wrist pain, swelling, and limitation of motion related to excessive load-bearing across the ulnar aspect of the wrist **(Fig. 28)**. The impaction between the ulnar head and the TFC complex and carpus produces a continuum of pathologic changes that are demonstrated by Palmer as type II TFCC lesions **(*see* Table 1 and Fig. 29)**. The changes broadly comprise of (in increasing order of severity) as:

- Degenerative tear of the TFC
- Chondromalacia of the lunate bone

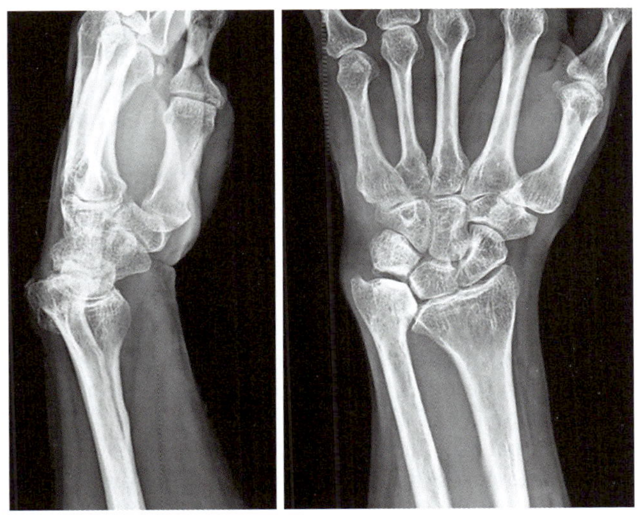

Fig. 28: Ulnocarpal impaction syndrome.

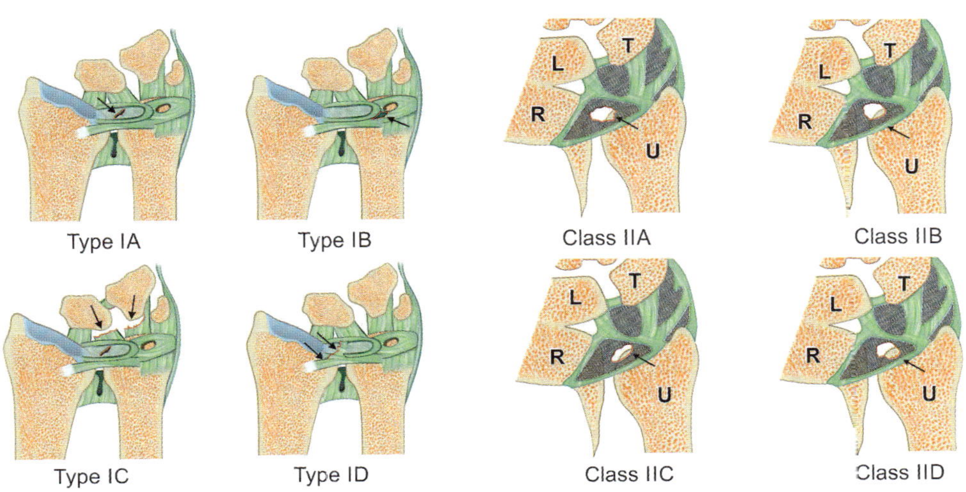

Fig. 29: Palmer classification of triangular fibrocartilage complex (TFCC) disorders.

- Progressive involvement of triquetrum and distal ulnar head
- Instability or tear of the LT ligament and finally
- Osteoarthritis of the ulnocarpal and DRUJ

Predisposing Factors

- Factors leading to increased length of ulna or dorsal radial tilt
    - Positive ulnar variance (but can as well occur with neutral or negative ulnar variance)
    - Malunion of the distal radius
    - Premature physeal closure of the distal radius
    - Previous radial head resection (in an unrecognized Essex-Lopresti fracture-dislocation)
    - Impaction fracture of the radial head
- Activities that cause excessive intermittent loading of the ulnar carpus
- Asymptomatic ulnocarpal impaction syndrome—this is rarely found where the patient is asymptomatic though radiologically all changes suggest impaction syndrome.

Clinical Manifestation

- Chronic or subacute ulnar wrist pain exacerbated by activity and relieved by rest.
- Swelling and limitation of forearm rotation and wrist motion.
- Firm grip, pronation, and ulnar deviation of the wrist that relatively cause dynamic positive ulna variance exacerbate the symptoms.

Imaging

Radiographic findings include:

- Subchondral sclerosis and cystic changes in the ulnar head, lunate bone, and proximal radial aspect of the triquetrum **(Fig. 28)**.
- Ulnocarpal osteoarthritis **(Fig. 28)**
- In subtle cases, the changes may not be present and in them recognition of the geographic nature of the abnormalities affecting the articular surfaces of the ulna, lunate and triquetrum is essential (MRI may be helpful).

The following etiological findings should be noted:

- Positive ulnar variance
- Neutral or negative variance
- Malunion of a distal radial fracture with residual radial shortening
- Abnormal dorsal tilt
- Premature physeal arrest of the distal radius
- Essex-Lopresti fracture or resection of the radial head may also be evident on conventional radiographs.

Magnetic resonance imaging is helpful in detecting occult disease that shows fibrillation of the joint cartilage of the ulnar head and ulnar carpus followed by bone hyperemia (low-signal intensity on T1-weighted images and high-signal intensity on T2-weighted images). In advanced stages, sclerotic changes appear as areas of low-signal intensity on both T1- and T2-weighted images. Magnetic resonance arthrography may be done to demonstrate the integrity of the TFC and LT ligament.

Differential Diagnosis

- Age-related degeneration
- Intraosseous ganglia (MRI helps in differential)
- True cysts (differentiated better by MRI)
- Vascular grooves (a vascular groove usually appears as a central proximal radiolucent defect that communicates with the radiolunate joint space)
- Kienböck's disease

Treatment

The determining factors for the type of intervention are:

- The amount of ulnar variance
- The Palmer lesion class **(*see* Fig. 29)**
- The shape of the sigmoid fossa and ulnar seat
- The presence of concomitant LT instability

A simple algorithm to understand the basic treatment options are:

- Palmer class IIA and IIB lesions (no TFC perforation)—an open wafer procedure or formal ulnar shortening (preferred).
- Palmer class IIC and IID lesions (TFCC perforated)—arthroscopic wafer procedure (causes destruction of articular cartilage of ulna so may not be as prudent as considered by many).
- Class IIE lesions—Darrach's procedure or Sauvé–Kapandji procedure. They all however produce convergent instability (ulna impingement syndrome; see later).
- Ulnar impaction due to Essex-Lopresti fracture is very difficult to treat in chronic instability so every attempt should be made to prevent its occurrence. Ulnar shortening should be avoided as it is more dynamic than static, and in any case, the radius will migrate proximally due to compromised IOM. Radial head replacement may be considered for these patients.

ULNOCARPAL IMPACTION SYNDROME SECONDARY TO ULNAR STYLOID NONUNION

Ulnar styloid fractures may be isolated injuries or more commonly occur in association with distal radius fractures **(Figs. 30A and B)**. Ulnar styloid nonunion is quite frequent and is often symptomatic (painful) in younger patients due to:

- The nonunited fragment may act as an irritative loose body.
- Ununited fragment may abut the ulnar carpus.
- A malaligned fibrous nonunion may cause impingement of the ECU tendon sheath.
- Associated TFCC perforation or complete rupture of the ulnar attachments of the TFCC and instability of the DRUJ.

Two types of nonunion of the ulnar styloid process have been described in terms of anatomic features and treatment options.

- *Type 1* is fracture only of the tip of ulnar styloid so the DRUJ is stable as ligamentous complexes attach only to the base of styloid.

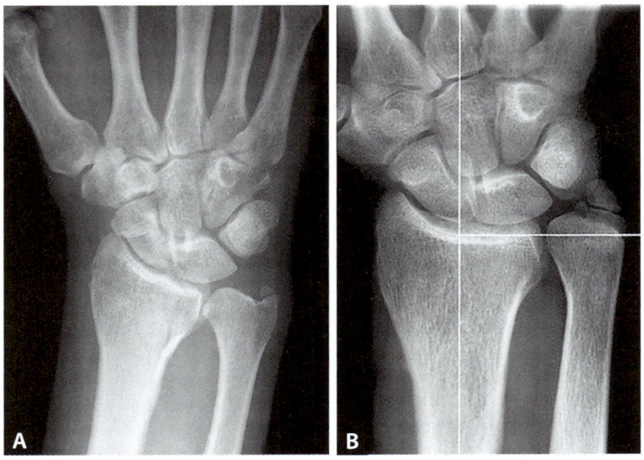

Figs. 30A and B: Possible ulnocarpal impaction due to nonunion of ulnar styloid type 1 (A) and type 2 (B) fractures. Note the developing ulna positive variant in both these patients approaching the carpal region. There is high likelihood of torn triangular fibrocartilage (TFC) in both.

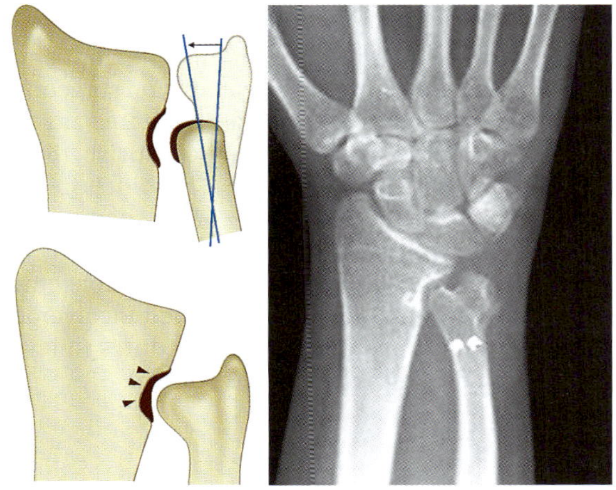

Fig. 31: Ulna impingement syndrome.

- *Type 2* is major disabling one as it is associated with avulsion of the ulnar attachment of the TFC complex (Palmer class IB lesion). There is DRUJ instability (subluxation/dislocation).

Radiologically the two types can be seen but MRI is the best modality for visualizing the integrity of the TFC complex and its ulnar attachments. It also reveals any associated chondromalacia of the ulnar carpus and degenerative changes.

Differential Diagnosis

The fractured fragment may be confused with accessory ossicles such as the lunula and os triangulare. Diagnostic arthroscopy is possibly the best investigation to guide treatment—loss of resilience of TFC (central disk) and loss of "trampoline effect" (bouncing back on hitting centrally) are the best indicator of the need to relocate the ulnar styloid at the anatomical location and reconstruction/repair of TFCC. Conversely if resilience is seen during arthroscopy and symptoms are significant then ulnar styloid can be removed (it indicates functional TFCC while styloid impingement as the cause of symptoms).

ULNAR IMPINGEMENT SYNDROME

This is not only distinct but mutually exclusive from the previously detailed ulnar abutment syndrome.

Ulnar impingement syndrome is caused by distal ulna "impingement" on the distal radius **(Fig. 31)** proximal to the sigmoid notch [due either to ulna shortening commonly or radial lengthening (rare)].

Etiology

The ulnar shortening often results from:

- Surgical procedures that involve resection of the distal ulna (Darrach's, Sauvé-Kapandji, matched ulnar resection, etc.)
- Prior wrist trauma
- Rheumatoid arthritis
- Correction of Madelung's deformity
- De novo cases of negative ulnar variance
- Premature fusion of the distal ulna

Radioulnar convergence then occurs due to shortened ulna by the combined effects of contraction of the extensor pollicis brevis, abductor pollicis longus and pronator quadratus muscles and the loss of the buttress effect of the radioulnar joint. This approximation of radius and ulna is often asymptomatic while in ulna impingement syndrome it causes pain and other symptoms.

The clinical manifestations of ulnar impingement syndrome are similar but much more severe than that of ulnar impaction syndrome. The symptoms increase markedly with pronosupination due to increased pressure of DRUJ on radius. In long standing cases, the patients additionally have grating sensation.

Radiology

- Ulnar impingement produces erosive cortical changes at the corresponding level of the radius (radial scalloping, **Fig. 31**).
- There is subchondral sclerosis of ulna. Degenerative changes appear in the form of deformation, deshapening, and loss of ulnar profile.
- MRI may help in confirming the diagnosis before radiological changes are visible and may help diagnose it early.

Treatment

- Aggressive ulnar shortening and stabilization by Breen and Jupiter or Bunnell-Boyes reconstruction (see above).
- Ulna head replacement (see above).
- Distraction lengthening of the ulna—using external fixation, restores the length discrepancy, however, will not be suitable in cases of settled arthritis.
- Radial shortening in early cases—where the DRUJ can be specifically relocated and stabilized by soft tissue procedures additionally (see above).

CONCLUSION

- Ulnar-sided wrist pain is a common complaint encountered in outpatient clinic of dedicated hand surgeons.
- Disorders of DRUJ are often neglected as being nonspecific pain; however, they comprise the most common cause of ulnar wrist pain. The joint is frequently involved in wrist trauma and becomes symptomatic in many cases managed suboptimally.
- Wrist arthroscopy is a good technique of management of TFCC disorders while chronic advanced involvement of the DRUJ needs open operative procedures to level the joint or provide alternative reconstruction.
- The wrist joint and extensor tendons are also frequently involved in rheumatoid arthritis to produce wrist pain or tendon ruptures causing disability. The management is often symptomatic for wrist pain or debridement/arthrodesis in unresponsive cases while tendon ruptures need tendon transfer to restore the motor.
- Ulna impaction and impingement syndrome comprise a less common cause of wrist or DRUJ pain. They are commonly a product of malunions following trauma or residue of inflammatory arthritis and need specific management once identified.

CHAPTER 115

Rheumatoid Hand

Manish Kumar Varshney

INTRODUCTION

Rheumatoid arthritis (RA) is a systemic autoimmune disease with an emerging genetic basis. Virtually any synovial joint of the body is affected with a characteristic involvement of the hand. Due to varied form of disease taking a monocyclic, polycyclic, or progressive form, the actual course a patient will take is not known and hence most patients have been seen to discontinue treatment. This leads to variable presentation of deformities and disabilities.

The early stages of rheumatoid affection of small joints of hands are characterized by active inflammation and initial involvement of tendons and intrinsic muscles (IMs). The deformities are subtle at this stage but joint symptoms are prominent. Tendon involvement may cause pain, "triggering" and difficulty in active finger flexion. After weeks, months, or years, the active inflammation usually decreases with subsidence in joint and tendon symptoms. IM spasm usually disappears. At this stage, there is a mixture of low-grade active inflammation and permanent deformity. The patients begin to learn with the disabilities and how to counter them with rehabilitation and skill development so much so that in a few patients, the hands become normal both in function and on clinical examination.

In most of the early-onset arthritis, however, and those with monocyclic disease with poor remission if at all permanent deformities may arise in the joints, the tendons, or the small muscles of the hands. In such patients, joints may become stiff by deformation or may become loose due to stretching or destructive processes in ligaments. There is often a mixture of rupture of ligaments, and subluxation or dislocation of joints, causing directional instability and stiffness in other direction. The tendons also contribute to functional loss by getting dislocated, stretched, or ruptured. IMs are not only weakened but also are often the site of contractures hampering joint movement and producing joint deformity. One can logically understand that a permuted combination of all these factors would result in infinite variations of presentation so that two cases are seldom alike.

GENERAL PERSPECTIVE OF HAND DEFORMITIES

The rheumatoid hand deformities can be grouped as to those occurring at wrist, metacarpophalangeal (MCP) joint and fingers. The hand characteristically has a Z-deformity with ulnar deviation of fingers at MCP joint while radial deviation at the wrist **(Figs. 1 and 2)**. The proximal phalanges sublux or dislocate palmarly, lying beneath the metacarpal heads.

- The palmar displacement of the proximal phalanges could occur from a combination of various causes like:
  - Migration/displacement of the long flexor tendons
  - Lax collateral ligaments of the MCP joint
  - Attenuation of the dorsoradial support system
  - Intrinsic muscles of hand undergo contracture or may be involved in spasm from joint inflammation
  - Destruction of the metacarpal heads
- Ulnar drift of the digits at MCP joints (it is a combination of ulnar shift, ulnar deviation, and volar dislocation, **Fig. 3**) involves several deforming factors in combination.
  - Synovitis of MCP joint produce capsular laxity, so normally a lateral movement that is not possible at MCP joint becomes prominent and up to 45° of lateral deviation can occur.

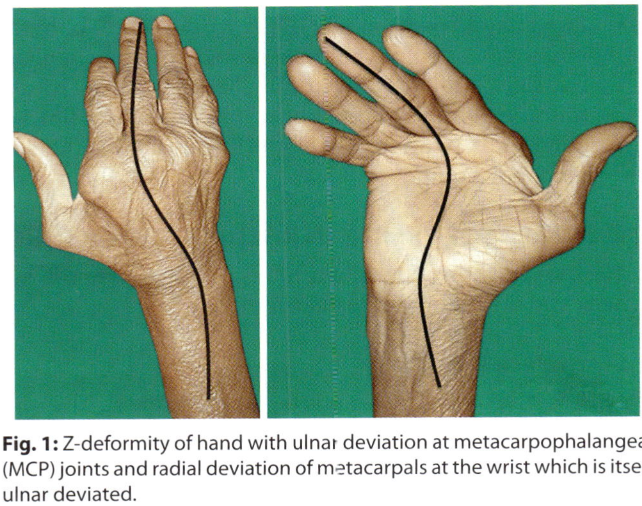

Fig. 1: Z-deformity of hand with ulnar deviation at metacarpophalangeal (MCP) joints and radial deviation of metacarpals at the wrist which is itself ulnar deviated.

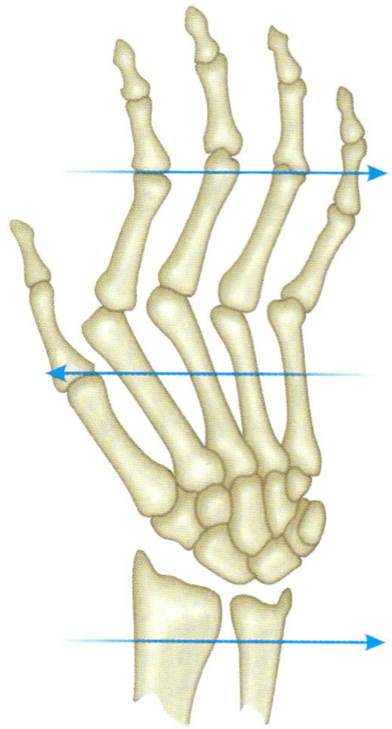

Fig. 2: Illustration of Z-deformity of hand and wrist: There is ulnar deviation at the metacarpophalangeal (MCP) joints and radial deviation of metacarpals at the wrist joint due to articular and soft tissue changes.

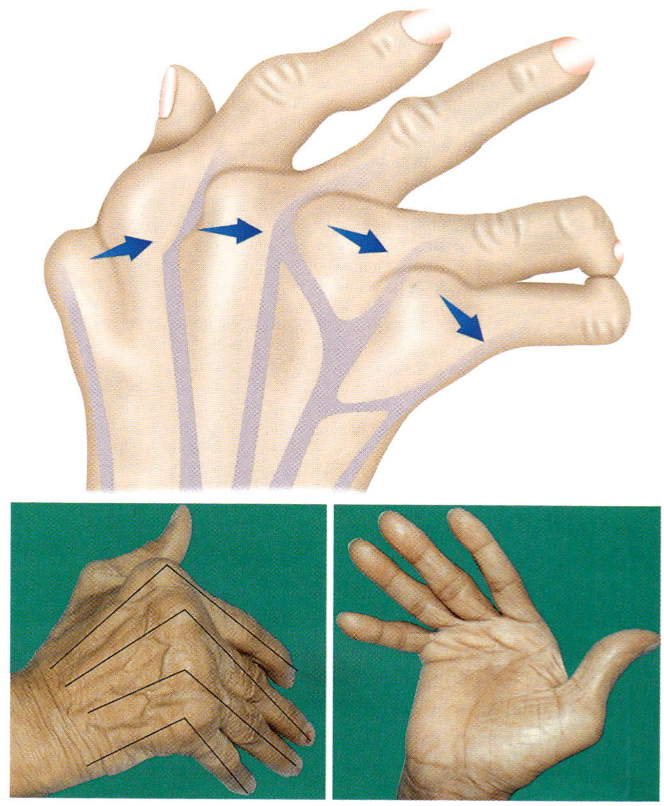

Fig. 3: Ulnar drift of fingers: Displacement of the extensor tendons occurs into the ulnar valleys between the metacarpal heads producing an ulnar moment of pull to the fingers.

  - The normal tendency of the fingers to move into slight ulnar angulation during full flexion (ulnar predominance of forces).
  - Ulnar displacement of the extensor tendons, due to various factors:
    - Synovitis in the radial extensor triangle
    - Stretching of the radial-sided transverse extensor fibers (sagittal bands)
  - Increased ulnar pull tag due to lost extensor power (following tendon subluxation)
  - An increased ulnar pull of the junctura tendinae
  - Intrinsic muscle tightness and a weakened dorsoradial support system
  - *Radial deviation at wrist:* Produces vectorial forces favoring ulnar deviation at MCP joint
- Rheumatoid involvement of the wrist leads to obligatory radial deviation of the metacarpals; the mechanism is not fully understood but may be due mainly to ulnar translocation and supination of the carpus. This produces abnormal vectorial force on the fingers pulling them into ulnar deviation.

FINGER DEFORMITY IN RHEUMATOID ARTHRITIS

The two most peculiar deformities of fingers are the swan neck and the boutonniére deformities.

Swan Neck Deformity

This is the most common finger deformity. The distal interphalangeal (DIP) joint is flexed and the proximal interphalangeal (PIP) joint is hyperextended [**(Figs. 4A and B)**, also termed recurvatum]. MCP flexion, although common in RA and other intrinsic-plus swan neck deformity (SND), need not be present. Hyperextension of the MCP joint and flexion at IP joint is termed SND of the thumb **(Figs. 5A and B)**. The term "SND" was specifically used by Laine in 1957 though the description has been given by authors in past as old as 300 years ago. The deformity gets its name due to close resemblance with swan neck. Deformity develops from inequilibrium of the factors that provide control over the digit. Three sets of muscles and tendons provide digital equilibrium and control:

1. *The extrinsic extensor group:* Extensor digitorum communis, extensor digiti minimi, and the extensor indicis. These insert to the extensor hood. They produce extension at the MCP joint and in concert with IMs also extend the PIP and DIP joints.
2. *The extrinsic flexor group:* Flexor digitorum profundus (FDP) and superficialis.
3. *The IMs:* Include the four lumbricals and the seven volar and dorsal interossei. The former insert onto the lateral extensor bands while the latter insert onto various sites in the MCP capsule and proximal phalangeal base, the extensor hood and the medial and lateral extensor bands.

Other structures that act in passively stabilizing the finger include: Fibrous joint capsule, the collateral ligaments, the volar plate, retinacular system, and including the ligament of Landsmeer. The latter also facilitates the rhythm of digital flexion and extension.

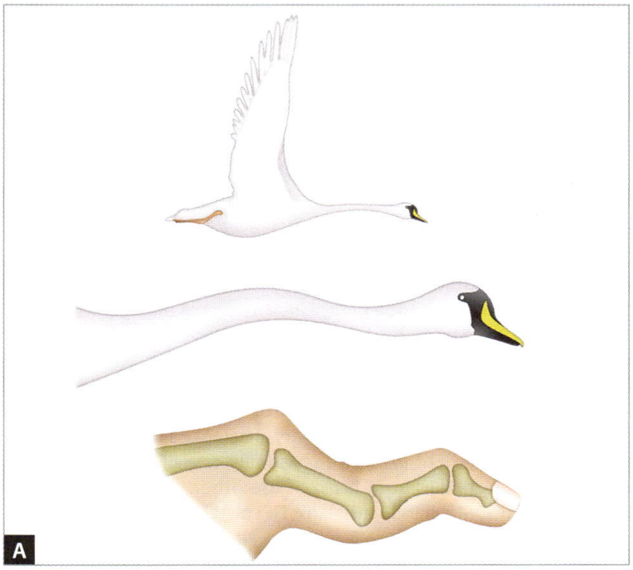
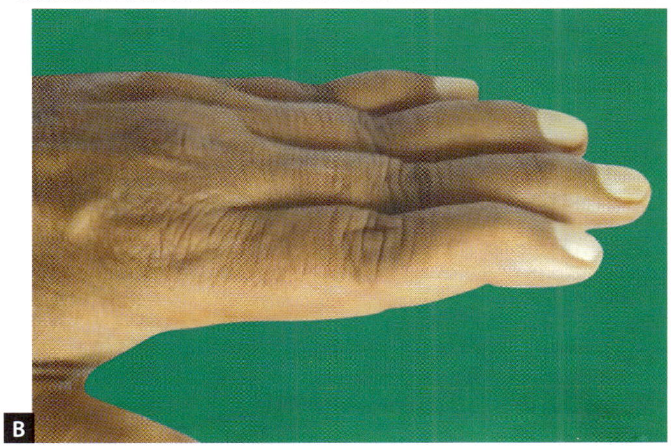

Figs. 4A and B: Swan neck deformity: The finger deformity resembles the neck of swan (A). There is flexion at the distal interphalangeal (DIP) but hyperextension at the proximal interphalangeal (PIP) joint (B).

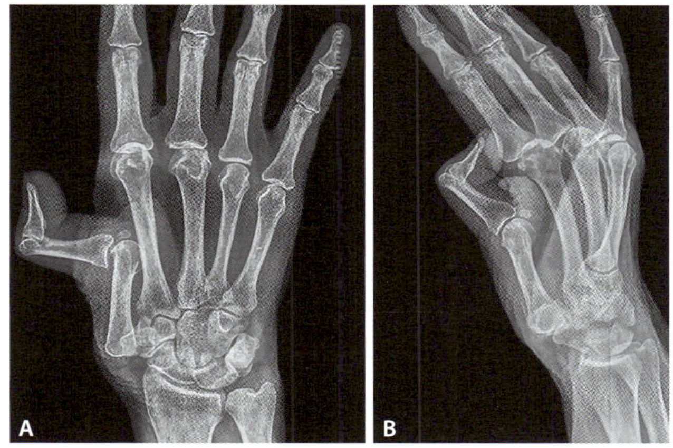

Figs. 5A and B: Swan neck deformity of thumb. The radiograph demonstrates the classical swan neck deformity of thumb with interphalangeal (IP) joint flexion (90°) and metacarpophalangeal (MCP) joint hyperextension (90°) appearing more or less dislocated.

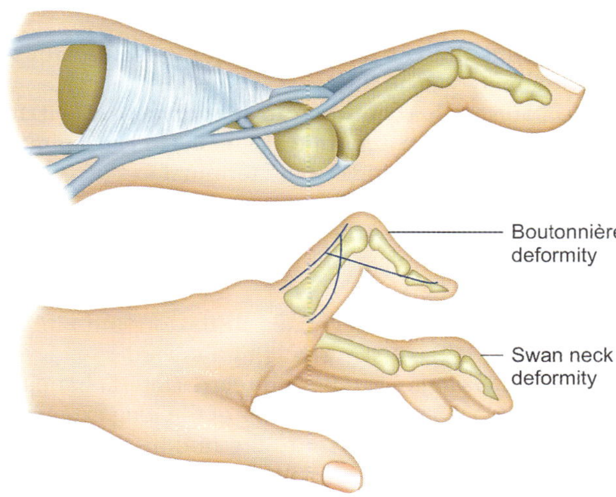

Fig. 6: Pathogenesis of the swan neck deformity. Proximal interphalangeal (PIP) hyperextension causes dorsal displacement of the lateral bands and laxity causing distal interphalangeal (DIP) flexion. Note the contrasting difference from boutonniere's deformity.

The IMs act as a functional unit with two major effects:

1. Flexion of the MCP joints by virtue of insertions into the base of the proximal phalanx volar to the axis of the MCP joint.
2. Extension of the PIP and DIP joints as the tendons cross dorsally and join the extensor apparatus over the PIP producing an extension moment at the PIP and DIP.

This dual flexor/extensor action of the IM is important mechanism for partial development of SND.

Pathomechanics of Development of Swan Neck Deformity

Zancolli has emphasized the fact that the two constituent deformities (PIP recurvatum and DIP flexion) are interrelated and are a logical consequence of the normal kinesiology of the digit. Any hyperextension of the PIP for any reason will secondarily produce flexion of the DIP. Conversely, a DIP flexion deformity produces hyperextension at PIP due to alteration of forces. The deformities also tend to vary equally in severity. The greater the recurvatum of the PIP, the greater is the flexion deformity of the DIP and vice-versa. Primary PIP hyperextension is more frequently a cause of SND as seen in RA.

Mechanisms that contribute to the secondary DIP flexion from a primary PIP hyperextension.

- *Proximal interphalangeal* recurvatum relaxes the normal tension on the lateral extensor bands. These hence move centrally and dorsally **(Figs. 6 and 7)**. In such a lax position the bands lose ability to extend the DIP, which hence drops into flexion.
- The FDP is pulled by recurvatum of the PIP causing prominent flexion of DIP by the law of maintaining constant length **(Figs. 7A and B)**.
- The mechanical advantage of FDP flexion at DIP produces equivalent mechanical disadvantage of the spiral oblique retinacular ligament (SORL) in extending the DIP.
- The last possible factor producing PIP recurvatum is the stretching of the capsule secondary to active synovitis or ruptured flexor digitorum superficialis (FDS) tendon,

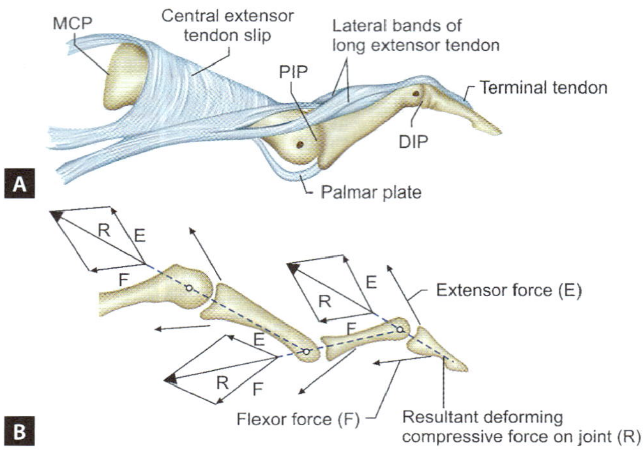

Figs. 7A and B: Swan neck deformity—pathomechanism and vectorial distribution of forces that maintain the deformity and prevent spontaneous correction. (DIP: distal interphalangeal; MCP: metacarpophalangeal; PIP: proximal interphalangeal)

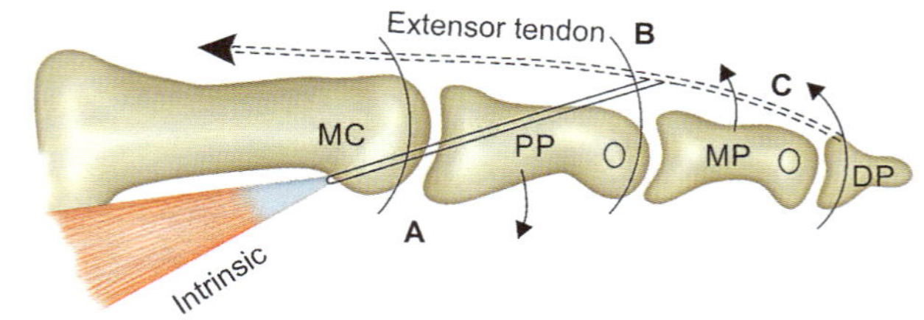

Fig. 8: Action of intrinsic and extrinsic muscles: The intrinsic muscles of hand lie volar to the metacarpophalangeal (MCP) joint axis and thus have primary flexion moment to this joint (A). The tendon of these intrinsic muscles crosses to dorsal side of proximal interphalangeal (PIP) joint axis and hence act to extend this joint (B). The intrinsic muscle tendon then joins the extensor apparatus of finger causing distal interphalangeal (DIP) joint extension (C). Flexion moment is created by the action of flexor digitorum profundus (FDP) at DIP and PIP by flexor digitorum superficialis (FDS) in the fingers. Normally the activity is balanced between these two groups but weakness of insufficiency of any one of them may tip the balance at respective joint in favor of the other. (MC: metacarpal; PP: proximal phalanx; MP: middle phalanx; DP: distal phalanx)

removing the restraint to PIP joint hyperextension (commonly seen in RA).

Mechanisms that contribute to development of SND from a primary DIP flexion deformity or "mallet finger," culminate in disruption or stretching of the terminal extensor tendon or the lateral extensor bands.

- In RA, DIP synovitis results in stretching/rupture of the extensor mechanism's terminal tendon attachment to the distal phalanx.
- Gradually, the DIP gets fixed in flexion and ability to extend the DIP is lost, resembling a mallet.
- *Distal interphalangeal* flexion relaxes lateral bands and thence concentrating the power of the long extensor on central slip that inserts into the middle phalanx. This produces PIP hyperextension.

Only for the sake of completion it should be mentioned here that the extensive work of Zancolli divides the causes of PIP hyperextension (commoner cause of SND in RA) into three types based on action of intrinsic and extrinsic hand muscle activity **(Fig. 8)**:

1. *Extrinsic type (not seen with RA):* Due to excess traction of the extrinsic extensor tendons (say with cerebral palsy, etc.) the central slip is tightened that inserts at the base of the middle phalanx. This produces an initially dynamic form of SND that appears only on wrist or MCP joint flexion. In these situations, it is impossible to flex the PIP with wrist flexed (positive extrinsic plus test).
2. *Intrinsic type:* Due to overactivity of IMs (intrinsic plus hand as in ischemic contracture, spasticity or tendon adhesions as in RA). Here the IMs oppose the extrinsic flexor muscles producing PIP hyperextension in the tug-of-war **(Fig. 9)**. The test for intrinsic plus deformities are positive here. The overactivity of intrinsics have led some authors to classify the SND into mobile, snapping, or fixed types based on condition of digital IMs.
3. *Articular type:* This is commonly seen in RA and is due secondary to weakening or destruction of normal stabilizing mechanisms of the PIP that prevent hyperextension.

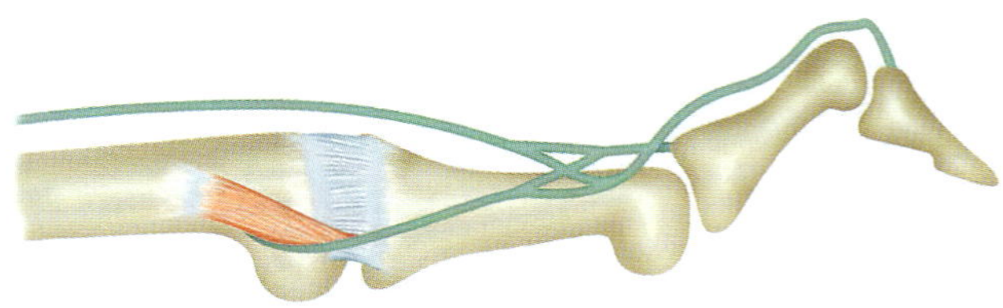

Fig. 9: Pathogenesis of the distal interphalangeal (DIP) flexion deformity in primary proximal interphalangeal (PIP) hyperextension. In intrinsic overactivity, the PIP is hyperextended causing slackening of the lateral bands and distal extensor apparatus and thus the DIP drops into flexion.

The latter two are the pathogenic mechanisms in RA that produce a primary hyperextension at the PIP followed by DIP flexion and hence complete SND.

Classification

From a management perspective the SND have been classified into four main types by Nalebuff.

1. *Type I:* PIP joints are flexible in all positions of hand and fingers.
2. *Type II:* PIP joint flexion is limited in certain positions.
    - When the MCP joints are extended or radially deviated, passive PIP joint flexion is limited while higher flexion is possible with MCP in flexion or ulnar deviation.
3. *Type III:* PIP joint flexion is limited in all positions due to contracture of the extensor mechanism, collateral ligaments and skin.
4. *Type IV:* PIP joints get stiff and show radiographic destruction.

Management

The management is best discussed on the basis of Nalebuff classification as follows:

Nalebuff type I deformity: Treatment focuses on correcting the PIP hyperextension and hence the DIP secondarily corrects.

- *Nonoperative:* Using silver rings (permit active PIP flexion and limit hyperextension of the PIP joint) or thermoplastic figure-of-8 splints.

- *Operative:*
  - Distal interphalangeal fusion along with PIP flexor tenodesis. Tenodesis is produced proximal to the A1 pulley by removing FDS from the sheath creating a flexion deformity at the PIP.
  - Spiral oblique retinacular ligament reconstruction ± dermodesis (removing elliptical skin wedge from volar aspect of the PIP and resuturing under tension).

Nalebuff type II deformity: The treatment here is focused on relieving the intrinsic tightness that is produced due to malposition of the finger at MCP.

- Surgical resection of the lateral bands is done through which the lumbricals produce deformity. Ulnar extensor aponeurosis release is also done to prevent ulnar subluxation of the tendons and reduce extensor tightness. Silicone arthroplasty is done in cases of severe involvement of the MCP joint.

Nalebuff type III deformity: The treatment focuses on restoration of passive motion to the PIP joint. The following measures help in achieving the goals:

- *Proximal interphalangeal joint manipulation:* By doing a dorsal skin release distal to PIP joint and leaving the scar to heal over 2–3 weeks.
- *Lateral band mobilization:* The lateral bands are freed from the central slip and PIP mobilized to full flexion completing the release passively.
- *Ancillary procedure:* Flexor tenolysis may be needed in above additionally to provide adequate motor power.

Nalebuff type IV deformity: Only salvage is possible for this type of deformity in the form of:

- *Arthrodesis*—of PIP joint is particularly useful for the index and middle fingers, because these digits need lateral stability when opposed to the thumb during pinch. Arthrodesis is also commonly done/preferred traditionally if concomitant MCP joint arthroplasty is being done (recently however arthroplasty has been favored concomitantly).
- *Arthroplasty*—is performed when the soft tissue and ligamentous support is adequate, especially for ring and small fingers, where mobility aids grasp.

Boutonnière Deformity

The deformity is converse to SND with the PIP joint flexed and the DIP and MP joints hyperextended **(Fig. 10)**. The abnormal finger posture in RA starts with PIP joint flexion that leads to the changes in the other joints.

Pathomechanics

- *Synovial proliferation due to RA in the PIP stretches and weakens the extensor mechanism:* Full extension cannot be achieved.
- Also the effusion and distended joint due to the synovitis forces joint to go into partial flexion (position of maximum capsular volume).
- Over time the lateral bands are displaced volarly and the SORL are shortened. SORL shortening causes DIP hyperextension.

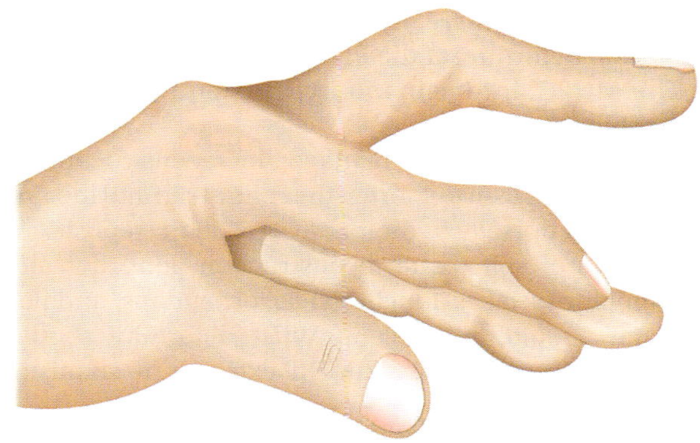

Fig. 10: Boutonniére deformity. There is flexion at proximal interphalangeal (PIP) and hyperextension at the distal interphalangeal (DIP) joint.

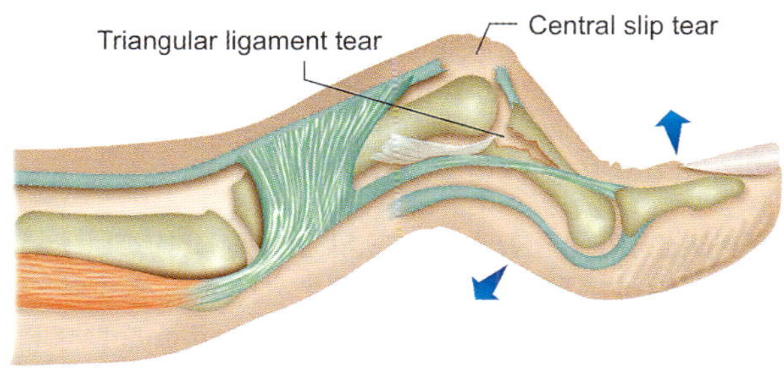

Fig. 11: Elson test mechanism: Rupture or incompetency of triangular ligament lets lateral bands to subluxate volarly. This causes proximal interphalangeal (PIP) joint flexion but a relative extension moment at the distal interphalangeal (DIP).

- The MCP joint hyperextends to compensate increasing PIP joint flexion.

Clinical Feature

Elson test: Bend PIP joint to 90° over a table top. Block middle phalanx and ask patient to extend finger. DIP should remain flaccid, if DIP extends, this indicates a central slip rupture. In boutonniére deformity incompetent triangular ligaments due to central slip rupture allow volar subluxation of lateral bands **(Fig. 11)**. With PIP extension the lateral bands will thus produce an extension moment at the DIP that is not seen in normal persons.

Management

There is specific classification of the boutonniere deformity and its management can be better discussed by grade of deformity (mild, moderate, and severe).

Mild Boutonnière deformity

- Minimal distortion of the joint positions and functional loss
- Slight extensor lag (10–15°) at the PIP joint
- Slight hyperextension at the DIP joint
- No involvement of the MCP joint

Mild deformity is usually corrected by extensor tenotomy (usually limited) to increase DIP joint flexion.

Moderate Boutonnière deformity

- Flexion deformity at the PIP joint increases to 30–40°
- The MCP joint begins to hyperextend (compensatory mechanism)

Moderate deformity is managed by reconstruction of the extensor mechanism to shorten the central slip and moving the lateral bands dorsally in their native position (repositioning). For success of soft tissue reconstruction good dorsal skin, smooth joint surfaces, functional flexor tendons, and flexible PIP joint should be present. Wrist deformity should be corrected before addressing the PIP extensor mechanism.

Severe Boutonniére deformity: In "severe boutonnière deformity", the PIP joint can no longer be passively extended. This stage is treated by fusion of the joint or arthroplasty. Fusion of the PIP joint is performed in a functional (flexed) position. Functional position of PIP flexion increases from the index finger (25°) to small finger (40°). PIP joint arthroplasty is acceptable option if the extensor mechanism is healthy enough to be repaired. As mentioned, for SND arthroplasty is useful for boutonniére deformities of the small and ring fingers to improve grip strength.

METACARPOPHALANGEAL JOINT INVOLVEMENT IN RHEUMATOID ARTHRITIS

It is helpful to describe rheumatoid involvement of MCP joint in progressive stages. The following Stirrat's modification of Nalebuff's classification is quite useful in planning surgical decisions on the basis of identified pathology:

- ***Early:*** Inflammation and swelling of MCP joint in the form of synovitis with little or no extension lag or deformity like ulnar deviation.
  - Pain is not a prominent feature
- ***Moderate:*** Radiologically demonstrable early erosions of metacarpal heads around erosions of collateral ligament.
  - Extensor tendon displacement, ulnar deviation of fingers, extension lag, or a combination of these (all/any deformity in initial stage only).
  - Pain present and constant but minimal to moderate.
- ***Late:*** Destruction of articular cartilage precluding instability and causing joint subluxation. Extension deficit or lag is prominent though mostly passively correctable. Prominent ulnar deviation and extensor tendon displacement.
  - Pain and disability prominent.
- ***Very late/advanced:*** Destruction of MCP joint associated with fixed palmar subluxation or dislocation of MCP joint. The deformities are prominent with severe and fixed ulnar deviation and ulnar and palmar displacement of the extensor tendons.
- Pain is definitely a prominent factor but functional disability is considerable.

The development of ulnar drift of fingers has been described previously. PIP joint flexion should be corrected before MCP joint soft tissue procedures or arthroplasty because achieving adequate MCP joint flexion while the PIP joint is also flexed is difficult. Wrist should also be balanced before performing the procedures on MCP joint. Ulnarly translocated wrist with supination and radial deviation of metacarpals places undue ulnarly angulating forces on the area in which rebalancing procedures are to be carried out. In late stages the joint is eroded with development of typical arthritic changes like cyst formation and loss of bony architecture **(Figs. 12A and B)**. The various methods for management of rheumatoid MCP joint affection are as follows:

- *Conservative management* by medications [disease-modifying antirheumatic drugs (DMARDs) or biologics] hardly improves established deformities but is the most important aspect in prevention of deformities.

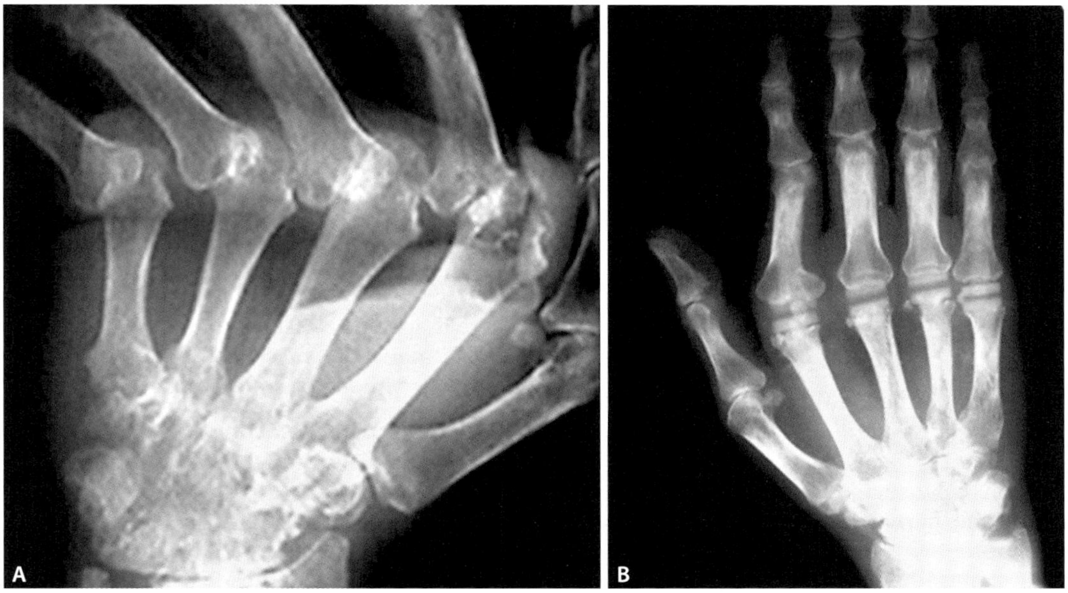

Figs. 12A and B: Arthritis of metacarpophalangeal joints in severe rheumatoid involvement. See this patient also has completely obscured carpal bones of the wrist (A). The best way to manage such severe bone erosions is perhaps arthroplasty of the joint (B) (different patient than in A).

- *Operative management:*
  - *Synovectomy:* Typically done for joint swellings not remitted by >6 months of medical therapy. Joint erosions should be absent.
  - *Extensor tendon relocation:* This is usually combined with synovectomy for patients who also demonstrate ulnar subluxation of the tendon and early ulnar drift. The extensor expansion is release from the ulnar aspect (tight side) while radial imbrication or tightening is done. Overtightening should be avoided to avoid loss of MCP flexion. This should be performed early in young patients with a stable disease (remission or partial remission). In a progressive disease, the procedure may ultimately fail. Patient should be counseled that though he may not be actively able to extend fingers, the procedure will relieve him from extensor lag at least.
  - *Intrinsic balancing:* This is done by release of IMs that relaxes the dorsal digital expansion. Crossed intrinsic transfer from ulnar side to radial side is another option taking not to excessively tension the dorsal expansion.
  - *Metacarpophalangeal joint replacement* **(Figs. 12A and B)** is by far the most popular method of restoring alignment and flexibility of MCP joint. The procedure is combined with ulnar extensor expansion release and tendon balancing. The metacarpal head and the base of proximal phalanx are cut perpendicular to the long axis. Shafts are reamed and the prosthesis is seated. The osteophytes and synovium should be debrided before prosthesis being fitted with using "no touch technique". Postoperatively the splints to maintain the finger position are provided for soft tissues to heal in good position and maintain the joints.

RHEUMATOID AFFECTION OF THE WRIST JOINT

The ulnar side of the wrist is most commonly affected producing distal radial ulnar joint (DRUJ) disruption and caput ulna syndrome (*see* Chapter on "Distal Radioulnar Joint Disorders and Ulnar Wrist Pain"). On the radial side, destructive process produces attenuation of the radioscaphocapitate ligament with rotatory subluxation of the scaphoid and ulnar translocation of the carpal bones (producing the characteristic radial deviated component of Z-deformity). In late cases, carpal coalition develops **(Figs. 12 and 13)** where the carpal bones lose distinctive boundaries and appear as a mass.

Treatment

Ideally, wrist should be managed before development of deformity at the joint but this is neglected most often. In most cases, wrist joint is addressed as a composite hand reconstruction plan where correction of finger deformities should follow wrist deformity correction.

- ***Synovectomy:*** It helps to control pain and reduce disease load. It may also help in reducing joint destruction if managed well in accordance with medical management.
- ***Distal radial ulnar joint destruction/subluxation*** (*see* Chapter on "Distal Radioulnar Joint Disorders and Ulnar Wrist Pain")
- ***Wrist fusion:*** This is a salvage procedure but a preferred option to sturdily balance the wrist. Functional loss due to arthrodesis still produces better results for function gained by the procedure and stability. This is hence a preferred option for composite hand and wrist reconstruction of late and neglected cases.
- Interposition arthroplasty has not been well-accepted by orthopedic community.
- ***Wrist arthroplasty (Fig. 14):*** This is a growing field and not many replacements have been done world over compared to large joint replacements. The primary reason is the late introduction of the implants and patients already spend so much on other joint replacements that this comes in later stage of reconstructive ladder, cost is also a deterrent.

Indications of total wrist "arthroplasty":

- The primary indication for total wrist arthroplasty is painful radiocarpal arthritis that is significantly impacting on function.
- The ultimate indication is when the contralateral wrist has already been fused; it is then desirable to retain

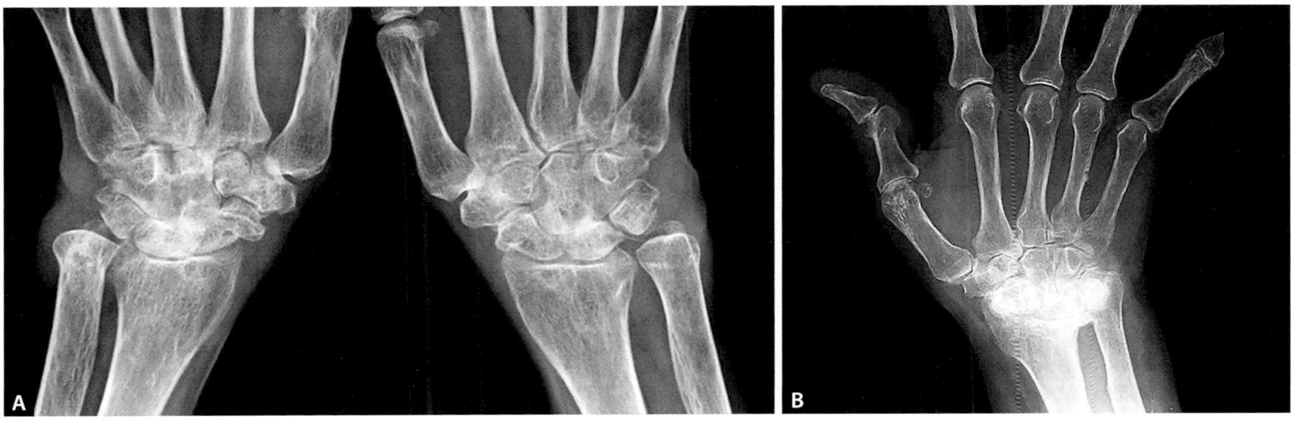

Figs. 13A and B: Wrist arthritis in rheumatoid arthritis (RA): There is involvement of both intercarpal joints and radiocarpal joints (A) causing symptoms and the bony outline has been obscured. In late stages (B) the carpals ultimately loose their outline and may appear as a single mass of bones so-called "carpal coalition".

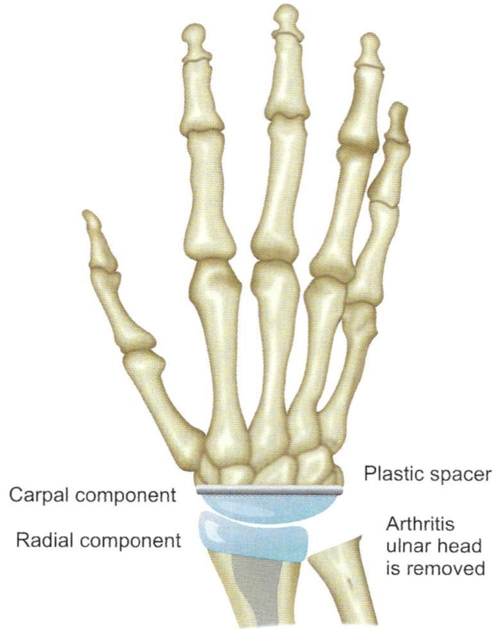

Fig. 14: Wrist arthroplasty: Total joint replacement with replacement of both the carpal and radial component.

motion in one wrist in order to improve overall function. It can correct deformity and address the degenerated parts of the joint.

Success of arthroplasty depends on bone stalk (often weak in RA), condition of tendons (frail in RA), and soft tissue around the wrist. The capsule is quite thin due to the disease process in RA so stability in motion of joint is always questionable. In the presence of soft tissue compromise arthroplasty may not be a good option in RA but otherwise (post-traumatic arthritis) it is a suitable option. In middle-aged patients with late-onset RA, the disease process is not severe enough to cause soft tissue damage where wrist arthroplasty can be successfully employed.

Contraindications:
- Infection
- Tendon disorders and ruptures
- Poor soft tissue envelope
- Poor bone stalk
- Charcot arthropathy (loss of innervation)
- Chronic subluxation
- Need of weight-bearing through the joint (assisted walk using crutches/walker, etc.)
- Involvement of contralateral wrist that also needs treatment (relative)

The implant design has changed since its introduction and currently we have third- and fourth-generation implants available for total wrist replacement. The first total wrist arthroplasty was performed by Gluck in 1890. This was not a true replacement and failed with infection (it was done in fact in a patient with tuberculosis of wrist).

- ***First-generation implants:*** Swanson flexible hinged silicone implant (1967); this was more of a spacer than a true implant. It failed quickly with typical silicone synovitis.
- ***Second-generation implants:*** This was true replacement arthroplasty and was a multicomponent design. It contained two components, a curved radial plate and flat carpal plate [fixed to metacarpal through inbuilt stem(s)] with an intervening mobile ball component made ultra-high molecular weight polyethylene (UHMWPE). The ball component is usually flat on the carpal plate while it is curved on radial aspect articulating with the concave UHMPE plate on radius (semiconstrained) mimicking the natural wrist movements.
- ***Third generation:*** These are like the second-generation implants but are characterized by minimal bone resection and avoiding fixation in metacarpal bones (there may be a restricted fixation in the second metacarpal). The implants are mostly unconstrained.
- ***Fourth generation:*** There is no definition available but the recently introduced pyrocarbon single component interposition arthroplasty or hemiarthroplasty has been mentioned as fourth-generation implants.

  Techniques vary with individual implants and are best read from the supportive literature.

Complications of the wrist arthroplasty:
- Periprosthetic lucency/osteolysis (more frequent on carpal side)
- Deep infection
- Dislocation
- Instability

The outcomes are compared with wrist fusion in most cases and with newer implants the short-term outcomes are not bad. There is around 95% survival with good function as assessed using functional assessment scores (DASH, PRIVE, etc.). These functional scores in fact score above that for wrist fusion. The main concern is the longevity and once that improves the total wrist arthroplasty may become the favored method of managing damaged wrist joints.

THUMB DEFORMITIES IN RHEUMATOID ARTHRITIS

Most of the patients with RA develop thumb deformities **(Figs. 15A and B)**. The forces causing deformities of the thumb are similar to finger deformities yet there are important differences. Synovial hypertrophy is a common pathway in development of deformities and joint destruction. Observation of umpteen patients with RA thumb involvement has led to characterization of six types of deformities classically but that does not usually finish the complexities encountered and a mixture or partial affection is also commonly seen. So, instead of boutonniére deformity with hyperextended distal digit it may fall into flexion due to associated tendon rupture producing a complex pattern. Functional effect of thumb affection is quite prominent and is due to thumb phylogenetically developing as an independent unit in humans. It has been likened to an organ in itself. Day-to-day activities such as buttoning, combing, and holding objects are all compromised.

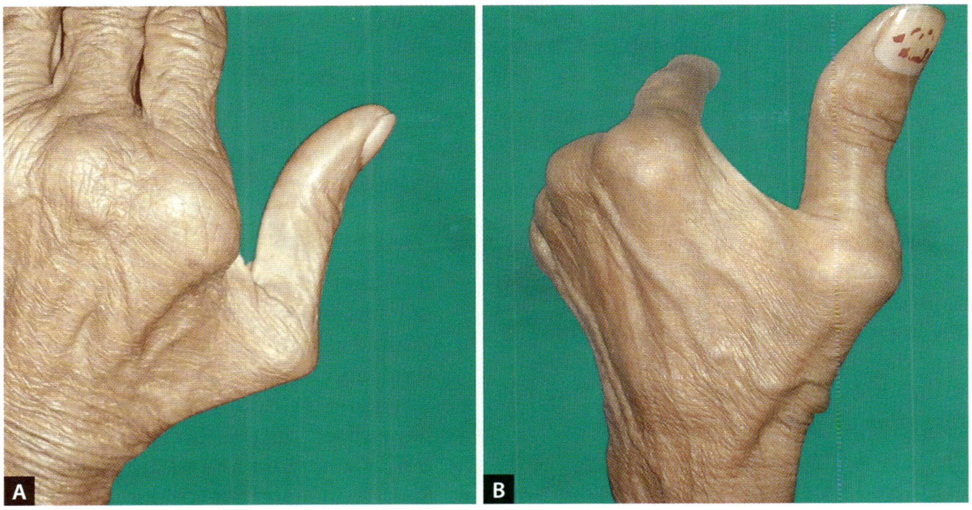

Figs. 15A and B: Thumb deformity in rheumatoid arthritis. The clinical pictures show typical boutonnisds deformity of the thumb.

TABLE 1: Nalebuff classification of thumb deformities in rheumatoid hand.

Type	*IP joint*	*MCP joint*	*CMC joint*
I (Boutonniére)	Hyperextended	Flexed	Not involved
II (Uncommon)	Hyperextended	Flexed	Flexed and ad ducted
III (Swan neck)	Flexed	Hyperextended	Subluxed, flexed, and adducted
IV (Gamekeeper's)	Not involved	Radial deviation at MCP, ulnar collateral liga-ment unstable	The joint is uninvolved (neither subluxed nor flexed or adducted)
V	Not involved	MCP primarily hyperextended due to volar plate instability	May or may not be involved
VI (Mutilated thumb, Ratliff addition)	Bone loss at any level	Bone loss at any level	Bone loss at any level

(CMC: carpometacarpal; IP: interphalangeal; MCP: metacarpophalangeal)

Classification and Pathogenesis of Thumb Deformities

The deformities have been grouped as mentioned before into six types where Nalebuff described five types of deformities and Ratliff described a sixth type **(Table 1)**.

Type I synovitis with dorsal hood disruption (due to stretching). The extensor pollicis longus (EPL) tendon subluxes ulnarly and is attenuated. Poor extension force at MCP joint produces volar subluxation of proximal phalanx base. Hyperextension of interphalangeal (IP) joint develops secondarily due to altered pull of intrinsics and EPL. There is loss of active MCP extension and during pinch the MCP joint always goes into flexion with hyperextension of the IP joint that keep increasing the deformity (progressive deformity). This is the most common deformity of thumb in RA. Other pathogenic mechanism for this deformity is rupture of EPL at wrist with IP joint hyperextension due to volar plate attenuation and flexor pollicis longus (FPL) rupture (IP hyperextension so can be primary also!).

Type II thumb deformity maintains the flexion at the MCP joint and hyperextension at the IP joint but there is additional metacarpal adduction due to carpometacarpal (CMC) joint involvement. CMC joint is often subluxed (flexion and adducted). As the patient attempts to open the first web space to grasp an object, the extension forces are transmitted to the MCP joint, resulting in the secondary hyperextension deformity of IP joint.

Type III thumb deformity is a progression of the uncommon type II deformity. The deformity results from progression of events resulting from CMC subluxation resulting in a SND and is the second most common type of thumb in RA. CMC joint synovitis initiates the dorsoradial subluxation and then dislocation of the first metacarpal base. The first metacarpal is hence adducted. This adduction combined with volar plate laxity results in hyperextension of the MP joint. Due to hyperextension at the MCP joint lateral bands are relatively shortened and this along with the pull of the FPL draws the distal phalanx into flexion completing swan neck.

Type IV deformity is analogous to gamekeeper's thumb. The MCP joint synovitis causes laxity and inefficiency of the ulnar collateral ligament. This often causes secondary adduction of the first metacarpal.

Type V deformity is identical to the type III deformity but without adduction of the first metacarpal. This is due to volar plate laxity causing primary MCP hyperextension and secondary IP joint flexion.

Type VI deformity involves bone destruction at isolated or multiple joints with subluxation and dislocation of the joints. The thumb is also shortened.

Treatment of Thumb Deformities

The treatment of specific deformities depends on the severity of disease in each involved joint and the type of deformity (as follows). In general, fixed joint deformities with bony destruction are usually more amenable to fusion than arthroplasty.

Type I deformity: MCP joint synovectomy + EPL rerouting in early cases. In late cases with 90–90 deformity, it is better to fuse the MCP joint or do an arthroplasty.

Type III (and type II) deformity: Metacarpal adduction correction is the focus of treatment of type III deformity (and type II also but is uncommon to see). Block arthrodesis to restore abduction of metacarpal (± CMC arthrodesis) is done that usually corrects the secondary deformities. If not then MCP hyperextension is corrected by capsulodesis, sesamoidesis, or arthrodesis (if fixed deformity or minimal active flexion is present) in a slightly flexed position.

Type IV deformity: It is managed by stabilizing the MCP joint and correcting the adduction contracture by Z-plasty. Ulnar collateral ligament reconstruction is done to stabilize the MCP joint, but if not possible then an arthrodesis usually helps (arthroplasty can be also considered). Thumb abduction can be efficiently done by the thenar muscles then.

Type V deformity: Best corrected by stabilization of the MCP joint by a capsulodesis, sesamoidesis, or fusion (if fixed deformity or minimal active flexion) in a slightly flexed position. Volar plate advancement is a good option or even arthroplasty is now being preferred.

Type VI deformity: Deformity is treated by fusion of the involved joints in functional position. Arthroplasty has no role at all. The IP joint should be fused at 0–20° of flexion.

CONCLUSION

- Rheumatoid arthritis commonly involves the small joint of hand and wrist. Due to numerous joints and relatively limited restraining structures destruction produced by synovitis causes frequent deformities.
- The type of deformity that specifically develops is dependent on the forces impressed by extrinsic and intrinsic tendons and subluxation of the reigns.
- Specific management options are available for correction of swan neck and boutonnière deformities depending on the stage of development of deformity and extent of involvement.
- Advanced destruction of MCP joint usually needs arthroplasty but destruction of wrist joint needs arthrodesis in view of the unavailable long-term results of arthroplasty of wrist joint.

CHAPTER 116

Infections of the Hand

Manish Kumar Varshney

INTRODUCTION

Hand, being used in varied ways and situations, is prone to trauma and infections. The hand comprises several spaces walled off by fibrous septae or synovial sheaths. The scope for expansion by inflammatory edema is very little, and thus infection in these spaces causes severe pain and toxemia. The infections range from cellulitis to surgically treatable necrotizing fasciitis and chronic infections. The subcutaneous tissue on the dorsum of the hand is more lax and hence edema of the dorsum of the hand is more prominent in palmar infections. The following are some of the infection categories that help in understanding the various types of infections of hand; categorization is done specifically with respect to the anatomical location, type of organism and discrete treatment needed.

- *Nail bed infections:*
  - Acute paronychia
  - Chronic paronychia
  - Subungual abscess
  - Felon
- Herpetic whitlow
- Flexor tenosynovitis
- *Hand space infections (deep space infections):*
  - Midpalmar space
  - Thenar
  - Hypothenar
- Cellulitis and lymphangitis
- Animal bites
- Human bites
- Septic arthritis and osteomyelitis
- *Systemic disease related infections:*
  - Diabetes mellitus
  - Intravenous drug abuse.

GENERAL PRINCIPLES OF TREATMENT OF HAND INFECTIONS

- ***Rest and elevation:*** Elevation will reduce the edema and prevent stiffness. All constricting rings on the fingers and bangles (in women and "kara" in men) should be removed. Following incision of an abscess, the hand should be kept elevated.
- ***Antibiotic treatment:*** Should be administered intravenously without delay. When cellulitis is present, antibiotics may be the sole treatment. The antibiotic of choice is first-generation cephalosporin. Antibiotics should be continued for 48 hours after pain and fever have subsided.
- ***Analgesia and anesthesia:*** Adequate analgesia should be administered and the operative procedure performed under a regional anesthesia (brachial block or ring block) and a tourniquet.
- ***Physiotherapy:*** Most essential part of therapy and for obtaining good function postoperatively.

COMPLICATIONS OF HAND INFECTIONS

- Osteomyelitis and necrosis of the terminal phalanx in pulp space infections.
- Infections of the tendon sheaths may produce sloughing of the flexor tendon.

NAIL BED INFECTIONS

A definition of the terms is appropriate to understand the various hand infection descriptions:

- ***Paronychium:*** Border tissue around the nail
- ***Nail bed:*** Germinal and sterile matrix beneath the nail plate and at its base
- ***Perionychium:*** Paronychium + nail bed
- ***Eponychium:*** The thin membrane distal to the nail wall at the base of the nail
- Paronychia is an infection of the lateral nail fold. It involves the soft tissue fold around the fingernail. The abscess is localized between the nail and nail bed.
- Eponychia is the infection of eponychial space.
- ***Run-around infection:*** Infection involving both the lateral folds and eponychium, i.e., a horseshoe-shaped infection around the nail except its tip.

Anatomy of Nail (Fig. 1)

The nail matrix (synonyms: matrix unguis, keratogenous membrane, nail matrix, and onychostroma) is the tissue (or germinal matrix) upon which the nail rests. It extends beneath the nail root and is richly supplied by nerves, lymph and blood vessels so it is highly pain sensitive and bleeds profusely on injury. Nail matrix is primarily responsible for formation of the nail by producing cells. The size, length, and thickness of the matrix, hence is a determinant of the shape (width and thickness) of nail however while the shape of the fingertip and distal phalanx bone determines if the nail plate would be flat, arched, or hooked. The nail matrix grows till it receives nutrition and remains healthy. The new nail plate cells emerge from the matrix pushing older nail plate cells forward. The older cells hence get compressed and flattened and become translucent partly revealing the highly vascular nature of matrix below in a pink hue. The lunula (the moon) is the visible part of the matrix appearing as a whitish crescent-shaped base of the visible nail. Lunula reduces as one course to ulnar fingers being the largest in the thumb and may be absent in little finger.

The nail bed or the skin below nail plate is composed of deeper dermis fixed to the bone containing capillaries and glands and the superficial epidermis just beneath the nail plate which moves forward with the plate. The epidermis and the dermis remain attached by tiny longitudinal "grooves" called the crests of nail matrix or "cristae matrices unguis". With aging the nail plate becomes thin and ridges more prominent. The nail sinus (sinus unguis) is the deep furrow into which the nail root is inserted. The nail root (radix unguis) is situated in nail sinus, i.e., the base of the nail embedded underneath the skin. Radix unguis develops from the nail matrix that is an actively growing tissue beneath. The nail plate that is the grossly visible part of nail is called the body of nail (corpus unguis). The body comprises mainly of the translucent keratin protein primarily composed of amino acids. Actually it is made of several layers of dead and flattened cells forming a strong but flexible material. Due to translucency, the nail plate appears pink as it immediately covers the underlying capillaries. The free margin or distal edge is called "margo liber". It is the anterior margin of nail that corresponds to the abrasive or cutting edge of the nail and varies in shape in different species—in humans, it is flat but in carnivores, it is often pointed into spikes. The free margin meets the epithelium of the fingertip at transition zone of hyponychium which is also known as the "quick". It is the epithelium located beneath the junction between the free edge and the skin of the fingertip and forms a seal that protects the nail bed. It is most resistant to infection. The tight seal between the nail plate and the hyponychium is called onychodermal band. It marks the end of nail bed. The eponychium (erroneously called the "proximal fold" or "cuticle") represents the small band of epithelium that extends from the posterior nail wall onto the base of the nail. It is the end of the proximal skin fold that folds back upon itself. The edge is made up of a layer of nonliving, almost invisible skin that sheds an epidermal layer of skin onto the newly formed nail plate called the cuticle. One can see cuticle as an edge that "rides out" on the posterior surface of the nail plate. The eponychium and cuticle both form a protective seal. The cuticle is formed by dead cells so may be removed during manicure but one should refrain from touching the eponychium formed of living cells. Covering the proximal band of the lunula is the projecting edge of the eponychium called perionyx. Covering the nail from sides and proximally are the overlapping cutaneous folds forming the nail wall (vallum unguis). The lateral margin (margo lateralis) of nail lies below the nail wall on both sides of the nail and the nail groove (sulcus matrices unguis) represents the cutaneous slits into which these lateral margins are embedded [into which the ingrowing nail pathologically grows as ingrowing toenail (IGTN)]. The paronychium is the border tissue around the nail.

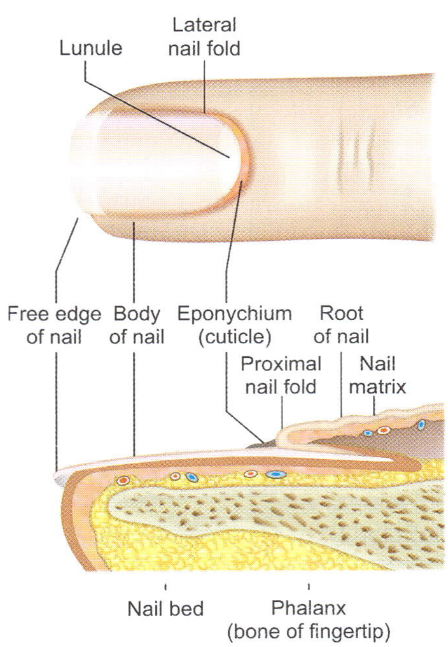

Fig. 1: Detailed anatomy of the finger nail.

Acute Paronychia

A paronychia (para-around, onukh-nail) is most common localized, superficial infection, or abscess of the paronychial tissues (perionychium-epidermis bordering the nails) of the hands **(Figs. 2A and B)** or, less commonly, the feet. The causative organism for most is usually *Staphylococcus aureus,* followed by streptococci and *Pseudomonas* organisms. Gram-negative organisms, herpes simplex virus, dermatophytes, and yeasts have also been reported

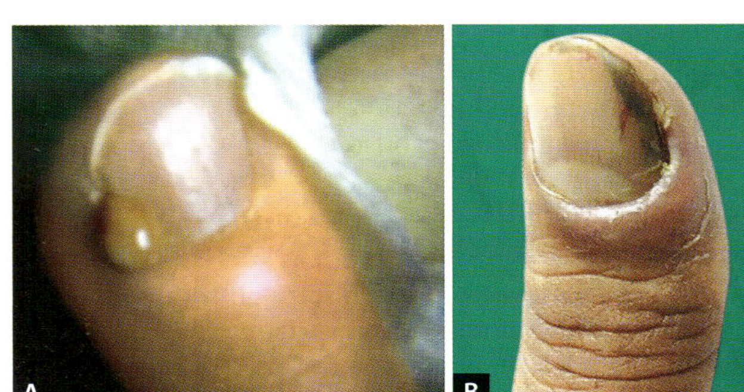

Figs. 2A and B: (A) Acute and (B) chronic paronychia.

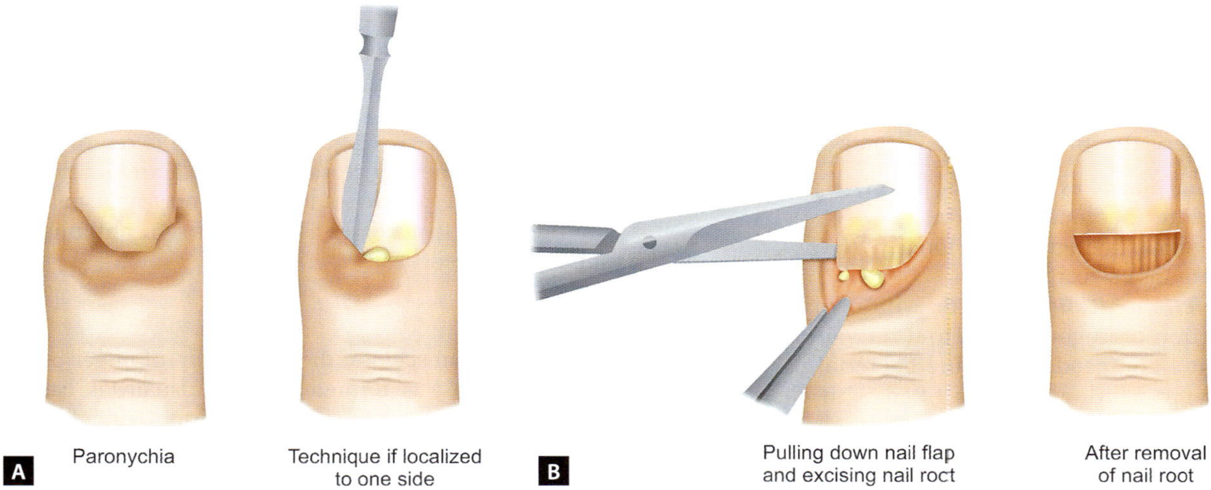

Figs. 3A and B: Paronychia treatment.

as causative agents. The infection usually occurs due to violation of the seal between the nail plate and nail fold as commonly occurs with hangnails, manicures, nail biting or sucking habit, and penetrating trauma. With the sucking habit in children the microbiology is often mixed comprising of aerobic and anaerobic organisms.

Presentation

Patients initially have classic signs of infection/inflammation such as erythema, tenderness, swelling, and warm region that is quite quickly followed (within 24 hours usually) by abscess formation giving classical presentation of fluctuance and local purulence at the nail margin. If untreated at this stage (which is often painful) the abscess may decompress to deeper tissues and involve other structures forming subungual abscess and destruction of nail-bed, causing pulp-space infection (felon—see below) or even osteomyelitis.

Treatment

Before the formation of abscess, warm water soaks and oral antibiotics covering broad spectrum of organisms (e.g., clindamycin or combination of amoxicillin-clavulanate potassium are instituted). Anaerobic coverage should be added in children having infection due to sucking habit. An incision is made where the abscess points or better entering the abscess cavity between the nail plate and nail fold with a scalpel **(Figs. 3A and B)**. Wick should be placed in the gap to prevent spontaneous closure and recurrence of the abscess that may be done without anesthesia. If there is subungual pus or some resistant infection occurs, part or whole of the nail should be removed by applying a relief incision at the base perpendicular to the nail fold.

Subungual Abscess

These form usually in association with the paronychia but may also arise de novo by infection seeding the vascular nail bed (say in infective endocarditis/septicemia).

Treatment

Removal of a portion of or the entire nail is the treatment of choice. The abscess is debrided while protecting the sterile and germinal matrices. Distal interphalangeal (DIP) is splinted and intermittent saline or antiseptic soaks may be given.

Chronic Paronychia

Chronic paronychia is usually nonsuppurative and is more difficult to treat. In chronic paronychia, the cuticle separates from the nail plate, leaving the region between the proximal nail fold and the nail plate vulnerable to infection **(Fig. 2B)**. It is commonly due to a fungal infection (*Candida albicans*) of the nail fold and seen specifically in persons constantly exposed to moist environments or otherwise due to contact dermatitis. The infections are often intermittent with characteristic thickening of the eponychial fold that also remains painful in general. Persons characteristically affected by chronic paronychia include homemakers, gardeners, housekeepers, bartenders, dish cleaners, and swimmers. Patients with diabetes and immunocompromised state are also predisposed.

Clinical Features

Chronic paronychia presents as swollen, red, boggy, and tender nail folds. Symptoms often intermittent are present for >6 weeks in a typical case. Pus formation and fluctuance is uncommon and erythema is much less than seen in acute paronychia. Inflammation is intermittent commonly exacerbating after exposure to water and appearing as pain and swelling. The nail plate changes are typical, it is thickened, discolored, and develops prominent transverse ridges. The underlying epidermis separates from the nail fold and the nail plate forming potential space that are then homed by various microbes and fungi like *Candida albicans*. These are revealed in a wet mount washed with potassium hydroxide from a scraping that demonstrate hyphae and clusters of grape-like yeast cells. Alternatively, a culture of the pus may show hyphae and fungal elements along with bacterial elements. *Candida albicans* is cultured from >90% cases of chronic paronychia. Other identified common pathogens include gram-negative rods and cocci, atypical mycobacteria that may also cause chronic paronychia.

Differential diagnosis for chronic paronychia:

- Dyshidrotic eczema
- Malignant subungual melanoma
- Squamous cell carcinoma
- ***Herpetic whitlow:*** Herpetic whitlow represents viral infection of fingertip pulp and the perionychium that is often confused with acute bacterial paronychia. In herpetic whitlow vesicles filled with clear fluid are grouped on an erythematous base characteristically. It is caused by herpes simplex virus 1 in >60% of cases while remaining cases are caused by herpes simplex virus 2.
- Psoriasis
- Bowen disease
- Kaposi sarcoma
- Metastatic cancer
- Pemphigus vulgaris
- Pyogenic granuloma
- Reiter disease

Treatment

Management primarily involves avoiding predisposing factors. Treatment with a combination of topical steroids and an antifungal agent is successful when there is no frank pus. Treatment of potential secondary bacterial infections with antibacterial solutions or ointments, acetic acid soaks (1:1 ratio of vinegar to water), or oral antibiotics may be necessary. Eponychial marsupialization (surgical treatment of choice) of the nail bed is done by removing crescent-shaped portion of the eponychial fold proximal to the distal edge of the eponychial fold without injuring the germinal matrix **(Fig. 4)**. Nail plate is removed only if severely deformed or grossly infected. Careful attention to hygiene, protective gloves to keep hand dry, usually clears the infection. Recurrence is common. An antifungal drug should be added.

Felon

A deep space abscess of the distal pulp of finger or thumb **(Figs. 5A to C)** is termed felon. It usually is caused by bacterial infection, but herpes virus (called herpetic whitlow) and, more rarely, fungi also can cause felons. The distal pulp space is walled off by fibrous septa at the level of

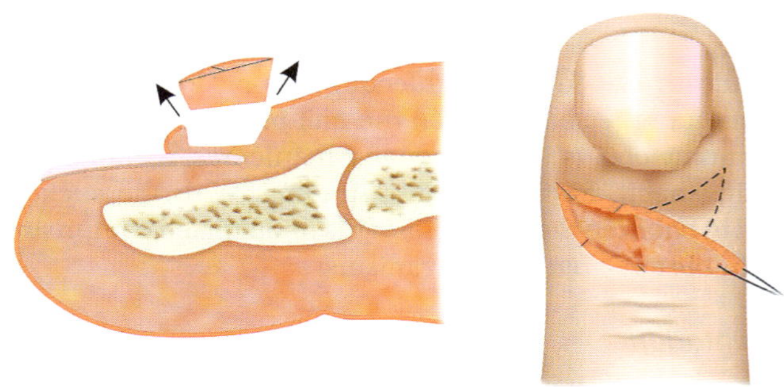

Fig. 4: Marsupialization of eponychium for chronic paronychia.

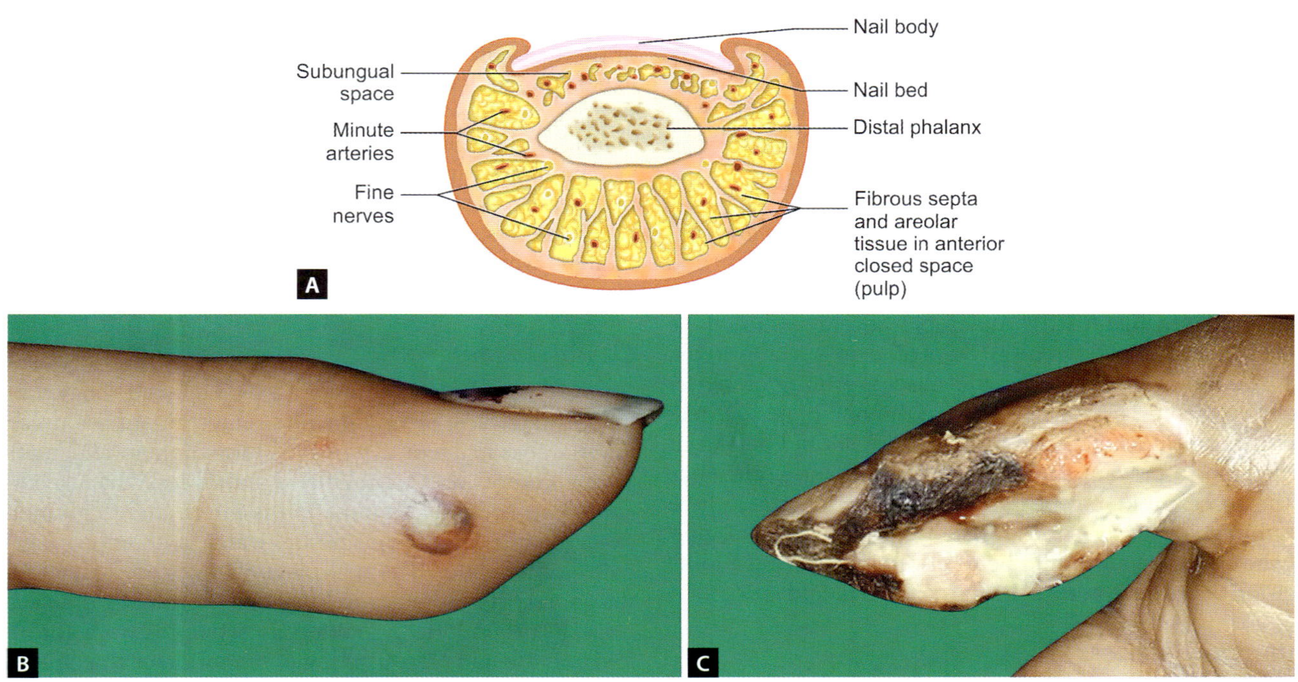

Figs. 5A to C: Felon is a deep space infection of distal pulp of finger. (A) There are several fibrous septa forming compartments in the pulp space. (B) Typical appearance of felon with swollen thumb distal pulp space and an imminent rupture point for pus in this case; (C) If the abscess is not drained early (<24 hours)—there are high chances of deep slough and necrosis formation.

the distal crease. These form small compartments separated by vertical 15–20 fibrous septa extending from skin to periosteum, filled with connective tissue and fat globules **(Figs. 5A to C)**. If unchecked, the infection can progress to produce a sinus, skin sloughing, or osteomyelitis and further to septic arthritis of the DIP joint or pyogenic tenosynovitis.

Pathophysiology

Felon is usually preceded by penetrating trauma. Splinters of glass, plywood, abrasions, and minor puncture wounds are the most common predisposing factors. Felon also may arise from the rupture of untreated paronychia into the volar pad of fingertip. Uncommon but iatrogenic cause of felons could be following finger-stick blood tests neither for hemoglobin estimation nor more commonly in diabetics for blood sugar estimation. The most common offending organism is *Staphylococcus aureus*. Diabetics in the habit of biting their fingernails have *Eikenella corrodens* reported in cultures.

Felon represents an urgency because if the pus pocket continues to expand, it may compress transiting blood vessels in the finger cutting off the fingertip circulation. This may cause wet gangrene of the distal part, and hence permanent damage to the finger. Also untreated felon can spread infection to underlying bone within the finger causing osteomyelitis that is quite recalcitrant **(Fig. 5C)**.

Diagnosis

It is usually evident clinically. Patient has history of injury in the area. Initially, it presents with cellulitis and severe throbbing pain. Tenderness, redness, firmness, and enlargement of the fingertip are all signs of a felon-containing tense abscess and are warning signs indicating the need of surgical evacuation. If there is small bubble-like cyst on the skin, called vesicles, and repeated episodes, it is a herpetic whitlow. Radiographs should be obtained for evaluating osteomyelitis (in order to prognosticate the patient).

Treatment

The initial treatment (<24 hours) is by antibiotics and rest. Give appropriate tetanus prophylaxis. If the symptoms are present for >48 hours, incision and evacuation of pus is treatment of choice **(Figs. 6A and B)**. Presence of throbbing pain is an indication of abscess formation. Pus is evacuated by "a unilateral longitudinal incision" (usually preferred but may have higher chances of ischemia and anesthesia by injuring one or both neurovascular bundles) over the most tender spot on the pulp or ideally performed on the noncontact surface of the involved digit. This includes the ulnar sides of the index and long fingers **(Fig. 6A)** and the radial sides of the ring finger, small finger, and thumb. Fish-mouth incision should be avoided (causes unstable painful fingertip). "A longitudinal central midline incision" is advocated to avoid skin slough, digital nerve injury, or creation of an unstable fat pad **(Fig. 6B)**. This incision is especially useful in the presence of a sinus track that can be incorporated within the incision. In any case, the following precautions are imperative:

- The incision should not cross the DIP joint to prevent formation of a flexion contracture at the DIP flexion crease.
- Probing is not carried out proximally to avoid extension of infection into the flexor tendon sheath.

Wick is placed to prevent premature closure of the incision and recurrence of abscess. Obtain cultures from the evacuated pus. Empiric antibiotic coverage with a first-generation cephalosporin or anti-staphylococcal penicillin usually is adequate treatment for an uncomplicated felon. This should be later changed to culture and sensitivity patterns. Especially one should look for methicillin-resistant *Staphylococcus aureus* (MRSA) or gram-negative organisms.

Potential complications of a felon and felon drainage include an anesthetic fingertip, a neuroma and an unstable finger pad.

BITE WOUNDS OF HAND

Bite wounds can be caused by human or animals bite. These are always contaminated. Animal bites are very common with most comprising of dog bites (90%) followed by cat bites (5%) and rest are from other pet/domestic animals and miscellaneous wild animals. Children are most susceptible to animal bites and it is the dominant hand that is frequently affected. The infection is polymicrobial in nature but less pathogenic to humans than flora of human bites. The predominant organisms are anaerobic (10:1) with a mixture of *Pasteurella species, Streptococcus,*

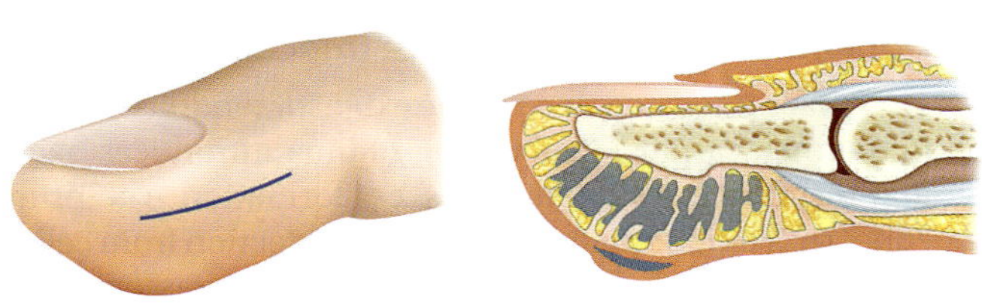

A

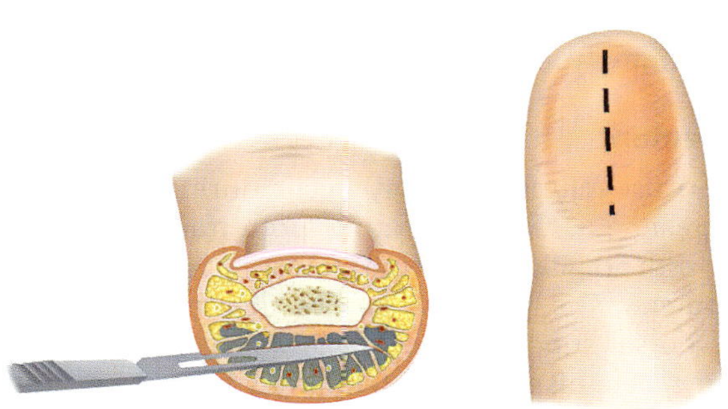

B

Figs. 6A and B: Drainage of pus from felon, usually unilateral incisions are preferred but some surgeons prefer a central midline incision to prevent skin slough and digital nerve injury (see text).

Staphylococcus, Moraxella, Neisseria, Proteus, Pseudomonas, Eikenella, Peptostreptococcus, Bacteroides, Fusobacterium, Propionibacterium, Veillonella, and *Actinomyces*. Cat-scratch disease is a specific condition that occurs after cat, dog, or monkey bite or scratch. The site develops erythematous lesion followed by a primary papule 3–5 days after injury. This is followed by adenopathy of the draining part 5–50 days later. *Afipia felis* and *Bartonella henselae* (gram-negative bacteria) have been implicated as causative pathogens. Usually self-limiting, the disease can also be managed by fluoroquinolones or macrolides.

Animal bite infections manifest as cellulitis, lymphangitis, and subsequently purulent drainage commonly. Most animal bites are deep-seated punctures rather than simple avulsions and deliver the pathogens deep into the wounds. Also the anaerobic environment is favored here. The infection potential of these bites is hence high. Arthropods and insect bites infrequently get infected. Snake bites are sharp but mainly deliver the venom that is essentially sterile. Still the snake oral flora resembles the fecal flora of its prey so there is always a potential for infection. The venom is inhibitory to the aerobic pathogens but not to the anaerobic ones.

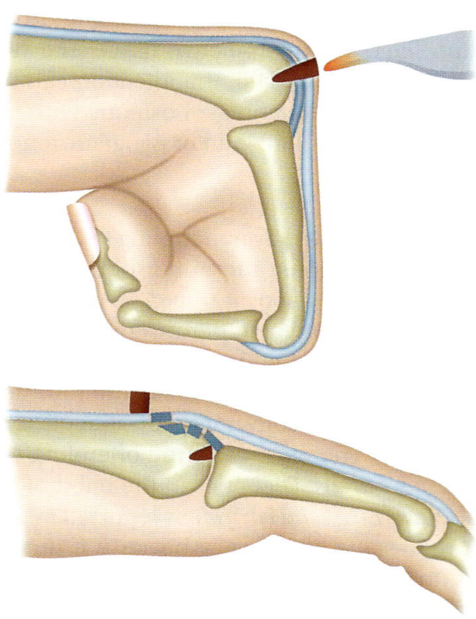

Fig. 7: Fight bite injuries: The skin mark from tooth injury is mostly misleading and the deep injury does not correspond to it by the time patient presents to the clinician. Underlying tissue hence appears normal to clinician missing the deep tendon or other structure injury. Also prolonged incision needs to be given for adequate wound toileting.

Treatment

Treatment is done through cleaning with a topical antiseptic agent in running water. Broad-spectrum antibiotic coverage should include a beta-lactam antibiotic (usually a cephalosporin) with beta-lactamase inhibitor along with fluoroquinolone. If infection of the wound has occurred, then surgical excision of the wound, thorough irrigation, and instillation of appropriate antibiotics are done and the wound is left open. When the infection has subsided, the wound is then closed. The surgical debridement as a primary measure is used for pyogenic tenosynovitis and osteomyelitis.

Human bites are classified into four types:
1. Self-inflicted
2. Traumatic amputations
3. Full-thickness bite wounds to the hand or digits
4. Clenched-fist (e.g., blow to the mouth producing a knuckle-tooth wound) injuries **(Fig. 7)**

The bacterial flora is same as described for animal bites while there is predominance of *Streptococcus* and *Staphylococcus spp.* and *Eikenella corrodens*. The latter is found commonly in the dental scrapings.

Management

Clenched fist injuries (as may occur during street fights) are interesting as the penetrating tooth track is effectively sealed with digital extension, creating a closed-space environment. The potential spaces that may be entered are the dorsal subcutaneous space between the skin and extensor mechanism, the subtendinous space between the extensor mechanism and joint capsule and the joint space itself but importantly the site of entry of all changes with the position of hand during examination with fingers extended. Bites seen within 24 hours should be treated with cleansing and local therapy, especially if there is no evidence of joint or tenosynovium penetration. Oral antibiotics should be added, commonly the combination of amoxicillin and clavulanic acid is used. Close follow-up with review at 12–24 hours should be done for spreading infection. Surgical debridement is done primarily for obvious infection (presenting late) or joint/tendon space penetration as the coverage with antibiotics is not sufficient at these places.

DEEP SPACE INFECTIONS

There are six spaces in hand which can become infected **(Fig. 8)**:
1. Dorsal subaponeurotic space
2. Web space
3. Midpalmar space
4. Thenar space
5. Hypothenar space
6. *Dorsal adductor space:* Potential space located dorsal to the adductor pollicis and palmar to the first dorsal interosseous.

Dorsal Subaponeurotic Space Infections

This space is located deep to the extensor tendons and dorsal to the metacarpals. Penetrating trauma introduces bacteria that result in infection and abscess formation. The primary concern is differentiating this serious infection from cellulitis and whenever in doubt one should do aggressive surgical debridement. Two dorsal longitudinal incisions (one over second metacarpal and the other between fourth and fifth metacarpal space) are preferred over a single incision to prevent tendon desiccation. Wounds are allowed to heal by secondary intention.

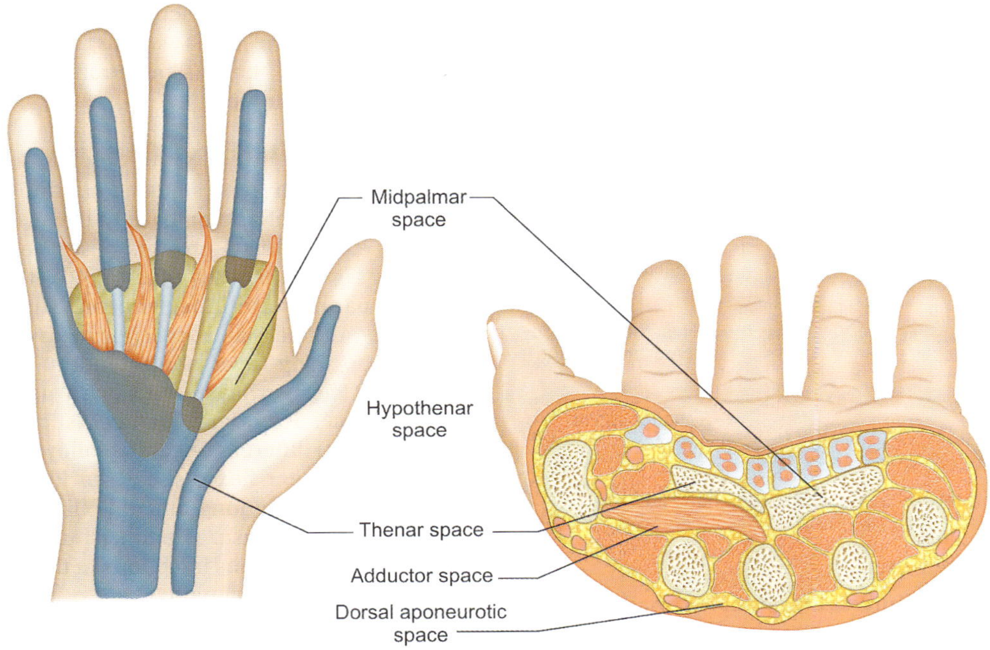

Fig. 8: Deep spaces of hand. In the illustration through axial section of hand and profile view are shown thenar space, adductor space, dorsal aponeurotic space, midpalmar space, and hypothenar space.

Web Space Infection (Collar-Button Abscess/ Hourglass Abscess) (Fig. 9)

There are three interdigital web spaces containing loose fat and communicate proximally along the lumbrical canals with the middle palmar space. Infection in any one of these spaces gives rise to a local swelling and swelling of the dorsum. The infection occurs through a crack in the skin between the fingers or from an infected blister, an open wound, or a palmar callus or from the adjacent subcutaneous area. An abscess subsequently develops and extends either volarly or usually dorsally to include the contiguous subcutaneous space of the dorsal hand. Severe pain and swelling is generally limited to the web space area and the distal palm. The fingers adjoining the space are abducted from each other. The maximum tenderness is over the palmar aspect of the web space.

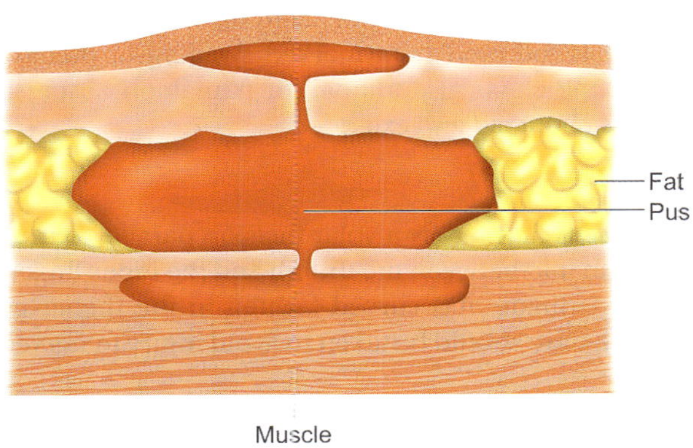

Fig. 9: Collar-button abscess.

Treatment

In the stage of cellulitis, infection is treated with antibiotics and elevation. Once the abscess forms, it is drained where it is pointing by a curved incision overlying the abscess on palmar aspect or a straight dorsal incision or a combination of both. After evacuation of pus, wound is dressed over polyethylene/silicone catheter (to allow drainage and saline irrigation for 24 hours) and *plaster of Paris* (POP) slab applied.

Midpalmar Space Infection

This space is bounded ventrally by flexor tendons and lumbricals and dorsally by volar fascia investing the second and third volar interossei and the third and fourth metacarpals. On the radial side, it is separated from the thenar space by a fibrous septum (midpalmar of oblique fascial septum) extending between the palmar fascia and the middle metacarpal. Distally, it extends to the level of the vertical septa of the palmar fascia, ending approximately 2 cm proximal to the web spaces or may communicate with them.

Infection can reach this space through various places including direct penetrating injury or rupture of flexor tenosynovitis of middle, ring, or small finger or a distal palmar abscess. The hand becomes swollen; the palm loses its concavity and becomes full (frog-hand).

Treatment

The space is drained by an incision commonly through the middle third of the distal palmar crease **(Fig. 10)** though various incisions have been described. The pus is evacuated and hand rested in plaster slab and elevated.

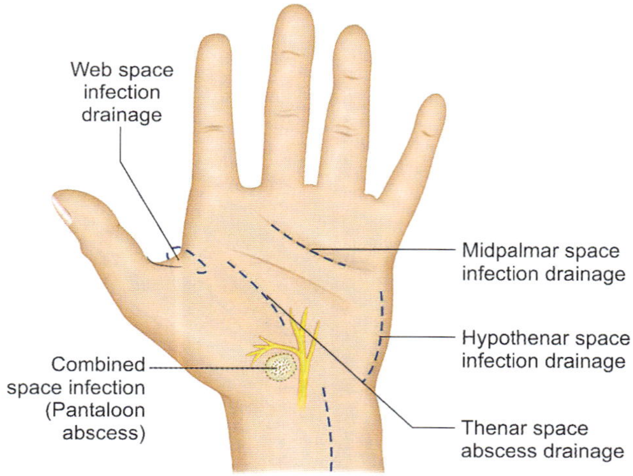

Fig. 10: Incisions for drainage of various hand abscess.

Thenar Space Infections

The thenar space is bound ventrally by the palmar fascia and dorsally by the transverse head of adductor pollicis. It is bordered ulnarly by the vertical midpalmar septum and radially by the adductor pollicis fascia. The infection occurs through penetrating injury or subcutaneous abscess of thumb or index finger or extension from infection of radial bursa. It is followed by a marked swelling of thenar area forming the classical dumbbell or pantaloon abscess. The thumb is abducted and extended.

Treatment

The space is drained by a volar incision parallel to the edge of the skin fold between the thumb and the index finger. The incision is made in a curved fashion in the thenar crease **(Fig. 10)**. Care should be taken to avoid injury to nerves and vessels.

Hypothenar Space

It contains the hypothenar muscles and is enclosed by their investing fascia. This space is located ulnar to midpalmar space and is bordered radially by a fibrous hypothenar septum coursing between the fifth metacarpal and palmar aponeurosis. The space can get infected from pyogenic tenosynovitis of the little finger (or ulnar bursa as they are contiguous) or penetrating injuries causing erythema, swelling, and throbbing pain.

Treatment

Volar longitudinal incision is used to drain the space followed by saline irrigation and antibiotic therapy.

FLEXOR TENOSYNOVITIS (PYOGENIC FLEXOR TENOSYNOVITIS OR SUPPURATIVE FLEXOR TENOSYNOVITIS)

It is a bacterial infection of the digital flexor sheath. Tenosynovitis is often caused by a penetrating injury in the flexor crease or by spread of a pulp space infection. It is the most fearsome of infections in hand. Most common causative organism is *S. aureus* and other organisms resemble the skin flora as penetrating injury is the most common mode of injury.

Anatomy of Digital Flexor Sheath

The flexor sheath represents a continuous longitudinal synovial pouch that originates at the level of the metacarpal neck and ends at distal phalanx base near the insertion of the *flexor digitorum profundus* (FDP). It has two layers—the outer parietal and inner visceral. The former develops distinctive annular and cruciform thickenings forming pulleys. The deep layer abuts tendon and is also called "epitenon". The two layers enclose a potential fluid-filled synovial space. There are characteristic features of digital flexor sheath of different fingers as follows:

- The little finger flexor sheath of FDP tendon (and on occasion, the ring, long, and index fingers) communicates with the ulnar bursa. The ulnar bursa extends proximal to the wrist level thus infections in these spaces may well spread to wrist proximally.
- Similarly the flexor sheath of the *flexor pollicis longus* (FPL) (to thumb) communicates with the radial bursa that also extends proximal to the wrist level.
- The flexor sheaths of ring and middle finger are usually isolated in most patients and do not communicate with other spaces.
- The radial and ulnar bursae communicate with each other at the level of the transverse carpal ligament through space of Parona (space between the pronator quadratus and the FDP tendons). Infection in any one of them may communicate to the other side when profuse and produce a "horseshoe abscess" (80% patients).

Clinical Features

Kanavel's four cardinal signs **(Figs. 11A and B)** are quite characteristic to diagnose pyogenic flexor tenosynovitis.

1. Semiflexed posture of involved finger in rest
2. Symmetric enlargement of the whole finger (sausage digit)
3. Excessive tenderness limited to the course of the sheath
4. Excruciating pain in extending the finger passively (the most dependable sign)

It causes a cylindrical swelling of the finger, which is kept semiflexed. Infection of the ulnar bursa causes edema of the whole hand with fullness above the flexor retinaculum. Infection of the radial bursa causes pain, swelling, and tenderness along the bursa. When the two bursae communicate through space of Parona there forms horseshoe abscess. The gliding mechanism of the tendon can be damaged or ischemic necrosis of the tendon may take place. If not treated early, it may lead to protracted tendon sheath infection or osteomyelitis. This may eventually lead to loss of finger and hand function. Depending on the duration of infection and tissue changes the pyogenic flexor tenosynovitis has been classified into three stages:

1. *Stage 1:* Increased fluid in sheath mainly serous exudate
2. *Stage 2:* Cloudy/purulent fluid, synovium may be granulomatous
3. *Stage 3:* Septic necrosis of the tendon, pulleys, or sheath

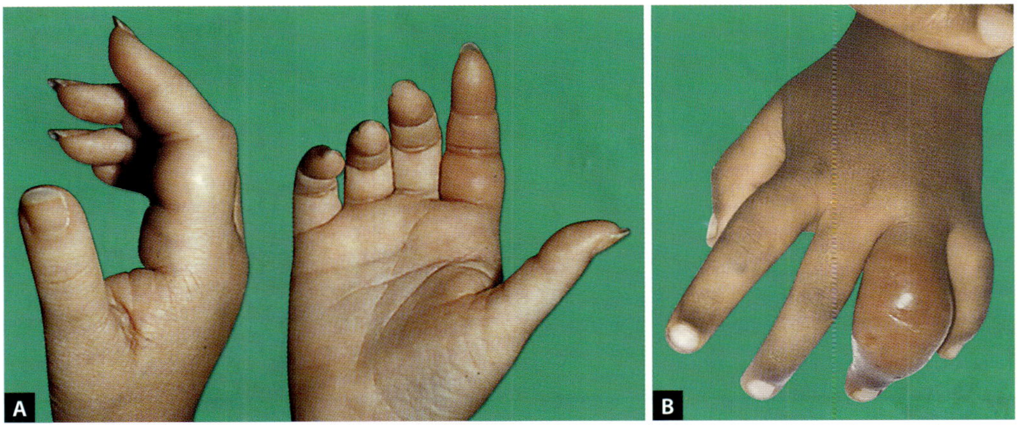

Figs. 11A and B: Flexor tenosynovitis: Kanavel's signs help to differentiate from abscess formation in finger.

Treatment

Treatment should be prompt and effective. The infection is treated conservatively with antibiotics if detected within first 24 hours. If this causes relief of pain, conservative treatment is continued else surgery is the treatment of choice.

Surgery

If signs and symptoms are not abating, decision to surgically drain the infection is taken. For stages 1 and 2, the incision is made classically through midlateral crease in case of index and little fingers where the entire sheath can be laid open. Pus is expressed from terminal part to over metacarpophalangeal joint. In case of middle or ring finger volar approach, a zig-zag incision (Brunner's) or a combination of midlateral incision in finger and a transverse incision in palm over the proximal end of the flexor tendon sheath can be made. The fibrous flexor sheath should not be completely incised along its whole length, but important pulleys should be left intact particularly A2 and A4 pulleys. After a thorough decompression, drain is put for 24 hours; hand is splinted, elevated, and treated by systemic antibiotics.

I prefer a two-incision approach (for middle and ring fingers) in which the A1 pulley is approached proximally through a preferred transverse incision at the level of the metacarpal head. After entering the sheath pus and debris is aspirated and a small infant feeding tube or 16-gauge suction catheter is passed up the sheath. Another palmar incision is made transversely distal to the A4 pulley in the finger and the sheath is irrigated using saline. I commonly use last wash with antibiotic before withdrawing the catheter back. Another catheter is then inserted and sutured to act as drain for next 24 hours. The radial and ulnar bursae are exposed through open technique. Horseshoe abscess is drained through both radial and ulnar bursae.

For stage 3, the treatment is more extensive with extensive debridement and patient should be counseled in advance for possible need of amputation, the decision of which is taken by two consultants after independent evaluation.

Physiotherapy

As soon as infection is controlled, favorable active movements of fingers can be started.

CONCLUSION

- Although small in size, the hand provides various potential sites for infection. Due to its important function in body and frequent use, hand is also subjected to injuries and hence infections.
- Infections in various parts of hand should be promptly identified and treated else loss of function and resulting disability is quite unacceptable.

CHAPTER 117

Tendon Injuries of Hand and Management

Manish Kumar Varshney

INTRODUCTION

Tendon injuries have been recognized since times immemorial. The understanding of tendons as a distinct structure from nerve took few decades to establish, and the management of injuries took serpentine turns and even U-turn over past centuries. The management is still evolving and now has reached to understanding of molecular levels; it is unsure whether a management perspective based on these advanced understanding of the tendon will crop up in future (say nanotechnology).

HISTORICAL PERSPECTIVE

It is interesting to know the poor understanding and mostly misunderstandings about tendons in past that slowly evolved into the current microscopic understanding of tendon structure and function. This gives a background understanding of the management evolution of tendon injuries also.

- Ancient literature refers tendon as “neurons” mistaking the structure for whitish cord-like structure. This was also partially attributed to misunderstanding of the Galen’s writing that pricking the tendon would cause twitching; however, he meant pricking the muscle will cause twitching through force transmitted across tendon.
- Galen advised not to suture tendons (primarily as he thought that pricking will damage the structure and cause twitching and convulsions!), though being the physician to gladiators he did suture tendons.
- Avicenna (Muslim physician, philosopher of the 11th century) has been described as the first surgeon recommending suturing the tendons (he was quite influenced by Galen’s work).
- Still considering the high influence of Galen, tenorrhaphy was not practiced universally.
- Galen’s influence finally received a blow and the dictum of not suturing tendons was abolished by two events:
  1. Meekren (1682) crushed tendon fibers and demonstrated that no pain or twitching occurs as propounded by Galen.
  2. Von Haller (1752) investigated the irritability and excitability of various tissues including tendon and concluded that it is a nonexcitable tissue, and there is no reason to not to suture tendons.
- John hunter (1767) evaluated the tendon healing process. This was followed by other studies but all were on canine Achilles tendon.
- Flexor tendon healing in the sheath was studied by Bier and Saloman and found poor healing of the tendons possibility related to hormonal influence and poor cellular response. They recommended leaving the defect and not suturing them.
- Bunnell (1934) additionally observed adhesion formation at the site where tendon pass through sheath that was more pronounced when sheath was left open or injured. He termed this zone as “no man’s land” (NML) in his text in 1948. NML was derived from the land outside city of London that was used for executions and also from the classical description of World War I where the lands between the frontline trenches of the two opposing armies would be fraught and soldiers ventured if at all with extreme caution. Bunnell however did “venture with extreme caution” in this NML of hand and stated the importance of no tension (by flexing the wrist), that improves the chances of healing.
- Boyes stated that the NML repairs frequently failed due to infection, excessive scarring, and flexion contracture caused by poorly placed incisions so recommended against it. This area has now been labeled zone II of flexor tendons.
- Exceptions are a rule in medicine so slowly reports were published for successful repair of tendons in NML or zone II by various authors and conditions for improving the success of repair were laid down.
- Kleinert’s classic presentation in 1967 American Society for Surgery of the Hand (ASSH) meet about primary repair of flexor tendons in NML proved to be the turning point to establish primary repair of flexor tendon in any area.
- Mode of healing has long been debated as to whether the tendon healing is an intrinsic process or extrinsic one.

The various findings by different investigators have been not in absolute congruence.

- ***Intrinsic tendon healing concept:*** Lindsay established that epitenon and later endotenon cell proliferation and migration are responsible for primary healing. This is later marred by proliferating collagen and its maturation. Importantly, this response occurs whether the sheath is present or absent so sheath plays minimal role if any. Lundborg also demonstrated complete tendon healing when tendon has been isolated from its sheath. This is further supported by studies that demonstrate healing of the tendon when placed in extracorporeal tissue culture environment.
- ***Extrinsic cellular influence and tendon healing:*** Potenza and Herte and Chow demonstrated that extrinsic synovial cells "seed" on to nonviable tendon segments and potentiated the healing process.

- As of current understandings, the following things are quite established from literature:
  - Peripheral adhesions are not essential to the tendon healing
  - Enhancing repair with strong suture materials
    - Multiple suture strands
    - Core and peripheral combinations
  - Atraumatic approach is the best yielding.
  - Early mobilization and role of tension to healing cells.

ANATOMICAL AND BIOMECHANICAL CONSIDERATIONS

Only the salient features of tendon anatomy and some description of terms will be done herewith. Tendon derives its name from Latin word *tendere*, meaning "to stretch"—the tendon serves to conduct tension. The property of stretch is conferred by collagen and elastin.

- Tendon is made-up of:
  - Cellular component—fibroblasts and spindle-shaped (production of collagen and extracellular matrix reorganization)
  - *Extracellular matrix:*
    - Water (60–80% of the wet weight)
    - Collagen (86% of dry weight)—type 1 collagen predominates. Five crosslinked collagen molecules form a microfibril, groups of which join to make subfibrils, and then ultimately larger fibrils **(Fig. 1)**.
    - Proteoglycans (1–5% of dry weight)
    - Elastin (2% of dry weight)
- Tendon fascicles are bound by endotenon (similar to endoneurium of nerves). Tendon as a whole is encased in epitenon. While the latter produces synovial fluid, the endotenon provides a route for vessels and nerves.
- The tendon can stretch from 9 to 35% of initial length before it breaks **(Fig. 2)**. The young's modulus of human tendon ranges from 1,200 MPa to 1,800 MPa.
- Tendon exhibits a unique viscoelastic nature demonstrated by:
  - ***Creep:*** Creep is the time-dependent elongation of tendon under a constant load. It is characterized by an initial large elongation followed by elongation in smaller increments. With continued cycling, there is a tendency of creep to continue elongating the tendon.
  - Stress relaxation is the concomitant decrease in load exhibited as the tissue is subjected to constant elongation.
- Elastic modulus of tendon is highest at maturity with increasing cross-sectional area while the same decreases after age due to decreased tendon collagen, proteoglycan, and water content.
- Contrary to the common tendon inflammation and tendinopathies seen in diabetics, glucose solution has been found to increase collagen crosslinking and increase in maximum load, elastic modulus, energy-to-yield, and toughness.
- Excursion of tendon is the distance that the tendon slides along its path. Brand identified three distinct terms to clarify muscle-tendon relationship:
  1. Potential excursion—resting fiber length of muscle independent of connective tissue restraints

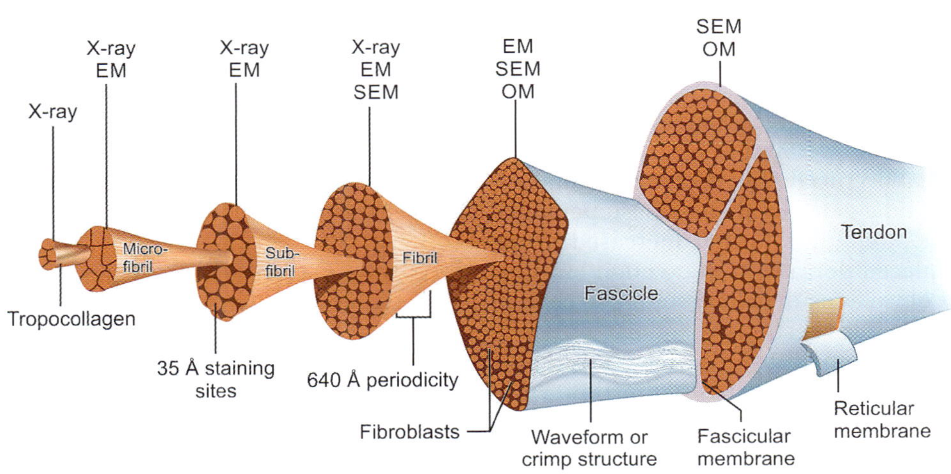

Fig. 1: Microarchitecture of collagen. Collagen molecules are arranged in progressively larger strands, coalescing into the structure of tendon.

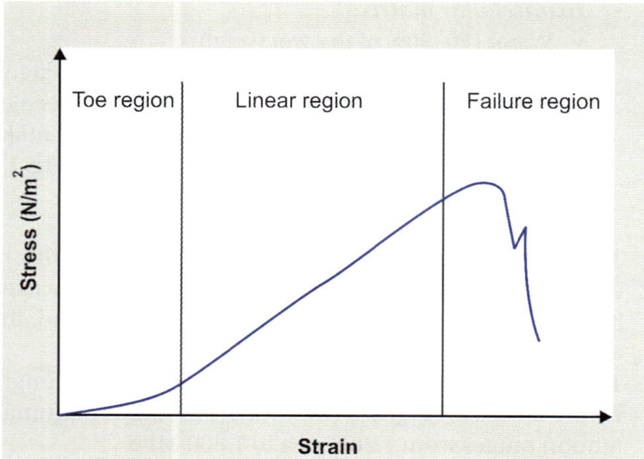

Fig. 2: Elastic modulus of tendon: A stress-strain curve of tendon in response to mechanical testing. Note the ramping toe region at the beginning of the curve.

2. Required excursion—maximum excursion required of a muscle in situ
3. Available excursion—maximum excursion of a muscle when freed from its insertion

- After flexor tendon repair, there is always a decrease in the repair strength. To allow for early tendon motion, hence the repair should be as strong as possible. It was supposed that the force for active motion should be limited to lower than 75 N. Currently, such strength is provided by meticulous multistrand repair (strands mean the number of suture filaments crossing the repair site) using locking large caliber sutures **(Fig. 3)**. Kessler repair gives strength of 20–30 N only and is liable to rupture with the early motion concept. But now it is becoming evident that the real strength of repair need not exceed 10 times the *in vitro* tendon forces of 2.4–3.8 N so that even two-strand repairs may be adequate by this dictum. To be more cautious till clarity emerges, four-strand repair should satisfy the currently known criteria/belief. There are various described techniques of tendon repair including:
    - ***Two-strand techniques:*** Bunnell (condemned), Mason-Allen, modified Kessler
    - ***Four-strand techniques:*** Strickland, Lee, Robertson, Becker, modified Becker and Locked cruciate (McLarney)
    - ***Six-strand techniques:*** Savage, Sandow, Lim
    - ***Eight-Strand technique:*** Silva
    - Tajima, Strickland, cruciate and Becker configuration all offer good time-zero (immediate postoperative) strength. The strength is further increased if the sutures are placed dorsally in the tendon but this has chances of violating the blood supply so central placement is adjudged best.
    - Augmenting the repair by placing continuous circumferential sutures increases the time-zero strength tremendously (15–20%). These sutures are placed in epitenon and also smoothens the tendon surface reducing the bulk in addition to providing the strength **(Figs. 4A and B)**.

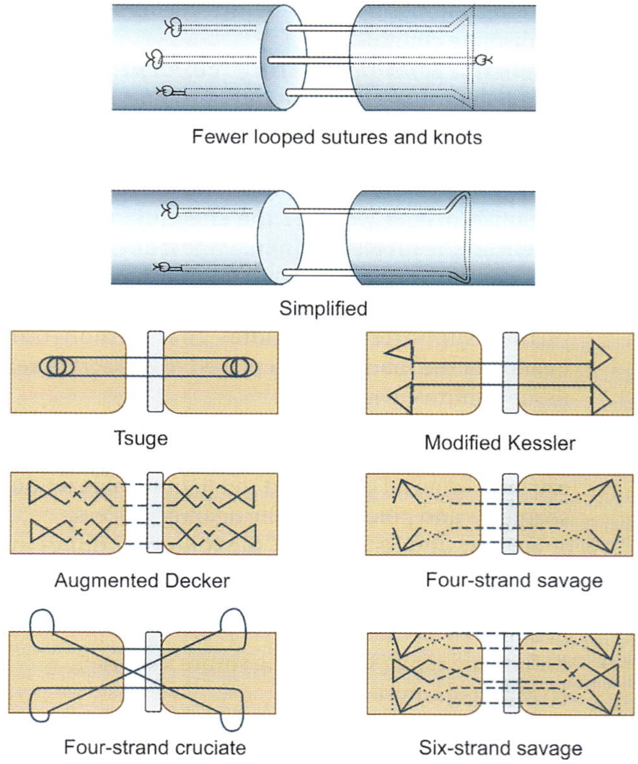

Fig. 3: Various methods of tendon suturing and repair—the "strands" of tendon repair.

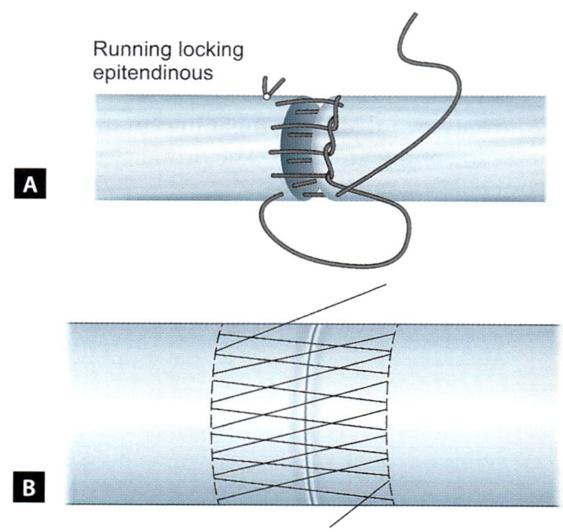

Figs. 4A and B: (A) Augmenting repair epitendinous suture, putting the fine sutures through epitenon in a continuous fashion; (B) The finalized repair.

- Effect of repair site gap on tendon healing—gaps as large as 3 mm do not have significant impact if repair is strong, but ideally no gaps should be left during primary repair. Gaps developing within 3 weeks at the repair site do however mar the ultimate healing and are associated with adhesion formation. Possibly these gaps develop due to poor strength of primary repair and hence the healing is affected as the tendon excursion may be nonuniform.

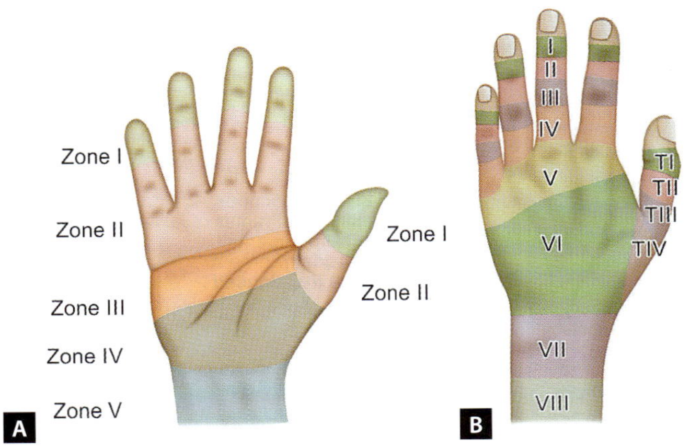

Figs. 5A and B: Various zones of tendon injury. (A) Flexor tendons; (B) Extensor tendons.

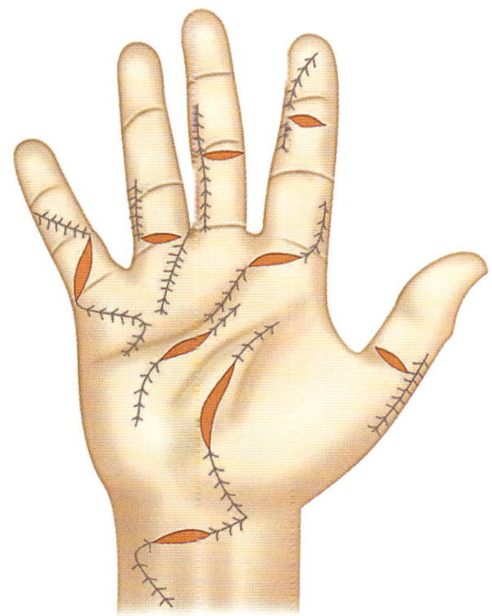

Fig. 6: Brunner incisions.

BOX 1: The guiding principles for placing incisions in fingers and hand.

- Avoid crossing flexion creases at right angles (to prevent later flexion contracture caused by scar).
- Protect the underlying neurovascular bundles from harm.
- As far as location of the incision is concerned, place the incision as close to the expected site of finding tendon and not always at the site of injury as if the injury occurred in flexed position, the distal stump would require great deal of exposure distally.
- Oblique Bruner incisions **(Fig. 6)** or straight midlateral incisions are best for exposure of structures.

Effect of Zone of Flexor Tendon

The synovial sheaths mark the various classically described zones for flexor tendons **(Figs. 5A and B)**:

- Zone I represents the region distal to the synovial sheath occupied only by flexor digitorum profundus (FDP) tendon. It is represented by insertion of FDP tendon at distal phalange to insertion of flexor digitorum superficialis (FDS) at middle phalanx.
- Zone II (NML) extends the length of the fibro-osseous sheath (insertion of FDS at middle phalanx to A1 pulley) of the digit occupied by both FDS and FDP. The tendons are nourished by synovial fluid within the sheath and through direct vascular inflow by way of the vincula dorsally. So repairs should avoid approaching the tendons dorsally **(Box 1)**.
- Zone III extends from the proximal aspect of the digital synovial sheath to the distal aspect of the transverse carpal ligament. For pinky finger, the zone III is considered to begin with A1 pulley as the sheath may be continuous in the palm.
- Zone IV (enemy territory) lies beneath the transverse carpal ligament—here it is easy to expose the tendons but repair often leads to cross adhesions. Also the presence of median nerve and closed space for tendon healing it is given the name of "enemy territory" as this will be the region where you would like your enemy to get injured—too sarcastic I know!
- Zone V is the area proximal to transverse carpal ligament—injuries here involve multiple structures and neurovascular contiguity/repair takes precedence. This region is often affected in crush injuries where extensive laceration of muscles has been colloquially called "spaghetti wrist/full house injuries".

CAUSES OF TENDON INJURIES

It may be mentioned here that spontaneous tendon discontinuity is named rupture (as happens in RA or due to malunited fractures), while injuries refer to direct tendon insult causing discontinuity. The common causes of tendon injuries of hand are:

- Cut injuries
- *Sports injuries:* Jersey finger and mallet finger
- Rheumatoid arthritis—flexor pollicis longus (FPL) (rupture) is the most common flexor tendon to be affected.
- Malunited fractures of distal radius or metacarpals causing attritional injury **(Fig. 7)**.
- Bite injury—commonly the extensor tendons are involved **(Fig. 8)**.

CLINICAL FEATURES

A tendon injury is present when the patient is unable to flex or extend the involved finger suddenly. One should enquire the mode of injury to detail:

- Type of tendon injury—cut/lacerated or crushed
- Possibility of contamination (tooth injuries and razor injuries)
- *Level of tendon injury:* This is impacted by the position of finger or hand at the time of injury. One must specifically ask the patient position of hand during injury.
    - Injury inflicted at finger flexion suggests that the level of wound; cut FDS and cut FDP will be different and is a favorable situation as "bunching" at repair is less likely with minimal chances of cross union and adhesions or mechanical block later during rehabilitation training.
    - An injury in extension would although make it easier to find the cut structure through smaller incision;

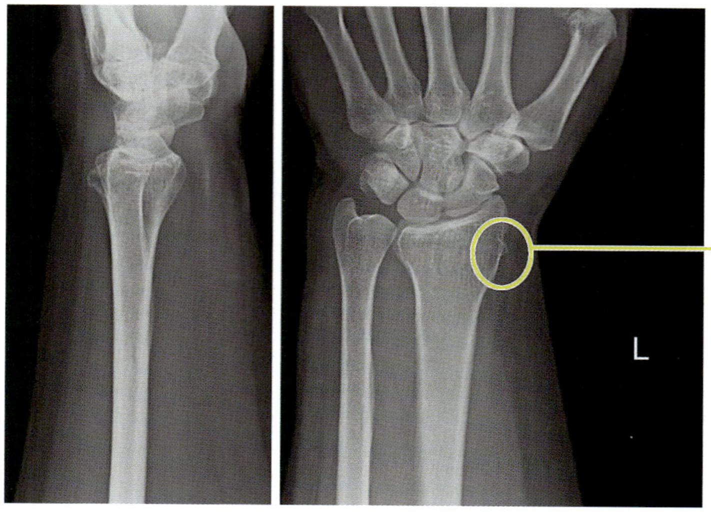

Fig. 7: This patient with distal radius fracture had attritional rupture of extensor pollicis longus (EPL) tendon.

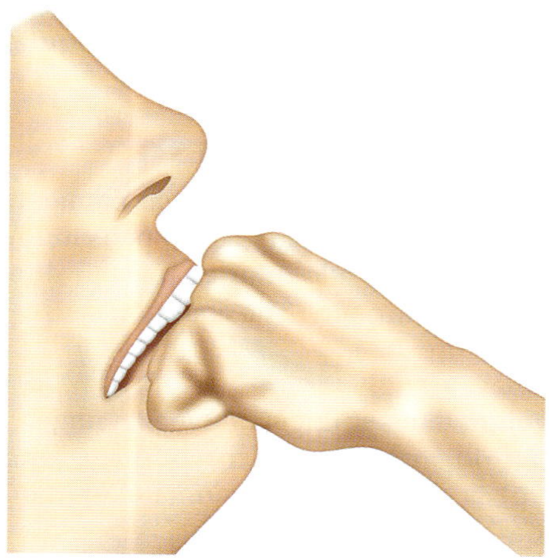

Fig. 8: Bite injuries/fight injuries causing extensor tendon injury commonly.

however, there are higher risk of healing process and tendons becoming one scar unit.

- Cut injury of both tendons in zone II will raise alarm for associated digital neurovascular injury.
- Cut injury at zone III often implicates injury to digital nerves and superficial arch injury.
- Cut flexor tendons except palmaris longus at zone IV should be explored for median nerve injury.
- Cut injury to flexor carpi ulnaris (FCU) often indicates ulnar neurovascular injury.

The following are the common signs variably present in patients depending on the mode of injury.

- Scar mark over palmar aspect of hand healed with primary/secondary intention.
- ***Loss of finger flexion cascade (Figs. 9A and B):*** When the wrist is allowed to drop free into extension, there is a passive tenodesis effect of long flexors that bring all four fingers into a smooth flexion cascade ("arcade") with incremental flexion from index to little finger. Also there is flexion at interphalangeal (IP) joint of thumb. Any break in this smooth transition indicates pathology (the interpretation is true for zone I–III injuries and some zone IV injuries):
  - A finger held with slight flexion at both IP joints but with a break in cascade indicates FDS injury.
  - A finger is straighter than others but there is slight flexion at proximal interphalangeal (PIP) joint indicates FDP injury.
  - A completely straight finger → injury to both FDP and FDS.
- Palpable gap at the injury site.
- Palpable nodule (of retracted tendon) proximal to injury site (commonly at A2 pulley or at FDS chiasm or in palm).
- Inability to actively flex the finger at PIP and distal interphalangeal (DIP) joints *(examine both for all injured fingers)*—importantly to make the diagnosis of concomitant FDP and FDS tendon rupture, passive motion of the finger must be present in the absence of active motion at the DIP and PIP joints.
- *Additional injury to digital nerve:* Loss of sensation distal to the injury site [cut injury to digital nerve(s)]: Loss of sweat and two-point discrimination.
- Flexor pollicis longus injury in rheumatoid arthritis: Patient is not able to actively flex the thumb IP joint.

MANAGEMENT OF FLEXOR TENDON INJURIES

Treatment of flexor tendon rupture varies with the degree of functional disability and the level of injury:

- ***Zone I flexor tendon injuries*** include injury to FDP tendon. Commonly the tendon is avulsed as in Rugby finger (Jersey finger), other mechanisms like cut or laceration can also occur. In partial flexion of hand, the Rugby finger is the most prominent finger. The FDP attachment to distal phalanx is weaker in ring finger than middle finger (Manske), so avulsions here are common. The FDP avulsion injuries have been classified into three types (Leddy and Packer):

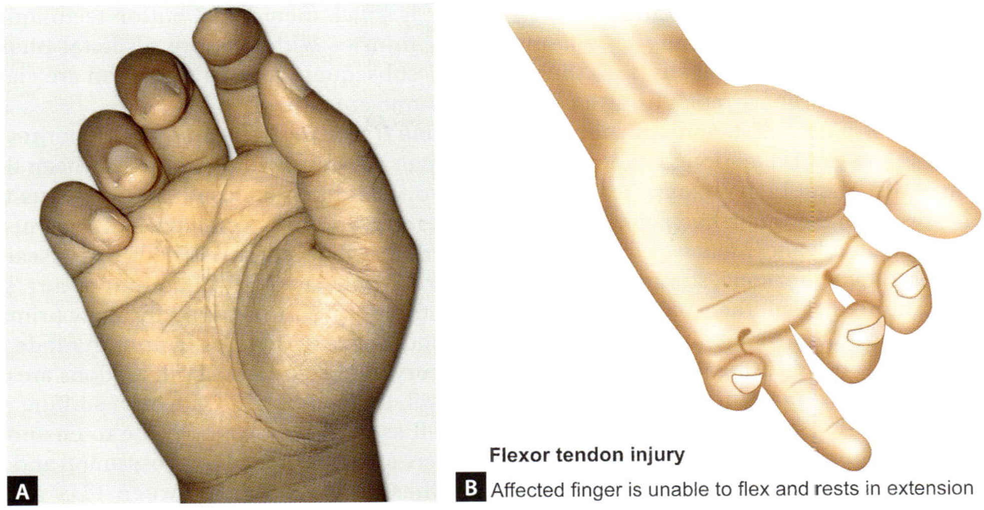

Figs. 9A and B: (A) Normal finger cascade—in a normal uninjured hand the fingers, a smooth cascade of flexion from index to little fingers; (B) In a tendon injury, the injured finger keeps straight due to loss of flexor tendon continuity.

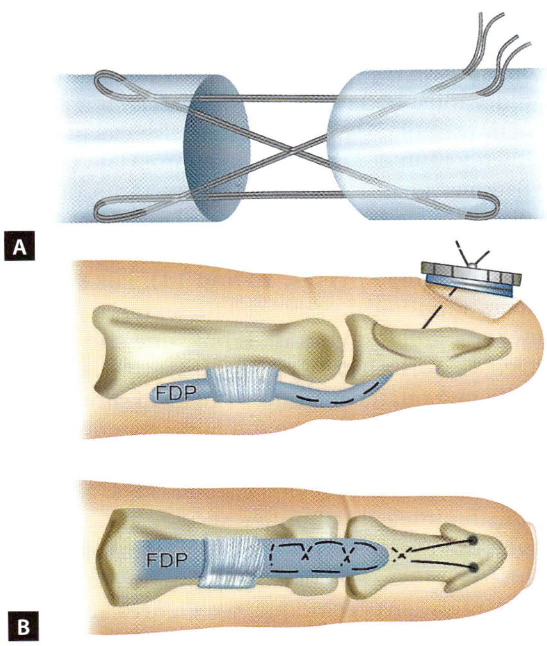

Figs. 10A and B: (A) Zone I treatment—perform an urgent repair using cruciate repair (B) of the flexor digitorum profundus (FDP) that can be protected by dorsal button.

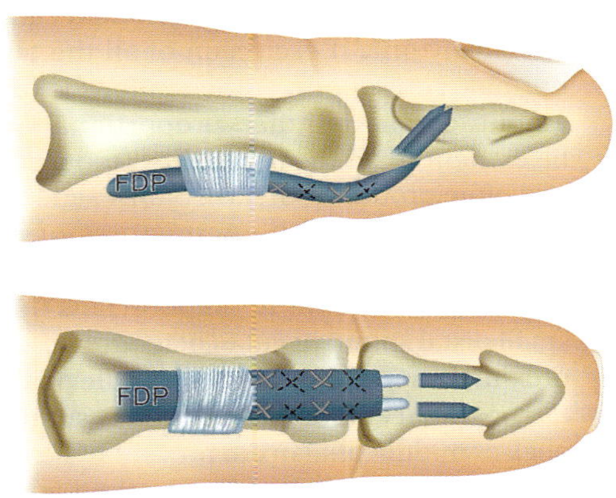

Fig. 11: Zone I injuries can now also be successfully managed by augmenting the repair in suture anchors (FDP: flexor digitorum profundus).

- *Type 1 (Proximal retraction of the tendon into the palm):* Urgent repair **(Figs. 10A and B)** needed due to rupture of both vincula causing tendon revascularization and hematoma in the flexor sheath increases chances of scar formation. There is high chance of tendon degeneration and myostatic contracture. Delay in diagnosis is often due to patient neglect as he finds the finger effortlessly moving at PIP joint. Immediate repair for acutely diagnosed cases include repair over a dorsal button **(Figs. 10A and B)** or suture anchors **(Fig. 11)**. The tendon insertion site is exposed distally using Brunner's incision, and the tendon is also proximally exposed in palm. The tendon is delivered over infant feeding tube passed retrogradely through the sheath. For delayed cases (>21 days) depending on the symptoms treatment is instituted.
    - For painful finger with nodule formation in palm—excise tendon.
    - Reconstruction of the tendon (often two stages) for functional need—high precision requiring jobs.
    - Fusion of DIP joint—disabled patients who need full cylindrical grip formation for functional demand.
    - No treatment—no troubling symptoms.
- *Type 2 injuries (Proximal retraction of the tendon till FDS decussation or PIP joint):* These are commonly seen. Long vinculum remains intact though the short one ruptures. Tendon length is preserved and contraction is rare. Delayed repair up to 3 months is possible as vascularity of tendon remains and often the tendon hypertrophies retaining its suture retaining

capability. For injuries caused by laceration, type 2 is the most common presentation and the tendon is seen at PIP joint. If enough distal stump is there (>7.5 mm), then perform primary repair using locked cruciate repair with 3-0 Ethibond, and epitendinous repair using 6-0 suture else do tendon to bone repair using suture anchors. About 1 cm proximal to tendon attachment is present in the watershed zone for FDP. Always remember that advancement >1 cm leads to *quadriga effect*. Sometimes for small stumps, one may bring the repair suture through the small stump and pass through bone to do dorsal repair using button. Then do epitendinous repair using 6-0 nylon. Other option is to suture the proximal stump to volar plate.

- Quadriga (Roman 4-horsed chariot—single driver holding reins to 4 horses, **Fig. 12**) syndrome was first described by Verdan in 1960. The common muscle belly of FDP to four fingers (and analogous EDS—extensor quadriga) limits independent function of flexor tendons (or extensor tendons) to individual finger. Also the muscle belly can contract effectively only if excursion of all the tendons is normal. Thus, if one of the tendons is fixed or its amplitude altered, then proportional effect will be evident in all the other slips (reduced flexion) and often produces forearm pain. Pseudoquadriga is produced by fixed contractures of IP joints. If quadriga effect is expected, then one may consider conversion to "superficialis finger". For small distal stump in cut FDP tendon in zone I, the proximal stump is sutured to middle phalanx, and the proximal end of distal stump is sutured to the neck of middle phalanx to prevent hyperextension deformity at DIP joint. The method is also used for nonreconstructible pulley in zone II with bowstringing of FDP.

- *Type 3 injuries (The tendon retracts only till A4 pulley):* These fortunate patients have a bony piece attached to the avulsed tendon end that gets caught at the pulley. Both vincula are intact and treatment by open reduction internal fixation (ORIF) suffices. If bone is small, then dorsal button technique is successful. Injuries with fracture of distal phalanx and then subsequent tendon retraction are classified type 3A and are rare.

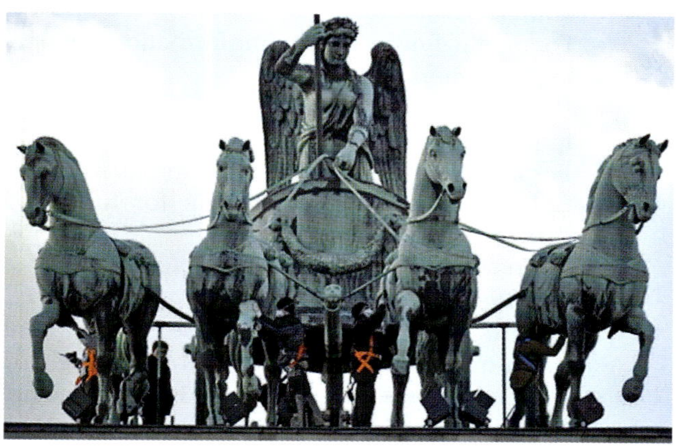

Fig. 12: Quadriga—the term is derived from Roman mythology of a chariot pulled by four horses dedicated to "Sun God".

- ***Zone II injuries:*** The reason for poor results of primary repair previously in this zone had been the enclosure of two tendons in a closed fibro-osseous tunnel marked by many important pulleys. This region when repaired with less than adequate skills cause scar and adhesion formation. The technique and suture materials have both improved to reasonably allow primary repair with good success. The most common mode of injury is cut injury of the tendon. If both tendons are cut at the same level, there are high chances of stuffing of the repair as well as increased volume due to ensuing edema. Also there are high chances of cross union and intertendinous adhesion formation between FDS and FDP. If only one of the tendons is injured, it may be left unrepaired with proper patient explanation and counseling. This especially holds true for FDS injury. Cut FDP is better repaired (I am biased). Partial lacerations up to even 90% of the tendon width heal spontaneously, but if the torn ends cause triggering then they may be trimmed. The injury must be repaired immediately, if associated with neurovascular damage is there, else elective repair scheduled within 2–3 days is also appropriate **(Fig. 13)**. I use Brunner's incisions and assess the status of A2 and A4 pulley. Open a flap through pulley to retrieve the cut ends of FDP tendon and perform a four-strand repair using cruciate repair **(Figs. 10 and 14)**. For FDS slips, I perform modified Kessler repair taking care not to narrow the Camper's chiasm. If only one slip of FDS is damaged, I leave it alone. If FDS is cut proximal to chiasm, I try to do up both the tendons in an ideal sitting, but if I find that the repair is getting too bulky then only repair the FDP. FDP tendon is then closed with epitendinous 6-0 nylon stitch in Lin-locking fashion **(Figs. 4A and B)**. Look for the integrity of pulley system. If A2 pulley is damaged then reconstruct it using dorsal retinaculum or palmaris longus tendon (using the Kleinert/Weilby shoelace interweave technique, see **Figures 15A to E** for other methods).
  - For delayed cases (>3 weeks), there is a high chance that the repair is not possible as the cut ends would have retracted, contracted, and hypertrophied. Tendon grafting is the best possible option in this scenario. This can be done as single stage or a double-stage technique. If the peritendinous tissue is healthy (not scarred and provide gliding) then I will do a single stage tendon grafting else do a two-stage grafting. Mostly for acute cases with intact pulley system single stage tendon graft using palmaris longus tendon or plantaris tendon if the former is absent suffices. There are a few prerequisites that must be fulfilled before tendon grafting procedure:
    - There should be no extensive scarring and hand should be supple. Passive joint movements should be nearly normal.

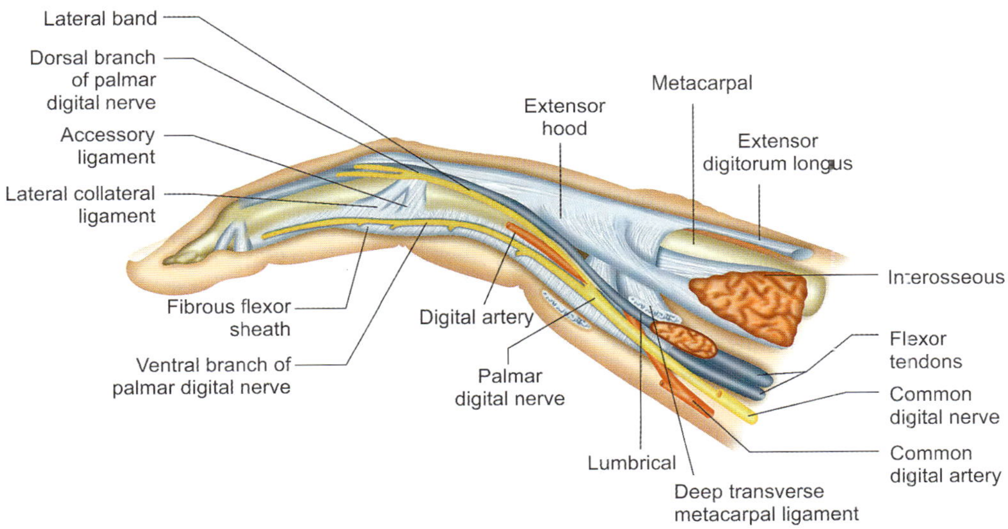

Fig. 13: Close association of neurovascular structures makes them vulnerable in cut injuries.

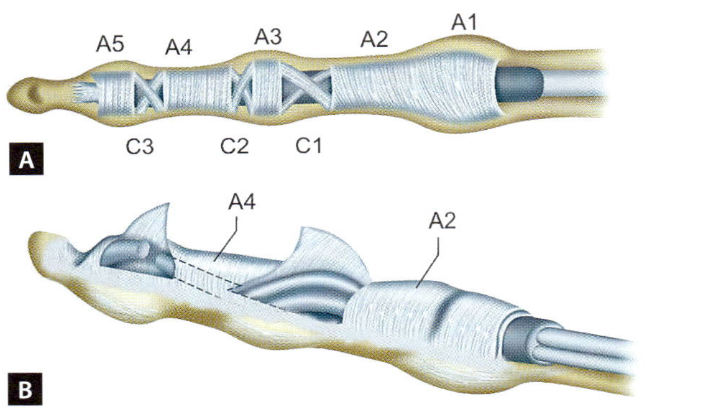

Figs. 14A and B: (A) Zone II—the anatomy is highly complex containing numerous important structures with tight spaces; (B) It is useful to raise "L-shaped" flaps instead of transverse or longitudinal incisions.

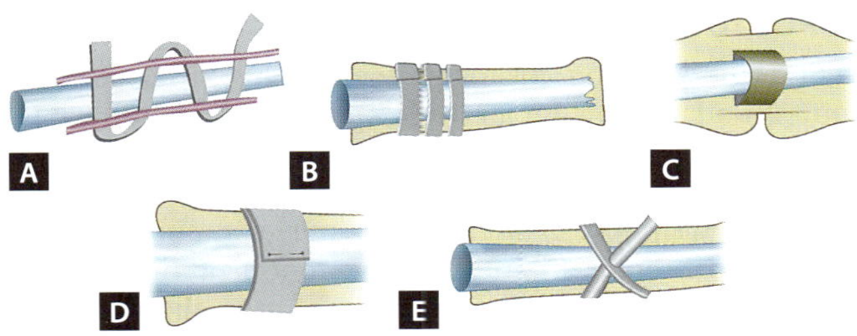

Figs. 15A to E: The various methods for pulley reconstruction. (A) The Kleinert/Weilby technique weaves a tendon through the "always-present fibrous rim" of the injured pulley; (B) The triple loop technique (synthesis of wide pulley); (C) The Karev technique involves incising the volar plate and sliding the tendon through "belt-loop"; (D) Lister's technique using the extensor retinaculum strip; (E) The loop and a half technique.

- Circulation should be adequate.
- At least one digital nerve of the finger should be intact.
- Cooperative patient
- Tubiana recommended some principles for a successful tendon grafting that hold true for both primary procedure and two-staged one but especially true for the former.
  - Only one tendon for one finger.
  - Do not sacrifice intact superficialis tendon.
  - Graft should be of smaller caliber.
  - Ends of tendon graft should be fixed away from tendon sheath.
  - Save as many pulleys as possible.
- *Two-stage tendon grafting:* If the tendon bed and peritendinous tissue are badly disrupted so that the gliding sheath for tendon is not available and/or pulley system is damaged, I will place a silicone sheath in place (as spacer) so that pseudosheath develops around it which will act as tendon sheath for the future graft preserving or reconstructing A2 and A4 pulley. It is often difficult for the surgeon to know beforehand the condition of flexor sheath (which is deemed normal in fresh cases). But if one finds excessive fibrosis, poor tendon bed or incompetent pulley, then it is better to do a two-staged procedure. One should preserve as much of the flexor sheath as possible in stage I. Stage II performed at least 3 months after; requires extrasynovial grafts from palmaris longus (present in 85% population) or plantaris (present in 93% population) or toe extensor passed through the formed tunnel using rail road technique. The formed pseudosheath should never be opened proximal to DIP joint. The tendon graft is attached to the distal end of silicone implant and pulled proximally into forearm wrist incision. The distal graft is secured to bone using suture anchors. The motor tendon graft is then sutured in the wrist wound using weaving technique.

- *Zone III–V injuries:* Injuries in this zone are mainly due to the cut or less commonly from crush injuries. Self-mutilation is much less a cause if at all. Proximity to neurovascular structures make them prone as associated injuries. Most commonly the ulnar artery injury is missed, so do perform Allen's test. FCU injuries in zone V are also often missed as are the FDS injuries in zone III.

- *Zone III:* Proximally distal transverse carpal ligament release helps. If the ulnar nerve is injured, then repair it (8–0 or 9–0 nylon with magnification) followed by palmar arterial arch injury (may be left unrepaired in a viable hand). Deliver the tendons into injured area and repair using any preferred four-strand techniques.
- *Zone IV:* The transverse carpal ligament is completely released. Tendons are identified and repaired individually. Try not to bulk up the repair. As the space is limited so repairs are limited to terminal digital flexors. I will repair FPL and index profundus independently while FDP to middle, ring, and little fingers are combined anatomically into single unit. Superficialis tendons to repair should be so chosen that they will not be in contact with any other tendon repair. I will keep the carpal ligament open.
- *Zone V:* Repair the individual units separately.

POSTOPERATIVE PROTOCOL

I find the Indiana protocol devised by Strickland for four-strand tendon repair with epitendinous suture best in rehabilitation and precise enough to cover most of the aspects **(Table 1)**. The regime has evolved from the classic description of Kleinert regime to mobilize flexor tendon post repair. Kleinert passive mobilization protocol involved the use of a protective splint with wrist and metacarpophalangeal (MCP) joints in flexion and IP joints in extension; whereby active extension was encouraged while flexion was passive using elastic rubber band **(Fig. 16)**. This slowly progressed to progressive resistive exercises. The observations made from the regime lead into further insights that improved our understanding of repair process and the opportunity to organize the rehabilitation program in a better way. The following are some of the key observations made from the Kleinert regime:

- Passive DIP extension with PIP and MCP joint flexion glides FDP away from FDS suture site.
- Passive PIP extension with DIP and MCP flexion glides both tendons away from wound.
- Combined MCP flexion and wrist extension produces the least tension on repaired site.
- Tendon loses its tensile strength in first 2 weeks and gliding function by 10 days.
- Work of flexion (resistance to tendon gliding) at 1 week is least for repairs protected for first 3 days compared to those mobilized immediately (during edema) or at 7 days.
- IP joint flexion is critical to preventing adhesion (it is difficult to determine in Kleinert regime if flexion is really occurring at IP joints or MCP joint only).
- Wrist joint with greatest moment arm for flexor tendons produces greatest tendon excursion so tenodesis exercises have been added to active exercises.

TREATMENT OF TENDON RUPTURES

Rheumatoid hand is the most common cause of spontaneous tendon ruptures followed by malunited fractures. Only

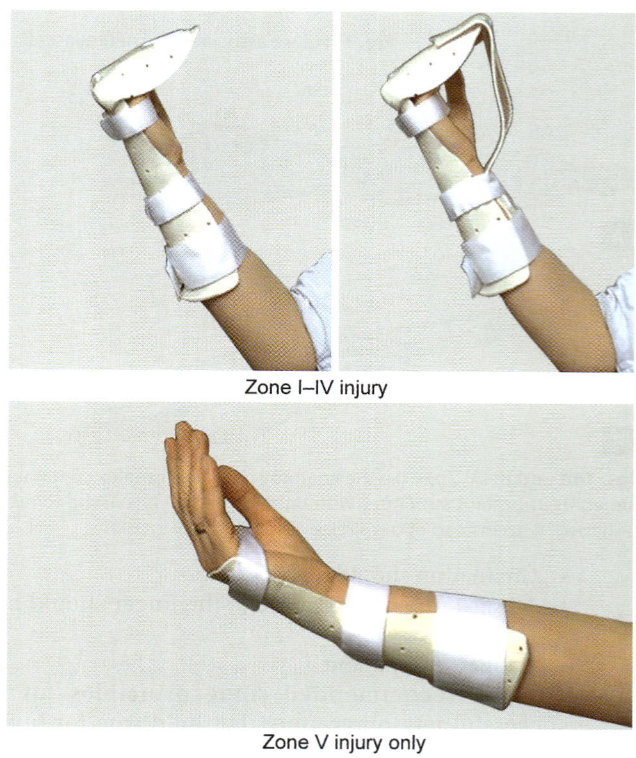

Fig. 16: Postoperative rehabilitation after tendon repair.

TABLE 1: Indiana protocol for flexor tendon repair.

0–3 days	*0–4 weeks*	*4 weeks*	*5 weeks*	*6 weeks*	*8 weeks*
• Dorsal blocking splint (DBS) with wrist in 20° and metacarpophalangeal (MCP) in 50° flexion • Tenodesis splint (TS) allowing 30° wrist extension and full wrist flexion, maintaining MCP in 50° flexion	• Passive distal interphalangeal (DIP) extension with proximal interphalangeal (PIP) and MCP flexion (DBS) (15 repetitions/2 hours) • Passive PIP extension with DIP and MCP flexion (DBS) (15 repetitions/2 hours) • Tenodesis exercises within hinged splint (TS) (15 repetitions/2 hours)	• Dorsal blocking splint removed during exercise • Tenodesis exercise continue (TS)	Active interphalangeal (IP) flexion with MCP extension followed by full digital extension	Blocking exercise if active tip to distal palmar crease >3 cm	• Progressive resistive exercises begin • Unrestricted use of hand at 14 weeks

the salient points will be highlighted here. Details can be obtained from dedicated texts on rheumatoid arthritis of hand.

- Rupture of the FDP alone may not require repair if the DIP joint remains stable, despite compromised active flexion. Aggressive attempts to repair may compromise the FDS tendon and result in finger stiffness especially the zone II ruptures.
- The treatment of most FDP ruptures is best done with arthrodesis at the DIP joint.
- FDS tendon rupture alone may be left as it is because the functional loss is minimal.
- Rupture of both the FDP and FDS tendons is better managed as FDP injury and done with tendon grafting, primary repairs usually yield poor results. Tendon grafting is best performed in stages in this setting (two-stage tendon reconstruction).
- In the wrist and palm, the ruptured tendon can be managed by tenodesis to adjacent tendon.
- For patients with severe disease, fusion of the PIP and DIP joints in a functional position may be preferred, especially the elderly population.

Extensor Tendon Ruptures

Commonly affected extensor tendons are the extensor pollicis longus (EPL), extensor digiti quinti, and extensor digiti communis (caput ulnae syndrome—*see* Chapter on "Distal Radioulnar Joint Disorders and Ulnar Wrist Pain"). Multiple extensor tendon ruptures are usually initiated by attrition of a single tendon and progress radially, frequently beginning with the small finger extensor. The most frequent sites for extensor tendon rupture are at the distal end of the ulna or at the Lister tubercle, which acts like a fulcrum for the EPL tendon.

- EPL tendon rupture may not significantly affect the thumb IP joint extension, because this motion is also controlled by the intrinsic muscles. Extension at the thumb MCP joint is usually reduced because the extensor pollicis brevis cannot compensate for deficient EPL function. Functional loss in younger patients and prevention of flexion contracture may be done successfully by tendon transfer (extensor indicis proprius to EPL or using the extensor carpi radialis longus).
- Small finger extension loss up to 30–40° is caused by extensor digiti quinti rupture and loss of extension more than this indicates concomitant extensor digitorum communis injury.

CONCLUSION

- Tendon injuries of hand have interested hand surgeons immensely as the management had been constantly evolving. Newer techniques of tendon repair have improved the outcome drastically as the newer methods afford better repair strength.
- The tendons are commonly divided into zones for ease of understanding the treatment protocols and repair methods that are common to a particular region.
- Associated digital nerve injury and injury to pulley should be always looked for and corrected to prevent morbidity.

CHAPTER 118

Volkmann's Ischemic Contracture

Manish Kumar Varshney

INTRODUCTION

Volkmann's ischemic contracture (VIC) is a condition which is characterized by ischemic necrosis of the structures in forearm (extending to lower arm and hand) and subsequent crippling contractures associated with varying degrees of neurologic deficit. The condition was first described by Richard van Volkmann in 1881, but his name was associated with the contracture later in 1889 by Hildebrand to describe the end result of any untreated/inadequately treated compartment syndrome. For all such contractures, he used the term Volkmann's contracture. The concept has evolved from its early stage misrecognition to being caused by neurologic injury (1860–1880) only; to being caused by increased interstitial pressure (1881–1900) and then as a sequel to compartment syndrome (1920s); to arterial ischemia (First World War) and finally to a disease caused by pressure applied from without or increased from within (combined effects). It was Holden who unified the concepts of ischemia arising either from increased pressure from within or from external pressure that broke down the Griffith's misleading argument of arterial ischemia that persisted for some 25 years as the basic cause since First World War. Holden also introduced the classification system after combining the two views. The following are the current recognized and agreed upon causes of VIC.

- Compartment syndrome is the basis of majority of the VIC that can develop from various causes (discussed elsewhere). The common causes of forearm compartment syndrome are:
  - Prolonged external compression
  - Internal bleeding (hemophilia) or fluid extravasation
  - Burns
  - Snake bites
  - Regional anesthesia (especially the intravenous regional anesthesia—Bier's block)
- The second most common recognized cause especially in children for VIC is the ischemic contracture following supracondylar fracture of humerus. Though terminally, it produces compartment like state but has a special mention due to frequent cause and distinctive vascular injury that needs specialty vascular intervention.
- The other major cause is the crush injuries and severe contusions of the forearm identified by Sir Thomas in 1909 very correctly.
- Uncommon causes:
  - Chronic infections
  - Congenital
  - Idiopathic

PATHOGENESIS

Whatever be the cause, VIC is the end result of prolonged ischemia of the muscles and nerves in an extremity. Muscles are the primary targets of ischemia while nerves are secondarily involved. Muscle undergoes necrosis, fibrosis and contracture while nerve injury causes further muscle dysfunction, sensory deficits or chronic pain. Muscles retain the electrical response up to 3 hours and tolerate ischemia up to 4 hours. Irreversible damage occurs nearly around 6–8 hours of ischemia. Nerves retain electrical activity up to 1 hour and undergo physiological dysfunction by 4 hours (neuropraxia). They also undergo irreversible damage by 6–8 hours of ischemia.

- Development of ischemia can be explained by the Rowland's arteriovenous gradient theory supported by Matsen as depicted by the following equation:

$$\text{Local blood flow} = (P_a - P_v)/R$$

Where, P_a is the local arterial pressure, P_v is the local venous pressure and R is the local vascular resistance. Blood flow will reduce if the arterial pressure decreases (reduced P_a, arterial occlusion/thrombosis/injury) or increased P_v (venous stasis) or increased R (compression bandage/increased interstitial pressure).

Following ischemic necrosis, if infection does not occur (aseptic), the process of contracture formation begins. The process is due to the action of the myofibroblast—a cell with fibroblast and smooth muscle characteristics distributed throughout granulation tissue. Contraction of myofibroblasts shrinks the necrosed tissue. This is followed by collagen deposition and cross-linking to maintain contraction. The flexor digitorum profundus (FDP) and flexor pollicis longus (FPL) muscles are most affected. In mild affections only a portion of the FDP undergoes necrosis (usually to the ring and long fingers). In severe contractures, all four digits are involved. With increasing severity, flexor digitorum superficialis (FDS) and pronator teres (PT) with wrist extensors are also involved. The characteristic distribution of ischemia and fibrotic pathological tissue can be explained by "the Seddon's ellipsoid infarct concept":

- Seddon described ischemic zone of injury usually following brachial artery injury that acquires ellipsoid shape **(Fig. 1)** which is in general different from conical ischemic zones observed in lung and liver ischemia.
- He described the "axial" oxygenation around anterior interosseous artery with center just above mid-forearm.
- So the middle thirds of muscles get most involved evolving in an ellipse with long axis along this region. He also noted that the center of muscle was most ischemic and the region was closest to the interosseous membrane (deeper aspect of forearm) while the peripheral parts escaped moderate reductions in main-line blood flow due to collateral circulation. In the modern unified concept of Holden one can view the ischemia as a global phenomenon affecting the muscles of forearm. As in developing and expanding osteosarcoma where the central cells get necrosed early due to loss of nutrition and blood supply, similarly in the growing sphere of ischemia the centrally lying muscles (FDP and FPL) get involved earlier and to a larger extent than the peripherally lying muscles (FDS and PT).
- Finally, hence the structures closest to the interosseous membrane are affected centrally.

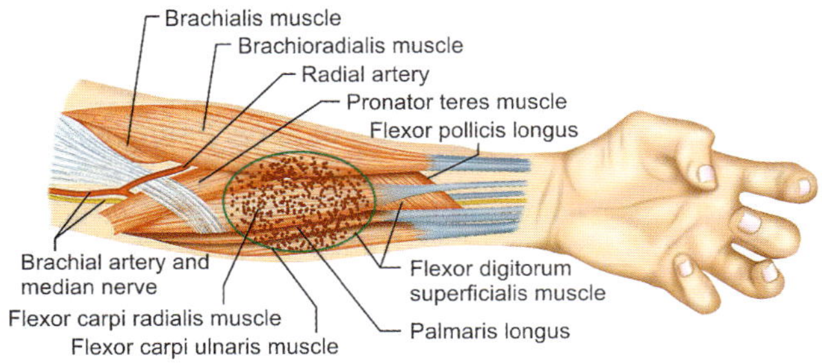

Fig. 1: Seddon ellipsoid.

- FDP and FPL lying on either side of vessel are the most severely affected muscles.
- Median nerve at the center is most affected in VIC whereas ulnar nerve being in periphery is variably involved.
- Necrotic muscle is colloquially termed "muscle sequestrum".
- Nerves are also affected latter by the continuing fibrosis and autoamputation from resulting contractions and hence most pathological specimens report their diameter being reduced to one-third of the original.

CLASSIFICATION OF VOLKMANN'S ISCHEMIC CONTRACTURE

- Bunnell classified VIC as simple or severe considering the involvement at the forearm and hand.
- Pedemonte (1948) classified the VIC into classic (favorable type) or useless hand depending on the possibilities of recovery with reconstructive procedure.
- Merle d'Aubigné (1955) also classified VIC into two types, one with claw hand and the other without.
- **Seddon** proposed classification according to increasing grades of involvement in 1956 and 1964, that was modified by **Tsuge** (pronounced "suj") in 1975 **(Fig. 2)** as follows:
  - **Mild or localized type** (Seddon described this as having diffuse but moderate ischemia without infarct and spontaneous recovery)
    - The deep flexor muscles are partly degenerated.
    - The fingers involved are most often the ring finger and the long finger. When the degree of muscle degeneration is more extensive, the little and index fingers may also be affected.
    - Joints are spared.
    - Sometimes, there is a contracture of the thumb.
    - Cord-like induration on the volar forearm.
    - There is usually no sensory disturbance but, if present, it is slight.
    - The tenodesis effect can be demonstrated (Volkmann's sign).
  - **Moderate or classic type** (Seddon described this as intense but localized muscle damage with typical muscular infarct with or without nerve lesion):
    - The degeneration involves nearly all of the deep flexor muscles to the fingers and the pollicis longus, with partial involvement of the FDS and wrist flexors leading to contracture.

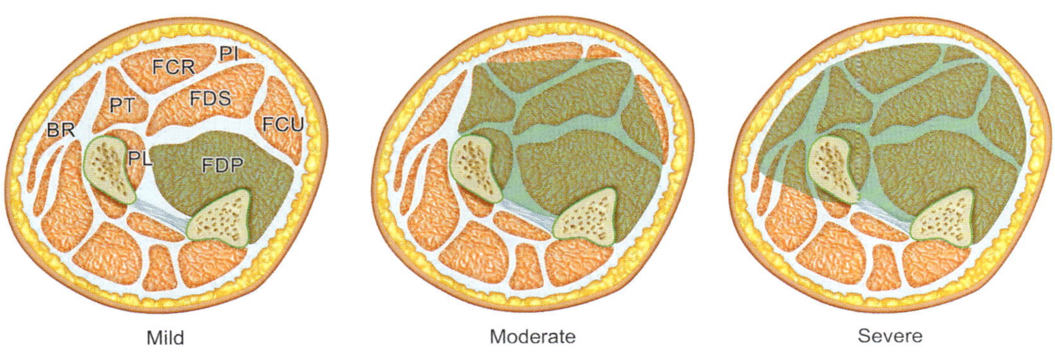

Fig. 2: Forearm cross-section of mild, moderate and severe types of involvement in VIC (Tsuge).

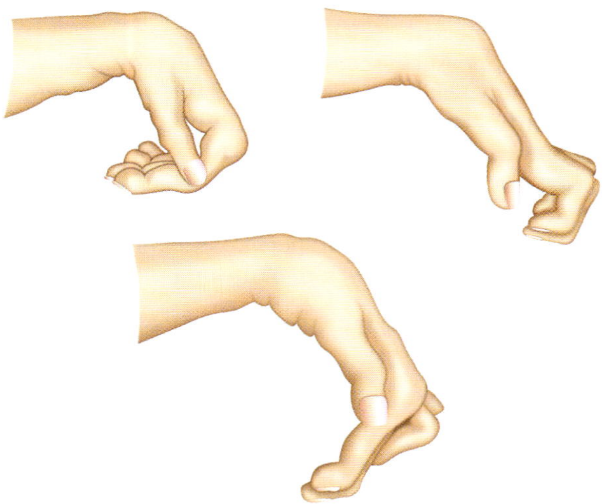

Fig. 3: Zancolli's types.

- Flexion contractures of all fingers and thumb and wrist.
- Neurologic signs are invariably present, most commonly involving the median nerve.

- **The severe type** (Seddon's widespread necrosis and fibrosis with severe paralysis and deformity):
  - Degeneration of all flexor muscles and partial involvement of the wrist extensor muscles. Extensor involvement is seen in 13% of all the patients seen.
  - The neurologic signs are severe.

- ***Zancolli (1975, Fig. 3):*** The Zancolli classification is based on the condition of intrinsic muscles of hand as it gives a rough idea of neurological involvement and deficits. It has been found that use of this classification leads to grouping of clinically discrete patients into same group despite obvious differences in pathology and requirement of management. The described pathology in Zancolli classification is true only of delayed presentations:
  - Normal intrinsic muscle type (type I, simple digital claw)—the contracture is limited to the forearm muscles.
    - Joints spared—no stiffness.
  - Paralytic intrinsic muscle type (type II, intrinsic claw hand).
    - Simple claw type—flexed position of wrist, contracture of the long flexor muscles of fingers.
    - Complicated claw type—severe intrinsic paralysis along with digital joint stiffness.
    - Totally rigid claw hand—flexed interphalangeal joints while metacarpophalangeal (MCP) joints stiff in extension.
  - Retracted intrinsic muscle type (type III, intrinsic contracture of the interosseous and/or thumb muscles)—fingers have typical posture due to intrinsic muscle contracture and retraction of the interossei. MCP joints are flexed while the interphalangeal joints are in extension. Distal interphalangeal flexed due to FDP contracture. Wrist is also flexed.

TABLE 1: Functional classification of the VIC-produced functional limitation (adapted and modified from Ultee et al. and Adu EJK).

	Possible values of total active range of movement that can serve as guide at		
Functional grade description	***Wrist***	***Fingers***	***Thumb***
Grade I: Symptomatic tightness but no limitation in range-of-motion or function	>90°	>160°	>40°
Grade II: Mild decrease in range-of-motion or mild impairment of function, but without significant impact on activities of daily living, no distortion of normal architecture	>70°	>140°	>30°
Grade III: Functional deficit noted with early changes in normal architecture of the site or part	>25°	>120°	>20°
Grade IV: Loss of function of the site or part	<25°	<120°	<20°

  - Combined type (type IV) usually a combination of type I and II.

- ***Functional classification (Table 1)***
- ***Holden's classification:*** This classification marked a breakthrough from the somehow developed misleading concept of ischemia as the sole cause of VIC during World War I.
  - *Level I:* Injury is proximal to the ischemia and later contracture, as in a brachial artery injury say by supracondylar fracture. These injuries if treated early result in Tsuge type 1 injuries but, if untreated, lead to moderate and then severe type depending on the evolution.
  - *Level II:* Ischemia is directly under the injury (pressure) usually produced by tight bandages and casts (classically reported by Volkmann)—these are moderate to severe types of Tsuge. These are commonly observed with unfortunate treatment from traditional bone setters.
- *Classification of the nerve lesions in VIC:* Ercetin et al. (1994) reported a classification of nerve lesions in three grades:
  1. *Grade 1:* A pearly white nerve without vasa vasorum.
  2. *Grade 2:* A constricted nerve section (hour-glass deformity).
  3. *Grade 3:* Continuation of the nerve is not detectable.

ASSESSMENT OF PATIENT

Detailed History

This may enlighten as to the cause and extent of damage. Supracondylar fractures result in moderate type of VIC most often. Treatment received is important modifiers to management like tight bandage, massage, quack treatment all increase the severity of ischemia.

Functional Evaluation/Examination

- The active and passive range-of-motion of all joints:
  - ***Volkmann's sign:*** Inability to actively extend fingers (at interphalangeal and/or MCP joints) without flexing wrist and passive extension of fingers is

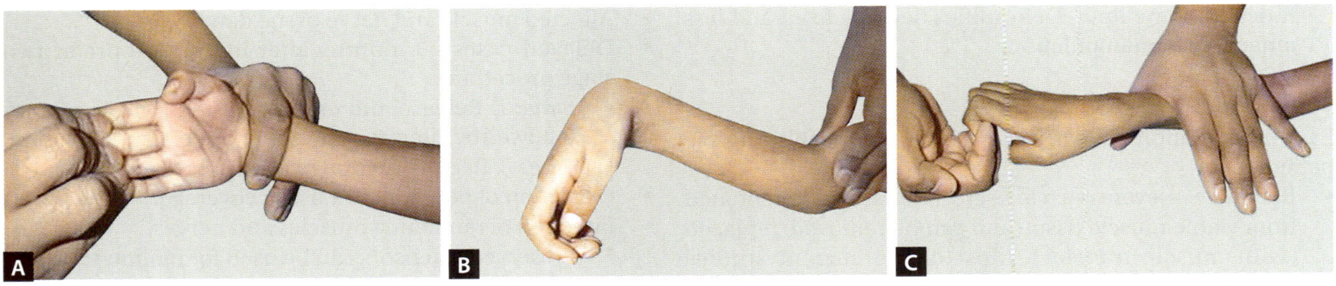

Figs. 4A to C: Volkmann's sign—with wrist flexed the fingers can be extended (A and B); however, it is virtually impossible to extend the finger completely with wrist extended (C).

possible only with wrist flexion (or conversely the wrist flexes with passive finger extension) this is a classical sign for type I VIC **(Figs. 4A to C)**.
  - In VIC type II (Zancolli), the fingers tend to extend when the wrist is flexed and hyperextension of the proximal phalanx is prevented (Bouvier's maneuver), though these are also the findings in a normal hand! Interphalangeal joints may not extend in patients with complicated claw hand (stiff joints).
  - For Volkmann's type III (Zancolli), characteristically the proximal interphalangeal joint flexion increases only after the MCP joints are passively flexed. This is true of all intrinsic contractures of the fingers. Passive extension of the MCP joint produces hyperextension of the PIP joint and flexion of the distal interphalangeal joint.
- Wrist flexion deformity
- Pronated forearm and wasting is also prominent.
- Flexed elbow
- Cord-like induration on the flexor side, extensors affected/spared
- Paresthesia or anesthesia in the hand and fingers
- Flexed and adducted thumb
- Claw hand
- Deformity and trophic changes due to ulnar and median nerve involvement

Additional Tests

- ***Radiology***: This is an essential test to be done for the following reasons:
  - *Radiographs of forearm and elbow in two projections:* To evaluate and understand the primary pathology (fracture type, location, status of union and nonunion, malunion, and degree of malunion).
  - To determine if anything is needed to be done to the fracture itself now.
  - Radiographs of the hand to determine joint subluxations and severity of flexion contracture/secondary changes in joints in long neglected cases (need joint procedures like fusion or capsulotomies in management).
- Electromyography can produce information concerning nerve function and nerve regeneration.
- Angiography is required for information regarding the vascular status—especially to know the caliber of vessels and the best place to do anastomosis in case if free-muscle transfer is needed. (It is important to note that angiogram should not be done as therapeutic measure in cases of suspected thrombosis as else the thrombus will get dislodged to cause blockade distally and one may lose hand).
- Determination of the severity and the extent of muscle damage in Volkmann's ischemic contracture by use of CT scan or MRI—MRI demonstrates fibrosis and the extent of loss of muscular tissue, but the operative technique, as yet, has not been altered by this information. I find specific use of MRI in determining the extent of damage in early cases presenting to us (2 days to few weeks) as if the involvement is severe, the trend is tilted to early intervention now. This "severe" involvement in late acute cases is difficult to judge clinically.

DIFFERENTIAL DIAGNOSIS

- Post-traumatic hematoma and resulting contracture.
- Osteomyelitis and muscle involvement either by intervention or disease process.
- Hemangioma of forearm muscles.
- Pseudo-VIC (tethering of muscle often FDP/FPL to healing fractures of radius or ulna or both). Other causes include adhesions around internal fixation, tendon rupture, crush injury and scarring secondary to infection. Myotenolysis or tenolyses cures the problem.
- Burns

TIMING OF INTERVENTION

(*See* also Chapter on "Compartment Syndrome") There has been no singleton guideline available as to when to intervene surgically. Instead, broadly there are two distinctive recommendations (quite contrarian in perspective with their own rationale) practiced variably by hand surgeons.

Classical View

Delay the intervention (Seddon advocated delay of at least 3 months; Tsuge advised waiting for at least 6 months but less than 1 year).

- Rationale—muscle tissue might spontaneously recover and intervention could possibly inflict more muscle damage. Necrotic region segregates completely and is demarcated. Final deformities are established.
- Problem—nerves become thinned as a result of fibrotic compression reducing their function as it acts like autoamputation. Joint stiffness develops reducing overall

function of the limb. Deformities become fixed and less amenable to manipulation.

Emerging View

Early intervention (as early as possible after stabilizing the patient):

- Rationale—severe muscle necrosis is easily differentiated from viable muscle tissue and can be removed/replaced (with muscle transfer). Most of the current studies do not advocate delay especially with severe cases and poor hand function (*see* Zancolli's classification). Prompt surgery is also needed in patients with neuralgia ("prolonged pain syndrome"). Excision of fibrotic tissue (causing compression of the nerve) and neurolysis resolves pain immediately.

TREATMENT OPTIONS

Often a variety of treatment options are used in combination. The following are the different methods deployed in customized combinations for management and functional improvement.

- ***Conservative***—consisting of a combination of exercises and orthoses for wrist, hand, and fingers. Stiffness of joints should at all times be prevented. Turnbuckle splint comes in handy to mobilize the fingers here.
- Excision of fibrous tissue:
  - Capsulotomy—needed if the fingers cannot be stretched after muscle sequestrum excision.
  - Neurolysis
  - Tenolysis
- ***Proximal "muscle slide" of Max Page***—there is now vehement opposition to this procedure due to the fact that a fibrotic tissue is in any case not going to provide contractile function in any position. Considering the logic, we also advise this procedure only when there is adequate muscle mass left that can provide contractile function else prefer reconstruction by tendon transfer.
- Tendon lengthening
- Tendon transfers
- Nerve grafting
- ***Free, vascularized, innervated musculocutaneous flaps:***
  - Gracilis muscle transfer—this has only 17% of the contractile force of forearm flexors and is more bulky, but the minimal donor site morbidity and consistent pedicle makes it the first choice.
  - Latissimus dorsi provides 33% of the contractile force and has longer pedicle and is the second choice (disadvantage due primarily to its bulk).
  - Rectus femoris is the third choice though it has good contractile force, and cross sectional area fit according to the region but donor site morbidity is obvious.

Determining Factors

All the above-mentioned options are not used in all patients and the choice of procedure(s) usually depends on the following determinants.

- Severity of the infarction and contracture.
- Affected muscle and nerve tissue damage.
- Delayed cases—3 months after injury. We prefer two stage procedure:
  - *Stage 1:* Release and excision of the fibrotic masses followed by intensive physiotherapy and mobilization.
  - *Stage 2:* Reconstruction of the lost function.
- Condition of potential soft tissue coverage.
- Function of remaining muscles and nerves.
  - Preserved extensors can be used for tendon transfer.

Over a period of time, I have realized that descriptions and categorization of the treatment methods based on the classification systems does not help anyone in complete understanding. The various procedures described above are adequate for discrete problems that are uniquely applied to individuals, either individually or in various combinations, so generalizations are not possible. How I proceed is as follows:

- Evaluate the extent of infarction clinically (range-of-motion, grip strength, sensation testing, classify—Tsuge)
- If mild or moderate, I assess the remaining hand function and put the patient on aggressive physiotherapy to stretch the contractures and promote functional rehabilitation simultaneously (no surgery initially). If the function does not improve or there is less than satisfactory function grade 3 or less **(*see* Table 1)** at 3 months then do surgical reconstruction for individual deficits (no generalization). Specifics can be read from below.
- If the function is poor to start with and there is severe contracture then there is nothing further to lose, and surgery should be considered for excision and reconstruction planning anyway (as a two-staged procedure, see the management of severe type for details). Also early surgery is done for:
  - Cases with severe involvement presenting early (acute or late acute cases) to preserve as much function we can by improving ischemia.
  - Cases with neuralgic pain.

For simplicity in understanding, a common guideline is still presented according to the two classification systems (Tsuge and Zancolli) commonly followed for VIC to only grab basics:

Based on Tsuge Classification

Mild Type

- Stretching and physiotherapy if adequate muscle mass is preserved. Correct wrist flexor contracture by releasing flexor carpi radialis (FCR) (more commonly affected) and flexor carpi ulnaris (FCU) (less common). If the contracture recurs then wrist arthrodesis is appropriate.
- Tendon transfer/lengthening when there is loss of muscle mass due contracture of FDP and FPL:
  - Z-plasty (of involved FDP, FPL tendons)—see below also (treatment based on Zancolli classification)
  - And/or "motorization of FDP" (this can be done to improve the power of FDP without or with preceding z-plasty)—it is commonly done by FDS to FDP transfer of Parkes where the distal cut tendons of FDP are attached proximally to FDS).

- For involvement of multiple tendon units (FDP 3rd and 4th, and partial FDS), prefer muscle slide operation (Page's operation) or less favorably proximal row carpectomy. Page's operation is successful if there is clinically good finger flexion available and may not require a good available muscle mass. Also there is no need to excise the muscle sequestrum while doing slide. The steps are as follows:
  - Use ulnar distal arm incision extending to the ulnar border of forearm up to wrist!
  - Mobilize ulnar nerve but do not devascularize it.
  - Flexor pronator mass is elevated off the medial epicondyle of humerus and preserve ulnar collateral ligament of elbow.
  - FCU, FDS, and FDP are elevated off the ulna, and interosseous membrane protecting the interosseous nerve and artery.
  - Keep checking the correction obtained at wrist and finger movements, often the dissection is continued till wrist to achieve acceptable correction.
  - Pronator release (interossei and pronator quadratus) is needed if the correction of fixed pronator deformity is not achieved.
  - Ulnar nerve is transposed at the conclusion of procedure.

Moderate Type (Classic Type)

Initial stretching and correction of wrist flexion contracture followed by:

- For preserved muscle mass—Muscle sliding operation (of Max Page) with neurolysis of median and ulnar nerve as neurological damage is characteristic of moderate type. Carpal tunnel release is done through a second approach. Again muscle slide is preferable only if finger movements are there else consider the following option.
- When there is no useful finger flexion left, or there is proximal skin problem then brachioradialis and extensor carpi radialis longus (ECRL) transfer to flexors (FPL and FDP respectively) and complete release of contracture and neurolysis is the usual option. Extensor indicis proprius (EIP) is used for thumb opposition.
- Sensation may be restored by nerve grafting.
- Other options are proximal row carpectomy or forearm shortening by 2–3 cm (Garre's operation).

Severe Type

There are two methods to handle the severe type:

1. I prefer a two-stage approach. Early excision of all necrotic tissue with complete neurolysis of ulnar and median nerves to give them fair chance to recover (at least 3 months). This is followed by aggressive mobilization of joints of wrist and hand to prevent deformity and retain mobility. Reconstruction is then done in second stage by tendon transfer as detailed previously for moderate type. If no tendons are available (due to extensor involvement) then Gracilis (muscle after expanding skin with tissue expanders) or latissimus dorsi/medial gastrocnemius (myocutaneous) free innervated muscle graft transfer is needed.
2. If facilities are available and expertise present then severe cases have reported good outcome with primary functional free-muscle transfers along with the debridement of necrotic tissue to make space. The radial/ulnar/brachial artery serves as a good donor and anterior interosseous nerve is used as a motor nerve donor. Muscle suture to medial epicondyle and distally to FPL and FDP. If extensor compartment is also involved then double free-muscle transfer is done.

   Treatment of delayed cases with severe involvement and poor initial function or unimproving function with aggressive physiotherapy usually involves one of the following two approaches:

   i. Combined procedure of flexor tenodesis with inter-metacarpal fusion to place thumb in opposition.
   ii. Non-salvageable (damn useless) limb can even be amputated—this is a better option I think rather than creating a functionally "dead" forearm.

Thumb functionality restoration may need some ancillary procedures in moderate and severe types:

- Release of first web space contracture (and EIP or extensor digiti minimi transfer for opposition as mentioned above).
- Intermetacarpal fusion with thumb in opposition.

Treatment based on Zancolli's Classification

1. *Type 1:*
   - The palmaris longus, retracted or paralyzed, is excised. Excision of the retracted infarcted or fibrotic muscles, and the functional reconstruction by tendon transfers and tendinous lengthening (excision reconstruction procedure) is done in following steps.
     - "Z" lengthening of the principal flexor tendons of the wrist (FCR and FCU) and the FPL.
     - Flexor digitorum sublimis tendons are excised completely to the limit of the forearm incision. The tendons of the FDP are partially excised at their musculotendinous junction, for use in tendon transfer.
     - The ECRL is transferred to the distal stumps of the FDP tendons.
     - Wrist flexor tendons are repaired.
   - For severe pronation contractures, excise the distal part of the PT muscle. The brachioradialis is a very efficient transfer to activate the FPL tendon.
2. *Type 2:* Better treated in two stages.
   i. *First stage*—the retracted muscles of the forearm are released.
   ii. *Second stage* is reconstruction of the intrinsic paralysis. The "lasso" procedure is most commonly employed. If there is claw hand with definitive interphalangeal stiffness, joint fusion in functional position is indicated.
3. *Type 3:* Forearm muscle contracture and contractures of the intrinsic muscles are corrected during the same

surgical procedure. It would be impossible to obtain digital function with contracted intrinsic muscles. Interossei are hence released (intrinsic release) depending on the severity of contracture.

- In mild cases with positive Bunnell's test, perform a distal intrinsic release—intrinsic lateral bands and triangular interosseous laminae excision.
- In severe cases with flexion contracture of the MCP joints and PIP joints
    - Perform dorsal capsular release.
    - Interosseous slide—muscle origin of all interossei are stripped subperiosteally from the proximal half of the metacarpals. Abductor digiti quinti and flexor digiti minimi tendons are transected.
    - The interosseous tendons are excised at the level of the neck of the metacarpal bones (proximal intrinsic release).

CONCLUSION

- Development of Volkmann's ischemic contracture is an unfortunate complication of a complication (compartment syndrome) not uncommonly seen in orthopedic injuries.
- Depending on the severity of ischemia the destruction of soft tissues including nerves takes place in the involved region. The best management is hence prevention of the ischemic injury by realizing it at the earliest.
- The surgeon should be hence very well versed with diagnosis of a compartment syndrome and should have low threshold for treatment if these is suspicion of same.
- The severe the VIC the greater is the disability. The aim of any treatment is limiting the functional deficit by maximizing the remaining function of the limb.

CHAPTER 119

Compressive and Entrapment Neuropathies of Upper Limb

Manish Kumar Varshney

INTRODUCTION

It is not uncommon to find patients with peripheral nerve compression in common day practice. Most common among the compression neuropathies is the compression of median nerve in the carpal tunnel and second in line is the compression of the ulnar nerve at the cubital tunnel. The radial nerve compression and anterior interosseous compression neuropathies are still rarer. Compression of a peripheral nerve predominantly affects the nerve in three ways:

- Hampering the intraneural blood flow and hence transport of oxygen and nutrients: Venous blood flow is reduced at 20–30 mm Hg. Frank ischemia develops at pressures of 60–80 mm Hg. Reduction in the blood flow interferes with maintenance of neural myelination and frequent compression episodes or prolonged compression is known to cause demyelination **(Fig. 1)**.
- Direct injury to axons also causes nerve dysfunction.
- Interfering with the axoplasmic flow altering the dispersion of metabolites within nerve: Axonal flow reduces by pressures as low as 50 mm Hg and complete conduction loss occurs at pressures of 130–150 mm Hg.

Pathophysiology of effect of compression on nerve: Often mild pressure reduces epineural blood flow → edema and fibrosis of nerve increases pressure on other fibers → further increase in pressure and axonal damage due to lost axoplasmic flow.

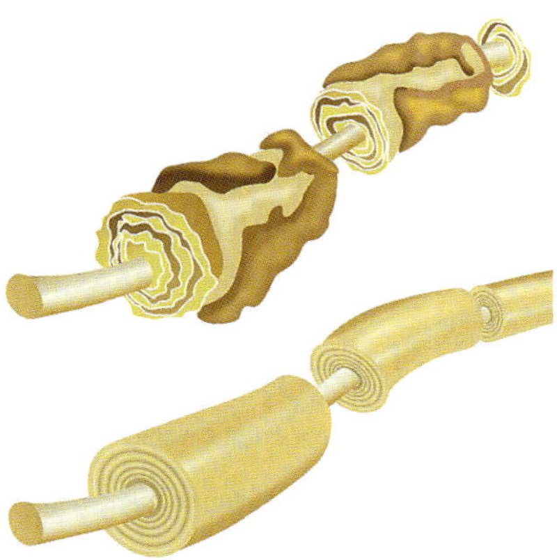

Fig. 1: Compression neuropathy: Demyelination due to prolonged compression and ensuing ischemia.

The following section describes the compression neuropathies of upper limb involving various nerves.

CARPAL TUNNEL SYNDROME

Carpal tunnel syndrome (CTS), the term first used by Kremer in 1953, was initially described by Brain in the year 1947 and George Phalen in 1950. It refers to the compression of median nerve at the wrist while passing through the carpal tunnel. CTS is one of the most common compressive neuropathies of the upper limb. Historically the evolution of CTS description (as varied pathologies, no unification) and knowledge has various lineages that can be partially explained to varied etiology and presentation of the condition. Isolated compression of median nerve has been described by Paget in 1854 as sequel to trauma but as a group, recognition of CTS took time. Herbert Galloway was the first to perform the carpal tunnel release (CTR) and Phalen was the first to use steroid injections for the treatment of CTS, even before the complete understanding of the pathogenesis of the disease. As our understanding and knowledge of pathogenesis of CTS is evolving there is increasing debate over the superiority of the treatment modalities like endoscopic carpal tunnel surgeries, and has instigated the revaluation of the role of vitamins and diuretics in the treatment of CTS.

Epidemiology

The exact epidemiology in Indian population is unknown; however, the incidence is 1–3.5 cases per 100,000 person years. Due to variability in presentation there seems to be an occult reservoir for the condition.

Anatomy, Pathoanatomy, and Pathophysiology

The carpal tunnel is formed by the carpal bones dorsally forming an arch and at the volar aspect the transverse carpal ligament (TCL). The TCL is a tough fibrous band which acts as a tie beam which converts the concave surface of the carpus into an osseofibrous tunnel **(Figs. 2A and B)**.

Medially it is attached to the pisiform and the hook of the hamate and laterally to the tubercle of the scaphoid and the trapezium's crest. The depth of the tunnel varies from 10 to 13 mm. Ten structures from the volar forearm pass through the carpal tunnel **(Figs. 2A and B)**:

- Eight flexor tendons to the fingers
- Flexor pollicis longus (FPL)
- The median nerve

The median nerve is the most superficial of the structures; it is closely applied to the posterior surface of the TCL **(Fig. 3)**. It may lie either in the center or just radial to the midline. At the distal edge of the TCL the median nerve gives six terminal branches, two common digital nerves, three proper digital nerves, and the recurrent motor branch. A number of variations for median nerve ramification have been identified that are described into four groups (with various subgroups) by Lanz **(Fig. 4)**. Among the four groups the group I (that deals with the course of the recurrent branch) is the most important. With regard to the relation between the thenar branch and the flexor retinaculum, Poisel described three subtypes:

1. 46% of thenar recurrent branches were extraligamentous.
2. 31% of them were subligamentous.
3. 23% were transligamentous **(Fig. 4)**.

Some of the variations that may influence the treatment and should be considered while planning for surgery include duplication of the thenar branch, palmaris profundus muscle, reverse palmaris longus, high division of the median nerve into forearm which is accompanied by accessory lumbrical muscle, and median artery.

Normal pressure within the carpal tunnel measures 2.5 mm Hg. An external compression of 20–30 mm Hg reduces the venule flow in the epineurium and the nerve gets edematous, and a pressure of >30 mm Hg diminishes the nerve conduction. It seems that with chronic compression pathologies higher pressure is needed to reproduce symptoms probably due to adaptation.

Etiopathogenesis

Carpal tunnel syndrome can develop acutely or have an insidious onset. Acute onset CTS is characterized by rapid

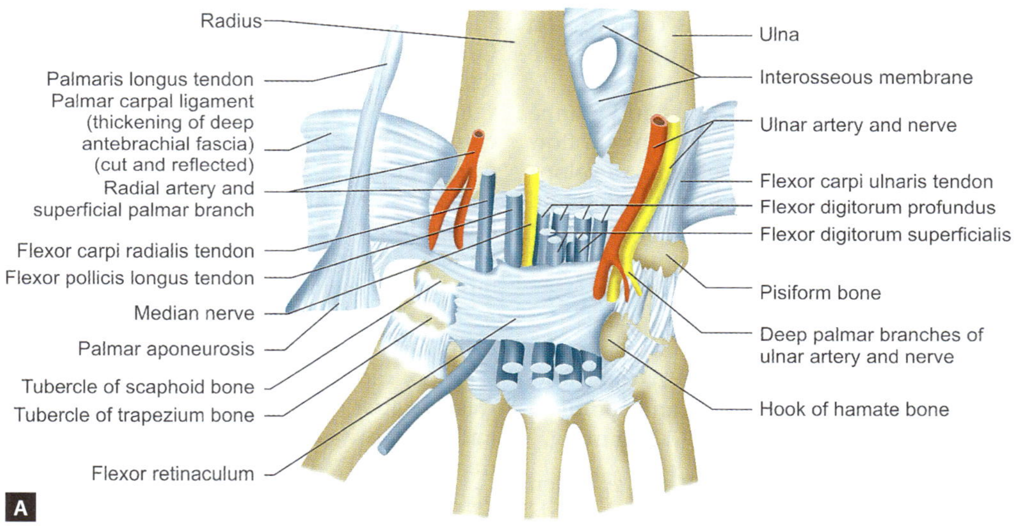

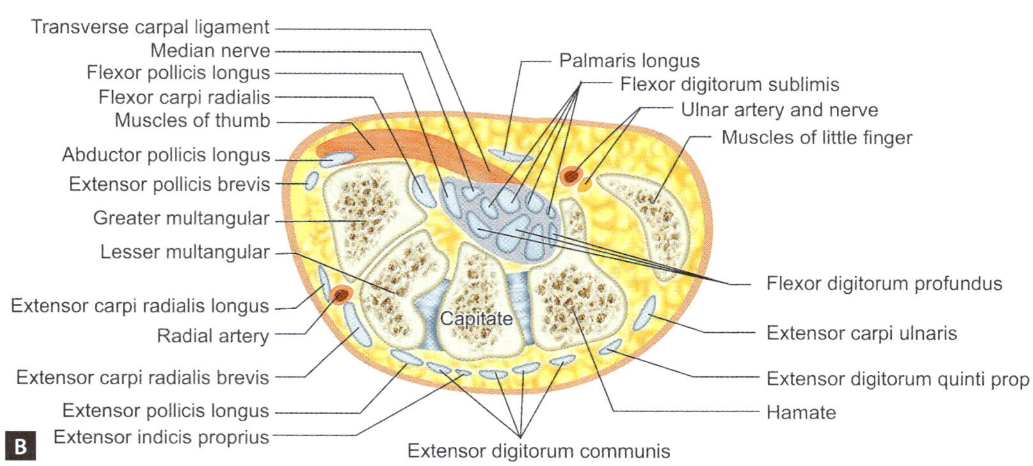

Figs. 2A and B: Carpal tunnel anatomy—the tunnel is formed by roofing of the carpal ligament across the carpal bones volarly that provides space for ten prominent structures passing through, (A) profile view; (B) axial cut section.

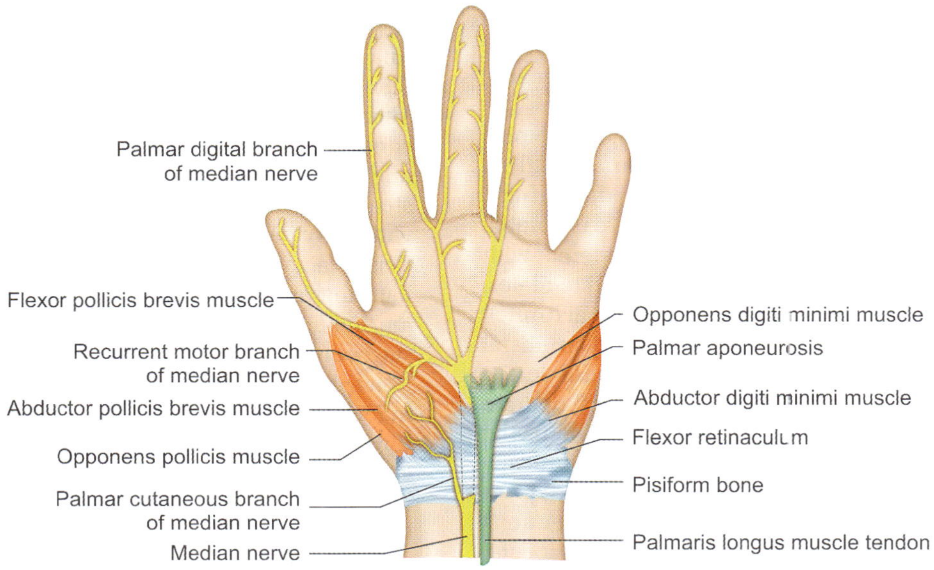

Fig. 3: Median nerve anatomy and relations in the carpal tunnel. Also shown is the distribution and branching pattern in a typical case.

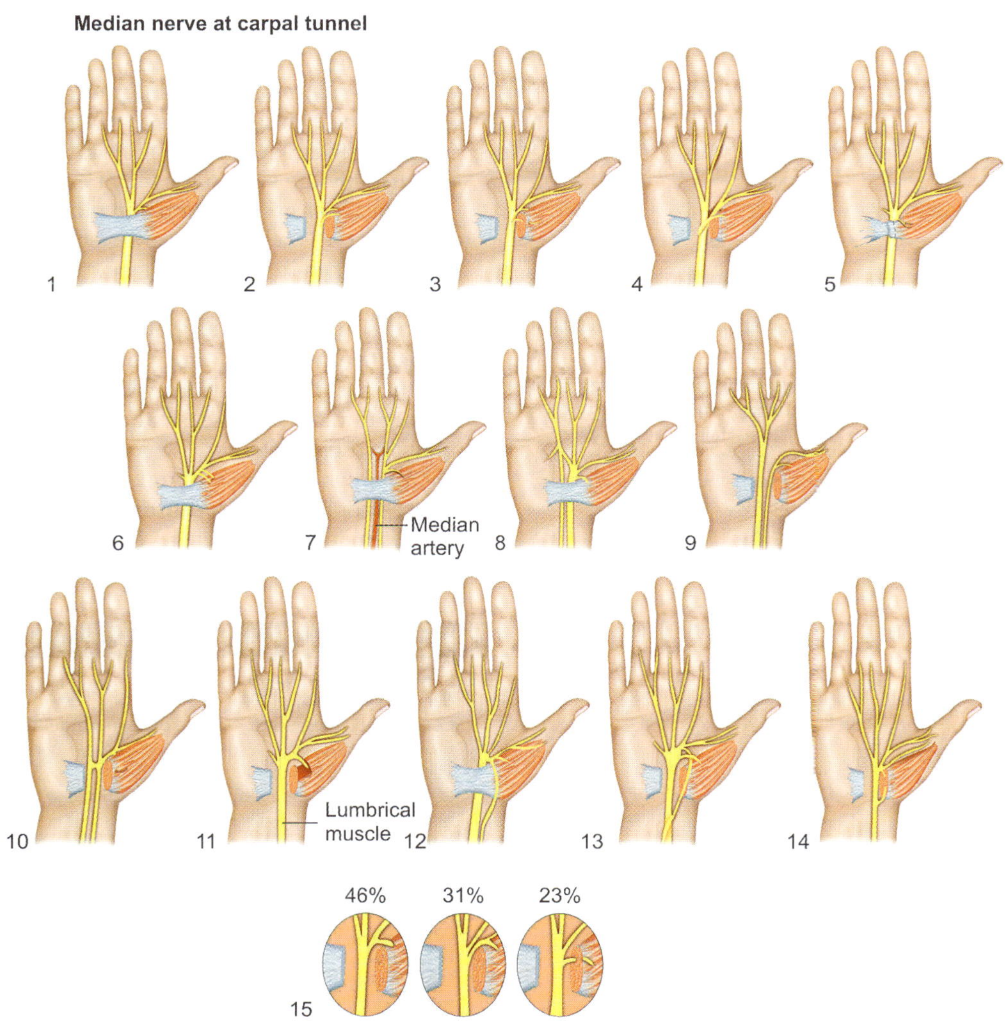

Fig. 4: Poisel subtypes for median nerve anatomical variations based on relation of thenar branch to flexor retinaculum.

and sustained increment in pressure in the carpal tunnel and requires urgent decompression. These factors are few but not uncommon and include, wrist trauma, infection, hematoma, and high pressure injections.

Most common presentation of CTS is chronic symptoms having varied pathology **(Table 1)**, and among these idiopathic one is the most common. In idiopathic variety, the exact cause is not identifiable, however, there is notable hypertrophy of fibrous tissue and chronic edema with minimal inflammation of the nerve. As compared to males, females are more commonly involved. In the carpal tunnel, the most common location of compression is 1 cm distal to proximal border of ligament which corresponds to the thickest part of the ligament. Anatomic factors operate locally and have in common the characteristic of behaving as space occupying lesions. Factors operating systemically either raise the interstitial pressure or may deposit pathological material that constricts the already tenuous space of the carpal tunnel. Pregnancy deserves special mention as the reported incidence is 20–45%. Symptoms typically develop during the third trimester, vary in severity and abate postpartum with nonsurgical treatment. The etiology of gestational CTS is unknown, but is thought to be due to fluid retention. Keyboarding and occupational exposure to vibration has also been symptomatically associated to CTS. Repetitive movements of the wrist and fingers are associated with exertional CTS. It has been shown experimentally that extremes of wrist flexion and extension is associated with increased pressure in the carpal tunnel.

TABLE 1: Causes of carpal tunnel syndrome.

Idiopathic	*Occupational (use of vibrating tools)*
Local anatomic: • Acute (fracture, crushing hand injury, hemorrhage, burn, median artery thrombosis, infection, and pregnancy) • *Distal radius malunion* • *Carpal canal stenosis* (deformity congenital or acquired) • *Anomalous structures* (palmaris profundus, proximal origin of a lumbrical, reversed palmaris longus, and anomalous branch of radial artery) • *Space occupying lesions* (ganglion, lipoma, fibroma, synovial sarcoma, neuroma, neurofibroma, neurilemmoma, and hemangioma)	*Systemic:* • Disorders affecting fluid balance (pregnancy, congestive heart failure, renal failure, acromegaly, and myxedema) • Endocrinopathy (diabetes mellitus, thyroid disease, and growth hormone) • Collagen and autoimmune diseases • Inflammatory conditions (scleroderma, dermatomyositis, tenovaginitis, rheumatoid arthritis, scleroderma, gout, etc.) • Amyloidosis • Polyneuropathy • Alcoholism • Myeloma • Obesity • Constitutional (advancing age and female gender) • Hemorrhagic conditions (hemophilia and anticoagulation) • Consequential forms (oral contraceptives, anticoagulants, and lack of vitamin B_6) • Congenital diseases (mucopolysaccharidosis and mucolipidosis)

Diagnosis

The diagnosis is mainly clinical, based on history and clinical examination.

- The most common symptom is "nocturnal acroparesthesia," consisting of a painful tingling and numbness in the thumb and one of the radial digits, which may even disturb sleep, however, daytime paresthesias may also occur with activities which involve extremes of wrist flexion. Certain activities or positions of the hands that may trigger paresthesias in daytime are pray position, the act of sewing, and holding the phone or a book while reading. In the initial stages of the disease the patients find it difficult to describe exact distribution of paresthesia, whereas aggravating maneuvers can aptly localize the paresthesia to the radial three digits and the radial side of the fourth digit. A self-completed Katz and Stirrat hand symptom diagram may be used to make a correct clinical diagnosis. The patients often describe shaking or flicking their wrists to relieve the paresthesia and pain ("flick sign").
- The most sensitive test for detecting early CTS is the Semmes-Weinstein monofilament test and probably vibrometry. These threshold tests reflect both sensory changes and decreases in sensory nerve function quite reliably and early. Innervation density tests (2-point discrimination and moving 2-point discrimination) correlate poorly due to subjective sensation and remain normal until all sensation has ceased.
- Carpal tunnel syndrome may involve both the limbs but usually the symptoms may be more in one hand. In chronic cases grip strength and pinch may diminish.
- Bilateral CTS is common; however, the symptoms may be more marked in one hand.
- There may be symptoms of autonomic dysfunction such as finger blanching, Raynaud's phenomenon, and subjective swelling of fingers.
- Thenar atrophy is a late sign often in neglected cases over a long duration of disease and patients often report less pain by this time!

A thorough physical examination should exclude the presence of double crush syndrome and CTS mimics **(Box 1)**. Spurling's maneuver is helpful in diagnosing cervical spine pathology along with other routine examination of cervical

BOX 1: Carpal tunnel syndrome mimics.

- Median nerve contusion
- Cervical syringomyelia
- Cervical radiculopathy (double-crush syndrome)
- Pronator syndrome
- Thoracic outlet syndrome
- Idiopathic brachial plexitis (Parsonage–Turner syndrome **(Box 2)**/ neuralgic amyotrophy)
- Intracranial neoplasm
- Multiple sclerosis
- Pancoast tumor
- Generalized neuropathy (diabetes/mononeuritis multiplex)
- Peripheral nerve tumor (schwannoma, hamartoma, etc.)
- Lower trunk brachial plexopathy
- Ulnar neuropathy
- Radial neuropathy
- Churg–Strauss syndrome

movements. Adson's test, Wright's hyperabduction maneuver, costoclavicular test, and assessment of blood flow help in excluding thoracic outlet syndrome and Raynaud's disease.

Various "provocative tests" for CTS have been described **(Table 2)**.

- *Tinel's sign:* An electric shock like or tingling sensation is felt in the distribution of median nerve after a firm but gentle tap on the median nerve at the TCL region. Truly speaking this has not been described for CTS as it is mainly a sign of regenerating sensory nerves after injury and should not be present for an ongoing damaging process.

BOX 2: Idiopathic brachial plexitis or Parsonage–Turner syndrome.

This was originally described by Drs Parsonage and Turner in 1948 (neurologists) from United Kingdom. It has an incidence of two to three cases or 100,000 population per year. The syndrome classically presents as pain in the region of shoulder followed by delayed weakness of muscles in the distribution of variably involved nerves from brachial plexus. Typically, the shoulder pain is present for several days to weeks preceding the muscle weakness. The typically affected nerves include axillary, suprascapular, dorsal scapular, and long thoracic nerves. Anterior and posterior interosseous nerves are also variably involved. Recovery is also variable and delayed and may take from several months to 2–3 years.

Pathophysiology of development of the syndrome is unclear but appears to be an autoimmune reaction to nerve tissue triggered by a viral illness or a vaccine or stress like surgery or trauma. It has been recently suggested that some mononeuropathies previously thought to be isolated compression syndromes have subtle findings of underlying inflammation suggestive of Parsonage–Turner syndrome; so, the incidence of disorder maybe higher than previously reported.

Clinically shoulder pain is present in more than three-fourths of the patients which is followed by multiple mononeuropathies or a complex pattern of weakness or uncommon brachial plexus involvement that needs careful evaluation. Electrodiagnostic studies and MRI imaging are very helpful in making ultimate diagnosis. MRI identifies T2 hyper intensities of brachial plexus or the involved peripheral nerves that is distinct from extrinsic compression as well as denervation changes in muscles in a patchy pattern.

The ***treatment*** has yet not been elucidated while experimentally steroids or immunoglobulins are commonly administered. There is no support to routine use of steroids in the treatment of idiopathic brachial plexitis. The recovery from disease may not begin until one year after the onset while it may slowly continue till two to three years after the disease sets in. There had been recommendation of surgical exploration and inter positional grafting or nerve transfer as a treatment strategy but its use remains more or less controversial, especially due to the favorable outcome in many patients with conservative treatment and also the unknown timing of surgical reconstruction if at all used.

- *Phalen's wrist hyperflexion test:* Paresthesia in the median nerve distribution on flexion of the wrist for 60 seconds **(Figs. 5A and B)**.
- Durkan's direct median nerve compression at TCL for 30 seconds (variously described as 15–120 seconds) also elicits similar response in a patient with CTS **(Fig. 6)**. Performing Durkan's after Phalen's might increase its sensitivity.
- *Reverse Phalen's test* **(Fig. 7)** has also been found positive and useful but in moderate to advanced compression predominantly.
- *Scratch collapse test* ***(Fig. 8)*** *or hierarchical scratch collapse test:* It is relatively a new provocative clinical test of nerve compression **(Table 2)**. The use of ethyl chloride allows for a hierarchical test which can even reveal additional sites of compression. In various studies it shows a sensitivity of 64% and specificity of 69% for diagnosing CTS.

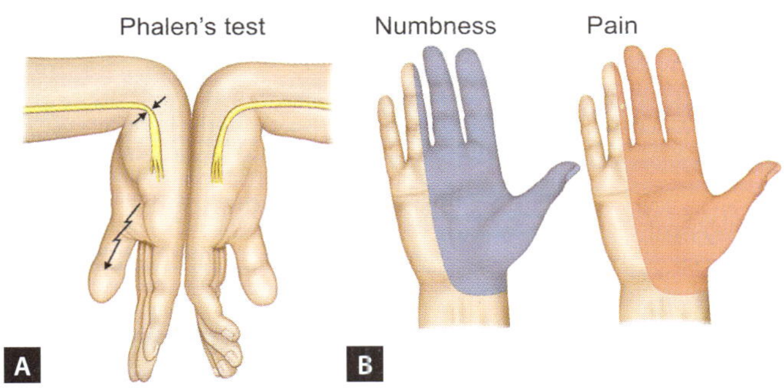

Figs. 5A and B: Phalen's test (A) produces paresthesia and pain (B) in median nerve distribution.

TABLE 2: Tests and signs for carpal tunnel syndrome.

Test/sign	*Method*	*Significance*	*Sensitivity*	*Specificity*
Tinel's sign	Percussion at wrist over carpal tunnel	Acceptable (+ Phalen's)	0.41	0.90
Phalen's test	Wrist hyperflexed at for 60 seconds	Acceptable (+ Tinel's)	0.59	0.93
Durkan's direct median nerve compression test	Manual pressure over carpal tunnel for 30 seconds	Acceptable (+ Tinel's)	0.42	0.99
Wrist extension (reverse Phalen'stest; pray position)	Active extension of wrist for 2 minutes	Acceptable (+ Tinel's)	0.55	0.96
Tourniquet test (Gilliat and Wilson)	Arm tourniquet inflated above systolic pressure for 60 seconds	Not significant	–	–
Closed fist sign	Making tight fist for 60 seconds	Significant only if at least one moresign positive	–	–
Hand elevation test	Hand elevated above head for 60 seconds	Not significant	–	–
Ames test	Make fist and ask to press the fists together	Identifies malingering if positive	–	–
Scratch collapse test	Sequential scratching the skin over the median nerve, with documenting of power of shoulder external rotation	Decrease in the power of external rotation signifies site of compression	0.64	0.69

Diagnostic Studies

Electrodiagnostic Testing

The goals of an electrodiagnostic examination are basically to:

- Localization of lesion
- Determine evidence of reinnervation or of ongoing axonal loss
- Find the type of fibers involved motor, sensory fibers, or both
- Define the extent of injury to neural tissue (axon loss, demyelination)
- Defining degree of axonal loss, the continuity of axon

Specific Diagnostic Criteria of CTS (Box 3)

The primary objective of nerve conduction velocity (NCV) in a suspected case of CTS is to confirm the diagnosis of compression of the median nerve at the wrist. Also it may help to rule out other causes of the symptoms such as plexopathies, radiculopathies, and other causes not evident from clinical examination. Neurophysiologic examination in the preoperative work-up of a CTS patient allows quantification of the severity and the type of nerve lesion; moreover, it can be of some value in litigation. It has been proposed that neurophysiological testing for CTS is more sensitive than routine clinical testing and may be positive

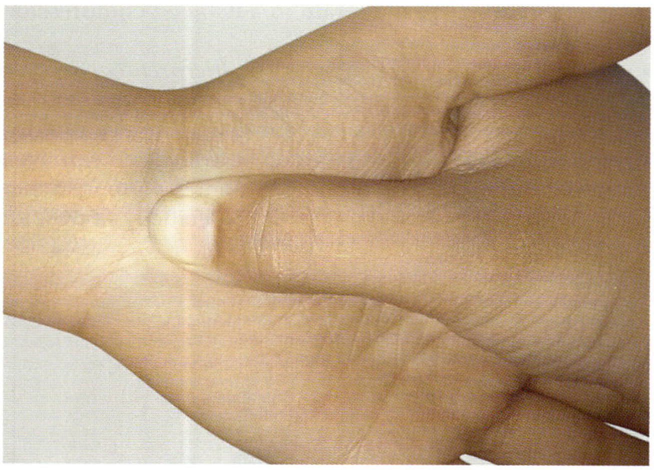

Fig. 6: Durkan's test (see text).

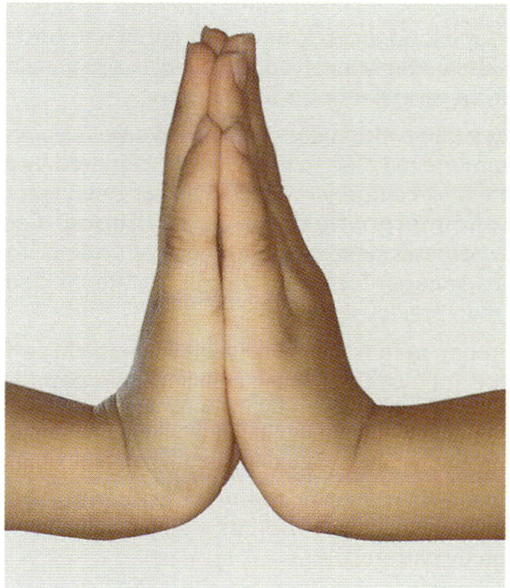

Fig. 7: Reverse Phalen's: It is actually "Namaskar posture" in exaggeration or a "Thai namaskar posture".

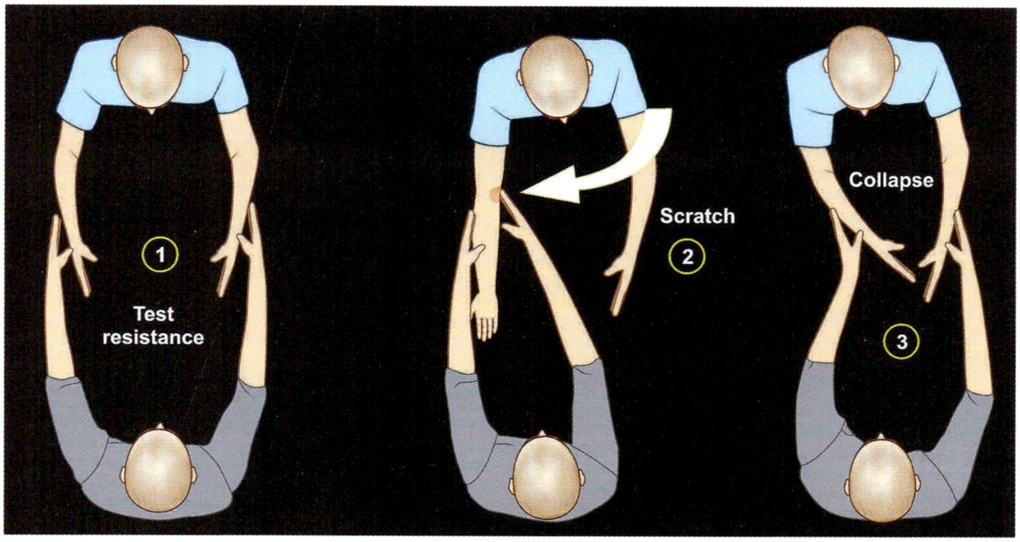

Fig. 8: The scratch collapse test is used for evaluation of compressive neuropathies but its true significance with respect to sensitivity and specificity is unknown. The examiner first tests the patient's ability to perform resisted bilateral shoulder external rotation (1). The suspected area of nerve compression is then lightly scratched (2) which results in transient weakness of same side shoulder external rotation demonstrable as collapse (3) during resisted external rotation. The test was classically described for cubital and carpal tunnel syndromes but it can also be used for radial tunnel syndrome, pronator teres syndrome, and other entrapment neuropathies. They originally described sensitivity and specificity of the test were in the range of 65–70% but over time it has been found that the test is no more sensitive than 30% and is the specificity is also around 60%. So one must exercise caution in the interpretation of its results.

in clinically silent patients. The phenomenon of increased excitability and generation of ectopic impulses in the initial CTS (irritative stage), discharge cannot be demonstrated and the test will be normal.

Imaging

Radiographs in standard anteroposterior and lateral projections are commonly ordered, carpal tunnel view are also sometimes ordered **(Fig. 9)** but are helpful only to identify and study cause of CTS due to:

- Trauma
- Arthritis
- Degenerative cases may show calcification at the carpal region in carpal tunnel view.

Magnetic resonance imaging (MRI) and ultrasonography have been shown to be of useful to a variable extent defining the pathology and also provides measurements of the canal size. Flattening of the nerve at the level of hook of hamate is a usual finding.

- Cross-sectional diameter ratio of median nerve at the level of pisiform and distal radius: In normal individuals it should be one, an increase in the diameter is diagnostic.
- Additional findings on MRI may be inflammation of other structures, fatty infiltration of median nerve, bursitis, and demonstration of neuroma or other space occupying lesions.

BOX 3: Diagnostic criteria for carpal tunnel syndrome (CTS) on electrodiagnostic study.

Evidence of sensory nerve fiber compression:
- Delayed or absent motor nerve sensory action potential (SAP), >3.4 ms
- Increased median-to-ulnar latency difference of the fourth finger SAP (>0.5 ms)

Evidence of motor nerve fiber compression:
- Prolonged distal motor latency (>4.2 ms)
- Denervation signs in the abductor pollicis brevis muscle

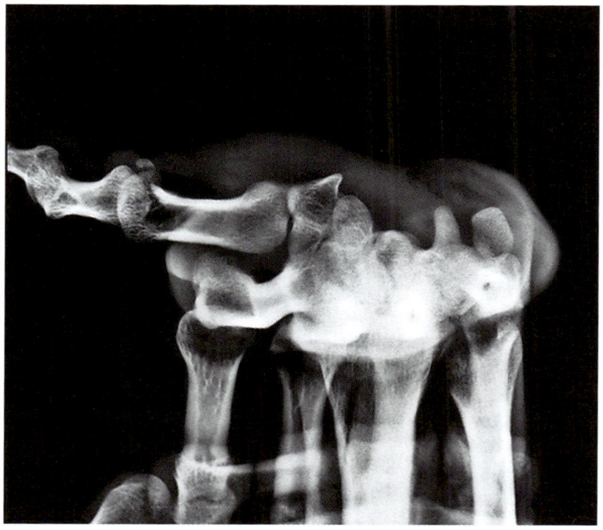

Fig. 9: Carpal tunnel view.

- Scarring
- Algodystrophy
- Inflammation
- Incomplete resection of ligament
- Real canal widening

Differential Diagnosis

The presentation is often vague and so varied (unclear description and poor communication) that the symptomatology may not fit with a diagnosis of CTS and quite often mimics other conditions **(*see* Box 1)**:

- Cervical spondylosis
- Rheumatoid arthritis (RA)
- Neural tumors
- Brachial plexopathy

Treatment

Treatment options for CTS range from:

- Nonsurgical measures
- Steroid injections
- Surgical CTR including endoscopic methods

The decision for specific modality relies on severity of nerve involvement judged by clinical examination and electrophysiological studies, chronicity of symptoms, and individual patient choices. Some factors have been recognized to affect the treatment outcome.

Prognostic Factors that Determine the Outcome of Treatment

Poor outcome is commonly seen in:

- Diabetics
- Patients with workman compensation act
- Patients who fail on steroid injections and wrist orthosis
- Patients with prolonged duration of symptoms (3–5 years), these often have thenar atrophy.

Ehlers–Danlos syndrome (EDS) has no bearing on the outcome of patients.

Splinting may be appropriate in initial disease or mild chronic symptoms. Surgical release is typically prescribed in acute CTS due to infection, trauma, or hematoma formation. Findings of evident denervation in typical symptoms confirmed by electrodiagnostic studies are primary candidates for surgical release.

Nonsurgical Measures

Splinting (Fig. 10), Activity Modification and Oral Medications

About 80% patients respond to wrist immobilization in night and intermittently during day within days.

- Particularly helpful in patients with positive Phalen's test or a positive fist test. It keeps the lumbricals out of the tunnel.
- The position of splint is debatable, it has been demonstrated that the pressure is lowest 2° ± 9° of extension and 2° ± 6° of ulnar deviation.

Ergonomic modifications may be of some help. Anti-inflammatory medications like nonsteroidal anti-inflammatory drugs (NSAIDs) and supplementation with pyridoxine (B6) and methylcobalamin for its neurotropic action may have a beneficial role. Oral steroids and diuretics are prescribed to lower the interstitial fluid pressure with documented benefit in some studies.

Local Corticosteroid Injections (Fig. 11)

The benefits and effectiveness of local steroids is controversial, the use has been empirical and little information is available at present regarding the dosage, site of injection, and number of repetitions.

The reported recurrence of symptoms after local corticosteroid injection has been demonstrated to range 8–100%. Some investigators have even found the benefit of injection to be similar to NSAIDs and splinting. Up to 3 months, the local injection with a steroid is better than oral steroids.

Adjunctive Measures

Laser therapy, local ultrasound therapy, and iontophoresis are variably been used but the benefits has been inconsistent.

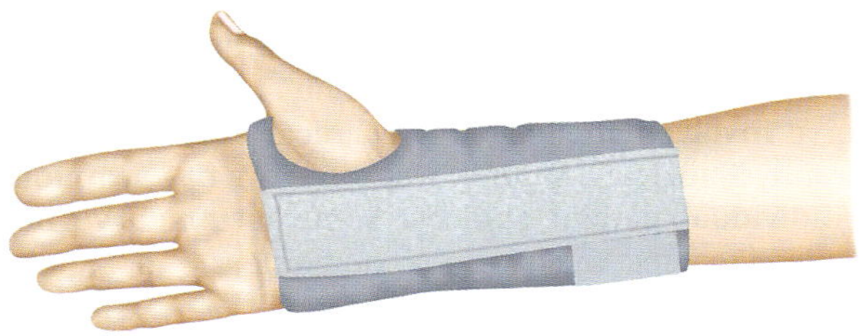

Fig. 10: Splinting for carpal tunnel syndrome—to maintain wrist extension or neutral position mostly in night.

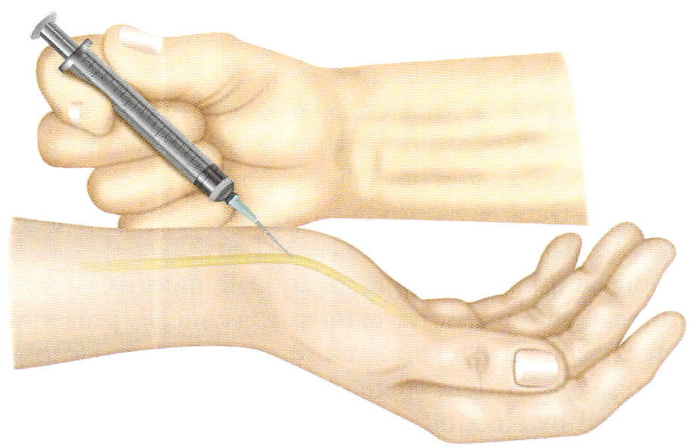

Fig. 11: Injection for carpal tunnel syndrome. The injection is given along the fourth ray entering proximally, progressing obliquely distally into the tunnel to hit the carpal bones.

Surgical Release

The various techniques of CTR or division of TCL described in literature are:

- Standard open CTR
- Mini-open CTR
- Endoscopic release
- Ultrasonography-guided release
- Thread CTR

Improvement in ultrasonographic visualization has aided in development of new techniques such as hydrodissection and CTR with thread device or retractable blade. These techniques are still evolving. Choice of method of release is mainly surgeon dependent and comfort of the surgeon (while advanced methods like endoscopic release may also have a marketing motive). The different methods have their own pros and cons. A number of methods have been developed so as to reduce recurrence rates, limit the postoperative weakness and to avoid complications.

Open Release

It is the most common used method for carpal tunnel decompression. Various authors have described different incisions although the shape of incisions varies **(Fig. 12)**, they commonly involve similar deep dissection releasing palmar fascia and splitting open the carpal ligament longitudinally. The proximal point for starting the incision is determined by flexing the fourth finger towards the distal wrist crease. The cutaneous incision line is ulnarly located with respect to the thenar crease and is located 2 mm ulnarly to the fourth ray **(Figs. 13A and B)**. It is important to keep the superficial and the deep dissection ulnarward so as to prevent injury to motor branch and palmar cutaneous nerve of median nerve. Some principles for the nerve release are as follows:

- Care is taken to prevent laceration to recurrent motor branch and palmar cutaneous branch of median nerve.
- Internal neurolysis, epineurotomy, and tenosynovectomy often initially performed commonly leads to skin adhesions, neurodermodesis phenomenon, and algoparesthesias. Hence, internal neurolysis has been definitively abandoned.
- Immediately after skin incision one should be extremely cautious for anomalies that cross over the same incision line.
- The sectioning of the TCL is performed in layers and is kept along the 4th ray.

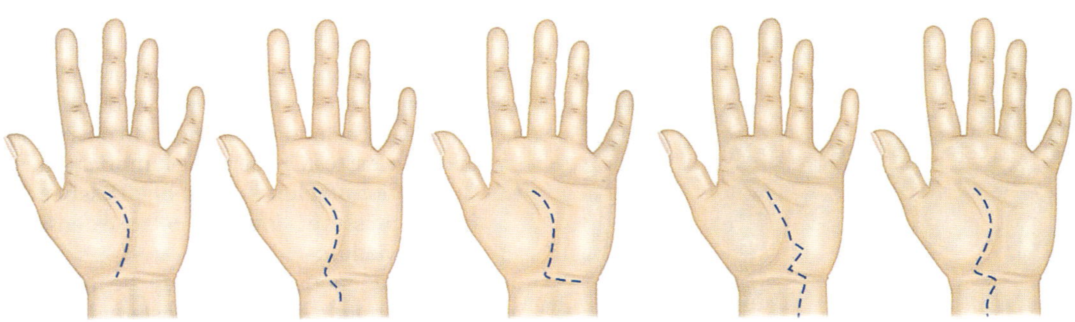

Fig. 12: Various described incisions for open carpal tunnel release.

- While sectioning the midpalmar adipose tissue one should also be extremely careful not to injure the superficial vascular arch.
- In majority of cases, there is hourglass constriction in the median nerve at the level of hook of hamate while occasionally there is marked compression of the nerve with ecchymosis.

An optimally done surgery satisfies the criteria of the three Es:

1. It has a limited impact on health care resources (*economy*).
2. It consists of methods that can be performed with few difficult surgical skills (*efficiency*).
3. It fairly accomplishes its goals of relief of symptoms and restoration of function (*effectiveness*).

Limited open CTR: Limited-incision CTR techniques similar to endoscopic surgery were developed to decrease palmar discomfort and hasten the return to activities. Modified instruments, light source, availability of magnification have led to development of this technique. A "palm-only" <2 cm mini-incision is used to release the TCL. Some authors have recommended both proximal and distal release.

Endoscopic Technique

In an attempt to reduce the complications of open release like scar tenderness and prolonged healing time endoscopic procedures were developed. Both single and dual portals **(Fig. 14)** have been described. In single portal technique, a portal placed midway between flexor carpi ulnaris (FCU)

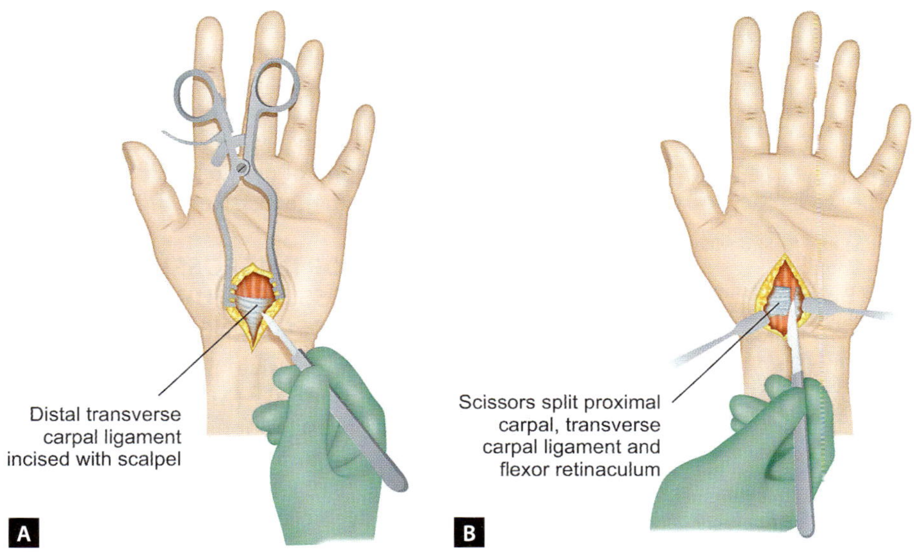

Figs. 13A and B: Open carpal tunnel release. I prefer to do the surgical release just ulnar to the midline of hand to preserve the thenar branch and also comfortably resuture the transverse carpal ligament, which will be otherwise difficult over the nerve directly. (A) Demonstrates the exposure of transverse carpal ligament and incising the distal portion of it under direct vision, I use number 10 scalpel itself to release the proximal part also by turning the cutting edge up (B).

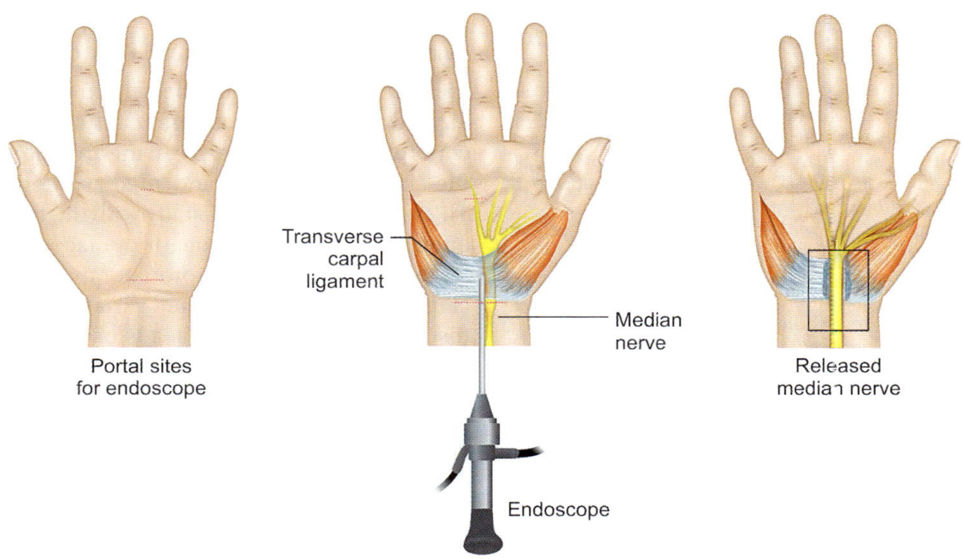

Fig. 14: Endoscopic carpal tunnel release using dual portals.

and flexor carpi radialis (FCR). With wrist extended and endoscopic blade assembly aligned to ring finger distal edge of ligament is identified and sectioned from distal to proximal in controlled fashion. Contraindications of endoscopic procedures include:

- Proliferative synovitis
- Stiffness of wrist joint
- Space occupying lesions in the tunnel that obliterate the view of canal

The American Academy of Orthopaedic Surgeons (AAOS) clinical practice guidelines (Adapted from publication in the AAOS journal) for the management of CTS are presented in **Box 4**.

BOX 4: The American Academy of Orthopaedic Surgeons (AAOS) clinical practice guidelines for management of carpal tunnel syndrome (CTS).

- Thenar atrophy is strongly associated with ruling-in the diagnosis of carpal tunnel syndrome in association with appropriate clinical setting.
- Individual signs or tests should not be relied upon making diagnosis of carpal tunnel syndrome, a combination of them increases reliability of the diagnosis.
- Provocative maneuver individually have poor or weak association with ruling-in or ruling-out carpal tunnel syndrome so a combination of them should be used.
- Hand-held nerve conduction study (NCS) device may be used for the diagnosis of carpal tunnel syndrome.
- MRI is not routinely needed for diagnosis of carpal tunnel syndrome and ultrasound may also not be routinely needed for diagnosis.
- Diagnostic questionnaires and/or electrodiagnostic studies could be used to aid the diagnosis of carpal tunnel syndrome.
- Body mass index (BMI) and high hand/wrist repetition rate are associated with the increased risk of developing CTS.
- Increased risk of developing CTS is associated with perimenopausal, wrist ratio/index, rheumatoid arthritis, psychosocial factors, distal upper extremity tendinopathies, gardening, assembly line work, computer work, vibration, tendonitis, and workplace forceful grip/exertion. There may be an association with dialysis, fibromyalgia, varicosis, and distal radius fracture. Race/ethnicity, hormone replacement therapy is not associated with increased or decreased risk of CTS. There is conflicting evidence with respect to diabetes, genetics, age, smoking, workplace, and wrist bending for causation of CTS.
- Physical activity/exercise is associated with a decreased risk of developing CTS.
- Immobilization (brace/splint/orthosis) should improve patient reported outcomes.
- The use of steroid (methylprednisolone) injection should improve patient reported outcomes.
- Magnet therapy has no role for the treatment of carpal tunnel syndrome.
- There is no benefit of oral treatments [diuretic, gabapentin, nonsteroidal anti-inflammatory drugs (NSAIDs), or pyridoxine] compared to placebo but oral steroids could improve patient reported outcomes.
- Ketoprofen phonophoresis could provide reduction in pain compared to placebo and therapeutic ultrasound might also be effective.
- Surgical release of the transverse carpal ligament should relieve symptoms and improve function.
- Endoscopic carpal tunnel release may be used based on possible short-term benefits.
- There is no benefit to routine inclusion of the following adjunctive techniques: epineurotomy, neurolysis, flexor tenosynovectomy, and lengthening/reconstruction of the flexor retinaculum (transverse carpal ligament).
- There is no benefit to routine postoperative immobilization after carpal tunnel release.

Source: The American Academy of Orthopaedic Surgeons (2016). Management of Carpal Tunnel Syndrome: Evidence-Based Clinical Practice Guideline. [online] Available from https://www.aaos.org/globalassets/quality-and-practice-resources/carpal-tunnel/management-of-carpal-tunnel-syndrome-7-31-19.pdf [Last accessed January, 2022].

Complications of Surgical Procedures

Commonly encountered complications are:

- Motor and/or palmar cutaneous branch injuries
- Hypertrophic scar formation and scar tenderness
- Pillar pain
- Injury to superficial palmar arch (more with endoscopic release)
- Tendon adhesions
- Infection
- Incomplete CTR
- Wound hematoma
- Reflex sympathetic dystrophy
- Weak grip strength
- Finger stiffness
- Laceration of ulnar artery (more with endoscopic release)
- Recurrence 7–20%
- Transient paresthesias (more with endoscopic release)

The two most common complications following open CTR are pillar pain and injury to the palmar cutaneous branch of median nerve while incomplete release is a common complication of endoscopic procedure. Comparatively recurrence of the disease is difficult to treat.

ANTERIOR INTEROSSEOUS NERVE COMPRESSIVE NEUROPATHY (ANTERIOR INTEROSSEOUS NERVE SYNDROME)

It is a compressive neuropathy involving the anterior interosseous nerve (AIN) manifesting as isolated motor deficit of muscles innervated by the nerve without any sensory symptoms. It was first described by Parsonage and Turner in 1948 who termed it "neuralgic amyotrophy". The compressive neuropathy is deemed as a syndrome now that has two specific presentations:

1. An acute self-resolving nontraumatic, inflammatory syndrome.
2. A chronic often traumatic compression that needs release commonly.

Anatomy of the Nerve and Pathoanatomy

Median nerve receives fibers from roots C6 to T1 and is formed in the axilla from branches of the medial and lateral cords of the brachial plexus. In the arm the nerve lies between the brachialis muscle and medial intermuscular septum. The nerve then passes distally with the brachial artery to the antecubital fossa underneath the lacertus fibrosus and the fascia covering the flexor-pronator mass near distal humerus **(Fig. 15)**. With a few reported variations the nerve continues distally between the two heads of pronator teres (PT) with a few reported variations. It gives four groups of branches [(1) To PT itself; (2) FCR, *flexor digitorum superficialis* (FDS), and palmaris longus; (3) AIN; and (4) FDS again]. The AIN arises from the posterolateral part of median nerve beneath the fibrous arch of FDS, approximately 4 cm distal to medial epicondyle. AIN is terminal motor branch of median nerve. AIN has motor innervation only (no sensory) while it lies between flexor digitorum profundus (FDP) and FPL on the

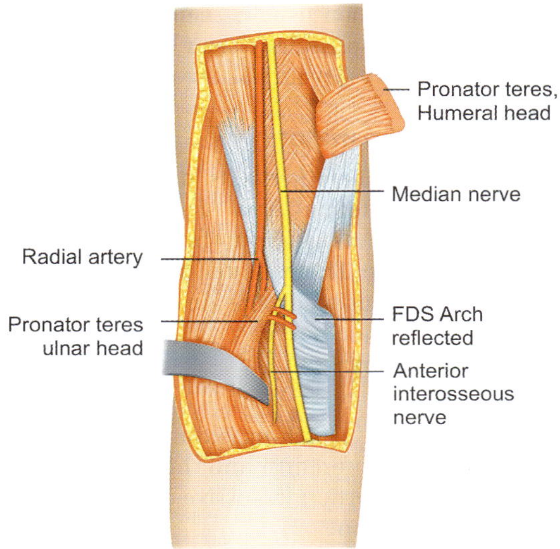

Fig. 15: Anterior interosseous nerve anatomy. (FDS: flexor digitorum superficialis)

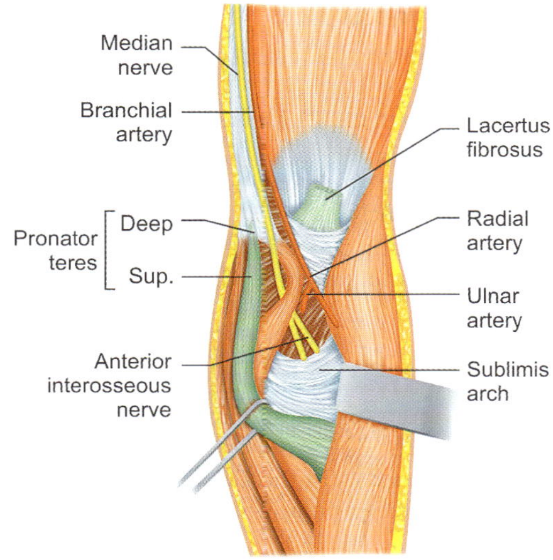

Fig. 16: Sites of anterior interosseous nerve compression.

BOX 5: The common sites of compression of median.

- The most common site and cause is where the nerve passes between the two heads of pronator teres (PT). The tendinous edge promulgating as a fibrous band of deep head of PT (underside of the humeral origin).
- Flexor digitorum profundus arcade
- Edge of lacertus fibrosus
- Anomalous structures:
  - Supracondylar spurring giving origin to the accessory bicipital aponeurosis
  - Accessory head of flexor pollicis longus (FPL) (Gantzer's muscle) this muscle is found in 66% of the limbs (possibly
  - Absence should be a variation!)
  - Palmaris profundus
  - Anomalous heads of PT
- Thrombosed ulnar radial or ulnar collateral vessels crossing the nerve near its origin.
- Other isolated reported causes include forearm mass (metastatic), polyarteritis nodosa, cytomegalovirus (CMV) infection, enlarged bursa, hereditary neuropathies with predisposition to the compressive neuropathies and intraepidural fascicular constriction.

interosseous membrane. The following are the muscle it innervates:

- Flexor pollicis longus
- Radial half of FDP (to index and middle finger)
- Few branches to PT
- Terminally to pronator quadratus

The potential sites of AIN entrapment in elbow and forearm are presented in **Box 5** and shown in **Figure 16**. The most common site and cause is where the nerve passes between the two heads of PT. The tendinous edge promulgating as a fibrous band of deep head of PT (underside of the humeral origin).

Etiology

Various causes can be attributed to the compression of AIN:

- Spontaneous compression
- Anatomic variations
- *Trauma*—supracondylar fractures (usually traction injury)
- Infections
- *Iatrogenic cause*—venipuncture, catheterization, etc., in cubital fossa
- Compartment syndrome and ensuing Volkmann ischemic contracture (VIC)

Clinical Presentation

Palsy of AIN accounts for the upper limb neuropathies. The palsy may be complete or incomplete. In a complete palsy, the following is usually observed.

- *Symptoms include:*
  - *Motor deficits only:* Patient with complete AIN palsy loses motor function of all the four muscles supplied by AIN. The patient is unable to flex the interphalangeal (IP) joint of the thumb and the distal interphalangeal (DIP) joint of the index and long fingers. A typical pinch attitude occurs where patient is unable to make a ring by bringing together the tips of thumb and index finger and rather it transforms into a "Peacock's eye".
  - Notion that no pain occurs is incorrect as these patients report pain after repetitive activity in proximal volar forearm. This is possibly due to fatigue and dyskinesia that prevails due to nonfunction of other muscles.
- *On physical examination, there is specifically include:*
  - Patient is unable to make the OK sign which tests for weakness of FDP and FPL. There may be weakness of grip and pinch, specifically thumb, index, and middle finger flexion. Weakness of pronator quadratus is difficult to elicit as it is a weaker pronating muscle than PT. But some weakness can be elicited after flexing the elbow.
  - Patients with a Martin-Gruber anastomosis may have incomplete paralysis.

Differential Diagnosis

- Partial median nerve lesion—so called pseudo-AIN syndrome
- Attritional rupture of FPL (seen in rheumatoids) test the tenodesis effect
- Parsonage-Turner syndrome—brachial plexopathy
- Cervical spondylosis
- Bilateral AIN signs caused by viral brachial neuritis—usually painful and pain precedes neural symptoms

Evaluation

Electromyography (EMG) includes:

- Helpful adjunct to clinical diagnosis and rule out differential diagnosis.
- Reveal abnormalities in the FPL and FDP of index and middle finger and pronator quadratus muscles (in 85% patients).
- Can define the severity of involvement and can also rule out more proximal lesion.

Treatment

- Nonoperative treatment is commonly effective for acute onset lesions while long-standing ones do not always improve with these measures. Empirically; observation, rest, and splinting in supination help if no organic lesion for compression is identified. Systemic disorders should be corrected (diabetes mellitus, alcoholism, and hypothyroidism). Additional vitamins like pyridoxine 100 mg for a few weeks (6–8 weeks) may be given.
- Operative indication is needed for surgical decompression of AIN in case nonoperative measures fail or if the cause of nerve compression is evident (supracondylar spur and forearm mass). The cause of compression should be relieved and surgical decompression is done by a long incision beginning 5 cm proximal to elbow near the supracondylar spur to medially along the biceps tendon in forearm and further 5 cm into forearm. The nerve is decompressed all along, while the following salient points during surgery should be borne in mind.
  - Cutaneous nerves should be preserved.
  - Nerve should be isolated from the brachial vessels and released from compressive lesions.
  - Excise the supracondylar spur and fibrous bands (ligament of Struthers, pronator band, lacertus fibrosus, etc.).
  - Preserve the branches to PT.
  - Interfascicular neurolysis may be necessary in some long-standing cases (resection and anastomosis is not recommended).

PRONATOR SYNDROME

It is a compression of median nerve between the two heads of pronator muscle at the level of elbow joint. Seyffarth first drew attention to pronator syndrome where he treated most patients conservatively. Apt description of pronator syndrome has been given by Johnson and Spinner. The syndrome is more common in women usually seen in 5th decade. The syndrome in males is especially seen in weight-lifters and body builders with well-developed forearm muscles.

Anatomy and Pathoanatomy

The anatomy of median nerve is described previously. Pathologically the potential sites of compression are the same as described for AIN syndrome but being more relevant for pronator syndrome. The potential sites of entrapment of AIN producing pronator syndrome are detailed in **Box 6**.

Clinical Presentation

- *Symptoms include:*
  - Insidious inset of aching pain in the volar aspect of the proximal forearm and the distal arm. Pain is increased by exertion, excessive use of extremity, and forceful pronation.
  - Paresthesias and hypoesthesias similar to CTS is present, but the difference being that it is more severe with pronation and supination rather than wrist flexion and also sensory loss over the distribution of palmar cutaneous branch of median nerve.
- *Physical examination includes:*
  - Tenderness on the median nerve in the proximal forearm
  - Weakness of the muscles supplied by median nerve
  - Provocative tests are specific for different sites of entrapment:
    - Positive Tinel's sign in the proximal anterior forearm that is usually present only after 4–5 months of compression
    - Resisted elbow flexion with forearm in supination (compression at bicipital aponeurosis)
    - Direct pressure over proximal pronator muscle increases paresthesias
    - Resisted forearm pronation with elbow flexed and gradually extended (compression at two heads of PT)
    - Resisted contraction of FDS to middle finger suggests compression at FDS fibrous arch.

BOX 6: The various sites for potential compression of anterior interosseous nerve (AIN) producing pronator syndrome.

- Fibrous bands between ulnar and humeral heads of pronator teres (PT) where the median nerve passes—most common cause of compression.
- *Thickened or tight bicipital aponeurosis (lacertus fibrosus):* Lacertus fibrosus syndrome is acute pronator syndrome after venipuncture or exercise (described by Swiggett and Ruby).
- *Supracondylar process:* Present in 1% of population. It is a residual osseous structure on distal humerus that gives rise to ligament of Struthers (this structure is different from arcade of Struthers which is a site of ulnar compression neuropathy in cubital tunnel syndrome). The ligament travels from tip of supracondylar process to medial epicondyle. The site is a rare point for compression.
- Flexor digitorum superficialis (FDS) aponeurotic arch
- *Honeymoon paralysis:* This is a transient compression of median nerve at elbow due to prolonged compression on forearm.
- Other uncommon causes of compression include compression due to casting (iatrogenic), hypertrophic PT, or its high origin, especially the humeral head, an anomalous insertion of the coracobrachialis muscle.

Diagnostic Studies

- *Radiographs:* It may reveal supracondylar process.
- *Electromyogram and NCV:* To exclude other sites of nerve entrapment.

Differential Diagnosis

- Carpal tunnel syndrome (the following points favor CTS):
  - Absence of pain over proximal volar forearm
  - Absence of sensory disturbances over the distribution of palmar cutaneous branch of the median nerve
  - Phalen's/Durkan's positive (Phalen's is positive however in 50% patients with pronator syndrome also)
  - *Ehlers-Danlos syndrome* is more useful in any case to differentiate CTS from pronator syndrome
- Cervical radiculopathy (the following points favor cervical root compression):
  - Pain localized in the C6 and C7 dermatomes with weakness of biceps and diminished biceps reflex
- Parsonage-Turner syndrome
- *Thoracic-outlet syndrome:* Symptoms in C8 and T1 distribution
- Medial epicondylitis

Treatment

- "Nonoperative" is effective in 50% of patients. The typical nonoperative treatment comprises rest, splinting and NSAIDs for 3–6 months but effect may be seen up to a year or later. The typical indication is mild-to-moderate symptoms in and otherwise untroubled patient. Patients experiencing progressive symptoms and those with trouble are not good candidates. Also in patients with less than satisfactory control of the symptoms operative treatment is indicated.
- "Operative treatment" involves surgical decompression of median nerve as detailed for AIN above. Typically the decompression of nerve is done simultaneously at all the possible compression sites. The operative treatment is effective in 90% patients.

CUBITAL TUNNEL SYNDROME

It is a compressive neuropathy of the ulnar nerve. The syndrome accounts for being the second most common entrapment neuropathy of upper extremity. Ulnar nerve compression at elbow was first described by Panas in 1878. The ulnar nerve has a typical vulnerable position at the elbow making it quite amenable to injury and compression due to various causes and structures. It is such a susceptible position that experienced surgeons have described the neural position as if the nerve is "asking for trouble" (Lundborg) at elbow. It is commonly seen that people play with the "funny bone" by directly hitting the nerve in superficial position.

Anatomy and Pathoanatomy

Anatomy of ulnar nerve: The ulnar nerve is one of the major terminal branches of the brachial plexus; it takes origin from the medial cord of the brachial plexus with a root value of C8 and T1. In the axilla, the nerve lies medial to axillary artery, from the axilla it enters the arm and stays between the axillary artery and vein. Near the insertion of coracobrachialis it pierces the medial intermuscular septum and enters the posterior compartment. The superior ulnar collateral artery joins ulnar nerve that then run together over the medial head of the triceps till cubital tunnel. The fibers of the nerve are arranged in layers with the sensory nerves for the hand lying superficially, followed by the intrinsic muscle nerves. The branches to the FDP and FCU lie deep against the ulnar collateral ligament.

Anatomy of cubital tunnel (Fig. 17): This tunnel connects the extensor surface of the upper brachium to the flexor surface of antibrachium. The cubital tunnel is a fibro-osseous tunnel that can be divided into three parts:

1. The entrance to the tunnel (posterior to the medial epicondyle)
2. The area of "Osborne's fascia" (the aponeurosis combining the two heads of FCU)
3. The muscle bellies of the FCU itself

The "anatomical boundaries" of cubital tunnel are:

- *Roof:* Formed by Osborne's fascia and Osborne's ligament (fibrous band from the medial epicondyle to the olecranon)
- *Floor:* Formed by ulnar groove of the medial epicondyle anteriorly in its first two parts with the posterior and oblique portions of the ulnar collateral ligament and elbow joint capsule in the third part
- *Walls:* Formed by medial epicondyle and olecranon

Pathophysiology

The shape of the cubital tunnel changes with elbow movements. As the elbow flexes the cubital tunnel converts from a round configuration to a flattened triangle (reducing the cross-sectional area by approximately 55%). Medial epicondyle is a fixed structure while for each 45° of forward flexion the olecranon moves forward some 5 mm. The combination of the above two of these phenomenon produces an elongation stretch of approximately 47 mm on the ulnar nerve from full extension to full flexion. This

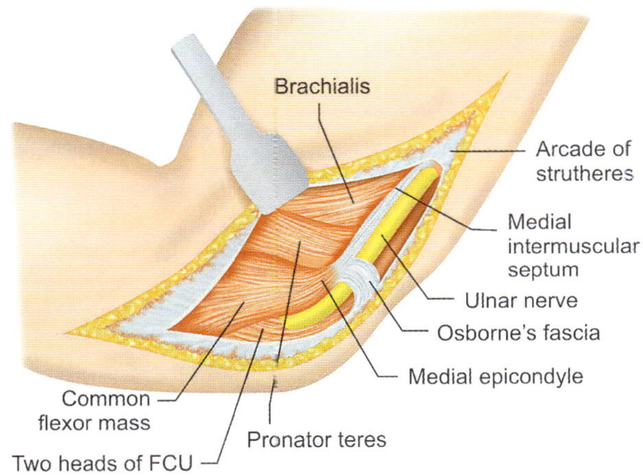

Fig. 17: Cubital tunnel anatomy. (FCU: flexor carpi ulnaris)

is divided into excursion of 13 mm and elongation of 23%. There is increase in the cubital tunnel pressure from 9 to 63 mm Hg with full flexion that substantially increases to 209 mm Hg with FCU contraction. The pressure increase can be partly dissipated by division of Osborne's fascia.

The common sites of entrapment are described in **Box 7** and shown in **Figure 18**.

Presentation

The findings are more common in a male that often reports paresthesia and other symptoms exaggerated by the elbow flexion (say cellphone use). Clinical diagnosis is based on careful evaluation of symptoms and signs. However, one should always borne in mind the anomalous communication from radial or median nerves. The dorsum of the hand may be supplied in its entirety by the superficial radial nerve, leading to an erroneous conclusion that the entrapment is distal. An anomalous communication between the ulnar and median nerves in the palm may lead to combined innervation of the third and fourth lumbricals (or solely by median nerve) thus preventing the onset of clawing.

BOX 7: The common sites for entrapment of ulnar nerve.

- Most common site for ulnar nerve compression is:
  - Between the two heads of flexor carpi ulnaris (FCU)/aponeurosis (most common site) followed by
  - *Arcade of Struthers:* In up to 70% of the population, a band of fascia extends from the medial head of the triceps (8–10 cm proximal to the medial epicondyle) to the medial intermuscular septum (arcade of Struthers). This may be a source of entrapment of the ulnar nerve followed by
  - Hiatus in medial intermuscular septum where the ulnar nerve pierces the septum to enter posterior compartment followed by
  - Location between Osborne's ligament and medial collateral ligament (MCL)
- Less common sites of compression (though important still) include:
  - Medial head of triceps
  - Medial epicondyle
  - Anconeus epitrochlearis (anomalous muscle from the medial olecranon to the medial epicondyle)
  - Fascial bands within FCU
  - Proximal edge of the flexor digitorum superficialis (FDS) aponeurosis
- Extrinsic and miscellaneous causes:
  - Fractures and nonunions
  - Cubitus varus or valgus deformities (tardy ulnar nerve palsy)
  - Osteophytes in the cubital tunnel
  - Heterotopic ossification
  - Tumors, cysts, and medial epicondylitis:
  - Burns
  - *Iatrogenic:* Fixation of intercondylar fractures and medial epicondyle fractures in malposition reducing the tunnel volume. Radial head excision produces lateral instability and tardy ulnar like phenomenon.

- ***Symptoms include:***
  - Sensory symptoms of small finger, ulnar half of ring finger, and ulnar dorsal hand (it is a localizing sign that can exclude compression in Guyon's canal)
  - *Night symptoms:* Due to flexion of the arm while sleeping, may even awaken the patient from sleep.
- ***Physical examination:*** The features are of high ulnar nerve palsy.
  - *Inspection and palpation:*
    - Atrophy of first web space and the interosseous muscles
    - Clawing of the ringing and fifth finger (**Fig. 19**, *see* anomalous connection/innervation by median nerve also): Benediction hand, this is less marked than in lower level ulnar nerve palsies (due to weakness of long flexors here). The clawing is due to loss of intrinsic muscles, especially the lumbricals that produce extension at the IP joint so there is flexion at the IP joints.
    - MCP joint hyperextension
    - Subluxation of ulnar nerve on the medial epicondyle during flexion of elbow.
  - *Sensory examination:*
    - *Hypoesthesia in ulnar 1½ digits and dorsal ulnar half of hand:* The latter is a localizing sign of high ulnar nerve palsy. The dorsal ulnar half of hand is supplied by sensory nerve that arises from ulnar nerve some 6 cm proximal to the wrist. If sensation in this area is spared then compression is likely distal (for example in Guyon's canal) while diminished sensation in dorsal ulnar hand would indicate proximal compression say in the cubital tunnel.
  - *Motor testing:*
    - Reduced strength/paralysis of deep head flexor pollicis brevis (FPB), adductor pollicis, all

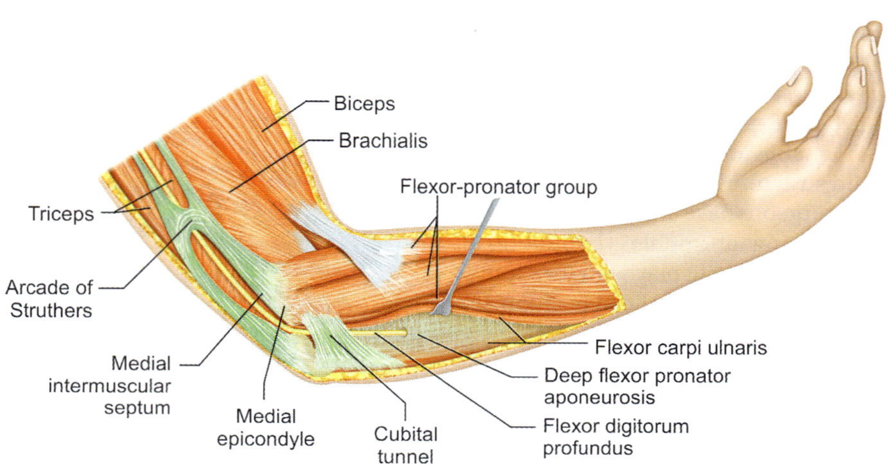

Fig. 18: Sites of entrapment of ulnar nerve.

hypothenar muscles, and 4th and 5th lumbricals and interossei. The following signs can be elicited utilizing this knowledge in a classic case.

- *Weak grasp:* Because of loss of flexion power of metacarpophalangeal (MCP) joint
- *Weak pinch:* Because of loss of adduction of thumb (as much as 70% of pinch strength is lost)
- *Froment's sign* **(Fig. 20)**: Compensatory flexion of thumb IP joint by FPL (supplied by AIN) during key pinch. It compensates for the loss of MCP joint flexion by adductor pollicis supplied by ulnar nerve. Adductor pollicis muscle normally acts as a MCP flexor, first metacarpal adductor, and IP extensor.
- *Earle and Valstou (cross your finger test)* **(Figs. 21A and B)**: Inability to cross the middle over index (testing volar interossei of first and dorsal interossei of second) or vice versa.

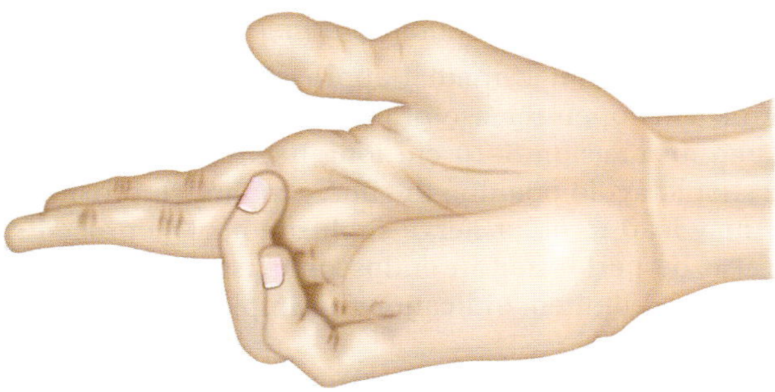

Fig. 19: Claw hand.

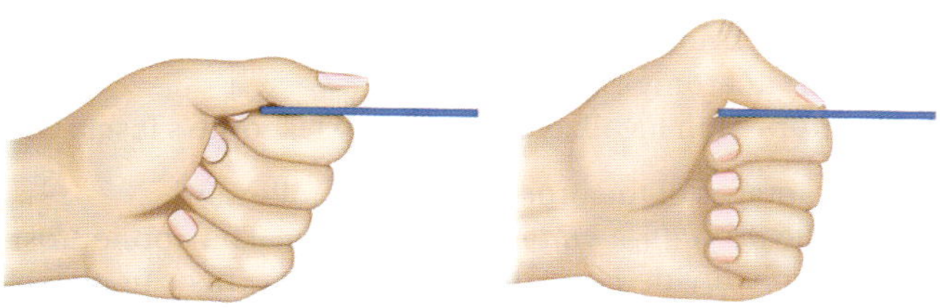

Fig. 20: Froment's sign.

- *Jeanne's sign:* An extension of thumb MCP joint hyperextension due to compensation and thumb adduction by extensor pollicis longus (EPL) supplied by radial nerve during key pinch. The EPL compensates for loss of IP extension and thumb adduction by adductor pollicis supplied by ulnar nerve.
- *Wartenberg's sign:* Persistent abduction and extension of small finger during attempted adduction, occurring secondary to weak third palmar interosseous and small finger lumbrical.
- *Brand sign:* Objects cannot be grasped and rather get pushed away due to fingers curling and rolling into the palm instead of flexing in integrated fashion. The MCP joint flexion starts normally simultaneously with IP joint flexion and completes before complete IP flexion. In ulnar nerve palsy, the MCP joint flexion does not start late until completion of IP joint flexion (Flat sign).
- *Masse's sign:* Flattening of palmar arch and loss of elevation of hand in ulnar direction due to weak opponens digiti quinti and decreased small finger MCP flexion.
- *Bunnell's "O" test:* Hyperextension at MCP joint and hyperflexion of IP joint making an "O" when the patient is asked to make pulp to pulp contact of thumb and index finger **(Fig. 22)**.

- *Extrinsic weakness:*
  - *Pollock's test:* Loss of flexion of distal IP joint of the ring and little finger—due to weakness of two ulnar FDPs
  - *Bowden and Napier:* Partial loss of wrist flexion with inability to perform power grip with a neutral wrist (due to paralysis of the FCU)
  - *Conversion of "X" crease to "Y" pattern of intersected crease:* Normally the little and ring fingers are flexed fully into the palm on closing the fist to give an X configuration to the folded creases of the little finger **(Figs. 23A and B)**. Loss of DIP flexion in ulnar nerve palsy converts the X configuration to a Y.

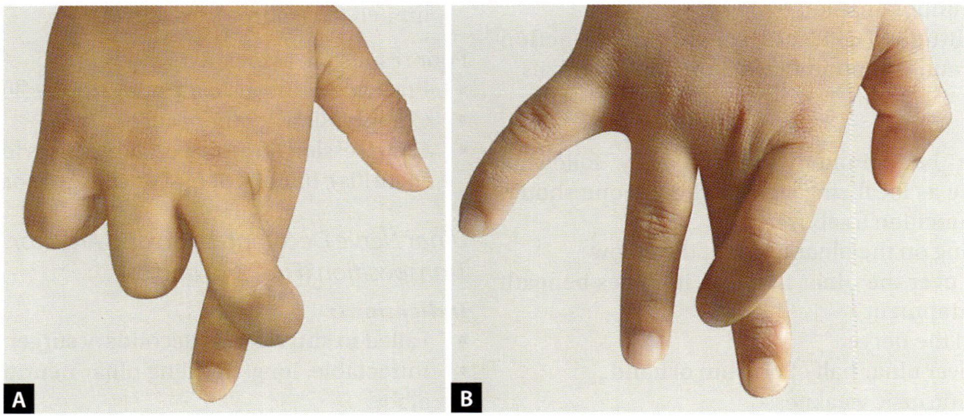

Figs. 21A and B: Earle and Valstou—the cross-over of middle over index (A) tests volar interossei of first and dorsal interossei of second. The reverse would help test (B) the dorsal interossei of the first and palmar interossei of second.

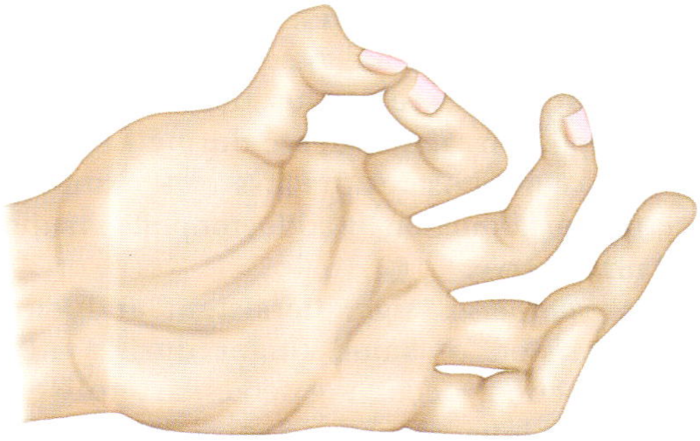

Fig. 22: Bunnell's "O" test.

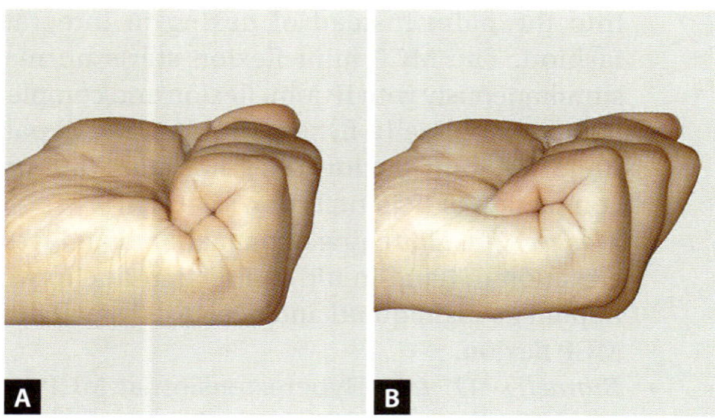

Figs. 23A and B: "X" sign of finger crease. In a normal fist the complete flexion of finger produces "X"-shaped impression (A) due to merging of creases, this changes to "Y" if there is extrinsic weakness (B).

- ***Provocative tests includes:***
  - Positive Tinel's sign over cubital tunnel
  - *Elbow flexion test:* An elbow flexion of >60 seconds reproduces symptoms
  - Direct compression of cubital tunnel exacerbates symptoms

Studies

Electromyogram/NCV

- Helpful to confirm the diagnosis and prognosis:
  - Nerve conduction velocity <48 m/s or difference on two sides of >10 m/s is suggestive
  - Distal motor and sensory latencies higher than normal or unobtainable
  - Low amplitudes (<50%) of sensory nerve action potentials and compound muscle action potentials

Diagnosis

A diagnosis can be commonly obtained by following findings that serve as localizing signs, although one should do thorough examination as above:

- Pain on pressing on the ulnar nerve at the elbow
- A Tinel's sign over the ulnar nerve as it passes beneath the area of entrapment
- Subluxation of the nerve
- Sensory loss over ulnar half of dorsum of hand
- Extrinsic and intrinsic weakness
- Reproduction of symptoms by holding the elbow fully flexed

Differential Diagnosis

- Cervical spondylosis
- Thoracic outlet syndrome
- Ulnar nerve entrapment at Guyon's canal
- Double crush phenomenon
- Systemic conditions diabetes and leprosy

Treatment

Nonoperative treatment involves NSAIDs, activity modification, and night-time elbow extension splinting (forearm in neutral rotation and an extended forearm of about 45°)

Operative treatment: The interventions can be grouped into three categories as follows:

1. In situ nerve decompression (simple decompression).
2. Anterior transposition (subcutaneous, intramuscular, or submuscular)
3. Medial epicondylectomy

In situ Decompression of Cubital Tunnel

This is done through medial approach under tourniquet control. This open release of cubital tunnel is performed through an incision 5–10 cm long beginning proximally. One should avoid opening the nerve too much proximally as it may lead to ulnar nerve subluxation. The procedure can also be performed in endoscopic assistance, but the experience is limited. Indications of simple decompression are:

- Mild symptoms and a short history
- Nonsubluxating nerve and symptoms not associated with varus or valgus deformity
- No prior evidence of injury or degenerative changes that distort anatomy
- Compression localized to be due to Osborne's fascia.

The advantages of the procedure are as follows:

- *Simple procedure and easy to perform:* The aponeurosis is simply divided over the ulnar nerve. This can also be performed under local anesthesia.
- Safe as the handling of ulnar nerve is minimal not interfering with the intrinsic and extrinsic blood supply.
- Prompt result if the site of compression of the nerve is limited to Osborne's fascia.

Poor results are associated with:

- Presence of intrinsic muscle atrophy (long duration)
- Compression at other causes
- Compression due to secondary causes [deformity at elbow (neuritis), tumors, or cyst as cause of compression, etc.]

Ulnar Nerve Decompression and Anterior Transposition (Figs. 24A and B)

Indications:

- Failed in situ release: Secondary surgery
- Intractable, long-standing ulnar neuritis localized to the elbow
- Throwing athlete
- Metabolic/granulomatous neuropathy

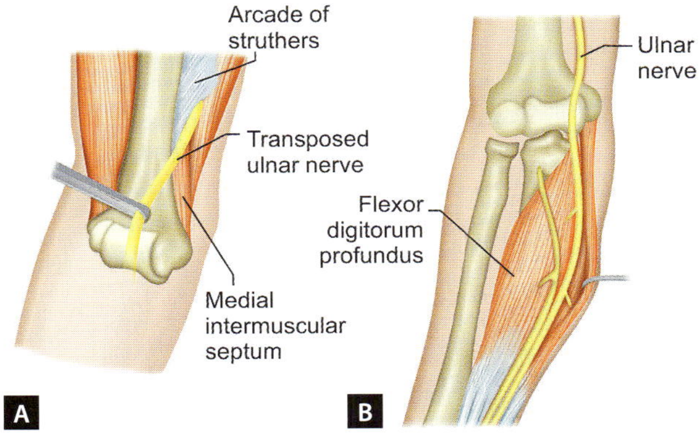

Figs. 24A and B: Transposition of ulnar nerve. The ulnar nerve is transposed anterior to the medial epicondyle (A) that can be placed beneath the skin or muscle or within the flexor pronator mass. The normal disposition of nerve posterior to the medial epicondyle is also shown for reference (B).

- Mobilization associated with nerve repair at the elbow
- Preventive
- Open reduction of intra-articular fractures
- Elbow reconstruction and arthroplasty.

The procedure can be performed in various ways

- *Subcutaneous:* The nerve is transposed anteriorly beneath the skin and subcutaneous fat after releasing the intermuscular septum proximally and freeing the nerve 6 cm proximally and 3–4 cm distally. Vascular supply should be preserved. The nerve is stabilized in position by suturing a flap of pronator muscle raised from the medial epicondyle to the anterior skin flap. This is the most commonly performed procedure and ironically preferred for severe nerve compressions.
- *Submuscular:* It places the nerve in an intermuscular interval, where nerves normally run. The neural bed prevents scarring and provides it the straightest route. The indication is mainly for recurrent cases. The flexor pronator muscle group is transected sharply; leaving a cuff of tissue on the medial epicondyle that is repaired after the nerve is transposed. This procedure is associated with the least recurrence rates but requires a bit more experience. It is commonly preferred by the experienced surgeons over subcutaneous transposition for moderate nerve compressions.
- *Intramuscular transposition:* The nerve is placed in the groove formed by splitting the muscle. The problem is same of rescarring and hence neural compression.

It is not very clear when to choose in situ decompression versus anterior transposition of ulnar nerve in the management of cubital tunnel syndrome. Both the procedures have their pros and cons and similar complication profile. Complications from both procedures include ulnar instability, infection, and medial antebrachial cutaneous nerve injury. The rates of these complications are higher with anterior transposition likely due to more extensive dissection needed for the surgery. Also, the rates of secondary surgery are higher with anterior transposition of ulnar nerve. This has led to increased adoption of in situ decompression rather than anterior transposition of ulnar nerve by the surgeons. Also, endoscopic techniques are being increasingly used due to favorable outcomes for symptom relief comparable to in situ decompression. It is suggested that anterior transposition is better done in patients where ulnar nerve subluxation or dislocation is apparent during clinical examination while patients with ulnar neuropathy without any evidence of active subluxation are better managed by in situ decompression.

Medial Epicondylectomy

Serves to decompress the nerve and also moves it anteriorly. Though theoretical advantages are many but the biggest problem is of creating valgus elbow instability. It has been found that only 19% of medial epicondyle can be resected without producing instability by O'Driscoll. So a complete epicondylectomy is to be combined with medial collateral ligament (MCL) reconstruction/repair. The technique could be specifically preferred for subluxating nerves and recurrent cases or very severe neural compression.

Complications of surgical decompression/transposition:

- *Recurrence:* Often due to inadequate decompression, perineural scarring, or tethering at various places. There is higher rate of recurrence than after CTR. This should be treated by extensive re-exploration, microsurgical neurolysis, and autogenous saphenous nerve wrapping.
- *Neuroma formation:* Branch of the medial antebrachial cutaneous nerve may get injured.

ULNAR TUNNEL SYNDROME

Direct compression of the ulnar nerve in the Guyon's canal. It is also known as handlebar palsy (seen in long distance cyclists who rest their hand on the cycle handle bar).

Anatomy

The ulnar nerve in forearm lies deep to the FCU. Distally it becomes more superficial as it crosses the myotendinous junction of FCU. Radially it is accompanied by the ulnar artery and FCU lies on the ulnar aspect as it progresses further and enters the ulnar canal/tunnel (Guyon's canal).

Guyon's canal: It is a 4 cm long structure starting at the proximal extent of the volar carpal ligament and ends at the arch of the hypothenar muscles. It was originally described in 1861 by a French urologist named Guyon which he recognized as a "loge" (French for "space") where ulnar nerve can get compressed. The boundaries and zones of the Guyon's canal are shown in **Figures 25A and B (Table 3)**. The ulnar canal contains the:

- *Bifurcation of ulnar nerve:* The ulnar nerve divides into the superficial sensory and deep motor branches **(Fig. 26)**. The deep branch supplies all the interosseous muscles and the third and fourth lumbricals, the hypothenar muscles and some thenar muscles [the adductor pollicis and the medial head (deep) of the FPB].
- Ulnar artery

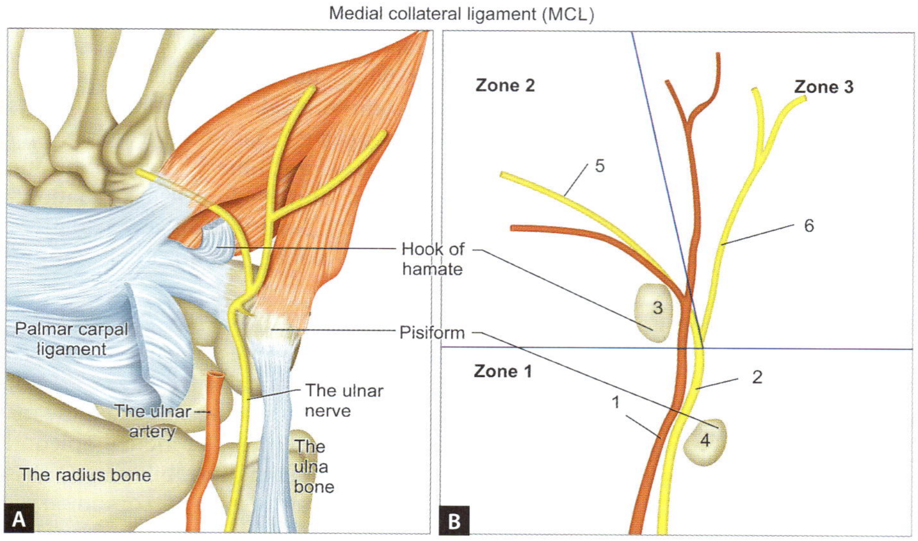

Figs. 25A and B: Guyon's canal anatomy (A) and the three zones (B) (1—ulnar artery; 2—ulnar nerve; 3—hook of hamate; 4—pisiform; 5—deep motor branch; 6—superficial sensory branch).

TABLE 3: Anatomical boundaries of Guyon's canal.

Boundaries of Guyon's canal				
Floor	Transverse carpal ligament, hypothenar muscles			
Roof	Volar carpal ligament			
Ulnar border	Pisiform and pisohamate ligament, abductor digiti minimi muscle belly			
Radial border	Hook of hamate			
Zones of Guyon's canal (Shea and McClain)				
	Location	***Boundaries***	***Common causes of compression***	***Symptoms***
Zone 1	Proximal to bifurcation of the nerve, it contains both the sensoryand motor fascicles (motor fascicles lie deeper to sensory)	Bound ulnarly by the FCU and the pisiform. Roof is formed by the volar carpal ligament. Floor is formed by the transverse carpal ligament	Ganglia and hook ofhamate fractures	Mixed motor andsensory
Zone 2	Surrounds deep motor branch. The deep motor branch passes through zone 2, around the hookof the hamate and then betweenthe pisohamate ligament and thefibrous arch of the flexor digiti minimi	Bound radially by the hook of the hamate, the transverse carpal ligament and the flexor digiti minimi muscle. Roof formed by palmaris brevis muscle and the fibrous arch of the hypothenar muscles. Ulnarly by the pisohamate and pisometacarpal ligaments. Floor is formed by triquetrohamate joint	Ganglia and hook ofhamate fractures	Motor only
Zone 3	Surrounds superficial sensory branch (the superficial sensory branch gives off branches to thepalmaris brevis)	Roof formed by palmaris brevis and the ulnarartery. Radially there is deep motor branch. Ulnarly bound by abductor digiti minimi muscle. Floor formed by hypothenar fascia	Ulnar artery thrombosisor aneurysm	Sensory only (ulnar aspect of the tip of thesmall finger serves as an autonomous zone of sensation for the superficial branch of theulnar nerve)

(FCU: flexor carpi ulnaris)

The various causes of ulnar tunnel syndrome are presented in **Box 8**.

Clinical Presentation

It depends on the location of compression in the canal

- Pure motor symptoms
- Pure sensory symptoms
- Mixed motor and sensory

In a mixed sensorimotor, palsy patients usually have pain in the wrist and paresthesias/numbness in ulnar one and a half. They also report loss of dexterity and a loss of control of the hand. Patients with hypothenar hammer syndrome have history of repeated use of hammer causing proximal superficial arch occlusion. They have pain, cold insensitivity, weakness, and numbness.

On physical examination, they have clawing of ring and little fingers because of loss of intrinsics flexing the MCPs and extending the IP joints. There may be tenderness at hook of hamate. The Allen test is performed to diagnose ulnar artery thrombosis or a palpable mass felt in the ulnar artery.

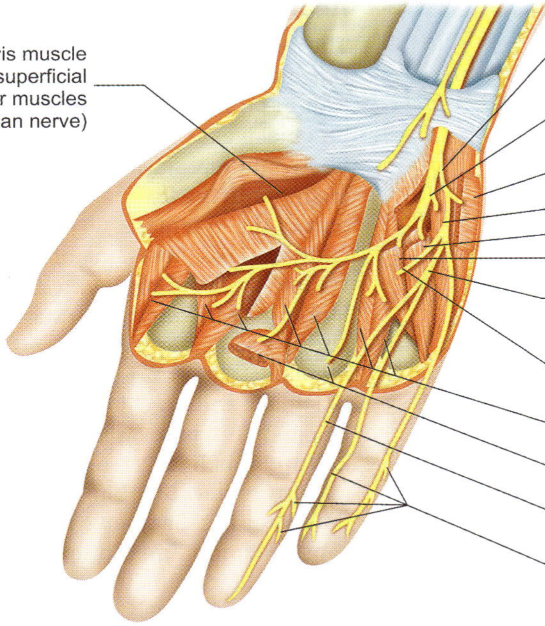

Fig. 26: The location of ulnar nerve and its branching pattern and muscles supplied by it along the course. Distal sensory supply by nerve is also shown.

BOX 8: The various causes of ulnar tunnel syndrome.

- *Anatomical (anomalies or malformations):*
  - Ganglion cyst: This is the most common cause in nontraumatic cases (86% of nontraumatic causes with combined sensory-motor palsy)
  - Lipoma and neurilemmoma
  - Fibrous band(s)
  - Accessory flexor digiti minimi, palmaris longus, and palmaris brevis hypertrophy (accessory palmaris brevis—palmaris brevis profundus)
  - Congenital bands
  - Pisiform-hamate coalition
- *Traumatic:*
  - Repetitive trauma
  - Nonunion or fracture of hook of hamate
  - Dislocation of pisiform
  - Handlebar palsy
- *Systemic:*
  - Diabetes
  - Alcoholism
  - Hypothyroidism
- Ulnar artery thrombosis (hypothenar hammer syndrome), aneurysm, and hemangioma
- Inflammatory arthritis
- Calcinosis (metastatic and scleroderma)
- Pigmented villonodular synovitis (PVNS)

Paralysis of the intrinsic muscles. The abductor digiti minimi may be spared when compression is in zone 2, because the motor branch to this muscle has already exited. It is important to note that abnormal sensation in the dorsal-ulnar hand and decreased power of FDP of fourth and fifth finger indicate a high-ulnar nerve palsy (proximal to ulnar tunnel). The common physical findings due to nerve compression in Guyon's canal are:

- *Clawing* of the ring and little finger that is more pronounced than cubital tunnel syndrome
- *Weakened grasp:* From loss of MCP joint flexion power
- *Weak pinch:* From loss of thumb adduction (as much as 70% of pinch strength is lost)
- *Froment's sign:* Compensatory thumb IP flexion by FPL (AIN) during key pinch
- *Jeanne's sign:* Compensatory thumb MCP hyperextension and thumb adduction by EPL supplied by radial nerve during key pinch. The EPL compensates for loss of IP extension and thumb adduction by adductor pollicis supplied by ulnar nerve.
- *Wartenberg's sign:* Persistent small finger abduction and extension during attempted adduction secondary to weak third palmar interosseous and small finger lumbrical.

Diagnostic Imaging

None of the studies establish diagnosis which is made clinically; they are mere adjuncts to know the cause. Plain radiographs may show hook of hamate fractures or other bony abnormalities. Also they help evaluate RA. MRI is useful to evaluate ganglion cysts and other soft tissue conditions known to produce ulnar nerve compression. MR angiography may additionally reveal aneurysms and thrombosis.

Differential Diagnosis

Cubital tunnel syndrome (high ulnar nerve palsy) differentiate by the presence of:

- Less clawing (due to involvement of long flexors also that remain weak to flex the joints)
- Positive elbow flexion test
- Motor deficit to ulnar-innervated extrinsic muscles
- Sensory deficit to ulnar half of dorsum of the hand
- Tinel's sign positive at the elbow

- Cervical spondylosis
- Thoracic outlet syndrome
- Pancoast tumor
- Charcot-Marie-Tooth disease
- Guillain-Barré syndrome

Treatment

The nonoperative management is indicated in mild symptoms and comprises of activity modification, NSAIDs, and splinting.

The operative treatment is needed for obvious disability due to clawed fingers, loss of power in pinch, and grasp. It is usually indicated for severe symptoms or failed nonoperative treatment. The operative treatment comprises of:

- *Local decompression:* Done for compression identified at the wrist joint not improving with conservative treatment. The decompression is done through an incision given in line with the radial aspect of ring finger. Decompression is done sequentially from zone 1 to 3. Ganglions and other masses are removed. Nonunion hook of hamate is excised. In case of arterial thrombosis or aneurysm reconstruction with autogenous vein graft is performed especially if the thrombosis extends beyond the common digital arteries.
- *Tendon transfers:* For correction of clawing and to restore power of pinch
  - Lasso procedure can correct the clawing deformity
  - Using the FDS of ring finger or *extensor carpi radialis brevis* (ECRB) to restore power pinch with smith transfer if the former has been used for Lasso.

RADIAL TUNNEL SYNDROME (SUPINATOR SYNDROME)

It is a compressive neuropathy of the radial nerve main trunk in the proximal forearm before/at/just after it splits into main trunk posterior interosseous neuropathy (PIN) and the minor trunk (sensory branch) which results in refractory lateral elbow and forearm symptoms (both sensory and motor). Compression of only sensory nerve [radial sensory nerve (RSN)] is called Wartenberg's syndrome (see below) while that of only motor component (PIN only is called PIN compression palsy) and are distinct entities. It should be mentioned at the outset that though there is PIN compression in both radial tunnel syndrome (RTS) and PIN compression syndrome but the motor symptoms are not very prominent in the former, as also evidenced by EMG studies.

Radial tunnel syndrome is possibly a misnomer and not a true representative of the compressive neuropathies for following reasons:

- Prominent focal tenderness
- Normal neurologic function
- No confirmatory electrodiagnostic evidence of nerve dysfunction

The description will be made still in context of the classical knowledge that helps to understand the other compression neuropathies of radial nerve (Wartenberg's and PIN compression). The syndrome is reported to occur in 2.97 per 100,000 people annually (reported incidence does not cater for patients not presenting to the physicians due to various reasons). It is more common in male manual laborers and bodybuilders.

Anatomy

The radial nerve anatomy is variable. It is the largest branch of brachial plexus that receives branches from all the roots (C5–8 and T1) and is the continuation of posterior divisions of the brachial plexus. The nerve is mixed with predominant motor fibers and few sensory nerve fibers. Radial nerve descends posterior to the first part of the axillary artery and the upper part of the brachial artery. The nerve passes anterior to the subscapularis, teres major and latissimus dorsi muscles. It then curves from the medial to lateral in a groove of the humerus with the profunda brachii, between the medial and lateral heads of the triceps. Travelling distally it pierces the lateral intermuscular septum, and lies between the brachialis and brachioradialis (BR) to the front of the lateral epicondyle, where it divides into a superficial (sensory) and a deep branch (PIN) in the radial tunnel. The radial tunnel (approximately 5 cm in length) originates near the level of the radiocapitellar joint where the nerve lies against the joint capsule continuing further to the distal border of supinator. The boundaries of the tunnel are as follows:

- Medial border is the brachialis muscle proximally and the biceps tendon distally
- Roof and lateral border of the tunnel is made by the extensor carpi radialis longus (ECRL) and the ECRB
- *Floor:* Capsule of radiocapitellar joint

Posterior interosseous neuropathy: It is the deepest branch of the radial nerve in the radial tunnel **(Fig. 27)**. It gives motor innervation to the muscles of extensor compartment of forearm. Approximately 3.5 cm distal to the radial head the nerve passes between the two heads of supinator muscle, the nerve then winds to the dorsal side of forearm and enters the middle of forearm (i.e., exit the supinator, at 7.5 cm distal to the radial head) positioned over the interosseous membrane in front of EPL. Here it forms a gangliform enlargement and supplies the muscles as filaments, still two main branches,

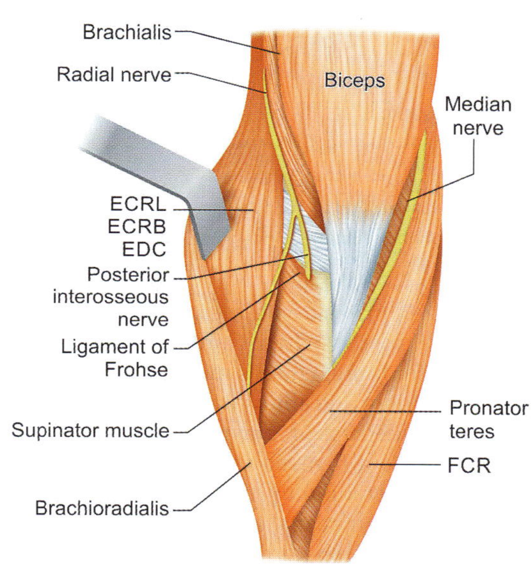

Fig. 27: Radial tunnel anatomy. (ECRB: extensor carpi radialis brevis; ECRL: extensor carpi radialis longus; EDC: extensor digitorum communis; FCR: flexor carpi radial)

the medial and lateral can be identified in 65% population). These branches have distinct motor supply (see below). Distal most continuation travels over interosseous membrane to supply sensory fibers to dorsal wrist capsule through 4th extensor compartment. Motor innervation is provided to:

- *Common extensors include:*
  - Extensor digitorum communis (EDC) (medial branch of PIN)
  - Extensor carpi radialis brevis (often from radial nerve, but can be from PIN)
  - Extensor digiti minimi/quinti (EDM) (medial branch of PIN)
  - Extensor carpi ulnaris (ECU) (medial branch of PIN)
- *Deep extensors include:*
  - Supinator
  - Abductor pollicis longus (APL) (lateral branch of PIN)
  - Extensor pollicis brevis (EPB) (lateral branch of PIN)
  - Extensor pollicis longus (lateral branch of PIN)
  - Extensor indicis proprius (EIP) (lateral branch of PIN)

The superficial RSN lies below the BR muscle in the forearm. The nerve pierces the fascia on the medial side of BR about 8 cm proximal to the tip of the radial styloid and then lies dorsal to the extensor tendons **(Fig. 28)**. RSN then divides into a medial and lateral branch with specific innervation:

- Lateral branch lies 1–3 cm radial to Lister's tubercle and supplies 1st and 2nd web space:
  - Dorsal radial hand
  - Dorsum of the radial 3.5 digits (to approximately the middle phalanx level)
- Medial branch passes within 2 cm of 1st dorsal compartment, directly over EPL and innervates:
  - The radial wrist (with some variable overlap from the lateral antebrachial cutaneous nerve)
  - Dorsolateral thumb

Etiology of Nerve Compression

Typically five potential sites of compression are recognized **(Box 9)**. There are various causes of nerve compression/injury at these sites as follows:

- Repetitive pronosupination movements as in industrial workers causing microtrauma
- Monteggia fracture dislocation and radial head fracture (with or without dislocation)
- Lesions compressing the nerve in the tunnel such as ganglion, neuromas, and lipomas
- Rheumatoid synovitis of radiocapitellar joint
- Iatrogenic while surgery on radial head/neck or replacement

There are commonly mentioned five potential sites of compression as follows:

1. Between the brachialis and BR
2. "Leash of Henry" are recurrent radial vessels that fan out across the PIN at the level of the radial neck causing **(Fig. 29)**
3. Distal border of supinator muscle at its edge
4. At the origin of ECRB or fibrous bands within ECRB
5. "Arcade of Frohse" that lies at the proximal edge of the superficial portion of the supinator.

BOX 9: The five potential sites for nerve compression in radial tunnel syndrome.

1. Between the brachialis and brachioradialis (BR)
2. "Leash of Henry" are recurrent radial vessels that fan out across the posterior interosseous neuropathy (PIN) at the level of the radial neck causing **(Fig. 29)**
3. Distal border of supinator muscle at its edge
4. At the origin of extensor carpi radialis brevis (ECRB) or fibrous bands within ECRB
5. "Arcade of Frohse" that lies at the proximal edge of the superficial portion of the supinator.

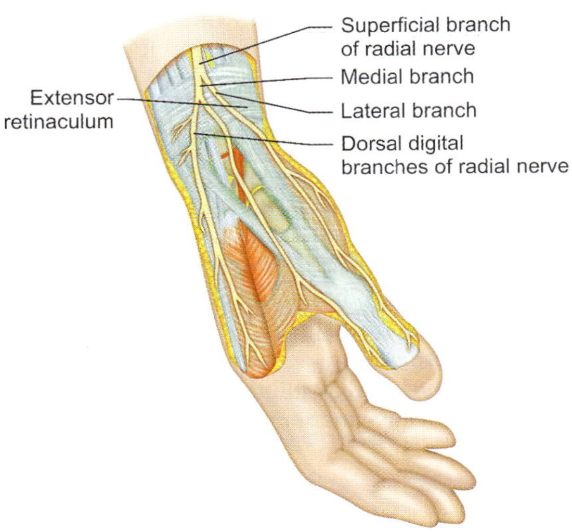

Fig. 28: The superficial branch of radial nerve as it emerges from beneath brachioradialis and further course in the hand.

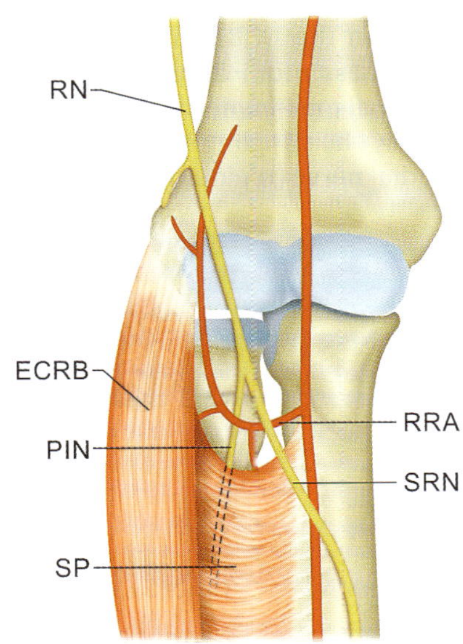

Fig. 29: Causes of radial nerve compression. (ECRB: extensor carpi radialis brevis; PIN: posterior interosseous nerve; RN: radial nerve; RRA: recurrent radial artery; SP: supinator; SRN: superficial radial nerve)

Presentation

The main complaint is pain in the forearm and wrist distal to the lateral epicondyle about 4–5 cm in the region of the mobile wad, the ECRL, ECRB, and BR and over the course of the radial nerve down the forearm (here the pain is usually an ache and has deep burning characteristic). The location of pain varies with the site of nerve compression—pain just distal to the lateral epicondyle of the elbow is due to compression at arcade of Frohse. The various characteristics of pain in PIN compression include:

- Presence of night pain and pain at rest
- Pain increases with activities requiring wrist extension and forearm pronation.

The patients report weakness with finger, wrist, and thumb movements and reduced endurance of affective hand for repetitive activity. The patient also has declined functional use of affective hand for activities of daily living (ADL). It should be re-emphasized that in PIN compression syndrome the sensory disturbances/abnormality are missing and the motor weakness is predominant symptom.

On "physical examination", atrophy can be noticed in the extensor compartment in long-standing cases. The typical examination findings are as follows:

- (Quick examination finding to identify PIN compression): Patient has pain and inability to extend the middle finger against resistance with elbow extended and forearm pronated with wrist neutral **(Fig. 30)**.
- There is tenderness over the region of the PIN in forearm 2 cm anterior and 4–5 cm distal to lateral epicondyle (area of arcade of Frohse) elicited by rolling fingers perpendicular to the PIN course over extensor muscles. The "rule of nines" test is particularly helpful for identifying RTS. The above region is palpated at nine different locations where the area of radial nerve can be identified in the plane between BR and ECRL while resisting the patient's effort to flex elbow with his hand in neutral position. Maximal site of tenderness in radial tunnel verses on the ECRB differentiates from tennis elbow. Tenderness more distally and medially would indicate proximal median nerve compression.
- Tinel's sign may elicit tingling along the course of sensory branch of radial nerve (uncommon).

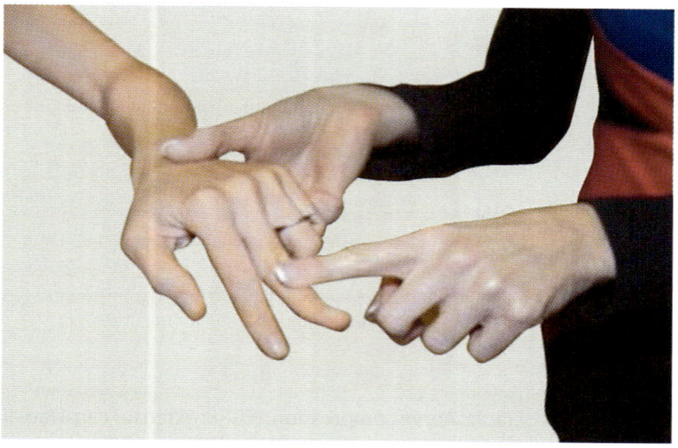

Fig. 30: Resisted middle finger extension.

- The extension of finger at MCP joints is typically weak (tested with wrist dorsiflexed passively).
- *Weakness of wrist extension (long-standing cases):* The patient is unable to extend wrist in ulnar deviation
  - The wrist will extend with radial deviation due to intact ECRL supplied by radial nerve but not in ulnar deviation (paralyzed/weak ECU supplied by PIN).
- *Provocative tests:*
  - Painful resisted supination: Compression at the Arcade of Frohse.
  - Painful resisted middle finger extension test: Compression at ECRB and BR.
- *Normal tenodesis test:* With passive wrist flexion the fingers extend at MCP, it differentiates from extensor tendon rupture (traumatic/inflammatory from RA).

Evaluation

- Radiographs are not diagnostic.
- Magnetic resonance imaging is helpful only for surgical planning of mass resection. Also, it may show thickened edge of ECRB, prominent radial recurrent vessels (leash of Henry), swelling of nerve, radiocapitellar lesions, and rheumatoid synovitis.
- *Electromyography/nerve conduction studies (NCS):* May help in differentiating close differentials. Hardly useful information with regard to RTS is obtained as the test is often negative.

Differential Diagnosis

- *Cervical spondylosis and radiculopathy:* Perform upper limb tension test 2 for radial nerve (ULNT2)
- Ganglion cyst of proximal radioulnar joint
- Intra-articular elbow pathology
- Brachial plexus compression
- Posterior interosseous nerve syndrome (only motor symptoms no sensory involvement)
- Lateral antebrachial nerve irritation or neuritis
- Anconeus/extensor compartment chronic compartment syndrome
- *Tennis elbow (coexists in 5% cases):*
  - Maximal tenderness at the ECRB
  - Pain with resisted wrist extension in radial deviation at the ECRB

Diagnosis of Radial Tunnel Syndrome

The following points help in making the diagnosis of RTS.

- Pain in lateral elbow and forearm (absent in PIN compression syndrome)
- *Paresthesias:* Numbness and/or tingling that also impairs the patient's fine motor control of affected digits
- Weakness of pinch and grip
- Typical tenderness
- Weakness of finger MCP joints
- Positive provocative maneuvers

Treatment

Goals of treatment include:

- Resolve symptoms and maximize pain relief
- Regain radial nerve glide without compression

- Regain independence with ADL.
  - Conservative and rehabilitative treatment comprises of activity modification, stretching, splinting, and medications (NSAIDs, neurotropic vitamins, and limited use of corticosteroids).
    - *Splinting:* Splinting of the wrist is done in extension (approximately 15°) primarily for night-time use. The splint is used commonly for 4–6 weeks continuously and the use is reduced over further 4 weeks if symptoms improve. If the symptoms do not improve with wrist extension then elbow flexion of 90° may be added.
    - *Activity modification:* Repetitive tasks identified to increase the symptoms and poor posture are corrected or avoided. Specifically repetitive work involving forces >1 kg more than 10 times per hour and activities involving constant elbow extension of 0–45° (with pronosupination of forearm) are avoided.
    - *Modalities:* Local ultrasonics, superficial heat, or cryotherapy is still inconclusive for effect but may be prescribed.
    - *Stretching/strengthening program and nerve gliding exercises:* Stretching of the functional muscle groups (not isolated muscles) and strengthening of muscles for improving muscle balance help in maintaining and improving the patient functional status. Nerve gliding exercises include depressing the shoulder, internally rotate the arm and flexion of the wrist followed by lateral cervical flexion to the contralateral side and then shoulder extension. This also stretches the nerve so it should not be overdone.
    - Local corticosteroid injection is given to facilitate the rehabilitation and improve symptoms. It also helps in subsiding any ensuing inflammation. Injections are given after ruling out a compressive mass lesion (lipoma or ganglion) in a patient with isolated tenderness distal to lateral epicondyle. They are often used as a second rung when patient shows minimal or no improvement with initial conservative methods.

"Poor prognostic factors" for conservative treatment (ideally patient should not be managed by conservative treatment if any/combination of the following are present):

- Severe muscle atrophy
- Severe pain [>8/10 on visual analog scale (VAS)]
- Patients who cannot tolerate NSAIDs
- Worsening neurological symptoms
- Compliance issues.

"Surgical decompression" is typically indicated for:

- Symptoms that persist for >3 months of nonoperative treatment or patients with worsening neurology identified in the first three weeks.
- The other definitive indication is a compressive mass detected on imaging.

Patients should be counseled that results are variable and that spontaneous recovery of motor function is seen in 50–95% of nontraumatic causes so that minority may not get any benefit. Also the symptoms may continue to improve for up to 18 months so they should have patience and stick to postoperative rehabilitation protocol.

Technique

The radial tunnel can be approached both anteriorly and posteriorly. The anterior approach is between the BR and biceps and is most popular. For dorsal approach various authors have used different planes to approach the radial nerve and are a bit complicated. The incision is placed along a line joining the lateral radial head to midwidth of the wrist. The planes described for dorsal approach include:

- Between ECRB and EDC
- Between BR and ECRL
- Transmuscular BR-splitting

By any method it is imperative to decompress with sequential release of:

- Fibrous bands connecting brachialis and BR
- Leash of Henry (ligate and cut)
- Fibrous edge of ECRB
- Arcade of Frohse (most important structure to be released)
- Distal edge of supinator
- Release radiocapitellar joint superficial bands

WARTENBERG'S SYNDROME

(Synonyms: Cheiralgia paresthetica, hand cuff neuropathy/neuropraxia, and wristlet watch neuritis)

Wartenberg's syndrome is the compressive neuropathy of the superficial RSN described first in 1926. Wartenberg called it cheiralgia (pain in hand) paresthetica. There are no motor deficits. This is an uncommon syndrome and contrary to RTS females are four times more commonly affected. The syndrome is commonly seen associated with De Quervain's disease in 20–50% patients.

Pathoanatomy of nerve compression: (Kindly see the detailed anatomy previously described in RTS). Various activities and normal or anomalous structures can produce Wartenberg's syndrome and are presented in **Box 10**.

Presentation

- The patient should be evaluated for any history of forearm fractures, trauma, wearing tight handcuffs, bracelets, tight wrist band, wristwatch band, or plaster cast.

BOX 10: The etiology for development of Wartenberg's syndrome.

- During forearm pronation there is a scissoring action of brachioradialis (BR) and extensor carpi radialis longus (ECRL) tendons which may cause superficial radial nerve (SRN) compression
- Fascial bands in the subcutaneous plane as the nerve exits about 8 cm proximal to the radial styloid
- Etiological causes (uncommon case reports):
  - Trauma (Colles' fracture and stretch injuries by bony spike)
  - Diabetes
  - Lipoma
  - Operative scars
  - Brachioradialis anatomic variations

- The symptoms include an ill-defined pain over dorsoradial hand with reluctant to wear watch, paresthesias, and numbness over dorsoradial forearm. Repetitive wrist flexion and ulnar deviation aggravates the symptoms and motor symptoms are conspicuously absent.
- *On examination:*
  - Tinel's sign positivity is the most common finding, over the superficial sensory radial nerve. It can be positive at the exit point of the nerve from forearm fascia (8–9 cm from radial styloid) or over the radial styloid or over both.
  - *Dellon's provocative test is positive:* Increased symptoms on wrist flexion, ulnar deviation and pronation for 1 minute **(Fig. 31)**.
  - Finkelstein test is positive in 96% of cases because of traction on the nerve.

Imaging

- Radiographs may demonstrate malunited fracture or spike.
- Electrodiagnostic tests are not of much help.

Differential Diagnosis

- De Quervain's tenosynovitis:
  - No increase in pain on wrist pronation
  - The symptoms are present with activity while in patients with RSN syndrome, the symptoms are also present at rest
- Lateral antebrachial cutaneous nerve neuritis
- Intersection syndrome

Treatment

- Nonoperative management is the prime modality and mostly effective and rarely surgical decompression or release is needed. The modalities used are rest, activity modification, NSAIDs, and wrist splints. Patient and treating surgeon should have patience as the symptoms are self-resolving.
- Additional modalities for peripheral nerve stimulation like pulsed low-intensity infrared laser or local ultrasonics may be selectively provided.
- Surgical decompression (done only after 6–8 months of aggressive treatment) is done via longitudinal incision volar to Tinel's sign (to protect the lateral antebrachial cutaneous nerve).

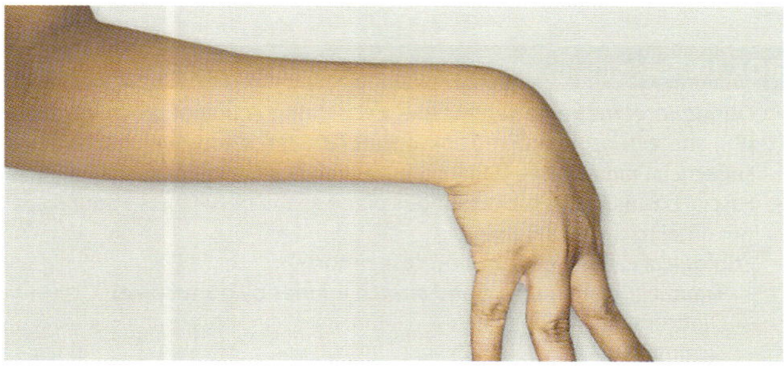

Fig. 31: Dellon's provocative maneuver for identifying Wartenberg's syndrome.

POSTERIOR INTEROSSEOUS NERVE COMPRESSION SYNDROME

First ever report of a PIN palsy was made in 1950 by Guillain and Courtellemont. It is a compressive neuropathy involving the posterior interosseous branch of the radial nerve (PIN) with only motor dysfunction and no sensory dysfunction. The anatomy and sites of compression are similar to that of RTS as described previously.

Etiology

Various causes of compression of the nerve have been reported.

- Lipomas
- Synovial chondromatosis
- Ganglia from anterior capsule of radioulnar joint
- Septic arthritis of elbow
- Pannus in RA
- Fibrous bands in muscle or anterior to capsule
- Vasculitis physical examination reveals weakness in the innervated muscles without any sensory involvement. Most of the provocative maneuvers as for RTS are negative while one should always check for tenodesis effect (to rule out tendon rupture).

Presentation

The patients typically present with dropped fingers and thumb. ECRL is preserved as it receives supply along with BR before the nerve enters radial tunnel. Partial lesions are seen that cause specific motor weakness:

- Predominant involvement of medial branch may cause weakness of the ECU, EDC, and extensor digiti minimi.
- Predominant compression of lateral branch may cause weakness of the EPB, APL, extensor indicis proprius, and EPL.

Imaging

- MRI is usually negative but may be indicated for identification of muscle changes in innervated group appearing as denervation edema/atrophy within the supinator/extensor. It may also reveal the cause of compression as mentioned above. It is intriguing to understand that despite proximal compression in RTS the EMG findings are not prominent.
- Electrodiagnostic studies includes: *Electromyography*/NCV should be performed where the EMG is usually positive due to deinnervation.

Differential Diagnosis

- Cervical radiculopathy at C6–7 with predominant motor symptoms
- Brachial plexopathy (partial involvement)

Treatment

The management is essentially same as that for the RTS except that the NSAIDs may not be needed due to absence of pain. Splinting is a more prominent part of management and the wrist-drop splint improvised to finger drop splint is needed that allows active flexion and passive extension of the IP joints. Nonoperative management is done for 4–6 months followed by surgical release of the nerve if there are no improvement or neurology progresses. Surgical release is also indicated in delayed cases with evident atrophy of muscles at presentation. The surgical release of the radial tunnel has been detailed above. Outcomes have improved over time and now currently the good reported outcomes stand at around 80%. Patient should be cautioned and counseled for delayed recovery seen after the procedure.

Lower success rate has been observed in the following groups:

- Workers compensation patients
- Associated with multiple entrapment neuropathies

CONCLUSION

- Entrapment neuropathies better called compression neuropathies are commonly seen in the practice of a hand and upper extremity clinician.
- It is imperative to realize that initial compression neuropathy later produces irreversible changes in the nerve and consequent dysfunction to produce disability, so early identification and rectification of the pathology is essential.
- To understand the causes and sites of compression the clinician should have thorough knowledge of the anatomy of involved nerves, only then will he be able to localize the pathology.
- Treatment mostly comprises decompression of the nerve if initial conservative trial fails. Surgical decompression is curative in most cases.

CHAPTER 120

Peripheral Nerve Injuries

Manish Kumar Varshney

INTRODUCTION

Peripheral nerves provide important connection between central nervous system (CNS) and peripheral body. Together these nerves form essential component of the peripheral nervous system and in human body there are 43 pairs of peripheral nerves. Injury to peripheral nerves is common as is seen in most crush or cut injuries. Unlike the CNS, peripheral nerves have ability to regenerate via a stereotyped process. This ability enables a surgeon to repair the nerves so that the communication can be re-established. It is thus imperative that one understands the anatomy of peripheral nerves well and the regenerative process. The concept that nerve function can be restored has been known since long, possibly the initial description was given by Paul of Aegina (625–690) who recommended approximation of nerve cut ends along with wound closure. This was later refined by eminent surgeons of the time to introduce concepts of epineural repair (Hueter, 1871) and secondary nerve repair (Nelaton, 1864). Since the descriptions, stress has always been laid down on producing tension-free repairs at the injury site.

ANATOMICAL CONSIDERATIONS

The peripheral nervous system (PNS) comprises of nerves and ganglion outside the brain and spinal cord. It acts as a relay center of sensory and motor impulses between the CNS and the internal organs, surface of body and the skeletal muscles. The nerves of PNS may be arbitrarily arranged in two groups: (1) the cerebrospinal group of nerves and (2) sympathetic system. These are, however, intricately intermingled and related to work in tandem.

- Cerebrospinal nerves (on either side)—43 in number (12 cranial and 31 spinal). They are concerned with the functions of the special and general senses and the voluntary movements of the body. Cranial nerves III–XII are also considered to be peripheral nerves.
- Sympathetic nerves are concerned with movements of the viscera, vasomotor activities and control the phenomena of secretion. Their axial "brain" is located in two rows of *central ganglia* situated on either side of the midline **(Fig. 1)**. These ganglia are closely connected with the spinal cord and the spinal nerves. The ganglia are joined to each other by vertical strands of nerve fibers constituting a pair of knotted cords—the *sympathetic trunks*. The sympathetic nerves ensuing from the ganglia form three great prevertebral plexuses which supply the thoracic, abdominal and pelvic viscera. These work intricately with the *peripheral ganglia* found in the walls of viscera.

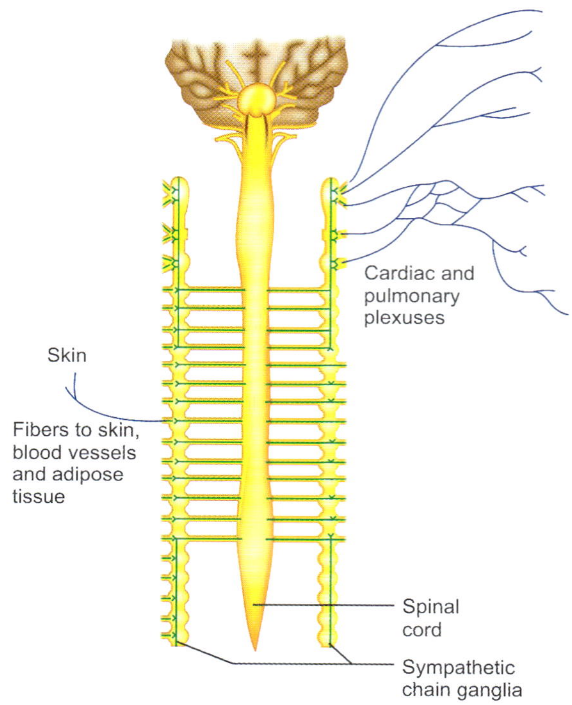

Fig. 1: The sympathetic chains extend from the brain to coccyx along the vertebral column on each side.

NEURON

The nerve cell and its processes is termed as *neuron*. Waldeyer formulated the theory (popularly known as "Neuron theory") that nervous system is built up of numerous neurons, "anatomically and genetically independent of one another". According to this theory (*Neuron theory*):

- The processes of one neuron only come into contact to the other and are never continuous—no continuity is seen between the neighboring neurons stained by Golgi method.
- Impulses are transmitted from one nerve cell to another through points of contact—the synapses.
- The synapse or synaptic membrane seems to allow nerve impulses to pass in one direction only, namely, from the terminals of the axis cylinder to the dendrons.
- Degenerative changes in nervous tissue as a result of disease, trauma or experiment never spread from one neuron to another and are limited to the individual neurons or groups of neurons, primarily affected.

Inferences from the *Neuron theory* have formulated the current concept of "the neurons being the units or structural elements of the nervous system". A newborn has all the neurons present in it which are present in an adult, they stop dividing before birth. All neurons gradually assume function after birth, not all are functional at birth. They are of various types according to morphology and number of processes **(Figs. 2A to E)**. Once the cell body of a neuron is destroyed, there is no indication of any regeneration possible.

The body of the nerve cell is known as the "cyton". It consists of a finely fibrillated reddish or yellowish-brown color protoplasmic material **(Fig. 3)**. To the cyton are attached small irregular processes called dendrites and a long axial cylinder fibril. The protoplasm of cyton contains the Nissl's granules which are peculiar angular granules, and stain deeply with methylene blue (basic dyes). They extend into the dendritic processes, but not into the axon (axis cylinder). There is small clear area at the point of exit of an axon from cyton is termed the "cone of origin" **(Fig. 3)**. The "Nissl's granules" gets "chromatolyzed" or disappear during various pathological and physiological processes like injury (Wallerian degeneration), fatigue or after prolonged stimulation of the nerve fibers connected with the cells. They are supposed to represent a store of nervous energy, and are absent or deficient in various mental diseases. The nucleus is large, well-defined and spherical containing a well-marked nucleolus. The cell bodies of peripheral neurons are often found grouped into clusters called ganglia that may be either motor or sensory.

- Sensory ganglia or posterior root ganglion is an oval swelling located on the dorsal roots of spinal nerves and on the roots of certain cranial nerves. The axons of posterior root ganglia neurons are known as the afferent neurons. Cell bodies of both somatic and visceral sensory neurons are located in the dorsal root ganglia, also known as the spinal ganglia. The sensory neurons making up these ganglia are unipolar (inverted teardrop) since, there are no synaptic contacts between neurons in a sensory ganglion. The cell bodies of sensory ganglia are slightly oval or round with concentric nuclei **(Figs. 2A to E)**. A single axon fiber arises from it which undergoes a T-shaped bifurcation, one branch of it goes to the periphery, and the other enters the CNS, i.e., the brain or the spinal cord.
- Motor ganglia are associated with neurons of the autonomic nervous system. Many motor ganglia are located in the sympathetic trunks (paravertebral ganglia, as mentioned earlier) stretching from the base of the skull to the coccyx, along each side of the vertebral column. The intermediolateral cell column of T1-L2 or sometimes L3 segments of the spinal cord contain cell bodies of visceral motor neurons and autonomic neurons of the sympathetic nervous system, whereas the cell bodies of visceral motoneurons of the parasympathetic nervous system are located in the cranial nerves nuclei of III, VII, IX and X, and in the intermediolateral cell column of the S2–S4 segments of the spinal cord. The cell bodies of motor ganglia are multipolar. The preganglionic fibers of the motor ganglia arises from the brain or the spinal cord and synapse in the ganglia with the multipolar cell bodies. The postganglionic axons from the motor ganglia end up in the target visceral organs.

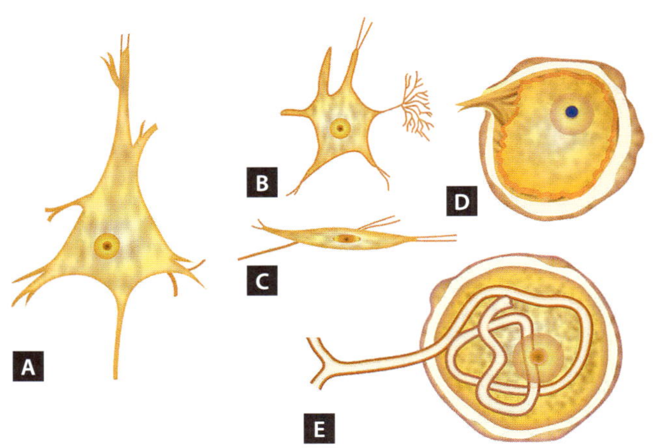

Figs. 2A to E: Various morphological forms of neurons. (A) Pyramidal cell; (B) Small multipolar cell—the axon is small and quickly divides into numerous branches; (C) Fusiform neuron; (D and E) Ganglion cells—note that the axon of sensory ganglion cells divide into T-shaped fashion into lateral and medial division.

Structure and Function of a Peripheral Nerve

Nerve is defined as a bundle of fibers that uses electrical and chemical signals to transmit sensory and motor information from one body part to another. A peripheral nerve (or parts like root, ramus, trunk, branch, etc.) is composed of orderly arrangements of the axonal and dendritic processes of many nerve cell bodies. Axons are arranged in bundles.

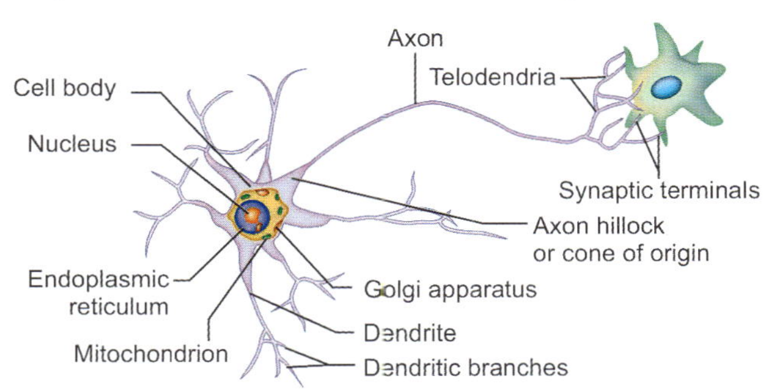

Fig. 3: The detailed anatomy of neuron.

A small bundle of such fibers enclosed in a tubular sheath (*perineurium*) is called a *funiculus* (termed by Sunderland, it is the smallest unit of nerve that can be manipulated surgically) and several such bundles form fascicles of variable sizes arranged together form a nerve **(Fig. 4)**. Depending on the number of fascicles present a nerve may be monofascicular (single fascicle), oligofascicular (few fascicles) or polyfascicular (many fascicles) **(Figs. 5A to C)**. These fasciculi are bound together in a common membranous investment or sheath of the whole nerve called *epineurium* **(Fig. 4)**. These fascicles are hence united together by the epineurium. Each bundle contains variable amount of nerve fibers. Horsley demonstrated certain myelinated fibers running in the epineurium and terminating in small *spheroidal tactile corpuscles* or *end-bulbs of Krause*. These nerve fibers, according to Marshall, are sensory and have been termed *nervi nervorum*. They are considered to have an important bearing upon certain neuralgic pains. The coverings of peripheral nerve are:

- *Epineurium* typically is what we see from eyes when we see a naked nerve and has two parts. The dense connective tissue portion makes the fibrous coat of the whole nerve. The loose connective tissue portion of epineurium fills the spaces between the bundles of nerve fibers. It also contains the blood supply of nerve (vasa nervorum). Bundles of types I and III collagen fibrils and elastic fibers are arranged in an undulated orientation along the epineurium. Epineurium represents analog of the dura mater from CNS. Damage to epineurium does not hamper physiological nerve conduction.
- *Perineurium* is an important structure physiologically and anatomically. It has several layers (1–15) of the flattened epithelial cells (the perineural epithelium) with basal lamina on both sides. The cells in the internal layer consist of single layer and are sealed with zonulae occludentes (singular—Zonula occludens) and desmosomes. In the intermediate zone there are 3–15 concentric layers of perineurial cells. Between layers of perineurial cells in the external zone are types I and II collagen fibrils and elastic fibers arranged in circumferential, oblique and longitudinal layers. Physiologically, any damage to perineurium is not compatible with nerve conduction. It provides the necessary milieu inside the nerve to conduct impulses. Perineurium surrounds primary bundles of nerve fibers. It represents the analog of the arachnoid membrane. Perineurium provides mechanical support to the nerve and is dense (increased number of perineural cells), where the nerve crosses joint for greater need of mechanical strength. It is also thickened at nerve bifurcations and branches.
- *Endoneurium* (analog of the pia mater) is the loose connective tissue between nerve fibers representing analog of the pia mater. It contains a basal layer of Schwann cells along with reticular tissue, blood capillaries, endoneural fluid, type I and type II collagen fibers (forming the so-called basement membrane), and endothelial cells sealed by zonula occludens (sort of maintains the "blood-brain barrier" of nerve). The basal lamina that surrounds each axon and its Schwann cells is made up of type IV collagen, laminin, fibronectin, and heparan sulfate.

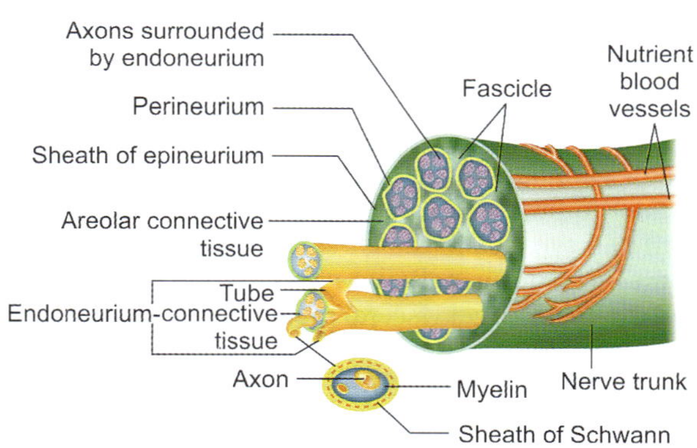

Fig. 4: Diagrammatic representation of the cross-section of a normal peripheral nerve demonstrating the connective tissue and nerve tissue components.

Individual nerve fibers (myelinated and unmyelinated) form nerve bundle. An individual nerve fiber is formed by axon of nervous cells and its coverings (myelin sheath and/or Schwann cells). Three classes of fibers are recognized in a peripheral nerve.

1. The motoneurones axons—they are myelinated (in majority).
2. Axons of ganglionic (multipolar) cells of vegetative ganglia (unmyelinated).
3. Axons of the pseudounipolar cells of spinal ganglia (myelinated).

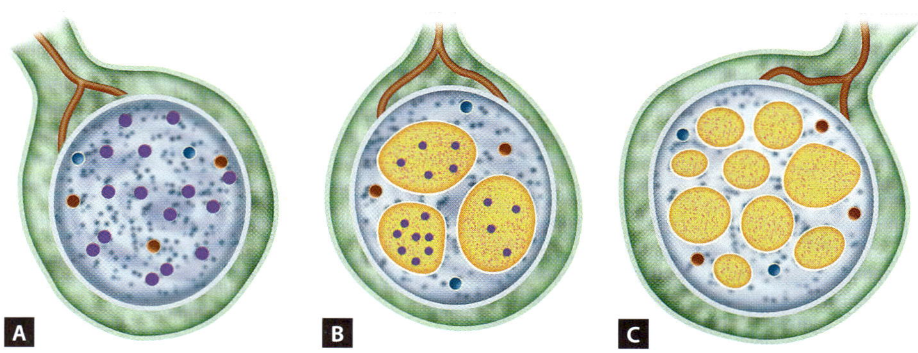

Figs. 5A to C: Schematic diagram of the three types of fascicular patterns: (A) Monofascicular; (B) Oligofascicular; (C) Polyfascicular.

The myelinated nerve fibers (medullated or white fibers) contain central axon (axial cylinder) are surrounded by a sheath of fatty material (staining black with osmic acid) that is known as *white substance of Schwann* or *medullary sheath* (myelin sheath) **(Figs. 6A and B)**. This is then enclosed in a delicate membrane called the *neurolemma, primitive sheath, or nucleated sheath of Schwann*. The endoneurium then wraps the whole structure completing the nerve fiber. During development, only axons that are 0.7 mm or larger in diameter are myelinated. Sensory and motor nerves contain both types of fibers in a ratio of 4:1, i.e., four unmyelinated and one myelinated. Unmyelinated fibers constitute 75% of cutaneous nerves and 50% of motor nerves. The medullary sheath and the neurolemma are absent at places, especially at the origin and termination of the nerve fiber.

- *Axon:* The axon (axis cylinder) is a direct prolongation of a nerve cell continuous throughout. It constitutes about one-half or one-third of the thickness of nerve fiber. Axon is made up of exceedingly fine fibrils which seem to break up at termination. These fibrils have been termed the *primitive fibrils of Schultze*. The axis cylinder is said by some scholars to be enveloped in a special reticular sheath (axolemma) separating it from the myelin sheath composed of a substance called *neurokeratin*.
- The *myelin sheath, medullary sheath or white matter of Schwann* is regarded as a lipid in a fluid state which insulates and protects the axon. Myelinated fibers when examined in the fresh condition frequently present a beaded or varicose appearance due to the oily matter collecting into drops. The extreme delicacy of the primitive sheath causes transudation of the fatty matter even on slight pressure which collects as drops of oil outside the membrane. It varies in thickness (2–14 mm) and this variation gives alteration in diameter of the nerve fibers. The medullary sheath is interrupted (unlike continuous axon) at regular intervals, giving to the fiber the appearance of constriction at these points: these are known as the *nodes of Ranvier*. The portion of nerve fiber between two nodes is called an *internodal segment* or simply *internodes*. The neurolemma or primitive sheath is not interrupted at the nodes, but passes over them as a continuous membrane. On treatment, with silver nitrate the reagent penetrates the neurolemma at the nodes that on exposure to light reduces to silver giving rise to the appearance of black crosses—*Ranvier's crosses* on the axon (unknown significance). Transverse lines may also be seen beyond the nodes and are termed *Frommann's lines*. Oblique clefts have been observed in the medullary sheath that divides the intermodal segment into irregular portions called *medullary segments, or segments of Lantermann*.
- The *Schwann cell membrane* (*neurolemma or primitive sheath)* is a delicate structureless membrane. The Schwann cells independently act as specialized satellite cells and are characterized at the electromicroscopic level by their double basement membrane. Situated in depressions in the white matter of Schwann are nuclei surrounded by a small amount of protoplasm. The nuclei bear a definite relation to the nodes of Ranvier—one nucleus generally lying in the center of each internode. The primitive sheath is absent from fibers found in the brain and spinal cord (CNS). The Schwann cells of myelinated fibers are different from the cells of unmyelinated fibers. Myelinating Schwann cells form a multilayered, membranous myelin sheath around axons (motor or sensory) and are evenly spaced along the length of the axon.

Unmyelinated fiber (non-medullated fibers, gray or gelatinous nerve fibers, fibers of Remak) on the other hand contains central axon surrounded by sheath of Schwann cell and endoneurium only. Unmyelinated nerves usually have several axons encircled by a single Schwann cell **(Figs. 6B and C)**. Each of these consists of an axon to which nuclei are applied at intervals. These nuclei are believed to be in connection with a delicate sheath corresponding with the neurolemma of the myelinated nerve fiber. The Schwann cells of unmyelinated nerves are called "ensheathing Schwann cells" or "Remak cells". They loosely ensheath multiple small diameter unmyelinated axons. The ensheathing Schwann cell's cytoplasmic processes segregate and surround axons and are not involved at all with the production of myelin. In external appearance the unmyelinated nerve fibers are semitransparent and gray or yellowish-gray. The individual fibers vary in size, generally averaging about half the size of the myelinated fibers. Unmyelinated fiber diameter has been measured in electron micrographs to be 0.2–3.0 mm.

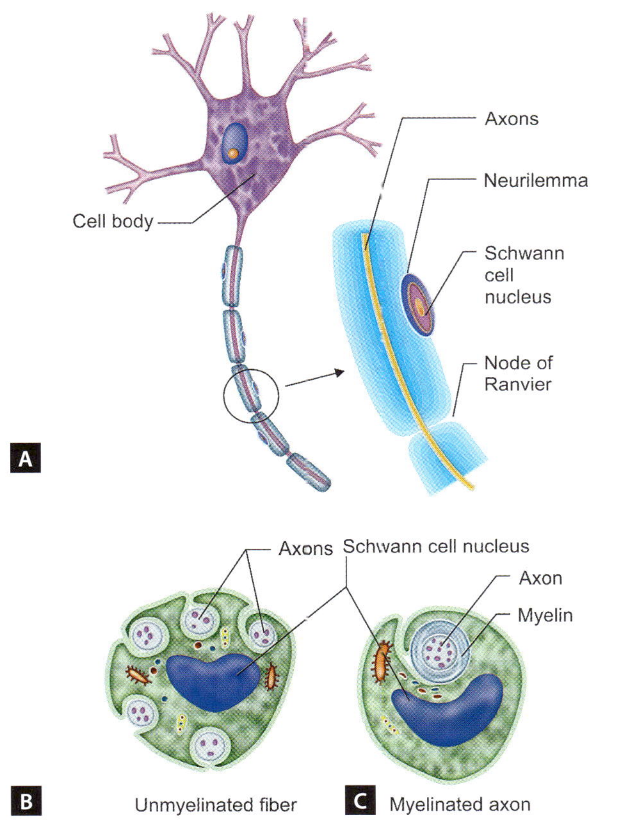

Figs. 6A to C: The illustration of myelinated axons (A). A single Schwann cell can envelop multiple unmyelinated axons (B) or concentrically wrap around an axon to form a myelinated fiber (C).

Gross Fascicle Organization of Nerve Structure

Nerve fibers are insulated and never coalesce, they pursue an uninterrupted course from the center to the periphery. However, the bundled funiculi have been seen to not pursue a perfectly insulated course, but they occasionally join with other funiculi proceeding in the same direction. This does not remain constant, but again branches are given from this conglomeration to join again other funiculi forming a "plexiform arrangement" within the nerve **(Fig. 7)**. This is the real structure and is quite different from the "cable" structure we often envisage in our minds from undergraduate anatomy. Cross-sectional morphometric studies have indicated that funicular anatomy changes every 0.5–15 mm. The cable arrangement of fascicles is seen only in the distal aspects of nerve. However, in these plexiform communications the individual nerve fibers do not coalesce, but merely pass from one sheath to another randomly, the fibers become intermixed, and again intermingle to pass on to the nerve fibers of another funiculus. Every peripheral nerve has two types of funiculi.

- *Simple funiculi:* The funiculi that contain fibers and serve solely a particular cutaneous area or muscle.
- *Compound funiculi:* The funiculi in which the axons coming of various in varying combinations and proportions. This feature allows for the integration of various funicular components that distribute to innervate specific anatomical regions. The clinical importance of this plexus formation can be noted as follows:
  - Organs innervated by compound funiculi may retain certain function in neural injury, unless complete transection of a nerve trunk has occurred.
  - If there is loss of neural tissue in a due course of a traumatic wound, funicular alignment and continuity may not be possible at the time of surgical repair. This entails the fact that if resection anastomosis has been planned one may not encounter matching geometry as the fascicles may have thinned or thickened due to branching or coalescence.

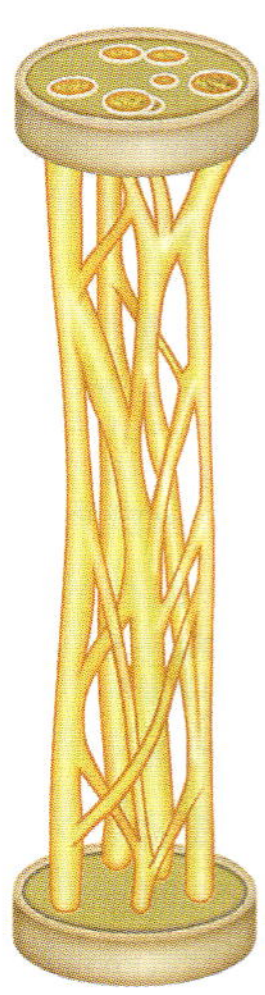

Fig. 7: Within an individual fascicle the axons repetitively divide and unite so that the disposition of axons change over the entire length of nerve. If a gap is hence coapted by end-to-end repair the axons will not be facing their cur ends and cross-connections are legible.

Similarly, in the formation of plexus the component nerves divide, then join, and again subdivide in such a complex manner that the individual funiculi become interlaced most intricately. The branches leaving plexus may contain fibers from all root components. In each case, however, the individual fibers remain separated, and distinct.

AXONAL TRANSPORT

This is the means of transport of substance within the axon. Several neurodegenerative diseases have been linked to defects in axonal transport. The axon terminal may be up to 3 feet distance from the cell body in large nerves and thus it depends on regulated axonal transport for growth and maintenance. Neurons have thus developed directional *fast axonal transport* (up to 410 mm/day) to deliver required substances (like neurotransmitters) in anterograde direction. There is also a *slow anterograde axonal transport* (1–6 mm/day) that helps to deliver cytoskeletal proteins like actin, tubulin, and microfilament that help to build the nerve tissue **(Fig. 8)**. Retrograde transport (first detected by the migration of poliovirus to cell bodies from periphery) is constant at 240 mm/day and allows return of spent neurotransmitter vesicles for recycling. Neuronal microtubules are the key to axonal transport and form the tracks that facilitate the transport.

- Microtubules are directionally oriented with their ± ends oriented toward the periphery.
- Plus-end directed fast anterograde traffic is operated by kinesin family ATPase motor molecules and is involved with movement of:
  - Synaptic vesicle precursors
  - Mitochondria
- Minus-end directed fast retrograde traffic is moved by dynein family motors and is involved with movement of:
  - Organelles
  - Clearing aggregated proteins
  - Signaling of neurotrophins
  - Stress indicators in response to environmental changes
- The rate of axonal regeneration after injury is similar to the rate of slow axonal transport of structural cytoskeletal proteins, approximating 1 mm/day. Axon stretching may speed the rate of slow axonal transport and neuron growth (inhibition of kinesin may accelerate axonal growth).

MYONEURAL JUNCTION (FIG. 9)

A single motor neuron may supply anything from ten to several thousand muscle fibers, the ratio depending on the degree of dexterity demanded of the particular muscle (the smaller the ratio, the finer the movement). In the voluntary muscle, the nerve after entering the sheath of the muscle, breaks up into fibers or bundles of fibers, which form plexuses, and gradually divide until a single nerve fiber enters a single muscular fiber. However, if the muscular fiber is long, more than one nerve fiber may enter it (rare). Within the muscular fiber the nerve terminates in a special expansion, called motor endplate of Kuhne.

The nerve fiber, on approaching the muscular fiber, loses its medullary sheath so that the neurolemma and

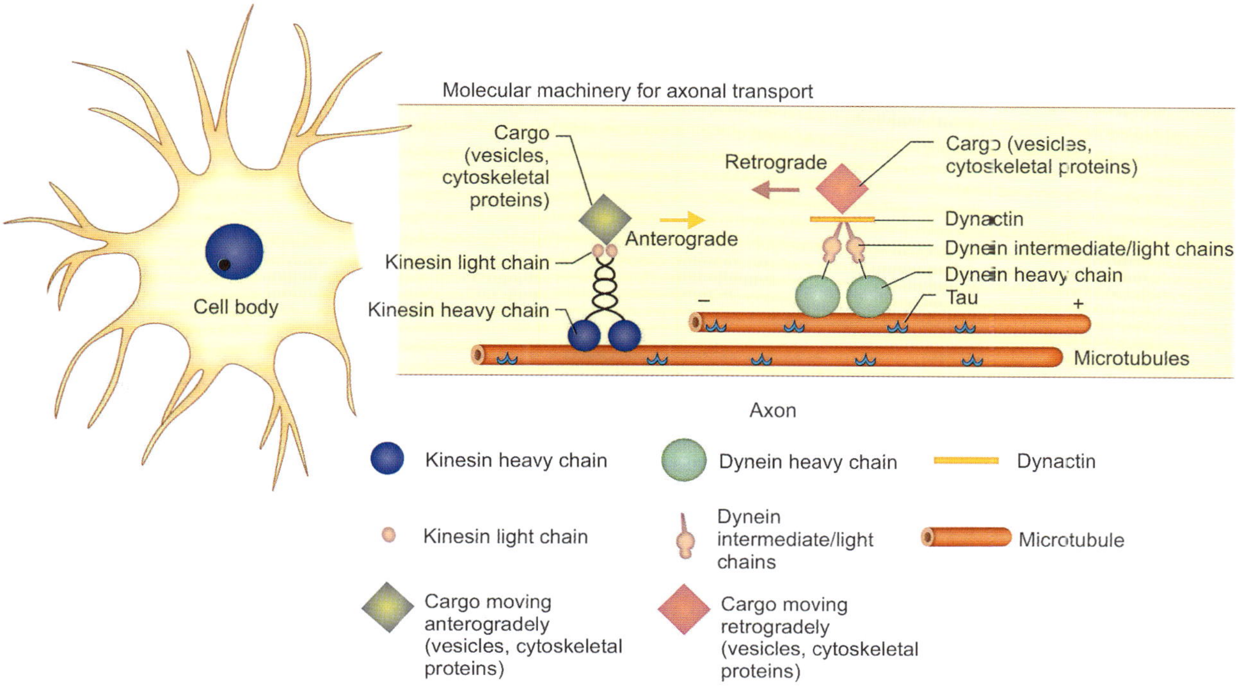

Fig. 8: Axonal transport.

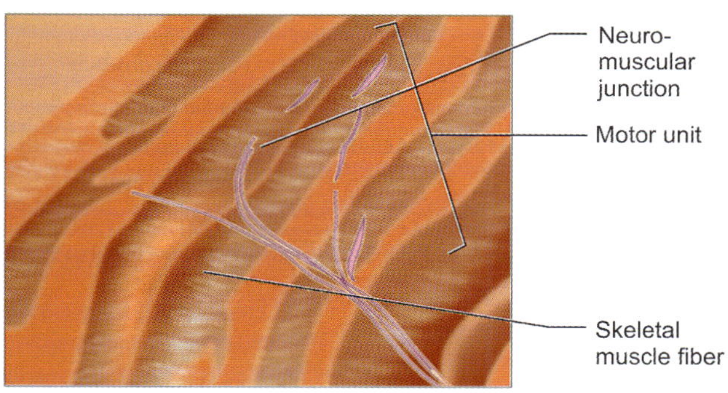

Fig. 9: Myoneural junction.

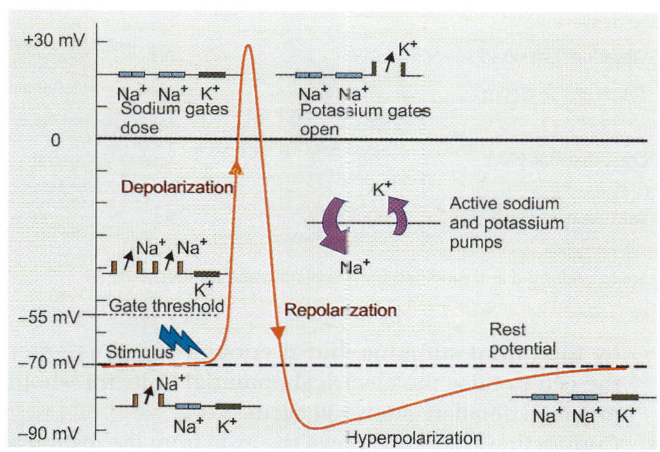

Fig. 10: Nerve action potential.

endoneurium becomes continuous with the sarcolemma of the muscle. Only the axon enters the muscular fiber. Axon then spreads out ramifying like the roots of a tree immediately beneath the sarcolemma and becomes imbedded in a layer of granular matter, containing a number of clear, oblong nuclei. The whole constituting an endplate from which the contractile wave of the muscular fiber is said to start.

Neuron Action Potential

The physics of action potential propagation were first proposed and studied by Hodgkin and Huxley in 1952. Action potential refers to the brief reversal of the electrical potential across a cell membrane **(Fig. 10)**. The change in potential generates impulse along the nerve that helps neurons transmit information. The following is a brief description of how this happens:

- The resting potential of nerve cell is –70 mV, and neurons are polarized in this resting state. Critical membrane potential is –55 mV above which the sodium channels open (conformational change).
- The sodium channels (different from voltage-gated fast channels) open in response to specific stimuli, viz. mechanical, chemical or thermal stimulation in sensory neurons, or neurotransmitter stimulation in motoneurons. This briefly elevates the action potential. If the stimuli is significant or strong enough to cause more than critical influx of the Na^+ ions then potential across membrane raises beyond the critical –55 mV. This causes sudden opening of voltage-gated fast sodium channels causing heavy influx of the sodium ions and complete depolarization.
- Potassium channels function opposite to the sodium ions. Although potassium (K^+) channels are also opened

TABLE 1: Different types of nerve fibers.

Neuron chief function	*Electrophysiological classification*	*Myelination*	*Sensory fiber classification*	*Adaptation rate*	*Diameter (mm)*	*Conduction velocity*	*Terminal/receptor*
Motor							
	Aa	Yes	–	–	12–20	72–120	Extrafusal muscle fiber
	Ag	Yes	–	–	2–8	12–48	Intrafusal muscle fiber
	B	Yes	–	–	1–3	6–18	Preganglionic autonomic fiber
	C	No	–	–	0.2–2	0.5–2	Postganglionic autonomic fiber
Sensory							
Muscle and joint proprioception							
Length and velocity of length change	Aa	Yes	Ia	Slow	13–20	80–120	Muscle spindle (intrafusal) nuclear bag (annulospiral ending)
Length and tension	Ab	Yes	II	Slow	6–12	35–75	Flower spray ending
Muscle force and tension	Aa	Yes	Ib	Slow	13–20	80–120	Golgi tendon organ
Joint position and movement		Yes	I	Slow			Ruffini ending
Cutaneous and deep mechanoreception							
Tapping (slow vibration up to 40 Hz)	Ab	Yes	II	Rapid	6–12	35–75	Meissner corpuscle
Motion, direction and velocity	Ab	Yes	II	Rapid and slow	6–12	35–75	Hair follicle
Vibration (fast up to 300 Hz)	Ab	Yes	II	Rapid	6–12	35–75	Pacinian corpuscle
Touch and pressure	Ab	Yes	II	Slow	6–12	35–75	Merkel disk
	Ab	Yes	II	Slow	6–12	35–75	Ruffini endings
Cold, thermal, pain	Ad	Yes/no	III		1–5	5–30	Thermoreceptors, nociceptive
Pain, heat	C	No	IV		0.2–1.5	0.5–2	Thermoreceptors, nociceptive

Source: Adapted and modified from Benjamin and Kimberly.

by the initial stimulus, but if enough Na^+ ions enter the cell to raise the electrical potential to its threshold potential depolarization will occur.

- Current flows passively down the axon from the resulting spreading local membrane depolarization by the opening of new voltage-activated Na^+ channels downstream.
- The voltage-activated potassium (K^+) channels open and previously open Na^+ channels inactivate which brings the membrane potential back toward the resting potential and even to a hyperpolarized state.
- An absolute refractory period occurs at the site of previous depolarization by inactivated Na^+ channels, thus delaying any subsequent action potentials. Some K^+ channels remain open.
- In larger axons, the insulating myelin sheath reduces current leakage across the plasma membrane. The ion channels are concentrated at nodes of Ranvier and current (depolarization) jumps from node to node called saltatory conduction.
- The compound action potential of nerve is seen in electrophysiological recordings.
- The conduction velocity is related to the size of the nerve fiber **(Table 1)**.
  - Large and small diameter myelinated axons conduct at a rate of approximately 6.0 and 4.6 m/sec/mm diameter respectively.
  - Unmyelinated fibers conducts at a rate of approximately 1.7 m/sec/mm diameter.

BLOOD-NERVE INTERFACE

The blood-nerve interface controls the environment within nerve to create compartment pressures (endoneurial fluid pressure at 2–3 mm Hg) that facilitate blood flow, maintain excitability and conduction properties. This essential milieu is actively maintained by perineurium (perineurial cells) and endothelial cells of endoneurial capillaries. The blood-nerve barrier is not present till 13th day of life when the clefts between endothelial cells are replaced by tight junctions. Endoneurial fluid is contiguous with cerebrospinal fluid of the subarachnoid space and flows at rate of 4–8 mm/hour in a proximodistal direction. Tight junctions between the innermost perineurial cells and between endothelial cells of endoneurial capillaries are permeable to small ions, but selectively permeable to larger, nonlipophilic molecules. The blood-nerve barrier is more permeable in spinal roots, dorsal root ganglia, and autonomic ganglia due to the presence of fenestrations and interendothelial cell clefts in root and ganglia capillaries. Ganglia have specialized needs for electrical conduction and chemical signaling explaining the lack of a blood-nerve barrier in them. This characteristic also explains the response and control of ganglion cells to circulating compounds, while sparing the CNS.

Injuries to endoneurial capillaries cause leakage of albumin and fluid into the endoneurial space increasing endoneurial pressure due to tight junctions of the perineurial cells preventing egress. This compresses the blood vessels and results in hypoperfusion and/or ischemia and injury to Schwann cells, axons and endothelial cells.

Biomechanical Properties of Peripheral Nerve

Peripheral nerves bear a vast array of mechanical stresses related to professional, recreational and daily activities. This is made possible by certain biomechanical properties of nerves as follows:

- The capacity of nerve to change its length, commonly measured as percent change in length or strain. The nerve has the capacity to stretch to accommodate for a modest increase in length (viscoelastic properties). With joint motions the nerve length increases or restores depending on the need. More than 8% elongation (limited traction) of nerve will diminish its microcirculation which, if persistent, will damage the nerve while more than 15% elongation (extreme stretch/traction) will disrupt axons.
- The capacity of the nerve to slide or glide relative to the surrounding interfacing tissue. The nerve has to glide toward the moving joint relative to the surrounding tissues when the nerve path is elongated (convergence of nerve movement).
- The capacity to tolerate increases in pressure or compression from the surrounding interfacing tissue (say the changes in carpal tunnel pressure with movements). Though pressure sensitivity varies greatly among nerves and even fiber types, but in general pressures more than 30 mm Hg cause paresthesias and praxia while pressures more than 60 mm Hg cause complete blockade of conduction (*see* carpal tunnel syndrome for more effects of pressure changes on nerve). Compression for 15 minutes produces numbness and tingling while pain sensitivity is lost after 30 minutes. Motor weakness is demonstrable after 45 minutes. Relief of compression causes intense paresthesias and pins and needles sensation for 5 minutes, if compression is relieved within 30 minutes. Motor recovery takes around 10 minutes.

PERIPHERAL NERVE INJURY

Peripheral nerves may get damaged by a variety of mechanisms that include, but are not restricted to stretching, ischemia (transient or complete), compression, crush, traction (pulling), laceration (traction to cause nerve discontinuity), cut (say iatrogenic) or burning (say by cautery).

Pathophysiology

The process of degeneration and regeneration [Wallerian degeneration (WD)] is also called anterograde degeneration, named after Augustus Volney Waller, an English neurophysiologist (1816–1870), who was the first to describe the degeneration of distal nerve stump after injury to neuron based on his observations in transected glossopharyngeal and hypoglossal nerves in 1850. This process is *not* apoptosis and has a specifically conserved pathway. At the outset it should be mentioned that a retrograde degeneration also occurs causing loss of Nissl's granules, chromatolysis, nucleolar swelling and swelling of the cell body which reverses, if the cell survives (the factors determining cell survival are discussed later). The proximal stump degenerates till nearest node of Ranvier from where new sprouts grow (2–5 sprouts within 6 hours). This retrograde change in nerve is referred to as "traumatic degeneration" **(Fig. 11)**. This is different from Wallerain degeneration which strictly refers to the anterograde degeneration. Wallerian degeneration is also seen in CNS and in neurodegenerative and demyelinating diseases [amyotrophic lateral sclerosis (ALS), Alzheimer's disease, Parkinson's disease (PD), Huntington's disease and glaucoma], suggesting a common triggering mechanism. The sequence of events can be summarized as follows:

- Within few hours of injury the axon remain excitable in rats, but in primates the axons may remain intact for days. The Na^+/Ca^{++} pump and the Na^+/K^+ ATPase remain functional. The lag between injury and degeneration may range from 24 hours to few days hence in humans, but it is for sure that the degeneration occurs.
- *Phase of granular disintegration:* Just a few hours after injury axons become swollen and their axoplasm is filled with an amorphous matrix (24–72 hours). During this period, the major cytoskeleton proteins (microtubules and neurofilaments) are being degraded by activation of ubiquitin-proteasome system (UPS) and calcium-dependent proteases, respectively. This phase is triggered by large influx of Ca^{++} ions attributed to reversal of the function of the plasma membrane Na^+/Ca^{++} exchanger as a consequence of dysfunction of the Na^+-K^+ ATPase. Increased intra-axonal Ca^{++} causes:
  - Disruption of mitochondrial oxidative phosphorylation
  - Excessive formation of free radicals
  - Activation of calpains, calcium-activated neutral cysteine proteases—causing cytoskeletal breakdown.
- By 72–96 hours the myelin lamellae are disrupted into small fragments known as myelin ovoids (bead-like pattern formation along the degenerating axon) described by Lubinska in 1977. This is the basic criterion used by investigators to define Wallerian degeneration in various studies.
- Within 96 hours after the injury, the Schwann cells from neurolemma synthesize growth factors which attract axonal sprouts to the distal end of the severed axon.

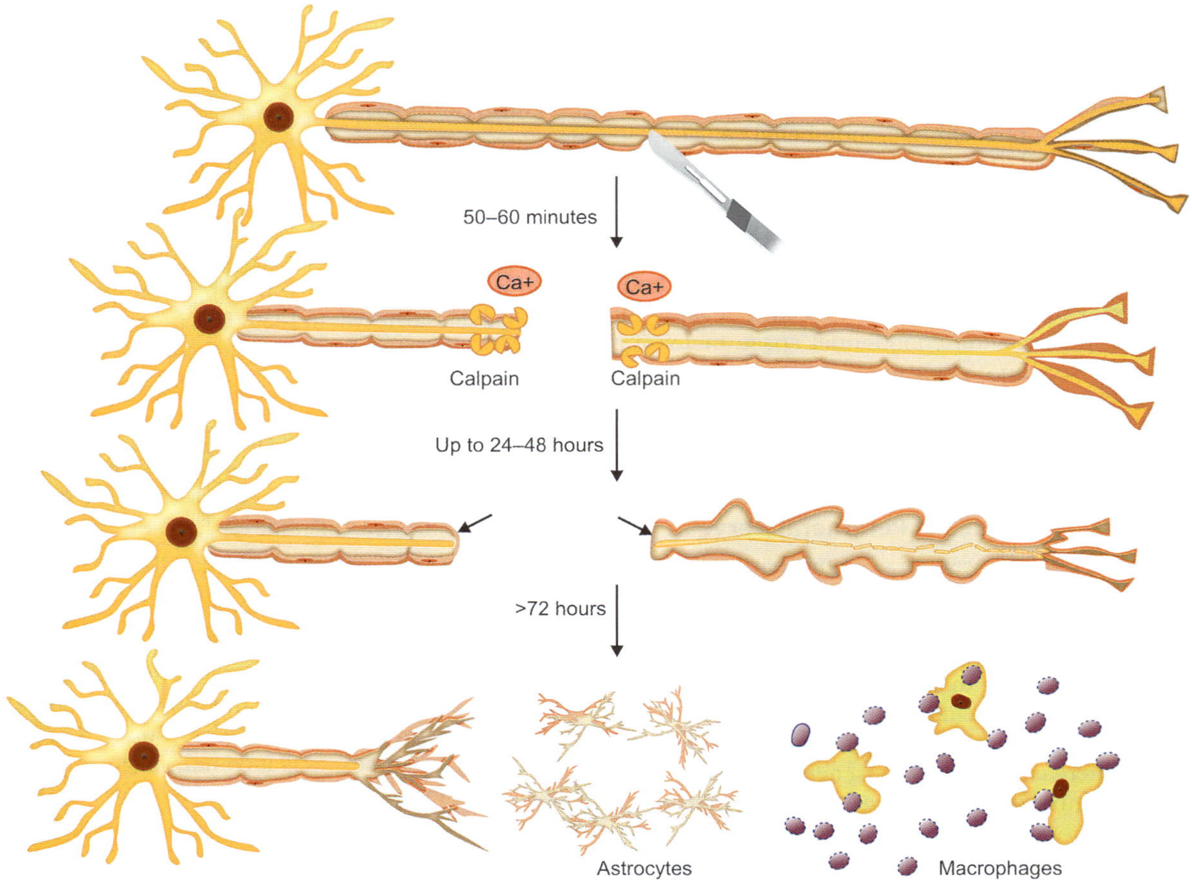

Fig. 11: Nerve response to injury.

These axonal sprouts originate at the proximal end of the severed axon. There is also increased phospholipase-A2 (PLA2) expression that is mediated by inflammatory mediators serving for complex pathway of chemotaxis and inflammation. The PLA2 expression returns to normal by 3 weeks whence the axonal regeneration commences.

- There is increased neuronal permeability by the breakdown of blood-neuron barrier. Neuronal permeability approaches four times the normal over a course of 4 days.
- Myelin and axonal debris are removed by resident and newly recruited inflammatory cells (monocytes/macrophages) and microglia (in the CNS) and by Schwann cells (in PNS). Schwann cells clear away the degraded myelin that contains axon-inhibitory proteins like myelin-associated glycoprotein (MAG) and oligodendrocyte-myelin glycoprotein (OMgp). This is important as without clearance the new axonal sprouts will not grow. The process is undertaken by:
  - *Immune cells:* Monocytes/macrophages, T and B lymphocytes, dendritic cells and neutrophils. The monocyte-macrophage system (both resident and recruited) works a great deal to remove myelin by "opsonization". The process is also facilitated by the breakdown of blood-nerve barrier so that circulating chemokines can stimulate the cells toward faster clearance.
  - *Resident non-neuronal cells:* Astrocytes and microglia in the CNS and Schwann cells in the PNS.
- The neurolemma of axons (the outermost layer of the neuron made of Schwann cells) does not degenerate and remains as a hollow tube. Immediately after axonal degeneration and fragmentation, Schwann cells in the PNS enter continuous cell division, degrade their own membrane and phagocytose myelin and axonal debris. In CNS, the oligodendrocytes undergo apoptosis (Schwann cells are absent from CNS) and are not involved in chemotaxis of inflammatory cells so the process is delayed there.
- If an axon sprout reaches the tube, it grows into it and advances about 1 mm/day (3 cm/month, Steindler). The tubes provide pathways for the sprouting (regenerating) axons to follow to muscles and skin (topographic sensitivity, discussed below in role of Schwann cells, **Figs. 12 and 13**). The Schwann cells then remyelinate, the newly formed axons which eventually reach and innervate the target tissue **(Fig. 12)**. In CNS, the microenvironment is often hostile to axonal regeneration due to exposure of myelin inhibitory proteins and secretion of inhibitory molecules such as chondroitin-sulfate proteoglycans which result in formation of astroglial scar. It is not

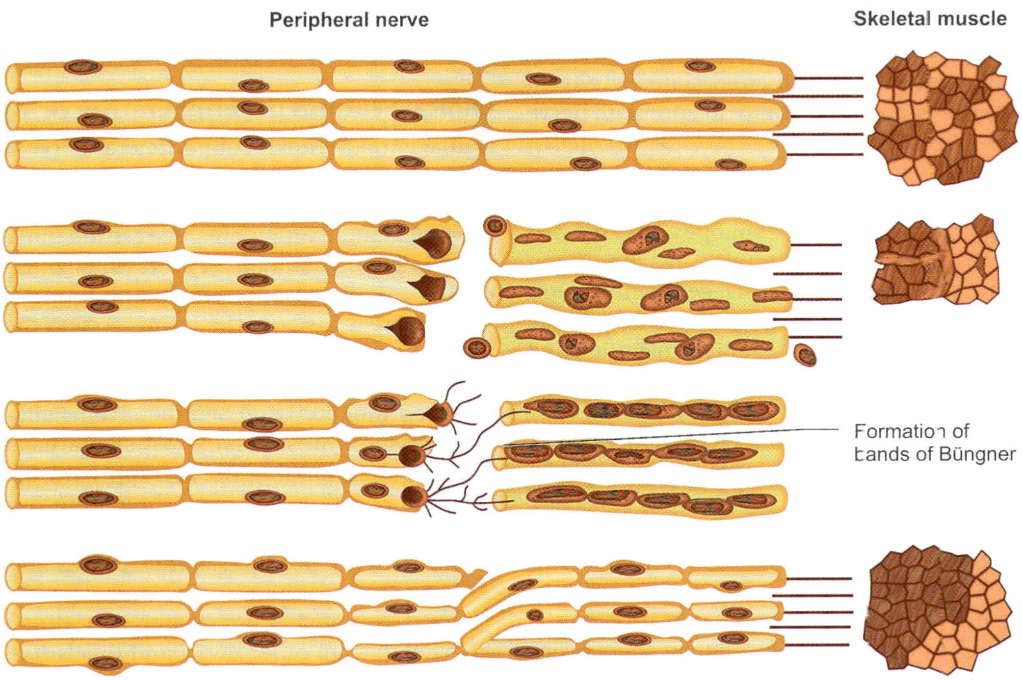

Fig. 12: Regeneration of the neural tubes and formation of cross-connections in the process. Kindly note that some topographic sensitivity is exhibited by the Schwann cells during the process.

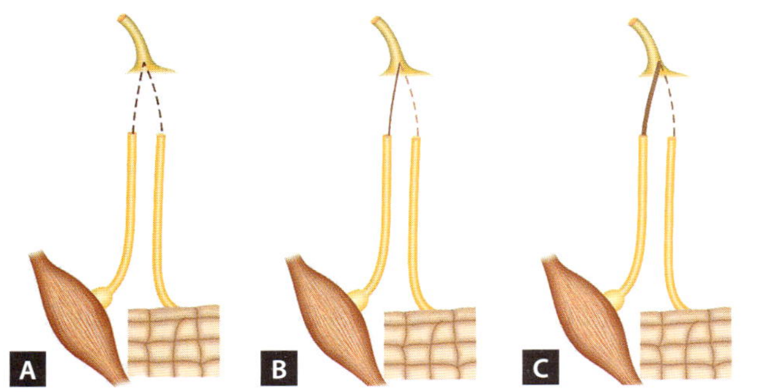

Figs. 13A to C: Schematic diagram representing the concept of preferential motor regeneration and neurotropism by contact guidance after an axonotomy of a mixed nerve. (A) After the nerve is damaged, the new nerve fiber sprout into Schwann cell tubes; (B) If motor axons regenerate into sensory cell tubes then they do not mature; (C) The motor axons developing into motor regenerating Schwann cell tubes establish connection by preferential facilitation.

universal that the axonal sprout will form the proximal stump and it survives. There is simultaneously change in the proximal stump of the cut neuron that may result in neuronal death. Whether the proximal stump survives and is stimulated to produce an axonal sprout or it dies is dependent on the retrograde flow of factors from the target areas. The retrograde transport of ciliary neurotrophic factor (CNTF), brain-derived neurotrophic factor (BDNF) and nerve growth factor (NGF) from target areas, promotes neuronal regeneration and prevent neuronal death, while activation of the signal transducer and activator of transcription 3 (STAT3) and its retrograde transport activates genes important for neuronal degeneration. Schwann cells produce laminins that are potent promoters of axonal regeneration particularly the laminin 2, laminin 8. The proximal neuron survival is also dependent on the production of trophic factors like IL-6 and NGF as above.

- The first responder (Role of Schwann cells)—immediately after injury the process of regeneration is dependent on Schwann cell that is the first responder. This also processes the initial degeneration to clean up the area for regeneration. The process by which a Schwann cell responds is as follows:
  - Gene expression is altered immediately after injury and cells stop producing myelin within 48 hours.
  - There is upregulation of regeneration-associated genes (GAP43, neurotrophic factors and their receptors, and neuregulin and its receptors) and Schwann cells begin to proliferate. This proliferation is at its peak at 4 days following injury.
  - Proliferating Schwann cells are confined to their basal lamina tubes where they align to form *bands of Büngner*. These provide a supportive substrate and growth factors for regenerating axons giving the regenerating nerve topographic sensitivity (reinnervation of correct muscle within motor system or correct patch of skin in sensory system).
  - *Contact guidance and neurotropism* ***(Figs. 13A to C)****:* Contact guidance refers to homing of the nerve sprouts to the empty tubes. It has been seen that the motor axonal sprouts migrate toward the motor Schwann cell tubes, while sensory to their specific tubes preferentially. There is a possible role of the cellular adhesion molecules (CAM) upregulation after axonotomy. Upregulation of glycoprotein L1, neural

cell adhesion molecule (NCAM) and N-cadherin is a consequence of Schwann cells transition from myelinated to unmyelinated state. The term "neurotropism" implies an ability to stimulate nerve maturation **(Figs. 13A to C)**. These include NGF, BDNF, neurotrophin-3, neurotrophin-4/5, etc. The human natural killer (HNK) cell glycan (3' sulfoglucuronyl β1, 3 galactoside) known as HNK-1 epitope and expressed on different cell adhesion molecules has been associated with proper targeting of regenerating motor axons. Neurotrophins bind to specialized high affinity tyrosine kinase receptors and stimulate migration and adhesion of axonal projections. They seem to play a major role in progression of axonal growth cone.

- Schwann cells perform a sentinel role in the PNS by expressing the toll-like receptors (TLRs). TLR3, TLR4 and TLR7 are constitutively expressed while TLR1 is upregulated after axonotomy. Endogenous TLR ligands liberated from disintegrating axons, bind TLRs found on Schwann cells and immune cells leading to activation of inflammatory cascades that are essential for promoting axon regeneration. Similar effect is also produced by P2 receptor ligands (e.g., purines).

Factors Affecting Wallerian Degeneration and the Effect of Slow Wallerian Degeneration Protein and Nicotinamide Mononucleotide Adenylyltransferase

- Rapid Wallerian degeneration requires the prodegenerative molecules SARM1 (sterile α and HEAT/Armadillo motif containing protein 1) and PHR1 (PAM-Highwire-Rpm-1 ubiquitin ligase).
- Nicotinamide mononucleotide adenylyltransferase 2 (NMNAT2) is essential for axon growth and survival.

Its loss from injured axons may activate Wallerian degeneration, explaining why NMNAT overexpression also rescues them. NMNATs and slow Wallerian degeneration protein (WLDS) which contains NMNAT1 delay Wallerian degeneration up to tenfold when overexpressed within axons. Loss of NMNAT2 causes WLDS-sensitive axon degeneration. Loss or deletion of SARM1 or PHR1 (aka MYCBP2) has a protective effect on nerve and delay Wallerian degeneration.

The initiation of Wallerian degeneration and its completion is dependent on fine balance of the prodegenerative and protective factors as mentioned above and is discrete for different locations of body and microenvironments.

Strategies based on Wallerian degeneration pathway to prevent axonal degeneration and promote regeneration have been employed in experimental models and should be shortly available to improve the outcome after neuronal injury. Various methods being evaluated are:

- Sodium or calcium channel blockers
- Calpain inhibition
- Administration of NGF, CNTF and BDNF
- Use of apoptotic and necrotic blockers
- Application of amyloid precursor protein (APP), neuregulin 1 (NRG1) and 2,4-dinitrophenol (DNP). The latter is an uncoupler of oxidative phosphorylation (so harmful), but at low concentrations it is a powerful neuroprotective agent.

Clinical Features of Peripheral Nerve Injury

Damage to an individual peripheral nerve is characterized by:

- *Motor:* Flaccid, atrophic paralysis of the muscles in its typical innervation area. Assess the pinch strength, grip strength (dynamometer), individual muscle function.
- Loss of all sensation, including proprioception, in the skin areas distal to the lesion. Assess the sensations by static and moving two-point discrimination (innervation density), vibrometer (more sensitive than two-point discrimination) and Semmes-Weinstein monofilaments (pressure thresholds). Most skin areas are innervated by an overlapping nerve supply from adjacent nerve branches, thus making it difficult in testing cutaneous sensations. *Autonomous zone* is the area exclusively (no other nerve has interference in this zone) supplied by nerve in question. While clinically testing for sensory loss a somewhat larger area is outlined that contains overlap from other nerve and this is *intermediate zone*. In actual there is still a larger area that can only be tested by blocking the other nerves; however, it is clinically irrelevant as it has predominant brain representation by other nerve, this is *maximal area*. Some diagnostic sensory areas have been however identified that help in localizing the nerve and confirming particular nerve involvement:
  - The radial sensory area is located on the back of the hand in first web space toward the thumb as a coin shaped region.
  - The median area is located at the tips of the index (autonomous) and middle fingers.
  - The ulnar nerve region is limited to the little finger volar ulnar aspect.
  - The musculocutaneous area is located on the medial aspect of the forearm.
  - The axillary nerve area (inconsistent) is located over the point of shoulder laterally (regiment badge area).
  - The femoral nerve region is broad anteromedial aspect of the thigh.
  - The lateral cutaneous nerve of thigh supplies the distal part of the lateral surface of the thigh.
  - The common peroneal area is represented as a vertical strip on the front of the ankle.
  - The deep peroneal nerve is located as a small area of first webspace of foot.
- There is a loss of both superficial and deep reflexes.
- In early stage fibrillations and fasciculations are present.
- *Tinel's sign (Tinel's-Hoffmann sign):* Paresthesia (*fornication*) experienced along the nerve distribution (*not at the percussion site*) on gentle percussion from distal to proximal over the nerve. It was described in 1917 by Jules Tinel to evaluate the nerve regeneration clinically by applying pressure (and not tapping/ percussion). The phenomenon was explained by Paul Hoffman later with tapping. The fornication is due to

bare young hyperexcitable unmyelinated sprouts from injured proximal end. It is a commonly relied sign in clinical practice and is done almost for any nerve that has sensory fibers (for obvious reasons sign should be absent in pure motor nerves). Most nerve are mixed so the sign is however present in nearly all common nerve injuries. Interpretation of the sign is made as follows:

- Advancing Tinel's can be used to calculate and gauge progression of recovery (spontaneous or following repair).
- Nonprogressing Tinel's indicates interruption of nerve regeneration.
- Static Tinel's at injury site and one present distally also indicates poor prognosis.
- Advancing Tinel's seen only in grades II and III (IV and V grades show it only after repair).

There are however a lot of fallacies that should be borne in mind when doing a Tinel's sign and making clinical judgment:

- Few sensory sprouts and partial regeneration may also give a false positive Tinel's sign while the clinical response is poor at the end. This gives a false sense of satisfaction that the nerve is regenerating when in reality the recovery is much less than optimal.
- No estimate of motor recovery should be made from Tinel's sign as it indicates sensory recovery from sensory sprouts.
- Single time estimation is also useless and needs to be regularly followed.
- Trophic lesions of the joints, muscles (atrophy), skin and nails are prominent in delayed presentations:
  - 1 month after denervation there is approximately 30% muscle atrophy.
  - By 2 months 50–60% of muscle mass is lost (number of fibers remain same only the mass reduces).
  - By 3 months 60–80% of the muscle mass is gone.
  - After 3 months equilibrium is reached and further detectable atrophy is minimal. Cross-sectional area diminishes 80–90% by 90 days.
- Reaction of degeneration is seen from 10 to 14 days after the injury, i.e. muscle does not respond to galvanic or faradic stimuli.
- Additional vasomotor changes may be present. Loss of sweating in the area can be demonstrated by ninhydrin test (that detects amino acids in the sweat).
- Loss of function—there is around 1% loss of function of the involved muscle for every 6 days of denervation.

Nerve Pinch or Stretch Syndromes

Nerve "pinch" or "stretch" syndromes are common in sports injuries. Various terms are used synonymously to describe these symptoms and include nerve compression, spinal dysarthria, nerve contusion, nerve root syndrome, nerve pinch syndrome, nerve stretch syndrome, radiculopathy, subluxation, or traumatic neuritis. Injury to the nerves of the neck and shoulder that cause a burning or stinging feeling are called *burners* or *stingers*. These syndromes are however described for almost all peripheral sensory nerves and are quite common in footballers. Due to stretch, the cervical nerves cause tingling, numbness in arm and fingers, and weakness may be noticed by some athletes. The cause is an athlete's head being forced to the opposite side while going in to make a tackle or block during football pulling the head away from shoulder and stretching the nerve or "spearing" (attempting to make a tackle while leading with the crown of the head). The athletes describe symptoms like sudden short sensation of electrical shock, warmth, etc., with the neck in flexion, but mostly the symptoms appear throughout the cranium, spine, pelvis and extremities in many sports. Nerve fibers may be stretched, partially torn, or ruptured but often the symptoms are short-lasting indicating only stretch. For long-lasting symptoms more than few hours, rest, anti-inflammatory medications and rehabilitation are begun. Sports should be discontinued till weakness has been recovered and symptoms subside fully. Some patients who repeatedly develop symptoms may have to unfortunately leave the sport altogether.

Any telescoping, hyperflexion, hyperextension, or hyper-rotational blow or force to the spine may result in a nerve "pinch" syndrome where pain may be local or extending distally. A nerve pinch syndrome may arise from a direct trauma (contusion and swelling), a protruded disk and subluxation which results in nerve compression, or a fracture (callus formation and associated post-traumatic adhesions). These are much more serious and need thorough work-up and treatment on the lines of identified pathology before any return to sport.

CLASSIFICATION OF NERVE INJURY (TABLE 2)

There are three main systems for classifying nerve injuries, Cohen's system (1941) popularized by Seddon in 1943, Sunderland in 1951, and Mackinnon in 1992. Apart from these there is also transient nerve palsy observed due to reversible compression over nerve commonly experienced as "sleeping foot" (*see* above in biomechanics). The latter is due to temporary ischemia and follows the events described above in biomechanical properties of nerve. Cohen (Seddon) described three basic progressively increasing damage to nerves **(Table 2)** to which Sunderland added two degrees in

TABLE 2: Classification of nerve injuries

Cohen/Seddon	*Sunderland*	*Description*
Neurapraxia	1	Local conduction block, variable myelin damage, no axonal discontinuity
Axonotmesis	2	Loss of axonal continuity, endoneurium intact, no conduction
	3	Loss of axonal and endoneurial continuity, perineurium intact, no conduction
	4	Loss of axonal, endoneurial and perineurial continuity, epineurium intact, no conduction
Neurotmesis	5	Epineurium also damaged—neural discontinuity with separation of ends, no conduction
	6	Mixed nerve damage along the nerve trunk, all types of nerve injuries seen 1–5, recovery is hence variable with nearly no recovery in combined types 4 and 5

between axonotmesis and neurotmesis **(Fig. 14)**. Mackinnon added the concept of mixed nerve injury.

- *Neurapraxia (Sunderland first-degree):*
  - No disruption of internal structure only a localized conduction block exists (physiological disruption with anatomical preservation)
  - Tinel's sign absent
  - Loss of function is often complete initially but recovery can be expected to be complete within 3–6 weeks or maximum up to 3 months
  - Nerve conduction velocity (NCV) shows increased latency.
- *Axonotmesis (Sunderland second-degree):*
  - Disruption of axons and Wallerian degeneration
  - Maintenance of gross architecture of the nerve
  - Tinel's sign positive as axonal regeneration occurs
  - For Seddon's classification there is no differentiation between partial or complete loss of axons but Sunderland classifies them further. For second-degree injury there is limited loss of axons and minimal endoneurial scarring will occur, so that the Tinel's will proceed distally.
  - Recovery should be complete.
- *Sunderland third- and fourth-grade neural disruption:*
  - *Third-degree:* Axonal injury is associated with endoneurial scarring. Nerve is in continuity. It yields the most variable ultimate clinical recovery. The Tinel's is characteristically positive both at the injury site (due to entangled regenerating axons in scar) and also proceeds distally due to retubulating axon regenerates. There is erroneous alignment of axons.

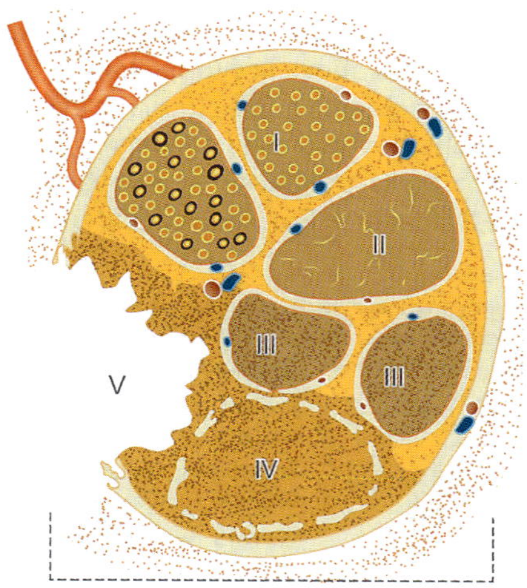

Fig. 14: Illustration depicting the six classes of nerve injury. Not numbered is the healthy fascicle. Neurapraxia (I) showing loss of axonal myelin. Axonotmesis—second-degree injury (II) with loss of myelin and axonal loss without any damage to the endoneurium. Third-degree injury (III). A fourth-degree injury (IV) represents damage to all portions of the nerve except epineurium. Fifth-degree injury or neurotmesis (V) encompasses nerve transection with damage even to epineurium. Microsurgical repair is essential for recovery after fifth-degree injury. (VI) Mixed nerve injury (sixth-degree injury) is a combination of various other degrees of nerve injury that results in neuroma in—continuity.

  - *Fourth-degree:* Nerve still in continuity, but at the level of injury there is complete scarring that no conduction will ever across. Scar prevents axonal regeneration into distal tubes. Tinel's sign is present at site of injury, but does not progress or proceed distally. Excision repair is the best option for treatment. These often result from severe stretch, traction, crush or nerve injection.
- *Neurotmesis (Sunderland fifth-degree,* ***Fig. 14****):*
  - There is complete transection of the nerve and anatomical interruption of continuity of all neural tissues. They may result from severe stretch resulting into avulsion, but often they are result of penetrating injury or iatrogenic nerve damage during dissection.
  - No spontaneous recovery expected without surgical intervention.
  - Electromyogram (EMG) shows fibrillation potentials (FP), and positive sharp waves (PSW) (2–3 weeks post injury).
- *Mackinnon's mixed injury (1992, colloquially called Sunderland's sixth-degree):*
  - This is a combination injury where the pattern of injury varies from fascicle to fascicle (among fascicles) and even along the length of the same fascicle.
  - There is often a "neuroma in continuity" (Mackinnon) that needs resection anastomosis.
  - Surgically the challenge is to protect good fascicles and correct the damaged ones.
  - Tinel's sign and recovery patterns differ according to pattern and severity of injury.
  - This nerve injury demonstrates variable recovery patterns.

DIAGNOSIS OF NERVE INJURY

- Clinical examination (discussed above)
- *Electrodiagnostic studies (EDS):* It comprise of electromyography (EMG), nerve conduction studies (NCS) and strength-duration curve.

Electromyography is a technique of recording the electrical activity within a striated muscle belly by inserting needle in it. The electrical signal generated by the muscle tissue is detected by an electrode which is further amplified and monitored by oscilloscope or a speaker or recorded in system. Alterations in this signal are seen in various neuromuscular diseases. The signal detected by EMG reflects actions of motor unit (a motor neuron branch and the muscles fibers innervated by it). The EMG is used to:

- Demonstrate quantitative or qualitative changes in electrical activity of the muscle motor units in the resting state.
- Changes in electrical activity following direct or indirect electrical stimulation, or during voluntary or reflex motor unit activation.
- It can also be used to evaluate nerve conduction velocity and nerve terminal conduction time.

There are two common ways of performing EMG either using three small monopolar needle electrodes or by coaxial/concentric electrodes. The latter has the advantage of sampling a smaller volume of tissue than the monopolar design. Commonly a record shows **(Fig. 15)**:

- A brief burst of electrical activity upon electrode insertion (normal in neutrally intact person). This activity is a result of sarcolemmal depolarization by electrode placement.
- After this quiescence should return (straight line) except for voluntary muscle contraction or passive limb movement. Normal muscle is electrically silent at rest (embryonic muscle show fibrillation till ≈ 6 weeks of fetal life).
- In neural, neuromuscular or muscular disease aberrant patterns are seen. Changes in frequency, amplitude, and character of electrical signals occur and/or bursts of spontaneous electrical activity without stimulation may be noted. These changes are usually related to specific disease processes that can be recognized.
- In peripheral nerve injury, denervation to a group or region of muscles occurs. The muscle fibers develop spontaneous electrical activity due to the loss of innervation 5–7 days after injury represented as complex bizarre repetitive discharges. This baseline activity continues for a variable period until either reinnervation happens or muscle fibrosis ultimately occurs producing either reversal to near normal pattern of activity (reinnervation) or complete absence of electrical activity due to muscle fibrosis.
- Fibrillation and fasciculation waves are commonly seen in neuromuscular injury.
    - Fibrillation potentials could be in the form of PSW)—monophasic waves with an initial positive deflection. These are frequently associated with denervation of tested muscles. They have characteristic appearance as above along with an irregular rate and rhythm. PSW are produced by lack of inhibitory "feedback" (stabilization) that nerves normally exert on muscle fibers to maintain quiescence during the resting phase. PSW produce sound of "claps of distant thunder". They are initiated by insertion of a needle electrode into a muscle belly, but electrical activity continues in excess of that associated with electrode insertion "the bizarre repetitive discharges" heard as "rain on a tin roof". On an oscilloscope they can be graded into increasing severity of four grades.
        - *Grade 1:* Rare occasional waves
        - *Grade 2:* Several
        - *Grade 3:* Abundant while
        - *Grade 4:* Innumerable filling the screen.
- *Endplate fibrillation potentials (EPFP):* These are closely associated with the end-plate region. The end-plates become unstable following denervation and this causes aberrant membrane potentials that are picked up as fibrillations. This is different from PSW waves and has an initial negative deflection in the end-plate region, while in other areas of the muscle an initial positive deflection is noted. EPFP are mainly monophasic or biphasic in configuration. They appear usually within 8–14 days post injury, but may take 21 days in some cases. It is to be noted that as long as viable denervated muscle fibers are present, fibrillations will occur. With reinnervation a marked decrease in fibrillation occurs 2 weeks prior to reappearance of motor unit action potentials (MUAP) of low magnitude. Polyphasic waves are also noted with reinnervation.
- Giant MUAP are seen in a partially denervated muscle, which is additionally reinnnervated by nearby nerve.
- There is decreased muscle recruitment with denervation.

EMG finding	Normal	Peripheral nerve injury/denervation
Insertional activity	Normal	Increased
Spontaneous activity		Fibrillation Positive wave
Motor unit potential	0.5–1.0 mV 5–10 msec	Large unit Limited recruitment
Interference pattern	Full	Reduced Fast firing rate

Fig. 15: Electromyography record.

NERVE CONDUCTION VELOCITY

Normal conduction velocity (NCV) in humans is approximately 50 m/sec (slightly more in sensory nerves). Motor nerve conduction velocity is more commonly measured although it is always better to measure both sensory and motor nerve velocities. Demyelization reduces conduction speed as is evident from the NCV in unmyelinated fibers that have nearly 10 m/sec of conduction velocity. Sunderland type I injury may show delay at the site of injury, but otherwise NCS and EMG is normal.

- Two sets of stimulating electrodes along the nerve trunk to be tested **(Fig. 16)**. A recording electrode is placed in a muscle belly known to be innervated by the nerve to be tested. After applying stimulus along the nerve evoked muscle depolarization is noted. When the nerve is stimulated at two different points the time difference between evoked potential can be determined. With a known distance between the two electrodes the velocity of conduction along the nerve trunk can now be determined.
- Incomplete nerve injury only slightly alters the results of EMG and NCV testing that may not be discernible. Reduced amplitude in evoked potentials and/or prolongation of the potential evoked from a point distal to the injury site may be noted (due to delayed conduction in the injured fascicle). After complete transection normal conduction in the distal stump is noted for 4–6 days postinjury.

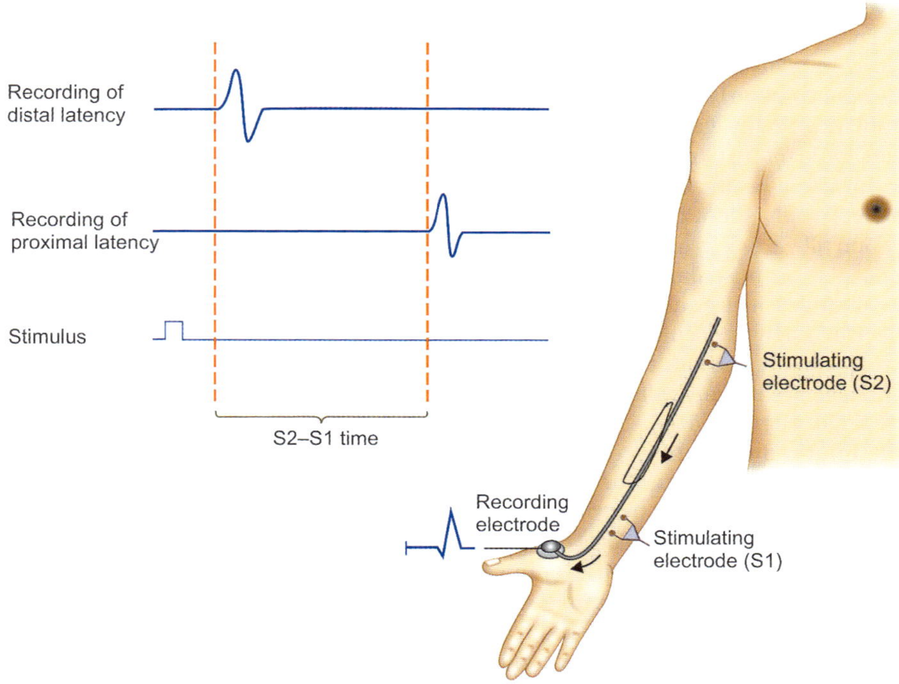

Fig. 16: Nerve conduction velocity.

STRENGTH-DURATION CURVE

A graph plotting the intensity of electrical stimulus to the length of time it must flow to produce response **(Fig. 17)**. The strength-duration curve was first discovered by G Weiss in 1901. The curve is defined by rheobase and chronaxie (the strength-duration time constant). These curves are used to identify various neurological diseases and pathologies.

- Rheobase (Rheos = current or flow; base = foundation): It is the minimal amount of stimulus strength that will produce a response (action potential or muscle contraction) when applied indefinitely (practically a few milliseconds–300 milliseconds). It is used to measure membrane excitability. Louis Lapicque coined the term "rheobase" in 1909.
- Chronaxie (chronos = time; axie = axis): It is the stimulation duration that yields a response when stimulus strength is set to exactly 2X rheobase. For two nerves that have same rheobase chronaxie gives an indication of relative excitability, this also holds true for sequential strength-duration curve plots done for neuropathic diseases **(Figs. 18A and B)**. It is evident by right shift in the curve (showing poorer excitability).
- F wave—stimulation of motor nerve and recording action potential from muscle supplied by it. The stimulus travels up the nerve to spinal cord then back to limb. It measures the conduction between nerve and spinal cord (others measure conduction within limb).
- H-reflex—in this case afferent impulse travels up the sensory nerve and travels down motor nerve to produce discharge.
- Upward kink in strength-duration curve indicates partial denervation.

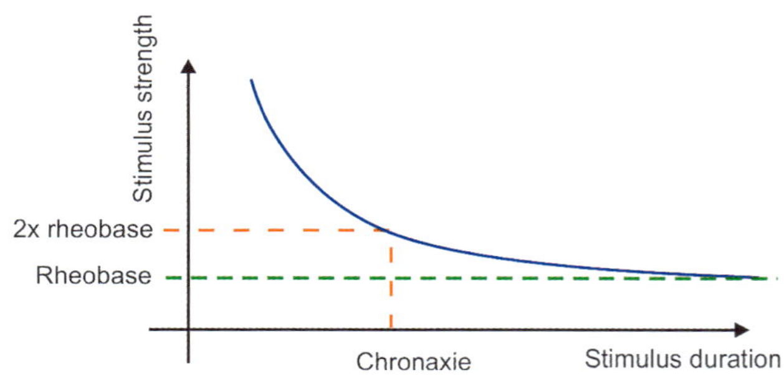

Fig. 17: Strength-duration curve.

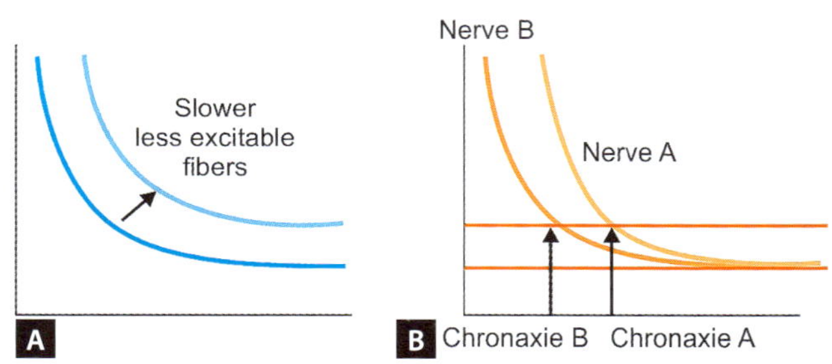

Figs. 18A and B: (A) The graph showing right shift of SDC suggesting reducing excitability of nerve (may occur with neuropathies) or demyelination; (B) At the same rheobase two nerves with different excitabilities show different chronaxie.

MANAGEMENT OF NERVE INJURY

Management of a clinically identified nerve injury depends on the type of injury (classification, complete/incomplete), associated injuries (fracture/crush/open injury/head injury), level of injury (stronger repair needed at mobile regions), availability of facilities and expertise, and duration of presentation.

The indications for primary open exploration and repair of a nerve are as follows:

- Nerve injury secondary to manipulation of fracture (absolute indication) that was previously absent. Here just assuming a simple traction injury may be criminal as most are due to compression of the nerve in the fracture site.
- *Open fractures:* These fractures have to be taken up for debridement and primary stabilization in operation theater based on the principles of management of open fractures. Here, the surgeon has a good chance to evaluate the nerve injury, explore them and others and possibly do a primary repair before edema or infection sets in. In cases of gross contamination, one may prefer to tag the gap separated nerves for wound to stabilize and do a secondary repair.
- Fractures in which satisfactory alignment is not possible by closed methods—obviously these fractures are taken-up in operation theater to be fixed primarily and simultaneous nerve injury should be explored and repaired.
- Fractures with associated vascular injury—again vascular exploration and repair will be a must so that the associated nerve injuries should be addressed.
- Patients with multiple trauma—this is a relative indication as extensive exploration may prolong the surgical time. Patients are managed on concept of damage control orthopedics (DCO) for quick stabilization of the injuries to prevent an ongoing tissue damage process. Proceed with nerve exploration only if it is easily assessable and good expertise is available that could make a remarkable difference between primary repair and secondary repair.

NERVE REPAIR (NEURORRHAPHY)

Nerve repair in partial nerve injuries is directed mainly at restoring continuity of the nerve with all of its elements. The principles of nerve repair are as follows:

- Preparation of the nerve stump and approximation of the stumps with no tension are essential, because blood supply to the nerve, especially intraneural, may be compromised. The tension at the repair site is assessed by one of the following methods (institutional practice):
  - Wilgis → take a single suture bite with 8–0 suture and if a knot cannot be tied without tension (or if it breaks) then there will be unacceptable tension at suture site (or a gap >4 cm).
  - Millesi → gap of more than or equals to 2.5 cm after keeping the limb in functional position indicates possibility of tension.
  - Elbow flexion more than 90° or wrist flexion more than 40° required for nerve approximation indicates tension at a repair site.
  - *Brooks:* If gap cannot be closed after adequately mobilizing the nerve.
- It is important to consider normal excursion of the nerve when the extremity is moving. The nerve will elongate with extension of the joints and repair may fail, so extremity should be moved through range of motion during repair itself.
- Lacerated fascicles must be dissected proximally and distally until adequate exposure is obtained for repair.
- Epineural vessels must be preserved, because they serve as an important guide for fascicular orientation during repair.

The various methods of nerve repair depending on time duration from injury are:

1. ***Primary repair***: Within hours, it is not always possible and though considered ideal may actually be suboptimal in the absence of skilled repair done often by junior surgeons. Also, there is a phenomenon of "conditioning effect" (discussed later) that may improve the chances of a delayed primary repair.
2. ***Delayed primary:*** Within 5–7 days. This is the common scenario, where the repair is undertaken as an elective procedure with all available tools and possibilities so is the clinically preferred scenario. It also takes the advantage of conditioning effect on nerves following an injury. "Conditioning effect" is based on the premises that a "primed" neuron will regenerate faster at its peak metabolic activity due to "conditioning effect". Conditioning effect presupposes that axons regenerate quickly, if they have been damaged previously.
3. ***Secondary:*** Any repair more than 7 days. This may be done in grossly contaminated wounds, delayed referrals or in polytrauma patients.

Technique or method of repair (neurorrhaphy) is based on the location of the injury and the type and size of the nerve. Surgical repair can be broadly divided into three types depending on the finer level at which repair are being done, although epineural is the most common method used by hand surgeons generally.

Epineural

This is the most common technique of nerve repair. A series of simple interrupted sutures are placed through the epineurium under low-power magnification **(Fig. 19)**. The epineurium is grasped and tensed with the Jeweler's forceps. Placement of sutures should be approximately

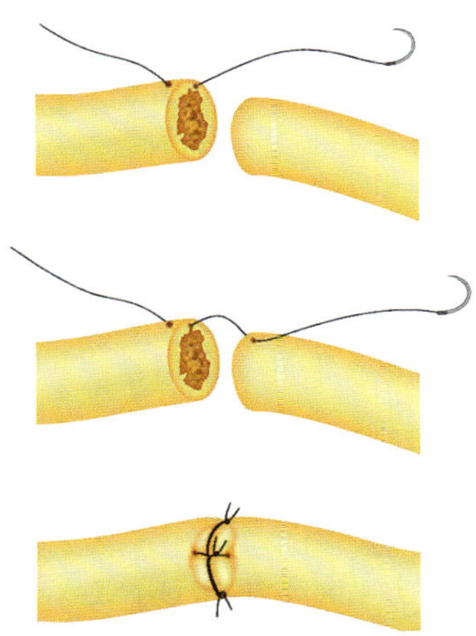

Fig. 19: Epineural repair: The sutures are carefully placed through the epineurium. It is useful to place all sutures through the nerve before tying so that suture tension can be controlled.

0.5–1.0 mm from edge. The suture material (3-0–5-0 Prolene often) is placed from the surface of the nerve to emerge just subepineurially. It is then brought out to the free edge and the process continued in the opposing nerve stump to begin subepineurially and emerge on the surface.

This completes one simple interrupted suture. The number of sutures required for adequate alignment of the stumps varies depending upon the diameter of the nerve. Optimal alignment is guided by epineural vessels. Smallest number of sutures possible is placed so that the inflammatory reaction is minimized. However, adequate alignment is paramount for the success of the surgical procedure. Often four equidistant sutures as suggested by Swaim provide sufficient strength for healing.

- *Epineurorrhaphy:* This means the stitches passed through the epineurium. Less time consuming, but higher chances of mismatch of the nerve ends.
- *Perineurorrhaphy:* This means the suturing is done through the perineurium. Improved nerve alignment, but slightly increased scarring.
- *Epiperineurorrhaphy:* The needle is passed through both the epineurium and perineurium. Strong coaptation and better alignment (preferred).
- *Interneural neurorrhaphy:* This is an alternative to epineural neurorrhaphy. It involves use of a double-armed suture material. Needle is centrally inserted into one of the two nerve stumps and directed down the longitudinal axis so that it emerges 180° from its counterpart. The suture is hence placed centrally increasing the chances of proper alignment with minimal injury. Each end of the nerve is sutured to a button through which slip sutures are passed and tied together **(Figs. 20A to C).** Stump rotation may be prevented by single epineural stitch.

Group Fascicular

Placement of one or two sutures of 10-0 suture material in the perineurium to anastomose individual funiculi has found favor in the past 10 years. This avoids lateral growth and allows best possible coaptation of the fascicles. Clinically, there have not been any demonstrable advantages of this technique over epineural neurorrhaphy. The technique can be improved with the use of simultaneous nerve stimulation.

- *Anchor funicular suture technique of Tsuge:* It uses both epineurial and funicular repair. A horizontal mattress suture is utilized to incorporate both the epineurium and perineurium, thereby aligning the major funiculi and also improves the holding strength by including the epineurium in the stitch. One of the major disadvantages of this technique is inability to achieve approximation in all the funiculi.

Fascicular (Funicular for Small Nerve, Fig. 21)

Individual fascicles are identified and sutured. This is even more precise but cumbersome.

Augmentation of Nerve Repair

Taking into consideration the sensitive issue of failure of nerve repair and resulting morbidity, various attempts at improving the success of primary repair have been done by experts. Though none have been shown to definitely improve the outcome but some may be selectively utilized to improve upon a suboptimal repair. The following are some of the reported methods.

- ***Neurorrhaphy using ensheathing materials:*** The disadvantages of standard repair methods are that connective tissue growth from neighboring regions occurs at the repair site and the nerve ends are also misguided peripherally. Many biologic and synthetic materials have been employed as an ensheathing cuff to shield the surgical site that can be incorporated with primary repair **(Fig. 22)**. These primarily prevent surrounding tissue to migrate into the repair site. The cross-sectional area of the cuff should be two to three times that of the nerve trunk. The length of the cuff should not exceed 8–10 mm. The following materials have been used:
    - Tantalum
    - Plasma clots
    - Gold films
    - Autografted and homografted blood vessels

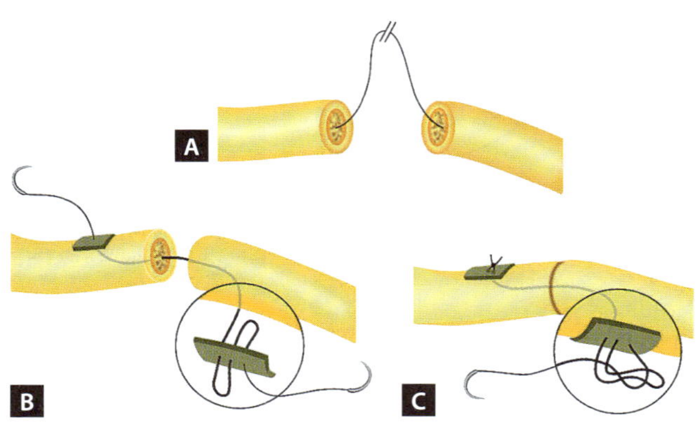

Figs. 20A to C: Intraneural neurorrhaphy: (A) The suture is placed along the center of the nerve trunk and (B) and is tied to silicone buttons or fascial tissue; (C) Simple knot is tied across.

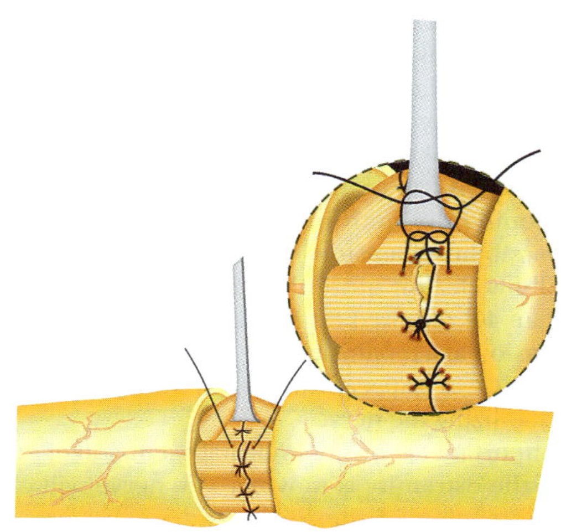

Fig. 21: Funicular repair—may be done in small nerves with few fascicles. The individual fascicles are sutured together.

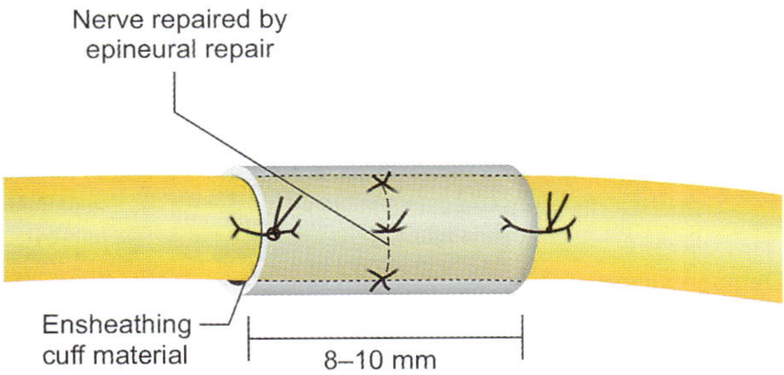

Fig. 22: Protection or augmentation of nerve repair using cuffing material.

- Muscle
- Surgicel
- Surgical tape
- Liquid plasticizers
- Collagen
- *Millipore membranes:* A pore size of 0.45 gun allows migration of extracellular fluid but not the tissue. The regeneration is hence augmented by "contact guidance" phenomenon.
- Silastic sheets and tubes.

- ***Fibrin clot augmentation of repair:***
  - Pure platelet rich plasma (PPRP) at the repair site
  - Stem cells at the repair site (? Value)
  - Application of trophic factors
  - Application of antibodies against neurotrophic factors (contra approach)
  - Mechanical stimulation of target musculature
  - Use of glycomimetic peptides like α-2, 8-Polysialic acid (PSA) mimetic peptides at the nerve repair site.

MANAGEMENT OF NERVE DEFECTS

In general indication for a primary, direct repair of a nerve is a defect of size approximately less than 2 cm and, if the defect is greater than 4 cm a repair is performed with a nerve graft. For defects between 2 cm and 4 cm, direct repair (with nerve mobilization) or grafting may be chosen on a case-by-case basis. The following methods are employed to address the issue and coapt the ends without undue tension (≈8% tension reduces venular flow and 10–15%—tension causes blood flow arrest):

- *Mobilization:* It is usually done proximally as distally most of the nerves thin down and gives branches so tethering effect is more pronounced distally. In general up to 4 cm of mobilization can be done. Mobilization more than 6–8 cm reduces perfusion. Distal nerve mobilization is also associated with increased collagen production and cross-linking. Eminent authors (Zachary) have but mobilized nerves extensively with good results—the median and ulnar nerves mobilized 7–9 cm and with anterior transposition an ulnar nerve gap of 13 cm were also filled.
- *Transposition:* The nerves are placed in position where the change in length effect resulting from joint motion is minimal and the nerves are relaxed like anterior transposition of ulnar nerve. Median nerve can also be transported anterior beneath pronator teres **(Fig. 23)**.

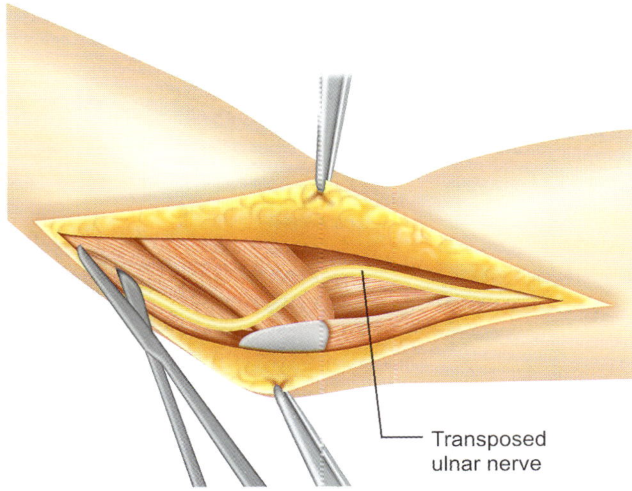

Fig. 23: Transposition of nerve—most commonly this technique is employed for ulnar nerve that is transposed anteriorly.

- *Limb positioning:* For upper limb placing the elbow in flexion (not more than 90°) and wrist in flexion (not more than 40°) for radial nerve repair helps. Limb can be then gradually extended.
- *Resection osteotomy:* If, for example, a nonunion is being addressed then the bone ends can be cut to provide better contact area and simultaneously this also relaxes the nerve by increasing the relative length. This also holds true for comminuted fractures.
- Nerve stretching and bulb suture (neuroma to glioma suture).
- Neuromatous neurotization (e.g., intercostal nerve for brachial plexus).
- *Nerve grafting:* Nerve grafting was first reported by Philipeaux and Vulpian in 1870. The first human allograft was reported in 1878 by Albert. This is a commonly employed technique to address nerve gaps. Fresh nerve grafts is the best choice. The nerve grafts can be harvested from various autogenous sites of body like:
  - Lateral cutaneous nerve of thigh
  - Medial brachial and antebrachial cutaneous nerve
  - Radial sensory nerve
  - Sural nerve (up to 40 cm of graft)
  - Lateral cutaneous nerve of forearm (up to 20 cm)
  - Terminal branch of PIN (for digital nerves).

The various options of grafting a nerve defect are:

- Trunk grafting using full-thickness segment of major nerve trunk (**Fig. 24**; disadvantage—central necrosis/ total graft dissolution). The nerve fascicle anatomy changes every 0.5–1 mm (discussed earlier) so chances of success are quite limited with this technique.
- Cable graft using multiple strands of cut nerve sewn at both ends (drawback—waste axons and ignores anatomic localization of function). This improves the chances of success as the fascicles are grafted by individual cable like grafts. It is also called interfascicular nerve graft (**Figs. 25A to E**, group fascicular nerve grafting)—described by Seddon.

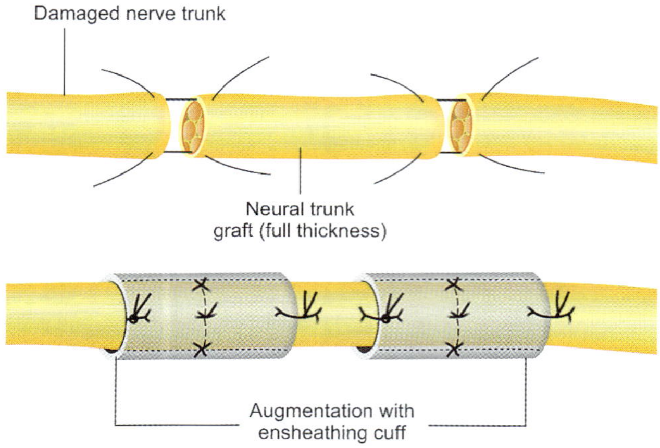

Fig. 24: Nerve grafting (trunk).

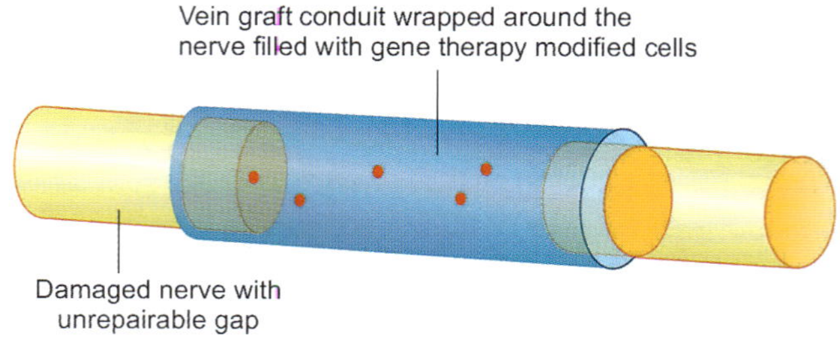

Fig. 26: Vein intersegmental graft for nerve repair. The graft can also be filled with stem cells (found ineffective) or modified with gene therapy (shown as dots here).

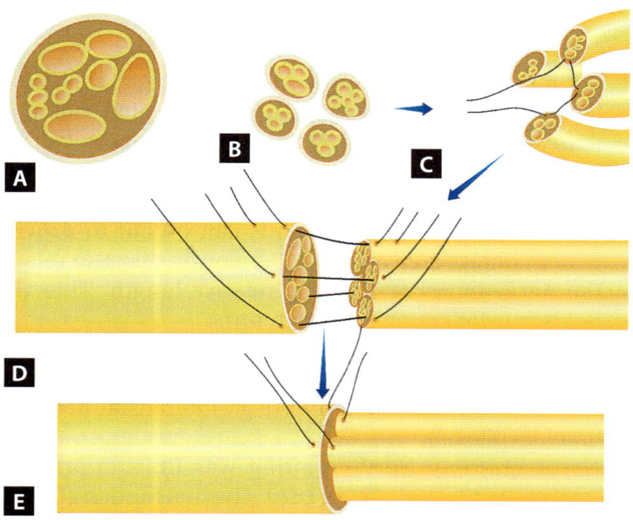

Figs. 25A to E: Interfascicular nerve grafting: (A) The cut nerve trunk is trimmed to uniformity; (B) The large fascicles are isolated somewhat; (C) Harvested nerve grafts are prepared in the form of cables and (D) approximated to the large fascicles isolated from nerve trunk; (E) Careful suturing under magnification is then done.

- Pedicle grafting often preferred for high combined ulnar and median nerve palsy where ulnar nerve is used as a pedicle graft to repair median nerve.
- Individual fascicular nerve grafting—often done for paucifascicular nerve e.g., ulnar nerve at elbow or for thin/terminal nerves, e.g., motor thenar branch of distal digital nerve.
- Free vascularized nerve graft
- Nerve crossing (ulnar → median)
- *Addition of non-neural tubes (e.g., vein segment):* Arterial segments have been used by Bungner in 1891 with success, but these are limited by ready availability of useable arterial segment always. Wrede described the first use of *vein* for repairing nerve lesions **(Fig. 26)**. The problem with them is that they tend to collapse. *Skeletal muscle* has been also used successfully by a handful of surgeons, but is not very popular as a nerve guide. These single component conduits can approximate the gaps up to 2.5–4 cm (critical defect repair limit) so further attempts were made to improve the method. Use of *multiple component tissue conduits* have been described like vein-filled with nerve or skeletal muscle tissue. The muscle vein combined conduits have been shown to be as good as autogenous nerve grafts. Interestingly they can be also shaped into Y-shaped structure to innervate two distal nerve stumps. Another advancement in the biological conduits is *addition of trophic factors or gene transfer* to improve the repair process. Bone marrow derived stem cells have been added to the vein-muscle conduits that seem to have a better repair capability. These advancements have improved the outcome of nerve gap repair to as close as using a nerve autograft and also have overcome the critical gap length limits that increased to 6 cm.
- *Biological conduits ± ?stem cells:* This is a further advancement that is still under infancy. The multiple component tissue components can be infected with adeno-associated viruses (AAV) to deliver specific molecules locally that is portend to enhance repair process.
- *Artificial conduits:* Lot of research and development of nanoarchitectures is underway to replace the biological conduits. Conduits of collagen, polyglycolic acid (PGA) and poly-L-lactic acid (PLLA) have been developed and are under study. The aligned nanofiber materials support a plethora of regenerating tissue including nerve cells. The presently available artificial systems of biomaterial nerve scaffolds mainly include hydrogel, self-assembly peptide, nanofibers and their combinations. Hydrogels like thermoresponsive xyloglucan hydrogel scaffolds functionalized through immobilization of poly-D-lysine were fabricated have been found to support differentiation of primary cortical neurons. 3D nerve scaffolds developed by blending of different polymers [like Poly (3-hydroxybutyrate-co-3- hydroxyvalerate) (PHBV) nanofibers cross-linked with chitosan] have already been studied in vivo. Further, strategies include electrosprayed micro/nanoparticles for nerve regeneration. Advanced regenerative strategies include developing conductive biomaterials and using electrical stimulation like Aligned poly(lactic-co-glycolic acid) (PLGA) nanofiber coated with polypyrrole (PPy). The PPy

or polyaniline coating allows development of conductive biomaterials which are able to enhance neurite extension with low electrical stimulation.

Factors affecting the success of nerve repair: Technical errors are the most common cause of failure of nerve repairs. The other causes are:

- *Type of nerve:* Pure motor or sensory has the best chance of recovery compared to mixed nerves.
- Younger patients have better recovery in least time.
- Proximal nerve injuries have poor chances of recovery as percentage cell death is quite high due to high metabolic demands.
- Gap defect in nerve have poor chances of recovery compared to direct repair.
- Clean vascular beds and absence of infection improves chances of recovery.
- *Delay between injury and repair:* Motor recovery has been reported for delay in nerve as long as 12 months (Suntherland). For sensory nerve this time delay is not known. In any case earlier the suture faster is the recovery.
- Associated injuries (like deep wounds/polytrauma) reduce chances of successful healing.
- *Condition of the nerve ends:* Lacerated ends may indicate tractional injury that may have occurred along the course of nerve unidentified. Clean cut ends are liable to recover much better.
- Neurogenic atrophy, fibrosis of denervated muscle, scar formation and wound contraction all lead to poor results.

SPECIAL SCENARIOS

Commonly closed nerve injuries say after a fracture is observed unless the fracture needs operative stabilization. These injuries can occur during the primary trauma or fracture, during the attempted reduction of the fracture, or during the surgical management of the fracture. Two common situations for nerve injuries with closed fractures are discussed here.

Fracture Shaft of Humerus

We will not discuss the brachial plexus injury with fracture dislocation or the axillary nerve injury with fracture proximal humerus (surgical neck fractures). The following discussion will be limited to the shaft humerus fracture that is classically associated with radial nerve palsy because of typical anterolateral angulation **(Fig. 27)**. Classically, the occurrence of the nerve injury during an attempt at reduction of a distal third spiral oblique humerus fracture has been termed a Holstein-Lewis injury. The features that make radial nerve susceptible to injury during midshaft and distal one-third fractures of the humerus include:

- Its location in the spiral groove on the posterior aspect of the midshaft of the humerus close to bone.
- Tethering of the nerve as it pierces the lateral intra-muscular septum to enter the anterior compartment.

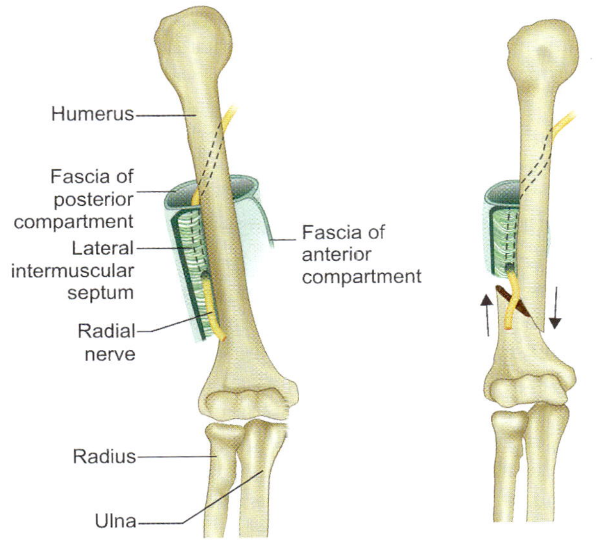

Fig. 27: Fracture shaft humerus and radial nerve injury: Diagrammatic illustration of the anatomy of radial nerve in relation to the shaft of the humerus. The radial nerve becomes relatively fixed as it pierces the intermuscular septum to enter the anterior compartment.

The factors are more pronounced when traction is applied or fracture angulates with a sharp lateral spike compressing the nerve.

The incidence of radial nerve palsies has been reported to be as high as 18% but in 90% of these injuries, nerve function returns by 4–5 months. This time for waiting return of function is logically derived. According to Steindler's formula, the nerve usually regenerates 1 mm/day or 3 cm in a month. Radial nerve injury often occurs 90–110 mm above the lateral condyle. Innervation of brachioradialis that originates 2 cm above the lateral condyle thus requires 70–90 mm of nerve regeneration. Considering the delay at neuromuscular junction of 1 month and a week delay at the nerve injury site for regeneration to begin, it will take 4–5 months' time for clinically detectable functional recovery of muscle. This implies that most radial nerve palsies are secondary to stretch or contusion. Laceration rate of 12% has been reported in the literature, but considering the fact that there is hardly any discernible difference between early and late repairs (functional outcome) it is better to wait for the recovery than explore the nerve. This saves many patients of unnecessary exploration. Acute nerve exploration is however indicated in:

- The palsy is associated with open humeral fractures.
- The palsy is associated with fractures requiring open reduction and internal fixation (displaced and non-reducible fractures. The fracture may be nonreducible due to nerve interposition itself).
- Fracture associated with vascular injury.
- The palsy occurs following an attempted reduction of the humerus shaft fracture.

While the surgeon is awaiting neurological recovery, the patient is encouraged to passively mobilize the joints of hand and wrist. Additionally, to maintain the wrist in extension **(Fig. 28)** for preventing any flexion contracture he can be given dynamic or static cock-up splint **(Fig. 29)**. Dynamic cock-up splint **(Fig. 30)** allows active flexion of the fingers and passive extension with static wrist extension. Static splints may additionally have option for passive finger extension.

Supracondylar Fracture of Humerus

The direction of displacement of the distal fragment determines which nerve will be injured by the sharp spike of proximal fragment. Radial nerve injury is associated with fractures in which the distal fragment is posteromedially displaced, whereas median nerve injuries are associated with fractures in which the distal fragment is posterolaterally displaced **(Figs. 31A and B)**. Although, the radial nerve had been the most frequently involved nerve in older studies it is the median nerve (the anterior interosseous nerve) which is injured much more commonly. Apart from acute injury median nerve can also get entrapped in the fracture callus during the healing phase. Ulnar nerve injury most frequently occurs iatrogenically during pinning **(Fig. 32)** or much less commonly with the flexion-type supracondylar fracture when the spike of the proximal fragment is directed posteriorly. Acute ulnar nerve injury has also been reported following medial condyle fractures of the humerus in children and is one of the relative indications for operative intervention. Tardy ulnar nerve palsies can be seen secondary to malunion or nonunion causing valgus deformity.

Most of these injuries are often not an indication for open exploration. However, prompt reduction of the fracture should be done. If the nerve injury is seen after reduction then it should be explored. Offending wire should be removed, if it causes ulnar nerve symptoms. Tardy ulnar nerve palsy is an indication of operative management.

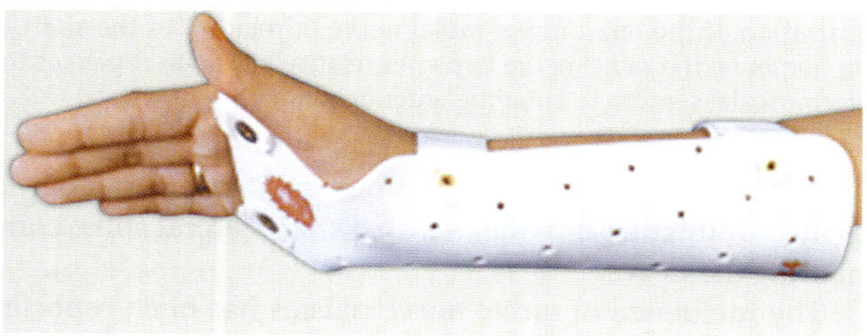

Fig. 28: Static dorsiflexion wrist splint.

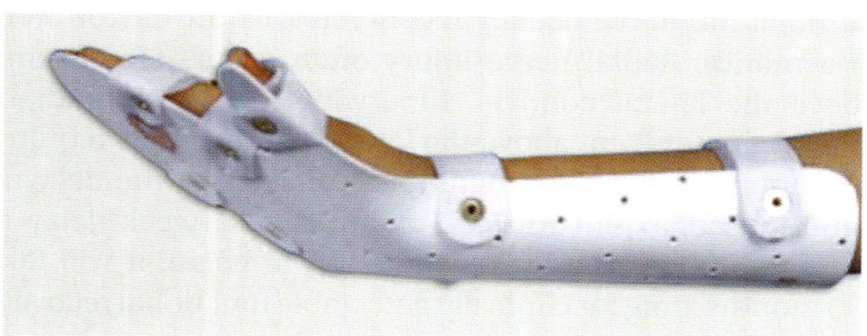

Fig. 29: Static wrist and finger cock-up splint.

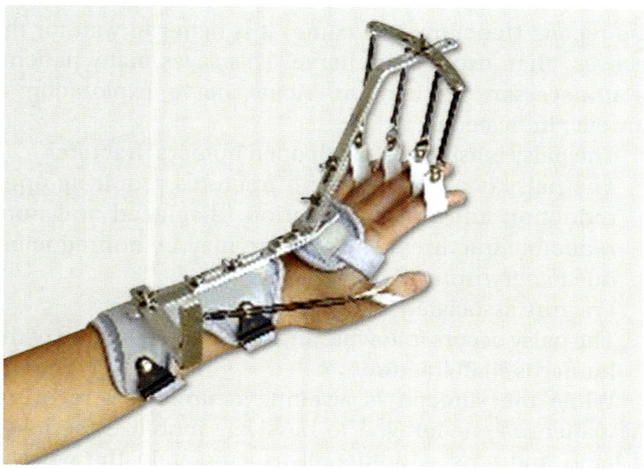

Fig. 30: Dynamic cock-up splint.

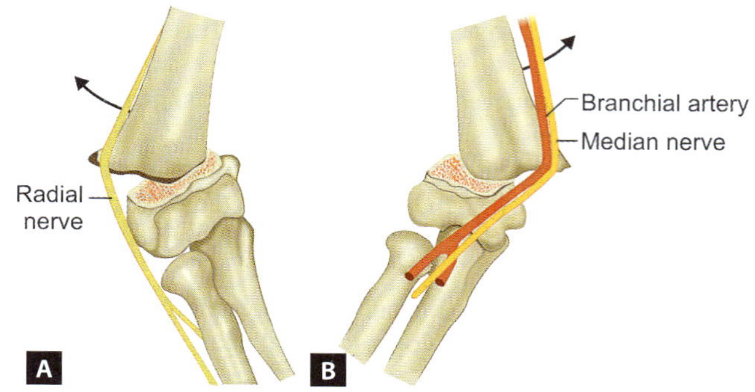

Figs. 31A and B: Supracondylar fractures of humerus and associated nerve injuries. (A) The neurovascular relationship of the supracondylar fracture explains that if the proximal spike penetrates the brachialis muscle laterally in a posteromedial fracture displacement → the radial nerve is prone to injury; (B) If the spike however penetrates anteromedially in a posterolateral fracture, the median nerve and brachial artery gets injured. Tethering by ulnar-sided supratrochlear artery fixes the brachial artery making it vulnerable to injury.

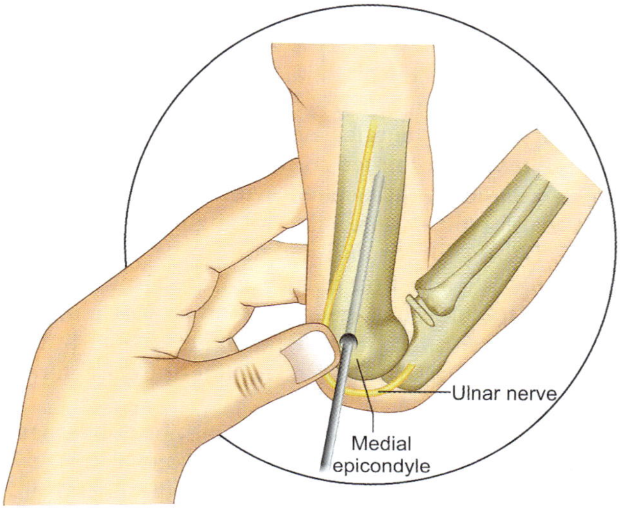

Fig. 32: Protecting ulnar nerve while pinning the fracture from medial side.

INJECTION NERVE PALSY

Injections into nerve directly may cause damage. There have been a number of instances of radial and sciatic nerve palsies following injections into the nerves. Brachial plexus palsy has also been reported following anesthetic blocks. Improper administration of injected medications or technique is usually the fault resulting in wide range of injury patterns and recovery. There are various ways (mostly theoretical) that have been proposed as the possible cause of nerve injury and these include:

- *Mechanical:*
  - Laceration—resulting from the needle entry into the nerve (large bore needles are likely to result into laceration).
  - Intraneural injection (this has been the most frequently sites reason). Intraneural injection produces syrinx and pressure on surrounding fascicles.
- *Vascular:*
  - *Acute ischemia:* Due to endoneural vasospasm or compression from the fluid.
  - *Hemorrhage:* Results from the damage to the neural vasculature and bleeding in the nerve structure.
- *Pressure:*
  - *Extraneural:* Deposition of medicine outside the nerve in a closed space causes external pressure.
  - *Intraneural:* Injecting the medicine into nerve itself causes increased pressure.
  - Compartment syndrome is produced, if the fluid does not extravasate fast and the nerve is then strangled.
- *Chemical:*
  - *Injection of neurotoxic solutions:* Drugs such as colchicine, tetracycline, bleomycin, certain vaccines (influenza), older diclofenac injections (containing fibrosing preservative), alcohol, phenol, etc. cause a lot of chemical neuritis that culminates into neural fibrosis and hence nerve damage. Progressive fibrosis causes internal amputation of the nerve fibers and complete damage.

The fibrosis is an important aspect in development of nerve damage due to injections. It may arise from toxic drugs, ischemic necrosis and collagen deposition, vascular injury, etc. The fibrosis resulting from direct injury may not involve the whole nerve, as such Millesi classified the fibrosis as follows that also has a therapeutic rationale:

- Epifascicular epineurium involved
- Interfascicular epineurium involved
- Endoneurium involved.

When used together with Sunderland system of nerve injury, if there is type A/B fibrosis in a patient with Sunderland degree I/II nerve injury, then the patient is a good case for neurolysis. It is imperative to understand that the fibrosis is progressive so earlier, the treatment is instilled better will be the supposed recovery. Neurolysis is an option for all early presenting cases up to 3 months (<3 weeks, they have best chance of recovery). Neurolysis will remove the ongoing constriction of the nerve fibers and relieve them of pressure.

There are various forms of *neurolysis* done to relieve the nerve pressure:

- *External neurolysis (Epineural):* It consists of freeing the nerve and injury sites from surrounding connective tissues or scar in a 360° fashion. This is adequate for nerve lesions where there is significant edema in fresh cases. Lying open the epineurium suffices as it reduces the pressure and re-establishes the blood flow.
- *Internal neurolysis:* It involves an internal dissection of the nerve, splitting it into at least its larger fascicles or sometimes groups of smaller fascicles, but maintaining their integrity.
  - *Perineural (interfascicular),* where the perineurium is dissected to exposed and lay open the fascicles. This is preferred in circumstances where an injury or a lesion in continuity is present that conducts a nerve action potential and the patient has severe pain.
  - *Endoneural:* Here the funicular dissection is also done for removing the fibrotic tissue that has penetrated deep within the nerve tissue. The risk of ensuing fibrosis with this extensive dissection is much more than the possible benefit by removing pathological tissue.
- *Hemicircumferential neurolysis:* This is an internal neurolysis (interfascicular) done for partial nerve lesion, with or without regeneration, as shown by preoperative and intraoperative electrical studies. Under these circumstances, a portion of the cross-section of the nerve may be more involved by injury and a secondary scar than the rest of the nerve.

Management of Old and Late Presenting Cases

Limb functional restoration has to be done for late and non-recoverable nerve injuries like delayed/late presentations of peripheral nerve injuries (>1 year), injection nerve palsies (>3 months), long standing brachial plexus palsies, gunshot injuries, extensive gaps between nerve ends that cannot be reconstructed, etc. Timing a reconstruction is difficult, but depends on individual case and surgeon reference. The reconstructive procedures fall into following categories:

- Skeletal stabilization
- Tendon transfers are usually done in cases where denervation has been present for more than a year. Moderate-to-severe atrophy of muscles is seen by 3 months, moderate to severe fibrosis seen by 11 months, beyond 3 years there is fragmentation and disintegration of muscle fibers; hence ideal reinnervation can be expected after 1–3 months, functional reinnervation up to 1 year and no reinnervation more than 3 years.
- Restoring sensibility of the limb

Skeletal stabilization is done before motor reconstruction as the motor units need a stable skeleton to work. Sensory restoration is done in the end. We will restrict ourselves to tendon transfers (motor reconstruction) in this section.

Tendon transfer is done to provide following functions:

- Replace a single joint motion that assists in grasp, pinch, or release.

- Eliminate a deforming force that may produce further functional limitations like claw hand deformity.
- Improve muscle balance for the best functional use.

Tendon transfer can be done only if certain conditions are met in a patient. These *prerequisites* should be established before surgery and the principles followed during surgery, else the results will be poor or suboptimal:

- *Correction of contractures:* All joints that the tendon is deemed to cross must be supple and passively mobilized. This maintains the expected range of motion after tendon transfer.
- *Adequate strength of the transferred tendon:*
    - 85% of power in the donor muscle is a must (Steindler)—described as good power.
    - Omer stated that a muscle loses at least one grade of strength after transfer so for useful postoperative movements four-fifths power (Lovett scale) is a must.
- *Straight line of pull:* No pulley is ideal or minimum number of pulleys should be required or made for tendon to act. Chances of adhesion and attritional rupture and ultimate failure of procedure are prominent, if pulleys are made.
- *One tendon-one function:* It is a dictum that one tendon should do only one function with effectiveness (but often accessory functions are availed by positioning the tendon).
- *Synergism:* Synergistic transfer should be preferred as much as possible; however, there are lots of violations of this rule.
- The muscle selected for transfer should have a work capacity equal to that of the antagonist muscle.
- *Expendable donor:* There should be no functional morbidity following use of a tendon, this is again mostly relative in the sense that there will always be a functional loss, but the functional gain should excel loss.
- Tissue should be in equilibrium (tissue equilibrium—termed by Steindler):
    - Soft tissue induration should subside.
    - No reaction in wounds.
    - Scars should be as soft as possible.
- *Patient equilibrium:*
    - Emotionally stable.
    - Compliant.
    - No reflex sympathetic dystrophy (RSD).
    - No chronic pain syndrome.
- Pass tendon below fascial planes/sheaths and not below incision line/scar (best between subcutaneous fat and fascial sheath):
    - Incisions should be transverse to the subcutaneous path of tendons.
    - Tendon junctions should be beneath the skin flaps and not at subcutaneous scars.
    - Fascial openings must be as large as possible for tendons that pass through them.
- Amplitude of transferred tendon should be as near to the original tendon for which the transfer is being done (33 mm for wrist movers, 70 mm for finger flexors, and 50 mm for finger extensors and the thumb extrinsic muscle tendons). For tendons that have low amplitude it can be improved by two ways:
    1. Converting a monoarticular muscle into bi-/multiarticular, e.g., flexor carpi ulnaris (FCU)/flexor carpi radialis (FCR) → extensor digitorum communis (EDC). The effective amplitude of motion is enhanced due to tenodesis effect by active volar flexion of wrist.
    2. Muscle release from surrounding tissue to improve sliding.
- Try preserving the nerve and vascular supply to muscle and vascular supply to tendon.
- Insertion of the tendon should be as close to the insertion of paralyzed tendon and at the same angle; if split transfers then keep both slips in same tension.
- The tension of transferred muscle must be adequate enough (not too slack that most of the contraction is taken up in generating tension; not too tight as to prevent passive positioning the wrist in resting position). Required excursion is the actual distance a tendon must move to produce a specific movement. Maintaining tension is a difficult aspect in tendon transfer and the following are a few ways to manage it:
    - Intraoperative muscle stimulation after tendon transfer (Omer and Vogel).
    - Intraoperative laser diffraction technique that measures sarcomere length change.
    - *Goldner (as communicated to Omer in personal communication):* Position the extremity and the recipient tendon in functional position and the transfer tendon in resting length. Traction is applied to the transferred tendon and distance is recorded in centimeters and marked. A point at 60% of the distance between resting and traction length is marked. This gives the position of transferred muscle at final insertion of tendon.
    - *Cooney:* It measured the distance that a muscle contracts after release from its normal insertion. This lost length is restored and some tension is added at final insertion to accommodate for the elasticity of surrounding tissues. It should be remembered that the final tension be always set with tourniquet deflated.
- Plan for restoring sensibility of distal organ before motor reconstruction.
- Arthrodesis/joint procedure should be done before tendon transfer.
- The disorder should be a nonprogressive one. Charcot-Marie-Tooth progressive muscular atrophy, cerebrovascular accidents produce nonstatic and variable muscle imbalance difficult to correct.
- Keep dissection to a minimum around the muscle to be transferred and achieve meticulous hemostasis to prevent adhesion formation.
- Pertinent explanation should be given to the patient and he should develop a "cerebral imprint" for the function to be reconstructed.

- Lastly keep the tendon transfer as simple as possible the more complex transfers have high chances of failure.

Early Tendon Transfers—"Internal Splints"

When a precise neurorrhaphy has been performed early in a patient selected tendon transfers may be performed early as internal splints to support partial function and prevent deformity, while awaiting the potential nerve recovery. These substitute also the function of external splints and immobilizers. The selected early tendon transfers (internal splints) enhance function while awaiting the return of nerve control and total muscle activity. The combined results of early tendon transfer plus the return from nerve repair often are better than those of either procedure separately by stimulating sensibility, reeducation and improving the coordination of residual muscle-tendon units.

Principles of early tendon transfer:

- Should not ↓ function in remaining hand
- Should not create deformity
- Should be phasic or capable of phasic conversion, e.g., Pronator teres (PT) → Extensor carpi radialis brevis (ECRB) transfer described by Burkhalter for radial nerve palsy or a wrist flexor in substitution for a finger extensor. A synergistic muscle-tendon unit will be able to use spinal reflex arcs and other autonomic feedback mechanisms to enhance re-education.

Indications

- Substitutes function during nerve regrowth eliminating the need of splintage.
- Helper following reinnervation → aiding power of normally innervated muscle or helping a suboptimally innervated muscle.
- Substitute in cases where results of repair are poor or nerve irreparable.

Common examples of early tendon transfers done for upper limb:

- Radial nerve palsy—Pronator teres to ECRB.
- Low median—extensor indicis proprius (EIP) to abductor pollicis brevis (APB) (and EPL for combined palsy) or flexor digitorum superficialis (FDS) ring to APB to improve thumb abduction.
- Low ulnar—FDS 3 (middle finger) to adductor pollicis (for thumb adduction) and additional slips to A2 pulley of 4 and 5 for metacarpophalangeal (MCP) flexion.

Individual Upper Limb Nerve Palsies of Upper Limb

Radial Nerve Palsy

The radial nerve may be damaged anywhere in its course from axilla to forearm. The nerve is formed in front of subscapularis muscle from posterior cord receiving components from all roots of brachial plexus (C5-T1) and follows the course as below:

It passes anterior to latissimus dorsi muscle → to enter the triangular space accompanied with profunda brachii artery → spirals around the posterior aspect of humerus into radial groove (not spiral groove; radial groove is few millimeter above spiral groove) where it is separated from bone by medial head of triceps (it is not in direct contact with bone here) coursing obliquely laterally → pierces the lateral intermuscular septum around 122 mm above lateral epicondyle (gets tethered at this point limiting its translation) → The nerve then enters into anterior compartment emerging beneath Brachioradialis → divides into two branches → the deep branch [posterior interosseous neuropathy (PIN)] pierces supinator muscle to emerge into extensor compartment of forearm → forms cauda equina of spinner 8 cm distal to elbow joint. So along the course the nerve supplies triceps, anconeus, radial half of brachialis, brachioradialis, extensor carpi radialis longus (ECRL), ECRB, supinator, EDC, extensor carpi ulnaris (ECU), extensor digiti minimi (EDM), abductor pollicis longus (APL), extensor pollicis brevis (EPB), extensor pollicis longus (EPL) and extensor indicis propolis (EIP) in that order.

For reconstruction purpose and clinical identification terminology has been developed to classify the nerve injuries into various levels as follows:

- *Complete radial nerve palsy (very high):* Triceps and all distal muscles supplied by the nerve paralyzed (injury in axillary region).
- *High radial nerve palsy:* Triceps and often anconeus spared, but rest all other distal muscles paralyzed (injury around radial groove till it pierces septum, typified by Holstein-Lewis injury).
- *Low radial nerve palsy:* BR and ECRL preserved [≡ posterior interosseous nerve (PIN) palsy as in high both bone forearm fractures, local penetrating injuries like bullet injury and iatrogenic injury during radial head/neck surgeries. ECRB in only 58% cases is supplied by PIN so it may also be spared in some cases].

Functional deficit produced by nerve injury at various levels include (numbers indicate the five digits, one is thumb while five is little finger):

- Inability to extend fingers (1, 2, 3, 4 and 5) (low) and wrist (low + high) **(Fig. 33)**.
- Inability to stabilize the wrist (wrist drop) and thumb (radial abduction of thumb) (low + high).
- Loss of grip strength (accessory forearm flexion) (high).
- Accessory forearm supination (very high).
- Accessory elbow flexion (high) there is mild weakness only as biceps is intact.
- Unstable CMC joint (low + high).
- Sensory loss (radial two-thirds dorsal sensation) (high and above).

The disabilities that need reconstruction for optimal functional gain are as not all listed above. The priority includes:

- Wrist extension
- Finger (MCP) extension
- Combination of thumb extension and abduction.

After following the prerequisites of tendon transfer surgeon can perform motor reconstruction using various options. Till the time patient awaits surgery wrist can be

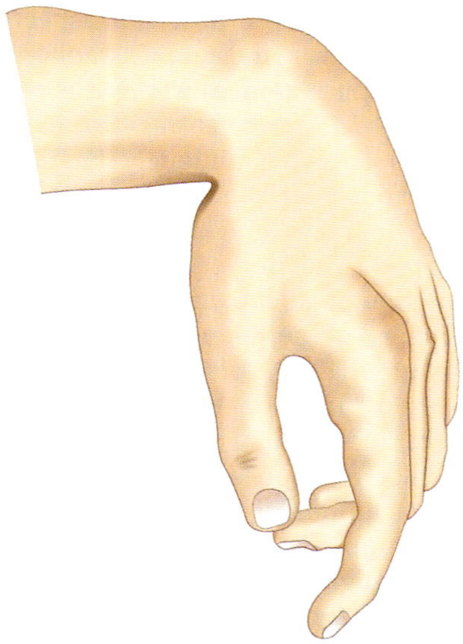

Fig. 33: Wrist and finger drop in high radial nerve palsy.

managed in extension using static or dynamic cock-up splint. The motors supplied by median and ulnar nerves are all available. The various methods have their own merits and utility. Surgeon must always check for the presence of PL before proceeding for surgery as this will change the reconstruction plan completely. The procedures described in literature for motor reconstruction following the radial nerve palsy are:

- *Jones transfer:* Quite a lot of transfers done around the wrist for radial nerve palsy have been colloquially named Jones transfer, but in reality the tendon transfers described by Jones have met lot of criticism and are seldom if ever done. Jones transfer (and modified one also) use both the primary wrist flexors causing unacceptable functional loss at the wrist (*see* principles of tendon transfer above).

Classical (1916):

1. PT → ECRL and ECRB
2. FCU → EDC III-IV
3. FCR → EPL, EDC II, EIP.

Classical (1921):

1. PT → ECRL and ECRB
2. FCU → EDC III–IV
3. FCR → EDC II, EIP, EPL, EPB, APL.

Modified jones: PT → ECRB and rest as above.

- *FCR transfer (of Starr; Brand; Tsuge):* This is the preferred transfer I would do in my patients. Additionally, I usually tend to improve the thumb proximal stability by tenodesing the EPL to EPB.
    1. PT → ECRB
    2. FCR → EDC II–V
    3. PL → rerouted APL.
- *Boyes transfer (superficialis transfer):* This is possibly the best alternative in cases with absent palmaris longus (PL). However, surgeon should be meticulous enough to create large interosseous window to avoid tethering the tendons and developing adhesions and protect the interosseous nerve and artery. Complete FCU transfer is also an alternative but less preferred.
    1. PT → ECRB
    2. FCR → APL and EPB
    3. FDS III → EDC II–V via interosseous membrane
    4. FDS IV → EIP; EPL via interosseous membrane.
- *FCU transfer (standard transfer, this is not modified Jones transfer):* This is the oldest described transfer for providing digital extension. The FCU is freed from fascial attachments to increase excursion, but mobilization is still limited by the innervation that enters muscle in its proximal 5 cm. EDM is included in transfer only if the EDC to little finger is absent. Classically, the FCU was itself used to motorize the EPL also but over time the practice was discouraged (one muscle one function).
    1. PT → ECRB
    2. FCU → EDC
    3. PL → rerouted EPL (the EPL is taken out of dorsal retinaculum (junction is made between PL and EPL in the region of snuff box). This gives a combination of abduction and extension force on thumb).

The disadvantage of FCU transfer is that there is slight radial deviation after the surgery and loss of the most powerful wrist flexor causes weakness of grip strength, this may be unacceptable to laborers.

Postoperatively, a POP slab or splint is applied to immobilize the forearm in 30° pronation, wrist in 45° of extension, MCP joints in 0° of extension, and the thumb in maximum extension and abduction. Six weeks after surgery the patient is explained the retraining and placed in a dynamic splint to obtain independent action for wrist and finger extension.

Median Nerve Palsy

Anatomical Consideration

Median nerve is formed from medial and lateral heads of medial and lateral cords respectively and enters arm in close relation to brachial artery. It receives components from C6-T1 roots. In the cubital fossa nerve lies lateral to brachialis tendon and passes between two heads of pronator teres → gives anterior interosseous nerve (AIN) → continues in forearm sandwiched between FDS and flexor digitorum profundus (FDP) → emerges just proximal to wrist between FDS and FCU→ passes through carpal tunnel → lies anterior and radial to FDS tendons → divides in hand into recurrent motor and sensory branches.

The median nerve supplies all flexors of forearm except the FCU and ulnar half FDP, i.e., PT, flexor carpi radialis (FCR), PL, FDS, FDP (lateral half), flexor pollicis longus (FPL), PQ, and "LOAF muscles"—first and second lumbrical, opponens pollicis, APB and FPB. Interesting anomalies of innervation have been noted between ulnar and median nerves and include:

- *Martin-Gruber anastomosis:* In proximal forearm between median/AIN and ulnar nerve providing additional intrinsic innervations.
- *Riche-Cannieu:* Motor deep ulnar branch with recurrent branch of median—complete/partial intrinsic innervations.

- Ulnar nerve always contains fibers from C8 and T1; additional C7 in 5–10% that supplies the FCU.
- FDP innervation may vary from all ulnar to all median.
- Dorsoulnar surface of hand may be innervated by radial nerve.

The median nerve is involved often in the region of elbow or forearm. Low median nerve palsy results from injuries in the distal third of the forearm or wrist. The following are the functional deficits resulting from the nerve injury based on its location.

1. Loss of thumb adduction, opposition, finger stabilization 1, 2 (low + high) (simian hand, **Fig. 34**)
2. Loss of thumb flexion (High)
3. Weakness of wrist and partial loss of finger flexion 2, 3 (high) (pointing index sign, **Fig. 35**)

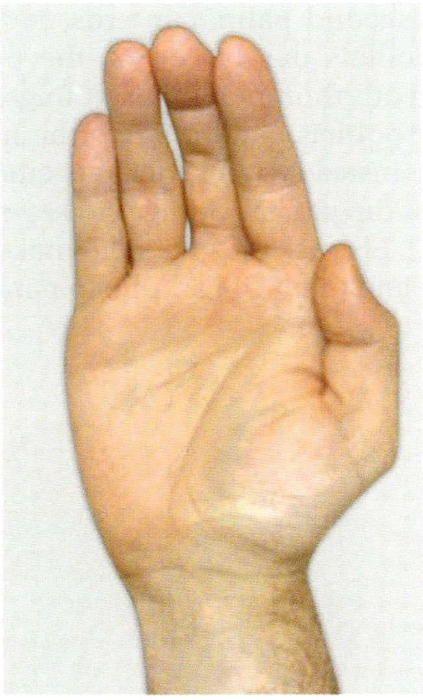

Fig. 34: Simian hand.

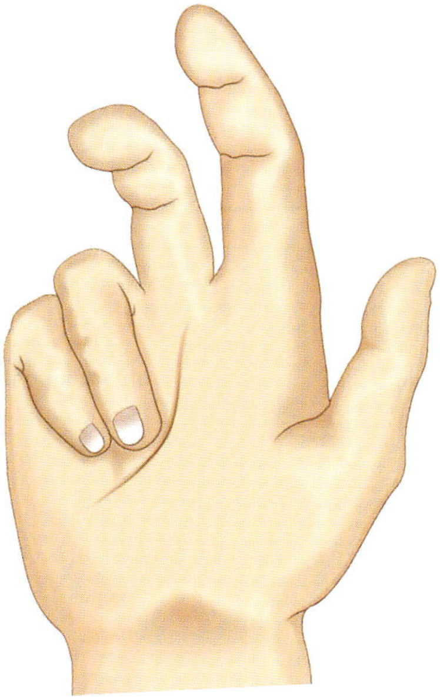

Fig. 35: Pointing index—when asked to make a fist the patient is unable to flex the index finger (and also sometimes the middle finger).

4. Forearm pronation (high)
5. Sensory loss (radial volar two-thirds hand).

Reconstruction of specific deficits in median nerve palsy can be done as mentioned later. It should be borne in mind that for any thumb reconstruction procedure first web space contracture is the biggest deterrent and should be released; also stability of MCP joint will prove a transfer successful else the procedure is bound to fail. For the sake of simplicity and basic understanding only the standard transfers with their details are included. Dedicated text can be referred for alternative transfers done and available in literature.

- *Thumb abduction (low or high palsy):* EIP to APB is the preferred transfer. The tendon is passed from the ulnar aspect of forearm using pisiform as pulley. The tendon can be attached either to the APB in isolated median palsy else in combined palsies the transfer should be done to the APB tendon and the EPL tendon over the proximal phalanx. If the MCP joint is unstable then arthrodesis is done.
- *For thumb flexion (high palsies):* BR transfer to FPL is good. The problem is mobilizing the BR through extensive dissection that should be done as clean as possible to achieve at least 5 cm of passive mobility.
- *Flexion 2, 3 digits (index and middle finger):* The easiest way is to tenodese the FDP 2 and 3 to FDP 4 and 5. The FDP of all fingers are pulled so that the finger tips get into a single transverse plane instead of the normal resting oblique alignment (cascading). The tendons are then tenodesed using double line of sutures to prevent tendon shifting during power grasp. In skilled people the index finger flexion is a separate requirement and this also holds true with the current world immense use of computers and gadgets. In this case, ECRL transfer to FDP 2 should be done while FDP 3 should be tenodesed as above.
- *Sensory reconstruction* is difficult and various techniques described are:
    - Neurocutaneous island flaps
    - Ulnar digital nerve translocation

Isolated Ulnar Nerve Palsy

Anatomical Consideration

Ulnar nerve is formed from medial cord receiving fibers from C8 and T1, rarely C7 also. The nerve runs inferomedial to axillary artery to continue behind brachial artery over triceps muscle → passes straight to posterior aspect of medial epicondyle in "ulnar groove" between medial epicondyle and olecranon process **(Fig. 36)** → passes between two heads of FCU [the so-called "cubital tunnel" better called humeroulnar aponeurosis **(Fig. 36)**] → remains deep to FCU overlying FDP muscle accompanied with ulnar artery → passes superficially; emerging beneath FCU to reach Guyon's canal at wrist.

The muscles supplied by the ulnar nerve include FCU, FDP 3 and 4, abductor digiti minimi, opponens digiti minimi, flexor digiti minimi, palmaris brevis, third and fourth lumbricals, all dorsal and palmar interosseous, flexor pollicis brevis (deep head), adductor pollicis.

Compared to the easier median nerve deficient hand reconstruction; the deficiencies resulting from ulnar nerve injury are difficult to reconstruct as the functional deficits are too many. This has logically led to umpteen number of transfers described for the ulnar nerve palsy. Also combined ulnar and median nerve palsies had been common (leprosy, etc.) that makes the reconstruction options even more complex and difficult due to limited number of motors available. Low ulnar nerve palsy mainly results in loss of intrinsic muscle function to hand due to injury in distal third forearm and/or wrist. The overall functional deficits resulting from isolated ulnar nerve palsy are as follows:

- Loss of grip strength (impairment of power grip is more than precise grasp) (high)
- Flexion of distal phalanx 4, 5 (high)
- Digital balance 4, 5 (high)
- Loss of finger function [flexion (partial), adduction, abduction] (high + low) there is loss of power flexion of the proximal phalanges and integration of MCP-IP motion. Normally, the fingers start flexion at DIP with simultaneous or just followed by (but in smaller amplitude) flexion at MCP joints. In ulnar nerve palsy the flexion at DIP is associated with MCP extension instead and the fingers curl-up in the palm instead of making a fist.
- Loss of thumb adduction and weakness of thumb flexion (high + low)
- Sensory loss (medial 11/2 digits—low; ulnar 1/3 volar—high)

On clinical examination some functional requirements can be assessed and treatment planned. Also distinction can be made between high and low ulnar nerve palsy.

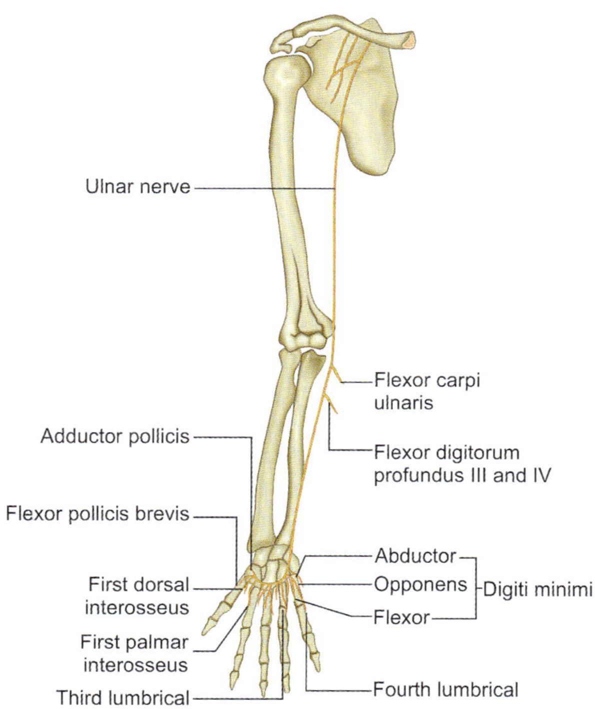

Fig. 36: The anatomical course of ulnar nerve in upper limb.

- *Ulnar claw hand* **(Fig. 37)**: It is the most characteristic deformity ascribed to ulnar nerve injury (as "pointing index" for median and "wrist drop" for radial nerve injury). This is due to loss of intrinsic function of flexion at the MCP joint while long flexor tendons flex the IP joints. The clawing is more apparent in low ulnar nerve palsy as the maintained basal tone of long flexors make the clawing prominent while in a high palsy even the long flexors are paralyzed so flexion at interphalangeal joint is less pronounced and is only due to tenodesis effect. Complete claw hand (involving all four fingers) results from combined median and ulnar nerve palsy.
- Look for wasting in first webspace (first dorsal interosseous)
- *Froment's sign (Book test)/Bunnell's O sign/newspaper sign* **(Figs. 38A and B)**: This tests for paralysis of first dorsal and second palmar interosseous muscle with adductor pollicis paralysis. Ask the patient to hold newspaper with thumb and flexed fingers. Due to lack of adductor pollicis patient flexes the interphalangeal and use FPL instead. Other trick movement to cover for deficit is that the patient changes to key-pinch grip (this is also weak). Else ask the patient to make a "Deer's eye" with thumb and index finger. Due to paralytic interossei

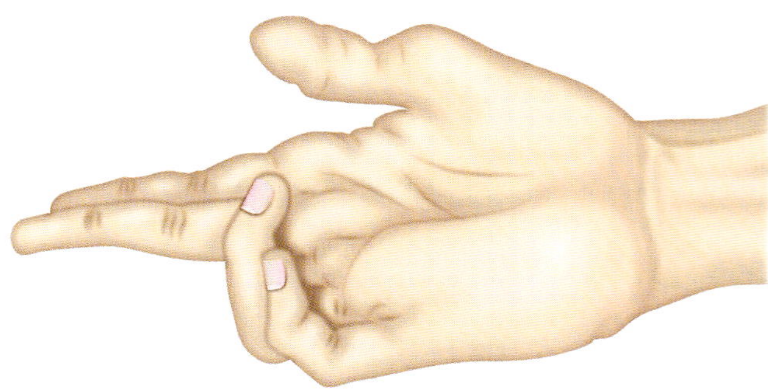

Fig. 37: Ulnar claw hand: The clawing of little and ring finger is much more prominent in lower ulnar nerve palsy.

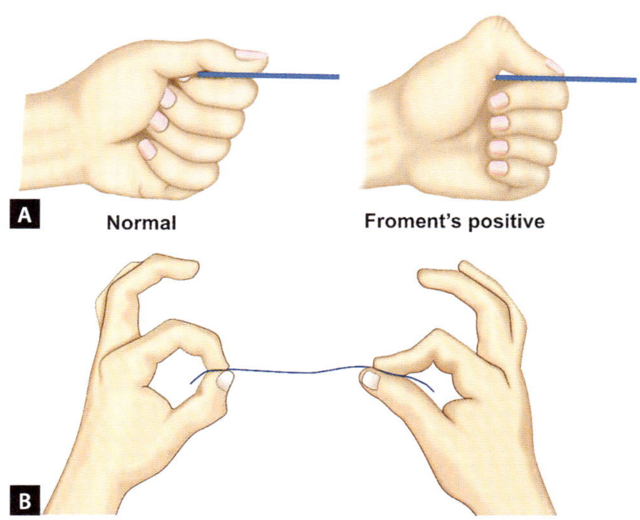

Figs. 38A and B: (A) Froment's sign; (B) Bunnell's O sign.

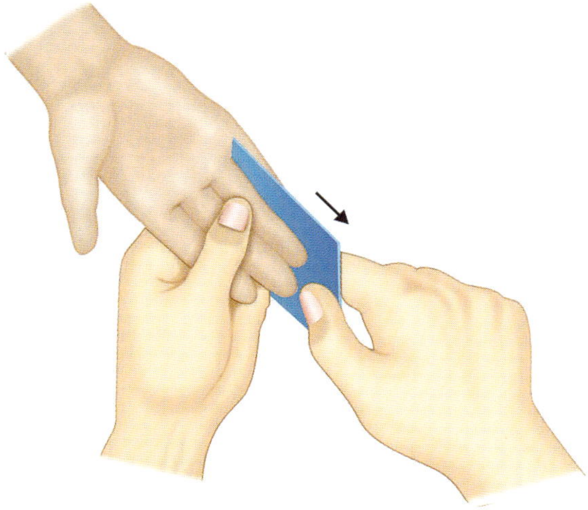

Fig. 39: The "Card test".

and adductor muscles the patient flexes the thumb, so that Deer's eye changes to "O" instead. Patient flexes thumb as a trick/compensatory maneuver.

- *Card test* ***(Fig. 39)****:* To test palmar interossei (PAD = palmar-adduct; DAB = dorsal-abduct)—ask the patient to adduct fingers and hold card as string as possible. The card slips out easily due to interossei paralysis.
- *Egawa test:* Patient is asked to abduct fingers against examiner's resistance palm facing downward.
- *Wartenberg's sign:* EDM unopposed by third palmar interossei. Ask the patient to push the abducted little fingers against each other. The little ginger on the paralyzed side is weak and gets adducted.
- *Jeanne's sign:* Loss of key pinch (adductor pollicis)
- *Bouvier's maneuver:* Passive block of MCP hyper-extension facilitates interphalangeal extension. This is an important test to decide if blocking hyperextension at the MCP will produce functionally improved grip.
- *Duchenne sign:* Loss of MCP flexion and instead hyper extension at the MCP joint.
- *Pitres-stut sign:* Inability to cross fingers, e.g., IF on MF tests Palmar interosseous of index and dorsal interosseous of middle finger.
- *Pitres-stut sign 2:* Inability to make cone with extended fingers
- *Pitres-stut test:* Inability to radial and ulnar deviate MF.
- Masse's sign: Intermetacarpal muscle wasting and loss of metacarpal arch.
- *Pollock sign:* Inability to flex DIP of RF and LF (paralysis of ulnar half of FDP)

The following are some commonly done motor transfers to address the requirements of low ulnar nerve palsied hand.

- *Thumb adduction:* ECRB transferred and attached to abductor tubercle (Smith/Boyes). In other scenario ECRB can be better attached to the APB insertion that additionally provides pronation for pinch. Tendon graft has to be used to accomplish the transfer which is done through third metacarpal space and passed volar to AP and deep to flexor tendons.
- *Metacarpophalangeal flexion with integrated IP flexion:* ECRL (Brown's 4 tailed; EF4) or FCR (if there is flexion contracture at wrist); tendon grafts are passed volar to transverse carpal ligament and attached to A2 pulley or radial band of dorsal apparatus.
- *Maintenance of palmar (transverse metacarpal) arch and adduction of little finger:* EDM tendon split and ulnar half transferred to radial collateral ligament of PP or radial band of dorsal apparatus of little finger. If the little finger is clawed and abducted then the tendon slip is inserted into A2 pulley of the flexor sheath.
- *Thumb-index finger "tip pinch":* Accessory slip of APL to first dorsal interosseous and MCP joint arthrodesis. If MCP joint already arthrodesed EPB may be transferred. This procedure does not increase the power, but only stabilizes the index finger.
- *Volar sensation:* Vascular nerve grafts or proximal medial digital nerve translocation to distal ulnar digital nerve.

For high ulnar nerve palsy in addition the following are done:

1. Wrist flexion (ulnar side) (*not frequently done*): FCR → FCU or PL → FCU.
2. *DIP flexion for RF and LF:* FDP of MF is tenodesed to FDP (RF and LF).
3. *Ulnar deviation:* For persons requiring strong wrist flexion we need ulnar deviation so that FCR can be transferred to the FCU attachment.

COMBINED NERVE PALSIES OF UPPER LIMB

Tendon transfers in combined nerve palsies are more complicated. These combined injuries are seen in situations such as VIC, Hansen's disease and brachial plexus lesions. These are summarized in **Table 3**. For combined low ulnar and median nerve palsy reconstruction of thumb is essential as without a stable thumb flexion contracture of the wrist will result due to constant use of flexed position to achieve functional tenodesis. For combined high ulnar and median nerve palsy sensory deficit reconstruction is more important and the limb will hardly be any useful for precision activities otherwise. Reconstructing just the finger flexion results in increased claw so intrinsic function should also be restored. Preventing the first webspace contracture is again a priority. In combined radial nerve (+ulnar/median) palsy although sensation is not such a big problem, but rehabilitation is difficult as reconstruction for both finger flexion and extension is done as is needed for thumb adduction and abduction. Worst situation results from combined high median and radial nerve palsy as even after best possible reconstruction (from the meager options available) the hand is no better than a prosthesis. Precision is lost and no useful motors that can give precision are left. Sensory reconstruction is also not that successful as the cerebral cortical orientation for these patients is not that successful.

TABLE 3: Management options for combined nerve palsies.

Needed function	***Preferred transfer***
Combined low median and ulnar nerve palsy:	
Thumb adduction (key pinch)	ECRB → APB tendon (see text)
Thumb abduction (opposition)	EIP → EPL tendon around pisiform pulley
Thumb-index tip punch	APL slip → dorsal interosseous tendon + arthrodesis MCP
Transverse metacarpal arch	EDM tendon split and transferred to A2 pulley or radial collateral ligament of little finger
Proximal phalanx flexion (MCP flexion)	ECRL to A2 pulley of fingers (using 4-tailed graft)
Ulnar hand sensibility	Superficial radial nerve translocation or neurocutaneous island
Combined high median and ulnar nerve palsy:	
Thumb adduction (key pinch)	ECRB → APB tendon (see text)
Thumb abduction (opposition)	EIP → EPL tendon around pisiform pulley
Thumb-index tip punch	APL slip → dorsal interosseous tendon + arthrodesis MCP
Transverse metacarpal arch	EDM tendon split and transferred to A2 pulley or radial collateral ligament of little finger
Proximal phalanx flexion (MCP flexion, power grip)	Tenodesis of all four digits with free tendon grafts to extensor apparatus or lateral bands. Else do capsulodesis of volar aspect of MCP
Thumb flexion (IP joint)	Brachioradialis to FPL transfer in forearm
Finger flexion (FDP function)	ECRL to all 4 tendons of FDP + tenodesis of DIP of 3, 4, 5 fingers
Wrist flexion	ECU to FCU transfer
Sensory reconstruction	Superficial radial nerve fillet flap to palm or superficial radial nerve translocation
Combined high ulnar and radial nerve palsy:	
Wrist extension	PT to ECRB
Thumb adduction	Split FDS to 3 (middle finger) to abductor tubercle
Claw fingers (4 and 5)	Other half of split FDS to A2 pulley
Thumb-index tip pinch	Arthrodesis of MCP joint of thumb
Wrist flexion	PL to FCU insertion
Finger and thumb extension	FDS 2,3 to EDC and EPL (through interosseous membrane)
Finger flexion	Tenodesis of FDP 3 to FDP 4 and 5
Volar sensitivity	Median digital nerve translocation
Combined median and radial palsy:	
Forearm pronation	Biceps brachii tendon rerouting around radius
Wrist extension and flexion	Wrist arthrodesis
Finger flexion	Tenodesis of FDP 4, 5 to FDP 2, 3
Finger and thumb extension	FCU to tendons of EDC and EPL
Thumb stability	MCP arthrodesis and tenodese APL tendon to radius
Opposition for thumb	Abductor digiti minimi (ADM) → APB insertion
Thumb flexion	Tenodesis of FPL across thumb IP joint
Radiovolar sensitivity	Ulnar digital nerve translocation

CONCLUSION

- Damage to peripheral nerves is common in limb trauma. Nerve injuries produce complete loss of function resulting in disability of the specific function served.
- Peripheral nerves have ability to regenerate themselves and hence the function can be restored if appropriate repair is undertaken.
- There are various methods to repair the nerves depending on the type of nerve, type of damage, delay, expertise of surgeon, etc. In any case treatment should be undertaken to provide best chance to the patient for obtaining his functional gain.
- In case nerve function cannot be restored, alternative ways of restoring function to the injured limb and minimizing disability to patient are resorted to which mainly comprises of tendon transfers. Thus, the surgeon should evaluate the lost function, function needed and importantly should restore the limb function in such a way that alternative disability is not produced.

SECTION

12

Miscellaneous Topics

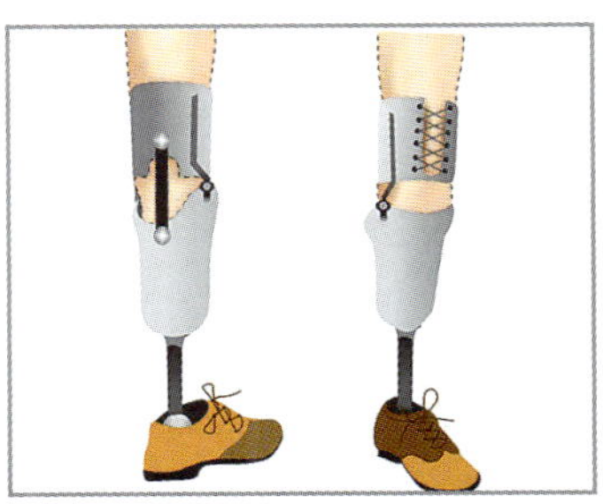

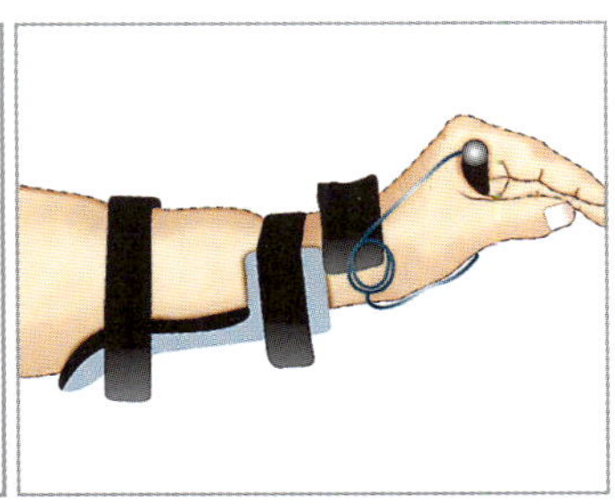

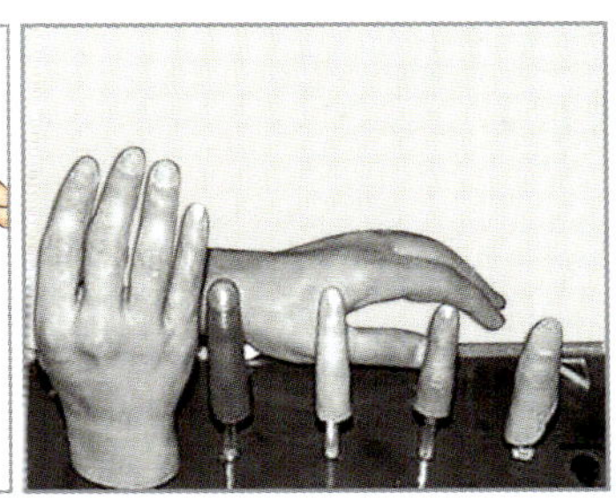

CHAPTER 121

Amputations and Rehabilitation

S Pavan

AMPUTATIONS

INTRODUCTION

"Amputation is a surgical procedure for removal of part or the whole of a limb". This procedure has been around for a long time. One of the earliest records of the procedure is in 1st century CE where use of cautery for large vessels (Celsus), first mention of ligatures and removal of gangrenous extremity through the viable tissue edge with a bone-cut shorter than the soft tissues are mentioned. Worldwide prevalence is difficult to estimate due to limited data from developing countries. The estimated number of people with major limb loss in the United States (no Indian data available) in 2005 was about 664,000 and for minor limb loss it was about 900,000 (Ziegler-Graham et al.). This number is expected to rise to about 58,000 per year by 2030 (Cutson and Bongiorni; Fletcher et al.) with most of it occurring in those aged 65 years and older (Clark et al.). In children, congenital deformity and trauma are the leading causes. In young adults' trauma and older population, vascular dysfunction is the main cause **(Figs. 1 and 2)**.

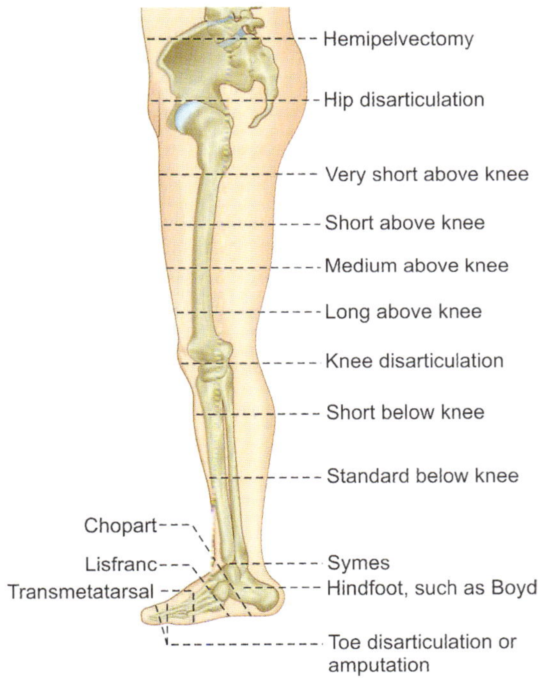

Fig. 1: Lower limb amputation levels.

INDICATIONS AND PRINCIPLES

We can group them into easy-to-remember format as follows:

- *Dead limb:* Ischemic limb, wet and dry gangrene, and frostbite.
- *Dying limb:* Traumatic nonreconstructable limb (crush injury), thermal trauma, electrical burns and vascular disorders like Berger's disease and generalized atherosclerosis.
- *Deadly limb:* Malignancy and acute spreading infections (necrotizing fasciitis and gas gangrene).
- *Damn useless:* Congenital deficiencies, poorly reconstructed limb following trauma or malignancy that are actually functionally hindering. Here, it is deemed that the prosthetic replacement will provide better function than the useless counterpart.
- *Damn painful: Complex regional pain syndrome* (CRPS) and neuropathic limb.
- *Damn nuisance:* Diabetic foot and neuropathic joint (Charcot's or Syphilis). Here the primary disease and its sequel are so dramatically unmanageable that it is better to part away the affected limb.

The only "absolute indication" for amputation is an ischemic limb where revascularization is not possible.

Amputation is ethically unacceptable and is usually the last resort measure for different ailments as it is associated with a high degree of morbidity and mortality along with psychological trauma. Thirty-day mortality rates range from 6.3% to 42.3%. Some studies report up to 25% mortality in patients with lower limb amputations within 2 months and nearly 40% within 1 year. The 1-year survival following lower limb amputation ranges from 50% to 80% depending on the amputation level. Therefore, the procedure should be performed by an experienced team keeping certain objectives and principles in mind.

Amputation is not a destructive procedure and should not be construed as a mutilating one instead it is a "reconstructive

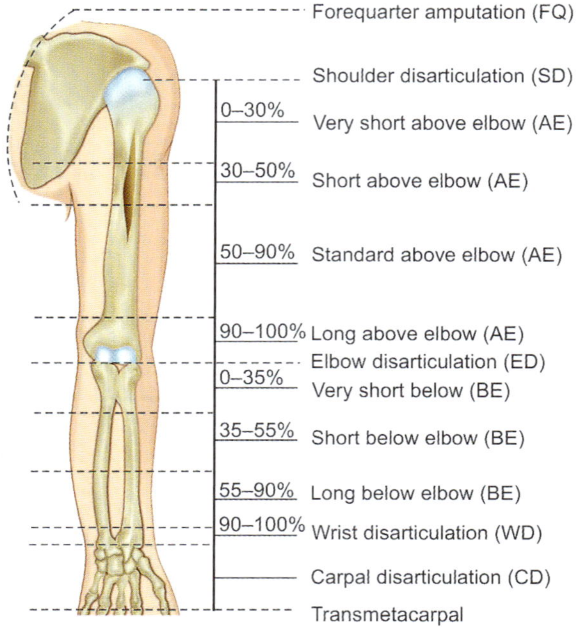

Fig. 2: Upper limb amputation levels.

procedure" that removes the incurable disease improving the function and reducing morbidity drastically. The amputation should provide a physiological end organ for further prosthetic fitting. Hence, the surgery should be done with the following objectives in mind.

- *Adequate length of stump:* Enough to get a reasonably good prosthetic fit
- Rapid tissue healing
- Maximum function of the residual limb
- Rehabilitation of the whole person

These objectives can be achieved by following certain "principles of amputation surgery" which can be broadly divided into surgical techniques, dressing techniques, immediate postoperative prosthesis and physiotherapy, pain management, and rehabilitation.

SURGICAL TECHNIQUE

- *Clean operative field:* The procedure should be performed through tissues that are not infected using all aseptic techniques. In case of open wounds, the surface through which the amputation plane will pass should be covered by healthy red granulation tissue or ideally should be fully healed.
- *Tourniquet:* Tourniquet should be used in all cases as it reduces surgical time, makes the surgery less traumatic and bloodless and makes identification of muscles, nerves, and vessels easier. In ischemic limbs though it can cause further hypoxic damage to already compromised tissues so they should be avoided. Ex-sanguination of limb before application of tourniquet should not be done in cases on malignancy and infection to prevent proximal dissemination.
- *Skin flap:* The greatest skin length possible should be maintained for muscle coverage and a tension-free closure. Skin should be mobile, sensate, and of adequate thickness. Scars adherent to underlying tissue and having redundant tissue and "dog ears" should be avoided. With modern day prosthesis, the location of the scar is not important but if possible, the following principles should be used:
  - *Equal anterior posterior flaps:* Above wrist, mid-thigh, and below knee.
  - *Long posterior flap (skewed flap):* Ischemic limbs, Syme's amputation, and toe amputations.
  - *Long anterior flap:* Below wrist and distal end femur.
  - *Racquet incision:* Hip and shoulder disarticulation, fore, and hind quarter amputations.
  - The other special types of flaps that can be used as per the condition of the limb are sagittal and skewed flaps.
  - *Free vascularized or Scandinavian flaps (equal medial and lateral flaps):* Sometimes, the local tissues are insufficient to provide adequate cover and in order to preserve the length of limb and avoid a more proximal amputation a free vascularized graft having skin, subcutaneous fat, and even muscle can be used. It is preferred for stump coverage over a split thickness graft as it is sensate and has a higher resistance to breakdown under the prostheses.
- *Muscles*: The muscles are divided just distal approximately 5 cm to the bone cut. Separation of muscles from overlying skin should be avoided as far as possible. Muscles are stabilized either by "myodesis" (i.e., muscle sutured through drill holes in bone) or by "myoplasty" (i.e., antagonistic muscle and fascia groups sutured together). Both these techniques should be done under appropriate tension and bulky muscles over stump should be avoided. In "cineplastic amputation" the muscles and tendons in the stump are arranged so that they can perform independent movements and communicate motion to a especially constructed prosthetic apparatus. This is done by forming a flap in form of a tube covered by skin through which a percutaneous endoscopic gastrostomy is inserted.
- *Nerves:* Nerves should be cut under tension and allowed to retract proximally to the end of the bone where there is no scar and tension. In this way, the chance of neuromas formation will be less and there will also be reduced potential for irritation and pain. Large nerves, which have vessels along with them should be tied.
- *Blood vessels:* Separation and tying of the larger arteries and veins individually prevents the formation of arteriovenous fistulas and aneurysms.
- *Bone:* Osteophytes or bone prominences around the joint that has been disarticulated are removed and filed. The edges are beveled to reduce irritation and pressure over the stump when a prosthesis is worn or direct weight is borne on the stump end. Diaphyseal transections can be covered with a local flexible osteoperiosteal graft to close the medullary canal and provide a better end bearing stump. This is known as osteoplasty.
- *Open amputations:* The amputation in which the stump is left open is called an open amputation. It is

always done in presence of established or potential infection. It is of two types—Open circular amputation also known as guillotine amputation or it can be an open amputation with flaps designed for closure but left open. In open circular amputation, the aim is to produce a slightly concave open cross-section with skin slightly longer than superficial muscle which is slightly longer than deep muscle and finally bone which is cut shortest. Skin traction applied postoperatively helps to prevent retraction of skin and muscles and after 6–8 weeks the scar is excised and final closure of stump is done. Skin traction should be avoided in ischemic limbs. In these limbs, a better plan is to invert the skin margin and suture this to underlying subcutaneous fascia at the base of the flaps with nonabsorbable sutures. The sutures can be removed and the margins unrolled at the time of secondary closure. This type of amputation is not generally recommended now except in cases of emergencies where the amputation needs to be performed with minimal shock and surgical time. Even in case of infection it is preferred to plan the open amputation in such a way that the flaps are designed at the time of the primary procedure, and then they can be closed as soon as wound condition permits without waiting for 6–8 weeks.

- *Revision amputation:* The same principles that are applied for primary amputation are also true for revision. When a primary amputation fails or is unsuitable for a prosthesis or does not serve the functional requirement of the patient, a revision is required. Out of these indications the advances in prosthetic devices have made limbs that were earlier difficult to fit, and fitable with a reasonably functional device. Pain is another cause for revision but there should be a clearly identified etiology. Some causes of pain that can be treated surgically are extra tissue, skin folds, painful scars, bony prominences or spurs, heterotopic ossification, unsuccessful myodesis, symptomatic neuromas, and chronic skin conditions like epidermoid cysts and skin breakdown or ulceration. Phantom pain does not respond well to surgical treatment.
- *Level of amputation:* As much of the limb that is consistent with good function should be preserved. At the same time care should be taken to perform the amputation through healthy tissue to avoid revisions which delay the rehabilitation of the patient. For above knee amputations usually a length of 18–20 cm is left below the greater trochanter. For below knee amputation minimum working length for prosthetic fitting is 9 cm so length >12 cm (ideally 15 cm) is required. Smaller stumps (<6 cm) are more of a pain due to improper prosthetic fitting and ultimately rely on hip muscles for mobilization so should be avoided. One quick guide is to make a limb 2.5 cm long from knee joint for every 30 cm of body height. For ischemic limbs, a higher level of 10–12.5 cm below the joint line is used because making limbs longer than this can interfere with prosthetic use and design. Above elbow amputations do well with arm length of 20 cm while below elbow amputations function well with length 15–18 cm distal to olecranon. There are various proposed advantages for adequately preserved limbs with "good length" stumps:
    - Ethically preserve as much tissue as possible
    - Higher acceptability and better compliance
    - Functionality is better with less energy consumption.

In any case, modern prosthetic fitting compensates short limb length and the current standard for level of amputation is status of vascularity at the deemed site of amputation. The assessment should be judged clinically and supplemented by investigation(s) as per institutional policy for minimizing wound-related complications.

Assessment of ischemic limb: The level of amputation that is chosen must have enough arterial supply to promote healing. This is determined by clinical criteria and vascular studies.

- *Clinical criteria:* Warm skin, hair growth, capillary filling and absence of dependent rubor and venous filling time of <25 seconds are indicators of a good vascular supply and a good potential to heal. A palpable pulse proximal to the chosen level of amputation will almost always give full healing. In reverse the absence of a palpable pulse does not always lead to failed wound healing but the revision rates may be higher.
- *Vascular studies:* The vascular assessment of the limb can be performed by various methods as follows:
    - *Arteriography:* Though invasive, it is the gold standard as good flow distally is an irrefutable sign of perfusion of all tissues.
    - *Doppler ultrasonography:* It is a study that can be used to calculate arterial pressure. A waveform is created, the area under which is a measure of flow. In some patients with peripheral vascular disease (PVD), calcified arteries may give false high readings. A measure of 70 mm Hg is thought to be required for wound healing.

The various parameters used at different places are as follows:

- *Ischemic index (II):* The ratio of pressure at the level chosen for amputation to the brachial systolic pressure. It should be 0.5 or greater for good wound healing.
- *Ankle-brachial index:* It is the ratio of pressure at the ankle level to the brachial systolic pressure. It should be 0.45 or more for good healing to take place beyond the ankle.
- *Toe-brachial index:* When an abnormally high ankle-brachial index or ABI is detected (>1.3) it is thought to be due plaque and calcification of the arteries due atherosclerosis commonly found in diabetic patients. In such cases, a "toe-brachial index" is performed. If it is below 0.65 it indicates reduced blood flow to the small vessels in the big toe.
- *Finger-brachial index:* Finger/Brachial index normal >0.75.
- *Wrist-brachial index:* Normal value >0.63.

Transcutaneous oxygen pressure: It is a noninvasive test which is supposed to be a reliable and sensitive indicator of wound healing. In this, the partial pressure of oxygen diffusing through the skin is measured. It can be measured at any place where the skin is intact and is a measure of the oxygen-delivering capacity. False low readings may be seen in areas of edema and cellulitis. The measurements are commonly made at the chest, above knee, below knee (10 cm proximal and distal to patella) and on dorsum of foot. Values less than 20 mm Hg indicate poor healing potential. Oxygen tension of at least 26 mm Hg result in good rate of successful healing and values >40 mm Hg indicate acceptable wound-healing potential. These values have around 88% sensitivity and an 84% specificity rate.

Plethysmography: Preceded ultrasound in the evaluation of lower extremity ischemia. Plethysmography is based on the detection of volume changes in the limb in response to arterial inflow. In addition to volume flow, the basic technology can be modified to produce pulse waveforms and determine digital pressures. Mercury strain gauge plethysmography, air plethysmography (pulse volume recordings), and photo-plethysmography all have been used clinically. But neither calf nor foot blood flows at rest differ between normal subjects and patients with even rather severe degrees of arterial insufficiency therefore have been replaced by other more accurate tests.

Fluorescein dye test: Skin perfusion can be assessed using fluorescein. Fluorescein sodium (4–8 mg/kg), a nonradioactive tracer dye, is injected and 20 minutes following the injection skin is observed under ultraviolet or blue light. Following intravenous injection, the dye distributes to all perfused tissues by diffusing across capillary walls. When excited by ultraviolet or blue light, fluorescein molecules fluoresce and well-perfused tissues which have acquired the dye appear yellow green. Unstained nonperfused tissues simply reflect the blue light. This can also be used intraoperative.

Laser: Induced fluorescence of indocyanine green (ICG) is a new method for evaluating skin perfusion, which is superior to conventional fluorescein angiography.

Radioactive xenon-133: Xenon-133 has gained wide acceptance as an indicator of the perfusion of various organs, including kidneys, brains, and heart. Several investigators have used the clearance from the skin of Xenon-133, intradermally or epicutaneously applied, to quantitate skin blood flow. Following injection the xenon activity is monitored using a gamma camera. Rate meters and strip chart recorders are then used to measure the washout of xenon-133 from the skin. A skin blood flow above 1 mL/100 g of tissue/min, measured with 133Xe is indicative of good vascularity.

Technetium-99m (^{99m}Tc) pyrophosphate bone scanning: It can be used in cases of burns, electric shocks, frostbite, etc. as a predictor of vascularity of the limb. This test has 94% sensitivity rate and a 100% specificity rate for marking viable tissues from nonviable tissues.

Near infrared spectroscopy: It is another noninvasive method that can be applied on skin flaps intraoperatively to assess perfusion. The ratio of oxyhemoglobin ($HgbO_2$) and deoxyhemoglobin (Hgb) is measured (StO_2) and a noninvasive, real-time measurement of tissue pO_2 is obtained. A spectroscope is used to take the measurements.

DRESSING TECHNIQUE

A good postoperative dressing ensures rapid tissue healing, relief from pain and good stump maturation without contractures.

There are four types of postoperative dressings:
1. Soft dressing
2. Semirigid dressing
3. Rigid dressing
4. Compressive bandage dressing

A good postoperative dressing has the following advantages:
- Ensures rapid tissue healing
- Relief from pain
- Good stump maturation without contractures

Rigid postoperative dressings in the form of postoperative slab or rarely casts are quite popular. They allow immediate postsurgical prosthesis to be worn and a more rapid rehabilitation. The disadvantages of rigid dressing are:
- It is technically more demanding.
- If applied wrongly can lead to ischemia of stump.
- It inhibits frequent stump inspection.
- Consumes OT time.

The application of rigid dressing follows the same principles that are used for cast application. Use of soft felt padding to protect bony prominences, protection of skin with stockinette, avoiding excessive pressure and ensuring a snug fit. A simple compression bandage is more forgiving in the inexperienced hand and wound inspection is easier **(Fig. 3)**.

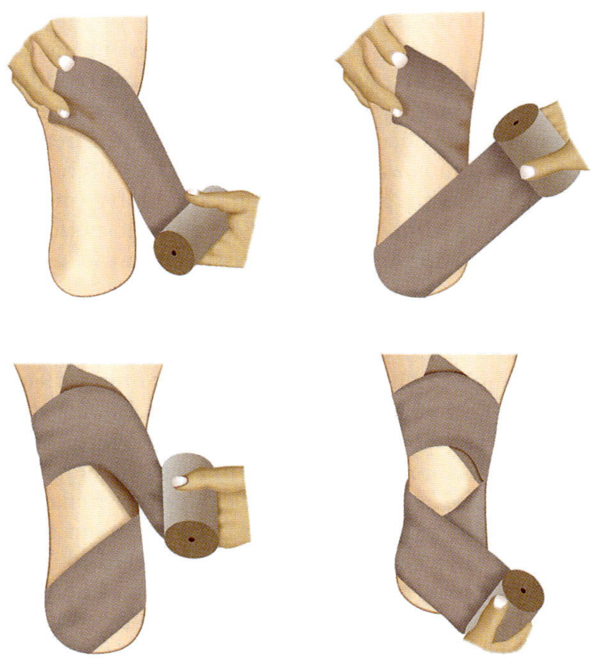

Fig. 3: Compression bandage.

IMMEDIATE POSTOPERATIVE PROSTHESIS AND PHYSIOTHERAPHY

Immediate postoperative prosthetic fitting has many advantages especially when it is done in combined care of prosthetist, rehabilitative medicine, and physiotherapist. This phase begins at the time of injury and continues until all wounds have successfully closed and are free of infection. The length of time spent in this phase varies depending on the extent of the patient's injury.

A very important part of this rehabilitation is the fitting of "pylon prosthesis". Pylon prosthesis is also called endoskeletal prosthesis which means the internal (endo-) structure of prosthesis and has no relation to osteointegrated prosthesis. The prosthesis used initially is made of plaster and is contoured proximally but resembles a plug fit. This socket is gradually replaced by a total-contact quadrilateral socket of plaster that is hand molded over the stump and elongated by a crutch and suspended by a waist belt and/or a shoulder strap. The initial period of standing is limited to minimal touch down weight bearing. The patient stands on a scale to get a feel of the pressure to apply. Usually around 20 pounds of pressure is encouraged. Pressure in excess of 40 pounds can compromise wound healing. This endoskeletal structure can be carried forward to provide or construct a definitive prosthesis. The advantages of pylon prosthesis are:

- Immediately after surgery limb elevation prevents edema.
- Active and passive limb mobilization to prevent contractures is started as soon as pain permits.
- Immediate upright posture and ambulation with support with fitting of temporary prosthesis is encouraged for both physiological and psychological wellbeing of the patient. This encourages early gait training and walking.
- When managing an amputee acutely, the rehabilitation goals are to promote healing of the residual limb wound; achieve independence in self-feeding, toileting and oral hygiene; and provide the client and family education on the rehabilitation process.
- Patients and family members are introduced to rehabilitative and prosthetic services in the early stage of this phase.
- Eases patient's and family member's fears, provides support throughout the grieving and recovery processes, and engages the patient and family with the rehabilitative team.
- The possible other advantages are:
  - Faster stump maturation due to edema subsidence and wound healing
  - Reduction of postoperative pain
  - May help to save knee joint in amputations done for peripheral vascular disease.

Immediate postoperative prosthetic fitting requires specialized cooperation between the surgeon, prosthetic specialist, and physical rehabilitation specialist. Amateur process can lead to unacceptable consequences:

- The prosthesis socket needs continuous refurbishment as it gets loosened with reduction in edema of the wound.
- The prosthesis is a bit heavy and not very esthetic looking; may impede walking and psychologically unacceptable.
- With a weak and loose cast, socket-pistoning effect may ensue on the stump consequently increasing edema and wound dehiscence.
- Interestingly with early fitting some authors have reported muscle atrophy due to differential stimulation of a group of muscles required for ambulation while inhibition of others.

PAIN MANAGEMENT

A common symptom after limb amputation is pain. It can be caused by multiple factors. It can be divided into immediate postoperative pain or a more chronic pain persisting for a long time after the amputation. This chronic pain includes residual limb pain or phantom limb pain. There may be musculoskeletal pain (low back, hip, and knee pain) due to altered biomechanics. Treatment is done by a combination of pharmacological and nonpharmacological means based on the type and severity of pain. Another cause of pain after amputations is bruising of the limb, chafing, or rubbing of the skin due to an ill-fitting prosthesis. Other common causes are ischemia, heterotopic ossification, or post-amputation neuromas.

Phantom Pain

The term "phantom limb" was first coined by American neurologist l Silas Weir Mitchell in 1871. It occurs in the missing or amputated part of the limb or some part of it.

- Phantom limb "sensation" occurs in almost all amputees. In many patients, this sensation will fade with time—and there is no pain experienced.
- This is distinguished from the syndrome of phantom limb pain: A chronic pain occurring in some smaller subset of patients. Some patients experience "jactitation"—distressing phantom limb pain with involuntary jerking of stump.

Phantom pain is experienced by approximately 30–40% of patients and may be constant in one-third of them (Desmond and MacLachlan). Abnormal sensations like tingling, warmth, cold, cramping, or constriction are felt by most amputees in the missing limb and sometimes may persist throughout life.

Pathophysiology

No single theory can explain the pathophysiology of phantom limb pain and all have some supporting data. The suspected causes are peripheral due to injury to nerve, spinal due to changes that take place in the spinal cord leading to abnormal sensation and central caused by some mechanism in the brain.

The peripheral causes that can lead to phantom sensations are regeneration of the injured nerves, changes in the ion channel at the injured site and neuroma formation.

Spinal: The loss of inputs to the spine from the amputated part leads to abnormal signals in the spinal cord called "deafferentation".

Central: Similar changes due to loss of input from the amputated limb take place in the cortex and thalamus, sometimes psychological changes like stress and depression may cause such pain. After loss of input from the amputated limb to the brain it tries to "re-wire" its existing pathways by growing new cells leading to functional reorganization of somatotopic maps in the primary somatosensory cortex. The process or reorganization starts immediately after the amputation and goes on for several years. The neurons that lose their original inputs start responding to stimulus from other body parts.

Treatment

Phantom sensation should be considered normal and treated only if it becomes disruptive to functional activities.

Nonsurgical Techniques

- Local therapy in form of relaxation techniques, massage of the amputation area, and biofeedback to reduce muscle tension.
- Nerve blocks, regional blocks, intrathecal or epidural opioids, sympathetic blocks and electrical nerve stimulators have also been tried with limited effectiveness. There is not a single technique that works all the time or even most of the time. More radical therapy has been suggested and undertaken which involves ablation of various parts of the nervous system—whether in the brain or spinal cord.
- The use of a mirror box in which the uninvolved side is visually reflected as the missing side, has been shown to decrease phantom limb pain in some cases by Dr Ramachandran and colleagues.

Surgical Techniques

- Removal of neuromas if identified as cause of pain.
- Deep brain stimulation is a surgical technique used to alleviate patients from phantom limb pain. Prior to surgery, patients undergo functional brain imaging techniques such as *positron emission tomography* (PET) scan and functional magnetic resonance imaging (MRI) to determine an appropriate trajectory of where pain is originating. This is followed by electrode implantation.

REHABILITATION

The rehabilitation is aimed to achieve specific goals in an amputee with regard to:

- Rapid wound healing
- Prevention of contractures
- Maintaining flexibility of the residual limb
- Restoring strength of residual limb
- Early return to ambulation and independent living

Rehabilitation after amputation is multidisciplinary and requires coordinated effort of multiple specialties. It aims to improve the individual's mobility and health and also their vocational capabilities. One classification of the process is Time, Place, and Type (TPT) framework which organizes the rehabilitation processes according to timing, place, and types of service (Steinman et al. 2008).

The timeline of rehabilitation denotes the start of the process of rehabilitation from the initial surgery till the rehabilitation process ends. It can even begin before surgery or the onset of disability in cases of planned amputations. Preoperatively, it consists of psychological support and explaining future services and requirements. In the immediate postoperative period, rehabilitation aims to prevent deconditioning and joint contractures. Later rehabilitation would consist of training, activities of daily living, and vocational training.

Place denotes where rehabilitation takes place and includes services given as inpatient, outpatient or at nursing homes or home. The area where the rehabilitation process takes is important to achieve a quality outcome. Environment modifications and architectural design are just as important as biomedical inputs because the mobility of an amputee is not only dependent on prosthetics but also on a friendly environment which facilitates their movement, like ramps, low floor buses, etc.

"Type" of rehabilitation approximates what is done for the patient. Type can either focus on the detailed or center more broadly on the integration of amputees into the society. This involves making their life more meaningful by making them active contributors to society by vocational training and return to physical and economical independent lives.

COMPLICATIONS OF AMPUTATION SURGERY

Like all other surgical procedures, amputations are met with complication and surprisingly they are common. Some complications are general surgical complications while a lot are unique to this disfiguring surgery. A lot I believe are possibly due to the fact that this surgery is performed not uncommonly by the junior most residents in the department and often unsupervised. There should be a rising concern to this fact and with proper acceptance of this surgery as a "reconstructive" procedure rather than a mutilating one, senior surgeons with adequate experience should at least supervise.

Early

- Wound hematoma
- Skin flap breakdown and wound dehiscence
- Proximal myonecrosis and wound extension especially in PVD patients
- Infection (especially in diabetics), one should be wary of clostridial infection secondary to perineal contamination.
- Neuralgic pain due to excessive pulling of nerves while transecting or formation of neuroma, wound pain, phantom sensation, and phantom pain
- *Skin complications:*
  - Skin maceration
  - Blisters
  - Abrasion

Late

- Phantom sensation and phantom pain
- Joint contracture and instability

- Pain due to pressure of ill-fitting socket causing impingement and neuroma
- Flabby and unstable soft tissue stump due to excessive soft tissue at stump or failure to perform myodesis
- *Skin complications:*
  - Verrucous hyperplasia
  - Fungal infection
  - Skin atrophy
  - Callosities
  - Follicular hyperkeratosis **(Fig. 4)**
  - Allergic reactions to material of cup or liner
- *Bone spur formation:* Due to periosteal bone formation
- Osteoporosis and fracture of bone

LOWER LIMB AMPUTATIONS

Toe Amputations

For the first and fifth toe, a racquet-shaped incision is given over medial or lateral border of foot with equal anterior and posterior flaps favoring the thick planter skin. If required part of metatarsal too can be removed through the same incision. The middle toes can be removed by a similar racquet incision placed on the dorsum of foot.

Ray Amputation

This involves removal of one or more of the metatarsals along with the toes. It is usually required for a tropic ulcer on the planter aspect. The incision is placed on dorsum of foot and the terminal part of the incision is made into racquet shape to include the ulcer. Dissection is carried dorsal to plantar wards.

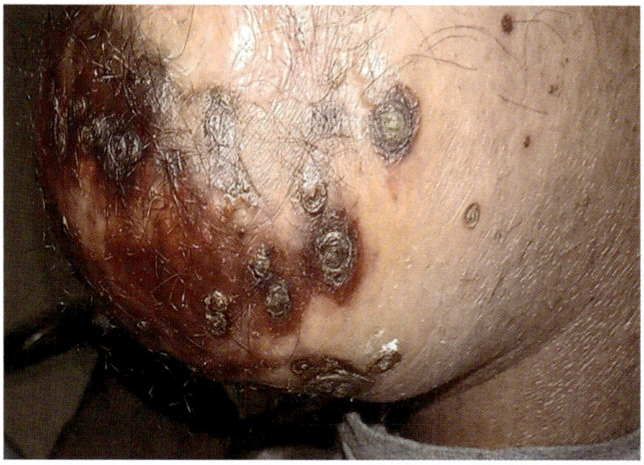

Fig. 4: The skin complications are not uncommon in amputation stump and may even arise several days after complete healing of the stump.

The removal of toes seldom causes any significant gait disturbance, except during fast walking where toe-off phase is lost. Removal of middle toes/ray may cause severe hallux valgus deformity. Squatting and tip toeing are severely affected. No special prosthetics are required except for shoe fillers.

Transmetatarsal Amptutation and Metatarsophalangeal Disarticulation

A long posterior and short anterior flap is made. The degree of gait disturbance depends on the level. The more proximal the level the greater is the gait disturbance. But, no special prosthesis is required except shoe fillers **(Figs. 5A and B)**.

Mid Foot Amputations

The Lisfranc amputation is carried out through the tarsometatarsal joints **(Fig. 6)**, whereas the Chopart amputation is a disarticulation through the talonavicular and calcaneocuboid joints **(Fig. 7)**. Both amputations sacrifice the insertions of the muscles that aid in the extension of the ankle joint; therefore, the anterior tibial tendon, the toe extensors, and the peroneal tendons must be reinserted into the tarsal bones. Even so, dorsiflexion of the ankle joints often is inadequate, requiring a transcutaneous Achilles tenotomy. These levels of amputations are less desirable than a transmetatarsal amputation, as the stump has a tendency to develop an equinus posture over time. The Chopart amputation is the highest level of amputation of the foot that allows the possibility of fitting with a shoe and shoe filler; however, frequently the patient prefers a formal prosthesis because the shoe is unstable.

AMPUTATIONS AROUND ANKLE

Boyd Amputation and Pirogoff Amputation

Both these amputation involve fusion of part of calcaneum to distal end of tibia to create a weight-bearing stump wherein the amputee can walk without prosthesis. In Boyd, the tuber of calcaneum is used **(Fig. 8)** and in Pirogoff, the anterior two-thirds of calcaneum is fused to the distal tibia. The heel pad is then shifted distally for weight-bearing. Posterior flap

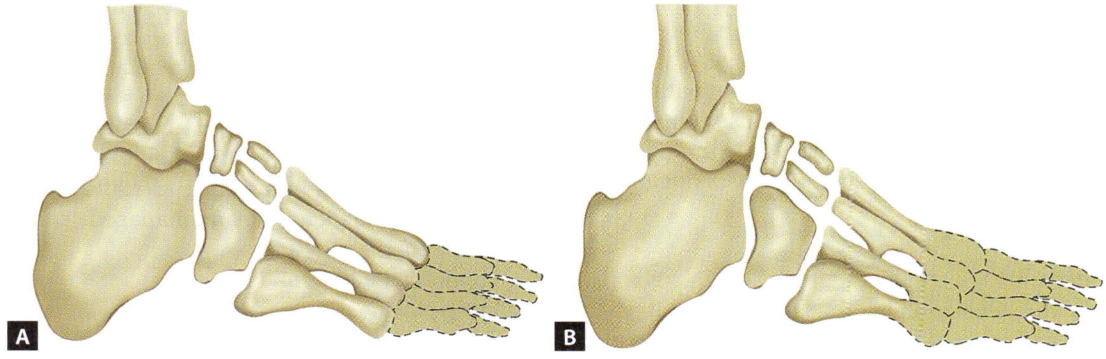

Figs. 5A and B: (A) Metatarsophalangeal disarticulation; (B) Transmetatarsal amputation.

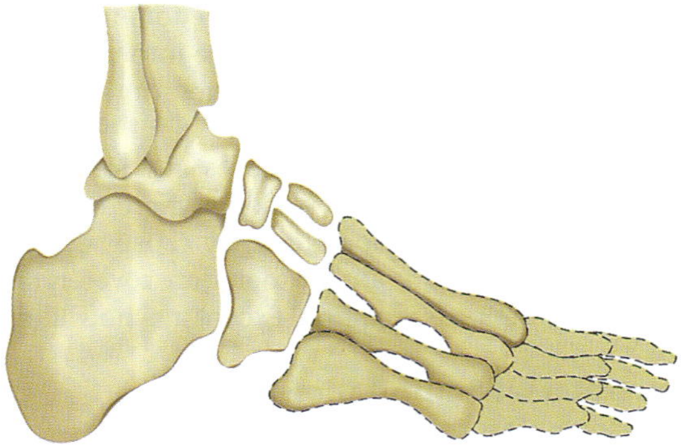

Fig. 6: Lisfranc amputation.

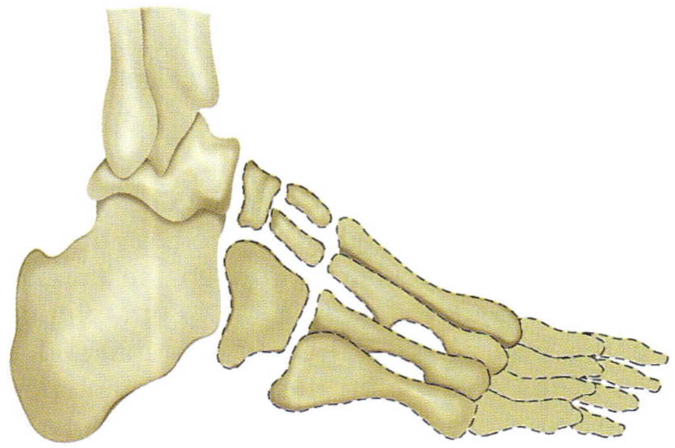

Fig. 7: Chopart amputation.

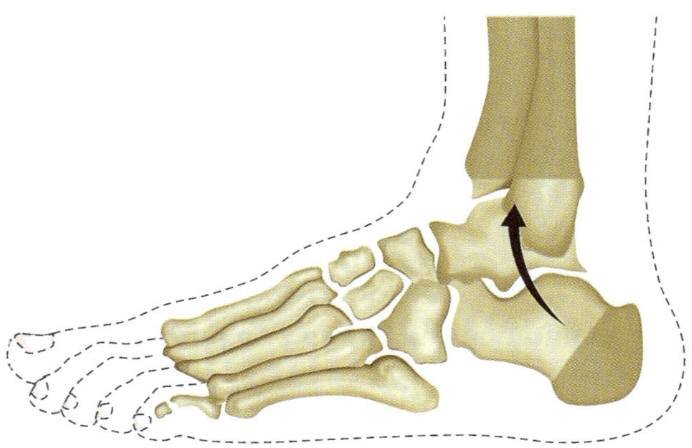

Fig. 8: Boyd amputation.

is designed longer and care is taken to preserve the posterior tibial vessels. The heel pad should be shifted along with the calcaneum avoiding undermining and finally a Steinmann pin is used to fix the calcaneum to the denuded undersurface of tibia. Both these amputations give a longer stump and the migration of heel pad which is a problem with Syme's amputation is prevented. But because of fusion involved it is technically more demanding. Of the two techniques, Boyd is the most common; Pirogoff's technique does not give any added advantage.

Symes Amputation

This involves disarticulation at the ankle joint. It is the amputation of choice in children as it leaves the distal tibial epiphysis intact. The anterior incision is at the level of the ankle joint and the posterior flap is kept longer so that the heel pad is mobilized anteriorly to the distal tibia. Anterior tibial vessels are ligated and care is taken not to damage the posterior tibial vessels. Calcaneum is removed by sharp dissection from the heel pad. The blood supply to the heel pad must be carefully preserved. Both the malleoli are resected at the level of the dome of talus. This cut must be taken parallel to the ground and not at 90° to the tibial plane. The heel pad is mobilized over distal stump of tibia and can be stabilized by one of the following methods:

- By attaching the extensor tendons to the flap
- By tying the flap to the bone by drilling holes
- By fixing the pad by K-wires
- By leaving a sliver of calcaneum attached which fuses to the tibia.

Skin tags left after the procedure should not be removed as it compromises the supply of the heel pad. They disappear as the stump matures. A special bulky prosthesis needs to be worn to accommodate the distal tibial flare. Though this prosthesis is not esthetic, it provides a better ambulation than a transtibial amputation.

"Sarmiento's modification" of Syme's amputation partially reduces this complication by trimming tibia 1.3 cm from the ankle joint thus reducing the distal radial flare.

Wagner's modification: In this, the amputation is carried out in two stages. In the first stage, only the disarticulation is done and the heel flap is closed over a drain. After the infection subsides then the malleoli are removed and final stump fashioned. The incidence of flap necrosis and infection is less with this two-stage procedure.

Symes amputations will not heal without palpable posterior artery pulse and in the past Syme's amputation was avoided in ischemic limbs because of the high rate of flap necrosis, but with the advent of newer imaging techniques like Doppler ultrasound measurement of segmental blood pressures, radioactive xenon clearance tests, and transcutaneous oxygen the success rate of the Syme's amputation in these limbs has significantly increased.

Transtibial Amputation

This is probably the most common amputation performed in the lower limb. The ideal site for this amputation is 12–17 cm from the upper end of tibia. A shorter stump makes prosthetic fitment difficult and knee function is reduced. Whereas a longer stump extending to the lower third of leg has greater chances of wound breakdown due to reduced vascularity though a longer stump would give better ambulation.

The skin incision is given about 4 cm from the site of intended bone section and equal anterior and posterior flaps are designed. Skin and fascia are elevated as one unit. The major neurovascular bundles are identified and ligated. Five nerves should be identified and managed:

1. Saphenous
2. Superficial peroneal
3. Deep peroneal
4. Tibial
5. Sural

Nerves should be drawn distally cleanly divided and allowed to retract back away from areas of scar, pressure, and vessels. Three major vessels should identify and ligated. The three major vascular bundles are:

1. Anterior tibial vessels
2. Posterior tibial vessels
3. Peroneal vessels

Muscles are cut proximally to the bone cut and the posterior muscles are attached to the anterior compartment muscles and the anterior periosteum of the tibia. Both myodesis and myoplasty can be used. Sharp bone ends of the tibia are beveled and the fibula is transected 1–2 cm higher than the tibia **(Fig. 9)**.

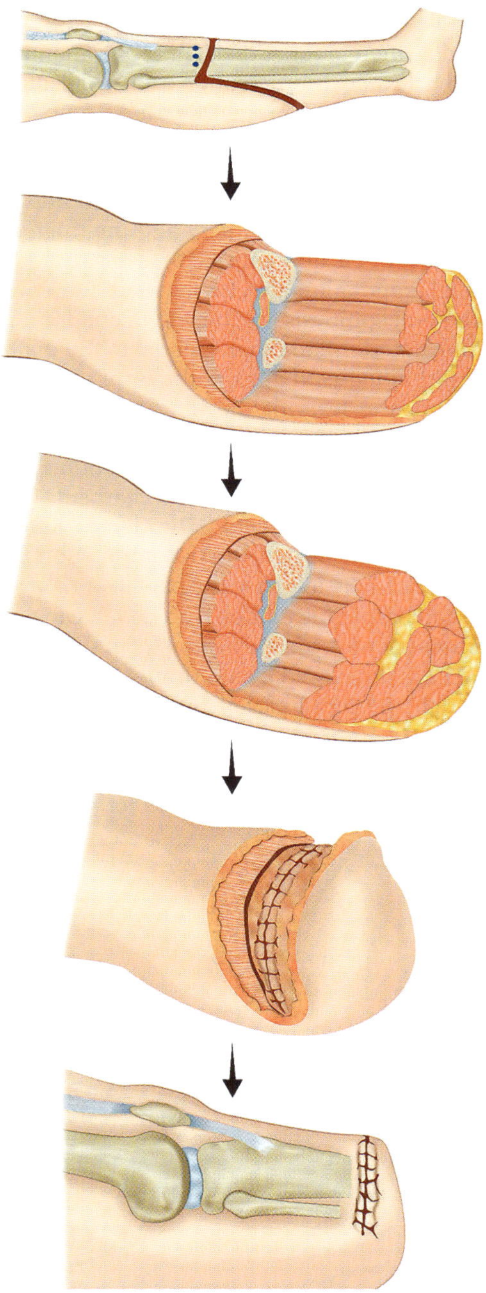

Fig. 9: Transtibial amputation.

In a short stump of 8.8 cm or less, it has been recommended that the entire fibula together with some of the muscle bulk be removed so that the stump may fit more easily into the prosthetic socket. The fibular head can be retained because the modern total-contact socket can obtain a better purchase on the short stump. Transecting the hamstring tendons to allow a short stump to fall deeper into the socket also may be considered.

"Osteoplasty" may be performed to convert the stump to an end-bearing stump. This has the theoretical advantage of better proprioception and gait and is best suited for nonischemic limbs in young vigorous patients. Various procedures are described, the most common being "Ertls" procedure. Technique developed by Dr Janos Ertl in Hungary in the 1920s and first described in the literature in 1939. The procedure is designed to seal the medullary cavity of the tibia and fibula to allow end weight-bearing. Two different techniques can be used to seal the medullary cavity:

1. *Periosteal sleeve:* This created by suturing the periosteum in a flap over the medullary canal and closing the muscle flap over it. A flap consisting of flakes of bone with periosteum from the posterior surface of the tibia is sutured over the tibial osteotomy. This periosteal pouch is filled with bone chips and bone slurry. The open end of fibula can also be sealed in the same way. Covering callous then develops over a few weeks and months.
2. *Bony wedge:* A wedge of bone is fashioned from removed fibula and a bony bridge is created between the tibia and fibula to enhance the end bearing capacity of the stump and to close the medullary canal **(Fig. 10)**. Both techniques can be performed with a long posterior, sagittal, or skewed flap incision.

A lot of modifications have been proposed for specific situations few are discussed below:

Burgess' modification: This is used for ischemic limb. It differs from a traditional amputation in that it is done at a higher level of 10–12 cm from joint line and a long posterior flap is fashioned consisting mainly of the lateral and medial

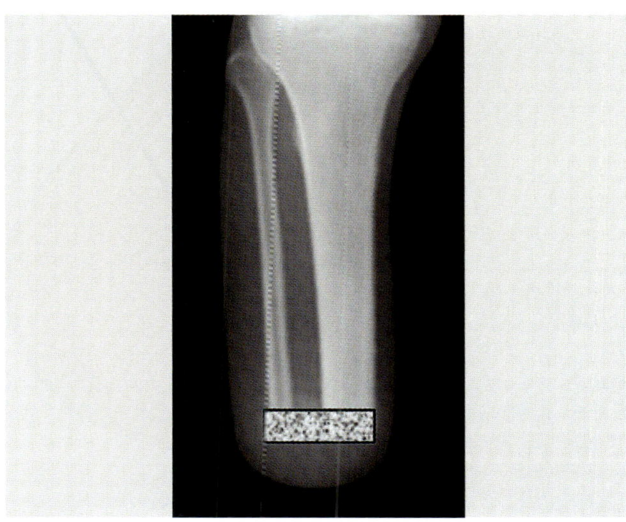

Fig. 10: Ertl's procedure.

gastrocnemius muscle and some soleus **(Fig. 11)**. Debulking the soleus muscle may be required. Tension myodesis is avoided.

Bruckner modification: This is a variation used for ischemic limb. Landmarks and skin incisions are equivalent to the Burgess technique. Fibula disarticulated proximally from the tibia and resected completely. Complete resection of the anterior and lateral compartment muscles and complete resection of the soleus muscle is done. The amputation flap is fashioned from the medial gastrocnemius and the lateral gastrocnemius may be used if required. Closure is same as Burgess.

Sagittal flap: This flap consists of semicircular medial and lateral flaps with apex 1 cm lateral to tibial crest. It was first described by Tracey in 1966. The "tibia" is transacted 13–15 cm from knee joint. At the level of tibial cut the inferior margin of flap measures 13–15 cm and is about quarter circumference of the calf. Laterally, the flap has the anterior and lateral muscles groups with overlying skin and medially it has the medial gastrocnemius and overlying skin. A myoplasty is performed over the end of tibia **(Fig. 12)**.

Skewed flap: The anterior junction of the two flaps is located about 2 cm from the tibial crest and then the posterior junction is fashioned 180° from the anterior junction. It was described by Robsinson et al. in 1982. The dimensions of the skin flaps remain the same as the sagittal technique. A muscle flap of gastrocnemius is used to cover the end of the tibia and fibula, and a myoplasty is performed with the periosteum and deep fascia anteriorly. These anteromedial and posterolateral flaps are closed in an oblique manner so that the scar line runs from anterolateral to posteromedial **(Fig. 13)**.

Medial and lateral flaps of equal length are fashioned in a fish-mouth fashion. Semicircular skin flaps with length one-fourth the circumference around the cut end of the tibia are made and the muscles are closed side-to-side over the cut bone ends **(Fig. 14)**.

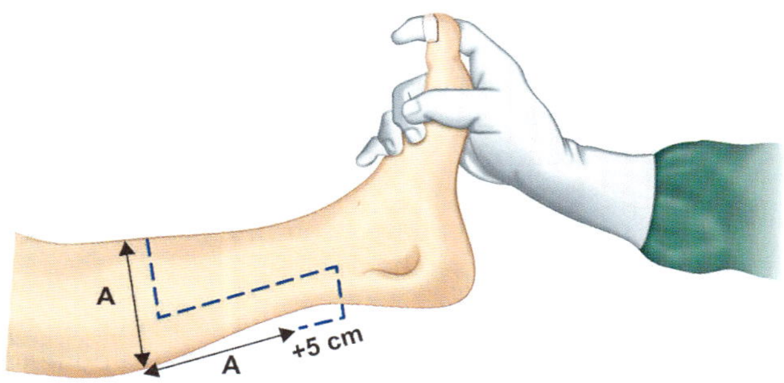

Fig. 11: Burgess technique for ischemic limb.

KNEE DISARTICULATION

In patients where a functional tibial amputation cannot be performed, a knee disarticulation is the procedure of choice. It provides an excellent weight-bearing stump and the distal femoral flare provides suspension to prosthesis. The creation of a long lever arm for muscles to act and stability while sitting for nonambulatory patients are additional benefits. It is relatively a vascular surgery and the thigh muscles are well preserved. Flexion contractures associated with short transtibial amputation are also avoided. Preservation of the distal femoral epiphysis is of benefit in children.

A long anterior flap roughly equal to the diameter of the knee is fashioned with apex at the level of tibial tuberosity and base at the level of the tibial condyles. The shorter posterior flap is half the anterior flap. Dissection is carried out anterior to posterior. The patellar tendon is cut as long as possible. Capsule and collateral ligaments are cut along with the "cruciate ligaments." The nerves and vessels are now identified and ligated and the amputation is competed. No attempt is made to excise the patella or to fuse it. Patellar tendon and hamstring tendons are tied to each other and to the remnant of the cruciate ligaments in the condylar notch and the flaps are closed over a drain **(Fig. 15)**. In case skin cover is tight, posterior part of femoral condyles is excised.

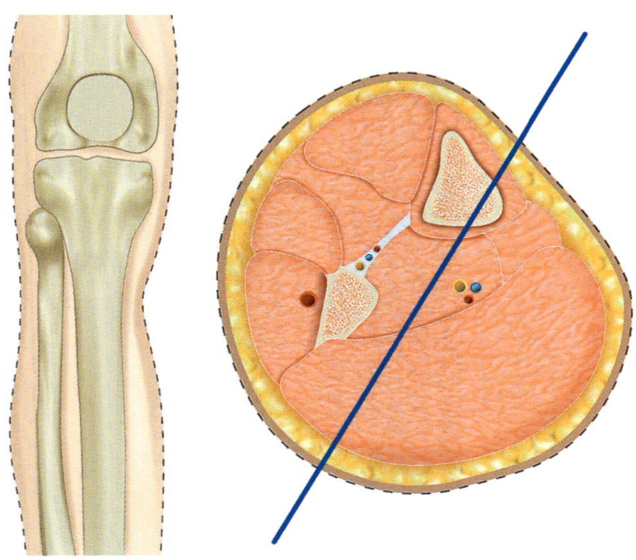

Fig. 12: Sagittal flaps.

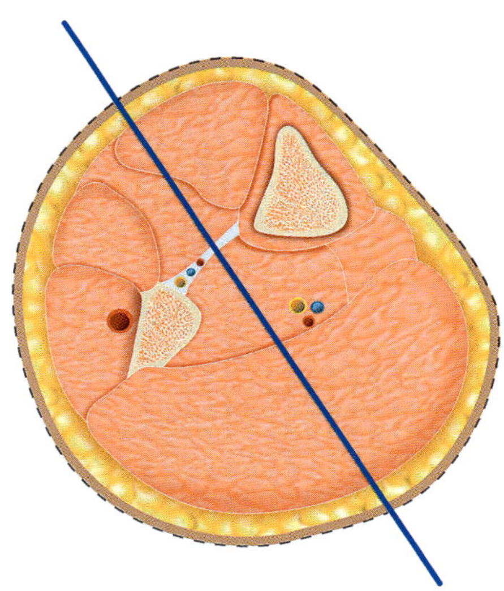

Fig. 13: Skew flaps.

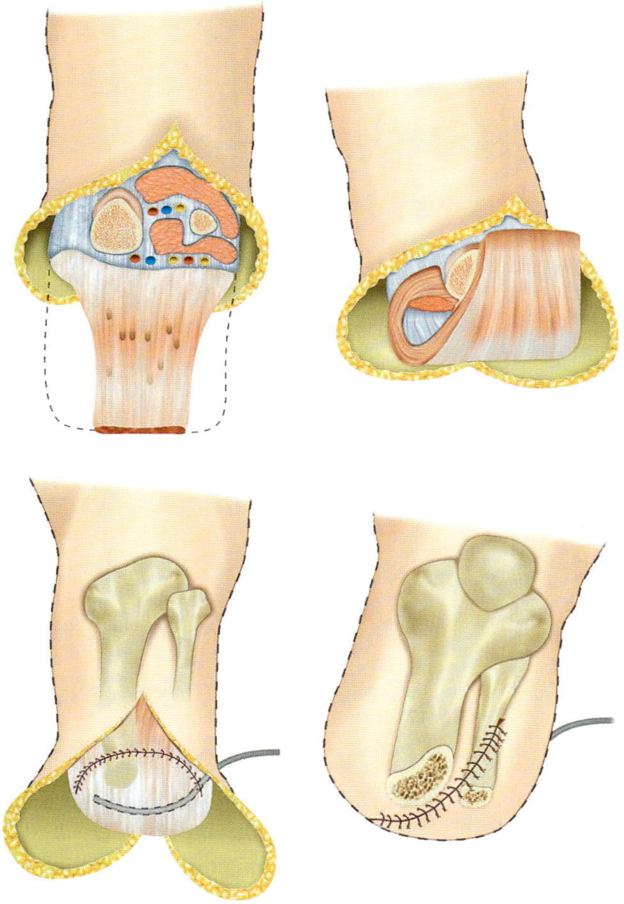

Fig. 14: Robb-Persson modification.

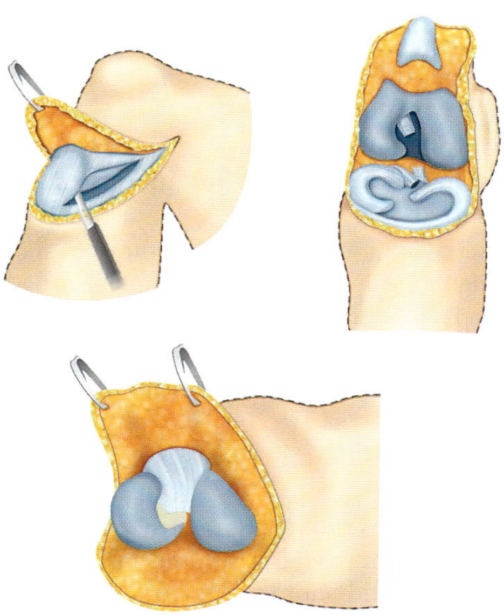

Fig. 15: Knee disarticulation.

Mazet and Hennessy modification: In this anterior, posterior, and lateral part of the femoral condyles are excised to make a less bulky stump. It has the following advantages:

- Easier skin closure in ischemic limbs
- Cosmetically better stump

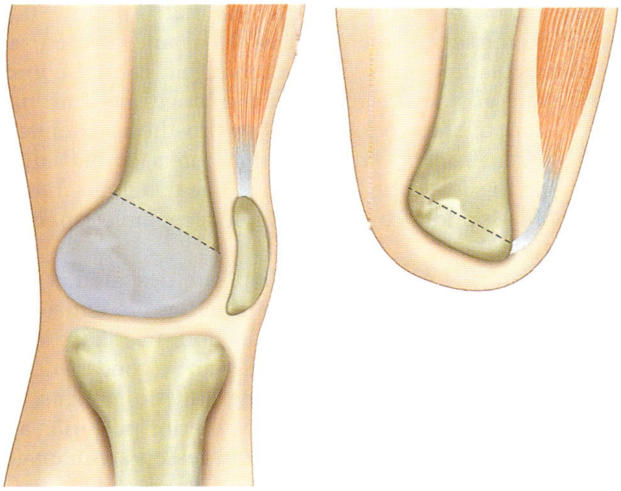

Fig. 16: Gritti-Stokes amputation.

- Application of a suction-type prosthesis that is easier to wear and remove and does not need removal for toileting.

Kjøble modification: A lateral flap that is one half the anteroposterior diameter of the knee in length and a medial flap that is 2–3 cm longer to allow adequate coverage of the large medial femoral condyle are fashioned. By constructing shorter medial and lateral flaps, this technique provides more frequent healing in ischemic limbs than techniques using long anterior and posterior flaps. The underlying tissues are closed as in standard knee disarticulation.

Klaes and Eigler modification: In this method, for closure of a knee disarticulation wound the posterior calf skin and gastrocnemius muscle bellies are used as an integral flap without destruction of the perforating vessels. In this padding of the distal part of the femur is done with the gastrocnemius muscle bellies. It preserves the blood supply that passes from the gastrocnemius muscle bellies to the skin through the perforators.

Gritti-Stokes modification: This is an alternative to knee disarticulation in ischemic limbs where the femur is cut at the level of the condyles or through the supracondylar region and the patella is mobilized and fused to the distal end femur to create an end-bearing stump **(Fig. 16)**. Gritti first described his amputation in 1857, while working in Milan, but he only performed it once and then on a corpse. The operation was modified and performed successfully on a number of patients by Stokes in 1870 but has never gained widespread acceptance as an amputation of choice for ischemia because of the commonly ensuing complications:

- Nonunion of the patella
- Painful stump and difficulties in fitting a satisfactory prosthesis

Transfemoral Amputation

This is done when the knee joint cannot be preserved. It can be supracondylar, long, medial, or short amputation. While planning the amputation as much of the femur as possible should be preserved as it provides a long lever arm for the attachment of thigh muscle. A femur that is shorter than 5 cm from the lesser trochanter works as and is fitted as a hip disarticulation as the short stump that cannot control above-knee prosthesis even with a hip hinge and waist belt. The conventional knee joint used in prosthesis extends to about 9–10 cm from the knee joint therefore a femoral stump longer that this leads the knee joint of the two limbs to be at different levels and is cosmetically not acceptable especially while sitting.

Equal anterior and posterior flaps are designed at least half the diameter of the thigh. The muscles are cut so that they retract to the level of the bone section. The sharp edges of the bone are smoothened with a rasp and a good myodesis or myoplasty is performed. In young athletic patients, the muscles are fixed by drilling holes on anterior, posterior, and medial aspect of femur. The nerves and vessels are managed in the usual manner.

Modification in ischemic limbs: Undermining of the skin is avoided and the skin along with anterior group of muscles is lifted as a myocutaenous flap to preserve the blood supply. Myodesis and tight myoplasty are avoided.

Gottschalk's modification: The level of amputation is 12.5 cm from the knee joint. A long medial flap is designed in the sagittal plane. The adductor magnus muscle is detached from the adductor tubercle and the nerves and vessels are managed in the usual manner.

The adductor magnus is then attached to the lateral, anterior, and posterior parts of the femoral stump using holes drilled in the femur. The quadriceps muscle is then taken over the adductor magnus muscle and attached to the posterior part of the femoral stump and the posterior muscles are attached to the posterior part of the adductor magnus **(Fig. 17)**.

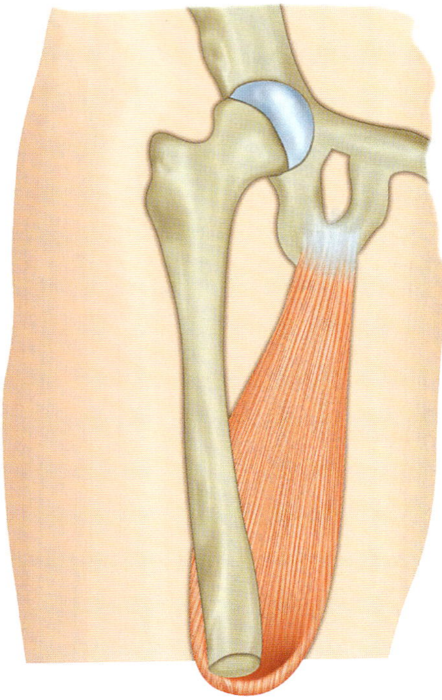

Fig. 17: Gottschalk's modification.

Osteomyoplasty: Similar to the Ertl's procedure in the tibia an osteomyoplasty can be performed in the femur by closing a periosteal sleeve over the open end of the femoral medullary canal thus closing the canal by new bone formation. The muscle flaps are taken over the periosteal sleeve. This creates a good end bearing stump.

HIP DISARTICULATION

This procedure is usually performed for tumors and rarely for massive trauma or ischemia. The procedure is performed in the lateral position with the limb draped free.

The incision: A racquet-shaped incision starting from the anterior superior iliac spine going along the inguinal ligament is used. On the medial aspect of the thigh, it is extended up to 5 cm from the origin of the adductor muscles then extended posteriorly about 5 cm from the ischial tuberosity. Laterally, the incision is carried up to 8 cm from the base of the greater trochanter and then extended to join the incision at the anterior superior iliac spine.

Management of vessels, muscles, and nerves includes:

- The femoral vessels are identified and ligated.
- The sartorius and the rectus femoris are detached from the anterior iliac spines.
- Pectineus is cut about 0.6 cm from the pubis and adductor and gracilis muscles from the pubis are also detached.
- The muscle plane between the pectineus and obturator externus and short external rotators of the hip is dissected to expose the branches of the obturator artery and it is ligated.
- The gluteus medius and minimus from the greater trochanter and iliopsoas tendon from the lesser trochanter are detached.
- The part of adductor magnus arising from the ischium and the hamstring muscles from the ischial tuberosity are detached.
- The fascia lata is cut in line with the skin incision and attachment of gluteus maximus from linea aspera and the short lateral rotator attachments to the femur are detached.
- The sciatic nerve is ligated and cut as it, many a times, contains feeding vessel that can cause significant hemorrhage.
- The capsule and ligament teres is cut to complete the amputation.
- The gluteal flap is brought anteriorly and the distal parts of the gluteal muscles are sutured to the origin of the pectineus and adductor muscles and skin is closed over drain.

Slocum's modification: This is also known as the "posterior flap technique". In this, a long posteromedial flap containing the gluteus maximus is taken anteriorly and sutured to the anterior margins of the incision.

A special type of prosthesis: Canadian hip prosthesis is used.

Hindquarter Amputation

The primary indication for hemipelvectomy, or hindquarter amputation, is the eradication of malignant tumors of the soft tissues or bone of the hip or pelvis. Occasionally, overwhelming infections such as gas gangrene or the consequences of trauma may require this operation. The standard hemipelvectomy employs a posterior or gluteal flap and disarticulates the symphysis pubis and sacroiliac joint and the ipsilateral limb. An extended hemipelvectomy includes resection of adjacent musculoskeletal structures, such as the sacrum or parts of the lumbar spine. In a conservative hemipelvectomy, the bony section divides the ilium above the acetabulum, preserving the crest of the ilium.

It is a traumatic procedure with a high intraoperative mortality (1–2%) and high morbidity (50–55%) rate. The patients' nutritional status needs to be optimized preoperatively and adequate (2,000–3,000 mL) of blood needs to be available.

Prosthetic fitting is difficult and relies on weight bearing on the uninvolved side. Depending on the location of the tumor, an anterior-flap or a posterior-flap technique can be used.

Preoperatively preparation consists of insertion of a ureteral catheter for identification of the ureter and a Foley catheter to drain the bladder.

The patient is operated in the lateral position, but the supports are kept loose to enable shift to a more prone or supine position intraoperatively. The involved extremity is draped free. Care should be taken to isolate the anus. It can alternatively be closed temporarily with a purse string suture.

Posterior-Flap Technique

This is done in three steps: (1) Anterior, (2) Perineal, and (3) Posterior.

1. For the anterior portion, the skin incision starts at the pubic tubercle and extends along the inguinal ligament to the anterior superior iliac spine. From here, it extends along the anterior part of the iliac crest up to mid ilium. The inguinal ligament and abdominal muscles are detached from the iliac crest and the space between the peritoneum and the iliacus muscle is developed. Then the inguinal ligament and rectus abdominus muscle are detached from the pubic bone. In men the spermatic cord is retracted medially to enter the space of Retzius and the bladder is retracted into the pelvis. The external iliac vessels are ligated and the femoral nerve is cut. This completes the anterior part.
2. For the perineal part, the hip is abducted and incision is extended vertically through the perineum to the ischial tuberosity. The pubic and the ischial rami are exposed and the adductor, hamstring, and perineal muscles originating from them, as well as the corpus cavernosum are detached. The pubic symphysis is then divided taking care to protect the urethra.
3. For the posterior part, the patient is rolled forward and the skin incision is completed by extending it from the ischial tuberosity laterally along the gluteal crease to the greater trochanter and then superiorly to join the anterior incision at the mid iliac crest. The "gluteus maximus" is exposed and its aponeurosis cut in line with the skin incision. Its femoral insertion is detached and it is lifted as a composite flap along with fat and skin proximally. The sciatic nerve is transected sharply and allowed to retract into pelvis. A gigli saw is passed through the greater sciatic notch and sacrotuberous, sacrospinous ligament, and ilium are divided just lateral to sacroiliac joint. For further extension, the sacroiliac joint can be disarticulated or even a part of sacrum can be removed. Next the innominate bone is rotated to isolate ligate and divide the obturator nerves and vessels. The external rotator muscles are divided close to the ischium and levator ani from close to its attachment to ischium and pubis.
4. *Closure*: The wound is closed by bringing anteriorly the posterior skin and muscle flap and suturing it to the lateral border of abdominal and rectus muscle anteriorly and to psoas and quadratus muscle posteriorly. A superficial and a deep negative suction drain are applied and a loose skin flap is closed.

Anterior-Flap Technique

The anterior-flap technique for hemipelvectomy as described by Larsen and Liang requires retention of the femoral nerve and vessels as well as the quadriceps musculature.

The anterior flap is created by starting the incision at the anterior superior iliac spine and extending it along the lateral aspect of the thigh to the level of the superior pole of the patella. It is then extended transversely across the quadriceps tendon and medially to the midline and subsequently proximal ward to the groin. A musculocutaneous flap is developed from lateral to medial by incising the deep fascia and transecting the quadriceps tendon horizontally. The quadriceps muscle is elevated from the femur, developing the dissection along the vastus medialis. The adductor canal is located and the sartorius muscle transected and ligated. The femoral vessels are ligated as far distally as possible so that their proximal ends remain with the musculocutaneous flap. Care should be taken not to damage the femoral vessels and nerve during further proximal dissection. The profunda femoris artery is ligated farther proximally. The hemipelvectomy is then completed as described previously, but exclude the posterior flap which is replaced by the anterior flap. Removal of the innominate bone can be made easier by osteotomy of the pubic rami rather than by disarticulation of the pubic symphysis.

Rotationplasty

As an alternative to amputation in cases of malignant tumors involving distal femur and proximal tibia as a limb salvage procedure various rotationplasties have been described. These are based on the principle of rotating the distal part of the lower limb by 180° so that the ankle joint functions like a knee joint and a below knee prosthesis can be used. It is especially useful in children where the growth potential of distal end tibia is preserved. These are modifications of the Van Ness rotationplasty which was described for congenital proximal femoral deficiencies.

Winkelmann classified rotationplasty into five groups, as follows:

1. Group AI—here the lesion is in the distal femur and requires resection of the distal femur, knee joint and proximal tibia. The lower leg is rotated 180° and the tibia is joined to the remaining femur **(Fig. 18A)**.
2. Group AII—here the lesion is in the proximal tibia requiring the resection of distal femur, knee joint, and proximal tibia. After 180° rotation, the distal tibia is joined to the distal femur **(Fig. 18B)**.
3. Group BI—the lesion is in the proximal femur but spares the hip joint and gluteal muscles. The upper femur and hip joint require resection. The distal femur is joined to the pelvis to make the knee function as the hip and the ankle as the knee **(Fig. 18C)**.
4. Group BII—the lesion is also in the proximal femur but involves the hip joint soft tissue. The entire hemipelvis requires resection. The femur is joined to the remaining ilium and the knee functions as a hip joint and the ankle functions as the knee **(Fig. 18D)**.
5. Group BIII—the lesion is in the mid femur, requiring the entire femur to be resected. The tibia is attached to pelvis with the help of an endoprosthesis **(Fig. 18E)**.

The basic principles of rotationplasty are as follows:

- The ankle and foot must be disease free.
- Adequate nerve supply to the foot and ankle
- Adequate blood supply to the foot and ankle must be restorable after resection.
- It must be possible to restore adequate muscle power to the ankle joint.
- Complete resection of the tumor must be possible while preserving the neurovascular structures.

The most commonly used rotationplasty is for lesion involving the distal femur. The skin incision is made in the shape of a rhombus with its long axis on the anterior surface and its two lateral points meeting on the posterior surface. If a biopsy scar is present it must be included in the incision and the incision must be about 5–10 cm longer than the intended bone resection.

The common peroneal, tibial, and sciatic nerves are identified and dissected away from the tumor. The femoral vessels are identified in the adductor canal and are similarly dissected distally. If the tumor involves the vessels, then part of the vessel is removed with the tumor and reconstructed later ensuring that the ischemia time does not exceed 2 hours.

The femur is transected with a healthy margin of 5 cm.

The tibia is transected just distal to the knee joint capsule in adults and distal to the proximal physis in children.

Frozen sections are taken to ensure adequate resection.

The limb is then rotated to 180° so that the peroneal and tibial nerves lie on the medial side and the femur is joined to the tibia with a compression plate. In adults, the ankle joint should be at the same level as the contralateral knee joint. In children, an estimate of the growth potential of the contralateral leg should be made using a green Anderson table and the ankle should be lower than the knee to compensate for this growth.

The muscles of the thigh are sutured to the leg fascia and skin is closed.

After adequate bone union a modified below knee prosthesis can be worn.

UPPER LIMB AMPUTATIONS

Upper-extremity amputations, excluding fingers, account for 15–20% of major extremity amputations. Acutely severed, crushed, or mangled limbs may require immediate amputation whereas irreversible brachial plexus injuries resulting in a flail, useless limb may come to amputation later. Most upper-extremity amputations are a result of trauma and most of these occur in men between the ages of 20 and 40 years. The loss of an upper extremity has more devastating consequences than the loss of a lower extremity. Upper-extremity amputations are most common in young male trauma victims, in whom the loss greatly affects function and self-image. Despite improvements in materials and design, long-term use of prosthetics by upper-extremity amputees is only about 50%. Most activities of daily living can be performed adequately with one limb, so most unilateral upper limb amputees do not use prosthesis. Prosthetic use is reduced in patients with higher levels of amputation, those with brachial plexus injury and when initiation of prosthetic limb rehabilitation is delayed. Prosthetic function is severely impaired at shoulder level and prostheses are used primarily as a holding device when performing activities with both hands.

HAND AMPUTATIONS

Principles of Finger Amputations

The key elements are to provide good skin sensation, joint mobility, and digital length with well-padded bony elements. Achieving supple soft tissue coverage of the ends of the thumb and fingers is essential. The chief functions to preserve are pinch and grasp. A careful assessment should be made of skin, tendon, nerve, bone, and joints. If three or more of these require special procedures, such as grafting of skin, suture of tendon or nerve, bony fixation, or closure of the joint, amputation should be considered because the function of the remaining fingers may be compromised by functionless finger. It may be wise to delay amputation if parts of the finger may be useful later in a reconstructive procedure. Skin, tendon graft, bone, segment of nerves, etc. from an otherwise useless digit can be employed as a free graft ("fillet" graft procedure). The tendon along with muscle of flexor digitorum sublimis or extensor indicis proprius can be transferred to improve function in an intact digit.

Certain principles must be followed to provide the patient with a painless and useful stump. Length of the volar skin flap should cover the volar surface and the exposed bones and should close with the dorsal flap but not under tension. Digital nerves should be separated out from the flap and cut about 6 mm proximal to the tip of the flap. Usually neuromas develop but if they are in padded areas they are less painful.

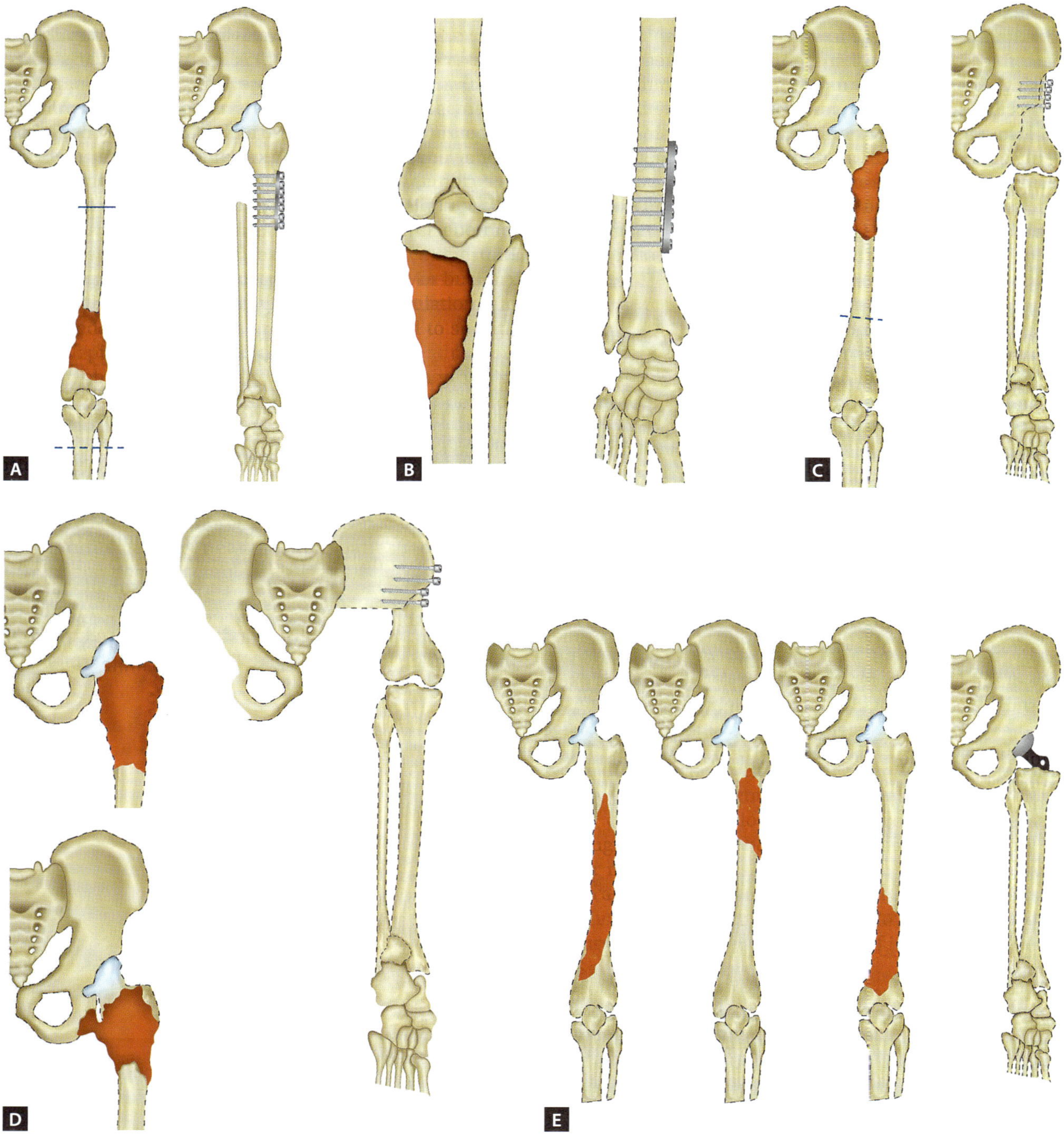

Figs. 18A to E: (A) Rotationplasty: Group AI; (B) Rotationplasty: Group AII; (C) Rotationplasty: Group BI; (D) Rotationplasty: Group BII; (E) Rotationplasty: Group BIII.

Wherever a classic flap is not possible a different shape of flap can be made but good padding for end of bones should be ensured. The tendons are cut and may retract proximally. At the level of the joint condyles should be tapered to prevent a club-like stump.

Finger Tip Amputation

If half of the nail is unsupported by the remaining distal phalanx, a nailbed ablation usually is indicated; otherwise, a hook nail may develop. In small children, fingertips commonly heal without grafts. Various types of flaps can be used to get coverage of the tip.

For small defects bone can be shortened to permit closure. Split thickness grafts should be avoided over finger tips as they are insensate and fragile. Full thickness grafts are preferable. Occasionally, the amputated part of the fingertip is recovered and replaced as a free graft or cap technique. This procedure requires removing bone debris and partially defatting the distal part before reattachment. The cap procedure is quite successful in both children and adults. These free composite grafts should be secured by a stent dressing tied over the end of the finger. For larger defects, various types of flap grafts can be used. They can be divided into local regional or distant grafts. Same finger grafts have the advantage of earlier mobility and function of the rest of the fingers is not compromised. Distal flaps can cover greater defects but can lead to stiffness and contractures of other fingers and should be avoided in persons over 50 years of age or who have a tendency to develop finger stiffness due to any other reason.

Local Finger Flaps

Kutler advancement flap: This is used when the pulp is compromised and the lateral hyponychial skin is uninjured. Two triangular flaps, one on each side of the finger, are raised with the apex of each directed proximally and centered in the mid lateral line of the digit. Their sides should each measure about 6 mm and their bases should measure about the same. The flaps are further developed by incising deeper toward the nail bed and volar pulp. A skin hook is used to handle the flaps and they are drawn distally after dividing the pulp just enough to allow the flap to be mobilized toward the finger tip. Excessive division of pulp distally should be avoided **(Fig. 19)**.

Atasoy advancement flap (V-Y advancement): When more of the pulp skin remains, then the Atasoy flap is used. A distally based triangular flap through the pulp is raised with the base of the triangle equal in width to the cut edge of the nail. It is a full-thickness flap with nerves and blood supply preserved. The vertical septa that hold the flap in place are cut and the flap advanced distally and sutured to the sterile matrix or nail. Defect on the volar surface is usually heals by secondary intention **(Fig. 20)**.

"Bipedicle dorsal flap" is used when the level of amputation is below the nail bed and it is desirable to retain length. If this flap is made wide then one of the pedicles can be divided, leaving one pedicle attached. The dissection is started at the margin of the skin and the skin and subcutaneous tissue is lifted from the dorsal surface. Proximally on the dorsal surface, a transverse incision is made to create a flap having supply from both pedicles and of enough length to cover the stump. The defect left by the flap is closed by a graft.

Volar advancement flap (Moberg): Like a dorsal flap a bipedicle volar flap too can be raised using the remnant pulp of the finger. It is mostly used for the thumb. After the debridement of the fingertip, make midlateral incisions dorsal to the neurovascular bundles and dissect the flap from the flexor tendon sheath mobilize the flap and advance it along with the neurovascular bundles. The advancement is helped by flexion of the interphalangeal joint of the thumb. If the flap is under tension, perform a transverse incision on the skin at the base of the flap. This results in a rectangular defect that needs a full-thickness skin graft. In the other fingers, the prospect of flap survival is increased by limiting the volar flap incision distal to the proximal interphalangeal joint **(Fig. 21)**.

Adipofascial turnover flap: It is used to cover defects on the dorsum of the finger just proximal to the nail bed. The

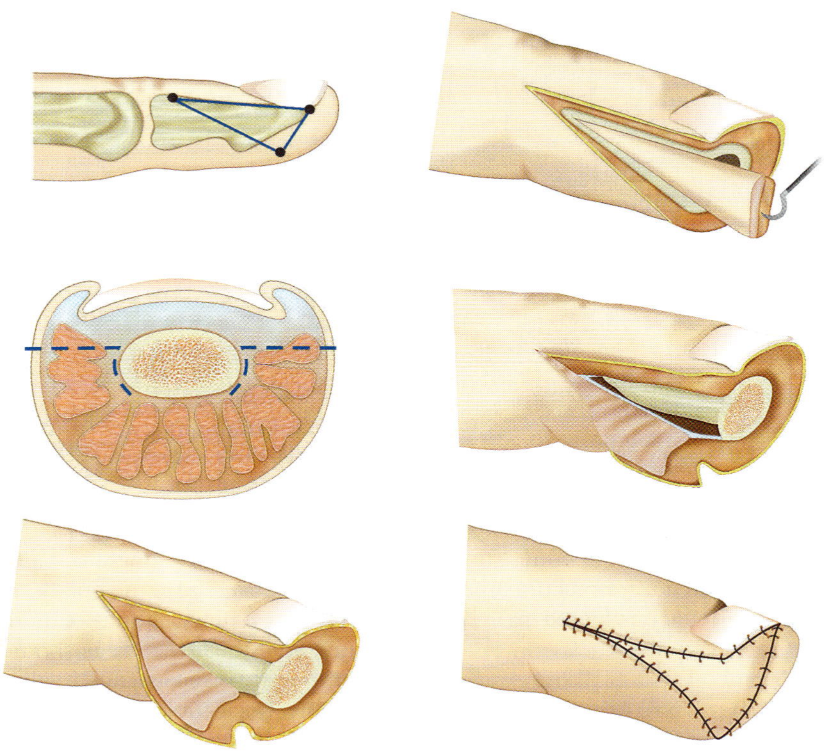

Fig. 19: Kutler advancement flap.

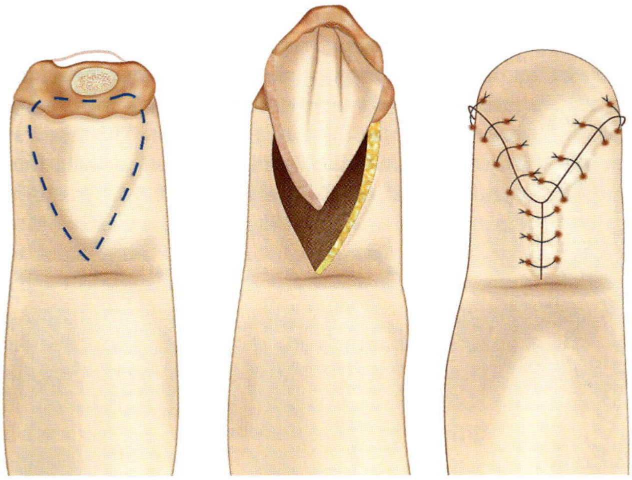

Fig. 20: Atasoy advancement flap (V-Y advancement).

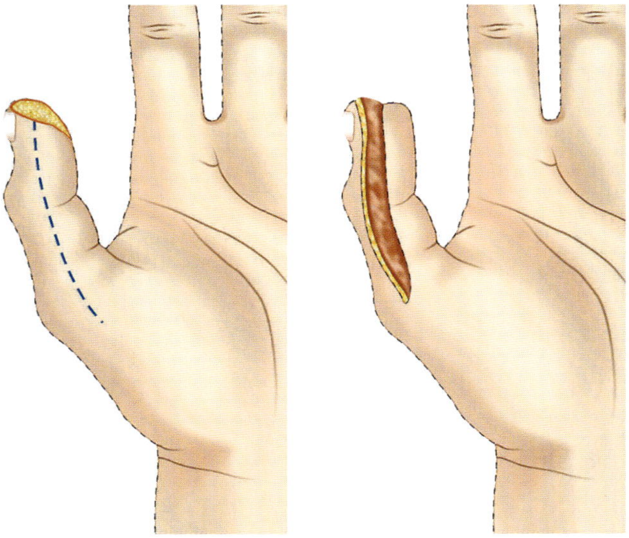

Fig. 21: Volar advancement flap (Moberg).

width of the flap is 2–4 mm wider than the traumatic defect. The base-to-length ratio should be 1:1.5–1:3. The flap base should be 0.5–1 cm in length and is made just proximal to the defect. The adipofascial flap is developed superficial to the extensor tendon paratenon from proximal to distal. The flap is detached proximally and along its sides to the flap base and flipped over and sutured distally. Suture over the turn over site is avoided to protect the vascular pedicle and the flap is covered with a split thickness graft.

Local neurovascular island flap: It can be antegrade or retrograde and can provide satisfactory padding and normal sensibility to the most important working surface of the digit.

Antegrade flaps are used for the volar surface of the digits. A midlateral incision is made on each side of the finger or thumb beginning distally at the defect and extending proximally to the level of the proximal interphalangeal joint or thumb interphalangeal joint. On each side, the neurovascular bundle is dissected till the required length of the flap and the flap is then separated by a transverse volar incision taking care to keep the neurovascular bundle intact. A second incision can be used to create a rectangular flap attached to both neurovascular bundles. The graft is then migrated distally to cover the defect or stump. Tension on the neurovascular bundles can be reduced by dissecting them more proximally or by flexing the distal interphalangeal (DIP) joint. The defect created on the volar surface of the finger is covered with a free full-thickness graft **(Fig. 22)**.

The retrograde homodigital island flap is well suited to cover dorsal and volar defects distally. The procedure relies on retrograde flow through the proper digital artery, supplying the proximal composite tissue. The vascular pedicle is exposed and the digital artery proximal to the flap is separated from the digital nerve. The artery is ligated distal to the flap and the flap can now be raised with its pedicle to cover the defect. About 1-cm section of pedicle is needed for adequate nourishment of the flap and to act as a pivot. The defect left behind is covered with a graft. A variation of this flap is to de-epithelialize it to reduce the bulk **(Fig. 23)**.

Ulnar hypothenar flap: This flap gets its supply retrograde from the distal part of the ulnar digital artery of the little finger over the hypothenar skin. Defects of the size 5 cm × 2 cm over the little finger can be covered. Sensation can be retained by joining the ulnar digital nerve with the sensory branch harvested with the flap. Dissection is carried out in such a way so as to include multiple vascular perforators in the flap and then dividing the ulnar palmar digital artery proximally. The point of pivot of the flap is at the level of the proximal interphalangeal joint, so turn over the flap and suture it loosely over the defect and cover the donor site with split thickness graft.

Regional Flaps

Thenar flaps: The index, middle, and ring finger pulp coverage can be accomplished by the use of the thenar flap **(Fig. 24)**.

Some tips include:

- On the thenar eminence outline a flap that, when raised, is large enough to cover the defect. The flap should be 50% more than the defect to create the pulp of finger. The length should not be more than twice the width.
- The base of the flap can be distal or proximal depending on whether the defect is on the volar or dorsal aspect. The thenar flap is raised to include most of the underlying fat.
- The flap should be handled with skin hooks to avoid crushing it even with small forceps.
- By gentle undermining of the skin border at the donor site, the defect can be closed directly. Hold the finger in the proper position by gauze and adhesive tape and splint the wrist. The flap is released at 3 weeks.

Caution the patient preoperatively that donor site tenderness and proximal interphalangeal joint flexion contractures can occur. Avoid keeping the flaps in place for >3 weeks.

For the little finger, a similar flap can also be raised from over the hypothenar eminence.

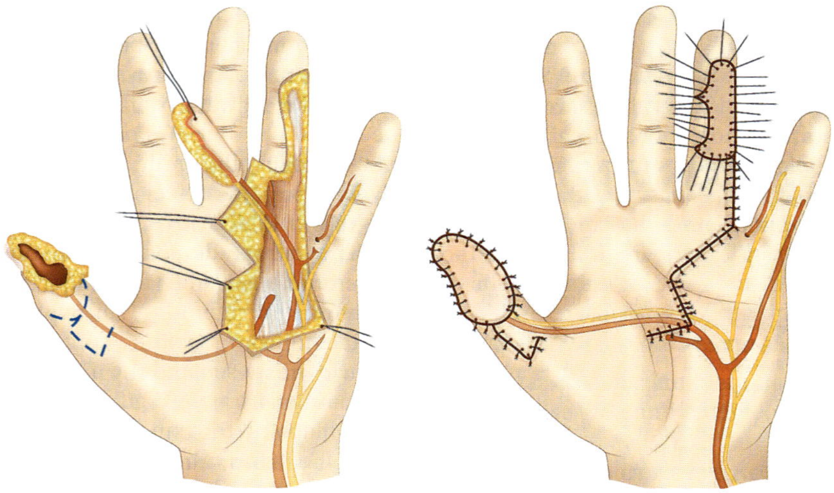

Fig. 22: Local neurovascular island flap.

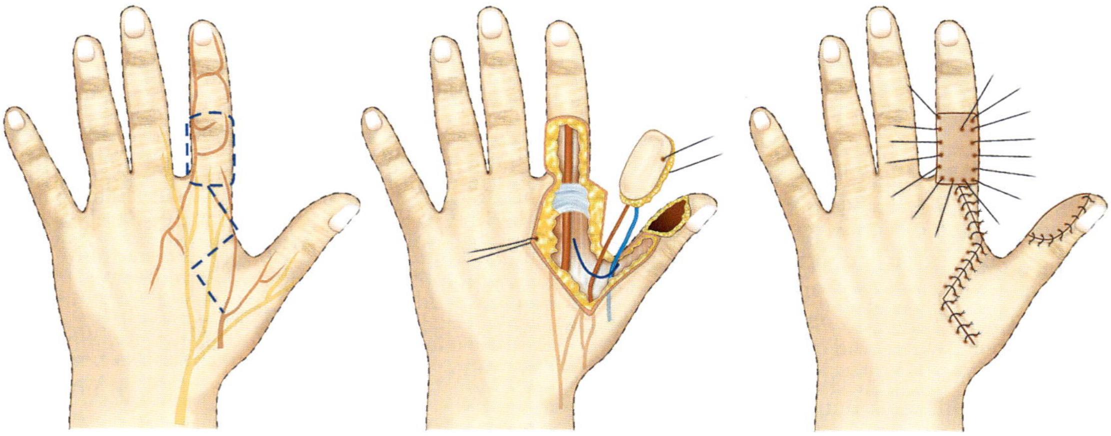

Fig. 23: Retrograde homodigital island flap.

Cross-finger flaps: These are useful for covering defects of the skin and other soft tissues on the volar surface of the finger when tendons and neurovascular structures are exposed **(Fig. 25)**. Some technical tips that could be of help during execution are detailed below:

- The edges of the defect are excised so that it is rectangular, with its longer side parallel to the long axis of the finger but not crossing skin creases. The injured finger is placed against the donor finger to determine where to locate the base of the proposed flap and to determine its size.
- The flap is raised from the donor finger through the skin and subcutaneous tissues, leaving its base attached to the side adjacent to the recipient finger. Flap should be of adequate size that is about 4–6 mm wider and longer than the defect to compensate for skin contracture later and also to provide enough bridge between the fingers. Another option is to raise the flap from one midlateral line to the other, without incising the volar surface on the donor finger.
- The skin and subcutaneous tissue is raised together and the skin distal to the DIP is avoided to prevent injury to the nail bed. The dorsal surface of the *proximal interphalangeal* (PIP) joint is also avoided unless more width is required.

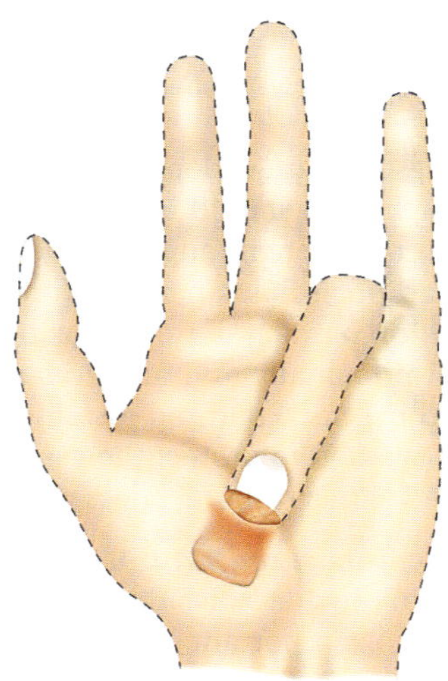

Fig. 24: Thenar flap.

- The flap can be further mobilized by dissecting the oblique fibers of the deep tissue attaching the skin to the extensor tendon and periosteum.
- The donor area and the area under bridge are covered with thick split graft from the forearm or thigh.

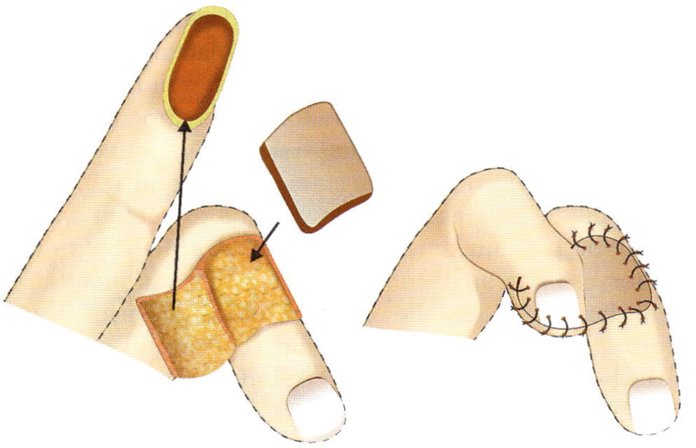

Fig. 25: Cross-finger flap.

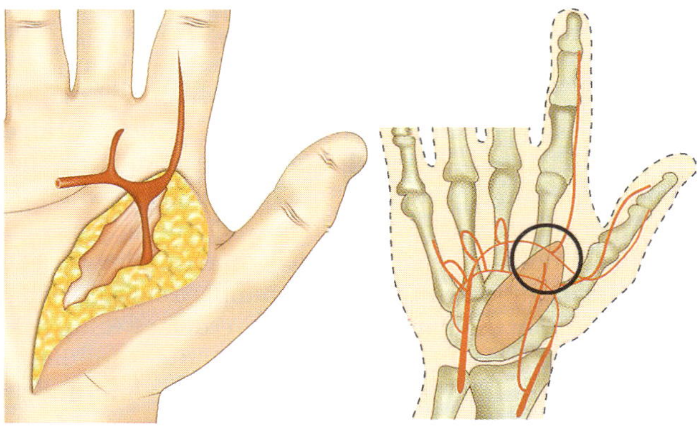

Fig. 26: Reverse thenar perforator flap.

- While suturing the flap in place tension transverse to the long axis of the finger should be avoided.

Palmar pivot flap:
- An axial pattern flap getting supply from subcutaneous transverse branches of the digital artery.
- Pivoted up to 90° from the proximal or the middle phalangeal segments to cover an adjacent defect.
- Coverage is from the PIP joint to the fingertip.
- Defect at the donor site is on the same digit and is filled with a skin graft.

Reverse thenar perforator flap: This flap is based on vascular supply from the perforating branches of the terminal part of the superficial palmar arch. It may also get supply from the superficial palmar branch of the radial artery. Flap sizes range from 1.5 cm × 3.0 cm to 2.5 cm × 6.5 cm. The donor site is repaired primarily. The reverse thenar perforator flap offers glabrous skin for defects of the palm, first web and index finger **(Fig. 26)**.

Distant Flaps

Groin flaps: The salient features of groin flaps are:
- Graft has sparse hair.
- Multiple vascular supply
- Large size
- Minimal morbidity at donor site
- Can be used to cover even bare bone.

Drawbacks

- Color may not match recipient site.
- In obsess patients, the flap harvested can be very thick.
- If scarring is present from previous inguinal surgeries, then the supplying vessel may be damaged.

The supply to the flap is from the superficial circumflex iliac branch of the femoral artery and the veins drain through the superficial inferior epigastric and superficial circumflex iliac veins **(Fig. 27)**.

The patient is positioned supine. To help to determine the central axis of the flap a Doppler probe may be used to identify and locate the course of the superficial circumflex iliac artery which lies usually about 2.5 cm distal and parallel to the inguinal ligament. The usual dimensions are about

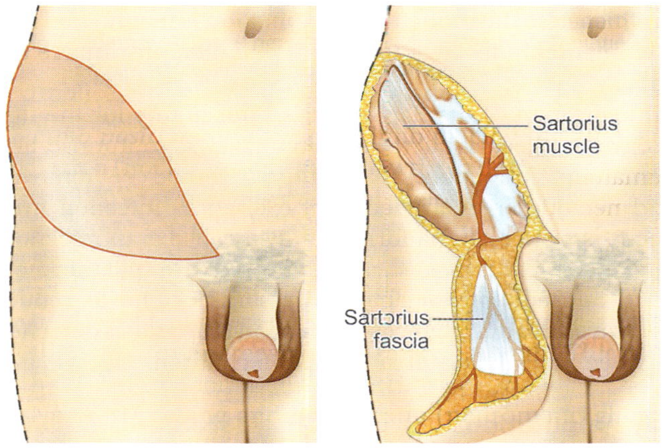

Fig. 27: Groin flap.

10 cm and a length extending about 5 cm posterolateral to the anterosuperior iliac spine. The skin and subcutaneous tissue are incised down to the deep fascia and the flap elevated in this plane. The superficial epigastric vessels are identified and ligated. The superficial circumflex iliac vessels must be kept within the flap. The dissection does not extend medial to the sartorius. The limb is positioned in such a way so as to avoid tension on the pedicle. Small defects at the donor site can be closed. For larger flaps, split thickness grafts can be used. Nonadherent gauze is applied to the suture lines and the axilla is padded to avoid maceration. Opening is created in the dressing to inspect the flap. The flap is detached after 2–3 weeks. In case, the flap appears to loose vascularity it can be reattached to donor site for 7–10 days and shifted to the recipient site again.

Random Pattern Abdominal Pedicle Flaps

Random pattern abdominal flaps to be applied to the hand have their base either distal, toward the superficial epigastric vessels, usually on the same side as the affected hand, or proximal, above the umbilicus toward the thoracoepigastric vessels, usually on the opposite side. Above umbilicus flaps should not be used in a patient with a "barrel chest" with chronic lung disease. Abdominal flaps obtained from areas above the umbilicus usually avoid the fat "storage areas".

If the flap is obtained from the infraumbilical area, the recipient grafted area usually increases in bulk, since the infraumbilical area skin adds fat.

The flap raised should be larger than the defect to allow for normal skin contraction and for the pedicle "bridge" between the abdomen and the defect. As a rule, the flap should be rectangular to avoid a circular outline when the flap is attached to the hand. Avoid making the flap too thick. Close the donor site defect by widely undermining the skin margins and suture them together, or apply a split-thickness skin graft. Apply the flap over the entire defect. Suture the edges of the flap to those of the defect and ensure that all the raw surfaces are covered. The position of the limb and the dressing should be in such a way so as to avoid tension on the flap and allow for easy inspection through the dressing. This may require marked pronation or supination of the forearm, in which case the pronation or supination is maintained by a Steinmann pin through the radius and ulna proximal to the wrist.

Inspection of the flap is carried out hourly for the first 2 days to check for tension, circulatory compromise and hematoma formation. Tight sutures should be removed and necrotic areas immediately excised as infection from necrosis or hematoma formation will cause graft rejection. The raw area thus created can be covered with split thickness graft. Subsequently regular redressing is done to reduce offensive odor and chances of infection. The graft is detached at 3 weeks in adults and in 2 weeks in children.

Ray Amputations

Index Ray

Imperfections of the index finger are poorly tolerated. When the index finger of an otherwise normal hand is compromised by loss of length especially if loss is at or proximal to the proximal PIP joint, then its removal is indicated. Amputation of the index finger may be accomplished by either metacarpophalangeal (MP) joint disarticulation or index ray resection. MP joint disarticulation preserves the breadth of the palm, which is helpful in stabilizing objects held with a cylindrical grip but presents an obtrusive prominence in the webspace. Ray resection narrows the palm and improves the appearance of the hand by achieving a broad, smooth webspace contour. The skin incision is designed to provide a supple webspace that will allow thumb mobility. If the wedge of skin removed is too large, the distance from thumb to middle metacarpal will be diminished and thumb abduction may be limited. Dissect skin flaps from the index digit, taking care to preserve flap innervation. Divide the extensor indicis proprius tendon from its insertion ulnar to the index communis tendon and tag it. Apply traction to the extensor digitorum communis tendon, divide it and allow it to retract. Osteotomize the index metacarpal obliquely through the proximal metaphysis dorsoradial proximally to volar-ulnar distally about 2 cm distal to its base preserving the insertion of the extensor carpi radialis longus and flexor carpi radialis tendons. Anchor the tendinous insertion of the first dorsal interosseous to the base of the proximal phalanx of the middle finger. Do not anchor it to the extensor tendon or its hood because this might cause intrinsic over pull. Divide the deep transverse metacarpal ligament adjacent to the middle finger. Identify the index flexor tendons, pull them distally, divide them, and allow them to retract proximally. Take care in dealing with the digital nerves: The radial nerve to the index finger must not be extensively mobilized. Sharply divide digital nerves and allow them to retract into the soft tissue without tension. The ultimate neuroma end of the nerves must be distanced from further trauma. Remove the index finger. Sew the extensor indicis proprius into the middle finger extensor digitorum communis tendon at the level of its insertion to enhance independence of middle-finger extension. Trim the first dorsal and first palmar interosseous muscles as necessary to ensure a smooth web-space contour. Close the skin flaps with the thumb in palmar and radial abduction **(Fig. 28)**.

Central Ray

Amputation of the middle or ring finger especially proximal to the PIP joint leaves an awkward space between the fingers making holding small objects in the hand difficult as they fall through this gap. To overcome this "ray" resection and reconstruction by either soft-tissue coaptation or ray transfer can be done. This closes the gap and improves the esthetic appearance of the hand. Both procedures narrow the palm and weaken grasp and cylindrical grip palmar stabilization.

Central Ray Resection and Soft-tissue Coaptation

A zigzag incision is made on the palmar surface overlying the metacarpal to be resected. A generous wedge of dorsal skin is removed. This provides a dermodesis, which will stabilize the digit. The entire metacarpal is resected subperiosteally. If the middle metacarpal is excised, the proximal insertion of the extensor carpi radialis and the origin of the adductor pollicis muscle are preserved. When the ring metacarpal is resected, the entire metacarpal base may be removed, allowing radial shift of the little metacarpal on the hamate. The deep motor branch of the ulnar nerve, which runs just palmar to the metacarpal, must be protected when excising the metacarpals. Identify and ligate the correct digital arteries.

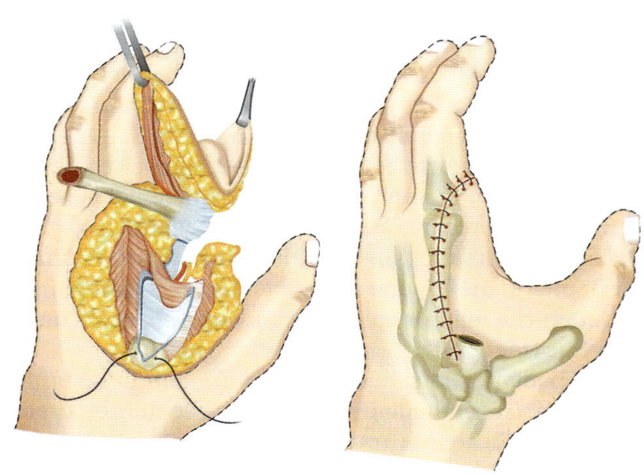

Fig. 28: Index ray amputation.

The correct digital nerves are divided distal to the common digital nerve bifurcation. Pull flexor and extensor tendons distally, divide them and allow them to retract proximally. Divide the interosseous and lumbrical tendons. A single continuous soft-tissue band, consisting of the palmar plate and the two adjacent deep transverse metacarpal ligaments is retained, each of which is firmly attached to adjacent digits. The metacarpal heads are pressed together and the digits adjacent to the resected metacarpal are fixed to one another by dividing the ligament-palmar plate complex and weaving the two segments together. Then securely suture the shortened ligament-palmar plate complex with interrupted sutures. The palmar skin incision is closed first. Observe the fingers with the wrist in both flexion and extension. Assess the extent of digital scissoring. If residual scissoring persists, excise further dorsal skin. Circumferential dressing and splinting maintains lateral metacarpal pressure and protects the ligament repair during the first 3 weeks after reconstruction **(Fig. 29)**.

Central Ray Resection and Ray Transposition

A palmar zigzag incision is made that converges over the middle third of the metacarpal to be resected. Resect a dorsal wedge of skin with its apex over the proximal third of the metacarpal. Recreation of a normal webspace contour between the retained digits is facilitated, if the skin of a single webspace is preserved and shifted intact to the new webspace. The digital nerves and vessels, the flexor and extensor tendons, the interossei, lumbricals, and the adductor pollicis are resected as in coaptation. To prevent nonunion of the bone-to-bone junction between transferred and recipient rays, the osteotomy is performed through the metaphyseal area to provide a large cancellous-to-cancellous surface for union. A transverse osteotomy is performed. The transferred ray is mobilized to allow transfer without tension. The interosseous muscle origins may need to be released. Suture the adductor pollicis origin to the ring metacarpal when the index ray is transposed to the middle position. Precisely fit the transferred ray onto the recipient base and secure with and plate. Ensure that rotational alignment has been preserved, that the digit is clinically straight and that the fingers do not overlap in flexion. A distal transversely placed Kirschner wire may be helpful in further stabilizing the transferred digit. Approximate the deep transverse metacarpal ligaments from the adjacent sides of the resected metacarpal. The ultimate length discrepancy between the little and middle fingers may be minimized if the osteotomy is performed more proximally in the metaphysis of the little finger than in the metaphysis of the ring-finger metacarpal.

Little-Finger Ray Resection

When amputation of the little finger at the MP joint level is required, consider ray resection because it has a better cosmetic appearance then a digit resection. For this reason, ray resection is recommended in sedentary patients or those particularly concerned about cosmesis. In patients who depend on the breadth of the palm to stabilize a hammer or other object with a cylindrical grip, removing the little-finger metacarpal will result in a significant loss of strength and every attempt should be made to preserve the fifth metacarpal in such cases.

Make a dorsoulnar incision to expose the little-finger metacarpal. Isolate and divide the extensor communis and extensor quinti tendons. Because the extensor carpi ulnaris inserts on the base of the little-finger metacarpal, disarticulation is avoided. Instead, divide the metacarpal obliquely through the tapering metaphysis. Divide the flexor tendons as well as the third palmar interosseous, lumbrical, and hypothenar muscle tendons. Trim the hypothenar muscles to create a smooth contour along the ulnar border of the hand **(Fig. 30)**. Alternatively, the metacarpal can be divided at the neck and then the cut obliquely tapered through the shaft to give better cosmesis.

Thumb Amputation

In partial amputation of the thumb reamputation at a more proximal level to obtain closure should not be done because the thumb should not be shortened and every attempt

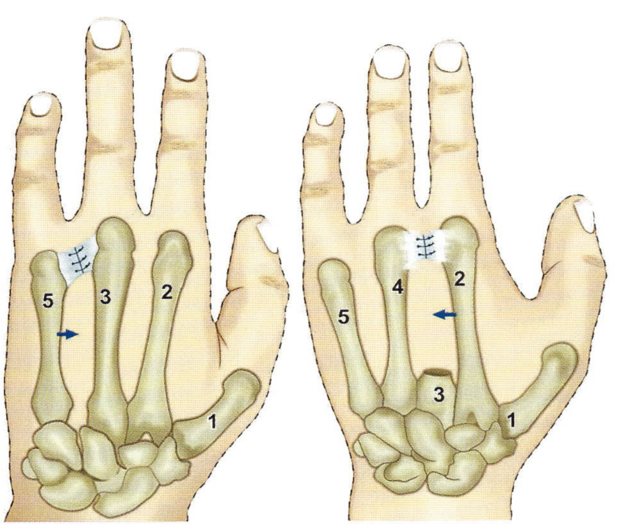

Fig. 29: Central ray resection and soft-tissue coaptation.

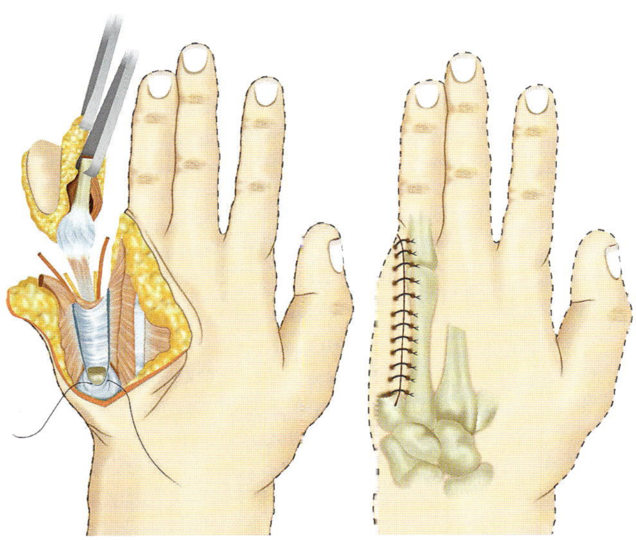

Fig. 30: Little-finger ray resection.

should be made to preserve its length. Various same fingers, regional or distal flaps as described earlier can be used. The flap required for coverage is taken it from the dorsum of the hand or the index or middle finger. This type of flap taken from the fingers is insensate but provides a stable pad for pinch grip. The volar surface of thumb should not be covered with abdominal flap as they do not have septae and tend to roll and shift under pressure.

When the level of amputation leaves a useful length of the proximal phalanx then the thumb web is made deeper with a Z-plasty.

For more proximal amputation, thumb reconstruction is required.

THUMB RECONSTRUCTION

The thumb is the single most important digit in the hand and its absence is considered to cause a disability of 40% for hand function. Therefore, a patient with partial or total absence of thumb should always be considered for reconstruction. Before any planning for surgery is made, however, several factors must be considered like:

- The remaining length
- The condition of the other digits
- The age and requirement of the patient
- The expertise of the surgeon
- The condition of the opposite hand. If the opposite thumb is normal, even for a totally absent thumb reconstruction is not mandatory.

A reconstructed thumb must fulfill the following requirements:

- It should be sensate enough to recognize objects and should be painless.
- The stability should be enough to allow pinch without deviation.
- The range of mobility should allow both flattening of hand and opposition.
- The length should be enough to allow the opposing digits to touch at the tips. If the remaining digits are short or stiff then greater than normal length may be required to achieve this.
- Cosmesis should be acceptable to the patient.

The following reconstructive procedures are possible:

- The thumb can be lengthened by a short bone graft or distraction osteoplasty.
- Sensibility can be restored by skin rotation flaps.
- Pollicizing of a digit.
- Microvascular free transfer of a toe to the hand.
- Osteoplastic technique with a bone graft and tube pedicle skin graft supplemented by a neurovascular pedicle.

For congenital or traumatic absence of the thumb, pollicization of the index finger is the most used technique. In case of congenital absence, reconstructive procedures usually are done after the first 1 year or 2 years of life.

Pollicization

Skin incision has to be individualized when skin along the radial border of the hand is scarred. The flap should be designed to bring the best skin to the web of hand skin grafting can be done dorsally and radially but should be avoided in the webspace. Digital artery integrity of index and middle finger should be evaluated. If it is insufficient, then vein graft from the radial artery in the anatomical snuff box to the digit must be planned.

The radial and ulnar index digital nerves and arteries must be identified and preserved. In adult pollicization, skeletal length is established by combining remaining thumb and index parts **(Fig. 31)**. The goal is to achieve a reconstructed thumb whose tip extends to about 75% of the length of the proximal phalanx of the middle finger.

- If the index is of normal length and the thumb basilar joint is absent, then rotated index metacarpal head is used as trapezium.
- When the trapezium and part of the thumb metacarpal remain, the entire index metacarpal and an appropriate portion of the proximal phalanx is resected and secured directly on top of the thumb metacarpal remnant.
- When the distal portion of the index has been damaged, an appropriate metacarpal length is retained to achieve a composite digit of proper length.
- The index MP joint is retained to provide thumb MP motion, while the PIP joint of the index will provide an interphalangeal joint for the reconstructed thumb.

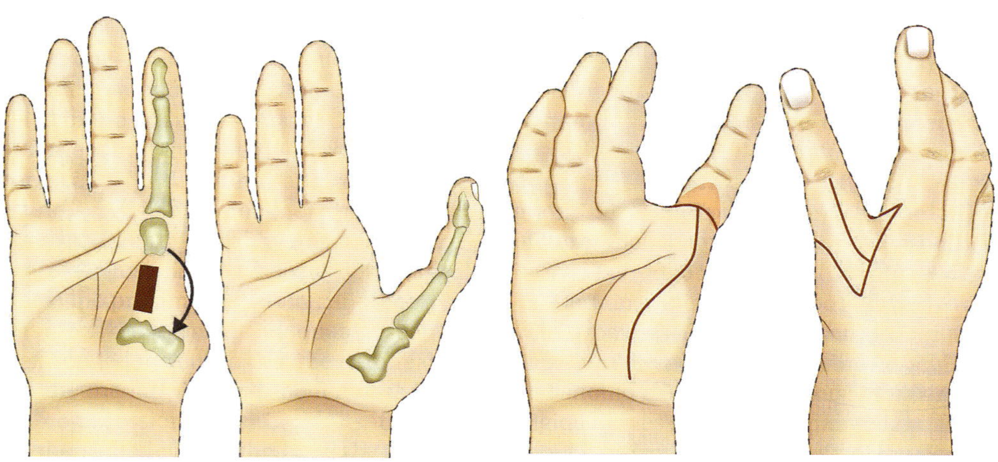

Fig. 31: Pollicization.

Musculotendinous rearrangement is done as follows:

- Advance the first dorsal and first palmar interossei insertions distally on the hood and shorten the extensor tendons.
- If the first dorsal interosseous muscle has been damaged, consider simultaneous opponensplasty tendon transfer.
- When the index digit is merely being moved radial ward without skeletal shortening extensor tendon shortening may not be required.
- In adult pollicization, the flexor tendons to the pollicized digit will not spontaneously shorten and readapt their optimal resting length as occurs in pediatric pollicization. Therefore, the tendon must be resected and shortened.

Amputations of Multiple Digits

In partial amputations of all fingers, preserving the remaining length of the digits become all the most important. In partial amputation of all fingers and the thumb, function can be improved by lengthening the digits relatively and by increasing their mobility. This is achieved by:

- Deepening the webspace between the fingers by z-plasty.
- If only first and fifth fingers are left, then improved function is achieved by osteotomizing their metacarpals and rotating the distal fragments toward each other.
- Division of the transverse metacarpal ligament between the fourth and fifth rays gives increased mobility to the rays thus improving function.
- Transposition of the second metacarpal to the first to increase its length and function is further improved by widening and deepening the first web.
- If only the thumb is left then phalangization of the fifth metacarpal (MC) is done. This consists of removing the fourth MC, osteotomizing, rotating, and separating the fifth MC from the palm. It can also be lengthened.
- When the thumb and all the fingers are lost at the level of the MC heads then phalangization of selected metacarpals can improve function. The second and fourth metacarpals are removed, this increases the range of motion of the fifth and first MC. Function is further improved by osteotomy and radial rotation and flexion of fifth MC. When the amputation is through the MC shafts, prehension is difficult to restore. In such cases, hook function can be given by flexion of the stump at the wrist.

Wrist Disarticulation

Transcarpal: At this level, supination and pronation of the forearm, as well as flexion and extension of the wrist, are preserved. When compared to more proximal amputations, the long lever arm increases the ease and power with which prosthesis can be used. However, prosthetic fitting is more difficult and requires a skilled prosthetist. Long palmer and short dorsal skin flaps in the ratio of 2:1 are fashioned. The long tendon of the extensor and flexor compartment are divided and allowed to retract into the forearm. The wrist flexors and extensors are identified and freed from their attachments. The median, ulnar, and filaments of radial nerve are transected sharply and allowed to retract into the forearm. The radial and ulnar arteries are ligated. The bone is cut with saw and rough ends are smoothened. The earlier identified wrist flexors and extensors are attached to the remaining carpal bones and wound closed over suction drain.

Disarticulation at wrist: Long palmer and short dorsal skin flaps in the ratio of 2:1 are fashioned. The incision starts 1.3 cm from the radial styloid and it is carried distally across the palm and curved proximally to end 1.3 cm from the ulnar styloid. The radial and ulnar arteries are ligated. The radial, median, and ulnar nerves are cut so that they retract well proximal into the forearm. Louis, Hunter, and Keatin described a technique to reduce pain by neuroma formation. They extended the dissection between the pronator teres and brachioradialis just distal to the elbow flexion crease and ligated the median, ulnar, and superficial radial nerves at this level. The neuroma formed at this site is away from the prosthetic wall or scar. All the tendons are cut and allowed to retract into the forearm. The disarticulation is completed. The radial and ulnar styloids are resected and edges of the bone made smooth. Care should be taken not to damage the distal radioulnar joint so that pronation and supination of the forearm is preserved and the joint does not become painful. The skin flap is closed directly over the bone **(Fig. 32)**.

Distal Forearm Amputation

In the upper limb, every attempt should be made to maintain as much of length as possible. But, the thin underlying structures and relative avascularity of the distal forearm do not provide adequate padding for the bony stump leading to wound problems. Thus, the best suited balance between lengths and wound healing is at the junction of the distal and middle third of the forearm **(Fig. 33A)**. Some amount of pronation and supination is possible in limbs with forearm amputations. Equal anterior and posterior flaps are made taking care to reflect the subcutaneous fat and fascia along with the skin. The length of flap is half the diameter of forearm at the level of amputation. The ulnar and radial arteries and the radial, ulnar and median nerves are managed similar to wrist disarticulation. The bone ends are cut and contoured to complete the amputation. The flap can be devised in two ways:

1. The first is to allow the muscles and tendons to retract into the forearm and only use the skin and fascia flap.
2. In younger patient, myoplastic closure can be done by fashioning an anterior flap of flexor digitorum sublimis and taking it across the bone ends and suturing it to the dorsal fascia and closing the skin over it. The entire anterior group of muscles should not be used as it makes the stump bulky **(Fig. 33B)**.

Proximal Forearm Amputation

A short stump having as little as even 4 cm of ulna is preferable to an above-elbow amputation. In individuals with tenuous soft tissue coverage for the stump Jones and Blair have described a salvage technique in which a free latissimus

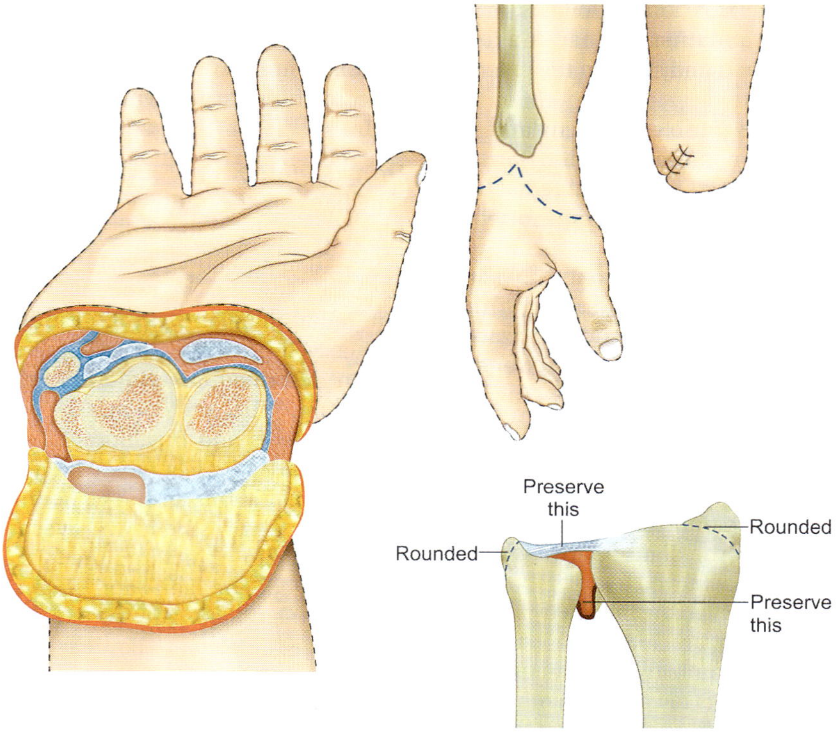

Fig. 32: Disarticulation at wrist.

dorsi flap is used, rather than resorting to an above-elbow amputation.

Equal anterior and posterior flaps are made. Skin along with fascia is reflected to the level of bone section. The nerves and vessels are managed as for distal forearm amputation. Muscle bellies are divided so that their edges are at the level of intended bone section. Excess muscles are trimmed. Radius and ulna are divided. The radius is divided proximal from the insertion of the biceps muscle and 2.5 cm of the tendon is resected and allowed to retract into the arm. This lengthens stump functionally and enhances prosthetic fitting. Flexion of the stump then is done by the brachialis muscle. Fascia and skin is closed over the stump. No studies have shown the necessity of myoplasty in forearm amputees.

"Krukenberg" described a technique that converts a forearm stump into a pincer that is motorized by the pronator teres muscle **(Fig. 33C)**. It is performed as a secondary procedure after a below elbow amputation.

Prerequisites are:

- Below elbow stump of at least 10 cm
- Sensate extremity
- Flexible elbow
- Mobile proximal radioulnar joint
- Working pronator teres
- Willingness to accept the cosmesis

Indications

- Inability to adapt to functional upper limb prosthesis
- Inability to afford prosthesis
- In blind persons where tactile function is important.

Procedure

Midline volar and dorsal incisions are taken in such a way that full thickness skin cover can be given over the opposing surfaces to ensure tactile sensation. Flexor digitorum sublimis is split into two and each half is attached to radius and ulna. Proximally the dissection is carried up to the cubital fossa taking care to preserve the pronator teres. The median nerve and ulnar nerve are cut and tied distal to the supply to flexor digitorum sublimis and flexor carpi ulnaris. The flexor digitorum profundus and flexor pollicis longus muscles are excised to reduce the bulk of the stump. On the dorsal aspect, dissection is carried out between the two heads of extensor digitorum communis and as in the volar surface the deep muscles are excised and discarded. The deepest structure the interosseous membrane is then divided up to the proximal radioulnar joint and the joint is subluxated to achieve as much opening up as possible. The longer the stump the greater opening can be obtained. The remaining muscles are attached to the bone and skin is closed without tension. Active exercises and training are started at 2–3 weeks.

Complications

- Skin necrosis
- Neuromas
- Scarring in the axilla of stump
- Inability to accept cosmetic appearance

Advantages

- Preservation of proprioception especially in blind persons.

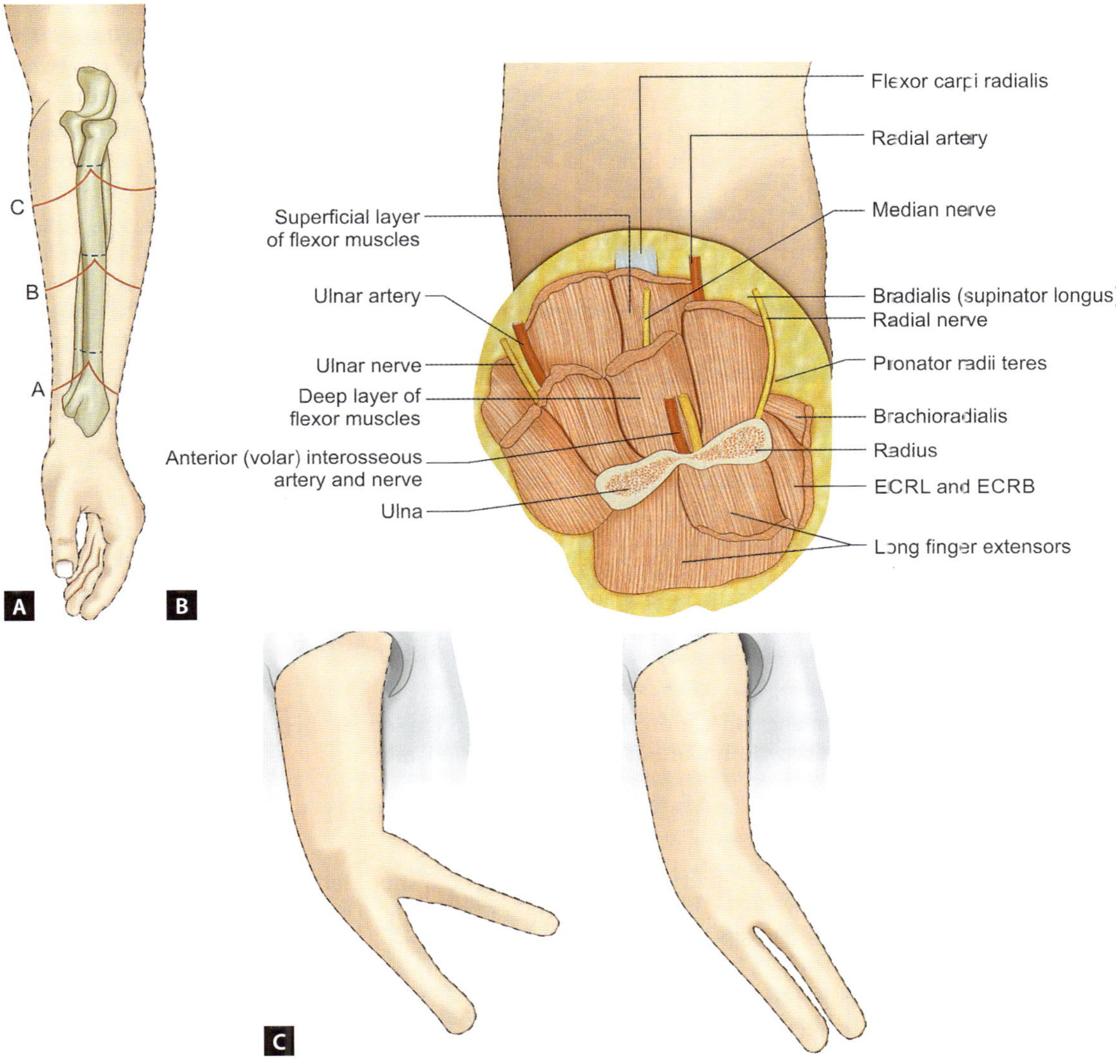

Figs. 33A to C: (A) Forearm amputation (Various levels of amputation, viz., distal, mid, and proximal); (B) Distal forearm amputation; (C) Krukenberg amputation.

- Better functional outcomes as compared to prosthesis
- Cost advantage in low income groups as expensive prosthesis is not required.
- If required prosthesis can still be used.

Disadvantages

- The chief disadvantage is the poor cosmetic outcome that most patients find unacceptable.
- Cannot be performed if adequate sensory and motor supply to provide proprioception and power are not there.

Elbow Disarticulation

It is preferred to more proximal amputation as the distal flare of humerus grabs the prosthetic stump better and transmits rotation of humerus.

Equal anterior and posterior flaps are made starting proximally at the level of the epicondyles and extending distally 2.5 cm from tip of olecranon and just distal to biceps insertion. The flexor attachment at the medial epicondyle is released. Proximal to the joint, the brachial artery is double ligated. Ulnar and medial nerves are cut so that they lie 2.5 cm proximal to the joint line. The tendons of the biceps and the brachialis are released from the radius and ulna and the radial nerve is cut in a similar manner. The extensor musculature arising from the lateral epicondyle is sectioned 6.3 cm from the joint line and the proximal part is retracted proximally. The posterior fascia along with the triceps tendon is cut at the level of the tip of olecranon and the amputation is completed by cutting the joint capsule. The triceps tendon is then brought anteriorly and attached to the remnant of biceps and brachialis tendon. The extensor muscle mass is carried medially and sutured to the remnant of the flexor muscle mass. The skin flaps are closed over the muscle flaps **(Fig. 34)**. A distal humeral osteotomy to create an anterior angulation of 45° can be added to the above procedure. This aids prosthesis fitting/reduces need for shoulder harness. A shortening supracondylar osteotomy

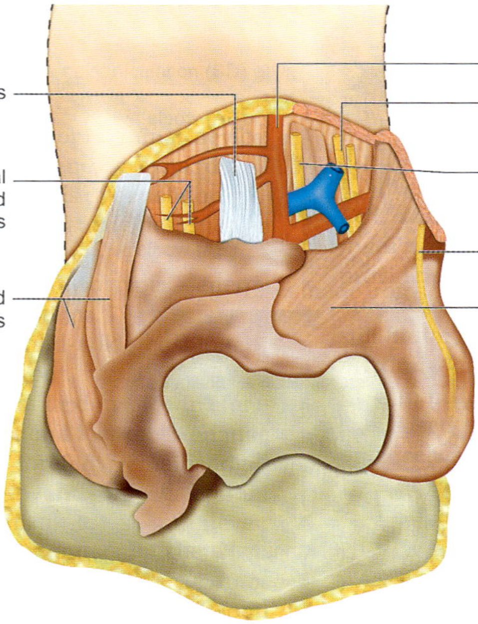

Fig. 34: Elbow disarticulation.

has also been described to provide space for a motorized elbow joint prosthesis so that both elbow joints are at the same level.

Transhumeral Amputation

This includes any amputation of the humerus from the supracondylar area to the level of the axillary fold. Amputations distal to supracondylar area like transcondylar amputation behave as and are fitted as an elbow disarticulation. Proximally, any amputation proximal to the axillary fold functions like a shoulder disarticulation. As in the knee the greatest length is desirable but the level of bone section should be at least 3.8 cm from the elbow for allowing an elbow lock mechanism to be fitted in the prosthesis. With amputations extending proximal to the axillary fold every attempt should be made to preserve the humeral head as it gives contour to the shoulder and better attachment to the prosthesis.

Supracondylar Amputation

Equal anterior and posterior flaps are made beginning at the level of the intended bone section. Brachial artery is ligated just proximal to the level of the intended bone section. The radial, ulnar, and median nerves are cut so that they retract proximally. The anterior groups of muscles are cut so that they retract and come to lie at the level of bone section. Triceps is detached from the olecranon and along with its fascia preserved as a long flap. The bone is cut 3.8 cm from the joint line and the trimmed triceps tendon is carried across the cut end and sutured to the fascia of the anterior musculature. Skin flaps are closed over drain **(Fig. 35)**.

For more proximal amputations through the shaft of humerus the technique and flaps remain the same. The triceps is cut 3–5 cm longer then the intended level of bone section and carried anteriorly to cover the cut end of the bone.

Amputation through Neck of Humerus

The patient is placed supine with a sandbag beneath the affected shoulder so that the back is at a 45° angle to the operating table. The skin incision begins anteriorly at the level of the coracoid process and is carried distally along the anterior border of the deltoid muscle to the insertion of the muscle and along the posterior border of the muscle to the posterior axillary fold. The two limbs of the incision are connected by a second incision that passes through the axilla. The cephalic vein in the deltopectoral groove is identified, ligated, and cut. The deltoid is separated from the pectoralis major and retracted laterally. The pectoralis major muscle is cut at its insertion and reflected medially. The interval between the pectoralis minor and coracobrachialis muscles is developed to expose the neurovascular bundle. The axillary artery and vein immediately inferior to the pectoralis minor are isolated doubly ligated and cut. The median, ulnar, radial, and musculocutaneous nerves are divided so that their ends retract well proximal to the pectoralis minor. The deltoid muscle is divided at its insertion and reflected superiorly together with the attached lateral skin flap. The teres major and latissimus dorsi muscles are divided near their insertions at the bicipital groove. The long and short heads of the biceps, the triceps, and the coracobrachialis are cut at a point proximally 2 cm distal to the level of intended bone section. The humerus is cut at the level of its neck. The long head of the triceps, both heads of the biceps, and the coracobrachialis are sutured over the end of the humerus. Swing the pectoralis major muscle laterally and suture it to the end of the bone. The lateral skin flap and underlying

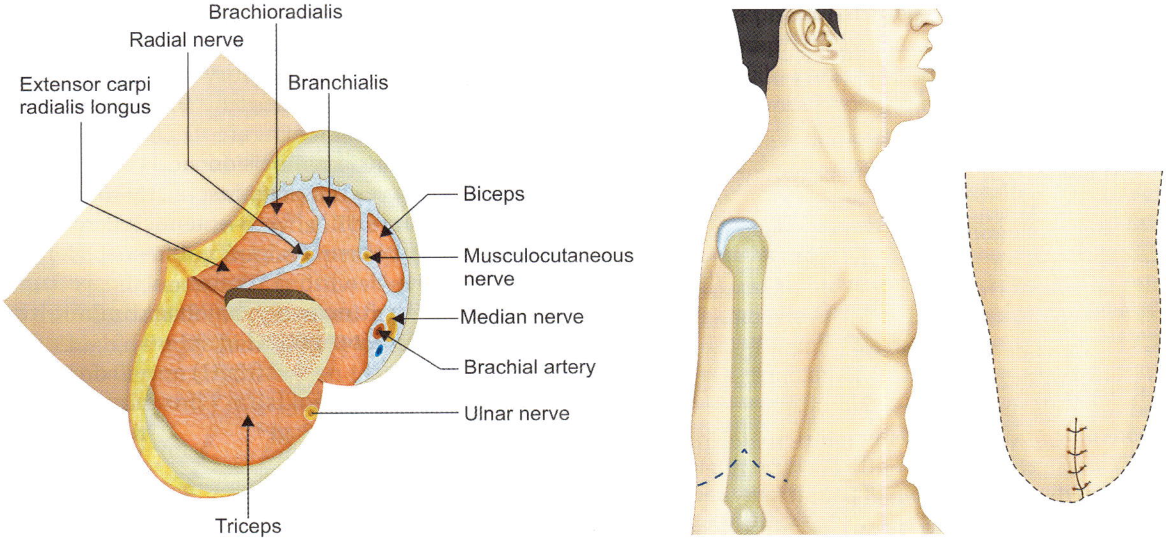

Fig. 35: Supracondylar amputation.

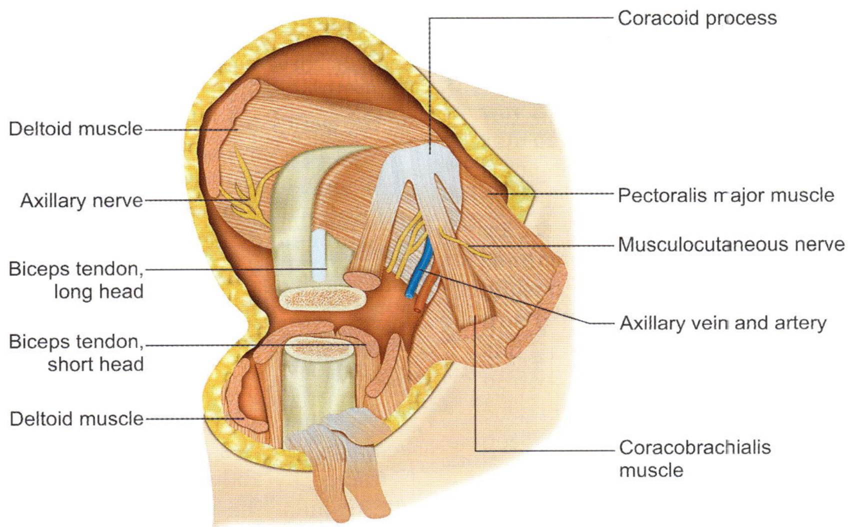

Fig. 36: Amputation through neck of humerus.

deltoid muscle are trimmed to allow accurate apposition of the skin edges and sutured with interrupted nonabsorbable material. Deep to the muscles and at the end of the bone, insert drains or plastic tubes for suction drainage **(Fig. 36)**.

Shoulder Disarticulation

The patient is supine with the shoulder at an angle of 45° to the table. The incision is begun at the coracoid process and proceeds distally along the anterior border of the deltoid up to its insertion. It is then continued along the posterior border of deltoid to meet the anterior incision in the axilla. The neurovascular bundle is identified in the interval between the coracobrachialis and the short head of the biceps and axillary artery and vein ligated and divided. The thoracoacromial artery is identified and treated in a similar manner. Allow the vessel to retract superiorly beneath the pectoralis minor muscle. The median, ulnar, radial, and musculocutaneous nerves are sharply divided and to retract into soft tissue. The deltoid is detached from its humeral insertion and retracted along with its overlying skin proximally. The coracobrachialis and short head of the biceps are released from their origin from the coracoid and the humeral insertion of the pectoralis major is also released. The arm is externally rotated and the anterior joint capsule and subscapularis muscle divided. The arm is then internally rotated and the short external rotators and the teres major divided. Finally, the triceps and inferior capsule are divided to remove the arm. Any unduly prominent acromion process is trimmed to give the shoulder a smooth contour. The muscle ends are sutured into the glenoid to fill dead space and the deltoid with its overlying skin inferiorly is brought and sutured to the margin of the posterior axilla, completing the procedure.

Forequarter Amputation Anterior Approach (Berger)

Also known as shoulder girdle amputation consists of removal of entire shoulder girdle/upper limb in interval between scapula and thoracic wall. It is classically indicated for malignant tumor involving upper humerus or shoulder joint. Atypical skin flaps often used and may require axillary skin grafts.

The incision is begun lateral to the clavicular insertion of the sternocleidomastoid muscle and extended distally along the clavicle to the acromioclavicular joint over the acromion to the spine of the scapula and posteriorly along the vertebral border of the scapula. The lower incision is begun at the middle third of the clavicle and proceeds distally to the deltopectoral groove and across the axilla horizontally and joins the first incision posteriorly at the spine of the scapula. The pectoralis major is released from the clavicle and the clavicle divided lateral to the insertion of the sternocleidomastoid. The clavicle is excised to the level of the acromioclavicular joint. The external jugular vein is ligated and the pectoralis major and minor released from their insertions, exposing the neurovascular bundle. The subclavian artery and veins are ligated. The components of the brachial plexus are sectioned and allowed to retract. The latissimus dorsi and axillary fascia is released from the humerus, allowing the limb to fall posteriorly. The arm is held across the chest and from superiorly to inferiorly the remaining muscles that fix the shoulder to the scapula are divided. The muscles that hold the scapula to the thorax are divided, starting with the trapezius and continuing through the omohyoid, levator scapulae, rhomboid major and minor, and serratus anterior. The arm and scapula are removed. The remaining muscles are sutured over the lateral chest wall and the skin flaps closed over suction drainage **(Figs. 37A to C)**.

Forequarter Amputation Posterior Approach (Little Wood)

The patient is placed in a lateral position in such a way as to permit anterior and posterior tilting. The posterior cervicoscapular incision is given first. It begins at the medial end of the clavicle and is extended laterally along its whole length, then over the acromion process to the posterior axillary fold. From here, it is extended along the axillary border of scapula till its inferior angle and then curved medially up to 5 cm from midline of the back. The skin and subcutaneous tissues are elevated, and the trapezius and latissimus dorsi muscles are divided close to the scapula. Using a hook the scapula is drawn away from the chest wall enabling the division of the levator scapulae and the rhomboids minor and major. Branches of the superficial cervical and descending scapular vessels are ligated. The serratus anterior is separated from the vertebral border of the scapula. At the medial end of the bone, the clavicle and subclavius muscle are divided. This allows the extremity to fall anteriorly, placing the neurovascular bundle under tension. The latter is found in the fibro-fatty tissue near the superior digitation of the serratus anterior. Divide the cords of the brachial plexus close to the spine and doubly ligate and divide the subclavian artery and vein. Care should be taken to avoid injury to the pleural dome. The omohyoid muscle is divided and the suprascapular vessels and external jugular vein are ligated and divided. The anterior pectoroaxillary incision starts at the middle of the clavicle and curves inferiorly just lateral to but parallel with the deltopectoral groove. It is extended across the anterior axillary fold and carried inferiorly and posteriorly to join the posterior incision at the lower third of the axillary border of the scapula. The pectoralis major and minor muscles are divided to remove the limb **(Fig. 38)**.

Tikhoff–Linberg Resection

The Tikhoff–Linberg resection is a limb-sparing surgery that involves removal of scapula, clavicle, and proximal humerus while preserving the arm. It is indicated in malignant tumors of the shoulder girdle which do not involve the neurovascular structures or the chest wall. It provides better functional and cosmetic outcomes than forequarter amputation.

It is done with the patient in lateral position and the arm draped free for manipulation. The approach is posterior with a curved incision to cover the entire tumor starting from tip of acromion suprolaterally and can be extended up to the paravertebral region or midline inferomedially. After raising medial and lateral skin flaps the trapezius muscle is detached from its attachment and raised to expose the supraspinatus muscle. The deltoid is also raised from its attachment to the scapula. The rhomboid major on the vertebral border, the latissimus dorsi on the inferior, the teres major and minor on the lateral border and the infraspinatus are identified. These are detached from the scapula starting with the latissimus dorsi from the inferior. This allows the inferior angle of scapula to be manipulated to give traction to the scapula and help removal of the rhomboids and levator scapulae muscles. The axillary contents can be explored and retracted by abducting the arm and applying traction on the scapula. The anterior structures are exposed through a deltopectoral approach. The pectoralis major is detached from the humerus and clavicle and reflected toward the sternum to expose the axilla, coracoid, brachial plexus, and anterior chest wall. Through the anterior incision short head of biceps and pectoralis major from the coracoid process are detached. Now the teres major and minor on the lateral border of scapula, the long head of triceps, the supra- and infraspinatus muscle and the serratus anterior are removed from the scapula. Lastly, the subscapularis is released. Part of the clavicle along with proximal humerus is now excised with the scapula. Soft-tissue reconstruction is done by suturing the deltoid and trapezius and teres and lattismus dorsi under tension.

Postoperative the arm is kept in a sling with pressure bandage to reduce swelling and elbow and hand movements are started within the sling. After above 2 weeks, the sling is discarded gradually and full range of motion exercises for elbow and wrist are started.

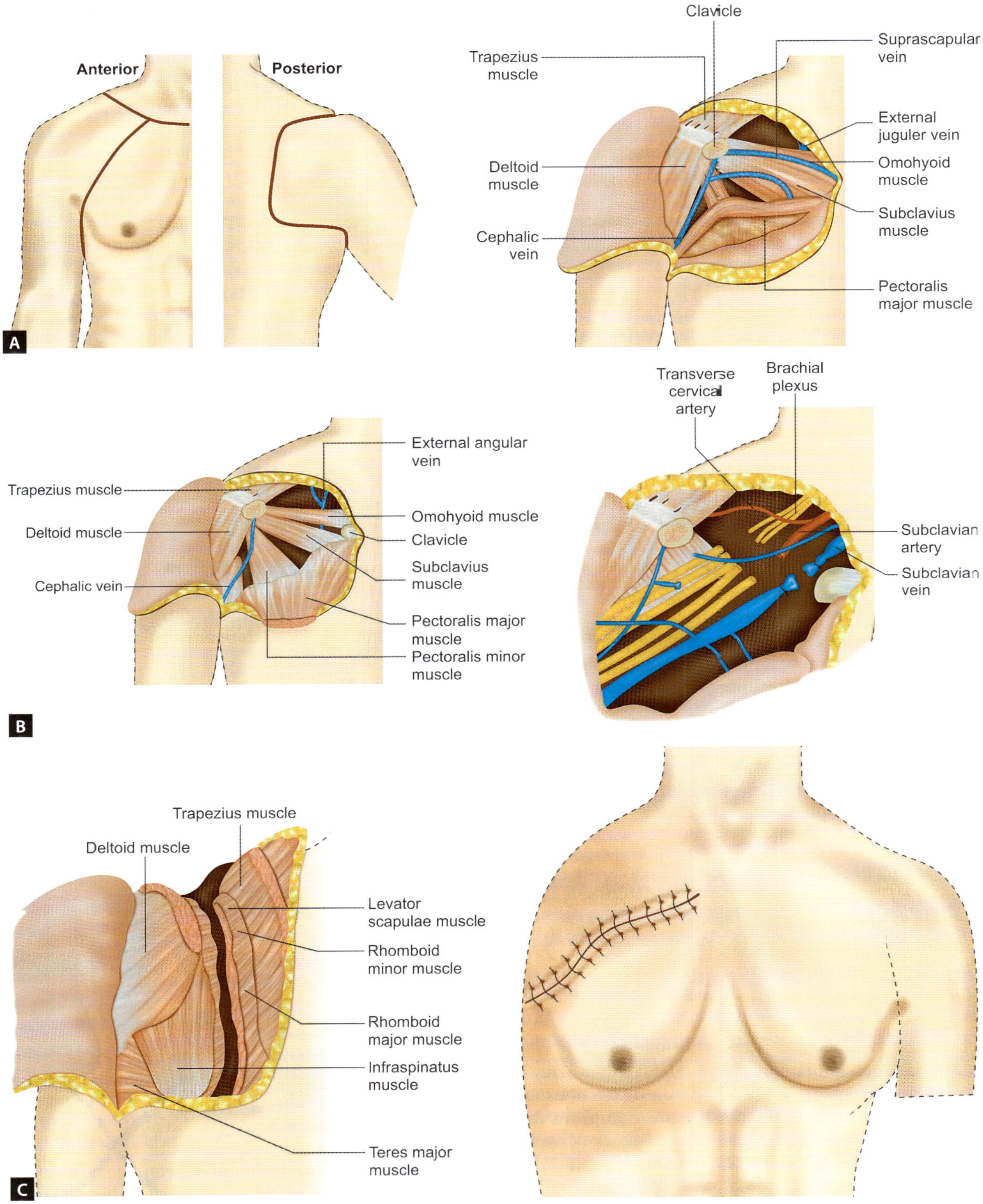

Figs. 37A to C: Forequarter amputation anterior approach (Berger).

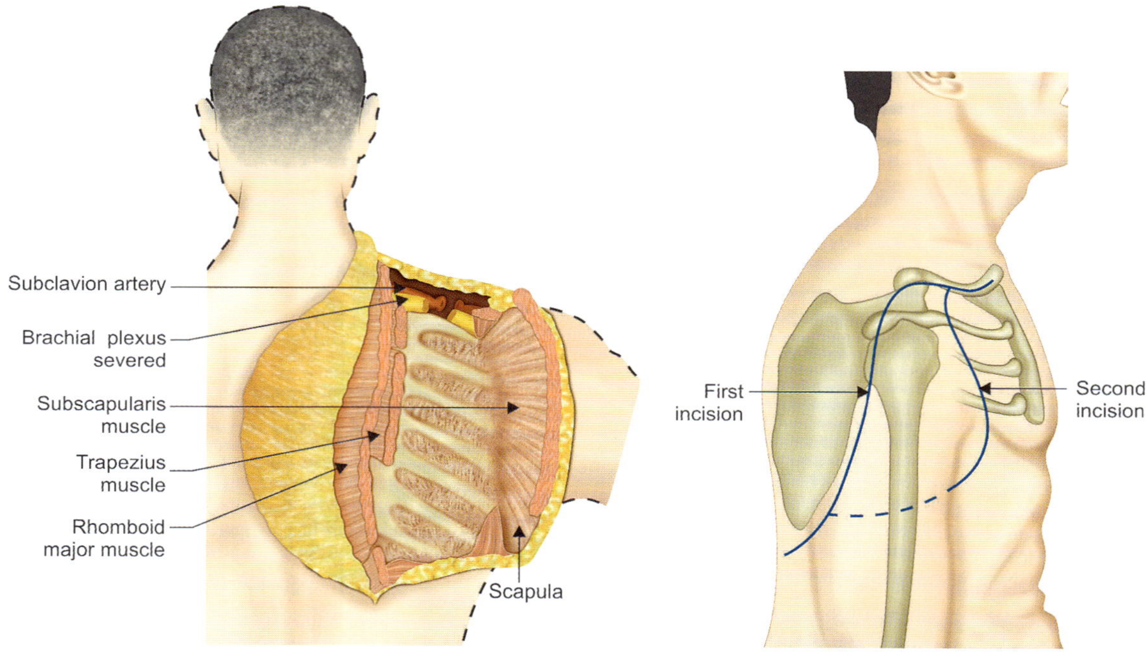

Fig. 38: Forequarter amputation posterior approach (Little wood).

PROSTHESES

INTRODUCTION

Prostheses are devices designed to replace the function or appearance of the missing limb. Whereas orthosis support, supplement, or augment the function of an existing limb.

Characteristic of a good prosthesis:

- Comfortable
- Convenient to do and remove
- Mechanically efficient and needing minimal maintenance
- Cosmetically acceptable
- Light weight and durable

While choosing prosthesis for a patient the following points must be taken into account:

- Level of amputation
- Condition of the residual limb
- Cognitive and neurological function of the patient
- Needs and vocation of the patient
- Financial resources
- Physical status. Which is assessed as follows:
    - A patient cannot ambulate safely either with or without assistance is classified as level 0 and usually in such patients a prosthesis cannot improve their mobility to a great extent.
    - A level 1 patient will have the ability to ambulate using a prosthesis but only on level surface and at a fixed speed. Typically, these are limited to activity around the household.
    - A level 2 patient can ambulate across and negotiate low level barriers such as curbs, stairs and limited uneven surfaces. They have some limited mobility around the community.
    - A level 3 patient can cross most environment barriers and also ambulate with varied speed. Their requirement for prosthesis may extend beyond simple locomotion to therapeutic exercise or vocational activity.
    - The level 4 patient is much more active and can do high impact activities and has high energy levels like children, active adults, and athletes.

LOWER LIMB PROSTHESIS

The lower limb prosthesis consists of the following parts (components):

- Socket (with or without liner)
- Suspension system
- Joint component (as needed)
- A connecting shank or pylon
- A prosthetic foot

The above components are fitted as per the level of amputation and requirement of the patient.

Socket

The socket is the bearing point and interface between the prosthesis and residual limb. It serves following purpose:

- It protects the residual limb.
- Transmits the forces during ambulation.

It is commonly made using a plaster mold of the residual limb. Computer-assisted technology can also be used to map the residual limb, manufacturing a socket directly from that data.

These are usually total contact sockets that prevent complications of earlier plug-fit design, like skin problems, chronic choke syndrome and ulceration.

The most common socket for transtibial amputations is the patellar tendon bearing (PTB) socket, where the predominant weight bearing is over the patellar tendon below the patella **(Fig. 39)**.

Total surface bearing (TSB): Transtibial sockets are now designed in which weight is distributed over many different areas, such as the anterior and posterior compartments and the medial tibial flair.

Variations: Patellar tendon bearing-supracondylar (PTB-SC) socket that has high medial and lateral sidewalls that extend above and over the femoral condyles, providing enhanced mediolateral stability and self-suspension **(Fig. 40)**.

Patellar tendon bearing-supracondylar-suprapatellar (PTB-SCSP) socket furthers the PTB-SC concept by also extending the anterior aspect so that the patella is enclosed within the socket. The PTB-SCSP socket gives additional stiffness to the mediolateral walls **(Fig. 41)**.

Both the above variations are especially useful for short residual stumps to improve varus/valgus control and to provide greater area for weight distribution.

A joint-and-corset system can also be used to take the weight bearing to the thigh and it is especially good for heavy-duty use **(Fig. 42)**.

Gel liners can be used with total surface weight-bearing (TSB) socket to distribute pressure uniformly over the stump. These require minimal modifications to the original cast mold of the stump.

Icelandic-Swedish-New York (ISNY) University PTB socket is a two-layered PTB socket with an inner thin, flexible, vacuum-formed plastic PTB socket and an outer rigid, carbon-fiber-reinforced and laminated frame for weight transmission.

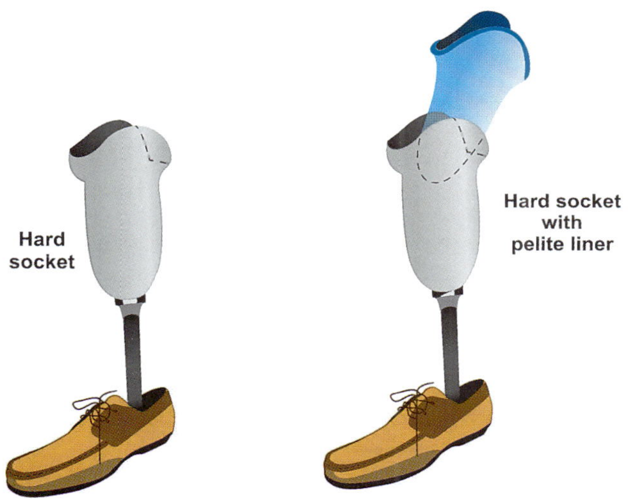

Fig. 39: Patellar tendon bearing (PTB) socket.

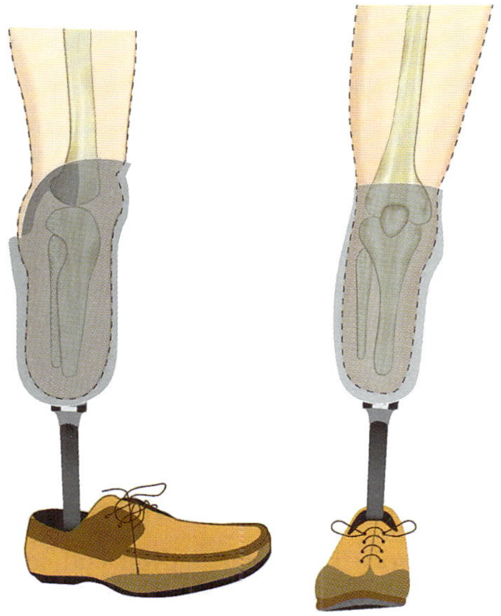

Fig. 41: Patellar tendon bearing-supracondylar suprapatellar (PTB-SCSP) socket.

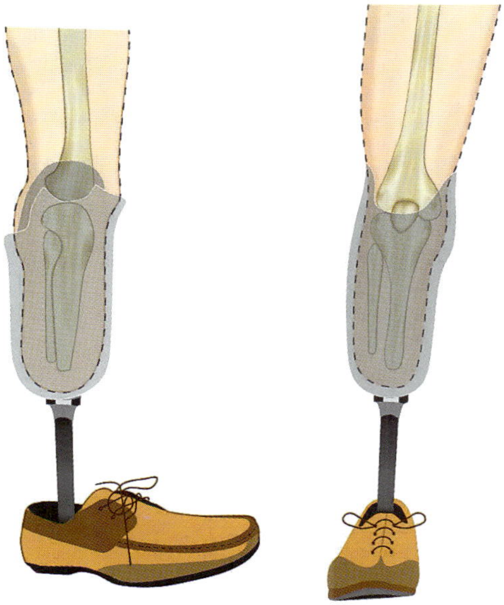

Fig. 40: Patellar tendon bearing-supracondylar (PTB-SC) socket.

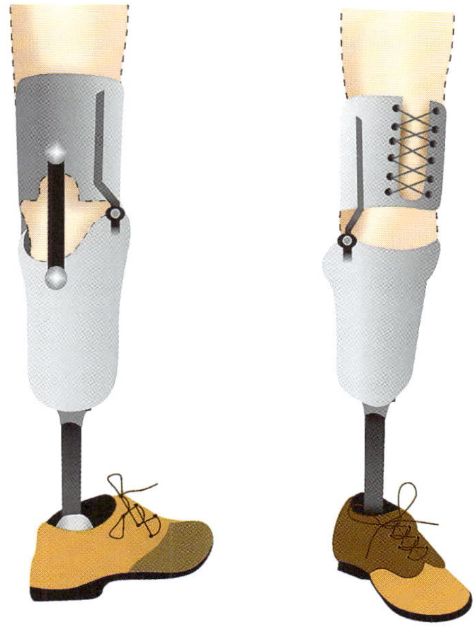

Fig. 42: Joint-and-corset system.

The most commonly used socket for transfemoral amputations is the ischial containment socket. It has a wide anteroposterior diameter and narrow mediolateral diameter. The narrow mediolateral fit is that it prevents abduction of the thigh stump during the stance phase especially in limbs where the adductors have not been anchored distally. The predominant weight-bearing is over the ischial tuberosity and a posterior rim is created parallel to the floor and when the patient walks he actually sits on the posterior wall of the prosthesis.

Suspension Systems

Suspension systems are required to prevent the prosthesis from falling off the residual limb.

Self-suspension: In this, the normal anatomical flare of the stump is used to provide suspension like use of malleolus flare in Symes, amputation or femoral condylar flare in knee disarticulation.

Suction suspension: Commonly used for transfemoral prosthesis. It consists of a close-fitting rigid socket with a one-way air valve at the distal end. The close fit creates a seal between the skin and the socket. When air is driven out from the distal end of the socket in weight bearing, a small negative pressure is created, which is strong enough to suspend the prosthesis. It is a light-weight system and provides good proprioceptive feedback but it does not tolerate much weight and requires frequent change as the volume and shape of the stump changes **(Fig. 43)**.

Another method to create vacuum is through a vacuum pump built into the prosthesis. It uses the vertical shock of the pylon to continually withdraw air from the sealed socket.

Suspension harness: The supracondylar cuff consisting of an adjustable strap encircling the thigh just over the femoral condyles can be used as a harness suspension system for a transtibial prosthesis **(Fig. 44)**.

The Silesian belt is used for transfemoral prosthesis, it is attached to the socket laterally, above the greater trochanter and wrapped around the opposite iliac crest. It does not control rotation very well but a single-axis hip joint can be integrated into the lateral socket wall and pelvic band can be used to control rotation **(Fig. 45)**.

The total elastic suspension (TES) belt is made from neoprene material. It slips over the outside of the prosthetic socket and surrounds the waist above the iliac crest to provide suspension. The TES belt provides better rotational control and is more commonly used **(Fig. 46)**.

The gel liner suction system, which uses a gel elastomeric liner, can also be used as a suspension system. The liner rolls onto the residual limb and is then inserted and locked

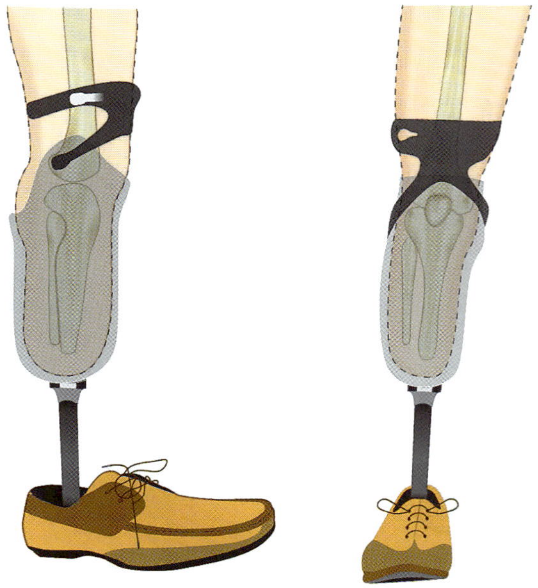

Fig. 44: Suspension harness.

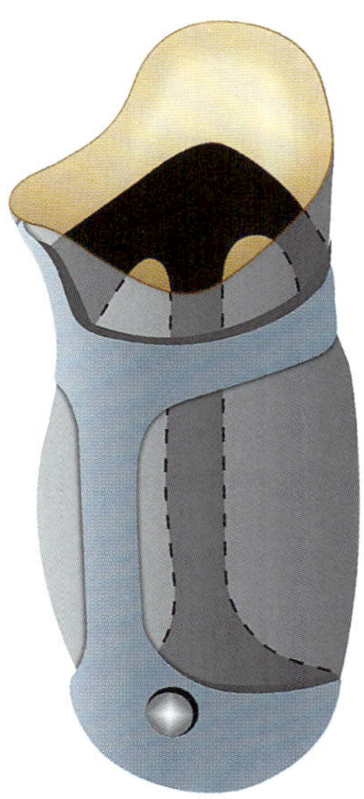

Fig. 43: Suction suspension.

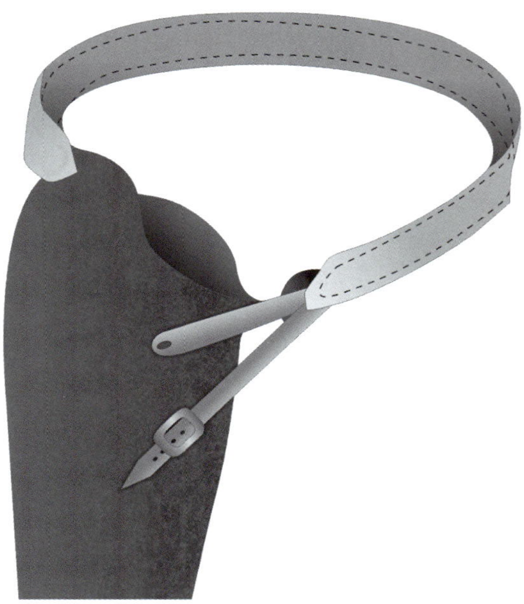

Fig. 45: Silesian belt.

into the socket. This suspension system provides improved cosmesis, cushions the residual limb, reduces shear between the residual limb and the socket and minimizes pistoning of the residual limb in the socket, but it causes heat buildup, skin problems, and decreased proprioception.

Disadvantages of harness systems:

- Pistoning
- Reduced comfort
- Heat
- Dermatitis and chafing

JOINTS

Knee

The most important joint in the lower limb prosthesis is the knee joint. A large variety of designs are available to suit various needs. It can be a simple hinge joint or a polycentric knee with multiple centers of rotation but polycentric knees are heavy, costly, and require high maintenance.

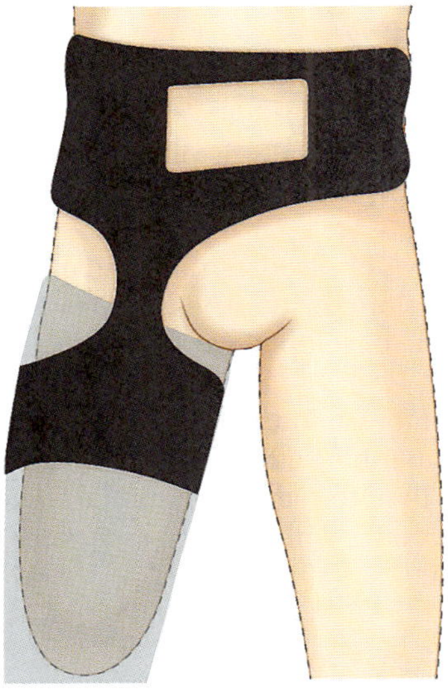

Fig. 46: The total elastic suspension (TES).

For stability during stance phase, various types of locking mechanisms are there for knee joint.

The most basic is the manual-locking knee which provides the most stability, but the gait is awkward and energy consuming. It is ideal for a hemiparetic residual limb and in heavy manual laborer.

The weight activated or safety knee produces friction and locks during extension and on weight bearing and automatically unlocks during swing phase when weight is removed **(Fig. 47)**. It allows for ambulation on uneven surfaces and is the ideal knee for geriatric patients and for patients with poor hip control. There is a delay in swing phase as complete unloading must occur for the knee to unlock. Patient with bilateral transfemoral amputations cannot use this as a bilateral delay in swing phase is not tolerated.

The hydraulic knee (pneumatic or oil) allows for variable friction during various phases of gait ranging from minimal during swing phase to maximum during stance phase. It provides for a more natural gait but requires more muscle control and is ideal for younger patients. The knee is heavy, costly, and requires high maintenance **(Fig. 48)**.

Microprocessor-based hydraulic knees are a further advancement which improve the timing and rate of change of friction of hydraulic and pneumatic knees. It leads to a more natural gait and minimal energy expenditure. Their greatest advantage is while climbing up and down stairs. They automatically adjust the rate of change of friction as the pace of walking changes allowing for greater speeds, e.g., Otto Bock C-Leg.

Microprocessor-based knees have been further improved by sensors that measure the angle and load on the knee up to 1,000 times per second and using a varying magnetic field bring about a change in friction in the knee by changing the

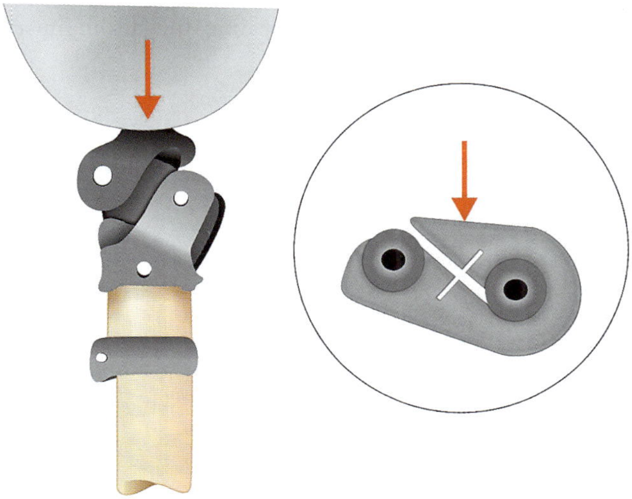

Fig. 47: Weight activated or safety knee.

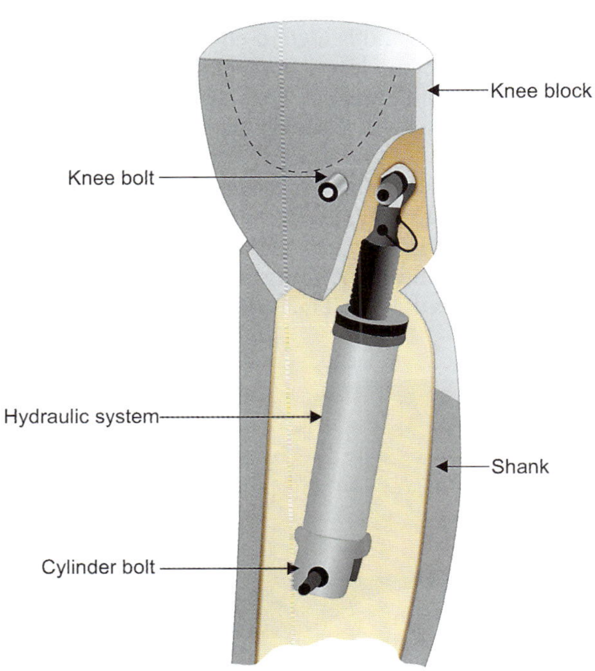

Fig. 48: Hydraulic knee.

viscosity of a special fluid in the knee, which is sensitive to magnetics fields, e.g., Rheo knee.

Ankle and Foot

The ankle function is part of the foot or terminal device. A separate ankle joint requires more energy expenditure and greater limb strength to control and is of benefit only in heavy-duty industrial work or specialized activities, such as mountain climbing, swimming, and rowing.

Ankle and foot systems can be of two types—energy returning and nonenergy-returning systems.

Nonenergy-returning feet are the solid-ankle, cushioned-heel (SACH) foot, and the single-axis foot.

The SACH foot allows ankle plantar flexion allowing for a smooth gait **(Fig. 49)**. It is a low-cost and low-maintenance foot for a sedentary patient. The forefoot remains rigid and provides an anterior lever arm and proprioception. It consumes more energy and is difficult to use on uneven surfaces.

Stationary attachment/flexible endoskeleton (SAFE) foot is another solid foot which is more mobile than a SACH foot. It has a flexible keel which allows some movement in frontal and transverse planes. It can be used on uneven surfaces.

Stored energy (STEN) foot has a three-piece wooden keel joined by two rubber plugs. The compression and recoil of the rubber plugs gives it some amount of energy return. The single-axis foot has additional passive plantar flexion and dorsiflexion, thus giving stability during the stance phase. It enhances knee stability but is heavier than SACH foot and requires more maintenance.

Energy-returning feet assist the body's natural biomechanics and cause less oxygen consumption. The multiaxis foot and the dynamic-response foot are some examples.

The multiaxis foot has inversion, eversion, and rotation in addition to plantar flexion and dorsiflexion; it is good for uneven terrain well and is a good choice for the individual with a minimal-to-moderate activity level. It is expensive and has greater maintenance cost. The greater latitude of movement makes it unstable in patients with decreased coordination.

The dynamic-response foot is the most advanced foot and used by young, active persons, and by athletic individuals. The forefoot acts like a spring, compressing in the stance phase and rebounding at toe-off. Some examples are the College Park Foot **(Fig. 50)**, the Otto Bock Dynamic Foot, the Flex Foot, the Seattle Foot, the Quantum Foot, and the Carbon Copy II.

Jaipur foot: It is an indigenous transtibial prosthesis created in 1968 by Dr PK Sethi and Ram Chandra Sharma at Department of Orthopedics at Sawai Man Singh Medical College, Jaipur, Rajasthan. It was created as a substitute for the SACH foot to suit certain local requirements and to reduce cost. The objectives were to create a low cost low maintenance prosthesis that was durable, waterproof, could be used without footwear, could be made from locally available material, and allow squatting and walking on uneven terrain.

The Jaipur foot is a nonarticulated foot-ankle assembly. It consists of three structural blocks. The forefoot and hindfoot are made of rubber and the ankle block is of light wood. These three blocks along with the toes are bound together and encapsulated in skin-colored compound **(Fig. 51)**. It permits the following range of motion:

- *Dorsiflexion:* 20–35°
- *Heel compression:* 8–2.8 mm
- *Pronation:* 26–29°
- *Supination:* 15–22°
- *Axial internal rotation:* 11–12°
- *Axial external rotation:* 4–8°

The socket was initially a plug fit design made from aluminum, but now it is made using a molded total contact sockets.

Though it is widely used in India and in other developing and under developed countries, it has not found wide acceptance in the developed world because of the following disadvantages:

- It is not available in international standard sizes.
- It is not compatible with designs of western limbs.
- It is heavier than the set international standards.
- It does not come with quality assurance and standard certification.

Hip Prosthesis

Disarticulation or hemipelvectomy prosthesis is the most difficult to fit and has very high rejection rates. The energy requirements to use such prostheses are as much as 200% of normal ambulation. At the same time, the lack of muscle

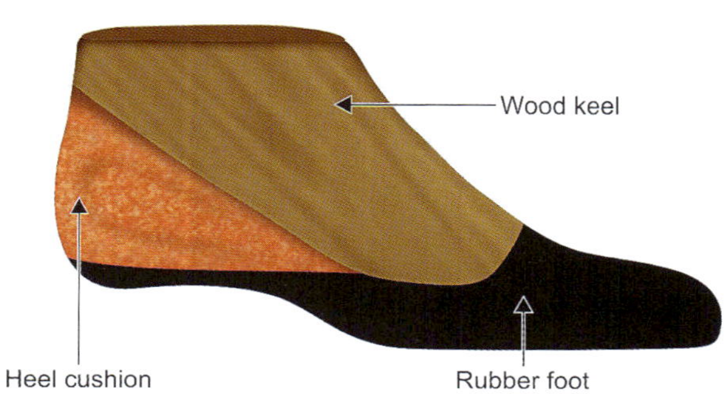

Fig. 49: Solid-ankle, cushioned-heel (SACH) foot.

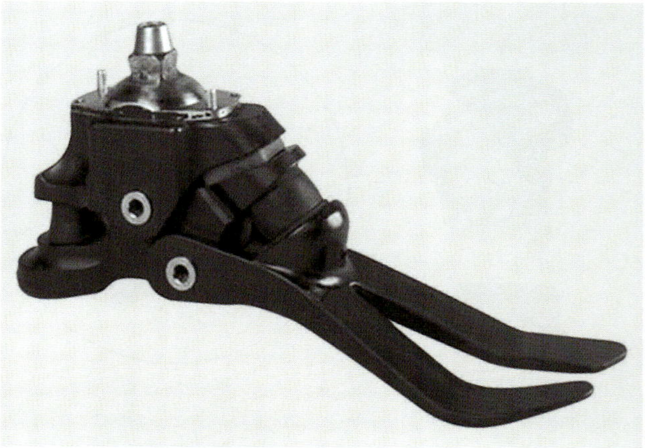

Fig. 50: Multiaxis foot (College Park Foot).

power at the hip, knee, and ankle/foot results in a fixed, slow cadence. Only those who develop sufficient balance to ambulate with a single cane are likely to wear such prosthesis. Those who remain dependent on dual canes or crutches for balance move much better without prosthesis, with no more energy expenditure than prosthesis. Such prosthesis is typically fitted to motivated and physiologically vigorous individuals.

One of the earliest designs was "the saucer-type prosthesis". The saucer type of prosthesis was essentially a standard above-knee leg with a saucer-shaped socket on top of the thigh. Suspension was by means of a single-axis joint and pelvic band. This type was most suitable for short-femur amputations. It could be used with a manual or semiautomatic lock.

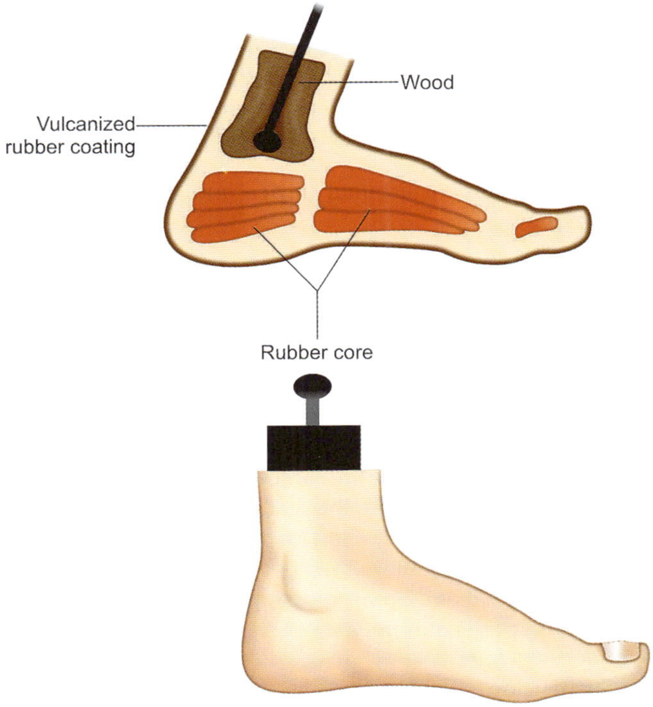

Fig. 51: The Jaipur foot.

The "tilting-table prosthesis" has a molded leather socket which is laterally placed for the hip joint. It fits the stump and is attached to the pelvis and shoulder with straps. A simple metal hinge joint connects it to the thigh section; this can have a semiautomatic lock. This type of prosthesis requires a large amount of pelvic thrust to propel it resulting in a vaulting gait.

McLaurin introduced a design in 1954 called the "Canadian" design. The prostheses has only unlocked joints and relies on biomechanics for stability during stance phase and the unlocked joints permit flexion at hip and knee during the swing phase.

Suspension during swing is provided by a molded plastic socket which covers the ischial tuberosity and the crest of the ilium. It also encases the contralateral pelvis thus providing mediolateral trunk stability. The hip joint is positioned anteriorly helping to achieve good stance-phase stability in addition to good swing-phase flexion provided by the nonlock design. The hip joint moves in a single axis and has an extension stop and extension assist.

The Canadian design requires that the prosthesis must be significantly short (1 cm+) to avoid forcing the amputee to vault for toe clearance. This can be overcome by the hip flexion bias system. At toe-off, kinetic energy from the coil spring is released and the prosthetic thigh is thrust forward. During stance phase, the coiled spring again collapses. This provides the amputee with a more normal-appearing gait and improves ground clearance. As a result, the prosthesis can be lengthened to a nearly level configuration. This must be combined with a stable locking safe knee to prevent the strong flexion that occurs at the knee as the spring coils **(Fig. 52)**.

The single-axis (constant-friction) knee remains the most widely utilized due to its light weight, low cost, and

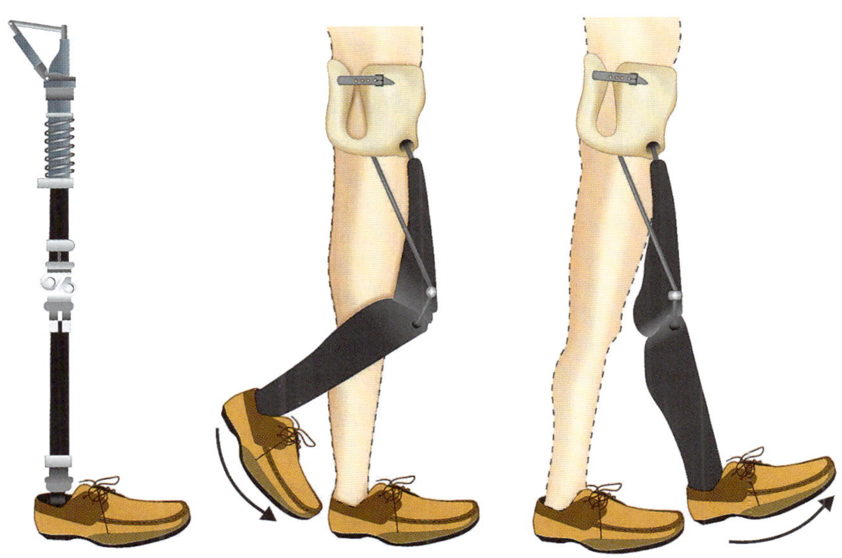

Fig. 52: Canadian hip prosthesis.

excellent durability. The friction-brake stance control (safety) knee is the second most frequently utilized component.

The SACH foot is the most common foot used with the hip prosthesis because of its inherent stability and durability.

A transverse-rotation unit or positional rotators or "turn-table attachment" can be installed above the knee mechanism, these devices permit the amputee to press a button and passively rotate the shank 90° or more for sitting comfort. They only facilitate sitting cross-legged upon the floor, permit easier entry into restaurant booths and other confined areas. It also makes for easier donning of the prosthesis.

In recent times, the Canadian hip prosthesis has been combined with more advanced hydraulic and micro-processor-controlled knees and multi-axis and energy returning ankle and foot systems to provide a more natural gait. This is especially important in young fit individuals who feel the need to have a faster gait than that provided by the traditional prosthesis.

Pylon or Shank

The pylon is a tube or shell that attaches the socket to the terminal device. It can be simple, static shells having an exoskeleton (soft foam contoured to match the other limb and covered with a hard, laminated shell) or an endoskeleton (an internal, metal frame with cosmetic soft covering). It can also be a dynamic device that allows axial rotation (turn-table attachment) and that absorbs, stores, and releases energy (spring loaded).

The above-mentioned parts are assembled as per the level of amputation and requirement of patient.

Below Knee Prosthesis

- *Socket:* Patellar tendon bearing-supracondylar (PTB-SC) socket
  - Patellar tendon bearing-supracondylar-suprapatellar (PTB-SCSP) socket
  - Gel liners can be used with total surface weight-bearing (TSB) socket.
  - *Suspension harness:* The supracondylar cuff
- *Shank:* Exoskeleton or endoskeleton with cosmetic covering
- *Foot:* The solid-ankle cushioned-heel (SACH) foot.
  - The single-axis foot
  - Stationary attachment/flexible endoskeleton (SAFE) foot
  - Stored energy (STEN) foot
  - The single-axis foot
  - The multiaxis foot
  - The dynamic-response foot

Above Knee Prosthesis

- *Socket:* The ischial containment socket
  - Suction suspension
  - The Silesian belt
  - The TES belt
- *Knee joint:*
  - Simple hinge joint
  - Polycentric knee
  - The manual-locking knee
  - Weight activated or safety knee
  - Hydraulic knee (pneumatic or oil)
  - Microprocessor based hydraulic knees

The shank and foot are same as that of a below knee prosthesis.

Upper Limb Prosthesis

Upper limb prosthesis can be broadly of the following types:

- Cosmetic prostheses
- Body-powered prostheses (Cable controlled)
- Externally powered prostheses (Myoelectric and switch-controlled prostheses)
- *Hybrid:*
  - Cable to elbow or terminal device and battery powered
  - Excursion to elbow and battery-powered terminal device
  - Excursion to terminal device and battery-powered elbow

Cosmetic Prostheses

These look natural, but they are difficult to keep clean, expensive and usually sacrifice function for increased cosmetic appearance.

Body-powered Prostheses

Body-powered prostheses are cable driven. They are durable and have better sensory feedback. They are less cosmetically pleasing than a myoelectrically controlled type and require grosser limb movement.

Conventional body-powered, upper extremity prosthesis has the following components:

- Socket
- Suspension
- Control-cable system
- Terminal device
- Components for any interposing joints as needed according to the level of amputation

Socket

The socket of upper extremity prosthesis has a dual-wall design. A rigid inner socket is fabricated to fit the patient's residual limb and the second, outer wall is added for cosmesis.

The inner liner can also have two components, a flexible gel material for greater comfort and a rigid frame, which is utilized for structural support and for attaching the necessary cables and joints as needed.

Suspension

As in lower limb the suspension systems can be divided into harness based, suction, and self-suspending socket based.

Of the above-mentioned systems the "harness based" ones are most common. A "Figure-of-8 strap" loops around the axilla on contralateral side and is used to anchors the harness and provides force for the suspension and control-cable. There are two straps—the anterior or superior; one is attached to the socket of a transhumeral prosthesis or to the intermediate Y-strap and triceps cuff of a transradial prosthesis. Whereas, the posterior or inferior strap is used to attach the control cable.

For heavier prosthesis suspension, an additional chest-strap suspension can be used **(Fig. 53)**.

For wrist elbow or transradial amputations. "Self-suspending sockets" like the "Munster socket" can be used. It is most commonly used with an externally powered, myoelectrically-controlled transradial prosthesis.

Like in the lower extremity a suction system using a one-way air valve and gel liner can be used to provide a "Suction suspension". As in the lower limb, they can be fitted only in a residual limb with no skin scarring. These used for the patient with a transhumeral amputation. They can also be used with a harness suspension to provide for a more secure suspension of the prosthesis.

Control-cable Mechanisms

Body-powered prosthetic limbs use cables to control a function. A single cable passing through a single housing can transfer movement from the humerus, shoulder, or chest to the terminal device **(Fig. 54)**. It activates a single prosthetic

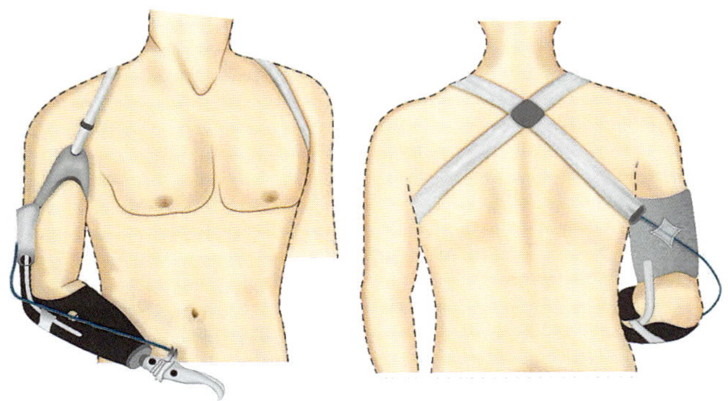

Fig. 53: Shoulder saddle.

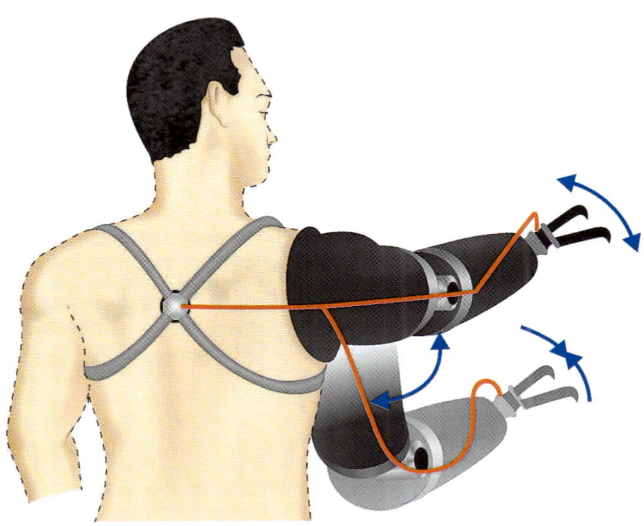

Fig. 54: Single-control cable.

component or function and is called a "Bowden cable system". One cable can be used to control two prosthetic functions by passing it through two separate cable housings, an arrangement known as "fair lead cable system". Two functions like flexion of the elbow and when the elbow is locked, movement of the terminal device can be accomplished.

Body movements that are used for prosthetic control via cables are:

- *Glenohumeral forward flexion*: It provides excellent power and reach and is good for activities away from midline.
- *Biscapular abduction (chest expansion), mutual protraction*: The force generated is weak but it is good for fine motor activities that are performed near the midline or close to the trunk of the body.
- *Glenohumeral depression/elevation, extension and abduction*: In transhumeral amputation, this movement can lock and unlock the elbow using a separate cable place anteriorly.
- An alternative is to use scapular elevation transmitted via a waist-belt or groin loop to achieve the same effect.

Terminal Device

The terminal device replicates five types of grip **(Fig. 55)**:

The "precision or pinch grip" is between the thumb and index finger used to pick a small object. The "tripod/palmer or three jaw chuck grip" uses the thumb against the index and middle finger. The "lateral grip or key pinch" uses the thumb against the lateral aspect of index finger as in turning a key in a lock. "Hook grip" is used to carry things with handles like a briefcase. Here, the DIP joint and PIP joint are flexed and the thumb is extended. "Spherical grip" uses the tips of thumb and all four fingers as in turning a door knob.

Passive Terminal Devices

Passive terminal devices can also be for both function and cosmesis **(Fig. 56)**.

A simple mitten used by an infant to facilitate crawling or ball holding or racquet-like devices used by adults for sports are some functional passive terminal devices. They are more cosmetic but less functional than active terminal devices.

Active Terminal Devices

Active devices are of two main categories: (1) Specialized function terminal devices (e.g., hook) and (2) Prosthetic hands. They can be cable or power operated.

Cable-operated active terminal devices like hooks or hands function by two types of mechanisms. If the device remains closed at rest using spring or cables, it is called voluntary opening mechanism. Movement by patient opens the device and relaxation closes it. The force that is generated and this can be varied by using different numbers of bands **(Fig. 57)**.

In a voluntary closing mechanism, the terminal device is open at rest. The patient uses motion to close the terminal device, grasping the desired object. It is usually heavier and less durable than a voluntary opening mechanism but offers better control of closing pressure and is more physiologic.

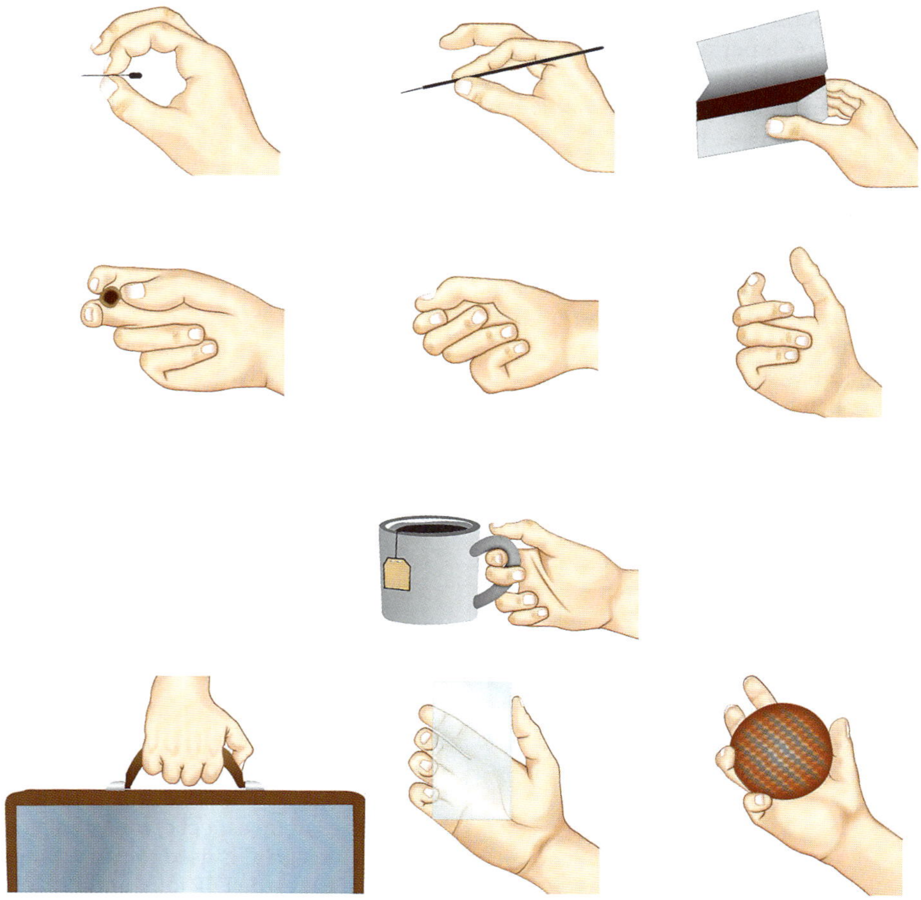

Fig. 55: Types of grips.

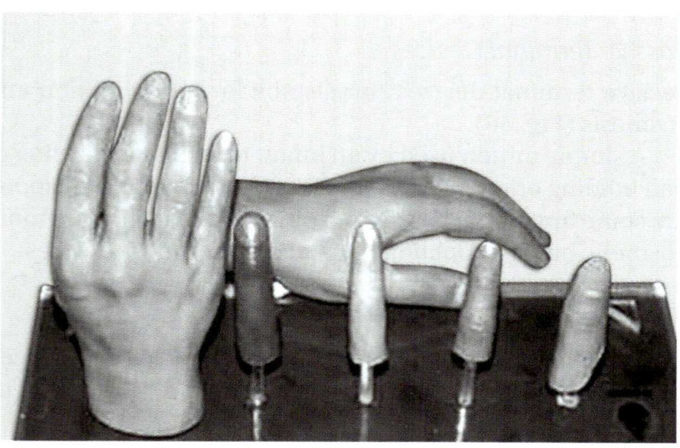

Fig. 56: Passive terminal devices.

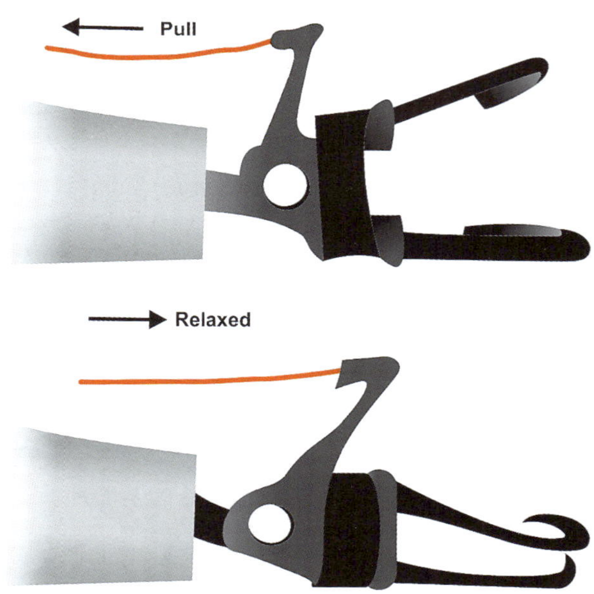

Fig. 57: Hook.

It requires sustained active effort and is needed to maintain closure to prevent dropping items. The amputee gets some sensory feedback with this type of terminal device.

A prosthetic hand is bulkier and heavier than a hook, but is more cosmetically pleasing. It can be powered by a cable or utilize external power.

Hook-style terminal devices provide only lateral pinch grip, whereas active hands provide a three-point chuck action. Many different options are available for terminal devices that address occupations, hobbies, and sports.

Multiarticulating prosthetic hands terminal devices are electrically powered and have more functionality than

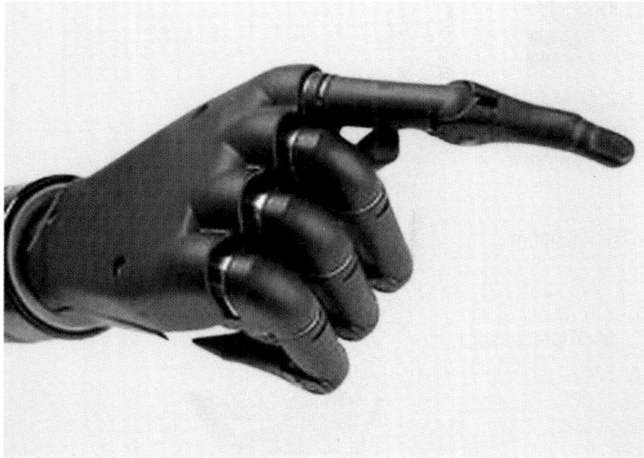

Fig. 58: Multiarticulating prosthetic hand.

other terminal device types **(Fig. 58)**. Grip, prehension, and positioning patterns can all be programed into the hand and are limited only by the number of control sites available. Grip force can be varied by increasing the electric signal to the hand. They are fragile and cannot be used for heavy-duty activities. Multiarticulating hand can be used for everyday tasks and a myoelectric hook or body-powered prosthesis with a hook for heavy-duty tasks.

COMPONENTS FOR INTERPOSING JOINTS

Wrist Units

It provides orientation of the terminal device. It can be positioned manually, by cable operation, or with external power. The wrist unit can be held steady by friction or mechanical lock. Of the two friction units are easier to position but unsuitable for heavy loads. The locking wrist unit can lock and thus lift heavier loads.

A quick-disconnect system with the wrist unit allows rapid and easy change of different types of terminal devices as required.

A wrist flexion unit provides an amputee improved function for midline activities, such as shaving, manipulating buttons, or performing perineal care. Multifunction wrist units combine the above functions.

Elbow Units

Elbow units are chosen based on the level of the amputation and the amount of residual function as supination and pronation of the forearm decrease as the site of amputation becomes more proximal. There are two types: (1) Flexible and (2) rigid.

Flexible elbow hinges are used for medium and long transradial amputations and wrist disarticulations. They help to translate any residual active pronation and supination to the terminal device.

Rigid elbow hinges are used in short transradial amputations, when the patient has no residual, active forearm pronation, and supination.

In patients with very short transradial, residual limbs or limited active elbow flexion, the use of step-up elbow hinges improves prosthetic function by increasing functional, active elbow motion. In this system, for the terminal device to move 2°, 1° of actual motion is required at elbow of the residual limb. The proprioceptive feedback is compromised.

Transhumeral prosthesis uses an internal locking elbow joint. This allows for 135° of flexion and can be locked into a number of preset flexed positions. A turntable is incorporated permitting internal or external rotation. Elbow flexion is facilitated with a spring lift to counter weight of forearm part of the prosthesis.

About 8–10 cm is needed to fit a standard elbow unit. For longer residual limb, the forearm section of the prosthesis needs to be lengthened to accommodate the lengthened arm section to allow the amputee to reach the midline or mouth. However, this results in difficulties when the patient tries to perform bimanual activities. In such cases, external elbow joints may be used, but they are not cosmetic or as durable as internal elbow joints.

Shoulder and Forequarter Units

Function is difficult to restore at the shoulder or forequarter level. This is due to the weight of the prosthetic components and the diminished overall function. A high amount of energy is required to use the prosthesis and unilateral amputees usually prefer cosmetic prosthesis.

EXTERNALLY POWERED PROSTHESES

Motors and batteries can be used to operate these prostheses and they provide better proximal function and better grip. Their disadvantages are that they are heavy, expensive, and difficult to maintain. Also have minimal sensory feedback.

These prostheses can be controlled by either "myoelectric or switch control".

In myoelectric control, muscle contractions are used as a signal to move the prosthesis. Surface electrodes are used to detect the electrical activity generated by muscle without gross movement taking place in the muscle **(Fig. 59)**.

Different switch systems exist:

- The two-site/two-function (dual-site) system has separate electrodes for separate prosthetic activity, such as flexion/extension or pronation/supination and is easier to control.
- But, when limited control sites are available on the residual limb a 1-site/2-function (single-site) device may be used. This system uses 1 electrode to control two functions of a paired activity (e.g., flexion and extension); the patient uses contractions of different strengths to differentiate between flexion and extension (e.g., a strong contraction opens the device and a weak contraction closes it).
- Sometimes multiple powered components on a single prosthesis must be controlled by a single switch, (e.g., terminal device, elbow activation) using sequential or multistate controller. The electrode function can be switched from one to another either by an external switch or by a brief contraction of the muscle.

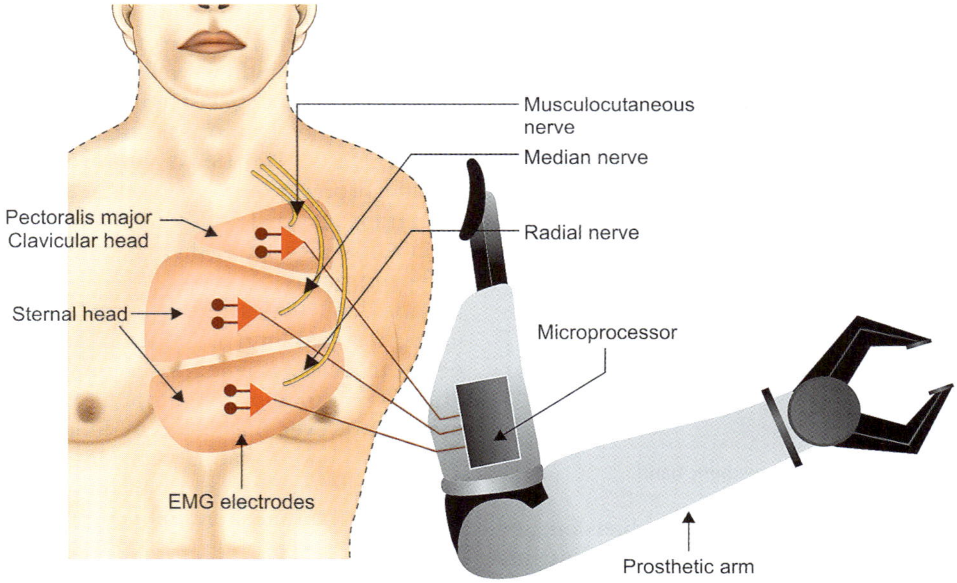

Fig. 59: Myoelectrically-controlled prosthesis. (EMG: electromyography)

- In "switch-controlled" prostheses, there are switches in the socket or in the suspension harness of the prosthesis. These switches are activated by the movement of a remnant part or by pull on harness. They are used in those patients who are unable to control myoelectric points or if such points are not available.
- The speed or force generated in the prosthesis can be varied by changing the intensity of muscle contraction.

ORTHOTICS

Orthotics are mechanical aids that are given to improve the function and to stabilize limbs. They are commonly used for neurologic problems, such as stroke, cerebral palsy, traumatic brain injury, spinal cord injury, multiple sclerosis, and peripheral nerve injury. Another common use is in arthritic conditions.

An orthosis serves the following functions:

- Stabilization of joints
- Prevention and correction of deformities
- To prevent unwanted and to promotes useful movement
- Provide rest

When used for lower limbs they are known as calipers. They are commonly classified based on the joints which they span and support. For example:

- Foot orthosis (FO), ankle orthosis (AO), knee orthosis (KO), and hip orthosis (HO)
- Ankle foot orthosis (AFO)
- Knee ankle foot orthosis (KAFO)

Orthosis spanning five or more segments are called compound orthosis.

Common materials used for orthosis are metals like steel or aluminum and plastics. Metals are heavy but more durable whereas plastic are lighter, cosmetic, and easier to mold. Usually an orthosis is a hybrid of these two materials. It can be made to fit from a plaster of Paris mold of the part or may be an off the shelf devise in different sizes.

The following are the main components of a lower limb orthosis:

Foot Orthosis

The shoe is a basic foot orthosis. It consists of the following parts:

Bottom: It includes:

- "Outsole" is the part that contacts with floor and is made of anti-skid material-like rubber.
- "Insole" is the part in contact with the foot and is made of soft material. It may be reinforced at the front middle or back part to give support to metatarsal head, arch or heel of foot. These two layers are usually separated by a compressible material.
- "Ball" is the anterior part of the bottom that corresponds to the metatarsal head. Heel is the posterior most part and the shank area is the intervening part. Based on the height, it can be of following types: Spring heel (3–5 mm), Oxford heel (19–25 mm), Military heel (31 mm), and Cuban heel (38 mm).

Upper: This is the part above the sole and consists of and anterior section (vamp) and posterior section (quarters). This part also has the tying laces **(Fig. 60)**.

Shoe attachments: These are used to attach the shoe to a proximal ankle joint. It can be directly attached to the sole of the shoe in form of a stirrup or a tube-like caliper inserted in the heel. Or, it can be incorporated into a shoe insert making interchange of shoes simpler.

Indications: It includes:

- Tendonitis (Tenosynovitis)
- Posterior tibial dysfunction (causing pes plano valgus deformity)
- Iliotibial band syndrome (where the cause is found to be excessive subtalar joint pronation)

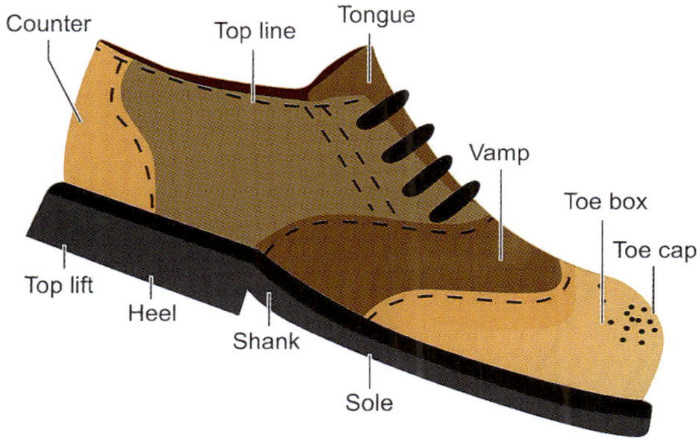

Fig. 60: Parts of shoe.

- Limb length discrepancy
- Bursitis
- Rheumatoid nodules
- Enthesopathy
- Soft-tissue atrophy
- Connective tissue disorders
- Hammer digit syndrome (Hammer toe, Mallet toe, overlapping toe, and claw toe)
- Plantar fasciitis (Heel spur syndrome)
- Equinus
- Sinus tarsi syndrome
- Tailor's bunion (Bunionette)
- Hallux abducto-valgus (Hallux valgus and bunion)
- Pes planus
- Metatarsalgia
- Freiberg's disease (Avascular necrosis of metatarsal head)
- Sesamoiditis
- Morton's neuroma

Ankle Orthosis

Ankle joint: These are single axis joints allowing only dorsi and planter flexion. Based on the degree of freedom allowed they can be classified as:

- No motion joint
- Free joints
- Adjustable joints where a lock allows the joint to be set at different angles
- Assisted joints where assistance to motion is provided by springs or elastic straps. They can be single action assisting only dorsiflexion or can be dual action assisting both dorsi and planter flexion **(Fig. 61)**.

Further control and stability of the ankle joint can be obtained by ankle controls like medial or lateral straps or bands, pads, and ankle stops or a complete solid ankle.

Calf Attachments

These give further stability to the ankle. They can be in form of:

Bar: Single or double places medial lateral or posterior.

Calf band: It can be metal with leather strap or purely soft-tissue strap.

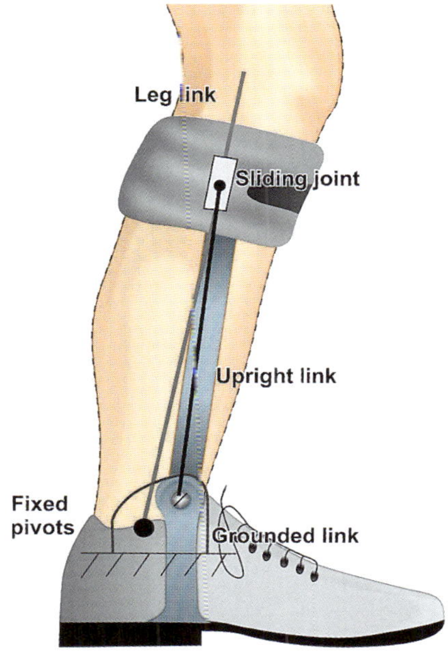

Fig. 61: Ankle foot orthosis (AFO).

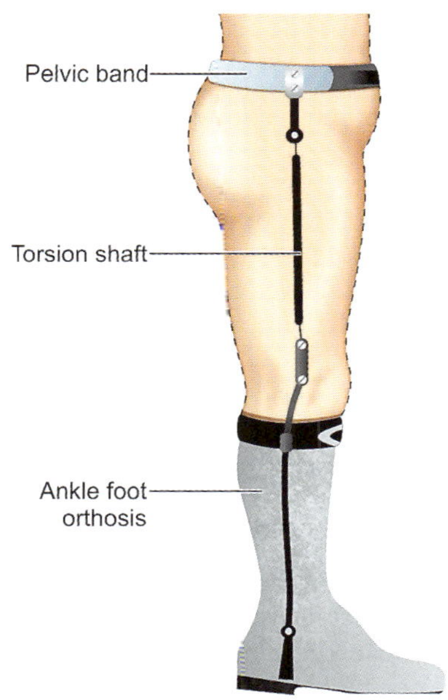

Fig. 62: Ankle foot orthosis (AFO) with torsion shaft.

Torsional shaft: Made of spring which is attached to shoe at one end and a pelvic band at the other end. It applies rotatory force to the lower limb and is used in scissor gait spasticity; toe in or out gait **(Fig. 62)**.

Patellar tendon bearing rim: It can replace the calf cuff and provide purchase from the patellar tendon **(Fig. 63)**.

Polyethylene AFO: It has three parts: Calf strap, calf shell, and shoe insert. It is commonly open from front and prevents dorsal and planter flexion. It has minimal control on varus and valgus.

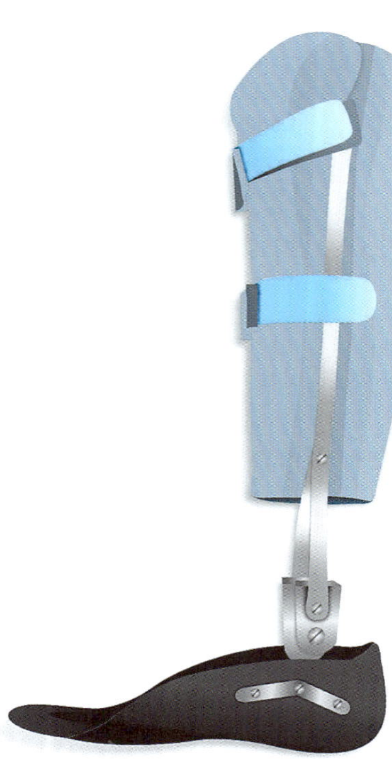

Fig. 63: Patellar bearing ankle foot orthosis.

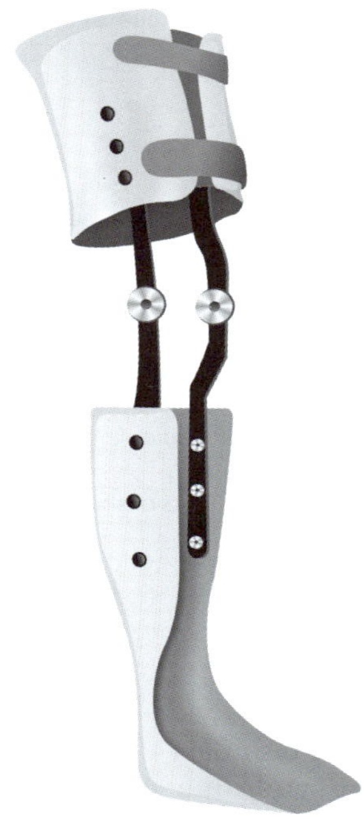

Fig. 64: Knee-ankle-foot orthosis (KAFO).

Indications

Ankle support for paralyzed legs:

- Night splint
- Prevention and treatment of plantar flexion contracture
- Achilles tendonitis treatment
- Stabilization of ankle
- To correct for muscle weakness as seen in cases of diseases such as peripheral neuropathy muscular dystrophy stroke, spinal cord injury, etc.
- To give rest to ankle and lower leg in cases of arthritis or fracture
- In some cases of abnormal gait to improve efficiency of walking

Knee-Ankle-Foot Orthosis (KAFO)

This is a proximal extension of the AFO spanning the knee joint. Uprights span the knee joints and the knee joint is stabilized by knee pads or hinge joints as per requirements. The uprights are held to the thigh with straps **(Fig. 64)**.

As with ankle joint, the knee joint can be fixed (monocentric or polycentric), free motion or adjustable. The locks in the knee can be spring loaded or gravity controlled which lock in upright position.

"Scott-Craig orthosis" is a KAFO designed for spinal cord injury patients. Here, the ankle joint is kept at 10° dorsiflexion causing the patient to lean forward slightly and counter balance is by hyperextension of hip. This causes center of gravity to come posterior to hip and anterior to fixed knee and ankle joint **(Fig. 65)**.

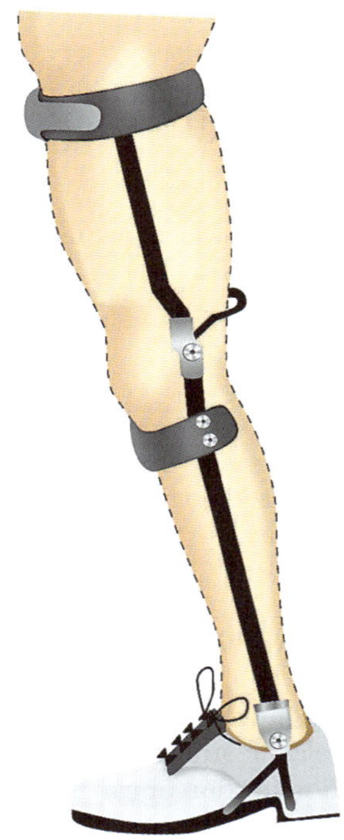

Fig. 65: Scott-Craig orthosis.

"Floor reaction orthosis" immobilizes the ankle in slight equinus. This causes the knee to go into extension when the forefoot is in contact with the ground. It is used in patients with knee extensor weakness and eliminates the need for a locked knee joint **(Fig. 66)**. It cannot be used bilaterally as bilateral equinus foot interferes with gait.

Indications: Used for knee instability caused by:

- Arthritic joints
- Bowleg
- Knock-knee
- Knee hyperextension
- Muscular weakness and paralysis

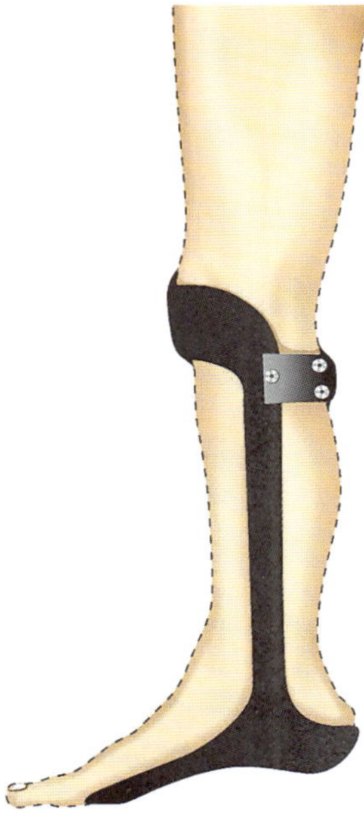

Fig. 66: Floor reaction orthosis.

Knee orthoses (KO): In the simplest form, it consists of two lateral bars and a thigh and calf cuffs. Single or double knee pads may be used to control knee. Strap may replace bar on one side if control is required only on one side **(Fig. 67)**.

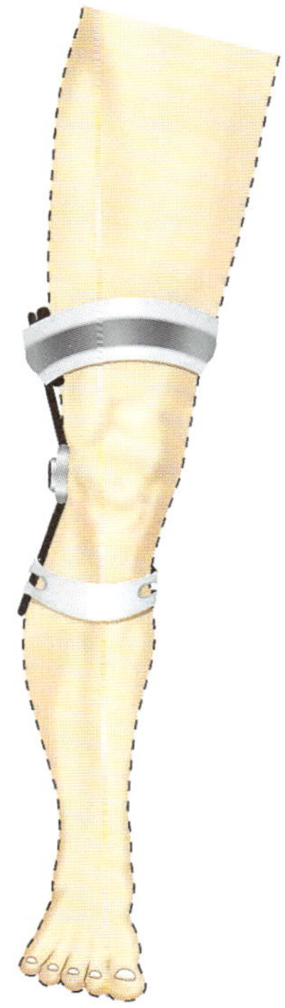

Fig. 67: Knee orthosis

Indications

Knee strains or sprains:

- Osteoarthritis
- Chondromalacia
- Osgood–Schlatter disease
- Subluxing patella
- Inflamed bursa
- Knee pain
- Patella femoral syndrome
- Knee flexion contractures
- Postsurgical after tendon and ligament repairs and total knee replacements

Hip Orthosis (Fig. 68)

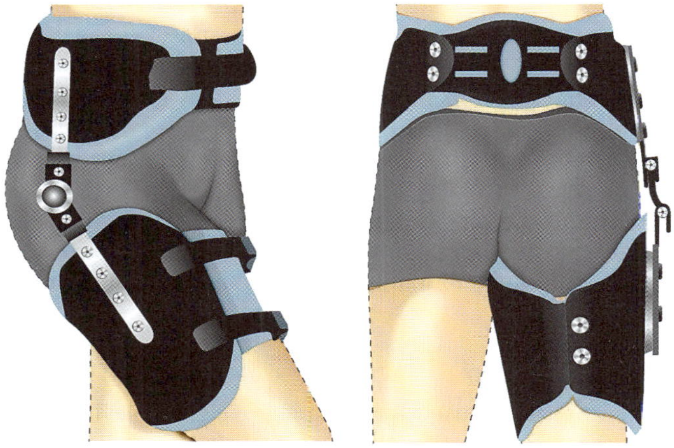

Fig. 68: Hip orthosis.

It has two parts—"hip joint" and "pelvic band". The pelvic band can be unilateral or bilateral.

Unilateral pelvic band covers the pelvis on the involved side below the iliac crest and above the greater trochanter, continues around the other side in the form of a belt.

Bilateral pelvic band cover the whole pelvis on both sides, beginning posterior to the anterior–superior iliac spine (AS1S), then curves downward and posteriorly to contact the most prominent portion of the buttocks and continues to overlie the sacrum. It gives better control.

Indications

Developmental dysplasia of the hip:

- Postoperative hip positioning
- Scissor gait
- To increase sitting balance
- Legg–Perthes disease

Hip Knee-ankle-foot Orthosis (HKAFO)

It consists of a hip joint and a pelvic band attached to the lateral upright of the KAFO. It has very high energy requirement **(Fig. 69)**.

The joint may be single axis hip joints allowing only flexion and extension and may lock to prevent flexion, while standing, whether locked or unlocked it limits mediolateral motion.

Double-axis hip joints allow lateral motion in addition to flexion and extension where adduction and rotation is desired.

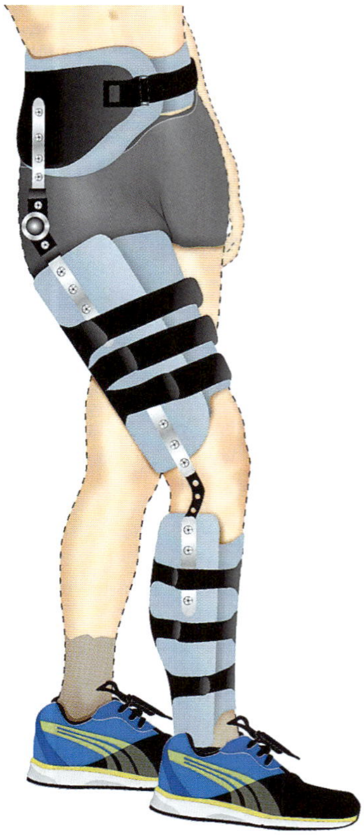

Fig. 69: Hip knee-ankle-foot orthosis (HKAFO).

Double position hip locks at both full extension and 90° of hip flexion. Useful in patients who have difficulty in maintaining the sitting position because of the spasticity of hip muscles.

Around the hip the following devices can be used for weight transfer: Ischial ring which is simple to fabricate and uses counterforce to maintain the ischial tuberosity on the ring.

Quadrilateral Brim

Patten-bottom is used for complete weight relieving with quadrilateral brim. Weight is transmitted directly by the orthoses from the ischial tuberosity to the Patten-bottom. Ankle joint is eliminated as lateral uprights extend distal to the shoe. Requires contralateral shoe lift **(Fig. 70)**.

Indications: Complete or partial loss of power in trunk and lower limb muscles usually after spinal trauma or other neurological disorder.
- Need to stabilize the body in upright position.

Upper Limb Orthoses

These can be static or dynamic. As in lower limb, they are classified as power the joints covered:
- *Clavicular and shoulder orthoses:*
  - *Figure-of-8-harness/clavicular brace:*
    - Used for fracture clavicle
    - As attachment for other assistive devices and prosthesis

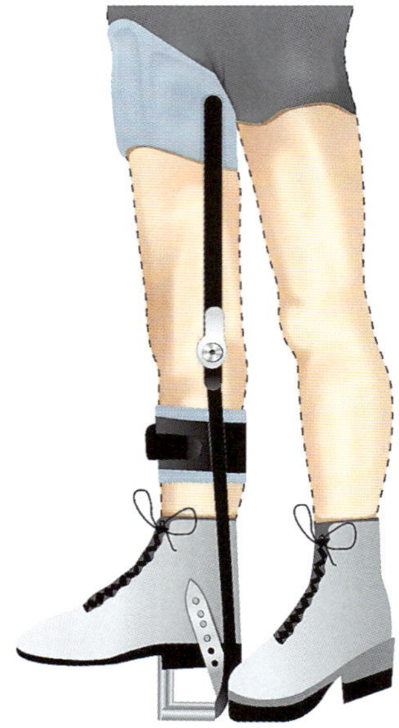

Fig. 70: Hip knee-ankle-foot orthosis (HKAFO) with patten bottom.

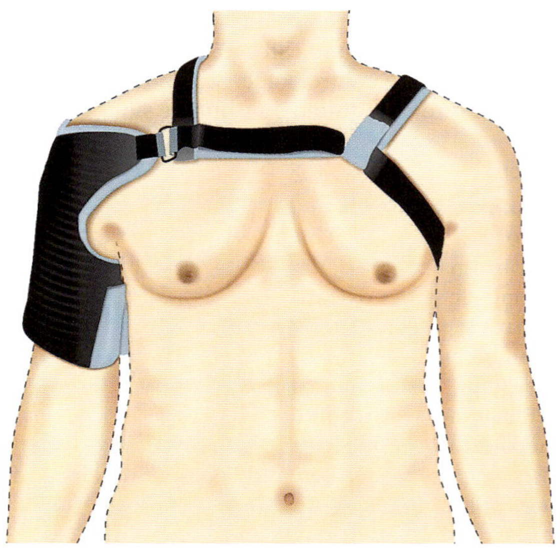

Fig. 71: Hemiplegic arm sling.

  - *Shoulder sling:* General purpose orthosis to provide rest to upper arm in cases of trauma or postoperative cases.
  - *Hemiplegic arm sling **(Fig. 71)**:* It is a especially designed shoulder harness to prevent shoulder subluxation in hemiplegic patients after stroke.
  - *Overhead sling suspension:* Used in proximal muscle weakness [amyotrophic lateral sclerosis (ALS), Guillian-Barré syndrome] to support the arm while performing various activities distal to the affected muscles.
- *Elbow orthoses:*
  - *Balanced forearm orthosis (Mobile arm support) **(Fig. 72)**:*

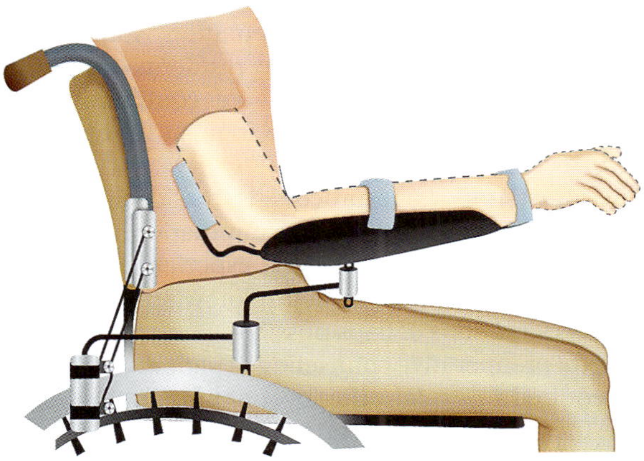

Fig. 72: Balanced forearm orthosis.

- Used in patients with partial C-4 weakness and inadequate elbow flexors and patients with C-5 lesions for enhanced arm placement.
- It provides a person with weak musculature the ability to move their arms in a horizontal plane and is attached to a wheel chair.

- *Posterior elbow splint:* Again a general purpose orthosis to provide rest to elbow wrist and forearm after trauma and surgery.
- *Dynamic elbow flexion orthosis* **(*Fig. 73*)**:
  - Any tissue joint contracture
  - Postsurgery
  - Post-trauma
  - Postarthroplasty
  - Joint inflammation
  - Muscle imbalance (Weak flexors)
  - Abnormal tone (Spasticity)
  - Shortening by scar tissues as in burn

- *Forearm-wrist orthoses:*
  - *Wrist cock-up splint:*
    - Wrist sprains
    - Carpal tunnel syndrome
    - Metacarpal fractures
    - Radial nerve palsy as a static splint
  - Wrist extension splint
  - *Ulnar gutter splint:*
    - Soft-tissue hand injuries to the fourth and fifth fingers
    - Fourth and fifth metacarpal fractures
    - Fractures of the fourth and fifth phalanges
    - Positioning for rheumatoid arthritis
- *Forearm-wrist-thumb orthoses* **(*Fig. 74*)** *and forearm-wrist-hand orthoses:*
  - *Maintenance of range of motion (ROM) in patients who have had burns:*
    - Rest to part in patients with arthritis
    - Serial static stretching in contractures
    - Stabilization of the thumb in opposition for three-point chuck pinch in patients with peripheral nerve lesions, spinal cord injury, upper motor neuron lesions and cerebrovascular disease
    - Immobilization in patients who have undergone tendon transfers or repairs

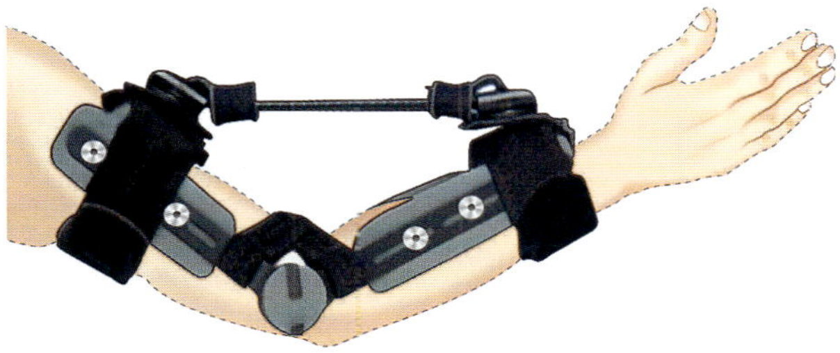

Fig. 73: Dynamic elbow flexion orthosis.

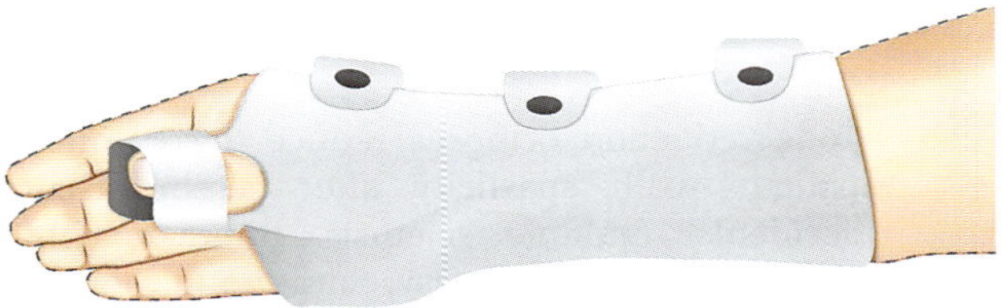

Fig. 74: Forearm-wrist-thumb orthoses.

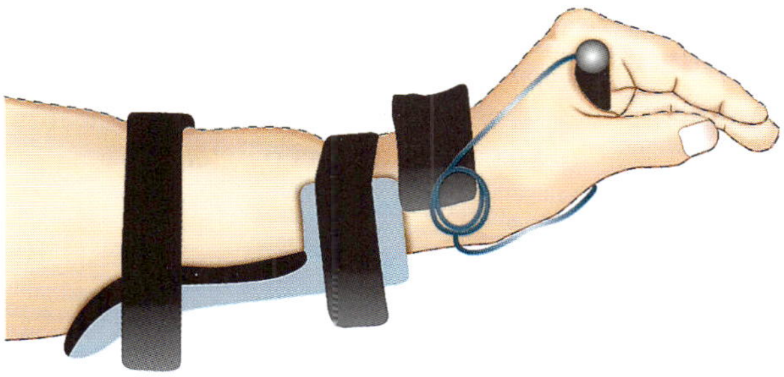

Fig. 75: The wrist-driven flexor hinge splint.

    - De Quervain's tenosynovitis
    - Median and ulnar nerve lesions
    - C5-6 spinal cord lesions
    - Wrist scaphoid or Bennett's fracture dislocation or thumb instability
- *Hand orthoses:*
  - *The static hand orthoses are used to correct the following deformities:*
    - Boutonnière deformities
    - Swan-neck deformities
    - Extensor tendon and collateral ligament repairs
    - Burns and contractures
    - Volkmann's ischemia
    - Nerve injuries and respective deformities (*see* Chapter on "Peripheral Nerve Injuries")
  - *Uses of dynamic hand orthoses:*
    - These devices are used with supports, cuffs, elastic threads, rubber bands, and hook applications for providing dynamic assistance to weak hand muscles after peripheral nerve injuries or spinal cord injuries.
  - *Upper extremity orthoses with special functions:*
    - The wrist-driven flexor hinge splint—used in spinal cord injury at C6-7 level. It has a spring to maintain pinch when wrist is relaxed **(Fig. 75)**.
    - Externally powered tenodesis orthosis **(Fig. 76)**. Uses motors to assist movements that are absent or weak.

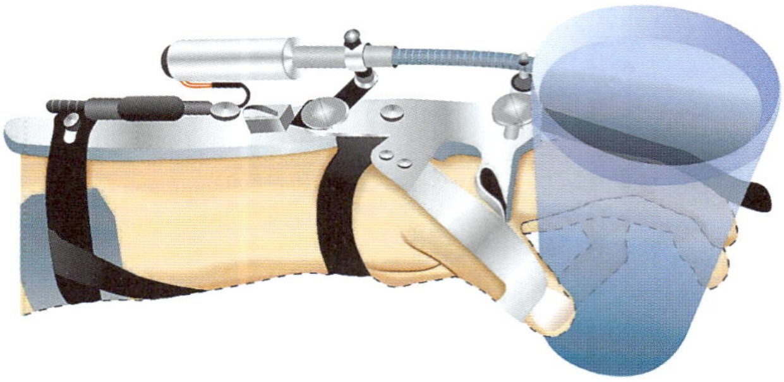

Fig. 76: Externally powered orthosis.

- Tone reduction orthoses reduce flexor tone in patients with spasticity after cerebrovascular accidents, multiple sclerosis, traumatic brain injury, and cerebral palsy. Some tone reduction orthoses include the Bobath splint, the cone splint, and the antispasticity ball splint.

CONCLUSION

- Amputation is a potentially mutilating and traumatic surgery both physically and psychologically.
- Optimal limb reconstruction is the most important aspect of successfully executed amputation surgery which cannot be delivered by a junior residents appropriately always. Amputation surgeries are commonly handed over to inexperienced residents in most set-ups which is incorrect.
- The most important process is the decision-making regarding the level and type of amputation.
- It should be done by the most experienced surgeon of the unit as it requires in-depth knowledge of anatomy, various variations of flaps possible.
- Careful preoperative counseling of patient and attendant is required to explain the level of amputation required and the potential loss of function.
- The expectation of the patient and his lifestyle plays a major role in decision-making process.
- A prosthesis may be preferred over a residual nonfunctional limb.
- Prosthetic technology too has progressed along with development of newer limb sparing surgeries.
- Newer computer-controlled prosthesis along with proprioception feedback have made near normal function possible.

CHAPTER 122

Replantation

S Pavan

INTRODUCTION

Factors that determine the success and indication of replantation are those factors that also affect the liability and expected function of the replanted part. The function regained would depend upon the type of injury, the level, age, and general condition of the patient. It would also depend on individual factors like level of motivation and the requirements of the patient. As the success of replantation is multifactorial it requires a large amount of clinical experience and should be conducted only by well-trained teams in tertiary care centers. The success of replantation is on the basis of restoration of viability and on functional outcome compared with primary amputation with early prosthetic fitting.

LEVEL OF AMPUTATION

In general, the more proximal the level the poorer is the outcome.

- As loss of thumb or multiple fingers causes severe disability, all such cases should be given high priority for replantation.
- The following levels have better functional outcomes:
    - Fingers distal to the flexor superficialis insertion
    - Amputation at the wrist level
    - Amputations at the level of the distal forearm
- The following levels have poor functional outcomes:
    - Zone II fingers proximal to insertion of flexor superficialis
    - Zone VI forearm amputations at the level of muscle belly
    - Amputation at the elbow level
- Replantation of the upper extremity at the proximal arm is attempted in order to preserve the elbow which allows for a forearm amputation and a below elbow prosthesis in case of failure.
- In children, replantation should be attempted in all levels of amputation because the functional outcomes are usually good.

MECHANISM OF INJURY

It is one the most predictive variables for successful replantation.

- There are higher success rates with replantation of guillotine versus avulsion amputations. The replantation of severely crushed and mangled body parts is contraindicated.
- *The red line sign or ribbon sign* is other contraindication because grafts cannot be used to re-establish flow outside the zone of injury in these circumstances. This red line on the vessels is caused by hematomas from transections of the branches off the proper digital vessels. A ribbon sign is seen in patients where the blood vessel was subjected to stretch and torsion. These vessels cannot successfully perfuse the replanted part, even after repair. When the ribbon sign is found to involve the length of both digital arteries, it is indicative of intimal injury up the length of the vessel, which is thrombogenic.

Other contraindications to replantation include:

- Amputations at multiple levels
- Patients who are mentally unstable

CONDITION OF THE VESSELS

The presence of arteriosclerotic plaques on the intima precludes functional patency following the anastomosis of small vessels. In patients with diabetes mellitus, may the diseased blood vessels would lessen the likelihood of the repaired vessels remaining patent. The arteries of such patients must be thoroughly evaluated under the microscope before reattachment.

The only absolute contraindication to replantation exists when associated injuries or preexisting illnesses preclude a prolonged and complex operation. In this circumstance, temporary ectopic implantation can be done for preservation of the amputated extremity elective replantation later.

TRANSPORT OF AMPUTATED PART

Amputated parts should always be retrieved and brought to the emergency department as they provide a valuable source of tissue, even if the part is not replantable. It should be cooled as soon as possible at the site. Cooling reduces metabolic acidosis, muscle autolysis and bacterial growth. Hemostatic control of the stump should be achieved with a compressive dressing, clamping and ligature of vessels should be avoided. Immersion of the amputated part in any solution or placing it directly on ice should be avoided. It should be wrapped in gauze soaked in saline, sealed in a plastic bag and the bag should be placed on ice.

The cut-off time for reliable implantation of digits is 12 hours if it has not been cooled and 24 hours if appropriate cooling has been done. This decreases to 6 and 12 hours, respectively, for major limb replantation at more proximal levels.

PREOPERATIVE PREPARATION

It is important to have a photograph of both parts for medico-legal protection. All other routine preoperative preparations that are required for any major surgery should be done. Proper counseling to patients and relatives is essential. The duration and type of rehabilitation required, the expected level of recovery of sensation, motion and function, and the failure rates should be clearly explained. Regional anesthesia is better because of the peripheral autonomic block, which increases vasodilation and peripheral blood flow and some inhalation anesthetics may result in vasospasm. The operating room should be kept warm at all times to diminish peripheral vasospasm.

ORDER OF REPLANTATION

The preparation of the amputated part can start before the patient is brought to the operating room:

- The part is irrigated to remove contamination.
- The neurovascular structures are identified and tagged with sutures to expedite identification later. Any requirement of nerve or vessel graft should be noted and this graft should be harvested before osteosynthesis in order to minimize warm ischemia time.
- Bone shortening should be done for tension-free nerve and vessel repairs. This should always be done on the amputated part to preserve maximum length of stump in case the replantation should fail.
- Once the patient is ready the next step is to tag the neurovascular structures as on the amputated part to facilitate identification of these structures when needed for repair later.
- Core sutures may also be taken over the tendons to make repair easier later on.
- The next step is to stabilize the limb by fixing the bone using K-wires/plates/nails as required.
- For digit replantation, the extensor tendons are repaired next, followed by the flexor tendons. In more proximal amputations with prolonged ischemia time, the vascular repair may take precedence.
- The next step is to reestablish the vascular supply by repairing the veins and arteries. This reduces the warm ischemia time. The veins are repaired first. A minimum of two and preferably three veins should be repaired, using grafts as required. The artery is repaired next. Again minimum one artery and preferably two should be repaired. If warm ischemia time is prolonged then artery may be repaired first. Tourniquet is released and the patency of the arterial anastomosis is assessed with the milk test, capillary refill test, and the pinprick bleeding test. If inadequate, then the vessel is bathed with papaverine, lidocaine, and warm irrigation solution. The hand can be placed in the dependent position to increase inflow pressure via gravity. At least 10 minutes of observation time is allowed for resolution of vasospasm. This is followed by reinspection of the anastomosis for thrombus and the repair is redone. Part of the thrombosed artery may need to be removed and replaced by a venous graft
- The next structures to be repaired are the nerves using the epineural technique. If the defect is <2 cm, a nerve conduit, such as unused vein graft or polyglycolic nerve tubes, can be used. For larger defects, donor nerve grafts like the medial antebrachial and posterior interosseous nerves are used.
- In the end, the skin is closed.
- In cases of multiple fingers, each finger is done at a time. Priority is given to the finger which contributes most to function and which has best chance of success. When multiple fingers are to be replanted, then each finger should be done one at a time to minimize the warm ischemia time.
- More proximal major replantations are usually done along with fasciotomies.

POSTOPERATIVE CARE AND OUTCOMES

- Limb and patient are kept warm to prevent vasospasm.
- Edema is reduced by keeping the limb at heart level.
- To prevent thrombus formation, aspirin, dextran, and heparin are used.
- Vascular flow to the replanted part can be further improved by giving sympathetic blocks.
- Periodic inspection, at hourly intervals initially, is done to check for signs of vascularity such as the color, capillary refill time, tissue turgor, and temperature.
- The patient is required to stop intake of tobacco and caffeine for 1 month.

The most common cause for replantation failure is arterial blockade. This blockade is seen by clinical signs such as reduced temperature, decreased tissue turgor, and a shortened capillary refill time. If the above signs appear then tight dressing and sutures are removed, elevation is decreased to improve blood flow by gravity, and a sympathetic block may be used. If there is no improvement, then surgical exploration may be required.

Venous congestion is less common. Clinical signs include oozing from the wound edges, prolonged capillary refill and increased tissue turgor. Again all tight bandages and sutures are removed and limb is elevated to reduce congestion. Surgical exploration is less successful. Overall, success rates for replantation approach are 80%.

CONCLUSION

- Replantation surgery is a high-skill surgery requiring expertise in microsurgery and organized setup for performing fine repairs that usually takes long times.
- Proper order of reconstruction should be followed, bearing in mind producing tension-free repairs.

CHAPTER 123

Robotics and Computers in Orthopedics

Manish Kumar Varshney

INTRODUCTION

Innovation has become norm in today's world and the public is constantly seeking the next revolutionary product or service. It is a constant endeavor among the scientific community to improve the available systems and techniques to maximally avoid errors and come over the limitations. This is usually achieved by improving the accuracy, durability and sophistication of existing techniques/instruments/implantation systems. Newer modalities are also used for marketing purpose and with growing awareness in digital social media, not only gaining a competitive edge but also a demand from patient pressurizes the surgeon to learn/use these technologies. Example is robotics and computers in orthopedics surgery. In orthopedics, nowadays they are mainly used for joint replacement surgeries but newer devices for spine fixation and management of complex fractures like pelvic fractures are also evolving. Computer-aided surgical tools range from an active robotic system capable of performing surgery autonomously to semiautomatic system that are assisted by surgeon control to passive or navigation systems that provide additional information during a procedure but do not perform the surgical action [the classical computer aided orthopedic surgery systems (CAOS)]. The surgeon controls the intervention but acts on information.

ROBOT is a term used for a machine that automatically carries out various tasks, requires little or no assistance from outside and can be programmable. "Robot" word is derived from Polish word "*robota*" which means *forced labor*. The inception of the concept of a machine doing manual labor for humans was already laid down in the Da Vinci's sketch book but the artificial intelligence (AI) to make it work was missing for long. The AI for engineering and medicine (or surgery) started blooming in 1956, which was ultimately fruitfully combined in 1985, whence neurosurgical biopsy was taken with the help of PUMA (Programmable Universal Manipulation Arm; Nokia) 260 robot. It is in 1992, when ROBODOC is introduced to world, for planning and performance of total hip replacement, the era of orthopedic robotic surgery began. Due to short-term promising radiological outcomes as compared to traditional procedures, robots are being used more often than before in the orthopedic surgery. Development of "neural networks" and fast computing has further lead to fast-paced incorporation of the technology and surgical advancements. The greatest improvement is coming in the field of "virtual AI" where the algorithms are designed for learning over a period of time. This learning can be supervised, unsupervised or reinforced learning. This will enable better bonding of the surgeon to 'his' robot and robot will learn the 'surgeon's' technique befriending him.

Robotic systems can be classified into three categories based on the manner in which the robot guides the procedure, viz.:

1. Passive
2. Haptic (technology that stimulates touch and proprioception senses; interacting with the surgeon) also called semi-active.
3. Autonomous system

In orthopedic surgery passive systems are not used. Example of such a passive system is the famous da Vinci surgical system (Intuitive Surgical) robot that is popular with urologists, gynecologists, and gastro-/oncosurgeons. Only athroscopic surgery was attempted using its robotic arm. The other two robotic systems are currently available for orthopedics and also under active competitive development. Haptic system requires surgeon's continuous input for efficiently performing and completing surgery. The surgeon uses or drives the robot to perform an operation. Autonomous systems differ from the above by having more independency. After the operative site is approached by the surgeon, he sets up the machine and then engages the robot, which completes the remaining task, without the help of a surgeon. In the haptic (semi-active) systems surgeon needs to move the robotic arm that is, however, limited by predefined border (in planning) beyond which the arm cannot be moved. Interestingly, some surgeons considered this a bit uncomfortable as there was a sudden stop so "boundary-controlled" systems were developed wherein semi-active robots the surgeon still moves the arm but the active end (like a burr) will stop working immediately when the border is crossed in space preventing over-cutting and damage. Additionally, in terms of the active involvement of the robot in performing surgery itself they can be classified into direct and indirect. In direct systems, the robot itself cuts the bone into desired final shape while in indirect systems it placed or facilitates jig placement to aid cutting by surgeon. The direct and indirect mechanisms may be combined in haptic or autonomous robots independently depending on the make of robot and its development algorithm so one can have systems like direct-autonomous, direct-haptic, indirect-haptic, indirect-boundary controlled and so on. Intuitively one would think that the haptic system would have been introduced first over which advancement into autonomous systems would have happened but the case is reverse for orthopedic surgery where first robot to be developed was autonomous system (ROBODOC) and then other entrants developed haptic systems!

Proposed advantages of robotic surgery include:
- Minimal invasive surgery (MIS) is possible.
- Implants can be placed more accurately.
- Radiologically, improved alignment of extremities.

ROBOTIC-ASSISTED ARTHROPLASTY SURGERY

Haptic Robotic Systems

The haptic systems provide feedback to the surgeon through some sort of auditory (beeps), tactile (vibratory) or visual (color change on screen) which guide as to completeness of the resection parameters preventing over resection and malpositioning. The surgeon is prevented from removing the bone outside the predefined area (as per preoperative planning) by either preventing the movement of the robotic arm (haptic) or "boundary-controlled" system that stops the burr as soon as the boundary of planned resection is exceeded.

Robotic arm interactive orthopedic system [RIO® from MAKO (Stryker)]: It is commercially available tactile systems for unicondylar knee replacement [MAKO surgicals acquired Acrobot systems and all its patents for knee replacement, that was merged with MAKO system (for total knee and total hip replacement (TKR and THR)]. So, the MAKO system caters to unicondylar knee replacement, TKR, and THR and is a semi-active haptic system that uses either a burr or a reamer or saw at its active end. But, it is a closed platform which is compatible with only Stryker hip and knee implants and not with other makes. As it is tactile system, surgeon's participation is must to complete unicompartmental knee replacement (UKR). Three-dimensional (3D) computer model of the knee is prepared with the use of computed tomography (CT) scans preoperatively, which forms the basis of preoperative planning. Based on this, surgeon will mark the bony surfaces of femur and tibia during operation. He merges the preoperative model into active anatomy of the knee. After taking the knee through a full range of motion, the flexion-extension gaps assessed, component size and implant placement finalized and a cutting zone is created for the robot. Preoperative planning and templating process forms the base for the system's algorithm. By viewing the 3D model of the knee on the monitor, the surgeon accurately manipulates the burr and resects the bone.

Forced controlled tip of the rotating burr cannot resect the bone outside the predefined cutting space. The safety system automatically stops the burr when the surgeon goes beyond the cutting zone. This feature also engages if the computer determines that the surgeon is resecting more bone than necessary.

The other example of semi-active system is Blue Belt's NAVIO that has been acquired by Smith and Nephew which was developed for UKR. It is also available for patellofemoral arthroplasty, femoroacetabular impingement (FAI) and now for total knee arthroplasty. It uses a burr at its active end but its advantage is that it is an open platform so it is compatible with various implants available in the market and not just Smith and Nephew. The other major advantage is that it is an image-free system and does not require any preoperative sophisticated imaging like CT scan etc. of the involved part/limb. The active end operates in two modes. The "exposure control" mode limits resection volume by modulating exposure of the cutting burr outside its protective sheath, and the "speed control" mode which limits the speed and ultimately stops the burr as it nears or exceeded the established cutting boundaries, respectively.

They have proposed advantages such as smaller incisions, short recovery and rehabilitation time, hence can be performed as an outpatient procedure, better American Knee Society (AKS) scores need large study for confirmation, improved tibiofemoral alignment and implant positioning within 2° of preoperative plan. The disadvantage is obviously the increased operating time.

Autonomous Robotic Systems

They differ from the tactile system by their independency. Autonomous robotic systems do not require surgeon's assistance. They can carry on and complete the surgery on their own, defined on the preset program. It is worth mentioned that a surgeon can immediately shut off the process with the help of the emergency switch. Currently, autonomous systems are still under investigation for use in orthopedic surgery.

ROBODOC (California): It is an autonomous robotic system, developed in 1980s and taken into surgical practice in 1992 for total hip arthroplasty (THA). This was developed as a joint collaboration between university of California—Davis and IBM Thomas Watson Research labs in New York. It was initially developed to ream the femoral canal for placement of cementless total hip stem and then advanced to TKR system. Though it became popular for a while in Germany due to its ability of good component positioning, it fell into disrepute because of safety concerns. The surgeon could start or stop the system but could not alter the course of robot operation in-between. The manual override would just shut the system and desired corrective alteration of the surgery was not possible. The ROBODOC is no longer available for clinical use and is taken over by ThinkSurgical that have launched a much more sophisticated and clinically used version the "T-Solution One". The CASPER (Computer-assisted Planning and Robotics, URS Ortho) system developed competing with the ROBODOC system initially but was removed from market completely due to high cost and complications like cut collateral ligaments.

Other examples inlcude:

- Mini bone-attached robotic system (MBARS) (Pittsburgh, Pennsylvania)—a hybrid semiautonomous robotic system which mounts on to the femur and completes the bony resection in total knee replacement (TKR).
- Praxiteles (France)—another similar robotic system developed in France.

ROBOTIC-ASSISTED SPINE SURGERY

The use of robotics in spine surgery has improved screw placement (spinal fixation/fusion) and has assisted in difficult cases like complex deformity correction requiring surgical resection of the spinal column, revision procedures and also surgical excision of intradural tumors. The first clinically useful robotics in the spine was done with the SpineAssist/Renaissance robot now "MAZOR-X" (MAZOR Robotics). It is a semi-active system that assists surgeon to perform surgical procedures such as drilling by positioning spinal instrumentation in correct position. The robot can be attached either to a predefined bony anatomic landmark like spinous process or can be mounted on a frame.

Another system is the ROSA robot that utilizes intra-operative imaging to provide guidance for pedicle screw placement and transforaminal lumbar interbody fusions (TLIF). Although one may expect improved pedicle screw placement and accuracy—this parameter has not been indisputably demonstrated, additionally other disadvantages like higher operative times and blood loss have limited the acceptance of robots in spine surgery.

ROBOTIC-ASSISTED TRAUMA AND REGIONAL ORTHOPEDIC SURGERY

Robots are being exploited for closed fracture reduction and accurate reconstruction using virtual 3D modeling and also in performing remote osteosynthesis surgery. The 3D technology assists with planning fracture reduction and intraoperative modification of the preplanned reduction. The results can be evaluated using intraoperative 3D imaging and further improved. This active feedback mechanism enables accurate intra-articular fracture reduction in minimally invasive manner. Remote surgery may be developed for creation of accurate entry point for femoral nail and assist in distal interlocking screws or bolt insertion. Robots can be used in warfare settings by providing critical acute surgical support and stabilization using telemedicine. Robots may help in shoulder surgery by negotiating the limited space available is arthroplasty in obese patients. It has been used in a limited manner in shoulder arthroscopy (da Vinci system). Future navigation may develop for placement of ankle arthroplasty implants.

ROBOTIC SURGERY: PITFALLS AND LIMITATIONS

- An alternative of robotic surgery in place of a conventional one is a costly option, until unless the institute has large volumes of surgery being performed routinely. Also, it constantly requires software upgradations and calibrations, making the option more expensive.
- Superiority and cost efficiency of robotic surgery in routine practice are yet to be demonstrated by long-term outcomes studies. Though some advantages such as short hospital stay, less blood loss, and greater accuracy are proposed.
  - As per dictum, total knee arthroplasty (TKA) is a soft-tissue operation where the bony cuts are supplementary. Bony anatomy can be well-identified by the robots, but the same is yet to be identified soft-tissue dissection by a robot.
  - Because of increased risk of infection, blood loss, neurological damage and perhaps an increased rate of litigation, the autonomous robotic system, the ROBODOC fell into disrepute.
  - Currently, high quality level I studies including Randomized Control Trials are not available for the use of robotic surgery in clinical practice.
  - The robotic surgery systems have promising short-term improvements at present, compared to their conventional counterpart. But, due to economic barriers and the lack of prospective, long-term, clinical outcome data, widespread adaptation of robotic surgery has still not occurred. However, there is a hope for robotic surgery to become more accessible as the technology continues to improve and let the world know how the ideal surgery should be performed.

ROLE OF COMPUTERS IN ORTHOPEDICS

"Computer" refers to a person computing/calculating using a mechanical device. The oldest computing devices included the abacus, the Antikythera mechanism (analog) and the slide rule. The computing methods were arithmetic's, Vedic mathematics, and the evolved binary calculations (the basis of present day computing). Punch cards were the oldest modern system that were employed to precisely guide large machines (textile) and then were used in computers. This was followed by magnetic tapes, cassettes, disks, then compact disks, digital disks, and finally current microstorage systems. The oldest digital computer that used vacuum tubes—the "electronic numerical integrator and calculator (ENIAC)" was the first general purpose computer but so cumbersome and uncomfortable that when it was started the lights of the whole city used to dim. This was followed by the use of transistors, integrated circuit (IC) and microprocessors that has now shifted to integrated/split microprocessors. Computers quite comfortably found their use in medicine albeit limited and were initially limited to data keeping and record management. There was fear among the then community that computers will make doctors obsolete (1963–1971). Use of computers in surgical specialties was discussed first in 1971. In 1979, Tracy et al. described using computers to diagnose gait disorders. CT then became a commonplace. Barmeir et al. described using CT to plan complicated total hip arthroplasty. With the declining fear of machines overtaking human brain and capabilities computers have found cosy place beside an orthopedic surgeon. They are being increasingly used as real-time intraoperative adjuncts in procedures described below:

- Minimally invasive total hip and total knee replacements
- Insertion of intramedullary locking screws
- Placement of cannulated hip screws
- Fixation of intertrochanteric femur fractures
- Placement of iliosacral screws
- Pelvic fracture fixation
- Placement of anterior cruciate ligament tunnels
- O-arm fluoroscopy.

The categorized use of computers in relevance to orthopedics can be put as follows:

Intraoperative assistance/planning:

- Computer-assisted orthopedic surgery (CAOS)
- Computer-guided joint replacement (navigation)
- Optotrak® system
- Hex Ilizarov
- Computer-assisted osteotomy.

Investigations:

- Computed tomography scans
- Magnetic resonance imaging (MRI)
- Positron emission tomography (PET) scans

Computers in orthopedic learning:

- Multicenter relay and communication intraoperatively and demonstrating surgical procedures
- Learning aids (Haptics)
- Simulating virtual surgeries

Computer-assisted Orthopedic Surgery and Navigation Systems

Computer-assisted orthopedic surgery (CAOS) and robotic surgery are both examples of computerized systems. The basic difference is that in CAOS the computers are utilized for real-time referencing, decision making, feedback, and checking the execution while in robotics a plan is preprepared and after registration of the therapeutic target the plan gets executed. Computer-assisted or computer navigation surgery systems, also called passive surgery systems, monitor progress and provide surgeons with data during procedures. The system is frequently used intraoperatively but has typical use pre- and postsurgery too. Not only in joint replacement the technology finds its use in spine surgery (pedicle screw fixation and anatomy), ligament reconstruction (commonly locating the anatomical landmarks and epicenter), complex fracture management (reconstruction and assessing fracture geometry—intraoperative CT scans) and acetabular reconstructions (iliosacral screws, long anterior column screw), etc., most of these are based on the premises of:

- Improving the planning and (now available rehearsing the surgery before actual procedure) to look for possible inconsistencies and faults.
- Improving accuracy of planned surgery.
- Handling compromised situations—like improving the consistency of surgery in minimally invasive spine surgery (MISS) procedures.
- Improving the undefined procedures such as the revision cases where most of the local landmarks are absent but overall alignment can be assessed by the computed systems. Most of the complicated fractures have comminution and the restoration of weight-bearing columns is indefinite that can be restored using the computed systems.

These systems are used during joint replacement surgery at various steps:

- Assessing joint irregularities and joint biomechanics.
- To monitor the accuracy of the bone cuts.
- Plan the component placement in advance.
- To make recommendations on ligament balancing (TKA), vertical and horizontal offsets (THA).
- Measure the intraoperative placement of the components in real-time.
- Assess the postoperative alignment/placement with respect to (wrt) preoperative plan.

The basic conceptual design for all CAOS modules is very similar. They all have three major components:

1. A therapeutic object [(TO), which is the target of the treatment].
2. A virtual object [(VO), which is the virtual representation in the planning and navigation computer]. In trauma systems, this is usually a fluoroscopy simulated model that may be in a 2-D (older) or 3-D format. In joint arthroplasty and spine surgery, virtual bone models are displayed. When the system uses a predefined VO then intraoperative registration has to be done (see later), but in systems that form a VO intraoperatively (time-consuming; as in robots) registration is automatic. The fluoroscopic based systems are especially intriguing and promising for spine surgery (using O-arm), long bone fractures and are also finding applications in total hip replacement.
3. A "navigator" links both objects. In robotic systems, the robot itself is the navigator, while in the navigated arthroplasty systems a position tracking device is used. Navigator is the central element of each CAOS system.

Navigator serves to establish a global, three-dimensional (3-D) coordinate system as a matrix in which the target is to be treated and localizes the current orientation of end-effectors (EEs) mathematically. EEs are commonly passive surgical instruments like the jigs, saw system, but they can also be semi-active (Navio and the MAKO systems) or active devices as in few robots. Most importantly the navigator transmits real-time positional information between the EEs, the TO, and the VO.

The navigation systems have several cameras to track surgical instrumentation, bony geometry, and alignment. The cameras are positioned above the patient and communicate with instruments and bony landmarks through light-emitting diodes (LEDs)/infrared rays. In each and every surgery and individualized CAOS system has to be established through coactions of navigator, TO, and VO that is done through three key procedural steps:

1. The first is the calibration of EEs (describe the EEs' geometry and shape) in the 3-D coordinate system of the

navigator. When an optical tracker is used, this is done via rigid attachment of three or more optical markers onto each EE.

2. The second process is registration, which aims to provide a geometrical transformation between the TO and the VO in order to display the end-effect's spatial and geometric localization with respect to the virtual representation on display. Registration is automatic in robotic systems but in most of CAOS it has to be done as a separate step. The geometrical transformation could be rigid or nonrigid. This registration is an algorithm based process that differs in different systems making them unique.
3. The third key ingredient is referencing. Referencing compensates for the relative motion of the navigator and/or the TO during the surgical actions. This is controlled by either attaching a so-called "dynamic reference bases (DRB)" holding three or more optical markers to the TO (like the tibial reference pins in older systems) or immobilizing the TO with respect to the navigator.

The surgeon always has the option to override the information given by the computer. The surgeon is not limited to "predefined cutting zones", as in robotic surgery. Despite its many recommended uses and advantages I personally consider this to be more of a useful tool for surgeons in the early learning curve. Later I find it useful only in revision cases or complex primary arthroplasty. Many authors have reported superior alignment of the femoral and tibial components, tibial slope and the mechanical axis using these passive surgery systems. But accuracy in restoring rotational alignment has been questioned while using computer navigation in TKA.

The commonly proposed advantages of computer-guided joint replacement surgery:

- Restore accurate limb alignment.
- Increase the survival of implanted joint (? Secondary to better placement).
- Constant guidance and monitoring during surgery [this is annoying initially and most often to experienced surgeons the system seems to give this "error" (I say) once every 5–6 surgeries and has to be shut down in middle].
- Reduce the risk of complications related to implant fitting.
- Secondary assistance/confirmation during MISS procedures.
- Decreased hospital stay—only later in the course when one is well-versed with the system and is performing MISS surgeries.
- Record keeping of the surgery for later analysis.
- No radiation during surgery.
- Intraoperative range of motion analysis to achieve maximum function.

Disadvantages:

- Increased blood loss
- Increased operative time
- Increased risk of general complications such as fat embolism, infection, atelectasis, etc., due to prolonged surgery.

The Optotrak® System

Developed at Northwestern University, Canada. The Optotrak® is a noncontact motion measurement system, which tracks small infrared (e.g., IRED) position sensors, which are attached to a subject, instead of reflective markers. It is most commonly used in osteotomy surgeries.

Hex Ilizarov

The Hexapod represents the kinematic mechanism that realizes the 3D movements by different lengths of the six distractors, connected to the two platforms. The Hexapod set for Ilizarov apparatus consists of six telescopic distraction rods of varying length from 105 mm to 240 mm, 6 Y adaptors, a measuring stick and the software. The center of rotation and angulation (CORA) is entered in relation to the center of the distal ring and the desired correction, entered into the computer. Rest will be done by the software which corrects the deformity by making appropriate adjustment in each plane. Malalignment test along three axes with six degrees of freedom forms the basis for this correction.

The software is very simple to use. All we need is the base data, which includes the upper and lower rings diameter, Y adaptors positions on each ring and the length of the distraction rods. This data is entered into the computer, based on which, the initial position of center of the upper ring in relation to the lower ring is shown by the program. According to the surgeons, input of the number of days and steps desired, the software displays a plan for correction, detailing the steps. All adjustments can be in three planes.

Uses

- Fracture treatment (especially compound fractures with bone loss)
- Correction of limb length disturbances
- Correction of rotational deformity with limb length correction can be done in a single set-up.

COMPUTER-AIDED ORTHOPEDIC LEARNING

(Possibly the book you are reading might become obsolete in future with advanced learning classrooms!)

Virtual reality (VR) has become a commonplace in our modern lifestyle. Immersive VR system generates another world in a computer that is channeled into the viewer through all his senses. VR training simulators let surgeons practice on virtual body tissue and get the same feedback they would experience in performing a real operation. The idea of using the VR system in orthopedics comes from efforts emanating from SGH, Singapore in connivance with School of Applied Science at Nanyang Technological University. In orthopedics still the immersive VR systems have not come in place. There are modified desktop VR orthopedic surgery training systems that help students in:

- Memorizing the techniques and respective tools and implants used for fixing fractures
- Choosing the most relevant technique for each case

- Learning how to put the implants in place, including exactly where and how deep to drill or cut the bone the proper insertion angle, and so on
- Acquiring "muscle memory" for the physical efforts applied to the tools and implants to avoid damaging the bones.

These systems lack in the "soft tissue" properties like dissection and having the feel of managing soft tissues and blood loss. This is as important I feel principally because bones are located centrally and exposure hence is an important aspect, also lot of functional outcome depends on soft-tissue management. To improve the systems and make them more realistic immersion needs to be added to the existing VR system. This is partially being achieved by:

- Realistic 3D geometric models with real-time function, behavior, and constraints.
- Real-time simulation including collision detection, sounds, etc.
- Virtual reality rendering and input techniques based on special hardware devices.
- Real-time 3D rendering
- Force feedback and tactile response using VR haptic devices.

Other methods of improving interaction and helping in training has emanated from use of worldwide web where live transmissions are carried out for the seminars, live surgeries and observers, students and residents can increase their learning simultaneously at various places. Innovative use of "Google Glasses®" intraoperatively also helps one to communicate with the peers or superiors during surgery for instant help. Such technologies have been made available with the modern computing and are still evolving.

CONCLUSION

- Orthopedics need exacting placement of implants for best outcome in terms of anatomic restoration of the bones and joints. As with most other fields, computers have slowly crept into the orthopedic faculty also and its use is gradually increasing.
- Adding of computers and navigation helps in providing the best chance of giving perfect placement of implants.
- The latest use of technology is in "conferencing"'the procedures for wider usage by incorporating the use of Internet.

CHAPTER 124

Lasers in Orthopedics

S Pavan

INTRODUCTION

Laser is an acronym for "light amplification by stimulated emission of radiation". The laser is a device that produces high-intensity light energy which is, (a) monochromatic—the light has a single wavelength, (b) coherent—the light waves are in phase with one another, and (c) directional.

The use of lasers in orthopedics can be divided into therapeutic and surgical.

THERAPEUTIC LASERS

The laser used in therapeutic is produced from laser diodes and is typically low energy (30–100 mW). The penetration into tissues depends on the wavelength. Shorter wavelengths (600–700 nm) are absorbed within a few millimeters by hemoglobin. Lasers with >1,000 nm wavelength penetrate better and are absorbed by water and fat. They act on tissues to give pain relief, resolve inflammation, and increase the speed quality and tensile strength of tissue repair. They can be used in pulsed or continuous phase.

Indications

- Fibromyalgia
- Myofascial pain
- Cervical neck pain
- Low back pain
- Joint pain
- Trigeminal neuralgia
- Rheumatoid arthritis
- Carpal tunnel syndrome
- Tendonitis
- Plantar fasciitis
- Bursitis
- Connective tissue injury
- Sprains
- Tendonitis
- Tendon ruptures

Contraindications

- Use around eye
- Within 6 months of radiotherapy
- Epilepsy
- Fever
- Malignant tumors
- Pregnancy

SURGICAL LASERS

These are high-energy lasers in the range of 10–60 W. Most surgical systems produce visible, near-infrared or infrared laser energy. For surgical applications, it is used to coagulate or ablate tissue. Laser systems have four basic components:

1. The laser medium—a solid, liquid, or gas that determines the wavelength of the laser. The standard media used in surgical lasers are CO_2 and argon gases, and yttrium-aluminum-garnet (YAG) crystals doped with heavy metals such as holmium (Ho), erbium (Er), thulium (Tm), and neodymium (Nd).
2. The resonator cavity—sandwiches the medium between two mirrors.
3. The excitation source that pumps high-energy electric or optical energy into the laser medium.
4. A cooling system—removes excess thermal energy.

The output can be in the form of continuous wave (CW) or pulsed. CW causes heat to be conducted to surrounding tissue and can produce large peripheral zones of thermal damage.

Pulsed laser systems produce high-intensity light over short time intervals. The time between pulses allows for dissipation of thermal energy and prevents excessive damage due to thermal conduction.

Surgical lasers act on tissues via three mechanisms:

1. ***Photothermal:*** Tissue ablation occurs by heating the tissues above 100°C with explosive release of the vaporized tissue contents. Heating tissues below the vaporization threshold produce thermal changes if collagen is heated above its phase transition temperature of 62°C.
2. ***Photochemical:*** Ablation by photons directly dissociates molecular bonds leading to nonthermal cutting of tissue. The so-called cold excimer lasers operate by this mechanism.

3. ***Photomechanical:*** The thermal energy and rapid expansion of vaporization contents create high pressure within the tissue causing shock waves that create damage at large distances from the site.

Some common types of lasers used in orthopedic surgery are—CO_2, neodymium:YAG (Nd:YAG), holmium:YAG (Ho: YAG), and the xenon chloride excimer laser.

CO_2 lasers are now no longer in use in orthopedic as they produce 10.6-μm light energy that cannot pass through standard optical fibers; therefore, they required large, cumbersome devices for light delivery to the joints. Also, the joint needs to be distended with gas.

The *Nd:YAG lasers* produce light (at 1.06 μm and 1.32 μm) that is readily transmitted through standard silica optical fibers but this light is absorbed only by pigmented or darkly stained tissue and not well absorbed by most intra-articular tissues. Because of its low tissue absorption, at high energies the light deeply coagulates tissue. Cutting effects vary significantly as more desiccation or charring of the tissue surface takes place. Functionally, a Nd:YAG laser causes necrosis of tissue to a depth > 1 cm before any apparent cutting effect. It has limited use as a cutting tool and has a low safety profile.

The *Ho: YAG laser* is the shorthand name for a family of solid-state lasers that use the doping element holmium in a laser crystal YAG and that emit energy at approximately 2.1 μm. The Ho:YAG laser is the most widely used arthroscopic laser system. It is readily transmitted down conventional optical fibers into low-profile handpieces. The Ho:YAG laser effectively cuts, coagulates, and ablates well-hydrated intra-articular tissues.

The *excimer laser* is a laser system that ablates and cuts tissues via nonthermal mechanisms using the photomechanical and photochemical effect of lasers. Tissue effects occur when ultraviolet light energy is absorbed by carbon-carbon double bonds of organic chromophores. Ultraviolet light energy cannot be transmitted down standard optical fibers. The 308-nanometer xenon chloride excimer laser can be delivered fiberoptically through nonflexible zirconia fluoride fibers. The system itself uses toxic gases as a laser medium. Excimer arthroscopic systems have limited use.

Uses of surgical lasers:

- Meniscectomy
- Lateral retinacular release
- Laser-induced capsular shift (tightening)
- Laser diskectomy
- Synovectomy
- Shoulder arthroscopic debridement
- Subacromial decompression
- Shoulder capsulorrhaphy—laser-assisted capsular shift

Certain other uses which are in the experimental stage:

- *Removal of polymethyl methacrylate (PMMA)*: PMMA strongly absorbs infrared and near-infrared light but these are produced by CO_2 lasers and cannot be passed through fiber optic systems. There is also extensive charring and desiccation of surrounding bone. Vaporization of PMMA produces highly toxic byproducts. Few surgeons currently use laser for cement removal.
- Laser osteotomy
- *Tissue welding*: Two techniques are used. First is to use low temperatures (62°C) to melt end of collagenous structures and fuse them. Second is photochemical technique, which uses light-activated chemicals to directly crosslink collagen of severed tissues.
- *Annealing:* The laser can thermally alter tissue if the energy striking the tissue is less than the tissue ablation threshold. At 62°C, collagen undergoes a phase transition from a triple helix to an amorphous gel. This process is called "annealing".
- *Biostimulation:* The theory is based on observations that low-level light energy increases cellular metabolism.
- *Photodynamic therapy:* Photodynamic therapy (PDT) is a treatment modality in which light-activated chemicals are used to treat pathologic conditions. In orthopedics, PDT has been evaluated for the treatment of inflammatory arthritis. The hypervascular proliferative synovium of rheumatoid arthritis can be targeted and destroyed with PDT. Photosensitizers are delivered systemically or via intra-articular injection.

PITFALLS

- There have been multiple reports of osteonecrosis following laser arthroscopy with either the Nd:YAG laser or the Ho:YAG laser systems.
- The laser produces extensive subchondral damage if used to drill into articular surfaces.
- Photoacoustic effects may produce damage in tissue remote from the laser site, especially if the laser is used in confined spaces.
- Thermal diffusion may occur between pulses and thermal damage may extend significantly greater distances within the tissue.
- Rather than minimizing damage, the laser when used in an unsafe manner can cause extensive damage.
- Though theoretical benefits exist, better clinical outcomes have not yet been clearly demonstrated over conventional mechanical techniques.

CONCLUSION

- Lasers have found good acceptance in other surgical faculties like urology and gastrointestinal surgeries. Their relevance and utility in orthopedics is limited, however.
- Lasers in orthopedics have been used in association with arthroscopic procedures but to a limited extent only, however, surgeon should be aware of the technical usage, principles, and complications associated with their use.

CHAPTER 125

Instruments and Implants

S Pavan, Manish Kumar Varshney

INTRODUCTION

Modern orthopedic surgery practice involves tremendous use of metallic implants for osteosynthesis and reconstruction. Proper knowledge and understanding of the surgical procedure involves a combination of soft tissue surgery and handling of implants. New and experienced orthopedic surgeons both need to know the various varieties of instruments available that may be of need in special situations and provide important bailout when stuck in nonconventional surgeries. A comprehensive attempt is made below to introduce and elaborate the various instruments and implants.

AWLS

They are used to penetrate bone and open bone canals to direct pin and nail insertions [Kuntscher's diamond pointed awl **(Fig. 1)** and bone awl with eye straight **(Fig. 2)**].

CHISELS/OSTEOTOMES/GOUGES

They are used to score, cut, scrape, clean, and sculpt bone. They differ in the type of tip. Osteotomes are beveled on both surfaces whereas chisels are beveled on one surface only. Gouges have a cupped tip to scoop out bone material.

Osteotomes are used to shape and sculpt bone, particularly cancellous bone, whereas chisels are used to cut a window in the bone cortex to allow harvesting of pure soft bone. Gouges scoop away strips of soft bone, especially in bone grafting. Osteotomes, chisels, and gouges are designed for use with a mallet. They are available in straight and curved types [Stille type chisel **(Fig. 3)**, Capener gouge **(Fig. 4)**, Stille gouge **(Fig. 5)**, Lambotte osteotome **(Fig. 6)**, Stille type osteotome **(Fig. 7)**, Hibbs osteotome **(Fig. 8)**].

BONE-HOLDING CLAMPS

They are used to hold, stabilize, rotate, reduce, and compress bone and to position bone screws and plates, and insert K-wire during trauma surgery. They come with some locking mechanism like ratchet or screw, which can be easily operated with one hand. Some models may have adjustable jaws or hinges. Narrow-jawed forceps do not compromise soft tissue and are better for hand and foot surgery, whereas broader-jawed instruments allow room for implant placement. A forceps that corresponds to bone size should be chosen as excessive forces may shatter the held bone [Lowman's bone-holding clamp **(Fig. 9)**, Fergusson bone-holding forceps **(Fig. 10)**, Heygroves' bone-holding forceps **(Fig. 11)**, Burn's bone-holding forceps **(Fig. 12)**, Farabeuf-Lambotte/lane bone-holding forceps **(Fig. 13)**, self-centering bone-holding forceps **(Fig. 14)**, and reduction forceps **(Fig. 15)**].

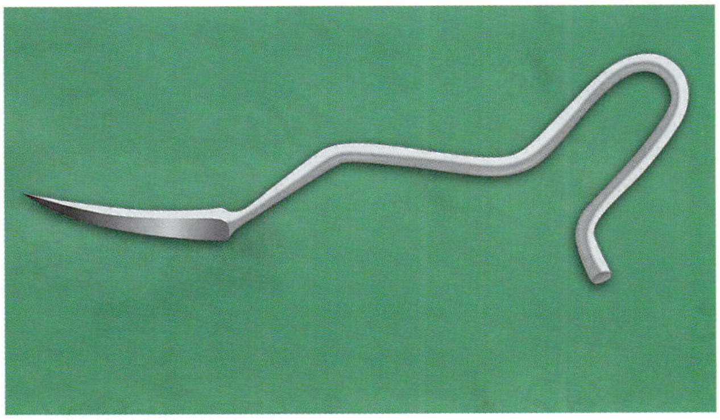

Fig. 1: Kuntscher's diamond pointed awl.

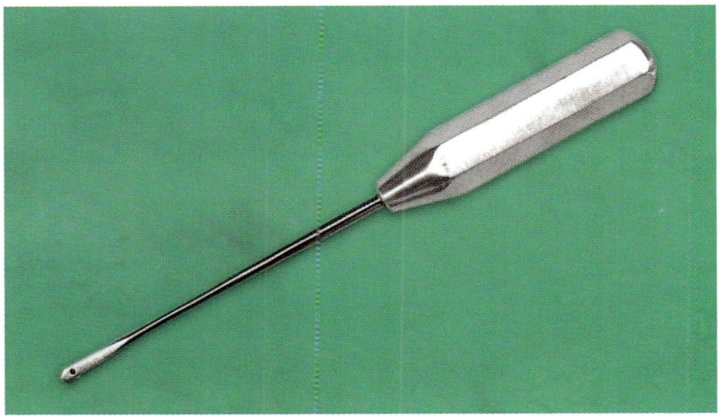

Fig. 2: Bone awl with eye straight.

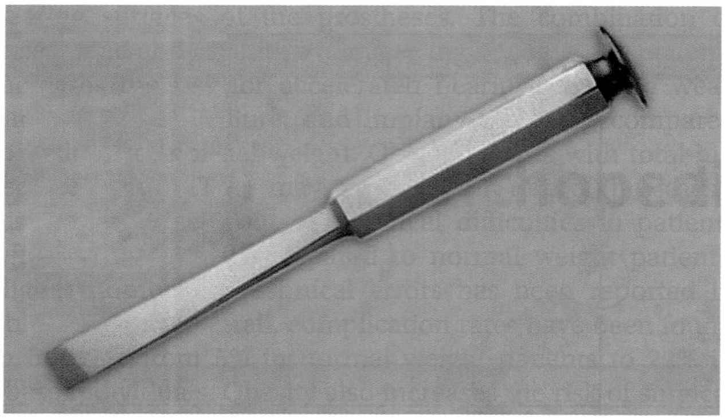

Fig. 3: Straight type chisel.

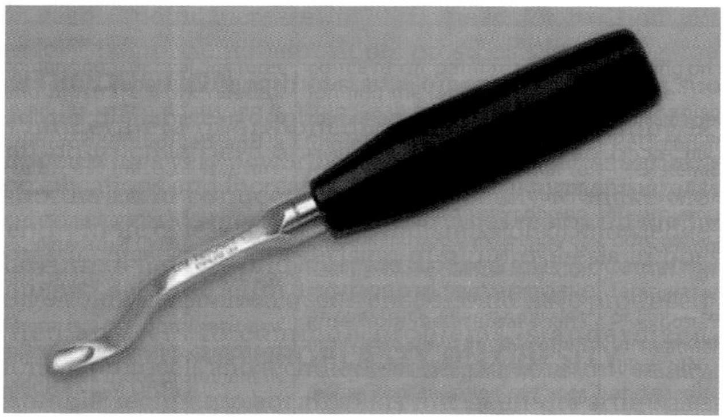

Fig. 4: Capener gouge.

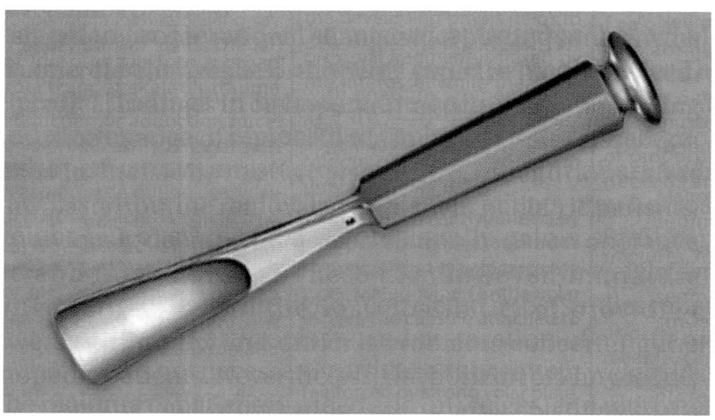

Fig. 5: Stille gouge.

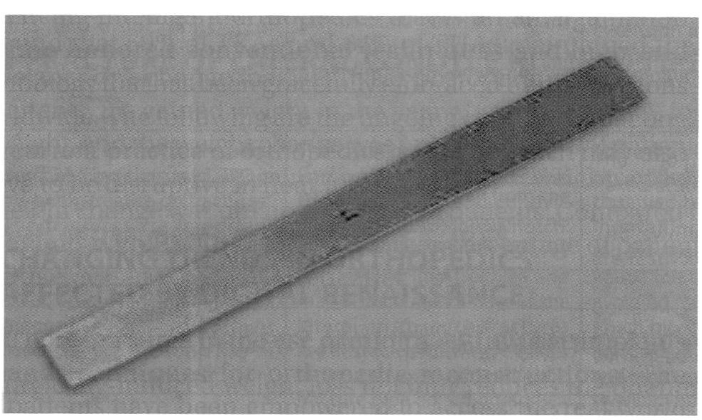

Fig. 6: Lambotte osteotome.

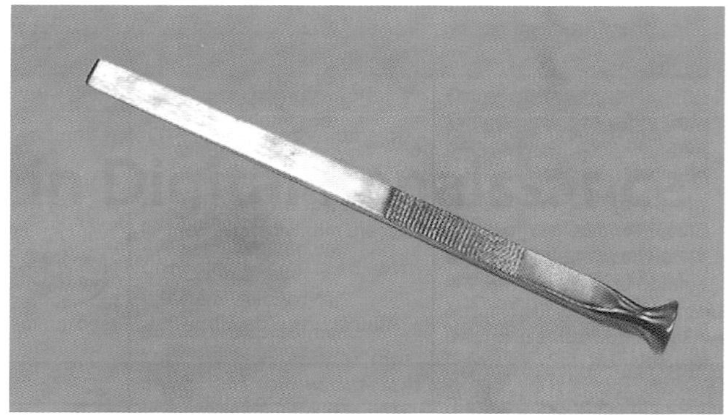

Fig. 7: Stille type osteotome.

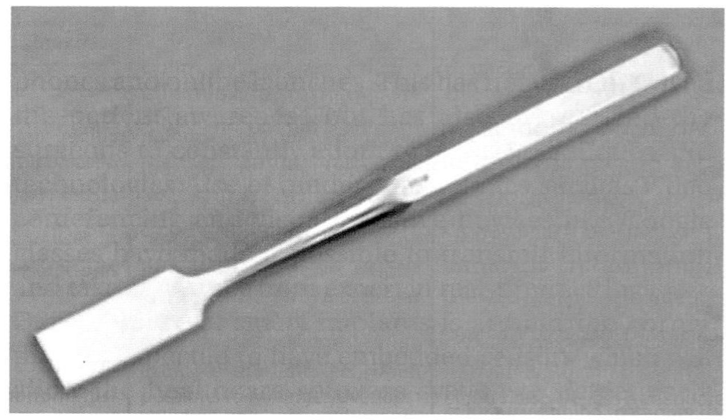

Fig. 8: Hibbs osteotome.

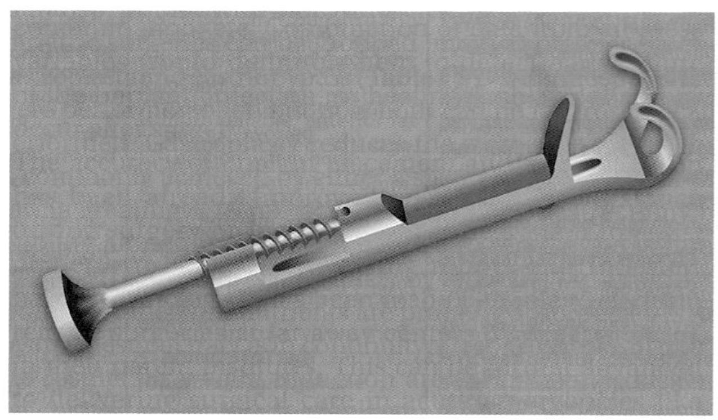

Fig. 9: Lowman's bone-holding clamp.

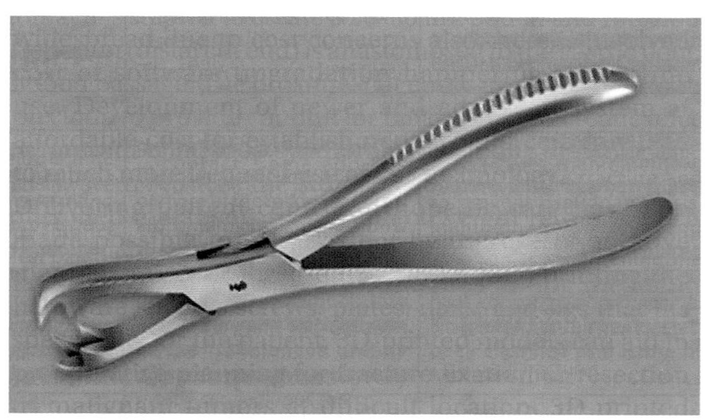

Fig. 10: Fergusson bone-holding forceps.

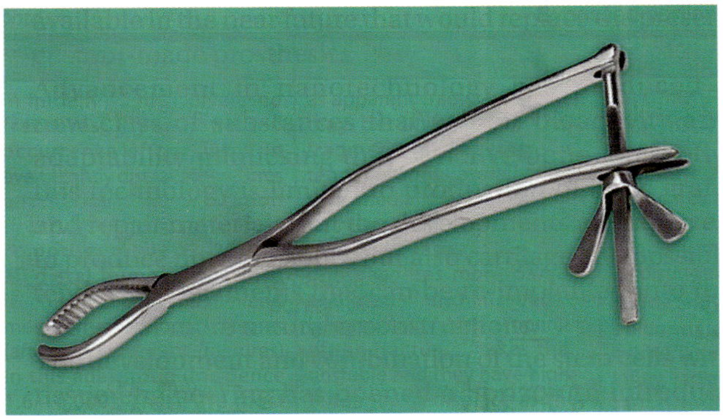

Fig. 11: Heygroves' bone-holding forceps.

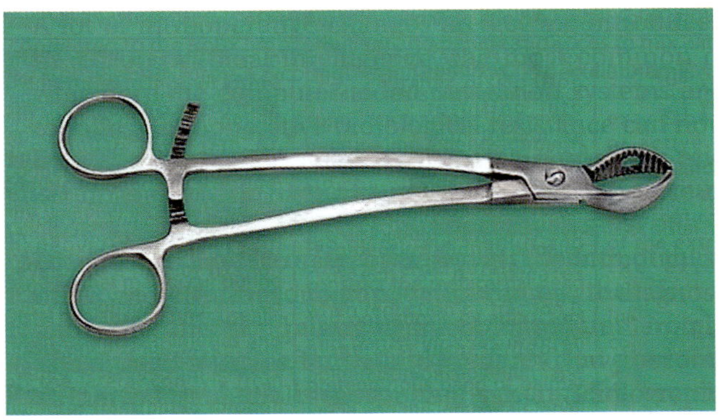

Fig. 12: Burn's bone-holding forceps.

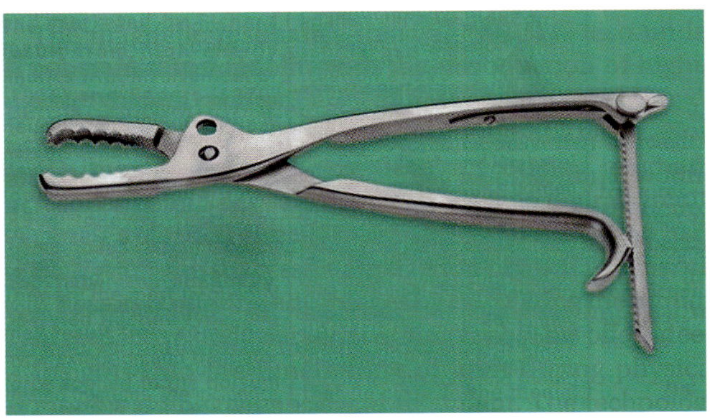

Fig. 13: Farabeuf-Lambotte bone-holding forceps.

BONE CUTTERS/NIBBLERS

Bone cutters are used to cut bone or to remove bone splinters. Bone nibblers or rongeurs are used to cut or remove small pieces of tissue or bone. They are available in straight and curved patterns, with a single-action or double-action joint. The double-action models provide much more power to the surgeon causing less hand fatigue. Rongeurs or nibblers have a hollowed, cup-like working end, while cutting forceps have beveled, scissor-like cutting edges [Liston-Stille/Tudor-Edward bone cutting forceps single action **(Fig. 16)**, Ruskin bone-cutting forceps double action **(Fig. 17)**, bone nibbler single action curved **(Fig. 18)**, Northfields-Sargent rongeur

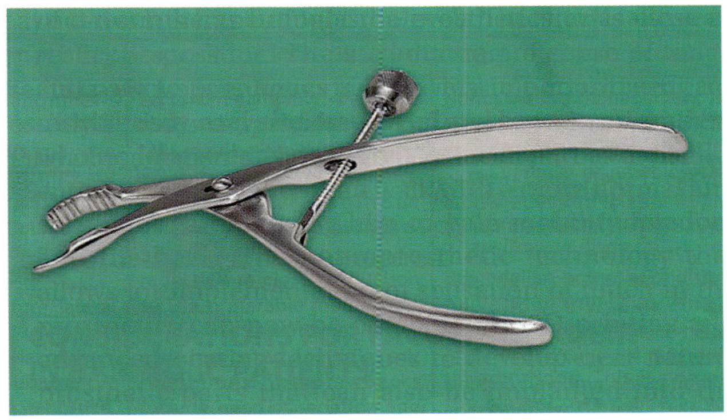

Fig. 14: Self-centering bone-holding forceps.

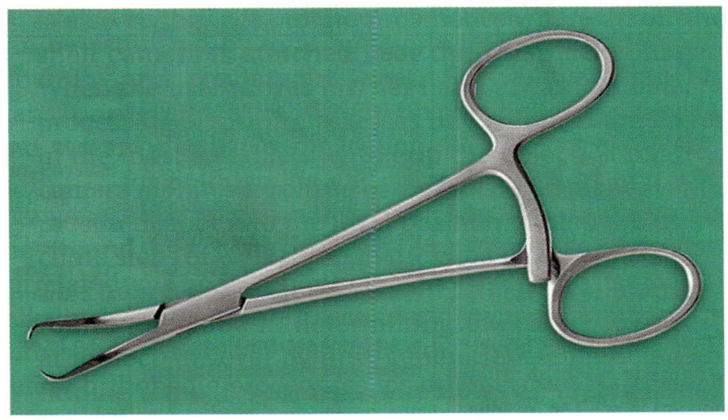

Fig. 15: Reduction forceps.

(Fig. 19), Leksell's rongeur **(Fig. 20)**, Stille-Ruskin rongeur **(Fig. 21)**].

PERIOSTEAL ELEVATORS

They are used to elevate and dissect bone, tissue, nerves, and to clean and scrape bone. They help to expose bone in fractures and other procedures. Periosteal elevators are used to strip portions of the periosteum covering the exterior surface of a bone [Doyen's periosteal elevator **(Fig. 22)** (right/left), Bristows/Jones periosteal elevator **(Fig. 23)**, Cobb's spinal elevator **(Fig. 24)**, Farabeuf rugine **(Fig. 25)**, and Key periosteal elevator **(Fig. 26)**].

CURETTES

Used to scrape, shape, and clean bone. To clear out cavities and abscess [Cone's spinal curette **(Fig. 27)**, Volkmann curette double ended **(Fig. 28)**, and cup curette **(Fig. 29)**].

RETRACTOR/LEVERS

There are of two types of retractors: hand-held and self-retaining. The first type requires constant holding and includes bone levers while the self-retaining type can be inserted and left unattended. Bone levers along with soft-tissue retraction can also be used to manipulate bone fragments to achieve reduction. The size and type used is determined by the task, including the depth of use. The smaller types are used generally on the surface to hold

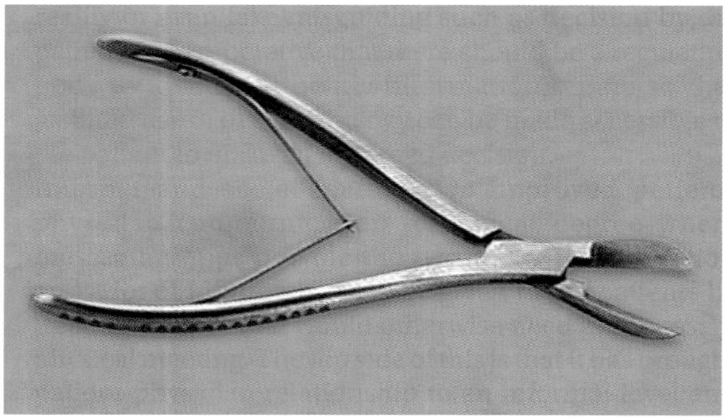

Fig. 16: Liston-Stille bone-cutting forceps single action.

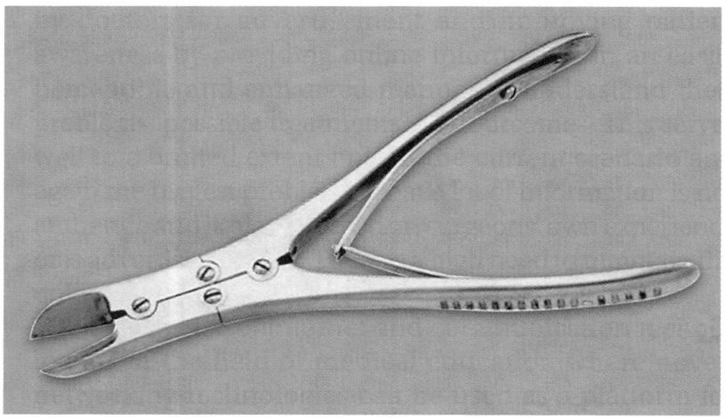

Fig. 17: Ruskin bone-cutting forceps double action.

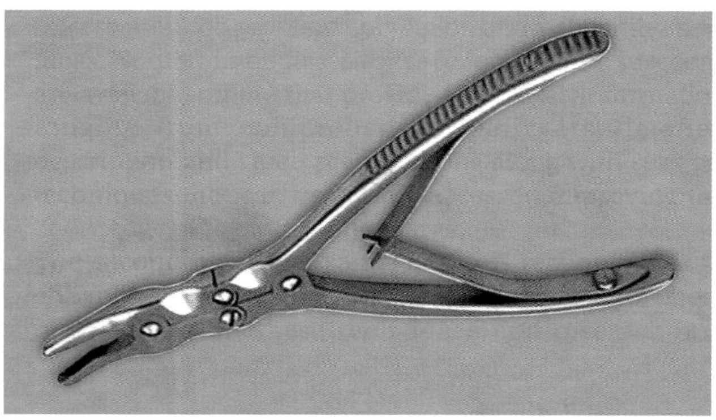

Fig. 18: Single action curved bone nibbler.

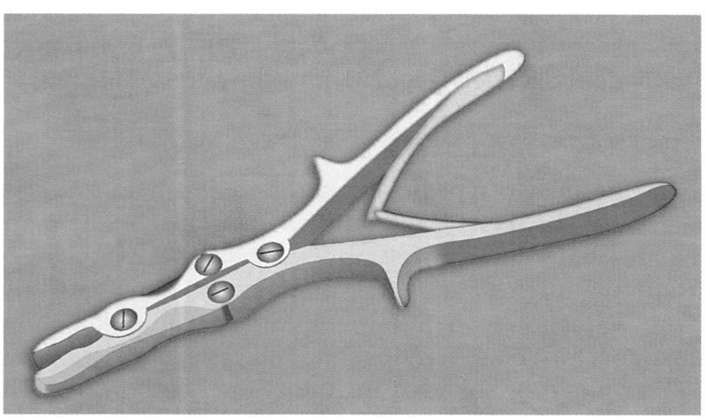

Fig. 19: Northfields-Sargent rongeur.

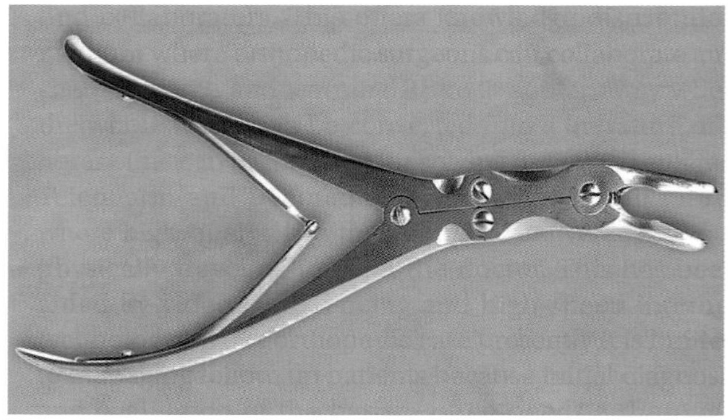

Fig. 20: Leksell's rongeur.

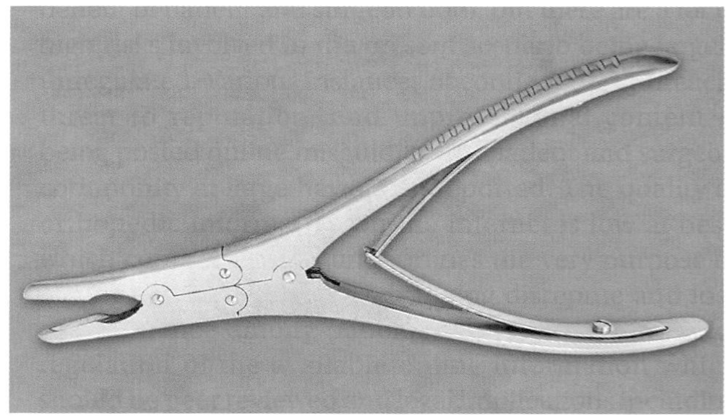

Fig. 21: Stille-Ruskin rongeur.

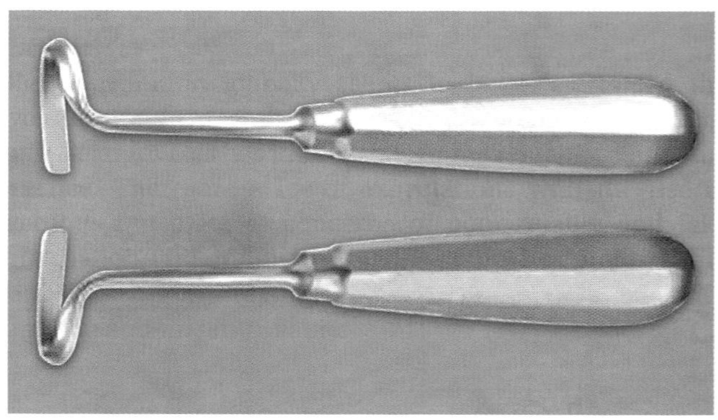

Fig. 22: Doyen's periosteal elevator.

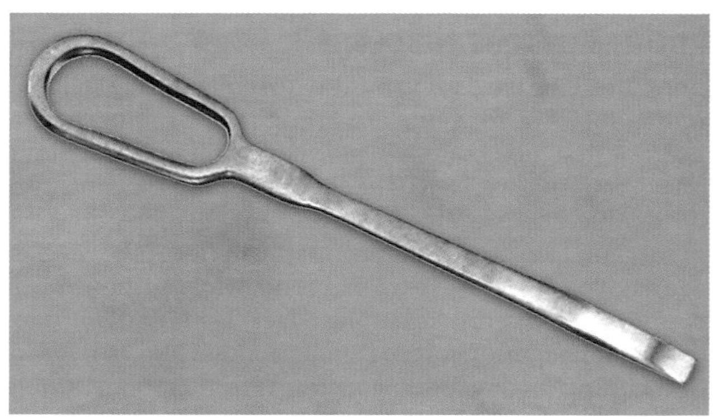

Fig. 23: Bristows periosteal elevator.

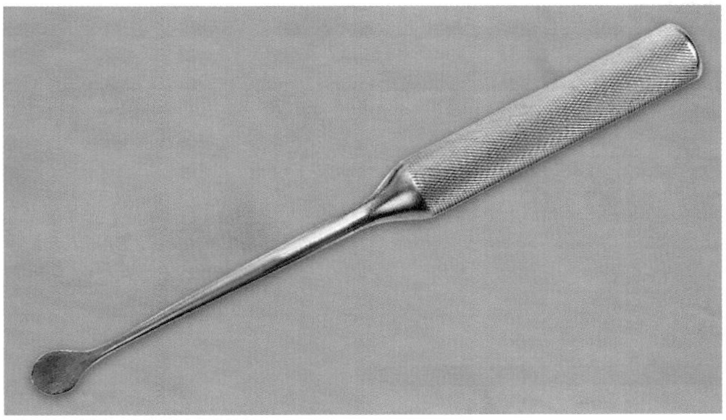

Fig. 24: Cobb's spinal elevator.

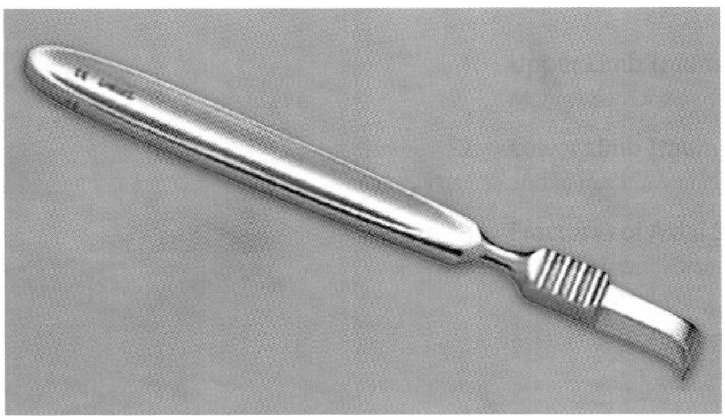

Fig. 25: Farabeuf rugine.

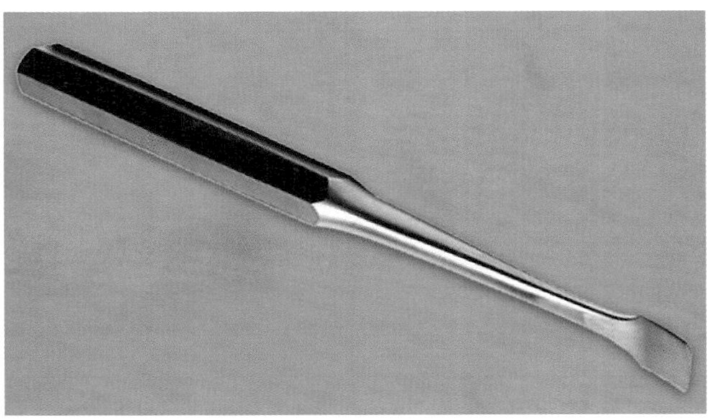

Fig. 26: Key periosteal elevator.

back skin and tissue, while the larger ones are designed to retract muscles, organs and bones. Position of the retractor should be changed frequently during surgery. Self-retaining retractors are set in a fixed position with adjustable ratchet lock handles. They help to minimize slippage. Some variations have curved or hinged handles to maximize visibility [Lane's/Trethowan bone lever **(Fig. 30)**, Smilie's knee joint retractor **(Fig. 31)**, Mayo Adson's laminectomy retractor **(Fig. 32)**, Love nerve root retractor **(Fig. 33)**, Senn-Miller double-ended retractor **(Fig. 34)**, mastoid retractor **(Fig. 35)**, Langenbeck right angle retractor **(Fig. 36)**, dura retractor **(Fig. 37)**, Hohmann retractor **(Fig. 38)**].

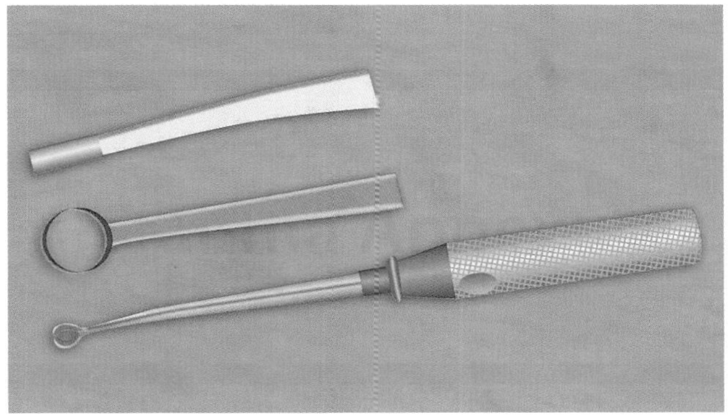

Fig. 27: Cone's spinal curette.

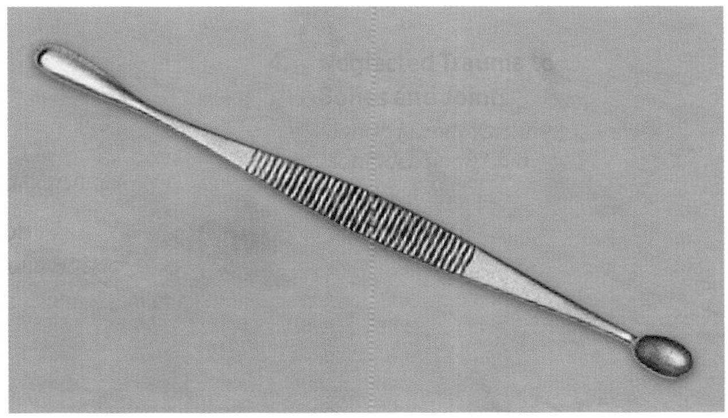

Fig. 28: Volkmann curette double ended.

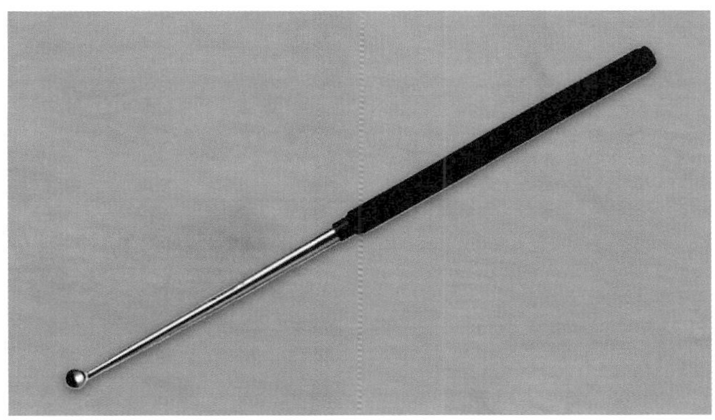

Fig. 29: Cup curette.

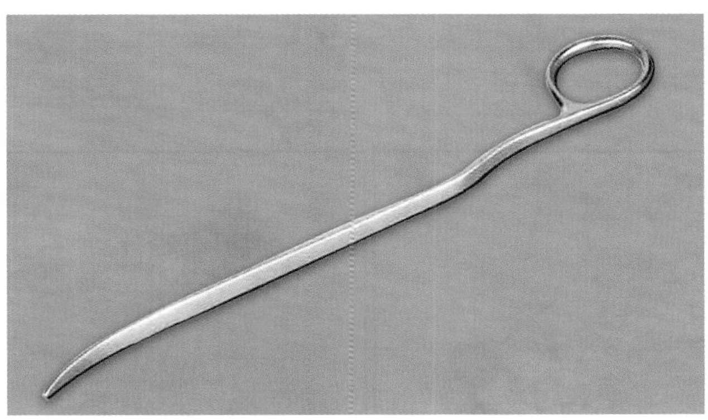

Fig. 30: Lane's bone lever.

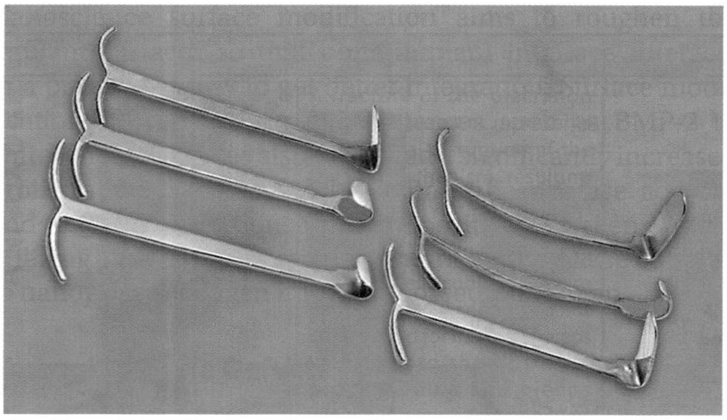

Fig. 31: Smilie's knee joint retractor.

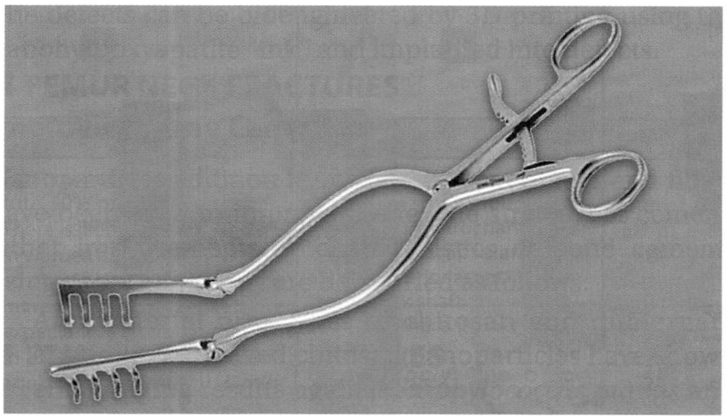

Fig. 32: Mayo Adson's laminectomy retractor.

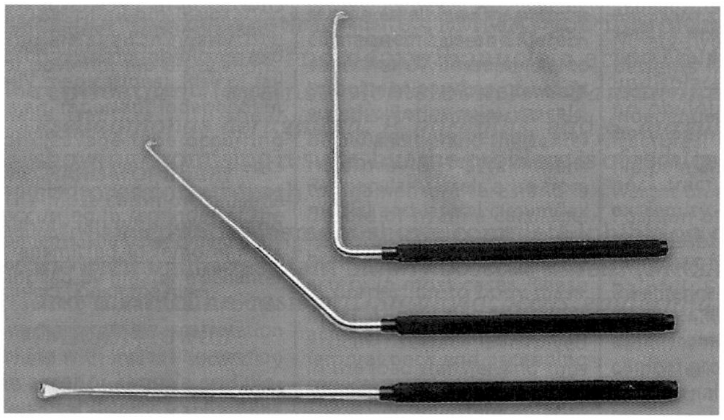

Fig. 33: Love nerve root retractor.

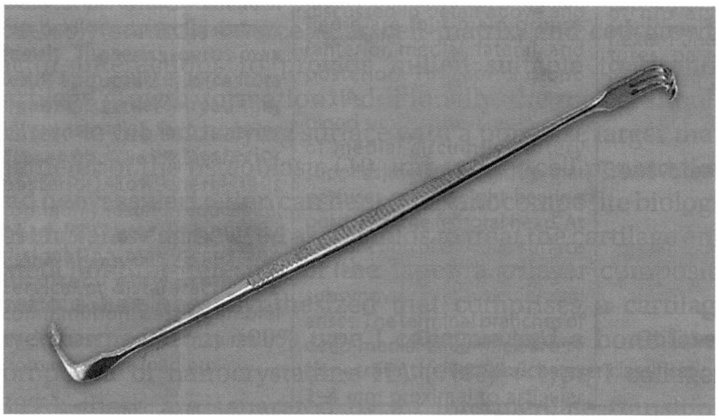

Fig. 34: Senn-Miller double-ended retractor.

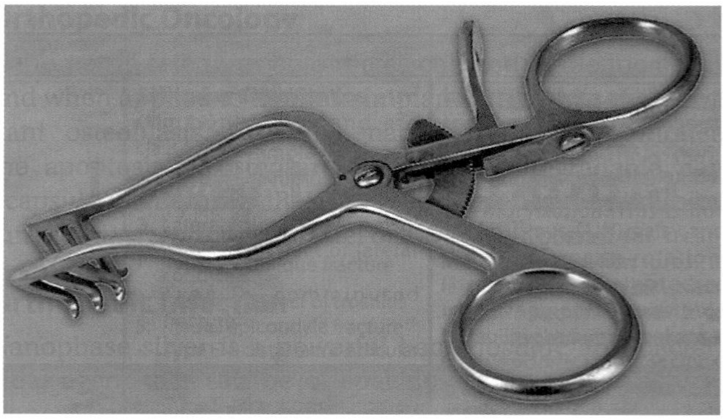

Fig. 35: Mastoid retractor.

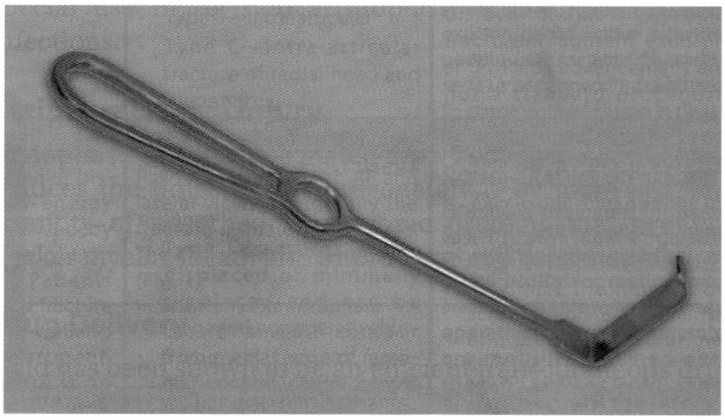

Fig. 36: Langenbeck right angle retractor.

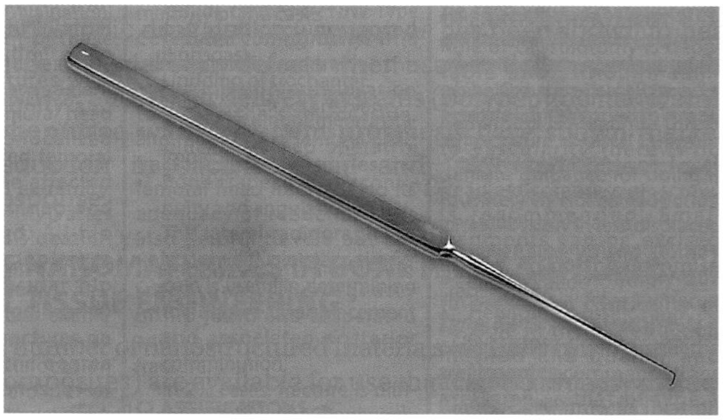

Fig. 37: Dura retractor.

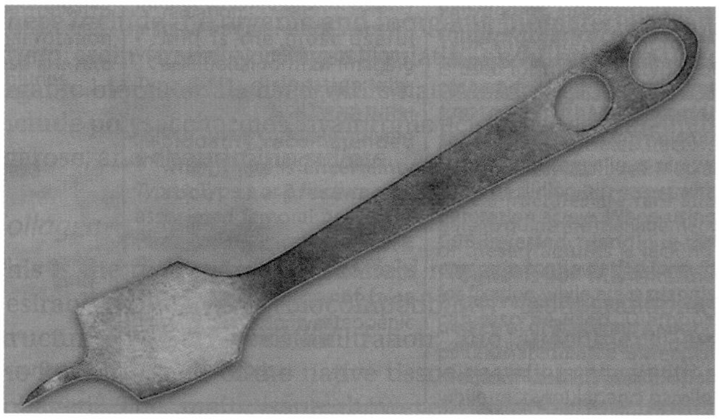

Fig. 38: Hohmann retractor.

CARTILAGE/TENDON INSTRUMENTS

They are used to retrieve, grasp, hold, cut, and separate cartilage and tendons. Used in trauma and reconstructive surgeries to repair or reattach torn tendon and cartilage [Martin's cartilage forceps **(Fig. 39)**, Sequestrum forceps **(Fig. 40)**, tendon-holding forceps **(Fig. 41)**, Caroll tendon-pulling forceps **(Fig. 42)**, Smillie's meniscus knife left/right point **(Fig. 43)**, and tendon stripper **(Fig. 44)**].

Spinal rongeurs: They are used to grasp or excise tissue, degenerated disk material or bone during spinal and neurological procedures. There can be different bite sizes and different angles up or down-cutting tips [disk punch upward **(Fig. 45)**, disk punch downward **(Fig. 46)**, disk punch straight **(Fig. 47)**, Kerrison's rongeur (up-cutting) **(Fig. 48)**, and Kerrison's rongeur (down-cutting) **(Fig. 49)**].

GENERAL INSTRUMENTS

Scissors: Used for dissecting and cutting tissues and material like thread, wire bandages, etc. The curved variety is preferred for dissecting, as they provide a better field of vision. Straight variety is used when a straight cut is needed, such as in sutures, nerves, and vessels. They can also use to spread and probe the area of incision [Metzenbaum scissors **(Fig. 50)** and Mayo scissors **(Fig. 51)**].

Forceps: Used to grasp, hold, or exert traction upon tissue or material. To clamp and restrict arteries or tissue and to

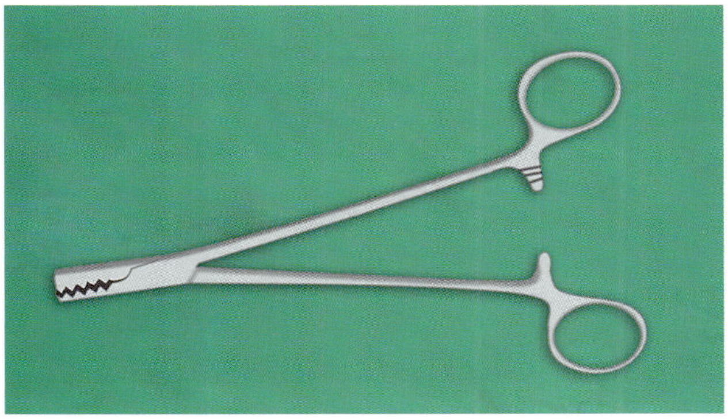

Fig. 39: Martin's cartilage forceps.

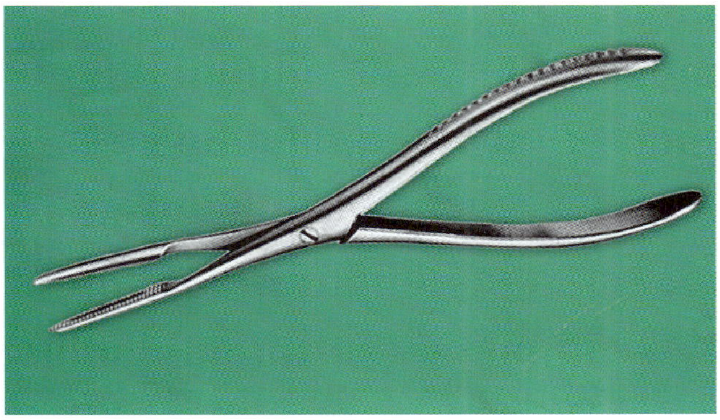

Fig. 40: Sequestrum forceps.

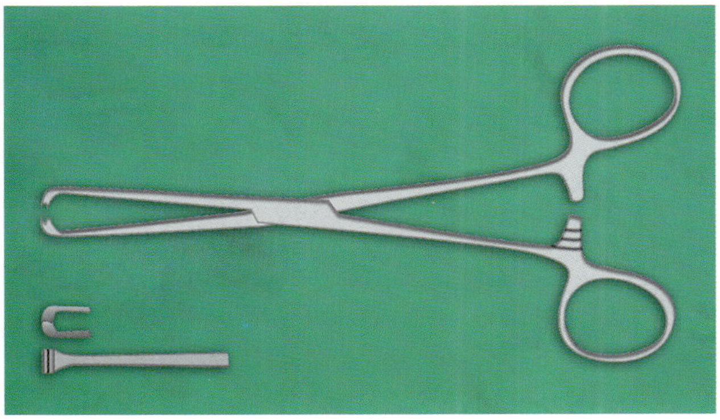

Fig. 41: Tendon-holding forceps.

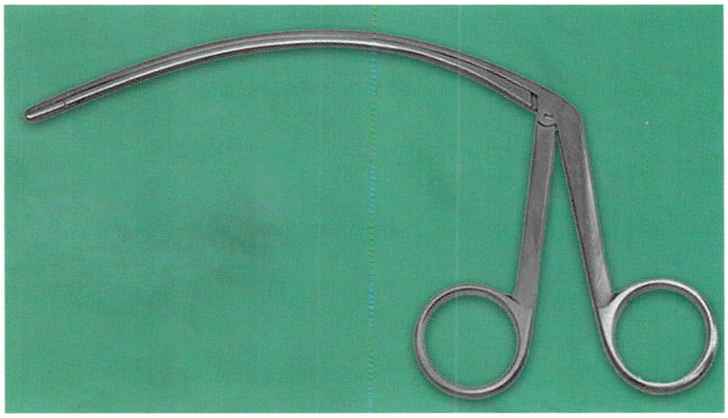

Fig. 42: Caroll tendon-pulling forceps.

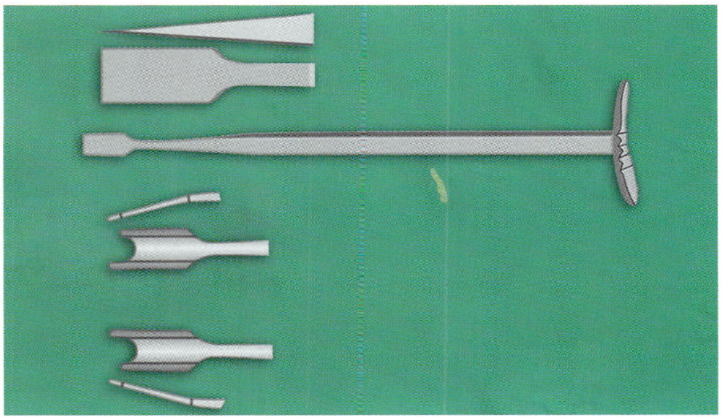

Fig. 43: Smillie's meniscus knife left/right point.

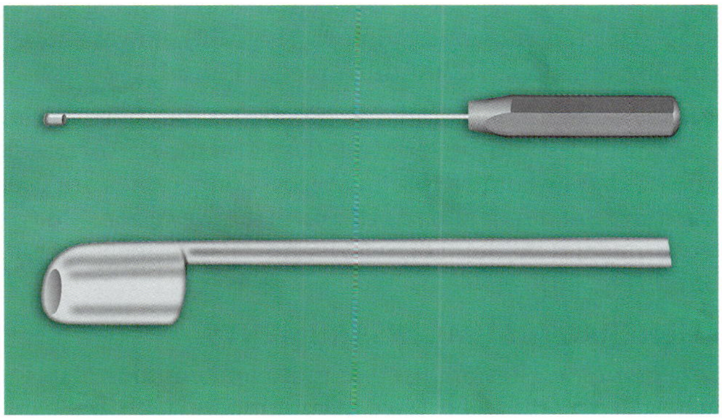

Fig. 44: Tendon stripper.

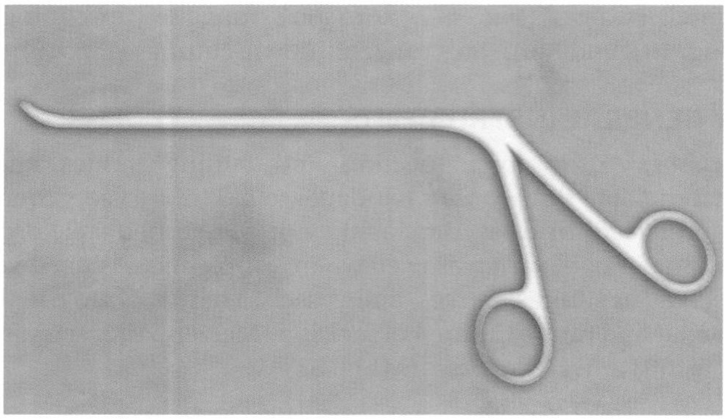

Fig. 45: Disk punch upward rongeur.

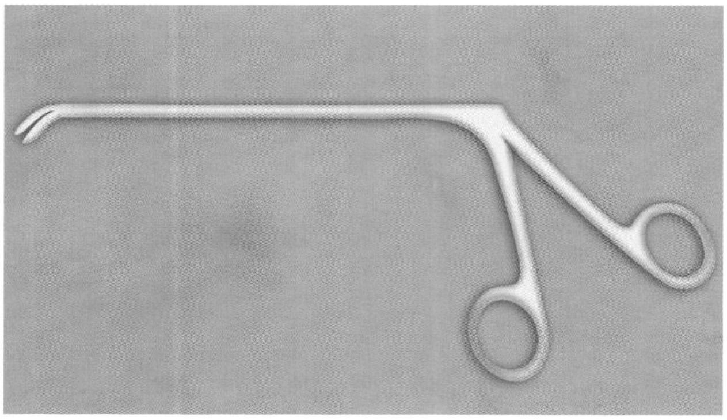

Fig. 46: Disk punch downward rongeur.

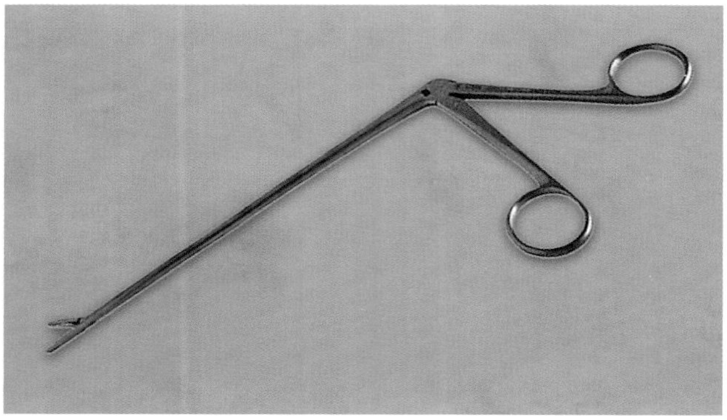

Fig. 47: Disk punch straight rongeur.

control the flow of blood. Dissection and probing of soft tissue [Halsted mosquito forceps **(Fig. 52)**, towel forceps **(Fig. 53)**, and dressing/thumb forceps **(Fig. 54)**].

Needle holders: Look similar to hemostats, but have thicker and shorter jaw and are grooved. Based on the size of needle to be held, they come in various sizes. Longer ones are used for suturing at depth and shorter ones for the surface [Mayo-Hegar needle holder **(Fig. 55)** and Olsen-Hegar needle holder **(Fig. 56)**].

GENERAL TRAUMA INSTRUMENTS

Plate benders: They are used to mold and contour plates to get best fit over the bone. Used in conjunction with malleable template to determine exact spot and degree of curvature

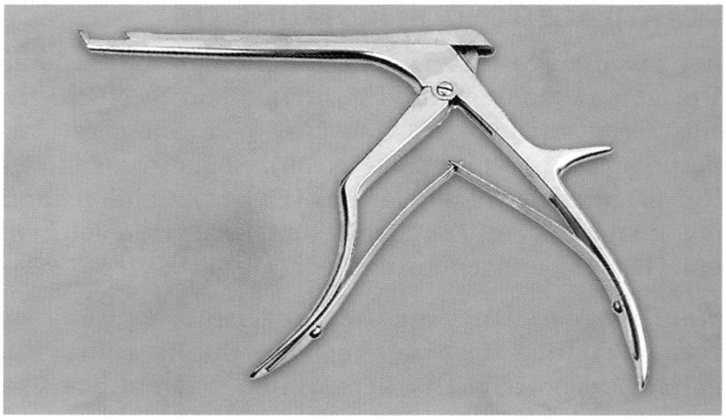

Fig. 48: Kerrison's rongeur (up-cutting).

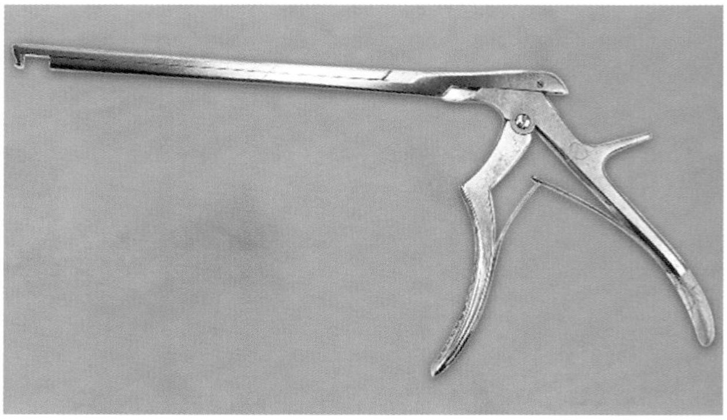

Fig. 49: Kerrison's rongeur (down-cutting).

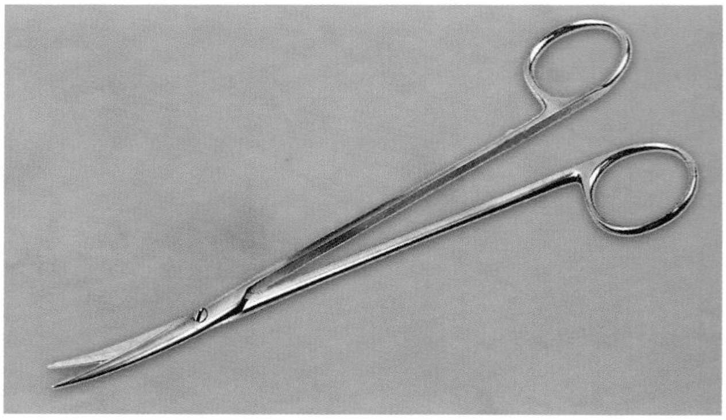

Fig. 50: Metzenbaum scissors.

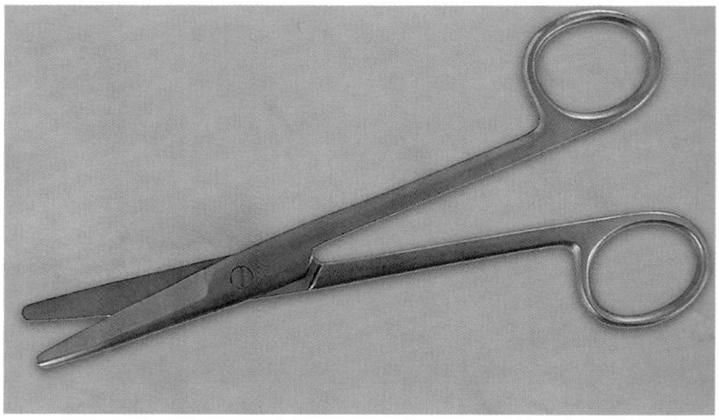

Fig. 51: Mayo scissors.

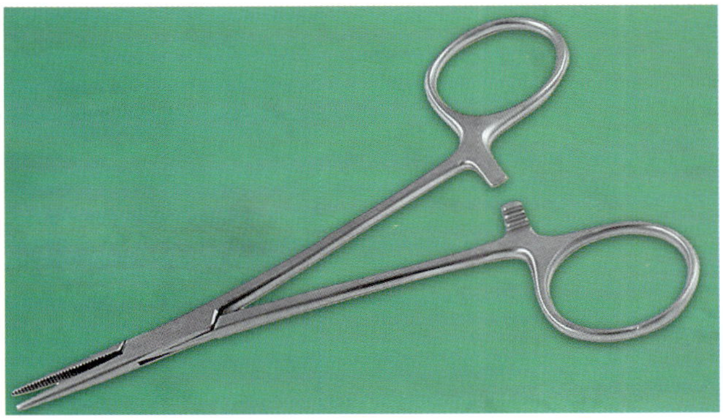

Fig. 52: Halsted mosquito forceps.

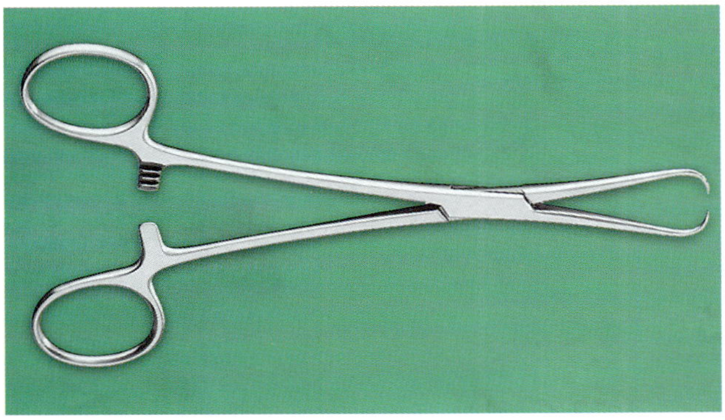

Fig. 53: Towel forceps.

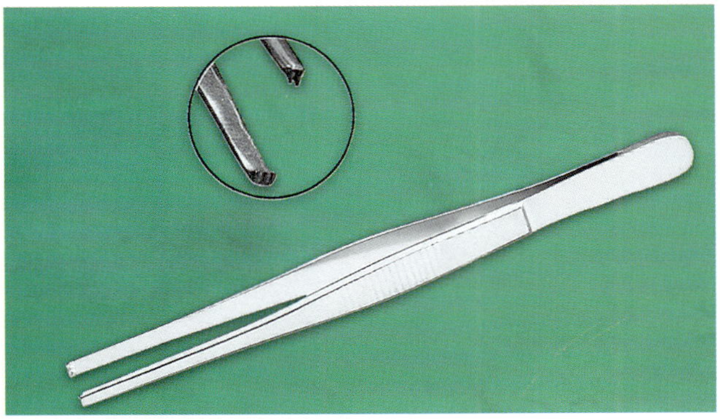

Fig. 54: Dressing/thumb forceps.

to be given. Use of plate benders over locking holes should be avoided [Roller type plate bender **(Fig. 57)** and plate-bending irons **(Fig. 58)**].

Charley's compression clamp (2 Pin) (Fig. 59): Used as an external fixator device to apply compression across arthrodesis or fracture sites.

Muller's compression device (Fig. 60): Used as an internal device along with a plate to apply compression or distraction across fracture site. It is removed after definite fixation of plate is done with screws.

Universal bone drill with chuck (Fig. 61): Used to insert K-Wires, guidewires, Steinmann pins, and rods. Also to make holes with drill bits for screw insertion.

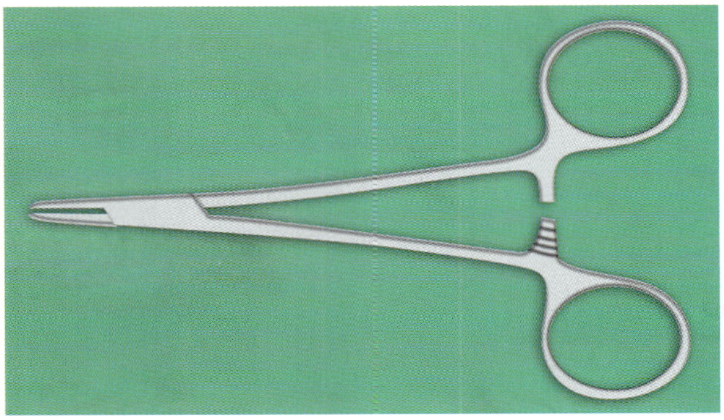

Fig. 55: Mayo-Hegar needle holder.

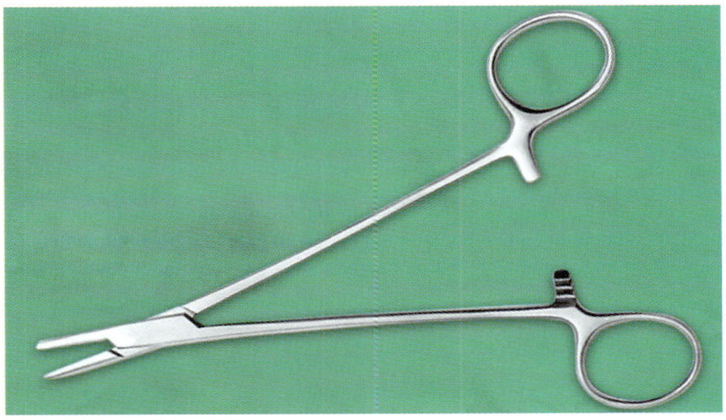

Fig. 56: Olsen-Hegar needle holder.

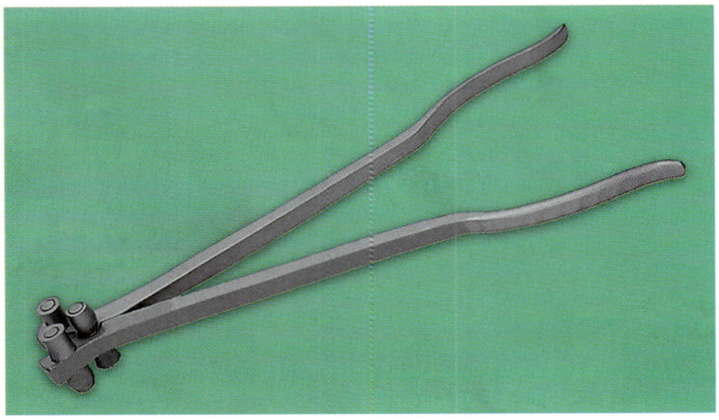

Fig. 57: Roller type plate bender.

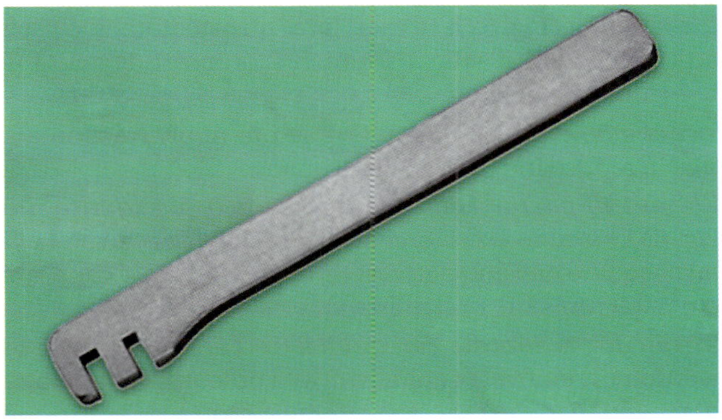

Fig. 58: Plate-bending irons.

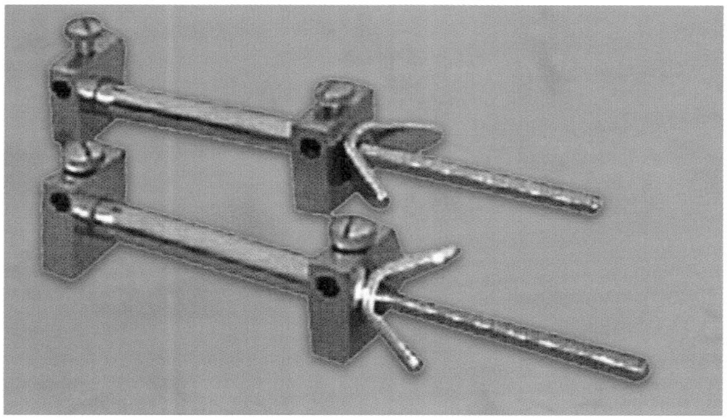

Fig. 59: Charley's compression clamp (2 pin).

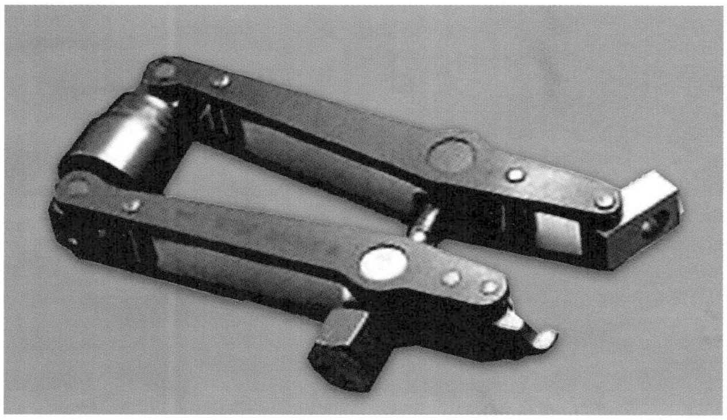

Fig. 60: Muller's compression device.

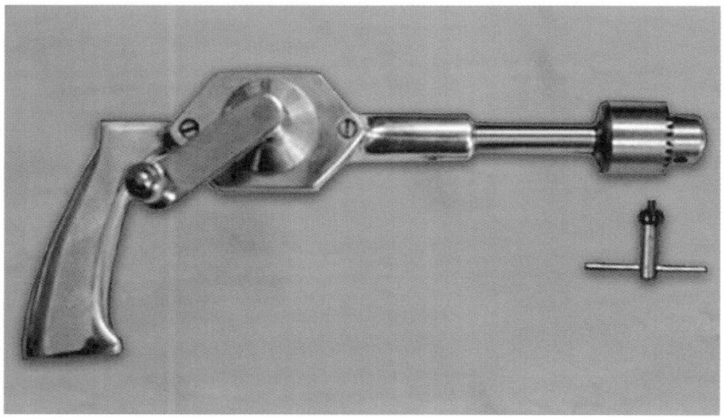

Fig. 61: Universal bone drill with chuck.

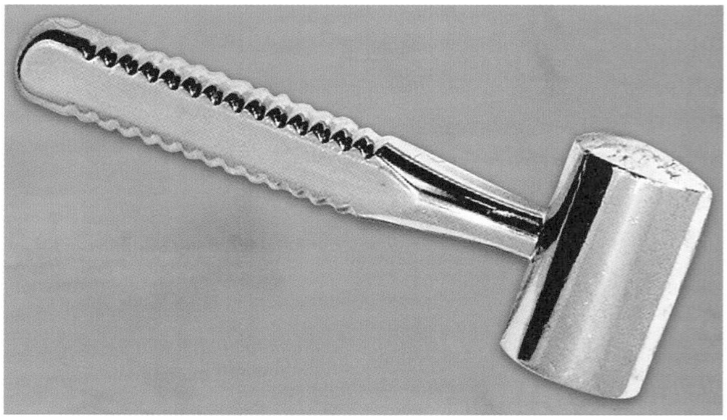

Fig. 62: Heath mallet.

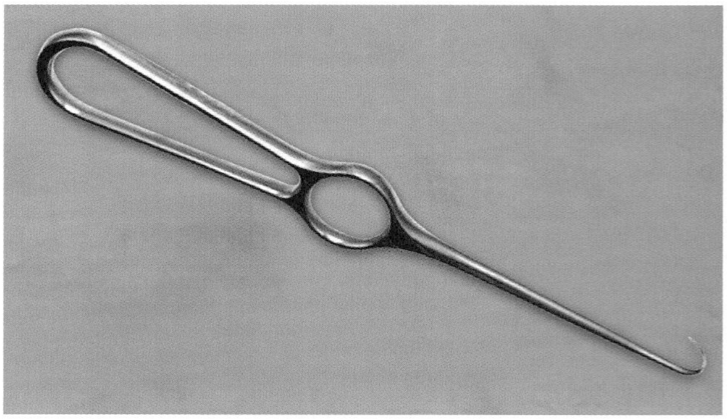

Fig. 63: Kocher's bone hook.

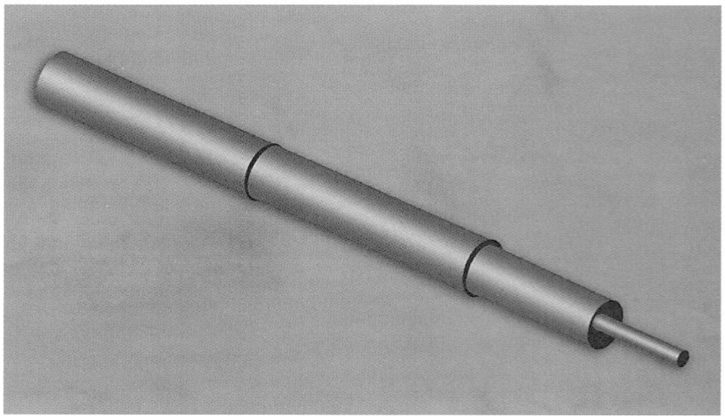

Fig. 64: "K" nail impactor.

Heath mallet (Fig. 62): To exert force on osteotomes, chisels, and gouges. To drive the instruments for inserting nails into the medullary canal.

Kocher's bone hook (Fig. 63): Used to apply traction and force to reduce fractures in large bones.

"K" nail impactor (Fig. 64) and punch for square nail (Fig. 65): Used to exert force with a mallet over the end of K nail or square nail and derive it through medullary canal and across fractures site to stabilize it.

Watson Jones handle for guidewire (Fig. 66): Used for insertion or removal of guidewire as a precursor to nailing.

Gigli saw wires and saw handle (Fig. 67) and amputation saw (Fig. 68): Used to cut bone in amputation. The Gigli

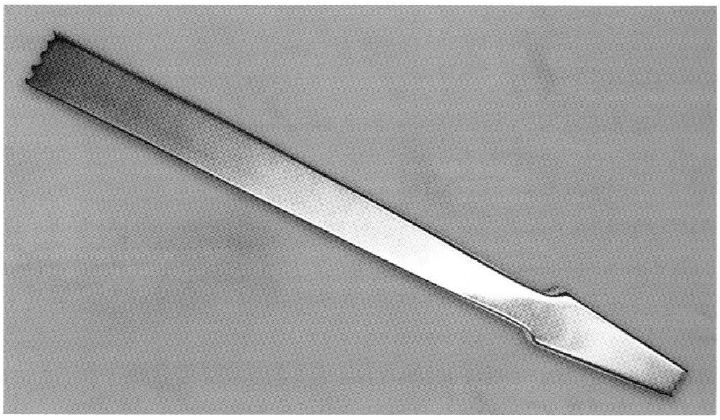

Fig. 65: Punch for square nail.

saw causes minimal tissue damage as compared to the amputation saw.

Bohler stirrup (Fig. 69): For applying skeletal traction for fracture reduction either in operation theater (OT) while fixing the fracture or bedside as temporary or permanent fracture immobilization.

Bone file/rasp (Fig. 70): To smooth, sculpt and clean bone particularly to smoothen end of amputated bone stump. They may have coarse or fine teeth and teeth may be forward or backward cutting.

Crutchfield tongs (Fig. 71): For applying traction on cervical spine and to immobilize the cervical spine. Can be used in OT during cervical spine surgery or bedside.

Murphy skid (Fig. 72): Used to reduce or deliver the femoral head during surgery.

Bone punch (Fig. 73): To wedge bone graft into place. Can also be used to elevate depressed segments of articular surface.

Wire cutter (Fig. 74): Used to cut wires and pins. Maximum cutting capacities are usually marked on each cutter and should not be exceeded. The cut should be taken in the center, avoid cutting on ends of cutting edge. When cutting, protect from flying particles.

Pliers with cutter (Fig. 75): Used in the implantation and removal of pins and wires. To store, pull, twist, cut and tighten wires, pins, and rods.

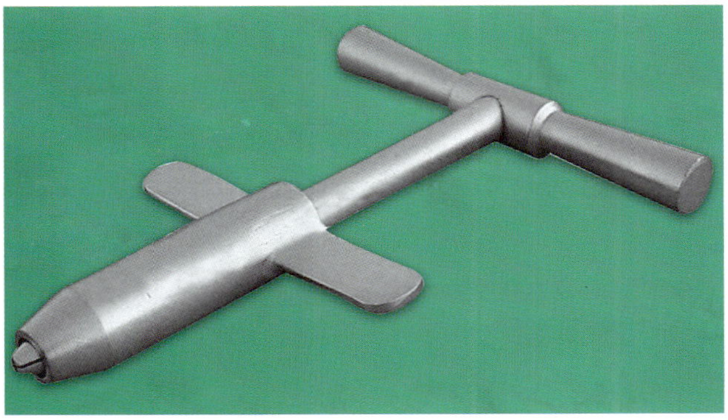

Fig. 66: Watson Jones handle for guidewire.

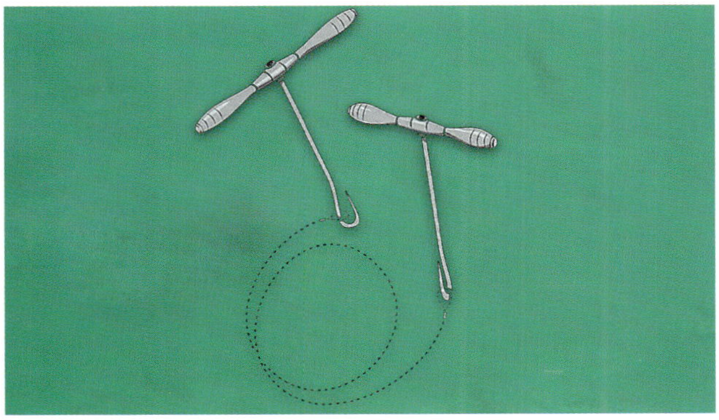

Fig. 67: Gigli saw wires.

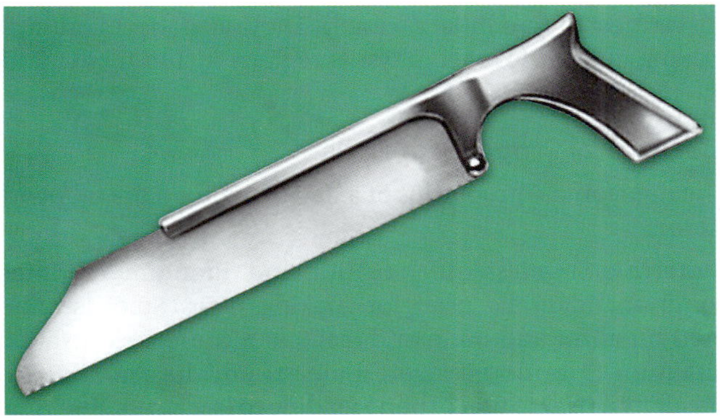

Fig. 68: Amputation saw.

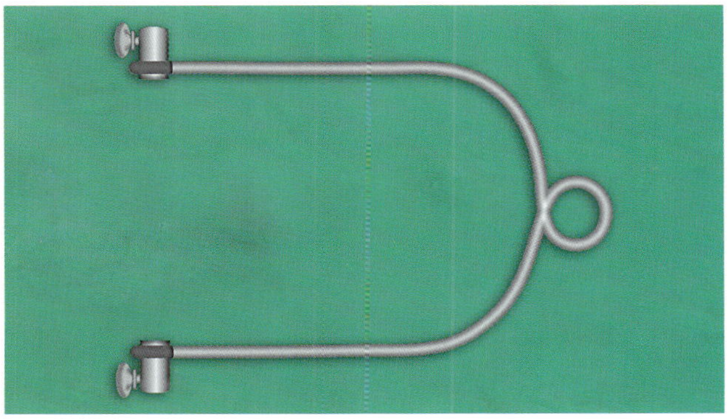

Fig. 69: Bohler stirrup.

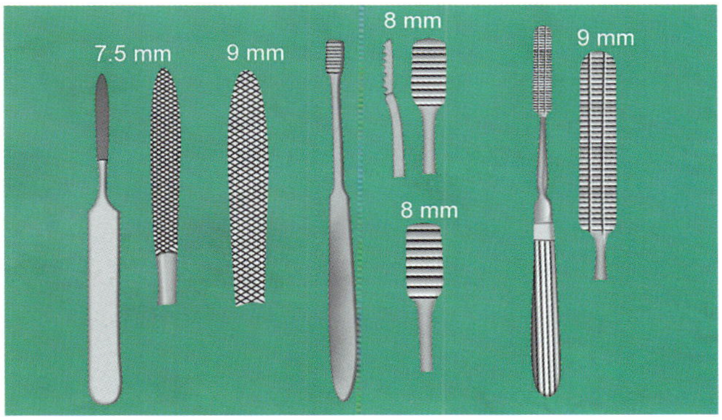

Fig. 70: Bone file/rasp.

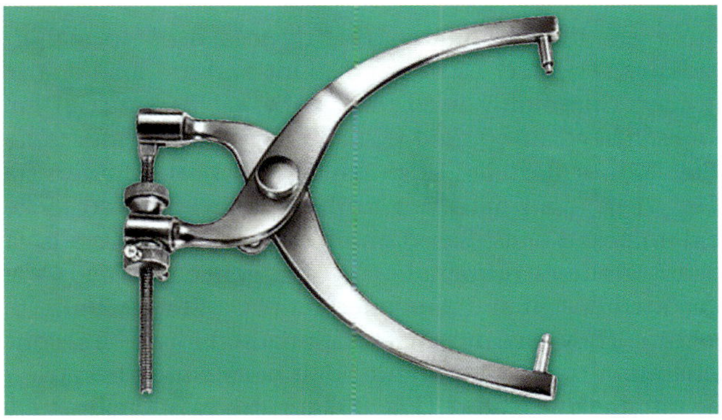

Fig. 71: Crutchfield tongs.

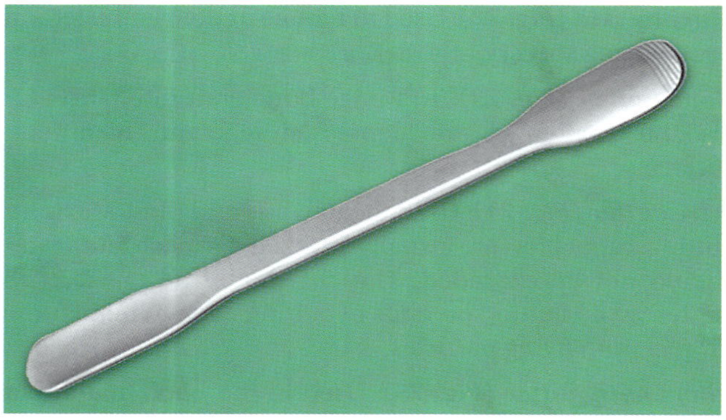

Fig. 72: Murphy skid.

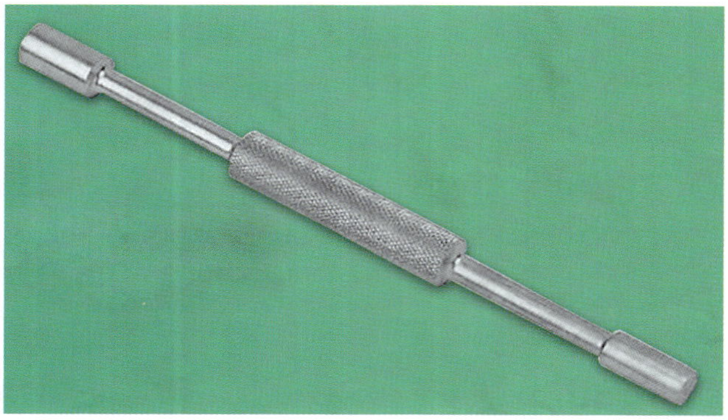

Fig. 73: Bone punch.

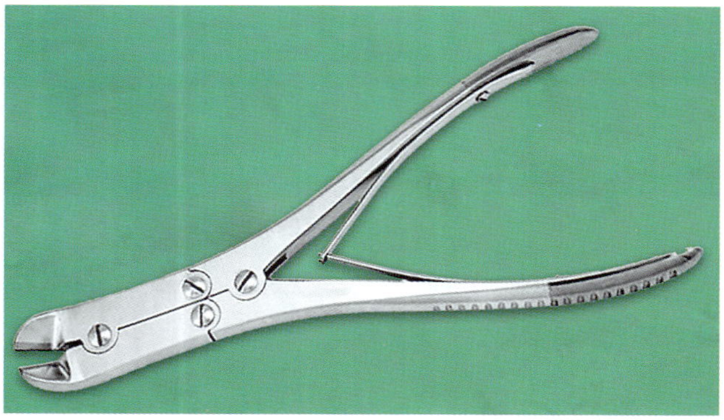

Fig. 74: Wire cutter.

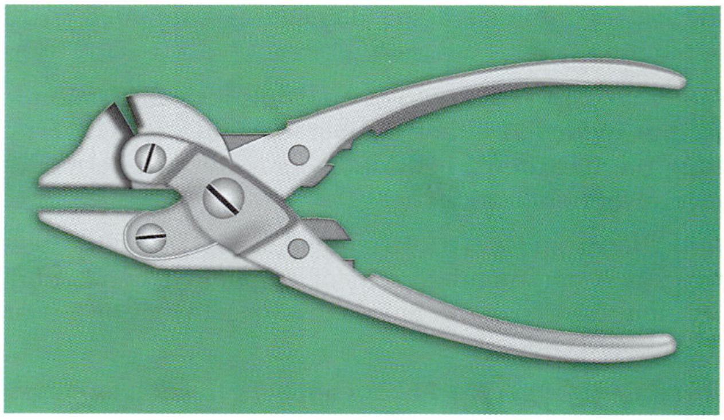

Fig. 75: Pliers with cutter.

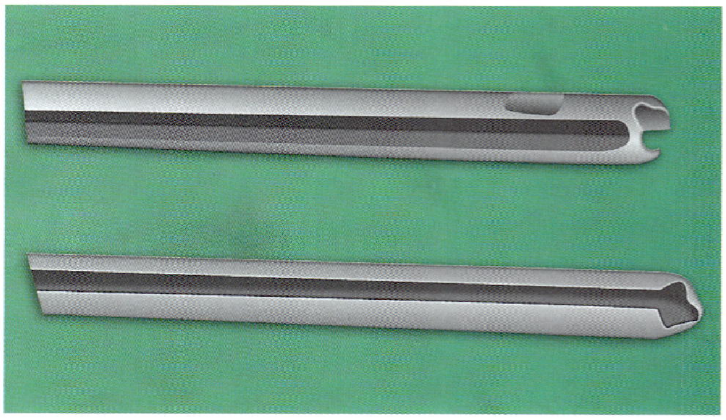

Fig. 76: K nail.

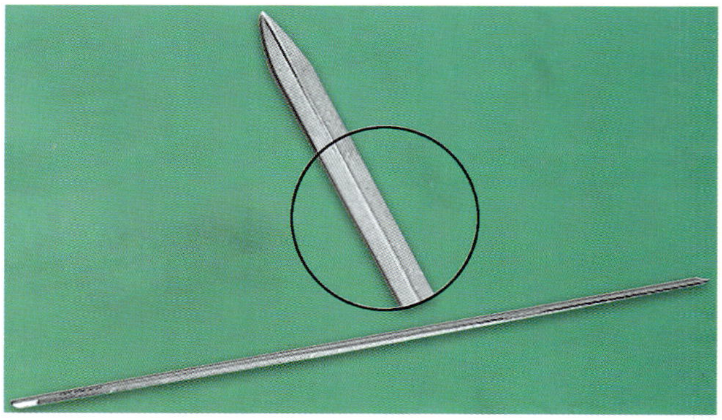

Fig. 77: Square nail.

NAILS

These are intramedullary (IM) devices used to stabilize fractures. They act as internal splint and are load sharing devices. Commonly used for diaphyseal fractures of long bones. They can be rigid [K nail **(Fig. 76)** and square nail **(Fig. 77)**] or flexible [TENS nail **(Fig. 78)** and Enders nail **(Fig. 79)**]. Rigid nails can further be divided into locked and unlocked nails. Based on modes of insertion, nails can be antegrade or retrograde. The first-generation nails were of slotted design and depended on close fit to stabilize the fracture. They gave minimal rotational stability. The second-generation nails were interlocking nails which because of the interlocking feature **(Fig. 80)** are also rotationally stable. The third-generation nails are designed to provide better fit by giving them double curvatures to mimic the natural curvatures of medullary canal. They also have multiple locking options for metaphyseal regions including dynamic interlocking slot.

Mechanical Property of Nails

The mechanical properties of a nail depend on the following factors:

Material: Stainless steel (316L) and titanium are most common materials used for making nails. Steel is stiffer than titanium and bone and leads to a more rigid fixation. Titanium is a more elastic material and has modulus of elasticity closer to that of bone leading to less stress shielding. It is also the preferred material for flexible nail systems.

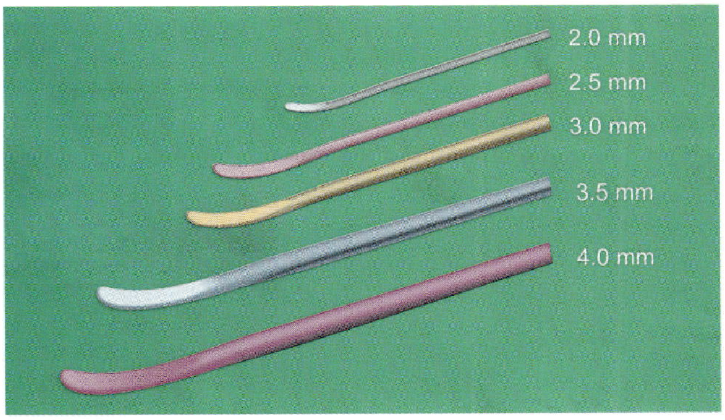

Fig. 78: TENS nail.

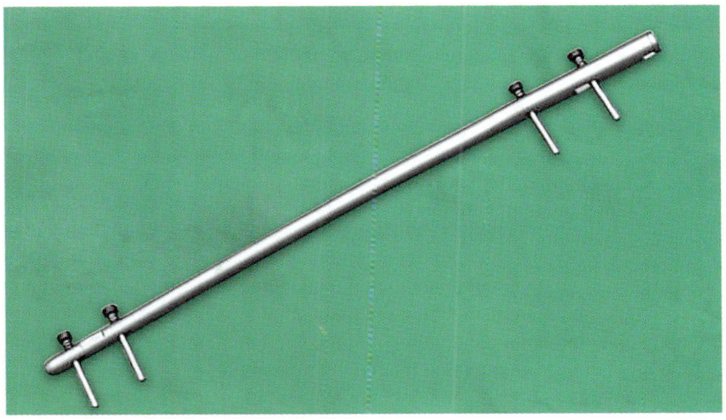

Fig. 80: Interlocking nail.

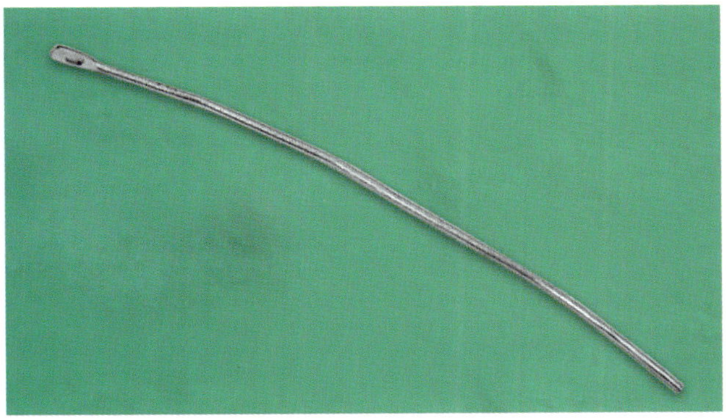

Fig. 79: Enders nail.

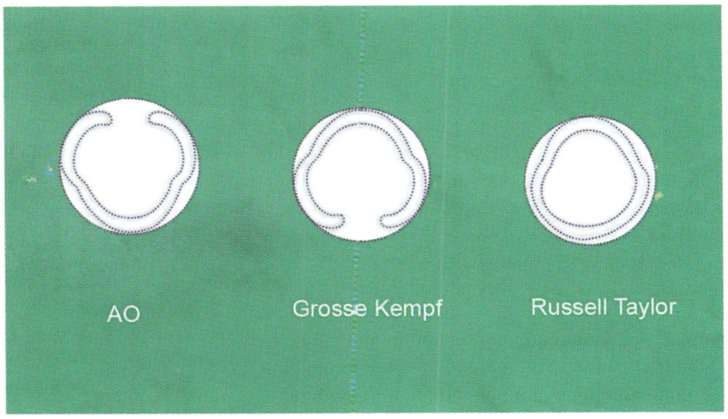

Fig. 81: Nail cross sections.

Cross-section: A variety of cross sections are available ranging from square to V to clover leaf. Presently, the most commonly used designs are AO, Russell Taylor, and Grosse Kempf **(Fig. 81)**. Clover leaf design resists bending most effectively but has less torsional stability. Slotted nails like the K nail have greatest rigidity when the slot is placed on the tensile side of the bone for shaft femur this is the anterolateral side.

Diameter: Torsion and bending resistance in a nail is proportional to the fourth power of its radius. In case of a cannulated nail, it is proportional to the difference to the fourth power in the inner and outer radius. When the radius is increased by a thicker wall or a greater diameter, rigidity increases. Increasing the diameter of an IM nail by 1 mm increases its rigidity by 30–45%.

Working length: The working length of the nail is that portion of the nail that is in contact with the bone proximal and distal to the fracture. It is this length that transmits load from one main fragment to the other. The longer this distance, the greater the flexion of the nail, and shorter the distance stiffer is the fixation. In case of unlocked nails, the length is determined by the contact between the nail and bone proximal and distal to the fracture. In case of unlocked nails like Kuntscher's nail, the stability and working length is determined by the three-point fixation between the bone and nail. The first point is at the proximal entry point, the second point is the point of maximal contact between nail and bone usually the isthmus, and the third point is in the distal cancellous part of the femur. In locked nails, this working length and three-point fixation is determined by the position of the locking screw along with the contact between the bone and nail **(Fig. 82)**. The working length is also determined by fracture pattern. It is shorter for transverse fractures and longer for comminuted or segmental fractures.

Curves: The normal femoral and tibial canals are not straight but curved in both planes. The design of nail must closely mimic these curves to maximize the contact between the bone and nail. Third-generation femoral nails are therefore curved both in anteroposterior and mediolateral planes **(Fig. 83)**. Similarly, tibial nails have an angulation of 11° in the proximal part known as angle of Herzog **(Fig. 84)**. The presence of these curves also reduces the force required to introduce the nail which reduces *hoop stress* which is the circumferential expansion stress on the bone as the nail is introduced, reducing the chances of splitting of bone while inserting nail.

Number and orientation of locking screws: Greater the number of locking screws, the stiffer is the fixation. Generally for transverse midshaft fractures one lock distal and one proximal is enough, whereas comminuted and segmental fractures require two locks on either side of fracture. If locking screws are inserted in different planes, the fixation is more stable.

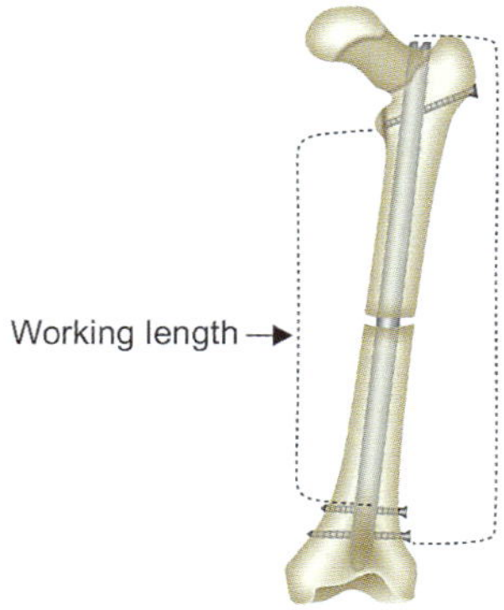

Fig. 82: Working length of nail.

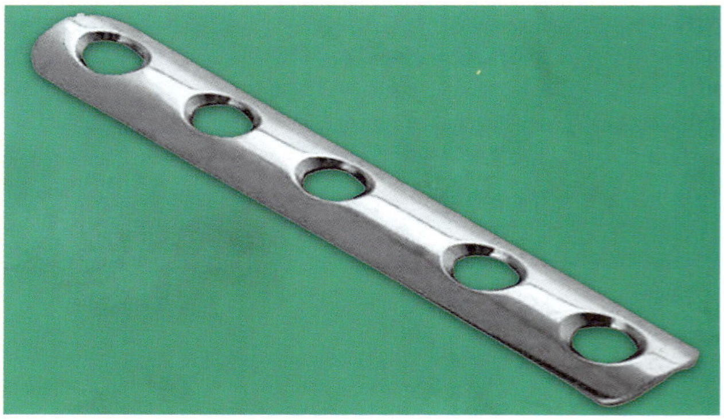

Fig. 85: One-third tubular plate.

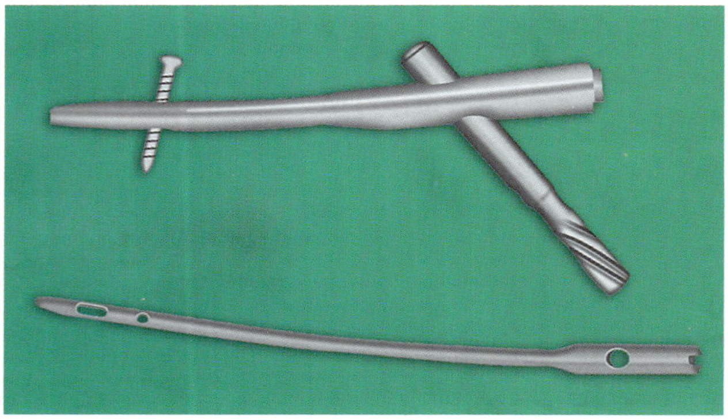

Fig. 83: Double-curved nail.

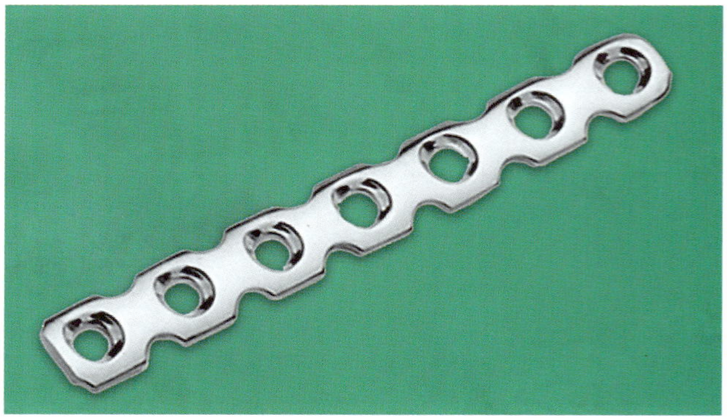

Fig. 86: Recon plates.

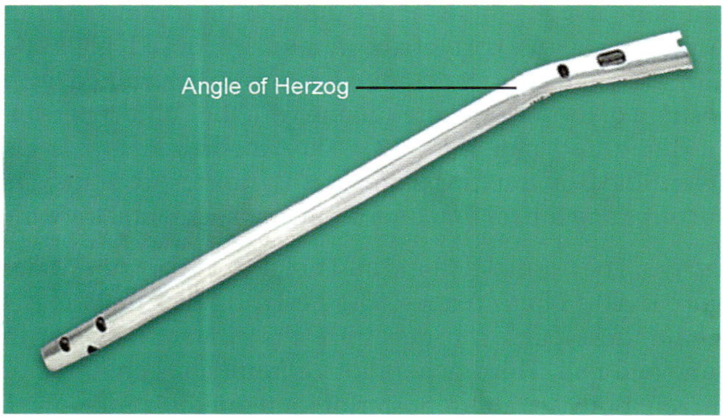

Fig. 84: Angle of Herzog.

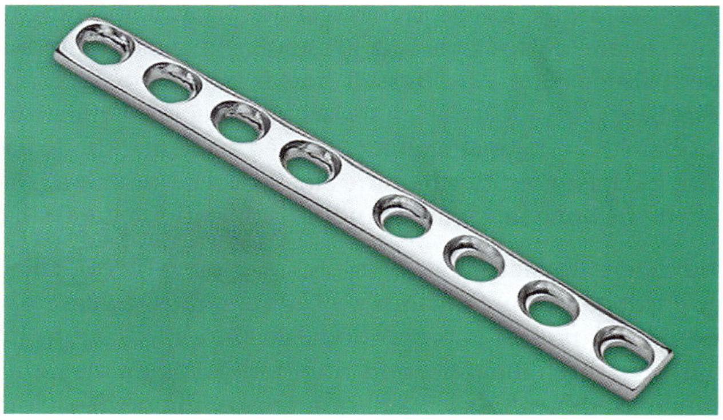

Fig. 87: Dynamic compression plate (DCP).

PLATES

These are system of fixation applied on the surface of the bone. Based on design, they are classified as:

One-third tubular plate (Fig. 85): They have the curve of one-third of the circumference of a cylinder. They are thin plates (1 mm thick and 9 mm wide) and are contoured to the shape of the bone. Used with 3.5 mm screws. Common sites of application are the lateral malleolus, the distal ulna, the olecranon, and the metatarsals.

Recon plates (Fig. 86): They are flat plates thicker than tubular plates (2.8 mm thick and 10 mm wide). They are characterized by presence of notches on the lateral edges which allow these plates to be contoured in all three dimensions. Commonly used with 3.5 mm screws, though smaller mini systems using 2 and 2.4 mm screw are also available for facial and hand bones. They also come with holes for locking screws. Common sites of application are pelvis, acetabulum, scapula, distal humerus, and proximal ulna.

Dynamic compression plate (DCP) (Fig. 87) and low contact dynamic compression plate (LCDCP) (Fig. 88): These are especially designed plates to apply axial compression. The 3.5 mm DCP is 3.3 mm thick and 10 mm wide and is used with 3.5 mm cortical screws, though 4 mm cancellous screws can also be used. The slots for the screws have a slope which allows the plate to slide when an eccentrically placed screw is tightened, leading to compression at the fracture site. The slope also permits oblique placement of screws allowing lag screws to be applied through the plate (7° in transverse plane and 40° in longitudinal plane). The LCDCP is similar in design but slightly broader (11 mm wide). It has cuts on the undersurface to minimize the plate bone contact and to preserve the periosteal blood supply. Common sites of application are forearm fractures, fibula, clavicle, and distal humerus.

The 4.5 mm DCP or LCDCP is used with 4.5 mm cortical screws and has similar design to the 3.5 mm DCP and LCDCP. It is broader and thicker and comes in two sizes—narrow (3.8 mm thick and 12 mm wide) and broad (4.8 mm thick and 16 mm wide). Common sites of application are humerus shaft, shaft femur, and tibia shaft.

Locking compression plates (LCP) (Fig. 89): These are 3.5 mm and 4.5 mm plates with especially designed holes that can be used in standard compression or neutral mode with cortical screws and can also accommodate locking screw that have special threads on the head that enable them to lock on to the plate leading to a more stable construct.

Precontoured or anatomical plates (Fig. 90): These are region-specific plates which are anatomically contoured to bone shape. They come with both combination holes like the LCP that can take both cortical and locking screws and with holes for only locking screws. The metaphyseal and juxta-articular part of the plate can also have variable angle locking holes that allow the locking screw to be placed at multiple angles through the same hole. Commonly used for juxta-articular fractures like distal radius and humerus, proximal and distal tibia, distal femur, clavicle.

Classification of Plates (Based on Function)

Neutralization plate (Fig. 91): It acts as a bridge between two main bone fragments. Does not produce compression at fracture site. It is used in conjunction with lag screws when butterfly fragments are reduced and fixed with lag screws. Can also be used alone across comminuted or segmental fractures whence it is called "bridge fixation".

Compression plate (Fig. 92): As the name suggests, it applies compression across the fracture site. It can be a DCP or LCDCP or even an ordinary plate with round holes used along with a compression device. A compression plate can apply two types of compression. Static compression is applied at the time of application of the plate. Dynamic compression is applied when the plate is applied on the tensile side of the bone where it acts as a tension band and converts physiological forces into compression across the fracture site. Compression plates are best suited for transverse or short oblique fractures.

Buttress plate (Fig. 93): This type of plate provides a buttress or wall to prevent collapse of the bone. The forces in a buttress plate are applied perpendicular to the surface of the bone.

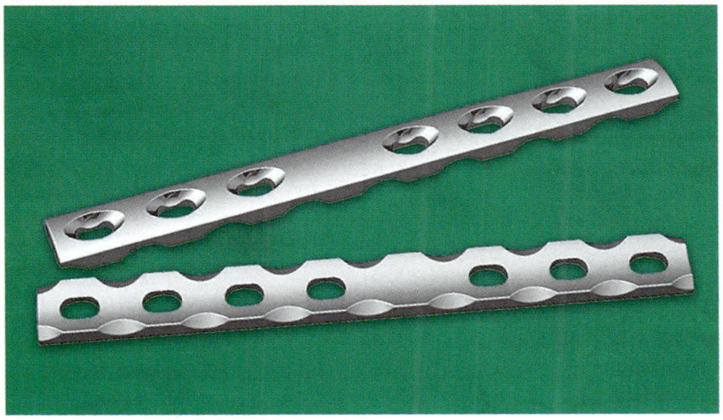

Fig. 88: Low contact dynamic compression plate (LCDCP).

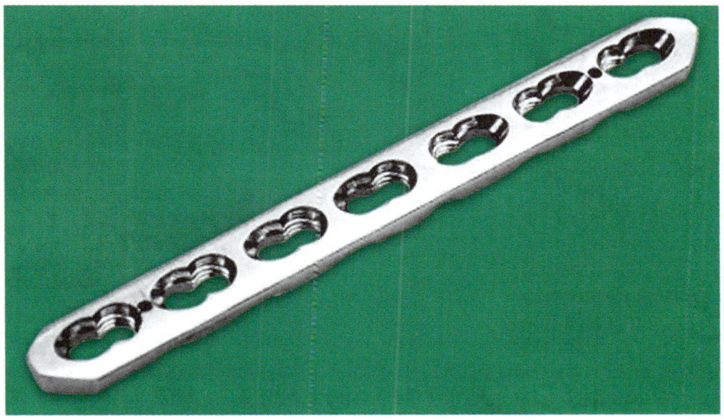

Fig. 89: Locking compression plates.

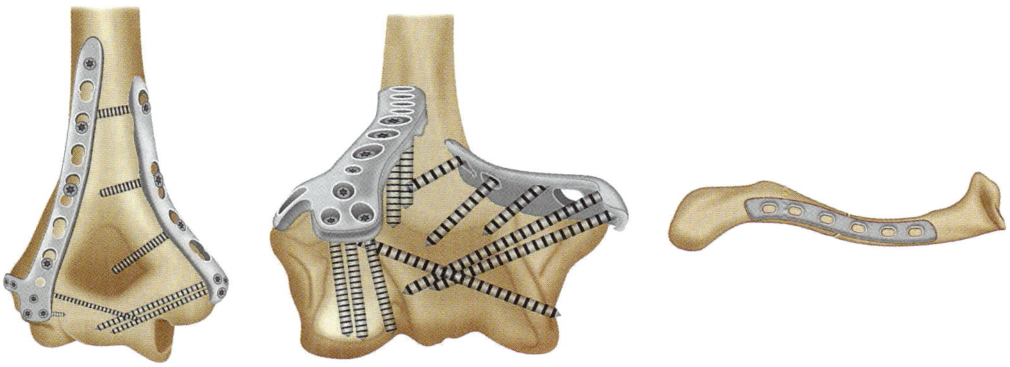

Fig. 90: Precontoured or anatomical plates.

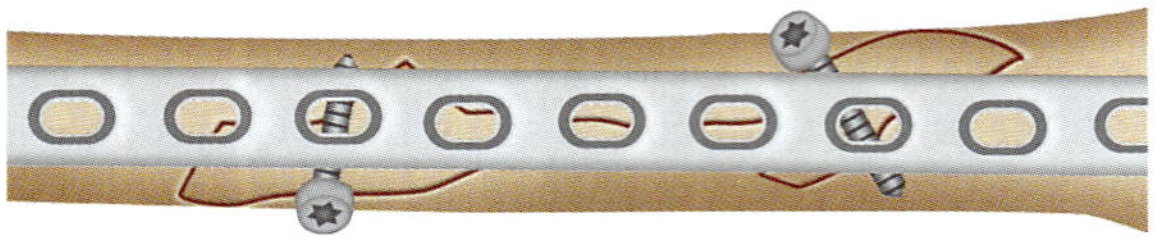

Fig. 91: Neutralization plate.

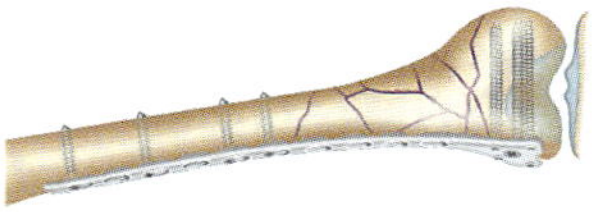

Fig. 94: Condylar plate.

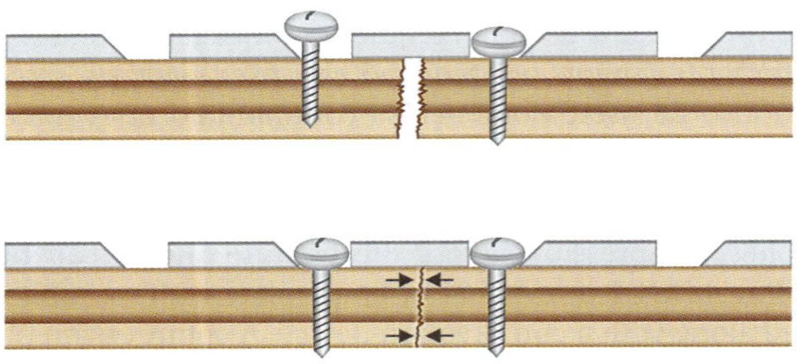

Fig. 92: Compression plate.

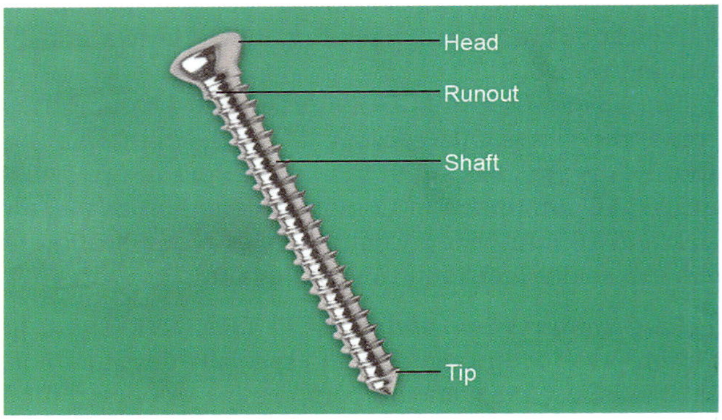

Fig. 95: Parts of a screw

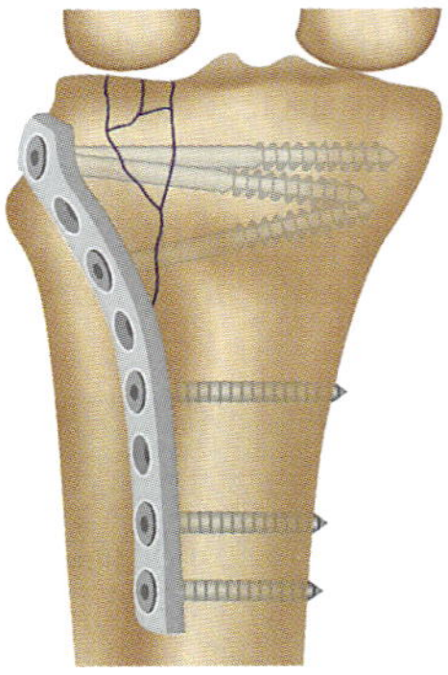

Fig. 93: Buttress plate.

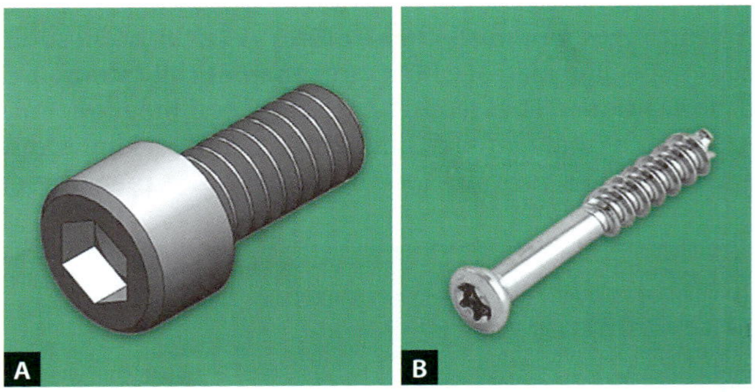

Figs. 96A and B: Types of screw heads: (A) AO/hexagonal screw head; (B) Star head.

It generally has a large surface area and is precontoured to snugly fit the bone surface to provide maximum surface contact. Common sites of application are distal radius and proximal tibia. An antiglide plate is a special type of buttress in where a one-third tubular plate is used to buttress a short oblique fracture commonly around lower lateral malleolus.

Condylar plate (Fig. 94): These are special function plates applied to distal femur and proximal tibia. These function as buttress plate for the intra-articular fractures and at the same time, bridge the metaphysis to the diaphysis thus also action as neutralizing plate. They can also be used to apply compression using compression device.

SCREW

As a fixation device, a screw can be used alone or with a plate. It converts torque applied on the head into tension along its axis. This tension along the axis can be applied in two ways. One is like a machine screw where the path of screw already has threads cut with a tap and the tension is created by elastic deformity of the screw itself. The cortical screw acts like a machine screw. Second is like a wood screw where the pilot hole is smaller than the screw and when a screw is inserted it compresses the surrounding tissue (cancellous bone) to create the required tension. A cancellous screw behaves like a wood screw and is inserted without tapping. Screws come in various sizes ranging from 7 mm to 1.5 mm. It has the following main parts **(Fig. 95)**:

Head: The head of the screw provides a mean to apply torque to the screw for insertion or removal and acts as a stop to apply compression. It has a recess for insertion of the screw driver on top and an undersurface also known as countersink which is hemispherical. The shape of the recess can vary from a simple slot as in a machine screw to a more complex star head screw. Two commonly used types are the hexagonal or AO head and the star head **(Figs. 96A and B)**. In a normal screw, the countersink is smooth and hemispherical. The hemispherical shape allows the screw to be inserted at an angle to the plate, if required. It also helps the screw to slide on the edges of a slope on the hole in DCP to provide compression. In locking screws, there are threads

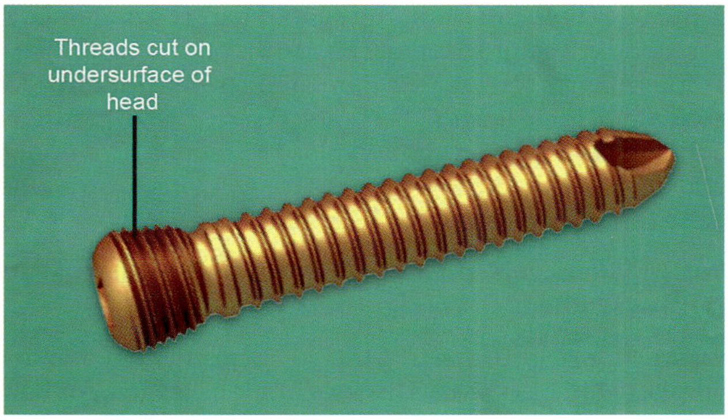

Fig. 97: Locking screw.

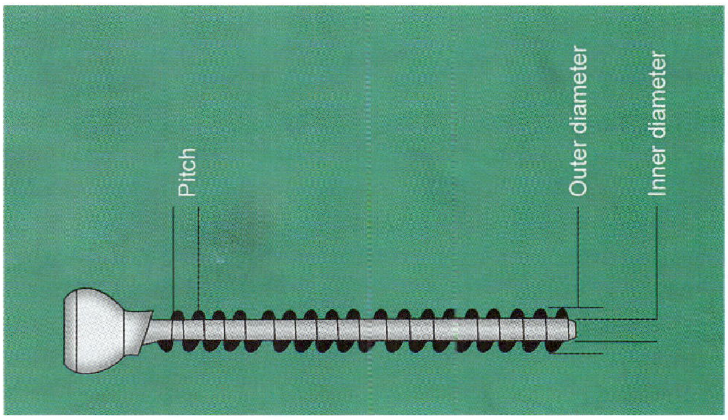

Fig. 98: Parts of screw.

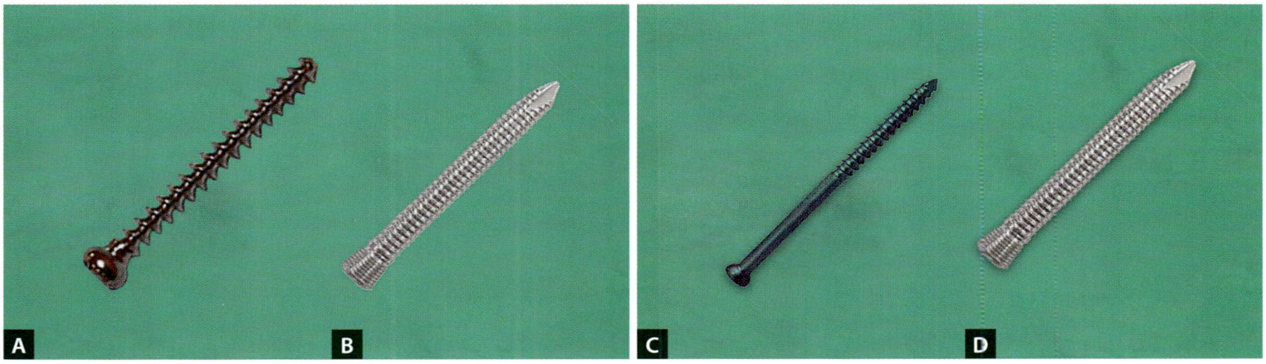

Figs. 99A to D: Types of screw tips: (A) Round tip; (B) Self-tapping tip; (C) Trocar tip; (D) Self-drilling self-tapping tip.

cut on the undersurface and the inner surface of the locking plate too has corresponding threads **(Fig. 97)**. When the locking screw is tightened, it locks on to the plate through these threads. Torque limiting screwdrivers must be used while tightening the locking screw to prevent cold fusion between the plate and screw making removal difficult.

Shaft: It is the part between the head and tip. Runout **(Fig. 95)** is the transition area between the head and shaft and is a region of significant stress concentration and breakage. The shaft can be fully threaded as in a cortical screw or partially threaded in case of malleolar screw.

The shaft has two diameters—the inner diameter without the thread and the outer with the thread **(Fig. 98)**. The breaking and torsional strength of a screw depends on its core diameter and strength of a screw varies with the cube of its diameter. Doubling root diameter will increase strength by a factor of eight. The outside diameter or thread diameter determines the pull-out strength of the screw. The larger the outer diameter, the greater is pull-out strength. Cancellous screws which are inserted into softer cancellous bone are therefore given larger thread diameter to improve the hold on the bone.

Pitch is the distance between the threads **(Fig. 98)**. It is also the distance traveled by the screw when it is given a full turn. It is also known as lead. Smaller the pitch, greater is the mechanical advantage. The pitch can be expressed in mm or threads per inch (cortical screw, 1.75 mm/40.5 tpi and cancellous screws, 2.75 mm/9.2 tpi).

The thread design may be in from of V where both sides have slanted profile or a buttress form where only one side has a slant. The buttress thread is less likely to loosen and offer greater pull-out strength in the longer run as the V thread produces sheer forces at the bone-thread junction leading to bone resorption.

Tip: The tip of the screw is basically of four types:

1. A non-self-tapping tip is rounded and requires the threads to be cut in the pilot hole with a tap for insertion **(Fig. 99A)**.
2. A self-tapping screw has a flute at the end which cuts its own thread as it is advanced into the bone and does not require prior tapping. It can be directly inserted into pilot hole. It reduces the time required for tapping and also ensures a snug fit of the screw. Cortical screws can have both rounded and self-tapping tips **(Fig. 99B)**.
3. Trocar or corkscrew tip is used in malleolar and cancellous screw. This tip cuts the threads by compression cancellous bone as it is advanced **(Fig. 99C)**.
4. Self-drilling self-tapping screws have a sharp tip and cut their own pilot hole as they are advanced. They do not require prior pilot hole to be drilled. They are usually used unicortically to prevent tissue irritation by the sharp tip **(Fig. 99D)**.

The *pilot hole* needed to insert a screw which can be drilled with a drill bit, K-Wire, or a burr. The size of pilot hole is always slightly smaller than the screw to be inserted allowing for threads to be tapped in the hole either with tap and self-tapping screws or by compression of cancellous bone (4.5/3.2–3.5/2.5–2.7/2.0–1.5/1).

Lagging or the lag screw is a technique used to apply compression across fracture site. The lag screw has purchase only on the distal fragment and it draws the two fragments together as it is tightened. The lag effect can be achieved by partially threaded screws where only the distal part of the screw is threaded or by overdrilling the proximal cortex to ensure that the proximal threads do not gain any purchase on it **(Fig. 100)**. For lag effect to happen the threaded portion of the partially threaded screw must lie entirely in the distal fragment.

Cannulated screws have an arrow hole drilled throughout their length and can be threaded over guidewire for precise placements. Usual sizes are 4 mm and 7 mm. They are available in 32 mm or 16 mm thread lengths **(Fig. 101)**.

Herbert screw (headless compression screw) is a special type of screw used which has dual threads of different diameter at both ends and the central part is smooth. Used for scaphoid fracture fixation **(Fig. 102)**.

Interference screws are cannulated screws fully threaded throughout their length. They are inserted into predrilled tunnels to hold tendon grafts in place by friction. Commonly used in anterior cruciate ligament (ACL) reconstruction. These can be bioabsorbable **(Fig. 103)**.

Plaster cutters and spreaders: For removing plaster of Paris (POP) or synthetic casts **(Fig. 104)**

Austin Moore prosthesis (AMP): Noncemented hemiarthroplasty hip prosthesis. Has fenestrations in stem for bony ingrowth (Thomson prosthesis cemented prosthesis without fenestrations) **(Fig. 105)**.

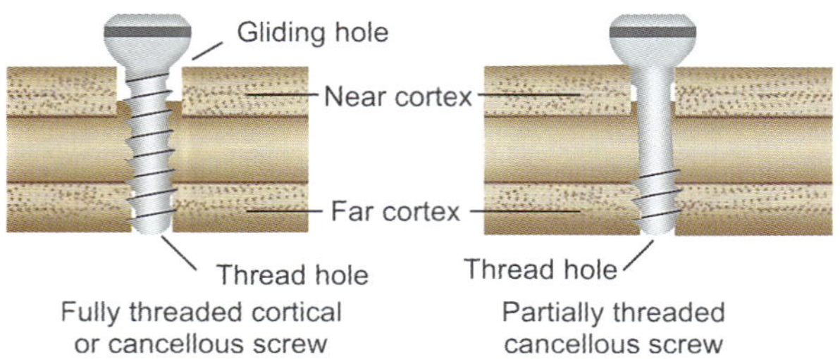

Fig. 100: Lag screw.

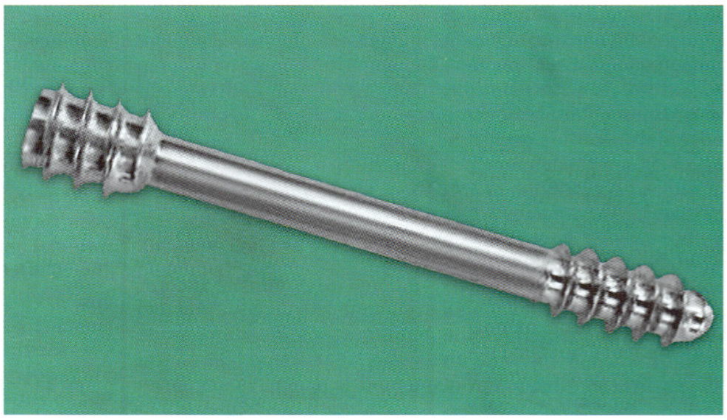

Fig. 102: Herbert screw.

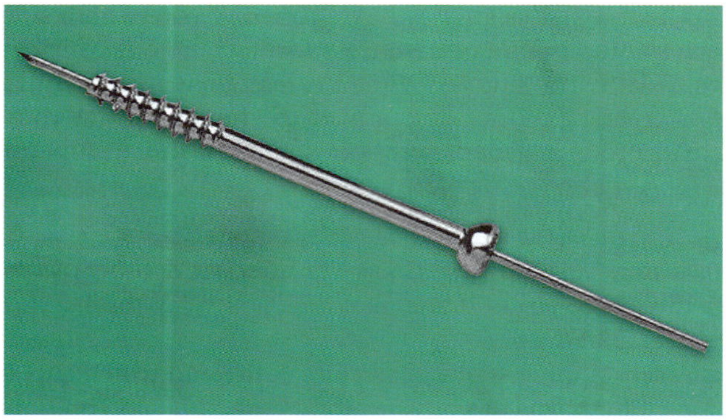

Fig. 101: Cannulated screws.

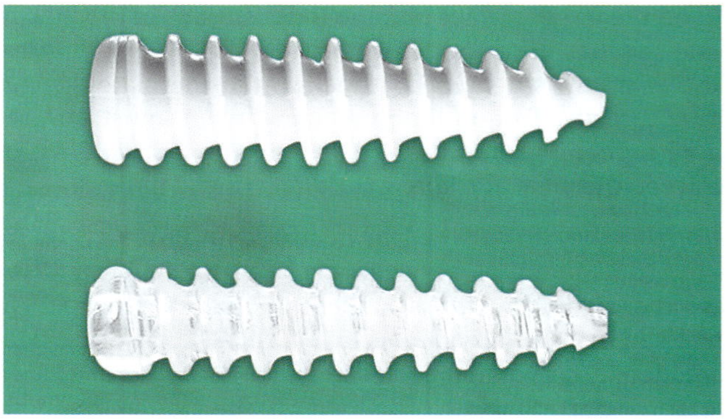

Fig. 103: Interference screws.

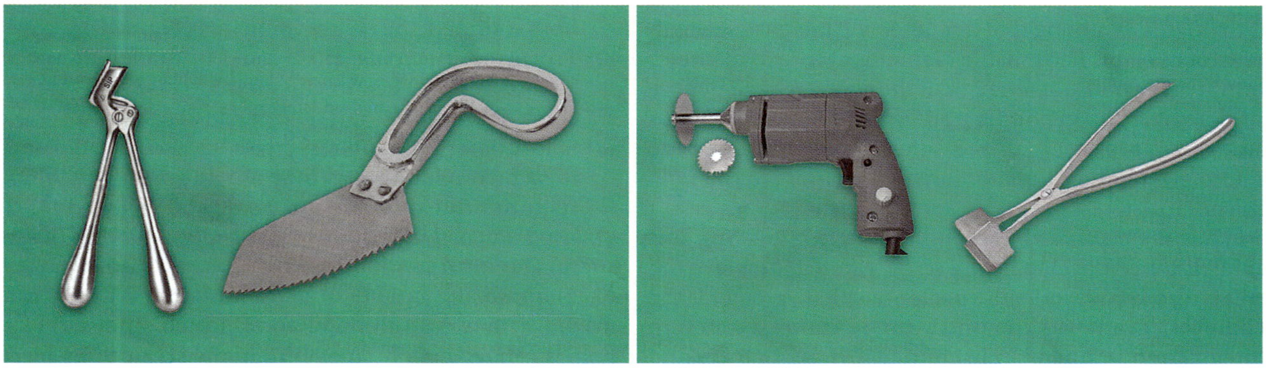

Fig. 104: Plaster cutters and spreaders.

Bipolar prosthesis: It is hemiarthroplasty hip prosthesis with an additional articulation between head and neck. Reduces the motion and wear between the metal head and acetabular cartilage. Can be both fenestrated and nonfenestrated **(Fig. 106)**.

Corkscrew head extractor: Used for removing head in hemi- or complete hip arthroplasty **(Fig. 107)**.

AMP measuring gauge: Used to determine the size of AMP/Thompson/bipolar prosthesis to be used after extracting head **(Fig. 108)**.

AMP rasp: Used to prepare the femoral canal for insertion of AMP/Thompson/bipolar prosthesis **(Fig. 109)**.

AMP impactor: Used to introduce the prosthesis into the femoral canal with mallet **(Fig. 110)**.

Charnley's hip retractor: A self-retaining retractor used for hip surgeries, especially arthroplasties **(Fig. 111)**.

Fixed angle osteotomy plates: Used to stabilize osteotomies done around the hip and knee joints for nonunion or deformity correction [Wainwright plate **(Figs. 112A and B)**, Kessel's plate **(Fig. 113)**, Muller osteotomy plate **(Fig. 114)**, and double-angle osteotomy plate **(Fig. 115)**].

Smith-Petersen (SP) nail and McLaughlin plate: Used to fix fracture neck of femur **(Fig. 116)**. The nail and plate are separate and attached to each other with a nut.

Jewett blade plate: Used to fix fracture neck of femur **(Fig. 117)**. It is single piece implant. It has a triflanged nail fixed to a plate. The angle between the blade and plate can be from 130 to 150°. No prior drilling is done; it is directly hammered over a guidewire and fixed to shaft femur with screws.

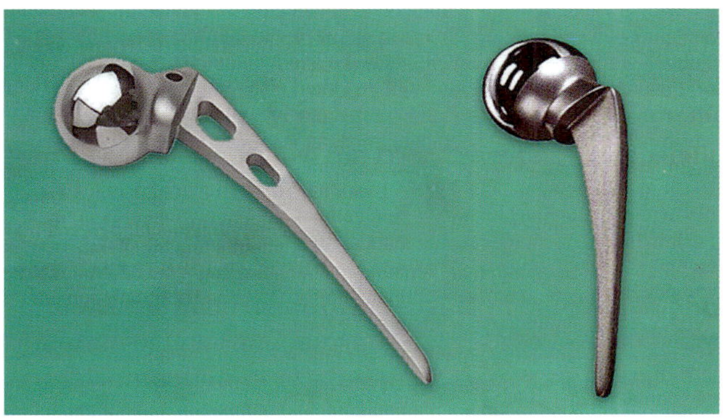

Fig. 105: Austin Moore and Thompson prosthesis.

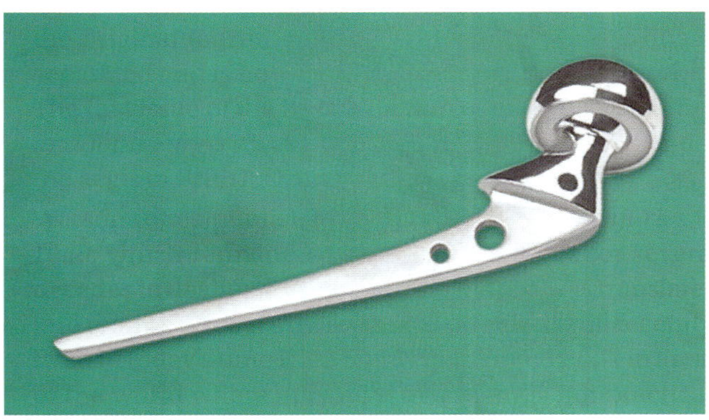

Fig. 106: Bipolar hip prosthesis.

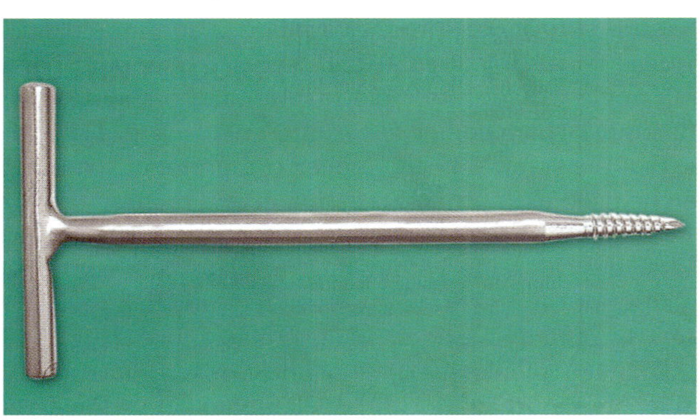

Fig. 107: Corkscrew head extractor.

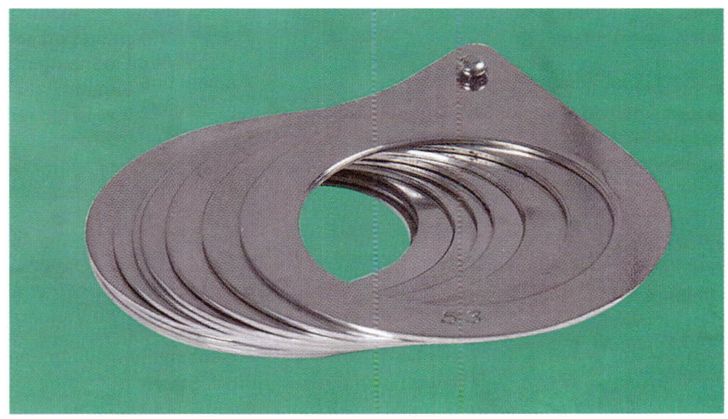

Fig. 108: AMP measuring gauge.

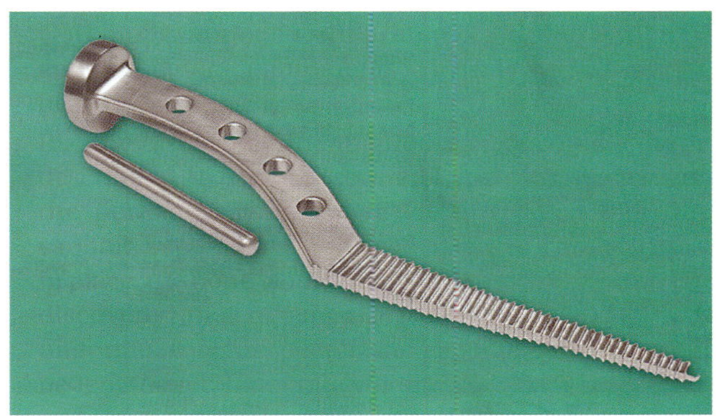

Fig. 109: AMP rasp

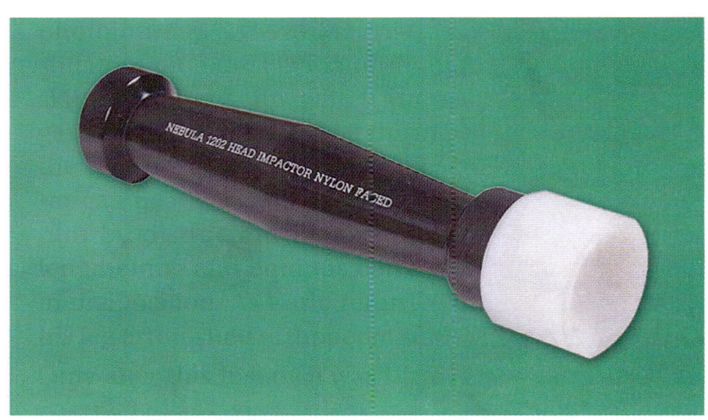

Fig. 110: AMP impactor.

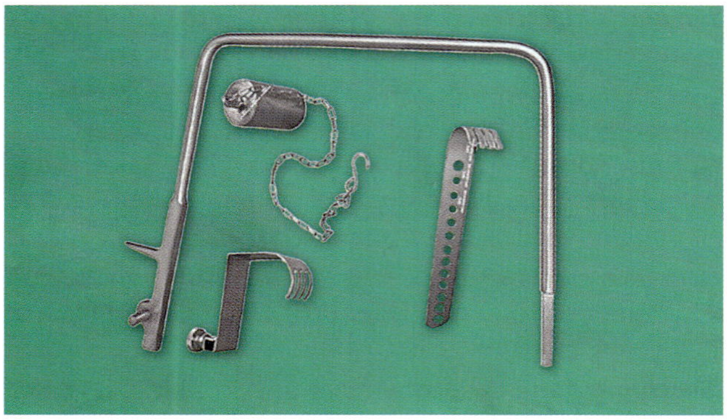

Fig. 111: Charnley's hip retractor.

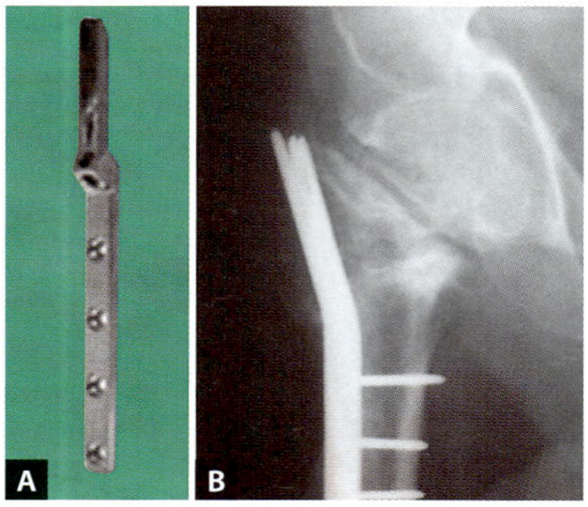

Figs. 112A and B: (A) Wainwright spline as used for (B) McMurray osteotomy.

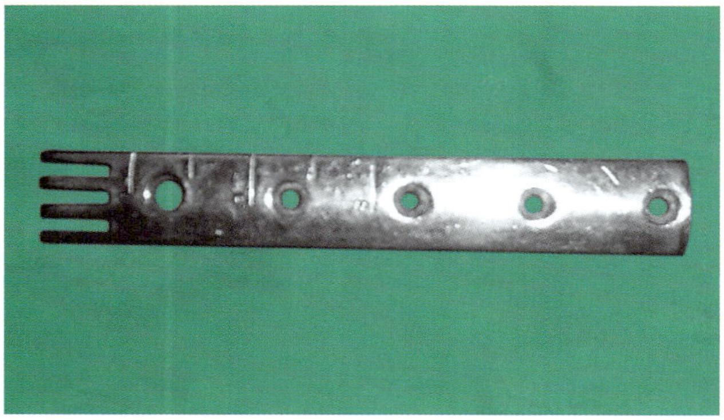

Fig. 113: Kessel's plate.

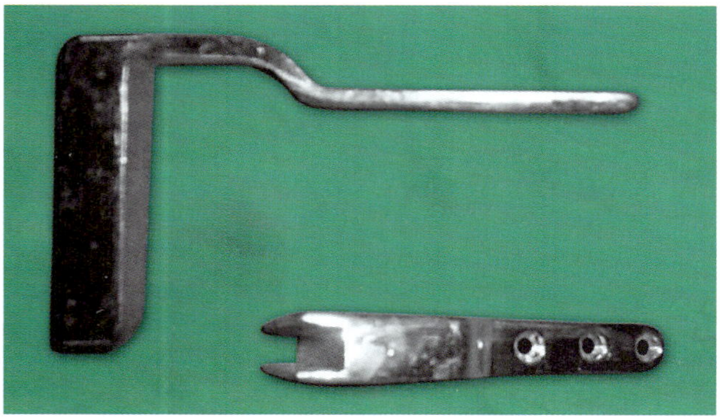

Fig. 114: Muller osteotomy plate.

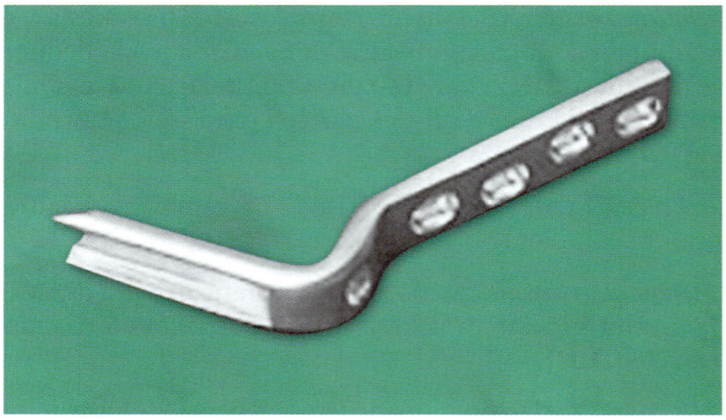

Fig. 115: Double-angle osteotomy plate.

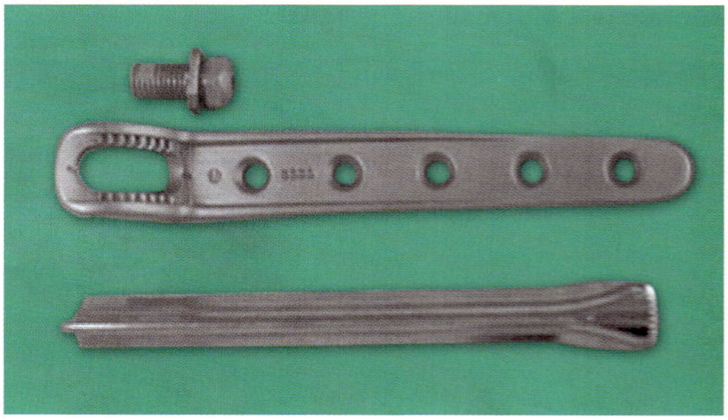

Fig. 116: Smith–Petersen (SP) nail and McLaughlin plate.

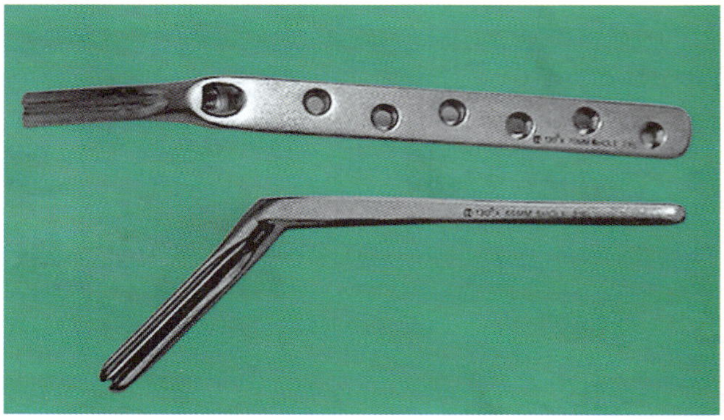

Fig. 117: Jewett blade plate.

Dynamic hip screw: Another implant used in the fixation of neck femur fractures. It consists of a plate and barrel with angle varying from 130 to 150°, and a sliding screw (12.5 mm) which comes in various lengths **(Fig. 118)**. The base of the screw takes a smaller compression screw that can be used to apply compression across the fracture site. The barrel and screw are slotted to prevent rotation and the screw can slide within the barrel to give controlled collapse of the fracture. The threaded guidewire (2.5/230 mm) is initially inserted using angle guide **(Fig. 119)** (usually 135° plate is used). Pilot hole is made with a special triple reamer that has three diameters, one for screw (8 mm), one for barrel (12.6 mm), and one for the base

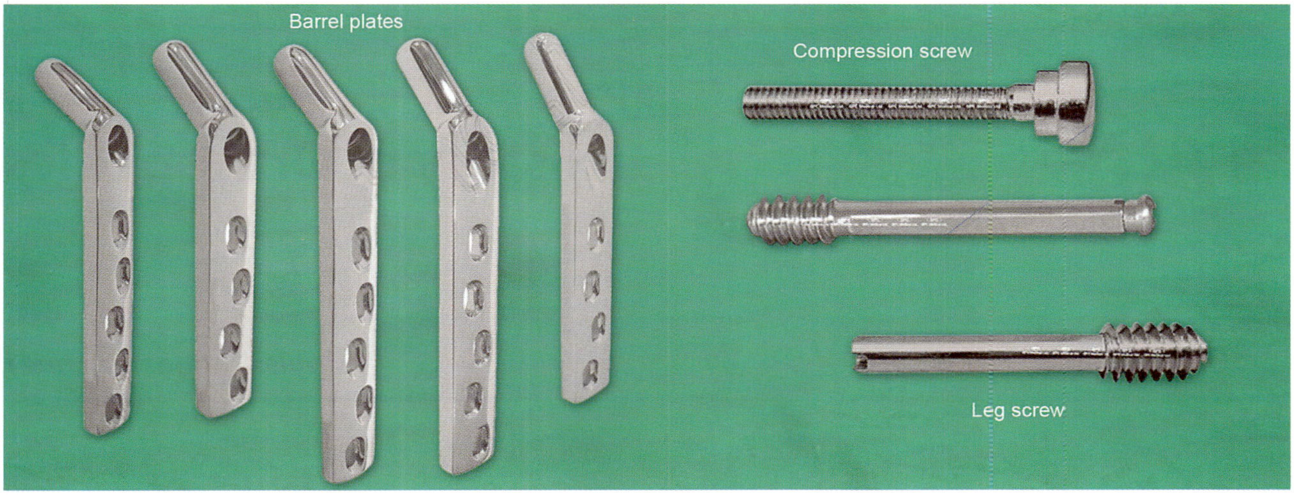

Fig. 118: Dynamic hip screw.

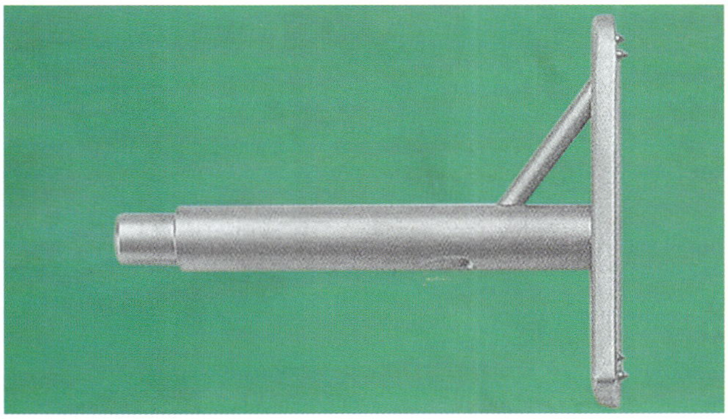

Fig. 119: Dynamic hip screw (DHS) angle guide.

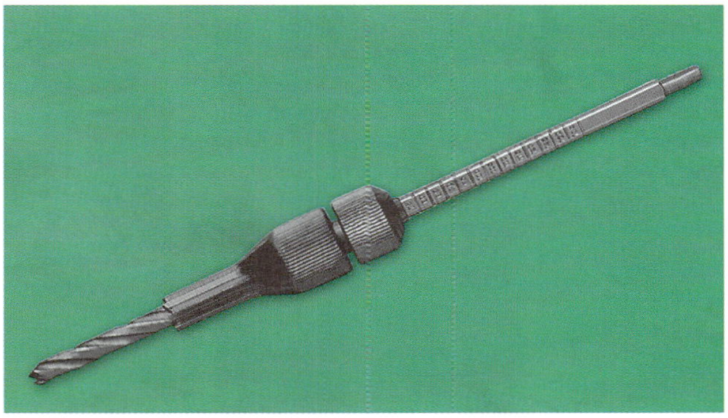

Fig. 120: Dynamic hip screw (DHS) triple reamer.

of the plate **(Fig. 120)**. Then a tap (12.5 mm) is used and then the screw is inserted into the neck. The barrel is then slid over the screw and fixed to the shaft. The smaller compression screw then can be used to apply compression across fracture site after reducing traction.

CONCLUSION

- Orthopedic surgeons have to deal with a variety of instruments and implantable devices. The surgery is performed as a team with scrub nurse, assistants and floor nurse. To communicate efficiently amongst the team members; universal language is needed. This entails good knowledge of the instruments and implants along with their nomenclature.
- The implantable devices are constantly undergoing upgradation and newer devices or modifications of older devices are regularly being introduced. One should keep abreast with the developments while also realizing the details of classical implants/instruments.

CHAPTER 126

History of Orthopedics

Manish Kumar Varshney

AMBROISE PARÉ (1510–1590)

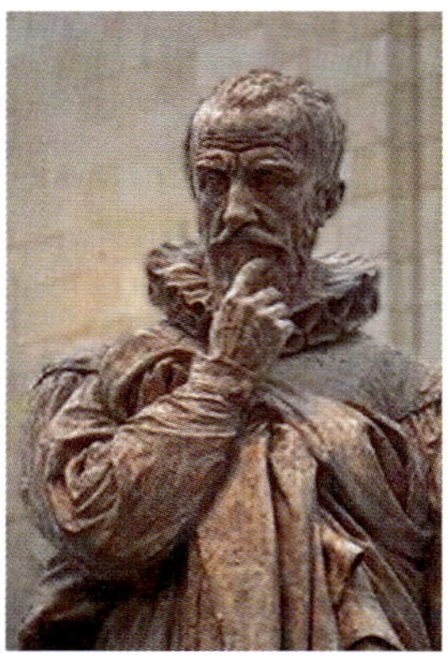

Early Life

- He was first apprenticed to a barber-surgeon in Paris.
- He initially served as a French barber surgeon for four kings of France, namely Henry II, Francis II, Charles IX and Henry III.
- Ambroise Paré was also a prominent personality in the progress made in the field of obstetrics in the middle of the 16th century.

Contribution

- Introduced the ligature of arteries instead of cauterization during amputation.
- He is considered the father of surgery and modern forensic pathology and has been a pioneer in various currently practiced/developed surgical techniques.
- Used tourniquet for his amputations.
- Described phantom pain.
- Books: The method of curing wounds caused by arquebus and firearms, Treatise on Surgery.
- Designed orthopedic boots **(Fig. 1)** for clubfoot, Paré's corset for scoliosis **(Figs. 2A and B)**.
- He revived the practice of podalic version in obstetrics.

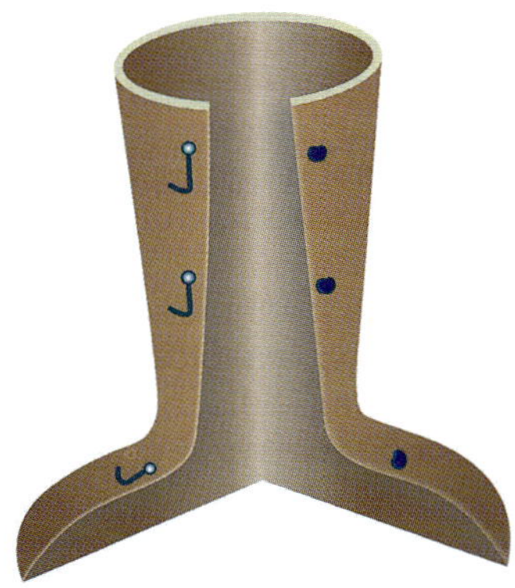

Fig. 1: Orthopedic boot.

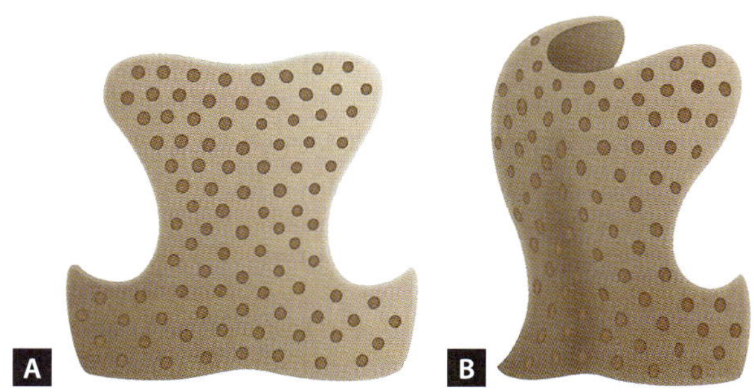

Figs. 2A and B: Paré's corset for scoliosis.

NICOLAS ANDRY (1658–1742)

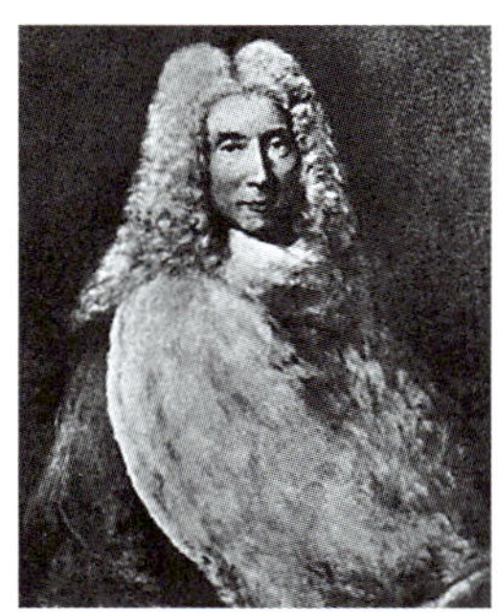

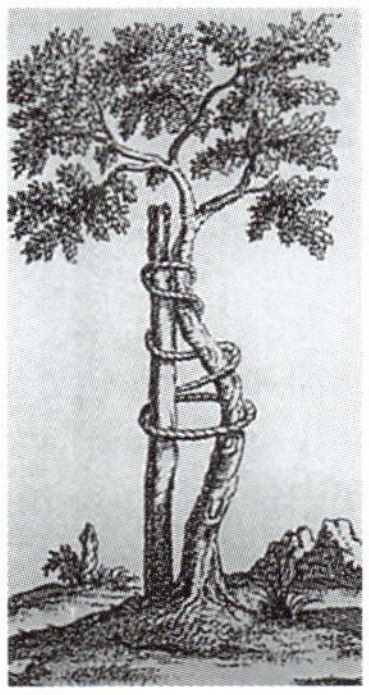

Fig. 3: Tree of Andry.

Early Life

- Nicolas Andry, a French medical doctor (Lyon 1658–Paris 1742) played a significant role in the early history of both parasitology and orthopedics.
- Gave the symbol Andry Tree **(Fig. 3)** (the crooked tree later became the symbol of numerous orthopedic societies around the world).
- Due to irony of fate (or what some call it the revenge of his contemporaries?), we are left with only one classic representation of Andry—the etching entitled "Homini verminoso" (Worm man), preserved in the French National Library.

Contribution

- Father of orthopedics and father of parasitology
- *Books:*
  1. *The generation of worms in the human body.* The different kinds and types of this disease and the ways of preventing and curing it.
  2. *L'Orthopédie* or *Orthopedia* (English) which teaches several ways of preventing and correcting deformities in children.

PERCIVALL POTT (1714–1788)

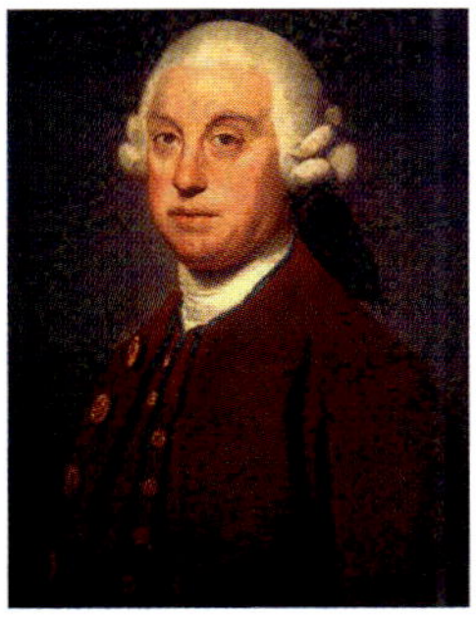

Early Life

- Born in Threadneedle Street of Cockney, England.
- At the tender age of 15 years, Pott got apprenticed to Edward Nourse, who was a surgeon at St Bartholomew's Hospital.
- He suffered a compound fracture of the ankle in 1756, when he was thrown from the horse, he was riding down the Old Kent Road to visit the Lock Hospital.

Contribution

- In 1775, Pott found the association between exposure to chimney soot and high incidence of scrotal cancer in chimney cleaners. This was the first occupational hazard linking to cancer.
- *Pott's disease of the spine*—tuberculosis of spine. He detailed the anterior spinal column involvement in disease process and noted that tuberculosis almost always affected the vertebral bodies and not the articular processes (though we know that they might be uncommonly involved). He also described Pott's paraplegia by severe destruction of the vertebrae that produced a sharp curvature of the spine, and finally a "useless state of the limbs".

Other named conditions on name of Percivall Pott:

- *Pott's classification of ankle fractures:* Pott classified ankle fractures based on the number of malleoli involved (uni-, bi-, trimalleolar fractures).
- *Pott's puffy tumor:* This is a rare infection and not a neoplasia per se. It arises from a subperiosteal extradural abscess commonly following frontal sinusitis, open trauma, cortical vein thrombosis, subdural empyema or middle ear disease.
- *Pott's lucid interval:* Pott also described the lucid interval that precedes the coma associated with an extradural hematoma.

JOHN HUNTER (1728–1793)

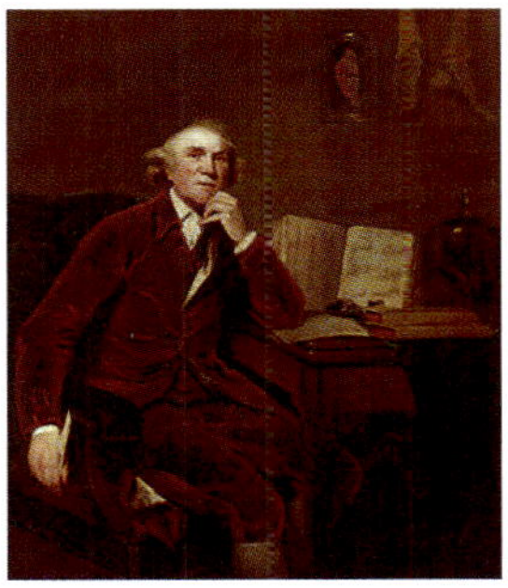

Early Life

- He was born in Scotland, and then moved to London to help his brother, William in running an anatomy school.
- Hunter maintained a huge collection of specimens based on his philosophy of "learning through observation". These specimens of skeleton and organs of various animals were displayed in an especially designed house constructed in Leicester Square.
- He also maintained an extensive menagerie housing collection of different animals like the zebra, jackals, goats, buffaloes, and built several laboratories in the house near Earl's Court in London to conduct research in animal anatomy.
- Many of his original specimens are now maintained in the Royal College of Surgeons in London in the Hunterian Museum.

Contribution

- He was the first to detail systematic surgical practice and was the Founder of Scientific Surgery.
- Hunterian Society of London was given its name in his honor.
- Due to his interest in collecting specimens the Hunterian Museum at the Royal College of Surgeons still retain his name.
- Discovered bone remodeling.
- Did studies on the repair and regeneration of bone, cartilage and tendon.
- Studied loose bodies in joints, pseudoarthrosis and fracture healing.

ABRAHAM COLLES (1773–1843)

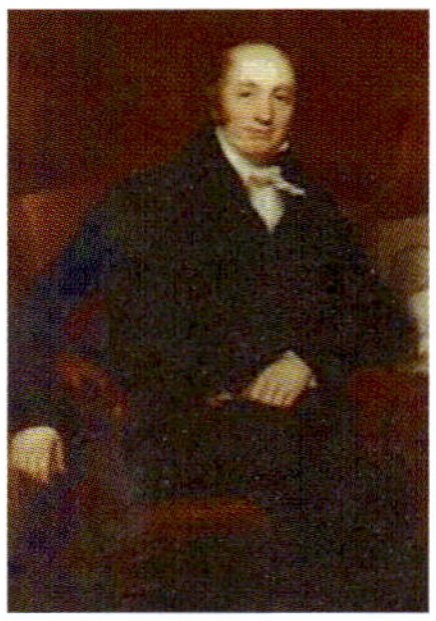

Early Life

- Abraham Colles was born at Kilkenny in Ireland.
- In an interesting incidence when Abraham was at Kilkenny College, there was a flood in destroying a local physician's house. Abraham incidentally found an anatomy book belonging to the doctor in a nearby field and came to return it to him. Realizing Abraham's interest in medicine, the physician let Abraham keep the book.
- In 1802, he was appointed professor of both anatomy/physiology and surgery at the Royal College of Surgeons (Ireland).
- He was later elected president in 1804 for the Royal College of Surgeons, Ireland, at the age of only 29 years, and again in 1830.
- Best known for his description of Colles' fracture in 1814. He became one of the most recognizable names in orthopedic surgery later.

Contribution

- *Colles' fracture:* In his classical paper, "On Fracture of the Carpal Extremity of the Radius" in 1814, when no X-rays were available, he had described accurately the classical deformity following the fracture of lower end of radius, which is known as Colles' fracture after him.
- *Colles' fascia:* In the perineum, the middle fascia of urogenital triangle, the attachment of which served to confine within strict limits extravasation of urine from a ruptured urethra is known as Colles' fascia.
- *Colles' ligament (reflected inguinal ligament):* It is the small triangular fascia that comprises tendinous fibers from lacunar ligament and inferior border of external inguinal ring passing upward and medially behind spermatic cord toward the linea alba, under cover of the external inguinal ring and superficial to inguinal aponeurotic falx.
- *Colles' law:* In 1837, Colles published a book entitled "Practical Observations", on the venereal disease and on the use of mercury. In a chapter, dealing with syphilis in infants, he made an observation that later came to known as Colles' law, which can be stated as, a child born of a mother, who is without any obvious syphilitic symptoms develops disease despite not being exposed to any infection after birth (in neonatal period). Within a few weeks this child will infect even the most healthy nurse who comes in child's contact, whether she suckles it or merely handles and dresses it. Despite this strong infectivity this child will never infect the mother, even though she suckles it, while it has venereal ulcer on lips and tongue.
- He could clearly observe the apparent immunity of the mother, but could not determine the cause as having acquired immunity by being infected in mild form. It was nearly 70 years later, that the Fritz Schaudinn, discovered *Spirochaeta pallida* and the serological test devised by Wassermann.

ANTONIUS MATHIJSEN (1805–1878)

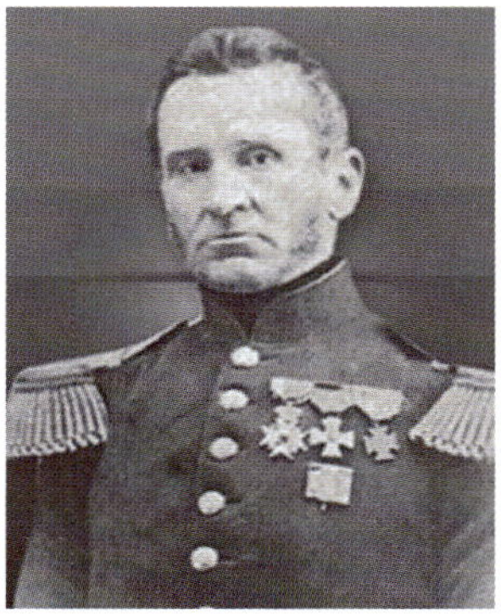

Early Life

Antonius Mathijsen was a Dutch military surgeon, who in 1851 invented the Plaster of Paris bandage, which has become so important in orthopedic practice.

Contribution

Plaster of Paris bandage.

HUGH OWEN THOMAS (1834–1891)

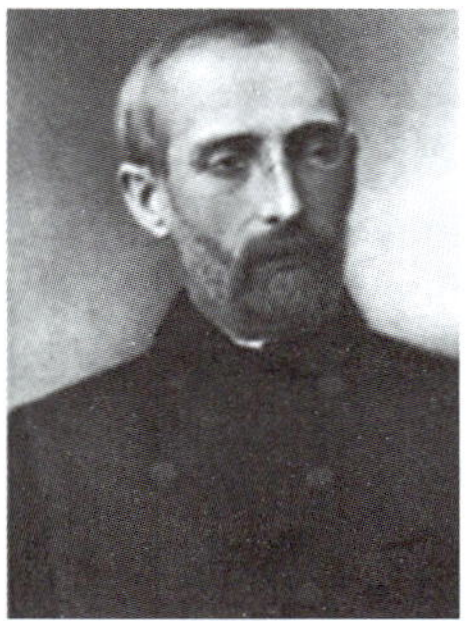

Early Life

- Hugh Owen Thomas is regarded as one of the great early pioneers of orthopedic surgery.
- He was born into a family steeped in the secrets of bone-setting. He was eldest of the five sons.
- He was the first medically qualified person in family, and he combined the conventional training with knowledge of bone-setting gained from his family in inheritance.
- Hugh got initial training first with his uncle, Dr Owen Roberts at St Asaph in North Wales for 4 years, and later he studied medicine at Edinburgh and University College, London. He qualified as MRCS in 1857.
- As an irony of fate his contribution to splinting of fractures and early fracture stabilization was never fully appreciated in his own lifetime. It was only when his nephew, Sir Robert Jones, used his splint extensively during the First World War showing the utility in reducing the compound fractures that would otherwise prove fatal from 1916 to 1918, did he got recognition. The mortality from compound fractures of the femur reduced from 87% to <8% in the period.

Contribution

- Thomas splint
- Thomas wrench for reducing fractures
- Cervical collar (Thomas collar) for tuberculosis of cervical spine
- Metatarsal bar
- Heel wedge
- Knee splint
- Osteoclast to break and reset bones
- Thomas test—first to demonstrate concealed flexion of hip joint and a way to unmask this.
- *Thomas's maneuver*, an orthopedic investigation for fracture of the hip joint
- In 1875, he wrote a book titled *Diseases of the Hip, Knee and Ankle Joints*.

SIR ROBERT JONES (1857–1933)

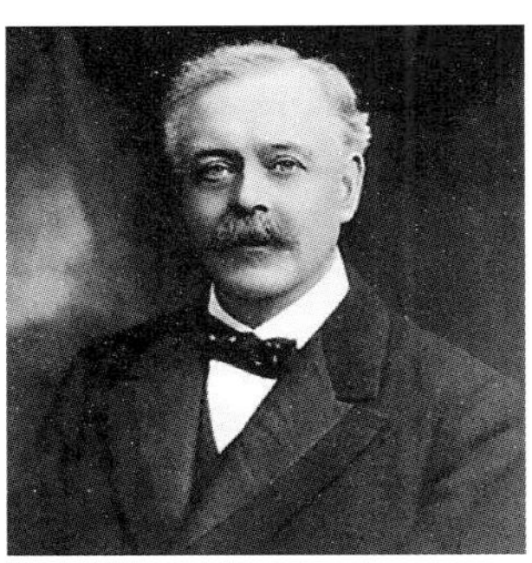

Early Life

- Jones was a nephew of the great Hugh Owen Thomas and became one of his apprentices in Liverpool. He completed his FRCS in 1889.
- Jones and his uncle were among the few surgeons interested in the treatment of fractures and practicing core orthopedics. Most other contemporary orthopedic surgery aimed at correcting deformity in children that was carried out by general surgeons.
- In 1888, Robert Jones was appointed surgeon to the Manchester Ship Canal Project, a 7-year project involving 20,000 workers.
- Sir Robert Jones' accomplishments during the World War were greatly appreciated and these facilitated his establishment of various societies including the British Orthopaedic Association in 1918.

Contribution

- In 1896, He published the first clinical use of X-ray, to locate a bullet in a wrist in The Lancet.
- At the end of his career, Sir Robert Jones published a paper entitled *Cure of the Crippled Children* with Robert Girdlestone from the University of Oxford.
- In 1915, he published book titled *Injuries of Joints* and his *Notes on Military Orthopaedics* in 1917.
- Robert Jones and Alfred Tubbe formed the British Orthopaedic Society on November 3rd, 1894.

THOMAS PORTER MCMURRAY (1888–1949)

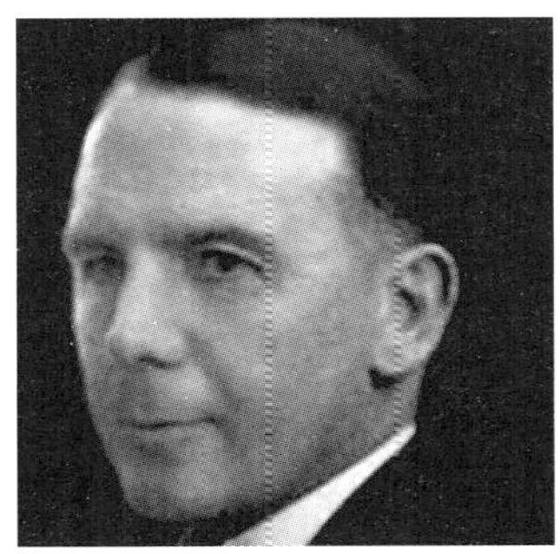

Early Life

- He was a staunch follower of Hugh Owen Thomas and also worked for Robert Jones.
- His operative dexterity was renowned, for he could remove an entire meniscus in 5 minutes and disarticulate a hip in 10 minutes.
- He introduced a test to identify tear in meniscus—McMurray's sign.

Contribution

- *McMurray's osteotomy:* This operation was named after him, as McMurray was the first to perform a displacement osteotomy, for nonunion of fractures of femoral neck and providing symptomatic relief in arthrosis of the hip (by shifting weight-bearing line), detailing the procedure and its utility in these conditions
- McMurray's sign for identifying meniscal tears.

WILLIS C CAMPBELL (1880–1941)

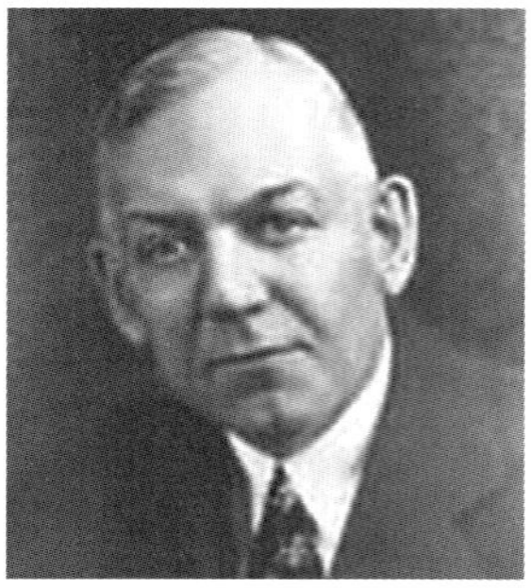

Early Life

Dr Willis C Campbell was born in Mississippi, in 1880. He became a medical graduate from University of Virginia (1904). Dr Campbell initially specialized in general surgery, anesthesia and pediatrics and later studied orthopedics in London and Vienna to start orthopedic practice in 1909. He became the Professor and Head of Department of Orthopedic Surgery in the University of Tennessee and served there till his death.

Contribution

- Campbell was the main advocate of interpositional arthroplasty at that time.
- He used a free autogenous transplant of fascia lata.
- Campbell was a key figure in bone grafting and performed inlay full thickness grafts, for nonunion bones fixed with screws of beef bone.
- *Publications: A monograph, Orthopedics of Childhood* in 1927; a textbook, *Orthopedic Surgery* in 1930; *Operative Orthopedics* in 1939.

GERHARD KÜNTSCHER (1900–1972)

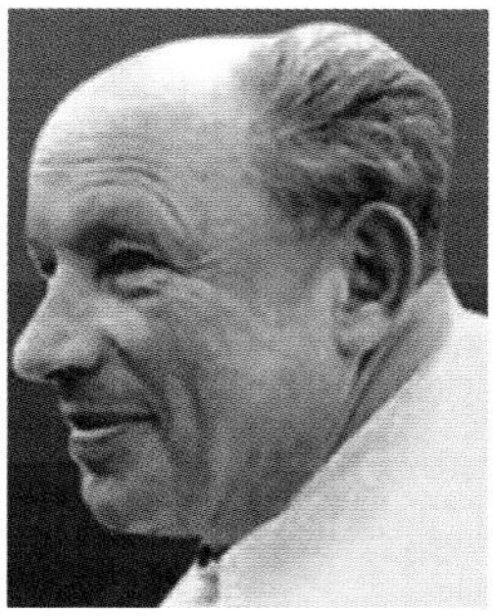

Early Life

- Gerhard Küntscher was born in Zwickau in 1900 and graduated from the School of Medicine in Jena (1926).
- He served in the German army, during the World War II in the Eastern front where he published his revolutionary procedure on intramedullary nailing for shaft femur fractures by initial reaming to enlarge the diameter to insert a large diameter nail and in turn give relatively rigid fixation. This allowed immediate weight-bearing and mobilization.
- He worked as a Chief Surgeon in German Military Hospital in Finland and then served in various hospitals in Germany to finally retire in 1965. His technique was ahead of the prevailing knowledge and methods, and even developed nailing technique for pertrochanteric fractures and intramedullary osteotomy.

Contribution

- Founder of modern intramedullary nailing
- Küntscher's nail
- Published more than 200 papers and 4 books.

MARTIN KIRSCHNER (1879–1942)

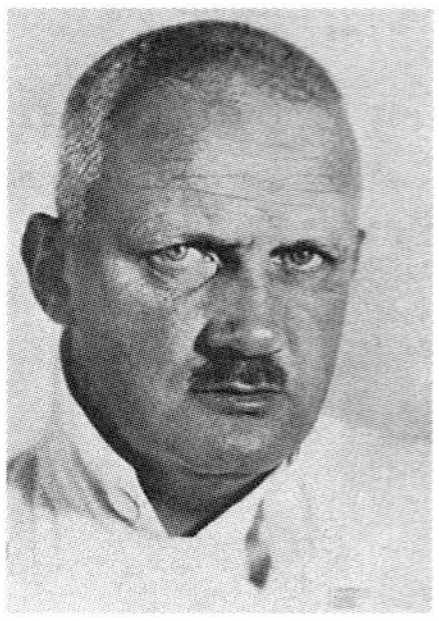

Early Life

- Born in Breslau, Germany
- Known for his method of fixation, in particular for Kirschner or K-wire.
- He also performed the first successful pulmonary embolectomy.

Contribution

- *Kirschner wire:* The K-wire was developed by Martin Kirschner who introduced the use of wire skeletal traction in 1909
- Kirschner's bloodlessness
- Method of making artificial esophagus
- Method of knee arthrotomy
- Kirschner-Perthes cuff.

SIR REGINALD WATSON-JONES (1902–1972)

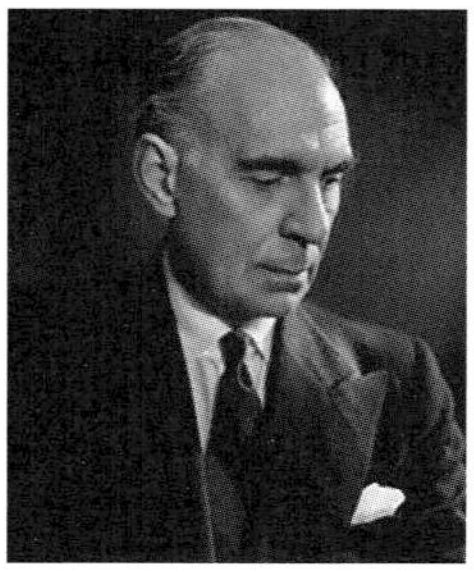

Early Life

- Watson-Jones interest in medicine developed after he suffered from typhoid, and he ultimately chose orthopedics after a hemangioma was removed from his leg.

- Sir Reginald Watson-Jones was trained initially by Sir Robert Jones. He was born in 1902. Though carrying the same surname he was not of the same family but he was both a student of Robert Jones and his advocate following Sir Robert's death.
- Early in his medical career Robert Jones recognized Reginald's talent and, in 1926, persuaded the Royal Liverpool Infirmary to appoint Watson-Jones as honorary assistant surgeon-in-charge of a new orthopedic department and fracture clinic. In order to distinguish himself from all the other Jones' in his home city of Liverpool, he hyphenated his name with his mother's maiden name in early 1930s. He gained the MCh(Orth) degree from Liverpool in 1926 and became FRCS in 1927.

Contribution

- He published his first paper in the Journal of Bone and Joint Surgery in the early 1930s and then at least three manuscripts every year were published later.
- In 1942, he established the Department of Orthopaedics and Accidents at the London Hospital.
- During World War, developed miners' rehabilitation in every coalfield in Britain.
- He was the main figure in independent publication— the *Journal of Bone and Joint Surgery (British)* due primarily to his intention of expanding the Journal of Bone and Joint Surgery to European nations so that it reaches as many researchers to contribute in it. The *Journal of Bone and Joint Surgery (British)* maintained close ties with the original journal until recently, until when it finally separated and is now named *The Bone and Joint journal.* The first issue of the British edition of the *Journal of Bone and Joint Surgery* was published in February 1948 under the aegis of British Orthopaedic Society.
- Watson jones published, *Fracture and Joint Injuries* in 1940, which remained a standard reference for several decades in dealing with fractures. This text was translated into many languages that retained popularity till recently. Even in today's time it is a highly demanded book in areas of the world where operative treatment is not practical. This text was lately usurped by the AO manual in the late 1950s and early 1960s.

AUSTIN T MOORE (1899–1963)

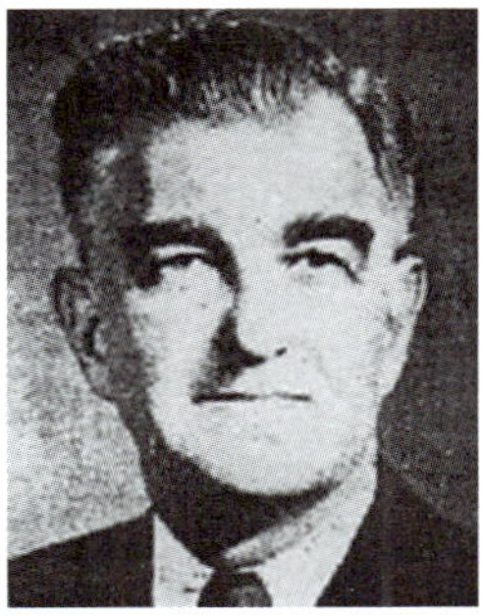

Contribution

- He performed the first metallic hip replacement. He was the first to replace the entire upper portion of the femur for the first time with a vitallium prosthesis.
- Over years, the design of the prosthesis improved and the procedure changed. Ultimately, one type of prosthesis called the Austin Moore prevailed which is still in use today.

GAVRIIL A ILIZAROV (1921–1992)

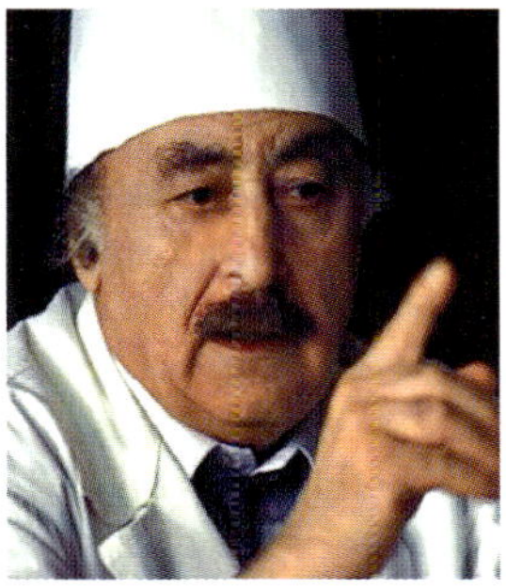

Early Life

- Ilizarov was born in the town of Belovezh, Polesie Voivodeship of Poland, to a Jewish family from the Dagestan region of the Russian Empire.
- He got educated (graduation) from the Simferopol Medical School. This was later moved during the war to the Soviet near east.
- During World War II, he was evacuated to Dolgovka, near Kurgan and ran a hospital single handed, where working conditions were primitive with no antibiotics and inadequate equipments. The operation room was heated with wood fire.
- Ilizarov discovered the method of corticotomy that he described as a carefully severed bone without damaging the periosteum around it. He envisaged that once carefully separated and the two halves of a bone are fixed in place, the bone would grow to fill the gap. He also later discovered that regenerating bone regrows at a fairly uniform rate across people and circumstances that could be lengthened indefinitely if one keeps the lengthening rate equal to the bone regeneration rate
- Ilizarov's popularity rose only after he treated an Italian photojournalist Carlo Mauri. Carlo was suffering from stiff nonunion tibia in malposition that he suffered while skiing accident, for which the then Italian surgeons gave up all hopes. In 1980 during the Cold War era, on the reference of a Russian colleague he agreed to visit Kurgan nearly 2,000 km east of Moscow. Ilizarov treated him by distraction for pseudoarthrosis healing, leg-lengthening and equinus correction for nonunion tibia in malposition. As Carlo returned to Italy, the healing of his leg astonished orthopedic surgeons of the region.

Only after this instance was Ilizarov's work realized and he was invited as a guest speaker at the AO Italy conference in 1981 popularizing his technique.

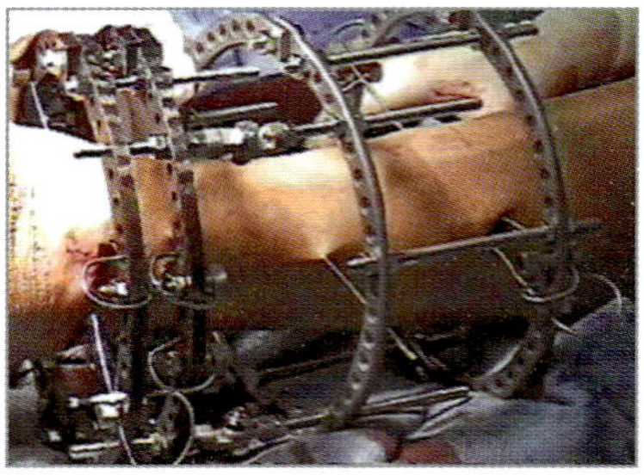

Fig. 4: Ilizarov method.

Contribution

- The experiments of GA Ilizarov led to the development of complete design of the renowned Ilizarov apparatus. This apparatus had the capability of holding a bone even if comminuted so meticulously in place, utilizing only a framework and pins through the bone that complete healing and regeneration is facilitated nearly always. The apparatus was also capable of healing bone defects by effective bone lengthening; by repeating lengthening procedure over time. This is done at the rate of the bone's regrowth (1 mm/day) and it is possible to extend a bone by a desired amount (ideally unlimited).
- The use of Ilizarov method is widespread **(Fig. 4)**.
- The North American Association for the Study and Application of the Methods of Ilizarov (ASAMI) includes over 200 surgeons.

SIR JOHN CHARNLEY (1911–1982)

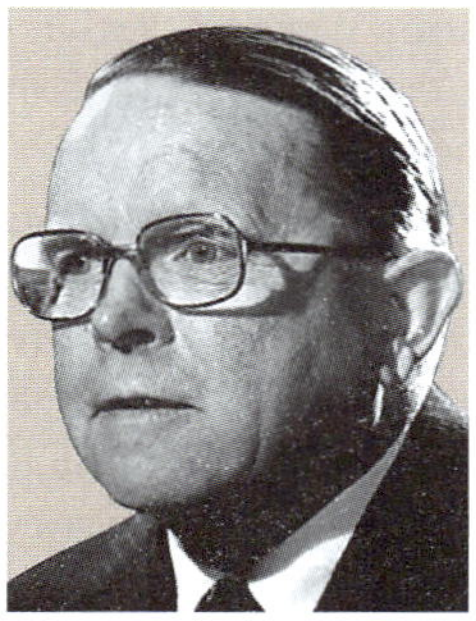

Early Life

- Sir John Charnley was born in Bury in Lancashire United Kingdom in August 1911 to a chemist father and mother trained as a nurse. He graduated from the medical school at the Victoria University of Manchester, where he qualified with Bachelor of Medicine and Bachelor of Science at the same time due to undaunted efforts and thirst of knowledge.
- He developed interest in study of cancer but was dissuaded by his teachers and so at 25 years of age he became a Fellow of the Royal College of Surgeons in London (Guy's Hospital). He was the youngest physician to receive that honor.
- He received training as a general surgeon at the Salford Royal Hospital and acquired excellent diagnostic and operative skills.
- He then returned to Manchester as resident casualty officer where in day he worked with various orthopedic surgeons but due to his thirst of surgical knowledge and experience, he used to do surgical emergencies in afternoon and night.
- Due to breakout of World War II in 1939, he joined the Royal Army Medical Corps from where he was transferred to many places finally resting under Dudley Buxton at Cairo. There his work was well recognized and he was made In-Charge of the New Orthopedic Workshop at the 2nd Orthopedic Center. He resigned from military and joined the Shaftesbury hospital as an orthopedics staff.

Contribution

- He created the "Wrightington center for hip surgery" and pioneered the concept of "low friction arthroplasty".
- In the 1960s, Sir John Charnley pioneered effective modern total hip arthroplasty introducing the concept of low-friction torque arthroplasty. He refined the procedure over next two decades working in concert with the commercial firm of Chas F Thackray Ltd (now a subsidiary of DePuy Synthes, a Johnson & Johnson Company).
- He was interested in bone union and worked a lot on principles of bone grafting. His method of bone grafting for delayed union is very popular (Phemister-Charnley subcortical cancellous bone-grafting).
- He stressed the importance of compression to achieve arthrodesis—Charnley compression arthrodesis and apparatus (clamp) splint.
- Charnley's retractor/spreader
- Charnley's hip prosthesis
- Charnley's bone curette and awl
- Published a book on conservative management of fractures in 1950.

CHAPTER 127

Emerging Terms and Concepts in Orthopedics

Manish Kumar Varshney

INTRODUCTION

With a growth in knowledge of molecular biology and its correlation with physiological and pathological processes, aggregation of concepts is occurring. This grouping concept seems more powerful in identifying and defining the processes rather than individual correlation. One of these is the use of orthobiologics—the term basically indicates the use of biological treatment modalities for functional and anatomical improvement and is a component of restorative medicine. Similarly, the term "metabolomics" is a grouping term where specific metabolites identified in the body serve to diagnose or prognosticate or target treatment for various diseases.

RESTORATIVE MEDICINE AND ORTHOBIOLOGICS

Restorative medicine is a new focus of evolving medical practice where trend has been shifted from symptomatic management of the disorder to biological restoration of function. Regenerative medicines including stem cell and bioprinting are included within restorative medicine. Orthobiologics are lately introduced term that encompasses use of biological substances to help musculoskeletal injuries to heal more quickly. Initially restricted to improvement of fracture healing; the term has now been extended to finding its use in enhancing the healing of injured cartilage, muscles tendons, and ligaments with identified substances that can do so. The effectors used in orthobiologics are made from substances that are naturally occur in the body. The strategy is to harness cells and proteins naturally found in the human biology (usually in higher than physiological concentration) help to support efficient/enhanced regrowth of injured tissues. It is interesting to note that most of these [like bone grafts, platelet-rich plasma, bone morphogenetic protein (BMP), etc.] were already in vogue for decades but only recently they have been grouped into fancy term "orthobiologics" by improvement in understanding the human biochemistry and biology. So, only the use of this term and not the knowledge of effector substances are new.

Orthobiologics use both cell-based therapies and biomaterials to enhance healing. By so, focusing on improved repair and regeneration current excitement has led to fast expansion in the field and research. The expected benefits of using orthobiologics in orthopedics are (not all of them universally agreed upon and may just be tentative in nature):

- Less invasive and possibly more effective at restoring function than large surgeries
- Improving the long-term health of patients suffering from disabling disorders and injuries
- Biological and natural alternatives to repair instead of artificial device implantation
- Reducing hospital visits and shortening stays
- Minimizing impact of degenerative diseases
- Most are outpatient day-care procedure requiring no overnight admission
- Recovery is more rapid.
- Much less financial liability

Origin of the Concept of Orthobiologics

After tissue injury or in chronic conditions, there is always an associated repair response aimed to restore the anatomy and function. This is basically affected by three closely connected constituents of matrix laydown, inoculation and homing of stem cells, and maintaining optimum balance of growth factors. The process is usually initiated by inflammatory response (that is mainly genetically controlled) that lasts for a variable period of time. The inflammatory process and further progress into healing response is controlled by sequential or simultaneous cytokines and growth factors presence/induction of which is controlled both genetically and by local environment. Many a times the inflammatory and/or fine-tuned repair process goes out of correct order. This happens due to the disruption of the fine balance interplayed by various cytokines and may arise due to deficiency or excess in any one of them. Genetic deficiency would lead to complete failure of the process in any stage. But more often than not it is the alteration in the fine balance of cytokine-mediated environment locally that is hampered. Ultimately, it causes incomplete/poor healing response and condition may persist as chronic (e.g., tendinopathies) or may change to another entity due to failure of biology (say a nonunion of bone). The three basic components of repair play their own roles—the matrix bridges the tissue gap, growth factors, and cytokines recruit cellular components involved in cleaning the area and developing the same to accept new tissue, stem cells are the precursor cells that build the new tissue for regeneration in the area. These are controlled by "soup" of numerous growth factors and cytokines that control each step and effect transition of one to another. If there is a deficiency of any one then the step may be incomplete or halted producing suboptimal or no healing. The purpose of orthobiologics is to supplement the inherent process of healing that ultimately produces complete response. This supplementation can be done in many ways including either individually providing matrix (synthetic bone graft) or matrix and growth factors [autologous bone grafts, three-dimensional (3D) bioprinting and genetic engineering], or stem cells (regenerative medicine) or growth factors (gene therapy and genetic engineering) or a combination of these.

As mentioned above, most of the orthobiologic products are natural substances that can be used to preserve and redirect the body repair process in our desired direction. Following are currently considered orthobiologics that would soon expand with continued search:

- *Bone grafts*: Both autologous and synthetic (*see* Chapter on "Fracture Repair, Bone Grafting, and Bone Banking").
- *Autologous blood*: This involves simply injecting the venous blood at the desired site like that for chronic tendinopathies (tennis elbow, Achilles insertional tendinosis, etc.) or to improve the strength of repair as in rotator cuff repair or Bankart's repair. This has also been sporadically used for sports-related ankle and foot injuries. The mechanism is unclear but possibly inducing inflammation and delivery of growth factors from limited cellular agents (platelets) may be involved. The results are variable and nonsubstantial.
- *Autologous conditioned serum*: It is a process to improve the concentration of interleukin-1 (IL-1) receptor antagonist in blood. The preparation involves incubation of 50 mL venous blood for 24 hours in 5% CO_2 in pH-neutralized environment with small glass beads. This is further centrifuged to obtain supernatant rich in growth factors [insulin-like growth factor (IGF), platelet-derived growth factor (PDGF), etc.]. Results so far for osteoarthritis of knee and lumbar radicular pain have not been very substantial.
- *Platelet-rich plasma (PRP, platelet-enriched plasma, platelet-rich concentrate, or autologous platelet gel)*: The basis of using the platelet concentrate obtained as autologous plasma fraction by centrifuging anticoagulated human blood is to capture the goodness of alpha-granules of platelet that are a rich source of numerous growth factors not limited to—PDGF, IGF, platelet factor-4 (PF4), IL, epidermal growth factor (EGF), vascular endothelial growth factor (VEGF), transforming growth factor (TGF) superfamily, platelet-derived endothelial growth factor (PDEGF), etc. The platelets are usually obtained by centrifugation into the inactive leukocyte-rich concentrate that can be further processed to deplete leukocytes by filtration and/or activate platelets by adding calcium chloride. Activated platelets are usually applied with thrombin in gel form at the desired site of action. Leukocyte rich or depleted makes no difference in the clinical results for orthobiological application. The platelet concentrate has been used for:
  - Lateral epicondylitis—can be considered as alternative to corticosteroid injections.
  - Rotator cuff repair—can be considered as adjuvant for surgical cuff repair—unclear efficacy.
  - *Knee osteoarthritis*: The results show no substantial benefit in late osteoarthritis of knee and have no logical reason for use also. Early osteoarthritis (Ahlback-1) may improve symptomatically with PRP injection—unknown value.
  - *Nonunion of long bones*: Some initial encouraging results fizzled out in uncertainty over study criteria and equivocal benefits. May be preferred to or added to bone marrow injections.
  - Achilles tendinopathy—may be considered as a failure to use of PRP, dismal results as only very few low-level supportive studies with no substantial benefit on record.
  - Patellar tendinopathy—not many studies to provide recommendation but some benefit reported in Jumper's knee.
  - Plantar fasciitis—equivocal results may consider alternative to steroid injections.
  - Shoulder osteoarthritis—unsubstantiated evidence suggests early improvement but long-term efficacy unknown.
- *Growth factors*: This is an emerging field in targeted drug delivery system which also utilizes the modalities like genetic engineering, stem cell therapy, and tissue bioprinting to deliver the required growth factors at a site considered deficient in them. TGF superfamily including BMP, use of VEGF, PDGF, etc. is coming up and is encouraging. It looks promising in terms of ideation and search is on to find the appropriate scaffolds for delivery system (*see* also Chapters on "Regenerative Medicine and Stem Cell Research in Orthopedics", "Electrospinning, Three-dimensional Printing and its Application in Orthopedics", and "Gene Therapy in Orthopedics"). Synthetic analogs of parathormone also fall into this group and has been found to enhance bone healing when given systemically.
- *Stem cells*—detailed with uses in Chapter on "Regenerative Medicine and Stem Cell Research in Orthopedics".

METABOLOMICS

The term "metabolomics" is again a newer term to the medical fraternity; but in reality the basis has been long known. We know that individual, physiological, and pathological processes have specific metabolites that may serve as a substrate or an end-product which can be measured. With increasing knowledge in the field, now we are able to "mark" the metabolites or a group of them to specific processes like a foot print or a fingerprint. Just this knowledge and systemic study of marker metabolites (fingerprint) that specific cellular processes leave behind is called metabolomics. More scientifically metabolomics can be defined as systematic, qualitative, and quantitative analysis of metabolites in an organism aimed to finding biomarkers and studying pathogenesis of physiology/diseases. Metabolites are highly stable end-products of specific pathways that serve as an important link between genotype and phenotype. A metabolome represents the whole group of metabolites specific to a given cellular process (usually directed genetically). Metabolome, hence, may be directly applied as a marker to disease diagnosis/prognosis/treatment/follow-up depending on the stage at which it is identified. It can be argued that the metabolite profile can also be determined using messenger ribonucleic acid (mRNA) gene expression (transcriptome) or proteomic analysis, but the difference lies in that with these the full set of gene products is determined not related only to the particular physiological process currently in action; but of all the physiological processes that the cell line is able to perform. We are, however, interested in knowing the current physiological process only so that the disease/pathology/physiology at the instant can be determined. This information will be revealed by metabolomics and not proteomics. One can think of it in a way that metabolome is a snapshot of genome, epigenome, transcriptome and proteome, and their interaction with environment at the given point of measurement. The most simplistic use of metabolomics was to use ants to analyze urine of a patient to determine, if he/she has diabetes.

Analyzing the metabolomes an online database has been created (METLIN) by the Siuzdak laboratory at the Scripps Research Institute that now contains more than 250,000 metabolites gathered from mass spectrometry, but the number of metabolomes is much less. The number of identified metabolomes for humans is lower than some other life forms due to the complexity in identification of the complete set by one single set of tests. Also it is difficult to identify a place where one should look at the metabolomes, urine for example, is easily analyzed but contains too many metabolites in different concentration that fail to characterize one single physiology. The characterization is further complicated by endogenous (produced by native cells), exogenous, or xenometabolites (like that of drugs or administered chemicals) and sometimes the metabolites themselves are substrates for downstream reactions making a hypercycle. Presently in orthopedics, the metabolomes are commonly searched in synovial fluid, serum/plasma, urine, synovial tissue, etc. by utilizing mass spectroscopy, secondary ion mass spectroscopy, and/or nuclear magnetic resonance (NMR) (high-resolution-magic-angle-spinning—NMR) spectroscopy. The following are some of the identified utility of metabolomics in orthopedics.

Osteoarthritis

Osteoarthritis is no longer a wear and tear disease only; a specific metabolic change has been reported in the patients that produce characteristic cartilage loss, subchondral sclerosis, and synovial membrane change. This entails that persons at risk for the development of osteoarthritis can be identified by metabolomics or the disease can be diagnosed early. The animal studies identified various metabolomes that may be characteristic for their species to identify "at risk" for the developments of the disease but recently human studies have also identified few. The ratio of branched-chain amino acid to histidine in synovial fluid may serve as a novel marker for the development of osteoarthritis. Synovial fluid analysis in human shows that levels of fructose and citrate are increased (suggestive of a hypoxic condition and high-energy requirements), reduced levels of malate (dysregulated energy production), reduction in O-acetylcarnitine, hexanoylcarnitine, N-phenylacetylglycine, and ethanolamine (related to higher fatty acid and lipid metabolism). Late stage of osteoarthritis has been linked to elevated levels of malate, ethanolamide, squalene, glycerol, myristic acid, oleic acid, lanosterol, heptadecanoic acid, and capric acid. During the metabolomics study of biomarkers for osteoarthritis, it has been substantiated that osteoarthritis is a heterogeneous disease. Metabolomically, osteoarthritis is currently distinguished into three metabolically distinct subgroups possibly linked to the differences in carnitine, lipid, and collagen metabolism. Also a systematic study of metabolites in patients with osteoarthritis was performed to analyze if there is any association to arthroplasty independent of age, sex, BMI, and cholesterol-lowering drugs. Two different factors were found to be significantly associated to ultimate the need of arthroplasty as a result of osteoarthritis. Factor 11 (e.g., linoleic acid) was found to be associated with arthroplasty of the hip while factor 22 (unsaturated fatty acids and degree of unsaturation) was linked to the need of arthroplasty irrespective of the site (hip/knee, etc.).

Bone Sarcoma

The use of metabolomics is helping not only in early detection but also improving the clinical efficiency of osteosarcoma chemotherapy. For diagnostic biomarker search, metabolomics combined with transcriptomics serve better than anyone alone. By various studies, it has been identified that in osteosarcoma, the metabolism of (TCA) (tricarboxylic citric acid) cycle, glycolysis, and lipid is downregulated while that of amino acids, glutathione, and polyamines are upregulated when identified in serum but analysis based on TAp73α (transactivation-proficient p73α) suggest upregulation of metabolisms of all—glycolysis, Krebs cycle, glutathione homeostasis, pentose phosphate pathway, purine, arginine-citrulline-NO serving as diagnostic biomarker. Tumors that metastasize to lungs are associated with upregulated metabolism of amino acids, TCA cycle, free fatty acids, sugars, and polyols. For treatment, upregulated metabolism of glycolysis, amino acids, acetyl-CoA, polyamine, and membrane phospholipids can be targeted. Chemoresistance has been correlated to upregulated choline, serine/glycine, and lipid metabolism. Soft-tissue sarcomas and liposarcomas have been also been screened for metabolomics studies.

Osteoporosis

Various amino acid metabolisms are current targets for early identification of persons at risk for osteoporosis those at risk of subsequent fractures and targeting treatment. Linoleic acid, oleic acid, arachidonic acid, and 11, 14-eicosadienoic acid are correlated to BMD of patients serving to identify the patients at risk for developing osteoporosis. Metabolism of arachidonic acid, octadecadienoic acid, valine, leucine, isoleucine, homocysteine, hydroxyproline, and 3-hydroxybutyric acid are commonly found to be elevated while that of docosahexaenoic acid, dodecanoic acid, and lysine are reduced. These are suggested to indicate higher fracture risk.

Ankylosing Spondylitis

Diagnosis of ankylosing spondylitis (AS) is commonly delayed till the clinical features are adequately developed beyond a threshold and disease progression prediction still remains elusive. Metabolomics have prospect to sort the issue. The pathological changes in AS have been correlated to (23S, 25R)-25-hydroxyvitamin D_3 26, 23-peroxylactone (vitamin D_3 metabolite) downregulation, also the ratio of this metabolite to that of vitamin D-binding protein is also corroborative. In a study, fecal metabolomes were studied and it was concluded that AS and rheumatoid arthritis are homologous diseases that cannot be distinguished based on fecal metabolome study. Both showed decreased metabolites of butyrate, propionate, methionine, and hypoxanthine while increased metabolites of taurine, methanol, fumarate, and tryptophan.

Prosthetic Joint Infection

In combination with transcriptomics, metabolomics can be utilized to identify infection and infecting organism. The studies are underway and some early encouraging results are reported in staphylococcal infections of implanted prosthesis.

CONCLUSION

Advances in medical research are exponentially expanding and specifically the smaller molecules forming the basis of disease are being increasingly realized. There is a wealth of accumulated data that needs to be organized to make sense in a way that diagnosis, prognosis, treatment, and follow-up can be eased and specifically directed. Newer terms will keep evolving and vocabulary enhancement has to keep pace with updated knowledge. Orthobiologics are under practice and updating with new research while metabolomics need quite sometimes to establish itself.

CHAPTER 128

Impact of Obesity and the Role of Bariatric Surgery in Lower Limb Joint Arthroplasty

Manish Kumar Varshney

INTRODUCTION

Obesity has been on a rise worldwide lately reaching epidemic proportions now. Morbid obesity [body mass index (BMI) > 40 kg/m^2] is also proportionately increasing. It is widely known that obesity accelerates the development of osteoarthritis of the knee and hip possibly through biomechanical alteration and systemic inflammatory changes. Biomechanically each kilogram of weight rise increases 2–3 N of force across each hip joint and 5–6 N of force across each knee joint. The prevalence of joint pain also increases with increasing BMI. Following higher incidence of degenerative joint disorders in obese they are also subjected to higher incidence of total joint arthroplasty. It is also not infrequent to see younger, heavier patients needing total knee joint arthroplasty (TJA). Obesity predisposes to higher risk of perioperative complications, such as poor wound healing, infection, respiratory complications, venous thromboembolism, need for revision joint surgery, prosthesis loosening, increased total cost of care, and prolonged hospital length of stay. The increased risks and complications preclude the utilization of TJA by surgeons in patients with a BMI of >40 kg/m^2. But, there are patients at extreme spectrum of obesity and joint disease who are so disabled to be unable to mobilize. Medical and noninvasive therapies are unlikely to improve function and quality of life for these patients. These patients are referred to tertiary medical centers. There is growing emphasis on value and outcomes over volume so there will be stringent screening and possibly higher denial rate for obese patients to undergo TJA. The only effective and durable treatment that remains for obesity is bariatric surgery. The patients lose 50–70% of their excess weight and 10–15 BMI points after stapled bariatric procedures. Maximal weight loss is seen 1–2 years after the bariatric procedure, and is usually maintained thereafter in most of the patients.

The safety profile of bariatric surgery has dramatically improved recently. Indications for bariatric surgery are prominently based upon BMI. Obese patients with a BMI ≥40 kg/m^2 are generally considered to be candidates for bariatric surgery. Obese patients with a BMI ≥35 kg/m^2 are also considered for bariatric surgery when comorbid disease such as diabetes, hypertension, sleep apnea, or severe osteoarthritis, is present. These patients otherwise also have a higher morbidity profile following TJA.

ALTERATION IN LOWER LIMB BIOMECHANICS DUE TO OBESITY

Loads across the hip and knee joints during normal activities of daily living are proportional to weight, with the knee experiencing consistently greater loads than the hip. In nonobese patients, during normal walking (4 km/h) the peak in vivo hip contact forces ranged between 2.1 and 2.9 times body weight (BW), with a mean of 2.4 BW. During stair climbing these loads ranged from 2.3 to 2.7 BW (mean ≈2.5 BW). Gait disturbance increase loads across joints while stumbling produces loads in excess of 8.7 BW. The normal tibiofemoral contact loads across the knee during walking and stair-climbing are higher than those measured in the hip. During walking these forces are approximately 3×BW demonstrating large peak tibiofemoral loads after heel-strike and a second peak of smaller magnitude before toe-off. Stair-climbing also results in higher forces with maximum mean forces ranging from 5.09 to 5.88 BW. In obese patients there are higher loads across the knee and lower loads across the hip compared to normal weight patients. In general obese individuals exhibit lower self-directed walking velocity, shorter stride lengths, longer times in stance phase, greater step widths measured in the frontal plane, and greater toe-out angles compared with normal weight patients. Lowering walking velocity is assumed to be an adaptive change to increased weight that results in lower joint moments (i.e., torques) in the hip, knee, and ankle. Increased toe-out angle may decrease knee adduction moments in normal gait to lower the load across the knee joint. High knee adduction moments correlate to the development of knee osteoarthritis.

JOINT ARTHROPLASTY OUTCOME IN OBESE PATIENTS

As the loads transmitted across hip and knee are proportional to the weight so it is quite logical to understand that in patients with TJA these elevated loads will be distributed across the bearing surfaces of the prostheses. The combination of excess load and repetitive joint cycling in obese TJA patients increases the risk for accelerated bearing surfacing wear, early prosthesis failure, and implant loosening compared to patients of normal weight. Obese patients with total hip replacements (THA) may have higher risk of prosthesis dislocation arising out of technical difficulties in patients with excessive BMI compared to normal weight patients. Higher number of technical errors has been reported in obese patients. Overall, complication rates have been found to increase from 5% in normal weight patients to 22% in obese individuals. Obesity also increases the risk of surgical site infections (including periprosthetic infections, rise from 0.4% in normal weight patients to 4.66% in obese), respiratory complications, thromboembolic events (1.5 times higher for each 5-point increase in BMI), need for revision joint surgery, component malposition, prosthesis loosening, total cost, and hospital length of stay. Comorbid conditions such as type II diabetes (doubles periprosthetic infection rates) and obstructive sleep apnea (increases the rate of serious complications and increased length of stay) further increases the perioperative morbidity. Some studies report up to three times increased need of revision of hip prosthesis in obese patients (BMI ≥ 40 kg/m^2) compared to nonobese.

IMPACT OF ARTHROPLASTY ON OBESITY

It was a misconception or a hyped propaganda for arthroplasty that after TJA increased activity would be helpful in reducing weight and as a consequence produce postoperative weight loss. This is so ingrained amongst patients too that sometimes they plead for TJA under the misconception that they would be able to lose weight if only they could just be mobile. The reported findings in literature are quite contrary. Patients undergoing either hip or knee replacement that had good orthopedic outcomes actually gained weight afterwards. Patients with a normal BMI and obese patients may not lose weight but overweight patients usually gain a significant amount of weight after surgery. The preoperative weight and postoperative weight are tightly correlated. Most studies report that a successful arthroplasty and restoration of a patient's mobility does not necessarily produce subsequent weight loss. The majority of patients instead add on weight, and ultimately there is overall net weight gain despite encouragement to lose weight. Not all report such dismal outcome, in a review by Inacio et al. for 20,060 TKAs and 10,572 THAs; the authors found that 69% of TKAs and 64% of THAs maintained their weight (<5% change in BMI) 1 year postoperatively. For TKA patients, 8% gained weight in the year after surgery, 14% lost weight, and the weight change was unknown in 9% of patients. For THA patients, 15% gained weight, 14% lost weight, and the weight change was unknown in 13% of patients. Compared to patients with BMI < 30 kg/m^2, a larger percentage of patients with elevated BMI lost weight after TJA.

BARIATRIC SURGERY AND ITS RELEVANT EFFECTS

Surgically-induced weight loss not only reduces the quantity of food consumed but also the amount of calories absorbed. Older procedures such as jejunoileal bypass were failure as they excessively reduced the surface area for absorption and produced complications such as diarrhea, nephrolithiasis, malabsorption syndrome, and cirrhosis. Presently, day-bariatric surgeries can be grouped into two broader types—gastroplasty and gastric bypass **(Table 1)**. During inception they were performed open but now both can be laparoscopically performed. Gastroplasty reduces the stomach volume that is commonly achieved by either a silicone ring placed in the cardia creating a 15 mL pouch or by sleeve gastrectomy by stapling along the greater curvature to reduce the volume by 25%. This induces early satiety by reducing the amount of food consumed but nutrients are properly absorbed as distal gastrointestinal tract is in continuity. Despite its ease of doing the results for weight reduction are variable in producing weight loss and failure is not uncommon. Gastric bypass, on the other hand, not only reduces the gastric volume but also limits absorption of nutrients **(Fig. 1)**. The proximal portion of stomach is stapled to create a 20–30 mL pouch and roux loop of jejunum (distal cut end) is anastomosed to the gastric pouch for food passage. The proximal cut end is anastomosed to the Roux loop to provide conduit for biliary and pancreatic juices and prevent blind loop syndrome completing the Roux-en-Y. This system reduces the stomach volume and also induces controlled malabsorption to effect weight reduction. The following are some of the consequences of bariatric surgery that one should be aware of while prescribing the faculty services.

TABLE 1: Types of bariatric surgery.

	Malabsorptive (Roux-en-Y)	*Restrictive (gastric banding/ sleeve gastrectomy)*
Mechanism	• Decreases volume of stomach • Reduces area of absorption	Decreases volume of stomach
Expected weight loss	Quite predictable	Unpredictable
Advantages	Predictable and significant weight reduction	• Ease of performance • Easier to reverse • Less metabolic derangements as the GIT is maintained in continuity
Disadvantages	• Malabsorption syndrome and nutrient deficiencies common—deficiency of iron, calcium, vitamin B_{12}, protein, and vitamin D are common • Wound healing complications and osteopenia seen frequently • Needs experience to perform surgery and manage complications	• Failure common • Weight loss is very unpredictable • Nutrient deficiency (less common) than malabsorptive procedures—iron, vitamin B_{12} and protein deficiency

Metabolic Consequences

Malabsorption produces nutritional deficiencies while in restrictive surgeries erratic food consumption also may

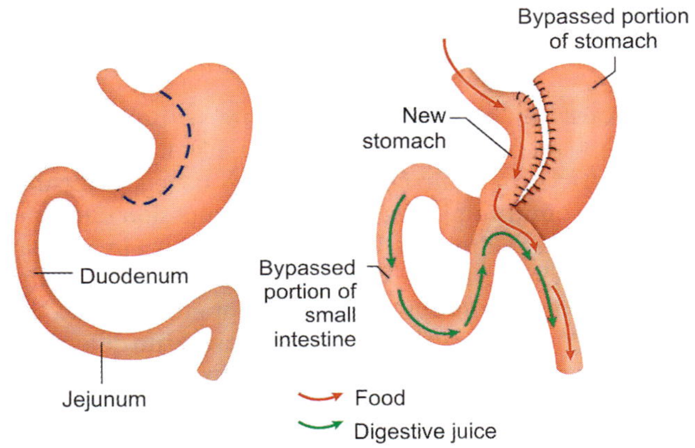

Fig. 1: The mini-gastric bypass in the form of Roux-en-Y. The small gastric pouch is anastomosed to the distal jejunal limb (Roux limb) and proximal is connected to the Roux limb for biliary and pancreatic juices to mix with food. The jejunum forms a Y-configuration deriving its peculiar name.

produce the same. Anemia due to iron and folic acid deficiency is common. Bypass surgery will limit the calcium and vitamin B_{12} absorption to a great extent as most of it is absorbed from duodenum that gets bypassed. Both of these thus need to be replaced in adequate amounts, the effect is though less pronounced after restrictive procedures. Protein deficiency is common after both procedures and produces muscle wasting there is also some amount of protein intolerance following both surgeries. Fat-soluble vitamins are also absorbed in limited amount following reduced bile salts.

Effect on Wound Healing

There is reduction in protein absorption and induction of a sort of catabolic state with erratic protein metabolism following bariatric surgery. Based on the studies on abdominal wound healing it has been found that there is significant reduction in the amount of hydroxyproline and other tissue proteins following this surgery. The elastic and collagen fibrils are irregular in structure all resulting in delaying wound healing and suboptimal wound healing (strength).

Effects on Bones and Fracture Repair

The malabsorption reduces bone mineral density (BMD) mediated by several factors such as reduced plasma leptin, ghrelin, and increased adiponectin. There is also reduction of estrogen in females that otherwise is trophic to bones. The reduction in BMD is proportional to weight reduction possibly because osteoporosis is a qualitative disorder that manifests quantitatively and bone quality is reduced in malabsorption and nutrient deficiency. The effect on fracture repair is unknown but hypovitaminosis and mineral deficiency is expected to retard the process.

Effect on Medications

The bioavailability of oral tablet and capsule preparations is expectedly reduced following reduced absorption surface area. Extended release and sustained release preparations may not reach therapeutic plasma levels. The effect is also seen for antibiotics so liquid preparations are preferred. Best is to use intravenous preparations where feasible considering the possibly already compromised renal and hepatic parameters in the obese patients. Nonsteroidal anti-inflammatory drugs (NSAIDs) have a detrimental effect following this procedure so usually centrally acting drugs such as acetaminophen or tramadol or tapentadol are preferred.

CONSIDERATIONS FOR FACULTY SURGERY IN BARIATRIC PATIENTS

Thorough preoperative evaluation is needed before embarking on major or even minor surgery in patients who have undergone bariatric surgery as metabolic alterations may compromise the critical functions. Protein deficiency can be estimated by total protein, total lymphocyte count, albumin, and prealbumin levels. Reduced albumin and transferrin levels are correlated with prosthetic joint infection and wound healing complications. Deficiency of vitamin A, B_{12}, C, folate, thiamine and minerals such as iron, zinc, manganese and magnesium and calcium would compromise the wound and bone healing. Zinc deficiency has been correlated with poor wound healing. Workup for osteomalacia (alkaline phosphatase, secondary hyperparathyroidism) with serum vitamin D and calcium levels should be done before orthopedic procedures for optimization if deficiency is detected.

Timing of Surgery after Bariatric Surgery

This issue is not fully agreed upon and no universal guidelines exist. Maximal weight loss and stabilization is reported at 2 years following bariatric surgery so logically this time-frame is generally mentioned in various studies, however, major orthopedic elective surgeries have been done as early as 6 months without undue complications. Studies specifically looking at 2 years as a time frame reported higher overall complications for surgeries performed within 2 years but difference may not be significant to reach statistical or practical conclusion.

IMPACT OF BARIATRIC SURGERY ON OSTEOARTHRITIC JOINTS

The bariatric surgery has been shown to effect joint pain, function, and osteoarthritis progression in the severely obese patients before arthroplasty. There is significant reduction of BMI after bariatric surgery reported in different studies beginning within 3 months and stabilizing till 1 year or more. There is also radiographic improvement of disease and clinically relevant improvement in pain and function. Site-specific pain like for knee and hip reduced both in frequency and intensity. The reduction is other painful musculoskeletal symptom, particularly concerning the cervical spine, lumbar spine, ankle, and foot are also remarkable. There is also less work-restricting knee and ankle pain overall following improved physical function, reduced knee stiffness, and improved range of motion.

BIOMECHANICS AFTER BARIATRIC SURGERY

Bariatric surgery also affects the kinematics and kinetics of joints following weight loss. Gait analysis to measure both ground reaction forces and three-dimensional kinematics of the lower extremities demonstrate significant decreases in step width in the frontal plane and peak moments (torques) around the hip and knee proportional to the amount of a patient's weight loss. Weight loss resulted in increased stride length and gait speed along with improvement in hip range of motion, maximal knee flexion, and ankle plantar flexion. There is general improvement in self-directed walking speed but no change in the fastest walking velocity. The patients also report subjective improvements in walking and stair climbing ability.

Ground reaction forces are highly correlated to body mass being proportionate to the body weight. The findings, however, revealed that ground reaction forces generally decrease with weight loss at lower gait velocities but they increase to levels beyond baseline measurements as the gait velocity increased. Low velocity and low-impact exercises are, hence, recommended after weight loss surgery.

ARTHROPLASTY OUTCOME IN PATIENTS TREATED WITH BARIATRIC SURGERY

Quite logically gathering from above that there is increased morbidity in obese patients and improvement following bariatric surgery would follow into recommendation of bariatric surgery before TJA as a strategy. The conclusion is, however, not so straightforward and the reports are mixed in outcome. The following are some of the studies done to look into the matter; however, most of the evidence is retrospective:

- McLawhorn et al. found that bariatric surgery 2 years before TKA can be a cost-effective treatment strategy compared to TKA alone in morbidly obese patients.
- Werner et al. analyzed the 90-day complication rates of TKA, comparing 11,294 morbidly obese patients to 219 morbidly obese patients (using a national database) who had bariatric surgery first. The latter group had half the rate of major complications and 40% fewer minor complications. This improvement, however, did not translate into reduction in complication rate to the level of nonobese controls.
- Parvizi et al. reported improved results after studying 20 patients with a mean BMI of 49 kg/m^2 who underwent bariatric surgery followed by lower extremity TJA. The BMI dropped to a mean of 29 kg/m^2, the cumulative Knee Society Score after TKA improved from 103.6 to 148.9, and the Harris hip score improved from 40 to 67.5 after THA.
- Kulkarni et al. identified 143 obese patients who underwent both bariatric surgery and TJA. Patients with bariatric surgery first were found to have significantly lower wound complications and re-admission rates.
- Severson et al. reported that patients with TJA >2 years after bariatric surgery had an anesthesia time that averaged 28 minutes shorter and operative time that averaged 39 minutes shorter but there were no differences observed in hospital stay or 90-day complication rates.
- Inacio et al. reported that bariatric surgery before TJA did not appear to reduce the frequency of complications, readmissions, deep surgical site infections, or revision following TJA. This study was purely a descriptive study.
- Martin et al. in a retrospective analysis reported that although patients receiving bariatric surgery reduced their BMI before TKA, there was an increased risk of reoperation in the bariatric group compared to the group matched to their prebariatric BMI, and there were no differences in complications, revision, or deep infection. The bariatric group had a higher risk of reoperation and revision TKA compared with patients who underwent TKA at an equivalent BMI, but the risks for complications and periprosthetic joint infection were not different.

CONCLUSION

Obesity has negative influence on both the development and progression of osteoarthritis and the outcomes of total joint arthroplasty. Weight loss improves body mechanics and joint kinetics and kinematics. Total joint arthroplasty is a reliable method for improving pain and joint function but by itself has no favorable influence on inducing weight loss. Although bariatric surgery reasonably reduces the complications associated with morbid obesity the approach is not completely hassle-free as secondary influence on metabolic changes might compromise some of the benefits. The current evidence for supporting bariatric surgery before total joint arthroplasty is gathered from retrospective studies reporting conflicting results. It is unclear as to when the elective surgeries can be done following initial bariatric surgery and one should do a thorough evaluation before taking major surgeries. Perioperative management should also be a team effort including various faculties managing the metabolic parameters and these should be communicated to the patient.

CHAPTER 129 Nanotechnology in Orthopedics

Manish Kumar Varshney

INTRODUCTION

Nanotechnology is a science dealing with objects functional on extremely small scale of the size from 1 to 100 nanometers. In 1959, Richard Feynman first introduced the concept of nanotechnology. The technology is based on two thoughts—one is to miniaturize the functional objects/machines so that they occupy less space and the other is basically an inspiration from living organisms where the molecular interactions taking place at miniature scale are able to produce directed functions (e.g., enzymatic actions). These objects for sheer size are referred to as nanomolecules. Despite the rationality in thought and the widespread interest, development encompasses a lot of hurdles and technology progress is not a straight path. As with quantum physics that does not follow the laws of particle physics, nanomolecules have unique chemical and physical properties that do not follow the laws of macromolecules/larger objects. Understanding the same is the primary reason for delay and limitation because control of these parameters has produced a new scientific field, experts of which are still evolving. The molecular interactions in human body occur at 4–400 atomic units measured in nanometers. Nanotechnology heralds to reproduce/produce/manipulate such processes on a scale of <100 nm by integration of nanoscopic materials into macro-/microscopic systems. In general, two approaches are used for nanoscience evolution, one uses the bottom-up approach where the simpler smaller elements are arranged in the designated patterns [e.g., in three-dimensional (3D) printing] to produce complex molecules and expected to have predefined function while the other approach is called the top-down approach where miniaturization comes to work and smaller and smaller objects are developed that can work similar to their larger predecessors. Nanophase describes conventional matter at very small sizes (<100 nm) but preserved atomic structure. At such small sizes, the physical properties behave in terms of quantum (in simple terms both wave + particle properties) physics instead of particle physics. The prominent characteristic exploited by biological systems for nanoparticles is its markedly enhanced surface area as we know that with reduction in size the surface area increases. Such large surface area provides for faster and much higher magnitude of reactions/processes to occur. So for orthopedic implants modified by nanotechnology, the interaction with bone cells and mesenchymal cells would enhance by multiple times. This is expected to produce better cell adsorption, differentiation, growth, and ultimately osseointegration and other desired properties.

GENERAL APPLICATIONS OF NANOTECHNOLOGY IN ORTHOPEDICS

Despite the limitations there are potential applications of nanotechnology that may be pertinent to the medical field for the resemblance to molecular mechanisms that occur at same scale. In orthopedics, the development of nanomedicine has currently focused on devices and implants for surface characteristics, molecular structure, bonding with bone, etc., while the typical clinical application is still limited to tissue-engineering, diagnostic aspects of musculoskeletal infection, and oncology. Therapeutic applications are still far away in orthopedic field. The current application of nanomedicine pertaining to orthopedics in nanoscale surface modification and tissue engineering is vastly expanding opening new horizons. If specific nanotopographical features are developed on implants that resemble biological surfaces, viz., type X collagen initiating endochondral ossification; complications such as loosening and implant subsidence may be ameliorated. The major focus of nanotechnology in orthopedics is to reduce the complications associated with operative procedures namely—aseptic loosening and periprosthetic osteolysis, infection, scar tissue formation, and management of bone defects; a spillover effect of technology is seen in cartilage regeneration, drug delivery system, etc.

The ***specific surface modifications*** presently studied include—nanophase ceramics [like nanophase hydroxyapatite (HA)], aluminum oxide and titanium dioxide, carbon, selenium, titanium, and nanocrystalline diamond. These are further supplemented by the use of fibronectin and vitronectin in a controlled manner that facilitates osteoblast activation, adhesion, and recruitment to a biomaterial. The currently used polished implants are smooth in nanoterms while the osseous inorganic phase has sizes of 50 nm × 25 nm × 4 nm; interaction of these produces fibrous interface.

Nanoscience surface modification aims to roughen the implant surfaces so that bone-implant interface interacts in a productive way to get better integration. Surface modification by conjugation of substances such as BMP-2 to chitosan membranes also produced a significantly increased proliferation of osteoblasts, alkaline phosphatase activity, and calcium deposition. Nanocomposites have been created utilizing the above-described nanoinorganic phase coupled to nanophase collagen improving osseointegration.

Managing Bone Defects

Nanocrystalline HA paste has been found to be efficient filler for bone defects. It has been used for filling distal radius defects and cavity after elevation of tibial plateau. The defects can be bioengineered by 3D printing using the nanohydroxyapatite "ink" and implanted into defects.

Improving Bone Cements

Nanoparticles addition in the form of nanotubes and fibers have been tried to improve the tensile strength of cement. Other improvements in characteristics of bone cements using nanotechnology are being tried as follows:

- Antibacterial properties of chitosan and quaternary ammonium-derived chitosan nanoparticles have shown encouraging results against *Staphylococcus aureus* and *S. epidermidis* with no significant cytotoxicity and pave way for further improvements.
- Silver ions and silver benzoate have been blended to polymethyl methacrylate (PMMA) for inhibiting bacterial enzymes and deoxyribonucleic acid (DNA) replication (against *Acinetobacter baumannii*, *Pseudomonas aeruginosa*, *P. mirabilis*, and *S. aureus*) showing promising results, but the problem is of reduced compression strength.
- Nanosilver-added cement shows complete inhibition of the methicillin-resistant *Staphylococcus aureus* (MRSA) and methicillin-resistant *Staphylococcus epidermidis* (MRSE) growth.

Cartilage Regeneration and Osteochondral Defects

The underlying basis is synthesis of 3D mirror scaffolds that precisely controls intercellular, cell-matrix, and cell-growth factor interactions to provide milieu suitable to hyaline cartilage growth/formation. Additionally, the matrix should adhere to the underlying surface with a pore size larger than diameter of the osteoblasts (10 μm) so that cell penetration and neovascularization can happen. Nanocomposite biological implants can be used as scaffolds to treat the cartilage and osteochondral defects. For the latter, a trilayer composite scaffold has been synthesized that comprises a cartilage layer formed from 100% type I collagen and a bone layer composed of nanocrystalline HA (70%) + type I collagen (30%); these are separated by an intermediate transition layer of collagen rich (60%) nanocrystalline HA (40%).

Orthopedic Oncology

Nanometric selenium potentiates chemotherapeutic agents and when applied to titanium implants, it inhibits the malignant osteoblasts. Similarly, nanocrystalline HA induces the apoptosis of osteosarcoma cells. Biodegradable nanocapsules containing siRNA targeting the oncogene inhibited tumor growth in mouse model of Ewing's sarcoma.

Orthopedic Infection

Nanophase silver is a powerful bacteriostatic and bactericidal agent that can be of specific use in open fractures. Nanophase silver deployed on surface of implants into titanium nanotubes is a strong bactericidal agent and also prevents bacterial adhesion for up to 30 days. This finds special use in revision arthroplasty and implant-related infections.

Peripheral Nerve Injury

Nanophase silver impregnated type I collagen significantly reduces the time to nerve regeneration by increasing the quantity of adsorbed neurotropic proteins that produce thicker myelin sheath and improves nerve conduction.

Drug Delivery

Gold has been shown to be an efficient transcutaneous drug delivery system for iontophoresis. Diclofenac administered with 30-nm gold nanoparticles produced marked anti-inflammatory properties than plain form in transcutaneous system. Nanophase poly-L-lactic acid (PLLA) is also a nanoscopic drug delivery system as has been shown to heal large calvarial bony defects when used as delivery system for BMP-2. Such drug delivery systems (polypeptide nanofilms) when used with total joint prosthesis have shown marked reduction in bacterial load and improved osteoblastic response.

NANOMATERIALS IN BONE AND CARTILAGE TISSUE ENGINEERING

A number of nanostructured materials (or their combination—composites) are available for use that can be broadly divided into natural and synthetic derived.

Natural Biomaterials

These include the organic and inorganic biomaterials both. The protein (mainly collagen), gelatin, and fibrin are usual organic biomaterials used while natural inorganic matrices include polysaccharides, hyaluronic acid, chitosan, alginate, agarose, and chondroitin sulfate.

Collagen

This is the most common scaffold material used due to its desirable properties (biocompatibility, biodegradability, structural integrity, cell infiltration, and attachment) and the fact that most of the native tissue matrix is made up of collagen. The main issue, however, is poor mechanical properties in loading. Type I collagen and recently type X collagen had been of interest to researchers. Type I collagen bears its desirable properties due to its property to bind integrins through RGD (arginine-glycine-aspartic acid) and non-RGD sites mediating cell migration, attachment, and proliferation. Type I collagen can act as a carrier for bone morphogenic protein (BMP) or bone sialoprotein (BSP) to enhance osteogenic properties. Collagens are produced by various procedures such as acid treatment, alkali treatment, proteolytic treatment in acidic environment (high yield), and dissolution-reconstitution procedure (produces collagen gel). Purified collagen and derivatives (injectable hydrogels, hydrogel membranes, films, sponges, scaffolds, microspheres, and nanospheres) have myriad of uses including neural repair, bladder repair, skin substitute, ligament, and tendon repair. Collagen gels containing mesenchymal stem cells (MSCs) have been used for cartilage regeneration also they can be used as ink in 3D printing of matrix scaffolds.

Gelatin

This is principally hydrolyzed form of collagen devoid of immunogenicity and pathogen transmission associated with collagen but has the integrin binding sites for cell adhesion and carboxylic acid groups that bind calcium. It is available as hydrogels and scaffolds having properties such as biocompatibility, biodegradability, no immunogenicity, and free from pathogen transmission.

Fibrin

Generally, it is derived from clotted blood. It can be used as glue (injectable hydrogel or scaffold) with bioactive molecules or MSCs. There is some suggestion that apart from biocompatibility and being biodegradable, there could be some enhancement in tissue formation.

Polysaccharides

These are usually bioactive oligosaccharides of which hyaluronic acid, chitosan, alginate, agarose, and chondroitin sulfate are commonly used.

Hyaluronic acid: This is a hydrophilic, biocompatible, biodegradable, nonimmunogenic glycosaminoglycan naturally produced by chondrocytes in cartilage and synoviocytes to provide viscoelasticity to joint fluid available for clinical use as injectable hydrogel and scaffold. Though nonimmunogenic by itself, its degradation products (by hyaluronidase) can induce chondrolysis. Its prominent effects are inhibition of fibronectic fragment-mediated chondrocytic chondrolysis, anti-inflammatory effects, inhibitory effects on prostaglandin synthesis, proteoglycan release, and degradation, rheological properties (improved synovial flow), and normalization of synthesis of hyaluronic acid. These are common benefits for its use as viscosupplementation agent in large joints.

Chitosan: It is partially deacetylated chitin having cationic nature of high charge density. It forms insoluble ionic and polyelectrolyte complexes with anionic polymers that can carry and interact with growth factors, adhesion proteins, and receptors. It has been used specifically as a carrier for MSCs being supportive to their attachment, proliferation, and viability.

Alginate: It is derived from brown algae or bacteria. It is a binary polymer [combination of (1-4)-linked β-D-mannuronic acid and R-L-guluronic acid]. Alginates have remarkable property of chelating divalent metal ions, such as calcium, magnesium, and barium and they are easy to prepare, support cellular elements, and have low cost of preparation. Alginate gels have been used extensively for studying the phenotype, organization, and turnover of chondrocytes or intervertebral disk cells and the differentiation of adipose-derived adult stem cells, and bone marrow-derived mesenchymal stem cells.

Agarose: Agarose gel is one of the most common systems used for in vitro studies and is basically composed of agarobiose repeat units. Homogeneous solution forms a gel when solution is cooled to 35° due to coilhelix transition. Cellular elements grown in agarose are stable with preserved phenotype and can respond to mechanical stimuli. It is cheap and easy to prepare.

Chondroitin sulfate: It is composed of chains of alternating sugars (N-acetylgalactosamine and glucuronic acid) forming a sulfated polysaccharide. It stimulates metabolic tissue response and has inflammatory property.

Artificial Materials

Because protein and polysaccharide matrices do not have compressive strength so artificial matrices are commonly used that may substitute for both soft and hard tissues. Biocompatibility is the major issue in selecting the artificial matrices. The following are some of the common artificial materials in use and the list is rapidly increasing:

Bioactive Ceramics

These materials have high cytocompatibility with bone cells. Bone tissue engineering has been done with alumina zirconia, titania, and calcium phosphate [{tricalcium phosphate (TCP), $Ca_3(PO_4)_2$}, hydroxyapatite {HA, $Ca_{10}(PO_4)_6(OH)_2$} and its derivatives].

Calcium phosphate: These have excellent osteoconductive properties and with growth factors they may also become osteoinductive or even osteogenic. They are incorporated in osseous tissues (bonding osteogenesis) and enhance tissue formation as the mineral phase of HA and tricalcium phosphate (β-TCP) ceramic is similar to natural bone. When bone accumulates on the ceramic, the new bone formation is similar to woven bone and is quickly remodeled into lamellar bone. The micropore structure is trophic to osteoblasts and other bone progenitor cells. This microstructural configuration amalgamates with native physiological processes that the whole tissue acts as a bioactive composite aligning with the bone tissue formative process. Rate of growth can be controlled by altering the crystallinity of HA and it has been seen that amorphous phase has greater and rapid resorption compared to crystalline phase. Nanophase ceramics, especially nanohydroxyapatite, offer high surface fraction of grain boundaries that enhance osteoblast functions (such as adhesion, proliferation, and differentiation) and adsorption of vitronectin (a protein well known to promote osteoblast adhesion) is remarkably increased. As β-TCP has very slow degradation kinetics its osteoconductivity is not impressive at physiological levels. "*Third generation biomaterials*" have, hence emerged where composites are used for supporting and stimulating cell and tissue growth. Bioactive glass has low bending strength and fracture toughness limiting its use and hence focus is being shifted to silicate bioceramics whose physiochemical properties can be altered to match mechanical strength, bioactivity, and degradation. The ***silicate bioceramics*** in study and clinical application include binary oxides (CaO-SiO_2, MgO-SiO_2), ternary oxides (MgOCaO-SiO_2, ZnO-CaO-SiO_2), and quaternary oxides (SrO-ZnO-CaO-SiO_2). ***Titania*** is a new interesting artificial matrix of research. It is basically the oxide layer that forms on titanium surfaces which is inherently very stable. Altering the micron size of titania has been shown to alter and enhance calcium deposition by osteoblasts so surface modification of titanium implants is the most topic in the field of implant-engineering. This is expected to produce implants that have enhanced osseointegration as use of titanium in operative orthopedics has risen drastically.

Biodegradable Polymers

Natural polymers are high-molecular weight compounds with complex structure that renders them less workable in laboratory as processes alter their structure and lose the biological characteristics. Synthetic polymers have ability to partly mimic the biological polymers and due to smaller size can be engineered to specific tissue needs. The commonly used polymers are polylactic acid (PLA, which is present in both L and D forms), polyglycolic acid (PGA), and their copolymer polylactic-co-glycolic acid (PLGA).

Polylactic-co-glycolic acid: This has been classically used as drug delivery system [*see* also Chapter on "Infections of Bone (Typical and Atypical) and Surgical Site Infection"]. The problems that may arise from use of synthetic polymers is their erratic degradation due to nonenzymatic hydrolysis (releasing less or excessive drug) and possible acute and/or chronic inflammatory response, potential localized pH decrease due to relative acidity of hydrolytically degraded by-products, retarded clearance rate, and limited biological function. By carefully controlling the chemical composition (the lactide/glycolide ratio), the crystallinity and molecular weight distribution, the scaffold degradation rate, and mechanical strength have been better controlled. In general, the hydrolytic degradation is directly proportional to molecular weight and inversely proportional to crystallinity. The polymer can be made more hydrophobic (reducing hydrolysis) by adding methyl group to PLA repeating unit. The PGA component improves proteoglycan synthesis necessary for cartilage regeneration. PLGA scaffolds are suitable for the chondrogenesis of human adipose-derived stem cells especially when chondrogenic factors such as TGF-β and dexamethasone are added to them.

Poly-ε-caprolactone (PCL): This is more suitable for long-term implantation as it degrades very slowly. It may be added in small amounts to PLGA scaffolds for chondrogenesis to improve the elasticity of the construct.

Polyglycerol sebacate (PGS): Its use is similar to PLGA.

Polyethylene glycol (PEG): This has been used in biomedical systems due to hydrophilic nature, readily polymerization and being biocompatible but it is not biodegradable. Due to its low molecular weight it is excreted as it is.

Hydrogels

In minimally invasive surgeries, it is highly desirable that the implanted substitute can be introduced in a minimally invasive manner and take on the shape of defect maintaining its microstructure for desired biological effect. Hydrogels have raised hope in this regard as they can be implanted by injections and then take on the desired shape. Adjuvants added to them help in biological tissue formation later. Hydrogels provide 3D polymeric networks that support cellular elements. The most commonly utilized materials are collagen, gelatin, chitosan, hyaluronic acid, alginates, PEG, PLGA, and polyvinyl alcohol. Chondrocyte impregnated hydrogels have been used in cartilage repair, however, they have not proven well for bone defect repair as hydrogels lack the ability to mineralize. Attempts are being made to coat the hydrogels with negatively charged subgroups and catalytic enzymes that can bond with mineral phase (calcium phosphate).

Nanocomposites

It is always a good idea to prepare and use composite materials (by combining two or more matrices) that can supplement each other reducing limitations and enhancing advantages. For chondrogenesis variable combination of fibrin glue, alginate, and hyaluronan have been used to modify various PLGA, PGA, PCL scaffolds for stabilization and growth of impregnated chondrocytes. Nanophase ceramics like nano-HA may be combined to collagen matrix to provide bone filler material. Similarly PLLA/HA and PLGA/HA scaffolds have been developed with improved properties. HA facilitates osteoblast seeding, prevents apoptosis, and allows better protein adsorption. Another approach is to generate apatite by biomimetic process in a simulated body fluid. The resulting carbonated HA is more similar to natural bone apatite (calcium deficient; Ca/P ratio = 1.5) compared to inorganic crystalline structure (Ca/P ratio = 1.67) and is expected to degrade faster than latter. Nanocomposites with HA nanofibers combined to α-TCP (not the β) show improved mechanical strength of porous composite scaffolds in some studies.

Nanofibers

The principal benefit of using nanofibers is high surface area to volume ratio offering better cell adhesion, proliferation, migration, and differentiation. Oriented nanofibrous polymeric scaffolds may closely resemble cartilage matrix supporting the hMSCs to transform and stabilize into mature chondrocytes. Such structures are possible by electrospinning and superficial layer of cartilage can be synthesized with impregnated chondrocytes or hMSCs that later develop into chondrocytes. The mechanism is not fully clear but possibly cell elongation induced by the aligned PCL nanofibers is expected to reorganize the cytoskeletal structures that regulate the cell morphology. Collagen type II synthesis is quite remarkable in nanofiber scaffolds. Nanofibers also facilitate cell adhesion by a process of selective adsorption of adhesion molecules like vitronectin and fibronectin. The improved microenvironment ultimately promotes Rac activation, a GTPase important in cell adhesion and signal transduction, and F-actin assembly and also expression of cartilage specific extracellular matrix genes such as aggrecan, collagen type II and IX, and cartilage oligomeric matrix proteins. These factors, hence, promote chondrogenesis. Large bone defects can be also addressed by developing microfiber approach. Self-assembling ***peptide-amphiphiles (PA)*** have been evaluated for osteogenic potential. Nanofiber PA molecules consist of peptide segment that has one domain facilitating formation of extended β-sheets (promotes the assembly of molecules into fibrous aggregates) and a second domain with amino acid residues (relevant for bioactivity). These self-assemble as fibers achieving micron sizes and nucleate *in vivo* HA crystals that resemble those in natural bone. In 3D-biomimetic system, these PA aggregates help in mineralization and bone defect filling in *in vitro* studies. ***Carbon nanotubes and nanofibers*** have attractive mechanical, electrical, thermal, optical, and structural properties and have been found to support osteoblastic cell adhesion. With increasing surface energy, the adhesion of smooth muscle cell, fibroblast, and chondrocyte was specifically retarded thus selective bone formation and deposition could be promoted as, for example, in nonunion.

SAFETY OF NANOTECHNOLOGY

The prime concern of any developing science is not just proving its efficacy but also to document its safety in clinical practice. Currently with the limited knowledge and study of nanoparticles and their impact on biological systems, they need proper study and audit before a large scale use. Nanoparticles have been found cytotoxic to lung and brain cells. In addition, the metabolism of these particles by liver, kidney, and in blood may induce oxidative stress.

CONCLUSION

- Nano-medicine is a specialized offshoot of nanotechnology that opens avenues for diagnostics, biomaterial and implant improvement and novel drug delivery systems by using molecular tools and knowledge of human body.
- Specific optimization of physiochemical properties of various biomaterials and implants have enabled improvement in properties like bio-integration, reduction in infection, improving toxicity profile and drug-delivery capabilities.
- Nanofabrication techniques such as lithography, electrospinning, polymer demixing, phase separation chemical etching and molecular self-assembly have produced myriads of biomaterials (both natural and artificial) that can be deployed to specific needs and usage. These can be discretely used for bone or cartilage or combined tissue engineering.
- Nanotechnology may evolve into disruptive science that would replace conventional approach to diagnostics and therapeutics but stringent regulatory and safety protocols need to be formulated to prevent its potential misuse.

CHAPTER 130

Orthopedics in Digital Renaissance

Manish Kumar Varshney

INTRODUCTION

The modern era of orthopedics to which we belong is equipped with a very powerful universal tool that has shrunk the borders and connected people globally to make the fraternity more or less "unity". The transmission of knowledge in the current digital world is very fast paced and is occurring in huge volumes. Such an occurrence should have produced unified answers to common problems, standardized treatment protocols and techniques, and provided universally acceptable regimens; but this has not been the true case and the evolutionary evidence being generated is at best confusing and changes within a matter of months to years without materializing or providing lasting answers. Only in a few situations, some rational changes like busting some myths and concrete changes in orthopedic practice have occurred. Such radical changes in orthopedic practice include shunning the routine change of scalpel blade for deep tissue dissection after skin incision, routine use of hip precautions after arthroplasty, routine removal of implant in pediatric patients, the previously deemed linear correlation between operative time and infection, etc. These are, however, miniature changes compared to the vast possibility of providing answers to complex and difficult problems concerning the orthopedic patients. Nevertheless, the horizon of knowledge, understanding, and cooperation is constantly enlarging so we would expect the digital age to provide practical answers to improve and simplify the orthopedic practice. We are currently practicing intelligent orthopedics that is an amalgamation of time honored conventional techniques and high-end technology that has been gracefully embraced by the surgeons worldwide. The following are the ongoing changes impacting the current practice of orthopedics, some of which may also prove to be disruptive in near future.

CHANGING TRENDS IN ORTHOPEDICS AFFECTED BY DIGITAL RENAISSANCE

- There is a surge in the use of minimally invasive implants and techniques for orthopedic reconstructions. The patients have been empowered to access the real world data and on the horizon technologies through smart phones and online launches. This has not only improved the patient awareness but has also pressurized the surgeons to constantly adopt to newer techniques and technologies. Use of modern techniques such as video conferencing and visual assistive devices like Google glasses have made it possible to transmit information and take assistance from expert in real-time settings.
- Development of smart implants is around the corner that are expected to have embedded sensors which will allow the healthcare software system to detect early problems, proactively treat them and also offer better care. The implant sensors are expected to measure loads, bacteria levels, temperature, motion, enzymes, pH, contamination, etc. Combination of data from all these variables would definitely help to detect early failure of the implant, infection, or healing problems that may occur after surgery.
- The accuracy of implant placement and reconstruction has been already improved by computer assistance during surgery or including a robotic system to assist or perform the surgery. Using robots and internet-based technology it has been made possible to perform remote surgeries at far away centers by experts sitting in their parent institutes. This can be further advanced to delivering surgical care in acute emergencies like warfare injuries where it is not always possible to provide expert care by physical presence of the surgeon. The adoption of this technology is fast increasing but is not widespread due to cost concerns also there is involved cost of software upgradation hampering its routine use. Development of newer and advanced system at affordable cost for establishments would certainly lead to much more frequent use of this technology.
- Delivering patient-centric orthopedic care has been made possible to some extent by the use of additive manufacturing or three-dimensional (3D) printing the hardware such as screws, plates, nails, and Jigs that fits specifically for the patient. 3D-printed models can aid in preoperative planning for fracture fixation or resection of malignant tumors at difficult location. 3D printed implants for joint reconstruction would also be made

available in the near future that would replace the present custom-made prosthesis.

- Advancement in nanotechnology has produced a new class of substances that exhibit bioactivity and adaptability mimicking that of native bone. Presently, this technology is limited to production of bone grafts and repair materials, but the developments are expected to produce not only bones but also cartilage and possibly tendons or ligaments that can be re-implanted into the patient for more natural reconstructions.
- The development and combination of the stem cells with tissue engineering has opened a horizon to introduce effective therapies for tissue healing that inherently have a low regenerative capacity. The typical examples being production of cartilage and native vascularized bone.
- A lot of intraoperative changes are getting introduced based on artificial intelligence, the most common of which are the computer-aided navigation systems and robotics. Intraoperative radiological resistance can now be also obtained through real-time fluoroscopy and 3D images which have virtually eliminated the use of computed tomography (CT) intraoperatively.
- Diagnostics has also seen a surge with the introduction of 3D and 4D ultrasonography that can easily diagnose tendon lesions or ruptures, ligament injuries, inflammation around muscles, bursa, and joints and have become an indispensable tool to the sports physician. Radiography has also changed from film screen radiography to digital radiography where the images can be directly shared electronically across platforms for cross reference. The magnetic resonance imaging (MRI) is also under constant development with the introduction of higher field strength such as 3 T, 7 T, and 9.4 T that have improved and enhance sensitivity and resolution of images. Now 4D imaging is also being developed using magnetic resonance and days are not far away when neural circuits can be uploaded directly into an MRI and stored as a hard disk. After the successful application of 3D CT scans, 4D CT scans is offering advantages by calculating the motion of respective body part concerning time. This offers deep insights into the functioning of joint during physical motion aiding diagnosis and treatment. The technology can be combined to development of custom-made prosthesis because it is not just the structure of the joint that needs to be reconstructed but the joint functions in varied ways in different individuals so specific functional reconstruction is also now being made possible by the use of this technology. The 4D scanning can detect smallest nonconformities and it will be of exceptional help in future for manufacturing of smart implants tools and devices.
- The advancements in artificial intelligence common nanotechnology and development of exciting new materials along with miniaturization, revolution has been brought about in development of orthosis and prosthetics. Mind control prosthetic arms that can move fingers, electronic gloves offering human-like features for prosthetic hand users, and development of e-dermis has brought the prosthetics to as close as reality as possible. The introduction of sense of touch and pain to prosthetics gives a very important feedback mechanism and the improved perception of patient who no longer considered the artificial part as a distinct entity. Now the patient can walk with a more normal and confident gait allowing him to gain mobility freedom and life back. The neuroprosthetic technology that allows for implementation of sensation of touch in the prosthetics can now be combined to 3D printing and advanced-coating techniques to develop near natural prosthetic parts that can also be implanted into the body. Implantable processes are already a realm but we are still some distance away from development of natural looking prosthetics. Use of artificial intelligence is also giving "eye" to the prosthetics where an off-the-shelf camera is attached near the wrist-facing fingers. When the user moves his/her hand toward an object, a processing algorithm assesses how to place the fingers in the most suitable way to grip the object. Similarly, a camera monitoring ahead of the foot could maneuver the prosthetic foot into the ideal position to help the user to climb steps or walk through tricky patch.
- The next level of development is close collaboration round the globe in determining the cause of diseases at molecular level by next-generation sequencing and finding remedies to most Therapies are being already developed at molecular level by devising specific humanoid antibodies and components that can help to control or cure the disease at the molecular level itself.

IMPROVING PATIENT CARE END EXPLOITING THE DIGITAL AGE BY DOCTORS IN ORTHOPEDICS

Social media offers an extension of physician's persona to online presence and the communication between patient and physician which has been expedited by the combination of internet and digital technology. The following are some of the ways in which this two-way communication or exploiting the digital world has improved the outreach of physicians to the patients as well as the patients have gained more access to the expert care.

- The various social networks and platforms such as Facebook, Twitter, Instagram, and a lot more are being used for prescribing over-the-counter drugs, patient education, creation of referrals, etc. These platforms are also being used for transmitting information and may serve as a source of inspiration for budding orthopedic surgeons.
- Orthopedic surgeons have a major following and are also being regarded as social media influencers in the community being very popular across social media platforms. Sports medicine orthopedic surgeons are most followed among all.
- The patients can select the doctors based on their social media presence along with a peer comparison to the locally available doctors. Although this is useful to some extent, but it has been found that a lot of information uploaded online is either unnecessary or a bit far from

reality or even fake misguiding such as decision by the patient. It is imperative that there should be a regulating body to upload authentic information online so that justified use of this technology can be made accessible to the patient to make an informed decision.

- Internet and social media have improved patient-physician communication to a great degree where messaging Apps provide the two-way communication and a lot of information can be given to the patients by treating doctors that would otherwise need unnecessary physical meeting. The flip side of this is that it has brought patient-physician relationship to an informal level and a lot of times there is unnecessary involvement of the physician in answering irrelevant questions.
- The social media platform is being increasingly used by doctors for advertisement and improving patient awareness by providing online information in an easily perceptible and enhanced manner to understand their problems, possible treatments, and outcomes. This serves well to a limited extent only in the current scenario and again the biggest problem is that a lot of information is not authentic and is biased based on surgeons' own experience or is advertising policy. There is a high need to maintain the online authenticity as much as we will do it offline.
- The biggest use of internet and communication technology is in the field of medical education where novel-networking technologies can be used as a platform for various purposes such as case presentations, communication for help in dealing with complicated and difficult cases, improving the peer review process, and exchanging information for problem solving or brain-storming new ideas. Numerous dedicated sites for orthopedic surgeons are available online that provide topic-wise information ranging from comprehensive policy to detailed description and video presentations along with surgical techniques that can be readily accessed improving the knowledge of the fraternity at large.
- The second biggest advantage of this technology is in enhancing physician-to-physician relationships where researchers can share their ideas and research and find collaborators. This offers knowledge distribution medium where orthopedic surgeons can collaborate and share research and learning. Time is not far away when the whole world will be converted into a literature or a library that can be assessed for solving difficult problems.
- Telehealth and telemedicine can become the future where high-quality healthcare can be delivered without physically traveling to meet the doctor. This has been aided by video conferencing and high-speed internet technology but for orthopedic care presently it is limited to managing follow-up patients because initial diagnosis and evaluation of the patient often needs a thorough physical examination that is of utmost importance.
- Although the digital technology is being exploited for the benefit of patient and surgeon both, but there are a lot of high risks involved in the present scenario being largely unregulated. Various instances of confidentiality breach, threat to reputation, and unprofessional content is being posted online misguiding the patient and surgeon community at large have been reported. The quality of orthopedic information on the internet is low at best, which contradicts and undermines the very purpose of having an online presence bringing disrepute and loss of confidence among patients. There should be strict regulation of the available online information which should be peer reviewed and legal implications including penalties such as fine should be deployed to improve the online content and its authenticity.

CONCLUSION

Digital evolution globally seems to have fast paced the evolution and research seemingly of benefit to the community at large. This has immensely influenced the orthopedic practice. There are a lot of expectations with the use of methods but a lot of concerns of poor quality and fake information and conflicting evidence are cropping up that should be tightly regulated before the misuse becomes rampant and uncontrollable.

Trauma Annexures

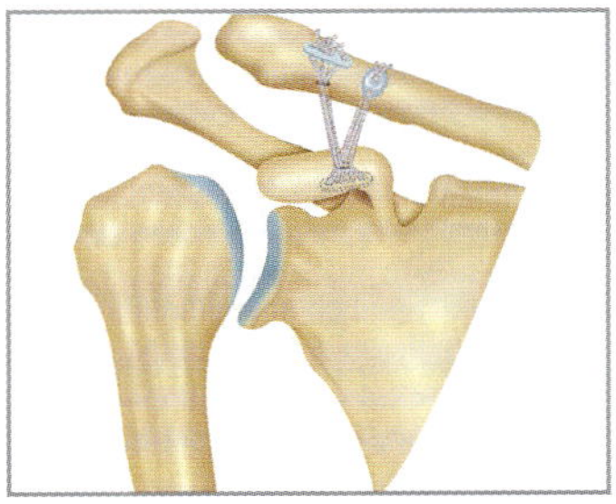

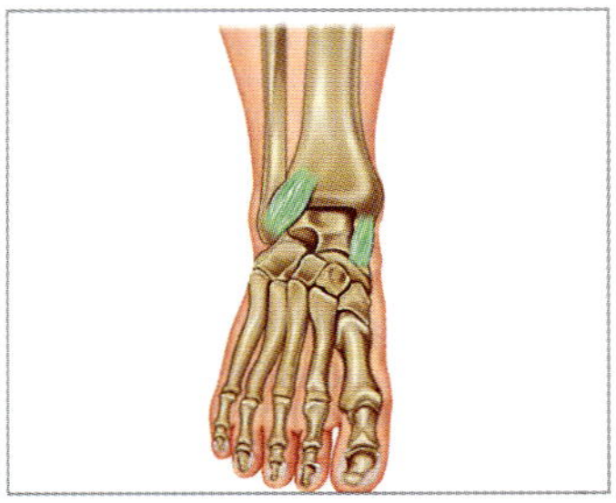

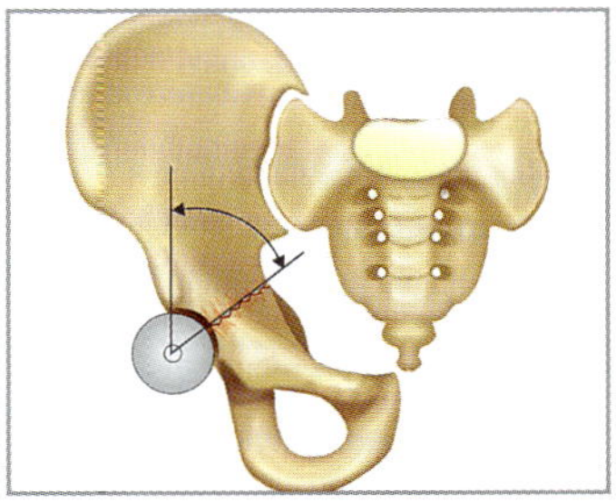

ANNEXURE

1 Upper Limb Trauma

Manish Kumar Varshney

CLAVICLE FRACTURES

Epidemiology	*Anatomy*	*Clinical Evaluation*	*Radiographic Evaluation*	*Treatment*
These comprise 2.6–5% of all the fractures (annual rate of 30 and 60 cases per 100,000 population) and nearly 44–66% of fractures around shoulder. The fracture is seen in all age groups (♂: ♀ = 3:1) mostly young active adults. Alcohol abuse has been linked to increased incidence of fracture clavicle. Middle-third fractures are most common accounting for 76% of all clavicle fractures occurring in teenagers mostly, the lateral end clavicle fractures occurring commonly in middle ages ($\bar{x}$ = 47 years) are second most common comprising 21% while medial third clavicle fracture ($\bar{x}$ = 59 years) comprises only around 3%. **MECHANISM OF INJURY** Most common cause is fall onto the affected shoulder (nearly 87%). Other mechanisms include direct impact—7%, falls onto an outstretched hand (FOOSH) accounting for 6% and rarely secondary to severe muscle contractions in epileptics or pathological fractures (neoplasia). Gunshot wounds, penetrating injuries and stress fractures, are still rare. Displacement results from the sternocleidomastoid (SCM) muscle pulling the medial fragment posterosuperiorly, while pectoralis and weight of arm pulling the lateral fragment inferomedially producing shoulder "ptosis". The displaced fragments may buttonhole through platysma precluding reduction and also predisposing to skin compromise.	[*clavicula* (L) = small key]. Uniquely, clavicle is the first bone to ossify (at 5th week of gestation) and the last one (sternal end ossification center) to fuse (at 22–25 years of age) and only long bone to have intramembranous only ossification. It is the only long bone to lie horizontally and has S-shape (the medial end convex forward and the lateral end concave forward). The lateral end of clavicle gives attachment to coracoclavicular (CC) ligaments inferiorly that has two components—the trapezoid and conoid ligaments. The conoid (medial) gives primary restraint to anterior and superior forces/displacement, while the trapezoid (lateral) is the major restraint to posterior displacement at the acromioclavicular (AC) joint overall giving vertical stability to the AC joint. Three muscles originate from (sternohyoid, pectoralis major, and deltoid) the clavicle, and three muscles insert (SCM), subclavius, trapezius) on it. Medial end is wide and rounded while lateral end is flat joined in middle by a tubular middle segment. The middle third is vulnerable to fracture due to change in configuration from lateral flat to broad medial; transmitting the forces in an uneven way concentrating them in thin center and also due to changed shape from lateral concave to medial convex giving torque to force; muscular cushion is also minimal in the center as also is any ligamentous support.	The most common presentation is splinting of the affected extremity with the arm adducted across the chest cradled by contralateral hand. Shortened shoulder distance, drooping shoulder. Swelling, ecchymosis, crepitus, and tenderness over the clavicle. Examine for neurovascular integrity distal to fracture (brachial plexus, subclavian/axillary vessel injury). Large swelling, extremity discoloration and swelling suggest venous injury. Look for overlying skin compromise, puncture or abrasion, latter suggests direct impact. Auscultate the chest for pneumothorax (apical lung injury). Tachypnea may be present as a result of pain and should not be confused with diminished breath sounds. **ASSOCIATED INJURIES** Up to 9% of patients with clavicle fractures have additional fractures, most commonly rib fractures. Other injuries include ipsilateral scapular fracture (floating shoulder), scapulothoracic dissociation, and vertebral fracture. Intrathoracic injuries include—pneumothorax, subclavian vessel injury (potentially life-threatening), axillary vessel injury, and internal jugular vein injury. Brachial plexus injuries are mostly associated with medial third clavicle fractures.	Standard expiration anteroposterior (AP) radiograph of both sides for assessing shortening (thorax–PA view is best for assessing shortening). A 45° cephalad/caudal tilt view (Quesana views) provides clear image without the overlap of the thorax (cephalad tilt) and facilitates superior-inferior displacement and AP displacement (caudal tilt). An apical oblique view (involved shoulder angled 45° toward the X-ray source, which is angled 20° cephalad) can be helpful in diagnosing minimally displaced fractures (children). Computed tomography (CT) scan useful for medial third fractures (differentiate from sternoclavicular (SC) dislocation, epiphyseal injury) evaluates displacement, comminution, shortening intra-articular extension (lateral third fractures). **CLASSIFICATIONS** **Descriptive** Displaced versus undisplaced, angulation, pattern (e.g., greenstick, oblique, and transverse), comminution, etc.—vague and not useful. **Allman (Fig. 1, similar to Neer's) Classification** *Group 1:* Fracture of middle one-third, most common *Group 2:* Fracture distal to CC ligament, nonunion common *Group 3:* Fractures of proximal end clavicle	**NONOPERATIVE** Most clavicle fractures [nondisplaced group 1, stable group 2 (types I, III, and IV), nondisplaced group III and pediatric distal clavicle fractures also) are treated successfully nonoperatively with simple immobilization in a sling or elbow support and analgesics till pain is bearable (2–3 weeks) followed by intermittent passive or assisted shoulder range of motion (ROM) exercises starting at 2–4 weeks and strengthening exercises by 6–10 weeks when the immobilization is completely taken off. Active ROM of the elbow, wrist, and hand should be performed at all times. Figure-of-eight bandage has fallen out-of-favor due to discomfort, skin problems, and frequent loosening precluding the very purpose of passive reduction. Clavicle braces may fare better. Passive reduction was aimed to raise the lateral fragment in an upward, outward, and backward direction while simultaneously depressing the medial fragment; but that frequently failed. Currently, the immobilization is aimed to support the shoulder girdle, maintain some degree of fracture reduction by supporting the elbow and countering downward pull of gravity, allowing the patient to use the ipsilateral hand and elbow. In significant number of longer-term studies and opinion of experts, no intervention is *NOT* the best option perhaps as nearly half of the patients suffer from sequelae. Complication of nonoperative treatment includes—malunion (shortening and deformity), nonunion (nearly 15% at 6 months fail to unite; predisposing factors—group II) comminuted

Contd...

Contd...

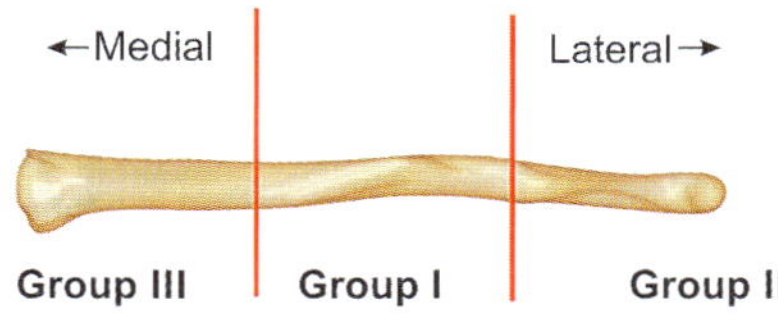

Fig. 1: Allman classification of clavicle fractures—descriptive illustration of classifying a left clavicle fracture.

Epidemiology	*Anatomy*	*Clinical Evaluation*	*Radiographic Evaluation*	*Treatment*
	The middle-third fractures displace with superior angulation, the medial end migrates superiorly due to pull of SCM, while the lateral end is pulled down by subclavius and intact CC ligaments. There is obligatory coupling of clavicle rotation with scapular motion and arm elevation, so one must not fix the AC joint by joint spanning methods of CC screws. This will restrict movement or hardware will ultimately fail. With respect to the thorax during elevation of the arm, the clavicle undergoes elevation of 11–15° and retraction of 15–29°. Also, there is 5–8° of rotation at the AC joint with forward elevation and abduction to 180°. *Functional and clinical importance:* The clavicle is the only bone strut connecting the shoulder and arm to the trunk and allowing the shoulder to function at optimal distance and strength. The medial and middle thirds provide protection to brachial plexus, subclavian and axillary vessels, and apex of lung. The vein is most medial followed by artery and brachial plexus lying most lateral. Vein may sit on the periosteum inferoposteriorly making it prone to injury by inadvertent drill bit passage or a long screw. Surgeon should always recheck, if screw length is >16 mm. Injury to subclavian vein may produce air embolism causing death. This complication is more common in late presentations or nonunion release where fragments or fibrous tissue may adhere to the neurovascular structures. One should release and clearly see the posteroinferior periosteum and protect the area. This anatomical description entails that, in medial thirds, superior to inferior trajectory for drilling is safe, while in middle thirds, anteroinferior to posterosuperior path would be safer. It is also safer to use positive pressure ventilation as added protection against air embolism or pneumothorax in case of venous injury.		**Craig Classification** *Group I:* Fracture of the middle third. Proximal and distal segments are secured by ligamentous and muscular attachments. *Group II:* Fracture of the distal third. This is subclassified according to the location of the CC ligaments relative to the fracture **(Fig. 2)**: *Type I*: Minimally displaced: Interligamentous fracture between the conoid and trapezoid or between the CC and AC ligaments; ligaments intact. *Type II*: Displaced secondary to a fracture medial to the CC ligaments: higher incidence of nonunion. IIA: Conoid and trapezoid attached to the distal segment. IIB: Conoid torn, trapezoid attached to the distal segment. *Type III*: Fracture into articular surface of the AC joint with no ligamentous injury: may be confused with first-degree AC joint separation. *Type IV*: Fractures in children, intact CC ligaments attached to periosteal sleeve, proximal fragment displaced *Type V*: Comminuted fractures, conoid and trapezoid ligaments remain attached to comminuted fragment. *Group III:* Fracture of the proximal third. Minimal displacement results, if the costoclavicular ligaments remain intact. It may represent epiphyseal injury in children and teenagers. Subgroups include: *Type I*: Minimal displacement *Type II*: Displaced—anterior displacement usually innocuous, posterior displacement may compromise airway and great vessels. *Type III*: Intra-articular *Type IV*: Epiphyseal separation *Type V*: Comminuted	fracture, vertical displacement >100%, or >2 cm separation or shortening >2 cm, old age females, smoking (strong association), severity of initial trauma, soft tissue interposition, refracture, inadequate period of immobilization), reduced shoulder strength and endurance, neurovascular compression from large callus, AC joint/SC joint arthritis (intra-articular fractures), and poor cosmesis. Shortening of clavicle where scapula is brought nearer to axial skeleton leads to loss of strength and poorer outcome. These along with symptomatic nonunion and malunion rates of 15–20% variously reported have rejuvinated interest in surgery for clavicle fractures. **OPERATIVE** The indications for operative treatment of fracture clavicle include: • Open fracture • Associated vascular compromise • Potential of skin compromise (tenting) • Displaced group I—displacement >100%, shortening >2 cm • Unstable group II fractures (types IIA, IIB, and V) • Posteriorly displaced group III fractures [keep Cardiovascular and Thoracic Surgery (CTVS) surgeon on hold] • Floating shoulder (clavicle fracture associated with scapular neck fracture) • Symptomatic nonunion • Relative—brachial plexus injury (>two-thirds recover), closed head injury, polytrauma, epilepsy, and failure to tolerate conservative management. Shortening (>2 cm) is the most debated topic but proponents say it leads to shoulder dysfunction and patient dissatisfaction due to shoulder ptosis with the resulting cosmetic deformity. Some discrepancy also exists over undisplaced group II fractures where it is considered that union will occur most of times with conservative management alone. **Methods of Open Reduction and Internal Fixation** Plate and screw osteosynthesis: 3.5-mm recon plate or anatomical locking compression plate (LCP) are the best choice positioned either superiorly or anteroinferiorly on clavicle. Former is a biomechanically stronger construct with higher load to failure even for comminuted fractures but is fraught with more neurovascular complications while drilling.

Contd...

Contd...

Epidemiology	*Anatomy*	*Clinical Evaluation*	*Radiographic Evaluation*	*Treatment*
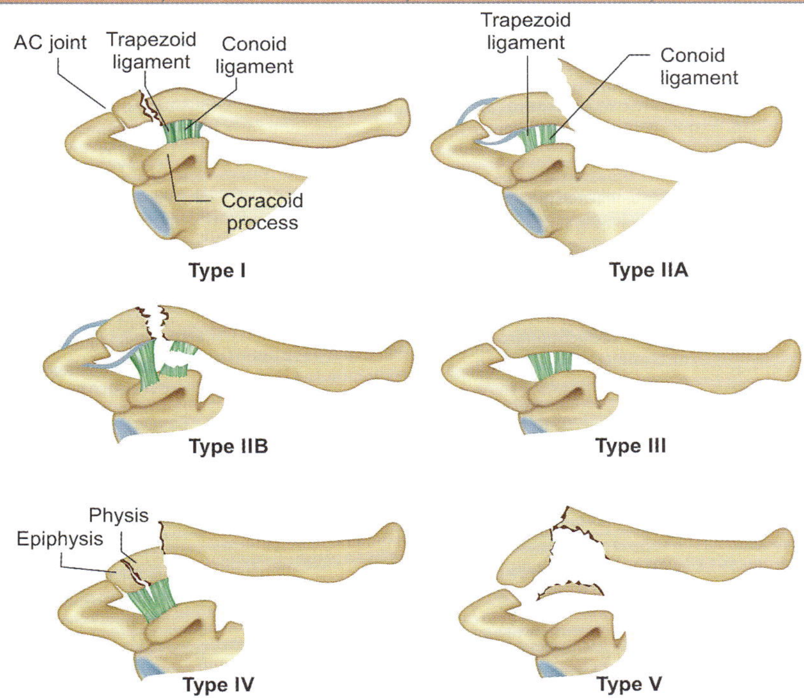 **Fig. 2:** Illustration for Craig group II fractures of clavicle.				Superior plate is also more prominent. Hook plates are not commonly used. It is recommended to use bicortical screws in medial and lateral thirds but unicortical screws in middle thirds for safer fixation (see anatomy also). Intramedullary screw/pin (Hagie pin, Rockwood pin)/nail (TENS)—to reduce the extensive exposure needed for plate and screw fixation. Difficult in Indian population due to narrow medullary canal and short-curved clavicles. Higher complication rate of implant migration and less secure fixation. Skin erosion at the hardware insertion site laterally is another concern. For reducible fractures, the nail is pushed retrograde but for open reduction and internal fixation (ORIF), it is placed in antegrade fashion through the lateral fragment and then in retrograde fashion into the medial fragment. For type II distal clavicle fractures, ligament reconstruction of ligament to reduce the medial fragment is important maneuver. This is accomplished by using either coracoclavicular fixation/reconstruction [Mersilene tape, suture anchors, endobutton, wires (tension band), or screws] or fixation across the AC joint, through the lateral fragment and into the medial fragment. ***Complications of surgical management include:*** Reoperation rate is very high (100% for intramedullary, 30% for plating) and mostly involves implant removal although that is not a complication per se. Taller patients have high rate of plate removal, especially if nonprecontoured plates are used. *Neurovascular injury (3%)*: Uncommon but results from penetration of drill or screw into vital structures or from subclavian thrombosis. • Hardware prominence nonunion (1–5%) • *Malunion*: Uncommon but may result in severely comminuted fracture/open fracture. • Unacceptable scar infection • Implant failure pneumothorax • Reactive shoulder effusion/pain and adhesive capsulitis • Complex regional pain syndrome (CRPS) • AC joint arthritis (distal third intra-articular fractures) • Numb patch below the scar due to cutaneous nerve injury

ACROMIOCLAVICULAR JOINT INJURY/SEPARATION

Epidemiology	*Anatomy*	*Clinical Evaluation*	*Radiographic Evaluation*	*Treatment*
Accounts for nearly 10–12% of shoulder girdle injuries. Active or athletic young adult males participating in contact athletic activities in the second decade of life are commonly affected. Most of the disruptions are incomplete (Types I and II) rather than complete in a ratio of 2:1. ♂:♀ = 5 to 10:1.	AC joint is a diarthrodial joint between lateral end of clavicle and acromion, with the bony ends covered by fibrocartilage. It is stabilized by four articular and two extra-articular ligaments (coracoacromial ligament is redundant for stability) and a meniscus inside along with the dynamic muscular support. Joint	The characteristic presenting feature is a downward sag of the shoulder and upper extremity with prominent lateral clavicle end and tenting of skin. Local tenderness can be elicited. Deformity can be pronounced by placing the upper extremity in a dependent position and even giving a downward pull to it.	Bilateral anteroposterior—radiographs for comparison of CC distance Scapular-Y, and axillary views help to diagnose type IV injury. Stress AP radiograph taken by tying weights (5–7 kg) strapped to the wrists is not of much help and painful so not recommended. This had been classically used to differentiate	The main goals of treatment irrespective of modality are to provide a pain-free shoulder with full ROM, normal strength, and no limitations in activities. **NONOPERATIVE** This is recommended for pseudodislocations, type I and II injuries and most type III injuries. Modalities include nonsteroidal

Contd...

Contd...

Epidemiology	Anatomy	Clinical Evaluation	Radiographic Evaluation	Treatment
MECHANISM OF INJURY *Direct:* Fall onto the adducted shoulder transmits force driving the acromion medial and inferior to the clavicle thus causing disruption of the AC joint. The downward displacement of the clavicle is primarily resisted through an interlocking of the SC and CC ligaments. *Indirect:* This is FOOSH injury where force is transmitted through the humeral head into AC articulation displacing the acromion superiorly. This is usually not associated with CC disruption.	width reduces from 1–3 mm in young age to <0.5 mm in the elderly. The joint may be inclined vertically or medially 50° making the joint both horizontally and vertically vulnerable. The horizontal stability of the AC joint is conferred by the AC ligaments (anterior, posterior, superior, and inferior) that strengthen capsule, whereas the vertical stability is maintained by the CC ligaments **(Fig. 3)**. The superior AC ligament confers 56% stability while posterior confers 25% resistance to posterior displacement. CC ligament has two parts—conoid and trapezoid, while the latter inserts 3 cm from end of clavicle and the former inserts 4.5 cm from end of clavicle in the posterior border. The conoid (medial) gives primary restraint to anterior and superior forces/displacement, while the trapezoid (lateral) provides restraint to posterior displacement at the AC joint. Overall AC ligaments are the primary restraints to posterior instability (89%) and also the posterior translation (68%). With increasing deformation, conoid ligament becomes primary restraint (62%) while AC ligaments still maintain the posterior stability. Trapezoid provides primary restraint to AC joint compression. The average CC distance is 1.1–1.3 cm that may be maintained in base of coracoid fractures but still mimic AC separation due to (pseudo-) CC disruption. The superior shoulder suspensory complex (SSSC) is a ligamento-osseous ring composed of the upper part of glenoid, the coracoid process, the CC ligament, the distal clavicle, the AC joint, and the acromial process.	Range of shoulder motion may be limited by pain. In standing or sitting position, stress the AC joint horizontally for AC ligament assessment and stress vertically for CC ligament assessment. Assess neurovascular status and possible associated other upper extremity injuries. *Paxinos test is perfromed by placing* thumb pressure at the posterior AC joint to elicit tenderness and instability. *Cross-arm adduction test:* The arm is elevated to 90° and then adducted across the chest with the elbow bent at approximately 90° to rest the hand on other shoulder. This cross-arm adduction produces pain specifically at the AC joint. *O'Brien's active compression test:* It helps to differentiate symptoms of AC joint arthrosis from intra-articular superior glenoid labrum (SLAP lesion). The test is performed with the arm elevated to 90°, elbow in extension, adduction of 10–15°, and a maximum pronation of the forearm with obligate internal rotation of the arm. The examiner applies a downward force resisted by the patient. Symptoms referred to the top of the shoulder indicate AC joint lesion. This can be confirmed by palpation of the AC joint. Symptoms referred to the anterior glenohumeral joint suggest labral or biceps injury. **ASSOCIATED INJURIES** Fractures of clavicle, acromion process, and coracoid process. Pneumothorax or pulmonary contusion may be associated with type VI AC separations.	grade III AC separations from partial grade I to II injuries but as mostly types I to III are all treated conservatively and due to possibility of false positive results, surgeons are questioning the radiograph. Instead, Zanca view is recommended performed by tilting the X-ray beam 10–15° toward the cephalic direction and using only 50% of the standard shoulder anteroposterior penetration. **CLASSIFICATIONS** This injury is classified depending on the degree and direction of displacement of the distal clavicle. **Rockwood Classification of AC Joint Injuries (Fig. 4)** Based on the degree and direction of displacement of the distal clavicle. *Type I:* Sprain of the AC ligament, intact joint capsule, intact CC ligament, deltoid, and trapezius. *Type II:* Rupture of the AC ligament and joint capsule, sprain of the CC ligament but intact CC interspace (<25% increase), minimal detachment of the deltoid and trapezius. *Type III:* Rupture of the AC ligament, joint capsule, and CC ligament; elevated clavicle (25–100% displacement); detachment of the deltoid and trapezius. *Type IV:* Posterior displacement of clavicle into the trapezius. Rupture of the AC ligament, joint capsule, and CC ligament; detachment of the deltoid and trapezius. *Type V:* Superior displacement of clavicle (>100%)	anti-inflammatory drugs (NSAIDs), ice therapy, activity modification, and complete rest (1 week for type-I, longer for type II and III). Simple sling or elbow support in brace would help. Physical therapy should then be started with both passive and active shoulder motion and contact sports and weight lifting only allowed once the patient is completely pain free and ROM is similar to uninjured shoulder. Warn patients that pain may persist for 6 months at AC joint and a significant minority (33%) may experience it till 6 years. For type III injury, the management is still controversial but significantly tilted to nonoperative having equivalent results as for type I or II injury. Cosmetic deformity, however, persists and functional improvement is nonlimiting (reduced power only of extreme activities such as bench press). To maximize function in high-demand athletes and overhead activity requiring jobs, some authors have advocated surgery for acute type III AC joint injuries in young patients. **OPERATIVE TREATMENT** Indicated for patients with type-III AC joint injuries for which nonsurgical treatment is unacceptable (see above) or had been unsuccessful as well as for medically stable patients with type-IV–VI AC joint injuries. A number of methods and modifications had been proposed but common to them are—anatomic reduction of the AC joint correcting superior displacement and anterior–posterior translation; direct repair (acute injury) or reconstruction (chronic injury) of the CC ligament,

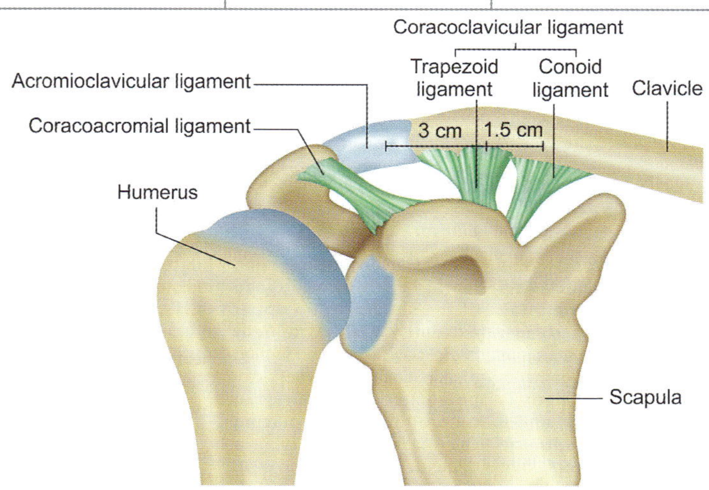

Fig. 3: Acromioclavicular joint anatomy with respect to disposition of ligaments.

Contd...

Contd...

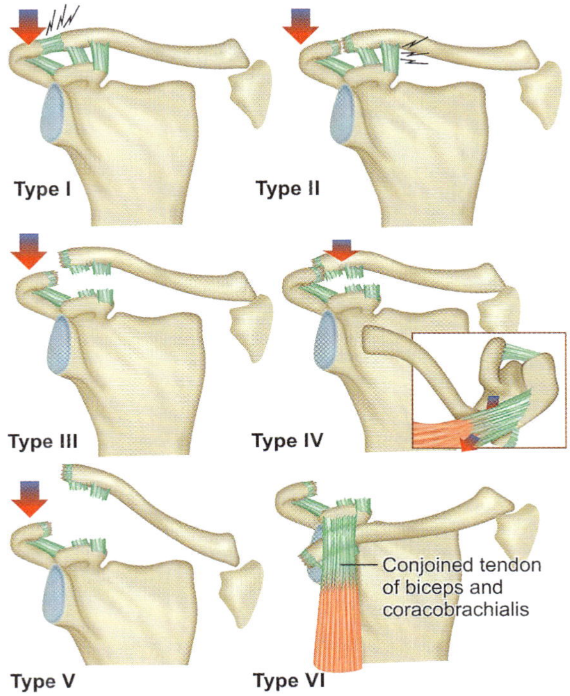

Fig. 4: Rockwood classification of six types of acromioclavicular joint disruption. Arrows depict the typical direction of force producing the injury pattern.

Epidemiology	*Anatomy*	*Clinical Evaluation*	*Radiographic Evaluation*	*Treatment*
	The displacement resulting in subcutaneous superior bony strut comprises the mid-shaft clavicle and the inferior bony strut is made by the junction of the lateral scapular body and the medial glenoid neck. Type III, IV, V, and VI AC separations comprise double disruptions of this complex where both the CC and AC ligaments are injured needing combined assessment and stabilization preferably. Inherently, the AC joint has minimal mobility and the fibrocartilaginous intra-articular disk demonstrates an age-related degeneration until it is essentially nonfunctional beyond the 4th decade. *Pediatric AC joint*: Here, the clavicle is encased in thick periosteum that also encompasses CC ligament while AC ligaments are separate, so it gets damaged more frequently.	**DIFFERENTIAL DIAGNOSIS** AC joint arthritis, intraarticular pathology, osteolysis of distal clavicle, degenerative instability of AC joint, rotator-cuff impingement, adhesive capsulitis, thoracic outlet syndrome, SLAP lesions, CRPS, fracture of lateral clavicle, coracoid fracture.	clavicle. Rupture of the AC ligament, joint capsule, and CC ligament; rupture of deltotrapezial fascia *Type VI (rare)*: Inferior displacement of clavicle into subcoracoid or subacromial position. Clavicle may lie behind the tendons of the biceps and coracobrachialis rupture of acromioclavicular ligament, joint capsule, and CC ligament. **Rockwood Classification of Pediatric Acromioclavicular Injuries** *Type I*: Stable clavicle; radiographically normal joint. *Type II*: Partial tear of the periosteal tube, allowing for some mobility of the distal clavicle; disrupted AC ligament. *Types III–VI*: Larger tear through the periosteal tube, allowing for greater clavicle mobility and gross instability with clavicle positioning; the CC ligament remains attached to the clavicle periosteal tube (pseudodislocation).	supplementation or protection of the CC ligament repair or reconstruction with synthetic material, rigid implant may be used to maintain AC joint stability during initial healing; repair of dynamic stabilizers (deltoid, trapezius); distal clavicular resection in patients with chronic acromioclavicular injuries where AC joint arthritis is present. *Resection of distal clavicle*: Simple resection is never recommended for AC joint injury; it should be combined with ligament reconstruction. *Repair of native ligaments*: This is possible for acute injuries that present within 7–10 days ideally, later ligaments become friable and may contract. Suture anchors are a good help but repairs are not very popular because of difficult access and inability to take sutures through ligament that has consistency like a painting brush. *Direct AC joint stabilization:* This appears to be the most logical treatment as radiological pathology is located here but it is actually a nonanatomical treatment. Mostly these methods are used to supplement CC repair/

Contd...

Contd...

Epidemiology	Anatomy	Clinical Evaluation	Radiographic Evaluation	Treatment

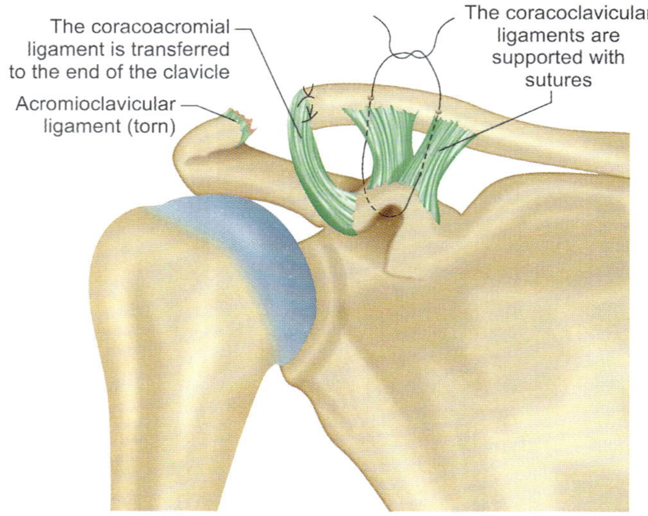

Fig. 5: Weaver–Dunn procedure for coracoclavicular ligament reconstruction. The coracoacromial ligament is transferred to the distal clavicle stabilizing the coracoclavicular gap and hence secondarily the acromioclavicular joint.

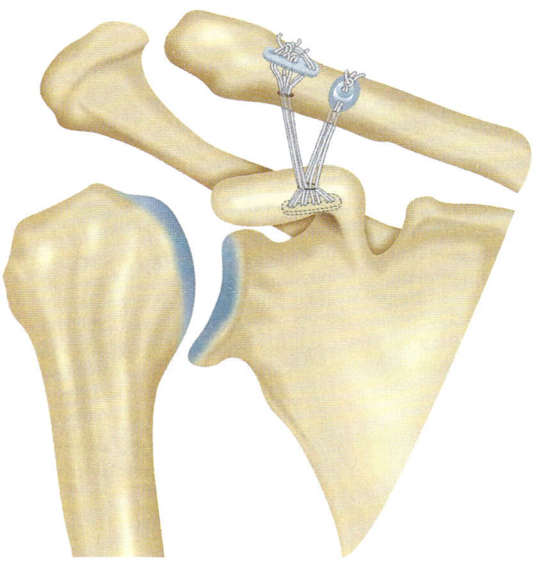

Fig. 6: Reconstruction of coracoclavicular ligament using endobuttons.

reconstruction. The methods include Bosworth screw fixation of CC region, AC joint fixation by tension band/wires, Hook plate fixation, etc. Rigid fixation prevents biological movements at AC joint as discussed in anatomy so it is not physiological.

CC ligament reconstruction:
These are the most preferred method(s) and so many modifications exist that it is difficult to list all here. Few of these are:

Weaver–Dunn procedure: Transfer of coracoacromial ligament to the distal clavicle to recreate CC ligament **(Fig. 5)**. Distal clavicle excision is needed. Added internal fixation needed as reconstruction has only 20% strength of native CC ligament. Arthroscopic modification is described. Augmentation with tendon or fascia auto-/allograft has also been described.

CC ligament reconstruction with biological tissue: Figure of eight or rectangular reconstruction of CC ligament using palmaris longus or other tendon or fascia lata. Reinforce with internal fixation. The reconstruction may be done only for conoid component or for both conoid and trapezoid components (anatomical).

CC reconstruction with sutures/tapes: This first commonly preferred for anatomical biligament reconstruction using endobutton **(Fig. 6)** and Mersilene tape. Suture/tapes are placed either around or through (preferred) clavicle and around the base of the coracoid, suture anchors may also be used. To prevent excess anterior translation of clavicle, the drill hole should be made in anterior thirds of bone for conoid portion. Simple cerclage around clavicle with suture or wire loops has chances of slippage and fracture of clavicle from attrition.

Complications of operative management:
- Coracoclavicular ossification
- Distal clavicle osteolysis
- AC arthritis
- Fracture of clavicle

STERNOCLAVICULAR JOINT DISRUPTION

Epidemiology	Anatomy	Clinical Evaluation	Radiographic Evaluation	Treatment
Injuries to the SC joint are rare accounting for nearly 3% of the injuries around shoulder girdle as reported in a large review and represents 1% of all dislocations in the body. Superior, anterior, and posterior dislocations **(Fig. 7)** of SC joint are reported but by far anterior traumatic dislocations are common.	The SC joint is a double arthrodial (double plane-saddle) joint with little intrinsic stability, formed by the medial end of clavicle, manubrium, and 1st rib cartilage. This joint in actual represents the only true articulation between the upper extremity and the axial skeleton. Intrinsic instability results from incongruously	Swelling, tenderness, and painful range of shoulder motion are usually present, with a variable change of the medial clavicular prominence, depending on the degree and direction of injury. The patient presents holding the injured limb across the trunk with the contralateral, uninjured arm/hand. SCM	The PA chest radiographs typically demonstrate asymmetry of the clavicles. Look also for the presence of pneumothorax. This is more helpful for anterior dislocation, especially if combined with panoramic view. *Oblique views:* Prevent distortion due to overlapping of clavicles.	In general, anterior dislocation is treated by closed reduction failing which still conservative treatment is commonly followed. For posterior dislocations, the initial treatment is closed reduction only if there is no neurovascular compromise failing which however ligament reconstruct for joint

Contd...

Contd...

Epidemiology	*Anatomy*	*Clinical Evaluation*	*Radiographic Evaluation*	*Treatment*
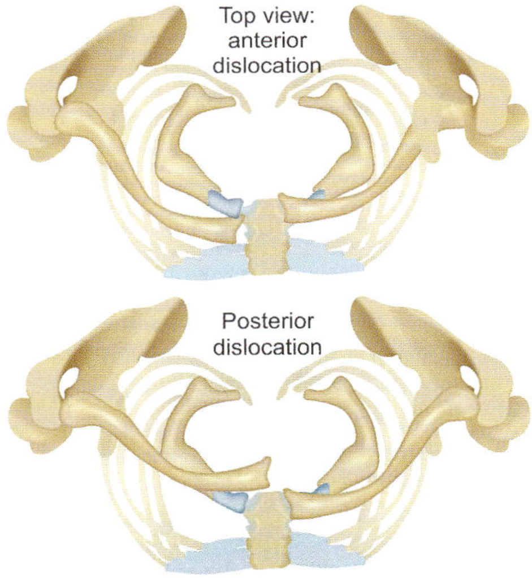 **Fig. 7:** The two types of sternoclavicular joint dislocations.				
MECHANISM OF INJURY **Traumatic** As the medial end of clavicle is the last bone to unite in body, so most injuries in patients <22–25 years are physeal injuries (Salter–Harris Type I or II) and true joint dislocations are extremely rare, further if any dislocation is seen it is usually in anterior direction and posterior displacements are still rare in children. *Direct (causing posterior dislocation):* Here, the posterior dislocations result from direct force applied to the anterior or anteromedial aspect of the clavicle that disrupts the strong posterior ligaments and push clavicle posteriorly into the mediastinum. Such an injury is less common and may occur in direct steering wheel impact injury or in athletes where they are pressed by other athletes falling directly on them lying supine or in run-over injury from vehicles or when a vehicle hits from front on an individual blocked by a wall/block behind. *Indirect (more common mechanism, causing anterior or posterior SC dislocation,* ***Figs. 8A and B****):* Here, the force is transmitted indirectly to the SC joint through clavicle from shoulder as in fall on an outstretched hand (FOOSH). Force applied from anterior or anterolateral aspect to the shoulder produces anterior SC dislocation, as the shoulder is pushed behind while clavicle levers the SC joint *anteriorly*	large surface of the clavicle (double) articulating with sternum; both are covered with fibrocartilage. Joint stability is derived mainly from the saddle-like configuration of the joint (convex vertically and concave anteroposteriorly), as well as from surrounding ligaments **(Fig. 9)**: The intra-articular fibrocartilage disk acts as shock absorber and its ligament attachment resist posteromedial displacement of the clavicle. The capsular ligaments (anterior, posterior) represent capsular thickenings and prevent superior displacement of the medial clavicle. They are the strongest structures stabilizing the joint. Posterior ligament is twice as thicker than the anterior. Posterosuperior capsule is tough enough to avulse bone before itself giving way. This part also maintains the lateral clavicle end up which was previously considered to be a function of trapezius. Posterior capsular ligament primary restraint to both anterior and posterior translation of the clavicle. The extra-articular costoclavicular (rhomboid) ligament is a short stout ligament that arises from the upper surface of the first rib and its chondrosternal junction to attach to the inferior surface of the medial clavicle. It primarily resists superior rotation (anterior fibers) and possibly lateral–superior displacement.	spasm may tilt patient's head toward the side of injury, this also reduces stress across SC joint. Pain is often poorly localized, and may be described as being in the neck or even jaw. Posterior dislocation may present in emergency with complaints of dyspnea, difficulty swallowing, or a choking sensation. *Waters test*: Localized lateral compression on shoulder exacerbates pain. Lying down supine is similarly nearly impossible in grade II to III injuries as protraction of scapula exacerbates pain, though this makes the deformity prominent. Neurovascular status must be assessed carefully. Especially look for venous congestion and evaluate distal pulses. Also, make a quick neurological examination for brachial plexus. The chest must be auscultated to ensure bilaterally symmetric breath sounds. **ASSOCIATED INJURIES** *(Associated with posterior dislocation, seen in 25% cases):* • Pneumothorax • Laceration of the superior vena cava • Venous congestion in the neck • Esophageal rupture • Subclavian artery compression • Carotid artery compression • Recurrent laryngeal nerve injury • Severe thoracic outlet syndrome	*Hobbs view:* In this 90° cephalocaudal lateral view, the patient leans over the plate, and the radiographic beam is angled behind the neck. *Serendipity view:* This is a bilateral view with the X-ray beam tilted 40° cephalically aimed at the manubrium allowing direct comparison of one side to another. With an anterior dislocation, the medial clavicle raises above the interclavicular line while it lies below in a posterior dislocation. *Computed tomography (CT) scan:* This is the investigation of choice to evaluate SC injuries. It differentiates fractures of the medial clavicle from SC dislocation as well as delineates minor joint subluxations. A contrast enhanced CT is most preferred technique for a suspected posterior dislocation because it can assess the direction of dislocation and the underlying vasculature and soft tissues. This may be combined with angiography/venography for vascular injury. **CLASSIFICATIONS** **Anatomic** Anterior versus posterior versus superior **Allman Classification of SC Joint Injury** *Grade I*: Sprain without ligament laxity or joint irregularity, ligamentous integrity maintained.	stabilization will be needed. For posterior dislocations that cause vascular compression or injury, open reduction and stabilization will be needed. **CONSERVATIVE MANAGEMENT** It is done for type I and II injuries—immobilize for few days to weeks in a sling along with analgesia and ice application. A clavicle strap, sling and swathe, or figure-of-eight bandage for 1 week, then sling immobilization for 4–6 weeks for grade II injuries. Closed reduction is recommended for al grade III injuries, if there is no emergent other indication (such as vascular compromise for posterior dislocations). Closed reduction usually fails due to local ligamentous injury and the cephalad pull of the sternocleidomastoid, soft tissue interposed at the fracture site, and the long lever arm of the upper extremity that tends to displace the medial end of the clavicle. *Anterior dislocations:* The conservative and operative management are both controversial as closed reduction is associated with a recurrence rate of between 21 and 100% and against operative management, the argument is the perceived fact that there is little if any impact of chronic anterior dislocation. What favors the operative management still is the fact that SC joint is an important link between axial skeleton and upper limb. Closed reduction may be accomplished using general anesthesia, or sedation and muscle relaxants

Contd...

Contd...

<table>
<tr><th>Epidemiology</th><th>Anatomy</th><th>Clinical Evaluation</th><th>Radiographic Evaluation</th><th>Treatment</th></tr>
<tr><td colspan="5">
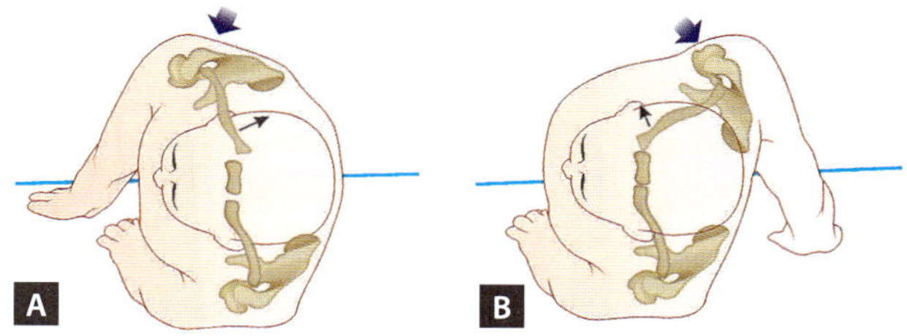

Figs. 8A and B: Mechanism of posterior (A) and anterior (B) sternoclavicular joint dislocations.

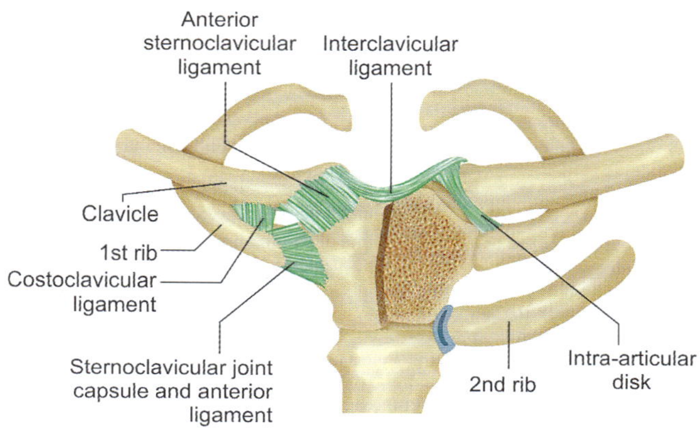

Fig. 9: Illustrated anatomy of the medial end clavicle articulation with the sternum (sternoclavicular joint).
</td></tr>
<tr>
<td>(like seesaw). The same force, if applied from a more posterior or posterolateral direction will lever the SC joint posteriorly acting through clavicle thereby producing a posterior SC dislocation. These injuries are seen in side-on vehicle collision or in athletes lying in oblique direction with other athletes falling onto them. Anteroinferior-directed force on ribcage produces surprisingly a posterosuperior SC dislocation as demonstrated in Bearn's vertical loading in cadaver specimens. Superior clavicle dislocation is reported rarely to result from direct downward force transmitted to shoulder lifting the medial clavicle up from lever action (like seesaw).

Atraumatic
Mostly result from generalized ligamentous laxity typically in young (<20 years) females but may also be seen in individuals without ligament laxity [developmental (congenital) dislocation, osteoarthritis, condensing osteitis hyperostosis, or infection]. Anterior dislocation will be apparent with elevation of the arm and reduce when the arm is returned to the side. Posterior spontaneous dislocation is very rare.</td>
<td>Posterior fibers resist inferior rotation and inferomedial dislocation. The primary function of the ligament is to provide a pivot for clavicle rotation rather than stability. The interclavicular ligament is a thickening of capsule connecting the two SC joints superiorly and has limited if any stabilizing role.

Movements
SC joint ROM is 60° of frontal plane elevation–depression, 20–30° of AP translation, 30–50° of rotation around its long axis and is possibly the most frequently moved joint of the long bones in the body. Within the first 90° of arm elevation, the clavicle elevates 4° for every 10° of arm elevation, with negligible motion after 90°.</td>
<td></td>
<td>Grade II: Subluxation with partial ligamentous disruption. There is moderate-to-strong pain with movement and palpation, and usually swelling over the joint. Anterior/posterior capsular ligaments may be torn but costoclavicular ligaments remain intact.
Grade III: Unstable joint, with complete ligamentous compromise. The ipsilateral shoulder may appear shortened and protracted.

Temporal Classification
Acute dislocation versus recurrent dislocation versus unreduced dislocation
Etiological classification:
Atraumatic versus traumatic</td>
<td>placing the patient supine with a roll between and underneath the scapulae (in early cases <5 days old). Direct, posteriorly directed pressure usually results in reduction. Postreduction provides a clavicle strap, sling, or figure-of-eight bandage for 4–6 weeks. A bulky anterior dressing with elastic tape may be applied to maintain reduction.
Posterior dislocations: I am a bit wary of conservative management for this dislocation as even if absent at initial presentation; problems/complications do creep in later. Even if inconspicuous, a posterior dislocation should be thoroughly investigated for presence of occult complication (such as vascular injury). Even if one attempts closed reduction do it under GA with vascular surgeon as standby. The success rate of closed reduction (abduction traction technique) is nearly two-thirds of the cases for acute dislocations. With patient supine and towel under the scapulae, apply traction to the arm first followed by extension of elbow and shoulder (Fig. 10).
Clavicle reduction can be assisted by towel clip pulling anteriorly. Usually, the reduction is stable and can be maintained by above techniques.</td>
</tr>
</table>

Contd...

Contd...

Epidemiology	*Anatomy*	*Clinical Evaluation*	*Radiographic Evaluation*	*Treatment*
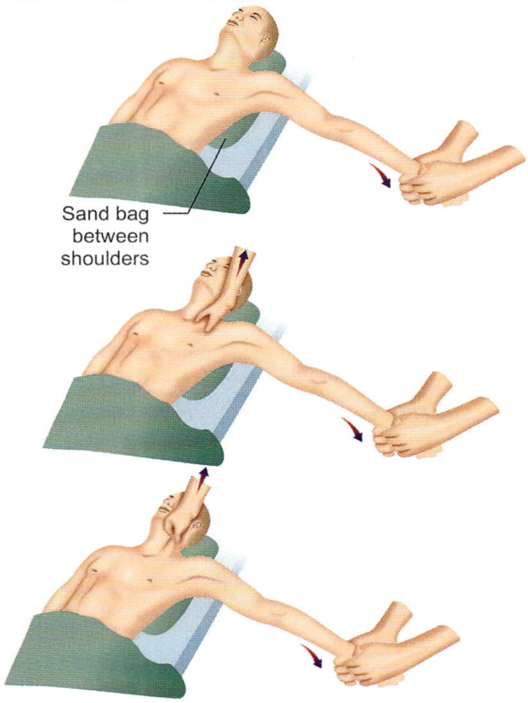 **Fig. 10:** Illustration demonstrating method of closed reduction for a posterior sternoclavicular joint dislocation.				*Physeal injuries*: Anterior dislocations/injuries are easy to reduce but difficult to maintain. They usually remodel well without much further treatment. Posterior dislocation should be attempted for closed reduction with above precautions. **SURGICAL MANAGEMENT** Proponents portend soft tissue interposition, difficulty in maintaining closed reduction, vascular compromise (posterior dislocations) and late cases necessitating reduction (unresolved closed reduction; anterior—cosmetic reasons, posterior—mediastinal compromise) to be the main indications of operating treatment. The aim is to achieve a stable and congruous SC articulation. Tenodesis, suture fixation, and ORIF have the highest percentage of excellent/good results in adults. Closed reduction of anterior dislocations usually fails due to complete loss of ligamentous support resulting from anterior periosteum disruption so along with nonabsorbable suture repair, one needs to necessarily repair the periosteum. For acute injury, suturing of SC ligaments and CC (costoclavicular) ligaments with/without suture anchor is recommended. For chronic symptomatic anterior SC dislocation, reconstruction of the anterior SC ligament is done using fascia lata or semitendinosus tendon (preferred) or medial portion of sternal head of SCM muscle. CC reconstruction can also be done for chronic dislocations using fascia lata, subclavius muscle transposition, or tenodesis of sternal head of SCM muscle. Balser plate fixation (akin to hook plate for AC joint stabilization) has been used by selective author only, tension band wiring (TBW) of SC joint, K-wire fixation, and resection of medial end of clavicle are not recommended due to high dissatisfactory results and complications. Maintain the limb with brace support for 3–6 weeks avoiding elevating the upper extremity above 60° for 4 weeks. **COMPLICATIONS (CONSERVATIVE/SURGICAL)** • Poor cosmesis (enlarged medial prominence) • Migration of hardware (into heart/artery) • Injury to mediastinal and deeper structures • Failure of hardware

SCAPULA FRACTURES AND INJURIES

Epidemiology

It is an uncommon injury and it represents some 3–5% of all shoulder girdle fractures and 0.4–1% of all fractures with an annual incidence of 10 per 100,000 population. The fractures are seen and commonly managed at level 1 trauma centers as most result from high-energy injuries where associated injuries and polytrauma/multiorgan are common.

The mean age of patients with fracture of the scapula is 35–45 years.

MECHANISM OF INJURY

Fractures of the scapula commonly occur from a high-energy blunt-force mechanism. Direct trauma occurs from a blow or fall as in motor vehicle accidents (scapula body fracture) or through direct trauma to the point of the shoulder (acromion, coracoid fracture).

Protection from impact is provided by the surrounding muscles and also the mobility of the scapula on the chest wall, further aiding in force dissipation. Direct high-energy impact can cause fracture of any part of scapula while indirect force via FOOSH impacting humeral head into glenoid causes fracture of glenoid and scapular neck. Avulsion fractures are uncommon resulting from muscle pull. Shoulder dislocation may cause a glenoid fracture.

Intrathoracic dislocation of the scapula is an extremely rare injury where the inferior angle of the scapula is locked in the intercostal space. Diagnosis is done by computed tomography.

Floating shoulder results from traumatic disruption of two or more components of the SSSC usually secondary to high-energy injury and needs operative treatment.

Scapulothoracic dislocation (StD) is traumatic disruption of the scapula from the posterior chest wall and is essentially similar to forequarter amputation. StD results from a violent traction and rotation force as in motor vehicle accidents. Diagnosis is suggested by lateral shift of scapula on a chest PA film.

Neurovascular compromise is quite common with brachial plexopathy seen in nearly all patients (80% complete, 15% partial) and injury to subclavian/axillary vessels in 88% cases. StD may be seen even in absence of any obvious bony injury. Four clinical types of StD are described:

Anatomy

This flat, triangular bone integrates the upper extremity to the axial skeleton by articulating with humerus (glenohumeral), clavicle (acromioclavicular), and thorax (scapulothoracic). The 18 muscles originating from scapular are responsible for six basic movements of the scapula: elevation, depression, upward rotation, downward rotation, protraction, and retraction.

The scapula as such is "suspended" from clavicle that serves as the sole connection between appendicular and axial skeleton for upper limb. The SSSC is a bone soft tissue ring formed by the glenoid process, coracoid process, CC ligaments, distal clavicle, acromioclavicular joint, and acromial process that is secured to trunk by bony struts. The superior strut is the middle-third clavicle **(Fig. 11)**. The inferior strut is the lateral scapular body and spine/glenoid neck. The SSSC has to be subdivided into three subunits depending on structure(s) involved leading to instability as follows:

1. The clavicular–AC joint: Acromion strut.
2. C4-linkage (clavicular-coracoclavicular ligamentous-coracoid linkage)
3. Junction of scapular body to its three processes

Double disruption means injury to SSSC at any two places of the complex. Significantly displaced double disruption produces unstable anatomy resulting in malunion, delayed union, or nonunion, subacromial impingement, weakness, shoulder ptosis, and discomfort. Shoulder ptosis results from dropping of shoulder and upper extremity that may compromise neurovascular structures and alter biomechanics ultimately leading to degenerative joint disease in long run. Floating shoulder is a specific subtype of double disruption that involves combined fracture of clavicle with glenoid neck fracture and was classically considered to be an unstable injury where one component destabilized the other. However, progressive release in anatomic specimens has identified that this combination of injury becomes unstable only if there is associated coracoacromial ligament and AC ligament disruption. Treatment of floating shoulder should aim at maintaining glenopolar angle >30°.

Clinical Evaluation

Full trauma evaluation is indicated with attention to airway, breathing, circulation, disability, and exposure. Patients present with ipsilateral upper extremity adducted against the body and protected from movement. There are swelling, ecchymosis, crepitus, and tenderness around girdle. Shoulder ROM is restricted particularly abduction. Compartment syndrome overlying the scapula is uncommon, but it must be ruled out in the presence of pain out of proportion to the apparent injury. *Comolli sign* is triangular swelling of the posterior thorax overlying the scapula suggestive of hematoma resulting in increased compartment pressures.

ASSOCIATED INJURIES

Due to high-energy nature of injury, 85–98% of scapula fractures occur in the presence of comorbid injuries. Patients with fractures of the scapula have commonly other injuries. Examine for the presence of associated injuries such as:

- Ipsilateral fractured ribs (injury to first rib is associated with increased mortality), clavicle, sternum, and humerus
- Pneumothorax (11–55% cases)
- Pulmonary contusion (11–54% cases)
- Brachial plexus injuries (serve as important prognostic indicator of outcome).
- Vascular avulsions
- *Spine injuries:* 20% lower cervical spine, 76% thoracic spine, and 4% lumbar spine
- Closed head injury, skull fracture, liver or splenic injury, pelvic ring injuries, and lower extremity injuries
- *Scapulothoracic dislocation* presents with massive swelling of the shoulder region with a pulseless arm. There is complete or partial neurological deficit according to the injury to brachial plexus. The patients need to be emergently managed else succumbing to the vascular injury and ensuing blood loss will result in rapid mortality.

Radiographic Evaluation

All patients with suspected scapular fractures should have dedicated AP perpendicular to the plane of the scapula), lateral scapular Y-view, and axillary (arm in 70–90° of abduction) radiographs of the shoulder performed. The Stryker notch view may be helpful for coracoid fractures, and the apical oblique view and West point lateral view are useful for glenoid rim fractures. Acromion fractures should not be confused to os acromiale (3% population). Perform CT scan for complex, displaced, or intra-articular fractures and I feel 3D-CT reconstruction is the single most useful radiological investigation for evaluation of scapula fractures.

CLASSIFICATIONS

Anatomic Classification (Zdravkovic and Damholt)

Type I: Scapula body.
Type II: Apophyseal fractures, including the acromion and coracoid
Type III: Fractures of the superolateral angle, including the scapular neck and glenoid.

Rüedi's Classification Modified by Euler and Habermeyer

A. Fractures of the body of scapula isolated or multifragmentary
B. Fractures of the process B1 spine, B2 coracoid, B3 acromion
C. Fractures of scapular neck C1 anatomical neck C2 surgical neck C3 surgical neck with:
   - Fracture clavicle and acromion
   - Torn CC and CA ligaments
D. Articular fractures D1 Glenoid rim D2 Glenoid fossa with:
   - Inferior glenoid fragment
   - Horizontal split of scapula
   - Coracoglenoid block formation
   - Comminuted fractures D3 scapula neck and body fracture
E. Fracture combination with humeral head fractures.

Goss Classification (modified from Ideberg, **Fig. 12**) of glenoid fracture

Type 1: Glenoid rim fractures
A—anterior rim
B—posterior rim.
Type 2: Glenoid fracture exits at lateral border of scapula.
Type 3: Glenoid fracture exits at superior border of scapula.
Type 4: Glenoid fracture exits at medial border of scapula.
Type 5: Combination fractures
A—types 2 and 4

Treatment

Most scapula fractures (>90%) are managed nonoperatively being nondisplaced/minimally displaced, by use of sling and beginning early range of shoulder motion. Malunion is the most common complication that may cause painful scapulothoracic movements later.

Surgical indications include:

- *Floating shoulder:* Double disruption of the superior scapula/shoulder suspensory complex (SSSC; including C4-linkage).
- Displaced intra-articular glenoid fractures involving >25% of the articular surface or intra-articular fractures with step of >5 mm (as articular cartilage is 5-mm thick and step-off more than this would expose subchondral bone).
- Scapular anatomical neck fractures with >40° angulation or 1 cm medial translation.
- Scapular neck fractures with an associated displaced clavicle fracture, if CC ligaments are disrupted or neck fragment is displaced (>40° angulation/>1 cm displacement).
- Scapular fractures with lateral column displacement
- Fractures of the acromion that impinge on the subacromial space.
- Fractures of the coracoid process that results in a functional acromioclavicular separation
- Comminuted fractures of the scapular spine

Fracture of body of scapula, rarely if ever needs fixation while displaced acromion fractures may be stabilized by dorsal tension banding in cases of subacromial impingement. Third-degree AC separation along with a significantly displaced coracoid fracture is an indication for ORIF of both injuries.

A variety of fixation techniques are reported for fixation of glenoid fractures including cannulated screws, various types of plates (usually recon plates), ± bone grafting, cerclage wiring, suture anchors or commonly a combination of these. Use of posterior approach (modified Judet approach) is the most common that commonly entails utilizing the internervous interval between infraspinatus and teres minor for fixation of glenoid fractures

Contd...

Contd...

Epidemiology	*Anatomy*	*Clinical Evaluation*	*Radiographic Evaluation*	*Treatment*
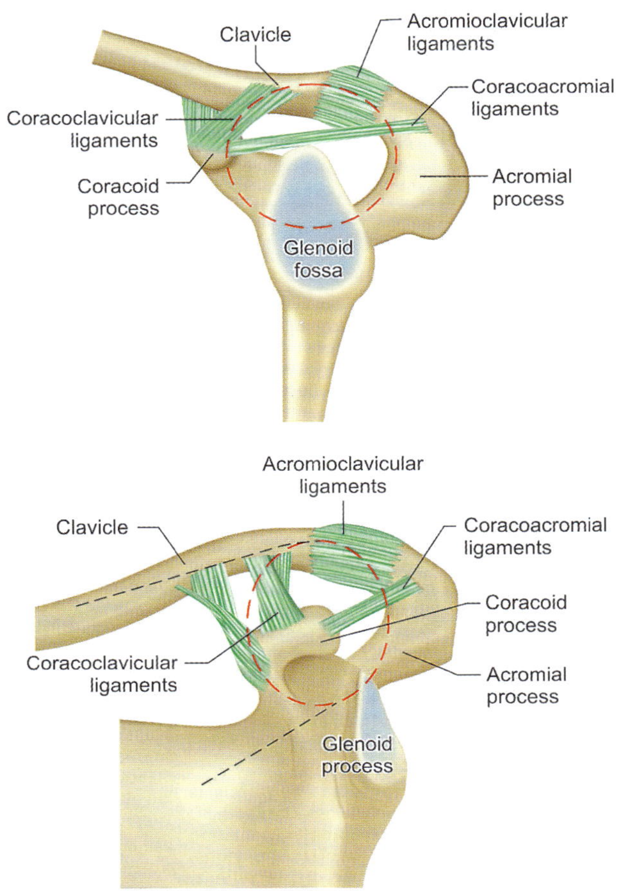 **Fig 11:** Diagrammatic representation of superior shoulder suspensory complex. 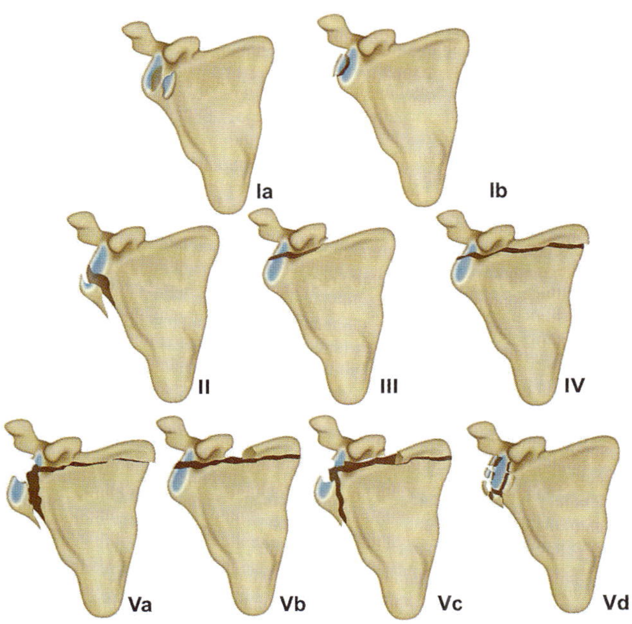 **Fig. 12:** Goss classification of scapular fractures (see text for details).			B—types 3 and 4 C—types 2, 3, and 4 D—comminuted. *Classification of acromial fractures (Kuhn et al.):* *Type I:* Minimally displaced *Type II:* Displaced but does not reduce the subacromial space *Type III:* Displaced with narrowing of the subacromial space *Classification of coracoid fractures (Ogawa et al.):* *Type I:* Proximal to the coracoclavicular ligament. *Type II:* Distal to the coracoclavicular ligament **OTA Classification of Scapula Fractures** Revised OTA classification for fractures of scapula has been presented in January, 2018. As a whole, the scapula has been assigned number '14" and subdivided into "A"—process fracture, "B"—body fracture, and "F"—fractures involving the glenoid fossa. The detailed description is as follows. *14A1:* Process, coracoid fracture *14A2:* Process, acromion fracture *14A3:* Process, spine fracture *14B1:* Body, fracture exits the body at 2 or less points *14B2:* Body, fracture exits the body at three or more points *14F0:* Glenoid fossa, through the extra-articular subchondral bone of the glenoid fossa (glenoid neck) *14F1:* Glenoid fossa, simple fracture *14F2:* Glenoid fossa, multi-fragmentary (three or more fracture lines)	(types 1b, 2, 3, 4, and 5) Anterior deltopectoral approach may be used for fixation of types 1a, 5b and some 2 and 3 fractures. If there is severe comminution of anterior glenoid fracture, then it is better excised and replaced by coracoid or iliac graft. If there is complex intra-articular scapular fracture, total reconstruction for scapula or glenoid is indicated. For fractures associated with SSSC injury, the reconstruction of latter usually takes precedence. Lax shoulder capsule would need capsular shift for restoring joint stability. Complications of ORIF include hardware failure, stiffness, infection and often weakness due to muscular/ rotator cuff injury. For patients of StD-associated neurological injury deserves special mention—Partial plexus injuries (uncommon) have good prognosis, and functional use of the extremity may be regained. Obtain electromyography at 3 weeks and myelography/MRI at 6 weeks. MRI demonstrates "empty sleeve sign". Nerve root avulsions and complete deficits have a poor prognosis. Severe injury to brachial plexus is an indication for primary above elbow amputation as the limb functions as a dead arm thence. For flail extremity, one may consider shoulder arthrodesis/ above elbow amputation. MRI scan/myelography demonstrating three or more pseudomeningoceles similarly indicates poor prognosis with flail extremity seen in 52%, early amputation needed in 21%, and death in 10%. Intrathoracic dislocation of scapula is treated by closed reduction and immobilization with a sling and swathe for 2 weeks, followed by progressive functional use of the shoulder and arm.

Contd...

Contd...

Epidemiology	Anatomy	Clinical Evaluation	Radiographic Evaluation	Treatment
Type I: Musculoskeletal injury alone *Type IIA:* Musculoskeletal injury with vascular disruption *Type IIB:* Musculoskeletal injury with neurologic impairment *Type III:* Musculoskeletal injury with both neurologic and vascular injury				

PROXIMAL HUMERUS FRACTURES

Epidemiology	Anatomy	Clinical Evaluation	Radiographic Evaluation	Treatment
These account for 4–5% of all fractures and represent third most common fracture in elderly (osteoporotic fracture, 70% of patients around 70 years of age, unimodal distribution) and it is the most common of all humerus fractures (45%) in adults. The fracture risk keeps steadily increasing with age. There is a 2:1 female-to-male ratio due to higher propensity for osteoporosis in former. Risk factors for this fracture are elderly patients, low BMD, impaired vision, poor balance, no history of hormone replacement therapy (HRT), smoking, >3 chronic illnesses, past history of previous fragility fracture. **MECHANISM OF INJURY** Most common mechanism (87% cases) is FOOSH from a standing height (low-energy fall) in elderly resulting from pathological processes of osteoporosis. The glenoid bone is much denser than metaphyseal proximal humerus, which gets impressed against the former acting as anvil. Intertuberosity fractures through the bicipital groove usually occur posterior to the groove. Fractures in younger patients result from high-energy trauma (motor vehicle accident) mostly; hence, they are associated with fracture-dislocations, significant soft tissue disruption, and often multiple injuries. *Uncommon mechanisms include:* *Excessive shoulder abduction* where the movement is blocked by greater tuberosity suddenly stressing forces at neck region and causing fracture. *Direct trauma* may cause greater tuberosity fractures. *Electrical shock or seizure* may cause violent contractions causing avulsion fractures. *Pathologic processes:* Malignant or benign processes in the proximal humerus.	The proximal humerus is retroverted at an average of 20° (high anatomical variance (6.7–47.5°) and inclined 130° relative to shaft. "Anatomical neck"— represents the physeal scar region of humeral head epiphysis while the "surgical neck" refers to the weak portion at the metaphyseal–diaphyseal junction. The shoulder is the most mobile joint of the body in terms of ROM at glenohumeral joint. Bony congruity at glenohumeral joint is minimal (unconstrained) and stability is typically provided by the capsuloligamentous structures (detailed elsewhere in text). Blood supply to proximal humerus is partly derived from anterior circumflex humeral artery through anterolateral ascending branch (along with biceps tendon in the groove) and arcuate artery. The arcuate artery is a continuation of the ascending branch of the anterior humeral circumflex. It enters the bicipital groove and supplies 34% of the head. The posterior circumflex humeral artery is now considered to be the main supply for humeral head—64% of the superior, posterior, and inferior aspects of humeral head. This is the reason why osteonecrosis is not very frequent despite disruption of anterior blood supply in 80% of fractures. Fractures of the anatomic neck have a poor prognosis because of the precarious vascular supply to humeral head epiphysis region that is a continuation from metaphyseal vascularity. Proximal humerus is divided into four osseous segments/ parts (vide radiographic evaluation). The displacing forces to parts are quite unique **(Fig. 13)**. The greater tuberosity displaced superiorly and posteriorly by the rotator cuff muscles. The greater tuberosity has attachments to the only external rotators (ER) of shoulder—infraspinatus	Patients present with involved upper extremity held close to the chest supported by contralateral hand due to pain. There is swelling and tenderness at proximal humerus region with painful ROM at shoulder and variable crepitus at fracture site. **ASSOCIATED INJURY** • Abdominal injury • Splenic injury • Pneumothorax • Axillary vessel injury (5–6%) from medially displaced head or shaft fragment • Suprascapular neuropathy • Musculocutaneous nerve injury • Brachial plexus injury. *Axillary nerve injury* (incidence 6–65%)—assess sensations over lateral aspect of proximal arm and deltoid function. This may be assessed by the presence of sensation on the lateral aspect of the proximal arm and deltoid function. Inferior translation of the distal fragment may result from deltoid atony that usually resolves by 4 weeks, but persistent atony indicates true axillary nerve injury. The axillary nerve courses just anteroinferior to the glenohumeral joint, traversing the quadrangular space. It is at particular risk for traction injury owing to fixation at the posterior cord and its proximity to the inferior capsule (during anterior dislocation and anterior fracture-dislocations). Skin compromise—0.2% *Chest injury:* Intrathoracic dislocation may occur with surgical neck fracture-dislocations; pneumothorax and hemothorax must be ruled out in the appropriate clinical setting. *Myositis ossificans:* This is uncommon and is associated with chronic unreduced fracture-dislocations and repeated attempts at closed reduction.	Trauma series—anteroposterior and lateral views in the scapular plane + axillary view. Axillary view best delineates glenoid articular fractures and dislocations, but it may be difficult to obtain due to pain. *Velpeau axillary:* Alternative to standard axillary view, if latter is not possible because of pain or if there is fear of fracture displacement, the patient may be left in the sling and leaned obliquely backward 45° over the cassette. The beam is directed caudally, orthogonal to the cassette, resulting in an axillary view with magnification. Internal and external rotation views in suspected Hill–Sachs lesion. Computed tomography is very helpful especially with 3D reconstruction in evaluating articular involvement, degree of fracture displacement, comminution assessment, impression fractures, and glenoid rim fractures. CT-based classification of displacement into posterior–medial (varus) impaction, lateral (valgus) impaction, isolated greater tuberosity, and anteromedial impaction may help in prognostication. Magnetic resonance imaging is generally not indicated for fracture management, but it may be used to assess rotator cuff integrity, if indicated. **CLASSIFICATION** Neer's four parts (Codman's division, **Fig. 14**): These are the greater and lesser tuberosities, humeral shaft, and humeral head (articular fragment). "Part" is considered as displaced, if there is >1 cm of fracture displacement or >45° of angulation. Greater tuberosity is an exception to this rule, requiring only 0.5 cm of displacement to be considered a part.	Aim: Acute—minimize pain and maximize shoulder function, definitive—restoration of pain-free functional ROM along with mandatory osteoporosis rehabilitation in indicated ones. Surgical and nonsurgical methods are both deployed successfully. In general, lower-demand elderly patients with significant comorbidities do well with conservative management to maximize shoulder function without undergoing risk associated with surgery. Predictors of poor outcome—alcohol abuse (poor compliance), smoking (nonunion), fragility, cognitive deficits, rotator cuff injuries, osteoporosis (loss of fixation), comminution and displacement, and delayed presentation. Minimally displaced fractures account for nearly 80% of proximal humerus fractures that can be managed conservatively by sling immobilization or swathe for comfort. Airplane splints and shoulder spica may counter some deforming forces but are poorly tolerated so not used. Stable fractures (minimal comminution, three or less fragments, absence of significant tuberosity displacement, cortical contact, relative impaction of the stem into the head, and no history of dislocation) are a good candidate for conservative management. "Pseudosubluxation" (due to deltoid atony, deltoid inhibition, neuropraxia, hemarthrosis, and rotator cuff dysfunction) does not mean unstable fracture. Near-normal outcome can be expected in only simple fractures, so proper counseling must be done. Conservative management does *not* always mean that fracture was/is simple; but it is indicated in specific circumstances. These patients should be followed frequently with reproducible

Contd...

Contd...

<table>
<tr><th>Epidemiology</th><th>Anatomy</th><th>Clinical Evaluation</th><th>Radiographic Evaluation</th><th>Treatment</th></tr>
<tr><td colspan="3">

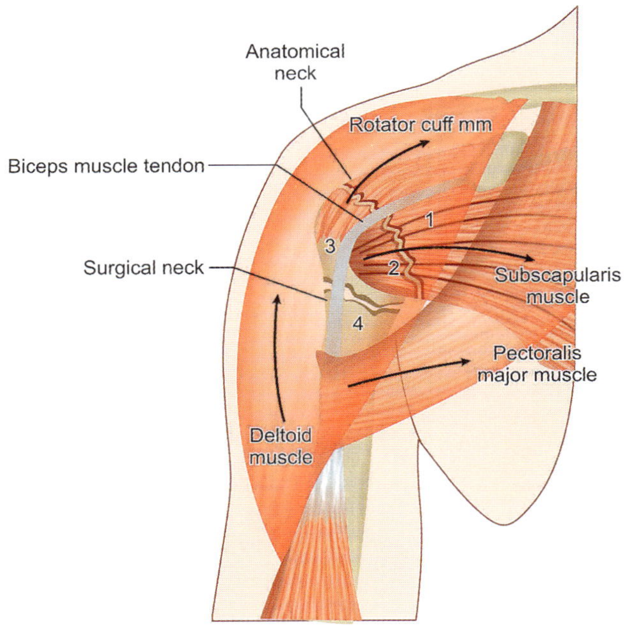

Fig. 13: Muscular attachments to the proximal humerus responsible for various displacements. The numbers depict the "parts" of humerus fracture (see text under radiology).

</td><td colspan="2">

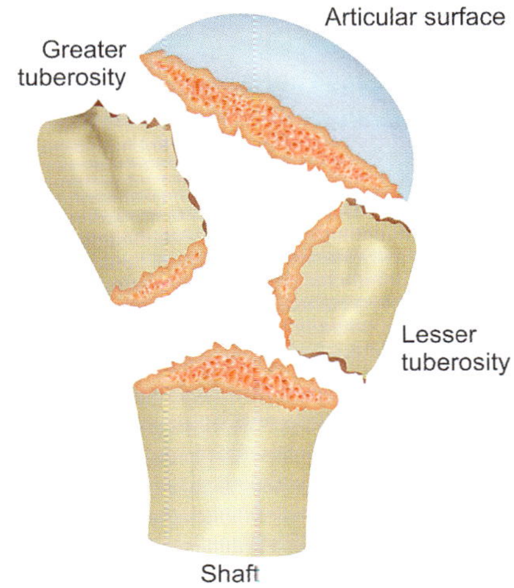

Fig. 14: Codman's four "parts" of proximal humerus fracture.

</td></tr>
<tr><td></td><td>

and the teres minor. These ER have to balance all the internal rotators namely subscapularis, teres major, latissimus dorsi, and pectoralis major. This is the reason why reconstruction of greater tuberosity is essential else if not fixed/replaced then it becomes equivalent to massive rotator cuff tear.

The lesser tuberosity—displaced medially by subscapularis.

The humeral shaft—displaced medially by the pectoralis major.

The deltoid insertion—abducts proximal fragment, if fracture is below it, else it causes elevation of the distal fragment up and impaction with head fragment.

Comminution of the medial metaphysis with preservation of metaphyseal beak of bone of <8 mm medially with the proximal head fragment has been associated with avascular necrosis.

</td><td></td><td>

Fracture types (modified Neer's—modification avoids use of roman numerals, **Fig. 15**) include:

One-part fractures: No displaced fragments regardless of number of fracture lines/fragments.

Two-part fractures: Any number of fractures/lines but one is displaced, viz., displaced anatomic neck or surgical neck or greater tuberosity or lesser tuberosity.

Three-part fractures: Three to four parts with displaced two parts relative to third (usually shaft).

Surgical (commonly)/anatomical (unlikely) neck with greater lesser tuberosity.

Four-part fractures: Fracture line involves four parts but three are displaced related to fourth.

Fracture dislocation.

Articular surface fracture—head splitting/articular impression fractures such as the Hill-Sachs lesion.

</td><td>

radiographs to detect loss of fracture reduction. Early shoulder motion may be instituted at 7–10 days, if the patient has a stable or impacted fracture.

Pendulum exercises are instructed initially followed by passive range-of-motion exercises. At 6 weeks, active range-of-motion exercises are started.

Resistive exercises are started at 12 weeks. Rapid improvement is seen till 6 months and then improvement continues till 2 years most gaining maximally by 1 year though.

Complications of nonoperative management—osteonecrosis—3–14% of three-part and 13–34% of four-part fractures [more in anatomic neck fracture, metaphyseal extension of head fragment <8 mm, and medial head disruption of >2 mm (Hertel criteria)].

Nonunion (1%): Especially in displaced two-part surgical neck fractures with soft tissue interposition. Other causes include excessive traction, severe fracture displacement, systemic disease, poor bone quality, and infection.

Stiffness: It may be minimized with an aggressive, supervised physical therapy regimen and

</td></tr>
</table>

Contd...

Contd...

Epidemiology	Anatomy	Clinical Evaluation	Radiographic Evaluation	Treatment

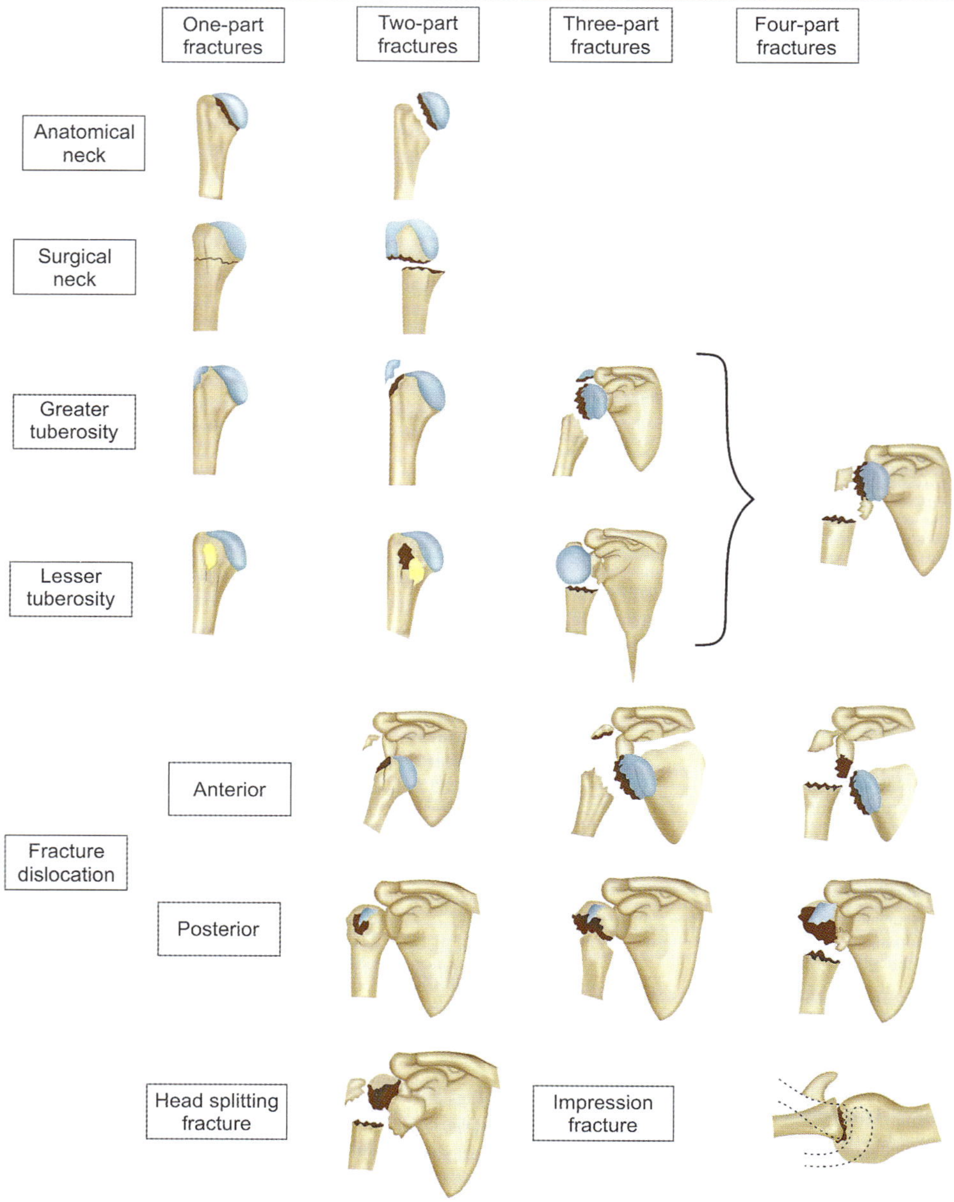

Fig. 15: Neer's classification for proximal humerus fracture.

may require open lysis of adhesions for recalcitrant cases. Malunion (worst is posterosuperior greater tuberosity malunion that increases the required force for deltoid and also causes impingement) and rotator cuff dysfunction.

Loss of function: Based on CT classification, lateral impaction has worst outcome. Outcome also worsens with posteromedial and greater tuberosity displacement. It is interesting to note that there is no definite correlation of AVN of humeral head to shoulder outcome scores presently in use.

General indications for **surgical management** are open fractures, significant displacement, and segmental injuries in patients who are healthy enough for surgery. Various tools to address specific fracture patterns and displacements include limited percutaneous fixation, open reduction internal fixation using standard or locked plating (anatomical or otherwise) techniques, intramedullary nails, osteo-suture fixation, bone grafting, and arthroplasty (hemiarthroplasty, total and reverse).

Isolated GT fractures: Prefer osteosuturing/transosseous-equivalent suturing else tension-band fixation or figure-of-eight construct.

Two- and three-part fractures: Closed reduction percutaneous pinning (done for displaced surgical neck fractures and valgus impacted fractures with intact medial hinge). Pinning contraindicated in medial comminution—prefer ORIF with locked plate osteosynthesis. ORIF preferred for displaced two-, three-, and four-part fractures, especially in younger patients. Outcomes are best, if tuberosity fragments (especially the greater tuberosity that has the only available external rotators (infraspinatus and teres minor attached) are reconstituted with anatomical reduction and one must avoid varus reduction (very high failure rates). Intramedullary nailing (Polarus/Telegraph nail) is done at select centers doing nailing as primary modality of fixation.

Reoperation rates of nailing are quite high. Difficult to really substantiate functional outcome between ORIF and conservative management using current scores. Reoperation rate is also significant after ORIF (loss of

Contd...

Contd...

Epidemiology	Anatomy	Clinical Evaluation	Radiographic Evaluation	Treatment
				reduction, loss of fixation, and stiffness). Advantage of ORIF—anatomic reduction, a decreased rate of malunion or nonunion, and the ability to begin early motion. **Four-part fractures and some comminuted/osteoporotic three-part fractures**—ORIF versus arthroplasty. ORIF preserves bone stock and avoids arthroplasty-related complications such as loosening and wear. Other complications of hemiarthroplasty-glenoid wear + subsequent failure of the rotator cuff with proximal humeral migration and pseudoparalysis. Randomized controlled trials report somewhat better functional outcomes following hemiarthroplasty compared to ORIF but no substantial improvement. The most important point against ORIF is high subsequent reoperation rate. *Anatomic neck fractures:* These are rare and difficult to treat by closed reduction. They require ORIF (younger patients) or prosthesis (e.g., shoulder hemiarthroplasty) and are associated with a high incidence of osteonecrosis. Best candidates for hemiarthroplasty—50–70 years physiologically young patients without metaphyseal comminution and nonreconstructible humeral head. Tuberosities should be intact with good calcar support. If there is preceding arthritis, then prefer total shoulder arthroplasty. Indications of reverse total shoulder arthroplasty are controversial and possibly include 3- or 4-part fractures in patients >70 years, nonconstructible tuberosities, presence of rotator cuff tear, pre-existing arthritis, and symptomatic malunion/nonunion.

HUMERAL SHAFT FRACTURES

Epidemiology	Anatomy	Clinical Evaluation	Radiographic Evaluation	Treatment
Fracture distal to pectoralis major insertion and proximal to supracondylar ridge is included in humeral shaft fractures. Common fracture accounts for 3–5% of all fractures in adults. It is seen in all ages but a bimodal hump in distribution. Younger patients (3rd decade) have high-energy injury while larger peak is seen in elderly (7th decade) group that usually suffer from	Humeral shaft is the region between surgical neck to supracondylar ridge beginning. It changes in anteroposterior cross-sectional shape from cylindrical to triangular from proximal to distal. The vascular supply comes from perforating branches of the brachial artery, with the main nutrient artery entering the medial humerus	Findings of fracture—pain, swelling, deformity, and shortening of the affected arm. A careful neurovascular examination is essential, with particular attention to radial nerve (radial nerve injury—20% incidence). Look for compartment syndrome in severe swelling. Vascular injury is an emergency—commonly involves brachial artery. Immediately repair and	AP and lateral radiographs (perpendicular) of the humerus including the shoulder and elbow joints on each view. Rotate the patient and not arm to obtain perpendicular view. Transthoracic lateral in case standard lateral not possible. Traction views for severe comminution and shortening. For pathological fractures, obtain MRI and/or CT scan as indicated.	*Goal:* To establish union with acceptable alignment and restore the function. **NONOPERATIVE** Usually followed, if acceptable reduction can be obtained in a cooperative and preferably upright and mobile patient with possible close supervision and follow-up. Most humeral shaft fractures (>90%) will heal with nonsurgical management.

Contd...

Contd...

Epidemiology	Anatomy	Clinical Evaluation	Radiographic Evaluation	Treatment
osteoporotic low-energy fractures seen in females. Open fractures are seen in 2–7% patients. **MECHANISM OF INJURY** *Direct (most common):* Direct trauma to the arm from a blow or road traffic accident à transverse or comminuted fractures. *Indirect:* FOOSH results in spiral or oblique fractures, especially in elderly patients. Very uncommonly, throwing injuries with extreme muscular contraction may cause humerus shaft fractures. Fracture pattern also varies with the type of force applied: Compressive load → proximal or distal humerus fracture. Bending load → transverse fractures of the humeral shaft. Torsional → spiral fractures of the humeral shaft. Torsional and bending → oblique fracture ± butterfly fragment. **Comminution an impact force**	distal to the midshaft. Also, the thick muscular cover of the humeral shaft provides periosteal supply. The radial nerve crosses the posterior aspect of the humerus in spiral groove 15 cm above lateral epicondyle (≈20 cm above medial epicondyle) adjacent to the posterior aspect of the humerus for a length of 6.5 cm. The nerve then pierces lateral intermuscular septum 10 cm proximal to the lateral epicondyle to reach anterior compartment. The musculotendinous attachments of the humerus (insertion—pectoralis major, deltoid, coracobrachialis; origin for—brachialis, triceps, brachioradialis) result in characteristic fracture displacements **(Fig. 16)**. • Fracture above the pectoralis insertion abduction and rotation of proximal fragment, neutral distal fragment. • Fracture below pectoralis insertion → adduction of proximal fragment and proximal migration and lateral translation of distal fragment. • Fracture below deltoid insertion → lateral angulation at fracture, abduction of proximal fragment.	establish vascular continuity, bone fixation is secondary and may follow vascular repair. Note for open fractures and intra-articular extensions of open fractures may be determined by ectopic intra-articular injection of saline looking for communication with the wound. Radial nerve injury commonly is seen with middle-third fractures especially those with a lateral bony spike (Holstein–Lewis type distal third spiral fracture). The radial nerve injury is seen in 11% of the cases. The risk factors include transverse/spiral fractures of middle and distal fifth's fracture. The nerve is commonly entrapped or lacerated as it passes through the intermuscular septum. Most injuries (70%), however, represent neurapraxias or partial injuries with intact perineurium and function usually returns within 3–4 months. Neurotmesis is more common in open fractures or gunshot injuries that need exploration. Injury may also occur following attempted reduction and current practice entails surgical exploration (urgent) + fixation of fracture in these cases. In cases initially conservatively managed, delayed surgical exploration is done at 3–4 months substantiated by no evidence of recovery clinically or on NCS. Late exploration is favored for giving the nerve "benefit of doubt" and also precise evaluation of a nerve lesion is possible. Brachioradialis is first to recover while extensor indices recover last. The associated fracture may unite by then and lastly the results of secondary nerve repair are as good as those of primary repair.	**CLASSIFICATIONS** ***Descriptive***—open versus closed versus pathological, fracture location (proximal/middle or lower one-third), metaphyseal extension or intra-articular extension. Geometry of fracture—transverse/oblique/spiral, comminution/segmental, angulation, displacement, and shortening. **OTA Classification** Bone number—1 Fracture location—2 Fracture pattern—simple (A), wedge (B), complex (C).	The recommended method is *coaptation splint* (extending to axilla from shoulder tip) followed by functional brace. The splint takes care of subsiding tissue edema minimizing loss of reduction. Apply valgus mold to counter varus displacement. Functional brace depends on hydrostatic soft tissue compression to affect and maintain fracture alignment while allowing motion of adjacent joints. It is applied from 2 cm distal to axilla extending to 2 cm proximal to humeral condyles without sling support for gravity-assisted reduction. Proximal extension may be used for upper-third fractures. Usually, it is given at 2 weeks (in younger patients or children may be even applied at 1 week or 10 days). Functional brace is continued for 8 weeks or till radiographic union. *Contraindications:* Open fractures, vascular injury, brachial plexus injury (not radial nerve injury), unreliable patient, loss of reduction. **Less than 20° of anterior angulation, 30° of varus/valgus angulation, and 3 cm of shortening are acceptable with conservative management.** Alternative to splint and bracing is use of hanging cast that utilizes gravity-assisted traction (weight of the cast and arm) to affect fracture reduction especially in displaced spiral or oblique midshaft humeral fractures with shortening. Transverse or short oblique fractures may distract and often go into nonunion so represent relative contraindications. After 2–3 weeks, it may be changed to functional brace. *Thoracobrachial immobilization* (Velpeau dressing): Usually done in elderly patients or children that do not tolerate other methods of treatment. It is indicated for minimally displaced or nondisplaced fractures that do not require reduction. Functional brace may be applied after 1–3 weeks and shoulder mobilization begun. *Shoulder spica cast*: Rarely, applied in a fracture pattern that necessitates significant abduction and external rotation of the upper extremity. Not favored because of difficulty in cast application, cast weight and bulkiness, skin irritation,

Contd...

Contd...

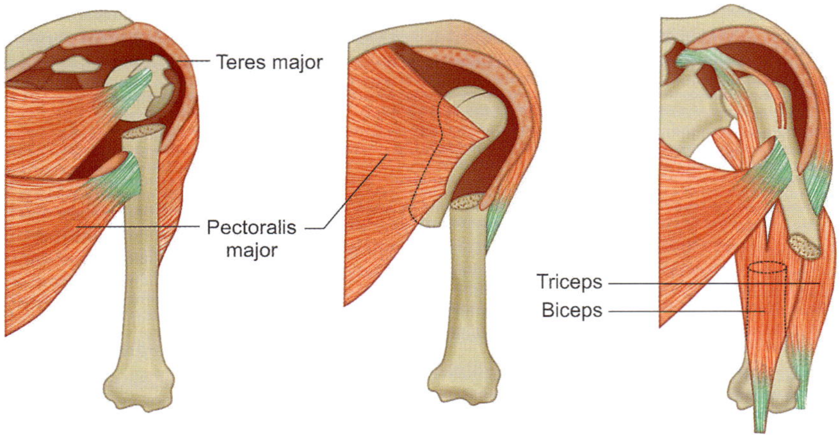

Fig. 16: Various displacements of humerus shaft fracture due to muscular attachments.

Epidemiology	Anatomy	Clinical Evaluation	Radiographic Evaluation	Treatment
				and patient discomfort. It was also uncommonly used to immobilize precarious fixation in osteoporotic nonunions before the availability of LCP. **OPERATIVE TREATMENT** *Indications:* • Polytrauma • Loss of reduction in closed method or irreducible fracture • Unacceptable reduction—soft tissue interposition precluding reduction • Malunion beyond acceptable parameters (Klenerman guidelines, see earlier for acceptable reduction) • Pathologic fracture • Associated vascular injury • Exploration of reduction attempted nerve injury • Floating elbow • Nonunion • Segmental fracture • Compartment syndrome • Intra-articular extension • Bilateral humeral fractures • Open fracture • Nerve injury in penetrating trauma • Transverse or short oblique fracture (relative) • Burns/soft tissue injury precluding bracing or cast management (relative) or obese patient. **Intramedullary nailing** of humeral shaft fractures is gaining popularity over plating as a treatment method. This is due to limited soft tissue dissection, preservation of fracture hematoma, and fragment vascularity, provides autograft, and is biomechanically superior. Antegrade and retrograde techniques can be both used for locked nails. Flexible intramedullary nailing is also described with transcutaneous electrical nerve stimulation (TENS) or rush nails but preferable in children only due to poor stability. The typical indications for nailing were: • Segmental and focal comminuted fractures • Fractures in osteoporotic bones • Pathological fractures. The indications have been extended to: • Transverse fractures and short oblique fractures • Fractures that need rapid immobilization as in multiple injury patients. Antegrade nail is associated with complication of shoulder pain, rotator cuff injury/impingement axillary nerve

Contd...

Contd...

Epidemiology	Anatomy	Clinical Evaluation	Radiographic Evaluation	Treatment
				injury and distally injury to lateral cutaneous nerve of forearm. There can be radial nerve injury during manipulation. Axillary nerve injury proximally usually occurs due to longer locking bolt that damages the nerve during internal rotation. Anteroposterior screws should be avoided proximally to prevent axillary nerve injury. Entry should be rotator cuff preserving to prevent complications. Distal coronal plane screws are avoided to prevent cutaneous nerve injury, radial nerve injury laterally or brachial artery injury medially. Distraction at fracture site is a concern as the IM canal narrows distally jamming the nail and causing distraction with further push to nail. Shoulder pain may occur due to adhesive capsulitis, rotator cuff lesion or nail protrusion (older nails—K-nails), choose a nail with lateral offset. Retrograde nailing requires prone position and is quite uncomfortable but the advantage is that distal locking screws are posteroanterior in the safe zone. **Plate fixation** has always been a preferred method of fixation since introduction by AO group. Compressed plating gave way to LCP that has also allowed minimally invasive percutaneous plate osteosynthesis (MIPPO) technique offsetting the disadvantage of extensive sift tissue dissection. Standard surgical approaches for plate fixation include: *Anterolateral approach*: → Proximal third and midshaft humeral shaft fractures. Can be extended proximally or distally. After retracting biceps, the brachialis is split. Anterior approach (not very common) Posterior approach → typically used for distal 1/4th fractures or fractures requiring radial nerve exploration. Disadvantage is inability to extend proximally for proximal humerus fractures. The muscular interval between the lateral and long heads of the triceps is utilized. **External fixation** is indicated in infected nonunions, Burn patients with fractures, Open fractures with extensive soft tissue loss. The complications include pin tract infection, neurovascular injury, and nonunion.

DISTAL HUMERUS

Epidemiology	*Anatomy*	*Clinical Evaluation*	*Radiographic Evaluation*	*Treatment*
Relatively uncommon in adults (0.5% of all fractures; one-third of all humerus fractures). Most are intercondylar fractures of the distal humerus. In pediatric population, extension-type supracondylar fractures of the distal humerus account for >80% of all distal humerus fractures. **MECHANISM OF INJURY** Intercondylar fracture usually results from high-energy trauma in adults as in side-swipe injuries. Most low-energy distal humeral fractures result from a simple fall in middle-aged and elderly female where elbow is struck directly. FOOSH injuries with hyperextension force on the distal humerus causes point concentration of forces at olecranon tip and results in comminuted fractures, if olecranon does not give way.	The distal humerus is considered to be a triangular structure of medial and lateral column connected distally by a tied-arch of metaphyseal bone. The medial column diverges from mid-humeral axis at 45° while lateral column diverges at 20°. The columns terminate at the epicondyles and are nonarticulating while the condyle (tied arch) is the articulating portion **(Fig. 17)**. Trochlea is covered by articular cartilage for 300° while capitellum is covered over 180°. The condyle comprises the capitellum (forming radiocapitellar articulation) and trochlea (ulnotrochlear articulation) that projects distally and anteriorly at an angle of 30–40° **(Fig. 18)**. The centers of the arcs of rotation of both articulations lie on the same horizontal axis congruent and anatomical reduction is a must while ORIF. Some other radiological parameters to keep in mind while reduction are: 4–8° of valgus of the trochlear axis compared with the longitudinal axis **(Fig. 18)**. The trochlear axis is also 3–8° externally rotated.	Signs and symptoms vary with degree of swelling and displacement; considerable swelling frequently occurs, rendering landmarks difficult to palpate. However, the normal relationship of the olecranon, medial, and lateral condyles should be maintained, roughly delineating an equilateral triangle. Crepitus with range of motion and gross instability may be present; although this is highly suggestive of fracture, no attempt should be made to elicit it because neurovascular compromise may result. A careful neurovascular evaluation is essential because the sharp, fractured end of the proximal fragment may impale or contuse the brachial artery, median nerve, or radial nerve. Serial neurovascular examinations with compartment pressure monitoring may be necessary with massive swelling; cubital fossa swelling may result in vascular impairment or the development of a volar compartment syndrome resulting in Volkmann ischemia.	Standard anteroposterior (AP) and lateral views of the elbow are obtained. Oblique radiographs may be done as necessary. Traction radiographs may be taken in comminuted fractures with significant deformity to understand the fracture geometry for fixation. Always look for intercondylar component in supracondylar fractures. Minimally displaced fractures may result in a decrease in the normal condylar shaft angle of 40° on the lateral radiograph. Also, fat pad signs (due to displacement of joint capsule) are helpful in identifying undisplaced fracture lines not readily evident on plain radiographs. Computed tomography may be utilized to delineate fracture fragments further. **CLASSIFICATIONS** ***OTA classification*** is frequently followed to report cases and series or for research purpose that can be seen from standard sources. ***Descriptive classification*** describes the involved anatomical region. Commonly following fractures are described:	The goals of treatment are anatomic reduction, stable internal fixation, restoration of articular axial alignment, early mobilization, and preservation of soft tissues. As the treatment differs for different fracture types so description will be provided individually below.

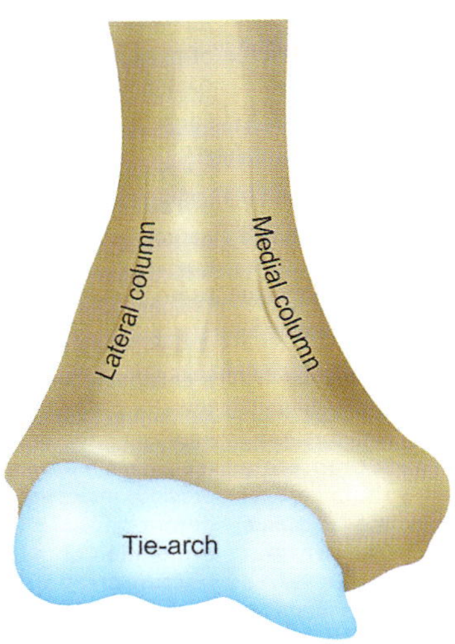

Fig. 17: Bony anatomy of distal humerus as represented by columns and tie-arch.

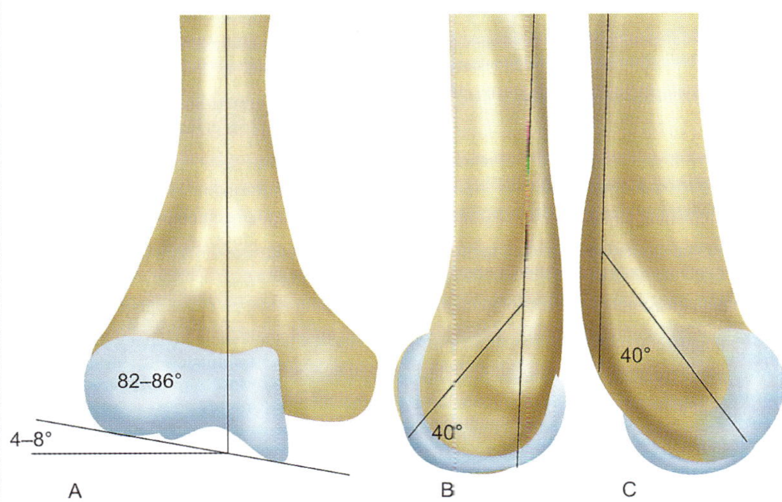

Fig. 18: The anatomical parameters of distal humerus osseous anatomy depicting valgus at the lateral humeral condyle and anterior disposition of distal humeral articular surface placing the capitellum and trochlea in front of the humerus shaft. The joint surface to shaft axis is 4–8° of valgus the A-carrying angle (A). The articular segment just forward from the line of the shaft at 40° and functions architecturally as the tie-arch at the point of maximum column divergence distally. The medial epicondyle is on the projected axis of the shaft, whereas the lateral epicondyle is projected slightly forward from the axis (B and C).

Contd...

Contd...

Epidemiology	*Anatomy*	*Clinical Evaluation*	*Radiographic Evaluation*	*Treatment*
			• Supracondylar fractures: – Extension-type – Flexion-type • Transcondylar fractures • Intercondylar fractures • Condylar fractures • Capitellum fractures • Trochlea fractures • Lateral epicondylar fractures • Medial epicondylar fractures • Fractures of the supracondylar process.	

SUPRACONDYLAR FRACTURES OF DISTAL HUMERUS (PEDIATRIC)

Epidemiology	*Anatomy*	*Clinical Evaluation*	*Radiographic Evaluation*	*Treatment*
As the fractures are uncommon in adults so the discussion is limited mostly to pediatric population. **EPIDEMIOLOGY** These commonly occur in children aged 5–10 years comprising 70% of elbow injuries (16% of all pediatric fractures). Most common age is 7±1 years. **MECHANISM OF INJURY** Children <3 years of age typically sustain the fracture following a fall from 3 feet. Older children sustain injury, following fall while playing say monkey bars or stairs. The fall is usually onto an outstretched hand with/without an abduction or adduction force. This produces hyperextension and associated extension type fracture. Flexion type fracture usually results from fall directly on the flexed elbow. This uncommon injury is frequently associated with open lesions as the sharp, proximal fragment pierces the triceps tendon and overlying skin.	The area of injury is usually a thin weak bone engulfed by olecranon and coronoid fossa. The area also contains many growth plates that weaken the tensile strength due to ongoing remodeling and flaring away of the medial and lateral columns reduces the aggregate strength of construct. Olecranon also provides a sharp edge fulcrum against which the counterforce causes concentration of forces resulting in easy fracture. In over 95% of cases, the distal fragment displaces posteriorly. Identification of the developing physis helps to determine the age **(Figs. 19A and B)** and also not to confuse with anatomy (remembered as CRITOE—1-4-5-8-9-10 for appearance) • Capitellum—1 year • Radial head—4 years • Internal epicondyle—5 years • Trochlea—5 years • Olecranon—8 years • External epicondyle—10 years	Note injury incidence, mechanism of fall, onset of pain (ischemia of muscles produces late-onset increased pain). Examine the distal neurovascular status—note both radial and ulnar pulses. In case of absent pulses note, the temperature and appearance of limb—should be warm and pink and note the capillary-filling time. Check radial, ulnar, and median nerves for motor and sensory function. Anterior pucker or dimpling indicates brachialis rupture by sharp proximal anterior fragment. Complete displacement is indicated by S-shaped deformity. Always look for signs of compartment syndrome—out of proportion pain (increased need of analgesics), out of proportion swelling, stretch pain more than usual in fractures, forearm tenderness, loss of respective compartment movements. Loss of pulses and capillary refill are not reliable. Obtain compartment pressures whenever there is doubt as associated median nerve injury would mask pain from compartment syndrome. **ASSOCIATED INJURY** Nerve injury—12–20% traumatic and 2–6% iatrogenic. Most common injury to anterior interosseous nerve (52%), radial nerve (32%) is second most commonly involved. Most of the deficits are neurapraxia that usually recover in 2–3 months → no improvement for 4–6 months are indication for exploration.	AP and lateral projection of the elbow and any other tender/deformed site on examination. Measure Baumann's angle (between humerus axis and lateral condyle growth plate, **Fig. 20**) for estimation of carrying angle (varus displacement increases Baumann's angle). Note the anterior humeral cortical line on lateral radiograph that passes through middle one-third of capitellum (in very young patients <3 years of age the line would pass anterior to the ossification center and not through it because the capitellar ossification begins from posterior to anterior). Note the fat pad sign—posterior is more reliable, anterior fat pad sign is called Sail sign. If no fracture line is visible but there is fat pad sign, then consider reimaging at 7–10 days. Oblique views better demonstrate isolated condyle fractures with intra-articular extension. **STAGING SYSTEM** ***(Gartland, Fig. 21):*** • Type I → nondisplaced fractures • Type II → displaced with angulation but intact posterior cortex – Type IIA—angulation only – Type IIB—with rotation • Type III → Completely displaced with no cortical contact. Some add two subtypes as A—without rotation and B—with rotation of the fragment. ***Modified Gartland*** classification divides type III into two subtypes and adds a fourth type as follows: Type IIIA—completely displaced posteromedially.	Initial splinting should be done with adequate padding in 20–30° of elbow flexion, splinting in full extension is contraindicated, as it may stretch the neurovascular structures over fracture site in displaced or unstable fractures. Conservative versus operative management depends on type of fracture as follows. Above elbow POP slab in 90° of elbow flexion or less is adequate for nondisplaced or minimally displaced fractures—type I, but if there is varus impaction with an increased Baumann angle (>10° of normal) then closed reduction and pinning are advised. For type II fractures, closed reduction and immobilization in 90° of elbow flexion is adequate. If >90° of flexion or less is needed, then percutaneous pinning should be considered to reduce risk of hyperflexion (Volkmann's contracture). For type III fractures, primary treatment recommended is closed reduction and percutaneous pinning, if neurovascular status is normal. For irreducible fractures open reduction is advised as is needed for all open supracondylar fractures. Usually, a compromised vessel over the sharp proximal fragment improves with reduction but if there is no improvement or the previous intact vascular status deteriorates then emergent exploration of the vessel and fracture fixation is needed. In this case, give priority to vascular repair. So, operative management is indicated in: • Open fractures • Type III fractures

Contd...

Contd...

Epidemiology	*Anatomy*	*Clinical Evaluation*	*Radiographic Evaluation*	*Treatment*
			Type IIIB—completely displaced posterolaterally. Type IV—multidirectional instability with circumferential periosteal disruption.	• Unstable type II fractures or irreducible fractures • Fractures that deteriorate for vascular or neurological status following reduction • Comminuted fractures that are likely to displace Remodeling potential of distal humerus is limited so varus/valgus angulation does not remodel well and persist till adulthood. This is one of the biases toward operative management for fractures that have impacted varus of 10° or more. Reduction maneuver involves generous traction in extension for 60–80 seconds and chacking the reduction in AP view. Coronal plane deformity is corrected by appropriate mediolateral force. Varus angulation is indicated by increased Baumann angle. Persistent coronal plane deformity is usually due to soft tissue interposition, e.g., in brachialis buttonholing and puckering due to fascia tethering. This is dealt by "milking maneuver" where brachialis is pushed (milked) by a firm persistent force pushing the muscle distally while maintaining the traction at elbow and thus allowing shaft fragment to retract back posteriorly. Once aligned in AP view, use double-thumb technique to correct extension and flex the elbow. Pronation (to tighten medial periosteal hinge) or supination is added, if there is medial or lateral tilt of the distal fragment, respectively. Placement of k-pins and their numbers are variable for each case but in general two pins for type 2, three pins for type 3, and four pins for type 4 are used. Pins should be as much spread at the fracture site as possible and may be passed across ossified portion of capitellum to maximize purchase. There is not much difference between lateral only or combined medial and lateral pinning but pins should be placed at a gap of 2 mm or more at the fracture site else they function as one pin only. One should avoid the temptation to avoid olecranon fossa as this actually provided four cortex purchase and superior fixation. The child will in any case not bend the elbow for 3–4 weeks following fixation whence the pins can be removed. Immobilize in 80° of flexion and need of >90° indicates unstable fixation/reduction.

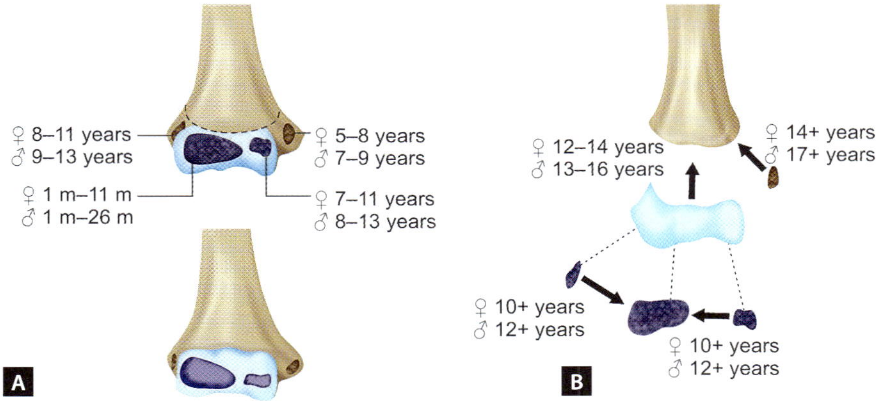

Figs. 19A and B: The age of appearance (A) and fusion (B) of ossification centers (sequence depicted by arrows) for various anatomical components of distal humerus.

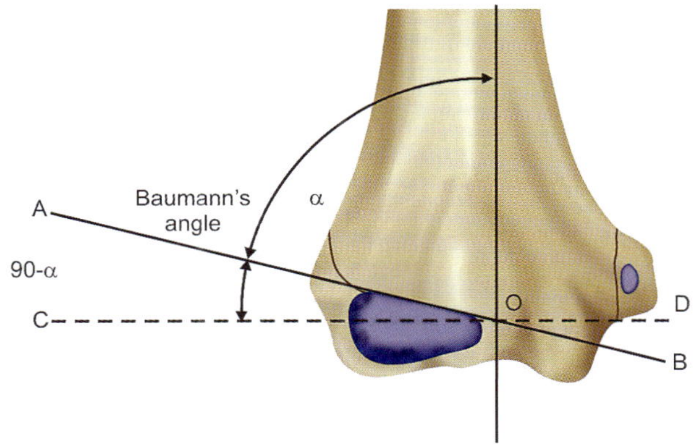

Fig. 20: Method for radiological estimation of Baumann's angle (normal value for Baumann's angle (humeral-capitellar angle is 72° ± 10°, but for individual estimation best is to measure from contralateral radiograph and any difference of >5° is abnormal).

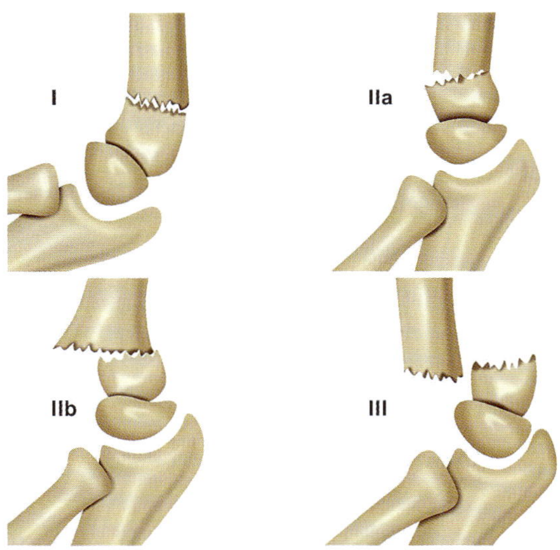

Fig. 21: Radiological classification of pediatric supracondylar fracture (Gartland).

Contd...

Contd...

Epidemiology	Anatomy	Clinical Evaluation	Radiographic Evaluation	Treatment
				Complications • Compartment syndrome • Nerve injury—iatrogenic 2–6%) • Cubitus varus • Nerve injury—ulnar common (iatrogenic) • Fishtail deformity due to resorption of trochlear ossification center. Vascular injury in supracondylar fractures and its management are quite debate with often the personal experience and preferences ruling over protocols and that is also not wholly incorrect. Vascular compromise is commonly seen in 5–12% patients that improve quickly in most with fracture reduction. Once perfusion improves, document with presence of pulses, good perfusion (capillary filling time), and temperature. If the pulses are absent but perfusion is good "pink pulseless hand" (no cold, clammy, and pale limb) then observation done at frequent intervals is the standard recommendation currently. Arteriogram is of little help so not recommended. Some studies suggest aggressive management with surgical exploration in pulseless pink hand. Individualized approach is hence advised for perfused pulseless limb. If perfusion is poor and pulses are still absent then vascular surgeon intervention should be done. Nerve injuries are seen in 10–20% cases depending on the direction of displacement. Posteromedial displacement produces radial nerve injury, posterolateral displacement would injure median nerve, while flexion-type injury would produce ulnar nerve injury. Most are "praxias" so nothing needs to be done actively unless the fracture is being explored for other reason (open fracture/vascular injury). Supracondylar factures are uncommon in adults and are commonly associated with comminution or some undisplaced intraocular fracture line. If the reduction is adequate by closed means, then posterior long-arm splint is placed in at least 90° of elbow flexion, with the forearm in neutral for 6 weeks or till radiographic healing. Chances of stiffness are high with prolonged immobilization. Operative management is commonly followed as there is frequent

Contd...

Contd...

Epidemiology	Anatomy	Clinical Evaluation	Radiographic Evaluation	Treatment
				loss of reduction and there are significant chances of stiff elbow with conservative management. Operative indications in adults are: • Displaced fracture • Vascular injury • Open fracture *Open reduction and internal fixation:* Plate fixation is used on each column, either in parallel or preferably set at 90°. Plate fixation is the procedure of choice, because this allows for early range of elbow motion. Total elbow replacement is considered in elderly patients that had good preinjury function and present with severely comminuted fracture of the distal humerus that cannot be reconstructed.

INTERCONDYLAR FRACTURE HUMERUS

Epidemiology	Anatomy	Clinical Evaluation	Radiographic Evaluation	Treatment
This is the most common distal humeral fracture making up of 30% of fractures of distal humerus in adults and 0.5–2% of all fractures. The incidence is rising with increased prevalence of osteoporosis. Most fractures are intra-articular and involve both medial and lateral columns. Bimodal distribution is seen where high-energy injuries are seen in younger people while low-energy injury is common mode of injury in elderly osteoporotic bones. **Comminution is common.** Fracture fragments are often displaced by unopposed muscle pull at the medial (flexor mass) and lateral (extensor mass) epicondyles, which rotate the articular surfaces. **MECHANISM OF INJURY** Force is directed against the posterior aspect of an elbow flexed >90°, thus driving the ulna into the trochlea.	Beside the bony anatomy described above, one should also remember the ligamentous anatomy (detailed in section on upper limb) as they should be preserved during reconstructions. Restoration of mediolateral length of the articular tie-arch is of utmost importance as is the preservation of the collateral ligaments. Reduction of length by overzealous compression would result in cramping of space for ulna to move and hence loss of movements. Expansion of length would always occur at the compromise of anatomical reduction so nonunion or failure of construct is a likely possibility.	The patient presents with swelling, ecchymosis, and deformity of the elbow. The swelling is usually proportionate to the energy of trauma. Comminuted fractures usually have more swelling. Blister formation is also common in high-energy injuries as injury to soft tissue component is also greater. Wait for a few days in such cases and attempt swelling reduction by conservative means, viz., PRICEM (protection, rest, immobilization, ice packs, elevation, medications, etc.). Manipulation should be avoided except one gentle attempt at reduction of fragments to restore functional length and fragment anatomy. Massage if done by quack would need further cooling off period before attempting surgery as chances of stiffness and ectopic bone formation are increased.	Obtain the standard AP and lateral projections, usually traction views are needed due to displacement and collapse. CT scans with 3D reconstruction and subtraction of radius and ulna reveal much better details of the fragments and displacements also the intra-articular comminution can be better judged and defined for reconstruction. For description and classification, the term condyles are changed to columns. The fractures are usually bicolumnar and unicolumnar fractures are uncommon (if at all the lateral column are commoner than medial). **CLASSIFICATIONS** **Reich Classification** "T" Type and "Y" type fractures. Riseborough and Radin classification (1969) of "T" type intercondylar fractures **(Figs. 22A to D)**: • Type 1—nondisplaced fracture • Type 2—displaced but without fragment rotation • Type 3—with fragment rotation • Type 4—severecomminution **Jupiter and Mehne Classification** (anatomical classification based on patterns): • "T" type—high and low • "Y" type • "H" type • Medial lambda • Lateral lambda pattern	Treatment is individualized based on patient age, bone quality, and degree of comminution. **NONOPERATIVE** It is uncommon to see this modality being pursued but is indicated for nondisplaced fractures, elderly low-demand patients with displaced fractures and patients in poor health. The options for management include: *Cast immobilization*: Not preferred due to inadequate fracture reduction and prolonged immobilization liable to stiffness. After brief immobilization supervised mobilization attempted. *"Bag of bones" technique*: The arm is placed in a collar and cuff with as much flexion as possible due to swelling; gravity helps in reduction followed by: *Traction with an olecranon pin*: Placed overhead to reduce swelling → limited axial control so malunion is common. **OPERATIVE** Open reduction and internal fixation is commonly preferred for a displaced reconstructible fracture. The aim is to restore both the articular congruity (rigid fixation by interfragmentary compression) and to secure the supracondylar component. Articular congruity is utmost

Contd...

Contd...

<table>
<tr><th>Epidemiology</th><th>Anatomy</th><th>Clinical Evaluation</th><th>Radiographic Evaluation</th><th>Treatment</th></tr>
<tr>
<td colspan="3">
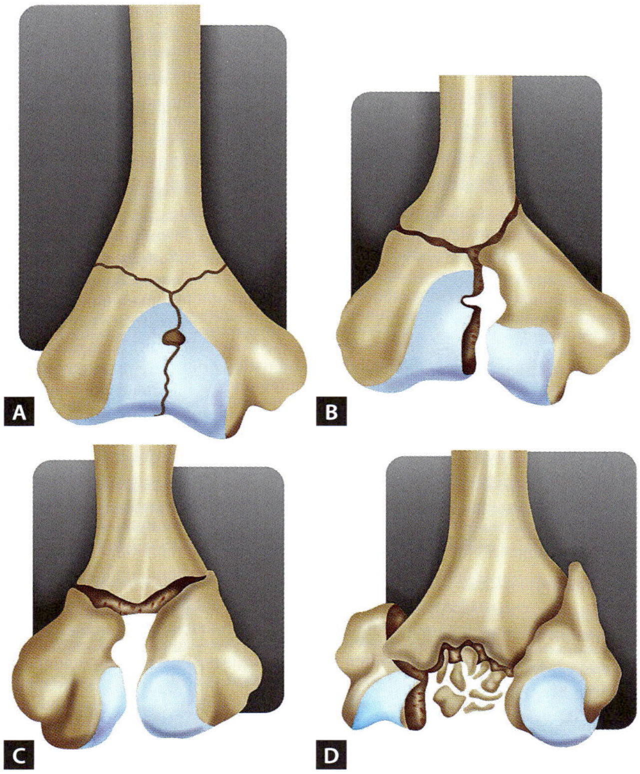

Figs. 22A to D: Riseborough and Radin classification of distal humerus fracture. (A) Type I undisplaced condylar fracture of the elbow; (B) Type II displaced but not rotated T-condylar fracture; (C) Type III displaced and rotated T-condylar fracture; (D) Type IV displaced, rotated, and comminuted condylar fracture.
</td>
<td>
Shearing injuries are also commonly seen and are classified into:
1. Capitellum and lateral trochlea
2. Lateral epicondyle
3. Posterior aspect of lateral condyle
4. Posterior aspect of trochlea
5. Medial epicondyle fracture
</td>
<td>
important—keep small 1.5 mm and 2 mm screws threaded k-wires and smooth pins for fixation of small fragments. Do not discard osteochondral fragments.
Methods of Fixation
• Interfragmentary screws: This has limited utility and has to be supplemented with POP slab usually.
• Dual plate fixation: Perpendicular construct is favored—one plate over medial column and another plate placed posterolaterally, 90° from the medial plate. Parallel LCP can also be applied as described by O'Driscoll. His principles are to maximize fixation in distal fragment and stabilize shaft to distal fragments. Every screw in distal fragment should pass through plate engaging the opposite fragment also fixed to plate. Maximize the number of screws in distal fragments and create a fixed angle construct.
• Total elbow arthroplasty (semiconstrained): Preferred in osteopenic bone with markedly comminuted fractures
The usual practice is to isolate the ulnar nerve during dissection (8 cm proximally to 6 cm below) and release of medial intermuscular septum followed by exposure of distal humerus using one of the below:
Alonso–Llames triceps sparing approach: Medial and lateral windows are developed by side of triceps and triceps erased subperiosteally from humerus. Done for limited extra-articular fractures.
Campbell triceps splitting approach: The triceps is split in the midline but approach is limited proximally by radial nerve.
Van Gordner approach: Distal tongue of triceps fascia is prepared in an inverted-V and rest as for triceps splitting approach. Better repairs extensor mechanism.
Bryan–Morrey approach: Medial approach raising triceps and extensor mechanism as a full subperiosteal sleeve off posterior humerus and ulna.
Triceps reflecting and anconeus pedicle (TRAP) approach of O'Driscoll: The extensor mechanism is raised with vascularized anconeus pedicle
</td>
</tr>
</table>

Contd...

Contd...

Epidemiology	*Anatomy*	*Clinical Evaluation*	*Radiographic Evaluation*	*Treatment*
				to act as dynamic stabilizer. The approach begins laterally in Kocher's interval (b/n ECU and anconeus) raisinganconeus from ulna preserving LCL and flap is continued with extensor mechanism (I raise with a sleeve of bone from olecranon) and triceps. Medially ulnar nerve is preserved. This raised tongue contains triceps, extensor mechanism, and anconeus. Olecranon osteotomy—preferred by many. Site of osteotomy is decided by either raising anconeus off laterally or medial capsular dissection to visualize trochlea. Chevron osteotomy is preferred as this enters in arearelatively devoid of articular cartilage. Incomplete osteotomy is completed by hand allowing interdigitation duringreplacement. Reflect the olecranon and triceps together to expose distal humerus. **COMPLICATIONS** • Elbow stiffness • Heterotopic ossification—1–3% • Nonunion—2–10% • Neuropathy (ulnar nerve)

CAPITELLUM FRACTURES

Epidemiology	*Anatomy*	*Clinical Evaluation*	*Radiographic Evaluation*	*Treatment*
This is a coronal shear fracture at the lateral distal articular surface of the humerus. These represent <1% of all elbow fractures and 6% of all distal humeral fractures with a slight female predilection. They occur in the coronal plane, parallel to the anterior humeral cortex. As there are minimal soft tissue attachments so fragment remains free and hence displacements are common. Comminution at the fracture line is also common. Displaced fragment or comminution in the joint space or the coronoid or radial fossae may result in a block to flexion. **MECHANISM OF INJURY** Usually results from low-energy FOOSH with the elbow in varying degrees of flexion. In this way, the forces are transmitted through the radial head onto the capitellum in a shearing manner causing the fracture. The other mechanism is during spontaneous reduction of posterolateral elbow dislocation.	Capitellum forms important articulation with radial head—the radiocapitellar joint, important for axial stability. The center of rotation of the capitellum is 12–15 mm anterior to the humeral shaft making it vulnerable to shearing fractures in the coronal plane. In females, the carrying angle is higher so forces are more laterally transferred. Osteoporosis may be an additional contributory factor. Being a part of radiocapitellar joint and secondary contributor to coronal plane elbow stability (see fortress concept in elbow section), the fracture of capitellum is commonly associated with other injuries such as: • Radial head fractures (20%) • Posterolateral dislocation of elbow • Lateral ulnar collateral ligament (LUCL) injury. • Injury to interosseous membrane • Essex-Lopresti lesion (DRUJ + interosseous membrane injury).	There are swelling and ecchymosis about the elbow and hemarthrosis. During ROM evaluation, a mechanical block to elbow flexion and painful pronosupination are usually present. EUA should be done preferably during the initial evaluation or at the time of surgical intervention. There is often laxity to valgus or varus stress. This indicates a more complex injury involving LUCL or lateral ligamentous complex tears. Management should be thence planned. Also, assess the distal radioulnar joint to rule-out concomitant Essex–Lopresti lesion.	Standard AP and lateral radiographs of elbow should be obtained. Lateral should be strict lateral else it is common to miss this fracture on lateral radiograph; also, AP radiograph misses the injury mostly. The capitellar injury is more complex than what it appears on the radiographs so obtaining a CT scan is best to demonstrate comminution and impaction. Appearance of double arc in the fractured fragment indicates significant associated trochlear chunk—a type-IV injury. **CLASSIFICATIONS (Bryan–Morrey with McKee modification, Figs. 23A to D)** *Type I (Hahn–Steinthal)*: Complete osseous capitellar fracture without any trochlear extension. *Type II (Kocher–Lorenz)*: Sliver fractures with only anterior osteochondral fracture fragment and only minimal subchondral bone remaining. May be missed even on a CT scan. Difficult to fix.	Management has evolved with better understanding of the injury. Complexity needs to be understood before initiating treatment plan with selecting approach, fixation methods, and prognostication. Operative management is the priority but prognosis is commonly guarded. **NONOPERATIVE** This is primarily used for nondisplaced fractures (<2 mm for types I-III) or for very low-demand ill patients with comorbidities. It consists of immobilization in a posterior splint at 90° of elbow flexion for 4–6 weeks followed by range of elbow motion. Capitellum should be reduced against radial head for optimal outcome. **OPERATIVE** The goal is anatomic restoration or articular congruity and open reduction + internal fixation is preferred modality. *Displaced (≥2 mm) type I–III fractures*: Using posterolateral or posterior approach, screws are placed from a posterior to anterior direction (alternatively,

Contd...

Contd...

Epidemiology	*Anatomy*	*Clinical Evaluation*	*Radiographic Evaluation*	*Treatment*
	The associated injuries are common with type II fractures (up to 50%) and the primary fracture is commonly missed, evident only on opening the joint.		*Type III (Broberg–Morrey fracture)*: Severely comminuted or compression fractures of capitellum with loss of anatomy. *Type IV (McKee modification)*: Coronal shear fracture with fracture line extending medially that includes significant chunk of trochlea. ***Dubberlay et al. classification:*** As most of capitellar fractures involve trochlea so this classification system is more helpful in these cases. *Type I:* Capitellum ± trochlear ridge *Type II:* Capitellum and trochlea (1 piece) *Type III:* Capitellum and trochlea (2 pieces): • *A*: No posterior column comminution • *B*: Posterior column comminution present	headless screws may be placed from anterior to posterior). Anterolateral internervous plane between brachialis (musculocutaneous nerve) and brachioradialis (radial nerve) or Kocher (anconeus and ECU) may be also used. Fixation should be stable enough to allow early range of elbow motion. Excision is indicated for severely comminuted type I fractures, nonreducible or nonfixable type III fractures and most type II fractures or in chronic missed fractures with limited range of elbow motion. Excision can also be done arthroscopically and for type II fractures chondroplasty may be attempted after excision of cartilage fragment. Proximal migration of the radius with distal radioulnar joint pain is uncommon. Excision is not advisable in the presence of associated elbow instability or with Essex–Lopresti lesion. *Type IV fractures*: These are better exposed by extensile lateral approach to address medial trochlear fragment and any associated radial head/neck fracture. Supplemental medial exposure may be also necessary—preserves the collateral ligaments. Fixation modalities include headless compression screws (Herbert or mini-Acutrek type) or minifragment screws sunk well below the articular cartilage. Place two or more divergent screws to control for fragment rotation. Supplemental k-wires (threaded) or bioabsorbable pins may be used for small capitellum or trochlea fragments. Ligament injury may need reconstruction by suture anchors. Total elbow arthroplasty may be considered for elderly patients with existing arthritis and if fracture fixation strength is deemed doubtful as in type III fractures or if there is associated gross elbow instability that cannot be otherwise restored. **COMPLICATIONS** Infection/instability loss of ROM—common • Nonunion • Heterotopic ossification Osteonecrosis of capitellum • Stiffness • Cubitus valgus and tardy ulnar nerve palsy • Ulnar neuropathy—due to incarceration of nerve in scar tissue around FCU/cubital tunnel in the healing process.

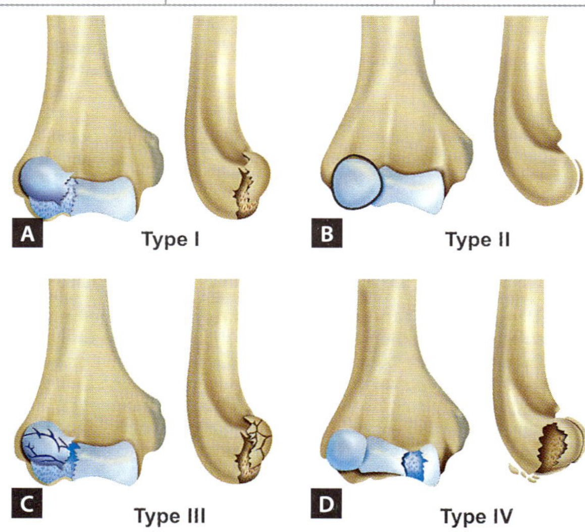

Figs. 23A to D: Bryan–Morrey with McKee modification for classifying capitellar fractures.

TROCHLEA FRACTURE (LAUGIER FRACTURE) AND MEDIAL EPICONDYLE FRACTURE

Epidemiology	*Anatomy*	*Clinical Evaluation*	*Radiographic Evaluation*	*Treatment*
Isolated shear fracture of trochlea: Trochlea fracture is an extremely rare injury otherwise this injury commonly accompanies elbow dislocation or capitellar or medial condyle fracture of humerus. Few case reports only exist for its description. The injury results from fall with possibly varus position of the elbow to redirect the radiocapitellar compressive forces to the ulnohumeral joint resulting in shear trochlear fracture. Reported literature varies widely for the position of elbow and extremity during fall. Both high-energy and low-energy injuries have been reported. *Medial epicondyle fracture*: These are more common (third most common elbow injuries) and represent around 12% of pediatric elbow fractures and 14% of distal humerus fractures. The peak age of occurrence is higher than lateral condyle fractures at around 11–12 years of age. The male to female ration is 4:1 where 50% are associated with elbow dislocation and in 15% cases, the fragment is incarcerated within the elbow joint. The mechanism of injury is a pull to the medial epicondylar epiphysis resulting from valgus forces on the elbow joint (FOOSH) and in others, the injury is a part of elbow dislocation where the attachments at the epicondyle shear the bone at physis. Direct injury is uncommon but forces parallel to physis applied eccentrically over medial epicondyle displaces it, as may occur while hitting an object medially with arm in motion. Chronic disruptions of the medial epicondyle may occur in repetitive sport injuries where valgus forces are applied on the bone such as little leaguers elbow (children) or Golfer's elbow (adults).	The trochlea is protected deep within elbow aloof from most of the forces sustained during fall. Compressive forces usually pass through the radiocapitellar joint due to carrying angle. As there is no soft tissue attachment to this articular region so displacing forces are also minimal. Osteochondral fracture fragments are also seen as with capitellar fractures. **Medial epicondyle fractures:** Medial epicondyle is the last ossification center to fuse to distal humerus, so physis remains open for a long time predisposing to failure at this level. The flexor–pronator mass and ulnar collateral ligament are attached to the medial epicondyle. The flexor–pronator mass includes pronator teres, flexor carpi ulnaris, palmaris longus, flexor digitorum superficialis, and flexor carpi ulnaris muscles. Traction at the medial epicondyle by forceful contractions (muscular) or static pulling on it (ligamentous) due to shear forces results in avulsion of the medial epicondyle causing a Salter–Harris type 1 injury pattern. The blood supply comes from inferior ulnar collateral artery anteriorly and superior and inferior ulnar collateral artery posteriorly that remain preserved in most of the cases even with dislocation. Open injuries are liable to disrupt them.	As for other fractures, the findings are swelling, pain, tenderness, limited ROM, and hemarthrosis. **Medial epicondyle fracture:** The patient presents with medial elbow pain usually following a trauma during sports while resisting valgus force at elbow joint. There is commonly prominent ecchymosis centered over the medial epicondyle and prominent valgus instability (tested if joint is not too painful). The presence of generalized swelling is more suggestive of larger injury complex like elbow dislocation. In that event look for lateral and anterior tenderness also indicating lateral complex and coronoid injuries. Always examine and document the status of ulnar nerve function in medial epicondyle injuries. The elbow should be taken through full ROM gently to identify block/locking from incarcerated fragment. **ASSOCIATED INJURY** Elbow dislocation and its accompanying injury components	AP views may show an irregularity at the ulnohumeral joint while lateral views may confuse this to capitellar fracture, as they are more common. CT scan is the best modality for diagnosis and characterization, displacement, and planning. **Medial epicondyle fracture:** Plain X-rays easily demonstrate the displaced fragment. Fragments appearing undisplaced on AP view are quite significantly displaced in sagittal plane anteriorly. It is better to evaluate with contralateral radiographs or if in doubt then use CT scan. Be cautious in children <7 years of age as in them, the epiphysis is itself not ossified so no displaced fragment can be seen instead only a medial soft tissue swelling will be observed. Absence of visualization of displaced fragment in older children should be carefully evaluated, as it is commonly mistaken to be ossification center of trochlea when actually it is incarcerated within the joint. Undisplaced fractures in older children would present with only soft tissue swelling, minimally displaced fractures just demonstrate a widened physis. Always look at the degree of displacement and its location. Elbow dislocation is indicated, if lateral condyle/coronoid injury/radial head fractures are seen. The fractures are classified more or less in a descriptive manner: **Papavasiliou Classification (Fig. 24)** • *Type 1*: Small avulsion [the medial humeral column line is continued on AP radiograph (Shentons line of humerus)], if it misses medial epicondyle then it indicates minimally displaced fracture. If the line contacts medial epicondyle but there is widening of physis then it indicates undisplaced fracture. • *Type 2*: Medial epicondyle displaced at the level of joint. • *Type 3*: Medial epicondyle displaced and incarcerated into elbow joint • *Type 4*: Associated with elbow dislocation	Operative management is best for all displaced fractures (≥2 mm). Undisplaced fractures (<2 mm) can be managed by above elbow posterior splint to immobilize the fracture keeping it well in contact against the olecranon and frequent follow-ups. The splint may be removed at 4–6 weeks and mobilization begun gradually. Operative management constitutes the mainstay due to inherent instability of the displaced fracture fragments. Medial approach is used to expose the joint and evaluate fracture configuration. After reduction, the fracture is fixed with headless compression screws or cancellous screws. If the fragment is large enough then cancellous screws can be passed from medial to lateral obliquely from nonarticular portion anteriorly to capitellar region posteriorly. For smaller fragments, Herbert screws or similar headless compression screws may be passed from anterior to posterior direction capitellar fractures (CF) and sunk beneath the cartilage. This offers possibly better fixation strength and stability, as it is perpendicular to fracture line. K-wires or smooth pins can be used for very small fragments that cannot be fixed with screws. Chondroplasty can be done, if there are articular fragments that were removed for nonfixability. **Complications** • Stiffness • Arthritis • Nonunion **Medial epicondyle fracture:** Nonoperative treatment is indicated for low-energy mechanism, minimally displaced fracture (some take up to 5 mm displacement as acceptable while some even do not accept 2-mm displacement!), elbow stable to valgus stress. The results of nonoperative treatment have been reported good even in largely displaced fractures undergoing fibrous union at ectopic places so surgery is not strongly favored by nontrauma, nonpediatric orthopedic surgeons. With pressure on more accurate management and stress on anatomical restorations, lot of surgeons are reporting interventional treatment of fractures displaced as less as 2 mm! The undisputed

Contd...

Contd...

Epidemiology	*Anatomy*	*Clinical Evaluation*	*Radiographic Evaluation*	*Treatment*
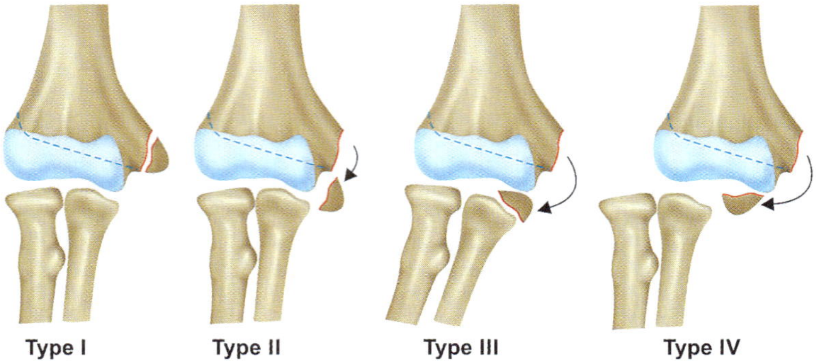 **Fig. 24:** The Papavasiliou classification of pediatric medial epicondyle fracture.			**Wilkins Classification** *Acute*: • Nondisplaced • Minimally displaced • Significantly displaced • Incarcerated within the joint *Chronic*: Associated with tension stress injuries ***Based on displacement:*** This is a gray area as most physicians follow different guidelines: • *Type I*: Undisplaced • *Type II*: Displaced less than or up to 5 mm (<2 mm is minimally displaced) • *Type III*: Displaced >5 mm	surgical indications include elbow displacement with incarcerated fragment and open injuries. Relative indications for surgery would be ulnar nerve injury, elbow instability, significantly displaced fractures (>5 mm for me!) and dominant arm injury in a professional overhead athlete. Nonoperative treatment includes placing the limb in above elbow POP slab with elbow at right angle and forearm in neutral rotation to promote fragment healing, prevent further displacement/instability/nonunion. This is done for 2–4 weeks followed by gradual mobilization. Surgical management is aimed at restoring stability, early mobilization and return of function, and promote fracture healing. Open reduction is better than closed one because targeting perfection is difficult closed. Reduction is aided by supine forearm, wrist flexion with an externally rotated shoulder. "Milking maneuver" to gradually proximally shift the fragment by an Esmarch bandage may be done by wrapping it from distal to proximal. Fractional lengthening of flexor–pronator mass may be additionally done, if still unreducible. Fixation may be done by K-wire, cannulated screw with/without washer, or suture anchor. **Complications** The complications of conservative treatment include elbow stiffness, instability, cubitus valgus, nonunion, and ulnar nerve neuropathy. Surgical treatment is additionally associated with: • Infection • Myositis ossificans • Radial nerve injury

FRACTURE OF LATERAL CONDYLE HUMERUS (PEDIATRIC)

Epidemiology	*Anatomy*	*Clinical Evaluation*	*Radiographic Evaluation*	*Treatment*
Historically, the fracture was first described by Stimson in 1883 in his book "treatise on fractures". The fractures are important for their high associated risk of nonunion/malunion and associated complications was recognized by Milch. Blount cautioned against the risk of later displacement even	The distal humerus in children is mostly cartilaginous and the physis of lateral condyle extends into trochlear notch. So lateral condyle fractures may extend into trochlea and may also contain a part of the lateral crista, such fractures are unstable (Milch type II). It is difficult to exactly identify the fracture type on radiographs	There is a history of fall usually on outstretched hand as observed by parents resulting in swelling and pain in the elbow region and the child keeps the extremity dropped avoiding movements and even touch by acquaintances. There is localized lateral elbow pain and tenderness associated with swelling, but an obvious	Standard AP, lateral, and oblique views are obtained of the affected extremity along with the other elbow for comparison. Internal oblique radiographs (must obtain) better demonstrate the fracture and displacement as the fragment is usually posterolateral. If the physis is mostly cartilaginous then	Treatment is aimed at ensuring healing of the fracture and to prevent pseudoarthrosis, malunion, deformities, and functional disorders. Displaced fractures (>2 mm displacement) have a uniformly poor outcome, if neglected, so this fracture has been classified as fracture of necessity.

Contd...

Contd...

Epidemiology	*Anatomy*	*Clinical Evaluation*	*Radiographic Evaluation*	*Treatment*
in initially slightly displaced fractures. Flynn reported occurrence of nonunion in even slightly displaced fractures and hence need of fixation *(fracture of necessity)*. They comprise nearly 12–20% of all distal humeral fractures in children and are the 2nd most common elbow fractures (after supracondylar fractures) in this age-group (incidence 1.6/10,000). These are most common in children around 6 years of age (range 5–10 years). Most of the fractures fall under Salter–Harris type-II or type-IV pattern. **MECHANISM OF INJURY** The fractures may result from a pull-off force or a push-off force to the lateral distal humerus. Pulling forces from eccentric contraction of common extensor muscle origin or from a varus force **(Fig. 25)** result in avulsion fracture of the lateral condyle that may occur during falls. Push-off forces are applied directly when there is a FOOSH mechanism of injury shearing off the lateral condyle from humerus transmitted through the elbow particularly in valgus.	as apparent fracture fragment may be smaller than real fragment. The fracture also tends to open laterally more than medially in lower stages of injury while as the force of injury increases the fracture line becomes more parallel and medial and lateral gaps become equal. Medial opening of the fractures makes them unstable and they have higher tendency to displace as they lose the cartilage hinge. Also, these fractures are purely intra-articular making them vulnerable to joint incongruity, if not treated with anatomical reduction. If articular surface is intact, then fracture is considered stable while in a complete fracture where the fracture line extends through the cartilage, the fracture is unstable and there are high chances of displacement. Fragment rotation is a major concern, as it indicates definitely unstable fracture. The rotation occurs in frontal plane first represented by obliteration of capitellum and then later along sagittal axis corresponding to intact lateral collateral ligament. Frontal plane rotation is usually at right angles while fragment may additionally flip by 180° along sagittal axis making a total rotation of 270° in complex geometry that should be understood while reducing the fracture. The vascularity of distal humeral metaphysis is vulnerable as the circulation is marred by various physeal cartilage plates. The lateral condyle is supplied by the common extensor origin posteriorly making it the dominating source of blood supply for this zone and should be preserved.	deformity or misalignment may not be obvious to the observer. Crepitus may be palpable and pain may be reproduced/accentuated with forced wrist extension. Clinically, the fracture needs to be distinguished from: Supracondylar fracture, lateral epicondyle injury (avulsion injury), lateral condylar physeal injury, radial head subluxation, radial head/neck fracture, elbow dislocations, and medial epicondylar fracture	an arthrogram may help to identify the lesion or an MRI may be preferred for its noninvasive nature. Presence of intact cartilaginous hinge changes the modality of treatment from open reduction to closed reduction so is a preferable modality in confusing situations. MRI is also indicated for delayed/nonunions. The drawbacks include need of sedation and higher cost. CT scan is rarely needed, if there is difficulty in identifying the fracture despite high suspicion. Else, CT scan may be used to determine the fracture gap as 2 mm is too less to ascertain on routine radiographs. When there is doubt, perform examination in anesthesia with arthrogram that also gives opportunity to simultaneously treat the patient. **CLASSIFICATIONS** **Milch Classification** divides the fracture based on the fracture line extension, but is less useful in guiding treatment **(Fig. 26)** Type I (uncommon)—fracture line lateral to trochlear groove (elbow is stable and less common fracture type). This results from push-off force causing shear/impaction injury and the fracture correlates with Salter–Harris type IV physeal injury. Type II—fracture line extends into trochlear groove (more common and unstable fracture pattern). This unstable fracture pattern results from "pull-off" forces from pull of ECRL/B and brachioradialis and results in Salter–Harris type II pattern fracture. **Jakob Classification (Fig. 27)** Stage 1—articular surface intact, <2 mm displacement Stage 2—articular surface disrupted Stage 3—fragment rotated **Weiss Classification** Type 1—<2 mm displacement indicating intact cartilage hinge. Risk of fracture displacement is much less, if displacement is <2 mm (Finnbogason et al.) Type 2—>2 mm but <4 mm displacement, mostly the cartilage is intact on an arthrogram Type 3—>4 mm displacement where the articular surface would be most likely disrupted on arthrogram	Nonoperative management is indicated only if the fracture has definite ≤2 mm displacement in all views (Song stage 1). Above elbow POP slab is applied in 90° of flexion else POP cast may be applied directly if swelling is less. Patient should be followed weekly for 3 weeks to detect displacement (20%) especially on internal oblique view. Immobilization is continued for 6 weeks usually followed by removal of slab/cast and gradual supervised mobilization over 2 weeks. Operative management includes closed reduction and percutaneous pinning (CRPP) for type 2 Weiss (stage 2 and some stage 3 Song) fractures or ORIF for type 3 Weiss fractures (most stage 3 and all stage 4/5 Song). In CRPP, the fracture fragment is pushed against the humerus by applying a force anteromedially and fixing by cross-pinning in a divergent fashion. Arthrogram is usually obtained intraoperatively to confirm cartilage continuity and joint congruity. Screw fixation may be done for a more rigid fixation with compression at fracture but screw has to be usually removed later and one must avoid olecranon fossa. The surgeon also should be experienced in the technique else surgical damage incurred is more. Open reduction internal fixation is the standard method of fixation for type 3 fractures and nonreducible fractures. Also, if arthrogram demonstrates joint incongruity in type 2 fractures, ORIF is better. Prefer approach between brachioradialis and triceps. The reduction is done under direct vision but sometimes due to plastic deformation, exact match may not be achieved at metaphysis. Check the intraarticular reduction and not reduction at metaphysis, as it is often inaccurate ("fool's gold"). Due to plastic deformation at the time of injury, avoid excessive dissection posteriorly and stay anterior to preserve blood supply. Do not put varus force or try varus reduction, as it displaces the fragment rather than helping. Fixation is usually done by two cross pins or a screw. Pins are placed percutaneous if will be removed

Contd...

Contd...

<table>
<tr><th>Epidemiology</th><th>Anatomy</th><th>Clinical Evaluation</th><th>Radiographic Evaluation</th><th>Treatment</th></tr>
<tr><td colspan="3">

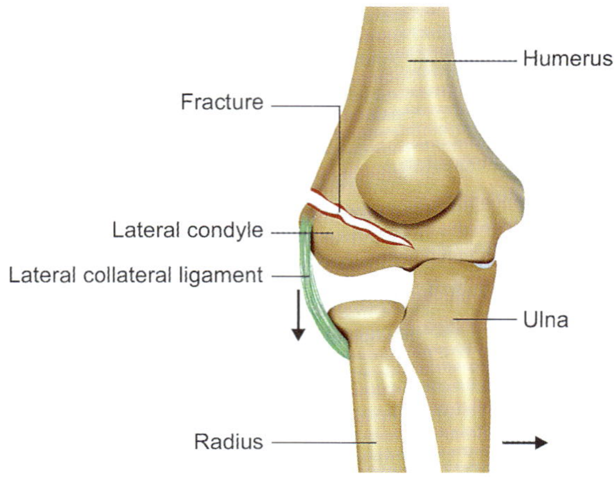

Fig. 25: Anatomical illustration of development of lateral condyle fracture resulting from varus producing force (pull-off type fracture), depicting how there could be lateral opening with an intact cartilage hinge. Once the fracture completes, the fracture lines become parallel with equal medial and lateral gaps.

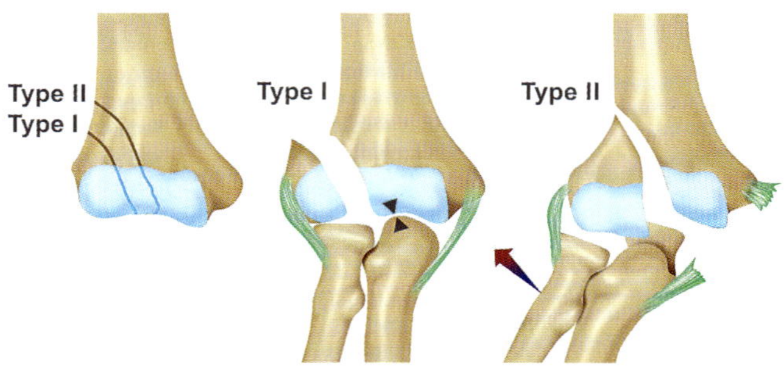

Fig. 26: The Milch classification of pediatric lateral condyle fracture.

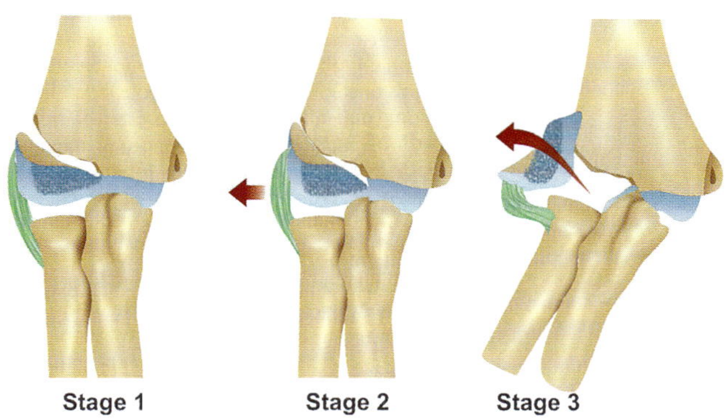

Fig. 27: The Jackob's stages of displacement of pediatric supracondylar fracture.

</td><td>

Song Classification (Fig. 28)
This classification also incorporates the medial and lateral fracture gaps to better guide treatment.

Stage 1—≤2 mm having limited fracture line within metaphysis in all views—stable fracture

Stage 2—≤2 mm with lateral gap in all views—?stability

Stage 3—≤2 mm with lateral gap as wide as medial one—unstable

Stage 4—>2 mm without fragment rotation on all views—unstable

Stage 5—>2 mm with fragment rotation—unstable

</td><td>

(preferred) at 4 weeks else bury them. Splint is applied posteriorly and pins taken out at 4 weeks while continuing splint for 2 more weeks.

COMPLICATIONS

- Stiffness—most common complication
- Nonunion—this occurs due to loss of precarious blood supply in a fracture distracted constantly by extensor pull and poor metaphyseal blood supply to distal humerus. The risk is high in nonoperated fractures. Treatment usually involves in-situ bone grafting and fixation instead of opening and freshening the fracture ends.
- Osteonecrosis—occurs after 1–3 years due to loss of blood supply posteriorly
- Malunion—commonly, a cubitus varus results (20%) in nondisplaced or minimally displaced fractures. Lateral overgrowth/spurring is possibly the most common deformity that occurs in 50% patients and is also responsible for cubitus varus appearance (*pseudocubitus varus*). This deformity is proportional to initial fracture displacement and is minimized, if the periosteum is aligned (counsel patient for its occurrence but innocuousness). In displaced fractures, cubitus valgus (10%) ± tardy ulnar nerve palsy results due to injury to the physis and lateral physeal arrest (bony bar formation or physis mismatch). Fishtail deformity may result from absorption of area between medial ossification center and lateral condyle ossification possibly due to loss of vascularity, which then fails to develop.

It may also result from arrest of the central physis and is then a cause of cubitus varus deformity. So, cubitus varus may result from lateral spur (pseudovariety), lateral physeal overgrowth, or from fish-tail deformity. Cubitus varus is often innocuous and also fish-tail deformity usually does not need surgical management. Significant deformities are managed by corrective

</td></tr>
</table>

Contd...

Contd...

Epidemiology	*Anatomy*	*Clinical Evaluation*	*Radiographic Evaluation*	*Treatment*

Stage	Degree of displacement	Fracture pattern	Radiograph views used as bas s	Stability
1	≤ 2 mm	Limited fracture line within the metaphysis	All 4 views	Stable
2	≤ 2 mm	Lateral gap	All 4 views	Indefinable
3	≤ 2 mm	Gap as wide laterally as medially	Any of 4 views	Unstable
4	> 2 mm	Without rotation of fragment	Any of 4 view	Unstable
5	> 2 mm	With rotation of fragment	Any of 4 view	Unstable

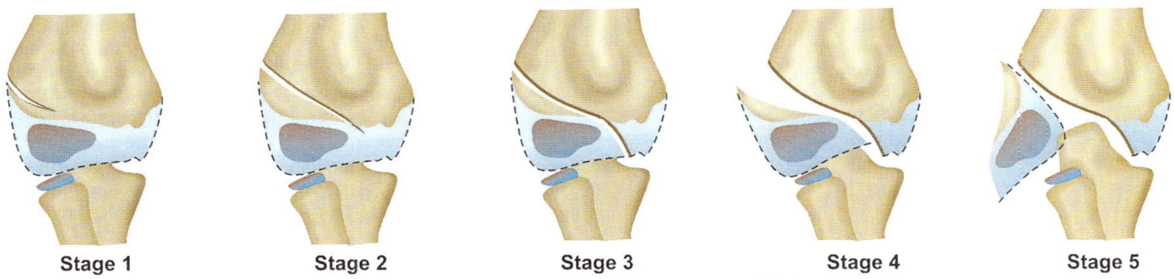

Fig. 28: Song et al. classification of pediatric supracondylar fracture.

Epidemiology	*Anatomy*	*Clinical Evaluation*	*Radiographic Evaluation*	*Treatment*
				osteotomy (for definitive indications) ± ulnar nerve transposition. • Tardy ulnar nerve palsy • Distal humeral growth arrest • Neglected fracture lateral condyle (>3 weeks old)—is a treatment dilemma, some consider it to be possibly better left alone and managed later by osteotomy while others aggressively fix them. There may be a role of fixation, if the fracture presents before hard callus formation (up to 4 weeks) while surgery should always be done under guarded prognosis. Fractures presenting later say after 6 weeks are better left alone.

OLECRANON FRACTURE

Epidemiology	*Anatomy*	*Clinical Evaluation*	*Radiographic Evaluation*	*Treatment*
Relatively common fracture around elbow (5% of all elbow fractures). Open fractures may be seen in 5–25% cases. As for most fractures, bimodal distribution is observed—younger individuals sustain high-energy trauma and older patients due to weak osteoporotic metaphyseal bones sustain fracture from a simple fall. **MECHANISM OF INJURY/ FRACTURE** • Direct blow/impact • FOOSH with elbow in flexion • Avulsion fracture • Stress fracture	There is high degree of congruity between trochlea and olecranon where the articulation is formed by the semilunar articular notch (greater sigmoid notch—smaller sigmoid notch is for radial head below) of ulna. The coronoid process marks the distal border of the greater sigmoid notch. This articulation allows motion in the flexion–extension axis. The greater sigmoid notch articular cartilage surface is interrupted by a transverse ridge known as the bare area. Posteriorly, the triceps tendon envelops the articular capsule before it inserts onto the olecranon.	There is pain, tenderness, and swelling. Deformity seen with associated injuries in the region. Palpable gap is present in displaced fractures with extensor lag against gravity at elbow in case of associated insufficiency of triceps tendon. ***Associated injuries*** are common and include: • Radial head fracture • Radial head dislocation (Monteggia variant) • Coronoid fracture • Lateral condyle fracture • Radial neck fracture • Supracondylar fracture • Ulnar nerve injury is seen in 2% of the cases.	AP and lateral views are obtained as standard while radiocapitellar view may be obtained for additional radial head/neck injuries. CT scan may be indicated for comminuted fractures for preoperative planning. **CLASSIFICATIONS** ***Colton classification*** • Nondisplaced—displacement does not increase with elbow flexion • Displaced avulsion fracture • Displaced oblique or transverse fracture • Displaced comminuted fracture • Fracture dislocation	***Nonoperative treatment***—undisplaced fractures or fractures in elderly low-demand patients can be managed nonoperatively in an above elbow splint applied in 45–90° of flexion for 4–6 weeks with movements begun thereafter. ***Operative treatment*** is indicated for all displaced fractures (>2 mm articular displacement) and for insufficiency of extensor mechanism. Tension band wiring (TBW) is the standard method of ORIF, long intramedullary screw can be used for pure transverse fractures. TBW does not provide rotational stability in comminuted fractures and

Contd...

Contd...

Epidemiology	*Anatomy*	*Clinical Evaluation*	*Radiographic Evaluation*	*Treatment*
	A fracture of the olecranon with displacement represents a functional disruption of the triceps mechanism, resulting in loss of active extension of the elbow. There can be persistent epiphyseal plates in adults (patella cubiti); these are usually bilateral and should not be confused for fracture. Triceps inserts onto the posterior proximal ulna and blends with periosteum. Anconeus inserts on the lateral aspect of olecranon. These muscles are responsible for displacement.		**Schatzker Classification (Fig. 29)** • Type A—simple transverse fracture = avulsion fractures • Type B—transverse impacted fracture • Type C—oblique fracture • Type D—comminuted fracture • Type E—distal extra-articular fracture • Type F—fracture dislocation **AO Classification** • Type A—extra-articular fracture • Type B—intra-articular • Type C—intra-articular fracture of radial head and olecranon **Mayo Classification (Fig. 30)** —possibly the most useful classification for treatment purpose • Type I fractures—non-displaced or minimally displaced and can be managed nonoperatively. • Subclassified as non-comminuted (A) or comminuted (B) • Type II—displaced without elbow instability and need operative fixation. Type IIA can be treated by TBW. Type IIB are comminuted and need plate fixation • Type III fractures are associated with ulnohumeral instability and need operative treatment.	has high chance of hardware removal. One may choose to engage anterior cortex to reduce chances of wire migration but overpenetration risks anterior interosseous (AIN) palsy and reduced forearm rotation. Displaced comminuted or multifragmentary unstable fractures are better managed by locked plate fixation. Dual plate (parallel) fixation has been proposed to avoid hardware-related complications of posterior plating. Plate fixation can be also done for fracture dislocations or Monteggia fracture. Fragment excision and triceps advancement are not a standard procedure but has been prescribed for nonunion of olecranon and for small articular fractures <20% of the joint surface in elderly osteoporotic bones where fixation has high chances of failure. Osteoporotic bones have poor implant purchase and hence fixation using suture anchors is a good interesting proposal but needs knowhow of thread management. Tension suturing using nonabsorbable heavy sutures is practiced by some but not popular. Overall, no technique is superior over other and all have high re-operation rates but, certainly plate fixation is much more costly than TBW. **COMPLICATIONS** • Hardware prominence • Stiffness • Infection • Pin migration • Heterotopic ossification • Synostosis development • Nonunion • AIN injury • Ulnar neuropathy • Loss of grip strength • Arthritis

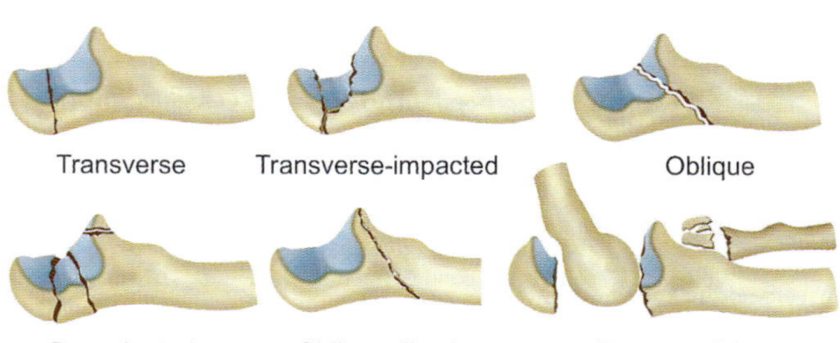

Fig. 29: Schatzker classification of olecranon fractures into six types.

Contd...

Contd...

Epidemiology	Anatomy	Clinical Evaluation	Radiographic Evaluation	Treatment

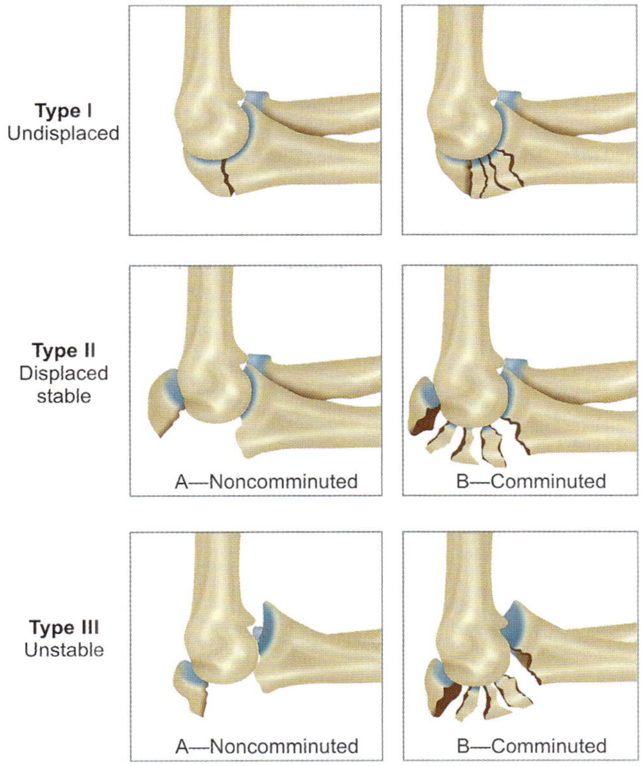

Fig. 30: Mayo classification of olecranon fractures.

RADIAL HEAD FRACTURES

Epidemiology	Anatomy	Clinical Evaluation	Radiographic Evaluation	Treatment
The fracture comprises 1.5–4% of all fractures and is the most common fracture of elbow region (33%). They usually occur in 20–40 years age group (75%) and are more common in females (twice as common). Female patients tend to be older and in older patients females largely outnumber males. **MECHANISM OF INJURY** *FOOSH:* When elbow is in extension and forearm pronated, there is maximal transmittance of force to the radial head (valgus-pronation stress) from wrist pushing radial head against capitellum. By itself, the fracture is commonly innocuous but there are a number of following associated injuries that should be taken into account, while planning fracture treatment. • Lateral collateral ligament (LCL) complex injury—most common associated injury • Medial collateral ligament injury and combined injury • Essex-Lopresti lesion (DRUJ + interosseous injury)	Radiocapitellar joint is a pivot joint that transmits 60% of load across at all angles of elbow flexion and is greatest in full extension. The capitellum and the radial head are reciprocally curved maintaining good congruity. The radial head is a "toffy"-shaped structure where the rim is also covered by articular cartilage due to its articulation with ulna lesser sigmoid notch. Here, a nonarticular portion of the radial head is a 90–110° arc from radial styloid to Lister's tubercle. This is the safe zone for hardware placement. Full rotation of the head of the radius requires accurate anatomic positioning in the lesser sigmoid notch. The radial head plays a role in valgus and longitudinal stability of the elbow. The radial head is a secondary restraint to valgus forces and comes into play in an MCL-deficient elbow when the center of varus-valgus rotation shifts laterally. More importantly, it prevents proximal migration of radius in	There are pain and tenderness over lateral aspect of elbow limiting the elbow and forearm motion especially the supination and pronation. Depending on displacement of the fracture fragments, there would be variable mechanical block to elbow and forearm motion especially pronosupination. The soft spot of elbow is obliterated and filled with hematoma. If permitted, evaluate the elbow stability for competency of LCL and MCL along with interosseous membrane (IM) and distal radioulnar Joint (DRUJ) stability. For IM competency, perform the radius pull test—a >3-mm translation indicates Essex-Lopresti lesion. For DRUJ, a sagittal plane translation of >50% indicates instability—compare from opposite side.	Anteroposterior and lateral elbow standard radiographs are obtained. Undisplaced/minimally displaced radial head fractures may demonstrate fat pad (supinator fat pad) sign. Also, posterior elbow fat pad (sail sign) is also an indication of radial head injury. Radiocapitellar view (Greenspan) better demonstrates the radial head anatomy by avoiding coronoid overlap. CT scan may better evaluate the fracture fragments and displacement. MRI evaluates the soft tissue better especially the collateral ligament sufficiency. **CLASSIFICATIONS** **Mason Classification** (modified by Hotchkiss and Broberg-Morrey, **Fig. 31**) • Type I ("chisel fracture")—nondisplaced or minimally displaced fracture, no mechanical block to rotations (<2 mm dislocation) • Type II—displaced (>2 mm) or angulated fracture, mechanical block to movements (>2 mm	*Aims:* Regaining the movements by removing block, stabilizing elbow, limiting the development of arthrosis later. *Conservative management* Mason type I fractures are amenable to nonoperative treatment with symptomatic immobilization in a posterior elbow splint in relative flexion until pain free, followed by range-of-motion and strengthening exercises. Aspiration of joint hematoma does not make much of a difference. It is recommended that mobilization be started early by 3 weeks or even earlier, if pain free. Management of type II isolated displaced, stable, partial articular fracture is highly debated. Currently, the literature reports equivalent results for both conservative and operative management of stable/unstable type II Mason-Johnston radial head fractures. Possibly significant mechanical block to ROM is an indication of fixation.

Contd...

Contd...

Epidemiology	Anatomy	Clinical Evaluation	Radiographic Evaluation	Treatment
• Coronoid fracture • Olecranon fracture • Osteochondral injury to capitellum • Terrible triad of Hotchkiss—elbow dislocation + radial head fracture + coronoid fracture • Fracture of carpal bones—scaphoid, triquetrum	association with interosseous membrane and competent DRUJ. Proximal migration of the radius can occur after radial head excision, if the interosseous ligament and DRUJ (TFCC tear) are disrupted (Essex–Lopresti lesion)—also called *longitudinal radioulnar dissociation*		dislocation and >30% radial head involved, Broberg-Morrey). Rinner added that if there is cortical contact between fragments then it is a stable fracture while if there is no cortical contact then it is unstable. • Type III—comminuted and displaced fracture with mechanical block to rotation • Type IIIA—fracture of entire radial neck with head completely separated from shaft • Type IIIB—articular fracture involving the entire head, consisting of >2 large fragments • Type IIIC—fracture with a tilted and impacted articular segment • Type IV (Johnston addition, 1962)—radial head fracture with elbow dislocation	*Mason type III*: It is recommended to reconstruct the radial head by ORIF, if up to three simple fragments are present and fixable. The osteosynthesis is done in the safe zone identified by either the Smith and Hotchkiss method or Caputo et al. method **(Fig. 32)**. Placement of implant beyond this zone would result in articular attrition arthritis of ulnar sigmoid notch and pain. For more than three fragments, the results of osteosynthesis are not very favorable and should be replaced by arthroplasty. It is difficult to comment on use of monopolar/bipolar, mono-block/modular, cemented/uncemented or material (pyrocarbon vs. metallic vs. poly) in view of evolving data. Kocher or Kaplan is the preferred exposure for radial head. So, indications of ORIF can be summarized as: • Mason type II with mechanical block • Up to three fragment comminution of Mason type III fracture • *Associated complex ipsilateral injuries*: For Essex–Lopresti lesion, it is recommended to address the TFCC simultaneously rather than just DRUJ stabilization with K-wire. • *Stable/unstable Mason type II*: ?? ORIF Fragment excision is usually not advisable, as it anyway causes instability, unless it cannot be fixed despite best of efforts. So, concepts of small free fragments <30% of articular surface to be excised and others to be preserved possibly does not hold true. Radial head resection—a nonanatomical treatment indicated only in low demand, sedentary patients without any associated destabilizing injuries (rare to find). There is a possibility to development of DRUJ instability and proximal radius migration if associated with Essex–Lopresti. Whenever done, err on the side of delaying the surgery by at least 4 weeks or more (preferably 3 months). *Type IV Mason and terrible triad injuries*: These need thorough evaluation of associated ligament and bony injuries. Restoration of ulnohumeral articulation is a priority along with elbow stability. So, fix olecranon/coronoid, repair/reconstruct LCL/MCL and if

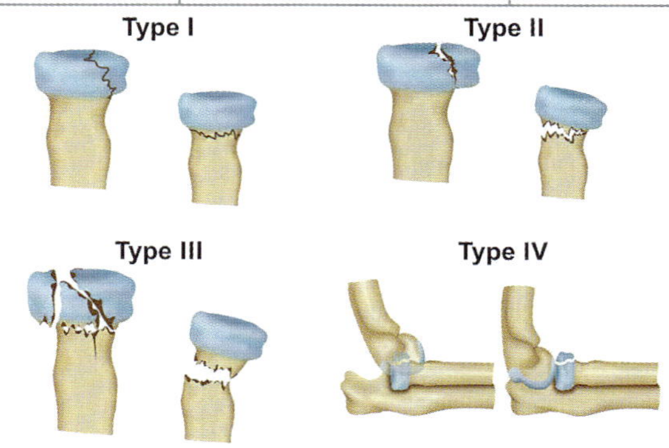

Fig. 31: Detailed Mason classification of distal radius fractures with modifications by Hotchkiss and Broberg–Morrey.

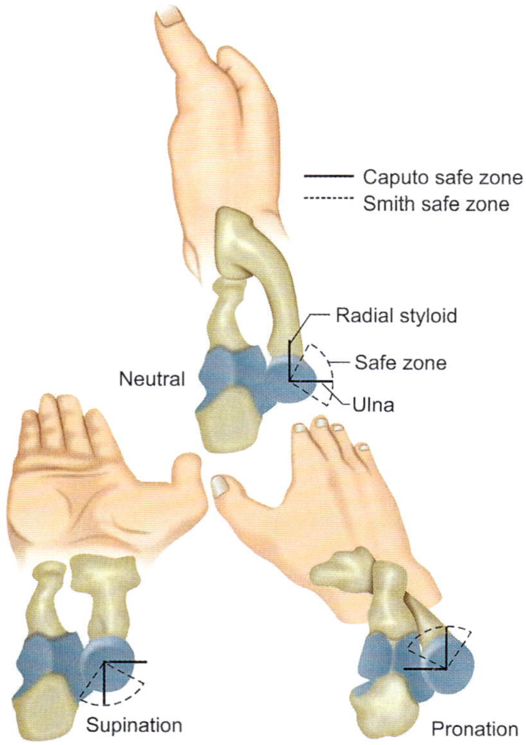

Fig. 32: The radial head is covered with articular cartilage all around but some part does not participate in articulation during range of motion (ROM) that may be plated safely. The nonarticular area of the radial head or the so-called safe zone for the application of internal fixation devices has been defined in various ways. Smith and Hotchkiss (discontinuous lines and zone) defined it based on lines bisecting the radial head made in full supination, full pronation, and neutral. Implants can be placed as far as halfway between the middle and posterior lines and a few millimeters beyond halfway between the middle and anterior lines. Caputo et al. (bold lines) recommended using the radial styloid and Lister tubercle as intraoperative guides to this safe zone, but this describes a slightly different zone.

Contd...

Contd...

Epidemiology	*Anatomy*	*Clinical Evaluation*	*Radiographic Evaluation*	*Treatment*
				osteosynthesis possible then ORIF for radial head else replace the same. **COMPLICATIONS** • Fracture displacement on conservative management—no change in management line with serial radiographs • PIN injury • Implant failure • Loss of pronosupination • Stiff elbow • Radiocapitellar arthritis • Nonunion • CRPS • Heterotopic ossification

MONTEGGIA FRACTURE DISLOCATION

Epidemiology	*Anatomy*	*Clinical Evaluation*	*Radiographic Evaluation*	*Treatment*
This is defined as injury to proximal third ulna with associated radial head dislocation/instability due to ligament injury. Various types and equivalent injuries have been described along with the use of terms such as Monteggia variants or Monteggia-like lesions all making the descriptions complicated and confusing. Giovanni Battista Monteggia described the lesion in preradiographic era (1814) by clinical examination. José Luis Bado in 1967 detailed Monteggia lesion and also described some related injuries that were termed equivalents; however, these equivalents are a matter of debate. The injury is seen commonly in children (4–10 years) while uncommon cases in adults are also reported. **MECHANISM OF INJURY** The injury results from FOOSH with forearm in hyperpronation. This position produces crossing of radius and ulna pushing proximal radius out of its ligamentous sleeve while also causing ulna fracture. Now, variable transfer of energy may sometimes cause radius fracture also and variable degree of hyperpronation and abduction/adduction forces might dislocate the radial head in different directions (anterior is most common). Concisely, the Monteggia equivalents are fractures that do not match the classic description of Bado types but have the same mechanism of injury.	Proximal radius articulates with the lesser sigmoid notch of ulna and is encased in a sleeve of fibrocartilaginous annular ligament. The ligament is attached to the edges of the sigmoid notch forming a near circular region for radial head to move. This is a pivot joint responsible for pronosupination movement in association with DRUJ. Laterally, support to this annular ligament is extended by musculotendinous and ligamentous structures to confer a reasonable stability. The PIN nerve embraces the radial neck before passing into the supinator, so with radial head dislocation neurapraxia of PIN is common.	There are pain and swelling at the elbow joint. Dislocated radial head is usually palpable in the elbow anteriorly and soft spot shows effusion. Loss of ROM at elbow occurs due to dislocation and pain. Ulnar bow is increased and tenderness is prominent at the ulna. Evaluate for PIN palsy—finger drop, weak thumb extension while maintained radial deviation of hand and wrist extension. Look also for associated olecranon injury, coronoid fracture, LCL injury, and terrible triad injury. The fracture is commonly associated with distal radius fracture in one-fourth of the cases.	Obtain the standard AP and lateral radiographs of the elbow joint, forearm, and wrist. One needs to know the age of appearance of radial head and olecranon epiphysis to discern the injury pattern (see CRITOE above). Also, one should be wary of the fact that ulna may just present with a greenstick type injury or plastic deformation. **CLASSIFICATION** Though the fracture was described by Giovanni Battista Monteggia (Bado type 1 in 1814), it is Bado who classified the fracture into four types that are commonly followed. In addition, Jupiter classified the type 2 into four subtypes. **Bado Classification (Fig. 33)** Type 1—anteriorly angulated fracture of proximal or middle-third ulna with anterior radial head dislocation. Type 2—posteriorly angulated fracture of proximal or middle-third ulna with posterior/posterolateral radial head dislocation. Type 3—fracture ulnar metaphysis distal to coronoid with lateral/anterolateral radial head dislocation. There is lateral angulation at the fracture. Inverted Bado type 3 is also described where the angulation is ulnar wards. Type 4—fracture of proximal or middle third ulna and radius with dislocation of radial head in any direction (commonly anterior).	**NONOPERATIVE** Nonoperative treatment is usually successful in children with type 1 and 3 injuries. The cast after reduction should be applied in supination and elbow flexion of 100° (type 1 and 3, while for type 2 if attempted then at 70°), reduction should be assessed for stability. The length of ulna should be restored else radial head dislocation is common with ensuing healing and bowing again of ulna. **OPERATIVE TREATMENT** There is usually a low threshold for operative reduction and realignment of ulna in view of poor prognosis for maintaining radial head reduction, if closed reduction is suboptimal. The indications are: • Unstable fracture or reduction • Open fractures • Comminuted fractures • Monteggia in adult patients This involves ORIF of the ulna shaft fracture and commonly the radial head relocates by itself. If radial head does not relocate then open reduction for radial head also needs to be performed. In proximal ulna, metaphyseal region locking recon plate gives better stability. Intramedullary fixation can be done for transverse fractures. For comminuted fractures, bone grafting should be considered. PIN neuropathy usually resolves in 3–4 months and observation only is advised for most cases.

Contd...

Contd...

Epidemiology	*Anatomy*	*Clinical Evaluation*	*Radiographic Evaluation*	*Treatment*
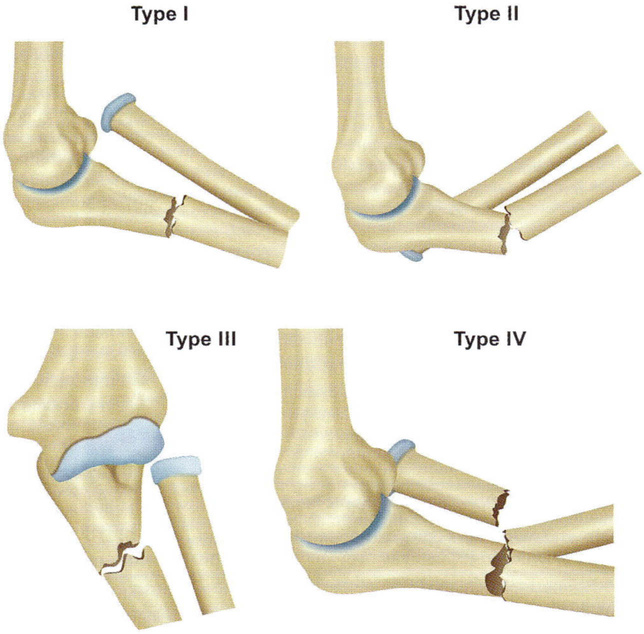 **Fig. 33:** The Bado classification of Monteggia fractures. Type 1 Bado is the classic fracture pattern described by Monteggia BG. Not depicted are the Monteggia equivalents. 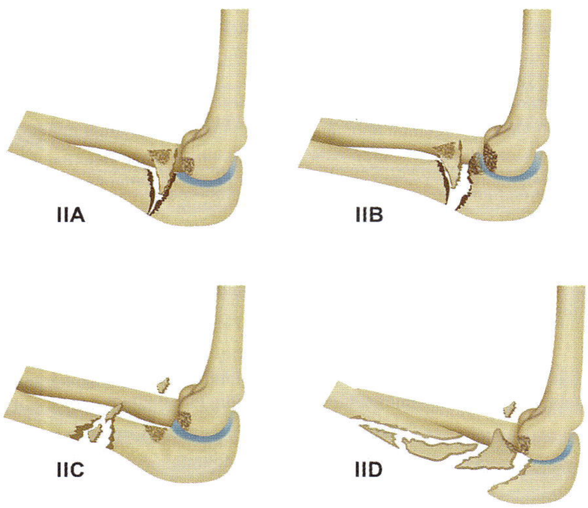 **Fig. 34:** Jupiter subclassification of type II Bado into four types.			**Jupiter Subclassification** of type 2 Bado **(Fig. 34)** Type 2A—coronoid level Type 2B—metadiaphyseal junction Type 2C—distal to coronoid Type 2D—fracture extending to distal half of ulna. "*Hybrid lesion of Monteggia*" is a fracture of metaphyseal region of ulna that extends into olecranon associated with anterior dislocation of radial head. Bado included most equivalents in type 1 but there has been immense controversy toward their recognition. For simplicity, some clarification is emerging. "Monteggia equivalents" are by definition fractures of ulna at any level conjoined with fracture of the neck or physeal or metaphyseal injury of proximal radius. Now, these "equivalents" can be displaced or nondisplaced and this distinction matters in terms of management and prognosis. "Displaced Monteggia equivalents" are those that have fracture of ulna at any level conjoined with displaced proximal radius injury (any direction) greater than first degree of Judet's classification (≥1° of displacement *ad axim*) The ulna fracture is frequently found in olecranon. Nondisplaced equivalents have any level ulna fracture with nondisplaced fracture of proximal radius. The displaced equivalents need aggressive and accurate reduction as their prognosis is poorer than classical Monteggia lesion while nondisplaced equivalents are commonly conservatively managed with good prognosis. Fracture that does not fall into the definition of Monteggia equivalents proposed above should not be described by using word "Monteggia" or its equivalent anywhere. These include pulled elbow syndrome (nursemaid elbow), isolated dislocation of proximal radius or head, fracture of ulna with dislocation of whole elbow, etc.	Neglected Monteggia presents with chronic radial head dislocation with persistent ulnar bow and needs ulnar osteotomy and relocation of radial head with procedures for further radial head stabilization such as Bell-Tawse (or its modification) procedure.

FRACTURE OF RADIUS AND ULNA SHAFT (BOTH BONE FOREARM FRACTURE)

Epidemiology	*Anatomy*	*Clinical Evaluation*	*Radiographic Evaluation*	*Treatment*
Fractures of both bones of forearm are more common in men than women. They are the second most common (after tibia) cause of open fractures. Higher incidence in males and higher percentage of open fracture is secondary to occurrence of this fracture in motor vehicle accidents, contact athletic sports, altercations/road rash, and falls from a height. It is a very common injury in pediatric patients accounting for 30–50% of all pediatric fractures. The majority of injuries are distal > middle thirds >> proximal thirds fracture. These are also most commonly complicated by open injuries at presentation and have high refracture rates after treatment. **MECHANISM OF INJURY** Direct trauma is common while protecting oneself from injury/assault. Indirect injury occurs in falls from height and athletic activities whence a person falls on the out-stretched hand.	The forearm acts as a continuous ring. Injury resulting in shortening of either radius or ulna would cause a fracture of the other forearm bone or a dislocation at the proximal or distal radioulnar joint. Isolated fracture of ulna (Nightstick injuries) is an exception. The ulna provides an axis around which the laterally bowed radius rotates effecting the supination and pronation. The ulna has wavy disposition where it is convex toward radius in the proximal thirds while it is concave in the distal thirds on AP profile projection creating a fusiform space. Factors leading to loss of the fusiform space between radius and ulna would cause variable loss in supination and pronation if anatomy is not restored. The interosseous membrane forms a fibrous articulation between radius and ulna extending for 3/4th of the forearm space **(Figs. 35A to C)**. The central band is approximately 3.5 cm wide running obliquely from its proximal origin on the radius to its distal insertion on the ulna. Incompetency of this central band alone will reduce stability by around 70%. It has been seen that the loss/block of forearm rotation in large parts is due to deformation of the interosseous membrane rather than a bony block. Remodeling potential is high in children so pediatric malreductions smoothen out with time. The remodeling potential is maximum in patients <8 years of age and fractures that are angulated in plane of movement (sagittal plane deformities) and fractures near to joints. The acceptable suboptimal reduction values in general are: Patient <8 years old: • 20° midshaft angulation • Bayonet apposition • No rotation Patient 8–12 years (F); or 14 years (M): • 10° midshaft angulation or 15° distal angulation • 50% translation • No rotation Patients >12 years(F); >14 years(M): Minimal displacement/angulation (treat like adult)	There is obvious deformity of the injured forearm with pain, swelling, and loss of hand and forearm function. Though not very common but evaluate for radial and ulnar nerve pulses, as well as median, radial, and ulnar nerve function. This is especially needed in penetrating and open injuries. Open injuries occur commonly on the side of ulna, as it is subcutaneous and with deformity, it is liable to break skin overlying it (internal compounding). High-energy injuries commonly disrupt soft tissue more than what is actually evident causing significant edema, now as forearm is a closed compartment, so development of compartment syndrome is also quite common. Look specifically for signs of compartment in both bone forearm fractures specifically excruciating, unremitting pain requiring incremental analgesics, tense forearm compartments, or pain out of proportion to injury on passive stretch of the fingers. Compartment pressure monitoring is best in this scenario else with strong suspicion, emergency fasciotomy can be done (see detailed discussion in Chapter on "Compartment Syndrome"). One should assess all three forearm compartments and carpal tunnel.	Standard AP and lateral views of the forearm with elbow and wrist joints. Oblique views are obtained as necessary for further fracture evaluation and identifying comminution. **CLASSIFICATIONS** One can either follow OTA classification or commonly descriptive classification is used defining the fracture in terms of closed versus open, location within forearm (dividing it into thirds or fourths), transverse/oblique/comminuted/segmental, multifragmented, displacement, angulation, rotations, etc. **OTA Classification** Diaphyseal fractures of radius and ulna: • Type A—simple fracture of ulna (A1), radius (A2), or both bones (A3) • Type B—wedge fracture of ulna (B1), radius (B2), or both bones (B3) • Type C—complex fractures. ***Pediatric forearm fractures:*** • *Plastic deformation*: – 2–15 years of age – Minimal deformity – Limited forearm rotation – Bowing of bone (but no cortex fractures) on X-rays with interosseous membrane irregularity. • *Greenstick fractures*: – One cortex fractured – Opposite cortex intact or undergoes plastic deformation – Usually rotational deformity • Complete (as for adults).	Nonoperative treatment was in practice till more than three decades ago with above elbow POP cast following manipulative reduction of the fracture. Supination or pronation to the forearm component was given depending on whether the fracture is in proximal or distal thirds but most common recommendation was to provide a long arm cast in neutral rotation with the elbow flexed to 90°. Loss of reduction and malunion were common and patient's limb was immobilized for 6–8 weeks. Isolated ulna fractures (*nightstick fractures—distal two-third*) may be treated with functional cast brace with good interosseous mold provided there is at least 50% contact between the fragments and <10° of angulation. Presently with advancements in operative management and following introduction of AO principles, operative management is the standard of care in adults barring a rare patient who is unfit for surgical management or in patients with undisplaced fractures. Operative management entails ORIF with plating as a standard procedure with uncommon surgeon preference to nailing. Indications include—displaced nightstick fractures, isolated all radial shaft fractures, all both bone forearm fractures, proximal third ulna shaft fractures, and open fractures. The fixation is done using compression plating [DCP is now obsolete and consensus is for limited contact DCP (LCDCP) which is slowly giving way to use of LCP even for fractures in nonosteoporotic bones]. Osteoporotic bones are fixed by LCP. In either case, the following principles must be followed: • Use separate approaches for radius [modified Henry distal third to half, dorsal (Thompson) for proximal thirds] and ulna (direct approach)—prevents radioulnar synostosis • Restore ulnar and radial lengths—fix the ulna first if both fractures simple, else fix the complex fracture first. The aim is to prevent subluxation of DRUJ or PRUJ. • Restore radial bow (essential for rotational function of the forearm)

Contd...

Contd...

Epidemiology	*Anatomy*	*Clinical Evaluation*	*Radiographic Evaluation*	*Treatment*
	Fractures of radius distal to the supinator muscle insertion but proximal to the pronator teres insertion results in supination of the proximal fragment owing to unopposed pull of the supinator and biceps brachii muscles. Fractures in middle-third of forearm result in neutral rotational alignment of the proximal fragment. Fractures distal to pronator teres insertion commonly go into pronation.			• Restore rotational alignment • Bone graft comminuted fractures where less than half of the circumference of bony contact is possible. Open fractures—follow the principles for management of open injuries—thorough wash, debridement, wound toileting, etc. Primary open reduction and internal fixation after debridement is usually possible, except in severe open or contaminated injuries where immediate wound cover is not possible. Early total care is effective approach and restores stability, limits dead space, and improves wound care. Bone grafting of open fractures for bone loss can be performed at first surgery itself if wound closure is possible or may be done later at the second surgery for delayed primary closure (6 weeks after injury). For extensive injuries to forearm causing bone and soft tissue loss or gross contamination, external fixation may be used initially till wound stabilizes. External fixator otherwise may also be used for infected nonunion or open elbow fracture-dislocations. Locked intramedullary nail fixation is done by select persons but its indications are unclear. It may be done for segmental fractures, open fractures with bone or soft tissue loss, pathologic fractures, and failed previous ORIF with plating. Nailing with straight nails causes loss of radial bow and may compromise rotations. The pediatric fractures are commonly nailed however. The surgical indications in pediatric forearm fractures include irreducible or unstable fractures (see acceptable safe deformities in anatomy), open fractures, fractures associated with vascular injury, polytrauma, floating elbow, and refracture. For younger children <12 years of age (female)/<14 years (male), closed reduction is the usual mainstay but they should be closely monitored (weekly for first 3 weeks) for redisplacement. Elastic intramedullary nailing is commonly used for nonreducible or redisplaced fractures. Less stable fracture is fixed first and is it generally acceptable to pin only one fracture, if stable. Avoid crossing the radial physis by using a mini-incision and

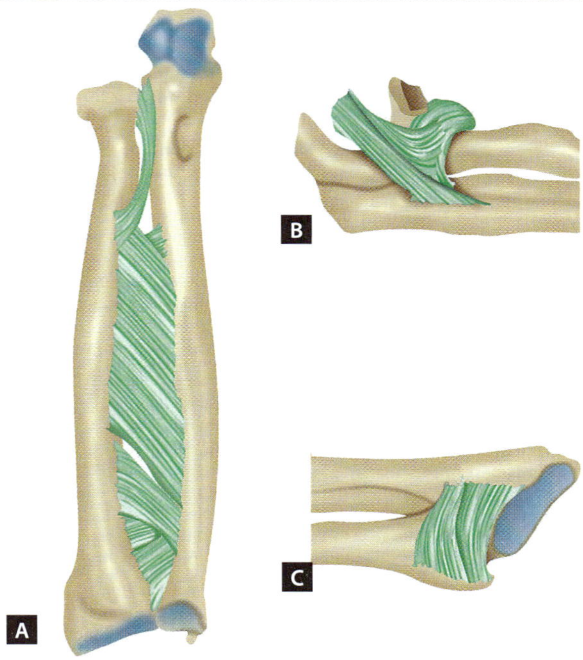

Figs. 35A to C: The illustration of forearm bones (A) with proximal radioulnar joint (B) and distal radioulnar joint (C).

Contd...

Contd...

Epidemiology	*Anatomy*	*Clinical Evaluation*	*Radiographic Evaluation*	*Treatment*
				protect EPL tendon in dorsal entry points else use a radial entry (protect sensory nerve). Olecranon apophysis is an acceptable entry point but consensus is growing toward proximal lateral ulna entry. In closed reduction, avoid more than three attempts or >10 minutes of traction to prevent compartment syndrome. ORIF with plating is usually done for older children (>12 years female or >14 years male) or in patients with comminuted unstable fractures. **COMPLICATIONS** • Infection—needs thorough debridement and wound toileting. Antibiotic coverage depending on wound culture has to be started. Deep infections need implant removal and temporary stabilization with external fixator, well-fixed implants with superficial infections may be retained. • *Nonunion and malunion:* Deformity correction, refixation, bone grafting commonly needed. • *Neurovascular injury:* Iatrogenic injury is uncommon but may definitely occur as the approach is quite in vicinity. Primary repair of nerves is indicated, if injured in surgery while vessel may be ligated, if unable to repair in case the other vessel is patent. • Volkmann ischemia. • Refracture—removing plates early (before 15 months), osteoporotic bones • *Post-traumatic radioulnar synostosis*: Uncommon (3–9%), if principles followed. The risk factors include: – Fracture of both bones at the same level (11% incidence) – Closed head injury – Surgical delay >2 weeks – Single incision for fixation of both bone forearm fractures – Penetration of the interosseous membrane by bone graft or screws, bone fragments, or surgical instruments – Crush injury – Infection. Surgical excision is needed if forearm rotations are limited. For proximal forearm synostosis, postoperative low-dose radiation may reduce recurrence.

FRACTURE OF RADIUS SHAFT AND GALEAZZI FRACTURE

Epidemiology	*Anatomy*	*Clinical Evaluation*	*Radiographic Evaluation*	*Treatment*
Radius fractures may occur isolated or in association with DRUJ injuries. Isolated fractures occur in the proximal third but distal third fractures are commonly associated with DRUJ disruption. The Galeazzi or Piedmont fracture occurring in radial diaphysis at the junction of the middle and distal thirds with distal radioulnar joint (DRUJ) disruption has been classically called the ***fracture of necessity*** because it requires open reduction and internal fixation to achieve a good result (other such fractures classically are fracture lateral condyle humerus in children, fracture neck femur in adults, fracture talus, fracture of scaphoid, and fractured odontoid). *Galeazzi variants*: Fracture occurring anywhere along the radius or both bones fracture with DRUJ disruption. A reverse Galeazzi fracture denotes a fracture of the distal ulna with associated disruption of the distal radioulnar joint. **MECHANISM OF INJURY** Direct trauma or indirect trauma (FOOSH) may cause radial shaft fractures in isolation (latter less common). Galeazzi fractures occur from direct trauma on dorsolateral aspect of the wrist or indirectly due to FOOSH with forearm pronated. Reverse Galeazzi fractures result from FOOSH with forearm supinated or pronated resulting in apex volar or dorsal angulation, respectively **(Figs. 36A and B)**. Proximal third radial shaft fracture is commonly associated with ulna fracture due to its location and soft tissue cover.	Vide anatomy of both bones forearm above and the anatomy of DRUJ discussed in detail in Chapter on "Distal Radioulnar Joint Disorders and Ulnar Wrist Pain". Extensor digiti minimi (EDM) tendon overlies the DRUJ so in dislocated joints that fail to reduce after radius fixation, this tendon is commonly found incarcerated within the joint.	Pain, swelling, and point tenderness over the fracture represent location of fracture. Elbow ROM and forearm rotations are evaluated—rare radial head dislocation may be noted in addition to the diaphyseal fracture. In Galeazzi fractures, there is typically wrist pain along with midline forearm pain that is exacerbated by stressing of the distal radioulnar joint. The ulna may become prominent dorsally in a DRUJ dislocation and in extreme cases, the ulna may come out of skin. In subluxations of the ulna head, a piano key sign would be elicited and is painful. There may be ulnar styloid tenderness due to associated ulna styloid fracture.	Standard AP and lateral radiographs of the forearm, elbow, and wrist should be obtained. The classic radiographic signs of distal radioulnar joint injury are: • Fracture at base of the ulnar styloid • Widened distal radioulnar joint on AP X-ray • Subluxed ulna on lateral X-ray • >5 mm radial shortening The fractures may be ***classified into two types:*** *Type I*: The radius fracture has apex volar angulation resulting from axial loading in supination with ulna displacement of ulna head volarly. *Type II*: The radius fracture has apex dorsal angulation due to loading in pronation with ulna head displaced dorsally.	**PROXIMAL RADIUS FRACTURE** Nondisplaced fractures may be managed in a above elbow POP cast. Failure of reduction or displacement during immobilization and loss of radial bow is an indication for ORIF. Displaced fractures are best managed by ORIF using a 3.5-mm dynamic compression plate. Galeazzi fracture needs to be always operated because of high chances of failure of closed method; unless the patient is too frail or unfit to undergo surgery. There is concentration of displacing forces in the region necessitating operative reduction and fixation. The deforming forces include—weight of the hand (causes dorsal angulation of the fracture and subluxation of the distal radioulnar joint). Pronator quadratus (tends to pronate the distal fragment pulling it proximally and volarly). Brachioradialis—pulls the distal fragment proximally causing shortening. Thumb extensors and abductors—again cause shortening and hence relaxation of the radial side ligaments causing failure of reduction despite immobilization of the wrist in ulnar deviation. Plate and screw fixation using LCDCP is the treatment of choice. An anterior modified Henry approach (interval between the flexor carpi radialis and the brachioradialis) is most commonly used and plate fixation volarly is usual practice, for middle thirds lateral (anterolateral) plate placement may be done (for tensile side fixation). The DRUJ commonly reduces with plating of radius and needs supplementary stabilization with transradioulnar K-wire stabilization in reduction and supination of forearm. Unreduced DRUJ results in dorsal instability and a dorsal capsulotomy may be needed to remove the incarcerated structures—EDM tendon, capsule, or TFC flap. Some people prefer POP immobilization (3–6 weeks) in supination for stable DRUJ, postoperatively. Remove pins by 6–8 weeks and begin mobilization. Capsular repair may be done in extensive lesions to facilitate early DRUJ recovery and optimal healing (undocumented).

Contd...

Contd...

Epidemiology	*Anatomy*	*Clinical Evaluation*	*Radiographic Evaluation*	*Treatment*
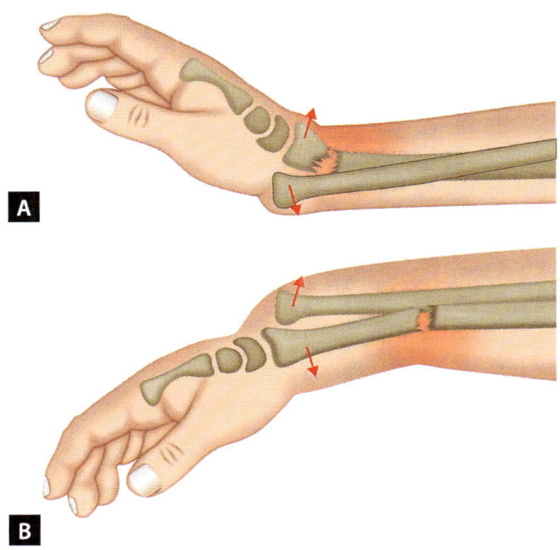 **Figs. 36A and B:** Illustration of distal radioulnar joint disruption causing instability in Galeazzi fracture dislocation pattern. The ulna head may be volarly displaced, if forces are transmitted in supination (A) or dorsally (B) if forces are transmitted with forearm in pronation.				**Complications** Malunion—following nonanatomic reduction/ fracture repair causes loss of supination and pronation and painful ROM. Reoperation with osteotomy, correction, and/or distal ulnar shortening, if there is ulnocarpal impaction. **NONUNION COMPARTMENT SYNDROME** Neurovascular injury — superficial radial nerve injury during exposure, posterior interosseous nerve injury (in the supinator) is at risk with proximal radius approaches. Recurrent dislocation occurs only if there is radial malreduction or incarcerated soft tissue in DRUJ that was not removed during reduction.

DISTAL RADIUS FRACTURE

Epidemiology	*Anatomy*	*Clinical Evaluation*	*Radiographic Evaluation*	*Treatment*
Most common fractures of upper extremity representing nearly one-sixth of all fractures treated in emergency departments (15% of all extremity fractures). In young population, commonly it occurs following high-energy injuries FOOSH or motor vehicle accidents, direct hit is not so common to cause the injury. Elderly patients comprise the majority, however, due to osteoporosis, which is the most important risk factor for this fracture along with tendency to fall. The fracture risk increases proportionately to the risk of hip fractures. Other risk factors in elderly patients include— • Female sex • White race • Family history • Early menopause • Previous osteoporotic fracture • Neurological conditions causing loss of balance **MECHANISM OF INJURY** Younger patient population—fall from height, motor vehicle accident, and athletic injuries. Elderly patients fracture distal radius from low-energy mechanisms—usually a simple fall from standing height. Overall, the most common mechanism of injury is a fall	Distal radius metaphysis is an expanded structure composed primarily of cancellous bone. The distal articular surface has a biconcave surface with two fossae for articulation with scaphoid and lunate bones. The sigmoid notch over ulnar aspect articulates with the distal ulna. The radius is surrounded by extensor tendons dorsally (EPL rupture is the most common tendon injury associated with Colles' fracture) and on volar aspect is the pronator quadratus (PQ) that separates the bone from flexor tendons. Distal to the distal attachment of PQ is a bony ridge called watershed line where the tendons are in close contact with the bone. Placing the hardware distal to this line may result in attrition wear of the tendons. Radius is primarily responsible for load transmission at wrist while ulna is important at elbow for the same. 80% of axial load passes through distal radius and rest through ulna and the triangular fibrocartilage complex (TFCC). Reversal of the normal volar tilt of distal radius shifts load onto the ulna and TFCC while much less load is borne by the distal radius in nonanatomical fashion—mostly passing dorsally then. Dividing the distal radius into	The wrist is typically swollen with ecchymosis, tenderness, and painful ROM. Deformity varies depending on the displacement of the hand in relation to the wrist—dinner fork in Colles or dorsal Barton fractures and garden spade in Smith-type or volar Barton fractures. Examine for **associated injuries:** Ipsilateral elbow and shoulder DRUJ and TFCC injury (40%) Ulnar styloid fracture Carpal injury—lunate/perilunate dislocation, scaphoid fracture, S-L dissociation (30%), and lunotriquetral ligament injury (15%) Neurovascular assessment—median nerve may get stretched owing to traction during forced hyperextension of the wrist, injury from sharp fracture fragments, hematoma compression causing increased carpal tunnel pressure. Take history for osteoporosis and make a point to assess the same for initiating secondary prophylaxis/treatment later.	Standard PA and lateral views of the wrist with oblique views as needed for fracture evaluation. Radiographs of other regions to evaluate symptoms, if necessary. It is a good practice to obtain contralateral wrist views to assess the normal ulnar variance and scapholunate angle. Computed tomography may be needed in multifragmentary and intra-articular fractures for treatment planning. MRI scan may be advised to assess the soft tissue structures at DRUJ and intercarpal or radiocarpal ligament injuries. In general, for distal radius, the normalized values for various parameters are as follows **(Figs. 37A and B)**: • *Radial inclination*: Mean 23° • (range, 13–30°) • *Radial length*: Mean 11 mm (range, 8–18 mm) • *Palmar (volar) tilt*: Mean 11–12° (range, 0–28°) Radiographic instability (Cooney et al.) is considered to exist when there is— 1. Significant comminution 2. Angular deformity (dorsal) >10° 3. Radial shortening >5 mm 4. Articular displacement >2 mm	For a good outcome, few things are essential in treatment that include—accurate articular reduction, restoration of wrist anatomy, and early mobilization to improve local biology and hand function. The factors having a bearing on treatment planning include: • Geometry of fracture and intra-articular extension, impaction, comminution, displacement, etc. • *Locoregional issues*: Quality of bone, soft tissue injury, and energy of injury • *Performance status of patient and general factors*: Physiologic patient age, lifestyle, occupation, hand dominance, associated medical conditions, associated injuries, and compliance. The acceptable radiographic parameters for reduction of displaced fracture distal radius include: • *Radial length*: Ideally, within 2–3 mm of the contralateral radius on AP view with ulnar variance = 0 mm • *Radial inclination*: <5° loss (ideally >15° should be maintained).

Contd...

Contd...

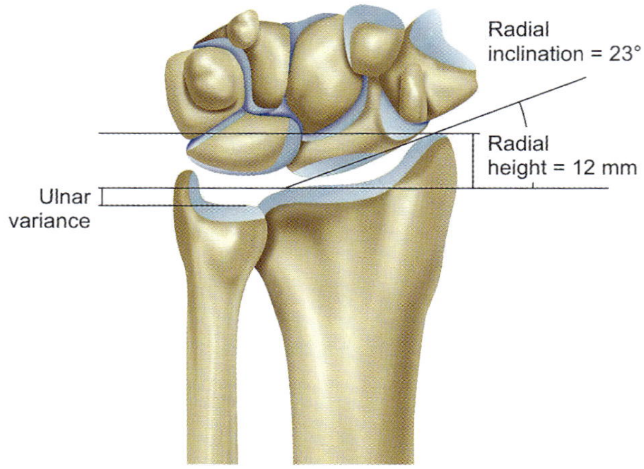

Fig. 37A: The various radiological parameters of distal radius that are commonly used to judge adequacy of reduction in management on anteroposterior.

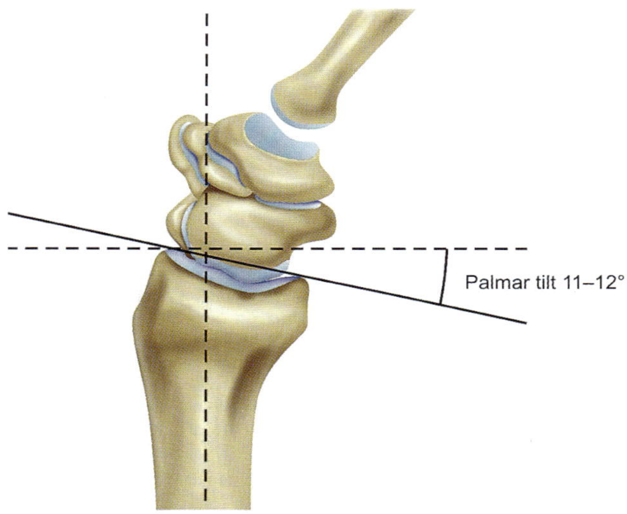

Fig. 37B: The various radiological parameters of distal radius that are commonly used to judge adequacy of reduction in management on lateral projections.

Epidemiology	***Anatomy***	***Clinical Evaluation***	***Radiographic Evaluation***	***Treatment***
onto outstretched hand with the wrist in dorsiflexion. With the exception of dorsal rim avulsion fractures. Hyperextension of wrist is the sole most common injury mechanism responsible for production of distal radius fractures (including volar Barton and Smith type fracture). The weak meta-physeodiaphyseal junction fails in dorsiflexion of the wrist between 40° and 90°, with lesser degrees of force required at smaller angles. Failure in volar tension results dorsal comminution due to cortical compression. With the application of bending moments, the radius initially fails in tension on the volar aspect, whereas same forces	three columns came in vogue in late 1990s where radial column is formed by scaphoid fossa with radial styloid, intermediate column is formed by lunate fossa and sigmoid notch. Ulnar column is formed by distal ulna and DRUJ (ulnar styloid, TFCC). Melone further divides the intermediate column into volar–ulnar and a dorsal–ulnar fragment. Most of the axial load is transmitted through intermediate column reconstruction of which is most important. The distal radius is also base for numerous ligamentous attachments that bind together the wrist joint and carpal bones. These also help in ligamentotaxis during closed reduction. The anatomy is		**CLASSIFICATIONS** Numerous classifications (>17) can be found in literature for classifying the distal radius fracture but only a few need to be familiar for treatment planning as none is universally superior. **Descriptive Classification** is most specific for an individual patient and should include parameters of: • Open versus closed • Intra versus extra-articular • Displacements—direction, degree of articular fragment • Angulations • Comminution—column-wise description • Loss of radial length Various classifications are, however, used for research purpose and reporting.	• *Palmar tilt:* Neutral tilt (0°) but should be within 20° of contralateral distal radius (confusing!) Comprehensively on a lateral view volar tilt should not exceed 20° and dorsal tilt should be <10° (ideally <5°) • Intra-articular step-off <1 mm and articular gap <2 mm There is a controversy as to the optimal radiological alignment restoration as many studies have found no definite clinical correlation of functional improvement versus radiological restoration. McQueen suggested that the carpal alignment after distal radius fracture has a dominating influence on ultimate outcome following treatment.

Contd...

Contd...

Epidemiology	*Anatomy*	*Clinical Evaluation*	*Radiographic Evaluation*	*Treatment*
acting reverse induce compression stresses on opposite cortex resulting in dorsal comminution. The vector always has some compression/axial direction causing impaction of the cancellous bone in metaphysis, which results in bone void despite reduction and is a major cause of instability in conservatively managed fractures along with dorsal comminution. In lesser degrees of dorsiflexion, the forces may have a predominant shearing component resulting in volar/dorsal shear intra-articular fractures. High-energy injuries (e.g., vehicular trauma) often result in displaced and highly comminuted unstable fractures to the distal radius with surrounding soft tissue injury (nerves/tendons). Sizable number of them may also be open fractures. A highly uncommon injury seen in older times was the radial styloid fracture occurring in isolation; due to the backfired engine turning handle that hit directly on to the wrist—the ***Chauffeur's fracture***. These days such an injury is mostly due to direct hit during fights, etc. Another fracture—***Hutchinson fracture***—is an avulsion fracture of the radial styloid with extrinsic ligaments remaining attached to the fractured fragment ± associated intercarpal ligament injury. In Hutchison's fracture, the scaphoid compresses against the distal radius in its fossa with the wrist in dorsiflexion and ulnar deviation. This would result in fracture of the entire	detailed elsewhere in Chapter on "Carpal Instability". There are some commonly used/misused terms for distal radius fractures eponymous **(Fig. 38)** to their initial describer and should be clarified. ***Colles' fracture*** Classically, it is the extra-articular fracture of distal radius occurring 2.5–4 cm from joint line without ulna side involvement causing dorsal angulation and shift, radial shift and tilt, shortening, and supination of distal fragment producing dinner fork deformity. Present usage of eponym, however, includes both extra- and intra-articular distal radius fractures ± ulna styloid fracture demonstrating various deformities. Most of the distal radius fractures are of this pattern resulting from a fall onto a hyperextended, radially deviated wrist with the forearm in pronation. Intra-articular component (present in nearly half of the patients) is commonly seen in younger patients as they commonly sustain higher-energy forces. In such cases, injuries to nerve, carpus, DRUJ, and distal ulna are more frequent. ***Smith fracture*** (reverse Colles fracture)—this is anatomically reverse of Colles in displacement where the distal fragment undergoes a volar tilt (apex dorsal angulation) resulting in garden spade deformity. The patient falls onto a flexed wrist with the forearm fixed in supination. Clinically, this is an unstable fracture pattern and needs open reduction and internal fixation because for stabilization.		**Frykman Classification**—based on the pattern of intra-articular involvement **(Fig. 39)**. *Type I:* Transverse metaphyseal fracture (irrespective of angulation)—both Colles' and Smith fractures are included *Type II:* type I + ulnar styloid fracture *Type III:* Fracture line enters radiocarpal joint—includes both volar and dorsal Barton fractures and Chauffeur/Hutchinson fracture *Type IV:* Type III + ulnar styloid fracture *Type V:* Fracture line enters the distal radioulnar joint but not radiocarpal joint *Type VI:* Type V + ulnar styloid fracture *Type VII:* Usually, a comminuted fracture with fracture line entering both the radiocarpal and radioulnar joints *Type VIII:* Type VII + ulnar styloid fracture **FERNANDEZ CLASSIFICATION** *Bending type:* One cortex of the metaphysis fails due to tensile stress (Colles' and Smith fractures), and the opposite cortex undergoes some comminution. *Shearing type:* Fracture of the joint surface: Barton's; reversed Barton's styloid process fracture, simple articular fracture *Compression type:* Fracture of the surface of the joint with impaction of subchondral and metaphyseal bone (die-punch); intra-articular comminuted fracture *Avulsion type:* Fracture of the ligament attachments to ulnar and radial styloid process; radiocarpal fracture-dislocation	To estimate carpal alignment in this method, the intersection point of two lines on the lateral radiograph is determined: one line is drawn parallel and through the middle of the radial shaft while the other is drawn through middle of and parallel to the capitate alignment. If the two lines intersect within the carpus, then the carpus is aligned. If the two lines intersect out of the capitate or lie parallel side-by-side, then the carpus is malaligned. **NONOPERATIVE MANAGEMENT** Every fracture unless undisplaced/contraindicated should be realigned, even if surgery is definite as realignment helps to limit postinjury swelling, limits secondary damage, gives some pain relief, and relieves compression on the median nerve. Classical indications for closed treatment include—extra-articular fracture with <5 mm radial shortening and/or <20° dorsal angulation compared to contralateral wrist. *Closed manipulation (under radiology control) and cast immobilization*: Simple cast immobilization without manipulation → Nondisplaced or minimally displaced fractures. Manipulate for realignment → Displaced fractures with a stable fracture pattern, which can be expected to unite within acceptable radiographic parameters, low-demand elderly patients with higher operative risk than functional gains

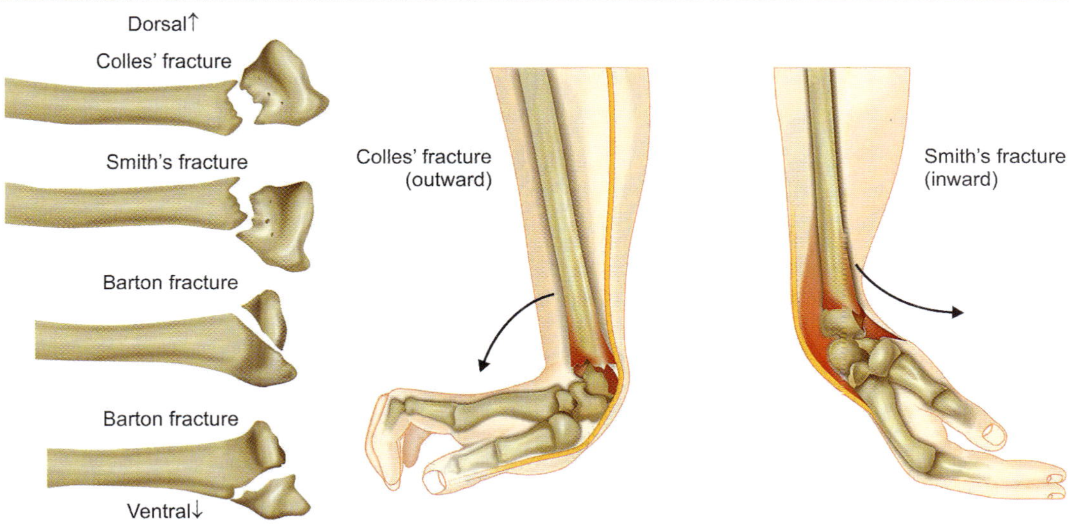

Fig. 38: The various eponymous distal radius fractures.

Contd...

Contd...

<table>
<tr><th>Epidemiology</th><th>Anatomy</th><th>Clinical Evaluation</th><th>Radiographic Evaluation</th><th>Treatment</th></tr>
<tr><td colspan="5">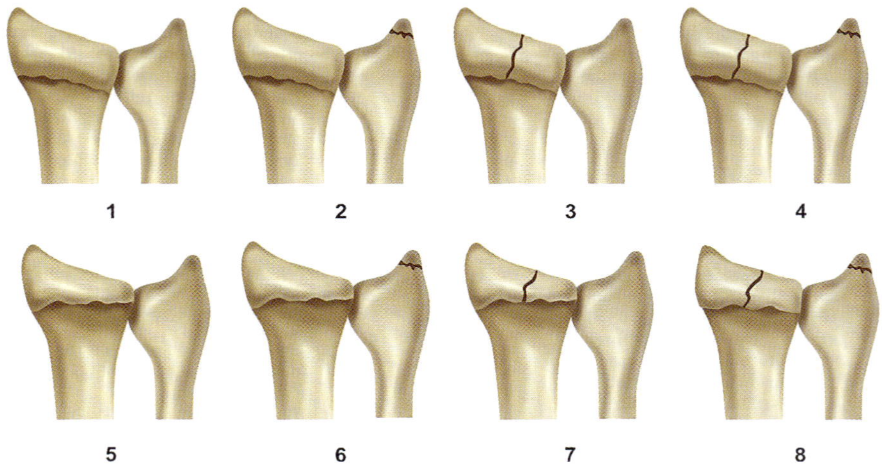
Fig. 39: The Frykman classification of distal radius fractures (see text for details).</td></tr>
<tr>
<td>styloid or only the dorsal or volar portion. The shear forces across intercarpal bones result in either S-L ligament injury (scapholunate dissociation) or fractured scaphoid (trans-scaphoperilunate dislocation).</td>
<td>Barton fracture:
This is a fracture-dislocation or subluxation of the wrist in which the dorsal or volar rim of the distal radius is displaced with the hand and carpus. Volar involvement is more common; however, Barton himself classically described dorsal fracture pattern.
Patient gives history of fall onto a dorsiflexed wrist with the forearm fixed in pronation. Being a shear pattern injury, the fractures are inherently unstable and require ORIF with a buttress plate to achieve stable, anatomic reduction.
Die-punch fracture (Fig. 41):
This is a depressed fracture of the articular surface of the distal radius at the lunate fossa. It results from axial weight transmission along the 2nd–3rd ray and lunate bone as in street fights. The outcome is bad with early onset arthritis, if treatment and elevation of the fracture fragment is not done.</td>
<td></td>
<td>Combination types: Usually, high-energy injuries and comminuted fractures
Melone Classification of intra-articular fractures (Fig. 40)
This is based on a consistent mechanism (lunate impaction injury).
Type I: Stable, without comminution
Type II: Unstable die-punch, dorsal, or volar
IIA: Reducible
IIB: Irreducible
Type III: Spike fracture; contused volar structures
Type IV: Split fracture; medial complex fractured with dorsal and palmar fragments displaced separately.
Type V: Explosion fracture; severe comminution with major soft tissue injury
One may prefer OTA/AO classification for research purpose available freely at respective websites.
Look carefully on the wrist for Gilula's lines and carpal bones individually to identify associated carpal injury.
Universal Classification
Type I: Extra-articular without deviation
Type II: Extra-articular with deviation
Type IIA: Reducible and stable
Type IIB: Reducible and unstable
Type IIC: Irreducible
Type III: Intra-articular without deviation
Type IV: Intra-articular with deviation
Type IVA: Reducible and stable
Type IVB: Reducible and unstable
Type IVC: Irreducible</td>
<td>Technique of closed reduction (dorsally tilted fracture): Use hematoma block ± supplemental IV sedation/Bier block, or conscious sedation
• Distal fragment hyperextension to unlock fragments → Traction (to separate fragments, minimize comminution and disimpaction) → Realignment in direction of radius → Reduce proximal fragment with pressure applied to the distal radius and position distal fragment by
Thumb pressure → apply well-molded long arm (sugar-tong) splint with the wrist in neutral to slight flexion (no hyperflexion (cotton-loader position) as was the older practice)
• Hyperflexion to maintain reduction increases carpal tunnel pressure and chances of median nerve compression and causes digital stiffness, also need of hyperflexion to maintain reduction indicates need of surgical stabilization. One can also apply POP cast instead of splint if there is no/minimal swelling but always leave the (MCP) joints free. Splint, if applied, should be changed to cast once swelling subsides without losing reduction.
(Note: Ideal forearm position, duration of immobilization, and need for a long arm cast all remain controversial as no superiority has been consistently demonstrated). Frequent radiographic examination is necessary to detect loss of reduction, maintain cast till union is demonstrated radiologically.</td>
</tr>
</table>

Contd...

Contd...

Epidemiology	*Anatomy*	*Clinical Evaluation*	*Radiographic Evaluation*	*Treatment*

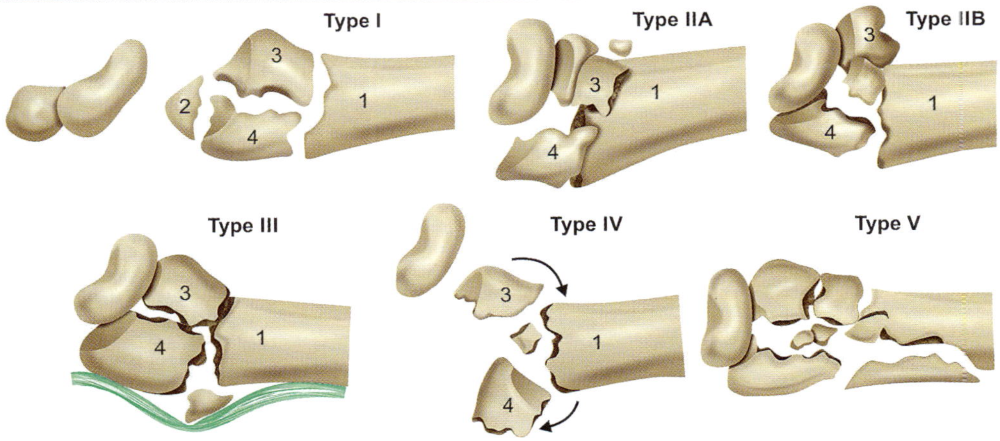

Fig. 40: The Melone classification for distal radius fracture. Arabic numerals depict the fragments—1 is radial shaft, 2 is radial styloid, 3 is palmar–ulnar fragment of intermediate column, 4 is dorsal ulnar fragment of intermediate column.

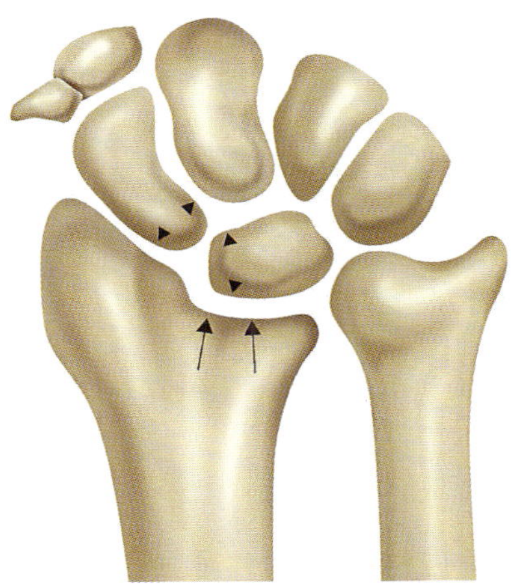

Fig. 41: Die-punch fracture of distal radius.

Redisplacement is a common problem and is associated with various factors (Lafontaine criteria):

- *Initial displacement of the fracture:* The greater the degree of displacement (particularly radial shortening), the more energy is imparted to the fracture resulting in a higher likelihood that closed treatment will be unsuccessful. Dorsal angulation >20°, volar displacement.
- *Age of the patient (actually bone quality):* Osteoporotic bones tend lose reduction and occur particularly late. Loss of radial height is most common causing ulnar impaction.
- The extent of metaphyseal comminution (the metaphyseal defect) → higher the comminution more are chances of displacement, dorsal comminution–dorsal angulation; circumferential comminution–loss of radial height

Associated ulnar fracture

- Displacement following closed treatment predicts instability of fracture. Repeat manipulation is less likely to result in a successful radiographic outcome and surgical management is indicated.

Complications of cast immobilization include—stiffness, RSD (CRPS/Sudeck's dystrophy), EPL rupture, and acute carpal tunnel syndrome.

OPERATIVE MANAGEMENT

The indications vary in institutes and with individuals but mostly include:

- High-energy injury
- Secondary loss of reduction
- Articular comminution, step-off, or gap
- Metaphyseal comminution or bone loss
- Loss of volar buttress with displacement
- DRUJ incongruity even after closed treatment

Relative indications are—dorsal angulation >20° compared to other wrist >5 mm radial shortening, Smith-type fracture

Operative Techniques

Percutaneous pinning: Maintains sagittal length/alignment in simpler fractures so indicated in extra-articular fractures or two-part intra-articular fractures where volar cortex is stable. It may also be used to supplement short arm casting or external fixation.

Contd...

Contd...

Epidemiology	Anatomy	Clinical Evaluation	Radiographic Evaluation	Treatment
				Trans-fracture pinning: Two or three Kirschner wires are placed across the fracture site (generally from the radial styloid) from the dorsoulnar side of the distal radial fragment directed proximally. Transulnar pinning has also been described but very uncommon. *Kapandji intrafocal pinning:* The K-wires are passed through fracture and used as joystick to reduce the fracture into position progressing them proximally intramedullary or impinging into the cortex. Here, the distal fragment is trapped (as in a basket of wires) and buttressed by K-wire disposition. A "basket" of wires is created by using dorsal and radial wires commonly and in very uncommon cases, a volar wire (high complication rate). The wires are levered to reduce fragment and stabilized in the position by passing wire intramedullary. Fixing in opposite cortex usually achieves less than optimal reduction. The method is relatively simple and inexpensive, and very effective, particularly in elderly patients. Pin migration and pin tract infection are common problems. *Rayhack technique:* The reduction is assisted arthroscopically for intra-articular fractures. *External fixation:* If used alone, achieving volar tilt is a concern so combined with percutaneous pinning. Both spanning and nonspanning external fixation are used. Reduction is primarily based on ligamentotaxis to restore radial length and radial inclination (assisted by K-wires). Fixator pins are placed in radial shaft (superficial radial nerve at risk of injury), and 2nd metacarpal. Alignment is achieved by distraction. Overdistraction should be avoided because it may result in finger stiffness. Supplemental dorsal K-wires are passed to achieve volar tilt under fluoroscopy. K-wires may be removed at 3–4 weeks, keeping fixator for 6–8 weeks. Nonspanning external fixation—has the advantage of sparing wrist joint and hence minimizing chances of stiffness. The distal fixator pins are placed in the large distal radius metaphyseal fragment distal to fracture line. McQueen advocated nonspanning fixator for better preservation of volar tilt, prevention of carpal malalignment possible gave better grip strength and hand function than spanning external fixation.

Contd...

Contd...

Epidemiology	Anatomy	Clinical Evaluation	Radiographic Evaluation	Treatment
				Complications of external fixation include—malunion, stiffness of wrist, RSD, pin-site infection, radial sensory nerve damage, and fracture through pin site. *Internal fixator*: These are temporary locked plate fixation used as internal fixators in severely comminuted fractures to maintain alignment. They are wrist spanning plates that maintain the distal radius and radiocarpal alignment until bony union and are removed at 3–4 months. They may be used in polytrauma patient where extensive reconstruction is not a priority as a replacement of external fixators. *Endomedullary fixation* devices temporarily attracted interest but no extensive use has been reported for specific indication or definitive use. *Open reduction and internal fixation*—typical indications for ORIF include multifragmentary fracture, die-punch fragment, Barton's fracture, volar buttress loss, meta-diaphyseal extension/comminution, and associated distal ulna shaft fracture. Dorsal plating, volar plating, and column fixation have their own proponents. *Dorsal plating (locked/buttress)*: Logically, this takes care of the dorsal displacement best by directly countering the displacement (provides buttress and reduces the compression side of fracture), also it avoids the neurovascular structures on the palmar side. But for its frequent extensor tendon irritation and attrition, it had fallen out of favor. Early plate removal or applying low-profile plates in association with column fixation are the way around. • Volar plating— both locked fixation and buttress modes are available. Buttress plating is done primarily for shear fracture of the volar lip without dorsal comminution. Volar locked plating is the mainstay of modern fixation, as it stabilizes even a dorsally comminuted fracture. The problem is irritation of both volar and extensor tendons (avoided by limiting the size of screws, using all locked screws, low-profile anatomical plates, and avoiding placement beyond watershed line). The best technique is reduction of all fragments and then applying plate in desired location; fixation to distal fragment first and then reducing

Contd...

Contd...

Epidemiology	Anatomy	Clinical Evaluation	Radiographic Evaluation	Treatment
				and fixing to proximal or proximal first fixation with later scrambling of fragments in reduced position are both time and energy consuming and often inaccurate. • The FPL rupture is the most common following volar plate fixation. Preventing failure of reduction involves subchondral placement of screws and engaging them in various directions by using variable angle locking. • Three-column fixation of distal radius fractures is based on the biomechanics proposed by Rikli where the distal radius and ulna are represented as a tricolumn strut having their own share of transmitting forces. Separate fixation plates are available for dorsal surface, volar locked anatomical plate, and radial styloid plate/tension band and emphasis is also given to ulnar side fixation. The concept is to reconstruct the three columns so that normal biomechanics may be restored. Quite extensive in approach as multiple incisions are used, this may be a logical approach to restore anatomy in young patients with extensively comminuted fractures or those with significant radial styloid fragment that needs separate care. Variable angle volar fixation screws may reduce the need for separate styloid fixation. *Adjunctive to primary fixation* may be needed in impacted fractures (bone grafting—autograft, allograft, or synthetic graft) or adjunctive K-wire fixation for smaller fragments. *Arthroscopically assisted intra-articular fracture reduction* is used by some preferentially. Difference in outcome is unclear. It may be beneficial in complex articular fractures without metaphyseal comminution especially die-punch fragments or centrally impacted fragments and fractures with evidence of substantial interosseous ligament or TFCC injury without large ulnar styloid base fracture. Fixation of ulna styloid fractures is still controversial but there may be some advantage to fixation of displaced fractures at the base of the ulna styloid.

Contd...

Contd...

Epidemiology	Anatomy	Clinical Evaluation	Radiographic Evaluation	Treatment
				COMPLICATIONS *Median nerve neuropathy*—most common neurological complication. Complete median nerve lesion with no improvement following fracture reduction requires surgical exploration. Median nerve dysfunction developing after reduction mandates release of the splint and positioning of the wrist in neutral position → no improvement (persistent or progressive paresthesias and weakness in thumb opposition), exploration and release of the carpal tunnel should be considered. Incomplete lesion in a fracture requiring operative intervention is a relative indication for carpal tunnel release. *Ulnar nerve neuropathy*—seen with DRUJ injuries *Malunion or nonunion:* This typically results from inadequate fracture reduction or stabilization. Extra-articular malunion → open wedge osteotomy; intra-articular malunion → either revise after 6 weeks or perform intra-articular osteotomy and lift the fragment if late; radial shortening (greatest loss of wrist function and associated arthrosis/ulnar impingement) → ulnar shortening/osteotomy and lift radius *Post-traumatic osteoarthritis:* This is a consequence of radiocarpal and radioulnar articular injury, thus emphasizing the need for anatomic restoration of the articular surface *Finger, wrist, and elbow stiffness:* This occurs especially with prolonged immobilization in a cast or with external fixation. Treat by aggressive occupational therapy to mobilize the digits and elbow while wrist immobilization, as well as a possible supervised therapy regimen once immobilization has been discontinued. *Tendon rupture/entrapment*—tendon disorders are possibly the most common complications following management. EPL rupture is most common following closed reduction or neglected fracture and commonly occurs as a late complication of distal radius fractures even in cases of minimally displaced injuries. Factors associated include degeneration of the tendon (vascular disruption of the tendon sheath), mechanical impingement (callus or sharp fragment). ECU/EDM entrapment commonly occurs in DRUJ injury. Dorsal

Contd...

Contd...

Epidemiology	Anatomy	Clinical Evaluation	Radiographic Evaluation	Treatment
				Complications *Symptomatic nonunion*: Usually occurs with hook of hamate fractures and are treated by excision of fragment. *Ulnar or median neuropathy*: May need surgical exploration and release. Malunion or irregular fragments may cause attritional wear of flexor tendons to the small finger.

METACARPAL AND PHALANGEAL FRACTURES AND JOINT DISLOCATIONS

Epidemiology	Anatomy	Clinical Evaluation	Radiographic Evaluation	Treatment
These are common injuries comprising 10% of all fractures and most are work related. Border digits are most commonly involved and a rough estimate of fracture prevalence is as follows: • Distal phalanx (45%) • Metacarpal (30%) • Proximal phalanx (15%) • Middle phalanx (10%) There is a predominance of injury seen in males compared to females more prominent in active age groups/work-related injuries (sports injuries in the early 3rd decade and workplace injuries in the 5th decade). **MECHANISM OF INJURY** Highly variable mechanism of injury result into a broad spectrum of skeletal trauma patterns. Axial load (jamming injuries) is seen in ball sports or sudden reaches made during everyday activities, such as to catch a falling object. This results in shearing articular fractures or metaphyseal compression fractures. (examine the whole extremity for associated injuries). Hitting a hard object (wall, floor, or street fight) with a closed fist may result in fracture of 4th or 5th metacarpal neck (Boxer's fracture). Diaphyseal fractures and joint dislocations occur from a bending moment, which can occur during ball handling sport or if the hand is trapped by an object and is unable to move with the rest of the arm. Individual digits can easily be caught in clothing, furniture, or workplace equipment to sustain torsional forces resulting in spiral fractures or more complex dislocation patterns.	*Metacarpals* are bowed, concave on palmar surface forming the longitudinal and transverse arches of the hand. The index and long-finger CMC joint is rigid with minimal to no movement during routine hand movements. The ring and small-finger CMC joint is flexible. Three palmar and four dorsal interosseous muscles arise from metacarpal shafts create deforming forces in fractured metacarpals, typically flexing the fracture (apex dorsal angulation). *Phalanges* Proximal phalanx fractures usually angulate into extension (apex volar) because the proximal fragment is flexed by the interossei while the distal fragment is extended by the central slip. Middle phalanx fractures are unpredictable. The *MCP joint* is surrounded by various ligamentotendinous structures that may incarcerate a dislocated joint. On the volar aspect, the capsule attached to the metacarpal proximally and proximal phalanx base distally is reinforced by strong volar plate. The deep transverse metacarpal and collateral ligaments provide protection radially, while ulnar side protection is given by extrinsic and intrinsic tendons along with the sagittal bands providing additional support thus preventing dislocation. In a dislocating joint, the volar plate remains attached to the deep transverse ligament while breaking away from the proximal metacarpal neck. This may incarcerate between the dislocating surfaces preventing reduction of the joint.	Note the following, as they have bearing on treatment: • Age • Hand dominance • Occupation • Systemic illnesses • *Mechanism of injury*: Crush, direct trauma, twist, tear, laceration, etc. • Time of injury (for open fractures) • Exposure to contamination • Treatment received • Financial issues • *Physical examination must record*: – Digital viability (capillary refill should be <2 seconds). – Neurologic status [documented by two-point discrimination (normal is 6 mm) and individual muscle testing] – Deformity – ROM – Malrotation at one bone segment is best represented by the alignment of the next more distal segment (best demonstrated when the intervening joint is flexed to 90°). Comparing *nail plate alignment is an inadequate method* of evaluating rotation. The *MCP joint dislocations* present with mild hyperextension and ulnar deviation attitude of the finger. There is severe tenderness and restricted movements at MCP joint of the index finger. The IP joints develop a mild flexed attitude with fairly free movements but due to pain and swelling, movements are restricted. Typical pathognomonic sign of complex dorsal MCP joint dislocation is puckering of the palmar skin with head of the metacarpal palpable underneath while dorsally there is a void.	Standard PA, lateral, and oblique radiographs of the affected digit or hand are obtained. Fractures of base of 5th metacarpal are best seen on radiographs in hand pronated 30° from a fully supinated (AP) position. A Robert-view radiograph with the hand in maximal pronation is helpful for visualizing intra-articular extension of an epibasilar fractures of 1st metacarpal. Evaluate injured digits, when possible, to minimize overlap. **CLASSIFICATION** Descriptive classification best describes individual injury as the patterns are varied and often complex to fit in a specific system. Report and record the following: • Open versus closed injury • Bone(s) involved • Location within bone • Fracture pattern—comminuted, transverse, spiral, and vertical split • Displacement and direction • Deformity (rotation and/or angulation) • Extra-articular versus intra-articular fracture • Stable versus unstable. *Open fractures*: The open fractures of hand are better reported as described by Swanson, Szabo, and Anderson system instead of Gustilo system. *Type I (infection rate 1.4%)*: Clean wound without significant contamination or delay in treatment and no systemic illness *Type II (infection rate 14%)*: One or more of the following— • Contamination (gross dirt/debris, human or animal bite, warm lake/river injury, barnyard injury) • Delay in treatment >24 hours	Regaining the hand function is a priority in managing hand fractures. The following are common methods employed for management of metacarpal and phalanges fractures (decide on individual basis): • Immediate motion—for undisplaced stable fractures • Temporary splinting—buddy strapping/splinting • CRIF produces less than perfect reduction preventing overt deformity, pin tract care needed • ORIF gives anatomical reduction but added risks of surgical complications • Immediate reconstruction—for combined bone and soft tissue complex injuries Fractures with segmental bone loss may be managed by maintaining length and stabilizing the soft tissues followed by definitive bone management (Masquelet technique can be helpful). **Metacarpal head fractures:** These include epiphyseal fractures, avulsion fractures from collateral ligaments, intra-articular head fractures, and boxer's fracture with articular extension. To preserve joint function and anatomy, open reduction is needed mostly with perfect reduction. For stable undisplaced fractures, James position of safe immobilization (POSI) is preferred (MCP flexion >70° and IP joint in extension, wrist in 30° of extension) followed by early ROM. Flexing the MCP to 90° and extending the IP joints produce intrinsic plus position that minimizes chances of stiffness and morbidity by tightening the MCP collaterals in maximum length **(Fig. 42)**.

Contd...

Contd...

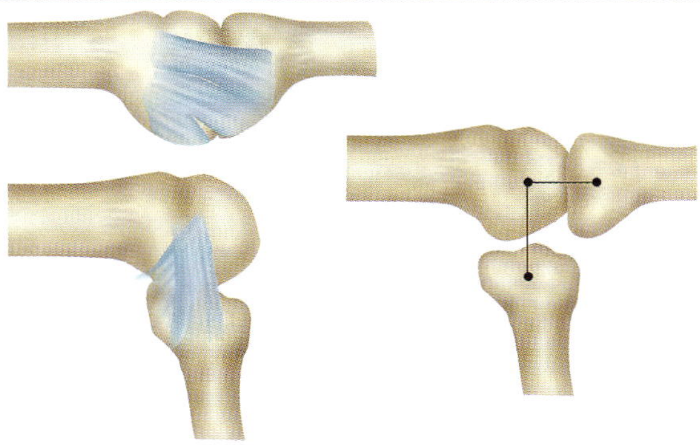

Fig. 42: Illustration depicting the position of collateral ligaments and their optimal lengthening with flexion of the metacarpophalangeal joint. This results from the "cam"-like volar projection of head of metacarpal resulting in higher volar offset of base phalanx in flexion causing lengthening of the ligament.

Epidemiology	*Anatomy*	*Clinical Evaluation*	*Radiographic Evaluation*	*Treatment*
Crushing injuries are seen in industrial settings or other physical labor (construction work) where heavy objects may fall crushing the bones with a combined bending, shearing, and torsional force to produce unique patterns of skeletal injury and associated soft tissue damage. Distal phalanx fractures usually result from crush injuries and are comminuted tuft fractures. The base fractures are usually avulsion injuries due to pull from long flexors (Jersey finger) or extensor slip attachment (mallet finger). The CMC joint dislocations result from high-energy injuries with involvement of associated structures, including neurovascular injury. Ulnar nerve is at risk in 5th CMC joint dislocation. ***MCP joint dislocations*** are commonly dorsal (phalanx displaced dorsally) resulting from hyperextension injury. Volar dislocations are rare and may result from combined hyperextension and translator force applied to the dorsum of proximal phalanx. It is seen in index finger most commonly followed by little finger, the ring and middle fingers are spared due to strong transverse metacarpal ligament and support from corner digits. Simple dislocation has no intervening structure while a complex dislocation (Farabeuf) results from volar plate/sesamoid interposition **(Figs. 43A and B)** preventing closed reduction and may involve Kaplan lesion (see anatomy).	Formation of Kaplan's complex needs further dissipation of energy resulting into buttonholing of the metacarpal volarly through various tight structures **(Figs. 43A and B)** making it impossible to reduce the dislocated joint by closed means as the structures further constrict the metacarpal head when reduction by traction is attempted. The flexor tendons on the ulnar side along with the pretendinous band of palmar fascia and the lumbricals radial ward form a tight constriction noose around the buttonholed metacarpal head preventing its reduction. From the volar aspect, the deep transverse metacarpal ligament may also form the part of noose (Murphy). It is important to note that in index finger, the flexor tendon displaces ulnarly and lumbrical displaces radially which tighten around metacarpal neck preventing reduction while in little finger, the flexor tendons and lumbrical displace radially and the abductor digiti minimi and flexor digiti minimi ulnarly preventing closed reduction		• Significant systemic illness, such as diabetes, hypertension, rheumatoid arthritis, hepatitis, or asthma The infection rate in type I injuries is not associated with primary internal fixation or immediate wound closure. Similarly, primary internal fixation is not associated with increased risk of infection in type II injuries. For type I injuries, primary wound closure is recommended while delayed closure is appropriate for type II injuries. First metacarpal base fractures can be extra-articular or intra-articular **(Fig. 44)**. The intra-articular fracture of base of 1st metacarpal is classified into two types: *Type I:* Bennett fracture—the oblique fracture line separates metacarpal base from single volar lip fragment that remains in place attached to the anterior oblique ligament. First metacarpal is pulled proximally by the abductor pollicis longus subluxating dorsally, radially, and proximally, producing a disruption of the first CMC joint **(Fig. 45)**. *Type II:* Rolando fracture—this is an intra-articular comminuted fracture where the fracture line results in two or more basal fragments and runs in a T, L, or Y shape. Thus, a bicondylar or multifragmentary fracture pattern is produced and shaft is separated from fragments at the epibasal region (metadiaphyseal disjunction). This is produced by a force greater than for Bennett fracture and may be considered a comminuted Bennett fracture. *MCP joint dislocations* are readily evident on radiographs—the pathognomonic sign of irreducible dislocation is appearance of a sesamoid in the joint space.	**Metacarpal neck fractures** There is dorsal angulation ± volar comminution. For 2nd and 3rd metacarpals, <10° of angulation is acceptable (less mobile) but for 4th—30° and for 5th—up to 50° is acceptable. Stable acceptable fractures may be splinted in James position (intrinsic plus position), while open/closed reduction and fixation (K-wires/condylar blade plate) is done for unstable fractures. For reduction, *Jahss technique* is commonly used **(Fig. 46)**—axial traction à followed by finger flexion at MCP → dorsal push from finger proximal phalanx to correct the deformity **Metacarpal shaft fractures** Acceptable upper limit for dorsal angulation is 10° for 2nd and 3rd while <20° for 4th and 5th. Proximal fractures tolerate less angulation. Rotational upper limit of acceptable deformity is 10° ≈ 1.5 cm overlap in clenched fist (to avoid "digital scissoring" rotation should be zero). Stable acceptable fractures can be immobilized in James POSI. Transverse fractures are inherently unstable. Unstable and displaced fractures are treated by closed/open reduction intramedullary K-wires, or/and plate fixation. Fracture base of 5th MC "Reverse Bennett's fracture" is the fracture dislocation of base of 5th metacarpal. The ECU pulls metacarpal proximally so stabilization utilizing closed/open reduction (traction, ulnar deviation, and radially directed pressure on the metacarpal shaft fragment) and percutaneous pinning is needed. **Fracture of base of 1st metacarpal** Extra-articular fractures (transverse/oblique) of base of thumb

Contd...

Contd...

Epidemiology	Anatomy	Clinical Evaluation	Radiographic Evaluation	Treatment

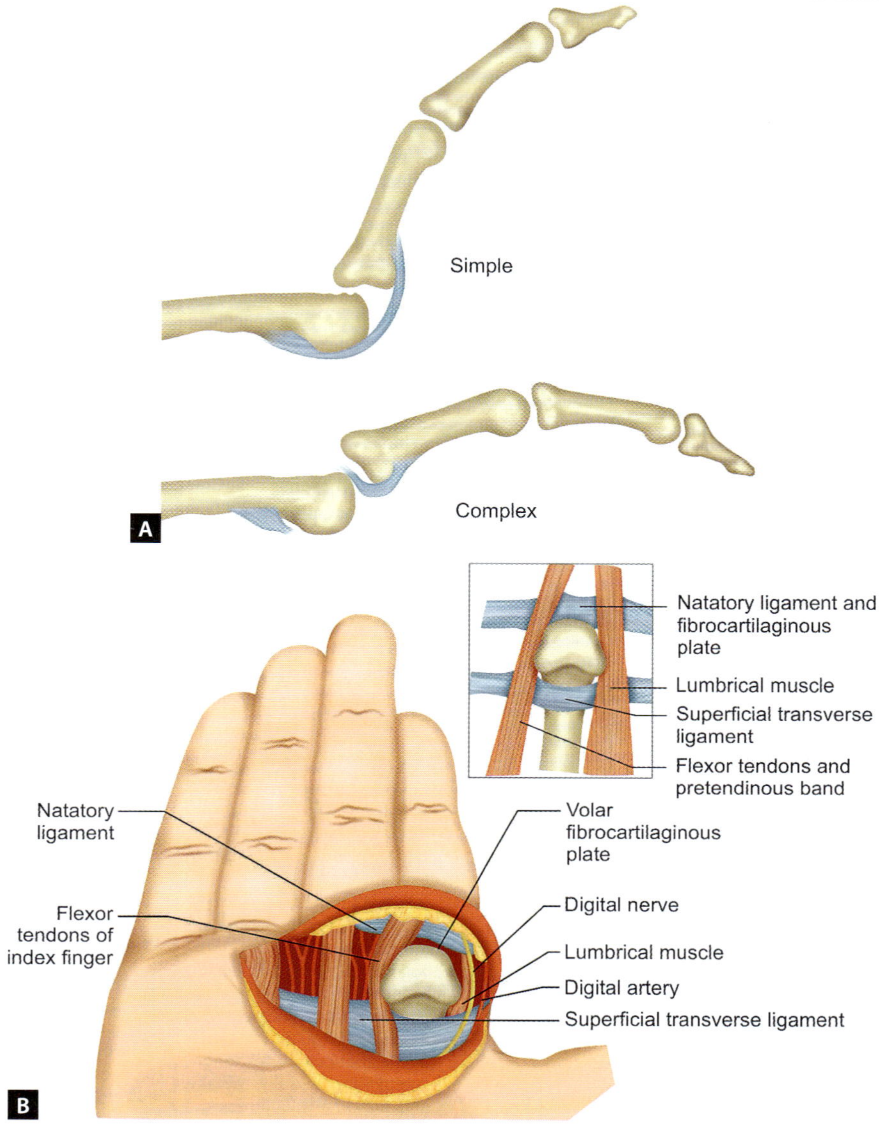

Figs. 43A and B: Dislocation of metacarpophalangeal joint, in complex dislocations the volar plate incarcerates within the joint preventing the reduction (A). Kaplan's complex may form with buttonholing of the metacarpal volarly preventing the joint reduction due to metacarpal head entrapment in a noose-like fashion by various structures (B).

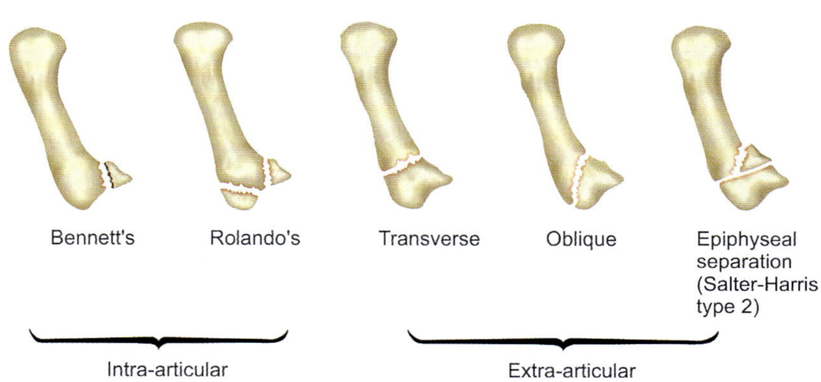

Fig. 44: The various types of 1st metacarpal base fractures.

Treatment (contd.):

metacarpal may be treated by CR and thumb spica immobilization else pinning may be done for unstable fractures.

Bennett's fracture needs reduction and stabilization (usually K-wires). Despite common belief and practice of abducting the metacarpal for reducing the fracture, contrarily the correct maneuver is traction → adduction into palm → pronation internal rotation and pushing the base into CMC joint. Bennett fragments involving >25% of the joint surface and those irreducible by closed techniques should be opened, reduced, and fixed internally.

Rolando fractures should be reduced for alignment and stabilized with K-wires. "Bag of bones" type fractures may be distracted and stabilized using distractor ± bone grafting. If pain persists later then arthrodesis or excision arthroplasty may be needed.

Other finger CMC joint dislocations in dorsal direction usually are unstable and need operative stabilization.

Fractures of proximal and middle phalanges

Extra-articular displaced fractures are reduced with finger trap axial traction and splinted.

Intra-articular condylar fractures need anatomical reduction and fixation. Severely comminuted fractures may undergo protected early mobilization.

Volar lip fractures of middle phalangeal base result in dorsal fracture subluxation/dislocation. Treatment is devised based on articular surface involvement. <30% articular surface involvement (usually occurs from hyperextension injury)—buddy strapping in reduced position. For >30% articular involvement—ORIF with anatomical articular surface reconstruction is needed. Volar plate arthroplasty may be done in comminuted or nonreconstructible fractures. If the joint is not subluxated then dorsal extension block splint may be used with immobilization.

Dorsal lip avulsion fractures are treated conservatively, if there is <1 mm displacement else ORIF should be done to prevent Boutonniere deformity.

Contd...

Contd...

Epidemiology	*Anatomy*	*Clinical Evaluation*	*Radiographic Evaluation*	*Treatment*
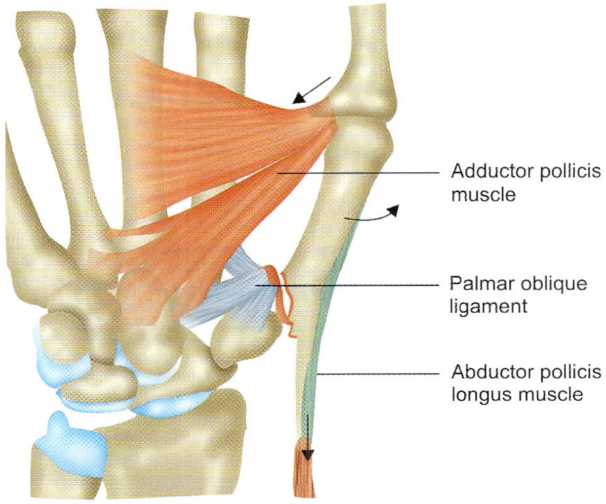 **Fig. 45:** The forces causing displacement in Bennett's fracture. 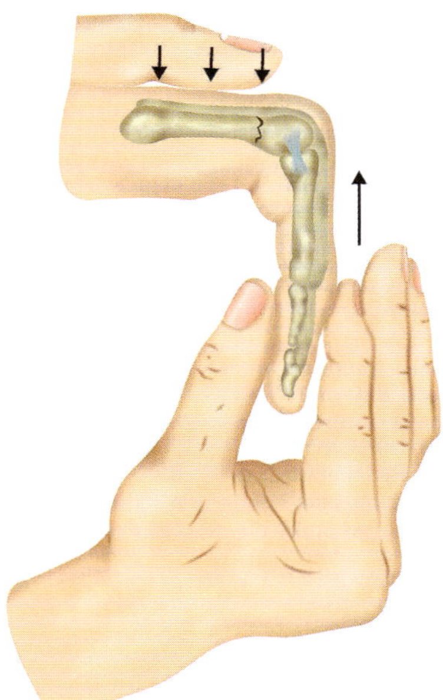 **Fig. 46:** Jahss technique of reduction of metacarpal neck subluxation/dislocation fractures for correcting apex dorsal angulation using the proximal phalanx as "joystick".				**MCP joint dislocations** Simple dislocations are reduced closed and splinted for few days to begin mobilization. Complex dislocations need open reduction using dorsal or volar (needs extensive release and A1 pulley with risk to neurovascular bundle) approach. In the dorsal approach, the capsule is incised longitudinally to expose the bones. Tight collateral ligaments may need release or retraction to look for volar plate that can be pushed volarly or need longitudinal incision to reduce the metacarpal head dorsally. Sometimes to reduce the metacarpal head, natatory ligaments and superficial transverse metacarpal ligaments may need to be released.

ANNEXURE 2

Lower Limb Trauma

Shafiq Hackla, Manish Kumar Varshney

FEMUR NECK FRACTURES

Epidemiology	*Anatomy*	*Clinical Evaluation*	*Radiographic Evaluation*	*Treatment*
Femoral neck fractures constitute 50% of all hip fractures. There is lifetime risk of 40–50% in women and 13–22% in men, so the incidence is likely to increase with increased life expectancy. It is more common in elderly females (>60 years age), white ethnicity, family history of osteoporotic fractures, alcohol abuse, smoking, chronic diseases such as diabetes, hyperthyroidism, renal disease, etc., medications (antileptics, antidepressant, proton-pump inhibitors, and HIV medications). Risk of fall is an important independent risk factor. **MECHANISM OF INJURY** The most common cause is simple fall with force being transmitted to femoral neck applied by greater trochanter resulting in fracture. Another mechanism is external rotation of leg with increasing tension in anterior capsule and iliofemoral ligament. As neck rotates, the head remains fixed and neck fracture occurs. The most common site is the weakest part of femoral neck just below the articular surface. Rarely, high-energy trauma with abducted hip results in neck fracture in younger patients (hip adduction causes fracture dislocation—posterior). Low-energy falls commonly result in subcapital fractures in elderly while higher energy falls cause transcervical or distal fractures ± comminution. Lastly, femoral neck stress fracture may result from repetitive loading.	Femoral neck connects femoral head to shaft through greater and lesser trochanter. It is entirely intracapsular except at the posterior aspect. Normal femur neck shaft angle is 130–135° and there is anteversion of 10 ± 7°. *Blood supply*: The blood supply of neck and head is important for high incidence of nonunion (*see* Chapter on "Nonunions and Malunions") and osteonecrosis in this region (*see* also Chapter on "Osteonecrosis and Osteochondrosis"). There are three important sources of blood supply: Retinacular vessels, intramedullary vessels, and ligamentum teres vessels. Retinacular vessels arise from medial and lateral circumflex femoral arteries, which are branches of profunda femoris artery in most cases. These vessels form extracapsular arterial ring at the base of femoral neck and ascending cervical vessels arise from this. The latter penetrate anterior capsule near base of neck at the level of intertrochanteric line. Inside the capsule these lay in the retinacular layer. There are four main groups (anterior, medial, lateral, and posterior). The lateral group is the main contributor of blood supply. The deep branch of medial circumflex artery supplies the lateral group that perfuses main weight-bearing portion of the femoral head. At the junction of articular surface of femoral head with neck, subsynovial intra-articular ring arises. The terminal branches of deep medial circumflex artery penetrate the femoral head 2–4 mm proximal to articular	Most patients will have history of simple, low-energy fall in elderly followed by inability to bear weight on the affected limb. Patients with valgus impacted fracture however may come walking to emergency department. In 2–3% cases, there is no history of trauma resulting in pathological fracture or a stress fracture. There is usually a history of prodromal symptoms in patients with stress fracture. Physical findings may be limited in undisplaced fractures with no obvious deformity and only painful range of hip motion. In displaced femoral neck fractures, the affected extremity is shortened and externally rotated. All hip ranges of movements are painful. Extracapsular hip fractures do not significantly differ from neck fractures on clinical grounds (the degree of external rotation is lesser in intracapsular femur neck fractures—the lesser toe of foot usually does not touch the couch). Anterior dislocation of hip also presents with flexion and external rotation deformity but these are rare injuries.	Plain radiographs with AP and lateral views will identify the fracture in majority of cases. The characteristic features are **(Fig. 1)**: • *Shenton's line disruption:* Loss of smooth contour from medial edge of femoral neck and inferior border of superior pubic ramus. • Lesser trochanter is more prominent (external rotation deformity). • Femur in flexion and external rotation (unopposed iliopsoas). • Upriding of trochanter. • Sclerosis in fracture plane. • Smudgy sclerosis from impaction. • Bone trabeculae discontinuity and angulation. • The lateral radiograph although difficult to acquire for pain is useful in determining the degree of displacement and associated posterior comminution. • In 2% cases, fracture is difficult to visualize, CT scan can identify the fracture more accurately but it exposes the patient to further radiation. • MRI is the most useful additional form of imaging in modern practice. MRI is the current additional modality recommended when there is uncertainty about the presence of fracture. • Bone scan can be used but is time-consuming, and there are high chances of false negative scan in osteopenic	**NONOPERATIVE TREATMENT** It can be considered in patients with poor chance of survival due to medical comorbidites or malignancy and in patients who declines operative treatment. Patients are mobilized in bed and then on walker with shoe raise as tolerated for pain. Stress fractures with valgus impaction of femoral neck can also be treated nonoperatively. **OPERATIVE TREATMENT** Role of capsulotomy is debatable and although tamponade from intracapsular hematoma is a definite threat to vascularity there is no definite guidance for doing it routinely in closed reduction cases. Possibly in less displaced fractures of young it may be indicated seemingly due to preserved continuity of capsule in them. Reduction method and quality and adequacy of fixation scores highly over time to fixation from injury. Fixation as early as possible is recommended to minimize complications of osteonecrosis and nonunion. *Undisplaced fractures*: Due to high chances of late displacement in these fractures (up to 50%) these fractures should be fixed with either cannulated cancellous screws (CCS) or sliding hip screw with derotation screw. When using CCS inverted triangle is the common configuration formed for fixation while erect triangle can also be used. Diamond configuration is good if there is posterior comminution while rectangular and parallel

Contd...

Contd...

Epidemiology	*Anatomy*	*Clinical Evaluation*	*Radiographic Evaluation*	*Treatment*
Associated injuries commonly include distal radius and proximal humerus fracture in elderly due to common mechanism of fall and osteoporosis. Femoral shaft fracture is seen in association in 2–5% of young patients with high energy trauma.	surface on posterio-superior aspect, that are at risk in subcapital displaced fractures. Artery of ligamentum teres arises from obturator artey or deep medial circumflex artery. Displaced femoral neck fracture damages these retinacular vessels risking vascularity to head.		bone if the investigation is carried within 72 hours of fall. **CLASSIFICATIONS** **Anatomical Classification (Figs. 2A to C)** *Subcapital*: Femoral head/neck junction—results in elderly from low energy fall. *Transcervical*: Midportion of femoral neck—these commonly result from higher energy injuries.	configurations have fallen out of favor. In an inverted triangle configuration, the first screw should be inferior along the calcar, the second should be posterior along the neck and the third should be superior at the tensile surface of the fracture while tightening should be done possibly anterosuperior (to maintain length as posteriorly there is comminution and tightening inferior first may result in varus), followed by inferior and lastly posterior screw. The reduction should be judged on anteroposterior (AP) and lateral views through Lowell S- or reverse S-shaped curve on both views. It is preferable to keep Garden alignment index of 160–180° on both views. Varus fixation is the biggest predictor of fixation failure.

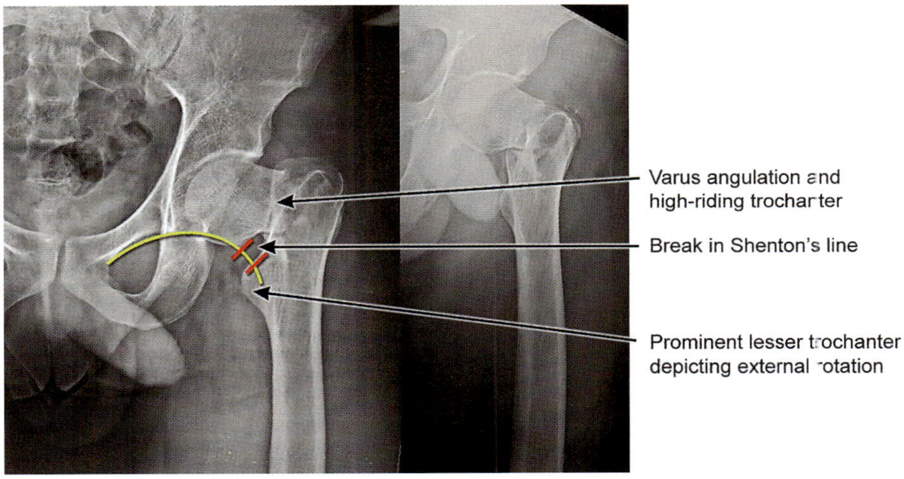

Fig. 1: The radiographic appearance of fracture neck of femur.

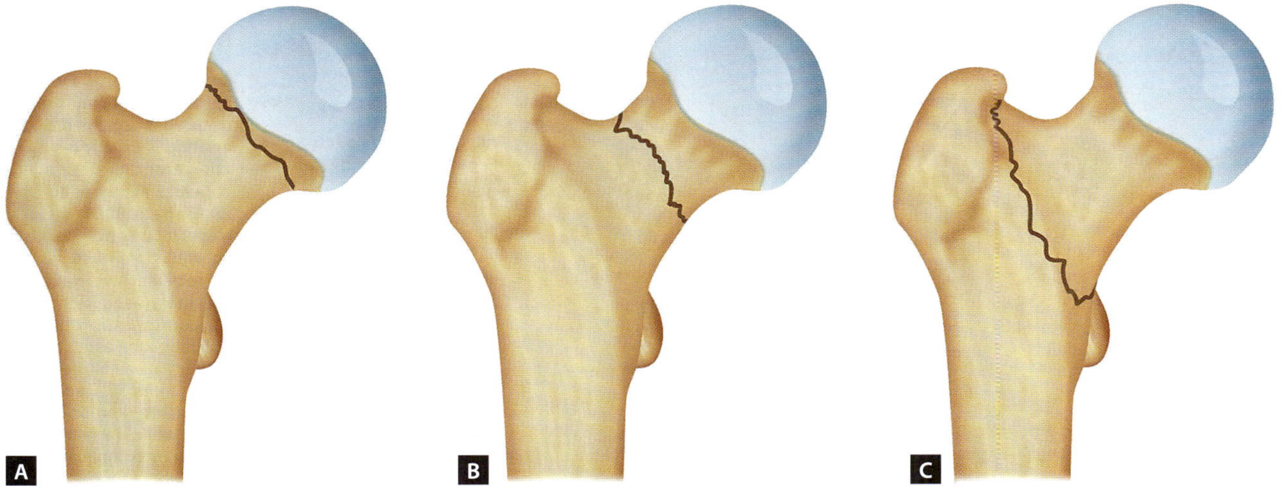

Figs. 2A to C: Anatomical classification for fracture neck of femur illustrating subcapital (A), transcervical (B), and basicervical (C) fractures.

Contd...

Contd...

Epidemiology	*Anatomy*	*Clinical Evaluation*	*Radiographic Evaluation*	*Treatment*
	After displaced fracture, revascularization of femoral head occurs by retained blood supply and ingrowth of vessels from metaphysis that takes time to establish hence variable degree of osteonecrosis is present.		*Basicervical*: Base of femoral neck. **Garden's Classification (Figs. 3A to D)** This classification is based on the degree of displacement on AP radiographs by determining the relationship of trabecular lines in the femoral head in the same orientation as those of acetabulum. Type 1 is valgus impacted subcapital fracture with incomplete lateral fracture line without breach of medial cortex. Type 2 is complete but undisplaced fracture and trabecular lines in the femoral head are collinear with that of acetabulum. Type 3 is incompletely displaced fracture of femoral neck. The trabecular lines of femoral neck are partially aligned with those of acetabulum. Type 4 is completely displaced fracture of femoral neck. The femoral neck externally rotates, so the trabecular lines in the neck are not collinear with those in the head. Types 1 and 2 are commonly called nondisplaced fractures while types 3 and 4 are considered displaced. **Pauwel Classification (Figs. 4A to C)** It is based on the angle the fracture forms with the horizontal plane. It was proposed that the classification would be the predictive of fixation failure or nonunion with increasing angle of fracture. Type 1 subtends an angle of <30°. Type 2 subtends an angle between 30 and 50°. Type 3 subtends an angle >50°. **AO/OTA Classification** Femoral neck is designated as 31B. 31B1 describes nondisplaced femoral neck fracture. 31B2 transcervical fracture and 31B3 describes displaced subcapital fracture. **Delbet Classification for Pediatric NOF Fracture (Figs. 5A to D)**—correlates with complications: Type 1—transepiphyseal fractures (90% risk of osteonecrosis). Type 2—transcervical fractures (50% risk of osteonecrosis).	*Displaced fractures:* Reduction and fixation of displaced fractures in patients younger than 60 years old (physiological age) with acceptable bone quality for osteosynthesis. Reduction can be done using Leadbetter technique in flexion (hip flexion to 90° (relaxes muscles) with adduction→traction and internal rotation (relaxes Y-ligament) to 45°→full flexion and adduction→slight abduction and full extension maintaining internal rotation. Check with heel-palm test—hold heels of both limbs in palm in adduction and internal rotation and release internal rotation to check for developing ER deformity, satisfactory if IR maintained. Reduction maneuver in extension is preferable for its simplicity—the Wellmerling technique (on a fracture table with leg in slight external rotation distract fracture by lengthening the affected leg by 1–2 cm. Place one forearm in the groin and the other beneath popliteal fossa and apply internal rotation while releasing the traction, simultaneously lift the knee with forearm in popliteal fossa and pushing below by the other forearm in groin). Maximum of two generous attempts at reduction are enough → proceed to open reduction if fails. Watson-Jones or Smith-Peterson approach may be used depending on surgeon preference. Either cannulated cancellous screw (Pauwel's type 1 and 2) or sliding hip screw (Pauwel's type 3) with short plate and derotation screw (debatable) can be used after gentle reduction of fracture in proper alignment. Performing valgus osteotomy primarily or using muscle pedicle bone grafting is usually a surgeon's choice and experience but concrete evidence to its use in management of acute fractures is not established. For reducible fractures, three or four screws have been routinely used. Read above for configuration of screws and reduction assessment. For higher Pauwel angle fractures varus collapse, uncontrolled neck shortening or nonunion (if collapse does not occur) are major complications that are reported variably but in significant patient population.

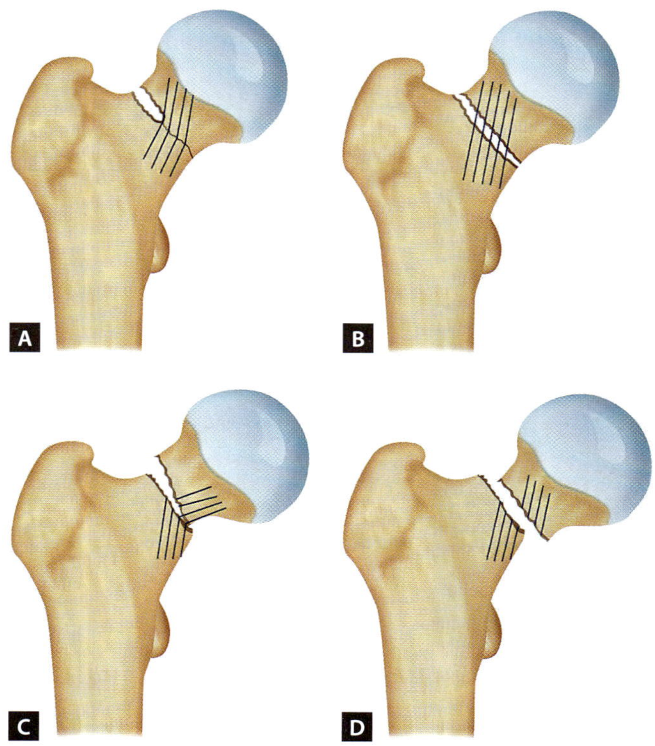

Figs. 3A to D: Garden's four types of fracture neck of femur (see text for description).

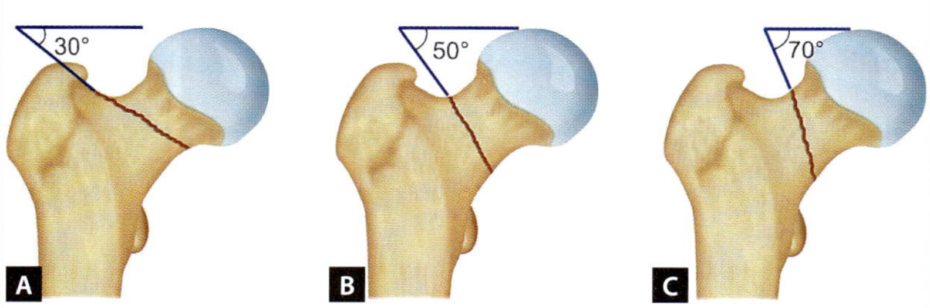

Figs. 4A to C: Pauwel's classification of fracture neck of femur based on fracture angle.

Contd...

Contd...

Epidemiology	Anatomy	Clinical Evaluation	Radiographic Evaluation	Treatment
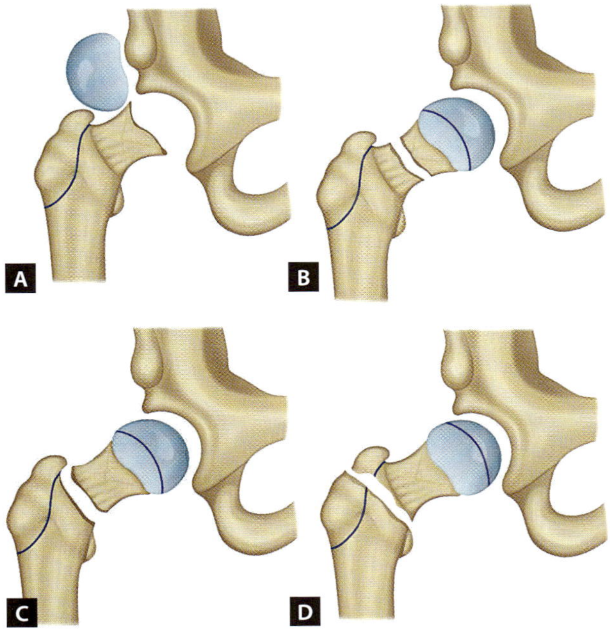 **Figs. 5A to D:** Delbet classification for fracture neck femur in pediatric age group (unfused femoral head epiphysis).			Type 3—basicervical cervico-trochanteric fractures (25% risk of osteonecrosis). Type 4—intertrochanteric fractures (10% risk of osteonecrosis).	DHS with anterotation screw is recommended in such cases and reasonably does well except for short stature patients and those with small femoral neck limiting optimal implant placement the implant obviously remains prominent. Controlled collapse is still an issue. Newer system like femoral neck system® has been developed that may resolve some of these limitations but widespread results and high-quality superiority trials are lacking. Complications are fixation failure, osteonecrosis of femoral head (16%), and nonunion (33%). The risk of nonunion increases with age where it is uncommon below 50 years of age while rises to 40% in patients in 70s. Poor outcomes in fracture displacements are >5 mm. **ARTHROPLASTY** It depends upon fracture characteristics and physiological age of patient. Older patients >65 years and those with poor bone quality to hold the fixation device sturdily should be treated with arthroplasty. The rates of reoperation are high in such patients with associated morbidity. Whether hemiarthoplasty or total hip arthoplasty is chosen is a matter of debate. The result of bipolar hemiarthroplasty is generally good in very elderly where life expectancy is <15 years and there is reduced demand on prosthesis. There are still high chances of painful hip (acetabular wear) following hemiarthroplasty and also revision is less rewarding. Total hip replacement (THR) is better option for patients with rheumatoid arthritis, relatively young (life expectancy >20 years, revision is more predictable), active, those on long-term steroids and chronic renal failure. Functional outcome of THR has been reported to be better than hemiarthroplasty albeit with slight increased risk of dislocation. Cemented stems have far better in reports. Prefer larger heads, bearing should have highly crosslinked poly to minimize wear rates (metal/ceramic possibly makes no difference). Summarizing the advantages of internal fixation over arthroplasty: • Native head retained

Contd...

Contd...

Epidemiology	Anatomy	Clinical Evaluation	Radiographic Evaluation	Treatment
				• Less surgical trauma • Reduced morbidity in frail elderly patients • Lesser surgical complications • Disadvantages of internal fixation • Risk of nonunion (33%) • Osteonecrosis (16%). Higher reoperation rates reported in literature (30–50%)—this is the prime reason for advocating arthroplasty even in relatively younger patients. Better functional outcomes and less residual pain after arthroplasty Disadvantages of arthroplasty: • Increased operative complications—infection (5%), hematoma formation (2%) • Risk of dislocation (2–4%) • Iatrogenic femur fracture • Periprosthetic fracture • Prosthetic loosening • Acetabular erosion with hemiarthroplasty. Overall complications include 30% mortality at 1 year, infection, deep vein thrombosis and pulmonary embolism, fixation failure, nonunion, osteonecrosis, prosthesis dislocation, and prosthesis loosening. Management in pediatric patients: Types 1, 2, and 3—nondisplaced/age up to 4 years → closed reduction and spica cast. Internal fixation (smooth pins/cannulated screw) for children >4 years and displaced fractures. Smooth pins are used for small/young children and need spica cast supplementation. Cannulated screw is good for older children and adolescents. Screw may cross the physis for stability else for short screw consider spica supplementation. Type 4 fracture—nondisplaced fractures till age 3–4 years → closed reduction and spica cast. Children up to 6 years → closed reduction, pin fixation and spica cast. Rigid internal fixation for children with displaced fractures in children >3 years, use closed/open reduction.

INTERTROCHANTERIC FRACTURES

Epidemiology	Anatomy	Clinical Evaluation	Radiographic Evaluation	Treatment
Pertrochanteric fractures involve those occurring in the region extending from	The main structural attachments to proximal femur include hip capsule, abductors,	The patients present with the history of pain and inability to ambulate after fall or other	Standard plain radiographs include AP of pelvis and AP and cross table lateral view	**NONOPERATIVE TREATMENT** It is considered only in nonambulatory patients

Contd...

Contd...

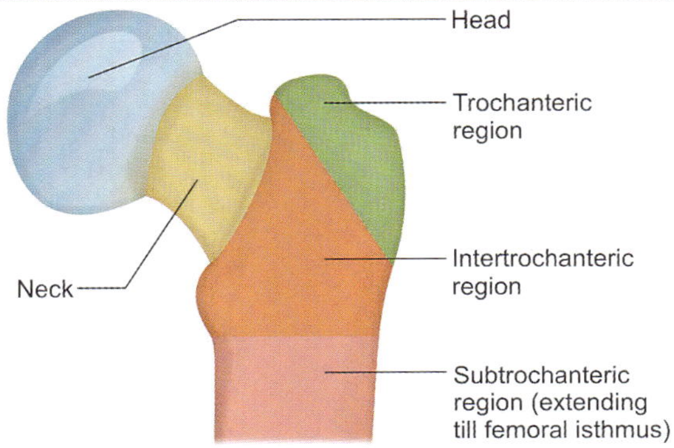

Fig. 6: The anatomical division of various regions of proximal femur.

Epidemiology	*Anatomy*	*Clinical Evaluation*	*Radiographic Evaluation*	*Treatment*
extracapsular basilar neck to region along lesser trochanter proximal to the development of medullary canal **(Fig. 6)**. Cooper described the fracture in 1951. Royal Whitman and Ledbetter developed reduction maneuvers. Jewett (1930) developed a nail for fixation of the fracture with a lateral plate. Earnest Roll (German) first used sliding screw and Pugh and Badgley introduced sliding nail with trephine tip in USA. Massie (1962) modified sliding devices to allow collapse and impaction of the fragments that was modified and marketed by Richard manufacturing company as DHS in 1966. Kuntscher (1966) and Enders (1970) introduced condylocephalic intramedullary fixation devices. Russel-Taylor developed intramedullary nail (1984) followed shortly by development of gamma nail by Halder and Williams (1992). They are the most frequently operated fracture type, and have higher postoperative fatality rate of all surgically treated fractures. The incidence is similar to intracapsular fracture neck femur with females outnumbering the males. Risk factors include elderly white females with a propensity to fall (forces must be concentrated around proximal femur minimally absorbed by soft tissues). Previous proximal humerus fractures and fractures of distal radius or vertebral osteoporotic fractures increase the risk of occurrence of proximal femoral fractures. Factors associated with increased mortality include male gender, operative delay of >2 days, age >85 years, ≥2 pre-existing medical conditions, and ASA grade III or IV.	flexors, and short external rotators. The displacement of fracture fragment is dependent on muscle attachment of respective fragments. The greater trochanter is abducted and externally rotated by gluteus medius and short external rotators and shaft is displaced medially and posteriorly by adductors and hamstrings resulting in shortening and coxa vara deformity. Calcar femorale is a dense bony strut present posteromedially in the proximal femur region that provides primary strength against varus angulation at the region. Separation of this region in a separate fragment or inability to restore the strut results in progressive varus angulation and failure with weight-bearing as it goes into varus collapse and retroversion. This makes it imperative to avoid a varus reduction in all. Also this entails that implants that can better handle varus moment will have better initial stability at the osteosynthesis, thus intramedullary implants that lie close to the medial wall (intramedullary implants) will have less varus moment to counter than the implants placed over lateral cortex (like dynamic hip screw plate construct). The rest of the proximal femur is composed of weak trabecular bone that serves elastic function in young while with aging osteoporosis causes dissolution of majority of this honeycomb structure leaving big voids in the trochanter, femoral neck, and head filled with fatty marrow. Only the tensile and some compressive trabeculae remain that serve to hold metal work used to fix these fractures.	injury. The pain is localized to proximal thigh and is exacerbated by passive or active attempts of hip flexion and rotation. Physical findings are shortening and external rotation deformity of the extremity. Classically, the external rotation deformity is more marked in intertrochanteric fractures compared to fracture of neck of femur. This is due to capsule that prevents excessive external rotation of distal fragment, but it is difficult on this basis only to differentiate between these two proximal femoral fractures. Pain with axial load (hitting on heel with fist or pushing along the leg) can be elicited in patients with occult fractures. Auscultation Lippman test is sensitive for detecting such fractures—place the bell of stethoscope on symphysis pubis and tap on patella of both extremities, reduced conduction from one extremity suggests intertrochanteric fracture.	of affected hip for diagnosis and preoperative planning. Fracture geometry may be better defined by traction views in internal rotation to aid in selection of internal fixation. CT or MRI scans are rarely required for displaced fractures but may be useful in establishing the diagnosis in nondisplaced fractures and atypical fractures from high energy trauma. MRI is preferred over CT or radionuclide scan due to higher sensitivity and specificity. **CLASSIFICATIONS** **Boyd and Griffin Classification (Fig. 7)** *Type 1*: Undisplaced fracture that extends along the intertrochanteric line (Two parts). *Type 2*: Posteromedial comminuted fractures with main fracture along the intertrochanteric line. *Type 3*: Fractures that extend distal to lesser trochanter or fracture lines run obliquely down from lateral to medial (Reverse obliquity type). *Type 4*: Fracture of trochanteric region or proximal shaft with fracture line in at least two planes. **Evans Classification (Figs. 8A to E)** It classifies the fracture on the basis of stability. *Type 1*: The fracture line that extends up from lesser trochanter to the greater trochanter. • Undisplaced • Displaced two-part fracture and reducible • Three-fragment fracture with posterolateral support. • Three-part fracture with lost medial support.	where life expectancy is <6 weeks, unresolvable medical condition that precludes surgical treatment, active infectious disease that precludes insertion of surgical implant or incomplete trochanteric fractures in selected patients. It includes good nursing care, attention to nutrition, and fluid homeostatsis and adequate pain suppression. General measures for prevention of bedsores, pulmonary and urinary complications, and deep vein thrombosis should be instituted. **Operative Treatment:** It should preferably be done within 24–48 hours (surgery within 48 hours reduced morbidity and mortality). Surgical implants used over time can be broadly divided into extramedullary and intramedullary implants. The plate and screw construct/nail construct with sliding mechanism had been the most popular extramedullary fixation with emerging intramedullary construct of a short or long nail with sliding screw. External fixation and arthroplasty are done in specific situations. *Dynamic hip screw:* It has been most commonly used device for both stable and unstable fractures historically, but is best suited for stable fractures only. It consists of lag screw and barrel plate with a sliding mechanism that allows controlled collapse of fracture fragments to impaction at the fracture site under weight-bearing. Derotation screw is commonly combined and prevents rotation of head fragment, but is not a routine. Tip-apex distance of Baumgartner is an important

Contd...

Contd...

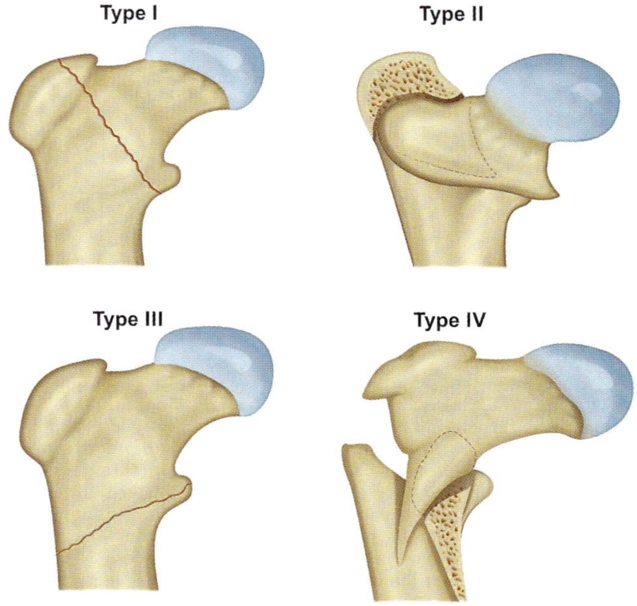

Fig. 7: Boyd and Griffin classification of intertrochanteric fractures.

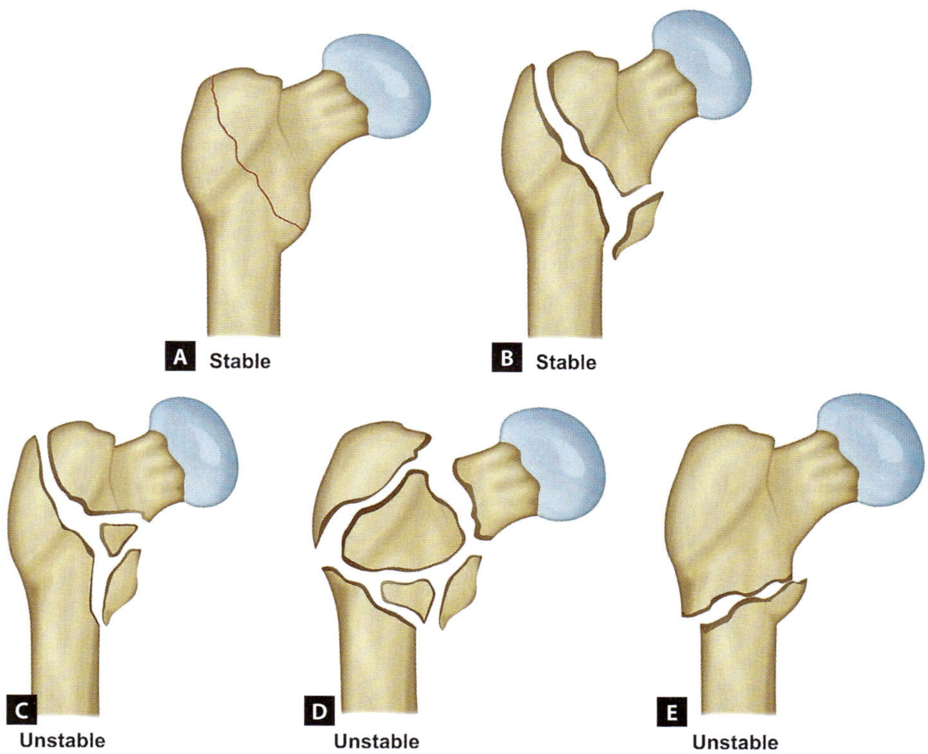

Figs. 8A to E: Evans classification for fracture intertrochanteric.

Epidemiology	*Anatomy*	*Clinical Evaluation*	*Radiographic Evaluation*	*Treatment*
MECHANISM OF INJURY Low energy falls from standing height is the most common cause of this fracture in elderly osteoporotic patients. High-energy trauma is relatively rare and occurs in young patients	Because of the poor hold and support to the implants there are high rates of failure. The failure is due to break in the implant-bone interface that has to resist a combination of rotational torque and		• Comminuted (four part or more) with separate posterolateral and medial fragments. Type 2: Reverse obliquity type.	predictor of DHS failure, a distance >25 mm or <10 mm predicts future failure. Excessive collapse may result in shortening, medialization of shaft and prominent implant. This can also be

Contd...

Contd...

Epidemiology	*Anatomy*	*Clinical Evaluation*	*Radiographic Evaluation*	*Treatment*
≈ 10% cases. In contrast to adduction/abduction during fall causing intracapsular fractures, falls with rotational components are more common with extracapsular hip fractures. Associated injuries include distal radius and proximal humerus fractures in low-energy fall. High-energy fractures are associated with ipsilateral extremity trauma, pelvic fractures, and head injury. Metastatic disease can present with pain in hip for several days and subsequent fracture with low energy mechanism or even no trauma sometimes.	compressive stress, which disengages the implant from bone resulting in migration and cut-out. This is the reason a variety of implants has been introduced for fixation of intertrochanteric fractures and are still under development.		**Russell Taylor Classification (Fig. 9)** *Type 1*: Fractures that do not extend to piriformis • Lesser trochanter is intact • Lesser trochanter is disrupted *Type 2*: Fractures that involve the piriformis fossa • Lesser trochanter is intact • Lesser trochanter is disrupted. **AO/OTA Classification** These fractures are classified as 31A. *31A1*: Simple two-part fracture. *31A2*: Fractures are comminuted with posteromedial comminution. Lateral cortex is intact. *31A3*: Fractures that extend across both medial and lateral cortex and include reverse obliquity type. Radiologically, the fractures with loss of lateral wall, posteromedial comminution, reverse obliquity type, and four parts or more are unstable types needing extra care while planning fixation.	used in combination with Dimon–Hughston osteotomy for unstable intertrochanteric fractures. *Medoff sliding plate:* It uses biaxial sliding hip screw. It has standard lag screw for compression along the femoral neck and coupled pair of sliding components in the shaft plate component that allows the fracture to also impact parallel to longitudinal axis of femur. Complications include varus angulation, shortening, loss of fixation, and implant failure. *Intramedullary hip screw nail construct*: These devices include impaction type nails (PFN, PFNA2, Kuntscher Y-nail), TFN, gamma nail, (single large lag screw in head) Recon nail (two screws in head) and InterTAN nail (integrated screws in head). These devices are most commonly indicated in pertrochanteric and subtrochanteric fractures, but also are implant of choice for unstable reverse oblique type fracture. Fractures with medial comminution can also be reliably fixed with long intramedullary component. These implants combine the feature of DHS and an intramedullary nail. The advantages of intramedullary implants over DHS include: • They can be inserted in a closed manner with limited fracture exposure. • There is decreased blood loss and less tissue damage. • It decreases abductor lever arm and consequently less chances of implant failure. • *Condylocephalic nails*—like Enders nail and TENS nail have been superseded

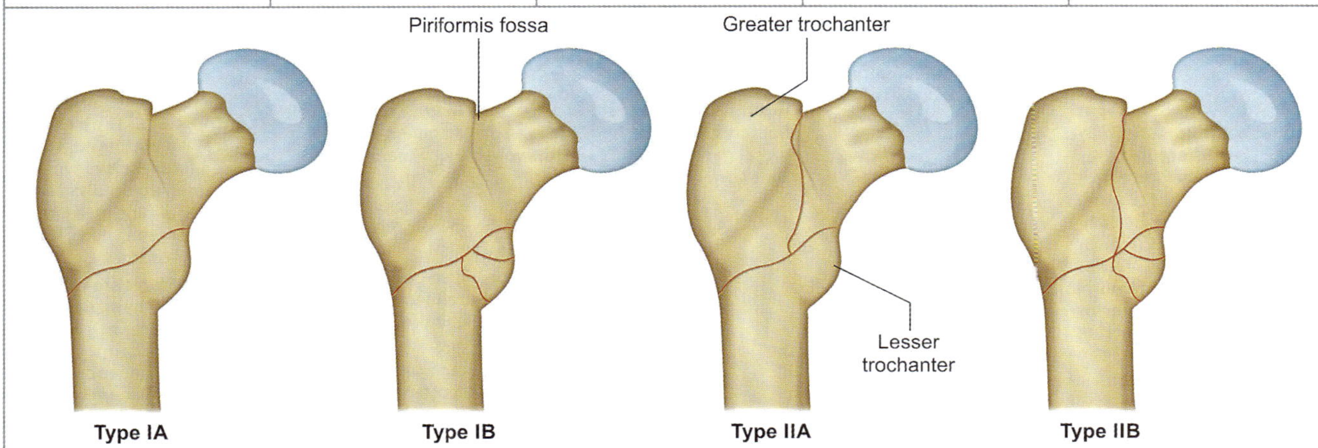

Fig. 9: Russell Taylor classification for fracture intertrochanteric region (see text for description).

Contd...

Contd...

Epidemiology	*Anatomy*	*Clinical Evaluation*	*Radiographic Evaluation*	*Treatment*
				by other devices but may be used if the entry for cephalomedullary nails preclude fixation. *External fixation:* This is not commonly used for treatment of these fractures. It is associated with pin tract infection, pin loosening, instability, and varus collapse. Classical indications include associated soft-tissue injury precluding other methods of fixation. *Arthroplasty:* It is indicated in severely comminuted trochantric fractures, pre-existing degenerative arthritis, neoplasia associated fractures, severe osteoprotic fractures (osteosynthesis may fail), and patients on dialysis. Cemented hemiarthoplasty with calcar replacements type is usually indicated in these cases. Always attempt greater trochanteric fixation onto shaft.

FEMORAL HEAD FRACTURES

Epidemiology	*Anatomy*	*Clinical Evaluation*	*Radiographic Evaluation*	*Treatment*
Femoral head fractures are almost always associated with hip dislocation. They occur in 5–15% of all hip dislocation and are seen in nearly 10% of posterior hip dislocations. There are two types of femoral head fracture with shear or cleavage type occurring in majority of the patients and indention or crush type occurring in reminder of the patients. The latter type mostly occurs in patients with anterior dislocation of the hip. **MECHANISM OF INJURY** These fractures are secondary to motor vehicle accidents with axial load transmitted proximally through the femur. If the thigh is in the neutral or adducted position, posterior dislocation with or without femoral head fractures may result. These fractures may result from counter force from ligamentum teres resulting in avulsion of fragment or cleavage by the posterior acetabular edge (shear fracture). Impacted femoral head fractures in anterior dislocation may occur due to direct blow from the acetabular margin.	Femoral head is composed mainly of dense trabecular bone. It is almost spherical and is covered all over by articular cartilage thickness of which varies from 4 mm superiorly to 3 mm inferiorly. Fovea centralis is a small ovoid depression just below and behind the center that provides attachment to ligamentum teres and is devoid of hyaline cartilage. Femoral head varies in size from 40 to 60 mm in diameter in proportion to body mass. Most of the femoral head articular surface is involved in the load transfer and thus damage to this surface may lead to the development of post-traumatic arthritis. So maintaining the anatomy is crucial. Blood supply to head is discussed in detail above and elsewhere.	The patients with femoral head fractures are usually the result of high-energy trauma and need formal trauma evaluation. Ninety-five percent of these patients have injuries that require inpatient management independent of femoral head fractures. There is localized hip pain and inability to bear weight on affected extremity. Position of extremity varies with associated dislocation (FADIR for posterior or FABER for anterior dislocation). Careful neurovascular examination is mandatory because of posterior hip dislocation leading to sciatic nerve injury and possible vascular compromise. ***Associated injury*** Hip dislocations, acetabular fractures, femoral shaft fractures, patella fractures, and knee ligamentous injuries.	*AP and Judet views of the pelvis*: Demonstrate the femoral head fractures and hip dislocation in majority of the cases. *Computed tomography*: It is usually performed after the reduction of hip dislocation to assess the size, location, and reduction of femoral head fracture. It demonstrates the femoral head fracture and its adequacy of reduction. It is also helpful to rule out the presence of intra-articular fragments, incongruity of hip joint, and associated acetabular or femoral neck fracture. **CLASSIFICATIONS** **Pipkin Classification (Fig. 10)** *Type 1*: Hip dislocation with the fracture of femoral head inferior to fovea capitis. Usually a small fragment does not involve weight-bearing portion. *Type 2:* Hip dislocation with fracture of femoral head superior to fovea capitis involving the weight-bearing portion. *Type 3*: Type 1 or 2 fracture with associated femoral neck fracture. High risk of osteonecrosis. *Type 4*: Type 1 or 2 fracture with associated acetabular fracture (usually posterior wall).	*Type 1 fractures*: These fractures occur in the nonweight-bearing surface. If reduction is adequate <1 mm step off and hip is stable, closed treatment is recommended else open reduction and internal fixation with small subarticlar screws (2.7 mm or 3.5 mm cortical screws or headless compression screw) is recommended. Small fragments can be excised if they do not compromise stability. *Type 2 fractures* involve the weight-bearing surface but the treatment recommendations are same as that of type 1 fractures. Reduction and fixation can be achieved through anterior (Smith Peterson) or posterior (Kocher Langenbeck) approach. Typically, anterior approach is used for these two types of fractures. Surgical dislocation of hip can also be used if there is no other associated fracture to be addressed. *Type 3 fractures* are rare and data to guide the management of these fractures is lacking. Prognosis for this fracture is poor and depends on the degree of displacement. Young patients are treated with open reduction and internal fixation

Contd...

Contd...

Epidemiology	***Anatomy***	***Clinical Evaluation***	***Radiographic Evaluation***	***Treatment***
			AO Classification It classifies the femoral head fractures into: • 31C Articular fracture, Head • 31C1 Split • 31C2 with depression • 31C3 with neck fracture	while older ones are treated with primary arthoplasty in view of poor results of osteosynthesis. *Type 4 fractures* are treated in tandem with acetabular fractures. The type of acetabular fracture dictates the surgical approach in these patients. The combination may be also treated with the surgical dislocation of hip. *Femoral head fracture with anterior dislocation*: These fractures are difficult to manage. Impaction fractures typically located on superior aspect of femoral head require no specific treatment. Displaced transchondral fractures that result in nonconcentric reduction require open reduction and internal fixation or excision depending on fragment size or location. **COMPLICATIONS** 1. *Osteonecrosis*: Patients with posterior hip dislocations with associated femoral head fractures are at high risk for developing osteonecrosis and degenerative arthritis. Type 3 injuries have poor prognosis among all. Patients with anterior hip dislocation develop osteonecrosis in 10% patients. Risk factors are delay in reduction and repeated reduction attempts.

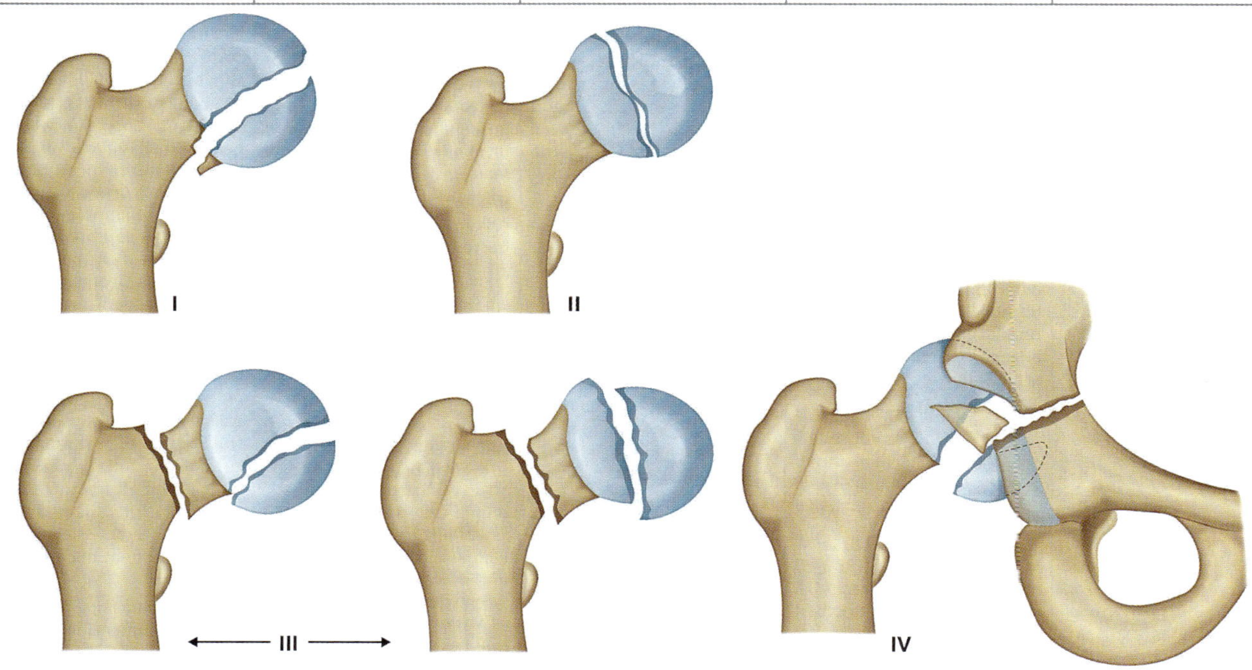

Fig. 10: Pipkin's classification for fracture of head of femur.

Contd...

Contd...

Epidemiology	*Anatomy*	*Clinical Evaluation*	*Radiographic Evaluation*	*Treatment*
				2. *Post-traumatic arthritis*: Multiple factors leading to post-traumatic osteoarthritis are transchondral fracture, indentation fracture >4 mm in depth and osteonecrosis.

SUBTROCHANTERIC FRACTURES

Epidemiology	*Anatomy*	*Clinical Evaluation*	*Radiographic Evaluation*	*Treatment*
Subtrochanteric fractures account for 10–30% of all hip fractures and they occur in all age groups. Anatomically, the subtrochanteric (ST) area is defined as 5 cm region from lesser trochanter onto shaft (some take up to 8 cm as the subtrochanteric region). Fractures beginning in intertrochanteric (IT) region and extending to ST area are classified as IT fractures with ST extension and not otherwise. **MECHANISM OF INJURY** • These fractures usually result due to either high energy or low energy mechanism. High-energy fractures occur in younger patients due to motor vehicle accidents, fall from height or gunshot wounds. Gunshot wounds account for 10% of higher energy ST fractures. • Elderly patients sustain these fractures through weakened bones due to minor fall. ST region is a frequent site for occurrence of pathological fractures accounting for 17–35% of all fractures especially in elderly. • Atypical bisphosphonate therapy associated fracture also occurs in ST region with low-energy trauma and is typically transverse ± small spike.	In general, fractures occurring in the area between lesser trochanter and the isthmus of femur are considered ST fractures despite the anatomical description of the region as a 5 cm region distal to lesser trochanter. The ST region is composed mainly of cortical bone, so there is less vascularity in this region and the potential for healing is diminished as compared to IT fractures. The ST region is subjected to high biomechanical stresses. The medial and posteromedial cortices are sites of high compressive stresses while lateral cortex experiences high tensile stress. These combined with smaller fragment proximally make adequate fixation challenging. The deforming forces on proximal fragment include abduction by glutei (medius and minimus), external rotation by short rotators and flexion by psoas muscle. The proximal fractures are more affected by these forces than distal fractures pulling it into flexion abduction and external rotation. The distal fragment is pulled proximally and into varus by the adductors **(Fig. 11)**. There is also shortening of the affected extremity due to pull of quadriceps and hamstrings muscle. The fracture of lesser trochanter results in less flexion and external rotation due to attachment of iliopsoas on lesser trochanter.	The patients usually present in emergency with history of high-energy trauma in younger patients. The patient has severe pain, is unable to move the extremity, unable to bear weight on the extremity and there is gross deformity and swelling of the proximal thigh. These patients should receive formal trauma assessment. There is abnormal mobility, crepitus and tenderness at the affected site. Neurovascular examination is performed to rule out associated injury. Elderly patients usually have trivial fall and gross weakening of the bones due to any underlying osteoporosis. Females are more affected than males. As ST region is a site of frequent metastasis and occurrence of pathological fracture a formal metastasis profile and work-up should be ordered to locate the primary malignancy. Always take a history for bisphosphonate/denosumab therapy in elderly low-energy trauma transverse ST fractures as there is a good association between the two. The following are the criteria to define an atypical femoral fracture: *Major criteria:* • Associated with no or minimal trauma, as in a fall from a standing height or less. • Fracture originates at the lateral cortex and is substantially transverse in its orientation, although it may become oblique as it crosses the medial femur. • Noncomminuted. • Complete fractures extend through both cortices and may be associated with a medial spike; incomplete fractures involve only the lateral cortex. • Localized periosteal or endosteal thickening of the lateral cortex is present at the fracture site.	An anteroposterior view of the entire pelvis and AP and lateral view of the affected hip with thigh should be obtained. Radiograph of the entire femur with knee should also be assessed to rule out associated injury. **CLASSIFICATIONS** **Fielding Classification (Fig. 12)** It is based on the level of the subtrochanteric region through which the fracture extends in relation to lesser trochanter. *Type 1*: Fracture at the level of lesser trochanter. *Type 2*: Fracture 2.5–5 cm below the lesser trochanter. *Type 3*: Fracture 5–7.5 cm below the lesser trochanter. **Shinsheimer Classification (Fig. 13)** This classification is based on the number of fracture lines and its location in relation to major bone fragments. It emphasizes the concept of posteromedial buttress support and also lays importance to the fact that the more distal a fracture is the more unstable it will be. *Grade I:* Undisplaced fracture or <2 mm of displacement of fracture fragments. *Grade II:* Two part fractures. *IIA*: Two part transverse femoral fracture. *IIB*: Two part spiral fracture with lesser trochanter attached to proximal fragment. *IIC*: Two part spiral fracture with lesser trochanter attached to distal fragment. *Grade III: Three part fractures* *IIIA*: Three part spiral fracture in which lesser trochanter is part of 3rd fragment, which has an inferior spike of cortex of varying length. Implant failures and nonunions are common. *IIIB*: Three part spiral fracture of proximal one-third of	**NONOPERATIVE** This is rarely recommended if ever with the exception of patients with poor surgical risk. The patient is placed in 90/90 position in a cumbersome hip spica cast. There is increased morbidity (Atelectasis, pneumonia, thromboembolic events, and bedsores) with this treatment itself due to increased chances of nonunion, malunion, stiffness of adjacent joints, and shortening of the limb. **OPERATIVE** It is the preferred modality of treatment for most ST fractures. There are different types of implants that can be used in these fractures. *Intramedullary implants:* These are most commonly used in the treatment of these fractures as it can be inserted in a minimally invasive manner (barring open reduction if needed), preserves vascularity and fracture hematoma. Other suggested advantages are shorter abductor lever arm and consequently less chances of implant failure, early weight bearing (nail is a load sharing implant) and reduced blood loss. Long intramedullary cephalomedullary nail is my personal favorite. Prerequisite is a fracture reduction by closed, miniopen or open method before passing the nail. One may use circlage wiring for spiked fragments that displace during nail placement. Centromedullary nails are used only when both trochanters are intact while cephalomedullary nail can be used for all fractures but especially for those having loss of posteromedial cortex and involvement of piriformis fossa. *Extramedullary implants:* Plate fixation—Indications for its use are Russell Taylor type IIA or IIB fractures, narrow medullary canal precluding stable intramedullary fixation,

Contd...

Contd...

Epidemiology	Anatomy	Clinical Evaluation	Radiographic Evaluation	Treatment
		Minor criteria: • Generalized increase in cortical thickness of the femoral diaphyses • Prodromal symptoms such as dull or aching pain in the groin or thigh • Bilateral incomplete or complete femoral diaphysis fractures	femur, with third part butterfly fragment. *Grade IV:* Comminuted fracture with four or more fragments. Implant failures and nonunions are common. *Grade V:* ST-IT fractures This group includes any ST fracture with extension through IT region.	pre-existing femoral shaft deformity, and associated displaced femoral neck fracture then would need open reduction. Proximal femoral locking plate or 95° fixed angle plate or dynamic condylar screw (DCS) with 95° barrel plate can all be used. Fractures with proximal extension which

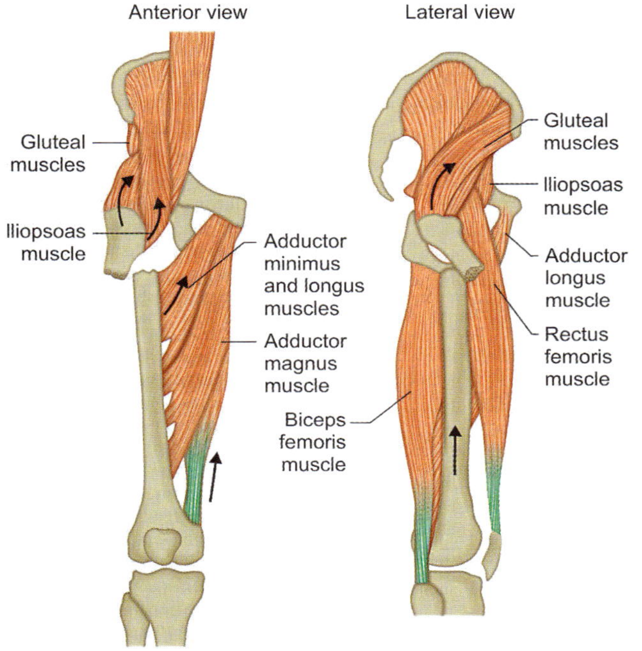

Fig. 11: Displacing muscular forces for fracture in subtrochanteric region.

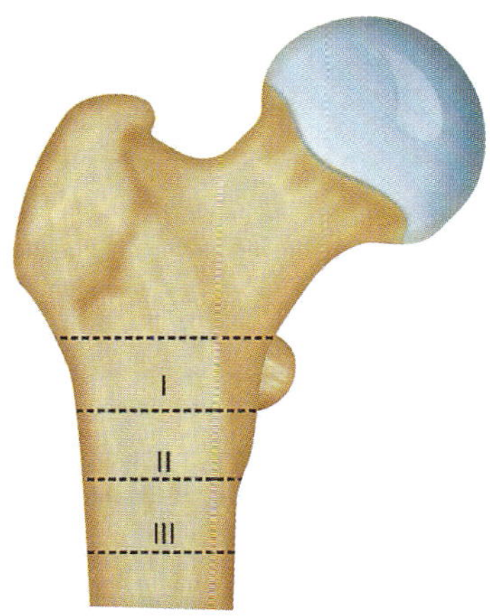

Fig. 12: The Fielding classification for subtrochanteric fractures. This is a pure anatomical classification that describes the position of major fracture line in reference to lesser trochanter.

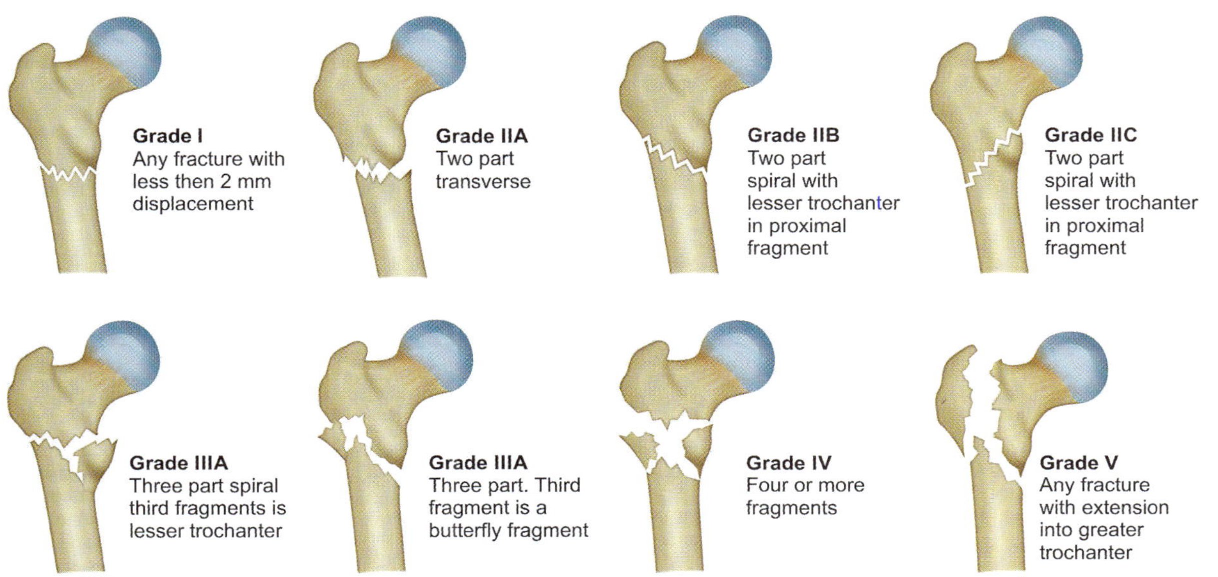

Fig. 13: The Seinsheimer classification for subtrochanteric fractures.

Contd...

Contd...

Epidemiology	*Anatomy*	*Clinical Evaluation*	*Radiographic Evaluation*	*Treatment*
		• Delayed fracture healing • Specifically excluded are fractures of the femoral neck, intertrochanteric fractures with spiral ST extension, pathological fractures associated with primary or metastatic bone tumors, and periprosthetic fractures.	**Russell Taylor Classification (Fig. 14)** This classification is based on the presence or absence of fracture involvement of piriformis fossa and lesser trochanter: *Type 1*: Fracture with intact piriformis fossa *A:* Lesser trochanter is attached to proximal fragment. *B:* Lesser trochanter is detached from proximal fragment. *Type 2*: Fracture that extends into piriformis fossa. *A*: Have a stable medial cortex. *B*: Have comminution of piriformis fossa and lesser trochanter associated with varying degree of femoral shaft comminution.	compromise the integrity of starting portal for a nail are best treated with these plates. Proximal femoral locking plates can be placed with either percutaneous or open technique based on fracture characteristics while this liberty is not available with blade plate that has to be placed open for mono-block angled nature of implant. A blade plate can be however placed using direct or indirect reduction technique and is useful in revision cases for its sturdiness and fixation strength. Angled blade plates work on the principle of tension band (lateral cortex tensile forces are converted into medial compressive ones) when the posteromedial cortex is restored. **COMPLICATIONS** 1. *Loss of fixation*: In DCS, it usually occurs due to screw cutout from femoral head in patients with osteoporotic bone or plate breakage (proximal femoral locked or angled blade plate) which is actually very common due to improper reduction of fracture or premature weight bearing. With interlocked nails, loss of fixation is due to failure to lock the device statically, comminution of the entry portal or use of small diameter nail. The nails usually fail by fatigue through lag screw hole in the nail. 2. *Nonunion*: Improper reduction or atypical fractures. 3. *Malunion*: Varus and/or recurvatum. Treatment recommendation based on Russell Taylor classification *IA*: Standard interlocking intramedullary (IM) nail *IB*: Recon intramedullay nail *IIA*: Hip screw or recon IM nail *IIB*: Hip screw with bone graft or recon IM nail. Bisphosphonate or denosumab associated fractures usually are treated by intramedullary nailing but risk of complications is higher in terms of iatrogenic fracture (brittle bone), increased risk of nonunion → needing revision surgery. There is an emerging role of teriparatide in managing these fractures especially to enhance healing.

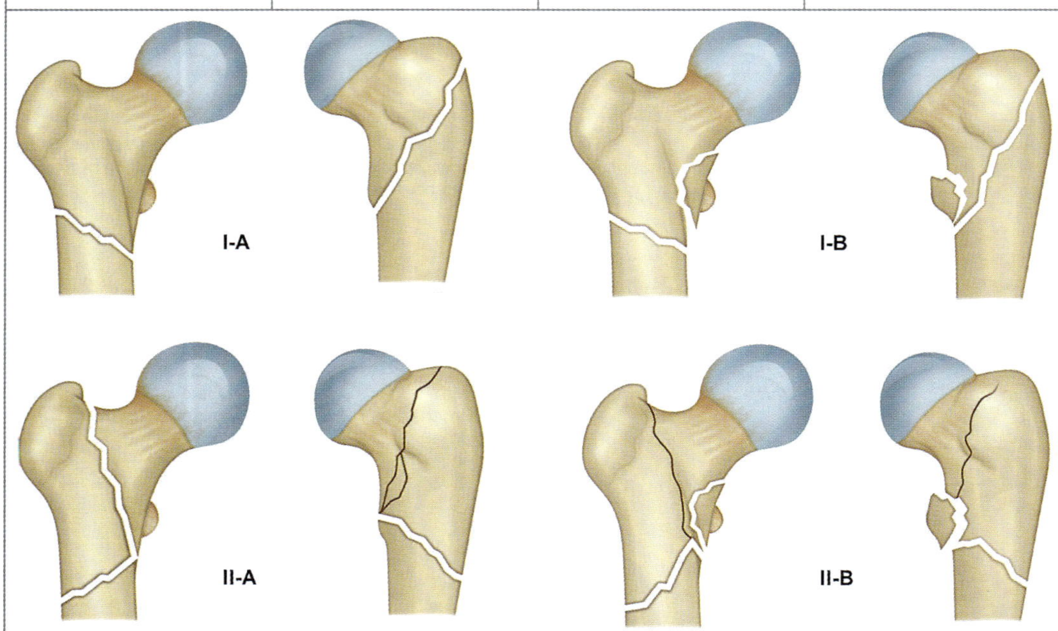

Fig. 14: The Russell Taylor classification for subtrochanteric fractures (kindly see text for details)

FRACTURE SHAFT OF FEMUR

Epidemiology	*Anatomy*	*Clinical Evaluation*	*Radiographic Evaluation*	*Treatment*
Fractures of the shaft of femur are among the most common fracture encountered in orthopedic practice. These fractures can cause prolonged morbidity and extensive disability unless treatment is appropriate. The incidence of femoral fractures is 30 per 100,000 per year. In younger age group, the fracture is more common in male patients while it is seen more commonly in females in older patients. There is bimodal distribution of these fractures—younger than 25 years and older than 65 years. **MECHANISM OF INJURY** Femoral shaft femur often results from high-energy trauma in young adults and may be associated with multiple system injuries. These fractures result from motor vehicle accident, fall from height, and gunshot injury. Fracture in elderly occurs due to low-energy fall commonly at metaphyseodiaphyseal areas. Fracture that is inconsistent with history of trauma should arouse suspicion of pathological fracture. Military recruits or runners having thigh pain after recent increased activity/training should be evaluated for pathological fracture. Bisphosphonates are known to cause insufficiency fractures in femur (see above).	Femur is the largest bone of the body and one of the principal load bearing bones of lower extremity. The bone is surrounded by largest mass of muscle divided into compartments as follows: *Anterior compartment:* It contains the quadriceps femoris, the sartorius, the psoas, the iliacus, and the pectineus, as well as the femoral artery, vein, and nerve, along with the lateral femoral cutaneous nerve. *Medial compartment:* It comprises the gracilis, the adductor brevis, longus and magnus, the obturator externus, the deep femoral artery and vein, and the obturator artery, vein, and nerve. *Posterior compartment:* It contains the hamstrings-semitendinosus, the semimembranosus, the biceps femoris and portion of the adductor magnus, perforating branches of the deep femoral artery, the sciatic nerve, and the posterior femoral cutaneous nerve. The diaphysis (portion excluding the proximal and distal metaphysis) is tubular throughout with a posterior linear strut of cortical bone—the linea aspera (rough line, it provides major attachment for fascia). The femur shaft has a notable anterior bow. The femur has abundant vascular supply predominantly perfused by profunda femoris artery. The nutrient artery usually enters along the linea aspera posteriorly along junction of upper and middle one-third following into endosteal circulation. The endosteal circulation supplies	Quite evidently there is gross deformity, swelling, pain, abnormal mobility and crepitus and shortening of the affected extremity. Distal neurovascular status should be carefully checked. These fractures usually result from high-energy trauma, so full trauma survey is required in these cases. Thorough examination of pelvis, hip, and knee should be performed. These fractures are associated with major blood loss into the thigh and hemodynamic status should be monitored and managed as needed. Open fractures are much less common due to significant muscle mass in thigh. Open fractures usually are associated with multiple other orthopedic injuries and other organ systems. ***Associated injuries*** are present in 5–15% of the patients that include trauma to spine, pelvis, and ipsilateral lower extremity injuries. Ligamentous and meniscal injuries of ipsilateral knee are present in 50% of patients with closed femur shaft fractures. Ipsilateral femoral neck fractures are seen in 2–6% cases and missed nearly 20% of the times. Polytrauma with associated abdominal visceral and pulmonary injuries are also common.	The AP and lateral view of the femur should be obtained. Also obtain the AP view of pelvis, hip, and knee and lateral view of hip and knee. CT scan may be needed in midshaft femoral fracture to identify associated femoral neck fracture if suspected. **Winquist and Hansen Classification of Comminution (Fig. 15)** *Type 0:* No comminution. *Type 1:* Comminuted fracture, in which small piece of bone has broken off not affecting fracture stability. *Type 2:* At least 50% contact of abutting cortices remain to prevent shortening and help to control rotation and in which sufficient proximal and distal cortical contact of nail is possible to prevent translation and shortening. *Type 3:* Comminuted fracture which has <50% of cortical contact or in which purchase of the nail would be poor in either proximal or distal fragment, allowing translation, rotation, and shortening. *Type 4:* Comminuted fracture in which circumferential buttress of bone has been lost and no fixed contact exists between major proximal and distal fragments to prevent shortening. This also includes segmental fractures with bone loss and no remaining contact between proximal and distal fragments. **AO/OTA Classification** It classifies the fractures as 32 which is further classified as: • 32-A (SIMPLE FRACTURE) – 32-A1: Spiral – 32-A2: Oblique >30° – 32-A3: Transverse <30°	The treatment of shaft femur fracture depends upon type of fracture, condition of bone, and quality of soft tissue and associated injuries. The goal of treatment is the restoration of length, alignment, and rotation and earlier rehabilitation of the limb and patients. **NONOPERATIVE** There are different methods like closed reduction and spica cast immobilization (pediatric patients till 3–4 years of age), skeletal traction and femoral cast bracing. This form of treatment is largely limited to adult patient with significant comorbidities that preclude operative management. Skeletal traction is also used as temporary measure to stabilize the fracture before surgery and to prevent fracture shortening. Disadvantages are knee stiffness, malunion, limb shortening, heterotopic ossification, prolonged hospitalization, and respiratory and skin complications. **OPERATIVE MANAGEMENT** It is the standard of care in femoral fractures. Early stabilization of femoral fractures appears to be particularly important in multiply injured patients. *Intramedullary nailing (antegrade):* It is the standard treatment of femoral shaft fractures. It should ideally be done within 24 hours of injury. The nailing can either be performed through closed or open technique and it can be either antegrade or retrograde. Closed intramedullary nailing maintains both fracture hematoma and the attached periosteum. Reaming of the medullary canal provides

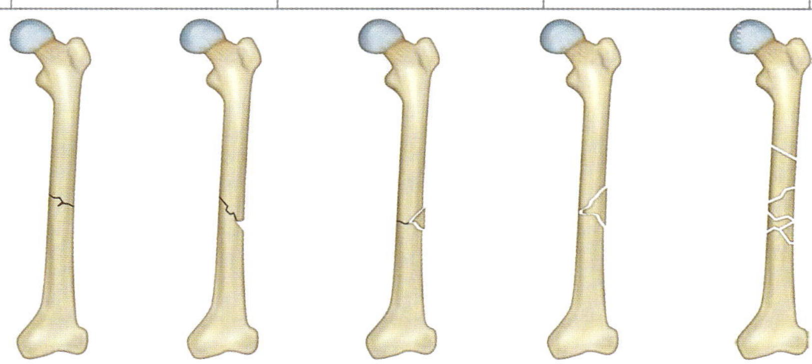

0 I II III IV

Fig. 15: Winquist classification for comminution in fracture shaft femur (See text for details).

Contd...

Contd...

Epidemiology	Anatomy	Clinical Evaluation	Radiographic Evaluation	Treatment
	the inner two-thirds to three-fourths of the cortical diameter, making the normal blood flow centrifugal. The periosteal circulation enters posteriorly for the most part along the linea aspera and is almost entirely directed in a circumferential direction, having little or no longitudinal spread. Periosteal circulation has been estimated to serve only the outer one-fourth to one-third of the cortex. However, the periosteal circulation is critical to fracture healing in the diaphysis. When a fracture is displaced, the sole medullary supply is disrupted and the periosteal vessels predominate as the vascular supply to the fracture site during early healing. In response to fracture, the periosteal vessels proliferate, while the endosteal circulation is restored much later. Therefore, the use of slotted nails may allow for enhanced return of endosteal neovascularization and a more normal blood flow pattern. The significance of periosteal blood flow in healing also emphasizes the importance of avoiding periosteal stripping especially along the linea aspera. Displacements of fragment depend on the level of the fracture manipulated by insertion and attachment of different muscles. The proximal segment of the femur is in flexion, abduction, and external rotation due to pull of glutei, ilipsoas, and short external rotators **(Figs. 16A and B)**. The adductors span most of the medial femur and produce an axial and varus force on the femur. Some of these medial forces are countered by the tension band effect of the fascia lata. The distal femur is under a flexing influence by the gastrocnemius.		• 32-B (WEDGE FRACTURE) – 32-B1: Spiral wedge – 32-B2: Bending wedge – 32-B3: Fragmented wedge • 32-C (COMPLEX FRACTURE) – 32-C1: Complex spiral – 32-C2: Complex segmental – 32-C3: Complex irregular	the osteoconductive and osteoinductive factors which help in achieving union at the fracture site. Intramedullary nailing results limited dissection, restoration of length and alignment even in comminuted fractures, rapid and early union, shorter hospital stay, rapid return of motion in all joints, prompt return to walking, and relatively short total disability time. Reaming enhances union rates, decreases time to union, and improves stability of fixation by allowing larger diameter nail. The effect of reaming on patients with multisystem trauma is controversial even today. The current consensus is that the immediate fixation of femoral fractures with reamed intramedullary nail does not increase the risk of clinically significant pulmonary complications. The ill-effects of medullary reaming can be decreased by using sharp reamers with deep cutting flutes and by using minimal force during reamer insertion. The open femoral fractures are treated with urgent debridement with irrigation and intravenous antibiotics. The femur is stabilized with statically locked nail in lower grade open injuries. The wound is then closed over suction drains if surgically clean. Massive open wounds or those grossly contaminated (type IIIC Gustilo) are left open and better covered with VAC dressing. Repeat debridements are performed until wound can be safely closed. **Technique** Surgery can be performed on a fracture table with patient either supine or in lateral position. Piriformis fossa or trochanteric entry portal can be used for gaining entry into the femoral shaft (depending on nail design—straight vs. spiral nail). All nails should be statically locked to maintain femoral length and to control rotation. Retrograde intramedullary nailing. It is indicated in following situations. 1. Morbidly obese patients 2. Patient with ipsilateral femoral neck and shaft fractures 3. Floating knee injuries 4. Multiply injured patient

Contd...

Contd...

Epidemiology	*Anatomy*	*Clinical Evaluation*	*Radiographic Evaluation*	*Treatment*
				5. Bilateral femoral shaft fracture fixation 6. Pregnant women 7. Periprosthetic fractures 8. Ipsilateral through knee amputation in a patient with an associated femoral shaft fracture. It is contraindicated in patients with restricted knee motion (<60°) and patella baja. *Plate fixation:* Currently, plating (4.5 mm broad LCP used through anterolateral approach) of the femoral shaft has fallen out of favor due to success, ease and better acceptable function with intramedullary nailing and high complications rate of plating. It may be selectively indicated in: 1. Patient with ipsilateral femoral neck and shaft fracture. 2. *Arterial injuries*: Vascular exploration needed/done. 3. Extremely narrow medullary canal in which nailing is not possible. 4. Fracture associated with proximal or distal extension into pertrochantric or condylar region respectively. 5. Highly comminuted fracture. 6. Using Masquelet technique for segmental bone loss or infected nonunion. The advantages are anatomic reduction and lack of additional trauma to remote location such as femoral neck or distal femur. The disadvantages are extensive surgical dissection, with resultant risk of increased blood loss, soft-tissue insult, and infection. As plate is a load sharing implant, there are higher chances of implant failure especially with premature weight-bearing. There are higher chances of delayed union and nonunion. *External fixation:* Its use has been limited to temporary fixation and DCO until patient is ready for definitive fixation (2–3 weeks later). The indications for its use are: 1. Massively contaminated fracture 2. Arterial injury that requires repair. The advantages are minimal trauma to soft tissue, procedure is rapid, no additional foreign material is introduced and allow the patient transfer while maintain skeletal stabilization.

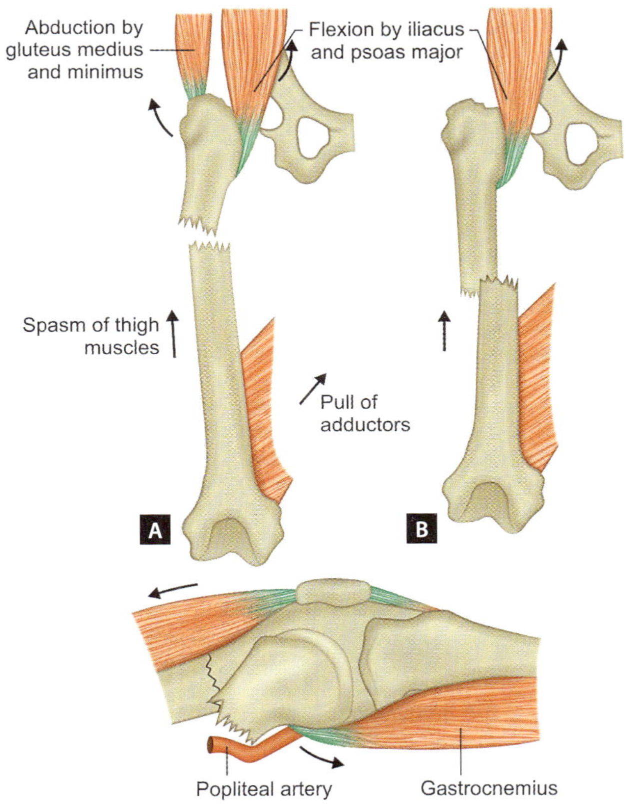

Figs. 16A and B: Displacing forces for fracture shaft of femur.

Contd...

Contd...

Epidemiology	Anatomy	Clinical Evaluation	Radiographic Evaluation	Treatment
				The disadvantages are pin tract infection (may preclude definitive fixation later), loss of knee motion, angular malunion, and femoral shortening and potential risk of infection. **COMPLICATIONS** 1. *Nerve injury*: It is rare, may occur due to traction or compression during surgery. 2. *Vascular injury*: Usually seen in distal one-third fractures due to tethering of femoral artery at adductor hiatus. 3. Compartment syndrome. 4. Heterotopic ossification seen in 25% but is rarely clinically significant. 5. Pudendal nerve injury (10%)—Seen with traction of fracture table. 6. Malunion and rotational malalignment—For determining the latter, use Jeanmart method (angle between a line drawn tangential to the femoral condyles and a line drawn through the axis of the femoral neck. Incidence is higher in proximal fractures and comminuted fractures (30%) than distal fractures. 7. Delayed union—Treatment is dynamization of nail ± bone grafting. 8. Nonunion is seen in <10%, the risk factors are postoperative use of nonsteroidal anti-inflammatory drugs (NSAIDs), smoking, and gap at the fracture site. 9. Infection—incidence <1%, treated by removal of nail and reaming of canal external fixation used if fracture not healed. 10. Weakness of quadriceps and hip abductors. 11. Iatrogenic fracture seen with antegrade nailing if starting point is 6 mm or more anterior to the intramedullary axis (though anterior starting point improves position of screws into femoral head). Overreaming canal by at least 5 mm also can cause fracture. 12. Mechanical axis deviation (MAD): Lengthening along the anatomical axis of the femur leads to lateral MAD. Shortening along the anatomical axis of the femur leads to medial MAD.

Contd...

Contd...

Epidemiology	*Anatomy*	*Clinical Evaluation*	*Radiographic Evaluation*	*Treatment*
				Ipsilateral femoral shaft and neck of femur fractures—these are special problems which can be tackled in one of following ways (in order of preference): Screws for neck + retrograde femur nailing Screws for neck + plating of the femur fracture DHS for femur neck + retrograde nail for shaft (overlapping plate in another plane–less preferred) Recon antegrade nail (femoral head screw option) if fracture undisplaced or anatomically reduced with closed method. Antegrade nailing with screw in miss-a-nail technique.

DISTAL FEMORAL FRACTURE

Epidemiology	*Anatomy*	*Clinical Evaluation*	*Radiographic Evaluation*	*Treatment*
Distal femur fractures account for about 7% of all femur fractures. These fractures often are unstable and comminuted. There is a bimodal distribution of these fractures where first peak is seen in young adolescent age group of 15–24 years and 2nd peak occurs in elderly women older than 65 years. The incidence of open fractures among these fractures is about 5–10%, more in younger population. **MECHANISM OF INJURY** The distal femur fractures usually occur as a result of high-energy trauma such as motor vehicle accidents or fall from height with severe axial load and varus, valgus, or rotational force. The elderly people with osteoporotic bones usually sustain minor slip or fall onto the flexed knee and sustain fractures that are usually spiral. Periprosthetic fractures in the region are getting more common following the increased prevalence of total knee arthroplasty.	The distal femur includes supracondylar and condylar regions in a trapezoidal configuration with base at the joint line. Supracondylar area is the distal 10–15 cm of the femur and is defined as the zone between femoral condyles and the junction of metaphysis with the femoral shaft (just distal to divarization of linea aspera into two popliteal ridges). The medial condyle extends more distally and is more convex than the lateral femoral condyle accounting for the physiological valgus of the femur (6–7°). Axial loading hence results in bending moment at the distal femur. When looked end-on, the anterior surface slopes downward from lateral to medial, the lateral wall inclines 10° and the medial wall inclines 25°. The posterior aspect of the condyles has a sagittal offset posterior to femoral diaphysis cortex. Muscular deforming forces of distal femur causing characteristic displacements, gastrocnemius extends the distal fragment causing posterior displacement and angulation **(Fig. 17)**. Quadriceps and hamstrings exert proximal traction resulting in the shortening of the lower extremity. Adductor magnus pulls the condyle medially producing varus at fracture. **BLOOD SUPPLY** Superior and inferior lateral genicular arteries supply the	The patient typically presents with a history of trauma and unable to ambulate with pain, swelling, and variable deformity in the lower thigh and knee. There is noticeable deformity and painful ROM of the knee. Full trauma survey should be done if there is high energy trauma. Neurovascular status is assessed. Unusual and tense swelling in the popliteal area with sign of pallor and lack of pulse should arise the suspicion of vascular injury. Examination of the ipsilateral hip, knee, leg, and ankle should be done for associated injuries. ***The common associated injuries are:*** • Knee ligament injuries • Meniscal injuries • Vascular injury • Nerve injury • Fracture shaft femur.	Standard AP and lateral views of knee with thigh should be obtained to know the fracture characteristics and the extent of the injury. 45° oblique and traction views may be helpful to further define the fracture morphology and intra-articular extension. CT scan is the preferred modality for evaluating complex intra-articular fractures and osteochondral lesions for preoperative planning. It is common to find Hoffa's fragments in "type C" AO fractures. MRI of the knee may be of value in evaluating associated ligamentous or meniscal injuries to the knee. Arteriography may be indicated in patients with dislocations of knee or suspected vascular injury. Half of the patients with knee dislocation presents with vascular injury. The incidence of vascular injury in isolated supracondylar fractures is 2–3%. **CLASSIFICATIONS** **Descriptive** Supracondylar/intercondylar, ± comminution ± intra-articular extension, open/closed, etc. **AO/OTA Classification (Fig. 18)** AO classify the distal femur fractures into group 33 which is further classified as extra-articular, partial articular, and intra-articular.	**NONOPERATIVE** It is indicated in stable undisplaced or incomplete fracture. The patient with underlying medical conditions precluding surgery or patients unwilling to undergo surgery or non-ambulatory patients are treated with hinged brace with early nonweight bearing mobilization out of the bed. The displaced fractures are treated with above knee cast for 6–12 weeks with acceptance of the residual deformity. Disadvantages are varus and internal rotation deformity, knee stiffness, and prolonged bed rest (and associated complications). **OPERATIVE TREATMENT** The operative treatment is indicated in all patients of displaced distal femur fractures. The goal of the treatment is anatomical restoration of the articular surface, maintenance of the femoral length and rotation, and early rehabilitation of the patient. The goals can be achieved with various osteosynthesis construct choices like use of screws only, plates and screws (varied constructs), intramedullary nail or external fixator. **Screws Only** This may be used for reconstruction of type B3 fractures after anatomical reduction. Else screws are a common adjunctive fixation for stabilizing the condylar fragments.

Contd...

Contd...

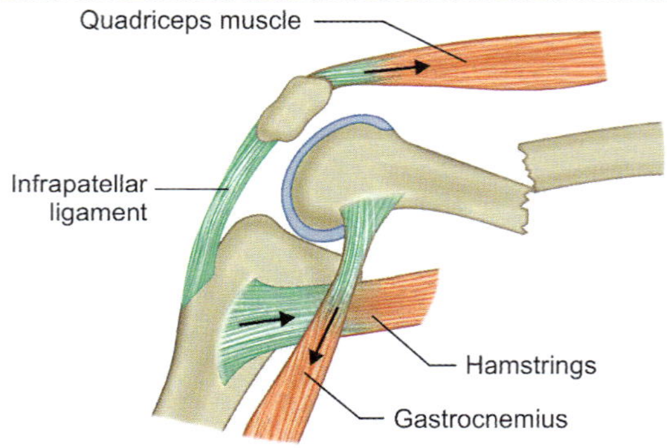

Fig. 17: The displacing forces on distal fragment in distal femoral fractures. The fragment is pulled into extension by gastrocnemius while hamstring tendons pull the tibia proximally along with quadriceps.

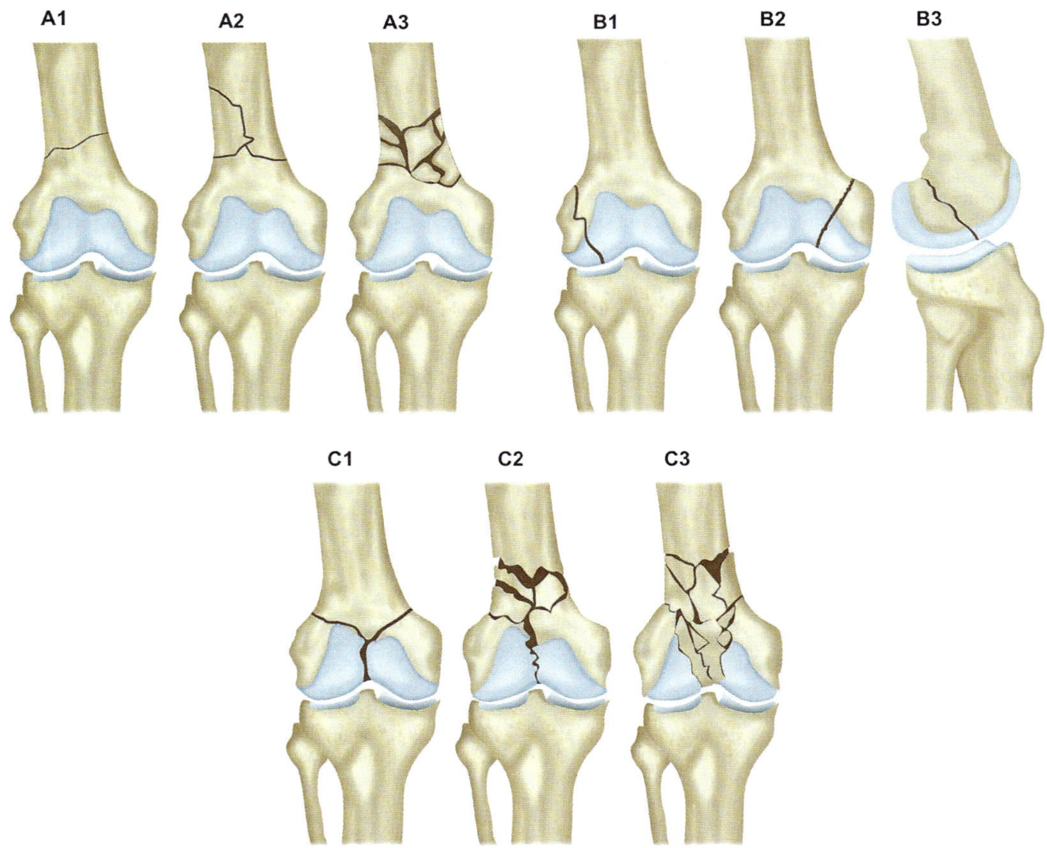

Fig. 18: The AO Foundation/Orthopedic Trauma Association (AO/OTA) classification for fractures of distal femur.

Epidemiology	*Anatomy*	*Clinical Evaluation*	*Radiographic Evaluation*	*Treatment*
	lateral femoral condyle while the medial femoral condyle is primarily supplied by superior medial genicular artery. The interosseous supply to lateral condyle consists of arcade of vessels with no obvious watershed zone while interosseous supply of medial femoral condyle consists of single nutrient artery with		A. Extra-articular • 33-A1: Simple • 33-A2: Metaphyseal wedge • 33-A3: Metaphyseal complex *Partial articular* • 33-B1: Sagittal fracture of lateral condyle • 33-B2: Sagittal fracture of medial condyle	**Plates and Screw** The condylar blade plate was one of the first devices to gain wide acceptability in treatment of these fractures. The blade plate provides stable fixation but it requires accurate insertion in three planes simultaneously. A minimum of 4 cm of uncomminuted bone in femoral condyles

Contd...

Contd...

Epidemiology	***Anatomy***	***Clinical Evaluation***	***Radiographic Evaluation***	***Treatment***
	wide watershed zone making it susceptible to osteonecrosis.		• 33-B3: Coronal split fracture (Hoffa's fracture) *Intra-articular* • 33-C1: Articular simple, metaphyseal simple • 33-C2: Articular simple, metaphyseal multi-fragmentary • 33-C3: Articular multi-fragmentary. **Neer Classification (Figs. 19A to C)** It classifies the distal femur fractures into three types: 1: Minimal displacement 2: Displaced condyles: A: Medial condyle displacement B: Lateral condyle displacement 3: Concomitant supracondylar and shaft fractures. **Seinsheimer** (1980) classified the fractures of the distal 3.5 inches of the femur into four types: 1. *Type I*: Nondisplaced fractures (<2 mm displacement). 2. *Type II*: Distal metaphyseal fractures (extra-articular). – II-A: 2 part fractures. – II-B: Comminuted fractures 3. *Type III*: Fractures involving the intercondylar notch in which one or both condyles are separate fragments. 4. *Type IV*: Intra-articular fractures. – IV-A: Medial condyle fracture. – IV-B: Lateral condyle fracture. – IV-C: Comminuted fractures. **CLASSIFICATION OF DISTAL FEMUR PERIPROSTHETIC FRACTURES [FOLLOWING TOTAL KNEE ARTHROPLASTY (TKA)]** **Lewis and Rorabeck Classification (Fig. 20)** • *Type I*—undisplaced fracture with fixed prosthesis. • *Type II*: Displaced fracture with fixed prosthesis. • *Type III*: Loose prosthesis, displaced nondisplaced fracture. **Su Classification (Fig. 21)** • *Type I*: Fracture line proximal to femoral prosthesis component (no extension distal to anterior shield). • *Type II*: Fracture starts at the level of prosthesis shield and extends proximal.	above intercondylar notch is necessary for successful fixation and is unsuitable for fractures with articular comminution, especially medial deficiency. Disadvantages are technical difficulty, inadequate fixation in osteoporotic bone, unintentional shortening, malalignment and varus collapse in medial deficiency and refracture after plate removal. *Dynamic condylar screw* This is technically easier to insert than blade plate. It allows freedom in flexion extension plane and it also allows interfragmentary compression at the fracture site. Disadvantages are minimum 4 cm of noncomminuted bone required above intercondylar notch, insertion of lag screw requires removal of large amount of bone which makes revision surgery difficult, poor rotational control than blade plate and device is bulky. The interfragmentary movement on the bones fixed with blade plate is greater than on the bones fixed by DCS when medial defect is present. *Anatomical condylar locking plate* It is indicated in AO type A and C fractures requiring plate osteosynthesis, becoming the modality of choice for fixation of these fractures now-a-days. Extra-articular and intra-articular condylar fractures, buttressing of comminuted distal femoral fractures, periprosthetic fractures, and treatment of distal femoral malunion can all be achieved with it. Fracture reduction before plate application is a prerequisite, reduction should not be attempted through plate. Anterolateral approach is commonly used to expose the fracture while parapatellar approaches may be needed for intra-articular comminution. These plates are fixed angle-locking plates which allows the screws lock to the plate and provide angular stability to the construct. Variable angle locking option is also available to position screw in dense safe bone and for management of periprosthetic fractures. Long elastic construct is recommended for comminuted fractures.

Contd...

Contd...

Epidemiology	Anatomy	Clinical Evaluation	Radiographic Evaluation	Treatment

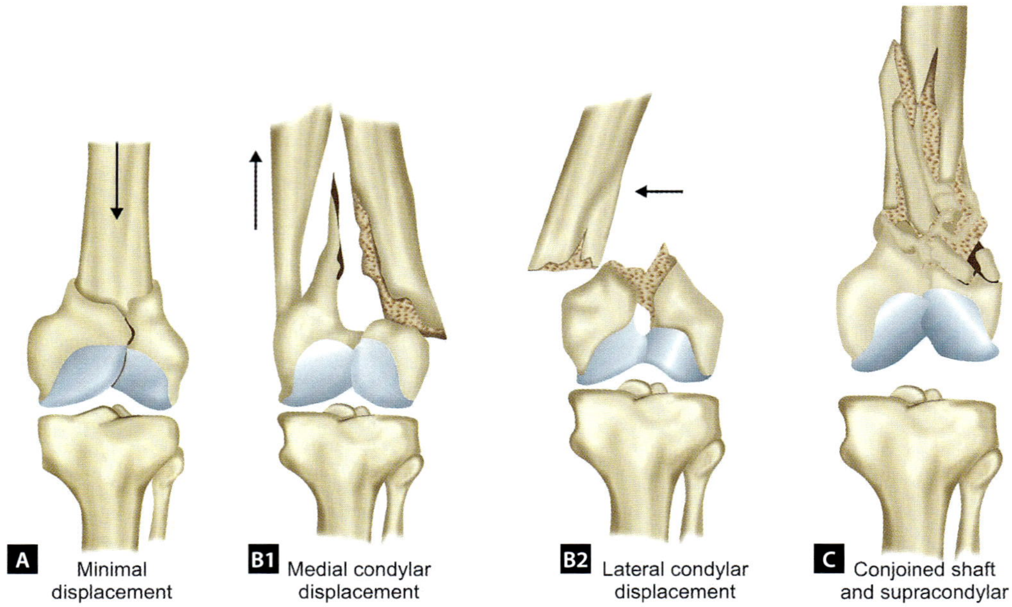

Figs. 19A to C: The Neer classification for distal femur fractures.

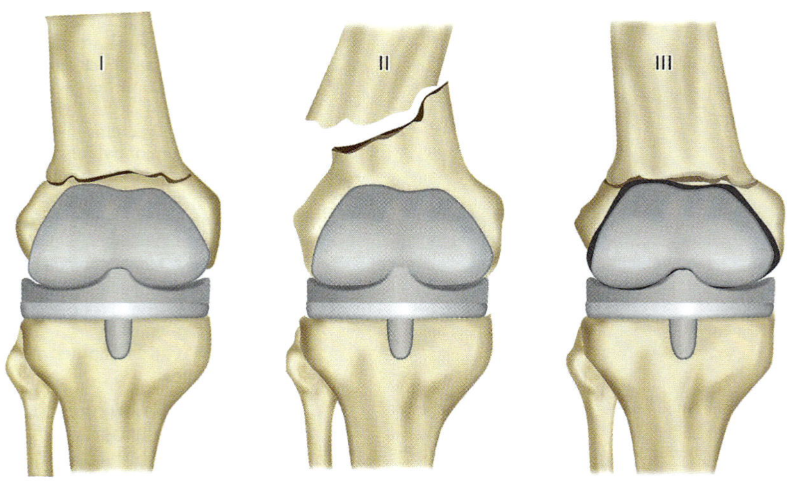

Fig. 20: Lewis and Rorabeck classification for knee periprosthetic femoral fractures.

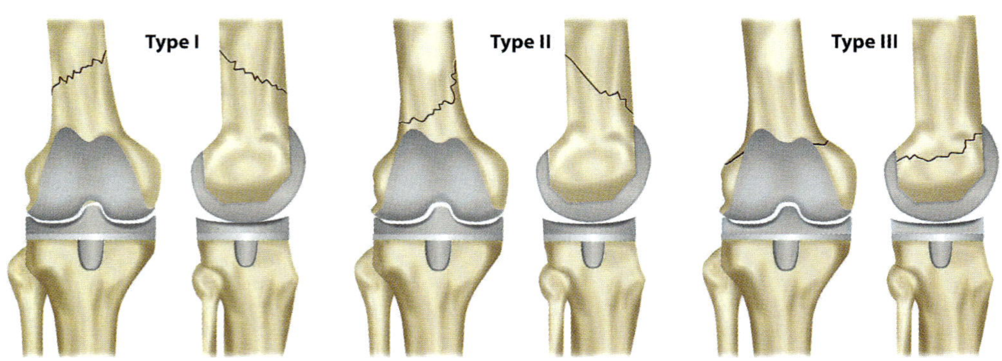

Fig. 21: Su classification for periprosthetic femoral fracture following total knee arthroplasty.

Contd...

Contd...

Epidemiology	Anatomy	Clinical Evaluation	Radiographic Evaluation	Treatment
			• *Type III*: All fracture elements/lines involve the segment below/distal to femoral prosthesis shield.	The advantages of these plates are that it mitigates the varus angulation that occurs with medial femoral defect and it may reduce the need for medial femoral plate. The plate may be also used in a minimally invasive plate osteosynthesis (MIPO) mode of fixation. *Condylar buttress plate* These plates are used for the fractures with articular comminution and in fractures with <4 cm of uncomminuted bone above intercondylar notch. The advantage is that the multiple holes in distal end of plate allow multiple screws into the comminuted fragments. Disadvantage is that the fracture with comminuted medial cortex, segmental bone loss, and very low transcondylar fracture may angulate into varus because of the movement at screw plate interface. The use of additional medial plate, double-plating with bone grafting, and locked dual plating has been recommended for these fractures. *Less invasive stabilization system* (LISS) This system uses locked screws and percutaneous fixation. This system is made of titanium, so it has higher elastic deformation than other system, placing it between rigid fixation and intramedullary nail. LISS relies on the reduction being achieved before implant fixation. It is also called internal-external fixator where placing the locking screw near and far from fracture site provides the greatest stability. The screw fixation is entirely unicortical in this system. **Intramedullary Nailing** The intramedullary nailing has now been increasingly used with improvement in design of condylar blade for osteoporotic bone. It is preferred for type A fractures with intact distal femur to fix with screws. Retrograde nail can also be used for type C1 and C2 fracture fixation. The suggested advantages are more biological fixation because it is a load-sharing implant, greater soft-tissue preservation, and less requirement of bone grafting. The disadvantages are that it provides less rigid fixation,

Contd...

Contd...

Epidemiology	Anatomy	Clinical Evaluation	Radiographic Evaluation	Treatment
				higher chances of implant failure due to toggle of nail. The hardware failure has been reported in 15% of cases and chances are increased if fracture is within 5 cm of subchondral bone. It can be prevented by delaying full weight bearing, driving the nail into subchondral bone, and using appropriate size nail. The nailing can be performed through antegrade or retrograde technique. Retrograde nailing is used most often because it is easier to insert and it allows improved distal fixation. The disadvantages are insult to knee joint and potential of knee sepsis. The retrograde nail should bypass the isthmus proximally. **External Fixation** It can be used as temporary or definitive fixation in severe open distal femoral fractures for later definitive fixation. The fracture with severe intercondylar comminution should be spanned by external fixator. Fractures associated with vascular injury are also treated with external fixator. *Arthroplasty* Distal femoral arthroplasty using a tumor or revision prosthesis is indicated in nonreconstructible fractures with pre-existing arthritic changes or where the osteosynthesis is highly likely to fail. The same may also be preferred in periprosthetic fractures where reconstruction is not possible or original implant has loosened/unstable. *Intramedullary nailing* The intramedullary nailing has now been increasingly used with improvement in design of condylar blade for osteoporotic bone. It is preferred for type A fractures with intact distal femur to fix with screws. Retrograde nail can also be used for type C1 and C2 fracture fixation. The suggested advantages are more biological fixation because it is a load sharing implant, greater soft-tissue preservation and less requirement of bone grafting. The disadvantages are that it provides less rigid fixation, higher chances of implant failure due to toggle of nail. The hardware failure has been reported in 15% of cases

Contd...

Contd...

Epidemiology	Anatomy	Clinical Evaluation	Radiographic Evaluation	Treatment
				and chances are increased if fracture is within 5 cm of subchondral bone. It can be prevented by delaying full weight bearing, driving the nail into subchondral bone, and using appropriate size nail. The nailing can be performed through antegrade or retrograde technique. Retrograde nailing is used most often because it is easier to insert and it allows improved distal fixation. The disadvantages are insult to knee joint and potential of knee sepsis. The retrograde nail should bypass the isthmus proximally. **External Fixation** It can be used as temporary or definitive fixation in severe open distal femoral fractures for later definitive fixation. The fracture with severe intercondylar comminution should be spanned by external fixator. Fractures associated with vascular injury are also treated with external fixator. **Arthroplasty** Distal femoral arthroplasty using a tumor or revision prosthesis is indicated in nonreconstructible fractures with pre-existing arthritic changes or where the osteosynthesis is highly likely to fail. The same may also be preferred in periprosthetic fractures where reconstruction is not possible or original implant has loosened/unstable.

PATELLA FRACTURES

Epidemiology	Anatomy	Clinical Evaluation	Radiographic Evaluation	Treatment
Patella fractures constitute 1% of all skeletal injuries. It mostly occurrs in age group of 20–50 years (males > female in ratio of 2:1). Patella sleeve fractures may be seen in pediatric population (8–10 years old). **MECHANISM OF INJURY** The patella can be fractured by direct or indirect trauma. *Direct trauma*: The direct trauma usually occurs due to fall on the anterior knee or striking of knee against the dashboard of motor vehicle. It may produce incomplete, simple, stellate or comminuted fracture patterns. The medial and lateral retinacular expansions are usually preserved due to which displacement is minimal and active knee extension may	Patella is the largest sesamoid bone of the body and has the thickest coverage of articular cartilage in the body. It is triangular in shape with superior base and inferior apex. It receives the insertion of quadriceps tendon on superior pole and inferior pole gives origin to patellar tendon. The medial and lateral retinacula are longitudinal expansions of extensor mechanism. The upper three-fourths of posterior surface of patella is articular while lower one-fourth is nonarticular. Articular cartilage is up to 1 cm thick. There are seven articular facets (detailed elsewhere). *Blood supply*: The patella is supplied by paired superior	Patient presents with a history of trauma and pain, swelling, tenderness of involved knee with limited or no ambulatory capability. Palpable defect is present if fracture is displaced or have concomitant retinacular tears. Active knee extension (or active straight leg raising test) should be evaluated to determine injury to extensor retinaculum. If it is limited by hemarthrosis, then it can be aided by decompression or pain may be relieved by intra-atricular lidocaine temporarily. Open wound may be the sign of open fracture. Saline load test can be used to ascertain whether open wound communicates with the joint or not.	Patella fractures should be radiographically evaluated with anteroposterior, lateral, and axial view. Transverse fractures are best seen on lateral view while vertical fractures, osteochondral fractures and articular incongruity are best seen on axial view. Computed tomography may be used to delineate the fracture patterns, marginal fractures, and osteochondral fractures. MRI may be indicated in a child who is unable to straighten the leg despite normal X-rays. **CLASSIFICATIONS** **Descriptive**—nondisplaced, displaced, or open closed fractures.	The initial treatment consists of splinting the extremity in extension or slight flexion and applying ice. **NONOPERATIVE TREATMENT** *Bostrom criteria*: Closed fracture with <3 mm of displacement and 2 mm of articular incongruity and intact extensor retinaculum can be treated nonoperatively. It can also be used for vertical fracture patterns. A cylinder cast or knee immobilizer is applied from ankle to groin for 4–6 weeks. Early weight bearing in extension is encouraged and progressed to full weight bearing as tolerated.

Contd...

Contd...

Epidemiology	*Anatomy*	*Clinical Evaluation*	*Radiographic Evaluation*	*Treatment*
be preserved. Abrasion or open injuries over knee are common. *Indirect trauma*: It usually occurs due to violent quadriceps contraction with knee in semi-flexed position. These fractures are transverse and may be associated with tears of medial and lateral retinacular expansions. There is variable degree of displacement due to which active knee extension is lost (extension lag). Most patellar fractures are caused by combination of direct and indirect mechanisms such as fall from height. The most significant effects are loss of continuity of extensor mechanism of knee and potential incongruity of patellofemoral articulations. Iatrogenic fracture patella may be seen in patellar tendon graft harvest for anterior cruciate ligament (ACL) reconstruction or rarely during TKA.	and inferior geniculate arteries which enters from anterior surface and forms the anastomotic patella ring. *Bipartite patella*: It is important to have a knowledge of bipartite patella as they mimic patella fractures and may get misrepresented. They represent unfused or incompletely fused secondary ossification centers of patella. Their incidence is about 1% and is much more common in women than men [approximately 9 times]. It occurs bilaterally in about 50% of cases and may be associated with nail-patella syndrome. Saupe described three types based on location of the fragment **(Fig. 22)**: *Type I*: Inferior pole *Type II*: Lateral margin *Type III*: Superolateral pole. They can be radiologically differentiated from fractures by their location, rounded borders, and presence on other knee also. As such they are incidental and in uncommon cases they may become painful following repetitive activities.	There may be associated injuries to pelvis, hip, thigh, legs, and ankle should be ruled out.	The patella fractures can also be classified on the basis of fracture patterns **(Fig. 23)** as undisplaced, transverse, lower or upper pole, stellate (multifragmentary undisplaced), comminuted displaced, vertical and osteochondral fracture. **AO/OTA** place patella fractures as group 34 which further divides into extra-articular, partial articular, and intra-articular **(Fig. 24)**. *A. Extra-articular* • 34-A1: Avulsion • 34-A2: Isolated body *B. Partial articular* • 34-B1.1: Vertical, lateral (noncomminuted) • 34-B1.2: Vertical, lateral (comminuted) • 34-B2.1: Vertical, medial (noncomminuted) • 34-B2.2: Vertical, medial (comminuted)	**OPERATIVE TREATMENT** Fractures with >3 mm displacement and 2 mm of articular incongruity, fractures associated with retinacular tears and open fractures are best treated operatively. The goal is restoration of articular incongruity and repair of extensor mechanism. There are different methods of treatment like tension band wiring, circlage wiring, screw fixation, partial patellectomy, and total patellectomy. **Wiring Techniques** These are used most often for transverse fracture. They can also be used for comminuted fracture if it is converted to transverse fracture by lag screw. The technique converts tensile forces into articular compressive forces.

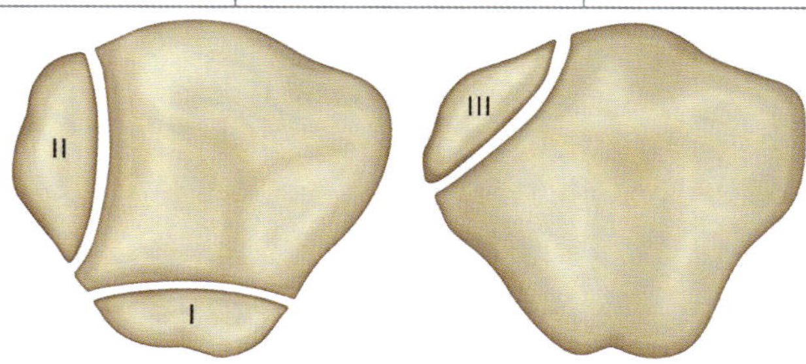

Fig. 22: The three types of bipartite patella based on location of the fragment.

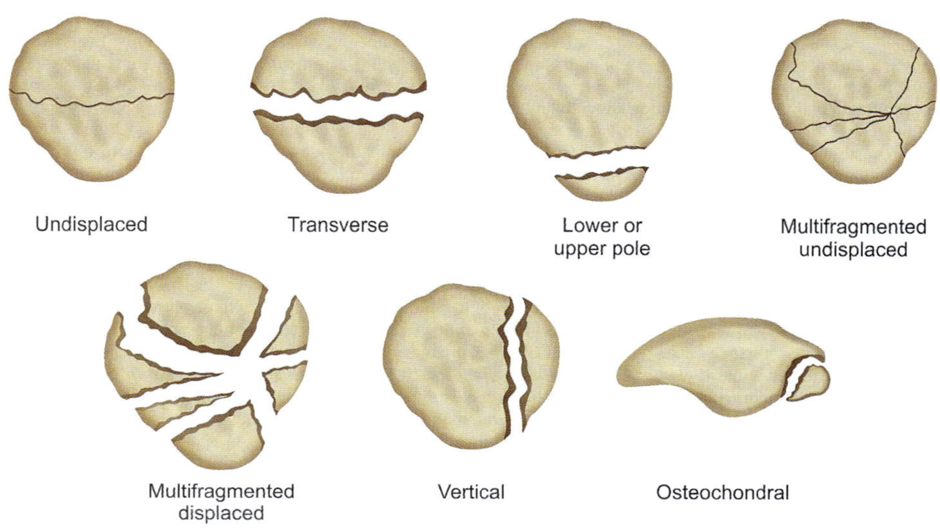

Fig. 23: The different patterns of patella fracture.

Contd...

Contd...

Epidemiology	***Anatomy***	***Clinical Evaluation***	***Radiographic Evaluation***	***Treatment***
			C. Complete articular • 34-C1.1/2: Transverse (middle/upper) • 34-C1.3: Transverse (lower) • 34-C2.1/2/3: Transverse plus second fragment • 34- C3.1/2/3: Complex pattern	The different options are tension band wiring, Magnusson wiring and Lotke anterior band wiring. Wiring through two cannulated longitudinal screws (Berg technique) has been found to be mechanically superior. Martin described a circumferential wire loop technique in which loop of stainless steel wire is threaded through soft tissue around patella and can be done percutaneously also. Schauwecker described a technique in which comminuted fracture is stabilized by screws and converted into bifragment fracture and then tension band wiring is done. Stainless steel wires are used most often but braided polyester and braided cable have also been used. Arthroscopic assisted percutaneous screw fixation has been described for displaced transverse fracture. **Plate Fixation** This has been found to be mechanically superior to tension wiring technique but not gained popularity due to implant prominence issues. Low-profile titanium mesh may be used as for maxillofacial surgery and has the advantage of multiple screw placement option and low profile preventing implant impingement. Now low-profile patella mesh plates are available that can be used to reconstruct comminuted fractures. **External Fixation** It has no universal acceptance and is not cosmetic also. I find its application only to gradually bring the fragments together in a patella nonunion. **Partial Patellectomy** It is indicated when there is comminuted fracture of superior or inferior pole of patella along with large normal patellar fragment. The comminuted fragment is hence removed and retained tendon is approximated with large nonabsorbable suture to the large fragment. The tendon is reattached as close to articular surface as possible. Perry also described a technique of partial patellectomy with figure of eight cable.

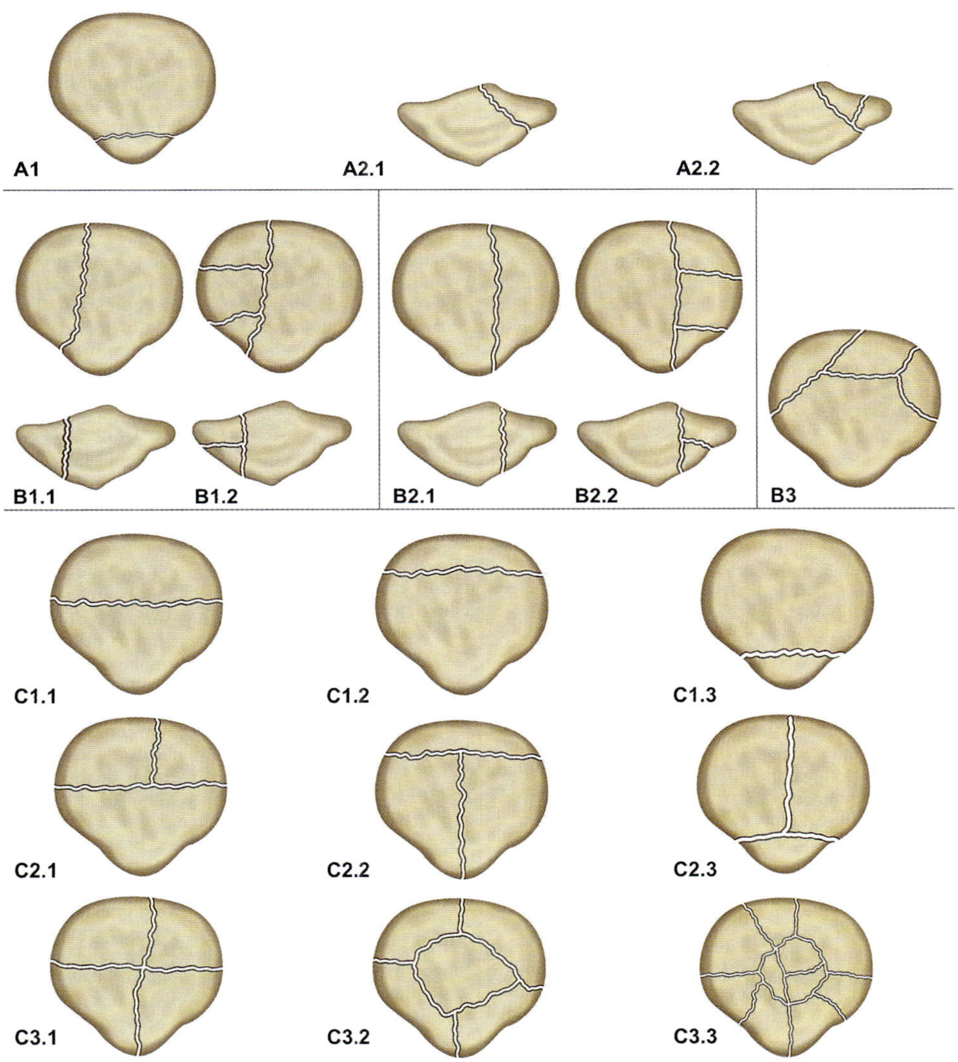

Fig. 24: The AO/OTA classification of patellar fractures.

Contd...

Contd...

Epidemiology	Anatomy	Clinical Evaluation	Radiographic Evaluation	Treatment
				Total Patellectomy It is indicated in fractures where severe comminution leaves no sizeable fragments that can be reconstructed/salvaged. **COMPLICATIONS** Postoperative infection, fixation failure, refracture (1–5%), nonunion (2%), osteonecrosis of proximal fragment. Post-traumatic osteoarthritis is present in >50% of patient in long-term studies, loss of knee motion, painful retained hardware, extensor lag, and patellar instability.

TIBIAL PLATEAU FRACTURES

Epidemiology	Anatomy	Clinical Evaluation	Radiographic Evaluation	Treatment
Tibial plateau fractures constitute 1% of all fractures and >50% of patients who sustain these fractures are aged 50 years or older. There is bimodal distribution with younger males in 40s affected by high-energy trauma while elderly females affected in 70s due to falls. There is high incidence of these fractures in females probably due to increased prevalence of osteoporosis. Lateral tibial plateau fractures are most common in 55–70% of cases while medial plateau fractures occur in 10–25% patients. Bicondylar fractures occur in 10–30% of the patients. Open fractures are seen in 1–3% of the patients. **MECHANISM OF INJURY** The fractures of tibial plateau usually occur due to valgus force with axial loading in majority and varus force in some. Motor vehicles accidents or bumper strike account for majority of these fractures in young and elderly patients with osteopenia suffer from these fractures after simple fall. Young adults with strong bone typically develop split fractures and associated ligamentous injury while older patients with osteopenia sustain split depression and pure depression fractures and lower rates of ligamentous injuries. Bicondylar fractures result from severe axial load in fully extended knee. Medial plateau fractures are associated with higher energy injury and are commonly associated with soft-tissue injuries such as	The knee is a complex joint where increased mobility is seen at the cost of stability. The tibial plateau is composed of articular surface of medial and lateral tibial plateau. The medial plateau is larger and is concave in both sagittal and coronal planes. Lateral tibial plateau is placed above medial plateau and is convex in both planes. It has 10° posteroinferior slope. Intercondylar eminence separates the two plateaus and is nonarticular. It provides attachment to cruciate ligaments. Menisci are present on both the plateaus. Medial articular surface and its condyle is stronger than lateral due to which fractures of lateral condyle are common. Also being convex the articulation with convex femoral condyle produces higher forces per unit area resulting in increased propensity to fracture. The medial tibial (concave) and medial femoral condyle (convex) are more congruent so force per unit area is dissipated on a larger surface giving some protection from fractures. The last reason for higher lateral condyle fractures is the normal knee joint physiological valgus alignment, so more compressive forces during acute trauma in a nonphysiological setting are passed through the same, despite 60% physiological load being transmitted through medial condyle. There is a revised three column concept **(Fig. 25)** of proximal tibia for management of the fractures. The tibial plateau is	Patients usually present with the history of trauma and painful, swollen knee with inability to bear weight. Soft tissue should be evaluated to rule out compartment syndrome especially in bicondylar fractures and if high-energy mechanism is involved. Neurovascular examination is also essential in high-energy trauma. Dislocation relocation injuries common in medial plateau fractures are associated with high risk of peroneal and popliteal injuries. Ligaments of knee should be checked and lateral collateral ligament injury is associated with high chances of neurovascular injury. Gentle stress testing can be performed with leg in extension to evaluate the ligamentous stability. **ASSOCIATED INJURY** Soft-tissue injury occurs in about 90% of patients. Articular depression > 6 mm and/or articular widening > 5 mm are associated with the existence of lateral meniscus, lateral collateral ligament (LCL) or posterior cruciate ligament injuries. Meniscal injuries occur in 67% of plateau fractures while 96% of cruciate and 85% of medial collateral ligament injuries occur in fracture dislocation patterns. Meniscal tears are commonly seen usually with >10 mm articular depression. Lateral meniscal tear is more common than medial and is usually associated with Schatzker type II fracture pattern while	AP, lateral, and oblique views should be obtained to evaluate these fractures. 40° oblique view in internal rotation (lateral plateau) and external rotation (medial plateau) should be used to assess these individual plateau fractures. Caudally tilted plateau view by 10–15° can be used to assess the articular step off and better visualizes tibial plateaus. Stress views can be used to detect the collateral ligaments injuries. Computed tomography is used for the assessment of the degree and size of depressed articular fragments as well as for preoperative planning. MRI is useful to evaluate the injuries to ligaments. **CLASSIFICATIONS** **Schatzker Classification (Fig. 26)** It only considers AP view to classify the fractures. It also helps to guide the fracture treatment but emerging concepts of posterolateral and posteromedial fragments is not addressed. • *Type 1:* Split fracture of lateral tibial plateau. • *Type 2:* Split depression fracture of lateral plateau. • *Type 3:* Pure central depression. • *Type 4:* Medial condyle fracture. • *Type 5:* Bicondylar fracture in which metaphysis and diaphysis retain continuity. • *Type 6:* Plateau fracture with the dissociation of metaphysis and diaphysis. **Hohl and Moore Tibial Plateau Fracture Classification** This classification actually	Goals of treatment are restoration of axial alignment, articular congruity, joint stability, and functional movements. Limb alignment and knee stability are most crucial, whereas non-anatomical reduction may be less important regarding functional results. The factors influencing treatment are degree of displacement and joint depression along with extent of soft-tissue injury. Two stage management is recommended for complex fractures and those with associated significant soft-tissue injury. Joint spanning fixator maintains the fragments and alignment by ligamentotaxis. Take good pinsite care as there is evidence for increased incidence of infection on conversion to definitive fixation. In general, ***nonoperative treatment*** may be advised for nonambulatory patients, surgically unfit patients and those with minimally displaced (<5 mm condylar widening) or minimally depressed (≤3 mm) fractures. If the depression is <4 mm, nonoperative treatment with a hinged knee brace and delayed weight bearing is instituted. Weight bearing should be delayed until fracture healing is evident generally 8–10 weeks. If the depression is 4–8 mm, then treatment depends upon patient's age and activity levels. In elderly and low demand patients, nonoperative treatment is recommended. Depression >8 mm is treated with operative

Contd...

Contd...

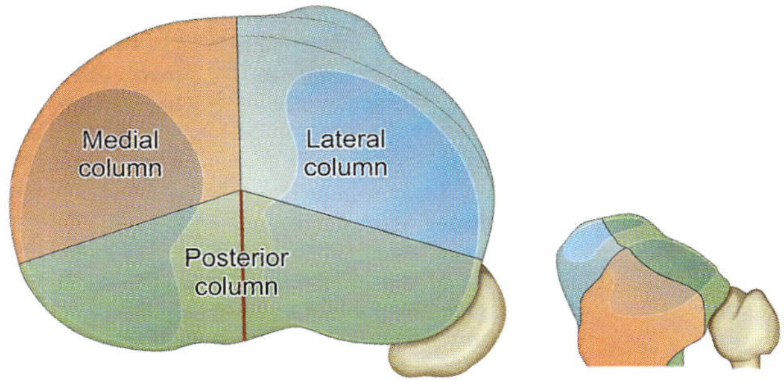

Fig. 25: The revised column concept of tibial plateau based on identification of fracture patterns outside the Schatzker classification and displacement pattern in comminuted fractures to guide fixation.

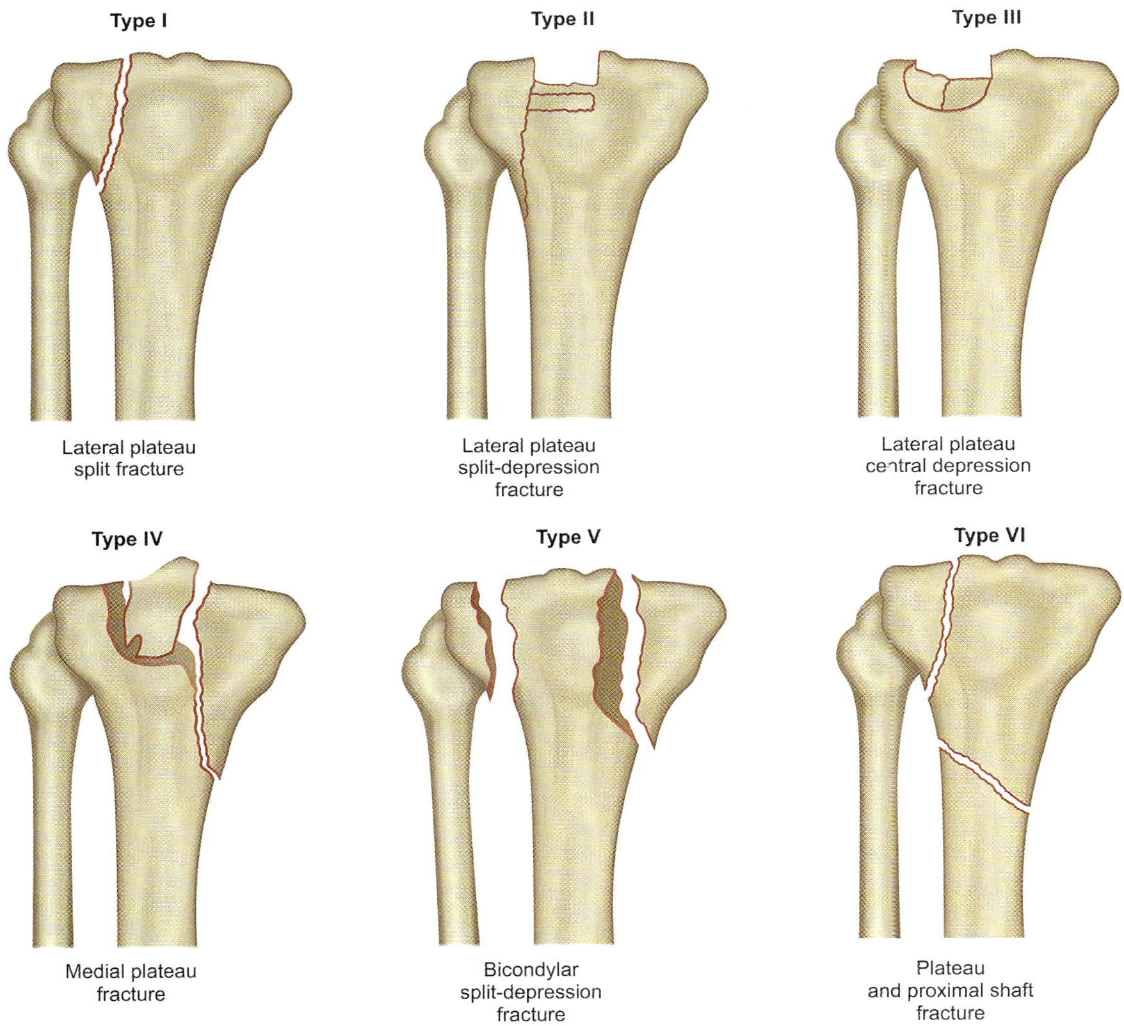

Fig. 26: The Schatzker classification of tibial plateau fractures.

Epidemiology	***Anatomy***	***Clinical Evaluation***	***Radiographic Evaluation***	***Treatment***
disruption of lateral collateral ligament, lesions of peroneal nerve, and damage to popliteal vessels. The fracture may also occur in association with TKA as a periprosthetic fracture.	divided into lateral column, medial column, and posterior column. The division is primarily based on observed fracture patterns and their mechanism of injury. The lateral column gives way in	medial meniscal tear is most commonly associated with Schatzker IV fractures. Arterial injuries are seen mostly with type IV or type VI injuries (but must be suspected in others also). These frequently	supplements to include fractures that are not covered in Schatzker classification and for fractures associated with knee instability or fracture-dislocations.	reduction of step-off. Other ***operative indications*** are: 1. Varus or valgus instability of >10° with knee flexed <20° 2. Open fractures 3. Associated compartment syndrome 4. Associated vascular injury

Contd...

Contd...

Epidemiology	Anatomy	Clinical Evaluation	Radiographic Evaluation	Treatment
	valgus + extension force, medial column fractures under a varus + extension force while the posterior column fractures in flexion. These columns need to be separately addressed for optimal osteosynthesis and outcome and can be individually buttressed.	involve traction induced intimal injuries presenting as thrombosis, rarely they present as transaction injuries secondary to laceration or avulsion. *Complex knee trauma:* These are injuries associated with significant damage to two or more of the following—soft-tissue envelope of knee, ligamentous stabilizers, meniscii and bony structures of the distal femur and proximal tibia. Presence of blisters are an important indication for impending/existing ischemia but do not necessarily indicate compartment syndrome. Usually the extremity is rested in a frame, cryotherapy with generous monitoring for signs of compartment syndrome and if compartment pressures are raised then management of the same takes priority. Hemorrhagic blisters (blood-filled blisters) are associated with higher degree of ischemia and muscle necrosis than clear blisters indication more severe injury so one must take caution.	• *Type 1*: Coronal split fracture (37%) in which fracture involves medial side and has fracture line running at 45° to the medial plateau in an oblique- coronal view. • *Type 2:* Entire condyle fracture may involve medial or lateral plateau. • *Type 3*: Rim avulsion fracture. • *Type 4*: Rim compression fracture. • *Type 5*: Four-part fracture. **AO Classification** It classifies the fracture into group 41: *A. Extra-articular* • 41-A1: Avulsion • 41-A2: Metaphyseal simple • 41-A3: Metaphyseal multi-fragmentary *B. Partial articular (≡ Schatzker i, ii, iii, iv)* • 41-B1: Pure split • 41-B2: Pure depression • 41-B3: Split depression *C. Complete articular (≡ Schatzker v, vi)* • 41-C1: Articular simple, metaphyseal simple • 41-C2: Articular simple, metaphyseal multifragmentary • 41-C3: Articular multifragmentary **COLUMN CONCEPT** for classification of tibial plateau fractures. "Column" involvement means breach in the cortex of the respective column. *"Zero column":* Pure articular depression. *"One-column" fracture:* Split and split depression types. Newly described posterior shear fractures. *"Two-column" fractures:* Anterolateral fractures with posterolateral articular depression and cortical breach. Anteromedial fragment + separate posteromedial fragment (type IV Schatzker). *"Three-column" fractures:* At least one independent articular fragment in each column—the type V and VI Schatzker fractures. Separate posterolateral fragment is commonly seen in complex fractures and usually inadequately addressed. **FOR PERIPROSTHETIC FRACTURES** **Lewis and Rorabeck Classification** is commonly	5. Metaphyseal-diaphyseal translation > 1 cm 6. Angular deformity of >10° in coronal or sagittal plane Operative treatment of plateau (simplified) can be described on the basis of Schatzker classification. • *Type 1:* These fractures can be fixed with two transverse cancellous screws. • *Type 2*: This fracture should be treated with open reduction, elevation of depressed plateau, bone grafting, fixation of fracture with buttress plating, and cancellous screw. • *Type 3*: In this fracture, articular fragment should be elevated, bone grafted, and lateral cortex is supported with the buttress plate. • *Type 4:* These fractures should be treated by open reduction and fixation with medial buttress plate and cancellous screw. • *Type 5:* Bicondylar fractures can be fixed with buttress plate and cancellous screw(s). The more displaced and comminuted condyle should be stabilized with buttress plate while less involved condyle is stabilized with cancellous screw. Small antiglide plate can also be used for less involved condyle. • *Type 6:* These fractures are usually comminuted and associated with swelling of the involved area. Hybrid fixator can be used if there is compartment syndrome or vascular injury and definitive management done later. Buttress plate and cancellous screw can also be used early if the soft tissue and fracture patterns allow. Usually bicondylar fracture fixation is done with a posteromedial buttress plate and lateral locked plate construct. Joint surface is restored with direct or indirect reduction. Posterolateral fixation may be added/done (three column fixation) using prone/supine posterolateral approach through fibular head osteotomy; if this region is not adequately captured in the two-column fixation and comprises large enough articular fragment that is compromising stability of osteosynthesis.

Contd...

Contd...

Epidemiology	*Anatomy*	*Clinical Evaluation*	*Radiographic Evaluation*	*Treatment*
			followed. However, Felix proposed a classification **(Fig. 27)** specifically for the proximal tibial periprosthetic fractures: • Type I—fracture tibial plateau with involvement of prosthesis implant interface • Type II—fracture of meta-diaphyseal transition • Type III—fracture distal to tibial component • Type IV—fracture of tibial tuberosity Subtypes—A: Stable prosthesis; B: Loose prosthesis; and C: Intraoperative fracture.	Arthroscopic assisted reduction can also be done but beware of creating a compartment syndrome if surgery is prolonged. Metaphyseal void is filled with autogenous or combined synthetic/autogenic bone graft. *Open fracture management:* It is better to put an external fixator if soft-tissue coverage is not possible immediately and let the soft-tissue edema settle with wound stabilization before definitive fixation. Both spanning and nonspanning fixator constructs can be used. Some simpler fractures may be amenable to external fixation and limited internal fixation where articular fragments could be reduced percutaneously. Lag screws are placed some 15 mm from the joint line. Use of a ring fixator is possibly better in this scenario as the wires are in tension and chances of pin-tract infection is much less. Fractures with impending compartment syndrome need to be managed on the lines of compartment syndrome. External fixator is the workhorse while ring-fixators also do well in the setting. If blisters are present but no

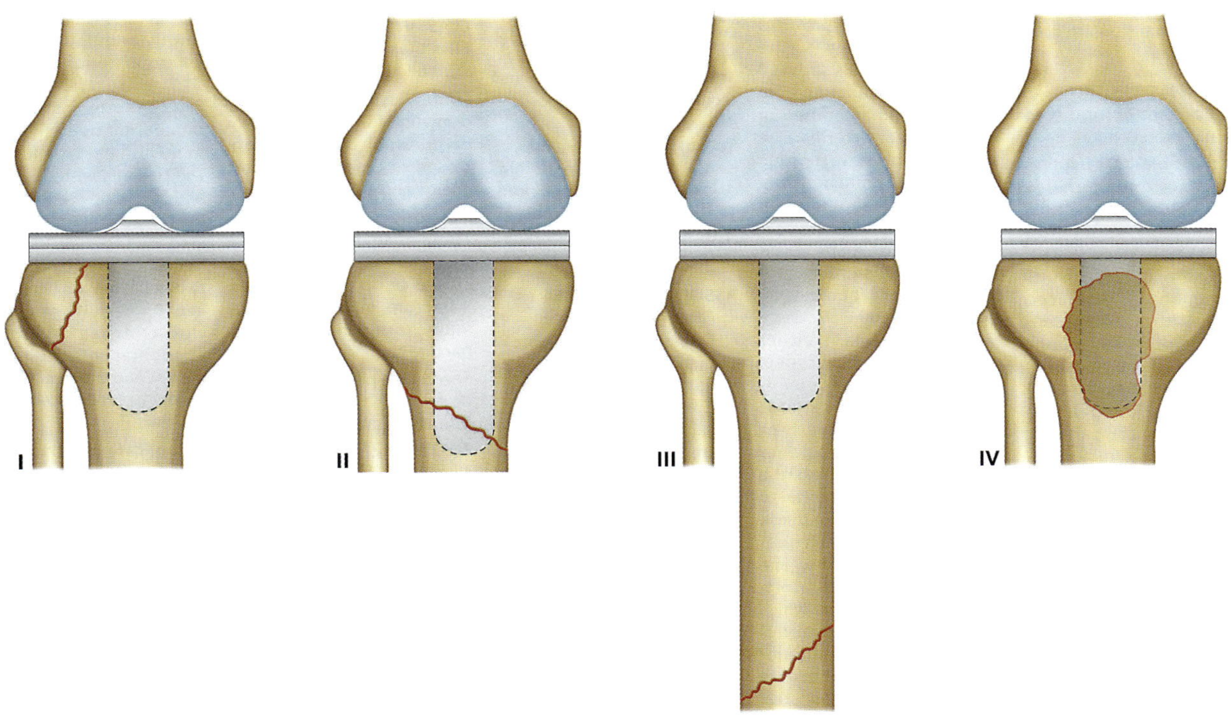

Fig. 27: Felix classification for tibial periprosthetic fractures following total knee arthroplasty.

Contd...

Contd...

Epidemiology	*Anatomy*	*Clinical Evaluation*	*Radiographic Evaluation*	*Treatment*
				evidence of compartment syndrome usually the definitive fixation is delayed for 7 days and more, but it is an individual call to treatment. Blood-filled blisters are associated with a worse outcome if operated early. **COMPLICATIONS** • Arthrofibrosis • Infection • Compartment syndrome • Malunion or nonunion • Post-traumatic osteoarthritis • Peroneal nerve injury • Popliteal vessel injury • Avascular necrosis of small articular fragment.

TIBIAL SHAFT FRACTURE

Epidemiology	*Anatomy*	*Clinical Evaluation*	*Radiographic Evaluation*	*Treatment*
Fractures of tibia and fibula are the most common long bone fractures (4% of all fractures seen). There are average 26 tibial diaphyseal fractures per 100,000 population. It is more common in adult males in second and third decade with an incidence of 109 per 100,000 population, about 5% of these fractures are segmental. In females, it occurs in slightly older age group. It is also the most common diaphyseal fracture which goes into nonunion. **MECHANISM OF INJURY** These fractures occur due to direct and indirect trauma. *Direct trauma:* Direct injury is usually due to high-energy motor vehicle accident, penetrating gun-shot injury, fall from height or jumps. This type of injury results in comminuted, displaced fractures with extensive soft-tissue compromise (± bone loss) and open wounds (Associated fibula fracture is at the same level). There are also high chances of compartment syndrome in these fractures. *Indirect trauma:* Twisting with foot fixed (torsional injury) and fall from low heights are the causes of these fractures. These fractures are usually spiral, nondisplaced with minimal comminution, and little soft-tissue damage. The associated fibula fracture is at a different level. *Stress fractures:* These fractures occur in long distance runners,	Tibia is long tubular bone with triangular cross section. It has subcutaneous anteromedial border. It is bounded by four fascial compartments which are extremely important in traumatic situation as internal bleeding in any can lead to compartment syndrome. **BLOOD SUPPLY** Tibia is supplied from periosteal vessels in four segments—the proximal and distal one-fifth and proximal and distal diaphysis. The proximal one-fifth is supplied by recurrent branches from tibialis anterior and posterior and genicular arteries. The proximal diaphysis is supplied by periosteal branches from tibialis anterior and posterior arteries. The distal diaphysis is supplied exclusively by tibialis anterior by a semicircular disposition of blood vessels meeting anteromedially. Distal one-fifth of tibia is either supplied through peroneal vessels or tibialis anterior or both via anastomosis around the ankle. The nutrient artery arises from posterior tibial artery that enters the posterolateral cortex distal to soleal line in the middle thirds. In intramedullary canal, it gives off three ascending and one descending branch which form endosteal vascular tree which anastomose with the periosteal vessels arising from anterior tibial artery. The distal third of tibia is supplied by periosteal anastomoses around the ankle with branches entering the	The patients present with history of trauma with pain, swelling, and deformity of the injured leg. The neurovascular status should be evaluated. Integrity of posterior tibial and dorsalis pedis artery with common peroneal nerve and tibial nerve should be checked and documented. Note for development of blisters indicating some degree of ischemia, and hemorrhagic blisters fare poorer. Open wounds should be thoroughly evaluated and classified (Oestern and Tscherne or Gustilo-Anderson system). Soft-tissue integrity and evidence of compartment syndrome should be checked. These fractures are associated with high incidence of knee ligamentous injuries. **ASSOCIATED INJURIES** • Fibular fracture • Extension into tibial plateau or plafond • Posterior malleolar fracture • Compartment syndrome (tibial shaft fractures are the most common cause of compartment syndrome of leg) • Knee ligamentous injury • Vascular injury—tibialis anterior/posterior. *Soft-tissue injury:* The soft-tissue injury may be classified by Oestern and Tscherne classification: • *Grade 0:* Injuries from indirect forces with negligible soft-tissue damage.	AP and lateral views of entire leg with visualization of knee and ankle should be obtained. Oblique views may be helpful to further characterize the fracture pattern. CT scan are generally not necessary but may be obtained if there is suspicion of articular extension. Technetium bone scanning and MRI may be useful in diagnosing stress fractures. **CLASSIFICATIONS** **Ellis Classification** of tibial shaft fracture: *Mild*: Displacement ≤50% diameter of shaft, no fragment or minimal comminution, closed or grade I open, low energy and helical fracture. *Moderate*: Deviation of 51–100% of shaft diameter, up to 1 fragment comminution, closed or up to open grade II fracture, moderate energy injury, transverse or oblique fracture line. *Severe*: Displacement 100% or more, ≥2 fragment comminution, any open grade, high-energy trauma, transverse or fragmented fracture. **AO Classification** AO classify the tibia fractures as 42 into simple (A), wedge (B) and complex (C) fractures *Simple fractures:* • 42-A1: Spiral • 42-A2: Oblique • 42-A3: Transverse *Wedge fractures* • 42-B1: Spiral wedge • 42-B2: Bending wedge • 42-B3: Fragmented wedge	The treatment of tibial shaft fractures continue to be refined. In the past, nonoperative treatment was used for closed, stable, isolated, and minimally displaced fractures caused by low-energy trauma and operative treatment for high-energy trauma having comminuted, displaced and unstable fractures. ***Trafton Recommendations:*** Trafton has suggested that the fractures with <5° of varus-valgus angulation, <10° of anteroposterior angulation, <10° of rotation and <15 mm of shortening should be treated nonoperatively, add to it Ellis mild type fractures. The patients with this criteria and stable, low-energy tibial fractures should be treated in long leg cast in 5–10° of knee flexion followed by conversion to patellar tendon bearing cast in 6–8 weeks. Weight bearing with crutches is permitted as soon as tolerated by the patient and progression to full weight bearing on seeing signs of union. **Complications of nonoperative cast management:** • Ankle stiffness (20%) • Angular deformity (10–55%) • Shortening of 1–1.5 cm (5–27%) • Loss of reduction (2.4–9.3%) **OPERATIVE TREATMENT** Nicoll indications of operative treatment: • Open fractures requiring complicated plastic surgery

Contd...

Contd...

Epidemiology	*Anatomy*	*Clinical Evaluation*	*Radiographic Evaluation*	*Treatment*
military recruits, ballet dancers, and sports persons. These fractures occur at metaphyseal diaphyseal junction in military recruits and middle third in ballet dancers. These fractures are insidious in onset and associated with sclerosis at the fracture site.	tibia through ligamentous attachments. When there is fracture of tibia, there is disruption of nutrient artery and the periosteal blood supply becomes dominant source of blood supply.	• *Grade I:* Superficial contusion/abrasion, simple fractures. • *Grade II:* Deep abrasions, muscle/skin contusion, direct trauma, impending compartment syndrome. • *Grade III:* Excessive skin contusion, crushed skin or destruction of muscle, subcutaneous degloving, acute compartment syndrome, and rupture of major blood vessel or nerve.	*Complex fractures* • 42-C1: Spiral • 42-C2: Segmental • 42-C3: Irregular **Gustil O Anderson Classification of Open Tibial Shaft Fracture** • *Type 1:* Open fractures have a clean wound < 1 cm long. • *Type 2:* Laceration is > 1 cm long (mild to moderate periosteal stripping) but is without extensive soft-tissue damage, skin flaps, or avulsions • *Type 3A:* Open fractures with extensive soft tissue lacerations (>5 cm) or flaps but maintain adequate soft-tissue coverage of bone or they result from high-energy trauma regardless of the size of wound. • *Type 3B:* Open fractures have extensive soft-tissue loss with periosteal stripping and bone exposure and usually are massively contaminated. Flap is required due to inadequate soft-tissue coverage (STSG does not count). • *Type 3C:* Open fractures with arterial injury that requires repair regardless of the size of soft-tissue wound. Severely comminuted fractures, segmental fractures, contaminated barnyard injuries, close range shotgun/high velocity gunshot injuries, and open fractures presenting over 24 hours from injury have all been included in type III injuries later.	• Floating knee injuries • Paraplegia with sensory loss • Segmental fracture with displaced central fragment • Gaps resulting from missing bone fragment. Bone and Johnson expanded the indication with internal fixation for bilateral tibial fractures, fractures with severe closed soft-tissue injury, fractures associated with compartment syndrome, vascular injury, and poly trauma. **Intramedullary Nailing** Intramedullary nailing is currently the preferred procedure for most type 1, 2, and 3A open and closed tibial shaft fractures. *Contraindications*: It is not recommended in patients with open physis, anatomical deformity, burns, wound over entry portal, and type 3C open fractures. *Advantages:* • It preserves the periosteal blood supply and soft-tissue sleeve around the fracture site. • It allows early motion of the adjacent joint. • The ability to lock the nail helps to control the length, rotation, and alignment in unstable fractures and fractures located in the proximal or distal third of tibial shaft. Reamed nailing is possibly better for closed fractures (SPRINT trial). Unreamed nailing is used in open tibial fractures. The proponents of this theory suggested that the insertion of reamed nail disturbs the cortical blood flow to greater extent than the unreamed, increasing the susceptibility to infection. Unreamed nailing results in shorter operative time, less blood loss, and less disruption of endosteal blood supply. Though SPRINT trial showed better rates of consolidation with undreamed nail the issue is not settled. Time limit for "definitively" managing the open injuries within 6 hours is debated and possibly makes no difference in terms of infection rates ("limit" of 6 hours originated from study on Guinea pigs by Friedrich (1898) where bacterial colonies replicated rapidly within 6 hours limiting

Contd...

Contd...

Epidemiology	Anatomy	Clinical Evaluation	Radiographic Evaluation	Treatment
				surgical success). What is agreed upon is that early debridement is a must and should be done as soon as possible and administering antibiotics at the earliest is the best preventive measure for infection. Infection rate is proportional to the severity of injury. With regard to wound closure the early dictum of delayed closure for grade III injuries is questioned as there is poor correlation between contaminating germs and ultimate infection so infection appears to be caused by hospital germs and this means early closure after debridement has a role. The concept is being supported by recent studies performing early would/flap closure even in grade III injuries if the wound bed is not grossly contaminated or stable after debridement. **Plating** Plate fixation is recommended for fractures extending into the metaphysis, periprosthetic diaphyseal fractures below the knee arthoplasty, patient in whom nailing cannot be done like narrow medullary canal/canal block and tibial shaft fractures associated with displaced intra-articular fractures. *Advantages*: It provides stable fixation, allows early motion of knee and ankle and maintains the length and alignment. *Disadvantages*: Excessive soft-tissue stripping which can lead to wound complications and infection. **Lag Screw Fixation** It is used for long oblique and spiral fractures that extend into the metaphysis. This technique is usually supplemented with external fixation or neutralization plate to stabilize the large butterfly fragment to one of the main fragments. **External Fixation** It is one of the most versatile tools in the management of open fractures type 3B and 3C, fractures complicated by the compartment syndrome, burns, vascular injury, and polytrauma patients especially with head injury. *Advantages*: It provides stable fixation, preserves soft tissue and bone vascularity, leaves wound accessible to further

Contd...

Contd...

Epidemiology	*Anatomy*	*Clinical Evaluation*	*Radiographic Evaluation*	*Treatment*
				care and causes little blood loss. It can also provide axial compression with weight bearing that stimulates fracture healing. *Disadvantages*: Pin site infection, pin loosening, malunion, joint stiffness, patient acceptance, delayed union, etc. **COMPLICATIONS** Malunion, nonunion, infection, stiffness of adjacent joint, anterior knee pain, hardware failure, neurovascular injury, compartment syndrome, fat embolism, reflex sympathetic dystrophy, claw toe deformity, peroneal nerve injury [minimally invasive plate osteosynthesis (MPPO) less invasive stablization system (LISS)].

TIBIAL PLAFOND (PILON) FRACTURE

Epidemiology	*Anatomy*	*Clinical Evaluation*	*Radiographic Evaluation*	*Treatment*
Tibial plafond fractures occur in 5–7% of all lower limb fractures. There is bimodal distribution of these fractures with peak incidence at 25 and 50 years of age. There is male predominance (57–65%) for these fractures. Women of older age with pre-existing osteoporosis sustain low-energy fractures while high-energy injuries occur in younger male patients. Open wounds are reported in approximately 20% patients. **MECHANISM OF INJURY** Tibial pilon fractures encompass a spectrum of injury from low-energy rotational trauma to high-energy axial compression force. **Low-energy Trauma** It usually occurs in sporting accidents or twisting injury in older patients. Mechanism is primarily torsion with varus or valgus stress. This results in a large fragment with minimal articular comminution. There is usually an associated short oblique or transverse fracture of fibula. **High-energy Trauma** It usually occurs in motor vehicle accidents or fall from height. There is axial force through the talus into the tibial plafond causing impaction of articular surfaces and a burst type fracture. This usually results in comminuted fracture	The term "tibial pilon" was first used by Destot who likened the pilon to pestle. The tibial pilon comprises anatomically the distal end of tibia including the articular surface. Proximally, it extends to approximately 8–10 cm from articular surface, where the triangular section of tibial diaphysis with its anterior crest changes direction forming metaphysis. The distal tibial articular surface is referred to as plafond which together with medial and lateral malleolus forms the mortise. The plafond expands into a quadrilateral surface and pyramid-shaped medial malleolus. Anatomically, three main regions are recognized that usually separate in high-energy injuries as separate fragments—the medial malleolus, posterolateral/Volkmann fragment and the anterolateral/Chaput fragment **(Fig. 28)**. The articular surface is concave in AP plane but convex in the lateral plane. It is wider anteriorly to allow congruence with Wedge-shaped talus. This provides for intrinsic stability in weight bearing. **BLOOD SUPPLY** Distal tibial metaphysis has extraosseous periosteal blood supply by the branches of anterior and posterior tibial arteries. Anterior tibial artery gives off several medial and lateral arterial	Patient is nonambulatory following trauma with pain, swelling, and gross deformity around the ankle and distal leg. Patients involved in high energy should be treated according to Advanced Trauma Life Support (ATLS) guidelines, full trauma survey, and secondary survey is needed. High-energy trauma is obvious on inspection while torsional mechanism has less obvious clinical signs. Extreme care should be taken in clinical examination to look for vascular or nerve injury and compartment syndrome requiring intervention. Note should also be made of skin integrity, necrosis, and fracture blisters. Soft-tissue damage should be assessed as significant damage to soft tissue occurs in these fractures. Poorly planned surgery or surgical incision would result in inadequate healing with wound necrosis and skin slough if not treated appropriately. Patient characteristics such as smoking, alcoholism, peripheral vascular disease or diabetes should also be noted as they affect treatment outcome. **ASSOCIATED INJURIES** There may be associated fractures of fibula (75%), calcaneum, talus, tibial plateau, pelvis, and vertebral fractures.	Standard radiographs include AP, lateral, and mortise view (leg internally rotated 15–20° so that X-ray is perpendicular to intermalleolar line) should be obtained. Computed tomography scans with 3D reconstruction are extremely useful to accurately define the fracture lines, size, and articular displacement of fracture fragment. They are also useful for operative planning of surgical incisions. Radiograph of contralateral side may also be obtained for preoperative planning. **CLASSIFICATIONS** **AO/OTA Classification** AO classify the distal tibia fractures as 43 into extra-articular (A), partial articular (B) and intra-articular (C) fractures *A. Extra-articular* • 43-A1: Metaphyseal simple • 43-A2: Metaphyseal wedge • 43-A3: Metaphyseal complex *B. Partial articular* • 43-B1: Pure split • 43-B2: Split depression • 43-B3: Multifragmentary depression *C. Intra-articular* • 43-C1: Articular simple, metaphyseal simple • 43-C2: Articular simple, metaphyseal multifragmentary • 43-C 3: Articular multifragmentary	The treatment of these fractures is very complex and depends upon multiple factors such as patient age and functional status, soft-tissue damage, degree of comminution, and articular involvement. The ultimate aim is to regain function and prevent development of arthritis which is seriously disabling. **NONOPERATIVE TREATMENT** It is indicated in undisplaced fracture (Ruedi type 1) and AO type A1, B1, C1, and severely comorbid patient. Patient is put on long leg cast for 6–8 weeks followed by fracture brace and ROM exercises. **OPERATIVE TREATMENT** It is indicated in all displaced fractures of tibial plafond. The goals are to restore anatomical articular surface, mechanical alignment, maintaining joint stability, achieving fracture union ultimately regaining function and pain-free weight bearing while avoiding the complications. **Open Reduction and Plate Fixation** Ruedi and Allgower used this technique which follows the AO principles of anatomical reduction and stable fixation. In this technique, fibula is stabilized first and then the articular surface of tibia is stabilized with K-wire.

Contd...

Contd...

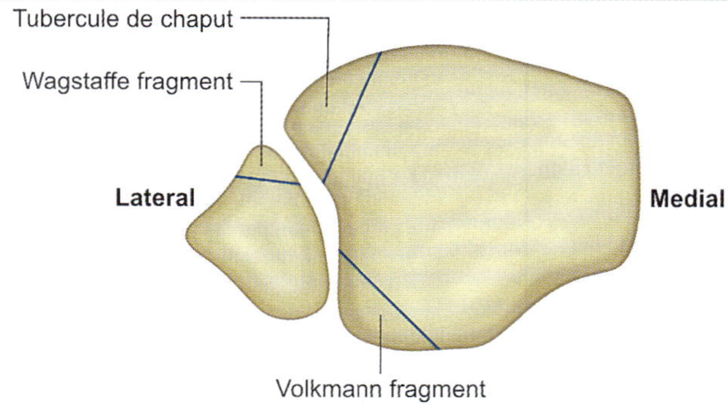

Fig. 28: The tibial pilon (Volkmann and Chaput) fragments as viewed from below.

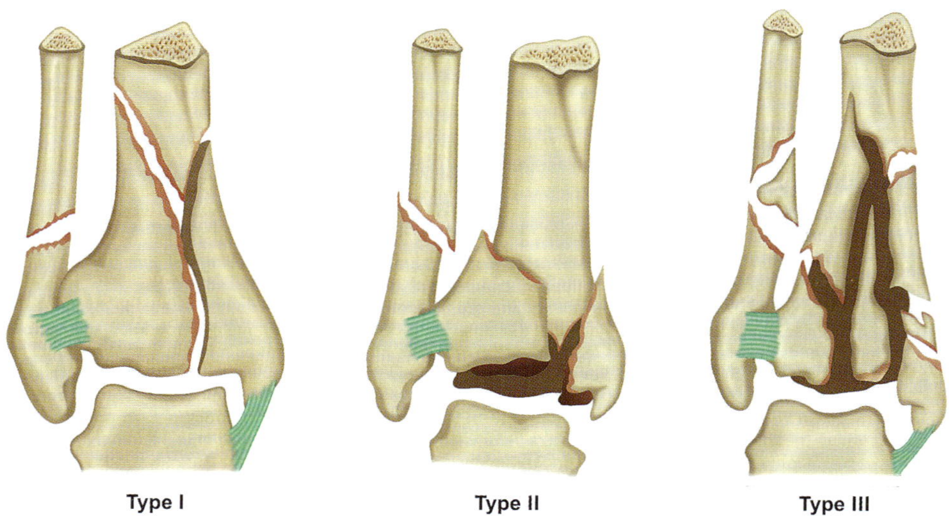

Fig. 29: The Ruedi-Allgower classification for tibial pilon fractures.

Epidemiology	*Anatomy*	*Clinical Evaluation*	*Radiographic Evaluation*	*Treatment*
of distal tibia with significant articular comminution. Plantar flexion or dorsiflexion of the ankle at the time of injury results in posterior or anterior plafond injury respectively. **Combined Compression and Shear Injury** The resultant vector of two forces determines the fracture pattern. *Pronation-dorsiflexion injury*: It produces oblique medial malleolus fracture, large anterior lip fracture, supra-articular fibular fracture, and posterior lip fracture. *Giachino fracture*: This fracture occurs due to external rotation, dorsiflexion, and abduction that produce oblique medial malleolar fracture and anterolateral tibial plafond fracture. There is little articular comminution and can be treated like ankle fractures.	branches that pass onto the surface of anterior distal tibial metaphysis. Posterior tibial artery supplies the posterior and medial surface of distal tibial metaphysis. It anastomoses with anterior tibial artery on medial surface. This extraosseous network is at risk during the injury process and also during the plate application.		**Ruedi-Allgower Classification (Fig. 29)** This classification is based on the severity of comminution and degree of articular displacement. It categorizes the plafond fracture into three types. 1. *Type I:* Nondisplaced cleavage fractures. 2. *Type II:* Cleavage type fracture with displacement of articular surface but minimal comminution. 3. *Type III:* Displaced fractures with significant articular comminution and metaphyseal impaction.	The metaphyseal defect is then filled with bone graft and fracture is stabilized with medial buttress plate. This technique was more frequently associated with wound breakdown and infection leading to search for other modalities of fixation. The introduction of locked plate osteosynthesis and low profile plates have improved the outcome of ORIF. Medial anatomical plates and anterolateral plates are both available with variable locking options. One should pay attention to the primary displacement pattern evident on CT reconstructions. Medial angulation with comminution of antero-/posterolateral column of tibia needs stabilization of the lateral column by anterolateral plate. Lateral angulation with medial main fragment/comminution needs medial column stabilization. Fibular fixation is an adjunct

Contd...

Contd...

Epidemiology	*Anatomy*	*Clinical Evaluation*	*Radiographic Evaluation*	*Treatment*
				for most of the comminuted fractures. Posterior fragment should also be addressed separately if present making the osteosynthesis bi-column or multicolumn fixation depending on the need assessed in planning (address all three fracture components—medial malleolus, Volkmann, and Chaput fragments). It should be remembered that despite best dissection, due to the traumatic nature of approach the chances of soft-tissue complications are high so definitive fixation can be safely postponed till edema subsides and wrinkles appear on the skin (7–14 days). *Minimally invasive plating technique* This technique is indicated in low-energy fractures with displaced large fragments, little comminution, and no diaphyseal extension. The fracture is reduced by ligamentotaxis and plating performed through limited incisions. **Two-stage Open Reduction and Internal Fixation** Due to complications of skin breakdown, two-stage protocol has been adopted. In first stage, fibular plating may be performed (it has been found that this makes no difference in the ultimate outcome but may induce specific wound complications so may be avoided) and then external fixator is placed, spanning the ankle. Or in emerging evidence just put an external fixator in stage 1. After the soft-tissue conditions improve and swelling decreases, tibial pilon reduction is done and low profile plate is applied. *Advantages:* • Better soft-tissue management and anatomical fibular and distal tibial realignment. • Anatomical reconstruction of articular surface under direct vision in second stage. *Disadvantages* • Need for large soft-tissue dissection initially and • Difficulty in obtaining reduction after 3 weeks. **External Fixation and Limited Internal Fixation** It is indicated in high-energy trauma Allgower type 2

Contd...

Contd...

Epidemiology	Anatomy	Clinical Evaluation	Radiographic Evaluation	Treatment
				fractures. In this technique, limited internal fixation of fibula and distal tibial articular surface is performed and supplemented by external fixator. This has unconfirmed role though sounding good it is actually a half-hearted approach to fracture management. **Spanning External Fixation** It is indicated to stabilize any fracture of distal tibia especially with soft-tissue compromise and fractures with diaphyseal extension. In this technique, two half pins are placed in tibia and one pin each is placed in talus and calcaneum. The fracture is reduced by distraction and ligamentotaxis. *Advantages:* Less soft-tissue dissection and no prominent implant in subcutaneous tissue reduces wound complica tions and infection. *Disadvantages:* Pin tract infection, pin loosening, poor reduction, loss of reduction, and ankle stiffness. **Hybrid External Fixation or Ring Fixator** It is indicated in comminuted fracture of tibial pilon with extensive soft-tissue compromise when no internal fixation can be done. It consists of tensioned wires connected to half pins in tibial diaphysis. The wire helps in the reduction of articular fragments. *Advantages:* It allows movements at ankle and subtalar joint which diminish the chances of ankle stiffness but fragment reduction is worse. External fixation in dynamic mode has been evaluated for definitive management by various studies and results have been variable. Possibly delayed ORIF or a two stage external fixator-ORIF is preferable for management. **Primary Arthrodesis** It is recommended in severely comminuted nonreconstructible fractures or fracture dislocations with complete talar dislocation and severe open injuries with extensive loss of cartilage from tibial and/or talar articular surfaces. **COMPLICATIONS** Soft-tissue necrosis, nonunion, malunion, infection, post-traumatic arthritis, tibial shortening, and ankle stiffness.

ANKLE FRACTURE

Epidemiology

Ankle fractures are common fractures in elderly patients and according to population based studies, its incidence is increasing from last 3–4 decades. The incidence of ankle fractures is approximately 187 per 100,000 population. Most ankle fractures are isolated malleolar fractures with bimalleolar fractures occurring in one-fourth of patients and trimalleolar fractures in 5–10% patients. Ankle fractures occur more commonly in middle age men while in women, it usually occurs after the age of 50 years. Diabetes and obesity are most common associated comorbidities in patients with ankle fractures.

Though ankle fractures are not considered fragility fractures but the highest incidence of these fractures occur in elderly women. Open ankle fractures account for 2% of ankle fractures.

These fractures result from low energy fall, sports injury, and twisting injury to ankle in elderly patients.

MECHANISM OF INJURY

Inversion stress to ankle is the most common cause of ankle fractures. It is because medial malleolus is shorter than lateral malleolus which allows the talus to invert more than evert and the deltoid ligaments stabilizing the ankle are stronger than lateral ligament. As a result, ankle is more stable and resistant to eversion injury than inversion injury. However, when eversion injury occurs, there is significant damage to bony and ligamentous structures. The mechanisms of malleolar fractures are best classified in Lauge–Hansen classification. They attempted to classify the ankle fractures on the basis of mechanism of injury and associated specific fracture pattern based on injury mechanism. It divides the fractures into four categories taking into account the position of foot at the time of injury and the direction of deforming force.

Supination-adduction (Fig. 31)

This occurs in 10– 20% of all malleolar fractures and it is the only pattern associated with medial displacement of talus.

Fracture components:

- Transverse avulsion type fracture of fibula below

Anatomy

Ankle joint is a hinge joint composed of articulation of tibia, fibula, and talus with associated ligamentous structure.

The expanded anteromedial end of tibia is called "medial malleous". Medial malleolus is divided into anterior and posterior colliculus by medial facet of talus. It serves as atachment site for superficial and deep deltoid ligaments.

The expanded distal end of fibula is called lateral malleolus, covered by articular cartilage on its medial aspect extending from level of the plafond distally. It serves as attachment site for the lateral ankle ligaments and syndesmotic ligaments **(Fig. 30)**.

DELTOID LIGAMENT

It provides support to medial side of ankle. It is divided into superficial and deep deltoid ligament.

Superficial ligament is divided into tibionavicular anteriorly, tibiocalcaneal ligament in the middle, and superficial tibiotalar ligament posteriorly.

The deep deltoid ligament are anterior and posterior deep tibiotalar ligament. These attach to undersurface of medial malleolus and body of talus. Both are intra-articular but extra-synovial. Posterior deep tibiotalar ligament is strongest of the all. All these ligaments resist valgus tilting of talus and secondary restraint against anterior translation of talus.

LATERAL COLLATERAL LIGAMENT

The lateral collateral ligament is divided into anterior talofibular, posterior talofibular, and calcaneofibular ligaments. Posterior talofibular ligament is strongest of these ligament. It arises anteriorly from digital fossa of fibula and inserts posteriorly to lateral tubercle of talus.

The lateral ligament resists varus tilting and anterior trans lation of talus.

Bifurcate ligament (calcaneocuboid and calcaneonavicular) is attached to anterior process of calcaneus.

SYNDESMOTIC LIGAMENT

These ligaments/structure reinforce distal tibia and fibula articulation and resist axial, rotational, and translational

Clinical Evaluation

The patient with inability to walk, bear weight on the extremity with pain, swelling, and variable deformity.

Soft-tissue injury should be checked and any evidence of open fractures and blisters should be noted.

The quality of surrounding tissue should also be assessed.

Neurovascular status should be checked and carefully documented.

Squeeze test should be performed to assess possible syndesmotic injury.

Fracture Variants

Maisonneuve fracture: Medial ankle injury with fracture of proximal third of fibula, seen in pronation external rotation type of injury.

Curbstone fracture: Avulsion fracture of posterior tibia by posterior tibiofibular ligament

Lefort-Wagstaffe fracture: Anterior fibular avulsion fracture by anterior tibiofibular ligament.

Tillaux fracture (or a Tillaux-Chaput avulsion fracture)—it is a Salter–Harris type III fracture through the anterolateral aspect of the distal tibial epiphysis. It occurs due to external rotation force.

Radiographic Evaluation

Standard AP, lateral, and mortise view of ankle should be obtained.

In AP view, the Weber-Shenton line should be a smooth curve without disruption (otherwise a fracture/disruption is indicated), a tibiofibular overlap of <10 mm and tibiofibular clear space >5 mm is abnormal and implies syndesmotic injury.

Talar tilt: Difference in the width of medial and lateral aspect of superior joint space of >2 mm indicates medial or lateral disruption.

Lateral View

The dome of talus should be centered under the tibia and congruous with the tibial plafond.

Posterior malleolar and talar avulsion fractures are detected by this view. ATFR (anterior tibiofibular ratio) is the ratio between anterior tibiofibular interval divided by fibular width measured 1 cm above the tibial plafond level may be a better measure of disruption (compare with normal side).

Mortise View

It is taken with the leg in 15° of internal rotation. On a mortise view, the medial joint space should be < 4 mm and the superior joint space should be within 2 mm medially of its width laterally. The parameters are however approximations only as sagittal movement of fibula also indicate T-F disruptions, poorly captured

Treatment

The goal of treatment is restoration of ankle joint congruity and maintenance of fibular length and alignment.

NONOPERATIVE TREATMENT

It is indicated in nondisplaced, stable fracture with intact syndesmosis and displaced fractures in which anatomical reduction of mortise is achieved by closed method.

The patient is put on short leg cast for 4–6 weeks. Serial radiographic evaluation is done to ensure maintenance of reduction and healing. The patient is allowed to bear weight when there are signs of healing.

OPERATIVE TREATMENT

Operative treatment is indicated in patients with displaced fractures.

1. Medial clear space > 4 mm
2. Tibiofibular overlap < 1 cm
3. Tibiofibular clear space > 5 mm
4. Talar tilt > 2 mm
5. Talar shift > 1 mm

Medial Malleolus

Displaced malleolar fractures are treated operatively because persistent displacement shifts the talus into varus. Larger displaced fragments can be fixed with 4 mm cannulated cancellous screw. Smaller fragments can be fixed with tension band wiring or one K-wire and one CCS screw construct. Vertical malleoli fractures are stabilized with two horizontal screws or antiglide plate.

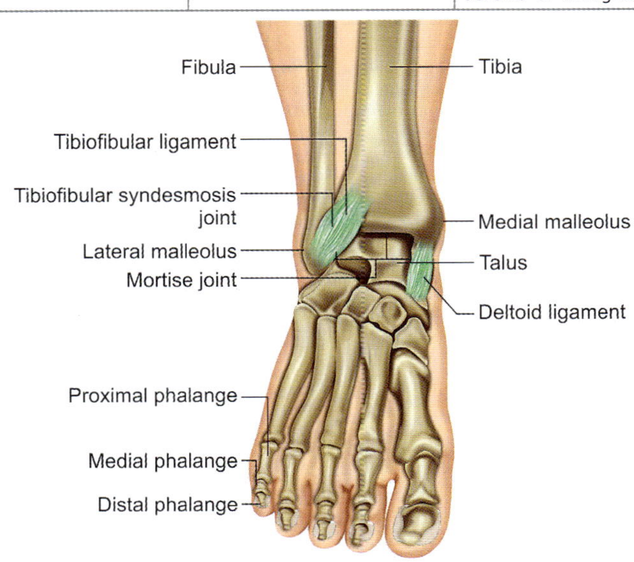

Fig. 30: The ligamentous supports for ankle joint.

Contd...

Contd...

Epidemiology	Anatomy	Clinical Evaluation	Radiographic Evaluation	Treatment
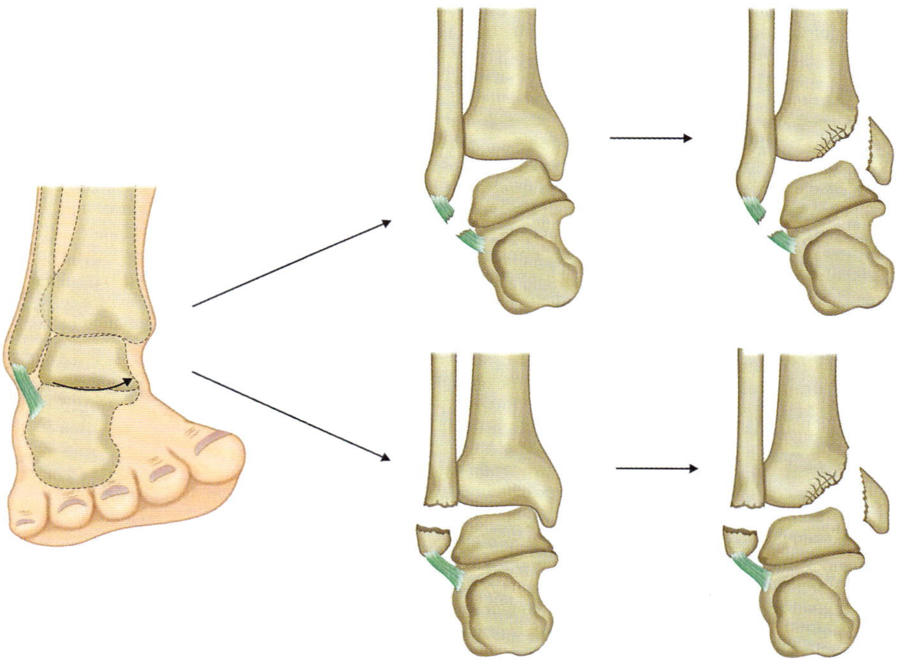 **Fig. 31:** The supination-adduction mechanism of injury. There is initially (I) either a fracture of lateral malleolus distally and/or rupture of calcaneofibular ligament followed by progression to oblique fracture of medial malleolus (II).				
the level of syndesmosis or disruption of lateral collateral ligament. • Vertical medial malleolar fracture **Supination-external Rotation (Fig. 32)** It is the most common injury pattern accounting for 40–75% fracture. There is: • Disruption of anterior tibiofibular ligament • Spiral oblique fracture of fibula which goes from antero-inferior to postero-superior. • Disruption of posterior tibiofibular ligament or fracture of posterior malleolus. • Transverse fracture of medial malleolus or rupture of deltoid ligament. **Pronation-abduction (Fig. 33)** It accounts for 5–20% of malleolar fractures. Injury components: • Transverse fracture of medial malleolus or rupture of deltoid ligament • Rupture of syndesmotic ligaments or avulsion fracture of their insertions • Spiral oblique fracture of fibula above the level of syndesmosis. **Pronation-external Rotation (Fig. 34)** • Transverse fracture of	force to maintain structural integrity of the mortise. There are four components at ankle mortise: 1. Anterior inferior tibiofibular ligament 2. Posterior inferior tibiofibular ligament 3. Transverse tibiofibular ligament 4. Interosseous ligament **BIOMECHANICS OF ANKLE JOINT** The normal range of ankle motion is 30° dorsiflexion and 45° plantarflexion. The axis of ankle flexion runs approximately 20° external rotation as compared to knee axis. Lateral talar shift of 1 mm decreases with decrease in surface contact forces by 40% and 3 mm results in >60% decrease.		by AP projections. With 7 mm anatomic diastasis, lateral malleolus may posteriorly displace 4–5 mm, whereas mortise view shows only 1–2 mm of displacement. Stress view, CT/MRI or arthroscopy better demonstrates this disruption. Medial clear space of >4 mm indicates lateral talar shift. Tibiofibular overlap should be >1 mm Talar shift should be < 1 mm. *Talocrural angle:* The angle formed by intermalleolar line and line parallel to distal tibial articular surface is called talocrural angle. It should be 83(±4) degree. Stress view may be used to identify the suspected ligamentous injuries and are possibly better than mortise view. Computed tomography to delineate the bony anatomy especially in patients with plafond fractures. MRI scan may be used to assess the occult cartilaginous, ligamentous, and tendinous injuries. **CLASSIFICATIONS** **Denis-Weber Classification (Figs. 35A to C)** This classification is based on the location and appearance of fibular fracture.	**Lateral Malleolus** Fibular fracture without medial malleolus are common and these fractures are usually treated nonoperatively unless there is fibular displacement of 2–3 mm. There is lateral displacement of talus. Axial loading of these fractures does not disturb the joint kinematics or cause talar displacement in some biomechanical studies, therefore operative or nonoperative of isolated lateral malleolus fracture does not affect the ultimate outcome. Lateral malleolus is usually stabilized by 3.5 mm one-third semitubular plate, fibular LCP, tension band wiring or single lag screw for smaller fragment. Long intramedullary screw, multiple lag screw also can be used depending upon the fracture pattern. **Bimalleolar Fracture** These fractures are usually displaced fractures. Fracture of both malleoli disrupts the stabilizing structures and alters the tibiotalar contact areas and joint kinematics. These fractures are treated operatively. Most fractures can be stabilized with plating of fibula and CCS screw or tension band wiring of medial malleolus.

Contd...

Contd...

Epidemiology	*Anatomy*	*Clinical Evaluation*	*Radiographic Evaluation*	*Treatment*

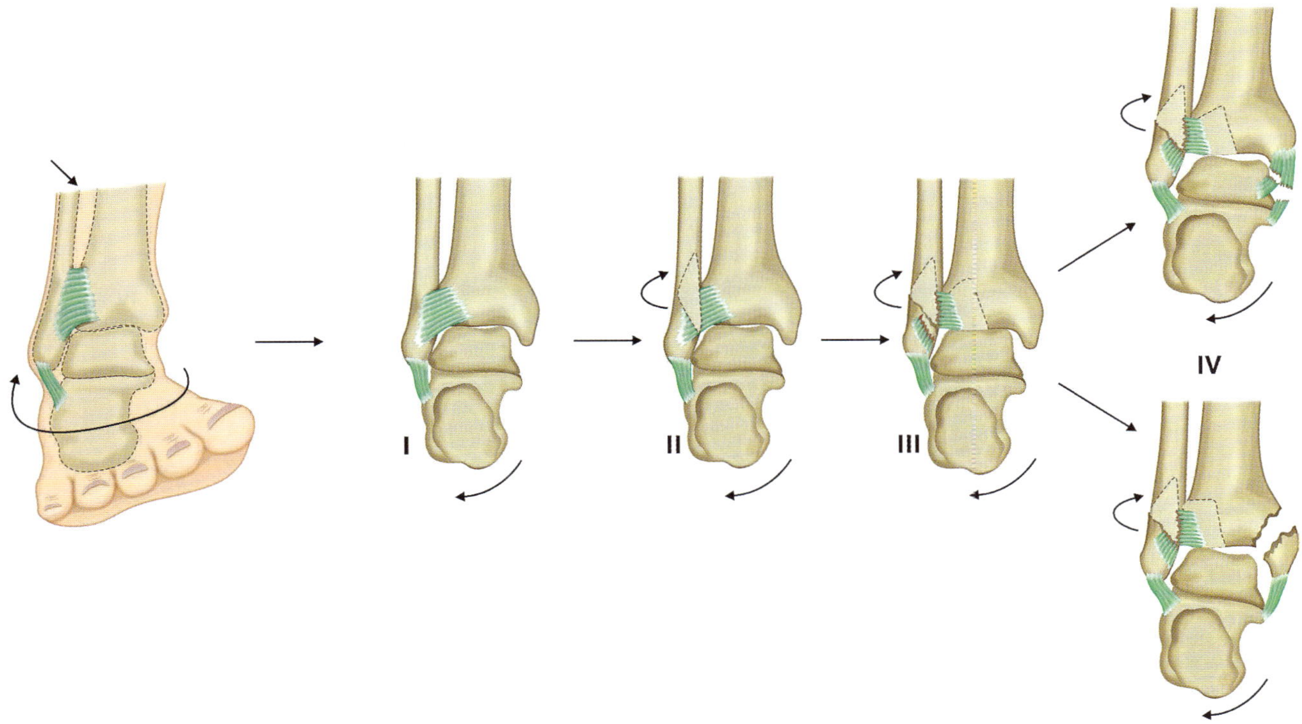

Fig. 32: The supination-external rotation mechanism of ankle injury. In stage I there is either anterior tibiofibular ligament rupture or Chaput fracture (tibia) or Wagstaffe fracture (fibula) that progresses to stage II of spiral oblique leteral malleolus fracture. Continuation of deforming force then produces posterior tibiofibular ligament tear and/or posterior malleolus fracture followed in stage IV by medial malleolus fracture.

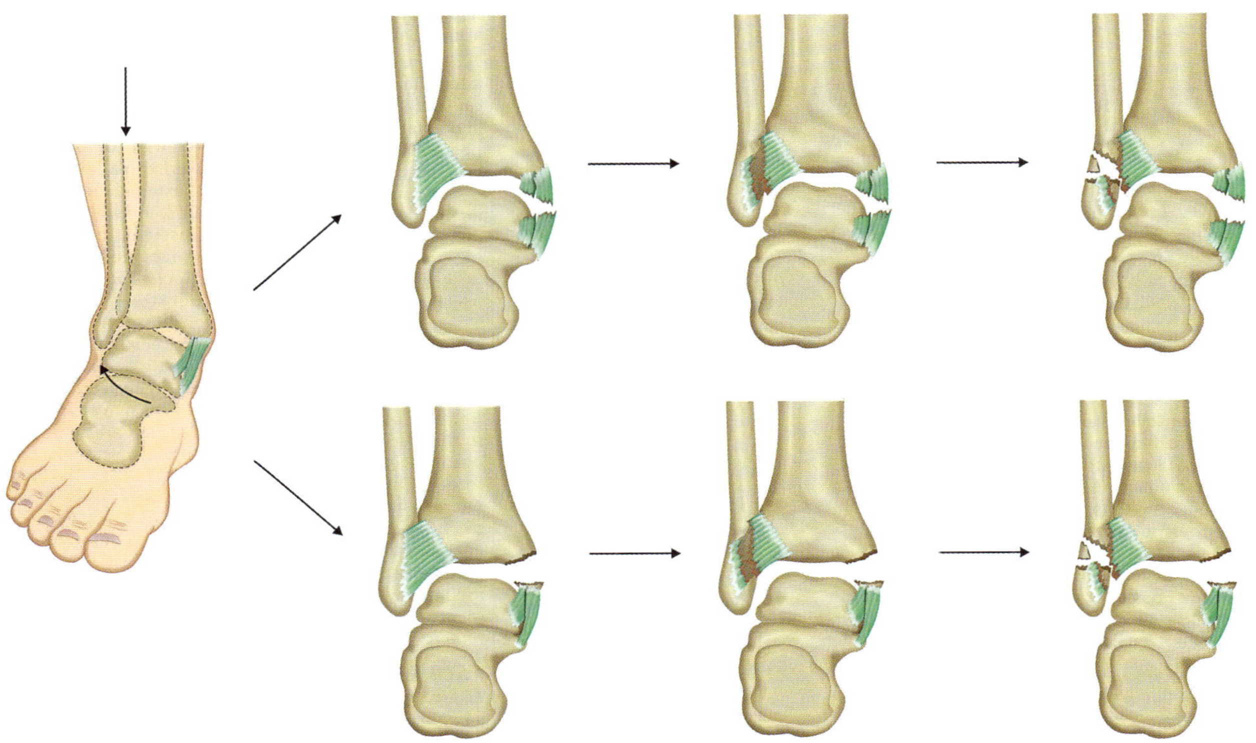

Fig. 33: The pronation-abduction mechanism involves either rupture of deltoid ligament or medial malleolus in stage I followed by posterior and anterior tibiofibular ligament and or Chaput/Wagstaffe fracture in stage II. This is followed by oblique lateral malleolus fracture (III).

Contd...

Contd...

Epidemiology	Anatomy	Clinical Evaluation	Radiographic Evaluation	Treatment

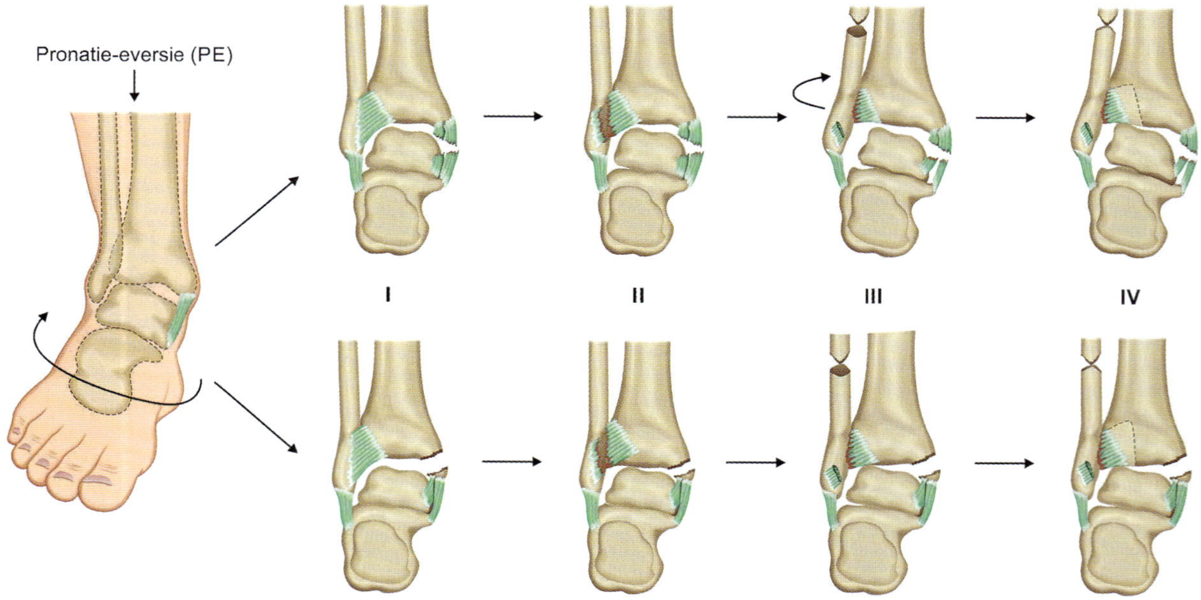

Fig. 34: The pronation-external rotation (eversion) injury mechanism. In stage I there is either deltoid ligament injury or medial malleolus fracture which is followed by injury to anterior tibiofibular ligament injury or Chaput fracture or Wagstaffe fracture. Further progression of injury produces fibular fracture at a higher level or Maisonneuve fracture.

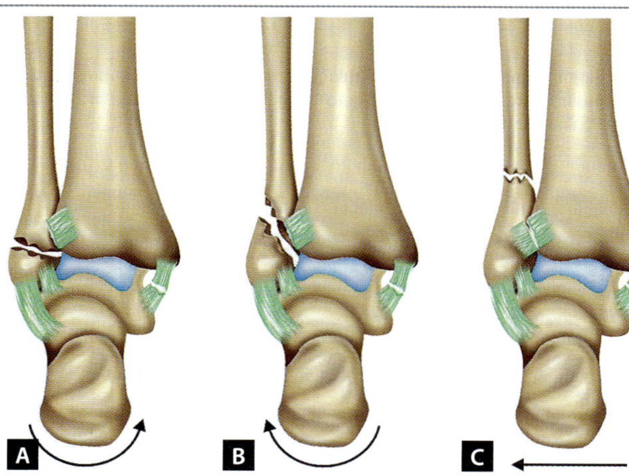

Figs. 35A to C: Denis-Weber system of classification of ankle injuries based on level of fibula fracture.

medial malleolus or disruption of deltoid ligament

- Disruption of anterior tibiofibular ligaments
- Short and oblique fracture of fibula above the level of syndesmosis running from anterosuperior to posteroinferior
- Rupture of posterior tibiofibular ligament or fracture of posterolateral tibia.

Pronation-dorsiflexion

Mechanism of injury has also been described where there is fracture of medial malleolus or deltoid ligament injury followed by anterior

Type A: Fracture of fibula below the level of syndesmosis with transverse fracture of fibula with or without oblique fracture of medial malleolus. It is produced by internal and adduction (Supination-adduction).

Type B: Oblique fracture of lateral malleolus beginning on anteromedial surface and extending proximally to posterolateral aspect. There may be associated rupture of anteroinferior tibiofibular ligament, fracture of medial malleolus or rupture of deltoid ligament. The injury is caused by external rotation of ankle (supination-external rotation).

Type C: The fracture of fibula above the level of syndesmosis which is divided into abduction injuries with oblique fracture of fibula proximal to the disrupted tibiofibular ligament, abduction-external rotation injuries with more proximal fracture of fibula and more extensive disruption of interosseous membrane. There may be associated fracture of medial malleolus, posterior malleolus or deltoid ligament rupture.

AO Classification

AO classify the ankle fracture as 44 which is further subclassified as infrasyndesmotic (A), trans-syndesmotic (B), and suprasyndesmotic (C).

Posterior Malleolus Fracture

Posterior malleolus fracture is usually caused by abduction or external rotation injury. The articular surface of tibia is displaced allowing posterior and lateral displacement and external rotation with supination of foot. It is associated with deltoid ligament rupture and lateral malleolus fracture. When it has three components, it is called trimalleolar fracture. 50° external rotation view (or a CT scan) is used for accurate assessment of the size and displacement of posterior malleolar fragment.

Operative treatment depends upon the size and displacement of the fragment. Fracture with >25–30% of articular surface involvement and >2–3 mm of articular step off or gap are to be treated with anatomical reduction and internal fixation. The fixation is usually achieved with a screw directed from posterior to anterior or CCS screw placed from anterior to posterior. Reduction can also be secured with a posteriorly placed buttress plate (my preference).

Syndesmotic Injury

The syndesmosis injury **(Fig. 36)** is usually caused by the fibular fracture above tibial plafond. Most

Contd...

Contd...

Epidemiology	*Anatomy*	*Clinical Evaluation*	*Radiographic Evaluation*	*Treatment*
tibiofibular ligament injury. Progression of injury leads to transverse fibula fracture above syndesmosis and then distal tibia articular (pilon) fracture.			*Infrasyndesmotic fibula fracture:* *44-A1:* Unifocal (isolated) lateral malleolus fracture or lateral collateral ligament injury *44-A2:* Lateral injury with medial malleolus fracture *44-A3:* Lateral injury with posteromedial fracture *Trans-syndesmotic fibula fracture:* *44-B1:* Lateral malleolus fracture at the level of syndesmosis *44-B2:* Lateral fracture with medial lesion *44-B3:* Lateral fracture with medial lesion and posterolateral tibia fracture *Suprasyndesmotic fibula fracture:* *44-C1:* Simple fibular shaft fracture *44-C2:* Multifragmentary fibular shaft fracture *44-C3:* Proximal fracture of fibula	common mechanism is pronation-external rotation, pronation-abduction or supination-external rotation. These forces cause the talus to abduct in the mortise leading to disruption of syndesmotic ligaments. The syndesmosis can be evaluated by squeeze test (Hopkin's) preoperatively and by external rotation stress test (external rotation/dorsiflexion of the foot with knee and hip flexed to 90°), cotton test (widening of the syndesmosis with lateral pull on the fibula) or the fibula translation (anterior-posterior drawer causes translation of fibula with tibia stabilized) intraoperatively. Anatomical restoration of syndesmosis is important. When medial injury is present, syndesmotic injury extending 4.5 cm above the ankle joint should be reduced. The treatment of injury between 3 and 4.5 cm is controversial and syndesmotic fixation of injury < 3 cm above the plafond is unnecessary. When no medial injury is present, disruption of syndesmosis does not cause ankle instability. Syndesmosis screw is placed 2–3 cm above the joint, parallel to joint surface, and angled 30° anteriorly so that it is perpendicular to tibiofibular joint. Dual screw fixation one within 2 cm from ankle joint and other above is generally recommended. 3.5 or 4.5 mm cortical screw can be used with three or four cortices purchased with foot dorsiflexed. There is controversy regarding the number of cortices to be purchased. There are different opinions regarding the timing of weight bearing and screw removal. Screw should never cause overtightening of the syndesmosis. Some of these complexities are reduced by flexible fixation for syndesmosis. **COMPLICATIONS** Nonunion, malunion, wound problems, infection, post-traumatic arthritis, reflex sympathetic dystrophy, tibiofibular synostosis, loss of fixation, hardware breakage, etc.

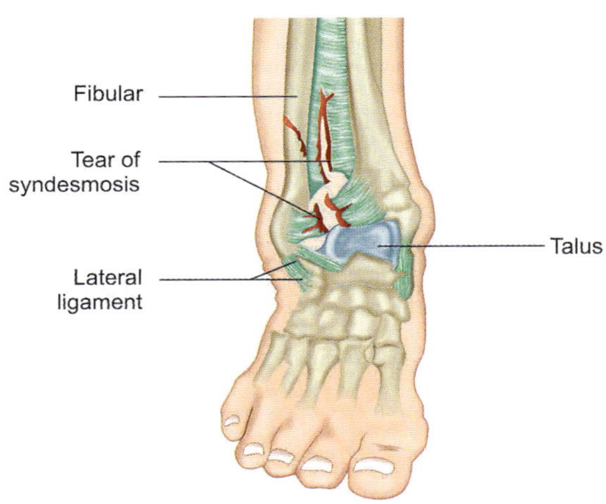

Fig. 36: The injury to syndesmosis is a common accompaniment to ankle injuries and accompanies fibular fracture above the tibial plafond level.

CALCANEUS FRACTURE

Epidemiology	Anatomy	Clinical Evaluation	Radiographic Evaluation	Treatment
Calcaneus is the most frequently fractured tarsal bone accounting for >60% of all tarsal fracture. Calcaneum fractures represent 2% of all fractures in adult. Extra-articular fractures do not involve the posterior facet or subtalar joint. They make up 25–30% of calcaneum fracture. Displaced intra-articular fractures comprise 60–75% of fracture and extra-articular fracture occurs in 30%. Anterior process fractures in 10–15%, tuberosity avulsion injuries in 10% of cases and sustentaculum tali rarely ever fractures as isolated injury. Open fractures are seen in 2–10% cases. The annual incidence is 11.5 per 100,000 population and 2.4 times more common in males than in females. The majority of fractures are sustained in falls from height (6 feet and above). Concomitant injuries to lower limb (13.2%) or spinal injuries (6.3%) are seen. Ninety percent of fractures occur in men between 21 and 45 years of age, majority being industrial workers. **MECHANISM OF INJURY** Twisting forces may be associated with extra-articular calcaneus fracture, especially anterior and medial process fracture. There is increased incidence of tuberosity avulsion fracture in diabetic patients. Anterior process fracture occurs with strong plantar flexion and inversion which tightens the bifurcate and interosseous ligament causing avulsion of bony fragment. Axial loading is the most common mechanism of calcaneus fracture. It occurs	Calcaneus is the largest tarsal bone. It forms the prominence of heel and is roughly cuboidal in shape. It is directed forward, upward, and laterally. It has six surfaces (anterior, posterior, superior, plantar, lateral. and medial surface) and three facets (anterior, middle, and posterior facet). The three facets are located on the anterior half of the superior articular surface that articulates with talus. Posterior facet is the largest and contains the weight bearing surface. The middle facet is located anteromedially on the sustentaculum tali. Sustentaculum tali is the medially oriented shelf like projection of bone. It supports the neck of talus medially and is attached to the talus by interosseous talocalcaneal and deltoid ligament and contains the middle articular facet on its superior aspect. **BLOOD SUPPLY** Calcaneus is supplied by calcaneal branches of deep peroneal and posterior tibial arteries.	The patient with this fracture typically presents with a history of fall or motor vehicle accident with pain, swelling, ecchymosis deformity of heel, and inability to bear weight. **Mondor sign:** Ecchymosis of heel that extends distally to the sole of the foot. It is pathognomonic for calcaneal fracture. Compartment syndrome of the foot is present in 10% of calcaneal fractures and may result in clawing of the lesser toes. Check for the signs of foot compartment syndrome like the paresthesia, pallor, diminished pulses or severe pain with passive flexion of toes. Blister may result from massive swelling usually within first 36 hours after injury. Distal neurovascular status should be checked. Squeeze the heel of patient's foot in the palm of the hand. Pain suggests calcaneal fracture. Open fractures should be thoroughly evaluated. **ASSOCIATED INJURIES** Extension of intra-articular fracture into calcaneocuboid joint. Bilateral calcaneus fractures are present in 5–10% cases. These fractures may be associated with lumbar spine fractures, pelvic fractures, fractures of proximal femur, basilar skull fractures, or tibial plateau fractures.	The standard radiographic evaluation in calcaneal fracture is lateral view of hindfoot, AP, and oblique view of foot, Harris axial view and in some cases Broden's view. Lateral view is used to assess the height loss and rotation of posterior facet. Loss of height is assessed by Bohler angle and Gissane angle **(Fig. 37)**. **Bohler angle:** It is the line drawn from the highest point of anterior process of calcaneus to the highest point of posterior facet and line drawn tangential from posterior facet to superior edge of the tuberosity. Normally, it is 20–40°. This angle decreases in calcaneal fracture suggesting that weight-bearing posterior facet has collapsed shifting body weight anteriorly. **Gissane critical angle:** It is formed by two cortical struts extending laterally, one along the lateral margin of posterior facet and another extending anterior to the beak of calcaneus. Normal angle is 105–135° and is visualized beneath the lateral process of talus. Increase in this angle suggests the collapse of posterior facet. AP and oblique views of foot assess the anterior process and calcaneocuboid joint. Harris axial view estimates the varus position of tuberosity and the width of the heel. It is obtained by maximally dorsiflexing the foot and angling the beam at 45° cephalad. *Broden view*: It is obtained by keeping the foot in neutral flexion and leg internally rotated 15–20°. The X-ray beam is then centered over the lateral malleolus and four	The goals of treatment of these fractures are restoration of congruency of posterior facet, restoration of calcaneus height and width, realignment of tuberosity into valgus position, decompression of the peroneal tendon. Extra-articular fractures are usually treated closed with closed reduction and casting, bulky Jones compression dressing and essex Lopresti pin fixation. Indications for nonoperative treatment: • Nondisplaced or minimally displaced intra- and extra-articular fractures • Sanders type 1 and type 4 intra-articular fractures • Patient older than 50–55 years with severe osteopenia, limited ambulatory abilities, and significant medical comorbidities • Patients with diabetes or insensate limb due to any cause. Anterior process fracture is commonly missed and may be confused with lateral ankle sprain (obtain lateral oblique view). They are classified into type 1—non-displaced fracture, type 2—displaced avulsion fracture, and type 3—Larger fragment involving calcaneocuboid joint. They may be managed by POP cast immobilization if nondisplaced or operated for fracture with >25% displacement of calcaneocuboid articulation on CT scan. ORIF with mini-fragment screws is commonly preferred. Excision of fragment isdone in delayed symptomatic nonunion. Calcaneal tuberosity fracture usually results from avulsion from violent pull of gastrosoleus

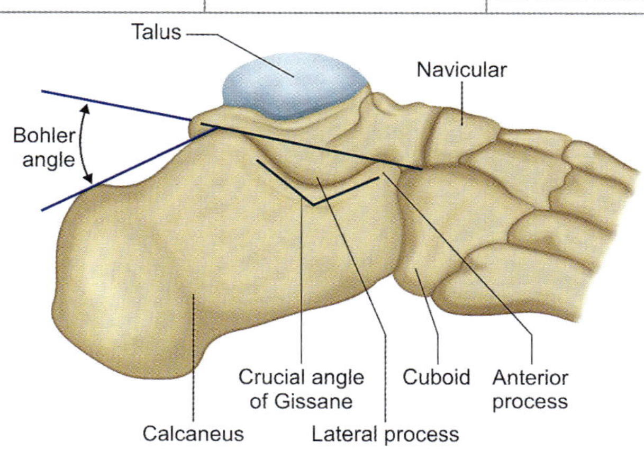

Fig. 37: Illustration showing the formation of critical angle of Gissane and the Bohler's angle.

Contd...

Contd...

Epidemiology	Anatomy	Clinical Evaluation	Radiographic Evaluation	Treatment
due to fall from height, motor vehicle accidents, and may be associated with lumbar, pelvic, or tibial plateau fracture. The contact of talus is situated lateral to weight-bearing axis of lower extremity. As axial load force is applied through posterior facet of calcaneus through the talus, shear forces are directed through posterior facet toward the medial wall of calcaneus. The ensuing fracture line extends from proximal medial aspect of calcaneal tuberosity through the anterolateral wall. The location of primary fracture line may be medial third, central third, or lateral third of posterior facet. As axial load force continues, two things happen: medial spike attached to sustentaculum is pushed further towardmedial heel skin and various secondary fracture lines occur in the region of posterior facet. Secondly, as talus pushes the posterior facet and underlying thalamic fragment into the body of calcaneus, it also pushes out the lateral wall, closing the space for peroneal tendon and occasionally abutting the fibula. As the force is removed, recoil of talus occurs leaving a depressed thalamic fragment and medial spike is retracted into the soft tissue. That is why, medial open fracture of the calcaneum requires deep dissection and debridement. On the basis of secondary fracture lines running through posterior facet Essex-Lopresti described two fracture patterns: 1. *Joint depression* ***(Fig. 38)***: The fracture line producing posterior facet fragment exits behind the posterior facet and anterior to the attachment of Achilles tendon is called joint depression fracture. 2. *Tongue type* ***(Fig. 39)***: Fracture line exits distal to the Achilles tendon insertion.			radiographs are made with tube angled 40°, 30°, 20°, and 10° toward the head of patient. 40° view shows the anterior portion and 10° view shows the posterior facet. It is used intraoperatively to assess reduction. *Computed tomography:* CT scans give detailed information. The semicoronal views give information about the articular surface of posterior facet, sustentaculum and shape of the heel. Axial view gives information about the calcaneocuboid joint, anteroinferior aspect of posterior facet and sustentaculum. **CLASSIFICATION** Extra-articular and intra-articular fractures Extra-articular fractures do not involve the posterior facet or subtalar joint. These are anterior process fracture, tuberosity fracture, sustentaculum fracture and body fracture not involving the subtalar joint. Intra-articular fracture has a primary fracture line running obliquely through the posterior facet and divides the calcaneus into anteromedial or sustentacular fragment and posterolateral or tuberosity fragment. The anteromedial fragment usually is noncomminuted and attached to the talus by deltoid and interosseous talocalcaneal ligament. Posterolateral fragment is usually comminuted and is displaced supero laterally resulting in incongruity of posterior facet and heel shortening and widening. Secondary fracture lines divide these fractures into joint depression and tongue type fracture on the basis of whether fracture line exits behind the posterior facet or through the tuberosity respectively. **Sander's Classification** This is based on the number of intra-articular fracture lines and their location on semi coronal CT images for intra-articular calacaneal fractures involving the posterior facet **(Fig. 40)**. The posterior facet is divided into three fracture lines (A, B, and C corresponding to lateral, central, and medial fracture lines on coronal images). *Type 1:* All fractures with <2 mm of displacement regardless of the number of fracture lines.	in diabetic or osteoporotic patients. Rarely, they occur by direct trauma. Three types are seen: type 1—Sleeve fracture in which a small piece of cortical bone is avulsed; type 2—Beak fracture with an oblique fracture line that exits close and posterior to posterior facet; and type 3—Infrabursal fracture in which there is an avulsion off the middle third of the posterior aspect of tuberosity. Surgery is indicated if gastrosoleus complex is incompetent, the avulsed fragment involves articular surface of joint or if posterior skin is at risk from displaced fragment. Usually, a screw or a lateral tension band wiring is used for fixation. Sustentaculum tali fractures are very rare and usually occur in association with ipsilateral foot and ankle fracture when heel is loaded in extreme foot inversion. Nondisplaced fractures are treated with short leg nonweight-bearing cast whereas ORIF is recommended in displaced fracture. Tarsal tunnel syndrome may result from displaced fragment or from nonunion of this fracture. Medial process fractures are again very rare and are commonly nondisplaced often resulting from loading of heel in valgus producing vertical shear fracture of medial process. POP cast for immobilization suffices for nondisplaced fractures while displaced fractures can be treated with close manipulation followed by casting, screw, or wire fixation. Operative management is prescribed commonly for displaced tongue-type fractures, Sanders Type II and III posterior facet displacement >2–3 mm, flattening of Bohler angle, large extra-articular fractures (>1 cm) with detachment of Achilles tendon and/or >2 mm displacement urgent if skin is compromised or other extra-articular fractures as above. Pin and Cast treatment is acceptable for minimally displaced tongue-type fractures with mild shortening. The Steinman pins are inserted from posterior superior tuberosity directing it inferiorly and distally, reducing the tongue fragment and fixing it. ORIF using plate fixation for calcaneum fractures should be done if the skin condition

Contd...

Contd...

Epidemiology	*Anatomy*	*Clinical Evaluation*	*Radiographic Evaluation*	*Treatment*

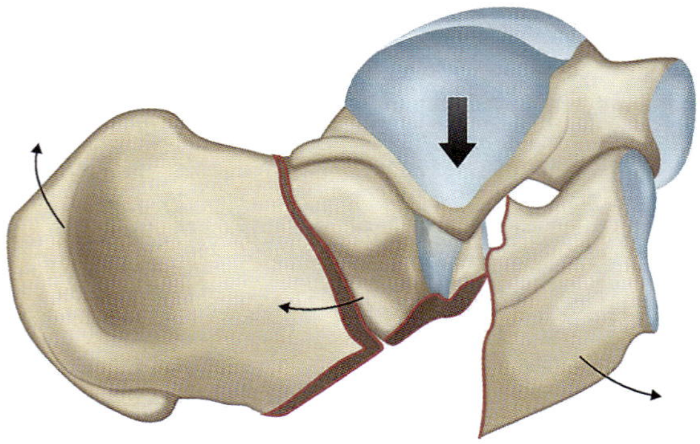

Fig. 38: The Joint depression type calcaneum fracture involves decrease in Gissane's critical angle.

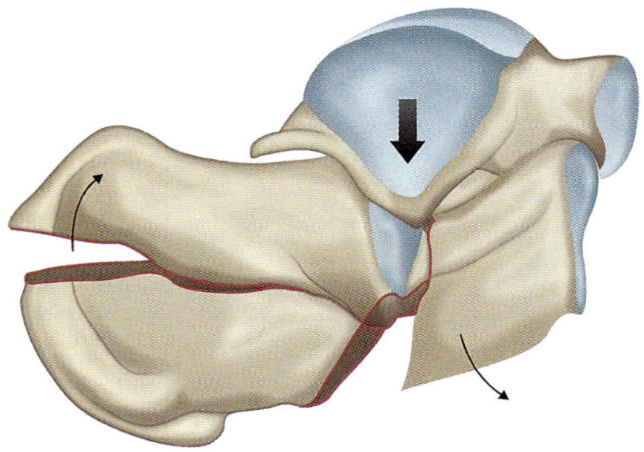

Fig. 39: The tongue-type calcaneum fracture where the fracture line exits posteriorly and typically leads to reduced Bohler angle.

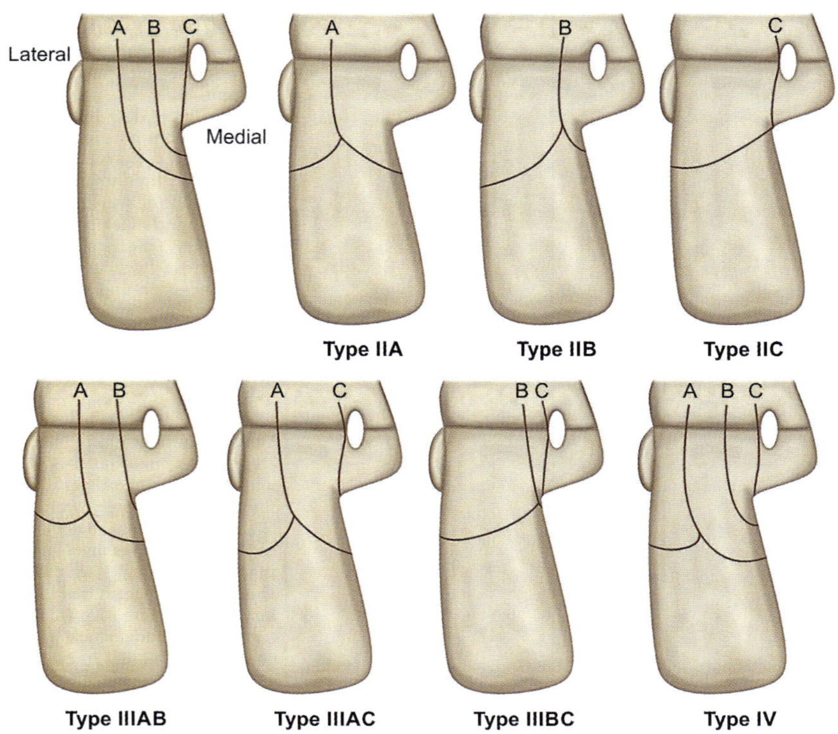

Fig. 40: The computed tomography based Sander's classification of calcaneal fractures (see text for details).

Contd...

Contd...

Epidemiology	*Anatomy*	*Clinical Evaluation*	*Radiographic Evaluation*	*Treatment*
			Type 2: Two-part fracture of posterior facet; further divided into: *2A:* One primary fracture line that courses through the lateral aspect of posterior facet *2B:* One primary fracture line that courses through the middle of posterior facet *2C:* One primary fracture line that courses through the medial aspect of posterior facet *Type 3:* Three-part fracture with centrally depressed fragment, further divided into: *3AB:* Two primary fracture lines, one coursing through the lateral aspect and another through the central aspect of posterior facet. *3AC:* Two primary fracture lines, one coursing through the lateral aspect and another through the medial aspect of posterior facet *3BC:* Two primary fracture lines, one coursing through the central aspect and another through the medial aspect of posterior facet. *Type 4:* Four-part intra-articular fracture with >2 mm displacement and is severely comminuted.	is good indicating stable soft-tissue injury. Usually, after 4–6 hours there is gross swelling that is associated with wound site complications if operated early. It is commonly recommended to wait for 10–14 days for swelling to subside and wrinkles to appear so that wound healing is optimized. Mostly an extensile L-shaped lateral incision is used with osteoperiosteal full thickness flaps that also provides access to the calcaneocuboid and subtalar joints. Good intra-articular visualization and restoring the congruity of subtalar joint are paramount. Correct varus malalignment and restore Bohler angle and calcaneal height. Low-profile lateral calcaneal locking plates are the preferred implants. Bone grafting is not absolutely necessary. Close the skin well without tension using fine sutures. Poor outcome is associated with elderly obese patients, manual labor, workmen compensation involvement, smokers, bilateral calcaneal fractures, multiple trauma, patients with vasculopathies. Primary subtalar arthrodesis is indicated in Sanders type IV as these are not usually amenable for ORIF. One may treat them initially in POP cast for consolidation if comminution is severe and perform arthrodesis later. **COMPLICATIONS** • Subtalar arthritis • Wound complications • Peroneal tendon irritation and impingement • Compartment syndrome • Damage to FHL • Malunion—Calcaneal malunion has been classified on CT scan into three types: 1. *Type 1:* Lateral exostosis with no subtalar arthritis. This is treated with lateral wall resection. 2. *Type 2:* Lateral exostosis with subtalar arthritis. This needs lateral wall excision and subtalar fusion. 3. *Type 3:* Lateral exostosis with subtalar arthritis and varus malunion. Treat with lateral wall resection, subtalar fusion ± valgus osteotomy.

TALUS FRACTURES

Epidemiology	*Anatomy*	*Clinical Evaluation*	*Radiographic Evaluation*	*Treatment*
Talus fractures comprise nearly 1% or less of all fractures and are second most tarsal bone fractures. Of all talar fractures neck of talus fractures are the most common comprising half of the injuries, body fractures account for 13–23% while lateral process fractures comprise nearly 10%. Head of talus is injured the least. The talar fractures have been brought into limelight by Anderson who reported fracture-dislocation in 18 cases coining the term "áviator's astragalus". **MECHANISM OF INJURY** The talus fractures result from high-energy injuries. Neck fractures result from axially transmitted force in forced dorsiflexion pushing the less dense bone of neck against the anterior tibial edge while body fractures occur in supination or pronation. In case of neck fractures if the applied force is not relieved a progression of injuries result into → interosseous talocalcaneal ligament disruption→posterior ankle ligament disruption→subtalar joint dislocation →dislocation of the talus from tibiotalar articulation ("aviator's astragalus"). If there is added supination (common) then the counter from medial malleolus results in medial neck comminution and rotatory displacement of head. Lateral process injuries result from forced dorsiflexion, inversion + external rotation (common in snow-boarding). Talar head fractures usually result from application of sudden dorsiflexion force on a plantarflexed foot while they may also be compressed by a hyperdorsiflexion force against the anterior tibial edge. The previous notion of neck fractures occurring commonly in aviators is incorrect instead it is more common in high-energy motor vehicle accidents where the pilot suddenly applies brakes forcing ankle into dorsiflexion.	The talus is the second largest tarsal bone covered mostly by articular cartilage. The superior aspect of body is trapezoidal, i.e., widest anteriorly, so its placement is secure within the ankle mortise in dorsiflexion. The articular medial wall is straight, while the lateral articular wall curves obliquely posteriorly meeting medial at the posterior tubercle. The neck of the talus faces medially approximately 10–44° with reference to the axis of talar body. The neck also deviates plantarward between 5 and 50°. The inferior middle, posterior, and anterior facets correspond to the calcaneal articular facets forming the subtalar joint. The tarsal sinus lies between middle and posterior facets opening medially as a funnel near medial malleolus. The talus has no muscle or tendinous attachments and is supported only by the joint capsules, ligaments, and synovial tissues. Ligaments provide stability by attaching the talus to tibia, fibula, calcaneus, and navicular. The tendon of FHL lies within the groove on posterior aspect held by a retinacular ligament. The spring (calcaneonavicular) ligament suspends the head like a sling. The blood vessels reach talus through the surrounding soft tissues, injury to which causes vascular compromise. **BLOOD SUPPLY** As per the works or Wildenauer, Mulfinger, and Trueta there is intraosseous and extraosseous arterial circulation. Only two-fifths of the talus can be perforated by vessels; the other three-fifths is covered by cartilage. The extraosseous blood supply of talus comes from posterior tibial, the anterior tibial, and the perforating peroneal arteries **(Fig. 41)**. Additional supply comes from the artery of the tarsal canal (a branch of the posterior tibial artery) and the artery of the tarsal sinus (a branch of the perforating peroneal artery) through an anastomotic sling inferior to the talus. The artery of the tarsal canal (main supply) supplies body through a deltoid ligament branch and through branches to the inferior talar neck. The head and neck are supplied	The patient presents with pain and swelling around ankle and foot following a high-energy injury. Lateral process fractures may present as ankle sprain. Tubercle fractures may be missed on a standard radiograph if undisplaced but the pain is specifically exacerbated by FHL flexion/extension movement. Neck fractures are usually prominent and need emergent if associated with subluxation or dislocation. **Associated Injury** • Thoracolumbar vertebral injuries • Neurovascular injury to posteromedial structures • Skin necrosis on dorsum of foot from compression by head fragment.	The radiological diagnosis is usually made on standard radiographs (AP, lateral, and mortise views) and a series of views for the foot (anteroposterior, lateral, and oblique). The view described by Canale and Kelly (radiograph in maximal equinus, 15° pronation with beam directed 75° cephalad from horizontal) especially is useful for evaluating medial aspect of the talar neck. Further fracture evaluation can be eased by true lateral view of the subtalar joint and the oblique view of the talus. Computed tomography in my opinion is the best modality for understanding fracture geometry as it cannot only detect fractures that are difficult to view on ordinary radiographs but also provides a good view of the talar joint congruence important for surgical planning. MRI serves an important role in estimating osteonecrosis of the talus, which is one of the most common and most feared complications of talar neck and body fractures. **CLASSIFICATIONS** **Anatomical Classification** • Lateral process fracture • Posterior process fracture • Talar head fracture • Talar body fracture • Talar neck fracture **Hawkin's Classification (Fig. 42)** for talar neck (Hawkins groups 1–3 were changed to "types" by Canale and Kelly and added type IV) • *Type I:* Nondisplaced fractures (fracture line enters the subtalar joint between the middle and posterior facets)—one of the three major sources of blood supply disrupted. • *Type II:* Subtalar dislocation, the posterior facet displaced posteriorly or calcaneus displaced medially. Two major blood supply disrupted. • *Type III*: Subtalar and tibiotalar dislocation. The body of talus dislocated posteriorly and medially between tibia and Achilles tendon. All three blood supply sources disrupted and two-thirds are open fractures-dislocations. • Type IV: Subtalar, tibiotalar, and talonavicular dislocation.	Treatment can be discussed for talar neck fractures and other fractures as a group. *Talar fractures other than neck fractures/fracture dislocation* Nonoperative treatment is followed for nondisplaced (≤2 mm) fractures of lateral process, posterior process, talar head, and body fractures. Commonly a below knee POP cast (or better a PTB cast) is applied for 6–10 weeks and molded for longitudinal arch. Operative treatment is indicated for displaced fractures (>2 mm displacement). The fragments are commonly fixed with k-wires/low head profile screws or screws buried within bone. Fixation of body fracture may need medial, lateral, or posterior malleolar osteotomy as may also be required for fixation of posteromedial fragment. Lateral approach through sinus tarsi is needed for lateral process fracture while posterolateral or posteromedial approach is needed for respective process fracture. Combined approach may be needed for body fracture. If the fragment is not fixable (comminuted, small) or there is nonunion then it may be excised. Lateral talocalcaneal ligament may become incompetent with excision of a fragment >1 cm. **Fractures of Talar Neck** All cases with subluxed or dislocated talus should be immediately reduced to prevent further vascular compromise. The goal of treatment is anatomical reduction. • For nondisplaced (Hawkins I) fractures below knee POP cast for 8–10 weeks suffice while all other fractures need ORIF. Regular follow-up is needed to identify early displacements. • Type II fractures—closed reduction is needed and after that unacceptable plantarflexion is needed to maintain reduction of head so surgery is indicated. Commonly a medial approach is used or alternatively anterolateral approach also allows reduction. Screws are placed just off the articular surface fixing the fracture. If lag screws are used then one needs to ensure that

Contd...

Contd...

Epidemiology	*Anatomy*	*Clinical Evaluation*	*Radiographic Evaluation*	*Treatment*
	by the dorsalis pedis artery and the artery of the tarsal sinus. (Detailed in Chapter on "Nonunions and Malunions"). Extensive intraosseous anastomoses are present throughout the talus helping it survive in severe injuries. Preservation of anyone of the three major extraosseous		**Classification of Body of Talus Fracture (Sneppen et al., Fig. 43)** • *Group I:* Transchondral dome fractures (horizontal, sagittal, or coronal fractures). • *Group II fracture:* Shear fracture	there is no comminution else impaction shortening may result. The screws can also be placed through posterolateral approach of Trillat. It is usual to combine the anteromedial with posterolateral approach, passing the screw (at least two screws, cannulated or soild core) from posterior to anterior.

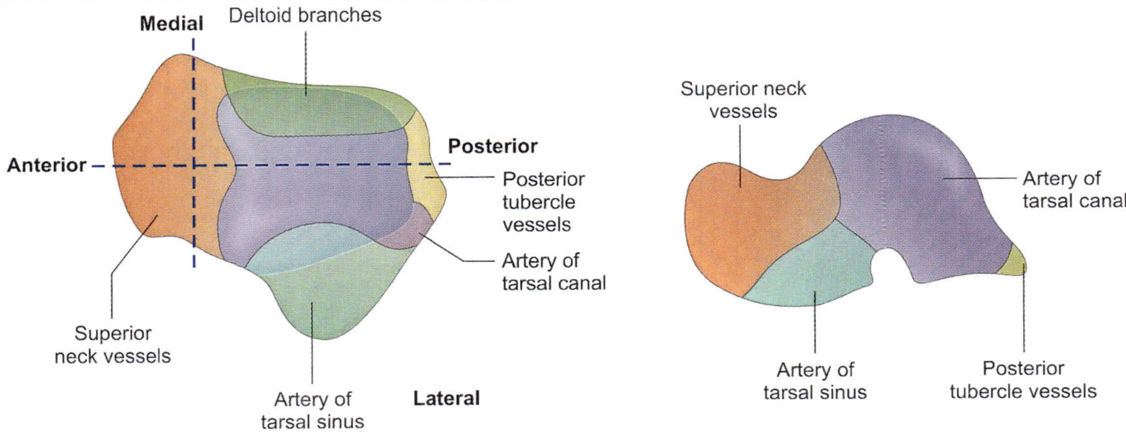

Fig. 41: The blood supply of the various anatomical parts of talus.

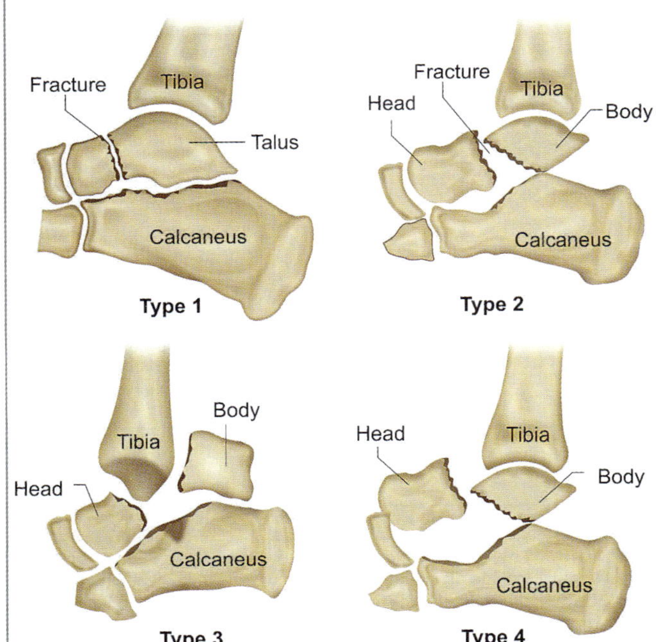

Fig. 42: The illustration for Hawkin's classification of talus fractures.

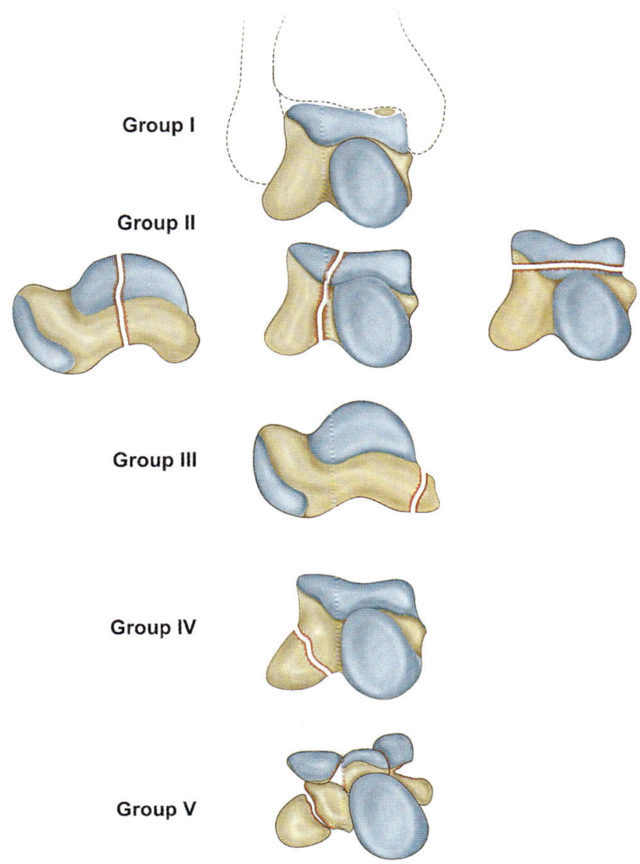

Fig. 43: The illustration representing the Sneppen classification for talus fractures.

Contd...

Contd...

Epidemiology	*Anatomy*	*Clinical Evaluation*	*Radiographic Evaluation*	*Treatment*
	sources can potentially allow adequate circulation via anastomotic channels.		• *Group III:* Posterior tubercle fracture • *Group IV:* Lateral process fracture • *Group V:* Crush fractures	In case of comminuted fractures it is better to place plate at the comminuted column while using a screw in neutralization mode. Plates offer a solid buttress as a bridging strut against collapse, supination or pronation of the fragments. • *Type III fractures*: After emergent reduction is imperative to reposition the body → that may be done by medial malleolus osteotomy (preserving the deltoid blood supply). In open fractures, it is better to debride, wash the site, and place a distractor while toggling the talar body in place with a pin. Fixation can be done as for type II fractures. If the body is totally extruded and wound is contaminated—it is better to discard the body fragment and plan a reconstruction by arthrodesis—usually in two stages. • *Type IV injuries:* These are managed like type III while considering the fact that there are high chances of additional osteonecrosis of head fragment. **COMPLICATIONS OF TALUS FRACTURES AND MANAGEMENT** *Osteonecrosis*: Seen with neck fractures commonly. Around 30% incidence and is associated with medial neck comminution and open fractures. Development of Hawkin's sign indicates revascularization with absorption of subchondral bone (osteonecrosis unlikely). *Post-traumatic arthritis*: It is the most common complication. Subtalar arthritis is seen in 50% cases while tibiotalar arthritis is seen in 33% cases. Talonavicular arthritis is also very common. *Varus malunion of the neck*: Due to medial comminution RSD, implant failure, and infection are other surgery related complications.

LISFRANC FRACTURE DISLOCATION

Epidemiology	*Anatomy*	*Clinical Evaluation*	*Radiographic Evaluation*	*Treatment*
These are uncommon injuries where there is disruption of the articulation between medial cuneiform and 2nd metatarsal base. These account for 0.2% of all fractures (most	Lisfranc joint complex (named after Jacques Lisfranc de Saint-Martin a French Napoleonic-era field army surgeon—not related to this injury but described Lisfranc amputation)	The patient presents with swelling (quite significant and may even mask bony deformity) and pain in the forefoot region. There may be forefoot shortening	The standard radiographs include AP, lateral, and oblique projections of the foot. CT scan may demonstrate additional injury to other metatarsal and tarsal bones. Normally on the	Stable anatomic alignment is the aim of management of these injuries. **NONOPERATIVE TREATMENT** It is indicated for minimally displaced or undisplaced injury

Contd...

Contd...

Epidemiology	*Anatomy*	*Clinical Evaluation*	*Radiographic Evaluation*	*Treatment*
common dislocations of foot) and are common in males in third decade resulting from commonly high-energy injuries or athletic activity. **MECHANISM OF INJURY** *Indirect injury:* The TMT joint disruption usually results from indirect rotational forces and axial load applied to the hyperplantar-flexed forefoot **(Fig. 44)**. The abduction moment applied to forefoot displaces the 2nd to 4th metatarsals dorsolaterally. *Direct injury:* Direct crush injury may also result in disruption of the articulation. Low-energy injuries may result in sprain of the ligament while higher-energy injuries result in complete ligament disruptions or osseo-ligamentous disruptions of the complex. Tarsometatarsal dislocation may also occur in Charcot's foot with minimal injury force.	is a combination of tarsometatarsal articulation, intermetatarsal articulation, and intertarsal articulation. The Lisfranc ligament is the most important stabilizer of second metatarsal and helps in maintaining the midfoot arch **(Fig. 45)**. The ligament is tightened with pronation and abduction of forefoot. The stability is reinforced by plantar ligaments between cuneiform and second to third metatarsals. The intermetatarsal ligament connects second to fifth metatarsal bases forming a group (first and second metatarsal bases are not connected by ligaments). The osseous stability is provided by articulation fitting of second metatarsal in the mortise created by medial cuneiform and middle cuneiform. Tendinous attachments to base of first metatarsal and plantar fascia provide stability against plantar dislocation of the metatarsal bases making it much less common than the dorsal dislocation. Dorsalis pedis artery with deep peroneal nerve crosses the joint superiorly and is at risk during Lisfranc dislocation.	and widening with plantar ecchymosis. One must look for possible forefoot compartment syndrome with this injury especially if closed. Open injuries are less common. Instability can be assessed by metatarsal displacement—if first and second metatarsals can be displaced medially and laterally it usually indicates global instability that would need fixation.	AP film, the medial border of the middle cuneiform aligns with the medial border of the second metatarsal. On 30° oblique view, the medial border of the lateral cuneiform aligns with the medial edge of the base of the third metatarsal and the medial border of the cuboid aligns with the medial edge of the fourth metatarsal. On strict lateral projection no metatarsal should lie superior or inferior to its respective tarsal bone. The "Fleck sign" is usually diagnostic of Lisfranc injury as it represents avulsion injury of Lisfranc ligament from the base of second metatarsal. Widening of the space between first and second ray or disruption of any of above associations represent an injury to the Lisfranc joint. **CLASSIFICATIONS** **Quenu and Kuss (Fig. 46):** It is based on direction of displacement at tarsometatarsal joint: *Homolateral:* This is lateral displacement of the first to fifth metatarsals, or of second to fifth metatarsals where the first MTP joint remains congruent. *Divergent:* There is lateral dislocation of the second to fifth metatarsals with medial dislocation of the first metatarsal. *Isolated:* This involves one or two metatarsals that dislocate dorsally in isolation.	patterns or in patients with surgical contraindication (poor medical status, dysvascular foot, Charcot's foot). The foot is placed in a splint and when swelling reduces POP cast is applied till healing. **OPERATIVE TREATMENT** This is indicated in unstable and or displaced fracture dislocation injuries. Surgery is commonly performed within 24 hours before the foot swelling becomes unmanageable or after the foot swelling subsides and wrinkles appear (10–14 days). Till then the foot may be elevated in splint and swelling reduced by controlled crepe bandage application. If anatomical reduction is obtained by closed reduction then the injury may be fixed with thick K-wires under C-arm guidance. Else if stable reduction is not obtained by closed method then open reduction is the preferred method (some prefer this to open straightaway). The tendons of tibialis anterior or peronei may interpose precluding reduction, these can be extruded using dorsal approach and after accurate reduction and confirmation under C-arm fixation can be done with K-wires or screw osteosynthesis or mini-fragment plate fixation. In general K-wires are sufficient for lateral column fixation (as they have some mobility so rigid fixation compromises arch resilience) while multiple cannulated screws

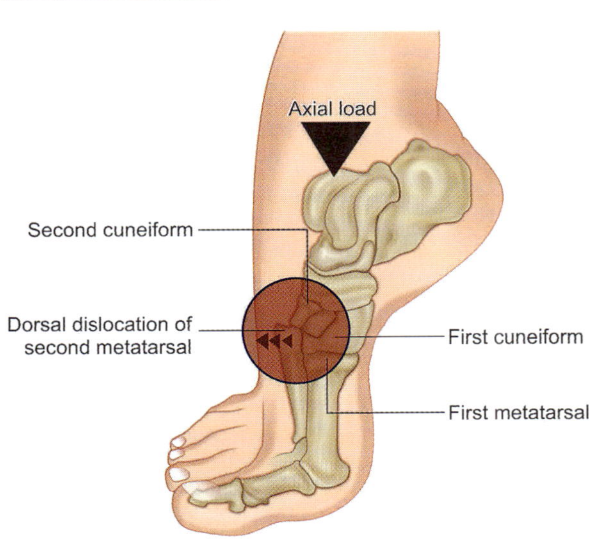

Fig. 44: The mechanism of sustaining the Lisfranc injury.

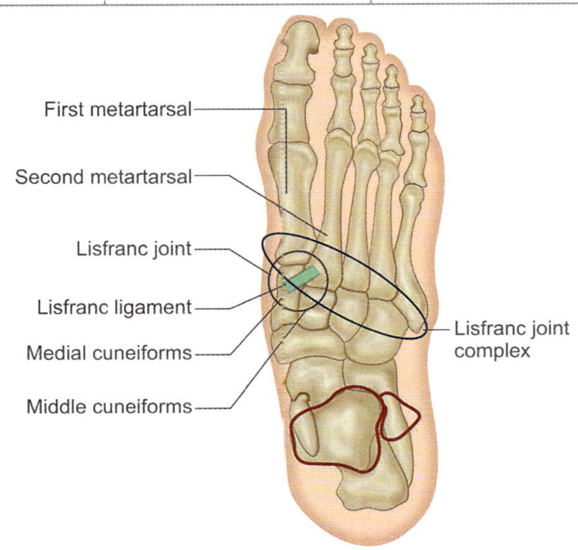

Fig. 45: Illustration for Lisfranc joint and the ligament that is the key injured element in Lisfranc injury.

Contd...

Contd...

Epidemiology	*Anatomy*	*Clinical Evaluation*	*Radiographic Evaluation*	*Treatment*
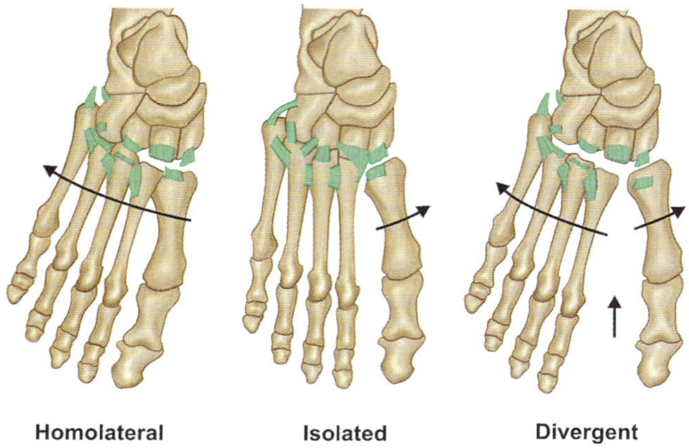 **Fig. 46:** The Quenu and Kuss classification for Lisfranc injury.			**Meyerson Classification (Fig. 47):** • *Type A:* Total incongruity of the TMT joint. • *Type B1:* Partial incongruity affecting the first ray in relative isolation (i.e., partial medial incongruity). • *Type B2:* Partial incongruity in which the displacement affects one or more of the lateral four metatarsals (i.e., partial lateral incongruity). • *Type C1 and C2:* A divergent pattern with partial or total displacement.	(preferable) provide best multidirectional stability for injury stabilization especially first to second metatarsal and tarsometatarsal stabilization. I prefer screw fixation between the medial cuneiform and the 2nd metatarsal to recreate the stability of Lisfranc ligament. Screws are also placed between the first metatarsal and the medial cuneiform, and between the second metatarsal and middle cuneiform. The fourth and fifth metatarsals (lateral column) can be reduced and pinned to the cuboid using K-wires. Due to concern of articular damage with screws, extra-articular fixation with plates is preferred by many. The disadvantage of plating is that it always needs an open fixation. The foot is supported in a splint for 6 weeks after surgery and K-wires removed at 6 weeks followed by support to foot in a rocker style shoe. Screws are removed at 4 months, but one should ensure that there is no loss of reduction after implants removal. External fixation may be done for fractures where tissue condition does not permit screw/plate placement. Primary medial two rays TMT arthrodesis is indicated in comminuted fractures that cannot be reconstructed or in neuropathic foot. Some tend to fix the comminuted injuries using a "Lisfranc screw" and dorsal plate. Midfoot arthrodesis may be done in progressive arch collapse or chronic Lisfranc injuries that produced midfoot arthrosis.
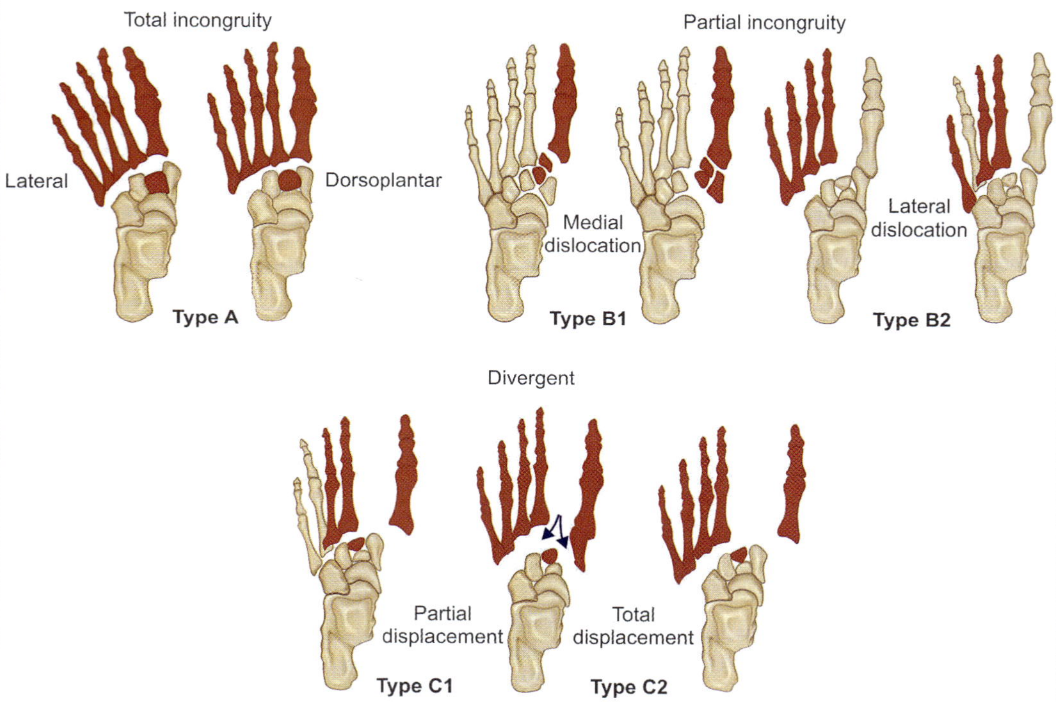 **Fig. 47:** The Meyerson classification for Lisfranc injury.				

ANNEXURE 3

Fractures of Axial Skeleton

Manish Kumar Varshney, Shafiq Hackla

PELVIS FRACTURE

Epidemiology	*Anatomy*	*Clinical Evaluation*	*Radiographic Evaluation*	*Treatment*
The incidence of pelvic fractures has been estimated to be 35 cases per 100,000 per year and ranges from low-energy osteoporotic fractures to high-energy disruption of the pelvic ring. Men suffer more of these injuries in younger age groups while older women suffer these more compared to elderly men. High-energy trauma typically occurs in younger patients while low energy falls result in fracture in older patients. The reported mortality in these fractures ranges from 10% to as high as 40% in some series of open pelvic fractures. Risk factors for increased mortality are high injury severity score, associated head and visceral injuries, hypotension, coagulopathy, and open pelvic fractures. **MECHANISM OF INJURY** High-energy trauma occurs due to motor vehicle accidents, pedestrian struck by moving high-speed vehicles, fall from height and crush injury. Low-energy injury results from sudden muscular contraction in young athletes, low-energy falls, and straddle type injury. Stable injury is one which can with stand normal physiological loads without deformation, occurs due to low-energy trauma and expected to heal uneventfully. Unstable injury is characterized by rotational and/or vertical instability and commonly result from high-energy trauma. These are commonly associated with injuries to major vessel and nerves of the pelvis, degloving injuries to surrounding soft tissue and injury to major viscera. The cause of early mortality is usually hemorrhagic shock or closed head injury while sepsis, gait abnormalities, or multiple organ dysfunctions result in late loss of life.	The pelvic ring is composed of sacrum and two innominate bones joined anteriorly at pubic symphysis and posteriorly at sacroiliac joint **(Figs. 1 and 2)**. The innominate bone is composed of ilium, ischium, and pubis. The pelvic brim is composed of greater or false pelvis and lesser or anatomically true pelvis. The stability to pelvis is provided by various ligaments **(Fig. 2)**: 1. *Sacrotuberous ligament:* It arises from posterolateral of sacrum and inserts into ischial tuberosity. It provides vertical stability to the pelvis. 2. *Sacrospinous ligament:* It runs from lateral margin of sacrum and coccyx and inserts into ischial spine. It provides rotational stability to the pelvis. 3. *Sacroiliac ligament:* There are anterior and posterior sacroiliac ligaments. Posterior sacroiliac ligaments are most important in maintaining the stability of the pelvis and serve as elastic tension band. 4. *Iliolumbar ligament:* It arises from transverse process of L4 and L5 and inserts into posterior iliac crest. 5. *Lumbosacral ligament:* It runs from transverse process of L5 to sacral ala. 6. *Symphyseal ligaments:* The stability of pelvis is determined by ligamentous structure in various planes. Anterior sacroiliac ligament, sacrospinous, and symphyseal ligament provide stability in external rotation. Vertical stability is provided by posterior sacroiliac and iliolumbar ligament. Intact pelvis provides protection to viscera and traversing neurovascular structures while the basin of pelvic floor supports the contents from sagging. Breach of pelvic floor provides seepage path to blood	Patient of pelvic trauma usually has history of high-energy trauma especially in younger patients. Advanced trauma life support (ATLS) protocol should be followed in these patients. Life-threatening injuries to head, chest, abdomen, and spine should be addressed initially. Assessment of all injuries to extremities and pelvis with careful assessment of distal neurovascular status. Scrotal, labial, and perineal hematoma is common and thigh ecchymosis may resultfrom pelvic floor injury. Pelvic instability may cause shortening of the affected side or marked external or internal rotation of the limb. Pelvic compression or distraction test should be performed only once to check for pelvic instability. Massive flank or buttock contusion is suggestive of significant bleeding. Palpation of posterior aspect may show large hematoma and fracture. Rectal examination (reduced rectal tone in lumbosacral plexus injury) in all and vaginal examination in women must be performed in all trauma patients with suspected pelvic injury. One should also evaluate the skin for internal (Morel-Lavallée lesion) external degloving. Morel-Lavallée lesion (first described by French physician Maurice Morel-Lavallée in the year 1853) precludes fixation of bony injuries and harbingers massive skin necrosis and infection if managed inappropriately. These are closed degloving injuries that occur from a shear force through subcutaneous plane causing disruption of capillaries cutting-off the blood supply to overlying dermis which is then left at mercy of horizontal dermal blood vessel network and oxygenation. In the created subcutaneous space between subcutaneous tissue and fascia from shear injury the hemolymph and necrotic fat collects. The effusion may take time	The standard trauma radiograph includes an anteroposterior (AP) view of the chest, lateral view of cervical spine, and AP view of the pelvis. Other views that help to evaluate the bony pelvic injuries are commonly done: 1. *Pennal inlet view:* It is taken with patient supine and tube angled caudad 40°. It shows anterior or posterior displacement of the sacroiliac joint and hemipelvis, sacrum, and internal rotation deformity of ilium and sacral impaction injuries. 2. *Pennal outlet view:* This is taken with patient supine and tube angled cephalad 40°. It shows the vertical displacement of hemipelvis, sacral fracture, flexion/extension of hemipelvis, and fracture of anterior pelvis. *Computed tomography:* It is useful for assessing the posterior pelvis and sacroiliac joint and has become a routine for evaluation of the injuries. *MRI scan:* It is useful for imaging of pelvic vascular structure and genitourinary system but still it has limited utility in imaging of pelvic trauma patients in an emergency set-up. *Stress radiographs (Push-pull radiographs):* It is performed under general anesthesia to test for vertical stability. Under radiographic control, examiner pushes up one extremity while pulling down on other. The maneuver is then reversed and maximal displacement between two films is determined. Cephlad displacement of >1 cm is defined as vertical instability. This is not a routine for evaluation and is contraindicated if there is hemodynamic instability or sacral fracture is in zone 2 or 3. **CLASSIFICATIONS** **Tile Classification (Fig. 3)** is based on forces acting on the pelvis:	**ACUTE PHASE** The acute management of unstable pelvic fracture involves combined approach of general surgeon, orthopedician, and anesthesiologists. *Circumferential pelvic binder:* It is bound around pelvis at the level of trochanter with internal rotation of lower limb and slight flexion of knees. It reduces pelvic volume, apposes raw bony cancellous fracture surfaces, and encourages tamponade. One should be cautious if there is hollow visceral injury (bladder, etc.) in pelvic fractures with internal rotation component as they may be further driven inward. *External fixator:* It can be used in acute phase to provide temporary pelvic stability or as definitive fixation in some cases. There are two types: Anterior external fixation using the universal clamp and rods and the C-Clamp pelvic fixator. *Anterior fixator:* Two 5 mm pins are placed in each iliac wing and compression of pelvic fracture achieved. This fixator is contraindicated in fractures of iliac wing and acetabulum. *Ganz C:* Clamp is most commonly used for immediate provisional fixation of pelvic fracture. It maintains pelvic stability while allowing access to abdomen and perineum. Significant posterior displacement is treated with these clamps. Patient with persistent hypotension after these remedies should be considered for arteriography. About 10% patients present with arterial injuries. These patients are treated with ancillary/definitive embolization. The role of angiography has not been substantiated and varies with institutional protocol but need of blood transfusion >0.5 units/h and abbreviated injury score ≥3 is a good indicator for angiography.

Contd...

Contd...

<table>
<tr><th>Epidemiology</th><th>Anatomy</th><th>Clinical Evaluation</th><th>Radiographic Evaluation</th><th>Treatment</th></tr>
<tr><td colspan="3">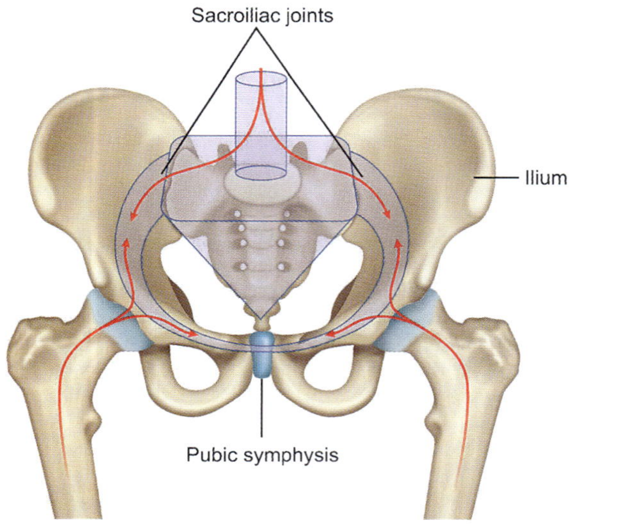

Fig. 1: The bony pelvic ring formed from ilium and sacral ala that helps in transmitting the load from spine to lower limbs.</td>
<td>A. Stable (posterior arch intact):
A1. Avulsion injury
A2. Iliac wing fracture
A3. Transverse sacrococcygeal fracture
B. Rotational unstable, vertically stable
B1. Open book fracture
B2. Lateral compression
B2-1. Ipsilateral anterior and posterior injury
B2-2. Bucket handle injury
B3. Bilateral injury
C. Unstable (posterior arch disruption):
C1. Unilateral
C1-1. Iliac fracture
C1-2. Sacroiliac fracture
C1-3. Sacrum fracture
C2. Bilateral (one side B and other side C)
C3. Bilateral injury
Young and Burgess Classification (Fig. 4)
This classification is based on mechanism of injury:
1. Lateral compression (LC): Laterally applied force that shortens the anterior sacroiliac, sacrospinous and sacrotuberous ligaments
Type 1: Sacral impaction on side of impact.
Type 2: Iliac wing fracture on side of impact.
Type 3: LC1 and LC2 injury on side of impact and contralateral open book injury.</td>
<td>Open pelvic fractures are very difficult to manage and there are high chances of mortality in these cases.
Faringer classified the open pelvic wounds into three zones which guide the decision regarding colostomy in these fractures. Open fractures involving zone 1 and some zone 2 fractures require diverting colostomy while zone 3 can be managed without colostomy. Fractures with large flap avulsion with ischemic pelvic tissue, and rectum and anus involvement are treated with diverting colostomy.
RESUSCITATIVE PHASE
Nonoperative Treatment
• Stable, nondisplaced fracture (Tile type A or LC1 and APC 1 type)
• Pubic diastasis <2.5 cm. These fractures can be treated nonoperatively with analgesics and early mobilization.
Operative Treatment
Indications:
• Open pelvic fractures
• Vertically unstable fracture or open book fracture
• Pubic diastasis >2.5 cm
• Limb length discrepancy >1.5 cm
• Tile type B and C fractures
• Pubic rami fractures with >2 cm displacement</td></tr>
<tr><td colspan="5">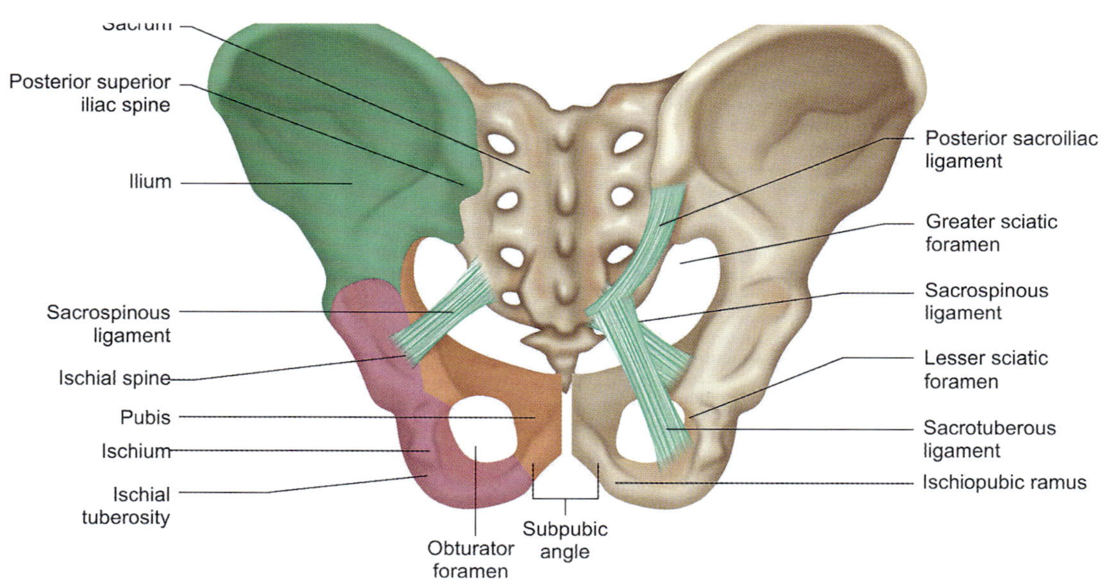

Fig. 2: The bones forming the pelvis and various ligaments stabilizing the structures.</td></tr>
</table>

Contd...

Contd...

Epidemiology	*Anatomy*	*Clinical Evaluation*	*Radiographic Evaluation*	*Treatment*
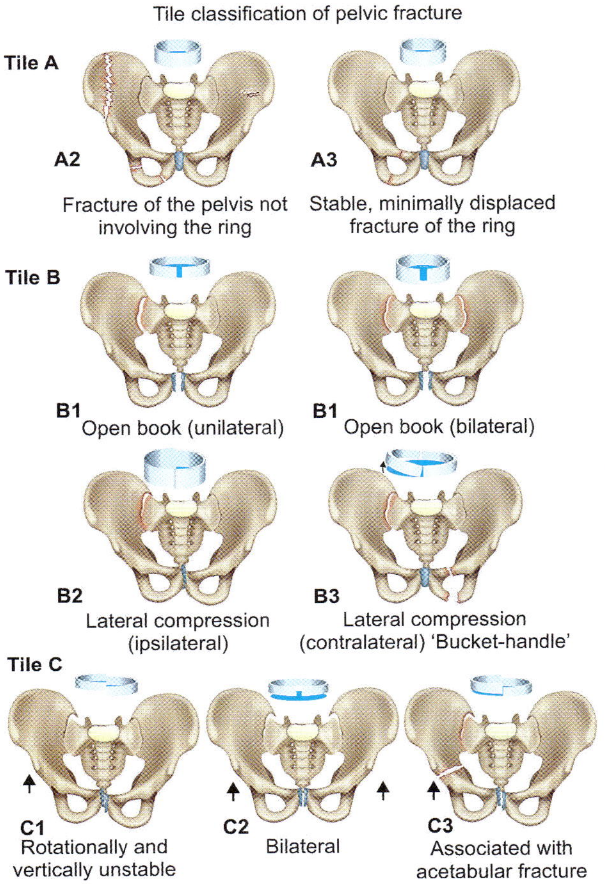 **Fig. 3:** Illustration depicting tile classification of pelvic ring, also shown are simplified ring structures demonstrating the disruptions.			2. *Anteroposterior compression (APC):* Anteriorly applied force that produces external rotation injuries, symphyseal diastasis or longitudinal rami fractures. *Type 1*: Intact posterior ligaments with <2.5 cm of symphyseal diastasis anteriorly. *Type 2:* More than 2.5 cm of symphyseal diastasis with disrupted anterior sacroiliac ligaments. *Type 3:* Complete disruption of anterior and posterior sacroiliac ligaments. It is completely unstable with highest rate of associated vascular injuries. 3. *Vertical shear:* Longitudinally applied forces caused by fall onto an externally lower extremity. There is vertical displacement anteriorly and posteriorly through sacroiliac joint. 4. *Combined mechanism:* Combination of other injury patterns, lateral compression with vertical shear is the most common.	*External fixator*: It is used as definitive treatment in anterior pelvic injuries (Tile type B or Burgess type LC2 or APC2). Contraindicated in type C injuries. *Anterior plating*: It is used as definitive fixation in APC-2 and APC-3 injuries. 3.5 mm recon plate is used. Dual plating of symphysis in Tile type C is done when posterior fixation is contraindicated by soft-tissue problems. **SACROILIAC FRACTURE** Sacroiliac fracture is classified as Tile type C injuries. The anterior injury is treated by anterior external fixator or plating of symphysis. The posterior injury is fixed by iliosacral screws from ilium to sacral body. Transiliac rods are inserted from outer aspect of one Ilium to other Ilium. Second rod is inserted 2.5 cm distal and parallel to first one.
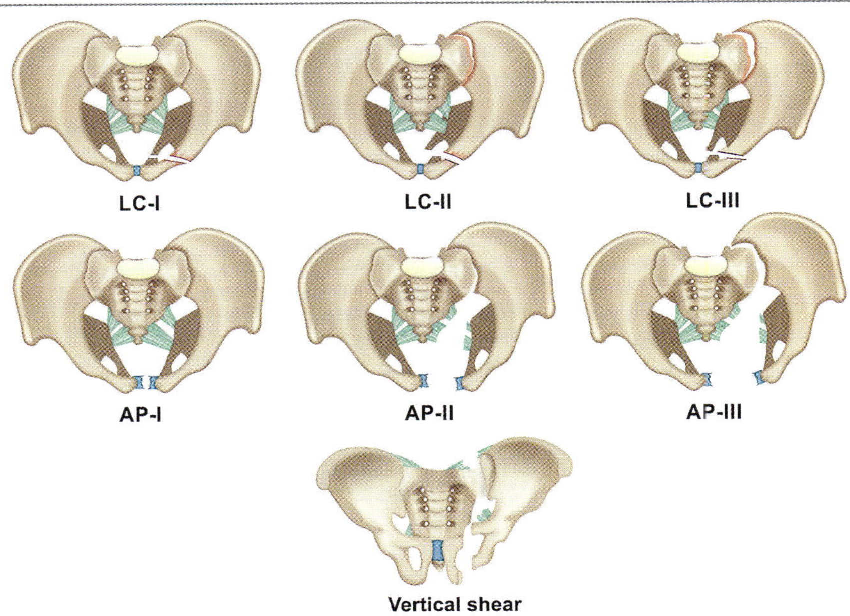 **Fig. 4:** The Young and Burgess classification of pelvic fractures. (AP: anteroposterior compression; LC: lateral compression)				

Contd...

Contd...

Epidemiology	Anatomy	Clinical Evaluation	Radiographic Evaluation	Treatment
In pediatric patients, with open triradiate cartilage the iliac wing being weaker than the elastic pelvic ligaments leads to failure of bone before pelvic ring disruption producing pubic rami and iliac wing fractures that rarely require surgical treatment.	into thighs resulting in massive blood loss in lack of tamponade. Pelvis also serves as the site of load transfer **(Fig. 1)** between the axial skeleton and the lower extremities by virtue of various ligamentous and muscle attachments. In view of the various transiting neural and vascular structures the management needs to be wholesome.	to collect and may later present as soft-tissue tumor. Ultrasonography of the lesion depends on the age of hematoma showing focal anechoic to isoechoic complex collection and may contain fat globules that appear as hyperechoic nodules all located superficial to muscle plane and deep to hypodermis. MRI is the investigation of choice demonstrating homogeneous hypointensity on T1-weighted (T1W) sequences and being hyperintense on T2-weighted (T2W) sequences. The Mellado and Bencardino MRI based classification is clinically not very helpful. The differential diagnosis of Morel-Lavallée lesion includes fat necrosis, coagulopathy-related hematoma, and early-stage myositis ossificans. The treatment usually consists of evacuation of hematoma and necrotic material while small acute lesions without capsule formation may be treated with compression. Once capsule is formed drainage and dermodesis with tetracycline or irritants like talc may be done. *Associated injuries:* • Chest injury • Long bone fractures • Urethral injury and bladder rupture • Sexual dysfunction • Head and abdominal injury • Spine fractures	**Bucholz Classification** *Group 1*: Displaced anterior ring injuries with minimally displaced, stable sacral fracture or incomplete tearing of sacroiliac joint. *Group 2*: Anterior injuries associated with rotational opening of sacroiliac joint with disruption of only anterior sacroiliac ligaments. *Group 3*: Complete disruption of anterior and posterior hemipelvis. *Pennal classification*: It classifies the fractures as anteroposterior compression, lateral compression, and vertical shear injuries.	Tension band plating of posterior iliac crest can also be done. For additional stability, some prefer anterior plating through anterior retroperitoneal approach. ***Displaced iliac wing fracture:*** Pelvic reconstruction plate as well as lag screw can be used as needed. Poor outcome following pelvic fractures is associated with: • SI joint incongruity of >1 cm • High grade of initial/residual displacement • Malunion causing leg length discrepancy >2 cm • Nonunion • Neurologic injury • Urethral injury **COMPLICATIONS** • Injury to L5 and S1 nerve root • Injury to iliac vessels • Screw malalignment • Infection • Thromboembolism • Malunion • Nonunion

ACETABULUM FRACTURE

Epidemiology	Anatomy	Clinical Evaluation	Radiographic Evaluation	Treatment
Acetabular fractures occur in approximately 3 per 100,000 population per year. These are usually resultant of high-energy trauma. Low-energy injuries may result from fall from standing height in elderly osteoporotic patients. **MECHANISM OF INJURY** High-energy trauma secondary to motor vehicle accidents or fall from height is the common mode of injury. The position of femoral head at the time of impact determines the type of fracture.	Letrounel and Judet have described acetabulum as two columns in an inverted Y-configuration supporting the acetabulum **(Fig. 5)**. Acetabulum is an incomplete hemispherical socket with inverted horse-shoe shaped articular surface surrounding the cotyloid fossa. Acetabulum extends into anterior and posterior column. Anterior column is made of anterior half acetabulum, anterior half of iliac crest, ischial spine and pubis and extends from Iliac crest to pubic symphysis. Posterior column extends from superior gluteal notch to ischial tuberosity and is made of posterior half of acetabulum, ishium, and dense bone-forming subchondral bone.	The patient usually sustains a high-energy trauma with involvement of multiple organ systems, therefore clinical assessment with attention to ATLS protocol must be followed in every case of suspected acetabular fracture, evaluating from head to toe. Assessment of neurovascular status is necessary because sciatic nerve is close to posterior wall of acetabulum and may be injured in up to 40% of the cases of posterior column fracture.	**RADIOGRAPHS** *AP view*: It should be evaluated systematically to look for continuity of iliopectineal line (anterior column), ilioischial line (Kohler's line; posterior column), tear drop, lines representing anterior and posterior walls of acetabulum and shenton line. **Judet Views (Figs. 6A and B)** There are two views: 1. *Iliac oblique view*: A bump is placed under the opposite buttock to rotate the pelvis externally about 45° and beam is focused perpendicular to body. It best demonstrates the posterior column, iliac wing, and anterior wall of the acetabulum.	Emergent relocation of any dislocation is imperative. **NONOPERATIVE TREATMENT** Nonoperative treatment of acetabular fracture can be judiciously advised in certain patients as follows: 1. Fracture with <2 mm displacement 2. Fracture with significant displacement (>2 mm) but in a nonweight-bearing region 3. Roof arc measurements >45° 4. Posterior wall fragment <20% 5. Secondary congruence without traction in a displaced both column fractures.

Contd...

Contd...

Epidemiology	Anatomy	Clinical Evaluation	Radiographic Evaluation	Treatment

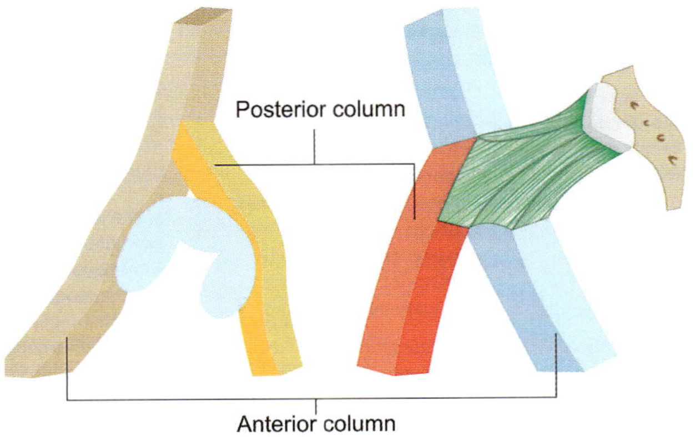

Fig. 5: The disposition of acetabulum in pelvic "columns". Acetabulum sits between the bony struts of anterior and posterior columns forming an inverted "Y".

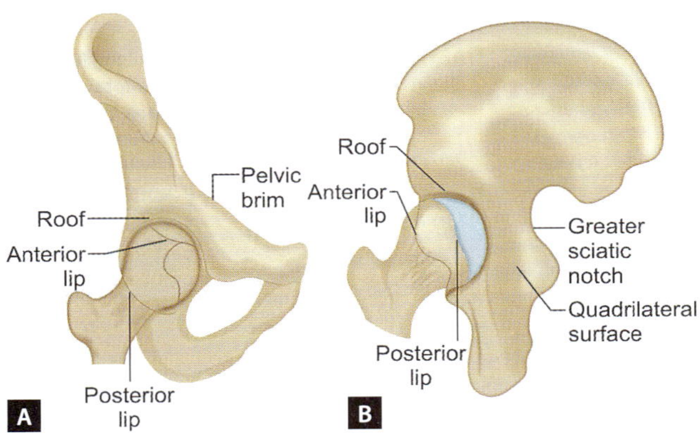

Figs. 6A and B: Line diagram for Judet obturator oblique view (A) showing the anterior column and posterior acetabular wall and iliac oblique view (B) demonstrating posterior column and quadrilateral surface.

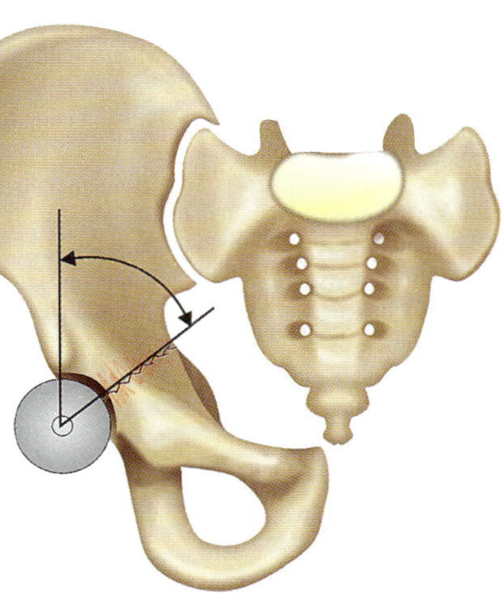

Fig. 7: The roof arc angle of Matta. Medial, anterior, and posterior roof arcs are measured on AP, obturator, and iliac oblique respectively. The arc is formed within the angle created by intersection of a line drawn vertically through the geometric center of acetabulum and another extended from the fracture line. The "roof arcs" demonstrate the amount of intact acetabular roof guiding treatment. The medial roof arc is commonly referred for planning as demonstrated here.

Radiographic Evaluation

2. *Obturator oblique view:* A bump is placed under the ipsilateral buttocks to rotate the pelvis internally about 45° and beam is directed perpendicular to the body. It shows the anterior column and posterior wall of the acetabulum.

Matta et al.* roof arc measurements *(Fig. 7) are used to quantify the acetabular dome after fracture (not applicable for bicolumn fractures and posterior wall fracture). These measurements are taken on three standard radiographic views.

Medial roof arc: Measured on AP view by drawing a vertical line through roof of acetabulum to its geometric center and second line through a point where fracture line intersects the roof of acetabulum to its geometric center. The angle formed is medial roof arc. Similarly, anterior and posterior roof arcs are measured on obturator and iliac oblique views. If roof arc measurement in displaced fracture is <45°, then operative treatment should be considered.

Spur sign: It is seen on obturator oblique view. In both column fracture, a fracture line divides the ilium, so the sacroiliac joint is not connected to any articular surface. On obturator oblique view, it shows the remaining portion of ilium still attached to the sacrum and is seen projected lateral to medially displaced acetabulum.

Gull-wing sign is seen in posterior wall fractures as a lateral spike protruding from acetabulum on an obturator oblique view.

Computed tomography: It is invaluable in the treatment of acetabular fractures. Axial cuts with 2 mm thickness are used. It gives us the detailed information about the size and position of fracture fragments, degree of comminution, status of joint, impaction fracture of acetabulum, and disruption of sacroiliac joint. Articular incongruity of >2 mm is considered unstable.

Treatment

6. Local soft-tissue problems like open wound in anticipated surgical field (Morel-Lavallée) lesion
7. Medical contraindication to surgery (comorbidities, elderly, bedridden, presence of DVT, etc.)
8. Elderly patients with osteoporotic bone

These patients are treated in nonweight-bearing for 6–12 weeks with gradual mobilization of the patient.

OPERATIVE TREATMENT

Surgery may be considered in physiologically stable patients with adequate soft-tissue envelope who present within 3 weeks from injury without incision site related complications. The common indications are:

1. Fracture with >2 mm of displacement.
2. Roof arc measurement <45° or subluxation of femoral head from a displaced acetabular fracture.
3. Posterior wall fracture with >50% involvement of the articular surface or clinical instability with hip flexion to >90°.

Open reduction and internal fixation (ORIF) of the acetabular fracture is commonly performed within 5–7 days of injury. The patients with open fracture, irreducible dislocation of hip, vascular compromise, and worsening neurological deficit must be treated urgently.

Madhu et al. had purposed that the associated fracture patterns should be treated within 5 days and elementary fracture pattern should be treated within 15 days of injury.

Kocher–Langenbach approach is used to treat posterior wall fractures while anterior wall fractures are mostly treated through modified Stoppa or ilioinguinal approach. Extensile approaches can be used to treat complicated fracture patterns. These approaches are extended iliofemoral approach, triradiate approach, and Reinert T approach. Column fixation, wall fixation or combined fixation can be done using different modalities. The commonly utilized ones are antegrade or retrograde column fixation with long screws or posterior column screws. Specific reconstruction bridge plating for column and wall, lag screws, spring/buttress plate, cable fixation in various combinations.

Contd...

Contd...

Epidemiology	*Anatomy*	*Clinical Evaluation*	*Radiographic Evaluation*	*Treatment*
Lower extremity in abduction and external rotation causes anterior column injury while internal rotation causes posterior column injury. Direct impact to greater trochanter causes transverse fracture of the acetabulum. Motor vehicle accident causes dashboard type of injury with degree of hip flexion determining the site and extent of posterior wall fracture.	Quadrilateral plate is a thin and flat plate forming lateral border of pelvic cavity and lies adjacent to medial wall of acetabulum. This plate is limiting factor in the type of fixation used. Acetabular dome is the weight-bearing surface of the acetabulum and is at the junction of anterior and posterior columns. Association of arteria corona magna (mortis) (described elsewhere) must be borne-in-mind while performing fixation.	Femoral nerve may be injured in anterior column injury although rarely. Injury to ipsilateral extremity particularly to proximal femur and knee in which posterior instability and patellar fracture are common should be checked.	**Judet-letournel Classification (Fig. 8)** It classifies the fracture into primary and associated fracture. Common age groups are mentioned in brackets. *Primary fracture:* 1. Anterior column (elderly) 2. Anterior wall 3. Posterior column 4. Posterior wall 5. Transverse fracture (young) *Associated fracture:* 1. Posterior column and posterior wall 2. Transverse and posterior wall fracture (young, most common associated fracture) 3. Anterior column/wall and posterior hemitransverse fracture (elderly) 4. T-type fracture (young) 5. Both column fracture (elderly).	**Complications** 1. *Imperfect reduction*: Both column fracture had highest chances and these lead to post-traumatic arthritis in future. 2. *Osteonecrosis*: It occurs more frequently in fractures with posterior dislocation and excessive fracture site exposure. It is usually apparent within 2 years of injury. 3. Infection occurs in 1–5% of patients. 4. Sciatic nerve palsy 5. Heterotopic ossification occurs in approximately 14–50% of patients with no prophylaxis. Posterior approach is mostly associated with this complication. Indomethacin and low-dose radiation have been shown to decrease the incidence of this complication 6. Thromboembolic complications occurred in 2–6% of patients. 7. Hematoma formation 8. Chondrolysis. Total hip arthroplasty is performed in patients with post-traumatic arthritis.

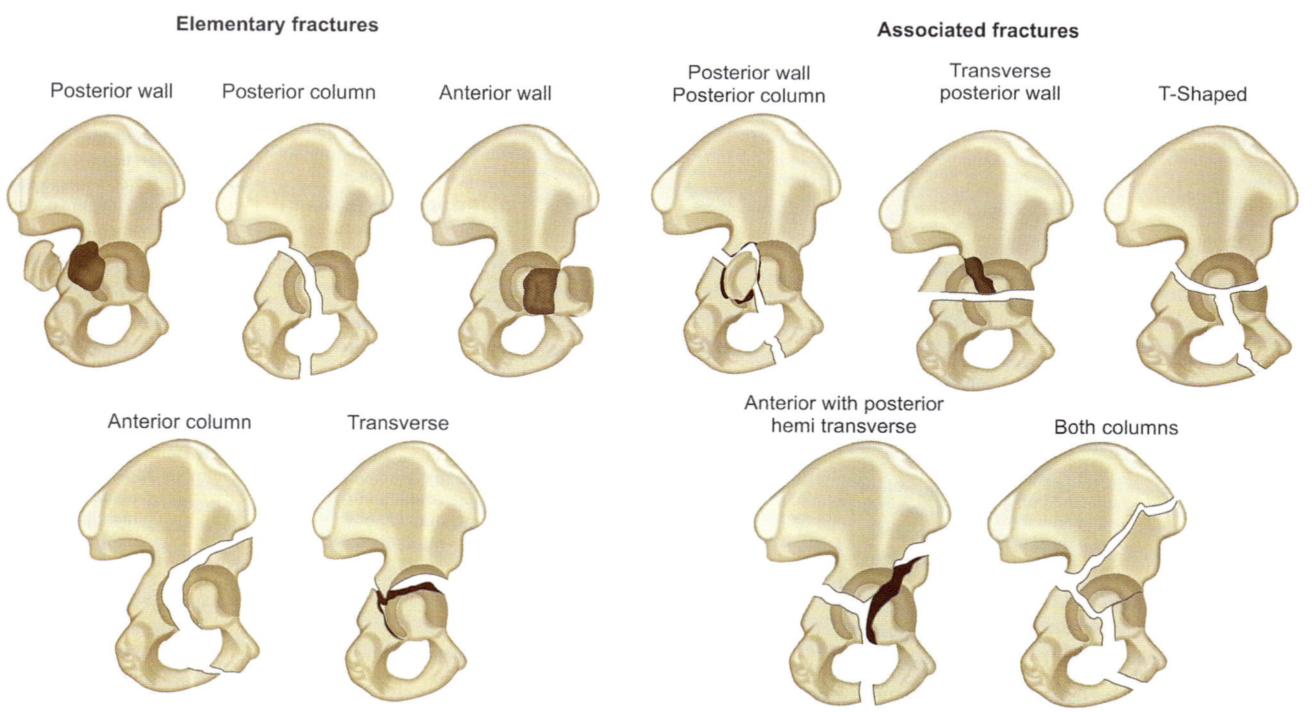

Fig. 8: The Letournel and Judet classification of acetabular fractures showing the elementary and associated types of acetabular fractures.

CERVICAL SPINE INJURY

Epidemiology	*Anatomy*	*Clinical Evaluation*	*Radiographic Evaluation*	*Treatment*
Cervical spine is injured in 2.4% of blunt trauma victims. The factors known to be associated with blunt cervical spine injury include age above 65 years, males and white ethnicity. There is no systematic data to define annual incidence but in general two peaks are seen one in 2nd–3rd decade in males and other in elderly females. Most common site of injury is the atlantoaxial region followed by C6–C7 level. The reported frequency of missed injuries in the cervical spine varies from 4% to 30%. *Mechanism of injury*: Mostly the injuries result from accidental falls, with motor vehicle/transport injuries. Cervical spine remains the most common level for spinal cord injury (SCI), representing 55% of all SCIs. In view of different characteristics of individual motion segments they are briefed individually. *Occipitocervical dissociation*: Usually a pedestrian injury (hit by motor vehicle) and common in children. *Atlas fractures*: These constitute 10% of all cervical spine fractures and are associated with other cervical spine injuries. Posterior arch fractures are commonly bilateral but mostly stable. Lateral mass fractures are usually unilateral and unstable if associated with ligament injury. Jefferson fracture (burst fracture of atlas) produces lateral displacement of both lateral masses but if the sum of lateral mass overhang is >6.9 mm on a coronal CT scan, then it indicates disruption of transverse ligament. *Atlantoaxial rotatory instability* commonly results from disruption of alar and transverse ligaments seen in association with other cervical injuries. These are commonly missed in pediatric patients and later present with torticollis and limited cervical movements. *Atlantodens instability* results from injury to the transverse ligament ± tectorial membrane/alar ligaments. It results commonly from flexion injury.	Cervical spine has seven vertebrae in which the upper two largely differ in characteristics. The vertebral bodies are small as they have less weight to carry and extensive joint surfaces for greater ROM. The cervical spine's range of motion is approximately 80° to 90° of flexion, 70° of extension, 20–45° of lateral flexion, and up to 90° of rotation to both sides. The occipitoatlantal joint supports the skull and supports minimal rotation while 25° of flexion-extension movement is allowed. The atlantoaxial joint just below it instead accounts for approximately 40–50% of cervical rotation. It also contributes 20° to the flexion-extension range of motion. The upper cervical spine (C1–2) and cranium are secured by external and internal ligaments **(Fig. 9)**. Atlanto-occipital, anterior atlanto-occipital, and anterior longitudinal ligaments support from outside. While the internal ligaments are: • Transverse ligament • Accessory ligament including apical ligament • Paired alar ligaments • Tectorial membrane (continuation of PLL) • Accessory atlantoaxial ligament The subaxial cervical spine can be studied into three column concept of Dennis. The anterior and middle column (vertebral body) provides support and stability along with intervertebral disks and the attachments of the ALL and PLL. The vertebral body carries two-thirds of the vertebral load. The posterior bony elements (lamina, facets, and spinous processes) provide attachments for the capsulo-ligamentous structures, viz., supraspinous and interspinous ligaments, ligamentum flavum, and facet capsules. These structures together make the posterior tension band. The facet joints provide the primary restraint against anterior subluxation. The transverse provides the conduit for the vertebral arteries bilaterally, beginning at C6.	Incidence of missed injuries is quite high and they contribute to significant number of patients with neurological compromise and permanent damage. The ATLS protocol should be followed in examining any suspected or overt cervical spine injury. Immobilize the spine in hard cervical collar and examine not only cervical but whole spine. Neurological examination includes evaluation of peripheral nerves and cranial nerves especially VI, VII, IX, X, XI, and XII. Blunt trauma injuries usually escape a standard evaluation and injuries like Hangman's fracture and SCIWORA (spinal cord injury without radiological abnormality) may be missed. Injury to vertebral artery (dissections, occlusions, transections, or pseudoaneurysms) produces diverse pattern like quadriplegia not specific to any cervical injury level, brainstem/cerebellar infarction, 5Ds (dysphagia, diplopia, dysarthria, drop attacks, and dizziness), 2Ns (nausea and nystagmus), 1T (Tinnitus) or a typical clinical picture of "Wallenberg syndrome". In Wallenberg syndrome, there is cranial nerve deficit of V, IX, X, and XI nerves + Horner's syndrome + ataxia + dysmetria and contralateral pain/temperature loss. The injury may be identified by digital subtraction arteriography or MR angiography. There is no specific injury pattern that results in vertebral artery injury as it has been seen with facet dislocations, vertebral body subluxations, transverse foramen fractures, and upper c-spine fractures all. According to American Association of Neurological Surgeons (AANS), the injuries are managed as follows: • Anticoagulation with intravenous heparin in patients with evidence of posterior circulation stroke. • Either observation or anticoagulation in patients with evidence of posterior circulation ischemia. • Observation of patients with no evidence of posterior circulation ischemia.	Standard radiographs of cervical spine in AP, lateral, and odontoid view are routine but should be supplanted with CT scan on a low threshold for suspected cervical spine injury. CT scan has far more sensitivity (99%) and specificity compared to radiographs (70% sensitivity). CT is especially sensitive to cervicothoracic injuries poorly visualized on radiographs. Evaluate the lordosis, disk space, vertebral body disposition and splaying of spinous process. Various radiographic parameters help to determine the atlanto-occipital subluxation. Powers ratio **(Fig. 10)** of >1 indicates anterior subluxation. Harris rule of 12s **(Fig. 11)** is also used to determine instability. Injury to other region of spine is present in 15–20% cases, so they also should be evaluated. **CLASSIFICATIONS** **Allen-ferguson Classification** This is based on major injury vector **(Fig. 12)** producing cervical injuries. The following common types are recognized and widely followed: • Compression-flexion • Compression-extension • Vertical-compression • Distraction-flexion • Distraction-extension • Lateral flexion **AO Classification** proposed three major types especially pertinent to subaxial spine. Three major groups are recognized: *Type A:* Compression only. *Type B:* Flexion-extension-distraction injury. *Type C:* Rotational injury. ***Moore et al.*** proposed a four-column based morphological approach. Four columns are recognized as follows: • Anterior column • Two lateral columns that include lateral mass and paired facets. • *Posterior column*: Posterior bony arch and supporting ligaments. Each column is then scored and complied for classifying the fracture.	Immobilization of cervical spine injuries is essential to prevent any deterioration or avoid further damage to the cord. Common management of specific injuries is briefed below: ***Atlanto-occipital dissociation*:** Traction is contraindicated and instead immobilization with halo-vest immediately after reduction is recommended. Obtain a CT scan to document reduction. Long-term stability is obtained with occipito-cervical (C2) fusion (Bohlman Wire, plate-screw construct or a screw-rod construct). ***Atlas fractures*:** Undisplaced or stable fractures can be immobilized in SOMI brace. Displaced or unstable fractures are treated with traction + bed rest for 4–6 weeks followed by halo-vest application or better a C1–2 transarticular screw fixation (Magerl technique) following reduction. Transoral reconstruction of C1 anterior ring and lateral masses is also described. ***Atlantoaxial rotatory instability:*** The aim is obtaining reduction by traction and then immobilization to maintain stability. Type I injuries are commonly immobilized in halo-vest, but in other unstable injuries open reduction and posterior stabilization is done by Gallie-type fusion, Magerl transarticular screws or Harms technique. In situ fusion may be done for late presenting cases. ***Odontoid fractures:*** Type I fractures are commonly immobilized in halo-vest. Type 2 fractures are prone to nonunion (up to 15–50%) and produce secondary instability so reduction and fixation are commonly practiced. Type III fractures have much better union rates. Nonunion is especially common in patients >65 years of age, smokers and those with angulation >10° so aggressive management is recommended. Transoral anterior odontoid screw fixation following reduction is commonly performed with a single screw.

Contd...

Contd...

Epidemiology	*Anatomy*	*Clinical Evaluation*	*Radiographic Evaluation*	*Treatment*

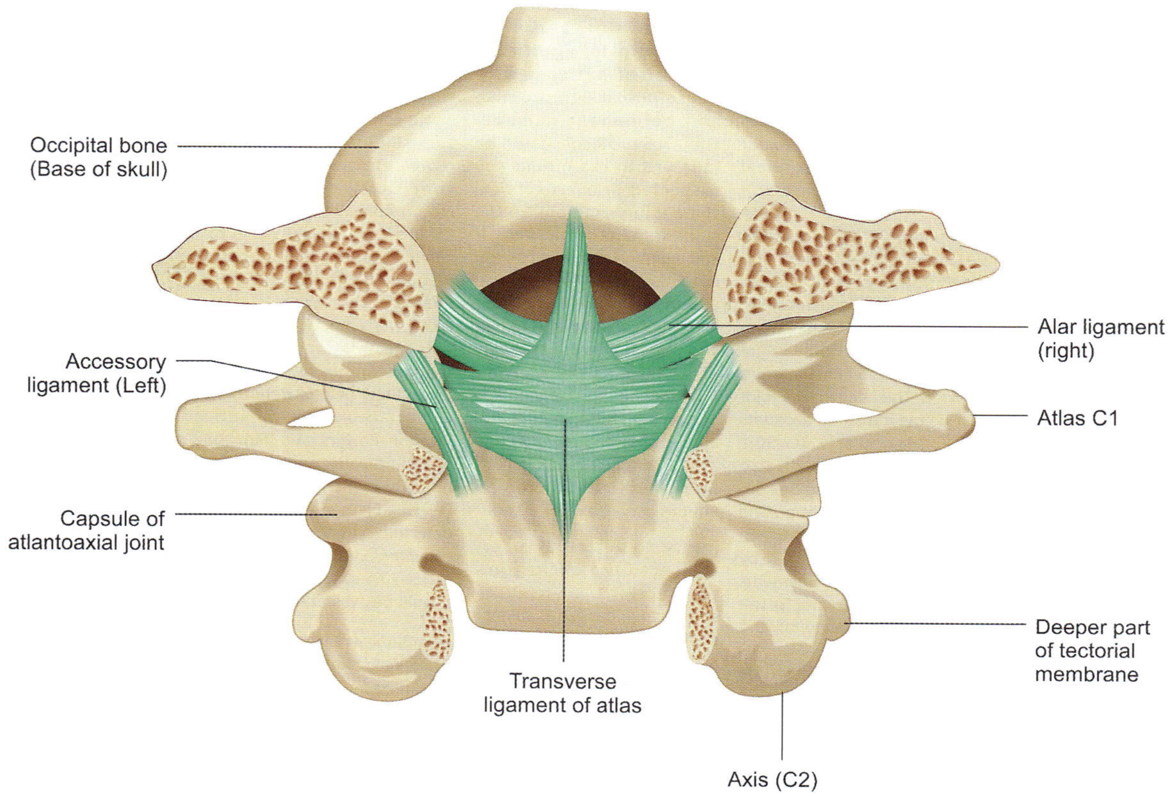

Fig. 9: The atlantoaxial articulation (view from behind after coronal section) and supporting ligaments for stabilization of occipitocervical region.

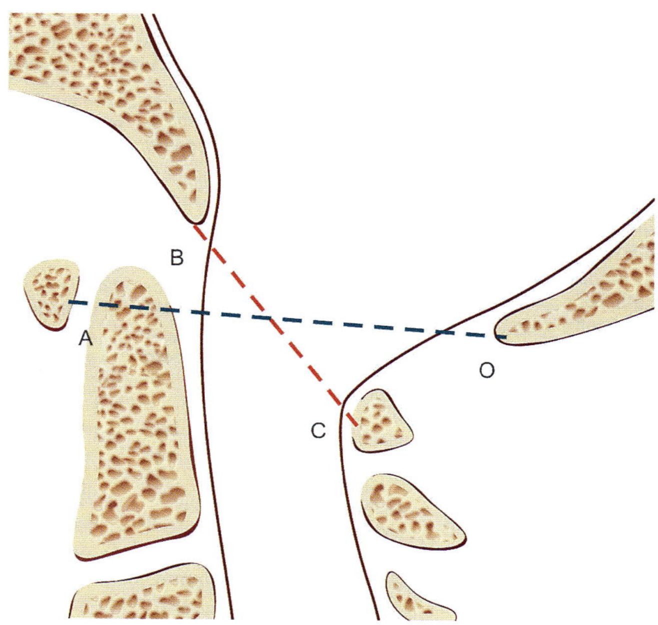

Fig. 10: The powers ratio (BC/AO) is measured as the ratio of the distance in the median (midsagittal) plane between the basion (B) and the posterior spinolaminar line of the atlas (C) and, opisthion (O) and the anterior arch of the atlas (A).

Contd...

Contd...

Epidemiology	Anatomy	Clinical Evaluation	Radiographic Evaluation	Treatment

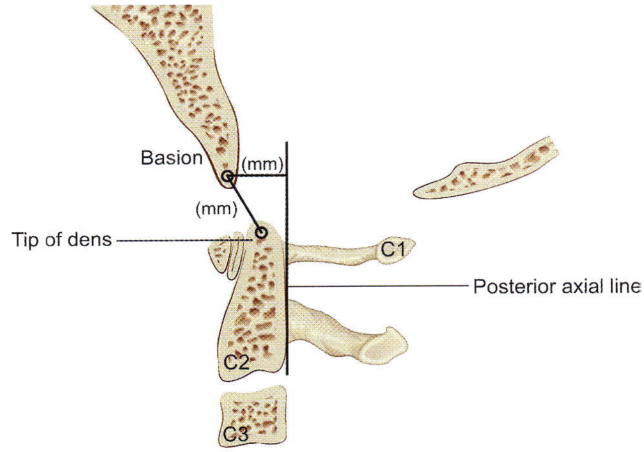

Fig. 11: The line diagram demonstrating the Harris rule of 12s. The basion-dens interval (BDI) and/or the basion-axis interval (BAI) measured in mm should not be <12.

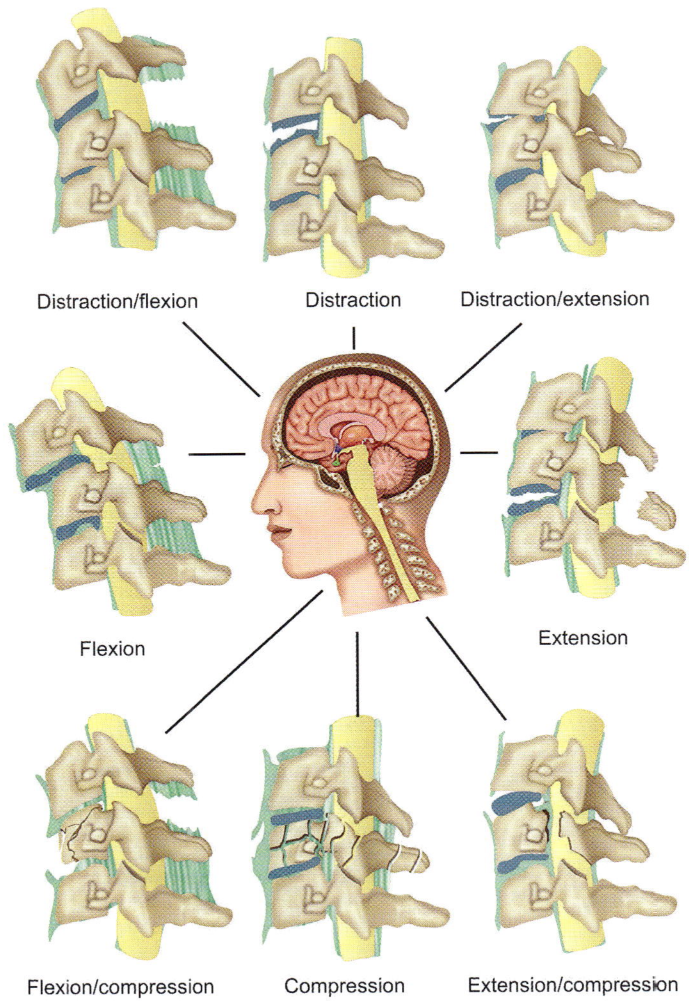

Fig. 12: The illustration demonstrating Allen–Ferguson mechanisms of cervical spine injury.

Contd...

Contd...

Epidemiology	Anatomy	Clinical Evaluation	Radiographic Evaluation	Treatment
Odontoid fractures represent 20% of cervical spine injury that may result from high-energy injury in younger patients or low-energy injury in elderly. Neurological damage is uncommon but may occur as incomplete involvement to quadriparesis. *Hangman's fracture (traumatic spondylolisthesis of axis)* result from high-energy trauma typically but the most common mechanism is hyperextension and axial loading. They are rarely associated with neurological deficits. *Subaxial (C3–C7) cervical spine trauma* result from various mechanisms (Allen and Ferguson classification): *Flexion-compression injuries*: In initial stages, this produces compression fracture while with increased severity triangular teardrop fracture or quadrangular fragment with posterior ligament complex tear results. This may produce posterior kyphosis and subluxation of vertebral body into spinal canal. *Flexion-distraction injuries:* Most common injury pattern. These produce posterior ligament sprain → tear → unilateral facet dislocation → bilateral facet dislocation. Neurological damage depends on extent of injury. *Vertical compression injury:* This is the most severe type of injury representing 9.7% of all subaxial cervical spine fractures. Axial force produces compression—burst fracture of body resulting in propulsion of posterior body fragment into canal. Flexion moment may lead to disruption of the ligament leading to unrestrained compression of the cord. *Extension (distraction-extension) injury pattern:* This mechanism produces → widened disk space → ALL disruption → posterior ligament injured and cephalad vertebral body displaced into canal. In DISH or ankylosing spondylosis, these can be potentially devastating.			**Occipitocervical Dissociation (Fig. 13) Classification** *Type I*: Anterior subluxation *Type II*: Vertical distraction >2 mm of atlanto-occipital joint *Type III*: Posterior dislocations **Classification of Atlas Fractures (Fig. 14)** *Type I:* Isolated posterior arch fracture *Type II:* Isolated anterior arch fracture *Type III:* Jefferson fracture; anterior and posterior arch fractures *Type IV:* Comminuted lateral arch fracture **Fielding Classification of Atlantoaxial Rotatory Instability (Fig. 15)** *Type I:* Rotatory fixation without anterior displacement of the atlas *Type II:* Rotatory fixation with anterior displacement of the atlas of 3–5 mm *Type III*: Rotatory fixation with anterior displacement greater than 5 mm *Type IV:* Rotatory fixation with posterior displacement **Anderson D'Alonzo Classification of Odontoid Fractures (Fig. 16)** *Type I:* Fracture of odontoid tip *Type II:* Fracture at junction of base and body of odontoid *Type III:* Fractures that extend into body of axis **Levine Modification of Effendi Classification of Hangman's Fractures (Fig. 17)** *Type I:* Bilateral pars fracture with a vertical fracture line (<3 mm of displacement and no angulation). *Type Ia (Starr and Eismont):* Fracture line passes through posterior body of C2 rather than the pars. *Type II:* Vertical fracture line with displacement of >3 mm and significant angulation. This is commonly associated with fracture of the anterior and superior endplate of C3.	It may not be appropriate if the fracture cannot be reduced, comminution present at the fracture, there is lysis or osteopenia at the fracture or of dens. In such patients posterior atlantoaxial fusion by Gallie-type wiring, Magerl trans-articular screw fixation or Harms fusion may be done. The latter procedures are also recommended for odontoid nonunion. ***Hangman's fractures:*** The type I/Ia injuries are commonly treated by collar immobilization/SOMI brace. Types II and IIa need reduction by traction and immobilization for 4–6 weeks. For fractures with <12° of angulation, halo-vest may be used for immobilization. Surgical stabilization can be achieved by transpedicular lag screws (does not address disk space pathology), anterior C2–3 arthrodesis (posterior instability persists), C2–3 rod construct. Some prefer to initially immobilize in halo reserving surgery for redisplacing fractures. Type III injuries are managed surgically by anterior fusion or posterior C2–3 lag screw/lateral mass screw rod construct. ***Cervical spine injury from C3–C7*** *Flexion compression injuries:* Initial management in halo-vest or surgical stabilization for unstable injuries that fail to maintain in halo-vest. Usually, an anterior corpectomy followed by column restoration with allograft and cage + plating is utilized but posterior fusion may be added for unstable fractures that do not achieve good stability by above methods. *Flexion-distraction injuries:* Facet dislocations need reduction by traction in an alert, awake patient. Traction is given commonly using crutch-field tongs, initially a weight of 10 pounds (5 kg) for atlanto-occipital region + 5 pounds for each cervical level is given and reduction assessed. Up to 140 pounds of traction can be given safely for reduction. If closed reduction fails (3–6 hours after trauma) or redislocation occurs, then open reduction is indicated using anterior or posterior approach followed by stabilization. If reduced then maintain with 20 pounds of weight. Operative stabilization fares better in maintaining reduction than nonoperative approach.

Contd...

Contd...

Epidemiology	*Anatomy*	*Clinical Evaluation*	*Radiographic Evaluation*	*Treatment*

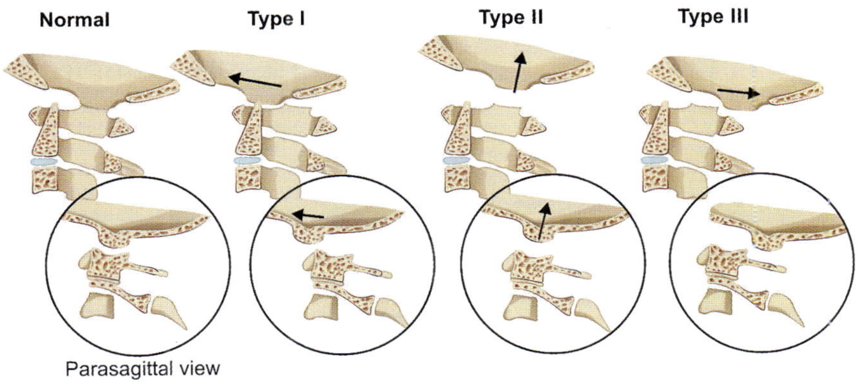

Fig. 13: The illustration demonstrating types of occipito-cervical dissociation.

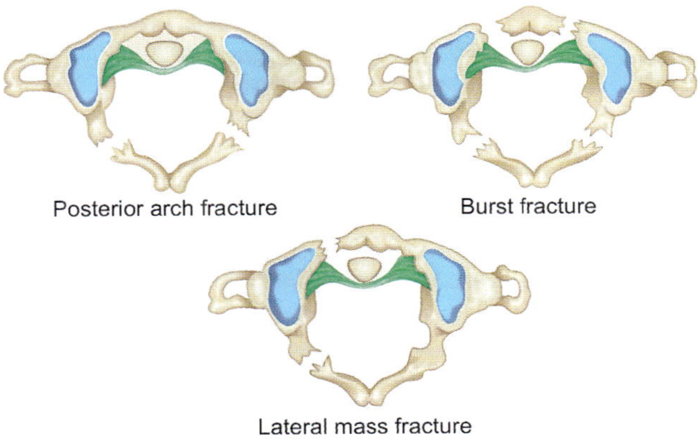

Fig. 14: Illustration depicting different patterns of atlas fracture.

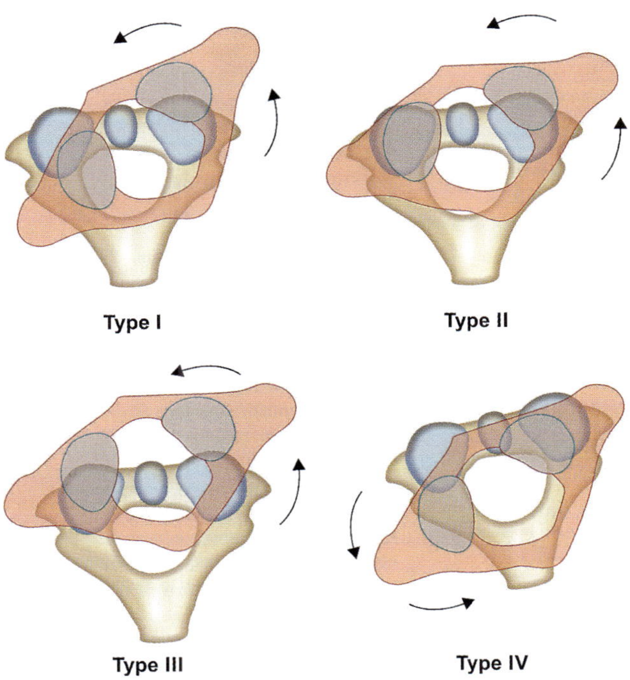

Fig. 15: Illustration of atlantoaxial rotatory instability (see text for details).

Contd...

Contd...

Epidemiology	*Anatomy*	*Clinical Features*	*Radiographic Evaluation*	*Treatment*
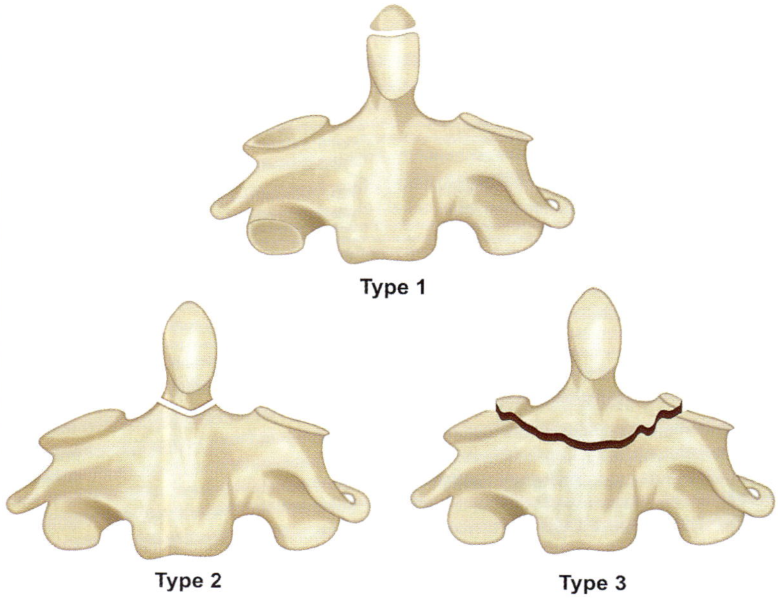 **Fig. 16:** Anderson D'Alonzo classification of odontoid fracture. 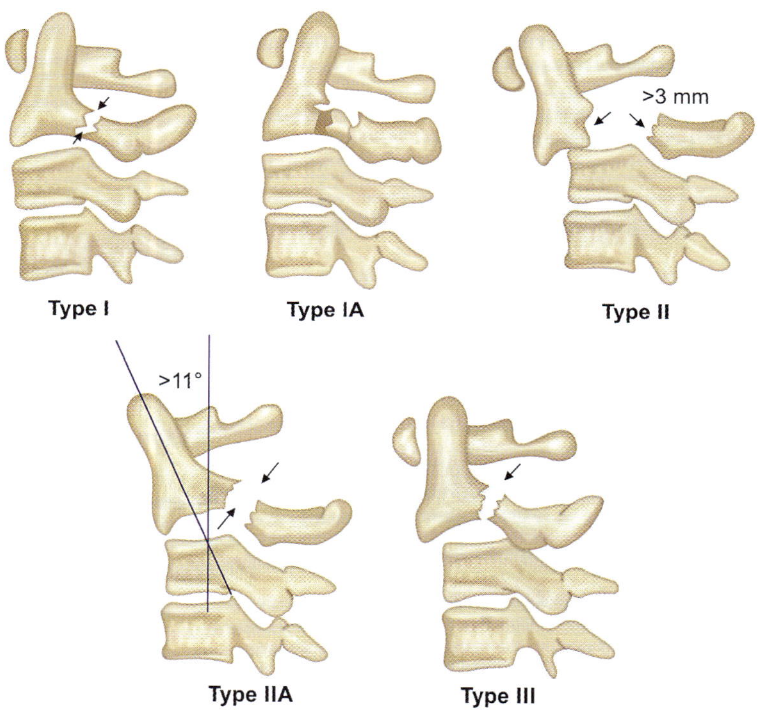 **Fig. 17:** The classification of different types of Hangman's fractures.			*Type IIa*: There is oblique fracture pattern of the pars, with no displacement but significant angulation (>11°). *A Type III fracture*: Same as Type I fracture but with bilateral C2–3 facet dislocations.	Facet fractures with <1 mm displacement can be managed with orthosis while larger facet fragments (>40% of absolute height of intact lateral mass) and displacement (>1 cm) are better managed by surgical stabilization. Anterior cervical discectomy and fusion (ACDF) with cage/plate is commonly performed. Posterior lateral mass screw fixation or facet/spinous process wiring can also be done adding one more fusion level. Posterior fusion has been found to be sturdier than anterior plating and the latter has been also reported to fail in a significant number of patients. *Vertical compression injuries*: These injuries are better managed surgically as anterior decompression and stabilization improves the lordosis and canal space than halo-traction immobilization. ***Distraction extension type I injuries*** can be managed by anterior plating to restore the anterior tension band but type II injuries better need a combined anterior and posterior approach (posterior first to obtain reduction). In patients with DISH or ankylosing spondylosis, operative management or halo-vest immobilization should be used.

THORACOLUMBAR SPINAL INJURY

Epidemiology

The usually quoted incidence of spinal injury is 64/100,000 population/year and is seen rising. In all of the thoracolumbar injuries 50–60% involve transitional zone (T11–L2), 25–40% are injuries to thoracic spine and 10–14% affect lower lumbar spine and sacrum. Thoracolumbar vertebral injuries are more common in men, especially between 20 and 40 years of age. Neurological injury is seen in one-third of the fractures at the thoracolumbar junction depending on the type of fracture. Due to frequent association of chest injury, abdominal, cardiovascular, long bone injuries, and head injury, the focus often shifts away from the spine injuries and 20% may get missed in this business.

MECHANISM OF INJURY

High-energy blunt trauma is the most common mode of injury to thoracolumbar spine. 65% of thoracolumbar fractures occur from motor vehicle injuries and falls from height, and rest being contributed by sports injuries and violence.

Anatomy

The thoracolumbar spine anatomy is detailed in Chapter on "Anatomy of the Spine and Spinal Cord". The Denis three column concept is illustrated in **Figure 18**.

Clinical Evaluation

The patient is evaluated following the ATLS guidelines and thorough survey of the body from head to toe. After initial stabilization evaluate the spine injury thoroughly. Axial and nonradiating back pain of stabbing or aching quality indicates spine injury. The patients with neurological injury report weakness, paresthesia or anesthesia below the injury level and urinary retention. After a careful log roll maneuver observe abrasions, tenderness, local kyphosis and a palpable gap in-between spinous processes. Record the neurological status as per standards of American Spinal Injury Association (ASIA) guidelines. As spinal cord ends at L1 lower border so injuries above this level result in upper motor neuron lesion while lower motor neuron lesions result below L2. Cauda equina type syndrome may be seen if multiple roots are involved together. Injuries of junctional spine (T12–L1) may produce conus medullaris syndrome characterized by damage to sacral innervations to the bowel and bladder with intact lumbar nerve roots.

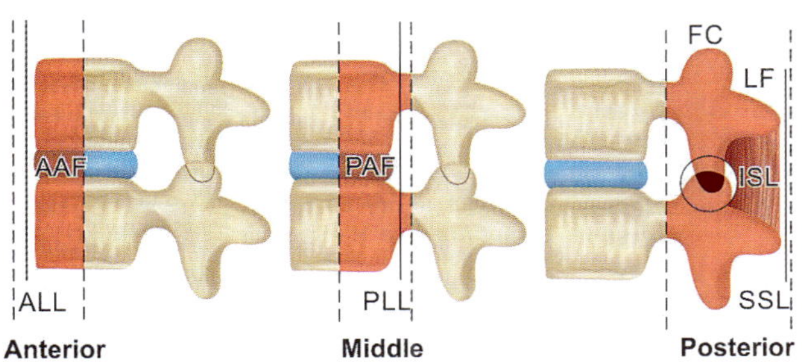

Fig. 18: The Denis three-column concept divides a spinal segment into three parts: anterior, middle, and posterior columns. The anterior column comprises the anterior longitudinal ligament (ALL) and the anterior half of the vertebral body along with anterior half of the disk; the middle column comprises the posterior half of the vertebral body along with the corresponding disk and the posterior longitudinal ligament (PLL); the posterior column comprises the pedicles, the facet joints with capsule (FC), ligamentum flavum (LF), and the supraspinous (SSL)/interspinous (ISL) ligaments.

Radiographic Evaluation

Standard AP and lateral radiographs are obtained to assess alignment, rotation, translation, angular deformity (kyphosis), loss of vertebral height, and widened interpedicular or interspinous distance. CT scan is a routine to assess the injuries further and detail planning. Burst fractures may be under-rated to compression injury only. MRI may be done for evaluation of disk space, ligament injury, status of cord and detecting noncont guous injury by screening. Missed injury(ies) at other place is (are) usually detected days after in 1/4th to half of the patients.

CLASSIFICATIONS

Denis Classification: Holdsworth two column concept was improved upon by Denis (following the Rene Louis' three-column system) by introduction of third "middle" column that was considered the key to stability (this is a conceptual column and not an anatomical one). Denis differentiated major and minor injuries. The *minor injuries* include transverse process fracture, articular process fracture, pars interarticularis fracture and spinous process fracture. *Major injuries* type **(Figs. 19A to D)**.

Compression fractures: Anterior column fracture with middle acting as a hinge. Posterior column may fail under tension. Intact middle column prevents subluxation of retropuls on.

Subtypes:

Type A: Both endplates involved.

Type B: Superior endplate involved.

Type C: Inferior endplate involved.

Type D: Anterior cortex buckled with both endplates intact.

Burst fracture: Both anterior and middle columns fail under axial load.

Subtypes:

Type A: Both endplates involved. Bone retropulsed into the canal.

Type B: Superior end-plate fracture under combined axial load and flexion.

Type C: Inferior endplate fracture.

Treatment

Medical management and stabilization of patient with initiation of measures for spinal cord injury takes precedence over surgical stabilization. SCI management has been detailed elsewhere. The management of thoracolumbar fractures can take non-operative or operative path depending on various parameters.

NONOPERATIVE MANAGEMENT

All stable thoracolumbar injuries without involvement of neurology are managed with thoracolumbar orthoses. There may be an increase in kyphosis during the course of management but up to 30° worsening has not been found to clinically deteriorate the results.

OPERATIVE MANAGEMENT

Operative management is indicated for all unstable thoracolumbar injuries (flexion distraction injuries, unstable burst fractures and fracture dislocations, AO type A4, B1, B2, B3, and C injuries, kyphosis >30°) that cannot be reliably stabilized by nonoperative measures and those injuries where involvement of neurology needs decompression (incomplete neurological deficit, progressive neurological deficit, and spinal cord compression) for deemed improvement in function. Surgical management also avoids the morbidity associated with conservative management in patients with polytrauma, obesity, and skin complications where early mobilization is needed. Ultimately an individual decision is needed weighing the benefits of surgical treatment against potential surgical morbidity. Timing of surgery is not fully agreed upon but early decompression has a role in better outcome compared to delayed decompression. Also progressive neurological deficit needs urgent decompression and stabilization.

Posterior short segment fixation (pedicle screw and rods) is the commonly performed surgery that intends to decompress and stabilize the involved segment.

Contd...

Contd...

<table>
<tr><th>Epidemiology</th><th>Anatomy</th><th>Clinical Evaluation</th><th>Radiographic Evaluation</th><th>Treatment</th></tr>
<tr><td colspan="5">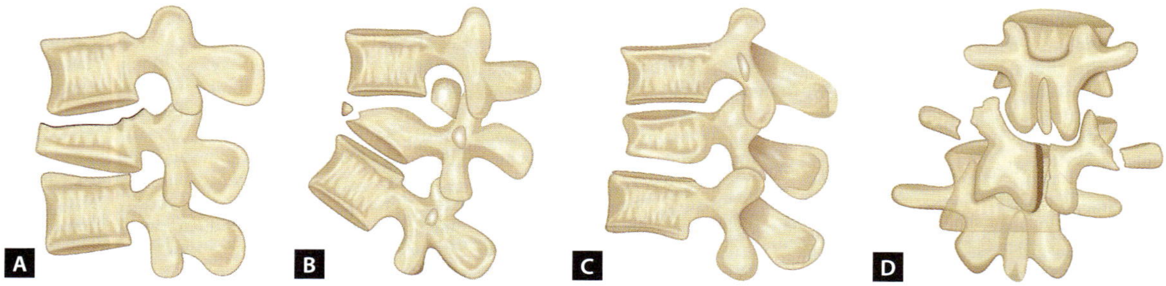
Figs. 19A to D: The different types of thoracolumbar spine injury according to Denis classification system. (A) Compression fracture; (B) Burst fracture; (C) Seat-belt injury; (D) Flexion-dislocation type.</td></tr>
<tr><td></td><td></td><td>Associated injuries like rib fractures, pneumohemothorax are quite common but may also involve cardiovascular system (great vessel injuries and hemopericardium) and rarely diaphragmatic rupture. Seat-belt injuries and flexion distraction injuries are often associated with intra-abdominal visceral injuries. Long bone fractures and head injuries are also common and can often lead to missed injuries of the spine.</td><td>Type D: Burst rotation due to axial load and rotation moment.
Type E: Burst lateral flexion, similar to lateral flexion but interpedicular distance increased.
Seatbelt type injury: Failure of both posterior and middle columns under hyperflexion and tension forces. Though there is damage to anterior cortex but the anterior hinge is intact. The spine is unstable under flexion but there is no subluxation.
Subtypes:
One-level injury: This is a chance fracture going through bone or a ligamentous disruption passing through posterior ligamentous complex and the intervertebral disk.
Two-level injury: The middle column is ruptured either through the bone or the disk. This injury pattern is comparable to Hangman's fracture.
Flexion-dislocations: They are failure of all three columns under compression, tension, rotation, or shear. It is similar to seatbelt-type injury with disrupted anterior hinge and some degree of dislocation is present.
Subtypes:
Flexion-rotation: Tension and rotation injury where posterior and middle columns are damaged in rotation and tension. Anterior column fractures under rotation or compression and rotation. The failure at the level of the middle and anterior columns may occur through the vertebral body or purely through the disk.</td><td>The disadvantages include instrumentation failure, pseudarthrosis, infection, risks of SCI, inadequate neurological decompression, insufficient correction of kyphosis, and the need for late instrumentation removal. For comminuted body fractures, additional anterior reconstruction may be needed to prevent implant failure. To avoid anterior additional surgery various measures have been proposed like intracorporeal bone grafting, vertebroplasty and kyphoplasty, intracorporeal filling with hydroxyapatite or calcium phosphate, use of cross-links, supplemental hook fixation at the levels of the screws and the addition of "intermediate" screw into the fractured vertebra.
Fracture dislocations are severe injuries needing more sturdy stabilization in the form of multilevel spinal fixation (two to three segments above and below the injury).
Anterior surgery is logically supported by the fact that 80% of weight is transmitted through anterior column. So in fractures where anterior column is significantly damaged (comminuted) this needs restoration, other indications include SCI by a retropulsed fragment that cannot be removed from posterior approach. Bone graft or cage strut is commonly deployed.
Combined (anterior and posterior) approach is indicated in burst fractures with significant kyphosis (>40°), >50% canal compromise and neurological deficit in the presence of spinal cord compression.</td></tr>
</table>

Contd...

Contd...

Epidemiology	*Anatomy*	*Clinical Evaluation*	*Radiographic Evaluation*	*Treatment*
			Flexion-distraction type is similar to seatbelt injury but there is disruption of both the posterior and middle columns under tension. There is annulus tear followed by ALL stripping during subluxation or dislocation. *Shear type fracture*: Dislocation results from extension injury disrupting ALL. Disk is torn from anterior to posterior translating upper segment over lower. In posteroanterior subtype, the upper segment displaces forward on lower. A floating posterior arch of upper segment may be left. Paraplegia is very common. In the anteroposterior subtype, the upper segment is displaced posteriorly on the lower one. **McAfee Classification** is a simplified classification system. **AO Classification:** It includes fracture morphology, neurological status, and patient-specific modifiers. *Type A:* Compression injury to vertebral body without posterior ligament complex injury. *Type B*: Tension band disruption, failure of anterior/posterior ligament constraints. *Type C*: Displacement/translational injuries. *Neurological status classification:* N1—no neurological injury N2—radicular symptoms/deficits N3—incomplete spinal cord injury (SCI)/cauda equina injury N4—complete SCI NX—unknown neurology **Thoracolumbar Injury Classification System (TLICS),** created by "The Spine Trauma Study Group," is based on three major injury characteristics—mechanism of injury, integrity of the PLC, and neurological status.	

SACRAL FRACTURES

Epidemiology	*Anatomy*	*Clinical Evaluation*	*Radiographic Evaluation*	*Treatment*
Fractures of the sacrum are commonly associated with pelvic ring injuries in up to 30–45% cases. Around one-fourth of these are associated with neurological injury. They are important to understand due to high rate of missing them in 75% cases where there is no neurological injury or even with neurological injury (1/2 of the cases). Neurological deficit may manifest as urinary/sexual dysfunction or rectal dysfunction and/or lower extremity neurological deficits. The fractures occur commonly in the young adults as a result of high-energy trauma while in elderly osteoporotic patients the fracture may occur even with low-energy injuries like a fall from standing height landing flat of back or buttocks or more commonly on one side.	Sacrum in an adult is a monoblock bone formed by fusion of five sacral vertebrae and contains four foramina that transmit sacral nerves. The foramina transmit S1–S4 nerve roots and are liable to injury during displaced fractures. The lower sacral nerve roots carry fibers for maintaining anal sphincter tone and voluntary action, perianal sensation, bulbocavernosus reflex and bladder control (detailed anatomy can be referred in Chapter on "Neurogenic Bladder").	Evaluation of pelvic ring injuries and visceral injuries takes precedence over sacral injuries. Patients have localized tenderness ± local bruise or ecchymosis. More commonly there is peripelvic pain. Vertically displaced fractures produce shortening of the extremity. Look additionally for neurological injury, bulbocavernosus reflex, anal sphincter tone (per rectal examination), soft tissues (Morel–Lavallee lesion), perineal injuries, pelvic ring stability, ipsilateral extremity—hip/knee injury, lumbar/thoracolumbar/cervical injuries.	AP projection of pelvis is highly insensitive in identifying sacral fractures. Inlet view demonstrates the sacral canal and S1 vertebra, outlet view gives true AP of sacrum but is often marred by soft-tissue shadows. Cross-table lateral is good in demonstrating sacral fractures but difficult to obtain and often has poor quality. Suspect sacrum injury if there is asymmetry of foramina (high), injury to transverse process injury to L4, and L5 vertebra (low). Obtain a CT scan in any case with pelvic injury as a diagnostic study of choice. **CLASSIFICATIONS (FIGS. 20A and B)** **Denis** classifies the sagittal fractures into three types and subtypes along sagittal plane. *Zone 1 injuries*: Fracture lateral to foramina. This is the most common injury and is associated with <5% incidence of neurological injury (mostly to L5). *Zone 2*: Fracture through foramina. Shear fractures are unstable and often associated with neurological injury. There is increased risk of nonunion and poor functional outcome. *Zone 3 injury:* Fracture is medial to foramina extending to spinal canal. They are associated with highest incidence of neurological injury—bowel, bladder dysfunction. These are subclassified onto four types as follows: *Type 1:* Only kyphotic angulation at the fracture site (no translation). *Type 2:* Kyphotic angulation with anterior translation of the distal sacrum. *Type 3:* Kyphotic angulation with complete offset of the fracture fragments. *Type 4:* Comminuted S1 segment, usually due to axial compression. ***Morphologically,*** the fractures are classified into H-shaped, T-shaped, U-shaped, and lambda-shaped fracture. Transverse sacral fractures have higher incidence of nerve dysfunction. U-type fractures result from axial loading and represent spino-pelvic dissociation. There is high incidence of neurological complications with this type of injury.	Most of the nondisplaced fractures (<1 cm) and fractures without neurological deficit are treated conservatively by rest and then protected weight-bearing beginning 6–8 weeks. ***Operative treatment*** is indicated in displaced fractures >1 cm displacement or those associated with neurological deficit. Other indications include soft-tissue compromise, persistent pain after nonoperative management, and fractures that displace with nonoperative management. In patients with neurological deficit, additional decompression is a must usually. ***Operative fixation techniques include:*** *Percutaneous screw fixation*—sacroiliac, trans-sacral, or trans-iliac trans-sacral screws are commonly placed for reducible sagittal plane fractures. Loss of reduction and malreduction may result if not perfect. L5 nerve root may be damaged. One should avoid the temptation to overcompress the fracture and failure is high in osteoporotic bones. *Posterior tension band plating* is a viable option in patients not suitable for percutaneous screw especially those with osteoporotic bones. *Iliosacral and lumbopelvic fixation* using pedicle screw in lumbar spine and iliac screws joined by longitudinal and transverse rods have highest stiffness and stability but needs experience.

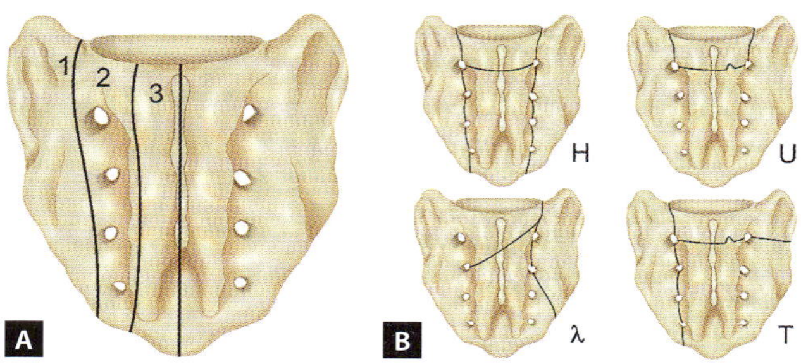

Figs. 20A and B: Illustration for classifications of sacral fracture: (A) Denis; (B) Morphological.

ANNEXURE 4

Neglected Trauma to Bones and Joints

Manish Kumar Varshney, Mohinder Singh Chib

Injuries lead to both mortality and morbidity worldwide. The rate is higher in developing countries because healthcare facilities are limited and far away from a greater percentage of population, less developed traveling facilities. Orthopedic injuries need early care and need a multispecialty approach. These injuries are usually treated by nonorthopedic doctors or quacks in developing countries. Also, nonspecialist persons treat them in rural areas as compared to urban areas where medical facilities are comparatively better. By the time a specialist doctor attends these patients, the status of fracture is either a malunion or nonunion. These may be superimposed by infection. Skin is scarred, adhered to underlying structures, muscle atrophied with developed/developing joint contractures.

A fracture gets neglected usually due to:

- Distracting injury like polytrauma that leads to bony injury being missed by the doctor or remains hidden or goes unnoticed (say head injury where patient is unable to talk about the injury).
- Wrong/missed diagnosis by the practitioner (usually quacks—now even more rampant due to unchecked government policies) where injury continues to be managed conservatively even in cases requiring fixation.
- Poor family support to carry patient to recognized facility.
- Frail, elderly, and too old a patient is often neglected to be carried to hospital or dedicated orthopedic care for "deemed" minor ailments by family.
- Prevailing practices in far-off closed communities/tribes to treat injuries by conventional methods.

The usual consequences of neglected injuries include:

- Distortion of the natural anatomy
- Pathological changes (like disuse osteoporosis) in bones and soft tissues (atrophy)
- Fibrous and capsular contractures occur around joints.
- The muscles get contracted.
- Possible impairment of neurovascular structures (prolonged shortening).

These often preclude closed reduction in most cases, and they need open reduction, threshold for which should be low. Various common neglected/delayed presentations, their related anatomy, and challenges to management are presented in **Table 1**.

TABLE 1: Various common neglected/delayed presentations, their related anatomy, and challenges to management.

Clavicle Malunion Clavicle malunion is very common and was previously considered to be of no significant clinical implication but more of radiological importance. But observing the patient symptomatology over so many years after clavicle malunion, various authors have described about its effects. Usually the patients are young and active in which significant shortening of clavicle length leads to biomechanical and clinical abnormalities. These lead to specific patient symptoms. ***Pathophysiology and clinical presentation:*** Clavicle shortening leads to: • Shortening of (resting length) muscles of rotator cuff. • Impairment of normal muscle function—never achieve maximal function/power. • Easy muscle fatigue. • Narrowing of thoracic outlet producing symptoms.   – Neurological and/or vascular symptoms develop due to nerves and/or vessels being compressed. The weight carrying capacity of the involved girdle also changes and there is abnormal shoulder appearance. Upper back pain is hence common in these patients. Abnormal scapular rhythm (scapular dyskinesia) causes spasm and scapular blade pain/interscapular fasciitis because the center of rotation of scapula gets shifted. Literature describes >2 cm shortening as cause of future problems (no validation to this figure but it is commonly accepted) which can be accentuated by shortening. ***Treatment:*** Patients having symptomatic malunion of clavicle have options of either to accept the deformity or to undergo corrective osteotomy. *Corrective osteotomy*: Performed almost exclusively in young patients with good bone quality. Length of both clavicles is measured radiographically. Standard approach to clavicle is made. Malunion site is identified. Recreating fracture with help of saw is done. Lengthening is avoided as it may lead to neurovascular injury due to stretching. Bone grafting is done to maintain length and promote healing. Definitive fixation is done with the help of plate.

Contd...

Contd...

Old Acromioclavicular (AC) Joint Dislocation

AC joint disruption injuries are uncommon but are very commonly missed due to other distracting injuries in polytrauma patients and otherwise also. Any of the six different types described for acute injury may be present.

Clinically, patients have pain, instability, decreased range of motion (ROM) at shoulder and a visible bony prominence.

Radiographs help in diagnosis of dislocation. Zanca views of both sides help in quantifying and comparing. For types IV, V, and VI, additional evaluation by CT scan and MRI may be done.

Treatment:

Patients with types I or II injury may have degenerative changes. Patients are given conservative treatment by mild analgesics, avoiding offending posture, and local steroid injection. If it fails then distal clavicle resection can be done in type I dislocations. It can be done either open or arthroscopically.

Surgical procedure for type II is different than type I. Only distal clavicle resection does not give relief as instability is there which needs capsular reconstruction.

Types III, IV, and V also are not treated only with a distal clavicle resection as length of clavicle will decrease without stability. Transferring attachment of coracoacromial ligament from acromion to the distal clavicle is needed along with CC stabilization.

Neglected Shoulder Dislocation

Shoulder is the most common joint to dislocate. Neglected old shoulder dislocations occur due to trauma, seizures, and under influence of alcohol or missed in polytrauma.

Clinical presentation: Pain and decreased ROM are the usual complaints. Loss of abduction is the most common complaint with restricted other movements of the joint. Patients having anterior dislocation have restricted internal rotation and vice versa. Associated tuberosity fractures and glenoid fractures are common.

Radiographic evaluation is done by anteroposterior (AP) and axillary views and AP in scapular glenoid plane. CT scan with three-dimensional (3D) reconstruction is needed to see for bony defects of humeral head or glenoid. MRI needed to look for viability of humeral head and status of labrum/rotator cuff and cuff muscles.

Pathoanatomy: Neviaser described a capsular bowstringing in which capsule becomes adherent to glenoid preventing closed reduction.

Commonly found in anterior shoulder dislocations are the typical Hill–Sachs lesion. In posterior dislocation, a reverse Hill–Sachs lesion is present in majority of cases.

Treatment options available are:

- *Benign neglect*: This is usually practiced in neglected posterior dislocation cases as in them the arm is closer to the body and hand reaches the face easily compared to the anterior type.
- *Closed reduction*: An initial trial is given keeping in mind age of patient, bone quality, duration of initial injury, and bone loss. Soft-tissue contractures and fibrous tissue filling the glenoid make the reduction procedure difficult. Gentle traction should be applied to prevent iatrogenic fractures due to osteopenia. General anesthesia leads to relaxation of surrounding muscles and aids in procedure. If reduced, the joint is immobilized for 6 weeks.
- *Open reduction*: It is performed when closed reduction fails. *The dictum is that neglected dislocations > 6 months old or having large bone defects of humeral head should be managed by replacement surgeries.* After open reduction, humeral head fixation is done to prevent re-dislocation. Various authors have given their techniques to do so **(Box 1)**.

In anterior dislocations, deltopectoral approach is used.

Difficulty arises in posterior dislocations as humeral head defect presents anteriorly leading to re-dislocations.

- *McLaughlin* recommended filling defect with subscapularis muscle.
- *Oyston, DePalma, and Schulz et al.* also recommended this.
- *Neer* modified this technique by taking lesser tuberosity along with subscapularis.
- *Chaudhuri et al.* recommended humeral derotational osteotomy in locked posterior dislocation which was performed by *Keppler et al.* through deltopectoral approach.
- *Rockwood* recommended posterior approach if bone defect < 15%.
- *Neviaser, Rowe, and Zarins* recommended superior approach.
- *Wilson, Mckeever, and McLaughlin* recommended anteromedial approach.

BOX 1: Prevention of re-dislocation after open reduction of neglected shoulder dislocation.

- **Wilson and Mckeever:** Inserting crossed K-wires from acromion to humeral head
- **Neviaser:** Swiss screw
- **Goga:** K-wires + transferring coracoid to glenoid
- **Rowe and Zarins:** No fixation needed. Immobilize with arm anterior to coronal plane of body

Arthroplasty of shoulder joint:

- Shoulder hemiarthroplasty is recommended as standard procedure by *Hawkins et al.* in those patients in whom duration is >6 months and defect is >45%.
- *Total shoulder replacement*: *Hawkins et al.* recommended this procedure in those patients in whom glenoid is destroyed with duration > 6 months and defect > 45%. Bone graft may be needed.

Proximal Humerus Fracture

Neglected cases of proximal humerus fractures go into malunion. Either head-neck relationship is disturbed due to malunion or tuberosities malunite which is well tolerated in elderly patients but is problematic to younger population.

Pathophysiology: As the shoulder biomechanics change due to the above said abnormal anatomy, it leads to shoulder pain, decreased range of movements (ROM) with weakness and easy fatiguability. Rotator cuff muscles are at a disadvantage due to malunion, and impingement also occurs due to decreased subacromial space.

Work-up: Three-dimensional CT scan is helpful in addition to radiographs to see for the malunited fragments and MRI shows any rotator cuff tear and impingement.

Treatment:

In older patients, conservative trial is given as they have low overall demand. For younger patient, the following attention is usually paid to:

Greater tuberosity fragment: This fragment retracts superiorly and posteriorly due to the muscle pull. Patient has weakness of abduction strength, and the bone fragment also leads to subacromial impingement. Surgery is done usually by deltoid splitting approach that gives direct visualization of greater tuberosity. The malunited fragment is osteotomized and fixed in position. Subacromial decompression is also done.

Lesser tuberosity: As subscapularis attaches to lesser tuberosity, weakness of internal rotation is there with subcoracoid impingement. To approach this fragment, a deltopectoral approach is done.

3- or 4-part fractures: If there is no osteonecrosis and deformity is less severe, osteotomy is the preferred option but as it is a complex 3D deformity in most of the cases, the only option left is a shoulder arthroplasty. The results of arthroplasty are inferior as compared to that in an acute fracture pattern. There is a very limited literature of reverse shoulder arthroplasty surgery in these neglected injuries.

Contd...

Contd...

Distal Humerus Fractures

These fractures are difficult to treat due to comminution, osteopenic bones, and the contour of bone fragments. The treating surgeon should have a 3D orientation of this area to understand the plate application and screw direction.

Pathophysiology: Nonunion is common in intra-articular distal humerus fractures as they are at epiphyseal level with precarious blood supply. Elbow ROM is painful and decreased. Patient has stiffness that hampers daily activities.

Work-up: Blood markers are done to see for signs of infection. Standard AP and lateral radiographs are needed. Oblique views are also needed to assess nonunion, but CT scan is the most useful modality.

Treatment:

Available options for management are:

- Open reduction and internal fixation (ORIF) + Bone grafting
- Conservative approach with physiotherapy and gaining functional range
- Arthrodesis
- Elbow arthroplasty

In young patients, the bone quality is better that is why ORIF is preferred. Further evaluation, e.g., number of previous procedures done, skin condition and scarring, number of small, comminuted fragments (their fixation is difficult), and dexterity is also done. If skin is scarred, then plastic surgeon help is sought, and surgery is done in two stages. In the first stage, full thickness skin graft is done and ORIF performed in the second stage. Bone loss is managed by cortical struts and cancellous bone is added to aid in union. Posterior approach is made and the need for olecranon osteotomy is decided intraoperatively. Fibrous tissues are excised but periosteal dissection is kept to a minimum.

If nonsalvageable then other methods of reconstruction are sought after.

Patients who are not fit for procedure or there is severe bone loss or in elderly patients (uncertain implant purchase) can be managed initially by bracing and gradually putting patient on a physiotherapy protocol thus achieving near functional ROM.

Elderly patients who are fit for surgery, but initial ORIF led to nonunion can be managed by elbow replacement as osteopenia will be there.

In infected nonunion cases, arthrodesis is a viable option as all other procedures cannot be undertaken in them.

Malunited Supracondylar Fractures *(Kindly also see Chapter on "Nonunions and Malunions" for detailed discussion)*

Pathoanatomy: It leads to cubitus varus or gunstock deformity. Varus is there in place of normal valgus at elbow. It is a 3D deformity formed by horizontal rotation, coronal tilt, and posterior displacement.

Pathophysiology: There is usually no functional complaints or decreased ROM, but the chief problem is mostly cosmetic appearance.

Clinically, the deformity can be measured with help of goniometer.

Work-up: Anteroposterior radiographs of both upper limbs in extension are taken. Baumann angle is measured by it. Crescent sign is seen. Metaphyseal diaphyseal angle also measured.

Treatment option is osteotomy.

Osteotomy can be either oblique osteotomy with derotation, medial opening, or lateral closing wedge.

- *Medial opening:* King and Secor
- *Lateral closing:* Voss et al., Hui et al., French, modified French by Bellemore et al.
- *Oblique osteotomy with derotation:* Amspacher and Messenbaugh

If done in children, osteotomy is fixed with K-wires and stainless-steel suture wires. In adults, distal humerus plates are used. Lateral closing wedge is usually done due to the advantages and the ease to perform. The wedge to be removed can be calculated from preoperative X-rays.

Kim et al. described a simple step cut osteotomy that can be used to correct cubitus varus as well as valgus.

Old Elbow Dislocation *(Kindly also see dedicated Chapters on "Stiff Elbow" and "The Unstable Elbow" for detailed discussion)*

Elbow is the second most common joint to dislocate in adults after shoulder and is the most common joint dislocation in children. Neglected injuries of elbow are common in developing countries. Mechanism of injury is fall on the outstretched hand. Most common type is a posterior dislocation.

Clinical presentation: Elbow is flexed in near full extension in most cases with inability to flex the elbow. Some patients have fixed flexed elbow with loss of movements. The initial presentation is totally dependent on initial injury. Pronation and supination are also restricted with pronation more affected than supination. Triceps tendon is prominent and shortened.

There is extensive myositis ossificans especially in brachialis. Muscles are shortened. Fibrosis around the joint and capsular thickening is also present. These make evaluation of elbow three-point relationship difficult. Forearm shortening is prominent.

Work-up: Standard AP and lateral views are needed. CT scan is particularly useful in finding malunited fracture fragments.

The available ***treatment options*** are:

- *Closed reduction*: If initial injury is <3 weeks then closed reduction should be attempted first as is described by *Allende and Freytes*. Manipulation should be gentle to prevent fractures and under general anesthesia so that complete relaxation of muscles occurs.
- *Open reduction*: As triceps is contracted and prevents reduction so it must be lengthened. *Speed* described a procedure of V-Y plasty of triceps and excision of fibrous tissue. Ulnar nerve should be released from the fibrous tissue and transposed anteriorly. Elbow is unstable after reduction and hence fixation with K wires as ulnohumeral or radiocapitellar fixation should be done.

There are a lot of variations and modifications practiced as follows:

- *Jupiter and Ring* used hinged external fixation after open reduction.
- *Hotchkiss* also described hinged external fixation in these cases.
- *Krishnamoorthy et al.* used medial and lateral incisions and did not lengthened triceps.
- *Arafiles* described collateral ligament reconstruction to prevent redislocation and instability. But, other authors with their experience described that suturing of collaterals is adequate. Most of their cases did not complain about instability.

If dislocation is older than 3 months then either arthrodesis or any form of arthroplasty is needed.

- Elbow arthrodesis
- Interpositional arthroplasty
- Total elbow replacement.

Lateral Condyle Nonunion

These are second most common fractures of the elbow in children. The most common near age of 6 years. As per majority of authors displaced fracture >3 weeks is termed as neglected lateral condyle fractures. This duration of 3 weeks is sometimes extended up to 6 weeks. A neglected fracture between 3 and 12 weeks is the gray area and no standard protocol is there for it. Authors describe surgery at this stage leads to stiffness, osteonecrosis of fragment due to dissection, and thus poor results.

Contd...

Contd...

But, some authors have advised ORIF in neglected cases with minimal dissection posteriorly and ulnar nerve transposition. Bone grafting is commonly needed to fill the remaining gap.

A lateral condyle fracture is designated as nonunion at 12 weeks. Gradually, it leads to cubitus valgus and tardy ulnar nerve palsy.

Pathoanatomy: Delay in fixation leads to fibrous tissue formation and open reduction at that time leads to extensive soft-tissue dissection that destroys blood supply to the fragment leading to avascular necrosis. Not operating this neglected fracture leads to cubitus valgus in future which is a progressive deformity and tardy ulnar nerve palsy may occur.

Clinically, there is some loss of motion at the elbow. The chief complaint is progressive valgus deformity that is cosmetically problematic. Ulnar nerve palsy is seen in long-standing cases especially with cubitus valgus deformity. Pain is an uncommon complaint. The three-point relationship is disturbed, and mobile lateral condyle fragment may be palpable. Due to fibrous type short-nonunion, it is difficult to elicit abnormal mobility in all. Lateral arm length shortening but maintained medial arm length strongly supports lateral condyle nonunion.

Work-up: Radiographs are the mainstay of initial evaluation and making diagnosis. 3D CT scan for planning osteotomy and treatment is recommended.

Treatment: In the absence of ulnar nerve symptoms, benign neglect is commonly practiced as there is minimal functional deficit but keep patients in close follow-up and explain them about the neurological complication in detail and how to identify it. Surgical intervention is performed near skeletal maturity or after skeletal maturity. The general considerations for operative procedure in late nonunion are:

- Surgeon should have experience in this type of surgeries.
- Displacement of fragment
- Minimal dissection especially posteriorly
- Adequate compression of fragment

The operative procedure commonly recommended for established nonunion with cubitus valgus deformity is osteotomy to correct deformity with anterior transposition of nerve. No attempt is made to treat the nonunion site. Lateral condyle fracture is classified into two types: Milch type I and II. In Milch type I, the cubitus valgus is mild and nonunion is seen early. In these cases, a closing wedge medial osteotomy described by *Speed* or opening wedge lateral osteotomy described by *Milch* is done. After osteotomy, bone graft is added and fixation done with K wires.

In Milch type II, due to severe displacement and rotation, simple opening lateral wedge osteotomy results in unacceptable medial prominence and unacceptable alignment of elbow as a whole. *Milch* described open wedge displacement osteotomy in them. In severe cases, *Kim et al.* described a step cut translational osteotomy and fixed it with a Y-shaped humeral plate. Apart from these standard procedures, various alternatives have also been described as follows:

- Two-stage procedure described by *Papandrea and Waters* in which screw fixation is done for fracture fragment and nerve transposition is done in first stage and osteotomy in the second stage.
- *Flynn and Richards* described small wedge-shaped graft to be applied at nonunion site with or without fixation.
- For early established nonunion in minimally displaced fractures, *Flynn and Jeffery* described bone grafting and fixation. Peg graft taken from proximal ulna. The fibrous union at nonunion site is not disturbed. Also, physis is not curetted and no fixation done across physis. Graft is placed in the metaphyseal region and screw placed across it without violating physis. Limb is immobilized for 12 weeks.

Old Neglected Monteggia Fracture Dislocation

It is an uncommon and neglected injury. The injury is either missed or inadequate treatment is given leading to nonanatomical reduction of ulna. As the ulna is shortened or angulated, it leads to a dislocated radial head.

Clinically, the patient has cubitus valgus and dislocated radial head. Elbow ROM is near normal, but rotations usually are decreased than normal. There may be elbow instability and associated nerve injuries (see Monteggia fracture in **Annexure 1**).

Work-up: Anteroposterior and lateral views of forearm are needed that should include elbow and wrist.

- McLaughlin line is a line drawn across radial shaft passing through the radial head and should bisect the capitellum in all views mainly lateral view.
- Mubarak line (Ulnar bow line) is line drawn along the posterior border of ulna and either bow should be absent or should be <1 mm. If more than that, it means old Monteggia is there.

Treatment options are divided into three types as per the level of radial head. The displaced radial head can be either at the level of radioulnar joint or within 1 cm to it or >1 cm from it.

- *Radial head at the level: Speed and Boyd* described this procedure. Boyd approach is made. Osteotomy of ulna is done at level of deformity. Radial head is reduced after removing fibrous tissue. This leads to angulation of ulna. Plate contoured and osteotomy fixed. Bone graft is added. Radial head usually is stable, and no fixation is needed.
- *Radial head within 1 cm:* Same approach is done. Bone graft added so that lengthening occurs, and radial head gets reduced. If unstable, radiocapitellar K-wire can be used.
- *Radial head >1 cm away:* As this much overlap needs gradual distraction of ulna. Ilizarov or mini rail fixator is used. Corticotomy is done and gradual lengthening is done till radial head can be reduced. Then, fixator is removed. Sling procedure is used to reconstruct the annular ligament and stabilize the radial head.
  - *Boyd* used slip of fascia from extensor aponeurosis.
  - *Bell Tawse* used central slip of triceps fascia.
  - *Lloyd Roberts* used lateral aspect of triceps fascia.

Neglected Both Bone Forearm Fractures

Neglected cases in adults lead to nonunion which are treated as per principles. In children, if adequate reduction is not done for that age or patient does not take treatment due to lack of facilities then forearm fractures lead to malunion.

Due to the growing age, at follow-up the magnitude of decreased ROM due to malunion may lessen and should be taken into account while treating the patient. Also, the level of initial fracture should be noted. Deformity in the plane of joint is acceptable near physis rather than at diaphysis.

Malunited fractures lead to visible deformity and decreased ROM, but significant issues are present in a small number of patients.

Time since injury if <5–6 weeks then osteoclasis can be done under general anesthesia. If it fails, then percutaneous methods are used. Multiple drilling at fracture aid in osteoclasis.

If significant callus has formed, then osteoclasis fails. Casting does not help in these cases. Also, elastic nailing is not possible as canal gets blocked from callus. Open reduction with plating remains the only option in these cases.

If fracture is united with malunion and significant time has passed, then regular follow-up with measurement of deformity and ROM is done. If it still fails to remodel, then corrective osteotomies are done but at a later stage. Usually, patients with decreased supination are the candidates for osteotomy as functional ROM is needed for activities of daily living.

Contd...

Contd...

Distal end Radius Malunion *(See also Chapters on "Carpal Instability" and "Nonunions and Malunions" for detailed discussion)*
In third world countries, these fractures usually are managed by quacks or bone setters and hence are neglected. As these are metaphyseal fractures, therefore these unite with malunion if not treated properly. Older patients tolerate deformity better as they are low demand patients.
Clinical presentation: Patients have pain, weakness in grip due to pain or mechanical factors, and decreased ROM, e.g., with dorsal malunion there is decreased wrist flexion and deformity.
Work-up: Anteroposterior and lateral X-rays are needed. CT scan is used to see for intra-articular fractures, distal radioulnar joint (DRUJ) instability/incongruence and 3D view of the distal radius as a whole.
Treatment options:
Osteotomy
Extra-articular osteotomy: Young and active patients are benefitted from it. This osteotomy changes the orientation of the joint making the joint kinematics better. Palmar tilt, radial inclination, radial length, rotational malalignment, and DRUJ incongruity are restored. Contraindications of the osteotomy are advanced arthritis, presence of CRPS, and osteoporosis.
For dorsal malunions, dorsal approach is made, and opening-wedge osteotomy is done. Irritation of tendons by implant is the disadvantage. Volar approach also can be done to perform dorsal opening-wedge osteotomy. Cavity filled with cancellous graft. Open wedge restores radial length and therefore is preferred. External fixator also can be used. Its advantage is easy removal of implant without hospitalization.
Volar malunion are corrected by approaching volarly. In these types of cases, supination is restricted. *Shea et al.* described a volar opening-wedge osteotomy.
Intra-articular osteotomy: Articular incongruity leads to poor long-term results. 3D CT scan helps in planning of these osteotomies. Indications for surgery are step off or gap > 2 mm, joint subluxation as in Barton's fracture. Both volar and dorsal approaches can be used. Osteotomy done by volar approach and joint visualized from dorsal approach by doing capsulotomy. Comminuted intra-articular fragments and die punch type fracture pattern cannot be treated by osteotomy and need fusion.
Wrist arthrodesis and replacement are the options when there is advanced wrist arthritis.

Old Metacarpophalangeal (MCP) Joint Dislocation ***(Also see Annexure 1)***
These are commonly missed in acute setting due to other severe and distracting injuries. Mechanism of injury is hyperextension at the joint leading to rupture of volar plate and capsule. Clinically, the joint is in a hyperextended state with loss of strength and stability of the involved digit. Commonly this is seen in index finger followed by thumb.
X-rays taken in two planes reveal the dislocation.
Treatment:
Closed reduction usually fails due to contractures developed due to long-standing dislocation. Damage to articular cartilage is also there. Buttonholing of metacarpal head also prevents reduction.
Kaplan lesion is a rare cause of irreducibility. The metacarpal head buttonholes volarly. Volar plate is struck between both the bone ends and prevents reduction. In these cases, traction is contraindicated as this leads to dislocation becoming irreducible by closed means.
Open reduction is done to reduce the dislocation. Both volar and dorsal approaches can be done to treat this. Dorsal approach is preferred as volar plate is visualized and released. Also, it prevents neurovascular damage. Both approaches may be needed in long-standing cases. Hyperextension is avoided in the immediate postoperative period.
If joint cartilage is damaged or arthritis is present, then joint fusion is done to get a stable and painless joint.

Hip Dislocation
In developing countries, neglected unreduced traumatic dislocations are common as compared to developed countries. Late presentation is due to nonavailability of healthcare facilities nearby, compromised healthcare facilities, and missed diagnosis.
Clinical presentation: The patient may be immobile due to loss of hip function or younger patients are seen walking on their dislocated hips with a limb!
Neglected hip dislocation can be anterior or posterior.
The movements of the hip joint are globally restricted with flexion, adduction, and internal deformity in posterior neglected dislocation. Shortening is marked and there is palpable globular/spherical swelling in the gluteal region posteriorly. There may be associated sciatic nerve injury and foot drop.
The deformities of acute anterior dislocation are seen in neglected cases.
Work-up: X-rays are done to confirm the diagnosis. Radiographs demonstrate dislocated hip joint with discontinuity in the Shenton's line and empty acetabulum. There is marked shortening with upriding of trochanters and internal rotation deformity (less prominent lesser trochanter). Myositis ossificans may be present. CT scan is done to see for associated acetabular and femoral head fractures. MRI evaluation is needed to demonstrate vascularity of femoral head and status of acetabular cavity.
Various ***treatment modalities*** available are:
- Attempting closed reduction
- Open reduction
- Heavy traction
- Intertrochanteric osteotomy
- Modified girdlestone arthroplasty
- Total hip replacement (THR) and bipolar replacement.

Closed reduction can be attempted in cases which are 3–6 weeks old, but failure rates are high along with associated complications of iatrogenic fractures.
Skeletal traction for a longer period is another option described in literature. *Gupta et al.* have described that weights up to 18 kg allow for reduction by overcoming capsular and muscular contractures. Patient is sedated and given muscle relaxants during the whole procedure. Then gradual abduction of hip with decreased traction is performed to accomplish reduction which usually occurs by 5th day when femoral head reaches at the level of acetabulum. If failure occurs by this technique or concentric reduction not achieved then open reduction is done.
Intertrochanteric osteotomy is done in neglected cases of anterior hip dislocation. *Aggarwal and Singh* described this procedure to correct deformity and to improve body biomechanics and balance.
Modified girdlestone arthroplasty described by *Nagi et al.* in which subcapital osteotomy was done and by manipulations the femoral neck is displaced into the acetabulum and skeletal traction given. This is no longer preferred now.
If head is not viable then replacement surgeries are the only option, but they also are difficult due to the shortening, contractures, and fibrous tissue obliterating acetabulum. Also, posterior lip of acetabulum usually is fractured and that leads to decreased support for the acetabular cup. In these cases, either ORIF of fractured fragment is done or excised femoral head is used as bone graft for support.

Contd...

Contd...

Neglected Femoral Neck Fractures *(See Chapter on "Nonunions and Malunions" for detailed discussion)*

Intertrochanteric malunion

Neglected trochanteric fractures are injuries of the elderly that cause mortality and morbidity in patients as they become bedridden. Fracture caused due to osteoporosis, falls due to poor vision and complicated by medical conditions, tendency for varus, and venous thromboembolism.

Pathoanatomy: Varus malunion leads to limp, shortened limb, and gluteal muscle insufficiency. It causes back pain due to increased forces around lumbar spine due to the deformity. Nonunion although rare but is possible due to shear forces across fracture site, intertrochanteric fractures with subtrochanteric extension or due to poorly performed DHS surgery where barrel plate resists further collapse, dynamic hip screw (DHS) screw abutting barrel before fracture collapse, unstable trochanteric cases, and presence of infection.

Clinically, patient has shortening, external rotation of lower extremity, wasting of thigh and gluteal muscles, greater trochanter at a higher level as compared to opposite side, and Trendelenburg gait.

Work-up: X-rays show coxa vara with malunion along with osteoporosis. CT scan may be used to evaluate operated cases or complex malunions planned for reconstruction.

Treatment:

Operative procedure is required in patients who have unacceptable deformity with shortening and pain that hampers activities of daily living.

- Valgus trochanteric osteotomy is the procedure of choice to correct coxa vara. *(Procedure explained in Chapter on "Osteotomies Around Hip Joint")*
- This osteotomy is especially preferred to improve hip function as it restores neck shaft angle and corrects shortening. Osteotomy is fixed with angled blade plate. Distal fragment is lateralized that compensates shortening and prevents Trendelenburg gait.
- Total hip replacement is done in patients with associated joint arthritis, poor bone stock, and failure of osteosynthesis.

Neglected Knee Dislocation

Knee is the largest joint in the body, but the bony surfaces are not congruent enough for stability and hence stability is provided by the muscles and ligaments across knee joint. Acute dislocations endanger neurovascular structures and frequently cause damage to ligaments. Neglected knee dislocations although rare but are encountered in developing countries. As in all neglected dislocations, adhesions are present that resist closed reduction.

Clinical presentation: The knee is mostly posteriorly dislocated with fixed flexion deformity. There is loss of extension movement and variable preserved flexion ROM. Commonly external rotation deformity is associated with dislocation. There is extensive posteriorly contracted soft tissues making closed reduction nearly impossible. Myositis ossificans may be variably present. Reflex sympathetic dystrophy (RSD) and nerve injury are variably present. Ligaments are commonly disrupted in these especially long-standing cases. With improved care most presentations involve patients who have spontaneously reduced knee after initial dislocation in high-energy trauma. There is no fixed deformity, but the knee is unstable due to ligament injury that involved more than two ligaments. Vascular injury should be carefully evaluated as popliteal vessels are commonly injured in them. Also evaluate the status of peroneal nerve. The movements are painful due to bone and soft-tissue contusion and in late cases the movements at knee are commonly restricted due to arthrofibrosis ± meniscal injury and displacement.

Work-up: The radiographs are the initial modalities that demonstrate various avulsion injuries for collateral ligament and may also show condylar fractures. Tibial spine fractures are also common. Best evaluation is done by MRI scan of the knee joint for global evaluation of ligaments and capsule. In late cases, >3 months old chondrolysis sets in along with arthrofibrosis compromising the success of preserving the native joint.

Pathoanatomy: Ligament injury of cruciates is commonly seen compromising the instability of knee if dislocation is already reduced. Stiff knee with fixed deformity is seen in unreduced dislocations, they have disrupted collaterals also in addition to cruciate injury. Displaced meniscus fragment usually prevents full movements of the knee joint.

Treatment options commonly available are:

- Open reduction (*Henshaw et al.*)—open arthrotomy, releasing of adhesions, and debridement and fixation with crossed Steinmann pins to maintain reduction. There is extensive chondrolysis. In long-term followed cases, ROM achieved is usually up to 45°. Anterior cruciate ligament (ACL) and the posterior cruciate ligament (PCL) reconstructions can be done to gain stability of knee and is usually done later.
- Ilizarov procedure where rings are applied, and gradual distraction is done to achieve reduction is another viable option.
- Total knee replacement (TKR)—neglected cases have chondrolysis, meniscal, and cruciate injuries. Open reduction does not give a near normal ROM and usually the joint becomes arthritic at an early stage. TKR is technically difficult in these cases as was described by *Petrie et al.* Constrained implant gives stability to the prosthesis as cruciates are torn. Intraoperatively, the knee is usually loose in flexion and tight in extension.
- Knee arthrodesis— this procedure gives inferior results to TKR but in a developing country like India where poverty, literacy levels, and heavy labor work are the reasons that this procedure is considered valid.

Tibial Plateau Fractures

Neglected proximal tibial fractures are uncommon. Malunion occurs due to iatrogenic causes and is comparatively common than nonunion at this site.

Pathoanatomy: Bone loss, osteoporosis, degenerative changes in joint, and inadequate soft-tissue coverage are the challenges that these neglected fractures pose. There is often associated meniscal and ligament injury that would need separate care after managing the bony abnormality.

Treatment options are:

- Open reduction and internal fixation for nonunion
- Corrective osteotomy for malunion if joint not degenerative
- Total knee replacement if joint is degenerative
- Knee arthrodesis.

Malunion: Tibial plateau malunion leads to extra-articular angulation or intra-articular malunion or both in combination. Angular malunion in any plane leads to cosmetic deformity and functional problem and increases osteoarthritis risk in future. For extra-articular malunion, osteotomies performed as in conventional axial skeleton deformities is done.

Intra-articular malunions are difficult to evaluate and treat. They lead to limb malalignment. For example, a malunited lateral plateau fracture with depression leads to valgus at knee.

Osteotomy: In an old malunited fracture when there is depression of condyle with minimally displaced fragment laterally then transverse subcondylar osteotomy without involving articular surface and filling gap with graft is done. But, in a young patient with recent malunion, recommended is oblique osteotomy going through the fracture and elevating the depressed surface. It is then fixed with buttress plate and bone graft added to it.

- Intra-articular osteotomy:
  Objective: To restore anatomy of joint surface of tibial plateau.
  Indication: Malunited tibial plateau fracture with significant intra-articular step/depression.
  Contraindications: Infection, soft-tissue compromise at the incision site, advanced knee osteoarthritis, associated internal derangements in the knee, e.g., meniscus tear/ligament tear.

Contd...

Contd...

Surgical technique: In case of lateral tibial plateau malunion where intra-articular osteotomy is planned, the malunion site is approached by lateral incision. Proximal fibular osteotomy is done. If necessary, callus is removed from malunion site. Intra-articular osteotomy of depressed fragment is done at the height of the malunion, and fragment aligned. It is then underplayed with bone graft and osteotomy fixed with plate.

- *Special attention to tibial slope*: There is sloping of tibial plateau which is inclined caudally posteriorly in relation to horizontal. Changes in tibial slope affect biomechanics of the knee joint. If osteotomy is opened more anteriorly than posteriorly (flexion type osteotomy) then the tibial slope increases and vice versa.
  No major change in rotation occurs during slope change. As preoperative evaluation in these neglected knee dislocations is done by MRI, damage to cruciate ligaments is kept in mind and slope changing is done accordingly. In PCL deficient cases, tibial slope is thus increased and decreased in ACL deficient knees. Increasing slope >10° should not be done as it leads to increased tension on ACL. Open-wedge osteotomy has the advantage of further adjusting the gap after osteotomy by further spreading or closing the gap. It also gives better control to adjust the slope.

Total knee replacement: In old malunion cases that lead to joint arthritis can be treated by replacement arthroplasty, but literature says the procedure is technically demanding and results inferior. Exposure is difficult due to malunited fragments and extensile approach is needed.

Nonunion: Nonunion of tibial plateau fractures is very rare. Type VI Schatzker fractures are more prone for nonunion especially when displaced or open type. These are managed by ORIF + bone grafting if joint is salvageable otherwise TKR or arthrodesis is considered. Ilizarov method is particularly helpful in managing these nonunion cases.

Neglected Dislocation and Injuries Around Ankle

Dislocation: Old dislocations of ankle without fracture are an exceedingly rare injury. These usually occur with bi- or tri-malleolar fractures. Neglected sprains lead to chronic ankle instability that are treated by ligament reconstruction.

Ankle fractures: They can be neglected in third world countries or in polytrauma patients. Subtle derangements in tibiotalar articulation lead to development of arthritis. Malunited fractures lead to significant morbidity in patients. X-rays in AP and lateral view are done. CT scan usually is needed to see for bony architecture.

Treatment options:

- *Osteotomy of the malleolus* (medial/lateral) and fixation—for medial malleolus malunion, osteotomy is done, and wedge-shaped graft inserted, and osteotomy is fixed. Lateral malleolar malunion leads to fibula maluniting with shortening and external rotation. It is osteotomized and lengthened with internal rotation to regain normal anatomy.
- *Supramalleolar osteotomy,* e.g., dome osteotomy—a bimalleolar fracture malunion leads to varus or valgus at ankle so this treatment method is done in these cases. Supramalleolar osteotomy is either of wedge type or dome type. Dome type is superior as it leads to near normal leg length and corrects multiaxial deformity.
- *Ankle arthrodesis*—in old cases with loss of joint cartilage and presence of arthritis, ankle should be arthrodesed. It is a preferred option in laborer's or those performing heavy work as it gives stability to ankle and joint becomes pain free.

Neglected Talar Fractures

It can malunite in varus or valgus. For varus type, triple arthrodesis is done. Valgus type which is more common can be treated with osteotomy + bone grafting + fixation. If osteonecrosis occurs, then *Blair* fusion is done.

Neglected Calcaneal Fractures

Like other neglected ankle injuries these can be missed or wrongly dealt conservatively when operative procedure was needed. Calcaneum fractures malunite and lead to difficulty walking especially when involving subtalar joint producing pain when walking on uneven surfaces. Loss of congruency in calcaneocuboid joint leads to midfoot pain. Broadening of heel which is a common complication of malunited calcaneal fracture leads to irritation and impingement of peroneal tendons.

Lateral and axial X-ray views are needed to evaluate malunion. CT scan helps to classify fracture type and involvement of subtalar joint.

Treatment:

Conservative: Soft shoes with padded heel and silicon heel pads can be tried for relief of pain.

Surgery:

- If isolated subtalar joint is involved, then subtalar arthrodesis is done.
- If along with subtalar, chopart joints are involved then triple arthrodesis is advocated.
- Peroneal impingement can be relieved by shaving off the lateral prominence of calcaneum.
- For malunited tuberosity fracture, osteotomy at malunited fracture is done to realign the fragment and then it is fixed.

Neglected Lisfranc Injuries

These injuries are common, frequently misdiagnosed, and mistreated leading to midfoot arthritis. These injuries range from mild sprain of ligamentous structures to frank dissociation of joints.

Anteroposterior and oblique views are needed to diagnose. CT scan gives 3D view of the deformity.

Treatment:

If there is no arthritis or fixed deformity, ORIF can be planned. Fixation with screws is necessary for rigid stabilization. If arthritic changes are present, then arthrodesis is the treatment of choice. 1st, 2nd, and 3rd tarsometatarsal joints are fused whereas in 4th and 5th joint a resection arthroplasty is done to maintain some physiological motion. Fusion is also recommended in Charcot arthropathy of Lisfranc joints.

Index

Page numbers followed by *b* refer to box, *f* refer to figure, *fc* refer to flowchart, and *t* refer to table.

A

D

F

H

J

K

L

M

P

S

T

W